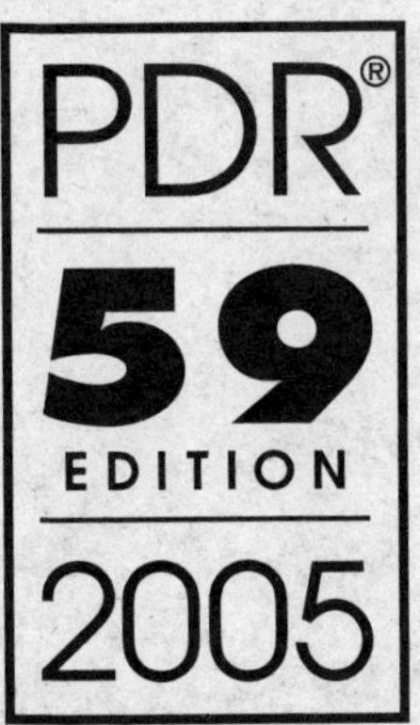

PHYSICIANS' DESK REFERENCE®

THOMSON™
PDR

ISBN: 1-56363-497-X

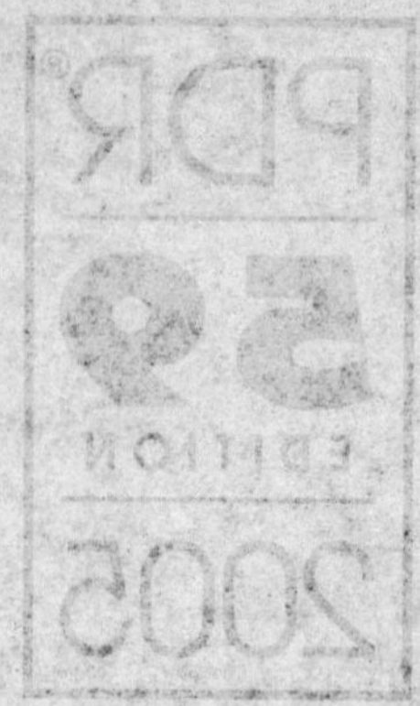

FOREWORD TO THE FIFTY-NINTH EDITION

PDR enters its fifty-ninth year offering a wider array of pharmaceutical reference options than ever before. Long available unabridged—in print, on CD-ROM, and via the Internet—*PDR* also provides essential prescribing information in other forms as well, detailed later in this foreword.

About This Book

Physicians' Desk Reference is published by Thomson PDR in cooperation with participating manufacturers. The *PDR* contains Food and Drug Administration (FDA)-approved labeling for drugs as well as prescription information provided by manufacturers for grandfathered drugs and other drugs marketed without FDA approval under current FDA policies. Some dietary supplements and other products are also included.

Each full-length entry provides you with an exact copy of the product's FDA-approved or other manufacturer-supplied labeling. Under the Federal Food, Drug and Cosmetic (FD&C) Act, a drug approved for marketing may be labeled, promoted, and advertised by the manufacturer for only those uses for which the drug's safety and effectiveness have been established. The Code of Federal Regulations Title 21 Section 201.100(d)(1) pertaining to labeling for prescription products requires that for *PDR* content "indications, effects, dosages, routes, methods, and frequency and duration of administration, and any relevant warnings, hazards, contraindications, side effects, and precautions" must be *"same in language and emphasis"* as the approved labeling for the products. The FDA regards the words *same in language and emphasis* as requiring VERBATIM use of the approved labeling providing such information. Furthermore, information that is emphasized in the approved labeling by the use of type set in a box, or in capitals, boldface, or italics, must be given the same emphasis in *PDR*.

The FDA has also recognized that the FD&C Act does not, however, limit the manner in which a physician may use an approved drug. Once a product has been approved for marketing, a physician may choose to prescribe it for uses or in treatment regimens or patient populations that are not included in approved labeling. The FDA also observes that accepted medical practice includes drug use that is not reflected in approved drug labeling. In the case of over-the-counter dietary supplements, it should be remembered that this information has not been evaluated by the Food and Drug Administration, and that such products are not intended to diagnose, treat, cure, or prevent any disease.

The function of the publisher is the compilation, organization, and distribution of this information. Each product description has been prepared by the manufacturer, and edited and approved by the manufacturer's medical department, medical director, and/or medical consultant. In organizing and presenting the material in *Physicians' Desk Reference*, the publisher does not warrant or guarantee any of the products described, or perform any independent analysis in connection with any of the product information contained herein. *Physicians' Desk Reference* does not assume, and expressly disclaims, any obligation to obtain and include any information other than that provided to it by the manufacturer. It should be understood that by making this material available, the publisher is not advocating the use of any product described herein, nor is the publisher responsible for misuse of a product due to typographical error. Additional information on any product may be obtained from the manufacturer.

Other Clinical Information Products from PDR

For complicated cases and special patient problems, there is no substitute for the in-depth data contained in *Physicians' Desk Reference.* But for those times when you need quick access to critical prescribing information, you'll want to consult the **PDR® Monthly Prescribing Guide™**, the essential drug reference designed specifically for use at the point of care. Distilled from the pages of *PDR*, this digest-sized reference presents the key facts on more than 2,000 drug formulations, including therapeutic class, indications and contraindications, warnings and precautions, pregnancy rating, drug interactions and side effects, and most importantly, adult and pediatric dosages. Each entry also gives the *PDR* page number to turn to for further information. In addition, a full-color insert of pill and product images allows you to correctly identify each product. Issued monthly, the guide is continuously updated with detailed descriptions of the latest drugs to receive FDA approval, as well as FDA-approved revisions to existing product information. You'll also find bulletins about major new developments in the pharmaceutical industry, an overview of important new agents nearing approval, and the latest clinical findings on common nutritional supplements. To learn more about this useful publication and to inquire about subscription rates, call 800-232-7379.

If you prefer to carry drug information with you on a handheld device like a Palm® or Pocket PC, consider **mobilePDR®**. This easy-to-use software allows you to retrieve in an instant concise summaries of the FDA-approved and other manufacturer-supplied labeling for 2,000 of the most frequently prescribed drugs, lets you run automatic interaction checks on multidrug regimens, and even alerts you to significant changes in drug labeling, usually within 24 to 48 hours of announcements. You can look up drugs by brand or generic name, by indication, and by therapeutic class. The drug interaction checker allows you to screen for interactions among as many as 32 drugs. The What's New feature provides daily alerts about drug recalls, labeling changes, new drug introductions, and so on. Our auto-update feature updates the content and the software, so upgrades are easy to manage. *mobilePDR®* works with both the Palm and Windows CE operating systems, and it's free to U.S.-based MDs, DOs, NPs, and PAs in full-time patient practice and to medical students and residents. Check it out today at www.PDR.net.

For those who prefer to view drug information on the Internet, **PDR.net** is the best online source for comprehensive FDA-approved and other manufacturer-supplied labeling information, as found in *PDR*. Updated monthly, this incredible resource allows you to look up drugs by brand or generic name, by key word, or by indication, side effect, contraindication, or manufacturer. The drug interaction checker allows you to screen for interactions among as many as 32 different drugs. The site provides an index that can be searched to find comparable drugs, and images of all products are included for easy identification. As an added benefit, *PDR.net* also gives users the option to order drug samples online. Finally, *PDR.net* hosts the download for *mobilePDR®*. At this one website, you get two great *PDR* products in one. In addition to all this, *PDR.net* provides links to such useful information as *Stedman's Medical Dictionary*, MEDLINE, online CME programs, clinical trials registries, evidence-based treatment decision tools, medical newsletters, Internet directories, online formularies, and the FDA's Medwatch. A wealth of information all in one place! Registration for *PDR.net* is free for U.S.-based MDs, DOs, NPs, and PAs in full-time patient practice as well as for medical students and residents. Visit www.PDR.net today to register.

For those times when all you need is quick confirmation of a particular dosage, you will want to have a copy of the **2005 PDR® Pharmacopoeia Pocket Dosing Guide**. Only slightly larger than an index card and a half inch thick, it fits easily into any pocket, and provides you with FDA-approved dosing recommendations for more than 1,500 drugs. Unlike other condensed drug references, the information is drawn almost exclusively from the FDA-approved drug labeling published in *Physicians' Desk Reference*. And its tabular presentation makes lookups a breeze. The *2005 PDR Pharmacopoeia Pocket Dosing Guide* is a tool you really can't afford to be without.

To help you counsel patients who use over-the-counter supplements, the **PDR® for Nutritional Supplements** offers the latest scientific consensus on hundreds of popular products, including amino acids, fatty acids, probiotics, phytoestrogens, phytosterols, over-the-counter hormones, and much more. Focused on the scientific evidence for each supplement's claims, this unique reference offers you today's most detailed, informed, and objective overview of a burgeoning new area in the field of self-treatment.

For counseling patients who favor herbal remedies, the newly updated **PDR® for Herbal Medicines Third Edition** provides you with the latest science-based assessment of more than 700 botanicals. Indexed by scientific and common names (as well as Western, Asian, and homeopathic indications), this volume also includes a Side Effects Index, a Drug/Herb Interactions Guide, an Herb Identification Guide with nearly 400 color photos, and a Safety Guide that lists herbs to be avoided during pregnancy and herbs to be used only under professional supervision. Although botanical products are not officially regulated or monitored in the United States, *PDR for Herbal Medicines* provides you with authoritative information—the findings of the German Regulatory Authority's expert committee on herbal medicines, Commission E.

To maximize the value of *PDR* itself, you'll also need a copy of the 2005 edition of the **PDR® Companion Guide**, a 1,700-page reference that augments *PDR* with nine unique decision-making tools:

- *Interactions Index* identifies pharmaceuticals and foods capable of interacting with a chosen medication.
- *Food Interactions Cross-Reference* lists drugs that may interact with a given dietary item.
- *Side Effects Index* pinpoints pharmaceuticals associated with each of 3,600 distinct adverse reactions.
- *Indications Index* presents a broad range of therapeutic options for any given diagnosis.
- *Off-Label Treatment Guide* lists medications routinely used—but never officially approved—for treatment of nearly 1,000 specific disorders.
- *Contraindications Index* lists drugs to avoid in the presence of any given medical condition.
- *International Drug Name Index* names the U.S. equivalents of some 15,000 foreign medications.
- *Generic Availability Guide* shows which forms and strengths of a brand-name drug are also available generically.
- *Imprint Identification Guide* enables you to establish the nature of any unknown tablet or capsule by matching its imprint against an exhaustive catalog of identifying codes.

PDR and its major companion volumes are also found in the ***PDR® Electronic Library*** on CD-ROM. This Windows-compatible disc provides users with a complete database of *PDR* prescribing information, electronically searchable for instant retrieval. A standard subscription includes *PDR's* sophisticated search software and an extensive file of chemical structures, illustrations, and full-color product photographs. Optional enhancements include the complete contents of *The Merck Manual Seventeenth Edition, Stedman's Medical Dictionary,* and *Stedman's Spellchecker.* For anyone who wants to run a fast double check on a proposed prescription, there's also the *PDR® Drug Interactions and Side Effects System* — sophisticated software capable of automatically screening a 20-drug regimen for conflicts, then proposing alternatives for any problematic medication. This unique decision-making tool comes free with the *PDR Electronic Library.* For more information on these or any other members of the growing family of *PDR* products, please call, toll-free, 1-800-232-7379 or fax 201-722-2680.

CONTENTS

MANUFACTURERS' INDEX

Listed in this index are all manufacturers participating in PHYSICIANS' DESK REFERENCE®. It is through their courtesy that PDR® is brought to the medical profession.

Each company's entry includes the address, phone, and fax number of its headquarters and regional offices, as well as contacts for inquiries, orders, and medical emergency information. Products with entries in the Product Information or Diagnostic Product Information sections are listed with their page numbers. Other products available from the manufacturer are listed following the described products.

If an entry in the index lists multiple page numbers, the first ones shown refer to photographs of the product, the last one to its prescribing information.

- **Bold page numbers** indicate full prescribing information.
- *Italic page numbers* signify partial information.
- The ◆ symbol marks drugs shown in the Product Identification Guide.
- The ▣ symbol means product information is located in *PDR For Nonprescription Drugs and Dietary Supplements*™.
- The ⊙ symbol means product information is located in *PDR For Ophthalmic Medicines*™.

AAI PHARMA **402**

2320 Scientific Park Drive
Wilmington, NC 28405

Direct Inquiries to:
(877) 263-6726
FAX: (866) 463-6726

Products Described:

ABBOTT LABORATORIES **303, 406**

100 Abbott Park Rd.
Abbott Park, IL 60064

Pharmaceutical Products Division--
Direct Inquiries to:
Customer Service:
(800) 255-5162
Technical Services:
(800) 441-4987
For Medical Information Contact:
Generally:
(800) 633-9110
Adverse experiences or side effects (for all Abbott drug products):
(800) 633-9110
Sales and Ordering:
(800) 255-5162

Products Described:

Other Products Available:

8.4% Sodium Bicarbonate Injection, 50 mEq in 50 mL Abboject or Fliptop Vial
5% Sodium Chloride
0.45% Sodium Chloride Injection, USP
0.9% Sodium Chloride Injection
0.9% Sodium Chloride Injection, USP (ADD-Vantage)
0.9% Sodium Chloride Injection, USP (Partial Fill)
0.45% Sodium Chloride Irrigation, USP (Aqualite)
0.9% Sodium Chloride Irrigation, USP (Flex and Aqualite)
Sodium Lactate Injection, USP, 1/6 Molar
Sodium Phosphate 45 mMoL
Sorbitol-Mannitol Irrigation (Flex & Aqualite)
Surbex 750 with Zinc Filmtab
Surbex with C Filmtab
Surbex-T Filmtab
Tham Solution
Theophylline in 5% Dextrose Injection (0.4, 0.8, 1.6, 2, 3.2, 4 mg/mL)
TPN Electrolytes
Tridione Dulcet Tablets
Tubocurarine Chloride Injection, USP
Ultane (Sevoflurane)
Ureaphil
Urologic G Irrigation (Aqualite)
Water for Injection Bacteriostatic 30 mL Fliptop
Water for Injection, Sterile, USP, Amps, Vial
Water for Irrigation, Sterile, USP (Flex and Aqualite)
Water for Respiratory Therapy, Sterile (Flex)
Zinc 10 mL (1 mg/1 mL)

ACTELION PHARMACEUTICALS U.S., INC. 304, 533
400 Shoreline Ct., Suite 200
S. San Francisco, CA 94080

Direct Inquiries to:
Actelion Medical Information
(866) 228-3546 (follow the prompts)

Products Described:
◆Tracleer Tablets.................. **304, 533**
◆Zavesca Capsules................ **304, 536**

AGOURON PHARMACEUTICALS, A PFIZER COMPANY
(See PFIZER INC.)

ALAMO PHARMACEUTICALS 304, 541
9 Campus Drive
Parsippany, NJ 07054

Direct Inquiries to:
(310) 859-7799
FAX: (310) 859-7755

Products Described:
◆Fazaclo Orally Disintegrating Tablets......................... **304, 541**

ALCON LABORATORIES, INC. 304, 546
Alcon Laboratories, Inc.
And its affiliates
Corporate Headquarters
6201 South Freeway
Fort Worth, TX 76134

Direct Inquiries to:
Pharmaceuticals/Consumer: (800) 451-3937
(Therapeutic Drugs/Lens Care)
Surgical: (800) 862-5266
(Instrumentation/Surgical Meds)
(817) 293-0450 (Main Switchboard)

Products Described:
Azopt Ophthalmic Suspension......... **546**
Betoptic S Ophthalmic Suspension..... **547**
Bion Tears Lubricant Eye Drops....... **547**
Ciloxan Ophthalmic Ointment.......... **548**
Ciloxan Ophthalmic Solution........... **548**
Cipro HC Otic Suspension............. **549**
◆Ciprodex Otic Suspension......... **304, 550**
Naphcon-A Ophthalmic Solution....... **552**
Patanol Ophthalmic Solution........... **552**
Tears Naturale Forte Lubricant Eye Drops.............................. **553**
Tears Naturale Free Lubricant Eye Drops.............................. **553**
TobraDex Ophthalmic Ointment....... **553**
TobraDex Ophthalmic Suspension..... **554**
Travatan Ophthalmic Solution......... **555**
Vigamox Ophthalmic Solution......... **556**

Other Products Available:
A.C.S. Closure System Needles and Sutures
Adsorbonac Ophthalmic Solution
Alcaine Ophthalmic Solution
Alcon Surgical System (Irrigation/Aspiration Kits; Phacoemulsification Kits)
Alomide Ophthalmic Solution
A-OK Ophthalmic Knives
Betaxon Ophthalmic Suspension
BSS and BSS Plus Irrigation Solution Administration Set
BSS Irrigation Solution (15 mL, 30 mL, 250 mL, 500 mL)
BSS Plus Irrigation Solution (250 mL, 500 mL)
Cellugel Ophthalmic Viscosurgical Device
Cetamide Ointment
Cetapred Ointment
Clearcut Dual Bevel Knives
Custom Pak Procedure Packs
Cyclogyl Ophthalmic Solution
Cystitomes & Cannulas
DuoVisc Viscoelastic System
Duratears Naturale Lubricant Eye Ointment
Econopred Plus Ophthalmic Suspension
Emadine Ophthalmic Solution
Enuclene Cleaning/Lubricating Solution for Artificial Eyes
Epinal Ophthalmic Solution
Eye Pak Surgical Drapes
Eye-Stream Eye Irrigating Solution
Flarex Ophthalmic Suspension
Fluorescite Injection
Greishaber Iris Retractors
I-Knife Ophthalmic Knife
Intraocular Lenses
Iopidine Ophthalmic Solution
Isopto Atropine Ophthalmic Solution
Isopto Carbachol Ophthalmic Solution
Isopto Carpine Ophthalmic Solution
Isopto Cetapred Ophthalmic Solution
Isopto Homatropine Ophthalmic Solution
Isopto Hyoscine Ophthalmic Solution
Isopto Tears Ophthalmic Solution
I-Spear Surgical Eye Sponge
Maxidex Ointment
Maxitrol Ointment
Maxitrol Suspension
Microsponge Surgical Eye Sponge
Miostat Intraocular Miotic Solution
Mydfrin Ophthalmic Solution
Mydriacyl Ophthalmic Solution
Naphcon Solution
Natacyn Ophthalmic Suspension
Ocucel Lint-Free Surgical Products
Optemp Sterile Disposable Cautery
Osmoglyn Oral Osmotic Agent
Pilopine HS Gel
Post-Operative Kits
ProShield Corneal Collagen Shield
ProVisc Ophthalmic Viscosurgical Device
PTG, Alcon Applanation Pneumatonograph
Schirmer Tear Test Strips
SofGuard Flexible Eye Shield
Steri-Units Single Dose Surgical Drops
Tetracaine Hydrochloride
Tobrex Ophthalmic Solution
Tobrex Ophthalmic Ointment
Ultra Tears Lubricant Eye Drops
Vexol Ophthalmic Suspension
Viscoat Ophthalmic Viscosurgical Device

ALLERGAN, INC. 304, 557
2525 Dupont Drive
P.O. Box 19534
Irvine, CA 92623-9534

Direct Inquiries to:
(714) 246-4500

Products Described:
◆Acular Ophthalmic Solution...... **304, 557**
◆Acular LS Ophthalmic Solution......................... **304, 557**
◆Acular PF Ophthalmic Solution......................... **304, 558**
◆Alphagan P Ophthalmic Solution......................... **304, 559**
◆Blephamide Ophthalmic Ointment........................ **304, 560**
◆Blephamide Ophthalmic Suspension...................... **304, 561**
Botox Purified Neurotoxin Complex... **562**
Elestat Ophthalmic Solution........... **565**
◆Lumigan Ophthalmic Solution...... **304, 565**
Polytrim Ophthalmic Solution......... **567**
◆Restasis Ophthalmic Emulsion..... **304, 566**
◆Zymar Ophthalmic Solution....... **304, 568**

Other Products Available:
Albalon Ophthalmic Solution
Alocril Ophthalmic Solution
Azelex Cream
Betagan Ophthalmic Solution
Bleph-10 Ophthalmic Solution
Elimite Cream
Epifrin Sterile Ophthalmic Solution
Fluoroplex Topical Cream
FML Forte Ophthalmic Suspension
FML Ophthalmic Ointment
FML Ophthalmic Suspension
FML-S Ophthalmic Suspension
Genoptic Ophthalmic Solution
HMS Ophthalmic Suspension
Ocufen Ophthalmic Solution
Ocuflox Ophthalmic Solution
Ophthetic Ophthalmic Solution
Poly-Pred Ophthalmic Suspension
Pred Forte Ophthalmic Suspension
Pred-G Ophthalmic Ointment
Pred-G Ophthalmic Suspension
Pred Mild Ophthalmic Suspension
Propine Ophthalmic Solution
Refresh Celluvisc Lubricant Eye Drops
Refresh Endura Lubricant Eye Drops
Refresh Liquigel Lubricant Eye Drops
Refresh Plus Lubricant Eye Drops
Refresh P.M. Lubricant Eye Ointment
Refresh Tears Lubricant Eye Drops

ALLERGAN SKIN CARE
(See ALLERGAN, INC.)

ALPHA THERAPEUTIC CORPORATION
(see GRIFOLS BIOLOGICALS, INC.)

ALPHARMA BRANDED PRODUCTS DIVISION 304, 569
One New England Avenue
Piscataway, NJ 08854

Direct Inquiries to:
Medical Affairs
(877) 4-KADIAN

Products Described:
◆Kadian Capsules................. **304, 569**

ALTO PHARMACEUTICALS, INC. 304, 573
P.O. Box 271150
Tampa, FL 33688-1150

Direct Inquiries to:
John J. Cullaro
(800) 330-2891

Products Described:
◆Zinc-220 Capsules............... **304, 573**

Other Products Available:
Amino-G Tablets
Tri-Enz Tablets

AMARIN PHARMACEUTICALS
(see VALEANT PHARMACEUTICALS INTERNATIONAL)

AMERICAN RED CROSS 573
National Headquarters
Biomedical Services
2025 E Street NW
Washington, DC 20006-5009

Direct Inquiries to:
Medical Affairs Department:
(800) 293-5023
FAX: (202) 303-0089
Customer Service Department:
(800) 261-5772
Please see the American Red Cross Plasma Services Website for Full Prescribing Information: plasmaservices.redcross.org

Products Described:
Albuminar 5% Solution................. *573*
Albuminar 25% Solution............... *573*
Albumin 5% Solution................... *573*
Albumin 25% Solution.................. *573*
Genarc.................................. *573*
Monarc-M............................... *573*
Panglobulin............................. *573*
Panglobulin NF......................... *573*
Polygam S/D............................ *573*

AMGEN INC. 304, 573
One Amgen Center Drive
Thousand Oaks, CA 91320-1799

For Medical Information Contact:
Global Medical Affairs
(800) 772-6436
FAX: (805) 480-1299
In Emergencies:
(800) 772-6436
After Hours and Weekends:
(800) 772-6436

Sales and Ordering:
Customer Service Department
(800) 282-6436
FAX: (800) 292-6436

Products Described:
◆Aranesp for Injection....... **304, 305, 573**
◆Enbrel for Injection.............. **305, 577**
◆Epogen for Injection............. **305, 582**
◆Kineret Injection.................. **305, 588**
◆Neulasta Injection................ **305, 590**
◆Neupogen for Injection........... **305, 592**
◆Sensipar Tablets.................. **305, 597**

ANDRX LABORATORIES, INC. 305, 600
411 Hackensack Avenue, 3rd Floor
Hackensack, NJ 07601

Direct Inquiries to:
(800) 595-1883

Products Described:
◆Altoprev Extended-Release Tablets............................. **305, 600**
Fortamet Extended-Release Tablets.... **605**

ARCO PHARMACEUTICALS, INC. 610
105 Orville Drive
Bohemia, NY 11716

Direct Inquiries to:
Professional Service Department
(631) 567-9500

Products Described:
Mega-B Tablets........................ **610**

Other Products Available:
Arco-Lase Tablets
Arco-Lase Plus Tablets
Arcoret Tablets
Arcoret w/Iron Tablets
Arcotinic Liquid
Arcotinic Tablets
C-B Time Capsules
C-B Time Liquid
Co-Gel Tablets
Megadose Tablets
Spantuss Liquid

ASTRAZENECA LP 305, 610
Wilmington, DE 19850-5437

For Product and Business Information, and Adverse Drug Experiences:
Information Center
(800) 236-9933

For Product Ordering:
Trade Customer Service
(800) 842-9920
www.astrazeneca-us.com

Products Described:
Astramorph/PF Injection, USP (Preservative-Free)................... *610*
◆Atacand Tablets.................. **305, 610**
◆Atacand HCT 16-12.5 Tablets.... **305, 612**
◆Atacand HCT 32-12.5 Tablets.... **305, 612**
◆EMLA Cream...................... *305, 615*
EMLA Anesthetic Disc................. *615*
◆Entocort EC Capsules............ *305, 615*
Foscavir Injection..................... *616*
◆Lexxel Tablets.................... *305, 616*
◆Naropin Injection................ **305, 616**
Nesacaine Injection................... *621*
Nesacaine-MPF Injection.............. *621*
◆Nexium Delayed-Release Capsules......................... **305, 621**
◆Plendil Extended-Release Tablets........................... *305, 625*
Polocaine Injection, USP.............. *625*
Polocaine-MPF Injection, USP........ *625*
◆Prilosec Delayed-Release Capsules........................... *305, 625*
◆Pulmicort Respules............... **305, 625**
◆Pulmicort Turbuhaler Inhalation Powder................... *305, 629*
◆Rhinocort Aqua Nasal Spray...... **306, 630**
◆Toprol-XL Tablets................ **306, 632**
Xylocaine 2% Jelly.................... *635*

Other Products Available:
Aquasol E
Citanest Solutions

ASTRAZENECA PHARMACEUTICALS LP 306, 635
1800 Concord Pike
Wilmington, DE 19850-5437 USA

For Product and Business Information, and Adverse Drug Experiences:
Information Center
(800) 236-9933

For Product Ordering:
Trade Customer Service
(800) 842-9920
www.astrazeneca-us.com

Products Described:
◆Accolate Tablets.................. **306, 635**
◆Arimidex Tablets................. **306, 637**
◆Casodex Tablets.................. **306, 642**
◆Cefotan for Injection............ *306, 644*
Cefotan Injection...................... *644*
◆Crestor Tablets................... **306, 644**
◆Diprivan Injectable Emulsion..... **306, 647**
◆Faslodex Injection............... **306, 653**
◆Iressa Tablets.................... **306, 656**
◆Merrem I.V....................... **306, 658**
◆Nolvadex Tablets................. **306, 662**
◆Seroquel Tablets................. **306, 662**
◆Tenormin I.V. Injection.......... *306, 667*
◆Tenormin Tablets................. *306, 667*
◆Zestoretic Tablets................ *306, 667*
◆Zestril Tablets................... *306, 667*
◆Zoladex........................... **306, 668**
Zoladex 3-month...................... **671**

AUXILIUM PHARMACEUTICALS, INC. 673
160 West Germantown Pike
Norristown, PA 19401

Direct Inquiries to:
(610) 239-1499

Products Described:
Testim 1% Gel......................... **673**

AVENTIS BEHRING
(see ZLB BEHRING)

AVENTIS PASTEUR INC. 755
Swiftwater, PA 18370

For Medical Information Contact:
Generally:
Medical Affairs
(800) VACCINE
(800) 822-2463
www.us.aventispasteur.com

Adverse Drug Experiences:
Pharmacovigilance Department
(570) 839-7187
(800) 822-2463

Sales and Ordering:
Aventis Pasteur Inc.
Customer Service
(800) VACCINE
(800) 822-2463
(570) 839-7187
www.vaccineshoppe.com

Products Described:
DAPTACEL ... 755
Menomune-A/C/Y/W-135 ... 760
YF-VAX ... 762

Other Products Available:
ActHIB
Diphtheria & Tetanus Toxoids Adsorbed USP (For Pediatric Use)
Fluzone
Fluzone Preservative-free: Pediatric Dose
Imogam Rabies - HT
IMOVAX Rabies
IPOL
JE-VAX
Tetanus and Diphtheria Toxoids Adsorbed For Adult Use
Tetanus Toxoid Adsorbed USP
Tetanus Toxoid for Booster Use Only
Tetanus Toxoid USP
TheraCys
TriHIBit
Tripedia
TYPHIM Vi

AVENTIS PHARMACEUTICALS INC. 306, 676
300 Somerset Corporate Boulevard
Bridgewater, NJ 08807-2854

Direct Inquiries to:
Customer Service
300 Somerset Corporate Boulevard
Bridgewater, NJ 08807-2854
(800) 207-8049

For Medical Information Contact:
Generally:
Medical Information Services
300 Somerset Corporate Boulevard
Bridgewater, NJ 08807-2854
(800) 633-1610

For Oncology Medical Information Contact:
(866) 662-6411

Products Described:
Allegra Capsules ... 676
◆Allegra Tablets ... 306, 676
◆Allegra-D Extended-Release Tablets ... 306, 678
◆Amaryl Tablets ... 307, 681
◆Anzemet Injection ... 307, 683
◆Anzemet Tablets ... 307, 686
Apidra Injection ... 688
◆Arava Tablets ... 307, 693
Cantil Tablets ... *676*
◆Claforan Sterile for Injection ... 307, 699
◆Clomid Tablets ... 307, 702
◆DDAVP Injection 4 mcg/mL ... 307, 704
◆DDAVP Nasal Spray ... 307, 705
◆DDAVP Tablets ... 307, 707
◆DiaBeta Tablets ... 307, 708
Hiprex Tablets ... *676*
◆Ketek Tablets ... 307, 710
◆Lantus Injection ... 307, 715
Lasix Tablets ... *676*
◆Lovenox Injection ... 307, 719
Nasacort HFA Inhalation Aerosol ... 726
◆Nasacort AQ Nasal Spray ... 307, 725
◆Nilandron Tablets ... 307, 729
◆Norpramin Tablets ... 307, 731
Priftin Tablets ... 732
◆Rifadin Capsules ... 307, 736
Rifadin IV ... 736
◆Rifamate Capsules ... 307, 739
◆Rifater Tablets ... 307, 740
◆Rilutek Tablets ... 307, 744
◆Taxotere Injection Concentrate ... 307, 746
Tenuate Tablets/Dospan ... *676*
◆Trental Tablets ... 307, 754

AXCAN PHARMA U.S. INC.
(See AXCAN SCANDIPHARM INC.)

AXCAN SCANDIPHARM INC. 307, 764
22 Inverness Center Parkway
Birmingham, AL 35242

Direct Inquiries to:
Customer Service
(800) 950-8085
FAX: (205) 991-8426

For Medical Information Contact:
Marie-Helen Doyon
(800) 565-3255
FAX: (450) 467-5857

Products Described:
Bentyl Capsules ... 764
Bentyl Injection ... 764
Bentyl Syrup ... 764
Bentyl Tablets ... 764
◆Canasa Rectal Suppositories ... 307, 765
Carafate Suspension ... 767
Carafate Tablets ... 768
◆Photofrin for Injection ... 307, 769
◆Ultrase Capsules ... 307, 775
◆Ultrase MT Capsules ... 307, 775
◆Urso 250 Tablets ... 307, 776
Viokase Powder ... 777
◆Viokase Tablets ... 307, 777

Other Products Available:
ADEKs Multivitamin Supplement
ADEKs Pediatric Drops
FLUTTER
SCANDICAL
SCANDISHAKE
SCANDISHAKE -- Lactose Free
SCANDISHAKE -- Sweetened with Aspartame

BALLAY PHARMACEUTICALS, INC. 778
P.O. Box 1356
Wimberley, TX 78676

Direct Inquiries to:
Terry Ballay, President
(512) 847-6458

Products Described:
Alacol DM Syrup ... 778
Balamine DM Oral Drops ... 779
Balamine DM Syrup ... 779
Baltussin ... *778*
Nortemp Suspension ... *778*

BARR LABORATORIES 311, 779
2 Quaker Road, P.O. Box 2900
Pomona, NY 10970

Direct Inquiries to:
(800) BARRLAB (227-7522)

Products Described:
◆Plan B Tablets ... 311, 779
◆Seasonale Tablets ... 311, 781

BAXTER HEALTHCARE CORPORATION ANESTHESIA & CRITICAL CARE 804
95 Spring Street
New Providence, NJ 07974

Direct Inquiries to:
Professional Services Department
(800) ANA-DRUG
(800) 262-3784

For Medical Emergencies Contact:
Paula Dimopoulos PharmD
Director Medical Affairs
(800) ANA-DRUG
(800) 262-3784

Sales and Ordering:
To place an order call or fax:
(800) 667-0959
FAX: (877) 702-3580

Products Described:
Brevibloc Concentrate ... 804
Brevibloc Injection ... 804
Brevibloc Double Strength Injection ... 804
Brevibloc Premixed Injection ... 804
Brevibloc Double Strength Premixed Injection ... 804
Dopram Injectable ... *808*
Enlon Injection ... *808*
Enlon-Plus Injection ... *808*
Ethrane Liquid for Inhalation ... *808*
Factrel ... *3438*
Forane Liquid for Inhalation ... *808*
Phenergan Injection ... *808*
Propofol Injectable Emulsion 1% ... *809*
Protopam Chloride for Injection, USP ... *809*
Revex Injection ... *809*
Robaxin Injectable ... *809*
Suprane Liquid for Inhalation ... 809

BAXTER HEALTHCARE CORPORATION 788
1 Baxter Way
Westlake Village, CA 91362

Direct Inquiries to:
Product Management
(800) 423-2090

For Medical Emergencies Contact:
Edward Gomperts, M.D.
Medical Director,
Baxter Healthcare Corporation:
(805) 372-3000

Manufacturing and Distribution:
Coagulation Products Distributed By:
Baxter Healthcare Corporation,
Westlake Village, CA 91362
(800) 423-2090

Plasma Expanders & Gamma Globulin Products Distributed By:
Baxter Healthcare Corporation,
Westlake Village, CA 91362
(800) 423-2090

Products Described:
Advate Injection ... 788
Aralast ... 791
Buminate 5% Solution, USP ... 793
Buminate 25% Solution, USP ... 794
Feiba VH ... 795
Gammagard S/D ... 797
Hemofil M ... 800
Recombinate ... 801

BAYER CORPORATION 307, 859
Pharmaceutical Division
Biological Products
Elkhart, IN 46515

For Clinical Communications Contact:
Director, Clinical Services
(800) 288-8371
(203) 812-6901

Adverse Drug Experiences:
(800) 288-8371

Products Described:
BayGam ... 859
BayHep B ... 860
BayRab ... 861
BayRho-D Full Dose ... 865
BayRho-D Mini-Dose ... 863
BayTet ... 868
◆Biltricide Tablets ... 308, 3424
◆Gamimune N, 10% Solvent/Detergent Treated ... 307, 869
Gamunex Immune Globulin I.V., 10% ... 872
Koāte-DVI ... 877
Kogenate FS ... 878
Plasbumin-5 ... 880
Plasbumin-25 ... 881
Plasmanate ... 882
Prolastin ... 883
Thrombate III ... 884

BAYER PHARMACEUTICALS CORPORATION 307, 813
400 Morgan Lane
West Haven, CT 06516

For Medical Information Contact:
Director, Clinical Services
(800) 288-8371
(203) 812-2000

Adverse Drug Experiences:
(888) 765-3203

Products Described:
◆Adalat CC Tablets ... 307, 813
◆Avelox I.V. ... 308, 815
◆Avelox Tablets ... 308, 815
◆Cipro I.V. ... 308, 827
◆Cipro I.V. Pharmacy Bulk Package ... 308, 833
◆Cipro Oral Suspension ... 308, 821
◆Cipro Tablets ... 308, 821
◆Cipro XR Tablets ... 308, 839
DTIC-Dome ... 844
◆Levitra Tablets ... 308, 845
◆Nimotop Capsules ... 308, 848
◆Precose Tablets ... 308, 850
◆Trasylol Injection ... 308, 853
◆Viadur Implant ... 308, 856

Other Products Available:
Dome-Paste Bandage (Unna's Boot)

BEACH PHARMACEUTICALS 308, 886
Division of Beach Products, Inc.
5220 S. Manhattan Avenue
Tampa, FL 33611

Direct Inquiries to:
Richard Stephen Jenkins
(813) 839-6565
FAX: (813) 837-2511

Manufacturing and Distribution:
201 Delaware Street
Greenville, SC 29605
(800) 845-8210

Products Described:
◆Beelith Tablets ... 308, 886
◆K-Phos M.F. Tablets ... *308, 886*
◆K-Phos Neutral Tablets ... 308, 886
◆K-Phos No. 2 Tablets ... *308, 886*
◆K-Phos Original (Sodium Free) Tablets ... 308, 887
◆Uroqid-Acid No. 2 Tablets ... 308, 887

BEDFORD LABORATORIES 888
A Division of Ben Venue Laboratories, Inc.
300 Northfield Road
Bedford, OH 44146

Direct Inquiries to:
Customer Service
(800) 562-4797
FAX: (440) 232-6264

For Medical Emergencies Contact:
Professional Services
(800) 521-5169

Products Described:
Adriamycin for Injection, USP ... 888
Adriamycin Injection, USP ... 888
Cerubidine for Injection ... 890
GlucaGen for Injection ... 892

Other Products Available:
Acetazolamide for Injection USP
Acyclovir for Injection USP
Adenosine Injection USP
Alprostadil Injection, USP
Amikacin Sulfate Injection, USP
Amiodarone Hydrochloride Injection
Atracurium Besylate Injection
Azathioprine Sodium for Injection, USP
Bleomycin for Injection USP
Bumetanide Injection, USP
Butorphanol Tartrate Injection, USP CIV
Caffeine and Sodium Benzoate Injection USP
Carboplatin Injection
Chloroprocaine Hydrochloride Injection, USP
Cisplatin Injection
Cladribine Injection
Colchicine Injection, USP
Cyclosporine Injection, USP
Cytarabine for Injection USP
Dacarbazine for Injection USP
Daunorubicin Hydrochloride Injection (Solution)
Dicyclomine Hydrochloride Injection
Dihydroergotamine Mesylate Injection USP
Diltiazem Hydrochloride Injection
Dipyridamole Injection
Dobutamine Injection USP
Doxapram Hydrochloride Injection USP
Doxycycline for Injection, USP
Enaliprilat Injection
Ephedrine Sulfate Injection, USP
Esmolol Hydrochloride Injection
Etomidate Injection
Etoposide Injection
Famotidine Injection
Fenoldopam Mesylate Injection USP
Floxuridine for Injection USP
Fluconazole Injection
Flumazenil Injection
Fluphenazine Decanoate Injection, USP
Haloperidol Decanoate Injection
Haloperidol Injection USP
Inamrinone Injection, USP
Ketamine Hydrochloride Injection, USP CIII
Ketorolac Tromethamine Injection USP
Labetalol Hydrochloride Injection USP
Leucovorin Calcium for Injection (Lyophilized)
Leucovorin Calcium Injection, USP (Solution)
Levocarnitine Injection, USP
Levothyroxine Sodium for Injection
Mesna Injection
Methotrexate Injection USP
Metoprolol Tartrate Injection
Midazolam Hydrochloride Injection CIV
Milrinone Lactate Injection
Mitomycin for Injection, USP
Norepinephrine Bitartrate Injection USP
Orphenadrine Citrate Injection USP
Paclitaxel Injection
Pamidronate Disodium Injection
Pamidronate Disodium for Injection
Papaverine Hydrochloride Injection, USP
Phentolamine Mesylate for Injection, USP
Polymyxin B for Injection
Prochlorperazine Edisylate Injection USP
Propranolol Hydrochloride Injection USP
Rifampin for Injection, USP
Terbutaline Sulfate Injection USP
Thiotepa for Injection, USP
Valproate Sodium Injection
Vecuronium Bromide for Injection
Vinblastine Sulfate for Injection, USP
Vinorelbine Tartrate Injection

BERLEX, INC. 308, 893
6 West Belt
Wayne, NJ 07470
www.Berlex.com

Direct Inquiries to:
(888) BERLEX-4

Products Described:
◆Betaseron for SC Injection ... 308, 893
◆Climara Transdermal System ... 308, 897
◆Climara Pro Transdermal System ... 308, 902
◆Finacea Gel ... 308, 907
Levlen 21 Tablets ... 908
◆Levlen 28 Tablets ... 308, 908
◆Levlite 28 Tablets ... 308, 908
◆Menostar Transdermal System ... 308, 917
◆Mirena Intrauterine System ... 309, 921
◆Refludan for Injection ... 309, 926
Tri-Levlen 21 Tablets ... 908
◆Tri-Levlen 28 Tablets ... 309, 908
◆Yasmin 28 Tablets ... 309, 930

Other Products Available:
Campath Ampules (See BERLEX INC., WA)
Fludara for Injection (See BERLEX INC., WA)

BERLEX, INC. 308, 938
1191 Second Ave, Suite 1100
Seattle, WA 98101-2120

Direct Inquiries to:
(888) BERLEX-4

Products Described:
Campath Ampules ...
◆Fludara for Injection
Leukine ...

BERNA PRODUCTS, CORP. **309, 947**
an Acambis Company
4216 Ponce de Leon Boulevard
Coral Gables, FL 33146

Direct Inquiries to:
Gregory Koppel
(305) 443-2900 Ext. 242
(800) 533-5899

For Medical Information Contact:
Generally:
Andres Murai, Jr.
(305) 443-2900
(800) 533-5899
In Emergencies:
Andres Murai, Jr.
(305) 443-2900
(800) 533-5899

Products Described:
◆Vivotif.......................... **309, 947**

BERTEK PHARMACEUTICALS INC.
(See MYLAN BERTEK PHARMACEUTICALS INC.)

BEUTLICH LP PHARMACEUTICALS **948**
1541 Shields Drive
Waukegan, IL 60085-8304

Direct Inquiries to:
(847) 473-1100
(800) 238-8542 (in U.S. and Canada)
FAX: (847) 473-1122
E-mail: beutlich@beutlich.com
www.beutlich.com

Products Described:
Hurricaine Topical Anesthetic Aerosol Spray, 2 oz. Wild Cherry ... *948*
Hurricaine Topical Anesthetic Aerosol Spray, 2oz. Wild Cherry with 200 Disposable Extension Tubes........................ *948*
Hurricaine Topical Anesthetic Gel: 1 oz. Wild Cherry, Fresh Mint, Pina Colada, Watermelon, 1/6 oz. Wild Cherry...................... *948*
Hurricaine Topical Anesthetic Liquid: 1 oz. Wild Cherry and Pina Colada .25 ml Swab Applicator Wild Cherry............ *948*
Hurricaine Topical Anesthetic Spray Kit.............................. *948*
Hurricaine 5 ml. Snap N Go Tubes.... *948*
Peridin-C Tablets........................ *949*

BIOGEN, INC. - DERMATOLOGY
(see BIOGEN IDEC)

BIOGEN IDEC **949**
14 Cambridge Center
Cambridge, MA 02142

Direct Inquiries to:
AMEVIVE Customer Service:
(866) 263-8483
FAX: (866) 420-8888
AVONEX Customer Service:
(800) 456-2255
FAX: (617) 679-8100
RITUXAN Customer Service:
(800) 821-8590
ZEVALIN Customer Service:
(877) 433-4332

Products Described:
Amevive................................ **949**
Avonex................................. **951**
Rituxan for Infusion................... **958**
Zevalin Injection...................... **960**

BIOGEN, INC. - NEUROLOGY
(see BIOGEN IDEC)

BIOGLAN PHARMACEUTICALS COMPANY **965**
7 Great Valley Parkway
Suite 301
Malvern, PA 19355

Direct Inquiries to:
Phone (888) 246-4526
FAX (610) 232-2020

Products Described:
Adoxa Tablets.......................... *965*
Solaraze Gel........................... *966*
Zonalon Cream.......................... *966*

BIOMARIN PHARMACEUTICAL **966**
...ays Blvd.

BIOVAIL PHARMACEUTICALS, INC. **968**
700 Route 202-206 North
Bridgewater, NJ 08807-0980

Direct Inquiries to:
(866) BIOVAIL
(866) 246-8245

Products Described:
Cardizem LA Extended Release Tablets.............................. **968**
Teveten Tablets........................ **970**
Teveten HCT Tablets.................... **972**
Zovirax Cream.......................... **976**
Zovirax Ointment....................... **977**

BLAINE PHARMACEUTICALS **978**
1717 Dixie Highway
Suite 700
Fort Wright, KY 41011

For Inquiries or Medical Information Contact:
(859) 344-9600
(800) 633-9353
FAX: (859) 344-9601
www.MagOx.com

Products Described:
Mag-Ox 400 Tablets..................... **978**
Uro-Mag Capsules....................... **978**

BLANSETT PHARMACAL CO., INC. **978**
P.O. Box 638
North Little Rock, AR 72115
www.blansett.com

Direct Inquiries to:
Customer Service
(501) 758-8635
FAX: (501) 758-5369

Direct ProctoFoam HC Inquiries to:
Schwarz Pharma
Professional Services
(800) 558-5114
FAX (262) 238-0311

Products Described:
Cortane-B Aqueous Ear Drops........ *978*
Cortane-B Otic Drops.................. *978*
Nalex A-12 Suspension................. *978*
Proctofoam-HC......................... *978*
Relagard Therapeutic Vaginal Gel..... *978*

Other Products Available:
B-Tuss
Cortane-B Lotion
Nalex DH Liquid
Nalex Expectorant
Nalex-A Liquid
NutraCare Chewables
Prolex DH Liquid
Prolex DM Liquid
Prolex-D Tablets
Prolex-PD Tablets

BOEHRINGER INGELHEIM PHARMACEUTICALS, INC. **309, 978**
A subsidiary of Boehringer Ingelheim Corporation
900 Ridgebury Road
P.O. Box 368
Ridgefield, CT 06877-0368

For Medical Information Contact:
(800) 542-6257
E-mail:
druginfo@rdg.boehringer-ingelheim.com

Products Described:
◆Aggrenox Capsules............. **309, 978**
◆Alupent Inhalation Aerosol....... **309, 982**
◆Atrovent Inhalation Aerosol....... **309, 982**
◆Atrovent Inhalation Solution..... **309, 984**
◆Atrovent Nasal Spray 0.03%..... **309, 985**
◆Atrovent Nasal Spray 0.06%..... **309, 986**
◆Catapres Tablets................ **309, 988**
◆Catapres-TTS.................... **309, 989**
◆Combivent Inhalation Aerosol.... **309, 991**
◆Flomax Capsules................. **309, 994**
◆Micardis Tablets................ **309, 997**
◆Micardis HCT Tablets............ **309, 999**
Mirapex Tablets..................... **1002**
◆Mobic Tablets................... **309, 1006**
◆Persantine Tablets.............. **309, 1009**
◆Spiriva HandiHaler.............. **309, 1010**
◆Viramune Oral Suspension....... **309, 1013**
◆Viramune Tablets................ **309, 1013**

BONE CARE INTERNATIONAL **309, 1019**
Bone Care Center
1600 Aspen Commons
Middleton, WI 53562

Direct Inquiries to:
Professional Services Department
(888) 389-4242
FAX: (608) 662-7870

Products Described:
◆Hectorol Capsules............. **309, 1019**
◆Hectorol Injection............. **309, 1021**

BRAINTREE LABORATORIES, INC. **309, 1023**
P.O. Box 850929
Braintree, MA 02185-0929

Direct Inquiries to:
Harry P. Keegan, President
(781) 843-2202

For Medical Information or Emergencies Contact:
Jack DiPalma, M.D.
(800) 874-6756

Products Described:
◆GoLYTELY and Pineapple Flavor GoLYTELY for Oral Solution...................... **309, 1023**
◆HalfLytely and Bisacodyl Tablets......................... **309, 1024**
◆MiraLax Powder for Oral Solution......................... **309, 1025**
◆NuLYTELY, Cherry Flavor, Lemon-Lime Flavor, and Orange Flavor NuLYTELY for Oral Solution............ **309, 1023**

BRISTOL-MYERS SQUIBB COMPANY **310, 1026**
P.O. Box 4500
Princeton, NJ 08543-4500
(609) 897-2000

For Medical Information Contact:
Generally:
Bristol-Myers Squibb Drug Information Department
P.O. Box 4500
Princeton, NJ 08543-4500
(800) 321-1335
Adverse Drug Experiences and Product Defects Reporting
call between 8:30 AM-4:30 PM EST:
(609) 818-3737

Sales and Ordering:
Orders may be placed by:

1. Calling your purchase orders toll-free between 8:30 AM-5:00 PM EST: (800) 631-5244

2. Mailing your purchase orders to: Bristol-Myers Squibb U.S. Pharmaceuticals Attn: Customer Service P.O. Box 5250 Princeton, NJ 08543-5250

3. Faxing your purchase orders to: (800) 523-2965

4. Transmitting computer-to-computer on the NWDA and UCS formats through Ordernet Services use: DEA # PE0048579

Products Described:
◆Abilify Tablets................ **310, 1026**
◆Avalide Tablets................ **310, 1030**
◆Avapro Tablets................. **310, 1034**
Cefzil for Oral Suspension........... **1037**
◆Cefzil Tablets................. **310, 1037**
Coumadin for Injection.............. **1039**
◆Coumadin Tablets............... **310, 1039**
◆Erbitux........................ **310, 1044**
◆Metaglip Tablets............... **310, 1047**
◆Plavix Tablets................. **310, 1052**
◆Pravachol Tablets.............. **310, 1055**
◆Reyataz Capsules............... **310, 1060**
◆Sustiva Capsules............... **310, 1069**
◆Tequin Injection............... **310, 1075**
◆Tequin Tablets................. **310, 1075**
◆Videx EC Capsules.............. **310, 1082**
◆Zerit Capsules................. **310, 1087**
◆Zerit for Oral Solution........ **310, 1087**

J. R. CARLSON LABORATORIES, INC. **1091**
15 College Drive
Arlington Heights, IL 60004-1985

Direct Inquiries to:
Customer Service
(847) 255-1600
FAX: (847) 255-1605
www.carlsonlabs.com

For Medical Emergencies Contact:
Customer Service
(847) 255-1600
FAX: (847) 255-1605

Products Described:
ACES Antioxidant Soft Gels......... *1091*
E-Gems Soft Gels.................. *1091*
Norwegian Cod Liver Oil........... *1091*
Super Omega-3 Softgels............ *1091*

CELGENE CORPORATION **310, 1092**
7 Powder Horn Drive
Warren, NJ 07059
(732) 271-1001
(800) 890-4619

Direct Inquiries to:
Customer Service:
(888) 4-CELGENE
(888) 423-5436
Medical Services:
(732) 805-3905
FAX: (732) 805-3671
Drug Safety:
(732) 805-3667
FAX: (732) 271-4115

Products Described:
◆Alkeran for Injection........... **310, 1092**
◆Alkeran Tablets................. **310, 1093**
◆Thalomid Capsules............... **310, 1095**

CELL THERAPEUTICS, INC. **310, 1099**
501 Elliott Avenue West
Seattle, WA 98119

Direct Medical Inquiries to:
Professional Services
(800) 715-0944
(510) 985-9750

Customer Service:
(888) 305-2289

Products Described:
◆Trisenox Injection.............. **310, 1099**

CELLTECH PHARMACEUTICALS, INC. **1102**
755 Jefferson Road
Rochester, NY 14623

Direct Inquiries to:
Customer Service Department
P.O. Box 31766
(585) 932-1950
Rochester, NY 14603
(888) 963-3382
(585 274-5300

For Medical Emergencies Contact:
(800) 932-1950 (24 hrs.)

Products Described:
Americaine Anesthetic Lubricant..... **1102**
Dipentum Capsules.................. **1103**
Gastrocrom Oral Concentrate........ **1104**
Ionamin Capsules................... **1105**
Metadate CD Capsules............... **1106**
Metadate ER Tablets................ **1109**
Pediapred Oral Solution............ **1110**
Semprex-D Capsules................. **1112**
Tussionex Pennkinetic Extended-Release Suspension...... **1114**
Zaroxolyn Tablets.................. **1115**

CENTEON L.L.C.
(See ZLB BEHRING)

CENTOCOR, INC. **310, 1117**
200 Great Valley Parkway
Malvern, PA 19355

Direct General Inquiries to:
(610) 651-6000
(888) 874-3083
FAX: (610) 651-6100

For Medical Emergencies Contact:
(800) 457-6399

For Medical Information/Adverse Experience Reporting Contact:
Medical Information
(800) 457-6399

Branch Office:
Centocor B.V.
Einsteinweg 92
2333 CB Leiden, The Netherlands

Products Described:
◆Remicade for IV Injection...... **310, 1117**

Other Products Available:
ReoPro Vials
Retavase Vials

CEPHALON, INC. **310, 1122**
145 Brandywine Parkway
West Chester, PA 19380

For Medical Information and Adverse Drug Experience/Product Complaint Reporting Contact:
(800) 896-5855
FAX: (610) 738-6669

Products Described:
◆Actiq.......................... **310, 1122**
◆Gabitril Tablets............... **310, 1126**
◆Provigil Tablets............... **311, 1131**

CETYLITE INDUSTRIES, INC. 311, 1136
9051 River Road
Pennsauken, NJ 08110-3293
Mailing Address:
P.O. Box 90006
Pennsauken, NJ 08110-0700

Direct Inquiries to:
Mr. Stanley L. Wachman, President
(856) 665-6111
(800) 257-7740
FAX: (856) 665-5408

Products Described:
◆Cetacaine Topical Anesthetic.... **311, 1136**

Other Products Available:
Cetylcide G Sterilant
Cetylcide II Germicidal Concentrate
Cetylite Airfresh Deodorizer
Cetylite Skin Screen Protective Skin Lotion
Protexin Oral Breath Spray
Release Antiadhesive
Ultrasonic Cleaner
Varnal Cavity Varnish
Zarosen Desensitizer

CHIRON CORPORATION 311, 1136
4560 Horton Street
Emeryville, CA 94608-2916

For Medical Information Contact:
Generally:
Drug Information Services:
(800) CHIRON-8 selection #2
(800) 244-7668 selection #2
FAX: (510) 923-3435
E-mail: drug_info@chiron.com
Adverse Event Reporting:
(800) CHIRON-8 selection #3
(800) 244-7668 selection #3
After Hours & Weekends:
(415) 487-8335

Sales and Ordering:
(800) CHIRON-8 selection #1
(800) 244-7668 selection #1
FAX: (510) 923-3434

Products Described:
Proleukin for Injection.............. **1136**
◆Rabies Vaccine RabAvert....... **311, 1140**
◆TOBI Solution for Inhalation.... **311, 1143**

CLAY-PARK LABS, INC. 1145
1700 Bathgate Avenue
Bronx, NY 10457

Direct Inquires to:
(800) 933-5550

Products Described:
Ammonium Lactate Cream, 12%..... *1145*
Ammonium Lactate Lotion, 12%..... *1145*
Antipyrine/Benzocaine Otic Drops ... *1145*
Betamethasone Dipropionate Cream USP, 0.05%.............. *1145*
etamethasone Dipropionate Lotion USP, 0.05%.............. *1145*
Clindamycin Phosphate Pledgets, 1%.............. *1145*
Desonide Cream 0.05%.............. *1145*
Desonide Ointment 0.05%.......... *1145*
Desoximetasone Cream USP, 0.25%.............. *1145*
Econazole Nitrate Cream 1%......... *1145*
Erythromycin Topical Solution USP, 2%.............. *1145*
Erythromycin-Benzoyl Peroxide Topical Gel.............. *1145*
Fluticasone Propionate Cream, 0.05%.............. *1145*
Fluticasone Propionate Ointment, 0.005%.............. *1145*
Gentamicin Sulfate Cream, USP..... *1145*
Gentamicin Sulfate Ointment, USP... *1145*
Hydrocortisone Acetate Suppositories, 25 mg.............. *1145*
Hydrocortisone Cream USP, 2.5%.... *1145*
Hydrocortisone Ointment USP, 2.5%.............. *1145*
Hydrocortisone Valerate Cream USP, 0.2%.............. *1145*
Ketoconazole Shampoo, 2%........... *1145*
Mometasone Furoate Ointment USP, 0.1%.............. *1145*
Mupirocin Ointment USP, 2%......... *1145*
Nystatin Cream, USP.............. *1145*
Nystatin Ointment, USP............ *1145*
Permethrin Cream, 5%.............. *1145*
Promethazine Hydrochloride Suppositories USP, 12.5 mg......... *1145*
Promethazine Hydrochloride Suppositories USP, 25 mg......... *1145*
Selenium Sulfide Lotion USP, 2.5%.............. *1145*
Triamcinolone Acetonide Cream USP, 0.025%.............. *1145*
Triamcinolone Acetonide Cream USP, 0.1%.............. *1145*
Triamcinolone Acetonide Cream USP, 0.5%.............. *1145*
Triamcinolone Acetonide Ointment USP, 0.025%.............. *1145*
Triamcinolone Acetonide Ointment USP, 0.1%.............. *1145*
Triamcinolone Acetonide Ointment USP, 0.5%.............. *1145*
Tridesilon 0.05% Cream.............. *1145*
Tridesilon 0.05% Ointment.......... *1145*
Trimethobenzamide Suppositories, 100 mg.............. *1145*
Trimethobenzamide Suppositories, 200 mg.............. *1145*

COLLAGENEX PHARMACEUTICALS, INC. 1146
41 University Drive, Ste. 200
Newtown, PA 18940

Direct Inquiries to:
(888) 339-5678

Products Described:
Pandel Cream, 0.1%................ **1146**
Periostat Tablets.................... **1147**

COLUMBIA LABORATORIES, INC. 311, 1148
354 Eisenhower Parkway
Second Floor- Plaza I
Livingston, NJ 07039

Direct Inquiries to:
(973) 994-3999
FAX: (973) 994-3001 or (973) 994-2771

Products Described:
◆Prochieve 4% Gel.............. **311, 1148**
◆Prochieve 8% Gel.............. **311, 1148**
◆Striant Mucoadhesive........... **311, 1150**

CONNETICS CORPORATION 311, 1153
3290 West Bayshore Road
Palo Alto, CA 94303

Direct Inquiries to:
(650) 843-2800
FAX: (650) 843-2899
www.connetics.com

For Medical Information Contact:
Medical Information Department
(877) 821-5337
FAX: (510) 595-8183
E-mail: medicalaffairs@connetics.com

Products Described:
Luxíq Foam **1153**
Olux Foam.............. **1154**
◆Soriatane Capsules.............. **311, 1156**

CPH INTERNATIONAL 1162
P.O. Box 11439
Oakland, CA 94611

For Medical Information Contact:
FAX: (510) 352-6009
The following products are available for export.

Direct Inquiries to:
CPH International Corp. P.O. Box 94611
Oakland, CA 94611
FAX: (510) 352-6009

Products Described:
Acrobin.............. *1162*
Catasod-Ocuxtra/Optigold/Macutein.. **1162**
Cinaplex.............. *1162*
Cynaxin/ATK-250/Artichin/Scokin.... *1162*
Fenaxin.............. *1162*
Immulein Tablets.............. *1162*
Multizyme/Superzyme Chewable/Neo-Prozyme/Absorpase. *1162*
NT-Kinase 500/Fibrinase.............. *1162*
Panemax.............. *1162*
Procirc/Ecotran/Ginko-Q/Ubigin-Q... *1162*
Reniply.............. *1162*
Snovar.............. *1162*
Tofipan.............. *1162*
Vasonamin.............. *1162*
Zizodal.............. *1162*

CUBIST PHARMACEUTICALS, INC. 311, 1163
65 Hayden Avenue
Lexington, MA 02421

Direct Inquiries to:
(866) RX-DAPTO
(866) 793-2786
FAX: (866) 305-2039

Products Described:
◆Cubicin for Injection.............. **311, 1163**

DAIICHI PHARMACEUTICAL CORPORATION 311, 1166
11 Philips Parkway
Montvale, NJ 07645

Direct Inquiries to:
(877) 324-4244 (877-DAIICHI)
FAX: (888) 727-5666

For Medical Emergencies and Product Information Contact:
Medical Services Department
(888) 727-2500
FAX: (888) 272-7979

Products Described:
◆Evoxac Capsules.............. **311, 1166**
◆Floxin Otic Singles.............. **311, 1169**
◆Floxin Otic Solution.............. **311, 1168**

DERMIK LABORATORIES 1170
1050 Westlakes Drive
Berwyn, PA 19312
(484) 595-2700
www.dermik.com

Direct Inquiries to:
Customer Service
Somerset Corporate Center, Blg. 3
300 Somerset Corporate Blvd.
Bridgewater, NJ 08807-2854
(800) 207-8049

For Medical Information Contact:
Medical Information Services
Somerset Corporate Center, Blg. 3
300 Somerset Corporate Blvd.
Bridgewater, NJ 08807-2854
(800) 633-1610

Products Described:
Benzaclin Topical Gel.............. **1170**
5 Benzagel Acne Gel.............. *1172*
10 Benzagel Acne Gel.............. *1172*
Benzamycin Pak Topical Gel......... *1172*
Benzamycin Topical Gel.............. *1172*
Carac Cream, 0.5%.............. **1172**
Dermatop Emollient Cream.......... *1174*
Dermatop Ointment.............. *1174*
Klaron Lotion 10%.............. **1175**
Noritate Cream, 1%.............. **1175**
Penlac Nail Lacquer, Topical Solution, 8%.............. **1176**
Psorcon E Emollient Cream.......... *1178*
Psorcon E Emollient Ointment....... *1178*
Sculptra.............. **3425**
Sulfacet-R Lotion.............. *1178*
Sulfacet-R Tint Free Lotion.......... *1178*
Vanamide Urea Cream, 40%......... *1178*
Vytone Cream 1%.............. *1179*

Other Products Available:
Benzagel Wash
Shepard's Skin Cream
Zetar Shampoo

DEY, L.P. 311, 1179
2751 Napa Valley Corporate Drive
Napa, CA 94558
(800) 755-5560
www.dey.com

Direct Inquiries to:
DEY, L.P.
(800) 755-5560

For Medical Information Contact:
Gerald L. Klein, M.D.
Vice President
Medical Affairs & Clinical Research
(800) 429-7751
FAX: (510) 595-8183

Products Described:
◆AccuNeb Inhalation Solution.... **311, 1179**
◆Albuterol Sulfate Inhalation Solution.............. *311, 1179*
Cromolyn Sodium Inhalation Solution USP.............. *1179*
◆Curosurf Intratracheal Suspension.............. **311, 1181**
◆DuoNeb Inhalation Solution..... **311, 1183**
EpiPen Auto-Injector.............. **1185**
EpiPen 2-Pak.............. *1179*
EpiPen Jr. Auto-Injector.............. **1185**
EpiPen Jr. 2-Pak.............. *1179*
EpiPen Trainer.............. *1179*
◆Ipratropium Bromide Inhalation Solution.............. *311, 1179*
Metaproterenol Sulfate Inhalation Solution USP.............. *1179*
Sodium Chloride Inhalation Solutions USP.............. *1179*
Sodium Chloride Solution.............. *1179*

DURAMED PHARMACEUTICALS, INC. 311, 1186
Subsidiary of Barr Pharmaceuticals, Inc.
P.O. Box 2900
2 Quaker Road
Pomona, NY 10970

Direct Inquiries to:
Customer Service
(800) 222-4043
Cenestin Medical Information
(877) 405-0369

Products Described:
◆Aygestin Tablets.............. **311, 1186**
◆Cenestin Tablets, 0.45mg, 0.625mg, 0.9mg, 1.25mg...... **311, 1187**
◆Cenestin Tablets, 0.3mg.......... **311, 1187**

ECR PHARMACEUTICALS 1192
Distributor of ECR Pharmaceuticals & Wm. P. Poythress Products
3969 Deep Rock Road
P.O. Box 71600
Richmond, VA 23255

Direct Inquiries to:
Professional Services Department
(804) 527-1950
FAX: (804) 527-1959

For Medical Emergencies Contact:
Professional Services Department
(804) 527-1950
FAX: (804) 527-1959

Products Described:
Anaplex DM Cough Syrup........... *1192*
Anaplex HD Cough Syrup........... *1192*
Bupap Tablets.............. *1192*
DEXPAK Taperpak Tablets.......... *1192*
Lodrane Liquid.............. *1192*
Lodrane Sustained Release Liquid.... *1192*
Lodrane D Sustained Release Liquid.............. *1192*
Lodrane 12-Hour Extended Release Tablets.............. *1192*
Lodrane 12 D Extended Release Tablets.............. *1192*
Lodrane 24 Extended Release Capsules.............. *1192*
Lodrane 24 D Extended Release Capsules.............. *1192*
Nasatab LA Tablets.............. *1192*
Panalgesic Gold Cream.............. *1192*
Panalgesic Gold Liniment.............. *1192*
Pneumotussin 2.5 Cough Syrup...... *1192*
Pneumotussin Tablets.............. *1192*

EISAI INC. 311, 1192
500 Frank W. Burr Boulevard
Teaneck, NJ 07666

Direct Inquiries to:
Eisai Medical Services
(888) 422-4743 (888) 4ACIPHE(X)
(888) 274-2378 (888) ARICEPT
FAX: (201) 287-9744

For Medical Emergencies Contact:
(24 hours/day, 7 days/week)
(888) 422-4743 (888) 4ACIPHE(X)
(888) 274-2378 (888) ARICEPT

Products Described:
◆Aciphex Tablets.............. **311, 1192**
◆Aricept Tablets.............. **311, 1197**
◆Zonegran Capsules.............. **311, 1200**

ELAN PHARMACEUTICALS 1204
7475 Lusk Blvd.
San Diego, CA 92121

For Medical Information Contact:
(888) NEURO-05
(888) 638-7605

To Report Adverse Events Contact:
(877) ELAN GSS
(877) 352-6477
Products described below are distributed by Elan Pharmaceuticals.

Products Described:
Azactam for Injection.............. **1204**
Maxipime for Injection.............. **1207**

ENDO PHARMACEUTICALS 311, 1212
100 Painters Drive
Chadds Ford, PA 19317
(800) 462-3636

Direct Inquiries to:
Customer Service
(800) 462-3636
FAX: (877) 329-3636

For Medical Information/Adverse Drug Experience Reporting Contact:
Product Information:
(800) 462-3636

Products Described:
Hycodan Syrup.............. **1212**
◆Hycodan Tablets.............. **311, 1212**
◆Hycomine Compound Tablets... **311, 1213**
Hycotuss Expectorant Syrup.......... **1215**
◆Lidoderm Patch.............. **311, 1215**
◆Moban Tablets.............. **311, 1217**
Narcan Injection.............. **1218**
Nubain Injection.............. **1220**
Numorphan Injection.............. **1221**
Numorphan Suppositories.............. **1221**
◆Percocet Tablets.............. **311, 1222**
◆Percodan Tablets.............. **311, 1223**
Symmetrel Syrup.............. **1224**
◆Symmetrel Tablets.............. **311, 1224**
◆Zydone Tablets.............. **312, 1226**

ENDO PHARMACEUTICALS 1212
100 Painters Drive
Chadds Ford, PA 19317
(800) 462-3636

Direct Inquiries to:
Customer Service
(800) 462-3636
FAX: (877) 329-3636

For Medical Information/Adverse Drug Experience Reporting Contact:
Product Information:
(800) 462-3636

ENDO GENERIC PRODUCTS

Carbidopa and Levodopa Tablets, USP.............. *1212*
Endocet Tablets CII, USP.............. *1212*
Endodan Tablets CII, USP.............. *1212*
Morphine Sulfate Extended-Release Tablets, CII...... *1212*

ENZON PHARMACEUTICALS, INC. 1228
685 Route 202/206
Bridgewater, NJ 08807

Direct Inquiries to:
(908) 541-8600
FAX: (908) 541-8680
www.enzon.com

For Medical Emergencies Contact:
(866) 792-5172
FAX: (866) 666-5062

Products Described:
Abelcet Injection 1228
Adagen Injection 1230
DepoCyt Injection 1231
Oncaspar 1233

ESI PHARMA, INC.
(See WYETH PHARMACEUTICALS)

ESP PHARMA 1235
2035 Lincoln Highway
Suite 2150
Edison, NJ 08817

Direct Inquiries to:
(732) 650-1377

Products Described:
I.V. Busulfex 1235
Cardene I.V. 1239
Ismo *1235*
Sectral *1235*
Tenex *1235*

EVERETT LABORATORIES, INC. 1241
29 Spring Street
West Orange, NJ 07052

Direct Inquiries to:
Professional Service Department
(973) 324-0200
FAX: (973) 324-0795

Products Described:
Cortic-ND Ear Drops *1241*
Renax Caplets *1241*
Strovite Advance Caplets *1241*
Trituss-A Drops *1241*
Vitafol-OB Caplets *1242*

Other Products Available:
Repan Tablets
Strovite Forte Caplets
Strovite Forte Syrup
Strovite Plus Caplets
Strovite Tablets
Trituss Syrup
Trituss-ER Caplets
Tussafed-EX Drops
Tussafed-EX Syrup
Tussafed-HC Syrup CIII
Tussafed-HCG Syrup
Tussall Syrup
Tussall-ER Tablets
Tusso-DF Syrup CIII
Vitafol Caplets
Vitafol Syrup

FAULDING LABORATORIES
(see ALPHARMA BRANDED PRODUCTS DIVISION)

FEI PRODUCTS LLC 312, 1242
825 Wurlitzer Drive
North Tonawanda, NY 14120

For General Information Contact:
(800) 322-4966

For Medical Inquiries/Emergencies Contact:
(877) 601-7163
www.paragard.com

Products Described:
◆ParaGard T 380A Intrauterine Copper Contraceptive 312, 1242

FERNDALE LABORATORIES, INC. 1245
780 West Eight Mile Road
Ferndale, MI 48220

Direct Inquiries to:
Dr. Michael Burns
(248) 548-0900
FAX: (248) 548-8427

For Medical Emergencies Contact:
Pravin M. Patel
(248) 548-0900
FAX: (248) 548-0708

Products Described:
Analpram HC Lotion 1245
Analpram HC Cream 1245
Clinac BPO 7 Gel USP 1246
Kronofed-A Kronocaps *1246*
Kronofed-A-Jr. Kronocaps *1246*
L.M.X.4 Cream 1246
L.M.X.5 Cream 1246
Locoid Cream 1247
Locoid Lipocream Cream 1247
Locoid Ointment 1247
Locoid Topical Solution 1247
Pramosone Cream 1% and 2.5% 1248
Pramosone Lotion 1% and 2.5% 1248
Pramosone Ointment 1% and 2.5% 1248
Prax Lotion *1249*
SBR-Lipocream *1249*

Other Products Available:
Detachol Adhesive Remover
Liqui-Doss
Mastisol Liquid Adhesive

FERRING PHARMACEUTICALS INC. 1249
400 Rella Boulevard
Suite 300
Suffern, NY 10901

Direct Inquiries to:
Ferring Pharmaceuticals Inc.
Customer Service Department
400 Rella Boulevard
Suite 300
Suffern, NY 10901
(888) FERRING (337-7464)

For Medical Emergencies Contact:
Ferring Pharmaceuticals Inc.
Professional Services Department
400 Rella Boulevard
Suite 300
Suffern, NY 10901
(800) 822-8214

Products Described:
Acthrel for Injection 3438
Bravelle for Intramuscular or Subcutaneous Injection 1249
Desmopressin Acetate Injection 1252
Desmopressin Acetate Rhinal Tube 1253
Novarel for Injection 1254
Repronex for Intramuscular and Subcutaneous Injection 1255

FIELDING PHARMACEUTICAL COMPANY
(See NOVAVAX, INC.)

FIRST HORIZON PHARMACEUTICAL CORPORATION 312, 1258
6195 Shiloh Road
Alpharetta, GA 30005

Direct Inquiries to:
Drug Safety Department
(800) 849-9707
(770) 442-9707

Products Described:
◆Nitrolingual Pumpspray 312, 1258
Ponstel Capsules 1259
Prenate Elite Tablets 1259
Robinul Forte Tablets *1260*
Robinul Tablets *1260*
Sular Tablets 1260
Tanafed DMX Suspension *1262*
Tanafed DP Suspension *1262*

C. B. FLEET CO., INC. 1262
4615 Murray Place
Lynchburg, VA 24502

Direct Inquiries to:
Joseph A. Kanapka, Ph.D.
Director of Product Safety
(434) 528-4000
FAX: (434) 522-8429

Products Described:
Fleet Bisacodyl Laxatives 1262
Fleet Enema 1263
Fleet Enema for Children 1263
Fleet Glycerin Laxatives 1262
Fleet Mineral Oil Enema 1263
Fleet Phospho-soda 1264
Fleet Phospho-soda ACCU-PREP 1264
Fleet Prep Kits 1265

FLEMING & COMPANY 1266
1733 Gilsinn Lane
Fenton, MO 63026

Direct Inquiries to:
Fleming & Company
(636) 343-8200
FAX: (636) 343-5322
www.flemingcompany.com
For product orders, call (800) 343-0164

Products Described:
Extendryl Chewable Tablets 1266
Extendryl Syrup 1266
Extendryl SR. & JR. Capsules 1266
Magonate Tablets and Liquid 1266
Nephrocaps 1266
Ocean Nasal Spray ▣
Rum-K Liquid *1266*

FOREST PHARMACEUTICALS, INC. 312, 1266
Subsidiary of FOREST LABORATORIES, INC.
13600 Shoreline Drive
St. Louis, MO 63045

Direct Inquiries to:
Professional Affairs Department
13600 Shoreline Drive
St. Louis, MO 63045
(800) 678-1605

Products Described:
◆Aerobid Inhaler System 312, 1266
◆Aerobid-M Inhaler System 312, 1266
◆AeroChamber Plus and AeroChamber Plus with Mask 312, 1268
◆Armour Thyroid Tablets *312, 1269*
◆Campral Tablets 312, 3428
◆Celexa Oral Solution 312, 1269
◆Celexa Tablets 312, 1269
◆Cervidil Vaginal Insert 312, 1273
Esgic Capsules *1275*
Esgic Tablets *1275*
◆Esgic-Plus Tablets *312, 1275*
Flumadine Syrup 1275
◆Flumadine Tablets 312, 1275
◆Infasurf Intratracheal Suspension 312, 1276
Levothroid Tablets 1278
◆Lexapro Oral Solution 312, 1282
◆Lexapro Tablets 312, 1282
◆Lorcet 10/650 Tablets *312, 1287*
◆Lorcet Plus Tablets *312, 1286*
Lorcet-HD Capsules *1286*
◆Monurol Sachet 312, 1287
◆Namenda Tablets 312, 1288
Namenda Titration Pak *1288*
◆Tessalon Capsules 312, 1291
◆Tessalon Perles 312, 1291
◆Thyrolar Tablets *312, 1292*
◆Tiazac Capsules 312, 1292

Other Products Available:
Banalg Hospital Strength Arthritic Pain Reliever
Banalg Liniment
Cebocap Capsules
Elixophyllin Elixir
Elixophyllin-GG Oral Solution
Elixophyllin-KI Elixir
Eudal SR Tablets
Feostat Tablets
Isochron Tablets
Kay Ciel Oral Solution
Kay Ciel Powder Packets
Nitrogard Tablets
TheoCap
Theochron Tablets

FUJISAWA HEALTHCARE, INC. 312, 1294
Three Parkway North
Deerfield, IL 60015-2548

For Medical Information Contact:
Generally:
Medical and Scientific Information
(800) 727-7003
In Emergencies:
Medical and Scientific Information
(800) 727-7003

Products Described:
◆Adenocard Injection 312, 1294
◆Adenoscan 312, 1296
◆AmBisome for Injection 312, 1297
◆Prograf Capsules and Injection 313, 1302
◆Protopic Ointment 313, 1307

GALDERMA LABORATORIES, L.P. 1310
14501 North Freeway
Fort Worth, TX 76177

Direct Inquiries to:
(800) 582-8225
8 a.m. to 5 p.m. Central (Monday through Friday)
www.galdermaUSA.com

Products Described:
Capex Shampoo 1310
Clindagel 1310
Clobex Shampoo 1313
Clobex Lotion 1311
Differin Cream 1315
Differin Gel 1316
Differin Solution/Pledgets 1317
MetroGel 1317
MetroLotion 1318
Rosanil Cleanser 1319
Solagé Solution 1319
Tri-Luma Cream 1322

GATE PHARMACEUTICALS 1324
A Division of TEVA PHARMACEUTICALS USA
650 Cathill Road
Sellersville, PA 18960

Direct Inquiries to:
1090 Horsham Road
P.O. Box 1090
North Wales, PA 19454
(800) 292-4283

Products Described:
Adipex-P Capsules 1324
Adipex-P Tablets 1324
Lofibra Capsules 1325
Orap Tablets 1328
Purinethol Tablets 1330

GENENTECH, INC. 313, 1332
1 DNA Way
South San Francisco, CA 94080-4990
(650) 225-1000
www.gene.com

For Medical Information Contact:
(800) 821-8590
www.gene.com/gene/contact/

For Customer Service Contact:
(800) 551-2231

For Reimbursement Support:
(888) 249-4918

Products Described:
◆Activase I.V. 313, 1332
◆Avastin IV *313*
◆Cathflo Activase 313, 1336
◆Herceptin I.V. 313, 1337
◆Nutropin for Injection 313, 1341
◆Nutropin AQ Injection 313, 1345
◆Nutropin AQ Pen 313, 1345
◆Nutropin AQ Pen Cartridge 313, 1345
◆Nutropin Depot *313*
◆Pulmozyme Inhalation Solution 313, 1348
◆Raptiva for Injection 313, 1350
◆Rituxan I.V. 313, 1354
◆TNKase I.V. 313, 1357
◆Xolair 313, 1359

GENZYME CORPORATION 313, 1362
500 Kendall Street
Cambridge, MA 02142

Direct Inquiries to:
(800) 745-4447
(617) 768-9000

Products Described:
Aldurazyme for Intravenous Infusion 1362
Cerezyme for Injection 1364
Fabrazyme for Intravenous Infusion 1365
◆Renagel Tablets 313, 1366
Thyrogen for Injection 1368

GILEAD SCIENCES, INC. 313, 1370
333 Lakeside Drive
Foster City, CA 94404

Direct Inquiries to:
Customer Service
(800) GILEAD5

For Medical Emergencies Contact:
Medical Information
(800) GILEAD5
FAX: (650) 522-5466

Products Described:
◆Emtriva Capsules 313, 1370
◆Hepsera Tablets 313, 1373
◆Truvada Tablets 313, 1376
◆Viread Tablets 313, 1381

GLAXOSMITHKLINE 313, 1386
Five Moore Drive
Research Triangle Park
North Carolina 27709
(919) 483-2100

For Medical Emergencies, Medical Information for Healthcare Professionals, and Consumer Inquiries, Contact:
(888) 825-5249
www.druginfo.gsk.com

Products Described:
◆Aclovate Cream 313, 1386
◆Aclovate Ointment 313, 1386
◆Advair Diskus 100/50 314, 1387
◆Advair Diskus 250/50 314, 1387
◆Advair Diskus 500/50 314, 1387
◆Agenerase Capsules 314, 1396
◆Agenerase Oral Solution 314, 1401
◆Albenza Tablets 314, 1406
◆Amerge Tablets 314, 1408
◆Amoxil Capsules 314, 1411
◆Amoxil Chewable Tablets 314, 1411
◆Amoxil for Oral Suspension 314, 1411
◆Amoxil Pediatric Drops for Oral Suspension 314, 1411
◆Amoxil Tablets 314, 1411
◆Ancef for Injection 314, 1415
Ancef Injection 1415
◆Argatroban Injection 314, 1417
◆Augmentin Chewable Tablets 314, 1421
◆Augmentin Powder for Oral Suspension 314, 1421
◆Augmentin Tablets 314, 1424
◆Augmentin XR Tablets 314, 1430
◆Augmentin ES-600 Powder for Oral Suspension 314, 1427
◆Avandamet Tablets 314, 1433
◆Avandia Tablets 314, 1438
◆Avodart Soft Gelatin Capsules 314, 1443
◆Bactroban Cream 314, 1446
◆Bactroban Nasal 314, 1446

◆Bactroban Ointment **315, 1447**
◆Beconase AQ Nasal Spray **315, 1448**
◆Ceftin for Oral Suspension **315, 1450**
◆Ceftin Tablets **315, 1450**
◆Combivir Tablets **315, 1454**
◆Coreg Tablets **315, 1457**
◆Cutivate Cream **315, 1461**
◆Cutivate Ointment **315, 1463**
◆Daraprim Tablets **315, 1464**
◆Dexedrine Spansule Capsules **315, 1465**
◆Dexedrine Tablets **315, 1465**
◆Digibind for Injection **315, 1466**
◆Dyazide Capsules **315, 1468**
◆Engerix-B Vaccine **315, 1470**
◆Epivir Oral Solution **315, 1473**
◆Epivir Tablets **315, 1473**
◆Epivir-HBV Oral Solution **315, 1477**
◆Epivir-HBV Tablets **315, 1477**
Epzicom Tablets **1481**
◆Eskalith Capsules **315, 1485**
◆Eskalith CR
Controlled-Release Tablets **315, 1485**
◆Flolan for Injection **315, 1487**
◆Flonase Nasal Spray **315, 1491**
Flovent HFA 44 mcg Inhalation
Aerosol **1497**
Flovent HFA 110 mcg Inhalation
Aerosol **1497**
Flovent HFA 220 mcg Inhalation
Aerosol **1497**
◆Flovent 44 mcg Inhalation
Aerosol **315, 1494**
◆Flovent 110 mcg Inhalation
Aerosol **315, 1494**
◆Flovent 220 mcg Inhalation
Aerosol **315, 1494**
◆Flovent Rotadisk 50 mcg **315, 1500**
◆Flovent Rotadisk 100 mcg **315, 1500**
◆Flovent Rotadisk 250 mcg **315, 1500**
◆Fortaz Injection **316, 1504**
◆Fortaz for Injection **316, 1504**
◆Havrix Vaccine **316, 1507**
◆Hycamtin for Injection **316, 1509**
◆Imitrex Injection **316, 1513**
◆Imitrex Nasal Spray **316, 1517**
◆Imitrex Tablets **316, 1521**
◆Infanrix Vaccine **316, 1526**
◆Lamictal Tablets **316, 1531**
◆Lamictal Chewable
Dispersible Tablets **316, 1531**
◆Lanoxicaps Capsules **316, 1540**
◆Lanoxin Injection **316, 1546**
◆Lanoxin Tablets **316, 1553**
◆Lanoxin Elixir Pediatric **316, 1543**
◆Lanoxin Injection Pediatric **316, 1550**
◆Leukeran Tablets **316, 1556**
◆Lexiva Tablets **316, 1558**
◆Lotronex Tablets **316, 1564**
◆Malarone Tablets **316, 1568**
◆Malarone Pediatric Tablets **316, 1568**
◆Mepron Suspension **316, 1572**
◆Myleran Tablets **316, 1576**
◆Navelbine Injection **316, 1578**
◆Oxistat Cream **316, 1582**
◆Oxistat Lotion **317, 1582**
◆Parnate Tablets **317, 1583**
◆Paxil CR Controlled-Release
Tablets **317, 1592**
◆Paxil Oral Suspension **317, 1585**
◆Paxil Tablets **317, 1585**
◆Pediarix Vaccine **317, 1599**
◆Relafen Tablets **317, 1604**
◆Relenza Rotadisk **317, 1606**
◆Requip Tablets **317, 1608**
◆Retrovir Capsules **317, 1612**
◆Retrovir IV Infusion **317, 1616**
◆Retrovir Syrup **317, 1612**
◆Retrovir Tablets **317, 1612**
◆Serevent Diskus **317, 1620**
◆Tabloid Tablets **317, 1624**
Tagamet Injection **1626**
Tagamet Liquid **1626**
◆Tagamet Tablets **317, 1626**
◆Temovate E Emollient **317, 1631**
◆Temovate Cream **317, 1629**
◆Temovate Gel **317, 1630**
◆Temovate Ointment **317, 1629**
◆Temovate Scalp Application **317, 1630**
◆Timentin ADD-Vantage **317, 1635**
◆Timentin IV Infusion **317, 1632**
◆Timentin Pharmacy Bulk
Package **317, 1639**
◆Trizivir Tablets **317, 1642**
◆Twinrix Vaccine **317, 1648**
◆Valtrex Caplets **317, 1650**
◆Ventolin HFA Inhalation
Aerosol **317, 1653**
◆Wellbutrin Tablets **317, 1655**
◆Wellbutrin SR
Sustained-Release Tablets **317, 1659**
◆Wellbutrin XL
Extended-Release Tablets **318, 1663**
◆Zantac 150 Tablets **318, 1670**
◆Zantac 300 Tablets **318, 1670**
◆Zantac 25 EFFERdose
Tablets **318, 1670**
◆Zantac 150 EFFERdose
Tablets **318, 1670**
◆Zantac Injection **318, 1668**
◆Zantac Injection Premixed **318, 1668**
◆Zantac Syrup **318, 1670**
◆Ziagen Oral Solution **318, 1673**
◆Ziagen Tablets **318, 1673**
◆Zinacef Injection **318, 1676**
◆Zinacef for Injection **318, 1676**
◆Zofran Injection **318, 1679**
◆Zofran Injection Premixed **318, 1679**
◆Zofran Oral Solution **318, 1684**
◆Zofran Tablets **318, 1684**
◆Zofran ODT Orally
Disintegrating Tablets **318, 1684**
◆Zovirax Capsules **318, 1687**
◆Zovirax for Injection **318, 1689**
◆Zovirax Suspension **318, 1687**
◆Zovirax Tablets **318, 1687**
◆Zyban Sustained-Release
Tablets **318, 1691**

GLAXOSMITHKLINE CONSUMER HEALTHCARE, L.P. 1697
P.O. Box 1467
Pittsburgh, PA 15230

Direct Inquiries to:
(800) 245-1040 weekdays

Products Described:
Commit Lozenges **1697**
Debrox Drops .... ▣
Ecotrin Enteric Coated Aspirin
Low, Regular and Maximum
Strength Tablets **1699**
Feosol Caplets **1700**
Feosol Tablets **1701**
Gaviscon Regular Strength Antacid
Tablets .... ▣
Gaviscon Extra Strength Antacid
Tablets .... ▣
Gaviscon Regular Strength Liquid
Antacid .... ▣
Gaviscon Extra Strength Liquid
Antacid .... ▣
Nicoderm CQ Patch **1701**
Nicorette Gum **1703**
Os-Cal 500, 500 + D, and 500
Chewable Tablets .... ▣
Tagamet HB 200 Tablets .... ▣
Tums Regular, Tums EX, and Tums
ULTRA Antacid/Calcium
Supplement Tablets .... ▣

GLENWOOD 318, 1705
111 Cedar Lane
Englewood, NJ 07631

Direct Inquiries to:
Professional Services Department
(800) 542-0772
(201) 569-0050
FAX: (201) 569-0250

For Medical Emergencies Contact:
Professional Services Department
(800) 542-0772
(201) 569-0050
FAX: (201) 569-0250

Products Described:
◆Potaba Capsules **318, 1705**
◆Potaba Envules **318, 1705**
◆Potaba Tablets **318, 1705**

Other Products Available:
Bar-Test
Calphosan Injection
Scleromate Injection
Yocon Tablets
Yodoxin Tablets

GORDON LABORATORIES 1706
6801 Ludlow Street
Upper Darby, PA 19082

Direct Inquiries to:
Customer Service
(610) 734-2011
FAX: (610) 734-2049
www.gordonlabs.com
E-mail: gordonlabs@worldnet.att.net

For Medical Emergencies Contact:
David Dercher
(610) 734-2011
FAX: (610) 734-2049

Products Described:
Gordochom Solution **1706**

Other Products Available:
Abscents Deodorizing Powder
Aloe Grande Creme & Lotion
Bromi-Lotion
Bromi-Talc
Bromi-Talc Plus
Calicylic Creme
Emollia-Creme & Lotion
Formadon
Forma-Ray
Gordobalm
Gordofilm
Gordomatic Crystals
Gordon's Boro-Packs
Gordon's No. Five Spray Foot Powder
Gordon's Urea 40%
Gordon's Vite A Creme & Lotion
Gordon's Vite E Creme
Gordo-Pool
Gormel Creme & Lotion
Mycomist
Potassium Hydroxide Solution 5%
Silver Nitrate Solutions 10%, 25%, 50%
Sodium Hydroxide 10%
Sorbidon Hydrate
Stik It
Tri-Chlor
Vita-Ray Creme

GRIFOLS BIOLOGICALS, INC. 1706
5555 Valley Boulevard
Los Angeles, CA 90032

Contacts:
Medical and Technical Assistance,
Reimbursement Assistance,
24-Hour Ordering, and Customer Service:
(888) GRIFOLS
Direct Inquiries:
(323) 225-2221
FAX: (323)227-7613
www.grifolsusa.com

Products Described:
Albutein 5% Solution *1706*
Albutein 25% Solution *1706*
Alphanate Solvent Detergent/Heat
Treated *1706*
AlphaNine SD Solvent Detergent
Treated/Virus Filtered *1707*
Flebogamma 5% **1707**
Human Albumin Grifols 20%
Solution *1706*
Human Albumin Grifols 25%
Solution *1706*
Profilnine SD Solvent Detergent
Treated *1707*

GUARDIAN LABORATORIES 1707
A Division of United-Guardian, Inc.
230 Marcus Boulevard
Hauppauge, NY 11788

Direct Inquiries to:
P.O. Box 18050
Hauppauge, NY 11788
(631) 273-0900
(800) 645-5566
FAX: (631) 273-0858
E-mail: evp@u-g.com
www.u-g.com

For Medical Information Contact:
Director of Medical Information
(631) 273-0900
(800) 645-5566

Products Described:
Clorpactin WCS-90 .... **1707**
Renacidin Irrigation *1707*

HEALTHPOINT, LTD. 318, 1707
3909 Hulen Street
Fort Worth, TX 76107

Direct Inquiries to:
(800) 441-8227

Products Described:
◆Accuzyme Debriding
Ointment **318, 1707**
◆Accuzyme Spray **319, 1708**
◆Panafil Ointment **319, 1708**
◆Panafil Spray **319, 1708**
◆Prudoxin Cream *319, 1709*
◆Xenaderm Ointment **319, 1709**

HEEL INC. 1709
10421 Research Road SE
Albuquerque, NM 87123

Direct Inquiries to:
Medical Department
(800) 621-7644
FAX: (800) 217-6934
www.HeelUSA.com

Products Described:
Traumeel Gel *1709*
Traumeel Injection Solution **1709**
Traumeel Ointment *1709*
Traumeel Oral Drops *1709*
Traumeel Oral Liquid in Vials *1709*
Traumeel Tablets *1709*

Other Products Available:
Engystol Tablets
Euphorbium Sinus Relief Nasal Spray
Galium-Heel Oral Drops
Gripp-Heel Tablets
Lymphomyosot Oral Drops
Lymphomyosot Tablets
Vertigoheel Liquid in Oral Vials
Vertigoheel Oral Drops
Zeel Ointment
Zeel Tablets

HEMISPHERX BIOPHARMA, INC. 319, 1710
One Penn Center
1617 JFK Boulevard
Philadelphia, PA 19103-1806

Direct Inquiries to:
(732) 249-3250 (Alferon N Injection)
or
(215) 988-0080

Products Described:
◆Alferon N Injection **319, 1710**

HIGH CHEMICAL CO. 1712
3901-A Nebraska Street
Levittown, PA 19056

Direct Inquiries to:
Nalin Parikh
(800) 447-8792
(877) SARAPIN
FAX: (215) 788-3148

Products Described:
Sarapin **1712**

HILL DERMACEUTICALS, INC. 1713
2650 So. Mellonville Avenue
Sanford, Florida 32773

Direct Inquiries to:
Rosario G. Ramirez, MD
(407) 323-1887
FAX: (407) 649-9213

Products Described:
Derma-Smoothe/FS Topical Oil *1713*

ICN PHARMACEUTICALS, INC.
(see VALEANT PHARMACEUTICALS INTERNATIONAL)

IDEC PHARMACEUTICALS CORPORATION
(see BIOGEN IDEC)

IMMUNOTEC RESEARCH LTD. 1713
292 Adrien Patenaude
Vaudreuil-Dorion (Quebec)
Canada J7V 5V5

Direct Inquiries to:
Immunotec Medical Corp.
(800) 440-6250

Products Described:
Immunocal Powder Sachets **1713**
ProNutra Protein Supplement **1713**

INTEGRITY PHARMACEUTICAL CORPORATION
(See XANODYNE PHARMACEUTICALS, INC.)

INTERCURE, INC. 1714
Parker Plaza
400 Kelby St.
Fort Lee, NJ 07024

Direct Inquiries to:
RESPeRATE support center
(877) 988-9388
www.resperate.com/md
supportmd@resperate.com

Products Described:
Resperate Device **1714**

INTERMUNE INC. 319, 1714
3280 Bayshore Blvd.
Brisbane, CA 94005

Direct Inquiries to:
For Medical Information Contact:
(888) 486-6411
FAX: (415) 466-2300
Corporate Offices:
(415) 466-2200

Products Described:
◆Actimmune **319, 1714**
◆Infergen **319, 1716**

INTERNATIONAL NUTRITION RESEARCH CENTER INC. 1719
7900 Los Pinos Circle
Coral Gables, FL 33143

Direct Inquiries to:
(305) 740-7480
FAX: (305) 740-7478

Products Described:
SON Formula Tablets **1719**

IVAX LABORATORIES, INC. 1720
4400 Biscayne Blvd., 9th Floor
Miami, FL 33137

Direct Inquiries to:
Ivax Laboratories, Inc.
(888) 482-9522
FAX: (305) 575-6221

Products Described:
Nasarel Nasal Spray **1720**
Qvar Inhalation Aerosol **1722**

JACOBUS PHARMACEUTICAL CO., INC. 1724
37 Cleveland Lane
P.O. Box 5290
Princeton, NJ 08540

Direct Inquiries to:
Professional Services
(609) 921-7447
FAX: (609) 799-1176

For Medical Emergencies Contact:
Medical Department
(609) 921-7447
FAX: (609) 799-1176

Products Described:
Dapsone Tablets USP **1724**
Paser Granules **1725**

JANSSEN PHARMACEUTICA PRODUCTS, L.P. 319, 1726
1125 Trenton-Harbourton Road
P.O. Box 200
Titusville, NJ 08560-0200
us.janssen.com

For Medical Information Contact:
Monday through Friday 9am-5pm EST:
(800) JANSSEN
FAX: (609) 730-3138
After Hours & Weekends:
(800) JANSSEN
Holidays:
Emergencies: (800) JANSSEN

Products Described:
◆Aciphex Tablets ... 319, 1726
◆Duragesic Transdermal System ... 319, 1731
◆Nizoral Tablets ... 319, 1735
◆Reminyl Oral Solution ... 319, 1736
◆Reminyl Tablets ... 319, 1736
◆Risperdal Consta Injection ... 319, 1747
◆Risperdal M-Tab Tablets ... 319, 1742
◆Risperdal Oral Solution ... 319, 1742
◆Risperdal Tablets ... 319, 1742
◆Sporanox Capsules ... 319, 1753
Sporanox Injection ... 1757
Sporanox Oral Solution ... 1761

JOHNSON & JOHNSON • MERCK CONSUMER PHARMACEUTICALS CO. 319, 1766
Consumer Pharmaceuticals Co.
Camp Hill Road
Fort Washington, PA 19034

Direct Inquiries to:
Consumer Relationship Center
Fort Washington, PA 19034
(800) 469-5268

For Medical Information Contact:
In Emergencies:
(800) 469-5268

Products Described:
Pepcid AC Chewable Tablets ... 1766
◆Pepcid AC Gelcaps ... 319, 1766
◆Pepcid AC Tablets ... 319, 1766
◆Maximum Strength Pepcid AC Tablets ... 319, 1766
◆Pepcid Complete Chewable Tablets ... 319, 1767

JONES PHARMA INCORPORATED
(See KING PHARMACEUTICALS, INC)

KEY PHARMACEUTICALS, INC.
(See SCHERING CORPORATION)

KING PHARMACEUTICALS, INC. 319, 1767
501 Fifth Street
Bristol, TN 37620

Direct Inquiries to:
Customer Service
(800) 776-3637
FAX: (423) 989-8786

To Report an Adverse Drug Experience:
(800) 546-4905
FAX: (423) 990-0519

Products Described:
Adrenalin Chloride Injection ... *1767*
◆Altace Capsules ... 319, 1767
◆Aplisol Injection ... 319, 1771
Bicillin L-A Injection ... 1772
Brevital Sodium for Injection, USP .. 1774
◆Coly-Mycin M Parenteral ... 319, 1776
Cortisporin Cream ... 1777
◆Cortisporin-TC Otic Suspension ... 319, 1778
Corzide 40/5 Tablets ... 1779
Corzide 80/5 Tablets ... 1779
◆Cytomel Tablets ... 319, 1781
◆Intal Inhaler ... 319, 1783
◆Levoxyl Tablets ... 319, 1785
Neosporin G.U. Irrigant Sterile ... 1789
Septra Suspension ... 1790
Septra Grape Suspension ... 1790
Septra Tablets ... 1790
Septra DS Tablets ... 1790
Silvadene Cream 1% ... 1792
◆Skelaxin Tablets ... 320, 1793
◆Sonata Capsules ... 320, 1793
◆Synercid I.V. ... 320, 1798
◆Thrombin-JMI ... 320, 1801
◆Triostat Injection ... 320, 1802

KOS PHARMACEUTICALS, INC. 320, 1804
One Cedar Brook Drive
Cranbury, NJ 08512

For Medical Information Contact:
Drug Information Services
(888) 454-7437

Products Described:
◆Advicor Tablets ... 320, 1804
◆Azmacort Inhalation Aerosol ... 320, 1808
◆Niaspan Extended-Release Tablets ... 320, 1810

KYOWA ENGINEERING SUNDORY 337, 1814
5-964 Nakamozu-Cho, Sakai-City
Osaka, Japan

Direct Inquiries to:
Customer Relations
81-72-257-8568
Osaka
FAX: 81-722-57-8655
www.sundory.co.jp

Products Described:
◆Sen-Sei-Ro Liquid Gold ... 337, 1814
◆Sen-Sei-Ro Liquid Royal ... 337, 1814
◆Sen-Sei-Ro Powder Gold ... 337, 1815

LANE LABS U.S.A., Inc. 1815
25 Commerce Drive
Allendale, NJ 07401

Direct Inquiries to:
(800) 526-3001

Products Described:
Nature's Lining Chewable Tablets ... *1815*

LIGAND PHARMACEUTICALS INCORPORATED 320, 1815
10275 Science Center Drive
San Diego, CA 92121

Direct Inquiries to:
(858) 550-7500
www.ligand.com
Customer Service:
(877) 454-4263
Medical Information:
(800) 964-5836
Reimbursement Support:
(877) 654-4263

Products Described:
◆Avinza Capsules ... 320, 1815
Ontak Vials ... 1819
Panretin Gel ... *1821*
◆Targretin Capsules ... 320, 1821
Targretin Gel ... *1824*

ELI LILLY AND COMPANY 320, 1824

For Medical Information Contact:
Customer Services
Lilly Corporate Center
Indianapolis, IN 46285
(800) 545-5979

Direct Inquiries to:
Lilly Corporate Center
Indianapolis, IN 46285
(317) 276-2000
www.lilly.com
Sales and Ordering:
(800) LILLY-RX

Products Described:
Alimta for Injection ... 1824
Capastat Sulfate for Injection ... 1828
Ceclor Pulvules ... 1829
Ceclor Suspension ... 1829
◆Cymbalta Delayed-Release Capsules ... 320, 3430
◆Evista Tablets ... 320, 1836
◆Forteo for Injection ... 320, 1840
Gemzar for Injection ... 1844
Glucagon for Injection Vials and Emergency Kit ... 1849
◆Humalog-Pen ... 320, 1852
◆Humalog Mix 75/25-Pen ... 320, 1854
Humatrope Vials and Cartridges ... 1856
Humulin 50/50, 100 Units ... 1860
Humulin 70/30 Pen ... 1861
Humulin L, 100 Units ... 1863
Humulin N, 100 Units ... 1864
Humulin R (U-500) ... 1868
Humulin R, 100 Units ... 1867
Humulin U, 100 Units ... 1870
Humulin N Pen ... 1865
Keflex Pulvules ... 1871
◆Prozac Pulvules and Liquid ... 320, 1873
◆Prozac Weekly Capsules ... *320*
◆ReoPro Vials ... 320, 1879
Seromycin Capsules ... 1883
◆Strattera Capsules ... 320, 1884
◆Symbyax Capsules ... 320, 1888
Vancocin HCl Pulvules ... 1896
◆Xigris Powder for Intravenous Infusion ... 320, 1897
◆Zyprexa Tablets ... 320, 1899
◆Zyprexa IntraMuscular ... 320, 1899
◆Zyprexa ZYDIS Orally Disintegrating Tablets ... 320, 1899

Other Products Available:
Cialis Tablets (See LILLY ICOS LLC.)
Quinidine Gluconate Injection, USP

LILLY ICOS LLC 320, 1906
c/o Eli Lilly and Company
Lilly Corporate Center
Indianapolis, IN 46285

Direct Inquiries to:
Lilly ICOS LLC
c/o Eli Lilly and Company
Lilly Corporate Center
Indianapolis, IN 46285
(317) 276-2000
www.cialis.com

For Medical Information Contact:
Lilly ICOS LLC 1-877-Cialis-1

Products Described:
◆Cialis Tablets ... 320, 1906

3M PHARMACEUTICALS 320, 1911
3M Center, Bldg. 275-6W-13
P.O. Box 33275
St. Paul, MN 55144
www.3M.com/pharma

For Medical Information Contact:
Drug Surveillance & Information
3M Pharmaceuticals
3M Center, Bldg. 275-6W-13
P.O. Box 33275
St. Paul, MN 55144
(800) 814-1795 (Aldara)
(800) 328-0255 (All other products)
In Emergencies:
(800) 328-0255 (all hours)

Commercial Customers:
Orders, Returns, Accounting
(800) 447-4537

Trade and Government:
(800) 328-6523

Products Described:
◆Aldara Cream, 5% ... 320, 1911
Alu-Cap Capsules ... *1916*
Calcium Disodium Versenate Injection ... 1916
◆Maxair Autohaler ... 321, 1917
◆MetroGel-Vaginal Gel ... 321, 1919
Minitran Transdermal Delivery System ... *1920*
Norflex Extended-Release Tablets ... 1921
Norflex Injection ... 1921
Norgesic Tablets ... *1921*
Norgesic Forte Tablets ... *1921*
◆Tambocor Tablets ... 321, 1921

MAGNA PHARMACEUTICALS, INC. 1924
11802 Brinley Avenue, Suite 201
Louisville, KY 40243

Direct Inquiries to:
Customer Service Department
Toll free (888) 206-5525
FAX: (502)254-9279
www.magnaweb.com

Products Described:
Sta-D Tablets ... *1924*
Staflex Caplets ... *1924*
Stagesic Capsules CIII ... *1924*
Stahist Tablets ... *1924*
Stamoist E Tablets ... *1924*
Statuss DM Syrup ... *1924*
Statuss Green Syrup CIII ... *1924*
Ztuss Expectorant Syrup CIII ... *1924*
Ztuss Tablets CIII ... *1924*
Ztuss ZT Caplets CIII ... *1924*
Z-Xtra Medicated Lotion ... *1924*

MALLINCKRODT INC. 321, 1924
A Division of Tyco/Healthcare
675 McDonnell Blvd.
P.O. Box 5840
St. Louis, MO 63134

Direct Inquiries to:
Medical Information
(888) 744-1414, option #2 then #1
Customer Service (Sales and Ordering)
(800) 325-8888
www.mallinckrodt.com

Products Described:
Acetaminophen and Codeine Phosphate Tablets, USP ... *1924*
Anafranil Capsules ... *1925*
Anexsia Tablets ... *1925*
Butalbital, Acetaminophen and Caffeine Tablets, USP ... *1924*
Depade Tablets ... *1925*
Dextroamphetamine Saccharate, Amphetamine Aspartate, Dextroamphetamine Sulfate, Amphetamine Sulfate Tablets ... *1924*
Dextroamphetamine Sulfate ER Capsules ... *1924*
Dextroamphetamine Sulfate Tablets, USP ... *1924*
Fluoxetine Capsules, USP ... *1924*
Fluoxetine Oral Solution, USP ... *1924*
Hydrocodone Bitartrate and Acetaminophen Capsules ... *1924*
Hydrocodone Bitartrate and Acetaminophen Oral Solution ... *1924*
Hydrocodone Bitartrate and Acetaminophen Tablets, USP ... *1924*
Hydromorphone Hydrochloride Tablets, USP ... *1924*
Meperidine Hydrochloride Tablets, USP ... *1924*
Methadose Oral Concentrate ... *1925*
Methadose Sugar-Free Oral Concentrate ... *1925*
Methadose Dispersible Tablets ... *1925*
Methadose Oral Tablets ... *1924*
Methylin Tablets ... *1924*
Methylin ER Tablets ... *1924*
Morphine Sulfate Extended-Release Tablets ... *1924*
Naltrexone Hydrochloride Tablets, USP ... *1924*
Oxycodone and Acetaminophen Capsules, USP ... *1924*
Oxycodone and Acetaminophen Tablets, USP ... *1924*
Oxycodone Hydrochloride Capsules ... *1924*
Oxycodone Hydrochloride Oral Concentrate Solution ... *1924*
Oxycodone Hydrochloride Oral Solution, USP ... *1924*
Oxycodone Hydrochloride Tablets, USP ... *1924*
Pamelor Capsules ... *1925*
Pamelor Oral Solution ... *1925*
Pemoline Chewable Tablets ... *1924*
Pemoline Tablets ... *1924*
Propoxyphene Napsylate and Acetaminophen Tablets, USP ... *1924*
◆Restoril Capsules ... *321, 1926*
Tofranil Tablets ... *1925*
◆Tofranil-PM Capsules ... *321, 1926*
Tramadol Hydrochloride Tablets ... *1924*
Tussizone-12 RF Suspension ... *1924*
Tussizone-12 RF Tablets ... *1924*

MARLYN NUTRACEUTICALS, INC. 1926
4404 E. Elwood Street
Phoenix, AZ 85040

Direct Inquiries to:
Joe Lehmann
4404 E. Elwood Street
Phoenix, AZ 85040
(800) 899-4499
In AZ: (480) 991-0200
E-mail: info@naturallyvitamins.com

Products Described:
Hep-Forte Capsules ... 1926
Marlyn Formula 50 Capsules ... 1927
Wobenzym Tablets ... 1927

McNEIL CONSUMER & SPECIALTY PHARMACEUTICALS 321, 1927
Division of McNeil-PPC, Inc.
Camp Hill Road
Fort Washington, PA 19034

Direct Inquiries to:
Consumer Relationship Center
Fort Washington, PA 19034
(800) 962-5357
For Concerta and Flexeril, Direct Inquiries to:
(888) 440-7903

Products Described:
◆Concerta Extended-Release Tablets ... 321, 1927
◆Flexeril Tablets ... 321, 1930
◆Maximum Strength Gas Aid Softgels ... 321, 1932
Imodium Capsules ... 1932
◆Imodium A-D Liquid and Caplets ... 321, 1933
◆Imodium Advanced Caplets and Chewable Tablets ... 321, 1933
◆Lactaid Extra Strength Caplets ... 321, 1934
◆Lactaid Original Strength Caplets ... 321, 1934
◆Lactaid Ultra Caplets and Chewable Tablets ... 321, 1934
◆Children's Motrin Oral Suspension and Chewable Tablets ... 321, 1938
◆Children's Motrin Cold Non-Staining Dye-Free Oral Suspension ... 321, 1938
Children's Motrin Dosing Chart ... 1939
◆Children's Motrin Cold Oral Suspension ... 321, 1938
◆Children's Motrin Non-Staining Dye-Free Oral Suspension ... 321, 1938
◆Motrin Cold & Sinus Caplets ... 321, 1937
◆Motrin Suspension, Oral Drops, Chewable Tablets, and Caplets ... 321, 1935
◆Infants' Motrin Concentrated Drops ... 321, 1938
◆Infants' Motrin Non-Staining Dye-Free Drops ... 321, 1938
◆Junior Strength Motrin Caplets and Chewable Tablets ... 321, 1938
◆Motrin IB Tablets, Caplets, and Gelcaps ... 321, 1934
◆Nizoral A-D Shampoo ... 321, 1940
◆Nizoral 2% Shampoo ... 321, 1939
◆Simply Cough Liquid ... 321, 1940
◆Simply Sleep Caplets ... 321, 1940
◆Simply Stuffy Liquid ... 321, 1941
◆St. Joseph 81 mg Aspirin ... 321, 1941
◆Tylenol 8 Hour Extended Release Geltabs and Caplets ... 322, 1943
◆Children's Tylenol Suspension Liquid and Meltaways ... 322, 1948
◆Children's Tylenol Plus Cold & Allergy ... 322, 1949
◆Children's Tylenol Plus Cold Nighttime Suspension Liquid ... 322, 1949

MDR FITNESS CORP. 1952
Medical Doctors' Research
14101 NW 4th Street
Sunrise, FL 33325

Direct Inquiries to:
(800) MDR-TABS, ext. 5111 or 5445
(800) 637-8227, ext. 5111 or 5445
www.mdri.com

Products Described:

Other Products Available:
AM/PM Slimming Factors
CardioTone Heart Formula
Cholest-Defense
Chondro-Pro Arthritis Formula
Cranberry Capsules
Fibromy Support
Healthy Tract
Longevit-E
Longevity Antioxidants
MDR Vital Factors
Nature's Antioxidant
Nite-Cal Calcium
Prostate Health Tabs
Stress Defense Performance Tabs
Triple Bio-Flavonoids
Vision Formula
Vitamin B-12 Liquid B Complex

MEAD JOHNSON & COMPANY 322, 1953
2400 W. Lloyd Expressway
Evansville, IN 47721-0001

Direct Inquiries to:
For Medical Information Contact:
FAX: (609) 897-6859
E-mail: drug.information@bms.com
In Emergencies:
(800) 321-1335
Adverse Event Experiences and Product Defects Reporting:
(866) 232-2557
Sales and Ordering:
(800) 457-3550

Products Described:

MEDICIS, THE DERMATOLOGY COMPANY 1957
8125 North Hayden Road
Scottsdale, AZ 85258

For Medical Information Contact:
Generally:
Medical Affairs Department
(602) 808-8800
FAX: (602) 808-0822
In Emergencies:
(602) 808-8800

Products Described:

MEDIMMUNE, INC. 322, 1963
One MedImmune Way
Gaithersburg, MD 20878

For Medical Information please contact:
(800) 949-3789 or (877) 633-4411

Adverse Drug Experience:
(800) 949-3789 or (877) 633-4411

In Emergencies:
24-hour emergency
(800) 949-3789 or (877) 633-4411

Sales and Ordering/Customer Services:
(800) 527-7130 or (877) 633-4411

Customer Support Network:
(877) 633-4411

Products Described:

MEDIMMUNE ONCOLOGY, INC. 1967
One Medimmune Way
Gaithersburg, MD 20878

Direct Inquiries to:
MedImmune Oncology, Inc.
(877) 633-4411

For Medical Information, Adverse Drug Experiences, Product Sales and Ordering and other inquiries, please contact:
Medimmune Oncology, Inc.
(877) 633-4411
For Emergencies, 24 hours
(877) 633-4411
www.medimmune.com

Products Described:

MEDIMMUNE VACCINES 322, 1970
One MedImmune Way
Gaithersburg, MD 20878

For Medical Information, please contact:
(877) 633-4411 or (800) 949-3789

Adverse Drug Experience:
(877) 633-4411 or (800) 949-3789

In Emergencies
24 Hour Emergencies:
(877) 633-4411 or (800) 949-3789

Sales and Ordering/Customer Services:
(877) FLUMIST

Customer Support Network
(877) 633-4411

Products Described:

MEDPOINTE PHARMACEUTICALS 322, 1973
MedPointe Healthcare Inc.
Somerset, NJ 08873

For Medical Information Contact:
Generally:
Medical Information
(800) 526-3840
After Hours and Weekend Emergencies:
(800) 526-3840

Sales and Ordering:

MedPointe Pharmaceuticals
MedPointe Healthcare Inc.
Somerset, NJ 08873

Products Described:

Other Products Available:
Butisol Sodium Elixir
Butisol Sodium Tablets
Depen Titratable Tablets
Doral Tablets
Felbatol Oral Suspension
Felbatol Tablets
Lufyllin Tablets
Lufyllin-400 Tablets
Lufyllin-EPG Tablets
Lufyllin-GG Elixir
Lufyllin-GG Tablets
Maltsupex Powder, Liquid, Tablets (in 2002 PDR for Nonprescription Drugs)
Miltown Tablets
Organidin NR Liquid
Organidin NR Tablets
Ryna Liquid
Ryna-C Liquid
Soma Compound Tablets
Soma Compound w/Codeine Tablets
Tussi-Organidin NR Liquid
Tussi-Organidin-S NR Liquid
Tussi-Organidin DM NR Liquid
Tussi-Organidin DM-S NR Liquid

MERCK & CO., INC. 323, 1984
P.O. Box 4 WP39-206
West Point, PA 19486-0004

For Medical Information Contact:
Generally:
Product and service information:
Call the Merck National Service Center, 8:00 AM to 7:00 PM (ET), Monday through Friday:
(800) NSC-MERCK
(800) 672-6372
FAX: (800) MERCK-68
FAX: (800) 637-2568
www.merckservices.com
Adverse Drug Experiences:
Call the Merck National Service Center, 8:00 AM to 7:00 PM (ET), Monday through Friday:
(800) NSC-MERCK
(800) 672-6372
Pregnancy Registries:
(800) 986-8999
In Emergencies:
24-hour emergency information for healthcare professionals:
(800) NSC-MERCK
(800) 672-6372

Sales and Ordering:
For product orders and direct account inquiries only, call the Order Management Center, 8:00 AM to 7:00 PM (ET), Monday through Friday:
(800) MERCK RX
(800) 637-2579

Products Described:

MERCK/SCHERING PLOUGH PHARMACEUTICALS 324, 2183
P.O. Box 1000
UG4B-75a
351 N. Sumneytown Pike
North Wales, PA 19454

For Product and Service Information, Medical Information, and Adverse Drug Experience Reporting:
Call Merck/Schering-Plough National Service Center
Monday through Friday, 8:00 AM to 7:00 PM (ET)
(866) 637-2501
FAX: (800) 637-2568

For 24-hour emergency information, health care professionals should call: Merck/Schering-Plough National Service Center at (866) 637-2501

For Product Ordering:
Call:
Order Management Center
Monday through Friday, 8:00 AM to 7:00 PM (ET)
(800) 637-2579

Products Described:

MERICON INDUSTRIES, INC. 2194
8819 N. Pioneer Road
Peoria, IL 61615

Direct Inquiries to:
William R. Connelly
(309) 693-2150
FAX: (309) 693-2158
E-mail: MONOCAL@aol.com
www.mericon-industries.com

Sales & Ordering:
(800) 242-6464

Products Described:

Other Products Available:
1% Tolnaftate Cream
Delacort 1% Lotion Rx
Ginkgo Biloba Extract 60 mg
Glucosamine Sulfate 500 mg
Hard Nails 2.5mg biotin
Hydrocortisone Cream 1%
Hydrocortisone Lotion 1%
Zinc Gluconate Lozenges
Zinc Oxide Ointment
Zinc Sulfate Tabs & Caps

MERZ PHARMACEUTICALS **2194**
Division of Merz, Inc.
4215 Tudor Lane (27410)
P.O. Box 18806
Greensboro, NC 27419

Direct Inquiries to:
Medical/Regulatory Affairs
(336) 856-2003
FAX: (336) 856-0107

For Medical Emergencies Contact:
Medical/Regulatory Affairs
(336) 856-2003
FAX: (336) 856-0107

Products Described:
Appearex Tablets **2194**
Eldertonic **2194**
Erygel Topical Gel **2195**
Mederma Gel **2195**
Naftin Cream **2195**
Naftin Gel **2196**
Nu-Iron 150 Capsules **2196**
Nu-Iron V Tablets **2196**
Sedapap Tablets 50 mg/650 mg **2197**

METHAPHARM, INC. **2198**
11772 West Sample Road
Suite 101
Coral Springs, Florida 33065

Direct Inquiries to:
(800) 287-7686
FAX: (877) 718-9222
E-mail: sales@methapharm.com
www.methapharm.com

Products Described:
Provocholine Powder for Inhalation *2198*

MGI PHARMA, INC. **337, 2198**
5775 West Old Shakopee Road
Suite 100
Bloomington, MN 55437-3174

For Medical Information Contact:
(800) 562-5580
FAX: (952) 346-4800
Customer Service
(800) 562-4531
FAX: (952) 346-4800

Products Described:
◆Aloxi Injection **337, 2198**
◆Hexalen Capsules **337, 2200**
◆Salagen Tablets **337, 2201**

MILLENNIUM PHARMACEUTICALS, INC. **324, 2203**
40 Landsdowne Street
Cambridge, MA 02139

Direct Inquiries to:
(800) 589-9005

Products Described:
◆Integrilin Injection **324, 2203**
◆Velcade for Injection **324, 2207**

MISSION PHARMACAL COMPANY **2211**
10999 IH 10 West, Suite 1000
San Antonio, TX 78230-1355

Direct Inquiries to:
P.O. Box 786099
San Antonio, TX 78278-6099
Toll Free: (800) 292-7364
(210) 696-8400
FAX: (210) 696-6010

For Medical Emergencies Contact:
Mary Ann Walter
(210) 696-8400
FAX: (210) 696-6010

Products Described:
Calcet Tablets *2211*
Calcet Plus Tablets *2211*
Calcibind Oral Powder *2211*
Citracal Caplets + D *2211*
Citracal 250 mg + D Tablets *2211*
Citracal Plus Tablets *2211*
Citracal Prenatal Rx Tablets **2211**
Citracal Tablets **2211**
Fosfree Tablets *2211*
Iromin-G Tablets *2211*
Lithostat Tablets *2212*
Mission Prenatal Tablets *2212*
Mission Prenatal F.A. Tablets *2212*
Mission Prenatal H.P. Tablets *2212*
Thera-Gesic Creme **2212**
Thera-Gesic Plus Creme *2212*
Thiola Tablets *2212*
Urocit-K Tablets **2212**

Other Products Available:
Compete

MONARCH PHARMACEUTICALS
(See KING PHARMACEUTICALS, INC)

MONTIFF, INC. **2213**
Don Tyson's Advanced Nutraceuticals
3205 Santa Monica Blvd.
Santa Monica, CA 90404

Direct Inquiries to:
Customer Service
(877) 820-4883
(310) 582-8938
FAX: (310) 582-8939
E-Mail: montiffinc@aol.com

Products Described:
All-Basic Capsules **2213**
ATP *2213*
B-Long *2213*
Calcium Plus *2213*
CO-Q 10 Plus *2213*
Gluca-Balance Capsules **2213**
Karno-Life *2213*
Neuro-Balance *2213*
Prost-8 Palmetto *2213*
Pure D-Phenyl-Relief *2213*
Pure L-Arginine HCl *2213*
Super Antioxidant Formula *2213*
Tryptophan *2213*
Ultra Carnitine *2213*
Vaso-Lene *2213*
Vita-Minz Plus *2213*

MYLAN BERTEK PHARMACEUTICALS INC. **324, 2228**
P.O. Box 14149
Research Triangle Park, NC 27709
(919) 991-9800

For Medical Information Contact:
Medical Services Department:
(888) 523-7835
(919) 993-5910

Sales and Ordering:
Customer Service
(888) 823-7835

Products Described:
◆Acticin Cream **324, 2228**
◆Amnesteem Capsules **324, 2229**
◆Apokyn Injection **324, 2235**
◆Avita Cream **324, 2239**
◆Avita Gel **324, 2241**
◆Clorpres Tablets **324, 2242**
Clozapine Tablets **2244**
Digitek Tablets **2248**
Granulex Aerosol **2251**
Kristalose for Oral Solution **2252**
◆Maxzide Tablets **324, 2252**
◆Maxzide-25 mg Tablets **324, 2252**
◆Mentax Cream **324, 2254**
Nitrek *2228*
◆Phenytek Capsules **324, 2255**
Sulfamylon Cream **2257**
Sulfamylon Topical Solution **2258**

Other Products Available:
Biobrane Temporary Burn Dressing
Flexzan Wound Dressing
Hydrocol Hydrocolloid Wound Dressing
Proderm
Sorbsan Wound Dressing

MYLAN PHARMACEUTICALS INC. **2213**
781 Chestnut Ridge Road
P.O. Box 4310
Morgantown, WV 26504-4310

Direct Inquiries to:
(804) 599-2595

For Medical Information Contact:
Clinical Research Department
(877) 446-3679
(877) 4INFO-RX

Sales and Ordering:
Sales Department
(800) RX-MYLAN

Products Described:
Acebutolol Hydrochloride Capsules *2213*
Acyclovir Capsules and Tablets *2213*
Albuterol Tablets *2213*
Allopurinol Tablets *2213*
Alprazolam Tablets *2213*
Amiloride Hydrochloride and Hydrochlorothiazide Tablets *2213*
Amitriptyline Hydrochloride Tablets *2213*
Atenolol Tablets *2213*
Atenolol and Chlorthalidone Tablets *2213*
Benazepril Hydrochloride Tablets *2213*
Benazepril Hydrochloride and Hydrochlorothiazide Tablets *2213*
Bisoprolol Fumarate and Hydrochlorothiazide Tablets *2213*
Bumetanide Tablets *2213*
Bupropion Hydrochloride Tablets *2213*
Buspirone Hydrochloride Tablets *2213*
Butorphanol Tartrate Nasal Spray *2213*
Captopril Tablets **2217**
Captopril and Hydrochlorothiazide Tablets *2213*
Carbidopa and Levodopa Extended-release Tablets *2213*
Cefaclor Powders for Oral Suspension *2213*
Chlordiazepoxide and Amitriptyline Hydrochloride Tablets *2213*
Chlorothiazide Tablets *2213*
Chlorpropamide Tablets *2213*
Chlorthalidone Tablets *2213*
Cimetidine Tablets *2213*
Ciprofloxacin Tablets, USP *2213*
Clomipramine Hydrochloride Capsules *2213*
Clonazepam Tablets *2213*
Clonidine Hydrochloride Tablets *2213*
Clorazepate Dipotassium Tablets *2213*
Clozapine Tablets *2213*
Cyclobenzaprine Hydrochloride Tablets *2213*
Cystagon Capsules *2213*
Diazepam Tablets *2213*
Diclofenac Potassium Tablets *2213*
Diclofenac Sodium Extended-release Tablets *2213*
Dicyclomine Hydrochloride Capsules and Tablets *2213*
Diltiazem Hydrochloride Extended-release Capsules (once-a-day) *2213*
Diltiazem Hydrochloride Extended-release Capsules (twice-a-day) *2213*
Diltiazem Hydrochloride Tablets *2213*
Diphenoxylate Hydrochloride and Atropine Sulfate Tablets *2213*
Doxazosin Mesylate Tablets *2213*
Doxepin Hydrochloride Capsules *2213*
Enalapril Maleate and Hydrochlorothiazide Tablets *2213*
Enalapril Maleate Tablets *2213*
Erythromycin Ethylsuccinate Tablets *2213*
Erythromycin Stearate Tablets *2213*
Estradiol Tablets and Transdermal System Patches *2213*
Estropipate Tablets *2213*
Etodolac Tablets *2213*
Etoposide Capsules *2213*
Famotidine Tablets *2213*
Fenoprofen Calcium Tablets *2213*
Flecainide Acetate Tablets *2213*
Fluoxetine Capsules *2213*
Fluphenazine Hydrochloride Tablets *2213*
Flurazepam Hydrochloride Capsules *2213*
Flurbiprofen Tablets *2213*
Fluvoxamine Maleate Tablets *2213*
Furosemide Tablets **2220**
Glipizide Tablets *2213*
Glyburide Tablets *2213*
Guanfacine Tablets *2213*
Haloperidol Tablets *2213*
Hydrochlorothiazide Capsules *2213*
Hydroxychloroquine Sulfate Tablets *2213*
Indapamide Tablets **2222**
Indomethacin Capsules *2213*
Ketoconazole Tablets *2213*
Ketoprofen Capsules *2213*
Ketoprofen Extended-release Capsules *2213*
Ketorolac Tromethamine Tablets *2213*
Levothyroxine Sodium Tablets *2213*
Lisinopril and Hydrochlorothiazide Tablets *2213*
Lisinopril Tablets *2213*
Loperamide Hydrochloride Capsules *2213*
Lorazepam Tablets *2213*
Lovastatin Tablets *2213*
Maprotiline Hydrochloride Tablets *2213*
Meclofenamate Sodium Capsules *2213*
Metformin Hydrochloride Tablets *2213*
Methotrexate Tablets *2213*
Methyclothiazide Tablets *2213*
Methyldopa Tablets *2213*
Methyldopa and Hydrochlorothiazide Tablets *2213*
Metolazone Tablets *2213*
Metoprolol Tartrate Tablets *2213*
Midodrine Hydrochloride Tablets *2213*
Mirtazapine Tablets *2213*
Nadolol Tablets **2224**
Naproxen Tablets *2213*
Naproxen Sodium Tablets *2213*
Nefazodone Hydrochloride Tablets *2213*
Nicardipine Hydrochloride Capsules *2213*
Nifedipine Extended-release Tablets *2213*
Nitrofurantoin Macrocrystals Capsules *2213*
Nitrofurantoin Monohydrate/ Macrocrystals Capsules *2213*
Nitroglycerin Transdermal System Patches *2213*
Nizatidine Capsules *2213*
Nortriptyline Hydrochloride Capsules *2213*
Omeprazole Delayed-release Capsules *2213*
Orphenadrine Citrate Extended-release Tablets *2213*
Orphenadrine Citrate, Aspirin and Caffeine Tablets *2213*
Oxaprozin Tablets *2213*
Paclitaxel Injection *2213*
Pentoxifylline Extended-release Tablets *2213*
Perphenazine and Amitriptyline Hydrochloride Tablets *2213*
Extended Phenytoin Sodium Capsules *2213*
Pindolol Tablets *2213*
Piroxicam Capsules *2213*
Prazosin Hydrochloride Capsules *2213*
Probenecid Tablets *2213*
Prochlorperazine Maleate Tablets *2213*
Propoxyphene Hydrochloride Capsules *2213*
Propoxyphene Hydrochloride, Aspirin and Caffeine Capsules *2213*
Propoxyphene Hydrochloride and Acetaminophen Tablets *2213*
Propoxyphene Napsylate and Acetaminophen Tablets *2213*
Propranolol Hydrochloride Tablets *2213*
Propranolol Hydrochloride and Hydrochlorothiazide Tablets *2213*
Selegiline Hydrochloride Capsules and Tablets *2213*
Sotalol Hydrochloride Tablets *2213*
Spironolactone Tablets *2213*
Spironolactone and Hydrochlorothiazide Tablets *2213*
Sulindac Tablets *2213*
Tamoxifen Citrate Tablets *2213*
Temazepam Capsules *2213*
Terazosin Hydrochloride Capsules *2213*
Tetracycline Hydrochloride Capsules *2213*
Thioridazine Hydrochloride Tablets **2225**
Thiothixene Capsules **2227**
Timolol Maleate Tablets *2213*
Tizanidine Hydrochloride Tablets *2213*
Tolazamide Tablets *2213*
Tolbutamide Tablets *2213*
Tolmetin Sodium Capsules and Tablets *2213*
Tramadol Hydrochloride Tablets *2213*
Triamterene and Hydrochlorothiazide Capsules and Tablets *2213*
Trifluoperazine Hydrochloride Tablets *2213*
Verapamil Hydrochloride Tablets *2213*
Verapamil Hydrochloride Extended-release Capsules and Tablets *2213*

NABI BIOPHARMACEUTICALS **324, 2258**
5800 Park of Commerce Blvd., NW
Boca Raton, FL 33487

For Medical Information Contact:
Generally:
Immunotherapy Customer Service
(800) 458-4244
(561) 989-5783
(800) 4-WINRHO (494-6746)
(800) 685-5579 - Medical
FAX: (561) 989-5722
In Emergencies:
Immunotherapy Customer Service
(800) 458-4244
(800) 4-WINRHO (494-6746)
FAX: (561) 989-5722

Products Described:
◆Aloprim for Injection **324, 2258**
◆Nabi-HB **324, 2261**
◆NovaPlus Nabi-HB *324*
◆PhosLo Gelcaps **324, 2261**
◆PhosLo Tablets **324, 2261**
◆WinRho SDF **324, 2263**

NOVARTIS CONSUMER HEALTH, INC. **324, 2266**
200 Kimball Drive
Parsippany, NJ 07054-0622

Direct Product Inquiries to:
Consumer & Professional Affairs
(800) 452-0051
FAX: (800) 635-2801
or write to:
445 State Street
Fremont, MI 49413-0001

Products Described:
Denavir Cream **2266**
Ex•Lax Milk of Magnesia ■
Ex•Lax Ultra Pills ■
Ex•Lax Regular Strength Laxative Pills ■
Ex•Lax Chocolated Laxative ■
Ex•Lax Maximum Strength Laxative Pills ■
Gas-X Extra Strength Softgels ■
Gas-X Extra Strength Antigas Chewable Tablets ■
Gas-X Maximum Strength Softgels ■
Gas-X Regular Strength Chewable Tablets ■
Gas-X with Maalox Extra Strength Chewable Tablets ■
Gas-X with Maalox Extra Strength Softgels ■
Lamisil AT Cream ■
Lamisil AT Spray Pump ■
Maalox Max Maximum Strength Antacid/Anti-Gas Liquid **2267**
Maalox Regular Strength Antacid/ Antigas Liquid **2267**
Quick Dissolve Maalox Max Maximum Strength Antacid/ Antigas Tablets **2268**
Quick Dissolve Maalox Regular Strength Antacid Tablets **2268**
Perdiem Overnight Relief Pills **2268**
Theraflu Cold & Cough Hot Liquid Medicine ■
Theraflu Cold & Sore Throat Hot Liquid Medicine ■
Theraflu Flu & Chest Congestion Non-Drowsy ■
Theraflu Flu & Sore Throat Hot Liquid Medicine ■
Theraflu Severe Cold & Cough Hot Liquid Medicine ■
Theraflu Severe Cold Caplets ■
Theraflu Severe Cold Hot Liquid Medicine ■
Theraflu Severe Cold Non-Drowsy Caplets ■
Theraflu Severe Cold Non-Drowsy Hot Liquid Medicine ■
◆Transderm Scōp Transdermal Therapeutic System **324, 2268**

Other Products Available:
Regular Strength Ascriptin Tablets
Maximum Strength Ascriptin Caplets
Prescription Strength Cruex Cream
Prescription Strength Cruex Spray Powder
Desenex Foot and Sneaker Spray Powder
Desenex Shake Powder
Desenex Spray Powder AF

PAR PHARMACEUTICAL, INC. 2578

One Ram Ridge Road
Spring Valley, NY 10977

Direct Inquiries to:
Customer Representative
(800) 828-9393
(845) 425-7100

Products Described:

PARKEDALE PHARMACEUTICALS

(See KING PHARMACEUTICALS, INC)

PARKE-DAVIS 329, 2578

A Division of Warner-Lambert Company LLC
A Pfizer Company
235 East 42nd Street
New York, NY 10017-5755
For updates to the product information listed below,
please check the Pfizer Web site,
http://www.pfizer.com,
or call (800) 438-1985.

For Medical Information Contact:
(800) 438-1985
24 hours a day, seven days a week

Distribution:
1855 Shelby Oaks Drive North
Memphis, TN 38134
(901) 387-5200

Customer Service
(800) 533-4535

Products Described:

Other Products Available:
Celontin Capsules
Cerebyx Injection
Dilantin Infatabs
Dilantin Kapseals
Dilantin-125 Oral Suspension
Lopid Tablets
Nardil Tablets
Nitrostat Tablets
Zarontin Capsules
Zarontin Syrup

PBM PHARMACEUTICALS, INC. 2594

204 North Main Street
Gordonsville, VA 22942

Direct Inquiries to:
Customer Service
(866) 366-6282
Fax: (302) 266-7556

Products Described:

PEDINOL PHARMACAL INC. 2594

30 Banfi Plaza North
Farmingdale, NY 11735

Direct Inquiries to:
Director of Professional Services
(631) 293-9500
E-mail: Info@Pedinol.com

Products Described:

Other Products Available:
Breezee Mist Foot Powder
Fungoid Tincture Topical Antifungal Treatment Kit
Hydrisalic Gel
Hydrisinol Creme
Hydrisinol Lotion
LazerCreme
Nail Scrub with Brush
Ostiderm Roll-On
Pedi-Pro Foot Powder
PNS Unna Boot
Sal-Acid Plasters
Salactic Film
Sal-Plant Gel
TI-Screen Sunscreens, Lotion, Sports Gel, Spray and Lip Protectant

PERSŌN & COVEY, INC. 2595

616 Allen Avenue
Glendale, CA 91221-5018

Direct Inquiries to:
(800) 423-2341
FAX: (818) 547-9821
E-mail: helpdesk@personandcovey.com

Products Described:

PFIZER INC. 329, 2596

235 East 42nd Street
New York, NY 10017-5755
For updates to the product information listed below,
please check the Pfizer Web site,
http://www.pfizer.com,
or call (800) 438-1985.

For Medical Information Contact:
(800) 438-1985
24 hours a day, seven days a week

Distribution:
1855 Shelby Oaks Drive North
Memphis, TN 38134
(901) 387-5200
Customer Service:
(800) 533-4535

Pfizer Companies Include:
Agouron Pharmaceuticals
(see PARKE-DAVIS)
(see PHARMACIA & UPJOHN)
(see G.D. SEARLE & CO.)

Products Described:

Other Products Available:
Antivert, Antivert/25, & Antivert/50 Tablets
Atarax Tablets & Syrup
Cardura Tablets
Diabinese Tablets
Feldene Capsules
Geocillin Tablets
Glucotrol Tablets
Pfizerpen for Injection
Procardia Capsules
Procardia XL Extended Release Tablets
Sinequan Capsules
Sinequan Oral Concentrate
Tao Capsules
Urobiotic-250 Capsules
Vibramycin Calcium Oral Suspension Syrup
Vibramycin Hyclate Capsules
Vibramycin Hyclate Intravenous
Vibramycin Monohydrate for Oral Suspension
Vibra-Tabs Film Coated Tablets
Vistaril Capsules
Vistaril Intramuscular Solution
Vistaril Oral Suspension

PHARMACEUTICAL ASSOCIATES, INC. 2692

A Subsidiary of Beach Products, Inc.
201 Delaware Street
Greenville, SC 29605

Direct Inquiries to:
Clete Harmon, Vice President, Q.A.
(800) 845-8210
(864) 277-7282
FAX: (864) 236-0116

Products Described:

PHARMACIA & UPJOHN 330, 2693
A division of Pfizer
235 East 42nd Street
New York, NY 10017-5755
For updates to the product information listed below,
please check the Pfizer Web site,
http://www.pfizer.com,
or call (800) 438-1985.

For Medical Information Contact:
(800) 438-1985
24 hours a day, seven days a week

Distribution:
1855 Shelby Oaks Drive North
Memphis, TN 38134
(901) 387-5200

Customer Service:
(800) 533-4535

Products Described:
◆Aromasin Tablets 330, 2693
◆Bextra Tablets 330, 2695
Camptosar Injection 2699
◆Caverject Impulse Injection 330, 2707
◆Cleocin HCl Capsules 330, 2710
Depo-Provera Contraceptive Injection 2716
Depo-Medrol Injectable Suspension 2712
Depo-Medrol Single-Dose Vial 2714
Depo-Provera Sterile Aqueous Suspension 2718
◆Detrol Tablets 330, 2720
◆Detrol LA Capsules 330, 2722
◆Dostinex Tablets 330, 2724
Ellence Injection 2726
Estring Vaginal Ring 2730
Fragmin Injection 2733
Genotropin Lyophilized Powder 2738
Idamycin PFS Injection 2741
Lunelle Monthly Injection 2743
◆Mirapex Tablets 330, 2749
R-Gene 10 for Intravenous Use 2753
Somavert Injection 2754
Trelstar Depot 2757
◆Vantin Tablets and Oral Suspension 330, 2758
Xalatan Sterile Ophthalmic Solution 2762
◆Xanax Tablets 330, 2763
◆Xanax XR Tablets 330, 2767
Zinecard for Injection 2771
Zyvox Injection 2773
Zyvox for Oral Suspension 2773
◆Zyvox Tablets 330, 2773

Other Products Available:
Aldactazide Tablets
Aldactone Tablets
Amphocin Injection
Ansaid Tablets
Atgam Sterile Solution
Azulfidine EN-tabs Tablets
Azulfidine Tablets
Calan Tablets
Calan SR Caplets
Caverject Sterile Powder
Cleocin Pediatric for Oral Solution, USP
Cleocin Phosphate Sterile Solution
Cleocin T Topical Gel
Cleocin T Topical Lotion
Cleocin T Topical Solution
Cleocin Vaginal Cream
Cleocin Vaginal Ovules
Colestid Tablets
Colestid/Flavored Colestid for Oral Suspension
Cortef Tablets
Cortisone Acetate Tablets, USP
Corvert Injection
Cyklokapron Tablets and Injection
Daypro Caplets
Deltasone Tablets
Demulen 1/35-28 Tablets
Demulen 1/50-28 Tablets
Depo-Estradiol Injectable Solution
Depo-Testadiol Injectable Solution
Depo-Testosterone Injectable Solution
Didrex Tablets
Dipentum Capsules
Emcyt Capsules
Flagyl 375 Capsules
Flagyl ER Tablets
Flagyl Tablets
Gelfilm Sterile Film
Gelfilm Sterile Ophthalmic Film
Gelfoam Sterile Powder
Gelfoam Sterile Sponge
Glynase PresTab Tablets
Glyset Tablets
Halcion Tablets
Hemabate Sterile Solution (Sales restricted to hospitals only)
Idamycin Injection
Lincocin Capsules
Lincocin Sterile Solution
Lomotil Liquid
Lomotil Tablets
Loniten Tablets
Medrol Tablets and Dosepak
Micronase Tablets
Mycobutin Capsules
Norpace Capsules
Norpace CR Capsules
Ogen Tablets
Ogen Vaginal Cream
Prepidil Gel
Prostin E2 Suppositories
Prostin VR Pediatric Sterile Solution
Provera Tablets
Solu-Cortef Sterile Powder
Solu-Medrol Sterile Powder
Tolinase Tablets
Trelstar LA
Trobicin Sterile Powder

PHARMANEX, LLC 2781
75 West Center Street
Provo, UT 84601

For Technical Information and Product Support:
(888) 742-7626
www.pharmanex.com

Products Described:
CordyMax Cs-4 Capsules 2781
Cortitrol Capsules 2781
Lifepak Capsules 2781
Optimum Omega Softgels 2782
Reishimax Capsules 2782
Tēgreen 97 Capsules 2782

POLYMEDICA PHARMACEUTICALS (U.S.A.), INC. 2782
11 State Street
Woburn, MA 01801

For Medical Emergencies Contact:
Peter M. Etzel or Patricia Collins
(781) 933-2020
FAX: (781) 933-7992

Products Described:
Anestacon Jelly *2782*
B & O Supprettes *2782*
Cystospaz Tablets *2782*
Urised Tablets *2782*

WILLIAM P. POYTHRESS COMPANY
(See ECR PHARMACEUTICALS)

PRAECIS PHARMACEUTICALS INCORPORATED 2782
830 Winter Street
Waltham, MA 02451-1420

For Corporate Headquarters:
(877) 772-3247
(781) 795-4100
Internet: www.praecis.com
General Inquiries: info@praecis.com

For Medical Information, Consumer Inquiries, Adverse Drug Experiences and Medical Emergencies
(866) 753-6294
E-mail: medinfo@praecis.com

For Ordering Information:
(866) 753-6294
www.plenaxis.com

Products Described:
Plenaxis for Injectable Suspension ... 2782

PRESUTTI LABORATORIES 2785
1685 Winnetka Circle
Rolling Meadows, IL 60008-1372

Direct Inquiries to:
(888) 405-7800
(847) 483-6050
FAX: (847) 788-9192

Products Described:
Tindamax 2785

PROCAPS LABORATORIES 2787
Formerly YourVitamins, Inc.
430 Parkson Road
Henderson, NV 89015

For Sales Inquiries:
(800) 800-1200 (weekdays)

For Product Information:
Research Department
(702) 564-9000 (weekdays)
www.cholox.com
PDR@cholox.com

Products Described:
Cholox 2787

PROCTER & GAMBLE 2788
(For Rx products, see Procter & Gamble Pharmaceuticals
or call 1-800-836-0658)
P.O. Box 599
Cincinnati, OH 45201
Consumer Relations
(800) 832-3064

For Medical Information Contact:
In Emergencies, call collect:
(513) 636-5107

Products Described:
Head & Shoulders Dandruff Shampoo 2788
Head & Shoulders Dandruff Shampoo Dry Scalp 2788
Head & Shoulders Intensive Treatment Dandruff and Seborrheic Dermatitis Shampoo 2788
Metamucil Capsules 2789
Metamucil Coarse Milled Orange Flavor Powder 2789
Metamucil Coarse Milled Unflavored Powder 2789
Metamucil Smooth Texture Orange Flavor Powder 2789
Metamucil Smooth Texture Sugar-Free Orange Flavor Powder 2789
Metamucil Smooth Texture Sugar-Free Unflavored Powder 2789
Metamucil Wafers, Apple Crisp and Cinnamon Spice Flavors 2789
Pepto-Bismol Original Liquid, Maximum Strength Liquid, Original and Cherry Tablets and Easy-To-Swallow Caplets 2790
Prilosec OTC Tablets 2791
ThermaCare Heat Wraps 2791
Vicks 44 Cough Relief 2792
Vicks 44D Cough & Head Congestion Relief 2792
Vicks 44E Cough & Chest Congestion Relief 2793
Pediatric Vicks 44e Cough & Chest Congestion Relief Liquid 2790
Vicks 44M Cough, Cold & Flu Relief 2793
Pediatric Vicks 44m Cough & Cold Relief 2790
Vicks Cough Drops, Menthol & Cherry Flavors 2791
Vicks DayQuil Multi-Symptom Cold/Flu Relief Liquid & LiquiCaps 2792
Children's Vicks NyQuil Cold/Cough Relief 2788
Vicks NyQuil Cough Liquid 2793
Vicks NyQuil LiquiCaps 2793
Vicks NyQuil Liquid 2793
Vicks Sinex 12-Hour Nasal Spray and Ultra Fine Mist for Sinus Relief 2794
Vicks Sinex Nasal Spray and Ultra Fine Mist for Sinus Relief 2794
Vicks Vapor Inhaler 2795
Vicks VapoRub Cream 2795
Vicks VapoRub Ointment 2795
Vicks VapoSteam 2795

PROCTER & GAMBLE PHARMACEUTICALS, INC. 330, 2795
Health Care Research Center
8700 Mason Montgomery Road
Mason, OH 45040-9462

Direct Inquiries to:
Customer Service
(800) 448-4878

For Medical Information Contact:
Generally:
Medical Communication Services
(800) 836-0658
FAX: (800) 438-0138
Or Write:
Procter & Gamble Pharmaceuticals, Inc.
Medical Communication Services
Health Care Research Center
P.O. Box 8006
Mason, OH 45040-8006
In Emergencies:
Medical Communications
(800) 836-0658
For Product Information:
www.pgpharma.com

Products Described:
◆Actonel Tablets 330, 2795
◆Asacol Delayed-Release Tablets 330, 2800
Dantrium Capsules 2802
Dantrium Intravenous 2803
◆Didronel Tablets 330, 2805

THE PURDUE FREDERICK COMPANY 330, 2806
One Stamford Forum
Stamford, CT 06901-3431

For Medical Information Contact:
(888) 726-7535
Adverse Drug Experiences:
(888) 726-7535
Customer Service:
(800) 877-5666
FAX: (800) 877-3210

Products Described:
Betadine Skin Cleanser 2806
Betadine Solution 2806
Betadine Surgical Scrub 2806
Betasept Surgical Scrub 2807
◆MS Contin Tablets 330, 2807
MSIR Oral Solution Concentrate 2809
◆MSIR Oral Tablets 330, 2809
Senokot Tablets 2811
Senokot-S Tablets 2811
◆Uniphyl 400 mg and 600 mg Tablets 331, 2812

PURDUE PHARMA L.P. 330, 2818
One Stamford Forum
Stamford, CT 06901-3431

For Medical Information Contact:
(888) 726-7535

Adverse Drug Experiences:
(888) 726-7535

Customer Service:
(800) 877-5666
FAX: (800) 877-3210

Products Described:
◆OxyContin Tablets 330, 2818
◆OxyFast Oral Concentrate Solution 331, 2822
◆OxyIR Capsules 331, 2822

PURDUE PHARMACEUTICAL PRODUCTS L.P. 331, 2824
One Stamford Forum
Stamford, CT 06901-3431

For Medical Inquiries Contact:
(888) 726-7535

Adverse Drug Experiences:
(888) 726-7535

Customer Service:
(800) 877-5666
FAX: (800) 877-3210

Products Described:
◆Spectracef Tablets 331, 2824
◆Uniphyl 400mg and 600mg Tablets 331, 2812

PURDUE PRODUCTS L.P. 2827
One Stamford Forum
Stamford, CT 06901-3431

For Medical Information Contact:
(888) 726-7535

Adverse Drug Experiences:
(888) 726-7535

Customer Service:
(800) 877-5666
FAX: (800) 877-3210

Products Described:
Colace Capsules 100 mg 2827
Colace Capsules 50 mg 2827
Colace Glycerin, USP 1.2 grams - Children and Infants 2827
Colace Glycerin, USP 2.1 grams - Adults and Children 2827
Colace Liquid 1% Solution 2828
Mineral Oil 2828
Peri-Colace Tablets 2828
Senokot Tablets 2811
Senokot-S Tablets 2811

QUESTCOR PHARMACEUTICALS, INC. 2828
3260 Whipple Road
Union City, CA 94587
www.questcor.com

Direct Inquiries to:
(510) 400-0700
FAX: (510) 400-0799

Products Described:
H.P. Acthar Gel *2828*
Ethamolin Injection, 5% *2828*
Glofil-125 Injection *2828*
Nascobal Gel *2828*

RECKITT BENCKISER PHARMACEUTICALS INC. 331, 2828
10710 Midlothian Turnpike, Suite 430
Richmond, VA 23235

For Medical Information/Emergencies:
Generally:
(877)782-6966
www.suboxone.com
Emergencies:
(804) 423-7089

Distribution:
Distribution Center
5051 Commerce Crossing
Louisville, KY 40229
Customer Service:
(866) 282-2107
FAX: (866) 282-2138

Products Described:
◆Buprenex Injectable 331, 2828
◆Suboxone Tablets 331, 2830
◆Subutex Tablets 331, 2830

RELIANT PHARMACEUTICALS 331, 2833
110 Allen Road
Liberty Corner, NJ 07938

Direct Inquiries to:
(908) 580-1200

Products Described:
◆Axid Oral Solution 331, 2833
◆DynaCirc CR Tablets 331, 2836
◆InnoPran XL Capsules 331, 2838
Lescol Capsules 2840
◆Lescol XL Tablets 331, 2840
◆Rythmol SR Capsules 331, 2844

ROCHE PHARMACEUTICALS 331, 2848
Roche Laboratories Inc.
340 Kingsland Street
Nutley, New Jersey 07110-1199

For Medical Information:
(including routine inquiries, adverse drug events and product complaints)
Call: (800) 526-6367
In Emergencies: 24-hour service
For the Medical Needs Program
Call: (800) 285-4484
Write: Professional Product Information

Order Fulfillment:
(800) 526-0625

Products Described:
◆Accutane Capsules.............. **331, 2848**
◆Anaprox Tablets.............. **331, 2874**
◆Anaprox DS Tablets.............. **331, 2874**
◆CellCept Capsules.............. **331, 2855**
CellCept Intravenous.............. **2855**
CellCept Oral Suspension.............. **2855**
◆CellCept Tablets.............. **331, 2855**
Copegus Tablets.............. **2862**
◆Cytovene Capsules.............. **331, 2866**
Cytovene-IV.............. **2866**
◆Demadex Tablets and Injection.............. **331, 2871**
◆EC-Naprosyn Delayed-Release Tablets...... **331, 2874**
◆Fortovase Capsules.............. **331, 2876**
Fuzeon Injection.............. **2882**
◆Hivid Tablets.............. **331, 2886**
◆Invirase Capsules.............. **331, 2890**
◆Klonopin Tablets.............. **331, 2895**
◆Klonopin Wafers.............. **331, 2895**
Kytril Injection.............. **2898**
Kytril Oral Solution.............. **2901**
◆Kytril Tablets.............. **331, 2901**
◆Lariam Tablets.............. **331, 2903**
Naprosyn Suspension.............. **2874**
◆Naprosyn Tablets.............. **331, 2874**
Pegasys.............. **2906**
◆Rocaltrol Capsules.............. **331, 2913**
Rocaltrol Oral Solution.............. **2913**
Rocephin Injectable Vials, ADD-Vantage, Galaxy, Bulk....... **2915**
Roferon-A Injection.............. **2918**
Romazicon Injection.............. **2923**
◆Tamiflu Capsules.............. **331, 2927**
Tamiflu Oral Suspension.............. **2927**
◆Ticlid Tablets.............. **331, 2929**
Toradol IM Injection, IV Injection... **2932**
◆Toradol Tablets.............. **331, 2932**
◆Valcyte Tablets.............. **332, 2936**
◆Vesanoid Capsules.............. **332, 2941**
◆Xeloda Tablets.............. **332, 2943**
◆Xenical Capsules.............. **332, 2951**
Zenapax for Injection.............. **2955**

Other Products Available:
Bumex Tablets
Cardene Capsules
Cardene SR Capsules
Fansidar Tablets
Gantrisin Pediatric Suspension

ROCHE PHARMACEUTICALS 331, 2957
Roche Products Inc.
Manati, Puerto Rico 00674

For Medical Information Contact:
Roche Laboratories Inc.
(800) 526-6367

Order Fulfillment:
Roche Laboratories Inc.
(800) 526-0625

Products Described:
◆Valium Tablets.............. **332, 2957**

ROMARK PHARMACEUTICALS 2958
A Division of Romark Laboratories L.C.
3000 Bayport Drive
Suite 200
Tampa, FL 33607

For Medical Information:
(877) 925-4642
FAX: (813) 282-9055

Products Described:
Alinia for Oral Suspension.............. **2958**

ROSS PRODUCTS DIVISION 332, 2960
Abbott Laboratories USA
Columbus, OH 43215-1724

Direct Inquiries to:
(800) 227-5767

Products Described:
Pediaflor Drops.............. *2965*
Pedialyte Oral Electrolyte Maintenance Solution.............. **2960**
PediaSure Enteral Formula.............. **2962**
PediaSure Formula.............. **2962**
Pediazole Suspension.............. **2960**
◆Survanta Intratracheal Suspension.............. **332, 2963**
Vi-Daylin ADC Vitamins Drops...... *2965*
Vi-Daylin ADC Vitamins + Iron Drops.............. *2965*
Vi-Daylin Multivitamin Drops....... *2965*
Vi-Daylin Multivitamin + Iron Drops.............. *2965*
Vi-Daylin Multivitamin Liquid....... *2965*
Vi-Daylin Multivitamin + Iron Liquid.............. *2965*
Vi-Daylin/F ADC Vitamins Drops With Fluoride.............. *2965*
Vi-Daylin/F ADC Vitamins + Iron Drops With Fluoride.............. *2965*
Vi-Daylin/F Multivitamin Drops With Fluoride.............. *2965*
Vi-Daylin/F Multivitamin + Iron Drops With Fluoride.............. *2965*

ROXANE LABORATORIES, INC. 2966
P.O. Box 16532
Columbus, OH 43216-6532

Direct Inquiries to:
Technical Product Information
P.O. Box 16532
Columbus, OH 43216-6532
(800) 962-8364

Products Described:
Acetylcysteine Solution USP......... *2966*
Alprazolam Intensol Oral Solution (Concentrate) CIV.............. *2966*
Azathioprine Tablets USP.............. *2966*
Butorphanol Tartrate Nasal Spray CIV.............. *2966*
Calcitriol Oral Solution.............. *2966*
Calcium Carbonate Oral Suspension (not USP).............. *2966*
Calcium Carbonate Tablets USP...... *2966*
Calcium Gluconate Tablets USP...... *2966*
Clotrimazole Troche.............. *2966*
Cocaine Hydrochloride Topical Solution CII.............. *2966*
Codeine Sulfate Tablets USP CII...... *2966*
Cromolyn Sodium Inhalation Solution USP.............. *2966*
Cyclophosphamide Tablets USP...... *2966*
Dexamethasone Intensol Oral Solution (Concentrate).............. *2966*
Dexamethasone Oral Solution........ *2966*
Dexamethasone Tablets USP........ *2966*
DHT Dihydrotachysterol Tablets USP.............. *2966*
DHT Intensol Oral Solution (Concentrate).............. *2966*
Diazepam Intensol Oral Solution (Concentrate) CIV.............. *2966*
Diazepam Oral Solution CIV......... *2966*
Diclofenac Sodium Delayed-Release Tablets USP...... *2966*
Digoxin Elixir USP.............. *2966*
Diphenoxylate Hydrochloride & Atropine Sulfate Oral Solution USP CV.............. *2966*
Dolophine Hydrochloride Tablets (Methadone Hydrochloride Tablets USP) CII.............. *2966*
Flecainide Acetate Tablets USP...... *2966*
Fluconazole Tablets.............. *2966*
Furosemide Oral Solution USP....... *2966*
Furosemide Tablets USP.............. *2966*
Hydromorphone Hydrochloride Tablets USP CII.............. *2966*
Ipratropium Bromide Nasal Spray.... *2966*
Lactulose Solution USP.............. *2966*
Leucovorin Calcium Tablets USP.... *2966*
Levorphanol Tartrate Tablets USP CII.............. *2966*
Lidocaine Viscous 2% USP.............. *2966*
Lidocaine Hydrochloride Topical Solution 4% USP.............. *2966*
Lithium Carbonate Capsules USP.... *2966*
Lithium Carbonate Extended Release Tablets USP.............. *2966*
Lithium Carbonate Tablets USP...... *2966*
Lithium Citrate Syrup USP.............. *2966*
Loperamide Hydrochloride Oral Solution.............. *2966*
Lorazepam Intensol Oral Concentrate USP CIV.............. *2966*
Megestrol Acetate Tablets USP....... *2966*
Megestrol Acetate Oral Suspension USP.............. *2966*
Meperidine Hydrochloride Syrup USP CII.............. *2966*
Meperidine Hydrochloride Tablets USP CII.............. *2966*
Mercaptopurine Tablets USP.............. *2966*
Methadone Hydrochloride Tablets USP CII.............. *2966*
Methadone Hydrochloride Intensol Oral Concentrate USP CII.............. *2966*
Methadone Hydrochloride Oral Solution USP CII.............. *2966*
Methotrexate Tablets USP.............. *2966*
Mexiletine Hydrochloride Capsules USP.............. *2966*
Midazolam Hydrochloride Syrup CIV.............. *2966*
Milk of Magnesia Concentrated (Lemon Flavored).............. *2966*
Mirtazapine Tablets.............. *2966*
Morphine Sulfate (Immediate Release) Oral Solution CII.............. *2966*
Morphine Sulfate (Immediate Release) Tablets CII.............. *2966*
Naproxen Oral Suspension USP...... *2966*
Oxycodone and Acetaminophen Capsules USP CII.............. *2966*
PredniSONE Intensol Oral Solution (Concentrate).............. *2966*
PredniSONE Oral Solution USP...... *2966*
PredniSONE Tablets USP.............. *2966*
Propantheline Bromide Tablets USP.............. *2966*
Propranolol Hydrochloride Oral Solution.............. *2966*
Pseudoephedrine Hydrochloride Tablets USP.............. *2966*
Roxicet Oral Solution CII.............. *2966*
Roxicet Tablets USP CII.............. *2966*
Roxicet 5/500 Caplets USP CII........ *2966*
Saliva Substitute.............. *2966*
Sodium Polystyrene Sulfonate Suspension USP.............. *2966*
Tamoxifen Citrate Tablets USP....... *2966*
Triazolam Tablets USP CIV.......... *2966*

SALIX PHARMACEUTICALS, INC. 332, 2966
8540 Colonnade Center Drive
Suite 501
Raleigh, NC 27615

Direct Inquiries to:
(866) 669-7597
FAX: (919) 862-1096
www.salix.com

For adverse events, product quality complaints and patient information requests:
Product Information Center
(800) 508-0024
FAX: (510) 595-8183
E-mail: salix@medcomsol.com

Products Described:
◆Azasan Tablets.............. **332, 2966**
◆Colazal Capsules.............. **332, 2968**
◆Xifaxan Tablets.............. **332, 2969**

SANDOZ PHARMACEUTICALS CORPORATION
(See NOVARTIS PHARMACEUTICALS CORPORATION)

SANGSTAT MEDICAL CORPORATION 2971
6300 Dumbarton Circle
Fremont, CA 94555

Direct Inquiries to:
Medical and Scientific Information
(877) 264-7828
Customer Service
(888) 764-7828

Products Described:
Thymoglobulin for Injection......... **2971**

SANKYO PHARMA INC. 337, 2973
Two Hilton Court
Parsippany, NJ 07054

Direct Inquiries to:
(877) 4-SANKYO
www.sankyopharma.com

Products Described:
◆Benicar Tablets.............. **337, 2973**
◆Benicar HCT Tablets.............. **337, 2975**
◆WelChol Tablets.............. **337, 2978**

SANOFI-SYNTHELABO INC. 332, 2980
90 Park Avenue
New York, NY 10016

Direct Inquiries to:
(212) 551-4000

For Medical Information Contact:
Product Information Services
(800) 446-6267

Sales and Ordering:
East Coast: (800) 223-1062
West Coast: (800) 223-5511

Products Described:
◆Ambien Tablets.............. **332, 2980**
Aralen Tablets.............. **2983**
◆Avapro Tablets.............. **332, 2985**
Demerol Syrup.............. **2987**
◆Demerol Tablets.............. **332, 2987**
◆Eligard 7.5 mg.............. **332, 2989**
◆Eligard 22.5 mg.............. **332, 2992**
◆Eligard 30 mg.............. **332, 2994**
Elitek.............. **2997**
Eloxatin for Injection.............. **2998**
◆Hyalgan Solution.............. **332, 3005**
◆Plaquenil Tablets.............. **332, 3008**
◆Plavix Tablets.............. **332, 3009**
Uroxatral Tablets.............. **3012**

Other Products Available:
Aralen Injection
Breonesin Capsules
Broncholate Syrup
Danocrine Capsules
Drisdol 50,000 Unit Capsules
Drisdol in Propylene Glycol
Hytakerol Capsules
Kayexalate Powder
Mytelase Chloride Caplets
NegGram Caplets
Neo-Synephrine Ophthalmic Solution
Pediacof Syrup
pHisoHex Cleanser
Poly-Histine Elixir
Primaquine Phosphate Tablets
Vitamin D, USP
Vitamins

SANTARUS INC 332, 3015
10590 West Ocean Air Drive
Suite 200
San Diego, CA 92130

Direct Inquiries to:
(888) 778-0887

FAX: (858) 314-5701

Products Described:
◆Zegerid Powder for Oral Solution.............. **332, 3015**

SANTEN INC.
(see VISTAKON PHARMACEUTICALS, LLC)

SAVIENT PHARMACEUTICALS, INC. 332, 3018
One Tower Center
Fourteenth Flour
East Brunswick, NJ 08816

For Medical or Reimbursement Information Contact:
(866) OXANDRIN or visit
www.oxandrin.com

For Product Ordering please call:
(800) 741-2698
FAX: (800) 741-2696

Products Described:
◆Delatestryl Injection.............. **332, 3018**
◆Oxandrin Tablets.............. **332, 3019**

SCANDIPHARM, INC.
(See AXCAN SCANDIPHARM INC.)

SCHERING CORPORATION 332, 3021
A wholly-owned subsidiary of Schering-Plough Corporation
Galloping Hill Road
Kenilworth, NJ 07033
(908) 298-4000

Direct Inquiries to:
(908) 298-4000

Customer Service:
(800) 222 7579
FAX: (908) 595-3729

For Medical Information Contact:
Schering Laboratories
Drug/Information Services
2000 Galloping Hill Road
Kenilworth, NJ 07033
(800) 526-4099
FAX: (973) 921-7228

Distribution:
Southeast Branch
20 Crest Ridge Drive
Suwanee, GA 30024
(770) 831-2900
Western Distribution Center
12125 Moya Blvd.
Reno, NV 89506-2600
(775) 677-2222
Eastern Distribution Center
3070 Route 22 West
Branchburg, NJ 08876-3598
(908) 595-3761

Products Described:
Clarinex Tablets.............. **3021**
Clarinex Reditabs Tablets.............. **3021**
Diprolene AF Cream 0.05%.............. **3023**
◆Elocon Cream 0.1%.............. **332, 3024**
◆Elocon Lotion 0.1%.............. *332*
◆Elocon Ointment 0.1%.............. **332, 3025**
Foradil Aerolizer.............. **3026**
Guanidine Hydrochloride Tablets..... **3030**
Integrilin Injection.............. **3031**
Intron A for Injection.............. **3035**
Nasonex Nasal Spray.............. **3044**
PEG-Intron Powder for Injection..... **3046**
Rebetol Capsules.............. **3053**
Rebetol Oral Solution.............. **3053**
Rebetron Combination Therapy...... **3058**
Ribavirin, USP Capsules.............. **3063**
Temodar Capsules.............. **3067**
Vytorin 10/10 Tablets.............. **3070**
Vytorin 10/20 Tablets.............. **3070**
Vytorin 10/40 Tablets.............. **3070**
Vytorin 10/80 Tablets.............. **3070**
Zetia Tablets.............. **3075**

SCHWARZ PHARMA, INC. 332, 3080
6140 W. Executive Drive
Mequon, WI 53092

For Medical Information Contact:
Medical and Drug Information
(262) 238-9994
(800) 558-5114

Products Described:
Colyte for Oral Solution.............. *3080*
◆Colyte with Flavor Packs for Oral Solution.............. **332, 3080**

◆Cortifoam Rectal Foam *332, 3081*
Dilatrate-SR Capsules *3081*
Edex Injection *3081*
◆Epifoam *332, 3082*
Kutrase Capsules *3082*
Ku-Zyme Capsules *3082*
Ku-Zyme HP Capsules *3082*
Levatol Tablets *3082*
Levbid Extended-Release Tablets *3082*
Levsin Drops *3082*
Levsin Elixir *3082*
Levsin Injection *3082*
Levsin Tablets *3082*
Levsin/SL Tablets *3082*
Levsinex Timecaps *3082*
Monoket Tablets *3083*
NuLev Orally Disintegrating Tablets *3083*
Parcopa Orally Disintegrating Tablets **3083**
ProctoCream-HC 2.5% *3085*
◆ProctoFoam-HC **332, 3085**
◆TriLyte with Flavor Packs for Oral Solution **333, 3086**
◆Uniretic Tablets **333, 3086**
Univasc Tablets **3090**
Verelan Capsules *3092*
◆Verelan PM Capsules **333, 3092**

Other Products Available:
Calciferol Drops
Codiclear DH Syrup
Codimal DH Syrup
Codimal DM Syrup
Codimal PH Syrup
Co-Gesic Tablets
Guaimax-D Extended-Release Tablets
Lactrase Capsules
ProctoFoam-NS (Non-Steroid)
Reglan Tablets
Robaxin Tablets
Robaxin-750 Tablets
Trichotine Powder

SCS PHARMACEUTICALS
(See PHARMACIA & UPJOHN)

G.D. SEARLE & CO. 333, 3095
A Division of Pfizer
235 East 42nd Street
New York, NY 10017-5755
For updates to the product information listed below,
please check the Pfizer Web site,
http://www.pfizer.com,
or call (800) 438-1985.

For Medical Information Contact:
(800) 438-1985
24 hours a day, seven days a week

Distribution:
1855 Shelby Oaks Drive North
Memphis, TN 38134
(901) 387-5200

Customer Service:
(800) 533-4535

Products Described:
◆Celebrex Capsules **333, 3095**
◆Covera-HS Tablets **333, 3099**

Other Products Available:
Arthrotec Tablets
Cytotec Tablets
Synarel Nasal Solution for Central Precocious Puberty
Synarel Nasal Solution for Endometriosis

SEPRACOR INC. 333, 3102
84 Waterford Drive
Marlborough, MA 01752

For Direct Inquiries to the Customer Assistance Center (CAC) Contact:
(888) 394-7377
FAX: (508) 357-7589
E-mail: CAC@sepracor.com
Or write to Sepracor CAC at the address above.

For Medical Information for Healthcare Professionals Contact:
(800) 739-0565

Products Described:
◆Xopenex Inhalation Solution **333, 3102**

SERONO, INC. 333, 3106
One Technology Place
Rockland, MA 02370

Direct Inquiries to:
Customer Service, Sales and Ordering
(888) 398-4567
(781) 982-9000

For Medical Information or to Report Adverse Drug Experiences Contact:
U.S. Medical Information or U.S. Product Surveillance at:
(888) 275-7376
(781) 982-9000
www.seronousa.com
www.howkidsgrow.com
www.novantrone.com
www.rebif.com
www.seronofertility.com
www.serostim.com
www.zorbtive.com

Products Described:
Cetrotide for Injection **3106**
Crinone 4% Gel **3108**
Crinone 8% Gel **3108**
Geref Diagnostic for Injection *3439*
Gonal-f for Injection *3112*
Gonal-f RFF for Injection *3115*
◆Gonal-f RFF Pen for Injection **333, 3112**
Novantrone for Injection Concentrate **3115**
◆Ovidrel Prefilled Syringe for Injection **333, 3120**
◆Rebif Prefilled Syringe for Injection **333, 3123**
Saizen for Injection *3126*
Serophene Tablets *3127*
Serostim for Injection *3127*
Zorbtive for Injection *3127*

SHIONOGI U.S.A. 3127
100 Campus Drive
Florham Park, NJ 07932

Direct Inquiries to:
(973) 966-6900
FAX (973) 966-2820

Products Described:
Cedax Capsules **3127**
Cedax Oral Suspension **3127**

SHIRE US INC. 333, 3131
One Riverfront Place
Newport, KY 41071-4570

Direct Inquiries to:
Customer Service
(800) 828-2088
(859) 669-8000
FAX: (859) 669-8420

For Medical Information Contact:
(800) 828-2088

Products Described:
◆Adderall Tablets **333, 3131**
◆Adderall XR Capsules **333, 3132**
◆Agrylin Capsules **333, 3134**
◆Carbatrol Capsules **333, 3136**
◆DextroStat Tablets **333, 3138**
◆Fareston Tablets **333, 3139**
◆Pentasa Capsules **333, 3141**
◆ProAmatine Tablets **333, 3142**

SIGMA-TAU PHARMACEUTICALS, INC. 3144
800 South Frederick Avenue, Suite 300
Gaithersburg, MD 20877

Direct Inquiries to:
(301) 948-1041
(800) 447-0169
FAX: (301) 948-3194

Products Described:
Carnitor Injection **3144**
Carnitor Tablets and Oral Solution **3146**
Matulane Capsules **3147**

SIRIUS LABORATORIES, INC. 3148
100 Fairway Drive
Suite 130
Vernon Hills, IL 60061

Direct Inquiries to:
Customer Service:
(866) 292-2108

For Medical Emergencies Contact:
(847) 968-2424

Products Described:
Avar Cleanser **3148**
Avar Gel **3148**
Avar Green **3148**
Avar-e Emollient Cream **3148**
Avar-e Green Cream **3148**
Nicomide Tablets **3149**
Psoriatec Cream **3149**

SKINMEDICA, INC. 3150
5909 Sea Lion Place
Suite H
Carlsbad, CA 92008

Direct Inquiries to:
(760) 448-3600
FAX (760) 448-3601
www.SkinMedica.com

Products Described:
Epiquin Micro Topical Cream **3150**
Epiquin Micro XD Topical Cream **3150**
Neobenz Micro Cream **3150**
Vaniqa Cream, 13.9% **3151**

SOLVAY PHARMACEUTICALS, INC. 333, 3153
901 Sawyer Road
Marietta, GA 30062
(770) 578-9000
FAX: (770) 578-5597
www.solvaypharmaceuticals-us.com

For Medical Information Contact:
Generally:
Medical Information Department
(800) 241-1643 #8

Sales and Ordering:
Orders may be placed by calling this toll free number:
(800) 241-1643 #1
FAX: (770) 578-5901
Mail orders should be sent to:
Solvay Pharmaceuticals
Order Entry Department
901 Sawyer Road
Marietta, GA 30062

Products Described:
◆Aceon Tablets (2 mg, 4 mg, 8 mg) **333, 3153**
◆Creon 5 Capsules **333, 3156**
◆Creon 10 Capsules **333, 3156**
◆Creon 20 Capsules **333, 3156**
◆Estratest Tablets **333, 3157**
◆Estratest H.S. Tablets **333, 3157**
◆Estrogel 0.06% **333, 3160**
◆Prometrium Capsules (100 mg, 200 mg) **333, 3165**
◆Rowasa Rectal Suspension Enema **333, 3168**

Other Products Available:
Lithobid Tablets

SOMERSET PHARMACEUTICALS, INC. 333, 3170
2202 North Westshore Boulevard, Suite 450
Tampa, FL 33607

For Medical Information Contact:
Generally:
Professional Services Department
(813) 288-0040
FAX: (813) 282-3804
In Emergencies:
(800) 892-8889
FAX: (813) 282-3804

Products Described:
◆Eldepryl Capsules **333, 3170**

STAR PHARMACEUTICALS, INC. 3172
1881 W. State Road 84 Suite 101
Fort Lauderdale, FL 33315

Direct Inquiries to:
Roseanne Branciforte R.PH., MBA, President
(954) 971-9704

Sales and Ordering:
(800) 845-7827
FAX: (954) 971-7718
www.starpharm.com
E-mail: info@starpharm.com

Products Described:
Aphrodyne Caplets *3172*
Prosed EC Tablets **3173**
Prosed/DS Tablets **3172**
Uro-KP-Neutral Caplets *3173*
Urolene Blue Tablets *3173*
Virilon Capsules *3173*

STIEFEL LABORATORIES, INC. 3173
255 Alhambra Circle
Coral Gables, FL 33134

BRANCH OFFICES:
New York
Route 145
Oak Hill, NY 12460
(518) 239-6901

Direct Inquiries to:
Professional Services Department
(888) STIEFEL

Products Described:
Brevoxyl-4 Cleansing Lotion **3174**
Brevoxyl-4 Creamy Wash **3174**
Brevoxyl-4 Gel **3173**
Brevoxyl-8 Cleansing Lotion **3174**
Brevoxyl-8 Creamy Wash **3174**
Brevoxyl-8 Gel **3173**
Claripel Cream **3174**
Clindets Pledgets **3175**
Clobevate Gel **3176**
Duac Topical Gel **3176**
LactiCare-HC Lotion, 2½% *3177*
Rosac Cream with Sunscreens **3178**
Sulfoxyl Lotion Regular *3178*
Sulfoxyl Lotion Strong *3178*

Other Products Available:
Acne-Aid Cleansing Bar
Brasivol Fine Facial Cleanser and Conditioner
DermaVite Dietary Supplement
Epilyt Lotion
Impruv Natural Repair Hypoallergenic Cream
LactiCare Lotion
Oilatum Cleansing Bar (Unscented)
Oilatum-AD Soap Free Cleansing Lotion
PanOxyl Aqua Gel
PanOxyl Bar 10
Polytar Shampoo
Polytar Soap
Salicylic Acid Cleansing Bar
Sarna Lotion
Sarna Sensitive Anti-Itch Lotion
Sarnol-HC Lotion
SAStid Salicylic Acid and Sulfur Soap
Sulfur Soap
Zeasorb Powder
Zeasorb-AF Lotion/Powder
Zeasorb-AF Powder
ZNP Bar

SUPERGEN, INC. 3178
4140 Dublin Boulevard, Suite 200
Dublin, CA 94568

For Placing Orders Contact:
Nipent: (800) 222-6883
Mitomycin: (800) 905-5474

For Customer Service Contact:
(800) 353-1075 ext. 184

For Medical or Drug Information Contact:
(888) 437-8737

For Corporate Headquarters:
(800) 353-1075

Products Described:
Mitomycin for Injection, USP *3178*
Nipent for Injection **3178**

SWISS BIOCEUTICAL INTERNATIONAL, LTD. 3181
2533 No. Carson Street, Suite 3573
Carson City, NV 89706

Direct Inquiries to:
Executive Director
(775) 841-7020
FAX: (775) 883-2384
www.imuplus.net

Products Described:
IMUPlus Formula **3181**

TAKEDA PHARMACEUTICALS AMERICA, INC. 334, 3181
475 Half Day Road
Lincolnshire, IL 60069

Direct Inquiries to:
Sales and Ordering:
Customer Service
(877) 5 TAKEDA
(877) 582-5332

For Medical Information Contact:
General:
(877) TAKEDA 7
(877) 825-3327
Adverse Drug Experiences:
(877) TAKEDA 7
(877) 825-3327

Products Described:
◆Actos Tablets **334, 3181**

TAP PHARMACEUTICALS INC. 334, 3186
Lake Forest, IL 60045

For Medical Information Contact:
(800) 622-2011 (LUPRON, PREVACID, PREVPAC and PREVACID NAPRAPAC)

Products Described:
◆Lupron Depot 3.75 mg **334, 3188**
◆Lupron Depot 7.5 mg **334, 3192**
◆Lupron Depot--3 Month 11.25 mg **334, 3193**
◆Lupron Depot--3 Month 22.5 mg **334, 3197**
◆Lupron Depot--4 Month 30 mg **334, 3198**
◆Lupron Depot-PED 7.5 mg, 11.25 mg and 15 mg **334, 3200**
◆Lupron Injection **334, 3186**
Lupron Injection Pediatric **3187**
◆Prevacid Delayed-Release Capsules **334, 3202**
◆Prevacid for Delayed-Release Oral Suspension **334, 3202**
◆Prevacid I.V. for Injection **334, 3208**
◆Prevacid NapraPAC 375 .... **334, 3211**
◆Prevacid NapraPAC 500 .... **334, 3211**
◆Prevacid SoluTab Delayed-Release Orally Disintegrating Tablets **334, 3202**
◆PREVPAC **334, 3215**

TARGACEPT, INC. **334, 3220**
200 East First Street, Suite 300
Winston-Salem, NC 27101

Direct Inquiries to:
(336) 480-2233

Products Described:
◆Inversine Tablets................**334, 3220**

TARO PHARMACEUTICALS U.S.A., INC. **3220**
5 Skyline Drive
Hawthorne, NY 10532

Direct Inquiries to:
(888) TARO-USA
www.taro.com

Products Described:
Acetazolamide Tablets USP.......... *3220*
Acetic Acid 2% Otic Solution with Hydrocortisone 1% USP........... *3220*
Alclometasone Dipropionate USP.... *3220*
Amcinonide Cream, Lotion.......... *3220*
Amiodarone HCl Tablets............ *3220*
Ammonium Lactate Cream, Lotion... *3220*
Betamethasone Dipropionate Cream, Gel........................ *3220*
Betamethasone Dipropionate Cream USP........................ *3220*
Betamethasone Valerate Cream USP............................ *3220*
Carbamazepine Oral Suspension..... *3220*
Carbamazepine Tablets (Chewable) USP............................ *3220*
Carbamazepine Tablets USP......... *3220*
Clobetasol Propionate Cream, Ointment, Gel, Solution USP....... *3220*
Clobetasol Propionate Cream (Emollient) USP.................. *3220*
Clomipramine Hydrochloride Capsules......................... *3220*
Clorazepate Dipotassium Tablets USP............................ *3220*
Clotrimazole Cream, Solution........ *3220*
Clotrimazole and Betamethasone Dipropionate Cream, Lotion USP.. *3220*
Desonide Cream, Ointment.......... *3220*
Desoximetasone Cream, Gel, Ointment USP.................... *3220*
Diflorasone Diacetate Cream, Ointment.......................... *3220*
Econazole Nitrate Cream............ *3220*
Enalapril Maleate and Hydrochlorothiazide Tablets USP.. *3220*
Enalapril Maleate Tablets USP....... *3220*
Etodolac Capsules, Tablets USP...... *3220*
Etodolac Extended-Release Tablets... *3220*
Etodolac Tablets, USP.............. *3220*
Fluconazole Tablets................. *3220*
Fluocinonide (Emulsified Base) Cream USP.................... *3220*
Fluocinonide Cream, Ointment, Gel, Solution USP................ *3220*
Fluouracil Topical Solution.......... *3220*
Fluticasone Cream, Ointment........ *3220*
Gentamicin Sulfate Cream, Ointment USP.................... *3220*
Hydrocortisone Cream, Lotion, Ointment USP.................... *3220*
Hydrocortisone Valerate Cream, Ointment USP.................... *3220*
Ketoconazole Capsules............... *3220*
Ketoconazole Tablets USP........... *3220*
Lidocaine Ointment USP............. *3220*
Nystatin and Triamcinolone Acetonide Cream, Ointment USP.. *3220*
Nystatin Cream USP................. *3220*
Phenytoin Suspension USP.......... *3220*
Terconazole Vaginal Cream.......... *3220*
Triamcinolone Acetonide Dental Paste USP...................... *3220*
Warfarin Sodium Tablets USP........ *3220*

TAROPHARMA **3220**
5 Skyline Drive
Hawthorne, NY 10532

Direct Inquiries to:
(800) 544-1449

Products Described:
Lustra............................ *3220*
Lustra-AF......................... *3220*
Ovide .5% Lotion................... *3220*
Primsol 50 mg Solution............. *3220*
Topicort .05% Gel.................. *3220*
Topicort .25% Cream................ *3220*
Topicort .25% Ointment............. *3220*
Topicort LP .05% Gel............... *3220*
U-cort 1% Cream................... *3220*

TEVA NEUROSCIENCE, INC. **334, 3221**
901 E. 104th Street, Suite 900
Kansas City, MO 64131

For Company Inquiries Contact:
(800) 221-4026

For Medical Information Contact:
(800) 887-8100

Products Described:
◆Copaxone for Injection..........**334, 3221**

THE MEDICINES COMPANY **322, 1955**
8 Campus Drive
Parsippany, NJ 07054

Direct Inquiries to:
(800) 264-4662

Products Described:
◆Angiomax for Injection.........**322, 1955**

THER-Rx CORPORATION **334, 3225**
13622 Lakefront Drive
St. Louis, MO 63045

Direct Inquiries to:
(314) 209-1517
FAX: (314) 770-0371

Products Described:
◆Chromagen Soft Gelatin Capsules.....................**334, 3225**
◆Chromagen FA Soft Gelatin Capsules.....................**334, 3225**
◆Chromagen Forte Soft Gelatin Capsules...............**334, 3225**
◆Gynazole-1 Vaginal Cream......**334, 3226**
◆Niferex Capsules...............**334, 3226**
◆Niferex-150 Capsules...........**334, 3227**
◆Niferex-150 Forte Capsules.....**334, 3227**
◆PreCare Chewable Tablets......**334, 3227**
◆PreCare Conceive Tablets.......**334, 3227**
◆PreCare Prenatal Caplets........**334, 3228**
◆PremesisRx Tablets.............**334, 3228**
◆PrimaCare AM Capsules........**334, 3228**
◆PrimaCare One Capsules........**334, 3229**
◆PrimaCare PM Tablets..........**334, 3228**
◆StrongStart Caplets.............**334, 3229**
◆StrongStart Chewable Tablets...**334, 3229**

TIBOTEC THERAPEUTICS **334, 3230**
430 Route 22 East
P.O. Box 6914
Bridgewater, NJ 08807

Direct Inquiries to:
(800) 325-7504
Prompt #1, Customer Service
Prompt #2, Medical Information
FAX (908) 526-9230

Products Described:
◆Doxil Injection.................**334, 3230**

UAD LABORATORIES
(See FOREST PHARMACEUTICALS, INC.)

UCB PHARMA, INC. **334, 3234**
1950 Lake Park Drive
Smyrna, GA 30080

Direct Inquiries to:
(800) 477-7877

For Medical Information Contact:
Medical Affairs Department
(800) 477-7877, option 9
FAX: (770) 970-8859

Products Described:
◆Keppra Oral Solution...........**334, 3234**
◆Keppra Tablets.................**334, 3234**
Lortab 2.5/500 Tablets.............**3240**
Lortab 5/500 Tablets...............**3240**
Lortab 7.5/500 Tablets.............**3240**
Lortab 10/500 Tablets..............**3240**
Lortab Elixir......................**3238**
Theo-24 Extended Release Capsules........................ *3241*
Trinsicon Capsules.................. *3242*
Vicon Forte Capsules............... *3242*

Other Products Available:
Corticaine Cream
Vicon-C Capsules

UNICITY NETWORK, INC. **3242**
The Make Life Better Company
1201 North 800 East
Orem, UT 84097

Direct Inquiries to:
(801) 226-2600
www.makelifebetter.com
science@unicity.com
Products of Unicity, The Make Life Better Company are distributed through independant distributors.

Products Described:
Cardio Essentials Capsules...........**3242**
CM Plex Cream......................**3242**
CM Plex Softgels...................**3242**
Life Health - Bios Life 2 Drink Mix..............................**3242**
Life Health - Core Health Supplement........................**3242**
Life Health - Daily Produce 24 Capsules..........................**3242**
Visutein Capsules...................**3243**

UNIMED PHARMACEUTICALS, INC. **335, 3243**
A Solvay Pharmaceuticals, Inc. Company
901 Sawyer Road
Marietta, GA 30062

Direct Inquiries to:
(770) 578-9000

Products Described:
◆Anadrol-50 Tablets.............**335, 3243**
◆AndroGel........................**335, 3244**
◆Marinol Capsules...............**335, 3248**

THE UPJOHN COMPANY
(See PHARMACIA & UPJOHN)

UPSHER-SMITH LABORATORIES, INC. **335, 3250**
6701 Evenstad Drive
Minneapolis, MN 55369

For Medical Information Contact:
Write: Professional Services Department
or call: (800) 654-2299
(during business hours-8 a.m. to 5 p.m. CST)

Products Described:
Amlactin AP Cream................ *3250*
◆Clenia Foaming Wash and Emollient Cream............ *335, 3250*
◆Folgard OS Tablets................. *335*
◆Folgard RX 2.2 Tablets......... *335, 3250*
Folgard Tablets...................... *3250*
Hemril-30 Suppositories............ *3250*
◆Jantoven Tablets...............**335, 3250**
◆Klor-Con M20/Klor-Con M10/Klor-Con M15 Tablets...**335, 3255**
Klor-Con/EF Tablets................. *3255*
◆Klor-Con 8/Klor-Con 10 Tablets...................... *335, 3255*
Klor-Con Powder.................... *3255*
Klor-Con/25 Powder................. *3255*
◆Pacerone Tablets...............**335, 3256**
◆Slo-Niacin Tablets............. *335, 3260*

Other Products Available:
Amantadine HCl Capsules
Androxy Tablets CIII
Baclofen Tablets
Benztropine Mesylate Tablets
Bisacodyl Uniserts Suppositories
Chlorpromazine HCl Tablets
Feratab Tablets
Ferrous Gluconate Tablets
Ferrous Sulfate Enteric Coated Tablets
Hemorrhoidal-HC Uniserts Suppositories (Hemril-HC)
Hexavitamin Tablets
Niacor Tablets
Oxybutynin Chloride Tablets
Pentoxil Tablets
Prevalite Powder
RMS Suppositories CII
Sorbitol Solution
Sorine Tablets
SSKI Solution
Stress Formula Tablets
Stress Formula Tablets/Zinc
Therapeutic B Complex with Vitamin C Caplets
Therapeutic Multivitamin Tablets
Therapeutic Multivitamin with Minerals Tablets
Valproic Acid Capsules
Zinc Sulfate Capsules

U.S. PHARMACEUTICAL CORPORATION **3260**
2401-C Mellon Court
Decatur, GA 30035
FAX: (404) 987-4806

MAILING ADDRESS:
2401-C Mellon Court
Decatur, GA 30035

Direct Inquiries to:
Allison Krebs-Bensch
Vice President
(770) 987-4745, or
Clayton W. Bishop
National Sales Manager, or
Peter J. Krebs, Ph.D., CFO
(770) 987-4746 or
www.uspco.com

Products Described:
Cenogen Ultra Capsules.............**3260**
Hemocyte Plus Capsules............ *3260*
Hemocyte Tablets................... *3260*
Hemocyte Plus Tabules.............. *3260*
Hemocyte-F Elixir.................. *3260*
Hemocyte-F Tablets................. *3261*
Medigesic Capsules................. *3261*
Norel DM Liquid.................... *3261*
Novasal Tablets.................... *3261*

USANA HEALTH SCIENCES, INC. **335, 3261**
3838 West Parkway Boulevard
Salt Lake City, UT 84120-6336

Direct Inquiries to:
Technical Services Department
(801) 954-7860
FAX: (801) 954-7658

Products Described:
Active Calcium Tablets..............**3261**
◆Chelated Mineral Tablets........**335, 3261**
CoQuinone Capsules.................**3261**
◆Mega Antioxidant Tablets.......**335, 3261**
Procosa II Tablets..................**3261**
◆Proflavanol 90 Tablets..........**335, 3261**

VALEANT PHARMACEUTICALS INTERNATIONAL **335, 3262**
3300 Hyland Avenue
Costa Mesa, CA 92626

For Medical Information Contact:
(800) 548-5100, Ext. 2286
FAX: (714) 641-7241

Products Described:
8-MOP Capsules.....................**3262**
Ancobon Capsules...................**3264**
◆Bontril PDM Tablets............ *335, 3265*
◆Bontril Slow-Release Capsules..................... *335, 3266*
◆Capital and Codeine Oral Suspension.................. *335, 3266*
Dalmane Capsules...................**3266**
Efudex Topical Cream...............**3267**
Efudex Topical Solutions............**3267**
Glyquin XM Cream..................**3268**
Librium Capsules....................**3268**
Mestinon Syrup.....................**3269**
◆Mestinon Tablets...............**335, 3269**
◆Mestinon Timespan Tablets.....**335, 3269**
◆Motofen Tablets................ *335, 3270*
Oxsoralen Lotion 1%................**3270**
◆Oxsoralen-Ultra Capsules.......**335, 3270**
◆Permax Tablets.................**335, 3273**
◆Phrenilin Tablets............... *335, 3276*
◆Phrenilin Forte Capsules........ *335, 3276*
◆Tasmar Tablets.................**335, 3276**
◆Testred Capsules, 10 mg........**335, 3281**
Virazole for Inhalation Solution......**3282**

Other Products Available:
Android Capsules, 10 mg
Benoquin Cream 20%
Eldopaque 2% Cream
Eldopaque Forte 4% Cream
Eldoquin 2% Cream
Eldoquin Forte 4% Cream
Fluorouracil Injection
Fototar Cream
Gly-Derm Product Line
Glyquin Cream
Insta-Glucose
Kinerase Product Line
Levo-Dromoran Injectable
Levo-Dromoran Tablets
Librax Capsules
Librium for Injection
Limbitrol Tablets
Limbitrol DS Tablets
NiteBite
Nolahist Tablets
Phrenilin with Caffeine and Codeine Capsules
Prostigmin Injectable
Prostigmin Tablets
RVPaque Cream
Solaquin 2% Cream
Solaquin Forte 4% Gel
Solaquin Forte 4% Cream
Tensilon Injectable
Vitadye Lotion

VISTAKON PHARMACEUTICALS, LLC **335, 3284**
7500 Centurion Parkway
Jacksonville, FL 32256

Direct Inquiries to:
(866) 427-6815

Products Described:
◆Alamast Ophthalmic Solution...**335, 3284**
◆Betimol Ophthalmic Solution...**335, 3285**
◆Quixin Ophthalmic Solution....**335, 3286**

VIVUS, INC. **335, 3287**
1172 Castro Street
Mountain View, CA 94040

Direct Inquiries to:
(888) 345-6873

For Medical Information or Emergencies Contact:
Medical Services Department @ VIVUS:
(650) 934-5200
FAX: (650) 934-5212

Products Described:
◆MUSE Urethral Suppository....**335, 3287**

WARNER CHILCOTT **3291**
100 Enterprise Drive
Rockaway, NJ 07866

Direct Inquiries to:

For Product Information Contact:
(800) 521-8813
www.warnerchilcott.com

For Medical Emergencies:
(800) 521-8813

For After Hours and Weekend Emergencies Contact:
(303) 739-1110

For All Other Inquiries:
(800) 521-8813
www.warnerchilcott.com

Products Described:

WATSON LABORATORIES, INC. 335, 3296

311 Bonnie Circle
Corona, CA 92880

Direct Inquiries to:
Customer Support Department
(800) 272-5525
FAX: (909) 898-6743

For Medical Information Contact:
(800) 272-5525

Products Described:

WELLSPRING PHARMACEUTICAL CORPORATION 336, 3305

1430 State Route 34
Neptune, NJ 07753-6807

Direct Inquiries to:
(732) 938-5885

Products Described:

WESTLAKE LABORATORIES, INC. 3307

24700 Center Ridge Road
Cleveland, OH 44145
www.westlake-labs.com

Direct Inquiries to:
Customer Service
(888) WSTLAKE (978-5253)
FAX: (440) 835-2177

Products Described:

Other Products Available:

Authia Cream
Bona-Bacillus Capsules
Coenzyme Q-10 Chewable Tablets
Dimersa
GFS-2000 Capsules
Glutanac Capsules
Glutanac Cream
Meregan A Crystals
Nutrision Capsules
Nutrisure OTC Tablets
Pantethine Capsules
Phosphatidyl-Serine Capsules
Total-E Softgels
Ultra G.I. Capsules
Ultra-Carotenoids Capsules
Ultra-Lipoic Forte Capsules
Uro-Pro Capsules

WINSTON LABORATORIES, INC. 336, 3308

100 Fairway Drive
Vernon Hills, IL 60061

Direct Inquiries to:
Customer Service:
(877) 260-6534
Sales and Ordering:
(877) 260-6534

Products Described:

WYETH PHARMACEUTICALS 336, 3308

Division of Wyeth
P.O. Box 8299
Philadelphia, PA 19101

For Product Information Contact:
(800) 934-5556

For Product Quality Contact:
(800) 999-9384

For Professional Services Contact:
(800) 395-9938

For Customer Service and Ordering Information Contact:
Pharmaceuticals and Vaccines: (800) 666-7248

For Patient Assistance Program Contact:
(800) 568-9938

For All Other Inquiries:
(610) 688-4400
www.wyeth.com

Products Described:

Other Products Available:

Ativan Tablets
Auralgan Otic Solution
Inderal Tablets
Inderide Tablets
Inderide LA Long-Acting Capsules
Isordil Oral Titradose Tablets
Isordil Sublingual Tablets
Lodine Capsules
Lodine Tablets
Lodine XL Extended-Release Tablets
Materna
Neptazane Tablets, USP (See PDR for Ophthalmic Medicines for Prescribing Information)
Oruvail Extended-Release Capsules
Reglan Tablets, USP
Robaxin
Robaxin-750

XANODYNE PHARMACEUTICALS, INC. 3418

7300 Turfway Road, Suite 300
Florence, Kentucky 41042

Direct Inquiries to:
(877) XANODYNE (877-926-6396)

Products Described:

ZLB BEHRING 3418

1020 First Avenue
King of Prussia, PA 19406-0901

Direct Inquiries to:
(610) 878-4000

For Medical Information Contact:
(800) 504-5434

Sales and Ordering:
Customer Support Center
(800) 683-1288
FAX: (610) 878-4888

Products Described:

HOW TO USE THE BRAND AND GENERIC NAME INDEX

This index lists every product alphabetically by both brand and generic name. Generic names are underlined; brand names are not.

Under each generic name, you will find a list of the brands that contain it. This enables you to find a particular product by either of its names. For example, "Indocin Oral Suspension" is listed once alphabetically and again under its generic name, indomethacin.

Each time a brand name appears, it is followed by the manufacturer's name and the page to consult for further information. Under a generic heading, all fully described brands are listed first, followed by those with only partial information. In each case, the brands are listed alphabetically.

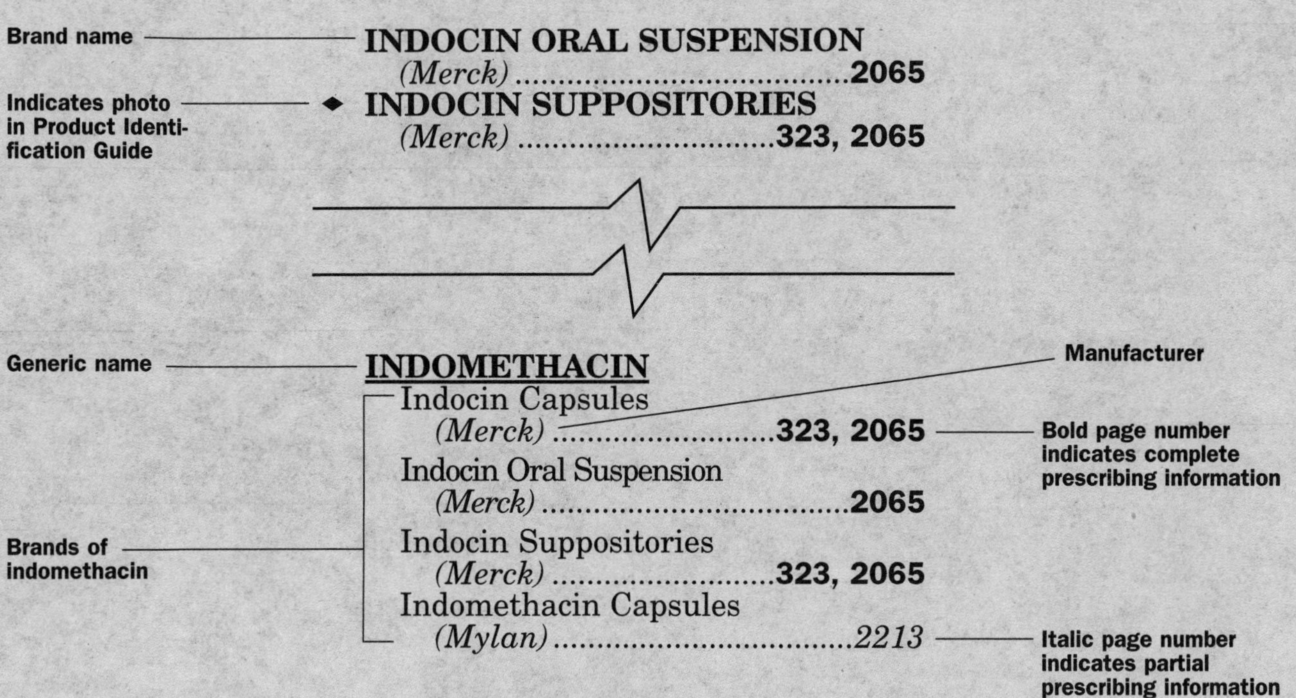

BRAND AND GENERIC NAME INDEX

This index includes all entries in the Product Information and Diagnostic Product Information sections. Products are listed alphabetically by both brand and generic name. Generic names are underlined; brand names are not. Under each generic name, you will find a list of the brands that contain it. This enables you to find a product by either of its names. For example, the brand Ativan appears once in the A's, and again under its generic name, lorazepam.

Each time a brand name appears, it is followed by the manufacturer's name and the page number to consult for further information. If multiple page numbers appear, the first ones refer to photos of the product, the last one to its prescribing information. Under a generic heading, all fully described brands are listed first, followed by those with only partial information.

- **Bold page numbers** indicate full prescribing information.
- *Italic page numbers* signify partial information.
- The ◆ symbol marks drugs shown in the Product Identification Guide.
- The 📖 symbol means product information is located in *PDR For Nonprescription Drugs and Dietary Supplements*™.
- The ⊙ symbol means product information is located in *PDR For Ophthalmic Medicines*™.

A

Levlen 28 Tablets *(Berlex)*. **308, 908**
Levlite 28 Tablets *(Berlex)*. **308, 908**
Lo/Ovral-28 Tablets *(Wyeth)*. **336, 3337**
NuvaRing *(Organon USA)*. **327, 2453**
Ortho Evra Transdermal System *(Ortho-McNeil)*. **328, 2515**
Ortho Tri-Cyclen Lo Tablets *(Ortho-McNeil)*. **328, 2533**
Ortho-Cept Tablets *(Ortho-McNeil)*. **328, 2508**
Ortho-Cyclen Tablets *(Ortho-McNeil)*. **328, 2526**
Ortho Tri-Cyclen Tablets *(Ortho-McNeil)*. **328, 2526**
Ovral-28 Tablets *(Wyeth)*. **336, 3352**
Seasonale Tablets *(Barr Labs)*. **311, 781**
Tri-Levlen 21 Tablets *(Berlex)*. **908**
Tri-Levlen 28 Tablets *(Berlex)*. **309, 908**
Triphasil-28 Tablets *(Wyeth)*. **337, 3407**
Yasmin 28 Tablets *(Berlex)*. **309, 930**
Brevicon Tablets *(Watson)*. *3299*
Femhrt Tablets *(Warner Chilcott)*. *3291*
Levora Tablets *(Watson)*. *3299*
Loestrin 21 1.5/30 Tablets *(Warner Chilcott)*. *3291*
Loestrin 21 1/20 Tablets *(Warner Chilcott)*. *3291*
Loestrin Fe 1.5/30 Tablets *(Warner Chilcott)*. *3291*
Loestrin Fe 1/20 Tablets *(Warner Chilcott)*. *3291*
Low-Ogestrel Tablets *(Watson)*. *3299*
Microgestin 1/20 Tablets *(Watson)*. *3299*
Microgestin 1.5/30 Tablets *(Watson)*. *3299*
Microgestin Fe 1/20 Tablets *(Watson)*. . . . *3299*
Microgestin Fe 1.5/30 Tablets *(Watson)*. *3299*
MonoNessa Tablets *(Watson)*. *3299*
Necon 0.5/35 Tablets *(Watson)*. *3299*
Necon 1/35 Tablets *(Watson)*. *3299*
Necon 10/11 Tablets *(Watson)*. *3299*
Necon 7/7/7 Tablets *(Watson)*. *3299*
Norinyl 1 + 35 Tablets *(Watson)*. *3299*
Ogestrel Tablets *(Watson)*. *3299*
Ovcon 35 Tablets *(Warner Chilcott)*. *3291*
Ovcon 50 Tablets *(Warner Chilcott)*. *3291*
TriNessa Tablets *(Watson)*. *3299*
Tri-Norinyl Tablets *(Watson)*. *3299*
Trivora-28 Tablets *(Watson)*. *3299*
Zovia 1/35E Tablets *(Watson)*. *3299*
Zovia 1/50E Tablets *(Watson)*. *3299*

ETHIONAMIDE
Trecator-SC Tablets *(Wyeth)*. **3406**

ETHOSUXIMIDE
Ethosuximide Syrup *(Pharmaceutical Associates)*. *2692*

ETHOTOIN
Peganone Tablets *(Ovation)*. **329, 2573**

ETHRANE LIQUID FOR INHALATION *(Baxter Anesthesia)*. . . *808*

ETHYL AMINOBENZOATE
(see under: **BENZOCAINE)**

ETHYNODIOL DIACETATE
Zovia 1/35E Tablets *(Watson)*. *3299*
Zovia 1/50E Tablets *(Watson)*. *3299*

ETHYOL FOR INJECTION *(MedImmune Oncology)*. **1967**

ETIDRONATE DISODIUM
Didronel Tablets *(Procter & Gamble Pharmaceuticals)*. **330, 2805**

ETODOLAC
Etodolac Capsules, Tablets USP *(Taro)*. . . *3220*
Etodolac Extended-Release Tablets *(Taro)*. *3220*
Etodolac Tablets *(Mylan)*. *2213*
Etodolac Tablets *(Par)*. *2578*
Etodolac Tablets, USP *(Taro)*. *3220*

ETONOGESTREL
NuvaRing *(Organon USA)*. **327, 2453**

ETOPOSIDE
Etoposide Capsules *(Mylan)*. *2213*

EUCALYPTUS, OIL OF
Vicks VapoRub Cream *(Procter & Gamble)*. **2795**
Vicks VapoRub Ointment *(Procter & Gamble)*. **2795**

◆ **EVISTA TABLETS** *(Lilly)*. **320, 1836**

◆ **EVOXAC CAPSULES** *(Daiichi)*. **311, 1166**

EX•LAX MILK OF MAGNESIA *(Novartis Consumer)*. . . . .

EX•LAX ULTRA PILLS *(Novartis Consumer)*. . . . .

◆ **EXELON CAPSULES** *(Novartis)*. **325, 2304**

EXELON ORAL SOLUTION *(Novartis)*. **2308**

EXEMESTANE
Aromasin Tablets *(Pharmacia & Upjohn)*. **330, 2693**

EX•LAX REGULAR STRENGTH LAXATIVE PILLS *(Novartis Consumer)*. . . . .

EX•LAX CHOCOLATED LAXATIVE *(Novartis Consumer)*. . . . .

EX•LAX MAXIMUM STRENGTH LAXATIVE PILLS *(Novartis Consumer)*. . . . .

EXTENDRYL CHEWABLE TABLETS *(Fleming)*. **1266**

EXTENDRYL SR. & JR. CAPSULES *(Fleming)*. **1266**

EXTENDRYL SYRUP *(Fleming)*. **1266**

EXTRA STRENGTH PRODUCTS ***(see base product name)***

EZ-CHAR PELLETS USP *(Paddock)*. *2576*

EZETIMIBE
Vytorin 10/10 Tablets *(Merck/Schering Plough)*. **2183**
Vytorin 10/10 Tablets *(Schering)*. **3070**
Vytorin 10/20 Tablets *(Merck/Schering Plough)*. **2183**
Vytorin 10/20 Tablets *(Schering)*. **3070**
Vytorin 10/40 Tablets *(Merck/Schering Plough)*. **2183**
Vytorin 10/40 Tablets *(Schering)*. **3070**
Vytorin 10/80 Tablets *(Merck/Schering Plough)*. **2183**
Vytorin 10/80 Tablets *(Schering)*. **3070**
Zetia Tablets *(Merck/Schering Plough)*. **324, 2189**
Zetia Tablets *(Schering)*. **3075**

F

FABRAZYME FOR INTRAVENOUS INFUSION *(Genzyme)*. **1365**

◆ **FACTIVE TABLETS** *(Ocient)*. . . **328, 2554**

FACTOR VIII (AHF, AHG)
Alphanate Solvent Detergent/Heat Treated *(Grifols)*. *1706*

FACTOR IX (HUMAN)
AlphaNine SD Solvent Detergent Treated/Virus Filtered *(Grifols)*. *1707*

FACTOR IX COMPLEX
Profilnine SD Solvent Detergent Treated *(Grifols)*. *1707*

FACTREL *(Baxter Anesthesia)*. *3438*

FAMCICLOVIR
Famvir Tablets *(Novartis)*. **2311**

FAMOTIDINE
Pepcid AC Chewable Tablets *(J&J • Merck)*. **1766**
Pepcid AC Gelcaps *(J&J • Merck)*. **319, 1766**
Pepcid AC Tablets *(J&J • Merck)*. **319, 1766**
Maximum Strength Pepcid AC Tablets *(J&J • Merck)*. **319, 1766**
Pepcid Complete Chewable Tablets *(J&J • Merck)*. **319, 1767**
Pepcid Injection *(Merck)*. **2111**
Pepcid Injection Premixed *(Merck)*. **2111**
Pepcid for Oral Suspension *(Merck)*. **2108**
Pepcid Tablets *(Merck)*. **323, 2108**
Famotidine Tablets *(Mylan)*. *2213*
Famotidine Tablets *(Par)*. *2578*

FAMVIR TABLETS *(Novartis)*. **2311**

◆ **FARESTON TABLETS** *(Shire US)*. **333, 3139**

◆ **FASLODEX INJECTION** *(AstraZeneca)*. **306, 653**

FATTY ACIDS
CM Plex Cream *(Unicity)*. **3242**
CM Plex Softgels *(Unicity)*. **3242**
Optimum Omega Softgels *(Pharmanex)*. **2782**
Super Omega-3 Softgels *(Carlson)*. *1091*

◆ **FAZACLO ORALLY DISINTEGRATING TABLETS** *(Alamo)*. **304, 541**

FEIBA VH *(Baxter Healthcare)*. **795**

FELODIPINE
Lexxel Tablets *(AstraZeneca LP)*. . . *305, 616*
Plendil Extended-Release Tablets *(AstraZeneca LP)*. *305, 625*

◆ **FEMARA TABLETS** *(Novartis)*. **325, 2314**

FEMHRT TABLETS *(Warner Chilcott)*. *3291*

FEMRING VAGINAL RING *(Warner Chilcott)*. *3291*

FEMTRACE TABLETS *(Warner Chilcott)*. **3293**

FENAXIN *(CPH)*. *1162*

FENOFIBRATE
Lofibra Capsules *(Gate)*. **1325**
Tricor Tablets *(Abbott)*. **303, 523**

FENOPROFEN CALCIUM
Fenoprofen Calcium Tablets *(Mylan)*. . . . *2213*

FENTANYL
Duragesic Transdermal System *(Janssen)*. **319, 1731**

FENTANYL CITRATE
Actiq *(Cephalon)*. **310, 1122**

FEOSOL CAPLETS *(GlaxoSmithKline Consumer)*. **1700**

FEOSOL TABLETS *(GlaxoSmithKline Consumer)*. **1701**

◆ **FERRLECIT INJECTION** *(Watson)*. **335, 3300**

FERROUS FUMARATE
Chromagen Forte Soft Gelatin Capsules *(Ther-Rx)*. **334, 3225**
StrongStart Caplets *(Ther-Rx)*. **334, 3229**
StrongStart Chewable Tablets *(Ther-Rx)*. **334, 3229**
Ferrous Fumarate Tablets *(Parke-Davis)*. *2578*
Hemocyte Plus Capsules *(U.S. Pharmaceutical)*. *3260*
Hemocyte Tablets *(U.S. Pharmaceutical)*. *3260*
Hemocyte Plus Tabules *(U.S. Pharmaceutical)*. *3260*
Hemocyte-F Tablets *(U.S. Pharmaceutical)*. *3261*
Loestrin Fe 1.5/30 Tablets *(Warner Chilcott)*. *3291*
Loestrin Fe 1/20 Tablets *(Warner Chilcott)*. *3291*
Microgestin Fe 1/20 Tablets *(Watson)*. . . . *3299*
Microgestin Fe 1.5/30 Tablets *(Watson)*. *3299*
NataChew Tablets *(Warner Chilcott)*. . . . *3291*
Trinsicon Capsules *(UCB)*. *3242*

FERROUS SULFATE
Feosol Tablets *(GlaxoSmithKline Consumer)*. **1701**
Ferrous Sulfate Liquid *(Pharmaceutical Associates)*. *2692*
Vi-Daylin/F ADC Vitamins + Iron Drops With Fluoride *(Ross)*. *2965*
Vi-Daylin/F Multivitamin + Iron Drops With Fluoride *(Ross)*. *2965*

FEXOFENADINE HYDROCHLORIDE
Allegra Capsules *(Aventis)*. **676**
Allegra Tablets *(Aventis)*. **306, 676**
Allegra-D Extended-Release Tablets *(Aventis)*. **306, 678**

FIBER
Life Health - Bios Life 2 Drink Mix *(Unicity)*. **3242**

FILGRASTIM
Neupogen for Injection *(Amgen)*. . . . **305, 592**

◆ **FINACEA GEL** *(Berlex)*. **308, 907**

FINASTERIDE
Propecia Tablets *(Merck)*. **323, 2130**
Proscar Tablets *(Merck)*. **323, 2133**

FIORICET TABLETS *(Watson)*. *3299*

FIORICET WITH CODEINE CAPSULES C-III *(Watson)*. *3299*

FIORINAL CAPSULES C-III *(Watson)*. *3299*

FIORINAL WITH CODEINE CAPSULES C-III *(Watson)*. *3299*

FLEBOGAMMA 5% *(Grifols)*. **1707**

FLECAINIDE ACETATE
Tambocor Tablets *(3M)*. **321, 1921**
Flecainide Acetate Tablets *(Mylan)*. *2213*
Flecainide Acetate Tablets *(Par)*. *2578*
Flecainide Acetate Tablets USP *(Roxane)*. *2966*

FLEET BISACODYL LAXATIVES *(Fleet)*. **1262**

FLEET ENEMA *(Fleet)*. **1263**

FLEET ENEMA FOR CHILDREN *(Fleet)*. **1263**

FLEET GLYCERIN LAXATIVES *(Fleet)*. **1262**

FLEET MINERAL OIL ENEMA *(Fleet)*. **1263**

FLEET PHOSPHO-SODA *(Fleet)*. . . . **1264**

FLEET PHOSPHO-SODA ACCU-PREP *(Fleet)*. **1264**

FLEET PREP KITS *(Fleet)*. **1265**

◆ **FLEXERIL TABLETS** *(McNeil Consumer)*. **321, 1930**

◆ **FLOLAN FOR INJECTION** *(GlaxoSmithKline)*. **315, 1487**

◆ **FLOMAX CAPSULES** *(Boehringer Ingelheim)*. **309, 994**

◆ **FLONASE NASAL SPRAY** *(GlaxoSmithKline)*. **315, 1491**

FLORICAL CAPSULES AND TABLETS *(Mericon)*. **2194**

FLOVENT HFA 44 MCG INHALATION AEROSOL *(GlaxoSmithKline)*. **1497**

FLOVENT HFA 110 MCG INHALATION AEROSOL *(GlaxoSmithKline)*. **1497**

FLOVENT HFA 220 MCG INHALATION AEROSOL *(GlaxoSmithKline)*. **1497**

◆ **FLOVENT 44 MCG INHALATION AEROSOL** *(GlaxoSmithKline)*. **315, 1494**

◆ **FLOVENT 110 MCG INHALATION AEROSOL** *(GlaxoSmithKline)*. **315, 1494**

◆ **FLOVENT 220 MCG INHALATION AEROSOL** *(GlaxoSmithKline)*. **315, 1494**

◆ **FLOVENT ROTADISK 50 MCG** *(GlaxoSmithKline)*. **315, 1500**

◆ **FLOVENT ROTADISK 100 MCG** *(GlaxoSmithKline)*. **315, 1500**

◆ **FLOVENT ROTADISK 250 MCG** *(GlaxoSmithKline)*. **315, 1500**

◆ **FLOXIN OTIC SINGLES** *(Daiichi)*. **311, 1169**

◆ **FLOXIN OTIC SOLUTION** *(Daiichi)*. **311, 1168**

FLOXIN TABLETS *(Ortho-McNeil)*. . **2495**

FLUCONAZOLE
Diflucan Injection *(Pfizer)*. **2605**
Diflucan Oral Suspension *(Pfizer)*. **2605**
Diflucan Tablets *(Pfizer)*. **329, 2605**
Fluconazole Tablets *(Roxane)*. *2966*
Fluconazole Tablets *(Taro)*. *3220*

FLUCYTOSINE
Ancobon Capsules *(Valeant)*. **3264**

◆ **FLUDARA FOR INJECTION** *(Berlex)*. **308, 940**

FLUDARABINE PHOSPHATE
Fludara for Injection *(Berlex)*. **308, 940**

FLUMADINE SYRUP *(Forest)*. **1275**

◆ **FLUMADINE TABLETS** *(Forest)*. **312, 1275**

FLUMAZENIL
Romazicon Injection *(Roche Laboratories)*. **2923**

◆ **FLUMIST VACCINE** *(Medimmune)*. **322, 1970**

FLUNISOLIDE
Aerobid Inhaler System *(Forest)*. . . **312, 1266**
Aerobid-M Inhaler System *(Forest)*. **312, 1266**
Nasarel Nasal Spray *(IVAX)*. **1720**

FLUOCINOLONE ACETONIDE
Capex Shampoo *(Galderma)*. **1310**
Tri-Luma Cream *(Galderma)*. **1322**
Derma-Smoothe/FS Topical Oil *(Hill)*. . . *1713*

FLUOCINONIDE
Fluocinonide (Emulsified Base) Cream USP *(Taro)*. *3220*
Fluocinonide Cream, Ointment, Gel, Solution USP *(Taro)*. *3220*

FLUOROURACIL
Carac Cream, 0.5% *(Dermik)*. **1172**
Efudex Topical Cream *(Valeant)*. **3267**
Efudex Topical Solutions *(Valeant)*. **3267**
Fluouracil Topical Solution *(Taro)*. *3220*

FLUOURACIL TOPICAL SOLUTION *(Taro)*. *3220*

FLUOXETINE
Fluoxetine Capsules *(Mylan)*. *2213*
Fluoxetine Oral Solution *(Par)*. *2578*

FLUOXETINE HYDROCHLORIDE
Prozac Pulvules and Liquid *(Lilly)*. **320, 1873**
Symbyax Capsules *(Lilly)*. **320, 1888**
Fluoxetine Capsules *(Par)*. *2578*
Fluoxetine Capsules, USP *(Mallinckrodt)*. *1924*
Fluoxetine HCl Tablets *(Par)*. *2578*
Fluoxetine Oral Solution USP *(Pharmaceutical Associates)*. *2692*
Fluoxetine Oral Solution, USP *(Mallinckrodt)*. *1924*
Prozac Weekly Capsules *(Lilly)*. *320*
Sarafem *(Warner Chilcott)*. *3291*

FLUPHENAZINE HYDROCHLORIDE
Fluphenazine HCl Tablets *(Par)*. *2578*
Fluphenazine Hydrochloride Elixir USP *(Pharmaceutical Associates)*. *2692*
Fluphenazine Hydrochloride Oral Solution USP (Concentrate) *(Pharmaceutical Associates)*. *2692*
Fluphenazine Hydrochloride Tablets *(Mylan)*. *2213*

FLURANDRENOLIDE
Cordran Lotion *(Watson)*. *3299*
Cordran Ointment *(Watson)*. *3299*
Cordran SP Cream *(Watson)*. *3299*
Cordran Tape *(Watson)*. *3299*

G

H

◆ **KLONOPIN TABLETS** *(Roche Laboratories)* 331, 2895

◆ **KLONOPIN WAFERS** *(Roche Laboratories)* 331, 2895

◆ **KLOR-CON M20/ KLOR-CON M10/ KLOR-CON M15 TABLETS** *(Upsher-Smith)* 335, 3255

K-LOR POWDER PACKETS *(Abbott)* 481

KLOR-CON/EF TABLETS *(Upsher-Smith)* *3255*

◆ **KLOR-CON 8/KLOR-CON 10 TABLETS** *(Upsher-Smith)* *335, 3255*

KLOR-CON POWDER *(Upsher-Smith)* *3255*

KLOR-CON/25 POWDER *(Upsher-Smith)* *3255*

KOĀTE-DVI *(Bayer Healthcare)* 877

KOGENATE FS *(Bayer Healthcare)* ... 878

◆ **K-PHOS M.F. TABLETS** *(Beach)* *308, 886*

◆ **K-PHOS NEUTRAL TABLETS** *(Beach)* 308, 886

◆ **K-PHOS NO. 2 TABLETS** *(Beach)* *308, 886*

◆ **K-PHOS ORIGINAL (SODIUM FREE) TABLETS** *(Beach)* 308, 887

KRISTALOSE FOR ORAL SOLUTION *(Mylan)* 2252

KRONOFED-A KRONOCAPS *(Ferndale)* *1246*

KRONOFED-A-JR. KRONOCAPS *(Ferndale)* *1246*

◆ **K-TAB FILMTAB TABLETS** *(Abbott)* 303, 482

KUTRASE CAPSULES *(Schwarz)* ... *3082*

KU-ZYME CAPSULES *(Schwarz)* *3082*

KU-ZYME HP CAPSULES *(Schwarz)* *3082*

KYTRIL INJECTION *(Roche Laboratories)* 2898

KYTRIL ORAL SOLUTION *(Roche Laboratories)* 2901

◆ **KYTRIL TABLETS** *(Roche Laboratories)* 331, 2901

L

L.M.X.4 CREAM *(Ferndale)* 1246

L.M.X.5 CREAM *(Ferndale)* 1246

LABETALOL HYDROCHLORIDE
- Labetalol HCl Tablets *(Watson)* *3296*

LACLOTION 12% LOTION *(Paddock)* 2576

LACRISERT STERILE OPHTHALMIC INSERT *(Merck)* 2074

◆ **LACTAID EXTRA STRENGTH CAPLETS** *(McNeil Consumer)* 321, 1934

◆ **LACTAID ORIGINAL STRENGTH CAPLETS** *(McNeil Consumer)* 321, 1934

◆ **LACTAID ULTRA CAPLETS AND CHEWABLE TABLETS** *(McNeil Consumer)* 321, 1934

LACTASE (BETA-D-GALACTOSIDASE)
- Lactaid Extra Strength Caplets *(McNeil Consumer)* 321, 1934
- Lactaid Original Strength Caplets *(McNeil Consumer)* 321, 1934
- Lactaid Ultra Caplets and Chewable Tablets *(McNeil Consumer)* 321, 1934

LACTIC ACID
- Lactinol Lotion *(Pedinol)* *2595*
- Lactinol-E Creme *(Pedinol)* *2595*

LACTICARE-HC LOTION, 2½% *(Stiefel)* *3177*

LACTINOL LOTION *(Pedinol)* *2595*

LACTINOL-E CREME *(Pedinol)* *2595*

LACTULOSE
- Kristalose for Oral Solution *(Mylan)* 2252
- Lactulose Solution *(Watson)* *3296*
- Lactulose Solution USP *(Pharmaceutical Associates)* *2692*
- Lactulose Solution USP *(Roxane)* *2966*

◆ **LAMICTAL TABLETS** *(GlaxoSmithKline)* 316, 1531

◆ **LAMICTAL CHEWABLE DISPERSIBLE TABLETS** *(GlaxoSmithKline)* 316, 1531

LAMISIL [AT] CREAM *(Novartis Consumer)* .... ▣

LAMISIL [AT] SPRAY PUMP *(Novartis Consumer)* .... ▣

◆ **LAMISIL TABLETS** *(Novartis)* 325, 2325

LAMIVUDINE
- Combivir Tablets *(GlaxoSmithKline)* 315, 1454
- Epivir Oral Solution *(GlaxoSmithKline)* 315, 1473
- Epivir Tablets *(GlaxoSmithKline)* 315, 1473
- Epivir-HBV Oral Solution *(GlaxoSmithKline)* 315, 1477
- Epivir-HBV Tablets *(GlaxoSmithKline)* 315, 1477
- Epzicom Tablets *(GlaxoSmithKline)* 1481
- Trizivir Tablets *(GlaxoSmithKline)* 317, 1642

LAMOTRIGINE
- Lamictal Tablets *(GlaxoSmithKline)* 316, 1531
- Lamictal Chewable Dispersible Tablets *(GlaxoSmithKline)* 316, 1531

◆ **LANOXICAPS CAPSULES** *(GlaxoSmithKline)* 316, 1540

◆ **LANOXIN INJECTION** *(GlaxoSmithKline)* 316, 1546

◆ **LANOXIN TABLETS** *(GlaxoSmithKline)* 316, 1553

◆ **LANOXIN ELIXIR PEDIATRIC** *(GlaxoSmithKline)* 316, 1543

◆ **LANOXIN INJECTION PEDIATRIC** *(GlaxoSmithKline)* 316, 1550

LANSOPRAZOLE
- Prevacid Delayed-Release Capsules *(TAP)* 334, 3202
- Prevacid for Delayed-Release Oral Suspension *(TAP)* 334, 3202
- Prevacid I.V. for Injection *(TAP)* ... 334, 3208
- Prevacid NapraPAC 375 *(TAP)* 334, 3211
- Prevacid NapraPAC 500 *(TAP)* 334, 3211
- Prevacid SoluTab Delayed-Release Orally Disintegrating Tablets *(TAP)* 334, 3202
- PREVPAC *(TAP)* 334, 3215

◆ **LANTUS INJECTION** *(Aventis)* 307, 715

◆ **LARIAM TABLETS** *(Roche Laboratories)* 331, 2903

LARONIDASE
- Aldurazyme for Intravenous Infusion *(Genzyme)* 1362

LASIX TABLETS *(Aventis)* *676*

LATANOPROST
- Xalatan Sterile Ophthalmic Solution *(Pharmacia & Upjohn)* 2762

LAZERFORMALYDE SOLUTION *(Pedinol)* *2595*

L-CARNITINE *(see under:* **LEVOCARNITINE)**

L-CARNOSINE
- Karno-Life *(Montiff)* *2213*
- Nature's Lining Chewable Tablets *(Lane)* *1815*

LEFLUNOMIDE
- Arava Tablets *(Aventis)* 307, 693

LEPIRUDIN
- Refludan for Injection *(Berlex)* 309, 926

◆ **LESCOL CAPSULES** *(Novartis)* 325, 2326

LESCOL CAPSULES *(Reliant)* 2840

LESCOL XL TABLETS *(Novartis)* ... 2326

◆ **LESCOL XL TABLETS** *(Reliant)* 331, 2840

LETROZOLE
- Femara Tablets *(Novartis)* 325, 2314

LEUCOVORIN CALCIUM
- Leucovorin Calcium Tablets USP *(Roxane)* *2966*

◆ **LEUKERAN TABLETS** *(GlaxoSmithKline)* 316, 1556

LEUKINE *(Berlex)* 942

LEUPROLIDE ACETATE
- Eligard 7.5 mg *(Sanofi-Synthelabo)* 332, 2989
- Eligard 22.5 mg *(Sanofi-Synthelabo)* 332, 2992
- Eligard 30 mg *(Sanofi-Synthelabo)* 332, 2994
- Lupron Depot 3.75 mg *(TAP)* 334, 3188
- Lupron Depot 7.5 mg *(TAP)* 334, 3192
- Lupron Depot--3 Month 11.25 mg *(TAP)* 334, 3193
- Lupron Depot--3 Month 22.5 mg *(TAP)* 334, 3197
- Lupron Depot--4 Month 30 mg *(TAP)* 334, 3198
- Lupron Depot-PED 7.5 mg, 11.25 mg and 15 mg *(TAP)* 334, 3200
- Lupron Injection *(TAP)* 334, 3186
- Lupron Injection Pediatric *(TAP)* 3187
- Viadur Implant *(Bayer)* 308, 856

LEUSTATIN INJECTION *(Ortho Biotech)* 2464

LEVALBUTEROL HYDROCHLORIDE
- Xopenex Inhalation Solution *(Sepracor)* 333, 3102

◆ **LEVA-PAK** *(Ortho-McNeil)* *328, 2501*

LEVAQUIN IN 5% DEXTROSE INJECTION *(Ortho-McNeil)* 2501

◆ **LEVAQUIN INJECTION** *(Ortho-McNeil)* 328, 2501

◆ **LEVAQUIN TABLETS** *(Ortho-McNeil)* 328, 2501

LEVATOL TABLETS *(Schwarz)* *3082*

LEVBID EXTENDED-RELEASE TABLETS *(Schwarz)* *3082*

LEVETIRACETAM
- Keppra Oral Solution *(UCB)* 334, 3234
- Keppra Tablets *(UCB)* 334, 3234

◆ **LEVITRA TABLETS** *(Bayer)* 308, 845

LEVLEN 21 TABLETS *(Berlex)* 908

◆ **LEVLEN 28 TABLETS** *(Berlex)* 308, 908

◆ **LEVLITE 28 TABLETS** *(Berlex)* 308, 908

LEVMETAMFETAMINE
- Vicks Vapor Inhaler *(Procter & Gamble)* 2795

LEVOCARNITINE
- Carnitor Injection *(Sigma-Tau)* 3144
- Carnitor Tablets and Oral Solution *(Sigma-Tau)* 3146

LEVODOPA
- Parcopa Orally Disintegrating Tablets *(Schwarz)* 3083
- Stalevo Tablets *(Novartis)* 326, 2369
- Carbidopa and Levodopa Extended-release Tablets *(Mylan)* *2213*
- Carbidopa and Levodopa Tablets, USP *(Endo Labs)* *1212*

LEVOFLOXACIN
- Levaquin in 5% Dextrose Injection *(Ortho-McNeil)* 2501
- Levaquin Injection *(Ortho-McNeil)* 328, 2501
- Levaquin Tablets *(Ortho-McNeil)* 328, 2501
- Quixin Ophthalmic Solution *(Vistakon)* 335, 3286

LEVONORGESTREL
- Alesse-28 Tablets *(Wyeth)* 336, 3308
- Climara Pro Transdermal System *(Berlex)* 308, 902
- Levlen 21 Tablets *(Berlex)* 908
- Levlen 28 Tablets *(Berlex)* 308, 908
- Levlite 28 Tablets *(Berlex)* 308, 908
- Mirena Intrauterine System *(Berlex)* 309, 921
- Plan B Tablets *(Barr Labs)* 311, 779
- Seasonale Tablets *(Barr Labs)* 311, 781
- Tri-Levlen 21 Tablets *(Berlex)* 908
- Tri-Levlen 28 Tablets *(Berlex)* 309, 908
- Triphasil-28 Tablets *(Wyeth)* 337, 3407
- Levora Tablets *(Watson)* *3299*
- Trivora-28 Tablets *(Watson)* *3299*

LEVORA TABLETS *(Watson)* *3299*

LEVORPHANOL TARTRATE
- Levorphanol Tartrate Tablets USP CII *(Roxane)* *2966*

LEVOTHROID TABLETS *(Forest)* ... 1278

LEVOTHYROXINE SODIUM
- Levothroid Tablets *(Forest)* 1278
- Levoxyl Tablets *(King)* 319, 1785
- Synthroid Tablets *(Abbott)* 303, 515
- Levothyroxine Sodium Tablets *(Mylan)* *2213*

◆ **LEVOXYL TABLETS** *(King)* 319, 1785

LEVSIN DROPS *(Schwarz)* *3082*

LEVSIN ELIXIR *(Schwarz)* *3082*

LEVSIN INJECTION *(Schwarz)* *3082*

LEVSIN TABLETS *(Schwarz)* *3082*

LEVSIN/SL TABLETS *(Schwarz)* *3082*

LEVSINEX TIMECAPS *(Schwarz)* ... *3082*

◆ **LEXAPRO ORAL SOLUTION** *(Forest)* 312, 1282

◆ **LEXAPRO TABLETS** *(Forest)* 312, 1282

◆ **LEXIVA TABLETS** *(GlaxoSmithKline)* 316, 1558

◆ **LEXXEL TABLETS** *(AstraZeneca LP)* *305, 616*

LIBRIUM CAPSULES *(Valeant)* 3268

LIDOCAINE
- L.M.X.4 Cream *(Ferndale)* 1246
- L.M.X.5 Cream *(Ferndale)* 1246
- Lidoderm Patch *(Endo Labs)* 311, 1215
- EMLA Cream *(AstraZeneca LP)* *305, 615*
- EMLA Anesthetic Disc *(AstraZeneca LP)* *615*
- Lidocaine Viscous 2% USP *(Roxane)* *2966*
- Lidocaine Ointment USP *(Taro)* *3220*

LIDOCAINE HYDROCHLORIDE
- Anestacon Jelly *(PolyMedica)* *2782*
- Lidocaine Hydrochloride Topical Solution 4% USP *(Roxane)* *2966*
- Xylocaine 2% Jelly *(AstraZeneca LP)* *635*

◆ **LIDODERM PATCH** *(Endo Labs)* 311, 1215

LIFE HEALTH - BIOS LIFE 2 DRINK MIX *(Unicity)* 3242

LIFE HEALTH - CORE HEALTH SUPPLEMENT *(Unicity)* 3242

LIFE HEALTH - DAILY PRODUCE 24 CAPSULES *(Unicity)* 3242

LIFEPAK CAPSULES *(Pharmanex)* 2781

LINEZOLID
- Zyvox Injection *(Pharmacia & Upjohn)* 2773
- Zyvox for Oral Suspension *(Pharmacia & Upjohn)* 2773
- Zyvox Tablets *(Pharmacia & Upjohn)* 330, 2773

LIOTHYRONINE SODIUM
- Cytomel Tablets *(King)* 319, 1781
- Triostat Injection *(King)* 320, 1802

LIOTRIX
- Thyrolar Tablets *(Forest)* *312, 1292*

LIPASE
- Kutrase Capsules *(Schwarz)* *3082*
- Ku-Zyme Capsules *(Schwarz)* *3082*
- Ku-Zyme HP Capsules *(Schwarz)* *3082*

◆ **LIPITOR TABLETS** *(Parke-Davis)* 329, 2585

LIPOIC ACID
- CoQuinone Capsules *(Usana)* 3261

LIPOLYTIC ENZYMES *(see under:* **LIPASE)**

LISINOPRIL
- Prinivil Tablets *(Merck)* 323, 2123
- Prinzide Tablets *(Merck)* 323, 2127
- Lisinopril and Hydrochlorothiazide Tablets *(Mylan)* *2213*
- Lisinopril/Hydrochlorothiazide Tablets *(Watson)* *3296*
- Lisinopril Tablets *(Mylan)* *2213*
- Lisinopril Tablets *(Par)* *2578*
- Lisinopril Tablets *(Watson)* *3296*
- Zestoretic Tablets *(AstraZeneca)* *306, 667*
- Zestril Tablets *(AstraZeneca)* *306, 667*

LISINOPRIL/ HYDROCHLOROTHIAZIDE TABLETS *(Watson)* *3296*

LITHIUM CARBONATE
- Eskalith Capsules *(GlaxoSmithKline)* 315, 1485
- Eskalith CR Controlled-Release Tablets *(GlaxoSmithKline)* 315, 1485
- Lithium Carbonate Capsules USP *(Roxane)* *2966*
- Lithium Carbonate Extended Release Tablets USP *(Roxane)* *2966*
- Lithium Carbonate Tablets USP *(Roxane)* *2966*

LITHIUM CITRATE
- Lithium Citrate Syrup USP *(Roxane)* *2966*

LITHOSTAT TABLETS *(Mission)* *2212*

LIVER PREPARATIONS
- Hep-Forte Capsules *(Marlyn)* 1926
- Trinsicon Capsules *(UCB)* *3242*

LOCOID CREAM *(Ferndale)* 1247

LOCOID LIPOCREAM CREAM *(Ferndale)* 1247

LOCOID OINTMENT *(Ferndale)* 1247

LOCOID TOPICAL SOLUTION *(Ferndale)* 1247

LODRANE LIQUID *(ECR)* *1192*

LODRANE SUSTAINED RELEASE LIQUID *(ECR)* *1192*

LODRANE D SUSTAINED RELEASE LIQUID *(ECR)* *1192*

LODRANE 12-HOUR EXTENDED RELEASE TABLETS *(ECR)* *1192*

LODRANE 12 D EXTENDED RELEASE TABLETS *(ECR)* *1192*

LODRANE 24 EXTENDED RELEASE CAPSULES *(ECR)* *1192*

LODRANE 24 D EXTENDED RELEASE CAPSULES *(ECR)* *1192*

LOESTRIN 21 1.5/30 TABLETS *(Warner Chilcott)* *3291*

LOESTRIN 21 1/20 TABLETS *(Warner Chilcott)* *3291*

SECTION 3

PRODUCT CATEGORY INDEX

This index lists products by prescribing category, allowing you to quickly and easily identify all agents with a given therapeutic use or mechanism of action. Categories are based on the latest medical terminology and are comprehensively cross-referenced. Included are all fully described products in both the Product Information and Diagnostic Product Information sections of PDR®.

If an entry in the index lists multiple page numbers, the first ones shown refer to photographs of the product, the last one to its prescribing information. The Quick-Reference Guide below gives you an overview of the categories.

PRODUCT CATEGORY QUICK-REFERENCE GUIDE

PRODUCT CATEGORY INDEX

Epzicom Tablets *(GlaxoSmithKline)*....... **1481**
Hivid Tablets *(Roche Laboratories)*................. **331, 2886**
Retrovir Capsules *(GlaxoSmithKline)*............. **317, 1612**
Retrovir IV Infusion *(GlaxoSmithKline)*............. **317, 1616**
Retrovir Syrup *(GlaxoSmithKline)*.. **317, 1612**
Retrovir Tablets *(GlaxoSmithKline)*............. **317, 1612**
Trizivir Tablets *(GlaxoSmithKline)*.. **317, 1642**
Truvada Tablets *(Gilead)*.......... **313, 1376**
Videx EC Capsules *(Bristol-Myers Squibb)*...................... **310, 1082**
Zerit Capsules *(Bristol-Myers Squibb)*...................... **310, 1087**
Zerit for Oral Solution *(Bristol-Myers Squibb)*.......... **310, 1087**
Ziagen Oral Solution *(GlaxoSmithKline)*............. **318, 1673**
Ziagen Tablets *(GlaxoSmithKline)*... **318, 1673**

NUCLEOTIDE ANALOGUE REVERSE TRANSCRIPTASE INHIBITORS

Truvada Tablets *(Gilead)*.......... **313, 1376**
Viread Tablets *(Gilead)*........... **313, 1381**

PROTEASE INHIBITORS

Agenerase Capsules *(GlaxoSmithKline)*............. **314, 1396**
Agenerase Oral Solution *(GlaxoSmithKline)*............. **314, 1401**
Crixivan Capsules *(Merck)*........ **323, 2021**
Fortovase Capsules *(Roche Laboratories)*................. **331, 2876**
Invirase Capsules *(Roche Laboratories)*................. **331, 2890**
Kaletra Capsules *(Abbott)*.......... **303, 483**
Kaletra Oral Solution *(Abbott)*....... **303, 483**
Lexiva Tablets *(GlaxoSmithKline)*... **316, 1558**
Norvir Soft Gelatin Capsules *(Abbott)*...................... **303, 500**
Norvir Oral Solution *(Abbott)*....... **303, 500**
Reyataz Capsules *(Bristol-Myers Squibb)*...................... **310, 1060**
Viracept Oral Powder *(Pfizer)*........... **2659**
Viracept Tablets *(Pfizer)*.......... **330, 2659**

AMEBICIDES

Aralen Tablets *(Sanofi-Synthelabo)*......... **2983**

ANTHELMINTICS

Albenza Tablets *(GlaxoSmithKline)*... **314, 1406**
Biltricide Tablets *(Bayer)*............ **308, 3424**
Mintezol Suspension *(Merck)*............. **2096**
Mintezol Chewable Tablets *(Merck)*... **323, 2096**
Stromectol Tablets *(Merck)*.......... **324, 2146**
Vermox Chewable Tablets *(McNeil Consumer)*..................... **322, 1952**

ANTIBIOTICS

AMINOGLYCOSIDES

Streptomycin Sulfate Injection *(Pfizer)*.... **2637**
TOBI Solution for Inhalation *(Chiron)*...................... **311, 1143**

β-LACTAM ANTIBIOTICS, MISCELLANEOUS

Azactam for Injection *(Elan)*............ **1204**
Invanz for Injection *(Merck)*............ **2069**
Mefoxin for Injection *(Merck)*........... **2081**
Mefoxin Premixed Intravenous Solution *(Merck)*.......................... **2084**
Merrem I.V. *(AstraZeneca)*.......... **306, 658**
Primaxin I.M. *(Merck)*................ **2116**
Primaxin I.V. *(Merck)*................. **2118**

CEPHALOSPORINS

Ancef for Injection *(GlaxoSmithKline)*............. **314, 1415**
Ancef Injection *(GlaxoSmithKline)*....... **1415**
Ceclor Pulvules *(Lilly)*................ **1829**
Ceclor Suspension *(Lilly)*............... **1829**
Cedax Capsules *(Shionogi)*............. **3127**
Cedax Oral Suspension *(Shionogi)*....... **3127**
Ceftin for Oral Suspension *(GlaxoSmithKline)*............. **315, 1450**
Ceftin Tablets *(GlaxoSmithKline)*... **315, 1450**
Cefzil for Oral Suspension *(Bristol-Myers Squibb)*............... **1037**
Cefzil Tablets *(Bristol-Myers Squibb)*...................... **310, 1037**
Claforan Sterile for Injection *(Aventis)*...................... **307, 699**
Fortaz Injection *(GlaxoSmithKline)*.. **316, 1504**
Fortaz for Injection *(GlaxoSmithKline)*............. **316, 1504**
Keflex Pulvules *(Lilly)*................ **1871**
Maxipime for Injection *(Elan)*........... **1207**
Omnicef Capsules *(Abbott)*.......... **303, 506**
Omnicef for Oral Suspension *(Abbott)*...................... **303, 506**
Rocephin Injectable Vials, ADD-Vantage, Galaxy, Bulk *(Roche Laboratories)*..................... **2915**
Spectracef Tablets *(Purdue Pharmaceutical)*.............. **331, 2824**
Vantin Tablets and Oral Suspension *(Pharmacia & Upjohn)*...................... **330, 2758**
Zinacef Injection *(GlaxoSmithKline)*............. **318, 1676**
Zinacef for Injection *(GlaxoSmithKline)*............. **318, 1676**

MACROLIDES & COMBINATIONS

Biaxin Filmtab Tablets *(Abbott)*...... **303, 408**
Biaxin Granules *(Abbott)*............ **303, 408**
Biaxin XL Filmtab Tablets *(Abbott)*.. **303, 408**
E.E.S. 200 Liquid *(Abbott)*............. **457**
E.E.S. 400 Liquid *(Abbott)*............. **457**
E.E.S. 400 Filmtab Tablets *(Abbott)*.. **303, 457**
E.E.S. Granules *(Abbott)*............... **457**
EryPed 200 & EryPed 400 *(Abbott)*....... **453**
EryPed Drops *(Abbott)*.................. **453**
EryPed Chewable Tablets *(Abbott)*........ **453**
Ery-Tab Tablets *(Abbott)*........... **303, 455**
Erythrocin Stearate Filmtab Tablets *(Abbott)*...................... **303, 460**
Erythromycin Base Filmtab Tablets *(Abbott)*.......................... **462**
Erythromycin Delayed-Release Capsules, USP *(Abbott)*.......... **303, 464**
PCE Dispertab Tablets *(Abbott)*...... **303, 511**
Pediazole Suspension *(Ross)*............ **2960**
PREVPAC *(TAP)*..................... **334, 3215**
Zithromax Capsules, 250 mg *(Pfizer)*..... **2672**
Zithromax for IV Infusion *(Pfizer)*....... **2677**
Zithromax for Oral Suspension, 1 g *(Pfizer)*.......................... **2672**
Zithromax for Oral Suspension, 300 mg, 600 mg, 900 mg, 1200 mg *(Pfizer)*..... **2665**
Zithromax Tablets, 250 mg, 500 mg *(Pfizer)*.............. **330, 2665**
Zithromax Tablets, 600 mg *(Pfizer)*...................... **330, 2672**
Zithromax Tri-Pak *(Pfizer)*............. **2665**
Zithromax Z-Pak *(Pfizer)*............... **2672**

MISCELLANEOUS ANTIBIOTICS

Cleocin HCl Capsules *(Pharmacia & Upjohn)*................... **330, 2710**
Coly-Mycin M Parenteral *(King)*... **319, 1776**
Cubicin for Injection *(Cubist)*...... **311, 1163**
Ketek Tablets *(Aventis)*............ **307, 710**
Seromycin Capsules *(Lilly)*............. **1883**
Synercid I.V. *(King)*.............. **320, 1798**
Vancocin HCl Pulvules *(Lilly)*........... **1896**
Zyvox Injection *(Pharmacia & Upjohn)*... **2773**
Zyvox for Oral Suspension *(Pharmacia & Upjohn)*......................... **2773**
Zyvox Tablets *(Pharmacia & Upjohn)*...................... **330, 2773**

PENICILLINS

Amoxil Capsules *(GlaxoSmithKline)*............. **314, 1411**
Amoxil Chewable Tablets *(GlaxoSmithKline)*............. **314, 1411**
Amoxil for Oral Suspension *(GlaxoSmithKline)*............. **314, 1411**
Amoxil Pediatric Drops for Oral Suspension *(GlaxoSmithKline)*... **314, 1411**
Amoxil Tablets *(GlaxoSmithKline)*.. **314, 1411**
Augmentin Chewable Tablets *(GlaxoSmithKline)*............. **314, 1421**
Augmentin Powder for Oral Suspension *(GlaxoSmithKline)*... **314, 1421**
Augmentin Tablets *(GlaxoSmithKline)*............. **314, 1424**
Augmentin XR Tablets *(GlaxoSmithKline)*............. **314, 1430**
Augmentin ES-600 Powder for Oral Suspension *(GlaxoSmithKline)*............. **314, 1427**
Bicillin L-A Injection *(King)*............ **1772**
PREVPAC *(TAP)*..................... **334, 3215**
Timentin ADD-Vantage *(GlaxoSmithKline)*............. **317, 1635**
Timentin IV Infusion *(GlaxoSmithKline)*............. **317, 1632**
Timentin Pharmacy Bulk Package *(GlaxoSmithKline)*............. **317, 1639**
Unasyn for Injection *(Pfizer)*........... **2644**
Zosyn *(Wyeth)*..................... **337, 3413**
Zosyn in Galaxy Containers *(Wyeth)*..... **3413**

QUINOLONES

Avelox I.V. *(Bayer)*................ **308, 815**
Avelox Tablets *(Bayer)*............. **308, 815**
Cipro I.V. *(Bayer)*................. **308, 827**
Cipro I.V. Pharmacy Bulk Package *(Bayer)*...................... **308, 833**
Cipro Oral Suspension *(Bayer)*...... **308, 821**
Cipro Tablets *(Bayer)*.............. **308, 821**
Cipro XR Tablets *(Bayer)*........... **308, 839**
Factive Tablets *(Ocient)*.......... **328, 2554**
Floxin Tablets *(Ortho-McNeil)*.......... **2495**
Levaquin in 5% Dextrose Injection *(Ortho-McNeil)*.......................... **2501**
Levaquin Injection *(Ortho-McNeil)*.. **328, 2501**
Levaquin Tablets *(Ortho-McNeil)*... **328, 2501**
Noroxin Tablets *(Merck)*........... **323, 2103**
Tequin Injection *(Bristol-Myers Squibb)*...................... **310, 1075**
Tequin Tablets *(Bristol-Myers Squibb)*...................... **310, 1075**

SULFONAMIDES & COMBINATIONS

Pediazole Suspension *(Ross)*............ **2960**
Septra Suspension *(King)*............... **1790**
Septra Grape Suspension *(King)*......... **1790**
Septra Tablets *(King)*.................. **1790**
Septra DS Tablets *(King)*............... **1790**

TETRACYCLINES

Dynacin Tablets *(Medicis)*.............. **1957**
Periostat Tablets *(CollaGenex)*.......... **1147**

ANTIFUNGALS

Abelcet Injection *(Enzon)*.............. **1228**
AmBisome for Injection *(Fujisawa)*... **312, 1297**
Ancobon Capsules *(Valeant)*............ **3264**
Cancidas for Injection *(Merck)*.......... **1999**
Diflucan Injection *(Pfizer)*.............. **2605**
Diflucan Oral Suspension *(Pfizer)*........ **2605**
Diflucan Tablets *(Pfizer)*........... **329, 2605**
Grifulvin V Tablets Microsize and Oral Suspension Microsize *(OrthoNeutrogena)*.............. **327, 2479**
Lamisil Tablets *(Novartis)*.......... **325, 2325**
Nizoral Tablets *(Janssen)*........... **319, 1735**
Sporanox Capsules *(Janssen)*........ **319, 1753**
Sporanox Injection *(Janssen)*............ **1757**
Sporanox Oral Solution *(Janssen)*........ **1761**
VFEND I.V. *(Pfizer)*................... **2647**
VFEND Oral Suspension *(Pfizer)*......... **2647**
VFEND Tablets *(Pfizer)*............ **329, 2647**

ANTIMALARIAL AGENTS

Aralen Tablets *(Sanofi-Synthelabo)*......... **2983**
Daraprim Tablets *(GlaxoSmithKline)*.. **315, 1464**
Lariam Tablets *(Roche Laboratories)*.. **331, 2903**
Malarone Tablets *(GlaxoSmithKline)*.. **316, 1568**
Malarone Pediatric Tablets *(GlaxoSmithKline)*.............. **316, 1568**
Plaquenil Tablets *(Sanofi-Synthelabo)*.. **332, 3008**

ANTITUBERCULOSIS AGENTS

Capastat Sulfate for Injection *(Lilly)*........ **1828**
Paser Granules *(Jacobus)*................ **1725**
Priftin Tablets *(Aventis)*................ **732**
Rifadin Capsules *(Aventis)*........... **307, 736**
Rifadin IV *(Aventis)*..................... **736**
Rifamate Capsules *(Aventis)*.......... **307, 739**
Rifater Tablets *(Aventis)*............. **307, 740**
Seromycin Capsules *(Lilly)*.............. **1883**
Streptomycin Sulfate Injection *(Pfizer)*...... **2637**
Trecator-SC Tablets *(Wyeth)*............. **3406**

ANTIVIRALS

Agenerase Capsules *(GlaxoSmithKline)*.............. **314, 1396**
Agenerase Oral Solution *(GlaxoSmithKline)*.............. **314, 1401**
Alferon N Injection *(Hemispherx)*..... **319, 1710**
Combivir Tablets *(GlaxoSmithKline)*.. **315, 1454**
Copegus Tablets *(Roche Laboratories)*...... **2862**
Crixivan Capsules *(Merck)*.......... **323, 2021**
Cytovene Capsules *(Roche Laboratories)*.................. **331, 2866**
Cytovene-IV *(Roche Laboratories)*......... **2866**
Emtriva Capsules *(Gilead)*.......... **313, 1370**
Epivir Oral Solution *(GlaxoSmithKline)*.............. **315, 1473**
Epivir Tablets *(GlaxoSmithKline)*..... **315, 1473**
Epivir-HBV Oral Solution *(GlaxoSmithKline)*.............. **315, 1477**
Epivir-HBV Tablets *(GlaxoSmithKline)*.............. **315, 1477**
Epzicom Tablets *(GlaxoSmithKline)*........ **1481**
Famvir Tablets *(Novartis)*................ **2311**
Flumadine Syrup *(Forest)*................ **1275**
Flumadine Tablets *(Forest)*.......... **312, 1275**
Fortovase Capsules *(Roche Laboratories)*.................. **331, 2876**
Hepsera Tablets *(Gilead)*........... **313, 1373**
Hivid Tablets *(Roche Laboratories)*... **331, 2886**
Infergen *(InterMune)*............... **319, 1716**
Intron A for Injection *(Schering)*........... **3035**
Invirase Capsules *(Roche Laboratories)*.................. **331, 2890**
Kaletra Capsules *(Abbott)*........... **303, 483**
Kaletra Oral Solution *(Abbott)*........ **303, 483**
Lexiva Tablets *(GlaxoSmithKline)*..... **316, 1558**
Norvir Soft Gelatin Capsules *(Abbott)*.. **303, 500**
Norvir Oral Solution *(Abbott)*........ **303, 500**
Pegasys *(Roche Laboratories)*............ **2906**
PEG-Intron Powder for Injection *(Schering)*.......................... **3046**
Rebetol Capsules *(Schering)*............. **3053**
Rebetol Oral Solution *(Schering)*......... **3053**
Rebetron Combination Therapy *(Schering)*.. **3058**
Relenza Rotadisk *(GlaxoSmithKline)*.. **317, 1606**
Rescriptor Tablets *(Pfizer)*.......... **329, 2629**
Retrovir Capsules *(GlaxoSmithKline)*.. **317, 1612**
Retrovir IV Infusion *(GlaxoSmithKline)*.............. **317, 1616**
Retrovir Syrup *(GlaxoSmithKline)*.... **317, 1612**
Retrovir Tablets *(GlaxoSmithKline)*... **317, 1612**
Reyataz Capsules *(Bristol-Myers Squibb)*.......................... **310, 1060**
Ribavirin, USP Capsules *(Schering)*........ **3063**
Roferon-A Injection *(Roche Laboratories)*... **2918**
Sustiva Capsules *(Bristol-Myers Squibb)*.......................... **310, 1069**
Symmetrel Syrup *(Endo Labs)*........... **1224**
Symmetrel Tablets *(Endo Labs)*...... **311, 1224**
Synagis Intramuscular Powder *(MedImmune)*.................. **322, 1965**
Synagis Intramuscular Solution *(MedImmune)*.................. **322, 1965**
Tamiflu Capsules *(Roche Laboratories)*.................. **331, 2927**
Tamiflu Oral Suspension *(Roche Laboratories)*.......................... **2927**
Trizivir Tablets *(GlaxoSmithKline)*.... **317, 1642**
Truvada Tablets *(Gilead)*........... **313, 1376**
Valcyte Tablets *(Roche Laboratories)*.. **332, 2936**
Valtrex Caplets *(GlaxoSmithKline)*.... **317, 1650**
Videx EC Capsules *(Bristol-Myers Squibb)*.......................... **310, 1082**
Viracept Oral Powder *(Pfizer)*............ **2659**
Viracept Tablets *(Pfizer)*........... **330, 2659**
Viramune Oral Suspension *(Boehringer Ingelheim)*........... **309, 1013**
Viramune Tablets *(Boehringer Ingelheim)*...................... **309, 1013**
Virazole for Inhalation Solution *(Valeant)*.... **3282**
Viread Tablets *(Gilead)*............ **313, 1381**
Zerit Capsules *(Bristol-Myers Squibb)*.......................... **310, 1087**
Zerit for Oral Solution *(Bristol-Myers Squibb)*.............. **310, 1087**
Ziagen Oral Solution *(GlaxoSmithKline)*.............. **318, 1673**
Ziagen Tablets *(GlaxoSmithKline)*..... **318, 1673**
Zovirax Capsules *(GlaxoSmithKline)*.. **318, 1687**
Zovirax for Injection *(GlaxoSmithKline)*.............. **318, 1689**
Zovirax Suspension *(GlaxoSmithKline)*.............. **318, 1687**
Zovirax Tablets *(GlaxoSmithKline)*.... **318, 1687**

LEPROSTATICS

Dapsone Tablets USP *(Jacobus)*........... **1724**

MISCELLANEOUS ANTI-INFECTIVES

Alinia for Oral Suspension *(Romark)*........ **2958**
Dapsone Tablets USP *(Jacobus)*........... **1724**
Daraprim Tablets *(GlaxoSmithKline)*.. **315, 1464**
Mepron Suspension *(GlaxoSmithKline)*.............. **316, 1572**
Xigris Powder for Intravenous Infusion *(Lilly)*................ **320, 1897**

URINARY ANTI-INFECTIVES & COMBINATIONS

Amoxil Capsules *(GlaxoSmithKline)*... **314, 1411**
Amoxil Chewable Tablets *(GlaxoSmithKline)*.............. **314, 1411**
Amoxil for Oral Suspension *(GlaxoSmithKline)*.............. **314, 1411**
Amoxil Pediatric Drops for Oral Suspension *(GlaxoSmithKline)*..... **314, 1411**
Amoxil Tablets *(GlaxoSmithKline)*.... **314, 1411**
Ancobon Capsules *(Valeant)*............. **3264**
Augmentin Tablets *(GlaxoSmithKline)*.............. **314, 1424**
Azactam for Injection *(Elan)*............. **1204**
Ceclor Pulvules *(Lilly)*................. **1829**
Ceclor Suspension *(Lilly)*............... **1829**
Ceftin for Oral Suspension *(GlaxoSmithKline)*.............. **315, 1450**
Ceftin Tablets *(GlaxoSmithKline)*..... **315, 1450**
Cipro I.V. *(Bayer)*.................. **308, 827**
Cipro I.V. Pharmacy Bulk Package *(Bayer)*.......................... **308, 833**
Cipro Oral Suspension *(Bayer)*........ **308, 821**
Cipro Tablets *(Bayer)*............... **308, 821**
Cipro XR Tablets *(Bayer)*............ **308, 839**
Claforan Sterile for Injection *(Aventis)*.. **307, 699**
Diflucan Injection *(Pfizer)*.............. **2605**
Diflucan Oral Suspension *(Pfizer)*......... **2605**
Diflucan Tablets *(Pfizer)*........... **329, 2605**
Dynacin Tablets *(Medicis)*............... **1957**
Floxin Tablets *(Ortho-McNeil)*........... **2495**
Fortaz Injection *(GlaxoSmithKline)*.... **316, 1504**
Fortaz for Injection *(GlaxoSmithKline)*.............. **316, 1504**
Invanz for Injection *(Merck)*............. **2069**
Keflex Pulvules *(Lilly)*................. **1871**
Levaquin in 5% Dextrose Injection *(Ortho-McNeil)*.......................... **2501**
Levaquin Injection *(Ortho-McNeil)*.... **328, 2501**
Levaquin Tablets *(Ortho-McNeil)*..... **328, 2501**
Maxipime for Injection *(Elan)*............ **1207**
Monurol Sachet *(Forest)*............ **312, 1287**
Neosporin G.U. Irrigant Sterile *(King)*...... **1789**
Noroxin Tablets *(Merck)*............ **323, 2103**
Primaxin I.V. *(Merck)*.................. **2118**
Prosed EC Tablets *(Star)*................ **3173**
Prosed/DS Tablets *(Star)*................ **3172**
Rocephin Injectable Vials, ADD-Vantage, Galaxy, Bulk *(Roche Laboratories)*...... **2915**
Septra Suspension *(King)*................ **1790**
Septra Grape Suspension *(King)*.......... **1790**
Septra Tablets *(King)*................... **1790**
Septra DS Tablets *(King)*................ **1790**
Tequin Injection *(Bristol-Myers Squibb)*.......................... **310, 1075**
Tequin Tablets *(Bristol-Myers Squibb)*.......................... **310, 1075**
Timentin ADD-Vantage *(GlaxoSmithKline)*.............. **317, 1635**
Timentin IV Infusion *(GlaxoSmithKline)*.............. **317, 1632**
Timentin Pharmacy Bulk Package *(GlaxoSmithKline)*.............. **317, 1639**
Uroqid-Acid No. 2 Tablets *(Beach)*..... **308, 887**
Vantin Tablets and Oral Suspension *(Pharmacia & Upjohn)*......... **330, 2758**
Zinacef Injection *(GlaxoSmithKline)*... **318, 1676**
Zinacef for Injection *(GlaxoSmithKline)*.............. **318, 1676**

ANTI-INFECTIVES, NON-SYSTEMIC

MISCELLANEOUS, ANTI-INFECTIVES, NON-SYSTEMIC

Xifaxan Tablets *(Salix)*............. **332, 2969**

SCABICIDES & PEDICULICIDES

(see under:
SKIN & MUCOUS MEMBRANE AGENTS
ANTI-INFECTIVES
SCABICIDES & PEDICULICIDES)

ANTI-INFLAMMATORY AGENTS

(see under:
ANALGESICS
NONSTEROIDAL ANTI-INFLAMMATORY DRUGS (NSAIDS)
SALICYLATES
ANTIRHEUMATIC AGENTS
GASTROINTESTINAL AGENTS
ANTI-INFLAMMATORY AGENTS
GOUT PREPARATIONS
HORMONES
GLUCOCORTICOIDS
NASAL PREPARATIONS
ANTI-INFLAMMATORY AGENTS
OPHTHALMIC PREPARATIONS
ANTI-INFLAMMATORY AGENTS
OTIC PREPARATIONS
ANTIBIOTIC & STEROID COMBINATIONS
RESPIRATORY AGENTS
ANTI-INFLAMMATORY AGENTS
SKIN & MUCOUS MEMBRANE AGENTS
STEROIDS & COMBINATIONS)

GLAUCOMA PREPARATIONS
(*see under:*
OPHTHALMIC PREPARATIONS
BETA ADRENERGIC BLOCKING AGENTS
CARBONIC ANHYDRASE INHIBITORS
MIOTICS
SYMPATHOMIMETICS & COMBINATIONS)

GLUCOSE ELEVATING AGENTS
(*see under:*
HORMONES
GLUCOSE ELEVATING AGENTS)

GONADOTROPIN INHIBITORS
(*see under:*
HORMONES
GONADOTROPIN INHIBITORS)

GONADOTROPIN RELEASING HORMONE (GNRH) ANALOGUES
(*see under:*
ANTINEOPLASTICS
HORMONAL AGONISTS/ANTAGONISTS
GONADOTROPIN RELEASING HORMONE (GNRH) ANALOGUES
HORMONES
GONADOTROPIN RELEASING HORMONES (GNRH)
GONADOTROPIN RELEASING HORMONE (GNRH) ANALOGUES)

GOUT PREPARATIONS

NONSTEROIDAL ANTI-INFLAMMATORY DRUGS (NSAIDS)
Anaprox Tablets (*Roche Laboratories*) 331, 2874
Anaprox DS Tablets (*Roche Laboratories*) 331, 2874
Clinoril Tablets (*Merck*) 323, 2004
Indocin Capsules (*Merck*) 323, 2065
Indocin Oral Suspension (*Merck*) 2065
Indocin Suppositories (*Merck*) 323, 2065
Naprosyn Suspension (*Roche Laboratories*) .. 2874
Naprosyn Tablets (*Roche Laboratories*) 331, 2874

H

HAIR GROWTH STIMULANTS
(*see under:*
SKIN & MUCOUS MEMBRANE AGENTS
HAIR GROWTH STIMULANTS)

HEAD LICE RELIEF
(*see under:*
SKIN & MUCOUS MEMBRANE AGENTS
ANTI-INFECTIVES
SCABICIDES & PEDICULICIDES)

HEMATINICS
(*see under:*
BLOOD MODIFIERS
HEMATINICS)

HEMORRHEOLOGIC AGENTS
(*see under:*
BLOOD MODIFIERS
HEMORRHEOLOGIC AGENTS)

HEMORRHOIDAL PREPARATIONS
(*see under:*
SKIN & MUCOUS MEMBRANE AGENTS
ANORECTAL PREPARATIONS)

HEMOSTATICS
(*see under:*
BLOOD MODIFIERS
HEMOSTATICS)

HERPES TREATMENT
(*see under:*
ANTI-INFECTIVE AGENTS, SYSTEMIC
ANTIVIRALS
OPHTHALMIC PREPARATIONS
ANTI-INFECTIVES
ANTIVIRALS
SKIN & MUCOUS MEMBRANE AGENTS
ANTI-INFECTIVES
ANTIVIRALS)

HISTAMINE (H_2) RECEPTOR ANTAGONISTS
(*see under:*
GASTROINTESTINAL AGENTS
HISTAMINE (H_2) RECEPTOR ANTAGONISTS)

HIV THERAPY
(*see under:*
AIDS/HIV ADJUNCT AGENTS
ANTI-INFECTIVE AGENTS, SYSTEMIC
AIDS ADJUNCT ANTI-INFECTIVES
AIDS CHEMOTHERAPEUTIC AGENTS)

HOMEOPATHIC REMEDIES

ANTI-INFLAMMATORY AGENTS
CM Plex Cream (*Unicity*) 3242
CM Plex Softgels (*Unicity*) 3242

HORMONES

ANABOLIC STEROIDS
Anadrol-50 Tablets (*Unimed*) 335, 3243
Oxandrin Tablets (*Savient*) 332, 3019

ANDROGEN & ESTROGEN COMBINATIONS
Estratest Tablets (*Solvay*) 333, 3157
Estratest H.S. Tablets (*Solvay*) 333, 3157

ANDROGENS
AndroGel (*Unimed*) 335, 3244
Delatestryl Injection (*Savient*) 332, 3018
Striant Mucoadhesive (*Columbia*) 311, 1150
Testim 1% Gel (*Auxilium*) 673
Testred Capsules, 10 mg (*Valeant*) 335, 3281

ANTIDIURETICS
(*see under:*
HORMONES
VASOPRESSIN & DERIVATIVES)

ANTINEOPLASTICS
(*see under:*
ANTINEOPLASTICS
HORMONAL AGONISTS/ANTAGONISTS)

CALCITONIN
Miacalcin Injection (*Novartis*) 2340
Miacalcin Nasal Spray (*Novartis*) 325, 2341

DIABETES AGENTS
(*see under:*
ANTIDIABETIC AGENTS)

ESTROGENS & COMBINATIONS
(*see also under:*
VAGINAL PREPARATIONS
ESTROGENS)
Cenestin Tablets, 0.45mg, 0.625mg, 0.9mg, 1.25mg (*Duramed*) 311, 1187
Cenestin Tablets, 0.3mg (*Duramed*) 311, 1187
Climara Transdermal System (*Berlex*) ... 308, 897
Climara Pro Transdermal System (*Berlex*) 308, 902
Estrasorb Topical Emulsion (*Novavax*) 326, 2406
Estring Vaginal Ring (*Pharmacia & Upjohn*) 2730
Estrogel 0.06% (*Solvay*) 333, 3160
Femtrace Tablets (*Warner Chilcott*) 3293
Menostar Transdermal System (*Berlex*) 308, 917
Premarin Intravenous (*Wyeth*) 336, 3363
Premarin Tablets (*Wyeth*) 336, 3366
Vagifem Tablets (*Novo Nordisk*) 2438
Vivelle Transdermal System (*Novartis*) 326, 2385
Vivelle-Dot Transdermal System (*Novartis*) 326, 2390

GLUCOCORTICOIDS
Decadron Tablets (*Merck*) 323, 2032
Decadron Phosphate Injection (*Merck*) 2034
Depo-Medrol Injectable Suspension (*Pharmacia & Upjohn*) 2712
Depo-Medrol Single-Dose Vial (*Pharmacia & Upjohn*) 2714
Hydrocortone Tablets (*Merck*) 323, 2058
Hydrocortone Phosphate Injection, Sterile (*Merck*) 2057
Orapred Oral Solution (*Biomarin*) 966
Pediapred Oral Solution (*Celltech*) 1110

GLUCOSE ELEVATING AGENTS
GlucaGen for Injection (*Bedford*) 892
Glucagon for Injection Vials and Emergency Kit (*Lilly*) 1849

GONADOTROPIN INHIBITORS
Eligard 7.5 mg (*Sanofi-Synthelabo*) ... 332, 2989
Eligard 22.5 mg (*Sanofi-Synthelabo*) .. 332, 2992
Eligard 30 mg (*Sanofi-Synthelabo*) 332, 2994
Lupron Depot 3.75 mg (*TAP*) 334, 3188
Lupron Depot 7.5 mg (*TAP*) 334, 3192
Lupron Depot--3 Month 11.25 mg (*TAP*) 334, 3193
Lupron Depot--3 Month 22.5 mg (*TAP*) 334, 3197
Lupron Depot--4 Month 30 mg (*TAP*) 334, 3198
Lupron Depot-PED 7.5 mg, 11.25 mg and 15 mg (*TAP*) 334, 3200
Lupron Injection (*TAP*) 334, 3186
Lupron Injection Pediatric (*TAP*) 3187
Plenaxis for Injectable Suspension (*Praecis*) 2782
Trelstar Depot (*Pharmacia & Upjohn*) 2757
Zoladex (*AstraZeneca*) 306, 668
Zoladex 3-month (*AstraZeneca*) 671

GONADOTROPIN RELEASING HORMONES (GNRH)

GONADOTROPIN RELEASING HORMONE (GNRH) ANALOGUES
Cetrotide for Injection (*Serono*) 3106
Eligard 7.5 mg (*Sanofi-Synthelabo*) 332, 2989
Eligard 22.5 mg (*Sanofi-Synthelabo*) 332, 2992
Eligard 30 mg (*Sanofi-Synthelabo*) .. 332, 2994
Lupron Depot 3.75 mg (*TAP*) 334, 3188
Lupron Depot 7.5 mg (*TAP*) 334, 3192
Lupron Depot--3 Month 11.25 mg (*TAP*) 334, 3193
Lupron Depot--3 Month 22.5 mg (*TAP*) 334, 3197
Lupron Depot--4 Month 30 mg (*TAP*) 334, 3198
Lupron Depot-PED 7.5 mg, 11.25 mg and 15 mg (*TAP*) 334, 3200
Lupron Injection (*TAP*) 334, 3186
Lupron Injection Pediatric (*TAP*) 3187
Trelstar Depot (*Pharmacia & Upjohn*) 2757
Zoladex (*AstraZeneca*) 306, 668
Zoladex 3-month (*AstraZeneca*) 671

GONADOTROPINS

CHORIONIC GONADOTROPIN
Novarel for Injection (*Ferring*) 1254

MENOTROPINS
Repronex for Intramuscular and Subcutaneous Injection (*Ferring*) 1255

UROFOLLITROPINS
Bravelle for Intramuscular or Subcutaneous Injection (*Ferring*) 1249

GROWTH HORMONE
Genotropin Lyophilized Powder (*Pharmacia & Upjohn*) 2738
Humatrope Vials and Cartridges (*Lilly*) 1856
Norditropin Cartridges (*Novo Nordisk*) 2418
Nutropin for Injection (*Genentech*) 313, 1341
Nutropin AQ Injection (*Genentech*) ... 313, 1345
Nutropin AQ Pen (*Genentech*) 313, 1345
Nutropin AQ Pen Cartridge (*Genentech*) 313, 1345

GROWTH HORMONE RECEPTOR ANTAGONIST
Somavert Injection (*Pharmacia & Upjohn*) .. 2754

PROGESTIN & ESTROGEN COMBINATIONS
Activella Tablets (*Novo Nordisk*) 2411
Alesse-28 Tablets (*Wyeth*) 336, 3308
CombiPatch Transdermal System (*Novartis*) 2285
Lo/Ovral-28 Tablets (*Wyeth*) 336, 3337
NuvaRing (*Organon USA*) 327, 2453
Ortho Evra Transdermal System (*Ortho-McNeil*) 328, 2515
Ortho Tri-Cyclen Lo Tablets (*Ortho-McNeil*) 328, 2533
Ortho-Cept Tablets (*Ortho-McNeil*) ... 328, 2508
Ortho-Cyclen Tablets (*Ortho-McNeil*) 328, 2526
Ortho Tri-Cyclen Tablets (*Ortho-McNeil*) 328, 2526
Ovral-28 Tablets (*Wyeth*) 336, 3352
Premphase Tablets (*Wyeth*) 336, 3375
Prempro Tablets (*Wyeth*) 336, 3375
Triphasil-28 Tablets (*Wyeth*) 337, 3407
Yasmin 28 Tablets (*Berlex*) 309, 930

PROGESTINS & COMBINATIONS
Aygestin Tablets (*Duramed*) 311, 1186
Crinone 4% Gel (*Serono*) 3108
Crinone 8% Gel (*Serono*) 3108
Mirena Intrauterine System (*Berlex*) 309, 921
Ortho Micronor Tablets (*Ortho-McNeil*) 328, 2524
Ovrette Tablets (*Wyeth*) 336, 3358
Prochieve 4% Gel (*Columbia*) 311, 1148
Prochieve 8% Gel (*Columbia*) 311, 1148
Prometrium Capsules (100 mg, 200 mg) (*Solvay*) 333, 3165

SOMATOSTATIN ANALOGUES
Sandostatin Injection (*Novartis*) 325, 2361
Sandostatin LAR Depot (*Novartis*) 325, 2363

THYROID PREPARATIONS

SYNTHETIC T3
Cytomel Tablets (*King*) 319, 1781
Triostat Injection (*King*) 320, 1802

SYNTHETIC T4
Levothroid Tablets (*Forest*) 1278
Levoxyl Tablets (*King*) 319, 1785
Synthroid Tablets (*Abbott*) 303, 515

VASOPRESSIN & DERIVATIVES
DDAVP Injection 4 mcg/mL (*Aventis*) .. 307, 704
DDAVP Nasal Spray (*Aventis*) 307, 705
DDAVP Tablets (*Aventis*) 307, 707
Desmopressin Acetate Injection (*Ferring*) ... 1252
Desmopressin Acetate Rhinal Tube (*Ferring*) 1253

HUMAN IMMUNODEFICIENCY VIRUS (HIV) THERAPY
(*see under:*
AIDS/HIV ADJUNCT AGENTS
ANTI-INFECTIVE AGENTS, SYSTEMIC
AIDS ADJUNCT ANTI-INFECTIVES
AIDS CHEMOTHERAPEUTIC AGENTS)

HYPERCALCEMIA MANAGEMENT
Aredia for Injection (*Novartis*) 324, 2274
Miacalcin Injection (*Novartis*) 2340
Sensipar Tablets (*Amgen*) 305, 597
Zometa for Intravenous Infusion (*Novartis*) 326, 2401

HYPERGLYCEMIC AGENTS
(*see under:*
HORMONES
GLUCOSE ELEVATING AGENTS)

HYPNOTICS
(*see under:*
SEDATIVES & HYPNOTICS)

HYPOCALCEMIA MANAGEMENT
Calcijex Injection (*Abbott*) 417
Rocaltrol Capsules (*Roche Laboratories*) 331, 2913
Rocaltrol Oral Solution (*Roche Laboratories*) 2913

HYPOGLYCEMIC AGENTS
(*see under:*
ANTIDIABETIC AGENTS)

HYPOLIPIDEMICS
(*see under:*
CARDIOVASCULAR AGENTS
ANTILIPIDEMIC AGENTS)

I

IMMUNE SERUMS
(*see under:*
BIOLOGICALS
IMMUNE SERUMS)

IMMUNE SYSTEM SUPPORT
(*see under:*
DIETARY SUPPLEMENTS
IMMUNE SYSTEM SUPPORT)

IMMUNOMODULATORS
(*see also under:*
ANTINEOPLASTICS
IMMUNOMODULATORS)

BLOOD MODIFIERS
COLONY STIMULATING FACTORS)
Alferon N Injection (*Hemispherx*) 319, 1710
Arava Tablets (*Aventis*) 307, 693
Avonex (*Biogen Idec*) 951
Betaseron for SC Injection (*Berlex*) 308, 893
Copaxone for Injection (*Teva Neuroscience*) 334, 3221
Infergen (*InterMune*) 319, 1716
Intron A for Injection (*Schering*) 3035
Pegasys (*Roche Laboratories*) 2906
PEG-Intron Powder for Injection (*Schering*) 3046
Rebetron Combination Therapy (*Schering*) .. 3058
Rebif Injection (*Pfizer*) 2623
Rebif Prefilled Syringe for Injection (*Serono*) 333, 3123
Roferon-A Injection (*Roche Laboratories*) ... 2918
Thalomid Capsules (*Celgene*) 310, 1095

IMMUNOSUPPRESSIVES
Azasan Tablets (*Salix*) 332, 2966
CellCept Capsules (*Roche Laboratories*) 331, 2855
CellCept Intravenous (*Roche Laboratories*) .. 2855
CellCept Oral Suspension (*Roche Laboratories*) 2855
CellCept Tablets (*Roche Laboratories*) 331, 2855
Gengraf Capsules (*Abbott*) 303, 466
MICRhoGAM Ultra-Filtered (*Ortho-Clinical*) 2486
Myfortic Tablets (*Novartis*) 325, 2343
Neoral Soft Gelatin Capsules (*Novartis*) 325, 2346
Neoral Oral Solution (*Novartis*) 325, 2346
Orthoclone OKT3 Sterile Solution (*Ortho Biotech*) 2466
Prograf Capsules and Injection (*Fujisawa*) 313, 1302
Rapamune Oral Solution and Tablets (*Wyeth*) 337, 3395
Sandimmune I.V. Ampuls for Infusion (*Novartis*) 325, 2358
Sandimmune Oral Solution (*Novartis*) 325, 2358
Sandimmune Soft Gelatin Capsules (*Novartis*) 325, 2358
Simulect for Injection (*Novartis*) 325, 2367
Thymoglobulin for Injection (*SangStat*) 2971
Zenapax for Injection (*Roche Laboratories*) 2955

IMPOTENCE AGENTS
(*see under:*
ERECTILE DYSFUNCTION THERAPY)

INSECT STING EMERGENCY KITS
(*see under:*
EMERGENCY KITS)

INSULIN REACTION
(*see under:*
HORMONES
GLUCOSE ELEVATING AGENTS)

INSULINS
(*see under:*
ANTIDIABETIC AGENTS
INSULINS)

ION EXCHANGE RESINS
(*see under:*
CARDIOVASCULAR AGENTS
ANTILIPIDEMIC AGENTS
BILE ACID SEQUESTRANTS)

IRON DEFICIENCY
(*see under:*
BLOOD MODIFIERS
HEMATINICS)

L

LAXATIVES
(*see under:*
GASTROINTESTINAL AGENTS
LAXATIVES)

LEAD POISONING
(*see under:*
ANTIDOTES
CHELATING AGENTS
LEAD)

LEPROSTATICS
(*see under:*
ANTI-INFECTIVE AGENTS, SYSTEMIC
LEPROSTATICS)

LEVOCARNITINE DEFICIENCY MANAGEMENT
Carnitor Injection (*Sigma-Tau*) 3144
Carnitor Tablets and Oral Solution (*Sigma-Tau*) 3146

LICE TREATMENTS
(*see under:*
SKIN & MUCOUS MEMBRANE AGENTS
ANTI-INFECTIVES
SCABICIDES & PEDICULICIDES)

LUBRICANTS
(*see under:*
OPHTHALMIC PREPARATIONS
ARTIFICIAL TEARS/LUBRICANTS & COMBINATIONS
SKIN & MUCOUS MEMBRANE AGENTS
EMOLLIENTS & MOISTURIZERS)

OSTEOPOROSIS PREPARATIONS

BISPHOSPHONATES
Actonel Tablets *(Procter & Gamble Pharmaceuticals)* ... 330, 2795
Fosamax Oral Solution *(Merck)* ... 2049
Fosamax Tablets *(Merck)* ... 323, 2049

HORMONAL AGENTS

CALCITONIN
Miacalcin Injection *(Novartis)* ... 2340
Miacalcin Nasal Spray *(Novartis)* ... 325, 2341

ESTROGENS & COMBINATIONS
Activella Tablets *(Novo Nordisk)* ... 2411
Climara Transdermal System *(Berlex)* ... 308, 897
Menostar Transdermal System *(Berlex)* ... 308, 917
Premarin Tablets *(Wyeth)* ... 336, 3366
Premphase Tablets *(Wyeth)* ... 336, 3375
Prempro Tablets *(Wyeth)* ... 336, 3375
Vivelle Transdermal System *(Novartis)* ... 326, 2385
Vivelle-Dot Transdermal System *(Novartis)* ... 326, 2390

MISCELLANEOUS HORMONAL AGENTS
Forteo for Injection *(Lilly)* ... 320, 1840

SELECTIVE ESTROGEN RECEPTOR MODULATORS
Evista Tablets *(Lilly)* ... 320, 1836

OTIC PREPARATIONS

ANTIBIOTIC & STEROID COMBINATIONS
Cipro HC Otic Suspension *(Alcon)* ... 549
Ciprodex Otic Suspension *(Alcon)* ... 304, 550
Cortisporin-TC Otic Suspension *(King)* ... 319, 1778

ANTIBIOTICS
Floxin Otic Singles *(Daiichi)* ... 311, 1169
Floxin Otic Solution *(Daiichi)* ... 311, 1168

OXYTOCICS
(see under:
VAGINAL PREPARATIONS
PROSTAGLANDINS)

P

PAIN RELIEVERS
(see under:
ANALGESICS)

PARASYMPATHOMIMETICS
Salagen Tablets *(MGI)* ... 337, 2201
Urecholine Injection *(Merck)* ... 2160
Urecholine Tablets *(Merck)* ... 324, 2160

PARKINSONISM DRUGS
(see under:
ANTIPARKINSONIAN AGENTS)

PARKINSON'S DISEASE
(see under:
ANTIPARKINSONIAN AGENTS)

PATENT DUCTUS ARTERIOSUS AGENTS
Indocin I.V. *(Merck)* ... 2068

PEDICULICIDES
(see under:
SKIN & MUCOUS MEMBRANE AGENTS
ANTI-INFECTIVES
SCABICIDES & PEDICULICIDES)

PHOSPHATE BINDERS
PhosLo Gelcaps *(Nabi)* ... 324, 2261
PhosLo Tablets *(Nabi)* ... 324, 2261
Renagel Tablets *(Genzyme)* ... 313, 1366

PHOSPHORUS PREPARATIONS
(see under:
DIETARY SUPPLEMENTS
MINERALS & ELECTROLYTES
PHOSPHORUS & COMBINATIONS)

PHOTOSENSITIZERS
(see under:
SKIN & MUCOUS MEMBRANE AGENTS
PHOTOSENSITIZING AGENTS)

PLASMA FRACTIONS, HUMAN
(see under:
BLOOD MODIFIERS
PLASMA FRACTIONS, HUMAN)

PLATELET INHIBITORS
(see under:
BLOOD MODIFIERS
ANTIPLATELET AGENTS)

PORPHYRIA AGENTS
Panhematin for Injection *(Ovation)* ... 329, 2573

POTASSIUM SUPPLEMENTS
(see under:
DIETARY SUPPLEMENTS
MINERALS & ELECTROLYTES
POTASSIUM & COMBINATIONS)

PROSTAGLANDINS
Cervidil Vaginal Insert *(Forest)* ... 312, 1273
Flolan for Injection *(GlaxoSmithKline)* ... 315, 1487
MUSE Urethral Suppository *(Vivus)* ... 335, 3287

PROSTATIC HYPERTROPHY MODIFIER
(see under:
URINARY TRACT AGENTS
BENIGN PROSTATIC HYPERPLASIA (BPH) THERAPY)

PROTEASE INHIBITORS
(see under:
ANTI-INFECTIVE AGENTS, SYSTEMIC
AIDS CHEMOTHERAPEUTIC AGENTS
PROTEASE INHIBITORS)

PROTON PUMP INHIBITORS
(see under:
GASTROINTESTINAL AGENTS
PROTON PUMP INHIBITORS)

PRURITUS MEDICATIONS
(see under:
ANTIHISTAMINES & COMBINATIONS
SKIN & MUCOUS MEMBRANE AGENTS
ANTIPRURITICS)

PSORIASIS AGENTS
(see under:
SKIN & MUCOUS MEMBRANE AGENTS
ANTIPSORIATIC AGENTS)

PSYCHOSTIMULANTS
(see under:
CENTRAL NERVOUS SYSTEM STIMULANTS)

PSYCHOTHERAPEUTIC AGENTS

ANTIANXIETY AGENTS

BENZODIAZEPINES & COMBINATIONS
Librium Capsules *(Valeant)* ... 3268
Tranxene T-TAB Tablets *(Ovation)* ... 329, 2574
Tranxene-SD Tablets *(Ovation)* ... 329, 2574
Tranxene-SD Half Strength Tablets *(Ovation)* ... 329, 2574
Valium Tablets *(Roche Products)* ... 332, 2957
Xanax Tablets *(Pharmacia & Upjohn)* ... 330, 2763

MISCELLANEOUS ANTIANXIETY AGENTS
Effexor XR Capsules *(Wyeth)* ... 336, 3326
Paxil Oral Suspension *(GlaxoSmithKline)* ... 317, 1585
Paxil Tablets *(GlaxoSmithKline)* ... 317, 1585
Zoloft Oral Concentrate *(Pfizer)* ... 2681
Zoloft Tablets *(Pfizer)* ... 330, 2681

ANTIDEPRESSANTS

MISCELLANEOUS ANTIDEPRESSANTS
Cymbalta Delayed-Release Capsules *(Eli Lilly)* ... 320, 3430
Effexor Tablets *(Wyeth)* ... 336, 3321
Effexor XR Capsules *(Wyeth)* ... 336, 3326
Wellbutrin Tablets *(GlaxoSmithKline)* ... 317, 1655
Wellbutrin SR Sustained-Release Tablets *(GlaxoSmithKline)* ... 317, 1659
Wellbutrin XL Extended-Release Tablets *(GlaxoSmithKline)* ... 318, 1663

MONOAMINE OXIDASE INHIBITORS (MAOI)
Parnate Tablets *(GlaxoSmithKline)* ... 317, 1583

SELECTIVE SEROTONIN REUPTAKE INHIBITORS (SSRI)
Celexa Oral Solution *(Forest)* ... 312, 1269
Celexa Tablets *(Forest)* ... 312, 1269
Lexapro Oral Solution *(Forest)* ... 312, 1282
Lexapro Tablets *(Forest)* ... 312, 1282
Paxil CR Controlled-Release Tablets *(GlaxoSmithKline)* ... 317, 1592
Paxil Oral Suspension *(GlaxoSmithKline)* ... 317, 1585
Paxil Tablets *(GlaxoSmithKline)* ... 317, 1585
Prozac Pulvules and Liquid *(Lilly)* ... 320, 1873
Zoloft Oral Concentrate *(Pfizer)* ... 2681
Zoloft Tablets *(Pfizer)* ... 330, 2681

TRICYCLIC ANTIDEPRESSANTS & COMBINATIONS
Norpramin Tablets *(Aventis)* ... 307, 731
Surmontil Capsules *(Odyssey)* ... 327, 2447
Vivactil Tablets *(Odyssey)* ... 327, 2449

ANTIPANIC AGENTS
Klonopin Tablets *(Roche Laboratories)* ... 331, 2895
Klonopin Wafers *(Roche Laboratories)* ... 331, 2895
Paxil CR Controlled-Release Tablets *(GlaxoSmithKline)* ... 317, 1592
Paxil Oral Suspension *(GlaxoSmithKline)* ... 317, 1585
Paxil Tablets *(GlaxoSmithKline)* ... 317, 1585
Prozac Pulvules and Liquid *(Lilly)* ... 320, 1873
Xanax Tablets *(Pharmacia & Upjohn)* ... 330, 2763
Xanax XR Tablets *(Pharmacia & Upjohn)* ... 330, 2767
Zoloft Oral Concentrate *(Pfizer)* ... 2681
Zoloft Tablets *(Pfizer)* ... 330, 2681

ANTIPSYCHOTIC AGENTS

MISCELLANEOUS ANTIPSYCHOTIC AGENTS
Abilify Tablets *(Bristol-Myers Squibb)* ... 310, 1026
Abilify Tablets *(Otsuka America)* ... 328, 2559
Clozapine Tablets *(Mylan)* ... 2244
Clozaril Tablets *(Novartis)* ... 324, 2280
Fazaclo Orally Disintegrating Tablets *(Alamo)* ... 304, 541
Geodon Capsules *(Pfizer)* ... 329, 2609
Geodon for Injection *(Pfizer)* ... 2609
Haldol Decanoate 50 Injection *(Ortho-McNeil)* ... 328, 2499
Haldol Decanoate 100 Injection *(Ortho-McNeil)* ... 328, 2499
Moban Tablets *(Endo Labs)* ... 311, 1217
Orap Tablets *(Gate)* ... 1328
Risperdal Consta Injection *(Janssen)* ... 319, 1747
Risperdal M-Tab Tablets *(Janssen)* ... 319, 1742
Risperdal Oral Solution *(Janssen)* ... 319, 1742
Risperdal Tablets *(Janssen)* ... 319, 1742
Seroquel Tablets *(AstraZeneca)* ... 306, 662
Thiothixene Capsules *(Mylan)* ... 2227
Zyprexa Tablets *(Lilly)* ... 320, 1899
Zyprexa IntraMuscular *(Lilly)* ... 320, 1899
Zyprexa ZYDIS Orally Disintegrating Tablets *(Lilly)* ... 320, 1899

PHENOTHIAZINES & COMBINATIONS
Thioridazine Hydrochloride Tablets *(Mylan)* ... 2225

BIPOLAR AGENTS
Depakote Tablets *(Abbott)* ... 303, 435
Eskalith Capsules *(GlaxoSmithKline)* ... 315, 1485
Eskalith CR Controlled-Release Tablets *(GlaxoSmithKline)* ... 315, 1485
Lamictal Tablets *(GlaxoSmithKline)* ... 316, 1531
Lamictal Chewable Dispersible Tablets *(GlaxoSmithKline)* ... 316, 1531
Risperdal M-Tab Tablets *(Janssen)* ... 319, 1742
Risperdal Oral Solution *(Janssen)* ... 319, 1742
Risperdal Tablets *(Janssen)* ... 319, 1742
Seroquel Tablets *(AstraZeneca)* ... 306, 662
Symbyax Capsules *(Lilly)* ... 320, 1888
Zyprexa Tablets *(Lilly)* ... 320, 1899
Zyprexa IntraMuscular *(Lilly)* ... 320, 1899
Zyprexa ZYDIS Orally Disintegrating Tablets *(Lilly)* ... 320, 1899

OBSESSIVE-COMPULSIVE DISORDER MANAGEMENT

SELECTIVE SEROTONIN REUPTAKE INHIBITORS (SSRI)
Paxil Oral Suspension *(GlaxoSmithKline)* ... 317, 1585
Paxil Tablets *(GlaxoSmithKline)* ... 317, 1585
Prozac Pulvules and Liquid *(Lilly)* ... 320, 1873
Zoloft Oral Concentrate *(Pfizer)* ... 2681
Zoloft Tablets *(Pfizer)* ... 330, 2681

PSYCHOSTIMULANTS
(see under:
CENTRAL NERVOUS SYSTEM STIMULANTS)

PSYCHOTROPICS
(see under:
PSYCHOTHERAPEUTIC AGENTS)

Q

QUINOLONES
(see under:
ANTI-INFECTIVE AGENTS, SYSTEMIC
ANTIBIOTICS
QUINOLONES
OPHTHALMIC PREPARATIONS
ANTI-INFECTIVES
QUINOLONES)

R

RENAL STONE PREVENTION
(see under:
URINARY TRACT AGENTS
CALCIUM OXALATE STONE PREVENTION)

RESINS, ION EXCHANGE
(see under:
CARDIOVASCULAR AGENTS
ANTILIPIDEMIC AGENTS
BILE ACID SEQUESTRANTS)

RESPIRATORY AGENTS
(see also under:
ANTIHISTAMINES & COMBINATIONS
NASAL PREPARATIONS)

ANTI-INFECTIVE AGENTS

CYSTIC FIBROSIS MANAGEMENT
(see also under:
CYSTIC FIBROSIS MANAGEMENT)

ANTI-INFLAMMATORY AGENTS

STEROIDAL ANTI-INFLAMMATORY AGENTS & COMBINATIONS
Advair Diskus 100/50 *(GlaxoSmithKline)* ... 314, 1387
Advair Diskus 250/50 *(GlaxoSmithKline)* ... 314, 1387
Advair Diskus 500/50 *(GlaxoSmithKline)* ... 314, 1387
Aerobid Inhaler System *(Forest)* ... 312, 1266
Aerobid-M Inhaler System *(Forest)* ... 312, 1266
Azmacort Inhalation Aerosol *(Kos)* ... 320, 1808
Flovent HFA 44 mcg Inhalation Aerosol *(GlaxoSmithKline)* ... 1497
Flovent HFA 110 mcg Inhalation Aerosol *(GlaxoSmithKline)* ... 1497
Flovent HFA 220 mcg Inhalation Aerosol *(GlaxoSmithKline)* ... 1497
Flovent 44 mcg Inhalation Aerosol *(GlaxoSmithKline)* ... 315, 1494
Flovent 110 mcg Inhalation Aerosol *(GlaxoSmithKline)* ... 315, 1494
Flovent 220 mcg Inhalation Aerosol *(GlaxoSmithKline)* ... 315, 1494
Flovent Rotadisk 50 mcg *(GlaxoSmithKline)* ... 315, 1500
Flovent Rotadisk 100 mcg *(GlaxoSmithKline)* ... 315, 1500
Flovent Rotadisk 250 mcg *(GlaxoSmithKline)* ... 315, 1500
Pulmicort Respules *(AstraZeneca LP)* ... 305, 625
Qvar Inhalation Aerosol *(IVAX)* ... 1722

ANTITUSSIVES

NARCOTIC ANTITUSSIVES & COMBINATIONS
Hycodan Syrup *(Endo Labs)* ... 1212
Hycodan Tablets *(Endo Labs)* ... 311, 1212
Hycomine Compound Tablets *(Endo Labs)* ... 311, 1213
Hycotuss Expectorant Syrup *(Endo Labs)* ... 1215
Tussionex Pennkinetic Extended-Release Suspension *(Celltech)* ... 1114

NON-NARCOTIC ANTITUSSIVES & COMBINATIONS
Alacol DM Syrup *(Ballay)* ... 778
Balamine DM Oral Drops *(Ballay)* ... 779
Balamine DM Syrup *(Ballay)* ... 779
Simply Cough Liquid *(McNeil Consumer)* ... 321, 1940
Tessalon Capsules *(Forest)* ... 312, 1291
Tessalon Perles *(Forest)* ... 312, 1291
Children's Tylenol Plus Cold & Cough Suspension Liquid and Chewable Tablets *(McNeil Consumer)* ... 322, 1949
Children's Tylenol Plus Flu *(McNeil Consumer)* ... 322, 1950
Concentrated Tylenol Infants' Drops Plus Cold and Cough *(McNeil Consumer)* ... 322, 1949
Tylenol Cold Day Non-Drowsy Caplets and Gelcaps *(McNeil Consumer)* ... 322, 1945
Tylenol Cold & Flu Severe Daytime Liquid *(McNeil Consumer)* ... 1946
Tylenol Cold & Flu Severe NightTime Liquid *(McNeil Consumer)* ... 1946
Tylenol Cold Severe Congestion Non-Drowsy Caplets *(McNeil Consumer)* ... 322, 1945
Tylenol Cold Night Time Caplets *(McNeil Consumer)* ... 322, 1945
Tylenol Flu Day Non-Drowsy Gelcaps *(McNeil Consumer)* ... 322, 1946
Vicks 44 Cough Relief *(Procter & Gamble)* ... 2792
Vicks 44D Cough & Head Congestion Relief *(Procter & Gamble)* ... 2792
Vicks 44E Cough & Chest Congestion Relief *(Procter & Gamble)* ... 2793
Pediatric Vicks 44e Cough & Chest Congestion Relief Liquid *(Procter & Gamble)* ... 2790
Vicks 44M Cough, Cold & Flu Relief *(Procter & Gamble)* ... 2793
Pediatric Vicks 44m Cough & Cold Relief *(Procter & Gamble)* ... 2790
Vicks Cough Drops, Menthol & Cherry Flavors *(Procter & Gamble)* ... 2791
Vicks DayQuil Multi-Symptom Cold/Flu Relief Liquid & LiquiCaps *(Procter & Gamble)* ... 2792
Children's Vicks NyQuil Cold/Cough Relief *(Procter & Gamble)* ... 2788
Vicks NyQuil Cough Liquid *(Procter & Gamble)* ... 2793
Vicks NyQuil LiquiCaps *(Procter & Gamble)* ... 2793
Vicks NyQuil Liquid *(Procter & Gamble)* ... 2793
Vicks VapoRub Cream *(Procter & Gamble)* ... 2795
Vicks VapoRub Ointment *(Procter & Gamble)* ... 2795
Vicks VapoSteam *(Procter & Gamble)* ... 2795

BRONCHODILATORS

ANTICHOLINERGICS
Atrovent Inhalation Aerosol *(Boehringer Ingelheim)* ... 309, 982
Atrovent Inhalation Solution *(Boehringer Ingelheim)* ... 309, 984
Spiriva HandiHaler *(Boehringer Ingelheim)* ... 309, 1010
Spiriva HandiHaler *(Pfizer)* ... 329, 2634

ANTICHOLINERGICS WITH SYMPATHOMIMETICS
Combivent Inhalation Aerosol *(Boehringer Ingelheim)* ... 309, 991
DuoNeb Inhalation Solution *(Dey)* ... 311, 1183

SYMPATHOMIMETICS & COMBINATIONS
AccuNeb Inhalation Solution *(Dey)* ... 311, 1179
Advair Diskus 100/50 *(GlaxoSmithKline)* ... 314, 1387
Advair Diskus 250/50 *(GlaxoSmithKline)* ... 314, 1387
Advair Diskus 500/50 *(GlaxoSmithKline)* ... 314, 1387
Alupent Inhalation Aerosol *(Boehringer Ingelheim)* ... 309, 982
EpiPen Auto-Injector *(Dey)* ... 1185
EpiPen Jr. Auto-Injector *(Dey)* ... 1185
Foradil Aerolizer *(Schering)* ... 3026
Maxair Autohaler *(3M)* ... 321, 1917

S

SKIN & MUCOUS MEMBRANE AGENTS—cont.

ANTIPRURITICS—cont.

Locoid Topical Solution *(Ferndale)* 1247
Luxíq Foam *(Connetics)* 1153
Olux Foam *(Connetics)* 1154
Pandel Cream, 0.1% *(CollaGenex)* 1146
Pramosone Cream 1% and 2.5% *(Ferndale)* 1248
Pramosone Lotion 1% and 2.5% *(Ferndale)* 1248
Pramosone Ointment 1% and 2.5% *(Ferndale)* 1248
Temovate E Emollient *(GlaxoSmithKline)* 317, 1631
Temovate Cream *(GlaxoSmithKline)* ... 317, 1629
Temovate Gel *(GlaxoSmithKline)* 317, 1630
Temovate Ointment *(GlaxoSmithKline)* 317, 1629
Temovate Scalp Application *(GlaxoSmithKline)* 317, 1630

ANTIPSORIATIC AGENTS

8-MOP Capsules *(Valeant)* 3262
Aclovate Cream *(GlaxoSmithKline)* ... 313, 1386
Aclovate Ointment *(GlaxoSmithKline)* 313, 1386
Amevive *(Biogen Idec)* 949
Clobex Shampoo *(Galderma)* 1313
Dovonex Cream 0.005% *(Warner Chilcott)* .. 3291
Dovonex Ointment 0.005% *(Warner Chilcott)* 3291
Dovonex Scalp Solution 0.005% *(Warner Chilcott)* 3292
Gengraf Capsules *(Abbott)* 303, 466
Neoral Soft Gelatin Capsules *(Novartis)* 325, 2346
Neoral Oral Solution *(Novartis)* 325, 2346
Oxsoralen-Ultra Capsules *(Valeant)* 335, 3270
Psoriatec Cream *(Sirius)* 3149
Raptiva for Injection *(Genentech)* 313, 1350
Soriatane Capsules *(Connetics)* 311, 1156
Temovate E Emollient *(GlaxoSmithKline)* 317, 1631
Temovate Cream *(GlaxoSmithKline)* ... 317, 1629
Temovate Gel *(GlaxoSmithKline)* 317, 1630
Temovate Ointment *(GlaxoSmithKline)* 317, 1629
Temovate Scalp Application *(GlaxoSmithKline)* 317, 1630

ANTISEBORRHEIC AGENTS

Capex Shampoo *(Galderma)* 1310
Head & Shoulders Dandruff Shampoo *(Procter & Gamble)* 2788
Head & Shoulders Dandruff Shampoo Dry Scalp *(Procter & Gamble)* 2788
Head & Shoulders Intensive Treatment Dandruff and Seborrheic Dermatitis Shampoo *(Procter & Gamble)* 2788
Locoid Cream *(Ferndale)* 1247
Locoid Ointment *(Ferndale)* 1247
Locoid Topical Solution *(Ferndale)* 1247
Nizoral A-D Shampoo *(McNeil Consumer)* 321, 1940
Plexion Cleanser *(Medicis)* 1962
Plexion SCT *(Medicis)* 1962
Plexion Topical Suspension *(Medicis)* 1962

BURN PREPARATIONS

Betadine Solution *(Purdue Frederick)* 2806
Silvadene Cream 1% *(King)* 1792
Sulfamylon Cream *(Mylan)* 2257
Sulfamylon Topical Solution *(Mylan)* 2258

CLEANSING AGENTS

Betadine Skin Cleanser *(Purdue Frederick)* .. 2806
Betadine Surgical Scrub *(Purdue Frederick)* 2806
Betasept Surgical Scrub *(Purdue Frederick)* 2807

DEODORANTS

Panafil Ointment *(Healthpoint)* 319, 1708
Panafil Spray *(Healthpoint)* 319, 1708

DEPIGMENTING AGENTS

Claripel Cream *(Stiefel)* 3174
Epiquin Micro Topical Cream *(Skinmedica)* .. 3150
Epiquin Micro XD Topical Cream *(Skinmedica)* 3150
Glyquin XM Cream *(Valeant)* 3268
Solagé Solution *(Galderma)* 1319
Tri-Luma Cream *(Galderma)* 1322

EMOLLIENTS & MOISTURIZERS

LAClotion 12% Lotion *(Paddock)* 2576

ENZYMES & COMBINATIONS

Accuzyme Debriding Ointment *(Healthpoint)* 318, 1707
Accuzyme Spray *(Healthpoint)* 319, 1708
Granulex Aerosol *(Mylan)* 2251
Panafil Ointment *(Healthpoint)* 319, 1708
Panafil Spray *(Healthpoint)* 319, 1708

HAIR GROWTH RETARDANTS

Vaniqa Cream, 13.9% *(Skinmedica)* 3151

HAIR GROWTH STIMULANTS

Propecia Tablets *(Merck)* 323, 2130

HEMOSTATICS

(see under:
BLOOD MODIFIERS
HEMOSTATICS
TOPICAL HEMOSTATICS)

KERATOLYTICS

(see also under:
SKIN & MUCOUS MEMBRANE AGENTS
WART PREPARATIONS)

MISCELLANEOUS SKIN & MUCOUS MEMBRANE AGENTS

Elidel Cream 1% *(Novartis)* 2302
Finacea Gel *(Berlex)* 308, 907
Protopic Ointment *(Fujisawa)* 313, 1307
Renova 0.02% Cream *(OrthoNeutrogena)* 327, 2480
Renova 0.05% Cream *(OrthoNeutrogena)* 327, 2482
Thalomid Capsules *(Celgene)* 310, 1095

MOUTH & THROAT PRODUCTS

ANTIFUNGALS

(see under:
SKIN & MUCOUS MEMBRANE AGENTS
ANTI-INFECTIVES
ANTIFUNGALS & COMBINATIONS)

COLD SORE PREPARATIONS

(see also under:
ANTI-INFECTIVE AGENTS, SYSTEMIC
ANTIVIRALS
SKIN & MUCOUS MEMBRANE AGENTS
ANTI-INFECTIVES
ANTIVIRALS)

DENTAL PREPARATIONS

(see also under:
DIETARY SUPPLEMENTS
MINERALS & ELECTROLYTES
FLUORIDE & COMBINATIONS)
Periostat Tablets *(CollaGenex)* 1147

LOZENGES & SPRAYS

Vicks Cough Drops, Menthol & Cherry Flavors *(Procter & Gamble)* 2791

SALIVA PRODUCTS

Evoxac Capsules *(Daiichi)* 311, 1166
Salagen Tablets *(MGI)* 337, 2201

PHOTOSENSITIZING AGENTS

8-MOP Capsules *(Valeant)* 3262
Oxsoralen Lotion 1% *(Valeant)* 3270
Oxsoralen-Ultra Capsules *(Valeant)* 335, 3270

SCAR TISSUE TREATMENT

Mederma Gel *(Merz)* 2195

SHAMPOOS

Capex Shampoo *(Galderma)* 1310
Clobex Shampoo *(Galderma)* 1313
Head & Shoulders Dandruff Shampoo *(Procter & Gamble)* 2788
Head & Shoulders Dandruff Shampoo Dry Scalp *(Procter & Gamble)* 2788
Head & Shoulders Intensive Treatment Dandruff and Seborrheic Dermatitis Shampoo *(Procter & Gamble)* 2788
Nizoral 2% Shampoo *(McNeil Consumer)* 321, 1939

STEROIDS & COMBINATIONS

Aclovate Cream *(GlaxoSmithKline)* ... 313, 1386
Aclovate Ointment *(GlaxoSmithKline)* 313, 1386
Analpram HC Lotion *(Ferndale)* 1245
Analpram HC Cream *(Ferndale)* 1245
Capex Shampoo *(Galderma)* 1310
Clobevate Gel *(Stiefel)* 3176
Clobex Shampoo *(Galderma)* 1313
Clobex Lotion *(Galderma)* 1311
Cutivate Cream *(GlaxoSmithKline)* 315, 1461
Cutivate Ointment *(GlaxoSmithKline)* 315, 1463
Diprolene AF Cream 0.05% *(Schering)* 3023
Elocon Cream 0.1% *(Schering)* 332, 3024
Elocon Ointment 0.1% *(Schering)* 332, 3025
Locoid Cream *(Ferndale)* 1247
Locoid Lipocream Cream *(Ferndale)* 1247
Locoid Ointment *(Ferndale)* 1247
Locoid Topical Solution *(Ferndale)* 1247
Luxíq Foam *(Connetics)* 1153
Olux Foam *(Connetics)* 1154
Pandel Cream, 0.1% *(CollaGenex)* 1146
Pramosone Cream 1% and 2.5% *(Ferndale)* 1248
Pramosone Lotion 1% and 2.5% *(Ferndale)* 1248
Pramosone Ointment 1% and 2.5% *(Ferndale)* 1248
ProctoFoam-HC *(Schwarz)* 332, 3085
Temovate E Emollient *(GlaxoSmithKline)* 317, 1631
Temovate Cream *(GlaxoSmithKline)* ... 317, 1629
Temovate Gel *(GlaxoSmithKline)* 317, 1630
Temovate Ointment *(GlaxoSmithKline)* 317, 1629
Temovate Scalp Application *(GlaxoSmithKline)* 317, 1630
Tri-Luma Cream *(Galderma)* 1322

VAGINAL PRODUCTS

(see under:
VAGINAL PREPARATIONS)

WART PREPARATIONS

Aldara Cream, 5% *(3M)* 320, 1911
Alferon N Injection *(Hemispherx)* 319, 1710

WET DRESSINGS

Betadine Solution *(Purdue Frederick)* 2806

WOUND CARE PRODUCTS

Accuzyme Debriding Ointment *(Healthpoint)* 318, 1707
Accuzyme Spray *(Healthpoint)* 319, 1708
Betadine Solution *(Purdue Frederick)* 2806
Granulex Aerosol *(Mylan)* 2251
Panafil Ointment *(Healthpoint)* 319, 1708
Panafil Spray *(Healthpoint)* 319, 1708
Silvadene Cream 1% *(King)* 1792
Xenaderm Ointment *(Healthpoint)* 319, 1709

SKIN BLEACHES

(see under:
SKIN & MUCOUS MEMBRANE AGENTS
DEPIGMENTING AGENTS)

SKIN CARE PRODUCTS

(see under:
SKIN & MUCOUS MEMBRANE AGENTS)

SLEEP AIDS

(see under:
SEDATIVES & HYPNOTICS)

SMOKING CESSATION AIDS

Commit Lozenges *(GlaxoSmithKline Consumer)* 1697
Nicoderm CQ Patch *(GlaxoSmithKline Consumer)* 1701
Nicorette Gum *(GlaxoSmithKline Consumer)* 1703
Zyban Sustained-Release Tablets *(GlaxoSmithKline)* 318, 1691

STEROIDS

(see under:
HORMONES
ANABOLIC STEROIDS
GLUCOCORTICOIDS
NASAL PREPARATIONS
ANTI-INFLAMMATORY AGENTS
STEROIDAL ANTI-INFLAMMATORY AGENTS
OPHTHALMIC PREPARATIONS
ANTI-INFLAMMATORY AGENTS
STEROIDAL ANTI-INFLAMMATORY AGENTS & COMBINATIONS
OTIC PREPARATIONS
ANTIBIOTIC & STEROID COMBINATIONS
RESPIRATORY AGENTS
ANTI-INFLAMMATORY AGENTS
STEROIDAL ANTI-INFLAMMATORY AGENTS & COMBINATIONS
SKIN & MUCOUS MEMBRANE AGENTS
STEROIDS & COMBINATIONS)

SULFONAMIDES

(see under:
ANTI-INFECTIVE AGENTS, SYSTEMIC
ANTIBIOTICS
SULFONAMIDES & COMBINATIONS
OPHTHALMIC PREPARATIONS
ANTI-INFECTIVES
SULFONAMIDES & COMBINATIONS)

SUPPLEMENTS

(see under:
DIETARY SUPPLEMENTS)

SYMPATHOMIMETICS

(see under:
NASAL PREPARATIONS
SYMPATHOMIMETICS & COMBINATIONS
OPHTHALMIC PREPARATIONS
SYMPATHOMIMETICS & COMBINATIONS
RESPIRATORY AGENTS
BRONCHODILATORS
SYMPATHOMIMETICS & COMBINATIONS
DECONGESTANTS & COMBINATIONS
DECONGESTANTS, EXPECTORANTS & COMBINATIONS)

T

THROAT LOZENGES

(see under:
SKIN & MUCOUS MEMBRANE AGENTS
MOUTH & THROAT PRODUCTS
LOZENGES & SPRAYS)

THROMBOLYTICS

(see under:
BLOOD MODIFIERS
THROMBOLYTIC AGENTS)

THYROID PREPARATIONS

(see under:
HORMONES
THYROID PREPARATIONS)

TOPICAL PREPARATIONS

(see under:
NASAL PREPARATIONS
OPHTHALMIC PREPARATIONS
OTIC PREPARATIONS
SKIN & MUCOUS MEMBRANE AGENTS
VAGINAL PREPARATIONS)

TOURETTE'S SYNDROME AGENTS

Orap Tablets *(Gate)* 1328

TRANQUILIZERS

(see under:
PSYCHOTHERAPEUTIC AGENTS
ANTIANXIETY AGENTS
ANTIPSYCHOTIC AGENTS)

TRICYCLIC ANTIDEPRESSANTS

(see under:
PSYCHOTHERAPEUTIC AGENTS
ANTIDEPRESSANTS
TRICYCLIC ANTIDEPRESSANTS & COMBINATIONS)

TUBERCULOSIS PREPARATIONS

(see under:
ANTI-INFECTIVE AGENTS, SYSTEMIC
ANTITUBERCULOSIS AGENTS)

U

URINARY TRACT AGENTS

(see also under:
ANTI-INFECTIVE AGENTS, SYSTEMIC
URINARY ANTI-INFECTIVES & COMBINATIONS)

ACIDIFIERS

K-Phos Neutral Tablets *(Beach)* 308, 886
K-Phos Original (Sodium Free) Tablets *(Beach)* 308, 887

ALKALINIZERS

Urocit-K Tablets *(Mission)* 2212

ANALGESICS & COMBINATIONS

Elmiron Capsules *(Ortho-McNeil)* 328, 2493
Prosed EC Tablets *(Star)* 3173
Prosed/DS Tablets *(Star)* 3172

ANTIBACTERIALS

Amoxil Capsules *(GlaxoSmithKline)* ... 314, 1411
Amoxil Chewable Tablets *(GlaxoSmithKline)* 314, 1411
Amoxil for Oral Suspension *(GlaxoSmithKline)* 314, 1411
Amoxil Pediatric Drops for Oral Suspension *(GlaxoSmithKline)* 314, 1411
Amoxil Tablets *(GlaxoSmithKline)* 314, 1411
Ancef for Injection *(GlaxoSmithKline)* 314, 1415
Ancef Injection *(GlaxoSmithKline)* 1415
Augmentin Chewable Tablets *(GlaxoSmithKline)* 314, 1421
Augmentin Powder for Oral Suspension *(GlaxoSmithKline)* 314, 1421
Augmentin Tablets *(GlaxoSmithKline)* 314, 1424
Azactam for Injection *(Elan)* 1204
Ceclor Pulvules *(Lilly)* 1829
Ceclor Suspension *(Lilly)* 1829
Ceftin for Oral Suspension *(GlaxoSmithKline)* 315, 1450
Ceftin Tablets *(GlaxoSmithKline)* 315, 1450
Cipro I.V. *(Bayer)* 308, 827
Cipro I.V. Pharmacy Bulk Package *(Bayer)* 308, 833
Cipro Oral Suspension *(Bayer)* 308, 821
Cipro Tablets *(Bayer)* 308, 821
Cipro XR Tablets *(Bayer)* 308, 839
Claforan Sterile for Injection *(Aventis)* .. 307, 699
Dynacin Tablets *(Medicis)* 1957
Floxin Tablets *(Ortho-McNeil)* 2495
Fortaz Injection *(GlaxoSmithKline)* 316, 1504
Fortaz for Injection *(GlaxoSmithKline)* 316, 1504
Invanz for Injection *(Merck)* 2069
Keflex Pulvules *(Lilly)* 1871
Levaquin in 5% Dextrose Injection *(Ortho-McNeil)* 2501
Levaquin Injection *(Ortho-McNeil)* 328, 2501
Levaquin Tablets *(Ortho-McNeil)* 328, 2501
Maxipime for Injection *(Elan)* 1207
Monurol Sachet *(Forest)* 312, 1287
Neosporin G.U. Irrigant Sterile *(King)* 1789
Noroxin Tablets *(Merck)* 323, 2103
Primaxin I.V. *(Merck)* 2118
Prosed EC Tablets *(Star)* 3173
Prosed/DS Tablets *(Star)* 3172
Rocephin Injectable Vials, ADD-Vantage, Galaxy, Bulk *(Roche Laboratories)* 2915
Septra Suspension *(King)* 1790
Septra Grape Suspension *(King)* 1790
Septra Tablets *(King)* 1790
Septra DS Tablets *(King)* 1790
Tequin Injection *(Bristol-Myers Squibb)* 310, 1075
Tequin Tablets *(Bristol-Myers Squibb)* 310, 1075
Timentin ADD-Vantage *(GlaxoSmithKline)* 317, 1635
Timentin IV Infusion *(GlaxoSmithKline)* 317, 1632
Timentin Pharmacy Bulk Package *(GlaxoSmithKline)* 317, 1639
Uroqid-Acid No. 2 Tablets *(Beach)* 308, 887
Vantin Tablets and Oral Suspension *(Pharmacia & Upjohn)* 330, 2758
Zinacef Injection *(GlaxoSmithKline)* ... 318, 1676
Zinacef for Injection *(GlaxoSmithKline)* 318, 1676
Zithromax for Oral Suspension, 300 mg, 600 mg, 900 mg, 1200 mg *(Pfizer)* 2665
Zithromax Tablets, 250 mg, 500 mg *(Pfizer)* 330, 2665
Zithromax Tri-Pak *(Pfizer)* 2665

ANTISPASMODICS

Detrol Tablets *(Pharmacia & Upjohn)* 330, 2720
Detrol LA Capsules *(Pharmacia & Upjohn)* 330, 2722
Ditropan XL Extended Release Tablets *(Ortho-McNeil)* 328, 2491
Oxytrol Transdermal System *(Watson)* 336, 3303
Prosed EC Tablets *(Star)* 3173
Prosed/DS Tablets *(Star)* 3172
Sanctura Tablets *(Odyssey)* 2445

BENIGN PROSTATIC HYPERPLASIA (BPH) THERAPY

Avodart Soft Gelatin Capsules *(GlaxoSmithKline)* 314, 1443
Flomax Capsules *(Boehringer Ingelheim)* 309, 994

Key to Controlled Substances Categories

Products listed with the symbols shown below are subject to the Controlled Substances Act of 1970. These drugs are categorized according to their potential for abuse. The greater the potential, the more severe the limitations on their prescription.

CATEGORY	INTERPRETATION
C-II	**HIGH POTENTIAL FOR ABUSE.** Use may lead to severe physical or psychological dependence. Prescriptions must be written in ink, or typewritten and signed by the practitioner. Verbal prescriptions must be confirmed in writing within 72 hours, and may be given only in a genuine emergency. No renewals are permitted.
C-III	**SOME POTENTIAL FOR ABUSE.** Use may lead to low-to-moderate physical dependence or high psychological dependence. Prescriptions may be oral or written. Up to 5 renewals are permitted within 6 months.
C-IV	**LOW POTENTIAL FOR ABUSE.** Use may lead to limited physical or psychological dependence. Prescriptions may be oral or written. Up to 5 renewals are permitted within 6 months.
C-V	**SUBJECT TO STATE AND LOCAL REGULATION.** Abuse potential is low; a prescription may not be required.

Key to FDA Use-in-Pregnancy Ratings

The U.S. Food and Drug Administration's use-in-pregnancy rating system weighs the degree to which available information has ruled out risk to the fetus against the drug's potential benefit to the patient. The ratings, and their interpretation, are as follows:

CATEGORY	INTERPRETATION
A	**CONTROLLED STUDIES SHOW NO RISK.** Adequate, well-controlled studies in pregnant women have failed to demonstrate a risk to the fetus in any trimester of pregnancy.
B	**NO EVIDENCE OF RISK IN HUMANS.** Adequate, well-controlled studies in pregnant women have not shown increased risk of fetal abnormalities despite adverse findings in animals, or, in the absence of adequate human studies, animal studies show no fetal risk. The chance of fetal harm is remote, but remains a possibility.
C	**RISK CANNOT BE RULED OUT.** Adequate, well-controlled human studies are lacking, and animal studies have shown a risk to the fetus or are lacking as well. There is a chance of fetal harm if the drug is administered during pregnancy; but the potential benefits may outweigh the potential risk.
D	**POSITIVE EVIDENCE OF RISK.** Studies in humans, or investigational or post-marketing data, have demonstrated fetal risk. Nevertheless, potential benefits from the use of the drug may outweigh the potential risk. For example, the drug may be acceptable if needed in a life-threatening situation or serious disease for which safer drugs cannot be used or are ineffective.
X	**CONTRAINDICATED IN PREGNANCY.** Studies in animals or humans, or investigational or post-marketing reports, have demonstrated positive evidence of fetal abnormalities or risk which clearly outweighs any possible benefit to the patient.

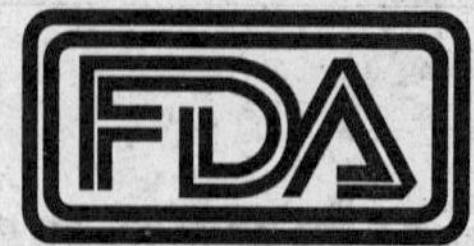

U.S. FOOD AND DRUG ADMINISTRATION

Medical Product Reporting Programs

MedWatch (24-hour service)....................800-332-1088
Reporting of problems with drugs, devices, biologics (except vaccines), medical foods, and dietary supplements.

Vaccine Adverse Event Reporting System (24-hour service)....................800-822-7967
Reporting of vaccine-related problems.

Mandatory Medical Device Reporting....................301-827-0360
Reporting required from user facilities regarding device-related deaths and serious injuries.

Veterinary Adverse Drug Reaction Program....................888-332-8387
Reporting of adverse drug events in animals.

Division of Drug Marketing, Advertising, and Communication (DDMAC)....................301-827-2828
Inquiries from health professionals regarding product promotion.

USP Medication Errors....................800-233-7767
Reporting of medication errors or near-errors to help avoid future problems through improvement in product names and packaging.

Information for Health Professionals

Center for Drug Evaluation and Research Drug Information Hotline....................301-827-4573
Information on human drugs including hormones.

Center for Biologics Office of Communications....................301-827-2000
Information on biological products including vaccines and blood.

Center for Devices and Radiological Health....................301-443-4190
Automated request for information on medical devices and radiation-emitting products.

Emergency Operations....................301-443-1240
Emergencies involving FDA-regulated products, tampering reports, and emergency Investigational New Drug requests.

Office of Orphan Products Development....................301-827-3666
Information on products for rare diseases.

General Information

General Consumer Inquiries....................888-463-6332
Consumer information on regulated products/issues.

Freedom of Information....................301-827-6500
Requests for publicly available FDA documents.

Office of Public Affairs....................301-827-6250
Interviews/press inquiries on FDA activities.

Center for Food Safety and Applied Nutrition....................888-723-3366
Information on food safety, seafood, dietary supplements, women's nutrition, and cosmetics.

Consumer Information Service, Center for Devices and Radiological Health....................301-443-4190
Information on medical devices, mammography facilities, and radiation-emitting products.

POISON CONTROL CENTERS

The American Association of Poison Control Centers (AAPCC) uses a single, nationwide emergency number to automatically link callers with their regional poison center. This toll-free number, **800-222-1222**, also works for **teletype lines (TTY)** for the hearing-impaired and **telecommunication devices (TTD)** for individuals who are deaf. However, a few local poison centers and the ASPCA/Animal Poison Control Center are not part of this nationwide system and continue to use separate numbers.

Most of the centers listed below are certified by the AAPCC. **Certified centers are marked by an asterisk after the name**. Each has to meet certain criteria. It must, for example, serve a large geographic area; it must be open 24 hours a day and provide direct-dial or toll-free access; it must be supervised by a medical director; and it must have registered pharmacists or nurses available to answer questions from the public.

Within each state, centers are listed alphabetically by city. Some state poison centers also list their original emergency numbers (including TTY/TDD) that only work within that state. For these listings, callers may use either the state number or the nationwide 800 number.

ALABAMA

BIRMINGHAM

Regional Poison Control Center, The Children's Hospital of Alabama (*)

1600 7th Ave. South
Birmingham, AL 35233-1711
Business: 205-939-9201
Emergency: 800-222-1222
800-292-6678 (AL)
www.chsys.org

TUSCALOOSA

Alabama Poison Center (*)

2503 Phoenix Dr.
Tuscaloosa, AL 35405
Business: 205-345-0600
Emergency: 800-222-1222
800-462-0800 (AL)
www.alapoisoncenter.org

ALASKA

JUNEAU

Alaska Poison Control System

Section of Community Health and EMS
410 Willoughby Ave., Room 109
Box 110616
Juneau, AK 99811-0616
Business: 907-465-3027
Emergency: 800-222-1222
www.chems.alaska.gov

(PORTLAND, OR)

**Oregon Poison Center (*)
Oregon Health Sciences University**

3181 SW Sam Jackson Park Rd.
CB550
Portland, OR 97239
Business: 503-494-8600
Emergency: 800-222-1222
www.oregonpoison.com

ARIZONA

PHOENIX

**Banner Poison Control Center (*)
Banner Good Samaritan Medical Center**

901 E. Willetta St.
Room 2701
Phoenix, AZ 85006
Business: 602-495-6360
Emergency: 800-222-1222
800-362-0101 (AZ)
602-253-3334 (AZ)
www.bannerpoisoncontrol.com

TUCSON

**Arizona Poison and Drug Information Center (*)
Arizona Health Sciences Center**

1501 N. Campbell Ave.
Room 1156
Tucson, AZ 85724
Business: 520-626-7899
Emergency: 800-222-1222

ARKANSAS

LITTLE ROCK

**Arkansas Poison and Drug Information Center
College of Pharmacy - UAMS**

4301 West Markham St.
Mail Slot 522-2
Little Rock, AR 72205-7122
Business: 501-686-5540
Emergency: 800-222-1222
800-376-4766 (AR)
TDD/TTY: 800-641-3805

ASPCA/ANIMAL POISON CONTROL CENTER

1717 South Philo Rd.
Suite 36
Urbana, IL 61802
Business: 217-337-5030
Emergency: 888-426-4435
800-548-2423
www.napcc.aspca.org

CALIFORNIA

FRESNO/MADERA

**California Poison Control System-Fresno/Madera Div.(*)
Children's Hospital of Central California**

9300 Valley Children's Place
MB 15
Madera, CA 93638-8762
Business: 559-622-2300
Emergency: 800-222-1222
800-876-4766 (CA)
TDD/TTY: 800-972-3323
www.calpoison.org

SACRAMENTO

**California Poison Control System-Sacramento Div.(*)
UC Davis Medical Center**

Room HSF 1024
2315 Stockton Blvd.
Sacramento, CA 95817
Business: 916-227-1400
Emergency: 800-222-1222
800-876-4766 (CA)
TDD/TTY: 800-972-3323
www.calpoison.org

SAN DIEGO

**California Poison Control System-San Diego Div. (*)
UC San Diego Medical Center**

200 West Arbor Dr.
San Diego, CA 92103-8925
Business: 858-715-6300
Emergency: 800-222-1222
800-876-4766 (CA)
TDD/TTY: 800-972-3323
www.calpoison.org

SAN FRANCISCO

**California Poison Control System-San Francisco Div.(*)
San Francisco General Hospital
University of California
San Francisco**

Box 1369
San Francisco, CA 94143-1369
Business: 415-502-6000
Emergency: 800-222-1222
800-876-4766 (CA)
TDD/TTY: 800-972-3323
www.calpoison.org

COLORADO

DENVER

Rocky Mountain Poison and Drug Center (*)

777 Bannock St.
Mail Code 0180
Denver CO 80204-4507
Business: 303-739-1100
Emergency: 800-222-1222
TDD/TTY: 303-739-1127 (CO)
www.RMPDC.org

CONNECTICUT

FARMINGTON

**Connecticut Regional Poison Control Center (*)
University of Connecticut Health Center**

263 Farmington Ave.
Farmington, CT 06030-5365
Business: 860-679-4540
Emergency: 800-222-1222
TDD/TTY: 866-218-5372
http://poisoncontrol.uchc.edu

DELAWARE

(PHILADELPHIA, PA)

**The Poison Control Center (*)
Children's Hospital of Philadelphia**

34th St. & Civic Center Blvd.
Philadelphia, PA 19104-4303
Business: 215-590-2003
Emergency: 800-222-1222
800-722-7112(DE)
TDD/TTY: 215-590-8789
www.poisoncontrol.chop.edu

DISTRICT OF COLUMBIA

WASHINGTON, DC

National Capital Poison Center (*)

3201 New Mexico Ave., NW
Suite 310
Washington, DC 20016
Business: 202-362-3867
Emergency: 800-222-1222
TDD/TTY: 202-362-8563
www.poison.org

FLORIDA

JACKSONVILLE

Florida Poison Information Center-Jacksonville (*)
SHANDS Hospital

655 West 8th St.
Jacksonville, FL 32209
Business: 904-244-4465
Emergency: 800-222-1222
http://fpicjax.org

MIAMI

Florida Poison Information Center-Miami (*)
University of Miami–Department of Pediatrics

P.O. Box 016960 (R-131)
Miami, FL 33101
Business: 305-585-5250
Emergency: 800-222-1222
www.miami.edu/poison-center

TAMPA

Florida Poison Information Center-Tampa (*)
Tampa General Hospital

P.O. Box 1289
Tampa, FL 33601-1289
Business: 813-844-7044
Emergency: 800-222-1222
www.poisoncentertampa.org

GEORGIA

ATLANTA

Georgia Poison Center (*)
Hughes Spalding Children's Hospital, Grady Health System

80 Jesse Hill Jr. Dr., SE
P.O. Box 26066
Atlanta, GA 30303-3050
Business: 404-616-9237
Emergency: 800-222-1222
404-616-9000
(Atlanta)
TDD: 404-616-9287
www.georgiapoisoncenter.org

HAWAII

(DENVER, CO)

Rocky Mountain Poison and Drug Center (*)

777 Bannock St.
Mail Code 0180
Denver CO 80204-4507
Business: 303-739-1100
Emergency: 800-222-1222
www.RMPDC.org

IDAHO

(DENVER, CO)

Rocky Mountain Poison & Drug Center (*)

777 Bannock St.
Mail Code 0180
Denver CO 80204-4507
Business: 303-739-1100
Emergency: 800-222-1222
www.RMPDC.org

ILLINOIS

CHICAGO

Illinois Poison Center (*)

222 South Riverside Plaza
Suite 1900
Chicago, IL 60606
Business: 312-906-6136
Emergency: 800-222-1222
TDD/TTY: 312-906-6185
www.illinoispoisoncenter.org

INDIANA

INDIANAPOLIS

Indiana Poison Control Center (*)
Clarian Health Partners Methodist Hospital

I-65 at 21st St.
Indianapolis, IN 46206-1367
Business: 317-962-2335
Emergency: 800-222-1222
800-382-9097
317-962-2323
(Indianapolis)
TTY: 317-962-2336
www.clarian.org/clinical/poisoncontrol

IOWA

SIOUX CITY

Iowa Statewide Poison Control Center
Iowa Health System and the University of Iowa Hospitals and Clinics

2910 Hamilton Blvd., Suite 101
Sioux City, IA 51104
Business: 712-279-3710
Emergency: 800-222-1222
712-277-2222 (IA)
www.iowapoison.org

KANSAS

KANSAS CITY

Mid-America Poison Control Center
University of Kansas Medical Center

3901 Rainbow Blvd.
Room B-400
Kansas City, KS 66160-7231
Business 913-588-6638
Emergency: 800-222-1222
800-332-6633 (KS)
TDD: 913-588-6639
www.kumc.edu/poison

KENTUCKY

LOUISVILLE

Kentucky Regional Poison Center (*)

PO Box 35070
Louisville, KY 40232-5070
Business: 502-629-7264
Emergency: 800-222-1222
502-589-8222
(Louisville)
www.krpc.com

LOUISIANA

MONROE

Louisiana Drug and Poison Information Center (*)
University of Louisiana at Monroe

700 University Ave.
Monroe, LA 71209-6430
Business: 318-342-3648
Emergency: 800-222-1222
www.lapcc.org

MAINE

PORTLAND

Northern New England Poison Center

Maine Medical Center
22 Bramhall St.
Portland, ME 04102
Business: 207-842-7220
Emergency: 800-222-1222
207-871-2879 (ME)
TDD/TTY: 877-299-4447 (ME)
207-871-2879 (ME)

MARYLAND

BALTIMORE

Maryland Poison Center (*)
University of Maryland at Baltimore
School of Pharmacy

20 North Pine St., PH 772
Baltimore, MD 21201
Business: 410-706-7604
Emergency: 800-222-1222
TDD: 410-706-1858
www.mdpoison.com

(WASHINGTON, DC)

National Capital Poison Center (*)

3201 New Mexico Ave., NW
Suite 310
Washington DC 20016
Business: 202-362-3867
Emergency: 800-222-1222
TDD/TTY: 202-362-8563 (MD)
www.poison.org

MASSACHUSETTS

BOSTON

Regional Center for Poison Control and Prevention (*)
(Serving Massachusetts and Rhode Island)

300 Longwood Ave.
Boston, MA 02115
Business: 617-355-6609
Emergency: 800-222-1222
TDD/TTY: 888-244-5313
www.maripoisoncenter.com

MICHIGAN

DETROIT

Regional Poison Control Center (*)
Children's Hospital of Michigan

4160 John R. Harper Professional Office Bldg.
Suite 616
Detroit, MI 48201
Business: 313-745-5335
Emergency: 800-222-1222
TDD/TTY: 800-356-3232
www.mitoxic.org/pcc

GRAND RAPIDS

DeVos Children's Hospital Regional Poison Center (*)

100 Michigan St., NE
Grand Rapids, MI 49503
Business: 616-391-3690
Emergency: 800-222-1222
http://poisoncenter.devoschildrens.org

MINNESOTA

MINNEAPOLIS

Minnesota Poison Control System (*) Hennepin County Medical Center

701 Park Ave.
Mail Code 820
Minneapolis, MN 55415
Business: 612-873-6000
Emergency: 800-222-1222
TTY: 612-904-4691
www.mnpoison.org

MISSISSIPPI

JACKSON

Mississippi Regional Poison Control Center, University of Mississippi Medical Center

2500 North State St.
Jackson, MS 39216
Business: 601-984-1675
Emergency: 800-222-1222

MISSOURI

ST. LOUIS

Missouri Regional Poison Center (*) Cardinal Glennon Children's Hospital

7980 Clayton Rd.
Suite 200
St. Louis, MO 63117
Business: 314-772-5200
Emergency: 800-222-1222
TDD/TTY: 314-612-5705
www.cardinalglennon.com

MONTANA

(DENVER, CO)

Rocky Mountain Poison and Drug Center (*)

777 Bannock St.
Mail Code 0180
Denver CO 80204-4507
Business: 303-739-1100
Emergency: 800-222-1222
TDD/TTY: 303-739-1127
www.RMPDC.org

NEBRASKA

OMAHA

The Poison Center (*) Children's Hospital

8200 Dodge St.
Omaha, NE 68114
Business: 402-955-5555
Emergency: 800-222-1222
www.poison-center.com

NEVADA

(DENVER, CO)

Rocky Mountain Poison and Drug Center (*)

777 Bannock St.
Mail Code 0180
Denver CO 80204-4507
Business: 303-739-1100
Emergency: 800-222-1222
www.RMPDC.org

(PORTLAND, OR)

Oregon Poison Center (*) Oregon Health Sciences University

3181 SW Sam Jackson Park Rd.
Portland, OR 97201
Business: 503-494-8600
Emergency: 800-222-1222
www.oregonpoison.com

NEW HAMPSHIRE

(PORTLAND, ME)

Northern New England Poison Center

Maine Medical Center
22 Bramhall St.
Portland, ME 04102
Business: 207-842-7220
Emergency: 800-222-1222

NEW JERSEY

NEWARK

New Jersey Poison Information and Education System (*) UMDNJ

65 Bergen St.
Newark, NJ 07101
Business: 973-972-9280
Emergency: 800-222-1222
TDD/TTY: 973-926-8008
www.njpies.org

NEW MEXICO

ALBUQUERQUE

New Mexico Poison and Drug Information Center (*)

MSC09-5080
1 University of New Mexico
Albuquerque, NM 87131-0001
Business: 505-272-4261
Emergency: 800-222-1222
http://HSC.UNM.edu/pharmacy/poison

NEW YORK

BUFFALO

Western New York Regional Poison Control Center (*) Children's Hospital of Buffalo

219 Bryant St.
Buffalo, NY 14222
Business: 716-878-7654
Emergency: 800-222-1222
www.fingerlakespoison.org

MINEOLA

Long Island Regional Poison and Drug Information Center (*) Winthrop University Hospital

259 First St.
Mineola, NY 11501
Business: 516-663-2650
Emergency: 800-222-1222
TDD: 516-747-3323 (Nassau)
516-924-8811 (Suffolk)
www.lirpdic.org

NEW YORK CITY

New York City Poison Control Center (*) NYC Dept. of Health

455 First Ave., Room 123
New York, NY 10016
Business: 212-447-8152
Emergency: 800-222-1222
(English) 212-340-4494
212-POISONS
(212-764-7667)

Emergency: 212-VENENOS
(Spanish) (212-836-3667)
TDD: 212-689-9014

ROCHESTER

Finger Lakes Regional Poison and Drug Information Center (*) University of Rochester Medical Center

601 Elmwood Ave.
Box 321
Rochester, NY 14642
Business: 585-273-4155
Emergency: 800-222-1222
TTY: 585-273-3854

SYRACUSE

Central New York Poison Center (*) SUNY Upstate Medical University

750 East Adams St.
Syracuse, NY 13210
Business: 315-464-7078
Emergency: 800-222-1222
www.cnypoison.org

NORTH CAROLINA

CHARLOTTE

Carolinas Poison Center (*) Carolinas Medical Center

PO Box 32861
Charlotte, NC 28232
Business: 704-395-3795
Emergency: 800-222-1222
TDD: 800-735-8262
TTY: 800-735-2962
www.ncpoisoncenter.org

NORTH DAKOTA

(MINNEAPOLIS, MN)

Minnesota Poison Control System (*) Hennepin County Medical Center

701 Park Ave.
Mail Code 820
Minneapolis, MN 55415
Business: 612-873-3144
Emergency: 800-222-1222
www.ndpoison.org

OHIO

CINCINNATI

Cincinnati Drug and Poison Information Center (*) Regional Poison Control System

3333 Burnet Ave.
Vernon Place, 3rd Floor
Cincinnati, OH 45229
Business: 513-636-5111
Emergency: 800-222-1222
TDD/TTY: 800-253-7955
www.cincinnatichildrens.org/dpic

CLEVELAND

Greater Cleveland Poison Control Center

11100 Euclid Ave.
MP 6007
Cleveland, OH 44106-6007
Business: 216-844-1573
Emergency: 800-222-1222
216-231-4455 (OH)

COLUMBUS

Central Ohio Poison Center (*)

700 Children's Dr.
Room L032
Columbus, OH 43205-2696
Business: 614-722-2635
Emergency: 614-228-1323
800-222-1222
937-222-2227
(Dayton region)
TTY: 614-228-2272
www.bepoisonsmart.com

OKLAHOMA

OKLAHOMA CITY

Oklahoma Poison Control Center (*) Children's Hospital at OU Medical Center

940 Northeast 13th St.
Room 3510
Oklahoma City, OK 73104
Business: 405-271-5062
Emergency: 800-222-1222
www.oklahomapoison.org

OREGON

PORTLAND

Oregon Poison Center (*) Oregon Health Sciences University

3181 S.W. Sam Jackson Park Rd., CB550
Portland, OR 97239
Business: 503-494-8600
Emergency: 800-222-1222
www.oregonpoison.com

PENNSYLVANIA

PHILADELPHIA

The Poison Control Center (*) Children's Hospital of Philadelphia

34th Street & Civic Center Blvd.
Philadelphia, PA 19104-4399
Business: 215-590-2003
Emergency: 800-222-1222
215-386-2100 (PA)
TDD/TTY: 215-590-8789
www.poisoncontrol.chop.edu

PITTSBURGH

Pittsburgh Poison Center (*) Children's Hospital of Pittsburgh

3705 Fifth Ave.
Pittsburgh, PA 15213
Business: 412-390-3300
Emergency: 800-222-1222
412-681-6669
www.chp.edu/clinical/03a_poison.php

PUERTO RICO

SANTURCE

San Jorge Children's Hospital Poison Center

258 San Jorge St.
Santurce, PR 00912
Business: 787-726-5660
Emergency: 800-222-1222
TTY: 787-641-1934
www.poisoncenter.net

RHODE ISLAND

(BOSTON, MA)

Regional Center for Poison Control and Prevention (*)
(Serving Massachusetts and Rhode Island)

300 Longwood Ave.
Boston, MA 02115
Business: 617-355-6609
Emergency: 800-222-1222
TDD/TTY: 888-244-5313
www.maripoisoncenter.com

SOUTH CAROLINA

COLUMBIA

Palmetto Poison Center (*) College of Pharmacy University of South Carolina

Columbia, SC 29208
Business: 803-777-7909
Drug Info: 800-777-7804
Emergency: 800-222-1222
803-777-1117 (SC)
www.pharm.sc.edu/PPS/pps.htm

SOUTH DAKOTA

(MINNEAPOLIS, MN)

Hennepin Regional Poison Center (*) Hennepin County Medical Center

701 Park Ave.
Minneapolis, MN 55415
Business: 612-873-6000
Emergency: 800-222-1222
TTY: 612-904-4691
www.mnpoison.org

SIOUX FALLS

Provides education only—Does not manage exposure cases.

Sioux Valley Poison Control Center (*)

1305 W. 18th St.
Box 5039
Sioux Falls, SD 57117-5039
Business: 605-333-6638
www.sdpoison.org

TENNESSEE

NASHVILLE

Tennessee Poison Center (*)

1161 21st Ave. South
501 Oxford House
Nashville, TN 37232-4632
Business: 615-936-0760
Emergency: 800-222-1222
www.poisonlifeline.org

TEXAS

AMARILLO

Texas Panhandle Poison Center (*) Northwest Texas Hospital

1501 S. Coulter Dr.
Amarillo, TX 79106
Business: 806-354-1630
Emergency: 800-222-1222
www.poisoncontrol.org

DALLAS

North Texas Poison Center (*) Texas Poison Center Network Parkland Health and Hospital System

5201 Harry Hines Blvd.
Dallas, TX 75235
Business: 214-589-0911
Emergency: 800-222-1222
www.poisoncontrol.org

EL PASO

West Texas Regional Poison Center (*) Thomason Hospital

4815 Alameda Ave.
El Paso, TX 79905
Business 915-534-3800
Emergency: 800-222-1222
www.poisoncontrol.org

GALVESTON

Southeast Texas Poison Center (*) The University of Texas Medical Branch

3.112 Trauma Bldg.
301 University Ave.
Galveston, TX 77555-1175
Business: 409-766-4403
Emergency: 800-222-1222
www.poisoncontrol.org

SAN ANTONIO

South Texas Poison Center (*) The University of Texas Health Science Center–San Antonio

7703 Floyd Curl Dr., MC 7849
San Antonio, TX 78229-3900
Business: 210-567-5762
Emergency: 800-222-1222
www.poisoncontrol.org

TEMPLE

Central Texas Poison Center (*) Scott & White Memorial Hospital

2401 South 31st St.
Temple, TX 76508
Business: 254-724-7401
Emergency: 800-222-1222
www.poisoncontrol.org

UTAH

SALT LAKE CITY

Utah Poison Control Center (*)

585 Komas Dr.
Suite 200
Salt Lake City, UT 84108
Business: 801-581-7504
Emergency: 800-222-1222
801-587-0600 (UT)
http://uuhsc.utah.edu/poison

VERMONT

(PORTLAND, ME)

Northern New England Poison Center

Maine Medical Center
22 Bramhall St.
Portland, ME 04102
Business: 207-842-7220
Emergency: 800-222-1222

VIRGINIA

CHARLOTTESVILLE

Blue Ridge Poison Center (*)
University of Virginia Health System

PO Box 800774
Charlottesville, VA 22908-0774
Business: 434-924-0347
Emergency: 800-222-1222
800-451-1428 (VA)
www.healthsystem.virginia.edu.brpc

RICHMOND

Virginia Poison Center (*)
Virginia Commonwealth University

P.O. Box 980522
Richmond, VA 23298-0522
Business: 804-828-4780
Emergency: 800-222-1222
804-828-9123
TDD/TTY: 804-828-9123

WASHINGTON

SEATTLE

Washington Poison Center (*)

155 NE 100th St.
Suite 400
Seattle, WA 98125-8011
Business: 206-517-2351
Emergency: 800-222-1222
206-526-2121 (WA)
TDD: 800-572-0638 (WA)
206-517-2394 (Seattle)
www.wapc.org

WEST VIRGINIA

CHARLESTON

West Virginia Poison Center (*)

3110 MacCorkle Ave. SE
Charleston, WV 25304
Business: 304-347-1212
Emergency: 800-222-1222
www.wvpoisoncontrol.org

WISCONSIN

MILWAUKEE

Children's Hospital of Wisconsin Statewide Poison Center

9000 W. Wisconsin Ave.
P.O. Box 1997, Mail Station 677A
Milwaukee, WI 53226
Business: 414-266-2000
Emergency: 800-222-1222
TDD/TTY: 414-964-3497
www.chw.org

WYOMING

(OMAHA, NE)

The Poison Center (*)
Children's Hospital

8200 Dodge St.
Omaha, NE 68114
Business: 402-955-5555
Emergency: 800-222-1222
www.poison-center.com

WEBSITE: www.vaers.org   E-MAIL: info@vaers.org   FAX: 1-877-721-0366

VAERS

VACCINE ADVERSE EVENT REPORTING SYSTEM

24 Hour Toll-Free Information 1-800-822-7967
P.O. Box 1100, Rockville, MD 20849-1100
PATIENT IDENTITY KEPT CONFIDENTIAL

For CDC/FDA Use Only
VAERS Number ____
Date Received ____

Patient Name: ____
Last First M.I.
Address ____
City State Zip
Telephone no. (____) ____

Vaccine administered by (Name): ____
Responsible Physician ____
Facility Name/Address ____
City State Zip
Telephone no. (____) ____

Form completed by (Name): ____
Relation to Patient ☐ Vaccine Provider ☐ Patient/Parent ☐ Manufacturer ☐ Other
Address *(if different from patient or provider)* ____
City State Zip
Telephone no. (____) ____

1. State
2. County where administered
3. Date of birth __/__/__ mm dd yy
4. Patient age
5. Sex ☐ M ☐ F
6. Date form completed __/__/__ mm dd yy

7. Describe adverse events(s) (symptoms, signs, time course) and treatment, if any

8. Check all appropriate:
- ☐ Patient died (date __/__/__ mm dd yy)
- ☐ Life threatening illness
- ☐ Required emergency room/doctor visit
- ☐ Required hospitalization (____days)
- ☐ Resulted in prolongation of hospitalization
- ☐ Resulted in permanent disability
- ☐ None of the above

9. Patient recovered ☐ YES ☐ NO ☐ UNKNOWN

10. Date of vaccination __/__/__ mm dd yy Time ____ AM PM

11. Adverse event onset __/__/__ mm dd yy Time ____ AM PM

12. Relevant diagnostic tests/laboratory data

13. Enter all vaccines given on date listed in no. 10

	Vaccine (type)	Manufacturer	Lot number	Route/Site	No. Previous Doses
a.					
b.					
c.					
d.					

14. Any other vaccinations within 4 weeks prior to the date listed in no. 10

	Vaccine (type)	Manufacturer	Lot number	Route/Site	No. Previous doses	Date given
a.						
b.						

15. Vaccinated at:
- ☐ Private doctor's office/hospital
- ☐ Public health clinic/hospital
- ☐ Military clinic/hospital
- ☐ Other/unknown

16. Vaccine purchased with:
- ☐ Private funds
- ☐ Public funds
- ☐ Military funds
- ☐ Other/unknown

17. Other medications

18. Illness at time of vaccination (specify)

19. Pre-existing physician-diagnosed allergies, birth defects, medical conditions (specify)

20. Have you reported this adverse event previously? ☐ No ☐ To health department ☐ To doctor ☐ To manufacturer

Only for children 5 and under

22. Birth weight ____ lb. ____ oz.
23. No. of brothers and sisters

21. Adverse event following prior vaccination (check all applicable, specify)

	Adverse Event	Onset Age	Type Vaccine	Dose no. in series
☐ In patient				
☐ In brother or sister				

Only for reports submitted by manufacturer/immunization project

24. Mfr./imm. proj. report no.
25. Date received by mfr./imm.proj.
26. 15 day report? ☐ Yes ☐ No
27. Report type ☐ Initial ☐ Follow-Up

Health care providers and manufacturers are required by law (42 USC 300aa-25) to report reactions to vaccines listed in the Table of Reportable Events Following Immunization. Reports for reactions to other vaccines are voluntary except when required as a condition of immunization grant awards.

Form VAERS-1(FDA)

"Fold in thirds, tape & mail — DO NOT STAPLE FORM"

NO POSTAGE NECESSARY IF MAILED IN THE UNITED STATES OR APO/FPO

BUSINESS REPLY MAIL

FIRST-CLASS MAIL PERMIT NO. 1895 ROCKVILLE, MD

POSTAGE WILL BE PAID BY ADDRESSEE

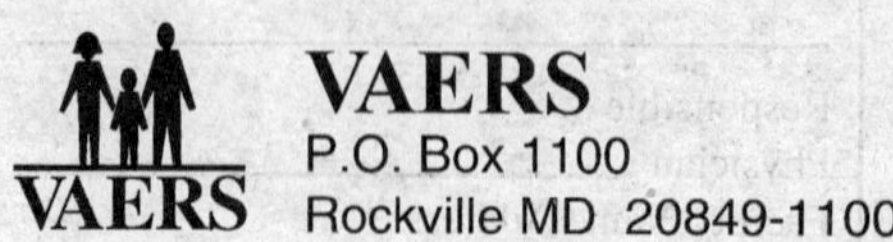

VAERS
P.O. Box 1100
Rockville MD 20849-1100

Fold

Fold

DIRECTIONS FOR COMPLETING FORM

(Additional pages may be attached if more space is needed.)

GENERAL

- Use a separate form for each patient. Complete the form to the best of your abilities. Items 3, 4, 7, 8, 10, 11, and 13 are considered essential and should be completed whenever possible. Parents/Guardians may need to consult the facility where the vaccine was administered for some of the information (such as manufacturer, lot number or laboratory data.)
- Refer to the Reportable Events Table (RET) for events mandated for reporting by law. Reporting for other serious events felt to be related but not on the RET is encouraged.
- Health care providers other than the vaccine administrator (VA) treating a patient for a suspected adverse event should notify the VA and provide the information about the adverse event to allow the VA to complete the form to meet the VA's legal responsibility.
- These data will be used to increase understanding of adverse events following vaccination and will become part of CDC Privacy Act System 09-20-0136, "Epidemiologic Studies and Surveillance of Disease Problems". Information identifying the person who received the vaccine or that person's legal representative will not be made available to the public, but may be available to the vaccinee or legal representative.
- Postage will be paid by addressee. Forms may be photocopied (must be front & back on same sheet).

SPECIFIC INSTRUCTIONS

Form Completed By: To be used by parents/guardians, vaccine manufacturers/distributors, vaccine administrators, and/or the person completing the form on behalf of the patient or the health professional who administered the vaccine.

Item 7: Describe the suspected adverse event. Such things as temperature, local and general signs and symptoms, time course, duration of symptoms, diagnosis, treatment and recovery should be noted.

Item 9: Check "YES" if the patient's health condition is the same as it was prior to the vaccine, "NO" if the patient has not returned to the pre-vaccination state of health, or "UNKNOWN" if the patient's condition is not known.

Item 10: and 11: Give dates and times as specifically as you can remember. If you do not know the exact time, please indicate "AM" or "PM" when possible if this information is known. If more than one adverse event, give the onset date and time for the most serious event.

Item 12: Include "negative" or "normal" results of any relevant tests performed as well as abnormal findings.

Item 13: List ONLY those vaccines given on the day listed in Item 10.

Item 14: List any other vaccines that the patient received within 4 weeks prior to the date listed in Item 10.

Item 16: This section refers to how the person who gave the vaccine purchased it, not to the patient's insurance.

Item 17: List any prescription or non-prescription medications the patient was taking when the vaccine(s) was given.

Item 18: List any short term illnesses the patient had on the date the vaccine(s) was given (i.e., cold, flu, ear infection).

Item 19: List any pre-existing physician-diagnosed allergies, birth defects, medical conditions (including developmental and/or neurologic disorders) for the patient.

Item 21: List any suspected adverse events the patient, or the patient's brothers or sisters, may have had to previous vaccinations. If more than one brother or sister, or if the patient has reacted to more than one prior vaccine, use additional pages to explain completely. For the onset age of a patient, provide the age in months if less than two years old.

Item 26: This space is for manufacturers' use only.

SECTION 4

PRODUCT IDENTIFICATION GUIDE

To aid in quick identification, this section provides full-color, actual-sized photographs of tablets and capsules. A variety of other dosage forms and packages are shown at less than actual size. In all, the guide contains some 2,400 photos.

Products in this section are arranged alphabetically by manufacturer. In some instances, not all dosage forms and sizes are pictured. If others are available, a † symbol precedes the product's name. Letters or numbers representing the manufacturer's identification code are followed by an asterisk.

For more information on any of the products in this section, please turn to the Product Information Section, or check directly with the manufacturer. The page number of each product's text entry appears with its photographs.

While every effort has been made to guarantee faithful reproduction of the photos in this section, changes in size, color, and design are always a possibility. Be sure to confirm a product's identity with the manufacturer or your pharmacist.

INDEX BY MANUFACTURER

This section is made possible through the courtesy of the manufacturers whose products appear on the following pages.

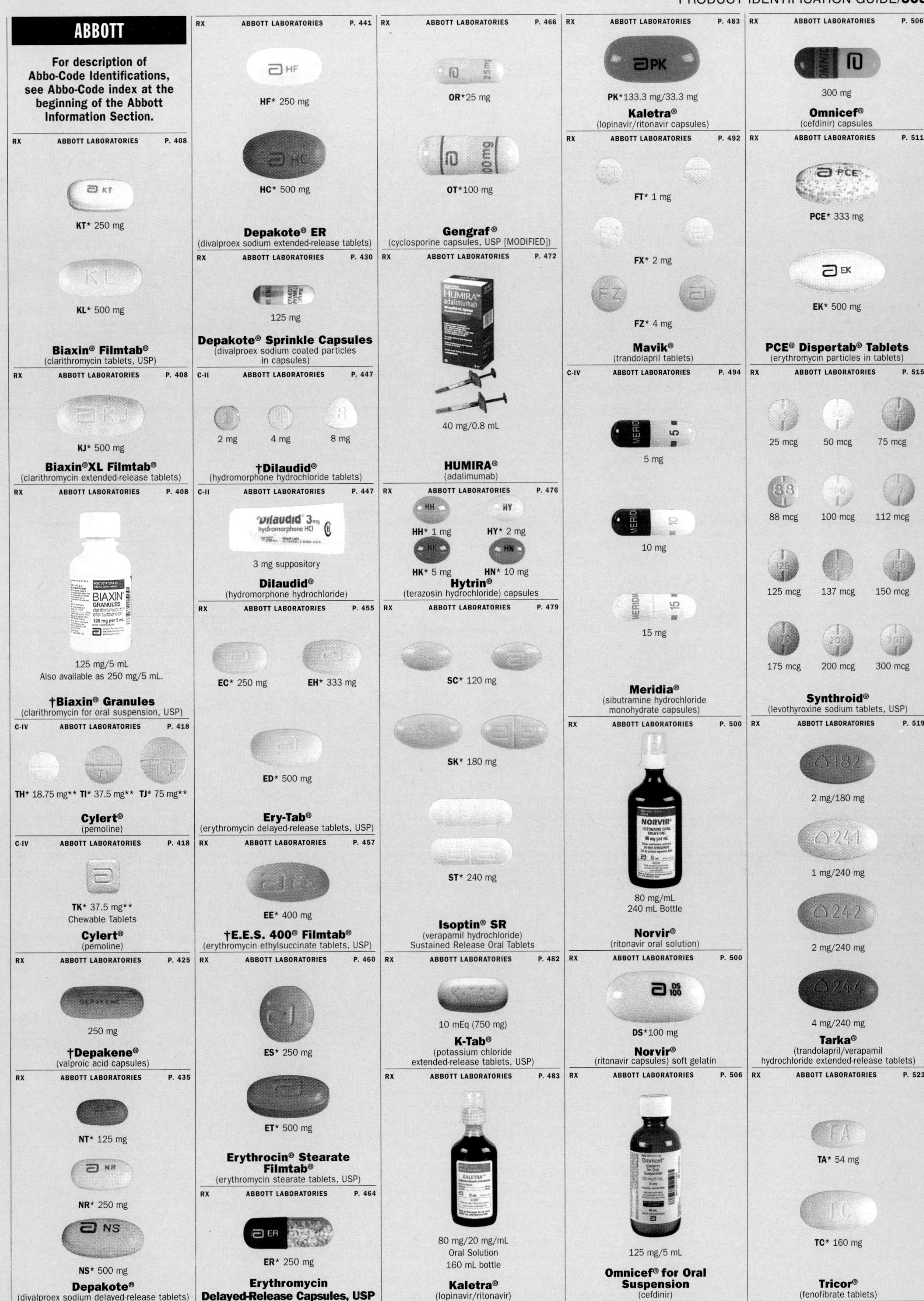

ABBOTT

For description of Abbo-Code Identifications, see Abbo-Code index at the beginning of the Abbott Information Section.

RX ABBOTT LABORATORIES P. 408

KT* 250 mg

KL* 500 mg

Biaxin® Filmtab®
(clarithromycin tablets, USP)

RX ABBOTT LABORATORIES P. 408

KJ* 500 mg

Biaxin®XL Filmtab®
(clarithromycin extended-release tablets)

RX ABBOTT LABORATORIES P. 408

125 mg/5 mL
Also available as 250 mg/5 mL.

†Biaxin® Granules
(clarithromycin for oral suspension, USP)

C-IV ABBOTT LABORATORIES P. 418

TH* 18.75 mg** **TI*** 37.5 mg** **TJ*** 75 mg**

Cylert®
(pemoline)

C-IV ABBOTT LABORATORIES P. 418

TK* 37.5 mg**
Chewable Tablets

Cylert®
(pemoline)

RX ABBOTT LABORATORIES P. 425

250 mg

†Depakene®
(valproic acid capsules)

RX ABBOTT LABORATORIES P. 435

NT* 125 mg

NR* 250 mg

NS* 500 mg

Depakote®
(divalproex sodium delayed-release tablets)

RX ABBOTT LABORATORIES P. 441

HF* 250 mg

HC* 500 mg

Depakote® ER
(divalproex sodium extended-release tablets)

RX ABBOTT LABORATORIES P. 430

125 mg

Depakote® Sprinkle Capsules
(divalproex sodium coated particles in capsules)

C-II ABBOTT LABORATORIES P. 447

2 mg 4 mg 8 mg

†Dilaudid®
(hydromorphone hydrochloride tablets)

C-II ABBOTT LABORATORIES P. 447

3 mg suppository

Dilaudid®
(hydromorphone hydrochloride)

RX ABBOTT LABORATORIES P. 455

EC* 250 mg **EH*** 333 mg

ED* 500 mg

Ery-Tab®
(erythromycin delayed-release tablets, USP)

RX ABBOTT LABORATORIES P. 457

EE* 400 mg

†E.E.S. 400® Filmtab®
(erythromycin ethylsuccinate tablets, USP)

RX ABBOTT LABORATORIES P. 460

ES* 250 mg

ET* 500 mg

Erythrocin® Stearate Filmtab®
(erythromycin stearate tablets, USP)

RX ABBOTT LABORATORIES P. 464

ER* 250 mg

Erythromycin Delayed-Release Capsules, USP

RX ABBOTT LABORATORIES P. 466

OR*25 mg

OT*100 mg

Gengraf®
(cyclosporine capsules, USP [MODIFIED])

RX ABBOTT LABORATORIES P. 472

40 mg/0.8 mL

HUMIRA®
(adalimumab)

RX ABBOTT LABORATORIES P. 476

HH* 1 mg **HY*** 2 mg

HK* 5 mg **HN*** 10 mg

Hytrin®
(terazosin hydrochloride) capsules

RX ABBOTT LABORATORIES P. 479

SC* 120 mg

SK* 180 mg

ST* 240 mg

Isoptin® SR
(verapamil hydrochloride)
Sustained Release Oral Tablets

RX ABBOTT LABORATORIES P. 482

10 mEq (750 mg)

K-Tab®
(potassium chloride extended-release tablets, USP)

RX ABBOTT LABORATORIES P. 483

80 mg/20 mg/mL
Oral Solution
160 mL bottle

Kaletra®
(lopinavir/ritonavir)

RX ABBOTT LABORATORIES P. 483

PK*133.3 mg/33.3 mg

Kaletra®
(lopinavir/ritonavir capsules)

RX ABBOTT LABORATORIES P. 492

FT* 1 mg

FX* 2 mg

FZ* 4 mg

Mavik®
(trandolapril tablets)

C-IV ABBOTT LABORATORIES P. 494

5 mg

10 mg

15 mg

Meridia®
(sibutramine hydrochloride monohydrate capsules)

RX ABBOTT LABORATORIES P. 500

80 mg/mL
240 mL Bottle

Norvir®
(ritonavir oral solution)

RX ABBOTT LABORATORIES P. 500

DS*100 mg

Norvir®
(ritonavir capsules) soft gelatin

RX ABBOTT LABORATORIES P. 506

125 mg/5 mL

Omnicef® for Oral Suspension
(cefdinir)

RX ABBOTT LABORATORIES P. 506

300 mg

Omnicef®
(cefdinir) capsules

RX ABBOTT LABORATORIES P. 511

PCE* 333 mg

EK* 500 mg

PCE® Dispertab® Tablets
(erythromycin particles in tablets)

RX ABBOTT LABORATORIES P. 515

25 mcg 50 mcg 75 mcg

88 mcg 100 mcg 112 mcg

125 mcg 137 mcg 150 mcg

175 mcg 200 mcg 300 mcg

Synthroid®
(levothyroxine sodium tablets, USP)

RX ABBOTT LABORATORIES P. 519

2 mg/180 mg

1 mg/240 mg

2 mg/240 mg

4 mg/240 mg

Tarka®
(trandolapril/verapamil hydrochloride extended-release tablets)

RX ABBOTT LABORATORIES P. 523

TA* 54 mg

TC* 160 mg

Tricor®
(fenofibrate tablets)

*Abbott Abbo-Code identification letters. Filmtab®-Film sealed tablets, Abbott. **Grooved tablets.

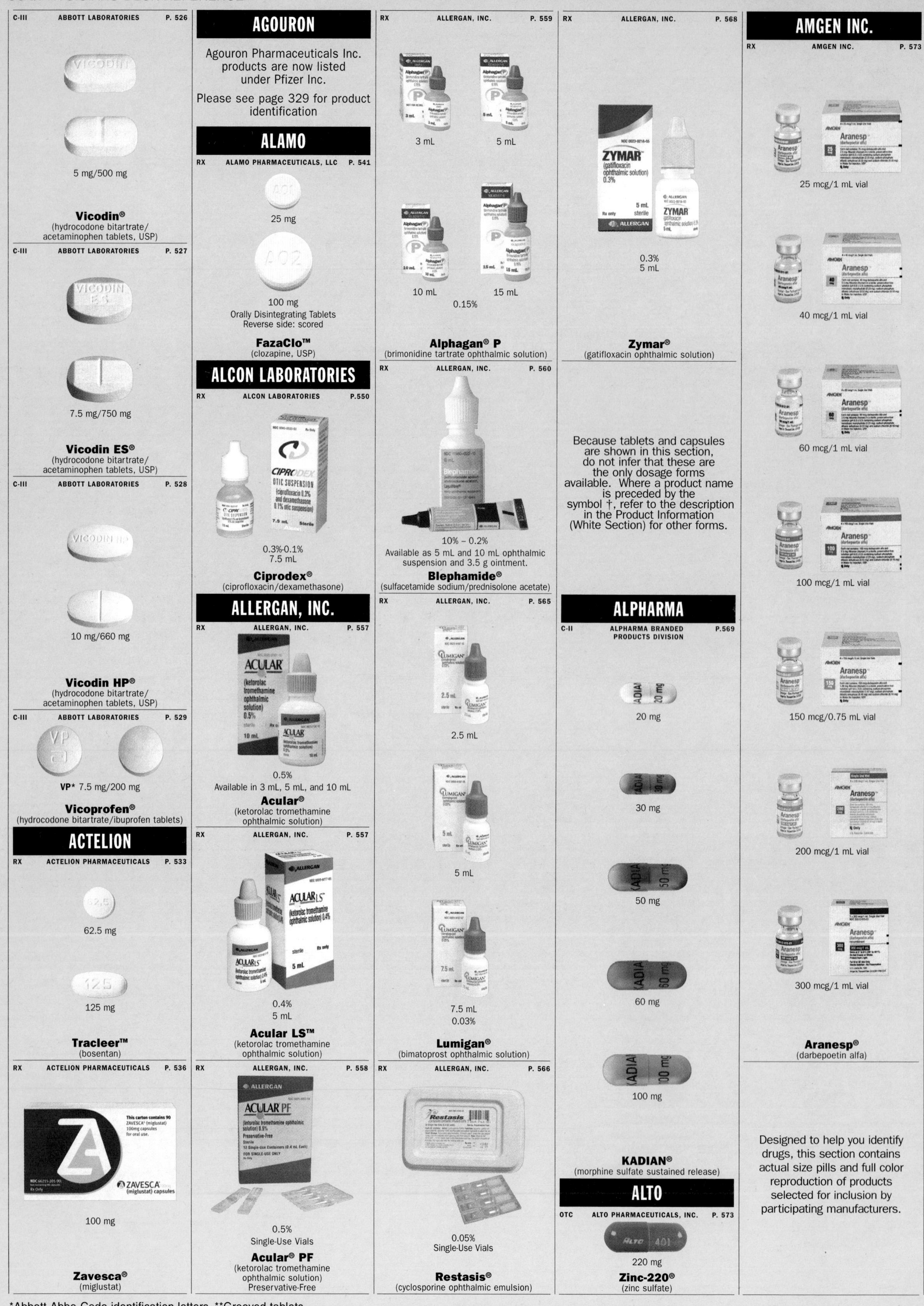
C-III ABBOTT LABORATORIES P. 526
5 mg/500 mg
Vicodin®
(hydrocodone bitartrate/ acetaminophen tablets, USP)
C-III ABBOTT LABORATORIES P. 527
7.5 mg/750 mg
Vicodin ES®
(hydrocodone bitartrate/ acetaminophen tablets, USP)
C-III ABBOTT LABORATORIES P. 528
10 mg/660 mg
Vicodin HP®
(hydrocodone bitartrate/ acetaminophen tablets, USP)
C-III ABBOTT LABORATORIES P. 529
VP* 7.5 mg/200 mg
Vicoprofen®
(hydrocodone bitartrate/ibuprofen tablets)
ACTELION
RX ACTELION PHARMACEUTICALS P. 533
62.5 mg
125 mg
Tracleer™
(bosentan)
RX ACTELION PHARMACEUTICALS P. 536
100 mg
Zavesca®
(miglustat)
AGOURON
Agouron Pharmaceuticals Inc. products are now listed under Pfizer Inc.
Please see page 329 for product identification
ALAMO
RX ALAMO PHARMACEUTICALS, LLC P. 541
25 mg
100 mg
Orally Disintegrating Tablets
Reverse side: scored
FazaClo™
(clozapine, USP)
ALCON LABORATORIES
RX ALCON LABORATORIES P.550
0.3%-0.1%
7.5 mL
Ciprodex®
(ciprofloxacin/dexamethasone)
ALLERGAN, INC.
RX ALLERGAN, INC. P. 557
0.5%
Available in 3 mL, 5 mL, and 10 mL
Acular®
(ketorolac tromethamine ophthalmic solution)
RX ALLERGAN, INC. P. 557
0.4%
5 mL
Acular LS™
(ketorolac tromethamine ophthalmic solution)
RX ALLERGAN, INC. P. 558
0.5%
Single-Use Vials
Acular® PF
(ketorolac tromethamine ophthalmic solution)
Preservative-Free
RX ALLERGAN, INC. P. 559
3 mL
5 mL
10 mL
15 mL
0.15%
Alphagan® P
(brimonidine tartrate ophthalmic solution)
RX ALLERGAN, INC. P. 560
10% – 0.2%
Available as 5 mL and 10 mL ophthalmic suspension and 3.5 g ointment.
Blephamide®
(sulfacetamide sodium/prednisolone acetate)
RX ALLERGAN, INC. P. 565
2.5 mL
5 mL
7.5 mL
0.03%
Lumigan®
(bimatoprost ophthalmic solution)
RX ALLERGAN, INC. P. 566
0.05%
Single-Use Vials
Restasis®
(cyclosporine ophthalmic emulsion)
RX ALLERGAN, INC. P. 568
0.3%
5 mL
Zymar®
(gatifloxacin ophthalmic solution)
Because tablets and capsules are shown in this section, do not infer that these are the only dosage forms available. Where a product name is preceded by the symbol †, refer to the description in the Product Information (White Section) for other forms.
ALPHARMA
C-II ALPHARMA BRANDED PRODUCTS DIVISION P.569
20 mg
30 mg
50 mg
60 mg
100 mg
KADIAN®
(morphine sulfate sustained release)
ALTO
OTC ALTO PHARMACEUTICALS, INC. P. 573
220 mg
Zinc-220®
(zinc sulfate)
AMGEN INC.
RX AMGEN INC. P. 573
25 mcg/1 mL vial
40 mcg/1 mL vial
60 mcg/1 mL vial
100 mcg/1 mL vial
150 mcg/0.75 mL vial
200 mcg/1 mL vial
300 mcg/1 mL vial
Aranesp®
(darbepoetin alfa)
Designed to help you identify drugs, this section contains actual size pills and full color reproduction of products selected for inclusion by participating manufacturers.

*Abbott Abbo-Code identification letters. **Grooved tablets.

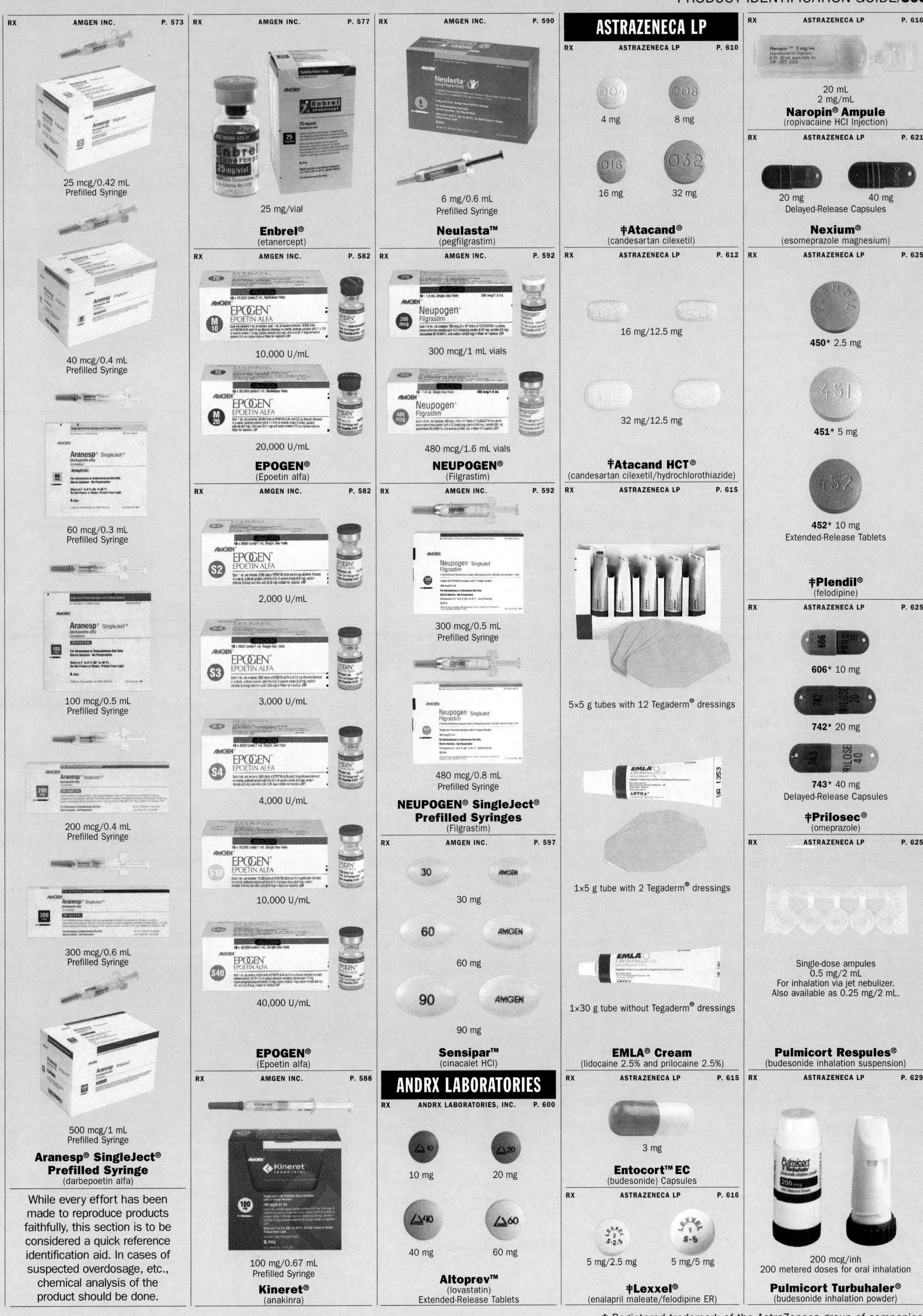

RX AMGEN INC. P. 573

25 mcg/0.42 mL
Prefilled Syringe

40 mcg/0.4 mL
Prefilled Syringe

60 mcg/0.3 mL
Prefilled Syringe

100 mcg/0.5 mL
Prefilled Syringe

200 mcg/0.4 mL
Prefilled Syringe

300 mcg/0.6 mL
Prefilled Syringe

500 mcg/1 mL
Prefilled Syringe

Aranesp® SingleJect® Prefilled Syringe
(darbepoetin alfa)

While every effort has been made to reproduce products faithfully, this section is to be considered a quick reference identification aid. In cases of suspected overdosage, etc., chemical analysis of the product should be done.

RX AMGEN INC. P. 577

25 mg/vial

Enbrel®
(etanercept)

RX AMGEN INC. P. 582

10,000 U/mL

20,000 U/mL

EPOGEN®
(Epoetin alfa)

RX AMGEN INC. P. 582

2,000 U/mL

3,000 U/mL

4,000 U/mL

10,000 U/mL

40,000 U/mL

EPOGEN®
(Epoetin alfa)

RX AMGEN INC. P. 588

100 mg/0.67 mL
Prefilled Syringe

Kineret®
(anakinra)

RX AMGEN INC. P. 590

6 mg/0.6 mL
Prefilled Syringe

Neulasta™
(pegfilgrastim)

RX AMGEN INC. P. 592

300 mcg/1 mL vials

480 mcg/1.6 mL vials

NEUPOGEN®
(Filgrastim)

RX AMGEN INC. P. 592

300 mcg/0.5 mL
Prefilled Syringe

480 mcg/0.8 mL
Prefilled Syringe

NEUPOGEN® SingleJect® Prefilled Syringes
(Filgrastim)

RX AMGEN INC. P. 597

30 mg

60 mg

90 mg

Sensipar™
(cinacalet HCl)

ANDRX LABORATORIES

RX ANDRX LABORATORIES, INC. P. 600

10 mg 20 mg

40 mg 60 mg

Altoprev™
(lovastatin)
Extended-Release Tablets

ASTRAZENECA LP

RX ASTRAZENECA LP P. 610

4 mg 8 mg

16 mg 32 mg

ǂAtacand®
(candesartan cilexetil)

RX ASTRAZENECA LP P. 612

16 mg/12.5 mg

32 mg/12.5 mg

ǂAtacand HCT®
(candesartan cilexetil/hydrochlorothiazide)

RX ASTRAZENECA LP P. 615

5×5 g tubes with 12 Tegaderm® dressings

1×5 g tube with 2 Tegaderm® dressings

1×30 g tube without Tegaderm® dressings

EMLA® Cream
(lidocaine 2.5% and prilocaine 2.5%)

RX ASTRAZENECA LP P. 615

3 mg

Entocort™ EC
(budesonide) Capsules

RX ASTRAZENECA LP P. 616

5 mg/2.5 mg 5 mg/5 mg

ǂLexxel®
(enalapril maleate/felodipine ER)

RX ASTRAZENECA LP P. 616

20 mL
2 mg/mL

Naropin® Ampule
(ropivacaine HCl Injection)

RX ASTRAZENECA LP P. 621

20 mg 40 mg
Delayed-Release Capsules

Nexium®
(esomeprazole magnesium)

RX ASTRAZENECA LP P. 625

450* 2.5 mg

451* 5 mg

452* 10 mg
Extended-Release Tablets

ǂPlendil®
(felodipine)

RX ASTRAZENECA LP P. 625

606* 10 mg

742* 20 mg

743* 40 mg
Delayed-Release Capsules

ǂPrilosec®
(omeprazole)

RX ASTRAZENECA LP P. 625

Single-dose ampules
0.5 mg/2 mL
For inhalation via jet nebulizer.
Also available as 0.25 mg/2 mL.

Pulmicort Respules®
(budesonide inhalation suspension)

RX ASTRAZENECA LP P. 629

200 mcg/inh
200 metered doses for oral inhalation

Pulmicort Turbuhaler®
(budesonide inhalation powder)

ǂ Registered trademark of the AstraZeneca group of companies.

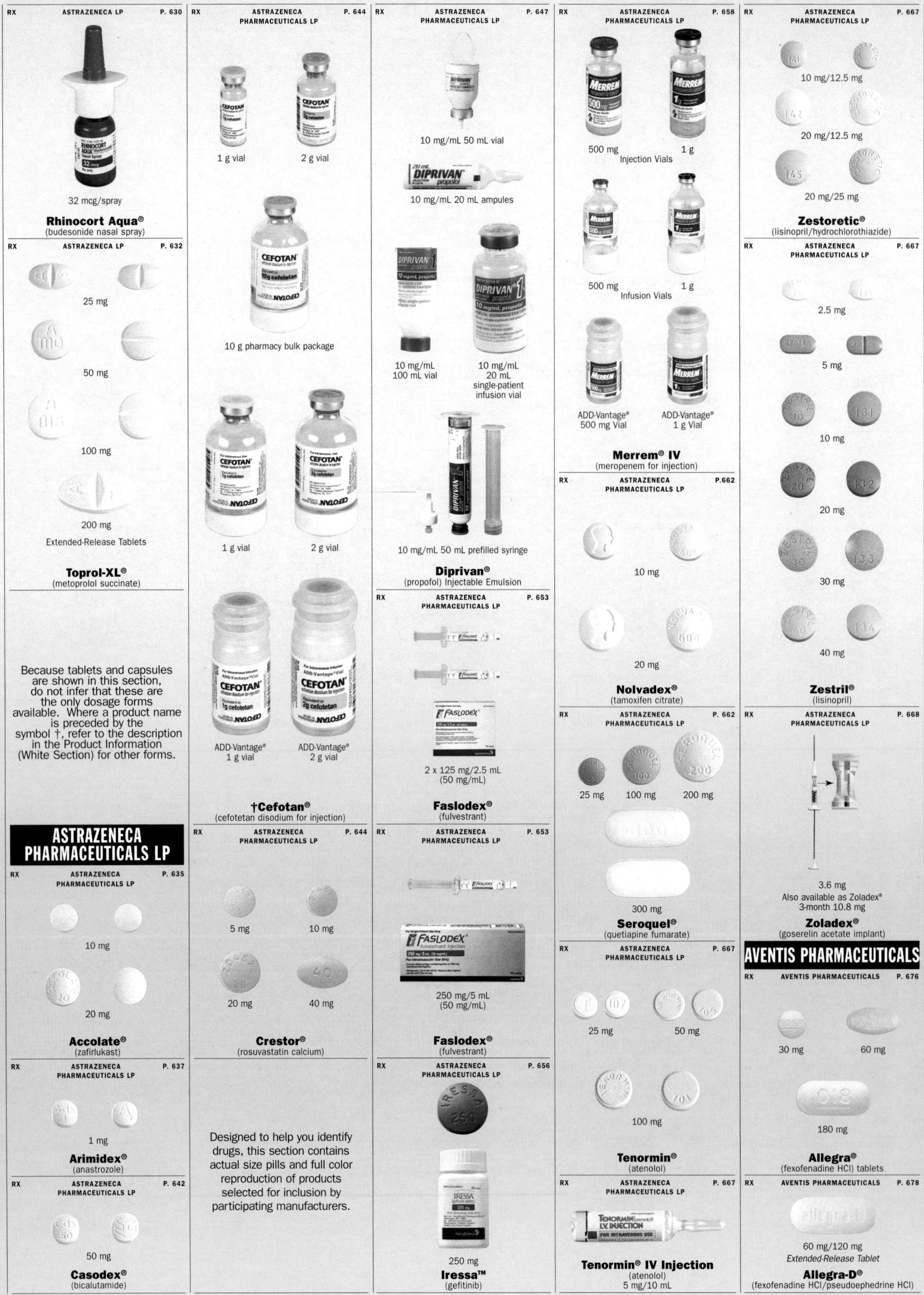

RX ASTRAZENECA LP P. 630

32 mcg/spray

Rhinocort Aqua®
(budesonide nasal spray)

RX ASTRAZENECA LP P. 632

25 mg

50 mg

100 mg

200 mg

Extended-Release Tablets

Toprol-XL®
(metoprolol succinate)

Because tablets and capsules are shown in this section, do not infer that these are the only dosage forms available. Where a product name is preceded by the symbol †, refer to the description in the Product Information (White Section) for other forms.

ASTRAZENECA PHARMACEUTICALS LP

RX ASTRAZENECA PHARMACEUTICALS LP P. 635

10 mg

20 mg

Accolate®
(zafirlukast)

RX ASTRAZENECA PHARMACEUTICALS LP P. 637

1 mg

Arimidex®
(anastrozole)

RX ASTRAZENECA PHARMACEUTICALS LP P. 642

50 mg

Casodex®
(bicalutamide)

RX ASTRAZENECA PHARMACEUTICALS LP P. 644

1 g vial 2 g vial

10 g pharmacy bulk package

1 g vial 2 g vial

ADD-Vantage® 1 g vial

ADD-Vantage® 2 g vial

†Cefotan®
(cefotetan disodium for injection)

RX ASTRAZENECA PHARMACEUTICALS LP P. 644

5 mg 10 mg

20 mg 40 mg

Crestor®
(rosuvastatin calcium)

Designed to help you identify drugs, this section contains actual size pills and full color reproduction of products selected for inclusion by participating manufacturers.

RX ASTRAZENECA PHARMACEUTICALS LP P. 647

10 mg/mL 50 mL vial

10 mg/mL 20 mL ampules

10 mg/mL 100 mL vial

10 mg/mL 20 mL single-patient infusion vial

10 mg/mL 50 mL prefilled syringe

Diprivan®
(propofol) Injectable Emulsion

RX ASTRAZENECA PHARMACEUTICALS LP P. 653

2 x 125 mg/2.5 mL (50 mg/mL)

Faslodex®
(fulvestrant)

RX ASTRAZENECA PHARMACEUTICALS LP P. 653

250 mg/5 mL (50 mg/mL)

Faslodex®
(fulvestrant)

RX ASTRAZENECA PHARMACEUTICALS LP P. 656

250 mg

Iressa™
(gefitinib)

RX ASTRAZENECA PHARMACEUTICALS LP P. 658

500 mg 1 g
Injection Vials

500 mg 1 g
Infusion Vials

ADD-Vantage® 500 mg Vial

ADD-Vantage® 1 g Vial

Merrem® IV
(meropenem for injection)

RX ASTRAZENECA PHARMACEUTICALS LP P.662

10 mg

20 mg

Nolvadex®
(tamoxifen citrate)

RX ASTRAZENECA PHARMACEUTICALS LP P. 662

25 mg 100 mg 200 mg

300 mg

Seroquel®
(quetiapine fumarate)

RX ASTRAZENECA PHARMACEUTICALS LP P. 667

25 mg 50 mg

100 mg

Tenormin®
(atenolol)

RX ASTRAZENECA PHARMACEUTICALS LP P. 667

Tenormin® IV Injection
(atenolol)
5 mg/10 mL

RX ASTRAZENECA PHARMACEUTICALS LP P. 667

10 mg/12.5 mg

20 mg/12.5 mg

20 mg/25 mg

Zestoretic®
(lisinopril/hydrochlorothiazide)

RX ASTRAZENECA PHARMACEUTICALS LP P. 667

2.5 mg

5 mg

10 mg

20 mg

30 mg

40 mg

Zestril®
(lisinopril)

RX ASTRAZENECA PHARMACEUTICALS LP P. 668

3.6 mg
Also available as Zoladex® 3-month 10.8 mg

Zoladex®
(goserelin acetate implant)

AVENTIS PHARMACEUTICALS

RX AVENTIS PHARMACEUTICALS P. 676

30 mg 60 mg

180 mg

Allegra®
(fexofenadine HCl) tablets

RX AVENTIS PHARMACEUTICALS P. 678

60 mg/120 mg
Extended-Release Tablet

Allegra-D®
(fexofenadine HCl/pseudoephedrine HCl)

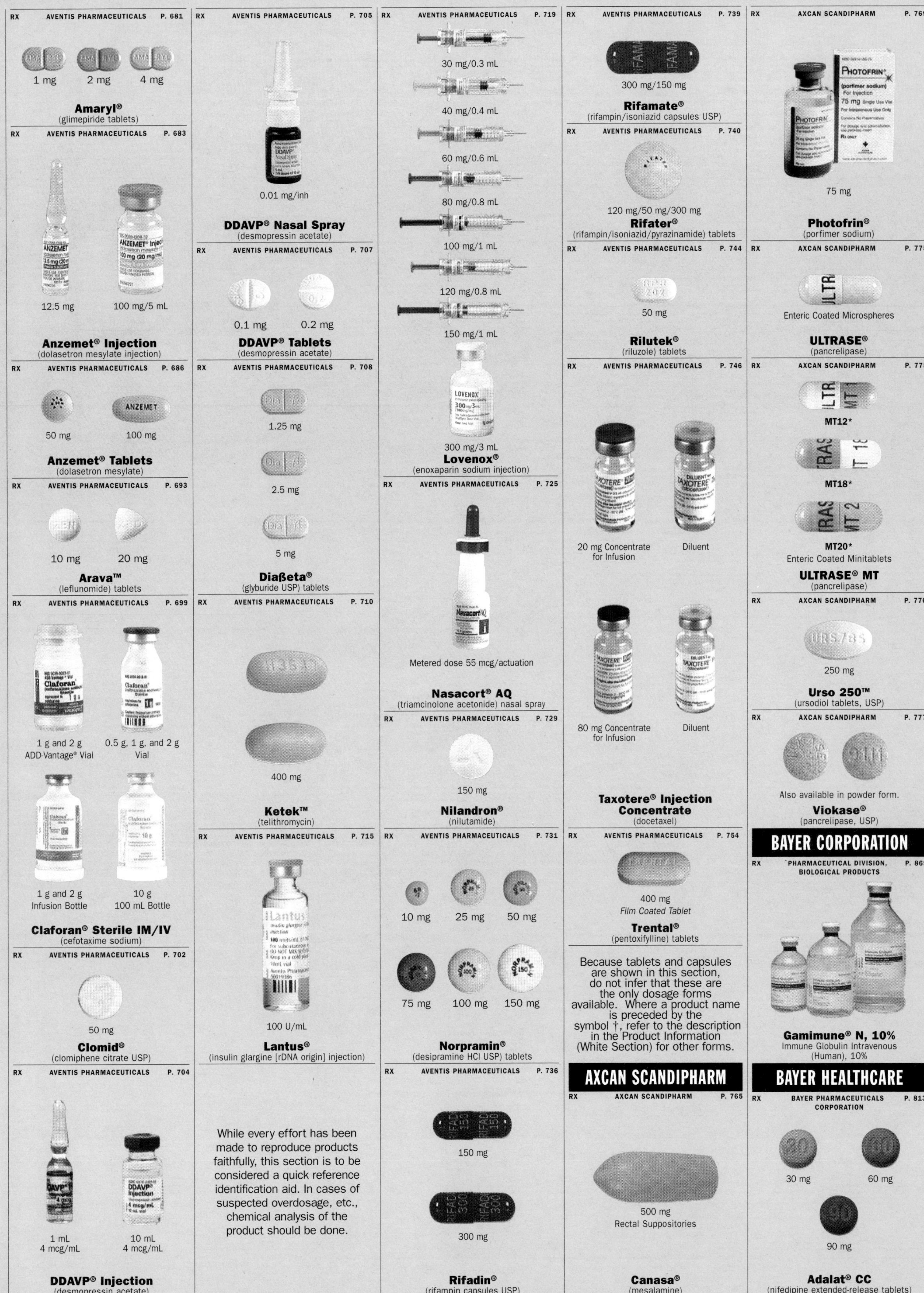
RX AVENTIS PHARMACEUTICALS P. 681
1 mg 2 mg 4 mg
Amaryl®
(glimepiride tablets)
RX AVENTIS PHARMACEUTICALS P. 683
12.5 mg 100 mg/5 mL
Anzemet® Injection
(dolasetron mesylate injection)
RX AVENTIS PHARMACEUTICALS P. 686
50 mg 100 mg
Anzemet® Tablets
(dolasetron mesylate)
RX AVENTIS PHARMACEUTICALS P. 693
10 mg 20 mg
Arava™
(leflunomide) tablets
RX AVENTIS PHARMACEUTICALS P. 699
1 g and 2 g ADD-Vantage® Vial
0.5 g, 1 g, and 2 g Vial
1 g and 2 g Infusion Bottle
10 g 100 mL Bottle
Claforan® Sterile IM/IV
(cefotaxime sodium)
RX AVENTIS PHARMACEUTICALS P. 702
50 mg
Clomid®
(clomiphene citrate USP)
RX AVENTIS PHARMACEUTICALS P. 704
1 mL 4 mcg/mL
10 mL 4 mcg/mL
DDAVP® Injection
(desmopressin acetate)
RX AVENTIS PHARMACEUTICALS P. 705
0.01 mg/inh
DDAVP® Nasal Spray
(desmopressin acetate)
RX AVENTIS PHARMACEUTICALS P. 707
0.1 mg 0.2 mg
DDAVP® Tablets
(desmopressin acetate)
RX AVENTIS PHARMACEUTICALS P. 708
1.25 mg
2.5 mg
5 mg
Diaßeta®
(glyburide USP) tablets
RX AVENTIS PHARMACEUTICALS P. 710
400 mg
Ketek™
(telithromycin)
RX AVENTIS PHARMACEUTICALS P. 715
100 U/mL
Lantus®
(insulin glargine [rDNA origin] injection)
While every effort has been made to reproduce products faithfully, this section is to be considered a quick reference identification aid. In cases of suspected overdosage, etc., chemical analysis of the product should be done.
RX AVENTIS PHARMACEUTICALS P. 719
30 mg/0.3 mL
40 mg/0.4 mL
60 mg/0.6 mL
80 mg/0.8 mL
100 mg/1 mL
120 mg/0.8 mL
150 mg/1 mL
300 mg/3 mL
Lovenox®
(enoxaparin sodium injection)
RX AVENTIS PHARMACEUTICALS P. 725
Metered dose 55 mcg/actuation
Nasacort® AQ
(triamcinolone acetonide) nasal spray
RX AVENTIS PHARMACEUTICALS P. 729
150 mg
Nilandron®
(nilutamide)
RX AVENTIS PHARMACEUTICALS P. 731
10 mg 25 mg 50 mg
75 mg 100 mg 150 mg
Norpramin®
(desipramine HCl USP) tablets
RX AVENTIS PHARMACEUTICALS P. 736
150 mg
300 mg
Rifadin®
(rifampin capsules USP)
RX AVENTIS PHARMACEUTICALS P. 739
300 mg/150 mg
Rifamate®
(rifampin/isoniazid capsules USP)
RX AVENTIS PHARMACEUTICALS P. 740
120 mg/50 mg/300 mg
Rifater®
(rifampin/isoniazid/pyrazinamide) tablets
RX AVENTIS PHARMACEUTICALS P. 744
50 mg
Rilutek®
(riluzole) tablets
RX AVENTIS PHARMACEUTICALS P. 746
20 mg Concentrate for Infusion
Diluent
80 mg Concentrate for Infusion
Diluent
Taxotere® Injection Concentrate
(docetaxel)
RX AVENTIS PHARMACEUTICALS P. 754
400 mg
Film Coated Tablet
Trental®
(pentoxifylline) tablets
Because tablets and capsules are shown in this section, do not infer that these are the only dosage forms available. Where a product name is preceded by the symbol †, refer to the description in the Product Information (White Section) for other forms.
AXCAN SCANDIPHARM
RX AXCAN SCANDIPHARM P. 765
500 mg
Rectal Suppositories
Canasa®
(mesalamine)
RX AXCAN SCANDIPHARM P. 769
75 mg
Photofrin®
(porfimer sodium)
RX AXCAN SCANDIPHARM P. 775
Enteric Coated Microspheres
ULTRASE®
(pancrelipase)
RX AXCAN SCANDIPHARM P. 775
MT12*
MT18*
MT20*
Enteric Coated Minitablets
ULTRASE® MT
(pancrelipase)
RX AXCAN SCANDIPHARM P. 776
250 mg
Urso 250™
(ursodiol tablets, USP)
RX AXCAN SCANDIPHARM P. 777
Also available in powder form.
Viokase®
(pancrelipase, USP)
BAYER CORPORATION
RX PHARMACEUTICAL DIVISION, BIOLOGICAL PRODUCTS P. 869
Gamimune® N, 10%
Immune Globulin Intravenous (Human), 10%
BAYER HEALTHCARE
RX BAYER PHARMACEUTICALS CORPORATION P. 813
30 mg 60 mg
90 mg
Adalat® CC
(nifedipine extended-release tablets)

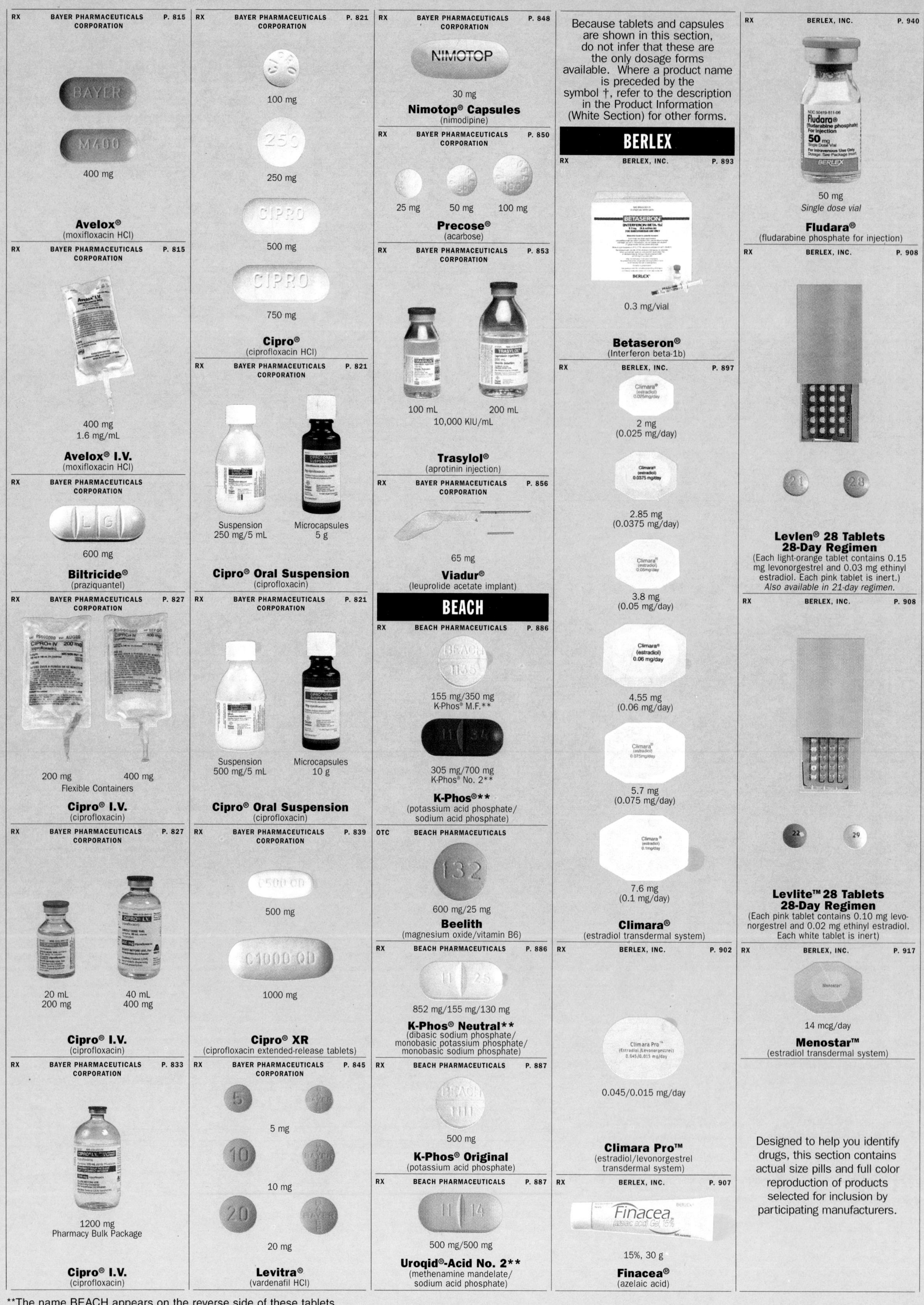

RX BAYER PHARMACEUTICALS CORPORATION P. 815

400 mg

Avelox®
(moxifloxacin HCl)

RX BAYER PHARMACEUTICALS CORPORATION P. 815

400 mg
1.6 mg/mL

Avelox® I.V.
(moxifloxacin HCl)

RX BAYER PHARMACEUTICALS CORPORATION

600 mg

Biltricide®
(praziquantel)

RX BAYER PHARMACEUTICALS CORPORATION P. 827

200 mg 400 mg
Flexible Containers

Cipro® I.V.
(ciprofloxacin)

RX BAYER PHARMACEUTICALS CORPORATION P. 827

20 mL 200 mg
40 mL 400 mg

Cipro® I.V.
(ciprofloxacin)

RX BAYER PHARMACEUTICALS CORPORATION P. 833

1200 mg
Pharmacy Bulk Package

Cipro® I.V.
(ciprofloxacin)

RX BAYER PHARMACEUTICALS CORPORATION P. 821

100 mg

250 mg

500 mg

750 mg

Cipro®
(ciprofloxacin HCl)

RX BAYER PHARMACEUTICALS CORPORATION P. 821

Suspension 250 mg/5 mL
Microcapsules 5 g

Cipro® Oral Suspension
(ciprofloxacin)

RX BAYER PHARMACEUTICALS CORPORATION P. 821

Suspension 500 mg/5 mL
Microcapsules 10 g

Cipro® Oral Suspension
(ciprofloxacin)

RX BAYER PHARMACEUTICALS CORPORATION P. 839

500 mg

1000 mg

Cipro® XR
(ciprofloxacin extended-release tablets)

RX BAYER PHARMACEUTICALS CORPORATION P. 845

5 mg

10 mg

20 mg

Levitra®
(vardenafil HCl)

RX BAYER PHARMACEUTICALS CORPORATION P. 848

30 mg

Nimotop® Capsules
(nimodipine)

RX BAYER PHARMACEUTICALS CORPORATION P. 850

25 mg 50 mg 100 mg

Precose®
(acarbose)

RX BAYER PHARMACEUTICALS CORPORATION P. 853

100 mL 200 mL
10,000 KIU/mL

Trasylol®
(aprotinin injection)

RX BAYER PHARMACEUTICALS CORPORATION P. 856

65 mg

Viadur®
(leuprolide acetate implant)

BEACH

RX BEACH PHARMACEUTICALS P. 886

155 mg/350 mg
K-Phos® M.F.**

305 mg/700 mg
K-Phos® No. 2**

K-Phos®**
(potassium acid phosphate/sodium acid phosphate)

OTC BEACH PHARMACEUTICALS

600 mg/25 mg

Beelith
(magnesium oxide/vitamin B6)

RX BEACH PHARMACEUTICALS P. 886

852 mg/155 mg/130 mg

K-Phos® Neutral**
(dibasic sodium phosphate/monobasic potassium phosphate/monobasic sodium phosphate)

RX BEACH PHARMACEUTICALS P. 887

500 mg

K-Phos® Original
(potassium acid phosphate)

RX BEACH PHARMACEUTICALS P. 887

500 mg/500 mg

Uroqid®-Acid No. 2**
(methenamine mandelate/sodium acid phosphate)

Because tablets and capsules are shown in this section, do not infer that these are the only dosage forms available. Where a product name is preceded by the symbol †, refer to the description in the Product Information (White Section) for other forms.

BERLEX

RX BERLEX, INC. P. 893

0.3 mg/vial

Betaseron®
(Interferon beta-1b)

RX BERLEX, INC. P. 897

2 mg
(0.025 mg/day)

2.85 mg
(0.0375 mg/day)

3.8 mg
(0.05 mg/day)

4.55 mg
(0.06 mg/day)

5.7 mg
(0.075 mg/day)

7.6 mg
(0.1 mg/day)

Climara®
(estradiol transdermal system)

RX BERLEX, INC. P. 902

0.045/0.015 mg/day

Climara Pro™
(estradiol/levonorgestrel transdermal system)

RX BERLEX, INC. P. 907

15%, 30 g

Finacea®
(azelaic acid)

RX BERLEX, INC. P. 940

50 mg
Single dose vial

Fludara®
(fludarabine phosphate for injection)

RX BERLEX, INC. P. 908

Levlen® 28 Tablets
28-Day Regimen
(Each light-orange tablet contains 0.15 mg levonorgestrel and 0.03 mg ethinyl estradiol. Each pink tablet is inert.)
Also available in 21-day regimen.

RX BERLEX, INC. P. 908

Levlite™ 28 Tablets
28-Day Regimen
(Each pink tablet contains 0.10 mg levonorgestrel and 0.02 mg ethinyl estradiol. Each white tablet is inert)

RX BERLEX, INC. P. 917

14 mcg/day

Menostar™
(estradiol transdermal system)

Designed to help you identify drugs, this section contains actual size pills and full color reproduction of products selected for inclusion by participating manufacturers.

**The name BEACH appears on the reverse side of these tablets.

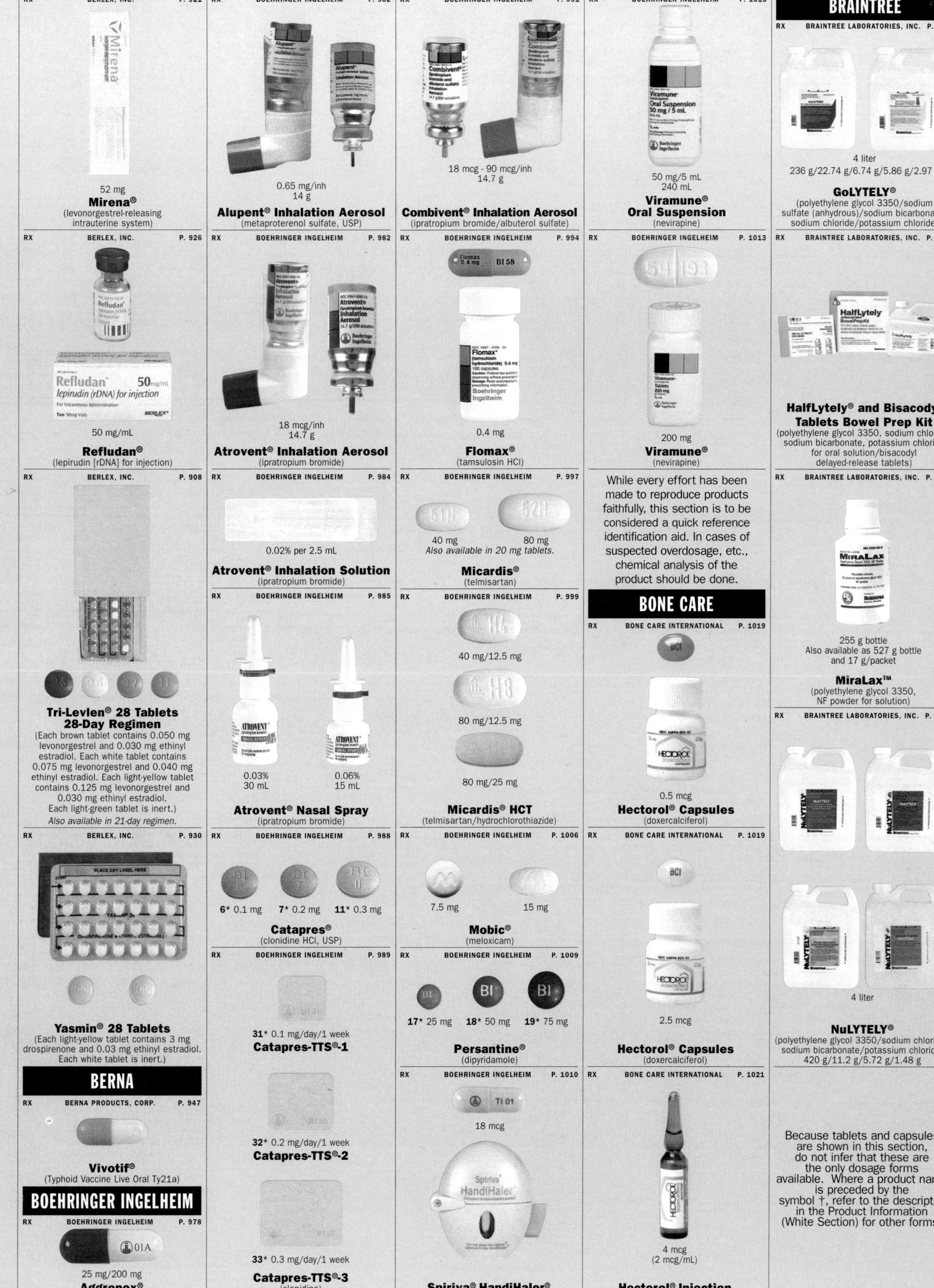

RX BERLEX, INC. P. 921

52 mg
Mirena®
(levonorgestrel-releasing intrauterine system)

RX BERLEX, INC. P. 926

50 mg/mL
Refludan®
(lepirudin [rDNA] for injection)

RX BERLEX, INC. P. 908

Tri-Levlen® 28 Tablets 28-Day Regimen
(Each brown tablet contains 0.050 mg levonorgestrel and 0.030 mg ethinyl estradiol. Each white tablet contains 0.075 mg levonorgestrel and 0.040 mg ethinyl estradiol. Each light-yellow tablet contains 0.125 mg levonorgestrel and 0.030 mg ethinyl estradiol. Each light-green tablet is inert.)
Also available in 21-day regimen.

RX BERLEX, INC. P. 930

Yasmin® 28 Tablets
(Each light-yellow tablet contains 3 mg drospirenone and 0.03 mg ethinyl estradiol. Each white tablet is inert.)

BERNA

RX BERNA PRODUCTS, CORP. P. 947

Vivotif®
(Typhoid Vaccine Live Oral Ty21a)

BOEHRINGER INGELHEIM

RX BOEHRINGER INGELHEIM P. 978

25 mg/200 mg
Aggrenox®
(aspirin/extended-release dipyridamole)

RX BOEHRINGER INGELHEIM P. 982

0.65 mg/inh
14 g
Alupent® Inhalation Aerosol
(metaproterenol sulfate, USP)

RX BOEHRINGER INGELHEIM P. 982

18 mcg/inh
14.7 g
Atrovent® Inhalation Aerosol
(ipratropium bromide)

RX BOEHRINGER INGELHEIM P. 984

0.02% per 2.5 mL
Atrovent® Inhalation Solution
(ipratropium bromide)

RX BOEHRINGER INGELHEIM P. 985

0.03% 30 mL
0.06% 15 mL
Atrovent® Nasal Spray
(ipratropium bromide)

RX BOEHRINGER INGELHEIM P. 988

6* 0.1 mg **7*** 0.2 mg **11*** 0.3 mg
Catapres®
(clonidine HCl, USP)

RX BOEHRINGER INGELHEIM P. 989

31* 0.1 mg/day/1 week
Catapres-TTS®-1

32* 0.2 mg/day/1 week
Catapres-TTS®-2

33* 0.3 mg/day/1 week
Catapres-TTS®-3
(clonidine)
Transdermal Therapeutic System

RX BOEHRINGER INGELHEIM P. 991

18 mcg - 90 mcg/inh
14.7 g
Combivent® Inhalation Aerosol
(ipratropium bromide/albuterol sulfate)

RX BOEHRINGER INGELHEIM P. 994

0.4 mg
Flomax®
(tamsulosin HCl)

RX BOEHRINGER INGELHEIM P. 997

40 mg 80 mg
Also available in 20 mg tablets.
Micardis®
(telmisartan)

RX BOEHRINGER INGELHEIM P. 999

40 mg/12.5 mg
80 mg/12.5 mg
80 mg/25 mg
Micardis® HCT
(telmisartan/hydrochlorothiazide)

RX BOEHRINGER INGELHEIM P. 1006

7.5 mg 15 mg
Mobic®
(meloxicam)

RX BOEHRINGER INGELHEIM P. 1009

17* 25 mg **18*** 50 mg **19*** 75 mg
Persantine®
(dipyridamole)

RX BOEHRINGER INGELHEIM P. 1010

18 mcg
Spiriva® HandiHaler®
(tiotropium bromide inhalation powder)

RX BOEHRINGER INGELHEIM P. 1013

50 mg/5 mL
240 mL
Viramune® Oral Suspension
(nevirapine)

RX BOEHRINGER INGELHEIM P. 1013

200 mg
Viramune®
(nevirapine)

While every effort has been made to reproduce products faithfully, this section is to be considered a quick reference identification aid. In cases of suspected overdosage, etc., chemical analysis of the product should be done.

BONE CARE

RX BONE CARE INTERNATIONAL P. 1019

0.5 mcg
Hectorol® Capsules
(doxercalciferol)

RX BONE CARE INTERNATIONAL P. 1019

2.5 mcg
Hectorol® Capsules
(doxercalciferol)

RX BONE CARE INTERNATIONAL P. 1021

4 mcg
(2 mcg/mL)
Hectorol® Injection
(doxercalciferol)

BRAINTREE

RX BRAINTREE LABORATORIES, INC. P. 1023

4 liter
236 g/22.74 g/6.74 g/5.86 g/2.97 g
GoLYTELY®
(polyethylene glycol 3350/sodium sulfate (anhydrous)/sodium bicarbonate/sodium chloride/potassium chloride)

RX BRAINTREE LABORATORIES, INC. P. 1024

HalfLytely® and Bisacodyl Tablets Bowel Prep Kit
(polyethylene glycol 3350, sodium chloride, sodium bicarbonate, potassium chloride for oral solution/bisacodyl delayed-release tablets)

RX BRAINTREE LABORATORIES, INC. P. 1025

255 g bottle
Also available as 527 g bottle and 17 g/packet
MiraLax™
(polyethylene glycol 3350, NF powder for solution)

RX BRAINTREE LABORATORIES, INC. P. 1023

4 liter
NuLYTELY®
(polyethylene glycol 3350/sodium chloride/sodium bicarbonate/potassium chloride)
420 g/11.2 g/5.72 g/1.48 g

Because tablets and capsules are shown in this section, do not infer that these are the only dosage forms available. Where a product name is preceded by the symbol †, refer to the description in the Product Information (White Section) for other forms.

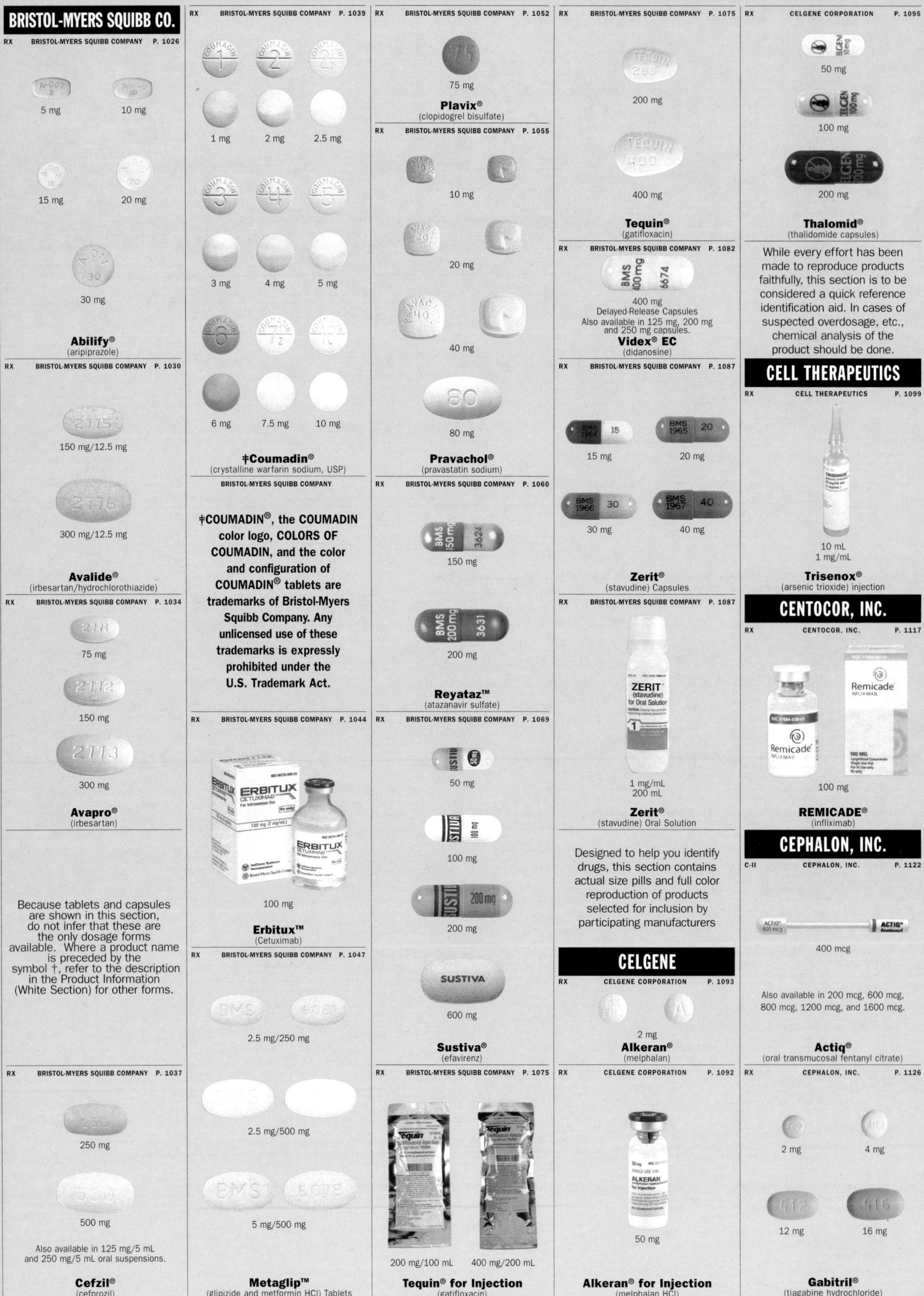
BRISTOL-MYERS SQUIBB CO.
RX BRISTOL-MYERS SQUIBB COMPANY P. 1026
5 mg
10 mg
15 mg
20 mg
30 mg
Abilify®
(aripiprazole)
RX BRISTOL-MYERS SQUIBB COMPANY P. 1030
150 mg/12.5 mg
300 mg/12.5 mg
Avalide®
(irbesartan/hydrochlorothiazide)
RX BRISTOL-MYERS SQUIBB COMPANY P. 1034
75 mg
150 mg
300 mg
Avapro®
(irbesartan)
Because tablets and capsules are shown in this section, do not infer that these are the only dosage forms available. Where a product name is preceded by the symbol †, refer to the description in the Product Information (White Section) for other forms.
RX BRISTOL-MYERS SQUIBB COMPANY P. 1037
250 mg
500 mg
Also available in 125 mg/5 mL and 250 mg/5 mL oral suspensions.
Cefzil®
(cefprozil)
RX BRISTOL-MYERS SQUIBB COMPANY P. 1039
1 mg
2 mg
2.5 mg
3 mg
4 mg
5 mg
6 mg
7.5 mg
10 mg
†Coumadin®
(crystalline warfarin sodium, USP)
BRISTOL-MYERS SQUIBB COMPANY
†COUMADIN®, the COUMADIN color logo, COLORS OF COUMADIN, and the color and configuration of COUMADIN® tablets are trademarks of Bristol-Myers Squibb Company. Any unlicensed use of these trademarks is expressly prohibited under the U.S. Trademark Act.
RX BRISTOL-MYERS SQUIBB COMPANY P. 1044
ERBITUX
CETUXIMAB
100 mg
Erbitux™
(Cetuximab)
RX BRISTOL-MYERS SQUIBB COMPANY P. 1047
2.5 mg/250 mg
2.5 mg/500 mg
5 mg/500 mg
Metaglip™
(glipizide and metformin HCl) Tablets
RX BRISTOL-MYERS SQUIBB COMPANY P. 1052
75 mg
Plavix®
(clopidogrel bisulfate)
RX BRISTOL-MYERS SQUIBB COMPANY P. 1055
10 mg
20 mg
40 mg
80 mg
Pravachol®
(pravastatin sodium)
RX BRISTOL-MYERS SQUIBB COMPANY P. 1060
150 mg
200 mg
Reyataz™
(atazanavir sulfate)
RX BRISTOL-MYERS SQUIBB COMPANY P. 1069
50 mg
100 mg
200 mg
600 mg
Sustiva®
(efavirenz)
RX BRISTOL-MYERS SQUIBB COMPANY P. 1075
200 mg/100 mL
400 mg/200 mL
Tequin® for Injection
(gatifloxacin)
RX BRISTOL-MYERS SQUIBB COMPANY P. 1075
200 mg
400 mg
Tequin®
(gatifloxacin)
RX BRISTOL-MYERS SQUIBB COMPANY P. 1082
400 mg
Delayed-Release Capsules
Also available in 125 mg, 200 mg and 250 mg capsules.
Videx® EC
(didanosine)
RX BRISTOL-MYERS SQUIBB COMPANY P. 1087
15 mg
20 mg
30 mg
40 mg
Zerit®
(stavudine) Capsules
RX BRISTOL-MYERS SQUIBB COMPANY P. 1087
ZERIT
(stavudine)
for Oral Solution
1 mg/mL
200 mL
Zerit®
(stavudine) Oral Solution
Designed to help you identify drugs, this section contains actual size pills and full color reproduction of products selected for inclusion by participating manufacturers
CELGENE
RX CELGENE CORPORATION P. 1093
2 mg
Alkeran®
(melphalan)
RX CELGENE CORPORATION P. 1092
ALKERAN
50 mg
Alkeran® for Injection
(melphalan HCl)
RX CELGENE CORPORATION P. 1095
50 mg
100 mg
200 mg
Thalomid®
(thalidomide capsules)
While every effort has been made to reproduce products faithfully, this section is to be considered a quick reference identification aid. In cases of suspected overdosage, etc., chemical analysis of the product should be done.
CELL THERAPEUTICS
RX CELL THERAPEUTICS P. 1099
10 mL
1 mg/mL
Trisenox®
(arsenic trioxide) injection
CENTOCOR, INC.
RX CENTOCOR, INC. P. 1117
Remicade
INFLIXIMAB
100 mg
REMICADE®
(infliximab)
CEPHALON, INC.
C-II CEPHALON, INC. P. 1122
ACTIQ
400 mcg
Also available in 200 mcg, 600 mcg, 800 mcg, 1200 mcg, and 1600 mcg.
Actiq®
(oral transmucosal fentanyl citrate)
RX CEPHALON, INC. P. 1126
2 mg
4 mg
12 mg
16 mg
Gabitril®
(tiagabine hydrochloride)

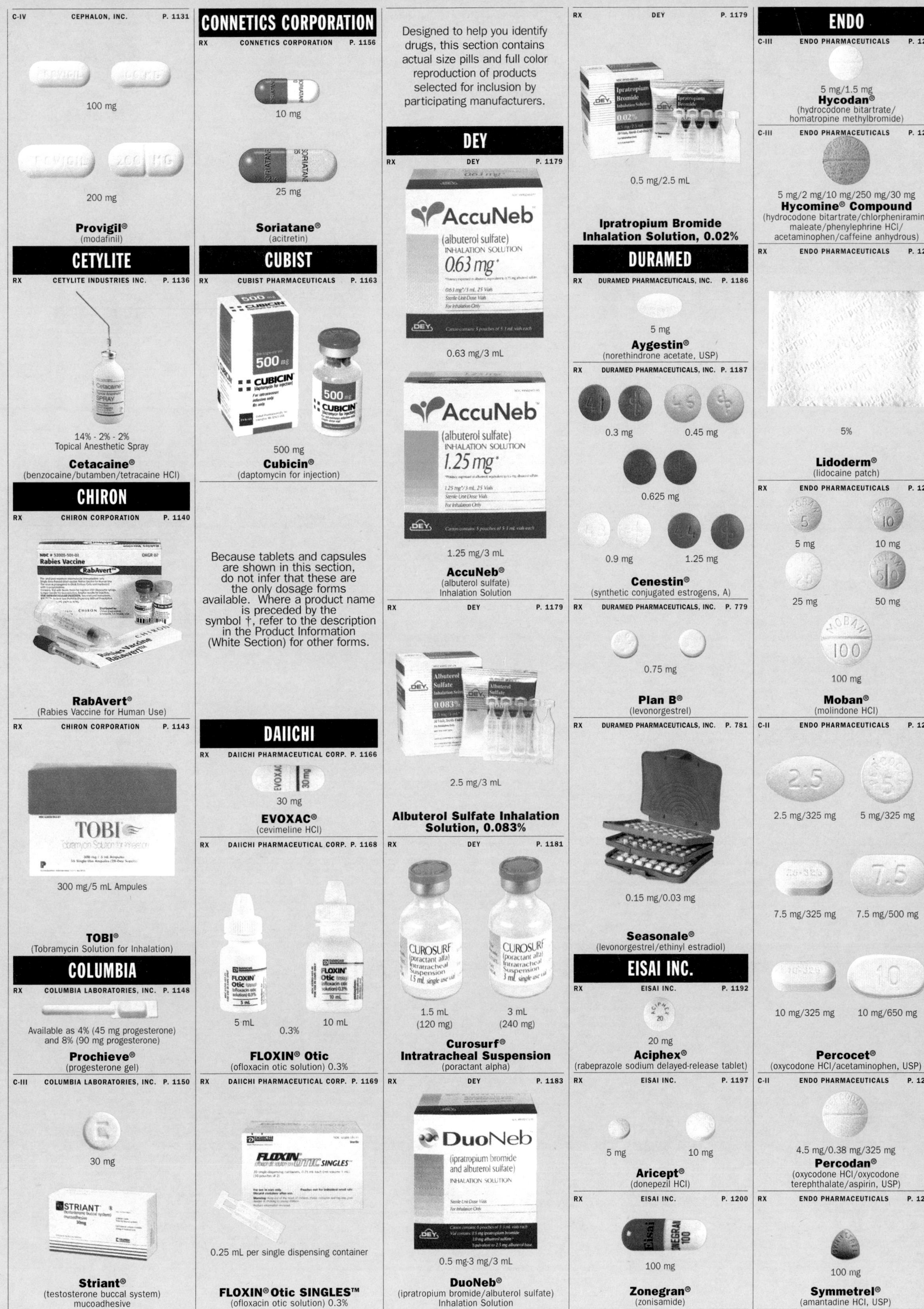
C-IV CEPHALON, INC. P. 1131
100 mg
200 mg
Provigil®
(modafinil)
CETYLITE
RX CETYLITE INDUSTRIES INC. P. 1136
14% - 2% - 2%
Topical Anesthetic Spray
Cetacaine®
(benzocaine/butamben/tetracaine HCl)
CHIRON
RX CHIRON CORPORATION P. 1140
RabAvert®
(Rabies Vaccine for Human Use)
RX CHIRON CORPORATION P. 1143
300 mg/5 mL Ampules
TOBI®
(Tobramycin Solution for Inhalation)
COLUMBIA
RX COLUMBIA LABORATORIES, INC. P. 1148
Available as 4% (45 mg progesterone) and 8% (90 mg progesterone)
Prochieve®
(progesterone gel)
C-III COLUMBIA LABORATORIES, INC. P. 1150
30 mg
Striant®
(testosterone buccal system) mucoadhesive
CONNETICS CORPORATION
RX CONNETICS CORPORATION P. 1156
10 mg
25 mg
Soriatane®
(acitretin)
CUBIST
RX CUBIST PHARMACEUTICALS P. 1163
500 mg
Cubicin®
(daptomycin for injection)
Because tablets and capsules are shown in this section, do not infer that these are the only dosage forms available. Where a product name is preceded by the symbol †, refer to the description in the Product Information (White Section) for other forms.
DAIICHI
RX DAIICHI PHARMACEUTICAL CORP. P. 1166
30 mg
EVOXAC®
(cevimeline HCl)
RX DAIICHI PHARMACEUTICAL CORP. P. 1168
5 mL
0.3%
10 mL
FLOXIN® Otic
(ofloxacin otic solution) 0.3%
RX DAIICHI PHARMACEUTICAL CORP. P. 1169
0.25 mL per single dispensing container
FLOXIN® Otic SINGLES™
(ofloxacin otic solution) 0.3%
Designed to help you identify drugs, this section contains actual size pills and full color reproduction of products selected for inclusion by participating manufacturers.
DEY
RX DEY P. 1179
AccuNeb
(albuterol sulfate)
INHALATION SOLUTION
0.63 mg*
0.63 mg/3 mL
AccuNeb
(albuterol sulfate)
INHALATION SOLUTION
1.25 mg*
1.25 mg/3 mL
AccuNeb®
(albuterol sulfate)
Inhalation Solution
RX DEY P. 1179
2.5 mg/3 mL
Albuterol Sulfate Inhalation Solution, 0.083%
RX DEY P. 1181
1.5 mL
(120 mg)
3 mL
(240 mg)
Curosurf®
Intratracheal Suspension
(poractant alpha)
RX DEY P. 1183
DuoNeb
(ipratropium bromide and albuterol sulfate)
INHALATION SOLUTION
0.5 mg-3 mg/3 mL
DuoNeb®
(ipratropium bromide/albuterol sulfate)
Inhalation Solution
RX DEY P. 1179
0.5 mg/2.5 mL
Ipratropium Bromide Inhalation Solution, 0.02%
DURAMED
RX DURAMED PHARMACEUTICALS, INC. P. 1186
5 mg
Aygestin®
(norethindrone acetate, USP)
RX DURAMED PHARMACEUTICALS, INC. P. 1187
0.3 mg
0.45 mg
0.625 mg
0.9 mg
1.25 mg
Cenestin®
(synthetic conjugated estrogens, A)
RX DURAMED PHARMACEUTICALS, INC. P. 779
0.75 mg
Plan B®
(levonorgestrel)
RX DURAMED PHARMACEUTICALS, INC. P. 781
0.15 mg/0.03 mg
Seasonale®
(levonorgestrel/ethinyl estradiol)
EISAI INC.
RX EISAI INC. P. 1192
20 mg
Aciphex®
(rabeprazole sodium delayed-release tablet)
RX EISAI INC. P. 1197
5 mg
10 mg
Aricept®
(donepezil HCl)
RX EISAI INC. P. 1200
100 mg
Zonegran®
(zonisamide)
ENDO
C-III ENDO PHARMACEUTICALS P. 1212
5 mg/1.5 mg
Hycodan®
(hydrocodone bitartrate/homatropine methylbromide)
C-III ENDO PHARMACEUTICALS P. 1213
5 mg/2 mg/10 mg/250 mg/30 mg
Hycomine® Compound
(hydrocodone bitartrate/chlorpheniramine maleate/phenylephrine HCl/acetaminophen/caffeine anhydrous)
RX ENDO PHARMACEUTICALS P. 1215
5%
Lidoderm®
(lidocaine patch)
RX ENDO PHARMACEUTICALS P. 1217
5 mg
10 mg
25 mg
50 mg
100 mg
Moban®
(molindone HCl)
C-II ENDO PHARMACEUTICALS P. 1222
2.5 mg/325 mg
5 mg/325 mg
7.5 mg/325 mg
7.5 mg/500 mg
10 mg/325 mg
10 mg/650 mg
Percocet®
(oxycodone HCl/acetaminophen, USP)
C-II ENDO PHARMACEUTICALS P. 1223
4.5 mg/0.38 mg/325 mg
Percodan®
(oxycodone HCl/oxycodone terephthalate/aspirin, USP)
RX ENDO PHARMACEUTICALS P. 1224
100 mg
Symmetrel®
(amantadine HCl, USP)

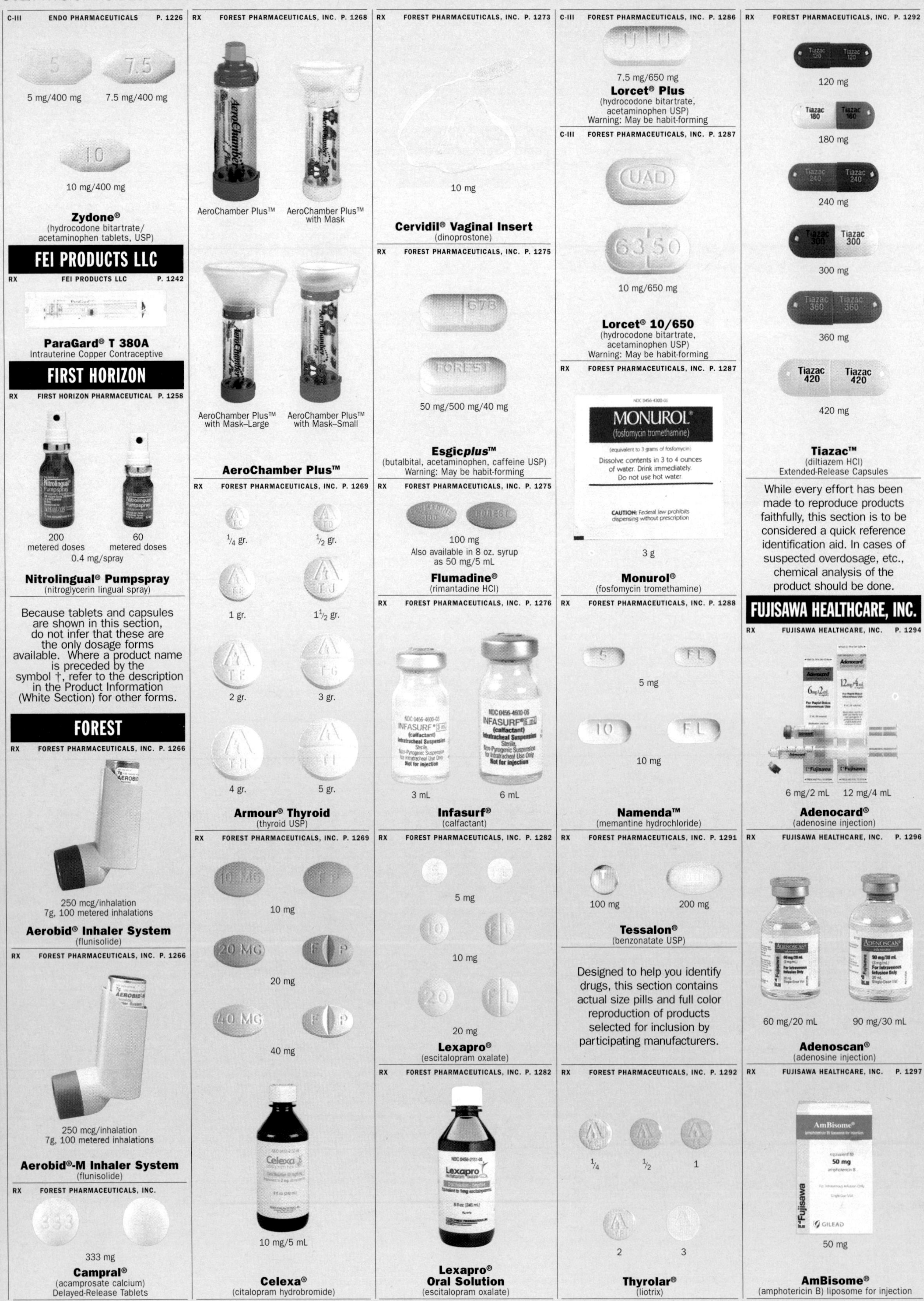

C-III ENDO PHARMACEUTICALS P. 1226

5 mg/400 mg 7.5 mg/400 mg

10 mg/400 mg

Zydone®
(hydrocodone bitartrate/ acetaminophen tablets, USP)

FEI PRODUCTS LLC

RX FEI PRODUCTS LLC P. 1242

ParaGard® T 380A
Intrauterine Copper Contraceptive

FIRST HORIZON

RX FIRST HORIZON PHARMACEUTICAL P. 1258

200 metered doses 60 metered doses
0.4 mg/spray

Nitrolingual® Pumpspray
(nitroglycerin lingual spray)

Because tablets and capsules are shown in this section, do not infer that these are the only dosage forms available. Where a product name is preceded by the symbol †, refer to the description in the Product Information (White Section) for other forms.

FOREST

RX FOREST PHARMACEUTICALS, INC. P. 1266

250 mcg/inhalation
7g, 100 metered inhalations

Aerobid® Inhaler System
(flunisolide)

RX FOREST PHARMACEUTICALS, INC. P. 1266

250 mcg/inhalation
7g, 100 metered inhalations

Aerobid®-M Inhaler System
(flunisolide)

RX FOREST PHARMACEUTICALS, INC.

333 mg

Campral®
(acamprosate calcium)
Delayed-Release Tablets

RX FOREST PHARMACEUTICALS, INC. P. 1268

AeroChamber Plus™ AeroChamber Plus™ with Mask

AeroChamber Plus™ with Mask–Large AeroChamber Plus™ with Mask–Small

AeroChamber Plus™

RX FOREST PHARMACEUTICALS, INC. P. 1269

1/4 gr. 1/2 gr.

1 gr. 1½ gr.

2 gr. 3 gr.

4 gr. 5 gr.

Armour® Thyroid
(thyroid USP)

RX FOREST PHARMACEUTICALS, INC. P. 1269

10 mg

20 mg

40 mg

10 mg/5 mL

Celexa®
(citalopram hydrobromide)

RX FOREST PHARMACEUTICALS, INC. P. 1273

10 mg

Cervidil® Vaginal Insert
(dinoprostone)

RX FOREST PHARMACEUTICALS, INC. P. 1275

50 mg/500 mg/40 mg

Esgic*plus*™
(butalbital, acetaminophen, caffeine USP)
Warning: May be habit-forming

RX FOREST PHARMACEUTICALS, INC. P. 1275

100 mg
Also available in 8 oz. syrup as 50 mg/5 mL

Flumadine®
(rimantadine HCl)

RX FOREST PHARMACEUTICALS, INC. P. 1276

3 mL 6 mL

Infasurf®
(calfactant)

RX FOREST PHARMACEUTICALS, INC. P. 1282

5 mg

10 mg

20 mg

Lexapro®
(escitalopram oxalate)

RX FOREST PHARMACEUTICALS, INC. P. 1282

Lexapro®
Oral Solution
(escitalopram oxalate)

C-III FOREST PHARMACEUTICALS, INC. P. 1286

7.5 mg/650 mg

Lorcet® Plus
(hydrocodone bitartrate, acetaminophen USP)
Warning: May be habit-forming

C-III FOREST PHARMACEUTICALS, INC. P. 1287

10 mg/650 mg

Lorcet® 10/650
(hydrocodone bitartrate, acetaminophen USP)
Warning: May be habit-forming

RX FOREST PHARMACEUTICALS, INC. P. 1287

3 g

Monurol®
(fosfomycin tromethamine)

RX FOREST PHARMACEUTICALS, INC. P. 1288

5 mg

10 mg

Namenda™
(memantine hydrochloride)

RX FOREST PHARMACEUTICALS, INC. P. 1291

100 mg 200 mg

Tessalon®
(benzonatate USP)

Designed to help you identify drugs, this section contains actual size pills and full color reproduction of products selected for inclusion by participating manufacturers.

RX FOREST PHARMACEUTICALS, INC. P. 1292

1/4 1/2 1

2 3

Thyrolar®
(liotrix)

RX FOREST PHARMACEUTICALS, INC. P. 1292

120 mg

180 mg

240 mg

300 mg

360 mg

420 mg

Tiazac™
(diltiazem HCl)
Extended-Release Capsules

While every effort has been made to reproduce products faithfully, this section is to be considered a quick reference identification aid. In cases of suspected overdosage, etc., chemical analysis of the product should be done.

FUJISAWA HEALTHCARE, INC.

RX FUJISAWA HEALTHCARE, INC. P. 1294

6 mg/2 mL 12 mg/4 mL

Adenocard®
(adenosine injection)

RX FUJISAWA HEALTHCARE, INC. P. 1296

60 mg/20 mL 90 mg/30 mL

Adenoscan®
(adenosine injection)

RX FUJISAWA HEALTHCARE, INC. P. 1297

50 mg

AmBisome®
(amphotericin B) liposome for injection

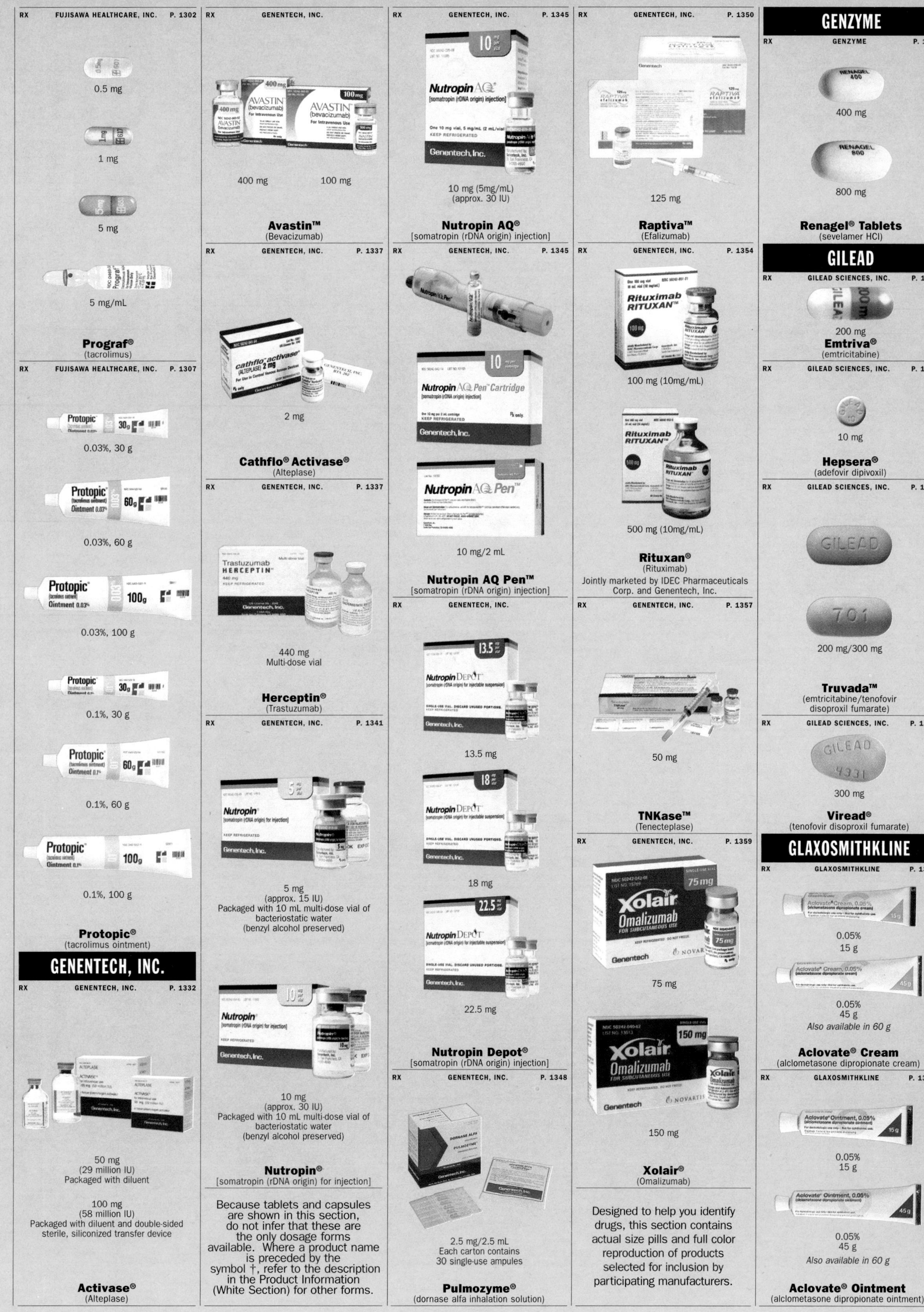

RX FUJISAWA HEALTHCARE, INC. P. 1302

0.5 mg

1 mg

5 mg

5 mg/mL

Prograf®
(tacrolimus)

RX FUJISAWA HEALTHCARE, INC. P. 1307

0.03%, 30 g

0.03%, 60 g

0.03%, 100 g

0.1%, 30 g

0.1%, 60 g

0.1%, 100 g

Protopic®
(tacrolimus ointment)

GENENTECH, INC.

RX GENENTECH, INC. P. 1332

50 mg
(29 million IU)
Packaged with diluent

100 mg
(58 million IU)
Packaged with diluent and double-sided sterile, siliconized transfer device

Activase®
(Alteplase)

RX GENENTECH, INC.

400 mg 100 mg

Avastin™
(Bevacizumab)

RX GENENTECH, INC. P. 1337

2 mg

Cathflo® Activase®
(Alteplase)

RX GENENTECH, INC. P. 1337

440 mg
Multi-dose vial

Herceptin®
(Trastuzumab)

RX GENENTECH, INC. P. 1341

5 mg
(approx. 15 IU)
Packaged with 10 mL multi-dose vial of bacteriostatic water
(benzyl alcohol preserved)

10 mg
(approx. 30 IU)
Packaged with 10 mL multi-dose vial of bacteriostatic water
(benzyl alcohol preserved)

Nutropin®
[somatropin (rDNA origin) for injection]

Because tablets and capsules are shown in this section, do not infer that these are the only dosage forms available. Where a product name is preceded by the symbol †, refer to the description in the Product Information (White Section) for other forms.

RX GENENTECH, INC. P. 1345

10 mg (5mg/mL)
(approx. 30 IU)

Nutropin AQ®
[somatropin (rDNA origin) injection]

RX GENENTECH, INC. P. 1345

10 mg/2 mL

Nutropin AQ Pen™
[somatropin (rDNA origin) injection]

RX GENENTECH, INC.

13.5 mg

18 mg

22.5 mg

Nutropin Depot®
[somatropin (rDNA origin) injection]

RX GENENTECH, INC. P. 1348

2.5 mg/2.5 mL
Each carton contains
30 single-use ampules

Pulmozyme®
(dornase alfa inhalation solution)

RX GENENTECH, INC. P. 1350

125 mg

Raptiva™
(Efalizumab)

RX GENENTECH, INC. P. 1354

100 mg (10mg/mL)

500 mg (10mg/mL)

Rituxan®
(Rituximab)
Jointly marketed by IDEC Pharmaceuticals Corp. and Genentech, Inc.

RX GENENTECH, INC. P. 1357

50 mg

TNKase™
(Tenecteplase)

RX GENENTECH, INC. P. 1359

75 mg

150 mg

Xolair®
(Omalizumab)

Designed to help you identify drugs, this section contains actual size pills and full color reproduction of products selected for inclusion by participating manufacturers.

GENZYME

RX GENZYME P. 1366

400 mg

800 mg

Renagel® Tablets
(sevelamer HCl)

GILEAD

RX GILEAD SCIENCES, INC. P. 1370

200 mg

Emtriva®
(emtricitabine)

RX GILEAD SCIENCES, INC. P. 1373

10 mg

Hepsera®
(adefovir dipivoxil)

RX GILEAD SCIENCES, INC. P. 1376

200 mg/300 mg

Truvada™
(emtricitabine/tenofovir disoproxil fumarate)

RX GILEAD SCIENCES, INC. P. 1381

300 mg

Viread®
(tenofovir disoproxil fumarate)

GLAXOSMITHKLINE

RX GLAXOSMITHKLINE P. 1386

0.05%
15 g

0.05%
45 g
Also available in 60 g

Aclovate® Cream
(alclometasone dipropionate cream)

RX GLAXOSMITHKLINE P. 1386

0.05%
15 g

0.05%
45 g
Also available in 60 g

Aclovate® Ointment
(alclometasone dipropionate ointment)

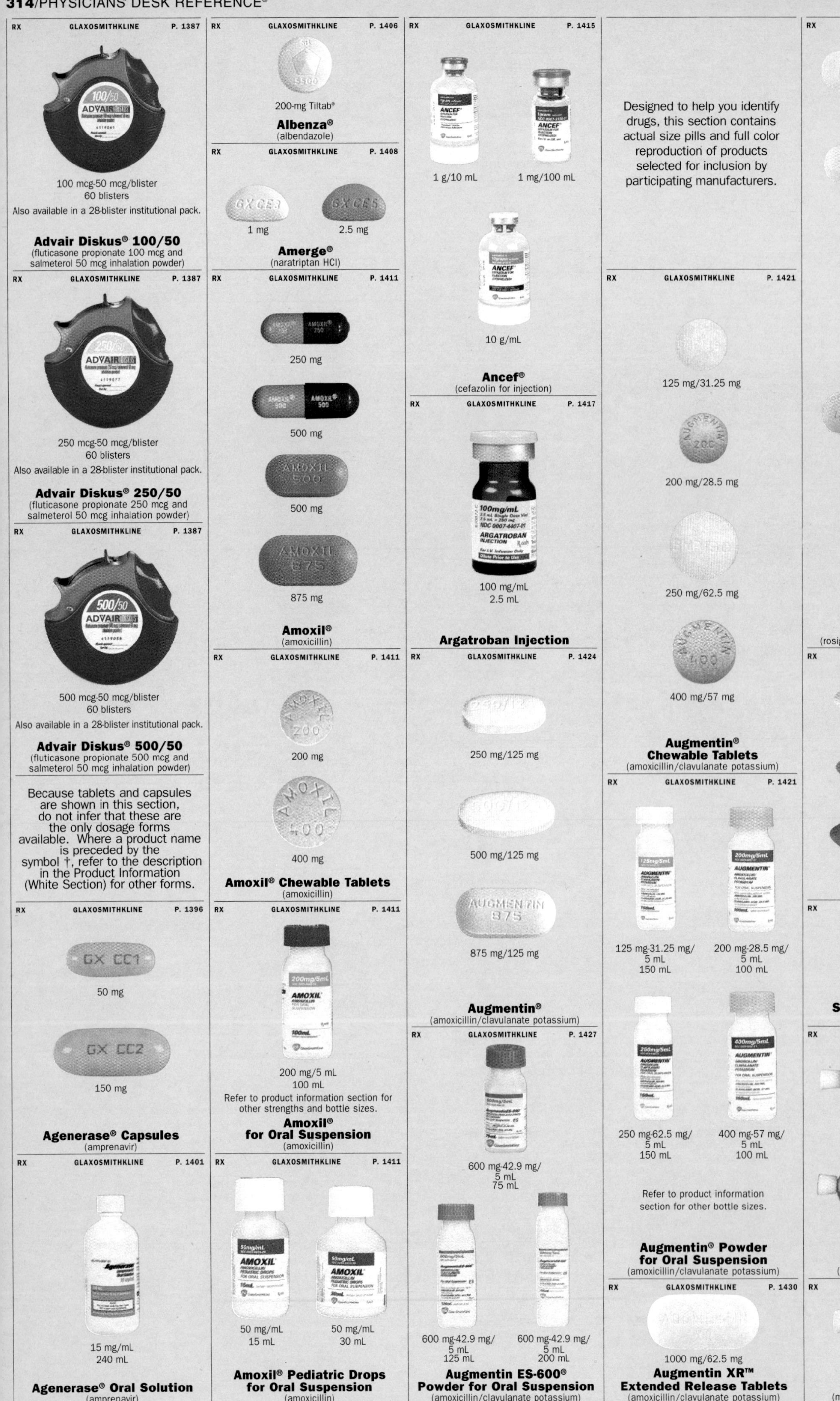

RX GLAXOSMITHKLINE P. 1387

100 mcg-50 mcg/blister
60 blisters
Also available in a 28-blister institutional pack.

Advair Diskus® 100/50
(fluticasone propionate 100 mcg and salmeterol 50 mcg inhalation powder)

RX GLAXOSMITHKLINE P. 1387

250 mcg-50 mcg/blister
60 blisters
Also available in a 28-blister institutional pack.

Advair Diskus® 250/50
(fluticasone propionate 250 mcg and salmeterol 50 mcg inhalation powder)

RX GLAXOSMITHKLINE P. 1387

500 mcg-50 mcg/blister
60 blisters
Also available in a 28-blister institutional pack.

Advair Diskus® 500/50
(fluticasone propionate 500 mcg and salmeterol 50 mcg inhalation powder)

Because tablets and capsules are shown in this section, do not infer that these are the only dosage forms available. Where a product name is preceded by the symbol †, refer to the description in the Product Information (White Section) for other forms.

RX GLAXOSMITHKLINE P. 1396

50 mg

150 mg

Agenerase® Capsules
(amprenavir)

RX GLAXOSMITHKLINE P. 1401

15 mg/mL
240 mL

Agenerase® Oral Solution
(amprenavir)

RX GLAXOSMITHKLINE P. 1406

200-mg Tiltab®

Albenza®
(albendazole)

RX GLAXOSMITHKLINE P. 1408

1 mg 2.5 mg

Amerge®
(naratriptan HCl)

RX GLAXOSMITHKLINE P. 1411

250 mg

500 mg

500 mg

875 mg

Amoxil®
(amoxicillin)

RX GLAXOSMITHKLINE P. 1411

200 mg

400 mg

Amoxil® Chewable Tablets
(amoxicillin)

RX GLAXOSMITHKLINE P. 1411

200 mg/5 mL
100 mL
Refer to product information section for other strengths and bottle sizes.

Amoxil® for Oral Suspension
(amoxicillin)

RX GLAXOSMITHKLINE P. 1411

50 mg/mL 15 mL

50 mg/mL 30 mL

Amoxil® Pediatric Drops for Oral Suspension
(amoxicillin)

RX GLAXOSMITHKLINE P. 1415

1 g/10 mL 1 mg/100 mL

10 g/mL

Ancef®
(cefazolin for injection)

RX GLAXOSMITHKLINE P. 1417

100 mg/mL
2.5 mL

Argatroban Injection

RX GLAXOSMITHKLINE P. 1424

250 mg/125 mg

500 mg/125 mg

875 mg/125 mg

Augmentin®
(amoxicillin/clavulanate potassium)

RX GLAXOSMITHKLINE P. 1427

600 mg-42.9 mg/
5 mL
75 mL

600 mg-42.9 mg/
5 mL
125 mL

600 mg-42.9 mg/
5 mL
200 mL

Augmentin ES-600® Powder for Oral Suspension
(amoxicillin/clavulanate potassium)

Designed to help you identify drugs, this section contains actual size pills and full color reproduction of products selected for inclusion by participating manufacturers.

RX GLAXOSMITHKLINE P. 1421

125 mg/31.25 mg

200 mg/28.5 mg

250 mg/62.5 mg

400 mg/57 mg

Augmentin® Chewable Tablets
(amoxicillin/clavulanate potassium)

RX GLAXOSMITHKLINE P. 1421

125 mg-31.25 mg/
5 mL
150 mL

200 mg-28.5 mg/
5 mL
100 mL

250 mg-62.5 mg/
5 mL
150 mL

400 mg-57 mg/
5 mL
100 mL

Refer to product information section for other bottle sizes.

Augmentin® Powder for Oral Suspension
(amoxicillin/clavulanate potassium)

RX GLAXOSMITHKLINE P. 1430

1000 mg/62.5 mg

Augmentin XR™ Extended Release Tablets
(amoxicillin/clavulanate potassium)

RX GLAXOSMITHKLINE P. 1433

1 mg/500 mg

2 mg/500 mg

2 mg/1000 mg

4 mg/500 mg

4 mg/1000 mg

Avandamet™
(rosiglitazone maleate/metformin HCl)

RX GLAXOSMITHKLINE P. 1438

2-mg Tiltab®

4-mg Tiltab®

8-mg Tiltab®

Avandia®
(rosiglitazone maleate)

RX GLAXOSMITHKLINE P. 1443

0.5 mg

Avodart™ Soft Gelatin Capsules
(dutasteride)

RX GLAXOSMITHKLINE P. 1446

2%
15 g

2%
30 g

Bactroban Cream®
(mupirocin calcium cream, 2%)

RX GLAXOSMITHKLINE P. 1446

2%
1 g

Bactroban Nasal®
(mupirocin calcium ointment, 2%)

RX GLAXOSMITHKLINE P. 1447

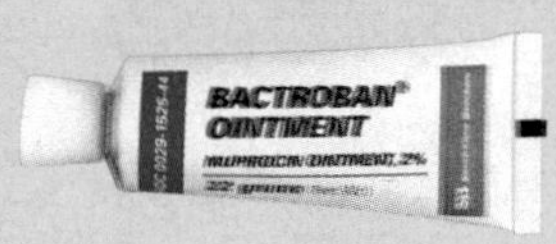

2%
22 g

Bactroban Ointment®
(mupirocin ointment, 2%)

While every effort has been made to reproduce products faithfully, this section is to be considered a quick reference identification aid. In cases of suspected overdosage, etc., chemical analysis of the product should be done.

RX GLAXOSMITHKLINE P. 1448

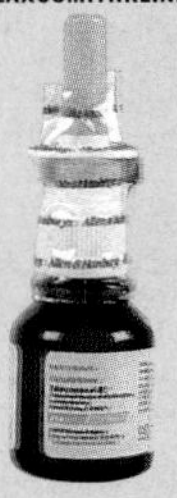

42 mcg/spray
25 g
180 metered sprays

Beconase AQ® Nasal Spray, 42 mcg
(beclomethasone dipropionate, monohydrate)

RX GLAXOSMITHKLINE P. 1450

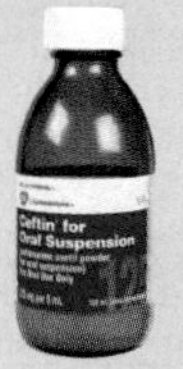

125 mg/5 mL
100 mL

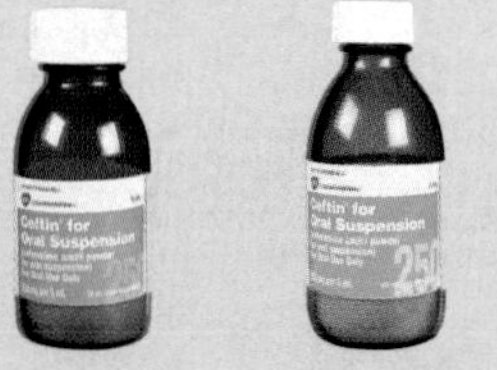

250 mg/5 mL
50 mL

250 mg/5 mL
100 mL

Ceftin® for Oral Suspension
(cefuroxime axetil powder for oral suspension)

RX GLAXOSMITHKLINE P. 1450

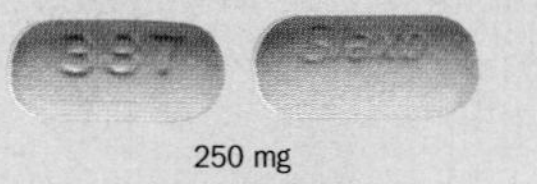

250 mg

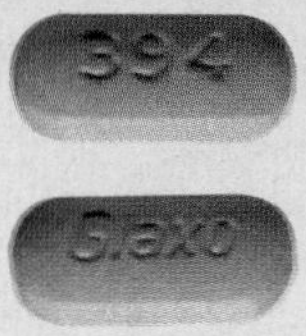

500 mg

Ceftin®
(cefuroxime axetil tablets)

RX GLAXOSMITHKLINE P. 1454

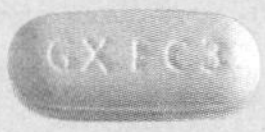

150 mg/300 mg

Combivir®
(lamivudine/zidovudine)

RX GLAXOSMITHKLINE P. 1457

3.125 mg Tiltab®

6.25 mg Tiltab®

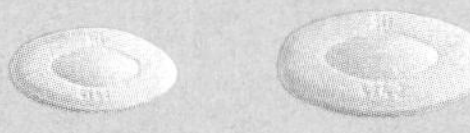

12.5 mg Tiltab®

25 mg Tiltab®

Coreg®
(carvedilol)

RX GLAXOSMITHKLINE P. 1461

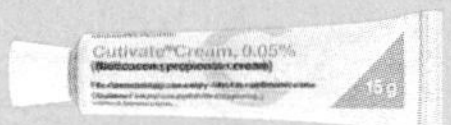

0.05%
15 g

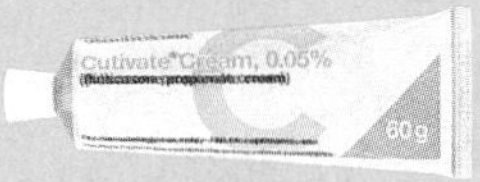

0.05%
60 g
Also available in 30 g

Cutivate® Cream
(fluticasone propionate cream)

RX GLAXOSMITHKLINE P. 1463

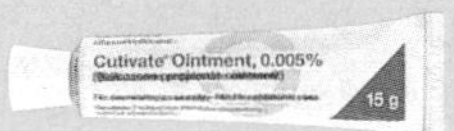

0.005%
15 g

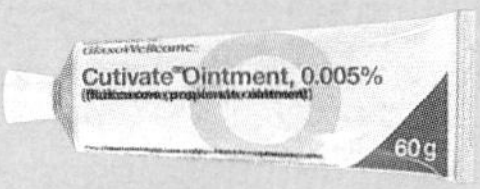

0.005%
60 g
Also available in 30 g

Cutivate® Ointment
(fluticasone propionate ointment)

RX GLAXOSMITHKLINE P. 1464

25 mg

Daraprim®
(pyrimethamine)

C-II GLAXOSMITHKLINE P. 1465

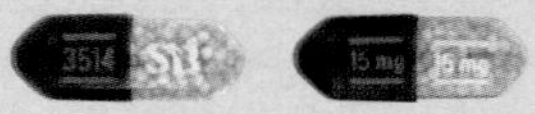

15-mg Spansule®
Also available as 5-mg Spansule® and 10-mg Spansule® capsules.

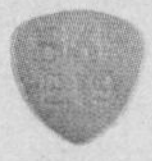

5 mg

Dexedrine®
(dextroamphetamine sulfate)

RX GLAXOSMITHKLINE P. 1466

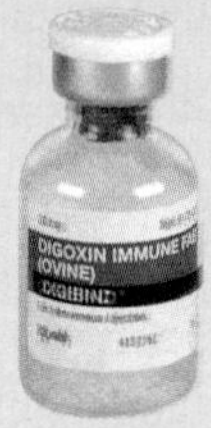

38 mg

Digibind® Digoxin Immune Fab
(ovine)

RX GLAXOSMITHKLINE P. 1468

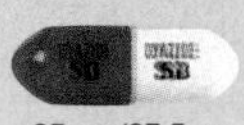

25 mg/37.5 mg

Dyazide®
(hydrochlorothiazide/triamterene)

RX GLAXOSMITHKLINE P. 1470

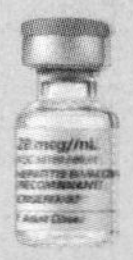

20 mcg/mL single-dose vial
Adult Dose

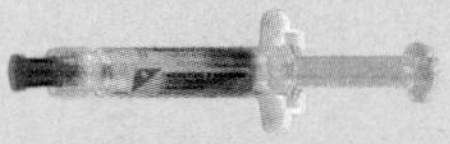

20 mcg/mL single-dose, prefilled, disposable Tip-Lok® syringe
Adult Dose

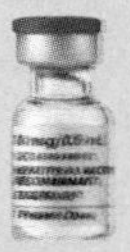

10 mcg/0.5 mL single-dose vial
Pediatric Dose/Adolescent Dose

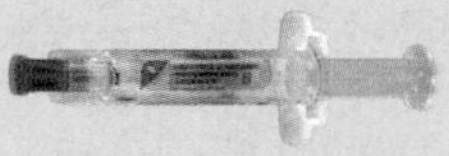

10 mcg/0.5 mL single-dose, prefilled, disposable Tip-Lok® syringe
Pediatric/Adolescent Dose

Also available in Pediatric/Adolescent Dose 10 mcg/0.5 mL single-dose, prefilled, disposable Tip-Lok® syringes with 5/8-inch 25-gauge SafetyGlide™ needles.

Engerix-B®
[Hepatitis B Vaccine (Recombinant)]

Because tablets and capsules are shown in this section, do not infer that these are the only dosage forms available. Where a product name is preceded by the symbol †, refer to the description in the Product Information (White Section) for other forms.

RX GLAXOSMITHKLINE P. 1473

150 mg

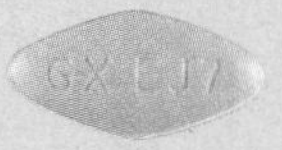

300 mg

Epivir®
(lamivudine tablets)

RX GLAXOSMITHKLINE P. 1473

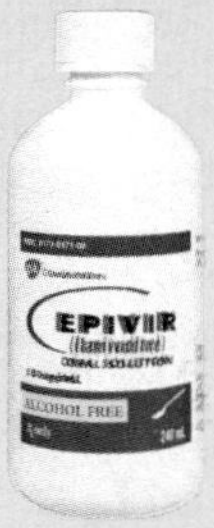

10 mg/ml
240 mL

Epivir® Oral Solution
(lamivudine oral solution)

RX GLAXOSMITHKLINE P. 1477

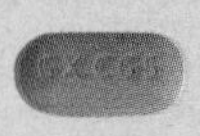

100 mg

Epivir-HBV®
(lamivudine)

RX GLAXOSMITHKLINE P. 1477

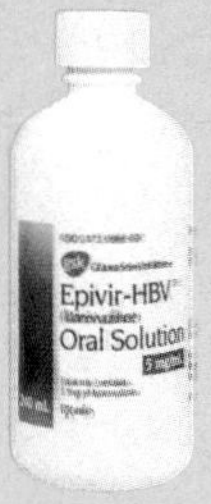

5 mg/mL
240 mL

Epivir-HBV® Oral Solution
(lamivudine)

RX GLAXOSMITHKLINE P. 1485

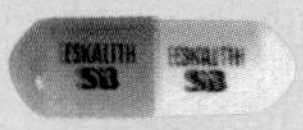

300 mg

Eskalith®
(lithium carbonate)

RX GLAXOSMITHKLINE P. 1485

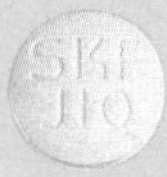

450 mg

Eskalith CR® Controlled-Release Tablets
(lithium carbonate)

RX GLAXOSMITHKLINE P. 1487

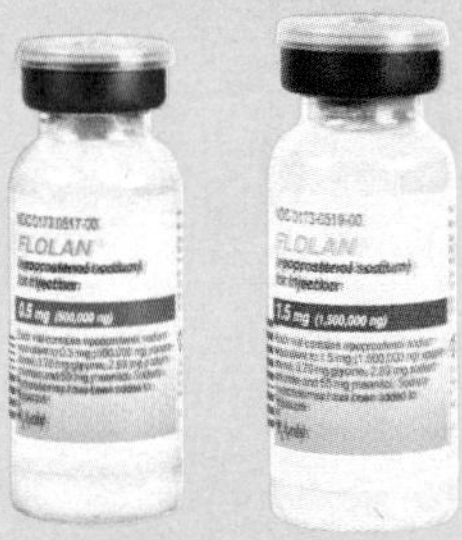

0.5 mg

1.5 mg

Flolan® for Injection
(epoprostenol sodium)

RX GLAXOSMITHKLINE P. 1491

50 mcg/spray
16 g
120 metered sprays

Flonase® Nasal Spray, 50 mcg
(fluticasone propionate)

RX GLAXOSMITHKLINE P. 1494

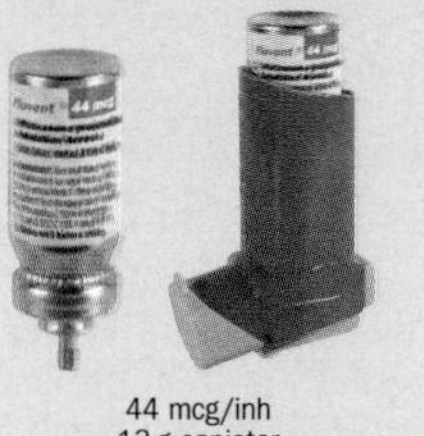

44 mcg/inh
13-g canister
120 metered inhalations
Also available in 7.9-g canister.

Flovent® 44 mcg Inhalation Aerosol
(fluticasone propionate, 44 mcg)

RX GLAXOSMITHKLINE P. 1494

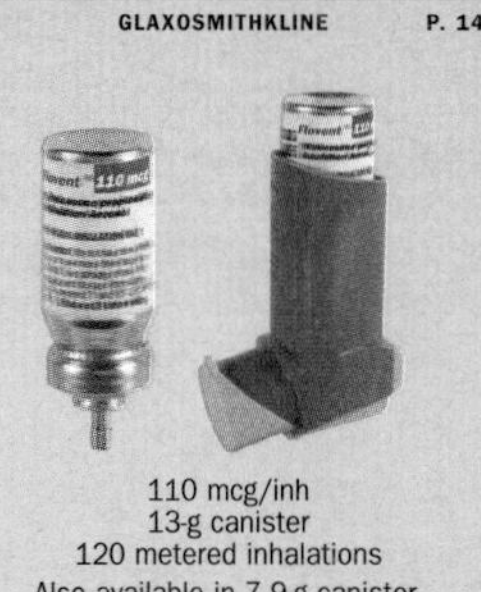

110 mcg/inh
13-g canister
120 metered inhalations
Also available in 7.9-g canister.

Flovent® 110 mcg Inhalation Aerosol
(fluticasone propionate, 110 mcg)

RX GLAXOSMITHKLINE P. 1494

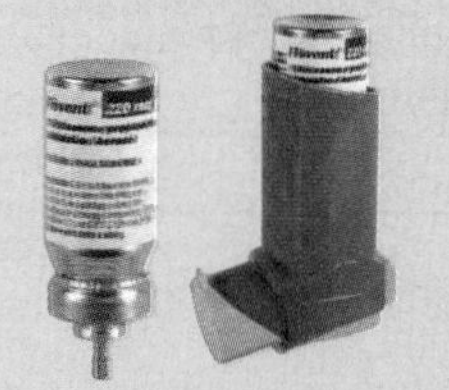

220 mcg/inh
13-g canister
120 metered inhalations
Also available in 7.9-g canister.

Flovent® 220 mcg Inhalation Aerosol
(fluticasone propionate, 220 mcg)

RX GLAXOSMITHKLINE P. 1500

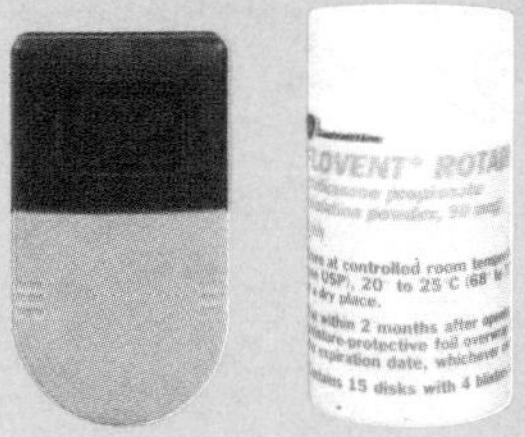

50 mcg/blister

Flovent® Rotadisk® 50 mcg
(fluticasone propionate inhalation powder, 50 mcg)

RX GLAXOSMITHKLINE P. 1500

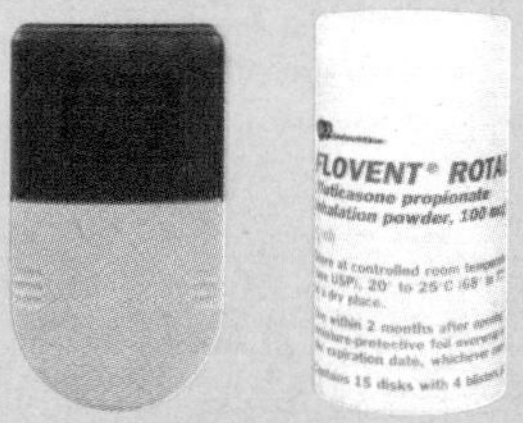

100 mcg/blister

Flovent® Rotadisk® 100 mcg
(fluticasone propionate inhalation powder, 100 mcg)

RX GLAXOSMITHKLINE P. 1500

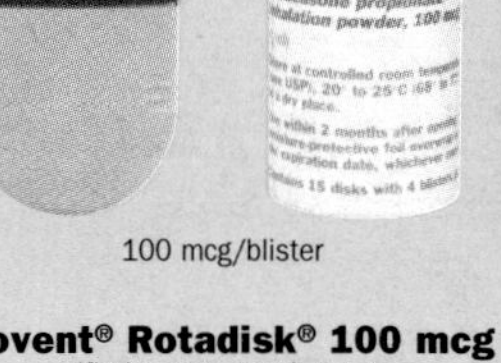

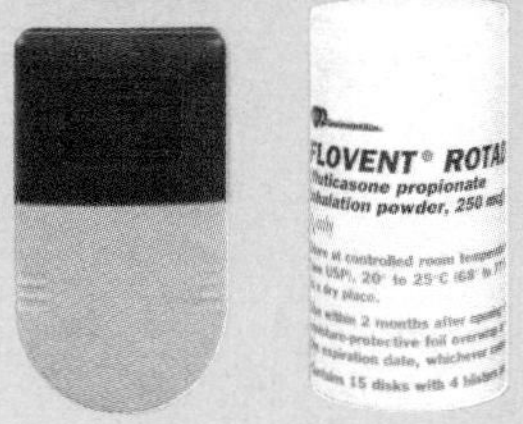

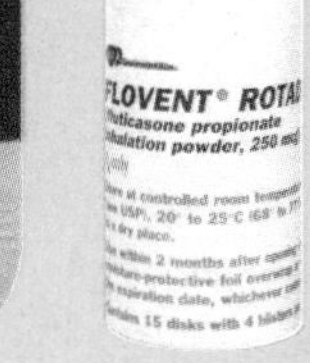

250 mcg/blister

Flovent® Rotadisk® 250 mcg
(fluticasone propionate inhalation powder, 250 mcg)

Designed to help you identify drugs, this section contains actual size pills and full color reproduction of products selected for inclusion by participating manufacturers.

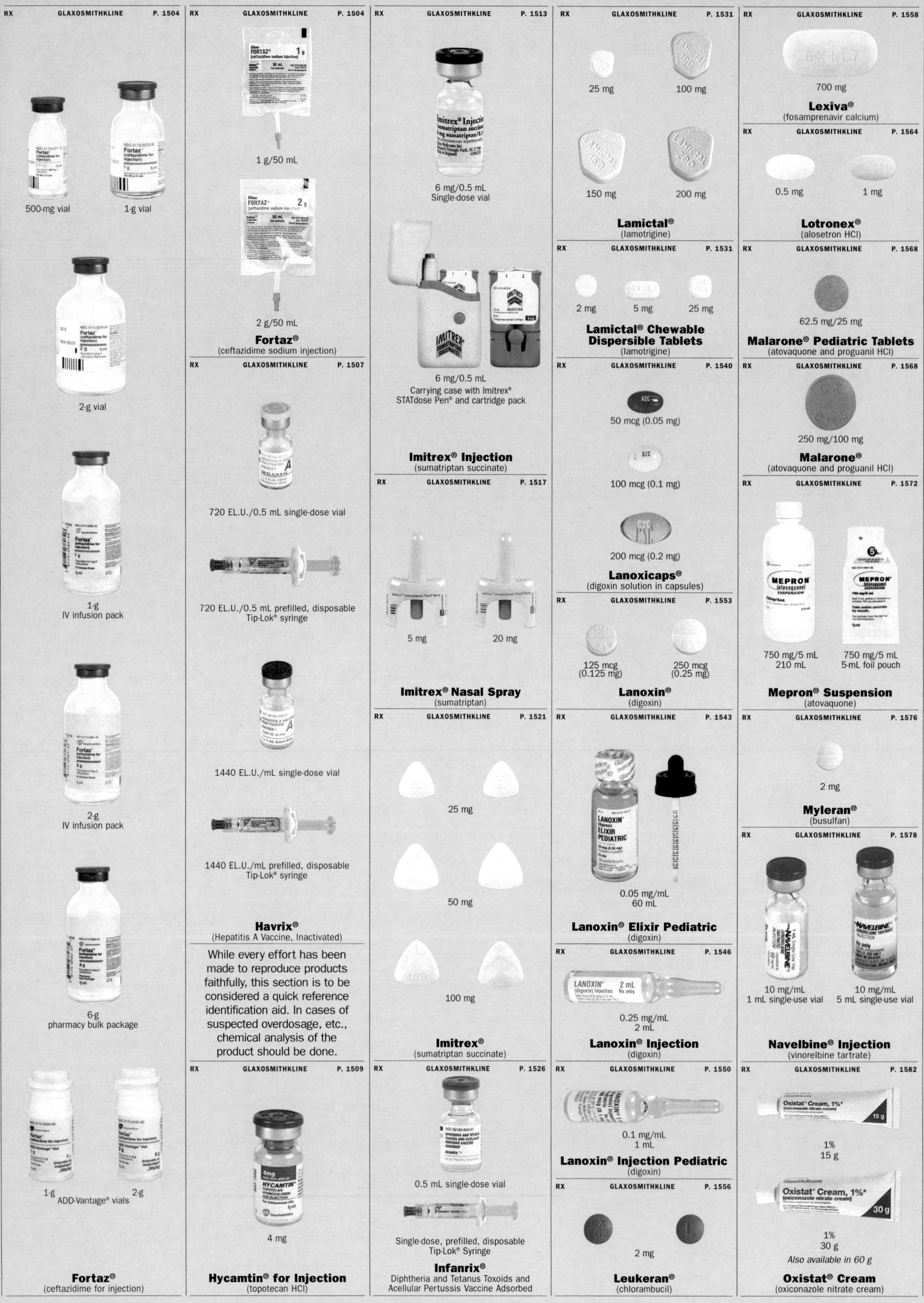

RX GLAXOSMITHKLINE P. 1504

500-mg vial
1-g vial
2-g vial
1-g IV infusion pack
2-g IV infusion pack
6-g pharmacy bulk package
1-g 2-g ADD-Vantage® vials

Fortaz®
(ceftazidime for injection)

RX GLAXOSMITHKLINE P. 1504

1 g/50 mL
2 g/50 mL

Fortaz®
(ceftazidime sodium injection)

RX GLAXOSMITHKLINE P. 1507

720 EL.U./0.5 mL single-dose vial
720 EL.U./0.5 mL prefilled, disposable Tip-Lok® syringe
1440 EL.U./mL single-dose vial
1440 EL.U./mL prefilled, disposable Tip-Lok® syringe

Havrix®
(Hepatitis A Vaccine, Inactivated)

While every effort has been made to reproduce products faithfully, this section is to be considered a quick reference identification aid. In cases of suspected overdosage, etc., chemical analysis of the product should be done.

RX GLAXOSMITHKLINE P. 1509

4 mg

Hycamtin® for Injection
(topotecan HCl)

RX GLAXOSMITHKLINE P. 1513

6 mg/0.5 mL
Single-dose vial
6 mg/0.5 mL
Carrying case with Imitrex® STATdose Pen® and cartridge pack

Imitrex® Injection
(sumatriptan succinate)

RX GLAXOSMITHKLINE P. 1517

5 mg
20 mg

Imitrex® Nasal Spray
(sumatriptan)

RX GLAXOSMITHKLINE P. 1521

25 mg
50 mg
100 mg

Imitrex®
(sumatriptan succinate)

RX GLAXOSMITHKLINE P. 1526

0.5 mL single-dose vial
Single-dose, prefilled, disposable Tip-Lok® Syringe

Infanrix®
Diphtheria and Tetanus Toxoids and Acellular Pertussis Vaccine Adsorbed

RX GLAXOSMITHKLINE P. 1531

25 mg
100 mg
150 mg
200 mg

Lamictal®
(lamotrigine)

RX GLAXOSMITHKLINE P. 1531

2 mg
5 mg
25 mg

Lamictal® Chewable Dispersible Tablets
(lamotrigine)

RX GLAXOSMITHKLINE P. 1540

50 mcg (0.05 mg)
100 mcg (0.1 mg)
200 mcg (0.2 mg)

Lanoxicaps®
(digoxin solution in capsules)

RX GLAXOSMITHKLINE P. 1553

125 mcg (0.125 mg)
250 mcg (0.25 mg)

Lanoxin®
(digoxin)

RX GLAXOSMITHKLINE P. 1543

0.05 mg/mL
60 mL

Lanoxin® Elixir Pediatric
(digoxin)

RX GLAXOSMITHKLINE P. 1546

0.25 mg/mL
2 mL

Lanoxin® Injection
(digoxin)

RX GLAXOSMITHKLINE P. 1550

0.1 mg/mL
1 mL

Lanoxin® Injection Pediatric
(digoxin)

RX GLAXOSMITHKLINE P. 1556

2 mg

Leukeran®
(chlorambucil)

RX GLAXOSMITHKLINE P. 1558

700 mg

Lexiva®
(fosamprenavir calcium)

RX GLAXOSMITHKLINE P. 1564

0.5 mg
1 mg

Lotronex®
(alosetron HCl)

RX GLAXOSMITHKLINE P. 1568

62.5 mg/25 mg

Malarone® Pediatric Tablets
(atovaquone and proguanil HCl)

RX GLAXOSMITHKLINE P. 1568

250 mg/100 mg

Malarone®
(atovaquone and proguanil HCl)

RX GLAXOSMITHKLINE P. 1572

750 mg/5 mL
210 mL
750 mg/5 mL
5-mL foil pouch

Mepron® Suspension
(atovaquone)

RX GLAXOSMITHKLINE P. 1576

2 mg

Myleran®
(busulfan)

RX GLAXOSMITHKLINE P. 1578

10 mg/mL
1 mL single-use vial
10 mg/mL
5 mL single-use vial

Navelbine® Injection
(vinorelbine tartrate)

RX GLAXOSMITHKLINE P. 1582

1%
15 g
1%
30 g
Also available in 60 g

Oxistat® Cream
(oxiconazole nitrate cream)

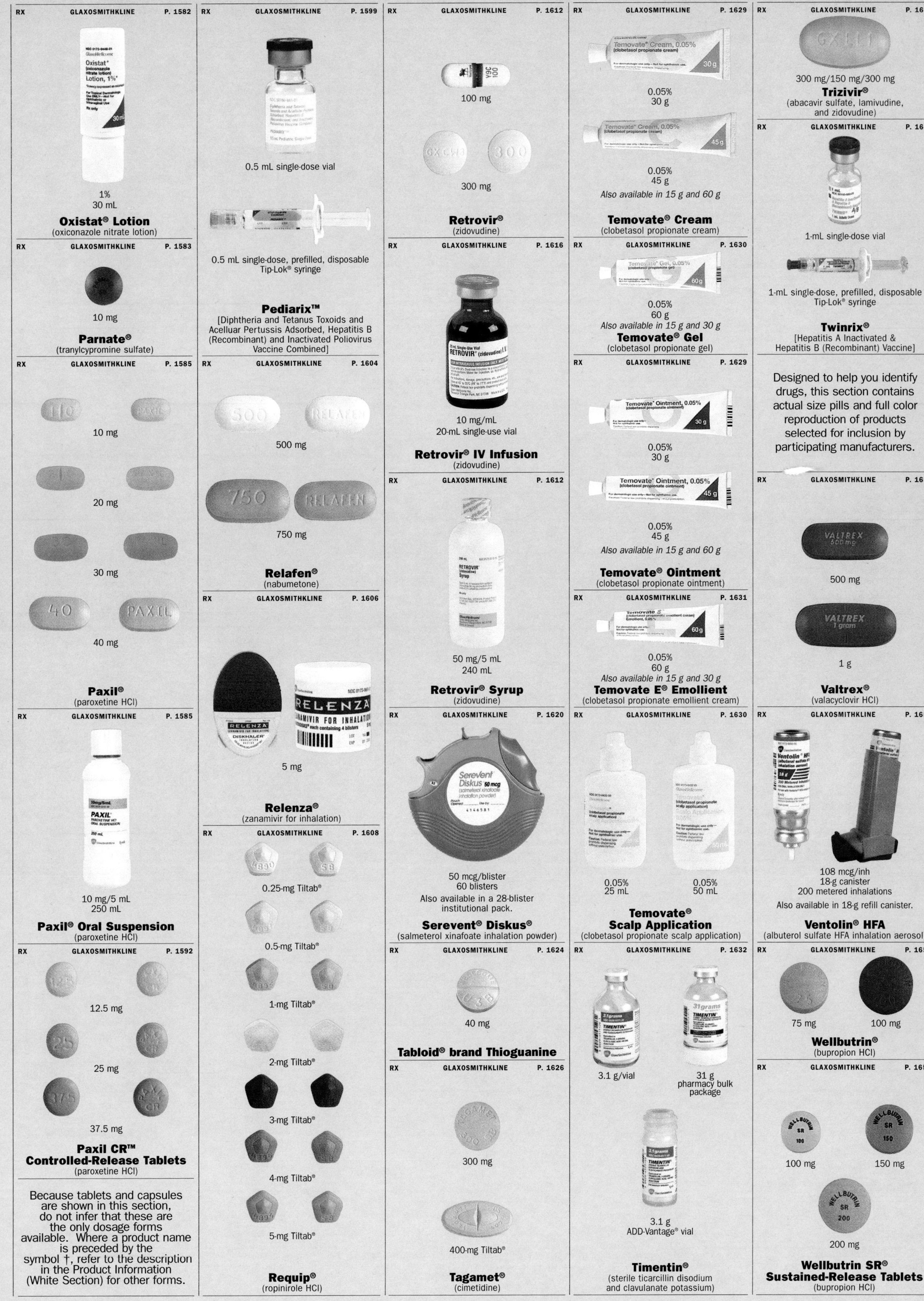

RX GLAXOSMITHKLINE P. 1582

1%
30 mL

Oxistat® Lotion
(oxiconazole nitrate lotion)

RX GLAXOSMITHKLINE P. 1583

10 mg

Parnate®
(tranylcypromine sulfate)

RX GLAXOSMITHKLINE P. 1585

10 mg

20 mg

30 mg

40 mg

Paxil®
(paroxetine HCl)

RX GLAXOSMITHKLINE P. 1585

10 mg/5 mL
250 mL

Paxil® Oral Suspension
(paroxetine HCl)

RX GLAXOSMITHKLINE P. 1592

12.5 mg

25 mg

37.5 mg

Paxil CR™
Controlled-Release Tablets
(paroxetine HCl)

Because tablets and capsules are shown in this section, do not infer that these are the only dosage forms available. Where a product name is preceded by the symbol †, refer to the description in the Product Information (White Section) for other forms.

RX GLAXOSMITHKLINE P. 1599

0.5 mL single-dose vial

0.5 mL single-dose, prefilled, disposable Tip-Lok® syringe

Pediarix™
[Diphtheria and Tetanus Toxoids and Acelluar Pertussis Adsorbed, Hepatitis B (Recombinant) and Inactivated Poliovirus Vaccine Combined]

RX GLAXOSMITHKLINE P. 1604

500 mg

750 mg

Relafen®
(nabumetone)

RX GLAXOSMITHKLINE P. 1606

5 mg

Relenza®
(zanamivir for inhalation)

RX GLAXOSMITHKLINE P. 1608

0.25-mg Tiltab®

0.5-mg Tiltab®

1-mg Tiltab®

2-mg Tiltab®

3-mg Tiltab®

4-mg Tiltab®

5-mg Tiltab®

Requip®
(ropinirole HCl)

RX GLAXOSMITHKLINE P. 1612

100 mg

300 mg

Retrovir®
(zidovudine)

RX GLAXOSMITHKLINE P. 1616

10 mg/mL
20-mL single-use vial

Retrovir® IV Infusion
(zidovudine)

RX GLAXOSMITHKLINE P. 1612

50 mg/5 mL
240 mL

Retrovir® Syrup
(zidovudine)

RX GLAXOSMITHKLINE P. 1620

50 mcg/blister
60 blisters
Also available in a 28-blister institutional pack.

Serevent® Diskus®
(salmeterol xinafoate inhalation powder)

RX GLAXOSMITHKLINE P. 1624

40 mg

Tabloid® brand Thioguanine

RX GLAXOSMITHKLINE P. 1626

300 mg

400-mg Tiltab®

Tagamet®
(cimetidine)

RX GLAXOSMITHKLINE P. 1629

0.05%
30 g

0.05%
45 g
Also available in 15 g and 60 g

Temovate® Cream
(clobetasol propionate cream)

RX GLAXOSMITHKLINE P. 1630

0.05%
60 g
Also available in 15 g and 30 g

Temovate® Gel
(clobetasol propionate gel)

RX GLAXOSMITHKLINE P. 1629

0.05%
30 g

0.05%
45 g
Also available in 15 g and 60 g

Temovate® Ointment
(clobetasol propionate ointment)

RX GLAXOSMITHKLINE P. 1631

0.05%
60 g
Also available in 15 g and 30 g

Temovate E® Emollient
(clobetasol propionate emollient cream)

RX GLAXOSMITHKLINE P. 1630

0.05%
25 mL

0.05%
50 mL

Temovate®
Scalp Application
(clobetasol propionate scalp application)

RX GLAXOSMITHKLINE P. 1632

3.1 g/vial

31 g
pharmacy bulk package

3.1 g
ADD-Vantage® vial

Timentin®
(sterile ticarcillin disodium and clavulanate potassium)

RX GLAXOSMITHKLINE P. 1642

300 mg/150 mg/300 mg

Trizivir®
(abacavir sulfate, lamivudine, and zidovudine)

RX GLAXOSMITHKLINE P. 1648

1-mL single-dose vial

1-mL single-dose, prefilled, disposable Tip-Lok® syringe

Twinrix®
[Hepatitis A Inactivated & Hepatitis B (Recombinant) Vaccine]

Designed to help you identify drugs, this section contains actual size pills and full color reproduction of products selected for inclusion by participating manufacturers.

RX GLAXOSMITHKLINE P. 1650

500 mg

1 g

Valtrex®
(valacyclovir HCl)

RX GLAXOSMITHKLINE P. 1653

108 mcg/inh
18-g canister
200 metered inhalations
Also available in 18-g refill canister.

Ventolin® HFA
(albuterol sulfate HFA inhalation aerosol)

RX GLAXOSMITHKLINE P. 1655

75 mg

100 mg

Wellbutrin®
(bupropion HCl)

RX GLAXOSMITHKLINE P. 1659

100 mg

150 mg

200 mg

Wellbutrin SR®
Sustained-Release Tablets
(bupropion HCl)

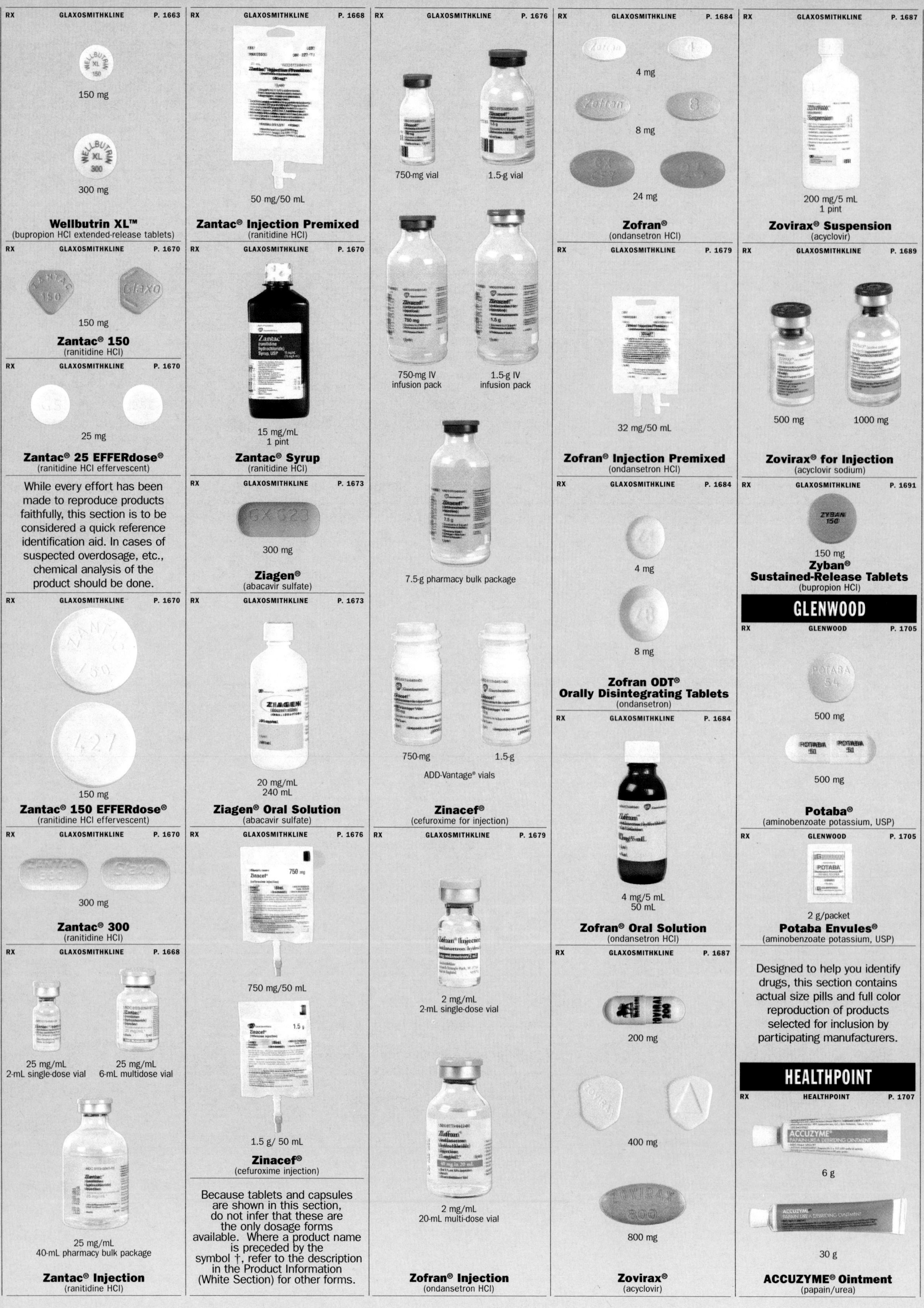

RX GLAXOSMITHKLINE P. 1663

150 mg

300 mg

Wellbutrin XL™
(bupropion HCl extended-release tablets)

RX GLAXOSMITHKLINE P. 1670

150 mg

Zantac® 150
(ranitidine HCl)

RX GLAXOSMITHKLINE P. 1670

25 mg

Zantac® 25 EFFERdose®
(ranitidine HCl effervescent)

While every effort has been made to reproduce products faithfully, this section is to be considered a quick reference identification aid. In cases of suspected overdosage, etc., chemical analysis of the product should be done.

RX GLAXOSMITHKLINE P. 1670

150 mg

Zantac® 150 EFFERdose®
(ranitidine HCl effervescent)

RX GLAXOSMITHKLINE P. 1670

300 mg

Zantac® 300
(ranitidine HCl)

RX GLAXOSMITHKLINE P. 1668

25 mg/mL
2-mL single-dose vial

25 mg/mL
6-mL multidose vial

25 mg/mL
40-mL pharmacy bulk package

Zantac® Injection
(ranitidine HCl)

RX GLAXOSMITHKLINE P. 1668

50 mg/50 mL

Zantac® Injection Premixed
(ranitidine HCl)

RX GLAXOSMITHKLINE P. 1670

15 mg/mL
1 pint

Zantac® Syrup
(ranitidine HCl)

RX GLAXOSMITHKLINE P. 1673

300 mg

Ziagen®
(abacavir sulfate)

RX GLAXOSMITHKLINE P. 1673

20 mg/mL
240 mL

Ziagen® Oral Solution
(abacavir sulfate)

RX GLAXOSMITHKLINE P. 1676

750 mg/50 mL

1.5 g/ 50 mL

Zinacef®
(cefuroxime injection)

Because tablets and capsules are shown in this section, do not infer that these are the only dosage forms available. Where a product name is preceded by the symbol †, refer to the description in the Product Information (White Section) for other forms.

RX GLAXOSMITHKLINE P. 1676

750-mg vial

1.5-g vial

750-mg IV
infusion pack

1.5-g IV
infusion pack

7.5-g pharmacy bulk package

750-mg

1.5-g

ADD-Vantage® vials

Zinacef®
(cefuroxime for injection)

RX GLAXOSMITHKLINE P. 1679

2 mg/mL
2-mL single-dose vial

2 mg/mL
20-mL multi-dose vial

Zofran® Injection
(ondansetron HCl)

RX GLAXOSMITHKLINE P. 1684

4 mg

8 mg

24 mg

Zofran®
(ondansetron HCl)

RX GLAXOSMITHKLINE P. 1679

32 mg/50 mL

Zofran® Injection Premixed
(ondansetron HCl)

RX GLAXOSMITHKLINE P. 1684

4 mg

8 mg

Zofran ODT®
Orally Disintegrating Tablets
(ondansetron)

RX GLAXOSMITHKLINE P. 1684

4 mg/5 mL
50 mL

Zofran® Oral Solution
(ondansetron HCl)

RX GLAXOSMITHKLINE P. 1687

200 mg

400 mg

800 mg

Zovirax®
(acyclovir)

RX GLAXOSMITHKLINE P. 1687

200 mg/5 mL
1 pint

Zovirax® Suspension
(acyclovir)

RX GLAXOSMITHKLINE P. 1689

500 mg

1000 mg

Zovirax® for Injection
(acyclovir sodium)

RX GLAXOSMITHKLINE P. 1691

150 mg

Zyban®
Sustained-Release Tablets
(bupropion HCl)

GLENWOOD

RX GLENWOOD P. 1705

500 mg

500 mg

Potaba®
(aminobenzoate potassium, USP)

RX GLENWOOD P. 1705

2 g/packet

Potaba Envules®
(aminobenzoate potassium, USP)

Designed to help you identify drugs, this section contains actual size pills and full color reproduction of products selected for inclusion by participating manufacturers.

HEALTHPOINT

RX HEALTHPOINT P. 1707

6 g

30 g

ACCUZYME® Ointment
(papain/urea)

RX HEALTHPOINT P. 1708

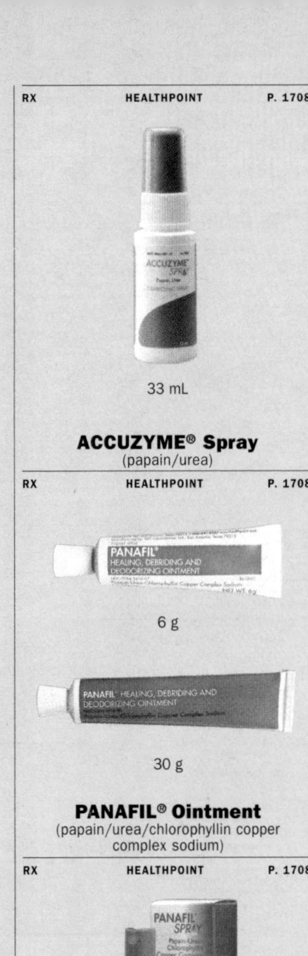

33 mL

ACCUZYME® Spray
(papain/urea)

RX HEALTHPOINT P. 1708

6 g

30 g

PANAFIL® Ointment
(papain/urea/chlorophyllin copper complex sodium)

RX HEALTHPOINT P. 1708

6 g
**Patent Pending

Panafil® Spray**
(papain/urea/chlorophyllin copper complex sodium)

RX HEALTHPOINT P. 1709

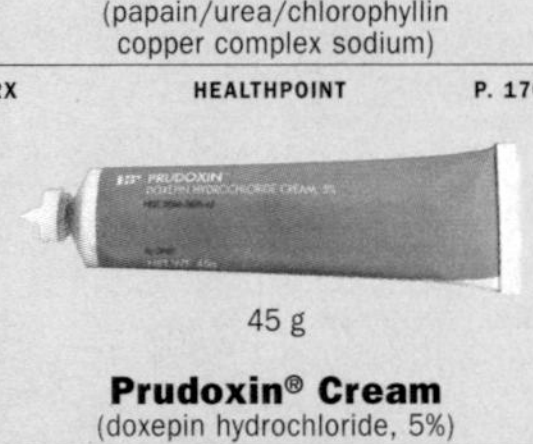

45 g

Prudoxin® Cream
(doxepin hydrochloride, 5%)

RX HEALTHPOINT P. 1709

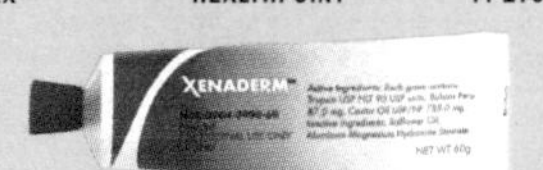

60 g

Xenaderm™ Ointment
(balsam peru/castor oil/trypsin)

While every effort has been made to reproduce products faithfully, this section is to be considered a quick reference identification aid. In cases of suspected overdosage, etc., chemical analysis of the product should be done.

HEMISPHERX BIOPHARMA

RX HEMISPHERX BIOPHARMA P. 1710

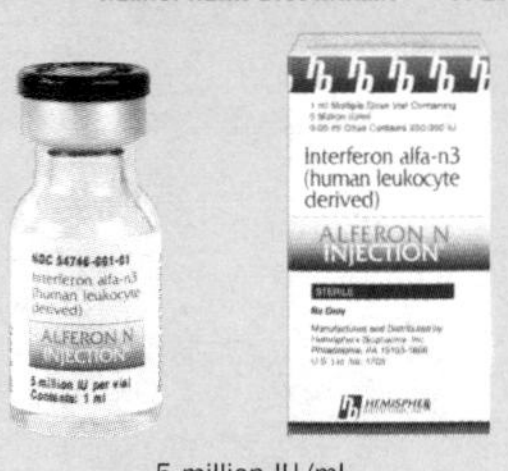

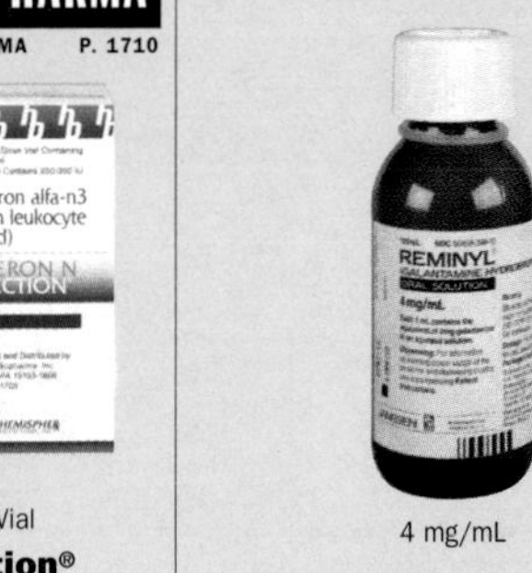

5 million IU/mL
1 mL Multiple Dose Vial

Alferon N Injection®
[Interferon alfa-n3 (human leukocyte derived)]

INTERMUNE

RX INTERMUNE, INC. P. 1714

100 mcg/0.5 mL

Actimmune®
(interferon gamma-1b)

RX INTERMUNE, INC. P. 1716

15 mcg/0.5 mL

Infergen®
(interferon alfacon-1)

Because tablets and capsules are shown in this section, do not infer that these are the only dosage forms available. Where a product name is preceded by the symbol †, refer to the description in the Product Information (White Section) for other forms.

JANSSEN

RX JANSSEN PHARMACEUTICA P. 1726

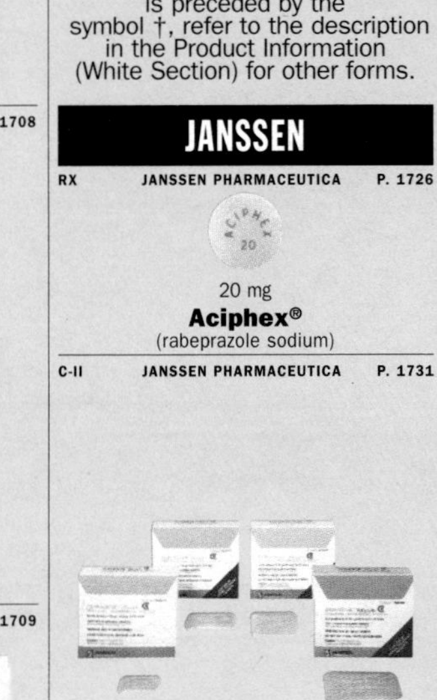

20 mg

Aciphex®
(rabeprazole sodium)

C-II JANSSEN PHARMACEUTICA P. 1731

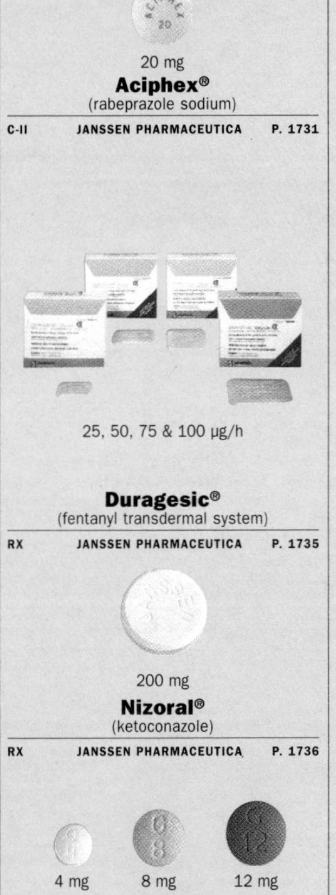

25, 50, 75 & 100 µg/h

Duragesic®
(fentanyl transdermal system)

RX JANSSEN PHARMACEUTICA P. 1735

200 mg

Nizoral®
(ketoconazole)

RX JANSSEN PHARMACEUTICA P. 1736

4 mg 8 mg 12 mg

Reminyl®
(galantamine HBr)

RX JANSSEN PHARMACEUTICA P. 1736

4 mg/mL

Reminyl®
(galantamine HBr oral solution)

RX JANSSEN PHARMACEUTICA P. 1447

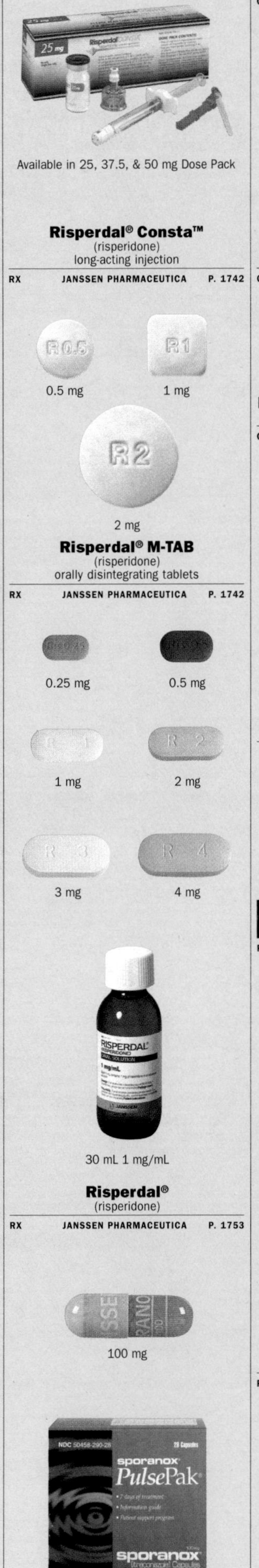

Available in 25, 37.5, & 50 mg Dose Pack

Risperdal® Consta™
(risperidone)
long-acting injection

RX JANSSEN PHARMACEUTICA P. 1742

0.5 mg 1 mg

2 mg

Risperdal® M-TAB
(risperidone)
orally disintegrating tablets

RX JANSSEN PHARMACEUTICA P. 1742

0.25 mg 0.5 mg

1 mg 2 mg

3 mg 4 mg

30 mL 1 mg/mL

Risperdal®
(risperidone)

RX JANSSEN PHARMACEUTICA P. 1753

100 mg

Each PulsePak® contains 28 x 100 mg capsules equivalent to 1 month therapy.

Sporanox®
(itraconazole)

J&J-MERCK CONSUMER

OTC J&J-MERCK CONSUMER P. 1766

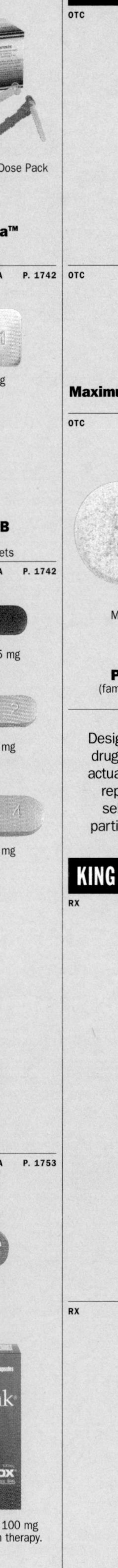

10 mg
Tablets and Gelcaps

Pepcid AC®
(famotidine)

OTC J&J-MERCK CONSUMER P. 1766

20 mg

Maximum Strength Pepcid AC®
(famotidine)

OTC J&J-MERCK CONSUMER P. 1767

10 mg/800 mg/165 mg
Mint and Berry Blend Flavor
Chewable Tablets

Pepcid® Complete
(famotidine/calcium carbonate/magnesium hydroxide)

Designed to help you identify drugs, this section contains actual size pills and full color reproduction of products selected for inclusion by participating manufacturers.

KING PHARMACEUTICALS

RX KING PHARMACEUTICALS P. 1767

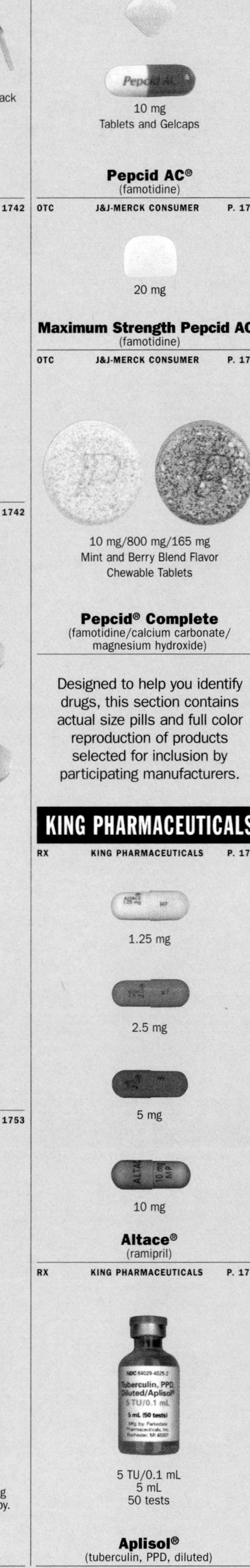

1.25 mg

2.5 mg

5 mg

10 mg

Altace®
(ramipril)

RX KING PHARMACEUTICALS P. 1771

5 TU/0.1 mL
5 mL
50 tests

Aplisol®
(tuberculin, PPD, diluted)

RX KING PHARMACEUTICALS P. 1776

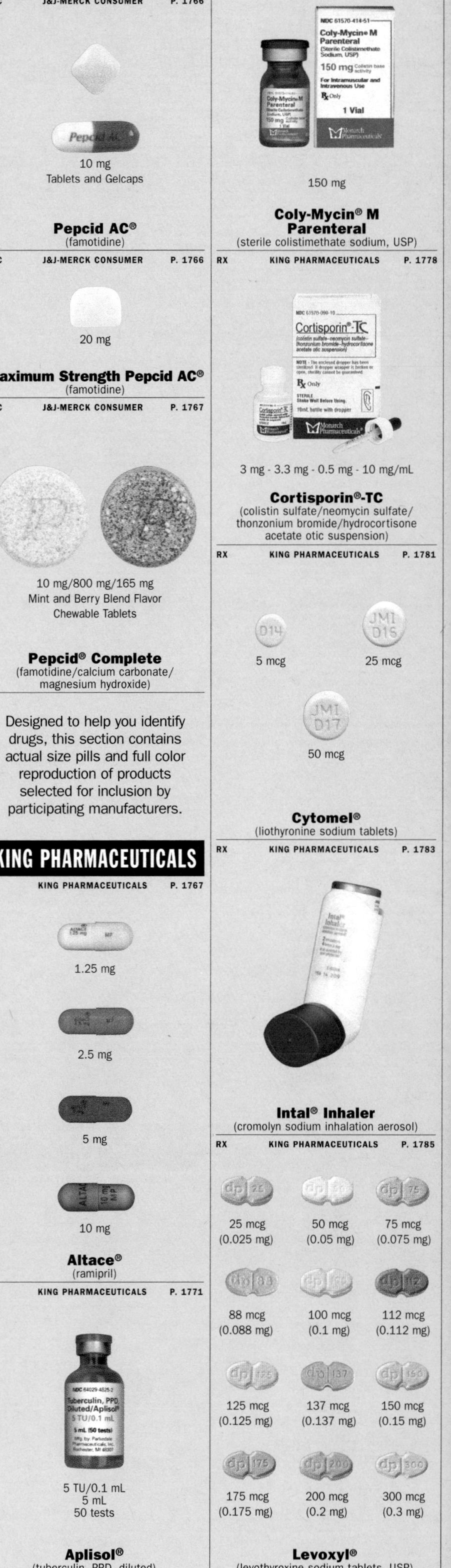

150 mg

Coly-Mycin® M Parenteral
(sterile colistimethate sodium, USP)

RX KING PHARMACEUTICALS P. 1778

3 mg - 3.3 mg - 0.5 mg - 10 mg/mL

Cortisporin®-TC
(colistin sulfate/neomycin sulfate/thonzonium bromide/hydrocortisone acetate otic suspension)

RX KING PHARMACEUTICALS P. 1781

5 mcg 25 mcg

50 mcg

Cytomel®
(liothyronine sodium tablets)

RX KING PHARMACEUTICALS P. 1783

Intal® Inhaler
(cromolyn sodium inhalation aerosol)

RX KING PHARMACEUTICALS P. 1785

25 mcg (0.025 mg) | 50 mcg (0.05 mg) | 75 mcg (0.075 mg)

88 mcg (0.088 mg) | 100 mcg (0.1 mg) | 112 mcg (0.112 mg)

125 mcg (0.125 mg) | 137 mcg (0.137 mg) | 150 mcg (0.15 mg)

175 mcg (0.175 mg) | 200 mcg (0.2 mg) | 300 mcg (0.3 mg)

Levoxyl®
(levothyroxine sodium tablets, USP)

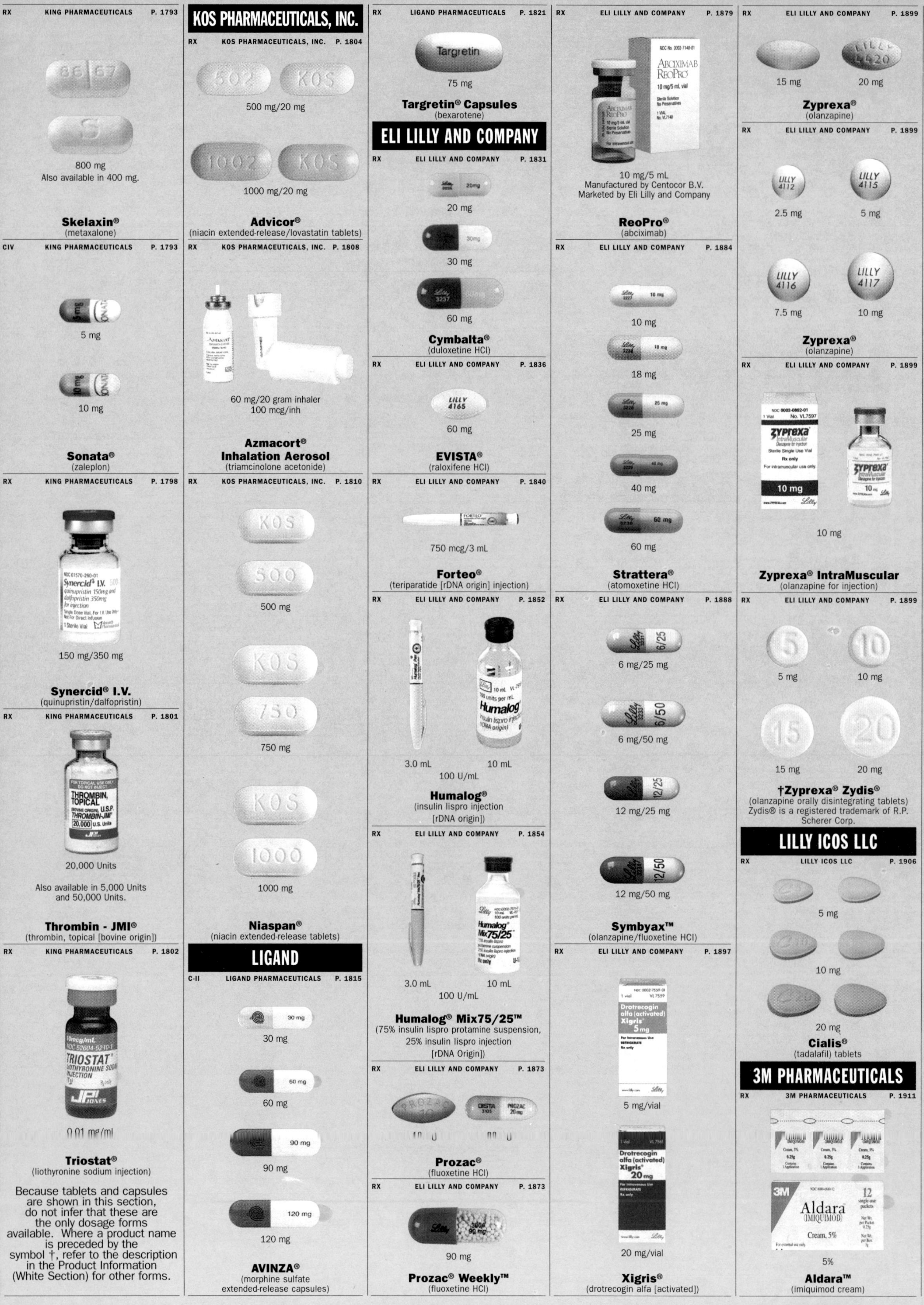

RX KING PHARMACEUTICALS P. 1793

800 mg
Also available in 400 mg.

Skelaxin®
(metaxalone)

CIV KING PHARMACEUTICALS P. 1793

5 mg

10 mg

Sonata®
(zaleplon)

RX KING PHARMACEUTICALS P. 1798

150 mg/350 mg

Synercid® I.V.
(quinupristin/dalfopristin)

RX KING PHARMACEUTICALS P. 1801

20,000 Units

Also available in 5,000 Units and 50,000 Units.

Thrombin - JMI®
(thrombin, topical [bovine origin])

RX KING PHARMACEUTICALS P. 1802

0.01 mg/ml

Triostat®
(liothyronine sodium injection)

Because tablets and capsules are shown in this section, do not infer that these are the only dosage forms available. Where a product name is preceded by the symbol †, refer to the description in the Product Information (White Section) for other forms.

KOS PHARMACEUTICALS, INC.

RX KOS PHARMACEUTICALS, INC. P. 1804

500 mg/20 mg

1000 mg/20 mg

Advicor®
(niacin extended-release/lovastatin tablets)

RX KOS PHARMACEUTICALS, INC. P. 1808

60 mg/20 gram inhaler
100 mcg/inh

Azmacort® Inhalation Aerosol
(triamcinolone acetonide)

RX KOS PHARMACEUTICALS, INC. P. 1810

500 mg

750 mg

1000 mg

Niaspan®
(niacin extended-release tablets)

LIGAND

C-II LIGAND PHARMACEUTICALS P. 1815

30 mg

60 mg

90 mg

120 mg

AVINZA®
(morphine sulfate extended-release capsules)

RX LIGAND PHARMACEUTICALS P. 1821

75 mg

Targretin® Capsules
(bexarotene)

ELI LILLY AND COMPANY

RX ELI LILLY AND COMPANY P. 1831

20 mg

30 mg

60 mg

Cymbalta®
(duloxetine HCl)

RX ELI LILLY AND COMPANY P. 1836

60 mg

EVISTA®
(raloxifene HCl)

RX ELI LILLY AND COMPANY P. 1840

750 mcg/3 mL

Forteo®
(teriparatide [rDNA origin] injection)

RX ELI LILLY AND COMPANY P. 1852

3.0 mL 10 mL
100 U/mL

Humalog®
(insulin lispro injection [rDNA origin])

RX ELI LILLY AND COMPANY P. 1854

3.0 mL 10 mL
100 U/mL

Humalog® Mix75/25™
(75% insulin lispro protamine suspension, 25% insulin lispro injection [rDNA Origin])

RX ELI LILLY AND COMPANY P. 1873

10 mg 20 mg

Prozac®
(fluoxetine HCl)

RX ELI LILLY AND COMPANY P. 1873

90 mg

Prozac® Weekly™
(fluoxetine HCl)

RX ELI LILLY AND COMPANY P. 1879

10 mg/5 mL
Manufactured by Centocor B.V.
Marketed by Eli Lilly and Company

ReoPro®
(abciximab)

RX ELI LILLY AND COMPANY P. 1884

10 mg

18 mg

25 mg

40 mg

60 mg

Strattera®
(atomoxetine HCl)

RX ELI LILLY AND COMPANY P. 1888

6 mg/25 mg

6 mg/50 mg

12 mg/25 mg

12 mg/50 mg

Symbyax™
(olanzapine/fluoxetine HCl)

RX ELI LILLY AND COMPANY P. 1897

5 mg/vial

20 mg/vial

Xigris®
(drotrecogin alfa [activated])

RX ELI LILLY AND COMPANY P. 1899

15 mg 20 mg

Zyprexa®
(olanzapine)

RX ELI LILLY AND COMPANY P. 1899

2.5 mg 5 mg

7.5 mg 10 mg

Zyprexa®
(olanzapine)

RX ELI LILLY AND COMPANY P. 1899

10 mg

Zyprexa® IntraMuscular
(olanzapine for injection)

RX ELI LILLY AND COMPANY P. 1899

5 mg 10 mg

15 mg 20 mg

†Zyprexa® Zydis®
(olanzapine orally disintegrating tablets)
Zydis® is a registered trademark of R.P. Scherer Corp.

LILLY ICOS LLC

RX LILLY ICOS LLC P. 1906

5 mg

10 mg

20 mg

Cialis®
(tadalafil) tablets

3M PHARMACEUTICALS

RX 3M PHARMACEUTICALS P. 1911

5%

Aldara™
(imiquimod cream)

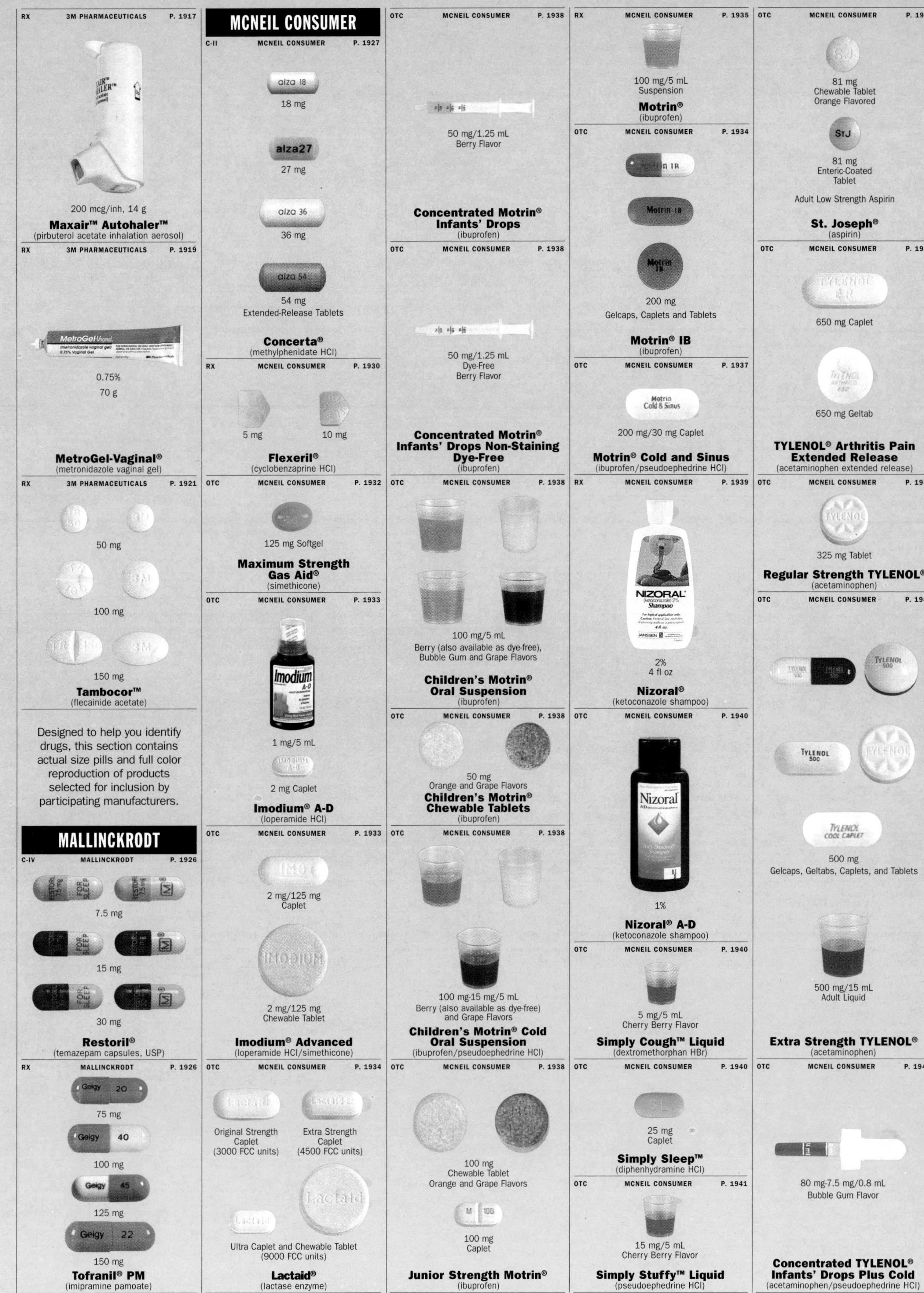

RX 3M PHARMACEUTICALS P. 1917

200 mcg/inh, 14 g

Maxair™ Autohaler™
(pirbuterol acetate inhalation aerosol)

RX 3M PHARMACEUTICALS P. 1919

0.75%
70 g

MetroGel-Vaginal®
(metronidazole vaginal gel)

RX 3M PHARMACEUTICALS P. 1921

50 mg

100 mg

150 mg

Tambocor™
(flecainide acetate)

Designed to help you identify drugs, this section contains actual size pills and full color reproduction of products selected for inclusion by participating manufacturers.

MALLINCKRODT

C-IV MALLINCKRODT P. 1926

7.5 mg

15 mg

30 mg

Restoril®
(temazepam capsules, USP)

RX MALLINCKRODT P. 1926

75 mg

100 mg

125 mg

150 mg

Tofranil® PM
(imipramine pamoate)

MCNEIL CONSUMER

C-II MCNEIL CONSUMER P. 1927

18 mg

27 mg

36 mg

54 mg
Extended-Release Tablets

Concerta®
(methylphenidate HCl)

RX MCNEIL CONSUMER P. 1930

5 mg 10 mg

Flexeril®
(cyclobenzaprine HCl)

OTC MCNEIL CONSUMER P. 1932

125 mg Softgel

Maximum Strength Gas Aid®
(simethicone)

OTC MCNEIL CONSUMER P. 1933

1 mg/5 mL

2 mg Caplet

Imodium® A-D
(loperamide HCl)

OTC MCNEIL CONSUMER P. 1933

2 mg/125 mg
Caplet

2 mg/125 mg
Chewable Tablet

Imodium® Advanced
(loperamide HCl/simethicone)

OTC MCNEIL CONSUMER P. 1934

Original Strength Caplet (3000 FCC units)

Extra Strength Caplet (4500 FCC units)

Ultra Caplet and Chewable Tablet
(9000 FCC units)

Lactaid®
(lactase enzyme)

OTC MCNEIL CONSUMER P. 1938

50 mg/1.25 mL
Berry Flavor

Concentrated Motrin® Infants' Drops
(ibuprofen)

OTC MCNEIL CONSUMER P. 1938

50 mg/1.25 mL
Dye-Free
Berry Flavor

Concentrated Motrin® Infants' Drops Non-Staining Dye-Free
(ibuprofen)

OTC MCNEIL CONSUMER P. 1938

100 mg/5 mL
Berry (also available as dye-free), Bubble Gum and Grape Flavors

Children's Motrin® Oral Suspension
(ibuprofen)

OTC MCNEIL CONSUMER P. 1938

50 mg
Orange and Grape Flavors

Children's Motrin® Chewable Tablets
(ibuprofen)

OTC MCNEIL CONSUMER P. 1938

100 mg-15 mg/5 mL
Berry (also available as dye-free) and Grape Flavors

Children's Motrin® Cold Oral Suspension
(ibuprofen/pseudoephedrine HCl)

OTC MCNEIL CONSUMER P. 1938

100 mg
Chewable Tablet
Orange and Grape Flavors

100 mg
Caplet

Junior Strength Motrin®
(ibuprofen)

RX MCNEIL CONSUMER P. 1935

100 mg/5 mL
Suspension

Motrin®
(ibuprofen)

OTC MCNEIL CONSUMER P. 1934

200 mg
Gelcaps, Caplets and Tablets

Motrin® IB
(ibuprofen)

OTC MCNEIL CONSUMER P. 1937

200 mg/30 mg Caplet

Motrin® Cold and Sinus
(ibuprofen/pseudoephedrine HCl)

RX MCNEIL CONSUMER P. 1939

2%
4 fl oz

Nizoral®
(ketoconazole shampoo)

OTC MCNEIL CONSUMER P. 1940

1%

Nizoral® A-D
(ketoconazole shampoo)

OTC MCNEIL CONSUMER P. 1940

5 mg/5 mL
Cherry Berry Flavor

Simply Cough™ Liquid
(dextromethorphan HBr)

OTC MCNEIL CONSUMER P. 1940

25 mg
Caplet

Simply Sleep™
(diphenhydramine HCl)

OTC MCNEIL CONSUMER P. 1941

15 mg/5 mL
Cherry Berry Flavor

Simply Stuffy™ Liquid
(pseudoephedrine HCl)

OTC MCNEIL CONSUMER P. 1941

81 mg
Chewable Tablet
Orange Flavored

81 mg
Enteric-Coated Tablet

Adult Low Strength Aspirin

St. Joseph®
(aspirin)

OTC MCNEIL CONSUMER P. 1943

650 mg Caplet

650 mg Geltab

TYLENOL® Arthritis Pain Extended Release
(acetaminophen extended release)

OTC MCNEIL CONSUMER P. 1943

325 mg Tablet

Regular Strength TYLENOL®
(acetaminophen)

OTC MCNEIL CONSUMER P. 1943

500 mg
Gelcaps, Geltabs, Caplets, and Tablets

500 mg/15 mL
Adult Liquid

Extra Strength TYLENOL®
(acetaminophen)

OTC MCNEIL CONSUMER P. 1949

80 mg-7.5 mg/0.8 mL
Bubble Gum Flavor

Concentrated TYLENOL® Infants' Drops Plus Cold
(acetaminophen/pseudoephedrine HCl)

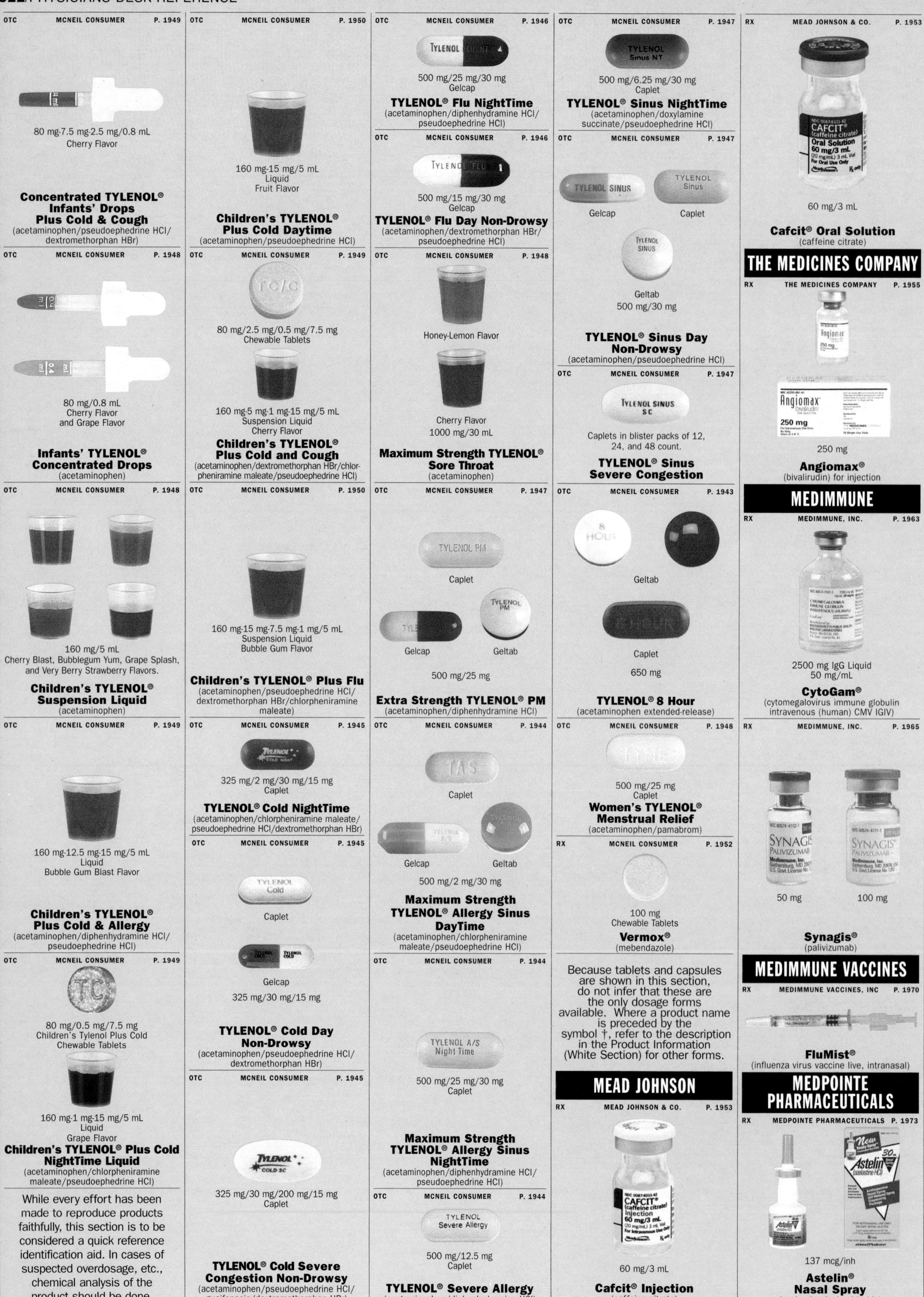

OTC MCNEIL CONSUMER P. 1949

80 mg-7.5 mg-2.5 mg/0.8 mL
Cherry Flavor

Concentrated TYLENOL® Infants' Drops Plus Cold & Cough
(acetaminophen/pseudoephedrine HCl/dextromethorphan HBr)

OTC MCNEIL CONSUMER P. 1948

80 mg/0.8 mL
Cherry Flavor
and Grape Flavor

Infants' TYLENOL® Concentrated Drops
(acetaminophen)

OTC MCNEIL CONSUMER P. 1948

160 mg/5 mL
Cherry Blast, Bubblegum Yum, Grape Splash, and Very Berry Strawberry Flavors.

Children's TYLENOL® Suspension Liquid
(acetaminophen)

OTC MCNEIL CONSUMER P. 1949

160 mg-12.5 mg-15 mg/5 mL
Liquid
Bubble Gum Blast Flavor

Children's TYLENOL® Plus Cold & Allergy
(acetaminophen/diphenhydramine HCl/pseudoephedrine HCl)

OTC MCNEIL CONSUMER P. 1949

80 mg/0.5 mg/7.5 mg
Children's Tylenol Plus Cold
Chewable Tablets

160 mg-1 mg-15 mg/5 mL
Liquid
Grape Flavor

Children's TYLENOL® Plus Cold NightTime Liquid
(acetaminophen/chlorpheniramine maleate/pseudoephedrine HCl)

While every effort has been made to reproduce products faithfully, this section is to be considered a quick reference identification aid. In cases of suspected overdosage, etc., chemical analysis of the product should be done.

OTC MCNEIL CONSUMER P. 1950

160 mg-15 mg/5 mL
Liquid
Fruit Flavor

Children's TYLENOL® Plus Cold Daytime
(acetaminophen/pseudoephedrine HCl)

OTC MCNEIL CONSUMER P. 1949

80 mg/2.5 mg/0.5 mg/7.5 mg
Chewable Tablets

160 mg-5 mg-1 mg-15 mg/5 mL
Suspension Liquid
Cherry Flavor

Children's TYLENOL® Plus Cold and Cough
(acetaminophen/dextromethorphan HBr/chlorpheniramine maleate/pseudoephedrine HCl)

OTC MCNEIL CONSUMER P. 1950

160 mg-15 mg-7.5 mg-1 mg/5 mL
Suspension Liquid
Bubble Gum Flavor

Children's TYLENOL® Plus Flu
(acetaminophen/pseudoephedrine HCl/dextromethorphan HBr/chlorpheniramine maleate)

OTC MCNEIL CONSUMER P. 1945

325 mg/2 mg/30 mg/15 mg
Caplet

TYLENOL® Cold NightTime
(acetaminophen/chlorpheniramine maleate/pseudoephedrine HCl/dextromethorphan HBr)

OTC MCNEIL CONSUMER P. 1945

Caplet

Gelcap
325 mg/30 mg/15 mg

TYLENOL® Cold Day Non-Drowsy
(acetaminophen/pseudoephedrine HCl/dextromethorphan HBr)

OTC MCNEIL CONSUMER P. 1945

325 mg/30 mg/200 mg/15 mg
Caplet

TYLENOL® Cold Severe Congestion Non-Drowsy
(acetaminophen/pseudoephedrine HCl/guaifenesin/dextromethorphan HBr)

OTC MCNEIL CONSUMER P. 1946

500 mg/25 mg/30 mg
Gelcap

TYLENOL® Flu NightTime
(acetaminophen/diphenhydramine HCl/pseudoephedrine HCl)

OTC MCNEIL CONSUMER P. 1946

500 mg/15 mg/30 mg
Gelcap

TYLENOL® Flu Day Non-Drowsy
(acetaminophen/dextromethorphan HBr/pseudoephedrine HCl)

OTC MCNEIL CONSUMER P. 1948

Honey-Lemon Flavor

Cherry Flavor
1000 mg/30 mL

Maximum Strength TYLENOL® Sore Throat
(acetaminophen)

OTC MCNEIL CONSUMER P. 1947

Caplet

Gelcap Geltab

500 mg/25 mg

Extra Strength TYLENOL® PM
(acetaminophen/diphenhydramine HCl)

OTC MCNEIL CONSUMER P. 1944

Caplet

Gelcap Geltab

500 mg/2 mg/30 mg

Maximum Strength TYLENOL® Allergy Sinus DayTime
(acetaminophen/chlorpheniramine maleate/pseudoephedrine HCl)

OTC MCNEIL CONSUMER P. 1944

500 mg/25 mg/30 mg
Caplet

Maximum Strength TYLENOL® Allergy Sinus NightTime
(acetaminophen/diphenhydramine HCl/pseudoephedrine HCl)

OTC MCNEIL CONSUMER P. 1944

500 mg/12.5 mg
Caplet

TYLENOL® Severe Allergy
(acetaminophen/diphenhydramine HCl)

OTC MCNEIL CONSUMER P. 1947

500 mg/6.25 mg/30 mg
Caplet

TYLENOL® Sinus NightTime
(acetaminophen/doxylamine succinate/pseudoephedrine HCl)

OTC MCNEIL CONSUMER P. 1947

Gelcap Caplet

Geltab
500 mg/30 mg

TYLENOL® Sinus Day Non-Drowsy
(acetaminophen/pseudoephedrine HCl)

OTC MCNEIL CONSUMER P. 1947

Caplets in blister packs of 12, 24, and 48 count.

TYLENOL® Sinus Severe Congestion

OTC MCNEIL CONSUMER P. 1943

Geltab

Caplet

650 mg

TYLENOL® 8 Hour
(acetaminophen extended-release)

OTC MCNEIL CONSUMER P. 1948

500 mg/25 mg
Caplet

Women's TYLENOL® Menstrual Relief
(acetaminophen/pamabrom)

RX MCNEIL CONSUMER P. 1952

100 mg
Chewable Tablets

Vermox®
(mebendazole)

Because tablets and capsules are shown in this section, do not infer that these are the only dosage forms available. Where a product name is preceded by the symbol †, refer to the description in the Product Information (White Section) for other forms.

MEAD JOHNSON

RX MEAD JOHNSON & CO. P. 1953

60 mg/3 mL

Cafcit® Injection
(caffeine citrate)

RX MEAD JOHNSON & CO. P. 1953

60 mg/3 mL

Cafcit® Oral Solution
(caffeine citrate)

THE MEDICINES COMPANY

RX THE MEDICINES COMPANY P. 1955

250 mg

Angiomax®
(bivalirudin) for injection

MEDIMMUNE

RX MEDIMMUNE, INC. P. 1963

2500 mg IgG Liquid
50 mg/mL

CytoGam®
(cytomegalovirus immune globulin intravenous (human) CMV IGIV)

RX MEDIMMUNE, INC. P. 1965

50 mg 100 mg

Synagis®
(palivizumab)

MEDIMMUNE VACCINES

RX MEDIMMUNE VACCINES, INC P. 1970

FluMist®
(influenza virus vaccine live, intranasal)

MEDPOINTE PHARMACEUTICALS

RX MEDPOINTE PHARMACEUTICALS P. 1973

137 mcg/inh

Astelin® Nasal Spray
(azelastine hydrochloride)

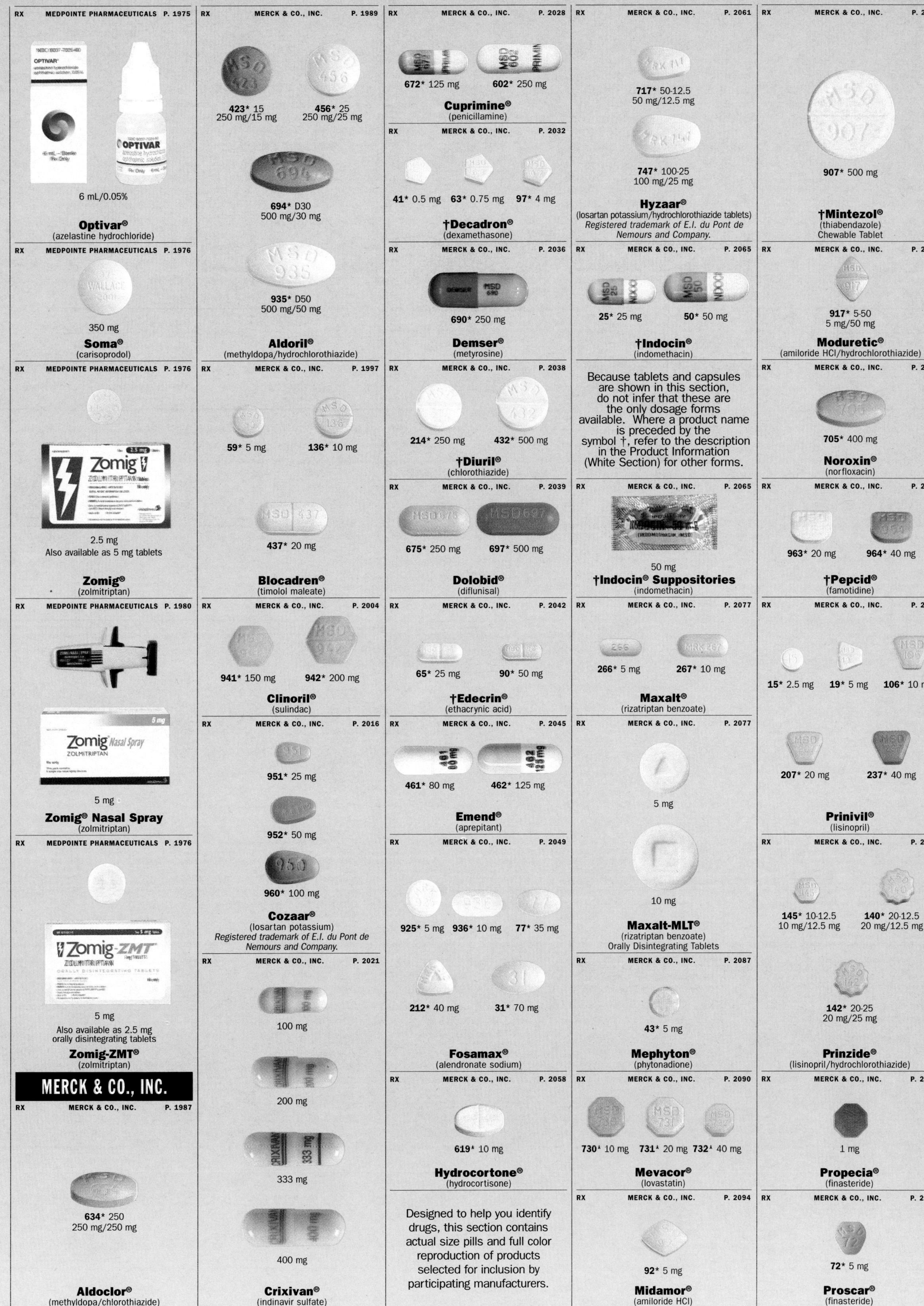

RX MEDPOINTE PHARMACEUTICALS P. 1975

6 mL/0.05%

Optivar®
(azelastine hydrochloride)

RX MEDPOINTE PHARMACEUTICALS P. 1976

350 mg

Soma®
(carisoprodol)

RX MEDPOINTE PHARMACEUTICALS P. 1976

2.5 mg
Also available as 5 mg tablets

Zomig®
(zolmitriptan)

RX MEDPOINTE PHARMACEUTICALS P. 1980

5 mg

Zomig® Nasal Spray
(zolmitriptan)

RX MEDPOINTE PHARMACEUTICALS P. 1976

5 mg
Also available as 2.5 mg orally disintegrating tablets

Zomig-ZMT®
(zolmitriptan)

MERCK & CO., INC.

RX MERCK & CO., INC. P. 1987

634* 250
250 mg/250 mg

Aldoclor®
(methyldopa/chlorothiazide)

RX MERCK & CO., INC. P. 1989

423* 15
250 mg/15 mg

456* 25
250 mg/25 mg

694* D30
500 mg/30 mg

935* D50
500 mg/50 mg

Aldoril®
(methyldopa/hydrochlorothiazide)

RX MERCK & CO., INC. P. 1997

59* 5 mg **136*** 10 mg

437* 20 mg

Blocadren®
(timolol maleate)

RX MERCK & CO., INC. P. 2004

941* 150 mg **942*** 200 mg

Clinoril®
(sulindac)

RX MERCK & CO., INC. P. 2016

951* 25 mg

952* 50 mg

960* 100 mg

Cozaar®
(losartan potassium)
Registered trademark of E.I. du Pont de Nemours and Company.

RX MERCK & CO., INC. P. 2021

100 mg

200 mg

333 mg

400 mg

Crixivan®
(indinavir sulfate)

RX MERCK & CO., INC. P. 2028

672* 125 mg **602*** 250 mg

Cuprimine®
(penicillamine)

RX MERCK & CO., INC. P. 2032

41* 0.5 mg **63*** 0.75 mg **97*** 4 mg

†Decadron®
(dexamethasone)

RX MERCK & CO., INC. P. 2036

690* 250 mg

Demser®
(metyrosine)

RX MERCK & CO., INC. P. 2038

214* 250 mg **432*** 500 mg

†Diuril®
(chlorothiazide)

RX MERCK & CO., INC. P. 2039

675* 250 mg **697*** 500 mg

Dolobid®
(diflunisal)

RX MERCK & CO., INC. P. 2042

65* 25 mg **90*** 50 mg

†Edecrin®
(ethacrynic acid)

RX MERCK & CO., INC. P. 2045

461* 80 mg **462*** 125 mg

Emend®
(aprepitant)

RX MERCK & CO., INC. P. 2049

925* 5 mg **936*** 10 mg **77*** 35 mg

212* 40 mg **31*** 70 mg

Fosamax®
(alendronate sodium)

RX MERCK & CO., INC. P. 2058

619* 10 mg

Hydrocortone®
(hydrocortisone)

Designed to help you identify drugs, this section contains actual size pills and full color reproduction of products selected for inclusion by participating manufacturers.

RX MERCK & CO., INC. P. 2061

717* 50-12.5
50 mg/12.5 mg

747* 100-25
100 mg/25 mg

Hyzaar®
(losartan potassium/hydrochlorothiazide tablets)
Registered trademark of E.I. du Pont de Nemours and Company.

RX MERCK & CO., INC. P. 2065

25* 25 mg **50*** 50 mg

†Indocin®
(indomethacin)

Because tablets and capsules are shown in this section, do not infer that these are the only dosage forms available. Where a product name is preceded by the symbol †, refer to the description in the Product Information (White Section) for other forms.

RX MERCK & CO., INC. P. 2065

50 mg

†Indocin® Suppositories
(indomethacin)

RX MERCK & CO., INC. P. 2077

266* 5 mg **267*** 10 mg

Maxalt®
(rizatriptan benzoate)

RX MERCK & CO., INC. P. 2077

5 mg

10 mg

Maxalt-MLT®
(rizatriptan benzoate)
Orally Disintegrating Tablets

RX MERCK & CO., INC. P. 2087

43* 5 mg

Mephyton®
(phytonadione)

RX MERCK & CO., INC. P. 2090

730* 10 mg **731*** 20 mg **732*** 40 mg

Mevacor®
(lovastatin)

RX MERCK & CO., INC. P. 2094

92* 5 mg

Midamor®
(amiloride HCl)

RX MERCK & CO., INC. P. 2096

907* 500 mg

†Mintezol®
(thiabendazole)
Chewable Tablet

RX MERCK & CO., INC. P. 2097

917* 5-50
5 mg/50 mg

Moduretic®
(amiloride HCl/hydrochlorothiazide)

RX MERCK & CO., INC. P. 2103

705* 400 mg

Noroxin®
(norfloxacin)

RX MERCK & CO., INC. P. 2108

963* 20 mg **964*** 40 mg

†Pepcid®
(famotidine)

RX MERCK & CO., INC. P. 2123

15* 2.5 mg **19*** 5 mg **106*** 10 mg

207* 20 mg **237*** 40 mg

Prinivil®
(lisinopril)

RX MERCK & CO., INC. P. 2127

145* 10-12.5
10 mg/12.5 mg

140* 20-12.5
20 mg/12.5 mg

142* 20-25
20 mg/25 mg

Prinzide®
(lisinopril/hydrochlorothiazide)

RX MERCK & CO., INC. P. 2130

1 mg

Propecia®
(finasteride)

RX MERCK & CO., INC. P. 2133

72* 5 mg

Proscar®
(finasteride)

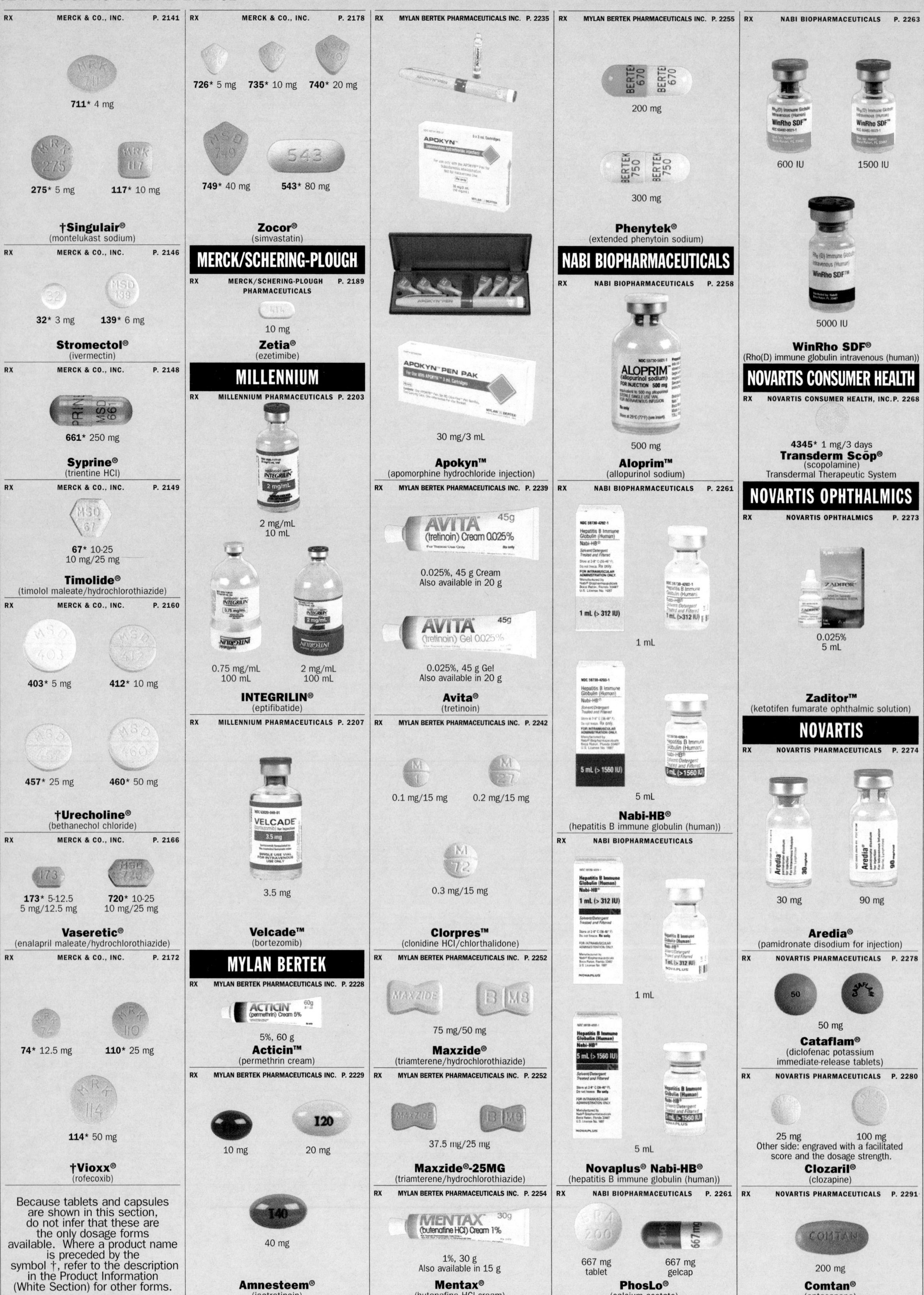

RX MERCK & CO., INC. P. 2141

711* 4 mg

275* 5 mg 117* 10 mg

†Singulair®
(montelukast sodium)

RX MERCK & CO., INC. P. 2146

32* 3 mg 139* 6 mg

Stromectol®
(ivermectin)

RX MERCK & CO., INC. P. 2148

661* 250 mg

Syprine®
(trientine HCl)

RX MERCK & CO., INC. P. 2149

67* 10-25
10 mg/25 mg

Timolide®
(timolol maleate/hydrochlorothiazide)

RX MERCK & CO., INC. P. 2160

403* 5 mg 412* 10 mg

457* 25 mg 460* 50 mg

†Urecholine®
(bethanechol chloride)

RX MERCK & CO., INC. P. 2166

173* 5-12.5
5 mg/12.5 mg

720* 10-25
10 mg/25 mg

Vaseretic®
(enalapril maleate/hydrochlorothiazide)

RX MERCK & CO., INC. P. 2172

74* 12.5 mg 110* 25 mg

114* 50 mg

†Vioxx®
(rofecoxib)

Because tablets and capsules are shown in this section, do not infer that these are the only dosage forms available. Where a product name is preceded by the symbol †, refer to the description in the Product Information (White Section) for other forms.

RX MERCK & CO., INC. P. 2178

726* 5 mg 735* 10 mg 740* 20 mg

749* 40 mg 543* 80 mg

Zocor®
(simvastatin)

MERCK/SCHERING-PLOUGH

RX MERCK/SCHERING-PLOUGH PHARMACEUTICALS P. 2189

10 mg

Zetia®
(ezetimibe)

MILLENNIUM

RX MILLENNIUM PHARMACEUTICALS P. 2203

2 mg/mL
10 mL

0.75 mg/mL
100 mL

2 mg/mL
100 mL

INTEGRILIN®
(eptifibatide)

RX MILLENNIUM PHARMACEUTICALS P. 2207

3.5 mg

Velcade™
(bortezomib)

MYLAN BERTEK

RX MYLAN BERTEK PHARMACEUTICALS INC. P. 2228

5%, 60 g

Acticin™
(permethrin cream)

RX MYLAN BERTEK PHARMACEUTICALS INC. P. 2229

10 mg 20 mg

40 mg

Amnesteem®
(isotretinoin)

RX MYLAN BERTEK PHARMACEUTICALS INC. P. 2235

30 mg/3 mL

Apokyn™
(apomorphine hydrochloride injection)

RX MYLAN BERTEK PHARMACEUTICALS INC. P. 2239

0.025%, 45 g Cream
Also available in 20 g

0.025%, 45 g Gel
Also available in 20 g

Avita®
(tretinoin)

RX MYLAN BERTEK PHARMACEUTICALS INC. P. 2242

0.1 mg/15 mg 0.2 mg/15 mg

0.3 mg/15 mg

Clorpres™
(clonidine HCl/chlorthalidone)

RX MYLAN BERTEK PHARMACEUTICALS INC. P. 2252

75 mg/50 mg

Maxzide®
(triamterene/hydrochlorothiazide)

RX MYLAN BERTEK PHARMACEUTICALS INC. P. 2252

37.5 mg/25 mg

Maxzide®-25MG
(triamterene/hydrochlorothiazide)

RX MYLAN BERTEK PHARMACEUTICALS INC. P. 2254

1%, 30 g
Also available in 15 g

Mentax®
(butenafine HCl cream)

RX MYLAN BERTEK PHARMACEUTICALS INC. P. 2255

200 mg

300 mg

Phenytek®
(extended phenytoin sodium)

NABI BIOPHARMACEUTICALS

RX NABI BIOPHARMACEUTICALS P. 2258

500 mg

Aloprim™
(allopurinol sodium)

RX NABI BIOPHARMACEUTICALS P. 2261

1 mL

5 mL

Nabi-HB®
(hepatitis B immune globulin (human))

RX NABI BIOPHARMACEUTICALS

1 mL

5 mL

Novaplus® Nabi-HB®
(hepatitis B immune globulin (human))

RX NABI BIOPHARMACEUTICALS P. 2261

667 mg
tablet

667 mg
gelcap

PhosLo®
(calcium acetate)

RX NABI BIOPHARMACEUTICALS P. 2263

600 IU 1500 IU

5000 IU

WinRho SDF®
(Rho(D) immune globulin intravenous (human))

NOVARTIS CONSUMER HEALTH

RX NOVARTIS CONSUMER HEALTH, INC. P. 2268

4345* 1 mg/3 days

Transderm Scōp®
(scopolamine)
Transdermal Therapeutic System

NOVARTIS OPHTHALMICS

RX NOVARTIS OPHTHALMICS P. 2273

0.025%
5 mL

Zaditor™
(ketotifen fumarate ophthalmic solution)

NOVARTIS

RX NOVARTIS PHARMACEUTICALS P. 2274

30 mg 90 mg

Aredia®
(pamidronate disodium for injection)

RX NOVARTIS PHARMACEUTICALS P. 2278

50 mg

Cataflam®
(diclofenac potassium immediate-release tablets)

RX NOVARTIS PHARMACEUTICALS P. 2280

25 mg 100 mg
Other side: engraved with a facilitated score and the dosage strength.

Clozaril®
(clozapine)

RX NOVARTIS PHARMACEUTICALS P. 2291

200 mg

Comtan®
(entacapone)

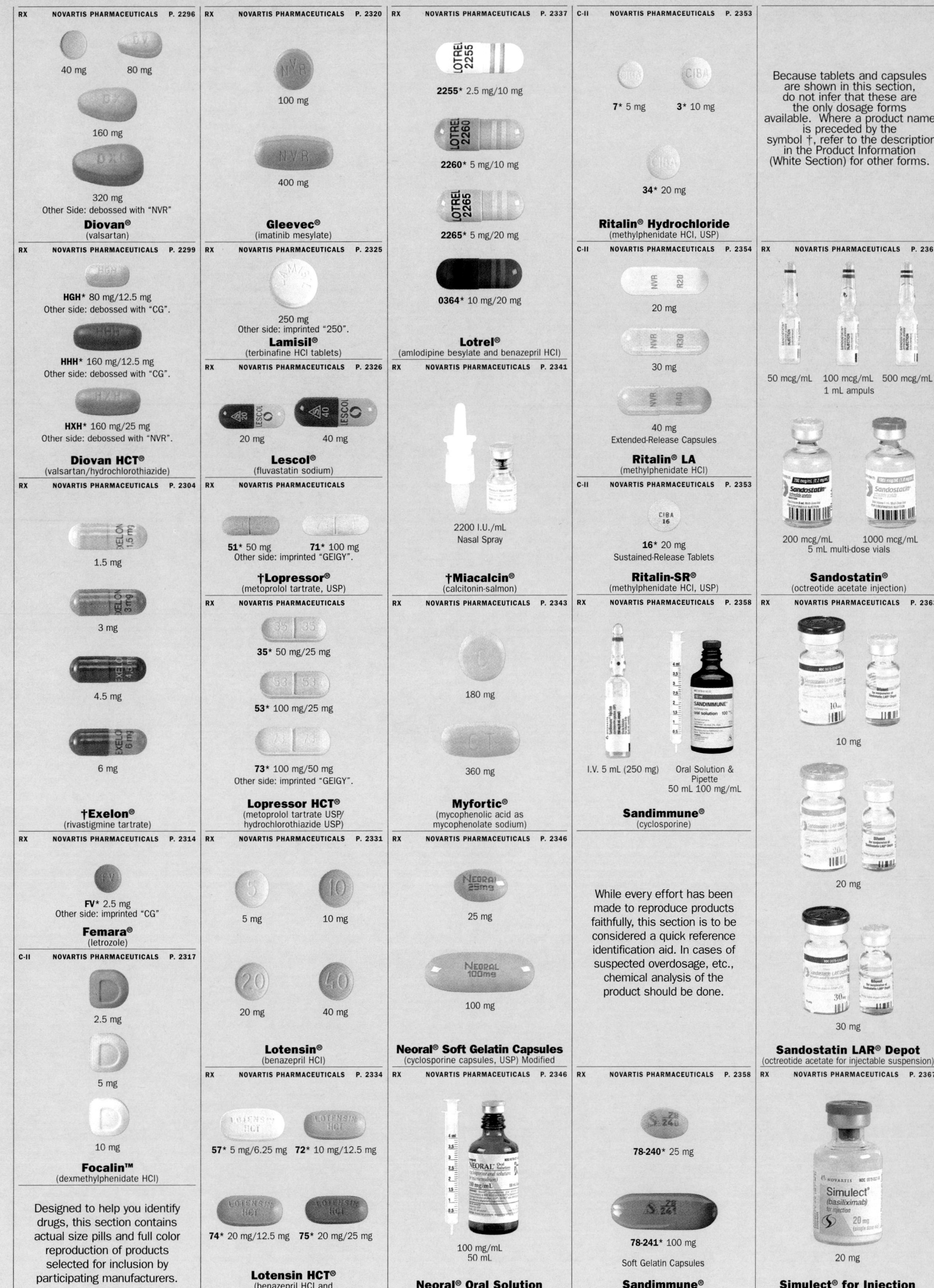

RX NOVARTIS PHARMACEUTICALS P. 2296

40 mg 80 mg

160 mg

320 mg
Other Side: debossed with "NVR"

Diovan®
(valsartan)

RX NOVARTIS PHARMACEUTICALS P. 2299

HGH* 80 mg/12.5 mg
Other side: debossed with "CG".

HHH* 160 mg/12.5 mg
Other side: debossed with "CG".

HXH* 160 mg/25 mg
Other side: debossed with "NVR".

Diovan HCT®
(valsartan/hydrochlorothiazide)

RX NOVARTIS PHARMACEUTICALS P. 2304

1.5 mg

3 mg

4.5 mg

6 mg

†Exelon®
(rivastigmine tartrate)

RX NOVARTIS PHARMACEUTICALS P. 2314

FV* 2.5 mg
Other side: imprinted "CG"

Femara®
(letrozole)

C-II NOVARTIS PHARMACEUTICALS P. 2317

2.5 mg

5 mg

10 mg

Focalin™
(dexmethylphenidate HCl)

Designed to help you identify drugs, this section contains actual size pills and full color reproduction of products selected for inclusion by participating manufacturers.

RX NOVARTIS PHARMACEUTICALS P. 2320

100 mg

400 mg

Gleevec®
(imatinib mesylate)

RX NOVARTIS PHARMACEUTICALS P. 2325

250 mg
Other side: imprinted "250".

Lamisil®
(terbinafine HCl tablets)

RX NOVARTIS PHARMACEUTICALS P. 2326

20 mg 40 mg

Lescol®
(fluvastatin sodium)

RX NOVARTIS PHARMACEUTICALS

51* 50 mg **71*** 100 mg
Other side: imprinted "GEIGY".

†Lopressor®
(metoprolol tartrate, USP)

RX NOVARTIS PHARMACEUTICALS

35* 50 mg/25 mg

53* 100 mg/25 mg

73* 100 mg/50 mg
Other side: imprinted "GEIGY".

Lopressor HCT®
(metoprolol tartrate USP/ hydrochlorothiazide USP)

RX NOVARTIS PHARMACEUTICALS P. 2331

5 mg 10 mg

20 mg 40 mg

Lotensin®
(benazepril HCl)

RX NOVARTIS PHARMACEUTICALS P. 2334

57* 5 mg/6.25 mg **72*** 10 mg/12.5 mg

74* 20 mg/12.5 mg **75*** 20 mg/25 mg

Lotensin HCT®
(benazepril HCl and hydrochlorothiazide USP)

RX NOVARTIS PHARMACEUTICALS P. 2337

2255* 2.5 mg/10 mg

2260* 5 mg/10 mg

2265* 5 mg/20 mg

0364* 10 mg/20 mg

Lotrel®
(amlodipine besylate and benazepril HCl)

RX NOVARTIS PHARMACEUTICALS P. 2341

2200 I.U./mL
Nasal Spray

†Miacalcin®
(calcitonin-salmon)

RX NOVARTIS PHARMACEUTICALS P. 2343

180 mg

360 mg

Myfortic®
(mycophenolic acid as mycophenolate sodium)

RX NOVARTIS PHARMACEUTICALS P. 2346

25 mg

100 mg

Neoral® Soft Gelatin Capsules
(cyclosporine capsules, USP) Modified

RX NOVARTIS PHARMACEUTICALS P. 2346

100 mg/mL
50 mL

Neoral® Oral Solution
(cyclosporine oral solution, USP) Modified

C-II NOVARTIS PHARMACEUTICALS P. 2353

7* 5 mg **3*** 10 mg

34* 20 mg

Ritalin® Hydrochloride
(methylphenidate HCl, USP)

C-II NOVARTIS PHARMACEUTICALS P. 2354

20 mg

30 mg

40 mg
Extended-Release Capsules

Ritalin® LA
(methylphenidate HCl)

C-II NOVARTIS PHARMACEUTICALS P. 2353

16* 20 mg
Sustained-Release Tablets

Ritalin-SR®
(methylphenidate HCl, USP)

RX NOVARTIS PHARMACEUTICALS P. 2358

I.V. 5 mL (250 mg)

Oral Solution & Pipette
50 mL 100 mg/mL

Sandimmune®
(cyclosporine)

While every effort has been made to reproduce products faithfully, this section is to be considered a quick reference identification aid. In cases of suspected overdosage, etc., chemical analysis of the product should be done.

RX NOVARTIS PHARMACEUTICALS P. 2358

78-240* 25 mg

78-241* 100 mg

Soft Gelatin Capsules

Sandimmune®
(cyclosporine capsules, USP)

Because tablets and capsules are shown in this section, do not infer that these are the only dosage forms available. Where a product name is preceded by the symbol †, refer to the description in the Product Information (White Section) for other forms.

RX NOVARTIS PHARMACEUTICALS P. 2361

50 mcg/mL 100 mcg/mL 500 mcg/mL
1 mL ampuls

200 mcg/mL 1000 mcg/mL
5 mL multi-dose vials

Sandostatin®
(octreotide acetate injection)

RX NOVARTIS PHARMACEUTICALS P. 2363

10 mg

20 mg

30 mg

Sandostatin LAR® Depot
(octreotide acetate for injectable suspension)

RX NOVARTIS PHARMACEUTICALS P. 2367

20 mg

Simulect® for Injection
(basiliximab)

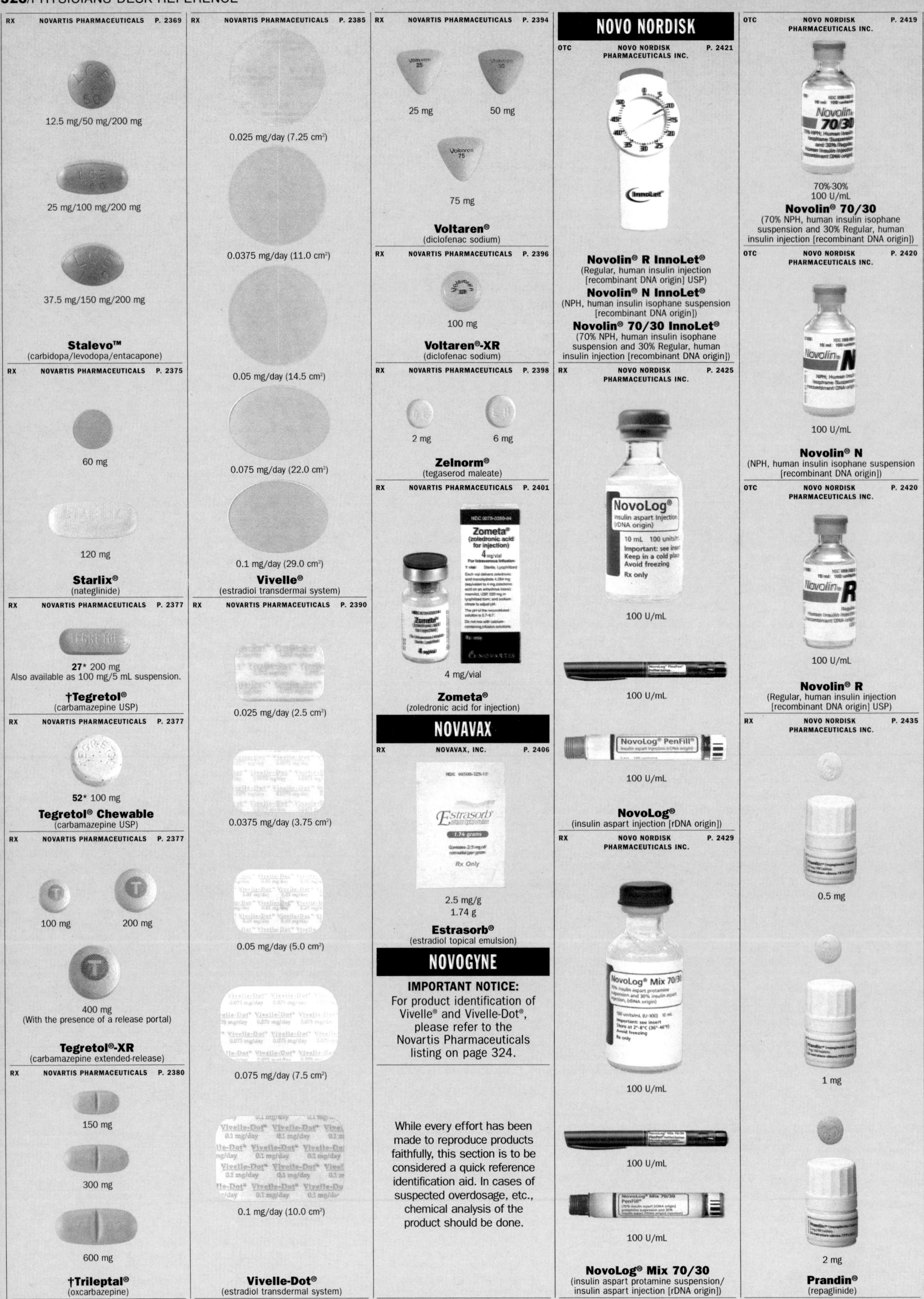

RX NOVARTIS PHARMACEUTICALS P. 2369

12.5 mg/50 mg/200 mg

25 mg/100 mg/200 mg

37.5 mg/150 mg/200 mg

Stalevo™
(carbidopa/levodopa/entacapone)

RX NOVARTIS PHARMACEUTICALS P. 2375

60 mg

120 mg

Starlix®
(nateglinide)

RX NOVARTIS PHARMACEUTICALS P. 2377

27* 200 mg
Also available as 100 mg/5 mL suspension.

†Tegretol®
(carbamazepine USP)

RX NOVARTIS PHARMACEUTICALS P. 2377

52* 100 mg

Tegretol® Chewable
(carbamazepine USP)

RX NOVARTIS PHARMACEUTICALS P. 2377

100 mg 200 mg

400 mg
(With the presence of a release portal)

Tegretol®-XR
(carbamazepine extended-release)

RX NOVARTIS PHARMACEUTICALS P. 2380

150 mg

300 mg

600 mg

†Trileptal®
(oxcarbazepine)

RX NOVARTIS PHARMACEUTICALS P. 2385

0.025 mg/day (7.25 cm²)

0.0375 mg/day (11.0 cm²)

0.05 mg/day (14.5 cm²)

0.075 mg/day (22.0 cm²)

0.1 mg/day (29.0 cm²)

Vivelle®
(estradiol transdermal system)

RX NOVARTIS PHARMACEUTICALS P. 2390

0.025 mg/day (2.5 cm²)

0.0375 mg/day (3.75 cm²)

0.05 mg/day (5.0 cm²)

0.075 mg/day (7.5 cm²)

0.1 mg/day (10.0 cm²)

Vivelle-Dot®
(estradiol transdermal system)

RX NOVARTIS PHARMACEUTICALS P. 2394

25 mg 50 mg

75 mg

Voltaren®
(diclofenac sodium)

RX NOVARTIS PHARMACEUTICALS P. 2396

100 mg

Voltaren®-XR
(diclofenac sodium)

RX NOVARTIS PHARMACEUTICALS P. 2398

2 mg 6 mg

Zelnorm®
(tegaserod maleate)

RX NOVARTIS PHARMACEUTICALS P. 2401

4 mg/vial

Zometa®
(zoledronic acid for injection)

NOVAVAX

RX NOVAVAX, INC. P. 2406

2.5 mg/g
1.74 g

Estrasorb®
(estradiol topical emulsion)

NOVOGYNE

IMPORTANT NOTICE:
For product identification of Vivelle® and Vivelle-Dot®, please refer to the Novartis Pharmaceuticals listing on page 324.

While every effort has been made to reproduce products faithfully, this section is to be considered a quick reference identification aid. In cases of suspected overdosage, etc., chemical analysis of the product should be done.

NOVO NORDISK

OTC NOVO NORDISK PHARMACEUTICALS INC. P. 2421

Novolin® R InnoLet®
(Regular, human insulin injection [recombinant DNA origin] USP)
Novolin® N InnoLet®
(NPH, human insulin isophane suspension [recombinant DNA origin])
Novolin® 70/30 InnoLet®
(70% NPH, human insulin isophane suspension and 30% Regular, human insulin injection [recombinant DNA origin])

RX NOVO NORDISK PHARMACEUTICALS INC. P. 2425

100 U/mL

100 U/mL

100 U/mL

NovoLog®
(insulin aspart injection [rDNA origin])

RX NOVO NORDISK PHARMACEUTICALS INC. P. 2429

100 U/mL

100 U/mL

100 U/mL

NovoLog® Mix 70/30
(insulin aspart protamine suspension/ insulin aspart injection [rDNA origin])

OTC NOVO NORDISK PHARMACEUTICALS INC. P. 2419

70%-30%
100 U/mL
Novolin® 70/30
(70% NPH, human insulin isophane suspension and 30% Regular, human insulin injection [recombinant DNA origin])

OTC NOVO NORDISK PHARMACEUTICALS INC. P. 2420

100 U/mL

Novolin® N
(NPH, human insulin isophane suspension [recombinant DNA origin])

OTC NOVO NORDISK PHARMACEUTICALS INC. P. 2420

100 U/mL

Novolin® R
(Regular, human insulin injection [recombinant DNA origin] USP)

RX NOVO NORDISK PHARMACEUTICALS INC. P. 2435

0.5 mg

1 mg

2 mg

Prandin®
(repaglinide)

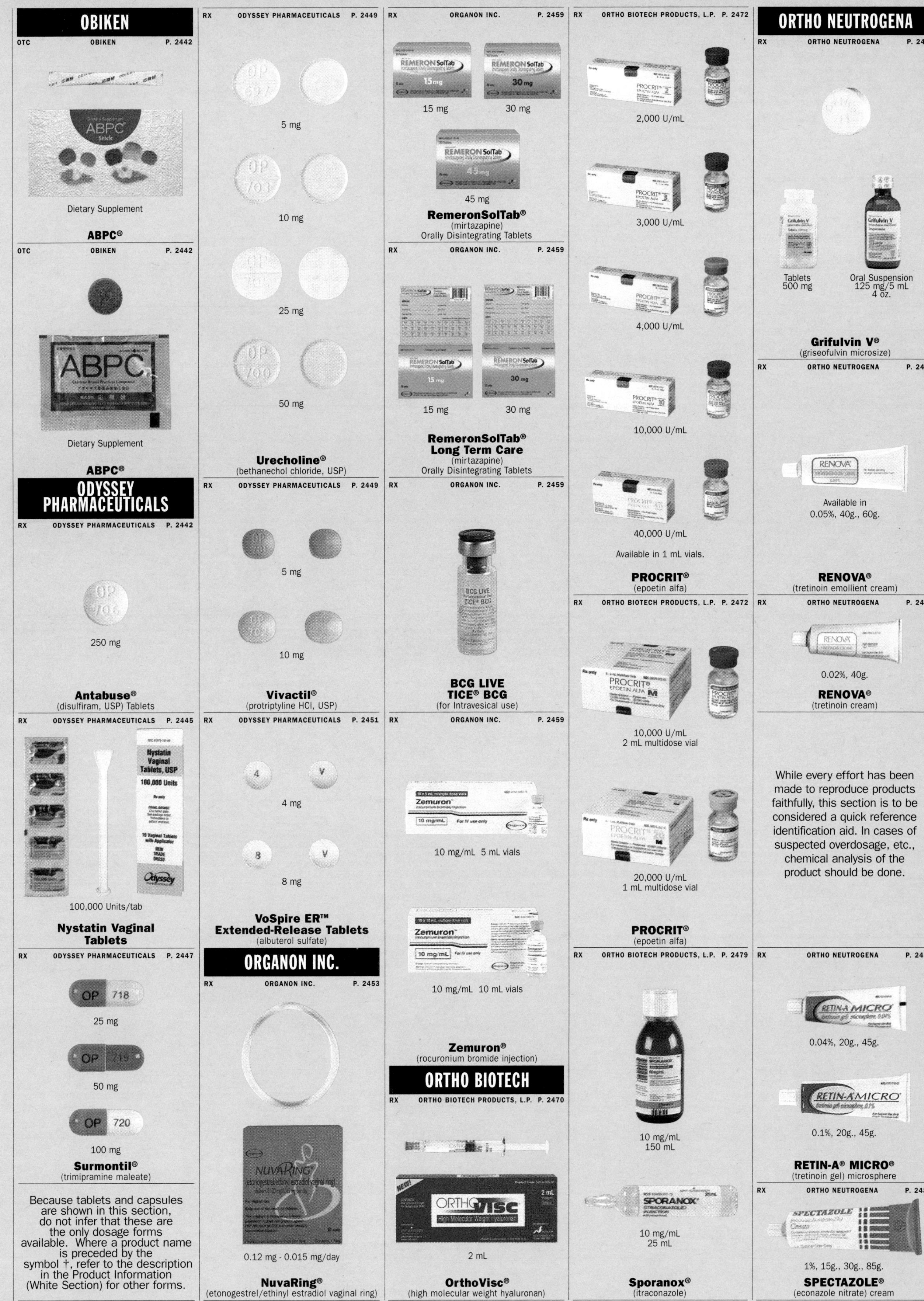

OBIKEN

OTC OBIKEN P. 2442

Dietary Supplement

ABPC®

OTC OBIKEN P. 2442

Dietary Supplement

ABPC®

ODYSSEY PHARMACEUTICALS

RX ODYSSEY PHARMACEUTICALS P. 2442

250 mg

Antabuse®
(disulfiram, USP) Tablets

RX ODYSSEY PHARMACEUTICALS P. 2445

100,000 Units/tab

Nystatin Vaginal Tablets

RX ODYSSEY PHARMACEUTICALS P. 2447

25 mg

50 mg

100 mg

Surmontil®
(trimipramine maleate)

Because tablets and capsules are shown in this section, do not infer that these are the only dosage forms available. Where a product name is preceded by the symbol †, refer to the description in the Product Information (White Section) for other forms.

RX ODYSSEY PHARMACEUTICALS P. 2449

5 mg

10 mg

25 mg

50 mg

Urecholine®
(bethanechol chloride, USP)

RX ODYSSEY PHARMACEUTICALS P. 2449

5 mg

10 mg

Vivactil®
(protriptyline HCl, USP)

RX ODYSSEY PHARMACEUTICALS P. 2451

4 mg

8 mg

VoSpire ER™ Extended-Release Tablets
(albuterol sulfate)

ORGANON INC.

RX ORGANON INC. P. 2453

0.12 mg - 0.015 mg/day

NuvaRing®
(etonogestrel/ethinyl estradiol vaginal ring)

RX ORGANON INC. P. 2459

15 mg 30 mg

45 mg

RemeronSolTab®
(mirtazapine)
Orally Disintegrating Tablets

RX ORGANON INC. P. 2459

15 mg 30 mg

RemeronSolTab® Long Term Care
(mirtazapine)
Orally Disintegrating Tablets

RX ORGANON INC. P. 2459

BCG LIVE TICE® BCG
(for Intravesical use)

RX ORGANON INC. P. 2459

10 mg/mL 5 mL vials

10 mg/mL 10 mL vials

Zemuron®
(rocuronium bromide injection)

ORTHO BIOTECH

RX ORTHO BIOTECH PRODUCTS, L.P. P. 2470

2 mL

OrthoVisc®
(high molecular weight hyaluronan)

RX ORTHO BIOTECH PRODUCTS, L.P. P. 2472

2,000 U/mL

3,000 U/mL

4,000 U/mL

10,000 U/mL

40,000 U/mL

Available in 1 mL vials.

PROCRIT®
(epoetin alfa)

RX ORTHO BIOTECH PRODUCTS, L.P. P. 2472

10,000 U/mL
2 mL multidose vial

20,000 U/mL
1 mL multidose vial

PROCRIT®
(epoetin alfa)

RX ORTHO BIOTECH PRODUCTS, L.P. P. 2479

10 mg/mL
150 mL

10 mg/mL
25 mL

Sporanox®
(itraconazole)

ORTHO NEUTROGENA

RX ORTHO NEUTROGENA P. 2479

Tablets
500 mg

Oral Suspension
125 mg/5 mL
4 oz.

Grifulvin V®
(griseofulvin microsize)

RX ORTHO NEUTROGENA P. 2482

Available in
0.05%, 40g., 60g.

RENOVA®
(tretinoin emollient cream)

RX ORTHO NEUTROGENA P. 2480

0.02%, 40g.

RENOVA®
(tretinoin cream)

While every effort has been made to reproduce products faithfully, this section is to be considered a quick reference identification aid. In cases of suspected overdosage, etc., chemical analysis of the product should be done.

RX ORTHO NEUTROGENA P. 2484

0.04%, 20g., 45g.

0.1%, 20g., 45g.

RETIN-A® MICRO®
(tretinoin gel) microsphere

RX ORTHO NEUTROGENA P. 2486

1%, 15g., 30g., 85g.

SPECTAZOLE®
(econazole nitrate) cream

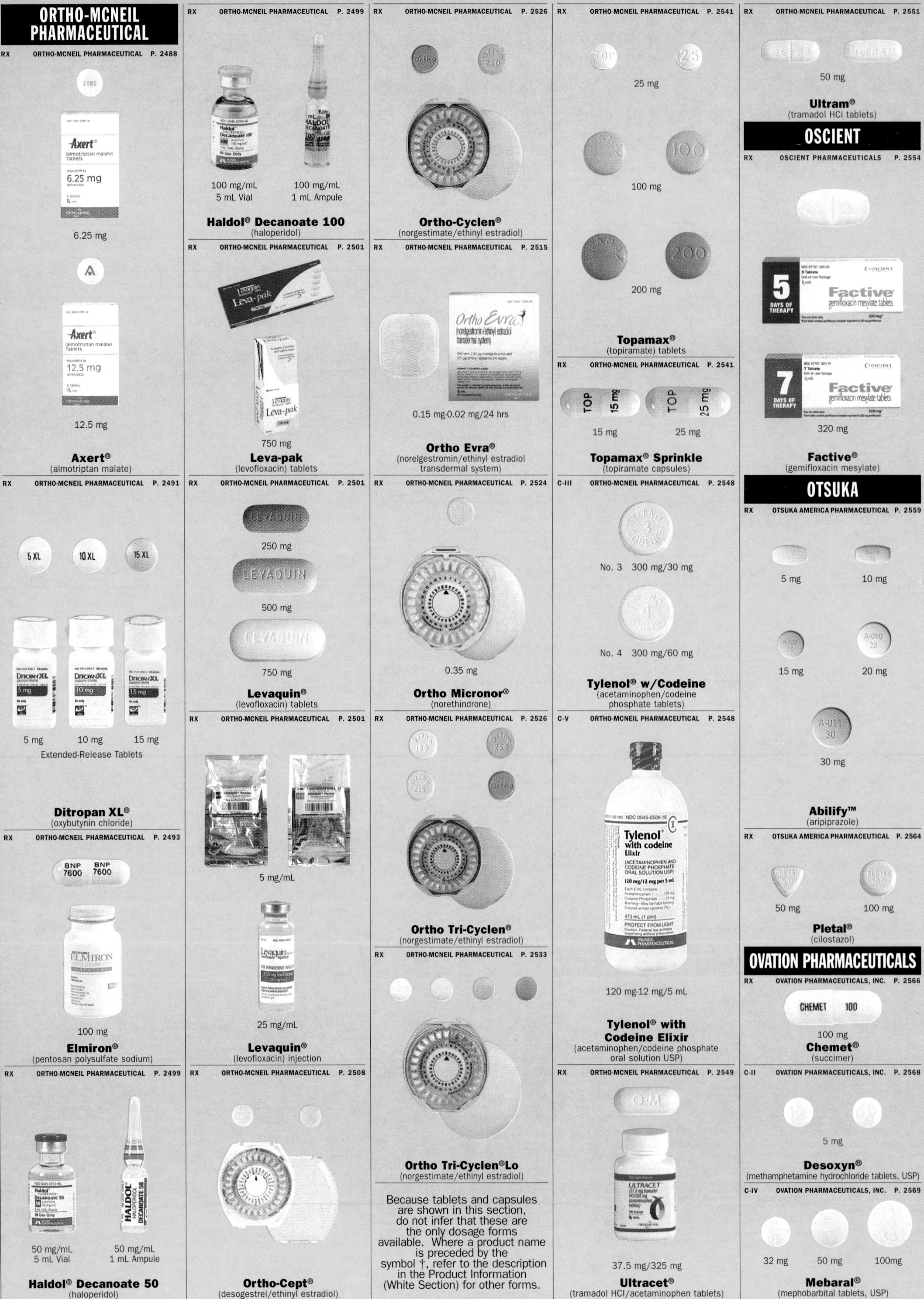

ORTHO-MCNEIL PHARMACEUTICAL
RX ORTHO-MCNEIL PHARMACEUTICAL P. 2488
6.25 mg
12.5 mg
Axert®
(almotriptan malate)
RX ORTHO-MCNEIL PHARMACEUTICAL P. 2491
5 mg 10 mg 15 mg
Extended-Release Tablets
Ditropan XL®
(oxybutynin chloride)
RX ORTHO-MCNEIL PHARMACEUTICAL P. 2493
BNP 7600
100 mg
Elmiron®
(pentosan polysulfate sodium)
RX ORTHO-MCNEIL PHARMACEUTICAL P. 2499
50 mg/mL 5 mL Vial
50 mg/mL 1 mL Ampule
Haldol® Decanoate 50
(haloperidol)
RX ORTHO-MCNEIL PHARMACEUTICAL P. 2499
100 mg/mL 5 mL Vial
100 mg/mL 1 mL Ampule
Haldol® Decanoate 100
(haloperidol)
RX ORTHO-MCNEIL PHARMACEUTICAL P. 2501
750 mg
Leva-pak
(levofloxacin) tablets
RX ORTHO-MCNEIL PHARMACEUTICAL P. 2501
250 mg
500 mg
750 mg
Levaquin®
(levofloxacin) tablets
RX ORTHO-MCNEIL PHARMACEUTICAL P. 2501
5 mg/mL
25 mg/mL
Levaquin®
(levofloxacin) injection
RX ORTHO-MCNEIL PHARMACEUTICAL P. 2508
Ortho-Cept®
(desogestrel/ethinyl estradiol)
RX ORTHO-MCNEIL PHARMACEUTICAL P. 2526
Ortho-Cyclen®
(norgestimate/ethinyl estradiol)
RX ORTHO-MCNEIL PHARMACEUTICAL P. 2515
0.15 mg-0.02 mg/24 hrs
Ortho Evra®
(norelgestromin/ethinyl estradiol transdermal system)
RX ORTHO-MCNEIL PHARMACEUTICAL P. 2524
0.35 mg
Ortho Micronor®
(norethindrone)
RX ORTHO-MCNEIL PHARMACEUTICAL P. 2526
Ortho Tri-Cyclen®
(norgestimate/ethinyl estradiol)
RX ORTHO-MCNEIL PHARMACEUTICAL P. 2533
Ortho Tri-Cyclen®Lo
(norgestimate/ethinyl estradiol)
Because tablets and capsules are shown in this section, do not infer that these are the only dosage forms available. Where a product name is preceded by the symbol †, refer to the description in the Product Information (White Section) for other forms.
RX ORTHO-MCNEIL PHARMACEUTICAL P. 2541
25 mg
100 mg
200 mg
Topamax®
(topiramate) tablets
RX ORTHO-MCNEIL PHARMACEUTICAL P. 2541
15 mg 25 mg
Topamax® Sprinkle
(topiramate capsules)
C-III ORTHO-MCNEIL PHARMACEUTICAL P. 2548
No. 3 300 mg/30 mg
No. 4 300 mg/60 mg
Tylenol® w/Codeine
(acetaminophen/codeine phosphate tablets)
C-V ORTHO-MCNEIL PHARMACEUTICAL P. 2548
120 mg-12 mg/5 mL
Tylenol® with Codeine Elixir
(acetaminophen/codeine phosphate oral solution USP)
RX ORTHO-MCNEIL PHARMACEUTICAL P. 2549
37.5 mg/325 mg
Ultracet®
(tramadol HCl/acetaminophen tablets)
RX ORTHO-MCNEIL PHARMACEUTICAL P. 2551
50 mg
Ultram®
(tramadol HCl tablets)
OSCIENT
RX OSCIENT PHARMACEUTICALS P. 2554
320 mg
Factive®
(gemifloxacin mesylate)
OTSUKA
RX OTSUKA AMERICA PHARMACEUTICAL P. 2559
5 mg 10 mg
15 mg 20 mg
30 mg
Abilify™
(aripiprazole)
RX OTSUKA AMERICA PHARMACEUTICAL P. 2564
50 mg 100 mg
Pletal®
(cilostazol)
OVATION PHARMACEUTICALS
RX OVATION PHARMACEUTICALS, INC. P. 2566
CHEMET 100
100 mg
Chemet®
(succimer)
C-II OVATION PHARMACEUTICALS, INC. P. 2568
5 mg
Desoxyn®
(methamphetamine hydrochloride tablets, USP)
C-IV OVATION PHARMACEUTICALS, INC. P. 2569
32 mg 50 mg 100mg
Mebaral®
(mephobarbital tablets, USP)

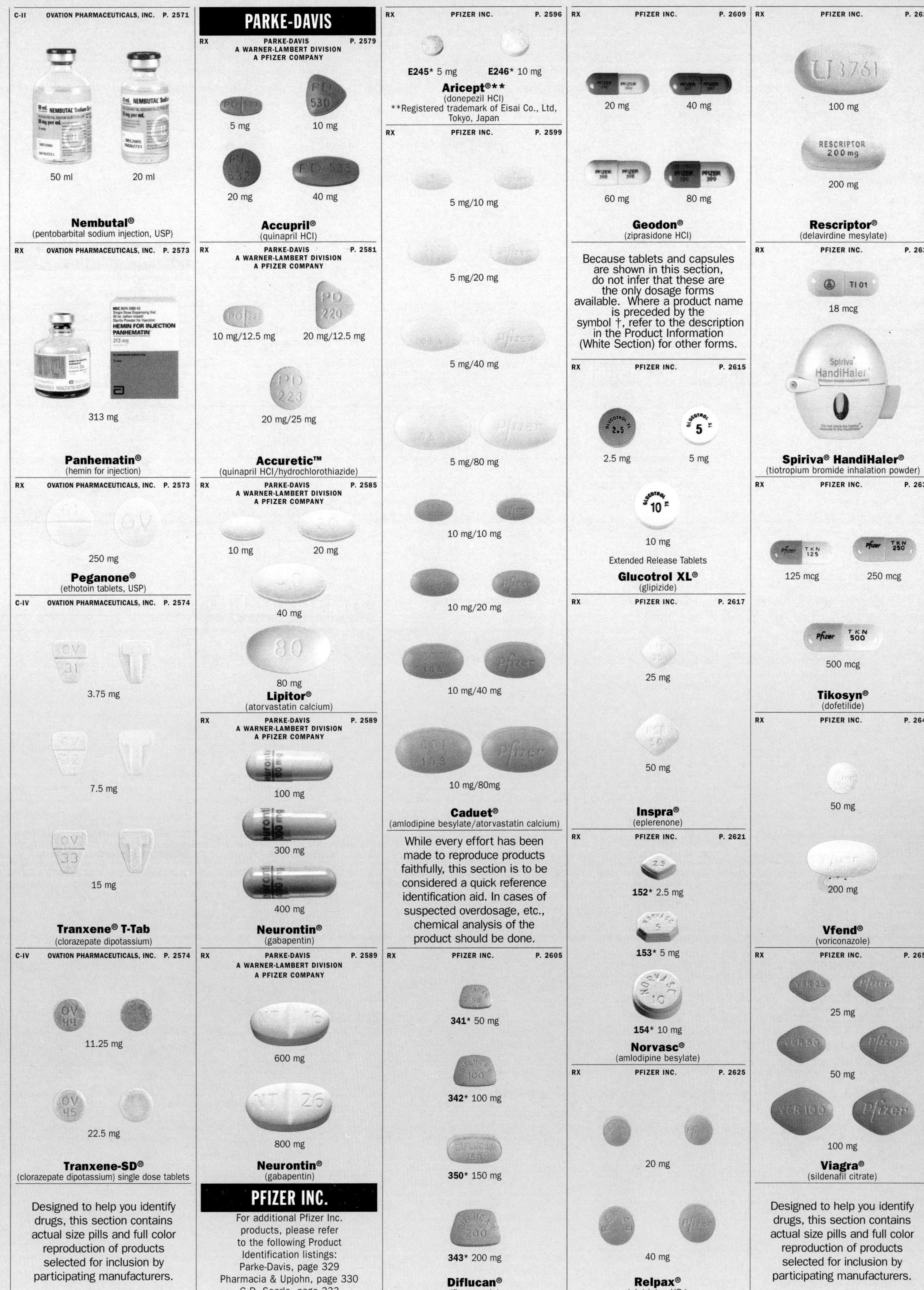

C-II OVATION PHARMACEUTICALS, INC. P. 2571

50 ml 20 ml

Nembutal®
(pentobarbital sodium injection, USP)

RX OVATION PHARMACEUTICALS, INC. P. 2573

313 mg

Panhematin®
(hemin for injection)

RX OVATION PHARMACEUTICALS, INC. P. 2573

250 mg

Peganone®
(ethotoin tablets, USP)

C-IV OVATION PHARMACEUTICALS, INC. P. 2574

3.75 mg

7.5 mg

15 mg

Tranxene® T-Tab
(clorazepate dipotassium)

C-IV OVATION PHARMACEUTICALS, INC. P. 2574

11.25 mg

22.5 mg

Tranxene-SD®
(clorazepate dipotassium) single dose tablets

Designed to help you identify drugs, this section contains actual size pills and full color reproduction of products selected for inclusion by participating manufacturers.

PARKE-DAVIS

RX PARKE-DAVIS A WARNER-LAMBERT DIVISION A PFIZER COMPANY P. 2579

5 mg 10 mg

20 mg 40 mg

Accupril®
(quinapril HCl)

RX PARKE-DAVIS A WARNER-LAMBERT DIVISION A PFIZER COMPANY P. 2581

10 mg/12.5 mg 20 mg/12.5 mg

20 mg/25 mg

Accuretic™
(quinapril HCl/hydrochlorothiazide)

RX PARKE-DAVIS A WARNER-LAMBERT DIVISION A PFIZER COMPANY P. 2585

10 mg 20 mg

40 mg

80 mg

Lipitor®
(atorvastatin calcium)

RX PARKE-DAVIS A WARNER-LAMBERT DIVISION A PFIZER COMPANY P. 2589

100 mg

300 mg

400 mg

Neurontin®
(gabapentin)

RX PARKE-DAVIS A WARNER-LAMBERT DIVISION A PFIZER COMPANY P. 2589

600 mg

800 mg

Neurontin®
(gabapentin)

PFIZER INC.

For additional Pfizer Inc. products, please refer to the following Product Identification listings:
Parke-Davis, page 329
Pharmacia & Upjohn, page 330
G.D. Searle, page 333

RX PFIZER INC. P. 2596

E245* 5 mg **E246*** 10 mg

Aricept®**
(donepezil HCl)
**Registered trademark of Eisai Co., Ltd, Tokyo, Japan

RX PFIZER INC. P. 2599

5 mg/10 mg

5 mg/20 mg

5 mg/40 mg

5 mg/80 mg

10 mg/10 mg

10 mg/20 mg

10 mg/40 mg

10 mg/80mg

Caduet®
(amlodipine besylate/atorvastatin calcium)

While every effort has been made to reproduce products faithfully, this section is to be considered a quick reference identification aid. In cases of suspected overdosage, etc., chemical analysis of the product should be done.

RX PFIZER INC. P. 2605

341* 50 mg

342* 100 mg

350* 150 mg

343* 200 mg

Diflucan®
(fluconazole)

RX PFIZER INC. P. 2609

20 mg 40 mg

60 mg 80 mg

Geodon®
(ziprasidone HCl)

Because tablets and capsules are shown in this section, do not infer that these are the only dosage forms available. Where a product name is preceded by the symbol †, refer to the description in the Product Information (White Section) for other forms.

RX PFIZER INC. P. 2615

2.5 mg 5 mg

10 mg

Extended Release Tablets

Glucotrol XL®
(glipizide)

RX PFIZER INC. P. 2617

25 mg

50 mg

Inspra®
(eplerenone)

RX PFIZER INC. P. 2621

152* 2.5 mg

153* 5 mg

154* 10 mg

Norvasc®
(amlodipine besylate)

RX PFIZER INC. P. 2625

20 mg

40 mg

Relpax®
(eletriptan HBr)

RX PFIZER INC. P. 2629

100 mg

200 mg

Rescriptor®
(delavirdine mesylate)

RX PFIZER INC. P. 2634

18 mcg

Spiriva® HandiHaler®
(tiotropium bromide inhalation powder)

RX PFIZER INC. P. 2639

125 mcg 250 mcg

500 mcg

Tikosyn®
(dofetilide)

RX PFIZER INC. P. 2647

50 mg

200 mg

Vfend®
(voriconazole)

RX PFIZER INC. P. 2656

25 mg

50 mg

100 mg

Viagra®
(sildenafil citrate)

Designed to help you identify drugs, this section contains actual size pills and full color reproduction of products selected for inclusion by participating manufacturers.

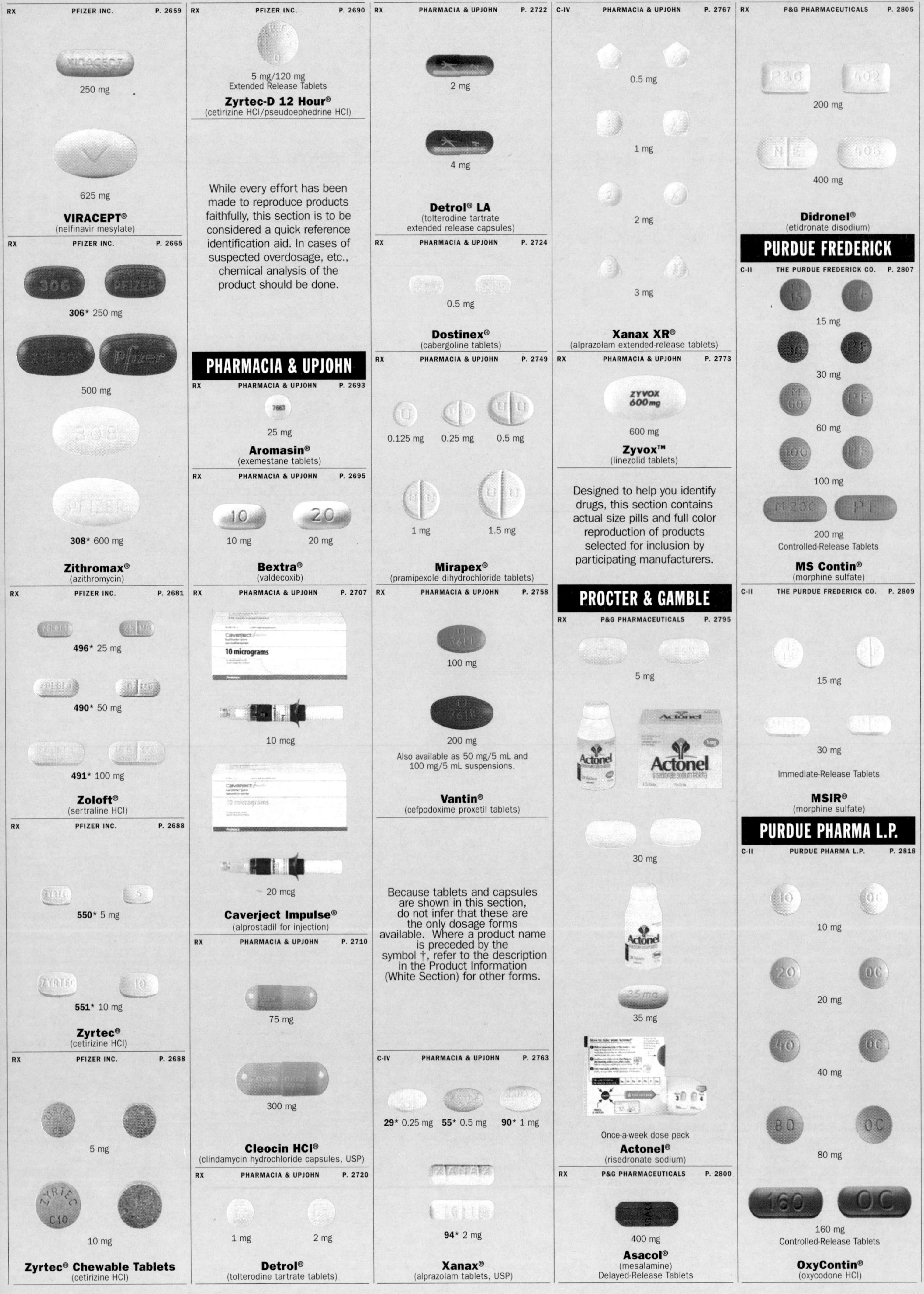

RX PFIZER INC. P. 2659

250 mg

625 mg

VIRACEPT®
(nelfinavir mesylate)

RX PFIZER INC. P. 2665

306* 250 mg

500 mg

308* 600 mg

Zithromax®
(azithromycin)

RX PFIZER INC. P. 2681

496* 25 mg

490* 50 mg

491* 100 mg

Zoloft®
(sertraline HCl)

RX PFIZER INC. P. 2688

550* 5 mg

551* 10 mg

Zyrtec®
(cetirizine HCl)

RX PFIZER INC. P. 2688

5 mg

10 mg

Zyrtec® Chewable Tablets
(cetirizine HCl)

RX PFIZER INC. P. 2690

5 mg/120 mg
Extended Release Tablets

Zyrtec-D 12 Hour®
(cetirizine HCl/pseudoephedrine HCl)

While every effort has been made to reproduce products faithfully, this section is to be considered a quick reference identification aid. In cases of suspected overdosage, etc., chemical analysis of the product should be done.

PHARMACIA & UPJOHN

RX PHARMACIA & UPJOHN P. 2693

25 mg

Aromasin®
(exemestane tablets)

RX PHARMACIA & UPJOHN P. 2695

10 mg 20 mg

Bextra®
(valdecoxib)

RX PHARMACIA & UPJOHN P. 2707

10 mcg

20 mcg

Caverject Impulse®
(alprostadil for injection)

RX PHARMACIA & UPJOHN P. 2710

75 mg

300 mg

Cleocin HCl®
(clindamycin hydrochloride capsules, USP)

RX PHARMACIA & UPJOHN P. 2720

1 mg 2 mg

Detrol®
(tolterodine tartrate tablets)

RX PHARMACIA & UPJOHN P. 2722

2 mg

4 mg

Detrol® LA
(tolterodine tartrate extended release capsules)

RX PHARMACIA & UPJOHN P. 2724

0.5 mg

Dostinex®
(cabergoline tablets)

RX PHARMACIA & UPJOHN P. 2749

0.125 mg 0.25 mg 0.5 mg

1 mg 1.5 mg

Mirapex®
(pramipexole dihydrochloride tablets)

RX PHARMACIA & UPJOHN P. 2758

100 mg

200 mg

Also available as 50 mg/5 mL and 100 mg/5 mL suspensions.

Vantin®
(cefpodoxime proxetil tablets)

Because tablets and capsules are shown in this section, do not infer that these are the only dosage forms available. Where a product name is preceded by the symbol †, refer to the description in the Product Information (White Section) for other forms.

C-IV PHARMACIA & UPJOHN P. 2763

29* 0.25 mg **55*** 0.5 mg **90*** 1 mg

94* 2 mg

Xanax®
(alprazolam tablets, USP)

C-IV PHARMACIA & UPJOHN P. 2767

0.5 mg

1 mg

2 mg

3 mg

Xanax XR®
(alprazolam extended-release tablets)

RX PHARMACIA & UPJOHN P. 2773

600 mg

Zyvox™
(linezolid tablets)

Designed to help you identify drugs, this section contains actual size pills and full color reproduction of products selected for inclusion by participating manufacturers.

PROCTER & GAMBLE

RX P&G PHARMACEUTICALS P. 2795

5 mg

30 mg

35 mg

Once-a-week dose pack

Actonel®
(risedronate sodium)

RX P&G PHARMACEUTICALS P. 2800

400 mg

Asacol®
(mesalamine)
Delayed-Release Tablets

RX P&G PHARMACEUTICALS P. 2805

200 mg

400 mg

Didronel®
(etidronate disodium)

PURDUE FREDERICK

C-II THE PURDUE FREDERICK CO. P. 2807

15 mg

30 mg

60 mg

100 mg

200 mg
Controlled-Release Tablets

MS Contin®
(morphine sulfate)

C-II THE PURDUE FREDERICK CO. P. 2809

15 mg

30 mg

Immediate-Release Tablets

MSIR®
(morphine sulfate)

PURDUE PHARMA L.P.

C-II PURDUE PHARMA L.P. P. 2818

10 mg

20 mg

40 mg

80 mg

160 mg
Controlled-Release Tablets

OxyContin®
(oxycodone HCl)

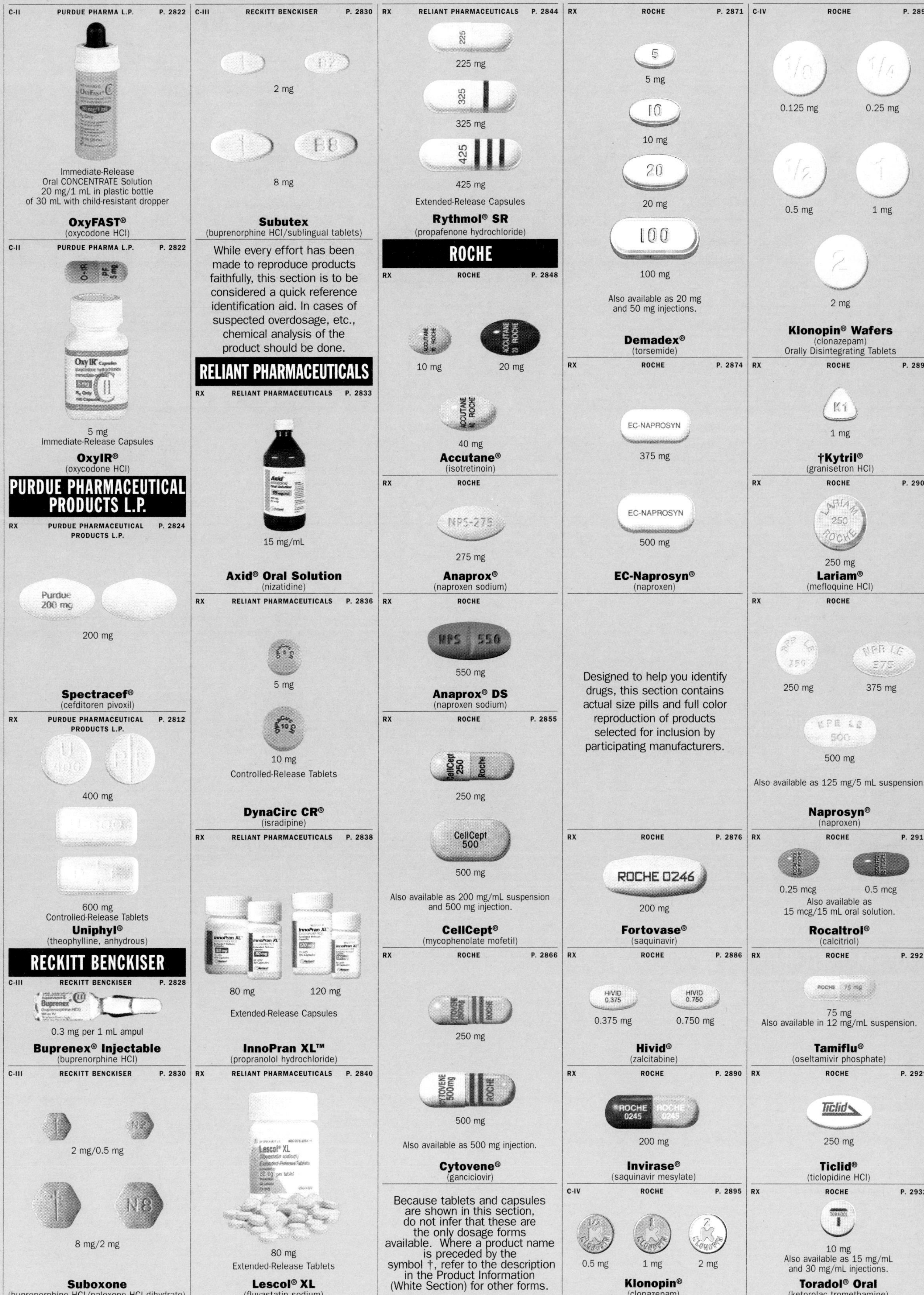

C-II PURDUE PHARMA L.P. P. 2822

Immediate-Release
Oral CONCENTRATE Solution
20 mg/1 mL in plastic bottle
of 30 mL with child-resistant dropper

OxyFAST®
(oxycodone HCl)

C-II PURDUE PHARMA L.P. P. 2822

5 mg
Immediate-Release Capsules

OxyIR®
(oxycodone HCl)

PURDUE PHARMACEUTICAL PRODUCTS L.P.

RX PURDUE PHARMACEUTICAL PRODUCTS L.P. P. 2824

200 mg

Spectracef®
(cefditoren pivoxil)

RX PURDUE PHARMACEUTICAL PRODUCTS L.P. P. 2812

400 mg

600 mg
Controlled-Release Tablets

Uniphyl®
(theophylline, anhydrous)

RECKITT BENCKISER

C-III RECKITT BENCKISER P. 2828

0.3 mg per 1 mL ampul

Buprenex® Injectable
(buprenorphine HCl)

C-III RECKITT BENCKISER P. 2830

2 mg/0.5 mg

8 mg/2 mg

Suboxone
(buprenorphine HCl/naloxone HCl dihydrate)

C-III RECKITT BENCKISER P. 2830

2 mg

8 mg

Subutex
(buprenorphine HCl/sublingual tablets)

While every effort has been made to reproduce products faithfully, this section is to be considered a quick reference identification aid. In cases of suspected overdosage, etc., chemical analysis of the product should be done.

RELIANT PHARMACEUTICALS

RX RELIANT PHARMACEUTICALS P. 2833

15 mg/mL

Axid® Oral Solution
(nizatidine)

RX RELIANT PHARMACEUTICALS P. 2836

5 mg

10 mg
Controlled-Release Tablets

DynaCirc CR®
(isradipine)

RX RELIANT PHARMACEUTICALS P. 2838

80 mg 120 mg

Extended-Release Capsules

InnoPran XL™
(propranolol hydrochloride)

RX RELIANT PHARMACEUTICALS P. 2840

80 mg
Extended-Release Tablets

Lescol® XL
(fluvastatin sodium)

RX RELIANT PHARMACEUTICALS P. 2844

225 mg

325 mg

425 mg

Extended-Release Capsules

Rythmol® SR
(propafenone hydrochloride)

ROCHE

RX ROCHE P. 2848

10 mg 20 mg

40 mg

Accutane®
(isotretinoin)

RX ROCHE

275 mg

Anaprox®
(naproxen sodium)

RX ROCHE

550 mg

Anaprox® DS
(naproxen sodium)

RX ROCHE P. 2855

250 mg

500 mg

Also available as 200 mg/mL suspension and 500 mg injection.

CellCept®
(mycophenolate mofetil)

RX ROCHE P. 2866

250 mg

500 mg

Also available as 500 mg injection.

Cytovene®
(ganciclovir)

Because tablets and capsules are shown in this section, do not infer that these are the only dosage forms available. Where a product name is preceded by the symbol †, refer to the description in the Product Information (White Section) for other forms.

RX ROCHE P. 2871

5 mg

10 mg

20 mg

100 mg

Also available as 20 mg and 50 mg injections.

Demadex®
(torsemide)

RX ROCHE P. 2874

375 mg

500 mg

EC-Naprosyn®
(naproxen)

Designed to help you identify drugs, this section contains actual size pills and full color reproduction of products selected for inclusion by participating manufacturers.

RX ROCHE P. 2876

200 mg

Fortovase®
(saquinavir)

RX ROCHE P. 2886

0.375 mg 0.750 mg

Hivid®
(zalcitabine)

RX ROCHE P. 2890

200 mg

Invirase®
(saquinavir mesylate)

C-IV ROCHE P. 2895

0.5 mg 1 mg 2 mg

Klonopin®
(clonazepam)

C-IV ROCHE P. 2895

0.125 mg 0.25 mg

0.5 mg 1 mg

2 mg

Klonopin® Wafers
(clonazepam)
Orally Disintegrating Tablets

RX ROCHE P. 2898

1 mg

†Kytril®
(granisetron HCl)

RX ROCHE P. 2903

250 mg

Lariam®
(mefloquine HCl)

RX ROCHE

250 mg 375 mg

500 mg

Also available as 125 mg/5 mL suspension.

Naprosyn®
(naproxen)

RX ROCHE P. 2913

0.25 mcg 0.5 mcg

Also available as 15 mcg/15 mL oral solution.

Rocaltrol®
(calcitriol)

RX ROCHE P. 2927

75 mg
Also available in 12 mg/mL suspension.

Tamiflu®
(oseltamivir phosphate)

RX ROCHE P. 2929

250 mg

Ticlid®
(ticlopidine HCl)

RX ROCHE P. 2932

10 mg
Also available as 15 mg/mL and 30 mg/mL injections.

Toradol® Oral
(ketorolac tromethamine)

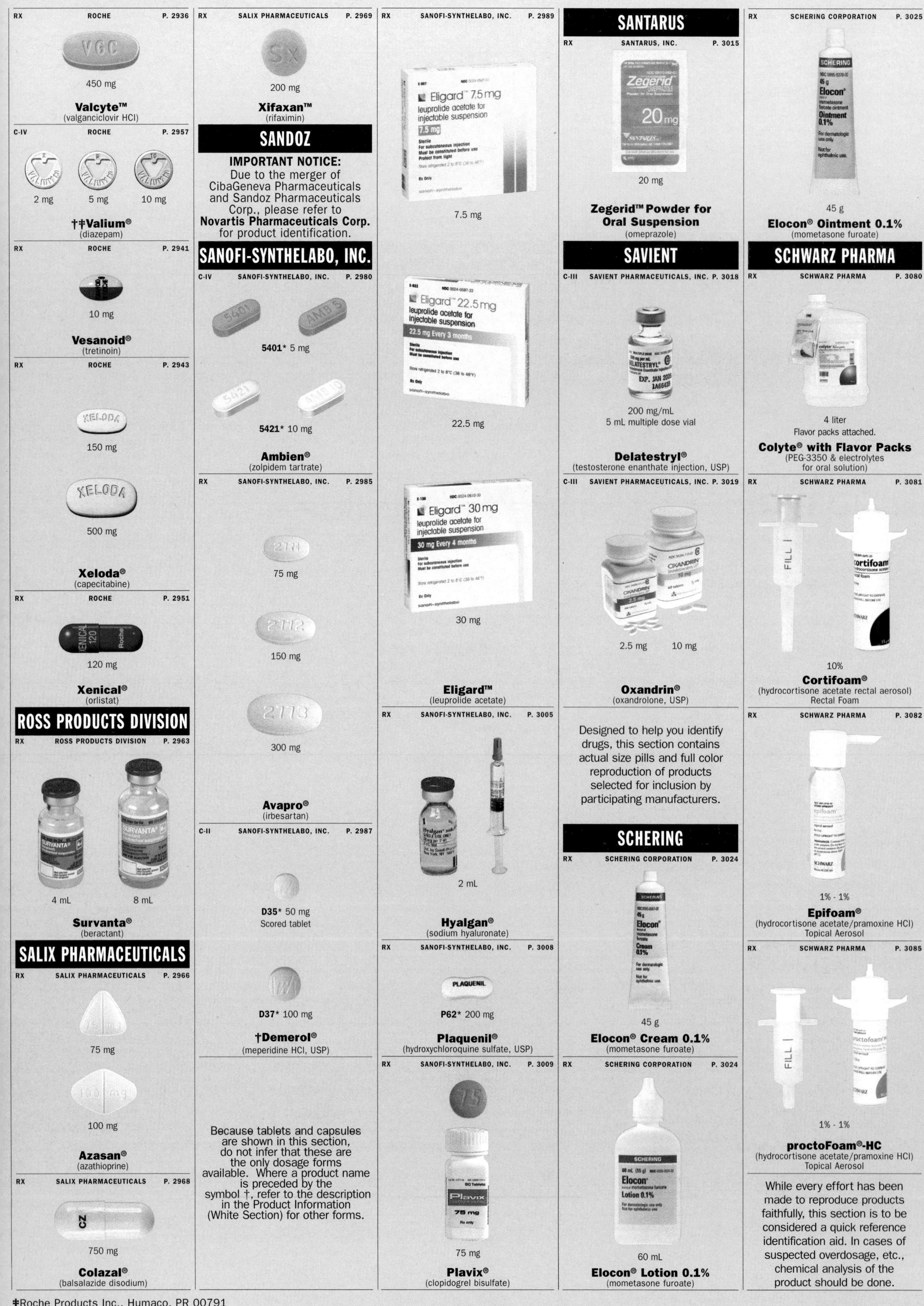

RX ROCHE P. 2936

450 mg

Valcyte™
(valganciclovir HCl)

C-IV ROCHE P. 2957

2 mg 5 mg 10 mg

†‡Valium®
(diazepam)

RX ROCHE P. 2941

10 mg

Vesanoid®
(tretinoin)

RX ROCHE P. 2943

150 mg

500 mg

Xeloda®
(capecitabine)

RX ROCHE P. 2951

120 mg

Xenical®
(orlistat)

ROSS PRODUCTS DIVISION

RX ROSS PRODUCTS DIVISION P. 2963

4 mL 8 mL

Survanta®
(beractant)

SALIX PHARMACEUTICALS

RX SALIX PHARMACEUTICALS P. 2966

75 mg

100 mg

Azasan®
(azathioprine)

RX SALIX PHARMACEUTICALS P. 2968

750 mg

Colazal®
(balsalazide disodium)

RX SALIX PHARMACEUTICALS P. 2969

200 mg

Xifaxan™
(rifaximin)

SANDOZ

IMPORTANT NOTICE:
Due to the merger of CibaGeneva Pharmaceuticals and Sandoz Pharmaceuticals Corp., please refer to **Novartis Pharmaceuticals Corp.** for product identification.

SANOFI-SYNTHELABO, INC.

C-IV SANOFI-SYNTHELABO, INC. P. 2980

5401* 5 mg

5421* 10 mg

Ambien®
(zolpidem tartrate)

RX SANOFI-SYNTHELABO, INC. P. 2985

75 mg

150 mg

300 mg

Avapro®
(irbesartan)

C-II SANOFI-SYNTHELABO, INC. P. 2987

D35* 50 mg
Scored tablet

D37* 100 mg

†Demerol®
(meperidine HCl, USP)

Because tablets and capsules are shown in this section, do not infer that these are the only dosage forms available. Where a product name is preceded by the symbol †, refer to the description in the Product Information (White Section) for other forms.

RX SANOFI-SYNTHELABO, INC. P. 2989

7.5 mg

22.5 mg

30 mg

Eligard™
(leuprolide acetate)

RX SANOFI-SYNTHELABO, INC. P. 3005

2 mL

Hyalgan®
(sodium hyaluronate)

RX SANOFI-SYNTHELABO, INC. P. 3008

P62* 200 mg

Plaquenil®
(hydroxychloroquine sulfate, USP)

RX SANOFI-SYNTHELABO, INC. P. 3009

75 mg

Plavix®
(clopidogrel bisulfate)

SANTARUS

RX SANTARUS, INC. P. 3015

20 mg

Zegerid™ Powder for Oral Suspension
(omeprazole)

SAVIENT

C-III SAVIENT PHARMACEUTICALS, INC. P. 3018

200 mg/mL
5 mL multiple dose vial

Delatestryl®
(testosterone enanthate injection, USP)

C-III SAVIENT PHARMACEUTICALS, INC. P. 3019

2.5 mg 10 mg

Oxandrin®
(oxandrolone, USP)

Designed to help you identify drugs, this section contains actual size pills and full color reproduction of products selected for inclusion by participating manufacturers.

SCHERING

RX SCHERING CORPORATION P. 3024

45 g

Elocon® Cream 0.1%
(mometasone furoate)

RX SCHERING CORPORATION P. 3024

60 mL

Elocon® Lotion 0.1%
(mometasone furoate)

RX SCHERING CORPORATION P. 3025

45 g

Elocon® Ointment 0.1%
(mometasone furoate)

SCHWARZ PHARMA

RX SCHWARZ PHARMA P. 3080

4 liter
Flavor packs attached.

Colyte® with Flavor Packs
(PEG-3350 & electrolytes for oral solution)

RX SCHWARZ PHARMA P. 3081

10%

Cortifoam®
(hydrocortisone acetate rectal aerosol)
Rectal Foam

RX SCHWARZ PHARMA P. 3082

1% - 1%

Epifoam®
(hydrocortisone acetate/pramoxine HCl)
Topical Aerosol

RX SCHWARZ PHARMA P. 3085

1% - 1%

proctoFoam®-HC
(hydrocortisone acetate/pramoxine HCl)
Topical Aerosol

While every effort has been made to reproduce products faithfully, this section is to be considered a quick reference identification aid. In cases of suspected overdosage, etc., chemical analysis of the product should be done.

‡Roche Products Inc., Humaco, PR 00791

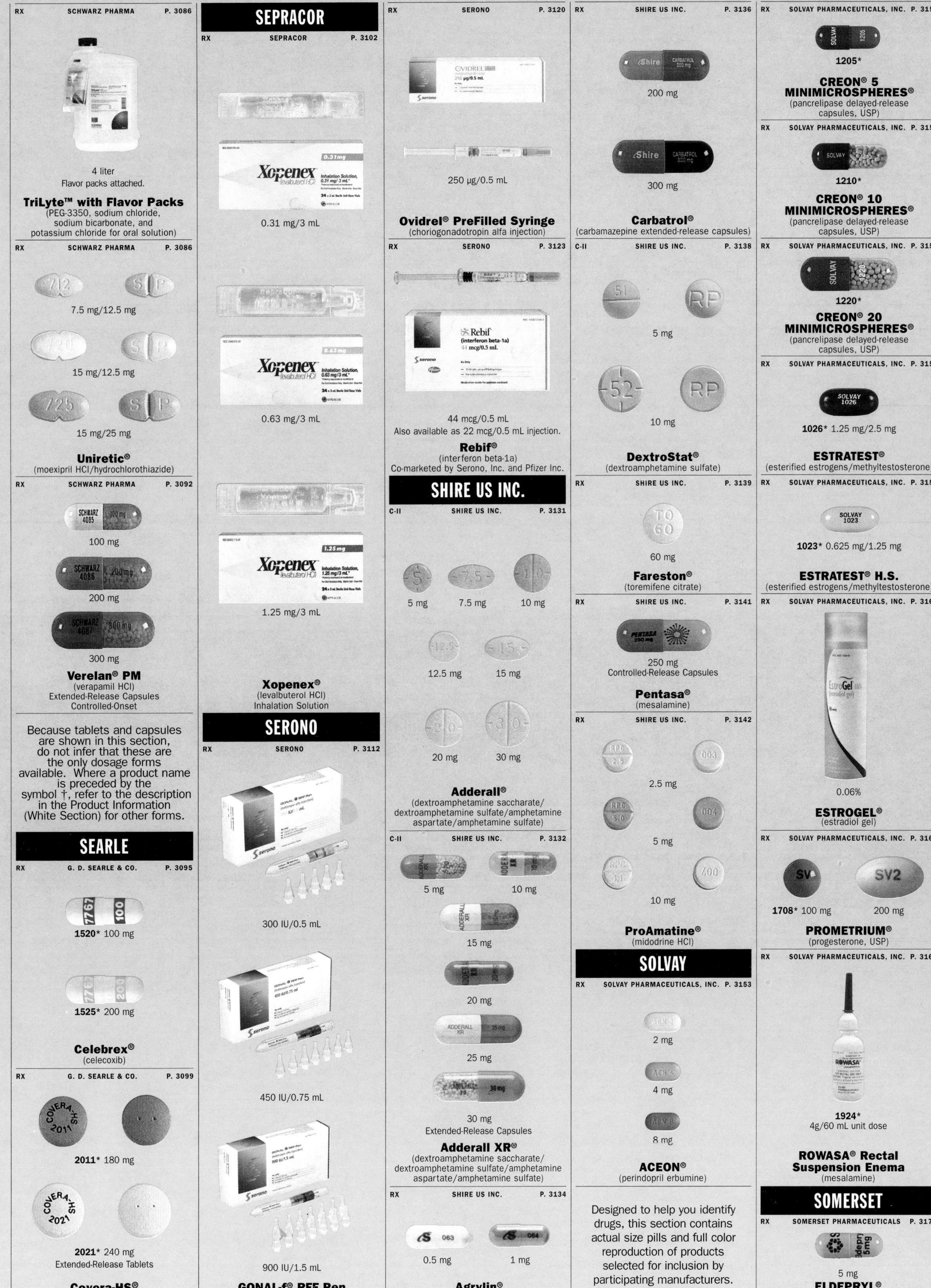

RX SCHWARZ PHARMA P. 3086

4 liter
Flavor packs attached.

TriLyte™ with Flavor Packs
(PEG-3350, sodium chloride, sodium bicarbonate, and potassium chloride for oral solution)

RX SCHWARZ PHARMA P. 3086

7.5 mg/12.5 mg

15 mg/12.5 mg

15 mg/25 mg

Uniretic®
(moexipril HCl/hydrochlorothiazide)

RX SCHWARZ PHARMA P. 3092

100 mg

200 mg

300 mg

Verelan® PM
(verapamil HCl)
Extended-Release Capsules
Controlled-Onset

Because tablets and capsules are shown in this section, do not infer that these are the only dosage forms available. Where a product name is preceded by the symbol †, refer to the description in the Product Information (White Section) for other forms.

SEARLE

RX G. D. SEARLE & CO. P. 3095

1520* 100 mg

1525* 200 mg

Celebrex®
(celecoxib)

RX G. D. SEARLE & CO. P. 3099

2011* 180 mg

2021* 240 mg
Extended-Release Tablets

Covera-HS®
(verapamil HCl)

SEPRACOR

RX SEPRACOR P. 3102

0.31 mg/3 mL

0.63 mg/3 mL

1.25 mg/3 mL

Xopenex®
(levalbuterol HCl)
Inhalation Solution

SERONO

RX SERONO P. 3112

300 IU/0.5 mL

450 IU/0.75 mL

900 IU/1.5 mL

GONAL-f® RFF Pen
(follitropin alfa injection)

RX SERONO P. 3120

250 µg/0.5 mL

Ovidrel® PreFilled Syringe
(choriogonadotropin alfa injection)

RX SERONO P. 3123

44 mcg/0.5 mL
Also available as 22 mcg/0.5 mL injection.

Rebif®
(interferon beta-1a)
Co-marketed by Serono, Inc. and Pfizer Inc.

SHIRE US INC.

C-II SHIRE US INC. P. 3131

5 mg 7.5 mg 10 mg

12.5 mg 15 mg

20 mg 30 mg

Adderall®
(dextroamphetamine saccharate/ dextroamphetamine sulfate/amphetamine aspartate/amphetamine sulfate)

C-II SHIRE US INC. P. 3132

5 mg 10 mg

15 mg

20 mg

25 mg

30 mg
Extended-Release Capsules

Adderall XR®
(dextroamphetamine saccharate/ dextroamphetamine sulfate/amphetamine aspartate/amphetamine sulfate)

RX SHIRE US INC. P. 3134

0.5 mg 1 mg

Agrylin®
(anagrelide HCl)

RX SHIRE US INC. P. 3136

200 mg

300 mg

Carbatrol®
(carbamazepine extended-release capsules)

C-II SHIRE US INC. P. 3138

5 mg

10 mg

DextroStat®
(dextroamphetamine sulfate)

RX SHIRE US INC. P. 3139

60 mg

Fareston®
(toremifene citrate)

RX SHIRE US INC. P. 3141

250 mg
Controlled-Release Capsules

Pentasa®
(mesalamine)

RX SHIRE US INC. P. 3142

2.5 mg

5 mg

10 mg

ProAmatine®
(midodrine HCl)

SOLVAY

RX SOLVAY PHARMACEUTICALS, INC. P. 3153

2 mg

4 mg

8 mg

ACEON®
(perindopril erbumine)

Designed to help you identify drugs, this section contains actual size pills and full color reproduction of products selected for inclusion by participating manufacturers.

RX SOLVAY PHARMACEUTICALS, INC. P. 3156

1205*

CREON® 5 MINIMICROSPHERES®
(pancrelipase delayed-release capsules, USP)

RX SOLVAY PHARMACEUTICALS, INC. P. 3156

1210*

CREON® 10 MINIMICROSPHERES®
(pancrelipase delayed-release capsules, USP)

RX SOLVAY PHARMACEUTICALS, INC. P. 3157

1220*

CREON® 20 MINIMICROSPHERES®
(pancrelipase delayed-release capsules, USP)

RX SOLVAY PHARMACEUTICALS, INC. P. 3157

1026* 1.25 mg/2.5 mg

ESTRATEST®
(esterified estrogens/methyltestosterone)

RX SOLVAY PHARMACEUTICALS, INC. P. 3157

1023* 0.625 mg/1.25 mg

ESTRATEST® H.S.
(esterified estrogens/methyltestosterone)

RX SOLVAY PHARMACEUTICALS, INC. P. 3160

0.06%

ESTROGEL®
(estradiol gel)

RX SOLVAY PHARMACEUTICALS, INC. P. 3165

1708* 100 mg 200 mg

PROMETRIUM®
(progesterone, USP)

RX SOLVAY PHARMACEUTICALS, INC. P. 3168

1924*
4g/60 mL unit dose

ROWASA® Rectal Suspension Enema
(mesalamine)

SOMERSET

RX SOMERSET PHARMACEUTICALS P. 3170

5 mg
ELDEPRYL®
(selegiline HCl)

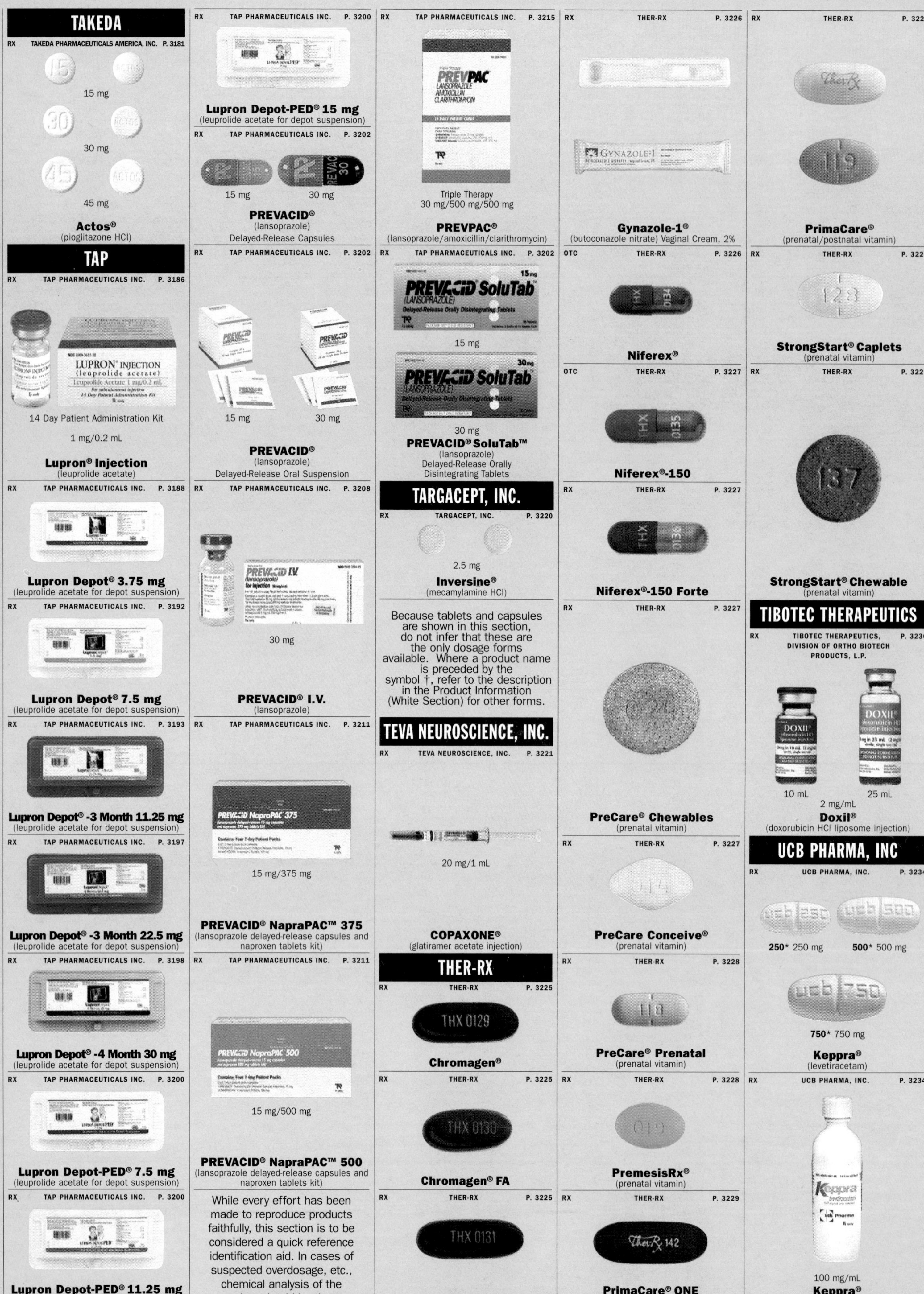

TAKEDA

RX TAKEDA PHARMACEUTICALS AMERICA, INC. P. 3181

15 mg

30 mg

45 mg

Actos®
(pioglitazone HCl)

TAP

RX TAP PHARMACEUTICALS INC. P. 3186

14 Day Patient Administration Kit

1 mg/0.2 mL

Lupron® Injection
(leuprolide acetate)

RX TAP PHARMACEUTICALS INC. P. 3188

Lupron Depot® 3.75 mg
(leuprolide acetate for depot suspension)

RX TAP PHARMACEUTICALS INC. P. 3192

Lupron Depot® 7.5 mg
(leuprolide acetate for depot suspension)

RX TAP PHARMACEUTICALS INC. P. 3193

Lupron Depot® -3 Month 11.25 mg
(leuprolide acetate for depot suspension)

RX TAP PHARMACEUTICALS INC. P. 3197

Lupron Depot® -3 Month 22.5 mg
(leuprolide acetate for depot suspension)

RX TAP PHARMACEUTICALS INC. P. 3198

Lupron Depot® -4 Month 30 mg
(leuprolide acetate for depot suspension)

RX TAP PHARMACEUTICALS INC. P. 3200

Lupron Depot-PED® 7.5 mg
(leuprolide acetate for depot suspension)

RX TAP PHARMACEUTICALS INC. P. 3200

Lupron Depot-PED® 11.25 mg
(leuprolide acetate for depot suspension)

RX TAP PHARMACEUTICALS INC. P. 3200

Lupron Depot-PED® 15 mg
(leuprolide acetate for depot suspension)

RX TAP PHARMACEUTICALS INC. P. 3202

15 mg 30 mg

PREVACID®
(lansoprazole)
Delayed-Release Capsules

RX TAP PHARMACEUTICALS INC. P. 3202

15 mg 30 mg

PREVACID®
(lansoprazole)
Delayed-Release Oral Suspension

RX TAP PHARMACEUTICALS INC. P. 3208

30 mg

PREVACID® I.V.
(lansoprazole)

RX TAP PHARMACEUTICALS INC. P. 3211

15 mg/375 mg

PREVACID® NapraPAC™ 375
(lansoprazole delayed-release capsules and naproxen tablets kit)

RX TAP PHARMACEUTICALS INC. P. 3211

15 mg/500 mg

PREVACID® NapraPAC™ 500
(lansoprazole delayed-release capsules and naproxen tablets kit)

While every effort has been made to reproduce products faithfully, this section is to be considered a quick reference identification aid. In cases of suspected overdosage, etc., chemical analysis of the product should be done.

RX TAP PHARMACEUTICALS INC. P. 3215

Triple Therapy
30 mg/500 mg/500 mg

PREVPAC®
(lansoprazole/amoxicillin/clarithromycin)

RX TAP PHARMACEUTICALS INC. P. 3202

15 mg

30 mg

PREVACID® SoluTab™
(lansoprazole)
Delayed-Release Orally Disintegrating Tablets

TARGACEPT, INC.

RX TARGACEPT, INC. P. 3220

2.5 mg

Inversine®
(mecamylamine HCl)

Because tablets and capsules are shown in this section, do not infer that these are the only dosage forms available. Where a product name is preceded by the symbol †, refer to the description in the Product Information (White Section) for other forms.

TEVA NEUROSCIENCE, INC.

RX TEVA NEUROSCIENCE, INC. P. 3221

20 mg/1 mL

COPAXONE®
(glatiramer acetate injection)

THER-RX

RX THER-RX P. 3225

Chromagen®

RX THER-RX P. 3225

Chromagen® FA

RX THER-RX P. 3225

Chromagen® Forte

RX THER-RX P. 3226

Gynazole-1®
(butoconazole nitrate) Vaginal Cream, 2%

OTC THER-RX P. 3226

Niferex®

OTC THER-RX P. 3227

Niferex®-150

RX THER-RX P. 3227

Niferex®-150 Forte

RX THER-RX P. 3227

PreCare® Chewables
(prenatal vitamin)

RX THER-RX P. 3227

PreCare Conceive®
(prenatal vitamin)

RX THER-RX P. 3228

PreCare® Prenatal
(prenatal vitamin)

RX THER-RX P. 3228

PremesisRx®
(prenatal vitamin)

RX THER-RX P. 3229

PrimaCare® ONE
(prenatal/postnatal vitamin)

RX THER-RX P. 3228

PrimaCare®
(prenatal/postnatal vitamin)

RX THER-RX P. 3229

StrongStart® Caplets
(prenatal vitamin)

RX THER-RX P. 3229

StrongStart® Chewable
(prenatal vitamin)

TIBOTEC THERAPEUTICS

RX TIBOTEC THERAPEUTICS, DIVISION OF ORTHO BIOTECH PRODUCTS, L.P. P. 3230

10 mL 25 mL
2 mg/mL

Doxil®
(doxorubicin HCl liposome injection)

UCB PHARMA, INC

RX UCB PHARMA, INC. P. 3234

250* 250 mg **500*** 500 mg

750* 750 mg

Keppra®
(levetiracetam)

RX UCB PHARMA, INC. P. 3234

100 mg/mL

Keppra®
(levetiracetam)

UNIMED

C-III UNIMED P. 3243

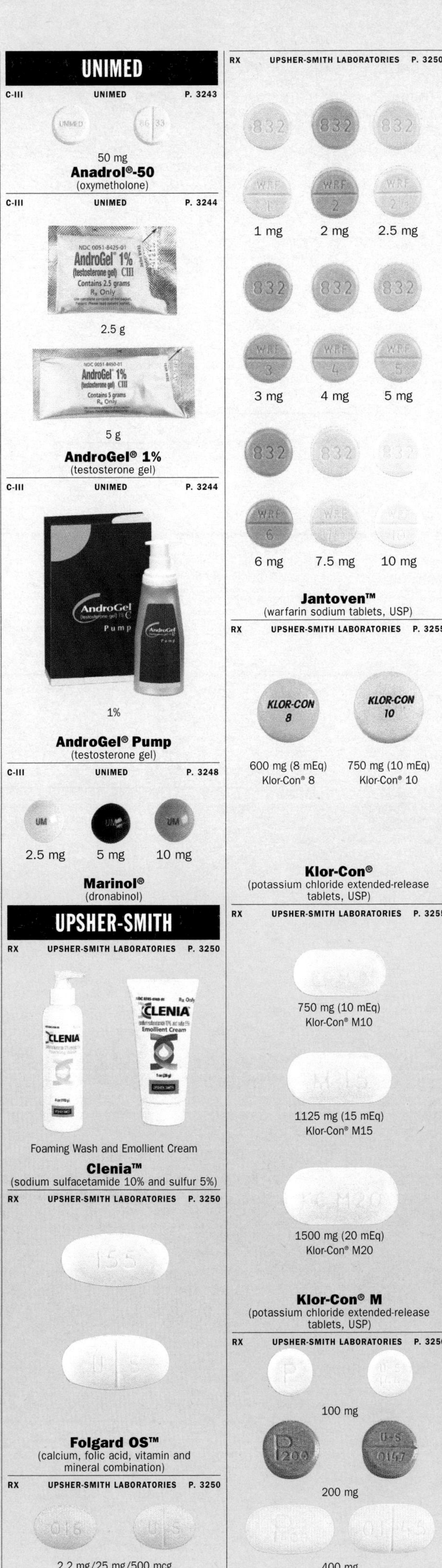

50 mg
Anadrol®-50
(oxymetholone)

C-III UNIMED P. 3244

2.5 g

5 g
AndroGel® 1%
(testosterone gel)

C-III UNIMED P. 3244

1%
AndroGel® Pump
(testosterone gel)

C-III UNIMED P. 3248

2.5 mg 5 mg 10 mg
Marinol®
(dronabinol)

UPSHER-SMITH

RX UPSHER-SMITH LABORATORIES P. 3250

Foaming Wash and Emollient Cream
Clenia™
(sodium sulfacetamide 10% and sulfur 5%)

RX UPSHER-SMITH LABORATORIES P. 3250

Folgard OS™
(calcium, folic acid, vitamin and mineral combination)

RX UPSHER-SMITH LABORATORIES P. 3250

2.2 mg/25 mg/500 mcg
Folgard Rx 2.2®
(folic acid/vitamin B-6/vitamin B-12)

RX UPSHER-SMITH LABORATORIES P. 3250

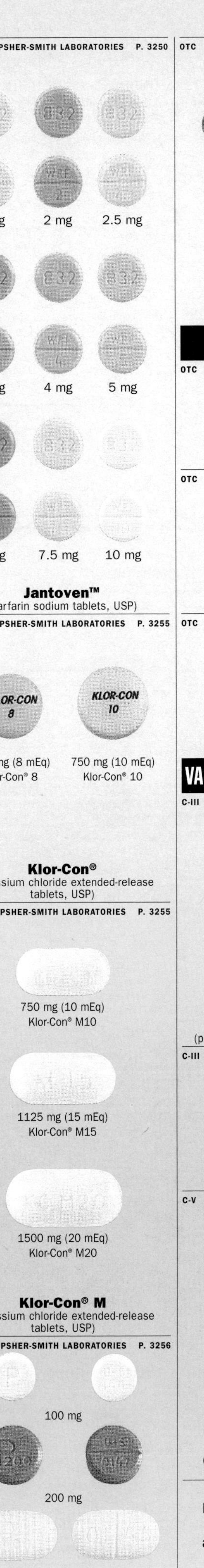

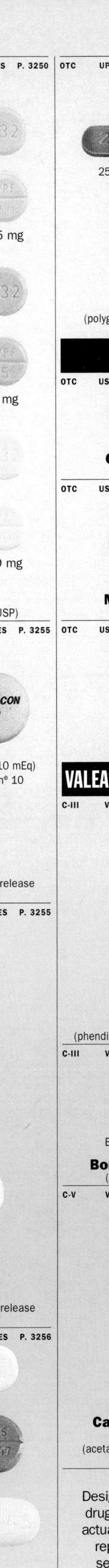

1 mg 2 mg 2.5 mg

3 mg 4 mg 5 mg

6 mg 7.5 mg 10 mg

Jantoven™
(warfarin sodium tablets, USP)

RX UPSHER-SMITH LABORATORIES P. 3255

600 mg (8 mEq) Klor-Con® 8
750 mg (10 mEq) Klor-Con® 10

Klor-Con®
(potassium chloride extended-release tablets, USP)

RX UPSHER-SMITH LABORATORIES P. 3255

750 mg (10 mEq)
Klor-Con® M10

1125 mg (15 mEq)
Klor-Con® M15

1500 mg (20 mEq)
Klor-Con® M20

Klor-Con® M
(potassium chloride extended-release tablets, USP)

RX UPSHER-SMITH LABORATORIES P. 3256

100 mg

200 mg

400 mg
Pacerone®
(amiodarone HCl tablets)

OTC UPSHER-SMITH LABORATORIES P. 3260

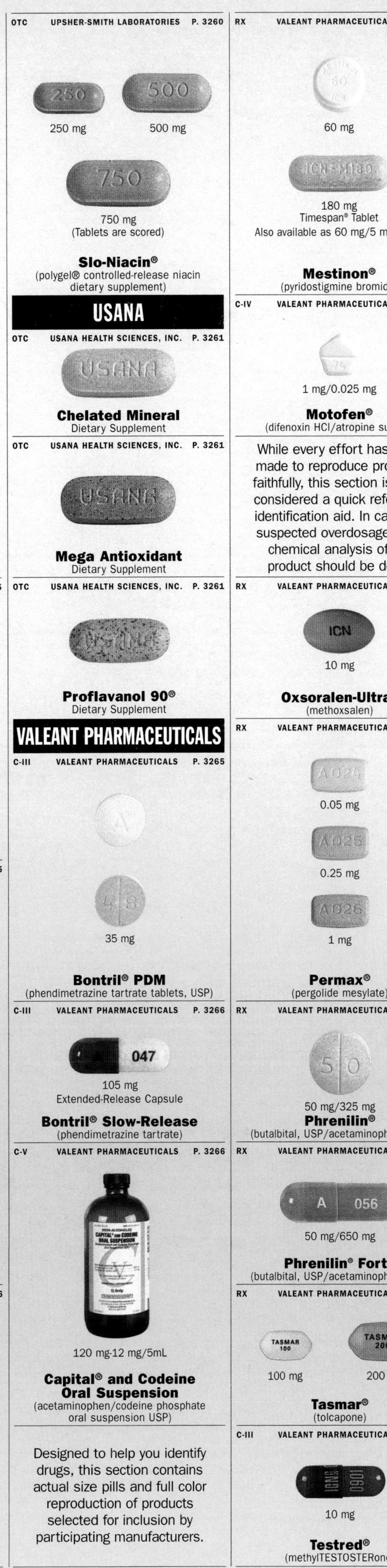

250 mg 500 mg

750 mg
(Tablets are scored)

Slo-Niacin®
(polygel® controlled-release niacin dietary supplement)

USANA

OTC USANA HEALTH SCIENCES, INC. P. 3261

Chelated Mineral
Dietary Supplement

OTC USANA HEALTH SCIENCES, INC. P. 3261

Mega Antioxidant
Dietary Supplement

OTC USANA HEALTH SCIENCES, INC. P. 3261

Proflavanol 90®
Dietary Supplement

VALEANT PHARMACEUTICALS

C-III VALEANT PHARMACEUTICALS P. 3265

35 mg

Bontril® PDM
(phendimetrazine tartrate tablets, USP)

C-III VALEANT PHARMACEUTICALS P. 3266

105 mg
Extended-Release Capsule
Bontril® Slow-Release
(phendimetrazine tartrate)

C-V VALEANT PHARMACEUTICALS P. 3266

120 mg-12 mg/5mL
Capital® and Codeine Oral Suspension
(acetaminophen/codeine phosphate oral suspension USP)

Designed to help you identify drugs, this section contains actual size pills and full color reproduction of products selected for inclusion by participating manufacturers.

RX VALEANT PHARMACEUTICALS P. 3269

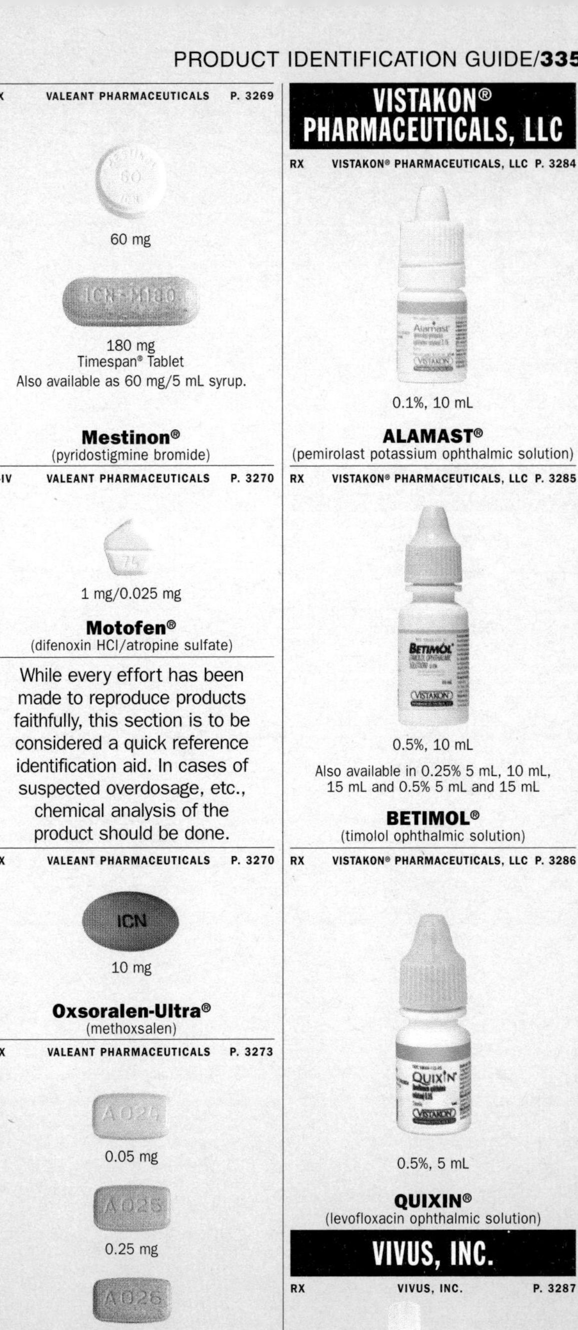

60 mg

180 mg
Timespan® Tablet
Also available as 60 mg/5 mL syrup.

Mestinon®
(pyridostigmine bromide)

C-IV VALEANT PHARMACEUTICALS P. 3270

1 mg/0.025 mg
Motofen®
(difenoxin HCl/atropine sulfate)

While every effort has been made to reproduce products faithfully, this section is to be considered a quick reference identification aid. In cases of suspected overdosage, etc., chemical analysis of the product should be done.

RX VALEANT PHARMACEUTICALS P. 3270

10 mg
Oxsoralen-Ultra®
(methoxsalen)

RX VALEANT PHARMACEUTICALS P. 3273

0.05 mg

0.25 mg

1 mg

Permax®
(pergolide mesylate)

RX VALEANT PHARMACEUTICALS P. 3276

50 mg/325 mg
Phrenilin®
(butalbital, USP/acetaminophen, USP)

RX VALEANT PHARMACEUTICALS P. 3276

50 mg/650 mg
Phrenilin® Forte
(butalbital, USP/acetaminophen, USP)

RX VALEANT PHARMACEUTICALS P. 3276

100 mg 200 mg
Tasmar®
(tolcapone)

C-III VALEANT PHARMACEUTICALS P. 3281

10 mg
Testred®
(methylTESTOSTERone)

VISTAKON® PHARMACEUTICALS, LLC

RX VISTAKON® PHARMACEUTICALS, LLC P. 3284

0.1%, 10 mL
ALAMAST®
(pemirolast potassium ophthalmic solution)

RX VISTAKON® PHARMACEUTICALS, LLC P. 3285

0.5%, 10 mL
Also available in 0.25% 5 mL, 10 mL, 15 mL and 0.5% 5 mL and 15 mL
BETIMOL®
(timolol ophthalmic solution)

RX VISTAKON® PHARMACEUTICALS, LLC P. 3286

0.5%, 5 mL
QUIXIN®
(levofloxacin ophthalmic solution)

VIVUS, INC.

RX VIVUS, INC. P. 3287

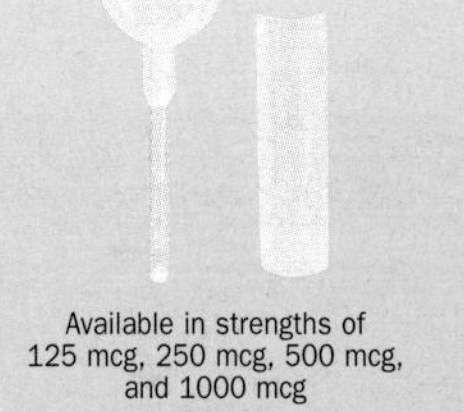

Available in strengths of 125 mcg, 250 mcg, 500 mcg, and 1000 mcg
MUSE®
Urethral Suppository (alprostadil)

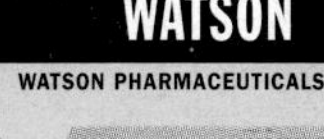

Because tablets and capsules are shown in this section, do not infer that these are the only dosage forms available. Where a product name is preceded by the symbol †, refer to the description in the Product Information (White Section) for other forms.

WATSON

RX WATSON PHARMACEUTICALS, INC. P. 3300

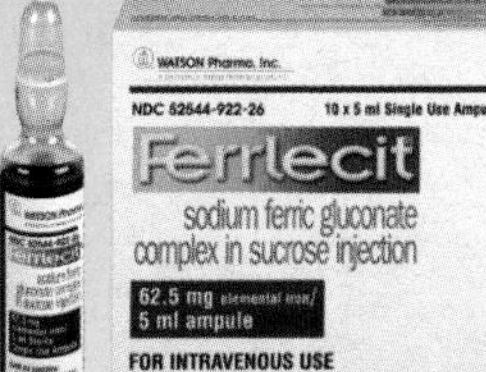

62.5 mg/5 mL
Ferrlecit®
(sodium ferric gluconate complex in sucrose injection)

RX WATSON PHARMACEUTICALS, INC. P. 3303

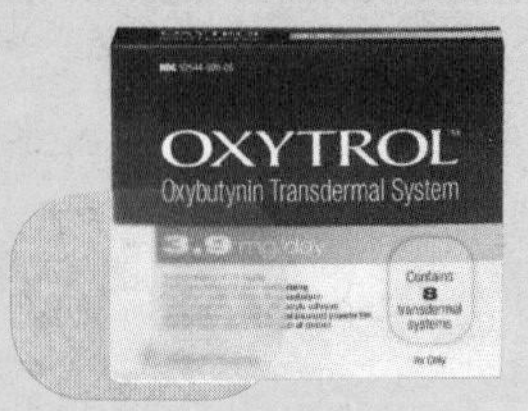

3.9 mg/day

Oxytrol®
(Oxybutynin Transdermal System)

WELLSPRING

RX WELLSPRING PHARMACEUTICAL CORP P. 3305

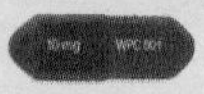

E33* 10 mg

Dibenzyline®
(phenoxybenzamine HCl)

RX WELLSPRING PHARMACEUTICAL CORP P. 3306

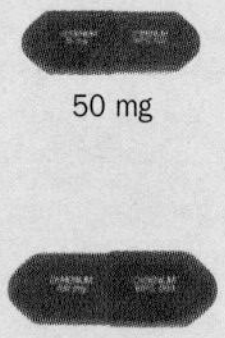

50 mg

100 mg

Dyrenium®
(triamterene)

Designed to help you identify drugs, this section contains actual size pills and full color reproduction of products selected for inclusion by participating manufacturers.

WINSTON

RX WINSTON LABORATORIES P. 3308

0.25%, 60 mg

Axsain™
(capsaicin, USP)

WYETH PHARMACEUTICALS

RX WYETH PHARMACEUTICALS P. 3308

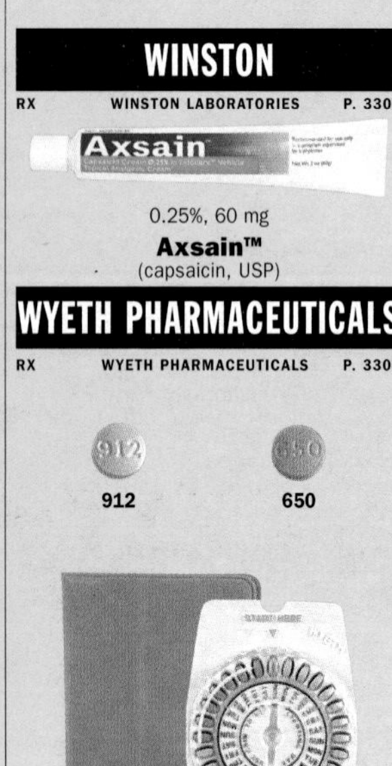

912 **650**

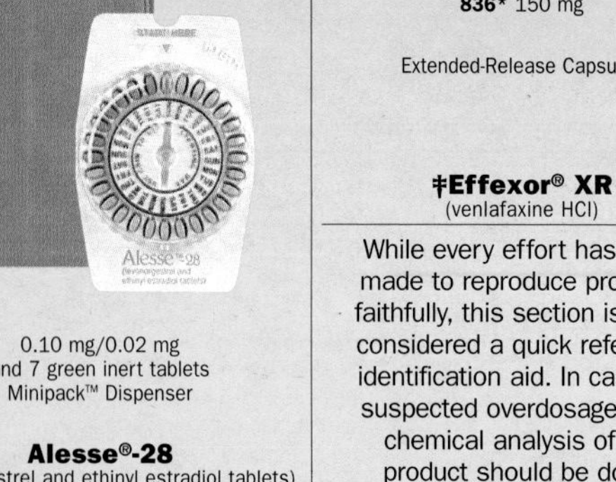

0.10 mg/0.02 mg
and 7 green inert tablets
Minipack™ Dispenser

Alesse®-28
(levonorgestrel and ethinyl estradiol tablets)

RX WYETH PHARMACEUTICALS P. 3318

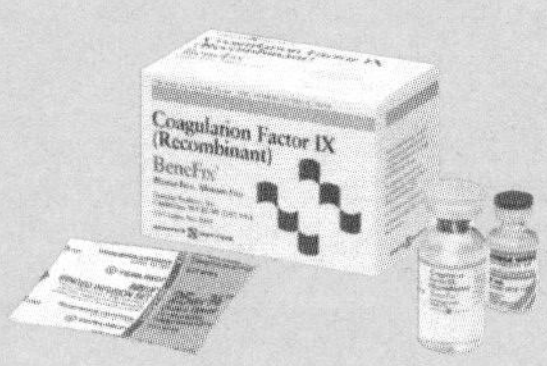

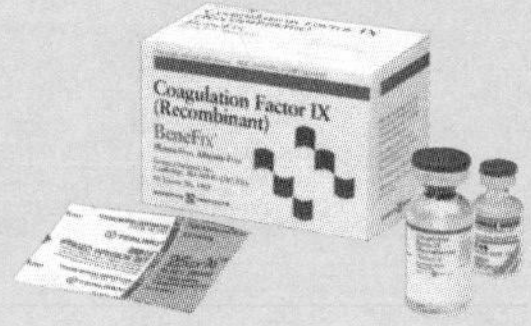

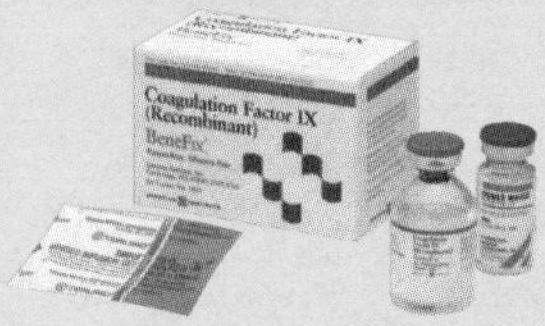

BeneFix®
(coagulation factor IX [recombinant])

RX WYETH PHARMACEUTICALS P. 3321

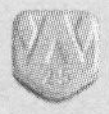

701** 25 mg

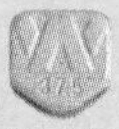

781** 37.5 mg

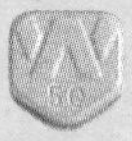

703** 50 mg

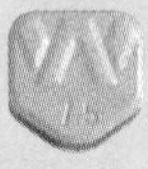

704** 75 mg

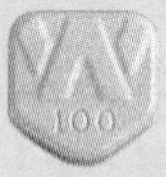

705** 100 mg

‡Effexor®
(venlafaxine HCl)

RX WYETH PHARMACEUTICALS P. 3326

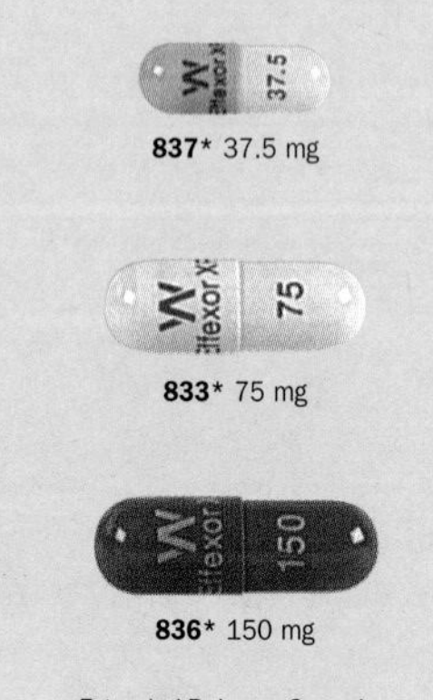

837* 37.5 mg

833* 75 mg

836* 150 mg

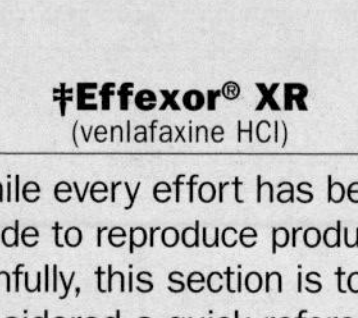

Extended-Release Capsules

‡Effexor® XR
(venlafaxine HCl)

While every effort has been made to reproduce products faithfully, this section is to be considered a quick reference identification aid. In cases of suspected overdosage, etc., chemical analysis of the product should be done.

RX WYETH PHARMACEUTICALS P. 3336

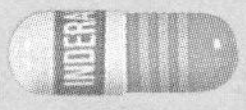

470* 60 mg

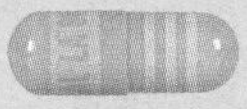

471* 80 mg

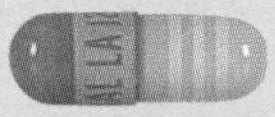

473* 120 mg

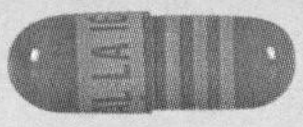

479* 160 mg

Long-Acting Capsules

‡Inderal® LA
(propranolol HCl)

RX WYETH PHARMACEUTICALS P. 3337

78** **486****

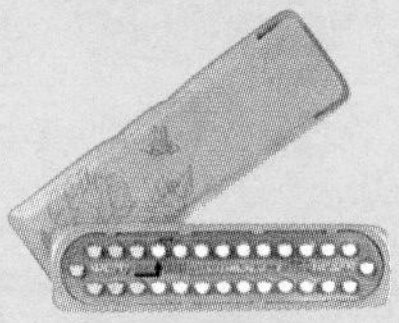

0.3 mg/0.03 mg
and 7 pink inert tablets
Pilpak® Dispenser

2514*

Lo/Ovral®-28
(norgestrel and ethinyl estradiol tablets)

RX WYETH PHARMACEUTICALS P. 3344

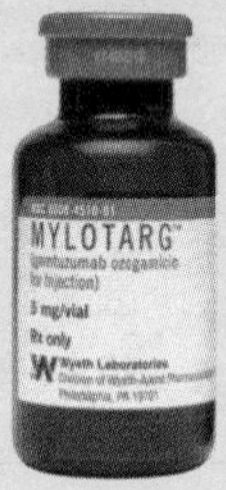

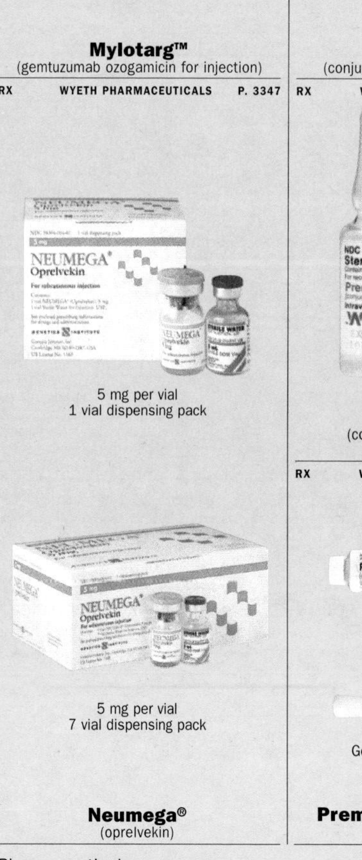

5 mg/vial

Mylotarg™
(gemtuzumab ozogamicin for injection)

RX WYETH PHARMACEUTICALS P. 3347

5 mg per vial
1 vial dispensing pack

5 mg per vial
7 vial dispensing pack

Neumega®
(oprelvekin)

RX WYETH PHARMACEUTICALS P. 3352

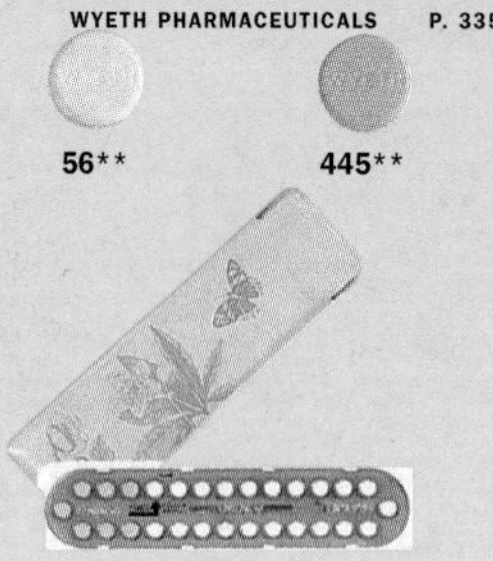

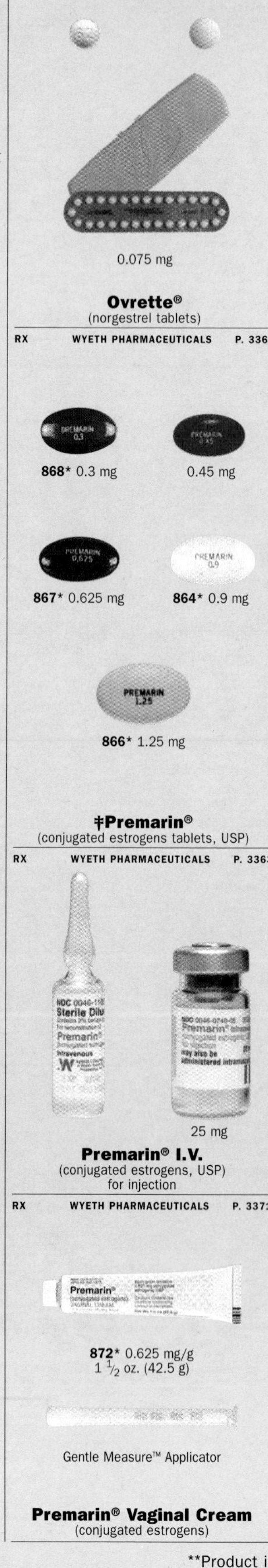

56** **445****

0.5 mg/0.05 mg
and 7 pink inert tablets

2511* Pilpak® Dispenser

Ovral®-28
(norgestrel and ethinyl estradiol tablets)

RX WYETH PHARMACEUTICALS P. 3358

0.075 mg

Ovrette®
(norgestrel tablets)

RX WYETH PHARMACEUTICALS P. 3363

868* 0.3 mg 0.45 mg

867* 0.625 mg **864*** 0.9 mg

866* 1.25 mg

‡Premarin®
(conjugated estrogens tablets, USP)

RX WYETH PHARMACEUTICALS P. 3363

25 mg

Premarin® I.V.
(conjugated estrogens, USP)
for injection

RX WYETH PHARMACEUTICALS P. 3371

872* 0.625 mg/g
1 $^1/_2$ oz. (42.5 g)

Gentle Measure™ Applicator

Premarin® Vaginal Cream
(conjugated estrogens)

RX WYETH PHARMACEUTICALS P. 3375

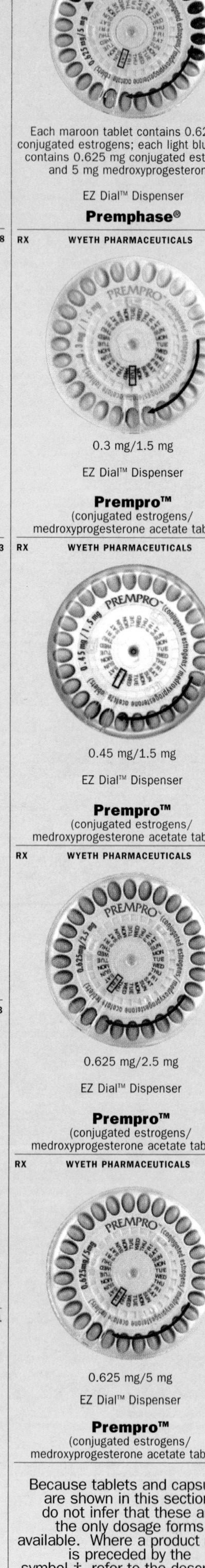

Each maroon tablet contains 0.625 mg conjugated estrogens; each light blue tablet contains 0.625 mg conjugated estrogens and 5 mg medroxyprogesterone.

EZ Dial™ Dispenser

Premphase®

RX WYETH PHARMACEUTICALS P. 3375

0.3 mg/1.5 mg

EZ Dial™ Dispenser

Prempro™
(conjugated estrogens/
medroxyprogesterone acetate tablets)

RX WYETH PHARMACEUTICALS P. 3375

0.45 mg/1.5 mg

EZ Dial™ Dispenser

Prempro™
(conjugated estrogens/
medroxyprogesterone acetate tablets)

RX WYETH PHARMACEUTICALS P. 3375

0.625 mg/2.5 mg

EZ Dial™ Dispenser

Prempro™
(conjugated estrogens/
medroxyprogesterone acetate tablets)

RX WYETH PHARMACEUTICALS P. 3375

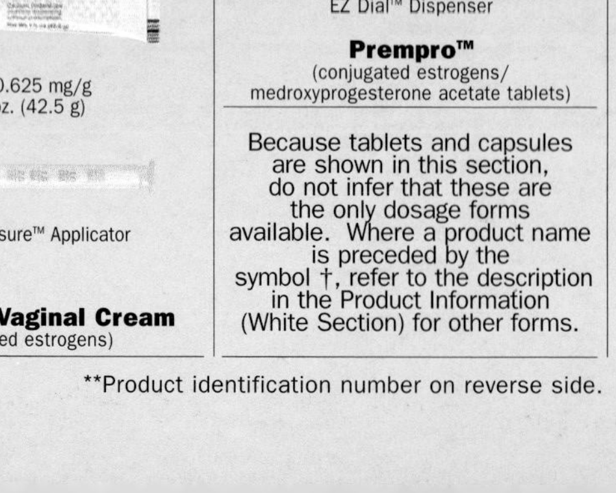

0.625 mg/5 mg

EZ Dial™ Dispenser

Prempro™
(conjugated estrogens/
medroxyprogesterone acetate tablets)

Because tablets and capsules are shown in this section, do not infer that these are the only dosage forms available. Where a product name is preceded by the symbol †, refer to the description in the Product Information (White Section) for other forms.

‡The appearance of these tablets and capsules is a trademark of Wyeth Pharmaceuticals.

**Product identification number on reverse side.

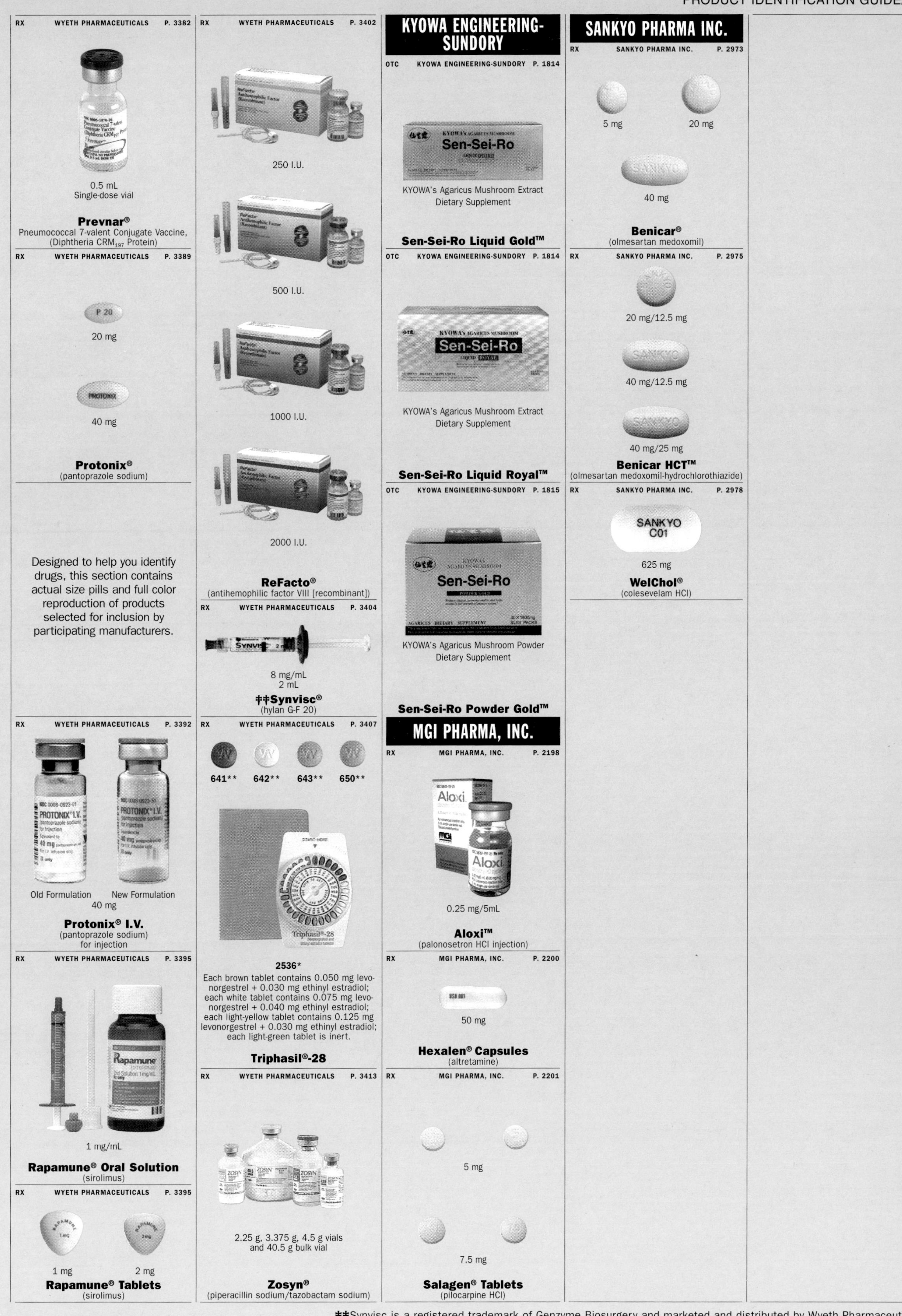

RX WYETH PHARMACEUTICALS P. 3382

0.5 mL
Single-dose vial

Prevnar®
Pneumococcal 7-valent Conjugate Vaccine, (Diphtheria CRM_{197} Protein)

RX WYETH PHARMACEUTICALS P. 3389

20 mg

40 mg

Protonix®
(pantoprazole sodium)

Designed to help you identify drugs, this section contains actual size pills and full color reproduction of products selected for inclusion by participating manufacturers.

RX WYETH PHARMACEUTICALS P. 3392

Old Formulation New Formulation
40 mg

Protonix® I.V.
(pantoprazole sodium)
for injection

RX WYETH PHARMACEUTICALS P. 3395

1 mg/mL

Rapamune® Oral Solution
(sirolimus)

RX WYETH PHARMACEUTICALS P. 3395

1 mg 2 mg

Rapamune® Tablets
(sirolimus)

RX WYETH PHARMACEUTICALS P. 3402

250 I.U.

500 I.U.

1000 I.U.

2000 I.U.

ReFacto®
(antihemophilic factor VIII [recombinant])

RX WYETH PHARMACEUTICALS P. 3404

8 mg/mL
2 mL

‡‡Synvisc®
(hylan G-F 20)

RX WYETH PHARMACEUTICALS P. 3407

641** 642** 643** 650**

2536*
Each brown tablet contains 0.050 mg levonorgestrel + 0.030 mg ethinyl estradiol; each white tablet contains 0.075 mg levonorgestrel + 0.040 mg ethinyl estradiol; each light-yellow tablet contains 0.125 mg levonorgestrel + 0.030 mg ethinyl estradiol; each light-green tablet is inert.

Triphasil®-28

RX WYETH PHARMACEUTICALS P. 3413

2.25 g, 3.375 g, 4.5 g vials and 40.5 g bulk vial

Zosyn®
(piperacillin sodium/tazobactam sodium)

KYOWA ENGINEERING-SUNDORY

OTC KYOWA ENGINEERING-SUNDORY P. 1814

KYOWA's Agaricus Mushroom Extract
Dietary Supplement

Sen-Sei-Ro Liquid Gold™

OTC KYOWA ENGINEERING-SUNDORY P. 1814

KYOWA's Agaricus Mushroom Extract
Dietary Supplement

Sen-Sei-Ro Liquid Royal™

OTC KYOWA ENGINEERING-SUNDORY P. 1815

KYOWA's Agaricus Mushroom Powder
Dietary Supplement

Sen-Sei-Ro Powder Gold™

MGI PHARMA, INC.

RX MGI PHARMA, INC. P. 2198

0.25 mg/5mL

Aloxi™
(palonosetron HCl injection)

RX MGI PHARMA, INC. P. 2200

50 mg

Hexalen® Capsules
(altretamine)

RX MGI PHARMA, INC. P. 2201

5 mg

7.5 mg

Salagen® Tablets
(pilocarpine HCl)

SANKYO PHARMA INC.

RX SANKYO PHARMA INC. P. 2973

5 mg 20 mg

40 mg

Benicar®
(olmesartan medoxomil)

RX SANKYO PHARMA INC. P. 2975

20 mg/12.5 mg

40 mg/12.5 mg

40 mg/25 mg

Benicar HCT™
(olmesartan medoxomil-hydrochlorothiazide)

RX SANKYO PHARMA INC. P. 2978

625 mg

WelChol®
(colesevelam HCl)

‡‡Synvisc is a registered trademark of Genzyme Biosurgery and marketed and distributed by Wyeth Pharmaceuticals.

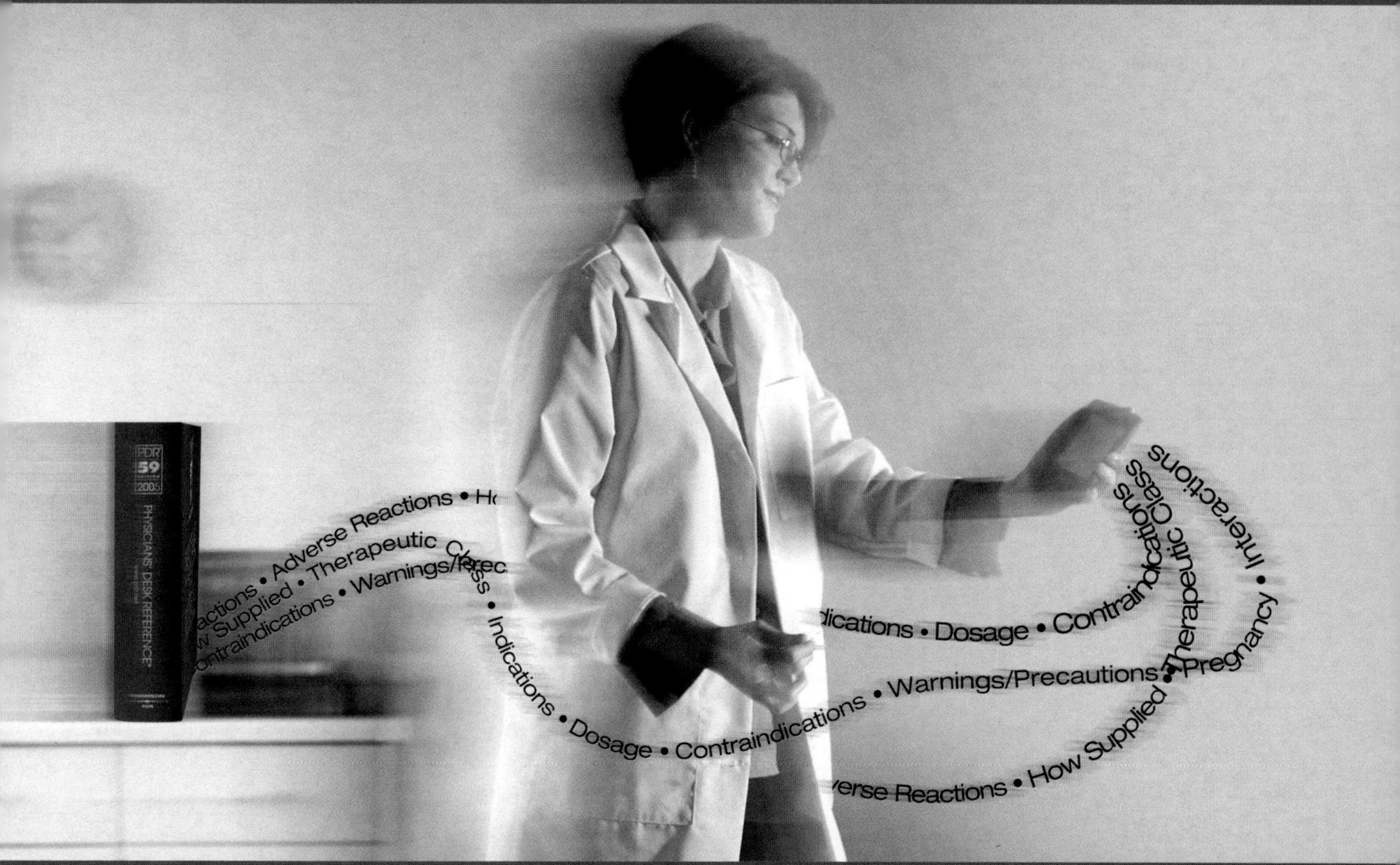

SECTION 5

PRODUCT INFORMATION

This section is made possible through the courtesy of the manufacturers whose products appear in it. The information concerning each product has been prepared, edited, and approved by the medical department, medical director, and/or medical counsel of its manufacturer.

When a product appearing in *Physicians' Desk Reference* has an official package circular, its description must be in full compliance with Food and Drug Administration (FDA) regulations pertaining to labeling for prescription drugs. These regulations require that in *PDR* "indications, effects, dosages, routes, methods, and frequency and duration of administration, and any relevant warnings, hazards, contraindications, side effects, and precautions" must be "*same in language and emphasis*" as those in the approved labeling for the product. The FDA regards the words "*same in language and emphasis*" as requiring VERBATIM use of the approved labeling providing such information. Furthermore, information in the approved labeling that is emphasized by the use of type set in a box or in capitals, boldface, or italics must be given the same emphasis in *PDR*.

For products that do not have official package circulars, the publisher has emphasized the necessity of describing such products comprehensively, so that physicians have access to all information essential for intelligent and informed decision making.

The product descriptions in *Physicians' Desk Reference* include all information made available to *PDR* by the manufacturer. The publisher does not warrant or guarantee any product, and does not perform any independent analysis of the information provided. Inclusion of a product in *PDR* does not represent an endorsement, and the publisher does not necessarily advocate the use of any product listed.

This edition of *Physicians' Desk Reference* contains the latest information available when the book went to press. As new drugs are released, and new research data and clinical findings become available throughout the year, the information in the *PDR* database is revised accordingly. These revisions are published twice annually in the *PDR* Supplements. To be certain that you have the most current data, always consult the supplements before prescribing or administering any product described in the following pages.

aaiPharma

**2320 SCIENTIFIC PARK DRIVE
WILMINGTON NC 28405**

Direct Inquiries to:
Phone: 1-877-263-6726
Fax: 1-866-463-6726

DARVOCET A500™ Ⓒ℞
[Dar-von]
(Propoxyphene Napsylate and Acetaminophen Tablets, USP)

DARVOCET-N® 50 and DARVOCET-N® 100
(Propoxyphene Napsylate and Acetaminophen Tablets, USP)

DARVON-N®
(Propoxyphene Napsylate Tablets, USP)

DARVON®
(Propoxyphene Hydrochloride Capsules, USP)

DARVON® Compound-65
(Propoxyphene Hydrochloride, Aspirin, and Caffeine Capsules, USP)

DESCRIPTION
Propoxyphene Hydrochloride, USP is an odorless, white crystalline powder with a bitter taste. It is freely soluble in water. Chemically, it is (2*S*, 3*R*)-(+)-4-(Dimethylamino)-3-methyl-1,2-diphenyl-2-butanol propionate (ester) hydrochloride, which can be represented by the accompanying structural formula. Its molecular weight is 375.94.

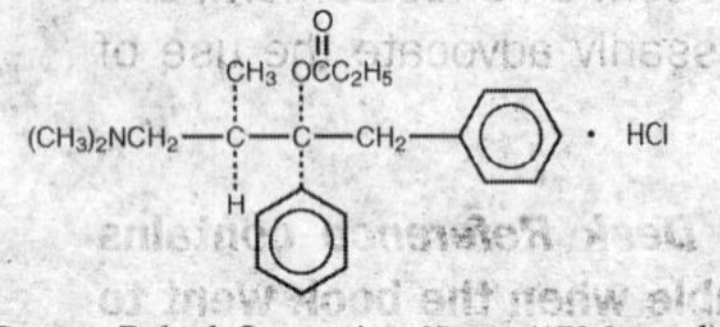

Each Darvon Pulvule® contains 65 mg (172.9 µmol) (No. 365) propoxyphene hydrochloride. It also contains FD&C Red No. 33, FD&C Yellow No. 6, gelatin, magnesium stearate, silicone, starch, titanium dioxide, and other inactive ingredients.
Each Darvon Compound-65 Pulvule contains 65 mg (172.9 µmol) propoxyphene hydrochloride, 389 mg (2,159 µmol) aspirin, and 32.4 mg (166.8 µmol) caffeine.
Darvon Compound-65 contains FD&C Red No. 3, FD&C Yellow No. 6, gelatin, glutamic acid hydrochloride, iron oxide, kaolin, silicone, titanium dioxide, and other inactive ingredients.
Propoxyphene Napsylate, USP is an odorless, white crystalline powder with a bitter taste. It is very slightly soluble in water and soluble in methanol, ethanol, chloroform, and acetone. Chemically, it is (α*S*, 1*R*)-α-[2-(Dimethylamino)-1-methylethyl]-α-phenylphenethyl propionate compound with 2-naphthalenesulfonic acid (1:1) monohydrate, which can be represented by the accompanying structural formula. Its molecular weight is 565.74.

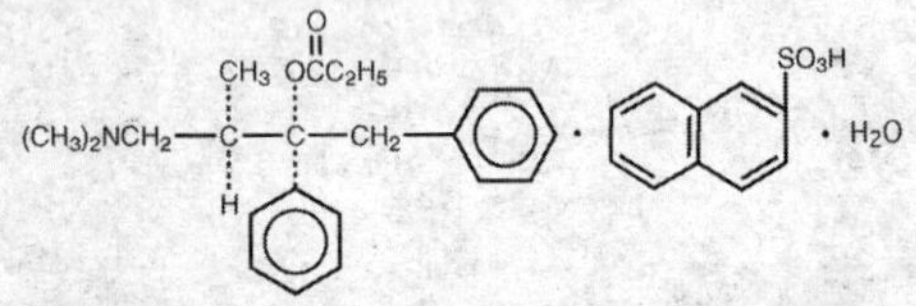

Propoxyphene napsylate differs from propoxyphene hydrochloride in that it allows more stable liquid dosage forms and tablet formulations. Because of differences in molecular weight, a dose of 100 mg (176.8 µmol) of propoxyphene napsylate is required to supply an amount of propoxyphene equivalent to that present in 65 mg (172.9 µmol) of propoxyphene hydrochloride.
Each tablet of Darvon-N contains 100 mg (176.8 µmol) propoxyphene napsylate. The tablet also contains cellulose, cornstarch, iron oxides, lactose, magnesium stearate, silicon dioxide, stearic acid, and titanium dioxide.
Each tablet of Darvocet-N 50 contains 50 mg (88.4 µmol) propoxyphene napsylate and 325 mg (2,150 µmol) acetaminophen.
Each tablet of Darvocet-N 100 contains 100 mg (176.8 µmol) propoxyphene napsylate and 650 mg (4,300 µmol) acetaminophen.
Each tablet of Darvocet-N also contains amberlite, cellulose, FD&CYellow No. 6, magnesium stearate, stearic acid, titanium dioxide, and other inactive ingredients.

CLINICAL PHARMACOLOGY
Propoxyphene is a centrally acting narcotic analgesic agent. Equimolar doses of propoxyphene hydrochloride or napsylate provide similar plasma concentrations. Following administration of 65, 130, or 195 mg of propoxyphene, the bioavailability of propoxyphene is equivalent to that of 100, 200, or 300 mg respectively of propoxyphene napsylate. Peak plasma concentrations of propoxyphene are reached in 2 to 2 1/2 hours. After a 65-mg oral dose of propoxyphene hydrochloride or a 100-mg oral dose of propoxyphene napsylate, peak plasma levels of 0.05 to 0.1 µg/mL are achieved. As shown in Figure 1, the napsylate salt tends to be absorbed more slowly than the hydrochloride. At or near therapeutic doses, this absorption difference is small when compared with that among subjects and among doses.
Figure 1. Mean plasma concentrations of propoxyphene in 8 human subjects following oral administration of 65 and 130 mg of the hydrochloride salt and 100 and 200 mg of the napsylate salt and in 7 given 195 mg of the hydrochloride and 300 mg of the napsylate salt.

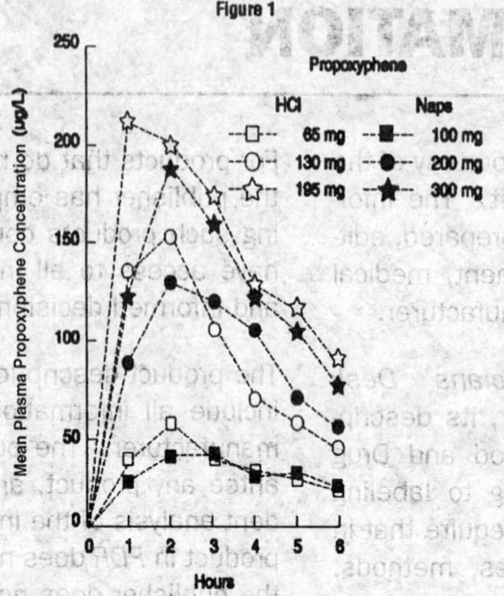

Because of this several hundredfold difference in solubility, the absorption rate of very large doses of the napsylate salt is significantly lower than that of equimolar doses of the hydrochloride.
Repeated doses of propoxyphene at 6-hour intervals lead to increasing plasma concentrations, with a plateau after the ninth dose at 48 hours.
Propoxyphene is metabolized in the liver to yield norpropoxyphene. Propoxyphene has a half-life of 6 to 12 hours, whereas that of norpropoxyphene is 30 to 36 hours.
Norpropoxyphene has substantially less central-nervous-system-depressant effect than propoxyphene but a greater local anesthetic effect, which is similar to that of amitriptyline and antiarrhythmic agents, such as lidocaine and quinidine.
In animal studies in which propoxyphene and norpropoxyphene were continuously infused in large amounts, intracardiac conduction time (PR and QRS intervals) was prolonged. Any intracardiac conduction delay attributable to high concentrations of norpropoxyphene may be of relatively long duration.

ACTIONS
Propoxyphene is a mild narcotic analgesic structurally related to methadone. The potency of propoxyphene hydrochloride and propoxyphene napsylate is from two thirds to equal that of codeine.
The combination of propoxyphene with a mixture of aspirin and caffeine produces greater analgesia than that produced by either propoxyphene or aspirin and caffeine administered alone.
Darvocet-N 50 and Darvocet-N 100 provide the analgesic activity of propoxyphene napsylate and the antipyretic-analgesic activity of acetaminophen.
The combination of propoxyphene and acetaminophen produces greater analgesia than that produced by either propoxyphene or acetaminophen administered alone.

INDICATION
These products are indicated for the relief of mild to moderate pain. Formulations containing either aspirin or acetaminophen are indicated for the relief of mild to moderate pain, either when pain is present alone or when it is accompanied by fever.

WARNINGS
- **Do not prescribe propoxyphene for patients who are suicidal or addiction-prone.**
- **Prescribe propoxyphene with caution for patients taking tranquilizers or antidepressant drugs and patients who use alcohol in excess.**
- **Tell your patients not to exceed the recommended dose and to limit their intake of alcohol.**

Propoxyphene products in excessive doses, either alone or in combination with other CNS depressants, including alcohol, are a major cause of drug-related deaths. Fatalities within the first hour of overdosage are not uncommon. In a survey of deaths due to overdosage conducted in 1975, in approximately 20% of the fatal cases, death occurred within the first hour (5% occurred within 15 minutes). Propoxyphene should not be taken in doses higher than those recommended by the physician. The judicious prescribing of propoxyphene is essential to the safe use of this drug. With patients who are depressed or suicidal, consideration should be given to the use of non-narcotic analgesics. Patients should be cautioned about the concomitant use of propoxyphene products and alcohol because of potentially serious CNS-additive effects of these agents. Because of its added depressant effects, propoxyphene should be prescribed with caution for those patients whose medical condition requires the concomitant administration of sedatives, tranquilizers, muscle relaxants, antidepressants, or other CNS-depressant drugs. Patients should be advised of the additive depressant effects of these combinations.
Many of the propoxyphene-related deaths have occurred in patients with previous histories of emotional disturbances or suicidal ideation or attempts as well as histories of misuse of tranquilizers, alcohol, and other CNS-active drugs. Some deaths have occurred as a consequence of the accidental ingestion of excessive quantities of propoxyphene alone or in combination with other drugs. Patients taking propoxyphene should be

CONTRAINDICATIONS
Hypersensitivity to propoxyphene, aspirin, caffeine or acetaminophen.

Drug Dependence—Propoxyphene, when taken in higher-than-recommended doses over long periods of time, can produce drug dependence characterized by psychic dependence and, less frequently, physical dependence and tolerance. Propoxyphene will only partially suppress the withdrawal syndrome in individuals physically dependent on morphine or other narcotics. The abuse liability of propoxyphene is qualitatively similar to that of codeine although quantitatively less, and propoxyphene should be prescribed with the same degree of caution appropriate to the use of codeine.
Usage in Ambulatory Patients—Propoxyphene may impair the mental and/or physical abilities required for the performance of potentially hazardous tasks, such as driving a car or operating machinery. The patient should be cautioned accordingly.
Warning: Reye Syndrome is a rare but serious disease which can follow flu or chicken pox in children and teenagers. While the cause of Reye Syndrome is unknown, some reports claim aspirin (or salicylates) may increase the risk of developing this disease.

PRECAUTIONS
General—Propoxyphene should be administered with caution to patients with hepatic or renal impairment since higher serum concentrations or delayed elimination may occur.
Salicylates should be used with extreme caution in the presence of peptic ulcer or coagulation abnormalities.
Drug Interactions—The CNS-depressant effect of propoxyphene is additive with that of other CNS depressants, including alcohol.
Salicylates may enhance the effect of anticoagulants and inhibit the uricosuric effect of uricosuric agents.
As is the case with many medicinal agents, propoxyphene may slow the metabolism of a concomitantly administered drug. Should this occur, the higher serum concentrations of that drug may result in increased pharmacologic or adverse effects of that drug. Such occurrences have been reported when propoxyphene was administered to patients on antidepressants, anticonvulsants, or warfarin-like drugs. Severe neurologic signs, including coma, have occurred with concurrent use of carbamazepine.
Usage in Pregnancy—Safe use in pregnancy has not been established relative to possible adverse effects on fetal development. Instances of withdrawal symptoms in the neonate have been reported following usage during pregnancy. Therefore, propoxyphene should not be used in pregnant women unless, in the judgment of the physician, the potential benefits outweigh the possible hazards. Aspirin does not appear to have teratogenic effects. However, prolonged pregnancy and labor with increased bleeding before and after delivery, decreased birth weight, and increased rate of stillbirth were reported with high blood salicylate levels. Because of possible adverse effects on the neonate and the potential for increased maternal blood loss, aspirin should be avoided during the last 3 months of pregnancy.
Usage in Nursing Mothers—Low levels of propoxyphene have been detected in human milk. In postpartum studies involving nursing mothers who were given propoxyphene, no adverse effects were noted in infants receiving mother's milk.
Usage in Pediatric Patients—Safety and effectiveness in pediatric patients have not been established.
Usage in the Elderly—The rate of propoxyphene metabolism may be reduced in some patients. Increased dosing interval should be considered.

ADVERSE REACTIONS
In a survey conducted in hospitalized patients, less than 1% of patients taking propoxyphene hydrochloride at recommended doses experienced side effects. The most frequently reported were dizziness, sedation, nausea, and vomiting. Some of these adverse reactions may be alleviated if the patient lies down.
Other adverse reactions include constipation, abdominal pain, skin rashes, lightheadedness, headache, weakness, euphoria, dysphoria, hallucinations and minor visual disturbances.
Propoxyphene therapy has been associated with abnormal liver function tests and, more rarely, with instances of reversible jaundice (including cholestatic jaundice). Liver dysfunction has been reported in association with both active

components of Darvocet-N 50 and Darvocet-N 100. Hepatic necrosis may result from acute overdose of acetaminophen (see Management of Overdosage). In chronic ethanol abusers, this has been reported rarely with short-term use of acetaminophen dosages of 2.5 to 10 g/day. Fatalities have occurred.

Renal papillary necrosis may result from chronic aspirin or acetaminophen use, particularly when the dosage is greater than recommended and when aspirin and acetaminophen are combined.

Subacute painful myopathy has occurred following chronic propoxyphene overdosage.

DOSAGE AND ADMINISTRATION

These products are given orally. For propoxyphene hydrochloride, the usual dose is 65 mg propoxyphene hydrochloride (with or without 389 mg aspirin, and 32.4 mg caffeine) every 4 hours as needed for pain. The maximum recommended dose of propoxyphene hydrochloride is 390 mg per day.

For propoxyphene napsylate, the usual dosage is 100 mg propoxyphene napsylate (with or without 650 mg acetaminophen) every 4 hours as needed for pain. The maximum recommended dose of propoxyphene napsylate is 600 mg per day.

Consideration should be given to a reduced total daily dosage in patients with hepatic or renal impairment.

MANAGEMENT OF OVERDOSAGE

In all cases of suspected overdosage, call your regional Poison Control Center to obtain the most up-to-date information about the treatment of overdose. This recommendation is made because, in general, information regarding the treatment of overdosage may change more rapidly than do package inserts.

Initial consideration should be given to the management of the CNS effects of propoxyphene overdosage. Resuscitative measures should be initiated promptly.

Symptoms of Propoxyphene Overdosage—The manifestations of acute overdosage with propoxyphene are those of narcotic overdosage. The patient is usually somnolent but may be stuporous or comatose and convulsing. Respiratory depression is characteristic. The ventilatory rate and/or tidal volume is decreased, which results in cyanosis and hypoxia. Pupils, initially pinpoint, may become dilated as hypoxia increases. Cheyne-Stokes respiration and apnea may occur. Blood pressure and heart rate are usually normal initially, but blood pressure falls and cardiac performance deteriorates, which ultimately results in pulmonary edema and circulatory collapse, unless the respiratory depression is corrected and adequate ventilation is restored promptly. Cardiac arrhythmias and conduction delay may be present. A combined respiratory-metabolic acidosis occurs owing to retained CO_2 (hypercapnia) and to lactic acid formed during anaerobic glycolysis. Acidosis may be severe if large amounts of salicylates have also been ingested. Death may occur.

Treatment of Propoxyphene Overdosage—Attention should be directed first to establishing a patent airway and restoring ventilation. Mechanically assisted ventilation, with or without oxygen, may be required, and positive pressure respiration may be desirable if pulmonary edema is present. The narcotic antagonist naloxone will markedly reduce the degree of respiratory depression, and 0.4 to 2 mg should be administered promptly, preferably intravenously. If the desired degree of counteraction with improvement in respiratory functions is not obtained, naloxone should be repeated at 2- to 3-minute intervals. The duration of action of the antagonist may be brief. If no response is observed after 10 mg of naloxone have been administered, the diagnosis of propoxyphene toxicity should be questioned. Naloxone may also be administered by continuous intravenous infusion.

Treatment of Propoxyphene Overdose in Pediatric Patients—The usual initial dose of naloxone in pediatric patients is 0.01 mg/kg body weight given intravenously. If this dose does not result in the desired degree of clinical improvement, a subsequent increased dose of 0.1 mg/kg body weight may be administered. If an IV route of administration is not available, naloxone may be administered IM or subcutaneously in divided doses. If necessary, naloxone can be diluted with Sterile Water for Injection.

Blood gases, pH, and electrolytes should be monitored in order that acidosis and any electrolyte disturbance present may be corrected promptly. Acidosis, hypoxia, and generalized CNS depression predispose to the development of cardiac arrhythmias. Ventricular fibrillation or cardiac arrest may occur and necessitate the full complement of cardiopulmonary resuscitation (CPR) measures. Respiratory acidosis rapidly subsides as ventilation is restored and hypercapnia eliminated, but lactic acidosis may require intravenous bicarbonate for prompt correction.

Electrocardiographic monitoring is essential. Prompt correction of hypoxia, acidosis, and electrolyte disturbance (when present) will help prevent these cardiac complications and will increase the effectiveness of agents administered to restore normal cardiac function.

In addition to the use of a narcotic antagonist, the patient may require careful titration with an anticonvulsant to control convulsions. Analeptic drugs (for example, caffeine or amphetamine) should not be used because of their tendency to precipitate convulsions.

General supportive measures, in addition to oxygen, include, when necessary, intravenous fluids, vasopressorinotropic compounds, and, when infection is likely, anti-infective agents. Gastric lavage may be useful, and activated charcoal can absorb a significant amount of ingested propoxyphene. Dialysis is of little value in poisoning due to propoxyphene. Efforts should be made to determine whether other agents, such as alcohol, barbiturates, tranquilizers, or other CNS depressants, were also ingested, since these increase CNS depression as well as cause specific toxic effects.

Symptoms of Salicylate Overdosage—Such symptoms include central nausea and vomiting, tinnitus and deafness, vertigo and headaches, mental dullness and confusion, diaphoresis, rapid pulse, and increased respiration and respiratory alkalosis.

Treatment of Salicylate Overdosage—When Darvon Compound-65 has been ingested, the clinical picture may be complicated by salicylism.

The treatment of acute salicylate intoxication includes minimizing drug absorption, promoting elimination through the kidneys, and correcting metabolic derangements affecting body temperature, hydration, acid-base balance, and electrolyte balance. The technique to be employed for eliminating salicylate from the bloodstream depends on the degree of drug intoxication.

If the patient is seen within 4 hours of ingestion, the stomach should be emptied by inducing vomiting or by gastric lavage as soon as possible.

The nomogram of Done is a useful prognostic guide in which the expected severity of salicylate intoxication is based on serum salicylate levels and the time interval between ingestion and taking the blood sample.

Exchange transfusion is most feasible for a small infant. Intermittent peritoneal dialysis is useful for cases of moderate severity in adults. Intravenous fluids alkalinized by the addition of sodium bicarbonate or potassium citrate are helpful. Hemodialysis with the artificial kidney is the most effective means of removing salicylate and is indicated for the very severe cases of salicylate intoxication.

Symptoms of Acetaminophen Overdosage—Shortly after oral ingestion of an overdose of acetaminophen and for the next 24 hours, anorexia, nausea, vomiting, diaphoresis, general malaise, and abdominal pain have been noted. The patient may then present no symptoms, but evidence of liver dysfunction may become apparent up to 72 hours after ingestion, with elevated serum transaminase and lactic dehydrogenese levels, an increase in serum bilirubin concentrations, and a prolonged prothrombin time. Death from hepatic failure may result 3 to 7 days after overdosage.

Acute renal failure may accompany the hepatic dysfunction and has been noted in patients who do not exhibit signs of fulminant hepatic failure. Typically, renal impairment is more apparent 6 to 9 days after ingestion of the overdose.

Treatment of Acetaminophen Overdose—Acetaminophen in massive overdosage may cause hepatic toxicity in some patients. In all cases of suspected overdose, immediately call your regional poison center or the Rocky Mountain Poison Center's toll-free number (800-525-6115) for assistance in diagnosis and for directions in the uses of N-acetylcysteine as an antidote.

In adults, hepatic toxicity has rarely been reported with acute overdoses of less than 10 g and fatalities with less than 15 g. Importantly, young children seem to be more resistant than adults to the hepatotoxic effect of an acetaminophen overdose. Despite this, the measures outlined below should be initiated in any adult or pediatric patient suspected of having ingested an acetaminophen overdose.

Because clinical and laboratory evidence of hepatic toxicity may not be apparent until 48 to 72 hours postingestion, liver function studies should be obtained initially and repeated at 24-hour intervals.

Consider emptying the stomach promptly by lavage or by induction of emesis with syrup of ipecac. Patients' estimates of the quantity of a drug ingested are notoriously unreliable. Therefore, if an acetaminophen overdose is suspected, a serum acetaminophen assay should be obtained as early as possible, but no sooner than 4 hours following ingestion. The antidote, N-acetylcysteine, should be administered as early as possible, and within 16 hours of the overdose ingestion for optimal results. Following recovery, there are no residual, structural, or functional hepatic abnormalities.

ANIMAL TOXICOLOGY

The acute lethal doses of the hydrochloride and napsylate salts of propoxyphene were determined in 4 species. The results shown in Figure 2 indicate that, on a molar basis, the napsylate salt is less toxic than the hydrochloride. This may be due to the relative insolubility and retarded absorption of propoxyphene napsylate.

Figure 2
ACUTE ORAL TOXICITY OF PROPOXYPHENE

Species	Propoxyphene Hydrochloride: LD_{50} (mg/kg ± SE) / LD_{50} (mmol/kg)	Propoxyphene Napsylate: LD_{50} (mg/kg ± SE) / LD_{50} (mmol/kg)
Mouse	282 ± 39 / 0.75	915 ± 163 / 1.62
Rat	230 ± 44 / 0.61	647 ± 95 / 1.14
Rabbit	ca 82 / 0.22	>183 / >0.32
Dog	ca 100 / 0.27	>183 / >0.32

Some indication of the relative insolubility and retarded absorption of propoxyphene napsylate was obtained by measuring plasma propoxyphene levels in 2 groups of 4 dogs following oral administration of equimolar doses of the 2 salts. As shown in Figure 3, the peak plasma concentration observed with propoxyphene hydrochloride was much higher than that obtained after administration of the napsylate salt.

Although none of the animals in this experiment died, 3 of the 4 dogs given propoxyphene hydrochloride exhibited convulsive seizures during the time interval corresponding to the peak plasma levels. The 4 animals receiving the napsylate salt were mildly ataxic but not acutely ill.

Figure 3. Plasma propoxyphene concentrations in dogs following large doses of the hydrochloride and napsylate salts.

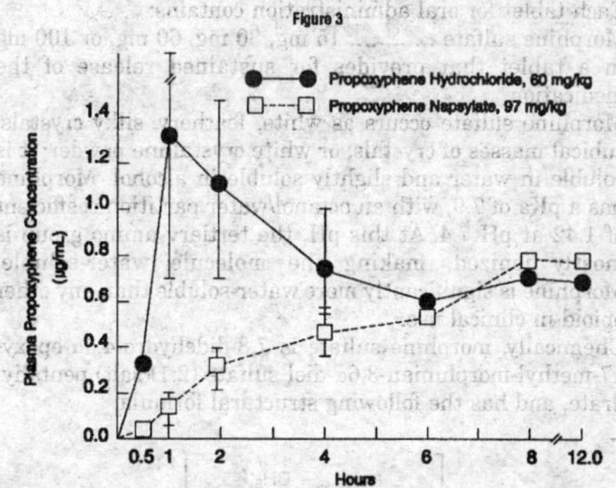

HOW SUPPLIED

Darvocet A500™ Tablets are available in:
The 100 mg/500 mg are available as dark orange, film coated, oval shaped tablets debossed "A500" on both sides.
Bottles of 100 Tablets NDC 66591-691-41

Darvocet-N® 50 Tablets are available in:
The 50 mg tablets are dark orange, capsule shaped, film coated, and imprinted with the script "Darvocet-N 50" on one side of the tablet, using edible black ink.
They are available as follows:
Bottles of 100 (RxPak*) NDC 66591-651-41

Darvocet-N® 100 Tablets are available in:
The 100 mg tablets are dark orange, capsule shaped, film coated, and imprinted with the script "Darvocet-N 100" on one side of the tablet, using edible black ink.
They are available as follows:
Bottles of 100 (RxPak*) NDC 66591-641-41
Bottles of 500 NDC 66591-641-51

Darvon-N® Tablets are available in:
The 100 mg tablets are buff colored, elliptical shaped, film coated, and imprinted with the script "Darvon-N 100" on one side of the tablet, using edible black ink.
They are available as follows:
Bottles of 100 (RxPak*) NDC 66591-631-41
Bottles of 500 NDC 66591-631-51

Darvon® Pulvules® are available in:
The 65 mg parabolic-shaped capsules are imprinted with the script "Lilly" and "H03" on the opaque pink cap and "Darvon" on the opaque pink body, using edible black ink.
They are available as follows:
Bottles of 100 (RxPak*) NDC 0002-0803-02 (PU0365)
Bottles of 500 NDC 0002-0803-03 (PU0365)
ID† 100 NDC 0002-0803-33 (PU0365)

Darvon® Compound-65 Pulvules® are available in:
The 65 mg parabolic-shaped capsules are imprinted with the script "Lilly" and "3111" on the opaque gray cap and "Darvon Comp 65" on the opaque red body, using edible black ink.
They are available as follows:
Bottles of 100 (RxPak*) NDC 0002-3111-02 (PU0369)
Bottles of 500 NDC 0002-3111-03 (PU0369)

*All RxPaks (prescription packages, Lilly) have safety closures.
† Identi-Dose® (unit dose medication, Lilly).

Store at 25°C (77°F); excursions are permitted to 15°-30°C (59°-86°F) [See USP Controlled Room Temperature]

CAUTION—Rx only

Literature revised June 2004.
Darvocet A500 manufactured by: Mikart, Inc.
Darvon, Darvon Compound 65, Darvon N, Darvocet-N50 & Darvocet-N100
manufactured by: Eli Lilly & Company, Inc.
Manufactured For:
aai Pharma®

Pulvules and Identi-Dose are registered trademarks of Eli Lilly and Company, Inc
Darvon, Darvon-N and Darvocet-N are registered trademarks of aaiPharma LLC
Darvocet A500 is a trademark of aaiPharma Inc

Continued on next page

ORAMORPH® SR Ⓒ℞

[ōr-ă-mōrf]

(MORPHINE SULFATE)
SUSTAINED RELEASE TABLETS
15 mg, 30 mg, 60 mg, 100 mg
℞ only

> **NOTE**
> THIS IS A SUSTAINED RELEASE DOSAGE FORM. PATIENT SHOULD BE INSTRUCTED TO SWALLOW THE TABLET AS A WHOLE; THE TABLET SHOULD NOT BE BROKEN IN HALF, NOR SHOULD IT BE CRUSHED OR CHEWED.
> THE SUSTAINED RELEASE OF MORPHINE FROM **ORAMORPH SR** SHOULD BE TAKEN INTO CONSIDERATION IN EVENT OF ADVERSE REACTIONS OR OVERDOSAGE.

DESCRIPTION

Each tablet for oral administration contains:
Morphine sulfate .... 15 mg, 30 mg, 60 mg, or 100 mg in a tablet that provides for sustained release of the medication.

Morphine sulfate occurs as white, feathery, silky crystals, cubical masses of crystals, or white crystalline powder; it is soluble in water and slightly soluble in alcohol. Morphine has a pKa of 7.9, with an octanol/water partition coefficient of 1.42 at pH 7.4. At this pH, the tertiary amino group is mostly ionized, making the molecule water-soluble. Morphine is significantly more water-soluble than any other opioid in clinical use.

Chemically, morphine sulfate is 7,8-didehydro-4,5α-epoxy-17-methyl-morphinian-3,6α-diol sulfate (2:1)(salt) pentahydrate, and has the following structural formula:

$[C_{17}H_{19}NO_3]_2 \cdot H_2SO_4 \cdot 5H_2O$

Each ORAMORPH SR Tablet contains 15 mg, 30 mg, 60 mg, or 100 mg Morphine Sulfate USP. Inactive ingredients: Lactose, Hydroxypropyl Methylcellulose, Colloidal Silicon Dioxide, and Stearic Acid.

CLINICAL PHARMACOLOGY

Morphine is the prototype of many narcotic drugs that interact predominantly with the opioid μ-receptor. These μ-binding sites are discretely distributed in the human brain, with high densities in the posterior amygdala, hypothalamus, thalamus, nucleus caudatus, putamen, and certain cortical areas. They are also found on the terminal axons of primary afferents within laminae I and II (substantia gelatinosa) of the spinal cord and in the spinal nucleus of the trigeminal nerve.

In clinical settings, morphine exerts its principal pharmacological effect on the central nervous system and gastrointestinal tract. Its primary actions of therapeutic value are analgesia and sedation. Morphine appears to increase the patient's tolerance for pain and to decrease discomfort, although the presence of the pain itself may still be recognized. In addition to analgesia, alterations in mood, euphoria and dysphoria, and drowsiness commonly occur.

Morphine depresses various respiratory centers, depresses the cough reflex, and constricts the pupils. Analgesically effective blood levels of morphine may cause nausea and vomiting directly by stimulating the chemoreceptor trigger zone, but nausea and vomiting are significantly more common in ambulatory than in recumbent patients, as is postural syncope.

Morphine increases the tone and decreases the propulsive contractions of the smooth muscle of the gastrointestinal tract. The resultant prolongation in gastrointestinal transit time is responsible for the constipating effect of morphine. Because morphine may increase biliary-tract pressure, some patients with biliary colic may experience worsening rather than relief of pain.

While morphine generally increases the tone of urinary-tract smooth muscle, the net effect tends to be variable, in some cases producing urinary urgency, in others, difficulty in urination.

In therapeutic doses, morphine does not usually exert major effects on the cardiovascular system. Some patients, however, exhibit a propensity to develop orthostatic hypotension and fainting. Rapid intravenous injection is more likely to precipitate a fall in blood pressure than oral dosing.

Morphine can cause histamine release, which appears to be responsible for dilation of cutaneous blood vessels, with resulting flushing of the face and neck, pruritus, and sweating.

PHARMACOKINETICS

ORAMORPH SR Tablets are a sustained release oral dosage form of morphine sulfate. Only about 40% of the administered dose reaches the central compartment because of first-pass effect (i.e., metabolism in the gut wall and liver). Once absorbed, morphine is distributed to skeletal muscle, kidneys, liver, intestinal tract, lungs, spleen and brain. Morphine also crosses the placental membrane and has been found in breast milk.

For all practical purposes, virtually all morphine is converted to glucuronide metabolites; only a small fraction (less than 5%) of absorbed morphine is demethylated. Among these glucuronide metabolites, morphine-3-glucuronide is present in the highest plasma concentration following oral administration; a smaller fraction is converted to morphine-6-glucuronide, which has the greater analgesic activity of these two metabolites.

The glucuronide system has a high capacity and is not easily saturated, even in disease. Therefore, the rate of delivery of morphine to the gut and liver does not influence the total and/or the relative quantities of the various metabolites formed.

The pharmacokinetic parameters following oral administration of ORAMORPH SR, presented in the table below, show considerable inter-subject variation, but are representative of average values reported in the literature. The volume of distribution (Vd) for morphine is 4 liters per kilogram (L/kg), and the terminal elimination half-life is approximately 2 to 4 hours.

[See table below]

Following the administration of conventional, immediate-release, oral morphine products, approximately 50% of the morphine, that will ever reach the central compartment, reaches it within 30 minutes. Following the administration of an equal amount of ORAMORPH SR to normal volunteers, however, 50% of absorption occurs, on average, after 1.5 hours.

A pharmacokinetic study in normal volunteers indicates that there is little to no effect on the systemic bioavailability of ORAMORPH SR when administered with food.

Although variation in the physico-mechanical properties of a formulation of an oral morphine drug product can affect both its absolute bioavailability and its absorption rate constant (k_a), morphine distribution and clearance are unchanged, as they are fundamental properties of morphine in the organism. However, in chronic use, the possibility of shifts in metabolite-to-parent drug ratios cannot be excluded.

When immediate-release oral morphine or ORAMORPH SR is given on a fixed dosing regimen, steady-state is achieved in about one to two days.

TABLE OF APPROXIMATE[1] AVERAGE PHARMACOKINETIC PARAMETERS FOLLOWING ORAL DOSING OF ORAMORPH SR

Pharmacokinetic Parameter (scientific notation) (unit)		**Dose of ORAMORPH SR**			
		Dose at 2 × 16 mg	**30 mg**	**60 mg**	**100 mg**
Bioavailability (oral compared to injectable)		**approximately 40%**			
Time-to-peak plasma concentration (T_{max}) (h)	mean (range)	3.7 (1-6)	3.8 (1-7)	3.8 (2-7)	3.6 (1.5-12)
Peak plasma concentration (C_{max}) (ng/mL) [single dose]	mean (range)	11.1 (6.5-16.2)	9.9 (5.0-18.6)	16.1 (10.0-25.3)	27.4 (14.1-46.1)
Volume of distribution(calculated from mean clearance and terminal half-life) [Vd(ß)] (L/kg)	mean	4 L/kg			

Dose metabolized = approximately 90%
Morphine metabolites (%) = morphine-3-glucuronide (55-75%), morphine-6-glucuronide (1-5%)

[1]Derived from pharmacokinetic studies in 24 normal volunteers

For a given dose and dosing interval, the Area-Under-the-Curve (AUC) and average blood concentration of morphine at steady-state (Css) will be independent of the type of oral formulation administered, as long as the formulations have the same absolute bioavailability. The absorption rate of a formulation will, however, affect the maximum (Cmax) and minimum (Cmin) plasma concentrations and the time between administration and their occurrence. For any fixed dose and dosing interval, ORAMORPH SR will have, at steady-state, a lower Cmax and a higher Cmin than conventional immediate-release morphine, which might be a therapeutic advantage in chronic pain control (see also PHARMACODYNAMICS).

The clearance of morphine occurs primarily as renal excretion of morphine-3-glucuronide. A small amount of the glucuronide conjugate is excreted in the bile, and there is some minor enterohepatic recycling; about 10% of the glucuronide conjugate is excreted in the feces. Because morphine is essentially metabolized in the liver, the effects of renal disease on morphine's clearance are not likely to be pronounced. As with any drug, however, caution should be taken to guard against unanticipated accumulation if renal and/or hepatic function is seriously impaired.

PHARMACODYNAMICS

In clinical settings, morphine's primary actions of therapeutic value are analgesia and sedation. Opiate analgesia involves at least three anatomical areas of the central nervous system: the periaqueductal-periventricular gray matter, the ventromedial medulla, and the spinal cord. Morphine appears to increase the patient's tolerance for pain, and to decrease the discomfort, although the presence of pain itself may still be recognized.

While there is considerable variability in the relationship between morphine blood concentration and analgesic response, effective analgesia probably will not occur below some minimum blood level in a given patient. The minimum effective blood level for analgesia will vary among patients, especially among patients who have been previously treated with potent μ-agonist opioids. Similarly, there is considerable variability in the relationship between morphine plasma concentration and untoward clinical responses, but higher concentrations are more likely to be toxic.

In contrast to immediate-release morphine, after dosing with ORAMORPH SR, the morphine blood levels show reduced fluctuation between peak and trough plasma levels; that means that they are more centered within the theoretical 'therapeutic window'. On the other hand, the reduced fluctuation in morphine plasma concentration might conceivably affect other phenomena, as for example, the rate of tolerance induction.

ORAMORPH SR is an analgesic intended for patients who require chronic morphine analgesia and who will have, in consequence, markedly different degrees of pharmacodynamic tolerance for opioid drugs. Morphine and similar opioids induce tolerance to their effects, so that a shortening of the duration of satisfactory analgesia may be the first sign of an increase in tolerance.

Once patients are started on morphine, the dose required for satisfactory analgesia will rise, with the rate of development of tolerance varying, depending on the patient's prior narcotic use, level of pain, degree of anxiety, use of other CNS-active drugs, circulatory status, total daily dose, and the dosing interval.

INDICATIONS AND USAGE

ORAMORPH SR is indicated for the relief of pain in patients who require opioid analgesics for more than a few days.

CONTRAINDICATIONS

ORAMORPH SR is contraindicated in patients with respiratory depression in the absence of resuscitative equipment, in patients with acute or severe bronchial asthma and in patients with known hypersensitivity to morphine.

ORAMORPH SR is contraindicated in any patient who has or is suspected of having a paralytic ileus.

WARNINGS

IMPAIRED RESPIRATION:

Respiratory depression is the chief hazard of all morphine preparations. Respiratory depression occurs more frequently in the elderly and debilitated patients, as well as in those suffering from conditions accompanied by hypoxia or hypercapnia when even moderate therapeutic doses may dangerously decrease pulmonary ventilation.

Morphine should be used with extreme caution in patients who have a decreased respiratory reserve (e.g., emphysema, severe obesity, kyphoscoliosis, or paralysis of the phrenic nerve). ORAMORPH SR should not be given in cases of chronic asthma, upper airway obstruction, or in any other chronic pulmonary disorder without due consideration of the known risk of acute respiratory failure following morphine administration in such patients.

DRUG ABUSE AND DEPENDENCE - CONTROLLED SUBSTANCE:

Morphine sulfate is a Schedule II narcotic under the United States Controlled Substance Act (21 U.S.C. 801-886).

Morphine is the most commonly cited prototype for narcotic substances that possess an addiction-forming or addiction-sustaining liability. A patient may be at risk for developing a dependence to morphine if used improperly or for overly long periods of time. As with all potent opioids which are μ-agonists, tolerance as well as psychological and physical dependence to morphine may develop irrespective of the route of administration (oral, intravenous, intramuscular,

intrathecal, or epidural). Individuals with a prior history of opioid or other substance abuse or dependence, being more apt to respond to euphorigenic and reinforcing properties of morphine, would be considered to be at greater risk.
Care must be taken to avert withdrawal symptoms when morphine is discontinued abruptly or upon administration of a narcotic antagonist.

PRECAUTIONS

General Precautions:
Selection of patients for treatment with ORAMORPH SR should be governed by the same principles that apply to the use of morphine or other potent opioid analgesics. Narcotic analgesics are drugs that have a narrow therapeutic index in the old, the sick, and the infirm, i.e., the very population in which their use is indicated. Physicians should individualize treatment with ORAMORPH SR in every case, weighing the need for analgesia against the risks of serious or fatal reactions to the drug.

Use in Patients with Increased Intracranial Pressure or with Head Injury:
ORAMORPH SR should be used with extreme caution in patients with increased intracranial pressure or with head injury. The respiratory depressant effects of morphine (increased pCO_2) may result in elevation of cerebrospinal fluid pressure and may thus be markedly exaggerated in the presence of head injury, other intracranial lesions, or a preexisting increased intracranial pressure. Morphine produces effects which may obscure neurologic signs of further increases in pressure in patients with head injuries. Pupillary changes (miosis), associated with morphine, may conceal the existence, extent, and course of intracranial pathology.

Use in Hepatic or Renal Disease:
The clearance of morphine may be reduced in patients with hepatic dysfunction, while the clearance of its metabolites may be decreased in renal dysfunction. This will be manifested by both a prolonged elimination half-life and the accumulation of levels of either morphine or its metabolites in excess of those produced in normals, with the potential for an increase of adverse effects (see WARNINGS and ADVERSE REACTIONS). These changes in morphine pharmacodynamics, in patients with hepatic or renal dysfunctions, should be considered when adjusting the dose and dosage intervals, taking also into account the slow-release character of ORAMORPH SR.

Drug Interactions:
Use with Other Central Nervous System Depressants:
The depressant effects of morphine are potentiated by the presence of other CNS depressants such as alcohol, sedatives, antihistaminics, or psychotropic drugs. Use of neuroleptics in conjunction with oral morphine may increase the risk of respiratory depression, hypotension and profound sedation or coma.
Interaction with Mixed Agonist/Antagonist Opioid Analgesics:
Agonist/antagonist analgesics (i.e., pentazocine, nalbuphine, butorphanol, or buprenorphine) should NOT be administered to patients who have received or are receiving a course of therapy with a pure opioid agonist analgesic. In these patients, the mixed agonist/antagonist may alter the analgesic effect or may precipitate withdrawal symptoms.

Carcinogenesis, Mutagenesis, Impairment of Fertility:
Studies of morphine sulfate in animals to evaluate the drug's carcinogenic and mutagenic potential or the effect on fertility have not been conducted.

Pregnancy:
Teratogenic Effects - Category C: There are no well-controlled studies in women, but marketing experience does not include any evidence of adverse effects on the fetus following routine (short-term) clinical use of morphine sulfate products. Although there is no clearly defined risk, such experience cannot exclude the possibility of infrequent or subtle damage to the human fetus.
ORAMORPH SR should be used in pregnant women only when clearly needed. (See also: PRECAUTIONS: Labor and Delivery, and DRUG ABUSE AND DEPENDENCE CONTROLLED SUBSTANCE.)

Nonteratogenic Effects:
Infants born from mothers who have been taking morphine chronically may exhibit withdrawal symptoms.

Labor and Delivery:
ORAMORPH SR is not recommended for use in women during and immediately prior to labor. Occasionally, opioid analgesics may prolong labor through actions which temporarily reduce the strength, duration and frequency of uterine contractions.
Neonates, whose mothers received opioid analgesics during labor, should be observed closely for signs of respiratory depression. A specific narcotic antagonist, naloxone, should be available for reversal of narcotic-induced respiratory depression in the neonate.

Nursing Mothers:
ORAMORPH SR should not be given to nursing mothers because morphine is excreted in maternal milk. Effects on the nursing infant are not known, but withdrawal symptoms can occur in breast-fed infants when maternal administration of morphine sulfate is stopped.

Pediatric Use:
ORAMORPH SR has not been evaluated in children. Its use in the pediatric population is, therefore, not recommended.

Use in the Aged:
The pharmacodynamic effects of morphine in the aged are more variable than in the younger population. Patients will vary widely in the effective initial dose, rate of development of tolerance, and the frequency and magnitude of associated adverse effects as the dose is increased. Individualization of doses must receive careful attention in elderly patients.

Information for Patients:
If clinically advisable, patients receiving ORAMORPH SR brand of morphine sulfate sustained release tablets, should be given the following instructions by the physician:

1. Morphine may produce psychological and/or physical dependence. For this reason, the dose of the drug should not be increased without consulting a physician.
2. Morphine may impair mental and/or physical ability required for the performance of potentially hazardous tasks (e.g., driving, operating machinery).
3. Morphine should not be taken with alcohol or other CNS depressants (sleep aids, tranquilizers) because additive effects, including CNS depression, may occur. A physician should be consulted if other prescription and/or over-the-counter medications are currently being used or are prescribed for future use.
4. For women of childbearing potential, who become or are planning to become pregnant, a physician should be consulted regarding analgesics and other drug use.

ADVERSE REACTIONS

NOTE: THE SUSTAINED RELEASE OF MORPHINE FROM ORAMORPH SR SHOULD BE TAKEN INTO CONSIDERATION IN THE EVENT OF OCCURRING ADVERSE REACTIONS.

Adverse reactions caused by morphine are essentially those observed with other opioid analgesics. They include the following *major hazards*: **respiratory depression**, and less frequently, **circulatory depression, apnea, shock** and **cardiac arrest** secondary to respiratory and/or circulatory depression.

Most Frequently Observed Reactions:
Constipation, nausea, vomiting, lightheadedness, dizziness, sedation, dysphoria, euphoria, and sweating. Some of these effects seem to be more prominent in ambulatory patients and in those not experiencing severe pain. Some adverse reactions in ambulatory patients may be alleviated if the patient is in a supine position.

Less Frequently Observed Reactions:
Body as a Whole: Edema, antidiuretic effect, chills, muscle tremor, muscle rigidity.
Cardiovascular: Flushing of the face, tachycardia, bradycardia, palpitation, faintness, syncope, hypotension, hypertension.
Gastrointestinal: Dry mouth, biliary tract spasm, laryngospasm, anorexia, diarrhea, cramps, taste alterations.
Genitourinary: Urine retention or hesitance, reduced libido and/or potency.
Nervous System: Weakness, headache, agitation, tremor, uncoordinated muscle movements, seizure, paresthesia, alterations of mood (nervousness, apprehension, depression, floating feelings), dreams, transient hallucination and disorientation, visual disturbances, insomnia, increased intracranial pressure.
Skin: Pruritus, urticaria and other skin rashes.
Special Senses: Blurred vision, nystagmus, diplopia, miosis.

DRUG ABUSE AND DEPENDENCE

Opioid analgesics may cause psychological and physical dependence (see WARNINGS). Physical dependence results in withdrawal symptoms in patients who abruptly discontinue the drug, or these symptoms may be precipitated through the administration of drugs with antagonistic activity, e.g., naloxone or mixed agonist/antagonist analgesics (pentazocine, etc.; see also OVERDOSAGE). Physical dependence usually does not occur, to a clinically significant degree, until several weeks of continued opioid usage. Tolerance, in which increasingly larger doses are required to produce the same degree of analgesia, is initially manifested by a shortened duration of analgesic effect and, subsequently, by decreases in the intensity of analgesia. In patients with chronic pain, as well as in opioid-tolerant cancer patients, the administration of ORAMORPH SR (morphine sulfate) should be guided by the degree of tolerance manifested. Physical dependence, per se, is not ordinarily a concern when one is dealing with opioid-tolerant patients whose pain and suffering is associated with an irreversible illness.
If ORAMORPH SR is abruptly discontinued, an abstinence syndrome may occur. Withdrawal symptoms, in patients dependent on morphine, begin shortly before the time of the next scheduled dose, reaching a peak at 36 to 72 hours after the last dose, and then slowly subside over a period of 7 to 10 days. Symptoms include yawning, sweating, lacrimation, rhinorrhea, restless sleep, dilated pupils, gooseflesh, irritability, tremor, nausea, vomiting, and diarrhea.
Treatment of the abstinence syndrome is primarily symptomatic and supportive, including maintenance of proper fluid and electrolyte balance. If withdrawal has inadvertently been precipitated in a patient who requires narcotics for pain management, the withdrawal syndrome can be terminated rapidly by the administration of an appropriate dose of a pure agonist opioid, such as morphine. The degree of physical dependence of a patient on ORAMORPH SR can be intentionally reduced by a gradual reduction of dosage and symptomatic treatment of withdrawal symptomatology.

OVERDOSAGE

NOTE: THE SUSTAINED RELEASE OF MORPHINE FROM **ORAMORPH SR** SHOULD BE TAKEN INTO CONSIDERATION IN THE EVENT OF AN OVERDOSAGE.

Overdosage of morphine is characterized by respiratory depression, with or without concomitant CNS depression. Since respiratory arrest may result either through direct depression of the respiratory center, or as the result of hypoxia, primary attention should be given to the establishment of adequate respiratory exchange through provision of a patent airway and institution of assisted, or controlled, ventilation. The narcotic antagonist, naloxone, is a specific antidote. An initial dose of 0.4 to 2 mg of naloxone should be administered intravenously, simultaneously with respiratory resuscitation. If the desired degree of counteraction and improvement in respiratory function is not obtained, naloxone may be repeated at 2 to 3 minute intervals. If no response is observed after 10 mg of naloxone has been administered, the diagnosis of narcotic-induced, or partial narcotic-induced, toxicity should be questioned. Intramuscular or subcutaneous administration may be used if the intravenous route is not available.
As the duration of effect of naloxone is considerably shorter than that of ORAMORPH SR, repeated administration may be necessary. Patients should be closely observed for evidence of renarcotization.

NOTE: In a individual physically dependent on opioids, administration of the usual dose of the antagonist will precipitate an acute withdrawal syndrome. The severity of the withdrawal syndrome produced will depend on the degree of physical dependence and the dose of the antagonist administered. Use of a narcotic antagonist in such a person should be avoided. If necessary to treat serious respiratory depression in a physically dependent patient, the antagonist should be administered with extreme care and by titration with smaller than usual doses of the antagonist.

When indicated, gut decontamination should be performed via emesis and/or activated charcoal (60 to 100 g in adults, 1 to 2 g/kg in children) with cathartic. Since ORAMORPH SR is a sustained release product, absorption may be expected to continue for many hours, particularly following an overdose, combined with decreased peristaltic activity of the gastrointestinal tract.
Supportive measures (including oxygen, vasopressors) should be employed in the management of circulatory shock and pulmonary edema accompanying overdose as indicated. Cardiac arrest or arrhythmias may require cardiac massage or defibrillation.

DOSAGE AND ADMINISTRATION

(See also: CLINICAL PHARMACOLOGY, WARNINGS and PRECAUTIONS sections.)
NOTE: ORAMORPH SR TABLET MUST BE SWALLOWED WHOLE. DO NOT BREAK THE TABLET IN HALF. DO NOT CRUSH OR CHEW. TAKING BROKEN, CHEWED OR CRUSHED TABLETS COULD LEAD TO THE RAPID RELEASE AND ABSORPTION OF A POTENTIALLY TOXIC DOSE OF MORPHINE.
ORAMORPH SR is intended for use in patients who require more than several days of continuous treatment with a potent opioid analgesic. The sustained release nature of the formulation allows it to be administered on a more convenient schedule than conventional immediate-release oral morphine products (see CLINICAL PHARMACOLOGY - PHARMACOKINETICS). However, ORAMORPH SR does not release morphine continuously over the course of a dosing interval. The administration of single doses of ORAMORPH SR on a q12h dosing schedule will result in peak and trough plasma levels similar to those following an identical daily dose of morphine administered using conventional oral formulations on a q4h regimen. If pain is not controlled for a full 12 hours, then the dosing interval should be shortened, but to no less than 8 hours.
As with any potent opioid, it is critical to adjust the dosing regimen for each patient individually, taking into account the patient's prior analgesic treatment experience. Attention should be given to the following in determining the initial dose of ORAMORPH SR, (1) the daily dose, potency and characteristics of a pure agonist, or mixed agonist-antagonist, the patient has been taking previously, (2) the reliability of the relative potency estimate to calculate the dose of morphine needed [N.B.: potency estimates may vary with the route of administration], (3) the fact that roughly only 40% of the morphine sulfate in ORAMORPH SR becomes available after pre-systemic metabolization in the intestinal wall and the liver, (4) the degree of opioid tolerance, and (5) the general condition and medical status of the patient.
The following dosing recommendations for ORAMORPH SR, therefore, can only be considered suggested approaches to the series of clinical decisions in the management of pain of an individual patient.

Continued on next page

Oramorph SR—Cont.

Conversion from Conventional Immediate-Release Oral Morphine to ORAMORPH SR:

A patient's daily morphine requirement is established by using the Daily Oral Morphine Requirement of the immediate-release formulation which gives the Daily Oral Morphine Requirement for ORAMORPH SR. Since ORAMORPH SR is given on an 'every 12 hour' schedule, the single dose of ORAMORPH SR is half of the Daily Oral Morphine Requirement. Dose and dosing interval is adjusted as needed (see discussion below). For initial conversion, the 30 mg tablet strength is recommended for patients with a daily morphine requirement of 120 mg or less.

Conversion from Parenteral Morphine or Other Opioid Analgesics (parenteral or oral) to ORAMORPH SR:

Because of uncertainty about relative estimates of opioid potency and cross tolerance, as well as intersubject variation, initial dosing regimens should be conservative, i.e., an underestimation of the 24-hour oral morphine requirement is preferred to an overestimate. To this end, initial individual doses of ORAMORPH SR should be estimated conservatively. In patients whose daily morphine requirements are expected to be less than or equal to 120 mg per day, the 30 mg tablet strength is recommended for the initial titration period. Once a stable dose regimen is reached, the patient can be converted to the 60 mg or 100 mg tablet strength, as appropriate.

Estimates of the relative potency of opioids are only approximate, and are influenced by route of administration, individual patient differences, and possibly, by the patient's medical condition. Consequently, it is difficult to recommend any precise rule for converting a patient to ORAMORPH SR directly. However, the following general points should be considered:

1. Parenteral to oral morphine ratio: Estimates of the oral-to-parenteral potency of morphine vary. Some authorities suggest that a dose of morphine only 3 times the daily parenteral morphine requirement may be sufficient in chronic use settings. (3 times the Daily Parenteral Morphine Requirement = the Daily Oral Morphine Requirement)
2. *Other parenteral or oral opioids to oral morphine:* Because of a lack of reliable relative potency assays, specific recommendations are not possible. In general, it is safer to underestimate the Total Daily Dose of ORAMORPH SR required and rely upon ad hoc supplementation to deal with inadequate analgesia (see discussion which follows).

Use of ORAMORPH SR as the First Opioid Analgesic:

There has been no systematic evaluation of ORAMORPH SR as an initial opioid analgesic in the management of pain. Because it may be more difficult to titrate a patient using a sustained release morphine, it is ordinarily advisable to begin treatment using an immediate release formulation.

Considerations in the Adjustment of Dosing Regimens:

Whatever the approach, if signs of excessive opioid effects are observed early in a dosing interval, the next dose should be reduced. If this adjustment leads to inadequate analgesia, i.e., 'breakthrough' pain occurs late in the dosing interval, the dosing interval may be shortened. Alternatively, a supplemental dose of a short-acting analgesic may be given. As experience is gained, adjustments can be made to obtain an appropriate balance between pain relief, opioid side effects and the convenience of the dosing schedule.

In adjusting dose requirements, it is recommended that the dosing interval never be extended beyond 12 hours, because the administration of very large single doses of ORAMORPH SR may lead to acute overdosage.

For patients with low daily morphine requirements, the 15 mg tablet should be used. In this regard, adjustment in dose should NOT be attempted by breaking or crushing the tablets. ORAMORPH SR tablets are intended to be swallowed whole.

Conversion from ORAMORPH SR to Parenteral Opioids:

When converting a patient from ORAMORPH SR to parenteral opioids, it is best to assume that the parenteral to oral potency relationship is high. NOTE THAT THIS IS THE CONVERSE OF THE STRATEGY USED WHEN THE DIRECTION OF CONVERSION IS FROM THE PARENTERAL TO ORAL FORMULATIONS. IN BOTH CASES, HOWEVER, THE AIM IS TO ESTIMATE THE NEW DOSE CONSERVATIVELY. For example, to estimate the required 24-hour dose of morphine for IM use, one could employ a conversion of 1 mg of morphine IM for every 6 mg of morphine as ORAMORPH SR. Of course, the IM 24-hour dose would have to be divided by six and administered on a q4h regimen. This approach is recommended because it is least likely to cause overdosage.

HOW SUPPLIED

ORAMORPH® SR (Morphine Sulfate)
Sustained Release Tablets
15 mg white tablets (Identified 54 782)
[Embossed with 15]
NDC 0054-8790-24: Unit dose, 25 tablets per card (reverse numbered), 4 cards per shipper.
NDC 0054-4790-25: Bottles of 100 tablets.
NDC 0054-4790-29: Bottles of 500 tablets.
30 mg white tablets (Identified 54 409)
[Embossed with 30]
NDC 0054-8805-24: Unit dose, 25 tablets per card (reverse numbered), 4 cards per shipper.
NDC 0054-4805-19: Bottles of 50 tablets.
NDC 0054-4805-25: Bottles of 100 tablets.
NDC 0054-4805-27: Bottles of 250 tablets.
60 mg white tablets (Identified 54 933)
[Embossed with 60]
NDC 0054-8792-11: Unit dose, 25 tablets per card (reverse numbered), 1 card per shipper.
NDC 0054-4792-25: Bottles of 100 tablets.
100 mg white tablets (Identified 54 862)
[Embossed with 100]
NDC 0054-8793-11: Unit dose, 25 tablets per card (reverse numbered), 1 card per shipper.
NDC 0054-4793-25: Bottles of 100 tablets.

DEA Order Form Required.

Dispense in a tight, light-resistant container.

Storage: ORAMORPH SR tablets should be stored in unopened containers at or below room temperature.

Federal law prohibits the transfer of this drug to any person other than the patient for whom it was prescribed.

Safety and Handling Instructions: ORAMORPH SR is supplied as tablets that pose little risk of direct exposure to health care personnel and should be handled and disposed of in accordance with hospital policy. Patients and their families should be instructed to dispose of ORAMORPH SR tablets, that are no longer needed, down the toilet.

4073305//02 **Revised May 2001**

Abbott Laboratories

Pharmaceutical Products Division
NORTH CHICAGO, IL 60064, U.S.A.

Pharmaceutical Products Division—
Direct Inquiries to:
Customer Service:
(800) 255-5162
Technical Services:
(800) 441-4987
For Medical Information Contact:
Generally:
(800) 633-9110
Adverse experiences or side effects (for all Abbott drug products):
(800) 633-9110
Sales and Ordering:
(800) 255-5162

ABBO-CODE™ INDEX

The Abbo-Code identification system provides positive identification of a drug and dosage strength. The following Abbott products are imprinted or debossed with an Abbo-Code designation:

PRODUCT	*ABBO-CODE*
Biaxin® Filmtab® Tablets (clarithromycin tablets, USP)	
250 mg	KT
500 mg	KL
Biaxin® XL Filmtab® Tablets (clarithromycin extended-release tablets)	
500 mg	KJ
Cefol® Filmtab® Tablets (B-complex vitamins with folic acid, vitamin E, and vitamin C)	NJ
Colchicine Tablets, USP	
0.6 mg	AF
Cylert® Tablets Ⓒ **(pemoline)**	
18.75 mg	TH
37.5 mg	TI
75 mg	TJ
37.5 mg Chewable	TK
Depakene® Capsules (valproic acid capsules, USP)	
250 mg	DEPAKENE
Depakote® ER Tablets (divalproex sodium EXTENDED-RELEASE tablets)	
500 mg	HC
250 mg	HF
Depakote® Sprinkle Capsules (divalproex sodium coated particles in capsules)	
125 mg	↑THIS END UP DEPAKOTE SPRINKLE 125 mg
Depakote® Tablets (divalproex sodium delayed-release tablets)	
125 mg	NT
250 mg	NR
500 mg	NS
Dilaudid® Tablets Ⓒ **(hydromorphone hydrochloride)**	
2 mg	2
4 mg	4
8 mg	8
E.E.S. 400® Filmtab® Tablets (erythromycin ethylsuccinate tablets, USP)	
400 mg erythromycin activity	EE
Ery-Tab® Enteric-Coated Tablets (erythromycin delayed-release tablets, USP)	
250 mg	EC
333 mg	EH
500 mg	ED
Erythrocin® Stearate Filmtab® Tablets (erythromycin stearate tablets, USP)	
250 mg erythromycin activity	ES
500 mg erythromycin activity	ET
Erythromycin Base Filmtab® Tablets (erythromycin tablets, USP)	
250 mg	EB
500 mg	EA
Erythromycin Delayed-release Capsules, USP	
250 mg	ER
Erythromycin Ethylsuccinate Tablets, USP	
400 mg erythromycin activity	74 ZE
Fero-Folic-500® Filmtab® Tablets (controlled-release iron, folic acid, and vitamin C)	AJ
Gengraf® Capsules (cyclosporine capsules, USP [MODIFIED])	
25 mg	OR 25 mg
100 mg	OT 100 mg
Hytrin® Capsules (terazosin hydrochloride capsules)	
1 mg	HH
2 mg	HY
5 mg	HK
10 mg	HN
Iberet-Folic-500® Filmtab® Tablets (controlled-release iron with vitamin C and B-complex including folic acid)	AK
Isoptin® SR Tablets (verapamil hydrochloride) sustained release oral tablets	
120 mg	SC
180 mg	SK
240 mg	ST
Kaletra® (lopinavir/ritonavir) capsules	
133.3 mg lopinavir/33.3 mg ritonavir	PK
K-Tab® Filmtab® Tablets (potassium chloride extended-release tablets, USP)	
10 mEq (750 mg)	K-TAB
Mavik® Tablets (trandolapril)	
1 mg	FT
2 mg	FX
4 mg	FZ
Meridia® Capsules Ⓒ **(sibutramine hydrochloride monohydrate)**	
5 mg	MERIDIA 5
10 mg	MERIDIA 10
15 mg	MERIDIA 15
Norvir® (ritonavir capsules) Soft Gelatin	
100 mg	DS 100
Omnicef® Capsules (cefdinir)	
300 mg	OMNICEF 300 mg
PCE® Dispertab® Tablets (erythromycin particles in tablets)	
333 mg	PCE
500 mg	EK
ProSom™ Tablets Ⓒ **(estazolam tablets)**	
1 mg	UC
2 mg	UD
Synthroid® Tablets (levothyroxine sodium tablets, USP)	
25 mcg (0.025 mg)	SYNTHROID 25
50 mcg (0.05 mg)	SYNTHROID 50
75 mcg (0.075 mg)	SYNTHROID 75
88 mcg (0.088 mg)	SYNTHROID 88
100 mcg (0.1 mg)	SYNTHROID 100
112 mcg (0.112 mg)	SYNTHROID 112
125 mcg (0.125 mg)	SYNTHROID 125
137 mcg (0.137 mg)	SYNTHROID 137
150 mcg (0.15 mg)	SYNTHROID 150
175 mcg (0.175 mg)	SYNTHROID 175
200 mcg (0.2 mg)	SYNTHROID 200
300 mcg (0.3 mg)	SYNTHROID 300
Tarka® Tablets (trandolapril/verapamil hydrochloride ER)	
2 mg/180 mg	182Δ
1 mg/240 mg	241Δ
2 mg/240 mg	242Δ
4 mg/240 mg	244Δ
Tricor® (fenofibrate tablets)	
54 mg	TA
160 mg	TC
Vicodin® Tablet	**VICODIN**
(hydrocodone bitartrate and acetaminophen tablets, USP)	
hydrocodone bitartrate	5 mg
acetaminophen	500 mg
Vicodin ES® Tablet	**VICODIN ES**
(hydrocodone bitartrate and acetaminophen tablets, USP)	
hydrocodone bitartrate	7.5 mg
acetaminophen	500 mg
Vicodin HP® Tablet	**VICODIN HP**
(hydrocodone bitartrate and acetaminophen tablets, USP)	
hydrocodone bitartrate	10 mg
acetaminophen	660 mg
Vicoprofen® Tablet	**VP**
(hydrocodone bitartrate and ibuprofen tablets)	
hydrocodone bitartrate	7.5 mg
ibuprofen	200 mg

ABBOKINASE® ℞

[ă bō kī′nās]
UROKINASE

DESCRIPTION

Abbokinase® (urokinase) is a thrombolytic agent obtained from human neonatal kidney cells grown in tissue culture. The principle active ingredient of Abbokinase® is the low molecular weight form of urokinase, and consists of an A chain of 2,000 daltons linked by a sulfhydryl bond to a B chain of 30,400 daltons. Abbokinase® is supplied as a sterile lyophilized white powder containing 250,000 IU urokinase per vial, mannitol (25 mg/vial), Albumin (Human) (250 mg/vial), and sodium chloride (50 mg/vial).

Following reconstitution with 5 mL of Sterile Water for Injection, USP, Abbokinase® is a clear, slightly straw-colored solution; each mL contains 50,000 IU of urokinase activity, 0.5% mannitol, 5% Albumin (Human), and 1% sodium chloride (pH range 6.0 to 7.5).

Thin translucent filaments may occasionally occur in reconstituted Abbokinase® vials (see **DOSAGE AND ADMINISTRATION**).

Abbokinase® is for intravenous infusion only.

Abbokinase® is produced from human neonatal kidney cells (see **WARNINGS**). No fetal tissue is used in the production of Abbokinase®. Kidney donations are obtained exclusively in the United States from neonates (birth to 28 days) for whom death has not been attributed to infectious causes and that have exhibited no evidence of an infectious disease based in part, on an examination of the maternal and neonatal donor medical records. The maternal and neonatal donor screening process also identifies specific risk factors for known infectious diseases and includes testing of sera for HBV, HCV, HIV-1, HIV-2, HTLV-I, HTLV-II, CMV, and EBV. Donors with sera testing positive or associated with other risk factors are excluded. During the manufacturing process, cells are tested at multiple stages for the presence of viruses using *in vitro* and *in vivo* tests that are capable of detecting a wide range of viruses. Cells are also screened for HPV using a DNA detection-based test and for reovirus using a polymerase chain reaction-based test. The manufacturing process used for this product has been validated in laboratory studies to inactivate and/or remove a diverse panel of spiked model enveloped and non-enveloped viruses, and includes purification steps and a heat treatment step (10 hours at 60°C in 2% sodium chloride). A single vial of Abbokinase® contains urokinase produced using cells derived from one or two donors.

CLINICAL PHARMACOLOGY

Urokinase is an enzyme (protein) produced by the kidney, and found in the urine. There are two forms of urokinase which differ in molecular weight but have similar clinical effects. Abbokinase® is the low molecular weight form. Abbokinase® acts on the endogenous fibrinolytic system. It converts plasminogen to the enzyme plasmin. Plasmin degrades fibrin clots as well as fibrinogen and some other plasma proteins.

Information about the pharmacokinetic properties in man is limited. Urokinase administered by intravenous infusion is rapidly cleared by the liver with an elimination half-life for biologic activity of 12.6 +/− 6.2 minutes and a distribution volume of 11.5 L. Small fractions of the administered dose are excreted in bile and urine. Although the pharmacokinetics of exogenously administered urokinase have not been characterized in patients with hepatic impairment, endogenous urokinase-type plasminogen activator plasma levels are elevated 2- to 4-fold in patients with moderate to severe cirrhosis.[1] Thus, reduced urokinase clearance in patients with hepatic impairment might be expected.

Intravenous infusion of Abbokinase® in doses recommended for lysis of pulmonary embolism is followed by increased fibrinolytic activity in the circulation. This effect disappears within a few hours after discontinuation, but a decrease in plasma levels of fibrinogen and plasminogen and an increase in the amount of circulating fibrin and fibrinogen degradation products may persist for 12-24 hours.[2] There is a lack of correlation between embolus resolution and changes in coagulation and fibrinolytic assay results.

Treatment with urokinase demonstrated more improvement on pulmonary angiography, lung perfusion scanning, and hemodynamic measurements within 24 hours than did treatment with heparin. Lung perfusion scanning showed no significant treatment-associated difference by day 7.[3]

Information based on patients treated with fibrinolytics for pulmonary embolus suggests that improvement in angiographic and lung perfusion scans is lessened when treatment is instituted more than several days (e.g., 4 to 6 days) after onset.[4]

INDICATIONS AND USAGE

Abbokinase® is indicated in adults:

- For the lysis of acute massive pulmonary emboli, defined as obstruction of blood flow to a lobe or multiple segments.
- For the lysis of pulmonary emboli accompanied by unstable hemodynamics, i.e., failure to maintain blood pressure without supportive measures.

The diagnosis should be confirmed by objective means, such as pulmonary angiography or non-invasive procedures such as lung scanning.

CONTRAINDICATIONS

The use of Abbokinase® is contraindicated in patients with a history of hypersensitivity to the product (see **WARNINGS** and **ADVERSE REACTIONS**).

Because thrombolytic therapy increases the risk of bleeding, Abbokinase® is contraindicated in the situations listed below (see **WARNINGS**).

- Active internal bleeding
- Recent (e.g., within two months) cerebrovascular accident
- Recent (e.g., within two months) intracranial or intraspinal surgery
- Recent trauma including cardiopulmonary resuscitation
- Intracranial neoplasm, arteriovenous malformation, or aneurysm
- Known bleeding diatheses
- Severe uncontrolled arterial hypertension

WARNINGS

Bleeding

The risk of serious bleeding is increased with use of Abbokinase®. Fatalities due to hemorrhage, including intracranial and retroperitoneal, have been reported in association with urokinase therapy.

Concurrent administration of Abbokinase® with other thrombolytic agents, anticoagulants, or agents inhibiting platelet function may further increase the risk of serious bleeding.

Abbokinase® therapy requires careful attention to all potential bleeding sites (including catheter insertion sites, arterial and venous puncture sites, cutdown sites, and other needle puncture sites).

Intramuscular injections and nonessential handling of the patient must be avoided during treatment with Abbokinase®. Venipunctures should be performed as infrequently as possible and with care to minimize bleeding.

Should an arterial puncture be necessary, upper extremity vessels are preferable. Direct pressure should be applied for at least 30 minutes, a pressure dressing applied, and the puncture site checked frequently for evidence of bleeding.

In the following conditions, the risk of bleeding may be increased and should be weighed against the anticipated benefits:

- Recent (within 10 days) major surgery, obstetrical delivery, organ biopsy, previous puncture of non-compressible vessels
- Recent (within 10 days) serious gastrointestinal bleeding
- High likelihood of a left heart thrombus, for example, mitral stenosis with atrial fibrillation
- Subacute bacterial endocarditis
- Hemostatic defects including those secondary to severe hepatic or renal disease
- Pregnancy
- Cerebrovascular disease
- Diabetic hemorrhagic retinopathy
- Any other condition in which bleeding might constitute a significant hazard or be particularly difficult to manage because of its location

When internal bleeding occurs, it may be more difficult to manage than that which occurs with conventional anticoagulant therapy. Should potentially serious spontaneous bleeding (not controllable by direct pressure) occur, the infusion of Abbokinase® should be terminated immediately, and measures to manage the bleeding implemented. Serious blood loss may be managed with volume replacement, including packed red blood cells. Dextran should not be used. When appropriate, fresh frozen plasma and/or cryoprecipitate may be considered to reverse the bleeding tendency.

Anaphylaxis and Other Infusion Reactions

Post-marketing reports of hypersensitivity reactions have included anaphylaxis (with rare reports of fatal anaphylaxis), bronchospasm, orolingual edema and urticaria (see **ADVERSE REACTIONS: Allergic Reactions**). There have also been reports of other infusion reactions which have included one or more of the following: fever and/or chills/rigors, hypoxia, cyanosis, dyspnea, tachycardia, hypotension, hypertension, acidosis, back pain, vomiting, and nausea. Reactions generally occurred within one hour of beginning

Abbokinase® infusion. Patients who exhibit reactions should be closely monitored and appropriate therapy instituted.

Infusion reactions generally respond to discontinuation of the infusion and/or administration of intravenous antihistamines, corticosteroids, or adrenergic agents.

Antipyretics which inhibit platelet function (aspirin and other non-steroidal anti-inflammatory agents) may increase the risk of bleeding and should not be used for treatment of fever.

Cholesterol Embolization

Cholesterol embolism has been reported rarely in patients treated with all types of thrombolytic agents; the true incidence is unknown. This serious condition, which can be lethal, is also associated with invasive vascular procedures (e.g., cardiac catheterization, angiography, vascular surgery) and/or anticoagulant therapy. Clinical features of cholesterol embolism may include livedo reticularis, "purple toe" syndrome, acute renal failure, gangrenous digits, hypertension, pancreatitis, myocardial infarction, cerebral infarction, spinal cord infarction, retinal artery occlusion, bowel infarction and rhabdomyolysis.

Product Source and Formulation with Albumin

Abbokinase® is made from human neonatal kidney cells grown in tissue culture. Products made from human source material may contain infectious agents, such as viruses, that can cause disease. The risk that Abbokinase® will transmit an infectious agent has been reduced by screening donors for prior exposure to certain viruses, by testing donors for the presence of certain current virus infections, by testing for certain viruses during manufacturing, and by inactivating and/or removing certain viruses during manufacturing (see **DESCRIPTION**). Despite these measures, Abbokinase® may carry a risk of transmitting infectious agents, including those that cause the Creutzfeldt-Jakob disease (CJD) or other diseases not yet known or identified; thus, the risk of transmission of infectious agents cannot be totally eliminated. A theoretical risk for transmission of Creutzfeldt-Jakob disease (CJD) is considered extremely remote.

This product is formulated in 5% albumin, a derivative of human blood. Based on effective donor screening and product manufacturing processes, albumin carries an extremely remote risk for transmission of viral diseases. A theoretical risk for transmission of Creutzfeldt-Jakob disease (CJD) also is considered extremely remote. No cases of transmission of viral diseases or CJD have ever been identified for albumin.

All infections thought by a physician possibly to have been transmitted by this product should be reported by the physician or other healthcare provider to Abbott Laboratories [1-800-441-4100].

PRECAUTIONS

General

Abbokinase® should be used in hospitals where the recommended diagnostic and monitoring techniques are available.

The clinical response and vital signs should be observed frequently during and following Abbokinase® infusion. Blood pressure should not be taken in the lower extremities to avoid dislodgement of possible deep vein thrombi.

Laboratory Tests

Before beginning thrombolytic therapy, obtain a hematocrit, platelet count, and an activated partial thromboplastin time (aPTT). If heparin has been given, it should be discontinued and the aPTT should be less than twice the normal control value before thrombolytic therapy is started.

Following the intravenous infusion of Abbokinase®, before (re)instituting anticoagulants, the aPTT should be less than twice the normal control value.

Results of coagulation tests and measures of fibrinolytic activity do not reliably predict either efficacy or risk of bleeding for patients receiving Abbokinase®.

Drug Interactions

Anticoagulants and agents that alter platelet function (such as aspirin, other non-steroidal anti-inflammatory agents, dipyridamole, and GP IIb/IIIa inhibitors) may increase the risk of serious bleeding.

Administration of Abbokinase® prior to, during, or after other thrombolytic agents may increase the risk of serious bleeding.

Because concomitant use of Abbokinase® with agents that alter coagulation, inhibit platelet function, or are thrombolytic may further increase the potential for bleeding complications, careful monitoring for bleeding is recommended.

The interaction of Abbokinase® with other drugs has not been studied and is not known.

Carcinogenicity

Adequate data are not available on the long-term potential for carcinogenicity in animals or humans.

Pregnancy

Pregnancy Category B: Reproduction studies have been performed in mice and rats at doses up to 1,000 times the human dose and have revealed no evidence of impaired fertility or harm to the fetus due to Abbokinase®. There are, however, no adequate and well-controlled studies in pregnant women. Because animal reproduction studies are not always predictive of human response, this drug should be used during pregnancy only if clearly needed.

Nursing Mothers

It is not known whether this drug is excreted in human milk. Because many drugs are excreted in human milk, caution should be exercised when Abbokinase® is administered to a nursing woman.

Pediatric Use

Safety and effectiveness in pediatric patients have not been established.

Geriatric Use

Clinical studies of Abbokinase® did not include sufficient numbers of subjects aged 65 and over to determine whether they respond differently from younger subjects. Abbokinase® should be used with caution in elderly patients.

ADVERSE REACTIONS

The most serious adverse reactions reported with Abbokinase® administration include fatal hemorrhage and anaphylaxis (see **WARNINGS**).

Bleeding

Bleeding is the most frequent adverse reaction associated with Abbokinase® and can be fatal (see **WARNINGS**).

In controlled clinical studies using a 12-hour infusion of urokinase for the treatment of pulmonary embolism (UPET and USPET),[3,5,6] bleeding resulting in at least a 5% decrease in hematocrit was reported in 52 of 141 urokinase-treated patients. Significant bleeding events requiring transfusion of greater than 2 units of blood were observed during the 14-day study period in 3 of 141 urokinase-treated patients in these studies. Multiple bleeding events may have occurred in an individual patient. Most bleeding occurred at sites of external incisions and vascular punc-

Continued on next page

Abbokinase—Cont.

ture, with lesser frequency in gastrointestinal, genitourinary, intracranial, retroperitoneal, and intramuscular sites.

Sources of Information on Adverse Reactions

There are limited well-controlled clinical studies performed using urokinase. The adverse reactions described in the following sections reflect both the clinical use of Abbokinase® in the general population and limited controlled study data. Because post-marketing reports of adverse reactions are voluntary and the population is of uncertain size, it is not always possible to reliably estimate the frequency of the reaction or establish a causal relationship to drug exposure.

Allergic Reactions

Rare cases of fatal anaphylaxis have been reported (see **WARNINGS**). In controlled clinical trials, allergic reaction was reported in 1 of 141 patients (<1%).

The following allergic-type reactions have been observed in clinical trials and/or post-marketing experience: bronchospasm, orolingual edema, urticaria, skin rash, and pruritus (see **WARNINGS**).

Infusion reaction symptoms include hypoxia, cyanosis, dyspnea, tachycardia, hypotension, hypertension, acidosis, fever and/or chills/rigors, back pain, vomiting, and nausea (see **WARNINGS**).

Other Adverse Reactions

Other adverse events occurring in patients receiving Abbokinase® therapy in clinical studies, regardless of causality, include myocardial infarction, recurrent pulmonary embolism, hemiplegia, stroke, decreased hematocrit, substernal pain, thrombocytopenia, and diaphoresis.

Additional adverse reactions reported from post-marketing experience include cardiac arrest, vascular embolization (cerebral and distal) including cholesterol emboli (see **WARNINGS**), cerebral vascular accident, pulmonary edema, reperfusion ventricular arrhythmias and chest pain. A cause and effect relationship has not been established.

Immunogenicity

The immunogenicity of Abbokinase® has not been studied.

DOSAGE AND ADMINISTRATION

ABBOKINASE® IS INTENDED FOR INTRAVENOUS INFUSION ONLY.

Abbokinase® treatment should be instituted soon after onset of pulmonary embolism. Delay in instituting therapy may decrease the potential for optimal efficacy (see **CLINICAL PHARMACOLOGY**).

Preparation

Abbokinase® contains no preservatives. Do not reconstitute until immediately before use. Any unused portion of the reconstituted material should be discarded.

Reconstitute Abbokinase® by aseptically adding 5 mL of Sterile Water for Injection, USP, to the vial. Abbokinase® should be reconstituted with Sterile Water for Injection, USP, without preservatives. Do not use Bacteriostatic Water for Injection, USP. After reconstituting, visually inspect each vial of Abbokinase® for discoloration and for the presence of particulate material. The solution should be pale and straw-colored; highly colored solutions should not be used.

Thin translucent filaments may occasionally occur in reconstituted Abbokinase® vials, but do not indicate any decrease in potency of this product. To minimize formation of filaments, avoid shaking the vial during reconstitution. Roll and tilt the vial to enhance reconstitution. The solution may be terminally filtered, for example through a 0.45 micron or smaller cellulose membrane filter. No other medication should be added to this solution.

Administration

Prior to infusing, dilute the reconstituted Abbokinase® with 0.9% Sodium Chloride Injection, USP or 5% Dextrose Injection, USP. The following table may be used as an aid in the preparation of Abbokinase® for administration.

[See table below]

Abbokinase® is administered using a constant infusion pump that is capable of delivering a total volume of 195 mL. A loading dose of 2,000 IU/lb (4,400 IU/kg) of Abbokinase® is given as the Abbokinase® 0.9% Sodium Chloride Injection, USP, or 5% Dextrose Injection, USP, admixture at a rate of 90 mL/hour over a period of 10 minutes. This is followed by a continuous infusion of 2,000 IU/lb/hr (4,400 IU/kg/hr) of Abbokinase® at a rate of 15 mL/hour for 12 hours. Since some Abbokinase® admixture will remain in the tubing at the end of an infusion pump delivery cycle, the following flush procedure should be performed to insure that the total dose of Abbokinase® is administered. A solution of 0.9% Sodium Chloride Injection, USP, or 5% Dextrose Injection, USP, approximately equal in amount to the volume of the tubing in the infusion set should be administered via the pump to flush the Abbokinase® admixture from the entire length of the infusion set. The pump should be set to administer the flush solution at the continuous rate of 15 mL/hour.

Anticoagulation After Terminating Abbokinase® Treatment

After infusing Abbokinase®, anticoagulation treatment is recommended to prevent recurrent thrombosis. Do not begin anticoagulation until the aPTT has decreased to *less than twice* the normal control value. If heparin is used, do not administer a loading dose of heparin. Treatment should be followed by oral anticoagulants.

HOW SUPPLIED

Abbokinase® is supplied as a sterile lyophilized preparation (NDC 0074-6109-05). Each vial contains 250,000 IU urokinase activity, 25 mg mannitol, 250 mg Albumin (Human), and 50 mg sodium chloride. Refrigerate Abbokinase® powder at 2° to 8°C (36° to 46°F) (see USP).

Dose Preparation-Pulmonary Embolism

Patient Weight (pounds)	Total Dose[a] Abbokinase® (IU)	Number of Vials of Abbokinase®	Volume of Abbokinase® After Reconstitution (mL)[b]	+	Volume of Diluent (mL)	=	Final Volume (mL)
81-90	2,250,000	9	45		150		195
91-100	2,500,000	10	50		145		195
101-110	2,750,000	11	55		140		195
111-120	3,000,000	12	60		135		195
121-130	3,250,000	13	65		130		195
131-140	3,500,000	14	70		125		195
141-150	3,750,000	15	75		120		195
151-160	4,000,000	16	80		115		195
161-170	4,250,000	17	85		110		195
171-180	4,500,000	18	90		105		195
181-190	4,750,000	19	95		100		195
191-200	5,000,000	20	100		95		195
201-210	5,250,000	21	105		90		195
211-220	5,500,000	22	110		85		195
221-230	5,750,000	23	115		80		195
231-240	6,000,000	24	120		75		195
241-250	6,250,000	25	125		70		195

	Loading Dose	Dose for 12-Hour Period
Infusion Rate:	15 mL/10 min[c]	15 mL/hr for 12 hrs

[a] Loading dose + dose administered during 12-hour period.
[b] After addition of 5 mL of Sterile Water for Injection, USP, per vial. (See Preparation.)
[c] Pump rate = 90 mL/hr

REFERENCES

1. Sato S, et al. Elevated Urokinase-Type Plasminogen Activator Plasma Levels Are Associated With Deterioration of Liver Function But Not With Hepatocellular Carcinoma. *J Gastroenterology*. 1994; 29: 745-750.
2. Bell WR. Thrombolytic Therapy: A Comparison Between Urokinase and Streptokinase. *Sem Thromb Hemost*. 1975; 2:1-13.
3. Sasahara AA, Hyers TM, Cole CM, et al. The Urokinase Pulmonary Embolism Trial. *Circulation*. 1973; 47 (suppl. 2): 1-108.
4. Daniels LB, Parker JA, Patel SR, Grodstein F, Goldhaber SZ. Relation of Duration of Symptoms With Response to Thrombolytic Therapy in Pulmonary Embolism. *Am J Cardiol*. 1997; 80:184-188.
5. Urokinase Pulmonary Embolism Trial Study Group: Urokinase-Streptokinase Embolism Trial. *JAMA*. 1974; 229: 1606-1613.
6. Sasahara AA, Bell WR, Simon TL, et al. The Phase II Urokinase-Streptokinase Pulmonary Embolism Trial. *Thrombos Diathes Haemorrh* (Stuttg). 1975; 33:464-476.

ABBOTT LABORATORIES, NORTH CHICAGO, IL 60064, USA

Reference 58-6978-R4-Rev. October, 2002

BIAXIN® FILMTAB® ℞

[*bī ax ən*]

(clarithromycin tablets, USP)

BIAXIN® XL FILMTAB®

(clarithromycin extended-release tablets)

BIAXIN® GRANULES

(clarithromycin for oral suspension, USP)

℞ only

To reduce the development of drug-resistant bacteria and maintain the effectiveness of BIAXIN and other antibacterial drugs, BIAXIN should be used only to treat or prevent infections that are proven or strongly suspected to be caused by bacteria.

DESCRIPTION

Clarithromycin is a semi-synthetic macrolide antibiotic. Chemically, it is 6-*0*-methylerythromycin. The molecular formula is $C_{38}H_{69}NO_{13}$, and the molecular weight is 747.96. The structural formula is:

Clarithromycin is a white to off-white crystalline powder. It is soluble in acetone, slightly soluble in methanol, ethanol, and acetonitrile, and practically insoluble in water.

BIAXIN is available as immediate-release tablets, extended-release tablets, and granules for oral suspension.

Each yellow oval film-coated immediate-release BIAXIN tablet (clarithromycin tablets, USP) contains 250 mg or 500 mg of clarithromycin and the following inactive ingredients:

250 mg tablets: hypromellose, hydroxypropyl cellulose, croscarmellose sodium, D&C Yellow No. 10, FD&C Blue No. 1, magnesium stearate, microcrystalline cellulose, povidone, pregelatinized starch, propylene glycol, silicon dioxide, sorbic acid, sorbitan monooleate, stearic acid, talc, titanium dioxide, and vanillin.

500 mg tablets: hypromellose, hydroxypropyl cellulose, colloidal silicon dioxide, croscarmellose sodium, D&C Yellow No. 10, magnesium stearate, microcrystalline cellulose, povidone, propylene glycol, sorbic acid, sorbitan monooleate, titanium dioxide, and vanillin.

Each yellow oval film-coated BIAXIN XL tablet (clarithromycin extended release tablets) contains 500 mg of clarithromycin and the following inactive ingredients: cellulosic polymers, D&C Yellow No. 10, lactose monohydrate, magnesium stearate, propylene glycol, sorbic acid, sorbitan monooleate, talc, titanium dioxide, and vanillin.

After constitution, each 5 mL of BIAXIN suspension (clarithromycin for oral suspension, USP) contains 125 mg or 250 mg of clarithromycin. Each bottle of BIAXIN granules contains 1250 mg (50 mL size), 2500 mg (50 and 100 mL sizes) or 5000 mg (100 mL size) of clarithromycin and the following inactive ingredients: carbomer, castor oil, citric acid, hypromellose phthalate, maltodextrin, potassium sorbate, povidone, silicon dioxide, sucrose, xanthan gum, titanium dioxide and fruit punch flavor.

CLINICAL PHARMACOLOGY

Pharmacokinetics:

Clarithromycin is rapidly absorbed from the gastrointestinal tract after oral administration. The absolute bioavailability of 250-mg clarithromycin tablets was approximately 50%. For a single 500-mg dose of clarithromycin, food slightly delays the onset of clarithromycin absorption, increasing the peak time from approximately 2 to 2.5 hours. Food also increases the clarithromycin peak plasma concentration by about 24%, but does not affect the extent of clarithromycin bioavailability. Food does not affect the onset of formation of the antimicrobially active metabolite, 14-OH clarithromycin or its peak plasma concentration but does slightly decrease the extent of metabolite formation, indicated by an 11% decrease in area under the plasma concentration-time curve (AUC). Therefore, BIAXIN tablets may be given without regard to food.

In nonfasting healthy human subjects (males and females), peak plasma concentrations were attained within 2 to 3 hours after oral dosing. Steady-state peak plasma clarithromycin concentrations were attained within 3 days and were approximately 1 to 2 µg/mL with a 250-mg dose administered every 12 hours and 3 to 4 µg/mL with a 500-mg dose administered every 8 to 12 hours. The elimination half-life of clarithromycin was about 3 to 4 hours with 250 mg administered every 12 hours but increased to 5 to 7 hours with 500 mg administered every 8 to 12 hours. The nonlinearity of clarithromycin pharmacokinetics is slight at the recommended doses of 250 mg and 500 mg administered every 8 to 12 hours. With a 250 mg every 12 hours dosing, the principal metabolite, 14-OH clarithromycin, attains a peak steady-state concentration of about 0.6 µg/mL and has an elimination half-life of 5 to 6 hours. With a 500 mg every 8 to 12 hours dosing, the peak steady-state concentration of 14-OH clarithromycin is slightly higher (up to 1 µg/mL), and its elimination half-life is about 7 to 9 hours. With any of these dosing regimens, the steady-state concentration of this metabolite is generally attained within 3 to 4 days.

After a 250-mg tablet every 12 hours, approximately 20% of the dose is excreted in the urine as clarithromycin, while after a 500-mg tablet every 12 hours, the urinary excretion of clarithromycin is somewhat greater, approximately 30%. In comparison, after an oral dose of 250 mg (125 mg/5 mL) suspension every 12 hours, approximately 40% is excreted in urine as clarithromycin. The renal clearance of clarithromycin is, however, relatively independent of the dose size and approximates the normal glomerular filtration rate. The major metabolite found in urine is 14-OH clarithromycin, which accounts for an additional 10% to 15% of the dose with either a 250-mg or a 500-mg tablet administered every 12 hours.

Steady-state concentrations of clarithromycin and 14-OH clarithromycin observed following administration of 500-mg doses of clarithromycin every 12 hours to adult patients with HIV infection were similar to those observed in healthy volunteers. In adult HIV-infected patients taking 500- or 1000-mg doses of clarithromycin every 12 hours, steady-state clarithromycin C_{max} values ranged from 2 to 4 µg/mL and 5 to 10 µg/mL, respectively.

The steady-state concentrations of clarithromycin in subjects with impaired hepatic function did not differ from those in normal subjects; however, the 14-OH clarithromycin concentrations were lower in the hepatically impaired subjects. The decreased formation of 14-OH clarithromycin was at least partially offset by an increase in renal clearance of clarithromycin in the subjects with impaired hepatic function when compared to healthy subjects.

The pharmacokinetics of clarithromycin was also altered in subjects with impaired renal function. (See **PRECAUTIONS** and **DOSAGE AND ADMINISTRATION**.)

Clarithromycin and the 14-OH clarithromycin metabolite distribute readily into body tissues and fluids. There are no data available on cerebrospinal fluid penetration. Because of high intracellular concentrations, tissue concentrations are higher than serum concentrations. Examples of tissue and serum concentrations are presented below.

CONCENTRATION
(after 250 mg q12h)

Tissue Type	Tissue (µg/g)	Serum (µg/mL)
Tonsil	1.6	0.8
Lung	8.8	1.7

Clarithromycin extended-release tablets provide extended absorption of clarithromycin from the gastrointestinal tract after oral administration. Relative to an equal total daily dose of immediate-release clarithromycin tablets, clarithromycin extended-release tablets provide lower and later steady-state peak plasma concentrations but equivalent 24-hour AUC's for both clarithromycin and its microbiologically-active metabolite, 14-OH clarithromycin. While the extent of formation of 14-OH clarithromycin following administration of BIAXIN XL tablets (2 × 500 mg once daily) is not affected by food, administration under fasting conditions is associated with approximately 30% lower clarithromycin AUC relative to administration with food. Therefore, BIAXIN XL tablets should be taken with food.

[See figure at top of next column]

In healthy human subjects, steady-state peak plasma clarithromycin concentrations of approximately 2 to

Clarithromycin Tissue Concentrations 2 hours after Dose (µg/mL)/(µg/g)

Treatment	N	antrum	fundus	N	mucus
Clarithromycin	5	10.48 ± 2.01	20.81 ± 7.64	4	4.15 ± 7.74
Clarithromycin + Omeprazole	5	19.96 ± 4.71	24.25 ± 6.37	4	39.29 ± 32.79

Steady-State Clarithromycin Plasma Concentration-Time Profiles

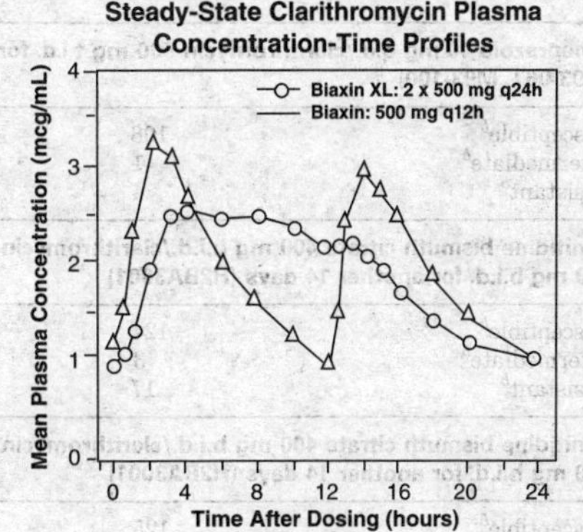

3 µg/mL were achieved about 5 to 8 hours after oral administration of 2 × 500 mg BIAXIN XL tablets once daily; for 14-OH clarithromycin, steady-state peak plasma concentrations of approximately 0.8 µg/mL were attained about 6 to 9 hours after dosing. Steady-state peak plasma clarithromycin concentrations of approximately 1 to 2 µg/mL were achieved about 5 to 6 hours after oral administration of a single 500 mg BIAXIN XL tablet once daily; for 14-OH clarithromycin, steady-state peak plasma concentrations of approximately 0.6 µg/mL were attained about 6 hours after dosing.

When 250-mg doses of clarithromycin as BIAXIN suspension were administered to fasting healthy adult subjects, peak plasma concentrations were attained around 3 hours after dosing. Steady-state peak plasma concentrations were attained in 2 to 3 days and were approximately 2 µg/mL for clarithromycin and 0.7 µg/mL for 14-OH clarithromycin when 250-mg doses of the clarithromycin suspension were administered every 12 hours. Elimination half-life of clarithromycin (3 to 4 hours) and that of 14-OH clarithromycin (5 to 7 hours) were similar to those observed at steady state following administration of equivalent doses of BIAXIN tablets.

For adult patients, the bioavailability of 10 mL of the 125-mg/5 mL suspension or 10 mL of the 250-mg/5 mL suspension is similar to a 250-mg or 500-mg tablet, respectively.

In children requiring antibiotic therapy, administration of 7.5 mg/kg q12h doses of clarithromycin as the suspension generally resulted in steady-state peak plasma concentrations of 3 to 7 µg/mL for clarithromycin and 1 to 2 µg/mL for 14-OH clarithromycin.

In HIV-infected children taking 15 mg/kg every 12 hours, steady-state clarithromycin peak concentrations generally ranged from 6 to 15 µg/mL.

Clarithromycin penetrates into the middle ear fluid of children with secretory otitis media.

CONCENTRATION
(after 7.5 mg/kg q12h for 5 doses)

Analyte	Middle Ear Fluid (µg/mL)	Serum (µg/mL)
Clarithromycin	2.5	1.7
14-OH Clarithromycin	1.3	0.8

In adults given 250 mg clarithromycin as suspension (n=22), food appeared to decrease mean peak plasma clarithromycin concentrations from 1.2 (± 0.4) µg/mL to 1.0 (± 0.4) µg/mL and the extent of absorption from 7.2 (± 2.5) hr•µg/mL to 6.5 (± 3.7) hr•µg/mL.

When children (n=10) were administered a single oral dose of 7.5 mg/kg suspension, food increased mean peak plasma clarithromycin concentrations from 3.6 (± 1.5) µg/mL to 4.6 (± 2.8) µg/mL and the extent of absorption from 10.0 (± 5.5) hr•µg/mL to 14.2 (± 9.4) hr•µg/mL.

Clarithromycin 500 mg every 8 hours was given in combination with omeprazole 40 mg daily to healthy adult males. The plasma levels of clarithromycin and 14-hydroxy-clarithromycin were increased by the concomitant administration of omeprazole. For clarithromycin, the mean C_{max} was 10% greater, the mean C_{min} was 27% greater, and the mean AUC_{0-8} was 15% greater when clarithromycin was administered with omeprazole than when clarithromycin was administered alone. Similar results were seen for 14-hydroxy-clarithromycin, the mean C_{max} was 45% greater, the mean C_{min} was 57% greater, and the mean AUC_{0-8} was 45% greater. Clarithromycin concentrations in the gastric tissue and mucus were also increased by concomitant administration of omeprazole.

[See table above]

For information about other drugs indicated in combination with BIAXIN, refer to the CLINICAL PHARMACOLOGY section of their package inserts.

Microbiology:

Clarithromycin exerts its antibacterial action by binding to the 50S ribosomal subunit of susceptible microorganisms resulting in inhibition of protein synthesis.

Clarithromycin is active *in vitro* against a variety of aerobic and anaerobic gram-positive and gram-negative microorganisms as well as most *Mycobacterium avium* complex (MAC) microorganisms.

Additionally, the 14-OH clarithromycin metabolite also has clinically significant antimicrobial activity. The 14-OH clarithromycin is twice as active against *Haemophilus influenzae* microorganisms as the parent compound. However, for *Mycobacterium avium* complex (MAC) isolates the 14-OH metabolite is 4 to 7 times less active than clarithromycin. The clinical significance of this activity against *Mycobacterium avium* complex is unknown.

Clarithromycin has been shown to be active against most strains of the following microorganisms both *in vitro* and in clinical infections as described in the **INDICATIONS AND USAGE** section:

Aerobic Gram-positive microorganisms

Staphylococcus aureus
Streptococcus pneumoniae
Streptococcus pyogenes

Aerobic Gram-negative microorganisms

Haemophilus influenzae
Haemophilus parainfluenzae
Moraxella catarrhalis

Other microorganisms

Mycoplasma pneumoniae
Chlamydia pneumoniae (TWAR)

Mycobacteria

Mycobacterium avium complex (MAC) consisting of:
Mycobacterium avium
Mycobacterium intracellulare

Beta-lactamase production should have no effect on clarithromycin activity.

NOTE: Most strains of methicillin-resistant and oxacillin-resistant staphylococci are resistant to clarithromycin.

Omeprazole/clarithromycin dual therapy; ranitidine bismuth citrate/clarithromycin dual therapy; omeprazole/clarithromycin/amoxicillin triple therapy; and lansoprazole/clarithromycin/amoxicillin triple therapy have been shown to be active against most strains of *Helicobacter pylori in vitro* and in clinical infections as described in the **INDICATIONS AND USAGE** section.

Helicobacter

Helicobacter pylori

Pretreatment Resistance

Clarithromycin pretreatment resistance rates were 3.5% (4/113) in the omeprazole/clarithromycin dual therapy studies (M93-067, M93-100) and 9.3% (41/439) in the omeprazole/clarithromycin/amoxicillin triple therapy studies (126, 127, M96-446). Clarithromycin pretreatment resistance was 12.6% (44/348) in the ranitidine bismuth citrate/clarithromycin b.i.d. versus t.i.d. clinical study (H2BA3001).

Clarithromycin pretreatment resistance rates were 9.5% (91/960) by E-test and 11.3% (12/106) by agar dilution in the lansoprazole/clarithromycin/amoxicillin triple therapy clinical trials (M93-125, M93-130, M93-131, M95-392, and M95-399).

Amoxicillin pretreatment susceptible isolates (<0.25 µg/mL) were found in 99.3% (436/439) of the patients in the omeprazole/clarithromycin/amoxicillin clinical studies (126, 127, M96-446). Amoxicillin pretreatment minimum inhibitory concentrations (MICs) > 0.25 µg/mL occurred in 0.7% (3/439) of the patients, all of whom were in the clarithromycin/amoxicillin study arm. Amoxicillin pretreatment susceptible isolates (< 0.25 µg/mL) occurred in 97.8% (936/957) and 98.0% (98/100) of the patients in the lansoprazole/clarithromycin/amoxicillin triple-therapy clinical trials by E-test and agar dilution, respectively. Twenty-one of the 957 patients (2.2%) by E-test and 2 of 100 patients (2.0%) by agar dilution had amoxicillin pretreatment MICs of > 0.25 µg/mL. Two patients had an unconfirmed pretreatment amoxicillin minimum inhibitory concentration (MIC) of > 256 µg/mL by E-test.

[See table at top of next page]

Patients not eradicated of *H. pylori* following omeprazole/clarithromycin, ranitidine bismuth citrate/clarithromycin, omeprazole/clarithromycin/amoxicillin, or lansoprazole/clarithromycin/amoxicillin therapy would likely have clarithromycin resistant *H. pylori* isolates. Therefore, for patients who fail therapy, clarithromycin susceptibility testing should be done, if possible. Patients with clarithromycin resistant *H. pylori* should not be treated with any of the following: omeprazole/clarithromycin dual therapy; ranitidine bismuth citrate/clarithromycin dual therapy; omeprazole/clarithromycin/amoxicillin triple therapy; lansoprazole/clarithromycin/amoxicillin triple therapy; or other regimens which include clarithromycin as the sole antimicrobial agent.

Continued on next page

Biaxin—Cont.

Amoxicillin Susceptibility Test Results and Clinical/Bacteriological Outcomes

In the omeprazole/clarithromycin/amoxicillin triple-therapy clinical trials, 84.9% (157/185) of the patients who had pretreatment amoxicillin susceptible MICs (< 0.25 µg/mL) were eradicated of *H. pylori* and 15.1% (28/185) failed therapy. Of the 28 patients who failed triple therapy, 11 had no post-treatment susceptibility test results, and 17 had post-treatment *H. pylori* isolates with amoxicillin susceptible MICs. Eleven of the patients who failed triple therapy also had post-treatment *H. pylori* isolates with clarithromycin resistant MICs.

In the lansoprazole/clarithromycin/amoxicillin triple-therapy clinical trials, 82.6% (195/236) of the patients that had pretreatment amoxicillin susceptible MICs (< 0.25 µg/mL) were eradicated of *H. pylori*. Of those with pretreatment amoxicillin MICs of > 0.25 µg/mL, three of six had the *H. pylori* eradicated. A total of 12.8% (22/172) of the patients failed the 10- and 14-day triple-therapy regimens. Post-treatment susceptibility results were not obtained on 11 of the patients who failed therapy. Nine of the 11 patients with amoxicillin post-treatment MICs that failed the triple-therapy regimen also had clarithromycin resistant *H. pylori* isolates.

The following *in vitro* data are available, **but their clinical significance is unknown**. Clarithromycin exhibits *in vitro* activity against most strains of the following microorganisms; however, the safety and effectiveness of clarithromycin in treating clinical infections due to these microorganisms have not been established in adequate and well-controlled clinical trials.

Aerobic Gram-positive microorganisms

Streptococcus agalactiae
Streptococci (Groups C, F, G)
Viridans group streptococci

Aerobic Gram-negative microorganisms

Bordetella pertussis
Legionella pneumophila
Pasteurella multocida

Anaerobic Gram-positive microorganisms

Clostridium perfringens
Peptococcus niger
Propionibacterium acnes

Anaerobic Gram-negative microorganisms

Prevotella melaninogenica (formerly *Bacteriodes melaninogenicus*)

Susceptibility Testing Excluding Mycobacteria and Helicobacter:

Dilution Techniques:

Quantitative methods are used to determine antimicrobial minimum inhibitory concentrations (MICs). These MICs provide estimates of the susceptibility of bacteria to antimicrobial compounds. The MICs should be determined using a standardized procedure. Standardized procedures are based on a dilution method[1] (broth or agar) or equivalent with standardized inoculum concentrations and standardized concentrations of clarithromycin powder. The MIC values should be interpreted according to the following criteria:

For testing *Staphylococcus* spp.

MIC (µg/mL)	Interpretation
≤ 2.0	Susceptible (S)
4.0	Intermediate (I)
≥ 8.0	Resistant (R)

For testing *Streptococcus* spp. including *Streptococcus pneumoniae*[a]

MIC (µg/mL)	Interpretation
≤ 0.25	Susceptible (S)
0.5	Intermediate (I)
≥ 1.0	Resistant (R)

[a] These interpretive standards are applicable only to broth microdilution susceptibility tests using cation-adjusted Mueller-Hinton broth with 2–5% lysed horse blood.

For testing *Haemophilus* spp.[b]

MIC (µg/mL)	Interpretation
≤ 8.0	Susceptible (S)
16.0	Intermediate (I)
≥ 32.0	Resistant (R)

[b] These interpretive standards are applicable only to broth microdilution susceptibility tests with *Haemophilus* spp. using Haemophilus Testing Medium (HTM).[1]

Note: When testing *Streptococcus* spp., including *Streptococcus pneumoniae*, susceptibility and resistance to clarithromycin can be predicted using erythromycin.

A report of "Susceptible" indicates that the pathogen is likely to be inhibited if the antimicrobial compound in the blood reaches the concentrations usually achievable. A report of "Intermediate" indicates that the result should be considered equivocal, and, if the microorganism is not fully susceptible to alternative, clinically feasible drugs, the test should be repeated. This category implies possible clinical applicability in body sites where the drug is physiologically concentrated or in situations where high dosage of drug can be used. This category also provides a buffer zone which prevents small uncontrolled technical factors from causing major discrepancies in interpretation. A report of "Resistant" indicates that the pathogen is not likely to be inhibited if the antimicrobial compound in the blood reaches the concentrations usually achievable; other therapy should be selected.

Clarithromycin Susceptibility Test Results and Clinical/Bacteriological Outcomes[a]

Clarithromycin Pretreatment Results		Clarithromycin Post-treatment Results				
		H. pylori negative - eradicated	*H. pylori* positive - not eradicated Post-treatment susceptibility results			
			S[b]	I[b]	R[b]	No MIC
Omeprazole 40 mg q.d./clarithromycin 500 mg t.i.d. for 14 days followed by omeprazole 20 mg q.d. for another 14 days (M93-067, M93-100)						
Susceptible[b]	108	72	1		26	9
Intermediate[b]	1				1	
Resistant[b]	4				4	
Ranitidine bismuth citrate 400 mg b.i.d./clarithromycin 500 mg t.i.d. for 14 days followed by ranitidine bismuth citrate 400 mg b.i.d. for another 14 days (H2BA3001)						
Susceptible[b]	124	98	4		14	8
Intermediate[b]	3	2				1
Resistant[b]	17	1			15	1
Ranitidine bismuth citrate 400 mg b.i.d./clarithromycin 500 mg b.i.d. for 14 days followed by ranitidine bismuth citrate 400 mg b.i.d. for another 14 days (H2BA3001)						
Susceptible[b]	125	106	1	1	12	5
Intermediate[b]	2	2				
Resistant[b]	20	1			19	
Omeprazole 20 mg b.i.d./clarithromycin 500 mg b.i.d./amoxicillin 1 g b.i.d. for 10 days (126, 127, M96-446)						
Susceptible[b]	171	153	7		3	8
Intermediate[b]						
Resistant[b]	14	4	1		6	3
Lansoprazole 30 mg b.i.d./clarithromycin 500 mg b.i.d./amoxicillin 1 g b.i.d. for 14 days (M95-399, M93-131, M95-392)						
Susceptible[b]	112	105				7
Intermediate[b]	3	3				
Resistant[b]	17	6			7	4
Lansoprazole 30 mg b.i.d./clarithromycin 500 mg b.i.d./amoxicillin 1 g b.i.d. for 10 days (M95-399)						
Susceptible[b]	42	40	1		1	
Intermediate[b]						
Resistant[b]	4	1			3	

[a] Includes only patients with pretreatment clarithromycin susceptibility tests
[b] Susceptible (S) MIC < 0.25 µg/mL, Intermediate (I) MIC 0.5–1.0 µg/mL, Resistant (R) MIC > 2 µg/mL

Standardized susceptibility test procedures require the use of laboratory control microorganisms to control the technical aspects of the laboratory procedures. Standard clarithromycin powder should provide the following MIC values:

Microorganism		MIC (µg/mL)
S. aureus	ATCC 29213	0.12 to 0.5
S. pneumoniae[c]	ATCC 49619	0.03 to 0.12
Haemophilus influenzae[d]	ATCC 49247	4 to 16

[c] This quality control range is applicable only to *S. pneumoniae* ATCC 49619 tested by a microdilution procedure using cation-adjusted Mueller-Hinton broth with 2–5% lysed horse blood.

[d] This quality control range is applicable only to *H. influenzae* ATCC 49247 tested by a microdilution procedure using HTM[1].

Diffusion Techniques:

Quantitative methods that require measurement of zone diameters also provide reproducible estimates of the susceptibility of bacteria to antimicrobial compounds. One such standardized procedure[2] requires the use of standardized inoculum concentrations. This procedure uses paper disks impregnated with 15-µg clarithromycin to test the susceptibility of microorganisms to clarithromycin.

Reports from the laboratory providing results of the standard single-disk susceptibility test with a 15-µg clarithromycin disk should be interpreted according to the following criteria:

For testing *Staphylococcus* spp.

Zone diameter (mm)	Interpretation
≥ 18	Susceptible (S)
14 to 17	Intermediate (I)
≤ 13	Resistant (R)

For testing *Streptococcus* spp. including *Streptococcus pneumoniae*[e]

Zone diameter (mm)	Interpretation
≥ 21	Susceptible (S)
17 to 20	Intermediate (I)
≤ 16	Resistant (R)

[e] These zone diameter standards only apply to tests performed using Mueller-Hinton agar supplemented with 5% sheep blood incubated in 5% CO_2.

For testing *Haemophilus* spp.[f]

Zone diameter (mm)	Interpretation
≥ 13	Susceptible (S)
11 to 12	Intermediate (I)
≤ 10	Resistant (R)

[f] These zone diameter standards are applicable only to tests with *Haemophilus* spp. using HTM[2].

Note: When testing *Streptococcus* spp., including *Streptococcus pneumoniae*, susceptibility and resistance to clarithromycin can be predicted using erythromycin.

Interpretation should be as stated above for results using dilution techniques. Interpretation involves correlation of the diameter obtained in the disk test with the MIC for clarithromycin.

As with standardized dilution techniques, diffusion methods require the use of laboratory control microorganisms that are used to control the technical aspects of the laboratory procedures. For the diffusion technique, the 15-µg clarithromycin disk should provide the following zone diameters in this laboratory test quality control strain:

Microorganism		Zone diameter (mm)
S. aureus	ATCC 25923	26 to 32
S. pneumoniae[g]	ATCC 49619	25 to 31
Haemophilus influenzae[h]	ATCC 49247	11 to 17

[g] This quality control range is applicable only to tests performed by disk diffusion using Mueller-Hinton agar supplemented with 5% defibrinated sheep blood.

[h] This quality control limit applies to tests conducted with *Haemophilius influenzae* ATCC 49247 using HTM[2].

***In vitro* Activity of Clarithromycin against Mycobacteria:**
Clarithromycin has demonstrated *in vitro* activity against *Mycobacterium avium* complex (MAC) microorganisms isolated from both AIDS and non-AIDS patients. While gene probe techniques may be used to distinguish *M. avium* species from *M. intracellulare*, many studies only reported results on *M. avium* complex (MAC) isolates.
Various *in vitro* methodologies employing broth or solid media at different pH's, with and without oleic acid-albumin-dextrose-catalase (OADC), have been used to determine clarithromycin MIC values for mycobacterial species. In general, MIC values decrease more than 16-fold as the pH of Middlebrook 7H12 broth media increases from 5.0 to 7.4. At pH 7.4, MIC values determined with Mueller-Hinton agar were 4- to 8-fold higher than those observed with Middlebrook 7H12 media. Utilization of oleic acid-albumin-dextrose-catalase (OADC) in these assays has been shown to further alter MIC values.
Clarithromycin activity against 80 MAC isolates from AIDS patients and 211 MAC isolates from non-AIDS patients was evaluated using a microdilution method with Middlebrook 7H9 broth. Results showed an MIC value of ≤ 4.0 μg/mL in 81% and 89% of the AIDS and non-AIDS MAC isolates, respectively. Twelve percent of the non-AIDS isolates had an MIC value ≤ 0.5 μg/mL. Clarithromycin was also shown to be active against phagocytized *M. avium* complex (MAC) in mouse and human macrophage cell cultures as well as in the beige mouse infection model.
Clarithromycin activity was evaluated against *Mycobacterium tuberculosis* microorganisms. In one study utilizing the agar dilution method with Middlebrook 7H10 media, 3 of 30 clinical isolates had an MIC of 2.5 μg/mL. Clarithromycin inhibited all isolates at > 10.0 μg/mL.

Susceptibility Testing for *Mycobacterium avium* Complex (MAC):
The disk diffusion and dilution techniques for susceptibility testing against gram-positive and gram-negative bacteria should not be used for determining clarithromycin MIC values against mycobacteria. *In vitro* susceptibility testing methods and diagnostic products currently available for determining minimum inhibitory concentration (MIC) values against *Mycobacterium avium* complex (MAC) organisms have not been standardized or validated. Clarithromycin MIC values will vary depending on the susceptibility testing method employed, composition and pH of the media, and the utilization of nutritional supplements. Breakpoints to determine whether clinical isolates of *M. avium* or *M. intracellulare* are susceptible or resistant to clarithromycin have not been established.

Susceptibility Test for *Helicobacter pylori*
The reference methodology for susceptibility testing of *H. pylori* is agar dilution MICs.[3] One to three microliters of an inoculum equivalent to a No. 2 McFarland standard ($1 \times 10^7 - 1 \times 10^8$ CFU/mL for *H. pylori*) are inoculated directly onto freshly prepared antimicrobial containing Mueller-Hinton agar plates with 5% aged defibrinated sheep blood (> 2-weeks old). The agar dilution plates are incubated at 35°C in a microaerobic environment produced by a gas generating system suitable for *Campylobacter* species. After 3 days of incubation, the MICs are recorded as the lowest concentration of antimicrobial agent required to inhibit growth of the organism. The clarithromycin and amoxicillin MIC values should be interpreted according to the following criteria:

Clarithromycin MIC (μg/mL)[i]	Interpretation
< 0.25	Susceptible (S)
0.5 – 1.0	Intermediate (I)
> 2.0	Resistant (R)

Amoxicillin MIC (μg/mL)[i,j]	Interpretation
< 0.25	Susceptible (S)

[i] These are tentative breakpoints for the agar dilution methodology, and they should not be used to interpret results obtained using alternative methods.
[j] There were not enough organisms with MICs > 0.25 μg/mL to determine a resistance breakpoint.

Standardized susceptibility test procedures require the use of laboratory control microorganisms to control the technical aspects of the laboratory procedures. Standard clarithromycin and amoxicillin powders should provide the following MIC values:
[See table above]

Microorganisms	Antimicrobial Agent	MIC (μg/mL)[k]
H. pylori ATCC 43504	Clarithromycin	0.015 – 0.12 μg/mL
H. pylori ATCC 43504	Amoxicillin	0.015 – 0.12 μg/mL

[k] These are quality control ranges for the agar dilution methodology and they should not be used to control test results obtained using alternative methods.

INDICATIONS AND USAGE

BIAXIN Filmtab (clarithromycin tablets, USP) and BIAXIN Granules (clarithromycin for oral suspension, USP) are indicated for the treatment of mild to moderate infections caused by susceptible strains of the designated microorganisms in the conditions as listed below:

Adults (BIAXIN Filmtab tablets and Granules for oral suspension):
Pharyngitis/Tonsillitis due to *Streptococcus pyogenes* (The usual drug of choice in the treatment and prevention of streptococcal infections and the prophylaxis of rheumatic fever is penicillin administered by either the intramuscular or the oral route. Clarithromycin is generally effective in the eradication of *S. pyogenes* from the nasopharynx; however, data establishing the efficacy of clarithromycin in the subsequent prevention of rheumatic fever are not available at present.)
Acute maxillary sinusitis due to *Haemophilus influenzae, Moraxella catarrhalis,* or *Streptococcus pneumoniae*
Acute bacterial exacerbation of chronic bronchitis due to *Haemophilus influenzae, Haemophilus parainfluenzae, Moraxella catarrhalis,* or *Streptococcus pneumoniae*
Community-Acquired Pneumonia due to *Haemophilus influenzae, Mycoplasma pneumoniae, Streptococcus pneumoniae,* or *Chlamydia pneumoniae* (TWAR)
Uncomplicated skin and skin structure infections due to *Staphylococcus aureus,* or *Streptococcus pyogenes* (Abscesses usually require surgical drainage.)
Disseminated mycobacterial infections due to *Mycobacterium avium,* or *Mycobacterium intracellulare*
BIAXIN (clarithromycin) Filmtab tablets in combination with amoxicillin and PREVACID (lansoprazole) or PRILOSEC (omeprazole) Delayed-Release Capsules, as triple therapy, are indicated for the treatment of patients with *H. pylori* infection and duodenal ulcer disease (active or five-year history of duodenal ulcer) to eradicate *H. pylori.*
BIAXIN Filmtab tablets in combination with PRILOSEC (omeprazole) capsules or TRITEC (ranitidine bismuth citrate) tablets are also indicated for the treatment of patients with an active duodenal ulcer associated with *H. pylori* infection. However, regimens which contain clarithromycin as the single antimicrobial agent are more likely to be associated with the development of clarithromycin resistance among patients who fail therapy. Clarithromycin-containing regimens should not be used in patients with known or suspected clarithromycin resistant isolates because the efficacy of treatment is reduced in this setting.
In patients who fail therapy, susceptibility testing should be done if possible. If resistance to clarithromycin is demonstrated, a non-clarithromycin-containing therapy is recommended. (For information on development of resistance see **Microbiology** section.) The eradication of *H. pylori* has been demonstrated to reduce the risk of duodenal ulcer recurrence.

Children (BIAXIN Filmtab tablets and Granules for oral suspension):
Pharyngitis/Tonsillitis due to *Streptococcus pyogenes*
Community-Acquired Pneumonia due to *Mycoplasma pneumoniae, Streptococcus pneumoniae,* or *Chlamydia pneumoniae* (TWAR)
Acute maxillary sinusitis due to *Haemophilus influenzae, Moraxella catarrhalis,* or *Streptococcus pneumoniae*
Acute otitis media due to *Haemophilus influenzae, Moraxella catarrhalis,* or *Streptococcus pneumoniae*
NOTE: For information on otitis media, see **CLINICAL STUDIES: Otitis Media.**
Uncomplicated skin and skin structure infections due to *Staphylococcus aureus,* or *Streptococcus pyogenes* (Abscesses usually require surgical drainage.)
Disseminated mycobacterial infections due to *Mycobacterium avium,* or *Mycobacterium intracellulare*

Adults (BIAXIN XL Filmtab tablets):
BIAXIN XL Filmtab (clarithromycin extended-release tablets) are indicated for the treatment of adults with mild to moderate infection caused by susceptible strains of the designated microorganisms in the conditions listed below:
Acute maxillary sinusitis due to *Haemophilus influenzae, Moraxella catarrhalis,* or *Streptococcus pneumoniae*
Acute bacterial exacerbation of chronic bronchitis due to *Haemophilus influenzae, Haemophilus parainfluenzae, Moraxella catarrhalis,* or *Streptococcus pneumoniae*
Community-Acquired Pneumonia due to *Haemophilus influenzae, Haemophilus parainfluenzae, Moraxella catarrhalis, Streptococcus pneumoniae, Chlamydia pneumoniae* (TWAR), or *Mycoplasma pneumoniae*
THE EFFICACY AND SAFETY OF BIAXIN XL IN TREATING OTHER INFECTIONS FOR WHICH OTHER FORMULATIONS OF BIAXIN ARE APPROVED HAVE NOT BEEN ESTABLISHED.

Prophylaxis:
BIAXIN Filmtab tablets and BIAXIN Granules for oral suspension are indicated for the prevention of disseminated *Mycobacterium avium* complex (MAC) disease in patients with advanced HIV infection.
To reduce the development of drug-resistant bacteria and maintain the effectiveness of BIAXIN and other antibacterial drugs, BIAXIN should be used only to treat or prevent infections that are proven or strongly suspected to be caused by susceptible bacteria. When culture and susceptibility information are available, they should be considered in selecting or modifying antibacterial therapy. In the absence of such data, local epidemiology and susceptibility patterns may contribute to the empiric selection of therapy.

CONTRAINDICATIONS

Clarithromycin is contraindicated in patients with a known hypersensitivity to clarithromycin, erythromycin, or any of the macrolide antibiotics.
Concomitant administration of clarithromycin with cisapride, pimozide, astemizole, or terfenadine is contraindicated. There have been post-marketing reports of drug interactions when clarithromycin and/or erythromycin are co-administered with cisapride, pimozide, astemizole, or terfenadine resulting in cardiac arrhythmias (QT prolongation, ventricular tachycardia, ventricular fibrillation, and torsades de pointes) most likely due to inhibition of metabolism of these drugs by erythromycin and clarithromycin. Fatalities have been reported.
For information about contraindications of other drugs indicated in combination with BIAXIN, refer to the CONTRAINDICATIONS section of their package inserts.

WARNINGS

CLARITHROMYCIN SHOULD NOT BE USED IN PREGNANT WOMEN EXCEPT IN CLINICAL CIRCUMSTANCES WHERE NO ALTERNATIVE THERAPY IS APPROPRIATE. IF PREGNANCY OCCURS WHILE TAKING THIS DRUG, THE PATIENT SHOULD BE APPRISED OF THE POTENTIAL HAZARD TO THE FETUS. CLARITHROMYCIN HAS DEMONSTRATED ADVERSE EFFECTS OF PREGNANCY OUTCOME AND/OR EMBRYO-FETAL DEVELOPMENT IN MONKEYS, RATS, MICE, AND RABBITS AT DOSES THAT PRODUCED PLASMA LEVELS 2 TO 17 TIMES THE SERUM LEVELS ACHIEVED IN HUMANS TREATED AT THE MAXIMUM RECOMMENDED HUMAN DOSES. (See PRECAUTIONS – *Pregnancy*.)
Pseudomembranous colitis has been reported with nearly all antibacterial agents, including clarithromycin, and may range in severity from mild to life threatening. Therefore, it is important to consider this diagnosis in patients who present with diarrhea subsequent to the administration of antibacterial agents.
Treatment with antibacterial agents alters the normal flora of the colon and may permit overgrowth of clostridia. Studies indicate that a toxin produced by *Clostridium difficile* is a primary cause of "antibiotic-associated colitis".
After the diagnosis of pseudomembranous colitis has been established, therapeutic measures should be initiated. Mild cases of pseudomembranous colitis usually respond to discontinuation of the drug alone. In moderate to severe cases, consideration should be given to management with fluids and electrolytes, protein supplementation, and treatment with an antibacterial drug clinically effective against *Clostridium difficile* colitis.
For information about warnings of other drugs indicated in combination with BIAXIN, refer to the WARNINGS section of their package inserts.

PRECAUTIONS

General: Prescribing BIAXIN in the absence of a proven or strongly suspected bacterial infection or a prophylactic indication is unlikely to provide benefit to the patient and increases the risk of the development of drug-resistant bacteria.
Clarithromycin is principally excreted via the liver and kidney. Clarithromycin may be administered without dosage adjustment to patients with hepatic impairment and normal renal function. However, in the presence of severe renal impairment with or without coexisting hepatic impairment, decreased dosage or prolonged dosing intervals may be appropriate.
Clarithromycin in combination with ranitidine bismuth citrate therapy is not recommended in patients with creatinine clearance less than 25 mL/min. (See **DOSAGE AND ADMINISTRATION**.)
Clarithromycin in combination with ranitidine bismuth citrate should not be used in patients with a history of acute porphyria.
For information about precautions of other drugs indicated in combination with BIAXIN, refer to the PRECAUTIONS section of their package inserts.
Information to Patients: Patients should be counseled that antibacterial drugs including BIAXIN should only be used to treat bacterial infections. They do not treat viral infections (e.g., the common cold). When BIAXIN is prescribed to treat a bacterial infection, patients should be told that although it is common to feel better early in the course of therapy, the medication should be taken exactly as directed. Skipping doses or not completing the full course of therapy may (1) decrease the effectiveness of the immediate treatment and (2) increase the likelihood that bacteria will develop resistance and will not be treatable by BIAXIN or other antibacterial drugs in the future.
BIAXIN may interact with some drugs; therefore patients should be advised to report to their doctor the use of any other medications.
BIAXIN tablets and oral suspension can be taken with or without food and can be taken with milk; however, BIAXIN XL tablets should be taken with food. Do **NOT** refrigerate the suspension.
Drug Interactions: Clarithromycin use in patients who are receiving theophylline may be associated with an increase of serum theophylline concentrations. Monitoring of serum theophylline concentrations should be considered for patients receiving high doses of theophylline or with baseline concentrations in the upper therapeutic range. In two studies in which theophylline was administered with clarithromycin (a theophylline sustained-release formulation was dosed at either 6.5 mg/kg or 12 mg/kg together

Continued on next page

Biaxin—Cont.

with 250 or 500 mg q12h clarithromycin), the steady-state levels of C_{max}, C_{min}, and the area under the serum concentration time curve (AUC) of theophylline increased about 20%.

Concomitant administration of single doses of clarithromycin and carbamazepine has been shown to result in increased plasma concentrations of carbamazepine. Blood level monitoring of carbamazepine may be considered.

When clarithromycin and terfenadine were coadministered, plasma concentrations of the active acid metabolite of terfenadine were threefold higher, on average, than the values observed when terfenadine was administered alone. The pharmacokinetics of clarithromycin and the 14-hydroxy-clarithromycin were not significantly affected by coadministration of terfenadine once clarithromycin reached steady-state conditions. Concomitant administration of clarithromycin with terfenadine is contraindicated. (See **CONTRAINDICATIONS**.)

Clarithromycin 500 mg every 8 hours was given in combination with omeprazole 40 mg daily to healthy adult subjects. The steady-state plasma concentrations of omeprazole were increased (C_{max}, AUC_{0-24}, and $T_{1/2}$ increases of 30%, 89%, and 34%, respectively), by the concomitant administration of clarithromycin. The mean 24-hour gastric pH value was 5.2 when omeprazole was administered alone and 5.7 when co-administered with clarithromycin.

Co-administration of clarithromycin with ranitidine bismuth citrate resulted in increased plasma ranitidine concentrations (57%), increased plasma bismuth trough concentrations (48%), and increased 14-hydroxy-clarithromycin plasma concentrations (31%). These effects are clinically insignificant.

Simultaneous oral administration of BIAXIN tablets and zidovudine to HIV-infected adult patients resulted in decreased steady-state zidovudine concentrations. When 500 mg of clarithromycin were administered twice daily, steady-state zidovudine AUC was reduced by a mean of 12% (n=4). Individual values ranged from a decrease of 34% to an increase of 14%. Based on limited data in 24 patients, when BIAXIN tablets were administered two to four hours prior to oral zidovudine, the steady-state zidovudine C_{max} was increased by approximately 2-fold, whereas the AUC was unaffected.

Simultaneous administration of BIAXIN tablets and didanosine to 12 HIV-infected adult patients resulted in no statistically significant change in didanosine pharmacokinetics.

Concomitant administration of fluconazole 200 mg daily and clarithromycin 500 mg twice daily to 21 healthy volunteers led to increases in the mean steady-state clarithromycin C_{min} and AUC of 33% and 18%, respectively. Steady-state concentrations of 14-OH clarithromycin were not significantly affected by concomitant administration of fluconazole.

Concomitant administration of clarithromycin and ritonavir (n=22) resulted in a 77% increase in clarithromycin AUC and a 100% decrease in the AUC of 14-OH clarithromycin. Clarithromycin may be administered without dosage adjustment to patients with normal renal function taking ritonavir. However, for patients with renal impairment, the following dosage adjustments should be considered. For patients with CL_{CR} 30 to 60 mL/min, the dose of clarithromycin should be reduced by 50%. For patients with $CL_{CR} < 30$ mL/min, the dose of clarithromycin should be decreased by 75%.

Spontaneous reports in the post-marketing period suggest that concomitant administration of clarithromycin and oral anticoagulants may potentiate the effects of the oral anticoagulants. Prothrombin times should be carefully monitored while patients are receiving clarithromycin and oral anticoagulants simultaneously.

Elevated digoxin serum concentrations in patients receiving clarithromycin and digoxin concomitantly have also been reported in post-marketing surveillance. Some patients have shown clinical signs consistent with digoxin toxicity, including potentially fatal arrhythmias. Serum digoxin concentrations should be carefully monitored while patients are receiving digoxin and clarithromycin simultaneously.

Erythromycin and clarithromycin are substrates and inhibitors of the 3A isoform subfamily of the cytochrome P450 enzyme system (CYP3A). Coadministration of erythromycin or clarithromycin and a drug primarily metabolized by CYP3A may be associated with elevations in drug concentrations that could increase or prolong both the therapeutic and adverse effects of the concomitant drug. Dosage adjustments may be considered, and when possible, serum concentrations of drugs primarily metabolized by CYP3A should be monitored closely in patients concurrently receiving clarithromycin or erythromycin.

The following are examples of some clinically significant CYP3A based drug interactions. Interactions with other drugs metabolized by the CYP3A isoform are also possible. Increased serum concentrations of carbamazepine and the active acid metabolite of terfenadine were observed in clinical trials with clarithromycin.

The following CYP3A based drug interactions have been observed with erythromycin products and/or with clarithromycin in postmarketing experience:

Antiarrhythmics: There have been postmarketing reports of torsades de pointes occurring with concurrent use of clarithromycin and quinidine or disopyramide. Electrocardiograms should be monitored for QTc prolongation during coadministration of clarithromycin with these drugs. Serum concentrations of these medications should also be monitored.

Ergotamine/dihydroergotamine: Concurrent use of erythromycin or clarithromycin and ergotamine or dihydroergotamine has been associated in some patients with acute ergot toxicity characterized by severe peripheral vasospasm and dysesthesia.

Triazolobenziodidiazepines (such as triazolam and alprazolam) and related benzodiazepines (such as midazolam): Erythromycin has been reported to decrease the clearance of triazolam and midazolam, and thus, may increase the pharmacologic effect of these benzodiazepines. There have been postmarketing reports of drug interactions and CNS effects (e.g., somnolence and confusion) with the concomitant use of clarithromycin and triazolam.

HMG-CoA Reductase Inhibitors: As with other macrolides, clarithromycin has been reported to increase concentrations of HMG-CoA reductase inhibitors (e.g., lovastatin and simvastatin). Rare reports of rhabdomyolysis have been reported in patients taking these drugs concomitantly.

Sildenafil (Viagra): Erythromycin has been reported to increase the systemic exposure (AUC) of sildenafil. A similar interaction may occur with clarithromycin; reduction of sildenafil dosage should be considered. (See Viagra package insert.)

There have been spontaneous or published reports of CYP3A based interactions of erythromycin and/or clarithromycin with cyclosporine, carbamazepine, tacrolimus, alfentanil, disopyramide, rifabutin, quinidine, methylprednisolone, cilostazol, and bromocriptine.

Concomitant administration of clarithromycin with cisapride, pimozide, astemizole, or terfenadine is contraindicated (see **CONTRAINDICATIONS**).

In addition, there have been reports of interactions of erythromycin or clarithromycin with drugs not thought to be metabolized by CYP3A including hexobarbital, phenytoin, and valproate.

Carcinogenesis, Mutagenesis, Impairment of Fertility:
The following *in vitro* mutagenicity tests have been conducted with clarithromycin:

Salmonella/Mammalian Microsomes Test
Bacterial Induced Mutation Frequency Test
In Vitro Chromosome Aberration Test
Rat Hepatocyte DNA Synthesis Assay
Mouse Lymphoma Assay
Mouse Dominant Lethal Study
Mouse Micronucleus Test

All tests had negative results except the *In Vitro* Chromosome Aberration Test which was weakly positive in one test and negative in another.

In addition, a Bacterial Reverse-Mutation Test (Ames Test) has been performed on clarithromycin metabolites with negative results.

Fertility and reproduction studies have shown that daily doses of up to 160 mg/kg/day (1.3 times the recommended maximum human dose based on mg/m^2) to male and female rats caused no adverse effects on the estrous cycle, fertility, parturition, or number and viability of offspring. Plasma levels in rats after 150 mg/kg/day were 2 times the human serum levels.

In the 150 mg/kg/day monkey studies, plasma levels were 3 times the human serum levels. When given orally at 150 mg/kg/day (2.4 times the recommended maximum human dose based on mg/m^2), clarithromycin was shown to produce embryonic loss in monkeys. This effect has been attributed to marked maternal toxicity of the drug at this high dose.

In rabbits, *in utero* fetal loss occurred at an intravenous dose of 33 mg/m^2, which is 17 times less than the maximum proposed human oral daily dose of 618 mg/m^2.

Long-term studies in animals have not been performed to evaluate the carcinogenic potential of clarithromycin.

Pregnancy: Teratogenic Effects. Pregnancy Category C.
Four teratogenicity studies in rats (three with oral doses and one with intravenous doses up to 160 mg/kg/day administered during the period of major organogenesis) and two in rabbits at oral doses up to 125 mg/kg/day (approximately 2 times the recommended maximum human dose based on mg/m^2) or intravenous doses of 30 mg/kg/day administered during gestation days 6 to 18 failed to demonstrate any teratogenicity from clarithromycin. Two additional oral studies in a different rat strain at similar doses and similar conditions demonstrated a low incidence of cardiovascular anomalies at doses of 150 mg/kg/day administered during gestation days 6 to 15. Plasma levels after 150 mg/kg/day were 2 times the human serum levels. Four studies in mice revealed a variable incidence of cleft palate following oral doses of 1000 mg/kg/day (2 and 4 times the recommended maximum human dose based on mg/m^2, respectively) during gestation days 6 to 15. Cleft palate was also seen at 500 mg/kg/day. The 1000 mg/kg/day exposure resulted in plasma levels 17 times the human serum levels. In monkeys, an oral dose of 70 mg/kg/day (an approximate equidose of the recommended maximum human dose based on mg/m^2) produced fetal growth retardation at plasma levels that were 2 times the human serum levels.

There are no adequate and well-controlled studies in pregnant women. Clarithromycin should be used during pregnancy only if the potential benefit justifies the potential risk to the fetus. (See **WARNINGS**.)

Nursing Mothers: It is not known whether clarithromycin is excreted in human milk. Because many drugs are excreted in human milk, caution should be exercised when clarithromycin is administered to a nursing woman. It is known that clarithromycin is excreted in the milk of lactating animals and that other drugs of this class are excreted in human milk. Preweaned rats, exposed indirectly via consumption of milk from dams treated with 150 mg/kg/day for 3 weeks, were not adversely affected, despite data indicating higher drug levels in milk than in plasma.

Pediatric Use: Safety and effectiveness of clarithromycin in pediatric patients under 6 months of age have not been established. The safety of clarithromycin has not been studied in MAC patients under the age of 20 months. Neonatal and juvenile animals tolerated clarithromycin in a manner similar to adult animals. Young animals were slightly more intolerant to acute overdosage and to subtle reductions in erythrocytes, platelets and leukocytes but were less sensitive to toxicity in the liver, kidney, thymus, and genitalia.

Geriatric Use: In a steady-state study in which healthy elderly subjects (age 65 to 81 years old) were given 500 mg every 12 hours, the maximum serum concentrations and area under the curves of clarithromycin and 14-OH clarithromycin were increased compared to those achieved in healthy young adults. These changes in pharmacokinetics parallel known age-related decreases in renal function. In clinical trials, elderly patients did not have an increased incidence of adverse events when compared to younger patients. Dosage adjustment should be considered in elderly patients with severe renal impairment.

ADVERSE REACTIONS

The majority of side effects observed in clinical trials were of a mild and transient nature. Fewer than 3% of adult patients without mycobacterial infections and fewer than 2% of pediatric patients without mycobacterial infections discontinued therapy because of drug-related side effects. Fewer than 2% of adult patients taking BIAXIN XL tablets discontinued therapy because of drug-related side effects.

The most frequently reported events in adults taking BIAXIN tablets (clarithromycin tablets, USP) were diarrhea (3%), nausea (3%), abnormal taste (3%), dyspepsia (2%), abdominal pain/discomfort (2%), and headache (2%). In pediatric patients, the most frequently reported events were diarrhea (6%), vomiting (6%), abdominal pain (3%), rash (3%), and headache (2%). Most of these events were described as mild or moderate in severity. Of the reported adverse events, only 1% was described as severe.

The most frequently reported events in adults taking BIAXIN XL (clarithromycin extended-release tablets) were diarrhea (6%), abnormal taste (7%), and nausea (3%). Most of these events were described as mild or moderate in severity. Of the reported adverse events, less than 1% were described as severe.

In the acute exacerbation of chronic bronchitis and acute maxillary sinusitis studies overall gastrointestinal adverse events were reported by a similar proportion of patients taking either BIAXIN tablets or BIAXIN XL tablets; however, patients taking BIAXIN XL tablets reported significantly less severe gastrointestinal symptoms compared to patients taking BIAXIN tablets. In addition, patients taking BIAXIN XL tablets had significantly fewer premature discontinuations for drug-related gastrointestinal or abnormal taste adverse events compared to BIAXIN tablets.

In community-acquired pneumonia studies conducted in adults comparing clarithromycin to erythromycin base or erythromycin stearate, there were fewer adverse events involving the digestive system in clarithromycin-treated patients compared to erythromycin-treated patients (13% vs 32%; p<0.01). Twenty percent of erythromycin-treated patients discontinued therapy due to adverse events compared to 4% of clarithromycin-treated patients.

In two U.S. studies of acute otitis media comparing clarithromycin to amoxicillin/potassium clavulanate in pediatric patients, there were fewer adverse events involving the digestive system in clarithromycin-treated patients compared to amoxicillin/potassium clavulanate-treated patients (21% vs 40%, p<0.001). One-third as many clarithromycin-treated patients reported diarrhea as did amoxicillin/potassium clavulanate-treated patients.

Post-Marketing Experience:
Allergic reactions ranging from urticaria and mild skin eruptions to rare cases of anaphylaxis, Stevens-Johnson syndrome and toxic epidermal necrolysis have occurred. Other spontaneously reported adverse events include glossitis, stomatitis, oral moniliasis, anorexia, vomiting, pancreatitis, tongue discoloration, thrombocytopenia, leukopenia, neutropenia, and dizziness. There have been reports of tooth discoloration in patients treated with BIAXIN. Tooth discoloration is usually reversible with professional dental cleaning. There have been isolated reports of hearing loss, which is usually reversible, occurring chiefly in elderly women. Reports of alterations of the sense of smell, usually in conjunction with taste perversion or taste loss have also been reported.

Transient CNS events including anxiety, behavioral changes, confusional states, convulsions, depersonalization, disorientation, hallucinations, insomnia, manic behavior, nightmares, psychosis, tinnitus, tremor, and vertigo have been reported during post-marketing surveillance. Events usually resolve with discontinuation of the drug.

Hepatic dysfunction, including increased liver enzymes, and hepatocellular and/or cholestatic hepatitis, with or without jaundice, has been infrequently reported with clarithromycin. This hepatic dysfunction may be severe and is usually reversible. In very rare instances, hepatic failure with fatal outcome has been reported and generally has been associated with serious underlying diseases and/or concomitant medications.

There have been rare reports of hypoglycemia, some of which have occurred in patients taking oral hypoglycemic agents or insulin.

There have been postmarketing reports of BIAXIN XL tablets in the stool, many of which have occurred in patients with anatomic (including ileostomy or colostomy) or functional gastrointestinal disorders with shortened GI transit times.

As with other macrolides, clarithromycin has been associated with QT prolongation and ventricular arrhythmias, including ventricular tachycardia and torsades de pointes.

Changes in Laboratory Values: Changes in laboratory values with possible clinical significance were as follows:

Hepatic—elevated SGPT (ALT) < 1%; SGOT (AST) < 1%; GGT < 1%; alkaline phosphatase <1%; LDH < 1%; total bilirubin < 1%

Hematologic—decreased WBC < 1%; elevated prothrombin time 1%

Renal—elevated BUN 4%; elevated serum creatinine < 1%

GGT, alkaline phosphatase, and prothrombin time data are from adult studies only.

OVERDOSAGE

Overdosage of clarithromycin can cause gastrointestinal symptoms such as abdominal pain, vomiting, nausea, and diarrhea.

Adverse reactions accompanying overdosage should be treated by the prompt elimination of unabsorbed drug and supportive measures. As with other macrolides, clarithromycin serum concentrations are not expected to be appreciably affected by hemodialysis or peritoneal dialysis.

DOSAGE AND ADMINISTRATION

BIAXIN® Filmtab® (clarithromycin tablets, USP) and BIAXIN® Granules (clarithromycin for oral suspension, USP) may be given with or without food. BIAXIN® XL Filmtab® (clarithromycin extended-release tablets) should be taken with food. BIAXIN® XL Filmtab® should be swallowed whole and not chewed, broken or crushed.

[See first table above]

H. pylori Eradication to Reduce the Risk of Duodenal Ulcer Recurrence

Triple therapy: BIAXIN/lansoprazole/amoxicillin

The recommended adult dose is 500 mg BIAXIN, 30 mg lansoprazole, and 1 gram amoxicillin, all given twice daily (q12h) for 10 or 14 days. (See **INDICATIONS AND USAGE** and **CLINICAL STUDIES** sections.)

Triple therapy: Biaxin/omeprazole/amoxicillin

The recommended adult dose is 500 mg BIAXIN, 20 mg omeprazole, and 1 gram amoxicillin, all given twice daily (q12h) for 10 days. (See **INDICATIONS AND USAGE** and **CLINICAL STUDIES** sections.) In patients with an ulcer present at the time of initiation of therapy, an additional 18 days of omeprazole 20 mg once daily is recommended for ulcer healing and symptom relief.

Dual therapy: BIAXIN/omeprazole

The recommended adult dose is 500 mg BIAXIN given three times daily (q8h) and 40 mg omeprazole given once daily (qAM) for 14 days. (See **INDICATIONS AND USAGE** and **CLINICAL STUDIES** sections.) An additional 14 days of omeprazole 20 mg once daily is recommended for ulcer healing and symptom relief.

Dual therapy: BIAXIN/ranitidine bismuth citrate

The recommended adult dose is 500 mg BIAXIN given twice daily (q12h) or three times daily (q8h) and 400 mg ranitidine bismuth citrate given twice daily (q12h) for 14 days. An additional 14 days of 400 mg twice daily is recommended for ulcer healing and symptom relief. BIAXIN and ranitidine bismuth citrate combination therapy is not recommended in patients with creatinine clearance less than 25 mL/min. (See **INDICATIONS AND USAGE** and **CLINICAL STUDIES** sections.)

Children - The usual recommended daily dosage is 15 mg/kg/day divided q12h for 10 days.

[See second table above]

Clarithromycin may be administered without dosage adjustment in the presence of hepatic impairment if there is normal renal function. However, in the presence of severe renal impairment (CR_{CL} < 30 mL/min), with or without coexisting hepatic impairment, the dose should be halved or the dosing interval doubled.

Mycobacterial infections:

Prophylaxis: The recommended dose of BIAXIN for the prevention of disseminated *Mycobacterium avium* disease is 500 mg b.i.d. In children, the recommended dose is 7.5 mg/kg b.i.d. up to 500 mg b.i.d. No studies of clarithromycin for MAC prophylaxis have been performed in pediatric populations and the doses recommended for prophylaxis are derived from MAC treatment studies in children. Dosing recommendations for children are in the table above.

Treatment: Clarithromycin is recommended as the primary agent for the treatment of disseminated infection due to *Mycobacterium avium* complex. Clarithromycin should be used in combination with other antimycobacterial drugs that have shown *in vitro* activity against MAC or clinical benefit in MAC treatment. (See **CLINICAL STUDIES**.) The recommended dose for mycobacterial infections in adults is 500 mg b.i.d. In children, the recommended dose is

ADULT DOSAGE GUIDELINES

Infection	BIAXIN Tablets Dosage (q12h)	BIAXIN Tablets Duration (days)	BIAXIN XL Tablets Dosage (q24h)	BIAXIN XL Tablets Duration (days)
Pharyngitis/Tonsillitis due to				
S. pyogenes	250 mg	10	—	—
Acute maxillary sinusitis due to	500 mg	14	2 × 500 mg	14
H. influenzae				
M. catarrhalis				
S. pneumoniae				
Acute exacerbation of chronic bronchitis due to				
H. influenzae	500 mg	7-14	2 × 500 mg	7
H. parainfluenzae	500 mg	7	2 × 500 mg	7
M. catarrhalis	250 mg	7-14	2 × 500 mg	7
S. pneumoniae	250 mg	7-14	2 × 500 mg	7
Community-Acquired Pneumonia due to				
H. influenzae	250 mg	7	2 × 500 mg	7
H. parainfluenzae	—	—	2 × 500 mg	7
M. catarrhalis	—	—	2 × 500 mg	7
S. pneumoniae	250 mg	7-14	2 × 500 mg	7
C. pneumoniae	250 mg	7-14	2 × 500 mg	7
M. pneumoniae	250 mg	7-14	2 × 500 mg	7
Uncomplicated skin and skin structure	250 mg	7-14	—	—
S. aureus				
S. pyogenes				

PEDIATRIC DOSAGE GUIDELINES

Based on Body Weight

Weight kg	Weight lbs	Dosing Calculated on 7.5 mg/kg q12h Dose (q12h)	125 mg/5 mL	250 mg/5 mL
9	20	62.5 mg	2.5 mL q12h	1.25 mL q12h
17	37	125 mg	5 mL q12h	2.5 mL q12h
25	55	187.5 mg	7.5 mL q12h	3.75 mL q12h
33	73	250 mg	10 mL q12h	5 mL q12h

Total volume after constitution	Clarithromycin concentration after constitution	Amount of water to be added*
50 mL	125 mg/5 mL	27 mL
100 mL	125 mg/5 mL	55 mL
50 mL	250 mg/5 mL	27 mL
100 mL	250 mg/5 mL	55 mL

* see instructions below.

7.5 mg/kg b.i.d. up to 500 mg b.i.d. Dosing recommendations for children are in the table above.

Clarithromycin therapy should continue for life if clinical and mycobacterial improvements are observed.

Constituting Instructions

The table below indicates the volume of water to be added when constituting:

[See third table above]

Add half the volume of water to the bottle and shake vigorously. Add the remainder of water to the bottle and shake. Shake well before each use. Oversize bottle provides shake space. Keep tightly closed. Do not refrigerate. After mixing, store at 15° to 30°C (59° to 86°F) and use within 14 days.

HOW SUPPLIED

BIAXIN® Filmtab® (clarithromycin tablets, USP) are supplied as yellow oval film-coated tablets in the following packaging sizes:

250 mg tablets: (imprinted in blue with the Abbott logo and Abbo-Code KT)

Bottles of 60 (**NDC** 0074-3368-60) and ABBO-PAC unit dose strip packages of 100 (**NDC** 0074-3368-11).

Store BIAXIN 250 mg tablets at controlled room temperature 15° to 30°C (59° to 86°F) in a well-closed container. Protect from light.

500 mg tablets: (debossed with the Abbott logo on one side and Abbo-Code KL on the opposite side)

Bottles of 60 (**NDC** 0074-2586-60) and ABBO-PAC unit dose strip packages of 100 (**NDC** 0074-2586-11).

Store BIAXIN 500 mg tablets at controlled room temperature 20° to 25°C (68° to 77°F) in a well-closed container.

BIAXIN® XL Filmtab® (clarithromycin extended-release tablets) are supplied as yellow oval film-coated 500 mg tablets debossed (on one side) with the Abbott logo and a two-letter Abbo-Code designation, KJ in the following packaging sizes:

500 mg tablets:

Bottles of 60 (**NDC** 0074-3165-60), ABBO-PAC unit dose strip packages of 100 (**NDC** 0074-3165-11), and BIAXIN® XL PAC carton of 4 blister packages 14 tablets each (**NDC** 0074-3165-41).

Store BIAXIN XL tablets at 20° to 25°C (68° to 77°F). Excursions permitted to 15° to 30°C (59° to 86°F). [See USP Controlled Room Temperature.]

BIAXIN® Granules (clarithromycin for oral suspension, USP) is supplied in the following strengths and sizes:

[See first table at top of next page]

Store BIAXIN granules for oral suspension at controlled room temperature 15° to 30°C (59° to 86°F) in a well-closed container. Do not refrigerate BIAXIN suspension.

CLINICAL STUDIES

Mycobacterial Infections

Prophylaxis:

A randomized, double-blind study (561) compared clarithromycin 500 mg b.i.d. to placebo in patients with CDC-defined AIDS and CD_4 counts <100 cells/µL. This study accrued 682 patients from November 1992 to January 1994, with a median CD_4 cell count at study entry of 30 cells/µL. Median duration of clarithromycin was 10.6 months vs. 8.2 months for placebo. More patients in the placebo arm than the clarithromycin arm discontinued prematurely from the study (75.6% and 67.4%, respectively). However, if premature discontinuations due to MAC or death are excluded, approximately equal percentages of patients on each arm (54.8% on clarithromycin and 52.5% on placebo) discontinued study drug early for other reasons. The study was designed to evaluate the following endpoints:

1. MAC bacteremia, defined as at least one positive culture for *M. avium* complex bacteria from blood or another normally sterile site.
2. Survival.
3. Clinically significant disseminated MAC disease, defined as MAC bacteremia accompanied by signs or symptoms of serious MAC infection, including fever, night sweats, weight loss, anemia, or elevations in liver function tests.

MAC bacteremia:

In patients randomized to clarithromycin, the risk of MAC bacteremia was reduced by 69% compared to placebo. The difference between groups was statistically significant (p<0.001). On an intent-to-treat basis, the one-year cumulative incidence of MAC bacteremia was 5.0% for patients randomized to clarithromycin and 19.4% for patients randomized to placebo. While only 19 of the 341 patients randomized to clarithromycin developed MAC, 11 of these cases were resistant to clarithromycin. The patients with resis-

Continued on next page

Biaxin—Cont.

tant MAC bacteremia had a median baseline CD_4 count of 10 cells/mm^3 (range 2 to 25 cells/mm^3). Information regarding the clinical course and response to treatment of the patients with resistant MAC bacteremia is limited. The 8 patients who received clarithromycin and developed susceptible MAC bacteremia had a median baseline CD_4 count of 25 cells/mm^3 (range 10 to 80 cells/mm^3). Comparatively, 53 of the 341 placebo patients developed MAC; none of these isolates were resistant to clarithromycin. The median baseline CD_4 count was 15 cells/mm^3 (range 2 to 130 cells/mm^3) for placebo patients that developed MAC.

Survival:
A statistically significant survival benefit was observed.

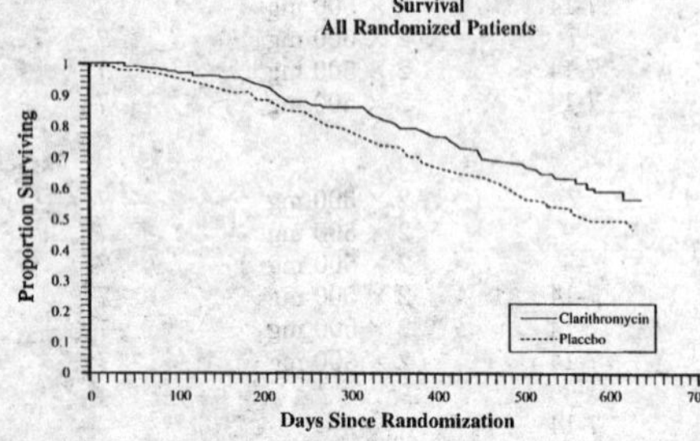

[See second table at right]
Since the analysis at 18 months includes patients no longer receiving prophylaxis the survival benefit of clarithromycin may be underestimated.

Clinically significant disseminated MAC disease:
In association with the decreased incidence of bacteremia, patients in the group randomized to clarithromycin showed reductions in the signs and symptoms of disseminated MAC disease, including fever, night sweats, weight loss, and anemia.

Safety:
In AIDS patients treated with clarithromycin over long periods of time for prophylaxis against *M. avium*, it was often difficult to distinguish adverse events possibly associated with clarithromycin administration from underlying HIV disease or intercurrent illness. Median duration of treatment was 10.6 months for the clarithromycin group and 8.2 months for the placebo group.
[See third table at right]
Among these events, taste perversion was the only event that had significantly higher incidence in the clarithromycin-treated group compared to the placebo-treated group.
Discontinuation due to adverse events was required in 18% of patients receiving clarithromycin compared to 17% of patients receiving placebo in this trial. Primary reasons for discontinuation in clarithromycin treated patients include headache, nausea, vomiting, depression and taste perversion.

Changes in Laboratory Values of Potential Clinical Importance:
In immunocompromised patients receiving prophylaxis against *M. avium*, evaluations of laboratory values were made by analyzing those values outside the seriously abnormal value (i.e., the extreme high or low limit) for the specified test.
[See fourth table at right]

Treatment:
Three randomized studies (500, 577, and 521) compared different dosages of clarithromycin in patients with CDC-defined AIDS and CD_4 counts <100 cells/µL. These studies accrued patients from May 1991 to March 1992. Study 500 was randomized, double-blind; Study 577 was open-label compassionate use. Both studies used 500 and 1000 mg b.i.d. doses; Study 500 also had a 2000 mg b.i.d. group. Study 521 was a pediatric study at 3.75, 7.5, and 15 mg/kg b.i.d. Study 500 enrolled 154 adult patients, Study 577 enrolled 469 adult patients, and Study 521 enrolled 25 patients between the ages of 1 to 20. The majority of patients had CD_4 cell counts <50/µL at study entry. The studies were designed to evaluate the following end points:

1. Change in MAC bacteremia or blood cultures negative for *M. avium*.
2. Change in clinical signs and symptoms of MAC infection including one or more of the following: fever, night sweats, weight loss, diarrhea, splenomegaly, and hepatomegaly.

The results for the 500 study are described below. The 577 study results were similar to the results of the 500 study. Results with the 7.5 mg/kg b.i.d. dose in the pediatric study were comparable to those for the 500 mg b.i.d. regimen in the adult studies.
Study 069 compared the safety and efficacy of clarithromycin in combination with ethambutol versus clarithromycin in combination with ethambutol and clofazimine for the treatment of disseminated MAC (dMAC) infection[4]. This 24-week study enrolled 106 patients with AIDS and dMAC, with 55 patients randomized to receive clarithromycin and ethambutol, and 51 patients randomized to receive clarithromycin, ethambutol, and clofazimine. Baseline characteristics between study arms were similar with the exception of median CFU counts being at least 1 log higher in the clarithromycin, ethambutol, and clofazimine arm.

Total volume after constitution	Clarithromycin concentration after constitution	Clarithromycin contents per bottle	NDC
50 mL	125 mg/5 mL	1250 mg	0074-3163-50
100 mL	125 mg/5 mL	2500 mg	0074-3163-13
50 mL	250 mg/5 mL	2500 mg	0074-3188-50
100 mL	250 mg/5 mL	5000 mg	0074-3188-13

	Mortality		Reduction in
	Placebo	Clarithromycin	Mortality on Clarithromycin
6 month	9.4%	6.5%	31%
12 month	29.7%	20.5%	31%
18 month	46.4%	37.5%	20%

Treatment-related* Adverse Event Incidence Rates (%) in Immunocompromised Adult Patients Receiving Prophylaxis Against *M. avium* Complex

Body System‡ Adverse Event	Clarithromycin (n = 339) %	Placebo (n = 339) %
Body as a Whole		
Abdominal pain	5.0%	3.5%
Headache	2.7%	0.9%
Digestive		
Diarrhea	7.7%	4.1%
Dyspepsia	3.8%	2.7%
Flatulence	2.4%	0.9%
Nausea	11.2%	7.1%
Vomiting	5.9%	3.2%
Skin & Appendages		
Rash	3.2%	3.5%
Special Senses		
Taste Perversion	8.0%	0.3%

* Includes those events possibly or probably related to study drug and excludes concurrent conditions.
‡ >2% Adverse Event Incidence Rates for either treatment group.

Percentage of Patients[(a)] Exceeding Extreme Laboratory Value in Patients Receiving Prophylaxis Against *M. avium* Complex

		Clarithromycin 500 mg b.i.d.		Placebo	
Hemoglobin	< 8 g/dL	4/118	3%	5/103	5%
Platelet Count	< 50 × 10^9/L	11/249	4%	12/250	5%
WBC Count	< 1 × 10^9/L	2/103	4%	0/95	0%
SGOT	> 5 × ULN[b]	7/196	4%	5/208	2%
SGPT	> 5 × ULN[b]	6/217	3%	4/232	2%
Alk. Phos.	> 5 × ULN[b]	5/220	2%	5/218	2%

[(a)] Includes only patients with baseline values within the normal range or borderline high (hematology variables) and within the normal range or borderline low (chemistry variables).
[(b)] ULN = Upper Limit of Normal

Mean Reductions in Log CFU from Baseline (After 4 Weeks of Therapy)

500 mg b.i.d. (N=35)	1000 mg b.i.d. (N=32)	2000 mg b.i.d. (N=26)	Four Drug Regimen (N=24)
1.5	2.3	2.3	1.4

Compared to prior experience with clarithromycin monotherapy, the two-drug regimen of clarithromycin and ethambutol was well tolerated and extended the time to microbiologic relapse, largely through suppressing the emergence of clarithromycin resistant strains. However, the addition of clofazimine to the regimen added no additional microbiologic or clinical benefit. Tolerability of both multidrug regimens was comparable with the most common adverse events being gastrointestinal in nature. Patients receiving the clofazimine-containing regimen had reduced survival rates; however, their baseline mycobacterial colony counts were higher. The results of this trial support the addition of ethambutol to clarithromycin for the treatment of initial dMAC infections but do not support adding clofazimine as a third agent.

MAC bacteremia:
Decreases in MAC bacteremia or negative blood cultures were seen in the majority of patients in all dose groups. Mean reductions in colony forming units (CFU) are shown below. Included in the table are results from a separate study with a four drug regimen[5] (ciprofloxacin, ethambutol, rifampicin, and clofazimine). Since patient populations and study procedures may vary between these two studies, comparisons between the clarithromycin results and the combination therapy results should be interpreted cautiously.
[See fifth table above]
Although the 1000 mg and 2000 mg b.i.d. doses showed significantly better control of bacteremia during the first four weeks of therapy, no significant differences were seen beyond that point. The percent of patients whose blood was sterilized as shown by one or more negative cultures at any time during acute therapy was 61% (30/49) for the 500 mg b.i.d. group and 59% (29/49) and 52% (25/48) for the 1000 and 2000 mg b.i.d. groups, respectively. The percent of patients who had 2 or more negative cultures during acute therapy that were sustained through study Day 84 was 25% (12/49) in both the 500 and 1000 mg b.i.d. groups and 8% (4/48) for the 2000 mg b.i.d. group. By Day 84, 23% (11/49), 37% (18/49), and 56% (27/48) of patients had died or discontinued from the study, and 14% (7/49), 12% (6/49), and 13% (6/48) of patients had relapsed in the 500, 1000, and 2000 mg b.i.d. dose groups, respectively. All of the isolates had an MIC < 8 µg/mL at pre-treatment. Relapse was almost always accompanied by an increase in MIC. The median time to first negative culture was 54, 41, and 29 days for the 500, 1000, and 2000 mg b.i.d. groups, respectively. The time to first decrease of at least 1 log in CFU count was significantly shorter with the 1000 and 2000 mg b.i.d. doses (median equal to 16 and 15 days, respectively) in comparison to the 500 mg b.i.d. group (median equal to 29 days). The median time to first positive culture or study discontinuation following the first negative culture was 43, 59 and 43 days for the 500, 1000, and 2000 mg b.i.d. groups, respectively.

Clinically significant disseminated MAC Disease:
Among patients experiencing night sweats prior to therapy, 84% showed resolution or improvement at some point during the 12 weeks of clarithromycin at 500 to 2000 mg b.i.d. doses. Similarly, 77% of patients reported resolution or improvement in fevers at some point. Response rates for clinical signs of MAC are given below:
[See first table at top of next page]
The median duration of response, defined as improvement or resolution of clinical signs and symptoms, was 2 to 6 weeks.
Since the study was not designed to determine the benefit of monotherapy beyond 12 weeks, the duration of response may be underestimated for the 25 to 33% of patients who continued to show clinical response after 12 weeks.

Survival:
Median survival time from study entry (Study 500) was 249 days at the 500 mg b.i.d. dose compared to 215 days with

the 1000 mg b.i.d. dose. However, during the first 12 weeks of therapy, there were 2 deaths in 53 patients in the 500 mg b.i.d. group versus 13 deaths in 51 patients in the 1000 mg b.i.d. group. The reason for this apparent mortality difference is not known. Survival in the two groups was similar beyond 12 weeks. The median survival times for these dosages were similar to recent historical controls with MAC when treated with combination therapies.[5]

Median survival time from study entry in Study 577 was 199 days for the 500 mg b.i.d. dose and 179 days for the 1000 mg b.i.d. dose. During the first four weeks of therapy, while patients were maintained on their originally assigned dose, there were 11 deaths in 255 patients taking 500 mg b.i.d. and 18 deaths in 214 patients taking 1000 mg b.i.d.

Safety:

The adverse event profiles showed that both the 500 and 1000 mg b.i.d. doses were well tolerated. The 2000 mg b.i.d. dose was poorly tolerated and resulted in a higher proportion of premature discontinuations.

In AIDS patients and other immunocompromised patients treated with the higher doses of clarithromycin over long periods of time for mycobacterial infections, it was often difficult to distinguish adverse events possibly associated with clarithromycin administration from underlying signs of HIV disease or intercurrent illness.

The following analyses summarize experience during the first 12 weeks of therapy with clarithromycin. Data are reported separately for Study 500 (randomized, double-blind) and Study 577 (open-label, compassionate use) and also combined. Adverse events were reported less frequently in Study 577, which may be due in part to differences in monitoring between the two studies. In adult patients receiving clarithromycin 500 mg b.i.d., the most frequently reported adverse events, considered possibly or probably related to study drug, with an incidence of 5% or greater, are listed below. Most of these events were mild to moderate in severity, although 5% (Study 500: 8%; Study 577: 4%) of patients receiving 500 mg b.i.d. and 5% (Study 500: 4%; Study 577: 6%) of patients receiving 1000 mg b.i.d. reported severe adverse events. Excluding those patients who discontinued therapy or died due to complications of their underlying non-mycobacterial disease, approximately 8% (Study 500: 15%; Study 577: 7%) of the patients who received 500 mg b.i.d. and 12% (Study 500: 14%; Study 577: 12%) of the patients who received 1000 mg b.i.d. discontinued therapy due to drug-related events during the first 12 weeks of therapy. Overall, the 500 and 1000 mg b.i.d. doses had similar adverse event profiles.

[See second table above]

A limited number of pediatric AIDS patients have been treated with clarithromycin suspension for mycobacterial infections. The most frequently reported adverse events, excluding those due to the patient's concurrent condition, were consistent with those observed in adult patients.

Changes in Laboratory Values:

In immunocompromised patients treated with clarithromycin for mycobacterial infections, evaluations of laboratory values were made by analyzing those values outside the seriously abnormal level (i.e., the extreme high or low limit) for the specified test.

[See third table above]

Otitis Media

In a controlled clinical study of acute otitis media performed in the United States, where significant rates of beta-lactamase producing organisms were found, clarithromycin was compared to an oral cephalosporin. In this study, very strict evaluability criteria were used to determine clinical response. For the 223 patients who were evaluated for clinical efficacy, the clinical success rate (i.e., cure plus improvement) at the post-therapy visit was 88% for clarithromycin and 91% for the cephalosporin.

In a smaller number of patients, microbiologic determinations were made at the pre-treatment visit. The following presumptive bacterial eradication/clinical cure outcomes (i.e., clinical success) were obtained:

U.S. Acute Otitis Media Study Clarithromycin vs. Oral Cephalosporin EFFICACY RESULTS

PATHOGEN	OUTCOME
S. pneumoniae	clarithromycin success rate, 13/15 (87%), control 4/5
*H. influenzae**	clarithromycin success rate, 10/14 (71%), control 3/4
M. catarrhalis	clarithromycin success rate, 4/5, control 1/1
S. pyogenes	clarithromycin success rate, 3/3, control 0/1
Overall	clarithromycin success rate, 30/37 (81%), control 8/11 (73%)

*None of the *H. influenzae* isolated pre-treatment was resistant to clarithromycin; 6% were resistant to the control agent.

Safety:

The incidence of adverse events in all patients treated, primarily diarrhea and vomiting, did not differ clinically or statistically for the two agents.

In two other controlled clinical trials of acute otitis media performed in the United States, where significant rates of beta-lactamase producing organisms were found, clarithromycin was compared to an oral antimicrobial agent that contained a specific beta-lactamase inhibitor. In these studies, very strict evaluability criteria were used to determine the clinical responses. In the 233 patients who were evaluated for clinical efficacy, the combined clinical success rate (i.e., cure and improvement) at the post-therapy visit was 91% for both clarithromycin and the control.

For the patients who had microbiologic determinations at the pre-treatment visit, the following presumptive bacterial eradication/clinical cure outcomes (i.e., clinical success) were obtained:

Two U.S. Acute Otitis Media Studies Clarithromycin vs. Antimicrobial/Beta-lactamase Inhibitor EFFICACY RESULTS

PATHOGEN	OUTCOME
S. pneumoniae	clarithromycin success rate, 43/51 (84%), control 55/56 (98%)
*H. influenzae**	clarithromycin success rate, 36/45 (80%), control 31/33 (94%)
M. catarrhalis	clarithromycin success rate, 9/10 (90%), control 6/6
S. pyogenes	clarithromycin success rate, 3/3, control 5/5
Overall	clarithromycin success rate, 91/109 (83%), control 97/100 (97%)

* Of the *H. influenzae* isolated pre-treatment, 3% were resistant to clarithromycin and 10% were resistant to the control agent.

Safety:

The incidence of adverse events in all patients treated, primarily diarrhea (15% vs. 38%) and diaper rash (3% vs. 11%) in young children, was clinically and statistically lower in the clarithromycin arm versus the control arm.

Duodenal Ulcer Associated with *H. pylori* Infection

Clarithromycin + Lansoprazole and Amoxicillin

H. pylori Eradication for Reducing the Risk of Duodenal Ulcer Recurrence:

Two U.S. randomized, double-blind clinical studies in patients with *H. pylori* and duodenal ulcer disease (defined as an active ulcer or history of an active ulcer within one year) evaluated the efficacy of clarithromycin in combination with lansoprazole and amoxicillin capsules as triple 14-day therapy for eradication of *H. pylori*. Based on the results of these studies, the safety and efficacy of the following eradication regimen were established:

Triple therapy: BIAXIN 500 mg b.i.d. + lansoprazole 30 mg b.i.d. + amoxicillin 1 gm b.i.d.

Treatment was for 14 days. *H. pylori* eradication was defined as two negative tests (culture and histology) at 4 to 6 weeks following the end of treatment.

The combination of BIAXIN (clarithromycin) plus lansoprazole and amoxicillin as triple therapy was effective in eradicating *H. pylori*. Eradication of *H. pylori* has been shown to reduce the risk of duodenal ulcer recurrence.

A randomized, double-blind clinical study performed in the U.S. in patients with *H. pylori* and duodenal ulcer disease (defined as an active ulcer or history of an ulcer within one year) compared the efficacy of clarithromycin in combination with lansoprazole and amoxicillin as triple therapy for 10 and 14 days. This study established that the 10-day triple therapy was equivalent to the 14-day triple therapy in eradicating *H. pylori*.

[See first table at top of next page]

Clarithromycin + Omeprazole and Amoxicillin Therapy

H. pylori Eradication for Reducing the Risk of Duodenal Ulcer Recurrence:

Three U.S., randomized, double-blind clinical studies in patients with *H. pylori* infection and duodenal ulcer disease (n = 558) compared clarithromycin plus omeprazole and amoxicillin to clarithromycin plus amoxicillin. Two studies (Studies 126 and 127) were conducted in patients with an active duodenal ulcer, and the third study (Study 446) was conducted in patients with a duodenal ulcer in the past 5 years, but without an ulcer present at the time of enrollment. The dosage regimen in the studies was clarithromycin 500 mg b.i.d. plus omeprazole 20 mg b.i.d. plus amoxicillin 1 gram b.i.d. for 10 days. In Studies 126 and 127, patients who took the omeprazole regimen also received an additional 18 days of omeprazole 20 mg q.d. Endpoints studied were eradication of *H. pylori* and duodenal ulcer healing (studies 126 and 127 only). *H. pylori* status was determined by CLOtest®, histology, and culture in all three studies. For a given patient, *H. pylori* was considered eradicated if at least two of these tests were negative, and none was positive. The combination of clarithromycin plus omeprazole and amoxicillin was effective in eradicating *H. pylori*.

Resolution of Fever / **Resolution of Night Sweats**

b.i.d. dose (mg)	% ever afebrile	% afebrile ≥6 weeks	b.i.d. dose (mg)	% ever resolving	% resolving ≥6 weeks
500	67%	23%	500	85%	42%
1000	67%	12%	1000	70%	33%
2000	62%	22%	2000	72%	36%

Weight Gain >3% / **Hemoglobin Increase >1 gm**

b.i.d. dose (mg)	% ever gaining	% gaining ≥6 weeks	b.i.d. dose (mg)	% ever increasing	% increasing ≥6 weeks
500	33%	14%	500	58%	26%
1000	26%	17%	1000	37%	6%
2000	26%	12%	2000	62%	18%

Treatment-related* Adverse Event Incidence Rates (%) in Immunocompromised Adult Patients During the First 12 Weeks of Therapy with 500 mg b.i.d. Clarithromycin Dose

Adverse Event	Study 500 (n=53)	Study 577 (n=255)	Combined (n=308)
Abdominal Pain	7.5	2.4	3.2
Diarrhea	9.4	1.6	2.9
Flatulence	7.5	0.0	1.3
Headache	7.5	0.4	1.6
Nausea	28.3	9.0	12.3
Rash	9.4	2.0	3.2
Taste Perversion	18.9	0.4	3.6
Vomiting	24.5	3.9	7.5

* Includes those events possibly or probably related to study drug and excludes concurrent conditions.

Percentage of Patients[a] Exceeding Extreme Laboratory Value Limits During First 12 Weeks of Treatment 500 mg b.i.d. Dose[b]

		Study 500	Study 577	Combined
BUN	>50 mg/dL	0%	<1%	<1%
Platelet Count	<50 × 10^9/L	0%	<1%	<1%
SGOT	>5 × ULN[c]	0%	3%	2%
SGPT	>5 × ULN[c]	0%	2%	1%
WBC	<1 × 10^9/L	0%	1%	1%

[a] Includes only patients with baseline values within the normal range or borderline high (hematology variables) and within the normal range or borderline low (chemistry variables)

[b] Includes all values within the first 12 weeks for patients who start on 500 mg b.i.d.

[c] ULN = Upper Limit of Normal

Continued on next page

Biaxin—Cont.

[See second table at right]

Safety:

In clinical trials using combination therapy with clarithromycin plus omeprazole and amoxicillin, no adverse reactions peculiar to the combination of these drugs have been observed. Adverse reactions that have occurred have been limited to those that have been previously reported with clarithromycin, omeprazole, or amoxicillin.

The most frequent adverse experiences observed in clinical trials using combination therapy with clarithromycin plus omeprazole and amoxicillin (n=274) were diarrhea (14%), taste perversion (10%), and headache (7%).

For information about adverse reactions with omeprazole or amoxicillin, refer to the ADVERSE REACTIONS section of their package inserts.

Clarithromycin + Omeprazole Therapy

Four randomized, double-blind, multi-center studies (067, 100, 812b, and 058) evaluated clarithromycin 500 mg t.i.d. plus omeprazole 40 mg q.d. for 14 days, followed by omeprazole 20 mg q.d. (067, 100, and 058) or by omeprazole 40 mg q.d. (812b) for an additional 14 days in patients with active duodenal ulcer associated with *H. pylori*. Studies 067 and 100 were conducted in the U.S. and Canada and enrolled 242 and 256 patients, respectively. *H. pylori* infection and duodenal ulcer were confirmed in 219 patients in Study 067 and 228 patients in Study 100. These studies compared the combination regimen to omeprazole and clarithromycin monotherapies. Studies 812b and 058 were conducted in Europe and enrolled 154 and 215 patients, respectively. *H. pylori* infection and duodenal ulcer were confirmed in 148 patients in Study 812b and 208 patients in Study 058. These studies compared the combination regimen to omeprazole monotherapy. The results for the efficacy analyses for these studies are described below.

Duodenal Ulcer Healing:

The combination of clarithromycin and omeprazole was as effective as omeprazole alone for healing duodenal ulcer.

[See third table at right]

Eradication of H. pylori Associated with Duodenal Ulcer:

The combination of clarithromycin and omeprazole was effective in eradicating *H. pylori.*

[See fourth table at right]

H. pylori eradication was defined as no positive test (culture or histology) at 4 weeks following the end of treatment, and two negative tests were required to be considered eradicated. In the per-protocol analysis, the following patients were excluded: dropouts, patients with major protocol violations, patients with missing *H. pylori* tests post-treatment, and patients that were not assessed for *H. pylori* eradication at 4 weeks after the end of treatment because they were found to have an unhealed ulcer at the end of treatment.

Ulcer recurrence at 6-months following the end of treatment was assessed for patients in whom ulcers were healed post-treatment.

[See first table at top of next page]

Thus, in patients with duodenal ulcer associated with *H. pylori* infection, eradication of *H. pylori* reduced ulcer recurrence.

Safety:

The adverse event profiles for the four studies showed that the combination of clarithromycin 500 mg t.i.d. and omeprazole 40 mg q.d. for 14 days, followed by omeprazole 20 mg q.d. (067, 100, and 058) or 40 mg q.d. (812b) for an additional 14 days was well tolerated. Of the 346 patients who received the combination, 12 (3.5%) patients discontinued study drug due to adverse events.

[See second table at top of next page]

Most of these events were mild to moderate in severity.

Changes in Laboratory Values:

Changes in laboratory values with possible clinical significance in patients taking clarithromycin and omeprazole were as follows:

Hepatic - elevated direct bilirubin <1%; GGT <1%; SGOT (AST) <1%; SGPT (ALT) <1%,

Renal - elevated serum creatinine <1%.

For information on omeprazole, refer to the ADVERSE REACTIONS section of the PRILOSEC package insert.

Clarithromycin + Ranitidine Bismuth Citrate Therapy

In a U.S. double-blind, randomized, multicenter, dose-comparison trial, ranitidine bismuth citrate 400 mg b.i.d. for 4 weeks plus clarithromycin 500 mg b.i.d. for the first 2 weeks was found to have an equivalent *H. pylori* eradication rate (based on culture and histology) when compared to ranitidine bismuth citrate 400 mg b.i.d. for 4 weeks plus clarithromycin 500 mg t.i.d. for the first 2 weeks. The intent-to-treat *H. pylori* eradication rates are shown below:

[See third table on next page]

H. pylori eradication was defined as no positive test at 4 weeks following the end of treatment. Patients must have had two tests performed, and these must have been negative to be considered eradicated of *H. pylori.* The following patients were excluded from the per-protocol analysis: patients not infected with *H. pylori* prestudy, dropouts, patients with major protocol violations, patients with missing *H. pylori* tests. Patients excluded from the intent-to-treat analysis included those not infected with *H. pylori* prestudy and those with missing *H. pylori* tests prestudy. Patients were assessed for *H. pylori* eradication (4 weeks following treatment) regardless of their healing status (at the end of treatment).

H. pylori Eradication Rates-Triple Therapy (BIAXIN/lansoprazole/amoxicillin)
Percent of Patients Cured [95% Confidence Interval]
(number of patients)

Study	Duration	Triple Therapy Evaluable Analysis*	Triple Therapy Intent-to-Treat Analysis#
M93-131	14 days	92† [80.0 - 97.7] (n = 48)	86† [73.3 - 93.5] (n = 55)
M95-392	14 days	86‡ [75.7 - 93.6] (n = 66)	83‡ [72.0 - 90.8] (n = 70)
M95-399¶	14 days	85 [77.0 - 91.0] (N = 113)	82 [73.9 - 88.1] (N = 126)
	10 days	84 [76.0 - 89.8] (N = 123)	81 [73.9 - 87.6] (N = 135)

* Based on evaluable patients with confirmed duodenal ulcer (active or within one year) and *H. pylori* infection at baseline defined as at least two of three positive endoscopic tests from CLOtest (Delta West LTD., Bentley, Australia), histology, and/or culture. Patients were included in the analysis if they completed the study. Additionally, if patients were dropped out of the study due to an adverse event related to the study drug, they were included in the analysis as evaluable failures of therapy.

\# Patients were included in the analysis if they had documented *H. pylori* infection at baseline as defined above and had a confirmed duodenal ulcer (active or within one year). All dropouts were included as failures of therapy.

† ($p<0.05$) versus BIAXIN/lansoprazole and lansoprazole/amoxicillin dual therapy.

‡ ($p<0.05$) versus BIAXIN/amoxicillin dual therapy.

¶ The 95% confidence interval for the difference in eradication rates, 10-day minus 14-day, is (-10.5, 8.1) in the evaluable analysis and (-9.7, 9.1) in the intent-to-treat analysis.

Per-Protocol and Intent-To-Treat H. pylori Eradication Rates
% of Patients Cured [95% Confidence Interval]

	Clarithromycin + omeprazole + amoxicillin		Clarithromycin + amoxicillin	
	Per-Protocol†	Intent-To-Treat‡	Per-Protocol†	Intent-To-Treat‡
Study 126	*77 [64, 86] (n = 64)	69 [57, 79] (n = 80)	43 [31, 56] (n = 67)	37 [27, 48] (n = 84)
Study 127	*78 [67, 88] (n = 65)	73 [61, 82] (n = 77)	41 [29, 54] (n = 68)	36 [26, 47] (n = 84)
Study M96-446	*90 [80, 96] (n = 69)	83 [74, 91] (n = 84)	32 [24, 44] (n = 93)	32 [23, 42] (n = 99)

† Patients were included in the analysis if they had confirmed duodenal ulcer disease (active ulcer studies 126 and 127; history of ulcer within 5 years, study M96-446) and *H. pylori* infection at baseline defined as at least two of three positive endoscopic tests from CLOtest®, histology, and/or culture. Patients were included in the analysis if they completed the study. Additionally, if patients dropped out of the study due to an adverse event related to the study drug, they were included in the analysis as failures of therapy. The impact of eradication on ulcer recurrence has not been assessed in patients with a past history of ulcer.

‡ Patients were included in the analysis if they had documented *H. pylori* infection at baseline and had confirmed duodenal ulcer disease. All dropouts were included as failures of therapy.

* $p < 0.05$ versus clarithromycin plus amoxicillin.

End-of-Treatment Ulcer Healing Rates
Percent of Patients Healed (n/N)

Study	Clarithromycin + Omeprazole	Omeprazole	Clarithromycin
U.S. Studies			
Study 100	94% (58/62)†	88% (60/68)	71% (49/69)
Study 067	88% (56/64)†	85% (55/65)	64% (44/69)
Non-U.S. Studies			
Study 058	99% (84/85)	95% (82/86)	N/A
Study 812b[1]	100% (64/64)	99% (71/72)	N/A

† $p<0.05$ for clarithromycin + omeprazole versus clarithromycin monotherapy.

[1] In Study 812b patients received omeprazole 40 mg daily for days 15 to 28.

H. pylori Eradication Rates (Per-Protocol Analysis) at 4 to 6 weeks
Percent of Patients Cured (n/N)

Study	Clarithromycin + Omeprazole	Omeprazole	Clarithromycin
U.S. Studies			
Study 100	64% (39/61)†‡	0% (0/59)	39% (17/44)
Study 067	74% (39/53)†‡	0% (0/54)	31% (13/42)
Non-U.S. Studies			
Study 058	74% (64/86)‡	1% (1/90)	N/A
Study 812b	83% (50/60)‡	1% (1/74)	N/A

† Statistically significantly higher than clarithromycin monotherapy ($p<0.05$).

‡ Statistically significantly higher than omeprazole monotherapy ($p<0.05$).

The relationship between *H. pylori* eradication and duodenal ulcer recurrence was assessed in a combined analysis of six U.S. randomized, double-blind, multicenter, placebo-controlled trials using ranitidine bismuth citrate with or without antibiotics. The results from approximately 650 U.S. patients showed that the risk of ulcer recurrence within 6 months of completing treatment was two times less likely in patients whose *H. pylori* infection was eradicated compared to patients in whom *H. pylori* infection was not eradicated.

Safety:

In clinical trials using combination therapy with clarithromycin plus ranitidine bismuth citrate, no adverse reactions peculiar to the combination of these drugs (using clarithromycin twice daily or three times a day) were observed. Adverse reactions that have occurred have been limited to those reported with clarithromycin or ranitidine bismuth citrate. (See **ADVERSE REACTIONS** section of the Tritec package insert.) The most frequent adverse experiences observed in clinical trials using combination therapy

Ulcer Recurrence at 6 months by *H. pylori* Status at 4-6 Weeks

	H. pylori Negative	*H. pylori* Positive
U.S. Studies		
Study 100		
Clarithromycin + Omeprazole	6% (2/34)	56% (9/16)
Omeprazole	- (0/0)	71% (35/49)
Clarithromycin	12% (2/17)	32% (7/22)
Study 067		
Clarithromycin + Omeprazole	38% (11/29)	50% (6/12)
Omeprazole	- (0/0)	67% (31/46)
Clarithromycin	18% (2/11)	52% (14/27)
Non-U.S.Studies		
Study 058		
Clarithromycin + Omeprazole	6% (3/53)	24% (4/17)
Omeprazole	0% (0/3)	55% (39/71)
Study 812b*		
Clarithromycin + Omeprazole	5% (2/42)	0% (0/7)
Omeprazole	0% (0/1)	54% (32/59)
***12-month recurrence rates:**		
Clarithromycin + Omeprazole	3% (1/40)	0% (0/6)
Omeprazole	0% (0/1)	67% (29/43)

Adverse Events with an Incidence of 3% or Greater

Adverse Event	Clarithromycin + Omeprazole (N = 346) % of Patients	Omeprazole (N = 355) % of Patients	Clarithromycin (N = 166) % of Patients*
Taste Perversion	15%	1%	16%
Nausea	5%	1%	3%
Headache	5%	6%	9%
Diarrhea	4%	3%	7%
Vomiting	4%	<1%	1%
Abdominal Pain	3%	2%	1%
Infection	3%	4%	2%

* Studies 067 and 100, only

H. pylori Eradication Rates in Study H2BA-3001

Analysis	RBC 400 mg + Clarithromycin 500 mg b.i.d.	RBC 400 mg + Clarithromycin 500 mg t.i.d.	95% CI Rate Difference
ITT	65% (122/188) [58%, 72%]	63% (122/195) [55%, 69%]	(-8%, 12%)
Per-Protocol	72% (117/162) [65%, 79%]	71% (120/170) [63%,77%]	(-9%, 12%)

with clarithromycin (500 mg three times a day) with ranitidine bismuth citrate (n = 329) were taste disturbance (11%), diarrhea (5%), nausea and vomiting (3%). The most frequent adverse experiences observed in clinical trials using combination therapy with clarithromycin (500 mg twice daily) with ranitidine bismuth citrate (n = 196) were taste disturbance (8%), nausea and vomiting (5%), and diarrhea (4%).

ANIMAL PHARMACOLOGY AND TOXICOLOGY

Clarithromycin is rapidly and well-absorbed with dose-linear kinetics, low protein binding, and a high volume of distribution. Plasma half-life ranged from 1 to 6 hours and was species dependent. High tissue concentrations were achieved, but negligible accumulation was observed. Fecal clearance predominated. Hepatotoxicity occurred in all species tested (i.e., in rats and monkeys at doses 2 times greater than and in dogs at doses comparable to the maximum human daily dose, based on mg/m^2). Renal tubular degeneration (calculated on a mg/m^2 basis) occurred in rats at doses 2 times, in monkeys at doses 8 times, and in dogs at doses 12 times greater than the maximum human daily dose. Testicular atrophy (on a mg/m^2 basis) occurred in rats at doses 7 times, in dogs at doses 3 times, and in monkeys at doses 8 times greater than the maximum human daily dose. Corneal opacity (on a mg/m^2 basis) occurred in dogs at doses 12 times and in monkeys at doses 8 times greater than the maximum human daily dose. Lymphoid depletion (on a mg/m^2 basis) occurred in dogs at doses 3 times greater than and in monkeys at doses 2 times greater than the maximum human daily dose. These adverse events were absent during clinical trials.

REFERENCES

1. National Committee for Clinical Laboratory Standards, Methods for Dilution Antimicrobial Susceptibility Tests for Bacteria that Grow Aerobically - Fourth Edition. Approved Standard NCCLS Document M7-A4, Vol. 17, No. 2, NCCLS, Wayne, PA, January, 1997.
2. National Committee for Clinical Laboratory Standards, Performance Standards for Antimicrobial Disk Susceptibility Tests - Sixth Edition. Approved Standard NCCLS Document M2-A6, Vol. 17, No. 1, NCCLS, Wayne, PA, January, 1997.
3. National Committee for Clinical Laboratory Standards. Summary Minutes, Subcommittee on Antimicrobial Susceptibility Testing, Tampa, FL. January 11-13, 1998.
4. Chaisson RE, et al. Clarithromycin and Ethambutol with or without Clofazimine for the Treatment of Bacteremic *Mycobacterium avium* Complex Disease in Patients with HIV Infection. *AIDS*. 1997;11:311-317.
5. Kemper CA, et al. Treatment of *Mycobacterium avium* Complex Bacteremia in AIDS with a Four-Drug Oral Regimen. *Ann Intern Med*. 1992;116:466-472.

Filmtab - Film-sealed tablets, Abbott

Ref.: 03-5328-R26 Revised December, 2003

Shown in Product Identification Guide, page 303

CALCIJEX® ℞

Calcitriol Injection
1 mcg/mL
℞ only

DESCRIPTION

Calcijex® (calcitriol injection) is synthetically manufactured calcitriol and is available as a sterile, isotonic, clear, colorless to yellow, aqueous solution for intravenous injection. Calcijex® is available in 1 mL ampuls. Each 1 mL contains calcitriol, 1 mcg; Polysorbate 20, 4 mg; sodium ascorbate 2.5 mg added. May contain hydrochloric acid and/or sodium hydroxide for pH adjustment. pH is 6.5 (5.9 to 7.0). Contains no more than 1 mcg/mL of aluminum.

Calcitriol is a crystalline compound which occurs naturally in humans. It is soluble in organic solvents but relatively insoluble in water.

Calcitriol is chemically designated (5Z,7E)-9, 10-secocholesta-5,7,10(19)-triene-1α,3β,25-triol and has the following structural formula:

Molecular Formula: $C_{27}H_{44}O_3$

The other names frequently used for calcitriol are 1α,25-dihydroxycholecalciferol, 1α,25-dihydroxyvitamin D_3, 1,25-DHCC, 1,25$(OH)_2D_3$ and 1,25-diOHC.

CLINICAL PHARMACOLOGY

Calcitriol is the active form of vitamin D_3 (cholecalciferol). The natural or endogenous supply of vitamin D in man mainly depends on ultraviolet light for conversion of 7-dehydrocholesterol to vitamin D_3 in the skin. Vitamin D_3 must be metabolically activated in the liver and the kidney before it is fully active on its target tissues. The initial transformation is catalyzed by a vitamin D_3-25-hydroxylase enzyme present in the liver, and the product of this reaction is 25-$(OH)D_3$ (calcifediol). The latter undergoes hydroxylation in the mitochondria of kidney tissue, and this reaction is activated by the renal 25-hydroxyvitamin D_3-1-α-hydroxylase to produce 1,25-$(OH)_2D_3$ (calcitriol), the active form of vitamin D_3.

The known sites of action of calcitriol are intestine, bone, kidney and parathyroid gland. Calcitriol is the most active known form of vitamin D_3 in stimulating intestinal calcium transport. In acutely uremic rats, calcitriol has been shown to stimulate intestinal calcium absorption. In bone, calcitriol, in conjunction with parathyroid hormone, stimulates resorption of calcium; and in the kidney, calcitriol increases the tubular reabsorption of calcium. *In vitro* and *in vivo* studies have shown that calcitriol directly suppresses secretion and synthesis of PTH. A vitamin D-resistant state may exist in uremic patients because of the failure of the kidney to adequately convert precursors to the active compound, calcitriol.

Calcitriol when administered by bolus injection is rapidly available in the blood stream. Vitamin D metabolites are known to be transported in blood, bound to specific plasma proteins. The pharmacologic activity of an administered dose of calcitriol is about 3 to 5 days. Two metabolic pathways for calcitriol have been identified, conversion to 1,24,25-$(OH)_3D_3$ and to calcitroic acid.

INDICATIONS AND USAGE

Calcijex® (calcitriol injection) is indicated in the management of hypocalcemia in patients undergoing chronic renal dialysis. It has been shown to significantly reduce elevated parathyroid hormone levels. Reduction of PTH has been shown to result in an improvement in renal osteodystrophy.

CONTRAINDICATIONS

Calcijex® (calcitriol injection) should not be given to patients with hypercalcemia or evidence of vitamin D toxicity.

WARNINGS

Since calcitriol is the most potent metabolite of vitamin D available, vitamin D and its derivatives should be withheld during treatment.

A non-aluminum phosphate-binding compound should be used to control serum phosphorus levels in patients undergoing dialysis.

Overdosage of any form of vitamin D is dangerous (see also **OVERDOSAGE**). Progressive hypercalcemia due to overdosage of vitamin D and its metabolites may be so severe as to require emergency attention. Chronic hypercalcemia can lead to generalized vascular calcification, nephrocalcinosis and other soft-tissue calcification. The serum calcium times phosphate (Ca × P) product should not be allowed to exceed 70. Radiographic evaluation of suspect anatomical regions may be useful in the early detection of this condition.

PRECAUTIONS

1. General

Excessive dosage of Calcijex® (calcitriol injection) induces hypercalcemia and in some instances hypercalciuria; therefore, early in treatment during dosage adjustment, serum calcium and phosphorus should be determined at least twice weekly. Should hypercalcemia develop, the drug should be discontinued immediately.

Calcijex® should be given cautiously to patients on digitalis, because hypercalcemia in such patients may precipitate cardiac arrhythmias.

2. Information for the Patient

The patient and his or her parents should be informed about adherence to instructions about diet and calcium supplementation and avoidance of the use of unapproved non-prescription drugs, including magnesium-containing antacids. Patients should also be carefully informed about the symptoms of hypercalcemia (see **ADVERSE REACTIONS**).

3. Essential Laboratory Tests

Serum calcium, phosphorus, magnesium and alkaline phosphatase and 24-hour urinary calcium and phosphorus should be determined periodically. During the initial phase of the medication, serum calcium and phosphorus should be determined more frequently (twice weekly).

Adynamic bone disease may develop if PTH levels are suppressed to abnormal levels. If biopsy is not being done for other (diagnostic) reasons, PTH levels may be used to indicate the rate of bone turnover. If PTH levels fall below recommended target range (1.5 to 3 times the upper limit of normal), in patients treated with Calcijex®, the Calcijex® dose should be reduced or therapy discontinued. Discontinuation of Calcijex® therapy may result in rebound effect, therefore, appropriate titration downward to a maintenance dose is recommended.

Continued on next page

Calcijex—Cont.

4. Drug Interactions
Magnesium-containing antacid and Calcijex® should not be used concomitantly, because such use may lead to the development of hypermagnesemia.

5. Carcinogenesis, Mutagenesis, Impairment of Fertility
Long-term studies in animals have not been conducted to evaluate the carcinogenic potential of Calcijex® (calcitriol injection). Calcitriol was not mutagenic *in vitro* in the Ames Test nor was oral calcitriol genotoxic *in vivo* in the Mouse Micronucleus Test. No significant effects on fertility and/or general reproductive performances were observed in a Segment I study in rats using oral calcitriol at doses of up to 0.3 mcg/kg.

6. Pregnancy: *Teratogenic Effects: Pregnancy Category C:* Calcitriol has been found to be teratogenic in rabbits when given orally at doses of 0.08 and 0.3 mcg/kg. All 15 fetuses in 3 litters at these doses showed external and skeletal abnormalities. However, none of the other 23 litters (156 fetuses) showed external and skeletal abnormalities compared with controls. Teratogenicity studies in rats at doses up to 0.45 mcg/kg orally showed no evidence of teratogenic potential. There are no adequate and well-controlled studies in pregnant women. Calcijex® should be used during pregnancy only if the potential benefit justifies the potential risk to the fetus.
Nonteratogenic Effects: In the rabbit, oral dosages of 0.3 mcg/kg/day administered on days 7 to 18 of gestation resulted in 19% maternal mortality, a decrease in mean fetal body weight and a reduced number of newborns surviving to 24 hours. A study of the effects on orally administered calcitriol on peri-and postnatal development in rats resulted in hypercalcemia in the offspring of dams given calcitriol at doses of 0.08 or 0.3 mcg/kg/day, hypercalcemia and hypophosphatemia in dams given calcitriol at a dose of 0.08 or 0.3 mcg/kg/day and increased serum urea nitrogen in dams given calcitriol at a dose of 0.3 mcg/kg/day. In another study in rats, maternal weight gain was slightly reduced at an oral dose of 0.3 mcg/kg/day administered on days 7 to 15 of gestation.
The offspring of a woman administered oral calcitriol at 17 to 36 mcg/day during pregnancy manifested mild hypercalcemia in the first 2 days of life which returned to normal at day 3.

7. Nursing Mothers
It is not known whether this drug is excreted in human milk. Because many drugs are excreted in human milk and because of the potential for serious adverse reactions in nursing infants from calcitriol, a decision should be made whether to discontinue nursing or to discontinue the drug, taking into account the importance of the drug to the mother.

8. Pediatric Use
The safety and effectiveness of Calcijex® were examined in a 12-week randomized, double-blind, placebo-controlled study of 35 pediatric patients, aged 13–18 years, with end-stage renal disease on hemodialysis. Sixty-six percent of the patients were male, 57% were African-American, and nearly all had received some form of vitamin D therapy prior to the study. The initial dose of Calcijex® was 0.5 mcg, 1.0 mcg, or 1.5 mcg, 3 times per week, based on baseline iPTH level of less than 500 pg/mL, 500–1000 pg/mL, or greater than 1000 pg/mL, respectively. The dose of Calcijex® was adjusted in 0.25 mcg increments based on the levels of serum iPTH, calcium, and Ca × P. The mean baseline levels of iPTH were 769 pg/mL for the 16 Calcijex®-treated patients and 897 pg/mL for the 19 placebo-treated subjects. The mean weekly dose of Calcijex® ranged from 1.0 mcg to 1.4 mcg. In the primary efficacy analysis, 7 of 16 (44%) subjects in the Calcijex® group had 2 consecutive 30% decreases from baseline iPTH compared with 3 of 19 (16%) patients in the placebo group (95% Cl for the difference between groups -6%, 62%). One Calcijex®-treated patient experienced transient hypercalcemia (>11.0 mg/dL), while 6 of 16 (38%) Calcijex®-treated patients vs. 2 of 19 (11%) placebo-treated patients experienced Ca × P >75.

9. Geriatric Use
Clinical studies of Calcijex® did not include sufficient numbers of subjects aged 65 and over to determine whether they respond differently from younger subjects. Other reported clinical experience has not identified differences in responses between the elderly and younger patients. In general, dose selection for an elderly patient should be cautious, usually starting at the low end of the dosage range, reflecting the greater frequency of decreased hepatic, renal, or cardiac function, and of concomitant disease or other drug therapy.

ADVERSE REACTIONS

Adverse effects of Calcijex® (calcitriol injection) are, in general, similar to those encountered with excessive vitamin D intake. The early and late signs and symptoms of vitamin D intoxication associated with hypercalcemia include:

1. Early
Weakness, headache, somnolence, nausea, vomiting, dry mouth, constipation, muscle pain, bone pain and metallic taste.

2. Late
Polyuria, polydipsia, anorexia, weight loss, nocturia, conjunctivitis (calcific), pancreatitis, photophobia, rhinorrhea, pruritus, hyperthermia, decreased libido, elevated BUN, albuminuria, hypercholesterolemia, elevated SGOT and SGPT, ectopic calcification, hypertension, cardiac arrhythmias and, rarely, overt psychosis.
Occasional mild pain on injection has been observed.

OVERDOSAGE

Administration of Calcijex® (calcitriol injection) to patients in excess of their requirements can cause hypercalcemia, hypercalciuria and hyperphosphatemia. High intake of calcium and phosphate concomitant with Calcijex® may lead to similar abnormalities.

1. Treatment of Hypercalcemia and Overdosage in Patients on Hemodialysis
General treatment of hypercalcemia (greater than 1 mg/dL above the upper limit of normal range) consists of immediate discontinuation of Calcijex® therapy, institution of a low calcium diet and withdrawal of calcium supplements. Serum calcium levels should be determined daily until normocalcemia ensues. Hypercalcemia usually resolves in two to seven days. When serum calcium levels have returned to within normal limits, Calcijex® therapy may be reinstituted at a dose 0.5 mcg less than prior therapy. Serum calcium levels should be obtained at least twice weekly after all dosage changes.
Persistent or markedly elevated serum calcium levels may be corrected by dialysis against a calcium-free dialysate.

2. Treatment of Accidental Overdosage of Calcitriol Injection
The treatment of acute accidental overdosage of Calcijex® should consist of general supportive measures. Serial serum electrolyte determinations (especially calcium), rate of urinary calcium excretion and assessment of electrocardiographic abnormalities due to hypercalcemia should be obtained. Such monitoring is critical in patients receiving digitalis. Discontinuation of supplemental calcium and low calcium diet are also indicated in accidental overdosage. Due to the relatively short duration of the pharmacological action of calcitriol, further measures are probably unnecessary. Should, however, persistent and markedly elevated serum calcium levels occur, there are a variety of therapeutic alternatives which may be considered, depending on the patients' underlying condition. These include the use of drugs such as phosphates and corticosteroids as well as measures to induce an appropriate forced diuresis. The use of peritoneal dialysis against a calcium-free dialysate has also been reported.

DOSAGE AND ADMINISTRATION

The optimal dose of Calcijex® (calcitriol injection) must be carefully determined for each patient.
The effectiveness of Calcijex® therapy is predicated on the assumption that each patient is receiving an adequate and appropriate daily intake of calcium. The RDA for calcium in adults is 800 mg. To ensure that each patient receives an adequate daily intake of calcium, the physician should either prescribe a calcium supplement or instruct the patient in proper dietary measures.
The recommended initial dose of Calcijex®, depending on the severity of the hypocalcemia and/or secondary hyperparathyroidism, is 1 mcg (0.02 mcg/kg) to 2 mcg administered three times weekly, approximately every other day. Doses as small as 0.5 mcg and as large as 4 mcg three times weekly have been used as an initial dose. If a satisfactory response is not observed, the dose may be increased by 0.5 to 1 mcg at two to four week intervals. During this titration period, serum calcium and phosphorus levels should be obtained at least twice weekly. If hypercalcemia or a serum calcium times phosphate product greater than 70 is noted, the drug should be immediately discontinued until these parameters are appropriate. Then, the Calcijex® dose should be reinitiated at a lower dose. Doses may need to be reduced as the PTH levels decrease in response to the therapy. Thus, incremental dosing must be individualized and commensurate with PTH, serum calcium and phosphorus levels. The following is a suggested approach in dose titration:

PTH Levels	Calcijex® Dose
the same or increasing	increase
decreasing by <30%	increase
decreasing by > 30%, < 60%	maintain
decreasing by > 60%	decrease
one and one-half to three times the upper limit of normal	maintain

Parenteral drug products should be inspected visually for particulate matter and discoloration prior to administration, whenever solution and container permit.
Discard unused portion.

HOW SUPPLIED

Calcijex® (calcitriol injection) is supplied as follows:

List	Container	Concentration	Fill
8110	Ampul	1 mcg/mL	1 mL

Protect from light.

Store at controlled room temperature 15° to 30°C (59° to 86°F).
Patent Pending.
Ref. 58-6661-R5-Rev. November, 2001

ABBOTT LABORATORIES, NORTH CHICAGO, IL 60064 USA

CYLERT® Ⓒ ℞

[cī'lert]
(Pemoline)
℞ only

CYLERT SHOULD NOT BE USED BY PATIENTS UNTIL THERE HAS BEEN A COMPLETE DISCUSSION OF THE RISKS AND BENEFITS OF CYLERT THERAPY AND WRITTEN INFORMED CONSENT HAS BEEN OBTAINED (SEE **PATIENT INFORMATION/CONSENT FORM**). A SUPPLY OF PATIENT INFORMATION/CONSENT FORMS AS PRINTED AT THE END OF THIS INSERT IS AVAILABLE, FREE OF CHARGE, BY CALLING (847) 937-7302. PERMISSION TO USE THE PATIENT INFORMATION/ CONSENT FORM BY PHOTOCOPY REPRODUCTION IS HEREBY GRANTED BY ABBOTT LABORATORIES.

Because of its association with life threatening hepatic failure, CYLERT should not ordinarily be considered as first line drug therapy for ADHD (see INDICATIONS AND USAGE). Because CYLERT provides an observable symptomatic benefit, patients who fail to show substantial clinical benefit within 3 weeks of completing dose titration, should be withdrawn from CYLERT therapy.
Since CYLERT's marketing in 1975, 15 cases of acute hepatic failure have been reported to the FDA. While the absolute number of reported cases is not large, the rate of reporting ranges from 4 to 17 times the rate expected in the general population. This estimate may be conservative because of under reporting and because the long latency between initiation of CYLERT treatment and the occurrence of hepatic failure may limit recognition of the association. If only a portion of actual cases were recognized and reported, the risk could be substantially higher.
Of the 15 cases reported as of December 1998, 12 resulted in death or liver transplantation, usually within four weeks of the onset of signs and symptoms of liver failure. The earliest onset of hepatic abnormalities occurred six months after initiation of CYLERT. Although some reports described dark urine and nonspecific prodromal symptoms (e.g., anorexia, malaise, and gastrointestinal symptoms), in other reports it was not clear if any prodromal symptoms preceded the onset of jaundice.
Treatment with CYLERT should be initiated only in individuals without liver disease and with normal baseline liver function tests. It is not clear if baseline and periodic liver function testing are predictive of these instances of acute liver failure; however it is generally believed that early detection of drug-induced hepatic injury along with immediate withdrawal of the suspect drug enhances the likelihood for recovery. Accordingly, the following liver monitoring program is recommended: Serum ALT (SGPT) levels should be determined at baseline, and every two weeks thereafter. If CYLERT therapy is discontinued and then restarted, liver function test monitoring should be done at baseline and reinitiated at the frequency above.
CYLERT should be discontinued if serum ALT (SGPT) is increased to a clinically significant level, or any increase ≥ 2 times the upper limit of normal, or if clinical signs and symptoms suggest liver failure (see PRECAUTIONS).
The physician who elects to use CYLERT should obtain written informed consent from the patient prior to initiation of CYLERT therapy (see PATIENT INFORMATION/CONSENT FORM).

DESCRIPTION

CYLERT (pemoline) is a central nervous system stimulant. Pemoline is structurally dissimilar to the amphetamines and methylphenidate.
It is an oxazolidine compound and is chemically identified as 2-amino-5-phenyl-2-oxazolin-4-one. Pemoline has the following structural formula:

NH_2 O N O

Pemoline is a white, tasteless, odorless powder, relatively insoluble (less than 1 mg/mL) in water, chloroform, ether, acetone, and benzene; its solubility in 95% ethyl alcohol is 2.2 mg/mL.

CYLERT (pemoline) is supplied as tablets containing 18.75 mg, 37.5 mg or 75 mg of pemoline for oral administration. CYLERT is also available as chewable tablets containing 37.5 mg of pemoline.

Inactive Ingredients

18.75 mg tablet: corn starch, gelatin, lactose, magnesium hydroxide, polyethylene glycol and talc.

37.5 mg tablet: corn starch, FD&C Yellow No. 6, gelatin, lactose, magnesium hydroxide, polyethylene glycol and talc.

37.5 mg chewable tablet: corn starch, FD&C Yellow No. 6, magnesium hydroxide, magnesium stearate, mannitol, polyethylene glycol, povidone, talc and artificial flavor.

75 mg tablet: corn starch, gelatin, iron oxide, lactose, magnesium hydroxide, polyethylene glycol and talc.

CLINICAL PHARMACOLOGY

CYLERT (pemoline) has a pharmacological activity similar to that of other known central nervous system stimulants; however, it has minimal sympathomimetic effects. Although studies indicate that pemoline may act in animals through dopaminergic mechanisms, the exact mechanism and site of action of the drug in man is not known.

There is neither specific evidence which clearly establishes the mechanism whereby CYLERT produces its mental and behavioral effects in children, nor conclusive evidence regarding how these effects relate to the condition of the central nervous system.

Pemoline is rapidly absorbed from the gastrointestinal tract. Approximately 50% is bound to plasma proteins. The serum half-life of pemoline is approximately 12 hours. Peak serum levels of the drug occur within 2 to 4 hours after ingestion of a single dose. Multiple dose studies in adults at several dose levels indicate that steady state is reached in approximately 2 to 3 days. In animals given radiolabeled pemoline, the drug was widely and uniformly distributed throughout the tissues, including the brain.

Pemoline is metabolized by the liver. Metabolites of pemoline include pemoline conjugate, pemoline dione, mandelic acid, and unidentified polar compounds. CYLERT is excreted primarily by the kidneys with approximately 50% excreted unchanged and only minor fractions present as metabolites.

CYLERT (pemoline) has a gradual onset of action. Using the recommended schedule of dosage titration, significant clinical benefit may not be evident until the third or fourth week of drug administration.

INDICATIONS AND USAGE

CYLERT (pemoline) is indicated in Attention Deficit Hyperactivity Disorder (ADHD). Because of its association with life threatening hepatic failure, CYLERT should not ordinarily be considered as first line therapy for ADHD (see **BOXED WARNING**).

CYLERT (pemoline) therapy should be part of a total treatment program which typically includes other remedial measures (psychological, educational, social) for a stabilizing effect in children with a behavioral syndrome characterized by the following group of developmentally inappropriate symptoms: moderate to severe distractibility, short attention span, hyperactivity, emotional lability, and impulsivity. The diagnosis of this syndrome should not be made with finality when these symptoms are only of comparatively recent origin. Nonlocalizing (soft) neurological signs, learning disability, and abnormal EEG may or may not be present, and a diagnosis of central nervous system dysfunction may or may not be warranted.

CONTRAINDICATIONS

CYLERT (pemoline) is contraindicated in patients with known hypersensitivity or idiosyncrasy to the drug. CYLERT should not be administered to patients with impaired hepatic function (see **BOXED WARNING** and **ADVERSE REACTIONS**).

WARNINGS

Decrements in the predicted growth (i.e., weight gain and/or height) rate have been reported with the long-term use of stimulants in children. Therefore, patients requiring long-term therapy should be carefully monitored.

PRECAUTIONS

General:

Clinical experience suggests that in psychotic children, administration of CYLERT may exacerbate symptoms of behavior disturbance and thought disorder.

CYLERT should be administered with caution to patients with significantly impaired renal function.

Information for Patients:

Patients should be informed that CYLERT therapy has been associated with liver abnormalities ranging from reversible liver function test increases that do not cause any symptoms to liver failure, which may result in death. Patients should be informed that the risk of liver failure in the general population is relatively rare; however patients taking CYLERT are at a greater risk of developing liver failure than that expected in the general population. At present, there is no way to predict who is likely to develop liver failure; however only patients without liver disease and with normal baseline liver function tests should initiate CYLERT therapy. Patients should be advised to follow their doctors directives for liver function tests prior to and during CYLERT therapy. Patients should be advised to be alert for signs of liver dysfunction (jaundice, anorexia, gastrointestinal complaints, malaise, etc.) and to report them to their doctor immediately if they should occur.

The physician who elects to use CYLERT should obtain written informed consent from patients prior to initiation of CYLERT therapy (see **PATIENT INFORMATION/CONSENT FORM**.)

Laboratory Tests:

Since CYLERT's market introduction, there have been reports of elevated liver enzymes associated with its use. Many of these patients had this increase detected several months after starting CYLERT. Most patients were asymptomatic, with the increase in liver enzymes returning to normal after CYLERT was discontinued.

Treatment with CYLERT should be initiated only in individuals without liver disease and with normal baseline liver function tests. It is not clear if baseline and periodic liver function testing are predictive of these instances of acute liver failure; however it is generally believed that early detection of drug-induced hepatic injury along with immediate withdrawal of the suspect drug enhances the likelihood for recovery. Accordingly, the following liver monitoring program is recommended.

Serum ALT (SGPT) levels should be determined at baseline, and every two weeks thereafter. If CYLERT therapy is discontinued and then restarted, liver function test monitoring should be done at baseline and reinitiated at the frequency above. CYLERT should be discontinued if serum ALT (SGPT) is increased to a clinically significant level, or any increase ≥ 2 times the upper limit of normal, or if clinical signs and symptoms suggest liver failure (see **BOXED WARNING**).

Drug Interactions:

The interaction of CYLERT (pemoline) with other drugs has not been studied in humans. Patients who are receiving CYLERT concurrently with other drugs, especially drugs with CNS activity, should be monitored carefully.

Decreased seizure threshold has been reported in patients receiving CYLERT concomitantly with *antiepileptic medications.*

Carcinogenesis:

Long-term studies have been conducted in rats with doses as high as 150 mg/kg/day for eighteen months. There was no significant difference in the incidence of any neoplasm between treated and control animals.

Mutagenesis:

Data are not available concerning long-term effects on mutagenicity in animals or humans.

Impairment of Fertility:

The results of studies in which rats were given 18.75 and 37.5 mg/kg/day indicated that pemoline did not affect fertility in males or females at those doses.

Pregnancy:

Teratogenic effects: Pregnancy Category B. Reproduction studies have been performed in rats and rabbits at doses of 18.75 and 37.5 mg/kg/day and have revealed no evidence of impaired fertility or harm to the fetus. There are, however, no adequate and well-controlled studies in pregnant women. Because animal reproduction studies are not always predictive of human response, this drug should be used during pregnancy only if clearly needed.

Nonteratogenic effects:

Studies in rats have shown an increased incidence of stillbirths and cannibalization when pemoline was administered at a dose of 37.5 mg/kg/day. Postnatal survival of offspring was reduced at doses of 18.75 and 37.5 mg/kg/day.

Nursing Mothers:

It is not known whether this drug is excreted in human milk. Because many drugs are excreted in human milk, caution should be exercised when CYLERT is administered to a nursing woman.

Pediatric Use:

Safety and effectiveness in children below the age of 6 years have not been established.

Long-term effects of CYLERT in children have not been established (see **WARNINGS**).

CNS stimulants, including pemoline, have been reported to precipitate motor and phonic tics and Tourette's syndrome. Therefore, clinical evaluation for tics and Tourette's syndrome in children and their families should precede use of stimulant medications.

Drug treatment is not indicated in all cases of ADHD and should be considered only in light of complete history and evaluation of the child. The decision to prescribe CYLERT (pemoline) should depend on the physician's assessment of the chronicity and severity of the child's symptoms and their appropriateness for his/her age.

Prescription should not depend solely on the presence of one or more of the behavioral characteristics.

Geriatric Use:

Clinical studies of CYLERT did not include sufficient numbers of subjects aged 65 and over to determine whether they respond differently from younger subjects. Other reported clinical experience has not identified differences in responses between the elderly and younger patients. In general, dose selection for an elderly patient should be cautious, usually starting at the low end of the dosing range, reflecting the greater frequency of decreased hepatic, renal, or cardiac function, and of concomitant disease or other drug therapy.

ADVERSE REACTIONS

The following are adverse reactions in decreasing order of severity within each category associated with CYLERT:

Hepatic: There have been reports of hepatic dysfunction, ranging from asymptomatic reversible increases in liver enzymes to hepatitis, jaundice and fatal hepatic failure, in patients taking CYLERT (see **BOXED WARNING** and **PRECAUTIONS**).

Hematopoietic: There have been isolated reports of aplastic anemia.

Central Nervous System: The following CNS effects have been reported with the use of CYLERT: convulsive seizures; literature reports indicate that CYLERT may precipitate attacks of Gilles de la Tourette syndrome; hallucinations; dyskinetic movements of the tongue, lips, face and extremities; abnormal oculomotor function including nystagmus and oculogyric crisis; mild depression; dizziness; increased irritability; headache; and drowsiness.

Insomnia is the most frequently reported side effect of CYLERT; it usually occurs early in therapy prior to an optimum therapeutic response. In the majority of cases it is transient in nature or responds to a reduction in dosage.

Gastrointestinal: Anorexia and weight loss may occur during the first weeks of therapy. In the majority of cases it is transient in nature; weight gain usually resumes within three to six months.

Nausea and stomach ache have also been reported.

Genitourinary: A case of elevated acid phosphatase in association with prostatic enlargement has been reported in a 63 year old male who was treated with CYLERT for sleepiness. The acid phosphatase normalized with discontinuation of CYLERT and was again elevated with rechallenge.

Miscellaneous: Suppression of growth has been reported with the long-term use of stimulants in children. (See **WARNINGS**.) Skin rash has been reported with CYLERT. If adverse reactions are of a significant or protracted nature, dosage should be reduced or the drug discontinued.

DRUG ABUSE AND DEPENDENCE

Controlled Substance: CYLERT is subject to control under DEA schedule IV.

Abuse: CYLERT failed to demonstrate a potential for self-administration in primates. However, the pharmacologic similarity of pemoline to other psychostimulants with known dependence liability suggests that psychological and/or physical dependence might also occur with CYLERT. There have been isolated reports of transient psychotic symptoms occurring in adults following the long-term misuse of excessive oral doses of pemoline. CYLERT should be given with caution to emotionally unstable patients who may increase the dosage on their own initiative.

OVERDOSAGE

Signs and symptoms of acute overdosage, resulting principally from overstimulation of the central nervous system and from excessive sympathomimetic effects, may include the following: vomiting, agitation, tremors, hyperreflexia, muscle twitching, convulsions (may be followed by coma), euphoria, confusion, hallucinations, delirium, sweating, flushing, headache, hyperpyrexia, tachycardia, hypertension and mydriasis. Consult with a Certified Poison Control Center regarding treatment for up-to-date guidance and advice. Treatment consists of appropriate supportive measures. The patient must be protected against self-injury and against external stimuli that would aggravate overstimulation already present. Gastric contents may be evacuated by gastric lavage. Other measures to detoxify the gut include administration of activated charcoal and a cathartic. Chlorpromazine has been reported in the literature to be useful in decreasing CNS stimulation and sympathomimetic effects. Efficacy of peritoneal dialysis or extracorporeal hemodialysis for CYLERT overdosage has not been established.

DOSAGE AND ADMINISTRATION

CYLERT (pemoline) is administered as a single oral dose each morning. The recommended starting dose is 37.5 mg/day. This daily dose should be gradually increased by 18.75 mg at one week intervals until the desired clinical response is obtained. The effective daily dose for most patients will range from 56.25 to 75 mg. The maximum recommended daily dose of pemoline is 112.5 mg.

Clinical improvement with CYLERT is gradual. Using the recommended schedule of dosage titration, significant benefit may not be evident until the third or fourth week of drug administration. Because CYLERT provides an observable symptomatic benefit, patients who fail to show substantial clinical benefit within 3 weeks of completing dose titration, should be withdrawn from CYLERT therapy.

Where possible, drug administration should be interrupted occasionally to determine if there is a recurrence of behavioral symptoms sufficient to require continued therapy.

HOW SUPPLIED

CYLERT (pemoline) is supplied as monogrammed, grooved tablets in three dosage strengths:

18.75 mg white tablets (imprinted with [Abbott logo] and the Abbo-Code TH),

Bottles of 100 .... (**NDC** 0074-6025-13).

37.5 mg orange-colored tablets (imprinted with [Abbott logo] and the Abbo-Code TI),

Bottles of 100 .... (**NDC** 0074-6057-13).

75 mg tan-colored tablets (imprinted with [Abbott logo] and the Abbo-Code TJ),

Bottles of 100 .... (**NDC** 0074-6073-13).

CYLERT (pemoline) Chewable is supplied as 37.5 mg monogrammed, grooved orange-colored tablets (imprinted with [Abbott logo] and the Abbo-Code TK),

Bottles of 100 .... (**NDC** 0074-6088-13).

Recommended Storage: Store below 86°F (30°C).

Continued on next page

Cylert—Cont.

PATIENT INFORMATION/CONSENT FORM

Cylert® (pemoline) should not be used by patients until there has been a complete discussion of the risks and benefits of Cylert therapy and written informed consent has been obtained.

IMPORTANT INFORMATION:

Cylert therapy has been associated with liver abnormalities ranging from reversible liver function test increases that do not cause any symptoms to liver failure, which may result in death. Therefore, you should have a full discussion of the risks and benefits of Cylert before beginning therapy.

PATIENT CONSENT:

My (son, daughter, ward) ________________________'s treatment with Cylert has been explained to me by Dr. ________________________.

The following points of information, among others, have been specifically discussed and explained and I have had the opportunity to ask any questions concerning this information.

1. I, ________________________ (Patient/Parent/Guardian's name), understand that Cylert is used to treat certain types of patients with the behavioral syndrome called attention deficit hyperactivity disorder (ADHD) and that I (my son/daugher/ward) am that type of patient.
   Initials: ____________
2. I understand that there is a risk that I (my son/daughter/ward) might develop liver failure, which may result in death, while taking Cylert. I understand that this could occur even after long-term therapy.
   Initials: ____________
3. I understand that I (my son/daughter/ward) should have blood taken to test liver function before Cylert is begun, and every two weeks from then on while taking Cylert. I understand that although the liver function tests may help detect if I (my son/daughter/ward) develop liver damage, it may do so only after significant, irreversible and potentially fatal damage has already occurred.
   Initials: ____________
4. I understand that if I (my son/daughter/ward) stop taking Cylert and then restart it at a later time (e.g., after summer vacation), I (my son/daughter/ward) should again have blood taken to test liver function before Cylert is restarted, and every two weeks from then on while taking Cylert.
   Initials: ____________
5. I understand that I should immediately report any unusual symptoms to the doctor and should be especially aware of persistent nausea, vomiting, fatigue, lethargy, loss of appetite, abdominal pain, dark urine, or yellowing of the skin or eyes.
   Initials: ____________

I now authorize Dr. ____________ to begin my (son/daughter/ward's) treatment with Cylert, or if treatment with Cylert has already begun, to continue this treatment.

____
Signature Date

____
Address

____
Telephone

PHYSICIAN STATEMENT:

I have fully explained to the patient (parent/guardian), ________________ the nature and purpose of treatment with Cylert and the potential risks associated with Cylert and the potential risks associated with that treatment. I have asked if he/she has any questions regarding this treatment or the associated risks and have answered these questions to the best of my ability.

____
Physician Signature

____
Date

NOTE TO PHYSICIAN: It is strongly recommended that you retain a completed copy of this informed consent form in your patient's records.

SUPPLY OF PATIENT INFORMATION/CONSENT FORMS: A supply of Patient Information/Consent Forms as printed above is available, free of charge, by calling (847) 937-7302. Permission to use the above Patient Information/Consent Form by photocopy reproduction is hereby granted by Abbott Laboratories.

ABBOTT LABORATORIES
NORTH CHICAGO, IL 60064, U.S.A.
(Nos. 6025, 6057, 6073, and 6088)
03-5228-R21-Rev. December, 2002

Shown in Product Identification Guide, page 303

DEPACON® ℞

[*dəp' ā-con*]

VALPROATE SODIUM INJECTION

BOX WARNING:

HEPATOTOXICITY:

HEPATIC FAILURE RESULTING IN FATALITIES HAS OCCURRED IN PATIENTS RECEIVING VALPROIC ACID AND ITS DERIVATIVES. EXPERIENCE HAS INDICATED THAT CHILDREN UNDER THE AGE OF TWO YEARS ARE AT A CONSIDERABLY INCREASED RISK OF DEVELOPING FATAL HEPATOTOXICITY, ESPECIALLY THOSE ON MULTIPLE ANTICONVULSANTS, THOSE WITH CONGENITAL METABOLIC DISORDERS, THOSE WITH SEVERE SEIZURE DISORDERS ACCOMPANIED BY MENTAL RETARDATION, AND THOSE WITH ORGANIC BRAIN DISEASE. WHEN DEPACON IS USED IN THIS PATIENT GROUP, IT SHOULD BE USED WITH EXTREME CAUTION AND AS A SOLE AGENT. THE BENEFITS OF THERAPY SHOULD BE WEIGHED AGAINST THE RISKS. ABOVE THIS AGE GROUP, EXPERIENCE IN EPILEPSY HAS INDICATED THAT THE INCIDENCE OF FATAL HEPATOTOXICITY DECREASES CONSIDERABLY IN PROGRESSIVELY OLDER PATIENT GROUPS.

THESE INCIDENTS USUALLY HAVE OCCURRED DURING THE FIRST SIX MONTHS OF TREATMENT. SERIOUS OR FATAL HEPATOTOXICITY MAY BE PRECEDED BY NON-SPECIFIC SYMPTOMS SUCH AS MALAISE, WEAKNESS, LETHARGY, FACIAL EDEMA, ANOREXIA, AND VOMITING. IN PATIENTS WITH EPILEPSY, A LOSS OF SEIZURE CONTROL MAY ALSO OCCUR. PATIENTS SHOULD BE MONITORED CLOSELY FOR APPEARANCE OF THESE SYMPTOMS. LIVER FUNCTION TESTS SHOULD BE PERFORMED PRIOR TO THERAPY AND AT FREQUENT INTERVALS THEREAFTER, ESPECIALLY DURING THE FIRST SIX MONTHS.

TERATOGENICITY:

VALPROATE CAN PRODUCE TERATOGENIC EFFECTS SUCH AS NEURAL TUBE DEFECTS (E.G., SPINA BIFIDA). ACCORDINGLY, THE USE OF VALPROATE PRODUCTS IN WOMEN OF CHILDBEARING POTENTIAL REQUIRES THAT THE BENEFITS OF ITS USE BE WEIGHED AGAINST THE RISK OF INJURY TO THE FETUS.

PANCREATITIS:

CASES OF LIFE-THREATENING PANCREATITIS HAVE BEEN REPORTED IN BOTH CHILDREN AND ADULTS RECEIVING VALPROATE. SOME OF THE CASES HAVE BEEN DESCRIBED AS HEMORRHAGIC WITH A RAPID PROGRESSION FROM INITIAL SYMPTOMS TO DEATH. CASES HAVE BEEN REPORTED SHORTLY AFTER INITIAL USE AS WELL AS AFTER SEVERAL YEARS OF USE. PATIENTS AND GUARDIANS SHOULD BE WARNED THAT ABDOMINAL PAIN, NAUSEA, VOMITING, AND/OR ANOREXIA CAN BE SYMPTOMS OF PANCREATITIS THAT REQUIRE PROMPT MEDICAL EVALUATION. IF PANCREATITIS IS DIAGNOSED, VALPROATE SHOULD ORDINARILY BE DISCONTINUED. ALTERNATIVE TREATMENT FOR THE UNDERLYING MEDICAL CONDITION SHOULD BE INITIATED AS CLINICALLY INDICATED. (See **WARNINGS** and **PRECAUTIONS**.)

DESCRIPTION

Valproate sodium is the sodium salt of valproic acid designated as sodium 2-propylpentanoate. Valproate sodium has the following structure:

$$\begin{matrix} CH_3-CH_2-CH_2 & & \\ & CH-C(=O)O^{\ominus} & Na^{\oplus} \\ CH_3-CH_2-CH_2 & & \end{matrix}$$

Valproate sodium has a molecular weight of 166.2. It occurs as an essentially white and odorless, crystalline, deliquescent powder.

DEPACON solution is available in 5 mL single-dose vials for intravenous injection. Each mL contains valproate sodium equivalent to 100 mg valproic acid, edetate disodium 0.40 mg, and water for injection to volume. The pH is adjusted to 7.6 with sodium hydroxide and/or hydrochloric acid. The solution is clear and colorless.

CLINICAL PHARMACOLOGY

DEPACON exists as the valproate ion in the blood. The mechanisms by which valproate exerts its therapeutic effects have not been established. It has been suggested that its activity in epilepsy is related to increased brain concentrations of gamma-aminobutyric acid (GABA).

Pharmacokinetics

Bioavailability

Equivalent doses of intravenous (IV) valproate and oral valproate products are expected to result in equivalent C_{max}, C_{min}, and total systemic exposure to the valproate ion when the IV valproate is administered as a 60 minute infusion. However, the rate of valproate ion absorption may vary with the formulation used. These differences should be of minor clinical importance under the steady state conditions achieved in chronic use in the treatment of epilepsy.

Administration of DEPAKOTE (divalproex sodium) tablets and IV valproate (given as a one hour infusion), 250 mg every 6 hours for 4 days to 18 healthy male volunteers resulted in equivalent AUC, C_{max}, C_{min} at steady state, as well as after the first dose. The T_{max} after IV DEPACON occurs at the end of the one hour infusion, while the T_{max} after oral dosing with DEPAKOTE occurs at approximately 4 hours. Because the kinetics of unbound valproate are linear, bioequivalence between DEPACON and DEPAKOTE up to the maximum recommended dose of 60 mg/kg/day can be assumed. The AUC and C_{max} resulting from administration of IV valproate 500 mg as a single one hour infusion and a single 500 mg dose of DEPAKENE syrup to 17 healthy male volunteers were also equivalent.

Patients maintained on valproic acid doses of 750 mg to 4250 mg daily (given in divided doses every 6 hours) as oral DEPAKOTE (divalproex sodium) alone (n=24) or with another stabilized antiepileptic drug [carbamazepine (n=15), phenytoin (n=11), or phenobarbital (n=1)], showed comparable plasma levels for valproic acid when switching from oral DEPAKOTE to IV valproate (1-hour infusion).

Eleven healthy volunteers were given single infusions of 1000 mg IV valproate over 5, 10, 30, and 60 minutes in a 4-period crossover study. Total valproate concentrations were measured; unbound concentrations were not measured. After the 5 minute infusions (mean rate of 2.8 mg/kg/min), mean C_{max} was 145 ± 32 µg/mL, while after the 60 minute infusions, mean C_{max} was 115 ± 8 µg/mL. Ninety to 120 minutes after infusion initiation, total valproate concentrations were similar for all 4 rates of infusion. Because protein binding is nonlinear at higher total valproate concentrations, the corresponding increase in unbound C_{max} at faster infusion rates will be greater.

Distribution

Protein Binding:

The plasma protein binding of valproate is concentration dependent and the free fraction increases from approximately 10% at 40 µg/mL to 18.5% at 130 µg/mL. Protein binding of valproate is reduced in the elderly, in patients with chronic hepatic diseases, in patients with renal impairment, and in the presence of other drugs (e.g., aspirin). Conversely, valproate may displace certain protein-bound drugs (e.g., phenytoin, carbamazepine, warfarin, and tolbutamide). (See **PRECAUTIONS, Drug Interactions** for more detailed information on the pharmacokinetic interactions of valproate with other drugs.)

CNS Distribution:

Valproate concentrations in cerebrospinal fluid (CSF) approximate unbound concentrations in plasma (about 10% of total concentration).

Metabolism

Valproate is metabolized almost entirely by the liver. In adult patients on monotherapy, 30–50% of an administered dose appears in urine as a glucuronide conjugate. Mitochondrial β-oxidation is the other major metabolic pathway, typically accounting for over 40% of the dose. Usually, less than 15–20% of the dose is eliminated by other oxidative mechanisms. Less than 3% of an administered dose is excreted unchanged in urine.

The relationship between dose and total valproate concentration is nonlinear; concentration does not increase proportionally with the dose, but rather, increases to a lesser extent due to saturable plasma protein binding. The kinetics of unbound drug are linear.

Elimination

Mean plasma clearance and volume of distribution for total valproate are 0.56 L/hr/1.73 m^2 and 11 L/1.73 m^2, respectively. Mean terminal half-life for valproate monotherapy after an intravenous infusion of 1000 mg was 16 ± 3.0 hours.

The estimates cited apply primarily to patients who are not taking drugs that affect hepatic metabolizing enzyme systems. For example, patients taking enzyme-inducing antiepileptic drugs (carbamazepine, phenytoin, and phenobarbital) will clear valproate more rapidly. Because of these changes in valproate clearance, monitoring of antiepileptic concentrations should be intensified whenever concomitant antiepileptics are introduced or withdrawn.

Special Populations

Effect of Age:

Neonates—Children within the first two months of life have a markedly decreased ability to eliminate valproate compared to older children and adults. This is a result of reduced clearance (perhaps due to delay in development of glucuronosyltransferase and other enzyme systems involved in valproate elimination) as well as increased volume of distribution (in part due to decreased plasma protein binding). For example, in one study, the half-life in children under 10 days ranged from 10 to 67 hours compared to a range of 7 to 13 hours in children greater than 2 months.

Children—Pediatric patients (i.e., between 3 months and 10 years) have 50% higher clearances expressed on weight (i.e., mL/min/kg) than do adults. Over the age of 10 years, children have pharmacokinetic parameters that approximate those of adults.

Elderly—The capacity of elderly patients (age range: 68 to 89 years) to eliminate valproate has been shown to be reduced compared to younger adults (age range: 22 to 26). Intrinsic clearance is reduced by 39%; the free fraction is increased by 44%. Accordingly, the initial dosage should be reduced in the elderly. (See **DOSAGE AND ADMINISTRATION**).

Effect of Gender:
There are no differences in the body surface area adjusted unbound clearance between males and females (4.8±0.17 and 4.7±0.07 L/hr per 1.73 m^2, respectively).
Effect of Race:
The effects of race on the kinetics of valproate have not been studied.
Effect of Disease:
Liver Disease—(See **BOXED WARNING**, **CONTRAINDICATIONS**, and **WARNINGS**). Liver disease impairs the capacity to eliminate valproate. In one study, the clearance of free valproate was decreased by 50% in 7 patients with cirrhosis and by 16% in 4 patients with acute hepatitis, compared with 6 healthy subjects. In that study, the half-life of valproate was increased from 12 to 18 hours. Liver disease is also associated with decreased albumin concentrations and larger unbound fractions (2 to 2.6 fold increase) of valproate. Accordingly, monitoring of total concentrations may be misleading since free concentrations may be substantially elevated in patients with hepatic disease whereas total concentrations may appear to be normal.
Renal Disease—A slight reduction (27%) in the unbound clearance of valproate has been reported in patients with renal failure (creatinine clearance < 10 mL/minute); however, hemodialysis typically reduces valproate concentrations by about 20%. Therefore, no dosage adjustment appears to be necessary in patients with renal failure. Protein binding in these patients is substantially reduced; thus, monitoring total concentrations may be misleading.

Plasma Levels and Clinical Effect

The relationship between plasma concentration and clinical response is not well documented. One contributing factor is the nonlinear, concentration dependent protein binding of valproate which affects the clearance of the drug. Thus, monitoring of total serum valproate cannot provide a reliable index of the bioactive valproate species.
For example, because the plasma protein binding of valproate is concentration dependent, the free fraction increases from approximately 10% at 40 µg/mL to 18.5% at 130 µg/mL. Higher than expected free fractions occur in the elderly, in hyperlipidemic patients, and in patients with hepatic and renal diseases.
Epilepsy:
The therapeutic range in epilepsy is commonly considered to be 50 to 100 µg/mL of total valproate, although some patients may be controlled with lower or higher plasma concentrations.
Equivalent doses of DEPACON and DEPAKOTE (divalproex sodium) yield equivalent plasma levels of the valproate ion (see **CLINICAL PHARMACOLOGY, Pharmacokinetics**).

Clinical Studies

The studies described in the following section were conducted with oral divalproex sodium products.

Epilepsy

The efficacy of DEPAKOTE (divalproex sodium) in reducing the incidence of complex partial seizures (CPS) that occur in isolation or in association with other seizure types was established in two controlled trials.
In one, multiclinic, placebo controlled study employing an add-on design (adjunctive therapy), 144 patients who continued to suffer eight or more CPS per 8 weeks during an 8 week period of monotherapy with doses of either carbamazepine or phenytoin sufficient to assure plasma concentrations within the "therapeutic range" were randomized to receive, in addition to their original antiepilepsy drug (AED), either DEPAKOTE or placebo. Randomized patients were to be followed for a total of 16 weeks. The following table presents the findings.

Adjunctive Therapy Study
Median Incidence of CPS per 8 Weeks

Add-on Treatment	Number of Patients	Baseline Incidence	Experimental Incidence
DEPAKOTE	75	16.0	8.9*
Placebo	69	14.5	11.5

*Reduction from baseline statistically significantly greater for DEPAKOTE than placebo at p ≤ 0.05 level.

Figure 1 presents the proportion of patients (X axis) whose percentage reduction from baseline in complex partial seizure rates was at least as great as that indicated on the Y axis in the adjunctive therapy study. A positive percent reduction indicates an improvement (i.e., a decrease in seizure frequency), while a negative percent reduction indicates worsening. Thus, in a display of this type, the curve for an effective treatment is shifted to the left of the curve for placebo. This figure shows that the proportion of patients achieving any particular level of improvement was consistently higher for DEPAKOTE than for placebo. For example, 45% of patients treated with DEPAKOTE had a ≥ 50% reduction in complex partial seizure rate compared to 23% of patients treated with placebo.
[See figure 1 at top of next column]
The second study assessed the capacity of DEPAKOTE to reduce the incidence of CPS when administered as the sole AED. The study compared the incidence of CPS among patients randomized to either a high or low dose treatment arm. Patients qualified for entry into the randomized comparison phase of this study only if 1) they continued to experience 2 or more CPS per 4 weeks during an 8 to 12

Figure 1

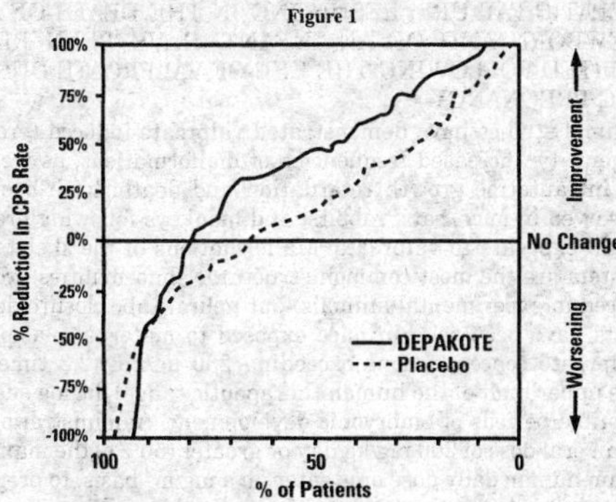

week long period of monotherapy with adequate doses of an AED (i.e., phenytoin, carbamazepine, phenobarbital, or primidone) and 2) they made a successful transition over a two week interval to DEPAKOTE. Patients entering the randomized phase were then brought to their assigned target dose, gradually tapered off their concomitant AED and followed for an interval as long as 22 weeks. Less than 50% of the patients randomized, however, completed the study. In patients converted to DEPAKOTE monotherapy, the mean total valproate concentrations during monotherapy were 71 and 123 µg/mL in the low dose and high dose groups, respectively.
The following table presents the findings for all patients randomized who had at least one post-randomization assessment.

Monotherapy Study
Median Incidence of CPS per 8 Weeks

Treatment	Number of Patients	Baseline Incidence	Randomized Phase Incidence
High dose DEPAKOTE	131	13.2	10.7*
Low dose DEPAKOTE	134	14.2	13.8

*Reduction from baseline statistically significantly greater for high dose than low dose at p ≤ 0.05 level.

Figure 2 presents the proportion of patients (X axis) whose percentage reduction from baseline in complex partial seizure rates was at least as great as that indicated on the Y axis in the monotherapy study. A positive percent reduction indicates an improvement (i.e., a decrease in seizure frequency), while a negative percent reduction indicates worsening. Thus, in a display of this type, the curve for a more effective treatment is shifted to the left of the curve for a less effective treatment. This figure shows that the proportion of patients achieving any particular level of reduction was consistently higher for high dose DEPAKOTE than for low dose DEPAKOTE. For example, when switching from carbamazepine, phenytoin, phenobarbital or primidone monotherapy to high dose DEPAKOTE monotherapy, 63% of patients experienced no change or a reduction in complex partial seizure rates compared to 54% of patients receiving low dose DEPAKOTE.

Figure 2

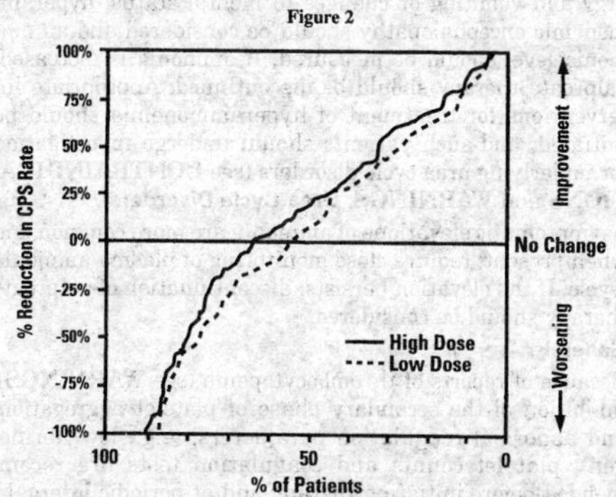

INDICATIONS AND USAGE

DEPACON is indicated as an intravenous alternative in patients for whom oral administration of valproate products is temporarily not feasible in the following conditions:
DEPACON is indicated as monotherapy and adjunctive therapy in the treatment of patients with complex partial seizures that occur either in isolation or in association with other types of seizures. DEPACON is also indicated for use as sole and adjunctive therapy in the treatment of patients with simple and complex absence seizures, and adjunctively in patients with multiple seizure types that include absence seizures.
Simple absence is defined as very brief clouding of the sensorium or loss of consciousness accompanied by certain generalized epileptic discharges without other detectable clinical signs. Complex absence is the term used when other signs are also present.
SEE **WARNINGS** FOR STATEMENT REGARDING FATAL HEPATIC DYSFUNCTION.

CONTRAINDICATIONS

VALPROATE SODIUM INJECTION SHOULD NOT BE ADMINISTERED TO PATIENTS WITH HEPATIC DISEASE OR SIGNIFICANT HEPATIC DYSFUNCTION.
Valproate sodium injection is contraindicated in patients with known hypersensitivity to the drug.
Valproate sodium injection is contraindicated in patients with known urea cycle disorders (see **WARNINGS**).

WARNINGS

Hepatotoxicity

Hepatic failure resulting in fatalities has occurred in patients receiving valproic acid. These incidents usually have occurred during the first six months of treatment. Serious or fatal hepatotoxicity may be preceded by non-specific symptoms such as malaise, weakness, lethargy, facial edema, anorexia, and vomiting. In patients with epilepsy, a loss of seizure control may also occur. Patients should be monitored closely for appearance of these symptoms. Liver function tests should be performed prior to therapy and at frequent intervals thereafter, especially during the first six months of valproate therapy. However, physicians should not rely totally on serum biochemistry since these tests may not be abnormal in all instances, but should also consider the results of careful interim medical history and physical examination.
Caution should be observed when administering valproate products to patients with a prior history of hepatic disease. Patients on multiple anticonvulsants, children, those with congenital metabolic disorders, those with severe seizure disorders accompanied by mental retardation, and those with organic brain disease may be at particular risk. Experience has indicated that children under the age of two years are at a considerably increased risk of developing fatal hepatotoxicity, especially those with the aforementioned conditions. When DEPACON is used in this patient group, it should be used with extreme caution and as a sole agent. The benefits of therapy should be weighed against the risks. Use of DEPACON has not been studied in children below the age of 2 years. Above this age group, experience with valproate products in epilepsy has indicated that the incidence of fatal hepatotoxicity decreases considerably in progressively older patient groups.
The drug should be discontinued immediately in the presence of significant hepatic dysfunction, suspected or apparent. In some cases, hepatic dysfunction has progressed in spite of discontinuation of drug.

Pancreatitis

Cases of life-threatening pancreatitis have been reported in both children and adults receiving valproate. Some of the cases have been described as hemorrhagic with rapid progression from initial symptoms to death. Some cases have occurred shortly after initial use as well as after several years of use. The rate based upon the reported cases exceeds that expected in the general population and there have been cases in which pancreatitis recurred after rechallenge with valproate. In clinical trials, there were 2 cases of pancreatitis without alternative etiology in 2416 patients, representing 1044 patient-years experience. Patients and guardians should be warned that abdominal pain, nausea, vomiting, and/or anorexia can be symptoms of pancreatitis that require prompt medical evaluation. If pancreatitis is diagnosed, valproate should ordinarily be discontinued. Alternative treatment for the underlying medical condition should be initiated as clinically indicated (see **BOXED WARNING**).

Urea Cycle Disorders (UCD)

Valproate sodium is contraindicated in patients with known urea cycle disorders.
Hyperammonemic encephalopathy, sometimes fatal, has been reported following initiation of valproate therapy in patients with urea cycle disorders, a group of uncommon genetic abnormalities, particularly ornithine transcarbamylase deficiency. Prior to the initiation of valproate therapy, evaluation for UCD should be considered in the following patients: 1) those with a history of unexplained encephalopathy or coma, encephalopathy associated with a protein load, pregnancy-related or postpartum encephalopathy, unexplained mental retardation, or history of elevated plasma ammonia or glutamine; 2) those with cyclical vomiting and lethargy, episodic extreme irritability, ataxia, low BUN, or protein avoidance; 3) those with a family history of UCD or a family history of unexplained infant deaths (particularly males); 4) those with other signs or symptoms of UCD. Patients who develop symptoms of unexplained hyperammonemic encephalopathy while receiving valproate therapy should receive prompt treatment (including discontinuation of valproate therapy) and be evaluated for underlying urea cycle disorders (see **CONTRAINDICATIONS** and **PRECAUTIONS**).

Somnolence in the Elderly

In a double-blind, multicenter trial of valproate in elderly patients with dementia (mean age = 83 years), doses were increased by 125 mg/day to a target dose of 20 mg/kg/day. A significantly higher proportion of valproate patients had somnolence compared to placebo, and although not statistically significant, there was a higher proportion of patients with dehydration. Discontinuations for somnolence were also significantly higher than with placebo. In some patients with somnolence (approximately one-half), there was associated reduced nutritional intake and weight loss. There was a trend for the patients who experienced these

Continued on next page

Depacon—Cont.

events to have a lower baseline albumin concentration, lower valproate clearance, and a higher BUN. In elderly patients, dosage should be increased more slowly and with regular monitoring for fluid and nutritional intake, dehydration, somnolence, and other adverse events. Dose reductions or discontinuation of valproate should be considered in patients with decreased food or fluid intake and in patients with excessive somnolence (see **DOSAGE AND ADMINISTRATION**).

Thrombocytopenia

The frequency of adverse effects (particularly elevated liver enzymes and thrombocytopenia [see **PRECAUTIONS**]) may be dose-related. In a clinical trial of DEPAKOTE as monotherapy in patients with epilepsy, 34/126 patients (27%) receiving approximately 50 mg/kg/day on average, had at least one value of platelets ≤ 75 x 10^9/L. Approximately half of these patients had treatment discontinued, with return of platelet counts to normal. In the remaining patients, platelet counts normalized with continued treatment. In this study, the probability of thrombocytopenia appeared to increase significantly at total valproate concentrations of ≥ 110 μg/mL (females) or ≥ 135 μg/mL (males). The therapeutic benefit which may accompany the higher doses should therefore be weighed against the possibility of a greater incidence of adverse effects.

Post-traumatic Seizures

A study was conducted to evaluate the effect of IV valproate in the prevention of post-traumatic seizures in patients with acute head injuries. Patients were randomly assigned to receive either IV valproate given for one week (followed by oral valproate products for either one or six months per random treatment assignment) or IV phenytoin given for one week (followed by placebo). In this study, the incidence of death was found to be higher in the two groups assigned to valproate treatment compared to the rate in those assigned to the IV phenytoin treatment group (13% vs 8.5%, respectively). Many of these patients were critically ill with multiple and/or severe injuries, and evaluation of the causes of death did not suggest any specific drug-related causation. Further, in the absence of a concurrent placebo control during the initial week of intravenous therapy, it is impossible to determine if the mortality rate in the patients treated with valproate was greater or less than that expected in a similar group not treated with valproate, or whether the rate seen in the IV phenytoin treated patients was lower than would be expected. Nonetheless, until further information is available, it seems prudent not to use DEPACON in patients with acute head trauma for the prophylaxis of post-traumatic seizures.

Usage In Pregnancy

ACCORDING TO PUBLISHED AND UNPUBLISHED REPORTS, VALPROIC ACID MAY PRODUCE TERATOGENIC EFFECTS IN THE OFFSPRING OF HUMAN FEMALES RECEIVING THE DRUG DURING PREGNANCY.

THERE ARE MULTIPLE REPORTS IN THE CLINICAL LITERATURE WHICH INDICATE THAT THE USE OF ANTIEPILEPSY DRUGS DURING PREGNANCY RESULTS IN AN INCREASED INCIDENCE OF BIRTH DEFECTS IN THE OFFSPRING. ALTHOUGH DATA ARE MORE EXTENSIVE WITH RESPECT TO TRIMETHADIONE, PARAMETHADIONE, PHENYTOIN, AND PHENOBARBITAL, REPORTS INDICATE A POSSIBLE SIMILAR ASSOCIATION WITH THE USE OF OTHER ANTIEPILEPSY DRUGS. THEREFORE, ANTIEPILEPSY DRUGS SHOULD BE ADMINISTERED TO WOMEN OF CHILDBEARING POTENTIAL ONLY IF THEY ARE CLEARLY SHOWN TO BE ESSENTIAL IN THE MANAGEMENT OF THEIR SEIZURES.

THE INCIDENCE OF NEURAL TUBE DEFECTS IN THE FETUS MAY BE INCREASED IN MOTHERS RECEIVING VALPROATE DURING THE FIRST TRIMESTER OF PREGNANCY. THE CENTERS FOR DISEASE CONTROL (CDC) HAS ESTIMATED THE RISK OF VALPROIC ACID EXPOSED WOMEN HAVING CHILDREN WITH SPINA BIFIDA TO BE APPROXIMATELY 1 TO 2%.

OTHER CONGENITAL ANOMALIES (E.G., CRANIOFACIAL DEFECTS, CARDIOVASCULAR MALFORMATIONS AND ANOMALIES INVOLVING VARIOUS BODY SYSTEMS), COMPATIBLE AND INCOMPATIBLE WITH LIFE, HAVE BEEN REPORTED. SUFFICIENT DATA TO DETERMINE THE INCIDENCE OF THESE CONGENITAL ANOMALIES IS NOT AVAILABLE.

THE HIGHER INCIDENCE OF CONGENITAL ANOMALIES IN ANTIEPILEPSY DRUG-TREATED WOMEN WITH SEIZURE DISORDERS CANNOT BE REGARDED AS A CAUSE AND EFFECT RELATIONSHIP. THERE ARE INTRINSIC METHODOLOGIC PROBLEMS IN OBTAINING ADEQUATE DATA ON DRUG TERATOGENICITY IN HUMANS; GENETIC FACTORS OR THE EPILEPTIC CONDITION ITSELF, MAY BE MORE IMPORTANT THAN DRUG THERAPY IN CONTRIBUTING TO CONGENITAL ANOMALIES.

PATIENTS TAKING VALPROATE MAY DEVELOP CLOTTING ABNORMALITIES. A PATIENT WHO HAD LOW FIBRINOGEN WHEN TAKING MULTIPLE ANTICONVULSANTS INCLUDING VALPROATE GAVE BIRTH TO AN INFANT WITH AFIBRINOGENEMIA WHO SUBSEQUENTLY DIED OF HEMORRHAGE. IF VALPROATE IS USED IN PREGNANCY, THE CLOTTING PARAMETERS SHOULD BE MONITORED CAREFULLY.

HEPATIC FAILURE, RESULTING IN THE DEATH OF A NEWBORN AND OF AN INFANT, HAVE BEEN REPORTED FOLLOWING THE USE OF VALPROATE DURING PREGNANCY.

Animal studies have demonstrated valproate-induced teratogenicity. Increased frequencies of malformations, as well as intrauterine growth retardation and death, have been observed in mice, rats, rabbits, and monkeys following prenatal exposure to valproate. Malformations of the skeletal system are the most common structural abnormalities produced in experimental animals, but neural tube closure defects have been seen in mice exposed to maternal plasma valproate concentrations exceeding 230 μg/mL (2.3 times the upper limit of the human therapeutic range) during susceptible periods of embryonic development. Administration of an oral dose of 200 mg/kg/day or greater (50% of the maximum human daily dose or greater on a mg/m^2 basis) to pregnant rats during organogenesis produced malformations (skeletal, cardiac, and urogenital) and growth retardation in the offspring. These doses resulted in peak maternal plasma valproate levels of approximately 340 μg/mL or greater (3.4 times the upper limit of the human therapeutic range or greater). Behavioral deficits have been reported in the offspring of rats given a dose of 200 mg/kg/day throughout most of pregnancy. An oral dose of 350 mg/kg/day (2 times the maximum human daily dose on a mg/m^2 basis) produced skeletal and visceral malformations in rabbits exposed during organogenesis. Skeletal malformations, growth retardation, and death were observed in rhesus monkeys following administration of an oral dose of 200 mg/kg/day (equal to the maximum human daily dose on a mg/m^2 basis) during organogenesis. This dose resulted in peak maternal plasma valproate levels of approximately 280 μg/mL (2.8 times the upper limit of the human therapeutic range).

The prescribing physician will wish to weigh the benefits of therapy against the risks in treating or counseling women of childbearing potential. If this drug is used during pregnancy, or if the patient becomes pregnant while taking this drug, the patient should be apprised of the potential hazard to the fetus.

Antiepilepsy drugs should not be discontinued abruptly in patients in whom the drug is administered to prevent major seizures because of the strong possibility of precipitating status epilepticus with attendant hypoxia and threat to life. In individual cases where the severity and frequency of the seizure disorder are such that the removal of medication does not pose a serious threat to the patient, discontinuation of the drug may be considered prior to and during pregnancy, although it cannot be said with any confidence that even minor seizures do not pose some hazard to the developing embryo or fetus.

Tests to detect neural tube and other defects using current accepted procedures should be considered a part of routine prenatal care in childbearing women receiving valproate.

PRECAUTIONS

Hepatic Dysfunction

See **BOXED WARNING**, **CONTRAINDICATIONS** and **WARNINGS**.

Pancreatitis

See **BOXED WARNING** and **WARNINGS**.

Hyperammonemia

Hyperammonemia has been reported in association with valproate therapy and may be present despite normal liver function tests. In patients who develop unexplained lethargy and vomiting or changes in mental status, hyperammonemic encephalopathy should be considered and an ammonia level should be measured. If ammonia is increased, valproate therapy should be discontinued. Appropriate interventions for treatment of hyperammonemia should be initiated, and such patients should undergo investigation for underlying urea cycle disorders (see **CONTRAINDICATIONS** and **WARNINGS: Urea Cycle Disorders**).

Asymptomatic elevations of ammonia are more common and when present, require close monitoring of plasma ammonia levels. If the elevation persists, discontinuation of valproate therapy should be considered.

General

Because of reports of thrombocytopenia (see **WARNINGS**), inhibition of the secondary phase of platelet aggregation, and abnormal coagulation parameters, (e.g., low fibrinogen), platelet counts and coagulation tests are recommended before initiating therapy and at periodic intervals. It is recommended that patients receiving DEPACON be monitored for platelet count and coagulation parameters prior to planned surgery. In a clinical trial of DEPAKOTE (divalproex sodium) as monotherapy in patients with epilepsy, 34/126 patients (27%) receiving approximately 50 mg/kg/day on average, had at least one value of platelets ≤ 75 × 10^9/L. Approximately half of these patients had treatment discontinued, with return of platelet counts to normal. In the remaining patients, platelet counts normalized with continued treatment. In this study, the probability of thrombocytopenia appeared to increase significantly at total valproate concentrations of ≥ 110 μg/mL (females) or ≥ 135 μg/mL (males). Evidence of hemorrhage, bruising, or a disorder of hemostasis/coagulation is an indication for reduction of the dosage or withdrawal of therapy.

Since DEPACON may interact with concurrently administered drugs which are capable of enzyme induction, periodic plasma concentration determinations of valproate and concomitant drugs are recommended during the early course of therapy. (See **PRECAUTIONS–Drug Interactions**).

Valproate is partially eliminated in the urine as a keto-metabolite which may lead to a false interpretation of the urine ketone test.

There have been reports of altered thyroid function tests associated with valproate. The clinical significance of these is unknown.

There are *in vitro* studies that suggest valproate stimulates the replication of the HIV and CMV viruses under certain experimental conditions. The clinical consequence, if any, is not known. Additionally, the relevance of these *in vitro* findings is uncertain for patients receiving maximally suppressive antiretroviral therapy.

Nevertheless, these data should be borne in mind when interpreting the results from regular monitoring of the viral load in HIV infected patients receiving valproate or when following CMV infected patients clinically.

Information for Patients

Patients and guardians should be warned that abdominal pain, nausea, vomiting, and/or anorexia can be symptoms of pancreatitis and, therefore, require further medical evaluation promptly.

Patients should be informed of the signs and symptoms associated with hyperammonemic encephalopathy (see **PRECAUTIONS—Hyperammonemia**) and be told to inform the prescriber if any of these symptoms occur.

Since DEPACON may produce CNS depression, especially when combined with another CNS depressant (e.g., alcohol), patients should be advised not to engage in hazardous activities, such as driving an automobile or operating dangerous machinery, until it is known that they do not become drowsy from the drug.

Drug Interactions

Effects of Co-Administered Drugs on Valproate Clearance

Drugs that affect the level of expression of hepatic enzymes, particularly those that elevate levels of glucuronosyltransferases, may increase the clearance of valproate. For example, phenytoin, carbamazepine, and phenobarbital (or primidone) can double the clearance of valproate. Thus, patients on monotherapy will generally have longer half-lives and higher concentrations than patients receiving polytherapy with antiepilepsy drugs.

In contrast, drugs that are inhibitors of cytochrome P450 isozymes, e.g., antidepressants, may be expected to have little effect on valproate clearance because cytochrome P450 microsomal mediated oxidation is a relatively minor secondary metabolic pathway compared to glucuronidation and beta-oxidation.

Because of these changes in valproate clearance, monitoring of valproate and concomitant drug concentrations should be increased whenever enzyme inducing drugs are introduced or withdrawn.

The following list provides information about the potential for an influence of several commonly prescribed medications on valproate pharmacokinetics. The list is not exhaustive nor could it be, since new interactions are continuously being reported.

Drugs for which a potentially important interaction has been observed:

Aspirin—A study involving the co-administration of aspirin at antipyretic doses (11 to 16 mg/kg) with valproate to pediatric patients (n=6) revealed a decrease in protein binding and an inhibition of metabolism of valproate. Valproate free fraction was increased 4-fold in the presence of aspirin compared to valproate alone. The β-oxidation pathway consisting of 2-E-valproic acid, 3-OH-valproic acid, and 3-keto valproic acid was decreased from 25% of total metabolites excreted on valproate alone to 8.3% in the presence of aspirin. Caution should be observed if valproate and aspirin are to be co-administered.

Felbamate—A study involving the co-administration of 1200 mg/day of felbamate with valproate to patients with epilepsy (n=10) revealed an increase in mean valproate peak concentration by 35% (from 86 to 115 μg/mL) compared to valproate alone. Increasing the felbamate dose to 2400 mg/day increased the mean valproate peak concentration to 133 μg/mL (another 16% increase). A decrease in valproate dosage may be necessary when felbamate therapy is initiated.

Meropenem— Subtherapeutic valproic acid levels have been reported when meropenem was coadministered.

Rifampin—A study involving the administration of a single dose of valproate (7 mg/kg) 36 hours after 5 nights of daily dosing with rifampin (600 mg) revealed a 40% increase in the oral clearance of valproate. Valproate dosage adjustment may be necessary when it is co-administered with rifampin.

Drugs for which either no interaction or a likely clinically unimportant interaction has been observed:

Antacids—A study involving the co-administration of valproate 500 mg with commonly administered antacids (Maalox, Trisogel, and Titralac—160 mEq doses) did not reveal any effect on the extent of absorption of valproate.

Chlorpromazine—A study involving the administration of 100 to 300 mg/day of chlorpromazine to schizophrenic patients already receiving valproate (200 mg BID) revealed a 15% increase in trough plasma levels of valproate.

Haloperidol—A study involving the administration of 6 to 10 mg/day of haloperidol to schizophrenic patients already receiving valproate (200 mg BID) revealed no significant changes in valproate trough plasma levels.

Cimetidine and Ranitidine—Cimetidine and ranitidine do not affect the clearance of valproate.

Effects of Valproate on Other Drugs

Valproate has been found to be a weak inhibitor of some P450 isozymes, epoxide hydrase, and glucuronyl transferases.

The following list provides information about the potential for an influence of valproate co-administration on the pharmacokinetics or pharmacodynamics of several commonly prescribed medications. The list is not exhaustive, since new interactions are continuously being reported.

Drugs for which a potentially important valproate interaction has been observed:

Amitriptyline/Nortriptyline—Administration of a single oral 50 mg dose of amitriptyline to 15 normal volunteers (10 males and 5 females) who received valproate (500 mg BID) resulted in a 21% decrease in plasma clearance of amitriptyline and a 34% decrease in the net clearance of nortriptyline. Rare postmarketing reports of concurrent use of valproate and amitriptyline resulting in an increased amitriptyline level have been received. Concurrent use of valproate and amitriptyline has rarely been associated with toxicity. Monitoring of amitriptyline levels should be considered for patients taking valproate concomitantly with amitriptyline. Consideration should be given to lowering the dose of amitriptyline/nortriptyline in the presence of valproate.

Carbamazepine/carbamazepine-10,11-Epoxide—Serum levels of carbamazepine (CBZ) decreased 17% while that of carbamazepine-10,11-epoxide (CBZ-E) increased by 45% upon co-administration of valproate and CBZ to epileptic patients.

Clonazepam—The concomitant use of valproic acid and clonazepam may induce absence status in patients with a history of absence type seizures.

Diazepam—Valproate displaces diazepam from its plasma albumin binding sites and inhibits its metabolism. Co-administration of valproate (1500 mg daily) increased the free fraction of diazepam (10 mg) by 90% in healthy volunteers (n=6). Plasma clearance and volume of distribution for free diazepam were reduced by 25% and 20%, respectively, in the presence of valproate. The elimination half-life of diazepam remained unchanged upon addition of valproate.

Ethosuximide—Valproate inhibits the metabolism of ethosuximide. Administration of a single ethosuximide dose of 500 mg with valproate (800 to 1600 mg/day) to healthy volunteers (n=6) was accompanied by a 25% increase in elimination half-life of ethosuximide and a 15% decrease in its total clearance as compared to ethosuximide alone. Patients receiving valproate and ethosuximide, especially along with other anticonvulsants, should be monitored for alterations in serum concentrations of both drugs.

Lamotrigine—In a steady-state study involving 10 healthy volunteers, the elimination half-life of lamotrigine increased from 26 to 70 hours with valproate co-administration (a 165% increase). The dose of lamotrigine should be reduced when co-administered with valproate. Serious skin reactions (such as Stevens-Johnson Syndrome and toxic epidermal necrolysis) have been reported with concomitant lamotrigine and valproate administration. See lamotrigine package insert for details on lamotrigine dosing with concomitant valproate administration.

Phenobarbital—Valproate was found to inhibit the metabolism of phenobarbital. Co-administration of valproate (250 mg BID for 14 days) with phenobarbital to normal subjects (n=6) resulted in a 50% increase in half-life and a 30% decrease in plasma clearance of phenobarbital (60 mg single-dose). The fraction of phenobarbital dose excreted unchanged increased by 50% in presence of valproate.

There is evidence for severe CNS depression, with or without significant elevations of barbiturate or valproate serum concentrations. All patients receiving concomitant barbiturate therapy should be closely monitored for neurological toxicity. Serum barbiturate concentrations should be obtained, if possible, and the barbiturate dosage decreased, if appropriate.

Primidone, which is metabolized to a barbiturate, may be involved in a similar interaction with valproate.

Phenytoin—Valproate displaces phenytoin from its plasma albumin binding sites and inhibits its hepatic metabolism. Co-administration of valproate (400 mg TID) with phenytoin (250 mg) in normal volunteers (n=7) was associated with a 60% increase in the free fraction of phenytoin. Total plasma clearance and apparent volume of distribution of phenytoin increased 30% in the presence of valproate. Both the clearance and apparent volume of distribution of free phenytoin were reduced by 25%.

In patients with epilepsy, there have been reports of breakthrough seizures occurring with the combination of valproate and phenytoin. The dosage of phenytoin should be adjusted as required by the clinical situation.

Tolbutamide—From *in vitro* experiments, the unbound fraction of tolbutamide was increased from 20% to 50% when added to plasma samples taken from patients treated with valproate. The clinical relevance of this displacement is unknown.

Warfarin—In an *in vitro* study, valproate increased the unbound fraction of warfarin by up to 32.6%. The therapeutic relevance of this is unknown; however, coagulation tests should be monitored if valproate therapy is instituted in patients taking anticoagulants.

Zidovudine—In six patients who were seropositive for HIV, the clearance of zidovudine (100 mg q8h) was decreased by 38% after administration of valproate (250 or 500 mg q8h); the half-life of zidovudine was unaffected.

Drugs for which either no interaction or a likely clinically unimportant interaction has been observed:

Acetaminophen—Valproate had no effect on any of the pharmacokinetic parameters of acetaminophen when it was concurrently administered to three epileptic patients.

Clozapine—In psychotic patients (n=11), no interaction was observed when valproate was co-administered with clozapine.

Lithium—Co-administration of valproate (500 mg BID) and lithium carbonate (300 mg TID) to normal male volunteers (n=16) had no effect on the steady-state kinetics of lithium.

Lorazepam—Concomitant administration of valproate (500 mg BID) and lorazepam (1 mg BID) in normal male volunteers (n=9) was accompanied by a 17% decrease in the plasma clearance of lorazepam.

Oral Contraceptive Steroids—Administration of a single-dose of ethinyloestradiol (50 µg)/levonorgestrel (250 µg) to 6 women on valproate (200 mg BID) therapy for 2 months did not reveal any pharmacokinetic interaction.

Carcinogenesis, Mutagenesis, Impairment of Fertility

Carcinogenesis

Valproic acid was administered orally to Sprague Dawley rats and ICR (HA/ICR) mice at doses of 80 and 170 mg/kg/day (approximately 10 to 50% of the maximum human daily dose on a mg/m^2 basis) for two years. A variety of neoplasms were observed in both species. The chief findings were a statistically significant increase in the incidence of subcutaneous fibrosarcomas in high dose male rats receiving valproic acid and a statistically significant dose-related trend for benign pulmonary adenomas in male mice receiving valproic acid. The significance of these findings for humans is unknown.

Mutagenesis

Valproate was not mutagenic in an *in vitro* bacterial assay (Ames test), did not produce dominant lethal effects in mice, and did not increase chromosome aberration frequency in an *in vivo* cytogenetic study in rats. Increased frequencies of sister chromatid exchange (SCE) have been reported in a study of epileptic children taking valproate, but this association was not observed in another study conducted in adults. There is some evidence that increased SCE frequencies may be associated with epilepsy. The biological significance of an increase in SCE frequency is not known.

Fertility

Chronic toxicity studies in juvenile and adult rats and dogs demonstrated reduced spermatogenesis and testicular atrophy at oral doses of 400 mg/kg/day or greater in rats (approximately equivalent to or greater than the maximum human daily dose on a mg/m^2 basis) and 150 mg/kg/day or greater in dogs (approximately 1.4 times the maximum human daily dose or greater on a mg/m^2 basis). Segment I fertility studies in rats have shown oral doses up to 350 mg/kg/day (approximately equal to the maximum human daily dose on a mg/m^2 basis) for 60 days to have no effect on fertility. THE EFFECT OF VALPROATE ON TESTICULAR DEVELOPMENT AND ON SPERM PRODUCTION AND FERTILITY IN HUMANS IS UNKNOWN.

Pregnancy

Pregnancy Category D: See **WARNINGS**.

Nursing Mothers

Valproate is excreted in breast milk. Concentrations in breast milk have been reported to be 1-10% of serum concentrations. It is not known what effect this would have on a nursing infant. Consideration should be given to discontinuing nursing when valproate is administered to a nursing woman.

Pediatric Use

Experience with oral valproate has indicated that pediatric patients under the age of two years are at a considerably increased risk of developing fatal hepatotoxicity, especially those with the aforementioned conditions (see **BOXED WARNING**). The safety of DEPACON has not been studied in individuals below the age of 2 years. If a decision is made to use DEPACON in this age group, it should be used with extreme caution and as a sole agent. The benefits of therapy should be weighed against the risks. Above the age of 2 years, experience in epilepsy has indicated that the incidence of fatal hepatotoxicity decreases considerably in progressively older patient groups.

Younger children, especially those receiving enzyme-inducing drugs, will require larger maintenance doses to attain targeted total and unbound valproic acid concentrations.

The variability in free fraction limits the clinical usefulness of monitoring total serum valproic acid concentrations. Interpretation of valproic acid concentrations in children should include consideration of factors that affect hepatic metabolism and protein binding.

No unique safety concerns were identified in the 35 patients age 2 to 17 years who received DEPACON in clinical trials.

The basic toxicology and pathologic manifestations of valproate sodium in neonatal (4-day old) and juvenile (14-day old) rats are similar to those seen in young adult rats. However, additional findings, including renal alterations in juvenile rats and renal alterations and retinal dysplasia in neonatal rats, have been reported. These findings occurred at 240 mg/kg/day, a dosage approximately equivalent to the human maximum recommended daily dose on a mg/m^2 basis. They were not seen at 90 mg/kg, or 40% of the maximum human daily dose on a mg/m^2 basis.

Geriatric Use

No patients above the age of 65 years were enrolled in double-blind prospective clinical trials of mania associated with bipolar illness. In a case review study of 583 patients, 72 patients (12%) were greater than 65 years of age. A higher percentage of patients above 65 years of age reported accidental injury, infection, pain, somnolence, and tremor. Discontinuation of valproate was occasionally associated with the latter two events. It is not clear whether these events indicate additional risk or whether they result from preexisting medical illness and concomitant medication use among these patients.

A study of elderly patients with dementia revealed drug related somnolence and discontinuation for somnolence (see **WARNINGS—Somnolence in the Elderly**).

The starting dose should be reduced in these patients, and dosage reductions or discontinuation should be considered in patients with excessive somnolence (see **DOSAGE AND ADMINISTRATION**).

No unique safety concerns were identified in the 21 patients > 65 years of age receiving DEPACON in clinical trials.

ADVERSE REACTIONS

The adverse events that can result from DEPACON use include all of those associated with oral forms of valproate. The following describes experience specifically with DEPACON. DEPACON has been generally well tolerated in clinical trials involving 111 healthy adult male volunteers and 352 patients with epilepsy, given at doses of 125 to 6000 mg (total daily dose). A total of 2% of patients discontinued treatment with DEPACON due to adverse events. The most common adverse events leading to discontinuation were 2 cases each of nausea/vomiting and elevated amylase. Other adverse events leading to discontinuation were hallucinations, pneumonia, headache, injection site reaction, and abnormal gait. Dizziness and injection site pain were observed more frequently at a 100 mg/min infusion rate than at rates up to 33 mg/min. At a 200 mg/min rate, dizziness and taste perversion occurred more frequently than at a 100 mg/min rate. The maximum rate of infusion studied was 200 mg/min.

Adverse events reported by at least 0.5% of all subjects/patients in clinical trials of DEPACON are summarized in Table 1.

Table 1
Adverse Events Reported During Studies of DEPACON

Body System/Event	N = 463
Body as a Whole	
Chest Pain	1.7%
Headache	4.3%
Injection Site Inflammation	0.6%
Injection Site Pain	2.6%
Injection Site Reaction	2.4%
Pain (unspecified)	1.3%
Cardiovascular	
Vasodilation	0.9%
Dermatologic	
Sweating	0.9%
Digestive System	
Abdominal Pain	1.1%
Diarrhea	0.9%
Nausea	3.2%
Vomiting	1.3%
Nervous System	
Dizziness	5.2%
Euphoria	0.9%
Hypesthesia	0.6%
Nervousness	0.9%
Paresthesia	0.9%
Somnolence	1.7%
Tremor	0.6%
Respiratory	
Pharyngitis	0.6%
Special Senses	
Taste Perversion	1.9%

In a separate clinical safety trial, 112 patients with epilepsy were given infusions of DEPACON (up to 15 mg/kg) over 5 to 10 minutes (1.5-3.0 mg/kg/min). The common adverse events (>2%) were somnolence (10.7%), dizziness (7.1%), paresthesia (7.1%), asthenia (7.1%), nausea (6.3%), and headache (2.7%). While the incidence of these adverse events was generally higher than in Table 1 (experience encompassing the standard, much slower infusion rates), e.g., somnolence (1.7%), dizziness (5.2%), paresthesia (0.9%), asthenia (0%), nausea (3.2%), and headache (4.3%), a direct comparison between the incidence of adverse events in the 2 cohorts cannot be made because of differences in patient populations and study designs.

Ammonia levels have not been systematically studied after IV valproate, so that an estimate of the incidence of hyperammonemia after IV DEPACON cannot be provided. Hyperammonemia with encephalopathy has been reported in 2 patients after infusions of DEPACON.

Epilepsy

Based on a placebo-controlled trial of adjunctive therapy for treatment of complex partial seizures, DEPAKOTE (divalproex sodium) was generally well tolerated with most adverse events rated as mild to moderate in severity. Intolerance was the primary reason for discontinuation in the DEPAKOTE-treated patients (6%), compared to 1% of placebo-treated patients.

Continued on next page

Depacon—Cont.

Table 2 lists treatment-emergent adverse events which were reported by ≥ 5% of DEPAKOTE-treated patients and for which the incidence was greater than in the placebo group, in the placebo-controlled trial of adjunctive therapy for treatment of complex partial seizures. Since patients were also treated with other antiepilepsy drugs, it is not possible, in most cases, to determine whether the following adverse events can be ascribed to DEPAKOTE alone, or the combination of DEPAKOTE and other antiepilepsy drugs.

Table 2
Adverse Events Reported by ≥ 5% of Patients Treated with DEPAKOTE During Placebo-Controlled Trial of Adjunctive Therapy for Complex Partial Seizures

Body System/Event	Depakote (%) (n = 77)	Placebo (%) (n = 70)
Body as a Whole		
Headache	31	21
Asthenia	27	7
Fever	6	4
Gastrointestinal System		
Nausea	48	14
Vomiting	27	7
Abdominal Pain	23	6
Diarrhea	13	6
Anorexia	12	0
Dyspepsia	8	4
Constipation	5	1
Nervous System		
Somnolence	27	11
Tremor	25	6
Dizziness	25	13
Diplopia	16	9
Amblyopia/Blurred Vision	12	9
Ataxia	8	1
Nystagmus	8	1
Emotional Lability	6	4
Thinking Abnormal	6	0
Amnesia	5	1
Respiratory System		
Flu Syndrome	12	9
Infection	12	6
Bronchitis	5	1
Rhinitis	5	4
Other		
Alopecia	6	1
Weight Loss	6	0

Table 3 lists treatment-emergent adverse events which were reported by ≥ 5% of patients in the high dose DEPAKOTE group, and for which the incidence was greater than in the low dose group, in a controlled trial of DEPAKOTE monotherapy treatment of complex partial seizures. Since patients were being titrated off another antiepilepsy drug during the first portion of the trial, it is not possible, in many cases, to determine whether the following adverse events can be ascribed to DEPAKOTE alone, or the combination of DEPAKOTE and other antiepilepsy drugs.

Table 3
Adverse Events Reported by ≥ 5% of Patients in the High Dose Group in the Controlled Trial of DEPAKOTE Monotherapy for Complex Partial Seizures[1]

Body System/Event	High Dose (%) (n = 131)	Low Dose (%) (n = 134)
Body as a Whole		
Asthenia	21	10
Digestive System		
Nausea	34	26
Diarrhea	23	19
Vomiting	23	15
Abdominal Pain	12	9
Anorexia	11	4
Dyspepsia	11	10
Hemic/Lymphatic System		
Thrombocytopenia	24	1
Ecchymosis	5	4
Metabolic/Nutritional		
Weight Gain	9	4
Peripheral Edema	8	3
Nervous System		
Tremor	57	19
Somnolence	30	18
Dizziness	18	13
Insomnia	15	9
Nervousness	11	7
Amnesia	7	4
Nystagmus	7	1
Depression	5	4
Respiratory System		
Infection	20	13
Pharyngitis	8	2
Dyspnea	5	1
Skin and Appendages		
Alopecia	24	13
Special Senses		
Amblyopia/Blurred Vision	8	4
Tinnitus	7	1

[1] Headache was the only adverse event that occurred in ≥ 5% of patients in the high dose group and at an equal or greater incidence in the low dose group.

The following additional adverse events were reported by greater than 1% but less than 5% of the 358 patients treated with DEPAKOTE in the controlled trials of complex partial seizures:

Body as a Whole: Back pain, chest pain, malaise.
Cardiovascular System: Tachycardia, hypertension, palpitation.
Digestive System: Increased appetite, flatulence, hematemesis, eructation, pancreatitis, periodontal abscess.
Hemic and Lymphatic System: Petechia.
Metabolic and Nutritional Disorders: SGOT increased, SGPT increased.
Musculoskeletal System: Myalgia, twitching, arthralgia, leg cramps, myasthenia.
Nervous System: Anxiety, confusion, abnormal gait, paresthesia, hypertonia, incoordination, abnormal dreams, personality disorder.
Respiratory System: Sinusitis, cough increased, pneumonia, epistaxis.
Skin and Appendages: Rash, pruritus, dry skin.
Special Senses: Taste perversion, abnormal vision, deafness, otitis media.
Urogenital System: Urinary incontinence, vaginitis, dysmenorrhea, amenorrhea, urinary frequency.

Other Patient Populations

Adverse events that have been reported with all dosage forms of valproate from epilepsy trials, spontaneous reports, and other sources are listed below by body system.

Gastrointestinal: The most commonly reported side effects at the initiation of therapy are nausea, vomiting, and indigestion. These effects are usually transient and rarely require discontinuation of therapy. Diarrhea, abdominal cramps, and constipation have been reported. Both anorexia with some weight loss and increased appetite with weight gain have also been reported. The administration of delayed-release divalproex sodium may result in reduction of gastrointestinal side effects in some patients using oral therapy.

CNS Effects: Sedative effects have occurred in patients receiving valproate alone but occur most often in patients receiving combination therapy. Sedation usually abates upon reduction of other antiepileptic medication. Tremor (may be dose-related), hallucinations, ataxia, headache, nystagmus, diplopia, asterixis, "spots before eyes", dysarthria, dizziness, confusion, hypesthesia, vertigo, incoordination, and parkinsonism have been reported with the use of valproate. Rare cases of coma have occurred in patients receiving valproate alone or in conjunction with phenobarbital. In rare instances encephalopathy with or without fever has developed shortly after the introduction of valproate monotherapy without evidence of hepatic dysfunction or inappropriately high plasma valproate levels. Although recovery has been described following drug withdrawal, there have been fatalities in patients with hyperammonemic encephalopathy, particularly in patients with underlying urea cycle disorders (see **WARNINGS—Urea Cycle Disorders** and **PRECAUTIONS**).

Several reports have noted reversible cerebral atrophy and dementia in association with valproate therapy.

Dermatologic: Transient hair loss, skin rash, photosensitivity, generalized pruritus, erythema multiforme, and Stevens-Johnson syndrome. Rare cases of toxic epidermal necrolysis have been reported including a fatal case in a 6 month old infant taking valproate and several other concomitant medications. An additional case of toxic epidermal necrosis resulting in death was reported in a 35 year old patient with AIDS taking several concomitant medications and with a history of multiple cutaneous drug reactions. Serious skin reactions have been reported with concomitant administration of lamotrigine and valproate (see **PRECAUTIONS-Drug Interactions**).

Psychiatric: Emotional upset, depression, psychosis, aggression, hyperactivity, hostility, and behavioral deterioration.

Musculoskeletal: Weakness.

Hematologic: Thrombocytopenia and inhibition of the secondary phase of platelet aggregation may be reflected in altered bleeding time, petechiae, bruising, hematoma formation, epistaxis, and frank hemorrhage (see **PRECAUTIONS—General** and **Drug Interactions**). Relative lymphocytosis, macrocytosis, hypofibrinogenemia, leukopenia, eosinophilia, anemia including macrocytic with or without folate deficiency, bone marrow suppression, pancytopenia, aplastic anemia, agranulocytosis, and acute intermittent porphyria.

Hepatic: Minor elevations of transaminases (e.g., SGOT and SGPT) and LDH are frequent and appear to be dose-related. Occasionally, laboratory test results include increases in serum bilirubin and abnormal changes in other liver function tests. These results may reflect potentially serious hepatotoxicity (see **WARNINGS**).

Endocrine: Irregular menses, secondary amenorrhea, breast enlargement, galactorrhea, and parotid gland swelling. Abnormal thyroid function tests (see **PRECAUTIONS**).

There have been rare spontaneous reports of polycystic ovary disease. A cause and effect relationship has not been established.

Pancreatic: Acute pancreatitis including fatalities (see **WARNINGS**).

Metabolic: Hyperammonemia (see **PRECAUTIONS**), hyponatremia, and inappropriate ADH secretion.

There have been rare reports of Fanconi's syndrome occurring chiefly in children.

Decreased carnitine concentrations have been reported although the clinical relevance is undetermined.

Hyperglycinemia has occurred and was associated with a fatal outcome in a patient with preexistent nonketotic hyperglycinemia.

Genitourinary: Enuresis and urinary tract infection.

Special Senses: Hearing loss, either reversible or irreversible, has been reported; however, a cause and effect relationship has not been established. Ear pain has also been reported.

Other: Allergic reaction, anaphylaxis, edema of the extremities, lupus erythematosus, bone pain, cough increased, pneumonia, otitis media, bradycardia, cutaneous vasculitis, fever, and hypothermia.

Mania

Although DEPACON has not been evaluated for safety and efficacy in the treatment of manic episodes associated with bipolar disorder, the following adverse events not listed above were reported by 1% or more of patients from two placebo-controlled clinical trials of DEPAKOTE (DIVALPROEX SODIUM) tablets.

Body as a Whole: Chills, neck pain, neck rigidity.
Cardiovascular System: Hypotension, postural hypotension, vasodilation.
Digestive System: Fecal incontinence, gastroenteritis, glossitis.
Musculoskeletal System: Arthrosis.
Nervous System: Agitation, catatonic reaction, hypokinesia, reflexes increased, tardive dyskinesia, vertigo.
Skin and Appendages: Furunculosis, maculopapular rash, seborrhea.
Special Senses: Conjunctivitis, dry eyes, eye pain.
Urogenital: Dysuria.

Migraine

Although DEPACON has not been evaluated for safety and efficacy in the prophylactic treatment of migraine headaches, the following adverse events not listed above were reported by 1% or more of patients from two placebo-controlled clinical trials of DEPAKOTE (DIVALPROEX SODIUM) tablets.

Body as a Whole: Face edema.
Digestive System: Dry mouth, stomatitis.
Urogenital System: Cystitis, metrorrhagia, and vaginal hemorrhage.

OVERDOSAGE

Overdosage with valproate may result in somnolence, heart block, and deep coma. Fatalities have been reported; however patients have recovered from valproate serum concentrations as high as 2120 µg/mL.

In overdose situations, the fraction of drug not bound to protein is high and hemodialysis or tandem hemodialysis plus hemoperfusion may result in significant removal of drug. General supportive measures should be applied with particular attention to the maintenance of adequate urinary output.

Naloxone has been reported to reverse the CNS depressant effects of valproate overdosage. Because naloxone could theoretically also reverse the antiepilepsy effects of valproate, it should be used with caution in patients with epilepsy.

DOSAGE AND ADMINISTRATION

DEPACON IS FOR INTRAVENOUS USE ONLY.

Use of DEPACON for periods of more than 14 days has not been studied. Patients should be switched to oral valproate products as soon as it is clinically feasible.

DEPACON should be administered as a 60 minute infusion (but not more than 20 mg/min) with the same frequency as the oral products, although plasma concentration monitoring and dosage adjustments may be necessary.

In one clinical safety study, approximately 90 patients with epilepsy and with no measurable plasma levels of valproate were given single infusions of DEPACON (up to 15 mg/kg and mean dose of 1184 mg) over 5-10 minutes (1.5-3.0 mg/kg/min). Patients generally tolerated the more rapid infusions well (see **ADVERSE REACTIONS**). This study was not designed to assess the effectiveness of these regimens. For pharmacokinetics with rapid infusions, see **CLINICAL PHARMACOLOGY, Pharmacokinetics—Bioavailability**.

Initial Exposure to Valproate:

The following dosage recommendations were obtained from studies utilizing oral divalproex sodium products.

Complex Partial Seizures: For adults and children 10 years of age or older.

Monotherapy (Initial Therapy): DEPACON has not been systematically studied as initial therapy. Patients should initiate therapy at 10 to 15 mg/kg/day. The dosage should be increased by 5 to 10 mg/kg/week to achieve optimal clinical response. Ordinarily, optimal clinical response is achieved at daily doses below 60 mg/kg/day. If satisfactory clinical response has not been achieved, plasma levels should be measured to determine whether or not they are in the usually accepted therapeutic range (50 to 100 µg/mL). No recommendation regarding the safety of valproate for use at doses above 60 mg/kg/day can be made.

The probability of thrombocytopenia increases significantly at total trough valproate plasma concentrations above 110 µg/mL in females and 135 µg/mL in males. The benefit of improved seizure control with higher doses should be weighed against the possibility of a greater incidence of adverse reactions.

Conversion to Monotherapy: Patients should initiate therapy at 10 to 15 mg/kg/day. The dosage should be increased by 5 to 10 mg/kg/week to achieve optimal clinical response. Ordinarily, optimal clinical response is achieved at daily doses below 60 mg/kg/day. If satisfactory clinical response has not been achieved, plasma levels should be measured to determine whether or not they are in the usually accepted therapeutic range (50-100 µg/mL). No recommendation regarding the safety of valproate for use at doses above 60 mg/kg/day can be made. Concomitant antiepilepsy drug (AED) dosage can ordinarily be reduced by approximately 25% every 2 weeks. This reduction may be started at initiation of DEPACON therapy, or delayed by 1 to 2 weeks if there is a concern that seizures are likely to occur with a reduction. The speed and duration of withdrawal of the concomitant AED can be highly variable, and patients should be monitored closely during this period for increased seizure frequency.

Adjunctive Therapy: DEPACON may be added to the patient's regimen at a dosage of 10 to 15 mg/kg/day. The dosage may be increased by 5 to 10 mg/kg/week to achieve optimal clinical response. Ordinarily, optimal clinical response is achieved at daily doses below 60 mg/kg/day. If satisfactory clinical response has not been achieved, plasma levels should be measured to determine whether or not they are in the usually accepted therapeutic range (50 to 100 µg/mL). No recommendation regarding the safety of valproate for use at doses above 60 mg/kg/day can be made. If the total daily dose exceeds 250 mg, it should be given in divided doses.

In a study of adjunctive therapy for complex partial seizures in which patients were receiving either carbamazepine or phenytoin in addition to DEPAKOTE (divalproex sodium), no adjustment of carbamazepine or phenytoin dosage was needed (see **CLINICAL STUDIES**). However, since valproate may interact with these or other concurrently administered AEDs as well as other drugs (see **Drug Interactions**), periodic plasma concentration determinations of concomitant AEDs are recommended during the early course of therapy (see **PRECAUTIONS—Drug Interactions**).

Simple and Complex Absence Seizures: The recommended initial dose is 15 mg/kg/day, increasing at one week intervals by 5 to 10 mg/kg/day until seizures are controlled or side effects preclude further increases. The maximum recommended dosage is 60 mg/kg/day. If the total daily dose exceeds 250 mg, it should be given in divided doses.

A good correlation has not been established between daily dose, serum concentrations, and therapeutic effect. However, therapeutic valproate serum concentrations for most patients with absence seizures is considered to range from 50 to 100 µg/mL. Some patients may be controlled with lower or higher serum concentrations (see **CLINICAL PHARMACOLOGY**).

As the DEPACON dosage is titrated upward, blood concentrations of phenobarbital and/or phenytoin may be affected (see **PRECAUTIONS**).

Antiepilepsy drugs should not be abruptly discontinued in patients in whom the drug is administered to prevent major seizures because of the strong possibility of precipitating status epilepticus with attendant hypoxia and threat to life.

Replacement Therapy:

When switching from oral valproate products, the total daily dose of DEPACON should be equivalent to the total daily dose of the oral valproate product (see **CLINICAL PHARMACOLOGY**), and should be administered as a 60 minute infusion (but not more than 20 mg/min) with the same frequency as the oral products, although plasma concentration monitoring and dosage adjustments may be necessary. Patients receiving doses near the maximum recommended daily dose of 60 mg/kg/day, particularly those not receiving enzyme-inducing drugs, should be monitored more closely. If the total daily dose exceeds 250 mg, it should be given in a divided regimen. There is no experience with more rapid infusions in patients receiving DEPACON as replacement therapy. However, the equivalence shown between DEPACON and oral valproate products (DEPAKOTE) at steady state was only evaluated in an every 6 hour regimen. Whether, when DEPACON is given less frequently (i.e., twice or three times a day), trough levels fall below those that result from an oral dosage form given via the same regimen, is unknown. For this reason, when DEPACON is given twice or three times a day, close monitoring of trough plasma levels may be needed.

General Dosing Advice

Dosing in Elderly Patients—Due to a decrease in unbound clearance of valproate and possibly a greater sensitivity to somnolence in the elderly, the starting dose should be reduced in these patients. Dosage should be increased more slowly and with regular monitoring for fluid and nutritional intake, dehydration, somnolence, and other adverse events. Dose reductions or discontinuation of valproate should be considered in patients with decreased food or fluid intake and in patients with excessive somnolence. The ultimate therapeutic dose should be achieved on the basis of both tolerability and clinical response (see **WARNINGS**).

Dose-Related Adverse Events—The frequency of adverse effects (particularly elevated liver enzymes and thrombocytopenia) may be dose-related. The probability of thrombocytopenia appears to increase significantly at total valproate concentrations of ≥ 110 µg/mL (females) or ≥ 135 µg/mL (males) (see **PRECAUTIONS**).

The benefit of improved therapeutic effect with higher doses should be weighed against the possibility of a greater incidence of adverse reactions.

Administration

Rapid infusion of DEPACON has been associated with an increase in adverse events. There is limited experience with infusion times of less than 60 minutes or rates of infusion > 20 mg/min in patients with epilepsy (see **ADVERSE REACTIONS**).

DEPACON should be administered intravenously as a 60 minute infusion, as noted above. It should be diluted with at least 50 mL of a compatible diluent. Any unused portion of the vial contents should be discarded.

Parenteral drug products should be inspected visually for particulate matter and discoloration prior to administration whenever solution and container permit.

Compatibility and Stability

DEPACON was found to be physically compatible and chemically stable in the following parenteral solutions for at least 24 hours when stored in glass or polyvinyl chloride (PVC) bags at controlled room temperature 15-30°C (59-86°F).

- dextrose (5%) injection, USP
- sodium chloride (0.9%) injection, USP
- lactated ringer's injection, USP

HOW SUPPLIED

DEPACON (valproate sodium injection), equivalent to 100 mg of valproic acid per mL, is a clear, colorless solution in 5 mL single-dose vials, available in trays of 10 vials (**NDC** 0074-1564-10).

Recommended storage: Store vials at controlled room temperature 15-30°C (59-86°F). No preservatives have been added. Unused portion of container should be discarded.

Revised: September, 2003

ABBOTT LABORATORIES
NORTH CHICAGO, IL 60064, U.S.A.
PRINTED IN U.S.A.

DEPAKENE® ℞

[dep 'a-kāne]

VALPROIC ACID
CAPSULES and SYRUP
℞ only

BOX WARNING:

HEPATOTOXICITY:

HEPATIC FAILURE RESULTING IN FATALITIES HAS OCCURRED IN PATIENTS RECEIVING VALPROIC ACID. EXPERIENCE HAS INDICATED THAT CHILDREN UNDER THE AGE OF TWO YEARS ARE AT A CONSIDERABLY INCREASED RISK OF DEVELOPING FATAL HEPATOTOXICITY, ESPECIALLY THOSE ON MULTIPLE ANTICONVULSANTS, THOSE WITH CONGENITAL METABOLIC DISORDERS, THOSE WITH SEVERE SEIZURE DISORDERS ACCOMPANIED BY MENTAL RETARDATION, AND THOSE WITH ORGANIC BRAIN DISEASE. WHEN DEPAKENE PRODUCTS ARE USED IN THIS PATIENT GROUP, THEY SHOULD BE USED WITH EXTREME CAUTION AND AS A SOLE AGENT. THE BENEFITS OF THERAPY SHOULD BE WEIGHED AGAINST THE RISKS. ABOVE THIS AGE GROUP, EXPERIENCE IN EPILEPSY HAS INDICATED THAT THE INCIDENCE OF FATAL HEPATOTOXICITY DECREASES CONSIDERABLY IN PROGRESSIVELY OLDER PATIENT GROUPS.

THESE INCIDENTS USUALLY HAVE OCCURRED DURING THE FIRST SIX MONTHS OF TREATMENT. SERIOUS OR FATAL HEPATOTOXICITY MAY BE PRECEDED BY NON-SPECIFIC SYMPTOMS SUCH AS MALAISE, WEAKNESS, LETHARGY, FACIAL EDEMA, ANOREXIA, AND VOMITING. IN PATIENTS WITH EPILEPSY, A LOSS OF SEIZURE CONTROL MAY ALSO OCCUR. PATIENTS SHOULD BE MONITORED CLOSELY FOR APPEARANCE OF THESE SYMPTOMS. LIVER FUNCTION TESTS SHOULD BE PERFORMED PRIOR TO THERAPY AND AT FREQUENT INTERVALS THEREAFTER, ESPECIALLY DURING THE FIRST SIX MONTHS.

TERATOGENICITY:

VALPROATE CAN PRODUCE TERATOGENIC EFFECTS SUCH AS NEURAL TUBE DEFECTS (E.G., SPINA BIFIDA). ACCORDINGLY, THE USE OF VALPROATE PRODUCTS IN WOMEN OF CHILDBEARING POTENTIAL REQUIRES THAT THE BENEFITS OF ITS USE BE WEIGHED AGAINST THE RISK OF INJURY TO THE FETUS.

PANCREATITIS:

CASES OF LIFE-THREATENING PANCREATITIS HAVE BEEN REPORTED IN BOTH CHILDREN AND ADULTS RECEIVING VALPROATE. SOME OF THE CASES HAVE BEEN DESCRIBED AS HEMORRHAGIC WITH A RAPID PROGRESSION FROM INITIAL SYMPTOMS TO DEATH. CASES HAVE BEEN REPORTED SHORTLY AFTER INITIAL USE AS WELL AS AFTER SEVERAL YEARS OF USE. PATIENTS AND GUARDIANS SHOULD BE WARNED THAT ABDOMINAL PAIN, NAUSEA, VOMITING, AND/OR ANOREXIA CAN BE SYMPTOMS OF PANCREATITIS THAT REQUIRE PROMPT MEDICAL EVALUATION. IF PANCREATITIS IS DIAGNOSED, VALPROATE SHOULD ORDINARILY BE DISCONTINUED. ALTERNATIVE TREATMENT FOR THE UNDERLYING MEDICAL CONDITION SHOULD BE INITIATED AS CLINICALLY INDICATED. (See **WARNINGS** and **PRECAUTIONS**.)

DESCRIPTION

DEPAKENE (valproic acid) is a carboxylic acid designated as 2-propylpentanoic acid. It is also known as dipropylacetic acid. Valproic acid has the following structure:

$$(CH_3-CH_2-CH_2)_2CH-C(=O)OH$$

Valproic acid (pKa 4.8) has a molecular weight of 144 and occurs as a colorless liquid with a characteristic odor. It is slightly soluble in water (1.3 mg/mL) and very soluble in organic solvents.

DEPAKENE capsules and syrup are antiepileptics for oral administration. Each soft elastic capsule contains 250 mg valproic acid. The syrup contains the equivalent of 250 mg valproic acid per 5 mL as the sodium salt.

Inactive Ingredients

250 mg capsules: corn oil, FD&C Yellow No. 6, gelatin, glycerin, iron oxide, methylparaben, propylparaben, and titanium dioxide.

Syrup: FD&C Red No. 40, glycerin, methylparaben, propylparaben, sorbitol, sucrose, water, and natural and artificial flavors.

CLINICAL PHARMACOLOGY

Pharmacodynamics

Valproic acid dissociates to the valproate ion in the gastrointestinal tract. The mechanisms by which valproate exerts its antiepileptic effects have not been established. It has been suggested that its activity in epilepsy is related to increased brain concentrations of gamma-aminobutyric acid (GABA).

Pharmacokinetics

Absorption/Bioavailability

Equivalent oral doses of DEPAKOTE (divalproex sodium) products and DEPAKENE (valproic acid) capsules deliver equivalent quantities of valproate ion systemically. Although the rate of valproate ion absorption may vary with the formulation administered (liquid, solid, or sprinkle), conditions of use (e.g., fasting or postprandial) and the method of administration (e.g., whether the contents of the capsule are sprinkled on food or the capsule is taken intact), these differences should be of minor clinical importance under the steady state conditions achieved in chronic use in the treatment of epilepsy.

However, it is possible that differences among the various valproate products in T_{max} and C_{max} could be important upon initiation of treatment. For example, in single dose studies, the effect of feeding had a greater influence on the rate of absorption of the DEPAKOTE tablet (increase in T_{max} from 4 to 8 hours) than on the absorption of the DEPAKOTE sprinkle capsules (increase in T_{max} from 3.3 to 4.8 hours).

While the absorption rate from the G.I. tract and fluctuation in valproate plasma concentrations vary with dosing regimen and formulation, the efficacy of valproate as an anticonvulsant in chronic use is unlikely to be affected. Experience employing dosing regimens from once-a-day to four-times-a-day, as well as studies in primate epilepsy models involving constant rate infusion, indicate that total daily systemic bioavailability (extent of absorption) is the primary determinant of seizure control and that differences in the ratios of plasma peak to trough concentrations between valproate formulations are inconsequential from a practical clinical standpoint.

Co-administration of oral valproate products with food and substitution among the various DEPAKOTE and DEPAKENE formulations should cause no clinical problems in the management of patients with epilepsy (see **DOSAGE AND ADMINISTRATION**). Nonetheless, any changes in dosage administration, or the addition or discontinuance of concomitant drugs should ordinarily be accompanied by close monitoring of clinical status and valproate plasma concentrations.

Distribution

Protein Binding:

The plasma protein binding of valproate is concentration dependent and the free fraction increases from approximately 10% at 40 µg/mL to 18.5% at 130 µg/mL. Protein binding of valproate is reduced in the elderly, in patients with chronic hepatic diseases, in patients with renal impairment, and in the presence of other drugs (e.g., aspirin). Conversely, valproate may displace certain protein-bound drugs (e.g., phenytoin, carbamazepine, warfarin, and tolbutamide). (See **PRECAUTIONS, Drug Interactions** for more detailed information on the pharmacokinetic interactions of valproate with other drugs.)

Continued on next page

Depakene—Cont.

CNS Distribution:
Valproate concentrations in cerebrospinal fluid (CSF) approximate unbound concentrations in plasma (about 10% of total concentration).
Metabolism
Valproate is metabolized almost entirely by the liver. In adult patients on monotherapy, 30-50% of an administered dose appears in urine as a glucuronide conjugate. Mitochondrial β-oxidation is the other major metabolic pathway, typically accounting for over 40% of the dose. Usually, less than 15-20% of the dose is eliminated by other oxidative mechanisms. Less than 3% of an administered dose is excreted unchanged in urine.
The relationship between dose and total valproate concentration is nonlinear; concentration does not increase proportionally with the dose, but rather, increases to a lesser extent due to saturable plasma protein binding. The kinetics of unbound drug are linear.
Elimination
Mean plasma clearance and volume of distribution for total valproate are 0.56 L/hr/1.73 m^2 and 11 L/1.73 m^2, respectively. Mean plasma clearance and volume of distribution for free valproate are 4.6 L/hr/1.73 m^2 and 92 L/1.73 m^2. Mean terminal half-life for valproate monotherapy ranged from 9 to 16 hours following oral dosing regimens of 250 to 1000 mg.
The estimates cited apply primarily to patients who are not taking drugs that affect hepatic metabolizing enzyme systems. For example, patients taking enzyme-inducing antiepileptic drugs (carbamazepine, phenytoin, and phenobarbital) will clear valproate more rapidly. Because of these changes in valproate clearance, monitoring of antiepileptic concentrations should be intensified whenever concomitant antiepileptics are introduced or withdrawn.
Special Populations
Effect of Age:
Neonates—Children within the first two months of life have a markedly decreased ability to eliminate valproate compared to older children and adults. This is a result of reduced clearance (perhaps due to delay in development of glucuronosyltransferase and other enzyme systems involved in valproate elimination) as well as increased volume of distribution (in part due to decreased plasma protein binding). For example, in one study, the half-life in children under 10 days ranged from 10 to 67 hours compared to a range of 7 to 13 hours in children greater than 2 months.
Children—Pediatric patients (i.e., between 3 months and 10 years) have 50% higher clearances expressed on weight (i.e., mL/min/kg) than do adults. Over the age of 10 years, children have pharmacokinetic parameters that approximate those of adults.
Elderly—The capacity of elderly patients (age range: 68 to 89 years) to eliminate valproate has been shown to be reduced compared to younger adults (age range: 22 to 26). Intrinsic clearance is reduced by 39%; the free fraction is increased by 44%. Accordingly, the initial dosage should be reduced in the elderly. (See **DOSAGE AND ADMINISTRATION**).
Effect of Gender:
There are no differences in the body surface area adjusted unbound clearance between males and females (4.8±0.17 and 4.7±0.07 L/hr per 1.73 m^2, respectively).
Effect of Race:
The effects of race on the kinetics of valproate have not been studied.
Effect of Disease:
Liver Disease—(See **BOXED WARNING, CONTRAINDICATIONS,** and **WARNINGS**). Liver disease impairs the capacity to eliminate valproate. In one study, the clearance of free valproate was decreased by 50% in 7 patients with cirrhosis and by 16% in 4 patients with acute hepatitis, compared with 6 healthy subjects. In that study, the half-life of valproate was increased from 12 to 18 hours. Liver disease is also associated with decreased albumin concentrations and larger unbound fractions (2 to 2.6 fold increase) of valproate. Accordingly, monitoring of total concentrations may be misleading since free concentrations may be substantially elevated in patients with hepatic disease whereas total concentrations may appear to be normal.
Renal Disease—A slight reduction (27%) in the unbound clearance of valproate has been reported in patients with renal failure (creatinine clearance < 10 mL/minute); however, hemodialysis typically reduces valproate concentrations by about 20%. Therefore, no dosage adjustment appears to be necessary in patients with renal failure. Protein binding in these patients is substantially reduced; thus, monitoring total concentrations may be misleading.

Plasma Levels and Clinical Effect
The relationship between plasma concentration and clinical response is not well documented. One contributing factor is the nonlinear, concentration dependent protein binding of valproate which affects the clearance of the drug. Thus, monitoring of total serum valproate cannot provide a reliable index of the bioactive valproate species.
For example, because the plasma protein binding of valproate is concentration dependent, the free fraction increases from approximately 10% at 40 µg/mL to 18.5% at 130 µg/mL. Higher than expected free fractions occur in the elderly, in hyperlipidemic patients, and in patients with hepatic and renal diseases.

Epilepsy:
The therapeutic range is commonly considered to be 50 to 100 µg/mL of total valproate, although some patients may be controlled with lower or higher plasma concentrations.

Clinical Trials

The studies described in the following section were conducted using DEPAKOTE (divalproex sodium) tablets.

Epilepsy
The efficacy of DEPAKOTE in reducing the incidence of complex partial seizures (CPS) that occur in isolation or in association with other seizure types was established in two controlled trials.
In one, multiclinic, placebo controlled study employing an add-on design (adjunctive therapy), 144 patients who continued to suffer eight or more CPS per 8 weeks during an 8 week period of monotherapy with doses of either carbamazepine or phenytoin sufficient to assure plasma concentrations within the "therapeutic range" were randomized to receive, in addition to their original antiepilepsy drug (AED), either DEPAKOTE or placebo. Randomized patients were to be followed for a total of 16 weeks. The following table presents the findings.

Adjunctive Therapy Study
Median Incidence of CPS per 8 Weeks

Add-on Treatment	Number of Patients	Baseline Incidence	Experimental Incidence
DEPAKOTE	75	16.0	8.9*
Placebo	69	14.5	11.5

* Reduction from baseline statistically significantly greater for DEPAKOTE than placebo at $p \leq 0.05$ level.

Figure 1 presents the proportion of patients (X axis) whose percentage reduction from baseline in complex partial seizure rates was at least as great as that indicated on the Y axis in the adjunctive therapy study. A positive percent reduction indicates an improvement (i.e., a decrease in seizure frequency), while a negative percent reduction indicates worsening. Thus, in a display of this type, the curve for an effective treatment is shifted to the left of the curve for placebo. This figure shows that the proportion of patients achieving any particular level of improvement was consistently higher for DEPAKOTE than for placebo. For example, 45% of patients treated with DEPAKOTE had a ≥50% reduction in complex partial seizure rate compared to 23% of patients treated with placebo.

Figure 1
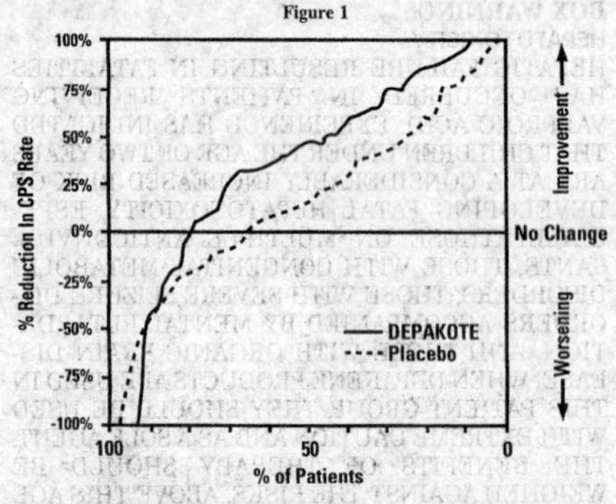

The second study assessed the capacity of DEPAKOTE to reduce the incidence of CPS when administered as the sole AED. The study compared the incidence of CPS among patients randomized to either a high or low dose treatment arm. Patients qualified for entry into the randomized comparison phase of this study only if 1) they continued to experience 2 or more CPS per 4 weeks during an 8 to 12 week long period of monotherapy with adequate doses of an AED (i.e., phenytoin, carbamazepine, phenobarbital, or primidone) and 2) they made a successful transition over a two week interval to DEPAKOTE. Patients entering the randomized phase were then brought to their assigned target dose, gradually tapered off their concomitant AED and followed for an interval as long as 22 weeks. Less than 50% of the patients randomized, however, completed the study. In patients converted to DEPAKOTE monotherapy, the mean total valproate concentrations during monotherapy were 71 and 123 µg/mL in the low dose and high dose groups, respectively.
The following table presents the findings for all patients randomized who had at least one post-randomization assessment.

Monotherapy Study
Median Incidence of CPS per 8 Weeks

Treatment	Number of Patients	Baseline Incidence	Randomized Phase Incidence
High dose DEPAKOTE	131	13.2	10.7*
Low dose DEPAKOTE	134	14.2	13.8

*Reduction from baseline statistically significantly greater for high dose than low dose at $p \leq 0.05$ level.

Figure 2 presents the proportion of patients (X axis) whose percentage reduction from baseline in complex partial seizure rates was at least as great as that indicated on the Y axis in the monotherapy study. A positive percent reduction indicates an improvement (i.e., a decrease in seizure frequency), while a negative percent reduction indicates worsening. Thus, in a display of this type, the curve for a more effective treatment is shifted to the left of the curve for a less effective treatment. This figure shows that the proportion of patients achieving any particular level of reduction was consistently higher for high dose DEPAKOTE than for low dose DEPAKOTE. For example, when switching from carbamazepine, phenytoin, phenobarbital or primidone monotherapy to high dose DEPAKOTE monotherapy, 63% of patients experienced no change or a reduction in complex partial seizure rates compared to 54% of patients receiving low dose DEPAKOTE.

Figure 2
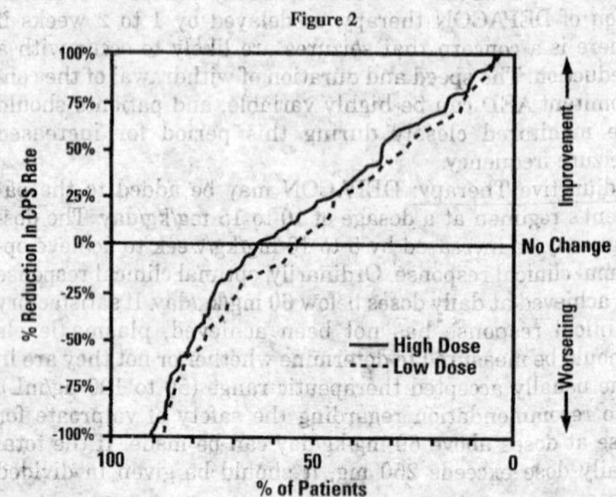

INDICATIONS AND USAGE

DEPAKENE (valproic acid) is indicated as monotherapy and adjunctive therapy in the treatment of patients with complex partial seizures that occur either in isolation or in association with other types of seizures. DEPAKENE (valproic acid) is indicated for use as sole and adjunctive therapy in the treatment of simple and complex absence seizures, and adjunctively in patients with multiple seizure types which include absence seizures.
Simple absence is defined as very brief clouding of the sensorium or loss of consciousness accompanied by certain generalized epileptic discharges without other detectable clinical signs. Complex absence is the term used when other signs are also present.
SEE **WARNINGS** FOR STATEMENT REGARDING FATAL HEPATIC DYSFUNCTION.

CONTRAINDICATIONS

VALPROIC ACID SHOULD NOT BE ADMINISTERED TO PATIENTS WITH HEPATIC DISEASE OR SIGNIFICANT HEPATIC DYSFUNCTION.
Valproic acid is contraindicated in patients with known hypersensitivity to the drug.
Valproic acid is contraindicated in patients with known urea cycle disorders (see **WARNINGS**).

WARNINGS

Hepatotoxicity
Hepatic failure resulting in fatalities has occurred in patients receiving valproic acid. These incidents usually have occurred during the first six months of treatment. Serious or fatal hepatotoxicity may be preceded by non-specific symptoms such as malaise, weakness, lethargy, facial edema, anorexia, and vomiting. In patients with epilepsy, a loss of seizure control may also occur. Patients should be monitored closely for appearance of these symptoms. Liver function tests should be performed prior to therapy and at frequent intervals thereafter, especially during the first six months. However, physicians should not rely totally on serum biochemistry since these tests may not be abnormal in all instances, but should also consider the results of careful interim medical history and physical examination. Caution should be observed when administering DEPAKENE (valproic acid) to patients with a prior history of hepatic disease. Patients on multiple anticonvulsants, children, those with congenital metabolic disorders, those with severe seizure disorders accompanied by mental retardation, and those with organic brain disease may be at particular risk. Experience has indicated that children under the age of two years are at a considerably increased risk of developing fatal hepatotoxicity, especially those with the aforementioned conditions. When DEPAKENE products are used in this patient group, they should be used with extreme caution and as a sole agent. The benefits of therapy should be weighed against the risks. Above this age group, experience has indicated that the incidence of fatal hepatotoxicity decreases considerably in progressively older patient groups.
The drug should be discontinued immediately in the presence of significant hepatic dysfunction, suspected or apparent. In some cases, hepatic dysfunction has progressed in spite of discontinuation of drug.

Pancreatitis
Cases of life-threatening pancreatitis have been reported in both children and adults receiving valproate. Some of the cases have been described as hemorrhagic with rapid progression from initial symptoms to death. Some cases have occurred shortly after initial use as well as after several

years of use. The rate based upon the reported cases exceeds that expected in the general population and there have been cases in which pancreatitis recurred after rechallenge with valproate. In clinical trials, there were 2 cases of pancreatitis without alternative etiology in 2416 patients, representing 1044 patient-years experience. Patients and guardians should be warned that abdominal pain, nausea, vomiting, and/or anorexia can be symptoms of pancreatitis that require prompt medical evaluation. If pancreatitis is diagnosed, valproate should ordinarily be discontinued. Alternative treatment for the underlying medical condition should be initiated as clinically indicated (see **BOXED WARNING**).

Urea Cycle Disorders (UCD)

Valproic acid is contraindicated in patients with known urea cycle disorders.

Hyperammonemic encephalopathy, sometimes fatal, has been reported following initiation of valproate therapy in patients with urea cycle disorders, a group of uncommon genetic abnormalities, particularly ornithine transcarbamylase deficiency. Prior to the initiation of valproate therapy, evaluation for UCD should be considered in the following patients: 1) those with a history of unexplained encephalopathy or coma, encephalopathy associated with a protein load, pregnancy-related or postpartum encephalopathy, unexplained mental retardation, or history of elevated plasma ammonia or glutamine; 2) those with cyclical vomiting and lethargy, episodic extreme irritability, ataxia, low BUN, or protein avoidance; 3) those with a family history of UCD or a family history of unexplained infant deaths (particularly males); 4) those with other signs or symptoms of UCD. Patients who develop symptoms of unexplained hyperammonemic encephalopathy while receiving valproate therapy should receive prompt treatment (including discontinuation of valproate therapy) and be evaluated for underlying urea cycle disorders (see **CONTRAINDICATIONS** and **PRECAUTIONS**).

Somnolence in the Elderly

In a double-blind, multicenter trial of valproate in elderly patients with dementia (mean age = 83 years), doses were increased by 125 mg/day to a target dose of 20 mg/kg/day. A significantly higher proportion of valproate patients had somnolence compared to placebo, and although not statistically significant, there was a higher proportion of patients with dehydration. Discontinuations for somnolence were also significantly higher than with placebo. In some patients with somnolence (approximately one-half), there was associated reduced nutritional intake and weight loss. There was a trend for the patients who experienced these events to have a lower baseline albumin concentration, lower valproate clearance, and a higher BUN. In elderly patients, dosage should be increased more slowly and with regular monitoring for fluid and nutritional intake, dehydration, somnolence, and other adverse events. Dose reductions or discontinuation of valproate should be considered in patients with decreased food or fluid intake and in patients with excessive somnolence (see **DOSAGE AND ADMINISTRATION**).

Thrombocytopenia

The frequency of adverse effects (particularly elevated liver enzymes and thrombocytopenia [see **PRECAUTIONS**]) may be dose-related. In a clinical trial of DEPAKOTE (divalproex sodium) as monotherapy in patients with epilepsy, 34/126 patients (27%) receiving approximately 50 mg/kg/day on average, had at least one value of platelets $\leq 75 \times 10^9$/L. Approximately half of these patients had treatment discontinued, with return of platelet counts to normal. In the remaining patients, platelet counts normalized with continued treatment. In this study, the probability of thrombocytopenia appeared to increase significantly at total valproate concentrations of ≥110 µg/mL (females) or ≥135 µg/mL (males). The therapeutic benefit which may accompany the higher doses should therefore be weighed against the possibility of a greater incidence of adverse effects.

Usage In Pregnancy

ACCORDING TO PUBLISHED AND UNPUBLISHED REPORTS, VALPROIC ACID MAY PRODUCE TERATOGENIC EFFECTS IN THE OFFSPRING OF HUMAN FEMALES RECEIVING THE DRUG DURING PREGNANCY. THERE ARE MULTIPLE REPORTS IN THE CLINICAL LITERATURE WHICH INDICATE THAT THE USE OF ANTIEPILEPTIC DRUGS DURING PREGNANCY RESULTS IN AN INCREASED INCIDENCE OF BIRTH DEFECTS IN THE OFFSPRING. ALTHOUGH DATA ARE MORE EXTENSIVE WITH RESPECT TO TRIMETHADIONE, PARAMETHADIONE, PHENYTOIN, AND PHENOBARBITAL, REPORTS INDICATE A POSSIBLE SIMILAR ASSOCIATION WITH THE USE OF OTHER ANTIEPILEPTIC DRUGS. THEREFORE, ANTIEPILEPSY DRUGS SHOULD BE ADMINISTERED TO WOMEN OF CHILDBEARING POTENTIAL ONLY IF THEY ARE CLEARLY SHOWN TO BE ESSENTIAL IN THE MANAGEMENT OF THEIR SEIZURES.

THE INCIDENCE OF NEURAL TUBE DEFECTS IN THE FETUS MAY BE INCREASED IN MOTHERS RECEIVING VALPROATE DURING THE FIRST TRIMESTER OF PREGNANCY. THE CENTERS FOR DISEASE CONTROL (CDC) HAS ESTIMATED THE RISK OF VALPROIC ACID EXPOSED WOMEN HAVING CHILDREN WITH SPINA BIFIDA TO BE APPROXIMATELY 1 TO 2%.

OTHER CONGENITAL ANOMALIES (E.G., CRANIOFACIAL DEFECTS, CARDIOVASCULAR MALFORMATIONS AND ANOMALIES INVOLVING VARIOUS BODY SYSTEMS), COMPATIBLE AND INCOMPATIBLE WITH LIFE, HAVE BEEN REPORTED. SUFFICIENT DATA TO DETERMINE THE INCIDENCE OF THESE CONGENITAL ANOMALIES IS NOT AVAILABLE.

THE HIGHER INCIDENCE OF CONGENITAL ANOMALIES IN ANTIEPILEPTIC DRUG-TREATED WOMEN WITH SEIZURE DISORDERS CANNOT BE REGARDED AS A CAUSE AND EFFECT RELATIONSHIP. THERE ARE INTRINSIC METHODOLOGIC PROBLEMS IN OBTAINING ADEQUATE DATA ON DRUG TERATOGENICITY IN HUMANS; GENETIC FACTORS OR THE EPILEPTIC CONDITION ITSELF, MAY BE MORE IMPORTANT THAN DRUG THERAPY IN CONTRIBUTING TO CONGENITAL ANOMALIES.

PATIENTS TAKING VALPROATE MAY DEVELOP CLOTTING ABNORMALITIES. A PATIENT WHO HAD LOW FIBRINOGEN WHEN TAKING MULTIPLE ANTICONVULSANTS INCLUDING VALPROATE GAVE BIRTH TO AN INFANT WITH AFIBRINOGENEMIA WHO SUBSEQUENTLY DIED OF HEMORRHAGE. IF VALPROATE IS USED IN PREGNANCY, THE CLOTTING PARAMETERS SHOULD BE MONITORED CAREFULLY.

HEPATIC FAILURE, RESULTING IN THE DEATH OF A NEWBORN AND OF AN INFANT, HAVE BEEN REPORTED FOLLOWING THE USE OF VALPROATE DURING PREGNANCY.

Animal studies have demonstrated valproate-induced teratogenicity. Increased frequencies of malformations, as well as intrauterine growth retardation and death, have been observed in mice, rats, rabbits, and monkeys following prenatal exposure to valproate. Malformations of the skeletal system are the most common structural abnormalities produced in experimental animals, but neural tube closure defects have been seen in mice exposed to maternal plasma valproate concentrations exceeding 230 µg/mL (2.3 times the upper limit of the human therapeutic range) during susceptible periods of embryonic development. Administration of an oral dose of 200 mg/kg/day or greater (50% of the maximum human daily dose or greater on a mg/m^2 basis) to pregnant rats during organogenesis produced malformations (skeletal, cardiac, and urogenital) and growth retardation in the offspring. These doses resulted in peak maternal plasma valproate levels of approximately 340 µg/mL or greater (3.4 times the upper limit of the human therapeutic range or greater). Behavioral deficits have been reported in the offspring of rats given a dose of 200 mg/kg/day throughout most of pregnancy. An oral dose of 350 mg/kg/day (approximately 2 times the maximum human daily dose on a mg/m^2 basis) produced skeletal and visceral malformations in rabbits exposed during organogenesis. Skeletal malformations, growth retardation, and death were observed in rhesus monkeys following administration of an oral dose of 200 mg/kg/day (equal to the maximum human daily dose on a mg/m^2 basis) during organogenesis. This dose resulted in peak maternal plasma valproate levels of approximately 280 µg/mL (2.8 times the upper limit of the human therapeutic range).

The prescribing physician will wish to weigh the benefits of therapy against the risks in treating or counseling women of childbearing potential. If this drug is used during pregnancy, or if the patient becomes pregnant while taking this drug, the patient should be apprised of the potential hazard to the fetus.

Antiepileptic drugs should not be discontinued abruptly in patients in whom the drug is administered to prevent major seizures because of the strong possibility of precipitating status epilepticus with attendant hypoxia and threat to life. In individual cases where the severity and frequency of the seizure disorder are such that the removal of medication does not pose a serious threat to the patient, discontinuation of the drug may be considered prior to and during pregnancy, although it cannot be said with any confidence that even minor seizures do not pose some hazard to the developing embryo or fetus.

Tests to detect neural tube and other defects using current accepted procedures should be considered a part of routine prenatal care in childbearing women receiving valproate.

PRECAUTIONS

Hepatic Dysfunction

See **BOXED WARNING**, **CONTRAINDICATIONS**, and **WARNINGS**.

Pancreatitis

See **BOXED WARNING** and **WARNINGS**.

Hyperammonemia

Hyperammonemia has been reported in association with valproate therapy and may be present despite normal liver function tests. In patients who develop unexplained lethargy and vomiting or changes in mental status, hyperammonemic encephalopathy should be considered and an ammonia level should be measured. If ammonia is increased, valproate therapy should be discontinued. Appropriate interventions for treatment of hyperammonemia should be initiated, and such patients should undergo investigation for underlying urea cycle disorders (see **CONTRAINDICATIONS** and **WARNINGS–Urea Cycle Disorders**).

Asymptomatic elevations of ammonia are more common and when present, require close monitoring of plasma ammonia levels. If the elevation persists, discontinuation of valproate therapy should be considered.

General

Because of reports of thrombocytopenia (see **WARNINGS**), inhibition of the secondary phase of platelet aggregation, and abnormal coagulation parameters, (e.g., low fibrinogen), platelet counts and coagulation tests are recommended before initiating therapy and at periodic intervals. It is recommended that patients receiving DEPAKENE (valproic acid) be monitored for platelet count and coagulation parameters prior to planned surgery. In a clinical trial of DEPAKOTE (divalproex sodium) as monotherapy in patients with epilepsy, 34/126 patients (27%) receiving approximately 50 mg/kg/day on average, had at least one value of platelets $\leq 75 \times 10^9$/L. Approximately half of these patients had treatment discontinued, with return of platelet counts to normal. In the remaining patients, platelet counts normalized with continued treatment. In this study, the probability of thrombocytopenia appeared to increase significantly at total valproate concentrations of ≥ 110 µg/mL (females) or ≥ 135 µg/mL (males). Evidence of hemorrhage, bruising, or a disorder of hemostasis/coagulation is an indication for reduction of the dosage or withdrawal of therapy.

Since valproate may interact with concurrently administered drugs which are capable of enzyme induction, periodic plasma concentration determinations of valproate and concomitant drugs are recommended during the early course of therapy (see **PRECAUTIONS—Drug Interactions**).

Valproate is partially eliminated in the urine as a keto-metabolite which may lead to a false interpretation of the urine ketone test.

There have been reports of altered thyroid function tests associated with valproate. The clinical significance of these is unknown.

There are *in vitro* studies that suggest valproate stimulates the replication of the HIV and CMV viruses under certain experimental conditions. The clinical consequence, if any, is not known. Additionally, the relevance of these *in vitro* findings is uncertain for patients receiving maximally suppressive antiretroviral therapy. Nevertheless, these data should be borne in mind when interpreting the results from regular monitoring of the viral load in HIV infected patients receiving valproate or when following CMV infected patients clinically.

Information for Patients

Patients and guardians should be warned that abdominal pain, nausea, vomiting, and/or anorexia can be symptoms of pancreatitis and, therefore, require further medical evaluation promptly.

Patients should be informed of the signs and symptoms associated with hyperammonemic encephalopathy (see **PRECAUTIONS—Hyperammonemia**) and be told to inform the prescriber if any of these symptoms occur.

Since DEPAKENE products may produce CNS depression, especially when combined with another CNS depressant (e.g., alcohol), patients should be advised not to engage in hazardous activities, such as driving an automobile or operating dangerous machinery, until it is known that they do not become drowsy from the drug.

Since DEPAKENE has been associated with certain types of birth defects, female patients of child-bearing age considering the use of DEPAKENE should be advised to read the **Patient Information Leaflet**, which appears as the last section of the labeling.

Drug Interactions

Effects of Co-Administered Drugs on Valproate Clearance

Drugs that affect the level of expression of hepatic enzymes, particularly those that elevate levels of glucuronosyltransferases, may increase the clearance of valproate. For example, phenytoin, carbamazepine, and phenobarbital (or primidone) can double the clearance of valproate. Thus, patients on monotherapy will generally have longer half-lives and higher concentrations than patients receiving polytherapy with antiepilepsy drugs.

In contrast, drugs that are inhibitors of cytochrome P450 isozymes, e.g., antidepressants, may be expected to have little effect on valproate clearance because cytochrome P450 microsomal mediated oxidation is a relatively minor secondary metabolic pathway compared to glucuronidation and beta-oxidation.

Because of these changes in valproate clearance, monitoring of valproate and concomitant drug concentrations should be increased whenever enzyme inducing drugs are introduced or withdrawn.

The following list provides information about the potential for an influence of several commonly prescribed medications on valproate pharmacokinetics. The list is not exhaustive nor could it be, since new interactions are continuously being reported.

Drugs for which a potentially important interaction has been observed:

Aspirin—A study involving the co-administration of aspirin at antipyretic doses (11 to 16 mg/kg) with valproate to pediatric patients (n=6) revealed a decrease in protein binding and an inhibition of metabolism of valproate. Valproate free fraction was increased 4-fold in the presence of aspirin compared to valproate alone. The β-oxidation pathway consisting of 2-E-valproic acid, 3-OH-valproic acid, and 3-keto valproic acid was decreased from 25% of total metabolites excreted on valproate alone to 8.3% in the presence of aspirin. Caution should be observed if valproate and aspirin are to be co-administered.

Felbamate—A study involving the co-administration of 1200 mg/day of felbamate with valproate to patients with epilepsy (n=10) revealed an increase in mean valproate peak concentration by 35% (from 86 to 115 µg/mL) compared to valproate alone. Increasing the felbamate dose to

Continued on next page

Depakene—Cont.

2400 mg/day increased the mean valproate peak concentration to 133 μg/mL (another 16% increase). A decrease in valproate dosage may be necessary when felbamate therapy is initiated.

Meropenem—Subtherapeutic valproic acid levels have been reported when meropenem was co-administered.

Rifampin—A study involving the administration of a single dose of valproate (7 mg/kg) 36 hours after 5 nights of daily dosing with rifampin (600 mg) revealed a 40% increase in the oral clearance of valproate. Valproate dosage adjustment may be necessary when it is co-administered with rifampin.

Drugs for which either no interaction or a likely clinically unimportant interaction has been observed:

Antacids—A study involving the co-administration of valproate 500 mg with commonly administered antacids (Maalox, Trisogel, and Titralac—160 mEq doses) did not reveal any effect on the extent of absorption of valproate.

Chlorpromazine—A study involving the administration of 100 to 300 mg/day of chlorpromazine to schizophrenic patients already receiving valproate (200 mg BID) revealed a 15% increase in trough plasma levels of valproate.

Haloperidol—A study involving the administration of 6 to 10 mg/day of haloperidol to schizophrenic patients already receiving valproate (200 mg BID) revealed no significant changes in valproate trough plasma levels.

Cimetidine and Ranitidine—Cimetidine and ranitidine do not affect the clearance of valproate.

Effects of Valproate on Other Drugs

Valproate has been found to be a weak inhibitor of some P450 isozymes, epoxide hydrase, and glucuronyltransferases.

The following list provides information about the potential for an influence of valproate co-administration on the pharmacokinetics or pharmacodynamics of several commonly prescribed medications. The list is not exhaustive, since new interactions are continuously being reported.

Drugs for which a potentially important valproate interaction has been observed:

Amitriptyline/Nortriptyline—Administration of a single oral 50 mg dose of amitriptyline to 15 normal volunteers (10 males and 5 females) who received valproate (500 mg BID) resulted in a 21% decrease in plasma clearance of amitriptyline and a 34% decrease in the net clearance of nortriptyline. Rare postmarketing reports of concurrent use of valproate and amitriptyline resulting in an increased amitriptyline level have been received. Concurrent use of valproate and amitriptyline has rarely been associated with toxicity. Monitoring of amitriptyline levels should be considered for patients taking valproate concomitantly with amitriptyline. Consideration should be given to lowering the dose of amitriptyline/nortriptyline in the presence of valproate.

Carbamazepine/carbamazepine-10,11-Epoxide—Serum levels of carbamazepine (CBZ) decreased 17% while that of carbamazepine-10,11-epoxide (CBZ-E) increased by 45% upon co-administration of valproate and CBZ to epileptic patients.

Clonazepam—The concomitant use of valproic acid and clonazepam may induce absence status in patients with a history of absence type seizures.

Diazepam—Valproate displaces diazepam from its plasma albumin binding sites and inhibits its metabolism. Co-administration of valproate (1500 mg daily) increased the free fraction of diazepam (10 mg) by 90% in healthy volunteers (n=6). Plasma clearance and volume of distribution for free diazepam were reduced by 25% and 20%, respectively, in the presence of valproate. The elimination half-life of diazepam remained unchanged upon addition of valproate.

Ethosuximide—Valproate inhibits the metabolism of ethosuximide. Administration of a single ethosuximide dose of 500 mg with valproate (800 to 1600 mg/day) to healthy volunteers (n=6) was accompanied by a 25% increase in elimination half-life of ethosuximide and a 15% decrease in its total clearance as compared to ethosuximide alone. Patients receiving valproate and ethosuximide, especially along with other anticonvulsants, should be monitored for alterations in serum concentrations of both drugs.

Lamotrigine—In a steady-state study involving 10 healthy volunteers, the elimination half-life of lamotrigine increased from 26 to 70 hours with valproate co-administration (a 165% increase). The dose of lamotrigine should be reduced when co-administered with valproate. Serious skin reactions (such as Stevens-Johnson Syndrome and toxic epidermal necrolysis) have been reported with concomitant lamotrigine and valproate administration. See lamotrigine package insert for details on lamotrigine dosing with concomitant valproate administration.

Phenobarbital—Valproate was found to inhibit the metabolism of phenobarbital. Co-administration of valproate (250 mg BID for 14 days) with phenobarbital to normal subjects (n=6) resulted in a 50% increase in half-life and a 30% decrease in plasma clearance of phenobarbital (60 mg single-dose). The fraction of phenobarbital dose excreted unchanged increased by 50% in presence of valproate.

There is evidence for severe CNS depression, with or without significant elevations of barbiturate or valproate serum concentrations. All patients receiving concomitant barbiturate therapy should be closely monitored for neurological toxicity. Serum barbiturate concentrations should be obtained, if possible, and the barbiturate dosage decreased, if appropriate.

Primidone, which is metabolized to a barbiturate, may be involved in a similar interaction with valproate.

Phenytoin—Valproate displaces phenytoin from its plasma albumin binding sites and inhibits its hepatic metabolism. Co-administration of valproate (400 mg TID) with phenytoin (250 mg) in normal volunteers (n=7) was associated with a 60% increase in the free fraction of phenytoin. Total plasma clearance and apparent volume of distribution of phenytoin increased 30% in the presence of valproate. Both the clearance and apparent volume of distribution of free phenytoin were reduced by 25%.

In patients with epilepsy, there have been reports of breakthrough seizures occurring with the combination of valproate and phenytoin. The dosage of phenytoin should be adjusted as required by the clinical situation.

Tolbutamide—From *in vitro* experiments, the unbound fraction of tolbutamide was increased from 20% to 50% when added to plasma samples taken from patients treated with valproate. The clinical relevance of this displacement is unknown.

Warfarin—In an *in vitro* study, valproate increased the unbound fraction of warfarin by up to 32.6%. The therapeutic relevance of this is unknown; however, coagulation tests should be monitored if DEPAKENE therapy is instituted in patients taking anticoagulants.

Zidovudine—In six patients who were seropositive for HIV, the clearance of zidovudine (100 mg q8h) was decreased by 38% after administration of valproate (250 or 500 mg q8h); the half-life of zidovudine was unaffected.

Drugs for which either no interaction or a likely clinically unimportant interaction has been observed:

Acetaminophen—Valproate had no effect on any of the pharmacokinetic parameters of acetaminophen when it was concurrently administered to three epileptic patients.

Clozapine—In psychotic patients (n=11), no interaction was observed when valproate was co-administered with clozapine.

Lithium—Co-administration of valproate (500 mg BID) and lithium carbonate (300 mg TID) to normal male volunteers (n=16) had no effect on the steady-state kinetics of lithium.

Lorazepam—Concomitant administration of valproate (500 mg BID) and lorazepam (1 mg BID) in normal male volunteers (n=9) was accompanied by a 17% decrease in the plasma clearance of lorazepam.

Oral Contraceptive Steroids—Administration of a single-dose of ethinyloestradiol (50 μg)/levonorgestrel (250 μg) to 6 women on valproate (200 mg BID) therapy for 2 months did not reveal any pharmacokinetic interaction.

Carcinogenesis, Mutagenesis, Impairment of Fertility

Carcinogenesis

Valproic acid was administered orally to Sprague Dawley rats and ICR (HA/ICR) mice at doses of 80 and 170 mg/kg/day (approximately 10 to 50% of the maximum human daily dose on a mg/m^2 basis) for two years. A variety of neoplasms were observed in both species. The chief findings were a statistically significant increase in the incidence of subcutaneous fibrosarcomas in high dose male rats receiving valproic acid and a statistically significant dose-related trend for benign pulmonary adenomas in male mice receiving valproic acid. The significance of these findings for humans is unknown.

Mutagenesis

Valproate was not mutagenic in an *in vitro* bacterial assay (Ames test), did not produce dominant lethal effects in mice, and did not increase chromosome aberration frequency in an *in vivo* cytogenetic study in rats. Increased frequencies of sister chromatid exchange (SCE) have been reported in a study of epileptic children taking valproate, but this association was not observed in another study conducted in adults. There is some evidence that increased SCE frequencies may be associated with epilepsy. The biological significance of an increase in SCE frequency is not known.

Fertility

Chronic toxicity studies in juvenile and adult rats and dogs demonstrated reduced spermatogenesis and testicular atrophy at oral doses of 400 mg/kg/day or greater in rats (approximately equivalent to or greater than the maximum human daily dose on a mg/m^2 basis) and 150 mg/kg/day or greater in dogs (approximately 1.4 times the maximum human daily dose or greater on a mg/m^2 basis). Segment I fertility studies in rats have shown oral doses up to 350 mg/kg/day (approximately equal to the maximum human daily dose on a mg/m^2 basis) for 60 days to have no effect on fertility. THE EFFECT OF VALPROATE ON TESTICULAR DEVELOPMENT AND ON SPERM PRODUCTION AND FERTILITY IN HUMANS IS UNKNOWN.

Pregnancy

Pregnancy Category D: See **WARNINGS**.

Nursing Mothers

Valproate is excreted in breast milk. Concentrations in breast milk have been reported to be 1-10% of serum concentrations. It is not known what effect this would have on a nursing infant. Consideration should be given to discontinuing nursing when valproic acid is administered to a nursing woman.

Pediatric Use

Experience has indicated that pediatric patients under the age of two years are at a considerably increased risk of developing fatal hepatotoxicity, especially those with the aforementioned conditions (see **BOXED WARNING**). When DEPAKENE is used in this patient group, it should be used with extreme caution and as a sole agent. The benefits of therapy should be weighed against the risks. Above the age of 2 years, experience in epilepsy has indicated that the incidence of fatal hepatotoxicity decreases considerably in progressively older patient groups.

Younger children, especially those receiving enzyme-inducing drugs, will require larger maintenance doses to attain targeted total and unbound valproic acid concentrations.

The variability in free fraction limits the clinical usefulness of monitoring total serum valproic acid concentrations. Interpretation of valproic acid concentrations in children should include consideration of factors that affect hepatic metabolism and protein binding.

The basic toxicology and pathologic manifestations of valproate sodium in neonatal (4-day old) and juvenile (14-day old) rats are similar to those seen in young adult rats. However, additional findings, including renal alterations in juvenile rats and renal alterations and retinal dysplasia in neonatal rats, have been reported. These findings occurred at 240 mg/kg/day, a dosage approximately equivalent to the human maximum recommended daily dose on a mg/m^2 basis. They were not seen at 90 mg/kg, or 40% of the maximum human daily dose on a mg/m^2 basis.

Geriatric Use

No patients above the age of 65 years were enrolled in double-blind prospective clinical trials of mania associated with bipolar illness. In a case review study of 583 patients, 72 patients (12%) were greater than 65 years of age. A higher percentage of patients above 65 years of age reported accidental injury, infection, pain, somnolence, and tremor. Discontinuation of valproate was occasionally associated with the latter two events. It is not clear whether these events indicate additional risk or whether they result from preexisting medical illness and concomitant medication use among these patients.

A study of elderly patients with dementia revealed drug related somnolence and discontinuation for somnolence (see **WARNINGS—Somnolence in the Elderly**). The starting dose should be reduced in these patients, and dosage reductions or discontinuation should be considered in patients with excessive somnolence (see **DOSAGE AND ADMINISTRATION**).

ADVERSE REACTIONS

Epilepsy

The data described in the following section were obtained using DEPAKOTE (divalproex sodium) tablets.

Based on a placebo-controlled trial of adjunctive therapy for treatment of complex partial seizures, DEPAKOTE was generally well tolerated with most adverse events rated as mild to moderate in severity. Intolerance was the primary reason for discontinuation in the DEPAKOTE-treated patients (6%), compared to 1% of placebo-treated patients.

Table 1 lists treatment-emergent adverse events which were reported by ≥ 5% of DEPAKOTE-treated patients and for which the incidence was greater than in the placebo group, in a placebo-controlled trial of adjunctive therapy for the treatment of complex partial seizures. Since patients were also treated with other antiepilepsy drugs, it is not possible, in most cases, to determine whether the following adverse events can be ascribed to DEPAKOTE alone, or the combination of DEPAKOTE and other antiepilepsy drugs.

Table 1
Adverse Events Reported by ≥ 5% of Patients Treated with DEPAKOTE During Placebo-Controlled Trial of Adjunctive Therapy for Complex Partial Seizures

Body System/Event	Depakote (%) (n = 77)	Placebo (%) (n = 70)
Body as a Whole		
Headache	31	21
Asthenia	27	7
Fever	6	4
Gastrointestinal System		
Nausea	48	14
Vomiting	27	7
Abdominal Pain	23	6
Diarrhea	13	6
Anorexia	12	0
Dyspepsia	8	4
Constipation	5	1
Nervous System		
Somnolence	27	11
Tremor	25	6
Dizziness	25	13
Diplopia	16	9
Amblyopia/Blurred Vision	12	9
Ataxia	8	1
Nystagmus	8	1
Emotional Lability	6	4
Thinking Abnormal	6	0
Amnesia	5	1
Respiratory System		
Flu Syndrome	12	9
Infection	12	6
Bronchitis	5	1
Rhinitis	5	4
Other		
Alopecia	6	1
Weight Loss	6	0

Table 2 lists treatment-emergent adverse events which were reported by ≥ 5% of patients in the high dose DEPAKOTE group, and for which the incidence was greater than in the low dose group, in a controlled trial of DEPAKOTE monotherapy treatment of complex partial seizures. Since patients were being titrated off another antiepilepsy drug during the first portion of the trial, it is not possible, in many cases, to determine whether the following adverse events can be ascribed to DEPAKOTE alone, or the combination of DEPAKOTE and other antiepilepsy drugs.

Table 2
Adverse Events Reported by ≥ 5% of Patients in the High Dose Group in the Controlled Trial of DEPAKOTE Monotherapy for Complex Partial Seizures[1]

Body System/Event	High Dose (%) (n = 131)	Low Dose (%) (n = 134)
Body as a Whole		
Asthenia	21	10
Digestive System		
Nausea	34	26
Diarrhea	23	19
Vomiting	23	15
Abdominal Pain	12	9
Anorexia	11	4
Dyspepsia	11	10
Hemic/Lymphatic System		
Thrombocytopenia	24	1
Ecchymosis	5	4
Metabolic/Nutritional		
Weight Gain	9	4
Peripheral Edema	8	3
Nervous System		
Tremor	57	19
Somnolence	30	18
Dizziness	18	13
Insomnia	15	9
Nervousness	11	7
Amnesia	7	4
Nystagmus	7	1
Depression	5	4
Respiratory System		
Infection	20	13
Pharyngitis	8	2
Dyspnea	5	1
Skin and Appendages		
Alopecia	24	13
Special Senses		
Amblyopia/Blurred Vision	8	4
Tinnitus	7	1

[1] Headache was the only adverse event that occurred in ≥ 5% of patients in the high dose group and at an equal or greater incidence in the low dose group.

The following additional adverse events were reported by greater than 1% but less than 5% of the 358 patients treated with DEPAKOTE in the controlled trials of complex partial seizures:

Body as a Whole: Back pain, chest pain, malaise.

Cardiovascular System: Tachycardia, hypertension, palpitation.

Digestive System: Increased appetite, flatulence, hematemesis, eructation, pancreatitis, periodontal abscess.

Hemic and Lymphatic System: Petechia.

Metabolic and Nutritional Disorders: SGOT increased, SGPT increased.

Musculoskeletal System: Myalgia, twitching, arthralgia, leg cramps, myasthenia.

Nervous System: Anxiety, confusion, abnormal gait, paresthesia, hypertonia, incoordination, abnormal dreams, personality disorder.

Respiratory System: Sinusitis, cough increased, pneumonia, epistaxis.

Skin and Appendages: Rash, pruritus, dry skin.

Special Senses: Taste perversion, abnormal vision, deafness, otitis media.

Urogenital System: Urinary incontinence, vaginitis, dysmenorrhea, amenorrhea, urinary frequency.

Other Patient Populations

Adverse events that have been reported with all dosage forms of valproate from epilepsy trials, spontaneous reports, and other sources are listed below by body system.

Gastrointestinal: The most commonly reported side effects at the initiation of therapy are nausea, vomiting, and indigestion. These effects are usually transient and rarely require discontinuation of therapy. Diarrhea, abdominal cramps, and constipation have been reported. Both anorexia with some weight loss and increased appetite with weight gain have also been reported. The administration of delayed-release divalproex sodium may result in reduction of gastrointestinal side effects in some patients.

CNS Effects: Sedative effects have occurred in patients receiving valproate alone but occur most often in patients receiving combination therapy. Sedation usually abates upon reduction of other antiepileptic medication. Tremor (may be dose-related), hallucinations, ataxia, headache, nystagmus, diplopia, asterixis, "spots before eyes", dysarthria, dizziness, confusion, hypesthesia, vertigo, incoordination, and parkinsonism have been reported with the use of valproate. Rare cases of coma have occurred in patients receiving valproate alone or in conjunction with phenobarbital. In rare instances encephalopathy with or without fever has developed shortly after the introduction of valproate monotherapy without evidence of hepatic dysfunction or inappropriately high plasma valproate levels. Although recovery has been described following drug withdrawal, there have been fatalities in patients with hyperammonemic encephalopathy, particularly in patients with underlying urea cycle disorders (see **WARNINGS—Urea Cycle Disorders** and **PRECAUTIONS**).

Several reports have noted reversible cerebral atrophy and dementia in association with valproate therapy.

Dermatologic: Transient hair loss, skin rash, photosensitivity, generalized pruritus, erythema multiforme, and Stevens-Johnson syndrome. Rare cases of toxic epidermal necrolysis have been reported including a fatal case in a 6 month old infant taking valproate and several other concomitant medications. An additional case of toxic epidermal necrosis resulting in death was reported in a 35 year old patient with AIDS taking several concomitant medications and with a history of multiple cutaneous drug reactions. Serious skin reactions have been reported with concomitant administration of lamotrigine and valproate (see **PRECAUTIONS—Drug Interactions**).

Psychiatric: Emotional upset, depression, psychosis, aggression, hyperactivity, hostility, and behavioral deterioration.

Musculoskeletal: Weakness.

Hematologic: Thrombocytopenia and inhibition of the secondary phase of platelet aggregation may be reflected in altered bleeding time, petechiae, bruising, hematoma formation, epistaxis, and frank hemorrhage (see **PRECAUTIONS—General** and **Drug Interactions**). Relative lymphocytosis, macrocytosis, hypofibrinogenemia, leukopenia, eosinophilia, anemia including macrocytic with or without folate deficiency, bone marrow suppression, pancytopenia, aplastic anemia, agranulocytosis, and acute intermittent porphyria.

Hepatic: Minor elevations of transaminases (e.g., SGOT and SGPT) and LDH are frequent and appear to be dose-related. Occasionally, laboratory test results include increases in serum bilirubin and abnormal changes in other liver function tests. These results may reflect potentially serious hepatotoxicity (see **WARNINGS**).

Endocrine: Irregular menses, secondary amenorrhea, breast enlargement, galactorrhea, and parotid gland swelling. Abnormal thyroid function tests (see **PRECAUTIONS**).

There have been rare spontaneous reports of polycystic ovary disease. A cause and effect relationship has not been established.

Pancreatic: Acute pancreatitis, including fatalities (see **WARNINGS**).

Metabolic: Hyperammonemia (see **PRECAUTIONS**), hyponatremia, and inappropriate ADH secretion.

There have been rare reports of Fanconi's syndrome occurring chiefly in children.

Decreased carnitine concentrations have been reported although the clinical relevance is undetermined.

Hyperglycinemia has occurred and was associated with a fatal outcome in a patient with preexistent nonketotic hyperglycinemia.

Genitourinary: Enuresis and urinary tract infection.

Special Senses: Hearing loss, either reversible or irreversible, has been reported; however, a cause and effect relationship has not been established. Ear pain has also been reported.

Other: Allergic reaction, anaphylaxis, edema of the extremities, lupus erythematosus, bone pain, cough increased, pneumonia, otitis media, bradycardia, cutaneous vasculitis, fever, and hypothermia.

Mania

Although DEPAKENE has not been evaluated for safety and efficacy in the treatment of manic episodes associated with bipolar disorder, the following adverse events not listed above were reported by 1% or more of patients from two placebo-controlled clinical trials of DEPAKOTE tablets.

Body as a Whole: Chills, neck pain, neck rigidity.

Cardiovascular System: Hypotension, postural hypotension, vasodilation.

Digestive System: Fecal incontinence, gastroenteritis, glossitis.

Musculoskeletal System: Arthrosis.

Nervous System: Agitation, catatonic reaction, hypokinesia, reflexes increased, tardive dyskinesia, vertigo.

Skin and Appendages: Furunculosis, maculopapular rash, seborrhea.

Special Senses: Conjunctivitis, dry eyes, eye pain.

Urogenital System: Dysuria.

Migraine

Although DEPAKENE has not been evaluated for safety and efficacy in the treatment of prophylaxis of migraine headaches, the following adverse events not listed above were reported by 1% or more of patients from two placebo-controlled clinical trials of DEPAKOTE tablets.

Body as a Whole: Face edema.

Digestive System: Dry mouth, stomatitis.

Urogenital System: Cystitis, metrorrhagia, and vaginal hemorrhage.

OVERDOSAGE

Overdosage with valproate may result in somnolence, heart block, and deep coma. Fatalities have been reported; however, patients have recovered from valproate levels as high as 2120 µg/mL.

In overdose situations, the fraction of drug not bound to protein is high and hemodialysis or tandem hemodialysis plus hemoperfusion may result in significant removal of drug. The benefit of gastric lavage or emesis will vary with the time since ingestion. General supportive measures should be applied with particular attention to the maintenance of adequate urinary output.

Naloxone has been reported to reverse the CNS depressant effects of valproate overdosage. Because naloxone could theoretically also reverse the antiepileptic effects of valproate, it should be used with caution in patients with epilepsy.

DOSAGE AND ADMINISTRATION

THE CAPSULES SHOULD BE SWALLOWED WITHOUT CHEWING TO AVOID LOCAL IRRITATION OF THE MOUTH AND THROAT.

DEPAKENE (valproic acid) is administered orally. DEPAKENE is indicated as monotherapy and adjunctive therapy in complex partial seizures in adults and pediatric patients down to the age of 10 years, and in simple and complex absence seizures. As the DEPAKENE dosage is titrated upward, concentrations of phenobarbital, carbamazepine, and/or phenytoin may be affected (see **PRECAUTIONS—Drug Interactions**).

Complex Partial Seizures: For adults and children 10 years of age or older.

Monotherapy (Initial Therapy): DEPAKENE has not been systematically studied as initial therapy. Patients should initiate therapy at 10 to 15 mg/kg/day. The dosage should be increased by 5 to 10 mg/kg/week to achieve optimal clinical response. Ordinarily, optimal clinical response is achieved at daily doses below 60 mg/kg/day. If satisfactory clinical response has not been achieved, plasma levels should be measured to determine whether or not they are in the usually accepted therapeutic range (50 to 100 µg/mL). No recommendation regarding the safety of valproate for use at doses above 60 mg/kg/day can be made.

The probability of thrombocytopenia increases significantly at total trough valproate plasma concentrations above 110 µg/mL in females and 135 µg/mL in males. The benefit of improved seizure control with higher doses should be weighed against the possibility of a greater incidence of adverse reactions.

Conversion to Monotherapy: Patients should initiate therapy at 10 to 15 mg/kg/day. The dosage should be increased by 5 to 10 mg/kg/week to achieve optimal clinical response. Ordinarily, optimal clinical response is achieved at daily doses below 60 mg/kg/day. If satisfactory clinical response has not been achieved, plasma levels should be measured to determine whether or not they are in the usually accepted therapeutic range (50-100 µg/mL). No recommendation regarding the safety of valproate for use at doses above 60 mg/kg/day can be made. Concomitant antiepilepsy drug (AED) dosage can ordinarily be reduced by approximately 25% every 2 weeks. This reduction may be started at initiation of DEPAKENE therapy, or delayed by 1 to 2 weeks if there is a concern that seizures are likely to occur with a reduction. The speed and duration of withdrawal of the concomitant AED can be highly variable, and patients should be monitored closely during this period for increased seizure frequency.

Adjunctive Therapy: DEPAKENE may be added to the patient's regimen at a dosage of 10 to 15 mg/kg/day. The dosage may be increased by 5 to 10 mg/kg/week to achieve optimal clinical response. Ordinarily, optimal clinical response is achieved at daily doses below 60 mg/kg/day. If satisfactory clinical response has not been achieved, plasma levels should be measured to determine whether or not they are in the usually accepted therapeutic range (50 to 100 µg/mL). No recommendation regarding the safety of valproate for use at doses above 60 mg/kg/day can be made. If the total daily dose exceeds 250 mg, it should be given in divided doses.

In a study of adjunctive therapy for complex partial seizures in which patients were receiving either carbamazepine or phenytoin in addition to DEPAKOTE tablets, no adjustment of carbamazepine or phenytoin dosage was needed (see **CLINICAL STUDIES**). However, since valproate may interact with these or other concurrently administered AEDs

Weight (Kg)	Weight (Lb)	Total Daily Dose (mg)	Number of Capsules or Teaspoonfuls of Syrup: Dose 1	Dose 2	Dose 3
10-24.9	22-54.9	250	0	0	1
25-39.9	55-87.9	500	1	0	1
40-59.9	88-131.9	750	1	1	1
60-74.9	132-164.9	1,000	1	1	2
75-89.9	165-197.9	1,250	2	1	2

Continued on next page

Depakene—Cont.

as well as other drugs (see **Drug Interactions**), periodic plasma concentration determinations of concomitant AEDs are recommended during the early course of therapy (see **PRECAUTIONS—Drug Interactions**).

Simple and Complex Absence Seizures: The recommended initial dose is 15 mg/kg/day, increasing at one week intervals by 5 to 10 mg/kg/day until seizures are controlled or side effects preclude further increases. The maximum recommended dosage is 60 mg/kg/day. If the total daily dose exceeds 250 mg, it should be given in divided doses.

A good correlation has not been established between daily dose, serum concentrations, and therapeutic effect. However, therapeutic valproate serum concentrations for most patients with absence seizures is considered to range from 50 to 100 µg/mL. Some patients may be controlled with lower or higher serum concentrations (see **CLINICAL PHARMACOLOGY**).

As the DEPAKENE dosage is titrated upward, blood concentrations of phenobarbital and/or phenytoin may be affected (see **PRECAUTIONS**).

Antiepilepsy drugs should not be abruptly discontinued in patients in whom the drug is administered to prevent major seizures because of the strong possibility of precipitating status epilepticus with attendant hypoxia and threat to life.

The following table is a guide for the initial daily dose of DEPAKENE (valproic acid) (15 mg/kg/day):

[See table at top of previous page]

General Dosing Advice

Dosing in Elderly Patients—Due to a decrease in unbound clearance of valproate and possibly a greater sensitivity to somnolence in the elderly, the starting dose should be reduced in these patients. Dosage should be increased more slowly and with regular monitoring for fluid and nutritional intake, dehydration, somnolence, and other adverse events. Dose reductions or discontinuation of valproate should be considered in patients with decreased food or fluid intake and in patients with excessive somnolence. The ultimate therapeutic dose should be achieved on the basis of both tolerability and clinical response (see **WARNINGS**).

Dose-Related Adverse Events—The frequency of adverse effects (particularly elevated liver enzymes and thrombocytopenia) may be dose-related. The probability of thrombocytopenia appears to increase significantly at total valproate concentrations of ≥ 110 µg/mL (females) or ≥ 135 µg/mL (males) (see **PRECAUTIONS**). The benefit of improved therapeutic effect with higher doses should be weighed against the possibility of a greater incidence of adverse reactions.

G.I. Irritation—Patients who experience G.I. irritation may benefit from administration of the drug with food or by slowly building up the dose from an initial low level.

HOW SUPPLIED

DEPAKENE (valproic acid) is available as orange-colored soft gelatin capsules of 250 mg valproic acid, bearing the trademark DEPAKENE for product identification, in bottles of 100 capsules (**NDC** 0074-5681-13), and as a red syrup containing the equivalent of 250 mg valproic acid per 5 mL as the sodium salt in bottles of 16 ounces (**NDC** 0074-5682-16). Store capsules at 59-77°F (15-25°C). Store syrup below 86°F (30°C).

Patient Information Leaflet

Important Information for Women Who Could Become Pregnant About the Use of DEPAKENE® (valproic acid)

Please read this leaflet carefully before you take DEPAKENE® (valproic acid) capsules and syrup. This leaflet provides a summary of important information about taking DEPAKENE® to women who could become pregnant. If you have any questions or concerns, or want more information about DEPAKENE®, contact your doctor or pharmacist.

Information For Women Who Could Become Pregnant

DEPAKENE® can be obtained only by prescription from your doctor. The decision to use DEPAKENE® is one that you and your doctor should make together, taking into account your individual needs and medical condition. **Before using DEPAKENE®, women who can become pregnant should consider the fact that DEPAKENE® has been associated with birth defects, in particular, with spina bifida and other defects related to failure of the spinal canal to close normally. Approximately 1 to 2% of children born to women with epilepsy taking DEPAKENE® in the first 12 weeks of pregnancy had these defects (based on data from the Centers for Disease Control, a U.S. agency based in Atlanta). The incidence in the general population is 0.1 to 0.2%.**

Information For Women Who Are Planning To Get Pregnant

- Women taking DEPAKENE® who are planning to get pregnant should discuss the treatment options with their doctor.

Information For Women Who Become Pregnant While Taking DEPAKENE®

- If you become pregnant while taking DEPAKENE®, you should contact your doctor immediately.

Other Important Information About DEPAKENE®

- DEPAKENE® capsules and syrup should be taken exactly as it is prescribed by your doctor to get the most benefits from DEPAKENE® and reduce the risk of side effects.
- If you have taken more than the prescribed dose of DEPAKENE®, contact your hospital emergency room or local poison center immediately.
- This medication was prescribed for your particular condition. Do not use it for another condition or give the drug to others.

Facts About Birth Defects

It is important to know that birth defects may occur even in children of individuals not taking any medications or without any additional risk factors.

This summary provides important information about the use of DEPAKENE® to women who could become pregnant. If you would like more information about the other potential risks and benefits of DEPAKENE®, ask your doctor or pharmacist to let you read the professional labeling and then discuss it with them. If you have any questions or concerns about taking DEPAKENE®, you should discuss them with your doctor.

Ref: 03-5294-R29
Revised: September, 2003
Manufactured by:
ABBOTT LABORATORIES
NORTH CHICAGO, IL 60064, U.S.A.
PRINTED IN U.S.A.

Shown in Product Identification Guide, page 303

DEPAKOTE® Sprinkle Capsules ℞

[dəp' ā-coat]

DIVALPROEX SODIUM
COATED PARTICLES IN CAPSULES
℞ only

BOX WARNING:

HEPATOTOXICITY:

HEPATIC FAILURE RESULTING IN FATALITIES HAS OCCURRED IN PATIENTS RECEIVING VALPROIC ACID AND ITS DERIVATIVES. EXPERIENCE HAS INDICATED THAT CHILDREN UNDER THE AGE OF TWO YEARS ARE AT A CONSIDERABLY INCREASED RISK OF DEVELOPING FATAL HEPATOTOXICITY, ESPECIALLY THOSE ON MULTIPLE ANTICONVULSANTS, THOSE WITH CONGENITAL METABOLIC DISORDERS, THOSE WITH SEVERE SEIZURE DISORDERS ACCOMPANIED BY MENTAL RETARDATION, AND THOSE WITH ORGANIC BRAIN DISEASE. WHEN DEPAKOTE IS USED IN THIS PATIENT GROUP, IT SHOULD BE USED WITH EXTREME CAUTION AND AS A SOLE AGENT. THE BENEFITS OF THERAPY SHOULD BE WEIGHED AGAINST THE RISKS. ABOVE THIS AGE GROUP, EXPERIENCE IN EPILEPSY HAS INDICATED THAT THE INCIDENCE OF FATAL HEPATOTOXICITY DECREASES CONSIDERABLY IN PROGRESSIVELY OLDER PATIENT GROUPS.

THESE INCIDENTS USUALLY HAVE OCCURRED DURING THE FIRST SIX MONTHS OF TREATMENT. SERIOUS OR FATAL HEPATOTOXICITY MAY BE PRECEDED BY NON-SPECIFIC SYMPTOMS SUCH AS MALAISE, WEAKNESS, LETHARGY, FACIAL EDEMA, ANOREXIA, AND VOMITING. IN PATIENTS WITH EPILEPSY, A LOSS OF SEIZURE CONTROL MAY ALSO OCCUR. PATIENTS SHOULD BE MONITORED CLOSELY FOR APPEARANCE OF THESE SYMPTOMS. LIVER FUNCTION TESTS SHOULD BE PERFORMED PRIOR TO THERAPY AND AT FREQUENT INTERVALS THEREAFTER, ESPECIALLY DURING THE FIRST SIX MONTHS.

TERATOGENICITY:

VALPROATE CAN PRODUCE TERATOGENIC EFFECTS SUCH AS NEURAL TUBE DEFECTS (E.G., SPINA BIFIDA). ACCORDINGLY, THE USE OF VALPROATE PRODUCTS IN WOMEN OF CHILDBEARING POTENTIAL REQUIRES THAT THE BENEFITS OF ITS USE BE WEIGHED AGAINST THE RISK OF INJURY TO THE FETUS.

PANCREATITIS:

CASES OF LIFE-THREATENING PANCREATITIS HAVE BEEN REPORTED IN BOTH CHILDREN AND ADULTS RECEIVING VALPROATE. SOME OF THE CASES HAVE BEEN DESCRIBED AS HEMORRHAGIC WITH A RAPID PROGRESSION FROM INITIAL SYMPTOMS TO DEATH. CASES HAVE BEEN REPORTED SHORTLY AFTER INITIAL USE AS WELL AS AFTER SEVERAL YEARS OF USE. PATIENTS AND GUARDIANS SHOULD BE WARNED THAT ABDOMINAL PAIN, NAUSEA, VOMITING, AND/OR ANOREXIA CAN BE SYMPTOMS OF PANCREATITIS THAT REQUIRE PROMPT MEDICAL EVALUATION. IF PANCREATITIS IS DIAGNOSED, VALPROATE SHOULD ORDINARILY BE DISCONTINUED. ALTERNATIVE TREATMENT FOR THE UNDERLYING MEDICAL CONDITION SHOULD BE INITIATED AS CLINICALLY INDICATED. (See **WARNINGS** and **PRECAUTIONS**.)

DESCRIPTION

Divalproex sodium is a stable co-ordination compound comprised of sodium valproate and valproic acid in a 1:1 molar relationship and formed during the partial neutralization of valproic acid with 0.5 equivalent of sodium hydroxide. Chemically it is designated as sodium hydrogen bis (2-propylpentanoate). Divalproex sodium has the following structure:

Divalproex sodium occurs as a white powder with a characteristic odor.

DEPAKOTE Sprinkle Capsules are for oral administration. DEPAKOTE Sprinkle Capsules contain specially coated particles of divalproex sodium equivalent to 125 mg of valproic acid in a hard gelatin capsule.

Inactive Ingredients

125 mg DEPAKOTE Sprinkle Capsules: cellulosic polymers, D&C Red No. 28, FD&C Blue No. 1, gelatin, iron oxide, magnesium stearate, silica gel, titanium dioxide, and triethyl citrate.

CLINICAL PHARMACOLOGY

Pharmacodynamics

Divalproex sodium dissociates to the valproate ion in the gastrointestinal tract. The mechanisms by which valproate exerts its therapeutic effects have not been established. It has been suggested that its activity in epilepsy is related to increased brain concentrations of gamma-aminobutyric acid (GABA).

Pharmacokinetics

Absorption/Bioavailability

Equivalent oral doses of DEPAKOTE (divalproex sodium) products and DEPAKENE (valproic acid) capsules deliver equivalent quantities of valproate ion systemically. Although the rate of valproate ion absorption may vary with the formulation administered (liquid, solid, or sprinkle), conditions of use (e.g., fasting or postprandial) and the method of administration (e.g., whether the contents of the capsule are sprinkled on food or the capsule is taken intact), these differences should be of minor clinical importance under the steady state conditions achieved in chronic use in the treatment of epilepsy.

However, it is possible that differences among the various valproate products in T_{max} and C_{max} could be important upon initiation of treatment. For example, in single dose studies, the effect of feeding had a greater influence on the rate of absorption of the tablet (increase in T_{max} from 4 to 8 hours) than on the absorption of the sprinkle capsules (increase in T_{max} from 3.3 to 4.8 hours).

While the absorption rate from the G.I. tract and fluctuation in valproate plasma concentrations vary with dosing regimen and formulation, the efficacy of valproate as an anticonvulsant in chronic use is unlikely to be affected. Experience employing dosing regimens from once-a-day to four-times-a-day, as well as studies in primate epilepsy models involving constant rate infusion, indicate that total daily systemic bioavailability (extent of absorption) is the primary determinant of seizure control and that differences in the ratios of plasma peak to trough concentrations between valproate formulations are inconsequential from a practical clinical standpoint.

Co-administration of oral valproate products with food and substitution among the various DEPAKOTE and DEPAKENE formulations should cause no clinical problems in the management of patients with epilepsy (see **DOSAGE AND ADMINISTRATION**). Nonetheless, any changes in dosage administration, or the addition or discontinuance of concomitant drugs should ordinarily be accompanied by close monitoring of clinical status and valproate plasma concentrations.

Distribution

Protein Binding:

The plasma protein binding of valproate is concentration dependent and the free fraction increases from approximately 10% at 40 µg/mL to 18.5% at 130 µg/mL. Protein binding of valproate is reduced in the elderly, in patients with chronic hepatic diseases, in patients with renal impairment, and in the presence of other drugs (e.g., aspirin). Conversely, valproate may displace certain protein-bound drugs (e.g., phenytoin, carbamazepine, warfarin, and tolbutamide). (See **PRECAUTIONS, Drug Interactions** for more detailed information on the pharmacokinetic interactions of valproate with other drugs.)

CNS Distribution:

Valproate concentrations in cerebrospinal fluid (CSF) approximate unbound concentrations in plasma (about 10% of total concentration).

Metabolism

Valproate is metabolized almost entirely by the liver. In adult patients on monotherapy, 30-50% of an administered dose appears in urine as a glucuronide conjugate. Mitochondrial β-oxidation is the other major metabolic pathway, typically accounting for over 40% of the dose. Usually, less than 15-20% of the dose is eliminated by other oxidative mechanisms. Less than 3% of an administered dose is excreted unchanged in urine.

The relationship between dose and total valproate concentration is nonlinear; concentration does not increase proportionally with the dose, but rather, increases to a lesser extent due to saturable plasma protein binding. The kinetics of unbound drug are linear.

Elimination
Mean plasma clearance and volume of distribution for total valproate are 0.56 L/hr/1.73 m^2 and 11 L/1.73 m^2, respectively. Mean plasma clearance and volume of distribution for free valproate are 4.6 L/hr/1.73 m^2 and 92 L/1.73 m^2. Mean terminal half-life for valproate monotherapy ranged from 9 to 16 hours following oral dosing regimens of 250 to 1000 mg.
The estimates cited apply primarily to patients who are not taking drugs that affect hepatic metabolizing enzyme systems. For example, patients taking enzyme-inducing antiepileptic drugs (carbamazepine, phenytoin, and phenobarbital) will clear valproate more rapidly. Because of these changes in valproate clearance, monitoring of antiepileptic concentrations should be intensified whenever concomitant antiepileptics are introduced or withdrawn.
Special Populations
Effect of Age:
Neonates - Children within the first two months of life have a markedly decreased ability to eliminate valproate compared to older children and adults. This is a result of reduced clearance (perhaps due to delay in development of glucuronosyltransferase and other enzyme systems involved in valproate elimination) as well as increased volume of distribution (in part due to decreased plasma protein binding). For example, in one study, the half-life in children under 10 days ranged from 10 to 67 hours compared to a range of 7 to 13 hours in children greater than 2 months.
Children - Pediatric patients (i.e., between 3 months and 10 years) have 50% higher clearances expressed on weight (i.e., mL/min/kg) than do adults. Over the age of 10 years, children have pharmacokinetic parameters that approximate those of adults.
Elderly - The capacity of elderly patients (age range: 68 to 89 years) to eliminate valproate has been shown to be reduced compared to younger adults (age range: 22 to 26). Intrinsic clearance is reduced by 39%; the free fraction is increased by 44%. Accordingly, the initial dosage should be reduced in the elderly. (See **DOSAGE AND ADMINISTRATION**).
Effect of Gender:
There are no differences in the body surface area adjusted unbound clearance between males and females (4.8±0.17 and 4.7±0.07 L/hr per 1.73 m^2, respectively).
Effect of Race:
The effects of race on the kinetics of valproate have not been studied.
Effect of Disease:
Liver Disease - (See **BOXED WARNING, CONTRAINDICATIONS**, and **WARNINGS**). Liver disease impairs the capacity to eliminate valproate. In one study, the clearance of free valproate was decreased by 50% in 7 patients with cirrhosis and by 16% in 4 patients with acute hepatitis, compared with 6 healthy subjects. In that study, the half-life of valproate was increased from 12 to 18 hours. Liver disease is also associated with decreased albumin concentrations and larger unbound fractions (2 to 2.6 fold increase) of valproate. Accordingly, monitoring of total concentrations may be misleading since free concentrations may be substantially elevated in patients with hepatic disease whereas total concentrations may appear to be normal.
Renal Disease - A slight reduction (27%) in the unbound clearance of valproate has been reported in patients with renal failure (creatinine clearance < 10 mL/minute); however, hemodialysis typically reduces valproate concentrations by about 20%. Therefore, no dosage adjustment appears to be necessary in patients with renal failure. Protein binding in these patients is substantially reduced; thus, monitoring total concentrations may be misleading.

Plasma Levels and Clinical Effect
The relationship between plasma concentration and clinical response is not well documented. One contributing factor is the nonlinear, concentration dependent protein binding of valproate which affects the clearance of the drug. Thus, monitoring of total serum valproate cannot provide a reliable index of the bioactive valproate species.
For example, because the plasma protein binding of valproate is concentration dependent, the free fraction increases from approximately 10% at 40 µg/mL to 18.5% at 130 µg/mL. Higher than expected free fractions occur in the elderly, in hyperlipidemic patients, and in patients with hepatic and renal diseases.
Epilepsy:
The therapeutic range in epilepsy is commonly considered to be 50 to 100 µg/mL of total valproate, although some patients may be controlled with lower or higher plasma concentrations.

CLINICAL STUDIES

Epilepsy
The efficacy of DEPAKOTE in reducing the incidence of complex partial seizures (CPS) that occur in isolation or in association with other seizure types was established in two controlled trials.
In one, multiclinic, placebo controlled study employing an add-on design (adjunctive therapy), 144 patients who continued to suffer eight or more CPS per 8 weeks during an 8 week period of monotherapy with doses of either carbamazepine or phenytoin sufficient to assure plasma concentrations within the "therapeutic range" were randomized to receive, in addition to their original antiepilepsy drug (AED), either DEPAKOTE or placebo. Randomized patients were to be followed for a total of 16 weeks. The following table presents the findings.

Adjunctive Therapy Study
Median Incidence of CPS per 8 Weeks

Add-on Treatment	Number of Patients	Baseline Incidence	Experimental Incidence
DEPAKOTE	75	16.0	8.9*
Placebo	69	14.5	11.5

*Reduction from baseline statistically significantly greater for DEPAKOTE than placebo at p ≤0.05 level.

Figure 1 presents the proportion of patients (X axis) whose percentage reduction from baseline in complex partial seizure rates was at least as great as that indicated on the Y axis in the adjunctive therapy study. A positive percent reduction indicates an improvement (i.e., a decrease in seizure frequency), while a negative percent reduction indicates worsening. Thus, in a display of this type, the curve for an effective treatment is shifted to the left of the curve for placebo. This figure shows that the proportion of patients achieving any particular level of improvement was consistently higher for DEPAKOTE than for placebo. For example, 45% of patients treated with DEPAKOTE had a ≥ 50% reduction in complex partial seizure rate compared to 23% of patients treated with placebo.

Figure 1

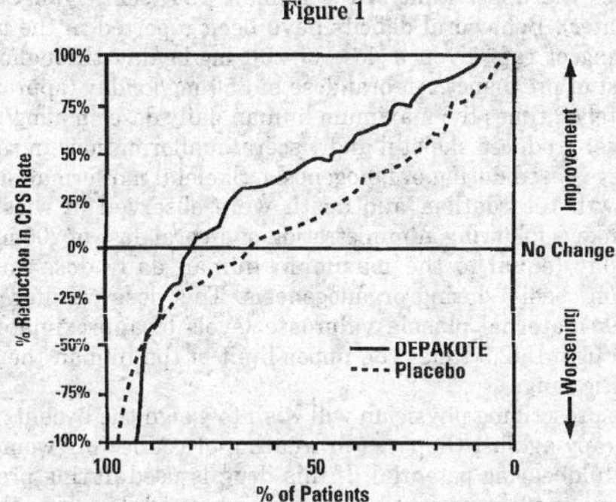

The second study assessed the capacity of DEPAKOTE to reduce the incidence of CPS when administered as the sole AED. The study compared the incidence of CPS among patients randomized to either a high or low dose treatment arm. Patients qualified for entry into the randomized comparison phase of this study only if 1) they continued to experience 2 or more CPS per 4 weeks during an 8 to 12 week long period of monotherapy with adequate doses of an AED (i.e., phenytoin, carbamazepine, phenobarbital, or primidone) and 2) they made a successful transition over a two week interval to DEPAKOTE. Patients entering the randomized phase were then brought to their assigned target dose, gradually tapered off their concomitant AED and followed for an interval as long as 22 weeks. Less than 50% of the patients randomized, however, completed the study. In patients converted to DEPAKOTE monotherapy, the mean total valproate concentrations during monotherapy were 71 and 123 µg/mL in the low dose and high dose groups, respectively.
The following table presents the findings for all patients randomized who had at least one post-randomization assessment.

Monotherapy Study
Median Incidence of CPS per 8 Weeks

Treatment	Number of Patients	Baseline Incidence	Randomized Phase Incidence
High dose			
DEPAKOTE	131	13.2	10.7*
Low dose			
DEPAKOTE	134	14.2	13.8

* Reduction from baseline statistically significantly greater for high dose than low dose at p ≤ 0.05 level.

Figure 2 presents the proportion of patients (X axis) whose percentage reduction from baseline in complex partial seizure rates was at least as great as that indicated on the Y axis in the monotherapy study. A positive percent reduction indicates an improvement (i.e., a decrease in seizure frequency), while a negative percent reduction indicates worsening. Thus, in a display of this type, the curve for a more effective treatment is shifted to the left of the curve for a less effective treatment. This figure shows that the proportion of patients achieving any particular level of reduction was consistently higher for high dose DEPAKOTE than for low dose DEPAKOTE. For example, when switching from carbamazepine, phenytoin, phenobarbital or primidone monotherapy to high dose DEPAKOTE monotherapy, 63% of patients experienced no change or a reduction in complex partial seizure rates compared to 54% of patients receiving low dose DEPAKOTE.
[See figure 2 at top of next column]

INDICATIONS AND USAGE

DEPAKOTE Sprinkle Capsules are indicated as monotherapy and adjunctive therapy in the treatment of patients

Figure 2

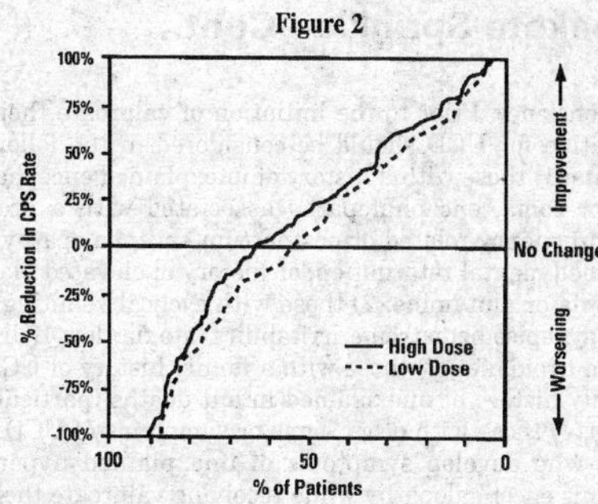

with complex partial seizures that occur either in isolation or in association with other types of seizure. DEPAKOTE Sprinkle Capsules are also indicated for use as sole and adjunctive therapy in the treatment of simple and complex absence seizures, and adjunctively in patients with multiple seizure types that include absence seizures.
Simple absence is defined as very brief clouding of the sensorium or loss of consciousness accompanied by certain generalized epileptic discharges without other detectable clinical signs. Complex absence is the term used when other signs are also present.
SEE **WARNINGS** FOR STATEMENT REGARDING FATAL HEPATIC DYSFUNCTION.

CONTRAINDICATIONS

DIVALPROEX SODIUM SHOULD NOT BE ADMINISTERED TO PATIENTS WITH HEPATIC DISEASE OR SIGNIFICANT HEPATIC DYSFUNCTION.
Divalproex sodium is contraindicated in patients with known hypersensitivity to the drug.
Divalproex sodium is contraindicated in patients with known urea cycle disorders (see **WARNINGS**).

WARNINGS

Hepatotoxicity
Hepatic failure resulting in fatalities has occurred in patients receiving valproic acid. These incidents usually have occurred during the first six months of treatment. Serious or fatal hepatotoxicity may be preceded by non-specific symptoms such as malaise, weakness, lethargy, facial edema, anorexia, and vomiting. In patients with epilepsy, a loss of seizure control may also occur. Patients should be monitored closely for appearance of these symptoms. Liver function tests should be performed prior to therapy and at frequent intervals thereafter, especially during the first six months. However, physicians should not rely totally on serum biochemistry since these tests may not be abnormal in all instances, but should also consider the results of careful interim medical history and physical examination.
Caution should be observed when administering DEPAKOTE products to patients with a prior history of hepatic disease. Patients on multiple anticonvulsants, children, those with congenital metabolic disorders, those with severe seizure disorders accompanied by mental retardation, and those with organic brain disease may be at particular risk. Experience has indicated that children under the age of two years are at a considerably increased risk of developing fatal hepatotoxicity, especially those with the aforementioned conditions. When DEPAKOTE is used in this patient group, it should be used with extreme caution and as a sole agent. The benefits of therapy should be weighed against the risks. Above this age group, experience in epilepsy has indicated that the incidence of fatal hepatotoxicity decreases considerably in progressively older patient groups.
The drug should be discontinued immediately in the presence of significant hepatic dysfunction, suspected or apparent. In some cases, hepatic dysfunction has progressed in spite of discontinuation of drug.
Pancreatitis
Cases of life-threatening pancreatitis have been reported in both children and adults receiving valproate. Some of the cases have been described as hemorrhagic with rapid progression from initial symptoms to death. Some cases have occurred shortly after initial use as well as after several years of use. The rate based upon the reported cases exceeds that expected in the general population and there have been cases in which pancreatitis recurred after rechallenge with valproate. In clinical trials, there were 2 cases of pancreatitis without alternative etiology in 2416 patients, representing 1044 patient-years experience. Patients and guardians should be warned that abdominal pain, nausea, vomiting, and/or anorexia can be symptoms of pancreatitis that require prompt medical evaluation. If pancreatitis is diagnosed, valproate should ordinarily be discontinued. Alternative treatment for the underlying medical condition should be initiated as clinically indicated (see **BOXED WARNING**).
Urea Cycle Disorders (UCD)
Divalproex sodium is contraindicated in patients with known urea cycle disorders.
Hyperammonemic encephalopathy, sometimes fatal, has been reported following initiation of valproate therapy in patients with urea cycle disorders, a group of uncommon genetic abnormalities, particularly ornithine transcarbamy-

Continued on next page

Depakote Sprinkle—Cont.

lase deficiency. Prior to the initiation of valproate therapy, evaluation for UCD should be considered in the following patients: 1) those with a history of unexplained encephalopathy or coma, encephalopathy associated with a protein load, pregnancy-related or postpartum encephalopathy, unexplained mental retardation, or history of elevated plasma ammonia or glutamine; 2) those with cyclical vomiting and lethargy, episodic extreme irritability, ataxia, low BUN, or protein avoidance; 3) those with a family history of UCD or a family history of unexplained infant deaths (particularly males); 4) those with other signs or symptoms of UCD. Patients who develop symptoms of unexplained hyperammonemic encephalopathy while receiving valproate therapy should receive prompt treatment (including discontinuation of valproate therapy) and be evaluated for underlying urea cycle disorders (see **CONTRAINDICATIONS** and **PRECAUTIONS**).

Somnolence in the Elderly

In a double-blind, multicenter trial of valproate in elderly patients with dementia (mean age = 83 years), doses were increased by 125 mg/day to a target dose of 20 mg/kg/day. A significantly higher proportion of valproate patients had somnolence compared to placebo, and although not statistically significant, there was a higher proportion of patients with dehydration. Discontinuations for somnolence were also significantly higher than with placebo. In some patients with somnolence (approximately one-half), there was associated reduced nutritional intake and weight loss. There was a trend for the patients who experienced these events to have a lower baseline albumin concentration, lower valproate clearance, and a higher BUN. In elderly patients, dosage should be increased more slowly and with regular monitoring for fluid and nutritional intake, dehydration, somnolence, and other adverse events. Dose reductions or discontinuation of valproate should be considered in patients with decreased food or fluid intake and in patients with excessive somnolence (see **DOSAGE AND ADMINISTRATION**).

Thrombocytopenia

The frequency of adverse effects (particularly elevated liver enzymes and thrombocytopenia [see **PRECAUTIONS**]) may be dose-related. In a clinical trial of DEPAKOTE (divalproex sodium) as monotherapy in patients with epilepsy, 34/126 patients (27%) receiving approximately 50 mg/kg/day on average, had at least one value of platelets $\leq$ 75 x 10^9/L. Approximately half of these patients had treatment discontinued, with return of platelet counts to normal. In the remaining patients, platelet counts normalized with continued treatment. In this study, the probability of thrombocytopenia appeared to increase significantly at total valproate concentrations of $\geq$ 110 μg/mL (females) or $\geq$ 135 μg/mL (males). The therapeutic benefit which may accompany the higher doses should therefore be weighed against the possibility of a greater incidence of adverse effects.

Usage In Pregnancy

ACCORDING TO PUBLISHED AND UNPUBLISHED REPORTS, VALPROIC ACID MAY PRODUCE TERATOGENIC EFFECTS IN THE OFFSPRING OF HUMAN FEMALES RECEIVING THE DRUG DURING PREGNANCY.

THERE ARE MULTIPLE REPORTS IN THE CLINICAL LITERATURE WHICH INDICATE THAT THE USE OF ANTIEPILEPTIC DRUGS DURING PREGNANCY RESULTS IN AN INCREASED INCIDENCE OF BIRTH DEFECTS IN THE OFFSPRING. ALTHOUGH DATA ARE MORE EXTENSIVE WITH RESPECT TO TRIMETHADIONE, PARAMETHADIONE, PHENYTOIN, AND PHENOBARBITAL, REPORTS INDICATE A POSSIBLE SIMILAR ASSOCIATION WITH THE USE OF OTHER ANTIEPILEPTIC DRUGS. THEREFORE, ANTIEPILEPSY DRUGS SHOULD BE ADMINISTERED TO WOMEN OF CHILDBEARING POTENTIAL ONLY IF THEY ARE CLEARLY SHOWN TO BE ESSENTIAL IN THE MANAGEMENT OF THEIR SEIZURES.

THE INCIDENCE OF NEURAL TUBE DEFECTS IN THE FETUS MAY BE INCREASED IN MOTHERS RECEIVING VALPROATE DURING THE FIRST TRIMESTER OF PREGNANCY. THE CENTERS FOR DISEASE CONTROL (CDC) HAS ESTIMATED THE RISK OF VALPROIC ACID EXPOSED WOMEN HAVING CHILDREN WITH SPINA BIFIDA TO BE APPROXIMATELY 1 TO 2%.

OTHER CONGENITAL ANOMALIES (E.G., CRANIOFACIAL DEFECTS, CARDIOVASCULAR MALFORMATIONS AND ANOMALIES INVOLVING VARIOUS BODY SYSTEMS), COMPATIBLE AND INCOMPATIBLE WITH LIFE, HAVE BEEN REPORTED. SUFFICIENT DATA TO DETERMINE THE INCIDENCE OF THESE CONGENITAL ANOMALIES IS NOT AVAILABLE.

THE HIGHER INCIDENCE OF CONGENITAL ANOMALIES IN ANTIEPILEPTIC DRUG-TREATED WOMEN WITH SEIZURE DISORDERS CANNOT BE REGARDED AS A CAUSE AND EFFECT RELATIONSHIP. THERE ARE INTRINSIC METHODOLOGIC PROBLEMS IN OBTAINING ADEQUATE DATA ON DRUG TERATOGENICITY IN HUMANS; GENETIC FACTORS OR THE EPILEPTIC CONDITION ITSELF, MAY BE MORE IMPORTANT THAN DRUG THERAPY IN CONTRIBUTING TO CONGENITAL ANOMALIES.

PATIENTS TAKING VALPROATE MAY DEVELOP CLOTTING ABNORMALITIES. A PATIENT WHO HAD LOW FIBRINOGEN WHEN TAKING MULTIPLE ANTICONVULSANTS INCLUDING VALPROATE GAVE BIRTH TO AN INFANT WITH AFIBRINOGENEMIA WHO SUBSEQUENTLY DIED OF HEMORRHAGE. IF VALPROATE IS USED IN PREGNANCY, THE CLOTTING PARAMETERS SHOULD BE MONITORED CAREFULLY.

HEPATIC FAILURE, RESULTING IN THE DEATH OF A NEWBORN AND OF AN INFANT, HAVE BEEN REPORTED FOLLOWING THE USE OF VALPROATE DURING PREGNANCY.

Animal studies have demonstrated valproate-induced teratogenicity. Increased frequencies of malformations, as well as intrauterine growth retardation and death, have been observed in mice, rats, rabbits, and monkeys following prenatal exposure to valproate. Malformations of the skeletal system are the most common structural abnormalities produced in experimental animals, but neural tube closure defects have been seen in mice exposed to maternal plasma valproate concentrations exceeding 230 μg/mL (2.3 times the upper limit of the human therapeutic range) during susceptible periods of embryonic development. Administration of an oral dose of 200 mg/kg/day or greater (50% of the maximum human daily dose or greater on a mg/m^2 basis) to pregnant rats during organogenesis produced malformations (skeletal, cardiac, and urogenital) and growth retardation in the offspring. These doses resulted in peak maternal plasma valproate levels of approximately 340 μg/mL or greater (3.4 times the upper limit of the human therapeutic range or greater). Behavioral deficits have been reported in the offspring of rats given a dose of 200 mg/kg/day throughout most of pregnancy. An oral dose of 350 mg/kg/day (approximately 2 times the maximum human daily dose on a mg/m^2 basis) produced skeletal and visceral malformations in rabbits exposed during organogenesis. Skeletal malformations, growth retardation, and death were observed in rhesus monkeys following administration of an oral dose of 200 mg/kg/day (equal to the maximum human daily dose on a mg/m^2 basis) during organogenesis. This dose resulted in peak maternal plasma valproate levels of approximately 280 μg/mL (2.8 times the upper limit of the human therapeutic range).

The prescribing physician will wish to weigh the benefits of therapy against the risks in treating or counseling women of childbearing potential. If this drug is used during pregnancy, or if the patient becomes pregnant while taking this drug, the patient should be apprised of the potential hazard to the fetus.

Antiepileptic drugs should not be discontinued abruptly in patients in whom the drug is administered to prevent major seizures because of the strong possibility of precipitating status epilepticus with attendant hypoxia and threat to life. In individual cases where the severity and frequency of the seizure disorder are such that the removal of medication does not pose a serious threat to the patient, discontinuation of the drug may be considered prior to and during pregnancy, although it cannot be said with any confidence that even minor seizures do not pose some hazard to the developing embryo or fetus.

Tests to detect neural tube and other defects using current accepted procedures should be considered a part of routine prenatal care in childbearing women receiving valproate.

PRECAUTIONS

Hepatic Dysfunction

See **BOXED WARNING**, **CONTRAINDICATIONS** and **WARNINGS**.

Pancreatitis

See **BOXED WARNING** and **WARNINGS**.

Hyperammonemia

Hyperammonemia has been reported in association with valproate therapy and may be present despite normal liver function tests. In patients who develop unexplained lethargy and vomiting or changes in mental status, hyperammonemic encephalopathy should be considered and an ammonia level should be measured. If ammonia is increased, valproate therapy should be discontinued. Appropriate interventions for treatment of hyperammonemia should be initiated, and such patients should undergo investigation for underlying urea cycle disorders (see **CONTRAINDICATIONS** and **WARNINGS—Urea Cycle Disorders**).

Asymptomatic elevations of ammonia are more common and when present, require close monitoring of plasma ammonia levels. If the elevation persists, discontinuation of valproate therapy should be considered.

General

Because of reports of thrombocytopenia (see **WARNINGS**), inhibition of the secondary phase of platelet aggregation, and abnormal coagulation parameters, (e.g., low fibrinogen), platelet counts and coagulation tests are recommended before initiating therapy and at periodic intervals. It is recommended that patients receiving DEPAKOTE be monitored for platelet count and coagulation parameters prior to planned surgery. In a clinical trial of DEPAKOTE as monotherapy in patients with epilepsy, 34/126 patients (27%) receiving approximately 50 mg/kg/day on average, had at least one value of platelets $\leq 75 \times 10^9$/L. Approximately half of these patients had treatment discontinued, with return of platelet counts to normal. In the remaining patients, platelet counts normalized with continued treatment. In this study, the probability of thrombocytopenia appeared to increase significantly at total valproate concentrations of $\geq$ 110 μg/mL (females) or $\geq$ 135 μg/mL (males). Evidence of hemorrhage, bruising, or a disorder of hemostasis/coagulation is an indication for reduction of the dosage or withdrawal of therapy.

Since DEPAKOTE may interact with concurrently administered drugs which are capable of enzyme induction, periodic plasma concentration determinations of valproate and concomitant drugs are recommended during the early course of therapy. (See **PRECAUTIONS - Drug Interactions.**)

Valproate is partially eliminated in the urine as a keto-metabolite which may lead to a false interpretation of the urine ketone test.

There have been reports of altered thyroid function tests associated with valproate. The clinical significance of these is unknown.

There are *in vitro* studies that suggest valproate stimulates the replication of the HIV and CMV viruses under certain experimental conditions. The clinical consequence, if any, is not known. Additionally, the relevance of these *in vitro* findings is uncertain for patients receiving maximally suppressive antiretroviral therapy. Nevertheless, these data should be borne in mind when interpreting the results from regular monitoring of the viral load in HIV infected patients receiving valproate or when following CMV infected patients clinically.

Information for Patients

Patients and guardians should be warned that abdominal pain, nausea, vomiting, and/or anorexia can be symptoms of pancreatitis and, therefore, require further medical evaluation promptly.

Patients should be informed of the signs and symptoms associated with hyperammonemic encephalopathy (see **PRECAUTIONS – Hyperammonemia**) and be told to inform the prescriber if any of these symptoms occur.

Since DEPAKOTE products may produce CNS depression, especially when combined with another CNS depressant (e.g., alcohol), patients should be advised not to engage in hazardous activities, such as driving an automobile or operating dangerous machinery, until it is known that they do not become drowsy from the drug.

The specially coated particles in DEPAKOTE Sprinkle Capsules have been observed in the stool, but this occurrence has not been associated with clinically significant effects.

Since DEPAKOTE Sprinkle Capsules has been associated with certain types of birth defects, female patients of childbearing age considering the use of DEPAKOTE Sprinkle Capsules should be advised to read the **Patient Information Leaflet**, which appears as the last section of the labeling.

Drug Interactions

Effects of Co-Administered Drugs on Valproate Clearance

Drugs that affect the level of expression of hepatic enzymes, particularly those that elevate levels of glucuronosyltransferases, may increase the clearance of valproate. For example, phenytoin, carbamazepine, and phenobarbital (or primidone) can double the clearance of valproate. Thus, patients on monotherapy will generally have longer half-lives and higher concentrations than patients receiving polytherapy with antiepilepsy drugs.

In contrast, drugs that are inhibitors of cytochrome P450 isozymes, e.g., antidepressants, may be expected to have little effect on valproate clearance because cytochrome P450 microsomal mediated oxidation is a relatively minor secondary metabolic pathway compared to glucuronidation and beta-oxidation.

Because of these changes in valproate clearance, monitoring of valproate and concomitant drug concentrations should be increased whenever enzyme inducing drugs are introduced or withdrawn.

The following list provides information about the potential for an influence of several commonly prescribed medications on valproate pharmacokinetics. The list is not exhaustive nor could it be, since new interactions are continuously being reported.

Drugs for which a potentially important interaction has been observed:

Aspirin - A study involving the co-administration of aspirin at antipyretic doses (11 to 16 mg/kg) with valproate to pediatric patients (n=6) revealed a decrease in protein binding and an inhibition of metabolism of valproate. Valproate free fraction was increased 4-fold in the presence of aspirin compared to valproate alone. The β-oxidation pathway consisting of 2-E-valproic acid, 3-OH-valproic acid, and 3-keto valproic acid was decreased from 25% of total metabolites excreted on valproate alone to 8.3% in the presence of aspirin. Caution should be observed if valproate and aspirin are to be co-administered.

Felbamate - A study involving the co-administration of 1200 mg/day of felbamate with valproate to patients with epilepsy (n=10) revealed an increase in mean valproate peak concentration by 35% (from 86 to 115 μg/mL) compared to valproate alone. Increasing the felbamate dose to 2400 mg/day increased the mean valproate peak concentration to 133 μg/mL (another 16% increase). A decrease in valproate dosage may be necessary when felbamate therapy is initiated.

Meropenem - Subtherapeutic valproic acid levels have been reported when meropenem was coadministered.

Rifampin - A study involving the administration of a single dose of valproate (7 mg/kg) 36 hours after 5 nights of daily dosing with rifampin (600 mg) revealed a 40% increase in the oral clearance of valproate. Valproate dosage adjustment may be necessary when it is co-administered with rifampin.

Drugs for which either no interaction or a likely clinically unimportant interaction has been observed:

Antacids - A study involving the co-administration of valproate 500 mg with commonly administered antacids

(Maalox, Trisogel, and Titralac - 160 mEq doses) did not reveal any effect on the extent of absorption of valproate.
Chlorpromazine - A study involving the administration of 100 to 300 mg/day of chlorpromazine to schizophrenic patients already receiving valproate (200 mg BID) revealed a 15% increase in trough plasma levels of valproate.
Haloperidol - A study involving the administration of 6 to 10 mg/day of haloperidol to schizophrenic patients already receiving valproate (200 mg BID) revealed no significant changes in valproate trough plasma levels.
Cimetidine and Ranitidine - Cimetidine and ranitidine do not affect the clearance of valproate.

Effects of Valproate on Other Drugs

Valproate has been found to be a weak inhibitor of some P450 isozymes, epoxide hydrase, and glucuronosyltransferases.
The following list provides information about the potential for an influence of valproate co-administration on the pharmacokinetics or pharmacodynamics of several commonly prescribed medications. The list is not exhaustive, since new interactions are continuously being reported.

Drugs for which a potentially important valproate interaction has been observed:

Amitriptyline/Nortriptyline - Administration of a single oral 50 mg dose of amitriptyline to 15 normal volunteers (10 males and 5 females) who received valproate (500 mg BID) resulted in a 21% decrease in plasma clearance of amitriptyline and a 34% decrease in the net clearance of nortriptyline. Rare postmarketing reports of concurrent use of valproate and amitriptyline resulting in an increased amitriptyline level have been received. Concurrent use of valproate and amitriptyline has rarely been associated with toxicity. Monitoring of amitriptyline levels should be considered for patients taking valproate concomitantly with amitriptyline. Consideration should be given to lowering the dose of amitriptyline/nortriptyline in the presence of valproate.
Carbamazepine/carbamazepine-10,11-Epoxide - Serum levels of carbamazepine (CBZ) decreased 17% while that of carbamazepine-10,11-epoxide (CBZ-E) increased by 45% upon co-administration of valproate and CBZ to epileptic patients.
Clonazepam - The concomitant use of valproic acid and clonazepam may induce absence status in patients with a history of absence type seizures.
Diazepam - Valproate displaces diazepam from its plasma albumin binding sites and inhibits its metabolism. Co-administration of valproate (1500 mg daily) increased the free fraction of diazepam (10 mg) by 90% in healthy volunteers (n=6). Plasma clearance and volume of distribution for free diazepam were reduced by 25% and 20%, respectively, in the presence of valproate. The elimination half-life of diazepam remained unchanged upon addition of valproate.
Ethosuximide - Valproate inhibits the metabolism of ethosuximide. Administration of a single ethosuximide dose of 500 mg with valproate (800 to 1600 mg/day) to healthy volunteers (n=6) was accompanied by a 25% increase in elimination half-life of ethosuximide and a 15% decrease in its total clearance as compared to ethosuximide alone. Patients receiving valproate and ethosuximide, especially along with other anticonvulsants, should be monitored for alterations in serum concentrations of both drugs.
Lamotrigine - In a steady-state study involving 10 healthy volunteers, the elimination half-life of lamotrigine increased from 26 to 70 hours with valproate co-administration (a 165% increase). The dose of lamotrigine should be reduced when co-administered with valproate. Serious skin reactions (such as Stevens-Johnson Syndrome and toxic epidermal necrolysis) have been reported with concomitant lamotrigine and valproate administration. See lamotrigine package insert for details on lamotrigine dosing with concomitant valproate administration.
Phenobarbital - Valproate was found to inhibit the metabolism of phenobarbital. Co-administration of valproate (250 mg BID for 14 days) with phenobarbital to normal subjects (n=6) resulted in a 50% increase in half-life and a 30% decrease in plasma clearance of phenobarbital (60 mg single-dose). The fraction of phenobarbital dose excreted unchanged increased by 50% in presence of valproate.
There is evidence for severe CNS depression, with or without significant elevations of barbiturate or valproate serum concentrations. All patients receiving concomitant barbiturate therapy should be closely monitored for neurological toxicity. Serum barbiturate concentrations should be obtained, if possible, and the barbiturate dosage decreased, if appropriate.
Primidone, which is metabolized to a barbiturate, may be involved in a similar interaction with valproate.
Phenytoin - Valproate displaces phenytoin from its plasma albumin binding sites and inhibits its hepatic metabolism. Co-administration of valproate (400 mg TID) with phenytoin (250 mg) in normal volunteers (n=7) was associated with a 60% increase in the free fraction of phenytoin. Total plasma clearance and apparent volume of distribution of phenytoin increased 30% in the presence of valproate. Both the clearance and apparent volume of distribution of free phenytoin were reduced by 25%.
In patients with epilepsy, there have been reports of breakthrough seizures occurring with the combination of valproate and phenytoin. The dosage of phenytoin should be adjusted as required by the clinical situation.
Tolbutamide - From *in vitro* experiments, the unbound fraction of tolbutamide was increased from 20% to 50% when added to plasma samples taken from patients treated with valproate. The clinical relevance of this displacement is unknown.
Warfarin - In an *in vitro* study, valproate increased the unbound fraction of warfarin by up to 32.6%. The therapeutic relevance of this is unknown; however, coagulation tests should be monitored if DEPAKOTE therapy is instituted in patients taking anticoagulants.
Zidovudine - In six patients who were seropositive for HIV, the clearance of zidovudine (100 mg q8h) was decreased by 38% after administration of valproate (250 or 500 mg q8h); the half-life of zidovudine was unaffected.

Drugs for which either no interaction or a likely clinically unimportant interaction has been observed:

Acetaminophen - Valproate had no effect on any of the pharmacokinetic parameters of acetaminophen when it was concurrently administered to three epileptic patients.
Clozapine - In psychotic patients (n=11), no interaction was observed when valproate was co-administered with clozapine.
Lithium - Co-administration of valproate (500 mg BID) and lithium carbonate (300 mg TID) to normal male volunteers (n=16) had no effect on the steady-state kinetics of lithium.
Lorazepam - Concomitant administration of valproate (500 mg BID) and lorazepam (1 mg BID) in normal male volunteers (n=9) was accompanied by a 17% decrease in the plasma clearance of lorazepam.
Oral Contraceptive Steroids - Administration of a single-dose of ethinyloestradiol (50 µg)/levonorgestrel (250 µg) to 6 women on valproate (200 mg BID) therapy for 2 months did not reveal any pharmacokinetic interaction.

Carcinogenesis, Mutagenesis, Impairment of Fertility

Carcinogenesis

Valproic acid was administered orally to Sprague Dawley rats and ICR (HA/ICR) mice at doses of 80 and 170 mg/kg/day (approximately 10 to 50% of the maximum human daily dose on a mg/m^2 basis) for two years. A variety of neoplasms were observed in both species. The chief findings were a statistically significant increase in the incidence of subcutaneous fibrosarcomas in high dose male rats receiving valproic acid and a statistically significant dose-related trend for benign pulmonary adenomas in male mice receiving valproic acid. The significance of these findings for humans is unknown.

Mutagenesis

Valproate was not mutagenic in an *in vitro* bacterial assay (Ames test), did not produce dominant lethal effects in mice, and did not increase chromosome aberration frequency in an *in vivo* cytogenetic study in rats. Increased frequencies of sister chromatid exchange (SCE) have been reported in a study of epileptic children taking valproate, but this association was not observed in another study conducted in adults. There is some evidence that increased SCE frequencies may be associated with epilepsy. The biological significance of an increase in SCE frequency is not known.

Fertility

Chronic toxicity studies in juvenile and adult rats and dogs demonstrated reduced spermatogenesis and testicular atrophy at oral doses of 400 mg/kg/day or greater in rats (approximately equivalent to or greater than the maximum human daily dose on a mg/m^2 basis) and 150 mg/kg/day or greater in dogs (approximately 1.4 times the maximum human daily dose or greater on a mg/m^2 basis). Segment I fertility studies in rats have shown oral doses up to 350 mg/kg/day (approximately equal to the maximum human daily dose on a mg/m^2 basis) for 60 days to have no effect on fertility. THE EFFECT OF VALPROATE ON TESTICULAR DEVELOPMENT AND ON SPERM PRODUCTION AND FERTILITY IN HUMANS IS UNKNOWN.

Pregnancy

Pregnancy Category D: See **WARNINGS**.

Nursing Mothers

Valproate is excreted in breast milk. Concentrations in breast milk have been reported to be 1-10% of serum concentrations. It is not known what effect this would have on a nursing infant. Consideration should be given to discontinuing nursing when divalproex sodium is administered to a nursing woman.

Pediatric Use

Experience has indicated that pediatric patients under the age of two years are at a considerably increased risk of developing fatal hepatotoxicity, especially those with the aforementioned conditions (see **BOXED WARNING**). When DEPAKOTE is used in this patient group, it should be used with extreme caution and as a sole agent. The benefits of therapy should be weighed against the risks. Above the age of 2 years, experience in epilepsy has indicated that the incidence of fatal hepatotoxicity decreases considerably in progressively older patient groups.
Younger children, especially those receiving enzyme-inducing drugs, will require larger maintenance doses to attain targeted total and unbound valproic acid concentrations.
The variability in free fraction limits the clinical usefulness of monitoring total serum valproic acid concentrations. Interpretation of valproic acid concentrations in children should include consideration of factors that affect hepatic metabolism and protein binding.
The basic toxicology and pathologic manifestations of valproate sodium in neonatal (4-day old) and juvenile (14-day old) rats are similar to those seen in young adult rats. However, additional findings, including renal alterations in juvenile rats and renal alterations and retinal dysplasia in neonatal rats, have been reported. These findings occurred at 240 mg/kg/day, a dosage approximately equivalent to the human maximum recommended daily dose on a mg/m^2 basis. They were not seen at 90 mg/kg, or 40% of the maximum human daily dose on a mg/m^2 basis.

Geriatric Use

No patients above the age of 65 years were enrolled in double-blind prospective clinical trials of mania associated with bipolar illness. In a case review study of 583 patients, 72 patients (12%) were greater than 65 years of age. A higher percentage of patients above 65 years of age reported accidental injury, infection, pain, somnolence, and tremor. Discontinuation of valproate was occasionally associated with the latter two events. It is not clear whether these events indicate additional risk or whether they result from preexisting medical illness and concomitant medication use among these patients.
A study of elderly patients with dementia revealed drug related somnolence and discontinuation for somnolence (see **WARNINGS—Somnolence in the Elderly**). The starting dose should be reduced in these patients, and dosage reductions or discontinuation should be considered in patients with excessive somnolence (see **DOSAGE AND ADMINISTRATION**).

ADVERSE REACTIONS

Epilepsy

Based on a placebo-controlled trial of adjunctive therapy for treatment of complex partial seizures, DEPAKOTE was generally well tolerated with most adverse events rated as mild to moderate in severity. Intolerance was the primary reason for discontinuation in the DEPAKOTE-treated patients (6%), compared to 1% of placebo-treated patients.
Table 1 lists treatment-emergent adverse events which were reported by ≥ 5% of DEPAKOTE-treated patients and for which the incidence was greater than in the placebo group, in the placebo-controlled trial of adjunctive therapy for treatment of complex partial seizures. Since patients were also treated with other antiepilepsy drugs, it is not possible, in most cases, to determine whether the following adverse events can be ascribed to DEPAKOTE alone, or the combination of DEPAKOTE and other antiepilepsy drugs.

Table 1
Adverse Events Reported by ≥ 5% of Patients Treated with DEPAKOTE During Placebo-Controlled Trial of Adjunctive Therapy for Complex Partial Seizures

Body System/Event	Depakote (%) (n = 77)	Placebo (%) (n = 70)
Body as a Whole		
Headache	31	21
Asthenia	27	7
Fever	6	4
Gastrointestinal System		
Nausea	48	14
Vomiting	27	7
Abdominal Pain	23	6
Diarrhea	13	6
Anorexia	12	0
Dyspepsia	8	4
Constipation	5	1
Nervous System		
Somnolence	27	11
Tremor	25	6
Dizziness	25	13
Diplopia	16	9
Amblyopia/Blurred Vision	12	9
Ataxia	8	1
Nystagmus	8	1
Emotional Lability	6	4
Thinking Abnormal	6	0
Amnesia	5	1
Respiratory System		
Flu Syndrome	12	9
Infection	12	6
Bronchitis	5	1
Rhinitis	5	4
Other		
Alopecia	6	1
Weight Loss	6	0

Table 2 lists treatment-emergent adverse events which were reported by ≥ 5% of patients in the high dose DEPAKOTE group, and for which the incidence was greater than in the low dose group, in a controlled trial of DEPAKOTE monotherapy treatment of complex partial seizures. Since patients were being titrated off another antiepilepsy drug during the first portion of the trial, it is not possible, in many cases, to determine whether the following adverse events can be ascribed to DEPAKOTE alone, or the combination of DEPAKOTE and other antiepilepsy drugs.

Continued on next page

Depakote Sprinkle—Cont.

Table 2
Adverse Events Reported by ≥ 5% of Patients in the High Dose Group in the Controlled Trial of DEPAKOTE Monotherapy for Complex Partial Seizures[1]

Body System/Event	High Dose (%) (n = 131)	Low Dose (%) (n = 134)
Body as a Whole		
Asthenia	21	10
Digestive System		
Nausea	34	26
Diarrhea	23	19
Vomiting	23	15
Abdominal Pain	12	9
Anorexia	11	4
Dyspepsia	11	10
Hemic/Lymphatic System		
Thrombocytopenia	24	1
Ecchymosis	5	4
Metabolic/Nutritional		
Weight Gain	9	4
Peripheral Edema	8	3
Nervous System		
Tremor	57	19
Somnolence	30	18
Dizziness	18	13
Insomnia	15	9
Nervousness	11	7
Amnesia	7	4
Nystagmus	7	1
Depression	5	4
Respiratory System		
Infection	20	13
Pharyngitis	8	2
Dyspnea	5	1
Skin and Appendages		
Alopecia	24	13
Special Senses		
Amblyopia/Blurred Vision	8	4
Tinnitus	7	1

[1] Headache was the only adverse event that occurred in ≥ 5% of patients in the high dose group and at an equal or greater incidence in the low dose group.

The following additional adverse events were reported by greater than 1% but less than 5% of the 358 patients treated with DEPAKOTE in the controlled trials of complex partial seizures:

Body as a Whole: Back pain, chest pain, malaise.
Cardiovascular System: Tachycardia, hypertension, palpitation.
Digestive System: Increased appetite, flatulence, hematemesis, eructation, pancreatitis, periodontal abscess.
Hemic and Lymphatic System: Petechia.
Metabolic and Nutritional Disorders: SGOT increased, SGPT increased.
Musculoskeletal System: Myalgia, twitching, arthralgia, leg cramps, myasthenia.
Nervous System: Anxiety, confusion, abnormal gait, paresthesia, hypertonia, incoordination, abnormal dreams, personality disorder.
Respiratory System: Sinusitis, cough increased, pneumonia, epistaxis.
Skin and Appendages: Rash, pruritus, dry skin.
Special Senses: Taste perversion, abnormal vision, deafness, otitis media.
Urogenital System: Urinary incontinence, vaginitis, dysmenorrhea, amenorrhea, urinary frequency.

Other Patient Populations

Adverse events that have been reported with all dosage forms of valproate from epilepsy trials, spontaneous reports, and other sources are listed below by body system.

Gastrointestinal: The most commonly reported side effects at the initiation of therapy are nausea, vomiting, and indigestion. These effects are usually transient and rarely require discontinuation of therapy. Diarrhea, abdominal cramps, and constipation have been reported. Both anorexia with some weight loss and increased appetite with weight gain have also been reported. The administration of delayed-release divalproex sodium may result in reduction of gastrointestinal side effects in some patients.

CNS Effects: Sedative effects have occurred in patients receiving valproate alone but occur most often in patients receiving combination therapy. Sedation usually abates upon reduction of other antiepileptic medication. Tremor (may be dose-related), hallucinations, ataxia, headache, nystagmus, diplopia, asterixis, "spots before eyes", dysarthria, dizziness, confusion, hypesthesia, vertigo, incoordination, and parkinsonism have been reported with the use of valproate. Rare cases of coma have occurred in patients receiving valproate alone or in conjunction with phenobarbital. In rare instances encephalopathy with or without fever has developed shortly after the introduction of valproate monotherapy without evidence of hepatic dysfunction or inappropriately high plasma valproate levels. Although recovery has been described following drug withdrawal, there have been fatalities in patients with hyperammonemic encephalopathy, particularly in patients with underlying urea cycle disorders (see **WARNINGS – Urea Cycle Disorders** and **PRECAUTIONS**).

Several reports have noted reversible cerebral atrophy and dementia in association with valproate therapy.

Dermatologic: Transient hair loss, skin rash, photosensitivity, generalized pruritus, erythema multiforme, and Stevens-Johnson syndrome. Rare cases of toxic epidermal necrolysis have been reported including a fatal case in a 6 month old infant taking valproate and several other concomitant medications. An additional case of toxic epidermal necrosis resulting in death was reported in a 35 year old patient with AIDS taking several concomitant medications and with a history of multiple cutaneous drug reactions. Serious skin reactions have been reported with concomitant administration of lamotrigine and valproate (see **PRECAUTIONS-Drug Interactions**).

Psychiatric: Emotional upset, depression, psychosis, aggression, hyperactivity, hostility, and behavioral deterioration.

Musculoskeletal: Weakness.

Hematologic: Thrombocytopenia and inhibition of the secondary phase of platelet aggregation may be reflected in altered bleeding time, petechia, bruising, hematoma formation, epistaxis, and frank hemorrhage (see **PRECAUTIONS - General** and **Drug Interactions**). Relative lymphocytosis, macrocytosis, hypofibrinogenemia, leukopenia, eosinophilia, anemia including macrocytic with or without folate deficiency, bone marrow suppression, pancytopenia, aplastic anemia, agranulocytosis and acute intermittent porphyria.

Hepatic: Minor elevations of transaminases (eg, SGOT and SGPT) and LDH are frequent and appear to be dose-related. Occasionally, laboratory test results include increases in serum bilirubin and abnormal changes in other liver function tests. These results may reflect potentially serious hepatotoxicity (see **WARNINGS**).

Endocrine: Irregular menses, secondary amenorrhea, breast enlargement, galactorrhea, and parotid gland swelling. Abnormal thyroid function tests (see **PRECAUTIONS**).

There have been rare spontaneous reports of polycystic ovary disease. A cause and effect relationship has not been established.

Pancreatic: Acute pancreatitis including fatalities (see **WARNINGS**).

Metabolic: Hyperammonemia (see **PRECAUTIONS**), hyponatremia, and inappropriate ADH secretion.

There have been rare reports of Fanconi's syndrome occurring chiefly in children.

Decreased carnitine concentrations have been reported although the clinical relevance is undetermined.

Hyperglycinemia has occurred and was associated with a fatal outcome in a patient with preexistent nonketotic hyperglycinemia.

Genitourinary: Enuresis and urinary tract infection.

Special Senses: Hearing loss, either reversible or irreversible, has been reported; however, a cause and effect relationship has not been established. Ear pain has also been reported.

Other: Allergic reaction, anaphylaxis, edema of the extremities, lupus erythematosus, bone pain, cough increased, pneumonia, otitis media, bradycardia, cutaneous vasculitis, fever, and hypothermia.

Mania

Although DEPAKOTE Sprinkle Capsules have not been evaluated for safety and efficacy in the treatment of manic episodes associated with bipolar disorder, the following adverse events not listed above were reported by 1% or more of patients from two placebo-controlled clinical trials of DEPAKOTE tablets.

Body as a Whole: Chills, neck pain, neck rigidity.
Cardiovascular System: Hypotension, postural hypotension, vasodilation.
Digestive System: Fecal incontinence, gastroenteritis, glossitis.
Musculoskeletal System: Arthrosis.
Nervous System: Agitation, catatonic reaction, hypokinesia, reflexes increased, tardive dyskinesia, vertigo.
Skin and Appendages: Furunculosis, maculopapular rash, seborrhea.
Special Senses: Conjunctivitis, dry eyes, eye pain.
Urogenital System: Dysuria.

Migraine

Although DEPAKOTE Sprinkle Capsules have not been evaluated for safety and efficacy in the treatment of prophylaxis of migraine headaches, the following adverse events not listed above were reported by 1% or more of patients from two placebo-controlled clinical trials of DEPAKOTE tablets.

Body as a Whole: Face edema.
Digestive System: Dry mouth, stomatitis.
Urogenital System: Cystitis, metrorrhagia, and vaginal hemorrhage.

OVERDOSAGE

Overdosage with valproate may result in somnolence, heart block, and deep coma. Fatalities have been reported; however patients have recovered from valproate levels as high as 2120 µg/mL.

In overdose situations, the fraction of drug not bound to protein is high and hemodialysis or tandem hemodialysis plus hemoperfusion may result in significant removal of drug. The benefit of gastric lavage or emesis will vary with the time since ingestion. General supportive measures should be applied with particular attention to the maintenance of adequate urinary output.

Naloxone has been reported to reverse the CNS depressant effects of valproate overdosage. Because naloxone could theoretically also reverse the antiepileptic effects of valproate, it should be used with caution in patients with epilepsy.

DOSAGE AND ADMINISTRATION

Epilepsy

DEPAKOTE Sprinkle Capsules are administered orally. DEPAKOTE is indicated as monotherapy and adjunctive therapy in complex partial seizures in adults and pediatric patients down to the age of 10 years, and in simple and complex absence seizures. As the DEPAKOTE dosage is titrated upward, concentrations of phenobarbital, carbamazepine, and/or phenytoin may be affected (see **PRECAUTIONS - Drug Interactions**).

Complex Partial Seizures: For adults and children 10 years of age or older.

Monotherapy (Initial Therapy): DEPAKOTE has not been systematically studied as initial therapy. Patients should initiate therapy at 10 to 15 mg/kg/day. The dosage should be increased by 5 to 10 mg/kg/week to achieve optimal clinical response. Ordinarily, optimal clinical response is achieved at daily doses below 60 mg/kg/day. If satisfactory clinical response has not been achieved, plasma levels should be measured to determine whether or not they are in the usually accepted therapeutic range (50 to 100 µg/mL). No recommendation regarding the safety of valproate for use at doses above 60 mg/kg/day can be made.

The probability of thrombocytopenia increases significantly at total trough valproate plasma concentrations above 110 µg/mL in females and 135 µg/mL in males. The benefit of improved seizure control with higher doses should be weighed against the possibility of a greater incidence of adverse reactions.

Conversion to Monotherapy: Patients should initiate therapy at 10 to 15 mg/kg/day. The dosage should be increased by 5 to 10 mg/kg/week to achieve optimal clinical response. Ordinarily, optimal clinical response is achieved at daily doses below 60 mg/kg/day. If satisfactory clinical response has not been achieved, plasma levels should be measured to determine whether or not they are in the usually accepted therapeutic range (50 - 100 µg/mL). No recommendation regarding the safety of valproate for use at doses above 60 mg/kg/day can be made. Concomitant antiepilepsy drug (AED) dosage can ordinarily be reduced by approximately 25% every 2 weeks. This reduction may be started at initiation of DEPAKOTE therapy, or delayed by 1 to 2 weeks if there is a concern that seizures are likely to occur with a reduction. The speed and duration of withdrawal of the concomitant AED can be highly variable, and patients should be monitored closely during this period for increased seizure frequency.

Adjunctive Therapy: DEPAKOTE may be added to the patient's regimen at a dosage of 10 to 15 mg/kg/day. The dosage may be increased by 5 to 10 mg/kg/week to achieve optimal clinical response. Ordinarily, optimal clinical response is achieved at daily doses below 60 mg/kg/day. If satisfactory clinical response has not been achieved, plasma levels should be measured to determine whether or not they are in the usually accepted therapeutic range (50 to 100 µg/mL). No recommendation regarding the safety of valproate for use at doses above 60 mg/kg/day can be made. If the total daily dose exceeds 250 mg, it should be given in divided doses.

In a study of adjunctive therapy for complex partial seizures in which patients were receiving either carbamazepine or phenytoin in addition to DEPAKOTE, no adjustment of carbamazepine or phenytoin dosage was needed (see **CLINICAL STUDIES**). However, since valproate may interact with these or other concurrently administered AEDs as well as other drugs (see **Drug Interactions**), periodic plasma concentration determinations of concomitant AEDs are recommended during the early course of therapy (see **PRECAUTIONS - Drug Interactions**).

Simple and Complex Absence Seizures: The recommended initial dose is 15 mg/kg/day, increasing at one week intervals by 5 to 10 mg/kg/day until seizures are controlled or side effects preclude further increases. The maximum recommended dosage is 60 mg/kg/day. If the total daily dose exceeds 250 mg, it should be given in divided doses.

A good correlation has not been established between daily dose, serum concentrations, and therapeutic effect. However, therapeutic valproate serum concentrations for most patients with absence seizures is considered to range from 50 to 100 µg/mL. Some patients may be controlled with lower or higher serum concentrations (see **CLINICAL PHARMACOLOGY**).

As the DEPAKOTE dosage is titrated upward, blood concentrations of phenobarbital and/or phenytoin may be affected (see **PRECAUTIONS**).

Antiepilepsy drugs should not be abruptly discontinued in patients in whom the drug is administered to prevent major seizures because of the strong possibility of precipitating status epilepticus with attendant hypoxia and threat to life.

In epileptic patients previously receiving DEPAKENE (valproic acid) therapy, DEPAKOTE Sprinkle Capsules should be initiated at the same daily dose and dosing schedule. After the patient is stabilized on DEPAKOTE Sprinkle Capsules, a dosing schedule of two or three times a day may be elected in selected patients.

General Dosing Advice

Dosing in Elderly Patients - Due to a decrease in unbound clearance of valproate and possibly a greater sensitivity to somnolence in the elderly, the starting dose should be reduced in these patients. Dosage should be increased more slowly and with regular monitoring for fluid and nutritional intake, dehydration, somnolence, and other adverse events. Dose reductions or discontinuation of valproate should be considered in patients with decreased food or fluid intake and in patients with excessive somnolence. The ultimate therapeutic dose should be achieved on the basis of both tolerability and clinical response (see **WARNINGS**).

Dose-Related Adverse Events - The frequency of adverse effects (particularly elevated liver enzymes and thrombocytopenia) may be dose-related. The probability of thrombocytopenia appears to increase significantly at total valproate concentrations of $\geq$ 110 μg/mL (females) or $\geq$ 135 μg/mL (males) (see **PRECAUTIONS**). The benefit of improved therapeutic effect with higher doses should be weighed against the possibility of a greater incidence of adverse reactions.

G.I. Irritation - Patients who experience G.I. irritation may benefit from administration of the drug with food or by slowly building up the dose from an initial low level.

Administration of Sprinkle Capsules - DEPAKOTE Sprinkle Capsules may be swallowed whole or may be administered by carefully opening the capsule and sprinkling the entire contents on a small amount (teaspoonful) of soft food such as applesauce or pudding. The drug/food mixture should be swallowed immediately (avoid chewing) and not stored for future use. Each capsule is oversized to allow ease of opening.

HOW SUPPLIED

DEPAKOTE Sprinkle Capsules (divalproex sodium coated particles in capsules), 125 mg, are white opaque and blue, and are supplied in bottles of 100 (**NDC** 0074-6114-13) and Abbo-Pac® unit dose packages of 100 (**NDC** 0074-6114-11).

Recommended storage: Store capsules below 77°F (25°C).

Patient Information Leaflet

Important Information for Women Who Could Become Pregnant About the Use of DEPAKOTE® Sprinkle Capsules (divalproex sodium coated particles in capsules)

Please read this leaflet carefully before you take DEPAKOTE® Sprinkle Capsules (divalproex sodium coated particles in capsules). This leaflet provides a summary of important information about taking DEPAKOTE Sprinkle Capsules to women who could become pregnant. If you have any questions or concerns, or want more information about DEPAKOTE Sprinkle Capsules, contact your doctor or pharmacist.

Information For Women Who Could Become Pregnant

DEPAKOTE Sprinkle Capsules can be obtained only by prescription from your doctor. The decision to use DEPAKOTE Sprinkle Capsules is one that you and your doctor should make together, taking into account your individual needs and medical condition.

Before using DEPAKOTE Sprinkle Capsules, women who can become pregnant should consider the fact that DEPAKOTE Sprinkle Capsules have been associated with birth defects, in particular, with spina bifida and other defects related to failure of the spinal canal to close normally. Approximately 1 to 2% of children born to women with epilepsy taking DEPAKOTE Sprinkle Capsules in the first 12 weeks of pregnancy had these defects (based on data from the Centers for Disease Control, a U.S. agency based in Atlanta). The incidence in the general population is 0.1 to 0.2%.

Information For Women Who Are Planning to Get Pregnant

- Women taking DEPAKOTE Sprinkle Capsules who are planning to get pregnant should discuss the treatment options with their doctor.

Information For Women Who Become Pregnant While Taking DEPAKOTE Sprinkle Capsules

- If you become pregnant while taking DEPAKOTE Sprinkle Capsules, you should contact your doctor immediately.

Other Important Information About DEPAKOTE Sprinkle Capsules

- DEPAKOTE Sprinkle Capsules should be taken exactly as it is prescribed by your doctor to get the most benefits from DEPAKOTE Sprinkle Capsules and reduce the risk of side effects.
- If you have taken more than the prescribed dose of DEPAKOTE Sprinkle Capsules, contact your hospital emergency room or local poison center immediately.
- This medication was prescribed for your particular condition. Do not use it for another condition or give the drug to others.

Facts About Birth Defects

It is important to know that birth defects may occur even in children of individuals not taking any medications or without any additional risk factors.

This summary provides important information about the use of DEPAKOTE Sprinkle Capsules to women who could become pregnant. If you would like more information about the other potential risks and benefits of DEPAKOTE Sprinkle Capsules, ask your doctor or pharmacist to let you read the professional labeling and then discuss it with them. If you have any questions or concerns about taking DEPAKOTE, you should discuss them with your doctor.

03-5283-R7

Revised: September, 2003

ABBOTT LABORATORIES
NORTH CHICAGO, IL 60064, U.S.A.
PRINTED IN U.S.A.

DEPAKOTE®
Sprinkle Capsules
DIVALPROEX SODIUM
COATED PARTICLES IN CAPSULES
Patient Information Guide
Administration Guide

DEPAKOTE® Sprinkle Capsules (divalproex sodium coated particles in capsules) may be swallowed whole or capsule contents may be sprinkled onto any soft food.

TO ADMINISTER WITH FOOD:

1 Hold the capsule so that the end marked "THIS END UP" is straight up. Although the capsule is oversized to help prevent spilling, it must be handled carefully.

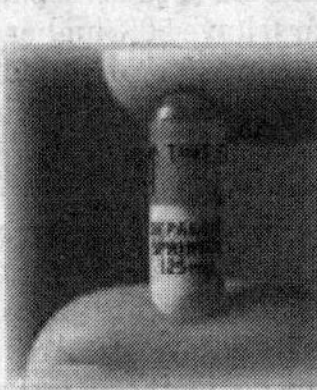

2 To open the capsule, hold it carefully, as shown here, and gently twist it apart. You may find it helpful to hold the capsule over the food to which you will be adding the sprinkles. If you spill *any* of the capsule contents it is important that you start over with a new capsule and a new portion of food.

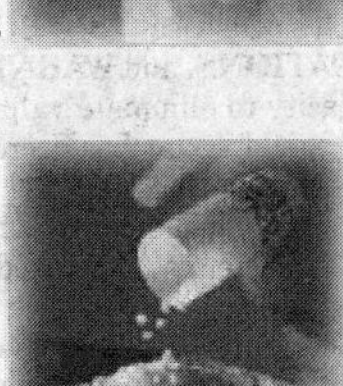

3 Place *all* the sprinkles onto a small amount (about a teaspoonful) of soft food such as applesauce or pudding. The reverse side of this sheet lists several serving suggestions.

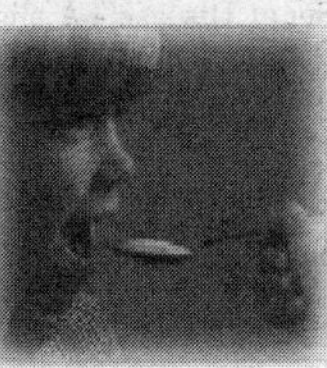

4 Make sure *all* of the sprinkle/food mixture is swallowed immediately. Chewing should be avoided. Fluid taken immediately after the sprinkle/food mixture will help make sure all sprinkles are swallowed. Never store any sprinkle/food mixture for future use.

Serving Suggestions

DEPAKOTE® Sprinkle Capsules (divalproex sodium coated particles in capsules) are designed to provide the medication your physician prescribed in a way that is more convenient for patients and their families. The flavorless sprinkles let the flavor of the food come through so that dosing time is pleasant for all concerned. Soft foods are appropriate for sprinkle dosing. Some examples include: applesauce, pudding, custard, yogurt, ice cream, and oatmeal. See reverse side for administration guidelines.

Make sure this medication is taken as your physician prescribed it. If you have any questions, please contact your physician or pharmacist. Keep all your physician appointments as scheduled. Make sure this and all other drugs are kept out of the reach of children.

Note:

The specially coated particles in DEPAKOTE Sprinkle Capsules have been observed in the stool, but this occurrence has not been associated with clinically significant effects. Ask your physician or pharmacist about possible side effects with Depakote Sprinkle Capsules.

Revised: September, 2003

ABBOTT LABORATORIES
NORTH CHICAGO, IL 60064, U.S.A.
PRINTED IN U.S.A.
Ref. 03-5283-R7

Shown in Product Identification Guide, page 303

DEPAKOTE® Tablets ℞

[*dəp 'ā-coat*]
DIVALPROEX SODIUM
DELAYED-RELEASE TABLETS
℞ only

BOX WARNING:
HEPATOTOXICITY:

HEPATIC FAILURE RESULTING IN FATALITIES HAS OCCURRED IN PATIENTS RECEIVING VALPROIC ACID AND ITS DERIVATIVES. EXPERIENCE HAS INDICATED THAT CHILDREN UNDER THE AGE OF TWO YEARS ARE AT A CONSIDERABLY INCREASED RISK OF DEVELOPING FATAL HEPATOTOXICITY, ESPECIALLY THOSE ON MULTIPLE ANTICONVULSANTS, THOSE WITH CONGENITAL METABOLIC DISORDERS, THOSE WITH SEVERE SEIZURE DISORDERS ACCOMPANIED BY MENTAL RETARDATION, AND THOSE WITH ORGANIC BRAIN DISEASE. WHEN DEPAKOTE IS USED IN THIS PATIENT GROUP, IT SHOULD BE USED WITH EXTREME CAUTION AND AS A SOLE AGENT. THE BENEFITS OF THERAPY SHOULD BE WEIGHED AGAINST THE RISKS. ABOVE THIS AGE GROUP, EXPERIENCE IN EPILEPSY HAS INDICATED THAT THE INCIDENCE OF FATAL HEPATOTOXICITY DECREASES CONSIDERABLY IN PROGRESSIVELY OLDER PATIENT GROUPS.

THESE INCIDENTS USUALLY HAVE OCCURRED DURING THE FIRST SIX MONTHS OF TREATMENT. SERIOUS OR FATAL HEPATOTOXICITY MAY BE PRECEDED BY NON-SPECIFIC SYMPTOMS SUCH AS MALAISE, WEAKNESS, LETHARGY, FACIAL EDEMA, ANOREXIA, AND VOMITING. IN PATIENTS WITH EPILEPSY, A LOSS OF SEIZURE CONTROL MAY ALSO OCCUR. PATIENTS SHOULD BE MONITORED CLOSELY FOR APPEARANCE OF THESE SYMPTOMS. LIVER FUNCTION TESTS SHOULD BE PERFORMED PRIOR TO THERAPY AND AT FREQUENT INTERVALS THEREAFTER, ESPECIALLY DURING THE FIRST SIX MONTHS.

TERATOGENICITY:

VALPROATE CAN PRODUCE TERATOGENIC EFFECTS SUCH AS NEURAL TUBE DEFECTS (E.G., SPINA BIFIDA). ACCORDINGLY, THE USE OF DEPAKOTE TABLETS IN WOMEN OF CHILDBEARING POTENTIAL REQUIRES THAT THE BENEFITS OF ITS USE BE WEIGHED AGAINST THE RISK OF INJURY TO THE FETUS. THIS IS ESPECIALLY IMPORTANT WHEN THE TREATMENT OF A SPONTANEOUSLY REVERSIBLE CONDITION NOT ORDINARILY ASSOCIATED WITH PERMANENT INJURY OR RISK OF DEATH (E.G., MIGRAINE) IS CONTEMPLATED. SEE WARNINGS, INFORMATION FOR PATIENTS.

AN INFORMATION SHEET DESCRIBING THE TERATOGENIC POTENTIAL OF VALPROATE IS AVAILABLE FOR PATIENTS.

PANCREATITIS:

CASES OF LIFE-THREATENING PANCREATITIS HAVE BEEN REPORTED IN BOTH CHILDREN AND ADULTS RECEIVING VALPROATE. SOME OF THE CASES HAVE BEEN DESCRIBED AS HEMORRHAGIC WITH A RAPID PROGRESSION FROM INITIAL SYMPTOMS TO DEATH. CASES HAVE BEEN REPORTED SHORTLY AFTER INITIAL USE AS WELL AS AFTER SEVERAL YEARS OF USE. PATIENTS AND GUARDIANS SHOULD BE WARNED THAT ABDOMINAL PAIN, NAUSEA, VOMITING, AND/OR ANOREXIA CAN BE SYMPTOMS OF PANCREATITIS THAT REQUIRE PROMPT MEDICAL EVALUATION. IF PANCREATITIS IS DIAGNOSED, VALPROATE SHOULD ORDINARILY BE DISCONTINUED. ALTERNATIVE TREATMENT FOR THE UNDERLYING MEDICAL CONDITION SHOULD BE INITIATED AS CLINICALLY INDICATED. (See **WARNINGS** and **PRECAUTIONS**.)

DESCRIPTION

Divalproex sodium is a stable co-ordination compound comprised of sodium valproate and valproic acid in a 1:1 molar relationship and formed during the partial neutralization of valproic acid with 0.5 equivalent of sodium hydroxide. Chemically it is designated as sodium hydrogen bis(2-propylpentanoate). Divalproex sodium has the following structure:

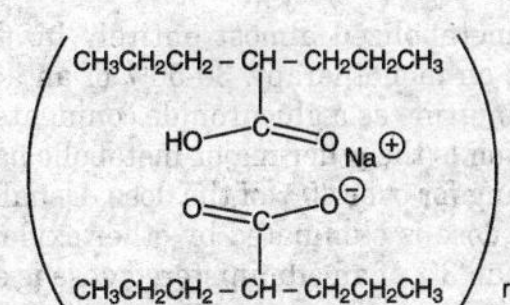

Divalproex sodium occurs as a white powder with a characteristic odor.

DEPAKOTE tablets are for oral administration. DEPAKOTE tablets are supplied in three dosage strengths containing divalproex sodium equivalent to 125 mg, 250 mg, or 500 mg of valproic acid.

Inactive Ingredients

DEPAKOTE tablets: cellulosic polymers, diacetylated monoglycerides, povidone, pregelatinized starch (contains corn starch), silica gel, talc, titanium dioxide, and vanillin.

In addition, individual tablets contain:

125 mg tablets: FD&C Blue No. 1 and FD&C Red No. 40.
250 mg tablets: FD&C Yellow No. 6 and iron oxide.
500 mg tablets: D&C Red No. 30, FD&C Blue No. 2, and iron oxide.

Continued on next page

Depakote Tablets—Cont.

CLINICAL PHARMACOLOGY

Pharmacodynamics

Divalproex sodium dissociates to the valproate ion in the gastrointestinal tract. The mechanisms by which valproate exerts its therapeutic effects have not been established. It has been suggested that its activity in epilepsy is related to increased brain concentrations of gamma-aminobutyric acid (GABA).

Pharmacokinetics

Absorption/Bioavailability

Equivalent oral doses of DEPAKOTE (divalproex sodium) products and DEPAKENE (valproic acid) capsules deliver equivalent quantities of valproate ion systemically. Although the rate of valproate ion absorption may vary with the formulation administered (liquid, solid, or sprinkle), conditions of use (e.g., fasting or postprandial) and the method of administration (e.g., whether the contents of the capsule are sprinkled on food or the capsule is taken intact), these differences should be of minor clinical importance under the steady state conditions achieved in chronic use in the treatment of epilepsy.

However, it is possible that differences among the various valproate products in T_{max} and C_{max} could be important upon initiation of treatment. For example, in single dose studies, the effect of feeding had a greater influence on the rate of absorption of the tablet (increase in T_{max} from 4 to 8 hours) than on the absorption of the sprinkle capsules (increase in T_{max} from 3.3 to 4.8 hours).

While the absorption rate from the G.I. tract and fluctuation in valproate plasma concentrations vary with dosing regimen and formulation, the efficacy of valproate as an anticonvulsant in chronic use is unlikely to be affected. Experience employing dosing regimens from once-a-day to four-times-a-day, as well as studies in primate epilepsy models involving constant rate infusion, indicate that total daily systemic bioavailability (extent of absorption) is the primary determinant of seizure control and that differences in the ratios of plasma peak to trough concentrations between valproate formulations are inconsequential from a practical clinical standpoint. Whether or not rate of absorption influences the efficacy of valproate as an antimanic or antimigraine agent is unknown.

Co-administration of oral valproate products with food and substitution among the various DEPAKOTE and DEPAKENE formulations should cause no clinical problems in the management of patients with epilepsy (see **DOSAGE AND ADMINISTRATION**). Nonetheless, any changes in dosage administration, or the addition or discontinuance of concomitant drugs should ordinarily be accompanied by close monitoring of clinical status and valproate plasma concentrations.

Distribution

Protein Binding:

The plasma protein binding of valproate is concentration dependent and the free fraction increases from approximately 10% at 40 µg/mL to 18.5% at 130 µg/mL. Protein binding of valproate is reduced in the elderly, in patients with chronic hepatic diseases, in patients with renal impairment, and in the presence of other drugs (e.g., aspirin). Conversely, valproate may displace certain protein-bound drugs (e.g., phenytoin, carbamazepine, warfarin, and tolbutamide). (See **PRECAUTIONS**, **Drug Interactions** for more detailed information on the pharmacokinetic interactions of valproate with other drugs.)

CNS Distribution:

Valproate concentrations in cerebrospinal fluid (CSF) approximate unbound concentrations in plasma (about 10% of total concentration).

Metabolism

Valproate is metabolized almost entirely by the liver. In adult patients on monotherapy, 30-50% of an administered dose appears in urine as a glucuronide conjugate. Mitochondrial β-oxidation is the other major metabolic pathway, typically accounting for over 40% of the dose. Usually, less than 15-20% of the dose is eliminated by other oxidative mechanisms. Less than 3% of an administered dose is excreted unchanged in urine.

The relationship between dose and total valproate concentration is nonlinear; concentration does not increase proportionally with the dose, but rather, increases to a lesser extent due to saturable plasma protein binding. The kinetics of unbound drug are linear.

Elimination

Mean plasma clearance and volume of distribution for total valproate are 0.56 L/hr/1.73 m^2 and 11 L/1.73 m^2, respectively. Mean plasma clearance and volume of distribution for free valproate are 4.6 L/hr/1.73 m^2 and 92 L/1.73 m^2. Mean terminal half-life for valproate monotherapy ranged from 9 to 16 hours following oral dosing regimens of 250 to 1000 mg.

The estimates cited apply primarily to patients who are not taking drugs that affect hepatic metabolizing enzyme systems. For example, patients taking enzyme-inducing antiepileptic drugs (carbamazepine, phenytoin, and phenobarbital) will clear valproate more rapidly. Because of these changes in valproate clearance, monitoring of antiepileptic concentrations should be intensified whenever concomitant antiepileptics are introduced or withdrawn.

Special Populations

Effect of Age:

Neonates - Children within the first two months of life have a markedly decreased ability to eliminate valproate compared to older children and adults. This is a result of reduced clearance (perhaps due to delay in development of glucuronosyltransferase and other enzyme systems involved in valproate elimination) as well as increased volume of distribution (in part due to decreased plasma protein binding). For example, in one study, the half-life in children under 10 days ranged from 10 to 67 hours compared to a range of 7 to 13 hours in children greater than 2 months.

Children - Pediatric patients (i.e., between 3 months and 10 years) have 50% higher clearances expressed on weight (i.e., mL/min/kg) than do adults. Over the age of 10 years, children have pharmacokinetic parameters that approximate those of adults.

Elderly - The capacity of elderly patients (age range: 68 to 89 years) to eliminate valproate has been shown to be reduced compared to younger adults (age range: 22 to 26). Intrinsic clearance is reduced by 39%; the free fraction is increased by 44%. Accordingly, the initial dosage should be reduced in the elderly. (See **DOSAGE AND ADMINISTRATION**).

Effect of Gender:

There are no differences in the body surface area adjusted unbound clearance between males and females (4.8±0.17 and 4.7±0.07 L/hr per 1.73 m^2, respectively).

Effect of Race:

The effects of race on the kinetics of valproate have not been studied.

Effect of Disease:

Liver Disease - (See **BOXED WARNING**, **CONTRAINDICATIONS**, and **WARNINGS**). Liver disease impairs the capacity to eliminate valproate. In one study, the clearance of free valproate was decreased by 50% in 7 patients with cirrhosis and by 16% in 4 patients with acute hepatitis, compared with 6 healthy subjects. In that study, the half-life of valproate was increased from 12 to 18 hours. Liver disease is also associated with decreased albumin concentrations and larger unbound fractions (2 to 2.6 fold increase) of valproate. Accordingly, monitoring of total concentrations may be misleading since free concentrations may be substantially elevated in patients with hepatic disease whereas total concentrations may appear to be normal.

Renal Disease - A slight reduction (27%) in the unbound clearance of valproate has been reported in patients with renal failure (creatinine clearance < 10 mL/minute); however, hemodialysis typically reduces valproate concentrations by about 20%. Therefore, no dosage adjustment appears to be necessary in patients with renal failure. Protein binding in these patients is substantially reduced; thus, monitoring total concentrations may be misleading.

Plasma Levels and Clinical Effect

The relationship between plasma concentration and clinical response is not well documented. One contributing factor is the nonlinear, concentration dependent protein binding of valproate which affects the clearance of the drug. Thus, monitoring of total serum valproate cannot provide a reliable index of the bioactive valproate species.

For example, because the plasma protein binding of valproate is concentration dependent, the free fraction increases from approximately 10% at 40 µg/mL to 18.5% at 130 µg/mL. Higher than expected free fractions occur in the elderly, in hyperlipidemic patients, and in patients with hepatic and renal diseases.

Epilepsy:

The therapeutic range in epilepsy is commonly considered to be 50 to 100 µg/mL of total valproate, although some patients may be controlled with lower or higher plasma concentrations.

Mania:

In placebo-controlled clinical trials of acute mania, patients were dosed to clinical response with trough plasma concentrations between 50 and 125 µg/mL (See **DOSAGE AND ADMINISTRATION**).

Clinical Trials

Mania

The effectiveness of DEPAKOTE for the treatment of acute mania was demonstrated in two 3-week, placebo controlled, parallel group studies.

(1) Study 1: The first study enrolled adult patients who met DSM-III-R criteria for Bipolar Disorder and who were hospitalized for acute mania. In addition, they had a history of failing to respond to or not tolerating previous lithium carbonate treatment. DEPAKOTE was initiated at a dose of 250 mg tid and adjusted to achieve serum valproate concentrations in a range of 50-100 µg/mL by day 7. Mean DEPAKOTE doses for completers in this study were 1118, 1525, and 2402 mg/day at days 7, 14, and 21, respectively. Patients were assessed on the Young Mania Rating Scale (YMRS; score ranges from 0-60), an augmented Brief Psychiatric Rating Scale (BPRS-A), and the Global Assessment Scale (GAS). Baseline scores and change from baseline in the week 3 endpoint (last-observation-carry-forward) analysis were as follows:

Study 1

YMRS Total Score

Group	Baseline[1]	BL to Wk 3[2]	Difference[3]
Placebo	28.8	+0.2	
DEPAKOTE	28.5	-9.5	9.7

BPRS-A Total Score

Group	Baseline[1]	BL to Wk 3[2]	Difference[3]
Placebo	76.2	+ 1.8	
DEPAKOTE	76.4	-17.0	18.8

GAS Score

Group	Baseline[1]	BL to Wk 3[2]	Difference[3]
Placebo	31.8	0.0	
DEPAKOTE	30.3	+18.1	18.1

[1] Mean score at baseline
[2] Change from baseline to week 3 (LOCF)
[3] Difference in change from baseline to week 3 endpoint (LOCF) between DEPAKOTE and placebo

DEPAKOTE was statistically significantly superior to placebo on all three measures of outcome.

(2) Study 2: The second study enrolled adult patients who met Research Diagnostic Criteria for manic disorder and who were hospitalized for acute mania. DEPAKOTE was initiated at a dose of 250 mg tid and adjusted within a dose range of 750-2500 mg/day to achieve serum valproate concentrations in a range of 40-150 µg/mL. Mean DEPAKOTE doses for completers in this study were 1116, 1683, and 2006 mg/day at days 7, 14, and 21, respectively. Study 2 also included a lithium group for which lithium doses for completers were 1312, 1869, and 1984 mg/day at days 7, 14, and 21, respectively. Patients were assessed on the Manic Rating Scale (MRS; score ranges from 11-63), and the primary outcome measures were the total MRS score, and scores for two subscales of the MRS, i.e., the Manic Syndrome Scale (MSS) and the Behavior and Ideation Scale (BIS). Baseline scores and change from baseline in the week 3 endpoint (last-observation-carry-forward) analysis were as follows:

Study 2

MRS Total Score

Group	Baseline[1]	BL to Day 21[2]	Difference[3]
Placebo	38.9	-4.4	
Lithium	37.9	-10.5	6.1
DEPAKOTE	38.1	-9.5	5.1

MSS Total Score

Group	Baseline[1]	BL to Day 21[2]	Difference[3]
Placebo	18.9	-2.5	
Lithium	18.5	-6.2	3.7
DEPAKOTE	18.9	-6.0	3.5

BIS Total Score

Group	Baseline[1]	BL to Day 21[2]	Difference[3]
Placebo	16.4	-1.4	
Lithium	16.0	-3.8	2.4
DEPAKOTE	15.7	-3.2	1.8

[1] Mean score at baseline
[2] Change from baseline to day 21 (LOCF)
[3] Difference in change from baseline to day 21 endpoint (LOCF) between DEPAKOTE and placebo and lithium and placebo

DEPAKOTE was statistically significantly superior to placebo on all three measures of outcome. An exploratory analysis for age and gender effects on outcome did not suggest any differential responsiveness on the basis of age or gender.

A comparison of the percentage of patients showing ≥ 30% reduction in the symptom score from baseline in each treatment group, separated by study, is shown in Figure 1.

Figure 1
Percentage of Patients Achieving ≥ 30% Reduction in Symptom Score From Baseline

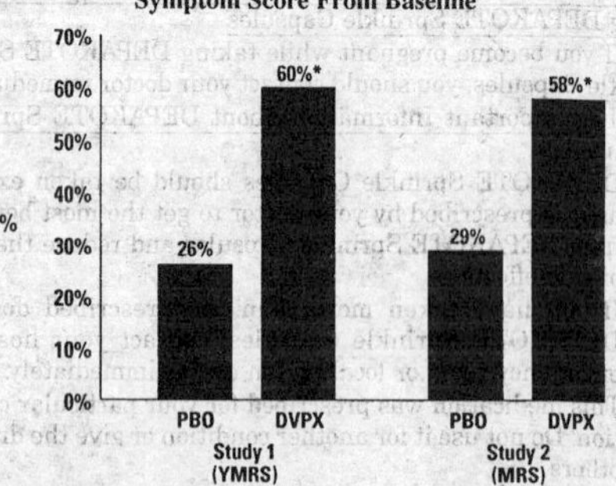

* $p < 0.05$
PBO = placebo, DVPX = DEPAKOTE

Migraine

The results of two multicenter, randomized, double-blind, placebo-controlled clinical trials established the effectiveness of DEPAKOTE in the prophylactic treatment of migraine headache.

Both studies employed essentially identical designs and recruited patients with a history of migraine with or without aura (of at least 6 months in duration) who were experiencing at least 2 migraine headaches a month during the 3 months prior to enrollment. Patients with cluster headaches were excluded. Women of childbearing potential were

excluded entirely from one study, but were permitted in the other if they were deemed to be practicing an effective method of contraception.
In each study following a 4-week single-blind placebo baseline period, patients were randomized, under double blind conditions, to DEPAKOTE or placebo for a 12-week treatment phase, comprised of a 4-week dose titration period followed by an 8-week maintenance period. Treatment outcome was assessed on the basis of 4-week migraine headache rates during the treatment phase.
In the first study, a total of 107 patients (24 M, 83 F), ranging in age from 26 to 73 were randomized 2:1, DEPAKOTE to placebo. Ninety patients completed the 8-week maintenance period. Drug dose titration, using 250 mg tablets, was individualized at the investigator's discretion. Adjustments were guided by actual/sham trough total serum valproate levels in order to maintain the study blind. In patients on DEPAKOTE doses ranged from 500 to 2500 mg a day. Doses over 500 mg were given in three divided doses (TID). The mean dose during the treatment phase was 1087 mg/day resulting in a mean trough total valproate level of 72.5 µg/mL, with a range of 31 to 133 µg/mL.
The mean 4-week migraine headache rate during the treatment phase was 5.7 in the placebo group compared to 3.5 in the DEPAKOTE group (see Figure 2). These rates were significantly different.
In the second study, a total of 176 patients (19 males and 157 females), ranging in age from 17 to 76 years, were randomized equally to one of three DEPAKOTE dose groups (500, 1000, or 1500 mg/day) or placebo. The treatments were given in two divided doses (BID). One hundred thirty-seven patients completed the 8-week maintenance period. Efficacy was to be determined by a comparison of the 4-week migraine headache rate in the combined 1000/1500 mg/day group and placebo group.
The initial dose was 250 mg daily. The regimen was advanced by 250 mg every 4 days (8 days for 500 mg/day group), until the randomized dose was achieved. The mean trough total valproate levels during the treatment phase were 39.6, 62.5, and 72.5 µg/mL in the DEPAKOTE 500, 1000, and 1500 mg/day groups, respectively.
The mean 4-week migraine headache rates during the treatment phase, adjusted for differences in baseline rates, were 4.5 in the placebo group, compared to 3.3, 3.0, and 3.3 in the DEPAKOTE 500, 1000, and 1500 mg/day groups, respectively, based on intent-to-treat results (see Figure 2). Migraine headache rates in the combined DEPAKOTE 1000/1500 mg group were significantly lower than in the placebo group.

Figure 2
Mean 4-week Migraine Rates

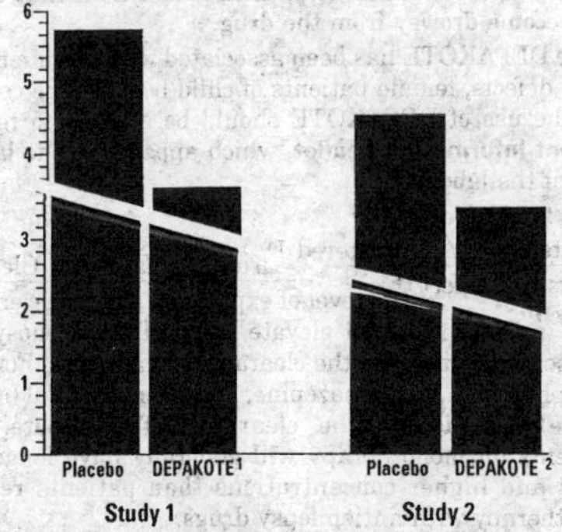

[1] Mean dose of DEPAKOTE was 1087 mg/day.
[2] Dose of DEPAKOTE was 500 or 1000 mg/day.

Epilepsy
The efficacy of DEPAKOTE in reducing the incidence of complex partial seizures (CPS) that occur in isolation or in association with other seizure types was established in two controlled trials.
In one, multiclinic, placebo controlled study employing an add-on design, (adjunctive therapy) 144 patients who continued to suffer eight or more CPS per 8 weeks during an 8 week period of monotherapy with doses of either carbamazepine or phenytoin sufficient to assure plasma concentrations within the "therapeutic range" were randomized to receive, in addition to their original antiepilepsy drug (AED), either DEPAKOTE or placebo. Randomized patients were to be followed for a total of 16 weeks. The following table presents the findings.

Adjunctive Therapy Study
Median Incidence of CPS per 8 Weeks

Add-on Treatment	Number of Patients	Baseline Incidence	Experimental Incidence
DEPAKOTE	75	16.0	8.9*
Placebo	69	14.5	11.5

*Reduction from baseline statistically significantly greater for DEPAKOTE than placebo at $p \leq 0.05$ level.

Figure 3 presents the proportion of patients (X axis) whose percentage reduction from baseline in complex partial seizure rates was at least as great as that indicated on the Y axis in the adjunctive therapy study. A positive percent reduction indicates an improvement (i.e., a decrease in seizure frequency), while a negative percent reduction indicates worsening. Thus, in a display of this type, the curve for an effective treatment is shifted to the left of the curve for placebo. This figure shows that the proportion of patients achieving any particular level of improvement was consistently higher for DEPAKOTE than for placebo. For example, 45% of patients treated with DEPAKOTE had a ≥ 50% reduction in complex partial seizure rate compared to 23% of patients treated with placebo.

Figure 3

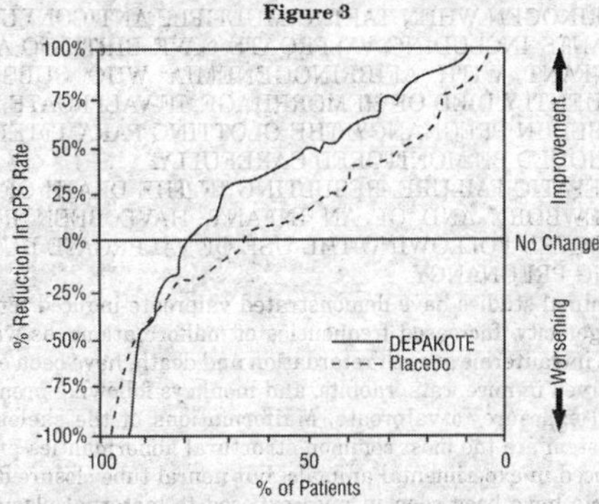

The second study assessed the capacity of DEPAKOTE to reduce the incidence of CPS when administered as the sole AED. The study compared the incidence of CPS among patients randomized to either a high or low dose treatment arm. Patients qualified for entry into the randomized comparison phase of this study only if 1) they continued to experience 2 or more CPS per 4 weeks during an 8 to 12 week long period of monotherapy with adequate doses of an AED (i.e., phenytoin, carbamazepine, phenobarbital, or primidone) and 2) they made a successful transition over a two week interval to DEPAKOTE. Patients entering the randomized phase were then brought to their assigned target dose, gradually tapered off their concomitant AED and followed for an interval as long as 22 weeks. Less than 50% of the patients randomized, however, completed the study. In patients converted to DEPAKOTE monotherapy, the mean total valproate concentrations during monotherapy were 71 and 123 µg/mL in the low dose and high dose groups, respectively.
The following table presents the findings for all patients randomized who had at least one post-randomization assessment.

Monotherapy Study
Median Incidence of CPS per 8 Weeks

Treatment	Number of Patients	Baseline Incidence	Randomized Phase Incidence
High dose DEPAKOTE	131	13.2	10.7*
Low dose DEPAKOTE	134	14.2	13.8

*Reduction from baseline statistically significantly greater for high dose than low dose at $p \leq 0.05$ level.

Figure 4 presents the proportion of patients (X axis) whose percentage reduction from baseline in complex partial seizure rates was at least as great as that indicated on the Y axis in the monotherapy study. A positive percent reduction indicates an improvement (i.e., a decrease in seizure frequency), while a negative percent reduction indicates worsening. Thus, in a display of this type, the curve for a more effective treatment is shifted to the left of the curve for a less effective treatment. This figure shows that the proportion of patients achieving any particular level of reduction was consistently higher for high dose DEPAKOTE than for low dose DEPAKOTE. For example, when switching from carbamazepine, phenytoin, phenobarbital or primidone monotherapy to high dose DEPAKOTE monotherapy, 63% of patients experienced no change or a reduction in complex partial seizure rates compared to 54% of patients receiving low dose DEPAKOTE.
[See figure at top of next column]

Figure 4

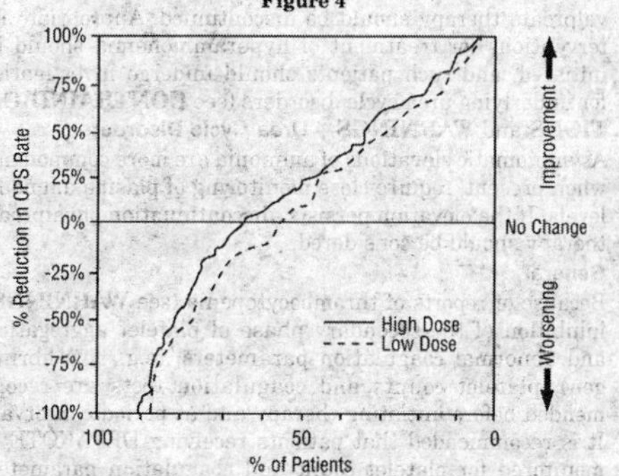

INDICATIONS AND USAGE

Mania
DEPAKOTE (divalproex sodium) is indicated for the treatment of the manic episodes associated with bipolar disorder. A manic episode is a distinct period of abnormally and persistently elevated, expansive, or irritable mood. Typical symptoms of mania include pressure of speech, motor hyperactivity, reduced need for sleep, flight of ideas, grandiosity, poor judgement, aggressiveness, and possible hostility. The efficacy of DEPAKOTE was established in 3-week trials with patients meeting DSM-III-R criteria for bipolar disorder who were hospitalized for acute mania (See **Clinical Trials** under **CLINICAL PHARMACOLOGY**).
The safety and effectiveness of DEPAKOTE for long-term use in mania, i.e., more than 3 weeks, has not been systematically evaluated in controlled clinical trials. Therefore, physicians who elect to use DEPAKOTE for extended periods should continually reevaluate the long-term usefulness of the drug for the individual patient.

Epilepsy
DEPAKOTE (divalproex sodium) is indicated as monotherapy and adjunctive therapy in the treatment of patients with complex partial seizures that occur either in isolation or in association with other types of seizures. DEPAKOTE (divalproex sodium) is also indicated for use as sole and adjunctive therapy in the treatment of simple and complex absence seizures, and adjunctively in patients with multiple seizure types that include absence seizures.
Simple absence is defined as very brief clouding of the sensorium or loss of consciousness accompanied by certain generalized epileptic discharges without other detectable clinical signs. Complex absence is the term used when other signs are also present.

Migraine
DEPAKOTE is indicated for prophylaxis of migraine headaches. There is no evidence that DEPAKOTE is useful in the acute treatment of migraine headaches. Because valproic acid may be a hazard to the fetus, DEPAKOTE should be considered for women of childbearing potential only after this risk has been thoroughly discussed with the patient and weighed against the potential benefits of treatment (see **WARNINGS - Usage In Pregnancy, PRECAUTIONS - Information for Patients**).
SEE **WARNINGS** FOR STATEMENT REGARDING FATAL HEPATIC DYSFUNCTION.

CONTRAINDICATIONS

DIVALPROEX SODIUM SHOULD NOT BE ADMINISTERED TO PATIENTS WITH HEPATIC DISEASE OR SIGNIFICANT HEPATIC DYSFUNCTION.
Divalproex sodium is contraindicated in patients with known hypersensitivity to the drug.
Divalproex sodium is contraindicated in patients with known urea cycle disorders (see **WARNINGS**).

WARNINGS

Hepatotoxicity
Hepatic failure resulting in fatalities has occurred in patients receiving valproic acid. These incidents usually have occurred during the first six months of treatment. Serious or fatal hepatotoxicity may be preceded by non-specific symptoms such as malaise, weakness, lethargy, facial edema, anorexia, and vomiting. In patients with epilepsy, a loss of seizure control may also occur. Patients should be monitored closely for appearance of these symptoms. Liver function tests should be performed prior to therapy and at frequent intervals thereafter, especially during the first six months. However, physicians should not rely totally on serum biochemistry since these tests may not be abnormal in all instances, but should also consider the results of careful interim medical history and physical examination. Caution should be observed when administering DEPAKOTE products to patients with a prior history of hepatic disease. Patients on multiple anticonvulsants, children, those with congenital metabolic disorders, those with severe seizure disorders accompanied by mental retardation, and those with organic brain disease may be at particular risk. Experience has indicated that children under the age of two years are at a considerably increased risk of developing fatal hepatotoxicity, especially those with the aforementioned conditions. When DEPAKOTE is used in this patient group, it should be used with extreme caution and as a sole agent. The benefits of therapy should be weighed against the risks. Above this age group, experience in epilepsy has indicated that the incidence of fatal hepatotoxicity decreases considerably in progressively older patient groups.
The drug should be discontinued immediately in the presence of significant hepatic dysfunction, suspected or apparent. In some cases, hepatic dysfunction has progressed in spite of discontinuation of drug.

Pancreatitis
Cases of life-threatening pancreatitis have been reported in both children and adults receiving valproate. Some of the cases have been described as hemorrhagic with rapid progression from initial symptoms to death. Some cases have occurred shortly after initial use as well as after several years of use. The rate based upon the reported cases exceeds that expected in the general population and there have been cases in which pancreatitis recurred after rechallenge with valproate. In clinical trials, there were 2 cases of pancreatitis without alternative etiology in 2416 patients, representing 1044 patient-years experience. Patients and guardians

Continued on next page

Depakote Tablets—Cont.

should be warned that abdominal pain, nausea, vomiting, and/or anorexia can be symptoms of pancreatitis that require prompt medical evaluation. If pancreatitis is diagnosed, valproate should ordinarily be discontinued. Alternative treatment for the underlying medical condition should be initiated as clinically indicated (see **BOXED WARNING**).

Urea Cycle Disorders (UCD)

Divalproex sodium is contraindicated in patients with known urea cycle disorders.

Hyperammonemic encephalopathy, sometimes fatal, has been reported following initiation of valproate therapy in patients with urea cycle disorders, a group of uncommon genetic abnormalities, particularly ornithine transcarbamylase deficiency. Prior to the initiation of valproate therapy, evaluation for UCD should be considered in the following patients: 1) those with a history of unexplained encephalopathy or coma, encephalopathy associated with a protein load, pregnancy- related or postpartum encephalopathy, unexplained mental retardation, or history of elevated plasma ammonia or glutamine; 2) those with cyclical vomiting and lethargy, episodic extreme irritability, ataxia, low BUN, or protein avoidance; 3) those with a family history of UCD or a family history of unexplained infant deaths (particularly males); 4) those with other signs or symptoms of UCD. Patients who develop symptoms of unexplained hyperammonemic encephalopathy while receiving valproate therapy should receive prompt treatment (including discontinuation of valproate therapy) and be evaluated for underlying urea cycle disorders (see **CONTRAINDICATIONS** and **PRECAUTIONS**).

Somnolence in the Elderly

In a double-blind, multicenter trial of valproate in elderly patients with dementia (mean age = 83 years), doses were increased by 125 mg/day to a target dose of 20 mg/kg/day. A significantly higher proportion of valproate patients had somnolence compared to placebo, and although not statistically significant, there was a higher proportion of patients with dehydration. Discontinuations for somnolence were also significantly higher than with placebo. In some patients with somnolence (approximately one-half), there was associated reduced nutritional intake and weight loss. There was a trend for the patients who experienced these events to have a lower baseline albumin concentration, lower valproate clearance, and a higher BUN. In elderly patients, dosage should be increased more slowly and with regular monitoring for fluid and nutritional intake, dehydration, somnolence, and other adverse events. Dose reductions or discontinuation of valproate should be considered in patients with decreased food or fluid intake and in patients with excessive somnolence (see **DOSAGE AND ADMINISTRATION**).

Thrombocytopenia

The frequency of adverse effects (particularly elevated liver enzymes and thrombocytopenia [see **PRECAUTIONS**]) may be dose-related. In a clinical trial of DEPAKOTE as monotherapy in patients with epilepsy, 34/126 patients (27%) receiving approximately 50 mg/kg/day on average, had at least one value of platelets ≤ 75 x 10^9/L. Approximately half of these patients had treatment discontinued, with return of platelet counts to normal. In the remaining patients, platelet counts normalized with continued treatment. In this study, the probability of thrombocytopenia appeared to increase significantly at total valproate concentrations of ≥ 110 µg/mL (females) or ≥ 135 µg/mL (males). The therapeutic benefit which may accompany the higher doses should therefore be weighed against the possibility of a greater incidence of adverse effects.

Usage In Pregnancy

ACCORDING TO PUBLISHED AND UN[illegible] PORTS, VALPROIC ACID M[illegible] [illegible]NPUBLISHED RE- GENIC EFFECTS IN [illegible] MAY PRODUCE TERATO- MALES RE[illegible] THE OFFSPRING OF HUMAN FE- TH[illegible] [illegible]CEIVING THE DRUG DURING PREGNANCY. [illegible]HERE AR[illegible] ARE MULTIPLE REPORTS IN THE CLINICAL LITERATURE WHICH INDICATE THAT THE USE OF ANTIEPILEPTIC DRUGS DURING PREGNANCY RESULTS IN AN INCREASED INCIDENCE OF BIRTH DEFECTS IN THE OFFSPRING. ALTHOUGH DATA ARE MORE EXTENSIVE WITH RESPECT TO TRIMETHADIONE, PARAMETHADIONE, PHENYTOIN, AND PHENOBARBITAL, REPORTS INDICATE A POSSIBLE SIMILAR ASSOCIATION WITH THE USE OF OTHER ANTIEPILEPTIC DRUGS. THEREFORE, ANTIEPILEPSY DRUGS SHOULD BE ADMINISTERED TO WOMEN OF CHILDBEARING POTENTIAL ONLY IF THEY ARE CLEARLY SHOWN TO BE ESSENTIAL IN THE MANAGEMENT OF THEIR SEIZURES.

THE INCIDENCE OF NEURAL TUBE DEFECTS IN THE FETUS MAY BE INCREASED IN MOTHERS RECEIVING VALPROATE DURING THE FIRST TRIMESTER OF PREGNANCY. THE CENTERS FOR DISEASE CONTROL (CDC) HAS ESTIMATED THE RISK OF VALPROIC ACID EXPOSED WOMEN HAVING CHILDREN WITH SPINA BIFIDA TO BE APPROXIMATELY 1 TO 2%.

OTHER CONGENITAL ANOMALIES (EG, CRANIOFACIAL DEFECTS, CARDIOVASCULAR MALFORMATIONS AND ANOMALIES INVOLVING VARIOUS BODY SYSTEMS), COMPATIBLE AND INCOMPATIBLE WITH LIFE, HAVE BEEN REPORTED. SUFFICIENT DATA TO DETERMINE THE INCIDENCE OF THESE CONGENITAL ANOMALIES IS NOT AVAILABLE.

THE HIGHER INCIDENCE OF CONGENITAL ANOMALIES IN ANTIEPILEPTIC DRUG-TREATED WOMEN WITH SEIZURE DISORDERS CANNOT BE REGARDED AS A CAUSE AND EFFECT RELATIONSHIP. THERE ARE INTRINSIC METHODOLOGIC PROBLEMS IN OBTAINING ADEQUATE DATA ON DRUG TERATOGENICITY IN HUMANS; GENETIC FACTORS OR THE EPILEPTIC CONDITION ITSELF, MAY BE MORE IMPORTANT THAN DRUG THERAPY IN CONTRIBUTING TO CONGENITAL ANOMALIES.

PATIENTS TAKING VALPROATE MAY DEVELOP CLOTTING ABNORMALITIES. A PATIENT WHO HAD LOW FIBRINOGEN WHEN TAKING MULTIPLE ANTICONVULSANTS INCLUDING VALPROATE GAVE BIRTH TO AN INFANT WITH AFIBRINOGENEMIA WHO SUBSEQUENTLY DIED OF HEMORRHAGE. IF VALPROATE IS USED IN PREGNANCY, THE CLOTTING PARAMETERS SHOULD BE MONITORED CAREFULLY.

HEPATIC FAILURE, RESULTING IN THE DEATH OF A NEWBORN AND OF AN INFANT, HAVE BEEN REPORTED FOLLOWING THE USE OF VALPROATE DURING PREGNANCY.

Animal studies have demonstrated valproate-induced teratogenicity. Increased frequencies of malformations, as well as intrauterine growth retardation and death, have been observed in mice, rats, rabbits, and monkeys following prenatal exposure to valproate. Malformations of the skeletal system are the most common structural abnormalities produced in experimental animals, but neural tube closure defects have been seen in mice exposed to maternal plasma valproate concentrations exceeding 230 µg/mL (2.3 times the upper limit of the human therapeutic range) during susceptible periods of embryonic development. Administration of an oral dose of 200 mg/kg/day or greater (50% of the maximum human daily dose or greater on a mg/m^2 basis) to pregnant rats during organogenesis produced malformations (skeletal, cardiac, and urogenital) and growth retardation in the offspring. These doses resulted in peak maternal plasma valproate levels of approximately 340 µg/mL or greater (3.4 times the upper limit of the human therapeutic range or greater). Behavioral deficits have been reported in the offspring of rats given a dose of 200 mg/kg/day throughout most of pregnancy. An oral dose of 350 mg/kg/day (approximately 2 times the maximum human daily dose on a mg/m^2 basis) produced skeletal and visceral malformations in rabbits exposed during organogenesis. Skeletal malformations, growth retardation, and death were observed in rhesus monkeys following administration of an oral dose of 200 mg/kg/day (equal to the maximum human daily dose on a mg/m^2 basis) during organogenesis. This dose resulted in peak maternal plasma valproate levels of approximately 280 µg/mL (2.8 times the upper limit of the human therapeutic range).

The prescribing physician will wish to weigh the benefits of therapy against the risks in treating or counseling women of childbearing potential. If this drug is used during pregnancy, or if the patient becomes pregnant while taking this drug, the patient should be apprised of the potential hazard to the fetus.

Antiepileptic drugs should not be discontinued abruptly in patients in whom the drug is administered to prevent major seizures because of the strong possibility of precipitating status epilepticus with attendant hypoxia and threat to life. In individual cases where the severity and frequency of the seizure disorder are such that the removal of medicati[illegible] does not pose a serious threat to the patient [illegible] [illegible]tion of the drug may be considered pri[illegible] [illegible] discontinuation of the drug may be considered [illegible] prior to and during pregnancy, although it cannot b[illegible] be said with any confidence that even minor sei[illegible] [illegible]zures do not pose some hazard to the developin[illegible] [illegible]s embryo or fetus.

Tests to detect neural tube and other defects using current accepted procedures should be considered a part of routine prenatal care in childbearing women receiving valproate.

PRECAUTIONS

Hepatic Dysfunction

See **BOXED WARNING, CONTRAINDICATIONS** and **WARNINGS**.

Pancreatitis

See **BOXED WARNING** and **WARNINGS**.

Hyperammonemia

Hyperammonemia has been reported in association with valproate therapy and may be present despite normal liver function tests. In patients who develop unexplained lethargy and vomiting or changes in mental status, hyperammonemic encephalopathy should be considered and an ammonia level should be measured. If ammonia is increased, valproate therapy should be discontinued. Appropriate interventions for treatment of hyperammonemia should be initiated, and such patients should undergo investigation for underlying urea cycle disorders (see **CONTRAINDICATIONS** and **WARNINGS – Urea Cycle Disorders**).

Asymptomatic elevations of ammonia are more common and when present, require close monitoring of plasma ammonia levels. If the elevation persists, discontinuation of valproate therapy should be considered.

General

Because of reports of thrombocytopenia (see **WARNINGS**), inhibition of the secondary phase of platelet aggregation, and abnormal coagulation parameters, (e.g., low fibrinogen), platelet counts and coagulation tests are recommended before initiating therapy and at periodic intervals. It is recommended that patients receiving DEPAKOTE be monitored for platelet count and coagulation parameters prior to planned surgery. In a clinical trial of DEPAKOTE as monotherapy in patients with epilepsy, 34/126 patients (27%) receiving approximately 50 mg/kg/day on average, had at least one value of platelets ≤ 75 x 10^9/L. Approximately half of these patients had treatment discontinued, with return of platelet counts to normal. In the remaining patients, platelet counts normalized with continued treatment. In this study, the probability of thrombocytopenia appeared to increase significantly at total valproate concentrations of ≥ 110 µg/mL (females) or ≥ 135 µg/mL (males). Evidence of hemorrhage, bruising, or a disorder of hemostasis/coagulation is an indication for reduction of the dosage or withdrawal of therapy.

Since DEPAKOTE may interact with concurrently administered drugs which are capable of enzyme induction, periodic plasma concentration determinations of valproate and concomitant drugs are recommended during the early course of therapy. (See **PRECAUTIONS - Drug Interactions.**)

Valproate is partially eliminated in the urine as a keto-metabolite which may lead to a false interpretation of the urine ketone test.

There have been reports of altered thyroid function tests associated with valproate. The clinical significance of these is unknown.

Suicidal ideation may be a manifestation of certain psychiatric disorders, and may persist until significant remission of symptoms occurs. Close supervision of high risk patients should accompany initial drug therapy.

There are *in vitro* studies that suggest valproate stimulates the replication of the HIV and CMV viruses under certain experimental conditions. The clinical consequence, if any, is not known. Additionally, the relevance of these *in vitro* findings is uncertain for patients receiving maximally suppressive antiretroviral therapy. Nevertheless, these data should be borne in mind when interpreting the results from regular monitoring of the viral load in HIV infected patients receiving valproate or when following CMV infected patients clinically.

Information for Patients

Patients and guardians should be warned that abdominal pain, nausea, vomiting, and/or anorexia can be symptoms of pancreatitis and, therefore, require further medical evaluation promptly.

Patients should be informed of the signs and symptoms associated with hyperammonemic encephalopathy (see **PRECAUTIONS – Hyperammonemia**) and be told to inform the prescriber if any of these symptoms occur.

Since DEPAKOTE products may produce CNS depression, especially when combined with another CNS depressant (eg, alcohol), patients should be advised not to engage in hazardous activities, such as driving an automobile or operating dangerous machinery, until it is known that they do not become drowsy from the drug.

Since DEPAKOTE has been associated with certain types of birth defects, female patients of child-bearing age considering the use of DEPAKOTE should be advised to read the **Patient Information Leaflet**, which appears as the last sec-tion of the labeling.

Drug Interactions

Effects of Co-Administered D[illegible] Drugs on Valproate Clearance: Drugs that affect th[illegible] the level of expression of hepatic enzymes, particul[illegible] [illegible]arly those that elevate levels of glucuronosyltransferases, may increase the clearance of valproate. For example, phenytoin, carbamazepine, and phenobarbital (or primidone) can double the clearance of valproate. Thus, patients on monotherapy will generally have longer half-lives and higher concentrations than patients receiving polytherapy with antiepilepsy drugs.

In contrast, drugs that are inhibitors of cytochrome P450 isozymes, e.g., antidepressants, may be expected to have little effect on valproate clearance because cytochrome P450 microsomal mediated oxidation is a relatively minor secondary metabolic pathway compared to glucuronidation and beta-oxidation.

Because of these changes in valproate clearance, monitoring of valproate and concomitant drug concentrations should be increased whenever enzyme inducing drugs are introduced or withdrawn.

The following list provides information about the potential for an influence of several commonly prescribed medications on valproate pharmacokinetics. The list is not exhaustive nor could it be, since new interactions are continuously being reported.

Drugs for which a potentially important interaction has been observed:

Aspirin—A study involving the co-administration of aspirin at antipyretic doses (11 to 16 mg/kg) with valproate to pediatric patients (n=6) revealed a decrease in protein binding and an inhibition of metabolism of valproate. Valproate free fraction was increased 4-fold in the presence of aspirin compared to valproate alone. The β-oxidation pathway consisting of 2-E-valproic acid, 3-OH-valproic acid, and 3-keto valproic acid was decreased from 25% of total metabolites excreted on valproate alone to 8.3% in the presence of aspirin. Caution should be observed if valproate and aspirin are to be co-administered.

Felbamate—A study involving the co-administration of 1200 mg/day of felbamate with valproate to patients with epilepsy (n=10) revealed an increase in mean valproate peak concentration by 35% (from 86 to 115 µg/mL) compared to valproate alone. Increasing the felbamate dose to 2400 mg/day increased the mean valproate peak concentra-

tion to 133 μg/mL (another 16% increase). A decrease in valproate dosage may be necessary when felbamate therapy is initiated.
Meropenem—Subtherapeutic valproic acid levels have been reported when meropenem was coadministered.
Rifampin—A study involving the administration of a single dose of valproate (7 mg/kg) 36 hours after 5 nights of daily dosing with rifampin (600 mg) revealed a 40% increase in the oral clearance of valproate. Valproate dosage adjustment may be necessary when it is co-administered with rifampin.
Drugs for which either no interaction or a likely clinically unimportant interaction has been observed:
Antacids—A study involving the co-administration of valproate 500 mg with commonly administered antacids (Maalox, Trisogel, and Titralac - 160 mEq doses) did not reveal any effect on the extent of absorption of valproate.
Chlorpromazine—A study involving the administration of 100 to 300 mg/day of chlorpromazine to schizophrenic patients already receiving valproate (200 mg BID) revealed a 15% increase in trough plasma levels of valproate.
Haloperidol—A study involving the administration of 6 to 10 mg/day of haloperidol to schizophrenic patients already receiving valproate (200 mg BID) revealed no significant changes in valproate trough plasma levels.
Cimetidine and Ranitidine—Cimetidine and ranitidine do not affect the clearance of valproate.
Effects of Valproate on Other Drugs:
Valproate has been found to be a weak inhibitor of some P450 isozymes, epoxide hydrase, and glucuronosyltransferases.
The following list provides information about the potential for an influence of valproate co-administration on the pharmacokinetics or pharmacodynamics of several commonly prescribed medications. The list is not exhaustive, since new interactions are continuously being reported.
Drugs for which a potentially important valproate interaction has been observed:
Amitriptyline/Nortriptyline—Administration of a single oral 50 mg dose of amitriptyline to 15 normal volunteers (10 males and 5 females) who received valproate (500 mg BID) resulted in a 21% decrease in plasma clearance of amitriptyline and a 34% decrease in the net clearance of nortriptyline. Rare postmarketing reports of concurrent use of valproate and amitriptyline resulting in an increased amitriptyline level have been received. Concurrent use of valproate and amitriptyline has rarely been associated with toxicity. Monitoring of amitriptyline levels should be considered for patients taking valproate concomitantly with amitriptyline. Consideration should be given to lowering the dose of amitriptyline/nortriptyline in the presence of valproate.
Carbamazepine/carbamazepine-10,11-Epoxide—Serum levels of carbamazepine (CBZ) decreased 17% while that of carbamazepine-10,11-epoxide (CBZ-E) increased by 45% upon co-administration of valproate and CBZ to epileptic patients.
Clonazepam—The concomitant use of valproic acid and clonazepam may induce absence status in patients with a history of absence type seizures.
Diazepam—Valproate displaces diazepam from its plasma albumin binding sites and inhibits its metabolism. Co-administration of valproate (1500 mg daily) increased the free fraction of diazepam (10 mg) by 90% in healthy volunteers (n=6). Plasma clearance and volume of distribution for free diazepam were reduced by 25% and 20%, respectively, in the presence of valproate. The elimination half-life of diazepam remained unchanged upon addition of valproate.
Ethosuximide—Valproate inhibits the metabolism of ethosuximide. Administration of a single ethosuximide dose of 500 mg with valproate (800 to 1600 mg/day) to healthy volunteers (n=6) was accompanied by a 25% increase in elimination half-life of ethosuximide and a 15% decrease in its total clearance as compared to ethosuximide alone. Patients receiving valproate and ethosuximide, especially along with other anticonvulsants, should be monitored for alterations in serum concentrations of both drugs.
Lamotrigine—In a steady-state study involving 10 healthy volunteers, the elimination half-life of lamotrigine increased from 26 to 70 hours with valproate co-administration (a 165% increase). The dose of lamotrigine should be reduced when co-administered with valproate. Serious skin reactions (such as Stevens-Johnson Syndrome and toxic epidermal necrolysis) have been reported with concomitant lamotrigine and valproate administration. See lamotrigine package insert for details on lamotrigine dosing with concomitant valproate administration.
Phenobarbital—Valproate was found to inhibit the metabolism of phenobarbital. Co-administration of valproate (250 mg BID for 14 days) with phenobarbital to normal subjects (n=6) resulted in a 50% increase in half-life and a 30% decrease in plasma clearance of phenobarbital (60 mg single-dose). The fraction of phenobarbital dose excreted unchanged increased by 50% in presence of valproate.
There is evidence for severe CNS depression, with or without significant elevations of barbiturate or valproate serum concentrations. All patients receiving concomitant barbiturate therapy should be closely monitored for neurological toxicity. Serum barbiturate concentrations should be obtained, if possible, and the barbiturate dosage decreased, if appropriate.
Primidone, which is metabolized to a barbiturate, may be involved in a similar interaction with valproate.
Phenytoin—Valproate displaces phenytoin from its plasma albumin binding sites and inhibits its hepatic metabolism. Co-administration of valproate (400 mg TID) with phenytoin (250 mg) in normal volunteers (n=7) was associated with a 60% increase in the free fraction of phenytoin. Total plasma clearance and apparent volume of distribution of phenytoin increased 30% in the presence of valproate. Both the clearance and apparent volume of distribution of free phenytoin were reduced by 25%.
In patients with epilepsy, there have been reports of breakthrough seizures occurring with the combination of valproate and phenytoin. The dosage of phenytoin should be adjusted as required by the clinical situation.
Tolbutamide—From *in vitro* experiments, the unbound fraction of tolbutamide was increased from 20% to 50% when added to plasma samples taken from patients treated with valproate. The clinical relevance of this displacement is unknown.
Warfarin—In an *in vitro* study, valproate increased the unbound fraction of warfarin by up to 32.6%. The therapeutic relevance of this is unknown; however, coagulation tests should be monitored if DEPAKOTE therapy is instituted in patients taking anticoagulants.
Zidovudine—In six patients who were seropositive for HIV, the clearance of zidovudine (100 mg q8h) was decreased by 38% after administration of valproate (250 or 500 mg q8h); the half-life of zidovudine was unaffected.
Drugs for which either no interaction or a likely clinically unimportant interaction has been observed:
Acetaminophen—Valproate had no effect on any of the pharmacokinetic parameters of acetaminophen when it was concurrently administered to three epileptic patients.
Clozapine—In psychotic patients (n=11), no interaction was observed when valproate was co-administered with clozapine.
Lithium—Co-administration of valproate (500 mg BID) and lithium carbonate (300 mg TID) to normal male volunteers (n=16) had no effect on the steady-state kinetics of lithium.
Lorazepam—Concomitant administration of valproate (500 mg BID) and lorazepam (1 mg BID) in normal male volunteers (n=9) was accompanied by a 17% decrease in the plasma clearance of lorazepam.
Oral Contraceptive Steroids—Administration of a single-dose of ethinyloestradiol (50 μg)/levonorgestrel (250 μg) to 6 women on valproate (200 mg BID) therapy for 2 months did not reveal any pharmacokinetic interaction.

Carcinogenesis, Mutagenesis, Impairment of Fertility

Carcinogenesis

Valproic acid was administered orally to Sprague Dawley rats and ICR (HA/ICR) mice at doses of 80 and 170 mg/kg/day (approximately 10 to 50% of the maximum human daily dose on a mg/m^2 basis) for two years. A variety of neoplasms were observed in both species. The chief findings were a statistically significant increase in the incidence of subcutaneous fibrosarcomas in high dose male rats receiving valproic acid and a statistically significant dose-related trend for benign pulmonary adenomas in male mice receiving valproic acid. The significance of these findings for humans is unknown.

Mutagenesis

Valproate was not mutagenic in an *in vitro* bacterial assay (Ames test), did not produce dominant lethal effects in mice, and did not increase chromosome aberration frequency in an *in vivo* cytogenetic study in rats. Increased frequencies of sister chromatid exchange (SCE) have been reported in a study of epileptic children taking valproate, but this association was not observed in another study conducted in adults. There is some evidence that increased SCE frequencies may be associated with epilepsy. The biological significance of an increase in SCE frequency is not known.

Fertility

Chronic toxicity studies in juvenile and adult rats and dogs demonstrated reduced spermatogenesis and testicular atrophy at oral doses of 400 mg/kg/day or greater in rats (approximately equivalent to or greater than the maximum human daily dose on a mg/m^2 basis) and 150 mg/kg/day or greater in dogs (approximately 1.4 times the maximum human daily dose or greater on a mg/m^2 basis). Segment I fertility studies in rats have shown doses up to 350 mg/kg/day (approximately equal to the maximum human daily dose on a mg/m^2 basis) for 60 days to have no effect on fertility. THE EFFECT OF VALPROATE ON TESTICULAR DEVELOPMENT AND ON SPERM PRODUCTION AND FERTILITY IN HUMANS IS UNKNOWN.

Pregnancy

Pregnancy Category D: See **WARNINGS**.

Nursing Mothers

Valproate is excreted in breast milk. Concentrations in breast milk have been reported to be 1-10% of serum concentrations. It is not known what effect this would have on a nursing infant. Consideration should be given to discontinuing nursing when divalproex sodium is administered to a nursing woman.

Pediatric Use

Experience has indicated that pediatric patients under the age of two years are at a considerably increased risk of developing fatal hepatotoxicity, especially those with the aforementioned conditions (see **BOXED WARNING**). When DEPAKOTE is used in this patient group, it should be used with extreme caution and as a sole agent. The benefits of therapy should be weighed against the risks. Above the age of 2 years, experience in epilepsy has indicated that the incidence of fatal hepatotoxicity decreases considerably in progressively older patient groups.
Younger children, especially those receiving enzyme-inducing drugs, will require larger maintenance doses to attain targeted total and unbound valproic acid concentrations.
The variability in free fraction limits the clinical usefulness of monitoring total serum valproic acid concentrations. Interpretation of valproic acid concentrations in children should include consideration of factors that affect hepatic metabolism and protein binding.
The safety and effectiveness of DEPAKOTE for the treatment of acute mania has not been studied in individuals below the age of 18 years.
The safety and effectiveness of DEPAKOTE for the prophylaxis of migraines has not been studied in individuals below the age of 16 years.
The basic toxicology and pathologic manifestations of valproate sodium in neonatal (4-day old) and juvenile (14-day old) rats are similar to those seen in young adult rats. However, additional findings, including renal alterations in juvenile rats and renal alterations and retinal dysplasia in neonatal rats, have been reported. These findings occurred at 240 mg/kg/day, a dosage approximately equivalent to the human maximum recommended daily dose on a mg/m^2 basis. They were not seen at 90 mg/kg, or 40% of the maximum human daily dose on a mg/m^2 basis.

Geriatric Use

No patients above the age of 65 years were enrolled in double-blind prospective clinical trials of mania associated with bipolar illness. In a case review study of 583 patients, 72 patients (12%) were greater than 65 years of age. A higher percentage of patients above 65 years of age reported accidental injury, infection, pain, somnolence, and tremor. Discontinuation of valproate was occasionally associated with the latter two events. It is not clear whether these events indicate additional risk or whether they result from preexisting medical illness and concomitant medication use among these patients.
A study of elderly patients with dementia revealed drug related somnolence and discontinuation for somnolence (see **WARNINGS-Somnolence in the Elderly**). The starting dose should be reduced in these patients, and dosage reductions or discontinuation should be considered in patients with excessive somnolence (see **DOSAGE AND ADMINISTRATION**).
There is insufficient information available to discern the safety and effectiveness of DEPAKOTE for the prophylaxis of migraines in patients over 65.

ADVERSE REACTIONS

Mania

The incidence of treatment-emergent events has been ascertained based on combined data from two placebo-controlled clinical trials of DEPAKOTE in the treatment of manic episodes associated with bipolar disorder. The adverse events were usually mild or moderate in intensity, but sometimes were serious enough to interrupt treatment. In clinical trials, the rates of premature termination due to intolerance were not statistically different between placebo, DEPAKOTE, and lithium carbonate. A total of 4%, 8% and 11% of patients discontinued therapy due to intolerance in the placebo, DEPAKOTE, and lithium carbonate groups, respectively.
Table 1 summarizes those adverse events reported for patients in these trials where the incidence rate in the DEPAKOTE-treated group was greater than 5% and greater than the placebo incidence, or where the incidence in the DEPAKOTE-treated group was statistically significantly greater than the placebo group. Vomiting was the only event that was reported by significantly ($p \leq 0.05$) more patients receiving DEPAKOTE compared to placebo.

Table 1
Adverse Events Reported by > 5% of DEPAKOTE-Treated Patients During Placebo-Controlled Trials of Acute Mania[1]

Adverse Event	DEPAKOTE (n=89)	Placebo (n=97)
Nausea	22%	15%
Somnolence	19%	12%
Dizziness	12%	4%
Vomiting	12%	3%
Asthenia	10%	7%
Abdominal Pain	9%	8%
Dyspepsia	9%	8%
Rash	6%	3%

[1] The following adverse events occurred at an equal or greater incidence for placebo than for DEPAKOTE: back pain, headache, constipation, diarrhea, tremor, and pharyngitis.

The following additional adverse events were reported by greater than 1% but not more than 5% of the 89 divalproex sodium-treated patients in controlled clinical trials:
Body as a Whole: Chest pain, chills, chills and fever, fever, neck pain, neck rigidity.
Cardiovascular System: Hypertension, hypotension, palpitations, postural hypotension, tachycardia, vasodilation.
Digestive System: Anorexia, fecal incontinence, flatulence, gastroenteritis, glossitis, periodontal abscess.
Hemic and Lymphatic System: Ecchymosis.
Metabolic and Nutritional Disorders: Edema, peripheral edema.

Continued on next page

Depakote Tablets—Cont.

Musculoskeletal System: Arthralgia, arthrosis, leg cramps, twitching.
Nervous System: Abnormal dreams, abnormal gait, agitation, ataxia, catatonic reaction, confusion, depression, diplopia, dysarthria, hallucinations, hypertonia, hypokinesia, insomnia, paresthesia, reflexes increased, tardive dyskinesia, thinking abnormalities, vertigo.
Respiratory System: Dyspnea, rhinitis.
Skin and Appendages: Alopecia, discoid lupus erythematosis, dry skin, furunculosis, maculopapular rash, seborrhea.
Special Senses: Amblyopia, conjunctivitis, deafness, dry eyes, ear pain, eye pain, tinnitus.
Urogenital System: Dysmenorrhea, dysuria, urinary incontinence.

Migraine

Based on two placebo-controlled clinical trials and their long term extension, DEPAKOTE was generally well tolerated with most adverse events rated as mild to moderate in severity. Of the 202 patients exposed to DEPAKOTE in the placebo-controlled trials, 17% discontinued for intolerance. This is compared to a rate of 5% for the 81 placebo patients. Including the long term extension study, the adverse events reported as the primary reason for discontinuation by ≥1% of 248 DEPAKOTE-treated patients were alopecia (6%), nausea and/or vomiting (5%), weight gain (2%), tremor (2%), somnolence (1%), elevated SGOT and/or SGPT (1%), and depression (1%).

Table 2 includes those adverse events reported for patients in the placebo-controlled trials where the incidence rate in the DEPAKOTE-treated group was greater than 5% and was greater than that for placebo patients.

Table 2
Adverse Events Reported by >5% of DEPAKOTE-Treated Patients During Migraine Placebo-Controlled Trials with a Greater Incidence Than Patients Taking Placebo[1]

Body System Event	Depakote (N = 202)	Placebo (N= 81)
Gastrointestinal System		
Nausea	31%	10%
Dyspepsia	13%	9%
Diarrhea	12%	7%
Vomiting	11%	1%
Abdominal pain	9%	4%
Increased appetite	6%	4%
Nervous System		
Asthenia	20%	9%
Somnolence	17%	5%
Dizziness	12%	6%
Tremor	9%	0%
Other		
Weight gain	8%	2%
Back pain	8%	6%
Alopecia	7%	1%

[1] The following adverse events occurred in at least 5% of DEPAKOTE-treated patients and at an equal or greater incidence for placebo than for DEPAKOTE: flu syndrome and pharyngitis.

The following additional adverse events were reported by greater than 1% but not more than 5% of the 202 divalproex sodium-treated patients in the controlled clinical trials:
Body as a Whole: Chest pain, chills, face edema, fever and malaise.
Cardiovascular System: Vasodilatation.
Digestive System: Anorexia, constipation, dry mouth, flatulence, gastrointestinal disorder (unspecified), and stomatitis.
Hemic and Lymphatic System: Ecchymosis.
Metabolic and Nutritional Disorders: Peripheral edema, SGOT increase, and SGPT increase.
Musculoskeletal System: Leg cramps and myalgia.
Nervous System: Abnormal dreams, amnesia, confusion, depression, emotional lability, insomnia, nervousness, paresthesia, speech disorder, thinking abnormalities, and vertigo.
Respiratory System: Cough increased, dyspnea, rhinitis, and sinusitis.
Skin and Appendages: Pruritus and rash.
Special Senses: Conjunctivitis, ear disorder, taste perversion, and tinnitus.
Urogenital System: Cystitis, metrorrhagia, and vaginal hemorrhage.

Epilepsy

Based on a placebo-controlled trial of adjunctive therapy for treatment of complex partial seizures, DEPAKOTE was generally well tolerated with most adverse events rated as mild to moderate in severity. Intolerance was the primary reason for discontinuation in the DEPAKOTE-treated patients (6%), compared to 1% of placebo-treated patients.

Table 3 lists treatment-emergent adverse events which were reported by ≥ 5% of DEPAKOTE-treated patients and for which the incidence was greater than in the placebo group, in the placebo-controlled trial of adjunctive therapy for treatment of complex partial seizures. Since patients were also treated with other antiepilepsy drugs, it is not possible, in most cases, to determine whether the following adverse events can be ascribed to DEPAKOTE alone, or the combination of DEPAKOTE and other antiepilepsy drugs.

Table 3
Adverse Events Reported by ≥ 5% of Patients Treated with DEPAKOTE During Placebo-Controlled Trial of Adjunctive Therapy for Complex Partial Seizures

Body System/Event	Depakote (%) (n = 77)	Placebo (%) (n = 70)
Body as a Whole		
Headache	31	21
Asthenia	27	7
Fever	6	4
Gastrointestinal System		
Nausea	48	14
Vomiting	27	7
Abdominal Pain	23	6
Diarrhea	13	6
Anorexia	12	0
Dyspepsia	8	4
Constipation	5	1
Nervous System		
Somnolence	27	11
Tremor	25	6
Dizziness	25	13
Diplopia	16	9
Amblyopia/Blurred Vision	12	9
Ataxia	8	1
Nystagmus	8	1
Emotional Lability	6	4
Thinking Abnormal	6	0
Amnesia	5	1
Respiratory System		
Flu Syndrome	12	9
Infection	12	6
Bronchitis	5	1
Rhinitis	5	4
Other		
Alopecia	6	1
Weight Loss	6	0

Table 4 lists treatment-emergent adverse events which were reported by ≥ 5% of patients in the high dose DEPAKOTE group, and for which the incidence was greater than in the low dose group, in a controlled trial of DEPAKOTE monotherapy treatment of complex partial seizures. Since patients were being titrated off another antiepilepsy drug during the first portion of the trial, it is not possible, in many cases, to determine whether the following adverse events can be ascribed to DEPAKOTE alone, or the combination of DEPAKOTE and other antiepilepsy drugs.

Table 4
Adverse Events Reported by ≥ 5% of Patients in the High Dose Group in the Controlled Trial of DEPAKOTE Monotherapy for Complex Partial Seizures[1]

Body System/Event	High Dose (%) (n = 131)	Low Dose (%) (n = 134)
Body as a Whole		
Asthenia	21	10
Digestive System		
Nausea	34	26
Diarrhea	23	19
Vomiting	23	15
Abdominal Pain	12	9
Anorexia	11	4
Dyspepsia	11	10
Hemic/Lymphatic System		
Thrombocytopenia	24	1
Ecchymosis	5	4
Metabolic/Nutritional		
Weight Gain	9	4
Peripheral Edema	8	3
Nervous System		
Tremor	57	19
Somnolence	30	18
Dizziness	18	13
Insomnia	15	9
Nervousness	11	7
Amnesia	7	4
Nystagmus	7	1
Depression	5	4
Respiratory System		
Infection	20	13
Pharyngitis	8	2
Dyspnea	5	1
Skin and Appendages		
Alopecia	24	13
Special Senses		
Amblyopia/Blurred Vision	8	4
Tinnitus	7	1

[1] Headache was the only adverse event that occurred in ≥ 5% of patients in the high dose group and at an equal or greater incidence in the low dose group.

The following additional adverse events were reported by greater than 1% but less than 5% of the 358 patients treated with DEPAKOTE in the controlled trials of complex partial seizures:
Body as a Whole: Back pain, chest pain, malaise.
Cardiovascular System: Tachycardia, hypertension, palpitation.
Digestive System: Increased appetite, flatulence, hematemesis, eructation, pancreatitis, periodontal abscess.
Hemic and Lymphatic System: Petechia.
Metabolic and Nutritional Disorders: SGOT increased, SGPT increased.
Musculoskeletal System: Myalgia, twitching, arthralgia, leg cramps, myasthenia.
Nervous System: Anxiety, confusion, abnormal gait, paresthesia, hypertonia, incoordination, abnormal dreams, personality disorder.
Respiratory System: Sinusitis, cough increased, pneumonia, epistaxis.
Skin and Appendages: Rash, pruritus, dry skin.
Special Senses: Taste perversion, abnormal vision, deafness, otitis media.
Urogenital System: Urinary incontinence, vaginitis, dysmenorrhea, amenorrhea, urinary frequency.

Other Patient Populations

Adverse events that have been reported with all dosage forms of valproate from epilepsy trials, spontaneous reports, and other sources are listed below by body system.

Gastrointestinal: The most commonly reported side effects at the initiation of therapy are nausea, vomiting, and indigestion. These effects are usually transient and rarely require discontinuation of therapy. Diarrhea, abdominal cramps, and constipation have been reported. Both anorexia with some weight loss and increased appetite with weight gain have also been reported. The administration of delayed-release divalproex sodium may result in reduction of gastrointestinal side effects in some patients.

CNS Effects: Sedative effects have occurred in patients receiving valproate alone but occur most often in patients receiving combination therapy. Sedation usually abates upon reduction of other antiepileptic medication. Tremor (may be dose-related), hallucinations, ataxia, headache, nystagmus, diplopia, asterixis, "spots before eyes", dysarthria, dizziness, confusion, hypesthesia, vertigo, incoordination, and parkinsonism have been reported with the use of valproate. Rare cases of coma have occurred in patients receiving valproate alone or in conjunction with phenobarbital. In rare instances encephalopathy with or without fever has developed shortly after the introduction of valproate monotherapy without evidence of hepatic dysfunction or inappropriately high plasma valproate levels. Although recovery has been described following drug withdrawal, there have been fatalities in patients with hyperammonemic encephalopathy, particularly in patients with underlying urea cycle disorders (see **WARNINGS – Urea Cycle Disorders** and **PRECAUTIONS**).

Several reports have noted reversible cerebral atrophy and dementia in association with valproate therapy.

Dermatologic: Transient hair loss, skin rash, photosensitivity, generalized pruritus, erythema multiforme, and Stevens-Johnson syndrome. Rare cases of toxic epidermal necrolysis have been reported including a fatal case in a 6 month old infant taking valproate and several other concomitant medications. An additional case of toxic epidermal necrosis resulting in death was reported in a 35 year old patient with AIDS taking several concomitant medications and with a history of multiple cutaneous drug reactions. Serious skin reactions have been reported with concomitant administration of lamotrigine and valproate (see**PRECAUTIONS - Drug Interactions**).

Psychiatric: Emotional upset, depression, psychosis, aggression, hyperactivity, hostility, and behavioral deterioration.

Musculoskeletal: Weakness.

Hematologic: Thrombocytopenia and inhibition of the secondary phase of platelet aggregation may be reflected in altered bleeding time, petechiae, bruising, hematoma formation, epistaxis, and frank hemorrhage (see **PRECAUTIONS - General** and **Drug Interactions**). Relative lymphocytosis, macrocytosis, hypofibrinogenemia, leukopenia, eosinophilia, anemia including macrocytic with or without folate deficiency, bone marrow suppression, pancytopenia, aplastic anemia, agranulocytosis, and acute intermittent porphyria.

Hepatic: Minor elevations of transaminases (eg, SGOT and SGPT) and LDH are frequent and appear to be dose-related. Occasionally, laboratory test results include increases in serum bilirubin and abnormal changes in other liver function tests. These results may reflect potentially serious hepatotoxicity (see **WARNINGS**).

Endocrine: Irregular menses, secondary amenorrhea, breast enlargement, galactorrhea, and parotid gland swelling. Abnormal thyroid function tests (see **PRECAUTIONS**).

There have been rare spontaneous reports of polycystic ovary disease. A cause and effect relationship has not been established.

Pancreatic: Acute pancreatitis including fatalities (see **WARNINGS**).

Metabolic: Hyperammonemia (see **PRECAUTIONS**), hyponatremia, and inappropriate ADH secretion.

There have been rare reports of Fanconi's syndrome occurring chiefly in children.

Decreased carnitine concentrations have been reported although the clinical relevance is undetermined.

Hyperglycinemia has occurred and was associated with a fatal outcome in a patient with preexistent nonketotic hyperglycinemia.

Genitourinary: Enuresis and urinary tract infection.

Special Senses: Hearing loss, either reversible or irreversible, has been reported; however, a cause and effect relationship has not been established. Ear pain has also been reported.

Other: Allergic reaction, anaphylaxis, edema of the extremities, lupus erythematosus, bone pain, cough increased, pneumonia, otitis media, bradycardia, cutaneous vasculitis, fever, and hypothermia.

OVERDOSAGE

Overdosage with valproate may result in somnolence, heart block, and deep coma. Fatalities have been reported; however patients have recovered from valproate levels as high as 2120 μg/mL.

In overdose situations, the fraction of drug not bound to protein is high and hemodialysis or tandem hemodialysis plus hemoperfusion may result in significant removal of drug. The benefit of gastric lavage or emesis will vary with the time since ingestion. General supportive measures should be applied with particular attention to the maintenance of adequate urinary output.

Naloxone has been reported to reverse the CNS depressant effects of valproate overdosage. Because naloxone could theoretically also reverse the antiepileptic effects of valproate, it should be used with caution in patients with epilepsy.

DOSAGE AND ADMINISTRATION

Mania

DEPAKOTE tablets are administered orally. The recommended initial dose is 750 mg daily in divided doses. The dose should be increased as rapidly as possible to achieve the lowest therapeutic dose which produces the desired clinical effect or the desired range of plasma concentrations. In placebo-controlled clinical trials of acute mania, patients were dosed to a clinical response with a trough plasma concentration between 50 and 125 μg/mL. Maximum concentrations were generally achieved within 14 days. The maximum recommended dosage is 60 mg/kg/day.

There is no body of evidence available from controlled trials to guide a clinician in the longer term management of a patient who improves during DEPAKOTE treatment of an acute manic episode. While it is generally agreed that pharmacological treatment beyond an acute response in mania is desirable, both for maintenance of the initial response and for prevention of new manic episodes, there are no systematically obtained data to support the benefits of DEPAKOTE in such longer-term treatment. Although there are no efficacy data that specifically address longer-term antimanic treatment with DEPAKOTE, the safety of DEPAKOTE in long-term use is supported by data from record reviews involving approximately 360 patients treated with DEPAKOTE for greater than 3 months.

Epilepsy

DEPAKOTE tablets are administered orally. DEPAKOTE is indicated as monotherapy and adjunctive therapy in complex partial seizures in adults and pediatric patients down to the age of 10 years, and in simple and complex absence seizures. As the DEPAKOTE dosage is titrated upward, concentrations of phenobarbital, carbamazepine, and/or phenytoin may be affected (see **PRECAUTIONS - Drug Interactions**).

Complex Partial Seizures: For adults and children 10 years of age or older.

Monotherapy (Initial Therapy): DEPAKOTE has not been systematically studied as initial therapy. Patients should initiate therapy at 10 to 15 mg/kg/day. The dosage should be increased by 5 to 10 mg/kg/week to achieve optimal clinical response. Ordinarily, optimal clinical response is achieved at daily doses below 60 mg/kg/day. If satisfactory clinical response has not been achieved, plasma levels should be measured to determine whether or not they are in the usually accepted therapeutic range (50 to 100 μg/mL). No recommendation regarding the safety of valproate for use at doses above 60 mg/kg/day can be made.

The probability of thrombocytopenia increases significantly at total trough valproate plasma concentrations above 110 μg/mL in females and 135 μg/mL in males. The benefit of improved seizure control with higher doses should be weighed against the possibility of a greater incidence of adverse reactions.

Conversion to Monotherapy: Patients should initiate therapy at 10 to 15 mg/kg/day. The dosage should be increased by 5 to 10 mg/kg/week to achieve optimal clinical response. Ordinarily, optimal clinical response is achieved at daily doses below 60 mg/kg/day. If satisfactory clinical response has not been achieved, plasma levels should be measured to determine whether or not they are in the usually accepted therapeutic range (50 - 100 μg/mL). No recommendation regarding the safety of valproate for use at doses above 60 mg/kg/day can be made. Concomitant antiepilepsy drug (AED) dosage can ordinarily be reduced by approximately 25% every 2 weeks. This reduction may be started at initiation of DEPAKOTE therapy, or delayed by 1 to 2 weeks if there is a concern that seizures are likely to occur with a reduction. The speed and duration of withdrawal of the concomitant AED can be highly variable, and patients should be monitored closely during this period for increased seizure frequency.

Adjunctive Therapy: DEPAKOTE may be added to the patient's regimen at a dosage of 10 to 15 mg/kg/day. The dosage may be increased by 5 to 10 mg/kg/week to achieve optimal clinical response. Ordinarily, optimal clinical response is achieved at daily doses below 60 mg/kg/day. If satisfactory clinical response has not been achieved, plasma levels should be measured to determine whether or not they are in the usually accepted therapeutic range (50 to 100 μg/mL). No recommendation regarding the safety of valproate for use at doses above 60 mg/kg/day can be made. If the total daily dose exceeds 250 mg, it should be given in divided doses.

In a study of adjunctive therapy for complex partial seizures in which patients were receiving either carbamazepine or phenytoin in addition to DEPAKOTE, no adjustment of carbamazepine or phenytoin dosage was needed (see **CLINICAL STUDIES**). However, since valproate may interact with these or other concurrently administered AEDs as well as other drugs (see **Drug Interactions**), periodic plasma concentration determinations of concomitant AEDs are recommended during the early course of therapy (see **PRECAUTIONS - Drug Interactions**).

Simple and Complex Absence Seizures: The recommended initial dose is 15 mg/kg/day, increasing at one week intervals by 5 to 10 mg/kg/day until seizures are controlled or side effects preclude further increases. The maximum recommended dosage is 60 mg/kg/day. If the total daily dose exceeds 250 mg, it should be given in divided doses.

A good correlation has not been established between daily dose, serum concentrations, and therapeutic effect. However, therapeutic valproate serum concentrations for most patients with absence seizures is considered to range from 50 to 100 μg/mL. Some patients may be controlled with lower or higher serum concentrations (see **CLINICAL PHARMACOLOGY**).

As the DEPAKOTE dosage is titrated upward, blood concentrations of phenobarbital and/or phenytoin may be affected (see **PRECAUTIONS**).

Antiepilepsy drugs should not be abruptly discontinued in patients in whom the drug is administered to prevent major seizures because of the strong possibility of precipitating status epilepticus with attendant hypoxia and threat to life.

In epileptic patients previously receiving DEPAKENE (valproic acid) therapy, DEPAKOTE tablets should be initiated at the same daily dose and dosing schedule. After the patient is stabilized on DEPAKOTE tablets, a dosing schedule of two or three times a day may be elected in selected patients.

Migraine

DEPAKOTE tablets are administered orally. The recommended starting dose is 250 mg twice daily. Some patients may benefit from doses up to 1000 mg/day. In the clinical trials, there was no evidence that higher doses led to greater efficacy.

General Dosing Advice

Dosing in Elderly Patients—Due to a decrease in unbound clearance of valproate and possibly a greater sensitivity to somnolence in the elderly, the starting dose should be reduced in these patients. Dosage should be increased more slowly and with regular monitoring for fluid and nutritional intake, dehydration, somnolence, and other adverse events. Dose reductions or discontinuation of valproate should be considered in patients with decreased food or fluid intake and in patients with excessive somnolence. The ultimate therapeutic dose should be achieved on the basis of both tolerability and clinical response (see **WARNINGS**).

Dose-Related Adverse Events—The frequency of adverse effects (particularly elevated liver enzymes and thrombocytopenia) may be dose-related. The probability of thrombocytopenia appears to increase significantly at total valproate concentrations of ≥ 110 μg/mL (females) or ≥ 135 μg/mL (males) (see **PRECAUTIONS**). The benefit of improved therapeutic effect with higher doses should be weighed against the possibility of a greater incidence of adverse reactions.

G.I. Irritation—Patients who experience G.I. irritation may benefit from administration of the drug with food or by slowly building up the dose from an initial low level.

HOW SUPPLIED

DEPAKOTE tablets (divalproex sodium delayed-release tablets) are supplied as:

125 mg salmon pink-colored tablets:
Bottles of 100 .... (**NDC** 0074-6212-13)
Abbo-Pac® unit dose packages of 100 .... (**NDC** 0074-6212-11).

250 mg peach-colored tablets:
Bottles of 100 .... (**NDC** 0074-6214-13)
Bottles of 500 .... (**NDC** 0074-6214-53)
Abbo-Pac® unit dose packages of 100 .... (**NDC** 0074-6214-11).

500 mg lavender-colored tablets:
Bottles of 100 .... (**NDC** 0074-6215-13)
Bottles of 500 .... (**NDC** 0074-6215-53)
Abbo-Pac® unit dose packages of 100 .... (**NDC** 0074-6215-11).

Recommended storage: Store tablets below 86°F (30°C).

Patient Information Leaflet

Important Information for Women Who Could Become Pregnant About the Use of DEPAKOTE® (divalproex sodium) Tablets

Please read this leaflet carefully before you take DEPAKOTE® (divalproex sodium) tablets. This leaflet provides a summary of important information about taking DEPAKOTE to women who could become pregnant. If you have any questions or concerns, or want more information about DEPAKOTE, contact your doctor or pharmacist.

Information For Women Who Could Become Pregnant

DEPAKOTE can be obtained only by prescription from your doctor. The decision to use DEPAKOTE is one that you and your doctor should make together, taking into account your individual needs and medical condition.

Before using DEPAKOTE, women who can become pregnant should consider the fact that DEPAKOTE has been associated with birth defects, in particular, with spina bifida and other defects related to failure of the spinal canal to close normally. Approximately 1 to 2% of children born to women with epilepsy taking DEPAKOTE in the first 12 weeks of pregnancy had these defects (based on data from the Centers for Disease Control, a U.S. agency based in Atlanta). The incidence in the general population is 0.1 to 0.2%.

Information For Women Who Are Planning to Get Pregnant

- Women taking DEPAKOTE who are planning to get pregnant should discuss the treatment options with their doctor.

Information For Women Who Become Pregnant While Taking DEPAKOTE

- If you become pregnant while taking DEPAKOTE you should contact your doctor immediately.

Other Important Information About DEPAKOTE Tablets

- DEPAKOTE tablets should be taken exactly as it is prescribed by your doctor to get the most benefits from DEPAKOTE and reduce the risk of side effects.
- If you have taken more than the prescribed dose of DEPAKOTE, contact your hospital emergency room or local poison center immediately.
- This medication was prescribed for your particular condition. Do not use it for another condition or give the drug to others.

Facts About Birth Defects

It is important to know that birth defects may occur even in children of individuals not taking any medications or without any additional risk factors.

This summary provides important information about the use of DEPAKOTE to women who could become pregnant. If you would like more information about the other potential risks and benefits of DEPAKOTE, ask your doctor or pharmacist to let you read the professional labeling and then discuss it with them. If you have any questions or concerns about taking DEPAKOTE, you should discuss them with your doctor.

Ref. 03-5292-R9

Revised: September, 2003

ABBOTT LABORATORIES

NORTH CHICAGO, IL 60064, U.S.A. PRINTED IN U.S.A.

Shown in Product Identification Guide, page 303

DEPAKOTE® ER ℞

[dĕp' ă-kōte]

(divalproex sodium)

EXTENDED-RELEASE TABLETS

℞ Only

BOX WARNING:

HEPATOTOXICITY:

HEPATIC FAILURE RESULTING IN FATALITIES HAS OCCURRED IN PATIENTS RECEIVING VALPROIC ACID AND ITS DERIVATIVES. EXPERIENCE HAS INDICATED THAT CHILDREN UNDER THE AGE OF TWO YEARS ARE AT A CONSIDERABLY INCREASED RISK OF DEVELOPING FATAL HEPATOTOXICITY, ESPECIALLY THOSE ON MULTIPLE ANTICONVULSANTS, THOSE WITH CONGENITAL METABOLIC DISORDERS, THOSE WITH SEVERE SEIZURE DISORDERS ACCOMPANIED BY MENTAL RETARDATION, AND THOSE WITH ORGANIC BRAIN DISEASE. WHEN DEPAKOTE IS USED IN THIS PATIENT GROUP, IT SHOULD BE USED WITH EXTREME CAUTION AND AS A SOLE AGENT. THE BENEFITS OF THERAPY SHOULD BE WEIGHED AGAINST THE RISKS. ABOVE THIS AGE GROUP, EXPERIENCE IN EPILEPSY HAS INDICATED THAT THE INCIDENCE OF FATAL HEPATOTOXICITY DECREASES CONSIDERABLY IN PROGRESSIVELY OLDER PATIENT GROUPS.

THESE INCIDENTS USUALLY HAVE OCCURRED DURING THE FIRST SIX MONTHS OF TREATMENT. SERIOUS OR FATAL HEPATOTOXICITY MAY BE PRECEDED BY NON-SPECIFIC SYMPTOMS SUCH AS MALAISE, WEAKNESS, LETHARGY, FACIAL EDEMA, ANOREXIA, AND VOMITING. IN PATIENTS WITH EPILEPSY, A LOSS OF SEIZURE CONTROL MAY ALSO OCCUR. PATIENTS SHOULD BE MONITORED CLOSELY FOR APPEARANCE OF THESE SYMPTOMS. LIVER FUNCTION TESTS SHOULD BE PERFORMED PRIOR TO THERAPY AND AT FREQUENT INTERVALS THEREAFTER, ESPECIALLY DURING THE FIRST SIX MONTHS.

TERATOGENICITY:

VALPROATE CAN PRODUCE TERATOGENIC EFFECTS SUCH AS NEURAL TUBE DEFECTS (E.G.,

Continued on next page

Depakote ER—Cont.

SPINA BIFIDA). ACCORDINGLY, THE USE OF DEPAKOTE TABLETS IN WOMEN OF CHILDBEARING POTENTIAL REQUIRES THAT THE BENEFITS OF ITS USE BE WEIGHED AGAINST THE RISK OF INJURY TO THE FETUS. THIS IS ESPECIALLY IMPORTANT WHEN THE TREATMENT OF A SPONTANEOUSLY REVERSIBLE CONDITION NOT ORDINARILY ASSOCIATED WITH PERMANENT INJURY OR RISK OF DEATH (E.G., MIGRAINE) IS CONTEMPLATED. SEE WARNINGS, INFORMATION FOR PATIENTS.

AN INFORMATION SHEET DESCRIBING THE TERATOGENIC POTENTIAL OF VALPROATE IS AVAILABLE FOR PATIENTS.

PANCREATITIS:

CASES OF LIFE-THREATENING PANCREATITIS HAVE BEEN REPORTED IN BOTH CHILDREN AND ADULTS RECEIVING VALPROATE. SOME OF THE CASES HAVE BEEN DESCRIBED AS HEMORRHAGIC WITH A RAPID PROGRESSION FROM INITIAL SYMPTOMS TO DEATH. CASES HAVE BEEN REPORTED SHORTLY AFTER INITIAL USE AS WELL AS AFTER SEVERAL YEARS OF USE. PATIENTS AND GUARDIANS SHOULD BE WARNED THAT ABDOMINAL PAIN, NAUSEA, VOMITING, AND/OR ANOREXIA CAN BE SYMPTOMS OF PANCREATITIS THAT REQUIRE PROMPT MEDICAL EVALUATION. IF PANCREATITIS IS DIAGNOSED, VALPROATE SHOULD ORDINARILY BE DISCONTINUED. ALTERNATIVE TREATMENT FOR THE UNDERLYING MEDICAL CONDITION SHOULD BE INITIATED AS CLINICALLY INDICATED. (See **WARNINGS** and **PRECAUTIONS**.)

DESCRIPTION

Divalproex sodium is a stable co-ordination compound comprised of sodium valproate and valproic acid in a 1:1 molar relationship and formed during the partial neutralization of valproic acid with 0.5 equivalent of sodium hydroxide. Chemically it is designated as sodium hydrogen bis(2-propylpentanoate). Divalproex sodium has the following structure:

$$\left[\begin{array}{c} CH_3CH_2CH_2-CH-CH_2CH_2CH_3 \\ | \\ HO-C=O \quad Na^{\oplus} \\ O=C-O^{\ominus} \\ | \\ CH_3CH_2CH_2-CH-CH_2CH_2CH_3 \end{array}\right]_n$$

Divalproex sodium occurs as a white powder with a characteristic odor.

DEPAKOTE ER 250 and 500 mg tablets are for oral administration. DEPAKOTE ER tablets contain divalproex sodium in a once-a-day extended-release formulation equivalent to 250 and 500 mg of valproic acid.

Inactive Ingredients

DEPAKOTE ER 250 and 500 mg tablets: FD&C Blue No. 1, hypromellose, lactose, microcrystalline cellulose, polyethylene glycol, potassium sorbate, propylene glycol, silicon dioxide, titanium dioxide, and triacetin.

In addition, 500 mg tablets contain iron oxide and polydextrose.

CLINICAL PHARMACOLOGY

Pharmacodynamics

Divalproex sodium dissociates to the valproate ion in the gastrointestinal tract. The mechanisms by which valproate exerts its therapeutic effects have not been established. It has been suggested that its activity in epilepsy is related to increased brain concentrations of gamma-aminobutyric acid (GABA).

Pharmacokinetics

Absorption/Bioavailability

The absolute bioavailability of DEPAKOTE ER tablets administered as a single dose after a meal was approximately 90% relative to intravenous infusion.

When given in equal total daily doses, the bioavailability of DEPAKOTE ER is less than that of DEPAKOTE (divalproex sodium delayed-release tablets). In five multiple-dose studies in healthy subjects (N=82) and in subjects with epilepsy (N=86), when administered under fasting and nonfasting conditions, DEPAKOTE ER given once daily produced an average bioavailability of 89% relative to an equal total daily dose of DEPAKOTE given BID, TID, or QID. The median time to maximum plasma valproate concentrations (C_{max}) after DEPAKOTE ER administration ranged from 4 to 17 hours. After multiple once-daily dosing of DEPAKOTE ER, the peak-to-trough fluctuation in plasma valproate concentrations was 10-20% lower than that of regular DEPAKOTE given BID, TID, or QID.

Conversion from DEPAKOTE to DEPAKOTE ER:

When DEPAKOTE ER is given in doses 8 to 20% higher than the total daily dose of DEPAKOTE, the two formulations are bioequivalent. In two randomized, crossover studies, multiple daily doses of DEPAKOTE were compared to 8 to 20% higher once-daily doses of DEPAKOTE ER. In these two studies, DEPAKOTE ER and DEPAKOTE regimens were equivalent with respect to area under the curve (AUC; a measure of the extent of bioavailability). Additionally, valproate C_{max} was lower, and C_{min} was either higher or not different, for DEPAKOTE ER relative to DEPAKOTE regimens (see following table).

[See table above]

Bioavailability of DEPAKOTE ER Tablets Relative to DEPAKOTE When DEPAKOTE ER Dose is 8 to 20% Higher

Study Population	Regimens DEPAKOTE ER vs. DEPAKOTE	Relative Bioavailability AUC_{24}	C_{max}	C_{min}
Healthy Volunteers (N=35)	1000 & 1500 mg DEPAKOTE ER vs. 875 & 1250 mg DEPAKOTE	1.059	0.882	1.173
Patients with epilepsy on concomitant enzyme-inducing antiepilepsy drugs (N=64)	1000 to 5000 mg DEPAKOTE ER vs. 875 to 4250 mg DEPAKOTE	1.008	0.899	1.022

Concomitant antiepilepsy drugs (topiramate, phenobarbital, carbamazepine, phenytoin, and lamotrigine were evaluated) that induce the cytochrome P450 isozyme system did not significantly alter valproate bioavailability when converting between DEPAKOTE and DEPAKOTE ER.

Distribution

Protein Binding:

The plasma protein binding of valproate is concentration dependent and the free fraction increases from approximately 10% at 40 µg/mL to 18.5% at 130 µg/mL. Protein binding of valproate is reduced in the elderly, in patients with chronic hepatic diseases, in patients with renal impairment, and in the presence of other drugs (e.g., aspirin). Conversely, valproate may displace certain protein-bound drugs (e.g., phenytoin, carbamazepine, warfarin, and tolbutamide) (see **PRECAUTIONS, Drug Interactions** for more detailed information on the pharmacokinetic interactions of valproate with other drugs).

CNS Distribution:

Valproate concentrations in cerebrospinal fluid (CSF) approximate unbound concentrations in plasma (about 10% of total concentration).

Metabolism

Valproate is metabolized almost entirely by the liver. In adult patients on monotherapy, 30-50% of an administered dose appears in urine as a glucuronide conjugate. Mitochondrial β-oxidation is the other major metabolic pathway, typically accounting for over 40% of the dose. Usually, less than 15-20% of the dose is eliminated by other oxidative mechanisms. Less than 3% of an administered dose is excreted unchanged in urine.

The relationship between dose and total valproate concentration is nonlinear; concentration does not increase proportionally with the dose, but rather, increases to a lesser extent due to saturable plasma protein binding. The kinetics of unbound drug are linear.

Elimination

Mean plasma clearance and volume of distribution for total valproate are 0.56 L/hr/1.73 m^2 and 11 L/1.73 m^2, respectively. Mean plasma clearance and volume of distribution for free valproate are 4.6 L/hr/1.73 m^2 and 92 L/1.73 m^2. Mean terminal half-life for valproate monotherapy ranged from 9 to 16 hours following oral dosing regimens of 250 to 1000 mg.

The estimates cited apply primarily to patients who are not taking drugs that affect hepatic metabolizing enzyme systems. For example, patients taking enzyme-inducing antiepileptic drugs (carbamazepine, phenytoin, and phenobarbital) will clear valproate more rapidly.

Special Populations

Effect of Age:

Pediatric—The valproate pharmacokinetic profile following administration of DEPAKOTE ER was characterized in a multiple-dose, non-fasting, open-label, multi-center study in children and adolescents. DEPAKOTE ER once-daily doses ranged from 250 to 1750 mg. Once-daily administration of DEPAKOTE ER in pediatric patients (10-17 years) produced plasma VPA concentration-time profiles similar to those that have been observed in adults.

Elderly—The capacity of elderly patients (age range: 68 to 89 years) to eliminate valproate has been shown to be reduced compared to younger adults (age range: 22 to 26 years). Intrinsic clearance is reduced by 39%; the free fraction is increased by 44%. Accordingly, the initial dosage should be reduced in the elderly (see **DOSAGE AND ADMINISTRATION**).

Effect of Gender:

There are no differences in the body surface area adjusted unbound clearance between males and females (4.8±0.17 and 4.7±0.07 L/hr per 1.73 m^2, respectively).

Effect of Race:

The effects of race on the kinetics of valproate have not been studied.

Effect of Disease:

Liver Disease—(see **BOXED WARNING, CONTRAINDICATIONS**, and **WARNINGS**). Liver disease impairs the capacity to eliminate valproate. In one study, the clearance of free valproate was decreased by 50% in 7 patients with cirrhosis and by 16% in 4 patients with acute hepatitis, compared with 6 healthy subjects. In that study, the half-life of valproate was increased from 12 to 18 hours. Liver disease is also associated with decreased albumin concentrations and larger unbound fractions (2 to 2.6 fold increase) of valproate. Accordingly, monitoring of total concentrations may be misleading since free concentrations may be substantially elevated in patients with hepatic disease whereas total concentrations may appear to be normal.

Renal Disease—A slight reduction (27%) in the unbound clearance of valproate has been reported in patients with renal failure (creatinine clearance < 10 mL/minute); however, hemodialysis typically reduces valproate concentrations by about 20%. Therefore, no dosage adjustment appears to be necessary in patients with renal failure. Protein binding in these patients is substantially reduced; thus, monitoring total concentrations may be misleading.

Plasma Levels and Clinical Effect

The relationship between plasma concentration and clinical response is not well documented. One contributing factor is the nonlinear, concentration dependent protein binding of valproate which affects the clearance of the drug. Thus, monitoring of total serum valproate cannot provide a reliable index of the bioactive valproate species.

For example, because the plasma protein binding of valproate is concentration dependent, the free fraction increases from approximately 10% at 40 µg/mL to 18.5% at 130 µg/mL. Higher than expected free fractions occur in the elderly, in hyperlipidemic patients, and in patients with hepatic and renal diseases.

Epilepsy:

The therapeutic range in epilepsy is commonly considered to be 50 to 100 µg/mL of total valproate, although some patients may be controlled with lower or higher plasma concentrations.

Clinical Trials

Migraine

The results of a multicenter, randomized, double-blind, placebo-controlled, parallel-group clinical trial demonstrated the effectiveness of DEPAKOTE ER in the prophylactic treatment of migraine headache. This trial recruited patients with a history of migraine headaches with or without aura occurring on average twice or more a month for the preceding three months. Patients with cluster or chronic daily headaches were excluded. Women of childbearing potential were allowed in the trial if they were deemed to be practicing an effective method of contraception.

Patients who experienced ≥2 migraine headaches in the 4-week baseline period were randomized in a 1:1 ratio to DEPAKOTE ER or placebo and treated for 12 weeks. Patients initiated treatment on 500 mg once daily for one week, and were then increased to 1000 mg once daily with an option to permanently decrease the dose back to 500 mg once daily during the second week of treatment if intolerance occurred. Ninety-eight of 114 DEPAKOTE ER-treated patients (86%) and 100 of 110 placebo-treated patients (91%) treated at least two weeks maintained the 1000 mg once daily dose for the duration of their treatment periods. Treatment outcome was assessed on the basis of reduction in 4-week migraine headache rate in the treatment period compared to the baseline period.

Patients (50 male, 187 female) ranging in age from 16 to 69 were treated with DEPAKOTE ER (N=122) or placebo (N=115). Four patients were below the age of 18 and 3 were above the age of 65. Two hundred and two patients (101 in each treatment group) completed the treatment period. The mean reduction in 4-week migraine headache rate was 1.2 from a baseline mean of 4.4 in the DEPAKOTE ER group, versus 0.6 from a baseline mean of 4.2 in the placebo group. The treatment difference was statistically significant (see Figure 1).

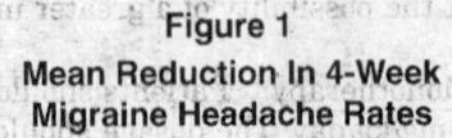

Figure 1

Mean Reduction In 4-Week Migraine Headache Rates

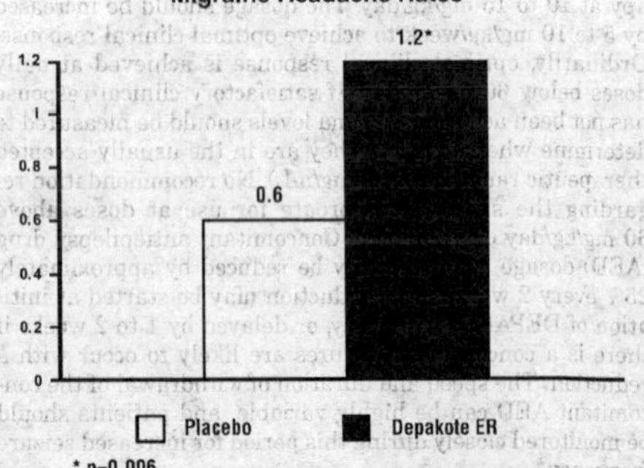

Epilepsy

The efficacy of DEPAKOTE reducing the incidence of complex partial seizures (CPS) that occur in isolation or in association with other seizure types was established in two controlled trials using DEPAKOTE (divalproex sodium delayed-release tablets).

In one, multiclinic, placebo controlled study employing an add-on design, (adjunctive therapy) using DEPAKOTE, 144 patients who continued to suffer eight or more CPS per 8 weeks during an 8 week period of monotherapy with doses of either carbamazepine or phenytoin sufficient to assure plasma concentrations within the "therapeutic range" were randomized to receive, in addition to their original antiepilepsy drug (AED), either DEPAKOTE or placebo. Randomized patients were to be followed for a total of 16 weeks. The following table presents the findings.

Adjunctive Therapy Study
Median Incidence of CPS per 8 Weeks

Add-on Treatment	Number of Patients	Baseline Incidence	Experimental Incidence
DEPAKOTE	75	16.0	8.9*
Placebo	69	14.5	11.5

*Reduction from baseline statistically significantly greater for DEPAKOTE than placebo at p ≤0.05 level.

Figure 2 presents the proportion of patients (X axis) whose percentage reduction from baseline in complex partial seizure rates was at least as great as that indicated on the Y axis in the adjunctive therapy study. A positive percent reduction indicates an improvement (i.e., a decrease in seizure frequency), while a negative percent reduction indicates worsening. Thus, in a display of this type, the curve for an effective treatment is shifted to the left of the curve for placebo. This figure shows that the proportion of patients achieving any particular level of improvement was consistently higher for DEPAKOTE than for placebo. For example, 45% of patients treated with DEPAKOTE had a ≥50% reduction in complex partial seizure rate compared to 23% of patients treated with placebo.

Figure 2

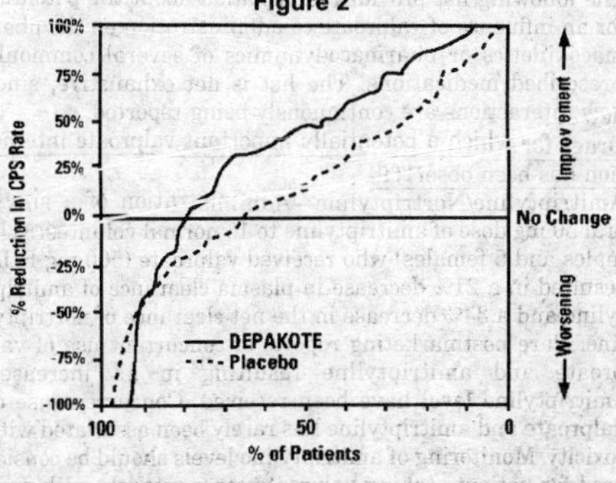

The second study assessed the capacity of DEPAKOTE to reduce the incidence of CPS when administered as the sole AED. The study compared the incidence of CPS among patients randomized to either a high or low dose treatment arm. Patients qualified for entry into the randomized comparison phase of this study only if 1) they continued to experience 2 or more CPS per 4 weeks during an 8 to 12 week long period of monotherapy with adequate doses of an AED (i.e., phenytoin, carbamazepine, phenobarbital, or primidone) and 2) they made a successful transition over a two week interval to DEPAKOTE. Patients entering the randomized phase were then brought to their assigned target dose, gradually tapered off their concomitant AED and followed for an interval as long as 22 weeks. Less than 50% of the patients randomized, however, completed the study. In patients converted to DEPAKOTE monotherapy, the mean total valproate concentrations during monotherapy were 71 and 123 µg/mL in the low dose and high dose groups, respectively.

The following table presents the findings for all patients randomized who had at least one post-randomization assessment.

Monotherapy Study
Median Incidence of CPS per 8 Weeks

Treatment	Number of Patients	Baseline Incidence	Randomized Phase Incidence
High dose DEPAKOTE	131	13.2	10.7*
Low dose DEPAKOTE	134	14.2	13.8

*Reduction from baseline statistically significantly greater for high dose than low dose at p ≤0.05 level.

Figure 3 presents the proportion of patients (X axis) whose percentage reduction from baseline in complex partial seizure rates was at least as great as that indicated on the Y axis in the monotherapy study. A positive percent reduction indicates an improvement (i.e., a decrease in seizure frequency), while a negative percent reduction indicates worsening. Thus, in a display of this type, the curve for a more effective treatment is shifted to the left of the curve for a less effective treatment. This figure shows that the proportion of patients achieving any particular level of reduction was consistently higher for high dose DEPAKOTE than for low dose DEPAKOTE. For example, when switching from carbamazepine, phenytoin, phenobarbital or primidone monotherapy to high dose DEPAKOTE monotherapy, 63% of patients experienced no change or a reduction in complex partial seizure rates compared to 54% of patients receiving low dose DEPAKOTE.

Figure 3

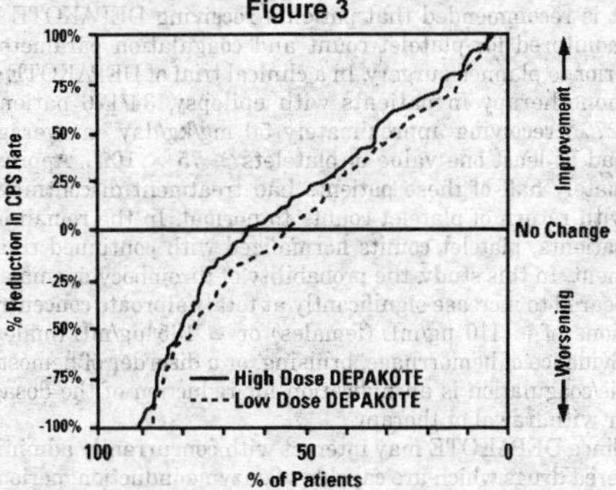

INDICATIONS AND USAGE

Migraine

DEPAKOTE ER is indicated for prophylaxis of migraine headaches in adults. There is no evidence that DEPAKOTE ER is useful in the acute treatment of migraine headaches. Because valproic acid may be a hazard to the fetus, DEPAKOTE ER should be considered for women of childbearing potential only after this risk has been thoroughly discussed with the patient and weighed against the potential benefits of treatment (see **WARNINGS—Usage In Pregnancy, PRECAUTIONS—Information for Patients**).

Epilepsy

DEPAKOTE ER is indicated as monotherapy and adjunctive therapy in the treatment of adults and children 10 years of age or older with complex partial seizures that occur either in isolation or in association with other types of seizures. DEPAKOTE ER is also indicated for use as sole and adjunctive therapy in the treatment of simple and complex absence seizures in adults and children 10 years of age or older, and adjunctively in adults and children 10 years of age or older with multiple seizure types that include absence seizures.

Simple absence is defined as very brief clouding of the sensorium or loss of consciousness accompanied by certain generalized epileptic discharges without other detectable clinical signs. Complex absence is the term used when other signs are also present.

SEE **WARNINGS** FOR STATEMENT REGARDING FATAL HEPATIC DYSFUNCTION.

CONTRAINDICATIONS

DIVALPROEX SODIUM SHOULD NOT BE ADMINISTERED TO PATIENTS WITH HEPATIC DISEASE OR SIGNIFICANT HEPATIC DYSFUNCTION.

Divalproex sodium is contraindicated in patients with known hypersensitivity to the drug.

Divalproex sodium is contraindicated in patients with known urea cycle disorders (see **WARNINGS**).

WARNINGS

Hepatotoxicity

Hepatic failure resulting in fatalities has occurred in patients receiving valproic acid. These incidents usually have occurred during the first six months of treatment. Serious or fatal hepatotoxicity may be preceded by non-specific symptoms such as malaise, weakness, lethargy, facial edema, anorexia, and vomiting. Patients should be monitored closely for appearance of these symptoms. Liver function tests should be performed prior to therapy and at frequent intervals thereafter, especially during the first six months. However, physicians should not rely totally on serum biochemistry since these tests may not be abnormal in all instances, but should also consider the results of careful interim medical history and physical examination. Caution should be observed when administering DEPAKOTE products to patients with a prior history of hepatic disease. Patients on multiple anticonvulsants, children, those with congenital metabolic disorders, those with severe seizure disorders accompanied by mental retardation, and those with organic brain disease may be at particular risk. Experience has indicated that children under the age of two years are at a considerably increased risk of developing fatal hepatotoxicity, especially those with the aforementioned conditions. Above this age group, experience in epilepsy has indicated that the incidence of fatal hepatotoxicity decreases considerably in progressively older patient groups.

The drug should be discontinued immediately in the presence of significant hepatic dysfunction, suspected or apparent. In some cases, hepatic dysfunction has progressed in spite of discontinuation of drug.

Pancreatitis

Cases of life-threatening pancreatitis have been reported in both children and adults receiving valproate. Some of the cases have been described as hemorrhagic with rapid progression from initial symptoms to death. Some cases have occurred shortly after initial use as well as after several years of use. The rate based upon the reported cases exceeds that expected in the general population and there have been cases in which pancreatitis recurred after rechallenge with valproate. In clinical trials, there were 2 cases of pancreatitis without alternative etiology in 2416 patients, representing 1044 patient-years experience. Patients and guardians should be warned that abdominal pain, nausea, vomiting, and/or anorexia can be symptoms of pancreatitis that require prompt medical evaluation. If pancreatitis is diagnosed, valproate should ordinarily be discontinued. Alternative treatment for the underlying medical condition should be initiated as clinically indicated (see **BOXED WARNING**).

Urea Cycle Disorders (UCD)

Divalproex sodium is contraindicated in patients with known urea cycle disorders.

Hyperammonemic encephalopathy, sometimes fatal, has been reported following initiation of valproate therapy in patients with urea cycle disorders, a group of uncommon genetic abnormalities, particularly ornithine transcarbamylase deficiency. Prior to the initiation of valproate therapy, evaluation for UCD should be considered in the following patients: 1) those with a history of unexplained encephalopathy or coma, encephalopathy associated with a protein load, pregnancy-related or postpartum encephalopathy, unexplained mental retardation, or history of elevated plasma ammonia or glutamine; 2) those with cyclical vomiting and lethargy, episodic extreme irritability, ataxia, low BUN, or protein avoidance; 3) those with a family history of UCD or a family history of unexplained infant deaths (particularly males); 4) those with other signs or symptoms of UCD. Patients who develop symptoms of unexplained hyperammonemic encephalopathy while receiving valproate therapy should receive prompt treatment (including discontinuation of valproate therapy) and be evaluated for underlying urea cycle disorders (see **CONTRAINDICATIONS** and **PRECAUTIONS**).

Somnolence in the Elderly

In a double-blind, multicenter trial of valproate in elderly patients with dementia (mean age = 83 years), doses were increased by 125 mg/day to a target dose of 20 mg/kg/day. A significantly higher proportion of valproate patients had somnolence compared to placebo, and although not statistically significant, there was a higher proportion of patients with dehydration. Discontinuations for somnolence were also significantly higher than with placebo. In some patients with somnolence (approximately one-half), there was associated reduced nutritional intake and weight loss. There was a trend for the patients who experienced these events to have a lower baseline albumin concentration, lower valproate clearance, and a higher BUN. In elderly patients, dosage should be increased more slowly and with regular monitoring for fluid and nutritional intake, dehydration, somnolence, and other adverse events. Dose reductions or discontinuation of valproate should be considered in patients with decreased food or fluid intake and in patients with excessive somnolence (see **DOSAGE AND ADMINISTRATION**).

Thrombocytopenia

The frequency of adverse effects (particularly elevated liver enzymes and thrombocytopenia [see **PRECAUTIONS** may be dose-related. In a clinical trial of DEPAKOTE (divalproex sodium) as monotherapy in patients with epilepsy, 34/126 patients (27%) receiving approximately 50 mg/kg/day on average, had at least one value of platelets ≤ 75 × 10^9/L. Approximately half of these patients had treatment discontinued, with return of platelet counts to normal. In the remaining patients, platelet counts normalized with continued treatment. In this study, the probability of thrombocytopenia appeared to increase significantly at total valproate concentrations of ≥ 110 µg/mL (females) or ≥ 135 µg/mL (males). The therapeutic benefit which may accompany the higher doses should therefore be weighed against the possibility of a greater incidence of adverse effects.

Usage In Pregnancy

ACCORDING TO PUBLISHED AND UNPUBLISHED REPORTS, VALPROIC ACID MAY PRODUCE TERATOGENIC EFFECTS IN THE OFFSPRING OF HUMAN FEMALES RECEIVING THE DRUG DURING PREGNANCY. THE DATA DESCRIBED BELOW WERE GAINED ALMOST EXCLUSIVELY FROM WOMEN WHO RECEIVED VALPROATE TO TREAT EPILEPSY. THERE ARE MULTIPLE REPORTS IN THE CLINICAL LITERATURE WHICH INDICATE THAT THE USE OF ANTIEPILEPTIC DRUGS DURING PREGNANCY RESULTS IN AN INCREASED INCIDENCE OF BIRTH DEFECTS IN THE OFFSPRING. ALTHOUGH DATA ARE MORE EXTENSIVE WITH RESPECT TO TRIMETHADIONE, PARAMETHADIONE, PHENYTOIN, AND PHENOBARBITAL, REPORTS INDICATE A POSSIBLE SIMILAR ASSOCIATION WITH THE USE OF OTHER ANTIEPILEPTIC DRUGS. THEREFORE, ANTIEPILEPSY DRUGS SHOULD BE ADMINISTERED TO WOMEN OF CHILDBEARING POTENTIAL ONLY IF THEY ARE CLEARLY SHOWN TO BE ESSENTIAL IN THE MANAGEMENT OF THEIR SEIZURES.

Continued on next page

Depakote ER—Cont.

THE INCIDENCE OF NEURAL TUBE DEFECTS IN THE FETUS MAY BE INCREASED IN MOTHERS RECEIVING VALPROATE DURING THE FIRST TRIMESTER OF PREGNANCY. THE CENTERS FOR DISEASE CONTROL (CDC) HAS ESTIMATED THE RISK OF VALPROIC ACID EXPOSED WOMEN HAVING CHILDREN WITH SPINA BIFIDA TO BE APPROXIMATELY 1 TO 2%.
OTHER CONGENITAL ANOMALIES (EG, CRANIOFACIAL DEFECTS, CARDIOVASCULAR MALFORMATIONS AND ANOMALIES INVOLVING VARIOUS BODY SYSTEMS), COMPATIBLE AND INCOMPATIBLE WITH LIFE, HAVE BEEN REPORTED. SUFFICIENT DATA TO DETERMINE THE INCIDENCE OF THESE CONGENITAL ANOMALIES IS NOT AVAILABLE.
THE HIGHER INCIDENCE OF CONGENITAL ANOMALIES IN ANTIEPILEPTIC DRUG-TREATED WOMEN WITH SEIZURE DISORDERS CANNOT BE REGARDED AS A CAUSE AND EFFECT RELATIONSHIP. THERE ARE INTRINSIC METHODOLOGIC PROBLEMS IN OBTAINING ADEQUATE DATA ON DRUG TERATOGENICITY IN HUMANS; GENETIC FACTORS OR THE EPILEPTIC CONDITION ITSELF, MAY BE MORE IMPORTANT THAN DRUG THERAPY IN CONTRIBUTING TO CONGENITAL ANOMALIES.
PATIENTS TAKING VALPROATE MAY DEVELOP CLOTTING ABNORMALITIES. A PATIENT WHO HAD LOW FIBRINOGEN WHEN TAKING MULTIPLE ANTICONVULSANTS INCLUDING VALPROATE GAVE BIRTH TO AN INFANT WITH AFIBRINOGENEMIA WHO SUBSEQUENTLY DIED OF HEMORRHAGE. IF VALPROATE IS USED IN PREGNANCY, THE CLOTTING PARAMETERS SHOULD BE MONITORED CAREFULLY.
HEPATIC FAILURE, RESULTING IN THE DEATH OF A NEWBORN AND OF AN INFANT, HAVE BEEN REPORTED FOLLOWING THE USE OF VALPROATE DURING PREGNANCY.
Animal studies have demonstrated valproate-induced teratogenicity. Increased frequencies of malformations, as well as intrauterine growth retardation and death, have been observed in mice, rats, rabbits, and monkeys following prenatal exposure to valproate. Malformations of the skeletal system are the most common structural abnormalities produced in experimental animals, but neural tube closure defects have been seen in mice exposed to maternal plasma valproate concentrations exceeding approximately 230 µg/mL (2.3 times the upper limit of the human therapeutic range for epilepsy) during susceptible periods of embryonic development. Administration of an oral dose of 200 mg/kg/day or greater (50% of the maximum human daily dose or greater on a mg/m^2 basis) to pregnant rats during organogenesis produced malformations (skeletal, cardiac, and urogenital) and growth retardation in the offspring. These doses resulted in peak maternal plasma valproate levels of approximately 340 µg/mL or greater (3.4 times the upper limit of the human therapeutic range for epilepsy or greater). Behavioral deficits have been reported in the offspring of rats given a dose of 200 mg/kg/day throughout most of pregnancy. An oral dose of 350 mg/kg/day (approximately 2 times the maximum human daily dose on a mg/m^2 basis) produced skeletal and visceral malformations in rabbits exposed during organogenesis. Skeletal malformations, growth retardation, and death were observed in rhesus monkeys following administration of an oral dose of 200 mg/kg/day (equal to the maximum human daily dose on a mg/m^2 basis) during organogenesis. This dose resulted in peak maternal plasma valproate levels of approximately 280 µg/mL (2.8 times the upper limit of the human therapeutic range for epilepsy).
The prescribing physician will wish to weigh the benefits of therapy against the risks in treating or counseling women of childbearing potential. If this drug is used during pregnancy, or if the patient becomes pregnant while taking this drug, the patient should be apprised of the potential hazard to the fetus.
Antiepileptic drugs should not be discontinued abruptly in patients in whom the drug is administered to prevent major seizures because of the strong possibility of precipitating status epilepticus with attendant hypoxia and threat to life. In individual cases where the severity and frequency of the seizure disorder are such that the removal of medication does not pose a serious threat to the patient, discontinuation of the drug may be considered prior to and during pregnancy, although it cannot be said with any confidence that even minor seizures do not pose some hazard to the developing embryo or fetus.
Tests to detect neural tube and other defects using current accepted procedures should be considered a part of routine prenatal care in childbearing women receiving valproate.

PRECAUTIONS

Hepatic Dysfunction
See **BOXED WARNING CONTRAINDICATIONS** and **WARNINGS.**
Pancreatitis
See **BOXED WARNING** and **WARNINGS.**
Hyperammonemia
Hyperammonemia has been reported in association with valproate therapy and may be present despite normal liver function tests. In patients who develop unexplained lethargy and vomiting or changes in mental status, hyperammonemic encephalopathy should be considered and an ammonia level should be measured. If ammonia is increased, valproate therapy should be discontinued. Appropriate interventions for treatment of hyperammonemia should be initiated, and such patients should undergo investigation for underlying urea cycle disorders (see **CONTRAINDICATIONS and WARNINGS—Urea Cycle Disorders**).
Asymptomatic elevations of ammonia are more common and when present, require close monitoring of plasma ammonia levels. If the elevation persists, discontinuation of valproate therapy should be considered.
General
Because of reports of thrombocytopenia (see **WARNINGS**), inhibition of the secondary phase of platelet aggregation, and abnormal coagulation parameters, (e.g., low fibrinogen), platelet counts and coagulation tests are recommended before initiating therapy and at periodic intervals. It is recommended that patients receiving DEPAKOTE be monitored for platelet count and coagulation parameters prior to planned surgery. In a clinical trial of DEPAKOTE as monotherapy in patients with epilepsy, 34/126 patients (27%) receiving approximately 50 mg/kg/day on average, had at least one value of platelets $\leq 75 \times 10^9$/L. Approximately half of these patients had treatment discontinued, with return of platelet counts to normal. In the remaining patients, platelet counts normalized with continued treatment. In this study, the probability of thrombocytopenia appeared to increase significantly at total valproate concentrations of ≥ 110 µg/mL (females) or ≥ 135 µg/mL (males). Evidence of hemorrhage, bruising, or a disorder of hemostasis/coagulation is an indication for reduction of the dosage or withdrawal of therapy.
Since DEPAKOTE may interact with concurrently administered drugs which are capable of enzyme induction, periodic plasma concentration determinations of valproate and concomitant drugs are recommended during the early course of therapy where clinically appropriate (see **PRECAUTIONS—Drug Interactions**).
Valproate is partially eliminated in the urine as a keto-metabolite which may lead to a false interpretation of the urine ketone test.
There have been reports of altered thyroid function tests associated with valproate. The clinical significance of these is unknown.
There are *in vitro* studies that suggest valproate stimulates the replication of the HIV and CMV viruses under certain experimental conditions. The clinical consequence, if any, is not known. Additionally, the relevance of these *in vitro* findings is uncertain for patients receiving maximally suppressive antiretroviral therapy. Nevertheless, these data should be borne in mind when interpreting the results from regular monitoring of the viral load in HIV infected patients receiving valproate or when following CMV infected patients clinically.
Information for Patients
Patients and guardians should be warned that abdominal pain, nausea, vomiting, and/or anorexia can be symptoms of pancreatitis and, therefore, require further medical evaluation promptly.
Patients should be informed of the signs and symptoms associated with hyperammonemic encephalopathy (see **PRECAUTIONS—Hyperammonemia**) and be told to inform the prescriber if any of these symptoms occur.
Since DEPAKOTE products may produce CNS depression, especially when combined with another CNS depressant (eg, alcohol), patients should be advised not to engage in hazardous activities, such as driving an automobile or operating dangerous machinery, until it is known that they do not become drowsy from the drug.
Since DEPAKOTE has been associated with certain types of birth defects, female patients of child-bearing age considering the use of DEPAKOTE ER should be advised to read the **Patient Information Leaflet**, which appears as the last section of the labeling.
Drug Interactions
Effects of Co-Administered Drugs on Valproate Clearance
Drugs that affect the level of expression of hepatic enzymes, particularly those that elevate levels of glucuronosyltransferases, may increase the clearance of valproate. For example, phenytoin, carbamazepine, and phenobarbital (or primidone) can double the clearance of valproate. Thus, patients on monotherapy will generally have longer half-lives and higher concentrations than patients receiving polytherapy with antiepilepsy drugs.
In contrast, drugs that are inhibitors of cytochrome P450 isozymes, e.g., antidepressants, may be expected to have little effect on valproate clearance because cytochrome P450 microsomal mediated oxidation is a relatively minor secondary metabolic pathway compared to glucuronidation and beta-oxidation.
Because of these changes in valproate clearance, monitoring of valproate and concomitant drug concentrations should be increased whenever enzyme inducing drugs are introduced or withdrawn.
The following list provides information about the potential for an influence of several commonly prescribed medications on valproate pharmacokinetics. The list is not exhaustive nor could it be, since new interactions are continuously being reported.
Drugs for which a potentially important interaction has been observed:
Aspirin—A study involving the co-administration of aspirin at antipyretic doses (11 to 16 mg/kg) with valproate to pediatric patients (n=6) revealed a decrease in protein binding and an inhibition of metabolism of valproate. Valproate free fraction was increased 4-fold in the presence of aspirin compared to valproate alone. The β-oxidation pathway consisting of 2-E-valproic acid, 3-OH-valproic acid, and 3-keto valproic acid was decreased from 25% of total metabolites excreted on valproate alone to 8.3% in the presence of aspirin. Whether or not the interaction observed in this study applies to adults is unknown, but caution should be observed if valproate and aspirin are to be co-administered.
Felbamate—A study involving the co-administration of 1200 mg/day of felbamate with valproate to patients with epilepsy (n=10) revealed an increase in mean valproate peak concentration by 35% (from 86 to 115 µg/mL) compared to valproate alone. Increasing the felbamate dose to 2400 mg/day increased the mean valproate peak concentration to 133 µg/mL (another 16% increase). A decrease in valproate dosage may be necessary when felbamate therapy is initiated.
Meropenem—Subtherapeutic valproic acid levels have been reported when meropenem was coadministered.
Rifampin—A study involving the administration of a single dose of valproate (7 mg/kg) 36 hours after 5 nights of daily dosing with rifampin (600 mg) revealed a 40% increase in the oral clearance of valproate. Valproate dosage adjustment may be necessary when it is co-administered with rifampin.
Drugs for which either no interaction or a likely clinically unimportant interaction has been observed:
Antacids—A study involving the co-administration of valproate 500 mg with commonly administered antacids (Maalox, Trisogel, and Titralac - 160 mEq doses) did not reveal any effect on the extent of absorption of valproate.
Chlorpromazine—A study involving the administration of 100 to 300 mg/day of chlorpromazine to schizophrenic patients already receiving valproate (200 mg BID) revealed a 15% increase in trough plasma levels of valproate.
Haloperidol—A study involving the administration of 6 to 10 mg/day of haloperidol to schizophrenic patients already receiving valproate (200 mg BID) revealed no significant changes in valproate trough plasma levels.
Cimetidine and Ranitidine—Cimetidine and ranitidine do not affect the clearance of valproate.
Effects of Valproate on Other Drugs
Valproate has been found to be a weak inhibitor of some P450 isozymes, epoxide hydrase, and glucuronyltransferases.
The following list provides information about the potential for an influence of valproate co-administration on the pharmacokinetics or pharmacodynamics of several commonly prescribed medications. The list is not exhaustive, since new interactions are continuously being reported.
Drugs for which a potentially important valproate interaction has been observed:
Amitriptyline/Nortriptyline—Administration of a single oral 50 mg dose of amitriptyline to 15 normal volunteers (10 males and 5 females) who received valproate (500 mg BID) resulted in a 21% decrease in plasma clearance of amitriptyline and a 34% decrease in the net clearance of nortriptyline. Rare postmarketing reports of concurrent use of valproate and amitriptyline resulting in an increased amitriptyline level have been received. Concurrent use of valproate and amitriptyline has rarely been associated with toxicity. Monitoring of amitriptyline levels should be considered for patients taking valproate concomitantly with amitriptyline. Consideration should be given to lowering the dose of amitriptyline/nortriptyline in the presence of valproate.
Carbamazepine/carbamazepine-10,11-Epoxide—Serum levels of carbamazepine (CBZ) decreased 17% while that of carbamazepine-10,11-epoxide (CBZ-E) increased by 45% upon co-administration of valproate and CBZ to epileptic patients.
Clonazepam—The concomitant use of valproic acid and clonazepam may induce absence status in patients with a history of absence type seizures.
Diazepam—Valproate displaces diazepam from its plasma albumin binding sites and inhibits its metabolism. Co-administration of valproate (1500 mg daily) increased the free fraction of diazepam (10 mg) by 90% in healthy volunteers (n=6). Plasma clearance and volume of distribution for free diazepam were reduced by 25% and 20%, respectively, in the presence of valproate. The elimination half-life of diazepam remained unchanged upon addition of valproate.
Ethosuximide—Valproate inhibits the metabolism of ethosuximide. Administration of a single ethosuximide dose of 500 mg with valproate (800 to 1600 mg/day) to healthy volunteers (n=6) was accompanied by a 25% increase in elimination half-life of ethosuximide and a 15% decrease in its total clearance as compared to ethosuximide alone. Patients receiving valproate and ethosuximide, especially along with other anticonvulsants, should be monitored for alterations in serum concentrations of both drugs.
Lamotrigine—In a steady-state study involving 10 healthy volunteers, the elimination half-life of lamotrigine increased from 26 to 70 hours with valproate co-administration (a 165% increase). The dose of lamotrigine should be reduced when co-administered with valproate. Serious skin reactions (such as Stevens-Johnson Syndrome and toxic epidermal necrolysis) have been reported with concomitant lamotrigine and valproate administration. See lamotrigine package insert for details on lamotrigine dosing with concomitant valporate administration.
Phenobarbital—Valproate was found to inhibit the metabolism of phenobarbital. Co-administration of valproate (250 mg BID for 14 days) with phenobarbital to normal sub-

jects (n=6) resulted in a 50% increase in half-life and a 30% decrease in plasma clearance of phenobarbital (60 mg single-dose). The fraction of phenobarbital dose excreted unchanged increased by 50% in presence of valproate.
There is evidence for severe CNS depression, with or without significant elevations of barbiturate or valproate serum concentrations. All patients receiving concomitant barbiturate therapy should be closely monitored for neurological toxicity. Serum barbiturate concentrations should be obtained, if possible, and the barbiturate dosage decreased, if appropriate.
Primidone, which is metabolized to a barbiturate, may be involved in a similar interaction with valproate.
Phenytoin—Valproate displaces phenytoin from its plasma albumin binding sites and inhibits its hepatic metabolism. Co-administration of valproate (400 mg TID) with phenytoin (250 mg) in normal volunteers (n=7) was associated with a 60% increase in the free fraction of phenytoin. Total plasma clearance and apparent volume of distribution of phenytoin increased 30% in the presence of valproate. Both the clearance and apparent volume of distribution of free phenytoin were reduced by 25%.
In patients with epilepsy, there have been reports of breakthrough seizures occurring with the combination of valproate and phenytoin. The dosage of phenytoin should be adjusted as required by the clinical situation.
Tolbutamide—From *in vitro* experiments, the unbound fraction of tolbutamide was increased from 20% to 50% when added to plasma samples taken from patients treated with valproate. The clinical relevance of this displacement is unknown.
Warfarin—In an *in vitro* study, valproate increased the unbound fraction of warfarin by up to 32.6%. The therapeutic relevance of this is unknown; however, coagulation tests should be monitored if DEPAKOTE therapy is instituted in patients taking anticoagulants.
Zidovudine—In six patients who were seropositive for HIV, the clearance of zidovudine (100 mg q8h) was decreased by 38% after administration of valproate (250 or 500 mg q8h); the half-life of zidovudine was unaffected.
Drugs for which either no interaction or a likely clinically unimportant interaction has been observed:
Acetaminophen—Valproate had no effect on any of the pharmacokinetic parameters of acetaminophen when it was concurrently administered to three epileptic patients.
Clozapine—In psychotic patients (n=11), no interaction was observed when valproate was co-administered with clozapine.
Lithium—Co-administration of valproate (500 mg BID) and lithium carbonate (300 mg TID) to normal male volunteers (n=16) had no effect on the steady-state kinetics of lithium.
Lorazepam—Concomitant administration of valproate (500 mg BID) and lorazepam (1 mg BID) in normal male volunteers (n=9) was accompanied by a 17% decrease in the plasma clearance of lorazepam.
Oral Contraceptive Steroids—Administration of a single-dose of ethinyloestradiol (50 μg)/levonorgestrel) (250 μg) to 6 women on valproate (200 mg BID) therapy for 2 months did not reveal any pharmacokinetic interaction.

Carcinogenesis, Mutagenesis, Impairment of Fertility

Carcinogenesis

Valproic acid was administered orally to Sprague Dawley rats and ICR (HA/ICR) mice at doses of 80 and 170 mg/kg/day (approximately 10 to 50% of the maximum human daily dose on a mg/m^2 basis) for two years. A variety of neoplasms were observed in both species. The chief findings were a statistically significant increase in the incidence of subcutaneous fibrosarcomas in high dose male rats receiving valproic acid and a statistically significant dose-related trend for benign pulmonary adenomas in male mice receiving valproic acid. The significance of these findings for humans is unknown.

Mutagenesis

Valproate was not mutagenic in an *in vitro* bacterial assay (Ames test), did not produce dominant lethal effects in mice, and did not increase chromosome aberration frequency in an *in vivo* cytogenetic study in rats. Increased frequencies of sister chromatid exchange (SCE) have been reported in a study of epileptic children taking valproate, but this association was not observed in another study conducted in adults. There is some evidence that increased SCE frequencies may be associated with epilepsy. The biological significance of an increase in SCE frequency is not known.

Fertility

Chronic toxicity studies in juvenile and adult rats and dogs demonstrated reduced spermatogenesis and testicular atrophy at oral doses of 400 mg/kg/day or greater in rats (approximately equivalent to or greater than the maximum human daily dose on a mg/m^2 basis) and 150 mg/kg/day or greater in dogs (approximately 1.4 times the maximum human daily dose or greater on a mg/m^2 basis). Segment I fertility studies in rats have shown oral doses up to 350 mg/kg/day (approximately equal to the maximum human daily dose on a mg/m^2 basis) for 60 days to have no effect on fertility. THE EFFECT OF VALPROATE ON TESTICULAR DEVELOPMENT AND ON SPERM PRODUCTION AND FERTILITY IN HUMANS IS UNKNOWN.

Pregnancy

Pregnancy Category D: see **WARNINGS**.

Nursing Mothers

Valproate is excreted in breast milk. Concentrations in breast milk have been reported to be 1–10% of serum concentrations. It is not known what effect this would have on a nursing infant. Consideration should be given to discontinuing nursing when divalproex sodium is administered to a nursing woman.

Pediatric Use

The safety and effectiveness of DEPAKOTE ER for the prophylaxis of migraine headaches in pediatric patients has not been established.
The safety and effectiveness of DEPAKOTE ER for the treatment of complex partial seizures, simple and complex absence seizures, and multiple seizure types that include absence seizures has not been established in pediatric patients under the age of 10 years.
Experience has indicated that pediatric patients under the age of two years are at a considerably increased risk of developing fatal hepatotoxicity, especially those with the aforementioned conditions (see **BOXED WARNING**). Above the age of 2 years, experience in epilepsy has indicated that the incidence of fatal hepatotoxicity decreases considerably in progressively older patient groups.
The basic toxicology and pathologic manifestations of valproate sodium in neonatal (4-day old) and juvenile (14-day old) rats are similar to those seen in young adult rats. However, additional findings, including renal alterations in juvenile rats and renal alterations and retinal dysplasia in neonatal rats, have been reported. These findings occurred at 240 mg/kg/day, a dosage approximately equivalent to the human maximum recommended daily dose on a mg/m^2 basis. They were not seen at 90 mg/kg, or 40% of the maximum human daily dose on a mg/m^2 basis.

Geriatric Use

Safety and effectiveness of DEPAKOTE ER in the prophylaxis of migraine patients over 65 have not been established.
No patients above the age of 65 years were enrolled in double-blind prospective clinical trials of mania associated with bipolar illness using DEPAKOTE (divalproex sodium delayed-release tablets). In a case review study of 583 patients using various valproate products, 72 patients (12%) were greater than 65 years of age. A higher percentage of patients above 65 years of age reported accidental injury, infection, pain, somnolence, and tremor. Discontinuation of valproate was occasionally associated with the latter two events. It is not clear whether these events indicate additional risk or whether they result from preexisting medical illness and concomitant medication use among these patients.
A study of elderly patients with dementia revealed drug related somnolence and discontinuation for somnolence (see **WARNINGS—Somnolence in the Elderly**). The starting dose should be reduced in these patients, and dosage reductions or discontinuation should be considered in patients with excessive somnolence (see **DOSAGE AND ADMINISTRATION**).

ADVERSE REACTIONS

Migraine

Based on the results of one multicenter, randomized, double-blind, placebo-controlled clinical trial, DEPAKOTE ER was well tolerated in the prophylactic treatment of migraine headache. Of the 122 patients exposed to DEPAKOTE ER in the placebo-controlled study, 8% discontinued for adverse events, compared to 9% for the 115 placebo patients.
Based on two placebo-controlled clinical trials and their long term extension, DEPAKOTE (divalproex sodium delayed-release tablets) was generally well tolerated with most adverse events rated as mild to moderate in severity. Of the 202 patients exposed to DEPAKOTE in the placebo-controlled trials, 17% discontinued for intolerance. This is compared to a rate of 5% for the 81 placebo patients. Including the long term extension study, the adverse events reported as the primary reason for discontinuation by ≥1% of 248 DEPAKOTE-treated patients were alopecia (6%), nausea and/or vomiting (5%), weight gain (2%), tremor (2%), somnolence (1%), elevated SGOT and/or SGPT (1%), and depression (1%).
Table 1 includes those adverse events reported for patients in the placebo-controlled trial where the incidence rate in the DEPAKOTE ER-treated group was greater than 5% and was greater than that for placebo patients.

Table 1
Adverse Events Reported by >5% of DEPAKOTE ER-Treated Patients During the Migraine Placebo-Controlled Trial with a Greater Incidence than Patients Taking Placebo[1]

Body System Event	Depakote ER (N=122)	Placebo (N=115)
Gastrointestinal System		
Nausea	15%	9%
Dyspepsia	7%	4%
Diarrhea	7%	3%
Vomiting	7%	2%
Abdominal Pain	7%	5%
Nervous System		
Somnolence	7%	2%
Other		
Infection	15%	14%

[1]The following adverse events occurred in greater than 5% of DEPAKOTE ER-treated patients and at a greater incidence for placebo than for DEPAKOTE ER: asthenia and flu syndrome.

The following additional adverse events were reported by greater than 1% but not more than 5% of DEPAKOTE ER-treated patients and with a greater incidence than placebo in the placebo-controlled clinical trial for migraine prophylaxis:
Body as a Whole: Accidental injury, viral infection.
Digestive System: Increased appetite, tooth disorder.
Metabolic and Nutritional Disorders: Edema, weight gain.
Nervous System: Abnormal gait, dizziness, hypertonia, insomnia, nervousness, tremor, vertigo.
Respiratory System: Pharyngitis, rhinitis.
Skin and Appendages: Rash.
Special Senses: Tinnitus.
Table 2 includes those adverse events reported for patients in the placebo-controlled trials where the incidence rate in the DEPAKOTE-treated group was greater than 5% and was greater than that for placebo patients.

Table 2
Adverse Events Reported by >5% of DEPAKOTE-Treated Patients During Migraine Placebo-Controlled Trials with a Greater Incidence than Patients Taking Placebo[1]

Body System Event	Depakote (N=202)	Placebo (N=81)
Gastrointestinal System		
Nausea	31%	10%
Dyspepsia	13%	9%
Diarrhea	12%	7%
Vomiting	11%	1%
Abdominal Pain	9%	4%
Increased Appetite	6%	4%
Nervous System		
Asthenia	20%	9%
Somnolence	17%	5%
Dizziness	12%	6%
Tremor	9%	0%
Other		
Weight Gain	8%	2%
Back Pain	8%	6%
Alopecia	7%	1%

[1]The following adverse events occurred in greater than 5% of DEPAKOTE-treated patients and at a greater incidence for placebo than for DEPAKOTE: flu syndrome and pharyngitis.

The following additional adverse events not referred to above were reported by greater than 1% but not more than 5% of DEPAKOTE-treated patients and with a greater incidence than placebo in the placebo-controlled clinical trials:
Body as a Whole: Chest pain.
Cardiovascular System: Vasodilatation.
Digestive System: Constipation, dry mouth, flatulence, stomatitis.
Hemic and Lymphatic System: Ecchymosis.
Metabolic and Nutritional Disorders: Peripheral edema.
Musculoskeletal System: Leg cramps.
Nervous System: Abnormal dreams, confusion, paresthesia, speech disorder, thinking abnormalities.
Respiratory System: Dyspnea, sinusitis.
Skin and Appendages: Pruritus.
Urogenital System: Metrorrhagia.

Epilepsy

Based on a placebo-controlled trial of adjunctive therapy for treatment of complex partial seizures, DEPAKOTE was generally well tolerated with most adverse events rated as mild to moderate in severity. Intolerance was the primary reason for discontinuation in the DEPAKOTE-treated patients (6%), compared to 1% of placebo-treated patients.
Table 3 lists treatment-emergent adverse events which were reported by ≥5% of DEPAKOTE-treated patients and for which the incidence was greater than in the placebo group, in the placebo-controlled trial of adjunctive therapy for treatment of complex partial seizures. Since patients were also treated with other antiepilepsy drugs, it is not possible, in most cases, to determine whether the following adverse events can be ascribed to DEPAKOTE alone, or the combination of DEPAKOTE and other antiepilepsy drugs.

Table 3
Adverse Events Reported by ≥ 5% of Patients Treated with DEPAKOTE During Placebo-Controlled Trial of Adjunctive Therapy for Complex Partial Seizures

Body System/Event	Depakote (%) (n = 77)	Placebo (%) (n = 70)
Body as a Whole		
Headache	31	21
Asthenia	27	7
Fever	6	4
Gastrointestinal System		
Nausea	48	14
Vomiting	27	7
Abdominal Pain	23	6
Diarrhea	13	6

Continued on next page

Depakote ER—Cont.

Anorexia	12	0
Dyspepsia	8	4
Constipation	5	1
Nervous System		
Somnolence	27	11
Tremor	25	6
Dizziness	25	13
Diplopia	16	9
Amblyopia/Blurred Vision	12	9
Ataxia	8	1
Nystagmus	8	1
Emotional Lability	6	4
Thinking Abnormal	6	0
Amnesia	5	1
Respiratory System		
Flu Syndrome	12	9
Infection	12	6
Bronchitis	5	1
Rhinitis	5	4
Other		
Alopecia	6	1
Weight Loss	6	0

Table 4 lists treatment-emergent adverse events which were reported by ≥5% of patients in the high dose DEPAKOTE group, and for which the incidence was greater than in the low dose group, in a controlled trial of DEPAKOTE monotherapy treatment of complex partial seizures. Since patients were being titrated off another antiepilepsy drug during the first portion of the trial, it is not possible, in many cases, to determine whether the following adverse events can be ascribed to DEPAKOTE alone, or the combination of DEPAKOTE and other antiepilepsy drugs.

Table 4
Adverse Events Reported by ≥ 5% of Patients in the High Dose Group in the Controlled Trial of DEPAKOTE Monotherapy for Complex Partial Seizures[1]

Body System/Event	High Dose (%) (n = 131)	Low Dow (%) (n = 134)
Body as a Whole		
Asthenia	21	10
Digestive System		
Nausea	34	26
Diarrhea	23	19
Vomiting	23	15
Abdominal Pain	12	9
Anorexia	11	4
Dyspepsia	11	10
Hemic/Lymphatic System		
Thrombocytopenia	24	1
Ecchymosis	5	4
Metabolic/Nutritional		
Weight Gain	9	4
Peripheral Edema	8	3
Nervous System		
Tremor	57	19
Somnolence	30	18
Dizziness	18	13
Insomnia	15	9
Nervousness	11	7
Amnesia	7	4
Nystagmus	7	1
Depression	5	4
Respiratory System		
Infection	20	13
Pharyngitis	8	2
Dyspnea	5	1
Skin and Appendages		
Alopecia	24	13
Special Senses		
Amblyopia/Blurred Vision	8	4
Tinnitus	7	1

[1]Headache was the only adverse event that occurred in ≥ 5% of patients in the high dose group and at an equal or greater incidence in the low dose group.

The following additional adverse events were reported by greater than 1% but less than 5% of the 358 patients treated with DEPAKOTE in the controlled trials of complex partial seizures:

Body as a Whole: Back pain, chest pain, malaise.
Cardiovascular System: Tachycardia, hypertension, palpitation.
Digestive System: Increased appetite, flatulence, hematemesis, eructation, pancreatitis, periodontal abscess.
Hemic and Lymphatic System: Petechia.
Metabolic and Nutritional Disorders: SGOT increased, SGPT increased.
Musculoskeletal System: Myalgia, twitching, arthralgia, leg cramps, myasthenia.
Nervous System: Anxiety, confusion, abnormal gait, paresthesia, hypertonia, incoordination, abnormal dreams, personality disorder.
Respiratory System: Sinusitis, cough increased, pneumonia, epistaxis.
Skin and Appendages: Rash, pruritus, dry skin.
Special Senses: Taste perversion, abnormal vision, deafness, otitis media.
Urogenital System: Urinary incontinence, vaginitis, dysmenorrhea, amenorrhea, urinary frequency.

Other Patient Populations

The following adverse events not listed previously were reported by greater than 1% of DEPAKOTE-treated patients and with a greater incidence than placebo in placebo-controlled trials of manic episodes associated with bipolar disorder:

Body as a Whole: Chills, chills and fever, drug level increased, neck rigidity.
Cardiovascular System: Arrhythmia, hypotension, postural hypotension.
Digestive System: Dysphagia, fecal incontinence, gastroenteritis, glossitis, gum hemorrhage, mouth ulceration.
Hemic and Lymphatic System: Anemia, bleeding time increased, leukopenia.
Metabolic and Nutritional Disorders: Hypoproteinemia.
Musculoskeletal System: Arthrosis.
Nervous System: Agitation, catatonic reaction, dysarthria, hallucinations, hypokinesia, psychosis, reflexes increased, sleep disorder, tardive dyskinesia.
Respiratory System: Hiccup.
Skin and Appendages: Discoid lupus erythematosis, erythema nodosum, furunculosis, maculopapular rash, seborrhea, sweating, vesiculobullous rash.
Special Senses: Conjunctivitis, dry eyes, eye disorder, eye pain, photophobia, taste perversion.
Urogenital System: Cystitis, menstrual disorder.

Adverse events that have been reported with all dosage forms of valproate from epilepsy trials, spontaneous reports, and other sources are listed below by body system.

Gastrointestinal: The most commonly reported side effects at the initiation of therapy are nausea, vomiting, and indigestion. These effects are usually transient and rarely require discontinuation of therapy. Diarrhea, abdominal cramps, and constipation have been reported. Both anorexia with some weight loss and increased appetite with weight gain have also been reported. In some patients, many of whom have functional or anatomic (including ileostomy or colostomy) gastrointestinal disorders with shortened GI transit times, there have been postmarketing reports of DEPAKOTE ER tablets in the stool.

CNS Effects: Sedative effects have occurred in patients receiving valproate alone but occur most often in patients receiving combination therapy. Sedation usually abates upon reduction of other antiepileptic medication. Tremor (may be dose-related), hallucinations, ataxia, headache, nystagmus, diplopia, asterixis, "spots before eyes", dysarthria, dizziness, confusion, hypesthesia, vertigo, incoordination, and parkinsonism have been reported with the use of valproate. Rare cases of coma have occurred in patients receiving valproate alone or in conjunction with phenobarbital. In rare instances encephalopathy with or without fever has developed shortly after the introduction of valproate monotherapy without evidence of hepatic dysfunction or inappropriately high plasma valproate levels. Although recovery has been described following drug withdrawal, there have been fatalities in patients with hyperammonemic encephalopathy, particularly in patients with underlying urea cycle disorders (see **WARNINGS—Urea Cycle Disorders** and **PRECAUTIONS**).

Several reports have noted reversible cerebral atrophy and dementia in association with valproate therapy.

Dermatologic: Transient hair loss, skin rash, photosensitivity, generalized pruritus, erythema multiforme, and Stevens-Johnson syndrome. Rare cases of toxic epidermal necrolysis have been reported including a fatal case in a 6 month old infant taking valproate and several other concomitant medications. An additional case of toxic epidermal necrosis resulting in death was reported in a 35 year old patient with AIDS taking several concomitant medications and with a history of multiple cutaneous drug reactions. Serious skin reactions have been reported with concomitant administration of lamotrigine and valproate (see **PRECAUTIONS—Drug Interactions**).

Psychiatric: Emotional Psychiatric: upset, depression, psychosis, aggression, hyperactivity, hostility, and behavioral deterioration.

Musculoskeletal: Weakness.

Hematologic: Thrombocytopenia and inhibition of the secondary phase of platelet aggregation may be reflected in altered bleeding time, petechiae, bruising, hematoma formation, epistaxis, and frank hemorrhage (see **PRECAUTIONS—General and Drug Interactions**). Relative lymphocytosis, macrocytosis, hypofibrinogenemia, leukopenia, eosinophilia, anemia including macrocytic with or without folate deficiency, bone marrow suppression, pancytopenia, aplastic anemia, agranulocytosis and acute intermittent porphyria.

Hepatic: Minor elevations of transaminases (eg, SGOT and SGPT) and LDH are frequent and appear to be dose-related. Occasionally, laboratory test results include increases in serum bilirubin and abnormal changes in other liver function tests. These results may reflect potentially serious hepatotoxicity (see **WARNINGS**).

Endocrine: Irregular menses, secondary amenorrhea, breast enlargement, galactorrhea, and parotid gland swelling. Abnormal thyroid function tests (see **PRECAUTIONS**).

There have been rare spontaneous reports of polycystic ovary disease. A cause and effect relationship has not been established.

Pancreatic: Acute pancreatitis including fatalities (see **WARNINGS**).

Metabolic: Hyperammonemia (see **PRECAUTIONS**), hyponatremia, and inappropriate ADH secretion.

There have been rare reports of Fanconi's syndrome occurring chiefly in children.

Decreased carnitine concentrations have been reported although the clinical relevance is undetermined.

Hyperglycinemia has occurred and was associated with a fatal outcome in a patient with preexistent nonketotic hyperglycinemia.

Genitourinary: Enuresis and urinary tract infection.

Special Senses: Hearing loss, either reversible or irreversible, has been reported; however, a cause and effect relationship has not been established. Ear pain has also been reported.

Other: Allergic reaction, anaphylaxis, edema of the extremities, lupus erythematosus, bone pain, cough increased, pneumonia, otitis media, bradycardia, cutaneous vasculitis, fever, and hypothermia.

OVERDOSAGE

Overdosage with valproate may result in somnolence, heart block, and deep coma. Fatalities have been reported; however patients have recovered from valproate levels as high as 2120 µg/mL.

In overdose situations, the fraction of drug not bound to protein is high and hemodialysis or tandem hemodialysis plus hemoperfusion may result in significant removal of drug. The benefit of gastric lavage or emesis will vary with the time since ingestion. General supportive measures should be applied with particular attention to the maintenance of adequate urinary output.

Naloxone has been reported to reverse the CNS depressant effects of valproate overdosage. Because naloxone could theoretically also reverse the antiepileptic effects of valproate, it should be used with caution in patients with epilepsy.

DOSAGE AND ADMINISTRATION

DEPAKOTE ER is an extended-release product intended for once-a-day oral administration. DEPAKOTE ER tablets should be swallowed whole and should not be crushed or chewed.

Migraine

DEPAKOTE ER is indicated for prophylaxis of migraine headaches in adults.

The recommended starting dose is 500 mg once daily for 1 week, thereafter increasing to 1000 mg once daily. Although doses other than 1000 mg once daily of DEPAKOTE ER have not been evaluated in patients with migraine, the effective dose range of DEPAKOTE (divalproex sodium delayed-release tablets) in these patients is 500-1000 mg/day. As with other valproate products, doses of DEPAKOTE ER should be individualized and dose adjustment may be necessary. If a patient requires smaller dose adjustments than that available with DEPAKOTE ER, DEPAKOTE should be used instead.

Epilepsy

DEPAKOTE ER is indicated as monotherapy and adjunctive therapy for complex partial seizures, and for simple and complex absence seizures in adult patients and pediatric patients 10 years of age or older. As the DEPAKOTE ER dosage is titrated upward, concentrations of phenobarbital, carbamazepine, and/or phenytoin may be affected (see **PRECAUTIONS—Drug Interactions**).

Complex Partial Seizures for adult patients and children 10 years of age or older:

Monotherapy (Initial Therapy): DEPAKOTE ER has not been systematically studied as initial therapy. Patients should initiate therapy at 10 to 15 mg/kg/day. The dosage should be increased by 5 to 10 mg/kg/week to achieve optimal clinical response. Ordinarily, optimal clinical response is achieved at daily doses below 60 mg/kg/day. If satisfactory clinical response has not been achieved, plasma levels should be measured to determine whether or not they are in the usually accepted therapeutic range (50 to 100 µg/mL). No recommendation regarding the safety of valproate for use at doses above 60 mg/kg/day can be made.

The probability of thrombocytopenia increases significantly at total trough valproate plasma concentrations above 110 µg/mL in females and 135 µg/mL in males. The benefit of improved seizure control with higher doses should be weighed against the possibility of a greater incidence of adverse reactions.

Conversion to Monotherapy: Patients should initiate therapy at 10 to 15 mg/kg/day. The dosage should be increased by 5 to 10 mg/kg/week to achieve optimal clinical response. Ordinarily, optimal clinical response is achieved at daily doses below 60 mg/kg/day. If satisfactory clinical response has not been achieved, plasma levels should be measured to determine whether or not they are in the usually accepted therapeutic range (50-100 µg/mL). No recommendation regarding the safety of valproate for use at doses above 60 mg/kg/day can be made. Concomitant antiepilepsy drug (AED) dosage can ordinarily be reduced by approximately 25% every 2 weeks. This reduction may be started at initiation of DEPAKOTE ER therapy, or delayed by 1 to 2 weeks if there is a concern that seizures are likely to occur with a reduction. The speed and duration of withdrawal of the concomitant AED can be highly variable, and patients should be monitored closely during this period for increased seizure frequency.

Adjunctive Therapy: DEPAKOTE ER may be added to the patient's regimen at a dosage of 10 to 15 mg/kg/day. The dosage may be increased by 5 to 10 mg/kg/week to achieve optimal clinical response. Ordinarily, optimal clinical response is achieved at daily doses below 60 mg/kg/day. If satisfactory clinical response has not been achieved, plasma levels should be measured to determine whether or not they are in the usually accepted therapeutic range (50 to 100 µg/mL). No recommendation regarding the safety of valproate for use at doses above 60 mg/kg/day can be made.
In a study of adjunctive therapy for complex partial seizures in which patients were receiving either carbamazepine or phenytoin in addition to DEPAKOTE, no adjustment of carbamazepine or phenytoin dosage was needed (see **CLINICAL STUDIES**). However, since valproate may interact with these or other concurrently administered AEDs as well as other drugs (see **Drug Interactions**), periodic plasma concentration determinations of concomitant AEDs are recommended during the early course of therapy (see **PRECAUTIONS—Drug Interactions**).

Simple and Complex Absence Seizures for adult patients and children 10 years of age or older:
The recommended initial dose is 15 mg/kg/day, increasing at one week intervals by 5 to 10 mg/kg/day until seizures are controlled or side effects preclude further increases. The maximum recommended dosage is 60 mg/kg/day.
A good correlation has not been established between daily dose, serum concentrations, and therapeutic effect. However, therapeutic valproate serum concentrations for most patients with absence seizures is considered to range from 50 to 100 µg/mL. Some patients may be controlled with lower or higher serum concentrations (see **CLINICAL PHARMACOLOGY**).
As the DEPAKOTE ER dosage is titrated upward, blood concentrations of phenobarbital and/or phenytoin may be affected (see **PRECAUTIONS**).
Antiepilepsy drugs should not be abruptly discontinued in patients in whom the drug is administered to prevent major seizures because of the strong possibility of precipitating status epilepticus with attendant hypoxia and threat to life.

Conversion from DEPAKOTE to DEPAKOTE ER:
In adult patients and pediatric patients 10 years of age or older with epilepsy previously receiving DEPAKOTE, DEPAKOTE ER should be administered once-daily using a dose 8 to 20% higher than the total daily dose of DEPAKOTE (Table 5). For patients whose DEPAKOTE total daily dose can not be directly converted to DEPAKOTE ER, consideration may be given at the clinician's discretion to increase the patient's DEPAKOTE total daily dose to the next higher dosage before converting to the appropriate total daily dose of DEPAKOTE ER.

Table 5
Dose Conversion

DEPAKOTE Total Daily Dose (mg)	**DEPAKOTE ER** (mg)
500*-625	750
750*-875	1000
1000*-1125	1250
1250-1375	1500
1500-1625	1750
1750	2000
1875-2000	2250
2125-2250	2500
2375	2750
2500-2750	3000
2875	3250
3000-3125	3500

*These total daily doses of DEPAKOTE cannot be directly converted to an 8 to 20% higher total daily dose of DEPAKOTE ER because the required dosing strengths of DEPAKOTE ER are not available. Consideration may be given at the clinician's discretion to increase the patient's DEPAKOTE total daily dose to the next higher dosage before converting to the appropriate total daily dose of DEPAKOTE ER.

There is insufficient data to allow a conversion factor recommendation for patients with DEPAKOTE doses above 3125 mg/day.
Plasma valproate C_{min} concentrations for DEPAKOTE ER on average are equivalent to DEPAKOTE, but may vary across patients after conversion. If satisfactory clinical response has not been achieved, plasma levels should be measured to determine whether or not they are in the usually accepted therapeutic range (50 to 100 µg/mL) (see **Pharmacokinetics**—Absorption/Bioavailability).

General Dosing Advice
Dosing in Elderly Patients—Due to a decrease in unbound clearance of valproate and possibly a greater sensitivity to somnolence in the elderly, the starting dose should be reduced in these patients. Starting doses in the elderly lower than 250 mg can only be achieved by the use of DEPAKOTE. Dosage should be increased more slowly and with regular monitoring for fluid and nutritional intake, dehydration, somnolence, and other adverse events. Dose reductions or discontinuation of valproate should be considered in patients with decreased food or fluid intake and in patients with excessive somnolence. The ultimate therapeutic dose should be achieved on the basis of both tolerability and clinical response (see **WARNINGS**).
Dose-Related Adverse Events—The frequency of adverse effects (particularly elevated liver enzymes and thrombocytopenia) may be dose-related. The probability of thrombocytopenia appears to increase significantly at total valproate concentrations of ≥ 110 µg/mL (females) or ≥ 135 µg/mL (males) (see **PRECAUTIONS**). The benefit of improved therapeutic effect with higher doses should be weighed against the possibility of a greater incidence of adverse reactions.
G.I. Irritation—Patients who experience G.I. irritation may benefit from administration of the drug with food or by initiating therapy with a lower dose of DEPAKOTE.
Compliance—Patients should be informed to take DEPAKOTE ER every day as prescribed. If a dose is missed it should be taken as soon as possible, unless it is almost time for the next dose. If a dose is skipped, the patient should not double the next dose.

HOW SUPPLIED

DEPAKOTE ER 250 mg is available as white ovaloid tablets with the corporate logo ⊐, and the Abbo-Code (HF). Each DEPAKOTE ER tablet contains divalproex sodium equivalent to 250 mg of valproic acid in the following package sizes:
Bottles of 60 .... (**NDC** 0074-3826-60).
Bottles of 100 .... (**NDC** 0074-3826-13).
Bottles of 500 .... (**NDC** 0074-3826-53).
ABBO-PAC unit dose packages of 100 . (**NDC** 0074-3826-11).
DEPAKOTE ER 500 mg is available as gray ovaloid tablets with the corporate logo ⊐, and the Abbo-Code HC. Each DEPAKOTE ER tablet contains divalproex sodium equivalent to 500 mg of valproic acid in the following packaging sizes:
Bottles of 100 .... (**NDC** 0074-7126-13).
Bottles of 500 .... (**NDC** 0074-7126-53).
ABBO-PAC unit dose packages of 100 . (**NDC** 0074-7126-11).
Recommended storage: Store tablets at 25°C (77°F); excursions permitted to 15–30°C (59–86°F) [see USP Controlled Room Temperature].
Revised: November, 2003
ABBOTT LABORATORIES
NORTH CHICAGO, IL 60064, U.S.A.

Patient Information Leaflet

Important Information for Women Who Could Become Pregnant
About the Use of DEPAKOTE® ER (divalproex sodium) Tablets

Please read this leaflet carefully before you take DEPAKOTE® ER (divalproex sodium) tablets. This leaflet provides a summary of important information about taking DEPAKOTE ER to women who could become pregnant. If you have any questions or concerns, or want more information about DEPAKOTE ER, contact your doctor or pharmacist.

Information For Women Who Could Become Pregnant
DEPAKOTE ER can be obtained only by prescription from your doctor. The decision to use DEPAKOTE ER is one that you and your doctor should make together, taking into account your individual needs and medical condition.
Before using DEPAKOTE ER, women who can become pregnant should consider the fact that DEPAKOTE has been associated with birth defects, in particular, with spina bifida and other defects related to failure of the spinal canal to close normally. Approximately 1 to 2% of children born to women with epilepsy taking DEPAKOTE in the first 12 weeks of pregnancy had these defects (based on data from the Centers for Disease Control, a U.S. agency based in Atlanta). The incidence in the general population is 0.1 to 0.2%.

Information For Women Who Are Planning To Get Pregnant
- Women taking DEPAKOTE ER who are planning to get pregnant should discuss the treatment options with their doctor

Information For Women Who Become Pregnant While Taking DEPAKOTE ER
- If you become pregnant while taking DEPAKOTE ER, you should contact your doctor immediately.

Other Important Information About DEPAKOTE ER Tablets
- DEPAKOTE ER tablets should be taken exactly as it is prescribed by your doctor to get the most benefits from DEPAKOTE ER and reduce the risk of side effects.
- If you have taken more than the prescribed dose of DEPAKOTE ER, contact your hospital emergency room or local poison center immediately.
- This medication was prescribed for your particular condition. Do not use it for another condition or give the drug to others.

Facts About Birth Defects
It is important to know that birth defects may occur even in children of individuals not taking any medications or without any additional risk factors.
This summary provides important information about the use of DEPAKOTE ER to women who could become pregnant. If you would like more information about the other potential risks and benefits of DEPAKOTE ER, ask your doctor or pharmacist to let you read the professional labeling and then discuss it with them. If you have any questions or concerns about taking DEPAKOTE ER, you should discuss them with your doctor.
03-5321-R6
Revised: November, 2003

ABBOTT LABORATORIES
NORTH CHICAGO, IL 60064, U.S.A.
PRINTED IN U.S.A.
Shown in Product Identification Guide, page 303

DILAUDID® Ⓒ℞
[dĭ-law-dĭd]
(hydromorphone hydrochloride)
℞ only

DESCRIPTION

DILAUDID (hydromorphone hydrochloride), a hydrogenated ketone of morphine, is an opioid analgesic. It is available in:
Ampules (for parenteral administration) containing:
1 mg, 2 mg, and 4 mg hydromorphone hydrochloride per mL with 0.2% sodium citrate, 0.2% citric acid solution. DILAUDID ampules are sterile.
Multiple Dose Vials (for parenteral administration) containing:
20 mL of solution. Each mL contains 2 mg hydromorphone hydrochloride and 0.5 mg edetate disodium with 1.8 mg methylparaben and 0.2 mg propylparaben as preservatives. Sodium hydroxide or hydrochloric acid is used for pH adjustment. DILAUDID multiple dose vials are sterile.
Color Coded Tablets (for oral administration) containing:
2 mg hydromorphone hydrochloride (orange tablet) and D&C red #30 Lake dye, D&C yellow #10 Lake dye, lactose, and magnesium stearate.
4 mg hydromorphone hydrochloride (yellow tablet) and D&C yellow #10 Lake dye, lactose, and magnesium stearate.
Suppositories (for rectal administration) containing:
3 mg hydromorphone hydrochloride in a cocoa butter base with silicon dioxide.
Non-Sterile Powder (for prescription compounding) containing hydromorphone hydrochloride. The chemical name of DILAUDID (hydromorphone hydrochloride) is 4,5α-epoxy-3-hydroxy-17-methylmorphinan-6-one hydrochloride. The structural formula is:

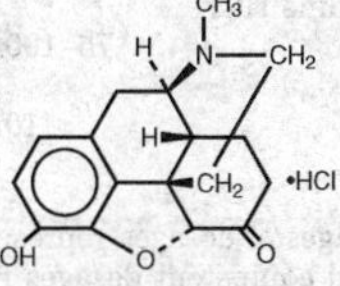

M.W. 321.8

CLINICAL PHARMACOLOGY

DILAUDID is an opioid analgesic; its principal therapeutic effect is relief of pain. The precise mechanism of action of DILAUDID and other opiates is not known, although it is believed to relate to the existence of opiate receptors in the central nervous system. There is no intrinsic limit to the analgesic effect of DILAUDID; like morphine, adequate doses will relieve even the most severe pain. Clinically, however, dosage limitations are imposed by the adverse effects, primarily respiratory depression, nausea, and vomiting, which can result from high doses.
DILAUDID has diverse additional actions. It may produce drowsiness, changes in mood and mental clouding, depress the respiratory center and the cough center, stimulate the vomiting center, produce pinpoint constriction of the pupil, enhance parasympathetic activity, elevate cerebrospinal fluid pressure, increase biliary pressure, produce transient hyperglycemia.
Generally, the analgesic action of parenterally administered DILAUDID is apparent within 15 minutes and usually remains in effect for more than five hours. The onset of action of oral DILAUDID is somewhat slower, with measurable analgesia occurring within 30 minutes.
In human plasma the half-life of a DILAUDID 4 mg tablet is 2.6 hours. In a random crossover study in six subjects, 4 mg of *oral* DILAUDID produced a mean concentration/time curve similar to that of 2 mg DILAUDID I.V., after the first hour.
The dosage of opioid analgesics like hydromorphone hydrochloride should be individualized for any given patient, since adverse events can occur at doses that may not provide complete freedom from pain (see **INDIVIDUALIZATION OF DOSAGE**).

INDIVIDUALIZATION OF DOSAGE

Safe and effective administration of opioid analgesics to patients with acute or chronic pain depends upon a comprehensive assessment of the patient. The nature of the pain (severity, frequency, etiology, and pathophysiology), as well as the concurrent medical status of the patient, will affect selection of the starting dosage.
In non-opioid-tolerant patients, therapy with hydromorphone hydrochloride is typically initiated at an oral dose of 2-4 mg every four hours, but elderly patients may require lower doses (see **PRECAUTIONS** - ***Geriatric Use***).
In patients receiving opioids, both the dose and duration of analgesia will vary substantially depending on the patient's opioid tolerance. The dose should be selected and adjusted so that at least 3–4 hours of pain relief may be achieved. In

Continued on next page

Dilaudid—Cont.

patients taking opioid analgesics, the starting dose of DILAUDID should be based on prior opioid usage. This should be done by converting the total daily usage of the previous opioid to an equivalent total daily dosage of oral DILAUDID using an equianalgesic table (see below). For opioids not in the table, first estimate the equivalent total daily usage of oral morphine, then use the table to find the equivalent total daily dosage of DILAUDID.

Once the total daily dosage of DILAUDID has been estimated, it should be divided into the desired number of doses. Since there is individual variation in response to different opioid drugs, only 1/2 to 2/3 of the estimated dose of DILAUDID calculated from equivalence tables should be given for the first few doses, then increased as needed according to the patient's response.

In chronic pain, doses should be administered around-the-clock. A supplemental dose of 5–15% of the total daily usage may be administered every two hours on an "as-needed" basis.

Periodic reassessment after the initial dosing is always required. If pain management is not satisfactory, and in the absence of significant opioid-induced adverse events, the hydromorphone dose may be increased gradually. If excessive opioid side effects are observed early in the dosing interval, the hydromorphone hydrochloride dose should be reduced. If this results in breakthrough pain at the end of the dosing interval, the dosing interval may need to be shortened. Dose titration should be guided more by the need for analgesia than the absolute dose of opioid employed.

OPIOID ANALGESIC EQUIVALENTS WITH APPROXIMATELY EQUIANALGESIC POTENCY*

Nonproprietary (Trade) Name	IM or SC Dose	ORAL Dose
Morphine sulfate	10mg	40–60mg
Hydromorphone HCl (DILAUDID)	1.3–2mg	6.5–7.5mg
Oxymorphone HCl (Numorphan)	1–1.1mg	6.6mg
Levorphanol tartrate (Levo-Dromoran)	2–2.3mg	4mg
Meperidine, pethidine HCl (Demerol)	75–100mg	300–400mg
Methadone HCl (Dolophine)	10mg	10–20mg

*Dosages, and ranges of dosages represented, are a compilation of estimated equipotent dosages from published references comparing opioid analgesics in cancer and severe pain.

INDICATIONS AND USAGE

DILAUDID is indicated for the relief of moderate to severe pain such as that due to:

- Surgery
- Cancer
- Trauma (soft tissue & bone)
- Biliary Colic
- Myocardial Infarction
- Burns
- Renal Colic

CONTRAINDICATIONS

DILAUDID is contraindicated in: patients with known hypersensitivity to hydromorphone, patients with respiratory depression in the absence of resuscitative equipment, and in patients with status asthmaticus. DILAUDID is also contraindicated for use in obstetrical analgesia.

WARNINGS

Impaired Respiration: Respiratory depression is the chief hazard of DILAUDID. Respiratory depression occurs most frequently in overdose situations, in the elderly, in the debilitated, and in those suffering from conditions accompanied by hypoxia or hypercapnia when even moderate therapeutic doses may dangerously decrease pulmonary ventilation. DILAUDID should be used with extreme caution in patients with chronic obstructive pulmonary disease or cor pulmonale, patients having a substantially decreased respiratory reserve, hypoxia, hypercapnia, or in patients with preexisting respiratory depression. In such patients, even usual therapeutic doses of opioid analgesics may decrease respiratory drive while simultaneously increasing airway resistance to the point of apnea.

Drug Dependence: DILAUDID is a Schedule II narcotic. DILAUDID can produce drug dependence of the morphine type and therefore have the potential for being abused. Psychic dependence, physical dependence and tolerance may develop upon repeated administration of DILAUDID, which should be prescribed and administered with the degree of caution appropriate to the use of morphine. Abrupt discontinuance in the administration of DILAUDID in patients who are physically dependent on opioids is likely to result in a withdrawal syndrome (see **DRUG ABUSE AND DEPENDENCE**).

Head Injury and Increased Intracranial Pressure: The respiratory depressant effects of DILAUDID with carbon dioxide retention and secondary elevation of cerebrospinal fluid pressure may be markedly exaggerated in the presence of head injury, other intracranial lesions or preexisting increase in intracranial pressure. Opioid analgesics including DILAUDID may produce effects which can obscure the clinical course and neurologic signs of further increase in intracranial pressure in patients with head injuries.

Hypotensive Effect: Opioid analgesics, including DILAUDID, may cause severe hypotension in an individual whose ability to maintain blood pressure has already been compromised by a depleted blood volume, or a concurrent administration of drugs such as phenothiazines or general anesthetics (see **PRECAUTIONS** - ***Drug Interactions***). Therefore, DILAUDID should be administered with caution to patients in circulatory shock, since vasodilation produced by the drug may further reduce cardiac output and blood pressure.

Sulfites: Contains sodium metabisulfite, a sulfite that may cause allergic-type reactions including anaphylactic symptoms and life-threatening or less severe asthmatic episodes in certain susceptible people. The overall prevalence of sulfite sensitivity in the general population is unknown and probably low. Sulfite sensitivity is seen more frequently in asthmatic than in nonasthmatic people.

PRECAUTIONS

Special Risk Patients: DILAUDID should be used with caution and the initial dose should be reduced in elderly or debilitated patients and those with impaired renal, pulmonary, or hepatic function; myxedema or hypothyroidism; adrenocortical insufficiency (e.g., Addison's disease); CNS depression or coma; toxic psychosis; prostatic hypertrophy or urethral stricture; gall bladder disease; acute alcoholism; delirium tremens; kyphoscoliosis or following gastrointestinal surgery. As with any opioid analgesic agent, the usual precautions should be observed and the possibility of respiratory depression should be kept in mind.

The administration of opioid analgesics, including DILAUDID, may obscure the diagnosis or clinical course of patients with acute abdominal conditions, and may aggravate preexisting convulsions in patients with convulsive disorders.

Reports of mild to severe seizures and myoclonus have been reported in severely compromised patients, administered high doses of parenteral hydromorphone, for cancer and severe pain. Opioid administration at very high doses is associated with seizures and myoclonus in a variety of diseases where pain control is the primary focus.

Cough Reflex: DILAUDID suppresses the cough reflex; as with all opioids, caution should be exercised when DILAUDID is used postoperatively and in patients with pulmonary disease.

Usage in Ambulatory Patients: DILAUDID may impair the mental and/or physical abilities required for the performance of potentially hazardous tasks such as driving a car or operating machinery; patients should be cautioned accordingly. DILAUDID may produce orthostatic hypotension in ambulatory patients. The addition of other CNS depressants to DILAUDID therapy may produce additive depressant effects, and DILAUDID should not be taken with alcohol.

Use in Biliary Surgery: Opioid analgesics, including DILAUDID, should also be used with caution in patients about to undergo surgery of the biliary tract since it may cause spasm of the sphincter of Oddi.

Use in Drug and Alcohol Dependent Patients: DILAUDID should be used with caution in patients with alcoholism and other drug dependencies due to the increased frequency of opioid tolerance, dependence, and the risk of addiction observed in these patient populations. Abuse of DILAUDID in combination with other CNS depressant drugs can result in serious risk to the patient.

Drug Interactions: Patients receiving other opioid analgesics, general anesthetics, phenothiazines, tranquilizers, sedative hypnotics, tricyclic antidepressants or other CNS depressants (including alcohol) concomitantly with DILAUDID may exhibit an additive CNS depression. When such combined therapy is contemplated, the dose of one or both agents should be reduced. Opioid analgesics, including DILAUDID, may enhance the action of neuromuscular blocking agents and produce an excessive degree of respiratory depression.

Parenteral Administration: The parenteral form of DILAUDID may be given intravenously, but the injection should be given very slowly. Rapid intravenous injection of opioid analgesics increases the possibility of side effects such as hypotension and respiratory depression.

Reports of mild to severe seizures and myoclonus have been reported in severely compromised patients, administered high doses of parenteral hydromorphone, for cancer and severe pain. Opioid administration at very high doses is associated with seizures and myoclonus in a variety of diseases where pain control is the primary focus.

Carcinogenesis, Mutagenesis, Impairment of Fertility: Animal carcinogenicity studies have not been performed with DILAUDID.

DILAUDID was not mutagenic in the *in vitro* Ames reverse mutation assay, in the *in vitro* chromosome aberration assay in human lymphocytes, or in the *in vivo* mouse bone marrow micronucleus test.

Fertility in male or female rats was not affected after daily oral administration at doses up to 7 mg/kg/day (41 mg/m^2). DILAUDID was dosed from 4 weeks prior to mating in males and 2 weeks prior to mating in females.

Pregnancy—Pregnancy Category C: Neither embryo-fetal toxicity nor teratogenic effects were observed following administration of DILAUDID at oral doses up to 7 mg/kg/day (41 mg/m^2) in rats from day 6 to day 17 of gestation and up to 25 mg/kg/day (315 mg/m^2) in rabbits from day 6 to day 20 of gestation.

Literature reports of hydromorphone hydrochloride administration to pregnant Syrian hamsters show that DILAUDID is teratogenic at a dose of 20 mg/kg which is 600 times the human dose. A maximal teratogenic effect (50% of fetuses affected) in the Syrian hamster was observed at a dose of 125 mg/kg (738 mg/m^2). There are no well-controlled studies in pregnant women. Hydromorphone hydrochloride is known to cross placental membranes. DILAUDID should be used in pregnant women only if the potential benefit justifies the potential risk to the fetus (see ***Labor and Delivery*** and **DRUG ABUSE AND DEPENDENCE**).

Nonteratogenic effects: Babies born to mothers who have been taking opioids regularly prior to delivery will be physically dependent. The withdrawal signs include irritability and excessive crying, tremors, hyperactive reflexes, increased respiratory rate, increased stools, sneezing, yawning, vomiting, and fever. The intensity of the syndrome does not always correlate with the duration of maternal opioid use or dose. There is no consensus on the best method of managing withdrawal. Approaches to the treatment of this syndrome have included supportive care and, when indicated, drugs such as paregoric or phenobarbital.

Labor and Delivery: DILAUDID is contraindicated in Labor and Delivery (see **CONTRAINDICATIONS**).

Nursing Mothers: Low levels of opioid analgesics have been detected in human milk. As a general rule, nursing should not be undertaken while a patient is receiving DILAUDID since it, and other drugs in this class, may be excreted in the milk.

Pediatric Use: Safety and effectiveness in children have not been established.

Geriatric Use: Clinical studies of DILAUDID did not include sufficient numbers of subjects aged 65 and over to determine whether they respond differently from younger subjects. Other reported clinical experience has not identified differences in responses between the elderly and younger patients. In general, dose selection for an elderly patient should be cautious, usually starting at the low end of the dosing range, reflecting the greater frequency of decreased hepatic, renal, or cardiac function, and of concomitant disease or other drug therapy.

ADVERSE REACTIONS

General and Central Nervous System: Sedation, drowsiness, mental clouding, lethargy, impairment of mental and physical performance, anxiety, fear, dysphoria, dizziness, psychic dependence, mood changes (nervousness, apprehension, depression, floating feelings, dreams), light-headedness, weakness, headache, agitation, tremor, uncoordinated muscle movements, muscle rigidity, paresthesia, muscle tremor, blurred vision, nystagmus, diplopia and miosis, transient hallucinations and disorientation, visual disturbances, insomnia, sweating, flushing, dysphoria, euphoria and increased intracranial pressure may occur.

Gastrointestinal System: Dry mouth, constipation, biliary tract spasm, ileus, anorexia, diarrhea, cramps, and taste alteration have been reported. Nausea and vomiting occur infrequently; they are more frequent in ambulatory than in recumbent patients. The antiemetic phenothiazines are useful in suppressing these effects; however, some phenothiazine derivatives seem to be antianalgesic and to increase the amount of opioid required to produce pain relief, while other phenothiazines reduce the amount of opioid required to produce a given level of analgesia. Prolonged administration of DILAUDID (hydromorphone hydrochloride) may produce constipation. Opiate agonist-induced increase in intraluminal pressure may endanger surgical anastomosis.

Cardiovascular System: Chills, shock, tachycardia, bradycardia, hypotension and hypertension have been reported. Circulatory depression, peripheral circulatory collapse and cardiac arrest have occurred after rapid intravenous injection. Orthostatic hypotension and fainting may occur if a patient stands up suddenly after receiving an injection of DILAUDID.

Genitourinary System: Ureteral spasm, antidiuretic effects, spasm of vesical sphincters and urinary retention or hesitancy have been reported.

Respiratory Depression: Bronchospasm and laryngospasm have been known to occur. DILAUDID produces dose-related respiratory depression by acting directly on brain stem respiratory centers. DILAUDID also affects centers that control respiratory rhythm, and may produce irregular and periodic breathing. If significant respiratory depression occurs, it may be antagonized by the use of naloxone hydrochloride (see **OVERDOSAGE**).

Dermatologic: Pruritis, urticaria, other skin rashes, and diaphoresis.

DRUG ABUSE AND DEPENDENCE

DILAUDID is a Schedule II narcotic. Psychic dependence, physical dependence, and tolerance may develop upon repeated administration of opioids; therefore DILAUDID should be prescribed and administered with caution. However, psychic dependence is unlikely to develop when DILAUDID is used for a short time for the treatment of pain. Physical dependence, the condition in which continued administration of the drug is required to prevent the appearance of a withdrawal syndrome, usually assumes clinically significant proportions only after several weeks of continued opioid use, although some mild degree of physical dependence may develop after a few days of opioid therapy. Withdrawal symptoms also may be precipitated in the patient with physical dependence by the administration of a drug with opioid antagonist activity, e.g., naloxone (see **OVERDOSAGE**). Tolerance, in which increasingly large doses are required in order to produce the same degree of analgesia, is manifested initially by a shortened duration of analgesic effect, and subsequently by decreases in the intensity of analgesia. The rate of development of tolerance varies among patients. In chronic pain patients, and in opioid-tolerant cancer patients, the dose of DILAUDID should be guided by the degree of tolerance manifested.

In chronic pain patients in whom opioid analgesics including DILAUDID are abruptly discontinued, a severe abstinence syndrome should be anticipated. This may be similar to the abstinence syndrome noted in patients who withdraw from heroin. The latter abstinence syndrome may be characterized by restlessness, lacrimation, rhinorrhea, yawning, perspiration, gooseflesh, restless sleep or "yen" and mydriasis during the first 24 hours. These symptoms may increase in severity and over the next 72 hours may be accompanied by increasing irritability, anxiety, weakness, twitching and spasms of muscles, kicking movements, severe backache, abdominal and leg pains, abdominal and muscle cramps, hot and cold flashes, insomnia, nausea, anorexia, vomiting, intestinal spasm, diarrhea, coryza and repetitive sneezing, increase in body temperature, blood pressure, respiratory rate and heart rate.

Because of excessive loss of fluids through sweating, or vomiting and diarrhea, patients experiencing the syndrome usually exhibit marked weight loss, dehydration, ketosis, and disturbances in acid-base balance. Cardiovascular collapse can occur. Without treatment most observable symptoms disappear in 5–14 days; however, there appears to be a phase of secondary or chronic abstinence, which may last for 2–6 months, characterized by insomnia, irritability, muscular aches, and autonomic instability.

In the treatment of physical dependence on DILAUDID, the patient may be detoxified by gradual reduction of the dosage, patient although this is unlikely to be necessary in the terminal cancer patient. If abstinence symptoms become severe, the patient may be detoxified with methadone. Temporary administration of tranquilizers and sedatives may aid in reducing patient anxiety. Gastrointestinal disturbances or dehydration should be treated accordingly.

OVERDOSAGE

Signs and Symptoms: Serious overdosage with DILAUDID is characterized by respiratory depression (a decrease in respiratory rate and/or tidal volume, Cheyne-Stokes respiration, cyanosis), extreme somnolence progressing to stupor or coma, skeletal muscle flaccidity, cold and clammy skin, constricted pupils, and sometimes bradycardia and hypotension. In severe overdosage, particularly by the intravenous route, apnea, circulatory collapse, cardiac arrest, and death may occur.

Treatment: Primary attention should be given to the reestablishment of adequate respiratory exchange through provision of a patent airway and institution of assisted or controlled ventilation. In cases of overdosage with oral DILAUDID, gastric lavage or induced emesis may be useful in removing unabsorbed drug from conscious patients. In unconscious patients with a secure airway, instill activated charcoal (30–100 g in adults, 1–2 g/kg in infants) via a nasogastric tube. A saline cathartic or sorbitol may be added to the first dose of activated charcoal.

Opioid-Tolerant Patient: Since tolerance to the respiratory and CNS depressant effects of opioids develops concomitantly with tolerance to their analgesic effects, serious respiratory depression due to an acute overdose is unlikely to be seen in opioid-tolerant patients receiving the usual therapeutic dosage of DILAUDID for chronic pain.

NOTE: In such an individual who is physically dependent on opioids, administration of the usual dose of an opioid antagonist will precipitate an acute withdrawal syndrome. The severity will depend on the degree of physical dependence and the dose of the antagonist administered. Use of an opioid antagonist should be reserved for cases where such treatment is clearly needed. If necessary to treat serious respiratory depression in the physically-dependent patient, the opioid antagonist should be administered with extreme care and by titration, using fractional (one fifth to one tenth) doses of the antagonist.

Non-Tolerant Patient: The opioid antagonist, naloxone, is a specific antidote against respiratory depression which may result from overdosage, or unusual sensitivity to DILAUDID. A dose of naloxone (usually given as a test dose of 0.4 mg, followed by up to 2.0 mg if needed) should be administered intravenously, if possible, simultaneously with respiratory resuscitation. The dose can be repeated in 3 minutes. Naloxone should not be administered in the absence of clinically significant respiratory or circulatory depression. Naloxone should be administered cautiously to persons who are known, or suspected to be physically dependent on DILAUDID (see **Opioid-Tolerant Patient**). In such cases, an abrupt or complete reversal of opioid effects may precipitate an acute abstinence syndrome. Since the duration of action of DILAUDID may exceed that of the antagonist, the patient should be kept under continued surveillance; repeated doses of the antagonist may be required to maintain adequate respiration. Apply other supportive measures when indicated.

Oxygen, intravenous fluids, vasopressors, and other supportive measures should be employed in the management of circulatory shock and pulmonary edema accompanying overdose as indicated. Cardiac arrest or arrhythmias may require cardiac massage or defibrillation.

DOSAGE AND ADMINISTRATION

Parenteral: The usual starting dose is 1-2 mg *subcutaneously* or *intramuscularly* every 4 to 6 hours as necessary for pain control. The dose should be adjusted according to the severity of pain, as well as the patient's underlying disease, age, and size. Patients with terminal cancer may be tolerant to opioid analgesics and may, therefore, require higher doses for adequate pain relief. Intravenous or subcutaneous administration is usually not painful. Should intravenous administration be necessary, the injection should be given ***slowly***, over at least 2 to 3 minutes, depending on the dose. A gradual increase in dose may be required if analgesia is inadequate, tolerance occurs, or if pain severity increases. The first sign of tolerance is usually a reduced duration of effect. NOTE: Parenteral drug products should be inspected visually for particulate matter and discoloration prior to administration, whenever solution and container permit. A slight yellowish discoloration may develop in DILAUDID ampules and multiple dose vials. No loss of potency has been demonstrated.

Oral: The usual oral dose is 2 mg every 4 to 6 hours as necessary. The dose must be individually adjusted according to severity of pain, patient response and patient size. More severe pain may require 4 mg or more every 4 to 6 hours. If the pain increases in severity, analgesia is not adequate or tolerance occurs, a gradual increase in dosage may be required. If pain is exceedingly severe, or if prompt response is desired, parenteral DILAUDID should be used initially in adequate amounts to control the pain.

Rectal: DILAUDID suppositories (3 mg) may provide longer duration of relief which could obviate additional medication during the sleeping hours. The usual adult dose is one (1) suppository inserted rectally every 6 to 8 hours or as directed by physician.

SAFETY AND HANDLING INSTRUCTIONS

DILAUDID poses little risk of direct exposure to health care personnel and should be handled and disposed of prudently in accordance with hospital or institutional policy. Patients and their families should be instructed to flush any DILAUDID that is no longer needed.

Access to abusable drugs such as DILAUDID presents an occupational hazard for addiction in the health care industry. Routine procedures for handling controlled substances developed to protect the public may not be adequate to protect health care workers. Implementation of more effective accounting procedures and measures to restrict access to drugs of this class (appropriate to the practice setting) may minimize the risk of self-administration by health care providers.

HOW SUPPLIED

Ampules: (One mL sterile solution for parenteral administration)

1 mg/mL ampules-Boxes of 10-
 NDC #0074-2332-11.

2 mg/mL ampules-Boxes of 10-
 NDC #0074-2333-11.
 Boxes of 25-
 NDC #0074-2333-26.

4 mg/mL ampules-Boxes of 10-
 NDC #0074-2334-11.

Multiple Dose Vials: (20 mL sterile solution for parenteral administration)

2 mg/mL-20 mL multiple dose vials-
 NDC #0074-2414-21.

Caution: The packaging (package) (vial stopper) of this product contains rubber latex which may cause allergic reactions.

Color Coded Tablets:

2 mg tablet (orange, debossed with the Abbott logo on one side and the number 2 on the opposite side)-Bottles of 100-
 NDC #0074-2415-14.
 Abbo-Pac® Unit Dose Packages of 100 (4 × 25)-
 NDC #0074-2415-12.
 Bottles of 500-NDC #0074-2415-54.

4 mg tablet (yellow, debossed with the Abbott logo on one side and the number 4 on the opposite side)-Bottles of 100-
 NDC #0074-2416-14.
 Abbo-Pac® Unit Dose Packages of 100 (4 × 25)-
 NDC #0074-2416-12.
 Bottles of 500-NDC #0074-2416-54.

Rectal Suppositories: 3 mg suppositories-Boxes of 6-
 NDC #0074-2451-07.

Non-Sterile Powder: For prescription compounding.
 15 grain vial-NDC #0074-2428-16.

STORAGE: Parenteral and oral dosage forms of DILAUDID should be stored at 25°C (77°F); excursions permitted to 15°–30°C (59°–86°F). [See USP Controlled Room Temperature]. Protect from light. DILAUDID suppositories should be stored in a refrigerator between 2°–8°C (36°–46°F).

A Schedule II Narcotic. DEA order form required.

Revised: February, 2003

Ref. 03-5258-R2

ABBOTT LABORATORIES
NORTH CHICAGO, IL 60064, U.S.A.

Shown in Product Identification Guide, page 303

DILAUDID-HP® INJECTION Ⓒ ℞

[*dī-lau-did*]

10 mg/mL

(hydromorphone hydrochloride)

℞ only

WARNING

DILAUDID-HP® (HIGH POTENCY) IS A HIGHLY CONCENTRATED SOLUTION OF HYDROMORPHONE INTENDED FOR USE IN OPIOID-TOLERANT PATIENTS. DO NOT CONFUSE DILAUDID-HP WITH STANDARD PARENTERAL FORMULATIONS OF DILAUDID OR OTHER OPIOIDS. OVERDOSE AND DEATH COULD RESULT.

DESCRIPTION

DILAUDID (hydromorphone hydrochloride), a hydrogenated ketone of morphine, is a opioid analgesic. HIGH POTENCY DILAUDID is available in AMBER ampules or single dose vials for intravenous (IV), subcutaneous (SC), or intramuscular (IM) administration. Each 1 mL of sterile solution contains 10 mg hydromorphone hydrochloride with 0.2% sodium citrate, and 0.2% citric acid solution.

It is also available as lyophilized DILAUDID for intravenous (IV), subcutaneous (SC), or intramuscular (IM) administration. Each single dose vial contains 250 mg sterile, lyophilized hydromorphone HCl to be reconstituted with 25 mL of Sterile Water for Injection USP to provide a solution containing 10 mg/mL.

The chemical name of of DILAUDID (hydromorphone hydrochloride) is 4,5α-epoxy-3-hydroxy-17-methylmorphinan-6-one hydrochloride. The structural formula is:

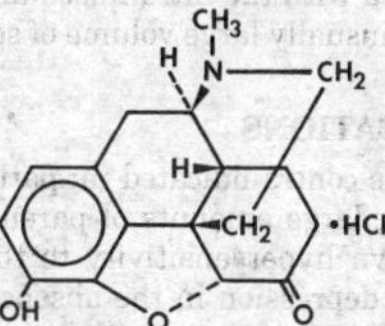

M.W. 321.8

CLINICAL PHARMACOLOGY

Many of the effects described below are common to the class of opioid analgesics. In some instances, data may not exist to demonstrate that DILAUDID-HP possesses similar or different effects than those observed with other opioid analgesics. However, in the absence of data to the contrary, it is assumed that DILAUDID-HP would possess these effects.

Central Nervous System: Opioid analgesics have multiple actions but exert their primary effects on the central nervous system and organs containing smooth muscle. The principal actions of therapeutic value are analgesia and sedation. A significant feature of the analgesia is that it occurs without loss of consciousness. Opioid analgesics also suppress the cough reflex and cause respiratory depression, mood changes, mental clouding, euphoria, dysphoria, nausea, vomiting and electroencephalographic changes. The precise mode of analgesic action of opioid analgesics is unknown. However, specific CNS opiate receptors have been identified. Opioid are believed to express their pharmacological effects by combining with these receptors.

Opioids depress the cough reflex by direct effect on the cough center in the medulla.

Opioids produce respiratory depression by direct effect on brain stem respiratory centers. The mechanism of respiratory depression also involves a reduction in the responsiveness of the brain stem respiratory centers to increases in carbon dioxide tension.

Opioids cause miosis. Pinpoint pupils are a common sign of opioid overdose but are not pathognomonic (e.g., pontine lesions of hemorrhagic or ischemic origin may produce similar findings) and marked mydriasis occurs when asphyxia intervenes.

Gastrointestinal Tract and Other Smooth Muscle: Gastric, biliary and pancreatic secretions are decreased by opioids. Opioids cause a reduction in motility associated with an increase in tone in the antrum portion of the stomach and duodenum. Digestion of food in the small intestine is delayed and propulsive contractions are decreased. Propulsive peristaltic waves in the colon are decreased, and tone may be increased to the point of spasm. The end result is constipation. Opioids can cause a marked increase in biliary tract pressure as a result of spasm of the sphincter of Oddi.

Cardiovascular System: Certain opioids produce peripheral vasodilation which may result in orthostatic hypotension. Release of histamine may occur with opioids and may contribute to drug-induced hypotension. Other manifestations of histamine release and/or peripheral vasodilation may include pruritis, flushing, and red eyes.

Effects on the myocardium after intravenous administration of opioids are not significant in normal persons, vary with different opioid analgesic agents and vary with the hemodynamic state of the patient, state of hydration and sympathetic drive.

PHARMACOKINETICS

In normal human volunteers hydromorphone hydrochloride is metabolized primarily in the liver. It is excreted primarily as the glucuronidated conjugate, with small amounts of parent drug and minor amounts of 6-hydroxy reduction metabolites.

Following intravenous administration of DILAUDID to normal volunteers, the mean half-life of elimination was 2.64 ± 0.88 hours. The mean volume of distribution was 91.5 liters, suggesting extensive tissue uptake. Hydromorphone hydrochloride is rapidly removed from the blood stream and distributed to skeletal muscle, kidneys, liver, intestinal tract, lungs, spleen and brain. Hydromorphone hydrochloride also crosses the placental membranes.

Continued on next page

Dilaudid-HP—Cont.

In terms of area under the analgesic time-effect curve, hydromorphone is approximately 8 times more potent than morphine (i.e., 1.3 mg of hydromorphone hydrochloride produces analgesia equal to that produced by 10 mg of morphine). After intramuscular administration, hydromorphone hydrochloride has a slightly more rapid onset and slightly shorter duration of action than morphine. The duration of DILAUDID analgesia in the non-tolerant patient with usual doses may be up to 4-5 hours. However, in tolerant subjects, duration will vary substantially depending on tolerance and dose. Dose should be adjusted so that 3-4 hours of pain relief may be achieved.

INDICATIONS AND USAGE

DILAUDID-HP is indicated for the relief of moderate-to-severe pain in opioid-tolerant patients who require larger than usual doses of opioids to provide adequate pain relief. Because DILAUDID-HP contains 10 mg of hydromorphone hydrochloride per mL, a smaller injection volume can be used than with other parenteral opioid formulations. Discomfort associated with the intramuscular or subcutaneous injection of an unusually large volume of solution can therefore be avoided.

CONTRAINDICATIONS

DILAUDID-HP is contraindicated in: patients who are not already receiving large amounts of parenteral opioids, patients with known hypersensitivity to the drug, patients with respiratory depression in the absence of resuscitative equipment, and in patients with status asthmaticus. DILAUDID-HP is also contraindicated for use in obstetrical analgesia.

WARNINGS - DRUG DEPENDENCE

DILAUDID is a Schedule II narcotic. DILAUDID-HP can produce drug dependence of the morphine type and therefore has the potential for being abused. Psychic dependence, physical dependence and tolerance may develop upon repeated administration of DILAUDID-HP, and it should be prescribed and administered with the same degree of caution appropriate for the use of morphine. Since DILAUDID-HP is indicated for use in patients who are already tolerant to and hence physically dependent on opioids, abrupt discontinuance in the administration of DILAUDID-HP is likely to result in a withdrawal syndrome. (see **DRUG ABUSE AND DEPENDENCE**).

Neonatal Withdrawal Syndrome: Infants born to mothers physically dependent on DILAUDID-HP will also be physically dependent and may exhibit respiratory difficulties and withdrawal symptoms. (see **DRUG ABUSE AND DEPENDENCE**).

Impaired Respiration: Respiratory depression is the chief hazard of DILAUDID-HP. Respiratory depression occurs most frequently in overdose situations, in the elderly, in the debilitated, and in those suffering from conditions accompanied by hypoxia or hypercapnia when even moderate therapeutic doses may dangerously decrease pulmonary ventilation.

DILAUDID-HP should be used with extreme caution in patients with chronic obstructive pulmonary disease or cor pulmonale, patients having a substantially decreased respiratory reserve, hypoxia, hypercapnia, or preexisting respiratory depression. In such patients even usual therapeutic doses of opioid analgesics may decrease respiratory drive while simultaneously increasing airway resistance to the point of apnea.

Head Injury and Increased Intracranial Pressure: The respiratory depressant effects of DILAUDID-HP with carbon dioxide retention and secondary elevation of cerebrospinal fluid pressure may be markedly exaggerated in the presence of head injury, other intracranial lesions, or preexisting increase in intracranial pressure. Opioid analgesics including DILAUDID-HP may produce effects which can obscure the clinical course and neurologic signs of further increase in pressure in patients with head injuries.

Hypotensive Effect: Opioid analgesics, including DILAUDID-HP, may cause severe hypotension in an individual whose ability to maintain his blood pressure has already been compromised by a depleted blood volume, or a concurrent administration of drugs such as phenothiazines or general anesthetics (see also **PRECAUTIONS—*Drug Interactions***). DILAUDID-HP may produce orthostatic hypotension in ambulatory patients.

DILAUDID-HP should be administered with caution to patients in circulatory shock, since vasodilation produced by the drug may further reduce cardiac output and blood pressure.

Sulfites: Contains sodium metabisulfite, a sulfite that may cause allergic-type reactions including anaphylactic symptoms and life-threatening or less severe asthmatic episodes in certain susceptible people. The overall prevalence of sulfite sensitivity in the general population is unknown and probably low. Sulfite sensitivity is seen more frequently in asthmatic than in nonasthmatic people.

PRECAUTIONS

General: Because of its high concentration, the delivery of precise doses of DILAUDID-HP may be difficult if low doses of hydromorphone are required. Therefore, DILAUDID-HP should be used only if the amount of hydromorphone required can be delivered accurately with this formulation.

Special Risk Patients: In general, opioids should be given with caution and the initial dose should be reduced in the elderly or debilitated and those with severe impairment of hepatic, pulmonary or renal function; myxedema or hypothyroidism; adrenocortical insufficiency (e.g., Addison's Disease); CNS depression or coma; toxic psychoses; prostatic hypertrophy or urethral stricture; gall bladder disease; acute alcoholism; delirium tremens; or kyphoscoliosis or following gastrointestinal surgery.

In the case of DILAUDID-HP, however, the patient is presumed to be receiving an opioid to which he or she exhibits tolerance and the initial dose of DILAUDID-HP selected should be estimated based on the relative potency of hydromorphone and the opioid previously used by the patient. (see **DOSAGE AND ADMINISTRATION**).

The administration of opioid analgesics including DILAUDID-HP may obscure the diagnosis or clinical course in patients with acute abdominal conditions and may aggravate preexisting convulsions in patients with convulsive disorders.

Reports of mild to severe seizures and myoclonus have been reported in severely compromised patients, administered high doses of parenteral hydromorphone, for cancer and severe pain. Opioid administration at very high doses is associated with seizures and myoclonus in a variety of diseases where pain control is the primary focus.

Use in Biliary Surgery: Opioid analgesics including DILAUDID-HP, should also be used with caution in patients about to undergo surgery of the biliary tract since it may cause spasm of the sphincter of Oddi.

Use in Drug and Alcohol Dependent Patients: DILAUDID-HP should be used with caution in patients with alcoholism and other drug dependencies due to the increased frequency of opioid tolerance, dependence, and the risk of addiction observed in these patient populations. Abuse of DILAUDID-HP in combination with other CNS depressant drugs can result in serious risk to the patient.

Drug Interactions: The concomitant use of other central nervous system depressants including sedatives or hypnotics, general anesthetics, phenothiazines, tranquilizers and alcohol may produce additive depressant effects. Respiratory depression, hypotension and profound sedation or coma may occur. When such combined therapy is contemplated, the dose of one or both agents should be reduced. Opioid analgesics, including DILAUDID-HP may enhance the action of neuromuscular blocking agents and produce an increased degree of respiratory depression.

Carcinogenesis, Mutagenesis, Impairment of Fertility: Animal carcinogenicity studies have not been performed with DILAUDID.

DILAUDID was not mutagenic in the *in vitro* Ames reverse mutation assay, in the *in vitro* chromosome aberration assay in human lymphocytes, or in the *in vivo* mouse bone marrow micronucleus test.

Fertility in male or female rats was not affected after daily oral administration at doses up to 7 mg/kg/day (41 mg/m^2). DILAUDID was dosed from 4 weeks prior to mating in males and 2 weeks prior to mating in females.

PREGNANCY–CATEGORY C:

Human: There are no well-controlled studies in women. Reports based on marketing experience do not identify any specific teratogenic risks following routine (short-term) clinical use. Although there is no clearly defined risk, such reports do not exclude the possibility of infrequent or subtle damage to the human fetus. DILAUDID-HP should be used in pregnant women only when clearly needed (see **Labor and Delivery** and **DRUG ABUSE AND DEPENDENCE**).

Animal: Neither embryo-fetal toxicity nor teratogenic effects were observed following administration of DILAUDID at oral doses up to 7 mg/kg/day (41 mg/m^2) in rats from day 6 to day 17 of gestation and up to 25 mg/kg/day (315 mg/m^2) in rabbits from day 6 to day 20 of gestation.

Literature reports of hydromorphone hydrochloride administration to pregnant Syrian hamsters show that DILAUDID is teratogenic at a dose of 20 mg/kg which is 600 times the human dose. A maximal teratogenic effect (50% of fetuses affected) in the Syrian hamster was observed at a dose of 125 mg/kg.

Nonteratogenic effects: Babies born to mothers who have been taking opoiods regularly prior to delivery will be physically dependent. The withdrawal signs include irritability and excessive crying, tremors, hyperactive reflexes, increased respiratory rate, increased stools, sneezing, yawning, vomiting, and fever. The intensity of the syndrome does not always correlate with the duration of maternal opioid use or dose. There is no consensus on the best method of managing withdrawal. Approaches to the treatment of this syndrome have included supportive care and, when indicated, drugs such as paregoric or phenobarbital.

Labor and Delivery: DILAUDID-HP is contraindicated in Labor and Delivery (see **CONTRAINDICATIONS**).

Nursing Mothers: Low levels of opioid analgesics have been detected in human milk. As a general rule, nursing should not be undertaken while a patient is receiving DILAUDID-HP since it, and other drugs in this class, may be excreted in the milk.

Pediatric Use: Safety and effectiveness have not been established.

Geriatric Use: Clinical studies of DILAUDID did not include sufficient numbers of subjects aged 65 and over to determine whether they respond differently from younger subjects. In general, dose selection for an elderly patient should be cautious, usually starting at the low end of the dosing range, reflecting the greater frequency of decreased hepatic, renal, or cardiac function, and of concomitant disease or other drug therapy. (see **PRECAUTIONS**).

ADVERSE REACTIONS

The adverse effects of DILAUDID-HP are similar to those of other opioid analgesics, and represent established pharmacological effects of the drug class. The major hazards include respiratory depression and apnea. To a lesser degree, circulatory depression, respiratory arrest, shock and cardiac arrest have occurred.

The most frequently observed adverse effects are lightheadedness, dizziness, sedation, nausea, vomiting, and sweating. These effects seem to be more prominent in ambulatory patients and in those not experiencing severe pain. Syncopal reactions and related symptoms in ambulatory patients may be alleviated if the patient lies down.

Less Frequently Observed with Opioid Analgesics:

General and CNS: Dysphoria, euphoria, weakness, headache, agitation, tremor, uncoordinated muscle movements, alterations of mood (nervousness, apprehension, depression, floating feelings, dreams), muscle rigidity, paresthesia, muscle tremor, blurred vision, nystagmus, diplopia and miosis, transient hallucinations* and disorientation, visual disturbances, insomnia and increased intracranial pressure may occur.

*Hallucinations, although unusual with pure agonist opioids, have been observed in one patient following both a 6 mg and a 4 mg DILAUDID-HP (hydromorphone hydrochloride) dose. However, the patient was receiving several concomitant medications during the second episode and a causal relationship cannot be established.

Cardiovascular: Flushing of the face, chills, tachycardia, bradycardia, palpitation, faintness, syncope, hypotension and hypertension have been reported.

Respiratory: Bronchospasm and laryngospasm have been known to occur.

Gastrointestinal: Dry mouth, constipation, biliary tract spasm, ileus anorexia, diarrhea, cramps and taste alterations have been reported.

Genitourinary: Urinary retention or hesitancy, and antidiuretic effects have been reported.

Dermatologic: Pruritis, urticaria, other skin rashes, wheal and flare over the vein with intravenous injection, and diaphoresis have been reported with opioid analgesics.

Other: In clinical trials, neither local tissue irritation nor induration was observed at the site of subcutaneous injection of DILAUDID-HP; pain at the injection site was rarely observed. However, local irritation and induration have been seen following parenteral injection of other opioid drug products.

DRUG ABUSE AND DEPENDENCE

DILAUDID-HP is a Schedule II narcotic, similar to morphine. Opioid analgesics may cause psychological and physical dependence (see **WARNINGS**). Physical dependence results in withdrawal symptoms in patients who abruptly discontinue the drug. Withdrawal symptoms may also be precipitated in the patient with physical dependence by the administration of a drug with opioid antagonist activity, e.g., naloxone (see **OVERDOSAGE**). Physical dependence usually does not occur to a clinically significant degree until after several weeks of continued opioid usage but it may become clinically detectable after as little as a week. Tolerance, in which increasingly large doses are required in order to produce the same degree of analgesia, is initially manifested by a shortened duration of analgesic effect, and subsequently, by decreases in the intensity of analgesia. In chronic pain patients, and in opioid-tolerant cancer patients, the dose of DILAUDID-HP should be guided by the degree of tolerance manifested.

In chronic pain patients in whom opioid analgesics including DILAUDID-HP are abruptly discontinued, a severe abstinence syndrome should be anticipated. This may be similar to the abstinence syndrome noted in patients who withdraw from heroin. The latter abstinence syndrome may be characterized by restlessness, lacrimation, rhinorrhea, yawning, perspiration, gooseflesh, restless sleep or "yen" and mydriasis during the first 24 hours. These symptoms may increase in severity and over the next 72 hours may be accompanied by increasing irritability, anxiety, weakness, twitching and spasms of muscles, kicking movements, severe backache, abdominal and leg pains, abdominal and muscle cramps, hot and cold flashes, insomnia, nausea, anorexia, vomiting, intestinal spasm, diarrhea, coryza and repetitive sneezing, increase in body temperature, blood pressure, respiratory rate and heart rate.

Because of excessive loss of fluids through sweating, or vomiting and diarrhea, patients experiencing the syndrome usually exhibit marked weight loss, dehydration, ketosis, and disturbances in acid-base balance. Cardiovascular collapse can occur. Without treatment, most observable symptoms disappear in 5-14 days; however, there appears to be a phase of secondary or chronic abstinence which may last for 2-6 months characterized by insomnia, irritability, muscular aches, and autonomic instability.

In the treatment of physical dependence on DILAUDID-HP, the patient may be detoxified by gradual reduction of the dosage, although this is unlikely to be necessary in the terminal cancer patient. If abstinence symptoms become severe, the patient may be given methadone. Temporary administration of tranquilizers and sedatives may aid in reducing patient anxiety. Gastrointestinal disturbances or dehydration should be treated accordingly.

OVERDOSAGE

Serious overdosage with DILAUDID-HP is characterized by respiratory depression, somnolence progressing to stupor or

STRONG ANALGESICS AND STRUCTURALLY RELATED DRUGS USED IN THE TREATMENT OF CANCER PAIN*

Nonproprietary (Trade) Names	IM OR SC ADMINISTRATION Dose, mg Equianalgesic to 10 mg of IM Morphine†	Duration Compared With Morphine
Morphine sulfate	10	Same
Papaveretum (Pantopon)	20	Same
Hydromorphone (DILAUDID) hydrochloride	1.3	Slightly Shorter
Oxymorphone (Numorphan) hydrochloride	1.1	Slightly Shorter
Nalbuphine (Nubain) hydrochloride	12	Same
Heroin, diamorphine hydrochloride (NA in U.S.)	4-5	Slightly Shorter
Levorphanol (Levo-Dromoran) tartrate	2.3	Same
Butorphanol (Stadol) tartrate	1.5-2.5	Same
Pentazocine (Talwin) lactate or hydrochloride	60	Shorter
Meperidine, pethidine (Demerol) hydrochloride	80	Shorter
Methadone (Dolophine) hydrochloride	10	Same

* From Beaver WT Management of cancer pain with parenteral medication. J. Am. Med. Assoc. 244:2653-2657 (1980).
† (In terms of the area under the analgesic time-effect curve.)

HIGH POTENCY:	10 mg/1 mL	*50 mg/5 mL	*500 mg/50 mL	*lyophilized 250 mg
	Box of 10 ampules	Box of 10 ampules	Single dose vial	Single dose vial
	NDC 0074-2453-11	NDC 0074-2453-27	NDC 0074-2453-51	NDC 0074-2455-31

*FOR USE IN THE PREPARATION OF LARGE VOLUME PARENTERAL SOLUTIONS

coma, skeletal muscle flaccidity, cold and clammy skin, constricted pupils, and sometimes bradycardia and hypotension. In serious overdosage, particularly following intravenous injection, apnea, circulatory collapse, cardiac arrest and death may occur.

In the treatment of overdosage primary attention should be given to the reestablishment of adequate respiratory exchange through provision of a patent airway and institution of assisted or controlled ventilation.

Opioid-Tolerant Patient: Since tolerance to the respiratory and CNS depressant effects of opioids develops concomitantly with tolerance to their analgesic effects, serious respiratory depression due to an acute overdose is unlikely to be seen in opioid-tolerant patients receiving DILAUDID-HP for chronic pain.

NOTE: In such an individual who is physically dependent on opioids, administration of the usual dose of the antagonist will precipitate an acute withdrawal syndrome. The severity will depend on the degree of physical dependence and the dose of the antagonist administered. Use of an opioid antagonist in such a person should be avoided. If necessary to treat serious respiratory depression in the physically dependent patient, the antagonist should be administered with extreme care and by titration with smaller than usual doses of the antagonist.

Non-Tolerant Patient: The opioid antagonist, naloxone, is a specific antidote against respiratory depression which may result from overdosage, or unusual sensitivity to DILAUDID-HP. A dose of naloxone (usually 0.4 to 2.0 mg) should be administered intravenously, if possible, simultaneously with respiratory resuscitation. The dose can be repeated in 3 minutes. Naloxone should not be administered in the absence of clinically significant respiratory or circulatory depression. Naloxone should be administered cautiously to persons who are known, or suspected to be physically dependent on DILAUDID-HP. In such cases, an abrupt or complete reversal of opioid effects may precipitate an acute abstinence syndrome.

Since the duration of action of DILAUDID-HP may exceed that of the antagonist, the patient should be kept under continued surveillance; repeated doses of the antagonist may be required to maintain adequate respiration. Apply other supportive measures when indicated.

Supportive measures (including oxygen, vasopressors) should be employed in the management of circulatory shock and pulmonary edema accompanying overdose as indicated. Cardiac arrest or arrhythmias may require cardiac massage or defibrillation.

DOSAGE AND ADMINISTRATION

Parenteral: DILAUDID-HP SHOULD BE GIVEN ONLY TO PATIENTS WHO ARE ALREADY RECEIVING LARGE DOSES OF OPIOIDS. DILAUDID-HP is indicated for relief of moderate-to-severe pain in opioid-tolerant patients. Thus, these patients will already have been treated with other opioid analgesics. If the patient is being changed from regular DILAUDID to DILAUDID-HP, similar doses should be used, depending on the patient's clinical response to the drug. If DILAUDID-HP is substituted for a different opioid analgesic, the following equivalency table should be used as a guide to determine the appropriate dose of DILAUDID-HP (hydromorphone hydrochloride).

[See table above]

In open clinical trials with DILAUDID-HP in patients with terminal cancer, doses ranged from 1-14 mg subcutaneously or intramuscularly; one patient received 30 mg subcutaneously on two occasions. In these trials, both subcutaneous and intramuscular injections of DILAUDID-HP were well-tolerated, with minimal pain and/or burning at the injection site. Mild erythema was rarely noted after intramuscular injection. There was no induration after either intramuscular or subcutaneous administration of DILAUDID-HP. Subcutaneous injections of DILAUDID-HP were particularly well accepted when administered with a short, 30 gauge needle.

Experience with administration of DILAUDID-HP by the intravenous route is limited. Should intravenous administration be necessary, the injection should be given slowly, over at least 2 to 3 minutes. The intravenous route is usually painless.

A gradual increase in dose may be required if analgesia is inadequate, tolerance occurs, or if pain severity increases. The first sign of tolerance is usually a reduced duration of effect.

NOTE: Parenteral drug products should be inspected visually for particulate matter and discoloration prior to administration, whenever solution and container permit. A slight yellowish discoloration may develop in DILAUDID-HP ampules. No loss of potency has been demonstrated. DILAUDID injection is physically compatible and chemically stable for at least 24 hours at 25°C protected from light in most common large volume parenteral solutions.

500 mg/50 mL Vial: To use this single dose presentation, do not penetrate the stopper with a syringe. Instead, remove both the aluminum flipseal and rubber stopper in a suitable work area such as under a laminar flow hood (or equivalent clean air compounding area). The contents may then be withdrawn for preparation of a single, large volume parenteral solution. Any unused portion should be discarded in an appropriate manner.

CAUTION: The packaging (vial stopper) of this product contains rubber latex which may cause allergic reactions.

Reconstitution of sterile lyophilized DILAUDID-HP 250mg: Reconstitute immediately prior to use with 25 mL of Sterile Water for Injection USP to provide a sterile solution containing 10 mg/mL.

SAFETY AND HANDLING INSTRUCTIONS:

DILAUDID-HP poses little risk of direct exposure to health care personnel and should be handled and disposed of prudently in accordance with hospital or institutional policy. Patients and their families should be instructed to flush any DILAUDID-HP that is no longer needed.

Access to abusable drugs such as DILAUDID-HP presents an occupational hazard for addiction in the health care industry. Routine procedures for handling controlled substances developed to protect the public may not be adequate to protect health care workers. Implementaiton of more effective accounting procedures and measures to restrict access to drugs of this class (appropriate to the practice setting) may minimize the risk of self-administration by health care providers.

HOW SUPPLIED

DILAUDID-HP *amber* ampules and single dose vials contain 10 mg hydromorphone hydrochloride per mL with 0.2% sodium citrate and 0.2% citric acid solution. No added preservative.

NOTE: DILAUDID-HP ampules are *amber* in color.

The lyophilized DILAUDID-HP Single Dose Vial contains 250 mg of sterile, lyophilized hydromorphone HCl.

[See second table above]

STORAGE: Store at 25°C (77°F); excursions permitted to 15°-30°C (59°-86°F). [See USP Controlled Room Temperature]. Protect from light.

A Schedule CII Narcotic. DEA Order Form Required.

Revised: February, 2003
58-7092-R2
ABBOTT LABORATORIES
NORTH CHICAGO, IL 60064, U.S.A.

DILAUDID® ORAL LIQUID and DILAUDID® 8 mg TABLETS

CII ℞

(hydromorphone hydrochloride)
(NOS. 2426 and 2452)
03-5259-R2-Rev. Feb., 2003
℞ only

DESCRIPTION

DILAUDID (hydromorphone hydrochloride), a hydrogenated ketone of morphine, is an opioid analgesic.

The chemical name of DILAUDID (hydromorphone hydrochloride) is 4,5α-epoxy-3-hydroxy-17-methylmorphinan-6-one hydrochloride. The structural formula is:

M.W. 321.8

Each 5 mL (1 teaspoon) of DILAUDID ORAL LIQUID contains 5 mg of hydromorphone hydrochloride. In addition, other ingredients include purified water, methylparaben, propylparaben, sucrose, and glycerin. DILAUDID ORAL LIQUID may contain traces of sodium metabisulfite.

Each DILAUDID 8 mg TABLET contains 8 mg hydromorphone hydrochloride. In addition, the tablets include lactose anhydrous, and magnesium stearate. DILAUDID 8 mg TABLET may contain traces of sodium metabisulfite.

CLINICAL PHARMACOLOGY

Many of the effects described below are common to this class of mu-opioid agonist analgesics. In some instances, data may not exist to distinguish the effects of DILAUDID ORAL LIQUID and DILAUDID 8 mg TABLETS from those observed with other opioid analgesics. However, in the absence of data to the contrary, it is assumed that DILAUDID ORAL LIQUID and DILAUDID 8 mg TABLETS would possess all the actions of mu-agonist opioids.

Central Nervous System: Opioid analgesics exert their primary effects on the central nervous system and organs containing smooth muscle. The principal actions of therapeutic value are analgesia and sedation. A significant feature of the analgesia is that it can occur without loss of consciousness. Opioid analgesics also suppress the cough reflex and may cause respiratory depression, mood changes, mental clouding, euphoria, dysphoria, nausea, vomiting and electroencephalographic changes.

The precise mode of analgesic action of opioid analgesics is unknown. However, specific CNS opiate receptors have been identified. Opioids are believed to express their pharmacological effects by combining with these receptors.

Opioids depress the cough reflex by direct effect on the cough center in the medulla.

Opioids depress the respiratory reflex by a direct effect on brain stem respiratory centers. The mechanism of respiratory depression also involves a reduction in the responsiveness of the brain stem respiratory centers to increases in carbon dioxide tension.

Opioids cause miosis. Pinpoint pupils are a common sign of opioid overdose but are not pathognomonic (e.g., pontine lesions of hemorrhagic or ischemic origin may produce similar findings) and marked mydriasis occurs with asphyxia.

Gastrointestinal Tract and Other Smooth Muscle: Gastric, biliary and pancreatic secretions are decreased by opioids. Opioids cause a reduction in motility associated with an increase in tone in the gastric antrum and duodenum. Digestion of food in the small intestine is delayed and propulsive contractions are decreased. Propulsive peristaltic waves in the colon are decreased, and tone may be increased to the point of spasm. The end result is constipation. Opioids can cause a marked increase in biliary tract pressure as a result of spasm of the sphincter of Oddi.

Cardiovascular System: Certain opioids produce peripheral vasodilation which may result in orthostatic hypotension. Release of histamine may occur with opioids and may contribute to drug-induced hypotension. Other manifestations of histamine release may include pruritus, flushing, and red eyes.

The dosage of opioid analgesics like hydromorphone hydrochloride should be individualized for any given patient,

Continued on next page

Dilaudid Oral Liquid/Tablets—Cont.

since adverse events can occur at doses that may not provide complete freedom from pain (see **INDIVIDUALIZATION OF DOSAGE**).

PHARMACOKINETICS:

The analgesic activity of DILAUDID (hydromorphone hydrochloride) is due to the parent drug, hydromorphone. Hydromorphone is rapidly absorbed from the gastrointestinal tract after oral administration and undergoes extensive first-pass metabolism. *In vivo* bioavailability following single-dose administration of the 8 mg tablet is approximately 24% (coefficient of variation 21%). Bioequivalence between the DILAUDID 8 mg TABLET and an equivalent dose of DILAUDID ORAL LIQUID has been demonstrated. Dose proportionality between DILAUDID 8 mg TABLET and other strength DILAUDID tablets (2 and 4 mg) has not been established.

Absorption: After oral administration of DILAUDID 8 mg liquid or tablets, peak plasma hydromorphone concentrations are generally attained within 1/2 to 1-hour.

[See table below]

Food effects: The effect on the rate and extent of absorption of DILAUDID tablet or oral liquid when given with food has not been studied.

Distribution: At therapeutic plasma levels, hydromorphone is approximately 8–19% bound to plasma proteins. After an intravenous bolus dose, the steady state of volume distribution [mean (%cv)] is 302.9 (32%) liters.

Metabolism: Hydromorphone is extensively metabolized via glucuronidation in the liver, with greater than 95% of the dose metabolized to hydromorphone-3-glucuronide along with minor amounts of 6-hydroxy reduction metabolites.

Elimination: Only a small amount of the hydromorphone dose is excreted unchanged in the urine. Most of the dose is excreted as hydromorphone-3-glucuronide along with minor amounts of 6-hydroxy reduction metabolites. The systemic clearance is approximately 1.96 (20%) liters/minute. The terminal elimination half-life of hydromorphone after an intravenous dose is about 2.3 hours.

Special Populations: Pediatrics: Pharmacokinetics of hydromorphone have not been evaluated in children.

Hepatic and renal impairment: The effects of hepatic and renal disease on the clearance of hydromorphone are unknown but caution should be taken to guard against possible accumulation if hepatic and/or renal functions are seriously impaired.

Pregnancy and nursing mothers: Hydromorphone crosses the placenta. Hydromorphone is also found in low levels in breast milk, and may cause respiratory compromise in newborns when administered during labor or delivery.

CLINICAL TRIALS

Analgesic effects of single doses of DILAUDID ORAL LIQUID administered to patients with post-surgical pain have been studied in double-blind controlled trials. In one study with 61 patients, both 5 mg and 10 mg of DILAUDID ORAL LIQUID provided significantly more analgesia than placebo. In another trial with 80 patients, 5 mg and 10 mg of DILAUDID ORAL LIQUID were compared to 30 mg and 60 mg of morphine sulfate oral liquid. The pain relief provided by 5 mg and 10 mg DILAUDID ORAL LIQUID was comparable to 30 mg and 60 mg oral morphine sulfate, respectively.

INDIVIDUALIZATION OF DOSAGE:

Safe and effective administration of opioid analgesics to patients with acute or chronic pain depends upon a comprehensive assessment of the patient. The nature of the pain (severity, frequency, etiology, and pathophysiology) as well as the concurrent medical status of the patient will affect selection of the starting dosage.

In non-opioid-tolerant patients, therapy with hydromorphone is typically initiated at an oral dose of 2–4 mg every four hours, but elderly patients may require lower doses (see **PRECAUTIONS**–***Geriatric Use***).

In patients receiving opioids, both the dose and duration of analgesia will vary substantially depending on the patient's opioid tolerance. The dose should be selected and adjusted so that at least 3–4 hours of pain relief may be achieved. In patients taking opioid analgesics, the starting dose of DILAUDID should be based on prior opioid usage. This should be done by converting the total daily usage of the previous opioid to an equivalent total daily dosage of oral DILAUDID using an equianalgesic table (see below). For opioids not in the table, first estimate the equivalent total daily usage of oral morphine, then use the table to find the equivalent total daily dosage of DILAUDID.

Once the total daily dosage of DILAUDID has been estimated, it should be divided into the desired number of doses. Since there is individual variation in response to different opioid drugs, only 1/2 to 2/3 of the estimated dose of DILAUDID calculated from equivalence tables should be given for the first few doses, then increased as needed according to the patient's response.

In chronic pain, doses should be administered around-the-clock. A supplemental dose of 5–15% of the total daily usage may be administered every two hours on an "as-needed" basis.

Periodic reassessment after the initial dosing is always required. If pain management is not satisfactory and in the absence of significant opioid-induced adverse events, the hydromorphone dose may be increased gradually. If excessive opioid side effects are observed early in the dosing interval, the hydromorphone dose should be reduced. If this results in breakthrough pain at the end of the dosing interval, the dosing interval may need to be shortened. Dose titration should be guided more by the need for analgesia than the absolute dose of opioid employed.

OPIOID ANALGESIC EQUIVALENTS WITH APPROXIMATELY EQUIANALGESIC POTENCY*

Nonproprietary (Trade) Name	IM or SC Dose	ORAL Dose
Morphine sulfate	10mg	40–60mg
Hydromorphone HCl (DILAUDID)	1.3–2mg	6.5–7.5mg
Oxymorphone HCl (Numorphan)	1–1.1mg	6.6mg
Levorphanol tartrate (Levo-Dromoran)	2–2.3mg	4 mg
Meperidine, pethidine HCl (Demerol)	75–100mg	300–400 mg
Methadone HCl (Dolophine)	10mg	10–20mg

*Dosages, and ranges of dosages represented, are a compilation of estimated equipotent dosages from published references comparing opioid analgesics in cancer and severe pain.

INDICATIONS AND USAGE

DILAUDID ORAL LIQUID and DILAUDID 8 mg TABLETS are indicated for the management of pain in patients where an opioid analgesic is appropriate.

CONTRAINDICATIONS

DILAUDID ORAL LIQUID and DILAUDID 8 mg TABLETS are contraindicated in: patients with known hypersensitivity to hydromorphone, patients with respiratory depression in the absence of resuscitative equipment, and in patients with status asthmaticus. DILAUDID ORAL LIQUID and DILAUDID 8 mg TABLETS are also contraindicated for use in obstetrical analgesia.

WARNINGS

Impaired Respiration: Respiratory depression is the chief hazard of DILAUDID ORAL LIQUID and DILAUDID 8 mg TABLETS. Respiratory depression occurs most frequently in overdose situations, in the elderly, in the debilitated, and in those suffering from conditions accompanied by hypoxia or hypercapnia when even moderate therapeutic doses may dangerously decrease pulmonary ventilation.

DILAUDID ORAL LIQUID and DILAUDID 8 mg TABLETS should be used with extreme caution in patients with chronic obstructive pulmonary disease or cor pulmonale, patients having a substantially decreased respiratory reserve, hypoxia, hypercapnia, or in patients with preexisting respiratory depression. In such patients even usual therapeutic doses of opioid analgesics may decrease respiratory drive while simultaneously increasing airway resistance to the point of apnea.

Drug Dependence: DILAUDID is a Schedule II narcotic. DILAUDID ORAL LIQUID and DILAUDID 8 mg TABLETS can produce drug dependence of the morphine type and therefore have the potential for being abused. Psychic dependence, physical dependence and tolerance may develop upon repeated administration of DILAUDID, which should be prescribed and administered with the degree of caution appropriate to the use of morphine. Abrupt discontinuance in the administration of DILAUDID ORAL LIQUID and DILAUDID 8 mg TABLETS in patients who are physically dependent on opioids is likely to result in a withdrawal syndrome (see **DRUG ABUSE AND DEPENDENCE**).

Neonatal Withdrawal Syndrome: Infants born to mothers physically dependent on DILAUDID will also be physically dependent and may exhibit respiratory difficulties and withdrawal symptoms. (see **DRUG ABUSE AND DEPENDENCE**).

Head Injury and Increased Intracranial Pressure: The respiratory depressant effects of DILAUDID ORAL LIQUID and DILAUDID 8 mg TABLETS with carbon dioxide retention and secondary elevation of cerebrospinal fluid pressure may be markedly exaggerated in the presence of head injury, other intracranial lesions, or preexisting increase in intracranial pressure. Opioid analgesics including DILAUDID ORAL LIQUID and DILAUDID 8 mg TABLETS (hydromorphone hydrochloride) may produce effects which can obscure the clinical course and neurologic signs of further increase in intracranial pressure in patients with head injuries.

Hypotensive Effect: Opioid analgesics, including DILAUDID ORAL LIQUID and DILAUDID 8 mg TABLETS, may cause severe hypotension in an individual whose ability to maintain blood pressure has already been compromised by a depleted blood volume, or a concurrent administration of drugs such as phenothiazines or general anesthetics (see **PRECAUTIONS**–***Drug Interactions***). Therefore, DILAUDID ORAL LIQUID and DILAUDID 8 mg TABLETS should be administered with caution to patients in circulatory shock, since vasodilation produced by the drug may further reduce cardiac output and blood pressure.

Sulfites: Contains sodium metabisulfite, a sulfite that may cause allergic-type reactions including anaphylactic symptoms and life-threatening or less severe asthmatic episodes in certain susceptible people. The overall prevalence of sulfite sensitivity in the general population is unknown and probably low. Sulfite sensitivity is seen more frequently in asthmatic than in nonasthmatic people.

PRECAUTIONS

Special Risk Patients: In general, opioids should be given with caution and the initial dose should be reduced in the elderly or debilitated and those with severe impairment of hepatic, pulmonary or renal functions; myxedema or hypothyroidism; adrenocortical insufficiency (e.g., Addison's Disease); CNS depression or coma; toxic psychoses; prostatic hypertrophy or urethral stricture; gall bladder disease; acute alcoholism; delirium tremens; kyphoscoliosis or following gastrointestinal surgery.

The administration of opioid analgesics including DILAUDID ORAL LIQUID and DILAUDID 8 mg TABLETS may obscure the diagnoses or clinical course in patients with acute abdominal conditions and may aggravate preexisting convulsions in patients with convulsive disorders. Reports of mild to severe seizures and myoclonus have been reported in severely compromised patients, administered high doses of parenteral hydromorphone, for cancer and severe pain. Opioid administration at very high doses is associated with seizures and myoclonus in a variety of diseases where pain control is the primary focus.

Use in Ambulatory Patients: DILAUDID ORAL LIQUID and DILAUDID 8 mg TABLETS may impair mental and/or physical ability required for the performance of potentially hazardous tasks (e.g. driving, operating machinery). Patients should be cautioned accordingly. DILAUDID may produce orthostatic hypotension in ambulatory patients. The addition of other CNS depressants to DILAUDID therapy may produce additive depressant effects, and DILAUDID should not be taken with alcohol.

Use in Biliary Surgery: Opioid analgesics, including DILAUDID ORAL LIQUID and DILAUDID 8 mg TABLETS, should also be used with caution in patients about to undergo surgery of the biliary tract since it may cause spasm of the sphincter of Oddi.

Use in Drug and Alcohol Dependent Patients: DILAUDID should be used with caution in patients with alcoholism and other drug dependencies due to the increased frequency of opioid tolerance, dependence, and the risk of addiction observed in these patient populations. Abuse of DILAUDID in combination with other CNS depressant drugs can result in serious risk to the patient.

Drug Interactions: The concomitant use of other central nervous system depressants including sedatives or hypnotics, general anesthetics, phenothiazines, tranquilizers and alcohol may produce additive depressant effects. Respiratory depression, hypotension and profound sedation or coma may occur. When such combined therapy is contemplated, the dose of one or both agents should be reduced. Opioid analgesics, including DILAUDID ORAL LIQUID and DILAUDID 8 mg TABLETS, may enhance the action of neuromuscular blocking agents and produce an excessive degree of respiratory depression.

Carcinogenesis, Mutagenesis, Impairment of Fertility: Animal carcinogenicity studies have not been performed with DILAUDID.

DILAUDID was not mutagenic in the *in vitro* Ames reverse mutation assay, in the *in vitro* chromosome aberration assay in human lymphocytes, or in the *in vivo* mouse bone marrow micronucleus test.

Fertility in male or female rats was not affected after daily oral administration at doses up to 7 mg/kg/day (41 mg/m^2). DILAUDID was dosed from 4 weeks prior to mating in males and 2 weeks prior to mating in females.

Pregnancy–Pregnancy Category C: Neither embryo-fetal toxicity nor teratogenic effects were observed following administration of DILAUDID at oral doses up to 7 mg/kg/day (41 mg/m^2) in rats from day 6 to day 17 of gestation and up to 25 mg/kg/day (315 mg/m^2) in rabbits from day 6 to day 20 of gestation.

Literature reports of hydromorphone hydrochloride administration to pregnant Syrian hamsters show that DILAUDID is teratogenic at a dose of 20 mg/kg which is 600 times the human dose. A maximal teratogenic effect (50% of fetuses affected) in the Syrian hamster was observed at a dose of 125 mg/kg (738 mg/m^2).

There are no well-controlled studies in women. Hydromorphone is known to cross placental membranes. DILAUDID ORAL LIQUID and DILAUDID 8 mg TABLETS should be used in pregnant women only if the potential benefit justifies the potential risk to the fetus (see ***Labor and Delivery*** and **DRUG ABUSE AND DEPENDENCE**).

Nonteratogenic effects: Babies born to mothers who have been taking opioids regularly prior to delivery will be physically dependent. The withdrawal signs include irritability

Mean (%cv)

Dosage Form	C_{max} (ng)	T_{max} (hrs)	AUC (ng*hr/mL)	$T_{1/2}$ (hrs)
8 mg Tablet	5.5 (33%)	0.74 (34%)	23.7 (28%)	2.6 (18%)
8 mg Oral Liquid	5.7 (31%)	0.73 (71%)	24.6 (29%)	2.8 (20%)

and excessive crying, tremors, hyperactive reflexes, increased respiratory rate, increased stools, sneezing, yawning, vomiting, and fever. The intensity of the syndrome does not always correlate with the duration of maternal opioid use or dose. There is no consensus on the best method of managing withdrawal. Approaches to the treatment of this syndrome have included supportive care and, when indicated, drugs such as paregoric or phenobarbital.

Labor and Delivery: DILAUDID ORAL LIQUID and DILAUDID 8 mg TABLETS are contraindicated in Labor and Delivery (see **CONTRAINDICATIONS**).

Nursing Mothers: Low levels of opioid analgesics have been detected in human milk. As a general rule, nursing should not be undertaken while a patient is receiving DILAUDID ORAL LIQUID and DILAUDID 8 mg TABLETS since it, and other drugs in this class, may be excreted in the milk.

Pediatric Use: Safety and effectiveness in children have not been established.

Geriatric Use: Clinical studies of DILAUDID did not include sufficient numbers of subjects aged 65 and over to determine whether they respond differently from younger subjects. In general, dose selection for an elderly patient should be cautious, usually starting at the low end of the dosing range, reflecting the greater frequency of decreased hepatic, renal, or cardiac function, and of concomitant disease or other drug therapy (see **INDIVIDUALIZATION OF DOSAGES** and **PRECAUTIONS**).

ADVERSE REACTIONS

The adverse effects of DILAUDID ORAL LIQUID and DILAUDID 8 mg TABLETS are similar to those of other opioid agonist analgesics, and represent established pharmacological effects of the drug class. The major hazards include respiratory depression and apnea. To a lesser degree, circulatory depression, respiratory arrest, shock and cardiac arrest have occurred.

The most frequently observed adverse effects are lightheadedness, dizziness, sedation, nausea, vomiting, sweating, flushing, dysphoria, euphoria, dry mouth, and pruritus. These effects seem to be more prominent in ambulatory patients and in those not experiencing severe pain. Syncopal reactions and related symptoms in ambulatory patients may be alleviated if the patient lies down.

Less Frequently Observed with Opioid Analgesics:

General and CNS: Weakness, headache, agitation, tremor, uncoordinated muscle movements, alterations of mood (nervousness, apprehension, depression, floating feelings, dreams), muscle rigidity, paresthesia, muscle tremor, blurred vision, nystagmus, diplopia and miosis, transient hallucinations and disorientation, visual disturbances, insomnia and increased intracranial pressure may occur.

Cardiovascular: Chills, tachycardia, bradycardia, palpitation, faintness, syncope, hypotension and hypertension have been reported.

Respiratory: Bronchospasm and laryngospasm have been known to occur.

Gastrointestinal: Constipation, biliary tract spasm, ileus, anorexia, diarrhea, cramps and taste alteration have been reported.

Genitourinary: Urinary retention or hesitancy, and antidiuretic effects have been reported.

Dermatologic: Urticaria, other skin rashes, and diaphoresis.

DRUG ABUSE AND DEPENDENCE

DILAUDID is a Schedule II narcotic, similar to morphine. Opioid analgesics may cause psychological and physical dependence (see **WARNINGS**). Physical dependence results in withdrawal symptoms in patients who abruptly discontinue the drug. Withdrawal symptoms also may be precipitated in the patient with physical dependence by the administration of a drug with opioid antagonist activity, e.g., naloxone (see **OVERDOSAGE**).

Physical dependence usually does not occur to a clinically significant degree until after several weeks of continued opioid usage, but it may become clinically detectable after as little as a week. Tolerance, in which increasingly larger doses are required in order to produce the same degree of analgesia, is initially manifested by a shortened duration of analgesic effect, and subsequently, by decreases in the intensity of analgesia. In chronic pain patients, and in opioid-tolerant cancer patients, the dose of DILAUDID ORAL LIQUID and DILAUDID 8 mg TABLETS should be guided by the degree of tolerance manifested.

In chronic pain patients in whom opioid analgesics including DILAUDID ORAL LIQUID and DILAUDID 8 mg TABLETS are abruptly discontinued, a severe abstinence syndrome should be anticipated. This may be similar to the abstinence syndrome noted in patients who withdraw from heroin. The latter abstinence syndrome may be characterized by restlessness, lacrimation, rhinorrhea, yawning, perspiration, gooseflesh, restless sleep or "yen" and mydriasis during the first 24 hours. These symptoms may increase in severity and over the next 72 hours may be accompanied by increasing irritability, anxiety, weakness, twitching and spasms of muscles, kicking movements, severe backache, abdominal and leg pains, abdominal and muscle cramps, hot and cold flashes, insomnia, nausea, anorexia, vomiting, intestinal spasm, diarrhea, coryza and repetitive sneezing, increase in body temperature, blood pressure, respiratory rate and heart rate.

Because of excessive loss of fluids through sweating, or vomiting and diarrhea, patients experiencing the syndrome usually exhibit marked weight loss, dehydration, ketosis, and disturbances in acid-base balance. Cardiovascular collapse can occur. Without treatment, most observable symptoms disappear in 5–14 days; however, there appears to be a phase of secondary or chronic abstinence which may last for 2–6 months characterized by insomnia, irritability, muscular aches, and autonomic instability.

In the treatment of physical dependence on DILAUDID ORAL LIQUID and DILAUDID 8 mg TABLETS, the patient may be detoxified by gradual reduction of the dosage, although this is unlikely to be necessary in the terminal cancer patient. If abstinence symptoms become severe, the patient may be detoxified with methadone. Temporary administration of tranquilizers and sedatives may aid in reducing patient anxiety. Gastrointestinal disturbances or dehydration should be treated accordingly.

OVERDOSAGE

Serious overdosage with DILAUDID ORAL LIQUID and DILAUDID 8 mg TABLETS is characterized by respiratory depression, somnolence progressing to stupor or coma, skeletal muscle flaccidity, cold and clammy skin, constricted pupils, and sometimes bradycardia and hypotension. In serious overdosage, particularly following intravenous injection, apnea, circulatory collapse, cardiac arrest and death may occur.

In the treatment of overdosage, primary attention should be given to the reestablishment of adequate respiratory exchange through provision of a patent airway and institution of assisted or controlled ventilation. A potentially serious oral ingestion, if recent, should be managed with gut decontamination. In unconscious patients with a secure airway, instill activated charcoal (30–100 g in adults, 1–2 g/kg in infants) via a nasogastric tube. A saline cathartic or sorbital may be added to the first dose of activated charcoal.

Opioid-Tolerant Patient: Since tolerance to the respiratory and CNS depressant effects of opioids develops concomitantly with tolerance to their analgesic effects, serious respiratory depression due to an acute overdose is unlikely to be seen in opioid-tolerant patients receiving the usual therapeutic dosage of DILAUDID ORAL LIQUID and DILAUDID 8 mg TABLETS for chronic pain.

NOTE: In such an individual who is physically dependent on opioids, administration of the usual dose of an opioid antagonist will precipitate an acute withdrawal syndrome. The severity will depend on the degree of physical dependence and the dose of the antagonist administered. Use of an opioid antagonist should be reserved for cases where such treatment is clearly needed. If necessary to treat serious respiratory depression in the physically-dependent patient, the opioid antagonist should be administered with extreme care and by titration, using fractional (one fifth to one tenth) doses of the antagonist.

Non-Tolerant Patient: The opioid antagonist, naloxone, is a specific antidote against respiratory depression which may result from overdosage, or unusual sensitivity to DILAUDID ORAL LIQUID and DILAUDID 8 mg TABLETS. A dose of naloxone (usually given as a test dose of 0.4 mg, followed by up to 2.0 mg if needed) should be administered intravenously, if possible, simultaneously with respiratory resuscitation. The dose can be repeated in 3 minutes. Naloxone should not be administered in the absence of clinically significant respiratory or circulatory depression. Naloxone should be administered cautiously to persons who are known, or suspected to be physically dependent on DILAUDID ORAL LIQUID and DILAUDID 8 mg TABLETS (see **Opioid-Tolerant Patient**). In such cases, an abrupt or complete reversal of narcotic effects may precipitate an acute abstinence syndrome. Since the duration of action of DILAUDID ORAL LIQUID and DILAUDID 8 mg TABLETS may exceed that of the antagonist, the patient should be kept under continued surveillance; repeated doses of the antagonist may be required to maintain adequate respiration. Apply other supportive measures when indicated.

Supportive measures (including oxygen, vasopressors) should be employed in the management of circulatory shock and pulmonary edema accompanying overdose as indicated. Cardiac arrest or arrhythmias may require cardiac massage or defibrillation.

DOSAGE AND ADMINISTRATION

DILAUDID ORAL LIQUID: The usual adult oral dosage of DILAUDID ORAL LIQUID is one-half (2.5 mL) in two teaspoonfuls (10 mL) (2.5 mg – 10 mg) every 3 to 6 hours as directed by the clinical situation. Oral dosages higher than the usual dosages may be required in some patients.

DILAUDID 8 mg TABLET: The usual starting dose for DILAUDID TABLETS is 2 mg to 4 mg, orally, every 4 to 6 hours. Appropriate use of the DILAUDID 8 mg TABLET must be decided by careful evaluation of each clinical situation.

A gradual increase in dose may be required if analgesia is inadequate, as tolerance develops, or if pain severity increases. The first sign of tolerance is usually a reduced duration of effect.

SAFETY AND HANDLING INSTRUCTIONS:

DILAUDID ORAL LIQUID and DILAUDID 8 mg TABLETS pose little risk of direct exposure to health care personnel and should be handled and disposed of prudently in accordance with hospital or institutional policy. Significant absorption from dermal exposure is unlikely; accidental dermal exposure to DILAUDID ORAL LIQUID should be treated by removal of any contaminated clothing and rinsing the affected area with cool water. Patients and their families should be instructed to flush any DILAUDID ORAL LIQUID and DILAUDID 8 mg TABLETS that are no longer needed.

Access to abusable drugs such as DILAUDID ORAL LIQUID and DILAUDID 8 mg TABLETS presents an occupational hazard for addiction in the health care industry. Routine procedures for handling controlled substances developed to protect the public may not be adequate to protect health care workers. Implementation of more effective accounting procedures and measures to restrict access to drugs of this class (appropriate to the practice setting) may minimize the risk of self-administration by health care providers.

HOW SUPPLIED

DILAUDID ORAL LIQUID is a clear, sweet, slightly viscous liquid. It is available in:

Bottles of 1 pint (473 mL) - NDC# 0074-2452-02

DILAUDID 8 mg TABLETS are white and triangular shaped, embossed with the number 8 on one side and bisected and embossed with a double ⊐ on the other side. They are available in:

Bottles of 100 - NDC# 0074-2426-14

STORAGE: Store at 25°C (77°F); excursions permitted to 15°–30°C (59°–86°F). [See USP Controlled Room Temperature]. Protect from light.

A schedule Ⓒ Narcotic. DEA Order Form Is Required.

Revised: February, 2003
Ref: 03-5259-R2
ABBOTT LABORATORIES
NORTH CHICAGO, IL 60064, U.S.A.

ERY-PED® ℞

[*erē ' ped*]

(ERYTHROMYCIN ETHYLSUCCINATE, USP)

℞ only

To reduce the development of drug-resistant bacteria and maintain the effectiveness of EryPed and other antibacterial drugs, EryPed should be used only to treat or prevent infections that are proven or strongly suspected to be caused by bacteria.

DESCRIPTION

Erythromycin is produced by a strain of *Saccharopolyspora erythraea* (formerly *Streptomyces erythraeus*) and belongs to the macrolide group of antibiotics. It is basic and readily forms salts with acids. The base, the stearate salt, and the esters are poorly soluble in water. Erythromycin ethylsuccinate is an ester of erythromycin suitable for oral administration. Erythromycin ethylsuccinate is known chemically as erythromycin 2′-(ethylsuccinate). The molecular formula is $C_{43}H_{75}NO_{16}$ and the molecular weight is 862.06. The structural formula is:

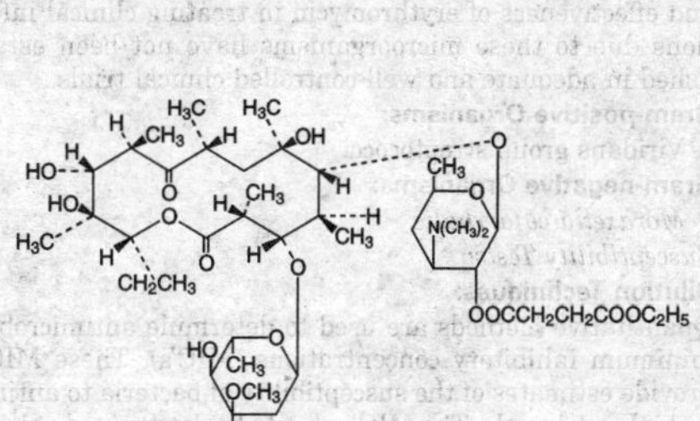

EryPed 200 and EryPed Drops (erythromycin ethylsuccinate for oral suspension) when reconstituted with water, forms a suspension containing erythromycin ethylsuccinate equivalent to 200 mg erythromycin per 5 mL (teaspoonful) or 100 mg per 2.5 mL (dropperful) with an appealing fruit flavor. EryPed 400 when reconstituted with water, forms a suspension containing erythromycin ethylsuccinate equivalent to 400 mg of erythromycin per 5 mL (teaspoonful) with an appealing banana flavor.

Fruit-flavored EryPed Chewable tablets are easily ingested and are particularly acceptable for the administration of antibiotic medication to young children who are unable to swallow regular tablets or in whom persuasion of a pleasant taste insures cooperation.

Each chewable tablet contains erythromycin ethylsuccinate equivalent to 200 mg of erythromycin and is scored for division into half-dose (100 mg) portions.

These products are intended primarily for pediatric use but can also be used in adults.

Inactive Ingredients:

EryPed 200, EryPed 400 and EryPed Drops: Caramel, polysorbate, sodium citrate, sucrose, xanthan gum and artificial flavors.

EryPed Chewable Tablets: Citric acid, confectioner's sugar (contains corn starch), magnesium aluminum silicate, magnesium stearate, sodium carboxymethylcellulose, sodium citrate and artificial flavor.

Continued on next page

Ery-Ped—Cont.

CLINICAL PHARMACOLOGY

Orally administered erythromycin ethylsuccinate suspension is readily and reliably absorbed under both fasting and nonfasting conditions.
Erythromycin diffuses readily into most body fluids. Only low concentrations are normally achieved in the spinal fluid, but passage of the drug across the blood-brain barrier increases in meningitis. In the presence of normal hepatic function, erythromycin is concentrated in the liver and excreted in the bile; the effect of hepatic dysfunction on excretion of erythromycin by the liver into the bile is not known. Less than 5 percent of the orally administered dose of erythromycin is excreted in active form in the urine.
Erythromycin crosses the placental barrier, but fetal plasma levels are low. The drug is excreted in human milk.
Microbiology:
Erythromycin acts by inhibition of protein synthesis by binding 50 *S* ribosomal subunits of susceptible organisms. It does not affect nucleic acid synthesis. Antagonism has been demonstrated *in vitro* between erythromycin and clindamycin, lincomycin, and chloramphenicol.
Many strains of *Haemophilus influenzae* are resistant to erythromycin alone but are susceptible to erythromycin and sulfonamides used concomitantly.
Staphylococci resistant to erythromycin may emerge during a course of therapy.
Erythromycin has been shown to be active against most strains of the following microorganisms, both *in vitro* and in clinical infections as described in the **INDICATIONS AND USAGE** section.

Gram-positive Organisms:
Corynebacterium diphtheriae
Corynebacterium minutissimum
Listeria monocytogenes
Staphylococcus aureus (resistant organisms may emerge during treatment)
Streptococcus pneumoniae
Streptococcus pyogenes

Gram-negative Organisms:
Bordetella pertussis
Legionella pneumophila
Neisseria gonorrhoeae

Other Microorganisms:
Chlamydia trachomatis
Entamoeba histolytica
Mycoplasma pneumoniae
Treponema pallidum
Ureaplasma urealyticum

The following *in vitro* data are available, **but their clinical significance is unknown.**
Erythromycin exhibits *in vitro* minimal inhibitory concentrations (MIC's) of 0.5 µg/mL or less against most (≥ 90%) strains of the following microorganisms; however, the safety and effectiveness of erythromycin in treating clinical infections due to these microorganisms have not been established in adequate and well-controlled clinical trials.

Gram-positive Organisms:
Viridans group streptococci

Gram-negative Organisms:
Moraxella catarrhalis

Susceptibility Tests:

Dilution Techniques:
Quantitative methods are used to determine antimicrobial minimum inhibitory concentrations (MIC's). These MIC's provide estimates of the susceptibility of bacteria to antimicrobial compounds. The MIC's should be determined using a standardized procedure. Standardized procedures are based on a dilution method[1] (broth or agar) or equivalent with standardized inoculum concentrations and standardized concentrations of erythromycin powder. The MIC values should be interpreted according to the following criteria:

MIC (µg/mL)	Interpretation
≤0.5	Susceptible (S)
1-4	Intermediate (I)
≥8	Resistant (R)

A report of "Susceptible" indicates that the pathogen is likely to be inhibited if the antimicrobial compound in the blood reaches the concentrations usually achievable. A report of "Intermediate" indicates that the result should be considered equivocal, and, if the microorganism is not fully susceptible to alternative, clinically feasible drugs, the test should be repeated. This category implies possible clinical applicability in body sites where the drug is physiologically concentrated or in situations where high dosage of drug can be used. This category also provides a buffer zone which prevents small uncontrolled technical factors from causing major discrepancies in interpretation. A report of "Resistant" indicates that the pathogen is not likely to be inhibited if the antimicrobial compound in the blood reaches the concentrations usually achievable; other therapy should be selected.
Standardized susceptibility test procedures require the use of laboratory control microorganisms to control the technical aspects of the laboratory procedures. Standard erythromycin powder should provide the following MIC values:

Microorganism	MIC (µg/mL)
S. aureus ATCC 29213	0.12-0.5
E. faecalis ATCC 22912	1-4

Diffusion Techniques:
Quantitative methods that require measurement of zone diameters also provide reproducible estimates of the susceptibility of bacteria to antimicrobial compounds. One such standardized procedure[2] requires the use of standardized inoculum concentrations. This procedure uses paper disks impregnated with 15-µg erythromycin to test the susceptibility of microorganisms to erythromycin.
Reports from the laboratory providing results of the standard single-disk susceptibility test with a 15-µg erythromycin disk should be interpreted according to the following criteria:

Zone Diameter (mm)	Interpretation
≥23	Susceptible (S)
14-22	Intermediate (I)
≤13	Resistant (R)

Interpretation should be as stated above for results using dilution techniques. Interpretation involves correlation of the diameter obtained in the disk test with the MIC for erythromycin.
As with standardized dilution techniques, diffusion methods require the use of laboratory control microorganisms that are used to control the technical aspects of the laboratory procedures. For the diffusion technique, the 15-µg erythromycin disk should provide the following zone diameters in these laboratory test quality control strains:

Microorganism	Zone Diameter (mm)
S. aureus ATCC 25923	22-30

INDICATIONS AND USAGE

To reduce the development drug-resistant bacteria and maintain the effectiveness of Ery-Ped and other antibacterial drugs, Ery-Ped should be used only to treat or prevent infections that are proven or strongly suspected to be caused by susceptible bacteria. When culture and susceptibility information are available, they should be considered in selecting or modifying antibacterial therapy. In the absence of such data, local epidemiology and susceptibility patterns may contribute to the empiric selection of therapy.
Ery-Ped is indicated in the treatment of infections caused by susceptible strains of the designated organisms in the diseases listed below:
Upper respiratory tract infections of mild to moderate degree caused by *Streptococcus pyogenes, Streptococcus pneumoniae,* or *Haemophilus influenzae* (when used concomitantly with adequate doses of sulfonamides, since many strains of *H. influenzae* are not susceptible to the erythromycin concentrations ordinarily achieved). (See appropriate sulfonamide labeling for prescribing information.)
Lower-respiratory tract infections of mild to moderate severity caused by *Streptococcus pneumoniae* or *Streptococcus pyogenes.*
Listeriosis caused by *Listeria monocytogenes.*
Pertussis (whooping cough) caused by *Bordetella pertussis.* Erythromycin is effective in eliminating the organism from the nasopharynx of infected individuals rendering them noninfectious. Some clinical studies suggest that erythromycin may be helpful in the prophylaxis of pertussis in exposed susceptible individuals.
Respiratory tract infections due to *Mycoplasma pneumoniae.*
Skin and skin structure infections of mild to moderate severity caused by *Streptococcus pyogenes* or *Staphylococcus aureus* (resistant staphylococci may emerge during treatment).
Diphtheria: Infections due to *Corynebacterium diphtheriae,* as an adjunct to antitoxin, to prevent establishment of carriers and to eradicate the organism in carriers.
Erythrasma: In the treatment of infections due to *Corynebacterium minutissimum.*
Intestinal amebiasis caused by *Entamoeba histolytica* (oral erythromycins only). Extraenteric amebiasis requires treatment with other agents.
Acute pelvic inflammatory disease caused by *Neisseria gonorrhoeae:* As an alternative drug in treatment of acute pelvic inflammatory disease caused by *N. gonorrhoeae* in female patients with a history of sensitivity to penicillin. Patients should have a serologic test for syphilis before receiving erythromycin as treatment of gonorrhea and a follow-up serologic test for syphilis after 3 months.
Syphilis caused by *Treponema pallidum:* Erythromycin is an alternate choice of treatment for primary syphilis in penicillin-allergic patients. In primary syphilis, spinal fluid examinations should be done before treatment and as part of follow-up after therapy.
Erythromycins are indicated for the treatment of the following infections caused by *Chlamydia trachomatis:* conjunctivitis of the newborn, pneumonia of infancy, and urogenital infections during pregnancy. When tetracyclines are contraindicated or not tolerated, erythromycin is indicated for the treatment of uncomplicated urethral, endocervical, or rectal infections in adults due to *Chlamydia trachomatis.*
When tetracyclines are contraindicated or not tolerated, erythromycin is indicated for the treatment of nongonococcal urethritis caused by *Ureaplasma urealyticum.*
Legionnaires' Disease caused by *Legionella pneumophila.* Although no controlled clinical efficacy studies have been conducted, *in vitro* and limited preliminary clinical data suggest that erythromycin may be effective in treating Legionnaires' Disease.

Prophylaxis:
Prevention of Initial Attacks of Rheumatic Fever: Penicillin is considered by the American Heart Association to be the drug of choice in the prevention of initial attacks of rheumatic fever (treatment of *Streptococcus pyogenes* infections of the upper respiratory tract, e.g., tonsillitis or pharyngitis). Erythromycin is indicated for the treatment of penicillin-allergic patients.[3] The therapeutic dose should be administered for 10 days.
Prevention of Recurrent Attacks of Rheumatic Fever: Penicillin or sulfonamides are considered by the American Heart Association to be the drugs of choice in the prevention of recurrent attacks of rheumatic fever. In patients who are allergic to penicillin and sulfonamides, oral erythromycin is recommended by the American Heart Association in the long-term prophylaxis of streptococcal pharyngitis (for the prevention of recurrent attacks of rheumatic fever).[3]

CONTRAINDICATIONS

Erythromycin is contraindicated in patients with known hypersensitivity to this antibiotic.
Erythromycin is contraindicated in patients taking terfenadine, astemizole, pimozide, or cisapride. (See **PRECAUTIONS** - *Drug Interactions.)*

WARNINGS

There have been reports of hepatic dysfunction, including increased liver enzymes, and hepatocellular and/or cholestatic hepatitis, with or without jaundice, occurring in patients receiving oral erythromycin products.
There have been reports suggesting that erythromycin does not reach the fetus in adequate concentration to prevent congenital syphilis. Infants born to women treated during pregnancy with oral erythromycin for early syphilis should be treated with an appropriate penicillin regimen.
Pseudomembranous colitis has been reported with nearly all antibacterial agents, including erythromycin, and may range in severity from mild to life threatening. Therefore, it is important to consider this diagnosis in patients who present with diarrhea subsequent to the administration of antibacterial agents.
Treatment with antibacterial agents alters the normal flora of the colon and may permit overgrowth of clostridia. Studies indicate that a toxin produced by *Clostridium difficile* is a primary cause of "antibiotic-associated colitis".
After the diagnosis of pseudomembranous colitis has been established, therapeutic measures should be initiated. Mild cases of pseudomembranous colitis usually respond to discontinuation of the drug alone. In moderate to severe cases, consideration should be given to management with fluids and electrolytes, protein supplementation, and treatment with an antibacterial drug clinically effective against *Clostridium difficile* colitis.
Rhabdomyolysis with or without renal impairment has been reported in seriously ill patients receiving erythromycin concomitantly with lovastatin. Therefore, patients receiving concomitant lovastatin and erythromycin should be carefully monitored for creatine kinase (CK) and serum transaminase levels. (See package insert for lovastatin.)

PRECAUTIONS

General: Prescribing Ery-Ped in the absence of a proven or strongly suspected bacterial infection or a prophylactic indication is unlikely to provide benefit to the patient and increases the risk of the development of drug-resistant bacteria.
Since erythromycin is principally excreted by the liver, caution should be exercised when erythromycin is administered to patients with impaired hepatic function. (See **CLINICAL PHARMACOLOGY** and **WARNINGS** sections.)
There have been reports that erythromycin may aggravate the weakness of patients with myasthenia gravis.
There have been reports of infantile hypertrophic pyloric stenosis (IHPS) occurring in infants following erythromycin therapy. In one cohort of 157 newborns who were given erythromycin for pertussis prophylaxis, seven neonates (5%) developed symptoms of non-bilious vomiting or irritability with feeding and were subsequently diagnosed as having IHPS requiring surgical pyloromyotomy. A possible dose-response effect was described with an absolute risk of IHPS of 5.1% for infants who took erythromycin for 8-14 days and 10% for infants who took erythromycin for 15-21 days.[4] Since erythromycin may be used in the treatment of conditions in infants which are associated with significant mortality or morbidity (such as pertussis or neonatal Chlamydia trachomatis infections), the benefit of erythromycin therapy needs to be weighed against the potential risk of developing IHPS. Parents should be informed to contact their physician if vomiting or irritability with feeding occurs.
Prolonged or repeated use of erythromycin may result in an overgrowth of nonsusceptible bacteria or fungi. If superinfection occurs, erythromycin should be discontinued and appropriate therapy instituted.

When indicated, incision and drainage or other surgical procedures should be performed in conjunction with antibiotic therapy.

Information for Patients: Patients should be counseled that antibacterial drugs including Ery-Ped should only be used to treat bacterial infections. They do not treat viral infections (e.g., the common cold). When Ery-Ped is prescribed to treat a bacterial infection, patients should be told that although it is common to feel better early in the course of therapy, the medication should be taken exactly as directed. Skipping doses or not completing the full course of therapy may (1) decrease the effectiveness of the immediate treatment and (2) increase the likelihood that bacteria will develop resistance and will not be treatable by Ery-Ped or other antibacterial drugs in the future.

Drug Interactions: Erythromycin use in patients who are receiving high doses of theophylline may be associated with an increase in serum theophylline levels and potential theophylline toxicity. In case of theophylline toxicity and/or elevated serum theophylline levels, the dose of theophylline should be reduced while the patient is receiving concomitant erythromycin therapy.

Concomitant administration of erythromycin and digoxin has been reported to result in elevated digoxin serum levels. There have been reports of increased anticoagulant effects when erythromycin and oral anticoagulants were used concomitantly. Increased anticoagulation effects due to interactions of erythromycin with various oral anticoagulants may be more pronounced in the elderly.

Erythromycin is a substrate and inhibitor of the 3A isoform subfamily of the cytochrome p450 enzyme system (CYP3A). Coadministration of erythromycin and a drug primarily metabolized by CYP3A may be associated with elevations in drug concentrations that could increase or prolong both the therapeutic and adverse effects of the concomitant drug. Dosage adjustments may be considered, and when possible, serum concentrations of drugs primarily metabolized by CYP3A should be monitored closely in patients concurrently receiving erythromycin.

The following are examples of some clinically significant CYP3A based drug interactions. Interactions with other drugs metabolized by the CYP3A isoform are also possible. The following CYP3A based drug interactions have been observed with erythromycin products in post-marketing experience:

Ergotamine/dihydroergotamine: Concurrent use of erythromycin and ergotamine or dihydroergotamine has been associated in some patients with acute ergot toxicity characterized by severe peripheral vasospasm and dysesthesia.

Triazolobenzodiazepines (such as triazolam and alprazolam) *and related benzodiazepines:* Erythromycin has been reported to decrease the clearance of triazolam and midazolam, and thus, may increase the pharmacologic effect of these benzodiazepines.

HMG-CoA Reductase Inhibitors: Erythromycin has been reported to increase concentrations of HMG-CoA reductase inhibitors (e.g., lovastatin and simvastatin). Rare reports of rhabdomyolysis have been reported in patients taking these drugs concomitantly.

Sildenafil (Viagra): Erythromycin has been reported to increase the systemic exposure (AUC) of sildenafil. Reduction of sildenafil dosage should be considered. (See Viagra package insert.)

There have been spontaneous or published reports of CYP3A based interactions of erythromycin with cyclosporine, carbamazepine, tacrolimus, alfentanil, disopyramide, rifabutin, quinidine, methylprednisolone, cilostazol, vinblastine, and bromocriptine.

Concomitant administration of erythromycin with cisapride, pimozide, astemizole, or terfenadine is contraindicated. (See **CONTRAINDICATIONS.**)

In addition, there have been reports of interactions of erythromycin with drugs not thought to be metabolized by CYP3A, including hexobarbital, phenytoin, and valproate.

Erythromycin has been reported to significantly alter the metabolism of the nonsedating antihistamines terfenadine and astemizole when taken concomitantly. Rare cases of serious cardiovascular adverse events, including electrocardiographic QT/QT_c interval prolongation, cardiac arrest, torsades de pointes, and other ventricular arrhythmias have been observed. (See **CONTRAINDICATIONS.**) In addition, deaths have been reported rarely with concomitant administration of terfenadine and erythromycin.

There have been post-marketing reports of drug interactions when erythromycin was coadministered with cisapride, resulting in QT prolongation, cardiac arrhythmias, ventricular tachycardia, ventricular fibrillation, and torsades de pointes most likely due to the inhibition of hepatic metabolism of cisapride by erythromycin. Fatalities have been reported. (See **CONTRAINDICATIONS.**)

Drug/Laboratory Test Interactions: Erythromycin interferes with the fluorometric determination of urinary catecholamines.

Carcinogenesis, Mutagenesis, Impairment of Fertility: Long-term (2-year) oral studies in rats with erythromycin ethylsuccinate and erythromycin base did not provide evidence of tumorigenicity. Mutagenicity studies have not been conducted. There was no apparent effect on male or female fertility in rats fed erythromycin (base) at levels up to 0.25% of diet.

Pregnancy: Teratogenic Effects. Pregnancy Category B: There is no evidence of teratogenicity or any other adverse effect on reproduction in female rats fed erythromycin base (up to 0.25% of diet) prior to and during mating, during gestation, and through weaning of two successive litters. There are, however, no adequate and well-controlled studies in pregnant women. Because animal reproduction studies are not always predictive of human response, this drug should be used during pregnancy only if clearly needed.

Labor and Delivery: The effect of erythromycin on labor and delivery is unknown.

Nursing Mothers: Erythromycin is excreted in human milk. Caution should be exercised when erythromycin is administered to a nursing woman.

Pediatric Use: See **INDICATIONS AND USAGE** and **DOSAGE AND ADMINISTRATION** sections.

ADVERSE REACTIONS

The most frequent side effects of oral erythromycin preparations are gastrointestinal and are dose-related. They include nausea, vomiting, abdominal pain, diarrhea and anorexia. Symptoms of hepatitis, hepatic dysfunction and/or abnormal liver function test results may occur. (See **WARNINGS** section.)

Onset of pseudomembranous colitis symptoms may occur during or after antibacterial treatment. (See **WARNINGS.**)

Erythromycin has been associated with QT prolongation and ventricular arrhythmias, including ventricular tachycardia and torsades de pointes.

Allergic reactions ranging from urticaria to anaphylaxis have occurred. Skin reactions ranging from mild eruptions to erythema multiforme, Stevens-Johnson syndrome, and toxic epidermal necrolysis have been reported rarely.

There have been rare reports pancreatitis and convulsions.

There have been isolated reports of reversible hearing loss occurring chiefly in patients with renal insufficiency and in patients receiving high doses of erythromycin.

OVERDOSAGE

In case of overdosage, erythromycin should be discontinued. Overdosage should be handled with the prompt elimination of unabsorbed drug and all other appropriate measures should be instituted.

Erythromycin is not removed by peritoneal dialysis or hemodialysis.

DOSAGE AND ADMINISTRATION

EryPed (erythromycin ethylsuccinate) oral suspensions and chewable tablets may be administered without regard to meals.

Children: Age, weight, and severity of the infection are important factors in determining the proper dosage. In mild to moderate infections, the usual dosage of erythromycin ethylsuccinate for children is 30 to 50 mg/kg/day in equally divided doses every 6 hours. For more severe infections this dosage may be doubled. If twice-a-day dosage is desired, one-half of the total daily dose may be given every 12 hours. Doses may also be given three times daily by administering one-third of the total daily dose every 8 hours.

The following dosage schedule is suggested for mild to moderate infections:

Body Weight	Total Daily Dose
Under 10 lbs	30-50 mg/kg/day 15-25 mg/lb/day
10 to 15 lbs	200 mg
16 to 25 lbs	400 mg
26 to 50 lbs	800 mg
51 to 100 lbs	1200 mg
over 100 lbs	1600 mg

Adults: 400 mg erythromycin ethylsuccinate every 6 hours is the usual dose. Dosage may be increased up to 4 g per day according to the severity of the infection. If twice-a-day dosage is desired, one-half of the total daily dose may be given every 12 hours. Doses may also be given three times daily by administering one-third of the total daily dose every 8 hours.

For adult dosage calculation, use a ratio of 400 mg of erythromycin activity as the ethylsuccinate to 250 mg of erythromycin activity as the stearate, base or estolate.

In the treatment of streptococcal infections, a therapeutic dosage of erythromycin ethylsuccinate should be administered for at least 10 days. In continuous prophylaxis against recurrences of streptococcal infections in persons with a history of rheumatic heart disease, the usual dosage is 400 mg twice a day.

For treatment of urethritis due to *C. trachomatis* or *U. urealyticum:* 800 mg three times a day for 7 days.

For treatment of primary syphilis: Adults: 48 to 64 g given in divided doses over a period of 10 to 15 days.

For intestinal amebiasis: Adults: 400 mg four times daily for 10 to 14 days. Children: 30 to 50 mg/kg/day in divided doses for 10 to 14 days.

For use in pertussis: Although optimal dosage and duration have not been established, doses of erythromycin utilized in reported clinical studies were 40 to 50 mg/kg/day, given in divided doses for 5 to 14 days.

For treatment of Legionnaires' Disease: Although optimal doses have not been established, doses utilized in reported clinical data were 1.6 to 4 g daily in divided doses.

For the EryPed 200 unit dose, reconstitute with 2.9 mL of water. For the EryPed 400 unit dose, reconstitute with 2.7 mL of water.

HOW SUPPLIED

EryPed 200 (erythromycin ethylsuccinate for oral suspension, USP) is supplied in bottles of 100 mL (**NDC** 0074-6302-13), 200 mL (**NDC** 0074-6302-53), and 5 mL unit dose ABBO-PAC® packages of 100 bottles (**NDC** 0074-6302-05).

EryPed 400 (erythromycin ethylsuccinate for oral suspension, USP) is supplied in bottles of 60 mL (**NDC** 0074-6305-60), 100 mL (**NDC** 0074-6305-13), 200 mL (**NDC** 0074-6305-53), and 5 mL unit dose ABBO-PAC packages of 100 bottles (**NDC** 0074-6305-05).

EryPed Drops (erythromycin ethylsuccinate for oral suspension) is supplied in 50 mL bottles (**NDC** 0074-6303-50).

EryPed Chewable (erythromycin ethylsuccinate tablets, USP) are fruit-flavored wafers containing activity equivalent to 200 mg of erythromycin and are available in packages of 40 (**NDC** 0074-6314-40). Each wafer is individually sealed in a blister package.

Recommended storage: Store EryPed Chewable below 86°F (30°C). Store EryPed 200, EryPed 400, and EryPed Drops, prior to mixing, below 86°F (30°C). After reconstitution, EryPed 200, EryPed 400, and EryPed Drops must be stored at or below 77°F (25°C) and used within 35 days; refrigeration is not required.

REFERENCES

1. National Committee for Clinical Laboratory Standards, *Method for Dilution Antimicrobial Susceptibility Tests for Bacteria that Grow Aerobically,* Third Edition. Approved Standard NCCLS Document M7-A3, Vol. 13, No. 25. NCCLS, Villanova, PA, December 1993.
2. National Committee for Clinical Laboratory Standards, *Performance Standards for Antimicrobial Disk Susceptibility Tests,* Fifth Edition. Approved Standard NCCLS Document M2-A5, Vol. 13, No. 24. NCCLS, Villanova, PA, December 1993.
3. Committee on Rheumatic Fever, Endocarditis, and Kawasaki Disease of the Council on Cardiovascular Disease in the Young, the American Heart Association: Prevention of Rheumatic Fever. *Circulation.* 78(4):1082-1086, October 1988.
4. Honein, M.A., et. al.: Infantile hypertrophic pyloric stenosis after pertussis prophylaxis with erythromycin: a case review and cohort study. The Lancet 1999; 354 (9196): 2101-5.

Revised: November, 2003
ABBOTT LABORATORIES
NORTH CHICAGO, IL 60064, U.S.A.
PRINTED IN U.S.A.

ERY-TAB® ℞

[*ē rē 'tab*]

(ERYTHROMYCIN DELAYED-RELEASE TABLETS, USP) ENTERIC-COATED

℞ only

03-5244-R5-Rev., August, 2003 (Nos. 6304, 6320, 6321)

To reduce the development of drug-resistant bacteria and maintain the effectiveness of ERY-TAB and other antibacterial drugs, ERY-TAB should be used only to treat or prevent infections that are proven or strongly suspected to be caused by bacteria.

DESCRIPTION

ERY-TAB (erythromycin delayed-release tablets) is an antibacterial product containing erythromycin base in a specially enteric-coated tablet to protect it from the inactivating effects of gastric acidity and to permit efficient absorption of the antibiotic in the small intestine. ERY-TAB tablets for oral administration are available in three dosage strengths, each white oval tablet containing either 250 mg, 333 mg, or 500 mg of erythromycin as the free base. ERY-TAB tablets comply with *USP Drug Release Test 1.*

Erythromycin is produced by a strain of *Saccharopolyspora erythraea* (formerly *Streptomyces erythraeus*) and belongs to the macrolide group of antibiotics. It is basic and readily forms salts with acids. Erythromycin is a white to off-white powder, slightly soluble in water, and soluble in alcohol, chloroform, and ether. Erythromycin is known chemically as (3R*, 4S*, 5S*, 6R*, 7R*, 9R*, 11R*, 12R*, 13S*, 14R*)-4-[(2,6-dideoxy-3-C-methyl-3-O-methyl-α-L-*ribo*-hexopyranosyl)oxy]-14-ethyl-7,12,13-trihydroxy-3,5,7,9,11,13-hexamethyl-6-[[3,4,6-trideoxy-3-(dimethylamino)-β-D-*xylo*-hexopyranosyl]oxy]oxacyclotetradecane-2,10-dione. The molecular formula is $C_{37}H_{67}NO_{13}$, and the molecular weight is 733.94. The structural formula is:

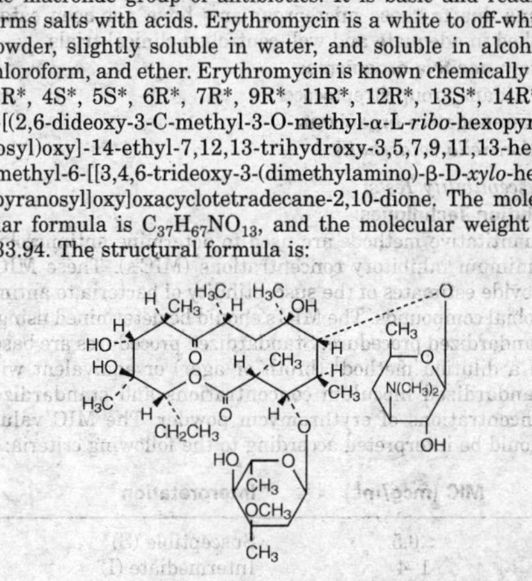

Continued on next page

Ery-Tab—Cont.

Inactive Ingredients
Ammonium hydroxide, colloidal silicon dioxide, croscarmellose sodium, crospovidone, diacetylated monoglycerides, hydroxypropyl cellulose, hypromellose, hypromellose phthalate, magnesium stearate, microcrystalline cellulose, povidone, propylene glycol, sodium citrate, sorbitan monooleate, talc, and titanium dioxide.

CLINICAL PHARMACOLOGY
Orally administered erythromycin base and its salts are readily absorbed in the microbiologically active form. Interindividual variations in the absorption of erythromycin are, however, observed, and some patients do not achieve optimal serum levels. Erythromycin is largely bound to plasma proteins. After absorption, erythromycin diffuses readily into most body fluids. In the absence of meningeal inflammation, low concentrations are normally achieved in the spinal fluid but the passage of the drug across the blood-brain barrier increases in meningitis. Erythromycin crosses the placental barrier, but fetal plasma levels are low. The drug is excreted in human milk. Erythromycin is not removed by peritoneal dialysis or hemodialysis.
In the presence of normal hepatic function, erythromycin is concentrated in the liver and is excreted in the bile; the effect of hepatic dysfunction on biliary excretion of erythromycin is not known. After oral administration, less than 5% of the administered dose can be recovered in the active form in the urine.
ERY-TAB tablets are coated with a polymer whose dissolution is pH dependent. This coating allows for minimal release of erythromycin in acidic environments, e.g. stomach. The tablets are designed for optimal drug release and absorption in the small intestine. In multiple-dose, steady-state studies, ERY-TAB tablets have demonstrated adequate drug delivery in both fasting and non-fasting conditions. Bioavailability data are available from Abbott Laboratories, Dept. 422.
Microbiology:
Erythromycin acts by inhibition of protein synthesis by binding 50 S ribosomal subunits of susceptible organisms. It does not affect nucleic acid synthesis. Antagonism has been demonstrated *in vitro* between erythromycin and clindamycin, lincomycin, and chloramphenicol.
Many strains of *Haemophilus influenzae* are resistant to erythromycin alone, but are susceptible to erythromycin and sulfonamides used concomitantly.
Staphylococci resistant to erythromycin may emerge during a course of erythromycin therapy.
Erythromycin has been shown to be active against most strains of the following microorganisms, both *in vitro* and in clinical infections as described in the **INDICATIONS AND USAGE** section.
Gram-positive organisms:
Corynebacterium diphtheriae
Corynebacterium minutissimum
Listeria monocytogenes
Staphylococcus aureus (resistant organisms may emerge during treatment)
Streptococcus pneumoniae
Streptococcus pyogenes
Gram-negative organisms:
Bordetella pertussis
Legionella pneumophila
Neisseria gonorrhoeae
Other microorganisms:
Chlamydia trachomatis
Entamoeba histolytica
Mycoplasma pneumoniae
Treponema pallidum
Ureaplasma urealyticum
The following *in vitro* data are available, **but their clinical significance is unknown.**
Erythromycin exhibits *in vitro* minimal inhibitory concentrations (MIC's) of 0.5 mcg/mL or less against most (≥ 90%) strains of the following microorganisms; however, the safety and effectiveness of erythromycin in treating clinical infections due to these microorganisms have not been established in adequate and well-controlled clinical trials.
Gram-positive organisms:
Viridans group streptococci
Gram-negative organisms:
Moraxella catarrhalis

Susceptibility Tests:
Dilution Techniques:
Quantitative methods are used to determine antimicrobial minimum inhibitory concentrations (MIC's). These MIC's provide estimates of the susceptibility of bacteria to antimicrobial compounds. The MIC's should be determined using a standardized procedure. Standardized procedures are based on a dilution method[1] (broth or agar) or equivalent with standardized inoculum concentrations and standardized concentrations of erythromycin powder. The MIC values should be interpreted according to the following criteria:

MIC (mcg/mL)	Interpretation
≤0.5	Susceptible (S)
1–4	Intermediate (I)
≥8	Resistant (R)

A report of "Susceptible" indicates that the pathogen is likely to be inhibited if the antimicrobial compound in the blood reaches the concentrations usually achievable. A report of "Intermediate" indicates that the result should be considered equivocal, and, if the microorganism is not fully susceptible to alternative, clinically feasible drugs, the test should be repeated. This category implies possible clinical applicability in body sites where the drug is physiologically concentrated or in situations where high dosage of drug can be used. This category also provides a buffer zone which prevents small uncontrolled technical factors from causing major discrepancies in interpretation. A report of "Resistant" indicates that the pathogen is not likely to be inhibited if the antimicrobial compound in the blood reaches the concentrations usually achievable; other therapy should be selected.
Standardized susceptibility test procedures require the use of laboratory control microorganisms to control the technical aspects of the laboratory procedures. Standard erythromycin powder should provide the following MIC values:

Microorganism	MIC (mcg/mL)
S. aureus ATCC 29213	0.12-0.5
E. faecalis ATCC 29212	1-4

Diffusion Techniques:
Quantitative methods that require measurement of zone diameters also provide reproducible estimates of the susceptibility of bacteria to antimicrobial compounds. One such standardized procedure[2] requires the use of standardized inoculum concentrations. This procedure uses paper disks impregnated with 15-mcg erythromycin to test the susceptibility of microorganisms to erythromycin.
Reports from the laboratory providing results of the standard single-disk susceptibility test with a 15-mcg erythromycin disk should be interpreted according to the following criteria:

Zone Diameter (mm)	Interpretation
≥23	Susceptible (S)
14–22	Intermediate (I)
≤13	Resistant (R)

Interpretation should be as stated above for results using dilution techniques. Interpretation involves correlation of the diameter obtained in the disk test with the MIC for erythromycin.
As with standardized dilution techniques, diffusion methods require the use of laboratory control microorganisms that are used to control the technical aspects of the laboratory procedures. For the diffusion technique, the 15-mcg erythromycin disk should provide the following zone diameters in these laboratory test quality control strains:

Microorganism	Zone Diameter (mm)
S. aureus ATCC 25923	22-30

INDICATIONS AND USAGE
To reduce the development of drug-resistant bacteria and maintain the effectiveness of ERY-TAB and other antibacterial drugs, ERY-TAB should be used only to treat or prevent infections that are proven or strongly suspected to be caused by susceptible bacteria. When culture and susceptibility information are available, they should be considered in selecting or modifying antibacterial therapy. In the absence of such data, local epidemiology and susceptibility patterns may contribute to the empiric selection of therapy.
ERY-TAB tablets are indicated in the treatment of infections caused by susceptible strains of the designated microorganisms in the diseases listed below:
Upper respiratory tract infections of mild to moderate degree caused by *Streptococcus pyogenes; Streptococcus pneumoniae; Haemophilus influenzae* (when used concomitantly with adequate doses of sulfonamides, since many strains of *H. influenzae* are not susceptible to the erythromycin concentrations ordinarily achieved). (See appropriate sulfonamide labeling for prescribing information.)
Lower respiratory tract infections of mild to moderate severity caused by *Streptococcus pyogenes* or *Streptococcus pneumoniae*.
Listeriosis caused by *Listeria monocytogenes*.
Respiratory tract infections due to *Mycoplasma pneumoniae*.
Skin and skin structure infections of mild to moderate severity caused by *Streptococcus pyogenes* or *Staphylococcus aureus* (resistant staphylococci may emerge during treatment).
Pertussis (whooping cough) caused by *Bordetella pertussis*. Erythromycin is effective in eliminating the organism from the nasopharynx of infected individuals, rendering them noninfectious. Some clinical studies suggest that erythromycin may be helpful in the prophylaxis of pertussis in exposed susceptible individuals.
Diphtheria: Infections due to *Corynebacterium diphtheriae*, as an adjunct to antitoxin, to prevent establishment of carriers and to eradicate the organism in carriers.
Erythrasma—In the treatment of infections due to *Corynebacterium minutissimum*.
Intestinal amebiasis caused by *Entamoeba histolytica* (oral erythromycins only). Extraenteric amebiasis requires treatment with other agents.
Acute pelvic inflammatory disease caused by *Neisseria gonorrhoeae:* Erythrocin® Lactobionate-I.V. (erythromycin lactobionate for injection, USP) followed by erythromycin base orally, as an alternative drug in treatment of acute pelvic inflammatory disease caused by *N. gonorrhoeae* in female patients with a history of sensitivity to penicillin. Patients should have a serologic test for syphilis before receiving erythromycin as treatment of gonorrhea and a follow-up serologic test for syphilis after 3 months.
Erythromycins are indicated for treatment of the following infections caused by *Chlamydia trachomatis*: conjunctivitis of the newborn, pneumonia of infancy, and urogenital infections during pregnancy. When tetracyclines are contraindicated or not tolerated, erythromycin is indicated for the treatment of uncomplicated urethral, endocervical, or rectal infections in adults due to *Chlamydia trachomatis*.
When tetracyclines are contraindicated or not tolerated, erythromycin is indicated for the treatment of nongonococcal urethritis caused by *Ureaplasma urealyticum*.
Primary syphilis caused by *Treponema pallidum*. Erythromycin (oral forms only) is an alternative choice of treatment for primary syphilis in patients allergic to the penicillins. In treatment of primary syphilis, spinal fluid should be examined before treatment and as part of the follow-up after therapy.
Legionnaires' Disease caused by *Legionella pneumophila*. Although no controlled clinical efficacy studies have been conducted, *in vitro* and limited preliminary clinical data suggest that erythromycin may be effective in treating Legionnaires' Disease.
Prophylaxis
Prevention of Initial Attacks of Rheumatic Fever—Penicillin is considered by the American Heart Association to be the drug of choice in the prevention of initial attacks of rheumatic fever (treatment of *Streptococcus pyogenes* infections of the upper respiratory tract e.g., tonsillitis, or pharyngitis).[3] Erythromycin is indicated for the treatment of penicillin-allergic patients. The therapeutic dose should be administered for ten days.
Prevention of Recurrent Attacks of Rheumatic Fever—Penicillin or sulfonamides are considered by the American Heart Association to be the drugs of choice in the prevention of recurrent attacks of rheumatic fever. In patients who are allergic to penicillin and sulfonamides, oral erythromycin is recommended by the American Heart Association in the long-term prophylaxis of streptococcal pharyngitis (for the prevention of recurrent attacks of rheumatic fever).[3]

CONTRAINDICATIONS
Erythromycin is contraindicated in patients with known hypersensitivity to this antibiotic.
Erythromycin is contraindicated in patients taking terfenadine, astemizole, pimozide, or cisapride. (See **PRECAUTIONS**—*Drug Interactions*.)

WARNINGS
There have been reports of hepatic dysfunction, including increased liver enzymes, and hepatocellular and/or cholestatic hepatitis, with or without jaundice, occurring in patients receiving oral erythromycin products.
There have been reports suggesting that erythromycin does not reach the fetus in adequate concentration to prevent congenital syphilis. Infants born to women treated during pregnancy with oral erythromycin for early syphilis should be treated with an appropriate penicillin regimen.
Rhabdomyolysis with or without renal impairment has been reported in seriously ill patients receiving erythromycin concomitantly with lovastatin. Therefore, patients receiving concomitant lovastatin and erythromycin should be carefully monitored for creatine kinase (CK) and serum transaminase levels. (See package insert for lovastatin.)
Pseudomembranous colitis has been reported with nearly all antibacterial agents, including erythromycin, and may range in severity from mild to life threatening. Therefore, it is important to consider this diagnosis in patients who present with diarrhea subsequent to the administration of antibacterial agents.
Treatment with antibacterial agents alters the normal flora of the colon and may permit overgrowth of clostridia. Studies indicate that a toxin produced by *Clostridium difficile* is a primary cause of "antibiotic-associated colitis".
After the diagnosis of pseudomembranous colitis has been established, therapeutic measures should be initiated. Mild cases of pseudomembranous colitis usually respond to discontinuation of the drug alone. In moderate to severe cases, consideration should be given to management with fluids and electrolytes, protein supplementation, and treatment with an antibacterial drug clinically effective against *Clostridium difficile* colitis.

PRECAUTIONS
Prescribing ERY-TAB in the absence of a proven or strongly suspected bacterial infection or a prophylactic indication is unlikely to provide benefit to the patient and increases the risk of the development of drug-resistant bacteria.
General: Since erythromycin is principally excreted by the liver, caution should be exercised when erythromycin is administered to patients with impaired hepatic function. (See **CLINICAL PHARMACOLOGY** and **WARNINGS**.)
There have been reports that erythromycin may aggravate the weakness of patients with myasthenia gravis.

There have been reports of infantile hypertrophic pyloric stenosis (IHPS) occurring in infants following erythromycin therapy. In one cohort of 157 newborns who were given erythromycin for pertussis prophylaxis, seven neonates (5%) developed symptoms of non-bilious vomiting or irritability with feeding and were subsequently diagnosed as having IHPS requiring surgical pyloromyotomy. A possible dose-response effect was described with an absolute risk of IHPS of 5.1% for infants who took erythromycin for 8-14 days and 10% for infants who took erythromycin for 15-21 days.[4] Since erythromycin may be used in the treatment of conditions in infants which are associated with significant mortality or morbidity (such as pertussis or neonatal Chlamydia trachomatis infections), the benefit of erythromycin therapy needs to be weighed against the potential risk of developing IHPS. Parents should be informed to contact their physician if vomiting or irritability with feeding occurs.

Prolonged or repeated use of erythromycin may result in an overgrowth of nonsusceptible bacteria or fungi. If superinfection occurs, erythromycin should be discontinued and appropriate therapy instituted.

When indicated, incision and drainage or other surgical procedures should be performed in conjunction with antibiotic therapy.

Information for Patients: Patients should be counseled that antibacterial drugs including ERY-TAB should only be used to treat bacterial infections. They do not treat viral infections (e.g., the common cold). When ERY-TAB is prescribed to treat a bacterial infection, patients should be told that although it is common to feel better early in the course of therapy, the medication should be taken exactly as directed. Skipping doses or not completing the full course of therapy may (1) decrease the effectiveness of the immediate treatment and (2) increase the likelihood that bacteria will develop resistance and will not be treatable by ERY-TAB or other antibacterial drugs in the future.

Drug Interactions: Erythromycin use in patients who are receiving high doses of theophylline may be associated with an increase in serum theophylline levels and potential theophylline toxicity. In case of theophylline toxicity and/or elevated serum theophylline levels, the dose of theophylline should be reduced while the patient is receiving concomitant erythromycin therapy.

Concomitant administration of erythromycin and digoxin has been reported to result in elevated digoxin serum levels.

There have been reports of increased anticoagulant effects when erythromycin and oral anticoagulants were used concomitantly. Increased anticoagulation effects due to interactions of erythromycin with oral anticoagulants may be more pronounced in the elderly.

Erythromycin is a substrate and inhibitor of the 3A isoform subfamily of the cytochrome p450 enzyme system (CYP3A). Coadministration of erythromycin and a drug primarily metabolized by CYP3A may be associated with elevations in drug concentrations that could increase or prolong both the therapeutic and adverse effects of the concomitant drug. Dosage adjustments may be considered, and when possible, serum concentrations of drugs primarily metabolized by CYP3A should be monitored closely in patients concurrently receiving erythromycin.

The following are examples of some clinically significant CYP3A based drug interactions. Interactions with other drugs metabolized by the CYP3A isoform are also possible. The following CYP3A based drug interactions have been observed with erythromycin products in post-marketing experience:

Ergotamine/dihydroergotamine: Concurrent use of erythromycin and ergotamine or dihydroergotamine has been associated in some patients with acute ergot toxicity characterized by severe peripheral vasospasm and dysesthesia.

Triazolobenzodiazepines (such as triazolam and alprazolam) *and related benzodiazepines:* Erythromycin has been reported to decrease the clearance of triazolam and midazolam, and thus, may increase the pharmacologic effect of these benzodiazepines.

HMG-CoA Reductase Inhibitors: Erythromycin has been reported to increase concentrations of HMG-CoA reductase inhibitors (e.g., lovastatin and simvastatin). Rare reports of rhabdomyolysis have been reported in patients taking these drugs concomitantly.

Sildenafil (Viagra): Erythromycin has been reported to increase the systemic exposure (AUC) of sildenafil. Reduction of sildenafil dosage should be considered. (See Viagra package insert.)

There have been spontaneous or published reports of CYP3A based interactions of erythromycin with cyclosporine, carbamazepine, tacrolimus, alfentanil, disopyramide, rifabutin, quinidine, methylprednisolone, cilostazol, vinblastine, and bromocriptine.

Concomitant administration of erythromycin with cisapride, pimozide, astemizole, or terfenadine is contraindicated. (See **CONTRAINDICATIONS.**)

In addition, there have been reports of interactions of erythromycin with drugs not thought to be metabolized by CYP3A, including hexobarbital, phenytoin, and valproate.

Erythromycin has been reported to significantly alter the metabolism of the nonsedating antihistamines terfenadine and astemizole when taken concomitantly. Rare cases of serious cardiovascular adverse events, including electrocardiographic QT/QT_c interval prolongation, cardiac arrest, torsades de pointes, and other ventricular arrhythmias have been observed. (See **CONTRAINDICATIONS.**) In addition, deaths have been reported rarely with concomitant administration of terfenadine and erythromycin.

There have been post-marketing reports of drug interactions when erythromycin was coadministered with cisapride, resulting in QT prolongation, cardiac arrhythmias, ventricular tachycardia, ventricular fibrillation, and torsades de pointes most likely due to the inhibition of hepatic metabolism of cisapride by erythromycin. Fatalities have been reported. (See **CONTRAINDICATIONS.**)

Drug/Laboratory Test interactions: Erythromycin interferes with the fluorometric determination of urinary catecholamines.

Carcinogenesis, Mutagenesis, Impairment of Fertility: Long-term (2-year) oral studies conducted in rats with erythromycin base did not provide evidence of tumorigenicity. Mutagenicity studies have not been conducted. There was no apparent effect on male or female fertility in rats fed erythromycin (base) at levels up to 0.25 percent of diet.

Pregnancy: Teratogenic effects. Pregnancy Category B: There is no evidence of teratogenicity or any other adverse effect on reproduction in female rats fed erythromycin base (up to 0.25 percent of diet) prior to and during mating, during gestation, and through weaning of two successive litters. There are, however, no adequate and well-controlled studies in pregnant women. Because animal reproduction studies are not always predictive of human response, this drug should be used during pregnancy only if clearly needed.

Labor and Delivery: The effect of erythromycin on labor and delivery is unknown.

Nursing Mothers: Erythromycin is excreted in human milk. Caution should be exercised when erythromycin is administered to a nursing woman.

Pediatric Use: See **INDICATIONS AND USAGE** and **DOSAGE AND ADMINISTRATION.**

ADVERSE REACTIONS

The most frequent side effects of oral erythromycin preparations are gastrointestinal and are dose-related. They include nausea, vomiting, abdominal pain, diarrhea and anorexia. Symptoms of hepatitis, hepatic dysfunction and/or abnormal liver function test results may occur. (See **WARNINGS.**)

Onset of pseudomembranous colitis symptoms may occur during or after antibacterial treatment. (See **WARNINGS.**)

Rarely, erythromycin has been associated with the production of ventricular arrhythmias, including ventricular tachycardia and torsades de pointes, in individuals with prolonged QT interval.

Allergic reactions ranging from urticaria to anaphylaxis have occurred. Skin reactions ranging from mild eruptions to erythema multiforme, Stevens-Johnson syndrome, and toxic epidermal necrolysis have been reported rarely.

There have been isolated reports of reversible hearing loss occurring chiefly in patients with renal insufficiency and in patients receiving high doses of erythromycin.

OVERDOSAGE

In case of overdosage, erythromycin should be discontinued. Overdosage should be handled with the prompt elimination of unabsorbed drug and all other appropriate measures should be instituted.

Erythromycin is not removed by peritoneal dialysis or hemodialysis.

DOSAGE AND ADMINISTRATION

In most patients, ERY-TAB (erythromycin delayed-release tablets) are well absorbed and may be given without regard to meals.

Adults: The usual dose is 250 mg four times daily in equally spaced doses. The 333 mg tablet is recommended if dosage is desired every 8 hours. If twice-a-day dosage is desired, the recommended dose is 500 mg every 12 hours. Dosage may be increased up to 4 g per day according to the severity of the infection. However, twice-a-day dosing is not recommended when doses larger than 1 g daily are administered.

Children: Age, weight, and severity of the infection are important factors in determining the proper dosage. The usual dosage is 30 to 50 mg/kg/day, in equally divided doses. For more severe infections, this dose may be doubled but should not exceed 4 g per day.

In the treatment of streptococcal infections of the upper respiratory tract (e.g., tonsillitis or pharyngitis), the therapeutic dosage of erythromycin should be administered for at least ten days.

The American Heart Association suggests a dosage of 250 mg of erythromycin orally, twice a day in long-term prophylaxis of streptococcal upper respiratory tract infections for the prevention of recurring attacks of rheumatic fever in patients allergic to penicillin and sulfonamides.[3]

Conjunctivitis of the newborn caused by *Chlamydia trachomatis:* Oral erythromycin suspension 50 mg/kg/day in 4 divided doses for at least 2 weeks.[3]

Pneumonia of infancy caused by *Chlamydia trachomatis:* Although the optimal duration of therapy has not been established, the recommended therapy is oral erythromycin suspension 50 mg/kg/day in 4 divided doses for at least 3 weeks.

Urogenital infections during pregnancy due to *Chlamydia trachomatis:* Although the optimal dose and duration of therapy have not been established, the suggested treatment is 500 mg of erythromycin by mouth four times a day or two erythromycin 333 mg tablets orally every 8 hours on an empty stomach for at least 7 days. For women who cannot tolerate this regimen, a decreased dose of one erythromycin 500 mg tablet orally every 12 hours, one 333 mg tablet orally every 8 hours or 250 mg by mouth four times a day should be used for at least 14 days.[5]

For adults with uncomplicated urethral, endocervical, or rectal infections caused by *Chlamydia trachomatis,* when tetracycline is contraindicated or not tolerated: 500 mg of erythromycin by mouth four times a day or two 333 mg tablets orally every 8 hours for at least 7 days.[5]

For patients with nongonococcal urethritis caused by *Ureaplasma urealyticum* when tetracycline is contraindicated or not tolerated: 500 mg of erythromycin by mouth four times a day or two 333 mg tablets orally every 8 hours for at least seven days.[5]

Primary syphilis: 30 to 40 g given in divided doses over a period of 10 to 15 days.

Acute pelvic inflammatory disease caused by *N. gonorrhoeae:* 500 mg Erythrocin Lactobionate-I.V. (erythromycin lactobionate for injection, USP) every 6 hours for 3 days, followed by 500 mg of erythromycin base orally every 12 hours, or 333 mg of erythromycin base orally every 8 hours for 7 days.

Intestinal amebiasis: Adults: 500 mg every 12 hours, 333 mg every 8 hours or 250 mg every 6 hours for 10 to 14 days. Children: 30 to 50 mg/kg/day in divided doses for 10 to 14 days.

Pertussis: Although optimal dosage and duration have not been established, doses of erythromycin utilized in reported clinical studies were 40 to 50 mg/kg/day, given in divided doses for 5 to 14 days.

Legionnaires' Disease: Although optimal dosage has not been established, doses utilized in reported clinical data were 1 to 4 grams daily in divided doses.

Preoperative Prophylaxis for Elective Colorectal Surgery: Listed below is an example of a recommended bowel preparation regimen. A proposed surgery time of 8:00 a.m. has been used.

Pre-op Day 3: Minimum residue or clear liquid diet. Bisacodyl, 1 tablet orally at 6:00 p.m.

Pre-op Day 2: Minimum residue or clear liquid diet. Magnesium sulfate, 30 mL, 50% solution (15g) orally at 10:00 a.m., 2:00 p.m. and 6:00 p.m. Enema at 7:00 p.m. and 8:00 p.m.

Pre-op Day 1: Clear liquid diet. Supplemental (IV) fluids as needed. Magnesium sulfate, 30 mL, 50% solution (15g) orally at 10:00 a.m. and 2:00 p.m. Neomycin sulfate (1.0g) and erythromycin base (two 500 mg tablets, three 333 mg tablets or four 250 mg tablets) orally at 1:00 p.m., 2:00 p.m. and 11:00 p.m. No enema.

Day of operation: Patient evacuates rectum at 6:30 a.m. for scheduled operation at 8:00 a.m.

HOW SUPPLIED

ERY-TAB (erythromycin delayed-release tablets, USP) are supplied as white oval enteric-coated tablets debossed on one side with the Abbott logo, [logo], and on the other side with a two letter Abbo-Code designation, EC for the 250 mg tablets, EH for the 333 mg tablets, and ED for the 500 mg tablets, in the following package sizes:

250 mg tablets: bottles of 100 (**NDC** 0074-6304-13), bottles of 500 (**NDC** 0074-6304-53), and Abbo-Pac ® unit dose packages of 100 (**NDC** 0074-6304-11).

333 mg tablets: bottles of 100 (**NDC** 0074-6320-13), bottles of 500 (**NDC** 0074-6320-53), and Abbo-Pac ® unit dose packages of 100 (**NDC** 0074-6320-11).

500 mg tablets: bottles of 100 (**NDC** 0074-6321-13), and Abbo-Pac ® unit dose packages of 100 (**NDC** 0074-6321-11).

Recommended Storage: Store below 86°F (30°C).

REFERENCES

1. National Committee for Clinical Laboratory Standards. *Methods for Dilution Antimicrobial Susceptibility Tests for Bacteria that Grow Aerobically,* Third Edition. Approved Standard NCCLS Document M7-A3, Vol. 13, No. 25 NCCLS, Villanova, PA, December 1993.
2. National Committee for Clinical Laboratory Standards, *Performance Standards for Antimicrobial Disk Susceptibility Tests,* Fifth Edition. Approved Standard NCCLS Document M2-A5, Vol. 13, No. 24 NCCLS, Villanova, PA, December 1993.
3. Committee on Rheumatic Fever, Endocarditis, and Kawasaki Disease of the Council on Cardiovascular Disease in the Young, the American Heart Association: Prevention of Rheumatic Fever. *Circulation.* 78(4):1082-1086, October 1988.
4. Honein, M.A., et. al.: Infantile hypertrophic pyloric stenosis after pertussis prophylaxis with erythromycin: a case review and cohort study. The Lancet 1999; 354 (9196): 2101-5.
5. Data on file, Abbott Laboratories.

333 mg and 500 mg tablets—U.S. Pat. No. 4,340,582

Revised: August, 2003
ABBOTT LABORATORIES
NORTH CHICAGO, IL 60064, U.S.A.
PRINTED IN U.S.A.

Shown in Product Identification Guide, page 303

E.E.S.® ℞
[ē-ē-s]
(ERYTHROMYCIN ETHYLSUCCINATE)
℞ only

To reduce the development of drug-resistant bacteria and maintain the effectiveness of E.E.S. and other antibacterial

Continued on next page

E.E.S.—Cont.

drugs, E.E.S. should be used only to treat or prevent infections that are proven or strongly suspected to be caused by bacteria.

DESCRIPTION

Erythromycin is produced by a strain of *Saccharopolyspora erythraea* (formerly *Streptomyces erythraeus*) and belongs to the macrolide group of antibiotics. It is basic and readily forms salts with acids. The base, the stearate salt, and the esters are poorly soluble in water. Erythromycin ethylsuccinate is an ester of erythromycin suitable for oral administration. Erythromycin ethylsuccinate is known chemically as erythromycin 2'-(ethylsuccinate). The molecular formula is $C_{43}H_{75}NO_{16}$ and the molecular weight is 862.06. The structural formula is:

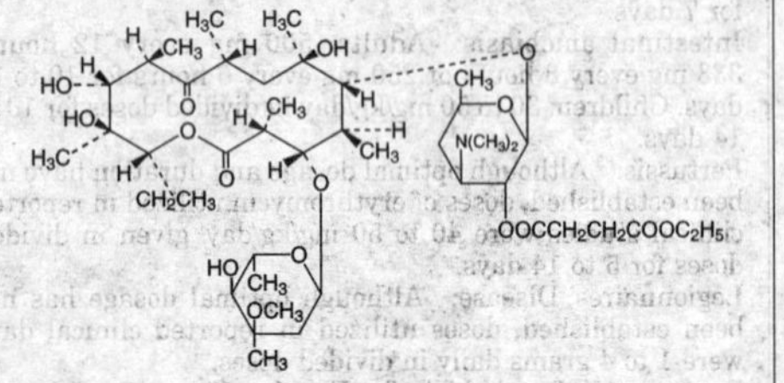

E.E.S. Granules are intended for reconstitution with water. Each 5-mL teaspoonful of reconstituted cherry-flavored suspension contains erythromycin ethylsuccinate equivalent to 200 mg of erythromycin.

The pleasant tasting, fruit-flavored liquids are supplied ready for oral administration.

E.E.S. 200 Liquid: Each 5-mL teaspoonful of fruit-flavored suspension contains erythromycin ethylsuccinate equivalent to 200 mg of erythromycin.

E.E.S. 400 Liquid: Each 5-mL teaspoonful of orange-flavored suspension contains erythromycin ethylsuccinate equivalent to 400 mg of erythromycin.

Granules and ready-made suspensions are intended primarily for pediatric use but can also be used in adults.

E.E.S. 400® Filmtab® Tablets: Each tablet contains erythromycin ethylsuccinate equivalent to 400 mg of erythromycin. The Filmtab® tablets are intended primarily for adults or older children.

Inactive Ingredients:

E.E.S. 200 Liquid: FD&C Red No. 40, methylparaben, polysorbate 60, propylparaben, sodium citrate, sucrose, water, xanthan gum and natural and artificial flavors.

E.E.S. 400 Liquid: D&C Yellow No. 10, FD&C Yellow No. 6, methylparaben, polysorbate 60, propylparaben, sodium citrate, sucrose, water, xanthan gum and natural and artificial flavors.

E.E.S. Granules: Citric acid, FD&C Red No. 3, magnesium aluminum silicate, sodium carboxymethylcellulose, sodium citrate, sucrose and artificial flavor.

E.E.S. 400 Filmtab Tablets: Cellulosic polymers, confectioner's sugar (contains corn starch), corn starch, D&C Red No. 30, D&C Yellow No. 10, FD&C Red No. 40, magnesium stearate, polacrilin potassium, polyethylene glycol, propylene glycol, sodium citrate, sorbic acid, and titanium dioxide.

CLINICAL PHARMACOLOGY

Orally administered erythromycin ethylsuccinate suspensions and Filmtab tablets are readily and reliably absorbed. Comparable serum levels of erythromycin are achieved in the fasting and nonfasting states.

Erythromycin diffuses readily into most body fluids. Only low concentrations are normally achieved in the spinal fluid, but passage of the drug across the blood-brain barrier increases in meningitis. In the presence of normal hepatic function, erythromycin is concentrated in the liver and excreted in the bile; the effect of hepatic dysfunction on excretion of erythromycin by the liver into the bile is not known. Less than 5 percent of the orally administered dose of erythromycin is excreted in active form in the urine.

Erythromycin crosses the placental barrier, but fetal plasma levels are low. The drug is excreted in human milk.

Microbiology:

Erythromycin acts by inhibition of protein synthesis by binding 50 *S* ribosomal subunits of susceptible organisms. It does not affect nucleic acid synthesis. Antagonism has been demonstrated *in vitro* between erythromycin and clindamycin, lincomycin, and chloramphenicol.

Many strains of *Haemophilus influenzae* are resistant to erythromycin alone but are susceptible to erythromycin and sulfonamides used concomitantly.

Staphylocci resistant to erythromycin may emerge during a course of therapy.

Erythromycin has been shown to be active against most strains of the following microorganisms, both *in vitro* and in clinical infections as described in the **INDICATIONS AND USAGE** section.

Gram-positive Organisms:

Corynebacterium diphtheriae
Corynebacterium minutissimum
Listeria monocytogenes
Staphylococcus aureus (resistant organisms may emerge during treatment)
Streptococcus pneumoniae
Streptococcus pyogenes

Gram-negative Organisms:

Bordetella pertussis
Legionella pneumophila
Neisseria gonorrhoeae

Other Microorganisms:

Chlamydia trachomatis
Entamoeba histolytica
Mycoplasma pneumoniae
Treponema pallidum
Ureaplasma urealyticum

The following *in vitro* data are available, **but their clinical significance is unknown.**

Erythromycin exhibits *in vitro* minimal inhibitory concentrations (MIC's) of 0.5 µg/mL or less against most (≥ 90%) strains of the following microorganisms; however, the safety and effectiveness of erythromycin in treating clinical infections due to these microorganisms have not been established in adequate and well controlled clinical trials.

Gram-positive Organisms:

Viridans group streptococci

Gram-negative Organisms:

Moraxella catarrhalis

Susceptibility Tests:

Dilution Techniques:

Quantitative methods are used to determine antimicrobial minimum inhibitory concentrations (MIC's). These MIC's provide estimates of the susceptibility of bacteria to antimicrobial compounds. The MIC's should be determined using a standardized procedure. Standardized procedures are based on a dilution method[1] (broth or agar) or equivalent with standardized inoculum concentrations and standardized concentrations of erythromycin powder. The MIC values should be interpreted according to the following criteria:

MIC (µg/mL)	Interpretation
≤0.5	Susceptible (S)
1-4	Intermediate (I)
≥8	Resistant (R)

A report of "Susceptible" indicates that the pathogen is likely to be inhibited if the antimicrobial compound in the blood reaches the concentrations usually achievable. A report of "Intermediate" indicates that the result should be considered equivocal, and, if the microorganism is not fully susceptible to alternative, clinically feasible drugs, the test should be repeated. This category implies possible clinical applicability in body sites where the drug is physiologically concentrated or in situations where high dosage of drug can be used. This category also provides a buffer zone which prevents small uncontrolled technical factors from causing major discrepancies in interpretation. A report of "Resistant" indicates that the pathogen is not likely to be inhibited if the antimicrobial compound in the blood reaches the concentrations usually achievable; other therapy should be selected.

Standardized susceptibility test procedures require the use of laboratory control microorganisms to control the technical aspects of the laboratory procedures. Standard erythromycin powder should provide the following MIC values:

Microorganism	MIC (µg/mL)
S. aureus ATCC 25923	0.12-0.5
E. faecalis ATCC 29212	1-4

Diffusion Techniques:

Quantitative methods that require measurement of zone diameters also provide reproducible estimates of the susceptibility of bacteria to antimicrobial compounds. One such standardized procedure[2] requires the use of standardized inoculum concentrations. This procedure uses paper disks impregnated with 15-µg erythromycin to test the susceptibility of microorganisms to erythromycin.

Reports from the laboratory providing results of the standard single-disk susceptibility test with a 15-µg erythromycin disk should be interpreted according to the following criteria:

Zone Diameter (mm)	Interpretation
≥23	Susceptible (S)
14-22	Intermediate (I)
≤13	Resistant (R)

Interpretation should be as stated above for results using dilution techniques. Interpretation involves correlation of the diameter obtained in the disk test with the MIC for erythromycin.

As with standardized dilution techniques, diffusion methods require the use of laboratory control microorganisms that are used to control the technical aspects of the laboratory procedures. For the diffusion technique, the 15-µg erythromycin disk should provide the following zone diameters in these laboratory test quality control strains:

Microorganism	Zone Diameter (mm)
S. aureus ATCC 25923	22-30

INDICATIONS AND USAGE

To reduce the development of drug-resistant bacteria and maintain the effectiveness of E.E.S® and other antibacterial drugs, E.E.S should be used only to treat or prevent infections that are proven or strongly suspected to be caused by susceptible bacteria. When culture and susceptibility information are available, they should be considered in selecting or modifying antibacterial therapy. In the absence of such data, local epidemiology and susceptibility patterns may contribute to the empiric selection of therapy.

E.E.S. is indicated in the treatment of infections caused by susceptible strains of the designated organisms in the diseases listed below:

Upper respiratory tract infections of mild to moderate degree caused by *Streptococcus pyogenes, Streptococcus pneumoniae,* or *Haemophilus influenzae* (when used concomitantly with adequate doses of sulfonamides, since many strains of *H. influenzae* are not susceptible to the erythromycin concentrations ordinarily achieved). (See appropriate sulfonamide labeling for prescribing information.)

Lower-respiratory tract infections of mild to moderate severity caused by *Streptococcus pneumoniae* or *Streptococcus pyogenes.*

Listeriosis caused by *Listeria monocytogenes.*

Pertussis (whooping cough) caused by *Bordetella pertussis.* Erythromycin is effective in eliminating the organism from the nasopharynx of infected individuals rendering them noninfectious. Some clinical studies suggest that erythromycin may be helpful in the prophylaxis of pertussis in exposed susceptible individuals.

Respiratory tract infections due to *Mycoplasma pneumoniae.*

Skin and skin structure infections of mild to moderate severity caused by *Streptococcus pyogenes* or *Staphylococcus aureus* (resistant staphylococci may emerge during treatment).

Diphtheria: Infections due to *Corynebacterium diphtheriae,* as an adjunct to antitoxin, to prevent establishment of carriers and to eradicate the organism in carriers.

Erythrasma: In the treatment of infections due to *Corynebacterium minutissimum.*

Intestinal amebiasis caused by *Entamoeba histolytica* (oral erythromycins only). Extraenteric amebiasis requires treatment with other agents.

Acute pelvic inflammatory disease caused by *Neisseria gonorrhoeae*: As an alternative drug in treatment of acute pelvic inflammatory disease caused by *N. gonorrhoeae* in female patients with a history of sensitivity to penicillin. Patients should have a serologic test for syphilis before receiving erythromycin as treatment of gonorrhea and a follow-up serologic test for syphilis after 3 months.

Syphilis caused by *Treponema pallidum*: Erythromycin is an alternate choice of treatment for primary syphilis in patients allergic to the penicillins. In treatment of primary syphilis, spinal fluid examinations should be done before treatment and as part of follow-up after therapy.

Erythromycins are indicated for the treatment of the following infections caused by *Chlamydia trachomatis*: conjunctivitis of the newborn, pneumonia of infancy, and urogenital infections during pregnancy. When tetracyclines are contraindicated or not tolerated, erythromycin is indicated for the treatment of uncomplicated urethral, endocervical, or rectal infections in adults due to *Chlamydia trachomatis.*

When tetracyclines are contraindicated or not tolerated, erythromycin is indicated for the treatment of nongonococcal urethritis caused by *Ureaplasma urealyticum.*

Legionnaires' Disease caused by *Legionella pneumophila.* Although no controlled clinical efficacy studies have been conducted, *in vitro* and limited preliminary clinical data suggest that erythromycin may be effective in treating Legionnaires' Disease.

Prophylaxis:

Prevention of Initial Attacks of Rheumatic Fever: Penicillin is considered by the American Heart Association to be the drug of choice in the prevention of initial attacks of rheumatic fever (treatment of *Streptococcus pyogenes* infections of the upper respiratory tract, e.g., tonsillitis or pharyngitis). Erythromycin is indicated for the treatment of penicillin-allergic patients.[3] The therapeutic dose should be administered for 10 days.

Prevention of Recurrent Attacks of Rheumatic Fever: Penicillin or sulfonamides are considered by the American Heart Association to be the drugs of choice in the prevention of recurrent attacks of rheumatic fever. In patients who are allergic to penicillin and sulfonamides, oral erythromycin is recommended by the American Heart Association in the long-term prophylaxis of streptococcal pharyngitis (for the prevention of recurrent attacks of rheumatic fever).[3]

CONTRAINDICATIONS

Erythromycin is contraindicated in patients with known hypersensitivity to this antibiotic.

Erythromycin is contraindicated in patients taking terfenadine, astemizole, pimozide, or cisapride. (See **PRECAUTIONS** - *Drug Interactions.*)

WARNINGS

There have been reports of hepatic dysfunction, including increased liver enzymes, and hepatocellular and/or cholestatic hepatitis, with or without jaundice, occurring in patients receiving oral erythromycin products.

There have been reports suggesting that erythromycin does not reach the fetus in adequate concentration to prevent congenital syphilis. Infants born to women treated during pregnancy with oral erythromycin for early syphilis should be treated with an appropriate penicillin regimen.

Pseudomembranous colitis has been reported with nearly all antibacterial agents, including erythromycin, and may range in severity from mild to life threatening. Therefore, it is important to consider this diagnosis in patients who present with diarrhea subsequent to the administration of antibacterial agents.

Treatment with antibacterial agents alters the normal flora of the colon and may permit overgrowth of clostridia. Studies indicate that a toxin produced by *Clostridium difficile* is a primary cause of "antibiotic-associated colitis".

After the diagnosis of pseudomembranous colitis has been established, therapeutic measures should be initiated. Mild cases of pseudomembranous colitis usually respond to discontinuation of the drug alone. In moderate to severe cases, consideration should be given to management with fluids and electrolytes, protein supplementation, and treatment with an antibacterial drug clinically effective against *Clostridium difficile* colitis.

Rhabdomyolysis with or without renal impairment has been reported in seriously ill patients receiving erythromycin concomitantly with lovastatin. Therefore, patients receiving concomitant lovastatin and erythromycin should be carefully monitored for creatine kinase (CK) and serum transaminase levels. (See package insert for lovastatin.)

PRECAUTIONS

General: Prescribing E.E.S. in the absence of a proven or strongly suspected bacterial infection or a prophylactic indication is unlikely to provide benefit to the patient and increases the risk of the development of drug-resistant bacteria.

Since erythromycin is principally excreted by the liver, caution should be exercised when erythromycin is administered to patients with impaired hepatic function. (See **CLINICAL PHARMACOLOGY** and **WARNINGS** sections.)

There have been reports that erythromycin may aggravate the weakness of patients with myasthenia gravis.

There have been reports of infantile hypertrophic pyloric stenosis (IHPS) occurring in infants following erythromycin therapy. In one cohort of 157 newborns who were given erythromycin for pertussis prophylaxis, seven neonates (5%) developed symptoms of non-bilious vomiting or irritability with feeding and were subsequently diagnosed as having IHPS requiring surgical pyloromyotomy. A possible dose-response effect was described with an absolute risk of IHPS of 5.1% for infants who took erythromycin for 8-14 days and 10% for infants who took erythromycin for 15-21 days.[4] Since erythromycin may be used in the treatment of conditions in infants which are associated with significant mortality or morbidity (such as pertussis or neonatal Chlamydia trachomatis infections), the benefit of erythromycin therapy needs to be weighed against the potential risk of developing IHPS. Parents should be informed to contact their physician if vomiting or irritability with feeding occurs.

Prolonged or repeated use of erythromycin may result in an overgrowth of nonsusceptible bacteria or fungi. If superinfection occurs, erythromycin should be discontinued and appropriate therapy instituted.

When indicated, incision and drainage or other surgical procedures should be performed in conjunction with antibiotic therapy.

Information for Patients: Patients should be counseled that antibacterial drugs including E.E.S. should only be used to treat bacterial infections. They do not treat viral infections (e.g., the common cold). When E.E.S. is prescribed to treat a bacterial infection, patients should be told that although it is common to feel better early in the course of therapy, the medication should be taken exactly as directed. Skipping doses or not completing the full course of therapy may (1) decrease the effectiveness of the immediate treatment and (2) increase the likelihood that bacteria will develop resistance and will not be treatable by E.E.S. or other antibacterial drugs in the future.

Drug Interactions: Erythromycin use in patients who are receiving high doses of theophylline may be associated with an increase in serum theophylline levels and potential theophylline toxicity. In case of theophylline toxicity and/or elevated serum theophylline levels, the dose of theophylline should be reduced while the patient is receiving concomitant erythromycin therapy.

Concomitant administration of erythromycin and digoxin has been reported to result in elevated digoxin serum levels.

There have been reports of increased anticoagulant effects when erythromycin and oral anticoagulants were used concomitantly. Increased anticoagulation effects due to interactions of erythromycin with various oral anticoagulants may be more pronounced in the elderly.

Erythromycin is a substrate and inhibitor of the 3A isoform subfamily of the cytochrome p450 enzyme system (CYP3A). Coadministration of erythromycin and a drug primarily metabolized by CYP3A may be associated with elevations in drug concentrations that could increase or prolong both the therapeutic and adverse effects of the concomitant drug. Dosage adjustments may be considered, and when possible, serum concentrations of drugs primarily metabolized by CYP3A should be monitored closely in patients concurrently receiving erythromycin.

The following are examples of some clinically significant CYP3A based drug interactions. Interactions with other drugs metabolized by the CYP3A isoform are also possible. The following CYP3A based drug interactions have been observed with erythromycin products in post-marketing experience:

Ergotamine/dihydroergotamine: Concurrent use of erythromycin and ergotamine or dihydroergotamine has been associated in some patients with acute ergot toxicity characterized by severe peripheral vasospasm and dysesthesia.

Triazolobenzodiazepines (such as triazolam and alprazolam) *and related benzodiazepines:* Erythromycin has been reported to decrease the clearance of triazolam and midazolam, and thus, may increase the pharmacologic effect of these benzodiazepines.

HMG-CoA Reductase Inhibitors: Erythromycin has been reported to increase concentrations of HMG-CoA reductase inhibitors (e.g., lovastatin and simvastatin). Rare reports of rhabdomyolysis have been reported in patients taking these drugs concomitantly.

Sildenafil (Viagra): Erythromycin has been reported to increase the systemic exposure (AUC) of sildenafil. Reduction of sildenafil dosage should be considered. (See Viagra package insert.)

There have been spontaneous or published reports of CYP3A based interactions of erythromycin with cyclosporine, carbamazepine, tacrolimus, alfentanil, disopyramide, rifabutin, quinidine, methylprednisolone, cilostazol, vinblastine, and bromocriptine.

Concomitant administration of erythromycin with cisapride, pimozide, astemizole, or terfenadine is contraindicated. (See **CONTRAINDICATIONS.**)

In addition, there have been reports of interactions of erythromycin with drugs not thought to be metabolized by CYP3A, including hexobarbital, phenytoin, and valproate.

Erythromycin has been reported to significantly alter the metabolism of the nonsedating antihistamines terfenadine and astemizole when taken concomitantly. Rare cases of serious cardiovascular adverse events, including electrocardiographic QT/QT$_c$ interval prolongation, cardiac arrest, torsades de pointes, and other ventricular arrhythmias have been observed. (See **CONTRAINDICATIONS.**) In addition, deaths have been reported rarely with concomitant administration of terfenadine and erythromycin.

There have been post-marketing reports of drug interactions when erythromycin is coadministered with cisapride, resulting in QT prolongation, cardiac arrhythmias, ventricular tachycardia, ventricular fibrillation, and torsades de pointes, most likely due to inhibition of hepatic metabolism of cisapride by erythromycin. Fatalities have been reported. (See **CONTRAINDICATIONS.**)

Drug/Laboratory Test Interactions: Erythromycin interferes with the fluorometric determination of urinary catecholamines.

Carcinogenesis, Mutagenesis, Impairment of Fertility: Long-term (2-year) oral studies in rats with erythromycin ethylsuccinate and erythromycin base did not provide evidence of tumorigenicity. Mutagenicity studies have not been conducted. There was no apparent effect on male or female fertility in rats fed erythromycin (base) at levels up to 0.25% of diet.

Pregnancy: Teratogenic Effects. Pregnancy Category B: There is no evidence of teratogenicity or any other adverse effect on reproduction in female rats fed erythromycin base (up to 0.25% of diet) prior to and during mating, during gestation, and through weaning of two successive litters. There are, however, no adequate and well-controlled studies in pregnant women. Because animal reproduction studies are not always predictive of human response, this drug should be used during pregnancy only if clearly needed.

Labor and Delivery: The effect of erythromycin on labor and delivery is unknown.

Nursing Mothers: Erythromycin is excreted in human milk. Caution should be exercised when erythromycin is administered to a nursing woman.

Pediatric Use: See **INDICATIONS AND USAGE** and **DOSAGE AND ADMINISTRATION** sections.

ADVERSE REACTIONS

The most frequent side effects of oral erythromycin preparations are gastrointestinal and are dose-related. They include nausea, vomiting, abdominal pain, diarrhea and anorexia. Symptoms of hepatitis, hepatic dysfunction and/or abnormal liver function test results may occur. (See **WARNINGS.**)

Onset of pseudomembranous colitis symptoms may occur during or after antibiotic treatment. (See **WARNINGS.**)

Erythromycin has been associated with QT prolongation and ventricular arrhythmias, including ventricular tachycardia and torsades de pointes.

Allergic reactions ranging from urticaria to anaphylaxis have occurred. Skin reactions ranging from mild eruptions to erythema multiforme, Stevens-Johnson syndrome, and toxic epidermal necrolysis have been reported rarely.

There have been rare reports of pancreatitis and convulsions.

There have been isolated reports of reversible hearing loss occurring chiefly in patients with renal insufficiency and in patients receiving high doses of erythromycin.

OVERDOSAGE

In case of overdosage, erythromycin should be discontinued. Overdosage should be handled with the prompt elimination of unabsorbed drug and all other appropriate measures should be instituted.

Erythromycin is not removed by peritoneal dialysis or hemodialysis.

DOSAGE AND ADMINISTRATION

Erythromycin ethylsuccinate suspensions and Filmtab tablets may be administered without regard to meals.

Children: Age, weight, and severity of the infection are important factors in determining the proper dosage. In mild to moderate infections the usual dosage of erythromycin ethylsuccinate for children is 30 to 50 mg/kg/day in equally divided doses every 6 hours. For more severe infections this dosage may be doubled. If twice-a-day dosage is desired, one-half of the total daily dose may be given every 12 hours. Doses may also be given three times daily by administering one-third of the total daily dose every 8 hours.

The following dosage schedule is suggested for mild to moderate infections:

Body Weight	Total Daily Dose
Under 10 lbs	30-50 mg/kg/day 15-25 mg/kg/q 12 h
10 to 15 lbs	200 mg
16 to 25 lbs	400 mg
26 to 50 lbs	800 mg
51 to 100 lbs	1200 mg
over 100 lbs	1600 mg

Adults: 400 mg erythromycin ethylsuccinate every 6 hours is the usual dose. Dosage may be increased up to 4 g per day according to the severity of the infection. If twice-a-day dosage is desired, one-half of the total daily dose may be given every 12 hours. Doses may also be given three times daily by administering one-third of the total daily dose every 8 hours.

For adult dosage calculation, use a ratio of 400 mg of erythromycin activity as the ethylsuccinate to 250 mg of erythromycin activity as the stearate, base or estolate.

In the treatment of streptococcal infections, therapeutic dosage of erythromycin ethylsuccinate should be administered for at least 10 days. In continuous prophylaxis against recurrences of streptococcal infections in persons with a history of rheumatic heart disease, the usual dosage is 400 mg twice a day.

For treatment of urethritis due to *C. trachomatis* or *U. urealyticum*: 800 mg three times a day for 7 days.

For treatment of primary syphilis: Adults: 48 to 64g given in divided doses over a period of 10 to 15 days.

For intestinal amebiasis: Adults: 400 mg four times daily for 10 to 14 days. Children: 30 to 50 mg/kg/day in divided doses for 10 to 14 days.

For use in pertussis: Although optimal dosage and duration have not been established, doses of erythromycin utilized in reported clinical studies were 40 to 50 mg/kg/day, given in divided doses for 5 to 14 days.

For treatment of Legionnaires' Disease: Although optimal doses have not been established, doses utilized in reported clinical data were those recommended above (1.6 to 4 g daily in divided doses.)

HOW SUPPLIED

E.E.S. 200 LIQUID (erythromycin ethylsuccinate oral suspension, USP) is supplied in 1 pint bottles (**NDC** 0074-6306-16) and in 100-mL bottles (**NDC** 0074-6306-13).

E.E.S. 400® LIQUID (erythromycin ethylsuccinate oral suspension, USP) is supplied in 1 pint bottles (**NDC** 0074-6373-16) and in 100-mL bottles (**NDC** 0074-6373-13).

Both liquid products require refrigeration to preserve taste until dispensed. Refrigeration by patient is not required if used within 14 days.

E.E.S. GRANULES (erythromycin ethylsuccinate for oral suspension, USP) is supplied in 100-mL (**NDC** 0074-6369-02) and 200-mL (**NDC** 0074-6369-10) size bottles.

E.E.S. 400 Filmtab tablets (erythromycin ethylsuccinate tablets, USP) 400 mg, are supplied as pink tablets imprinted with the Abbott logo, and two letter Abbo-Code designation, EE, in bottles of 100 (**NDC** 0074-5729-13), 500 (**NDC** 0074-5729-53) and 1000 (**NDC** 0074-5729-19) and in ABBO-PAC unit dose strip packages of 100 (**NDC** 0074-5729-11).

Recommended storage: Store tablets below 86°F (30°C).

Store granules, prior to mixing, below 86°F (30°C). After mixing, refrigerate and use within 10 days.

REFERENCES

1. National Committee for Clinical Laboratory Standards, *Methods for Dilution Antimicrobial Susceptibility Tests for Bacteria that Grow Aerobically*, Third Edition. Approved Standard NCCLS Document M7-A3, Vol. 13, No. 25. NCCLS, Villanova, PA, December 1993.
2. National Committee for Clinical Laboratory Standards, *Performance Standards for Antimicrobial Disk Suscepti-*

Continued on next page

E.E.S.—Cont.

bility Tests, Fifth Edition. Approved Standard NCCLS Document M2-A5, Vol. 13, No. 24. NCCLS, Villanova, PA, December 1993.
3. Committee on Rheumatic Fever, Endocarditis, and Kawasaki Disease of the Council on Cardiovascular Disease in the Young, the American Heart Association: Prevention of Rheumatic Fever. *Circulation*. 78(4): 1082-1086, October 1988.
4. Honein, M.A., et. al.: Infantile hypertrophic pyloric stenosis after pertussis prophylaxis with erythromycin: a case review and cohort study. The Lancet 1999; 354 (9196): 2101-5.

Filmtab—Film-sealed tablets, Abbott.

Revised: November, 2003
Ref. 03-5300-R22
ABBOTT LABORATORIES
NORTH CHICAGO, IL 60064, U.S.A.
PRINTED IN U.S.A.

Shown in Product Identification Guide, page 303

ERYTHROCIN® STEARATE ℞

[*ur-ith-ro-cin*]
ERYTHROMYCIN STEARATE
TABLETS, USP
Filmtab® Tablets
℞ only

To reduce the development of drug-resistant bacteria and maintain the effectiveness of ERYTHROCIN STEARATE Filmtab tablets and other antibacterial drugs, ERYTHROCIN STEARATE Filmtab tablets should be used only to treat or prevent infections that are proven or strongly suspected to be caused by bacteria.

DESCRIPTION

ERYTHROCIN STEARATE Filmtab tablets (erythromycin stearate tablets, USP) are an antibacterial product containing the stearate salt of erythromycin in a unique film coating.

Erythromycin is produced by a strain of *Saccharopolyspora erythraea* (formerly *Streptomyces erythraeus*) and belongs to the macrolide group of antibiotics. It is basic and readily forms salts with acids. Erythromycin is a white to off-white powder, slightly soluble in water, and soluble in alcohol, chloroform, and ether. Erythromycin stearate is known chemically as erythromycin octadecanoate. The molecular formula of erythromycin stearate is $C_{37}H_{67}NO_{13}•C_{18}H_{36}O_2$, and the molecular weight is 1018.43. The structural formula is:

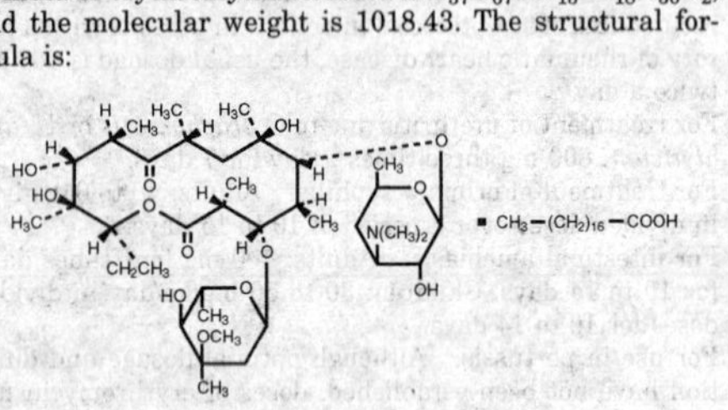

Inactive Ingredients:

250 mg tablet: Cellulosic polymers, corn starch, D&C Red No. 7, polacrilin potassium, polyethylene glycol, povidone, propylene glycol, sodium carboxymethylcellulose, sodium citrate, sorbic acid, sorbitan monooleate and titanium dioxide.

500 mg tablet: Cellulosic polymers, corn starch, FD&C Red No. 3, magnesium hydroxide, polacrilin potassium, povidone, propylene glycol, sorbitan monooleate, titanium dioxide and vanillin.

CLINICAL PHARMACOLOGY

Orally administered erythromycin base and its salts are readily absorbed in the microbiologically active form. Interindividual variations in the absorption of erythromycin are, however, observed, and some patients do not achieve optimal serum levels. Erythromycin is largely bound to plasma proteins. After absorption, erythromycin diffuses readily into most body fluids. In the absence of meningeal inflammation, low concentrations are normally achieved in the spinal fluid but the passage of the drug across the blood-brain barrier increases in meningitis. Erythromycin crosses the placental barrier, but fetal plasma levels are low. The drug is excreted in human milk. Erythromycin is not removed by peritoneal dialysis or hemodialysis.

In the presence of normal hepatic function, erythromycin is concentrated in the liver and is excreted in the bile; the effect of hepatic dysfunction on biliary excretion of erythromycin is not known. After oral administration, less than 5% of the administered dose can be recovered in the active form in the urine.

Orally administered ERYTHROCIN STEARATE tablets are readily and reliably absorbed. Optimal serum levels of erythromycin are reached when the drug is taken in the fasting state or immediately before meals.

Microbiology:

Erythromycin acts by inhibition of protein synthesis by binding 50 S ribosomal subunits of susceptible organisms. It does not affect nucleic acid synthesis. Antagonism has been demonstrated *in vitro* between erythromycin and clindamycin, lincomycin, and chloramphenicol.

Many strains of *Haemophilus influenzae* are resistant to erythromycin alone, but are susceptible to erythromycin and sulfonamides used concomitantly.

Staphylococci resistant to erythromycin may emerge during a course of erythromycin therapy. Erythromycin has been shown to be active against most strains of the following microorganisms, both *in vitro* and in clinical infections as described in the **INDICATIONS AND USAGE** section.

Gram-positive organisms:
Corynebacterium diphtheriae
Corynebacterium minutissimum
Listeria monocytogenes
Staphylococcus aureus (resistant organisms may emerge during treatment)
Streptococcus pneumoniae
Streptococcus pyogenes

Gram-negative organisms:
Bordetella pertussis
Legionella pneumophila
Neisseria gonorrhoeae

Other microorganisms:
Chlamydia trachomatis
Entamoeba histolytica
Mycoplasma pneumoniae
Treponema pallidum
Ureaplasma urealyticum

The following *in vitro* data are available, **but their clinical significance is unknown.**

Erythromycin exhibits *in vitro* minimal inhibitory concentrations (MIC's) of 0.5 µg/mL or less against most (≥ 90%) strains of the following microorganisms; however, the safety and effectiveness of erythromycin in treating clinical infections due to these microorganisms have not been established in adequate and well-controlled clinical trials.

Gram-positive organisms:
Viridans group streptococci

Gram-negative organisms:
Moraxella catarrhalis

Susceptibility Tests:

Dilution Techniques:

Quantitative methods are used to determine antimicrobial minimum inhibitory concentrations (MIC's). These MIC's provide estimates of the susceptibility of bacteria to antimicrobial compounds. The MIC's should be determined using a standardized procedure. Standardized procedures are based on a dilution method[1] (broth or agar) or equivalent with standardized inoculum concentrations and standardized concentrations of erythromycin powder. The MIC values should be interpreted according to the following criteria:

MIC (µg/mL)	Interpretation
≤0.5	Susceptible (S)
1–4	Intermediate (I)
≥8	Resistant (R)

A report of "Susceptible" indicates that the pathogen is likely to be inhibited if the antimicrobial compound in the blood reaches the concentrations usually achievable. A report of "Intermediate" indicates that the result should be considered equivocal, and, if the microorganism is not fully susceptible to alternative, clinically feasible drugs, the test should be repeated. This category implies possible clinical applicability in body sites where the drug is physiologically concentrated or in situations where high dosage of drug can be used. This category also provides a buffer zone which prevents small uncontrolled technical factors from causing major discrepancies in interpretation. A report of "Resistant" indicates that the pathogen is not likely to be inhibited if the antimicrobial compound in the blood reaches the concentrations usually achievable; other therapy should be selected.

Standardized susceptibility test procedures require the use of laboratory control microorganisms to control the technical aspects of the laboratory procedures. Standard erythromycin powder should provide the following MIC values:

Microorganism	MIC (µg/mL)
S. aureus ATCC 29213	0.12–0.5
E. faecalis ATCC 29212	1–4

Diffusion Techniques:

Quantitative methods that require measurement of zone diameters also provide reproducible estimates of the susceptibility of bacteria to antimicrobial compounds. One such standardized procedure[2] requires the use of standardized inoculum concentrations. This procedure uses paper disks impregnated with 15-µg erythromycin to test the susceptibility of microorganisms to erythromycin.

Reports from the laboratory providing results of the standard single-disk susceptibility test with a 15-µg erythromycin disk should be interpreted according to the following criteria:

Zone Diameter (mm)	Interpretation
≥23	Susceptible (S)
14–22	Intermediate (I)
≤13	Resistant (R)

Interpretation should be as stated above for results using dilution techniques. Interpretation involves correlation of the diameter obtained in the disk test with the MIC for erythromycin.

As with standardized dilution techniques, diffusion methods require the use of laboratory control microorganisms that are used to control the technical aspects of the laboratory procedures. For the diffusion technique, the 15-µg erythromycin disk should provide the following zone diameters in these laboratory test quality control strains:

Microorganism	Zone Diameter (mm)
S. aureus ATCC 25923	22–30

INDICATIONS AND USAGE

To reduce the development of drug-resistant bacteria and maintain the effectiveness of ERYTHROCIN STEARATE Filmtab tablets and other antibacterial drugs, ERYTHROCIN STEARATE Filmtab tablets should be used only to treat or prevent infections that are proven or strongly suspected to be caused by susceptible bacteria. When culture and susceptibility information are available, they should be considered in selecting or modifying antibacterial therapy. In the absence of such data, local epidemiology and susceptibility patterns may contribute to the empiric selection of therapy.

ERYTHROCIN STEARATE tablets are indicated in the treatment of infections caused by susceptible strains of the designated microorganisms in the diseases listed below:

Upper respiratory tract infections of mild to moderate degree caused by *Streptococcus pyogenes; Streptococcus pneumoniae; Haemophilus influenzae* (when used concomitantly with adequate doses of sulfonamides, since many strains of *H. influenzae* are not susceptible to the erythromycin concentrations ordinarily achieved). (See appropriate sulfonamide labeling for prescribing information.)

Lower respiratory tract infections of mild to moderate severity caused by *Streptococcus pyogenes* or *Streptococcus pneumoniae*.

Listeriosis caused by *Listeria monocytogenes*.

Respiratory tract infections due to *Mycoplasma pneumoniae*.

Skin and skin structure infections of mild to moderate severity caused by *Streptococcus pyogenes* or *Staphylococcus aureus* (resistant staphylococci may emerge during treatment).

Pertussis (whooping cough) caused by *Bordetella pertussis*. Erythromycin is effective in eliminating the organism from the nasopharynx of infected individuals, rendering them noninfectious. Some clinical studies suggest that erythromycin may be helpful in the prophylaxis of pertussis in exposed susceptible individuals.

Diphtheria: Infections due to *Corynebacterium diphtheriae*, as an adjunct to antitoxin, to prevent establishment of carriers and to eradicate the organism in carriers.

Erythrasma—In the treatment of infections due to *Corynebacterium minutissimum*.

Intestinal amebiasis caused by *Entamoeba histolytica* (oral erythromycins only). Extraenteric amebiasis requires treatment with other agents.

Acute pelvic inflammatory disease caused by *Neisseria gonorrhoeae*: Erythrocin® Lactobionate-I.V. (erythromycin lactobionate for injection, USP) followed by erythromycin base orally, as an alternative drug in treatment of acute pelvic inflammatory disease caused by *N. gonorrhoeae* in female patients with a history of sensitivity to penicillin. Patients should have a serologic test for syphilis before receiving erythromycin as treatment of gonorrhea and a follow-up serologic test for syphilis after 3 months.

Erythromycins are indicated for treatment of the following infections caused by *Chlamydia trachomatis*: conjunctivitis of the newborn, pneumonia of infancy, and urogenital infections during pregnancy. When tetracyclines are contraindicated or not tolerated, erythromycin is indicated for the treatment of uncomplicated urethral, endocervical, or rectal infections in adults due to *Chlamydia trachomatis*.

When tetracyclines are contraindicated or not tolerated, erythromycin is indicated for the treatment of nongonococcal urethritis caused by *Ureaplasma urealyticum*.

Primary syphilis caused by *Treponema pallidum*. Erythromycin (oral forms only) is an alternative choice of treatment for primary syphilis in patients allergic to the penicillins. In treatment of primary syphilis, spinal fluid should be examined before treatment and as part of the follow-up after therapy.

Legionnaires' Disease caused by *Legionella pneumophila*. Although no controlled clinical efficacy studies have been conducted, *in vitro* and limited preliminary clinical data suggest that erythromycin may be effective in treating Legionnaires' Disease.

Prophylaxis

Prevention of Initial Attacks of Rheumatic Fever–Penicillin is considered by the American Heart Association to be the drug of choice in the prevention of initial attacks of rheumatic fever (treatment of *Streptococcus pyogenes* infections of the upper respiratory tract e.g., tonsillitis, or pharyngitis).[3] Erythromycin is indicated for the treatment of penicillin-allergic patients. The therapeutic dose should be administered for ten days.

Prevention of Recurrent Attacks of Rheumatic Fever–Penicillin or sulfonamides are considered by the American Heart Association to be the drugs of choice in the prevention of recurrent attacks of rheumatic fever. In patients who are allergic to penicillin and sulfonamides, oral erythromycin is recommended by the American Heart Association in the long-term prophylaxis of streptococcal pharyngitis (for the prevention of recurrent attacks of rheumatic fever).[3]

CONTRAINDICATIONS

Erythromycin is contraindicated in patients with known hypersensitivity to this antibiotic.

Erythromycin is contraindicated in patients taking terfenadine, astemizole, pimozide or cisapride. (See **PRECAUTIONS**-*Drug Interactions*.)

WARNINGS

There have been reports of hepatic dysfunction, including increased liver enzymes, and hepatocellular and/or cholestatic hepatitis, with or without jaundice, occurring in patients receiving oral erythromycin products.

There have been reports suggesting that erythromycin does not reach the fetus in adequate concentration to prevent congenital syphilis. Infants born to women treated during pregnancy with oral erythromycin for early syphilis should be treated with an appropriate penicillin regimen.

Rhabdomyolysis with or without renal impairment has been reported in seriously ill patients receiving erythromycin concomitantly with lovastatin. Therefore, patients receiving concomitant lovastatin and erythromycin should be carefully monitored for creatine kinase (CK) and serum transaminase levels. (See package insert for lovastatin.)

Pseudomembranous colitis has been reported with nearly all antibacterial agents, including erythromycin, and may range in severity from mild to life threatening. Therefore, it is important to consider this diagnosis in patients who present with diarrhea subsequent to the administration of antibacterial agents.

Treatment with antibacterial agents alters the normal flora of the colon and may permit overgrowth of clostridia. Studies indicate that a toxin produced by *Clostridium difficile* is a primary cause of "antibiotic-associated colitis".

After the diagnosis of pseudomembranous colitis has been established, therapeutic measures should be initiated. Mild cases of pseudomembranous colitis usually respond to discontinuation of the drug alone. In moderate to severe cases, consideration should be given to management with fluids and electrolytes, protein supplementation, and treatment with an antibacterial drug clinically effective against *Clostridium difficile* colitis.

PRECAUTIONS

General: Prescribing ERYTHROCIN STEARATE Filmtab tablets in the absence of a proven or strongly suspected bacterial infection or a prophylactic indication is unlikely to provide benefit to the patient and increases the risk of the development of drug-resistant bacteria. Since erythromycin is principally excreted by the liver, caution should be exercised when erythromycin is administered to patients with impaired hepatic function. (See **CLINICAL PHARMACOLOGY** and **WARNINGS**.)

There have been reports that erythromycin may aggravate the weakness of patients with myasthenia gravis.

There have been reports of infantile hypertrophic pyloric stenosis (IHPS) occurring in infants following erythromycin therapy. In one cohort of 157 newborns who were given erythromycin for pertussis prophylaxis, seven neonates (5%) developed symptoms of non-bilious vomiting or irritability with feeding and were subsequently diagnosed as having IHPS requiring surgical pyloromyotomy. A possible dose-response effect was described with an absolute risk of IHPS of 5.1% for infants who took erythromycin for 8–14 days and 10% for infants who took erythromycin for 15–21 days.[4] Since erythromycin may be used in the treatment of conditions in infants which are associated with significant mortality or morbidity (such as pertussis or neonatal Chlamydia trachomatis infections), the benefit of erythromycin therapy needs to be weighed against the potential risk of developing IHPS. Parents should be informed to contact their physician if vomiting or irritability with feeding occurs.

Prolonged or repeated use of erythromycin may result in an overgrowth of nonsusceptible bacteria or fungi. If superinfection occurs, erythromycin should be discontinued and appropriate therapy instituted.

When indicated, incision and drainage or other surgical procedures should be performed in conjunction with antibiotic therapy.

Information for Patients: Patients should be counseled that antibacterial drugs including ERYTHROCIN STEARATE Filmtab tablets should only be used to treat bacterial infections. They do not treat viral infections (e.g., the common cold). When ERYTHROCIN STEARATE Filmtab tablets is prescribed to treat a bacterial infection, patients should be told that although it is common to feel better early in the course of therapy, the medication should be taken exactly as directed. Skipping doses or not completing the full course of therapy may (1) decrease the effectiveness of the immediate treatment and (2) increase the likelihood that bacteria will develop resistance and will not be treatable by ERYTHROCIN STEARATE Filmtab tablets or other antibacterial drugs in the future.

Drug Interactions: Erythromycin use in patients who are receiving high doses of theophylline may be associated with an increase in serum theophylline levels and potential theophylline toxicity. In case of theophylline toxicity and/or elevated serum theophylline levels, the dose of theophylline should be reduced while the patient is receiving concomitant erythromycin therapy.

Concomitant administration of erythromycin and digoxin has been reported to result in elevated digoxin serum levels.

There have been reports of increased anticoagulant effects when erythromycin and oral anticoagulants were used concomitantly. Increased anticoagulation effects due to interactions of erythromycin with oral anticoagulants may be more pronounced in the elderly.

Erythromycin is a substrate and inhibitor of the 3A isoform subfamily of the cytochrome p450 enzyme system (CYP3A). Coadministration of erythromycin and a drug primarily metabolized by CYP3A may be associated with elevations in drug concentrations that could increase or prolong both the therapeutic and adverse effects of the concomitant drug. Dosage adjustments may be considered, and when possible, serum concentrations of drugs primarily metabolized by CYP3A should be monitored closely in patients concurrently receiving erythromycin.

The following are examples of some clinically significant CYP3A based drug interactions. Interactions with other drugs metabolized by the CYP3A isoform are also possible. The following CYP3A based drug interactions have been observed with erythromycin products in post-marketing experience:

Ergotamine/dihydroergotamine: Concurrent use of erythromycin and ergotamine or dihydroergotamine has been associated in some patients with acute ergot toxicity characterized by severe peripheral vasospasm and dysesthesia.

Triazolobenzodiazepines (such as triazolam and alprazolam) *and related benzodiazepines*: Erythromycin has been reported to decrease the clearance of triazolam and midazolam, and thus, may increase the pharmacologic effect of these benzodiazepines.

HMG-CoA Reductase Inhibitors: Erythromycin has been reported to increase concentrations of HMG-CoA reductase inhibitors (e.g., lovastatin and simvastatin). Rare reports of rhabdomyolysis have been reported in patients taking these drugs concomitantly.

Sildenafil (Viagra): Erythromycin has been reported to increase the systemic exposure (AUC) of sildenafil. Reduction of sildenafil dosage should be considered. (See Viagra package insert.)

There have been spontaneous or published reports of CYP3A based interactions of erythromycin with cyclosporine, carbamazepine, tacrolimus, alfentanil, disopyramide, rifabutin, quinidine, methylprednisolone, cilostazol, vinblastine, and bromocriptine.

Concomitant administration of erythromycin with cisapride, pimozide, astemizole, or terfenadine is contraindicated. (See **CONTRAINDICATIONS**.)

In addition, there have been reports of interactions of erythromycin with drugs not thought to be metabolized by CYP3A, including hexobarbital, phenytoin, and valproate.

Erythromycin has been reported to significantly alter the metabolism of the nonsedating antihistamines terfenadine and astemizole when taken concomitantly. Rare cases of serious cardiovascular adverse events, including electrocardiographic QT/QT_c interval prolongation, cardiac arrest, torsades de pointes, and other ventricular arrhythmias, have been observed. (See **CONTRAINDICATIONS**.) In addition, deaths have been reported rarely with concomitant administration of terfenadine and erythromycin.

There have been post-marketing reports of drug interactions when erythromycin was coadministered with cisapride, resulting in QT prolongation, cardiac arrhythmias, ventricular tachycardia, ventricular fibrillation, and torsades de pointes, most likely due to the inhibition of hepatic metabolism of cisapride by erythromycin. Fatalities have been reported. (See **CONTRAINDICATIONS**).

Drug/Laboratory Test interactions: Erythromycin interferes with the fluorometric determination of urinary catecholamines.

Carcinogenesis, Mutagenesis, Impairment of Fertility: Long-term (2-year) oral studies conducted in rats with erythromycin base did not provide evidence of tumorigenicity. Mutagenicity studies have not been conducted. There was no apparent effect on male or female fertility in rats fed erythromycin (base) at levels up to 0.25 percent of diet.

Pregnancy: Teratogenic effects. Pregnancy Category B: There is no evidence of teratogenicity or any other adverse effect on reproduction in female rats fed erythromycin base (up to 0.25 percent of diet) prior to and during mating, during gestation, and through weaning of two successive litters. There are, however, no adequate and well-controlled studies in pregnant women. Because animal reproduction studies are not always predictive of human response, this drug should be used during pregnancy only if clearly needed.

Labor and Delivery: The effect of erythromycin on labor and delivery is unknown.

Nursing Mothers: Erythromycin is excreted in human milk. Caution should be exercised when erythromycin is administered to a nursing woman.

Pediatric Use: See **INDICATIONS AND USAGE** and **DOSAGE AND ADMINISTRATION**.

ADVERSE REACTIONS

The most frequent side effects of oral erythromycin preparations are gastrointestinal and are dose related. They include nausea, vomiting, abdominal pain, diarrhea and anorexia. Symptoms of hepatitis, hepatic dysfunction and/or abnormal liver function test results may occur. (See **WARNINGS**.)

Onset of pseudomembranous colitis symptoms may occur during or after antibacterial treatment. (See **WARNINGS**.)

Erythromycin has been associated with QT prolongation and ventricular arrhythmias, including ventricular tachycardia and torsades de pointes.

Allergic reactions ranging from urticaria to anaphylaxis have occurred. Skin reactions ranging from mild eruptions to erythema multiforme, Stevens-Johnson syndrome, and toxic epidermal necrolysis have been reported rarely.

There have been rare reports of pancreatitis and convulsions.

There have been isolated reports of reversible hearing loss occurring chiefly in patients with renal insufficiency and in patients receiving high doses of erythromycin.

OVERDOSAGE

In case of overdosage, erythromycin should be discontinued. Overdosage should be handled with the prompt elimination of unabsorbed drug and all other appropriate measures should be instituted.

Erythromycin is not removed by peritoneal dialysis or hemodialysis.

DOSAGE AND ADMINISTRATION

Optimal serum levels of erythromycin are reached when ERYTHROCIN STEARATE (erythromycin stearate) is taken in the fasting state or immediately before meals.

Adults: The usual dosage is 250 mg every 6 hours; or 500 mg every 12 hours. Dosage may be increased up to 4 g per day according to the severity of the infection. However, twice-a-day dosing is not recommended when doses larger than 1 g daily are administered.

Children: Age, weight, and severity of the infection are important factors in determining the proper dosage. The usual dosage is 30 to 50 mg/kg/day, in equally divided doses. For more severe infections this dosage may be doubled but should not exceed 4 g per day.

In the treatment of streptococcal infections of the upper respiratory tract (e.g., tonsillitis or pharyngitis), the therapeutic dosage of erythromycin should be administered for at least ten days.

The American Heart Association suggests a dosage of 250 mg of erythromycin orally, twice a day in long-term prophylaxis of streptococcal upper respiratory tract infections for the prevention of recurring attacks of rheumatic fever in patients allergic to penicillin and sulfonamides.[3]

Conjunctivitis of the newborn caused by *Chlamydia trachomatis:* Oral erythromycin suspension 50 mg/kg/day in 4 divided doses for at least 2 weeks.[3]

Pneumonia of infancy caused by *Chlamydia trachomatis:* Although the optimal duration of therapy has not been established, the recommended therapy is oral erythromycin suspension 50 mg/kg/day in 4 divided doses for at least 3 weeks.

Urogenital infections during pregnancy due to *Chlamydia trachomatis:* Although the optimal dose and duration of therapy have not been established, the suggested treatment is 500 mg of erythromycin by mouth four times a day or two erythromycin 333 mg tablets orally every 8 hours on an empty stomach for at least 7 days. For women who cannot tolerate this regimen, a decreased dose of one erythromycin 500 mg tablet orally every 12 hours, one 333 mg tablet orally every 8 hours or 250 mg by mouth four times a day should be used for at least 14 days.[5]

For adults with uncomplicated urethral, endocervical, or rectal infections caused by *Chlamydia trachomatis*, when tetracycline is contraindicated or not tolerated: 500 mg of erythromycin by mouth four times a day or two 333 mg tablets orally every 8 hours for at least 7 days.[5]

For patients with nongonococcal urethritis caused by *Ureaplasma urealyticum* when tetracycline is contraindicated or not tolerated: 500 mg of erythromycin by mouth four times a day or two 333 mg tablets orally every 8 hours for at least seven days.[5]

Primary syphilis: 30 to 40 g given in divided doses over a period of 10 to 15 days.

Acute pelvic inflammatory disease caused by *N. gonorrhoeae*: 500 mg Erythrocin Lactobionate-I.V. (erythromycin lactobionate for injection, USP) every 6 hours for 3 days, followed by 500 mg of erythromycin base orally every 12 hours, or 333 mg of erythromycin base orally every 8 hours for 7 days.

Intestinal amebiasis: Adults: 500 mg every 12 hours, 333 mg every 8 hours or 250 mg every 6 hours for 10 to 14 days. Children: 30 to 50 mg/kg/day in divided doses for 10 to 14 days.

Pertussis: Although optimal dosage and duration have not been established, doses of erythromycin utilized in reported clinical studies were 40 to 50 mg/kg/day, given in divided doses for 5 to 14 days.

Legionnaires' Disease: Although optimal dosage has not been established, doses utilized in reported clinical data were 1 to 4 g daily in divided doses.

HOW SUPPLIED

ERYTHROCIN STEARATE Filmtab Tablets (erythromycin stearate tablets, USP) are supplied in the following strengths and packages.

Continued on next page

Erythrocin Stearate—Cont.

ERYTHROCIN STEARATE Filmtab, 250 mg pink tablets imprinted with the corporate logo and the Abbo-Code designation ES:

Bottles of 100 .... (**NDC** 0074-6346-20)
Bottles of 500 .... (**NDC** 0074-6346-53)
Bottles of 1000 .... (**NDC** 0074-6346-19)
ABBO-PAC® unit dose strip packages
of 100 tablets .... (**NDC** 0074-6346-38)

ERYTHROCIN STEARATE Filmtab, 500 mg pink tablets imprinted with the corporate logo and the Abbo-Code designation ET:

Bottles of 100 .... (**NDC** 0074-6316-13)

Recommended Storage: Store below 86°F (30°C).

REFERENCES

1. National Committee for Clinical Laboratory Standards. *Methods for Dilution Antimicrobial Susceptibility Tests for Bacteria that Grow Aerobically,* Third Edition. Approved Standard NCCLS Document M7-A3, Vol. 13, No. 25 NCCLS, Villanova, PA, December 1993.
2. National Committee for Clinical Laboratory Standards, *Performance Standards for Antimicrobial Disk Susceptibility Tests,* Fifth Edition. Approved Standard NCCLS Document M2-A5, Vol. 13, No. 24 NCCLS, Villanova, PA, December 1993.
3. Committee on Rheumatic Fever, Endocarditis, and Kawasaki Disease of the Council on Cardiovascular Disease in the Young, the American Heart Association: Prevention of Rheumatic Fever. *Circulation.* 78(4):1082–1086, October 1988.
4. Honein, M.A., et. al.: Infantile hypertrophic pyloric stenosis after pertussis prophylaxis with erythromycin: a case review and cohort study. The Lancet 1999; 354 (9196): 2101–5.
5. Data on file, Abbott Laboratories.

FILMTAB—Film-sealed tablets, Abbott.
03-5298-R15
Revised: September, 2003
ABBOTT LABORATORIES
NORTH CHICAGO, IL 60064, U.S.A.

Shown in Product Identification Guide, page 303

ERYTHROMYCIN ℞

[ur-ith-ro-my-cin]
Base Filmtab®
ERYTHROMYCIN TABLETS, USP
℞ only
(Nos. 6326 and 6227)
03-5245-R5-Rev. July, 2003

To reduce the development of drug-resistant bacteria and maintain the effectiveness of Erythromycin Base Filmtab tablets and other antibacterial drugs, Erythromycin Base Filmtab tablets would be used only to treat or prevent infections that are proven or strongly suspected to be caused by bacteria.

DESCRIPTION

Erythromycin Base Filmtab (erythromycin tablets, USP) is an antibacterial product containing erythromycin, USP, in a unique, nonenteric film coating for oral administration. Erythromycin Base Filmtab tablets are available in two strengths containing either 250 mg or 500 mg of erythromycin base.

Erythromycin is produced by a strain of *Saccharopolyspora erythraea* (formerly *Streptomyces erythraeus*) and belongs to the macrolide group of antibiotics. It is basic and readily forms salts with acids. Erythromycin is a white to off-white powder, slightly soluble in water, and soluble in alcohol, chloroform, and ether. Erythromycin is known chemically as (3R*, 4S*, 5S*, 6R*, 7R*, 9R*, 11R*, 12R*, 13S*, 14R*)-4-[(2,6-dideoxy-3-C-methyl-3-O-methyl-α-L-*ribo*-hexopyranosyl)oxy]-14-ethyl-7,12,13-trihydroxy-3,5,7,9,11,13-hexamethyl-6-[[3,4,6-trideoxy-3-(dimethylamino)-β-D-*xylo*-hexopyranosyl]oxy]oxacyclotetradecane-2,10-dione. The molecular formula is $C_{37}H_{67}NO_{13}$, and the molecular weight is 733.94. The structural formula is:

Inactive Ingredients:

Colloidal silicon dioxide, croscarmellose sodium, crospovidone, D&C Red No. 30 Aluminum Lake, hydroxypropyl cellulose, hypromellose, hydroxypropyl methylcellulose phthalate, magnesium stearate, microcrystalline cellulose, povidone, polyethylene glycol, propylene glycol, sodium citrate, sodium hydroxide, sorbic acid, sorbitan monooleate, talc, and titanium dioxide.

CLINICAL PHARMACOLOGY

Orally administered erythromycin base and its salts are readily absorbed in the microbiologically active form. Individual variations in the absorption of erythromycin are, however, observed, and some patients do not achieve optimal serum levels. Erythromycin is largely bound to plasma proteins. After absorption, erythromycin diffuses readily into most body fluids. In the absence of meningeal inflammation, low concentrations are normally achieved in the spinal fluid but the passage of the drug across the blood-brain barrier increases in meningitis. Erythromycin crosses the placental barrier, but fetal plasma levels are low. The drug is excreted in human milk. Erythromycin is not removed by peritoneal dialysis or hemodialysis.

In the presence of normal hepatic function, erythromycin is concentrated in the liver and is excreted in the bile; the effect of hepatic dysfunction on biliary excretion of erythromycin is not known. After oral administration, less than 5% of the administered dose can be recovered in the active form in the urine.

Optimal blood levels are obtained when Erythromycin Base Filmtab tablets are given in the fasting state (at least 1/2 hour and preferably 2 hours before meals). Bioavailability data are available from Abbott Laboratories, Dept. 42W.

Microbiology:

Erythromycin acts by inhibition of protein synthesis by binding 50 S ribosomal subunits of susceptible organisms. It does not affect nucleic acid synthesis. Antagonism has been demonstrated *in vitro* between erythromycin and clindamycin, lincomycin, and chloramphenicol.

Many strains of *Haemophilus influenzae* are resistant to erythromycin alone, but are susceptible to erythromycin and sulfonamides used concomitantly.

Staphylococci resistant to erythromycin may emerge during a course of erythromycin therapy. Erythromycin has been shown to be active against most strains of the following microorganisms, both *in vitro* and in clinical infections as described in the **INDICATIONS AND USAGE** section.

Gram-positive organisms:

Corynebacterium diphtheriae
Corynebacterium minutissimum
Listeria monocytogenes
Staphylococcus aureus (resistant organisms may emerge during treatment)
Streptococcus pneumoniae
Streptococcus pyogenes

Gram-negative organisms:

Bordetella pertussis
Legionella pneumophila
Neisseria gonorrhoeae

Other microorganisms:

Chlamydia trachomatis
Entamoeba histolytica
Mycoplasma pneumoniae
Treponema pallidum
Ureaplasma urealyticum

The following *in vitro* data are available, **but their clinical significance is unknown.**

Erythromycin exhibits *in vitro* minimal inhibitory concentrations (MIC's) of 0.5 µg/mL or less against most (≥90%) strains of the following microorganisms; however, the safety and effectiveness of erythromycin in treating clinical infections due to these microorganisms have not been established in adequate and well-controlled clinical trials.

Gram-positive organisms:

Viridans group streptococci

Gram-negative organisms:

Moraxella catarrhalis

Susceptibility Tests:

Dilution Techniques:

Quantitative methods are used to determine antimicrobial minimum inhibitory concentrations (MIC's). These MIC's provide estimates of the susceptibility of bacteria to antimicrobial compounds. The MIC's should be determined using a standardized procedure. Standardized procedures are based on a dilution method[1] (broth or agar) or equivalent with standardized inoculum concentrations and standardized concentrations of erythromycin powder. The MIC values should be interpreted according to the following criteria:

MIC (µg/mL)	Interpretation
≤0.5	Susceptible (S)
1-4	Intermediate (I)
≥8	Resistant (R)

A report of "Susceptible" indicates that the pathogen is likely to be inhibited if the antimicrobial compound in the blood reaches the concentrations usually achievable. A report of "Intermediate" indicates that the result should be considered equivocal, and, if the microorganism is not fully susceptible to alternative, clinically feasible drugs, the test should be repeated. This category implies possible clinical applicability in body sites where the drug is physiologically concentrated or in situations where high dosage of drug can be used. This category also provides a buffer zone which prevents small uncontrolled technical factors from causing major discrepancies in interpretation. A report of "Resistant" indicates that the pathogen is not likely to be inhibited if the antimicrobial compound in the blood reaches the concentrations usually achievable; other therapy should be selected.

Standardized susceptibility test procedures require the use of laboratory control microorganisms to control the technical aspects of the laboratory procedures. Standard erythromycin powder should provide the following MIC values:

Microorganism	MIC (µg/mL)
S. aureus ATCC 29213	0.12-0.5
E. faecalis ATCC 29212	1-4

Diffusion Techniques:

Quantitative methods that require measurement of zone diameters also provide reproducible estimates of the susceptibility of bacteria to antimicrobial compounds. One such standardized procedure[2] requires the use of standardized inoculum concentrations. This procedure uses paper disks impregnated with 15-µg erythromycin to test the susceptibility of microorganisms to erythromycin.

Reports from the laboratory providing results of the standard single-disk susceptibility test with a 15-µg erythromycin disk should be interpreted according to the following criteria:

Zone Diameter (mm)	Interpretation
≥23	Susceptible (S)
14-22	Intermediate (I)
≤13	Resistant (R)

Interpretation Interpretation should be as stated above for results using dilution techniques. Interpretation involves correlation of the diameter obtained in the disk test with the MIC for erythromycin.

As with standardized dilution techniques, diffusion methods require the use of laboratory control microorganisms that are used to control the technical aspects of the laboratory procedures. For the diffusion technique, the 15-µg erythromycin disk should provide the following zone diameters in these laboratory test quality control strains:

Microorganism	Zone Diameter (mm)
S. aureus ATCC 25923	22-30

INDICATIONS AND USAGE

To reduce the development of drug-resistant bacteria and maintain the effectiveness ofErythromycin Base Filmtab tablets and other antibacterial drugs, Erythromycin Base Filmtab tablets should be used only to treat or prevent infections that are proven or strongly suspected to be caused by susceptible bacteria. When culture and susceptibility information are available, they should be considered in selecting or modifying antibacterial therapy. In the absence of such data, local epidemiology and susceptibility patterns may contribute to the empiric selection of therapy.

Erythromycin Base Filmtab tablets are indicated in the treatment of infections caused by susceptible strains of the designated microorganisms in the diseases listed below:

Upper respiratory tract infections of mild to moderate degree caused by *Streptococcus pyogenes; Streptococcus pneumoniae; Haemophilus influenzae* (when used concomitantly with adequate doses of sulfonamides, since many strains of *H. influenzae* are not susceptible to the erythromycin concentrations ordinarily achieved). (See appropriate sulfonamide labeling for prescribing information.)

Lower respiratory tract infections of mild to moderate severity caused by *Streptococcus pyogenes* or *Streptococcus pneumoniae.*

Listeriosis caused by *Listeria monocytogenes.*

Respiratory tract infections due to *Mycoplasma pneumoniae.*

Skin and skin structure infections of mild to moderate severity caused by *Streptococcus pyogenes* or *Staphylococcus aureus* (resistant staphylococci may emerge during treatment).

Pertussis (whooping cough) caused by *Bordetella pertussis.* Erythromycin is effective in eliminating the organism from the nasopharynx of infected individuals, rendering them noninfectious. Some clinical studies suggest that erythromycin may be helpful in the prophylaxis of pertussis in exposed susceptible individuals.

Diphtheria: Infections due to *Corynebacterium diphtheriae,* as an adjunct to antitoxin, to prevent establishment of carriers and to eradicate the organism in carriers.

Erythrasma—In the treatment of infections due to *Corynebacterium minutissimum.*

Intestinal amebiasis caused by *Entamoeba histolytica* (oral erythromycins only). Extraenteric amebiasis requires treatment with other agents.

Acute pelvic inflammatory disease caused by *Neisseria gonorrhoeae:* Erythrocin® Lactobionate-I.V. (erythromycin lactobionate for injection, USP) followed by erythromycin base orally, as an alternative drug in treatment of acute pelvic inflammatory disease caused by *N. gonorrhoeae* in female patients with a history of sensitivity to penicillin. Patients should have a serologic test for syphilis before receiving erythromycin as treatment of gonorrhea and a follow-up serologic test for syphilis after 3 months.

Erythromycins are indicated for treatment of the following infections caused by *Chlamydia trachomatis:* conjunctivitis of the newborn, pneumonia of infancy, and urogenital infections during pregnancy. When tetracyclines are contraindi-

cated or not tolerated, erythromycin is indicated for the treatment of uncomplicated urethral, endocervical, or rectal infections in adults due to *Chlamydia trachomatis*.[3]
When tetracyclines are contraindicated or not tolerated, erythromycin is indicated for the treatment of nongonococcal urethritis caused by *Ureaplasma urealyticum*.[3]
Primary syphilis caused by *Treponema pallidum*. Erythromycin (oral forms only) is an alternative choice of treatment for primary syphilis in patients allergic to the penicillins. In treatment of primary syphilis, spinal fluid should be examined before treatment and as part of the follow-up after therapy.
Legionnaires' Disease caused by *Legionella pneumophila*. Although no controlled clinical efficacy studies have been conducted, *in vitro* and limited preliminary clinical data suggest that erythromycin may be effective in treating Legionnaires' Disease.

Prophylaxis

Prevention of Initial Attacks of Rheumatic Fever—Penicillin is considered by the American Heart Association to be the drug of choice in the prevention of initial attacks of rheumatic fever (treatment of *Streptococcus pyogenes* infections of the upper respiratory tract e.g., tonsillitis, or pharyngitis).[3] Erythromycin is indicated for the treatment of penicillin-allergic patients. The therapeutic dose should be administered for ten days.
Prevention of Recurrent Attacks of Rheumatic Fever—Penicillin or sulfonamides are considered by the American Heart Association to be the drugs of choice in the prevention of recurrent attacks of rheumatic fever. In patients who are allergic to penicillin and sulfonamides, oral erythromycin is recommended by the American Heart Association in the long-term prophylaxis of streptococcal pharyngitis (for the prevention of recurrent attacks of rheumatic fever).[3]

CONTRAINDICATIONS

Erythromycin is contraindicated in patients with known hypersensitivity to this antibiotic.
Erythromycin is contraindicated in patients taking terfenadine, astemizole, pimozide, or cisapride. (See **PRECAUTIONS**—*Drug Interactions*.)

WARNINGS

There have been reports of hepatic dysfunction, including increased liver enzymes, and hepatocellular and/or cholestatic hepatitis, with or without jaundice, occurring in patients receiving oral erythromycin products.
There have been reports suggesting that erythromycin does not reach the fetus in adequate concentration to prevent congenital syphilis. Infants born to women treated during pregnancy with oral erythromycin for early syphilis should be treated with an appropriate penicillin regimen.
Rhabdomyolysis with or without renal impairment has been reported in seriously ill patients receiving erythromycin concomitantly with lovastatin. Therefore, patients receiving concomitant lovastatin and erythromycin should be carefully monitored for creatine kinase (CK) and serum transaminase levels. (See package insert for lovastatin.)
Pseudomembranous colitis has been reported with nearly all antibacterial agents, including erythromycin, and may range in severity from mild to life threatening. Therefore, it is important to consider this diagnosis in patients who present with diarrhea subsequent to the administration of antibacterial agents.
Treatment with antibacterial agents alters the normal flora of the colon and may permit overgrowth of clostridia. Studies indicate that a toxin produced by *Clostridium difficile* is a primary cause of "antibiotic-associated colitis".
After the diagnosis of pseudomembranous colitis has been established, therapeutic measures should be initiated. Mild cases of pseudomembranous colitis usually respond to discontinuation of the drug alone. In moderate to severe cases, consideration should be given to management with fluids and electrolytes, protein supplementation, and treatment with an antibacterial drug clinically effective against *Clostridium difficile* colitis.

PRECAUTIONS

Prescribing Erythromycin Base Filmtab tablets in the absence of a proven or strongly suspected bacterial infection or a prophylactic indication is unlikely to provide benefit to the patient and increases the risk of the development of drug-resistant bacteria.
General: Since erythromycin is principally excreted by the liver, caution should be exercised when erythromycin is administered to patients with impaired hepatic function. (See **CLINICAL PHARMACOLOGY** and **WARNINGS**.)
There have been reports that erythromycin may aggravate the weakness of patients with myasthenia gravis.
There have been reports of infantile hypertrophic pyloric stenosis (IHPS) occurring in infants following erythromycin therapy. In one cohort of 157 newborns who were given erythromycin for pertussis prophylaxis, seven neonates (5%) developed symptoms of non-bilious vomiting or irritability with feeding and were subsequently diagnosed as having IHPS requiring surgical pyloromyotomy. A possible dose-response effect was described with an absolute risk of IHPS of 5.1% for infants who took erythromycin for 8-14 days and 10% for infants who took erythromycin for 15-21 days.[4] Since erythromycin may be used in the treatment of conditions in infants which are associated with significant mortality or morbidity (such as pertussis or neonatal Chlamydia trachomatis infections), the benefit of erythromycin therapy needs to be weighed against the potential risk of developing IHPS. Parents should be informed to contact their physician if vomiting or irritability with feeding occurs.
Prolonged or repeated use of erythromycin may result in an overgrowth of nonsusceptible bacteria or fungi. If superinfection occurs, erythromycin should be discontinued and appropriate therapy instituted.
When indicated, incision and drainage or other surgical procedures should be performed in conjunction with antibiotic therapy.
Information for Patients: Patients should be counseled that antibacterial drugs including Erythromycin Base Filmtab tablets should only be used to treat bacterial infections. They do not treat viral infections (e.g., the common cold). When Erythromycin Base Filmtab tablets is prescribed to treat a bacterial infection, patients should be told that although it is common to feel better early in the course of therapy, the medication should be taken exactly as directed. Skipping doses or not completing the full course of therapy may (1) decrease the effectiveness of the immediate treatment and (2) increase the likelihood that bacteria will develop resistance and will not be treatable by Erythromycin Base Filmtab tablets or other antibacterial drugs in the future.
Drug Interactions: Erythromycin use in patients who are receiving high doses of theophylline may be associated with an increase in serum theophylline levels and potential theophylline toxicity. In case of theophylline toxicity and/or elevated serum theophylline levels, the dose of theophylline should be reduced while the patient is receiving concomitant erythromycin therapy.
Concomitant administration of erythromycin and digoxin has been reported to result in elevated digoxin serum levels.
There have been reports of increased anticoagulant effects when erythromycin and oral anticoagulants were used concomitantly. Increased anticoagulation effects due to interactions of erythromycin with oral anticoagulants may be more pronounced in the elderly.
Erythromycin is a substrate and inhibitor of the 3A isoform subfamily of the cytochrome p450 enzyme system (CYP3A). Coadministration of erythromycin and a drug primarily metabolized by CYP3A may be associated with elevations in drug concentrations that could increase or prolong both the and adverse effects of the concomitant drug. Dosage adjustments may be considered, and when possible, serum concentrations of drugs primarily metabolized by CYP3A should be monitored closely in patients concurrently receiving erythromycin.
The following are examples of some clinically significant CYP3A based drug interactions. Interactions with other drugs metabolized by the CYP3A isoform are also possible. The following CYP3A based drug interactions have been observed with erythromycin products in post-marketing experience:
Ergotamine/dihydroergotamine: Concurrent use of erythromycin and ergotamine or dihydroergotamine has been associated in some patients with acute ergot toxicity characterized by severe peripheral vasospasm and dysesthesia.
Triazolobenzodiazepines (such as triazolam and alprazolam) *and related benzodiazepines:* Erythromycin has been reported to decrease the clearance of triazolam and midazolam and, thus, may increase the pharmacologic effect of these benzodiazepines.
HMG-CoA Reductase Inhibitors: Erythromycin has been reported to increase concentrations of HMG-CoA reductase inhibitors (e.g., lovastatin and simvastatin). Rare reports of rhabdomyolysis have been reported in patients taking these drugs concomitantly.
Sildenafil (Viagra): Erythromycin has been reported to increase the systemic exposure (AUC) of sildenafil. Reduction of sildenafil dosage should be considered. (See Viagra package insert.)
There have been spontaneous or published reports of CYP3A based interactions of erythromycin with cyclosporine, carbamazepine, tacrolimus, alfentanil, disopyramide, rifabutin, quinidine, methylprednisolone, cilostazol, vinblastine, and bromocriptine.
Concomitant administration of erythromycin with cisapride, pimozide, astemizole, or terfenadine is contraindicated. (See **CONTRAINDICATIONS**.)
In addition, there have been reports of interactions of erythromycin with drugs not thought to be metabolized by CYP3A, including hexobarbital, phenytoin, and valproate.
Erythromycin has been reported to significantly alter the metabolism of the nonsedating antihistamines terfenadine and astemizole when taken concomitantly. Rare cases of serious cardiovascular adverse events, including electrocardiographic QT/QT_c interval prolongation, cardiac arrest, torsades de pointes, and other ventricular arrhythmias, have been observed. (See **CONTRAINDICATIONS**.) In addition, deaths have been reported rarely with concomitant administration of terfenadine and erythromycin.
There have been post-marketing reports of drug interactions when erythromycin was coadministered with cisapride, resulting in QT prolongation, cardiac arrhythmias, ventricular tachycardia, ventricular fibrillation, and torsades de pointes, most likely due to the inhibition of hepatic metabolism of cisapride by erythromycin. Fatalities have been reported. (See **CONTRAINDICATIONS**).
Drug/Laboratory Test interactions: Erythromycin interferes with the fluorometric determination of urinary catecholamines.
Carcinogenesis, Mutagenesis, Impairment of Fertility: Long-term (2-year) oral studies conducted in rats with erythromycin base did not provide evidence of tumorigenicity. Mutagenicity studies have not been conducted. There was no apparent effect on male or female fertility in rats fed erythromycin (base) at levels up to 0.25 percent of diet.
Pregnancy: Teratogenic effects. Pregnancy Category B: There is no evidence of teratogenicity or any other adverse effect on reproduction in female rats fed erythromycin base (up to 0.25 percent of diet) prior to and during mating, during gestation, and through weaning of two successive litters. There are, however, no adequate and well-controlled studies in pregnant women. Because animal reproduction studies are not always predictive of human response, this drug should be used during pregnancy only if clearly needed.
Labor and Delivery: The effect of erythromycin on labor and delivery is unknown.
Nursing Mothers: Erythromycin is excreted in human milk. Caution should be exercised when erythromycin is administered to a nursing woman.
Pediatric Use: See **INDICATIONS AND USAGE** and **DOSAGE AND ADMINISTRATION**.

ADVERSE REACTIONS

The most frequent side effects of oral erythromycin preparations are gastrointestinal and are dose-related. They include nausea, vomiting, abdominal pain, diarrhea and anorexia. Symptoms of hepatitis, hepatic dysfunction and/or abnormal liver function test results may occur. (See **WARNINGS**.)
Onset of pseudomembranous colitis symptoms may occur during or after antibacterial treatment. (See **WARNINGS**.)
Rarely, erythromycin has been associated with the production of ventricular arrhythmias, including ventricular tachycardia and torsades de pointes, in individuals with prolonged QT interval.
Allergic reactions ranging from urticaria to anaphylaxis have occurred. Skin reactions ranging from mild eruptions to erythema multiforme, Stevens-Johnson syndrome, and toxic epidermal necrolysis have been reported rarely.
There have been isolated reports of reversible hearing loss occurring chiefly in patients with renal insufficiency and in patients receiving high doses of erythromycin.

OVERDOSAGE

In case of overdosage, erythromycin should be discontinued. Overdosage should be handled with the prompt elimination of unabsorbed drug and all other appropriate measures should be instituted.
Erythromycin is not removed by peritoneal dialysis or hemodialysis.

DOSAGE AND ADMINISTRATION

Optimal blood levels are obtained when Erythromycin Base Filmtab tablets are given in the fasting state (at least 1/2 hour and preferably 2 hours before meals).
Adults: The usual dosage of Erythromycin Base Filmtab is one 250 mg tablet four times daily in equally spaced doses or one 500 mg tablet every 12 hours. Dosage may be increased up to 4 g per day according to the severity of the infection. However, twice-a-day dosing is not recommended when doses larger than 1 g daily are administered.
Children: Age, weight, and severity of the infection are important factors in determining the proper dosage. The usual dosage is 30 to 50 mg/kg/day, in equally divided doses. For more severe infections this dosage may be doubled but should not exceed 4 g per day.
In the treatment of streptococcal infections of the upper respiratory tract (e.g., tonsillitis or pharyngitis), the therapeutic dosage of erythromycin should be administered for at least ten days.
The American Heart Association suggests a dosage of 250 mg of erythromycin orally, twice a day in long-term prophylaxis of streptococcal upper respiratory tract infections for the prevention of recurring attacks of rheumatic fever in patients allergic to penicillin and sulfonamides.[3]
Conjunctivitis of the newborn caused by *Chlamydia trachomatis:* Oral erythromycin suspension 50 mg/kg/day in 4 divided doses for at least 2 weeks.[3]
Pneumonia of infancy caused by *Chlamydia trachomatis:* Although the optimal duration of therapy has not been established, the recommended therapy is oral erythromycin suspension 50 mg/kg/day in 4 divided doses for at least 3 weeks.
Urogenital infections during pregnancy due to *Chlamydia trachomatis:* Although the optimal dose and duration of therapy have not been established, the suggested treatment is 500 mg of erythromycin by mouth four times a day on an empty stomach for at least 7 days. For women who cannot tolerate this regimen, a decreased dose of one erythromycin 500 mg tablet orally every 12 hours or 250 mg by mouth four times a day should be used for at least 14 days.[5]
For adults with uncomplicated urethral, endocervical, or rectal infections caused by *Chlamydia trachomatis,* when tetracycline is contraindicated or not tolerated: 500 mg of erythromycin by mouth four times a day for at least 7 days.[5]
For patients with nongonococcal urethritis caused by *Ureaplasma urealyticum* when tetracycline is contraindicated or not tolerated: 500 mg of erythromycin by mouth four times a day for at least seven days.[5]
Primary syphilis: 30 to 40 g given in divided doses over a period of 10 to 15 days.

Continued on next page

Erythromycin Base Filmtab—Cont.

Acute pelvic inflammatory disease caused by *N. gonorrhoeae:* 500 mg Erythrocin® Lactobionate-I.V. (erythromycin lactobionate for injection, USP) every 6 hours for 3 days, followed by 500 mg of erythromycin base orally every 12 hours for 7 days.
Intestinal amebiasis: Adults: 500 mg every 12 hours or 250 mg every 6 hours for 10 to 14 days. Children: 30 to 50 mg/kg/day in divided doses for 10 to 14 days.
Pertussis: Although optimal dosage and duration have not been established, doses of erythromycin utilized in reported clinical studies were 40 to 50 mg/kg/day, given in divided doses for 5 to 14 days.
Legionnaires' Disease: Although optimal dosage has not been established, doses utilized in reported clinical data were 1 to 4 g daily in divided doses.

HOW SUPPLIED

Erythromycin Base Filmtab tablets (erythromycin tablets, USP) are supplied as pink, unscored oval tablets in the following strengths and packages.
250 mg tablets (debossed with ▭ and EB):
Bottles of 100 .... (**NDC** 0074-6326-13);
Bottles of 500 .... (**NDC** 0074-6326-53);
ABBO-PAC® unit dose strip packages
of 100 tablets .... (**NDC** 0074-6326-11).
500 mg tablets (debossed with ▭ and EA):
Bottles of 100 .... (**NDC** 0074-6227-13).
Recommended Storage: Store below 86°F (30°C). Keep tightly closed.

REFERENCES

1. National Committee for Clinical Laboratory Standards. *Methods for Dilution Antimicrobial Susceptibility Tests for Bacteria that Grow Aerobically,* Third Edition. Approved Standard NCCLS Document M7-A3, Vol. 13, No. 25 NCCLS, Villanova, PA, December 1993.
2. National Committee for Clinical Laboratory Standards, *Performance Standards for Antimicrobial Disk Susceptibility Tests,* Fifth Edition. Approved Standard NCCLS Document M2-A5, Vol. 13, No. 24 NCCLS, Villanova, PA, December 1993.
3. Committee on Rheumatic Fever, Endocarditis, and Kawasaki Disease of the Council on Cardiovascular Disease in the Young, the American Heart Association: Prevention of Rheumatic Fever. *Circulation.* 78(4):1082-1086, October 1988.
4. Honein, M.A. et. al.: Infantile hypertrophic pyloric stenosis after pertussis prophylaxis with erythromycin: a case review and cohort study. *The Lancet* 1999; 354 (9196): 2101-5.
5. Data on file, Abbott Laboratories.

FILMTAB—Film-sealed tablets, Abbott.
03-5245-R5
Revised: July, 2003
ABBOTT LABORATORIES
NORTH CHICAGO, IL 60064, U.S.A.
PRINTED IN U.S.A.

ERYTHROMYCIN DELAYED-RELEASE CAPSULES, USP ℞

℞ only

To reduce the development of drug-resistant bacteria and maintain the effectiveness of Erythromycin Delayed-release Capsules and other antibacterial drugs, Erythromycin Delayed-release Capsules should be used only to treat or prevent infections that are proven or strongly suspected to be caused by bacteria.

DESCRIPTION

Erythromycin Delayed-release Capsules contain enteric-coated pellets of erythromycin base for oral administration. Each Erythromycin Delayed-release Capsule contains 250 milligrams of erythromycin base.

Inactive Ingredients:

Cellulosic polymers, citrate ester, D&C Red No. 30, D&C Yellow No. 10, magnesium stearate and povidone. The capsule shell contains FD&C Blue No. 1, FD&C Red No. 3, gelatin, and titanium dioxide.
Erythromycin is produced by a strain of *Saccharopolyspora erythaea* (formerly *Streptomyces erythraeus*) and belongs to the macrolide group of antibiotics. It is basic and readily forms salts with acids but it is the base is microbiologically active. Erythromycin base is (3R*, 4S*, 5S*, 6R*, 7R*, 9R*, 11R*, 12R*, 13S*, 14R*)-4-[(2,6-Dideoxy-3-C-methyl-3-O-methyl-α-L-*ribo*-hexopyranosyl)oxy]-14-ethyl-7,12,13-trihydroxy-3,5,7,9,11,13-hexamethyl-6-[[3,4,6-trideoxy-3-(dimethylamino)-β-D-*xylo*-hexopyranosyl]oxy]oxacyclotetradecane-2,10-dione. The structural formula is:
[See chemical structure at top of next column]

CLINICAL PHARMACOLOGY

Orally administered erythromycin base and its salts are readily absorbed in the microbiologically active form. Interindividual variations in the absorption of erythromycin are, however, observed, and some patients do not achieve acceptable serum levels. Erythromycin is largely bound to plasma proteins, and the freely dissociating bound fraction after administration of erythromycin base represents 90% of the total erythromycin absorbed. After absorption, erythromycin

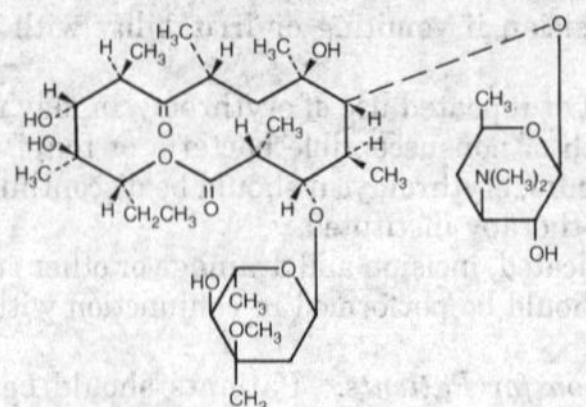

$C_{37}H_{67}NO_{13}$ MW 734

diffuses readily into most body fluids. In the absence of meningeal inflammation, low concentrations are normally achieved in the spinal fluid, but the passage of the drug across the blood-brain barrier increases in meningitis.
The drug is excreted in human milk. The drug crosses the placental barrier, but plasma levels are low. Erythromycin is not removed by peritoneal dialysis or hemodialysis.
In the presence of normal hepatic function erythromycin is concentrated in the liver and is excreted in the bile; the effect of hepatic dysfunction on biliary excretion of erythromycin is not known. After oral administration, less than 5% of the administered dose can be recovered in the active form in the urine.
The enteric coating of pellets in Erythromycin Delayed-release Capsules protects the erythromycin base from inactivation by gastric acidity. Because of their small size and enteric coating, the pellets readily pass intact from the stomach to the small intestine and dissolve efficiently to allow absorption of erythromycin in a uniform manner. After administration of a single dose of a 250 mg Erythromycin Delayed-release Capsule, peak serum levels in the range of 1.13 to 1.68 mcg/mL are attained in approximately 3 hours and decline to 0.30-0.42 mcg/mL in 6 hours. Optimal conditions for stability in the presence of gastric secretion and for complete absorption are attained when erythromycin is taken on an empty stomach.

Microbiology:

Erythromycin acts by inhibition of protein synthesis by binding 50 *S* ribosomal subunits of susceptible organisms. It does not affect nucleic acid synthesis. Antagonism has been demonstrated *in vitro* between erythromycin and clindamycin, lincomycin, and chloramphenicol.
Many strains of *Haemophilus influenzae* are resistant to erythromycin alone but are susceptible to erythromycin and sulfonamides used concomitantly.
Staphylococci resistant to erythromycin may emerge during a course of therapy.
Erythromycin has been shown to be active against most strains of the following microorganisms, both *in vitro* and in clinical infections as described in the **INDICATIONS AND USAGE** section.

Gram-positive Organisms:
Corynebacterium diphtheriae
Corynebacterium minutissimum
Listeria monocytogenes
Staphylococcus aureus (resistant organisms may emerge during treatment)
Streptococcus pneumoniae
Streptococcus pyogenes

Gram-negative Organisms:
Bordetella pertussis
Legionella pneumophila
Neisseria gonorrhoeae

Other Microorganisms:
Chlamydia trachomatis
Entamoeba histolytica
Mycoplasma pneumoniae
Treponema pallidum
Ureaplasma urealyticum

Susceptibility Tests:

Dilution Techniques:
Quantitative methods are used to determine antimicrobial minimum inhibitory concentrations (MIC's). These MIC's provide estimates of the susceptibility of bacteria to antimicrobial compounds. The MIC's should be determined using a standardized procedure. Standardized procedures are based on a dilution method[1] (broth or agar) or equivalent with standardized inoculum concentrations and standardized concentrations of erythromycin powder. The MIC values should be interpreted according to the following criteria:

MIC (µg/mL)	Interpretation
≤0.5	Susceptible (S)
1-4	Intermediate (I)
≥8	Resistant (R)

A report of "Susceptible" indicates that the pathogen is likely to be inhibited if the antimicrobial compound in the blood reaches the concentrations usually achievable. A report of "Intermediate" indicates that the result should be considered equivocal, and, if the microorganism is not fully susceptible to alternative, clinically feasible drugs, the test should be repeated. This category implies possible clinical applicability in body sites where the drug is physiologically concentrated or in situations where high dosage of drug can be used. This category also provides a buffer zone which prevents small uncontrolled technical factors from causing major discrepancies in interpretation. A report of "Resistant" indicates that the pathogen is not likely to be inhibited if the antimicrobial compound in the blood reaches the concentrations usually achievable; other therapy should be selected.
Standardized susceptibility test procedures require the use of laboratory control microorganisms to control the technical aspects of the laboratory procedures. Standard erythromycin powder should provide the following MIC values:

Microorganism	MIC (µg/mL)
S. aureus ATCC 29213	0.12-0.5

Diffusion Techniques:

Quantitative methods that require measurement of zone diameters also provide reproducible estimates of the susceptibility of bacteria to antimicrobial compounds. One such standardized procedure[2] requires the use of standardized inoculum concentrations. This procedure uses paper disks impregnated with 15-µg erythromycin to test the susceptibility of microorganisms to erythromycin.
Reports from the laboratory providing results of the standard single-disk susceptibility test with a 15-µg erythromycin disk should be interpreted according to the following criteria:

Zone Diameter (mm)	Interpretation
≥23	Susceptible (S)
14-22	Intermediate (I)
≤13	Resistant (R)

Interpretation should be as stated above for results using dilution techniques. Interpretation involves correlation of the diameter obtained in the disk test with the MIC for erythromycin.
As with standardized dilution techniques, diffusion methods require the use of laboratory control microorganisms that are used to control the technical aspects of the laboratory procedures. For the diffusion technique, the 15-µg erythromycin disk should provide the following zone diameters in these laboratory test quality control strains:

Microorganism	Zone Diameter (mm)
S. aureus ATCC 25923	22-30

INDICATIONS AND USAGE

To reduce the development of drug-resistant bacteria and maintain the effectiveness of Erythromycin Delayed-release Capsules and other antibacterial drugs, Erythromycin Delayed-release Capsules should be used only to treat or prevent infections that are proven or strongly suspected to be caused by susceptible bacteria. When culture and susceptibility information are available, they should be considered in selecting or modifying antibacterial therapy.
In the absence of such data, local epidemiology and susceptibility patterns may contribute to the empiric selection of therapy.
Erythromycin is indicated in the treatment of infections caused by susceptible strains of the designated microorganisms in the diseases listed below:
Upper respiratory tract infections of mild to moderate degree caused by *Streptococcus pyogenes, Streptococcus pneumoniae,* or *Haemophilus influenzae* (when used concomitantly with adequate doses of sulfonamides, since many strains of *H. influenzae* are not susceptible to the erythromycin concentrations ordinarily achieved). (See appropriate sulfonamide labeling for prescribing information.)
Lower-respiratory tract infections of mild to moderate severity caused by *Streptococcus pneumoniae* or *Streptococcus pyogenes.*
Listeriosis caused by *Listeria monocytogenes.*
Pertussis (whooping cough) caused by *Bordetella pertussis.* Erythromycin is effective in eliminating the organism from the nasopharynx of infected individuals rendering them noninfectious. Some clinical studies suggest that erythromycin may be helpful in the prophylaxis of pertussis in exposed susceptible individuals.
Respiratory tract infections due to *Mycoplasma pneumoniae.*
Skin and skin structure infections of mild to moderate severity caused by *Streptococcus pyogenes* or *Staphylococcus aureus* (resistant staphylococci may emerge during treatment).
Diphtheria: Infections due to *Corynebacterium diphtheria,* as an adjunct to antitoxin, to prevent establishment of carriers and to eradicate the organism in carriers.
Erythrasma: In the treatment of infections due to *Corynebacterium minutissimum.*
Syphilis caused by *Treponema pallidum*: Erythromycin is an alternate choice of treatment for primary syphilis in penicillin-allergic patients. In treatment of primary syphilis, spinal fluid examinations should be done before treatment and as part of follow-up after therapy.
Intestinal amebiasis caused by *Entamoeba histolytica* (oral erythromycins only). Extraenteric amebiasis requires treatment with other agents.
Acute pelvic inflammatory disease caused by *Neisseria gonorrhoeae*: Erythromycin lactobionate for injection, USP followed by erythromycin base orally as an alternative drug in treatment of acute pelvic inflammatory disease caused by

N. gonorrhoeae in female patients with a history of sensitivity to penicillin. Patients should have a serologic test for syphilis before receiving erythromycin as treatment of gonorrhea and a follow-up serologic test for syphilis after 3 months.

Erythromycins are indicated for the treatment of the following infections caused by *Chlamydia trachomatis*: conjunctivitis of the newborn, pneumonia of infancy, and urogenital infections during pregnancy. When tetracyclines are contraindicated or not tolerated, erythromycin is indicated for the treatment of uncomplicated urethral, endocervical, or rectal infections in adults due to *Chlamydia trachomatis*.

When tetracyclines are contraindicated or not tolerated, erythromycin is indicated for the treatment of nongonococcal urethritis caused by *Ureaplasma urealyticum*.

Legionnaires' Disease caused by *Legionella pneumophila*. Although no controlled clinical efficacy studies have been conducted, *in vitro* and limited preliminary clinical data suggest that erythromycin may be effective in treating Legionnaires' Disease.

Prophylaxis:

Prevention of Initial Attacks of Rheumatic Fever: Penicillin is considered by the American Heart Association to be the drug of choice in the prevention of initial attacks of rheumatic fever (treatment of *Streptococcus pyogenes* infections of the upper respiratory tract, e.g., tonsillitis or pharyngitis). Erythromycin is indicated for the treatment of penicillin-allergic patients.[3] The therapeutic dose should be administered for 10 days.

Prevention of Recurrent Attacks of Rheumatic Fever: Penicillin or sulfonamides are considered by the American Heart Association to be the drugs of choice in the prevention of recurrent attacks of rheumatic fever. In patients who are allergic to penicillin and sulfonamides, oral erythromycin is recommended by the American Heart Association in the long-term prophylaxis of streptococcal pharyngitis (for the prevention of recurrent attacks of rheumatic fever).[3]

CONTRAINDICATIONS

Erythromycin is contraindicated in patients with known hypersensitivity to this antibiotic.

Erythromycin is contraindicated in patients taking terfenadine, astemizole, pimozide, or cisapride. (See **PRECAUTIONS-Drug Interactions.**)

WARNINGS

There have been reports of hepatic dysfunction, including increased liver enzymes, and hepatocellular and/or cholestatic hepatitis, with or without jaundice, occurring in patients receiving oral erythromycin products.

There have been reports suggesting that erythromycin does not reach the fetus in adequate concentration to prevent congenital syphilis. Infants born to women treated during pregnancy with oral erythromycin for early syphilis should be treated with an appropriate penicillin regimen.

Rhabdomyolysis with or without renal impairment has been reported in seriously ill patients receiving erythromycin concomitantly with lovastatin. Therefore, patients receiving concomitant lovastatin and erythromycin should be carefully monitored for creatine kinase (CK) and serum transaminase levels. (See package insert for lovastatin.)

Pseudomembranous colitis has been reported with nearly all antibacterial agents, including erythromycin, and may range in severity from mild to life threatening. Therefore, it is important to consider this diagnosis in patients who present with diarrhea subsequent to the administration of antibacterial agents.

Treatment with antibacterial agents alters the normal flora of the colon and may permit overgrowth of clostridia. Studies indicate that a toxin produced by *Clostridium difficile* is one primary cause of "antibiotic-associated colitis".

After the diagnosis of pseudomembranous colitis has been established, therapeutic measures should be initiated. Mild cases of pseudomembranous colitis usually respond to drug discontinuation alone. In moderate to severe cases, consideration should be given to management with fluids and electrolytes, protein supplementation, and treatment with an antibacterial drug clinically effective against *Clostridium difficile colitis*.

PRECAUTIONS

Prescribing Erythromycin Delayed-release Capsules in the absence of a proven or strongly suspected bacterial infection or a prophylactic indication is unlikely to provide benefit to the patient and increases the risk of the development of drug-resistant bacteria.

General: Since erythromycin is principally excreted by the liver, caution should be exercised when erythromycin is administered to patients with impaired hepatic function. (See **CLINICAL PHARMACOLOGY** and **WARNINGS.**)

There have been reports that erythromycin may aggravate the weakness of patients with myasthenia gravis.

There have been reports of infantile hypertrophic pyloric stenosis (IHPS) occurring in infants following erythromycin therapy. In one cohort of 157 newborns who were given erythromycin for pertussis prophylaxis, seven neonates (5%) developed symptoms of non-bilious vomiting or irritability with feeding and were subsequently diagnosed as having IHPS requiring surgical pyloromyotomy. A possible dose-response effect was described with an absolute risk of IHPS of 5.1% for infants who took erythromycin for 8-14 days and 10% for infants who took erythromycin for 15-21 days.[4]

Since erythromycin may be used in the treatment of conditions in infants which are associated with significant mortality or morbidity (such as pertussis or neonatal Chlamydia trachomatis infections), the benefit of erythromycin therapy needs to be weighed against the potential risk of developing IHPS. Parents should be informed to contact their physician if vomiting or irritability with feeding occurs.

Prolonged or repeated use of erythromycin may result in an overgrowth of nonsusceptible bacteria or fungi. If superinfection occurs, erythromycin should be discontinued and appropriate therapy instituted.

When indicated, incision and drainage or other surgical procedures should be performed in conjunction with antibiotic therapy.

Information for Patients: Patients should be counseled that antibacterial drugs including Erythromycin Delayed-release Capsules should only be used to treat bacterial infections. They do not treat viral infections (e.g., the common cold). When Erythromycin Delayed-release Capsules is prescribed to treat a bacterial infection, patients should be told that although it is common to feel better early in the course of therapy, the medication should be taken exactly as directed.

Skipping doses or not completing the full course of therapy may (1) decrease the effectiveness of the immediate treatment and (2) increase the likelihood that bacteria will develop resistance and will not be treatable by Erythromycin Delayed-release Capsules or other antibacterial drugs in the future.

Drug Interactions: Erythromycin use in patients who are receiving high doses of theophylline may be associated with an increase in serum theophylline levels and potential theophylline toxicity. In case of theophylline toxicity and/or elevated serum theophylline levels, the dose of theophylline should be reduced while the patient is receiving concomitant erythromycin therapy.

Concomitant administration of erythromycin and digoxin has been reported to result in elevated digoxin serum levels.

There have been reports of increased anticoagulant effects when erythromycin and oral anticoagulants were used concomitantly. Increased anticoagulation effects due to interactions of erythromycin with various oral anticoagulants may be more pronounced in the elderly.

Erythromycin is a substrate and inhibitor of the 3A isoform subfamily of the cytochrome P450 enzyme system (CYP3A). Coadministration of erythromycin and a drug primarily metabolized by CYP3A may be associated with elevations in drug concentrations that could increase or prolong both the therapeutic and adverse effects of the concomitant drug. Dosage adjustments may be considered, and when possible, serum concentrations of drugs primarily metabolized by CYP3A should be monitored closely in patients concurrently receiving erythromycin.

The following are examples of some clinically significant CYP3A based drug interactions. Interactions with other drugs metabolized by the CYP3A isoform are also possible. The following CYP3A based drug interactions have been observed with erythromycin products in post-marketing experience:

Ergotamine/dihydroergotamine: Concurrent use of erythromycin and ergotamine or dihydroergotamine has been associated in some patients with acute ergot toxicity characterized by severe peripheral vasospasm and dysesthesia.

Triazolobenzodiazepines (such as triazolam and alprazolam) *and related benzodiazepines*: Erythromycin has been reported to decrease the clearance of triazolam and midazolam, and thus, may increase the pharmacologic effect of these benzodiazepines.

HMG-CoA Reductase Inhibitors: Erythromycin has been reported to increase concentrations of HMG-CoA reductase inhibitors (e.g., lovastatin and simvastatin). Rare reports of rhabdomyolysis have been reported in patients taking these drugs concomitantly.

Sildenafil (Viagra): Erythromycin has been reported to increase the systemic exposure (AUC) of sildenafil. Reduction of sildenafil dosage should be considered. (See Viagra package insert.)

There have been spontaneous or published reports of CYP3A based interactions of erythromycin with cyclosporine, carbamazepine, tacrolimus, alfentanil, disopyramide, rifabutin, quinidine, methylprednisolone, cilostazol, vinblastine, and bromocriptine.

Concomitant administration of erythromycin with cisapride, pimozide, astemizole, or terfenadine is contraindicated. (See **CONTRAINDICATIONS.**)

In addition, there have been reports of interactions of erythromycin with drugs not thought to be metabolized by CYP3A, including hexobarbital, phenytoin, and valproate.

Erythromycin has been reported to significantly alter the metabolism of the nonsedating antihistamines terfenadine and astemizole when taken concomitantly. Rare cases of serious cardiovascular adverse events, including electrocardiographic QT/QTc interval prolongation, cardiac arrest, torsades de pointes, and other ventricular arrhythmias have been observed. (See **CONTRAINDICATIONS.**) In addition, deaths have been reported rarely with concomitant administration of terfenadine and erythromycin.

There have been post-marketing reports of drug interactions when erythromycin was coadministered with cisapride, resulting in QT prolongation, cardiac arrhythmias, ventricular tachycardia, ventricular fibrillation, and torsades de pointes most likely due to the inhibition of hepatic metabolism of cisapride by erythromycin. Fatalities have been reported. (See **CONTRAINDICATIONS.**)

Drug/Laboratory Test interactions: Erythromycin interferes with the fluorometric determination of urinary catecholamines.

Carcinogenesis, Mutagenesis, Impairment of Fertility: Long-term (2-year) oral studies conducted in rats with erythromycin ethylsuccinate and erythromycin base did not provide evidence of tumorigenicity. Mutagenicity studies have not been conducted. There was no apparent effect on male or female fertility in rats fed erythromycin (base) at levels up to 0.25 percent of diet.

Pregnancy: *Teratogenic effects. Pregnancy Category B:* There is no evidence of teratogenicity or any other adverse effect on reproduction in female rats fed erythromycin base (up to 0.25 percent of diet) prior to and during mating, during gestation, and through weaning of two successive litters. There are, however, no adequate and well-controlled studies in pregnant women. Because animal reproduction studies are not always predictive of human response, this drug should be used during pregnancy only if clearly needed.

Labor and Delivery: The effect of erythromycin on labor and delivery is unknown.

Nursing Mothers: Erythromycin is excreted in human milk. Caution should be exercised when erythromycin is administered to a nursing woman.

Pediatric Use: See **INDICATIONS AND USAGE** and **DOSAGE AND ADMINISTRATION** sections.

ADVERSE REACTIONS

The most frequent side effects of oral erythromycin preparations are gastrointestinal and are dose-related. They include nausea, vomiting, abdominal pain, diarrhea and anorexia. Symptoms of hepatitis, hepatic dysfunction and/or abnormal liver function test results may occur. Onset of pseudomembranous colitis symptoms may occur during or after antibacterial treatment. (See **WARNINGS.**)

Erythromycin has been associated with QT prolongation and ventricular arrhythmias, including ventricular tachycardia and torsades de pointes.

Allergic reactions ranging from urticaria to anaphylaxis have occurred. Skin reactions ranging from mild eruptions to erythema multiforme, Stevens-Johnson syndrome, and toxic epidermal necrolysis have been reported rarely.

There have been rare reports of pancreatitis and convulsions.

There have been isolated reports of reversible hearing loss occurring chiefly in patients with renal insufficiency and in patients receiving high doses of erythromycin.

OVERDOSAGE

In case of overdosage, erythromycin should be discontinued. Overdosage should be handled with the prompt elimination of unabsorbed drug and all other appropriate measures.

Erythromycin is not removed by peritoneal dialysis or hemodialysis.

DOSAGE AND ADMINISTRATION

Erythromycin is well absorbed and may be given without regard to meals. Optimum blood levels are obtained in a fasting state (administration at least one half hour and preferably two hours before or after a meal); however, blood levels obtained upon administration of enteric-coated erythromycin products in the presence of food are still above minimal inhibitory concentrations (MICs) of most organisms for which erythromycin is indicated.

ADULTS: The usual dose is 250 mg every 6 hours taken one hour before meals. If twice-a-day dosage is desired, the recommended dose is 500 mg every 12 hours. Dosage may be increased up to 4 grams per day, according to the severity of infection. Twice-a-day dosing is not recommended when doses larger than 1 gram daily are administered.

CHILDREN: Age, weight, and severity of the infection are important factors in determining the proper dosage. The usual dosage is 30 to 50 mg/kg/day, in divided doses. For the treatment of more severe infections, this dose may be doubled.

Streptococcal infections: A therapeutic dosage of oral erythromycin should be administered for at least 10 days. For continuous prophylaxis against recurrences of streptococcal infections in persons with a history of rheumatic heart disease, the dose is 250 mg twice a day.

Primary syphilis: 30 to 40 grams given in divided doses over a period of 10-15 days.

Intestinal amebiasis: 250 mg four times daily for 10 to 14 days for adults; 30 to 50 mg/kg/day in divided doses for 10 to 14 days for children.

Legionnaires' Disease: Although optimal doses have not been established, doses utilized in reported clinical data were those recommended above (1 to 4 grams daily in divided doses).

Urogenital infections during pregnancy due to *Chlamydia trachomatis*: Although the optimal dose and duration of therapy have not been established, the suggested treatment is erythromycin 500 mg, by mouth, 4 times a day on an empty stomach for at least 7 days. For women who cannot tolerate this regimen, a decreased dose of 250 mg, by mouth, 4 times a day should be used for at least 14 days.

For adults with uncomplicated urethral, endocervical, or rectal infections caused by *Chlamydia trachomatis* in whom tetracyclines are contraindicated or not tolerated: 500 mg, by mouth, 4 times a day for at least 7 days.

Pertussis: Although optimum dosage and duration of therapy have not been established, doses of erythromycin utilized in reported clinical studies were 40-50 mg/kg/day, given in divided doses for 5 to 14 days.

Continued on next page

Erythromycin Delayed-Rel.—Cont.

Nongonococcal urethritis due to *Ureaplasma urealyticum*: When tetracycline is contraindicated or not tolerated: 500 mg of erythromycin, orally, four times daily for at least 7 days.
Acute pelvic inflammatory disease due to *N. gonorrhoeae*: 500 mg IV of erythromycin lactobionate for injection, USP every 6 hours for 3 days followed by 250 mg of erythromycin, orally every 6 hours for 7 days.

HOW SUPPLIED

Erythromycin Delayed-release Capsules, USP, are clear and opaque maroon capsules bearing the corporate logo and Abbo-Code ER with pink and yellow particles containing 250 mg of erythromycin supplied in bottles of 100 (**NDC** 0074-6301-13) and 500 (**NDC** 0074-6301-53).
Recommended Storage: Store below 86°F (30°C). Protect from moisture and excessive heat.

REFERENCES

1. National Committee for Clinical Laboratory Standards. *Methods for Dilution Antimicrobial Susceptibility Tests for Bacteria that Grow Aerobically*, Third Edition. Approved Standard NCCLS Document M7-A3, Vol. 13, No. 25 NCCLS, Villanova, PA, December 1993.
2. National Committee for Clinical Laboratory Standards, *Performance Standards for Antimicrobial Disk Susceptibility Tests*, Fifth Edition. Approved Standard NCCLS Document M2-A5, Vol. 13, No. 24 NCCLS, Villanova, PA, December 1993.
3. Committee on Rheumatic Fever , Endocarditis, and Kawasaki Disease of the Council on Cardiovascular Disease in the Young, the American Heart Association: Prevention of Rheumatic Fever. Special Report *Circulation*. 78(4): 1082-1086, October 1988.
4. Honein, M.A., et. al.: Infantile hypertrophic pyloric stenosis after pertussis prophylaxis with erythromycin: a case review and cohort study. The Lancet 1999; 354 (9196): 2101-5.

03-5261-R5-Revised August, 2003
ABBOTT LABORATORIES
NORTH CHICAGO,IL 60064, U.S.A.
PRINTED IN U.S.A.

Shown in Product Identification Guide, page 303

GENGRAF® Capsules ℞

[jĕn-grăf]
(cyclosporine capsules, USP [MODIFIED])
℞ only

> **WARNING**
> Only physicians experienced in the management of systemic immunosuppressive therapy for the indicated disease should prescribe Gengraf® (cyclosporine capsules, USP **[MODIFIED]**). At doses used in solid organ transplantation, only physicians experienced in immunosuppressive therapy and management of organ transplant recipients should prescribe Gengraf®. Patients receiving the drug should be managed in facilities equipped and staffed with adequate laboratory and supportive medical resources. The physician responsible for maintenance therapy should have complete information requisite for the follow-up of the patient.
> Gengraf®, a systemic immunosuppressant, may increase the susceptibility to infection and the development of neoplasia. In kidney, liver, and heart transplant patients Gengraf® may be administered with other immunosuppressive agents. Increased susceptibility to infection and the possible development of lymphoma and other neoplasms may result from the increase in the degree of immunosuppression in transplant patients.

> Gengraf® (cyclosporine capsules, USP **[MODIFIED]**) has increased bioavailability in comparison to Sandimmune®* (cyclosporine capsules, USP **[NON-MODIFIED]**). Gengraf® and Sandimmune®* are not bioequivalent and cannot be used interchangeably without physician supervision. For a given trough concentration, cyclosporine exposure will be greater with Gengraf® than with Sandimmune®*. If a patient who is receiving exceptionally high doses of Sandimmune®* is converted to Gengraf®, particular caution should be exercised. Cyclosporine blood concentrations should be monitored in transplant and rheumatoid arthritis patients taking Gengraf® to avoid toxicity due to high concentrations. Dose adjustments should be made in transplant patients to minimize possible organ rejection due to low concentrations. Comparison of blood concentrations in the published literature with blood concentrations obtained using current assays must be done with detailed knowledge of the assay methods employed.

> **For Psoriasis Patients (*see also* Boxed WARNINGS *above*)**
> Psoriasis patients previously treated with PUVA and to a lesser extent, methotrexate or other immunosuppressive agents, UVB, coal tar, or radiation therapy, are at an increased risk of developing skin malignancies when taking Gengraf® (cyclosporine capsules, USP **[MODIFIED]**).
> Cyclosporine, the active ingredient in Gengraf®, in recommended dosages, can cause systemic hypertension and nephrotoxicity. The risk increases with increasing dose and duration of cyclosporine therapy. Renal dysfunction, including structural kidney damage, is a potential consequence of cyclosporine, and therefore, renal function must be monitored during therapy.

DESCRIPTION

Gengraf® (cyclosporine capsules, USP **[MODIFIED]**) is a modified oral formulation of cyclosporine that forms an aqueous dispersion in an aqueous environment.
Cyclosporine, the active principle in Gengraf®, is a cyclic polypeptide immunosuppressant agent consisting of 11 amino acids. It is produced as a metabolite by the fungus species *Aphanocladium album*.
Chemically, cyclosporine is designated as [R-[R*, R*-(E)]]-cyclic-(L-alanyl-D-alanyl-*N*-methyl-L-leucyl-*N*-methyl-L-leucyl-*N*-methyl-L-valyl-3-hydroxy-*N*,4-dimethyl-L-2-amino-6-octenoyl-L-α-amino-butyryl-*N*-methylglycyl-*N*-methyl-L-leucyl-L-valyl-*N*-methyl-L-leucyl).
Gengraf® Capsules (cyclosporine capsules, USP **[MODIFIED]**) are available in 25 mg and 100 mg strengths.
Each 25 mg capsule contains: cyclosporine, 25 mg, alcohol, USP, absolute, 12.8% v/v (10.1% wt/vol.).
Each 100 mg capsule contains: cyclosporine, 100 mg, alcohol, USP, absolute, 12.8% v/v (10.1% wt/vol.).
Inactive Ingredients: FD&C Blue No. 2, gelatin NF, polyethylene glycol NF, polyoxyl 35 castor oil NF, polysorbate 80 NF, propylene glycol USP, sorbitan monooleate NF, titanium dioxide.
The chemical structure for cyclosporine USP is:

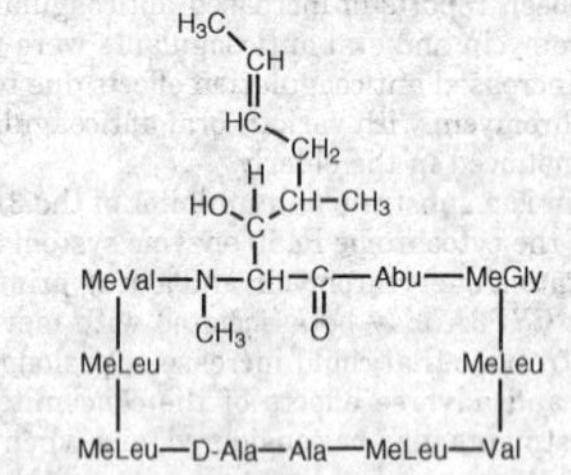

$C_{62}H_{111}N_{11}O_{12}$ Mol. Wt. 1202.64

CLINICAL PHARMACOLOGY

Cyclosporine is a potent immunosuppressive agent that in animals prolongs survival of allogeneic transplants involving skin, kidney, liver, heart, pancreas, bone marrow, small intestine, and lung. Cyclosporine has been demonstrated to suppress some humoral immunity and to a greater extent, cell-mediated immune reactions such as allograft rejection, delayed hypersensitivity, experimental allergic encephalomyelitis, Freund's adjuvant arthritis, and graft vs. host disease in many animal species for a variety of organs.
The effectiveness of cyclosporine results from specific and reversible inhibition of immunocompetent lymphocytes in the G_0- and G_1-phase of the cell cycle. T-lymphocytes are preferentially inhibited. The T-helper cell is the main target, although the T-suppressor cell may also be suppressed. Cyclosporine also inhibits lymphokine production and release including interleukin-2.
No effects on phagocytic function (changes in enzyme secretions, chemotactic migration of granulocytes, macrophage migration, carbon clearance *in vivo*) have been detected in animals. Cyclosporine does not cause bone marrow suppression in animal models or man.

Pharmacokinetics: The immunosuppressive activity of cyclosporine is primarily due to parent drug. Following oral administration, absorption of cyclosporine is incomplete. The extent of absorption of cyclosporine is dependent on the individual patient, the patient population, and the formulation. Elimination of cyclosporine is primarily biliary with only 6% of the dose (parent drug and metabolites) excreted in urine. The disposition of cyclosporine from blood is generally biphasic, with a terminal half-life of approximately 8.4 hours (range 5 to 18 hours). Following intravenous administration, the blood clearance of cyclosporine (assay: HPLC) is approximately 5 to 7 mL/min/kg in adult recipients of renal or liver allografts. Blood cyclosporine clearance appears to be slightly slower in cardiac transplant patients.
The Gengraf® Capsules (cyclosporine capsules, USP **[MODIFIED]**) and Gengraf® Oral Solution (cyclosporine oral solution, USP **[MODIFIED]**) are bioequivalent.
The relationship between administered dose and exposure (area under the concentration versus time curve, AUC) is linear within the therapeutic dose range. The intersubject variability (total, % CV) of cyclosporine exposure (AUC) when cyclosporine **(MODIFIED)** or cyclosporine **(NON-MODIFIED)** is administered ranges from approximately 20% to 50% in renal transplant patients. This intersubject variability contributes to the need for individualization of the dosing regimen for optimal therapy (*see DOSAGE AND ADMINISTRATION*). Intrasubject variability of AUC in renal transplant recipients (% CV) was 9%–21% for cyclosporine **(MODIFIED)** and 19%–26% for cyclosporine **(NON-MODIFIED)**. In the same studies, intrasubject variability of trough concentrations (% CV) was 17%–30% for cyclosporine **(MODIFIED)** and 16%-38% for cyclosporine **(NON-MODIFIED)**.

Absorption: Cyclosporine **(MODIFIED)** has increased bioavailability compared to cyclosporine **(NON-MODIFIED)**. The absolute bioavailability of cyclosporine administered as Sandimmune®* (cyclosporine **[NON-MODIFIED]**) is dependent on the patient population, estimated to be less than 10% in liver transplant patients and as great as 89% in some renal transplant patients. The absolute bioavailability of cyclosporine administered as cyclosporine **(MODIFIED)** has not been determined in adults. In studies of renal transplant, rheumatoid arthritis and psoriasis patients, the mean cyclosporine AUC was approximately 20% to 50% greater and the peak blood cyclosporine concentration (C_{max}) was approximately 40% to 106% greater following administration of cyclosporine **(MODIFIED)** compared to following administration of cyclosporine **(NON-MODIFIED)**. The dose normalized AUC in *de novo* liver transplant patients administered cyclosporine **(MODIFIED)** 28 days after transplantation was 50% greater and C_{max} was 90% greater than in those patients administered cyclosporine **(NON-MODIFIED)**. AUC and C_{max} are also increased cyclosporine **(MODIFIED)** relative to cyclosporine **(NON-MODIFIED)** in heart transplant patients, but data are very limited. Although the AUC and C_{max} values are higher on cyclosporine **(MODIFIED)** relative to cyclosporine **(NON-MODIFIED)**, the pre-dose trough concentrations (dose-normalized) are similar for the two formulations.
Following oral administration of cyclosporine **(MODIFIED)**, the time to peak blood cyclosporine concentration (T_{max}) ranged from 1.5 to 2.0 hours. The administration of food with cyclosporine **(MODIFIED)** decreases the cyclosporine AUC and C_{max}. A high fat meal (669 kcal, 45 grams fat) consumed within one-half hour before cyclosporine **(MODIFIED)** administration decreased the AUC by 13% and C_{max} by 33%. The effects of a low fat meal (667 kcal, 15 grams fat) were similar.
The effect of T-tube diversion of bile on the absorption of cyclosporine from cyclosporine **(MODIFIED)** was investigated in eleven *de novo* liver transplant patients. When the patients were administered cyclosporine **(MODIFIED)** with and without T-tube diversion of bile, very little difference in absorption was observed, as measured by the change in maximal cyclosporine blood concentrations from pre-dose values with the T-tube closed relative to when it was open: 6.9±41% (range −55% to 68%).
[See first table at top of next page]

Distribution: Cyclosporine is distributed largely outside the blood volume. The steady state volume of distribution during intravenous dosing has been reported as 3–5 L/kg in solid organ transplant recipients. In blood, the distribution is concentration dependent. Approximately 33%–47% is in plasma, 4%–9% in lymphocytes, 5%–12% in granulocytes, and 41%–58% in erythrocytes. At high concentrations, the binding capacity of leukocytes and erythrocytes becomes saturated. In plasma, approximately 90% is bound to proteins, primarily lipoproteins. Cyclosporine is excreted in human milk (*see PRECAUTIONS, Nursing Mothers*).

Metabolism: Cyclosporine is extensively metabolized by the cytochrome P-450 III-A enzyme system in the liver, and to a lesser degree in the gastrointestinal tract, and the kidney. The metabolism of cyclosporine can be altered by the coadministration of a variety of agents (*see PRECAUTIONS, Drug Interactions*). At least 25 metabolites have been identified from human bile, feces, blood, and urine. The biological activity of the metabolites and their contributions to toxicity are considerably less than those of the parent compound. The major metabolites (M1, M9, and M4N) result from oxidation at the 1-beta, 9-gamma, and 4-N-demethylated positions, respectively. At steady state following the oral administration of cyclosporine **(NON-MODIFIED)**, the mean AUCs for blood concentrations of M1, M9 and M4N are about 70%, 21%, and 7.5% of the AUC for blood cyclosporine concentrations, respectively. Based on blood concentration data from stable renal transplant patients (13 patients administered cyclosporine **(MODIFIED)** and cyclosporine **(NON-MODIFIED)** in a crossover study), and bile concentration data from *de novo* liver transplant patients (4 administered cyclosporine **(MODIFIED)**, 3 administered cyclosporine **(NON-MODIFIED)**, the percentage of dose present as M1, M9, and M4N metabolites is similar when either cyclosporine **(MODIFIED)** or cyclosporine **(NON-MODIFIED)** is administered.

Excretion: Only 0.1% of a cyclosporine dose is excreted unchanged in the urine. Elimination is primarily biliary with only 6% of the dose (parent drug and metabolites) excreted in the urine. Neither dialysis nor renal failure alter cyclosporine clearance significantly.

Drug Interactions: (*see PRECAUTIONS, Drug Interactions*). When diclofenac or methotrexate was co-administered with cyclosporine in rheumatoid arthritis patients, the AUC of diclofenac and methotrexate, each was significantly increased (*see PRECAUTIONS, Drug Interactions*). No clinically significant pharmacokinetic interactions occurred between cyclosporine and aspirin, ketoprofen, piroxicam, or indomethacin.

Special Population: ***Pediatric Population:*** Pharmacokinetic data from pediatric patients administered cyclosporine **(MODIFIED)** or cyclosporine **(NON-MODIFIED)** are very limited. In 15 renal transplant patients aged 3-16 years, cyclosporine whole blood clearance after IV administration of cyclosporine **(NON-MODIFIED)** was 10.6±3.7 mL/min/kg (assay: Cyclo-trac specific RIA). In a study of 7 renal transplant patients aged 2–16, the cyclosporine clearance ranged from 9.8 to 15.5 mL/min/kg. In 9 liver transplant patients aged 0.6 to 5.6 years, clearance was 9.3±5.4 mL/min/kg (assay: HPLC).

In the pediatric population, cyclosporine **(MODIFIED)** also demonstrates an increased bioavailability as compared to cyclosporine **(NON-MODIFIED)**. In 7 liver *de novo* transplant patients aged 1.4 to 10 years, the absolute bioavailability of cyclosporine **(MODIFIED)** was 43% (range 30% to 68%) and for cyclosporine **(NON-MODIFIED)** in the same individuals absolute bioavailability was 28% (range 17% to 42%).

[See second table at right]

Geriatric Population: Comparison of single dose data from both normal elderly volunteers (N=18, mean age 69 years) and elderly rheumatoid arthritis patients (N=16, mean age 68 years) to single dose data in young adult volunteers (N=16, mean age 26 years) showed no significant difference in the pharmacokinetic parameters.

CLINICAL TRIALS

Rheumatoid Arthritis: The effectiveness of cyclosporine **(NON-MODIFIED)** and cyclosporine **(MODIFIED)** in the treatment of severe rheumatoid arthritis was evaluated in five clinical studies involving a total of 728 cyclosporine treated patients and 273 placebo treated patients.

A summary of the results is presented for the "responder" rates per treatment group, with a responder being defined as a patient having *completed* the trial with a 20% improvement in the tender and the swollen joint count and a 20% improvement in 2 of 4 of investigator global, patient global, disability, and erythrocyte sedimentation rates (ESR) for the Studies 651 and 652 and 3 of 5 of investigator global, patient global, disability, visual analog pain, and ESR for Studies 2008, 654, and 302.

Study 651 enrolled 264 patients with active rheumatoid arthritis with at least 20 involved joints, who had failed at least one major RA drug, using a 3:3:2 randomization to one of the following three groups: (1) cyclosporine dosed at 2.5–5 mg/kg/day, (2) methotrexate at 7.5–15 mg/week, or (3) placebo. Treatment duration was 24 weeks. The mean cyclosporine dose at the last visit was 3.1 mg/kg/day. See Graph below.

Study 652 enrolled 250 patients with active RA with >6 active painful or tender joints who had failed at least one major RA drug. Patients were randomized using a 3:3:2 randomization to 1 of 3 treatment arms: (1) 1.5–5 mg/kg/day of cyclosporine, (2) 2.5–5 mg/kg/day of cyclosporine, and (3) placebo. Treatment duration was 16 weeks. The mean cyclosporine dose for group 2 at the last visit was 2.92 mg/kg/day. See Graph below.

Study 2008 enrolled 144 patients with active RA and >6 active joints who had unsuccessful treatment courses of aspirin and gold or Penicillamine. Patients were randomized to one of two treatment groups: (1) cyclosporine 2.5–5 mg/kg/day with adjustments after the first month to achieve a target trough level and (2) placebo. Treatment duration was 24 weeks. The mean cyclosporine dose at the last visit was 3.63 mg/kg/day. See Graph below.

Study 654 enrolled 148 patients who remained with active joint counts of 6 or more despite treatment with maximally tolerated methotrexate doses for at least three months. Patients continued to take their current dose of methotrexate and were randomized to receive, in addition, one of the following medications: (1) cyclosporine 2.5 mg/kg/day with dose increases of 0.5 mg/kg/day at weeks 2 and 4 if there was no evidence of toxicity and further increases of 0.5 mg/kg/day at weeks 8 and 16 if a <30% decrease in active joint count occurred without any significant toxicity; dose decreases could be made at any time for toxicity or (2) placebo. Treatment duration was 24 weeks. The mean cyclosporine dose at the last visit was 2.8 mg/kg/day (range: 1.3-4.1). See Graph below.

Study 302 enrolled 299 patients with severe active RA, 99% of whom were unresponsive or intolerant to at least one prior major RA drug. Patients were randomized to 1 of 2 treatment groups (1) cyclosporine **(MODIFIED)** and (2) cyclosporine **(NON-MODIFIED)**, both of which were started at 2.5 mg/kg/day and increased after 4 weeks for inefficacy in increments of 0.5 mg/kg/day to a maximum of 5 mg/kg/day and decreased at any time for toxicity. Treatment duration was 24 weeks. The mean cyclosporine dose at the last visit was 2.91 mg/kg/day (range: 0.72-5.17) for cyclosporine **(MODIFIED)** and 3.27 mg/kg/day (range: 0.73-5.68) for cyclosporine **(NON-MODIFIED)**. See Graph below.

[See graphic above]

INDICATIONS AND USAGE

Kidney, Liver and Heart Transplantation: Gengraf® (cyclosporine capsules, USP **[MODIFIED]**) is indicated for the prophylaxis of organ rejection in kidney, liver, and heart allogeneic transplants. Cyclosporine **(MODIFIED)** has been used in combination with azathioprine and corticosteroids.

Rheumatoid Arthritis: Gengraf® (cyclosporine capsules, USP **[MODIFIED]**) is indicated for the treatment of patients with severe active, rheumatoid arthritis where the disease has not adequately responded to methotrexate. Gengraf® can be used in combination with methotrexate in rheumatoid arthritis patients who do not respond adequately to methotrexate alone.

Psoriasis: Gengraf® (cyclosporine capsules, USP **[MODIFIED]**) is indicated for the treatment of *adult, nonimmunocompromised* patients with severe (i.e., extensive and/or disabling), recalcitrant, plaque psoriasis who have failed to respond to at least one systemic therapy (e.g., PUVA, retinoids, or methotrexate) or in patients for whom other systemic therapies are contraindicated, or cannot be tolerated.

While rebound rarely occurs, most patients will experience relapse with Gengraf® as with other therapies upon cessation of treatment.

Pharmacokinetic Parameters (mean ± SD)

Patient Population	Dose/day[1] (mg/d)	Dose/weight (mg/kg/d)	AUC[2] (ng•hr/mL)	C_{max} (ng/mL)	Trough[3] (ng/mL)	CL/F (mL/min)	CL/F (mL/min/kg)
De novo renal transplant[4] Week 4 (N=37)	597±174	7.95±2.81	8772±2089	1802±428	361±129	593±204	7.8±2.9
Stable renal transplant[4] (N=55)	344±122	4.10±1.58	6035±2194	1333±469	251±116	492±140	5.9±2.1
De novo liver transplant[5] Week 4 (N=18)	458±190	6.89±3.68	7187±2816	1555±740	268±101	577±309	8.6±5.7
De novo rheumatoid arthritis[6] (N=23)	182±55.6	2.37±0.36	2641±877	728±263	96.4±37.7	613±196	8.3±2.8
De novo psoriasis[6] Week 4 (N=18)	189±69.8	2.48±0.65	2324±1048	655±186	74.9±46.7	723±186	10.2±3.9

[1]Total daily dose was divided into two doses administered every 12 hours.
[2]AUC was measured over one dosing interval.
[3]Trough concentration was measured just prior to the morning cyclosporine (**MODIFIED**) dose, approximately 12 hours after the previous dose.
[4]Assay: TDx specific monoclonal fluorescence polarization immunoassay.
[5]Assay: Cyclo-trac specific monoclonal radioimmunoassay.
[6]Assay: INCSTAR specific monoclonal radioimmunoassay.

Pediatric Pharmacokinetic Parameters (mean ± SD)

Patient Population	Dose/day (mg/d)	Dose/weight (mg/kg/d)	AUC[1] (ng•hr/mL)	C_{max} (ng/mL)	CL/F (mL/min)	CL/F (mL/min/kg)
Stable liver transplant[2]						
Age 2–8, Dosed TID (N=9)	101±25	5.95±1.32	2163±801	629±219	285±94	16.6±4.3
Age 8–15, Dosed BID (N=8)	188±55	4.96±2.09	4272±1462	975±281	378±80	10.2±4.0
Stable liver transplant[3]						
Age 3, Dosed BID (N=1)	120	8.33	5832	1050	171	11.9
Age 8–15, Dosed BID (N=5)	158±55	5.51±1.91	4452±2475	1013±635	328±121	11.0±1.9
Stable renal transplant[3]						
Age 7–15, Dosed BID (N=5)	328±83	7.37±4.11	6922±1988	1827±487	418±143	8.7±2.9

[1]AUC was measured over one dosing interval.
[2]Assay: Cyclo-trac specific monoclonal radioimmunoassay.
[3]Assay: TDx specific monoclonal fluorescence polarization immunoassay.

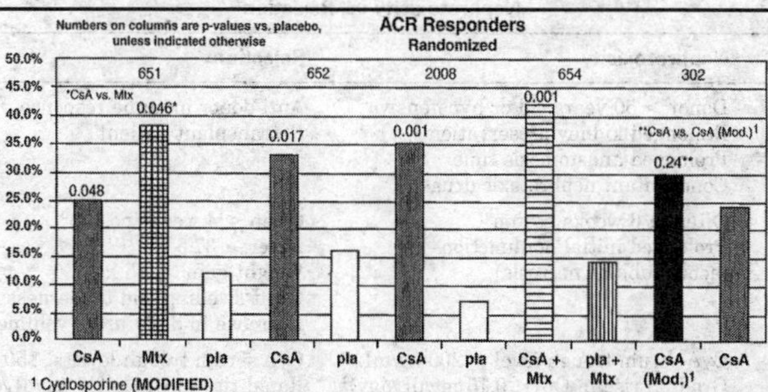

CONTRAINDICATIONS

General: Gengraf® (cyclosporine capsules, USP **[MODIFIED]**) is contraindicated in patients with a hypersensitivity to cyclosporine or to any of the ingredients of the formulation.

Rheumatoid Arthritis: Rheumatoid arthritis patients with abnormal renal function, uncontrolled hypertension or malignancies should not receive Gengraf® (cyclosporine capsules, USP **[MODIFIED]**).

Psoriasis: Psoriasis patients who are treated with Gengraf® (cyclosporine capsules, USP **[MODIFIED]**) should not receive concomitant PUVA or UVB therapy, methotrexate or other immunosuppressive agents, coal tar or radiation therapy. Psoriasis patients with abnormal renal function, uncontrolled hypertension, or malignancies should not receive Gengraf®.

WARNINGS *(see also Boxed WARNINGS)*.

All Patients: Cyclosporine, the active ingredient of Gengraf® (cyclosporine capsules, USP **[MODIFIED]**), can cause nephrotoxicity and hepatotoxicity. The risk increases with increasing doses of cyclosporine. Renal dysfunction including structural kidney damage is a potential consequence of Gengraf® and therefore renal function must be monitored during therapy. **Care should be taken in using cyclosporine with nephrotoxic drugs (see *PRECAUTIONS*).**

Patients receiving Gengraf® require frequent monitoring of serum creatinine (*see Special Monitoring under DOSAGE AND ADMINISTRATION*). Elderly patients should be monitored with particular care, since decreases in renal function also occur with age. If patients are not properly monitored and doses are not properly adjusted, cyclosporine therapy can be associated with the occurrence of structural kidney damage and persistent renal dysfunction.

An increase in serum creatinine and BUN may occur during Gengraf® therapy and reflect a reduction in the glomerular filtration rate. Impaired renal function at any time requires close monitoring, and frequent dosage adjustment may be indicated. The frequency and severity of serum creatinine elevations increase with dose and duration of cyclosporine therapy. These elevations are likely to become more pronounced without dose reduction or discontinuation.

Because Gengraf® (cyclosporine capsules, USP [MODIFIED]) is not bioequivalent to Sandimmune®* (cyclosporine [NON-MODIFIED]), conversion from Gengraf® to Sandimmune®* (cyclosporine [NON-MODIFIED]) using a 1:1 ratio (mg/kg/day) may result in lower cyclosporine blood concentrations. Conversion from Gengraf® to Sandimmune®* (cyclosporine [NON-MODIFIED]) should be made with increased monitoring to avoid the potential of underdosing.

Kidney, Liver, and Heart Transplant: Cyclosporine, the active ingredient of Gengraf® (cyclosporine capsules, USP **[MODIFIED]**), can cause nephrotoxicity and hepatotoxicity when used in high doses. It is not unusual for serum creatinine and BUN levels to be elevated during cyclosporine therapy. These elevations in renal transplant patients do not necessarily indicate rejection, and each patient must be fully evaluated before dosage adjustment is initiated.

Based on the historical cyclosporine **(NON-MODIFIED)** experience with oral solution, nephrotoxicity associated with cyclosporine had been noted in 25% of cases of renal transplantation, 38% of cases of cardiac transplantation, and 37% of cases of liver transplantation. Mild nephrotoxicity was generally noted 2–3 months after renal transplant and consisted of an arrest in the fall of the pre-operative elevations of BUN and creatinine at a range of 35–45 mg/dL and 2.0–2.5 mg/dL respectively. These elevations were often responsive to cyclosporine dosage reduction.

More overt nephrotoxicity was seen early after transplantation and was characterized by a rapidly rising BUN and cre-

Continued on next page

Gengraf—Cont.

atinine. Since these events are similar to renal rejection episodes, care must be taken to differentiate between them. This form of nephrotoxicity is usually responsive to cyclosporine dosage reduction.

Although specific diagnostic criteria which reliably differentiate renal graft rejection from drug toxicity have not been found, a number of parameters have been significantly associated with one or the other. It should be noted however, that up to 20% of patients may have simultaneous nephrotoxicity and rejection.

[See table below]

A form of a cyclosporine-associated nephropathy is characterized by serial deterioration in renal function and morphologic changes in the kidneys. From 5% to 15% of transplant recipients who have received cyclosporine will fail to show a reduction in rising serum creatinine despite a decrease or discontinuation of cyclosporine therapy. Renal biopsies from these patients will demonstrate one or several of the following alterations: tubular vacuolization, tubular microcalcifications, peritubular capillary congestion, arteriolopathy, and a striped form of interstitial fibrosis with tubular atrophy. Though none of these morphologic changes is entirely specific, a diagnosis of cyclosporine-associated structural nephrotoxicity requires evidence of these findings.

When considering the development of cyclosporine-associated nephropathy, it is noteworthy that several authors have reported an association between the appearance of interstitial fibrosis and higher cumulative doses or persistently high circulating trough levels of cyclosporine. This is particularly true during the first 6 post-transplant months when the dosage tends to be highest and when, in kidney recipients, the organ appears to be most vulnerable to the toxic effects of cyclosporine. Among other contributing factors to the development of interstitial fibrosis in these patients are prolonged perfusion time, warm ischemia time, as well as episodes of acute toxicity, and acute and chronic rejection. The reversibility of interstitial fibrosis and its correlation to renal function have not yet been determined. Reversibility of arteriolopathy has been reported after stopping cyclosporine or lowering the dosage.

Impaired renal function at any time requires close monitoring, and frequent dosage adjustment may be indicated.

In the event of severe and unremitting rejection, when rescue therapy with pulse steroids and monoclonal antibodies fail to reverse the rejection episode, it may be preferable to switch to alternative immunosuppressive therapy rather than increase the Gengraf® dose to excessive levels.

Occasionally patients have developed a syndrome of thrombocytopenia and microangiopathic hemolytic anemia which may result in graft failure. The vasculopathy can occur in the absence of rejection and is accompanied by avid platelet consumption within the graft as demonstrated by Indium 111 labeled platelet studies. Neither the pathogenesis nor the management of this syndrome is clear. Though resolution has occurred after reduction or discontinuation of cyclosporine and 1) administration of streptokinase and heparin or 2) plasmapheresis, this appears to depend upon early detection with Indium 111 labeled platelet scans (*see ADVERSE REACTIONS*).

Significant hyperkalemia (sometimes associated with hyperchloremic metabolic acidosis) and hyperuricemia have been seen occasionally in individual patients.

Hepatotoxicity associated with cyclosporine use had been noted in 4% of cases of renal transplantation, 7% of cases of cardiac transplantation, and 4% of cases of liver transplantation. This was usually noted during the first month of therapy when high doses of cyclosporine were used and consisted of elevations of hepatic enzymes and bilirubin. The chemistry elevations usually decreased with a reduction in dosage.

As in patients receiving other immunosuppressants, those patients receiving cyclosporine are at increased risk for development of lymphomas and other malignancies, particularly those of the skin. The increased risk appears related to the intensity and duration of immunosuppression rather than to the use of specific agents. Because of the danger of oversuppression of the immune system resulting in increased risk of infection or malignancy, a treatment regimen containing multiple immunosuppressants should be used with caution.

There have been reports of convulsions in adult and pediatric patients receiving cyclosporine, particularly in combination with high dose methylprednisolone.

Encephalopathy has been described both in post-marketing reports and in the literature. Manifestations include impaired consciousness, convulsions, visual disturbances (including blindness), loss of motor function, movement disorders and psychiatric disturbances. In many cases, changes in the white matter have been detected using imaging techniques and pathologic specimens. Predisposing factors such as hypertension, hypomagnesemia, hypocholesterolemia, high-dose corticosteroids, high cyclosporine blood concentrations, and graft-versus-host disease have been noted in many but not all of the reported cases. The changes in most cases have been reversible upon discontinuation of cyclosporine, and in some cases improvement was noted after reduction of dose. It appears that patients receiving liver transplant are more susceptible to encephalopathy than those patients receiving kidney transplant.

Care should be taken in using cyclosporine with nephrotoxic drugs (*see PRECAUTIONS*).

Rheumatoid Arthritis: Cyclosporine nephropathy was detected in renal biopsies of six out of 60 (10%) rheumatoid arthritis patients after the average treatment duration of 19 months. Only one patient, out of these 6 patients, was treated with a dose ≤4 mg/kg/day. Serum creatinine improved in all but one patient after discontinuation of cyclosporine. The "maximal creatinine increase" appears to be a factor in predicting cyclosporine nephropathy.

There is a potential, as with other immunosuppressive agents, for an increase in the occurrence of malignant lymphomas with cyclosporine. It is not clear whether the risk with cyclosporine is greater than that in Rheumatoid Arthritis patients or in Rheumatoid Arthritis patients on cytotoxic treatment for this indication. Five cases of lymphoma were detected: four in a survey of approximately 2,300 patients treated with cyclosporine for rheumatoid arthritis, and another case of lymphoma was reported in a clinical trial. Although other tumors (12 skin cancers, 24 solid tumors of diverse types, and 1 multiple myeloma) were also reported in this survey, epidemiologic analyses did not support a relationship to cyclosporine other than for malignant lymphomas.

Patients should be thoroughly evaluated before and during Gengraf® (cyclosporine capsules, USP **[MODIFIED]**) treatment for the development of malignancies. Moreover, use of Gengraf® therapy with other immunosuppressive agents may induce an excessive immunosuppression which is known to increase the risk of malignancy.

Psoriasis: (*see also Boxed WARNINGS for Psoriasis*). Since cyclosporine is a potent immunosuppressive agent with a number of potentially serious side effects, the risks and benefits of using Gengraf® (cyclosporine capsules, USP **[MODIFIED]**) should be considered before treatment of patients with psoriasis. Cyclosporine, the active ingredient in Gengraf®, can cause nephrotoxicity and hypertension (*see PRECAUTIONS*) and the risk increases with increasing dose and duration of therapy. Patients who may be at increased risk such as those with abnormal renal function, uncontrolled hypertension or malignancies, should not receive Gengraf®.

Renal dysfunction is a potential consequence of Gengraf®, therefore renal function must be monitored during therapy. Patients receiving Gengraf® require frequent monitoring of serum creatinine (*see Special Monitoring under DOSAGE AND ADMINISTRATION*). Elderly patients should be monitored with particular care, since decreases in renal function also occur with age. If patients are not properly monitored and doses are not properly adjusted, cyclosporine therapy can cause structural kidney damage and persistent renal dysfunction.

An increase in serum creatinine and BUN may occur during Gengraf® therapy and reflects a reduction in the glomerular filtration rate.

Kidney biopsies from 86 psoriasis patients treated for a mean duration of 23 months with 1.2–7.6 mg/kg/day of cyclosporine showed evidence of cyclosporine nephropathy in 18/86 (21%) of the patients. The pathology consisted of renal tubular atrophy and interstitial fibrosis. On repeat biopsy of 13 of these patients maintained on various dosages of cyclosporine for a mean of 2 additional years, the number with cyclosporine induced nephropathy rose to 26/86 (30%). The majority of patients (19/26) were on a dose of ≥5.0 mg/kg/day (the highest recommended dose is 4 mg/kg/day). The patients were also on cyclosporine for greater than 15 months (18/26) and/or had a clinically significant increase in serum creatinine for greater than 1 month (21/26). Creatinine levels returned to normal range in 7 of 11 patients in whom cyclosporine therapy was discontinued.

There is an increased risk for the development of skin and lymphoproliferative malignancies in cyclosporine-treated psoriasis patients. The relative risk of malignancies is comparable to that observed in psoriasis patients treated with other immunosuppressive agents.

Tumors were reported in 32 (2.2%) of 1439 psoriasis patients treated with cyclosporine worldwide from clinical trials. Additional tumors have been reported in 7 patients in cyclosporine postmarketing experience. Skin malignancies were reported in 16 (1.1%) of these patients; all but 2 of them had previously received PUVA therapy. Methotrexate was received by 7 patients. UVB and coal tar have been used by 2 and 3 patients, respectively. Seven patients had either a history of previous skin cancer or a potentially predisposing lesion was present prior to cyclosporine exposure. Of the 16 patients with skin cancer, 11 patients had 18 squamous cell carcinomas and 7 patients had 10 basal cell carcinomas.

There were two lymphoproliferative malignancies; one case of non-Hodgkin's lymphoma which required chemotherapy, and one case of mycosis fungoides which regressed spontaneously upon discontinuation of cyclosporine. There were four cases of benign lymphocytic infiltration: 3 regressed spontaneously upon discontinuation of cyclosporine, while the fourth regressed despite continuation of the drug. The remainder of the malignancies, 13 cases (0.9%), involved various organs.

Nephrotoxicity vs. Rejection

Parameter	Nephrotoxicity	Rejection
History	Donor > 50 years old or hypotensive Prolonged kidney preservation Prolonged anastomosis time Concomitant nephrotoxic drugs	Anti-donor immune response Retransplant patient
Clinical	Often > 6 weeks postop[b] Prolonged initial nonfunction (acute tubular necrosis)	Often < 4 weeks postop[b] Fever > 37.5°C Weight gain > 0.5 kg Graft swelling and tenderness Decrease in daily urine volume > 500 mL (or 50%)
Laboratory	CyA serum trough level > 200 ng/mL Gradual rise in Cr (< 0.15 mg/dL/day)[a] Cr plateau < 25% above baseline BUN/Cr ≥ 20	CyA serum trough level < 150 ng/mL Rapid rise in Cr (> 0.3 mg/dL/day)[a] Cr > 25% above baseline BUN/Cr < 20
Biopsy	Arteriolopathy (medial hypertrophy[a], hyalinosis, nodular deposits, intimal thickening, endothelial vacuolization, progressive scarring) Tubular atrophy, isometric vacuolization, isolated calcifications Minimal edema Mild focal infiltrates[c] Diffuse interstitial fibrosis, often striped form	Endovasculitis[c] (proliferation[a], intimal arteritis[b], necrosis, sclerosis) Tubulitis with RBC[b] and WBC[b] casts, some irregular vacuolization Interstitial edema[c] and hemorrhage[b] Diffuse moderate to severe mononuclear infiltrates[d] Glomerulitis (mononuclear cells)[c]
Aspiration Cytology	CyA deposits in tubular and endothelial cells Fine isometric vacuolization of tubular cells	Inflammatory infiltrate with mononuclear phagocytes, macrophages, lymphoblastoid cells, and activated T-cells These strongly express HLA-DR antigens
Urine Cytology	Tubular cells with vacuolization and granularization	Degenerative tubular cells, plasma cells, and lymphocyturia > 20% of sediment
Manometry	Intracapsular pressure < 40 mm Hg[b]	Intracapsular pressure > 40 mm Hg[b]
Ultrasonography	Unchanged graft cross sectional area	Increase in graft cross sectional area AP diameter ≥ Transverse diameter
Magnetic Resonance Imagery	Normal appearance	Loss of distinct corticomedullary junction, swelling image intensity of parachyma approaching that of psoas, loss of hilar fat
Radionuclide Scan	Normal or generally decreased perfusion Decrease in tubular function (^{131} I-hippuran) > decrease in perfusion (^{99m} Tc DTPA)	Patchy arterial flow Decrease in perfusion > decrease in tubular function Increased uptake of Indium 111 labeled platelets or Tc-99m in colloid
Therapy	Responds to decreased cyclosporine	Responds to increased steroids or antilymphocyte globulin

[a]p < 0.05, [b]p < 0.01, [c]p < 0.001, [d]p < 0.0001

Patients should not be treated concurrently with cyclosporine and PUVA or UVB, other radiation therapy, or other immunosuppressive agents, because of the possibility of excessive immunosuppression and the subsequent risk of malignancies (*see CONTRAINDICATIONS*). Patients should also be warned to protect themselves appropriately when in the sun, and to avoid excessive sun exposure. Patients should be thoroughly evaluated before and during treatment for the presence of malignancies remembering that malignant lesions may be hidden by psoriatic plaques. Skin lesions not typical of psoriasis should be biopsied before starting treatment. Patients should be treated with Gengraf® (cyclosporine capsules, USP **[MODIFIED]**) only after complete resolution of suspicious lesions, and only if there are no other treatment options (*see Special Monitoring for Psoriasis Patients*).

PRECAUTIONS

General: ***Hypertension:*** Cyclosporine is the active ingredient of Gengraf® (cyclosporine capsules, USP **[MODIFIED]**). Hypertension is a common side effect of cyclosporine therapy which may persist (*see ADVERSE REACTIONS and DOSAGE AND ADMINISTRATION for monitoring recommendations*). Mild or moderate hypertension is encountered more frequently than severe hypertension and the incidence decreases over time. In recipients of kidney, liver, and heart allografts treated with cyclosporine, antihypertensive therapy may be required (*see Special Monitoring of Rheumatoid Arthritis and Psoriasis Patients*). However, since cyclosporine may cause hyperkalemia, potassium-sparing diuretics should not be used. While calcium antagonists can be effective agents in treating cyclosporine-associated hypertension, they can interfere with cyclosporine metabolism (*see PRECAUTIONS, Drug Interactions*).

Vaccination: During treatment with cyclosporine, vaccination may be less effective; and the use of live attenuated vaccines should be avoided.

Special Monitoring of Rheumatoid Arthritis Patients: Before initiating treatment, a careful physical examination, including blood pressure measurements (on at least two occasions) and two creatinine levels to estimate baseline should be performed. Blood pressure and serum creatinine should be evaluated every 2 weeks during the initial 3 months and then monthly if the patient is stable. It is advisable to monitor serum creatinine and blood pressure always after an increase of the dose of nonsteroidal anti-inflammatory drugs and after initiation of new nonsteroidal anti-inflammatory drug therapy during Gengraf® (cyclosporine capsules, USP **[MODIFIED]**) treatment. If co-administered with methotrexate, CBC and liver function tests are recommended to be monitored monthly (*see also PRECAUTIONS, General, Hypertension*).

In patients who are receiving cyclosporine, the dose of Gengraf® should be decreased by 25%–50% if hypertension occurs. If hypertension persists, the dose of Gengraf® should be further reduced or blood pressure should be controlled with antihypertensive agents. In most cases, blood pressure has returned to baseline when cyclosporine was discontinued.

In placebo-controlled trials of rheumatoid arthritis patients, systolic hypertension (defined as an occurrence of two systolic blood pressure readings >140 mmHg) and diastolic hypertension (defined as two diastolic blood pressure readings >90 mmHg) occurred in 33% and 19% of patients treated with cyclosporine, respectively. The corresponding placebo rates were 22% and 8%.

Special Monitoring for Psoriasis Patients: Before initiating treatment, a careful dermatological and physical examination, including blood pressure measurements (on at least two occasions) should be performed. Since Gengraf® (cyclosporine capsules, USP **[MODIFIED]**) is an immunosuppressive agent, patients should be evaluated for the presence of occult infection on their first physical examination and for the presence of tumors initially, and throughout treatment with Gengraf®. Skin lesions not typical for psoriasis should be biopsied before starting Gengraf®. Patients with malignant or premalignant changes of the skin should be treated with Gengraf® only after appropriate treatment of such lesions and if no other treatment option exists.

Baseline laboratories should include serum creatinine (on two occasions), BUN, CBC, serum magnesium, potassium, uric acid, and lipids.

The risk of cyclosporine nephropathy is reduced when the starting dose is low (2.5 mg/kg/day), the maximum dose does not exceed 4.0 mg/kg/day, serum creatinine is monitored regularly while cyclosporine is administered, and the dose of Gengraf® is decreased when the rise in creatinine is greater than or equal to 25% above the patients pretreatment level. The increase in creatinine is generally reversible upon timely decrease of the dose of Gengraf® or its discontinuation.

Serum creatinine and BUN should be evaluated every 2 weeks during the initial 3 months of therapy and then monthly if the patient is stable. If the serum creatinine is greater than or equal to 25% above the patient's pretreatment level, serum creatinine should be repeated within two weeks. If the change in serum creatinine remains greater than or equal to 25% above baseline, Gengraf® should be reduced by 25%–50%. If at **any time** the serum creatinine increases by greater than or equal to 50% above pretreatment level, Gengraf® should be reduced by 25%–50%. Gengraf® should be discontinued if reversibility (within 25% of baseline) of serum creatinine is not achievable after two dosage modifications. It is advisable to monitor serum creatinine after an increase of the dose of nonsteroidal anti-inflammatory drug and after initiation of new nonsteroidal anti-inflammatory therapy during Gengraf® treatment.

Antibiotics	*Antineoplastics*	*Anti-inflammatory Drugs*	*Gastrointestinal Agents*
gentamicin	melphalan	azapropazon	cimetidine
tobramycin		diclofenac	ranitidine
vancomycin	*Antifungals*	naproxen	
trimethoprim with sulfamethoxazole	amphotericin B	sulindac	*Immunosuppressives*
	ketoconazole	colchicine	tacrolimus

Blood pressure should be evaluated every 2 weeks during the initial 3 months of therapy and then monthly if the patient is stable, or more frequently when dosage adjustments are made. Patients without a history of previous hypertension before initiation of treatment with Gengraf®, should have the drug reduced by 25%–50% if found to have sustained hypertension. If the patient continues to be hypertensive despite multiple reductions of Gengraf®, then Gengraf® should be discontinued. For patients with treated hypertension, before the initiation of Gengraf® therapy, their medication should be adjusted to control hypertension while on Gengraf®. Gengraf® should be discontinued if a change in hypertension management is not effective or tolerable.

CBC, uric acid, potassium, lipids, and magnesium should also be monitored every 2 weeks for the first 3 months of therapy, and then monthly if the patient is stable or more frequently when dosage adjustments are made. Gengraf® dosage should be reduced by 25%–50% for any abnormality of clinical concern.

In controlled trials of cyclosporine in psoriasis patients, cyclosporine blood concentrations did not correlate well with either improvement or with side effects such as renal dysfunction.

Information for Patients: Patients should be advised that any change of cyclosporine formulation should be made cautiously and only under physician supervision because it may result in the need for a change in dosage.

Patients should be informed of the necessity of repeated laboratory tests while they are receiving cyclosporine. Patients should be advised of the potential risks during pregnancy and informed of the increased risk of neoplasia. Patients should also be informed of the risk of hypertension and renal dysfunction.

Patients should be advised that during treatment with cyclosporine, vaccination may be less effective and the use of live attenuated vaccines should be avoided.

Patients should be advised to take Gengraf® on a consistent schedule with regard to time of day and relation to meals. Grapefruit and grapefruit juice affect metabolism, increasing blood concentration of cyclosporine, thus should be avoided.

Laboratory Tests: In all patients treated with cyclosporine, renal and liver functions should be assessed repeatedly by measurement of serum creatinine, BUN, serum bilirubin, and liver enzymes. Serum lipids, magnesium, and potassium should also be monitored. Cyclosporine blood concentrations should be routinely monitored in transplant patients (*see DOSAGE AND ADMINISTRATION, Blood Concentration Monitoring in Transplant Patients*), and periodically monitored in rheumatoid arthritis patients.

Drug Interactions: All of the individual drugs cited below are well substantiated to interact with cyclosporine. In addition, concomitant non-steroidal anti-inflammatory drugs, particularly in the setting of dehydration, may potentiate renal dysfunction.

Drugs That May Potentiate Renal Dysfunction

[See table above]

Drugs That Alter Cyclosporine Concentrations: Compounds that decrease cyclosporine absorption such as orlistat should be avoided. Cyclosporine is extensively metabolized by cytochrome P-450 3A. Substances that inhibit this enzyme could decrease metabolism and increase cyclosporine concentrations. Substances that are inducers of cytochrome P-450 activity could increase metabolism and decrease cyclosporine concentrations. Monitoring of circulating cyclosporine concentrations and appropriate Gengraf® (cyclosporine capsules, USP **[MODIFIED]**) dosage adjustment are essential when these drugs are used concomitantly (see *DOSAGE AND ADMINISTRATION, Blood Concentration Monitoring*).

Drugs That Increase Cyclosporine Concentrations

Calcium Channel Blockers	*Antibiotics*	*Other Drugs*
diltiazem	clarithromycin	allopurinol
nicardipine	erythromycin	bromocriptine
verapamil	quinupristin/dalfopristin	danazol
		metoclopramide
		colchicine
		amiodarone
Antifungals	*Glucocorticoids*	
fluconazole	methylprednisolone	
itraconazole		
ketoconazole		

The HIV protease inhibitors (e.g., indinavir, nelfinavir, ritonavir, and saquinavir) are known to inhibit cytochrome P-450 3A and thus could potentially increase the concentrations of cyclosporine, however no formal studies of the interaction are available. Care should be exercised when these drugs are administered concomitantly.

Grapefruit and grapefruit juice affect metabolism, increasing blood concentrations of cyclosporine, thus should be avoided.

Drugs/Dietary Supplements That Decrease Cyclosporine Concentrations

Antibiotics	*Anticonvulsants*	*Other Drugs*
nafcillin	carbamazepine	octreotide
rifampin	phenobarbital	ticlopidine
	phenytoin	orlistat
		St. John's Wort

There have been reports of a serious drug interaction between cyclosporine and the herbal dietary supplement, St. John's Wort. This interaction has been reported to produce a marked reduction in the blood concentrations of cyclosporine, resulting in subtherapeutic levels, rejection of transplant organs, and graft loss.

Rifabutin is known to increase the metabolism of other drugs metabolized by the cytochrome P-450 system. The interaction between rifabutin and cyclosporine has not been studied. Care should be exercised when these two drugs are administered concomitantly.

Nonsteroidal Anti-inflammatory Drug (NSAID) Interactions: Clinical status and serum creatinine should be closely monitored when cyclosporine is used with nonsteroidal anti-inflammatory agents in rheumatoid arthritis patients (*see WARNINGS*).

Pharmacodynamic interactions have been reported to occur between cyclosporine and both naproxen and sulindac, in that concomitant use is associated with additive decreases in renal function, as determined by ^{99m}Tc-diethylenetriaminepentaacetic acid (DTPA) and (*p*-aminohippuric acid) PAH clearances. Although concomitant administration of diclofenac does not affect blood levels of cyclosporine, it has been associated with approximate doubling of diclofenac blood levels and occasional reports of reversible decreases in renal function. Consequently, the dose of diclofenac should be in the lower end of the therapeutic range.

Methotrexate Interaction: Preliminary data indicate that when methotrexate and cyclosporine were co-administered to rheumatoid arthritis patients (N=20), methotrexate concentrations (AUCs) were increased approximately 30% and the concentrations (AUCs) of its metabolite, 7-hydroxy methotrexate, were decreased by approximately 80%. The clinical significance of this interaction is not known. Cyclosporine concentrations do not appear to have been altered (N=6).

Other Drug Interactions: Reduced clearance of prednisolone, digoxin, and lovastatin has been observed when these drugs are administered with cyclosporine. In addition, a decrease in the apparent volume of distribution of digoxin has been reported after cyclosporine administration. Severe digitalis toxicity has been seen within days of starting cyclosporine in several patients taking digoxin. Cyclosporine should not be used with potassium-sparing diuretics because hyperkalemia can occur.

During treatment with cyclosporine, vaccination may be less effective. The use of live vaccines should be avoided.

Myositis has occurred with concomitant lovastatin, frequent gingival hyperplasia with nifedipine, and convulsions with high dose methylprednisolone.

Psoriasis patients receiving other immunosuppressive agents or radiation therapy (including PUVA and UVB) should not receive concurrent cyclosporine because of the possibility of excessive immunosuppression.

For additional information on Cyclosporine Drug Interactions please contact Abbott Laboratories Medical Information Department at 1-800-633-9110.

Carcinogenesis, Mutagenesis, and Impairment of Fertility: Carcinogenicity studies were carried out in male and female rats and mice. In the 78-week mouse study, evidence of a statistically significant trend was found for lymphocytic lymphomas in females, and the incidence of hepatocellular carcinomas in mid-dose males significantly exceeded the control value. In the 24-month rat study, pancreatic islet cell adenomas significantly exceeded the control rate in the low dose level. Doses used in the mouse and rat studies were 0.01 to 0.16 times the clinical maintenance dose (6 mg/kg). The hepatocellular carcinomas and pancreatic islet cell adenomas were not dose related. Published reports indicate the co-treatment of hairless mice with UV irradiation and cyclosporine or other immunosuppressive agents shorten the time to skin tumor formation compared to UV irradiation alone.

Cyclosporine was not mutagenic in appropriate test systems. Cyclosporine has not been found to be mutagenic/genotoxic in the Ames Test, the V79-HGPRT Test, the micronucleus test in mice and Chinese hamsters, the chromosome-aberration tests in Chinese hamster bone-marrow, the mouse dominant lethal assay, and the DNA-repair test in sperm from treated mice. A recent study analyzing sister chromatid exchange (SCE) induction by cyclosporine using human lymphocytes *in vitro* gave indication of a positive effect (i.e., induction of SCE), at high concentrations in this system.

No impairment in fertility was demonstrated in studies in male and female rats.

Continued on next page

Gengraf—Cont.

Widely distributed papillomatosis of the skin was observed after chronic treatment of dogs with cyclosporine at 9 times the human initial psoriasis treatment dose of 2.5 mg/kg, where doses are expressed on a body surface area basis. This papillomatosis showed a spontaneous regression upon discontinuation of cyclosporine.

An increased incidence of malignancy is a recognized complication of immunosuppression in recipients of organ transplants and patients with rheumatoid arthritis and psoriasis. The most common forms of neoplasms are non-Hodgkin's lymphoma and carcinomas of the skin. The risk of malignancies in cyclosporine recipients is higher than in the normal, healthy population but similar to that in patients receiving other immunosuppressive therapies. Reduction or discontinuance of immunosuppression may cause the lesions to regress.

In psoriasis patients on cyclosporine, development of malignancies, especially those of the skin has been reported *(see WARNINGS)*. Skin lesions not typical for psoriasis should be biopsied before starting cyclosporine treatment. Patients with malignant or premalignant changes of the skin should be treated with cyclosporine only after appropriate treatment of such lesions and if no other treatment option exists.

Pregnancy: ***Pregnancy Category C.*** Cyclosporine was not teratogenic in appropriate test systems. Only at dose levels toxic to dams, were adverse effects seen in reproduction studies in rats. Cyclosporine has been shown to be embryo- and fetotoxic in rats and rabbits following oral administration at maternally toxic doses. Fetal toxicity was noted in rats at 0.8 and rabbits at 5.4 times the transplant doses in humans of 6.0 mg/kg, where dose corrections are based on body surface area. Cyclosporine was embryo- and fetotoxic as indicated by increased pre- and postnatal mortality and reduced fetal weight together with related skeletal retardation.

There are no adequate and well-controlled studies in pregnant women. Gengraf® (cyclosporine capsules, USP **[MODIFIED]**) should be used during pregnancy only if the potential benefit justifies the potential risk to the fetus.

The following data represent the reported outcomes of 116 pregnancies in women receiving cyclosporine during pregnancy, 90% of whom were transplant patients, and most of whom received cyclosporine throughout the entire gestational period. The only consistent patterns of abnormality were premature birth (gestational period of 28 to 36 weeks) and low birth weight for gestational age. Sixteen fetal losses occurred. Most of the pregnancies (85 of 100) were complicated by disorders; including, pre-eclampsia, eclampsia, premature labor, abruptio placentae, oligohydramnios, Rh incompatibility and fetoplacental dysfunction. Pre-term delivery occurred in 47%. Seven malformations were reported in 5 viable infants and in 2 cases of fetal loss. Twenty-eight percent of the infants were small for gestational age. Neonatal complications occurred in 27%. Therefore, the risks and benefits of using Gengraf® during pregnancy should be carefully weighed.

Because of the possible disruption of maternal-fetal interaction, the risk/benefit ratio of using Gengraf® in psoriasis patients during pregnancy should carefully be weighed with serious consideration for discontinuation of Gengraf®.

Nursing Mothers: Since cyclosporine is excreted in human milk, breast-feeding should be avoided.

Pediatric Use: Although no adequate and well-controlled studies have been completed in children, transplant recipients as young as one year of age have received cyclosporine **(MODIFIED)** with no unusual adverse effects. The safety and efficacy of cyclosporine **(MODIFIED)** treatment in pediatric patients with juvenile rheumatoid arthritis or psoriasis below the age of 18 have not been established.

Geriatric Use: In rheumatoid arthritis clinical trials with cyclosporine, 17.5% of patients were age 65 or older. These patients were more likely to develop systolic hypertension on therapy, and more likely to show serum creatinine rises ≥50% above the baseline after 3–4 months of therapy.

ADVERSE REACTIONS

Kidney, Liver, and Heart Transplantation: The principal adverse reactions of cyclosporine therapy are renal dysfunction, tremor, hirsutism, hypertension, and gum hyperplasia. Hypertension, which is usually mild to moderate, may occur in approximately 50% of patients following renal transplantation and in most cardiac transplant patients.

Glomerular capillary thrombosis has been found in patients treated with cyclosporine and may progress to graft failure. The pathologic changes resembled those seen in the hemolytic-uremic syndrome and include thrombosis of the renal microvasculature, with platelet-fibrin thrombi occluding glomerular capillaries and afferent arterioles, microangiopathic hemolytic anemia, thrombocytopenia, and decreased renal function. Similar findings have been observed when other immunosuppressives have been employed post-transplantation.

Hypomagnesemia has been reported in some, but not all, patients exhibiting convulsions while on cyclosporine therapy. Although magnesium-depletion studies in normal subjects suggest that hypomagnesemia is associated with neurologic disorders, multiple factors, including hypertension, high dose methylprednisolone, hypocholesterolemia, and nephrotoxicity associated with high plasma concentrations of cyclosporine appear to be related to the neurological manifestations of cyclosporine toxicity.

Body System	Adverse Reactions	Randomized Kidney Patients: Cyclosporine (NON-MODIFIED) (N=227) %	Randomized Kidney Patients: Azathioprine (N=228) %	Cyclosporine Patients Cyclosporine, (NON-MODIFIED): Kidney (N=705) %	Cyclosporine Patients Cyclosporine, (NON-MODIFIED): Heart (N=112) %	Cyclosporine Patients Cyclosporine, (NON-MODIFIED): Liver (N=75) %
Genitourinary	Renal Dysfunction	32	6	25	38	37
Cardiovascular	Hypertension	26	18	13	53	27
	Cramps	4	<1	2	<1	0
Skin	Hirsutism	21	<1	21	28	45
	Acne	6	8	2	2	1
Central Nervous System	Tremor	12	0	21	31	55
	Convulsions	3	1	1	4	5
	Headache	2	<1	2	15	4
Gastrointestinal	Gum Hyperplasia	4	0	9	5	16
	Diarrhea	3	<1	3	4	8
	Nausea/Vomiting	2	<1	4	10	4
	Hepatotoxicity	<1	<1	4	7	4
	Abdominal Discomfort	<1	0	<1	7	0
Autonomic Nervous System	Paresthesia	3	0	1	2	1
	Flushing	<1	0	4	0	4
Hematopoietic	Leukopenia	2	19	<1	6	0
	Lymphoma	<1	0	1	6	1
Respiratory	Sinusitis	<1	0	4	3	7
Miscellaneous	Gynecomastia	<1	0	<1	4	3

Infectious Complications in Historical Randomized Studies in Renal Transplant Patients Using Cyclosporine (NON-MODIFIED)

Complication	Cyclosporine Treatment (N=227) % of Complications	Azathioprine with Steroids* (N=228) % of Complications
Septicemia	5.3	4.8
Abscesses	4.4	5.3
Systemic Fungal Infection	2.2	3.9
Local Fungal Infection	7.5	9.6
Cytomegalovirus	4.8	12.3
Other Viral Infections	15.9	18.4
Urinary Tract Infections	21.1	20.2
Wound and Skin Infections	7.0	10.1
Pneumonia	6.2	9.2

*Some patients also received ALG.

In controlled studies, the nature, severity and incidence of the adverse events that were observed in 493 transplanted patients treated with cyclosporine **(MODIFIED)** were comparable with those observed in 208 transplanted patients who received cyclosporine **(NON-MODIFIED)** in these same studies when the dosage of the two drugs was adjusted to achieve the same cyclosporine blood trough concentrations.

Based on the historical experience with cyclosporine **(NON-MODIFIED)**, the following reactions occurred in 3% or greater of 892 patients involved in clinical trials of kidney, heart, and liver transplants.

[See first table above]

Among 705 kidney transplant patients treated with cyclosporine oral solution **(NON-MODIFIED)** in clinical trials, the reason for treatment discontinuation was renal toxicity in 5.4%, infection in 0.9%, lack of efficacy in 1.4%, acute tubular necrosis in 1.0%, lymphoproliferative disorders in 0.3%, hypertension in 0.3%, and other reasons in 0.7% of the patients.

The following reactions occurred in 2% or less of cyclosporine **(NON-MODIFIED)**-treated patients: allergic reactions, anemia, anorexia, confusion, conjunctivitis, edema, fever, brittle fingernails, gastritis, hearing loss, hiccups, hyperglycemia, muscle pain, peptic ulcer, thrombocytopenia, tinnitus.

The following reactions occurred rarely: anxiety, chest pain, constipation, depression, hair breaking, hematuria, joint pain, lethargy, mouth sores, myocardial infarction, night sweats, pancreatitis, pruritus, swallowing difficulty, tingling, upper GI bleeding, visual disturbance, weakness, weight loss.

[See second table above]

Rheumatoid Arthritis: The principal adverse reactions associated with the use of cyclosporine in rheumatoid arthritis are renal dysfunction (*see WARNINGS*), hypertension (*see PRECAUTIONS*), headache, gastrointestinal disturbances and hirsutism/hypertrichosis.

In rheumatoid arthritis patients treated in clinical trials within the recommended dose range, cyclosporine therapy was discontinued in 5.3% of the patients because of hypertension and in 7% of the patients because of increased creatinine. These changes are usually reversible with timely dose decrease or drug discontinuation. The frequency and severity of serum creatinine elevations increase with dose and duration of cyclosporine therapy. These elevations are likely to become more pronounced without dose reduction or discontinuation.

The following adverse events occurred in controlled clinical trials:

[See table at top of next page]

In addition, the following adverse events have been reported in 1% to <3% of the rheumatoid arthritis patients in the cyclosporine treatment group in controlled clinical trials.

Autonomic Nervous System: dry mouth, increased sweating;

Body as a Whole: allergy, asthenia, hot flushes, malaise, overdose, procedure NOS*, tumor NOS*, weight decrease, weight increase;

Cardiovascular: abnormal heart sounds, cardiac failure, myocardial infarction, peripheral ischemia;

Central and Peripheral Nervous System: hypoesthesia, neuropathy, vertigo;

Endocrine: goiter;

Gastrointestinal: constipation, dysphagia, enanthema, eructation, esophagitis, gastric ulcer, gastritis, gastroenteritus, gingival bleeding, glossitis, peptic ulcer, salivary gland enlargement, tongue disorder, tooth disorder;

Infection: abscess, bacterial infection, cellulitis, folliculitis, fungal infection, herpes simplex, herpes zoster, renal abscess, moniliasis, tonsillitis, viral infection;

Hematologic: anemia, epistaxis, leukopenia, lymphadenopathy;

Liver and Biliary System: bilirubinemia;

Metabolic and Nutritional: diabetes mellitus, hyperkalemia, hyperuricemia, hypoglycemia;

Musculoskeletal System: arthralgia, bone fracture, bursitis, joint dislocation, myalgia, stiffness, synovial cyst, tendon disorder;

Neoplasms: breast fibroadenosis, carcinoma;

Psychiatric: anxiety, confusion, decreased libido, emotional lability, impaired concentration, increased libido, nervousness, paroniria, somnolence;

Reproductive (Female): breast pain, uterine hemorrhage;

Respiratory System: abnormal chest sounds, bronchospasm;

Skin and Appendages: abnormal pigmentation, angioedema, dermatitis, dry skin, eczema, nail disorder, pruritus, skin disorder, urticaria;

Special Senses: abnormal vision, cataract, conjunctivitis, deafness, eye pain, taste perversion, tinnitus, vestibular disorder;

Urinary System: abnormal urine, hematuria, increased BUN, micturition urgency, nocturia, polyuria, pyelonephritis, urinary incontinence.

*NOS = Not Otherwise Specified.

Psoriasis: The principal adverse reactions associated with the use of cyclosporine in patients with psoriasis are renal dysfunction, headache, hypertension, hypertriglyceridemia, hirsutism/hypertrichosis, paresthesia or hyperesthesia, influenza-like symptoms, nausea/vomiting, diarrhea, abdominal discomfort, lethargy, and musculoskeletal or joint pain.

In psoriasis patients treated in U.S. controlled clinical studies within the recommended dose range, cyclosporine therapy was discontinued in 1.0% of the patients because of hypertension and in 5.4% of the patients because of increased creatinine. In the majority of cases, these changes were reversible after dose reduction or discontinuation of cyclosporine.

There has been one reported death associated with the use of cyclosporine in psoriasis. A 27 year old male developed renal deterioration and was continued on cyclosporine. He had progressive renal failure leading to death.

Cyclosporine (MODIFIED)/Cyclosporine (NON-MODIFIED) Rheumatoid Arthritis
Percentage of Patients with Adverse Events ≥ 3% in any Cyclosporine Treated Group

		Studies 651 + 652 + 2008	Study 302	Study 654	Study 654	Study 302	Studies 651 + 652 + 2008
Body System	Preferred Term	Cyclosporine (NON-MODIFIED)† (N=269)	Cyclosporine (NON-MODIFIED) (N=155)	Methotrexate & Cyclosporine (NON-MODIFIED) (N=74)	Methotrexate & Placebo (N=73)	Cyclosporine (MODIFIED) (N=143)	Placebo (N=201)
Autonomic Nervous System Disorders	Flushing	2%	2%	3%	0%	5%	2%
Body As A Whole - General Disorders	Accidental Trauma	0%	1%	10%	4%	4%	0%
	Edema NOS*	5%	14%	12%	4%	10%	<1%
	Fatigue	6%	3%	8%	12%	3%	7%
	Fever	2%	3%	0%	0%	2%	4%
	Influenza-like symptoms	<1%	6%	1%	0%	3%	2%
	Pain	6%	9%	10%	15%	13%	4%
	Rigors	1%	1%	4%	0%	3%	1%
Cardiovascular Disorders	Arrhythmia	2%	5%	5%	6%	2%	1%
	Chest Pain	4%	5%	1%	1%	6%	1%
	Hypertension	8%	26%	16%	12%	25%	2%
Central and Peripheral Nervous System Disorders	Dizziness	8%	6%	7%	3%	8%	3%
	Headache	17%	23%	22%	11%	25%	9%
	Migraine	2%	3%	0%	0%	3%	1%
	Paresthesia	8%	7%	8%	4%	11%	1%
	Tremor	8%	7%	7%	3%	13%	4%
Gastrointestinal System Disorders	Abdominal Pain	15%	15%	15%	7%	15%	10%
	Anorexia	3%	3%	1%	0%	3%	3%
	Diarrhea	12%	12%	18%	15%	13%	8%
	Dyspepsia	12%	12%	10%	8%	8%	4%
	Flatulence	5%	5%	5%	4%	4%	1%
	Gastrointestinal Disorder NOS*	0%	2%	1%	4%	4%	0%
	Gingivitis	4%	3%	0%	0%	0%	1%
	Gum Hyperplasia	2%	4%	1%	3%	4%	1%
	Nausea	23%	14%	24%	15%	18%	14%
	Rectal Hemorrhage	0%	3%	0%	0%	1%	1%
	Stomatitis	7%	5%	16%	12%	6%	8%
	Vomiting	9%	8%	14%	7%	6%	5%
Hearing and Vestibular Disorders	Eat Disorders NOS*	0%	5%	0%	0%	1%	0%
Metabolic and Nutritional Disorders	Hypomagnesemia	0%	4%	0%	0%	6%	0%
Musculoskeletal System Disorders	Arthropathy	0%	5%	0%	1%	4%	0%
	Leg Cramps/Involuntary Muscle Contractions	2%	11%	11%	3%	12%	1%
Psychiatric Disorders	Depression	3%	6%	3%	1%	1%	2%
	Insomnia	4%	1%	1%	0%	3%	2%
Renal	Creatinine elevations ≥30%	43%	39%	55%	19%	48%	13%
	Creatinine elevations ≥50%	24%	18%	26%	8%	18%	3%
Reproductive Disorders, Female	Leukorrhea	1%	0%	4%	0%	1%	0%
	Menstrual Disorder	3%	2%	1%	0%	1%	1%
Respiratory System Disorders	Bronchitis	1%	3%	1%	0%	1%	3%
	Coughing	5%	3%	5%	7%	4%	4%
	Dyspnea	5%	1%	3%	3%	1%	2%
	Infection NOS*	9%	5%	0%	7%	3%	10%
	Pharyngitis	3%	5%	5%	6%	4%	4%
	Pneumonia	1%	0%	4%	0%	1%	1%
	Rhinitis	0%	3%	11%	10%	1%	0%
	Sinusitis	4%	4%	8%	4%	3%	3%
	Upper Respiratory Tract	0%	14%	23%	15%	13%	0%
Skin and Appendages Disorders	Alopecia	3%	0%	1%	1%	4%	4%
	Bullous Eruption	1%	0%	4%	1%	1%	1%
	Hypertrichosis	19%	17%	12%	0%	15%	3%
	Rash	7%	12%	10%	7%	8%	10%
	Skin Ulceration	1%	1%	3%	4%	0%	2%
Urinary System Disorders	Dysuria	0%	0%	11%	3%	1%	2%
	Micturition Frequency	2%	4%	3%	1%	2%	2%
	NPN, Increased	0%	19%	12%	0%	18%	0%
	Urinary Tract Infection	0%	3%	5%	4%	3%	0%
Vascular (Extracardiac) Disorders	Pupura	3%	4%	1%	1%	2%	0%

† Includes patients in 2.5 mg/kg/day dose group only. *NOS = Not Otherwise Specified.

Frequency and severity of serum creatinine increases with dose and duration of cyclosporine therapy. These elevations are likely to become more pronounced and may result in irreversible renal damage without dose reduction or discontinuation.

[See table at top of next page]

The following events occurred in 1% to less than 3% of psoriasis patients treated with cyclosporine:

Body as a Whole: fever, flushes, hot flushes; ***Cardiovascular:*** chest pain; ***Central and Peripheral Nervous System:*** appetite increased, insomnia, dizziness, nervousness, vertigo; ***Gastrointestinal:*** abdominal distention, constipation, gingival bleeding; ***Liver and Biliary System:*** hyperbilirubinemia; ***Neoplasms:*** skin malignancies [squamous cell (0.9%) and basal cell (0.4%) carcinomas]; ***Reticuloendothelial:*** platelet, bleeding, and clotting disorders, red blood cell disorder; ***Respiratory:*** infection, viral and other infection; ***Skin and Appendages:*** acne, folliculitis, keratosis, pruritus, rash, dry skin; ***Urinary System:*** micturition frequency; ***Vision:*** abnormal vision.

Mild hypomagnesemia and hyperkalemia may occur but are asymptomatic. Increases in uric acid may occur and attacks of gout have been rarely reported. A minor and dose related hyperbilirubinemia has been observed in the absence of hepatocellular damage. Cyclosporine therapy may be associated with a modest increase of serum triglycerides or cholesterol. Elevations of triglycerides (>750 mg/dL) occur in about 15% of psoriasis patients; elevations of cholesterol (>300 mg/dL) are observed in less than 3% of psoriasis patients. Generally these laboratory abnormalities are reversible upon dose reduction or discontinuation of cyclosporine.

OVERDOSAGE

There is a minimal experience with cyclosporine overdosage. Forced emesis can be of value up to 2 hours after administration of Gengraf® (cyclosporine capsules, USP **[MODIFIED]**). Transient hepatotoxicity and nephrotoxicity may occur which should resolve following drug withdrawal. General supportive measures and symptomatic treatment should be followed in all cases of overdosage. Cyclosporine is not dialyzable to any great extent, nor is it cleared well by charcoal hemoperfusion. The oral dosage at which half of experimental animals are estimated to die is 31 times, 39 times and >54 times the human maintenance dose for transplant patients (6 mg/kg; corrections based on body surface area) in mice, rats, and rabbits.

DOSAGE AND ADMINISTRATION

Gengraf® (cyclosporine capsules, USP [MODIFIED]) has increased bioavailability in comparison to Sandimmune®* (cyclosporine [NON-MODIFIED]). Gengraf® and Sandimmune®* (cyclosporine [NON-MODIFIED]) are not bioequivalent and cannot be used interchangeably without physician supervision.

The daily dose of Gengraf® (cyclosporine capsules, USP **[MODIFIED]**) should always be given in two divided doses (BID). It is recommended that Gengraf® be administered on a consistent schedule with regard to time of day and relation to meals. Grapefruit and grapefruit juice affect metabolism, increasing blood concentration of cyclosporine, thus should be avoided.

Newly Transplanted Patients: The initial oral dose of Gengraf® (cyclosporine capsules, USP **[MODIFIED]**) can be given 4–12 hours prior to transplantation or be given postoperatively. The initial dose of Gengraf® varies depending on the transplanted organ and the other immunosuppressive agents included in the immunosuppressive protocol. In newly transplanted patients, the initial oral dose of Gengraf® is the same as the initial oral dose of cyclosporine (**NON-MODIFIED**). Suggested initial doses are available from the results of a 1994 survey of the use of cyclosporine (**NON-MODIFIED**) in U.S. transplant centers. The mean ± SD initial doses were 9±3 mg/kg/day for renal transplant patients (75 centers), 8±4 mg/kg/day for liver transplant patients (30 centers), and 7±3 mg/kg/day for heart transplant patients (24 centers). Total daily doses were divided into two equal daily doses. The Gengraf® dose is subsequently adjusted to achieve a pre-defined cyclosporine blood concentra-

Continued on next page

Gengraf—Cont.

tion (*see DOSAGE AND ADMINISTRATION, Blood Concentration Monitoring in Transplant Patients, below*). If cyclosporine trough blood concentrations are used, the target range is the same for Gengraf® as for cyclosporine (**NON-MODIFIED**). Using the same trough concentration target range for Gengraf® as for cyclosporine (**NON-MODIFIED**) results in greater cyclosporine exposure when Gengraf® is administered (*see CLINICAL PHARMACOLOGY, Pharmacokinetics, Absorption*). Dosing should be titrated based on clinical assessments of rejection and tolerability. Lower Gengraf® doses may be sufficient as maintenance therapy. Adjunct therapy with adrenal corticosteroids is recommended initially. Different tapering dosage schedules of prednisone appear to achieve similar results. A representative dosage schedule based on the patient's weight started with 2 mg/kg/day for the first 4 days tapered to 1 mg/kg/day by 1 week, 0.6 mg/kg/day by 2 weeks, 0.3 mg/kg/day by 1 month, and 0.15 mg/kg/day by 2 months and thereafter as a maintenance dose. Steroid doses may be further tapered on an individualized basis depending on status of patient and function of graft. Adjustments in dosage of prednisone must be made according to the clinical situation.

Conversion from Sandimmune®* (cyclosporine [NON-MODIFIED]) to Gengraf® (cyclosporine capsules, USP [MODIFIED]) in Transplant Patients: In transplanted patients who are considered for conversion to Gengraf® from Sandimmune®* (cyclosporine [**NON-MODIFIED**]), Gengraf® should be started with the same daily dose as was previously used with Sandimmune®* (cyclosporine [**NON-MODIFIED**]) (1:1 dose conversion). The Gengraf® dose should subsequently be adjusted to attain the pre-conversion cyclosporine blood trough concentration. Using the same trough concentration target range for Gengraf® as for Sandimmune®* (cyclosporine [**NON-MODIFIED**]) results in greater cyclosporine exposure when Gengraf® is administered (*see CLINICAL PHARMACOLOGY, Pharmacokinetics, Absorption*). Patients with suspected poor absorption of Sandimmune®* (cyclosporine [**NON-MODIFIED**]) require different dosing strategies (*see DOSAGE AND ADMINISTRATION, Transplant Patients with Poor Absorption of Sandimmune®* (cyclosporine [NON-MODIFIED]), below*). In some patients, the increase in blood trough concentration is more pronounced and may be of clinical significance.

Until the blood trough concentration attains the pre-conversion value, it is strongly recommended that the cyclosporine blood trough concentration be monitored every 4 to 7 days after conversion to Gengraf®. In addition, clinical safety parameters such as serum creatinine and blood pressure should be monitored every two weeks during the first two months after conversion. If the blood trough concentrations are outside the desired range and/or if the clinical safety parameters worsen, the dosage of Gengraf® must be adjusted accordingly.

Transplant Patients with Poor Absorption of Sandimmune®* (cyclosporine [NON-MODIFIED]): Patients with lower than expected cyclosporine blood trough concentrations in relation to the oral dose of Sandimmune®* (cyclosporine [**NON-MODIFIED**]) may have poor or inconsistent absorption of cyclosporine from Sandimmune®* (cyclosporine [**NON-MODIFIED**]). After conversion to Gengraf® (cyclosporine capsules, USP [**MODIFIED**]), patients tend to have higher cyclosporine concentrations. **Due to the increase in bioavailability of cyclosporine following conversion to Gengraf®, the cyclosporine blood trough concentration may exceed the target range. Particular caution should be exercised when converting patients to Gengraf® at doses greater than 10 mg/kg/day.** The dose of Gengraf® should be titrated individually based on cyclosporine trough concentrations, tolerability, and clinical response. In this population the cyclosporine blood trough concentration should be measured more frequently, at least twice a week (daily, if initial dose exceeds 10 mg/kg/day) until the concentration stabilizes within the desired range.

Rheumatoid Arthritis: The initial dose of Gengraf® (cyclosporine capsules, USP [**MODIFIED**]) is 2.5 mg/kg/day, taken twice daily as a divided (BID) oral dose. Salicylates, nonsteroidal anti-inflammatory agents, and oral corticosteroids may be continued (*see WARNINGS and PRECAUTIONS: Drug Interactions*). Onset of action generally occurs between 4 and 8 weeks. If insufficient clinical benefit is seen and tolerability is good (including serum creatinine less than 30% above baseline), the dose may be increased by 0.5–0.75 mg/kg/day after 8 weeks and again after 12 weeks to a maximum of 4 mg/kg/day. If no benefit is seen by 16 weeks of therapy, Gengraf® therapy should be discontinued.

Dose decreases by 25%–50% should be made at any time to control adverse events, e.g., hypertension elevations in serum creatinine (30% above patient's pretreatment level) or clinically significant laboratory abnormalities (*see WARNINGS and PRECAUTIONS*).

If dose reduction is not effective in controlling abnormalities or if the adverse event or abnormality is severe, Gengraf® should be discontinued. The same initial dose and dosage range should be used if Gengraf® is combined with the recommended dose of methotrexate. Most patients can be treated with Gengraf® doses of 3 mg/kg/day or below when combined with methotrexate doses of up to 15 mg/week (*see CLINICAL PHARMACOLOGY, Clinical Trials*).

There is limited long-term treatment data. Recurrence of rheumatoid arthritis disease activity is generally apparent within four weeks after stopping cyclosporine.

Adverse Events Occurring in 3% or More of Psoriasis Patients in Controlled Clinical Trials

Body System*	Preferred Term	Cyclosporine (MODIFIED) (N=182)	Cyclosporine (NON-MODIFIED) (N=185)
Infection or Partial Infection		24.7%	24.3%
	Influenza-like Symptoms	9.9%	8.1%
	Upper Respiratory Tract Infections	7.7%	11.3%
Cardiovascular System		28.0%	25.4%
	Hypertension**	27.5%	25.4%
Urinary System		24.2%	16.2%
	Increased Creatinine	19.8%	15.7%
Central and Peripheral Nervous System		26.4%	20.5%
	Headache	15.9%	14.0%
	Paresthesia	7.1%	4.8%
Musculoskeletal System		13.2%	8.7%
	Arthralgia	6.0%	1.1%
Body As a Whole - General		29.1%	22.2%
	Pain	4.4%	3.2%
Metabolic and Nutritional		9.3%	9.7%
Reproductive, Female		8.5% (4 of 47 females)	11.5% (6 of 52 females)
Resistance Mechanism		18.7%	21.1%
Skin and Appendages		17.6%	15.1%
	Hypertrichosis	6.6%	5.4%
Respiratory System		5.0%	6.5%
	Bronchospasm, Coughing, Dyspnea, Rhinitis	5.0%	4.9%
Psychiatric		5.0%	3.8%
Gastrointestinal System		19.8%	28.7%
	Abdominal Pain	2.7%	6.0%
	Diarrhea	5.0%	5.9%
	Dyspepsia	2.2%	3.2%
	Gum Hyperplasia	3.8%	6.0%
	Nausea	5.5%	5.9%
White cell and RES		4.4%	2.7%

* Total percentage of events within the system.
** Newly occurring hypertension = SBP ≥160 mm Hg and/or DBP ≥90 mm Hg.

Psoriasis: The initial dose of Gengraf® (cyclosporine capsules, USP [**MODIFIED**]) should be 2.5 mg/kg/day. Gengraf® should be taken twice daily, as a divided (1.25 mg/kg BID) oral dose. Patients should be kept at that dose for at least 4 weeks, barring adverse events. If significant clinical improvement has not occurred in patients by that time, the patient's dosage should be increased at 2 week intervals. Based on patient response, dose increases of approximately 0.5 mg/kg/day should be made to a maximum of 4 mg/kg/day.

Dose decreases by 25%-50% should be made at any time to control adverse events, e.g., hypertension, elevations in serum creatinine (≥25% above the patient's pretreatment level), or clinically significant laboratory abnormalities.

If dose reduction is not effective in controlling abnormalities, or if the adverse event or abnormality is severe, Gengraf® should be discontinued (*see PRECAUTIONS, Special Monitoring of Psoriasis Patients*).

Patients generally show some improvement in the clinical manifestations of psoriasis in 2 weeks. Satisfactory control and stabilization of the disease may take 12–16 weeks to achieve. Results of a dose-titration clinical trial with Gengraf® indicate that an improvement of psoriasis by 75% or more (based on PASI) was achieved in 51% of the patients after 8 weeks and in 79% of the patients after 16 weeks. Treatment should be discontinued if satisfactory response cannot be achieved after 6 weeks at 4 mg/kg/day or the patient's maximum tolerated dose. Once a patient is adequately controlled and appears stable the dose of Gengraf® should be lowered, and the patient treated with the lowest dose that maintains an adequate response (this should not necessarily be total clearing of the patient). In clinical trials, cyclosporine doses at the lower end of the recommended dosage range were effective in maintaining a satisfactory response in 60% of the patients. Doses below 2.5 mg/kg/day may also be equally effective.

Upon stopping treatment with cyclosporine, relapse will occur in approximately six weeks (50% of the patients) to 16 weeks (75% of the patients). In the majority of patients rebound does not occur after cessation of treatment with cyclosporine. Thirteen cases of transformation of chronic plaque psoriasis to more severe forms of psoriasis have been reported. There were 9 cases of pustular and 4 cases of erythrodermic psoriasis. Long term experience with Gengraf® in psoriasis patients is limited and continuous treatment for extended periods greater than one year is not recommended. Alternation with other forms of treatment should be considered in the long term management of patients with this life long disease.

Blood Concentration Monitoring in Transplant Patients: Transplant centers have found blood concentration monitoring of cyclosporine to be an essential component of patient management. Of importance to blood concentration analysis are the type of assay used, the transplanted organ, and other immunosuppressant agents being administered. While no fixed relationship has been established, blood concentration monitoring may assist in the clinical evaluation of rejection and toxicity, dose adjustments, and the assessment of compliance.

Various assays have been used to measure blood concentrations of cyclosporine. Older studies using a non-specific assay often cited concentrations that were roughly twice those of the specific assays. Therefore, comparison between concentrations in the published literature and an individual patient concentration using current assays must be made with detailed knowledge of the assay methods employed. Current assay results are also not interchangeable and their use should be guided by their approved labeling. A discussion of the different assay methods is contained in *Annals of Clinical Biochemistry* 1994;31:420-446. While several assays and assay matrices are available, there is a consensus that parent-compound-specific assays correlate best with clinical events. Of these, HPLC is the standard reference, but the monoclonal antibody RIAs and the monoclonal antibody FPIA offer sensitivity, reproducibility, and convenience. Most clinicians base their monitoring on trough cyclosporine concentrations. *Applied Pharmacokinetics, Principles of Therapeutic Drug Monitoring* (1992) contains a broad discussion of cyclosporine pharmacokinetics and drug monitoring techniques. Blood concentration monitoring is not a replacement for renal function monitoring or tissue biopsies.

HOW SUPPLIED

Gengraf® Capsules (cyclosporine capsules, USP [MODIFIED])

25 mg

Oval, white imprinted in blue, the corporate logo ⊡, 25 mg, and the Abbo-Code OR.

Packages of 30 unit-dose blisters. (**NDC** 0074-6463-32).

100 mg

Oval, white, with two blue stripes, imprinted in blue, the corporate logo ⊡, 100 mg, and Abbo-Code OT.

Packages of 30 unit-dose blisters. (**NDC** 0074-6479-32).

Store and Dispense: In the original unit-dose container at controlled room temperature 15°–30°C (59°–86°F). (See USP).

---

*Sandimmune® is a registered trademark of Novartis Pharmaceuticals Corporation.

Manufactured by: Abbott Laboratories North Chicago, IL 60064, U.S.A.
Distributed by: SangStat Medical Corporation Fremont, CA 94555, U.S.A.
03-5242-R4
Revised: January, 2003
ABBOTT LABORATORIES
NORTH CHICAGO, IL 60064, U.S.A.
SANGSTAT
The Transplant Company®
Fremont, CA 94555, U.S.A.

Shown in Product Identification Guide, page 303

HUMIRA® ℞

[*hew-mĭ-ră*]
(adalimumab)

℞ only

> **WARNING**
> **RISK OF INFECTIONS**
> **Cases of tuberculosis (frequently disseminated or extrapulmonary at clinical presentation) have been observed in patients receiving HUMIRA.**

Patients should be evaluated for latent tuberculosis infection with a tuberculin skin test. Treatment of latent tuberculosis infection should be initiated prior to therapy with HUMIRA.

DESCRIPTION

HUMIRA (adalimumab) is a recombinant human IgG1 monoclonal antibody specific for human tumor necrosis factor (TNF). HUMIRA was created using phage display technology resulting in an antibody with human derived heavy and light chain variable regions and human IgG1 : κ constant regions. HUMIRA is produced by recombinant DNA technology in a mammalian cell expression system and is purified by a process that includes specific viral inactivation and removal steps. It consists of 1330 amino acids and has a molecular weight of approximately 148 kilodaltons.

HUMIRA is supplied in single-use, 1 mL pre-filled glass syringes as a sterile, preservative-free solution for subcutaneous administration. The solution of HUMIRA is clear and colorless, with a pH of about 5.2. Each syringe delivers 0.8 mL (40 mg) of drug product. Each 0.8 mL of HUMIRA contains 40 mg adalimumab, 4.93 mg sodium chloride, 0.69 mg monobasic sodium phosphate dihydrate, 1.22 mg dibasic sodium phosphate dihydrate, 0.24 mg sodium citrate, 1.04 mg citric acid monohydrate, 9.6 mg mannitol, 0.8 mg polysorbate 80 and Water for Injection, USP. Sodium hydroxide added as necessary to adjust pH.

CLINICAL PHARMACOLOGY

General

Adalimumab binds specifically to TNF-alpha and blocks its interaction with the p55 and p75 cell surface TNF receptors. Adalimumab also lyses surface TNF expressing cells *in vitro* in the presence of complement. Adalimumab does not bind or inactivate lymphotoxin (TNF-beta). TNF is a naturally occurring cytokine that is involved in normal inflammatory and immune responses. Elevated levels of TNF are found in the synovial fluid of rheumatoid arthritis patients and play an important role in both the pathologic inflammation and the joint destruction that are hallmarks of rheumatoid arthritis.

Adalimumab also modulates biological responses that are induced or regulated by TNF, including changes in the levels of adhesion molecules responsible for leukocyte migration (ELAM-1, VCAM-1, and ICAM-1 with an IC_{50} of $1–2 \times 10^{-10}$M).

Pharmacodynamics

After treatment with HUMIRA, a rapid decrease in levels of acute phase reactants of inflammation (C-reactive protein (CRP) and erythrocyte sedimentation rate (ESR)) and serum cytokines (IL-6) was observed compared to baseline in patients with rheumatoid arthritis. Serum levels of matrix metalloproteinases (MMP-1 and MMP-3) that produce tissue remodeling responsible for cartilage destruction were also decreased after HUMIRA administration.

Pharmacokinetics

The maximum serum concentration (C_{max}) and the time to reach the maximum concentration (T_{max}) were 4.7 ± 1.6 μg/mL and 131 ± 56 hours respectively, following a single 40 mg subcutaneous administration of HUMIRA to healthy adult subjects. The average absolute bioavailability of adalimumab estimated from three studies following a single 40 mg subcutaneous dose was 64%. The pharmacokinetics of adalimumab were linear over the dose range of 0.5 to 10.0 mg/kg following a single intravenous dose.

The single dose pharmacokinetics of adalimumab were determined in several studies with intravenous doses ranging from 0.25 to 10 mg/kg. The distribution volume (V_{ss}) ranged from 4.7 to 6.0 L. The systemic clearance of adalimumab is approximately 12 mL/hr. The mean terminal half-life was approximately 2 weeks, ranging from 10 to 20 days across studies. Adalimumab concentrations in the synovial fluid from five rheumatoid arthritis patients ranged from 31-96% of those in serum.

Adalimumab mean steady-state trough concentrations of approximately 5 μg/mL and 8 to 9 μg/mL, were observed without and with methotrexate (MTX) respectively. The serum adalimumab trough levels at steady state increased approximately proportionally with dose following 20, 40 and 80 mg every other week and every week subcutaneous dosing. In long-term studies with dosing more than two years, there was no evidence of changes in clearance over time.

Population pharmacokinetic analyses revealed that there was a trend toward higher apparent clearance of adalimumab in the presence of anti-adalimumab antibodies, and lower clearance with increasing age in patients aged 40 to >75 years.

Minor increases in apparent clearance were also predicted in patients receiving doses lower than the recommended dose and in patients with high rheumatoid factor or CRP concentrations. These increases are not likely to be clinically important.

No gender-related pharmacokinetic differences were observed after correction for a patient's body weight. Healthy volunteers and patients with rheumatoid arthritis displayed similar adalimumab pharmacokinetics.

No pharmacokinetic data are available in patients with hepatic or renal impairment.

HUMIRA has not been studied in children.

Drug Interactions

MTX reduced adalimumab apparent clearance after single and multiple dosing by 29% and 44% respectively.

Table 1: ACR Responses in Placebo-Controlled Trials (Percent of Patients)

	Study II Monotherapy (26 weeks)			Study III Methotrexate Combination (24 and 52 weeks)	
Response	Placebo N=110	HUMIRA 40 mg every other week N=113	HUMIRA 40 mg weekly N=103	Placebo/MTX N=200	HUMIRA/MTX 40 mg every other week N=207
ACR20					
Month 6	19%	46%*	53%*	30%	63%*
Month 12	NA	NA	NA	24%	59%*
ACR50					
Month 6	8%	22%*	35%*	10%	39%*
Month 12	NA	NA	NA	10%	42%*
ACR70					
Month 6	2%	12%*	18%*	3%	21%*
Month 12	NA	NA	NA	5%	23%*

*p<0.01, HUMIRA vs. placebo

Table 2: Components of ACR Response in Studies II and III

Parameter (median)	Study II Placebo N=110		Study II HUMIRA[a] N=113		Study III Placebo/MTX N=200		Study III HUMIRA[a]/MTX N=207	
	Baseline	Wk 26	Baseline	Wk 26	Baseline	Wk 24	Baseline	Wk 24
Number of tender joints (0-68)	35	26	31	16*	26	15	24	8*
Number of swollen joints (0-66)	19	16	18	10*	17	11	18	5*
Physician global assessment[b]	7.0	6.1	6.6	3.7*	6.3	3.5	6.5	2.0*
Patient global assessment[b]	7.5	6.3	7.5	4.5*	5.4	3.9	5.2	2.0*
Pain[b]	7.3	6.1	7.3	4.1*	6.0	3.8	5.8	2.1*
Disability index (HAQ)[c]	2.0	1.9	1.9	1.5*	1.5	1.3	1.5	0.8*
CRP (mg/dL)	3.9	4.3	4.6	1.8*	1.0	0.9	1.0	0.4*

[a] 40 mg HUMIRA administered every other week
[b] Visual analogue scale; 0 = best, 10 = worst
[c] Disability Index of the Health Assessment Questionnaire[2]; 0 = best, 3 = worst, measures the patient's ability to perform the following: dress/groom, arise, eat, walk, reach, grip, maintain hygiene, and maintain daily activity
*p<0.001, HUMIRA vs. placebo, based on mean change from baseline

CLINICAL STUDIES

The efficacy and safety of HUMIRA were assessed in four randomized, double-blind studies in patients ≥ age 18 with active rheumatoid arthritis diagnosed according to American College of Rheumatology (ACR) criteria. Patients had at least 6 swollen and 9 tender joints. HUMIRA was administered subcutaneously in combination with MTX (12.5 to 25 mg, Studies I and III) or as monotherapy (Study II) or with other disease-modifying anti-rheumatic drugs (DMARDs) (Study IV).

Study I evaluated 271 patients who had failed therapy with at least one but no more than four DMARDs and had inadequate response to MTX. Doses of 20, 40 or 80 mg of HUMIRA or placebo were given every other week for 24 weeks.

Study II evaluated 544 patients who had failed therapy with at least one DMARD. Doses of placebo, 20 or 40 mg of HUMIRA were given as monotherapy every other week or weekly for 26 weeks.

Study III evaluated 619 patients who had an inadequate response to MTX. Patients received placebo, 40 mg of HUMIRA every other week with placebo injections on alternate weeks, or 20 mg of HUMIRA weekly for up to 52 weeks. Study III had an additional primary endpoint at 52 weeks of inhibition of disease progression (as detected by X-ray results).

Study IV assessed safety in 636 patients who were either DMARD-naive or were permitted to remain on their pre-existing rheumatologic therapy provided that therapy was stable for a minimum of 28 days. Patients were randomized to 40 mg of HUMIRA or placebo every other week for 24 weeks.

The percent of HUMIRA treated patients achieving ACR 20, 50 and 70 responses in Studies II and III are shown in Table 1.

[See table 1 above]

The results of Study I were similar to Study III; patients receiving HUMIRA 40 mg every other week in Study I also achieved ACR 20, 50 and 70 response rates of 65%, 52% and 24%, respectively, compared to placebo responses of 13%, 7% and 3% respectively, at 6 months (p<0.01).

The results of the components of the ACR response criteria for Studies II and III are shown in Table 2. Improvement was seen in all components and was maintained to week 52.

[See table 2 above]

The time course of ACR 20 response for Study III is shown in Figure 1. In Study III, 85% of patients with ACR 20 responses at week 24 maintained the response at 52 weeks.

The time course of ACR 20 response for Study I and Study II were similar.

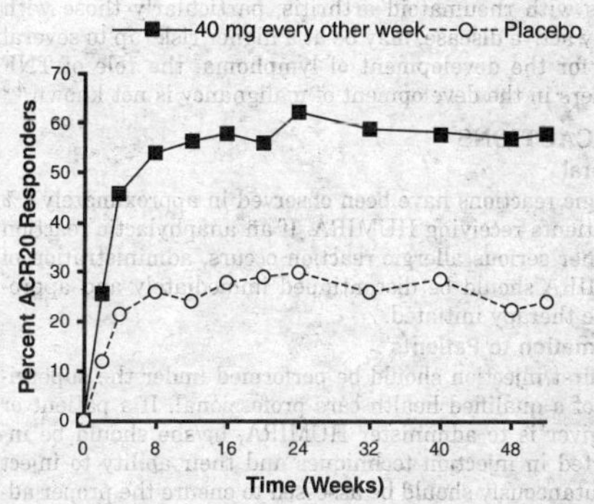

Figure 1: Study III ACR 20 Responses over 52 Weeks

In Study IV, 53% of patients treated with HUMIRA 40 mg every other week plus standard of care had an ACR 20 response at week 24 compared to 35% on placebo plus standard of care (p<0.001). No unique adverse reactions related to the combination of HUMIRA (adalimumab) and other DMARDs were observed.

In all four studies, HUMIRA showed significantly greater improvement than placebo in the disability index of Health Assessment Questionnaire (HAQ) from baseline to the end of study, and significantly greater improvement than placebo in the health-outcomes as assessed by The Short Form Health Survey (SF 36). Improvement was seen in both the Physical Component Summary (PCS) and the Mental Component Summary (MCS).

Radiographic Response

In Study III, structural joint damage was assessed radiographically and expressed as change in Total Sharp Score (TSS) and its components, the erosion score and Joint Space Narrowing (JSN) score, at month 12 compared to baseline. At baseline, the median TSS was approximately 55 in the

Continued on next page

Humira—Cont.

placebo and 40 mg every other week groups. The results are shown in Table 3. HUMIRA/MTX treated patients demonstrated less radiographic progression than patients receiving MTX alone.
[See table 3 below]

INDICATIONS AND USAGE

HUMIRA is indicated for reducing signs and symptoms and inhibiting the progression of structural damage in adult patients with moderately to severely active rheumatoid arthritis who have had an inadequate response to one or more DMARDs. HUMIRA can be used alone or in combination with MTX or other DMARDs.

CONTRAINDICATIONS

HUMIRA should not be administered to patients with known hypersensitivity to HUMIRA or any of its components.

WARNINGS

SERIOUS INFECTIONS AND SEPSIS, INCLUDING FATALITIES, HAVE BEEN REPORTED WITH THE USE OF TNF BLOCKING AGENTS INCLUDING HUMIRA. MANY OF THE SERIOUS INFECTIONS HAVE OCCURRED IN PATIENTS ON CONCOMITANT IMMUNOSUPPRESSIVE THERAPY THAT, IN ADDITION TO THEIR RHEUMATOID ARTHRITIS, COULD PREDISPOSE THEM TO INFECTIONS. TUBERCULOSIS AND INVASIVE OPPORTUNISTIC FUNGAL INFECTIONS HAVE BEEN OBSERVED IN PATIENTS TREATED WITH TNF BLOCKING AGENTS INCLUDING HUMIRA.

TREATMENT WITH HUMIRA SHOULD NOT BE INITIATED IN PATIENTS WITH ACTIVE INFECTIONS INCLUDING CHRONIC OR LOCALIZED INFECTIONS. PATIENTS WHO DEVELOP A NEW INFECTION WHILE UNDERGOING TREATMENT WITH HUMIRA SHOULD BE MONITORED CLOSELY. ADMINISTRATION OF HUMIRA SHOULD BE DISCONTINUED IF A PATIENT DEVELOPS A SERIOUS INFECTION. PHYSICIANS SHOULD EXERCISE CAUTION WHEN CONSIDERING THE USE OF HUMIRA IN PATIENTS WITH A HISTORY OF RECURRENT INFECTION OR UNDERLYING CONDITIONS WHICH MAY PREDISPOSE THEM TO INFECTIONS, OR PATIENTS WHO HAVE RESIDED IN REGIONS WHERE TUBERCULOSIS AND HISTOPLASMOSIS ARE ENDEMIC (see PRECAUTIONS - Tuberculosis and ADVERSE REACTIONS - Infections). THE BENEFITS AND RISKS OF HUMIRA TREATMENT SHOULD BE CAREFULLY CONSIDERED BEFORE INITIATION OF HUMIRA THERAPY.

Neurologic Events

Use of TNF blocking agents, including HUMIRA, has been associated with rare cases of exacerbation of clinical symptoms and/or radiographic evidence of demyelinating disease. Prescribers should exercise caution in considering the use of HUMIRA in patients with preexisting or recent-onset central nervous system demyelinating disorders.

Malignancies

Lymphomas have been observed in patients treated with TNF blocking agents including HUMIRA. In clinical trials, patients treated with HUMIRA had a higher incidence of lymphoma than the expected rate in the general population (see **ADVERSE REACTIONS-Malignancies**). While patients with rheumatoid arthritis, particularly those with highly active disease, may be at a higher risk (up to several fold) for the development of lymphoma, the role of TNF blockers in the development of malignancy is not known.[4,5]

PRECAUTIONS

General

Allergic reactions have been observed in approximately 1% of patients receiving HUMIRA. If an anaphylactic reaction or other serious allergic reaction occurs, administration of HUMIRA should be discontinued immediately and appropriate therapy initiated.

Information to Patients

The first injection should be performed under the supervision of a qualified health care professional. If a patient or caregiver is to administer HUMIRA, he/she should be instructed in injection techniques and their ability to inject subcutaneously should be assessed to ensure the proper administration of HUMIRA (see **HUMIRA, PATIENT INFORMATION LEAFLET**). A puncture-resistant container for disposal of needles and syringes should be used. Patients or caregivers should be instructed in the technique as well as proper syringe and needle disposal, and be cautioned against reuse of these items.

Tuberculosis

As observed with other TNF blocking agents, tuberculosis associated with the administration of HUMIRA in clinical trials has been reported (see **WARNINGS**). While cases were observed at all doses, the incidence of tuberculosis reactivations was particularly increased at doses of HUMIRA that were higher than the recommended dose. All patients recovered after standard antimicrobial therapy. No deaths due to tuberculosis occurred during the clinical trials.

Before initiation of therapy with HUMIRA, patients should be evaluated for active or latent tuberculosis infection with a tuberculin skin test. If latent infection is diagnosed, appropriate prophylaxis in accordance with the Centers for Disease Control and Prevention guidelines[6] should be instituted. Patients should be instructed to seek medical advice if signs/symptoms (e.g., persistent cough, wasting/weight loss, low grade fever) suggestive of a tuberculosis infection occur.

Immunosuppression

The possibility exists for TNF blocking agents, including HUMIRA, to affect host defenses against infections and malignancies since TNF mediates inflammation and modulates cellular immune responses. In a study of 64 patients with rheumatoid arthritis treated with HUMIRA, there was no evidence of depression of delayed-type hypersensitivity, depression of immunoglobulin levels, or change in enumeration of effector T- and B-cells and NK-cells, monocyte/macrophages, and neutrophils. The impact of treatment with HUMIRA on the development and course of malignancies, as well as active and/or chronic infections is not fully understood (see **WARNINGS, ADVERSE REACTIONS, Infections and Malignancies**). The safety and efficacy of HUMIRA in patients with immunosuppression have not been evaluated.

Immunizations

No data are available on the effects of vaccination in patients receiving HUMIRA. Live vaccines should not be given concurrently with HUMIRA. No data are available on the secondary transmission of infection by live vaccines in patients receiving HUMIRA.

Autoimmunity

Treatment with HUMIRA may result in the formation of autoantibodies and, rarely, in the development of a lupus-like syndrome. If a patient develops symptoms suggestive of a lupus-like syndrome following treatment with HUMIRA, treatment should be discontinued (see **ADVERSE REACTIONS, Autoantibodies**).

Drug Interactions

HUMIRA has been studied in rheumatoid arthritis patients taking concomitant MTX (see **CLINICAL PHARMACOLOGY: Drug Interactions**). The data do not suggest the need for dose adjustment of either HUMIRA or MTX.

Carcinogenesis, Mutagenesis, and Impairment of Fertility

Long-term animal studies of HUMIRA have not been conducted to evaluate the carcinogenic potential or its effect on fertility. No clastogenic or mutagenic effects of HUMIRA were observed in the *in vivo* mouse micronucleus test or the *Salmonella-Escherichia coli* (Ames) assay, respectively.

Pregnancy

Pregnancy Category B—An embryo-fetal perinatal developmental toxicity study has been performed in cynomolgus monkeys at dosages up to 100 mg/kg (266 times human AUC when given 40 mg subcutaneous with MTX every week or 373 times human AUC when given 40 mg subcutaneous without MTX) and has revealed no evidence of harm to the fetuses due to adalimumab. There are, however, no adequate and well-controlled studies in pregnant women. Because animal reproduction and developmental studies are not always predictive of human response, HUMIRA (adalimumab) should be used during pregnancy only if clearly needed.

Nursing Mothers

It is not known whether adalimumab is excreted in human milk or absorbed systemically after ingestion. Because many drugs and immunoglobulins are excreted in human milk, and because of the potential for serious adverse reactions in nursing infants from HUMIRA, a decision should be made whether to discontinue nursing or to discontinue the drug, taking into account the importance of the drug to the mother.

Pediatric Use

Safety and effectiveness of HUMIRA in pediatric patients have not been established.

Geriatric Use

A total of 519 patients 65 years of age and older, including 107 patients 75 years and older, received HUMIRA in clinical studies. No overall difference in effectiveness was observed between these subjects and younger subjects. The frequency of serious infection and malignancy among HUMIRA treated subjects over age 65 was higher than for those under age 65. Because there is a higher incidence of infections and malignancies in the elderly population in general, caution should be used when treating the elderly.

ADVERSE REACTIONS

General

The most serious adverse reactions were (see **WARNINGS**):
- Serious Infections
- Neurologic Events
- Malignancies

The most common adverse reaction with HUMIRA was injection site reactions. In placebo-controlled trials, 20% of patients treated with HUMIRA developed injection site reactions (erythema and/or itching, hemorrhage, pain or swelling), compared to 14% of patients receiving placebo. Most injection site reactions were described as mild and generally did not necessitate drug discontinuation.

The proportion of patients who discontinued treatment due to adverse events during the double-blind, placebo-controlled portion of Studies I, II, III and IV was 7% for patients taking HUMIRA and 4% for placebo-treated patients. The most common adverse events leading to discontinuation of HUMIRA were clinical flare reaction (0.7%), rash (0.3%) and pneumonia (0.3%).

Because clinical trials are conducted under widely varying and controlled conditions, adverse reaction rates observed in clinical trials of a drug cannot be directly compared to rates in the clinical trials of another drug and may not predict the rates observed in a broader patient population in clinical practice.

Infections

In placebo-controlled trials, the rate of infection was 1 per patient year in the HUMIRA treated patients and 0.9 per patient year in the placebo-treated patients. The infections consisted primarily of upper respiratory tract infections, bronchitis and urinary tract infections. Most patients continued on HUMIRA after the infection resolved. The incidence of serious infections was 0.04 per patient year in HUMIRA treated patients and 0.02 per patient year in placebo-treated patients. Serious infections observed included pneumonia, septic arthritis, prosthetic and post-surgical infections, erysipelas, cellulitis, diverticulitis, and pyelonephritis (see **WARNINGS**).

Thirteen cases of tuberculosis, including miliary, lymphatic, peritoneal, and pulmonary were reported in clinical trials. Most of the cases of tuberculosis occurred within the first eight months after initiation of therapy and may reflect recrudescence of latent disease. Six cases of invasive opportunistic infections caused by histoplasma, aspergillus, and nocardia were also reported in clinical trials (see **WARNINGS**).

Malignancies

Among 2468 rheumatoid arthritis patients treated in clinical trials with HUMIRA for a median of 24 months, 48 malignancies of various types were observed, including 10 patients with lymphoma. The Standardized Incidence Ratio (SIR) (ratio of observed rate to age-adjusted expected frequency in the general population) for malignancies was 1.0 (95% CI, 0.7, 1.3) and for lymphomas was 5.4 (95% CI, 2.6, 10.0). An increase of up to several fold in the rate of lymphomas has been reported in the rheumatoid arthritis patient population[4], and may be further increased in patients with more severe disease activity[5] (see **WARNINGS-Malignancies**). The other malignancies observed during use of HUMIRA were breast, colon-rectum, uterine-cervical, prostate, melanoma, gallbladder-bile ducts, and other carcinomas.

Autoantibodies

In the controlled trials, 12% of patients treated with HUMIRA and 7% of placebo-treated patients that had negative baseline ANA titers developed positive titers at week 24. One patient out of 2334 treated with HUMIRA developed clinical signs suggestive of new-onset lupus-like syndrome. The patient improved following discontinuation of therapy. No patients developed lupus nephritis or central nervous system symptoms. The impact of long-term treatment with HUMIRA on the development of autoimmune diseases is unknown.

Immunogenicity

Patients in Studies I, II, and III were tested at multiple time points for antibodies to adalimumab during the 6 to 12 month period. Approximately 5% (58 of 1,062) of adult rheumatoid arthritis patients receiving HUMIRA developed low-titer antibodies to adalimumab at least once during treatment, which were neutralizing *in vitro*. Patients treated with concomitant MTX had a lower rate of antibody development than patients on HUMIRA monotherapy (1% versus 12%). No apparent correlation of antibody development to adverse events was observed. With monotherapy, patients receiving every other week dosing may develop antibodies more frequently than those receiving weekly dosing. In patients receiving the recommended dosage of 40 mg every other week as monotherapy, the ACR 20 response was lower among antibody-positive patients than among antibody-negative patients. The long-term immunogenicity of HUMIRA is unknown.

The data reflect the percentage of patients whose test results were considered positive for antibodies to adalimumab in an ELISA assay, and are highly dependent on the sensitivity and specificity of the assay. Additionally the observed

Table 3: Radiographic Mean Changes Over 12 Months in Study III

	Placebo/MTX	HUMIRA/MTX 40 mg every other week	Placebo/MTX-HUMIRA/MTX (95% Confidence Interval*)	P-value**
Total Sharp score	2.7	0.1	2.6 (1.4, 3.8)	<0.001
Erosion score	1.6	0.0	1.6 (0.9, 2.2)	<0.001
JSN score	1.0	0.1	0.9 (0.3, 1.4)	0.002

*95% confidence intervals for the differences in change scores between MTX and HUMIRA.
**Based on rank analysis

incidence of antibody positivity in an assay may be influenced by several factors including sample handling, timing of sample collection, concomitant medications, and underlying disease. For these reasons, comparison of the incidence of antibodies to adalimumab with the incidence of antibodies to other products may be misleading.

Other Adverse Reactions

The data described below reflect exposure to HUMIRA in 2334 patients, including 2073 exposed for 6 months, 1497 exposed for greater than one year and 1380 in adequate and well-controlled studies (Studies I, II, III, and IV). HUMIRA was studied primarily in placebo-controlled trials and in long-term follow up studies for up to 36 months duration. The population had a mean age of 54 years, 77% were female, 91% were Caucasian and had moderately to severely active rheumatoid arthritis. Most patients received 40 mg HUMIRA every other week.

Table 4 summarizes events reported at a rate of at least 5% in patients treated with HUMIRA 40 mg every other week compared to placebo and with an incidence higher than placebo. Adverse event rates in patients treated with HUMIRA 40 mg weekly were similar to rates in patients treated with HUMIRA 40 mg every other week.

Table 4: Adverse Events Reported by ≥5% of Patients Treated with HUMIRA During Placebo-Controlled Period of Rheumatoid Arthritis Studies

Adverse Event (Preferred Term)	HUMIRA 40 mg subcutaneous Every Other Week (N=705) Percentage	Placebo (N=690) Percentage
Respiratory		
Upper respiratory infection	17	13
Sinusitis	11	9
Flu syndrome	7	6
Gastrointestinal		
Nausea	9	8
Abdominal pain	7	4
Laboratory Tests*		
Laboratory test abnormal	8	7
Hypercholesterolemia	6	4
Hyperlipidemia	7	5
Hematuria	5	4
Alkaline phosphatase increased	5	3
Other		
Injection site pain	12	12
Headache	12	8
Rash	12	6
Accidental injury	10	8
Injection site reaction**	8	1
Back pain	6	4
Urinary tract infection	8	5
Hypertension	5	3

* Laboratory test abnormalities were reported as adverse events in European trials

** Does not include erythema and/or itching, hemorrhage, pain or swelling

Other Adverse Events

Other infrequent serious adverse events occurring at an incidence of less than 5% in patients treated with HUMIRA were:

Body As A Whole: Fever, infection, pain in extremity, pelvic pain, sepsis, surgery, thorax pain, tuberculosis reactivated

Cardiovascular System: Arrhythmia, atrial fibrillation, cardiovascular disorder, chest pain, congestive heart failure, coronary artery disorder, heart arrest, hypertensive encephalopathy, myocardial infarct, palpitation, pericardial effusion, pericarditis, syncope, tachycardia, vascular disorder

Collagen Disorder: Lupus erythematosus syndrome

Digestive System: Cholecystitis, cholelithiasis, esophagitis, gastroenteritis, gastrointestinal disorder, gastrointestinal hemorrhage, hepatic necrosis, vomiting

Endocrine System: Parathyroid disorder

Hemic And Lymphatic System: Agranulocytosis, granulocytopenia, leukopenia, lymphoma like reaction, pancytopenia, polycythemia

Metabolic And Nutritional Disorders: Dehydration, healing abnormal, ketosis, paraproteinemia, peripheral edema

Musculo–Skeletal System: Arthritis, bone disorder, bone fracture (not spontaneous), bone necrosis, joint disorder, muscle cramps, myasthenia, pyogenic arthritis, synovitis, tendon disorder

Neoplasia: Adenoma, carcinomas such as breast, gastrointestinal, skin, urogenital, and others; lymphoma and melanoma.

Nervous System: Confusion, multiple sclerosis, paresthesia, subdural hematoma, tremor

Respiratory System: Asthma, bronchospasm, dyspnea, lung disorder, lung function decreased, pleural effusion, pneumonia

Skin And Appendages: Cellulitis, erysipelas, herpes zoster

Special Senses: Cataract

Thrombosis: Thrombosis leg

Urogenital System: Cystitis, kidney calculus, menstrual disorder, pyelonephritis

OVERDOSAGE

The maximum tolerated dose of HUMIRA has not been established in humans. Multiple doses up to 10 mg/kg have been administered to patients in clinical trials without evidence of dose-limiting toxicities. In case of overdosage, it is recommended that the patient be monitored for any signs or symptoms of adverse reactions or effects and appropriate symptomatic treatment instituted immediately.

DOSAGE AND ADMINISTRATION

The recommended dose of HUMIRA for adult patients with rheumatoid arthritis is 40 mg administered every other week as a subcutaneous injection. MTX, glucocorticoids, salicylates, nonsteroidal anti-inflammatory drugs (NSAIDs), analgesics or other DMARDs may be continued during treatment with HUMIRA. Some patients not taking concomitant MTX may derive additional benefit from increasing the dosing frequency of HUMIRA to 40 mg every week.

HUMIRA is intended for use under the guidance and supervision of a physician. Patients may self-inject HUMIRA if their physician determines that it is appropriate and with medical follow-up, as necessary, after proper training in injection technique.

The solution in the syringe should be carefully inspected visually for particulate matter and discoloration prior to subcutaneous administration. If particulates and discolorations are noted, the product should not be used. HUMIRA does not contain preservatives; therefore, unused portions of drug remaining from the syringe should be discarded. NOTE: The needle cover of the syringe contains dry rubber (latex), which should not be handled by persons sensitive to this substance.

Patients using the pre-filled syringes should be instructed to inject the full amount in the syringe (0.8 mL), which provides 40 mg of HUMIRA, according to the directions provided in the Patient Information Leaflet.

Injection sites should be rotated and injections should never be given into areas where the skin is tender, bruised, red or hard (see **PATIENT INFORMATION LEAFLET**).

Instructions For Activating the Needle Stick Device: Cartons for institutional use contain a syringe and needle with a needle protection device (see **HOW SUPPLIED**). To activate the needle stick protection device after injection, hold the syringe in one hand and, with the other hand, slide the outer protective shield over the exposed needle until it locks into place.

Storage and Stability

Do not use beyond the expiration date on the container. HUMIRA must be refrigerated at 2-8° C (36-46° F). DO NOT FREEZE. Protect the pre-filled syringe from exposure to light. Store in original carton until time of administration.

HOW SUPPLIED

HUMIRA® (adalimumab) is supplied in pre-filled syringes as a preservative-free, sterile solution for subcutaneous administration. The following packaging configurations are available:

Patient Use Syringe Carton

HUMIRA is dispensed in a carton containing two alcohol preps and two dose trays. Each dose tray consists of a single-use, 1 mL pre-filled glass syringe with a fixed 27 gauge ½ inch needle, providing 40 mg (0.8 mL) of HUMIRA. **The NDC number is 0074-3799-02.**

Institutional Use Syringe Carton

Each carton contains two alcohol preps and one dose tray. Each dose tray consists of a single-use, 1 mL pre-filled glass syringe with a fixed 27 gauge ½ inch needle (with a needle stick protection device) providing 40 mg (0.8 mL) of HUMIRA. **The NDC number is 0074-3799-01.**

REFERENCES

1. Arnett FC, Edworthy SM, Bloch DA, et. al. The American Rheumatology Association 1987 Revised Criteria for the Classification of Rheumatoid Arthritis. Arthritis Rheum 1988; 31:315-24.
2. Ramey DR, Fries JF, Singh G. The Health Assessment Questionnaire 1995 - Status and Review. In: Spilker B, ed. "Quality of Life and Pharmacoeconomics in Clinical Trials." 2nd ed. Philadelphia, PA. Lippincott-Raven 1996.
3. Ware JE, Gandek B. Overview of the SF-36 Health Survey and the International Quality of Life Assessment (IQOLA) Project. J Clin Epidemiol 1998; 51(11):903-12.
4. Mellemkjaer L, Linet MS, Gridley G, et al. Rheumatoid Arthritis and Cancer Risk. European Journal of Cancer 1996; 32A (10): 1753-1757.
5. Baecklund E, Ekbom A, Sparen P, et al. Disease Activity and Risk of Lymphoma in Patients With Rheumatoid Arthritis: Nested Case-Control Study. BMJ 1998; 317: 180-181.
6. Centers for Disease Control and Prevention. Targeted Tuberculin Testing and Treatment of Latent Tuberculosis Infection. MMWR 2000; 49(No. RR-6):26-38.

03-5318-R5
Revised: December, 2003
ABBOTT LABORATORIES
NORTH CHICAGO, IL 60064, U.S.A.
PRINTED IN U.S.A.
U.S. Govt. Lic. No. 0043

HUMIRA®
(adalimumab)
Patient Information

Read this leaflet carefully before you start taking HUMIRA (**hu-mare-ah**). You should also read this leaflet each time you get your prescription refilled, in case something has changed. The information in this leaflet does not take the place of talking with your doctor before you start taking this medicine and at check ups. Talk to your doctor if you have any questions about your treatment with HUMIRA.

What is HUMIRA?

HUMIRA is a medicine that is used in people with moderate to severe rheumatoid arthritis (RA). RA is an inflammatory disease of the joints. People with RA are usually given other medicines for their disease before they are given HUMIRA. HUMIRA is for people with RA who have not responded well enough to these other medicines.

How does HUMIRA work?

HUMIRA is a medicine called a *TNF blocker*, that is a type of protein that blocks the action of a substance your body makes called TNF-alpha. TNF-alpha (tumor necrosis factor alpha) is made by your body's immune system. People with RA have too much of it in their bodies. The extra TNF-alpha in your body can attack normal healthy body tissues and cause inflammation especially in the tissues in your bones, cartilage, and joints. HUMIRA helps reduce the signs and symptoms of RA (such as pain and swollen joints) and may help prevent further damage to your bones and joints. HUMIRA can block the damage that too much TNF-alpha can cause, and it can also lower your body's ability to fight infections. Taking HUMIRA can make you more prone to getting infections or make any infection you have worse.

Who should not take HUMIRA?

You should not take HUMIRA if you have an allergy to any of the ingredients in HUMIRA (sodium phosphate, sodium citrate, citric acid, mannitol, and polysorbate 80). The needle cover on the pre-filled syringe contains dry natural rubber. Tell your doctor if you have any allergies to rubber or latex.

Before you start taking HUMIRA you should tell your doctor if you have or have had any of the following:

- Any kind of infection including an infection that is in only one place in your body (such as an open cut or sore), or an infection that is in your whole body (such as the flu). Having an infection could put you at risk for serious side effects from HUMIRA. If you are unsure, please ask your doctor.
- A history of infections that keep coming back or other conditions that might increase your risk of infections.
- If you have ever had tuberculosis (TB), or if you have been in close contact with someone who has had tuberculosis. If you develop any of the symptoms of tuberculosis (a dry cough that doesn't go away, weight loss, fever, night sweats) call your doctor right away. Your doctor will need to examine you for TB and perform a skin test.
- If you experience any numbness or tingling or have ever had a disease that affects your nervous system like multiple sclerosis.
- If you are scheduled to have major surgery.
- If you are scheduled to be vaccinated for anything.

If you are not sure or have any questions about any of this information, ask your doctor.

What important information do I need to know about side effects with HUMIRA?

Any medicine can have side effects. Like all medicines that affect your immune system, HUMIRA can cause serious side effects. The possible serious side effects include:

Serious infections: There have been rare cases where patients taking HUMIRA or other TNF-blocking agents have developed serious infections, including tuberculosis (TB) and infections caused by bacteria or fungi. Some patients have died when the bacteria that cause infections have spread throughout their body (sepsis).

Nervous system diseases: There have been rare cases of disorders that affect the nervous system of people taking HUMIRA or other TNF blockers. Signs that you could be experiencing a problem affecting your nervous system include: numbness or tingling, problems with your vision, weakness in your legs and dizziness.

Malignancies: There have been very rare cases of certain kinds of cancer in patients taking HUMIRA or other TNF blockers. People with more serious RA that have had the disease for a long time may have a higher than average risk of getting a kind of cancer that affects the lymph system, called lymphoma. If you take HUMIRA or other TNF blockers, your risk may increase.

Lupus-like symptoms: Some patients have developed lupus-like symptoms that got better after their treatment was stopped. If you have chest pains that do not go away,

Continued on next page

Humira—Cont.

shortness of breath, joint pain or a rash on your cheeks or arms that is sensitive to the sun, call your doctor right away. Your doctor may decide to stop your treatment.

Allergic reactions: If you develop a severe rash, swollen face or difficulty breathing while taking HUMIRA, call your doctor right away.

What are the other more common side effects with HUMIRA?

Many patients experience a reaction where the injection was given. These reactions are usually mild and include redness, rash, swelling, itching or bruising. Usually, the rash will go away within a few days. If the skin around the area where you injected HUMIRA still hurts or is swollen, try using a towel soaked with cold water on the injection site. If you have pain, redness or swelling around the injection site that doesn't go away within a few days or gets worse, call your doctor right away. Other side effects are upper respiratory infections (sinus infections), headache and nausea.

Can I take HUMIRA if I am pregnant or breast-feeding?

HUMIRA has not been studied in pregnant women or nursing mothers, so we don't know what the effects are on pregnant women or nursing babies. You should tell your doctor if you are pregnant, become pregnant or are thinking about becoming pregnant.

Can I take HUMIRA if I am taking other medicines for my RA or other conditions?

Yes, you can take other medicines provided your doctor has prescribed them, or has told you it is ok to take them while you are taking HUMIRA. It is important that you tell your doctor about any other medicines you are taking for other conditions (for example, high blood pressure medicine) before you start taking HUMIRA.

You should also tell your doctor about any over-the-counter drugs, herbal medicines and vitamin and mineral supplements you are taking.

You should not take HUMIRA with other TNF blockers. If you have questions, ask your doctor.

How do I take HUMIRA?

You take HUMIRA by giving yourself an injection under the skin once every other week, or more frequently (every week) if your doctor tells you to. If you accidentally take more HUMIRA than you were told to take, you should call your doctor. Make sure you have been shown how to inject HUMIRA before you do it yourself. You can call your doctor or the HUMIRA Patient Resource Center at 1-800-4HUMIRA (448-6472) if you have any questions about giving yourself an injection. Someone you know can also help you with your injection. Remember to take this medicine just as your doctor has told you and do not miss any doses.

What should I do if I miss a dose of HUMIRA?

If you forget to take HUMIRA when you are supposed to, inject the next dose right away. Then, take your next dose when your next scheduled dose is due. This will put you back on schedule.

Is one time better than another for taking HUMIRA?

Always follow your doctor's instructions about when and how often to take HUMIRA. To help you remember when to take HUMIRA, you can mark your calendar ahead of time with the stickers provided in the back of the patient information booklet. For other information and ideas you can enroll in a patient support program by calling the HUMIRA Patient Resource Center at 1-800-4HUMIRA (448-6472).

What do I need to do to prepare and give an injection of HUMIRA?

1) Setting up for an injection

- Find a clean flat working surface.
- Remove one dose tray containing a pre-filled syringe of HUMIRA from the refrigerator. Do not use a pre-filled syringe that is frozen or if it has been left in direct sunlight.

You will need the following items for each dose:

- A dose tray containing a pre-filled syringe of HUMIRA with a fixed needle
- 1 alcohol prep

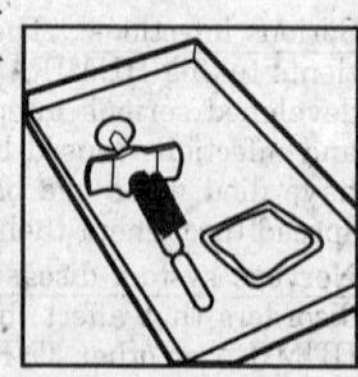

If you do not have all of the pieces you need to give yourself an injection, call your pharmacist. Use only the items provided in the box your HUMIRA comes in.

- Check and make sure the name HUMIRA appears on the dose tray and pre-filled syringe label.
- Check the expiration date on the dose tray label and pre-filled syringe to make sure the date has not passed. Do not use a pre-filled syringe if the date has passed.
- Make sure the liquid in the pre-filled syringe is clear and colorless. Do not use a pre-filled syringe if the liquid is cloudy or discolored or has flakes or particles in it.
- Have a puncture proof container nearby for disposing of used needles and syringes.

FOR YOUR PROTECTION, IT IS IMPORTANT THAT YOU FOLLOW THESE INSTRUCTIONS.

2) Choosing and preparing an injection site

- Wash your hands thoroughly
- Choose a site on the front of your thighs or your abdomen. If you choose your abdomen, you should avoid the area 2 inches around your navel.

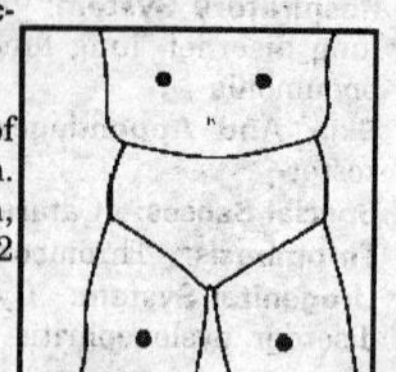

- Choose a different site each time you give yourself an injection. Each new injection should be given at least one inch from a site you used before. Do **NOT** inject into areas where the skin is tender, bruised, red or hard or where you have scars or stretch marks.
- You may find it helpful to keep notes on the location of previous injections.
- Wipe the site where HUMIRA is to be injected with an alcohol prep, using a circular motion. Do NOT touch this area again until you are ready to inject.

3) How to prepare your HUMIRA dose for injection with a Pre-filled Syringe

- Hold the syringe upright with the needle facing down. Check to make sure that the amount of liquid in the syringe is the same or close to the 0.8 mL line shown on the pre-filled syringe. The top of the liquid may be curved. If the syringe does not have the correct amount of liquid, DO NOT USE THAT SYRINGE. Call your pharmacist.
- Remove the needle cover taking care not to touch the needle with your fingers or allow it to touch any surface.
- Turn the syringe so the needle is facing up and slowly push the plunger in to push the air in the syringe out through the needle. If a small drop of liquid comes out of the needle that is ok.

4) Injecting HUMIRA

- With your other hand, gently pinch the cleaned area of skin and hold it firmly. Hold the syringe like a pencil at about a 45° angle to the skin.
- With a quick, short, "dart-like" motion, push the needle into the skin.

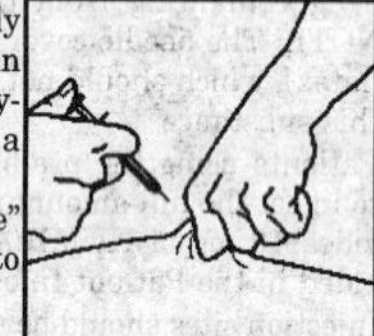

- After the needle is in, let go of the skin. Pull back slightly on the plunger, if blood appears in the syringe it means that you have entered a blood vessel. Do not inject HUMIRA. Withdraw the needle and repeat the steps to choose and clean a new injection site. DO NOT use the same syringe; discard it in your puncture proof container. If no blood appears, slowly push the plunger all the way in until all of the HUMIRA is injected.
- When the syringe is empty, remove the needle from the skin keeping it at the same angle it was when it was inserted.
- Press a cotton ball over the injection site and hold it for 10 seconds. Do **NOT** rub the injection site. If you have slight bleeding, do not be alarmed.
- Dispose of the syringe immediately.

5) Disposing of syringes and needles

You should always check with your healthcare provider for instructions on how to properly dispose of used needles and syringes. You should follow any special state or local laws regarding the proper disposal of needles and syringes. **DO NOT throw the needle or syringe in the household trash or recycle.**

- Place the used needles and syringes in a container made specially for disposing of used syringes and needles (called a "Sharps" container), or a hard plastic container with a screw-on cap or metal container with a plastic lid labeled *"Used Syringes"*. Do not use glass or clear plastic containers.
- Always keep the container out of the reach of children.
- When the container is about two-thirds full, tape the cap or lid down so it does not come off and dispose of it as instructed by your doctor, nurse or pharmacist. DO NOT THROW THE CONTAINER IN THE HOUSEHOLD TRASH OR RECYCLE.
- Used preps may be placed in the trash, unless otherwise instructed by your doctor, nurse or pharmacist. The dose tray and cover may be recycled.

HOW DO I STORE HUMIRA?

Store at 2°C–8°C/36–46°F (in a refrigerator) in the original container until it is used. Protect from light. DO NOT FREEZE HUMIRA. Refrigerated HUMIRA remains stable until the expiration date printed on the pre-filled syringe. If you need to take it with you, such as when traveling, store it in a cool carrier with an ice pack and protect it from light. Keep HUMIRA, injection supplies, and all other medicines out of the reach of children.

Revised: December, 2003

ABBOTT LABORATORIES

NORTH CHICAGO, IL 60064, U.S.A.

PRINTED IN U.S.A.

Shown in Product Identification Guide, page 303

HYTRIN® ℞

(terazosin hydrochloride)

Capsules

DESCRIPTION

HYTRIN (terazosin hydrochloride), an alpha-1-selective adrenoceptor blocking agent, is a quinazoline derivative represented by the following chemical name and structural formula: (RS)-Piperazine, 1-(4-amino-6,7-dimethoxy-2-quinazolinyl)-4-[(tetra-hydro-2-furanyl)carbonyl]-, monohydrochloride, dihydrate.

$\cdot HCl \cdot 2H_2O$

Terazosin hydrochloride is a white, crystalline substance, freely soluble in water and isotonic saline and has a molecular weight of 459.93. HYTRIN capsules (terazosin hydrochloride capsules) for oral ingestion are supplied in four dosage strengths containing terazosin hydrochloride equivalent to 1 mg, 2 mg, 5 mg, or 10 mg of terazosin.

Inactive Ingredients:

1 mg capsules: gelatin, glycerin, iron oxide, methylparaben, mineral oil, polyethylene glycol, povidone, propylparaben, titanium dioxide, and vanillin.

2 mg capsules: D&C yellow No. 10, gelatin, glycerin, methylparaben, mineral oil, polyethylene glycol, povidone, propylparaben, titanium dioxide, and vanillin.

5 mg capsules: D&C red No. 28, FD&C red No. 40, gelatin, glycerin, methylparaben, mineral oil, polyethylene glycol, povidone, propylparaben, titanium dioxide, and vanillin.

10 mg capsules: FD&C blue No. 1, gelatin, glycerin, methylparaben, mineral oil, polyethylene glycol, povidone, propylparaben, titanium dioxide, and vanillin.

CLINICAL PHARMACOLOGY

Pharmacodynamics:

A. Benign Prostatic Hyperplasia (BPH)

The symptoms associated with BPH are related to bladder outlet obstruction, which is comprised of two underlying components: a static component and a dynamic component. The static component is a consequence of an increase in prostate size. Over time, the prostate will continue to enlarge. However, clinical studies have demonstrated that the size of the prostate does not correlate with the severity of BPH symptoms or the degree of urinary obstruction. The dynamic component is a function of an increase in smooth muscle tone in the prostate and bladder neck, leading to constriction of the bladder outlet. Smooth muscle tone is mediated by sympathetic nervous stimulation of alpha-l adrenoceptors, which are abundant in the prostate, prostatic capsule and bladder neck. The reduction in symptoms and improvement in urine flow rates following administration of terazosin is related to relaxation of smooth muscle produced by blockade of alpha-l adrenoceptors in the bladder neck and prostate. Because there are relatively few alpha-l adrenoceptors in the bladder body, terazosin is able to reduce the bladder outlet obstruction without affecting bladder contractility.

Terazosin has been studied in 1222 men with symptomatic BPH. In three placebo-controlled studies, symptom evaluation and uroflowmetric measurements were performed approximately 24 hours following dosing. Symptoms were quantified using the Boyarsky Index. The questionnaire evaluated both obstructive (hesitancy, intermittency, terminal dribbling, impairment of size and force of stream, sensation of incomplete bladder emptying) and irritative (nocturia, daytime frequency, urgency, dysuria) symptoms by rating each of the 9 symptoms from 0-3, for a total score of 27 points. Results from these studies indicated that terazosin statistically significantly improved symptoms and peak urine flow rates over placebo as follows:

[See table at top of next page]

In all three studies, both symptom scores and peak urine flow rates showed statistically significant improvement from baseline in patients treated with terazosin from week 2 (or the first clinic visit) and throughout the study duration.

Analysis of the effect of terazosin on individual urinary symptoms demonstrated that compared to placebo, terazosin significantly improved the symptoms of hesitancy, intermittency, impairment in size and force of urinary stream, sensation of incomplete emptying, terminal dribbling, daytime frequency and nocturia.

Global assessments of overall urinary function and symptoms were also performed by investigators who were blinded to patient treatment assignment. In studies 1 and 3, patients treated with terazosin had a significantly ($p \leq 0.001$) greater overall improvement compared to placebo treated patients.

In a short term study (Study 1), patients were randomized to either 2, 5 or 10 mg of terazosin or placebo. Patients randomized to the 10 mg group achieved a statistically significant response in both symptoms and peak flow rate compared to placebo (Figure 1).

[See figure 1 at top of next column]

In a long-term, open-label, non-placebo controlled clinical trial, 181 men were followed for 2 years and 58 of these men

Figure 1
Study 1

Mean Change in Total Symptom Score from Baseline+ **Mean Increase in Peak Flow Rate (mL/sec) from Baseline+**

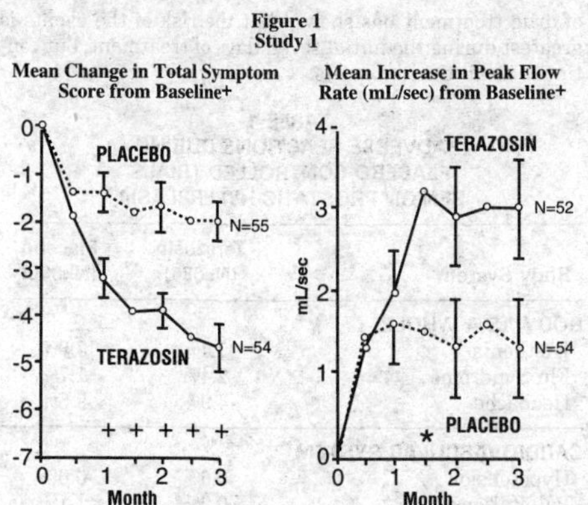

+ for baseline values see above table
* p ≤ 0.05, compared to placebo group

were followed for 30 months. The effect of terazosin on urinary symptom scores and peak flow rates was maintained throughout the study duration (Figures 2 and 3):

Figure 2
Mean Change in Total Symptom Score from Baseline Long-Term, Open-Label, Non-Placebo Controlled Study (N=494)

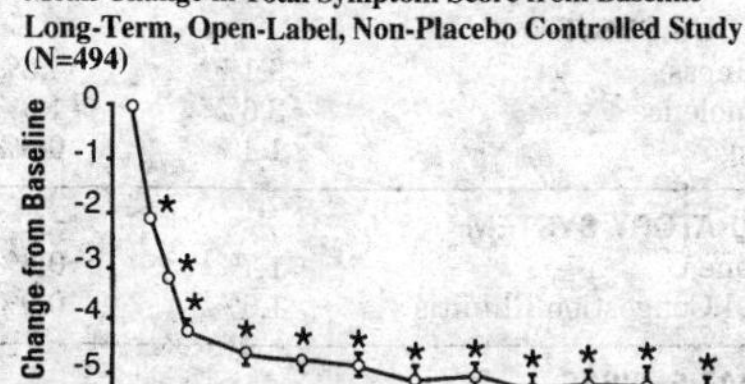

* p ≤ 0.05 vs. baseline
mean baseline = 10.7

Figure 3
Mean Change in Peak Flow Rate from Baseline Long-Term, Open-Label, Non-Placebo Controlled Study (N=494)

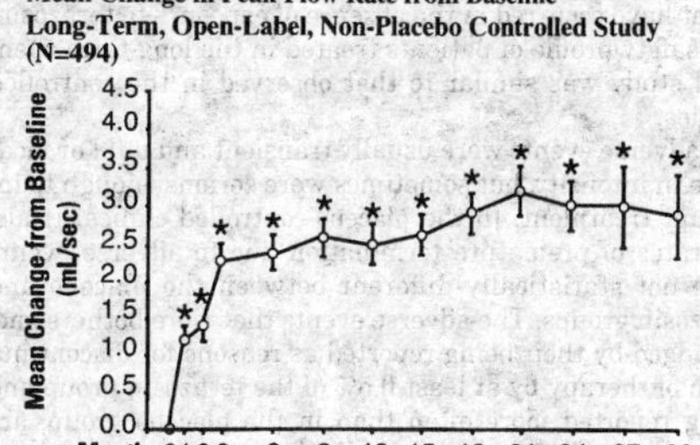

* p ≤ 0.05 vs. baseline
mean baseline = 9.9

In this long-term trial, both symptom scores and peak urinary flow rates showed statistically significant improvement suggesting a relaxation of smooth muscle cells.

Although blockade of alpha-1 adrenoceptors also lowers blood pressure in hypertensive patients with increased peripheral vascular resistance, terazosin treatment of normotensive men with BPH did not result in a clinically significant blood pressure lowering effect:

Mean Changes in Blood Pressure from Baseline to Final Visit in all Double-Blind, Placebo-Controlled Studies

		Normotensive Patients DBP ≤ 90 mm Hg		Hypertensive Patients DBP > 90 mm Hg	
	Group	**N**	**Mean Change**	**N**	**Mean Change**
SBP (mm Hg)	**Placebo**	293	-0.1	45	-5.8
	Terazosin	519	-3.3*	65	-14.4*
DBP (mm Hg)	**Placebo**	293	+0.4	45	-7.1
	Terazosin	519	-2.2*	65	-15.1*

*p ≤ 0.05 vs. placebo

B. Hypertension

In animals, terazosin causes a decrease in blood pressure by decreasing total peripheral vascular resistance. The vasodilatory hypotensive action of terazosin appears to be produced mainly by blockade of alpha-1 adrenoceptors. Terazosin decreases blood pressure gradually within 15 minutes following oral administration.

Patients in clinical trials of terazosin were administered once daily (the great majority) and twice daily regimens with total doses usually in the range of 5-20 mg/day, and

	Symptom Score (Range 0-27)			Peak Flow Rate (mL/sec)		
	N	**Mean Baseline**	**Mean Change (%)**	**N**	**Mean Baseline**	**Mean Change (%)**
Study 1 (10 mg)[a] **Titration to fixed dose (12 wks)**						
Placebo	55	9.7	-2.3 (24)	54	10.1	+1.0 (10)
Terazosin	54	10.1	-4.5 (45)*	52	8.8	+3.0 (34)*
Study 2 (2, 5, 10, 20 mg)[b] **Titration to response (24 wks)**						
Placebo	89	12.5	-3.8 (30)	88	8.8	+1.4 (16)
Terazosin	85	12.2	-5.3 (43)*	84	8.4	+2.9 (35)*
Study 3 (1, 2, 5, 10 mg)[c] **Titration to response (24 wks)**						
Placebo	74	10.4	-1.1 (11)	74	8.8	+1.2 (14)
Terazosin	73	10.9	-4.6 (42)*	73	8.6	+2.6 (30)*

[a] Highest dose 10 mg shown.
[b] 23% of patients on 10 mg, 41% of patients on 20 mg.
[c] 67% of patients on 10 mg.
* Significantly (p ≤ 0.05) more improvement than placebo.

had mild (about 77%, diastolic pressure 95-105 mmHg) or moderate (23%, diastolic pressure 105-115 mmHg) hypertension. Because terazosin, like all alpha antagonists, can cause unusually large falls in blood pressure after the first dose or first few doses, the initial dose was 1 mg in virtually all trials, with subsequent titration to a specified fixed dose or titration to some specified blood pressure end point (usually a supine diastolic pressure of 90 mmHg).

Blood pressure responses were measured at the end of the dosing interval (usually 24 hours) and effects were shown to persist throughout the interval, with the usual supine responses 5-10 mmHg systolic and 3.5-8 mmHg diastolic greater than placebo. The responses in the standing position tended to be somewhat larger, by 1-3 mmHg, although this was not true in all studies. The magnitude of the blood pressure responses was similar to prazosin and less than hydrochlorothiazide (in a single study of hypertensive patients). In measurements 24 hours after dosing, heart rate was unchanged.

Limited measurements of peak response (2-3 hours after dosing) during chronic terazosin administration indicate that it is greater than about twice the trough (24 hour) response, suggesting some attenuation of response at 24 hours, presumably due to a fall in blood terazosin concentrations at the end of the dose interval. This explanation is not established with certainty, however, and is not consistent with the similarity of blood pressure response to once daily and twice daily dosing and with the absence of an observed dose-response relationship over a range of 5-20 mg, i.e., if blood concentrations had fallen to the point of providing less than full effect at 24 hours, a shorter dosing interval or larger dose should have led to increased response.

Further dose response and dose duration studies are being carried out. Blood pressure should be measured at the end of the dose interval; if response is not satisfactory, patients may be tried on a larger dose or twice daily dosing regimen. The latter should also be considered if possibly blood pressure-related side effects, such as dizziness, palpitations, or orthostatic complaints, are seen within a few hours after dosing.

The greater blood pressure effect associated with peak plasma concentrations (first few hours after dosing) appears somewhat more position-dependent (greater in the erect position) than the effect of terazosin at 24 hours and in the erect position there is also a 6-10 beat per minute increase in heart rate in the first few hours after dosing. During the first 3 hours after dosing 12.5% of patients had a systolic pressure fall of 30 mmHg or more from supine to standing, or standing systolic pressure below 90 mmHg with a fall of at least 20 mmHg, compared to 4% of a placebo group.

There was a tendency for patients to gain weight during terazosin therapy. In placebo-controlled monotherapy trials, male and female patients receiving terazosin gained a mean of 1.7 and 2.2 pounds respectively, compared to losses of 0.2 and 1.2 pounds respectively in the placebo group. Both differences were statistically significant.

During controlled clinical trials, patients receiving terazosin monotherapy had a small but statistically significant decrease (a 3% fall) compared to placebo in total cholesterol and the combined low-density and very-low-density lipoprotein fractions. No significant changes were observed in high-density lipoprotein fraction and triglycerides compared to placebo.

Analysis of clinical laboratory data following administration of terazosin suggested the possibility of hemodilution based on decreases in hematocrit, hemoglobin, white blood cells, total protein and albumin. Decreases in hematocrit and total protein have been observed with alpha-blockade and are attributed to hemodilution.

Pharmacokinetics:

Terazosin hydrochloride administered as HYTRIN capsules is essentially completely absorbed in man. Administration of capsules immediately after meals had a minimal effect on the extent of absorption. The time to reach peak plasma concentration however, was delayed by about 40 minutes. Terazosin has been shown to undergo minimal hepatic first-pass metabolism and nearly all of the circulating dose is in the form of parent drug. The plasma levels peak about one hour after dosing, and then decline with a half-life of approximately 12 hours. In a study that evaluated the effect of age on terazosin pharmacokinetics, the mean plasma half-lives were 14.0 and 11.4 hours for the age group ≥70 years and the age group of 20-39 years, respectively. After oral administration the plasma clearance was decreased by 31.7% in patients 70 years of age or older compared to that in patients 20-39 years of age.

The drug is 90-94% bound to plasma proteins and binding is constant over the clinically observed concentration range. Approximately 10% of an orally administered dose is excreted as parent drug in the urine and approximately 20% is excreted in the feces. The remainder is eliminated as metabolites. Impaired renal function had no significant effect on the elimination of terazosin, and dosage adjustment of terazosin to compensate for the drug removal during hemodialysis (approximately 10%) does not appear to be necessary. Overall, approximately 40% of the administered dose is excreted in the urine and approximately 60% in the feces. The disposition of the compound in animals is qualitatively similar to that in man.

INDICATIONS AND USAGE

HYTRIN (terazosin hydrochloride) is indicated for the treatment of symptomatic benign prostatic hyperplasia (BPH). There is a rapid response, with approximately 70% of patients experiencing an increase in urinary flow and improvement in symptoms of BPH when treated with HYTRIN. The long-term effects of HYTRIN on the incidence of surgery, acute urinary obstruction or other complications of BPH are yet to be determined.

HYTRIN is also indicated for the treatment of hypertension. It can be used alone or in combination with other antihypertensive agents such as diuretics or beta-adrenergic blocking agents.

CONTRAINDICATIONS

HYTRIN capsules are contraindicated in patients known to be hypersensitive to terazosin hydrochloride.

WARNINGS

Syncope and "First-dose" Effect:

HYTRIN capsules, like other alpha-adrenergic blocking agents, can cause marked lowering of blood pressure, especially postural hypotension, and syncope in association with the first dose or first few days of therapy. A similar effect can be anticipated if therapy is interrupted for several days and then restarted. Syncope has also been reported with other alpha-adrenergic blocking agents in association with rapid dosage increases or the introduction of another antihypertensive drug. Syncope is believed to be due to an excessive postural hypotensive effect, although occasionally the syncopal episode has been preceded by about of severe supraventricular tachycardia with heart rates of 120-160 beats per minute. Additionally, the possibility of the contribution of hemodilution to the symptoms of postural hypotension should be considered.

To decrease the likelihood of syncope or excessive hypotension, treatment should always be initiated with a 1 mg dose of terazosin, given at bedtime. The 2 mg, 5 mg and 10 mg capsules are not indicated as initial therapy. Dosage should then be increased slowly, according to recommendations in the Dosage and Administration section and additional antihypertensive agents should be added with caution. The patient should be cautioned to avoid situations, such as driving or hazardous tasks, where injury could result should syncope occur during initiation of therapy.

In early investigational studies, where increasing single doses up to 7.5 mg were given at 3 day intervals, tolerance to the first dose phenomenon did not necessarily develop and the "first-dose" effect could be observed at all doses. Syncopal episodes occurred in 3 of the 14 subjects given terazosin at doses of 2.5, 5 and 7.5 mg, which are higher than the recommended initial dose; in addition, severe orthostatic hypotension (blood pressure falling to 50/0 mmHg) was seen in two others and dizziness, tachycardia, and lightheadedness occurred in most subjects. These adverse effects all occurred within 90 minutes of dosing.

In three placebo-controlled BPH studies 1, 2, and 3 (see CLINICAL PHARMACOLOGY), the incidence of postural hypotension in the terazosin treated patients was 5.1%, 5.2%, and 3.7% respectively.

Continued on next page

Hytrin—Cont.

In multiple dose clinical trials involving nearly 2000 hypertensive patients treated with terazosin, syncope was reported in about 1% of patients. Syncope was not necessarily associated only with the first dose.

If syncope occurs, the patient should be placed in a recumbent position and treated supportively as necessary. There is evidence that the orthostatic effect of terazosin is greater, even in chronic use, shortly after dosing. The risk of the events is greatest during the initial seven days of treatment, but continues at all time intervals.

Priapism:

Rarely, (probably less than once in every several thousand patients) terazosin and other α_1-antagonists have been associated with priapism (painful penile erection, sustained for hours and unrelieved by sexual intercourse or masturbation). Two or three dozen cases have been reported. Because this condition can lead to permanent impotence if not promptly treated, patients must be advised about the seriousness of the condition (see **PRECAUTIONS: Information for Patients**).

PRECAUTIONS

General:

Prostatic Cancer

Carcinoma of the prostate and BPH cause many of the same symptoms. These two diseases frequently co-exist. Therefore, patients thought to have BPH should be examined prior to starting HYTRIN therapy to rule out the presence of carcinoma of the prostate.

Orthostatic Hypotension

While syncope is the most severe orthostatic effect of terazosin (see Warnings), other symptoms of lowered blood pressure, such as dizziness, lightheadedness and palpitations, were more common and occurred in some 28% of patients in clinical trials of hypertension. In BPH clinical trials, 21% of the patients experienced one or more of the following: dizziness, hypotension, postural hypotension, syncope, and vertigo. Patients with occupations in which such events represent potential problems should be treated with particular caution.

Information for Patients (see Patient Package Insert):

Patients should be made aware of the possibility of syncopal and orthostatic symptoms, especially at the initiation of therapy, and to avoid driving or hazardous tasks for 12 hours after the first dose, after a dosage increase and after interruption of therapy when treatment is resumed. They should be cautioned to avoid situations where injury could result should syncope occur during initiation of terazosin therapy. They should also be advised of the need to sit or lie down when symptoms of lowered blood pressure occur, although these symptoms are not always orthostatic, and to be careful when rising from a sitting or lying position. If dizziness, lightheadedness, or palpitations are bothersome they should be reported to the physician, so that dose adjustment can be considered.

Patients should also be told that drowsiness or somnolence can occur with terazosin, requiring caution in people who must drive or operate heavy machinery.

Patients should be advised about the possibility of priapism as a result of treatment with HYTRIN and other similar medications. Patients should know that this reaction to HYTRIN is extremely rare, but that if it is not brought to immediate medical attention, it can lead to permanent erectile dysfunction (impotence).

Laboratory Tests:

Small but statistically significant decreases in hematocrit, hemoglobin, white blood cells, total protein and albumin were observed in controlled clinical trials. These laboratory findings suggested the possibility of hemodilution. Treatment with terazosin for up to 24 months had no significant effect on prostate specific antigen (PSA) levels.

Drug Interactions:

In controlled trials, terazosin has been added to diuretics, and several beta-adrenergic blockers; no unexpected interactions were observed. Terazosin has also been used in patients on a variety of concomitant therapies; while these were not formal interaction studies, no interactions were observed. Terazosin has been used concomitantly in at least 50 patients on the following drugs or drug classes: 1) analgesic/anti-inflammatory (e.g., acetaminophen, aspirin, codeine, ibuprofen, indomethacin); 2) antibiotics (e.g., erythromycin, trimethoprim and sulfamethoxazole); 3) anticholinergic/sympathomimetics (e.g., phenylephrine hydrochloride, phenylpropanolamine hydrochloride, pseudoephedrine hydrochloride); 4) antigout (e.g., allopurinol); 5) antihistamines (e.g., chlorpheniramine); 6) cardiovascular agents (e.g., atenolol, hydrochlorothiazide, methyclothiazide, propranolol); 7) corticosteroids; 8) gastrointestinal agents (e.g., antacids); 9) hypoglycemics; 10) sedatives and tranquilizers (e.g., diazepam).

Use with Other Drugs:

In a study (n=24) where terazosin and verapamil were administered concomitantly, terazosin's mean AUC_{0-24} increased 11% after the first verapamil dose and after 3 weeks of verapamil treatment it increased by 24% with associated increases in C_{max} (25%) and C_{min} (32%) means. Terazosin mean T_{max} decreased from 1.3 hours to 0.8 hours after 3 weeks of verapamil treatment. Statistically significant differences were not found in the verapamil level with and without terazosin. In a study (n=6) where terazosin and captopril were administered concomitantly, plasma disposition of captopril was not influenced by concomitant administration of terazosin and terazosin maximum plasma concentrations increased linearly with dose at steady-state after administration of terazosin plus captopril (see Dosage and Administration).

Carcinogenesis, Mutagenesis, Impairment of Fertility:

Terazosin was devoid of mutagenic potential when evaluated *in vivo* and *in vitro* (the Ames test, *in vivo* cytogenetics, the dominant lethal test in mice, *in vivo* Chinese hamster chromosome aberration test and V79 forward mutation assay).

Terazosin, administered in the feed to rats at doses of 8, 40, and 250 mg/kg/day (70, 350, and 2100 mg/M^2/day), for two years, was associated with a statistically significant increase in benign adrenal medullary tumors of male rats exposed to the 250 mg/kg dose. This dose is 175 times the maximum recommended human dose of 20 mg (12 mg/M^2). Female rats were unaffected. Terazosin was not oncogenic in mice when administered in feed for 2 years at a maximum tolerated dose of 32 mg/kg/day (110 mg/M^2; 9 times the maximum recommended human dose). The absence of mutagenicity in a battery of tests, of tumorigenicity of any cell type in the mouse carcinogenicity assay, of increased total tumor incidence in either species, and of proliferative adrenal lesions in female rats, suggests a male rat species-specific event. Numerous other diverse pharmaceutical and chemical compounds have also been associated with benign adrenal medullary tumors in male rats without supporting evidence for carcinogenicity in man.

The effect of terazosin on fertility was assessed in a standard fertility/reproductive performance study in which male and female rats were administered oral doses of 8, 30 and 120 mg/kg/day. Four of 20 male rats given 30 mg/kg (240 mg/M^2; 20 times the maximum recommended human dose) and five of 19 male rats given 120 mg/kg (960 mg/M^2; 80 times the maximum recommended human dose) failed to sire a litter. Testicular weights and morphology were unaffected by treatment. Vaginal smears at 30 and 120 mg/kg/day, however, appeared to contain less sperm than smears from control matings and good correlation was reported between sperm count and subsequent pregnancy.

Oral administration of terazosin for one or two years elicited a statistically significant increase in the incidence of testicular atrophy in rats exposed to 40 and 250 mg/kg/day (29 and 175 times the maximum recommended human dose), but not in rats exposed to 8 mg/kg/day (> 6 times the maximum recommended human dose). Testicular atrophy was also observed in dogs dosed with 300 mg/kg/day (> 500 times the maximum recommended human dose) for three months but not after one year when dosed with 20 mg/kg/day (38 times the maximum recommended human dose). This lesion has also been seen with Minipress®, another (marketed) selective-alpha-1 blocking agent.

Pregnancy:

Teratogenic effects: Pregnancy Category C. Terazosin was not teratogenic in either rats or rabbits when administered at oral doses up to 280 and 60 times, respectively, the maximum recommended human dose. Fetal resorptions occurred in rats dosed with 480 mg/kg/day, approximately 280 times the maximum recommended human dose. Increased fetal resorptions, decreased fetal weight and an increased number of supernumerary ribs were observed in offspring of rabbits dosed with 60 times the maximum recommended human dose. These findings (in both species) were most likely secondary to maternal toxicity. There are no adequate and well-controlled studies in pregnant women and the safety of terazosin in pregnancy has not been established. HYTRIN is not recommended during pregnancy unless the potential benefit justifies the potential risk to the mother and fetus.

Nonteratogenic effects: In a peri- and post-natal development study in rats, significantly more pups died in the group dosed with 120 mg/kg/day (> 75 times the maximum recommended human dose) than in the control group during the three-week postpartum period.

Nursing Mothers:

It is not known whether terazosin is excreted in breast milk. Because many drugs are excreted in breast milk, caution should be exercised when terazosin is administered to a nursing woman.

Pediatric Use:

Safety and effectiveness in children have not been determined.

ADVERSE REACTIONS

Benign Prostatic Hyperplasia

The incidence of treatment-emergent adverse events has been ascertained from clinical trials conducted worldwide. All adverse events reported during these trials were recorded as adverse reactions. The incidence rates presented below are based on combined data from six placebo-controlled trials involving once-a-day administration of terazosin at doses ranging from 1 to 20 mg. Table 1 summarizes those adverse events reported for patients in these trials when the incidence rate in the terazosin group was at least 1% and was greater than that for the placebo group, or where the reaction is of clinical interest. Asthenia, postural hypotension, dizziness, somnolence, nasal congestion/rhinitis, and impotence were the only events that were significantly ($p \leq 0.05$) more common in patients receiving terazosin than in patients receiving placebo. The incidence of urinary tract infection was significantly lower in the patients receiving terazosin than in patients receiving placebo. An analysis of the incidence rate of hypotensive adverse events (see PRECAUTIONS) adjusted for the length of drug treatment has shown that the risk of the events is greatest during the initial seven days of treatment, but continues at all time intervals.

TABLE 1
ADVERSE REACTIONS DURING PLACEBO-CONTROLLED TRIALS BENIGN PROSTATIC HYPERPLASIA

Body System	Terazosin (N=636)	Placebo (N=360)
BODY AS A WHOLE		
†Asthenia	7.4%*	3.3%
Flu Syndrome	2.4%	1.7%
Headache	4.9%	5.8%
CARDIOVASCULAR SYSTEM		
Hypotension	0.6%	0.6%
Palpitations	0.9%	1.1%
Postural Hypotension	3.9%*	0.8%
Syncope	0.6%	0.0%
DIGESTIVE SYSTEM		
Nausea	1.7%	1.1%
METABOLIC AND NUTRITIONAL DISORDERS		
Peripheral Edema	0.9%	0.3%
Weight Gain	0.5%	0.0%
NERVOUS SYSTEM		
Dizziness	9.1%*	4.2%
Somnolence	3.6%*	1.9%
Vertigo	1.4%	0.3%
RESPIRATORY SYSTEM		
Dyspnea	1.7%	0.8%
Nasal Congestion/Rhinitis	1.9%*	0.0%
SPECIAL SENSES		
Blurred Vision/Amblyopia	1.3%	0.6%
UROGENITAL SYSTEM		
Impotence	1.6%*	0.6%
Urinary Tract Infection	1.3%	3.9%*

† Includes weakness, tiredness, lassitude and fatigue.
* $p \leq 0.05$ comparison between groups.

Additional adverse events have been reported, but these are, in general, not distinguishable from symptoms that might have occurred in the absence of exposure to terazosin. The safety profile of patients treated in the long-term open-label study was similar to that observed in the controlled studies.

The adverse events were usually transient and mild or moderate in intensity, but sometimes were serious enough to interrupt treatment. In the placebo-controlled clinical trials, the rates of premature termination due to adverse events were not statistically different between the placebo and terazosin groups. The adverse events that were bothersome, as judged by their being reported as reasons for discontinuation of therapy by at least 0.5% of the terazosin group and being reported more often than in the placebo group, are shown in Table 2.

TABLE 2
DISCONTINUATION DURING PLACEBO-CONTROLLED TRIALS BENIGN PROSTATIC HYPERPLASIA

Body System	Terazosin (N=636)	Placebo (N=360)
BODY AS A WHOLE		
Fever	0.5%	0.0%
Headache	1.1%	0.8%
CARDIOVASCULAR SYSTEM		
Postural Hypotension	0.5%	0.0%
Syncope	0.5%	0.0%
DIGESTIVE SYSTEM		
Nausea	0.5%	0.3%
NERVOUS SYSTEM		
Dizziness	2.0%	1.1%
Vertigo	0.5%	0.0%
RESPIRATORY SYSTEM		
Dyspnea	0.5%	0.3%
SPECIAL SENSES		
Blurred Vision/Amblyopia	0.6%	0.0%
UROGENITAL SYSTEM		
Urinary Tract Infection	0.5%	0.3%

Hypertension

The prevalence of adverse reactions has been ascertained from clinical trials conducted primarily in the United States. All adverse experiences (events) reported during these trials were recorded as adverse reactions. The prevalence rates presented below are based on combined data from fourteen placebo-controlled trials involving once-a-day administration of terazosin, as monotherapy or in combination with other antihypertensive agents, at doses ranging from 1 to 40 mg. Table 3 summarizes those adverse experiences reported for patients in these trials where the prevalence rate in the terazosin group was at least 5%, where the prevalence rate for the terazosin group was at least 2% and was greater than the prevalence rate for the placebo group, or where the reaction is of particular interest. Asthenia, blurred vision, dizziness, nasal congestion, nausea, peripheral edema, palpitations and somnolence were the only symptoms that were significantly ($p \leq 0.05$) more common in patients receiving terazosin than in patients receiving placebo. Similar adverse reaction rates were observed in placebo-controlled monotherapy trials.

TABLE 3
ADVERSE REACTIONS DURING PLACEBO-CONTROLLED TRIALS HYPERTENSION

Body System	Terazosin (N=859)	Placebo (N=506)
BODY AS A WHOLE		
†Asthenia	11.3%*	4.3%
Back Pain	2.4%	1.2%
Headache	16.2%	15.8%
CARDIOVASCULAR SYSTEM		
Palpitations	4.3%*	1.2%
Postural Hypotension	1.3%	0.4%
Tachycardia	1.9%	1.2%
DIGESTIVE SYSTEM		
Nausea	4.4%*	1.4%
METABOLIC AND NUTRITIONAL DISORDERS		
Edema	0.9%	0.6%
Peripheral Edema	5.5%*	2.4%
Weight Gain	0.5%	0.2%
MUSCULOSKELETAL SYSTEM		
Pain–Extremities	3.5%	3.0%
NERVOUS SYSTEM		
Depression	0.3%	0.2%
Dizziness	19.3%*	7.5%
Libido Decreased	0.6%	0.2%
Nervousness	2.3%	1.8%
Paresthesia	2.9%	1.4%
Somnolence	5.4%*	2.6%
RESPIRATORY SYSTEM		
Dyspnea	3.1%	2.4%
Nasal Congestion	5.9%*	3.4%
Sinusitis	2.6%	1.4%
SPECIAL SENSES		
Blurred Vision	1.6%*	0.0%
UROGENITAL SYSTEM		
Impotence	1.2%	1.4%

† Includes weakness, tiredness, lassitude and fatigue.
* Statistically significant at p=0.05 level.

Additional adverse reactions have been reported, but these are, in general, not distinguishable from symptoms that might have occurred in the absence of exposure to terazosin. The following additional adverse reactions were reported by at least 1% of 1987 patients who received terazosin in controlled or open, short- or long-term clinical trials or have been reported during marketing experience: *Body as a Whole:* chest pain, facial edema, fever, abdominal pain, neck pain, shoulder pain; *Cardiovascular System:* arrhythmia, vasodilation; *Digestive System:* constipation, diarrhea, dry mouth, dyspepsia, flatulence, vomiting; *Metabolic/Nutritional Disorders:* gout; *Musculoskeletal System:* arthralgia, arthritis, joint disorder, myalgia; *Nervous System:* anxiety, insomnia; *Respiratory System:* bronchitis, cold symptoms, epistaxis, flu symptoms, increased cough, pharyngitis, rhinitis; *Skin and Appendages:* pruritus, rash, sweating; *Special Senses:* abnormal vision, conjunctivitis, tinnitus; *Urogenital System:* urinary frequency, urinary incontinence primarily reported in postmenopausal women, urinary tract infection.

The adverse reactions were usually mild or moderate in intensity but sometimes were serious enough to interrupt treatment. The adverse reactions that were most bothersome, as judged by their being reported as reasons for discontinuation of therapy by at least 0.5% of the terazosin group and being reported more often than in the placebo group, are shown in Table 4.

TABLE 4
DISCONTINUATIONS DURING PLACEBO-CONTROLLED TRIALS HYPERTENSION

Body System	Terazosin (N=859)	Placebo (N=506)
BODY AS A WHOLE		
Asthenia	1.6%	0.0%
Headache	1.3%	1.0%
CARDIOVASCULAR SYSTEM		
Palpitations	1.4%	0.2%
Postural Hypotension	0.5%	0.0%
Syncope	0.5%	0.2%
Tachycardia	0.6%	0.0%
DIGESTIVE SYSTEM		
Nausea	0.8%	0.0%
METABOLIC AND NUTRITIONAL DISORDERS		
Peripheral Edema	0.6%	0.0%
NERVOUS SYSTEM		
Dizziness	3.1%	0.4%
Paresthesia	0.8%	0.2%
Somnolence	0.6%	0.2%
RESPIRATORY SYSTEM		
Dyspnea	0.9%	0.6%
Nasal Congestion	0.6%	0.0%
SPECIAL SENSES		
Blurred Vision	0.6%	0.0%

Post-marketing Experience
Post-marketing experience indicates that in rare instances patients may develop allergic reactions, including anaphylaxis, following administration of terazosin hydrochloride. There have been reports of priapism and thrombocytopenia during post-marketing surveillance. Atrial fibrillation has been reported.

OVERDOSAGE

Should overdosage of HYTRIN lead to hypotension, support of the cardiovascular system is of first importance. Restoration of blood pressure and normalization of heart rate may be accomplished by keeping the patient in the supine position. If this measure is inadequate, shock should first be treated with volume expanders. If necessary, vasopressors should then be used and renal function should be monitored and supported as needed. Laboratory data indicate that terazosin is 90-94% protein bound; therefore, dialysis may not be of benefit.

DOSAGE AND ADMINISTRATION

If HYTRIN administration is discontinued for several days, therapy should be reinstituted using the initial dosing regimen.

Benign Prostatic Hyperplasia:
Initial Dose:
1 mg at bedtime is the starting dose for all patients, and this dose should not be exceeded as an initial dose. Patients should be closely followed during initial administration in order to minimize the risk of severe hypotensive response.

Subsequent Doses:
The dose should be increased in a stepwise fashion to 2 mg, 5 mg, or 10 mg once daily to achieve the desired improvement of symptoms and/or flow rates. Doses of 10 mg once daily are generally required for the clinical response. Therefore, treatment with 10 mg for a minimum of 4–6 weeks may be required to assess whether a beneficial response has been achieved. Some patients may not achieve a clinical response despite appropriate titration. Although some additional patients responded at a 20 mg daily dose, there was an insufficient number of patients studied to draw definitive conclusions about this dose. There are insufficient data to support the use of higher doses for those patients who show inadequate or no response to 20 mg daily. **If terazosin administration is discontinued for several days or longer, therapy should be reinstituted using the initial dosing regimen.**

Use with Other Drugs:
Caution should be observed when HYTRIN is administered concomitantly with other antihypertensive agents, especially the calcium channel blocker verapamil, to avoid the possibility of developing significant hypotension. When using HYTRIN and other antihypertensive agents concomitantly, dosage reduction and retitration of either agent may be necessary (see Precautions).

Hypertension:
The dose of HYTRIN and the dose interval (12 or 24 hours) should be adjusted according to the patient's individual blood pressure response. The following is a guide to its administration:

Initial Dose:
1 mg at bedtime is the starting dose for all patients, and this dose should not be exceeded. This initial dosing regimen should be strictly observed to minimize the potential for severe hypotensive effects.

Subsequent Doses:
The dose may be slowly increased to achieve the desired blood pressure response. The usual recommended dose range is 1 mg to 5 mg administered once a day; however, some patients may benefit from doses as high as 20 mg per day. Doses over 20 mg do not appear to provide further blood pressure effect and doses over 40 mg have not been studied. Blood pressure should be monitored at the end of the dosing interval to be sure control is maintained throughout the interval. It may also be helpful to measure blood pressure 2-3 hours after dosing to see if the maximum and minimum responses are similar, and to evaluate symptoms such as dizziness or palpitations which can result from excessive hypotensive response. If response is substantially diminished at 24 hours an increased dose or use of a twice daily regimen can be considered. **If terazosin administration is discontinued for several days or longer, therapy should be reinstituted using the initial dosing regimen.** In clinical trials, except for the initial dose, the dose was given in the morning.

Use With Other Drugs: (see above)

HOW SUPPLIED

HYTRIN capsules (terazosin hydrochloride capsules) are available in four dosage strengths:

1 mg grey capsules (imprinted with ⊐ and the Abbo-Code HH):
Bottles of 100 .... (**NDC** 0074-3805-13),
Abbo-Pac® unit dose strip packages
of 100 capsules .... (**NDC** 0074-3805-11).

2 mg yellow capsules (imprinted with ⊐ and the Abbo-Code HY):
Bottles of 100 .... (**NDC** 0074-3806-13),
Abbo-Pac® unit dose strip packages
of 100 capsules .... (**NDC** 0074-3806-11).

5 mg red capsules (imprinted with ⊐ and the Abbo-Code HK):
Bottles of 100 .... (**NDC** 0074-3807-13),
Abbo-Pac® unit dose strip packages
of 100 capsules .... (**NDC** 0074-3807-11).

10 mg blue capsules (imprinted with ⊐ and the Abbo-Code HN):
Bottles of 100 .... (**NDC** 0074-3808-13),
Abbo-Pac® unit dose strip packages
of 100 capsules .... (**NDC** 0074-3808-11).

Recommended storage: Store at controlled room temperature between 20-25°C (68-77°F). See USP. Protect from light and moisture.

Revised: February, 2001
Ref.: 03-5105
ABBOTT LABORATORIES
NORTH CHICAGO, IL 60064, U.S.A.

Shown in Product Identification Guide, page 303

ISOPTIN® SR ℞
(verapamil HCl)
Sustained Release Oral Tablets

DESCRIPTION

ISOPTIN® SR (verapamil hydrochloride) is a calcium ion influx inhibitor (slow channel blocker or calcium ion antagonist). ISOPTIN SR is available for oral administration as light green, capsule shaped, scored, film-coated tablets containing 240 mg verapamil hydrochloride, as light pink, oval shaped, scored, film-coated tablets containing 180 mg verapamil hydrochloride, and as light violet, oval shaped, film-coated tablets containing 120 mg verapamil hydrochloride. The tablets are designed for sustained release of the drug in the gastrointestinal tract, sustained release characteristics are not altered when the tablet is divided in half.

The structural formula of verapamil HCl is given below:

$C_{27}H_{38}N_2O_4 \cdot HCl$ M.W. 491.08

Benzeneacetronitrile, α[3-[[2-(3,4-dimethoxyphenyl) ethyl] methylamino] propyl]-3,4-dimethoxy-α-(1-methylethyl) hydrochloride

Verapamil HCl is an almost white, crystalline powder, practically free of odor, with a bitter taste. It is soluble in water, chloroform and methanol. Verapamil HCl is not chemically related to other cardioactive drugs.

In addition to verapamil HCl, the ISOPTIN SR tablet contains the following ingredients: alginate, hypromellose, magnesium stearate, microcrystalline cellulose, polyethylene glycol, polyvinyl pyrrolidone, talc, and titanium dioxide. The following are the color additives per tablet strength:

Strength (mg)	Color Additive(s)
120	Iron Oxide
180	Iron Oxide
240	D&C yellow #10 Lake dye, and FD&C blue #2 Lake dye

CLINICAL PHARMACOLOGY

ISOPTIN (verapamil HCl) is a calcium ion influx inhibitor (slow channel blocker or calcium ion antagonist) that exerts its pharmacologic effects by modulating the influx of ionic calcium across the cell membrane of the arterial smooth muscle as well as in conductile and contractile myocardial cells.

Mechanism of Action
Essential Hypertension
ISOPTIN exerts antihypertensive effects by decreasing systemic vascular resistance, usually without orthostatic decreases in blood pressure or reflex tachycardia; bradycardia (rate less than 50 beats/min) is uncommon (1.4%). During isometric or dynamic exercise ISOPTIN does not alter sys-

Continued on next page

Isoptin SR—Cont.

tolic cardiac function in patients with normal ventricular function. ISOPTIN does not alter total serum calcium levels. However, one report suggested that calcium levels above the normal range may alter the therapeutic effect of ISOPTIN.

Other Pharmacological Actions of ISOPTIN Include the Following

ISOPTIN (verapamil HCl) dilates the main coronary arteries and coronary arterioles, both in normal and ischemic regions, and is a potent inhibitor of coronary artery spasm, whether spontaneous or ergonovine-induced. This property increases myocardial oxygen delivery in patients with coronary artery spasm, and is responsible for the effectiveness of ISOPTIN in vasospastic (Prinzmetal's or variant) as well as unstable angina at rest. Whether this effect plays any role in classical effort angina is not clear, but studies of exercise tolerance have not shown an increase in the maximum exercise rate-pressure product, a widely accepted measure of oxygen utilization. This suggests that, in general, relief of spasm or dilation of coronary arteries is not an important factor in classical angina.

ISOPTIN regularly reduces the total systemic resistance (afterload) against which the heart works both at rest and at a given level of exercise by dilating peripheral arterioles. Electrical activity through the AV node depends, to a significant degree, upon calcium influx through the slow channel. By decreasing the influx of calcium, ISOPTIN prolongs the effective refractory period within the AV node and slows AV conduction in a rate-related manner.

Normal sinus rhythm is usually not affected, but in patients with sick sinus syndrome, ISOPTIN may interfere with sinus node impulse generation and may induce sinus arrest or sinoatrial block. Atrioventricular block can occur in patients without preexisting conduction defects (see WARNINGS).

ISOPTIN does not alter the normal atrial action potential or intraventricular conduction time, but depresses amplitude, velocity of depolarization and conduction in depressed atrial fibers. ISOPTIN may shorten the antegrade effective refractory period of accessory bypass tracts. Acceleration of ventricular rate and/or ventricular fibrillation has been reported in patients with atrial flutter or atrial fibrillation and a coexisting accessory AV pathway following administration of verapamil (see WARNINGS).

ISOPTIN has a local anesthetic action that is 1.6 times that of procaine on an equimolar basis. It is not known whether this action is important at the doses used in man.

Pharmacokinetics and Metabolism: With the immediate release formulation, more than 90% of the orally administered dose of ISOPTIN is absorbed. Because of rapid biotransformation of verapamil during its first pass through the portal circulation, bioavailability ranges from 20% to 35%. Peak plasma concentrations are reached between 1 and 2 hours after oral administration. Chronic oral administration of 120 mg of ISOPTIN every 6 hours resulted in plasma levels of verapamil ranging from 125 to 400 ng/mL with higher values reported occasionally. A nonlinear correlation between the verapamil dose administered and verapamil plasma levels does exist.

In early dose titration with verapamil a relationship exists between verapamil plasma concentrations and the prolongation of the PR interval. However, during chronic administration this relationship may disappear. The mean elimination half-life in single dose studies ranged from 2.8 to 7.4 hours. In these same studies, after repetitive dosing, the half-life increased to a range from 4.5 to 12.0 hours (after less than 10 consecutive doses given 6 hours apart). Half-life of verapamil may increase during titration. No relationship has been established between the plasma concentration of verapamil and a reduction in blood pressure.

Aging may affect the pharmacokinetics of verapamil. Elimination half-life may be prolonged in the elderly.

In multiple dose studies under fasting conditions the bioavailability measured by AUC of ISOPTIN SR was similar to ISOPTIN immediate release; rates of absorption were, of course, different. In a randomized, single-dose, crossover study using healthy volunteers, administration of 240 mg ISOPTIN SR with food produced peak plasma verapamil concentrations of 79 ng/mL, time to peak plasma verapamil concentrations of 7.71 hours, and AUC (0–24 hr) of 841 ng-hr/mL. When ISOPTIN SR was administered to fasting subjects, peak plasma verapamil concentration was 164 ng/mL; time to peak plasma verapamil concentration was 5.21 hours; and AUC (0–24 hr) was 1,478 ng-hr/mL. Similar results were demonstrated for plasma norverapamil. Food thus produces decreased bioavailability (AUC) but a narrower peak to trough ratio. Good correlation of dose and response is not available, but controlled studies of ISOPTIN SR have shown effectiveness of doses similar to the effective doses of ISOPTIN (immediate release).

In healthy man, orally administered ISOPTIN undergoes extensive metabolism in the liver. Twelve metabolites have been identified in plasma; all except norverapamil are present in trace amounts only. Norverapamil can reach steady-state plasma concentrations approximately equal to those of verapamil itself. The cardiovascular activity of norverapamil appears to be approximately 20% that of verapamil. Approximately 70% of an administered dose is excreted as metabolites in the urine and 16% or more in the feces within 5 days. About 3% to 4% is excreted in the urine as unchanged drug. Approximately 90% is bound to plasma proteins. In patients with hepatic insufficiency, metabolism of immediate release verapamil is delayed and elimination half-life prolonged up to 14 to 16 hours (see PRECAUTIONS); the volume of distribution is increased and plasma clearance reduced to about 30% of normal. Verapamil clearance values suggest that patients with liver dysfunction may attain therapeutic verapamil plasma concentrations with one-third of the oral daily dose required for patients with normal liver function.

After four weeks of oral dosing (120 mg q.i.d.), verapamil and norverapamil levels were noted in the cerebrospinal fluid with estimated partition coefficient of 0.06 for verapamil and 0.04 for norverapamil.

In ten healthy males, administration of oral verapamil (80 mg every 8 hours for 6 days) and a single oral dose of ethanol (0.8 g/kg) resulted in a 17% increase in mean peak ethanol concentrations (106.45 ± 21.40 to 124.23 ± 24.74 mg•hr/dL) compared to placebo. The area under the blood ethanol concentration versus time curve (AUC over 12 hours) increased by 30% (365.67 ± 93.52 to 475.07 ± 97.24 mg•hr/dL). Verapamil AUCs were positively correlated (r=0.71) to increased ethanol blood AUC values. (See PRECAUTIONS: Drug Interactions.)

Hemodynamics and Myocardial Metabolism:

ISOPTIN reduces afterload and myocardial contractility. Improved left ventricular diastolic function in patients with IHSS and those with coronary heart disease has also been observed with ISOPTIN therapy. In most patients, including those with organic cardiac disease, the negative inotropic action of ISOPTIN is countered by reduction of afterload and cardiac index is usually not reduced. However, in patients with severe left ventricular dysfunction (e.g., pulmonary wedge pressure above 20 mmHg or ejection fraction less than 30%), or in patients taking beta-adrenergic blocking agents or other cardiodepressant drugs, deterioration of ventricular function may occur (see DRUG INTERACTIONS).

Pulmonary Function: ISOPTIN does not induce bronchoconstriction and hence, does not impair ventilatory function.

INDICATIONS AND USAGE

ISOPTIN SR (verapamil HCl) is indicated for the management of essential hypertension.

CONTRAINDICATIONS

Verapamil HCl is contraindicated in:

1. Severe left ventricular dysfunction (see WARNINGS)
2. Hypotension (systolic pressure less than 90 mmHg) or cardiogenic shock
3. Sick sinus syndrome (except in patients with a functioning artificial ventricular pacemaker)
4. Second- or third-degree AV block (except in patients with a functioning artificial ventricular pacemaker).
5. Patients with atrial flutter or atrial fibrillation and an accessory bypass tract (e.g., Wolff-Parkinson-White, Lown-Ganong-Levine syndromes). (see WARNINGS).
6. Patients with known hypersensitivity to verapamil hydrochloride.

WARNINGS

Heart Failure: Verapamil has a negative inotropic effect which, in most patients, is compensated by its afterload reduction (decreased systemic vascular resistance) properties without a net impairment of ventricular performance. In clinical experience with 4,954 patients, 87 (1.8%) developed congestive heart failure or pulmonary edema. Verapamil should be avoided in patients with severe left ventricular dysfunction (e.g., ejection fraction less than 30%, or moderate to severe symptoms of cardiac failure) and in patients with any degree of ventricular dysfunction if they are receiving a beta adrenergic blocker (see DRUG INTERACTIONS). Patients with milder ventricular dysfunction should, if possible, be controlled with optimum doses of digitalis and/or diuretics before verapamil treatment (Note interactions with digoxin under: PRECAUTIONS).

Hypotension: Occasionally, the pharmacologic action of verapamil may produce a decrease in blood pressure below normal levels which may result in dizziness or symptomatic hypotension. The incidence of hypotension observed in 4,954 patients enrolled in clinical trials was 2.5%. In hypertensive patients, decreases in blood pressure below normal are unusual. Tilt table testing (60 degrees) was not able to induce orthostatic hypotension.

Elevated Liver Enzymes: Elevations of transaminases with and without concomitant elevations in alkaline phosphatase and bilirubin have been reported. Such elevations have sometimes been transient and may disappear even in the face of continued verapamil treatment. Several cases of hepatocellular injury related to verapamil have been proven by rechallenge; half of these had clinical symptoms (malaise, fever, and/or right upper quadrant pain) in addition to elevations of SGOT, SGPT and alkaline phosphatase. Periodic monitoring of liver function in patients receiving verapamil is therefore prudent.

Accessory Bypass Tract (Wolff-Parkinson-White or Lown-Ganong-Levine): Some patients with paroxysmal and/or chronic atrial fibrillation or atrial flutter and a coexisting accessory AV pathway have developed increased antegrade conduction across the accessory pathway bypassing the AV node, producing a very rapid ventricular response or ventricular fibrillation after receiving intravenous verapamil (or digitalis). Although a risk of this occurring with oral verapamil has not been established, such patients receiving oral verapamil may be at risk and its use in these patients is contraindicated (see CONTRAINDICATIONS). Treatment is usually DC-cardioversion. Cardioversion has been used safely and effectively after oral ISOPTIN.

Atrioventricular Block: The effect of verapamil on AV conduction and the SA node may cause asymptomatic first-degree AV block and transient bradycardia, sometimes accompanied by nodal escape rhythms. PR interval prolongation is correlated with verapamil plasma concentrations, especially during the early titration phases of therapy. Higher degrees of AV block, however, were infrequently (0.8%) observed. Marked first-degree block or progressive development to second- or third-degree AV block requires a reduction in dosage or, in rare instances, discontinuation of verapamil HCl and institution of appropriate therapy depending upon the clinical situation.

Patients with Hypertrophic Cardiomyopathy (IHSS): In 120 patients with hypertrophic cardiomyopathy (most of them refractory or intolerant to propranolol) who received therapy with verapamil at doses up to 720 mg/day, a variety of serious adverse effects were seen. Three patients died in pulmonary edema; all had severe left ventricular outflow obstruction and a past history of left ventricular dysfunction. Eight other patients had pulmonary edema and/or severe hypotension; abnormally high (greater than 20 mmHg) pulmonary wedge pressure and a marked left ventricular outflow obstruction were present in most of these patients. Concomitant administration of quinidine (see DRUG INTERACTIONS) preceded the severe hypotension in 3 of the 8 patients (2 of whom developed pulmonary edema). Sinus bradycardia occurred in 11% of the patients, second-degree AV block in 4% and sinus arrest in 2%. It must be appreciated that this group of patients had a serious disease with a high mortality rate. Most adverse effects responded well to dose reduction and only rarely did verapamil have to be discontinued.

PRECAUTIONS

General

Use in Patients with Impaired Hepatic Functions: Since verapamil is highly metabolized by the liver, it should be administered cautiously to patients with impaired hepatic function. Severe liver dysfunction prolongs the elimination half-life of immediate release verapamil to about 14 to 16 hours; hence, approximately 30% of the dose given to patients with normal liver function should be administered to these patients. Careful monitoring for abnormal prolongation of the PR interval or other signs of excessive pharmacologic effects (see OVERDOSAGE) should be carried out.

Use in Patients with Attenuated (Decreased) Neuromuscular Transmission: It has been reported that verapamil decreases neuromuscular transmission in patients with Duchenne's muscular dystrophy, prolongs recovery from the neuromuscular blocking agent vecuronium, and causes a worsening of myasthenia gravis. It may be necessary to decrease the dosage of verapamil when it is administered to patients with attenuated neuromuscular transmission.

Use in Patients with Impaired Renal Function: About 70% of an administered dose of verapamil is excreted as metabolites in the urine. Verapamil is not removed by hemodialysis. Until further data are available, verapamil should be administered cautiously to patients with impaired renal function. These patients should be carefully monitored for abnormal prolongation of the PR interval or other signs of overdosage (see OVERDOSAGE).

Drug Interactions

Cytochrome inducers/inhibitors: *In vitro* metabolic studies indicate that verapamil is metabolized by cytochrome P450 CYP3A4, CYP1A2, CYP2C8, CYP2C9 and CYP2C18. Clinically significant interactions have been reported with inhibitors of CYP3A4 (e.g. erythromycin, ritonavir) causing elevation of plasma levels of verapamil while inducers of CYP3A4 (e.g. rifampin) have caused a lowering of plasma levels of verapamil, therefore, patients should be monitored for drug interactions.

Aspirin: In a few reported cases, coadministration of verapamil with aspirin has led to increased bleeding time greater than observed with aspirin alone.

Grapefruit juice: The intake of grapefruit juice may increase drug levels of verapamil.

Beta Blockers: Concomitant therapy with beta-adrenergic blockers and verapamil may result in additive negative effects on heart rate, atrioventricular conduction, and/or cardiac contractility. The combination of sustained-release verapamil and beta-adrenergic blocking agents has not been studied. However, there have been reports of excessive bradycardia and AV block, including complete heart block, when the combination has been used for the treatment of hypertension. For hypertensive patients, the risks of combined therapy may outweigh the potential benefits. The combination should be used only with caution and close monitoring.

Asymptomatic bradycardia (36 beats/min) with a wandering atrial pacemaker has been observed in a patient receiving concomitant timolol (a beta-adrenergic blocker) eyedrops and oral verapamil.

A decrease in metoprolol and propranolol clearance has been observed when either drug is administered concomitantly with verapamil. A variable effect has been seen when verapamil and atenolol were given together.

Digitalis: Clinical use of verapamil in digitalized patients has shown the combination to be well tolerated if digoxin doses are properly adjusted. Chronic verapamil treatment can increase serum digoxin levels by 50 to 75% during the first week of therapy, and this can result in digitalis toxicity. In patients with hepatic cirrhosis the influence of verapamil on digoxin kinetics is magnified. Verapamil may reduce total body clearance and extrarenal clearance of digitoxin by 27% and 29%, respectively. Maintenance and digitalization doses should be reduced when verapamil is administered, and the patient should be carefully monitored to avoid over- or underdigitalization. Whenever overdigitalization is suspected, the daily dose of digitalis should be reduced or temporarily discontinued. Upon discontinuation of ISOPTIN (verapamil HCl), the patient should be reassessed to avoid underdigitalization.

Antihypertensive Agents: Verapamil administered concomitantly with oral antihypertensive agents (e.g., vasodilators, angiotensin-converting enzyme inhibitors, diuretics, beta blockers) will usually have an additive effect on lowering blood pressure. Patients receiving these combinations should be appropriately monitored. Concomitant use of agents that attenuate alpha-adrenergic function with verapamil may result in a reduction in blood pressure that is excessive in some patients. Such an effect was observed in one study following the concomitant administration of verapamil and prazosin.

Antiarrhythmic Agents

Disopyramide: Until data on possible interactions between verapamil and disopyramide phosphate are obtained, disopyramide should not be administered within 48 hours before or 24 hours after verapamil administration.

Flecainide: A study of healthy volunteers showed that the concomitant administration of flecainide and verapamil may have additive effects on myocardial contractility, AV conduction, and repolarization. Concomitant therapy with flecainide and verapamil may result in additive negative inotropic effect and prolongation of atrioventricular conduction.

Quinidine: In a small number of patients with hypertrophic cardiomyopathy (IHSS), concomitant use of verapamil and quinidine resulted in significant hypotension. Until further data are obtained, combined therapy of verapamil and quinidine in patients with hypertrophic cardiomyopathy should probably be avoided.

The electrophysiological effects of quinidine and verapamil on AV conduction were studied in 8 patients. Verapamil significantly counteracted the effects of quinidine on AV conduction. There has been a report of increased quinidine levels during verapamil therapy.

Nitrates: Verapamil has been given concomitantly with short- and long-acting nitrates without any undesirable drug interactions. The pharmacologic profile of both drugs and the clinical experience suggest beneficial interactions.

Other

Alcohol: Verapamil has been found to significantly inhibit ethanol elimination resulting in elevated blood ethanol concentrations that may prolong the intoxicating effects of alcohol. (See CLINICAL PHARMACOLOGY, Pharmacokinetics and Metabolism).

Cimetidine: The interaction between cimetidine and chronically administered verapamil has not been studied. Variable results on clearance have been obtained in acute studies of healthy volunteers; clearance of verapamil was either reduced or unchanged.

Lithium: Increased sensitivity to the effects of lithium (neurotoxicity) has been reported during concomitant verapamil-lithium therapy; lithium levels have been observed sometimes to increase, sometimes to decrease, and sometimes to be unchanged. Patients receiving both drugs must be monitored carefully.

Carbamazepine: Verapamil may increase carbamazepine concentrations during combined therapy. This may produce carbamazepine side effects such as diplopia, headache, ataxia, or dizziness.

Rifampin: Therapy with rifampin may markedly reduce oral verapamil bioavailability.

Phenobarbital: Phenobarbital therapy may increase verapamil clearance.

Cyclosporine: Verapamil therapy may increase serum levels of cyclosporine.

Theophylline: Verapamil therapy may inhibit the clearance and increase the plasma levels of theophylline.

Inhalation Anesthetics: Animal experiments have shown that inhalation anesthetics depress cardiovascular activity by decreasing the inward movement of calcium ions. When used concomitantly, inhalation anesthetics and calcium antagonists, such as verapamil, should each be titrated carefully to avoid excessive cardiovascular depression.

Neuromuscular Blocking Agents: Clinical data and animal studies suggest that verapamil may potentiate the activity of neuromuscular blocking agents (curare-like and depolarizing). It may be necessary to decrease the dose of verapamil and/or the dose of the neuromuscular blocking agent when the drugs are used concomitantly.

Carcinogenesis, Mutagenesis, Impairment of Fertility: An 18–month toxicity study in rats, at a low multiple (6 fold) of the maximum recommended human dose, and not the maximum tolerated dose, did not suggest a tumorigenic potential. There was no evidence of a carcinogenic potential of verapamil administered in the diet of rats for two years at doses of 10, 35, and 120 mg/kg per day or approximately 1×, 3.5×, and 12×, respectively, the maximum recommended human daily dose (480 mg per day or 9.6 mg/kg/day).

Verapamil was not mutagenic in the Ames test in 5 test strains at 3 mg per plate, with or without metabolic activation.

Studies in female rats at daily dietary doses up to 5.5 times (55 mg/kg/day) the maximum recommended human dose did not show impaired fertility. Effects on male fertility have not been determined.

Pregnancy: Pregnancy Category C. Reproduction studies have been performed in rabbits and rats at oral doses up to 1.5 (15 mg/kg/day) and 6 (60 mg/kg/day) times the human oral daily dose, respectively, and have revealed no evidence of teratogenicity. In the rat, however, this multiple of the human dose was embryocidal and retarded fetal growth and development, probably because of adverse maternal effects reflected in the reduced weight gains of the dams. This oral dose has also been shown to cause hypotension in rats. There are no adequate and well-controlled studies in pregnant women. Because animal reproduction studies are not always predictive of human response, this drug should be used during pregnancy only if clearly needed. Verapamil crosses the placental barrier and can be detected in umbilical vein blood at delivery.

Labor and Delivery: It is not known whether the use of verapamil during labor or delivery has immediate or delayed adverse effects on the fetus, or whether it prolongs the duration of labor or increases the need for forceps delivery or other obstetric intervention. Such adverse experiences have not been reported in the literature, despite a long history of use of verapamil in Europe in the treatment of cardiac side effects of beta-adrenergic agonist agents used to treat premature labor.

Nursing Mothers: Verapamil is excreted in human milk. Because of the potential for adverse reactions in nursing infants for verapamil, nursing should be discontinued while verapamil is administered.

Pediatric Use: Safety and efficacy of ISOPTIN tablets in pediatric patients below the age of 18 years have not been established.

Animal Pharmacology and/or Animal Toxicology: In chronic animal toxicology studies verapamil caused lenticular and/or suture line changes at 30 mg/kg/day or greater and frank cataracts at 62.5 mg/kg/day or greater in the beagle dog but not the rat. Development of cataracts due to verapamil has not been reported in man.

ADVERSE REACTIONS

Serious adverse reactions are uncommon when verapamil therapy is initiated with upward dose titration within the recommended single and total daily dose. See WARNINGS for discussion of heart failure, hypotension, elevated liver enzymes, AV block, and rapid ventricular response. Reversible (upon discontinuation of verapamil) non-obstructive, paralytic ileus has been infrequently reported in association with the use of verapamil. The following reactions to orally administered verapamil occurred at rates greater than 1.0% or occurred at lower rates but appeared clearly drug-related in clinical trials in 4,954 patients.

Constipation	7.3%	Fatigue	1.7%
Dizziness	3.3%	Dyspnea	1.4%
Nausea	2.7%	Bradycardia(HR <50/min)	1.4%
Hypotension	2.5%	AV Block-total (1°, 2°, 3°)	1.2%
Headache	2.2%	2° and 3°	0.8%
Edema	1.9%	Rash	1.2%
CHF/ Pulmonary Edema	1.8%	Flushing	0.6%
Elevated Liver Enzymes (see WARNING)			

In clinical trials related to the control of ventricular response in digitalized patients who had atrial fibrillation or atrial flutter, ventricular rates below 50/min at rest occurred in 15% of patients and asymptomatic hypotension occurred in 5% of patients.

The following reactions, reported in 1.0% or less of patients, occurred under conditions (open trials, marketing experience) where a causal relationship is uncertain; they are listed to alert the physician to a possible relationship.

Cardiovascular: angina pectoris, atrioventricular dissociation, chest pain, claudication, myocardial infarction, palpitations, purpura (vasculitis), syncope.

Digestive System: diarrhea, dry mouth, gastrointestinal distress, gingival hyperplasia.

Hemic and Lymphatic: ecchymosis or bruising.

Nervous System: cerebrovascular accident, confusion, equilibrium disorders, insomnia, muscle cramps, paresthesia, psychotic symptoms, shakiness, somnolence, extrapyramidal symptoms.

Skin: arthralgia and rash, exanthema, hair loss, hyperkeratosis, maculae, sweating, urticaria, Stevens-Johnson syndrome, erythema multiforme.

Special Senses: blurred vision, tinnitus.

Urogenital: gynecomastia, impotence, galactorrhea/hyperprolactinemia, increased urination, spotty menstruation.

Treatment of Acute Cardiovascular Adverse Reactions: The frequency of cardiovascular adverse reactions that require therapy is rare, hence, experience with their treatment is limited. Whenever severe hypotension or complete AV block occurs following oral administration of verapamil, the appropriate emergency measures should be applied immediately, e.g., intravenously administered isoproterenol HCl, norepinephrine bitartrate, atropine sulfate (all in the usual doses), or calcium gluconate (10% solution). In patients with hypertrophic cardiomyopathy (IHSS), alpha-adrenergic agents (phenylephrine HCl, metaraminol bitartrate or methoxamine HCl) should be used to maintain blood pressure, and isoproterenol and norepinephrine should be avoided. If further support is necessary, (dopamine HCl or dobutamine HCl) may be administered. Actual treatment and dosage should depend on the severity of the clinical situation and the judgment and experience of the treating physician.

OVERDOSAGE

Overdose with verapamil may lead to pronounced hypotension, bradycardia, and conduction system abnormalities (e.g., junctional rhythm with AV dissociation and high degree AV block, including asystole). Other symptoms secondary to hypoperfusion (e.g., metabolic acidosis, hyperglycemia, hyperkalemia, renal dysfunction, and convulsions) may be evident.

Treat all verapamil overdoses as serious and maintain observation for at least 48 hours [especially ISOPTIN® SR (verapamil hydrochloride)] preferably under continuous hospital care. Delayed pharmacodynamic consequences may occur with the sustained released formulation. Verapamil is known to decrease gastrointestinal transit time.

In overdose, tablets of ISOPTIN SR have occasionally been reported to form concretions within the stomach or intestines. These concretions have not been visible on plain radiographs of the abdomen, and no medical means of gastrointestinal emptying is of proven efficacy in removing them. Endoscopy might reasonably be considered in cases of massive overdose when symptoms are unusually prolonged.

Treatment of overdosage should be supportive. Beta adrenergic stimulation or parenteral administration of calcium solutions may increase calcium ion flux across the slow channel, and have been used effectively in treatment of deliberate overdosage with verapamil. Continued treatment with large doses of calcium may produce a response. In a few reported cases, overdose with calcium channel blockers that was initially refractory to atropine became more responsive to this treatment when the patients received large doses (close to 1 gram/hour for more than 24 hours) of calcium chloride. Verapamil cannot be removed by hemodialysis. Clinically significant hypotensive reactions or high degree AV block should be treated with vasopressor agents or cardiac pacing, respectively. Asystole should be handled by the usual measures including cardiopulmonary resuscitation.

DOSAGE AND ADMINISTRATION

Essential Hypertension

The dose of ISOPTIN SR should be individualized by titration and the drug should be administered with food. Initiate therapy with 180 mg of sustained-release verapamil HCl, ISOPTIN SR, given in the morning. Lower, initial doses of 120 mg a day may be warranted in patients who may have an increased response to verapamil (e.g., the elderly or small people etc.). Upward titration should be based on therapeutic efficacy and safety evaluated weekly and approximately 24 hours after the previous dose. The antihypertensive effects of ISOPTIN SR are evident within the first week of therapy.

If adequate response is not obtained with 180 mg of ISOPTIN SR, the dose may be titrated upward in the following manner:

a) 240 mg each morning,
b) 180 mg each morning plus 180 mg each evening, or 240 mg each morning plus 120 mg each evening
c) 240 mg every twelve hours.

When switching from immediate release ISOPTIN to ISOPTIN SR, the total daily dose in milligrams may remain the same.

HOW SUPPLIED

ISOPTIN® SR 240 mg tablets are supplied as light green, capsule shaped, scored, film-coated tablets containing 240 mg of verapamil hydrochloride. The tablet is embossed with a double Abbott logo on one side and "ST" on the other side. ISOPTIN® SR 180 mg tablets are supplied as light pink, oval shaped, scored, film-coated tablets containing 180 mg of verapamil hydrochloride. The tablet is embossed with a double Abbott logo on one side, and "SK" on the other side. The ISOPTIN® SR 120 mg tablets are supplied as light violet, oval shaped, film-coated tablets containing 120 mg of verapamil hydrochloride. The tablet is embossed with the Abbott logo on one side and "SC" on the other side.

240 mg (light green)-	Bottle of 100- NDC #0074-1625-14
	Bottle of 500- NDC #0074-1625-54
180 mg (light pink)-	Bottle of 100- NDC #0074-1486-14
120 mg (light violet)-	Bottle of 100- NDC #0074-1149-14

Storage: Store at 25°C (77°F); excursions permitted to 15°–30°C (59°–86°F) [see USP Controlled Room Temperature].

Protect from light and moisture.

Dispense in a tight, light-resistant container as defined in the USP.

Revised: July, 2003
Ref. 03-5276-R2
ABBOTT LABORATORIES
NORTH CHICAGO, IL 60064, U.S.A.

Shown in Product Identification Guide, page 303

K–LOR™ 20 mEq. ℞
[k 'lor]
(Potassium Chloride for Oral Solution, USP)

DESCRIPTION

Natural fruit-flavored K-LOR (potassium chloride for oral solution, USP) is an oral potassium supplement offered in

Continued on next page

K-Lor—Cont.

individual packets as a powder for reconstitution. Each packet of K-LOR 20 mEq powder contains potassium 20 mEq and chloride 20 mEq provided by potassium chloride 1.5 g.
K-LOR powder is an electrolyte replenisher. The chemical name is potassium chloride, and the structural formula is KCl. Potassium chloride, USP, occurs as a white, granular powder or as colorless crystals. It is odorless and has a saline taste. Its solutions are neutral to litmus. It is freely soluble in water and insoluble in alcohol.

Inactive Ingredients

FD&C Yellow No. 6, maltodextrin (contains corn derivative), malic acid, saccharin, silica gel and natural flavoring.

CLINICAL PHARMACOLOGY

Potassium ion is the principal intracellular cation of most body tissues. Potassium ions participate in a number of essential physiological processes including the maintenance of intracellular tonicity, the transmission of nerve impulses, the contraction of cardiac, skeletal and smooth muscle, and the maintenance of normal renal function.
The intracellular concentration of potassium is approximately 150 to 160 mEq per liter. The normal adult plasma concentration is 3.5 to 5 mEq per liter. An active ion transport system maintains this gradient across the plasma membrane.
Potassium is a normal dietary constituent and under steady state conditions the amount of potassium absorbed from the gastrointestinal tract is equal to the amount excreted in the urine. The usual dietary intake of potassium is 50 to 100 mEq per day.
Potassium depletion will occur whenever the rate of potassium loss through renal excretion and/or loss from the gastrointestinal tract exceeds the rate of potassium intake. Such depletion usually develops as a consequence of therapy with diuretics, primary or secondary hyperaldosteronism, diabetic ketoacidosis, or inadequate replacement of potassium in patients on prolonged parenteral nutrition. Depletion can develop rapidly with severe diarrhea, especially if associated with vomiting. Potassium depletion due to these causes is usually accompanied by a concomitant loss of chloride and is manifested by hypokalemia and metabolic alkalosis. Potassium depletion may produce weakness, fatigue, disturbances of cardiac rhythm (primarily ectopic beats), prominent U-waves in the electrocardiogram, and, in advanced cases, flaccid paralysis and/or impaired ability to concentrate urine.
If potassium depletion associated with metabolic alkalosis cannot be managed by correcting the fundamental cause of the deficiency, e.g., where the patient requires long term diuretic therapy, supplemental potassium in the form of high potassium food or potassium chloride may restore normal potassium levels.
In rare circumstances, (e.g., patients with renal tubular acidosis), potassium depletion may be associated with metabolic acidosis and hyperchloremia. In such patients potassium replacement should be accomplished with potassium salts other than the chloride, such as potassium bicarbonate, potassium citrate, potassium acetate, or potassium gluconate.

INDICATIONS AND USAGE

1. For the treatment of patients with hypokalemia with or without metabolic alkalosis, in digitalis intoxication, and in patients with hypokalemic familial periodic paralysis. If hypokalemia is the result of diuretic therapy, consideration should be given to the use of a lower dose of diuretic, which may be sufficient without leading to hypokalemia.
2. For the prevention of hypokalemia in patients who would be at particular risk if hypokalemia were to develop, e.g., digitalized patients or patients with significant cardiac arrhythmias.

The use of potassium salts in patients receiving diuretics for uncomplicated essential hypertension is often unnecessary when such patients have a normal dietary pattern, and when low doses of the diuretic are used. Serum potassium should be checked periodically, however, and, if hypokalemia occurs, dietary supplementation with potassium-containing foods may be adequate to control milder cases. In more severe cases, and if dose adjustment of the diuretic is ineffective or unwarranted, supplementation with potassium salts may be indicated.

CONTRAINDICATIONS

Potassium supplements are contraindicated in patients with hyperkalemia since a further increase in serum potassium concentration in such patients can produce cardiac arrest. Hyperkalemia may complicate any of the following conditions: chronic renal failure, systemic acidosis such as diabetic acidosis, acute dehydration, extensive tissue breakdown as in severe burns, adrenal insufficiency, or the administration of a potassium-sparing diuretic, e.g., spironolactone, triamterene, or amiloride (see OVERDOSAGE).
K-LOR (potassium chloride for oral solution) is contraindicated in patients with known hypersensitivity to any ingredient in this product.

WARNINGS

Hyperkalemia (See OVERDOSAGE)
In patients with impaired mechanisms for excreting potassium, the administration of potassium salts can produce hyperkalemia and cardiac arrest. This occurs most commonly in patients given potassium intravenously, but may also occur in patients given potassium orally. Potentially fatal hyperkalemia can develop rapidly and can be asymptomatic. The use of potassium salts in patients with chronic renal disease, or any other condition which impairs potassium excretion, requires particularly careful monitoring of the serum potassium concentration and appropriate dosage adjustment.
Interaction with Potassium-Sparing Diuretics
Hypokalemia should not be treated by the concomitant administration of potassium salts and a potassium-sparing diuretic, e.g., spironolactone, triamterene, or amiloride, since the simultaneous administration of these agents can produce severe hyperkalemia.
Interaction with Angiotensin Converting Enzyme Inhibitors
Angiotensin converting enzyme (ACE) inhibitors (e.g., captopril, enalapril) will produce some potassium retention by inhibiting aldosterone production. Potassium supplements should be given to patients receiving ACE inhibitors only with close monitoring
Metabolic Acidosis
Hypokalemia in patients with metabolic acidosis should be treated with an alkalinizing potassium salt such as potassium bicarbonate, potassium citrate, potassium acetate or potassium gluconate.

PRECAUTIONS

General: The diagnosis of potassium depletion is ordinarily made by demonstrating hypokalemia in a patient with a clinical history suggesting some cause for potassium depletion. In interpreting the serum potassium level, the physician should bear in mind that acute alkalosis *per se* can produce hypokalemia in the absence of a deficit in total body potassium, while acute acidosis *per se* can increase the serum potassium concentration to within the normal range even in the presence of a reduced total body potassium. The treatment of potassium depletion, particularly in the presence of cardiac disease, renal disease, or acidosis, requires careful attention to acid-base balance and appropriate monitoring of serum electrolytes, the electrocardiogram, and the clinical status of the patient.
Information for Patients: Physicians should consider reminding the patient of the following:
To dilute each packet of powder in $^{1}/_{2}$ glassful of water or other liquid and take each dose after a meal.
To take this medicine following the frequency and amount prescribed by the physician. This is especially important if the patient is also taking diuretics and/or digitalis preparations.
Laboratory Tests: When blood is drawn for analysis of plasma potassium it is important to recognize that artifactual elevations can occur after improper venipuncture technique or as a result of *in vitro* hemolysis of the sample.
Drug Interactions: Potassium-sparing diuretics, angiotensin converting enzyme inhibitors (see WARNINGS).
Carcinogenesis, Mutagenesis, Impairment of Fertility: Carcinogenicity, mutagenicity and fertility studies in animals have not been performed. Potassium is a normal dietary constituent.
Pregnancy Category C: Animal reproduction studies have not been conducted with K-LOR powder. It is unlikely that potassium supplementation that does not lead to hyperkalemia would have an adverse effect on the fetus or would affect reproductive capacity.
Nursing Mothers: The normal potassium ion content of human milk is about 13 mEq per liter. Since oral potassium becomes part of the body potassium pool, as long as body potassium is not excessive, the contribution of potassium chloride supplementation should have little or no effect on the level in human milk.
Pediatric Use: Safety and effectiveness in children have not been established.

ADVERSE REACTIONS

One of the most severe adverse effects is hyperkalemia (see CONTRAINDICATIONS, WARNINGS and OVERDOSAGE).
The most common adverse reactions to oral potassium salts are nausea, vomiting, flatulence, abdominal pain/discomfort, and diarrhea. These symptoms are due to irritation of the gastrointestinal tract and are best managed by diluting the preparation further, taking the dose with meals, or reducing the amount taken at one time.
Skin rash has been reported rarely.

OVERDOSAGE

The administration of oral potassium salts to persons with normal excretory mechanisms for potassium rarely causes serious hyperkalemia. However, if excretory mechanisms are impaired or if intravenous administration is too rapid, potentially fatal hyperkalemia can result (see CONTRAINDICATIONS and WARNINGS). It is important to recognize that hyperkalemia is usually asymptomatic and may be manifested only by an increased serum potassium concentration (6.5–8.0 mEq/L) and characteristic electrocardiographic changes (peaking of T-waves, loss of P-waves, depression of S-T segments, and prolongation of the QT intervals). Late manifestations include muscle paralysis and cardiovascular collapse from cardiac arrest (9–12 mEq/L).
Treatment measures for hyperkalemia include the following:

1. Elimination of foods and medications containing potassium and of any agents with potassium-sparing properties;
2. Intravenous administration of 300 to 500 ml/hr of 10% dextrose solution containing 10–20 units of crystalline insulin per 1,000 ml;
3. Correction of acidosis, if present, with intravenous sodium bicarbonate;
4. Use of exchange resins, hemodialysis, or peritoneal dialysis.

In treating hyperkalemia, it should be recalled that in patients who have been stabilized on digitalis, lowering the serum potassium concentration too rapidly can produce digitalis toxicity.

DOSAGE AND ADMINISTRATION

The usual dietary potassium intake by the average adult is 50 to 100 mEq per day. Potassium depletion sufficient to cause hypokalemia usually requires the loss of 200 or more mEq of potassium from the total body store.
Dosage must be adjusted to the individual needs of each patient. The dose for the prevention of hypokalemia is typically in the range of 20 mEq per day. Doses of 40–100 mEq per day or more are used for the treatment of potassium depletion. Dosage should be divided if more than 20 mEq per day is given such that no more than 20 mEq is given in a single dose. The dose should be taken after a meal.
K-LOR 20 mEq powder provides 20 mEq of potassium chloride.
Each 20 mEq (one K-LOR mEq packet) of potassium should be dissolved in at least 4 oz (approximately $^{1}/_{2}$ glassful) cold water or juice. This preparation, like other potassium supplements, must be properly diluted to avoid the possibility of gastrointestinal irritation.

HOW SUPPLIED

K-LOR 20 mEq (Potassium Chloride for Oral Solution, USP) is supplied in cartons of 30 packets (**NDC** 0074-3611-01), and in cartons of 100 packets (**NDC** 0074-3611-02). Each packet contains potassium, 20 mEq, and chloride, 20 mEq, provided by potassium chloride, 1.5 g.
Revised: June, 1994
Ref. 13-2184-5/R26

K-Tab® ℞

[*k 'tăb*]
(Potassium Chloride Extended-Release Tablets, USP)
℞ only

DESCRIPTION

K-TAB (potassium chloride extended-release tablets) is a solid oral dosage form of potassium chloride containing 750 mg of potassium chloride, USP, equivalent to 10 mEq of potassium in a film-coated (not enteric-coated), wax matrix tablet. This formulation is intended to slow the release of potassium so that the likelihood of a high localized concentration of potassium chloride within the gastrointestinal tract is reduced. The expended inert, porous, wax/polymer matrix is not absorbed and may be excreted intact in the stool.
K-TAB tablets are an electrolyte replenisher. The chemical name is potassium chloride, and the structural formula is KCl. Potassium chloride, USP, occurs as a white, granular powder or as colorless crystals. It is odorless and has a saline taste. Its solutions are neutral to litmus. It is freely soluble in water and insoluble in alcohol.

Inactive Ingredients

Castor oil, cellulosic polymers, colloidal silicon dioxide, D&C Yellow No. 10, magnesium stearate, paraffin, polyvinyl acetate, titanium dioxide, vanillin and vitamin E.

CLINICAL PHARMACOLOGY

Potassium ion is the principal intracellular cation of most body tissues. Potassium ions participate in a number of essential physiological processes including the maintenance of intracellular tonicity, the transmission of nerve impulses, the contraction of cardiac, skeletal, and smooth muscle, and the maintenance of normal renal function.
The intracellular concentration of potassium is approximately 150 to 160 mEq per liter. The normal adult plasma concentration is 3.5 to 5 mEq per liter. An active ion transport system maintains this gradient across the plasma membrane.
Potassium is a normal dietary constituent and under steady state conditions the amount of potassium absorbed from the gastrointestinal tract is equal to the amount excreted in the urine. The usual dietary intake of potassium is 50 to 100 mEq per day.
Potassium depletion will occur whenever the rate of potassium loss through renal excretion and/or loss from the gastrointestinal tract exceeds the rate of potassium intake. Such depletion usually develops as a consequence of therapy with diuretics, primary or secondary hyperaldosteronism, diabetic ketoacidosis, or inadequate replacement of potassium in patients on prolonged parenteral nutrition. Depletion can develop rapidly with severe diarrhea, especially if associated with vomiting. Potassium depletion due to these causes is usually accompanied by a concomitant loss of chloride and is manifested by hypokalemia and metabolic alkalosis. Potassium depletion may produce weakness, fatigue, disturbances of cardiac rhythm (primarily ectopic beats), prominent U-waves in the electrocardiogram, and, in advanced cases, flaccid paralysis and/or impaired ability to concentrate urine.
If potassium depletion associated with metabolic alkalosis cannot be managed by correcting the fundamental cause of

the deficiency, e.g., where the patient requires long term diuretic therapy, supplemental potassium in the form of high potassium food or potassium chloride may restore normal potassium levels.

In rare circumstances, (e.g., patients with renal tubular acidosis) potassium depletion may be associated with metabolic acidosis and hyperchloremia. In such patients potassium replacement should be accomplished with potassium salts other than the chloride, such as potassium bicarbonate, potassium citrate, potassium acetate, or potassium gluconate.

INDICATIONS AND USAGE

BECAUSE OF REPORTS OF INTESTINAL AND GASTRIC ULCERATION AND BLEEDING WITH CONTROLLED-RELEASE POTASSIUM CHLORIDE PREPARATIONS, THESE DRUGS SHOULD BE RESERVED FOR THOSE PATIENTS WHO CANNOT TOLERATE OR REFUSE TO TAKE LIQUID OR EFFERVESCENT POTASSIUM PREPARATIONS, OR FOR PATIENTS WITH WHOM THERE IS A PROBLEM OF COMPLIANCE WITH THESE PREPARATIONS.

1. For the treatment of patients with hypokalemia with or without metabolic alkalosis, in digitalis intoxication, and in patients with hypokalemic familial periodic paralysis. If hypokalemia is the result of diuretic therapy, consideration should be given to the use of a lower dose of diuretic, which may be sufficient without leading to hypokalemia.
2. For the prevention of hypokalemia in patients who would be at particular risk if hypokalemia were to develop, e.g., digitalized patients or patients with significant cardiac arrhythmias.

The use of potassium salts in patients receiving diuretics for uncomplicated essential hypertension is often unnecessary when such patients have a normal dietary pattern, and when low doses of the diuretic are used. Serum potassium should be checked periodically, however, and, if hypokalemia occurs, dietary supplementation with potassium-containing foods may be adequate to control milder cases. In more severe cases and if dose adjustment of the diuretic is ineffective or unwarranted supplementation with potassium salts may be indicated.

CONTRAINDICATIONS

Potassium supplements are contraindicated in patients with hyperkalemia since a further increase in serum potassium concentration in such patients can produce cardiac arrest. Hyperkalemia may complicate any of the following conditions: chronic renal failure, systemic acidosis such as diabetic acidosis, acute dehydration, extensive tissue breakdown as in severe burns, adrenal insufficiency, or the administration of potassium-sparing diuretic, e.g., spironolactone, triamterene, or amiloride (see OVERDOSAGE).

K-TAB tablets are contraindicated in patients with known hypersensitivity to any ingredient in this product.

Controlled-release formulations of potassium chloride have produced esophageal ulceration in certain cardiac patients with esophageal compression due to an enlarged left atrium. Potassium supplementation, when indicated in such patients, should be given as a liquid preparation.

All solid oral dosage forms of potassium chloride are contraindicated in any patient in whom there is structural, pathological, e.g., diabetic gastroparesis, or pharmacologic (use of anticholinergic agents or other agents with anticholinergic properties at sufficient doses to exert anticholinergic effects) cause for arrest or delay in tablet passage through the gastrointestinal tract.

WARNINGS

Hyperkalemia (see OVERDOSAGE)

In patients with impaired mechanisms for excreting potassium, the administration of potassium salts can produce hyperkalemia and cardiac arrest. This occurs most commonly in patients given potassium intravenously, but may also occur in patients given potassium orally. Potentially fatal hyperkalemia can develop rapidly and can be asymptomatic. The use of potassium salts in patients with chronic renal disease, or any other condition which impairs potassium excretion, requires particularly careful monitoring of the serum potassium concentration and appropriate dosage adjustment.

Interaction with Potassium-Sparing Diuretics

Hypokalemia should not be treated by the concomitant administration of potassium salts and a potassium-sparing diuretic, e.g., spironolactone, triamterene, or amiloride, since the simultaneous administration of these agents can produce severe hyperkalemia.

Interaction with Angiotensin Converting Enzyme Inhibitors

Angiotensin converting enzyme (ACE) inhibitors (e.g., captopril, enalapril) will produce some potassium retention by inhibiting aldosterone production. Potassium supplements should be given to patients receiving ACE inhibitors only with close monitoring.

Gastrointestinal Lesions

Solid oral dosage forms of potassium chloride can produce ulcerative and/or stenotic lesions of the gastrointestinal tract. Based on spontaneous adverse reaction reports, enteric-coated preparations of potassium chloride are associated with an increased frequency of small bowel lesions (40-50 per 100,000 patient years) compared to sustained-release wax matrix formulations (less than one per 100,000 patient years). Because of the lack of extensive marketing experience with microencapsulated products, a comparison between such products and wax matrix or enteric-coated products is not available. K-TAB tablets consist of a wax matrix formulated to provide a controlled rate of release potassium chloride and thus to minimize the possibility of a high local concentration of potassium near the gastrointestinal wall.

Prospective trials have been conducted in normal human volunteers in which the upper gastrointestinal tract was evaluated by endoscopic inspection before and after one week of solid oral potassium chloride therapy. The ability of this model to predict events occuring in usual clinical practice is unknown. Trials which approximated usual clinical practice did not reveal any clear differences between the wax matrix and microencapsulated dosage forms. In contrast, there was a higher incidence of gastric and duodenal lesions in subjects receiving a high dose of a wax matrix controlled-release formulation under conditions which did not resemble usual or recommended clinical practice, i.e., 96 mEq per day in divided doses of potassium chloride administered, to fasted patients in the presence of an anticholinergic drug to delay gastric emptying. The upper gastrointestinal lesions observed by endoscopy were asymptomatic and were not accompanied by evidence of bleeding (hemoccult testing). The relevance of these findings to the usual conditions, i.e., nonfasting, no anticholinergic agent, and smaller doses, under which controlled-release potassium chloride products are used is uncertain. Epidemiologic studies have not identified an elevated risk, compared to microencapsulated products, for upper gastrointestinal lesions in patients receiving wax matrix formulations. K-TAB tablets should be discontinued immediately and the possibility of ulceration, obstruction or perforation considered if severe vomiting, abdominal pain, distention, or gastrointestinal bleeding occurs.

Metabolic Acidosis

Hypokalemia in patients with metabolic acidosis should be treated with an alkalinizing potassium salt such as potassium bicarbonate, potassium citrate, potassium acetate, or potassium gluconate.

PRECAUTIONS

General: The diagnosis of potassium depletion is ordinarily made by demonstrating hypokalemia in a patient with a clinical history suggesting some cause for potassium depletion. In interpreting the serum potassium level, the physician should bear in mind that acute alkalosis *per se* can produce hypokalemia in the absence of a deficit in total body potassium, while acute acidosis *per se* can increase the serum potassium concentration to within the normal range even in the presence of a reduced total body potassium. The treatment of potassium depletion, particularly in the presence of cardiac disease, renal disease, or acidosis, requires careful attention to acid-base balance and appropriate monitoring of serum electrolytes, the electrocardiogram, and the clinical status of the patient.

Information for Patients: Physicians should consider reminding the patient of the following:

To take each dose with meals and with a full glass of water or other liquid.

To take this medicine following the frequency and amount prescribed by the physician. This is especially important if the patient is also taking diuretics and/or digitalis preparations.

To check with the physician if there is trouble swallowing tablets or if the tablets seem to stick in the throat.

To check with the physician at once if tarry stools or other evidence of gastrointestinal bleeding is noticed.

To take each dose without crushing, chewing or sucking the tablets.

Laboratory Tests: When blood is drawn for analysis of plasma potassium it is important to recognize that artifactual elevations can occur after improper venipuncture technique or as a result of *in vitro* hemolysis of the sample.

Drug Interactions: Potassium-sparing diuretics, angiotensin converting enzyme inhibitors (see WARNINGS).

Carcinogenesis, Mutagenesis, Impairment of Fertility: Carcinogenicity, mutagenicity and fertility studies in animals have not been performed. Potassium is a normal dietary constituent.

Pregnancy Category C: Animal reproduction studies have not been conducted with K-TAB tablets. It is unlikely that potassium supplementation that does not lead to hyperkalemia would have an adverse effect on the fetus or would affect reproductive capacity.

Nursing Mothers: The normal potassium ion content of human milk is about 13 mEq per liter. Since oral potassium becomes part of the body potassium pool, as long as body potassium is not excessive, the contribution of potassium chloride supplementation should have little or no effect on the level in human milk.

Pediatric Use: Safety and effectiveness in children have not been established.

Geriatric Use: Clinical Studies of K-Tab tablets did not include sufficient numbers of subjects aged 65 and over to determine whether they respond differently from younger subjects. Other reported clinical experience has not identified differences in responses between the elderly and younger patients. In general, dose selection for an elderly patient should be cautious, usually starting at the low end of the dosing range, reflecting the greater frequency of decreased heptatic, renal or cardiac function, and of concomitant disease or other drug therapy.

This drug is known to be substantially excreted by the kidney, and the risk of toxic reactions to this drug may be greater in patients with impaired renal function. Because elderly patients are more likely to have decreased renal function, care should be taken in dose selection, and it may be useful to monitor renal function.

ADVERSE REACTIONS

One of the most severe adverse effects is hyperkalemia (see CONTRAINDICATIONS, WARNINGS, and OVERDOSAGE). There also have been reports of upper and lower gastrointestinal conditions including obstruction, bleeding, ulceration, and perforation (see CONTRAINDICATIONS and WARNINGS).

The most common adverse reactions to oral potassium salts are nausea, vomiting, flatulence, abdominal pain/discomfort, and diarrhea. These symptoms are due to irritation of the gastrointestinal tract and are best managed by taking the dose with meals, or reducing the amount taken at one time.

Skin rash has been reported rarely.

OVERDOSAGE

The administration of oral potassium salts to persons with normal excretory mechanisms for potassium rarely causes serious hyperkalemia. However, if excretory mechanisms are impaired or if intravenous administration is too rapid, potentially fatal hyperkalemia can result (see CONTRAINDICATIONS and WARNINGS). It is important to recognize that hyperkalemia is usually asymptomatic and may be manifested only by an increased serum potassium concentration (6.5-8.0 mEq/L) and characteristic electrocardiographic changes (peaking of T-waves, loss P-waves, depression of S-T segments, and prolongation of QT intervals). Late manifestations include muscle paralysis and cardiovascular collapse from cardiac arrest (9-12 mEq/L).

Treatment measures for hyperkalemia include the following:

1. Elimination of foods and medications containing potassium and of any agents with potassium-sparing properties;
2. Intravenous administration of 300 to 500 mL/hr of 10% dextrose solution containing 10-20 units of crystalline insulin per 1,000 mL;
3. Correction of acidosis, if present, with intravenous sodium bicarbonate;
4. Use of exchange resins, hemodialysis, or peritoneal dialysis.

In treating hyperkalemia, it should be recalled that in patients who have been stabilized on digitalis, lowering the serum potassium concentration too rapidly can produce digitalis toxicity.

The extended release feature means that absorption and toxic effects may be delayed for hours. Consider standard measures to remove any unabsorbed drug.

DOSAGE AND ADMINISTRATION

The usual dietary potassium intake by the average adult is 50 to 100 mEq per day. Potassium depletion sufficient to cause hypokalemia usually requires the loss of 200 or more mEq of potassium from the total body store.

Dosage must be adjusted to the individual needs of each patient. The dose for the prevention of hypokalemia is typically in the range of 20 mEq per day. Doses of 40-100 mEq per day or more are used for the treatment of potassium depletion. Dosage should be divided if more than 20 mEq per day is given such that no more than 20 mEq is given in a single dose.

K-TAB tablets provide 10 mEq of potassium chloride.

K-TAB tablets should be taken with meals and with a glass of water or other liquid. This product should not be taken on an empty stomach because of its potential for gastric irritation (see WARNINGS).

NOTE: K-TAB tablets are to be swallowed whole without crushing, chewing or sucking the tablets.

HOW SUPPLIED

K-TAB (potassium chloride extended-release tablets, USP) contains 750 mg of potassium chloride (equivalent to 10 mEq). K-TAB tablets are provided as yellow, ovaloid, extended-release Filmtab® tablets in bottles of 100 (**NDC** 0074-7804-13), 1000 (**NDC** 0074-7804-19) and 5000 (**NDC** 0074-7804-59) and in ABBO-PAC® unit dose packages of 100 (**NDC** 0074-7804-11).

Recommended storage: Store below 86°F (30°C).

Revised: August, 2003

Filmtab—Film-sealed tablets, Abbott

Ref. 03-5288-R16-Rev. August, 2003

Shown in Product Identification Guide, page 303

KALETRA® ℞

[*kuh-LEE-tra*]

(lopinavir/ritonavir) capsules

(lopinavir/ritonavir) oral solution

℞ only

DESCRIPTION

KALETRA (lopinavir/ritonavir) is a co-formulation of lopinavir and ritonavir. Lopinavir is an inhibitor of the HIV protease. As co-formulated in KALETRA, ritonavir inhibits the CYP3A-mediated metabolism of lopinavir, thereby providing increased plasma levels of lopinavir.

Continued on next page

Kaletra—Cont.

Lopinavir is chemically designated as [1S-[1R*,(R*), 3R*, 4R*]]-N-[4-[[(2,6-dimethylphenoxy)acetyl]amino]-3-hydroxy-5-phenyl-1-(phenylmethyl)pentyl]tetrahydro-alpha-(1-methylethyl)-2-oxo-1(2H)-pyrimidineacetamide. Its molecular formula is $C_{37}H_{48}N_4O_5$, and its molecular weight is 628.80. Lopinavir has the following structural formula:

Ritonavir is chemically designated as 10-Hydroxy-2-methyl-5-(1-methylethyl)-1- [2-(1-methylethyl)-4-thiazolyl]-3,6-dioxo-8,11-bis(phenylmethyl)-2,4,7,12-tetraazatridecan-13-oic acid, 5-thiazolylmethyl ester, [5S-(5R*,8R*,10R*,11R*)]. Its molecular formula is $C_{37}H_{48}N_6O_5S_2$ and its molecular weight is 720.95. Ritonavir has the following structural formula:

Lopinavir is a white to light tan powder. It is freely soluble in methanol and ethanol, soluble in isopropanol and practically insoluble in water.

KALETRA capsules are available for oral administration in a strength of 133.3 mg lopinavir and 33.3 mg ritonavir with the following inactive ingredients: FD&C Yellow No. 6, gelatin, glycerin, oleic acid, polyoxyl 35 castor oil, propylene glycol, sorbitol special, titanium dioxide, and water.

KALETRA oral solution is available for oral administration as 80 mg lopinavir and 20 mg ritonavir per milliliter with the following inactive ingredients: Acesulfame potassium, alcohol, artificial cotton candy flavor, citric acid, glycerin, high fructose corn syrup, Magnasweet-110 flavor, menthol, natural & artificial vanilla flavor, peppermint oil, polyoxyl 40 hydrogenated castor oil, povidone, propylene glycol, saccharin sodium, sodium chloride, sodium citrate, and water.

KALETRA oral solution contains 42.4% alcohol (v/v).

CLINICAL PHARMACOLOGY

Microbiology

Mechanism of action: Lopinavir, an inhibitor of the HIV protease, prevents cleavage of the Gag-Pol polyprotein, resulting in the production of immature, non-infectious viral particles.

Antiviral activity in vitro: The *in vitro* antiviral activity of lopinavir against laboratory HIV strains and clinical HIV isolates was evaluated in acutely infected lymphoblastic cell lines and peripheral blood lymphocytes, respectively. In the absence of human serum, the mean 50% effective concentration (EC_{50}) of lopinavir against five different HIV-1 laboratory strains ranged from 10-27 nM (0.006-0.017 μg/mL, 1 μg/mL = 1.6 μM) and ranged from 4-11 nM (0.003-0.007 μg/mL) against several HIV-1 clinical isolates (n=6). In the presence of 50% human serum, the mean EC_{50} of lopinavir against these five laboratory strains ranged from 65-289 nM (0.04-0.18 μg/mL), representing a 7- to 11-fold attenuation. Combination drug activity studies with lopinavir and other protease inhibitors or reverse transcriptase inhibitors have not been completed.

Resistance: HIV-1 isolates with reduced susceptibility to lopinavir have been selected *in vitro*. The presence of ritonavir does not appear to influence the selection of lopinavir-resistant viruses *in vitro*.

The selection of resistance to KALETRA in antiretroviral treatment naive patients has not yet been characterized. In a Phase III study of 653 antiretroviral treatment naive patients (Study 863), plasma viral isolates from each patient on treatment with plasma HIV >400 copies/mL at Week 24, 32, 40 and/or 48 were analyzed. No evidence of resistance to KALETRA was observed in 37 evaluable KALETRA-treated patients (0%). Evidence of genotypic resistance to nelfinavir, defined as the presence of the D30N and/or L90M mutation in HIV protease, was observed in 25/76 (33%) of evaluable nelfinavir-treated patients. The selection of resistance to KALETRA in antiretroviral treatment naive pediatric patients (Study 940) appears to be consistent with that seen in adult patients (Study 863).

Resistance to KALETRA has been noted to emerge in patients treated with other protease inhibitors prior to KALETRA therapy. In Phase II studies of 227 antiretroviral treatment naive and protease inhibitor experienced patients, isolates from 4 of 23 patients with quantifiable (>400 copies/mL) viral RNA following treatment with KALETRA for 12 to 100 weeks displayed significantly reduced susceptibility to lopinavir compared to the corresponding baseline viral isolates. Three of these patients had previously received treatment with a single protease inhibitor (nelfinavir, indinavir, or saquinavir) and one patient had received treatment with multiple protease inhibitors (indinavir, saquinavir and ritonavir). All four of these patients had at least 4 mutations associated with protease inhibitor resistance immediately prior to KALETRA therapy. Following viral rebound, isolates from these patients all contained additional mutations, some of which are recognized to be associated with protease inhibitor resistance. However, there are insufficient data at this time to identify lopinavir-associated mutational patterns in isolates from patients on KALETRA therapy. The assessment of these mutational patterns is under study.

Cross-resistance — Preclinical Studies: Varying degrees of cross-resistance have been observed among HIV protease inhibitors. Little information is available on the cross-resistance of viruses that developed decreased susceptibility to lopinavir during KALETRA therapy.

The *in vitro* activity of lopinavir against clinical isolates from patients previously treated with a single protease inhibitor was determined. Isolates that displayed >4-fold reduced susceptibility to nelfinavir (n=13) and saquinavir (n=4), displayed <4-fold reduced susceptibility to lopinavir. Isolates with >4-fold reduced susceptibility to indinavir (n=16) and ritonavir (n=3) displayed a mean of 5.7- and 8.3-fold reduced susceptibility to lopinavir, respectively. Isolates from patients previously treated with two or more protease inhibitors showed greater reductions in susceptibility to lopinavir, as described in the following paragraph.

Clinical Studies — Antiviral activity of KALETRA in patients with previous protease inhibitor therapies: The clinical relevance of reduced *in vitro* susceptibility to lopinavir has been examined by assessing the virologic response to KALETRA therapy, with respect to baseline viral genotype and phenotype, in 56 NNRTI-naive patients with HIV RNA >1000 copies/mL despite previous therapy with at least two protease inhibitors selected from nelfinavir, indinavir, saquinavir and ritonavir (Study 957). In this study, patients were initially randomized to receive one of two doses of KALETRA in combination with efavirenz and nucleoside reverse transcriptase inhibitors. The EC_{50} values of lopinavir against the 56 baseline viral isolates ranged from 0.5- to 96-fold higher than the wild-type EC_{50}. Fifty-five percent (31/56) of these baseline isolates displayed a >4-fold reduced susceptibility to lopinavir. These 31 isolates had a mean reduction in lopinavir susceptibility of 27.9-fold. Table 1 shows the 48 week virologic response (HIV RNA <400 and <50 copies) according to susceptibility and number of genotypic mutations at baseline in 50 evaluable patients enrolled in the study (957) described above. Because this was a select patient population and the sample size was small, the data depicted in Table 1 do not constitute definitive clinical susceptibility breakpoints. Additional data are needed to determine clinically significant breakpoints for KALETRA.

Table 1: HIV RNA Response at Week 48 by baseline KALETRA susceptibility and by number of protease inhibitor-associated mutations[1]

Lopinavir susceptibility[2] at baseline	HIV RNA < 400 copies/mL (%)	HIV RNA < 50 copies/mL (%)
<10 fold	25/27 (93%)	22/27 (81%)
>10 and <40 fold	11/15 (73%)	9/15 (60%)
≥40 fold	2/8 (25%)	2/8 (25%)
Number of protease inhibitor mutations at baseline		
Up to 5	21/23 (91%)[3]	19/23 (83%)
>5	17/27 (63%)	14/27 (52%)

[1] Lopinavir susceptibility was determined by recombinant phenotypic technology performed by Virologic; genotype also performed by Virologic

[2] Fold change in susceptibility from wild type

[3] Thirteen of the 23 patient isolates contained PI mutations at positions 82, 84, and/or 90

There are insufficient data at this time to identify lopinavir-associated mutational patterns in isolates from patients on KALETRA therapy. Further studies are needed to assess the association between specific mutational patterns and virologic response rates.

Table 2: Drug Interactions: Pharmacokinetic Parameters for Lopinavir in the Presence of the Co-administered Drug (See Precautions, Table 9 for Recommended Alterations in Dose or Regimen)

Co-administered Drug	Dose of Co-administered Drug (mg)	Dose of KALETRA (mg)	n	Ratio (in combination with co-administered drug) of Lopinavir Pharmacokinetic Parameters (90% CI); No Effect = 1.00 C_{max}	AUC	C_{min}
Amprenavir	750 BID, 10 d	400/100 BID, 21 d	12	0.72 (0.65, 0.79)	0.62 (0.56, 0.70)	0.43 (0.34, 0.56)
Atorvastatin	20 QD, 4 d	400/100 BID, 14 d	12	0.90 (0.78, 1.06)	0.90 (0.79, 1.02)	0.92 (0.78, 1.10)
Efavirenz[1]	600 QHS, 9 d	400/100 BID, 9 d	11, 7*	0.97 (0.78, 1.22)	0.81 (0.64, 1.03)	0.61 (0.38, 0.97)
Ketoconazole	200 single dose	400/100 BID, 16 d	12	0.89 (0.80, 0.99)	0.87 (0.75, 1.00)	0.75 (0.55, 1.00)
Nelfinavir	1000 BID, 10 d	400/100 BID, 21 d	13	0.79 (0.70, 0.89)	0.73 (0.63, 0.85)	0.62 (0.49, 0.78)
Nevirapine	200 BID, steady-state (>1 yr)[2]	400/100 BID, steady-state (>1 yr)	22, 19*	0.81 (0.62, 1.05)	0.73 (0.53, 0.98)	0.49 (0.28, 0.74)
	7 mg/kg or 4 mg/kg QD, 2 wk; BID 1 wk[3]	300/75 mg/m[2] BID, 3 wk	12, 15*	0.86 (0.64, 1.16)	0.78 (0.56, 1.09)	0.45 (0.25, 0.81)
Pravastatin	20 QD, 4 d	400/100 BID, 14 d	12	0.98 (0.89, 1.08)	0.95 (0.85, 1.05)	0.88 (0.77, 1.02)
Rifabutin	150 QD, 10 d	400/100 BID, 20 d	14	1.08 (0.97, 1.19)	1.17 (1.04, 1.31)	1.20 (0.96, 1.65)
Rifampin	600 QD, 10 d	400/100 BID, 20 d	22	0.45 (0.40, 0.51)	0.25 (0.21, 0.29)	0.01 (0.01, 0.02)
	600 QD, 14 d	800/200 BID, 9d[4]	10	1.02 (0.85, 1.23)	0.84 (0.64, 1.10)	0.43 (0.19, 0.96)
	600 QD, 14 d	400/400 BID, 9 d[5]	9	0.93 (0.81, 1.07)	0.98 (0.81, 1.17)	1.03 (0.68, 1.56)
				Co-administration of KALETRA and rifampin is not recommended (See **PRECAUTIONS**: Tables 8 and 9)		
Ritonavir[2]	100 BID, 3-4 wk	400/100 BID, 3-4 wk	8, 21*	1.28 (0.94, 1.76)	1.46 (1.04, 2.06)	2.16 (1.29, 3.62)

All interaction studies conducted in healthy, HIV-negative subjects unless otherwise indicated.

[1] The pharmacokinetics of ritonavir are unaffected by concurrent efavirenz.

[2] Study conducted in HIV-positive adult subjects.

[3] Study conducted in HIV-positive pediatric subjects ranging in age from 6 months to 12 years.

[4] Titrated to 800/200 BID as 533/133 BID × 1 d, 667/167 BID × 1 d, then 800/200 BID × 7 d, compared to 400/100 BID × 10 days alone.

[5] Titrated to 400/400 BID as 400/200 BID × 1 d, 400/300 BID × 1 d, then 400/400 BID × 7 d, compared to 400/100 BID × 10 days alone.

*Parallel group design; n for KALETRA + co-administered drug, n for KALETRA alone.

Pharmacokinetics

The pharmacokinetic properties of lopinavir co-administered with ritonavir have been evaluated in healthy adult volunteers and in HIV-infected patients; no substantial differences were observed between the two groups. Lopinavir is essentially completely metabolized by CYP3A. Ritonavir inhibits the metabolism of lopinavir, thereby increasing the plasma levels of lopinavir. Across studies, administration of KALETRA 400/100 mg BID yields mean steady-state lopinavir plasma concentrations 15- to 20-fold higher than those of ritonavir in HIV-infected patients. The plasma levels of ritonavir are less than 7% of those obtained after the ritonavir dose of 600 mg BID. The *in vitro* antiviral EC_{50} of lopinavir is approximately 10-fold lower than that of ritonavir. Therefore, the antiviral activity of KALETRA is due to lopinavir.

Figure 1 displays the mean steady-state plasma concentrations of lopinavir and ritonavir after KALETRA 400/100 mg BID with food for 3 weeks from a pharmacokinetic study in HIV-infected adult subjects (n=19).

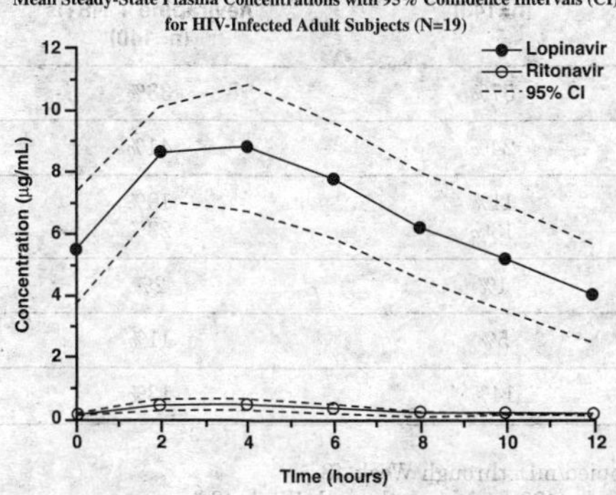

Figure 1:
Mean Steady-State Plasma Concentrations with 95% Confidence Intervals (CI) for HIV-Infected Adult Subjects (N=19)

Absorption: In a pharmacokinetic study in HIV-positive subjects (n=19), multiple dosing with 400/100 mg KALETRA BID with food for 3 weeks produced a mean ± SD lopinavir peak plasma concentration (C_{max}) of 9.8 ± 3.7 µg/mL, occurring approximately 4 hours after administration. The mean steady-state trough concentration prior to the morning dose was 7.1 ± 2.9 µg/mL and minimum concentration within dosing interval was 5.5 ± 2.7 µg/mL. Lopinavir AUC over a 12 hour dosing interval averaged 92.6 ± 36.7 µg•h/mL. The absolute bioavailability of lopinavir co-formulated with ritonavir in humans has not been established. Under nonfasting conditions (500 kcal, 25% from fat), lopinavir concentrations were similar following administration of KALETRA co-formulated capsules and liquid. When administered under fasting conditions, both the mean AUC and C_{max} of lopinavir were 22% lower for the KALETRA liquid relative to the capsule formulation.

Effects of Food on Oral Absorption: Administration of a single 400/100 mg dose of KALETRA capsules with a moderate fat meal (500-682 kcal, 23 to 25% calories from fat) was associated with a mean increase of 48 and 23% in lopinavir AUC and C_{max}, respectively, relative to fasting. For KALETRA oral solution, the corresponding increases in lopinavir AUC and C_{max} were 80 and 54%, respectively. Relative to fasting, administration of KALETRA with a high fat meal (872 kcal, 56% from fat) increased lopinavir AUC and C_{max} by 97 and 43%, respectively, for capsules, and 130 and 56%, respectively, for oral solution. To enhance bioavailability and minimize pharmacokinetic variability KALETRA should be taken with food.

Distribution: At steady state, lopinavir is approximately 98-99% bound to plasma proteins. Lopinavir binds to both alpha-1-acid glycoprotein (AAG) and albumin; however, it has a higher affinity for AAG. At steady state, lopinavir protein binding remains constant over the range of observed concentrations after 400/100 mg KALETRA BID, and is similar between healthy volunteers and HIV-positive patients.

Metabolism: *In vitro* experiments with human hepatic microsomes indicate that lopinavir primarily undergoes oxidative metabolism. Lopinavir is extensively metabolized by the hepatic cytochrome P450 system, almost exclusively by the CYP3A isozyme. Ritonavir is a potent CYP3A inhibitor which inhibits the metabolism of lopinavir, and therefore increases plasma levels of lopinavir. A ^{14}C-lopinavir study in humans showed that 89% of the plasma radioactivity after a single 400/100 mg KALETRA dose was due to parent drug. At least 13 lopinavir oxidative metabolites have been identified in man. Ritonavir has been shown to induce metabolic enzymes, resulting in the induction of its own metabolism. Pre-dose lopinavir concentrations decline with time during multiple dosing, stabilizing after approximately 10 to 16 days.

Elimination: Following a 400/100 mg ^{14}C-lopinavir/ritonavir dose, approximately 10.4 ± 2.3% and 82.6 ± 2.5% of an administered dose of ^{14}C-lopinavir can be accounted for in urine and feces, respectively, after 8 days. Unchanged lopinavir accounted for approximately 2.2 and 19.8% of the administered dose in urine and feces, respectively. After multiple dosing, less than 3% of the lopinavir dose is excreted unchanged in the urine. The apparent oral clearance (CL/F) of lopinavir is 5.98 ± 5.75 L/hr (mean ± SD, N=19).

Table 3: Drug Interactions: Pharmacokinetic Parameters for Co-administered Drug in the Presence of KALETRA (See Precautions, Table 9 for Recommended Alterations in Dose or Regimen)

Co-administered Drug	Dose of Co-administered Drug (mg)	Dose of KALETRA (mg)	n	Ratio (in combination with KALETRA/alone) of Co-administered Drug Pharmacokinetic Parameters (90% CI); No Effect = 1.00		
				C_{max}	AUC	C_{min}
Amprenavir[1]	750 BID, 10 d combo vs. 1200 BID, 14 d alone	400/100 BID, 21 d	11	1.12 (0.91, 1.39)	1.72 (1.41, 2.09)	4.57 (3.51, 5.95)
Atorvastatin	20 QD, 4 d	400/100 BID, 14 d	12	4.67 (3.35, 6.51)	5.88 (4.69, 7.37)	2.28 (1.91, 2.71)
Desipramine[2]	100 single dose	400/100 BID, 10 d	15	0.91 (0.84, 0.97)	1.05 (0.96, 1.16)	N/A
Efavirenz	600 QHS, 9 d	400/100 BID, 9 d	11, 12*	0.91 (0.72, 1.15)	0.84 (0.62, 1.15)	0.84 (0.58, 1.20)
Ethinyl Estradiol	35 µg QD, 21 d (Ortho Novum®)	400/100 BID, 14 d	12	0.59 (0.52, 0.66)	0.58 (0.54, 0.62)	0.42 (0.36, 0.49)
Indinavir[1]	600 BID, 10 d combo nonfasting vs. 800 TID, 5 d alone fasting	400/100 BID, 15 d	13	0.71 (0.63, 0.81)	0.91 (0.75, 1.10)	3.47 (2.60, 4.64)
Ketoconazole	200 single dose	400/100 BID, 16 d	12	1.13 (0.91, 1.40)	3.04 (2.44, 3.79)	N/A
Methadone	5 single dose	400/100 BID, 10 d	11	0.55 (0.48, 0.64)	0.47 (0.42, 0.53)	N/A
Nelfinavir[1]	1000 BID, 10 d combo vs. 1250 BID, 14 d alone	400/100 BID, 21 d	13	0.93 (0.82, 1.05)	1.07 (0.95, 1.19)	1.86 (1.57, 2.22)
M8 metabolite				2.36 (1.91, 2.91)	3.46 (2.78, 4.31)	7.49 (5.85, 9.58)
Nevirapine	200 QD, 14 d; BID, 6 d	400/100 BID, 20 d	5, 6*	1.05 (0.72, 1.52)	1.08 (0.72, 1.64)	1.15 (0.71, 1.86)
Norethindrone	1 QD, 21 d (Ortho Novum®)	400/100 BID, 14 d	12	0.84 (0.75, 0.94)	0.83 (0.73, 0.94)	0.68 (0.54, 0.85)
Pravastatin	20 QD, 4 d	400/100 BID, 14 d	12	1.26 (0.87, 1.83)	1.33 (0.91, 1.94)	N/A
Rifabutin	150 QD, 10 d; combo vs. 300 QD, 10 d; alone	400/100 BID, 10 d	12	2.12 (1.89, 2.38)	3.03 (2.79, 3.30)	4.90 (3.18, 5.76)
25-*O*-desacetyl rifabutin				23.6 (13.7, 25.3)	47.5 (29.3, 51.8)	94.9 (74.0, 122)
Rifabutin + 25-*O*-desacetyl rifabutin[3]				3.46 (3.07, 3.91)	5.73 (5.08, 6.46)	9.53 (7.56, 12.01)
Saquinavir[1]	800 BID, 10 d combo vs. 1200 TID, 5 d alone,	400/100 BID, 15 d	14	6.34 (5.32, 7.55)	9.62 (8.05, 11.49)	16.74 (13.73, 20.42)
	1200 BID, 5 d combo vs. 1200 TID, 5 d alone	400/100 BID, 20 d	10	6.44 (5.59, 7.41)	9.91 (8.28, 11.86)	16.54 (10.91, 25.08)

All interaction studies conducted in healthy, HIV-negative subjects unless otherwise indicated.
[1] Ratio of parameters for amprenavir, indinavir, nelfinavir, and saquinavir are not normalized for dose.
[2] Desipramine is a probe substrate for assessing effects on CYP2D6-mediated metabolism.
[3] Effect on the dose-normalized sum of rifabutin parent and 25-O-desacetyl rifabutin active metabolite.
*Parallel group design; n for KALETRA + co-administered drug, n for co-administered drug alone.
N/A=not available.

Special Populations:

Gender, Race and Age: Lopinavir pharmacokinetics have not been studied in elderly patients. No gender related pharmacokinetic differences have been observed in adult patients. No clinically important pharmacokinetic differences due to race have been identified.

Pediatric Patients: The pharmacokinetics of KALETRA 300/75 mg/m^2 BID and 230/57.5 mg/m^2 BID have been studied in a total of 53 pediatric patients, ranging in age from 6 months to 12 years. The 230/57.5 mg/m^2 BID regimen without nevirapine and the 300/75 mg/m^2 BID regimen with nevirapine provided lopinavir plasma concentrations similar to those obtained in adult patients receiving the 400/100 mg BID regimen (without nevirapine).

The mean steady-state lopinavir AUC, C_{max}, and C_{min} were 72.6 ± 31.1 µg•h/mL, 8.2 ± 2.9 and 3.4 ± 2.1 mg/mL respectively after KALETRA 230/57.5 mg/m^2 BID without nevirapine (n=12), and were 85.8 ± 36.9 µg•h/mL, 10.0 ± 3.3 and 3.6 ± 3.5 µg/mL, respectively, after 300/75 mg/m^2 BID with nevirapine (n=12). The nevirapine regimen was 7 mg/kg BID (6 months to 8 years) or 4 mg/kg BID (>8 years).

Renal Insufficiency: Lopinavir pharmacokinetics have not been studied in patients with renal insufficiency; however, since the renal clearance of lopinavir is negligible, a decrease in total body clearance is not expected in patients with renal insufficiency.

Hepatic Impairment: Lopinavir is principally metabolized and eliminated by the liver. Although KALETRA has not been studied in patients with hepatic impairment, lopinavir concentrations may be increased in these patients (see **PRECAUTIONS**).

Drug-Drug Interactions: See also **CONTRAINDICATIONS, WARNINGS** and **PRECAUTIONS: Drug Interactions.**

KALETRA is an inhibitor of the P450 isoform CYP3A *in vitro*. Co-administration of KALETRA and drugs primarily metabolized by CYP3A may result in increased plasma concentrations of the other drug, which could increase or prolong its therapeutic and adverse effects (see **CONTRAINDICATIONS**).

KALETRA does not inhibit CYP2D6, CYP2C9, CYP2C19, CYP2E1, CYP2B6 or CYP1A2 at clinically relevant concentrations.

KALETRA has been shown *in vivo* to induce its own metabolism and to increase the biotransformation of some drugs metabolized by cytochrome P450 enzymes and by glucuronidation.

Continued on next page

Kaletra—Cont.

KALETRA is metabolized by CYP3A. Drugs that induce CYP3A activity would be expected to increase the clearance of lopinavir, resulting in lowered plasma concentrations of lopinavir. Although not noted with concurrent ketoconazole, co-administration of KALETRA and other drugs that inhibit CYP3A may increase lopinavir plasma concentrations.

Drug interaction studies were performed with KALETRA and other drugs likely to be co-administered and some drugs commonly used as probes for pharmacokinetic interactions. The effects of co-administration of KALETRA on the AUC, C_{max} and C_{min} are summarized in Table 2 (effect of other drugs on lopinavir) and Table 3 (effect of KALETRA on other drugs). The effects of other drugs on ritonavir are not shown since they generally correlate with those observed with lopinavir (if lopinavir concentrations are decreased, ritonavir concentrations are decreased) unless otherwise indicated in the table footnotes. For information regarding clinical recommendations, see Table 9 in **PRECAUTIONS**.

[See table 2 at top of page 484]
[See table 3 at top of previous page]

INDICATIONS AND USAGE

KALETRA is indicated in combination with other antiretroviral agents for the treatment of HIV-infection. This indication is based on analyses of plasma HIV RNA levels and CD_4 cell counts in controlled studies of KALETRA of 48 weeks duration and in smaller uncontrolled dose-ranging studies of KALETRA of 72 weeks duration.

Description of Clinical Studies

Patients Without Prior Antiretroviral Therapy

Study 863: KALETRA BID + stavudine + lamivudine compared to nelfinavir TID + stavudine + lamivudine

Study 863 is an ongoing, randomized, double-blind, multicenter trial comparing treatment with KALETRA (400/100 mg BID) plus stavudine and lamivudine versus nelfinavir (750 mg TID) plus stavudine and lamivudine in 653 antiretroviral treatment naive patients. Patients had a mean age of 38 years (range: 19 to 84), 57% were Caucasian, and 80% were male. Mean baseline CD_4 cell count was 259 cells/mm^3 (range: 2 to 949 cells/mm^3) and mean baseline plasma HIV-1 RNA was 4.9 log_{10} copies/mL (range: 2.6 to 6.8 log_{10} copies/mL).

Treatment response and outcomes of randomized treatment are presented in Figure 2 and Table 4, respectively.

Figure 2: Virologic Response Through Week 48, Study 863*†

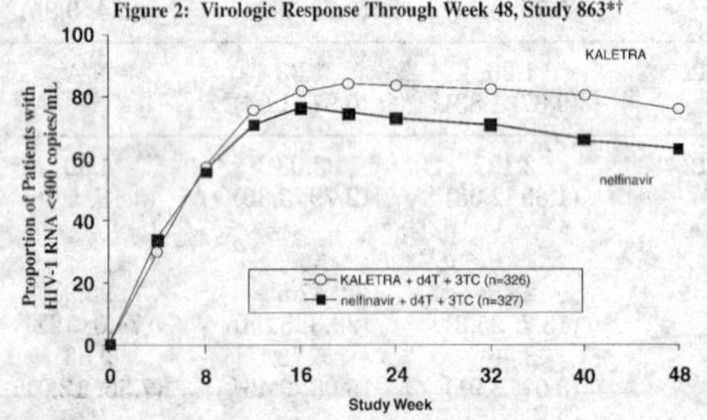

* Roche AMPLICOR HIV-1 MONITOR Assay.
† Responders at each visit are patients who had achieved and maintained HIV-1 RNA <400 copies/mL without discontinuation by that visit.

Table 4: Outcomes of Randomized Treatment Through Week 48 (Study 863)

Outcome	KALETRA +d4T + 3TC (N=326)	Nelfinavir +d4T + 3TC (N=327)
Responder*[1]	75%	62%
Virologic failure[2]	9%	25%
Rebound	7%	15%
Never suppressed through Week 48	2%	9%
Death	2%	1%
Discontinued due to adverse event	4%	4%
Discontinued for other reasons[3]	10%	8%

*Corresponds to rates at Week 48 in Figure 2.
[1] Patients achieved and maintained confirmed HIV RNA <400 copies/mL through Week 48.
[2] Includes confirmed viral rebound and failure to achieve confirmed <400 copies/mL through Week 48.
[3] Includes lost to follow-up, patient's withdrawal, non-compliance, protocol violation and other reasons. Overall discontinuation through week 48, including patients who discontinued subsequent to virologic failure, was 17% in the KALETRA arm and 24% in the nelfinavir arm.

Through 48 weeks of therapy, there was a statistically significantly higher proportion of patients in the KALETRA arm compared the nelfinavir arm with HIV RNA <400 copies/mL (75% vs. 62%, respectively) and HIV RNA <50 copies/mL (67% vs. 52%, respectively). Treatment response by baseline HIV RNA level subgroups is presented in Table 5.

Table 5: Proportion of Responders Through Week 48 by Baseline Viral Load (Study 863)

Baseline Viral Load (HIV-1 RNA copies/mL)	KALETRA +d4T + 3TC			Nelfinavir +d4T+ 3TC		
	<400 copies/mL[1]	<50 copies/mL[2]	n	<400 copies/mL[1]	<50 copies/mL[2]	n
<30,000	74%	71%	82	79%	72%	87
≥30,000 to <100,000	81%	73%	79	67%	54%	79
≥100,000 to <250,000	75%	64%	83	60%	47%	72
≥250,000	72%	60%	82	44%	33%	89

[1] Patients achieved and maintained confirmed HIV RNA <400 copies/mL through Week 48.
[2] Patients achieved HIV RNA <50 copies/mL at Week 48.

[See table 5 above]

Through 48 weeks of therapy, the mean increase from baseline in CD_4 cell count was 207 cells/mm^3 for the KALETRA arm and 195 cells/mm^3 for the nelfinavir arm.

Patients with Prior Antiretroviral Therapy

Study 888: KALETRA BID + nevirapine + NRTIs compared to investigator-selected protease inhibitor(s) + nevirapine + NRTIs.

Study 888 is a randomized, open-label, multicenter trial comparing treatment with KALETRA (400/100 mg BID) plus nevirapine and nucleoside reverse transcriptase inhibitors versus investigator-selected protease inhibitor(s) plus nevirapine and nucleoside reverse transcriptase inhibitors in 288 single protease inhibitor-experienced, non-nucleoside reverse transcriptase inhibitor (NNRTI)-naive patients. Patients had a mean age of 40 years (range: 18 to 74), 68% were Caucasian, and 86% were male. Mean baseline CD_4 cell count was 322 cells/mm^3 (range: 10 to 1059 cells/mm^3) and mean baseline plasma HIV-1 RNA was 4.1 log_{10} copies/mL (range: 2.6 to 6.0 log_{10} copies/mL).

Treatment response and outcomes of randomized treatment through Week 48 are presented in Figure 3 and Table 6, respectively.

Table 6. Outcomes of Randomized Treatment Through Week 48 (Study 888)

Outcome	KALETRA + nevirapine + NRTIs (n=148)	Investigator-Selected Protease Inhibitor(s) + nevirapine + NRTIs (n=140)
Responder*[1]	57%	33%
Virologic Failure[2]	24%	41%
Rebound	11%	19%
Never suppressed through Week 48	13%	23%
Death	1%	2%
Discontinued due to adverse events	5%	11%
Discontinued for other reasons[3]	14%	13%

*Corresponds to rates at Week 48 in Figure 3.
[1] Patients achieved and maintained confirmed HIV RNA <400 copied/mL, through Week 48.
[2] Includes confirmed viral rebound and failure to achieve confirmed <400 copies/mL through Week 48.
[3] Includes lost to follow-up, patient's withdrawal, non-compliance, protocol violation and other reasons.

Figure 3: Virologic Response Through Week 48, Study 888*†

KALETRA
ISPI
Proportion of Patients with HIV-1 RNA <400 copies/mL
Study Week
KALETRA + NVP + NRTIs (n=148)
Investigator-selected protease inhibitor(s) [ISPI] + NVP + NRTIs (n=140)

* Roche AMPLICOR HIV-1 MONITOR Assay.
† Responders at each visit are patients who had achieved and maintained HIV-1 RNA <400 copies/mL without discontinuation by that visit.

[See table 6 above]

Through 48 weeks of therapy, there was a statistically significantly higher proportion patients in the KALETRA arm compared to the investigator-selected protease inhibitor(s) arm with HIV RNA <400 copies/mL (57% vs. 33%, respectively).

Through 48 weeks of therapy, the mean increase from baseline in CD_4 cell count was 111 cells/mm^3 for the KALETRA arm and 112 cells/mm^3 for the investigator-selected protease inhibitor(s) arm.

Other Studies

Study 720: KALETRA BID + stavudine + lamivudine
Study 765: KALETRA BID + nevirapine + NRTIs

Study 720 (patients without prior antiretroviral therapy) and study 765 (patients with prior protease inhibitor therapy) are randomized, blinded, multi-center trials evaluating treatment with KALETRA at up to three dose levels (200/100 mg BID [720 only], 400/100 mg BID, and 400/200 mg BID). Patients in study 720 had a mean age of 35 years, 70% were Caucasian, and 96% were male, while patients in study 765 had a mean age of 40 years, 73% were Caucasian, and 90% were male. Mean (range) baseline CD_4 cell counts for patients in study 720 and study 765 were 338 (3-918) and 372 (72-807) cells/mm^3, respectively. Mean (range) baseline plasma HIV-1 RNA levels for patients in study 720 and study 765 were 4.9 (3.3 to 6.3) and 4.0 (2.9 to 5.8) log_{10} copies/mL, respectively.

Through 72 weeks of treatment, for patients randomized to the 400/100 mg BID dose of KALETRA, the proportion of patients with plasma HIV-1 RNA <400 (<50) copies/mL was 80% (78%) in study 720 [n=51] and 75% (58%) in study 765 [n=36]. The corresponding mean increase in CD_4 cell count was 256 cells/mm^3 for study 720 and 174 cells/mm^3 for study 765. At 72 weeks, 13 patients (13%) had discontinued study 720 for any reason, including four discontinuations (4%) secondary to adverse events or laboratory abnormalities with one of these discontinuations (1%) being attributed to a KALETRA adverse event. In study 765, 13 patients (19%) had discontinued the study for any reason at 72 weeks, including six discontinuations (9%) secondary to adverse events or laboratory abnormalities with three of these discontinuations (4%) being attributed to KALETRA adverse events.

CONTRAINDICATIONS

KALETRA is contraindicated in patients with known hypersensitivity to any of its ingredients, including ritonavir.

Co-administration of KALETRA is contraindicated with drugs that are highly dependent on CYP3A for clearance and for which elevated plasma concentrations are associated with serious and/or life-threatening events. These drugs are listed in Table 7.

Table 7: Drugs That Are Contraindicated With KALETRA

Drug Class	Drugs Within Class That Are Contraindicated With KALETRA
Antihistamines	Astemizole, Terfenadine
Ergot Derivatives	Dihydroergotamine, Ergonovine, Ergotamine, Methylergonovine
GI motility agent	Cisapride
Neuroleptic	Pimozide
Sedative/hypnotics	Midazolam, Triazolam

WARNINGS

ALERT: Find out about medicines that should NOT be taken with KALETRA. This statement is included on the product's bottle label.

Drug Interactions

KALETRA is an inhibitor of the P450 isoform CYP3A. Co-administration of KALETRA and drugs primarily metabolized by CYP3A may result in increased plasma concentrations of the other drug that could increase or prolong its therapeutic and adverse effects (see **Pharmacokinetics: Drug-Drug Interactions, CONTRAINDICATIONS — Table 7: Drugs That Are Contraindicated With KALETRA, PRECAUTIONS — Table 8: Drugs That Should Not Be Co-administered With KALETRA and Table 9: Established and Other Potentially Significant Drug Interactions**).

Particular caution should be used when prescribing sildenafil in patients receiving KALETRA. Co-administration of KALETRA with sildenafil is expected to substantially increase sildenafil concentrations and may result in an increase in sildenafil-associated adverse events including hypotension, syncope, visual changes and prolonged erection (see **PRECAUTIONS: Drug Interactions** and the complete prescribing information for sildenafil).

Concomitant use of KALETRA with lovastatin or simvastatin is not recommended. Caution should be exercised if HIV protease inhibitors, including KALETRA, are used concurrently with other HMG-CoA reductase inhibitors that are also metabolized by the CYP3A4 pathway (e.g., atorvastatin). The risk of myopathy, including rhabdomyolysis may be increased when HIV protease inhibitors, including KALETRA, are used in combination with these drugs.

Concomitant use of KALETRA and St. John's wort (hypericum perforatum), or products containing St. John's wort, is not recommended. Co-administration of protease inhibitors, including KALETRA, with St. John's wort is expected to substantially decrease protease inhibitor concentrations and may result in sub-optimal levels of lopinavir and lead to loss of virologic response and possible resistance to lopinavir or to the class of protease inhibitors.

Pancreatitis

Pancreatitis has been observed in patients receiving KALETRA therapy, including those who developed marked triglyceride elevations. In some cases, fatalities have been observed. Although a causal relationship to KALETRA has not been established, marked triglyceride elevations is a risk factor for development of pancreatitis (see **PRECAUTIONS — Lipid Elevations**). Patients with advanced HIV disease may be at increased risk of elevated triglycerides and pancreatitis, and patients with a history of pancreatitis may be at increased risk for recurrence during KALETRA therapy.

Pancreatitis should be considered if clinical symptoms (nausea, vomiting, abdominal pain) or abnormalities in laboratory values (such as increased serum lipase or amylase values) suggestive of pancreatitis should occur. Patients who exhibit these signs or symptoms should be evaluated and KALETRA and/or other antiretroviral therapy should be suspended as clinically appropriate.

Diabetes Mellitus/Hyperglycemia

New onset diabetes mellitus, exacerbation of pre-existing diabetes mellitus, and hyperglycemia have been reported during postmarketing surveillance in HIV-infected patients receiving protease inhibitor therapy. Some patients required either initiation or dose adjustments of insulin or oral hypoglycemic agents for treatment of these events. In some cases, diabetic ketoacidosis has occurred. In those patients who discontinued protease inhibitor therapy, hyperglycemia persisted in some cases. Because these events have been reported voluntarily during clinical practice, estimates of frequency cannot be made and a causal relationship between protease inhibitor therapy and these events has not been established.

PRECAUTIONS

Hepatic Impairment and Toxicity

KALETRA is principally metabolized by the liver; therefore, caution should be exercised when administering this drug to patients with hepatic impairment, because lopinavir concentrations may be increased. Patients with underlying hepatitis B or C or marked elevations in transaminases prior to treatment may be at increased risk for developing further transaminase elevations or hepatic decompensation. There have been postmarketing reports of hepatic dysfunction, including some fatalities. These have generally occurred in patients with advanced HIV disease taking multiple concomitant medications in the setting of underlying chronic hepatitis or cirrhosis. A causal relationship with KALETRA therapy has not been established. Increased AST/ALT monitoring should be considered in these patients, especially during the first several months of KALETRA treatment.

Resistance/Cross-resistance

Various degrees of cross-resistance among protease inhibitors have been observed. The effect of KALETRA therapy on the efficacy of subsequently administered protease inhibitors is under investigation (see **MICROBIOLOGY**).

Hemophilia

There have been reports of increased bleeding, including spontaneous skin hematomas and hemarthrosis, in patients with hemophilia type A and B treated with protease inhibitors. In some patients additional factor VIII was given. In more than half of the reported cases, treatment with protease inhibitors was continued or reintroduced. A causal relationship between protease inhibitor therapy and these events has not been established.

Fat Redistribution

Redistribution/accumulation of body fat including central obesity, dorsocervical fat enlargement (buffalo hump), peripheral wasting, facial wasting, breast enlargement, and "cushingoid appearance" have been observed in patients receiving antiretroviral therapy. The mechanism and long-term consequences of these events are currently unknown. A causal relationship has not been established.

Lipid Elevations

Treatment with KALETRA has resulted in large increases in the concentration of total cholesterol and triglycerides

Continued on next page

Table 8: Drugs That Should Not Be Co-administered With KALETRA

Drug Class: Drug Name	Clinical Comment
Antihistamines: astemizole, terfenadine	CONTRAINDICATED due to potential for serious and/or life-threatening reactions such as cardiac arrhythmias.
Antimycobacterial: rifampin	May lead to loss of virologic response and possible resistance to KALETRA or to the class of protease inhibitors or other co-administered antiretroviral agents (see Table 9 for further details).
Ergot Derivatives: dihydroergotamine, ergonovine, ergotamine, methylergonovine	CONTRAINDICATED due to potential for serious and/or life-threatening reactions such as acute ergot toxicity characterized by peripheral vasospasm and ischemia of the extremities and other tissues.
GI Motility Agent: cisapride	CONTRAINDICATED due to potential for serious and/or life-threatening reactions such as cardiac arrhythmias.
Herbal Products: St. John's wort (hypericum perforatum)	May lead to loss of virologic response and possible resistance to KALETRA or to the class of protease inhibitors.
HMG-CoA Reductase Inhibitors: lovastatin, simvastatin	Potential for serious reactions such as risk of myopathy including rhabdomyolysis.
Neuroleptic: pimozide	CONTRAINDICATED due to the potential for serious and/or life-threatening reactions such as cardiac arrhythmias.
Sedative/Hypnotics: midazolam, triazolam	CONTRAINDICATED due to potential for serious and/or life-threatening reactions such as prolonged or increased sedation or respiratory depression.

Table 9: Established and Other Potentially Significant Drug Interactions: Alteration in Dose or Regimen May Be Recommended Based on Drug Interaction Studies or Predicted Interaction (See CLINICAL PHARMACOLOGY for Magnitude of Interaction, Tables 2 and 3)

Concomitant Drug Class: Drug Name	Effect on Concentration of lopinavir or Concomitant Drug	Clinical Comment
	HIV-Antiviral Agents	
Non-nucleoside Reverse Transcriptase Inhibitors: efavirenz*, nevirapine*	↓ Lopinavir	A dose increase of KALETRA to 533/133 mg (4 capsules or 6.5 mL) twice daily taken with food is recommended when used in combination with efavirenz or nevirapine (see **DOSAGE AND ADMINISTRATION**). NOTE: Efavirenz and nevirapine induce the activity of CYP3A and thus have the potential to decrease plasma concentrations of other protease inhibitors when used in combination with KALETRA.
Non-nucleoside Reverse Transcriptase Inhibitor: delavirdine	↑ Lopinavir	Appropriate doses of the combination with respect to safety and efficacy have not been established.
Nucleoside Reverse Transcriptase Inhibitor: didanosine		It is recommended that didanosine be administered on an empty stomach; therefore, didanosine should be given one hour before or two hours after KALETRA (given with food).
HIV-Protease Inhibitor: amprenavir*	↑ Amprenavir (amprenavir 750 mg BID + KALETRA procudes ↑ AUC, similar C_{max} ↑ C_{min} relative to amprenavir 1200 mg BID ↓ Lopinavir	Increase KALETRA dose to 533/133 mg and decrease amprenavir dose to amprenavir 750 mg BID, when co-administered. (see **DOSAGE AND ADMINISTRATION**and **CLINICAL PHARMACOLOGY**: Tables 2 and 3). Appropriate doses of the combination of fosamprenavir and KALETRA have not been established.
HIV-Protease Inhibitor: indinavir*	↑ Indinavir (indinavir 600 mg BID + KALETRA produces similar AUC, ↓ C_{max}, ↑ C_{min} relative to indinavir 800 mg TID	Decrease indinavir dose to 600 mg BID, when co-administered with KALETRA 400/100 mg BID (see **CLINICAL PHARMACOLOGY**: Table 3).
HIV-Protease Inhibitor: nelfinavir*	↑ Nelfinavir (nelfinavir 1000 mg BID + KALETRA produces similar AUC, similar C_{max}, ↑ C_{min} relative to nelfinavir 1250 mg BID) ↑ M8 metabolite of nelfinavir ↓ Lopinavir	Increase KALETRA dose to 533/133 mg and decrease nelfinavir dose to 1000 mg BID, when co-administered. (see **DOSAGE AND ADMINISTRATION** and **CLINICAL PHARMACOLOGY**: Tables 2 and 3).

(Table continued on next page)

Kaletra—Cont.

(see **ADVERSE REACTIONS** — Table 11). Triglyceride and cholesterol testing should be performed prior to initiating KALETRA therapy and at periodic intervals during therapy. Lipid disorders should be managed as clinically appropriate. See **PRECAUTIONS Table 9: Established and Other Potentially Significant Drug Interactions** for additional information on potential drug interactions with KALETRA and HMG-CoA reductase inhibitors.

Information for Patients

A statement to patients and health care providers is included on the product's bottle label: **"ALERT: Find out about medicines that should NOT be taken with KALETRA."** A Patient Package Insert (PPI) for KALETRA is available for patient information.

Patients should be told that sustained decreases in plasma HIV RNA have been associated with a reduced risk of progression to AIDS and death. Patients should remain under the care of a physician while using KALETRA. Patients should be advised to take KALETRA and other concomitant antiretroviral therapy every day as prescribed. KALETRA must always be used in combination with other antiretroviral drugs. Patients should not alter the dose or discontinue therapy without consulting with their doctor. If a dose of KALETRA is missed patients should take the dose as soon as possible and then return to their normal schedule. However, if a dose is skipped the patient should not double the next dose.

Patients should be informed that KALETRA is not a cure for HIV infection and that they may continue to develop opportunistic infections and other complications associated with HIV disease. The long-term effects of KALETRA are unknown at this time. Patients should be told that there are currently no data demonstrating that therapy with KALETRA can reduce the risk of transmitting HIV to others through sexual contact.

KALETRA may interact with some drugs; therefore, patients should be advised to report to their doctor the use of any other prescription, non-prescription medication or herbal products, particularly St. John's wort.

Patients taking didanosine should take didanosine one hour before or two hours after KALETRA.

Patients receiving sildenafil should be advised that they may be at an increased risk of sildenafil-associated adverse events including hypotension, visual changes, and sustained erection, and should promptly report any symptoms to their doctor.

Patients receiving estrogen-based hormonal contraceptives should be instructed that additional or alternate contraceptive measures should be used during therapy with KALETRA.

KALETRA should be taken with food to enhance absorption.

Patients should be informed that redistribution or accumulation of body fat may occur in patients receiving antiretroviral therapy and that the cause and long term health effects of these conditions are not known at this time.

Drug Interactions

KALETRA is an inhibitor of CYP3A (cytochrome P450 3A) both *in vitro* and *in vivo*. Co-administration of KALETRA and drugs primarily metabolized by CYP3A (e.g., dihydropyridine calcium channel blockers, HMG-CoA reductase inhibitors, immunosuppressants and sildenafil) may result in increased plasma concentrations of the other drugs that could increase or prolong their therapeutic and adverse effects (see **Table 9: Established and Other Potentially Significant Drug Interactions**). Agents that are extensively metabolized by CYP3A and have high first pass metabolism appear to be the most susceptible to large increases in AUC (>3-fold) when co-administered with KALETRA.

KALETRA does not inhibit CYP2D6, CYP2C9, CYP2C19, CYP2E1, CYP2B6 or CYP1A2 at clinically relevant concentrations.

KALETRA has been shown *in vivo* to induce its own metabolism and to increase the biotransformation of some drugs metabolized by cytochrome P450 enzymes and by glucuronidation.

KALETRA is metabolized by CYP3A. Co-administration of KALETRA and drugs that induce CYP3A may decrease lopinavir plasma concentrations and reduce its therapeutic effect (see Table 9: **Established and Other Potentially Significant Drug Interactions**). Although not noted with concurrent ketoconazole, co-administration of KALETRA and other drugs that inhibit CYP3A may increase lopinavir plasma concentrations.

Drugs that are contraindicated and not recommended for co-administration with KALETRA are included in **Table 8: Drugs That Should Not Be Co-administered With KALETRA**. These recommendations are based on either drug interaction studies or predicted interactions due to the expected magnitude of interaction and potential for serious events or loss of efficacy.

[See table 8 at top of previous page]

[See table 9 on pages 487 through 489]

Other Drugs:

Drug interaction studies reveal no clinically significant interaction between KALETRA and desipramine (CYP2D6 probe), pravastatin, stavudine or lamivudine.

Based on known metabolic profiles, clinically significant drug interactions are not expected between KALETRA and fluvastatin, dapsone, trimethoprim/sulfamethoxazole, azithromycin, erythromycin, or fluconazole.

Zidovudine and Abacavir: KALETRA induces glucuronidation; therefore, KALETRA has the potential to reduce zidovudine and abacavir plasma concentrations. The clinical significance of this potential interaction is unknown.

Carcinogenesis, Mutagenesis and Impairment of Fertility

Long-term carcinogenicity studies of KALETRA in animal systems have not been completed.

Carcinogenicity studies in mice and rats have been carried out on ritonavir. In male mice, at levels of 50, 100 or 200 mg/kg/day, there was a dose dependent increase in the incidence of both adenomas and combined adenomas and carcinomas in the liver. Based on AUC measurements, the exposure at the high dose was approximately 4-fold for males that of the exposure in humans with the recommended therapeutic dose (400/100 mg KALETRA BID). There were no carcinogenic effects seen in females at the dosages tested. The exposure at the high dose was approximately 9-fold for the females that of the exposure in humans. In rats dosed at levels of 7, 15 or 30 mg/kg/day there were no carcinogenic effects. In this study, the exposure at the high dose was approximately 0.7-fold that of the exposure in humans with the 400/100 mg KALETRA BID regimen. Based on the exposures achieved in the animal studies, the significance of the observed effects is not known.

Table 9 *(cont.)*: Established and Other Potentially Significant Drug Interactions: Alteration in Dose or Regimen May Be Recommended Based on Drug Interaction Studies or Predicted Interaction (See CLINICAL PHARMACOLOGY for Magnitude of Interaction, Tables 2 and 3)

Concomitant Drug Class: Drug Name	Effect on Concentration of lopinavir or Concomitant Drug	Clinical Comment
	HIV-Antiviral Agents (cont.)	
HIV-Protease Inhibitor: saquinavir*	↑ Saquinavir (saquinavir 800 mg BID + KALETRA) produces ↑ AUC, ↑ C_{max}, ↑ C_{min} relative to saquinavir 1200 mg TID)	Decrease saquinavir dose to 800 mg BID, when co-administered with KALETRA 400/100 mg BID (see **CLINICAL PHARMACOLOGY**: Table 3).
HIV-Protease Inhibitor: ribonavir*	↑ Lopinavir	Appropriate doses of additional ritonavir in combination with KALETRA with respect to safety and efficacy have not been established.
	Other Agents	
Antiarrhythmics: amiodarone, bepridil, lidocaine (systemic), and quinidine	↑ Antiarrhythmics	Caution is warranted and therapeutic concentration monitoring is recommended for antiarrhythmics when co-administered with KALETRA, if available.
Anticoagulant: warfarin		Concentrations of warfarin may be affected. It is recommended that INR (international normalized ratio) be monitored.
Anticonvulsants: carbamazepine, phenobarbital, phenytoin	↓ Lopinavir	Use with caution. KALETRA may be less effective due to decreased lopinavir plasma concentrations in patients taking these agents concomitantly.
Anti-infective: clarithromycin	↑ Clarithromycin	For patients with renal impairment, the following dosage adjustments should be considered: •For patients with CL_{CR} 30 to 60 mL/min the dose of clarithromycin should be reduced by 50%. •For patients with CL_{CR} <30 mL/min the dose of clarithromycin should be decreased by 75%. No dose adjustment for patients with normal renal function is necessary.
Antifungals: ketoconazole*, itraconazole	↑ Ketoconazole ↑ Itraconazole	High doses of ketoconazole or itraconazole (>200 mg/day) are not recommended.
Antimycobacterial: rifabutin*	↑ Rifabutin and rifabutin metabolite	Dosage reduction of rifabutin by at least 75% of the usual dose of 300 mg/day is recommended (i.e., a maximum dose of 150 mg every other day or three times per week). Increased monitoring for adverse events is warranted in patients receiving the combination. Further dosage reduction of rifabutin may be necessary.
Antimycobacterial: Rifampin	↓ Lopinavir	May lead to loss of virologic response and possible resistance to KALETRA or to the class of protease inhibitors or other co-administered antiretroviral agents. A study evaluated combination of rifampin 600 mg QD, with KALETRA 800/200 mg BID or KALETRA 400/100 mg + ritonavir 300 mg BID. Pharmacokinetic and safety results from this study do not allow for a dose recommendation. Nine subjects (28%) experienced a ≥ grade 2 increase in ALT/AST, of which seven (21%) prematurely discontinued study per protocol. Based on the study design, it is not possible to determine whether the frequency or magnitude of the ALT/AST elevations observed is higher than what would be seen with rifampin alone. (see **CLINICAL PHARMACOLOGY** for magnitude of interaction, Table 2).
Antiparasitic: atovaquone	↓ Atovaquone	Clinical significance is unknown; however, increase in atovaquone doses may be needed.
Calcium Channel Blockers, Dihydropyridine: e.g, felodipine, nifedipine, nicardipine	↑ Dihydropyridine calcium channel blockers	Caution is warranted and clinical monitoring of patients is recommended.
Corticosteroid: Dexamethasone	↓ Lopinavir	Use with caution. KALETRA may be less effective due to decreased lopinavir plasma concentrations in patients taking these agents concomitantly.
Disulfiram/ metronidazole		KALETRA oral solution contains alcohol, which can produce disulfiram-like reactions when co-administered with disulfiram or other drugs that produce this reaction (e.g., metronidazole).

(Table continued on next page)

Table 9 *(cont.)*: Established and Other Potentially Significant Drug Interactions: Alteration in Dose or Regimen May Be Recommended Based on Drug Interaction Studies or Predicted Interaction (See CLINICAL PHARMACOLOGY for Magnitude of Interaction, Tables 2 and 3)

Concomitant Drug Class: Drug Name	Effect on Concentration of lopinavir or Concomitant Drug	Clinical Comment
	Other Agents (cont.)	
Erectile Dysfunction Agent: sidenafil	↑ Sidenafil	Use with caution at reduced doses of 25 mg every 48 hours with increased monitoring for adverse events.
HMG-CoA Reductase Inhibitors: atorvastatin*	↑ Atorvastatin	Use lowest possible dose of atorvastatin with careful monitoring, or consider other HMG-CoA reductase inhibitors such as pravastatin or fluvastatin in combination with KALETRA.
Immunosuppressants: cyclosporine, tacrolimus, rapamycin	↑ Immuno-suppressants	Therapeutic concentration monitoring is recommended for immunosuppressant agents when co-administered with KALETRA.
Nacrotic Analgesic: Methadone*	↓ Methadone	Dosage of methadone may need to be increased when co-administered with KALETRA.
Oral Contraceptive: ethinyl estradiol*	↓ Ethinyl estradiol	Alternative or additional contraceptive measures should be used when estrogen-based oral contraceptives and KALETRA are co-administered.

* See **CLINICAL PHARMACOLOGY** for Magnitude of Interaction, Tables 2 and 3

Table 10: Percentage of Patients with Selected Treatment-Emergent[1] Adverse Events of Moderate or Severe Intensity Reported in ≥ 2% of Adult Patients

	Study 863		Study 888		Other Studies	
	Antiretroviral-Naive Patients 48 Weeks		Protease Inhibitor-Experienced Patients 48 Weeks		Study 720 (72 Weeks)	Study 957[3] and Study 765[4] (48-72 Weeks)
	KALETRA 400/100 mg BID + d4T + 3TC (N=326)	Nelfinavir 750 mg TID + d4T + 3TC (N=327)	KALETRA 400/100 mg BID + NVP + NRTIs (N=148)	Investigator-selected protease inhibitor(s) + NVP + NRTIs (N=140)	KALETRA BID[2] + d4T + 3TC (N=84)	KALETRA BID + NNRTI + NRTIs (N=127)
Body as a Whole						
Abdominal Pain	4%	3%	2%	2%	5%	2%
Asthenia	4%	3%	3%	6%	7%	8%
Chills	0%	<1%	2%	0%	1%	0%
Fever	<1%	<1%	2%	1%	0%	2%
Headache	2%	2%	2%	3%	7%	2%
Digestive System						
Anorexia	1%	<1%	1%	3%	0%	0%
Diarrhea	16%	17%	7%	9%	24%	18%
Dyspepsia	2%	<1%	1%	1%	1%	0%
Dysphagia	0%	0%	2%	1%	1%	0%
Flatulence	2%	1%	1%	2%	1%	2%
Nausea	7%	5%	7%	16%	15%	4%
Vomiting	2%	2%	4%	12%	5%	2%
Nervous System						
Depression	1%	2%	1%	2%	0%	2%
Insomnia	2%	1%	0%	2%	2%	2%
Skin and Appendages						
Rash	1%	2%	2%	1%	4%	2%

[1] Includes adverse events of possible, probable or unknown relationship to study drug.
[2] Includes adverse event data from dose group I (400/100 mg BID only [N=16]) and dose group II (400/100 mg BID) [N=35]) and 400/200 mg BID [N=33]). Within dosing groups, moderate to severe nausea of probable/possible relationship to KALETRA occurred at a higher rate in the 400/200 mg dose arm compared to the 400/100 mg dose arm in group II.
[3] Includes adverse event data from patients receiving 400/100 mg BID (n=29) or 533/133 mg BID (n=28) for 48 weeks. Patients received KALETRA in combination with NRTIs and efavirenz.
[4] Includes adverse event data from patients receiving 400/100 mg BID (n=36) or 400/200 mg BID (n=34) for 72 weeks. Patients received KALETRA in combination with NRTIs and nevirapine.

However, neither lopinavir nor ritonavir was found to be mutagenic or clastogenic in a battery of *in vitro* and *in vivo* assays including the Ames bacterial reverse mutation assay using *S. typhimurium* and *E. coli*, the mouse lymphoma assay, the mouse micronucleus test and chromosomal aberration assays in human lymphocytes.

Lopinavir in combination with ritonavir at a 2:1 ratio produced no effects on fertility in male and female rats at levels of 10/5, 30/15 or 100/50 mg/kg/day. Based on AUC measurements, the exposures in rats at the high doses were approximately 0.7-fold for lopinavir and 1.8-fold for ritonavir of the exposures in humans at the recommended therapeutic dose (400/100 mg BID).

Pregnancy

Pregnancy Category C: No treatment-related malformations were observed when lopinavir in combination with ritonavir was administered to pregnant rats or rabbits. Embryonic and fetal developmental toxicities (early resorption, decreased fetal viability, decreased fetal body weight, increased incidence of skeletal variations and skeletal ossification delays) occurred in rats at a maternally toxic dosage (100/50 mg/kg/day). Based on AUC measurements, the drug exposures in rats at 100/50 mg/kg/day were approximately 0.7-fold for lopinavir and 1.8-fold for ritonavir for males and females that of the exposures in humans at the recommended therapeutic dose (400/100 mg BID). In a peri- and postnatal study in rats, a developmental toxicity (a decrease in survival in pups between birth and postnatal day 21) occurred at 40/20 mg/kg/day and greater.

No embryonic and fetal developmental toxicities were observed in rabbits at a maternally toxic dosage (80/40 mg/kg/day). Based on AUC measurements, the drug exposures in rabbits at 80/40 mg/kg/day were approximately 0.6-fold for lopinavir and 1.0-fold for ritonavir that of the exposures in humans at the recommended therapeutic dose (400/100 mg BID). There are, however, no adequate and well-controlled studies in pregnant women. KALETRA should be used during pregnancy only if the potential benefit justifies the potential risk to the fetus.

Antiretroviral Pregnancy Registry: To monitor maternal-fetal outcomes of pregnant women exposed to KALETRA, an Antiretroviral Pregnancy Registry has been established. Physicians are encouraged to register patients by calling 1-800-258-4263.

Nursing Mothers: The Centers for Disease Control and Prevention recommend that HIV-infected mothers not breast-feed their infants to avoid risking postnatal transmission of HIV. Studies in rats have demonstrated that lopinavir is secreted in milk. It is not known whether lopinavir is secreted in human milk. Because of both the potential for HIV transmission and the potential for serious adverse reactions in nursing infants, mothers should be instructed **not to breast-feed if they are receiving KALETRA.**

Geriatric Use

Clinical studies of KALETRA did not include sufficient numbers of subjects aged 65 and over to determine whether they respond differently from younger subjects. In general, appropriate caution should be exercised in the administration and monitoring of KALETRA in elderly patients reflecting the greater frequency of decreased hepatic, renal, or cardiac function, and of concomitant disease or other drug therapy.

Pediatric Use

The safety and pharmacokinetic profiles of KALETRA in pediatric patients below the age of 6 months have not been established. In HIV-infected patients age 6 months to 12 years, the adverse event profile seen during a clinical trial was similar to that for adult patients. The evaluation of the antiviral activity of KALETRA in pediatric patients in clinical trials is ongoing.

Study 940 is an ongoing open-label, multicenter trial evaluating the pharmacokinetic profile, tolerability, safety and efficacy of KALETRA oral solution containing lopinavir 80 mg/mL and ritonavir 20 mg/mL in 100 antiretroviral naive (44%) and experienced (56%) pediatric patients. All patients were non-nucleoside reverse transcriptase inhibitor naive. Patients were randomized to either 230 mg lopinavir/57.5 mg ritonavir per m^2 or 300 mg lopinavir/75 mg ritonavir per m^2. Naive patients also received lamivudine and stavudine. Experienced patients received nevirapine plus up to two nucleoside reverse transcriptase inhibitors. Safety, efficacy and pharmacokinetic profiles of the two dose regimens were assessed after three weeks of therapy in each patient. After analysis of these data, all patients were continued on the 300 mg lopinavir/75 mg ritonavir per m^2 dose. Patients had a mean age of 5 years (range 6 months to 12 years) with 14% less than 2 years. Mean baseline CD_4 cell count was 838 cells/mm^3 and mean baseline plasma HIV-1 RNA was 4.7 $\log_{10}$ copies/mL.

Through 48 weeks of therapy, the proportion of patients who achieved and sustained an HIV RNA < 400 copies/mL was 80% for antiretroviral naive patients and 71% for antiretroviral experienced patients. The mean increase from baseline in CD_4 cell count was 404 cells/mm^3 for antiretroviral naive and 284 cells/mm^3 for antiretroviral experienced patients treated through 48 weeks. At 48 weeks, two patients (2%) had prematurely discontinued the study. One antiretroviral naive patient prematurely discontinued secondary to an adverse event attributed to KALETRA, while one antiretroviral experienced patient prematurely discontinued secondary to an HIV-related event.

Dose selection for patients 6 months to 12 years of age was based on the following results. The 230/57.5 mg/m^2 BID regimen without nevirapine and the 300/75 mg/m^2 BID regimen with nevirapine provided lopinavir plasma concentrations similar to those obtained in adult patients receiving the 400/100 mg BID regimen (without nevirapine).

ADVERSE REACTIONS

Adults:

Treatment-Emergent Adverse Events: KALETRA has been studied in 701 patients as combination therapy in Phase I/II and Phase III clinical trials. The most common adverse event associated with KALETRA therapy was diarrhea, which was generally of mild to moderate severity. Rates of discontinuation of randomized therapy due to adverse events were 5.8% in KALETRA-treated and 4.9% in nelfinavir-treated patients in Study 863.

Drug related clinical adverse events of moderate or severe intensity in ≥ 2% of patients treated with combination ther-

Continued on next page

Kaletra—Cont.

apy for up to 48 weeks (Phase III) and for up to 72 weeks (Phase I/II) are presented in Table 10. For other information regarding observed or potentially serious adverse events, please see **WARNINGS** and **PRECAUTIONS**.

[See table 10 on previous page]

Treatment-emergent adverse events occurring in less than 2% of adult patients receiving KALETRA in all phase II/III clinical trials and considered at least possibly related or of unknown relationship to treatment with KALETRA and of at least moderate intensity are listed below by body system.

Body as a Whole: Abdomen enlarged, allergic reaction, back pain, chest pain, chest pain substernal, cyst, drug interaction, drug level increased, face edema, flu syndrome, hypertrophy, infection bacterial, malaise, and viral infection.

Cardiovascular System: Atrial fibrillation, deep vein thrombosis, hypertension, migraine, palpitation, thrombophlebitis, varicose vein, and vasculitis.

Digestive System: Cholangitis, cholecystitis, constipation, dry mouth, enteritis, enterocolitis, eructation, esophagitis, fecal incontinence, gastritis, gastroenteritis, hemorrhagic colitis, increased appetite, jaundice, mouth ulceration, pancreatitis, sialadenitis, stomatitis, and ulcerative stomatitis.

Endocrine System: Cushing's syndrome, diabetes mellitus, and hypothyroidism.

Hemic and Lymphatic System: Anemia, leukopenia, and lymphadenopathy.

Metabolic and Nutritional Disorders: Avitaminosis, dehydration, edema, glucose tolerance decreased, lactic acidosis, obesity, peripheral edema, weight gain, and weight loss.

Musculoskeletal System: Arthralgia, arthrosis and myalgia.

Nervous System: Abnormal dreams, agitation, amnesia, anxiety, apathy, ataxia, confusion, convulsion, dizziness, dyskinesia, emotional lability, encephalopathy, facial paralysis, hypertonia, libido decreased, neuropathy, paresthesia, peripheral neuritis, somnolence, thinking abnormal, and tremor.

Respiratory System: Asthma, bronchitis, dyspnea, lung edema, pharyngitis, rhinitis, and sinusitis.

Skin and Appendages: Acne, alopecia, dry skin, eczema, exfoliative dermatitis, furunculosis, maculopapular rash, nail disorder, pruritis, seborrhea, skin benign neoplasm, skin discoloration, skin ulcer, and sweating.

Special Senses: Abnormal vision, eye disorder, otitis media, taste perversion, and tinnitus.

Urogenital System: Abnormal ejaculation, gynecomastia, hypogonadism male, kidney calculus, and urine abnormality.

Post-Marketing Experience: The following adverse reactions have been reported during post-marketing use of KALETRA. Because these reactions are reported voluntarily from a population of unknown size, it is not possible to reliably estimate their frequency or establish a causal relationship to KALETRA exposure.

Body as a whole: Redistribution/accumulation of body fat has been reported (see **PRECAUTIONS, Fat Redistribution**).

Cardiovascular: Bradyarrhythmias.

Laboratory Abnormalities: The percentages of adult patients treated with combination therapy with Grade 3-4 laboratory abnormalities are presented in Table 11.

[See table 11 at right]

Pediatrics:

Treatment-Emergent Adverse Events: KALETRA has been studied in 100 pediatric patients 6 months to 12 years of age. The adverse event profile seen during a clinical trial was similar to that for adult patients.

Taste aversion, vomiting, and diarrhea were the most commonly reported drug related adverse events of any severity in pediatric patients treated with combination therapy including KALETRA for up to 48 weeks in Study 940. A total of 8 children experienced moderate or severe adverse events at least possibly related to KALETRA. Rash (reported in 3%) was the only drug-related clinical adverse event of moderate to severe intensity observed in ≥ 2% of children enrolled.

Laboratory Abnormalities: The percentages of pediatric patients treated with combination therapy including KALETRA with Grade 3-4 laboratory abnormalities are presented in Table 12.

Table 12: Grade 3-4 Laboratory Abnormalities Reported in ≥ 2% of Pediatric Patients

Variable	Limit[1]	KALETRA BID + RTIs (N=100)
Chemistry	High	
Sodium	>149 mEq/L	3%
Total bilirubin	≥3.0 × ULN	3%
SGOT/AST	>180 U/L	8%
SGPT/ALT	>215 U/L	7%
Total cholesterol	>300 mg/dL	3%
Amylase	>2.5 × ULN	7%[2]
Chemistry	Low	
Sodium	<130 mEq/L	3%
Hematology	Low	
Platelet Count	< 50 × 10^9/L	4%
Neutrophils	< 0.40 × 10^9/L	2%

[1] ULN = upper limit of the normal range.

[2] Subjects with Grade 3-4 amylase confirmed by elevations in pancreatic amylase.

Table 11: Grade 3-4 Laboratory Abnormalities Reported in ≥ 2% of Adult Patients

		Study 863		Study 888		Other Studies	
		Antiretroviral-Naive Patients 48 Weeks		Protease Inhibitor-Experienced Patients 48 Weeks		Study 720 (72 Weeks)	Study 957[3] and Study 765[4] (48-72 Weeks)
Variable	Limit[1]	KALETRA 400/100 mg BID + d4T + 3TC (N=326)	Nelfinavir 750 mg TID + d4T + 3TC (N=327)	KALETRA 400/100 mg BID + NVP + NRTIs (N=148)	Investigator-selected protease inhibitor(s) + NVP + NRTIs (N=140)	KALETRA BID[2] + d4T + 3TC (N=84)	KALETRA BID + NNRTI + NRTIs (N=127)
Chemistry	High						
Glucose	>250 mg/dL	2%	2%	1%	2%	2%	5%
Uric Acid	>12 mg/dL	2%	2%	0%	1%	4%	1%
Total Bilirubin	>3.48 mg/dL	<1%	0%	1%	3%	1%	0%
SGOT/AST	>180 U/L	2%	4%	5%	11%	10%	6%
SGPT/ALT	>215 U/L	4%	4%	6%	13%	8%	10%
GGT	>300 U/L	N/A	N/A	N/A	N/A	4%	28%
Total Cholesterol	>300 mg/dL	9%	5%	20%	21%	14%	33%
Triglycerides	>750 mg/dL	9%	1%	25%	21%	11%	32%
Amylase	>2 × ULN	3%	2%	4%	8%	5%	6%
Chemistry	Low						
Inorganic Phosphorus	<1.5 mg/dL	0%	0%	1%	0%	0%	2%
Hematology	Low						
Neutrophils	0.75 × 10^9/L	1%	3%	1%	2%	2%	4%

[1] ULN = upper limit of the normal range; N/A = Not Applicable.

[2] Includes clinical laboratory data from dose group I (400/100 mg BID only [N=16]) and dose group II (400/100 mg BID [N=35] and 400/200 mg BID [N=33]).

[3] Includes clinical laboratory data from patients receiving 400/100 mg BID (n=29) or 533/133 mg BID (n=28) for 48 weeks. Patients received KALETRA in combination with NRTIs and efavirenz.

[4] Includes clinical laboratory data from patients receiving 400/100 mg BID (n=36) or 400/200 mg BID (n=34) for 72 weeks. Patients received KALETRA in combination with NRTIs and nevirapine.

Weight (kg)	Dose (mg/kg)*	Volume of oral solution BID (80 mg lopinavir/ 20 mg ritonavir per mL)
Without nevirapine, efavirenz or amprenavir		
7 to <15 kg	12 mg/kg BID	
7 to 10 kg		1.25 mL
>10 to <15 kg		1.75 mL
15 to 40 kg	10 mg/kg BID	
15 to 20 kg		2.25 mL
>20 to 25 kg		2.75 mL
>25 to 30 kg		3.5 mL
>30 to 35 kg		4.0 mL
>35 to 40 kg		4.75 mL
>40 kg	Adult dose	5 mL (or 3 capsules)

*Dosing based on the lopinavir component of lopinavir/ritonavir solution (80 mg/20 mg per mL).

OVERDOSAGE

KALETRA oral solution contains 42.4% alcohol (v/v). Accidental ingestion of the product by a young child could result in significant alcohol-related toxicity and could approach the potential lethal dose of alcohol.

Human experience of acute overdosage with KALETRA is limited. Treatment of overdose with KALETRA should consist of general supportive measures including monitoring of vital signs and observation of the clinical status of the patient. There is no specific antidote for overdose with KALETRA. If indicated, elimination of unabsorbed drug should be achieved by emesis or gastric lavage. Administration of activated charcoal may also be used to aid in removal of unabsorbed drug. Since KALETRA is highly protein bound, dialysis is unlikely to be beneficial in significant removal of the drug.

DOSAGE AND ADMINISTRATION

Adults

The recommended dosage of KALETRA is 400/100 mg (3 capsules or 5.0 mL) twice daily taken with food.

Concomitant therapy: Efavirenz nevirapine, amprenavir or nelfinavir: A dose increase of KALETRA to 533/133 mg (4 capsules or 6.5 mL) twice daily taken with food is recommended when used in combination with efavirenz, nevirapine, amprenavir or nelfinavir (see **CLINICAL PHARMACOLOGY—Drug Interactions** and/or **PRECAUTIONS—**Table 9).

Pediatric Patients

In children 6 months to 12 years of age, the recommended dosage of KALETRA oral solution is 12/3 mg/kg for those 7 to <15 kg and 10/2.5 mg/kg for those 15 to 40 kg (approximately equivalent to 230/57.5 mg/m^2) twice daily taken with food, up to a maximum dose of 400/100 mg in children >40 kg (5.0 mL or 3 capsules) twice daily. **It is preferred that the prescriber calculate the appropriate milligram dose for each individual child ≤12 years old and determine the corresponding volume of solution or number of capsules.** However, as an alternative, the following table contains dosing guidelines for KALETRA oral solution based on body weight. When possible, dose should be administered using a calibrated dosing syringe.

[See second table above]

Note: Use adult dosage recommendation for children >12 years of age.

Concomitant therapy: Efavirenz, nevirapine or amprenavir: A dose increase of KALETRA oral solution to 13/3.25 mg/kg for those 7 to <15 kg and 11/2.75 mg/kg for those 15 to 45 kg (approximately equivalent to 300/75 mg/m^2) twice daily taken with food, up to a maximum dose of 533/133 mg in children >45 kg twice daily is recommended when used in combination with efavirenz, nevirapine amprenavir in children 6 months to 12 years of age. The following table contains dosing guidelines for KALETRA oral solution based on body weight, when used in combination with efavirenz, ne-

Weight (kg)	Dose (mg/kg)*	Volume of oral solution BID (80 mg lopinavir/ 20 mg ritonavir per mL)
With nevirapine, efavirenz or amprenavir		
7 to <15 kg	13 mg/kg BID	
7 to 10 kg		1.5 mL
>10 to <15 kg		2.0 mL
15 to 45 kg	11 mg/kg BID	
15 to 20 kg		2.5 mL
>20 to 25 kg		3.25 mL
>25 to 30 kg		4.0 mL
>30 to 35 kg		4.5 mL
>35 to 40 kg		5.0 mL (or 3 capsules)
>40 to 45 kg		5.75 mL
>45 kg	Adult dose	6.5 mL (or 4 capsules)

*Dosing based on the lopinavir component of lopinavir/ritonavir solution (80 mg/20 mg per mL).

virapine or amprenavir in children (see **CLINICAL PHARMACOLOGY-Drug Interactions** and/or **PRECAUTIONS-**Table 9).
[See table above]
Note: Use adult dosage recommendation for children >12 years of age.

HOW SUPPLIED

KALETRA (lopinavir/ritonavir) capsules are orange soft gelatin capsules imprinted with the corporate logo and the Abbo-Code PK. KALETRA is available as 133.3 mg lopinavir/33.3 mg ritonavir capsules in the following package sizes:
Bottles of 180 capsules each .... (**NDC** 0074-3959-77)
Recommended storage: Store KALETRA soft gelatin capsules at 36°F-46°F (2°C-8°C) until dispensed. Avoid exposure to excessive heat. For patient use, refrigerated KALETRA capsules remain stable until the expiration date printed on the label. If stored at room temperature up to 77°F (25°C), capsules should be used within 2 months.
KALETRA (lopinavir/ritonavir) oral solution is a light yellow to orange colored liquid supplied in amber-colored multiple-dose bottles containing 400 mg lopinavir/100 mg ritonavir per 5 mL (80 mg lopinavir/20 mg ritonavir per mL) packaged with a marked dosing cup in the following size:
160 mL bottle .... (**NDC** 0074-3956-46)
Recommended storage: Store KALETRA oral solution at 36°F-46°F (2°C-8°C) until dispensed. Avoid exposure to excessive heat. For patient use, refrigerated KALETRA oral solution remains stable until the expiration date printed on the label. If stored at room temperature up to 77°F (25°C), oral solution should be used within 2 months.
03-5341-R10-Rev. February, 2004
ABBOTT LABORATORIES
NORTH CHICAGO, IL 60064 U.S.A.
PRINTED IN U.S.A.

KALETRA®
(lopinavir/ritonavir) capsules
(lopinavir/ritonavir) oral solution

ALERT: Find out about medicines that should NOT be taken with KALETRA. Please also read the section "MEDICINES YOU SHOULD NOT TAKE WITH KALETRA."

Patient Information
KALETRA®
(kuh-LEE-tra)
Generic Name: lopinavir/ritonavir
(lop-IN-uh-veer/rit-ON-uh-veer)

Read this leaflet carefully before you start taking KALETRA. Also, read it each time you get your KALETRA prescription refilled, in case something has changed. This information does not take the place of talking with your doctor when you start this medicine and at check ups. Ask your doctor if you have any questions about KALETRA.
Before taking your medicine, make sure you have received the correct medicine. Compare the name above with the name on your bottle and the appearance of your medicine with the description provided below. Contact your pharmacist immediately if you believe dispensing error has occurred.

What is KALETRA and how does it work?
KALETRA is a combination of two medicines. They are lopinavir and ritonavir. KALETRA is a type of medicine called an HIV (human immunodeficiency virus) protease (PRO-tee-ase) inhibitor. KALETRA is always used in combination with other anti-HIV medicines to treat people with human immunodeficiency virus (HIV) infection. KALETRA is for adults and for children age 6 months and older.
HIV infection destroys CD_4 (T) cells, which are important to the immune system. After a large number of T cells are destroyed, acquired immune deficiency syndrome (AIDS) develops.
KALETRA blocks HIV protease, a chemical which is needed for HIV to multiply. KALETRA reduces the amount of HIV in your blood and increases the number of T cells. Reducing the amount of HIV in the blood reduces the chance of death or infections that happen when your immune system is weak (opportunistic infections).

Does KALETRA cure HIV or AIDS?
KALETRA does not cure HIV infection or AIDS. The long-term effects of KALETRA are not known at this time. People taking KALETRA may still get opportunistic infections or other conditions that happen with HIV infection. Some of these conditions are pneumonia, herpes virus infections, and *Mycobacterium avium* complex (MAC) infections.

Does KALETRA reduce the risk of passing HIV to others?
KALETRA does not reduce the risk of passing HIV to others through sexual contact or blood contamination. Continue to practice safe sex and do not use or share dirty needles.

How should I take KALETRA?
- You should stay under a doctor's care when taking KALETRA. Do not change your treatment or stop treatment without first talking with your doctor.
- You must take KALETRA every day exactly as your doctor prescribed it. The dose of KALETRA may be different for you than for other patients. Follow the directions from your doctor, exactly as written on the label.
- Dosing in adults (including children 12 years of age and older): The usual dose for adults is 3 capsules (400/100 mg) or 5.0 mL of the oral solution twice a day (morning and night), in combination with other anti-HIV medicines.
- Dosing in children from 6 months to 12 years of age: Children from 6 months to 12 years of age can also take KALETRA. The child's doctor will decide the right dose based on the child's weight.
- Take KALETRA with food to help it work better.
- Do not change your dose or stop taking KALETRA without first talking with your doctor.
- When your KALETRA supply starts to run low, get more from your doctor or pharmacy. This is very important because the amount of virus in your blood may increase if the medicine is stopped for even a short time. The virus may develop resistance to KALETRA and become harder to treat.
- Be sure to set up a schedule and follow it carefully.
- Only take medicine that has been prescribed specifically for you. Do not give KALETRA to others or take medicine prescribed for someone else.

What should I do if I miss a dose of KALETRA?
It is important that you do not miss any doses. If you miss a dose of KALETRA, take it as soon as possible and then take your next scheduled dose at its regular time. If it is almost time for your next dose, do not take the missed dose. Wait and take the next dose at the regular time. Do not double the next dose.

What happens if I take too much KALETRA?
If you suspect that you took more than the prescribed dose of this medicine, contact your local poison control center or emergency room immediately.
As with all prescription medicines, KALETRA should be kept out of the reach of young children. KALETRA liquid contains a large amount of alcohol. If a toddler or young child accidentally drinks more than the recommended dose of KALETRA, it could make him/her sick from too much alcohol. Contact your local poison control center or emergency room immediately if this happens.

Who should not take KALETRA?
Together with your doctor, you need to decide whether KALETRA is right for you.
- Do not take KALETRA if you are taking certain medicines. These could cause serious side effects that could cause death. Before you take KALETRA, you must tell your doctor about all the medicines you are taking or are planning to take. These include other prescription and non-prescription medicines and herbal supplements.

For more information about medicines you should not take with KALETRA, please read the section titled "MEDICINES YOU SHOULD NOT TAKE WITH KALETRA."
- Do not take KALETRA if you have an allergy to KALETRA or any of its ingredients, including ritonavir or lopinavir.

Can I take KALETRA with other medications?*
KALETRA may interact with other medicines, including those you take without a prescription. You must tell your doctor about all the medicines you are taking or planning to take before you take KALETRA.

MEDICINES YOU SHOULD NOT TAKE WITH KALETRA:
- Do not take the following medicines with KALETRA because they can cause serious problems or death if taken with KALETRA.
  — Dihydroergotamine, ergonovine, ergotamine and methylergonovine such as Cafergot®, Migranal®, D.H.E. 45®, Ergotrate Maleate, Methergine, and others
  — Halcion® (triazolam)
  — Hismanal® (astemizole)
  — Orap® (pimozide)
  — Propulsid® (cisapride)
  — Seldane® (terfenadine)
  — Versed® (midazolam)
- Do not take KALETRA with rifampin, also known as Rimactane®, Rifadin®, Rifater®, or Rifamate®. Rifampin may lower the amount of KALETRA in your blood and make it less effective.
- Do not take KALETRA with St. John's wort (hypericum perforatum), an herbal product sold as a dietary supplement, or products containing St. John's wort. Talk with your doctor if you are taking or planning to take St. John's wort. Taking St. John's wort may decrease KALETRA levels and lead to increased viral load and possible resistance to KALETRA or cross-resistance to other anti-HIV medicines.
- Do not take KALETRA with the cholesterol-lowering medicines Mevacor® (lovastatin) or Zocor® (simvastatin) because of possible serious reactions. There is also an increased risk of drug interactions between KALETRA and Lipitor® (atorvastatin); talk to your doctor before you take any of these cholesterol-reducing medicines with KALETRA.

Medicines that require dosage adjustments:
It is possible that your doctor may need to increase or decrease the dose of other medicines when you are also taking KALETRA. Remember to tell your doctor all medicines you are taking or plan to take.
Before you take Viagra® (sildenafil) with KALETRA, talk to your doctor about problems these two medicines can cause when taken together. You may get increased side effects of VIAGRA, such as low blood pressure, vision changes, and penis erection lasting more than 4 hours. If an erection lasts longer than 4 hours, get medical help right away to avoid permanent damage to your penis. Your doctor can explain these symptoms to you.
- If you are taking oral contraceptives ("the pill") to prevent pregnancy, you should use an additional or different type of contraception since KALETRA may reduce the effectiveness of oral contraceptives.
- Efavirenz (Sustiva™) nevirapine (Viramune®), Agenerase (amprenavir) and Viracept (nelfinavir) may lower the amount of KALETRA in your blood. Your doctor may increase your dose of KALETRA if you are also taking efavirenz, nevirapine, amprenavir or nelfinavir.
- If you are taking Mycobutin® (rifabutin), your doctor will lower the dose of Mycobutin.
- **A change in therapy should be considered if you are taking KALETRA with:**
  Phenobarbital
  Phenytoin (Dilantin® and others)
  Carbamazepine (Tegretol® and others)
  These medicines may lower the amount of KALETRA in your blood and make it less effective.
- **Other Special Considerations:**
  KALETRA oral solution contains alcohol. Talk with your doctor if you are taking or planning to take metronidazole or disulfiram. Severe nausea and vomiting can occur.
- **If you are taking both didanosine (Videx®) and KALETRA:**
  Didanosine (Videx®) should be taken one hour before or two hours after KALETRA.

What are the possible side effects of KALETRA?
- This list of side effects is **not** complete. If you have questions about side effects, ask your doctor, nurse, or pharmacist. You should report any new or continuing symptoms to your doctor right away. Your doctor may be able to help you manage these side effects.
- The most commonly reported side effects of moderate severity that are thought to be drug related are: abdominal pain, abnormal stools (bowel movements), diarrhea, feeling weak/tired, headache, and nausea. Children taking KALETRA may sometimes get a skin rash.
- Blood tests in patients taking KALETRA may show possible liver problems. People with liver disease such as Hepatitis B and Hepatitis C who take KALETRA may have worsening liver disease. Liver problems including death have occurred in patients taking KALETRA. In studies, it is unclear if KALETRA caused these liver problems because some patients had other illnesses or were taking other medicines.
- Some patients taking KALETRA can develop serious problems with their pancreas (pancreatitis), which may cause death. You have a higher chance of having pancreatitis if you have had it before. Tell your doctor if you have nausea, vomiting, or abdominal pain. These may be signs of pancreatitis.
- Some patients have large increases in triglycerides and cholesterol. The long-term chance of getting complications such as heart attacks or stroke due to increases in triglycerides and cholesterol caused by protease inhibitors is not known at this time.
- Diabetes and high blood sugar (hyperglycemia) occur in patients taking protease inhibitors such as KALETRA. Some patients had diabetes before starting protease inhibitors, others did not. Some patients need changes in their diabetes medicine. Others needed new diabetes medicine.
- Changes in body fat have been seen in some patients taking antiretroviral therapy. These changes may include increased amount of fat in the upper back and neck ("buffalo hump"), breast, and around the trunk. Loss of fat from the legs, arms and face may also happen. The cause and long term health effects of these conditions are not known at this time.
- Some patients with hemophilia have increased bleeding with protease inhibitors.

Continued on next page

Kaletra—Cont.

- There have been other side effects in patients taking KALETRA. However, these side effects may have been due to other medicines that patients were taking or to the illness itself. Some of these side effects can be serious.

What should I tell my doctor before taking KALETRA?

- *If you are pregnant or planning to become pregnant:* The effects of KALETRA on pregnant women or their unborn babies are not known.
- *If you are breast-feeding:* Do not breast-feed if you are taking KALETRA. You should not breast-feed if you have HIV. If you are a woman who has or will have a baby, talk with your doctor about the best way to feed your baby. You should be aware that if your baby does not already have HIV, there is a chance that HIV can be transmitted through breast-feeding.
- *If you have liver problems:* If you have liver problems or are infected with Hepatitis B or Hepatitis C, you should tell your doctor before taking KALETRA.
- *If you have diabetes:* Some people taking protease inhibitors develop new or more serious diabetes or high blood sugar. Tell your doctor if you have diabetes or an increase in thirst or frequent urination.
- *If you have hemophilia:* Patients taking KALETRA may have increased bleeding.

How do I store KALETRA?

- Keep KALETRA and all other medicines out of the reach of children.
- Refrigerated KALETRA capsules and oral solution remain stable until the expiration date printed on the label. If stored at room temperature up to 77°F (25°C), KALETRA capsules and oral solution should be used within 2 months.
- Avoid exposure to excessive heat.

Do not keep medicine that is out of date or that you no longer need. Be sure that if you throw any medicine away, it is out of the reach of children.

General advice about prescription medicines:

Talk to your doctor or other health care provider if you have any questions about this medicine or your condition. Medicines are sometimes prescribed for purposes other than those listed in a Patient Information Leaflet. If you have any concerns about this medicine, ask your doctor. Your doctor or pharmacist can give you information about this medicine that was written for health care professionals. Do not use this medicine for a condition for which it was not prescribed. Do not share this medicine with other people.

* The brands listed are trademarks of their respective owners and are not trademarks of Abbott Laboratories. The makers of these brands are not affiliated with and do not endorse Abbott Laboratories or its products.

03-5341-R10
Revised: February, 2004
ABBOTT LABORATORIES
NORTH CHICAGO, IL 60064 U.S.A.
PRINTED IN U.S.A.

Shown in Product Identification Guide, page 303

MAVIK® ℞
(Trandolapril Tablets)
Rx only

USE IN PREGNANCY
When used in pregnancy during the second and third trimesters, ACE inhibitors can cause injury and even death to the developing fetus. When pregnancy is detected, MAVIK® should be discontinued as soon as possible. See WARNINGS, Fetal/Neonatal Morbidity and Mortality.

DESCRIPTION

Trandolapril is the ethyl ester prodrug of a nonsulfhydryl angiotensin converting enzyme (ACE) inhibitor, trandolaprilat. Trandolapril is chemically described as (2S,3aR,7aS)-1-[(S)-N-[(S)-1-Carboxy-3-phenylpropyl]alanyl] hexahydro-2-indolinecarboxylic acid, 1-ethyl ester. Its empirical formula is $C_{24}H_{34}N_2O_5$ and its structural formula is

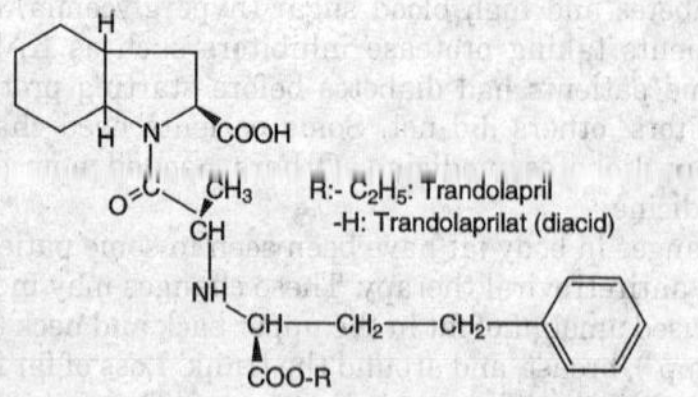

R:- C_2H_5: Trandolapril
-H: Trandolaprilat (diacid)

M.W.=430.54
Melting Point=125°C

Trandolapril is a colorless, crystalline substance that is soluble (>100 mg/mL) in chloroform, dichloromethane, and methanol. MAVIK tablets contain 1 mg, 2 mg, or 4 mg of trandolapril for oral administration. Each tablet also contains corn starch, croscarmellose sodium, hypromellose, iron oxide, lactose, povidone, sodium stearyl fumarate.

CLINICAL PHARMACOLOGY

Mechanism of Action:

Trandolapril is deesterified to the diacid metabolite, trandolaprilat, which is approximately eight times more active as an inhibitor of ACE activity. ACE is a peptidyl dipeptidase that catalyzes the conversion of angiotensin I to the vasoconstrictor, angiotensin II. Angiotensin II is a potent peripheral vasoconstrictor that also stimulates secretion of aldosterone by the adrenal cortex and provides negative feedback for renin secretion. The effect of trandolapril in hypertension appears to result primarily from the inhibition of circulating and tissue ACE activity thereby reducing angiotensin II formation, decreasing vasoconstriction, decreasing aldosterone secretion, and increasing plasma renin. Decreased aldosterone secretion leads to diuresis, natriuresis, and a small increase of serum potassium. In controlled clinical trials, treatment with MAVIK alone resulted in mean increases in potassium of 0.1 mEq/L. (See **PRECAUTIONS**.)

ACE is identical to kininase II, an enzyme that degrades bradykinin, a potent peptide vasodilator; whether increased levels of bradykinin play a role in the therapeutic effect of trandolapril remains to be elucidated.

While the principal mechanism of antihypertensive effect is thought to be through the renin-angiotensin-aldosterone system, trandolapril exerts antihypertensive actions even in patients with low-renin hypertension. MAVIK was an effective antihypertensive in all races studied. Both black patients (usually a predominantly low-renin group) and non-black patients responded to 2 to 4 mg of MAVIK.

Pharmacokinetics and Metabolism:

Pharmacokinetics—Trandolapril's ACE-inhibiting activity is primarily due to its diacid metabolite, trandolaprilat. Cleavage of the ester group of trandolapril, primarily in the liver, is responsible for conversion. Absolute bioavailability after oral administration of trandolapril is about 10% as trandolapril and 70% as trandolaprilat. After oral trandolapril under fasting conditions, peak trandolapril levels occur at about one hour and peak trandolaprilat levels occur between 4 and 10 hours. The elimination half lives of trandolapril and trandolaprilat are about 6 and 10 hours, respectively, but, like all ACE inhibitors, trandolaprilat also has a prolonged terminal elimination phase, involving a small fraction of administered drug, probably representing binding to plasma and tissue ACE. During multiple dosing of trandolapril, there is no significant accumulation of trandolaprilat. Food slows absorption of trandolapril, but does not affect AUC or C_{max} of trandolaprilat or C_{max} of trandolapril.

Metabolism and Excretion—After oral administration of trandolapril, about 33% of parent drug and metabolites are recovered in urine, mostly as trandolaprilat, with about 66% in feces. The extent of the absorbed dose which is biliary excreted has not been determined. Plasma concentrations (C_{max} and AUC of trandolapril and C_{max} trandolaprilat) are dose proportional over the 1–4 mg range, but the AUC of trandolaprilat is somewhat less than dose proportional. In addition to trandolaprilat, at least 7 other metabolites have been found, principally glucuronides or deesterification products.

Serum protein binding of trandolapril is about 80%, and is independent of concentration. Binding of trandolaprilat is concentration-dependent, varying from 65% at 1000 ng/mL to 94% at 0.1 ng/mL, indicating saturation of binding with increasing concentration.

The volume of distribution of trandolapril is about 18 liters. Total plasma clearances of trandolapril and trandolaprilat after approximately 2 mg IV doses are about 52 liters/hour and 7 liters/hour respectively. Renal clearance of trandolaprilat varies from 1–4 liters/hour, depending on dose.

Special populations:

Pediatric—Trandolapril pharmacokinetics have not been evaluated in patients <18 years of age.

Geriatric and Gender—Trandolapril pharmacokinetics have been investigated in the elderly (> 65 years) and in both genders. The plasma concentration of trandolapril is increased in elderly hypertensive patients, but the plasma concentration of trandolaprilat and inhibition of ACE activity are similar in elderly and young hypertensive patients. The pharmacokinetics of trandolapril and trandolaprilat and inhibition of ACE activity are similar in male and female elderly hypertensive patients.

Race—Pharmacokinetic differences have not been evaluated in different races.

Renal Insufficiency—Compared to normal subjects, the plasma concentrations of trandolapril and trandolaprilat are approximately 2-fold greater and renal clearance is reduced by about 85% in patients with creatinine clearance below 30 ml/min and in patients on hemodialysis. Dosage adjustment is recommended in renally impaired patients. (See **DOSAGE ADMINISTRATION**.)

Hepatic Insufficiency—Following oral administration in patients with mild to moderate alcoholic cirrhosis, plasma concentrations of trandolapril and trandolaprilat were, respectively, 9-fold and 2-fold greater than in normal subjects, but inhibition of ACE activity was not affected. Lower doses should be considered in patients with hepatic insufficiency. (See **DOSAGE AND ADMINISTRATION**.)

Drug Interactions—Trandolapril did not affect the plasma concentration (pre-dose and 2 hours post-dose) of oral digoxin (0.25 mg). Coadministration of trandolapril and cimetidine led to an increase of about 44% in C_{max} for trandolapril, but no difference in the pharmacokinetics of trandolaprilat or in ACE inhibition. Coadministration of trandolapril and furosemide led to an increase of about 25% in the renal clearance of trandolaprilat, but no effect was seen on the pharmacokinetics of furosemide or trandolaprilat or on ACE inhibition.

Pharmacodynamics and Clinical Effects:

A single 2-mg dose of MAVIK produces 70 to 85% inhibition of plasma ACE activity at 4 hours with about 10% decline at 24 hours and about half the effect manifest at 8 days. Maximum ACE inhibition is achieved with a plasma trandolaprilat concentration of 2 ng/mL. ACE inhibition is a function of trandolaprilat concentration, not trandolapril concentration. The effect of trandolapril on exogenous angiotensin I was not measured.

Hypertension:

Four placebo-controlled dose response studies were conducted using once-daily oral dosing of MAVIK in doses from 0.25 to 16 mg per day in 827 black and non-black patients with mild to moderate hypertension. The minimal effective once-daily dose was 1 mg in non-black patients and 2 mg in black patients. Further decreases in trough supine diastolic blood pressure were obtained in non-black patients with higher doses, and no further response was seen with doses above 4 mg (up to 16 mg). The antihypertensive effect diminished somewhat at the end of the dosing interval, but trough/peak ratios are well above 50% for all effective doses. There was a slightly greater effect on the diastolic pressure, but no difference on systolic pressure with b.i.d. dosing. During chronic therapy, the maximum reduction in blood pressure with any dose is achieved within one week. Following 6 weeks of monotherapy in placebo-controlled trials in patients with mild to moderate hypertension, once-daily doses of 2 to 4 mg lowered supine or standing systolic/diastolic blood pressure 24 hours after dosing by an average 7–10/4–5 mmHg below placebo responses in non-black patients. Once-daily doses of 2 to 4 mg lowered blood pressure 4–6/3–4 mmHg in black patients. Trough to peak ratios for effective doses ranged from 0.5 to 0.9. There were no differences in response between men and women, but responses were somewhat greater in patients under 60 than in patients over 60 years old. Abrupt withdrawal of MAVIK has not been associated with a rapid increase in blood pressure.

Administration of MAVIK to patients with mild to moderate hypertension results in a reduction of supine, sitting and standing blood pressure to about the same extent without compensatory tachycardia.

Symptomatic hypotension is infrequent, although it can occur in patients who are salt- and/or volume-depleted. (See **WARNINGS**.) Use of MAVIK in combination with thiazide diuretics gives a blood pressure lowering effect greater than that seen with either agent alone, and the additional effect of trandolapril is similar to the effect of monotherapy.

Heart Failure Post Myocardial Infarction or Left Ventricular Dysfunction Post Myocardial Infarction:

The Trandolapril Cardiac Evaluation (TRACE) Trial was a Danish, 27-center, double-blind, placebo controlled, parallel-group study of the effect of trandolapril on all-cause mortality in stable patients with echocardiographic evidence of left ventricular dysfunction 3 to 7 days after a myocardial infarction. Subjects with residual ischemia or overt heart failure were included. Patients tolerant of a test dose of 1 mg trandolapril were randomized to placebo (n=873) or trandolapril (n=876) and followed for 24 months. Among patients randomized to trandolapril, who began treatment on 1 mg, 62% were successfully titrated to a target dose of 4 mg once daily over a period of weeks. The use of trandolapril was associated with a 16% reduction in the risk of all-cause mortality (p=0.042), largely cardiovascular mortality. Trandolapril was also associated with a 20% reduction in the risk of progression of heart failure (p=0.047), defined by a time-to-first-event analysis of death attributed to heart failure, hospitalization for heart failure, or requirement for open-label ACE inhibitor for the treatment of heart failure. There was no significant effect of treatment on other endpoints: subsequent hospitalization, incidence of recurrent myocardial infarction, exercise tolerance, ventricular function, ventricular dimensions, or NYHA class.

The population in TRACE was entirely Caucasian and had less usage than would be typical in a U.S. population of other post-infarction interventions: 42% thrombolysis, 16% beta-adrenergic blockade, and 6.7% PTCA or CABG during the entire period of follow-up. Blood pressure control, especially in the placebo group, was poor: 47 to 53% of patients randomized to placebo and 32 to 40% of patients randomized to trandolapril had blood pressures >140/95 at 90-day follow-up visits.

INDICATIONS AND USAGE

Hypertension:

MAVIK is indicated for the treatment of hypertension. It may be used alone or in combination with other antihypertensive medication such as hydrochlorothiazide.

In considering the use of MAVIK, it should be noted that in controlled trials ACE inhibitors (for which adequate data are available) cause a higher rate of angioedema in black than in non-black patients. (See **Warnings: Angioedema**.)

When using MAVIK, consideration should be given to the fact that another angiotensin converting enzyme inhibitor, captopril, has caused agranulocytosis, particularly in patients with renal impairment or collagen-vascular disease. Available data are insufficient to show that MAVIK does not have a similar risk. (See **WARNINGS.**)

Heart Failure Post Myocardial Infarction or Left-Ventricular Dysfunction Post Myocardial Infarction:

MAVIK is indicated in stable patients who have evidence of left-ventricular systolic dysfunction (identified by wall motion abnormalities) or who are symptomatic from congestive heart failure within the first few days after sustaining acute myocardial infarction. Administration of trandolapril to Caucasian patients has been shown to decrease the risk of death (principally cardiovascular death) and to decrease the risk of heart failure-related hospitalization (See **CLINICAL PHARMACOLOGY, Heart Failure or Left-Ventricular Dysfunction Post Myocardial Infarction** for details of the survival trial.)

CONTRAINDICATIONS

MAVIK is contraindicated in patients who are hypersensitive to this product and in patients with a history of angioedema related to previous treatment with an ACE inhibitor.

WARNINGS

Anaphylactoid and Possibly Related Reactions:

Presumably because angiotensin converting enzyme inhibitors affect the metabolism of eicosanoids and polypeptides, including endogenous bradykinin, patients receiving ACE inhibitors, including MAVIK, may be subject to a variety of adverse reactions, some of them serious.

Anaphylactoid Reactions During Desensitization—Two patients undergoing desensitizing treatment with hymenoptera venom while receiving ACE inhibitors sustained life-threatening anaphylactoid reactions. In the same patients, these reactions did not occur when ACE inhibitors were temporarily withheld, but they reappeared when the ACE inhibitors were inadvertently readministered.

Anaphylactoid Reactions During Membrane Exposure—Anaphylactoid reactions have been reported in patients dialyzed with high-flux membranes and treated concomitantly with an ACE inhibitor. Anaphylactoid reactions have also been reported in patients undergoing low-density lipoprotein apheresis with dextran sulfate absorption.

Head and Neck Angioedema:

Angioedema of the face, extremities, lips, tongue, glottis, and larynx has been reported in patients treated with ACE inhibitors including MAVIK. Symptoms suggestive of angioedema or facial edema occurred in 0.13% of MAVIK-treated patients. Two of the four cases were life-threatening and resolved without treatment or with medication (corticosteroids). Angioedema associated with laryngeal edema can be fatal. If laryngeal stridor or angioedema of the face, tongue or glottis occurs, treatment with MAVIK should be discontinued immediately, the patient treated in accordance with accepted medical care and carefully observed until the swelling disappears. In instances where swelling is confined to the face and lips, the condition generally resolves without treatment; antihistamines may be useful in relieving symptoms. **Where there is involvement of the tongue, glottis, or larynx, likely to cause airway obstruction, emergency therapy, including but not limited to subcutaneous epinephrine solution 1:1,000 (0.3 to 0.5 mL) should be promptly administered.** (See **PRECAUTIONS: Information for Patients** and **ADVERSE REACTIONS.**)

Intestinal Angioedema: Intestinal angioedema has been reported in patients treated with ACE inhibitors. These patients presented with abdominal pain (with or without nausea or vomiting); in some cases there was no prior history of facial angioedema and C-1 esterase levels were normal. The angioedema was diagnosed by procedures including abdominal CT scan or ultrasound, or at surgery, and symptoms resolved after stopping the ACE inhibitor. Intestinal angioedema should be included in the differential diagnosis of patients on ACE inhibitors presenting with abdominal pain.

Hypotension:

MAVIK can cause symptomatic hypotension. Like other ACE inhibitors, MAVIK has only rarely been associated with symptomatic hypotension in uncomplicated hypertensive patients. Symptomatic hypotension is most likely to occur in patients who have been salt- or volume-depleted as a result of prolonged treatment with diuretics, dietary salt restriction, dialysis, diarrhea, or vomiting. Volume and/or salt depletion should be corrected before initiating treatment with MAVIK. (See **PRECAUTIONS: Drug Interactions,** and **ADVERSE REACTIONS.**) In controlled and uncontrolled studies, hypotension was reported as an adverse event in 0.6% of patients and led to discontinuations in 0.1% of patients.

In patients with concomitant congestive heart failure, with or without associated renal insufficiency, ACE inhibitor therapy may cause excessive hypotension, which may be associated with oliguria or azotemia, and rarely, with acute renal failure and death. In such patients, MAVIK therapy should be started at the recommended dose under close medical supervision. These patients should be followed closely during the first 2 weeks of treatment and, thereafter, whenever the dosage of MAVIK or diuretic is increased. (See **DOSAGE AND ADMINISTRATION.**) Care in avoiding hypotension should also be taken in patients with ischemic heart disease, aortic stenosis, or cerebrovascular disease.

If symptomatic hypotension occurs, the patient should be placed in the supine position and, if necessary, normal saline may be administered intravenously. A transient hypotensive response is not a contraindication to further doses; however, lower doses of MAVIK or reduced concomitant diuretic therapy should be considered.

Neutropenia/Agranulocytosis:

Another ACE inhibitor, captopril, has been shown to cause agranulocytosis and bone marrow depression rarely in patients with uncomplicated hypertension, but more frequently in patients with renal impairment, especially if they also have a collagen-vascular disease such as systemic lupus erythematosus or scleroderma. Available data from clinical trials of trandolapril are insufficient to show that trandolapril does not cause agranulocytosis at similar rates. As with other ACE inhibitors, periodic monitoring of white blood cell counts in patients with collagen-vascular disease and/or renal disease should be considered.

Hepatic Failure:

ACE inhibitors rarely have been associated with a syndrome of cholestatic jaundice, fulminant hepatic necrosis, and death. The mechanism of this syndrome is not understood. Patients receiving ACE inhibitors who develop jaundice should discontinue the ACE inhibitor and receive appropriate medical follow-up.

Fetal/Neonatal Morbidity and Mortality:

ACE inhibitors can cause fetal and neonatal morbidity and death when administered to pregnant women. Several dozen cases have been reported in the world literature. When pregnancy is detected, ACE inhibitors should be discontinued as soon as possible.

The use of ACE inhibitors during the second and third trimesters of pregnancy has been associated with fetal and neonatal injury, including hypotension, neonatal skull hypoplasia, anuria, reversible or irreversible renal failure, and death. Oligohydramnios has also been reported, presumably resulting from decreased fetal renal function; oligohydramnios in this setting has been associated with fetal limb contractures, craniofacial deformation, and hypoplastic lung development. Prematurity, intrauterine growth retardation, and patent ductus arteriosus have also been reported, although it is not clear whether these occurrences were due to the ACE inhibitor exposure.

These adverse effects do not appear to have resulted from intrauterine ACE-inhibitor exposure that has been limited to the first trimester. Mothers whose embryos and fetuses are exposed to ACE inhibitors only during the first trimester should be so informed. Nonetheless, when patients become pregnant, physicians should make every effort to discontinue the use of trandolapril as soon as possible.

Rarely (probably less often than once in every thousand pregnancies), no alternative to ACE inhibitors will be found. In these rare cases, the mothers should be apprised of the potential hazards to their fetuses, and serial ultrasound examinations should be performed to assess the intra-amniotic environment.

If oligohydramnios is observed, trandolapril should be discontinued unless it is considered life-saving for the mother. Contraction stress testing (CST), a non-stress test (NST), or biophysical profiling (BPP) may be appropriate, depending upon the week of pregnancy.

Patients and physicians should be aware, however, that oligohydramnios may not appear until after the fetus has sustained irreversible injury.

Infants with histories of *in utero* exposure to ACE inhibitors should be closely observed for hypotension, oliguria, and hyperkalemia. If oliguria occurs, attention should be directed toward support of blood pressure and renal perfusion. Exchange transfusions or dialysis may be required as a means of reversing hypotension and/or substituting for disordered renal function.

Doses of 0.8 mg/kg/day (9.4 mg/m^2/day) in rabbits, 1000 mg/kg/day (7000 mg/m^2/day) in rats, and 25 mg/kg/day (295 mg/m^2/day) in cynomolgus monkeys did not produce teratogenic effects. These doses represent 10 and 3 times (rabbits), 1250 and 2564 times (rats), and 312 and 108 times (monkeys) the maximum projected human dose of 4 mg based on body-weight and body-surface-area, respectively assuming a 50 kg woman.

PRECAUTIONS

General

Impaired Renal Function:

As a consequence of inhibiting the renin-angiotensin-aldosterone system, changes in renal function may be anticipated in susceptible individuals. In patients with severe heart failure whose renal function may depend on the activity of the renin-angiotensin-aldosterone system, treatment with ACE inhibitors, including MAVIK® (trandolapril), may be associated with oliguria and/or progressive azotemia and rarely with acute renal failure and/or death.

In hypertensive patients with unilateral or bilateral renal artery stenosis, increases in blood urea nitrogen and serum creatinine have been observed in some patients following ACE inhibitor therapy. These increases were almost always reversible upon discontinuation of the ACE inhibitor and/or diuretic therapy. In such patients, renal function should be monitored during the first few weeks of therapy.

Some hypertensive patients with no apparent preexisting renal vascular disease have developed increases in blood urea and serum creatinine, usually minor and transient, especially when ACE inhibitors have been given concomitantly with a diuretic. This is more likely to occur in patients with preexisting renal impairment. Dosage reduction and/or discontinuation of any diuretic and/or the ACE inhibitor may be required.

Evaluation of hypertensive patients should always include assessment of renal function. (See **DOSAGE AND ADMINISTRATION.**)

Hyperkalemia and potassium-sparing diuretics:

In clinical trials, hyperkalemia (serum potassium > 6.00 mEq/L) occurred in approximately 0.4% of hypertensive patients receiving MAVIK. In most cases, elevated serum potassium levels were isolated values, which resolved despite continued therapy. None of these patients were discontinued from the trials because of hyperkalemia. Risk factors for the development of hyperkalemia include renal insufficiency, diabetes mellitus, and the concomitant use of potassium-sparing diuretics, potassium supplements, and/or potassium-containing salt substitutes, which should be used cautiously, if at all, with MAVIK. (See **PRECAUTIONS: Drug Interactions.**)

Cough:

Presumably due to the inhibition of the degradation of endogenous bradykinin, persistent nonproductive cough has been reported with all ACE inhibitors, always resolving after discontinuation of therapy. ACE inhibitor-induced cough should be considered in the differential diagnosis of cough. In controlled trials of trandolapril, cough was present in 2% of trandolapril patients and 0% of patients given placebo. There was no evidence of a relationship to dose.

Surgery/anesthesia:

In patients undergoing major surgery or during anesthesia with agents that produce hypotension, MAVIK will block angiotensin II formation secondary to compensatory renin release. If hypotension occurs and is considered to be due to this mechanism, it can be corrected by volume expansion.

INFORMATION FOR PATIENTS

Angioedema:

Angioedema, including laryngeal edema, may occur at any time during treatment with ACE inhibitors, including MAVIK. Patients should be so advised and told to report immediately any signs or symptoms suggesting angioedema (swelling of face, extremities, eyes, lips, tongue, difficulty in swallowing or breathing) and to stop taking the drug until they have consulted with their physician. (See **WARNINGS** and **ADVERSE REACTIONS.**)

Symptomatic Hypotension:

Patients should be cautioned that light-headedness can occur, especially during the first days of MAVIK therapy, and should be reported to a physician. If actual syncope occurs, patients should be told to stop taking the drug until they have consulted with their physician (See **WARNINGS.**)

All patients should be cautioned that inadequate fluid intake, excessive perspiration, diarrhea, or vomiting, resulting in reduced fluid volume, may precipitate an excessive fall in blood pressure with the same consequences of light-headedness and possible syncope.

Patients planning to undergo any surgery and/or anesthesia should be told to inform their physician that they are taking an ACE inhibitor that has a long duration of action.

Hyperkalemia:

Patients should be told not to use potassium supplements or salt substitutes containing potassium without consulting their physician. (See **PRECAUTIONS.**)

Neutropenia:

Patients should be told to report promptly any indication of infection (e.g., sore throat, fever) which could be a sign of neutropenia.

Pregnancy:

Female patients of childbearing age should be told about the consequences of second- and third-trimester exposure to ACE inhibitors, and they should also be told that these consequences do not appear to have resulted from intrauterine ACE-inhibitor exposure that has been limited to the first trimester. These patients should be asked to report pregnancies to their physicians as soon as possible.

NOTE: As with many other drugs, certain advice to patients being treated with MAVIK is warranted. This information is intended to aid in the safe and effective use of this medication. It is not a disclosure of all possible adverse or intended effects.

DRUG INTERACTIONS

Concomitant diuretic therapy:

As with other ACE inhibitors, patients on diuretics, especially those on recently instituted diuretic therapy, may experience an excessive reduction of blood pressure after initiation of therapy with MAVIK. The possibility of exacerbation of hypotensive effects with MAVIK may be minimized by either discontinuing the diuretic or cautiously increasing salt intake prior to initiation of treatment with MAVIK. If it is not possible to discontinue the diuretic, the starting dose of trandolapril should be reduced. (See **DOSAGE AND ADMINISTRATION.**)

Agents increasing serum potassium:

Trandolapril can attenuate potassium loss caused by thiazide diuretics and increase serum potassium when used alone. Use of potassium-sparing diuretics (spironolactone, triamterene, or amiloride), potassium supplements, or potassium-containing salt substitutes concomitantly with ACE inhibitors can increase the risk of hyperkalemia. If concomitant use of such agents is indicated, they should be used with caution and with appropriate monitoring of serum potassium. (See **PRECAUTIONS.**)

Lithium:

Increased serum lithium levels and symptoms of lithium toxicity have been reported in patients receiving concomitant lithium and ACE inhibitor therapy. These drugs should

Continued on next page

Mavik—Cont.

be coadministered with caution, and frequent monitoring of serum lithium levels is recommended. If a diuretic is also used, the risk of lithium toxicity may be increased.

Other:
No clinically significant interaction has been found between trandolaprilat and food, cimetidine, digoxin, or furosemide. The anticoagulant effect of warfarin was not significantly changed by trandolapril.

Carcinogenesis, Mutagenesis, Impairment of Fertility:
Long-term studies were conducted with oral trandolapril administered by gavage to mice (78 weeks) and rats (104 and 106 weeks). No evidence of carcinogenic potential was seen in mice dosed up to 25 mg/kg/day (85 mg/m^2/day) or rats dosed up to 8 mg/kg/day (60 mg/m^2/day). These doses are 313 and 32 times (mice), and 100 and 23 times (rats) the maximum recommended human daily dose (MRHDD) of 4 mg based on body-weight and body-surface-area, respectively assuming a 50 kg individual. The genotoxic potential of trandolapril was evaluated in the microbial mutagenicity (Ames) test, the point mutation and chromosome aberration assays in Chinese hamster V79 cells, and the micronucleus test in mice. There was no evidence of mutagenic or clastogenic potential in these *in vitro* and *in vivo* assays.

Reproduction studies in rats did not show any impairment of fertility at doses up to 100 mg/kg/day (710 mg/m^2/day) of trandolapril, or 1250 and 260 times the MRHDD on the basis of body-weight and body-surface-area, respectively.

Pregnancy
Pregnancy Categories C (first trimester) and D (second and third trimesters): (See WARNINGS, Fetal/Neonatal Morbidity and Mortality.)

Nursing Mothers:
Radiolabeled trandolapril or its metabolites are secreted in rat milk. MAVIK should not be administered to nursing mothers.

Geriatric Use:
In placebo-controlled studies of MAVIK, 31.1% of patients were 60 years and older, 20.1% were 65 years and older, and 2.3% were 75 years and older. No overall differences in effectiveness or safety were observed between these patients and younger patients. (Greater sensitivity of some older individual patients cannot be ruled out).

Pediatric Use:
The safety and effectiveness of MAVIK in pediatric patients have not been established.

ADVERSE REACTIONS

The safety experience in U.S. placebo-controlled trials included 1067 hypertensive patients, of whom 831 received MAVIK. Nearly 200 hypertensive patients received MAVIK for over one year in open-label trials. In controlled trials, withdrawals for adverse events were 2.1% on placebo and 1.4% on MAVIK. Adverse events considered at least possibly related to treatment occurring in 1% of MAVIK-treated patients and more common on MAVIK than placebo, pooled for all doses, are shown below, together with the frequency of discontinuation of treatment because of these events.

ADVERSE EVENTS IN PLACEBO-CONTROLLED HYPERTENSION TRIALS
Occurring at 1% or greater

	MAVIK (N=832) % Incidence (% Discontinuance)	PLACEBO (N=237) % Incidence (% Discontinuance)
Cough	1.9 (0.1)	0.4 (0.4)
Dizziness	1.3 (0.2)	0.4 (0.4)
Diarrhea	1.0 (0.0)	0.4 (0.0)

Headache and fatigue were all seen in more than 1% of MAVIK-treated patients but were more frequently seen on placebo. Adverse events were not usually persistent or difficult to manage.

Left Ventricular Dysfunction Post Myocardial Infarction:
Adverse reactions related to MAVIK occurring at a rate greater than that observed in placebo-treated patients with left ventricular dysfunction, are shown below. The incidences represent the experiences from the TRACE study. The follow-up time was between 24 and 50 months for this study.

Percentage of Patients with Adverse Events Greater Than Placebo Placebo-Controlled (TRACE) Mortality Study

Adverse Event	Trandolapril N=876	Placebo N=873
Cough	35	22
Dizziness	23	17
Hypotension	11	6.8
Elevated serum uric acid	15	13
Elevated BUN	9.0	7.6
PICA or CABG	7.3	6.1
Dyspepsia	6.4	6.0
Syncope	5.9	3.3
Hyperkalemia	5.3	2.8
Bradycardia	4.7	4.4
Hypocalcemia	4.7	3.9
Myalgia	4.7	3.1
Elevated creatinine	4.7	2.4
Gastritis	4.2	3.6
Cardiogenic shock	3.8	<2
Intermittent claudication	3.8	<2
Stroke	3.3	3.2
Asthenia	3.3	2.6

Clinical adverse experiences possibly or probably related or of uncertain relationship to therapy occurring in 0.3% to 1.0% (except as noted) of the patients treated with MAVIK (with or without concomitant calcium ion antagonist or diuretic) in controlled or uncontrolled trials (N=1134) and less frequent, clinically significant events seen in clinical trials or post-marketing experience (the rarer events are in italics) include (listed by body system):

General Body Function: chest pain.
Cardiovascular: AV first degree block, bradycardia, edema, flushing, hypotension, palpitations.
Central Nervous System: drowsiness, insomnia, paresthesia, vertigo.
Dermatologic: pruritus, rash, pemphigus.
Eye, Ear, Nose, Throat: epistaxis, throat inflammation, upper respiratory tract infection.
Emotional, Mental, Sexual States: anxiety, impotence, decreased libido.
Gastrointestinal: abdominal distention, abdominal pain/cramps, constipation, dyspepsia, diarrhea, vomiting, *pancreatitis.*
Hemopoietic: *decreased leukocytes, decreased neutrophils.*
Metabolism and Endocrine: *increased creatinine, increased potassium*, increased SGPT (ALT).
Musculoskeletal System: extremity pain, muscle cramps, gout.
Pulmonary: dyspnea.
Angioedema: Angioedema has been reported in 4 (0.13%) patients receiving MAVIK in U.S. and foreign studies. Angioedema associated with laryngeal edema may be fatal. If angioedema of the face, extremities, lips, tongue, glottis, and/or larynx occurs, treatment with MAVIK should be discontinued and appropriate therapy instituted immediately. (See **WARNINGS.**)
Hypotension: In hypertensive patients, symptomatic hypotension occurred in 0.6% and near syncope occurred in 0.2%. Hypotension or syncope was a cause for discontinuation of therapy in 0.1% of hypertensive patients.
Fetal/Neonatal Morbidity and Mortality: (See **WARNINGS, Fetal Neonatal Morbidity and Mortality.**)
Cough: (See **PRECAUTIONS, Cough.**)

Clinical Laboratory Test Findings

Hematology: (See **WARNINGS.**) Low white blood cells, low neutrophils, low lymphocytes, thrombocytopenia.
Serum Electrolytes: Hyperkalemia (See **PRECAUTIONS,**) hyponatremia.
Creatinine and Blood Urea Nitrogen: Increases in creatinine levels occurred in 1.1% of patients receiving MAVIK alone and 7.3% of patients treated with MAVIK, a calcium ion antagonist and a diuretic. Increases in blood urea nitrogen levels occurred in 0.6% of patients receiving MAVIK alone and 1.4% of patients receiving MAVIK, a calcium ion antagonist, and a diuretic. None of these increases required discontinuation of treatment. Increases in these laboratory values are more likely to occur in patients with renal insufficiency or those pretreated with a diuretic and, based on experience with other ACE inhibitors, would be expected to be especially likely in patients with renal artery stenosis. (See **PRECAUTIONS** and **WARNINGS.**)
Liver Function Tests: Occasional elevation of transaminases at the rate of 3X upper normals occurred in 0.8% of patients and persistent increase in bilirubin occurred in 0.2% of patients. Discontinuation for elevated liver enzymes occurred in 0.2% of patients.
Other: Another potentially important adverse experience, eosinophilic pneumonitis, has been attributed to other ACE inhibitors.

OVERDOSAGE

No data are available with respect to overdosage in humans. The oral LD_{50} of trandolapril in mice was 4875 mg/Kg in males and 3990 mg/Kg in females. In rats, an oral dose of 5000 mg/Kg caused low mortality (1 male out of 5; 0 females). In dogs, an oral dose of 1000 mg/Kg did not cause mortality and abnormal clinical signs were not observed. In humans the most likely clinical manifestation would be symptoms attributable to severe hypotension.

Laboratory determinations of serum levels of trandolapril and its metabolites are not widely available, and such determinations have, in any event, no established role in the management of trandolapril overdose. No data are available to suggest that physiological maneuvers (e.g., maneuvers to change the pH of the urine) might accelerate elimination of trandolapril and its metabolites. Trandolaprilat is removed by hemodialysis. Angiotensin II could presumably serve as a specific antagonist antidote in the setting of trandolapril overdose, but angiotensin II is essentially unavailable outside of scattered research facilities. Because the hypotensive effect of trandolapril is achieved through vasodilation and effective hypovolemia, it is reasonable to treat trandolapril overdose by infusion of normal saline solution.

DOSAGE AND ADMINISTRATION

Hypertension:
The recommended initial dosage of MAVIK for patients not receiving a diuretic is 1 mg once daily in non-black patients and 2 mg in black patients. Dosage should be adjusted according to the blood pressure response. Generally, dosage adjustments should be made at intervals of at least 1 week. Most patients have required dosages of 2 to 4 mg once daily. There is little clinical experience with doses above 8 mg.

Patients inadequately treated with once-daily dosing at 4 mg may be treated with twice-daily dosing. If blood pressure is not adequately controlled with MAVIK monotherapy, a diuretic may be added.

In patients who are currently being treated with a diuretic, symptomatic hypotension occasionally can occur following the initial dose of MAVIK. To reduce the likelihood of hypotension, the diuretic should, if possible, be discontinued two to three days prior to beginning therapy with MAVIK®. (See **WARNINGS.**) Then, if blood pressure is not controlled with MAVIK alone, diuretic therapy should be resumed. If the diuretic cannot be discontinued, an initial dose of 0.5 mg MAVIK should be used with careful medical supervision for several hours until blood pressure has stabilized. The dosage should subsequently be titrated (as described above) to the optimal response. (See **WARNINGS, PRECAUTIONS,** and **DRUG INTERACTIONS.**)

Concomitant administration of MAVIK with potassium supplements, potassium salt substitutes, or potassium sparing diuretics can lead to increases of serum potassium. (See **PRECAUTIONS.**)

Heart Failure Post Myocardial Infarction or Left-Ventricular Dysfunction Post Myocardial Infarction:
The recommended starting dose is 1 mg, once daily. Following the initial dose, all patients should be titrated (as tolerated) toward a target dose of 4 mg, once daily. If a 4 mg dose is not tolerated, patients can continue therapy with the greatest tolerated dose.

Dosage Adjustment in Renal Impairment or Hepatic Cirrhosis:
For patients with a creatinine clearance <30 mL/min. or with hepatic cirrhosis, the recommended starting dose, based on clinical and pharmacokinetic data, is 0.5 mg daily. Patients should subsequently have their dosage titrated (as described above) to the optimal response.

HOW SUPPLIED

MAVIK® (trandolapril tablets) are supplied as follows:

1 mg tablet – salmon colored, round shaped, scored, compressed tablets, with ᗡ on one side and Abbo-Code identification letters FT on the other side.
NDC 0074-2278-13 - bottles of 100
NDC 0074-2278-11 - unit dose packs of 100

2 mg tablet – yellow colored, round shaped, compressed tablets with ᗡ on one side and Abbo-Code identification letters FX on the other side.
NDC 0074-2279-13 - bottles of 100
NDC 0074-2279-11 - unit dose packs of 100

4 mg tablet – rose colored, round shaped, compressed tablets, with ᗡ on one side and Abbo-Code identification letters FZ on the other side.
NDC 0074-2280-13 - bottles of 100
NDC 0074-2280-11 - unit dose packs of 100

Dispense in well-closed container with safety closure.

Storage: Store at controlled room temperature: 20–25°C (68–77°F) see USP.

Revised: July, 2003
Ref.: 03-5264-R2
Abbott Laboratories
North Chicago, IL 60064, U.S.A. PRINTED IN U.S.A.

Shown in Product Identification Guide, page 303

MERIDIA® Ⓒ℞

(sibutramine hydrochloride monohydrate)
Capsules
℞ only

DESCRIPTION

MERIDIA® (sibutramine hydrochloride monohydrate) is an orally administered agent for the treatment of obesity. Chemically, the active ingredient is a racemic mixture of the (+) and (-) enantiomers of cyclobutanemethanamine, 1-(4-chlorophenyl)-*N,N*-dimethyl-α-(2-methylpropyl)-, hydrochloride, monohydrate, and has an empirical formula of $C_{17}H_{29}Cl_2NO$. Its molecular weight is 334.33.

The structural formula is shown below:

Sibutramine hydrochloride monohydrate is a white to cream crystalline powder with a solubility of 2.9 mg/mL in pH 5.2 water. Its octanol:water partition coefficient is 30.9 at pH 5.0.

Each MERIDIA capsule contains 5 mg, 10 mg, and 15 mg of sibutramine hydrochloride monohydrate. It also contains as inactive ingredients: lactose monohydrate, NF; microcrystalline cellulose, NF; colloidal silicon dioxide, NF; and magnesium stearate, NF in a hard-gelatin capsule [which contains titanium dioxide, USP; gelatin; FD&C Blue No. 2 (5- and 10-mg capsules only); D&C Yellow No. 10 (5- and 15-mg capsules only), and other inactive ingredients].

CLINICAL PHARMACOLOGY

Mode of Action
Sibutramine produces its therapeutic effects by norepinephrine, serotonin and dopamine reuptake inhibition.

Sibutramine and its major pharmacologically active metabolites (M_1 and M_2) do not act via release of monoamines.

Pharmacodynamics

Sibutramine exerts its pharmacological actions predominantly via its secondary (M_1) and primary (M_2) amine metabolites. The parent compound, sibutramine, is a potent inhibitor of serotonin (5-hydroxytryptamine, 5-HT) and norepinephrine reuptake *in vivo*, but not *in vitro*. However, metabolites M_1 and M_2 inhibit the reuptake of these neurotransmitters both *in vitro* and *in vivo*.

In human brain tissue, M_1 and M_2 also inhibit dopamine reuptake *in vitro*, but with ~3-fold lower potency than for the reuptake inhibition of serotonin or norepinephrine.

Potencies of Sibutramine, M_1 and M_2 as *In Vitro* Inhibitors of Monoamine Reuptake in Human Brain

Potency to Inhibit Monoamine Reuptake (K_i;nM)

	Serotonin	Norepinephrine	Dopamine
Sibutramine	298	5451	943
M_1	15	20	49
M_2	20	15	45

A study using plasma samples taken from sibutramine-treated volunteers showed monoamine reuptake inhibition of norepinephrine > serotonin > dopamine; maximum inhibitions were norepinephrine = 73%, serotonin = 54% and dopamine = 16%.

Sibutramine and its metabolites (M_1 and M_2) are not serotonin, norepinephrine or dopamine releasing agents. Following chronic administration of sibutramine to rats, no depletion of brain monoamines has been observed.

Sibutramine, M_1 and M_2 exhibit no evidence of anticholinergic or antihistaminergic actions. In addition, receptor binding profiles show that sibutramine, M_1 and M_2 have low affinity for serotonin ($5\text{-}HT_1$, $5\text{-}HT_{1A}$, $5\text{-}HT_{1B}$, $5\text{-}HT_{2A}$, $5\text{-}HT_{2C}$), norepinephrine (β, β_1, β_3, α_1 and α_2), dopamine (D_1 and D_2), benzodiazepine, and glutamate (NMDA) receptors. These compounds also lack monoamine oxidase inhibitory activity *in vitro* and *in vivo*.

Pharmacokinetics

Absorption

Sibutramine is rapidly absorbed from the GI tract (T_{max} of 1.2 hours) following oral administration and undergoes extensive first-pass metabolism in the liver (oral clearance of 1750 L/h and half-life of 1.1 h) to form the pharmacologically active mono- and di-desmethyl metabolites M_1 and M_2. Peak plasma concentrations of M_1 and M_2 are reached within 3 to 4 hours. On the basis of mass balance studies, on average, at least 77% of a single oral dose of sibutramine is absorbed. The absolute bioavailability of sibutramine has not been determined.

Distribution

Radiolabeled studies in animals indicated rapid and extensive distribution into tissues: highest concentrations of radiolabeled material were found in the eliminating organs, liver and kidney. *In vitro*, sibutramine, M_1 and M_2 are extensively bound (97%, 94% and 94%, respectively) to human plasma proteins at plasma concentrations seen following therapeutic doses.

Metabolism

Sibutramine is metabolized in the liver principally by the cytochrome P450($3A_4$) isoenzyme, to desmethyl metabolites, M_1 and M_2. These active metabolites are further metabolized by hydroxylation and conjugation to pharmacologically inactive metabolites, M_5 and M_6. Following oral administration of radiolabeled sibutramine, essentially all of the peak radiolabeled material in plasma was accounted for by unchanged sibutramine (3%), M_1 (6%), M_2 (12%), M_5 (52%), and M_6 (27%).

M_1 and M_2 plasma concentrations reached steady-state within four days of dosing and were approximately two-fold higher than following a single dose. The elimination half-lives of M_1 and M_2, 14 and 16 hours, respectively, were unchanged following repeated dosing.

Excretion

Approximately 85% (range 68-95%) of a single orally administered radiolabeled dose was excreted in urine and feces over a 15-day collection period with the majority of the dose (77%) excreted in the urine. Major metabolites in urine were M_5 and M_6; unchanged sibutramine, M_1, and M_2 were not detected. The primary route of excretion for M_1 and M_2 is hepatic metabolism and for M_5 and M_6 is renal excretion.

Summary of Pharmacokinetic Parameters

[See first table above]

Effect of Food

Administration of a single 20 mg dose of sibutramine with a standard breakfast resulted in reduced peak M_1 and M_2 concentrations (by 27% and 32%, respectively) and delayed the time to peak by approximately three hours. However, the AUCs of M_1 and M_2 were not significantly altered.

Special Populations

Geriatric: Plasma concentrations of M_1 and M_2 were similar between elderly (ages 61 to 77 yr) and young (ages 19 to 30 yr) subjects following a single 15-mg oral sibutramine dose. Plasma concentrations of the inactive metabolites M_5 and M_6 were higher in the elderly; these differences are not likely to be of clinical significance. In general, dose selection for an elderly patient should be cautious, reflecting the greater frequency of decreased hepatic, renal, or cardiac function, and of concomitant disease or other drug therapy.

Mean (% CV) and 95% Confidence Intervals of Pharmacokinetic Parameters (Dose = 15 mg)

Study Population	C_{max} (ng/mL)	T_{max} (h)	AUC† (ng*h/mL)	T½ (h)
Metabolite M_1				
Target Population:				
Obese Subjects	4.0 (42)	3.6 (28)	25.5 (63)	—
(n=18)	3.2-4.8	3.1-4.1	18.1-32.9	
Special Population:				
Moderate Hepatic	2.2 (36)	3.3 (33)	18.7 (65)	—
Impairment (n=12)	1.8-2.7	2.7-3.9	11.9-25.5	
Metabolite M_2				
Target Population:				
Obese Subjects	6.4 (28)	3.5 (17)	92.1 (26)	17.2 (58)
(n=18)	5.6-7.2	3.2-3.8	81.2-103	12.5-21.8
Special Population:				
Moderate Hepatic	4.3 (37)	3.8 (34)	90.5 (27)	22.7 (30)
Impairment (n=12)	3.4-5.2	3.1-4.5	76.9-104	18.9-26.5

† Calculated only up to 24 hr for M_1

Mean Weight Loss (lbs) in the Six-Month and One-Year Trials

Study/Patient Group	Placebo (n)	MERIDIA (mg) 5 (n)	10 (n)	15 (n)	20 (n)
Study 1					
All patients*	2.0	6.6	9.7	12.1	13.6
	(142)	(148)	(148)	(150)	(145)
Completers**	2.9	8.1	12.1	15.4	18.0
	(84)	(103)	(95)	(94)	(89)
Early responders***	8.5	13.0	16.0	18.2	20.1
	(17)	(60)	(64)	(73)	(76)
Study 2					
All patients*	3.5		9.8	14.0	
	(157)		(154)	(152)	
Completers**	4.8		13.6	15.2	
	(76)		(80)	(93)	
Early responders***	10.7		18.2	18.8	
	(24)		(57)	(76)	
Study 3****					
All patients*	15.2		28.4		
	(78)		(81)		
Completers**	16.7		29.7		
	(48)		(60)		
Early responders***	21.5		33.0		
	(22)		(46)		

* Data for all patients who received study drug and who had any post-baseline measurement (last observation carried forward analysis).

** Data for patients who completed the entire 6-month (Study 1) or one-year period of dosing and have data recorded for the month 6 (Study 1) or month 12 visit.

*** Data for patients who lost at least 4 lbs in the first 4 weeks of treatment and completed the study.

**** Weight loss data shown describe changes in weight from the pre-VLCD; mean weight loss during the 4-week VLCD was 16.9 lbs for sibutramine and 16.3 lbs for placebo.

Pediatric: The safety and effectiveness of MERIDIA in pediatric patients under 16 years old have not been established.

Gender: Pooled pharmacokinetic parameters from 54 young, healthy volunteers (37 males and 17 females) receiving a 15-mg oral dose of sibutramine showed the mean C_{max} and AUC of M_1 and M_2 to be slightly (≤19% and ≤36%, respectively) higher in females than males. Somewhat higher steady-state trough plasma levels were observed in female obese patients from a large clinical efficacy trial. However, these differences are not likely to be of clinical significance. Dosage adjustment based upon the gender of a patient is not necessary (see "**DOSAGE AND ADMINISTRATION**").

Race: The relationship between race and steady-state trough M_1 and M_2 plasma concentrations was examined in a clinical trial in obese patients. A trend towards higher concentrations in Black patients over Caucasian patients was noted for M_1 and M_2. However, these differences are not considered to be of clinical significance.

Renal Insufficiency: The effect of renal disease has not been studied. However, since sibutramine and its active metabolites M_1 and M_2 are eliminated by hepatic metabolism, renal disease is unlikely to have a significant effect on their disposition. Elimination of the inactive metabolites M_5 and M_6, which are renally excreted, may be affected in this population. MERIDIA should not be used in patients with severe renal impairment.

Hepatic Insufficiency: In 12 patients with moderate hepatic impairment receiving a single 15-mg oral dose of sibutramine, the combined AUCs of M_1 and M_2 were increased by 24% compared to healthy subjects while M_5 and M_6 plasma concentrations were unchanged. The observed differences in M_1 and M_2 concentrations do not warrant dosage adjustment in patients with mild to moderate hepatic impairment. MERIDIA should not be used in patients with severe hepatic dysfunction.

CLINICAL STUDIES

Observational epidemiologic studies have established a relationship between obesity and the risks for cardiovascular disease, non-insulin dependent diabetes mellitus (NIDDM), certain forms of cancer, gallstones, certain respiratory disorders, and an increase in overall mortality. These studies suggest that weight loss, if maintained, may produce health benefits for some patients with chronic obesity who may also be at risk for other diseases.

The long-term effects of MERIDIA Capsules on the morbidity and mortality associated with obesity have not been established. Weight loss was examined in 11 double-blind, placebo-controlled obesity trials (BMI range across all studies 27-43) with study durations of 12 to 52 weeks and doses ranging from 1 to 30 mg once daily. Weight was significantly reduced in a dose-related manner in sibutramine-treated patients compared to placebo over the dose range of 5 to 20 mg once daily. In two 12-month studies, maximal weight loss was achieved by 6 months and statistically significant weight loss was maintained over 12 months. The amount of placebo-subtracted weight loss achieved on MERIDIA was consistent across studies.

Analysis of the data in three long-term (≥6 months) obesity trials indicates that patients who lose at least 4 pounds in the first 4 weeks of therapy with a given dose of MERIDIA are most likely to achieve significant long-term weight loss on that dose of MERIDIA. Approximately 60% of such patients went on to achieve a placebo-subtracted weight loss of ≥5% of their initial body weight by month 6. Conversely, of those patients on a given dose of MERIDIA who did not lose at least 4 pounds in the first 4 weeks of therapy, approximately 80% did not go on to achieve a placebo-subtracted weight loss of ≥5% of their initial body weight on that dose by month 6.

Significant dose-related reductions in waist circumference, an indicator of intra-abdominal fat, have also been observed over 6 and 12 months in placebo-controlled clinical trials. In a 12-week placebo-controlled study of non-insulin dependent diabetes mellitus patients randomized to placebo or 15 mg per day of MERIDIA, Dual Energy X-Ray Absorptiometry (DEXA) assessment of changes in body composition showed that total body fat mass decreased by 1.8 kg in the MERIDIA group versus 0.2 kg in the placebo group (p<0.001). Similarly, truncal (android) fat mass decreased by 0.6 kg in the MERIDIA group versus 0.1 kg in the placebo group (p<0.01). The changes in lean mass, fasting blood sugar, and HbA_1 were not statistically significantly different between the two groups.

Continued on next page

Meridia—Cont.

Eleven double-blind, placebo-controlled obesity trials with study durations of 12 to 52 weeks have provided evidence that MERIDIA does not adversely affect glycemia, serum lipid profiles, or serum uric acid in obese patients. Treatment with MERIDIA (5 to 20 mg once daily) is associated with mean increases in blood pressure of 1 to 3 mm Hg and with mean increases in pulse rate of 4 to 5 beats per minute relative to placebo. These findings are similar in normotensives and in patients with hypertension controlled with medication. Those patients who lose significant (≥ 5% weight loss) amounts of weight on MERIDIA tend to have smaller increases in blood pressure and pulse rate (see "**WARNINGS**").

In Study 1, a 6-month, double-blind, placebo-controlled study in obese patients, Study 2, a 1-year, double-blind, placebo-controlled study in obese patients, and Study 3, a 1-year, double-blind, placebo-controlled study in obese patients who lost at least 6 kg on a 4-week very low calorie diet (VLCD), MERIDIA produced significant reductions in weight, as shown below. In the two 1-year studies, maximal weight loss was achieved by 6 months and statistically significant weight loss was maintained over 12 months.

[See second table at top of previous page]

Maintenance of weight loss with Meridia® (sibutramine hydrochloride monohydrate) was examined in a 2-year, double-blind, placebo-controlled trial. After a 6-month run-in phase in which all patients received sibutramine 10 mg (mean weight loss, 26 lbs.), patients were randomized to sibutramine (10 to 20 mg, 352 patients) or placebo (115 patients). The mean weight loss from initial body weight to endpoint was 21 lbs. and 12 lbs. for sibutramine and placebo patients, respectively. A statistically significantly ($p<0.001$) greater proportion of sibutramine treated patients, 75%, 62%, and 43%, maintained at least 80% of their initial weight loss at 12, 18, and 24 months, respectively, compared with the placebo group (38%, 23%, and 16%). Also 67%, 37%, 17%, and 9% of sibutramine treated patients compared with 49%, 19%, 5%, and 3% of placebo patients lost ≥5%, ≥10%, ≥15%, and ≥20%, respectively, of their initial body weight at endpoint. From endpoint to the post-study follow-up visit (about 1 month), weight regain was approximately 4 lbs for the sibutramine patients and approximately 2 lbs for the placebo patients.

MERIDIA (sibutramine hydrochloride monohydrate) induced weight loss has been accompanied by beneficial changes in serum lipids that are similar to those seen with nonpharmacologically-mediated weight loss. A combined, weighted analysis of the changes in serum lipids in 11 placebo-controlled obesity studies ranging in length from 12 to 52 weeks is shown below for the last observation carried forward (LOCF) analysis.

[See first table above]

MERIDIA induced weight loss has been accompanied by reductions in serum uric acid.

Certain centrally-acting weight loss agents that cause release of serotonin from nerve terminals have been associated with cardiac valve dysfunction. The possible occurrence of cardiac valve disease was specifically investigated in two studies. In one study 2-D and color Doppler echocardiography were performed on 210 patients (mean age, 54 years) receiving MERIDIA 15 mg or placebo daily for periods of 2 weeks to 16 months (mean duration of treatment, 7.6 months). In patients without a prior history of valvular heart disease, the incidence of valvular heart disease was 3/132 (2.3%) in the sibutramine treatment group (all three cases were mild aortic insufficiency) and 2/77 (2.6%) in the placebo treatment group (one case of mild aortic insufficiency and one case of severe aortic insufficiency). In another study, 25 patients underwent 2-D and color Doppler echocardiography before treatment with MERIDIA and again after treatment with MERIDIA 5 to 30 mg daily for three months; there were no cases of valvular heart disease.

The effect of sibutramine 15 mg once daily on measures of 24-hour blood pressure was evaluated in a 12-week placebo-controlled study. Twenty-six male and female, primarily Caucasian individuals with an average BMI of 34 kg/m^2 and an average age of 39 years underwent 24-hour ambulatory blood pressure monitoring (ABPM). The mean changes from baseline to Week 12 in various measures of ABPM are shown in the following table.

[See second table above]

INDICATIONS AND USAGE

MERIDIA is indicated for the management of obesity, including weight loss and maintenance of weight loss, and should be used in conjunction with a reduced calorie diet. MERIDIA is recommended for obese patients with an initial body mass index ≥30 kg/m^2, or ≥27 kg/m^2 in the presence of other risk factors (e.g., hypertension, diabetes, dyslipidemia).

Below is a chart of Body Mass Index (BMI) based on various heights and weights.

BMI is calculated by taking the patient's weight, in kg, and dividing by the patient's height, in meters, squared. Metric conversions are as follows: pounds ÷ 2.2 = kg; inches × 0.0254 = meters.

[See figure at top of next column]

CONTRAINDICATIONS

MERIDIA is contraindicated in patients receiving monoamine oxidase inhibitors (MAOIs) (see "**WARNINGS**").

Combined Analysis (11 Studies) of Percentage Change in Serum Lipids (N) - LOCF

Category	TG	CHOL	LDL-C	HDL-C
All Placebo	0.53 (475)	-1.53 (475)	-0.09 (233)	-0.56 (248)
<5% Weight Loss	4.52 (382)	-0.42 (382)	-0.70 (205)	-0.71 (217)
≥5% Weight Loss	-15.30 (92)	-6.23 (92)	-6.19 (27)	0.94 (30)
All Sibutramine	-8.75 (1164)	-2.21 (1165)	-1.85 (642)	4.13 (664)
<5% Weight Loss	-0.54 (547)	0.17 (548)	-0.37 (320)	3.19 (331)
≥5% Weight Loss	-16.59 (612)	-4.87 (612)	-4.56 (317)	4.68 (328)

Baseline mean values:
Placebo: TG 187 mg/dL; CHOL 221 mg/dL; LDL-C 140 mg/dL; HDL-C 47 mg/dL
Sibutramine: TG 172 mg/dL; CHOL 215 mg/dL; LDL-C 140 mg/dL; HDL-C 47 mg/dL

Parameter	Systolic			Diastolic		
mm Hg	Placebo n=12	Sibutramine		Placebo	Sibutramine	
		15 mg n=14	20 mg n=16		15 mg n=12	20 mg n=16
Daytime	0.2	3.9	4.4	0.5	5.0	5.7
Nighttime	-0.3	4.1	6.4	-1.0	4.3	5.4
Early am	-0.9	9.4	5.3	-3.0	6.7	5.8
24-hour mean	-0.1	4.0	4.7	0.1	5.0	5.6

Normal diurnal variation of blood pressure was maintained.

BMI		25	26	27	28	29	30	31	32	33	34	35	40
		WEIGHT (lbs)											
	4'10"	119	124	129	134	138	143	149	153	158	163	167	191
	4'11"	124	128	133	138	143	148	154	158	164	169	173	198
	5'	128	133	138	143	148	153	159	164	169	175	179	204
	5'1"	132	137	143	148	153	158	165	169	175	180	185	211
	5'2"	136	142	147	153	158	164	170	175	181	186	191	218
H	5'3"	141	146	152	158	163	169	175	181	187	192	197	225
	5'4"	145	151	157	163	169	174	181	187	193	199	204	232
E	5'5"	150	156	162	168	174	180	187	193	199	205	210	240
	5'6"	155	161	167	173	179	186	192	199	205	211	216	247
I	5'7"	159	166	172	178	185	191	198	205	211	218	223	255
	5'8"	164	171	177	184	190	197	204	211	218	224	230	262
G	5'9"	169	176	182	189	196	203	210	217	224	231	236	270
	5'10"	174	181	188	195	202	207	216	223	230	237	243	278
H	5'11"	179	186	193	200	208	215	222	230	237	244	250	286
	6'	184	191	199	206	213	221	228	236	244	251	258	294
T	6'1"	189	197	204	212	219	227	236	243	251	258	265	302
	6'2"	194	202	210	218	225	233	241	250	258	265	272	311
	6'3"	200	208	216	224	232	240	248	256	264	272	279	319

MERIDIA is contraindicated in patients with hypersensitivity to sibutramine or any of the inactive ingredients of MERIDIA.

MERIDIA is contraindicated in patients who have a major eating disorder (anorexia nervosa or bulimia nervosa).

MERIDIA is contraindicated in patients taking other centrally acting appetite suppressant drugs.

WARNINGS

Blood Pressure and Pulse

MERIDIA SUBSTANTIALLY INCREASES BLOOD PRESSURE IN SOME PATIENTS. REGULAR MONITORING OF BLOOD PRESSURE IS REQUIRED WHEN PRESCRIBING MERIDIA.

In placebo-controlled obesity studies, MERIDIA 5 to 20 mg once daily was associated with mean increases in systolic and diastolic blood pressure of approximately 1 to 3 mm Hg relative to placebo, and with mean increases in pulse rate relative to placebo of approximately 4 to 5 beats per minute. Larger increases were seen in some patients, particularly when therapy with MERIDIA was initiated at the higher doses (see table below). In pre-marketing placebo-controlled obesity studies, 0.4% of patients treated with MERIDIA were discontinued for hypertension (SBP ≥ 160 mm Hg or DBP ≥ 95 mm Hg), compared with 0.4% in the placebo group, and 0.4% of patients treated with MERIDIA were discontinued for tachycardia (pulse rate ≥ 100 bpm), compared with 0.1% in the placebo group. Blood pressure and pulse should be measured prior to starting therapy with MERIDIA and should be monitored at regular intervals thereafter. For patients who experience a sustained increase in blood pressure or pulse rate while receiving MERIDIA, either dose reduction or discontinuation should be considered. MERIDIA should be given with caution to those patients with a history of hypertension (see "**DOSAGE AND ADMINISTRATION**"), and should not be given to patients with uncontrolled or poorly controlled hypertension.

Percent Outliers in Studies 1 and 2

Dose (mg)	% Outliers*		
	SBP	DBP	Pulse
Placebo	9	7	12
5	6	20	16
10	12	15	28
15	13	17	24
20	14	22	37

*Outlier defined as increase from baseline of ≥15 mm Hg for three consecutive visits (SBP), ≥10 mm Hg for three consecutive visits (DBP), or pulse ≥10 bpm for three consecutive visits.

Potential Interaction With Monoamine Oxidase Inhibitors

MERIDIA is a norepinephrine, serotonin and dopamine reuptake inhibitor and should not be used concomitantly with MAOIs (see "**PRECAUTIONS**", Drug Interactions subsection). There should be at least a 2-week interval after stopping MAOIs before commencing treatment with MERIDIA. Similarly, there should be at least a 2-week interval after stopping MERIDIA before starting treatment with MAOIs.

Concomitant Cardiovascular Disease

Treatment with MERIDIA has been associated with increases in heart rate and/or blood pressure. Therefore, MERIDIA should not be used in patients with a history of coronary artery disease, congestive heart failure, arrhythmias, or stroke.

Glaucoma

Because MERIDIA can cause mydriasis, it should be used with caution in patients with narrow angle glaucoma.

Miscellaneous

Organic causes of obesity (e.g., untreated hypothyroidism) should be excluded before prescribing MERIDIA.

PRECAUTIONS

Pulmonary Hypertension

Certain centrally-acting weight loss agents that cause release of serotonin from nerve terminals have been associated with pulmonary hypertension (PPH), a rare but lethal disease. In pre-marketing clinical studies, no cases of PPH have been reported with MERIDIA® (sibutramine hydrochloride monohydrate) Capsules. Because of the low incidence of this disease in the underlying population, however, it is not known whether or not MERIDIA may cause this disease.

Seizures

During premarketing testing, seizures were reported in <0.1% of MERIDIA treated patients. MERIDIA should be used cautiously in patients with a history of seizures. It should be discontinued in any patient who develops seizures.

Bleeding

There have been reports of bleeding in patients taking sibutramine. While a causal relationship is unclear, caution is advised in patients predisposed to bleeding events and those taking concomitant medications known to affect hemostasis or platelet function.

Gallstones

Weight loss can precipitate or exacerbate gallstone formation.

Renal/Hepatic Dysfunction

Patients with severe renal impairment or severe hepatic dysfunction have not been systematically studied; MERIDIA should therefore not be used in such patients.

Interference With Cognitive and Motor Performance

Although sibutramine did not affect psychomotor or cognitive performance in healthy volunteers, any CNS active drug has the potential to impair judgment, thinking or motor skills.

Information For Patients

Physicians should instruct their patients to read the patient package insert before starting therapy with MERIDIA and to reread it each time the prescription is renewed.

Physicians should also discuss with their patients any part of the package insert that is relevant to them. In particular, the importance of keeping appointments for follow-up visits should be emphasized.

Patients should be advised to notify their physician if they develop a rash, hives, or other allergic reactions.

Patients should be advised to inform their physicians if they are taking, or plan to take, any prescription or over-the-counter drugs, especially weight-reducing agents, decongestants, antidepressants, cough suppressants, lithium, dihydroergotamine, sumatriptan (Imitrex®), or tryptophan, since there is a potential for interactions.

Patients should be reminded of the importance of having their blood pressure and pulse monitored at regular intervals.

Drug Interactions

CNS Active Drugs: The use of MERIDIA in combination with other CNS-active drugs, particularly serotonergic agents, has not been systematically evaluated. Consequently, caution is advised if the concomitant administration of MERIDIA with other centrally-acting drugs is indicated (see "**CONTRAINDICATIONS**" and "**WARNINGS**").

In patients receiving monoamine oxidase inhibitors (MAOIs) (e.g., phenelzine, selegiline) in combination with serotonergic agents (e.g., fluoxetine, fluvoxamine, paroxetine, sertraline, venlafaxine), there have been reports of serious, sometimes fatal, reactions ("serotonin syndrome;" see below). Because MERIDIA inhibits serotonin reuptake, MERIDIA should not be used concomitantly with a MAOI (see "**CONTRAINDICATIONS**"). At least 2 weeks should elapse between discontinuation of a MAOI and initiation of treatment with MERIDIA. Similarly, at least 2 weeks should elapse between discontinuation of MERIDIA and initiation of treatment with a MAOI.

The rare, but serious, constellation of symptoms termed "serotonin syndrome" has also been reported with the concomitant use of selective serotonin reuptake inhibitors and agents for migraine therapy, such as Imitrex® (sumatriptan succinate) and dihydroergotamine, certain opioids, such as dextromethorphan, meperidine, pentazocine and fentanyl, lithium, or tryptophan. Serotonin syndrome has also been reported with the concomitant use of two serotonin reuptake inhibitors. The syndrome requires immediate medical attention and may include one or more of the following symptoms: excitement, hypomania, restlessness, loss of consciousness, confusion, disorientation, anxiety, agitation, motor weakness, myoclonus, tremor, hemiballismus, hyperreflexia, ataxia, dysarthria, incoordination, hyperthermia, shivering, pupillary dilation, diaphoresis, emesis, and tachycardia.

Because MERIDIA inhibits serotonin reuptake, in general, it should not be administered with other serotonergic agents such as those listed above. However, if such a combination is clinically indicated, appropriate observation of the patient is warranted.

Drugs That May Raise Blood Pressure and/or Heart Rate: Concomitant use of MERIDIA and other agents that may raise blood pressure or heart rate have not been evaluated. These include certain decongestants, cough, cold, and allergy medications that contain agents such as ephedrine, or pseudoephedrine. Caution should be used when prescribing MERIDIA to patients who use these medications.

Drugs That Inhibit Cytochrome P450($3A_4$) Metabolism: *In vitro* studies indicated that the cytochrome P450($3A_4$)-mediated metabolism of sibutramine was inhibited by ketoconazole and to a lesser extent by erythromycin. Clinical interaction trials were conducted on these substrates. The potential for such interactions is described below.

Ketoconazole: Concomitant administration of 200 mg doses of ketoconazole twice daily and 20 mg sibutramine once daily for 7 days in 12 uncomplicated obese subjects resulted in moderate increases in AUC and C_{max} of 58% and 36% for M_1 and of 20% and 19% for M_2, respectively.

Erythromycin: The steady-state pharmacokinetics of sibutramine and metabolites M_1 and M_2 were evaluated in 12 uncomplicated obese subjects following concomitant administration of 500 mg of erythromycin three times daily and 20 mg of sibutramine once daily for 7 days. Concomitant erythromycin resulted in small increases in the AUC (less than 14%) for M_1 and M_2. A small reduction in C_{max} for M_1 (11%) and a slight increase in C_{max} for M_2 (10%) were observed.

Cimetidine: Concomitant administration of cimetidine 400 mg twice daily and sibutramine 15 mg once daily for 7 days in 12 volunteers resulted in small increases in combined (M_1 and M_2) plasma C_{max} (3.4%) and AUC (7.3%); these differences are unlikely to be of clinical significance.

Alcohol: In a double-blind, placebo-controlled, crossover study in 19 volunteers, administration of a single dose of ethanol (0.5 mL/kg) together with 20 mg of sibutramine resulted in no psychomotor interactions of clinical significance between alcohol and sibutramine. However, the concomitant use of MERIDIA and excess alcohol is not recommended.

Oral Contraceptives: The suppression of ovulation by oral contraceptives was not inhibited by MERIDIA. In a crossover study, 12 healthy female volunteers on oral steroid contraceptives received placebo in one period and 15 mg sibutramine in another period over the course of 8 weeks. No clinically significant systemic interaction was observed; therefore, no requirement for alternative contraceptive precautions are needed when patients taking oral contraceptives are concurrently prescribed sibutramine.

Drugs Highly Bound to Plasma Proteins: Although sibutramine and its active metabolites M_1 and M_2 are extensively bound to plasma proteins (≥94%), the low therapeutic concentrations and basic characteristics of these compounds make them unlikely to result in clinically significant protein binding interactions with other highly protein bound drugs such as warfarin and phenytoin. *In vitro* protein binding interaction studies have not been conducted.

Carcinogenesis, Mutagenesis, Impairment of Fertility

Carcinogenicity

Sibutramine was administered in the diet to mice (1.25, 5 or 20 mg/kg/day) and rats (1, 3, or 9 mg/kg/day) for two years

	Obese Patients in Placebo-Controlled Studies	
	MERIDIA® (n = 2068)	Placebo (n = 884)
BODY SYSTEM Adverse Event	% Incidence	% Incidence
BODY AS A WHOLE:		
Headache	30.3	18.6
Back pain	8.2	5.5
Flu syndrome	8.2	5.8
Injury accident	5.9	4.1
Asthenia	5.9	5.3
Abdominal pain	4.5	3.6
Chest pain	1.8	1.2
Neck pain	1.6	1.1
Allergic reaction	1.5	0.8
CARDIOVASCULAR SYSTEM		
Tachycardia	2.6	0.6
Vasodilation	2.4	0.9
Migraine	2.4	2.0
Hypertension/increased blood pressure	2.1	0.9
Palpitation	2.0	0.8
DIGESTIVE SYSTEM		
Anorexia	13.0	3.5
Constipation	11.5	6.0
Increased appetite	8.7	2.7
Nausea	5.9	2.8
Dyspepsia	5.0	2.6
Gastritis	1.7	1.2
Vomiting	1.5	1.4
Rectal disorder	1.2	0.5
METABOLIC & NUTRITIONAL		
Thirst	1.7	0.9
Generalized edema	1.2	0.8
MUSCULOSKELETAL SYSTEM		
Arthralgia	5.9	5.0
Myalgia	1.9	1.1
Tenosynovitis	1.2	0.5
Joint disorder	1.1	0.6
NERVOUS SYSTEM		
Dry mouth	17.2	4.2
Insomnia	10.7	4.5
Dizziness	7.0	3.4
Nervousness	5.2	2.9
Anxiety	4.5	3.4
Depression	4.3	2.5
Paresthesia	2.0	0.5
Somnolence	1.7	0.9
CNS stimulation	1.5	0.5
Emotional lability	1.3	0.6
RESPIRATORY SYSTEM		
Rhinitis	10.2	7.1
Pharyngitis	10.0	8.4
Sinusitis	5.0	2.6
Cough increase	3.8	3.3
Laryngitis	1.3	0.9
SKIN & APPENDAGES		
Rash	3.8	2.5
Sweating	2.5	0.9
Herpes simplex	1.3	1.0
Acne	1.0	0.8
SPECIAL SENSES		
Taste perversion	2.2	0.8
Ear disorder	1.7	0.9
Ear pain	1.1	0.7
UROGENITAL SYSTEM		
Dysmenorrhea	3.5	1.4
Urinary tract infection	2.3	2.0
Vaginal monilia	1.2	0.5
Metrorrhagia	1.0	0.8

generating combined maximum plasma AUC's of the two major active metabolites equivalent to 0.4 and 16 times, respectively, those following a daily human dose of 15 mg. There was no evidence of carcinogenicity in mice or in female rats. In male rats there was a higher incidence of benign tumors of the testicular interstitial cells; such tumors are commonly seen in rats and are hormonally mediated. The relevance of these tumors to humans is not known.

Mutagenicity

Sibutramine was not mutagenic in the Ames test, *in vitro* Chinese hamster V79 cell mutation assay, *in vitro* clastogenicity assay in human lymphocytes or micronucleus assay in mice. Its two major active metabolites were found to have equivocal bacterial mutagenic activity in the Ames test. However, both metabolites gave consistently negative results in the *in vitro* Chinese hamster V79 cell mutation assay, *in vitro* clastogenicity assay in human lymphocytes, *in vitro* DNA-repair assay in HeLa cells, micronucleus assay in mice and *in vivo* unscheduled DNA-synthesis assay in rat hepatocytes.

Impairment of Fertility

In rats, there were no effects on fertility at doses generating combined plasma AUC's of the two major active metabolites up to 32 times those following a human dose of 15 mg. At 13 times the human combined AUC, there was maternal toxicity, and the dams' nest-building behavior was impaired, leading to a higher incidence of perinatal mortality; there was no effect at approximately 4 times the human combined AUC.

Pregnancy

Teratogenic Effects-Pregnancy Category C

Radiolabeled studies in animals indicated that tissue distribution was unaffected by pregnancy, with relatively low transfer to the fetus. In rats, there was no evidence of teratogenicity at doses of 1, 3, or 10 mg/kg/day generating combined plasma AUC's of the two major active metabolites up to approximately 32 times those following the human dose of 15 mg. In rabbits dosed at 3, 15, or 75 mg/kg/day, plasma AUC's greater than approximately 5 times those following the human dose of 15 mg caused maternal toxicity. At markedly toxic doses, Dutch Belted rabbits had a slightly higher than control incidence of pups with a broad short snout, short rounded pinnae, short tail and, in some, shorter thickened long bones in the limbs; at comparably high doses in New Zealand White rabbits, one study showed a slightly higher than control incidence of pups with cardiovascular anomalies while a second study showed a lower incidence than in the control group.

No adequate and well controlled studies with MERIDIA have been conducted in pregnant women. The use of MERIDIA during pregnancy is not recommended. Women of childbearing potential should employ adequate contraception while taking MERIDIA. Patients should be advised to notify their physician if they become pregnant or intend to become pregnant during therapy.

Continued on next page

Meridia—Cont.

Nursing Mothers
It is not known whether sibutramine or its metabolites are excreted in human milk. MERIDIA is not recommended for use in nursing mothers. Patients should be advised to notify their physician if they are breast-feeding.

Pediatric Use
The safety and effectiveness of MERIDIA in pediatric patients under 16 years of age have not been established.

Geriatric Use
Clinical studies of MERIDIA did not include sufficient numbers of patients aged 65 and over to determine whether they respond differently from younger patients. In general, dose selection for an elderly patient should be cautious, reflecting the greater frequency of decreased hepatic, renal, or cardiac function, and of concomitant disease or other drug therapy. Pharmacokinetics in elderly patients are discussed in "**CLINICAL PHARMACOLOGY**."

ADVERSE REACTIONS

In placebo-controlled studies, 9% of patients treated with MERIDIA (n=2068) and 7% of patients treated with placebo (n=884) withdrew for adverse events.

In placebo-controlled studies, the most common events were dry mouth, anorexia, insomnia, constipation and headache. Adverse events in these studies occurring in ≥1% of MERIDIA treated patients and more frequently than in the placebo group are shown in the following table.

[See table at top of previous page]

The following additional adverse events were reported in ≥ 1% of all patients who received MERIDIA in controlled and uncontrolled pre-marketing studies.

Body as a Whole: fever.
Digestive System: diarrhea, flatulence, gastroenteritis, tooth disorder.
Metabolic and Nutritional: peripheral edema.
Musculoskeletal System: arthritis.
Nervous System: agitation, leg cramps, hypertonia, thinking abnormal.
Respiratory System: bronchitis, dyspnea.
Skin and Appendages: pruritus.
Special Senses: amblyopia.
Urogenital System: menstrual disorders.

Other Adverse Events

Clinical Studies

Seizures: Convulsions were reported as an adverse event in three of 2068 (0.1%) MERIDIA treated patients and in none of 884 placebo-treated patients in placebo-controlled premarketing obesity studies. Two of the three patients with seizures had potentially predisposing factors (one had a prior history of epilepsy; one had a subsequent diagnosis of brain tumor). The incidence in all subjects who received MERIDIA (three of 4,588 subjects) was less than 0.1%.

Ecchymosis/Bleeding Disorders: Ecchymosis (bruising) was observed in 0.7% of MERIDIA treated patients and in 0.2% of placebo-treated patients in pre-marketing placebo-controlled obesity studies. One patient had prolonged bleeding of a small amount which occurred during minor facial surgery. MERIDIA may have an effect on platelet function due to its effect on serotonin uptake.

Interstitial Nephritis: Acute interstitial nephritis (confirmed by biopsy) was reported in one obese patient receiving MERIDIA during pre-marketing studies. After discontinuation of the medication, dialysis and oral corticosteroids were administered; renal function normalized. The patient made a full recovery.

Altered Laboratory Findings: Abnormal liver function tests, including increases in AST, ALT, GGT, LDH, alkaline phosphatase and bilirubin, were reported as adverse events in 1.6% of MERIDIA-treated obese patients in placebo-controlled trials compared with 0.8% of placebo patients. In these studies, potentially clinically significant values (total bilirubin ≥2 mg/dL; ALT, AST, GGT, LDH, or alkaline phosphatase ≥3x upper limit of normal) occurred in 0% (alkaline phosphatase) to 0.6% (ALT) of the MERIDIA treated patients and in none of the placebo-treated patients. Abnormal values tended to be sporadic, often diminished with continued treatment, and did not show a clear dose-response relationship.

Postmarketing Reports
Voluntary reports of adverse events temporally associated with the use of MERIDIA are listed below. It is important to emphasize that although these events occurred during treatment with MERIDIA, they may have no causal relationship with the drug. Obesity itself, concurrent disease states/risk factors, or weight reduction may be associated with an increased risk for some of these events.

Psychiatric: Cases of depression, suicidal ideation and suicide have been reported rarely in patients on sibutramine treatment. However, a relationship has not been established between the occurrence of depression and/or suicidal ideation and the use of sibutramine. If depression occurs during treatment with sibutramine, further evaluation may be necessary.

Hypersensitivity: Allergic hypersensitivity reactions ranging from mild skin eruptions and urticaria to angioedema and anaphylaxis have been reported (see "**CONTRAINDICATIONS**" and "**PRECAUTIONS-Information For Patients**", and other reports of allergic reactions listed below).

Other: Abnormal dreams, abnormal ejaculation, abnormal gait, abnormal vision, alopecia, amnesia, anaphylactic shock, anaphylactoid reaction, anemia, anger, angina pectoris, arthrosis, atrial fibrillation, blurred vision, bursitis, cerebrovascular accident, chest pressure, chest tightness, cholecystitis, cholelithiasis, concentration impaired, confusion, congestive heart failure, depression aggravated, dermatitis, dry eye, duodenal ulcer, epistaxis, eructation, eye pain, facial edema, gastrointestinal hemorrhage, Gilles de la Tourette's syndrome, goiter, heart arrest, heart rate decreased, hematuria, hyperglycemia, hyperthyroidism, hypesthesia, hypoglycemia, hypothyroidism, impotence, increased intraocular pressure, increased salivation, increased urinary frequency, intestinal obstruction, leukopenia, libido decreased, libido increased, limb pain, lymphadenopathy, manic reaction, micturition difficulty, mood changes, mouth ulcer, myocardial infarction, nasal congestion, nightmares, otitis externa, otitis media, petechiae, photosensitivity (eyes), photosensitivity (skin), respiratory disorder, serotonin syndrome, short term memory loss, speech disorder, stomach ulcer, sudden unexplained death, supraventricular tachycardia, syncope, thrombocytopenia, tinnitus, tongue edema, torsade de pointes, transient ischemic attack, tremor, twitch, urinary retention, urticaria, vascular headache, ventricular tachycardia, ventricular extrasystoles, ventricular fibrillation, vertigo, yawn.

DRUG ABUSE AND DEPENDENCE

Controlled Substance
MERIDIA is controlled in Schedule IV of the Controlled Substances Act (CSA).

Abuse and Physical and Psychological Dependence
Physicians should carefully evaluate patients for history of drug abuse and follow such patients closely, observing them for signs of misuse or abuse (e.g., drug development of tolerance, incrementation of doses, drug seeking behavior).

OVERDOSAGE

Human Experience
Three cases of overdose have been reported with MERIDIA. The first was in a 2-year-old child of one patient who ingested up to eight 10 mg capsules. No complications were observed during the overnight hospitalization, and the child was discharged the following day with no sequela. The second report was in a 30-year-old male in a depression study who ingested approximately 100 mg of sibutramine in an attempt to commit suicide. The patient suffered no adverse effects or ECG abnormalities post-ingestion. The third report was in the 45-year-old husband of a patient in an obese dyslipidemic study. He ingested 400 mg of his wife's drug supply and was hospitalized for observation; a heart rate of 120 bpm was noted. He was discharged the next day with no apparent sequelae.

Overdose Management
There is no specific antidote to MERIDIA. Treatment should consist of general measures employed in the management of overdosage: an airway should be established; cardiac and vital sign monitoring is recommended; general symptomatic and supportive measures should be instituted. Cautious use of β-blockers may be indicated to control elevated blood pressure or tachycardia. The benefits of forced diuresis and hemodialysis are unknown.

DOSAGE AND ADMINISTRATION

The recommended starting dose of MERIDIA is 10 mg administered once daily with or without food. If there is inadequate weight loss, the dose may be titrated after four weeks to a total of 15 mg once daily. The 5 mg dose should be reserved for patients who do not tolerate the 10 mg dose. Blood pressure and heart rate changes should be taken into account when making decisions regarding dose titration (see "**PRECAUTIONS**").

Doses above 15 mg daily are not recommended. In most of the clinical trials, MERIDIA was given in the morning.

Analysis of numerous variables has indicated that approximately 60% of patients who lose at least 4 pounds in the first 4 weeks of treatment with a given dose of MERIDIA in combination with a reduced-calorie diet lose at least 5% (placebo-subtracted) of their initial body weight by the end of 6 months to 1 year of treatment on that dose of MERIDIA. Conversely, approximately 80% of patients who do not lose at least 4 pounds in the first 4 weeks of treatment with a given dose of MERIDIA do not lose at least 5% (placebo-subtracted) of their initial body weight by the end of 6 months to 1 year of treatment on that dose. If a patient has not lost at least 4 pounds in the first 4 weeks of treatment, the physician should consider reevaluation of therapy which may include increasing the dose or discontinuation of MERIDIA.

The safety and effectiveness of MERIDIA, as demonstrated in double-blind, placebo-controlled trials, have not been determined beyond 2 years at this time.

HOW SUPPLIED

MERIDIA® (sibutramine hydrochloride monohydrate) Capsules contain 5 mg, 10 mg, or 15 mg sibutramine hydrochloride monohydrate and are supplied as follows:

5 mg, NDC 0074-2456-13, blue/yellow capsules imprinted with "MERIDIA" on the cap and "-5-" on the body, in bottles of 100 capsules.

10 mg, NDC 0074-2457-13, blue/white capsules imprinted with "MERIDIA" on the cap and "-10-" on the body, in bottles of 100 capsules.

15 mg, NDC 0074-2458-13, yellow/white capsules imprinted with "MERIDIA" on the cap and "-15-" on the body, in bottles of 100 capsules.

Storage: Store at 25°C (77°F); excursions permitted to 15°-30°C (59°-86°F) [see USP controlled room temperature]. Protect capsules from heat and moisture. Dispense in a tight, light-resistant container as defined in USP.

Manufactured by Abbott Laboratories
North Chicago, IL 60064, U.S.A.
or
for Abbott Laboratories
by BASF Corporation,
Mount Olive, NJ 07828, U.S.A.
Product of United Kingdom

IMITREX is a registered trademark of Glaxo Group Limited.

Sibutramine is covered by US Patent Nos. 4,746,680; 4,929,629; and 5,436,272.

Printed in USA
Revised: October, 2003
03-5309-R4

ABBOTT LABORATORIES
NORTH CHICAGO, IL60064, U.S.A.

MERIDIA® Ⓒ

(sibutramine hydrochloride monohydrate) Capsules

PATIENT INFORMATION

IMPORTANT PATIENT INFORMATION. READ THIS PATIENT INFORMATION CAREFULLY AND COMPLETELY BEFORE YOU START TAKING MERIDIA AND REREAD IT EACH TIME THE PRESCRIPTION IS RENEWED. CONTACT YOUR DOCTOR IMMEDIATELY IF YOU HAVE ANY QUESTIONS OR CONCERNS. SAVE THIS PATIENT INFORMATION SHEET FOR FUTURE REFERENCE.

Patient information about MERIDIA® (sibutramine hydrochloride monohydrate) Capsules.

MERIDIA capsules come in three strengths: 5 mg, 10 mg, and 15 mg.

What is MERIDIA?
MERIDIA is an oral prescription medication used for the medical management of obesity, including weight loss and the maintenance of weight loss. MERIDIA can only be prescribed by a medical doctor.

MERIDIA comes in three different strength capsules (5 mg, 10 mg, and 15 mg). The recommended initial starting dose of MERIDIA is one 10 mg capsule per day. Your doctor will determine the starting dose that is best for you.

How does MERIDIA work?
MERIDIA works by affecting appetite control centers in the brain.

In medical studies in overweight people, MERIDIA, along with a reduced calorie diet, produced significant reductions in body weight.

MERIDIA should be used as part of a comprehensive weight-loss program, supervised by your doctor, that includes a reduced calorie diet and appropriate physical activity.

How long does it take for MERIDIA to work?
Every person will respond differently to MERIDIA when used as part of a comprehensive weight-loss program. You may be able to lose 4 or more pounds of body weight in the first month you take MERIDIA. If you find that you do not lose at least 4 pounds during the first month, you should notify your doctor so he or she can re-evaluate your situation. Your doctor may wish to change your dose of MERIDIA.

Most people who lose weight on MERIDIA lose it in the first 6 months of treatment. Scientific studies that lasted two years have shown that many people who lost weight and remained on MERIDIA therapy maintained their weight loss.

Who should take MERIDIA?
A weight-loss program that includes a reduced calorie diet and appropriate physical activity may be adequate in some patients. You should discuss with your doctor whether MERIDIA should be added to such a program.

MERIDIA is recommended for overweight people with an initial body mass index (BMI) of 30 or higher, or for overweight people with a BMI of 27 or higher if they have medical risk factors such as high blood pressure, diabetes, or high cholesterol. Your doctor can determine your BMI and will decide if you meet these criteria.

How and when should I take MERIDIA?
Follow your doctor's instructions on how and when to take MERIDIA.

Your doctor will recommend that you take one (1) MERIDIA capsule a day.

You can take MERIDIA on an empty stomach or after a meal.

What if I miss a dose?
If you forget to take a dose of MERIDIA, do not take an extra capsule to "make up" for the dose you forgot.

How long should I take MERIDIA?
Your doctor will determine how long you should take MERIDIA. Follow your doctor's advice.

The safety and effectiveness of MERIDIA have not been determined beyond two (2) years at this time.

Who should not take MERIDIA?
MERIDIA should not be taken by people who:

1. **HAVE UNCONTROLLED OR POORLY CONTROLLED HIGH BLOOD PRESSURE BECAUSE MERIDIA SUBSTANTIALLY INCREASES BLOOD PRESSURE IN SOME PATIENTS.**
2. Are taking prescription medicines called monoamine oxidase inhibitors (MAOIs) for depression, Parkinson's Disease, or any other disorder (for example: Eldepryl®, Parnate®, Nardil®).

3. Are taking other weight loss medications that act on the brain (for example: phentermine). This includes prescription and over-the-counter medications and herbal products.
4. Have had prior allergic reactions to MERIDIA or sibutramine.
5. Have a diagnosis of coronary artery disease and/or who have angina pectoris (heart-related chest pain).
6. Have arrhythmias (irregular heart beats).
7. Have had a prior heart attack.
8. Have a diagnosis of congestive heart failure.
9. Have severe liver or kidney disease.
10. Have had a stroke or symptoms of a stroke (transient ischemic attacks [TIAs]).
11. Are pregnant or planning to become pregnant.
12. Are breast-feeding their infants.
13. Are suffering from a major eating disorder (anorexia nervosa or bulimia nervosa).
14. Are under 16 years of age.

If you have any concerns or questions about whether or not you should take MERIDIA, talk to your doctor.

IMPORTANT: It is very important that you make sure that your primary care doctor and all your other health care providers know what medications you take and what medical conditions and allergies you have.

What medical conditions or information should I tell my doctor?

It is important that you tell your doctor all about your medical history, whether you are taking or have taken weight loss drugs in the past, current medical problems, current symptoms, what other medications you take or have taken (prescription and over-the-counter medicines and herbal products) and any prior allergies to medicines.

It is important to make sure your doctor knows if you have heart disease of any kind, high blood pressure, migraine headaches, Parkinson's Disease, prior strokes, prior transient ischemic attacks (TIAs), thyroid disorders, osteoporosis, gallstones, liver disease, kidney disease, history of a major eating disorder (anorexia nervosa or bulimia nervosa) or any other medical problem.

It is important to make sure your doctor knows if you have had depression or are taking prescription medications for depression. The use of MERIDIA in a patient with depression may require extra caution.

You should tell your doctor if you are taking medications that regulate the neurotransmitter serotonin in the brain (for example: Prozac®, Zoloft®, Effexor®, Luvox®, Paxil®, or Zyban®).

It is important to tell your doctor if you have had seizures (epilepsy or convulsions). The use of MERIDIA in a patient with seizures may require extra caution.

It is important to tell your doctor if you have glaucoma. The use of MERIDIA in a patient with glaucoma may require extra caution.

It is important to tell your doctor if you are taking any medications that may increase your risk of bleeding (e.g. aspirin, clopidogrel, ticlopidine, warfarin). The use of MERIDIA in patients taking medications that may increase the risk of bleeding may require extra caution. Signs of bleeding may include bruising, nose bleeds, and gum bleeding.

What about physician follow-up visits?

You should make sure you see your doctor as directed for regular follow-up visits, during which your doctor can follow your body weight, and carefully monitor your overall health as you try to lose weight and maintain weight loss.

What medications can cause problems if taken at the same time I take MERIDIA?

You cannot take MERIDIA if you are taking prescription medicines called monoamine oxidase inhibitors (MAOIs). It is especially important to make sure you tell your doctor if you are taking MAOIs which are sometimes used to treat depression or Parkinson's Disease (for example: Eldepryl®, Nardil®, Parnate®). This is very important because serious, sometimes even fatal, reactions can occur if MERIDIA is taken at the same time MAOIs are taken.

If you are currently taking an MAOI, your doctor will want you to stop taking it for at least two (2) full weeks before starting you on MERIDIA.

If you are currently taking MERIDIA, your doctor will want you to stop taking it for at least two (2) full weeks before starting you on an MAOI.

It is important to tell your doctor if you are taking any medications that may increase your risk of bleeding such as aspirin, clopidogrel, ticlopidine or warfarin.

MERIDIA should not be taken if you are taking other weight-loss medications that act on the brain (for example: phentermine). This includes both prescription and over-the-counter medications and herbal products.

In addition to the above, a rare, but serious, medical syndrome called the "serotonin syndrome" has been reported in patients when medications like MERIDIA are taken along with other drugs that may alter serotonin activity such as: drugs for depression (for example: Celexa®, Lexapro®, Desyrel®, Effexor®, Eldepryl®, Remeron®, Serzone®, Wellbutrin®, Nardil®, Parnate®, Paxil®, Prozac®, Zoloft®, Ludiomil®, Adapin®, Asendin®, Elavil®, Etrafon®, Limbitrol®, Norpramin®, Pamelor®, Sinequan®, Surmontil®, Tofranil®, Triavil®, Vivactil®, Luvox®, Anafranil®), drugs for migraine headache therapy (Amerge®, Axert®, Frova®, Imitrex®, Maxalt®, Zomig®) and Migranal®, (dihydroergotamine), certain pain medications such as Demerol® (meperidine), Duragesic® (fentanyl), and Talwin® (pentazocine); the cough suppressant dextromethorphan found in many cough medicines; lithium; and the amino acid tryptophan. The syndrome requires immediate medical attention and may include one or more of the following symptoms: restlessness, loss of consciousness, confusion, disorientation, anxiety, agitation, weakness, tremor, incoordination, fever, shivering, sweating, vomiting and increased heart rate. Note: This may not be a complete list of medications. Check with your doctor or pharmacist before starting any new medications. It is important to make sure your doctor knows you are taking these medicines before you take MERIDIA.

The metabolism of MERIDIA may be inhibited by ketoconazole (an anti-fungal medicine) and to a lesser degree erythromycin (an antibiotic medicine). You need to make sure your doctor knows you are taking these medicines before you take MERIDIA. If, while taking MERIDIA, your doctor decides to put you on ketoconazole or erythromycin, you should remind him or her that you are also on MERIDIA.

Many over-the-counter cough and cold remedies, as well as certain allergy products and decongestants, contain medicines such as phenylpropanolamine, ephedrine, or pseudoephedrine that may increase blood pressure or heart rate. Before taking these medications on your own, you should check with your doctor to make sure it is all right to take these medicines if you are already taking MERIDIA. Your doctor may advise you to take a certain type of cough, cold, decongestant or allergy medicine that will not interact with MERIDIA.

When should I call my doctor?

It is important that you call your doctor immediately if you experience any symptoms or feelings that make you concerned about your health or a possible drug side effect. Let your doctor advise you on your concerns. If you experience any of the following symptoms, stop taking MERIDIA and notify your doctor immediately: trouble breathing, shortness of breath, chest pain, angina, rapid heart beats over 100 beats a minute, pounding or irregular heart beats, restlessness, lightheadedness, blackout spells, disorientation, depression, mental confusion, anxiety, nervousness, tremors, loss of muscle coordination, muscle stiffness or muscle rigidity, high fever, pain in the eyes, dilated pupils, shivering, sweating, abdominal pain, nausea or vomiting, or other symptoms that concern you.

Is MERIDIA a controlled substance?

Yes, MERIDIA is a controlled substance in Schedule IV of the Controlled Substances Act (CSA).

What weight-loss results have been observed with MERIDIA?

Patients treated with MERIDIA while on a reduced calorie diet, showed a significant weight-loss during the first 6 months of treatment, and significant weight loss was maintained for one year. In one 12-month study, the average weight loss in patients taking MERIDIA, 10 mg daily, was about 10 lbs. and in those taking 15 mg daily was about 14 lbs. The average weight loss in persons on only a reduced calorie diet was 3½ lbs.

What are some of the more common side effects of MERIDIA?

MERIDIA, like all medications, may cause side effects. In studies the most common side effects were: dry mouth, constipation, loss of appetite, and insomnia (inability to fall asleep). Other side effects that may occur include: headache, increased sweating, an increase in blood pressure, and an increase in heart rate. These side effects are generally mild, and have usually not caused people to stop taking MERIDIA. If you develop a symptom that you think might be a side effect, stop taking MERIDIA and notify your doctor immediately so he or she can advise you on what to do.

Can MERIDIA affect blood pressure or heart rate?

MERIDIA SUBSTANTIALLY INCREASES BLOOD PRESSURE IN SOME PATIENTS. REGULAR MONITORING OF BLOOD PRESSURE IS REQUIRED WHEN TAKING MERIDIA.

On average, small increases in blood pressure and small increases in heart rate were seen in overweight people who took MERIDIA in scientifically controlled studies. You should make sure you see your doctor as directed for regular follow-up visits. Your blood pressure and pulse should be measured prior to starting therapy with MERIDIA and should be monitored at regular intervals thereafter. If you experience an increase in blood pressure or heart rate while taking MERIDIA, your doctor may decide to decrease the dose or discontinue MERIDIA.

If you have high blood pressure that is controlled by medication or diet, your doctor may choose to prescribe MERIDIA for you as part of a comprehensive weight-management program. MERIDIA should not be taken by people who have uncontrolled or poorly controlled high blood pressure.

Are there any severe side effects?

Certain weight-loss drugs have been associated with pulmonary hypertension (PPH), a rare but sometimes fatal disease. In clinical studies, no cases of PPH have been reported with MERIDIA. Because this disease is so rare, however, it is not known whether or not MERIDIA may cause this disease.

The first symptom of PPH is usually shortness of breath. If you experience new or worsening shortness of breath, or if you experience chest pain, fainting, or swelling of your feet, ankles, or legs, stop taking MERIDIA, and notify your doctor immediately.

Does MERIDIA cause damage to the heart valves?

Certain weight-loss drugs have been associated with cardiac valve dysfunction (heart valve disease). Patients in two studies were examined by doctors who used cardiac ultrasound testing to carefully look at heart valve structure and function. In one study, 25 patients were examined before treatment with MERIDIA and again after three months of treatment. None of the patients had heart valve disease. In another study, patients who had received either MERIDIA or placebo (sugar pills) for periods of two weeks to 16 months were examined. Three out of 132 patients (2.3%) who had taken MERIDIA and two out of 77 patients (2.6%) who had taken placebo were found to have heart valve disease. You should discuss this further with your doctor.

Will MERIDIA change the way I need to take my nutritional supplements?

Non-drug nutritional supplements, like vitamins, minerals and amino acids (with the exception of tryptophan) can be used along with MERIDIA. You should make sure your doctor knows what nutritional supplements you are taking and why you are taking them. You should not take MERIDIA if you are taking tryptophan. You should not use herbal or over-the-counter weight-loss products while taking MERIDIA.

What about drinking alcoholic beverages?

MERIDIA may increase the sedative effects of alcohol. It is important that you let your doctor know how often, and what type of alcoholic beverages you drink. Your doctor can advise you best as to whether you should drink alcoholic beverages while on MERIDIA.

What about drinking coffee, tea and caffeinated beverages?

MERIDIA can be safely taken with moderate use of coffee, tea or caffeinated beverages. You should check with your doctor to make sure that you do not have a medical condition that can be aggravated by these beverages independent of being on MERIDIA. You should check with your doctor if you consume a great deal of caffeinated beverages or use over-the-counter pills that contain caffeine.

What if I develop allergic reactions?

Stop taking MERIDIA and notify your doctor immediately if you develop a skin rash, hives or other allergic reactions.

What if I am pregnant or nursing?

MERIDIA should not be used by pregnant women or nursing mothers. You should notify your doctor immediately if you become pregnant or plan to become pregnant.

What about sexual activity and potential pregnancy?

Women of child bearing potential should use an effective birth control method while taking MERIDIA. Check with your doctor to make sure you are on a medically safe and effective birth control method while taking MERIDIA.

Will MERIDIA affect the effectiveness of birth control pills?

No.

What about driving a car or dangerous work activities?

MERIDIA should not interfere with your ability to drive your car. However, you should be on the alert for any signs of fatigue, sedation, or lack of alertness. You should be very careful about using alcohol before you drive as MERIDIA may increase the sedative effects of alcohol.

MERIDIA was studied in healthy people and did not affect their coordination or impair their judgment. However, MERIDIA has the potential to impair judgment, thinking, coordination or motor skills. You should check with your doctor if you have any questions with regard to your work and the use of MERIDIA.

How should I keep and use MERIDIA?

MERIDIA should be stored at normal room temperature (about 60 to 85°F). Never leave MERIDIA in hot or moist places.

It is important to keep MERIDIA in a safe area where children cannot get it.

If your child swallows MERIDIA, immediately speak with your doctor and/or take your child to the emergency room for immediate medical attention. If you are unable to reach a doctor or emergency room, call the poison control center at 1-800-764-7661.

Never take more MERIDIA than prescribed by your doctor. You should never share MERIDIA with a friend.

SAVE THIS PATIENT INFORMATION SHEET ON MERIDIA. YOU SHOULD KEEP THIS SHEET TO REFER BACK TO FROM TIME TO TIME. KEEP IT IN A SAFE PLACE WHERE YOU CAN FIND IT. YOU MAY WISH TO BRING THIS SHEET WITH YOU EVERY TIME YOU VISIT YOUR DOCTOR. IT MAY HELP YOU WITH YOUR DISCUSSIONS WITH YOUR DOCTOR.

The brands listed, with the exception of MERIDIA, are trademarks of their respective owners and are not trademarks of Abbott Laboratories. The makers of these brands are not affiliated with and do not endorse Abbott Laboratories or its products.

Sibutramine is covered by US Patent Nos 4,746,680; 4,929,629; and 5,436,272.

This patient information sheet is intended for information only. It is not a substitute for your doctor's instructions. Notify your doctor immediately of any questions or concerns. Never take extra doses of MERIDIA.

For additional information on MERIDIA and weight management, please talk with your doctor, nurse, pharmacist, other health care professional or call 1-800-633-9110.

Revised: October, 2003

Continued on next page

Meridia—Cont.

03-5309-R4
Manufactured by Abbott Laboratories
North Chicago, IL 60064, U.S.A.
or
for Abbott Laboratories
by BASF Corporation,
Mount Olive, NJ 07828, U.S.A.
Product of United Kingdom
ABBOTT LABORATORIES
NORTH CHICAGO, IL 60064, U.S.A.
Printed in USA

Shown in Product Identification Guide, page 303

NORVIR® ℞

[*nŏr-vĭr*]
(ritonavir capsules) Soft Gelatin
(ritonavir oral solution)
℞ only

WARNING
CO-ADMINISTRATION OF NORVIR WITH CERTAIN NONSEDATING ANTIHISTAMINES, SEDATIVE HYPNOTICS, ANTIARRHYTHMICS, OR ERGOT ALKALOID PREPARATIONS MAY RESULT IN POTENTIALLY SERIOUS AND/OR LIFE-THREATENING ADVERSE EVENTS DUE TO POSSIBLE EFFECTS OF NORVIR ON THE HEPATIC METABOLISM OF CERTAIN DRUGS. SEE **CONTRAINDICATIONS** AND **PRECAUTIONS** SECTIONS.

DESCRIPTION

NORVIR (ritonavir) is an inhibitor of HIV protease with activity against the Human Immunodeficiency Virus (HIV). Ritonavir is chemically designated as 10-Hydroxy-2-methyl-5-(1-methylethyl)-1-[2-(1-methylethyl)-4-thiazolyl]-3,6-dioxo-8,11-bis(phenylmethyl)-2,4,7,12-tetraazatridecan-13-oic acid, 5-thiazolylmethyl ester, [5S-(5R*,8R*,10R*,11R*)]. Its molecular formula is $C_{37}H_{48}N_6O_5S_2$, and its molecular weight is 720.95. Ritonavir has the following structural formula:

Ritonavir is a white-to-light-tan powder. Ritonavir has a bitter metallic taste. It is freely soluble in methanol and ethanol, soluble in isopropanol and practically insoluble in water.

NORVIR soft gelatin capsules are available for oral administration in a strength of 100 mg ritonavir with the following inactive ingredients: Butylated hydroxytoluene, ethanol, gelatin, iron oxide, oleic acid, polyoxyl 35 castor oil, and titanium dioxide.

NORVIR oral solution is available for oral administration as 80 mg/mL of ritonavir in a peppermint and caramel flavored vehicle. Each 8-ounce bottle contains 19.2 grams of ritonavir. NORVIR oral solution also contains ethanol, water, polyoxyl 35 castor oil, propylene glycol, anhydrous citric acid to adjust pH, saccharin sodium, peppermint oil, creamy caramel flavoring, and FD&C Yellow No. 6.

CLINICAL PHARMACOLOGY

Microbiology

Mechanism of action: Ritonavir is a peptidomimetic inhibitor of both the HIV-1 and HIV-2 proteases. Inhibition of HIV protease renders the enzyme incapable of processing the *gag-pol* polyprotein precursor which leads to production of non-infectious immature HIV particles.

Antiviral activity *in vitro*: The activity of ritonavir was assessed *in vitro* in acutely infected lymphoblastoid cell lines and in peripheral blood lymphocytes. The concentration of drug that inhibits 50% (EC_{50}) of viral replication ranged from 3.8 to 153 nM depending upon the HIV-1 isolate and the cells employed. The average EC_{50} for low passage clinical isolates was 22 nM (n=13). In MT_4 cells, ritonavir demonstrated additive effects against HIV-1 in combination with either zidovudine (ZDV) or didanosine (ddI). Studies which measured cytotoxicity of ritonavir on several cell lines showed that >20 μM was required to inhibit cellular growth by 50% resulting in an *in vitro* therapeutic index of at least 1000.

Resistance: HIV-1 isolates with reduced susceptibility to ritonavir have been selected *in vitro*. Genotypic analysis of these isolates showed mutations in the HIV protease gene at amino acid positions 84 (Ile to Val), 82 (Val to Phe), 71 (Ala to Val), and 46 (Met to Ile). Phenotypic (n=18) and genotypic (n=44) changes in HIV isolates from selected patients treated with ritonavir were monitored in phase I/II trials over a period of 3 to 32 weeks. Mutations associated with the HIV viral protease in isolates obtained from 41 patients appeared to occur in a stepwise and ordered fashion; in sequence, these mutations were position 82 (Val to Ala/Phe), 54 (Ile to Val), 71 (Ala to Val/Thr), and 36 (Ile to Leu), followed by combinations of mutations at an additional 5 specific amino acid positions. Of 18 patients for which both phenotypic and genotypic analysis were performed on free virus isolated from plasma, 12 showed reduced susceptibility to ritonavir *in vitro*. All 18 patients possessed one or more mutations in the viral protease gene. The 82 mutation appeared to be necessary but not sufficient to confer phenotypic resistance. Phenotypic resistance was defined as a ≥5-fold decrease in viral sensitivity *in vitro* from baseline. The clinical relevance of phenotypic and genotypic changes associated with ritonavir therapy has not been established.

Cross-resistance to other antiretrovirals: Among protease inhibitors variable cross-resistance has been recognized. Serial HIV isolates obtained from six patients during ritonavir therapy showed a decrease in ritonavir susceptibility *in vitro* but did not demonstrate a concordant decrease in susceptibility to saquinavir *in vitro* when compared to matched baseline isolates. However, isolates from two of these patients demonstrated decreased susceptibility to indinavir *in vitro* (8-fold). Isolates from 5 patients were also tested for cross-resistance to amprenavir and nelfinavir; isolates from 2 patients had a decrease in susceptibility to nelfinavir (12- to 14-fold), and none to amprenavir. Cross-resistance between ritonavir and reverse transcriptase inhibitors is unlikely because of the different enzyme targets involved. One ZDV-resistant HIV isolate tested *in vitro* retained full susceptibility to ritonavir.

Pharmacokinetics

The pharmacokinetics of ritonavir have been studied in healthy volunteers and HIV-infected patients (CD_4 ≥ 50 cells/μL). See Table 1 for ritonavir pharmacokinetic characteristics.

Absorption: The absolute bioavailability of ritonavir has not been determined. After a 600 mg dose of oral solution, peak concentrations of ritonavir were achieved approximately 2 hours and 4 hours after dosing under fasting and non-fasting (514 KCal; 9% fat, 12% protein, and 79% carbohydrate) conditions, respectively.

Effect of Food on Oral Absorption: When the oral solution was given under non-fasting conditions, peak ritonavir concentrations decreased 23% and the extent of absorption decreased 7% relative to fasting conditions. Dilution of the oral solution, within one hour of administration, with 240 mL of chocolate milk, Advera® or Ensure® did not significantly affect the extent and rate of ritonavir absorption. After a single 600 mg dose under non-fasting conditions, in two separate studies, the soft gelatin capsule (n=57) and oral solution (n=18) formulations yielded mean ± SD areas under the plasma concentration-time curve (AUCs) of 121.7 ± 53.8 and 129.0 ± 39.3 μg•h/mL, respectively. Relative to fasting conditions, the extent of absorption of ritonavir from the soft gelatin capsule formulation was 13% higher when administered with a meal (615 KCal; 14.5% fat, 9% protein, and 76% carbohydrate).

Metabolism: Nearly all of the plasma radioactivity after a single oral 600 mg dose of ^{14}C-ritonavir oral solution (n=5) was attributed to unchanged ritonavir. Five ritonavir metabolites have been identified in human urine and feces. The isopropylthiazole oxidation metabolite (M-2) is the major metabolite and has antiviral activity similar to that of parent drug; however, the concentrations of this metabolite in plasma are low. *In vitro* studies utilizing human liver microsomes have demonstrated that cytochrome P450 3A (CYP3A) is the major isoform involved in ritonavir metabolism, although CYP2D6 also contributes to the formation of M-2.

Elimination: In a study of five subjects receiving a 600 mg dose of ^{14}C-ritonavir oral solution, 11.3 ± 2.8% of the dose was excreted into the urine, with 3.5 ± 1.8% of the dose excreted as unchanged parent drug. In that study, 86.4 ± 2.9% of the dose was excreted in the feces with 33.8 ± 10.8% of the dose excreted as unchanged parent drug. Upon multiple dosing, ritonavir accumulation is less than predicted from a single dose possibly due to a time and dose-related increase in clearance.

[See table 1 above]

Table 1
Ritonavir Pharmacokinetic Characteristics

Parameter	n	Values (Mean ± SD)
C_{max} SS†	10	11.2 ± 3.6 μg/mL
C_{trough} SS†	10	3.7 ± 2.6 μg/mL
V_β/F‡	91	0.41 ± 0.25 L/kg
$t_{1/2}$		3 – 5 h
CL/F SS†	10	8.8 ± 3.2 L/h
CL/F‡	91	4.6 ± 1.6 L/h
CL_R	62	<0.1 L/h
RBC/Plasma Ratio		0.14
Percent Bound*		98 to 99%

† SS = steady state; patients taking ritonavir 600 mg q12h.
‡ Single ritonavir 600 mg dose.
* Primarily bound to human serum albumin and alpha-1 acid glycoprotein over the ritonavir concentration range of 0.01 to 30 μg/mL.

Special Populations:

Gender, Race and Age: No age-related pharmacokinetic differences have been observed in adult patients (18 to 63 years). Ritonavir pharmacokinetics have not been studied in older patients. A study of ritonavir pharmacokinetics in healthy males and females showed no statistically significant differences in the pharmacokinetics of ritonavir. Pharmacokinetic differences due to race have not been identified.

Pediatric Patients: The pharmacokinetic profile of ritonavir in pediatric patients below the age of 2 years has not been established. Steady-state pharmacokinetics were evaluated in 37 HIV-infected patients ages 2 to 14 years receiving doses ranging from 250 mg/m^2 b.i.d. to 400 mg/m^2 b.i.d. Across dose groups, ritonavir steady-state oral clearance (CL/F/m^2) was approximately 1.5 times faster in pediatric patients than in adult subjects. Ritonavir concentrations obtained after 350 to 400 mg/m^2 twice daily in pediatric patients were comparable to those obtained in adults receiving 600 mg (approximately 330 mg/m^2) twice daily.

Renal Insufficiency: Ritonavir pharmacokinetics have not been studied in patients with renal insufficiency, however, since renal clearance is negligible, a decrease in total body clearance is not expected in patients with renal insufficiency.

Hepatic Insufficiency: Dose-normalized steady-state ritonavir concentrations in subjects with mild hepatic insufficiency (400 mg BID, n=6) were similar to those in control subjects dosed with 500 mg BID. Dose-normalized steady-state ritonavir exposures in subjects with moderate hepatic impairment (400 mg BID, n=6) were about 40% lower than those in subjects with normal hepatic function (500 mg BID, n=6). Protein binding of ritonavir was not statistically significantly affected by mild or moderately impaired hepatic function. No dose adjustment is recommended in patients with mild or moderate hepatic impairment. However, health care providers should be aware of potential for lower ritonavir concentrations in patients with moderate hepatic impairment and should monitor patient response carefully. Ritonavir has not been studied in patients with severe hepatic impairment.

Drug-Drug Interactions: See also **CONTRAINDICATIONS, WARNINGS**, and **PRECAUTIONS: Drug Interactions.**

Tables 2 and 3 summarize the effects on AUC and C_{max}, with 95% confidence intervals (95% CI), of co-administration of ritonavir with a variety of drugs. For information about clinical recommendations see **PRECAUTIONS-Drug Interactions.**

[See tables 2 and 3 on next page]

INDICATIONS AND USAGE

NORVIR is indicated in combination with other antiretroviral agents for the treatment of HIV-infection. This indication is based on the results from a study in patients with advanced HIV disease that showed a reduction in both mortality and AIDS-defining clinical events for patients who received NORVIR either alone or in combination with nucleoside analogues. Median duration of follow-up in this study was 13.5 months.

Description of Clinical Studies

The activity of NORVIR as monotherapy or in combination with nucleoside analogues has been evaluated in 1446 patients enrolled in two double-blind, randomized trials.

Advanced Patients with Prior Antiretroviral Therapy

Study 247 was a randomized, double-blind trial (with open-label follow-up) conducted in HIV-infected patients with at least nine months of prior antiretroviral therapy and baseline CD_4 cell counts ≤ 100 cells/μL. NORVIR 600 mg b.i.d. or placebo was added to each patient's baseline antiretroviral therapy regimen, which could have consisted of up to two approved antiretroviral agents. The study accrued 1090 patients, with mean baseline CD_4 cell count at study entry of 32 cells/μL. After the clinical benefit of NORVIR therapy was demonstrated, all patients were eligible to switch to open-label NORVIR for the duration of the follow-up period. Median duration of double-blind therapy with NORVIR and placebo was 6 months. The median duration of follow-up through the end of the open-label phase was 13.5 months for patients randomized to NORVIR and 14 months for patients randomized to placebo.

The cumulative incidence of clinical disease progression or death during the double-blind phase of Study 247 was 26% for patients initially randomized to NORVIR compared to

42% for patients initially randomized to placebo. This difference in rates was statistically significant (see Figure 1). [See figure 1 at top of third column]

The cumulative mortality through the end of the open-label follow-up phase for patients enrolled in Study 247 was 18% for patients initially randomized to NORVIR compared to 26% for patients initially randomized to placebo. This difference in rates was statistically significant (see Figure 2). Since the analysis at the end of the open-label phase includes patients in the placebo arm who were switched from

Table 2: Drug Interactions: Pharmacokinetic Parameters for Ritonavir in the Presence of the Co-administered Drug (See Precautions, Table 6 for Recommended Alterations in the Dose or Regimen)

Co-administered Drug	Dose of Co-administered Drug (mg)	Dose of NORVIR (mg)	n	AUC % (95% CI)	C_{max} (95% CI)
Clarithromycin	500 q12h, 4 d	200 q8h, 4 d	22	↑ 12% (2, 23%)	↑ 15% (2, 28%)
Didanosine	200 q12h, 4 d	600 q12h, 4 d	12	↔	↔
Fluconazole	400 single dose, day 1; 200 daily, 4 d	200 q6h, 4 d	8	↑ 12% (5, 20%)	↑ 15% (7, 22%)
Fluoxetine	30 q12h, 8 d	600 single dose, 1 d	16	↑ 19% (7, 34%)	↔
Ketoconazole	200 daily, 7 d	500 q12h, 10 d	12	↑ 18% (-3, 52%)	↑ 10% (-11, 36%)
Rifampin	600 or 300 daily, 10 d	500 q12h, 20 d	7, 9*	↓ 35% (7, 55%)	↓ 25% (-5, 46%)
Zidovudine	200 q8h, 4 d	300 q6h, 4 d	10	↔	↔

Table 3: Drug Interactions: Pharmacokinetic Parameters for Co-administered Drug in the Presence of NORVIR (See Precautions, Table 6 for Recommended Alterations in Dose or Regimen)

Co-administered Drug	Dose of Co-administered Drug (mg)	Dose of NORVIR (mg)	n	AUC % (95% CI)	C_{max} (95% CI)
Alprazolam	1, single dose	500 q12h, 10 d	12	↓ 12% (-5, 30%)	↓ 16% (5, 27%)
Clarithromycin 14–OH clarithromycin metabolite	500 q12h, 4 d	200 q8h, 4 d	22	↑ 77% (56, 103%) ↓ 100%	↑ 31% (15, 51%) ↓ 99%
Desipramine 2–OH desipramine metabolite	100, single dose	500 q12h, 12 d	14	↑ 145% (103, 211%) ↓ 15% (3, 26%)	↑ 22% (12, 35%) ↓ 67% (62, 72%)
Didanosine	200 q12h, 4 d	600 q12h, 4 d	12	↓ 13% (0, 23%)	↓ 16% (5, 26%)
Ethinyl estradiol	50 µg single dose	500 q12h, 16 d	23	↓ 40% (31, 49%)	↓ 32% (24, 39%)
Indinavir[1] Day 14 Day 15	400 q12h, 15 d	400 q12h, 15 d	10	 ↑ 6% (-14, 29%) ↓ 7% (-25, 16%)	 ↓ 51% (40, 61%) ↓ 62% (52, 70%)
Ketoconazole	200 daily, 7 d	500 q12h, 10 d	12	↑ 3.4-fold (2.8, 4.3X)	↑ 55% (40, 72%)
Meperidine Normeperidine metabolite	50 oral single dose	500 q12h, 10 d	8 6	↓ 62% (59, 65%) ↑ 47% (-24, 345%)	↓ 59% (42, 72%) ↑ 87% (42, 147%)
Methadone[2]	5, single dose	500 q12h, 15 d	11	↓ 36% (16, 52%)	↓ 38% (28, 46%)
Rifabutin 25-O-desacetyl rifabutin metabolite	150 daily, 16 d	500 q12h, 10 d	5, 11*	↑ 4-fold (2.8, 6.1X) ↑ 35-fold (25, 78X)	↑ 2.5-fold (1.9, 3.4X) ↑ 16-fold (14, 20X)
Saquinavir[3]	400 BID steady-state	400 BID steady-state	7	↑ 17-fold (9, 31X)	↑ 14-fold (7, 28X)
Sildenafil	100, single dose	500 BID, 8 d	28	↑ 11-fold	↑ 4-fold
Sulfamethoxazole[4]	800, single dose	500 q12h, 12 d	15	↓ 20% (16, 23%)	↔
Theophylline	3 mg/kg q8h, 15 d	500 q12h, 10 d	13, 11*	↓ 43% (42, 45%)	↓ 32% (29, 34%)
Trimethoprim[4]	160, single dose	500 q12h, 12 d	15	↑ 20% (3, 43%)	↔
Warfarin S-Warfarin R-Warfarin	5, single dose	400 q12h, 12d	12	 ↑ 9% (-17, 44%)[5] ↓ 33% (-38, -27%)[5]	 ↓ 9% (-16, -2%)[5] ↔
Zidovudine	200 q8h, 4 d	300 q6h, 4 d	9	↓ 25% (15, 34%)	↓ 27% (4, 45%)

1 Ritonavir and indinavir were coadministered for 15 days; Day 14 doses were administered after a 15%-fat breakfast (757 Kcal) and 9%-fat evening snack (236 Kcal), and Day 15 doses were administered after a 15%-fat breakfast (757 Kcal) and 32%-fat dinner (815 Kcal). Indinavir C_{min} was also increased 4-fold. Effects were assessed relative to an indinavir 800 mg q8h regimen under fasting conditions.

2 Effects were assessed on a dose-normalized comparison to a methadone 20 mg single dose.

3 Comparison to a standard saquinavir HGC 600 mg t.i.d. regimen (n=114). Saquinavir C_{min} was 0.48 ± 0.36 µg/mL for 400/400 mg BID compared to below quantifiable limits for Saquinavir HGC 600 mg TID.

4 Sulfamethoxazole and trimethoprim taken as single combination tablet.

5 90% CI presented for R- and S-warfarin AUC and C_{max} ratios.

↑ Indicates increase.

↓ Indicates decrease.

↔ Indicates no change.

* Parallel group design; entries are subjects receiving combination and control regimens, respectively.

Figure 1
Time to Disease Progression or Death During the Double-Blind Phase of Study 247

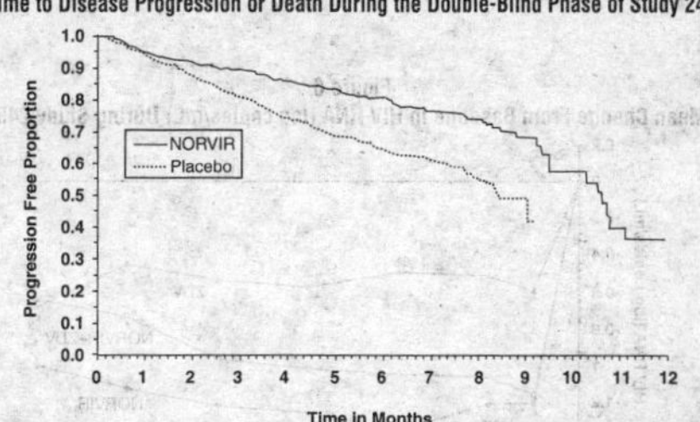

placebo to NORVIR therapy, the survival benefit of NORVIR cannot be precisely estimated.

Figure 2
Survival of Patients by Randomized Treatment Regimen in Study 247

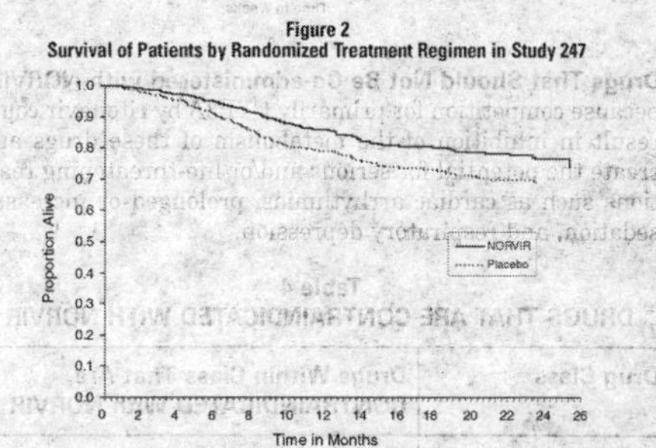

Figures 3 and 4 summarize the mean change from baseline for CD_4 cell count and plasma HIV RNA (copies/mL), respectively, during the first 24 weeks for the double-blind phase of Study 247.

Figure 3
Mean Change From Baseline in CD_4 Cell Count (cells/µL) During the Double-Blind Phase of Study 247

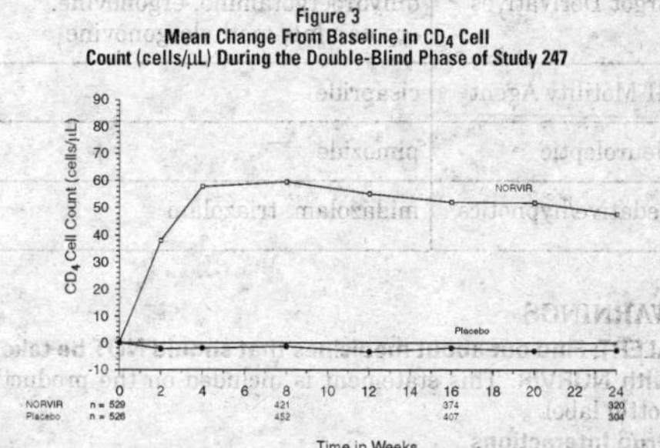

Figure 4
Mean Change From Baseline in HIV RNA (log copies/mL) During the Double-Blind Phase of Study 247

Patients Without Prior Antiretroviral Therapy

In Study 245, 356 antiretroviral-naive HIV-infected patients (mean baseline CD_4 = 364 cells/µL) were randomized to receive either NORVIR 600 mg b.i.d., zidovudine 200 mg t.i.d., or a combination of these drugs. Figures 5 and 6 summarize the mean change from baseline for CD_4 cell count and plasma HIV RNA (copies/mL), respectively, during the first 24 weeks for the double-blind phase of Study 245.

Figure 5
Mean Change From Baseline in CD_4 Cell Count (cells/µL) During Study 245

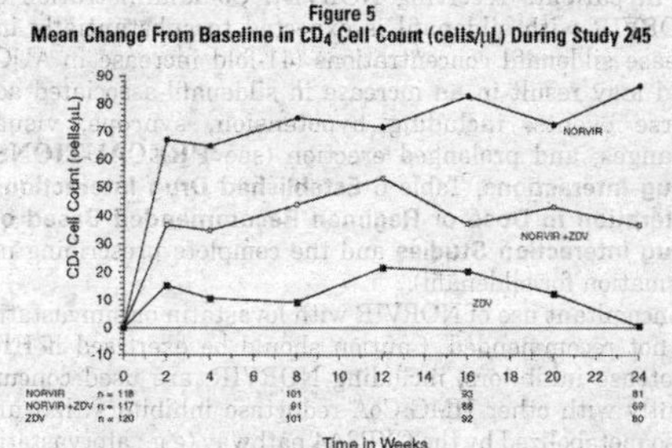

[See figure 6 at top of next column]

CONTRAINDICATIONS

NORVIR is contraindicated in patients with known hypersensitivity to ritonavir or any of its ingredients.

Co-administration of NORVIR is contraindicated with the drugs listed in Table 4 (also see **PRECAUTIONS** Table 5:

Continued on next page

Norvir—Cont.

Figure 6
Mean Change From Baseline in HIV RNA (log copies/mL) During Study 245

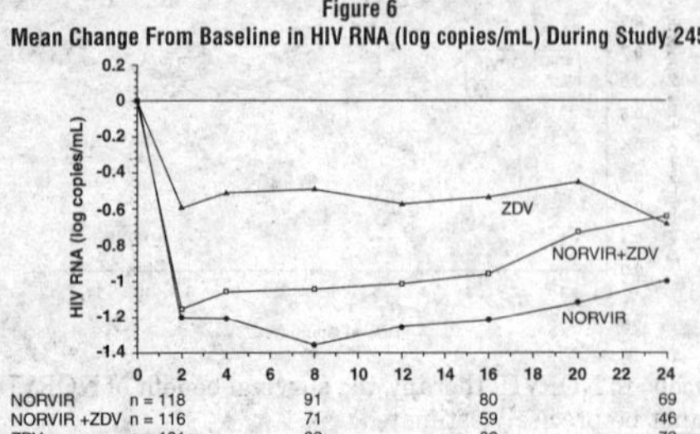

Drugs That Should Not Be Co-administered with NORVIR) because competition for primarily CYP3A by ritonavir could result in inhibition of the metabolism of these drugs and create the potential for serious and/or life-threatening reactions such as cardiac arrhythmias, prolonged or increased sedation, and respiratory depression.

Table 4
DRUGS THAT ARE CONTRAINDICATED WITH NORVIR

Drug Class	Drugs Within Class That Are CONTRAINDICATED With NORVIR
Antiarrhythmics	amiodarone, bepridil, flecainide, propafenone, quinidine
Antihistamines	astemizole, terfenadine
Ergot Derivatives	dihydroergotamine, ergonovine, ergotamine, methylergonovine
GI Motility Agent	cisapride
Neuroleptic	pimozide
Sedative/hypnotics	midazolam, triazolam

WARNINGS

ALERT: Find out about medicines that should NOT be taken with NORVIR. This statement is included on the product's bottle label.

Drug Interactions

Ritonavir is an inhibitor of cytochrome P450 3A (CYP3A) both *in vitro* and *in vivo*. Ritonavir also inhibits CYP2D6 *in vitro*, but to a lesser extent than CYP3A. Co-administration of ritonavir and drugs primarily metabolized by CYP3A or CYP2D6 may result in increased plasma concentrations of other drugs that could increase or prolong its therapeutic and adverse effects (see **Pharmacokinetics: Drug-Drug Interactions, CONTRAINDICATIONS** – Table 4 **Drugs That Are Contraindicated with NORVIR, PRECAUTIONS** – Table 5 **Drugs That Should Not Be Co-administered with NORVIR,** Table 6 **Established Drug Interactions and** Tables 7 and 8 **Predicted Drug Interactions: Use with Caution**).

The magnitude of the interactions and therapeutic consequences between ritonavir and the drugs listed in Tables 7 and 8 **Predicted Drug Interactions: Use With Caution** cannot be predicted with any certainty. When co-administering ritonavir with any agent listed in Tables 7 and 8 **Predicted Drug Interactions: Use With Caution,** special attention is warranted. Refer to **PRECAUTIONS**: **Established Drug Interactions** and **Predicted Drug Interactions** for additional information.

Cardiac and neurologic events have been reported with ritonavir when co-administered with disopyramide, mexiletine, nefazodone, fluoxetine and beta blockers. The possibility of drug interaction cannot be excluded.

Particular caution should be used when prescribing sildenafil in patients receiving NORVIR. Co-administration of NORVIR with sildenafil is expected to substantially increase sildenafil concentrations (11-fold increase in AUC) and may result in an increase in sildenafil-associated adverse events, including hypotension, syncope, visual changes, and prolonged erection (see **PRECAUTIONS: Drug Interactions,** Table 6 **Established Drug Interactions: Alteration in Dose or Regimen Recommended Based on Drug Interaction Studies** and the complete prescribing information for sildenafil).

Concomitant use of NORVIR with lovastatin or simvastatin is not recommended. Caution should be exercised if HIV protease inhibitors, including NORVIR, are used concurrently with other HMG-CoA reductase inhibitors that are also metabolized by the CYP3A4 pathway (e.g., atorvastatin or cerivastatin). The risk of myopathy including rhabdomyolysis may be increased when HIV protease inhibitors, including NORVIR, are used in combination with these drugs.

Concomitant use of NORVIR, and St. John's wort (hypericum perforatum) or products containing St. John's wort is not recommended. Coadministration of protease inhibitors, including NORVIR, with St. John's wort is expected to substantially decrease protease inhibitor concentrations and may result in sub-optimal levels of NORVIR and lead to loss of virologic response and possible resistance to NORVIR or to the class of protease inhibitors.

Allergic Reactions

Allergic reactions including urticaria, mild skin eruptions, bronchospasm, and angioedema have been reported. Rare cases of anaphylaxis and Stevens-Johnson syndrome have also been reported.

Hepatic Reactions

Hepatic transaminase elevations exceeding 5 times the upper limit of normal, clinical hepatitis, and jaundice have occurred in patients receiving NORVIR alone or in combination with other antiretroviral drugs (see Table 10). There may be an increased risk for transaminase elevations in patients with underlying hepatitis B or C. Therefore, caution should be exercised when administering NORVIR to patients with pre-existing liver diseases, liver enzyme abnormalities, or hepatitis. Increased AST/ALT monitoring should be considered in these patients, especially during the first three months of NORVIR treatment.

There have been postmarketing reports of hepatic dysfunction, including some fatalities. These have generally occurred in patients taking multiple concomitant medications and/or with advanced AIDS.

Pancreatitis

Pancreatitis has been observed in patients receiving NORVIR therapy, including those who developed hypertriglyceridemia. In some cases fatalities have been observed. Patients with advanced HIV disease may be at increased risk of elevated triglycerides and pancreatitis.

Pancreatitis should be considered if clinical symptoms (nausea, vomiting, abdominal pain) or abnormalities in laboratory values (such as increased serum lipase or amylase values) suggestive of pancreatitis should occur. Patients who exhibit these signs or symptoms should be evaluated and NORVIR therapy should be discontinued if a diagnosis of pancreatitis is made.

Diabetes Mellitus/Hyperglycemia

New onset diabetes mellitus, exacerbation of pre-existing diabetes mellitus, and hyperglycemia have been reported during postmarketing surveillance in HIV-infected patients receiving protease inhibitor therapy. Some patients required either initiation or dose adjustments of insulin or oral hypoglycemic agents for treatment of these events. In some cases, diabetic ketoacidosis has occurred. In those patients who discontinued protease inhibitor therapy, hyperglycemia persisted in some cases. Because these events have been reported voluntarily during clinical practice, estimates of frequency cannot be made and a causal relationship between protease inhibitor therapy and these events has not been established.

PRECAUTIONS

General

Ritonavir is principally metabolized by the liver. Therefore, caution should be exercised when administering this drug to patients with impaired hepatic function (see **WARNINGS** and **CLINICAL PHARMACOLOGY**: Hepatic Insufficiency).

Resistance/Cross-resistance

Varying degrees of cross-resistance among protease inhibitors have been observed. Continued administration of ritonavir therapy following loss of viral suppression may increase the likelihood of cross-resistance to other protease inhibitors (see **MICROBIOLOGY**).

Hemophilia

There have been reports of increased bleeding, including spontaneous skin hematomas and hemarthrosis, in patients with hemophilia type A and B treated with protease inhibitors. In some patients additional factor VIII was given. In more than half of the reported cases, treatment with protease inhibitors was continued or reintroduced. A causal relationship has not been established.

Fat Redistribution

Redistribution/accumulation of body fat including central obesity, dorsocervical fat enlargement (buffalo hump), peripheral wasting, facial wasting, breast enlargement, and "cushingoid appearance" have been observed in patients receiving antiretroviral therapy. The mechanism and long-term consequences of these events are currently unknown. A causal relationship has not been established.

Lipid Disorders

Treatment with NORVIR therapy alone or in combination with saquinavir has resulted in substantial increases in the concentration of total triglycerides and cholesterol. Triglyceride and cholesterol testing should be performed prior to initiating NORVIR therapy and at periodic intervals during therapy. Lipid disorders should be managed as clinically appropriate. See **PRECAUTIONS** Tables 5 and 7 for additional information on potential drug interactions with NORVIR and HMG CoA reductase inhibitors.

Information For Patients

A statement to patients and health care providers is included on the product's bottle label: **ALERT: Find out about medicines that should NOT be taken with NORVIR.** A Patient Package Insert (PPI) for Norvir is available for patient information.

Patients should be informed that NORVIR is not a cure for HIV infection and that they may continue to acquire illnesses associated with advanced HIV infection, including opportunistic infections.

Patients should be told that the long-term effects of NORVIR are unknown at this time. They should be informed that NORVIR therapy has not been shown to reduce the risk of transmitting HIV to others through sexual contact or blood contamination.

Patients should be advised to take NORVIR with food, if possible.

Patients should be informed to take NORVIR every day as prescribed. Patients should not alter the dose or discontinue NORVIR without consulting their doctor. If a dose is missed, patients should take the next dose as soon as possible. However, if a dose is skipped, the patient should not double the next dose.

Patients should be informed that redistribution or accumulation of body fat may occur in patients receiving antiretroviral therapy and that the cause and long term health effects of these conditions are not known at this time.

NORVIR may interact with some drugs; therefore, patients should be advised to report to their doctor the use of any other prescription, non-prescription medication or herbal products, particularly St. John's wort.

Laboratory Tests

Ritonavir has been shown to increase triglycerides, cholesterol, SGOT (AST), SGPT (ALT), GGT, CPK, and uric acid. Appropriate laboratory testing should be performed prior to initiating NORVIR therapy and at periodic intervals or if any clinical signs or symptoms occur during therapy. For comprehensive information concerning laboratory test alterations associated with nucleoside analogues, physicians should refer to the complete product information for each of these drugs.

Drug Interactions

Ritonavir has been found to be an inhibitor of cytochrome P450 3A (CYP3A) both *in vitro* and *in vivo* (Table 3). Agents that are extensively metabolized by CYP3A and have high first pass metabolism appear to be the most susceptible to large increases in AUC (>3-fold) when co-administered with ritonavir. Ritonavir also inhibits CYP2D6 to a lesser extent. Co-administration of substrates of CYP2D6 with ritonavir could result in increases (up to 2-fold) in the AUC of the other agent, possibly requiring a proportional dosage reduction. Ritonavir also appears to induce CYP3A as well as other enzymes, including glucuronosyl transferase, CYP1A2, and possibly CYP2C9.

Drugs that are contraindicated specifically due to the expected magnitude of interaction and potential for serious adverse events are listed both in **CONTRAINDICATIONS** Table 4 and under **Drugs That Should Not Be Co-administered with NORVIR** in Table 5.

Those drug interactions that have been established based on drug interaction studies are listed with the pharmacokinetic results in **CLINICAL PHARMACOLOGY,** Tables 2 and 3. The clinical recommendations based on the results of these studies are listed in Table 6 **Established Drug Interactions: Alteration in Dose or Regimen Recommended Based on Drug Interaction Studies.**

A systematic review of over 200 medications prescribed to HIV-infected patients was performed to identify potential drug interactions with ritonavir.[2] There are a number of agents in which CYP3A or CYP2D6 partially contribute to the metabolism of the agent. In these cases, the magnitude of the interaction and therapeutic consequences cannot be predicted with any certainty.

When co-administering ritonavir with calcium channel blockers, immunosuppressants, some HMG-CoA reductase inhibitors (see **WARNINGS, Drug Interactions**), some steroids, or other substrates of CYP3A, or most antidepressants, certain antiarrhythmics, and some narcotic analgesics which are partially mediated by CYP2D6 metabolism, it is possible that substantial increases in concentrations of these other agents may occur, possibly requiring a dosage reduction (>50%); examples are listed in Table 7 **Predicted Drug Interactions: Use With Caution, Dose Decrease May Be Needed.**

When co-administering ritonavir with any agent having a narrow therapeutic margin, such as anticoagulants, anticonvulsants, and antiarrhythmics, special attention is warranted. With some agents, the metabolism may be induced, resulting in decreased concentrations (see Table 8 **Predicted Drug Interactions: Use With Caution, Dose Increase May Be Needed**).

Table 5
Drugs That Should Not Be Co-administered with NORVIR

Drug Class: Drug Name	Clinical Comment
Antiarrhythmics: amiodarone, bepridil, flecainide, propafenone, quinidine	CONTRAINDICATED due to potential for serious and/or life threatening reactions such as cardiac arrhythmias.
Antihistamines: astemizole, terfenadine	CONTRAINDICATED due to potential for serious and/or life-threatening reactions such as cardiac arrhythmias.
Ergot Derivatives: dihydroergotamine, ergonovine, ergotamine, methylergonivine	CONTRAINDICATED due to potential for serious and/or life-threatening reactions such as acute ergot toxicity characterized by vasospasm and ischemia of the extremities and other tissues including the central nervous system.

GI Motility Agent: cisapride	CONTRAINDICATED due to potential for serious and/or life-threatening reactions such as cardiac arrhythmias.
Herbal Products: St. John's wort (hypericum perforatum)	May lead to loss of virologic response and possible resistance to NORVIR or to the class of protease inhibitors.
HMG-CoA Reductase Inhibitors: lovastatin, simvastatin	Potential for serious reactions such as risk of myopathy including rhabdomyolysis.
Neuroleptic: pimozide	CONTRAINDICATED due to the potential for serious and/or life-threatening reactions such as cardiac arrhythmias.
Sedative/hypnotics: midazolam, triazolam	CONTRAINDICATED due to potential for serious and/or life-threatening reactions such as prolonged or increased sedation or respiratory depression.

[See table 6 at right]

Table 7: Predicted Drug Interactions: Use With Caution, Dose Decrease of Coadministered Drug May Be Needed (see WARNINGS)

Examples of Drugs in Which Plasma Concentrations May Be Increased By Co-Administration With NORVIR

Drug Class	Examples of Drugs
Analgesics, narcotic	tramadol, propoxyphene
Antiarrhythmics	disopyramide, lidocaine, mexilitine
Anticonvulsants	carbamazepine, clonazepam, ethosuximide
Antidepressants	bupropion, nefazodone, selective serotonin reuptake inhibitors (SSRIs), tricyclics
Antiemetics	dronabinol
Antifungals	itraconazole
Antiparasitics	quinine
β-blockers	metoprolol, timolol
Calcium channel blockers	diltiazem, nifedipine, verapamil
Hypolipidemics, HMG CoA reductase inhibitors[1]	atorvastatin[2]
Immunosuppressants	cyclosporine, tacrolimus, sirolimus (rapamycin)
Neuroleptics	perphenazine, risperidone, thioridazine
Sedative/hypnotics	clorazepate, diazepam, estazolam, flurazepam, zolpidem
Steroids	dexamethasone, fluticasone, prednisone
Stimulants	methamphetamine

[1] Coadministration with lovastatin and simvastatin is not recommended (see **WARNINGS, Drug Interactions**).
[2] Use lowest possible dose of atorvastatin with careful monitoring or consider HMG-CoA reductase inhibitor such as pravastatin or fluvastatin.

Table 8: Predicted Drug Interactions: Use With Caution, Dose Increase of Coadministered Drug May Be Needed (see WARNINGS)

Examples of Drugs in Which Plasma Concentrations May Be Decreased By Co-Administration With NORVIR

Anticonvulsants	phenytoin, divalproex, lamotrigine
Antiparasitics	atovaquone

Table 6: Established Drug Interactions: Alteration in Dose or Regimen Recommended Based on Drug Interaction Studies (see CLINICAL PHARMACOLOGY, Tables 2 and 3 for Magnitude or Interaction)

Concomitant Drug Class: Drug Name	Effect on Concentration of Ritonavir or Concomitant Drug	Clinical Comment
		HIV-Antiviral Agents
HIV Protease Inhibitor: indinavir	When co-administered with reduced doses of indinavir and ritonavir ↑ indinavir (↔ AUC, ↓ C_{max}, ↑ C_{min})	Alterations in concentrations are noted when reduced doses of indinavir are co-administered with NORVIR. Appropriate doses for this combination, with respect to efficacy and safety, have not been established
HIV Protease Inhibitor: saquinavir	When co-administered with reduced doses of saquinavir and ritonavir ↑ saquinavir (↑ AUC, ↑ C_{max}, ↑ C_{min})	When used in combination therapy for up to 24 weeks, doses of 400 mg b.i.d. of ritonavir and saquinavir were better tolerated than the higher doses of the combination. Saquinavir plasma concentrations achieved with Invirase® (saquinavir mesylate) (400 mg b.i.d.) and ritonavir (400 mg b.i.d.) are similar to those achieved with Fortovase™ (saquinavir) (400 mg b.i.d.) and ritonavir (400 mg b.i.d.)
Nucleoside Reverse Transcriptase Inhibitor: didanosine		Dosing of didanosine and ritonavir should be separated by 2.5 hours to avoid formulation incompatibility
		Other Agents
Anesthetic: meperidine	↓ meperidine/ ↑ normeperidine (metabolite)	Dosage increase and long-term use of meperidine with ritonavir are not recommended due to the increased concentrations of the metabolite normeperidine which has both analgesic activity and CNS stimulant activity (e.g., seizures)
Antialcoholics: disulfiram/metronidazole		Ritonavir formulations contain alcohol, which can produce disulfiram-like reactions when co-administered with disulfiram or other drugs that produce this reaction (e.g., metronidazole)
Anticoagulant: warfarin	↓ R-warfarin ↓ ↑ S-warfarin	Initial frequent monitoring of the INR during ritonavir and warfarin coadministration is indicated.
Antidepressant: desipramine	↑ desipramine	Dosage reduction and concentration monitoring of desipramine is recommended
Antifungal: ketoconazole	↑ ketoconazole	High doses of ketoconazole (>200 mg/day) are not recommended
Anti-infective: clarithromycin	↑ clarithromycin	For patients with renal impairment the following dosage adjustments should be considered: •For patients with CL_{CR} 30 to 60 mL/min the dose of clarithromycin should be reduced by 50%. •For patients with CL_{CR} <30 mL/min the dose of clarithromycin should be decreased by 75%. No dose adjustment for patients with normal renal function is necessary.
Antimycobacterial: rifabutin	↑ rifabutin and rifabutin metabolite	Dosage reduction of rifabutin by at least three-quarters of the usual dose of 300 mg/day is recommended (e.g., 150 mg every other day or three times a week). Further dosage reduction may be necessary
Antimycobacterial: rifampin	↓ ritonavir	May lead to loss of virologic response. Alternate antimycobacterial agents such as rifabutin should be considered (see Antimycobacterial: rifabutin, for dose reduction recommendations)
Bronchodilator: theophylline	↓ theophylline	Increased dosage of theophylline may be required; therapeutic monitoring should be considered
Erectile Dysfunction: sildenafil	↑ sildenafil	Sildenafil should not exceed a maximum single dose of 25 mg in a 48-hour period in patients receiving concomitant ritonavir therapy (see **WARNINGS**)
Narcotic Analgesic: methadone	↓ methadone	Dosage increase of methadone may be considered
Oral Contraceptive: ethinyl estradiol	↓ ethinyl estradiol	Dosage increase or alternate contraceptive measures should be considered

Carcinogenesis and Mutagenesis

Carcinogenicity studies in mice and rats have been carried out on ritonavir. In male mice, at levels of 50, 100 or 200 mg/kg/day, there was a dose dependent increase in the incidence of both adenomas and combined adenomas and carcinomas in the liver. Based on AUC measurements, the exposure at the high dose was approximately 0.3-fold for males that of the exposure in humans with the recommended therapeutic dose (600 mg BID). There were no carcinogenic effects seen in females at the dosages tested. The exposure at the high dose was approximately 0.6-fold for the females that of the exposure in humans. In rats dosed at levels of 7, 15 or 30 mg/kg/day there were no carcinogenic effects. In this study, the exposure at the high dose was approximately 6% that of the exposure in humans with the recommended therapeutic dose. Based on the exposures achieved in the animal studies, the significance of the observed effects is not known. However, ritonavir was found to be negative for mutagenic or clastogenic activity in a battery of *in vitro* and *in vivo* assays including the Ames bacterial reverse mutation assay using *S. typhimurium* and *E. coli*, the mouse lymphoma assay, the mouse micronucleus test and chromosomal aberration assays in human lymphocytes.

Pregnancy, Fertility, and Reproduction

Pregnancy Category B: Ritonavir produced no effects on fertility in rats at drug exposures approximately 40% (male) and 60% (female) of that achieved with the proposed therapeutic dose. Higher dosages were not feasible due to hepatic toxicity.

No treatment-related malformations were observed when ritonavir was administered to pregnant rats or rabbits. Developmental toxicity observed in rats (early resorptions, decreased fetal body weight and ossification delays and developmental variations) occurred at a maternally toxic dosage at an exposure equivalent to approximately 30% of that achieved with the proposed therapeutic dose. A slight increase in the incidence of cryptorchidism was also noted in rats at an exposure approximately 22% of that achieved with the proposed therapeutic dose.

Developmental toxicity observed in rabbits (resorptions, decreased litter size and decreased fetal weights) also

Continued on next page

Norvir—Cont.

occurred at a maternally toxic dosage equivalent to 1.8 times the proposed therapeutic dose based on a body surface area conversion factor.

There are, however, no adequate and well-controlled studies in pregnant women. Because animal reproduction studies are not always predictive of human response, this drug should be used during pregnancy only if clearly needed.

***Antiretroviral Pregnancy Registry*:** To monitor maternal-fetal outcomes of pregnant women exposed to NORVIR, an Antiretroviral Pregnancy Registry has been established. Physicians are encouraged to register patients by calling 1-800-258-4263.

Nursing Mothers: The Centers for Disease Control and Prevention recommend that HIV-infected mothers not breast-feed their infants to avoid risking postnatal transmission of HIV. It is not known whether ritonavir is secreted in human milk. Because of both the potential for HIV transmission and the potential for serious adverse reactions in nursing infants, mothers should be instructed **not to breast-feed if they are receiving NORVIR.**

Pediatric Use

The safety and pharmacokinetic profile of ritonavir in pediatric patients below the age of 2 years have not been established. In HIV-infected patients age 2 to 16 years, the adverse event profile seen during a clinical trial and post-marketing experience was similar to that for adult patients. The evaluation of the antiviral activity of ritonavir in pediatric patients in clinical trials is ongoing.

Geriatric Use

Clinical studies of NORVIR did not include sufficient numbers of subjects aged 65 and over to determine whether they respond differently from younger subjects. In general, dose selection for an elderly patient should be cautious, usually starting at the low end of the dosing range, reflecting the greater frequency of decreased hepatic, renal or cardiac function, and of concomitant disease or other drug therapy.

ADVERSE REACTIONS

The safety of NORVIR alone and in combination with nucleoside analogues was studied in 1270 patients. Table 9 lists treatment-emergent adverse events (at least possibly related and of at least moderate intensity) that occurred in 2% or greater of patients receiving NORVIR alone or in combination with nucleosides in Study 245 or Study 247 and in combination with saquinavir in ongoing study 462. In that study, 141 protease inhibitor-naive, HIV-infected patients with mean baseline CD_4 of 300 cells/µL were randomized to one of four regimens of NORVIR + saquinavir, including NORVIR 400 mg b.i.d. + saquinavir 400 mg b.i.d. Overall the most frequently reported clinical adverse events, other than asthenia, among patients receiving NORVIR were gastrointestinal and neurological disturbances including nausea, diarrhea, vomiting, anorexia, abdominal pain, taste perversion, and circumoral and peripheral paresthesias. Similar adverse event profiles were reported in patients receiving ritonavir in other trials.

[See table 9 below]

Adverse events occurring in less than 2% of patients receiving NORVIR in all phase II/phase III studies and considered at least possibly related or of unknown relationship to treatment and of at least moderate intensity are listed below by body system.

Body as a Whole: Abdomen enlarged, accidental injury, allergic reaction, back pain, cachexia, chest pain, chills, facial edema, facial pain, flu syndrome, hormone level altered, hypothermia, kidney pain, neck pain, neck rigidity, pelvic pain, photosensitivity reaction, and substernal chest pain.

Cardiovascular System: Cardiovascular disorder, cerebral ischemia, cerebral venous thrombosis, hypertension, hypotension, migraine, myocardial infarct, palpitation, peripheral vascular disorder, phlebitis, postural hypotension, tachycardia and vasospasm.

Digestive System: Abnormal stools, bloody diarrhea, cheilitis, cholestatic jaundice, colitis, dry mouth, dysphagia, eructation, esophageal ulcer, esophagitis, gastritis, gastroenteritis, gastrointestinal disorder, gastrointestinal hemorrhage, gingivitis, hepatic coma, hepatitis, hepatomegaly, hepatosplenomegaly, ileus, liver damage, melena, mouth ulcer, pancreatitis, pseudomembranous colitis, rectal disorder, rectal hemorrhage, sialadenitis, stomatitis, tenesmus, thirst, tongue edema, and ulcerative colitis.

Endocrine System: Adrenal cortex insufficiency and diabetes mellitus.

Hemic and Lymphatic System: Acute myeloblastic leukemia, anemia, ecchymosis, leukopenia, lymphadenopathy, lymphocytosis, myeloproliferative disorder, and thrombocytopenia.

Metabolic and Nutritional Disorders: Albuminuria, alcohol intolerance, avitaminosis, BUN increased, dehydration, edema, enzymatic abnormality, glycosuria, gout, hypercholesteremia, peripheral edema, and xanthomatosis.

Musculoskeletal System: Arthritis, arthrosis, bone disorder, bone pain, extraocular palsy, joint disorder, leg cramps, muscle cramps, muscle weakness, myositis, and twitching.

Nervous System: Abnormal dreams, abnormal gait, agitation, amnesia, aphasia, ataxia, coma, convulsion, dementia, depersonalization, diplopia, emotional lability, euphoria, grand mal convulsion, hallucinations, hyperesthesia, hyperkinesia, hypesthesia, incoordination, libido decreased, manic reaction, nervousness, neuralgia, neuropathy, paralysis, peripheral neuropathic pain, peripheral neuropathy, peripheral sensory neuropathy, personality disorder, sleep disorder, speech disorder, stupor, subdural hematoma, tremor, urinary retention, vertigo, and vestibular disorder.

Respiratory System: Asthma, bronchitis, dyspnea, epistaxis, hiccup, hypoventilation, increased cough, interstitial pneumonia, larynx edema, lung disorder, rhinitis, and sinusitis.

Skin and Appendages: Acne, contact dermatitis, dry skin, eczema, erythema multiforme, exfoliative dermatitis, folliculitis, fungal dermatitis, furunculosis, maculopapular rash, molluscum contagiosum, onychomycosis, pruritus, psoriasis, pustular rash, seborrhea, skin discoloration, skin disorder, skin hypertrophy, skin melanoma, urticaria, and vesiculobullous rash.

Special Senses: Abnormal electro-oculogram, abnormal electroretinogram, abnormal vision, amblyopia/blurred vision, blepharitis, conjunctivitis, ear pain, eye disorder, eye pain, hearing impairment, increased cerumen, iritis, parosmia, photophobia, taste loss, tinnitus, uveitis, visual field defect, and vitreous disorder.

Urogenital System: Acute kidney failure, breast pain, cystitis, dysuria, hematuria, impotence, kidney calculus, kidney failure, kidney function abnormal, kidney pain, menorrhagia, penis disorder, polyuria, urethritis, urinary frequency, urinary tract infection, and vaginitis.

Post-Marketing Experience: The following adverse events have been reported during post-marketing use of NORVIR. Because these reactions are reported voluntarily from a population of unknown size, it is not possible to reliably estimate their frequency or establish a causal relationship to NORVIR exposure.

Body as a whole: Dehydration, usually associated with gastrointestinal symptoms, and sometimes resulting in hypotension, syncope, or renal insufficiency has been reported. Syncope, orthostatic hypotension, and renal insufficiency have also been reported without known dehydration. Co-administration of ritonavir with ergotamine or dihydroergotamine has been associated with acute ergot toxicity characterized by vasospasm and ischemia of the extremities and other tissues including the central nervous system. Redistribution/accumulation of body fat has been reported (see **PRECAUTIONS, Fat Redistribution**).

Cardiovascular System: Cardiac and neurologic events have been reported when ritonavir has been co-administered with disopyramide, mexiletine, nefazodone, fluoxetine, and beta blockers. The possibility of drug interaction cannot be excluded.

Endocrine System: Cushing's syndrome and adrenal suppression have been reported when ritonavir, primarily at higher doses, has been co-administered with fluticasone propionate.

Hemic and Lyphatic System: There have been reports of increased bleeding in patients with hemophilia A or B (see **PRECAUTIONS, Hemophilia**).

Nervous System: There have been postmarketing reports of seizure. Also, see *Cardiovascular System*.

Laboratory Abnormalities

Table 10 shows the percentage of patients who developed marked laboratory abnormalities.

[See table 10 at top of next page]

OVERDOSAGE

Acute Overdosage

Human Overdose Experience: Human experience of acute overdose with NORVIR is limited. One patient in clinical trials took NORVIR 1500 mg/day for two days. The patient reported paresthesias which resolved after the dose was decreased. A post-marketing case of renal failure with eosinophilia has been reported with ritonavir overdose.

The approximate lethal dose was found to be greater than 20 times the related human dose in rats and 10 times the related human dose in mice.

Table 9
Percentage of Patients with Treatment-Emergent Adverse Events[1] of Moderate or Severe Intensity Occurring in ≥ 2% of Patients Receiving NORVIR

	Study 245 Naive Patients[2]			Study 247 Advanced Patients[3]		Study 462 PI-Naive Patients[4]
Adverse Events	NORVIR + ZDV n=116	NORVIR n=117	ZDV n=119	NORVIR n=541	Placebo n=545	NORVIR + Saquinavir n=141
Body as a Whole						
Abdominal Pain	5.2	6.0	5.9	8.3	5.1	2.1
Asthenia	28.4	10.3	11.8	15.3	6.4	16.3
Fever	1.7	0.9	1.7	5.0	2.4	0.7
Headache	7.8	6.0	6.7	6.5	5.7	4.3
Malaise	5.2	1.7	3.4	0.7	0.2	2.8
Pain (unspecified)	0.9	1.7	0.8	2.2	1.8	4.3
Cardiovascular						
Syncope	0.9	1.7	0.8	0.6	0.0	2.1
Vasodilation	3.4	1.7	0.8	1.7	0.0	3.5
Digestive						
Anorexia	8.6	1.7	4.2	7.8	4.2	4.3
Constipation	3.4	0.0	0.8	0.2	0.4	1.4
Diarrhea	25.0	15.4	2.5	23.3	7.9	22.7
Dyspepsia	2.6	0.0	1.7	5.9	1.5	0.7
Fecal Incontinence	0.0	0.0	0.0	0.0	0.0	2.8
Flatulence	2.6	0.9	1.7	1.7	0.7	3.5
Local Throat Irritation	0.9	1.7	0.8	2.8	0.4	1.4
Nausea	46.6	25.6	26.1	29.8	8.4	18.4
Vomiting	23.3	13.7	12.6	17.4	4.4	7.1
Metabolic and Nutritional						
Weight Loss	0.0	0.0	0.0	2.4	1.7	0.0
Musculoskeletal						
Arthralgia	0.0	0.0	0.0	1.7	0.7	2.1
Myalgia	1.7	1.7	0.8	2.4	1.1	2.1
Nervous						
Anxiety	0.9	0.0	0.8	1.7	0.9	2.1
Circumoral Paresthesia	5.2	3.4	0.0	6.7	0.4	6.4
Confusion	0.0	0.9	0.0	0.6	0.6	2.1
Depression	1.7	1.7	2.5	1.7	0.7	7.1
Dizziness	5.2	2.6	3.4	3.9	1.1	8.5
Insomnia	3.4	2.6	0.8	2.0	1.8	2.8
Paresthesia	5.2	2.6	0.0	3.0	0.4	2.1
Peripheral Paresthesia	0.0	6.0	0.8	5.0	1.1	5.7
Somnolence	2.6	2.6	0.0	2.4	0.2	0.0
Thinking Abnormal	2.6	0.0	0.8	0.9	0.4	0.7
Respiratory						
Pharyngitis	0.9	2.6	0.0	0.4	0.4	1.4
Skin and Appendages						
Rash	0.9	0.0	0.8	3.5	1.5	0.7
Sweating	3.4	2.6	1.7	1.7	1.1	2.8
Special Senses						
Taste Perversion	17.2	11.1	8.4	7.0	2.2	5.0
Urogenital						
Nocturia	0.0	0.0	0.0	0.2	0.0	2.8

[1] Includes those adverse events at least possibly related to study drug or of unknown relationship and excludes concurrent HIV conditions.
[2] The median duration of treatment for patients randomized to regimens containing NORVIR in Study 245 was 9.1 months.
[3] The median duration of treatment for patients randomized to regimens containing NORVIR in Study 247 was 9.4 months.
[4] The median duration of treatment for patients in ongoing Study 462 was 48 weeks.

Table 10
Percentage of Patients, by Study and Treatment Group, with Chemistry and Hematology Abnormalities Occurring in > 3% of Patients Receiving NORVIR

			Study 245 Naive Patients		Study 247 Advanced Patients		Study 462 PI-Naive Patients
Variable	**Limit**	**NORVIR + ZDV**	**NORVIR**	**ZDV**	**NORVIR**	**Placebo**	**NORVIR + Saquinavir**
Chemistry	High						
Cholesterol	>240 mg/dL	30.7	44.8	9.3	36.5	8.0	65.2
CPK	>1000 IU/L	9.6	12.1	11.0	9.1	6.3	9.9
GGT	>300 IU/L	1.8	5.2	1.7	19.6	11.3	9.2
SGOT (AST)	>180 IU/L	5.3	9.5	2.5	6.4	7.0	7.8
SGPT (ALT)	>215 IU/L	5.3	7.8	3.4	8.5	4.4	9.2
Triglycerides	>800 mg/dL	9.6	17.2	3.4	33.6	9.4	23.4
Triglycerides	>1500 mg/dL	1.8	2.6	-	12.6	0.4	11.3
Triglycerides Fasting	>1500 mg/dL	1.5	1.3	-	9.9	0.3	-
Uric Acid	>12 mg/dL	-	-	-	3.8	0.2	1.4
Hematology	Low						
Hematocrit	<30%	2.6	-	0.8	17.3	22.0	0.7
Hemoglobin	<8.0 g/dL	0.9	-	-	3.8	3.9	-
Neutrophils	$\leq 0.5 \times 10^9$/L	-	-	-	6.0	8.3	-
RBC	$<3.0 \times 10^{12}$/L	1.8	-	5.9	18.6	24.4	-
WBC	$<2.5 \times 10^9$/L	-	0.9	6.8	36.9	59.4	3.5

[1] ULN = upper limit of the normal range.
- Indicates no events reported.

Pediatric Dosage Guidelines[1]

Body Surface Area* (m^2)	Twice Daily Dose 250 mg/m^2	Twice Daily Dose 300 mg/m^2	Twice Daily Dose 350 mg/m^2	Twice Daily Dose 400 mg/m^2
0.25	0.8 mL (62.5 mg)	0.9 mL (75 mg)	1.1 mL (87.5 mg)	1.25 mL (100 mg)
0.50	1.6 mL (125 mg)	1.9 mL (150 mg)	2.2 mL (175 mg)	2.5 mL (200 mg)
1.00	3.1 mL (250 mg)	3.75 mL (300 mg)	4.4 mL (350 mg)	5 mL (400 mg)
1.25	3.9 mL (312.5 mg)	4.7 mL (375 mg)	5.5 mL (437.5 mg)	6.25 mL (500 mg)
1.50	4.7 mL (375 mg)	5.6 mL (450 mg)	6.6 mL (525 mg)	7.5 mL (600 mg)

*Body surface area can be calculated with the following equation: $\text{BSA (m}^2) = \sqrt{\dfrac{\text{Ht (cm)} \times \text{Wt (kg)}}{3600}}$

Management of Overdosage
NORVIR oral solution contains 43% alcohol by volume. Accidental ingestion of the product by a young child could result in significant alcohol-related toxicity and could approach the potential lethal dose of alcohol.
Treatment of overdose with NORVIR consists of general supportive measures including monitoring of vital signs and observation of the clinical status of the patient. There is no specific antidote for overdose with NORVIR. If indicated, elimination of unabsorbed drug should be achieved by emesis or gastric lavage; usual precautions should be observed to maintain the airway. Administration of activated charcoal may also be used to aid in removal of unabsorbed drug. Since ritonavir is extensively metabolized by the liver and is highly protein bound, dialysis is unlikely to be beneficial in significant removal of the drug. A Certified Poison Control Center should be consulted for up-to-date information on the management of overdose with NORVIR.

DOSAGE AND ADMINISTRATION

NORVIR is administered orally. It is recommended that NORVIR be taken with meals if possible. Patients may improve the taste of NORVIR oral solution by mixing with chocolate milk, Ensure®, or Advera® within one hour of dosing. The effects of antacids on the absorption of ritonavir have not been studied.

Adults
Recommended Dosage: The recommended dosage of ritonavir is 600 mg twice daily by mouth. Use of a dose titration schedule may help to reduce treatment-emergent adverse events while maintaining appropriate ritonavir plasma levels. Ritonavir should be started at no less than 300 mg twice daily and increased at 2 to 3 day intervals by 100 mg twice daily.
Concomitant Therapy: If saquinavir and ritonavir are used in combination, the dosage of saquinavir should be reduced to 400 mg twice daily. The optimum dosage of NORVIR (400 mg or 600 mg twice daily), in combination with saquinavir, has not been determined; however, the combination regimen was better tolerated in patients who received NORVIR 400 mg twice daily.

Pediatric Patients
Ritonavir should be used in combination with other antiretroviral agents (see **General Dosing Guidelines**). The recommended dosage of ritonavir is 400 mg/m^2 twice daily by mouth and should not exceed 600 mg twice daily. Ritonavir should be started at 250 mg/m^2 and increased at 2 to 3 day intervals by 50 mg/m^2 twice daily. If patients do not tolerate 400 mg/m^2 twice daily due to adverse events, the highest tolerated dose may be used for maintenance therapy in combination with other antiretroviral agents, however, alternative therapy should be considered. When possible, dose should be administered using a calibrated dosing syringe. [See second table above]

General Dosing Guidelines
Patients should be aware that frequently observed adverse events, such as mild to moderate gastrointestinal disturbances and paraesthesias, may diminish as therapy is continued. In addition, patients initiating combination regimens with NORVIR and nucleosides may improve gastrointestinal tolerance by initiating NORVIR alone and subsequently adding nucleosides before completing two weeks of NORVIR monotherapy.

HOW SUPPLIED

NORVIR (ritonavir capsules) soft gelatin are white capsules imprinted with the corporate logo [logo], 100 and the Abbo-Code DS, available in the following package size:
Bottles of 120 capsules each .... (**NDC** 0074-6633-22).
Recommended storage: Store soft gelatin capsules in the refrigerator between 36-46°F (2-8°C) until dispensed. Refrigeration of NORVIR soft gelatin capsules by the patient is recommended, but not required if used within 30 days and stored below 77°F (25°C). Protect from light. Avoid exposure to excessive heat.
NORVIR (ritonavir oral solution) is an orange-colored liquid, supplied in amber-colored, multi-dose bottles containing 600 mg ritonavir per 7.5 mL marked dosage cup (80 mg/mL) in the following size:
240 mL bottles .... (**NDC** 0074-1940-63).
Recommended storage: Store NORVIR oral solution at room temperature 68°F to 77°F (20°C to 25°C). Do not refrigerate. Shake well before each use. Use by product expiration date.
Product should be stored and dispensed in the original container.
Avoid exposure to excessive heat. Keep cap tightly closed.

REFERENCES

1. Sewester CS. Calculations. In: Drug Facts and Comparisons. St. Louis, MO: J.B. Lippincott Co; January, 1997: xix.
2. Bertz RJ and Granneman GR. Use of *in vitro* and *in vivo* data to estimate the likelihood of metabolic pharmacokinetic interactions. *Clin Pharmacokinet* 1997; 32(3):210-258.

(Nos. 1940 and 6633)
03-5311-R18-Rev. October, 2003
ABBOTT LABORATORIES
NORTH CHICAGO, IL
60064, U.S.A.

NORVIR®
(ritonavir capsules) Soft Gelatin
(ritonavir oral solution)

ALERT: Find out about medicines that should NOT be taken with NORVIR. Please also read the section "MEDICINES YOU SHOULD NOT TAKE WITH NORVIR."

Patient Information
NORVIR®
(Nor-veer)
Generic Name: ritonavir
(rit-ON-uh-veer)

Please read this leaflet carefully before you start taking NORVIR. Also, read it each time you get your NORVIR prescription refilled, just in case something has changed. Remember that this information does not take the place of careful discussions with your doctor when you start this medication and at check ups.
You should remain under a doctor's care when taking NORVIR and you should not change or stop treatment without first talking with your doctor.
You should tell your doctor about any medicine you are taking or planning to take because taking NORVIR with some medications can result in serious or life-threatening problems.
Talk to your doctor if you have any questions about NORVIR. Your doctor or pharmacist can also give you more information about NORVIR.

What is NORVIR and how does it work?
NORVIR is in a class of medicines called the HIV protease (PRO-tee-ase) inhibitors. NORVIR is used in combination with other anti-HIV medicines to treat people with human immunodeficiency virus (HIV) infection. NORVIR is for adults and for children age 2 years and older.
HIV infection leads to the destruction of CD_4 (T) cells, which are important to the immune system. After a large number of CD_4 (T) cells have been destroyed, acquired immune deficiency syndrome (AIDS) develops.
NORVIR blocks HIV protease, a chemical which is needed for HIV to multiply. NORVIR reduces the amount of HIV in your blood and increases the number of CD_4 (T) cells. Patients who took NORVIR in clinical studies had significant reductions in both death and AIDS defining diseases; however NORVIR may not have these effects in all patients.

Does NORVIR cure HIV or AIDS?
NORVIR does not cure HIV infection or AIDS. The long-term effects of NORVIR are not known at this time. People taking NORVIR may still get opportunistic infections or other conditions that happen with HIV infection. Some of these conditions are pneumonia, herpes virus infections, and *Mycobacterium avium* complex (MAC) infections.

Does NORVIR reduce the risk of passing HIV to others?
NORVIR does not reduce the risk of passing HIV to others through sexual contact or blood contamination. Continue to practice safe sex and do not use or share dirty needles.

How should I take NORVIR?
- You should stay under a doctor's care when taking NORVIR. Do not change your treatment or stop treatment without first talking with your doctor.
- It is very important that you take NORVIR every day exactly as your doctor prescribed it.
- The usual dose for adults is six 100 mg capsules or 7.5 mL of the oral solution twice a day (morning and night), in combination with other anti-HIV medicines.
- The dosing of NORVIR may be different for you than for other patients. Follow the directions from your doctor, exactly as written on the label.
- Children from 2 to 16 years of age can also take NORVIR. The child's doctor will decide the right dose based on the child's height and weight.
- Take NORVIR with food if possible.
- NORVIR Oral Solution is peppermint/caramel flavored. You can take it alone, or improve the taste by mixing it with 8 ounces of chocolate milk, Ensure®, or Advera®. NORVIR Oral Solution should be taken within 1 hour if mixed with these items. Ask your doctor, nurse or pharmacist about other ways to improve the taste of NORVIR Oral Solution.
- Do not change or stop taking NORVIR without first talking with your health care provider.
- When your NORVIR supply starts to run low, get more from your doctor or pharmacy. This is very important because the amount of virus in your blood may increase if the medicine is stopped for even a short time. The virus may develop resistance to NORVIR and become harder to treat.
- Be sure to set up a schedule and follow it carefully.
- Only take medicine that has been prescribed specifically for you. Do not give NORVIR to others or take medicine prescribed for someone else.

What should I do if I miss a dose of NORVIR?
It is important that you do not miss any doses. If you miss a dose of NORVIR, take it as soon as possible and then take your next scheduled dose at its regular time. If it is almost time for your next dose, wait and take the next dose at the regular time. Do not double the next dose.

What happens if I take too much NORVIR?
If you think that you took more than the prescribed dose of this medicine, contact your local poison control center or emergency room immediately.
As with all prescription medicines, NORVIR should be kept out of the reach of young children. NORVIR liquid contains a large amount of alcohol. If a toddler or young child accidentally drinks more than the recommended dose of NORVIR, it could make him/her sick from too much alcohol. Contact your local poison control center or emergency room immediately if this happens.

Continued on next page

Norvir—Cont.

Who should not take NORVIR?
Together with your doctor, you need to decide whether NORVIR is right for you.

- Do not take NORVIR if you are taking certain medicines. These could cause serious side effects that could cause death. Before you take NORVIR, you must tell your doctor about all the medicines you are taking or are planning to take. These include other prescription and nonprescription medicines and herbal supplements.

For more information about medicines you should not take with NORVIR, please read the section "MEDICINES YOU SHOULD NOT TAKE WITH NORVIR."

- Do not take NORVIR if you have had a serious allergic reaction to NORVIR or any of its ingredients.

Can I take NORVIR with other medications?*
NORVIR may interact with other medicines, including those you take without a prescription. You must tell your doctor about all the medicines you are taking or are planning to take.

MEDICINES YOU SHOULD NOT TAKE WITH NORVIR.

- *Do not take the following medicines with NORVIR because they can cause serious or life-threatening problems such as irregular heartbeat, breathing difficulties or excessive sleepiness could occur:*
  Cordarone® (amiodarone)
  Ergotamine, ergonovine, methylergonovine, and dihydroergotamine such as Cafergot®, Migranal®, D.H.E 45®, and others
  Halcion® (triazolam)
  Hismanal® (astemizole)
  Orap® (pimozide)
  Propulsid® (cisapride)
  Quinidine, also known as Quinaglute®, Cardioquin®, Quinidex®, and others
  Rythmol® (propafenone)
  Seldane® (terfenadine)
  Tambocor® (flecainide)
  Vascor® (bepridil)
  Versed® (midazolam)
- Do not take NORVIR with St. John's wort (hypericum perforatum), an herbal product sold as a dietary supplement or products containing St. John's wort. Talk with your doctor if you are taking or are planning to take St. John's wort. Taking St. John's wort may decrease NORVIR levels and lead to increased viral load and possible resistance to NORVIR or cross-resistance to other antiretroviral medicines.
- Do not take NORVIR with the cholesterol-lowering medicines Mevacor® (lovastatin) or Zocor® (simvastatin) because of possible serious reactions. There is also an increased risk of drug interactions between NORVIR and Lipitor® (atorvastatin); talk to your doctor before you take any of these cholesterol-reducing medicines with NORVIR.

Medicines that may require dosage adjustments:
It is possible that your doctor may need to increase or decrease the dose of other medicines when you are also taking NORVIR. Remember to tell your doctor all medicines you are taking or plan to take.

- The following medicines require dose reduction if taken with NORVIR:
  If you are taking Viagra® (sildenafil), your doctor may lower your dose of Viagra.

Before you take Viagra with NORVIR, talk to your doctor about possible drug interactions and side effects. If you take Viagra and NORVIR together, you may be at risk of side effects of Viagra such as low blood pressure, visual changes, and penile erection lasting more than 4 hours. If an erection lasts longer than 4 hours, you should get medical help immediately to avoid permanent damage to your penis. Your doctor can explain these symptoms to you.

- If you are taking Oral contraceptives ("the pill") to prevent pregnancy, your doctor should increase the dose or you should use a different type of contraception since NORVIR may reduce the effectiveness of oral contraceptives.
- If you are taking Mycobutin® (rifabutin), your doctor will lower the dose of Mycobutin.
- **Other Special Considerations:**
  NORVIR oral solution contains alcohol. Talk with your doctor if you are taking or planning to take metronidazole or disulfiram. Severe nausea and vomiting can occur.
- **If you are taking both didanosine (Videx) and NORVIR:**
  Didanosine and NORVIR should be separated by at least 2.5 hours.
- Rifampin, also known as Rimactane®, Rifadin®, Rifater®, or Rifamate®, may reduce blood levels of NORVIR. Be sure to tell your doctor if you are taking rifampin.

What are the possible side effects of NORVIR?

- This list of side effects is **not** complete. If you have questions about side effects, ask your doctor, nurse, or pharmacist. You should report any new or continuing symptoms to your doctor right away. Your doctor may be able to help you manage these side effects.
- The most commonly reported side effects are: feeling weak/tired, nausea, vomiting, diarrhea, loss of appetite, abdominal pain, changes in taste, tingling feeling or numbness in hands or feet or around the lips, headache, and dizziness.
- Blood tests in patients taking NORVIR may show possible liver problems. People with liver disease such as Hepatitis B and Hepatitis C who take NORVIR may have worsening liver disease. Liver problems including rare cases of death have occurred in patients taking NORVIR. It is unclear if NORVIR caused these liver problems because some patients had other illnesses or were taking other medicines.
- Some patients taking NORVIR can develop serious problems with their pancreas (pancreatitis) which may cause death. Tell your doctor if you have nausea, vomiting, or abdominal pain. These may be signs of pancreatitis.
- Some patients have large increases in triglycerides and cholesterol. The long-term chance of getting complications such as heart attacks or stroke due to increases in triglycerides and cholesterol caused by protease inhibitors is not known at this time.
- Diabetes and high blood sugar (hyperglycemia) have occurred in patients taking protease inhibitors. Some patients had diabetes before starting protease inhibitors, others did not. Some patients need changes in their diabetes medication. Others needed new diabetes medication.
- Changes in body fat have been seen in some patients taking antiretroviral therapy. These changes may include increased amount of fat in the upper back and neck ("buffalo hump"), breast and around the trunk. Loss of fat from the legs, arms and face may also happen. The cause and long term health effects of these conditions are not known at this time.
- Some patients with hemophilia have increased bleeding with protease inhibitors.
- Allergic reactions ranging from mild to severe have occurred in patients taking NORVIR.

There have been other side effects noted in patients receiving NORVIR; however, these side effects may have been due to other medicines that patients were taking or to the illness itself. Some of these side effects can be serious. If you have questions about side effects, ask your doctor, nurse, or pharmacist. You should report any new or persistent symptoms to your doctor immediately.

What should I tell my doctor before taking NORVIR?

- *If you are pregnant or planning to become pregnant:* The effects of NORVIR on pregnant women or their unborn babies are not known.
- *If you are breast-feeding:* Do not breast-feed if you are taking NORVIR. You should not breast-feed if you have HIV. If you are a woman who has or will have a baby, talk with your doctor about the best way to feed your baby. You should be aware that if your baby does not already have HIV, there is a chance that HIV can be transmitted through breast-feeding.
- *If you have liver problems:* If you have liver problems or are infected with Hepatitis B or Hepatitis C, you should tell your doctor before taking NORVIR.
- *If you have diabetes:* Some people taking protease inhibitors develop new or more serious diabetes or high blood sugar. Be sure to tell your doctor if you have diabetes or an increase in thirst and/or frequent urination.
- *If you have hemophilia:* Some people with hemophilia have had increased bleeding. It is not known whether the protease inhibitors caused these problems. Be sure to tell your doctor if you have hemophilia types A and B.

How do I store NORVIR?

- Keep NORVIR and all other medicines out of the reach of children.
- Store NORVIR Oral Solution at room temperature. Do not refrigerate NORVIR Oral Solution. Avoid exposing NORVIR Oral Solution to excessive heat or cold.
- Refrigeration of NORVIR soft gelatin capsules by the patient is recommended, but not required if used within 30 days and stored below 77°F (25°C). Avoid exposing NORVIR soft gelatin capsules to excessive heat or cold.
- Store NORVIR soft gelatin capsules and NORVIR Oral Solution in the original container.
- Shake NORVIR Oral Solution well before each use.
- Use NORVIR Oral Solution by the expiration date on the bottle.

Do not keep medicine that is out of date or that you no longer need. Be sure that if you throw any medicine away, it is out of the reach of children.

General advice about prescription medicines:
Talk to your doctor or other health care provider if you have any questions about this medicine or your condition. Medicines are sometimes prescribed for purposes other than those listed in a Patient Information Leaflet. If you have any concerns about this medicine, ask your doctor. Your doctor or pharmacist can give you information about this medicine that was written for health care professionals. Do not use this medicine for a condition for which it was not prescribed. Do not share this medicine with other people.

*The brands listed are trademarks of their respective owners and are not trademarks of Abbott Laboratories. The makers of these brands are not affiliated with and do not endorse Abbott Laboratories or its products.

03-5311-R18

Revised: October, 2003

ABBOTT LABORATORIES
NORTH CHICAGO, IL 60064, U.S.A.

PRINTED IN U.S.A.

Shown in Product Identification Guide, page 303

OMNICEF® ℞
(cefdinir) capsules
[omnē-sĕf]

OMNICEF®
(cefdinir) for oral suspension

To reduce the development of drug-resistant bacteria and maintain the effectiveness of OMNICEF and other antibacterial drugs, OMNICEF should be used only to treat or prevent infections that are proven or strongly suspected to be caused by bacteria.

DESCRIPTION

OMNICEF® (cefdinir) capsules and OMNICEF® (cefdinir) for oral suspension contain the active ingredient cefdinir, an extended-spectrum, semisynthetic cephalosporin, for oral administration. Chemically, cefdinir is [6R-[6α,7β (Z)]]-7-[[(2-amino-4-thiazolyl)(hydroxyimino)acetyl]amino]-3-ethenyl-8-oxo-5-thia-1-azabicyclo[4.2.0]oct-2-ene-2-carboxylic acid. Cefdinir is a white to slightly brownish-yellow solid. It is slightly soluble in dilute hydrochloric acid and sparingly soluble in 0.1 M pH 7.0 phosphate buffer. The empirical formula is $C_{14}H_{13}N_5O_5S_2$ and the molecular weight is 395.42. Cefdinir has the structural formula shown below:

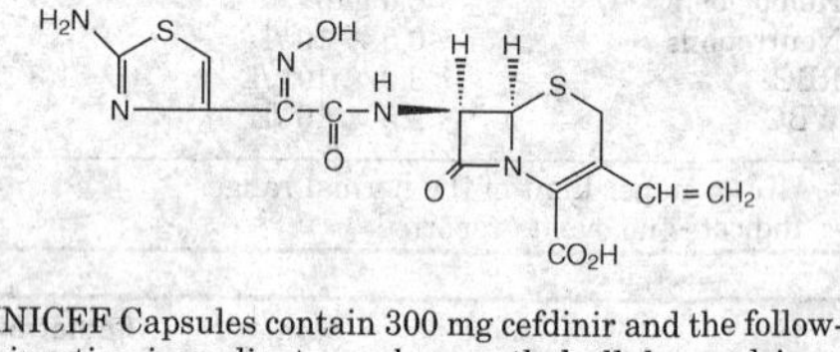

OMNICEF Capsules contain 300 mg cefdinir and the following inactive ingredients: carboxymethylcellulose calcium, NF; polyoxyl 40 stearate, NF; magnesium stearate, NF; and silicon dioxide, NF. The capsule shells contain FD&C Blue #1; FD&C Red #40; D&C Red #28; titanium dioxide, NF; gelatin, NF; and sodium lauryl sulfate, NF.

OMNICEF for Oral Suspension, after reconstitution, contains 125 mg cefdinir per 5 mL and the following inactive ingredients: sucrose, NF; citric acid, USP; sodium citrate, USP; sodium benzoate, NF; xanthan gum, NF; guar gum, NF; artificial strawberry and cream flavors; silicon dioxide, NF; and magnesium stearate, NF.

CLINICAL PHARMACOLOGY

Pharmacokinetics and Drug Metabolism

Absorption:

Oral Bioavailability: Maximal plasma cefdinir concentrations occur 2 to 4 hours postdose following capsule or suspension administration. Plasma cefdinir concentrations increase with dose, but the increases are less than dose-proportional from 300 mg (7 mg/kg) to 600 mg (14 mg/kg). Following administration of suspension to healthy adults, cefdinir bioavailability is 120% relative to capsules. Estimated bioavailability of cefdinir capsules is 21% following administration of a 300 mg capsule dose, and 16% following administration of a 600 mg capsule dose. Estimated absolute bioavailability of cefdinir suspension is 25%.

Effect of Food: Although the rate (C_{max}) and extent (AUC) of cefdinir absorption from the capsules are reduced by 16% and 10%, respectively, when given with a high-fat meal, the magnitude of these reductions is not likely to be clinically significant. Therefore, cefdinir may be taken without regard to food.

Cefdinir Capsules: Cefdinir plasma concentrations and pharmacokinetic parameter values following administration of single 300- and 600-mg oral doses of cefdinir to adult subjects are presented in the following table:

Mean (±SD) Plasma Cefdinir Pharmacokinetic Parameter Values Following Administration of Capsules to Adult Subjects

Dose	C_{max} (μg/mL)	t_{max} (hr)	AUC (μg•hr/mL)
300 mg	1.60 (0.55)	2.9 (0.89)	7.05 (2.17)
600 mg	2.87 (1.01)	3.0 (0.66)	11.1 (3.87)

Cefdinir Suspension: Cefdinir plasma concentrations and pharmacokinetic parameter values following administration of single 7- and 14-mg/kg oral doses of cefdinir to pediatric subjects (age 6 months–12 years) are presented in the following table:

Mean (±SD) Plasma Cefdinir Pharmacokinetic Parameter Values Following Administration of Suspension to Pediatric Subjects

Dose	C_{max} (μg/mL)	t_{max} (hr)	AUC (μg•hr/mL)
7 mg/kg	2.30 (0.65)	2.2 (0.6)	8.31 (2.50)
14 mg/kg	3.86 (0.62)	1.8 (0.4)	13.4 (2.64)

Multiple Dosing: Cefdinir does not accumulate in plasma following once- or twice-daily administration to subjects with normal renal function.

Distribution: The mean volume of distribution (Vd_{area}) of cefdinir in adult subjects is 0.35 L/kg (±0.29); in pediatric subjects (age 6 months–12 years), cefdinir Vd_{area} is 0.67 L/kg (±0.38). Cefdinir is 60% to 70% bound to plasma proteins in both adult and pediatric subjects; binding is independent of concentration.

Skin Blister: In adult subjects, median (range) maximal blister fluid cefdinir concentrations of 0.65 (0.33-1.1) and 1.1 (0.49-1.9) µg/mL were observed 4 to 5 hours following administration of 300- and 600-mg doses, respectively. Mean (±SD) blister C_{max} and AUC (0-∞) values were 48% (±13) and 91% (±18) of corresponding plasma values.

Tonsil Tissue: In adult patients undergoing elective tonsillectomy, respective median tonsil tissue cefdinir concentrations 4 hours after administration of single 300- and 600-mg doses were 0.25 (0.22-0.46) and 0.36 (0.22-0.80) µg/g. Mean tonsil tissue concentrations were 24% (±8) of corresponding plasma concentrations.

Sinus Tissue: In adult patients undergoing elective maxillary and ethmoid sinus surgery, respective median sinus tissue cefdinir concentrations 4 hours after administration of single 300- and 600-mg doses were <0.12 (<0.12-0.46) and 0.21 (<0.12-2.0) µg/g. Mean sinus tissue concentrations were 16% (±20) of corresponding plasma concentrations.

Lung Tissue: In adult patients undergoing diagnostic bronchoscopy, respective median bronchial mucosa cefdinir concentrations 4 hours after administration of single 300- and 600-mg doses were 0.78 (<0.06-1.33) and 1.14 (<0.06-1.92) µg/mL, and were 31% (±18) of corresponding plasma concentrations. Respective median epithelial lining fluid concentrations were 0.29 (<0.3-4.73) and 0.49 (<0.3-0.59) µg/mL, and were 35% (±83) of corresponding plasma concentrations.

Middle Ear Fluid: In 14 pediatric patients with acute bacterial otitis media, respective median middle ear fluid cefdinir concentrations 3 hours after administration of single 7- and 14-mg/kg doses were 0.21 (<0.09-0.94) and 0.72 (0.14-1.42) µg/mL. Mean middle ear fluid concentrations were 15% (±15) of corresponding plasma concentrations.

CSF: Data on cefdinir penetration into human cerebrospinal fluid are not available.

Metabolism and Excretion: Cefdinir is not appreciably metabolized. Activity is primarily due to parent drug. Cefdinir is eliminated principally via renal excretion with a mean plasma elimination half-life ($t_{1/2}$) of 1.7 (±0.6) hours. In healthy subjects with normal renal function, renal clearance is 2.0 (±1.0) mL/min/kg, and apparent oral clearance is 11.6 (±6.0) and 15.5 (±5.4) mL/min/kg following doses of 300- and 600-mg, respectively. Mean percent of dose recovered unchanged in the urine following 300- and 600-mg doses is 18.4% (±6.4) and 11.6% (±4.6), respectively. Cefdinir clearance is reduced in patients with renal dysfunction (see **Special Populations:** *Patients with Renal Insufficiency*).

Because renal excretion is the predominant pathway of elimination, dosage should be adjusted in patients with markedly compromised renal function or who are undergoing hemodialysis (see **DOSAGE AND ADMINISTRATION**).

Special Populations:

Patients with Renal Insufficiency: Cefdinir pharmacokinetics were investigated in 21 adult subjects with varying degrees of renal function. Decreases in cefdinir elimination rate, apparent oral clearance (CL/F), and renal clearance were approximately proportional to the reduction in creatinine clearance (CL_{cr}). As a result, plasma cefdinir concentrations were higher and persisted longer in subjects with renal impairment than in those without renal impairment. In subjects with CL_{cr} between 30 and 60 mL/min, C_{max} and $t_{1/2}$ increased by approximately 2-fold and AUC by approximately 3-fold. In subjects with CL_{cr} <30 mL/min, C_{max} increased by approximately 2-fold, $t_{1/2}$ by approximately 5-fold, and AUC by approximately 6-fold. Dosage adjustment is recommended in patients with markedly compromised renal function (creatinine clearance ≤30 mL/min; see **DOSAGE AND ADMINISTRATION**).

Hemodialysis: Cefdinir pharmacokinetics were studied in 8 adult subjects undergoing hemodialysis. Dialysis (4 hours duration) removed 63% of cefdinir from the body and reduced apparent elimination $t_{1/2}$ from 16 (±3.5) to 3.2 (±1.2) hours. Dosage adjustment is recommended in this patient population (see **DOSAGE AND ADMINISTRATION**).

Hepatic Disease: Because cefdinir is predominantly renally eliminated and not appreciably metabolized, studies in patients with hepatic impairment were not conducted. It is not expected that dosage adjustment will be required in this population.

Geriatric Patients: The effect of age on cefdinir pharmacokinetics after a single 300-mg dose was evaluated in 32 subjects 19 to 91 years of age. Systemic exposure to cefdinir was substantially increased in older subjects (N=16), C_{max} by 44% and AUC by 86%. This increase was due to a reduction in cefdinir clearance. The apparent volume of distribution was also reduced, thus no appreciable alterations in apparent elimination $t_{1/2}$ were observed (elderly: 2.2 ± 0.6 hours vs young: 1.8 ± 0.4 hours). Since cefdinir clearance has been shown to be primarily related to changes in renal function rather than age, elderly patients do not require dosage adjustment unless they have markedly compromised renal function (creatinine clearance <30 mL/min, see *Patients with Renal Insufficiency*, above).

Gender and Race: The results of a meta-analysis of clinical pharmacokinetics (N=217) indicated no significant impact of either gender or race on cefdinir pharmacokinetics.

Microbiology

As with other cephalosporins, bactericidal activity of cefdinir results from inhibition of cell wall synthesis. Cefdinir is stable in the presence of some, but not all, β-lactamase enzymes. As a result, many organisms resistant to penicillins and some cephalosporins are susceptible to cefdinir.

Cefdinir has been shown to be active against most strains of the following microorganisms, both *in vitro* and in clinical infections as described in **INDICATIONS AND USAGE.**

Aerobic Gram-Positive Microorganisms:

Staphylococcus aureus (including β-lactamase producing strains)

NOTE: Cefdinir is inactive against methicillin-resistant staphylococci.

Streptococcus pneumoniae (penicillin-susceptible strains only)

Streptococcus pyogenes

Aerobic Gram-Negative Microorganisms:

Haemophilus influenzae (including β-lactamase producing strains)

Haemophilus parainfluenzae (including β-lactamase producing strains)

Moraxella catarrhalis (including β-lactamase producing strains)

The following *in vitro* data are available, **but their clinical significance is unknown.**

Cefdinir exhibits *in vitro* minimum inhibitory concentrations (MICs) of 1 µg/mL or less against (≥90%) strains of the following microorganisms; however, the safety and effectiveness of cefdinir in treating clinical infections due to these microorganisms have not been established in adequate and well-controlled clinical trials.

Aerobic Gram-Positive Microorganisms:

Staphylococcus epidermidis (methicillin-susceptible strains only)

Streptococcus agalactiae

Viridans group streptococci

NOTE: Cefdinir is inactive against *Enterococcus* and methicillin-resistant *Staphylococcus* species.

Aerobic Gram-Negative Microorganisms:

Citrobacter diversus

Escherichia coli

Klebsiella pneumoniae

Proteus mirabilis

NOTE: Cefdinir is inactive against *Pseudomonas* and *Enterobacter* species.

Susceptibility Tests:

Dilution Techniques: Quantitative methods are used to determine antimicrobial minimum inhibitory concentrations (MICs). These MICs provide estimates of the susceptibility of bacteria to antimicrobial compounds. The MICs should be determined using a standardized procedure. Standardized procedures are based on a dilution method[1] (broth or agar) or equivalent with standardized inoculum concentrations and standardized concentrations of cefdinir powder. The MIC values should be interpreted according to the following criteria:

For organisms other than *Haemophilus* spp. and *Streptococcus* spp:

MIC (µg/mL)	Interpretation
≤1	Susceptible (S)
2	Intermediate (I)
≥4	Resistant (R)

For *Haemophilus* spp:[a]

MIC (µg/mL)	Interpretation[b]
≤1	Susceptible (S)

[a] These interpretive standards are applicable only to broth microdilution susceptibility tests with *Haemophilus* spp. using *Haemophilus* Test Medium (HTM).[1]

[b] The current absence of data on resistant strains precludes defining any results other than "Susceptible." Strains yielding MIC results suggestive of a "nonsusceptible" category should be submitted to a reference laboratory for further testing.

For *Streptococcus* spp:

Streptococcus pneumoniae that are susceptible to penicillin (MIC ≤0.06 µg/mL), or streptococci other than *S. pneumoniae* that are susceptible to penicillin (MIC ≤0.12 µg/mL), can be considered susceptible to cefdinir. Testing of cefdinir against penicillin-intermediate or penicillin-resistant isolates is not recommended. Reliable interpretive criteria for cefdinir are not available.

A report of "Susceptible" indicates that the pathogen is likely to be inhibited if the antimicrobial compound in the blood reaches the concentration usually achievable. A report of "Intermediate" indicates that the result should be considered equivocal, and, if the microorganism is not fully susceptible to alternative, clinically feasible drugs, the test should be repeated. This category implies possible clinical applicability in body sites where the drug is physiologically concentrated or in situations where high dosage of drug can be used. This category also provides a buffer zone which prevents small uncontrolled technical factors from causing major discrepancies in interpretation. A report of "Resistant" indicates that the pathogen is not likely to be inhibited if the antimicrobial compound in the blood reaches the concentrations usually achievable; other therapy should be selected.

Standardized susceptibility test procedures require the use of laboratory control microorganisms to control the technical aspects of laboratory procedures. Standard cefdinir powder should provide the following MIC values:

Microorganism	MIC Range (µg/mL)
Escherichia coli ATCC 25922	0.12-0.5
Haemophilus influenzae ATCC 49766[c]	0.12-0.5
Staphylococcus aureus ATCC 29213	0.12-0.5

[c] This quality control range is applicable only to *H. influenzae* ATCC 49766 tested by a broth microdilution procedure using HTM.

Diffusion Techniques: Quantitative methods that require measurement of zone diameters also provide reproducible estimates of the susceptibility of bacteria to antimicrobial compounds. One such standardized procedure[2] requires the use of standardized inoculum concentrations. This procedure uses paper disks impregnated with 5-µg cefdinir to test the susceptibility of microorganisms to cefdinir.

Reports from the laboratory providing results of the standard single-disk susceptibility test with a 5-µg cefdinir disk should be interpreted according to the following criteria:

For organisms other than *Haemophilus* spp. and *Streptococcus* spp:[d]

Zone Diameter (mm)	Interpretation
≥20	Susceptible (S)
17-19	Intermediate (I)
≤16	Resistant (R)

[d] Because certain strains of *Citrobacter, Providencia,* and *Enterobacter* spp. have been reported to give false susceptible results with the cefdinir disk, strains of these genera should not be tested and reported with this disk.

For *Haemophilus* spp:[e]

Zone Diameter (mm)	Interpretation[f]
≥20	Susceptible (S)

[e] These zone diameter standards are applicable only to tests with *Haemophilus* spp. using HTM.[2]

[f] The current absence of data on resistant strains precludes defining any results other than "Susceptible." Strains yielding results suggestive of a "nonsusceptible" category should be submitted to a reference laboratory for further testing.

For *Streptococcus* spp:

Isolates of *Streptococcus pneumoniae* should be tested against a 1-µg oxacillin disk. Isolates with oxacillin zone sizes ≥20 mm are susceptible to penicillin and can be considered susceptible to cefdinir. Streptococci other than *S. pneumoniae* should be tested with a 10-unit penicillin disk. Isolates with penicillin zone sizes ≥28 mm are susceptible to penicillin and can be considered susceptible to cefdinir.

As with standardized dilution techniques, diffusion methods require the use of laboratory control microorganisms to control the technical aspects of laboratory procedures. For the diffusion technique, the 5-µg cefdinir disk should provide the following zone diameters in these laboratory quality control strains:

Organism	Zone Diameter (mm)
Escherichia coli ATCC 25922	24-28
Haemophilus influenzae ATCC 49766[g]	24-31
Staphylococcus aureus ATCC 25923	25-32

[g] This quality control range is applicable only to testing of *H. influenzae* ATCC 49766 using HTM.

INDICATIONS AND USAGE

To reduce the development of drug-resistant bacteria and maintain the effectiveness of OMNICEF and other antibacterial drugs, OMNICEF should be used only to treat or prevent infections that are proven or strongly suspected to be caused by susceptible bacteria. When culture and susceptibility information are available, they should be considered in selecting or modifying antibacterial therapy. In the absence of such data, local epidemiology and susceptibility patterns may contribute to the empiric selection of therapy.

OMNICEF (cefdinir) capsules and OMNICEF (cefdinir) for oral suspension are indicated for the treatment of patients with mild to moderate infections caused by susceptible strains of the designated microorganisms in the conditions listed below.

Adults and Adolescents

Community-Acquired Pneumonia caused by *Haemophilus influenzae* (including β-lactamase producing strains), *Hae-*

Continued on next page

Omnicef—Cont.

mophilus parainfluenzae (including β-lactamase producing strains), *Streptococcus pneumoniae* (penicillin-susceptible strains only), and *Moraxella catarrhalis* (including β-lactamase producing strains) (see **CLINICAL STUDIES**).

Acute Exacerbations of Chronic Bronchitis caused by *Haemophilus influenzae* (including β-lactamase producing strains), *Haemophilus parainfluenzae* (including β-lactamase producing strains), *Streptococcus pneumoniae* (penicillin-susceptible strains only), and *Moraxella catarrhalis* (including β-lactamase producing strains).

Acute Maxillary Sinusitis caused by *Haemophilus influenzae* (including β-lactamase producing strains), *Streptococcus pneumoniae* (penicillin-susceptible strains only), and *Moraxella catarrhalis* (including β-lactamase producing strains).

NOTE: For information on use in pediatric patients, See **Pediatric Use** and **DOSAGE AND ADMINISTRATION.**

Pharyngitis/Tonsillitis caused by *Streptococcus pyogenes* (see **CLINICAL STUDIES**).

NOTE: Cefdinir is effective in the eradication of *S. pyogenes* from the oropharynx. Cefdinir has not, however, been studied for the prevention of rheumatic fever following *S. pyogenes* pharyngitis/tonsillitis. Only intramuscular penicillin has been demonstrated to be effective for the prevention of rheumatic fever.

Uncomplicated Skin and Skin Structure Infections caused by *Staphylococcus aureus* (including β-lactamase producing strains) and *Streptococcus pyogenes*.

Pediatric Patients

Acute Bacterial Otitis Media caused by *Haemophilus influenzae* (including β-lactamase producing strains), *Streptococcus pneumoniae* (penicillin-susceptible strains only), and *Moraxella catarrhalis* (including β-lactamase producing strains).

Pharyngitis/Tonsillitis caused by *Streptococcus pyogenes* (see **CLINICAL STUDIES**).

NOTE: Cefdinir is effective in the eradication of *S. pyogenes* from the oropharynx. Cefdinir has not, however, been studied for the prevention of rheumatic fever following *S. pyogenes* pharyngitis/tonsillitis. Only intramuscular penicillin has been demonstrated to be effective for the prevention of rheumatic fever.

Uncomplicated Skin and Skin Structure Infections caused by *Staphylococcus aureus* (including β-lactamase producing strains) and *Streptococcus pyogenes*.

CONTRAINDICATIONS

OMNICEF (cefdinir) is contraindicated in patients with known allergy to the cephalosporin class of antibiotics.

WARNINGS

BEFORE THERAPY WITH OMNICEF (CEFDINIR) IS INSTITUTED, CAREFUL INQUIRY SHOULD BE MADE TO DETERMINE WHETHER THE PATIENT HAS HAD PREVIOUS HYPERSENSITIVITY REACTIONS TO CEFDINIR, OTHER CEPHALOSPORINS, PENICILLINS, OR OTHER DRUGS. IF CEFDINIR IS TO BE GIVEN TO PENICILLIN-SENSITIVE PATIENTS, CAUTION SHOULD BE EXERCISED BECAUSE CROSS-HYPERSENSITIVITY AMONG β-LACTAM ANTIBIOTICS HAS BEEN CLEARLY DOCUMENTED AND MAY OCCUR IN UP TO 10% OF PATIENTS WITH A HISTORY OF PENICILLIN ALLERGY. IF AN ALLERGIC REACTION TO CEFDINIR OCCURS, THE DRUG SHOULD BE DISCONTINUED. SERIOUS ACUTE HYPERSENSITIVITY REACTIONS MAY REQUIRE TREATMENT WITH EPINEPHRINE AND OTHER EMERGENCY MEASURES, INCLUDING OXYGEN, INTRAVENOUS FLUIDS, INTRAVENOUS ANTIHISTAMINES, CORTICOSTEROIDS, PRESSOR AMINES, AND AIRWAY MANAGEMENT, AS CLINICALLY INDICATED.

Pseudomembranous colitis has been reported with nearly all antibacterial agents, including cefdinir, and may range in severity from mild-to-life-threatening. Therefore, it is important to consider this diagnosis in patients who present with diarrhea subsequent to the administration of antibacterial agents.

Treatment with antibacterial agents alters the normal flora of the colon and may permit overgrowth of clostridia. Studies indicate that a toxin produced by *Clostridium difficile* is a primary cause of "antibiotic-associated colitis."

After the diagnosis of pseudomembranous colitis has been established, appropriate therapeutic measures should be initiated. Mild cases of pseudomembranous colitis usually respond to drug discontinuation alone. In moderate to severe cases, consideration should be given to management with fluids and electrolytes, protein supplementation, and treatment with an antibacterial drug clinically effective against *Clostridium difficile*.

PRECAUTIONS

General

Prescribing OMNICEF in the absence of a proven or strongly suspected bacterial infection or a prophylactic indication is unlikely to provide benefit to the patient and increases the risk of the development of drug-resistant bacteria.

As with other broad-spectrum antibiotics, prolonged treatment may result in the possible emergence and overgrowth of resistant organisms. Careful observation of the patient is essential. If superinfection occurs during therapy, appropriate alternative therapy should be administered.

LABORATORY VALUE CHANGES OBSERVED WITH CEFDINIR CAPSULES US TRIALS IN ADULT AND ADOLESCENT PATIENTS (N=3841)

Incidence ≥ 1%	↑ Urine leukocytes	2%
	↑ Urine protein	2%
	↑ Gamma-glutamyltransferase[a]	1%
	↓ Lymphocytes, ↑ Lymphocytes	1%, 0.2%
	↑ Microhematuria	1%
Incidence <1% but >0.1%	↑ Glucose[a]	0.9%
	↑ Urine glucose	0.9%
	↑ White blood cells, ↓ White blood cells	0.9%, 0.7%
	↑ Alanine aminotransferase (ALT)	0.7%
	↑ Eosinophils	0.7%
	↑ Urine specific gravity, ↓ Urine specific gravity[a]	0.6%, 0.2%
	↓ Bicarbonate[a]	0.6%
	↑ Phosphorus, ↓ Phosphorus[a]	0.6%, 0.3%
	↑ Aspartate aminotransferase (AST)	0.4%
	↑ Alkaline phosphatase	0.3%
	↑ Blood urea nitrogen (BUN)	0.3%
	↓ Hemoglobin	0.3%
	↑ Polymorphonuclear neutrophils (PMNs), ↓ PMNs	0.3%, 0.2%
	↑ Bilirubin	0.2%
	↑ Lactate dehydrogenase[a]	0.2%
	↑ Platelets	0.2%
	↑ Potassium[a]	0.2%
	↑ Urine pH[a]	0.2%

[a] N<3841 for these parameters

Cefdinir, as with other broad-spectrum antimicrobials (antibiotics), should be prescribed with caution in individuals with a history of colitis.

In patients with transient or persistent renal insufficiency (creatinine clearance <30 mL/min), the total daily dose of OMNICEF should be reduced because high and prolonged plasma concentrations of cefdinir can result following recommended doses (see **DOSAGE AND ADMINISTRATION**).

Information for Patients

Patients should be counseled that antibacterial drugs including OMNICEF should only be used to treat bacterial infections. They do not treat viral infections (e.g., the common cold). When OMNICEF is prescribed to treat a bacterial infection, patients should be told that although it is common to feel better early in the course of therapy, the medication should be taken exactly as directed. Skipping doses or not completing the full course of therapy may (1) decrease the effectiveness of the immediate-treatment and (2) increase the likelihood that bacteria will develop resistance and will not be treatable by OMNICEF or other antibacterial drugs in the future.

Antacids containing magnesium or aluminum interfere with the absorption of cefdinir. If this type of antacid is required during OMNICEF therapy, OMNICEF should be taken at least 2 hours before or after the antacid.

Iron supplements, including multivitamins that contain iron, interfere with the absorption of cefdinir. If iron supplements are required during OMNICEF therapy, OMNICEF should be taken at least 2 hours before or after the supplement.

Iron-fortified infant formula does not significantly interfere with the absorption of cefdinir. Therefore, OMNICEF for Oral Suspension can be administered with iron-fortified infant formula.

Diabetic patients and caregivers should be aware that the oral suspension contains 2.86 g of sucrose per teaspoon.

Drug Interactions

Antacids: (aluminum- or magnesium-containing): Concomitant administration of 300-mg cefdinir capsules with 30 mL Maalox® TC suspension reduces rate (C_{max}) and extent (AUC) of absorption by approximately 40%. Time to reach C_{max} is also prolonged by 1 hour. There are no significant effects on cefdinir pharmacokinetics if the antacid is administered 2 hours before or 2 hours after cefdinir. If antacids are required during OMNICEF therapy, OMNICEF should be taken at least 2 hours before or after the antacid.

Probenecid: As with other β-lactam antibiotics, probenecid inhibits the renal excretion of cefdinir, resulting in an approximate doubling in AUC, a 54% increase in peak cefdinir plasma levels, and a 50% prolongation in the apparent elimination $t_{1/2}$.

Iron Supplements and Foods Fortified With Iron: Concomitant administration of cefdinir with a therapeutic iron supplement containing 60 mg of elemental iron (as $FeSO_4$) or vitamins supplemented with 10 mg of elemental iron reduced extent of absorption by 80% and 31%, respectively. If iron supplements are required during OMNICEF therapy, OMNICEF should be taken at least 2 hours before or after the supplement.

The effect of foods highly fortified with elemental iron (primarily iron-fortified breakfast cereals) on cefdinir absorption has not been studied.

Concomitantly administered iron-fortified infant formula (2.2 mg elemental iron/6 oz) has no significant effect on cefdinir pharmacokinetics. Therefore, OMNICEF for Oral Suspension can be administered with iron-fortified infant formula.

There have been reports of reddish stools in patients receiving cefdinir. In many cases, patients were also receiving iron-containing products. The reddish color is due to the formation of a nonabsorbable complex between cefdinir or its breakdown products and iron in the gastrointestinal tract.

Drug/Laboratory Test Interactions

A false-positive reaction for ketones in the urine may occur with tests using nitroprusside, but not with those using nitroferricyanide. The administration of cefdinir may result in a false-positive reaction for glucose in urine using Clinitest®, Benedict's solution, or Fehling's solution. It is recommended that glucose tests based on enzymatic glucose oxidase reactions (such as Clinistix® or Tes-Tape®) be used. Cephalosporins are known to occasionally induce a positive direct Coombs' test.

Carcinogenesis, Mutagenesis, Impairment of Fertility

The carcinogenic potential of cefdinir has not been evaluated. No mutagenic effects were seen in the bacterial reverse mutation assay (Ames) or point mutation assay at the hypoxanthineguanine phosphoribosyltransferase locus (HGPRT) in V79 Chinese hamster lung cells. No clastogenic effects were observed *in vitro* in the structural chromosome aberration assay in V79 Chinese hamster lung cells or *in vivo* in the micronucleus assay in mouse bone marrow. In rats, fertility and reproductive performance were not affected by cefdinir at oral doses up to 1000 mg/kg/day (70 times the human dose based on mg/kg/day, 11 times based on mg/m²/day).

Pregnancy - Teratogenic Effects

Pregnancy Category B: Cefdinir was not teratogenic in rats at oral doses up to 1000 mg/kg/day (70 times the human dose based on mg/kg/day, 11 times based on mg/m²/day) or in rabbits at oral doses up to 10 mg/kg/day (0.7 times the human dose based on mg/kg/day, 0.23 times based on mg/m²/day). Maternal toxicity (decreased body weight gain) was observed in rabbits at the maximum tolerated dose of 10 mg/kg/day without adverse effects on offspring. Decreased body weight occurred in rat fetuses at ≥100 mg/kg/day, and in rat offspring at ≥32 mg/kg/day. No effects were observed on maternal reproductive parameters or offspring survival, development, behavior, or reproductive function. There are, however, no adequate and well-controlled studies in pregnant women. Because animal reproduction studies are not always predictive of human response, this drug should be used during pregnancy only if clearly needed.

Labor and Delivery

Cefdinir has not been studied for use during labor and delivery.

Nursing Mothers

Following administration of single 600-mg doses, cefdinir was not detected in human breast milk.

Pediatric Use

Safety and efficacy in neonates and infants less than 6 months of age have not been established. Use of cefdinir for the treatment of acute maxillary sinusitis in pediatric patients (age 6 months through 12 years) is supported by evidence from adequate and well-controlled studies in adults and adolescents, the similar pathophysiology of acute sinusitis in adult and pediatric patients, and comparative pharmacokinetic data in the pediatric population.

Geriatric Use

Efficacy is comparable in geriatric patients and younger adults. While cefdinir has been well-tolerated in all age groups, in clinical trials geriatric patients experienced a lower rate of adverse events, including diarrhea, than younger adults. Dose adjustment in elderly patients is not necessary unless renal function is markedly compromised (see **DOSAGE AND ADMINISTRATION**).

ADVERSE EVENTS

Clinical Trials - OMNICEF Capsules (Adult and Adolescent Patients):

In clinical trials, 5093 adult and adolescent patients (3841 US and 1252 non-US) were treated with the recommended dose of cefdinir capsules (600 mg/day). Most adverse events were mild and self-limiting. No deaths or permanent disabilities were attributed to cefdinir. One hundred forty-seven of 5093 (3%) patients discontinued medication due to adverse events thought by the investigators to be possibly, probably, or definitely associated with cefdinir therapy. The discontinuations were primarily for gastrointestinal disturbances, usually diarrhea or nausea. Nineteen of 5093 (0.4%) patients were discontinued due to rash thought related to cefdinir administration.

In the US, the following adverse events were thought by the investigators to be possibly, probably, or definitely related to cefdinir capsules in clinical trials (N = 3841 cefdinir-treated patients):

ADVERSE EVENTS ASSOCIATED WITH CEFDINIR CAPSULES US TRIALS IN ADULT AND ADOLESCENT PATIENTS (N=3841)[a]

Incidence ≥1%	Diarrhea	15%
	Vaginal moniliasis	4% of women
	Nausea	3%
	Headache	2%
	Abdominal pain	1%
	Vaginitis	1% of women
Incidence <1% but >0.1%	Rash	0.9%
	Dyspepsia	0.7%
	Flatulence	0.7%
	Vomiting	0.7%
	Abnormal stools	0.3%
	Anorexia	0.3%
	Constipation	0.3%
	Dizziness	0.3%
	Dry Mouth	0.3%
	Asthenia	0.2%
	Insomnia	0.2%
	Leukorrhea	0.2% of women
	Moniliasis	0.2%
	Pruritus	0.2%
	Somnolence	0.2%

[a] 1733 males, 2108 females

The following laboratory value changes of possible clinical significance, irrespective of relationship to therapy with cefdinir, were seen during clinical trials conducted in the US:

[See table at top of previous page]

Clinical Trials - OMNICEF for Oral Suspension (Pediatric Patients):

In clinical trials, 2289 pediatric patients (1783 US and 506 non-US) were treated with the recommended dose of cefdinir suspension (14 mg/kg/day). Most adverse events were mild and self-limiting. No deaths or permanent disabilities were attributed to cefdinir. Forty of 2289 (2%) patients discontinued medication due to adverse events considered by the investigators to be possibly, probably, or definitely associated with cefdinir therapy. Discontinuations were primarily for gastrointestinal disturbances, usually diarrhea. Five of 2289 (0.2%) patients were discontinued due to rash thought related to cefdinir administration.

In the US, the following adverse events were thought by investigators to be possibly, probably, or definitely related to cefdinir suspension in multiple-dose clinical trials (N=1783 cefdinir-treated patients):

[See first table above]

NOTE: In both cefdinir- and control-treated patients, rates of diarrhea and rash were higher in the youngest pediatric patients. The incidence of diarrhea in cefdinir-treated patients ≤2 years of age was 17% (95/557) compared with 4% (51/1226) in those >2 years old. The incidence of rash (primarily diaper rash in the younger patients) was 8% (43/557) in patients ≤2 years of age compared with 1% (8/1226) in those >2 years old.

The following laboratory value changes of possible clinical significance, irrespective of relationship to therapy with cefdinir, were seen during clinical trials conducted in the US:

[See second table above]

Postmarketing Experience

The following adverse experiences and altered laboratory tests, regardless of their relationship to cefdinir, have been reported during extensive postmarketing experience, beginning with approval in Japan in 1991: Stevens-Johnson syndrome, toxic epidermal necrolysis, exfoliative dermatitis, erythema multiforme, erythema nodosum, conjunctivitis, stomatitis, acute hepatitis, cholestasis, fulminant hepatitis, hepatic failure, jaundice, increased amylase, shock, anaphylaxis, facial and laryngeal edema, feeling of suffocation, acute enterocolitis, bloody diarrhea, hemorrhagic colitis, melena, pseudomembranous colitis, pancytopenia, granulocytopenia, leukopenia, thrombocytopenia, idiopathic thrombocytopenic purpura, hemolytic anemia, acute respiratory failure, asthmatic attack, drug-induced pneumonia, eosinophilic pneumonia, idiopathic interstitial pneumonia, fever, acute renal failure, nephropathy, bleeding tendency, coagulation disorder, disseminated intravascular coagulation, upper GI bleed, peptic ulcer, ileus, loss of consciousness, allergic vasculitis, possible cefdinir-diclofenac interaction, cardiac failure, chest pain, myocardial infarction, hypertension, involuntary movements, and rhabdomyolysis.

Cephalosporin Class Adverse Events

The following adverse events and altered laboratory tests have been reported for cephalosporin-class antibiotics in general:

ADVERSE EVENTS ASSOCIATED WITH CEFDINIR SUSPENSION US TRIALS IN PEDIATRIC PATIENTS (N = 1783)[a]

Incidence ≥ 1%	Diarrhea	8%
	Rash	3%
	Vomiting	1%
Incidence <1% but >0.1%	Cutaneous moniliasis	0.9%
	Abdominal pain	0.8%
	Leukopenia[b]	0.3%
	Vaginal moniliasis	0.3% of girls
	Vaginitis	0.3% of girls
	Abnormal stools	0.2%
	Dyspepsia	0.2%
	Hyperkinesia	0.2%
	Increased AST[b]	0.2%
	Maculopapular rash	0.2%
	Nausea	0.2%

[a] 977 males, 806 females

[b] Laboratory changes were occasionally reported as adverse events.

LABORATORY VALUE CHANGES OF POSSIBLE CLINICAL SIGNIFICANCE OBSERVED WITH CEFDINIR SUSPENSION US TRIALS IN PEDIATRIC PATIENTS (N = 1783)

Incidence ≥1%	↑ Lymphocytes, ↓ Lymphocytes	2%, 0.8%
	↑ Alkaline phosphatase	1%
	↓ Bicarbonate[a]	1%
	↑ Eosinophils	1%
	↑ Lactate dehydrogenase	1%
	↑ Platelets	1%
	↑ PMNs, ↓ PMNs	1%, 1%
	↑ Urine protein	1%
Incidence <1% but >0.1%	↑ Phosphorus, ↓ Phosphorus	0.9%, 0.4%
	↑ Urine pH	0.8%
	↓ White blood cells, ↑ White blood cells	0.7%, 0.3%
	↓ Calcium[a]	0.5%
	↓ Hemoglobin	0.5%
	↑ Urine leukocytes	0.5%
	↑ Monocytes	0.4%
	↑ AST	0.3%
	↑ Potassium[a]	0.3%
	↑ Urine specific gravity, ↓ Urine specific gravity	0.3%, 0.1%
	↓ Hematocrit[a]	0.2%

[a] N = 1387 for these parameters.

Adults and Adolescents (Age 13 Years and Older)

Type of Infection	Dosage	Duration
Community-Acquired Pneumonia	300 mg q12h	10 days
Acute Exacerbations of Chronic Bronchitis	300 mg q12h or 600 mg q24h	5 to 10 days 10 days
Acute Maxillary Sinusitis	300 mg q12h or 600 mg q24h	10 days 10 days
Pharyngitis/Tonsillitis	300 mg q12h or 600 mg q24h	5 to 10 days 10 days
Uncomplicated Skin and Skin Structure Infections	300 mg q12h	10 days

Pediatric Patients (Age 6 Months Through 12 Years)

Type of Infection	Dosage	Duration
Acute Bacterial Otitis Media	7 mg/kg q12h or 14 mg/kg q24h	5 to 10 days 10 days
Acute Maxillary Sinusitis	7 mg/kg q12h or 14 mg/kg q24h	10 days 10 days
Pharyngitis/Tonsillitis	7 mg/kg q12h or 14 mg/kg q24h	5 to 10 days 10 days
Uncomplicated Skin and Skin Structure Infections	7 mg/kg q12h	10 days

Allergic reactions, anaphylaxis, Stevens-Johnson syndrome, erythema multiforme, toxic epidermal necrolysis, renal dysfunction, toxic nephropathy, hepatic dysfunction including cholestasis, aplastic anemia, hemolytic anemia, hemorrhage, false-positive test for urinary glucose, neutropenia, pancytopenia, and agranulocytosis.

Pseudomembranous colitis symptoms may begin during or after antibiotic treatment (see **WARNINGS**).

Several cephalosporins have been implicated in triggering seizures, particularly in patients with renal impairment when the dosage was not reduced (see **DOSAGE AND ADMINISTRATION** and **OVERDOSAGE**). If seizures associated with drug therapy occur, the drug should be discontinued. Anticonvulsant therapy can be given if clinically indicated.

OVERDOSAGE

Information on cefdinir overdosage in humans is not available. In acute rodent toxicity studies, a single oral 5600-mg/kg dose produced no adverse effects. Toxic signs and symptoms following overdosage with other β-lactam antibiotics have included nausea, vomiting, epigastric distress, diarrhea, and convulsions. Hemodialysis removes cefdinir from the body. This may be useful in the event of a serious toxic reaction from overdosage, particularly if renal function is compromised.

DOSAGE AND ADMINISTRATION

(see **INDICATIONS AND USAGE** for Indicated Pathogens)

Continued on next page

Omnicef—Cont.

Capsules
The recommended dosage and duration of treatment for infections in adults and adolescents are described in the following chart; the total daily dose for all infections is 600 mg. Once-daily dosing for 10 days is as effective as BID dosing. Once-daily dosing has not been studied in pneumonia or skin infections; therefore, OMNICEF Capsules should be administered twice daily in these infections. OMNICEF Capsules may be taken without regard to meals.
[See third table at top of previous page]

Powder for Oral Suspension
The recommended dosage and duration of treatment for infections in pediatric patients are described in the following chart; the total daily dose for all infections is 14 mg/kg, up to a maximum dose of 600 mg per day. Once-daily dosing for 10 days is as effective as BID dosing. Once-daily dosing has not been studied in skin infections; therefore, OMNICEF for Oral Suspension should be administered twice daily in this infection. OMNICEF for Oral Suspension may be administered without regard to meals.
[See fourth table at top of previous page]
[See first table at right]

Patients With Renal Insufficiency
For adult patients with creatinine clearance <30 mL/min, the dose of cefdinir should be 300 mg given once daily. Creatinine clearance is difficult to measure in outpatients. However, the following formula may be used to estimate creatinine clearance (CL_{cr}) in adult patients. For estimates to be valid, serum creatinine levels should reflect steady-state levels of renal function.

Males: $$CL_{cr} = \frac{(\text{weight})\ (140 - \text{age})}{(72)\ (\text{serum creatinine})}$$

Females: $$CL_{cr} = 0.85 \times \text{above value}$$

where creatinine clearance is in mL/min, age is in years, weight is in kilograms, and serum creatinine is in mg/dL.[3] The following formula may be used to estimate creatinine clearance in pediatric patients:

$$CL_{cr} = K \times \frac{\text{body length or height}}{\text{serum creatinine}}$$

where K=0.55 for pediatric patients older than 1 year[4] and 0.45 for infants (up to 1 year)[5].
In the above equation, creatinine clearance is in mL/min/1.73 m^2, body length or height is in centimeters, and serum creatinine is in mg/dL.
For pediatric patients with a creatinine clearance of <30 mL/min/1.73 m^2, the dose of cefdinir should be 7 mg/kg (up to 300 mg) given once daily.

Patients on Hemodialysis
Hemodialysis removes cefdinir from the body. In patients maintained on chronic hemodialysis, the recommended initial dosage regimen is a 300-mg or 7-mg/kg dose every other day. At the conclusion of each hemodialysis session, 300 mg (or 7 mg/kg) should be given. Subsequent doses (300 mg or 7 mg/kg) are then administered every other day.

Directions for Mixing Omnicef for Oral Suspension

Final Concentration	Final Volume (mL)	Amount of Water	Directions
125 mg/5 mL	60 100	38 mL 63 mL	Tap bottle to loosen powder, then add water in 2 portions. Shake well after each aliquot.

After mixing, the suspension can be stored at room temperature (25°C/77°F). The container should be kept tightly closed, and the suspension should be shaken well before each administration. The suspension may be used for 10 days, after which any unused portion must be discarded.

HOW SUPPLIED

OMNICEF Capsules, containing 300 mg cefdinir, as lavender and turquoise capsules imprinted with the product name, are available as follows:
60 Capsules/Bottle **NDC** 0074-3769-60
OMNI-PAC™ carton of 3 unit-of-use, 5-day,
10-capsule blister cards **NDC** 0074-3769-30
OMNICEF for Oral Suspension is a cream-colored powder formulation that, when reconstituted as directed, contains 125 mg cefdinir/5 mL. The reconstituted suspension has a cream color and strawberry flavor. The powder is available as follows:
60-mL bottles **NDC** 0074-3771-60
100-mL bottles **NDC** 0074-3771-13
Store the capsules and unsuspended powder at 25°C (77°F); excursions permitted to 15°-30°C (59°-86°F) [see USP Controlled Room Temperature]. Once reconstituted, the oral suspension can be stored at controlled room temperature for 10 days.

CLINICAL STUDIES

Community-Acquired Bacterial Pneumonia
In a controlled, double-blind study in adults and adolescents conducted in the US, cefdinir BID was compared with cefaclor 500 mg TID. Using strict evaluability and microbiologic/clinical response criteria 6 to 14 days posttherapy, the following clinical cure rates, presumptive microbiologic eradication rates, and statistical outcomes were obtained:
[See second table above]
In a second controlled, investigator-blind study in adults and adolescents conducted primarily in Europe, cefdinir BID was compared with amoxicillin/clavulanate 500/125 mg TID. Using strict evaluability and clinical response criteria 6 to 14 days posttherapy, the following clinical cure rates, presumptive microbiologic eradication rates, and statistical outcomes were obtained:
[See third table above]

Streptococcal Pharyngitis/Tonsillitis
In four controlled studies conducted in the US, cefdinir was compared with 10 days of penicillin in adult, adolescent, and pediatric patients. Two studies (one in adults and adolescents, the other in pediatric patients) compared 10 days of cefdinir QD or BID to penicillin 250 mg or 10 mg/kg QID. Using strict evaluability and microbiologic/clinical response criteria 5 to 10 days posttherapy, the following clinical cure rates, microbiologic eradication rates, and statistical outcomes were obtained:
[See fourth table above]
Two studies (one in adults and adolescents, the other in pediatric patients) compared 5 days of cefdinir BID to 10 days of penicillin 250 mg or 10 mg/kg QID. Using strict evaluability and microbiologic/clinical response criteria 4 to 10 days posttherapy, the following clinical cure rates, microbiologic eradication rates, and statistical outcomes were obtained:
[See fifth table above]

OMNICEF FOR ORAL SUSPENSION PEDIATRIC DOSAGE CHART

Weight	125 mg/5 mL
9 kg/20 lbs	2.5 mL (½ tsp) q12h or 5 mL (1 tsp) q24h
18 kg/40 lbs	5 mL (1 tsp) q12h or 10 mL (2 tsp) q24h
27 kg/60 lbs	7.5 mL (1½ tsp) q12h or 15 mL (3 tsp) q24h
36 kg/80 lbs	10 mL (2 tsp) q12h or 20 mL (4 tsp) q24h
≥ 43 kg[a]/95 lbs	12 mL (2½ tsp) q12h or 24 mL (5 tsp) q24h

[a] Pediatric patients who weigh ≥43 kg should receive the maximum daily dose of 600 mg.

US Community-Acquired Pneumonia Study
Cefdinir vs Cefaclor

	Cefdinir BID	Cefaclor TID	Outcome
Clinical Cure Rates	150/187 (80%)	147/186 (79%)	Cefdinir equivalent to control
Eradication Rates			
Overall	177/195 (91%)	184/200 (92%)	Cefdinir equivalent to control
S. pneumoniae	31/31 (100%)	35/35 (100%)	
H. influenzae	55/65 (85%)	60/72 (83%)	
M. catarrhalis	10/10 (100%)	11/11 (100%)	
H. parainfluenzae	81/89 (91%)	78/82 (95%)	

European Community-Acquired Pneumonia Study
Cefdinir vs Amoxicillin/Clavulanate

	Cefdinir BID	Amoxicillin/ Clavulanate TID	Outcome
Clinical Cure Rates	83/104 (80%)	86/97 (89%)	Cefdinir not equivalent to control
Eradication Rates			
Overall	85/96 (89%)	84/90 (93%)	Cefdinir equivalent to control
S. pneumoniae	42/44 (95%)	43/44 (98%)	
H. influenzae	26/35 (74%)	21/26 (81%)	
M. catarrhalis	6/6 (100%)	8/8 (100%)	
H. parainfluenzae	11/11 (100%)	12/12 (100%)	

Pharyngitis/Tonsillitis Studies
Cefdinir (10 days) vs Penicillin (10 days)

Study	Efficacy Parameter	Cefdinir QD	Cefdinir BID	Penicillin QID	Outcome
Adults/ Adolescents	Eradication of *S. pyogenes*	192/210 (91%)	199/217 (92%)	181/217 (83%)	Cefdinir superior to control
	Clinical Cure Rates	199/210 (95%)	209/217 (96%)	193/217 (89%)	Cefdinir superior to control
Pediatric Patients	Eradication of *S. pyogenes*	215/228 (94%)	214/227 (94%)	159/227 (70%)	Cefdinir superior to control
	Clinical Cure Rates	222/228 (97%)	218/227 (96%)	196/227 (86%)	Cefdinir superior to control

Pharyngitis/Tonsillitis Studies
Cefdinir (5 days) vs Penicillin (10 days)

Study	Efficacy Parameter	Cefdinir BID	Penicillin QID	Outcome
Adults/ Adolescents	Eradication of *S. pyogenes*	193/218 (89%)	176/214 (82%)	Cefdinir equivalent to control
	Clinical Cure Rates	194/218 (89%)	181/214 (85%)	Cefdinir equivalent to control
Pediatric Patients	Eradication of *S. pyogenes*	176/196 (90%)	135/193 (70%)	Cefdinir superior to control
	Clinical Cure Rates	179/196 (91%)	173/193 (90%)	Cefdinir equivalent to control

REFERENCES

1. National Committee for Clinical Laboratory Standards. Methods for Dilution Antimicrobial Susceptibility Tests for Bacteria That Grow Aerobically, 4th ed. Approved Standard, NCCLS Document M7-A4, Vol 17(2). NCCLS, Villanova, PA, Jan 1997.
2. National Committee for Clinical Laboratory Standards. Performance Standards for Antimicrobial Disk Susceptibility Tests, 6th ed. Approved Standard, NCCLS Document M2-A6, Vol 17(1). NCCLS, Villanova, PA, Jan 1997.
3. Cockcroft DW, Gault MH. Prediction of creatinine clearance from serum creatinine. Nephron, 1976;16:31-41.

4. Schwartz GJ, Haycock GB, Edelmann CM, Spitzer A. A simple estimate of glomerular filtration rate in children derived from body length and plasma creatinine. Pediatrics 1976;58:259-63.
5. Schwartz GJ, Feld LG, Langford DJ. A simple estimate of glomerular filtration rate in full-term infants during the first year of life. J Pediatrics 1984;104:849-54.

℞ **only**
Ref.: 03-5331-Rev. Jan., 2004
(Nos. 3769, 3771)
TM-Trademark

Manufactured by:
CEPH International Corporation
Carolina, Puerto Rico 00986
For:
Abbott Laboratories
North Chicago, IL 60064
Under License of:
Fujisawa Pharmaceutical Co., Ltd.
Osaka, Japan
Shown in Product Identification Guide, page 303

PCE® ℞

[p-c-ē]
(erythromycin particles in tablets)
Dispertab® Tablets
℞ **only**

To reduce the development of drug-resistant bacteria and maintain the effectiveness of PCE and other antibacterial drugs, PCE should be used only to treat or prevent infections that are proven or strongly suspected to be caused by bacteria.

DESCRIPTION

PCE (erythromycin particles in tablets) is an antibacterial product containing specially coated erythromycin base particles for oral administration. The coating protects the antibiotic from the inactivating effects of gastric acidity and permits efficient absorption of the antibiotic in the small intestine. PCE is available in two strengths containing either 333 mg or 500 mg of erythromycin base. PCE 500 mg tablets contain no synthetic dyes or artificial colors.
Erythromycin is produced by a strain of *Saccharopolyspora erythraea* (formerly *Streptomyces erythraeus*) and belongs to the macrolide group of antibiotics. It is basic and readily forms salts with acids. Erythromycin is a white to off-white powder, slightly soluble in water, and soluble in alcohol, chloroform, and ether. Erythromycin is known chemically as (3R*, 4S*, 5S*, 6R*, 7R*, 9R*, 11R*, 12R*, 13S*, 14R*)-4-[(2,6-dideoxy-3-C-methyl-3-O-methyl-α-L-*ribo*hexopyranosyl)oxy]-14-ethyl-7,12,13-trihydroxy-3,5,7,9,11,13-hexamethyl-6-[[3,4,6-trideoxy-3-(dimethylamino)-β-D-*xylo*-hexopyranosyl]oxy]oxacyclotetradecane-2,10-dione. The molecular formula is $C_{37}H_{67}NO_{13}$, and the molecular weight is 733.94. The structural formula is:

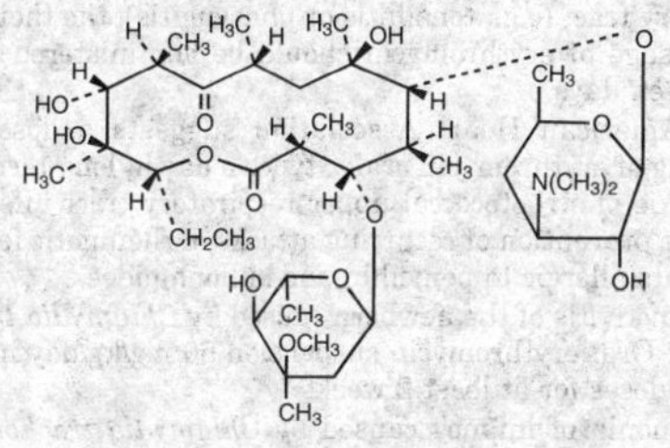

Inactive Ingredients:
PCE 333 mg tablets: Cellulosic polymers, citrate ester, colloidal silicon dioxide, D&C Red No. 30, hydrogenated vegetable oil wax, lactose, magnesium stearate, microcrystalline cellulose, povidone, propylene glycol, sodium starch glycolate, stearic acid and vanillin.
PCE 500 mg tablets: Cellulosic polymers, citrate ester, colloidal silicon dioxide, crospovidone, hydrogenated vegetable oil wax, iron oxide, microcrystalline cellulose, polyethylene glycol, povidone, propylene glycol, stearic acid, talc, titanium dioxide and vanillin.

CLINICAL PHARMACOLOGY

Orally administered erythromycin base and its salts are readily absorbed in the microbiologically active form. Interindividual variations in the absorption of erythromycin are, however, observed, and some patients do not achieve optimal serum levels. Erythromycin is largely bound to plasma proteins. After absorption, erythromycin diffuses readily into most body fluids. In the absence of meningeal inflammation, low concentrations are normally achieved in the spinal fluid but the passage of the drug across the blood-brain barrier increases in meningitis. Erythromycin crosses the placental barrier, but fetal plasma levels are low. The drug is excreted in human milk. Erythromycin is not removed by peritoneal dialysis or hemodialysis.
In the presence of normal hepatic function, erythromycin is concentrated in the liver and is excreted in the bile; the effect of hepatic dysfunction on biliary excretion of erythromycin is not known. After oral administration, less than 5% of the administered dose can be recovered in the active form in the urine.
The erythromycin particles in PCE tablets are coated with a polymer whose dissolution is pH dependent. This coating allows for minimal release of erythromycin in acidic environments, e.g. stomach. This delivery system is designed for optimal drug release and absorption in the small intestine. In multiple-dose, steady-state studies, PCE tablets have demonstrated rapid and generally adequate drug delivery in both fasting and nonfasting conditions. However, the presence of food results in lower blood levels, and optimal blood levels are obtained when PCE tablets are given in the fasting state (at least 1/2 hour and preferably 2 hours before meals). Bioavailability data are available from Abbott Laboratories, Dept. 4PI.

Microbiology:
Erythromycin acts by inhibition of protein synthesis by binding 50 S ribosomal subunits of susceptible organisms. It does not affect nucleic acid synthesis. Antagonism has been demonstrated *in vitro* between erythromycin and clindamycin, lincomycin, and chloramphenicol.
Many strains of *Haemophilus influenzae* are resistant to erythromycin alone, but are susceptible to erythromycin and sulfonamides used concomitantly.
Staphylococci resistant to erythromycin may emerge during a course of erythromycin therapy.
Erythromycin has been shown to be active against most strains of the following microorganisms, both *in vitro* and in clinical infections as described in the **INDICATIONS AND USAGE** section.

Gram-positive organisms:
Corynebacterium diphtheriae
Corynebacterium minutissimum
Listeria monocytogenes
Staphylococcus aureus (resistant organisms may emerge during treatment)
Streptococcus pneumoniae
Streptococcus pyogenes

Gram-negative organisms:
Bordetella pertussis
Legionella pneumophila
Neisseria gonorrhoeae

Other microorganisms:
Chlamydia trachomatis
Entamoeba histolytica
Mycoplasma pneumoniae
Treponema pallidum
Ureaplasma urealyticum

The following *in vitro* data are available, **but their clinical significance is unknown.**
Erythromycin exhibits *in vitro* minimal inhibitory concentrations (MIC's) of 0.5 µg/mL or less against most (≥ 90%) strains of the following microorganisms; however, the safety and effectiveness of erythromycin in treating clinical infections due to these microorganisms have not been established in adequate and well-controlled clinical trials.

Gram-positive organisms:
Viridans group streptococci

Gram-negative organisms:
Moraxella catarrhalis

Susceptibility Tests:
Dilution Techniques:
Quantitative methods are used to determine antimicrobial minimum inhibitory concentrations (MIC's). These MIC's provide estimates of the susceptibility of bacteria to antimicrobial compounds. The MIC's should be determined using a standardized procedure. Standardized procedures are based on a dilution method[1] (broth or agar) or equivalent with standardized inoculum concentrations and standardized concentrations of erythromycin powder. The MIC values should be interpreted according to the following criteria:

MIC (µg/mL)	Interpretation
≤0.5	Susceptible (S)
1–4	Intermediate (I)
≥8	Resistant (R)

A report of "Susceptible" indicates that the pathogen is likely to be inhibited if the antimicrobial compound in the blood reaches the concentrations usually achievable. A report of "Intermediate" indicates that the result should be considered equivocal, and, if the microorganism is not fully susceptible to alternative, clinically feasible drugs, the test should be repeated. This category implies possible clinical applicability in body sites where the drug is physiologically concentrated or in situations where high dosage of drug can be used. This category also provides a buffer zone which prevents small uncontrolled technical factors from causing major discrepancies in interpretation. A report of "Resistant" indicates that the pathogen is not likely to be inhibited if the antimicrobial compound in the blood reaches the concentrations usually achievable; other therapy should be selected.
Standardized susceptibility test procedures require the use of laboratory control microorganisms to control the technical aspects of the laboratory procedures. Standard erythromycin powder should provide the following MIC values:

Microorganism	MIC (µg/mL)
S. aureus ATCC 29213	0.12–0.5
E. faecalis ATCC 29212	1–4

Diffusion Techniques:
Quantitative methods that require measurement of zone diameters also provide reproducible estimates of the susceptibility of bacteria to antimicrobial compounds. One such standardized procedure[2] requires the use of standardized inoculum concentrations. This procedure uses paper disks impregnated with 15-µg erythromycin to test the susceptibility of microorganisms to erythromycin.
Reports from the laboratory providing results of the standard single-disk susceptibility test with a 15-µg erythromycin disk should be interpreted according to the following criteria:

Zone Diameter (mm)	Interpretation
≥23	Susceptible (S)
14–22	Intermediate (I)
≤13	Resistant (R)

Interpretation should be as stated above for results using dilution techniques. Interpretation involves correlation of the diameter obtained in the disk test with the MIC for erythromycin.
As with standardized dilution techniques, diffusion methods require the use of laboratory control microorganisms that are used to control the technical aspects of the laboratory procedures. For the diffusion technique, the 15-µg erythromycin disk should provide the following zone diameters in these laboratory test quality control strains:

Microorganism	Zone Diameter (mm)
S. aureus ATCC 25923	22–30

INDICATIONS AND USAGE

To reduce the development of drug-resistant bacteria and maintain the effectiveness of PCE and other antibacterial drugs, PCE should be used only to treat or prevent infections that are proven or strongly suspected to be caused by susceptible bacteria. When culture and susceptibility information are available, they should be considered in selecting or modifying antibacterial therapy. In the absence of such data, local epidemiology and susceptibility patterns may contribute to the empiric selection of therapy.
PCE tablets are indicated in the treatment of infections caused by susceptible strains of the designated microorganisms in the diseases listed below:
Upper respiratory tract infections of mild to moderate degree caused by *Streptococcus pyogenes; Streptococcus pneumoniae; Haemophilus influenzae* (when used concomitantly with adequate doses of sulfonamides, since many strains of *H. influenzae* are not susceptible to the erythromycin concentrations ordinarily achieved). (See appropriate sulfonamide labeling for prescribing information.)
Lower respiratory tract infections of mild to moderate severity caused by *Streptococcus pyogenes* or *Streptococcus pneumoniae*.
Listeriosis caused by *Listeria monocytogenes*.
Respiratory tract infections due to *Mycoplasma pneumoniae*.
Skin and skin structure infections of mild to moderate severity caused by *Streptococcus pyogenes* or *Staphylococcus aureus* (resistant staphylococci may emerge during treatment).
Pertussis (whooping cough) caused by *Bordetella pertussis*. Erythromycin is effective in eliminating the organism from the nasopharynx of infected individuals, rendering them noninfectious. Some clinical studies suggest that erythromycin may be helpful in the prophylaxis of pertussis in exposed susceptible individuals.
Diphtheria: Infections due to *Corynebacterium diphtheriae*. as an adjunct to antitoxin, to prevent establishment of carriers and to eradicate the organism in carriers.
Erythrasma—In the treatment of infections due to *Corynebacterium minutissimum*.
Intestinal amebiasis caused by *Entamoeba histolytica* (oral erythromycins only). Extraenteric amebiasis requires treatment with other agents.
Acute pelvic inflammatory disease caused by *Neisseria gonorrhoeae*: Erythrocin® Lactobionate-I.V. (erythromycin lactobionate for injection, USP) followed by erythromycin base orally, as an alternative drug in treatment of acute pelvic inflammatory disease caused by *N. gonorrhoeae* in female patients with a history of sensitivity to penicillin. Patients should have a serologic test for syphilis before receiving erythromycin as treatment of gonorrhea and a follow-up serologic test for syphilis after 3 months.
Erythromycins are indicated for treatment of the following infections caused by *Chlamydia trachomatis*: conjunctivitis of the newborn, pneumonia of infancy, and urogenital infections during pregnancy. When tetracyclines are contraindicated or not tolerated, erythromycin is indicated for the treatment of uncomplicated urethral, endocervical, or rectal infections in adults due to *Chlamydia trachomatis*.
When tetracyclines are contraindicated or not tolerated, erythromycin is indicated for the treatment of nongonococcal urethritis caused by *Ureaplasma urealyticum*.
Primary syphilis caused by *Treponema pallidum*. Erythromycin (oral forms only) is an alternative choice of treatment

Continued on next page

PCE—Cont.

for primary syphilis in patients allergic to the penicillins. In treatment of primary syphilis, spinal fluid should be examined before treatment and as part of the follow-up after therapy.

Legionnaires' Disease caused by *Legionella pneumophila*. Although no controlled clinical efficacy studies have been conducted, *in vitro* and limited preliminary clinical data suggest that erythromycin may be effective in treating Legionnaires' Disease.

Prophylaxis

Prevention of Initial Attacks of Rheumatic Fever—Penicillin is considered by the American Heart Association to be the drug of choice in the prevention of initial attacks of rheumatic fever (treatment of *Streptococcus pyogenes* infections of the upper respiratory tract e.g., tonsillitis, or pharyngitis).[3] Erythromycin is indicated for the treatment of penicillin-allergic patients. The therapeutic dose should be administered for ten days.

Prevention of Recurrent Attacks of Rheumatic Fever—Penicillin or sulfonamides are considered by the American Heart Association to be the drugs of choice in the prevention of recurrent attacks of rheumatic fever. In patients who are allergic to penicillin and sulfonamides, oral erythromycin is recommended by the American Heart Association in the long-term prophylaxis of streptococcal pharyngitis (for the prevention of recurrent attacks of rheumatic fever).[3]

CONTRAINDICATIONS

Erythromycin is contraindicated in patients with known hypersensitivity to this antibiotic.

Erythromycin is contraindicated in patients taking terfenadine, astemizole, pimozide, or cisapride. (See **PRECAUTIONS**-*Drug Interactions.*)

WARNINGS

There have been reports of hepatic dysfunction, including increased liver enzymes, and hepatocellular and/or cholestatic hepatitis, with or without jaundice, occurring in patients receiving oral erythromycin products.

There have been reports suggesting that erythromycin does not reach the fetus in adequate concentration to prevent congenital syphilis. Infants born to women treated during pregnancy with oral erythromycin for early syphilis should be treated with an appropriate penicillin regimen.

Rhabdomyolysis with or without renal impairment has been reported in seriously ill patients receiving erythromycin concomitantly with lovastatin. Therefore, patients receiving concomitant lovastatin and erythromycin should be carefully monitored for creatine kinase (CK) and serum transaminase levels. (See package insert for lovastatin.)

Pseudomembranous colitis has been reported with nearly all antibacterial agents, including erythromycin, and may range in severity from mild to life threatening. Therefore, it is important to consider this diagnosis in patients who present with diarrhea subsequent to the administration of antibacterial agents.

Treatment with antibacterial agents alters the normal flora of the colon and may permit overgrowth of clostridia. Studies indicate that a toxin produced by *Clostridium difficile* is a primary cause of "antibiotic-associated colitis".

After the diagnosis of pseudomembranous colitis has been established, therapeutic measures should be initiated. Mild cases of pseudomembranous colitis usually respond to discontinuation of the drug alone. In moderate to severe cases, consideration should be given to management with fluids and electrolytes, protein supplementation, and treatment with an antibacterial drug clinically effective against *Clostridium difficile* colitis.

PRECAUTIONS

General: Prescribing PCE in the absence of a proven or strongly suspected bacterial infection or a prophylactic indication is unlikely to provide benefit to the patient and increases the risk of the development of drug-resistant bacteria.

Since erythromycin is principally excreted by the liver, caution should be exercised when erythromycin is administered to patients with impaired hepatic function. (See **CLINICAL PHARMACOLOGY** and **WARNINGS.**)

There have been reports that erythromycin may aggravate the weakness of patients with myasthenia gravis.

There have been reports of infantile hypertrophic pyloric stenosis (IHPS) occurring in infants following erythromycin therapy. In one cohort of 157 newborns who were given erythromycin for pertussis prophylaxis, seven neonates (5%) developed symptoms of non-bilious vomiting or irritability with feeding and were subsequently diagnosed as having IHPS requiring surgical pyloromyotomy. A possible dose-response effect was described with an absolute risk of IHPS of 5.1% for infants who took erythromycin for 8–14 days and 10% for infants who took erythromycin for 5–21 days.[4] Since erythromycin may be used in the treatment of conditions in infants which are associated with significant mortality or morbidity (such as pertussis or neonatal Chlamydia trachomatis infections), the benefit of erythromycin therapy needs to be weighed against the potential risk of developing IHPS. Parents should be informed to contact their physician if vomiting or irritability with feeding occurs.

Prolonged or repeated use of erythromycin may result in an overgrowth of nonsusceptible bacteria or fungi. If superinfection occurs, erythromycin should be discontinued and appropriate therapy instituted.

When indicated, incision and drainage or other surgical procedures should be performed in conjunction with antibiotic therapy.

Information for Patients: Patients should be counseled that antibacterial drugs including PCE should only be used to treat bacterial infections. They do not treat viral infections (e.g., the common cold). When PCE is prescribed to treat a bacterial infection, patients should be told that although it is common to feel better early in the course of therapy, the medication should be taken exactly as directed. Skipping doses or not completing the full course of therapy may (1) decrease the effectiveness of the immediate treatment and (2) increase the likelihood that bacteria will develop resistance and will not be treatable by PCE or other antibacterial drugs in the future.

Drug Interactions: Erythromycin use in patients who are receiving high doses of theophylline may be associated with an increase in serum theophylline levels and potential theophylline toxicity. In case of theophylline toxicity and/or elevated serum theophylline levels, the dose of theophylline should be reduced while the patient is receiving concomitant erythromycin therapy.

Concomitant administration of erythromycin and digoxin has been reported to result in elevated digoxin serum levels.

There have been reports of increased anticoagulant effects when erythromycin and oral anticoagulants were used concomitantly. Increased anticoagulation effects due to interactions of erythromycin with oral anticoagulants may be more pronounced in the elderly.

Erythromycin is a substrate and inhibitor of the 3A isoform subfamily of the cytochrome p450 enzyme system (CYP3A). Coadministration of erythromycin and a drug primarily metabolized by CYP3A may be associated with elevations in drug concentrations that could increase or prolong both the therapeutic and adverse effects of the concomitant drug. Dosage adjustments may be considered, and when possible, serum concentrations of drugs primarily metabolized by CYP3A should be monitored closely in patients concurrently receiving erythromycin.

The following are examples of some clinically significant CYP3A based drug interactions. Interactions with other drugs metabolized by the CYP3A isoform are also possible. The following CYP3A based drug interactions have been observed with erythromycin products in post-marketing experience:

Ergotamine/dihydroergotamine: Concurrent use of erythromycin and ergotamine or dihydroergotamine has been associated in some patients with acute ergot toxicity characterized by severe peripheral vasospasm and dysesthesia.

Triazolobenzodiazepines (such as triazolam and alprazolam) *and related benzodiazepines:* Erythromycin has been reported to decrease the clearance of triazolam and midazolam, and thus, may increase the pharmacologic effect of these benzodiazepines.

HMG-CoA Reductase Inhibitors: Erythromycin has been reported to increase concentrations of HMG-CoA reductase inhibitors (e.g., lovastatin and simvastatin). Rare reports of rhabdomyolysis have been reported in patients taking these drugs concomitantly.

Sildenafil (Viagra): Erythromycin has been reported to increase the systemic exposure (AUC) of sildenafil. Reduction of sildenafil dosage should be considered. (See Viagra package insert.)

There have been spontaneous or published reports of CYP3A based interactions of erythromycin with cyclosporine, carbamazepine, tacrolimus, alfentanil, disopyramide, rifabutin, quinidine, methylprednisolone, cilostazol, vinblastine, and bromocriptine.

Concomitant administration of erythromycin with cisapride, pimozide, astemizole, or terfenadine is contraindicated. (See **CONTRAINDICATIONS.**)

In addition, there have been reports of interactions of erythromycin with drugs not thought to be metabolized by CYP3A, including hexobarbital, phenytoin, and valproate.

Erythromycin has been reported to significantly alter the metabolism of the nonsedating antihistamines terfenadine and astemizole when taken concomitantly. Rare cases of serious cardiovascular adverse events, including electrocardiographic QT/QT_c interval prolongation, cardiac arrest, torsades de pointes, and other ventricular arrhythmias, have been observed. (See **CONTRAINDICATIONS.**) In addition, deaths have been reported rarely with concomitant administration of terfenadine and erythromycin.

There have been post-marketing reports of drug interactions when erythromycin was coadministered with cisapride, resulting in QT prolongation, cardiac arrhythmias, ventricular tachycardia, ventricular fibrillation, and torsades de pointes, most likely due to the inhibition of hepatic metabolism of cisapride by erythromycin. Fatalities have been reported. (See **CONTRAINDICATIONS.**)

Drug/Laboratory Test interactions: Erythromycin interferes with the fluorometric determination of urinary catecholamines.

Carcinogenesis, Mutagenesis, Impairment of Fertility: Long-term (2-year) oral studies conducted in rats with erythromycin base did not provide evidence of tumorigenicity. Mutagenicity studies have not been conducted. There was no apparent effect on male or female fertility in rats fed erythromycin (base) at levels up to 0.25 percent of diet.

Pregnancy: Teratogenic effects. Pregnancy Category B: There is no evidence of teratogenicity or any other adverse effect on reproduction in female rats fed erythromycin base (up to 0.25 percent of diet) prior to and during mating, during gestation, and through weaning of two successive litters. There are, however, no adequate and well-controlled studies in pregnant women. Because animal reproduction studies are not always predictive of human response, this drug should be used during pregnancy only if clearly needed.

Labor and Delivery: The effect of erythromycin on labor and delivery is unknown.

Nursing Mothers: Erythromycin is excreted in human milk. Caution should be exercised when erythromycin is administered to a nursing woman.

Pediatric Use: See **INDICATIONS AND USAGE** and **DOSAGE AND ADMINISTRATION**.

ADVERSE REACTIONS

The most frequent side effects of oral erythromycin preparations are gastrointestinal and are dose-related. They include nausea, vomiting, abdominal pain, diarrhea and anorexia. Symptoms of hepatitis, hepatic dysfunction and/or abnormal liver function test results may occur. (See **WARNINGS.**)

Onset of pseudomembranous colitis symptoms may occur during or after antibacterial treatment. (See **WARNINGS.**)

Erythromycin has been associated with QT prolongation and ventricular arrhythmias, including ventricular tachycardia and torsades de pointes.

Allergic reactions ranging from urticaria to anaphylaxis have occurred. Skin reactions ranging from mild eruptions to erythema multiforme, Stevens-Johnson syndrome, and toxic epidermal necrolysis have been reported rarely.

There have been rare reports of pancreatitis and convulsions.

There have been isolated reports of reversible hearing loss occurring chiefly in patients with renal insufficiency and in patients receiving high doses of erythromycin.

OVERDOSAGE

In case of overdosage, erythromycin should be discontinued. Overdosage should be handled with the prompt elimination of unabsorbed drug and all other appropriate measures should be instituted.

Erythromycin is not removed by peritoneal dialysis or hemodialysis.

DOSAGE AND ADMINISTRATION

In most patients, PCE tablets are well absorbed and may be dosed orally without regard to meals. However, optimal blood levels are obtained when either PCE 333 mg or PCE 500 mg tablets are given in the fasting state (at least 1/2 hour and preferably 2 hours before meals).

Adults: The usual dosage of PCE is one 333 mg tablet every 8 hours or one 500 mg tablet every 12 hours. Dosage may be increased up to 4 g per day according to the severity of the infection. However, twice-a-day dosing is not recommended when doses larger than 1 g daily are administered.

Children: Age, weight, and severity of the infection are important factors in determining the proper dosage. The usual dosage is 30 to 50 mg/kg/day, in equally divided doses. For more severe infections this dosage may be doubled but should not exceed 4 g per day.

In the treatment of streptococcal infections of the upper respiratory tract (e.g., tonsillitis or pharyngitis), the therapeutic dosage of erythromycin should be administered for at least ten days.

The American Heart Association suggests a dosage of 250 mg of erythromycin orally, twice a day in long-term prophylaxis of streptococcal upper respiratory tract infections for the prevention of recurring attacks of rheumatic fever in patients allergic to penicillin and sulfonamides.[3]

Conjunctivitis of the newborn caused by *Chlamydia trachomatis*: Oral erythromycin suspension 50 mg/kg/day in 4 divided doses for at least 2 weeks.[3]

Pneumonia of infancy caused by *Chlamydia trachomatis*: Although the optimal duration of therapy has not been established, the recommended therapy is oral erythromycin suspension 50 mg/kg/day in 4 divided doses for at least 3 weeks.

Urogenital infections during pregnancy due to *Chlamydia trachomatis*: Although the optimal dose and duration of therapy have not been established, the suggested treatment is 500 mg of erythromycin by mouth four times a day or two erythromycin 333 mg tablets orally every 8 hours on an empty stomach for at least 7 days. For women who cannot tolerate this regimen, a decreased dose of one erythromycin 500 mg tablet orally every 12 hours, one 333 mg tablet orally every 8 hours or 250 mg by mouth four times a day should be used for at least 14 days.[5]

For adults with uncomplicated urethral, endocervical, or rectal infections caused by *Chlamydia trachomatis*, when tetracycline is contraindicated or not tolerated: 500 mg of erythromycin by mouth four times a day or two 333 mg tablets orally every 8 hours for at least 7 days.[5]

For patients with nongonococcal urethritis caused by *Ureaplasma urealyticum* when tetracycline is contraindicated or not tolerated: 500 mg of erythromycin by mouth four times a day or two 333 mg tablets orally every 8 hours for at least seven days.[5]

Primary syphilis: 30 to 40 g given in divided doses over a period of 10 to 15 days.

Acute pelvic inflammatory disease caused by *N. gonorrhoeae*: 500 mg Erythrocin Lactobionate-I.V. (erythromycin lactobionate for injection, USP) every 6 hours for 3 days, followed by 500 mg of erythromycin base orally every 12 hours, or 333 mg of erythromycin base orally every 8 hours for 7 days.

Intestinal amebiasis: Adults: 500 mg every 12 hours, 333 mg every 8 hours or 250 mg every 6 hours for 10 to 14 days. Children: 30 to 50 mg/kg/day in divided doses for 10 to 14 days.
Pertussis: Although optimal dosage and duration have not been established, doses of erythromycin utilized in reported clinical studies were 40 to 50 mg/kg/day, given in divided doses for 5 to 14 days.
Legionnaires' Disease: Although optimal dosage has not been established, doses utilized in reported clinical data were 1 to 4 g daily in divided doses.

HOW SUPPLIED

PCE (erythromycin particles in tablets) is supplied as unscored, ovaloid, Dispertab® tablets in the following strengths and packages.
333 mg, pink-speckled white (imprinted with [logo] and PCE):
Bottles of 60 .... (**NDC** 0074-6290-60).
500 mg, white (imprinted with [logo] and EK):
Bottles of 100 .... (**NDC** 0074-3389-13).
Recommended Storage: Store below 86°F (30°C).

REFERENCES

1. National Committee for Clinical Laboratory Standards. *Methods for Dilution Antimicrobial Susceptibility Tests for Bacteria that Grow Aerobically*, Third Edition. Approved Standard NCCLS Document M7-A3, Vol. 13, No. 25 NCCLS, Villanova, PA, December 1993.
2. National Committee for Clinical Laboratory Standards, *Performance Standards for Antimicrobial Disk Susceptibility Tests*, Fifth Edition. Approved Standard NCCLS Document M2-A5, Vol. 13, No. 24 NCCLS, Villanova, PA, December 1993.
3. Committee on Rheumatic Fever, Endocarditis, and Kawasaki Disease of the Council on Cardiovascular Disease in the Young, the American Heart Association: Prevention of Rheumatic Fever. *Circulation*. 78(4):1082-1086, October 1988.
4. Honein, M.A., et. al.: Infantile hypertrophic pyloric stenosis after pertussis prophylaxis with erythromycin: a case review and cohort study. The Lancet 1999; 354 (9196): 2101–5.
5. Data on file, Abbott Laboratories.

Ref. 03-5324-R9
Revised: November, 2003
PCE 333 mg: U.S. Pat. No. 4,874,614.
PCE 500 mg: U.S. Pat. No. 4,874,614 and 5,009,897.
ABBOTT LABORATORIES
NORTH CHICAGO, IL 60064, U.S.A.
PRINTED IN U.S.A.

PROSOM™ Ⓒ℞

[*prō-som*]
(estazolam tablets)

DESCRIPTION

ProSom (estazolam), a triazolobenzodiazepine derivative, is an oral hypnotic agent. Estazolam occurs as a fine, white, odorless powder that is soluble in alcohol and practically insoluble in water. The chemical name for estazolam is 8-chloro-6-phenyl-4H-s-triazolo[4,3-α] [1,4]benzodiazepine. The empirical formula is $C_{16}H_{11}ClN_4$. The structural formula is represented as follows:

ProSom tablets are scored and contain either 1 mg or 2 mg of estazolam.
Inactive Ingredients: colloidal silicon dioxide, lactose, povidone, stearic acid, and sodium starch glycolate.
In addition, the 2 mg tablets contain FD&C Red No. 40.

CLINICAL PHARMACOLOGY

Pharmacokinetics

Absorption
ProSom tablets have been found to be equivalent in absorption to an orally administered solution of estazolam. In healthy subjects who received up to three times the recommended dose of ProSom, peak estazolam plasma concentrations occurred within two hours after dosing (range 0.5 to 6.0 hours) and were proportional to the administered dose, suggesting linear pharmacokinetics over the dosage range tested.
Distribution
Independent of concentration, estazolam in plasma is 93% protein bound.
Metabolism
Estazolam is extensively metabolized. Only two metabolites (1-oxo-estazolam & 4-hydroxy-estazolam) were detected in human plasma up to 18 hrs.
The pharmacologic activity of estazolam is primarily from the parent drug. The elimination of the parent drug takes place via hepatic metabolism of estazolam to hydroxylated and other metabolites that are eliminated largely in the urine both free and conjugated. In humans, greater than 70% of a single dose of estazolam was recovered in the urine as metabolites. Less than 5% of a 2 mg dose of estazolam was excreted unchanged in the urine, with only 4% of the dose appearing in the feces. The principal urinary excretion product is an unidentified metabolite, presumed to be a metabolic product of 4-hydroxy-estazolam, accounting for at least 27% of the administered dose. 4-hydroxy-estazolam is the major metabolite in plasma, with concentrations approaching 12% of those of the parent eight hours after administration. Urinary 4-hydroxy-estazolam and 1-oxo-estazolam account for 11.9% and 4.4% of the dose respectively. *In vitro* studies with human liver microsomes indicate that the biotransformation of estazolam to the major circulating metabolite 4-hydroxy-estazolam is mediated by cytochrome P450 3A (CYP3A). While 4-hydroxy-estazolam and the lesser metabolite, 1-oxo-estazolam, have some pharmacologic activity, their low potencies and low concentrations preclude any significant contribution to the hypnotic effect of ProSom.
Elimination
The range of estimates for the mean elimination half-life of estazolam varied from 10 to 24 hours. Radiolabel mass balance studies indicate that the main route of excretion is via the kidneys. After 5 days, 87% of the administered radioactivity was excreted in human urine. Less than 4% of the dose was excreted unchanged. Eleven metabolites were found in urine. Four metabolites were identified as 1-oxo-estazolam, 4'-hydroxy-estazolam, 4-hydroxy-estazolam, and benzophenone, as free metabolites and glucuronides. The predominant metabolite in urine (17% of the administered dose) has not been identified, but is likely to be a metabolite of 4-hydroxy-estazolam.

Special Populations:
In a small study (N=8) using various doses in older subjects (59 to 68 years), peak estazolam concentrations were found to be similar to those observed in younger subjects with a mean elimination half-life of 18.4 hours (range 13.5 to 34.6 hours). The influence of hepatic or renal impairment on the pharmacokinetics of estazolam has not been studied.
Pediatrics: The pharmacokinetics of estazolam have not been studied in pediatric patients.
Race: The influence of race on the pharmacokinetics of estazolam has not been studied.
Gender: The gender-effect on the pharmacokinetics of estazolam has not been investigated.
Cigarette Smoking: The clearance of benzodiazepines is accelerated in smokers compared to nonsmokers, and there is evidence that this occurs with estazolam. This decrease in half-life, presumably due to enzyme induction by smoking, is consistent with other drugs with similar hepatic clearance characteristics. In all subjects and at all doses, the mean elimination half-life appeared to be independent of the dose.
Drug-Drug Interaction: The metabolism of estazolam to the major circulating metabolite 4-hydroxy-estazolam is catalyzed by CYP3A. While no *in vivo* drug-drug interaction studies were conducted between estazolam and inhibitors/inducers of CYP3A, compounds that are potent CYP3A inhibitors (such as ketoconazole, itraconazole, nefazodone, fluvoxamine, and erythromycin) would be expected to increase plasma estazolam concentrations and CYP3A inducers (such as carbamazepine, phenytoin, rifampin and barbiturates) would be expected to decrease estazolam concentrations.
Drug Interaction with Fluoxetine: A multiple-dose study was conducted to assess the effect of fluoxetine 20 mg BID on the pharmacokinetics of estazolam 2 mg QHS after seven days. The pharmacokinetics of estazolam (C_{max} and AUC) were not affected during multiple-dose fluoxetine, suggesting no clinically significant pharmacokinetic interaction.
The Ability of Estazolam to Induce or Inhibit Human Enzyme Systems: The results from *in vitro* human liver microsomal studies suggest that at therapeutic concentrations, estazolam has no significant inhibitory effect on the major human cytochrome P450 enzyme activities (i.e., CYP1A2, CYP2A6, CYP2C9, CYP2C19, CYP2D6, CYP2E1, and CYP3A). The ability of estazolam to induce human hepatic enzyme systems has not been determined.

Pharmacodynamics
Postulated relationship between elimination rate of benzodiazepine hypnotics and their profile of common untoward effects: The type and duration of hypnotic effects and the profile of unwanted effects during administration of benzodiazepine drugs may be influenced by the biologic half-life of administered drug and any active metabolites formed. If half-lives are long, drug or metabolites may accumulate during periods of nightly administration and may be associated with impairments of cognitive and/or motor performance during waking hours; the possibility of interaction with other psychoactive drugs or alcohol will be increased. In contrast, if half-lives are short, drug and metabolites will be cleared before the next dose is ingested, and carry-over effects related to excessive sedation or CNS depression should be minimal or absent. However, during nightly use for an extended period, pharmacodynamic tolerance or adaptation to some effects of benzodiazepine hypnotics may develop. If the drug has a short elimination half-life, it is possible that a relative deficiency of the drug or its active metabolites (ie, in relationship to the receptor site) may occur at some point in the interval between each night's use. This sequence of events may account for two clinical findings reported to occur after several weeks of nightly use of rapidly eliminated benzodiazepine hypnotics, namely, increased wakefulness during the last third of the night and increased daytime anxiety in selected patients.

CLINICAL STUDIES

Controlled Trials Supporting Efficacy: In three 7-night, double-blind, parallel-group trials comparing estazolam 1 mg and/or 2 mg with placebo in adult outpatients with chronic insomnia, estazolam 2 mg was consistently superior to placebo in subjective measures of sleep induction (latency) and sleep maintenance (duration, number of awakenings, depth and quality of sleep); estazolam 1 mg was similarly superior to placebo on all measures of sleep maintenance, however, it significantly improved sleep induction in only one of two studies. In a similarly designed trial comparing estazolam 0.5 mg and 1 mg with placebo in geriatric outpatients with chronic insomnia, only the 1 mg estazolam dose was consistently superior to placebo in sleep induction (latency) and in only one measure of sleep maintenance (ie, duration of sleep).
In a single-night, double-blind, parallel-group trial comparing estazolam 2 mg and placebo in patients admitted for elective surgery and requiring sleep medications, estazolam was superior to placebo in subjective measures of sleep induction and maintenance.
In a 12-week, double-blind, parallel-group trial including a comparison of estazolam 2 mg and placebo in adult outpatients with chronic insomnia, estazolam was superior to placebo in subjective measures of sleep induction (latency) and maintenance (duration, number of awakenings, total wake time during sleep) at week 2, but produced consistent improvement over 12 weeks only for sleep duration and total wake time during sleep. Following withdrawal at week 12, rebound insomnia was seen at the first withdrawal week, but there was no difference between drug and placebo by the second withdrawal week in all parameters except latency, for which normalization did not occur until the fourth withdrawal week.
Adult outpatients with chronic insomnia were evaluated in a sleep laboratory trial comparing four doses of estazolam (0.25, 0.50, 1.0 and 2.0 mg) and placebo, each administered for 2 nights in a crossover design. The higher estazolam doses were superior to placebo in most EEG measures of sleep induction and maintenance, especially at the 2 mg dose, but only for sleep duration in subjective measures of sleep.

INDICATIONS AND USAGE

ProSom (estazolam) is indicated for the short-term management of insomnia characterized by difficulty in falling asleep, frequent nocturnal awakenings, and/or early morning awakenings. Both outpatient studies and a sleep laboratory study have shown that ProSom administered at bedtime improved sleep induction and sleep maintenance (see **CLINICAL PHARMACOLOGY**).
Because insomnia is often transient and intermittent, the prolonged administration of ProSom is generally neither necessary nor recommended. Since insomnia may be a symptom of several other disorders, the possibility that the complaint may be related to a condition for which there is a more specific treatment should be considered.
There is evidence to support the ability of ProSom to enhance the duration and quality of sleep for intervals up to 12 weeks (see **CLINICAL PHARMACOLOGY**).

CONTRAINDICATIONS

Benzodiazepines may cause fetal damage when administered during pregnancy. An increased risk of congenital malformations associated with the use of diazepam and chlordiazepoxide during the first trimester of pregnancy has been suggested in several studies. Transplacental distribution has resulted in neonatal CNS depression and also withdrawal phenomena following the ingestion of therapeutic doses of a benzodiazepine hypnotic during the last weeks of pregnancy.
ProSom is contraindicated in pregnant women. If there is a likelihood of the patient becoming pregnant while receiving ProSom she should be warned of the potential risk to the fetus and instructed to discontinue the drug prior to becoming pregnant. The possibility that a woman of childbearing potential is pregnant at the time of institution of therapy should be considered.
Estazolam is contraindicated with ketoconazole and itraconazole, since these medications significantly impair oxidative metabolism mediated by CYP3A (see **WARNINGS** and **PRECAUTIONS**: Drug Interactions).

WARNINGS

ProSom, like other benzodiazepines, has CNS depressant effects. For this reason, patients should be cautioned against engaging in hazardous occupations requiring complete mental alertness, such as operating machinery or driving a motor vehicle, after ingesting the drug, including potential impairment of the performance of such activities that may occur the day following ingestion of ProSom. Patients should also be cautioned about possible combined effects with alcohol and other CNS depressant drugs.
As with all benzodiazepines, amnesia, paradoxical reactions (eg, excitement, agitation, etc.), and other adverse behavioral effects may occur unpredictably.
There have been reports of withdrawal signs and symptoms of the type associated with withdrawal from CNS depressant drugs following the rapid decrease or the abrupt discontinuation of benzodiazepines (see **DRUG ABUSE AND DEPENDENCE**).

Continued on next page

ProSom—Cont.

Estazolam Interaction with Drugs that Inhibit Metabolism via Cytochrome P450 3A (CYP3A): The metabolism of estazolam to the major circulating metabolite 4-hydroxy-estazolam and the metabolism of other triazolobenzodiazepines is catalyzed by CYP3A. Consequently, estazolam should be avoided in patients receiving ketoconazole and itraconazole, which are very potent inhibitors of CYP3A (see **CONTRAINDICATIONS**). With drugs inhibiting CYP3A to a lesser, but still significant degree, estazolam should be used only with caution and consideration of appropriate dosage reduction. The following are examples of drugs known to inhibit the metabolism of other related benzodiazepines, presumably through inhibition of CYP3A: nefazodone, fluvoxamine, cimetidine, diltiazem, isoniazide, and some macrolide antibiotics.

While no *in vivo* drug-drug interaction studies were conducted between estazolam and inducers of CYP3A, compounds that are potent CYP3A inducers (such as carbamazepine, phenytoin, rifampin, and barbiturates) would be expected to decrease estazolam concentrations.

PRECAUTIONS

General: Impaired motor and/or cognitive performance attributable to the accumulation of benzodiazepines and their active metabolites following several days of repeated use at their recommended doses is a concern in certain vulnerable patients (eg, those especially sensitive to the effects of benzodiazepines or those with a reduced capacity to metabolize and eliminate them) (see **DOSAGE AND ADMINISTRATION**).

Elderly or debilitated patients and those with impaired renal or hepatic function should be cautioned about these risks and advised to monitor themselves for signs of excessive sedation or impaired conditions.

ProSom appears to cause dose-related respiratory depression that is ordinarily not clinically relevant at recommended doses in patients with normal respiratory function. However, patients with compromised respiratory function may be at risk and should be monitored appropriately. As a class, benzodiazepines have the capacity to depress respiratory drive; there are insufficient data available, however, to characterize their relative potency in depressing respiratory drive at clinically recommended doses.

As with other benzodiazepines, ProSom should be administered with caution to patients exhibiting signs or symptoms of depression. Suicidal tendencies may be present in such patients and protective measures may be required. Intentional overdosage is more common in this group of patients; therefore, the least amount of drug that is feasible should be prescribed for the patient at any one time.

Information for Patients: To assure the safe and effective use of ProSom, the following information and instructions should be given to patients:

1. Inform your physician about any alcohol consumption and medicine you are taking now, including drugs you may buy without a prescription. Alcohol should not be used during treatment with hypnotics.
2. Inform your physician if you are planning to become pregnant, if you are pregnant, or if you become pregnant while you are taking this medicine.
3. You should not take this medicine if you are nursing, as the drug may be excreted in breast milk.
4. Until you experience the way this medicine affects you, do not drive a car, operate potentially dangerous machinery, or engage in hazardous occupations requiring complete mental alertness after taking this medicine.
5. Since benzodiazepines may produce psychological and physical dependence, you should not increase the dose before consulting your physician. In addition, since the abrupt discontinuation of ProSom may be associated with temporary sleep disturbances, you should consult your physician before abruptly discontinuing doses of 2 mg per night or more.

Laboratory Tests: Laboratory tests are not ordinarily required in otherwise healthy patients. When treatment with ProSom is protracted, periodic blood counts, urinalyses, and blood chemistry analyses are advisable.

Drug Interactions: If ProSom is given concomitantly with other drugs acting on the central nervous system, careful consideration should be given to the pharmacology of all agents. The action of the benzodiazepines may be potentiated by anticonvulsants, antihistamines, alcohol, barbiturates, monoamine oxidase inhibitors, narcotics, phenothiazines, psychotropic medications, or other drugs that produce CNS depression. Smokers have an increased clearance of benzodiazepines as compared to nonsmokers; this was seen in studies with estazolam (see **CLINICAL PHARMACOLOGY**).

While no *in vivo* drug-drug interaction studies were conducted between estazolam and inducers of CYP3A, compounds that are potent CYP3A inducers (such as carbamazepine, phenytoin, rifampin, and barbiturates) would be expected to decrease estazolam concentrations.

Estazolam Interaction with Drugs that Inhibit Metabolism via Cytochrome P450 3A (CYP3A): The metabolism of estazolam to the major circulating metabolite 4-hydroxy-estazolam and the metabolism of other triazolobenzodiazepines is catalyzed by CYP3A. Consequently, estazolam should be avoided in patients receiving ketoconazole and itraconazole, which are very potent inhibitors of CYP3A (see **CONTRINDICATIONS**). With drugs inhibiting CYP3A to a lesser, but still significant degree, estazolam should be used only with caution and consideration of appropriate dosage reduction. The following are examples of drugs known to inhibit the metabolism of other related benzodiazepines, presumably through inhibition of CYP3A: nefazodone, fluvoxamine, cimetidine, diltiazem, isoniazide, and some macrolide antibiotics.

Drug Interaction with Fluoxetine: A multiple-dose study was conducted to assess the effect of fluoxetine 20 mg BID on the pharmacokinetics of estazolam 2 mg QHS after seven days. The pharmacokinetics of estazolam (C_{max} and AUC) were not affected during multiple-dose fluoxetine, suggesting no clinically significant pharmacokinetic interaction.

Estazolam Interaction with Other Drugs that are Metabolized by Cytochrome P450 (CYP): At clinically relevant concentrations, *in vitro* studies indicate that estazolam (0.6μM) was not inhibitory towards the major cytochrome P450 isoforms CYP1A2, CYP2A6, CYP2C9, CYP2C19, CYP2D6, CYP2E1, and CYP3A. Therefore, based on these *in vitro* data, estazolam is very unlikely to inhibit the biotransformation of other drugs metabolized by these CYP isoforms.

Carcinogenesis, Mutagenesis, Impairment of Fertility: Two-year carcinogenicity studies were conducted in mice and rats at dietary doses of 0.8, 3, and 10 mg/kg/day and 0.5, 2, and 10 mg/kg/day, respectively. Evidence of tumorigenicity was not observed in either study. Incidence of hyperplastic liver nodules increased in female mice given the mid- and high-dose levels. The significance of such nodules in mice is not known at this time.

In vitro and *in vivo* mutagenicity tests including the Ames test, DNA repair in *B. subtilis, in vivo* cytogenetics in mice and rats, and the dominant lethal test in mice did not show a mutagenic potential for estazolam.

Fertility in male and female rats was not affected by doses up to 30 times the usual recommended human dose.

Pregnancy:

1. Teratogenic Effects: Pregnancy Category X (see **CONTRAINDICATIONS**).
2. Nonteratogenic Effects: The child born of a mother taking benzodiazepines may be at some risk for withdrawal symptoms during the postnatal period. Neonatal flaccidity has been reported in an infant born of a mother who received benzodiazepines during pregnancy.

Labor and Delivery: ProSom has no established use in labor or delivery.

Nursing Mothers: Human studies have not been conducted; however, studies in lactating rats indicate that estazolam and/or its metabolites are secreted in the milk. The use of ProSom in nursing mothers is not recommended.

Pediatric Use: Safety and effectiveness in pediatric patients below the age of 18 have not been established.

Geriatric Use: Approximately 18% of individuals participating in the premarketing clinical trials of ProSom were 60 years of age or older. Overall, the adverse event profile did not differ substantively from that observed in younger individuals. Care should be exercised when prescribing benzodiazepines to small or debilitated elderly patients (see **DOSAGE AND ADMINISTRATION**).

ADVERSE REACTIONS

Commonly Observed: The most commonly observed adverse events associated with the use of ProSom, not seen at an equivalent incidence among placebo-treated patients were somnolence, hypokinesia, dizziness, and abnormal coordination.

Associated with Discontinuation of Treatment: Approximately 3% of 1277 patients who received ProSom in US premarketing clinical trials discontinued treatment because of an adverse clinical event. The only event commonly associated with discontinuation, accounting for 1.3% of the total, was somnolence.

Incidence in Controlled Clinical Trials: The table below enumerates adverse events that occurred at an incidence of 1% or greater among patients with insomnia who received ProSom in 7-night, placebo-controlled trials. Events reported by investigators were classified into standard dictionary (COSTART) terms to establish event frequencies. Event frequencies reported were not corrected for the occurrence of these events at baseline. The frequencies were obtained from data pooled across six studies: ProSom, N=685; placebo, N=433. The prescriber should be aware that these figures cannot be used to predict the incidence of side effects in the course of usual medical practice in which patient characteristics and other factors differ from those that prevailed in these six clinical trials. Similarly, the cited frequencies cannot be compared with figures obtained from other clinical investigators involving related drug products and uses, since each group of drug trials was conducted under a different set of conditions. However, the cited figures provide the physician with a basis of estimating the relative contribution of drug and nondrug factors to the incidence of side effects in the population studied.

[See table below]

INCIDENCE OF ADVERSE EXPERIENCES IN PLACEBO-CONTROLLED CLINICAL TRIALS
(Percentage of Patients Reporting)

Body System/ Adverse Event*	ProSom (N=685)	Placebo (N=433)
Body as a Whole		
Headache	16	27
Asthenia	11	8
Malaise	5	5
Lower extremity pain	3	2
Back pain	2	2
Body pain	2	2
Abdominal pain	1	2
Chest pain	1	1
Digestive System		
Nausea	4	5
Dyspepsia	2	2
Musculoskeletal System		
Stiffness	1	—
Nervous System		
Somnolence	42	27
Hypokinesia	8	4
Nervousness	8	11
Dizziness	7	3
Coordination abnormal	4	1
Hangover	3	2
Confusion	2	—
Depression	2	3
Dream abnormal	2	2
Thinking abnormal	2	1
Respiratory System		
Cold symptoms	3	5
Pharyngitis	1	2
Skin and Appendages		
Pruritus	1	—

*Events reported by at least 1% of ProSom patients.

Other Adverse Events:

During clinical trials conducted by Abbott, some of which were not placebo-controlled, ProSom was administered to approximately 1300 patients. Untoward events associated with this exposure were recorded by clinical investigators using terminology of their own choosing. To provide a meaningful estimate of the proportion of individuals experiencing adverse events, similar types of untoward events must be grouped into a smaller number of standardized event categories. In the tabulations that follow, a standard COSTART dictionary terminology has been used to classify reported adverse events. The frequencies presented, therefore, represent the proportion of the 1277 individuals exposed to ProSom who experienced an event of the type cited on at least one occasion while receiving ProSom. All reported events are included except those already listed in the previous table, those COSTART terms too general to be informative, and those events where a drug cause was remote. Events are further classified within body system categories and enumerated in order of decreasing frequency using the following definitions: frequent adverse events are defined as those occurring on one or more occasions in at least 1/100 patients; infrequent adverse events are those occurring in 1/100 to 1/1000 patients; rare events are those occurring in less than 1/1000 patients. It is important to emphasize that, although the events reported did occur during treatment with ProSom, they were not necessarily caused by it.

Body as a Whole — Infrequent: allergic reaction, chills, fever, neck pain, upper extremity pain; Rare: edema, jaw pain, swollen breast.

Cardiovascular System — Infrequent: flushing, palpitation; Rare: arrhythmia, syncope.

Digestive System — Frequent: constipation, dry mouth; Infrequent: decreased appetite, flatulence, gastritis, increased appetite, vomiting; Rare: enterocolitis, melena, ulceration of the mouth.

Endocrine System — Rare: thyroid nodule.
Hematologic and Lymphatic System — Rare: leukopenia, purpura, swollen lymph nodes.
Metabolic/Nutritional Disorders — Infrequent: thirst; Rare: increased SGOT, weight gain, weight loss.
Musculoskeletal System — Infrequent: arthritis, muscle spasm, myalgia; Rare: arthralgia.
Nervous System — Frequent: anxiety; Infrequent: agitation, amnesia, apathy, emotional lability, euphoria, hostility, paresthesia, seizure, sleep disorder, stupor, twitch; Rare: ataxia, circumoral paresthesia, decreased libido, decreased reflexes, hallucinations, neuritis, nystagmus, tremor.
Minor changes in EEG patterns, usually low-voltage fast activity, have been observed in patients during ProSom therapy or withdrawal and are of no known clinical significance.
Respiratory System — Infrequent: asthma, cough, dyspnea, rhinitis, sinusitis; Rare: epistaxis, hyperventilation, laryngitis.
Skin and Appendages — Infrequent: rash, sweating, urticaria; Rare: acne, dry skin.
Special Senses — Infrequent: abnormal vision, ear pain, eye irritation, eye pain, eye swelling, perverse taste, photophobia, tinnitus; Rare: decreased hearing, diplopia, scotomata.
Urogenital System — Infrequent: frequent urination, menstrual cramps, urinary hesitancy, urinary urgency, vaginal discharge/itching; Rare: hematuria, nocturia, oliguria, penile discharge, urinary incontinence.
Postintroduction Reports — Voluntary reports of non-US postmarketing experience with estazolam have included rare occurrences of photosensitivity, Stevens-Johnson syndrome, and agranulocytosis. Because of the uncontrolled nature of these spontaneous reports, a causal relationship to estazolam treatment has not been determined.

DRUG ABUSE AND DEPENDENCE

Controlled Substance: ProSom tablets are a controlled substance in Schedule IV.
Abuse and Dependence: Withdrawal symptoms similar to those noted with sedatives/hypnotics and alcohol have occurred following the abrupt discontinuation of drugs in the benzodiazepine class. The symptoms can range from mild dysphoria and insomnia to a major syndrome that may include abdominal and muscle cramps, vomiting, sweating, tremors, and convulsions.
Although withdrawal symptoms are more commonly noted after the discontinuation of higher than therapeutic doses of benzodiazepines, a proportion of patients taking benzodiazepines chronically at therapeutic doses may become physically dependent on them. Available data, however, cannot provide a reliable estimate of the incidence of dependency or the relationship of the dependency to dose and duration of treatment. There is some evidence to suggest that gradual reduction of dosage will attenuate or eliminate some withdrawal phenomena. In most instances, withdrawal phenomena are relatively mild and transient; however, life-threatening events (eg, seizures, delirium, etc.) have been reported.
Gradual withdrawal is the preferred course for any patient taking benzodiazepines for a prolonged period. Patients with a history of seizures, regardless of their concomitant antiseizure drug therapy, should not be withdrawn abruptly from benzodiazepines.
Individuals with a history of addiction to or abuse of drugs or alcohol should be under careful surveillance when receiving benzodiazepines because of the risk of habituation and dependence to such patients.

OVERDOSAGE

As with other benzodiazepines, experience with ProSom indicates that manifestations of overdosage include somnolence, respiratory depression, confusion, impaired coordination, slurred speech, and ultimately, coma. Patients have recovered from overdosage as high as 40 mg. As in the management of intentional overdose with any drug, the possibility should be considered that multiple agents may have been taken.
Gastric evacuation, either by the induction of emesis, lavage, or both, should be performed immediately. Maintenance of adequate ventilation is essential. General supportive care, including frequent monitoring of the vital signs and close observation of the patient, is indicated. Fluids should be administered intravenously to maintain blood pressure and encourage diuresis. The value of dialysis in treatment of benzodiazepine overdose has not been determined. The physician may wish to consider contacting a Poison Control Center for up-to-date information on the management of hypnotic drug product overdose.
Flumazenil, a specific benzodiazepine receptor antagonist, is indicated for the complete or partial reversal of the sedative effects of benzodiazepines and may be used in situations when an overdose with a benzodiazepine is known or suspected. Prior to the administration of flumazenil, necessary measures should be instituted to secure airway, ventilation, and intravenous access. Flumazenil is intended as an adjunct to, not as a substitute for, proper management of benzodiazepine overdose. Patients treated with flumazenil should be monitored for resedation, respiratory depression, and other residual benzodiazepine effects for an appropriate period after treatment. **The prescriber should be aware of a risk of seizure in association with flumazenil treatment, particularly in long-term benzodiazepine users and in cyclic antidepressant overdose.** The complete flumazenil package insert including CONTRAINDICATIONS, WARNINGS, and PRECAUTIONS should be consulted prior to use.

DOSAGE AND ADMINISTRATION

The recommended initial dose for adults is 1 mg at bedtime; however, some patients may need a 2 mg dose. In healthy elderly patients, 1 mg is also the appropriate starting dose, but increases should be initiated with particular care. In small or debilitated older patients, a starting dose of 0.5 mg, while only marginally effective in the overall elderly population, should be considered.

HOW SUPPLIED

ProSom tablets are scored tablets supplied as:
ProSom Tablets 1 mg white tablets bearing the Abbott logo and UC (Abbo-Code).
Bottles of 100 .... (**NDC** 0074-3735-13)
ProSom Tablets 2 mg pink tablets bearing the Abbott logo and UD (Abbo-Code).
Bottles of 100 .... (**NDC** 0074-3736-13)
Recommended storage: Store below 86°F (30°C).
Revised: January, 2004
Ref. 03-5333-R9
ABBOTT LABORATORIES
NORTH CHICAGO, IL 60064, U.S.A.
PRINTED IN U.S.A.

SYNTHROID® ℞
(levothyroxine sodium tablets, USP)
℞ only

DESCRIPTION

SYNTHROID® (levothyroxine sodium tablets, USP) contain synthetic crystalline L-3,3′,5,5′-tetraiodothyronine sodium salt [levothyroxine (T_4) sodium]. Synthetic T_4 is identical to that produced in the human thyroid gland. Levothyroxine (T_4) sodium has an empirical formula of $C_{15}H_{10}I_4N\ NaO_4 \bullet H_2O$, molecular weight of 798.86 g/mol (anhydrous), and structural formula as shown:

Inactive Ingredients: acacia, confectioner's sugar (contains corn starch), lactose monohydrate, magnesium stearate, povidone, and talc. The following are the color additives by tablet strength:

Strength (mcg)	Color additive(s)
25	FD&C Yellow No. 6 Aluminum Lake
50	None
75	FD&C Red No. 40 Aluminum Lake, FD&C Blue No. 2 Aluminum Lake
88	FD&C Blue No. 1 Aluminum Lake, FD&C Yellow No. 6 Aluminum Lake, D&C Yellow No. 10 Aluminum Lake
100	D&C Yellow No. 10 Aluminum Lake, FD&C Yellow No. 6 Aluminum Lake
112	D&C Red No. 27 & 30 Aluminum Lake
125	FD&C Yellow No. 6 Aluminum Lake, FD&C Red No. 40 Aluminum Lake, FD&C Blue No. 1 Aluminum Lake
137	FD&C Blue No. 1 Aluminum Lake
150	FD&C Blue No. 2 Aluminum Lake
175	FD&C Blue No. 1 Aluminum Lake, D&C Red No. 27 & 30 Aluminum Lake
200	FD&C Red No. 40 Aluminum Lake
300	D&C Yellow No. 10 Aluminum Lake, FD&C Yellow No. 6 Aluminum Lake, FD&C Blue No. 1 Aluminum Lake

CLINICAL PHARMACOLOGY

Thyroid hormone synthesis and secretion is regulated by the hypothalamic-pituitary-thyroid axis. Thyrotropin-releasing hormone (TRH) released from the hypothalamus stimulates secretion of thyrotropin-stimulating hormone, TSH, from the anterior pituitary. TSH, in turn, is the physiologic stimulus for the synthesis and secretion of thyroid hormones, L-thyroxine (T_4) and L-triiodothyronine (T_3), by the thyroid gland. Circulating serum T_3 and T_4 levels exert a feedback effect on both TRH and TSH secretion. When serum T_3 and T_4 levels increase, TRH and TSH secretion decrease. When thyroid hormone levels decrease, TRH and TSH secretion increase.
The mechanisms by which thyroid hormones exert their physiologic actions are not completely understood, but it is thought that their principal effects are exerted through control of DNA transcription and protein synthesis. T_3 and T_4 diffuse into the cell nucleus and bind to thyroid receptor proteins attached to DNA. This hormone nuclear receptor complex activates gene transcription and synthesis of messenger RNA and cytoplasmic proteins.
Thyroid hormones regulate multiple metabolic processes and play an essential role in normal growth and development, and normal maturation of the central nervous system and bone. The metabolic actions of thyroid hormones include augmentation of cellular respiration and thermogenesis, as well as metabolism of proteins, carbohydrates and lipids. The protein anabolic effects of thyroid hormones are essential to normal growth and development.
The physiological actions of thyroid hormones are produced predominantly by T_3, the majority of which (approximately 80%) is derived from T_4 by deiodination in peripheral tissues.
Levothyroxine, at doses individualized according to patient response, is effective as replacement or supplemental therapy in hypothyroidism of any etiology, except transient hypothyroidism during the recovery phase of subacute thyroiditis.
Levothyroxine is also effective in the suppression of pituitary TSH secretion in the treatment or prevention of various types of euthyroid goiters, including thyroid nodules, Hashimoto's thyroiditis, multinodular goiter and, as adjunctive therapy in the management of thyrotropin-dependent well-differentiated thyroid cancer (see **INDICATIONS AND USAGE, PRECAUTIONS,** and **DOSAGE AND ADMINISTRATION**).

Pharmacokinetics

Absorption—Absorption of orally administered T_4 from the gastrointestinal (GI) tract ranges from 40% to 80%. The majority of the levothyroxine dose is absorbed from the jejunum and upper ileum. The relative bioavailability of SYNTHROID tablets, compared to an equal nominal dose of oral levothyroxine sodium solution, is approximately 93%. T_4 absorption is increased by fasting, and decreased in malabsorption syndromes and by certain foods such as soybean infant formula. Dietary fiber decreases bioavailability of T_4. Absorption may also decrease with age. In addition, many drugs and foods affect T_4 absorption (see **PRECAUTIONS, Drug Interactions** and **Drug-Food Interactions**).
Distribution—Circulating thyroid hormones are greater than 99% bound to plasma proteins, including thyroxine-binding globulin (TBG), thyroxine-binding prealbumin (TBPA), and albumin (TBA), whose capacities and affinities vary for each hormone. The higher affinity of both TBG and TBPA for T_4 partially explains the higher serum levels, slower metabolic clearance, and longer half-life of T_4 compared to T_3. Protein-bound thyroid hormones exist in reverse equilibrium with small amounts of free hormone. Only unbound hormone is metabolically active. Many drugs and physiologic conditions affect the binding of thyroid hormones to serum proteins (see **PRECAUTIONS, Drug Interactions** and **Drug-Laboratory Test Interactions**). Thyroid hormones do not readily cross the placental barrier (see **PRECAUTIONS, Pregnancy**).
Metabolism—T_4 is slowly eliminated (see **Table 1**). The major pathway of thyroid hormone metabolism is through sequential deiodination. Approximately eighty-percent of circulating T_3 is derived from peripheral T_4 by monodeiodination. The liver is the major site of degradation for both T_4 and T_3, with T_4 deiodination also occurring at a number of additional sites, including the kidney and other tissues. Approximately 80% of the daily dose of T_4 is deiodinated to yield equal amounts of T_3 and reverse T_3 (rT_3). T_3 and rT_3 are further deiodinated to diiodothyronine. Thyroid hormones are also metabolized via conjugation with glucuronides and sulfates and excreted directly into the bile and gut where they undergo enterohepatic recirculation.
Elimination—Thyroid hormones are primarily eliminated by the kidneys. A portion of the conjugated hormone reaches the colon unchanged and is eliminated in the feces. Approximately 20% of T_4 is eliminated in the stool. Urinary excretion of T_4 decreases with age.
[See table 1 at top of next page]

INDICATIONS AND USAGE

Levothyroxine sodium is used for the following indications:
Hypothyroidism—As replacement or supplemental therapy in congenital or acquired hypothyroidism of any etiology, except transient hypothyroidism during the recovery phase of subacute thyroiditis. Specific indications include: primary (thyroidal), secondary (pituitary), and tertiary (hypothalamic) hypothyroidism and subclinical hypothyroidism. Primary hypothyroidism may result from functional deficiency, primary atrophy, partial or total congenital absence of the thyroid gland, or from the effects of surgery, radiation, or drugs, with or without the presence of goiter.
Pituitary TSH Suppression—In the treatment or prevention of various types of euthyroid goiters (see **WARNINGS** and **PRECAUTIONS**), including thyroid nodules (see **WARNINGS** and **PRECAUTIONS**), subacute or chronic lymphocytic thyroiditis (Hashimoto's thyroiditis), multinodular goiter (see **WARNINGS** and **PRECAUTIONS**) and, as an adjunct to surgery and radioiodine therapy in the management of thyrotropin-dependent well-differentiated thyroid cancer.

Continued on next page

Synthroid—Cont.

CONTRAINDICATIONS

Levothyroxine is contraindicated in patients with untreated subclinical (suppressed serum TSH level with normal T_3 and T_4 levels) or overt thyrotoxicosis of any etiology and in patients with acute myocardial infarction. Levothyroxine is contraindicated in patients with uncorrected adrenal insufficiency since thyroid hormones may precipitate an acute adrenal crisis by increasing the metabolic clearance of glucocorticoids (see **PRECAUTIONS**). SYNTHROID is contraindicated in patients with hypersensitivity to any of the inactive ingredients in SYNTHROID tablets (See **DESCRIPTION, Inactive Ingredients**).

WARNINGS

WARNING: Thyroid hormones, including SYNTHROID, either alone or with other therapeutic agents, should not be used for the treatment of obesity or for weight loss. In euthyroid patients, doses within the range of daily hormonal requirements are ineffective for weight reduction. Larger doses may produce serious or even life threatening manifestations of toxicity, particularly when given in association with sympathomimetic amines such as those used for their anorectic effects.

Levothyroxine sodium should not be used in the treatment of male or female infertility unless this condition is associated with hypothyroidism.

In patients with nontoxic diffuse goiter or nodular thyroid disease, particularly the elderly or those with underlying cardiovascular disease, levothyroxine sodium therapy is contraindicated if the serum TSH level is already suppressed due to the risk of precipitating overt thyrotoxicosis (see **CONTRAINDICATIONS**). If the serum TSH level is not suppressed, SYNTHROID should be used with caution in conjunction with careful monitoring of thyroid function for evidence of hyperthyroidism and clinical monitoring for potential associated adverse cardiovascular signs and symptoms of hyperthyroidism.

PRECAUTIONS

General

Levothyroxine has a narrow therapeutic index. Regardless of the indication for use, careful dosage titration is necessary to avoid the consequences of over- or under-treatment. These consequences include, among others, effects on growth and development, cardiovascular function, bone metabolism, reproductive function, cognitive function, emotional state, gastrointestinal function, and on glucose and lipid metabolism. Many drugs interact with levothyroxine sodium necessitating adjustments in dosing to maintain therapeutic response (see **Drug Interactions**).

Effects on bone mineral density—In women, long-term levothyroxine sodium therapy has been associated with increased bone resorption, thereby decreasing bone mineral density, especially in post-menopausal women on greater than replacement doses or in women who are receiving suppressive doses of levothyroxine sodium. The increased bone resorption may be associated with increased serum levels and urinary excretion of calcium and phosphorous, elevations in bone alkaline phosphatase and suppressed serum parathyroid hormone levels. Therefore, it is recommended that patients receiving levothyroxine sodium be given the minimum dose necessary to achieve the desired clinical and biochemical response.

Patients with underlying cardiovascular disease—Exercise caution when administering levothyroxine to patients with cardiovascular disorders and to the elderly in whom there is an increased risk of occult cardiac disease. In these patients, levothyroxine therapy should be initiated at lower doses than those recommended in younger individuals or in patients without cardiac disease (see **WARNINGS**; **PRECAUTIONS, Geriatric Use; and DOSAGE AND ADMINISTRATION**). If cardiac symptoms develop or worsen, the levothyroxine dose should be reduced or withheld for one week and then cautiously restarted at a lower dose. Overtreatment with levothyroxine sodium may have adverse cardiovascular effects such as an increase in heart rate, cardiac wall thickness, and cardiac contractility and may precipitate angina or arrhythmias. Patients with coronary artery disease who are receiving levothyroxine therapy should be monitored closely during surgical procedures, since the possibility of precipitating cardiac arrhythmias may be greater in those treated with levothyroxine. Concomitant administration of levothyroxine and sympathomimetic agents to patients with coronary artery disease may precipitate coronary insufficiency.

Patients with nontoxic diffuse goiter or nodular thyroid disease—Exercise caution when administering levothyroxine to patients with nontoxic diffuse goiter or nodular thyroid disease in order to prevent precipitation of thyrotoxicosis (see **WARNINGS**). If the serum TSH is already suppressed, levothyroxine sodium should not be administered (see **CONTRAINDICATIONS**).

Table 1: Pharmacokinetic Parameters of Thyroid Hormones in Euthyroid Patients

Hormone	Ratio in Thyroglobulin	Biologic Potency	$t_{1/2}$ (days)	Protein Binding (%)[2]
Levothyroxine (T_4)	10–20	1	6–7[1]	99.96
Liothyronine (T_3)	1	4	≤ 2	99.5

[1] 3 to 4 days in hyperthyroidism, 9 to 10 days in hypothyroidism
[2] Includes TBG, TBPA, and TBA

Associated endocrine disorders

Hypothalamic/pituitary hormone deficiencies—In patients with secondary or tertiary hypothyroidism, additional hypothalamic/pituitary hormone deficiencies should be considered, and, if diagnosed, treated (see **PRECAUTIONS, Autoimmune polyglandular syndrome** for adrenal insufficiency).

Autoimmune polyglandular syndrome—Occasionally, chronic autoimmune thyroiditis may occur in association with other autoimmune disorders such as adrenal insufficiency, pernicious anemia, and insulin-dependent diabetes mellitus. Patients with concomitant adrenal insufficiency should be treated with replacement glucocorticoids prior to initiation of treatment with levothyroxine sodium. Failure to do so may precipitate an acute adrenal crisis when thyroid hormone therapy is initiated, due to increased metabolic clearance of glucocorticoids by thyroid hormone. Patients with diabetes mellitus may require upward adjustments of their antidiabetic therapeutic regimens when treated with levothyroxine (see **PRECAUTIONS, Drug Interactions**).

Other associated medical conditions

Infants with congenital hypothyroidism appear to be at increased risk for other congenital anomalies, with cardiovascular anomalies (pulmonary stenosis, atrial septal defect, and ventricular septal defect) being the most common association.

Information for Patients

Patients should be informed of the following information to aid in the safe and effective use of SYNTHROID:

1. Notify your physician if you are allergic to any foods or medicines, are pregnant or intend to become pregnant, are breast-feeding or are taking any other medications, including prescription and over-the-counter preparations.
2. Notify your physician of any other medical conditions you may have, particularly heart disease, diabetes, clotting disorders, and adrenal or pituitary gland problems. Your dose of medications used to control these other conditions may need to be adjusted while you are taking SYNTHROID. If you have diabetes, monitor your blood and/or urinary glucose levels as directed by your physician and immediately report any changes to your physician. If you are taking anticoagulants (blood thinners), your clotting status should be checked frequently.
3. Use SYNTHROID only as prescribed by your physician. Do not discontinue or change the amount you take or how often you take it, unless directed to do so by your physician.
4. The levothyroxine in SYNTHROID is intended to replace a hormone that is normally produced by your thyroid gland. Generally, replacement therapy is to be taken for life, except in cases of transient hypothyroidism, which is usually associated with an inflammation of the thyroid gland (thyroiditis).
5. Take SYNTHROID as a single dose, preferably on an empty stomach, one-half to one hour before breakfast. Levothyroxine absorption is increased on an empty stomach.
6. It may take several weeks before you notice an improvement in your symptoms.
7. Notify your physician if you experience any of the following symptoms: rapid or irregular heartbeat, chest pain, shortness of breath, leg cramps, headache, nervousness, irritability, sleeplessness, tremors, change in appetite, weight gain or loss, vomiting, diarrhea, excessive sweating, heat intolerance, fever, changes in menstrual periods, hives or skin rash, or any other unusual medical event.
8. Notify your physician if you become pregnant while taking SYNTHROID. It is likely that your dose of SYNTHROID will need to be increased while you are pregnant.
9. Notify your physician or dentist that you are taking SYNTHROID prior to any surgery.
10. Partial hair loss may occur rarely during the first few months of SYNTHROID therapy, but this is usually temporary.
11. SYNTHROID should not be used as a primary or adjunctive therapy in a weight control program.
12. Keep SYNTHROID out of the reach of children. Store SYNTHROID away from heat, moisture, and light.

Laboratory Tests

General

The diagnosis of hypothyroidism is confirmed by measuring TSH levels using a sensitive assay (second generation assay sensitivity ≤ 0.1 mIU/L or third generation assay sensitivity ≤ 0.01 mIU/L) and measurement of free-T_4.

The adequacy of therapy is determined by periodic assessment of appropriate laboratory tests and clinical evaluation. The choice of laboratory tests depends on various factors including the etiology of the underlying thyroid disease, the presence of concomitant medical conditions, including pregnancy, and the use of concomitant medications (see **PRECAUTIONS, Drug Interactions and Drug-Laboratory Test Interactions**). Persistent clinical and laboratory evidence of hypothyroidism despite an apparent adequate replacement dose of SYNTHROID may be evidence of inadequate absorption, poor compliance, drug interactions, or decreased T_4 potency of the drug product.

Adults

In adult patients with primary (thyroidal) hypothyroidism, serum TSH levels (using a sensitive assay) alone may be used to monitor therapy. The frequency of TSH monitoring during levothyroxine dose titration depends on the clinical situation but it is generally recommended at 6–8 week intervals until normalization. For patients who have recently initiated levothyroxine therapy and whose serum TSH has normalized or in patients who have had their dosage or brand of levothyroxine changed, the serum TSH concentration should be measured after 8–12 weeks. When the optimum replacement dose has been attained, clinical (physical examination) and biochemical monitoring may be performed every 6–12 months, depending on the clinical situation, and whenever there is a change in the patient's status. It is recommended that a physical examination and a serum TSH measurement be performed at least annually in patients receiving SYNTHROID (see **WARNINGS, PRECAUTIONS**, and **DOSAGE AND ADMINISTRATION**).

Pediatrics

In patients with congenital hypothyroidism, the adequacy of replacement therapy should be assessed by measuring both serum TSH (using a sensitive assay) and total- or free- T_4. During the first three years of life, the serum total- or free-T_4 should be maintained at all times in the upper half of the normal range. While the aim of therapy is to also normalize the serum TSH level, this is not always possible in a small percentage of patients, particularly in the first few months of therapy. TSH may not normalize due to a resetting of the pituitary-thyroid feedback threshold as a result of *in utero* hypothyroidism. Failure of the serum T_4 to increase into the upper half of the normal range within 2 weeks of initiation of SYNTHROID therapy and/or of the serum TSH to decrease below 20 mU/L within 4 weeks should alert the physician to the possibility that the child is not receiving adequate therapy. Careful inquiry should then be made regarding compliance, dose of medication administered, and method of administration prior to raising the dose of SYNTHROID.

The recommended frequency of monitoring of TSH and total or free T_4 in children is as follows: at 2 and 4 weeks after the initiation of treatment; every 1–2 months during the first year of life; every 2–3 months between 1 and 3 years of age; and every 3 to 12 months thereafter until growth is completed. More frequent intervals of monitoring may be necessary if poor compliance is suspected or abnormal values are obtained. It is recommended that TSH and T_4 levels, and a physical examination, if indicated, be performed 2 weeks after any change in SYNTHROID dosage. Routine clinical examination, including assessment of mental and physical growth and development, and bone maturation, should be performed at regular intervals (see **PRECAUTIONS, Pediatric Use and DOSAGE AND ADMINISTRATION**).

Secondary (pituitary) and tertiary (hypothalamic) hypothyroidism

Adequacy of therapy should be assessed by measuring serum free-T_4 levels, which should be maintained in the upper half of the normal range in these patients.

Drug Interactions

Many drugs affect thyroid hormone pharmacokinetics and metabolism (e.g., absorption, synthesis, secretion, catabolism, protein binding, and target tissue response) and may alter the therapeutic response to SYNTHROID. In addition, thyroid hormones and thyroid status have varied effects on the pharmacokinetics and actions of other drugs. A listing of drug-thyroidal axis interactions is contained in Table 2.

The list of drug-thyroidal axis interactions in Table 2 may not be comprehensive due to the introduction of new drugs that interact with the thyroidal axis or the discovery of previously unknown interactions. The prescriber should be aware of this fact and should consult appropriate reference sources (e.g., package inserts of newly approved drugs, medical literature) for additional information if a drug-drug interaction with levothyroxine is suspected.

Table 2: Drug-Thyroidal Axis Interactions

Drug or Drug Class	Effect
Drugs that may reduce TSH secretion—the reduction is not sustained; therefore, hypothyroidism does not occur	
Dopamine/Dopamine Agonists Glucocorticoids Octreotide	Use of these agents may result in a transient reduction in TSH secretion when administered at the following doses: Dopamine (≥ 1 mcg/kg/min); Glucocorticoids (hydrocortisone ≥ 100 mg/day or equivalent); Octreotide (> 100 mcg/day).
Drugs that alter thyroid hormone secretion	
Drugs that may decrease thyroid hormone secretion, which may result in hypothyroidism	
Aminoglutethimide Amiodarone Iodide (including iodine-containing radiographic contrast agents) Lithium Methimazole Propylthiouracil (PTU) Sulfonamides Tolbutamide	Long-term lithium therapy can result in goiter in up to 50% of patients, and either subclinical or overt hypothyroidism, each in up to 20% of patients. The fetus, neonate, elderly and euthyroid patients with underlying thyroid disease (e.g., Hashimoto's thyroiditis or with Grave's disease previously treated with radioiodine or surgery) are among those individuals who are particularly susceptible to iodine-induced hypothyroidism. Oral cholecystographic agents and amiodarone are slowly excreted, producing more prolonged hypothyroidism than parenterally administered iodinated contrast agents. Long-term aminoglutethimide therapy may minimally decrease T_4 and T_3 levels and increase TSH, although all values remain within normal limits in most patients.
Drugs that may increase thyroid hormone secretion, which may result in hyperthyroidism	
Amiodarone Iodide (including iodine-containing radiographic contrast agents)	Iodide and drugs that contain pharmacologic amounts of iodide may cause hyperthyroidism in euthyroid patients with Grave's disease previously treated with antithyroid drugs or in euthyroid patients with thyroid autonomy (e.g., multinodular goiter or hyperfunctioning thyroid adenoma). Hyperthyroidism may develop over several weeks and may persist for several months after therapy discontinuation. Amiodarone may induce hyperthyroidism by causing thyroiditis.
Drugs that may decrease T_4 absorption, which may result in hypothyroidism	
Antacids — Aluminum & Magnesium Hydroxides — Simethicone Bile Acid Sequestrants — Cholestyramine — Colestipol Calcium Carbonate Cation Exchange Resins — Kayexalate Ferrous Sulfate Sucralfate	Concurrent use may reduce the efficacy of levothyroxine by binding and delaying or preventing absorption, potentially resulting in hypothyroidism. Calcium carbonate may form an insoluble chelate with levothyroxine, and ferrous sulfate likely forms a ferric-thyroxine complex. Administer levothyroxine at least 4 hours apart from these agents.
Drugs that may alter T_4 and T_3 serum transport – but FT_4 concentration remains normal; and therefore, the patient remains euthyroid	
Drugs that may increase serum TBG concentration	**Drugs that may decrease serum TBG concentration**
Clofibrate Estrogen-containing oral contraceptives Estrogens (oral) Heroin / Methadone 5-Fluorouracil Mitotane Tamoxifen	Androgens / Anabolic Steroids Asparaginase Glucocorticoids Slow-Release Nicotinic Acid
Drugs that may cause protein-binding site displacement	
Furosemide (> 80 mg IV) Heparin Hydantoins Non Steroidal Anti-Inflammatory Drugs — Fenamates — Phenylbutazone Salicylates (> 2 g/day)	Administration of these agents with levothyroxine results in an initial transient increase in FT_4. Continued administration results in a decrease in serum T_4 and normal FT_4 and TSH concentrations and, therefore, patients are clinically euthyroid. Salicylates inhibit binding of T_4 and T_3 to TBG and transthyretin. An initial increase in serum FT_4 is followed by return of FT_4 to normal levels with sustained therapeutic serum salicylate concentrations, although total-T_4 levels may decrease by as much as 30%.
Drugs that may alter T_4 and T_3 metabolism	
Drugs that may increase hepatic metabolism, which may result in hypothyroidism	
Carbamazepine Hydantoins Phenobarbital Rifampin	Stimulation of hepatic microsomal drug-metabolizing enzyme activity may cause increased hepatic degradation of levothyroxine, resulting in increased levothyroxine requirements. Phenytoin and carbamazepine reduce serum protein binding of levothyroxine, and total- and free- T_4 may be reduced by 20% to 40%, but most patients have normal serum TSH levels and are clinically euthyroid.
Drugs that may decrease T_4 5′-deiodinase activity	
Amiodarone Beta-adrenergic antagonists — (e.g., Propranolol > 160 mg/day) Glucocorticoids — (e.g., Dexamethasone ≥ 4 mg/day) Propylthiouracil (PTU)	Administration of these enzyme inhibitors decreases the peripheral conversion of T_4 to T_3, leading to decreased T_3 levels. However, serum T_4 levels are usually normal but may occasionally be slightly increased. In patients treated with large doses of propranolol (> 160 mg/day), T_3 and T_4 levels change slightly, TSH levels remain normal, and patients are clinically euthyroid. It should be noted that actions of particular beta-adrenergic antagonists may be impaired when the hypothyroid patient is converted to the euthyroid state. Short-term administration of large doses of glucocorticoids may decrease serum T_3 concentrations by 30% with minimal change in serum T_4 levels. However, long-term glucocorticoid therapy may result in slightly decreased T_3 and T_4levels due to decreased TBG production (see above).
Miscellaneous	
Anticoagulants (oral) — Coumarin Derivatives — Indandione Derivatives	Thyroid hormones appear to increase the catabolism of vitamin K-dependent clotting factors, thereby increasing the anticoagulant activity of oral anticoagulants. Concomitant use of these agents impairs the compensatory increases in clotting factor synthesis. Prothrombin time should be carefully monitored in patients taking levothyroxine and oral anticoagulants and the dose of anticoagulant therapy adjusted accordingly.
Antidepressants — Tricyclics (e.g., Amitriptyline) — Tetracyclics (e.g., Maprotiline) — Selective Serotonin Reuptake Inhibitors (SSRIs; e.g., Sertraline)	Concurrent use of tri/tetracyclic antidepressants and levothyroxine may increase the therapeutic and toxic effects of both drugs, possibly due to increased receptor sensitivity to catecholamines. Toxic effects may include increased risk of cardiac arrhythmias and CNS stimulation; onset of action of tricyclics may be accelerated. Administration of sertraline in patients stabilized on levothyroxine may result in increased levothyroxine requirements.
Antidiabetic Agents — Biguanides — Meglitinides — Sulfonylureas — Thiazolidinediones — Insulin	Addition of levothyroxine to antidiabetic or insulin therapy may result in increased antidiabetic agent or insulin requirements. Careful monitoring of diabetic control is recommended, especially when thyroid therapy is started, changed, or discontinued.
Cardiac Glycosides	Serum digitalis glycoside levels may be reduced in hyperthyroidism or when the hypothyroid patient is converted to the euthyroid state. Therapeutic effect of digitalis glycosides may be reduced.
Cytokines — Interferon-α — Interleukin-2	Therapy with interferon-α has been associated with the development of antithyroid microsomal antibodies in 20% of patients and some have transient hypothyroidism, hyperthyroidism, or both. Patients who have antithyroid antibodies before treatment are at higher risk for thyroid dysfunction during treatment. Interleukin-2 has been associated with transient painless thyroiditis in 20% of patients. Interferon-β and -γ have not been reported to cause thyroid dysfunction.
Growth Hormones — Somatrem — Somatropin	Excessive use of thyroid hormones with growth hormones may accelerate epiphyseal closure. However, untreated hypothyroidism may interfere with growth response to growth hormone.
Ketamine	Concurrent use may produce marked hypertension and tachycardia; cautious administration to patients receiving thyroid hormone therapy is recommended.
Methylxanthine Bronchodilators — (e.g., Theophylline)	Decreased theophylline clearance may occur in hypothyroid patients; clearance returns to normal when the euthyroid state is achieved.
Radiographic Agents	Thyroid hormones may reduce the uptake of ^{123}I, ^{131}I, and ^{99m}Tc.
Sympathomimetics	Concurrent use may increase the effects of sympathomimetics or thyroid hormone. Thyroid hormones may increase the risk of coronary insufficiency when sympathomimetic agents are administered to patients with coronary artery disease.
Chloral Hydrate Diazepam Ethionamide Lovastatin Metoclopramide 6-Mercaptopurine Nitroprusside Para-aminosalicylate sodium Perphenazine Resorcinol (excessive topical use) Thiazide Diuretics	These agents have been associated with thyroid hormone and/or TSH level alterations by various mechanisms.

Oral anticoagulants—Levothyroxine increases the response to oral anticoagulant therapy. Therefore, a decrease in the dose of anticoagulant may be warranted with correction of the hypothyroid state or when the SYNTHROID dose is increased. Prothrombin time should be closely monitored to permit appropriate and timely dosage adjustments (see **Table 2**).

Continued on next page

Synthroid—Cont.

Digitalis glycosides—The therapeutic effects of digitalis glycosides may be reduced by levothyroxine. Serum digitalis glycoside levels may be decreased when a hypothyroid patient becomes euthyroid, necessitating an increase in the dose of digitalis glycosides (see **Table 2**).

Drug-Food Interactions—Consumption of certain foods may affect levothyroxine absorption thereby necessitating adjustments in dosing. Soybean flour (infant formula), cotton seed meal, walnuts, and dietary fiber may bind and decrease the absorption of levothyroxine sodium from the GI tract.

Drug-Laboratory Test Interactions—Changes in TBG concentration must be considered when interpreting T_4 and T_3 values, which necessitates measurement and evaluation of unbound (free) hormone and/or determination of the free T_4 index (FT_4I). Pregnancy, infectious hepatitis, estrogens, estrogen-containing oral contraceptives, and acute intermittent porphyria increase TBG concentrations. Decreases in TBG concentrations are observed in nephrosis, severe hypoproteinemia, severe liver disease, acromegaly, and after androgen or corticosteroid therapy (see also **Table 2**). Familial hyper- or hypo-thyroxine binding globulinemias have been described, with the incidence of TBG deficiency approximating 1 in 9000.

Carcinogenesis, Mutagenesis, and Impairment of Fertility—Animal studies have not been performed to evaluate the carcinogenic potential, mutagenic potential or effects on fertility of levothyroxine. The synthetic T_4 in SYNTHROID is identical to that produced naturally by the human thyroid gland. Although there has been a reported association between prolonged thyroid hormone therapy and breast cancer, this has not been confirmed. Patients receiving SYNTHROID for appropriate clinical indications should be titrated to the lowest effective replacement dose.

Pregnancy—Category A—Studies in women taking levothyroxine sodium during pregnancy have not shown an increased risk of congenital abnormalities. Therefore, the possibility of fetal harm appears remote. SYNTHROID should not be discontinued during pregnancy and hypothyroidism diagnosed during pregnancy should be promptly treated.

Hypothyroidism during pregnancy is associated with a higher rate of complications, including spontaneous abortion, pre-eclampsia, stillbirth and premature delivery. Maternal hypothyroidism may have an adverse effect on fetal and childhood growth and development. During pregnancy, serum T_4 levels may decrease and serum TSH levels increase to values outside the normal range. Since elevations in serum TSH may occur as early as 4 weeks gestation, pregnant women taking SYNTHROID should have their TSH measured during each trimester. An elevated serum TSH level should be corrected by an increase in the dose of SYNTHROID. Since postpartum TSH levels are similar to preconception values, the SYNTHROID dosage should return to the pre-pregnancy dose immediately after delivery. A serum TSH level should be obtained 6–8 weeks postpartum.

Thyroid hormones cross the placental barrier to some extent as evidenced by levels in cord blood of athyreotic fetuses being approximately one-third maternal levels. Transfer of thyroid hormone from the mother to the fetus, however, may not be adequate to prevent *in utero* hypothyroidism.

Nursing Mothers—Although thyroid hormones are excreted only minimally in human milk, caution should be exercised when SYNTHROID is administered to a nursing woman. However, adequate replacement doses of levothyroxine are generally needed to maintain normal lactation.

Pediatric Use

General

The goal of treatment in pediatric patients with hypothyroidism is to achieve and maintain normal intellectual and physical growth and development.

The initial dose of levothyroxine varies with age and body weight (see **DOSAGE AND ADMINISTRATION, Table 3**). Dosing adjustments are based on an assessment of the individual patient's clinical and laboratory parameters (see **PRECAUTIONS, Laboratory Tests**).

In children in whom a diagnosis of permanent hypothyroidism has not been established, it is recommended that levothyroxine administration be discontinued for a 30-day trial period, but only after the child is at least 3 years of age. Serum T_4 and TSH levels should then be obtained. If the T_4 is low and the TSH high, the diagnosis of permanent hypothyroidism is established, and levothyroxine therapy should be reinstituted. If the T_4 and TSH levels are normal, euthyroidism may be assumed and, therefore, the hypothyroidism can be considered to have been transient. In this instance, however, the physician should carefully monitor the child and repeat the thyroid function tests if any signs or symptoms of hypothyroidism develop. In this setting, the clinician should have a high index of suspicion of relapse. If the results of the levothyroxine withdrawal test are inconclusive, careful follow-up and subsequent testing will be necessary.

Since some more severely affected children may become clinically hypothyroid when treatment is discontinued for 30 days, an alternate approach is to reduce the replacement dose of levothyroxine by half during the 30-day trial period. If, after 30 days, the serum TSH is elevated above 20 mU/L, the diagnosis of permanent hypothyroidism is confirmed, and full replacement therapy should be resumed. However, if the serum TSH has not risen to greater than 20 mU/L, levothyroxine treatment should be discontinued for another 30-day trial period followed by repeat serum T_4 and TSH testing.

The presence of concomitant medical conditions should be considered in certain clinical circumstances and, if present, appropriately treated (see **PRECAUTIONS**).

Congenital Hypothyroidism (see **PRECAUTIONS, Laboratory Tests and DOSAGE AND ADMINISTRATION**)

Rapid restoration of normal serum T_4 concentrations is essential for preventing the adverse effects of congenital hypothyroidism on intellectual development as well as on overall physical growth and maturation. Therefore, SYNTHROID therapy should be initiated immediately upon diagnosis and is generally continued for life.

During the first 2 weeks of SYNTHROID therapy, infants should be closely monitored for cardiac overload, arrhythmias, and aspiration from avid suckling.

The patient should be monitored closely to avoid undertreatment or overtreatment. Undertreatment may have deleterious effects on intellectual development and linear growth. Overtreatment has been associated with craniosynostosis in infants, and may adversely affect the tempo of brain maturation and accelerate the bone age with resultant premature closure of the epiphyses and compromised adult stature.

Acquired Hypothyroidism in Pediatric Patients

The patient should be monitored closely to avoid undertreatment and overtreatment. Undertreatment may result in poor school performance due to impaired concentration and slowed mentation and in reduced adult height. Overtreatment may accelerate the bone age and result in premature epiphyseal closure and compromised adult stature.

Treated children may manifest a period of catch-up growth, which may be adequate in some cases to normalize adult height. In children with severe or prolonged hypothyroidism, catch-up growth may not be adequate to normalize adult height.

Geriatric Use

Because of the increased prevalence of cardiovascular disease among the elderly, levothyroxine therapy should not be initiated at the full replacement dose (see **WARNINGS, PRECAUTIONS**, and **DOSAGE AND ADMINISTRATION**).

ADVERSE REACTIONS

Adverse reactions associated with levothyroxine therapy are primarily those of hyperthyroidism due to therapeutic overdosage (see **PRECAUTIONS** and **OVERDOSAGE**). They include the following:

General: fatigue, increased appetite, weight loss, heat intolerance, fever, excessive sweating;

Central nervous system: headache, hyperactivity, nervousness, anxiety, irritability, emotional lability, insomnia;

Musculoskeletal: tremors, muscle weakness;

Cardiovascular: palpitations, tachycardia, arrhythmias, increased pulse and blood pressure, heart failure, angina, myocardial infarction, cardiac arrest;

Respiratory: dyspnea;

Gastrointestinal: diarrhea, vomiting, abdominal cramps and elevations in liver function tests;

Dermatologic: hair loss, flushing;

Endocrine: decreased bone mineral density;

Reproductive: menstrual irregularities, impaired fertility.

Pseudotumor cerebri and slipped capital femoral epiphysis have been reported in children receiving levothyroxine therapy. Overtreatment may result in craniosynostosis in infants and premature closure of the epiphyses in children with resultant compromised adult height.

Seizures have been reported rarely with the institution of levothyroxine therapy.

Inadequate levothyroxine dosage will produce or fail to ameliorate the signs and symptoms of hypothyroidism.

Hypersensitivity reactions to inactive ingredients have occurred in patients treated with thyroid hormone products. These include urticaria, pruritus, skin rash, flushing, angioedema, various GI symptoms (abdominal pain, nausea, vomiting and diarrhea), fever, arthralgia, serum sickness and wheezing. Hypersensitivity to levothyroxine itself is not known to occur.

OVERDOSAGE

The signs and symptoms of overdosage are those of hyperthyroidism (see **PRECAUTIONS** and **ADVERSE REACTIONS**). In addition, confusion and disorientation may occur. Cerebral embolism, shock, coma, and death have been reported. Seizures have occurred in a child ingesting 18 mg of levothyroxine. Symptoms may not necessarily be evident or may not appear until several days after ingestion of levothyroxine sodium.

Treatment of Overdosage

Levothyroxine sodium should be reduced in dose or temporarily discontinued if signs or symptoms of overdosage occur.

Acute Massive Overdosage—This may be a life-threatening emergency, therefore, symptomatic and supportive therapy should be instituted immediately. If not contraindicated (e.g., by seizures, coma, or loss of the gag reflex), the stomach should be emptied by emesis or gastric lavage to decrease gastrointestinal absorption. Activated charcoal or cholestyramine may also be used to decrease absorption. Central and peripheral increased sympathetic activity may be treated by administering β-receptor antagonists, e.g. propranolol, provided there are no medical contraindications to their use. Provide respiratory support as needed; control congestive heart failure and arrhythmia; control fever, hypoglycemia, and fluid loss as necessary. Large doses of antithyroid drugs (e.g., methimazole or propylthiouracil) followed in one to two hours by large doses of iodine may be given to inhibit synthesis and release of thyroid hormones. Glucocorticoids may be given to inhibit the conversion of T_4 to T_3. Plasmapheresis, charcoal hemoperfusion and exchange transfusion have been reserved for cases in which continued clinical deterioration occurs despite conventional therapy. Because T_4 is highly protein bound, very little drug will be removed by dialysis.

DOSAGE AND ADMINISTRATION

General Principles

The goal of replacement therapy is to achieve and maintain a clinical and biochemical euthyroid state. The goal of suppressive therapy is to inhibit growth and/or function of abnormal thyroid tissue. The dose of SYNTHROID (levothyroxine sodium tablets, USP) that is adequate to achieve these goals depends on a variety of factors including the patient's age, body weight, cardiovascular status, concomitant medical conditions, including pregnancy, concomitant medications, and the specific nature of the condition being treated (see **WARNINGS** and **PRECAUTIONS**). Hence, the following recommendations serve only as dosing guidelines. Dosing must be individualized and adjustments made based on periodic assessment of the patient's clinical response and laboratory parameters (see **PRECAUTIONS, Laboratory Tests**).

SYNTHROID is administered as a single daily dose, preferably one-half to one-hour before breakfast. SYNTHROID should be taken at least 4 hours apart from drugs that are known to interfere with its absorption (see **PRECAUTIONS, Drug Interactions**).

Due to the long half-life of levothyroxine, the peak therapeutic effect at a given dose of levothyroxine sodium may not be attained for 4–6 weeks.

Caution should be exercised when administering SYNTHROID to patients with underlying cardiovascular disease, to the elderly, and to those with concomitant adrenal insufficiency (see **PRECAUTIONS**).

Specific Patient Populations

Hypothyroidism in Adults and in Children in Whom Growth and Puberty are Complete (see **WARNINGS** and **PRECAUTIONS, Laboratory Tests**)

Therapy may begin at full replacement doses in otherwise healthy individuals less than 50 years old and in those older than 50 years who have been recently treated for hyperthyroidism or who have been hypothyroid for only a short time (such as a few months). The average full replacement dose of levothyroxine sodium is approximately 1.7 mcg/kg/day (e.g., **100–125 mcg/day** for a 70 kg adult). Older patients may require less than 1 mcg/kg/day. Levothyroxine sodium doses greater than 200 mcg/day are seldom required. An inadequate response to daily doses ≥ 300 mcg/day is rare and may indicate poor compliance, malabsorption, and/or drug interactions.

For most patients older than 50 years or for patients under 50 years of age with underlying cardiac disease, an initial starting dose of **25–50 mcg/day** of levothyroxine sodium is recommended, with gradual increments in dose at 6–8 week intervals, as needed. The recommended starting dose of levothyroxine sodium in elderly patients with cardiac disease is **12.5–25 mcg/day**, with gradual dose increments at 4–6 week intervals. The levothyroxine sodium dose is generally adjusted in 12.5–25 mcg increments until the patient with primary hypothyroidism is clinically euthyroid and the serum TSH has normalized.

In patients with severe hypothyroidism, the recommended initial levothyroxine sodium dose is **12.5–25 mcg/day** with increases of 25 mcg/day every 2–4 weeks, accompanied by clinical and laboratory assessment, until the TSH level is normalized.

In patients with secondary (pituitary) or tertiary (hypothalamic) hypothyroidism, the levothyroxine sodium dose should be titrated until the patient is clinically euthyroid and the serum free- T_4 level is restored to the upper half of the normal range.

Pediatric Dosage—Congenital or Acquired Hypothyroidism (see **PRECAUTIONS, Laboratory Tests**)

General Principles

In general, levothyroxine therapy should be instituted at full replacement doses as soon as possible. Delays in diagnosis and institution of therapy may have deleterious effects on the child's intellectual and physical growth and development.

Undertreatment and overtreatment should be avoided (see **PRECAUTIONS, Pediatric Use**).

SYNTHROID may be administered to infants and children who cannot swallow intact tablets by crushing the tablet and suspending the freshly crushed tablet in a small amount (5–10 mL or 1–2 teaspoons) of water. This suspension can be administered by spoon or dropper. **DO NOT STORE THE SUSPENSION.** Foods that decrease absorption of levothyroxine, such as soybean infant formula, should not be used for administering levothyroxine sodium tablets (see **PRECAUTIONS, Drug-Food Interactions**).

Newborns

The recommended starting dose of levothyroxine sodium in newborn infants is **10–15 mcg/kg/day**. A lower starting dose (e.g., 25 mcg/day) should be considered in infants at risk for cardiac failure, and the dose should be increased in 4–6 weeks as needed based on clinical and laboratory response

Strength (mcg)	Color	NDC # for bottles of 100	NDC # for bottles of 1000	NDC # for unit dose cartons of 100
25	orange	0074-4341-13	0074-4341-19	—
50	white	0074-4552-13	0074-4552-19	0074-4552-11
75	violet	0074-5182-13	0074-5182-19	0074-5182-11
88	olive	0074-6594-13	0074-6594-19	—
100	yellow	0074-6624-13	0074-6624-19	0074-6624-11
112	rose	0074-9296-13	0074-9296-19	—
125	brown	0074-7068-13	0074-7068-19	0074-7068-11
137	turquoise	0074-3727-13	0074-3727-19	—
150	blue	0074-7069-13	0074-7069-19	0074-7069-11
175	lilac	0074-7070-13	0074-7070-19	—
200	pink	0074-7148-13	0074-7148-19	0074-7148-11
300	green	0074-7149-13	0074-7149-19	—

to treatment. In infants with very low (< 5 mcg/dL) or undetectable serum T_4 concentrations, the recommended initial starting dose is **50 mcg/day** of levothyroxine sodium.

Infants and Children

Levothyroxine therapy is usually initiated at full replacement doses, with the recommended dose per body weight decreasing with age (see **Table 3**). However, in children with chronic or severe hypothyroidism, an initial dose of **25 mcg/day** of levothyroxine sodium is recommended with increments of 25 mcg every 2–4 weeks until the desired effect is achieved.

Hyperactivity in an older child can be minimized if the starting dose is one-fourth of the recommended full replacement dose, and the dose is then increased on a weekly basis by an amount equal to one-fourth the full-recommended replacement dose until the full recommended replacement dose is reached.

Table 3: Levothyroxine Sodium Dosing Guidelines for Pediatric Hypothyroidism

AGE	Daily Dose Per Kg Body Weight[a]
0–3 months	10–15 mcg/kg/day
3–6 months	8–10 mcg/kg/day
6–12 months	6–8 mcg/kg/day
1–5 years	5–6 mcg/kg/day
6–12 years	4–5 mcg/kg/day
>12 years but growth and puberty incomplete	2–3 mcg/kg/day
Growth and puberty complete	1.7 mcg/kg/day

[a] The dose should be adjusted based on clinical response and laboratory parameters (**see PRECAUTIONS, Laboratory Tests and Pediatric Use**).

Pregnancy—Pregnancy may increase levothyroxine requirements (see **PREGNANCY**).

Subclinical Hypothyroidism—If this condition is treated, a lower levothyroxine sodium dose (e.g., **1 mcg/kg/day**) than that used for full replacement may be adequate to normalize the serum TSH level. Patients who are not treated should be monitored yearly for changes in clinical status and thyroid laboratory parameters.

TSH Suppression in Well-differentiated Thyroid Cancer and Thyroid Nodules—The target level for TSH suppression in these conditions has not been established with controlled studies. In addition, the efficacy of TSH suppression for benign nodular disease is controversial. Therefore, the dose of SYNTHROID used for TSH suppression should be individualized based on the specific disease and the patient being treated.

In the treatment of well-differentiated (papillary and follicular) thyroid cancer, levothyroxine is used as an adjunct to surgery and radioiodine therapy. Generally, TSH is suppressed to <0.1 mU/L, and this usually requires a levothyroxine sodium dose of **greater than 2 mcg/kg/day**. However, in patients with high-risk tumors, the target level for TSH suppression may be <0.01 mU/L.

In the treatment of benign nodules and nontoxic multinodular goiter, TSH is generally suppressed to a higher target (e.g., 0.1 to either 0.5 or 1.0 mU/L) than that used for the treatment of thyroid cancer. Levothyroxine sodium is contraindicated if the serum TSH is already suppressed due to the risk of precipitating overt thyrotoxicosis (see **CONTRAINDICATIONS, WARNINGS** and **PRECAUTIONS**).

Myxedema Coma—Myxedema coma is a life-threatening emergency characterized by poor circulation and hypometabolism, and may result in unpredictable absorption of levothyroxine sodium from the gastrointestinal tract. Therefore, oral thyroid hormone drug products are not recommended to treat this condition. Thyroid hormone products formulated for intravenous administration should be administered.

HOW SUPPLIED

SYNTHROID® (levothyroxine sodium tablets, USP) are round, color coded, scored and debossed with "SYNTHROID" on one side and potency on the other side. They are supplied as follows:

[See table above]

Storage Conditions

Store at 25°C (77°F); excursions permitted to 15°–30°C (59°–86°F) [see USP Controlled Room Temperature]. SYNTHROID tablets should be protected from light and moisture.

(Nos. 4341, 4552, 5182, 6594, 6624, 9296, 7068, 3727, 7069, 7070, 7148, 7149)

Revised: July, 2002

03-5194-R1

ABBOTT LABORATORIES

NORTH CHICAGO, IL 60064, U.S.A.

Shown in Product Identification Guide, page 303

TARKA® ℞

(Trandolapril/Verapamil Hydrochloride ER Tablets)

USE IN PREGNANCY

When used in pregnancy during the second and third trimesters, ACE inhibitors can cause injury and even death to the developing fetus. When pregnancy is detected, TARKA® should be discontinued as soon as possible. **See WARNINGS, Fetal/Neonatal Morbidity and Mortality.**

DESCRIPTION

TARKA® (trandolapril/verapamil hydrochloride ER) combines a slow release formulation of a calcium channel blocker, verapamil hydrochloride, and an immediate release formulation of an angiotensin converting enzyme inhibitor, trandolapril.

Verapamil Component—Verapamil hydrochloride is chemically described as benzeneacetonitrile, α[3-[[2-(3,4-dimethoxyphenyl) ethyl] methylamino] propyl]-3,4-dimethoxy-α-(1-methylethyl) hydrochloride. Its empirical formula is $C_{27}H_{38}N_2O_4$ HCl and its structural formula is:

$$CH_3O-C_6H_3(OCH_3)-C(CH(CH_3)_2)(C{\equiv}N)-CH_2-CH_2-CH_2-N(CH_3)-CH_2-CH_2-C_6H_3(OCH_3)_2 \cdot HCl$$

Verapamil hydrochloride is an almost white crystalline powder, with a molecular weight of 491.08. It is soluble in water, chloroform, and methanol. It is practically free of odor, with a bitter taste.

Trandolapril Component—Trandolapril is the ethyl ester prodrug of a nonsulfhydryl angiotensin converting enzyme (ACE) inhibitor, trandolaprilat. It is chemically described as (2S,3aR,7aS)-1-[(S)-N-[(S)-Carboxy-3-phenylpropyl]alanyl] hexahydro-2-indolinecarboxylic acid, 1-ethyl ester. Its empirical formula is $C_{24}H_{34}N_2O_5$ and its structural formula is:

[See chemical structure at top of next column]

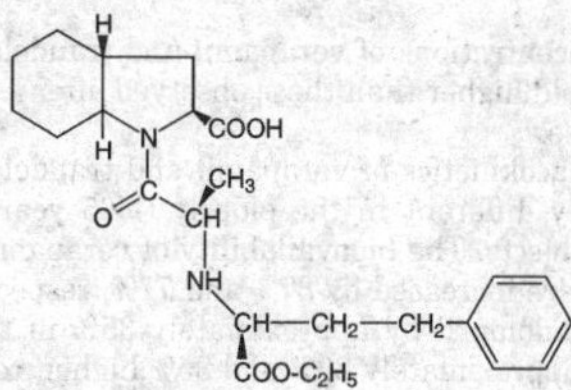

Trandolapril is a colorless, crystalline substance with a molecular weight of 430.54. It is soluble (>100 mg/mL) in chloroform, dichloromethane, and methanol.

TARKA tablets are formulated for oral administration, containing verapamil hydrochloride as a controlled release formulation and trandolapril as an immediate release formulation. The tablet strengths are trandolapril 2 mg/verapamil hydrochloride ER 180 mg, trandolapril 1 mg/verapamil hydrochloride ER 240 mg, trandolapril 2 mg/verapamil hydrochloride ER 240 mg, and trandolapril 4 mg/verapamil hydrochloride ER 240 mg. The tablets also contain the following ingredients: corn starch, dioctyl sodium sulfosuccinate, ethanol, hydroxypropyl cellulose, hypromellose, lactose, magnesium stearate, microcrystalline cellulose, polyethylene glycol, povidone, purified water, silicon dioxide, sodium alginate, sodium stearyl fumarate, synthetic iron oxides, talc, and titanium dioxide.

CLINICAL PHARMACOLOGY

Verapamil hydrochloride and trandolapril have been used individually and in combination for the treatment of hypertension. For the four dosing strengths, the antihypertensive effect of the combination is approximately additive to the individual components.

Verapamil Component—Verapamil is a calcium channel blocker that exerts its pharmacologic effects by modulating the influx of ionic calcium across the cell membrane of the arterial smooth muscle as well as in conductile and contractile myocardial cells. Verapamil exerts antihypertensive effects by decreasing systemic vascular resistance, usually without orthostatic decreases in blood pressure or reflex tachycardia. During isometric or dynamic exercise, verapamil does not alter systolic cardiac function in patients with normal ventricular function. Verapamil does not alter total serum calcium levels.

Trandolapril Component—Trandolapril is de-esterified to its diacid metabolite, trandolaprilat. Both inhibit angiotensin-converting enzyme (ACE) in human subjects and in animals. Trandolaprilat is about 8 times more potent than trandolapril. ACE is a peptidyl dipeptidase that catalyzes the conversion of angiotensin I to the vasoconstrictor, angiotensin II. Angiotensin II also stimulates aldosterone secretion by the adrenal cortex.

Inhibition of ACE results in decreased plasma angiotensin II, which leads to decreased vasopressor activity and to decreased aldosterone secretion. The latter decrease may result in a small increase of serum potassium. In controlled clinical trials, treatment with TARKA resulted in mean increases in potassium of 0.1 mEq/L (see **PRECAUTIONS**). Removal of angiotensin II negative feedback on renin secretion leads to increased plasma renin activity (PRA).

ACE is identical to kininase II, an enzyme that degrades bradykinin. Whether increased levels of bradykinin, a potent vasodepressor peptide, play a role in the therapeutic effect of TARKA remains to be elucidated.

While the mechanism through which trandolapril lowers blood pressure is believed to be primarily suppression of the renin-angiotensin-aldosterone system, trandolapril has an antihypertensive effect even in patients with low renin hypertension. Trandolapril is an effective antihypertensive in all races studied. Both black patients (usually a predominantly low renin group) and non-black patients respond to 2 to 4 mg of trandolapril.

Pharmacokinetics and Metabolism: *TARKA*—Following a single oral dose of TARKA in healthy subjects, peak plasma concentrations are reached within 0.5–2 hours for trandolapril and within 4–15 hours for verapamil. Peak plasma concentrations of the active desmethyl metabolite of verapamil, norverapamil, are reached within 5–15 hours. Cleavage of the ester group converts trandolapril to its active diacid metabolite, trandolaprilat, which reaches peak plasma concentrations within 2–12 hours. The pharmacokinetics of trandolapril and trandolaprilat are not altered when trandolapril is administered in combination with verapamil, compared to monotherapy. The AUC and C_{max} for both verapamil and norverapamil are increased when 240 mg of controlled release verapamil is administered concomitantly with 4 mg trandolapril. The increase in C_{max} is 54 and 30% and the AUC is increased by 65 and 32% for verapamil and norverapamil, respectively. Administration of TARKA 4/240 (4 mg trandolapril and 240 mg verapamil hydrochloride ER) with a high-fat meal does not alter the bioavailability of trandolapril whereas verapamil peak concentrations and area under the curve (AUC) decrease 37% and 28%, respectively. Food thus decreases verapamil bioavailability and the time to peak plasma concentration for both verapamil and norverapamil are delayed by approximately 7 hours. Both optical isomers of verapamil are similarly affected.

Trandolaprilat has an effective elimination half-life of approximately 10 hours but like all ACE inhibitors, it has a prolonged terminal elimination half-life. The terminal half-life of verapamil is 6–11 hours. Steady-state plasma concentrations of the two components are achieved after about a week of once-daily dosing of TARKA. At steady-state,

Continued on next page

Tarka—Cont.

plasma concentrations of verapamil and trandolaprilat are up to two-fold higher than those observed after a single oral TARKA dose.
The pharmacokinetics of verapamil and trandolaprilat are significantly different in the elderly (≥65 years) than in younger subjects. The bioavailability of verapamil and norverapamil are increased by 87% and 77%, respectively, and that of trandolapril by approximately 35% in the elderly. AUCs are approximately 80% and 35% higher, respectively.
Verapamil Component—With the immediate release formulation, more than 90% of the orally administered dose is absorbed with peak plasma concentrations of verapamil observed 1 to 2 hours after dosing. A delayed rate but similar extent of absorption is observed for the sustained release formulation when compared to the immediate release formulation. Because of the rapid biotransformation of verapamil during its first pass through the portal circulation, absolute bioavailability ranges from 20% to 35%. A nonlinear correlation exists between verapamil dose and plasma concentrations.
In early dose titration with verapamil, a relationship exists between plasma concentrations of verapamil and prolongation of the PR interval. However, during chronic administration, this relationship may disappear. No relationship has been established between the plasma concentration of verapamil and reduction in blood pressure.
In healthy subjects, orally administered verapamil undergoes extensive metabolism in the liver. Twelve metabolites have been identified in plasma; all except norverapamil are present in trace amounts only. Approximately 70% of an administered dose is excreted as metabolites in the urine and 16% or more in the feces within 5 days. Urinary excretion of unchanged drug is about 3% to 4% of the dose. Verapamil is approximately 90% bound to plasma proteins.
In patients with hepatic insufficiency, verapamil clearance is decreased about 30% and the elimination half-life is prolonged up to 14 to 16 hours (see **PRECAUTIONS**). In patients with liver dysfunction, a dosage adjustment may be required. In the elderly (≥65 years), verapamil clearance is reduced resulting in increases in elimination half-life.
Trandolapril Component—Following oral administration of trandolapril, the absolute bioavailability of trandolapril is approximately 10% as trandolapril and 10% as trandolaprilat. Plasma concentrations of trandolaprilat but not trandolapril increase in proportion with dose. Plasma concentrations of trandolaprilat decline in a triphasic manner. The more prolonged terminal elimination phase probably represents a small fraction of dose saturably bound to ACE. After an oral radiolabeled dose of trandolapril, excretion of trandolapril and metabolites account for 33% of the dose in the urine and about 66% in the feces. Less than 1% of the dose is excreted in the urine as unchanged drug. Serum protein binding of trandolapril is about 80%, and is independent of concentration. Binding of trandolaprilat is concentration-dependent, varying from 65% at 1000 ng/mL to 94% at 0.1 ng/mL, indicating saturation of binding with increasing concentration.
Compared to normal subjects, the plasma concentrations of trandolapril and trandolaprilat are approximately 2-fold greater and renal clearance is reduced by about 85% in patients with creatinine clearance below 30 mL/min and in patients on hemodialysis. Dosage adjustment is recommended in renally impaired patients. (See **DOSAGE AND ADMINISTRATION**).
Following oral administration in patients with mild to moderate alcoholic cirrhosis, plasma concentrations of trandolapril and trandolaprilat were, respectively, 9-fold and 2-fold greater than in normal subjects, but inhibition of ACE activity was not affected. Lower doses should be considered in patients with hepatic insufficiency. (see **DOSAGE AND ADMINISTRATION**).
Pharmacodynamics: *TARKA*—Verapamil does not interfere with ACE inhibition by trandolapril. Trandolapril does not alter the effect of verapamil on intra-cardiac conduction.
Verapamil Component—Verapamil dilates the main coronary arteries and coronary arterioles, both in normal and ischemic regions, and is a potent inhibitor of coronary artery spasm. This property increases myocardial oxygen delivery in patients with coronary artery spasm, and is responsible for the effectiveness of verapamil in vasospastic (Prinzmetal's or variant) as well as unstable angina at rest. Verapamil regularly reduces the total systemic resistance (afterload) by dilating peripheral arterioles. By decreasing the influx of calcium, verapamil prolongs the effective refractory period within the AV node and slows AV conduction in a rate-related manner.
Normal sinus rhythm is usually not affected, but in patients with sick sinus syndrome, verapamil may interfere with sinus node impulse generation and may induce sinus arrest or sinoatrial block. Atrioventricular block can occur in patients without preexisting conduction defects (see **WARNINGS**).
Verapamil does not alter the normal atrial action potential or intraventricular conduction time, but depresses amplitude, velocity of depolarization and conduction in depressed atrial fibers. Verapamil may shorten the antegrade effective refractory period of accessory bypass tracts. Acceleration of ventricular rate and/or ventricular fibrillation has been reported in patients with atrial flutter or atrial fibrillation and a coexisting accessory AV pathway following administration of verapamil (see **WARNINGS**).
Hemodynamics and Myocardial Metabolism: Verapamil reduces afterload and myocardial contractility. Improved left ventricular diastolic function in patients with idiopathic hypertrophic subaortic stenosis (IHSS) and those with coronary heart disease has also been observed with verapamil therapy. In most patients, including those with organic cardiac disease, the negative inotropic action of verapamil is countered by a reduction of afterload and cardiac index is usually not reduced. However, in patients with severe left ventricular dysfunction (e.g., pulmonary wedge pressure about 20 mmHg or ejection fraction less than 30%), or in patients taking beta-adrenergic blocking agents or other cardio-depressant drugs, deterioration of ventricular function may occur (see **DRUG INTERACTIONS**).
Pulmonary Function: Verapamil does not induce bronchoconstriction and hence, does not impair ventilatory function.
Trandolapril Component—After a single 2 mg dose of trandolapril, inhibition of ACE activity reaches a maximum (70–85%) at 4 hours with about 1% decline at 24 hours. Eight days after dosing, ACE inhibition is still 40%.
Four placebo-controlled dose response studies were conducted using once daily oral dosing of trandolapril in doses from 0.25 to 16 mg per day in 827 black and non-black patients with mild to moderate hypertension. The minimal effective once daily dose was 1.0 mg in non-black patients and 2.0 mg in black patients. Further decreases in trough supine diastolic blood pressure were obtained in non-black patients with higher doses, and no further response was seen with doses above 4 mg (up to 16 mg). The antihypertensive effect diminished somewhat at the end of the dosing interval.
During chronic therapy, the maximum reduction in blood pressure with any dose is achieved within one week. Following 6 weeks of monotherapy in placebo-controlled trials in patients with mild to moderate hypertension, once daily doses of 2 to 4 mg lowered supine or standing systolic/diastolic blood pressure 24 hours after dosing by an average 7–10/4–5 mmHg below placebo responses in non-black patients. Once daily doses of 2 to 4 mg lowered blood pressures 4–6/3–4 mmHg below placebo responses in black patients.

CLINICAL STUDIES

In controlled clinical trials, once daily doses of TARKA, trandolapril 4 mg/verapamil HCl ER 240 mg or trandolapril 2 mg/verapamil HCl ER 180 mg, decreased placebo-corrected seated pressure (systolic/diastolic) 24 hours after dosing by about 7–12/6–8 mmHg. Each of the components of TARKA added to the antihypertensive effect. Treatment effects were consistent across age groups (<65, ≥65 years), and gender (male, female).
Blood pressure reductions were significantly greater for the TARKA 4/240 combination than for either of the components used alone.
The antihypertensive effects of TARKA have continued during therapy for at least 1 year.

INDICATIONS AND USAGE

TARKA is indicated for the treatment of hypertension.
This fixed combination drug is not indicated for the initial therapy of hypertension (see DOSAGE and ADMINISTRATION).
In using TARKA, consideration should be given to the fact that an angiotensin converting enzyme inhibitor, captopril, has caused agranulocytosis, particularly in patients with renal impairment or collagen vascular disease, and that available data are insufficient to show that trandolapril does not have similar risk (see **WARNINGS: Neutropenia/Agranulocytosis**).

CONTRAINDICATIONS

TARKA is contraindicated in patients who are hypersensitive to any ACE inhibitor or verapamil.
Because of the verapamil component, TARKA is contraindicated in:

1. Severe left ventricular dysfunction (see **WARNINGS**).
2. Hypotension (systolic pressure less than 90 mmHg) or cardiogenic shock.
3. Sick sinus syndrome (except in patients with a functioning artificial ventricular pacemaker).
4. Second- or third-degree AV block (except in patients with a functioning artificial ventricular pacemaker).
5. Patients with atrial flutter or atrial fibrillation and an accessory bypass tract (e.g. Wolff-Parkinson-White, Lown-Ganong-Levine syndromes) (see **WARNINGS**).

Because of the trandolapril component, TARKA is contraindicated in patients with a history of angioedema related to previous treatment with an angiotensin converting enzyme (ACE) inhibitor.

WARNINGS

Heart Failure: *Verapamil Component*—Verapamil has a negative inotropic effect which, in most patients, is compensated by its afterload reduction (decreased systemic vascular resistance) properties without a net impairment of ventricular performance. In clinical experience with 4,954 patients, 87 (1.8%) developed congestive heart failure or pulmonary edema. Verapamil should be avoided in patients with severe left ventricular dysfunction (e.g., ejection fraction less than 30%, pulmonary wedge pressure above 20 mmHg, or severe symptoms of cardiac failure) and in patients with any degree of ventricular dysfunction if they are receiving a beta adrenergic blocker (see **DRUG INTERACTIONS**). Patients with milder ventricular dysfunction should, if possible, be controlled with optimum doses of digitalis and/or diuretics before verapamil treatment (Note interactions with digoxin under: **PRECAUTIONS**).
Trandolapril Component—Trandolapril, as an ACE inhibitor, may cause excessive hypotension in patients with congestive heart failure (see **WARNINGS, Hypotension**).
Hypotension: *Verapamil Component*—Occasionally, the pharmacologic action of verapamil may produce a decrease in blood pressure below normal levels which may result in dizziness or symptomatic hypotension.
Trandolapril Component—Trandolapril can cause symptomatic hypotension. Like other ACE inhibitors, trandolapril has only rarely been associated with symptomatic hypotension in uncomplicated hypertensive patients. Symptomatic hypotension is most likely to occur in patients who are salt- or volume-depleted as a result of prolonged treatment with diuretics, dietary salt restriction, dialysis, diarrhea, or vomiting. Volume and/or salt depletion should be corrected before initiating treatment with trandolapril (see **PRECAUTIONS, Drug Interactions**, and **ADVERSE REACTIONS**).
In controlled studies, hypotension was observed in 0.6% of patients receiving any combination of trandolapril and verapamil HCl ER.
In patients with concomitant congestive heart failure, with or without associated renal insufficiency, ACE inhibitor therapy may cause excessive hypotension, which may be associated with oliguria or azotemia, and, rarely, with acute renal failure and death (see **DOSAGE AND ADMINISTRATION**).
If symptomatic hypotension occurs, the patient should be placed in the supine position and, if necessary, normal saline may be administered intravenously. A transient hypotensive response is not a contraindication to further doses; however, lower doses of verapamil HCl ER and/or trandolapril or reduced concomitant diuretic therapy should be considered.
Elevated Liver Enzymes/Hepatic Failure:
Verapamil Component—Elevations of transaminases with and without concomitant elevations in alkaline phosphatase and bilirubin have been reported. Such elevations have sometimes been transient and may disappear even in the face of continued verapamil treatment. Several cases of hepatocellular injury related to verapamil have been proven by rechallenge; half of these had clinical symptoms (malaise, fever, and/or right upper quadrant pain) in addition to elevations of SGOT, SGPT, and alkaline phosphatase.
Trandolapril Component—ACE inhibitors rarely have been associated with a syndrome of cholestatic jaundice, fulminant hepatic necrosis, and death. The mechanism of this syndrome is not understood. Patients receiving ACE inhibitors who develop jaundice should discontinue the ACE inhibitor and receive appropriate medical follow-up.
Liver abnormalities were noted in 3.2% of patients taking any of several combinations of trandolapril/verapamil doses. Periodic monitoring of liver function in patients taking TARKA is therefore prudent.
Accessory Bypass Tract (Wolff-Parkinson-White or Lown-Ganong-Levine Syndromes):
Verapamil Component—Some patients with paroxysmal and/or chronic atrial fibrillation or atrial flutter and a coexisting accessory AV pathway have developed increased antegrade conduction across the accessory pathway bypassing the AV node, producing a very rapid ventricular response or ventricular fibrillation after receiving intravenous verapamil (or digitalis). Although a risk of this occurring with oral verapamil has not been established, such patients receiving oral verapamil may be at risk and its use in these patients is contraindicated (see **CONTRAINDICATIONS**). Treatment is usually DC-cardioversion. Cardioversion has been used safely and effectively after oral verapamil.
Atrioventricular Block:
Verapamil Component—The effect of verapamil on AV conduction and the SA node may lead to asymptomatic first-degree AV block and transient bradycardia, sometimes accompanied by nodal escape rhythms. PR interval prolongation is correlated with verapamil plasma concentrations, especially during the early titration phases of therapy. Higher degrees of AV block, however, were infrequently (0.8%) observed. Marked first-degree block or progressive development to second- or third-degree AV block requires a reduction in dosage or, in rare instances, discontinuation of verapamil HCl and institution of appropriate therapy depending upon the clinical situation.
Patients with Hypertrophic Cardiomyopathy (IHSS):
Verapamil Component—In 120 patients with hypertrophic cardiomyopathy (most of them refractory or intolerant to propranolol) who received therapy with verapamil at doses up to 720 mg/day, a variety of serious adverse effects were seen. Three patients died in pulmonary edema; all had severe left ventricular outflow obstruction and a past history of left ventricular dysfunction. Eight other patients had pulmonary edema and/or severe hypotension; abnormally high (over 20 mmHg) capillary wedge pressure and a marked left ventricular outflow obstruction were present in most of these patients. Sinus bradycardia occurred in 11% of the patients, second-degree AV block in 4% and sinus arrest in 2%. It must be appreciated that this group of patients had a serious disease with a high mortality rate. Most adverse effects responded well to dose reduction and only rarely did verapamil have to be discontinued.
Anaphylactoid and Possibly Related Reactions:
Presumably because angiotensin-converting enzyme inhibitors affect the metabolism of eicosanoids and polypeptides, including endogenous bradykinin, patients receiving ACE inhibitors, including trandolapril may be subject to a variety of adverse reactions, some of them serious.

Angioedema:
Angioedema of the face, extremities, lips, tongue, glottis, and larynx has been reported in patients treated with ACE inhibitors including trandolapril. Symptoms suggestive of angioedema or facial edema occurred in 0.13% of trandolapril-treated patients. Two of the four cases were life-threatening and resolved without treatment or with medication (corticosteroids). Angioedema associated with laryngeal edema can be fatal. If laryngeal stridor or angioedema of the face, tongue or glottis occurs, treatment with TARKA should be discontinued immediately, the patient treated in accordance with accepted medical care and carefully observed until the swelling disappears. In instances where swelling is confined to the face and lips, the condition generally resolves without treatment; antihistamines may be useful in relieving symptoms. **Where there is involvement of the tongue, glottis, or larynx, likely to cause airway obstruction, emergency therapy, including but not limited to subcutaneous epinephrine solution 1:1,000 (0.3 to 0.5 mL) should be promptly administered.** (see **PRECAUTIONS: Information for Patients** and **ADVERSE REACTIONS**).

Anaphylactoid Reactions During Desensitization: Two patients undergoing desensitizing treatment with hymenoptera venom while receiving ACE inhibitors sustained life-threatening anaphylactoid reactions. In the same patients, these reactions did not occur when ACE inhibitors were temporarily withheld, but they reappeared when the ACE inhibitors were inadvertently readministered.

Anaphylactoid Reactions During Membrane Exposure: Anaphylactoid reactions have been reported in patients dialyzed with high-flux membranes and treated concomitantly with an ACE inhibitor. Anaphylactoid reactions have also been reported in patients undergoing low-density lipoprotein apheresis with dextran sulfate absorption.

Neutropenia/Agranulocytosis:
Trandolapril Component—Another ACE inhibitor, captopril, has been shown to cause agranulocytosis and bone marrow depression rarely in patients with uncomplicated hypertension, but more frequently in patients with renal impairment, especially if they also have a collagen-vascular disease such as systemic lupus erythematosus or scleroderma. Available data from clinical trials of trandolapril or TARKA are insufficient to show that trandolapril does not cause agranulocytosis at similar rates. As with other ACE inhibitors, periodic monitoring of white blood cell counts in patients with collagen-vascular disease and/or renal disease should be considered.

Fetal/Neonatal Morbidity and Mortality:
Trandolapril Component—ACE inhibitors can cause fetal and neonatal morbidity and death when administered to pregnant women. Several dozen cases have been reported in the world literature. When pregnancy is detected, ACE inhibitors should be discontinued as soon as possible.

The use of ACE inhibitors during the second and third trimesters of pregnancy has been associated with fetal and neonatal injury, including hypotension, neonatal skull hypoplasia, anuria, reversible or irreversible renal failure, and death. Oligohydramnios has also been reported, presumably resulting from decreased fetal renal function; oligohydramnios in this setting has been associated with fetal limb contractures, craniofacial deformation, and hypoplastic lung development. Prematurity, intrauterine growth retardation, and patent ductus arteriosus have also been reported, although it is not clear whether these occurrences were due to the ACE-inhibitor exposure.

These adverse effects do not appear to have resulted from intrauterine ACE-inhibitor exposure that has been limited to the first trimester. Mothers whose embryos and fetuses are exposed to ACE inhibitors only during the first trimester should be so informed. Nonetheless, when patients become pregnant, physicians should make every effort to discontinue the use of TARKA as soon as possible.

Rarely (probably less often than once in every thousand pregnancies), no alternative to ACE inhibitors will be found. In these rare cases, the mothers should be apprised of the potential hazards to their fetuses, and serial ultrasound examinations should be performed to assess the intra-amniotic environment.

If oligohydramnios is observed, TARKA should be discontinued unless it is considered life-saving for the mother. Contraction stress testing (CST), a non-stress test (NST), or biophysical profiling (BPP) may be appropriate, depending upon the week of pregnancy. Patients and physicians should be aware, however, that oligohydramnios may not appear until after the fetus has sustained irreversible injury.

Infants with histories of in utero exposure to ACE inhibitors should be closely observed for hypotension, oliguria, and hyperkalemia. If oliguria occurs, attention should be directed toward support of blood pressure and renal perfusion. Exchange transfusion or dialysis may be required as a means of reversing hypotension and/or substituting for disordered renal function.

Trandolapril in doses of 0.8 mg/kg/day in rabbits, 100.0 mg/kg/day in rats, and 25 mg/kg/day in cynomolgus monkeys (10, 1,250, and 312 times the maximum projected human dose, respectively, assuming a 50 kg woman) did not produce teratogenic effects.

PRECAUTIONS

Use in Patients with Impaired Hepatic Function:
TARKA has not been evaluated in subjects with impaired hepatic function.

Verapamil Component—Since verapamil is highly metabolized by the liver, it should be administered cautiously to patients with impaired hepatic function. Severe liver dysfunction prolongs the elimination half-life of immediate release verapamil to about 14 to 16 hours; hence, approximately 30% of the dose given to patients with normal liver function should be administered to these patients.

Careful monitoring for abnormal prolongation of the PR interval or other signs of excessive pharmacologic effects (see **OVERDOSAGE**) should be carried out.

Trandolapril Component—Trandolapril and trandolaprilat concentrations increase in patients with impaired liver function.

Use in Patients with Impaired Renal Function:
TARKA has not been evaluated in patients with impaired renal function.

Verapamil Component—About 70% of an administered dose of verapamil is excreted as metabolites in the urine. Verapamil is not removed by hemodialysis. Until further data are available, verapamil should be administered cautiously to patients with impaired renal function. These patients should be carefully monitored for abnormal prolongation of the PR interval or other signs of overdosage (see **OVERDOSAGE**).

Trandolapril Component—As a consequence of inhibiting the renin-angiotensin-aldosterone system, changes in renal function may be anticipated in susceptible individuals. In patients with severe heart failure whose renal function may depend on the activity of the renin-angiotensin-aldosterone system, treatment with ACE inhibitors, including trandolapril, may be associated with oliguria and/or progressive azotemia and rarely with acute renal failure and/or death.

In hypertensive patients with unilateral or bilateral renal artery stenosis, increases in blood urea nitrogen and serum creatinine have been observed in some patients following ACE inhibitor therapy. These increases were almost always reversible upon discontinuation of the ACE inhibitor and/or diuretic therapy. In such patients, renal function should be monitored during the first few weeks of therapy.

Some hypertensive patients with no apparent pre-existing renal vascular disease have developed increases in blood urea and serum creatinine, usually minor and transient, especially when ACE inhibitors have been given concomitantly with a diuretic. This is more likely to occur in patients with pre-existing renal impairment. Dosage reduction and/or discontinuation of any diuretic and/or the ACE inhibitor may be required.

Evaluation of hypertensive patients should always include assessment of renal function (see **DOSAGE AND ADMINISTRATION**).

Use in Patients with Attenuated (Decreased) Neuromuscular Transmission:
Verapamil Component—It has been reported that verapamil decreases neuromuscular transmission in patients with Duchenne's muscular dystrophy, and that verapamil prolongs recovery from the neuromuscular blocking agent vecuronium. It may be necessary to decrease the dosage of verapamil when it is administered to patients with attenuated neuromuscular transmission. (See **PRECAUTIONS—Surgery/Anesthesia**.)

Hyperkalemia and potassium-sparing diuretics:
Trandolapril Component—In clinical trials, hyperkalemia (serum potassium > 6.00 mEq/L) occurred in approximately 0.4 percent of hypertensive patients receiving trandolapril and in 0.8% of patients receiving a dose of trandolapril (0.5–8 mg) in combination with a dose of verapamil SR (120–240 mg). In most cases, elevated serum potassium levels were isolated values, which resolved despite continued therapy. None of these patients were discontinued from the trials because of hyperkalemia. Risk factors for the development of hyperkalemia include renal insufficiency, diabetes mellitus, and the concomitant use of potassium-sparing diuretics, potassium supplements, and/or potassium-containing salt substitutes, which should be used cautiously, if at all, with trandolapril (see **PRECAUTIONS, Drug Interactions**).

Cough:
Presumably due to the inhibition of the degradation of endogenous bradykinin, persistent nonproductive cough has been reported with all ACE inhibitors, always resolving after discontinuation of therapy. ACE inhibitor-induced cough should be considered in the differential diagnosis of cough. In controlled trials of trandolapril, cough was present in 2% of trandolapril patients and 0% of patients given placebo. There was no evidence of a relationship to dose.

Surgery/anesthesia:
Trandolapril Component—In patients undergoing major surgery or during anesthesia with agents that produce hypotension, trandolapril will block angiotensin II formation secondary to compensatory renin release. If hypotension occurs and is considered to be due to this mechanism, it can be corrected by volume expansion. (See **PRECAUTIONS—Use in Patients with Attenuated (Decreased) Neuromuscular Transmission.**)

Drug Interactions:
Digitalis: Clinical use of verapamil in digitalized patients has shown the combination to be well tolerated if digoxin doses are properly adjusted. Chronic verapamil treatment can increase serum digoxin levels by 50 to 75% during the first week of therapy, and this can result in digoxin toxicity. In patients with hepatic cirrhosis, the influence of verapamil on digoxin kinetics is magnified. Verapamil may reduce total body clearance and extrarenal clearance of digitoxin by 27% and 29%, respectively. Maintenance digoxin doses should be reduced when verapamil is administered, and the patient should be carefully monitored to avoid over- or under-digitalization. Whenever overdigitalization is suspected, the daily dose of digoxin should be reduced or temporarily discontinued. Upon discontinuation of any verapamil-containing regime including TARKA® (trandolapril/verapamil hydrochloride ER), the patient should be reassessed to avoid underdigitalization. Neither trandolapril nor its metabolites have been found to interact with digoxin.

Lithium: Increased sensitivity to the effects of lithium (neurotoxicity) has been reported during concomitant verapamil-lithium therapy with either no change or an increase in serum lithium levels. Increased serum lithium levels and symptoms of lithium toxicity have been reported in patients receiving concomitant lithium and ACE inhibitor therapy. TARKA and lithium should be coadministered with caution, and frequent monitoring of serum lithium levels is recommended. If a diuretic is also used, the risk of lithium toxicity may be increased.

Cimetidine: The interaction between cimetidine and chronically administered verapamil has not been studied. Variable results on clearance have been obtained in acute studies of healthy volunteers; clearance of verapamil was either reduced or unchanged. Neither trandolapril nor its metabolites have been found to interact with cimetidine.

Beta Blockers: *Verapamil Component*—Concomitant therapy with beta-adrenergic blockers and verapamil may result in additive negative effects on heart rate, atrioventricular conduction, and/or cardiac contractility. The use of verapamil in combination with a beta-blocker should be used only with caution, and close monitoring.

Asymptomatic bradycardia (36 beats/min) with a wandering atrial pacemaker has been observed in a patient receiving concomitant timolol (a beta-adrenergic blocker) eyedrops and oral verapamil.

Antiarrhythmic Agents:
Verapamil Component—Disopyramide—Data on possible interactions between verapamil and disopyramide phosphate are not available. Therefore, disopyramide should not be administered within 48 hours before or 24 hours after verapamil administration.

Flecainide—A study of healthy volunteers showed that the concomitant administration of flecainide and verapamil may have additive effects on myocardial contractility, AV conduction, and repolarization. Concomitant therapy with flecainide and verapamil may result in additive negative inotropic effect and prolongation of atrioventricular conduction.

Quinidine—In a small number of patients with hypertrophic cardiomyopathy (IHSS), concomitant use of verapamil and quinidine resulted in significant hypotension. Until further data are obtained, combined therapy of verapamil and quinidine in patients with hypertrophic cardiomyopathy should probably be avoided.

The electrophysiological effects of quinidine and verapamil on AV conduction were studied in 8 patients. Verapamil significantly counteracted the effects of quinidine on AV conduction. There has been a report of increased quinidine levels during verapamil therapy.

Nitrates—Verapamil has been given concomitantly with short- and long-acting nitrates without any undesirable drug interactions. The pharmacologic profile of both drugs and the clinical experience suggest beneficial interactions.

Other: *Verapamil Component*—Carbamazepine—Verapamil may increase carbamazepine concentrations during combined therapy. This may produce carbamazepine side effects such as diplopia, headache, ataxia, or dizziness.

Rifampin—Therapy with rifampin may markedly reduce oral verapamil bioavailability.

Phenobarbital—Phenobarbital therapy may increase verapamil clearance.

Cyclosporin—Verapamil therapy may increase serum levels of cyclosporin.

Theophylline—Verapamil therapy may inhibit the clearance and increase the plasma levels of theophylline.

Inhalation Anesthetics—Animal experiments have shown that inhalation anesthetics depress cardiovascular activity by decreasing the inward movement of calcium ions. When used concomitantly, inhalation anesthetics and calcium antagonists, such as verapamil, should be titrated carefully to avoid excessive cardiovascular depression.

Neuromuscular Blocking Agents—Clinical data and animal studies suggest that verapamil may potentiate the activity of neuromuscular blocking agents (curare-like and depolarizing). It may be necessary to decrease the dose of verapamil and/or the dose of the neuromuscular blocking agent when the drugs are used concomitantly.

Concomitant diuretic therapy:
Trandolapril Component—As with other ACE inhibitors, patients on diuretics, especially those on recently instituted diuretic therapy, may occasionally experience an excessive reduction of blood pressure after initiation of therapy with TARKA. The possibility of exacerbation of hypotensive effects with TARKA may be minimized by either discontinuing the diuretic or cautiously increasing salt intake prior to initiation of treatment with TARKA. If it is not possible to discontinue the diuretic, the starting dose of TARKA should be reduced (see **DOSAGE AND ADMINISTRATION**).

Continued on next page

Tarka—Cont.

Agents increasing serum potassium:
Trandolapril can attenuate potassium loss caused by thiazide diuretics and increase serum potassium when used alone. Use of potassium-sparing diuretics (spironolactone, triamterene, or amiloride), potassium supplements, or potassium-containing salt substitutes concomitantly with ACE inhibitors can increase the risk of hyperkalemia. If concomitant use of such agents is indicated, they should be used with caution and with appropriate monitoring of serum potassium. (See **PRECAUTIONS**.)
Other: *Trandolapril Component*—Neither trandolapril nor its metabolites have been found to interact with furosemide or nifedipine. The anticoagulant effect of warfarin was not significantly changed by trandolapril.
Carcinogenesis, Mutagenesis, Impairment of Fertility:
Verapamil Component—An 18-month toxicity study in rats, at a low multiple (6 fold) of the maximum recommended human dose, and not the maximum tolerated dose, did not suggest a tumorigenic potential. There was no evidence of a carcinogenic potential of verapamil administered in the diet of rats for two years at doses of 10, 35, and 120 mg/kg per day or approximately 1×, 3.5×, and 12×, respectively, the maximum recommended human daily dose (480 mg per day or 9.6 mg/kg/day).
Verapamil was not mutagenic in the Ames test in 5 test strains at 3 mg per plate, with or without metabolic activation.
Studies in female rats at daily dietary doses up to 5.5 times (55 mg/kg/day) the maximum recommended human dose did not show impaired fertility. Effects on male fertility have not been determined.
Long-term studies were conducted with oral trandolapril administered by gavage to mice (78 weeks) and rats (104 and 106 weeks). No evidence of carcinogenic potential was seen in mice dosed up to 25 mg/kg/day (85 mg/m^2/day) or rats dosed up to 8 mg/kg/day (60 mg/m^2/day). These doses are 313 and 32 times (mice), and 100 and 23 times (rats) the maximum recommended human daily dose (MRHDD) of 4 mg based on body-weight and body-surface-area, respectively assuming a 50 kg individual. The genotoxic potential of trandolapril was evaluated in the microbial mutagenicity (Ames) test, the point mutation and chromosome aberration assays in Chinese hamster V79 cells, and the micronucleus test in mice. There was no evidence of mutagenic or clastogenic potential in these *in vitro* and *in vivo* assays.
Reproduction studies in rats did not show any impairment of fertility at doses up to 100 mg/kg/day (710 mg/m^2/day) of trandolapril, or 1250 and 260 times the MRHDD on the basis of body-weight and body-surface-area, respectively.
Pregnancy: Pregnancy Categories C (first trimester) and D (second and third trimesters). See WARNINGS, Fetal/Neonatal Morbidity and Mortality.
Nursing Mothers: Verapamil is excreted in human milk. Radiolabeled trandolapril or its metabolites are secreted in rat milk. TARKA should not be administered to nursing mothers.
Geriatric Use: In placebo-controlled studies, where 23% of patients receiving TARKA were 65 years and older, and 2.4% were 75 years and older, no overall differences in effectiveness or safety were observed between these patients and younger patients. However, greater sensitivity of some older individual patients cannot be ruled out.
Pediatric Use: The safety and effectiveness of TARKA in children below the age of 18 have not been established.
Animal Pharmacology and/or Animal Toxicology: In chronic animal toxicology studies, verapamil caused lenticular and/or suture line changes at 30 mg/kg/day or greater and frank cataracts at 62.5 mg/kg/day or greater in the beagle dog but not the rat. Development of cataracts due to verapamil has not been reported in man.

ADVERSE REACTIONS

TARKA has been evaluated in over 1,957 subjects and patients. Of these, 541 patients, including 23% elderly patients, participated in U.S. controlled clinical trials, and 251 were studied in foreign controlled clinical trials. In clinical trials with TARKA, no adverse experiences peculiar to this combination drug have been observed. Adverse experiences that have occurred have been limited to those that have been previously reported with verapamil or trandolapril.
TARKA has been evaluated for long-term safety in 272 patients treated for 1 year or more. Adverse experiences were usually mild and transient.
Discontinuation of therapy because of adverse events in U.S. placebo-controlled hypertension studies was required in 2.6% and 1.9% of patients treated with TARKA and placebo, respectively.
Adverse experiences occurring in 1% or more of the 541 patients in placebo-controlled hypertension trials who were treated with a range of trandolapril (0.5–8 mg) and verapamil (120–240 mg) combinations are shown below.
[See table below]
Other clinical adverse experiences possibly, probably, or definitely related to drug treatment occurring in 0.3% or more of patients treated with trandolapril/verapamil combinations with or without concomitant diuretic in controlled or uncontrolled trials (N=990) and less frequent, clinically significant events (in italics) include the following:
Cardiovascular: angina, *AV block second degree, bundle branch block*, edema, flushing, hypotension, *myocardial infarction*, palpitations, premature ventricular contractions, nonspecific ST-T changes, near syncope, tachycardia.
Central Nervous System: drowsiness, *hypesthesia, insomnia, loss of balance, paresthesia, vertigo.*
Dermatologic: pruritus, rash.
Emotional, Mental, Sexual States: anxiety, impotence, *abnormal mentation.*
Eye, Ear, Nose, Throat: epistaxis, tinnitus, upper respiratory tract infection, *blurred vision.*
Gastrointestinal: diarrhea, dyspepsia, dry mouth, nausea.
General Body Function: chest pain, malaise, weakness.
Genitourinary: endometriosis, hematuria, nocturia, polyuria, proteinuria.
Hemopoietic: decreased leukocytes, *decreased neutrophils.*
Musculoskeletal System: arthralgias/myalgias, *gout (increased uric acid).*
Pulmonary: dyspnea.
Angioedema: Angioedema has been reported in 3 (0.15%) patients receiving TARKA in U.S. and foreign studies (N=1,957). Angioedema associated with laryngeal edema may be fatal. If angioedema of the face, extremities, lips, tongue, glottis, and/or larynx occurs, treatment with TARKA should be discontinued and appropriate therapy instituted immediately (see **WARNINGS**).
Hypotension: (See **WARNINGS**). In hypertensive patients, hypotension occurred in 0.6% and near syncope occurred in 0.1%. Hypotension or syncope was a cause for discontinuation of therapy in 0.4% of hypertensive patients.
Treatment of Acute Cardiovascular Adverse Reactions: The frequency of cardiovascular adverse reactions which require therapy is rare, hence, experience with their treatment is limited. Whenever severe hypotension or complete AV block occur following oral administration of TARKA (verapamil component), the appropriate emergency measures should be applied immediately, e.g., intravenously administered isoproterenol HCl, levarterenol bitartrate, atropine (all in the usual doses), or calcium gluconate (10% solution). In patients with hypertrophic cardiomyopathy (IHSS), alpha-adrenergic agents (phenylephrine, metaraminol bitartrate or methoxamine) should be used to maintain blood pressure, and isoproterenol and levarterenol should be avoided. If further support is necessary, inotropic agents (dopamine or dobutamine) may be administered. Actual treatment and dosage should depend on the severity and the clinical situation and the judgment and experience of the treating physician.
Fetal/Neonatal Morbidity and Mortality: See **WARNINGS, Fetal Neonatal Morbidity and Mortality.**
Other adverse experiences (in addition to those in table and listed above) that have been reported with the individual components are listed below.
Verapamil Component:
Cardiovascular: (See **WARNINGS.**) CHF/pulmonary edema, AV block 3°, atrioventricular dissociation, claudication, purpura (vasculitis), syncope.
Digestive System: gingival hyperplasia. Reversible, (upon discontinuation of verapamil) nonobstructive, paralytic ileus has been infrequently reported in association with the use of verapamil.
Hemic and Lymphatic: ecchymosis or bruising.
Nervous System: cerebrovascular accident, confusion, psychotic symptoms, shakiness, somnolence.
Skin: exanthema, hair loss, hyperkeratosis, maculae, sweating, urticaria, Stevens-Johnson syndrome, erythema multiform.
Urogenital: gynecomastia, galactorrhea/hyperprolactinemia, increased urination, spotty menstruation.
Trandolapril Component:
Emotional, Mental, Sexual States: decreased libido.
Gastrointestinal: pancreatitis.
Clinical Laboratory Test Findings
Hematology: (See **WARNINGS.**) Low white blood cells, low neutrophils, low lymphocytes, low platelets.
Serum Electrolytes: Hyperkalemia (See **PRECAUTIONS**), hyponatremia.
Renal Function Tests: Increases in creatinine and blood urea nitrogen levels occurred in 1.1 percent and 0.3 percent, respectively, of patients receiving TARKA with or without hydrochlorothiazide therapy. None of these increases required discontinuation of treatment. Increases in these laboratory values are more likely to occur in patients with renal insufficiency or those pretreated with a diuretic and, based on experience with other ACE inhibitors, would be expected to be especially likely in patients with renal artery stenosis. (See **PRECAUTIONS** and **WARNINGS.**)
Liver function tests: Elevations of liver enzymes (SGOT, SGPT, LDH, and alkaline phosphatase) and/or serum bilirubin occurred. Discontinuation for elevated liver enzymes occurred in 0.9 percent of patients. (See **WARNINGS.**)

OVERDOSAGE

No specific information is available on the treatment of overdosage with TARKA.
Verapamil Component—Overdose with verapamil may lead to pronounced hypotension, bradycardia, and conduction system abnormalities (e.g., junctional rhythm with AV dissociation and high degree AV block, including asystole). Other symptoms secondary to hypoperfusion (e.g., metabolic acidosis, hyperglycemia, hyperkalemia, renal dysfunction, and convulsions) may be evident.
Treat all verapamil overdoses as serious and maintain observation for at least 48 hours, preferably under continuous hospital care. Delayed pharmacodynamic consequences may occur with the sustained release formulation. Verapamil is known to decrease gastrointestinal transit time. In cases of overdose, tablets of ISOPTIN SR have occasionally been reported to form concretions within the stomach or intestines. These concretions have not been visible on plain radiographs of the abdomen, and no medical means of gastrointestinal emptying is of proven efficacy in removing them. Endoscopy might reasonably be considered in cases of overdose when symptoms are unusually prolonged. Verapamil cannot be removed by hemodialysis.
Treatment of overdosage should be supportive. Beta adrenergic stimulation or parenteral administration of calcium solutions may increase calcium ion flux across the slow channel, and have been used effectively in treatment of deliberate overdosage with verapamil. The following measures may be considered:
Bradycardia and conduction system abnormalities: Atropine, isoproterenol, and cardiac pacing.
Hypotension: Intravenous fluids, vasopressors (e.g., dopamine, dobutamine), calcium solutions (e.g., 10% calcium chloride solution)
Cardiac failures: Inotropic agents (e.g., isoproterenol, dopamine, dobutamine), diuretics. Asystole should be handled by the usual measures including cardiopulmonary resuscitation.
Trandolapril Component—The oral LD_{50} of trandolapril in mice was 4875 mg/kg in males and 3990 mg/kg in females. In rats, an oral dose of 5000 mg/kg caused low mortality (1 male out of 5; 0 females). In dogs, an oral dose of 1000 mg/kg did not cause mortality and abnormal clinical signs were not observed.
In humans, the most likely clinical manifestation would be symptoms attributable to severe hypotension. Laboratory determinations of serum levels of trandolapril and its metabolites are not widely available, and such determinations have, in any event, no established role in the management of trandolapril overdose. No data are available to suggest that physiological maneuvers (e.g., maneuvers to change pH of the urine) might accelerate elimination of trandolapril and its metabolites. It is not known if trandolapril or trandolaprilat can be usefully removed from the body by hemodialysis.
Angiotensin II could presumably serve as a specific antagonist antidote in the setting of trandolapril overdose, but an-

ADVERSE EVENTS OCCURRING IN ≥ 1% OF TARKA® PATIENTS IN U.S. PLACEBO-CONTROLLED TRIALS

	TARKA (N=541) % Incidence (% Discontinuance)	PLACEBO (N=206) % Incidence (% Discontinuance)
AV Block First Degree	3.9 (0.2)	0.5 (0.0)
Bradycardia	1.8 (0.0)	0.0 (0.0)
Bronchitis	1.5 (0.0)	0.5 (0.0)
Chest Pain	2.2 (0.0)	1.0 (0.0)
Constipation	3.3 (0.0)	1.0 (0.0)
Cough	4.6 (0.0)	2.4 (0.0)
Diarrhea	1.5 (0.2)	1.0 (0.0)
Dizziness	3.1 (0.0)	1.9 (0.5)
Dyspnea	1.3 (0.4)	0.0 (0.0)
Edema	1.3 (0.0)	2.4 (0.0)
Fatigue	2.8 (0.4)	2.4 (0.0)
Headache(s)+	8.9 (0.0)	9.7 (0.5)
Increased Liver Enzymes*	2.8 (0.2)	1.0 (0.0)
Nausea	1.5 (0.2)	0.5 (0.0)
Pain Extremity(ies)	1.1 (0.2)	0.5 (0.0)
Pain Back+	2.2 (0.0)	2.4 (0.0)
Pain Joint(s)	1.7 (0.0)	1.0 (0.0)
Upper Respiratory Tract Infection(s)+	5.4 (0.0)	7.8 (0.0)
Upper Respiratory Tract Congestion+	2.4 (0.0)	3.4 (0.0)

* Also includes increase in SGPT, SGOT, Alkaline Phosphatase
+ Incidence of adverse events is higher in Placebo group than TARKA patients

giotensin II is essentially unavailable outside of scattered research facilities. Because the hypotensive effect of trandolapril is achieved through vasodilation and effective hypovolemia, it is reasonable to treat trandolapril overdose by infusion of normal saline solution.

DOSAGE AND ADMINISTRATION

The recommended usual dosage range of trandolapril for hypertension is 1 to 4 mg per day administered in a single dose or two divided doses. The recommended usual dosage range of Isoptin-SR for hypertension is 120 to 480 mg per day administered in a single dose or two divided doses.

The hazards (see **WARNINGS**) of trandolapril are generally independent of dose; those of verapamil are a mixture of dose-dependent phenomena (primarily dizziness, AV block, constipation) and dose-independent phenomena, the former much more common than the latter. Therapy with any combination of trandolapril and verapamil will thus be associated with both sets of dose-independent hazards. The dose-dependent side effects of verapamil have not been shown to be decreased by the addition of trandolapril nor visa versa. Rarely, the dose-independent hazards of trandolapril are serious. To minimize dose-independent hazards, it is usually appropriate to begin therapy with TARKA only after a patient has either (a) failed to achieve the desired antihypertensive effect with one or the other monotherapy at its respective maximally recommended dose and shortest dosing interval, or (b) the dose of one or the other monotherapy cannot be increased further because of dose-limiting side effects.

Clinical trials with TARKA have explored only once-a-day doses. The antihypertensive effect and or adverse effects of adding 4 mg of trandolapril once-a-day to a dose of 240 mg Isoptin-SR administered twice-a-day has not been studied, nor have the effects of adding as little of 180 mg Isoptin-SR to 2 mg trandolapril administered twice-a-day been evaluated. Over the dose range of Isoptin-SR 120 to 240 mg once-a-day and trandolapril 0.5 to 8 mg once-a-day, the effects of the combination increase with increasing doses of either component.

Replacement therapy: For convenience, patients receiving trandolapril (up to 8 mg) and verapamil (up to 240 mg) in separate tablets, administered once-a-day, may instead wish to receive tablets of TARKA containing the same component doses.

TARKA should be administered with food.

HOW SUPPLIED

TARKA 2/180 mg tablets are supplied as pink, oval, film-coated tablets containing 2 mg trandolapril in an immediate release form and 180 mg verapamil hydrochloride in a sustained release form. The tablet is embossed with a triangle and 182 on one side and plain on the other side.

NDC 0074-3287-13 — bottles of 100

TARKA 1/240 mg tablets are supplied as white, oval, film-coated tablets containing 1 mg trandolapril in an immediate release form and 240 mg verapamil hydrochloride in a sustained release form. The tablet is embossed with a triangle and 241 on one side and plain on the other side.

NDC 0074-3288-13 — bottles of 100

TARKA 2/240 mg tablets are supplied as gold, oval, film-coated tablets containing 2 mg trandolapril in an immediate release form and 240 mg verapamil hydrochloride in a sustained release form. The tablet is embossed with a triangle and 242 on one side and plain on the other side.

NDC 0074-3289-13 — bottles of 100

TARKA 4/240 mg tablets are supplied as reddish-brown, oval, film-coated tablets containing 4 mg trandolapril in an immediate release form and 240 mg verapamil hydrochloride in a sustained release form. The tablet is embossed with a triangle and 244 on one side and plain on the other side.

NDC 0074-3290-13 — bottles of 100

Dispense in well-closed container with safety closure.

Storage: Store at 15°–25°C (59°–77°F) see USP.

Ref. 03-5279-R2

Revised: July, 2003

ABBOTT LABORATORIES

NORTH CHICAGO, IL 60064, U.S.A.

Shown in Product Identification Guide, page 303

TRICOR® ℞

[tri cŏr]

(fenofibrate tablets)

DESCRIPTION

TRICOR (fenofibrate tablets), is a lipid regulating agent available as tablets for oral administration. Each tablet contains 54 mg or 160 mg of fenofibrate. The chemical name for fenofibrate is 2-[4-(4-chlorobenzoyl) phenoxy]-2-methyl-propanoic acid, 1-methylethyl ester with the following structural formula:

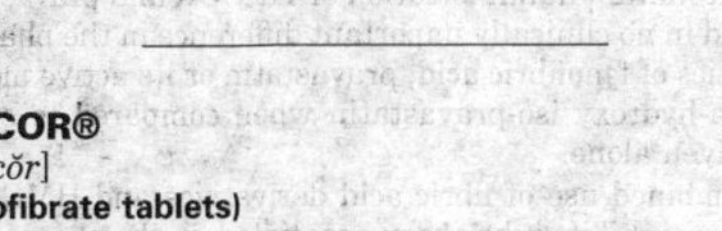

The empirical formula is $C_{20}H_{21}O_4Cl$ and the molecular weight is 360.83; fenofibrate is insoluble in water. The melting point is 79–82°C. Fenofibrate is a white solid which is stable under ordinary conditions.

Inactive Ingredients: Each tablet contains colloidal silicon dioxide, crospovidone, lactose monohydrate, lecithin, microcrystalline cellulose, polyvinyl alcohol, povidone, sodium lauryl sulfate, sodium stearyl fumarate, talc, titanium dioxide, and xanthan gum. In addition, individual tablets contain:

54 mg tablets: D&C Yellow No. 10, FD&C Yellow No. 6, FD&C Blue No. 2.

Table 1
Mean Percent Change in Lipid Parameters at End of Treatment†

Treatment Group	Total-C	LDL-C	HDL-C	TG
Pooled Cohort				
Mean baseline lipid values (n=646)	306.9 mg/dL	213.8 mg/dL	52.3 mg/dL	191.0 mg/dL
All FEN (n=361)	−18.7%*	−20.6%*	+11.0%*	−28.9%*
Placebo (n=285)	−0.4%	−2.2%	+0.7%	+7.7%
Baseline LDL-C > 160 mg/dL and TG < 150 mg/dL (Type IIa)				
Mean baseline lipid values (n=334)	307.7 mg/dL	227.7 mg/dL	58.1 mg/dL	101.7 mg/dL
All FEN (n=193)	−22.4%*	−31.4%*	+9.8%*	−23.5%*
Placebo (n=141)	+0.2%	−2.2%	+2.6%	+11.7%
Baseline LDL-C > 160 mg/dL and TG ≥ 150 mg/dL (Type IIb)				
Mean baseline lipid values (n=242)	312.8 mg/dL	219.8 mg/dL	46.7 mg/dL	231.9 mg/dL
All FEN (n=126)	−16.8%*	−20.1%*	+14.6%*	−35.9%*
Placebo (n=116)	−3.0%	−6.6%	+2.3%	+0.9%

†Duration of study treatment was 3 to 6 months.
*p= <0.05 vs. Placebo

CLINICAL PHARMACOLOGY

A variety of clinical studies have demonstrated that elevated levels of total cholesterol (total-C), low density lipoprotein cholesterol (LDL-C), and apolipoprotein B (apo B), an LDL membrane complex, are associated with human atherosclerosis. Similarly, decreased levels of high density lipoprotein cholesterol (HDL-C) and its transport complex, apolipoprotein A (apo AI and apo AII) are associated with the development of atherosclerosis. Epidemiologic investigations have established that cardiovascular morbidity and mortality vary directly with the level of total-C, LDL-C, and triglycerides, and inversely with the level of HDL-C. The independent effect of raising HDL-C or lowering triglycerides (TG) on the risk of cardiovascular morbidity and mortality has not been determined.

Fenofibric acid, the active metabolite of fenofibrate, produces reductions in total cholesterol, LDL cholesterol, apolipoprotein B, total triglycerides and triglyceride rich lipoprotein (VLDL) in treated patients. In addition, treatment with fenofibrate results in increases in high density lipoprotein (HDL) and apoproteins apoAI and apoAII.

The effects of fenofibric acid seen in clinical practice have been explained *in vivo* in transgenic mice and *in vitro* in human hepatocyte cultures by the activation of peroxisome proliferator activated receptor α (PPARα). Through this mechanism, fenofibrate increases lipolysis and elimination of triglyceride-rich particles from plasma by activating lipoprotein lipase and reducing production of apoprotein C-III (an inhibitor of lipoprotein lipase activity). The resulting fall in triglycerides produces an alteration in the size and composition of LDL from small, dense particles (which are thought to be atherogenic due to their susceptibility to oxidation), to large buoyant particles. These larger particles have a greater affinity for cholesterol receptors and are catabolized rapidly. Activation of PPARα also induces an increase in the synthesis of apoproteins A-I, A-II and HDL-cholesterol.

Fenofibrate also reduces serum uric acid levels in hyperuricemic and normal individuals by increasing the urinary excretion of uric acid.

Pharmacokinetics/Metabolism

Plasma concentrations of fenofibric acid after administration of 54 mg and 160 mg tablets are equivalent under fed conditions to 67 and 200 mg capsules, respectively.

Absorption

The absolute bioavailability of fenofibrate cannot be determined as the compound is virtually insoluble in aqueous media suitable for injection. However, fenofibrate is well absorbed from the gastrointestinal tract. Following oral administration in healthy volunteers, approximately 60% of a single dose of radiolabelled fenofibrate appeared in urine, primarily as fenofibric acid and its glucuronate conjugate, and 25% was excreted in the feces. Peak plasma levels of fenofibric acid occur within 6 to 8 hours after administration.

The absorption of fenofibrate is increased when administered with food. With fenofibrate tablets, the extent of absorption is increased by approximately 35% under fed as compared to fasting conditions.

Distribution

In healthy volunteers, steady-state plasma levels of fenofibric acid were shown to be achieved within 5 days of dosing and did not demonstrate accumulation across time following multiple dose administration. Serum protein binding was approximately 99% in normal and hyperlipidemic subjects.

Metabolism

Following oral administration, fenofibrate is rapidly hydrolyzed by esterases to the active metabolite, fenofibric acid; no unchanged fenofibrate is detected in plasma.

Fenofibric acid is primarily conjugated with glucuronic acid and then excreted in urine. A small amount of fenofibric acid is reduced at the carbonyl moiety to a benzhydrol metabolite which is, in turn, conjugated with glucuronic acid and excreted in urine.

In vivo metabolism data indicate that neither fenofibrate nor fenofibric acid undergo oxidative metabolism (e.g., cytochrome P450) to a significant extent.

Excretion

After absorption, fenofibrate is mainly excreted in the urine in the form of metabolites, primarily fenofibric acid and fenofibric acid glucuronide. After administration of radiolabelled fenofibrate, approximately 60% of the dose appeared in the urine and 25% was excreted in the feces.

Fenofibric acid is eliminated with a half-life of 20 hours, allowing once daily administration in a clinical setting.

Special Populations

Geriatrics

In elderly volunteers 77–87 years of age, the oral clearance of fenofibric acid following a single oral dose of fenofibrate was 1.2 L/h, which compares to 1.1 L/h in young adults. This indicates that a similar dosage regimen can be used in the elderly, without increasing accumulation of the drug or metabolites.

Pediatrics

TRICOR has not been investigated in adequate and well-controlled trials in pediatric patients.

Gender

No pharmacokinetic difference between males and females has been observed for fenofibrate.

Race

The influence of race on the pharmacokinetics of fenofibrate has not been studied, however fenofibrate is not metabolized by enzymes known for exhibiting inter-ethnic variability. Therefore, inter-ethnic pharmacokinetic differences are very unlikely.

Renal insufficiency

In a study in patients with severe renal impairment (creatinine clearance <50 mL/min), the rate of clearance of fenofibric acid was greatly reduced, and the compound accumulated during chronic dosage. However, in patients having moderate renal impairment (creatinine clearance of 50 to 90 mL/min), the oral clearance and the oral volume of distribution of fenofibric acid are increased compared to healthy adults (2.1 L/h and 95 L versus 1.1 L/h and 30 L, respectively). Therefore, the dosage of TRICOR should be minimized in patients who have severe renal impairment, while no modification of dosage is required in patients having moderate renal impairment.

Hepatic insufficiency

No pharmacokinetic studies have been conducted in patients having hepatic insufficiency.

Drug-drug interactions

In vitro studies using human liver microsomes indicate that fenofibrate and fenofibric acid are not inhibitors of cytochrome (CYP) P450 isoforms CYP3A4, CYP2D6, CYP2E1, or CYP1A2. They are weak inhibitors of CYP2C19 and CYP2A6, and mild-to-moderate inhibitors of CYP2C9 at therapeutic concentrations.

Potentiation of coumarin-type anticoagulants has been observed with prolongation of the prothrombin time/INR.

Bile acid sequestrants have been shown to bind other drugs given concurrently. Therefore, fenofibrate should be taken at least 1 hour before or 4–6 hours after a bile acid binding resin to avoid impeding its absorption (see WARNINGS and PRECAUTIONS).

Clinical Trials

Hypercholesterolemia (Heterozygous Familial and Nonfamilial) and Mixed Dyslipidemia (Fredrickson Types IIa and IIb)

The effects of fenofibrate at a dose equivalent to 160 mg TRICOR per day were assessed from four randomized, placebo-controlled, double-blind, parallel-group studies including patients with the following mean baseline lipid val-

Continued on next page

Tricor—Cont.

ues: total-C 306.9 mg/dL; LDL-C 213.8 mg/dL; HDL-C 52.3 mg/dL; and triglycerides 191.0 mg/dL. TRICOR therapy lowered LDL-C, Total-C, and the LDL-C/HDL-C ratio. TRICOR therapy also lowered triglycerides and raised HDL-C (see Table 1).

[See table 1 at top of previous page]

In a subset of the subjects, measurements of apo B were conducted. TRICOR treatment significantly reduced apo B from baseline to endpoint as compared with placebo (−25.1% vs. 2.4%, p<0.0001, n=213 and 143 respectively).

Hypertriglyceridemia (Fredrickson Type IV and V)

The effects of fenofibrate on serum triglycerides were studied in two randomized, double-blind, placebo-controlled clinical trials[1] of 147 hypertriglyceridemic patients (Fredrickson Types IV and V). Patients were treated for eight weeks under protocols that differed only in that one entered patients with baseline triglyceride (TG) levels of 500 to 1500 mg/dL, and the other TG levels of 350 to 500 mg/dL. In patients with hypertriglyceridemia and normal cholesterolemia with or without hyperchylomicronemia (Type IV/V hyperlipidemia), treatment with fenofibrate at dosages equivalent to 160 mg TRICOR per day decreased primarily very low density lipoprotein (VLDL) triglycerides and VLDL cholesterol. Treatment of patients with Type IV hyperlipoproteinemia and elevated triglycerides often results in an increase of low density lipoprotein (LDL) cholesterol (see Table 2).

[See table 2 at right]

The effect of TRICOR on cardiovascular morbidity and mortality has not been determined.

INDICATIONS AND USAGE

Treatment of Hypercholesterolemia

TRICOR is indicated as adjunctive therapy to diet to reduce elevated LDL-C, Total-C, Triglycerides and Apo B, and to increase HDL-C in adult patients with primary hypercholesterolemia or mixed dyslipidemia (Fredrickson Types IIa and IIb). Lipid-altering agents should be used in addition to a diet restricted in saturated fat and cholesterol when response to diet and non-pharmacological interventions alone has been inadequate (see National Cholesterol Education Program [NCEP] Treatment Guidelines, below).

Treatment of Hypertriglyceridemia

TRICOR is also indicated as adjunctive therapy to diet for treatment of adult patients with hypertriglyceridemia (Fredrickson Types IV and V hyperlipidemia). Improving glycemic control in diabetic patients showing fasting chylomicronemia will usually reduce fasting triglycerides and eliminate chylomicronemia thereby obviating the need for pharmacologic intervention.

Markedly elevated levels of serum triglycerides (e.g. > 2,000 mg/dL) may increase the risk of developing pancreatitis. The effect of TRICOR therapy on reducing this risk has not been adequately studied.

Drug therapy is not indicated for patients with Type I hyperlipoproteinemia, who have elevations of chylomicrons and plasma triglycerides, but who have normal levels of very low density lipoprotein (VLDL). Inspection of plasma refrigerated for 14 hours is helpful in distinguishing Types I, IV and V hyperlipoproteinemia[2].

The initial treatment for dyslipidemia is dietary therapy specific for the type of lipoprotein abnormality. Excess body weight and excess alcoholic intake may be important factors in hypertriglyceridemia and should be addressed prior to any drug therapy. Physical exercise can be an important ancillary measure. Diseases contributory to hyperlipidemia, such as hypothyroidism or diabetes mellitus should be looked for and adequately treated. Estrogen therapy, thiazide diuretics and beta-blockers, are sometimes associated with massive rises in plasma triglycerides, especially in subjects with familial hypertriglyceridemia. In such cases, discontinuation of the specific etiologic agent may obviate the need for specific drug therapy of hypertriglyceridemia.

The use of drugs should be considered only when reasonable attempts have been made to obtain satisfactory results with non-drug methods. If the decision is made to use drugs, the patient should be instructed that this does not reduce the importance of adhering to diet. (See WARNINGS and PRECAUTIONS).

Fredrickson Classification of Hyperlipoproteinemias

Type	Lipoprotein Elevated	Lipid Elevation Major	Lipid Elevation Minor
I (rare)	chylomicrons	TG	↑↔C
IIa	LDL	C	–
IIb	LDL, VLDL	C	TG
III (rare)	IDL	C, TG	–
IV	VLDL	TG	↑↔C
V (rare)	chylomicrons, VLDL	TG	↑↔

C=cholesterol
TG=triglycerides
LDL=low density lipoprotein
VLDL=very low density lipoprotein
IDL=intermediate density lipoprotein

[See second table above]

After the LDL-C goal has been achieved, if the TG is still >200 mg/dL, non HDL-C (total-C minus HDL-C) becomes a secondary target of therapy. Non-HDL-C goals are set 30 mg/dL higher than LDL-C goals for each risk category.

Table 2
Effects of TRICOR in Patients With Fredrickson Type IV/V Hyperlipidemia

Study 1	Placebo				TRICOR			
Baseline TG levels 350 to 499 mg/dL	N	Baseline (Mean)	Endpoint (Mean)	% Change (Mean)	N	Baseline (Mean)	Endpoint (Mean)	% Change (Mean)
Triglycerides	28	449	450	−0.5	27	432	223	−46.2*
VLDL Triglycerides	19	367	350	2.7	19	350	178	−44.1*
Total Cholesterol	28	255	261	2.8	27	252	227	−9.1*
HDL Cholesterol	28	35	36	4	27	34	40	19.6*
LDL Cholesterol	28	120	129	12	27	128	137	14.5
VLDL Cholesterol	27	99	99	5.8	27	92	46	−44.7*

Study 2	Placebo				TRICOR			
Baseline TG levels 500 to 1500 mg/dL	N	Baseline (Mean)	Endpoint (Mean)	% Change (Mean)	N	Baseline (Mean)	Endpoint (Mean)	% Change (Mean)
Triglycerides	44	710	750	7.2	48	726	308	−54.5*
VLDL Triglycerides	29	537	571	18.7	33	543	205	−50.6*
Total Cholesterol	44	272	271	0.4	48	261	223	−13.8*
HDL Cholesterol	44	27	28	5.0	48	30	36	22.9*
LDL Cholesterol	42	100	90	−4.2	45	103	131	45.0*
VLDL Cholesterol	42	137	142	11.0	45	126	54	−49.4*

* = p<0.05 vs. Placebo

NCEP Treatment Guidelines: LDL-C Goals and Cutpoints for Therapeutic Lifestyle Changes and Drug Therapy in Different Risk Categories

Risk Category	LDL Goal (mg/dL)	LDL Level at Which to Initiate Therapeutic Lifestyle Changes (mg/dL)	LDL Level at which to Consider Drug Thereapy (mg/dL)
CHD[†] or CHD risk equivalents (10-years risk >20%)	<100	≥100	≥130 (100–129:drug optional)[††]
2+ Risk Factors (10-years risk ≤20%)	<130	≥130	10-year risk 10%–20%:≥130 10-Year risk <10%: ≥160
0–1 Risk Factor [†††]	<160	≥160	≥190 (160–189: LDL-lowering drug optional)

† CHD = coronary heart disease
†† Some authorities recommend use of LDL-lowering drugs in this category if an LDL-C level of <100 mg/dL cannot be achieved by therapeutic lifestyle changes. Others prefer use of drugs that primarily modify triglycerides and HDL-C, e.g., nicotinic acid or fibrate. Clinical judgement also may call for deferring drug therapy in this subcategory.
††† Almost all people with 0–1 risk factor have 10-year risk <10%; thus, 10-year risk assessment in people with 0–1 risk factor is not necessary.

CONTRAINDICATIONS

TRICOR is contraindicated in patients who exhibit hypersensitivity to fenofibrate.

TRICOR is contraindicated in patients with hepatic or severe renal dysfunction, including primary biliary cirrhosis, and patients with unexplained persistent liver function abnormality.

TRICOR is contraindicated in patients with preexisting gallbladder disease (see WARNINGS).

WARNINGS

Liver Function: Fenofibrate at doses equivalent to 107 mg to 160 mg TRICOR per day has been associated with increases in serum transaminases [AST (SGOT) or ALT (SGPT)]. In a pooled analysis of 10 placebo-controlled trials, increases to > 3 times the upper limit of normal occurred in 5.3% of patients taking fenofibrate versus 1.1% of patients treated with placebo.

When transaminase determinations were followed either after discontinuation of treatment or during continued treatment, a return to normal limits was usually observed. The incidence of increases in transaminases related to fenofibrate therapy appear to be dose related. In an 8-week dose-ranging study, the incidence of ALT or AST elevations to at least three times the upper limit of normal was 13% in patients receiving dosages equivalent to 107 mg to 160 mg TRICOR per day and was 0% in those receiving dosages equivalent to 54 mg or less TRICOR per day, or placebo. Hepatocellular, chronic active and cholestatic hepatitis associated with fenofibrate therapy have been reported after exposures of weeks to several years. In extremely rare cases, cirrhosis has been reported in association with chronic active hepatitis.

Regular periodic monitoring of liver function, including serum ALT (SGPT) should be performed for the duration of therapy with TRICOR, and therapy discontinued if enzyme levels persist above three times the normal limit.

Cholelithiasis: Fenofibrate, like clofibrate and gemfibrozil, may increase cholesterol excretion into the bile, leading to cholelithiasis. If cholelithiasis is suspected, gallbladder studies are indicated. TRICOR therapy should be discontinued if gallstones are found.

Concomitant Oral Anticoagulants: Caution should be exercised when anticoagulants are given in conjunction with TRICOR because of the potentiation of coumarin-type anticoagulants in prolonging the prothrombin time/INR. The dosage of the anticoagulant should be reduced to maintain the prothrombin time/INR at the desired level to prevent bleeding complications. Frequent prothrombin time/INR determinations are advisable until it has been definitely determined that the prothrombin time/INR has stabilized.

Concomitant HMG-CoA Reductase Inhibitors: The combined use of TRICOR and HMG-CoA reductase inhibitors should be avoided unless the benefit of further alterations in lipid levels is likely to outweigh the increased risk of this drug combination.

In a single-dose drug interaction study in 23 healthy adults the concomitant administration of TRICOR and pravastatin resulted in no clinically important difference in the pharmacokinetics of fenofibric acid, pravastatin or its active metabolite 3a-hydroxy iso-pravastatin when compared to either drug given alone.

The combined use of fibric acid derivatives and HMG-CoA reductase inhibitors has been associated, in the absence of a marked pharmacokinetic interaction, in numerous case reports, with rhabdomyolysis, markedly elevated creatine kinase (CK) levels and myoglobinuria, leading in a high proportion of cases to acute renal failure.

The use of fibrates alone, including TRICOR, may occasionally be associated with myositis, myopathy, or rhabdomyolysis. Patients receiving TRICOR and complaining of muscle pain, tenderness, or weakness should have prompt medical evaluation for myopathy, including serum creatine kinase level determination. If myopathy/myositis is suspected or diagnosed, TRICOR therapy should be stopped.

Mortality: The effect of TRICOR on coronary heart disease morbidity and mortality and non-cardiovascular mortality has not been established.

Other Considerations: In the Coronary Drug Project, a large study of post myocardial infarction of patients treated for 5 years with clofibrate, there was no difference in mortality seen between the clofibrate group and the placebo group. There was however, a difference in the rate of cholelithiasis and cholecystitis requiring surgery between the two groups (3.0% vs. 1.8%).

Because of chemical, pharmacological, and clinical similarities between TRICOR (fenofibrate tablets), Atromid-S (clofibrate), and Lopid (gemfibrozil), the adverse findings in 4 large randomized, placebo-controlled clinical studies with these other fibrate drugs may also apply to TRICOR.

In a study conducted by the World Health Organization (WHO), 5000 subjects without known coronary artery disease were treated with placebo or clofibrate for 5 years and followed for an additional one year. There was a statistically significant, higher age-adjusted all-cause mortality in the clofibrate group compared with the placebo group (5.70% vs. 3.96%, p=<0.01). Excess mortality was due to a 33% increase in non-cardiovascular causes, including malignancy, post-cholecystectomy complications, and pancreatitis. This appeared to confirm the higher risk of gallbladder disease seen in clofibrate-treated patients studied in the Coronary Drug Project.

The Helsinki Heart Study was a large (n=4081) study of middle-aged men without a history of coronary artery disease. Subjects received either placebo or gemfibrozil for 5 years, with a 3.5 year open extension afterward. Total mortality was numerically higher in the gemfibrozil randomization group but did not achieve statistical significance (p=0.19, 95% confidence interval for relative risk G:P=.91–1.64). Although cancer deaths trended higher in the gemfibrozil group (p=0.11), cancers (excluding basal cell carcinoma) were diagnosed with equal frequency in both study groups. Due to the limited size of the study, the relative risk of death from any cause was not shown to be different than that seen in the 9 year follow-up data from World Health Organization study (RR=1.29). Similarly, the numerical excess of gallbladder surgeries in the gemfibrozil group did not differ statistically from that observed in the WHO study.

A secondary prevention component of the Helsinki Heart Study enrolled middle-aged men excluded from the primary prevention study because of known or suspected coronary heart disease. Subjects received gemfibrozil or placebo for 5 years. Although cardiac deaths trended higher in the gemfibrozil group, this was not statistically significant (hazard ratio 2.2, 95% confidence interval: 0.94–5.05). The rate of gallbladder surgery was not statistically significant between study groups, but did trend higher in the gemfibrozil group, (1.9% vs. 0.3%, p=0.07). There was a statistically significant difference in the number of appendectomies in the gemfibrozil group (6/311 vs. 0/317, p=0.029).

PRECAUTIONS

Initial therapy: Laboratory studies should be done to ascertain that the lipid levels are consistently abnormal before instituting TRICOR therapy. Every attempt should be made to control serum lipids with appropriate diet, exercise, weight loss in obese patients, and control of any medical problems such as diabetes mellitus and hypothyroidism that are contributing to the lipid abnormalities. Medications known to exacerbate hypertriglyceridemia (beta-blockers, thiazides, estrogens) should be discontinued or changed if possible prior to consideration of triglyceride-lowering drug therapy.

Continued therapy: Periodic determination of serum lipids should be obtained during initial therapy in order to establish the lowest effective dose of TRICOR. Therapy should be withdrawn in patients who do not have an adequate response after two months of treatment with the maximum recommended dose of 160 mg per day.

Pancreatitis: Pancreatitis has been reported in patients taking fenofibrate, gemfibrozil, and clofibrate. This occurrence may represent a failure of efficacy in patients with severe hypertriglyceridemia, a direct drug effect, or a secondary phenomenon mediated through biliary tract stone or sludge formation with obstruction of the common bile duct.

Hypersensitivity Reactions: Acute hypersensitivity reactions including severe skin rashes requiring patient hospitalization and treatment with steroids have occurred very rarely during treatment with fenofibrate, including rare spontaneous reports of Stevens-Johnson syndrome, and toxic epidermal necrolysis. Urticaria was seen in 1.1 vs 0%, and rash in 1.4 vs 0.8% of fenofibrate and placebo patients respectively in controlled trials.

Hematologic Changes: Mild to moderate hemoglobin, hematocrit, and white blood cell decreases have been observed in patients following initiation of fenofibrate therapy. However, these levels stabilize during long-term administration. Extremely rare spontaneous reports of thrombocytopenia and agranulocytosis have been received during post-marketing surveillance outside of the U.S. Periodic blood counts are recommended during the first 12 months of TRICOR administration.

Skeletal muscle: The use of fibrates alone, including TRICOR, may occasionally be associated with myopathy. Treatment with drugs of the fibrate class has been associated on rare occasions with rhabdomyolysis, usually in patients with impaired renal function. Myopathy should be considered in any patient with diffuse myalgias, muscle tenderness or weakness, and/or marked elevations of creatine phosphokinase levels.

Patients should be advised to report promptly unexplained muscle pain, tenderness or weakness, particularly if accompanied by malaise or fever. CPK levels should be assessed in patients reporting these symptoms, and fenofibrate therapy should be discontinued if markedly elevated CPK levels occur or myopathy is diagnosed.

BODY SYSTEM Adverse Event	Fenofibrate* (N=439)	Placebo (N=365)
BODY AS A WHOLE		
Abdominal Pain	4.6%	4.4%
Back Pain	3.4%	2.5%
Headache	3.2%	2.7%
Asthenia	2.1%	3.0%
Flu Syndrome	2.1%	2.7%
DIGESTIVE		
Liver Function Tests Abnormal	7.5%**	1.4%
Diarrhea	2.3%	4.1%
Nausea	2.3%	1.9%
Constipation	2.1%	1.4%
METABOLIC AND NUTRITIONAL DISORDERS		
SGPT Increased	3.0%	1.6%
Creatine Phosphokinase Increased	3.0%	1.4%
SGOT Increased	3.4%**	0.5%
RESPIRATORY		
Respiratory Disorder	6.2%	5.5%
Rhinitis	2.3%	1.1%

* Dosage equivalent to 200 mg TRICOR
** Significantly different from Placebo

Drug Interactions

Oral Anticoagulants: CAUTION SHOULD BE EXERCISED WHEN COUMARIN ANTICOAGULANTS ARE GIVEN IN CONJUNCTION WITH TRICOR. THE DOSAGE OF THE ANTICOAGULANTS SHOULD BE REDUCED TO MAINTAIN THE PROTHROMBIN TIME/INR AT THE DESIRED LEVEL TO PREVENT BLEEDING COMPLICATIONS. FREQUENT PROTHROMBIN TIME/INR DETERMINATIONS ARE ADVISABLE UNTIL IT HAS BEEN DEFINITELY DETERMINED THAT THE PROTHROMBIN TIME/INR HAS STABILIZED.

HMG-CoA reductase inhibitors: The combined use of TRICOR and HMG-CoA reductase inhibitors should be avoided unless the benefit of further alterations in lipid levels is likely to outweigh the increased risk of this drug combination (see WARNINGS).

Resins: Since bile acid sequestrants may bind other drugs given concurrently, patients should take TRICOR at least 1 hour before or 4–6 hours after a bile acid binding resin to avoid impeding its absorption.

Cyclosporine: Because cyclosporine can produce nephrotoxicity with decreases in creatinine clearance and rises in serum creatinine, and because renal excretion is the primary elimination route of fibrate drugs including TRICOR, there is a risk that an interaction will lead to deterioration. The benefits and risks of using TRICOR with immunosuppressants and other potentially nephrotoxic agents should be carefully considered, and the lowest effective dose employed.

Carcinogenesis, Mutagenesis, Impairment of Fertility: In a 24-month study in rats (10, 45, and 200 mg/kg; 0.3, 1, and 6 times the maximum recommended human dose on the basis of mg/meter^2 of surface area), the incidence of liver carcinoma was significantly increased at 6 times the maximum recommended human dose in males and females. A statistically significant increase in pancreatic carcinomas occurred in males at 1 and 6 times the maximum recommended human dose; there were also increases in pancreatic adenomas and benign testicular interstitial cell tumors at 6 times the maximum recommended human dose in males. In a second 24-month study in a different strain of rats (doses of 10 and 60 mg/kg; 0.3 and 2 times the maximum recommended human dose based on mg/meter^2 surface area), there were significant increases in the incidence of pancreatic acinar adenomas in both sexes and increases in interstitial cell tumors of the testes at 2 times the maximum recommended human dose.

A comparative carcinogenicity study was done in rats comparing three drugs: fenofibrate (10 and 70 mg/kg; 0.3 and 1.6 times the maximum recommended human dose), clofibrate (400 mg/kg; 1.6 times the human dose), and gemfibrozil (250 mg/kg; 1.7 times the human dose) (multiples based on mg/meter^2 surface area). Pancreatic acinar adenomas were increased in males and females on fenofibrate; hepatocellular carcinoma and pancreatic acinar adenomas were increased in males and hepatic neoplastic nodules in females treated with clofibrate; hepatic neoplastic nodules were increased in males and females treated with gemfibrozil while testicular interstitial cell tumors were increased in males on all three drugs.

In a 21-month study in mice at doses of 10, 45, and 200 mg/kg (approximately 0.2, 0.7 and 3 times the maximum recommended human dose on the basis of mg/meter^2 surface area), there were statistically significant increases in liver carcinoma at 3 times the maximum recommended human dose in both males and females. In a second 18-month study at the same doses, there was a significant increase in liver carcinoma in male mice and liver adenoma in female mice at 3 times the maximum recommended human dose.

Electron microscopy studies have demonstrated peroxisomal proliferation following fenofibrate administration to the rat. An adequate study to test for peroxisome proliferation in humans has not been done, but changes in peroxisome morphology and numbers have been observed in humans after treatment with other members of the fibrate class when liver biopsies were compared before and after treatment in the same individual.

Fenofibrate has been demonstrated to be devoid of mutagenic potential in the following tests: Ames, mouse lymphoma, chromosomal aberration and unscheduled DNA synthesis.

Pregnancy Category C: Fenofibrate has been shown to be embryocidal and teratogenic in rats when given in doses 7 to 10 times the maximum recommended human dose and embryocidal in rabbits when given at 9 times the maximum recommended human dose (on the basis of mg/meter^2 surface area). There are no adequate and well-controlled studies in pregnant women. Fenofibrate should be used during pregnancy only if the potential benefit justifies the potential risk to the fetus.

Administration of 9 times the maximum recommended human dose of fenofibrate to female rats before and throughout gestation caused 100% of dams to delay delivery and resulted in a 60% increase in post-implantation loss, a decrease in litter size, a decrease in birth weight, a 40% survival of pups at birth, a 4% survival of pups as neonates, and a 0% survival of pups to weaning, and an increase in spina bifida.

Administration of 10 times the maximum recommended human dose to female rats on days 6–15 of gestation caused an increase in gross, visceral and skeletal findings in fetuses (domed head/hunched shoulders/rounded body/abnormal chest, kyphosis, stunted fetuses, elongated sternal ribs, malformed sternebrae, extra foramen in palatine, misshapen vertebrae, supernumerary ribs).

Administration of 7 times the maximum recommended human dose to female rats from day 15 of gestation through weaning caused a delay in delivery, a 40% decrease in live births, a 75% decrease in neonatal survival, and decreases in pup weight, at birth as well as on days 4 and 21 postpartum.

Administration of 9 and 18 times the maximum recommended human dose to female rabbits caused abortions in 10% of dams at 9 times and 25% of dams at 18 times the maximum recommended human dose and death of 7% of fetuses at 18 times the maximum recommended human dose.

Nursing mothers: Fenofibrate should not be used in nursing mothers. Because of the potential for tumorigenicity seen in animal studies, a decision should be made whether to discontinue nursing or to discontinue the drug.

Pediatric Use: Safety and efficacy in pediatric patients have not been established.

Geriatric Use: Fenofibric acid is known to be substantially excreted by the kidney, and the risk of adverse reactions to this drug may be greater in patients with impaired renal function. Because elderly patients are more likely to have decreased renal function, care should be taken in dose selection.

ADVERSE REACTIONS

CLINICAL: Adverse events reported by 2% or more of patients treated with fenofibrate during the double-blind, placebo-controlled trials, regardless of causality, are listed in the table above. Adverse events led to discontinuation of treatment in 5.0% of patients treated with fenofibrate and in 3.0% treated with placebo. Increases in liver function tests were the most frequent events, causing discontinuation of fenofibrate treatment in 1.6% of patients in double-blind trials.

[See table above]

Additional adverse events reported by three or more patients in placebo-controlled trials or reported in other controlled or open trials, regardless of causality are listed below.

BODY AS A WHOLE: Chest pain, pain (unspecified), infection, malaise, allergic reaction, cyst, hernia, fever, photosensitivity reaction, and accidental injury.

CARDIOVASCULAR SYSTEM: Angina pectoris, hypertension, vasodilatation, coronary artery disorder, electrocardiogram abnormal, ventricular extrasystoles, myocardial infarct, peripheral vascular disorder, migraine, varicose vein, cardiovascular disorder, hypotension, palpitation, vascular

Continued on next page

Tricor—Cont.

disorder, arrhythmia, phlebitis, tachycardia, extrasystoles, and atrial fibrillation.

DIGESTIVE SYSTEM: Dyspepsia, flatulence, nausea, increased appetite, gastroenteritis, cholelithiasis, rectal disorder, esophagitis, gastritis, colitis, tooth disorder, vomiting, anorexia, gastrointestinal disorder, duodenal ulcer, nausea and vomiting, peptic ulcer, rectal hemorrhage, liver fatty deposit, cholecystitis, eructation, gamma glutamyl transpeptidase, and diarrhea.

ENDOCRINE SYSTEM: Diabetes mellitus

HEMIC AND LYMPHATIC SYSTEM: Anemia, leukopenia, ecchymosis, eosinophilia, lymphadenopathy, and thrombocytopenia.

METABOLIC AND NUTRITIONAL DISORDERS: Creatinine increased, weight gain, hypoglycemia, gout, weight loss, edema, hyperuricemia, and peripheral edema.

MUSCULOSKELETAL SYSTEM: Myositis, myalgia, arthralgia, arthritis, tenosynovitis, joint disorder, arthrosis, leg cramps, bursitis, and myasthenia.

NERVOUS SYSTEM: Dizziness, insomnia, depression, vertigo, libido decreased, anxiety, paresthesia, dry mouth, hypertonia, nervousness, neuralgia, and somnolence.

RESPIRATORY SYSTEM: Pharyngitis, bronchitis, cough increased, dyspnea, asthma, allergic pulmonary alveolitis, pneumonia, laryngitis, and sinusitis.

SKIN AND APPENDAGES: Rash, pruritus, eczema, herpes zoster, urticaria, acne, sweating, fungal dermatitis, skin disorder, alopecia, contact dermatitis, herpes simplex, maculopapular rash, nail disorder, and skin ulcer.

SPECIAL SENSES: Conjunctivitis, eye disorder, amblyopia, ear pain, otitis media, abnormal vision, cataract specified, and refraction disorder.

UROGENITAL SYSTEM: Urinary frequency, prostatic disorder, dysuria, abnormal kidney function, urolithiasis, gynecomastia, unintended pregnancy, vaginal moniliasis, and cystitis.

OVERDOSAGE

There is no specific treatment for overdose with TRICOR. General supportive care of the patient is indicated, including monitoring of vital signs and observation of clinical status, should an overdose occur. If indicated, elimination of unabsorbed drug should be achieved by emesis or gastric lavage; usual precautions should be observed to maintain the airway. Because fenofibrate is highly bound to plasma proteins, hemodialysis should not be considered.

DOSAGE AND ADMINISTRATION

Patients should be placed on an appropriate lipid-lowering diet before receiving TRICOR, and should continue this diet during treatment with TRICOR. TRICOR tablets should be given with meals, thereby optimizing the bioavailability of the medication.

For the treatment of adult patients with primary hypercholesterolemia or mixed hyperlipidemia, the initial dose of TRICOR is 160 mg per day.

For adult patients with hypertriglyceridemia, the initial dose is 54 to 160 mg per day. Dosage should be individualized according to patient response, and should be adjusted if necessary following repeat lipid determinations at 4 to 8 week intervals. The maximum dose is 160 mg per day.

Treatment with TRICOR should be initiated at a dose of 54 mg/day in patients having impaired renal function, and increased only after evaluation of the effects on renal function and lipid levels at this dose. In the elderly, the initial dose should likewise be limited to 54 mg/day.

Lipid levels should be monitored periodically and consideration should be given to reducing the dosage of TRICOR if lipid levels fall significantly below the targeted range.

HOW SUPPLIED

TRICOR® (fenofibrate tablets) is available in two strengths:

54 mg yellow tablets, imprinted with ⊐ and Abbo-Code identification letters "TA", available in bottles of 90 (**NDC** 0074-4009-90).

160 mg white tablets, imprinted with ⊐ and Abbo-Code identification letters "TC", available in bottles of 90 (**NDC** 0074-4013-90).

Storage

Store at controlled room temperature, 15–30°C (59–86°F). Keep out of the reach of children. Protect from moisture.

Manufactured for Abbott Laboratories, North Chicago, IL 60064, U.S.A. by Laboratoires Fournier, S.A., 21300 Chenôve, France

REFERENCES

1. GOLDBERG AC, *et al.* Fenofibrate for the Treatment of Type IV and V Hyperlipoproteinemias: A Double-Blind, Placebo-Controlled Multicenter US Study. *Clinical Therapeutics,* 11, pp. 69–83, 1989.
2. NIKKILA EA. Familial Lipoprotein Lipase Deficiency and Related Disorders of Chylomicron Metabolism. In Stanbury J.B., *et al.* (eds.): *The Metabolic Basis of Inherited Disease,* 5th edition, McGraw-Hill, 1983, Chap. 30, pp. 622–642.
3. BROWN WV, *et al.* Effects of Fenofibrate on Plasma Lipids: Double-Blind, Multicenter Study In Patients with Type IIA or IIB Hyperlipidemia. *Arteriosclerosis.* 6, pp. 670–678, 1986.

Revised: February, 2003

Ref.: 03-5240-R2

ABBOTT LABORATORIES

NORTH CHICAGO, IL 60064, USA

VICODIN® Ⓒ ℞

(hydrocodone bitartrate and acetaminophen tablets, USP)

5 mg/500 mg

℞ only

DESCRIPTION

Hydrocodone bitartrate and acetaminophen is supplied in tablet form for oral administration.

Hydrocodone bitartrate is an opioid analgesic and antitussive and occurs as fine, white crystals or as a crystalline powder. It is affected by light. The chemical name is: 4,5α-epoxy-3-methoxy-17-methylmorphinan-6-one tartrate (1:1) hydrate (2:5). It has the following structural formula:

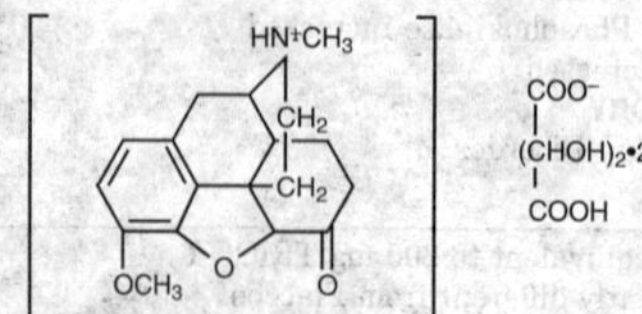

$C_{18}H_{21}NO_3 \bullet C_4H_6O_6 \bullet 2\frac{1}{2}H_2O$ M.W. 494.50

Acetaminophen, 4′-hydroxyacetanilide, a slightly bitter, white, odorless, crystalline powder, is a non-opiate, non-salicylate analgesic and antipyretic. It has the following structural formula:

NHCOCH3

OH

$C_8H_9NO_2$ M.W. 151.16

Each VICODIN tablet contains:

Hydrocodone Bitartrate	5 mg
Acetaminophen	500 mg

In addition each tablet contains the following inactive ingredients: colloidal silicon dioxide, starch, croscarmellose sodium, dibasic calcium phosphate, magnesium stearate, microcrystalline cellulose, povidone, and stearic acid.

Meets USP Dissolution Test 2.

CLINICAL PHARMACOLOGY

Hydrocodone is a semisynthetic narcotic analgesic and antitussive with multiple actions qualitatively similar to those of codeine. Most of these involve the central nervous system and smooth muscle. The precise mechanism of action of hydrocodone and other opiates is not known, although it is believed to relate to the existence of opiate receptors in the central nervous system. In addition to analgesia, narcotics may produce drowsiness, changes in mood and mental clouding.

The analgesic action of acetaminophen involves peripheral influences, but the specific mechanism is as yet undetermined. Antipyretic activity is mediated through hypothalmic heat regulating centers. Acetaminophen inhibits prostaglandin synthetase. Therapeutic doses of acetaminophen have negligible effects on the cardiovascular or respiratory systems; however, toxic doses may cause circulatory failure and rapid, shallow breathing.

Pharmacokinetics: The behavior of the individual components is described below.

Hydrocodone: Following a 10mg oral dose of hydrocodone administered to five adult male subjects, the mean peak concentration was 23.6 ± 5.2ng/mL. Maximum serum levels were achieved at 1.3 ± 0.3 hours and the half-life was determined to be 3.8 ± 0.3 hours. Hydrocodone exhibits a complex pattern of metabolism including O-demethylation, N-demethylation and 6-keto reduction to the corresponding 6-α- and 6-β–hydroxy- metabolites. See OVERDOSAGE for toxicity information.

Acetaminophen: Acetaminophen is rapidly absorbed from the gastrointestinal tract and is distributed throughout most body tissues. The plasma half-life is 1.25 to 3 hours, but may be increased by liver damage and following overdosage. Elimination of acetaminophen is principally by liver metabolism (conjugation) and subsequent renal excretion of metabolites. Approximately 85% of an oral dose appears in the urine within 24 hours of administration, most as the glucuronide conjugate, with small amounts of other conjugates and unchanged drug. See OVERDOSAGE for toxicity information.

INDICATIONS AND USAGE

VICODIN tablets are indicated for the relief of moderate to moderately severe pain.

CONTRAINDICATIONS

This product should not be administered to patients who have previously exhibited hypersensitivity to hydrocodone or acetaminophen.

Patients known to be hypersensitive to other opioids may exhibit cross-sensitivity to hydrocodone.

WARNINGS

Respiratory Depression: At high doses or in sensitive patients, hydrocodone may produce dose-related respiratory depression by acting directly on the brain stem respiratory center. Hydrocodone also affects the center that controls respiratory rhythm, and may produce irregular and periodic breathing.

Head Injury and Increased Intracranial Pressure: The respiratory depressant effects of narcotics and their capacity to elevate cerebrospinal fluid pressure may be markedly exaggerated in the presence of head injury, other intracranial lesions or a preexisting increase in intracranial pressure. Furthermore, narcotics produce adverse reactions which may obscure the clinical course of patients with head injuries.

Acute Abdominal Conditions: The administration of narcotics may obscure the diagnosis or clinical course of patients with acute abdominal conditions.

PRECAUTIONS

General:

Special Risk Patients: As with any narcotic analgesic agent, VICODIN Tablets should be used with caution in elderly or debilitated patients and those with severe impairment of hepatic or renal function, hypothyroidism, Addison's disease, prostatic hypertrophy or urethral stricture. The usual precautions should be observed and the possibility of respiratory depression should be kept in mind.

Cough Reflex: Hydrocodone suppresses the cough reflex; as with all narcotics, caution should be exercised when VICODIN Tablets are used postoperatively and in patients with pulmonary disease.

Information for Patients: Hydrocodone, like all narcotics, may impair the mental and/or physical abilities required for the performance of potentially hazardous tasks such as driving a car or operating machinery; patients should be cautioned accordingly.

Alcohol and other CNS depressants may produce an additive CNS depression, when taken with this combination product, and should be avoided.

Hydrocodone may be habit forming. Patients should take the drug only for as long as it is prescribed, in the amounts prescribed, and no more frequently than prescribed.

Laboratory Tests: In patients with severe hepatic or renal disease, effects of therapy should be monitored with serial liver and/or renal function tests.

Drug Interactions: Patients receiving other narcotic analgesics, antihistamines, antipsychotics, antianxiety agents, or other CNS depressants (including alcohol) concomitantly with VICODIN Tablets may exhibit an additive CNS depression. When combined therapy is contemplated, the dose of one or both agents should be reduced.

The use of MAO inhibitors or tricyclic antidepressants with hydrocodone preparations may increase the effect of either the antidepressant or hydrocodone.

Drug/Laboratory Test Interactions: Acetaminophen may produce false-positive test results for urinary 5-hydroxyindoleacetic acid.

Carcinogenesis, Mutagenesis, Impairment of Fertility: No adequate studies have been conducted in animals to determine whether hydrocodone or acetaminophen have a potential for carcinogenesis, mutagenesis, or impairment of fertility.

Pregnancy:

Teratogenic Effects: Pregnancy Category C. There are no adequate and well-controlled studies in pregnant women. VICODIN Tablets should be used during pregnancy only if the potential benefit justifies the potential risk to the fetus.

Nonteratogenic Effects: Babies born to mothers who have been taking opioids regularly prior to delivery will be physically dependent. The withdrawal signs include irritability and excessive crying, tremors, hyperactive reflexes, increased respiratory rate, increased stools, sneezing, yawning, vomiting, and fever. The intensity of the syndrome does not always correlate with the duration of maternal opioid use or dose. There is no consensus on the best method of managing withdrawal.

Labor and Delivery: As with all narcotics, administration of VICODIN Tablets to the mother shortly before delivery may result in some degree of respiratory depression in the newborn, especially if higher doses are used.

Nursing Mothers: Acetaminophen is excreted in breast milk in small amounts, but the significance of its effects on nursing infants is not known. It is not known whether hydrocodone is excreted in human milk. Because many drugs are excreted in human milk and because of the potential for serious adverse reactions in nursing infants from hydrocodone and acetaminophen, a decision should be made whether to discontinue nursing or to discontinue the drug, taking into account the importance of the drug to the mother.

Pediatric Use: Safety and effectiveness in the pediatric population have not been established.

Geriatric Use: Clinical studies of VICODIN® (hydrocodone bitartrate 5 mg and acetaminophen 500 mg) did not include sufficient numbers of subjects aged 65 and over to determine whether they respond differently from younger subjects. Other reported clinical experience has not identified differences in responses between the elderly and younger patients. In general, dose selection for an elderly patient should be cautious, usually starting at the low end of the dosing range, reflecting the greater frequency of decreased hepatic, renal, or cardiac function, and of concomitant disease or other drug therapy.

ADVERSE REACTIONS

The most frequently reported adverse reactions include: lightheadedness, dizziness, sedation, nausea and vomiting.

These effects seem to be more prominent in ambulatory than in nonambulatory patients and some of these adverse reactions may be alleviated if the patient lies down.
Other adverse reactions include:
Central Nervous System: Drowsiness, mental clouding, lethargy, impairment of mental and physical performance, anxiety, fear, dysphoria, psychic dependence, mood changes.
Gastrointestinal System: Prolonged administration of VICODIN Tablets may produce constipation.
Genitourinary System: Ureteral spasm, spasm of vesical sphincters and urinary retention have been reported with opiates.
Respiratory Depression: Hydrocodone bitartrate may produce dose-related respiratory depression by acting directly on the brain stem respiratory center. (see OVERDOSAGE).
Special Senses: Very rare cases of hearing impairment or loss have been reported in patients predominantly receiving very high doses of hydrocodone/acetaminophen for long periods of time.
Dermatological: Skin rash, pruritus.
The following adverse drug events may be borne in mind as potential effects of acetaminophen: allergic reactions, rash, thrombocytopenia, agranulocytosis.
Potential effects of high dosage are listed in the OVERDOSAGE section.

DRUG ABUSE AND DEPENDENCE

Controlled Substance: VICODIN Tablets are classified as a Schedule Ⓒⅲ controlled substance.
Abuse and Dependence: Psychic dependence, physical dependence, and tolerance may develop upon repeated administration of narcotics; therefore, VICODIN Tablets should be prescribed and administered with caution. However, psychic dependence is unlikely to develop when VICODIN Tablets are used for a short time for the treatment of pain.
Physical dependence, the condition in which continued administration of the drug is required to prevent the appearance of a withdrawal syndrome, assumes clinically significant proportions only after several weeks of continued narcotic use, although some mild degree of physical dependence may develop after a few days of narcotic therapy. Tolerance, in which increasingly large doses are required in order to produce the same degree of analgesia, is manifested initially by a shortened duration of analgesic effect, and subsequently by decreases in the intensity of analgesia. The rate of development of tolerance varies among patients.

OVERDOSAGE

Following an acute overdosage, toxicity may result from hydrocodone or acetaminophen.
Signs and Symptoms:
Hydrocodone: Serious overdose with hydrocodone is characterized by respiratory depression (a decrease in respiratory rate and/or tidal volume, Cheyne-Stokes respiration, cyanosis), extreme somnolence progressing to stupor or coma, skeletal muscle flaccidity, cold and clammy skin, and sometimes bradycardia and hypotension. In severe overdosage, apnea, circulatory collapse, cardiac arrest and death may occur.
Acetaminophen: In acetaminophen overdosage: dose-dependent, potentially fatal hepatic necrosis is the most serious adverse effect. Renal tubular necrosis, hypoglycemic coma, and thrombocytopenia may also occur.
Early symptoms following a potentially hepatotoxic overdose may include: nausea, vomiting, diaphoresis and general malaise. Clinical and laboratory evidence of hepatic toxicity may not be apparent until 48 to 72 hours post-ingestion.
In adults, hepatic toxicity has rarely been reported with acute overdoses of less than 10 grams and fatalities with less than 15 grams.
Treatment: A single or multiple overdose with hydrocodone and acetaminophen is a potentially lethal polydrug overdose, and consultation with a regional poison control center is recommended.
Immediate treatment includes support of cardiorespiratory function and measures to reduce drug absorption. Vomiting should be induced mechanically, or with syrup of ipecac, if the patient is alert (adequate pharyngeal and laryngeal reflexes). Oral activated charcoal (1 g/kg) should follow gastric emptying. The first dose should be accompanied by an appropriate cathartic. If repeated doses are used, the cathartic might be included with alternate doses as required. Hypotension is usually hypovolemic and should respond to fluids. Vasopressors and other supportive measures should be employed as indicated. A cuffed endo-tracheal tube should be inserted before gastric lavage of the unconscious patient and, when necessary, to provide assisted respiration.
Meticulous attention should be given to maintaining adequate pulmonary ventilation. In severe cases of intoxication, peritoneal dialysis, or preferably hemodialysis may be considered. If hypoprothrombinemia occurs due to acetaminophen overdose, vitamin K should be administered intravenously.
Naloxone, a narcotic antagonist, can reverse respiratory depression and coma associated with opioid overdose. Naloxone hydrochloride 0.4 mg to 2 mg is given parenterally. Since the duration of action of hydrocodone may exceed that of the naloxone, the patient should be kept under continuous surveillance and repeated doses of the antagonist should be administered as needed to maintain adequate respiration. A narcotic antagonist should not be administered in the absence of clinically significant respiratory or cardiovascular depression.
If the dose of acetaminophen may have exceeded 140 mg/kg, acetylcysteine should be administered as early as possible. Serum acetaminophen levels should be obtained, since levels four or more hours following ingestion help predict acetaminophen toxicity. Do not await acetaminophen assay results before initiating treatment. Hepatic enzymes should be obtained initially, and repeated at 24-hour intervals.
Methemoglobinemia over 30% should be treated with methylene blue by slow intravenous administration.
The toxic dose for adults for acetaminophen is 10 g.

DOSAGE AND ADMINISTRATION

Dosage should be adjusted according to the severity of the pain and the response of the patient. However, it should be kept in mind that tolerance to hydrocodone can develop with continued use and that the incidence of untoward effects is dose related.
The usual adult dosage is one or two tablets every four to six hours as needed for pain. The total daily dosage should not exceed 8 tablets.

HOW SUPPLIED

VICODIN® is supplied as white, capsule-shaped tablets containing 5 mg hydrocodone bitartrate and 500 mg acetaminophen, bisected on one side and debossed with "VICODIN" on the other.
Bottles of 100—NDC 0074-1949-14.
Bottles of 500—NDC 0074-1949-54.
Hospital Unit Dose Package-100 tablets
(4×25 tablets)—NDC 0074-1949-12.
Storage: Store at 25°C (77°F); excursions permitted to 15°–30°C (59°–86°F). [See USP Controlled Room Temperature].
Dispense in a tight, light-resistant container as defined in the USP.
A Schedule Ⓒⅲ controlled drug substance.

Ref. 03-5216
Revised: June, 2002
ABBOTT LABORATORIES
NORTH CHICAGO, IL 60064, U.S.A.
PRINTED IN U.S.A.
Shown in Product Identification Guide, page 303

VICODIN ES® TABLETS Ⓒⅲ ℞

(hydrocodone bitartrate and acetaminophen tablets, USP)
7.5 mg/750 mg
℞ only

DESCRIPTION

Hydrocodone bitartrate and acetaminophen is supplied in tablet form for oral administration.
Hydrocodone bitartrate is an opioid analgesic and antitussive and occurs as fine, white crystals or as a crystalline powder. It is affected by light. The chemical name is: 4,5α-epoxy-3-methoxy-17-methylmorphinan-6-one tartrate (1:1) hydrate (2:5). It has the following structural formula:

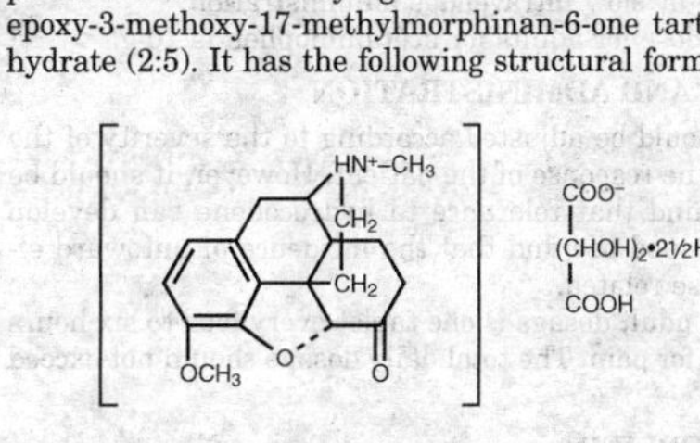

$C_{18}H_{21}NO_3 \cdot C_4H_6O_6 \cdot 2\frac{1}{2}H_2O$ M.W.=494.50

Acetaminophen, 4'-hydroxyacetanilide, a slightly bitter, white, odorless, crystalline powder, is a non-opiate, non-salicylate analgesic and antipyretic. It has the following structural formula:

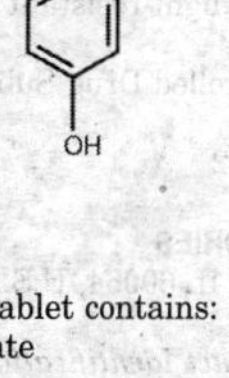

$C_8H_9NO_2$ M.W.151.16

Each VICODIN ES Tablet contains:

Hydrocodone Bitartrate	7.5 mg
Acetaminophen	750 mg

In addition each tablet contains the following inactive ingredients: Colloidal silicon dioxide, pregelatinized starch, magnesium stearate, croscarmellose sodium povidone, and stearic acid.
Meets USP Dissolution Test 2.

CLINICAL PHARMACOLOGY

Hydrocodone is a semisynthetic narcotic analgesic and antitussive with multiple actions qualitatively similar to those of codeine. Most of these involve the central nervous system and smooth muscle. The precise mechanism of action of hydrocodone and other opiates is not known, although it is believed to relate to the existence of opiate receptors in the central nervous system. In addition to analgesia, narcotics may produce drowsiness, changes in mood and mental clouding.
The analgesic action of acetaminophen involves peripheral influences, but the specific mechanism is as yet undetermined. Antipyretic activity is mediated through hypothalmic heat regulating centers. Acetaminophen inhibits prostaglandin synthetase. Therapeutic doses of acetaminophen have negligible effects on the cardiovascular or respiratory systems; however, toxic doses may cause circulatory failure and rapid, shallow breathing.
Pharmacokinetics: The behavior of the individual components is described below.
Hydrocodone: Following a 10mg oral dose of hydrocodone administered to five adult male subjects, the mean peak concentration was 23.6 ± 5.2ng/mL. Maximum serum levels were achieved at 1.3 ± 0.3 hours and the half-life was determined to be 3.8 ± 0.3 hours. Hydrocodone exhibits a complex pattern of metabolism including O-demethylation, N-demethylation and 6-keto reduction to the corresponding 6-α- and 6-β- hydroxy- metabolites. See OVERDOSAGE for toxicity information.
Acetaminophen: Acetaminophen is rapidly absorbed from the gastrointestinal tract and is distributed throughout most body tissues. The plasma half-life is 1.25 to 3 hours, but may be increased by liver damage and following overdosage. Elimination of acetaminophen is principally by liver metabolism (conjugation) and subsequent renal excretion of metabolites. Approximately 85% of an oral dose appears in the urine within 24 hours of administration, most as the glucuronide conjugate, with small amounts of other conjugates and unchanged drug. See OVERDOSAGE for toxicity information.

INDICATIONS AND USAGE

VICODIN ES Tablets are indicated for the relief of moderate to moderately severe pain.

CONTRAINDICATIONS

This product should not be administered to patients who have previously exhibited hypersensitivity to hydrocodone or acetaminophen.
Patients known to be hypersensitive to other opioids may exhibit cross-sensitivity to hydrocodone.

WARNINGS

Respiratory Depression: At high doses or in sensitive patients, hydrocodone may produce dose-related respiratory depression by acting directly on the brain stem respiratory center. Hydrocodone also affects the center that controls respiratory rhythm, and may produce irregular and periodic breathing.
Head Injury and Increased Intracranial Pressure: The respiratory depressant effects of narcotics and their capacity to elevate cerebrospinal fluid pressure may be markedly exaggerated in the presence of head injury, other intracranial lesions or a preexisting increase in intracranial pressure. Furthermore, narcotics produce adverse reactions which may obscure the clinical course of patients with head injuries.
Acute Abdominal Conditions: The administration of narcotics may obscure the diagnosis or clinical course of patients with acute abdominal conditions.

PRECAUTIONS

General:
Special Risk Patients: As with any narcotic analgesic agent, VICODIN ES Tablets should be used with caution in elderly or debilitated patients and those with severe impairment of hepatic or renal function, hypothyroidism, Addison's disease, prostatic hypertrophy or urethral stricture. The usual precautions should be observed and the possibility of respiratory depression should be kept in mind.
Cough Reflex: Hydrocodone suppresses the cough reflex; as with all narcotics, caution should be exercised when VICODIN ES Tablets are used postoperatively and in patients with pulmonary disease.
Information for Patients: Hydrocodone, like all narcotics, may impair the mental and/or physical abilities required for the performance of potentially hazardous tasks such as driving a car or operating machinery; patients should be cautioned accordingly.
Alcohol and other CNS depressants may produce an additive CNS depression, when taken with this combination product, and should be avoided.
Hydrocodone may be habit forming. Patients should take the drug only for as long as it is prescribed, in the amounts prescribed, and no more frequently than prescribed.
Laboratory Tests: In patients with severe hepatic or renal disease, effects of therapy should be monitored with serial liver and/or renal function tests.
Drug Interactions: Patients receiving other narcotic analgesics, antihistamines, antipsychotics, antianxiety agents, or other CNS depressants (including alcohol) concomitantly with VICODIN ES Tablets may exhibit an additive CNS depression. When combined therapy is contemplated, the dose of one or both agents should be reduced.
The use of MAO inhibitors or tricyclic antidepressants with hydrocodone preparations may increase the effect of either the antidepressant or hydrocodone.
Drug/Laboratory Test Interactions: Acetaminophen may produce false-positive test results for urinary 5-hydroxyindoleacetic acid.

Continued on next page

Vicodin ES—Cont.

Carcinogenesis, Mutagenesis, Impairment of Fertility: No adequate studies have been conducted in animals to determine whether hydrocodone or acetaminophen have a potential for carcinogenesis, mutagenesis, or impairment of fertility.

Pregnancy:

Teratogenic Effects: Pregnancy Category C. There are no adequate and well-controlled studies in pregnant women. VICODIN ES Tablets should be used during pregnancy only if the potential benefit justifies the potential risk to the fetus.

Nonteratogenic Effects: Babies born to mothers who have been taking opioids regularly prior to delivery will be physically dependent. The withdrawal signs include irritability and excessive crying, tremors, hyperactive reflexes, increased respiratory rate, increased stools, sneezing, yawning, vomiting, and fever. The intensity of the syndrome does not always correlate with the duration of maternal opioid use or dose. There is no consensus on the best method of managing withdrawal.

Labor and Delivery: As with all narcotics, administration of VICODIN ES Tablets to the mother shortly before delivery may result in some degree of respiratory depression in the newborn, especially if higher doses are used.

Nursing Mothers: Acetaminophen is excreted in breast milk in small amounts, but the significance of its effects on nursing infants is not known. It is not known whether hydrocodone is excreted in human milk. Because many drugs are excreted in human milk and because of the potential for serious adverse reactions in nursing infants from hydrocodone and acetaminophen, a decision should be made whether to discontinue nursing or to discontinue the drug, taking into account the importance of the drug to the mother.

Pediatric Use: Safety and effectiveness in the pediatric population have not been established.

Geriatric Use: Clinical studies of VICODIN ES® (hydrocodone bitartrate 7.5 mg and acetaminophen 750 mg) did not include sufficient numbers of subjects aged 65 and over to determine whether they respond differently from younger subjects. Other reported clinical experience has not identified differences in responses between the elderly and younger patients. In general, dose selection for an elderly patient should be cautious, usually starting at the low end of the dosing range, reflecting the greater frequency of decreased hepatic, renal, or cardiac function, and of concomitant disease or other drug therapy.

ADVERSE REACTIONS

The most frequently reported adverse reactions include: lightheadedness, dizziness, sedation, nausea and vomiting. These effects seem to be more prominent in ambulatory than in nonambulatory patients and some of these adverse reactions may be alleviated if the patient lies down.

Other adverse reactions include:

Central Nervous System: Drowsiness, mental clouding, lethargy, impairment of mental and physical performance, anxiety, fear, dysphoria, psychic dependence, mood changes.

Gastrointestinal System: Prolonged administration of VICODIN ES Tablets may produce constipation.

Genitourinary System: Ureteral spasm, spasm of vesical sphincters and urinary retention have been reported with opiates.

Respiratory Depression: Hydrocodone bitartrate may produce dose-related respiratory depression by acting directly on the brain stem respiratory center. (see OVERDOSAGE).

Special Senses: Very rare cases of hearing impairment or loss have been reported in patients predominantly receiving very high doses of hydrocodone/acetaminophen for long periods of time.

Dermatological: Skin rash, pruritus.

The following adverse drug events may be borne in mind as potential effects of acetaminophen: allergic reactions, rash, thrombocytopenia, agranulocytosis.

Potential effects of high dosage are listed in the OVERDOSAGE section.

DRUG ABUSE AND DEPENDENCE

Controlled Substance: VICODIN ES Tablets are classified as a Schedule ⓒIII controlled substance.

Abuse and Dependence: Psychic dependence, physical dependence, and tolerance may develop upon repeated administration of narcotics; therefore, VICODIN ES Tablets should be prescribed and administered with caution. However, psychic dependence is unlikely to develop when VICODIN ES Tablets are used for a short time for the treatment of pain.

Physical dependence, the condition in which continued administration of the drug is required to prevent the appearance of a withdrawal syndrome, assumes clinically significant proportions only after several weeks of continued narcotic use, although some mild degree of physical dependence may develop after a few days of narcotic therapy. Tolerance, in which increasingly large doses are required in order to produce the same degree of analgesia, is manifested initially by a shortened duration of analgesic effect, and subsequently by decreases in the intensity of analgesia. The rate of development of tolerance varies among patients.

OVERDOSAGE

Following an acute overdosage, toxicity may result from hydrocodone or acetaminophen.

Signs and Symptoms:

Hydrocodone: Serious overdose with hydrocodone is characterized by respiratory depression (a decrease in respiratory rate and/or tidal volume, Cheyne-Stokes respiration, cyanosis), extreme somnolence progressing to stupor or coma, skeletal muscle flaccidity, cold and clammy skin, and sometimes bradycardia and hypotension. In severe overdosage, apnea, circulatory collapse, cardiac arrest and death may occur.

Acetaminophen: In acetaminophen overdosage: dose-dependent, potentially fatal hepatic necrosis is the most serious adverse effect. Renal tubular necrosis, hypoglycemic coma, and thrombocytopenia may also occur.

Early symptoms following a potentially hepatotoxic overdose may include: nausea, vomiting, diaphoresis and general malaise. Clinical and laboratory evidence of hepatic toxicity may not be apparent until 48 to 72 hours post-ingestion.

In adults, hepatic toxicity has rarely been reported with acute overdoses of less than 10 grams and fatalities with less than 15 grams.

Treatment: A single or multiple overdose with hydrocodone and acetaminophen is a potentially lethal polydrug overdose, and consultation with a regional poison control center is recommended.

Immediate treatment includes support of cardiorespiratory function and measures to reduce drug absorption. Vomiting should be induced mechanically, or with syrup of ipecac, if the patient is alert (adequate pharyngeal and laryngeal reflexes). Oral activated charcoal (1 g/kg) should follow gastric emptying. The first dose should be accompanied by an appropriate cathartic. If repeated doses are used, the cathartic might be included with alternate doses as required. Hypotension is usually hypovolemic and should respond to fluids. Vasopressors and other supportive measures should be employed as indicated. A cuffed endo-tracheal tube should be inserted before gastric lavage of the unconscious patient and, when necessary, to provide assisted respiration.

Meticulous attention should be given to maintaining adequate pulmonary ventilation. In severe cases of intoxication, peritoneal dialysis, or preferably hemodialysis may be considered. If hypoprothrombinemia occurs due to acetaminophen overdose, vitamin K should be administered intravenously.

Naloxone, a narcotic antagonist, can reverse respiratory depression and coma associated with opioid overdose. Naloxone hydrochloride 0.4 mg to 2 mg is given parenterally. Since the duration of action of hydrocodone may exceed that of the naloxone, the patient should be kept under continuous surveillance and repeated doses of the antagonist should be administered as needed to maintain adequate respiration. A narcotic antagonist should not be administered in the absence of clinically significant respiratory or cardiovascular depression.

If the dose of acetaminophen may have exceeded 140 mg/kg, acetylcysteine should be administered as early as possible. Serum acetaminophen levels should be obtained, since levels four or more hours following ingestion help predict acetaminophen toxicity. Do not await acetaminophen assay results before initiating treatment. Hepatic enzymes should be obtained initially, and repeated at 24-hour intervals.

Methemoglobinemia over 30% should be treated with methylene blue by slow intravenous administration.

The toxic dose for adults for acetaminophen is 10 g.

DOSAGE AND ADMINISTRATION

Dosage should be adjusted according to the severity of the pain and the response of the patient. However, it should be kept in mind that tolerance to hydrocodone can develop with continued use and that the incidence of untoward effects is dose related.

The usual adult dosage is one tablet every four to six hours as needed for pain. The total daily dosage should not exceed 5 tablets.

HOW SUPPLIED

White, oval-shaped, faceted edged tablet bisected on one side and imprinted with "VICODIN ES" on the other side.

Bottles of 100-NDC #0074-1973-14

Bottles of 500-NDC #0074-1973-54

Hospital Unit Dosage Package — 100 tablets (4×25 tablets) — NDC #0074-1973-12.

Storage: Store at 25°C (77°F); excursions permitted to 15°-30°C (59°-86°F). [See USP Controlled Room Temperature].

Dispense in a tight, light-resistant container as defined in the USP.

A Schedule ⓒIII Controlled Drug Substance.

Revised: March, 2002

Ref. 03-5191-R2

ABBOTT LABORATORIES

NORTH CHICAGO, IL 60064, U.S.A.

PRINTED IN U.S.A.

Shown in Product Identification Guide, page 304

VICODIN HP® ⓒIII ℞

[*vī'kō-dĭn*]

(hydrocodone bitartrate and acetaminophen tablets, USP)

10 mg/660 mg

Rx only

DESCRIPTION

Hydrocodone bitartrate and acetaminophen is supplied in tablet form for oral administration.

Hydrocodone bitartrate is an opioid analgesic and antitussive and occurs as fine, white crystals or as a crystalline powder. It is affected by light. The chemical name is 4,5α-epoxy-3-methoxy-17-methylmorphinan-6-one tartrate (1:1) hydrate (2:5). It has the following structural formula:

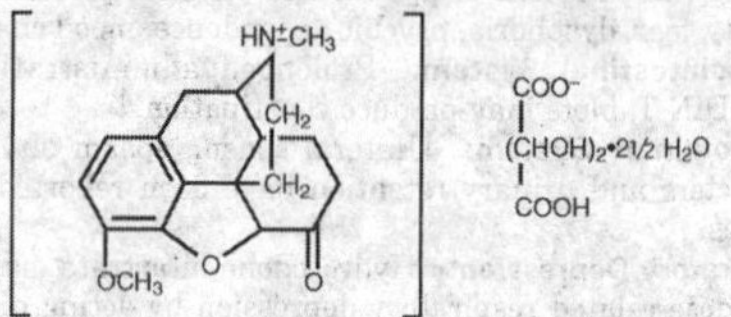

$C_{18}H_{21}NO_3 \cdot C_4H_6O_6 \cdot 2\frac{1}{2} H_2O$ M.W.= 494.50

Acetaminophen, 4'-hydroxyacetanilide, a slightly bitter, white, odorless, crystalline powder, is a non-opiate, non-salicylate analgesic and antipyretic. It has the following structural formula:

NHCOCH₃

OH

$C_8H_9NO_2$ M.W.= 151.17

Each VICODIN HP Tablet contains:

Hydrocodone Bitartrate	10 mg
Acetaminophen	660 mg

In addition each tablet contains the following inactive ingredients: colloidal silicon dioxide, croscarmellose sodium, magnesium stearate, microcrystalline cellulose, povidone, pregelatinized starch, and stearic acid.

Meets USP Dissolution Test 2.

CLINICAL PHARMACOLOGY

Hydrocodone is a semisynthetic narcotic analgesic and antitussive with multiple actions qualitatively similar to those of codeine. Most of these involve the central nervous system and smooth muscle. The precise mechanism of action of hydrocodone and other opiates is not known, although it is believed to relate to the existence of opiate receptors in the central nervous system. In addition to analgesia, narcotics may produce drowsiness, changes in mood and mental clouding.

The analgesic action of acetaminophen involves peripheral influences, but the specific mechanism is as yet undetermined. Antipyretic activity is mediated through hypothalamic heat regulating centers. Acetaminophen inhibits prostaglandin synthetase. Therapeutic doses of acetaminophen have negligible effects on the cardiovascular or respiratory systems; however, toxic doses may cause circulatory failure and rapid, shallow breathing.

Pharmacokinetics: The behavior of the individual components is described below.

Hydrocodone: Following a 10 mg oral dose of hydrocodone administered to five adult male subjects, the mean peak concentration was 23.6 ± 5.2ng/mL. Maximum serum levels were achieved at 1.3 ± 0.3 hours and the half-life was determined to be 3.8 ± 0.3 hours. Hydrocodone exhibits a complex pattern of metabolism including O-demethylation, N-demethylation and 6-keto reduction to the corresponding 6-α- and 6-β- hydroxy- metabolites. See OVERDOSAGE for toxicity information.

Acetaminophen: Acetaminophen is rapidly absorbed from the gastrointestinal tract and is distributed throughout most body tissues. The plasma half-life is 1.25 to 3 hours, but may be increased by liver damage and following overdosage. Elimination of acetaminophen is principally by liver metabolism (conjugation) and subsequent renal excretion of metabolites. Approximately 85% of an oral dose appears in the urine within 24 hours of administration, most as the glucuronide conjugate, with small amounts of other conjugates and unchanged drug. See OVERDOSAGE for toxicity information.

INDICATIONS AND USAGE

VICODIN HP Tablets are indicated for the relief of moderate to moderately severe pain.

CONTRAINDICATIONS

This product should not be administered to patients who have previously exhibited hypersensitivity to hydrocodone or acetaminophen.

Patients known to be hypersensitive to other opioids may exhibit cross-sensitivity to hydrocodone.

WARNINGS

Respiratory Depression: At high doses or in sensitive patients, hydrocodone may produce dose-related respiratory depression by acting directly on the brain stem respiratory center. Hydrocodone also affects the center that controls respiratory rhythm, and may produce irregular and periodic breathing.

Head Injury and Increased Intracranial Pressure: The respiratory depressant effects of narcotics and their capacity to elevate cerebrospinal fluid pressure may be markedly exaggerated in the presence of head injury, other intracranial lesions or a preexisting increase in intracranial pressure. Fur-

thermore, narcotics produce adverse reactions which may obscure the clinical course of patients with head injuries.
Acute Abdominal Conditions: The administration of narcotics may obscure the diagnosis or clinical course of patients with acute abdominal conditions.

PRECAUTIONS

General:
Special Risk Patients: As with any narcotic analgesic agent, VICODIN HP Tablets should be used with caution in elderly or debilitated patients, and those with severe impairment of hepatic or renal function, hypothyroidism, Addison's disease, prostatic hypertrophy or urethral stricture. The usual precautions should be observed and the possibility of respiratory depression should be kept in mind.
Cough Reflex: Hydrocodone suppresses the cough reflex; as with all narcotics, caution should be exercised when VICODIN HP Tablets are used postoperatively and in patients with pulmonary disease.
Information for Patients: Hydrocodone, like all narcotics, may impair the mental and/or physical abilities required for the performance of potentially hazardous tasks such as driving a car or operating machinery; patients should be cautioned accordingly.
Alcohol and other CNS depressants may produce an additive CNS depression, when taken with this combination product, and should be avoided.
Hydrocodone may be habit forming. Patients should take the drug only for as long as it is prescribed, in the amounts prescribed, and no more frequently than prescribed.
Laboratory Tests: In patients with severe hepatic or renal disease, effects of therapy should be monitored with serial liver and/or renal function tests.
Drug Interactions: Patients receiving narcotics, antihistamines, antipsychotics, antianxiety agents, or other CNS depressants (including alcohol) concomitantly with VICODIN HP Tablets may exhibit an additive CNS depression. When combined therapy is contemplated, the dose of one or both agents should be reduced.
The use of MAO inhibitors or tricyclic antidepressants with hydrocodone preparations may increase the effect of either the antidepressant or hydrocodone.
Drug/Laboratory Test Interactions: Acetaminophen may produce false-positive test results for urinary 5-hydroxyindoleacetic acid.
Carcinogenesis, Mutagenesis, Impairment of Fertility: No adequate studies have been conducted in animals to determine whether hydrocodone or acetaminophen have a potential for carcinogenesis, mutagenesis, or impairment of fertility.
Pregnancy:
Teratogenic Effects: Pregnancy Category C. There are no adequate and well-controlled studies in pregnant women. VICODIN HP Tablets should be used during pregnancy only if the potential benefit justifies the potential risk to the fetus.
Nonteratogenic Effects: Babies born to mothers who have been taking opioids regularly prior to delivery will be physically dependent. The withdrawal signs include irritability and excessive crying, tremors, hyperactive reflexes, increased respiratory rate, increased stools, sneezing, yawning, vomiting, and fever. The intensity of the syndrome does not always correlate with the duration of maternal opioid use or dose. There is no consensus on the best method of managing withdrawal.
Labor and Delivery: As with all narcotics, administration of VICODIN HP Tablets to the mother shortly before delivery may result in some degree of respiratory depression in the newborn, especially if higher doses are used.
Nursing Mothers: Acetaminophen is excreted in breast milk in small amounts, but the significance of its effects on nursing infants is not known. It is not known whether hydrocodone is excreted in human milk.
Because many drugs are excreted in human milk and because of the potential for serious adverse reactions in nursing infants from hydrocodone and acetaminophen, a decision should be made whether to discontinue nursing or to discontinue the drug, taking into account the importance of the drug to the mother.
Pediatric Use: Safety and effectiveness in the pediatric population have not been established.
Geriatric Use: Clinical studies of VICODIN HP® (hydrocodone bitartrate and acetaminophen 10 mg/660 mg) did not include sufficient numbers of subjects aged 65 and over to determine whether they respond differently from younger subjects. Other reported clinical experience has not identified differences in responses between the elderly and younger patients. In general, dose selection for an elderly patient should be cautious, usually starting at the low end of the dosing range, reflecting the greater frequency of decreased hepatic, renal, or cardiac function, and of concomitant disease or other drug therapy.

ADVERSE REACTIONS

The most frequently reported adverse reactions are lightheadedness, dizziness, sedation, nausea and vomiting. These effects seem to be more prominent in ambulatory than in nonambulatory patients, and some of these adverse reactions may be alleviated if the patient lies down.
Other adverse reactions include:
Central Nervous System: Drowsiness, mental clouding, lethargy, impairment of mental and physical performance, anxiety, fear, dysphoria, psychic dependence, mood changes.
Gastrointestinal System: Prolonged administration of VICODIN HP Tablets may produce constipation.
Genitourinary System: Ureteral spasm, spasm of vesical sphincters and urinary retention have been reported with opiates.
Respiratory Depression: Hydrocodone bitartrate may produce dose-related respiratory depression by acting directly on the brain stem respiratory centers (see OVERDOSAGE).
Special Senses: Very rare cases of hearing impairment or loss have been reported in patients predominantly receiving very high doses of hydrocodone/acetaminophen for long periods of time.
Dermatological: Skin rash, pruritus.
The following adverse drug events may be borne in mind as potential effects of acetaminophen: allergic reactions, rash, thrombocytopenia, agranulocytosis.
Potential effects of high dosage are listed in the OVERDOSAGE section.

DRUG ABUSE AND DEPENDENCE

Controlled Substance: VICODIN HP Tablets are classified as a Schedule Ⓒⅲ controlled substance.
Abuse and Dependence: Psychic dependence, physical dependence, and tolerance may develop upon repeated administration of narcotics; therefore, VICODIN HP Tablets should be prescribed and administered with caution. However, psychic dependence is unlikely to develop when VICODIN HP Tablets are used for a short time for the treatment of pain.
Physical dependence, the condition in which continued administration of the drug is required to prevent the appearance of a withdrawal syndrome, assumes clinically significant proportions only after several weeks of continued narcotic use, although some mild degree of physical dependence may develop after a few days of narcotic therapy. Tolerance, in which increasingly large doses are required in order to produce the same degree of analgesia, is manifested initially by a shortened duration of analgesic effect, and subsequently by decreases in the intensity of analgesia. The rate of development of tolerance varies among patients.

OVERDOSAGE

Following an acute overdosage, toxicity may result from hydrocodone or acetaminophen.
Signs and Symptoms:
Hydrocodone: Serious overdose with hydrocodone is characterized by respiratory depression (a decrease in respiratory rate and/or tidal volume, Cheyne-Stokes respiration, cyanosis), extreme somnolence progressing to stupor or coma, skeletal muscle flaccidity, cold and clammy skin, and sometimes bradycardia and hypotension. In severe overdosage, apnea, circulatory collapse, cardiac arrest and death may occur.
Acetaminophen: In acetaminophen overdosage: dose-dependent, potentially fatal hepatic necrosis is the most serious adverse effect. Renal tubular necrosis, hypoglycemic coma, and thrombocytopenia may also occur.
Early symptoms following a potentially hepatotoxic overdose may include: nausea, vomiting, diaphoresis and general malaise. Clinical and laboratory evidence of hepatic toxicity may not be apparent until 48 to 72 hours post-ingestion.
In adults, hepatic toxicity has rarely been reported with acute overdoses of less than 10 grams, or fatalities with less than 15 grams.
Treatment: A single or multiple overdose with hydrocodone and acetaminophen is a potentially lethal polydrug overdose, and consultation with a regional poison control center is recommended.
Immediate treatment includes support of cardiorespiratory function and measures to reduce drug absorption. Vomiting should be induced mechanically, or with syrup of ipecac, if the patient is alert (adequate pharyngeal and laryngeal reflexes). Oral activated charcoal (1 g/kg) should follow gastric emptying. The first dose should be accompanied by an appropriate cathartic. If repeated doses are used, the cathartic might be included with alternate doses as required. Hypotension is usually hypovolemic and should respond to fluids. Vasopressors and other supportive measures should be employed as indicated. A cuffed endo-tracheal tube should be inserted before gastric lavage of the unconscious patient and, when necessary, to provide assisted respiration.
Meticulous attention should be given to maintaining adequate pulmonary ventilation. In severe cases of intoxication, peritoneal dialysis, or preferably hemodialysis may be considered. If hypoprothrombinemia occurs due to acetaminophen overdose, vitamin K should be administered intravenously.
Naloxone, a narcotic antagonist, can reverse respiratory depression and coma associated with opioid overdose. Naloxone hydrochloride 0.4 mg to 2 mg is given parenterally. Since the duration of action of hydrocodone may exceed that of the naloxone, the patient should be kept under continuous surveillance and repeated doses of the antagonist should be administered as needed to maintain adequate respiration. A narcotic antagonist should not be administered in the absence of clinically significant respiratory or cardiovascular depression.
If the dose of acetaminophen may have exceeded 140 mg/kg, acetylcysteine should be administered as early as possible. Serum acetaminophen levels should be obtained, since levels four or more hours following ingestion help predict acetaminophen toxicity. Do not await acetaminophen assay results before initiating treatment. Hepatic enzymes should be obtained initially, and repeated at 24-hour intervals.
Methemoglobinemia over 30% should be treated with methylene blue by slow intravenous administration.
The toxic dose for adults for acetaminophen is 10 g.

DOSAGE AND ADMINISTRATION

Dosage should be adjusted according to severity of pain and the response of the patient. However, it should be kept in mind that tolerance to hydrocodone can develop with continued use and that the incidence of untoward effects is dose related.
The usual adult dosage is one tablet every four to six hours as needed for pain. The total daily dosage should not exceed 6 tablets.

HOW SUPPLIED

VICODIN HP® (hydrocodone bitartrate and acetaminophen, 10 mg/660 mg) is supplied as a white, oval-shaped, tablet bisected on one side and debossed with "VICODIN HP" on the other side.
Bottles of 100-NDC #0074-2274-14
Bottles of 500-NDC #0074-2274-54
Storage: Store at 25°C (77°F); excursions permitted to 15°-30°C (59°-86°F). [see USP Controlled Room Temperature].
Dispense in a tight, light-resistant container as defined in the USP.
A Schedule Ⓒⅲ Controlled Drug Substance.
©Abbott
Ref. 03-5164
Revised: November, 2001
Abbott Laboratories
North Chicago, IL 60064, U.S.A.
Shown in Product Identification Guide, page 304

VICOPROFEN® Ⓒⅲ ℞

(hydrocodone bitartrate and ibuprofen tablets)
7.5 mg/200 mg
℞ only

DESCRIPTION

Each VICOPROFEN® tablet contains:

Hydrocodone Bitartrate, USP	7.5 mg
Ibuprofen, USP	200 mg

VICOPROFEN is supplied in a fixed combination tablet form for oral administration. VICOPROFEN combines the opioid analgesic agent, hydrocodone bitartrate, with the nonsteroidal anti-inflammatory (NSAID) agent, ibuprofen.
Hydrocodone bitartrate is a semisynthetic and centrally acting opioid analgesic. Its chemical name is: 4,5 α-epoxy-3-methoxy-17-methylmorphinan-6-one tartrate (1:1) hydrate (2:5). Its chemical formula is:
$C_{18}H_{21}NO_3 \bullet C_4H_6O_6 \bullet 2\frac{1}{2}H_2O$, and the molecular weight is 494.50. Its structural formula is:

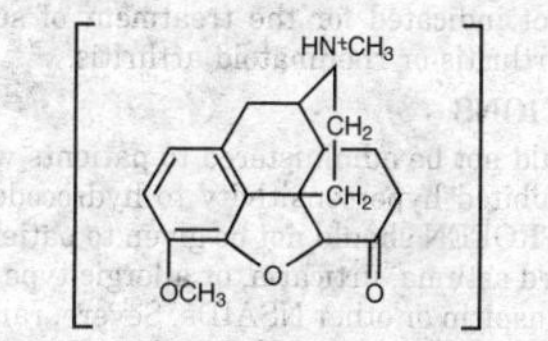

Ibuprofen is a nonsteroidal anti-inflammatory drug with analgesic and antipyretic properties. Its chemical name is: (±)-2-(*p*-isobutylphenyl) propionic acid. Its chemical formula is: $C_{13}H_{18}O_2$, and the molecular weight is 206.29. Its structural formula is:

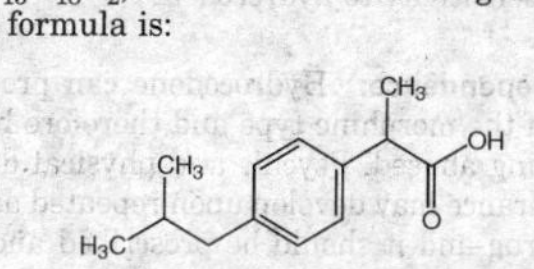

Inactive ingredients in VICOPROFEN tablets include: colloidal silicon dioxide, corn starch, croscarmellose sodium, hypromellose, magnesium stearate, microcrystalline cellulose, polyethylene glycol, polysorbate 80, and titanium dioxide.

CLINICAL PHARMACOLOGY

Hydrocodone component: Hydrocodone is a semisynthetic opioid analgesic and antitussive with multiple actions qualitatively similar to those of codeine. Most of these involve the central nervous system and smooth muscle. The precise mechanism of action of hydrocodone and other opioids is not known, although it is believed to relate to the existence of opiate receptors in the central nervous system. In addition to analgesia, opioids may produce drowsiness, changes in mood, and mental clouding.
Ibuprofen component: Ibuprofen is a non-steroidal anti-inflammatory agent that possesses analgesic and antipyretic activities. Its mode action, like that of other NSAIDs, is not completely understood, but may be related to inhibition of cyclooxygenase activity and prostaglandin synthesis. Ibuprofen is a peripherally acting analgesic. Ibuprofen does not have any known effects on opiate receptors.
Pharmacokinetics:
Absorption: After oral dosing with the VICOPROFEN tablet, a peak hydrocodone plasma level of 27 ng/mL is achieved at 1.7 hours, and a peak ibuprofen plasma level of

Continued on next page

Vicoprofen—Cont.

30 mcg/mL is achieved at 1.8 hours. The effect of food on the absorption of either component from the VICOPROFEN tablet has not been established.

Distribution: Ibuprofen is highly protein-bound (99%) like most other non-steroidal anti-inflammatory agents. Although the extent of protein binding of hydrocodone in human plasma has not been definitely determined, structural similarities to related opioid analgesics suggest that hydrocodone is not extensively protein bound. As most agents in the 5-ring morphinan group of semi-synthetic opioids bind plasma protein to a similar degree (range 19% [hydromorphone] to 45% [oxycodone]), hydrocodone is expected to fall within this range.

Metabolism: Hydrocodone exhibits a complex pattern of metabolism, including *O*-demethylation, *N*-demethylation, and 6-keto reduction to the corresponding 6-α-and 6-β-hydroxy metabolites. Hydromorphone, a potent opioid, is formed from the *O*-demethylation of hydrocodone and contributes to the total analgesic effect of hydrocodone. The *O*- and *N*-demethylation processes are mediated by separate P-450 isoenzymes: CYP2D6 and CYP3A4, respectively.

Ibuprofen is present in this product as a racemate, and following absorption it undergoes interconversion in the plasma from the R-isomer to the S-isomer. Both the R- and S- isomers are metabolized to two primary metabolites: (+)-2-4′-(2hydroxy-2-methyl-propyl) phenyl propionic acid and (+)-2-4′-(2carboxypropyl) phenyl propionic acid, both of which circulate in the plasma at low levels relative to the parent.

Elimination: Hydrocodone and its metabolites are eliminated primarily in the kidneys, with a mean plasma half-life of 4.5 hours. Ibuprofen is excreted in the urine, 50% to 60% as metabolites and approximately 15% as unchanged drug and conjugate. The plasma half-life is 2.2 hours.

Special Populations: No significant pharmacokinetic differences based on age or gender have been demonstrated. The pharmacokinetics of hydrocodone and ibuprofen from VICOPROFEN has not been evaluated in children.

Renal Impairment: The effect of renal insufficiency on the pharmacokinetics of the VICOPROFEN dosage form has not been determined.

CLINICAL STUDIES

In single-dose studies of post surgical pain (abdominal, gynecological, orthopedic), 940 patients were studied at doses of one or two tablets. VICOPROFEN produced greater efficacy than placebo and each of its individual components given at the same dose. No advantage was demonstrated for the two-tablet dose.

INDICATIONS AND USAGE

VICOPROFEN tablets are indicated for the short-term (generally less than 10 days) management of acute pain. VICOPROFEN is not indicated for the treatment of such conditions as osteoarthritis or rheumatoid arthritis.

CONTRAINDICATIONS

VICOPROFEN should not be administered to patients who previously have exhibited hypersensitivity to hydrocodone or ibuprofen. VICOPROFEN should not be given to patients who have experienced asthma, urticaria, or allergic-type reactions after taking aspirin or other NSAIDs. Severe, rarely fatal, anaphylactic-like reactions to NSAIDs have been reported in such patients (see WARNINGS - Anaphylactoid Reactions, and PRECAUTIONS - Pre-existing Asthma).

Patients known to be hypersensitive to other opioids may exhibit cross-sensitivity to hydrocodone.

WARNINGS

Abuse and Dependence: Hydrocodone can produce drug dependence of the morphine type and therefore has the potential for being abused. Psychic and physical dependence as well as tolerance may develop upon repeated administration of this drug and it should be prescribed and administered with the same degree of caution as other narcotic drugs (see DRUG ABUSE AND DEPENDENCE).

Respiratory Depression: At high doses or in opioid-sensitive patients, hydrocodone may produce dose-related respiratory depression by acting directly on the brain stem respiratory centers. Hydrocodone also affects the center that controls respiratory rhythm, and may produce irregular and periodic breathing.

Head Injury and Increased Intracranial Pressure: The respiratory depressant effects of opioids and their capacity to elevate cerebrospinal fluid pressure may be markedly exaggerated in the presence of head injury, intracranial lesions or a pre-existing increase in intracranial pressure. Furthermore, opioids produce adverse reactions which may obscure the clinical course of patients with head injuries.

Acute Abdominal Conditions: The administration of opioids may obscure the diagnosis or clinical course of patients with acute abdominal conditions.

Gastrointestinal (GI) Effects - Risk of GI Ulceration, Bleeding and Perforation: Serious gastrointestinal toxicity, such as inflammation, bleeding, ulceration, and perforation of the stomach, small intestine or large intestine, can occur at any time, with or without warning symptoms, in patients treated with nonsteroidal anti-inflammatory drugs (NSAIDs). Minor upper GI problems, such as dyspepsia, are common and may also occur at any time during NSAID therapy. Therefore, physicians and patients should remain alert for ulceration and bleeding even in the absence of previous GI tract symptoms. Patients should be informed about the signs and/or symptoms of serious GI toxicity and what steps to take if they occur. The utility of periodic laboratory monitoring has not been demonstrated, nor has it been adequately assessed. Only one in five patients, who develop a serious upper GI adverse event of NSAID therapy, is symptomatic. Even short term therapy is not without risk. NSAIDs should be prescribed with extreme caution in those with a prior history of ulcer disease or gastrointestinal bleeding. Most spontaneous reports of fatal GI events are in elderly or debilitated patients and therefore special care should be taken in treating this population. To minimize the potential risk for an adverse GI event, the lowest effective dose should be used for the shortest possible duration. For high risk patients, alternate therapies that do not involve NSAIDs should be considered.

Studies have shown that patients with a prior history of peptic ulcer disease and/or gastrointestinal bleeding and who use NSAIDs, have a greater than 10-fold risk for developing a GI bleed than patients with neither of these risk factors. In addition to a past history of ulcer disease, pharmaco-epidemiological studies have identified several other co-therapies or co-morbid conditions that may increase the risk for GI bleeding such as: treatment with oral corticosteroids, treatment with anticoagulants, longer duration of NSAID therapy, smoking, alcoholism, older age, and poor general health status.

Anaphylactoid Reactions: Anaphylactoid reactions may occur in patients without known prior exposure to VICOPROFEN. VICOPROFEN should not be given to patients with the aspirin triad. The triad typically occurs in asthmatic patients who experience rhinitis with or without nasal polyps, or who exhibit severe, potentially fatal bronchospasm after taking aspirin or other NSAIDs. Fatal reactions to NSAIDs have been reported in such patients (see CONTRAINDICATIONS and PRECAUTIONS - Pre-existing Asthma). Emergency help should be sought when anaphylactoid reaction occurs.

Advanced Renal Disease: In cases with advanced kidney disease, treatment with VICOPROFEN is not recommended. If NSAID therapy, however, must be initiated, close monitoring of the patient's kidney function is advisable (see PRECAUTIONS - Renal Effects).

Pregnancy: As with other NSAID-containing products, VICOPROFEN should be avoided in late pregnancy because it may cause premature closure of the ductus arteriosus.

PRECAUTIONS

General Precautions

Special Risk Patients: As with any opioid analgesic agent, VICOPROFEN tablets should be used with caution in elderly or debilitated patients, and those with severe impairment of hepatic or renal function, hypothyroidism, Addison's disease, prostatic hypertrophy or urethral stricture. The usual precautions should be observed and the possibility of respiratory depression should be kept in mind.

Cough Reflex: Hydrocodone suppresses the cough reflex; as with opioids, caution should be exercised when VICOPROFEN is used postoperatively and in patients with pulmonary disease.

Effect on Diagnostic Signs: The antipyretic and anti-inflammatory activity of ibuprofen may reduce fever and inflammation, thus diminishing their utility as diagnostic signs in detecting complications of presumed noninfectious, noninflammatory painful conditions.

Hepatic Effects: As with other NSAIDs, ibuprofen has been reported to cause borderline elevations of one or more liver enzymes; this may occur in up to 15% of patients. These abnormalities may progress, may remain essentially unchanged, or may be transient with continued therapy. Notable (3 times the upper limit of normal) elevations of SGPT (ALT) or SGOT (AST) occurred in controlled clinical trials in less than 1% of patients. A patient with symptoms and/or signs suggesting liver dysfunction, or in whom an abnormal liver test has occurred, should be evaluated for evidence of the development of more severe hepatic reactions while on therapy with VICOPROFEN. Severe hepatic reactions, including jaundice and cases of fatal hepatitis, have been reported with ibuprofen as with other NSAIDs. Although such reactions are rare, if abnormal liver tests persist or worsen, if clinical signs and symptoms consistent with liver disease develop, or if systemic manifestations occur (e.g. eosinophilia, rash, etc.), VICOPROFEN should be discontinued.

Renal Effects: Caution should be used when initiating treatment with VICOPROFEN in patients with considerable dehydration. It is advisable to rehydrate patients first and then start therapy with VICOPROFEN. Caution is also recommended in patients with pre-existing kidney disease (see WARNINGS - Advanced Renal Disease).

As with other NSAIDs, long-term administration of ibuprofen has resulted in renal papillary necrosis and other renal pathologic changes. Renal toxicity has also been seen in patients in which renal prostaglandins have a compensatory role in the maintenance of renal perfusion. In these patients, administration of a nonsteroidal anti-inflammatory drug may cause a dose-dependent reduction in prostaglandin formation and, secondarily, in renal blood flow, which may precipitate overt renal decompensation. Patients at greatest risk of this reaction are those with impaired renal function, heart failure, liver dysfunction, those taking diuretics and ACE inhibitors, and the elderly. Discontinuation of nonsteroidal anti-inflammatory drug therapy is usually followed by recovery to the pretreatment state.

Ibuprofen metabolites are eliminated primarily by the kidneys. The extent to which the metabolites may accumulate in patients with renal failure has not been studied. Patients with significantly impaired renal function should be more closely monitored.

Hematological Effects: Ibuprofen, like other NSAIDs, can inhibit platelet aggregation but the effect is quantitatively less and of shorter duration than that seen with aspirin. Ibuprofen has been shown to prolong bleeding time in normal subjects. Because this prolonged bleeding effect may be exaggerated in patients with underlying hemostatic defects, VICOPROFEN should be used with caution in persons with intrinsic coagulation defects and those on anticoagulant therapy.

Anemia is sometimes seen in patients receiving NSAIDs, including ibuprofen. This may be due to fluid retention, GI loss, or an incompletely described effect upon erythropoiesis.

Fluid Retention and Edema: Fluid retention and edema have been reported in association with ibuprofen; therefore, the drug should be used with caution in patients with a history of cardiac decompensation, hypertension or heart failure.

Pre-existing Asthma: Patients with asthma may have aspirin-sensitive asthma. The use of aspirin in patients with aspirin-sensitive asthma has been associated with severe bronchospasm, which may be fatal. Since cross-reactivity between aspirin and other NSAIDs has been reported in such aspirin-sensitive patients, VICOPROFEN should not be administered to patients with this form of aspirin sensitivity and should be used with caution in patients with pre-existing asthma.

Aseptic Meningitis: Aseptic meningitis with fever and coma has been observed on rare occasions in patients on ibuprofen therapy. Although it is probably more likely to occur in patients with systemic lupus erythematosus and related connective tissue diseases, it has been reported in patients who do not have an underlying chronic disease. If signs or symptoms of meningitis develop in a patient on VICOPROFEN, the possibility of its being related to ibuprofen should be considered.

Information for Patients

VICOPROFEN® (hydrocodone bitartrate 7.5 mg and ibuprofen 200 mg), like other opioid-containing analgesics, may impair mental and/or physical abilities required for the performance of potentially hazardous tasks such as driving a car or operating machinery; patients should be cautioned accordingly.

Alcohol and other CNS depressants may produce an additive CNS depression, when taken with this combination product, and should be avoided.

VICOPROFEN may be habit-forming. Patients should take the drug only for as long as it is prescribed, in the amounts prescribed, and no more frequently than prescribed.

VICOPROFEN, like other drugs containing ibuprofen, is not free of side effects. The side effects of these drugs can cause discomfort and, rarely, there are more serious side effects, such as gastrointestinal bleeding, which may result in hospitalization and even fatal outcomes. Patients should be instructed to report any signs and symptoms of gastrointestinal bleeding, blurred vision or other eye symptoms, skin rash, weight gain, or edema.

Laboratory Tests

A decrease in hemoglobin may occur during VICOPROFEN therapy, and elevations of liver enzymes may be seen in a small percentage of patients during VICOPROFEN therapy (see PRECAUTIONS - Hematological Effects and PRECAUTIONS - Hepatic Effects).

In patients with severe hepatic or renal disease, effects of therapy should be monitored with liver and/or renal function tests.

Drug Interactions

ACE-inhibitors: Reports suggest that NSAIDs may diminish the antihypertensive effect of ACE-inhibitors. This interaction should be given consideration in patients taking VICOPROFEN concomitantly with ACE-inhibitors.

Anticholinergics: The concurrent use of anticholinergics with hydrocodone preparations may produce paralytic ileus.

Antidepressants: The use of MAO inhibitors or tricyclic antidepressants with VICOPROFEN may increase the effect of either the antidepressant or hydrocodone.

Aspirin: As with other products containing NSAIDs, concomitant administration of VICOPROFEN and aspirin is not generally recommended because of the potential of increased adverse effects.

CNS Depressants: Patients receiving other opioids, antihistamines, antipsychotics, antianxiety agents, or other CNS depressants (including alcohol) concomitantly with VICOPROFEN may exhibit an additive CNS depression. When combined therapy is contemplated, the dose of one or both agents should be reduced.

Furosemide: Ibuprofen has been shown to reduce the natriuretic effect of furosemide and thiazides in some patients. This response has been attributed to inhibition of renal prostaglandin synthesis. During concomitant therapy with VICOPROFEN the patient should be observed closely for signs of renal failure (see PRECAUTIONS - Renal Effects), as well as diuretic efficacy.

Lithium: Ibuprofen has been shown to elevate plasma lithium concentration and reduce renal lithium clearance. This effect has been attributed to inhibition of renal prostaglandin synthesis by ibuprofen. Thus, when VICOPROFEN and lithium are administered concurrently, patients should be observed for signs of lithium toxicity.

Methotrexate: Ibuprofen, as well as other NSAIDs, has been reported to competitively inhibit methotrexate accumulation in rabbit kidney slices. This may indicate that ibuprofen could enhance the toxicity of methotrexate. Caution should be used when VICOPROFEN is administered concomitantly with methotrexate.

Warfarin: The effects of warfarin and NSAIDs on GI bleeding are synergistic, such that users of both drugs together have a risk of serious GI bleeding higher than users of either drug alone.

Carcinogenicity, Mutagenicity, and Impairment of Fertility

The carcinogenic and mutagenic potential of VICOPROFEN has not been investigated. The ability of VICOPROFEN to impair fertility has not been assessed.

Pregnancy: Pregnancy Category C.

Teratogenic Effects: VICOPROFEN, administered to rabbits at 95 mg/kg (5.72 and 1.9 times the maximum clinical dose based on body weight and surface area, respectively), a maternally toxic dose, resulted in an increase in the percentage of litters and fetuses with any major abnormality and an increase in the number of litters and fetuses with one or more nonossified metacarpals (a minor abnormality). VICOPROFEN, administered to rats at 166 mg/kg (10.0 and 1.66 times the maximum clinical dose based on body weight and surface area, respectively), a maternally toxic dose, did not result in any reproductive toxicity. There are no adequate and well-controlled studies in pregnant women. VICOPROFEN should be used during pregnancy only if the potential benefit justifies the potential risk to the fetus.

Nonteratogenic Effects: Because of the known effects of nonsteroidal anti-inflammatory drugs on the fetal cardiovascular system (closure of the ductus arteriosus), use during pregnancy (particularly late pregnancy) should be avoided. Babies born to mothers who have been taking opioids regularly prior to delivery will be physically dependent. The withdrawal signs include irritability and excessive crying, tremors, hyperactive reflexes, increased respiratory rate, increased stools, sneezing, yawning, vomiting, and fever. The intensity of the syndrome does not always correlate with the duration of maternal opioid use or dose. There is no consensus on the best method of managing withdrawal.

Labor and Delivery

As with other drugs known to inhibit prostaglandin synthesis, an increased incidence of dystocia and delayed parturition occurred in rats. Administration of VICOPROFEN is not recommended during labor and delivery.

Nursing Mothers

It is not known whether hydrocodone is excreted in human milk. In limited studies, an assay capable of detecting 1 mcg/mL did not demonstrate ibuprofen in the milk of lactating mothers. However, because of the limited nature of the studies, and the possible adverse effects of prostaglandin-inhibiting drugs on neonates, VICOPROFEN is not recommended for use in nursing mothers.

Pediatric Use

The safety and effectiveness of VICOPROFEN in pediatric patients below the age of 16 have not been established.

Geriatric Use

In controlled clinical trials there was no difference in tolerability between patients < 65 years of age and those ≥ 65, apart from an increased tendency of the elderly to develop constipation. However, because the elderly may be more sensitive to the renal and gastrointestinal effects of nonsteroidal anti-inflammatory agents as well as possible increased risk of respiratory depression with opioids, extra caution and reduced dosages should be used when treating the elderly with VICOPROFEN.

ADVERSE REACTIONS

VICOPROFEN was administered to approximately 300 pain patients in a safety study that employed dosages and a duration of treatment sufficient to encompass the recommended usage (see DOSAGE AND ADMINISTRATION). Adverse event rates generally increased with increasing daily dose. The event rates reported below are from approximately 150 patients who were in a group that received one tablet of VICOPROFEN an average of three to four times daily. The overall incidence rates of adverse experiences in the trials were fairly similar for this patient group and those who received the comparison treatment, acetaminophen 600 mg with codeine 60 mg.

The following lists adverse events that occurred with an incidence of 1% or greater in clinical trials of VICOPROFEN, without regard to the causal relationship of the events to the drug. To distinguish different rates of occurrence in clinical studies, the adverse events are listed as follows:

name of adverse event = less than 3%

adverse events marked with an asterisk * = 3% to 9%

adverse event rates over 9% are in parentheses.

Body as a Whole: Abdominal pain*; Asthenia*; Fever; Flu syndrome; Headache (27%); Infection*; Pain.

Cardiovascular: Palpitations; Vasodilation.

Central Nervous System: Anxiety*; Confusion; Dizziness (14%); Hypertonia; Insomnia*; Nervousness*; Paresthesia; Somnolence (22%); Thinking abnormalities.

Digestive: Anorexia; Constipation (22%); Diarrhea*; Dry mouth*; Dyspepsia (12%); Flatulence*; Gastritis; Melena; Mouth ulcers; Nausea (21%); Thirst; Vomiting*.

Metabolic and Nutritional Disorders: Edema*.

Respiratory: Dyspnea; Hiccups; Pharyngitis; Rhinitis.

Skin and Appendages: Pruritus*; Sweating*.

Special Senses: Tinnitus.

Urogenital: Urinary frequency.

Incidence less than 1%

Body as a Whole: Allergic reaction.

Cardiovascular: Arrhythmia; Hypotension; Tachycardia.

Central Nervous System: Agitation; Abnormal dreams; Decreased libido; Depression; Euphoria; Mood changes; Neuralgia; Slurred speech; Tremor, Vertigo.

Digestive: Chalky stool; "Clenching teeth"; Dysphagia; Esophageal spasm; Esophagitis; Gastroenteritis; Glossitis; Liver enzyme elevation.

Metabolic and Nutritional: Weight decrease.

Musculoskeletal: Arthralgia; Myalgia.

Respiratory: Asthma; Bronchitis; Hoarseness; Increased cough; Pulmonary congestion; Pneumonia; Shallow breathing; Sinusitis.

Skin and Appendages: Rash; Urticaria.

Special Senses: Altered vision; Bad taste; Dry eyes.

Urogenital: Cystitis; Glycosuria; Impotence; Urinary incontinence; Urinary retention.

DRUG ABUSE AND DEPENDENCE

Controlled Substance: VICOPROFEN Tablets are a Schedule III controlled substance.

Abuse: Psychic dependence, physical dependence, and tolerance may develop upon repeated administration of opioids; therefore, VICOPROFEN Tablets should be prescribed and administered with the same degree of caution appropriate to use of other oral narcotic medications.

Dependence: Physical dependence, the condition in which continued administration of the drug is required to prevent the appearance of a withdrawal syndrome, assumes clinically significant proportions only after several weeks of continued opioid use, although a mild degree of physical dependence may develop after a few days of opioid therapy. Tolerance, in which increasingly large doses are required in order to produce the same degree of analgesia, is manifested initially by a shortened duration of analgesic effect, and subsequently by decreases in the intensity of analgesia. The rate of development of tolerance varies among patients. However, psychic dependence is unlikely to develop when VICOPROFEN Tablets are used for a short time for the treatment of acute pain.

OVERDOSAGE

Following an acute overdosage, toxicity may result from hydrocodone and/or ibuprofen.

Signs and Symptoms:

Hydrocodone component: Serious overdose with hydrocodone is characterized by respiratory depression (a decrease in respiratory rate and/or tidal volume, Cheyne-Stokes respiration, cyanosis) extreme somnolence progressing to stupor or coma, skeletal muscle flaccidity, cold and clammy skin, and sometimes bradycardia and hypotension. In severe overdosage, apnea, circulatory collapse, cardiac arrest and death may occur.

Ibuprofen component: Symptoms include gastrointestinal irritation with erosion and hemorrhage or perforation, kidney damage, liver damage, heart damage, hemolytic anemia, agranulocytosis, thrombocytopenia, aplastic anemia, and meningitis. Other symptoms may include headache, dizziness, tinnitus, confusion, blurred vision, mental disturbances, skin rash, stomatitis, edema, reduced retinal sensitivity, corneal deposits, and hyperkalemia.

Treatment:

Primary attention should be given to the re-establishment of adequate respiratory exchange through provision of a patent airway and the institution of assisted or controlled ventilation. Naloxone, a narcotic antagonist, can reverse respiratory depression and coma associated with opioid overdose or unusual sensitivity to opioids, including hydrocodone. Therefore, an appropriate dose of naloxone hydrochloride should be administered intravenously with simultaneous efforts at respiratory resuscitation. Since the duration of action of hydrocodone may exceed that of the naloxone, the patient should be kept under continuous surveillance and repeated doses of the antagonist should be administered as needed to maintain adequate respiration. Supportive measures should be employed as indicated. Gastric emptying may be useful in removing unabsorbed drug. In cases where consciousness is impaired it may be inadvisable to perform gastric lavage. If gastric lavage is performed, little drug will likely be recovered if more than an hour has elapsed since ingestion. Ibuprofen is acidic and is excreted in the urine; therefore, it may be beneficial to administer alkali and induce diuresis. In addition to supportive measures the use of oral activated charcoal may help to reduce the absorption and reabsorption of ibuprofen. Dialysis is not likely to be effective for removal of ibuprofen because it is very highly bound to plasma proteins.

DOSAGE AND ADMINISTRATION

For the short-term (generally less than 10 days) management of acute pain, the recommended dose of VICOPROFEN is one tablet every 4 to 6 hours, as necessary. Dosage should not exceed 5 tablets in a 24-hour period. It should be kept in mind that tolerance to hydrocodone can develop with continued use and that the incidence of untoward effects is dose related.

The lowest effective dose or the longest dosing interval should be sought for each patient, especially in the elderly. After observing the initial response to therapy with VICOPROFEN, the dose and frequency of dosing should be adjusted to suit the individual patient's need, without exceeding the total daily dose recommended.

HOW SUPPLIED

VICOPROFEN® tablets are available as:

White film-coated round convex tablets, engraved with "VP" over [Abbott logo] on one side and plain on the other side.

Bottles of 100-NDC 0074-2277-14

Bottles of 500-NDC 0074-2277-54

Hospital Unit Dosage Package-100 tablets

(4×25 tablets)-NDC 0074-2277-12

Storage: Store at 25°C (77°F); excursions permitted to 15°-30°C (59°-86°F). [See USP Controlled Room Temperature].

Dispense in a tight, light-resistant container.

A Schedule Ⓒⅲ Narcotic.

©Abbott

Revised: July, 2003

Ref.: 03-5280-R2

ABBOTT LABORATORIES

NORTH CHICAGO, IL 60064, U.S.A. PRINTED IN U.S.A.

Shown in Product Identification Guide, page 304

ZEMPLAR®

[*zĕm-plər*]

(paricalcitol injection)

Fliptop Vial

℞ only

DESCRIPTION

Zemplar® (paricalcitol injection) is a synthetically manufactured vitamin D analog. It is available as a sterile, clear, colorless, aqueous solution for intravenous injection. Each mL contains paricalcitol, 5 mcg; propylene glycol, 30% (v/v); and alcohol, 20% (v/v).

Paricalcitol is a white powder chemically designated as 19-nor-1α,3β,25-trihydroxy-9,10-secoergosta-5(Z),7(E),22(E)-triene and has the following structural formula:

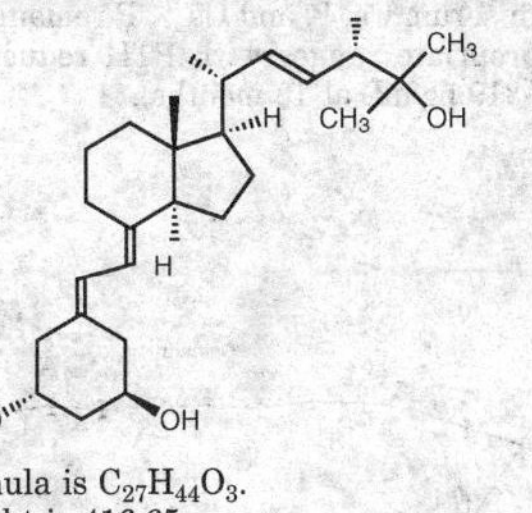

Molecular formula is $C_{27}H_{44}O_3$.

Molecular weight is 416.65.

CLINICAL PHARMACOLOGY

Mechanism of Action

Paricalcitol is a synthetic vitamin D analog. Vitamin D and paricalcitol have been shown to reduce parathyroid hormone (PTH) levels.

Pharmacokinetics

Distribution

The pharmacokinetics of paricalcitol have been studied in patients with chronic renal failure (CRF) requiring hemodialysis. Zemplar® is administered as an intravenous bolus injection. Within two hours after administering doses ranging from 0.04 to 0.24 mcg/kg, concentrations of paricalcitol decreased rapidly; thereafter, concentrations of paricalcitol declined log-linearly with a mean half-life of about 15 hours. No accumulation of paricalcitol was observed with multiple dosing.

Elimination

In healthy subjects, plasma radioactivity after a single 0.16 mcg/kg intravenous bolus dose of ^{3}H-paricalcitol (n=4) was attributed to parent drug. Paricalcitol was eliminated primarily by hepatobiliary excretion, as 74% of the radioactive dose was recovered in feces and only 16% was found in urine.

Metabolism

Several unknown metabolites were detected in both the urine and feces, with no detectable paricalcitol in the urine. These metabolites have not been characterized and have not been identified. Together, these metabolites contributed 51% of the urinary radioactivity and 59% of the fecal radioactivity. *In vitro* plasma protein binding of paricalcitol was extensive (>99.9%) and nonsaturable over the concentration range of 1 to 100 ng/mL.

Paricalcitol Pharmacokinetic Characteristics in CRF Patients (0.24 mcg/kg dose)

Parameter	n	Values (Mean ± SD)
C_{max} (5 min. after bolus)	6	1850 ± 664 (pg/mL)
$AUC_{0-\infty}$	5	27382 ± 8230 (pg•hr/mL)
CL	5	0.72 ± 0.24 (L/hr)
V_{ss}	5	6 ± 2 (L)

Laboratory Tests

In placebo-controlled studies, paricalcitol reduced serum total alkaline phosphatase levels.

Special Populations

Paricalcitol pharmacokinetics have not been investigated in geriatric or pediatric populations, or for drug-drug interactions. Pharmacokinetics were not gender-dependent.

The disposition of paricalcitol was compared in patients with mild (n=5) and moderate (n=5) hepatic impairment (as indicated by the Child-Pugh method) and subjects with normal hepatic function (n=10). Following administration of a

Continued on next page

Zemplar—Cont.

single dose, the pharmacokinetics of unbound paricalcitol were similar across hepatic function groups. Paricalcitol binding to plasma proteins was very high in all hepatic function groups (mean values >99.7%). The protein binding of paricalcitol was decreased in subjects with moderate (but not mild) hepatic impairment; total paricalcitol concentrations tended to be lower for subjects with moderate hepatic impairment compared to the other two hepatic function groups. No dosing adjustment is required in patients with mild and moderate hepatic impairment. The influence of severe hepatic impairment on the pharmacokinetics of paricalcitol has not been evaluated.

Clinical Studies

In three 12-week, placebo-controlled, phase 3 studies in chronic renal failure patients on dialysis, the dose of Zemplar® was started at 0.04 mcg/kg 3 times per week. The dose was increased by 0.04 mcg/kg every 2 weeks until intact parathyroid hormone (iPTH) levels were decreased at least 30% from baseline or a fifth escalation brought the dose to 0.24 mcg/kg, or iPTH fell to less than 100 pg/mL, or the Ca × P product was greater than 75 within any 2 week period, or serum calcium became greater than 11.5 mg/dL at any time.

Patients treated with Zemplar® achieved a mean iPTH reduction of 30% within 6 weeks. In these studies, there was no significant difference in the incidence of hypercalcemia or hyperphosphatemia between Zemplar® and placebo-treated patients. The results from these studies are as follows:

[See table above]

A long-term, open-label safety study of 164 CRF patients (mean dose of 7.5 mcg three times per week), demonstrated that mean serum Ca, P, and Ca × P remained within clinically appropriate ranges with PTH reduction (mean decrease of 319 pg/mL at 13 months).

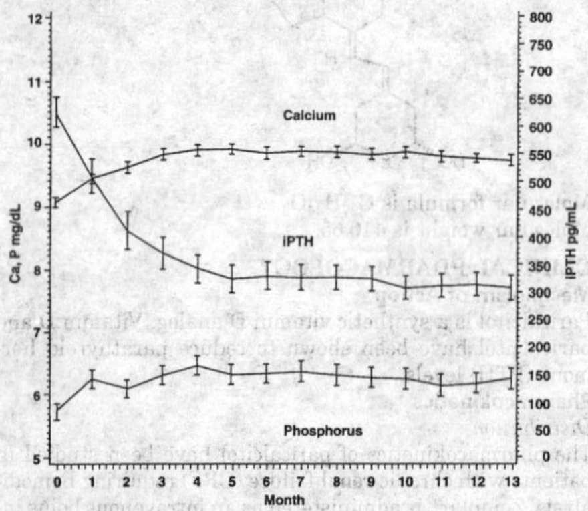

INDICATIONS AND USAGE

Zemplar® is indicated for the prevention and treatment of secondary hyperparathyroidism associated with chronic renal failure. Studies in patients with chronic renal failure show that Zemplar® suppresses PTH levels with no significant difference in the incidence of hypercalcemia or hyperphosphatemia when compared to placebo. However, the serum phosphorus, calcium and calcium × phosphorus product (Ca × P) may increase when Zemplar® is administered.

CONTRAINDICATIONS

Zemplar® should not be given to patients with evidence of vitamin D toxicity, hypercalcemia, or hypersensitivity to any ingredient in this product (see **PRECAUTIONS, General**).

WARNINGS

Acute overdose of Zemplar® may cause hypercalcemia, and require emergency attention. During dose adjustment, serum calcium and phosphorus levels should be monitored closely (e.g., twice weekly). If clinically significant hypercalcemia develops, the dose should be reduced or interrupted. Chronic administration of Zemplar® may place patients at risk of hypercalcemia, elevated Ca × P product, and metastatic calcification. Signs and symptoms of vitamin D intoxication associated with hypercalcemia include:

Early

Weakness, headache, somnolence, nausea, vomiting, dry mouth, constipation, muscle pain, bone pain, and metallic taste.

Late

Anorexia, weight loss, conjunctivitis (calcific), pancreatitis, photophobia, rhinorrhea, pruritus, hyperthermia, decreased libido, elevated BUN, hypercholesterolemia, elevated AST and ALT, ectopic calcification, hypertension, cardiac arrhythmias, somnolence, death, and rarely, overt psychosis.

Treatment of patients with clinically significant hypercalcemia consists of immediate dose reduction or interruption of Zemplar® therapy and includes a low calcium diet, withdrawal of calcium supplements, patient mobilization, attention to fluid and electrolyte imbalances, assessment of electrocardiographic abnormalities (critical in patients receiving digitalis), and hemodialysis or peritoneal dialysis

	Group (No. of Pts.)	Baseline Mean (Range)	Mean (SE) Change From Baseline to Final Evaluation
PTH (pg/mL)	Zemplar® (n=40)	783 (291–2076)	−379 (43.7)
	placebo (n=38)	745 (320–1671)	−69.6 (44.8)
Alkaline Phosphatase (U/L)	Zemplar® (n=31)	150 (40–600)	−41.5 (10.6)
	placebo (n=34)	169 (56–911)	+2.6 (10.1)
Calcium (mg/dL)	Zemplar® (n=40)	9.3 (7.2–10.4)	+0.47 (0.1)
	placebo (n=38)	9.1 (7.8–10.7)	+0.02 (0.1)
Phosphorus (mg/dL)	Zemplar® (n=40)	5.8 (3.7–10.2)	+0.47 (0.3)
	placebo (n=38)	6.0 (2.8–8.8)	−0.47 (0.3)
Calcium × Phosphorus Product	Zemplar® (n=40)	54 (32–106)	+7.9 (2.2)
	placebo (n=38)	54 (26–77)	−3.9 (2.3)

against a calcium-free dialysate, as warranted. Serum calcium levels should be monitored frequently until normocalcemia ensues.

Phosphate or vitamin D-related compounds should not be taken concomitantly with Zemplar®.

PRECAUTIONS

General: Digitalis toxicity is potentiated by hypercalcemia of any cause, so caution should be applied when digitalis compounds are prescribed concomitantly with Zemplar®. Adynamic bone lesions may develop if PTH levels are suppressed to abnormal levels.

Information for the Patient: The patient should be instructed that, to ensure effectiveness of Zemplar® therapy, it is important to adhere to a dietary regimen of calcium supplementation and phosphorus restriction. Appropriate types of phosphate-binding compounds may be needed to control serum phosphorus levels in patients with chronic renal failure (CRF), but excessive use of aluminum containing compounds should be avoided. Patients should also be carefully informed about the symptoms of elevated calcium

Essential Laboratory Tests: During the initial phase of medication, serum calcium and phosphorus should be determined frequently (e.g., twice weekly). Once dosage has been established, serum calcium and phosphorus should be measured at least monthly. Measurements of serum or plasma PTH are recommended every 3 months. An intact PTH (iPTH) assay is recommended for reliable detection of biologically active PTH in patients with CRF. During dose adjustment of Zemplar®, laboratory tests may be required more frequently.

Drug Interactions: Specific interaction studies were not performed. Digitalis toxicity is potentiated by hypercalcemia of any cause, so caution should be applied when digitalis compounds are prescribed concomitantly with Zemplar®.

Carcinogenesis, Mutagenesis, Impairment of Fertility: In a 104-week carcinogenicity study in CD-1 mice, an increased incidence of uterine leiomyoma and leiomyosarcoma was observed at subcutaneous doses of 1 to 10 mcg/kg (< 1 to 3 times the maximum recommended human weekly dose of 0.72 mcg/kg, based on body surface area, mg/m^2). The incidence rate of uterine leiomyoma was significantly different than the control group at the highest dose of 10 mcg/kg. In a 104-week carcinogenicity study in rats, there was an increased incidence of benign adrenal pheochromocytoma at subcutaneous doses of 0.15 to 1.5 mcg/kg (≤ 1 times the maximum recommended human weekly dose of 0.72 mcg/kg, based on body surface area, mg/m^2). The increased incidence of pheochromocytomas in rats may be related to the alteration of calcium homeostasis by paricalcitol. In carcinogenicity studies in rats and mice, paricalcitol did not affect the incidences of tumors apart from benign rodent-specific lesions related to the effects of chronic hypercalcemia.

Paricalcitol did not exhibit genetic toxicity *in vitro* with or without metabolic activation in the microbial mutagenesis assay (Ames Assay), mouse lymphoma mutagenesis assay (L5178Y), or a human lymphocyte cell chromosomal aberration assay. There was also no evidence of genetic toxicity in an *in vivo* mouse micronucleus assay. Zemplar® had no effect on fertility (male or female) in rats at intravenous doses up to 20 mcg/kg/dose [equivalent to 13 times the highest recommended human dose (0.24 mcg/kg) based on surface area, mg/m^2].

Pregnancy: *Pregnancy Category C.* Paricalcitol has been shown to cause minimal decreases in fetal viability (5%) when administered daily to rabbits at a dose 0.5 times the 0.24 mcg/kg human dose (based on surface area, mg/m^2) and when administered to rats at a dose 2 times the 0.24 mcg/kg human dose (based on plasma levels of exposure). At the highest dose tested (20 mcg/kg 3 times per week in rats, 13 times the 0.24 mcg/kg human dose based on surface area), there was a significant increase of the mortality of newborn rats at doses that were maternally toxic (hypercalcemia). No other effects on offspring development were observed. Paricalcitol was not teratogenic at the doses tested.

There are no adequate and well-controlled studies in pregnant women. Zemplar® should be used during pregnancy only if the potential benefit justifies the potential risk to the fetus.

Nursing Mothers: It is not known whether paricalcitol is excreted in human milk. Because many drugs are excreted in human milk, caution should be exercised when Zemplar® is administered to a nursing woman.

Pediatric Use: Safety and efficacy of Zemplar® in pediatric patients have not been established.

Geriatric Use: Of the 40 patients receiving Zemplar® in the three phase 3 placebo-controlled CRF studies, 10 patients were 65 years or over. In these studies, no overall differences in efficacy or safety were observed between patients 65 years or older and younger patients.

ADVERSE REACTIONS

Zemplar® has been evaluated for safety in clinical studies in 454 CRF patients. In four, placebo-controlled, double-blind, multicenter studies, discontinuation of therapy due to any adverse event occurred in 6.5% of 62 patients treated with Zemplar® (dosage titrated as tolerated, see **CLINICAL PHARMACOLOGY, Clinical Studies**) and 2.0% of 51 patients treated with placebo for one to three months. Adverse events occurring with greater frequency in the Zemplar® group at a frequency of 2% or greater, regardless of causality, are presented in the following table:

Adverse Event Incidence Rates for All Treated Patients In All Placebo-Controlled Studies

Adverse Event	Zemplar® (n=62)%	Placebo (n=51)%
Overall	71	78
Body as a Whole		
Chills	5	0
Feeling unwell	3	0
Fever	5	2
Flu	5	4
Sepsis	5	2
Cardiovascular System		
Palpitation	3	0
Digestive System		
Dry mouth	3	2
Gastrointestinal bleeding	5	2
Nausea	13	8
Vomiting	8	4
Metabolic and Nutritional Disorders		
Edema	7	0
Nervous System		
Light-headedness	5	2
Respiratory System		
Pneumonia	5	0

A patient who reported the same medical term more than once was counted only once for that medical term.

Safety parameters (changes in mean Ca, P, Ca × P) in an open-label safety study up to 13 months in duration support the long-term safety of Zemplar® in this patient population.

Adverse Events during post-marketing experience: Taste perversion, such as metallic taste, and allergic reactions, such as rash, urticaria and pruritus rarely have been reported.

OVERDOSAGE

Overdosage of Zemplar® may lead to hypercalcemia (see **WARNINGS**).

DOSAGE AND ADMINISTRATION

The currently accepted target range for iPTH levels in CRF patients is no more than 1.5 to 3 times the non-uremic upper limit of normal.

The recommended initial dose of Zemplar® is 0.04 mcg/kg to 0.1 mcg/kg (2.8 – 7 mcg) administered as a bolus dose no more frequently than every other day at any time during dialysis. Doses as high as 0.24 mcg/kg (16.8 mcg) have been safely administered.

If a satisfactory response is not observed, the dose may be increased by 2 to 4 mcg at 2- to 4-week intervals. During any dose adjustment period, serum calcium and phosphorus levels should be monitored more frequently, and if an elevated calcium level or a Ca × P product greater than 75 is noted, the drug dosage should be immediately reduced or interrupted until these parameters are normalized. Then, Zemplar® should be reinitiated at a lower dose. Doses may need to be decreased as the PTH levels decrease in response to therapy. Thus, incremental dosing must be individualized.
The following table is a suggested approach in dose titration:

Suggested Dosing Guidelines

PTH Level	Zemplar® Dose
the same or increasing	increase
decreasing by <30%	increase
decreasing by >30%, <60%	maintain
decreasing by >60%	decrease
one and one-half to three times upper limit of normal	maintain

The influence of mild to moderately impaired hepatic function on paricalcitol pharmacokinetics is sufficiently small that no dosing adjustment is required.
Parenteral drug products should be inspected visually for particulate matter and discoloration prior to administration whenever solution and container permit.
Discard unused portion.

HOW SUPPLIED

Zemplar® (paricalcitol injection) 5 mcg/mL is supplied as 1 and 2 mL single-dose Fliptop Vials.

List No.	Volume/ Container	Concentration	Total Content
1658	1 mL/Fliptop Vial	5 mcg/mL	5 mcg
1658	2 mL/Fliptop Vial	5 mcg/mL	10 mcg

Store at 25°C (77°F). Excursions permitted to 15°–30°C (59°–86°F).
U.S. patents: 5,246,925; 5,587,497
Ref. 58-6995
Revised: March, 2003

ABBOTT LABORATORIES, NORTH CHICAGO, IL 60064, USA

Actelion Pharmaceuticals US, Inc.

5000 SHORELINE CT., SUITE 200
S. SAN FRANCISCO, CA 94080

Direct Inquiries to:
Actelion Medical Information
866-228-3546
(follow the prompts)

TRACLEER® ℞
[trək' lēr]
BOSENTAN TABLETS
62.5 mg and 125 mg film-coated tablets

Use of TRACLEER® requires attention to two significant concerns: 1) potential for serious liver injury, and 2) potential damage to a fetus.

WARNING: Potential liver injury
TRACLEER® causes at least 3-fold (upper limit of normal; ULN) elevation of liver aminotransferases (ALT and AST) in about 11% of patients, accompanied by elevated bilirubin in a small number of cases. Because these changes are a marker for potential serious liver injury, serum aminotransferase levels must be measured prior to initiation of treatment and then monthly (see WARNINGS: Potential Liver Injury and DOSAGE AND ADMINISTRATION). To date, in a setting of close monitoring, elevations have been reversible, within a few days to 9 weeks, either spontaneously or after dose reduction or discontinuation, and without sequelae.
Elevations in aminotransferases require close attention (see DOSAGE AND ADMINISTRATION). TRACLEER® should generally be avoided in patients with elevated aminotransferases (> 3 × ULN) at baseline because monitoring liver injury may be more difficult. If liver aminotransferase elevations are accompanied by clinical symptoms of liver injury (such as nausea, vomiting, fever, abdominal pain, jaundice, or unusual lethargy or fatigue) or increases in bilirubin ≥ 2 × ULN, treatment should be stopped. There is no experience with the re-introduction of TRACLEER® in these circumstances.

CONTRAINDICATION: Pregnancy
TRACLEER® (bosentan) is very likely to produce major birth defects if used by pregnant women, as this effect has been seen consistently when it is administered to animals (see CONTRAINDICATIONS). Therefore, pregnancy must be excluded before the start of treatment with TRACLEER® and prevented thereafter by the use of a reliable method of contraception. Hormonal contraceptives, including oral, injectable and implantable contraceptives should not be used as the sole means of contraception because these may not be effective in patients receiving TRACLEER® (see Precautions: Drug Interactions). Monthly pregnancy tests should be obtained.
Because of potential liver injury and in an effort to make the chance of fetal exposure to TRACLEER® (bosentan) as small as possible, TRACLEER® may be prescribed only through the TRACLEER® Access Program by calling 1 866 228 3546. Adverse events can also be reported directly via this number.

Table 1 Effects of bosentan on 6-minute walk distance

	BREATHE-1			Study 351	
	Bosentan 125 mg b.i.d. (n = 74)	*Bosentan 250 mg b.i.d. (n = 70)*	Placebo (n = 69)	Bosentan 125 mg b.i.d. (n = 21)	Placebo (n =11)
Baseline	*326 ± 73*	*333 ± 75*	344 ± 76	360 ± 86	355 ± 82
End point	*353 ± 115*	*379 ± 101*	336 ± 129	431 ± 66	350 ± 147
Change from baseline	*27 ± 75*	*46 ± 62*	-8 ± 96	70 ± 56	-6 ± 121
Placebo - substracted	*35[(a)]*	*54[(b)]*		76[(c)]	

Distance in meters: mean ± standard deviation. Changes are to week 16 for BREATHE-1 and to week 12 for Study 351.
[(a)]p=0.01; by Wilcoxon
[(b)]p=0.0001 for 250 mg; by Wilcoxon
[(c)]p=0.02 by Student's t-test.

DESCRIPTION

Bosentan is the first of a new drug class, an endothelin receptor antagonist.
TRACLEER® (bosentan) belongs to a class of highly substituted pyrimidine derivatives, with no chiral centers. It is designated chemically as 4-tert-butyl-N-[6-(2-hydroxy-ethoxy)-5-(2-methoxy-phenoxy)-[2,2′]-bipyrimidin-4-yl]-benzenesulfonamide monohydrate and has the following structural formula:

Bosentan has a molecular weight of 569.64 and a molecular formula of $C_{27}H_{29}N_5O_6S \bullet H_2O$. Bosentan is a white to yellowish powder. It is poorly soluble in water (1.0 mg/100 ml) and in aqueous solutions at low pH (0.1 mg/100 ml at pH 1.1 and 4.0; 0.2 mg/100 ml at pH 5.0). Solubility increases at higher pH values (43 mg/100 ml at pH 7.5). In the solid state, bosentan is very stable, is not hygroscopic and is not light sensitive.
TRACLEER® is available as 62.5 mg and 125 mg film-coated tablets for oral administration, and contains the following excipients: corn starch, pregelatinized starch, sodium starch glycolate, povidone, glyceryl behenate, magnesium stearate, hydroxypropylmethylcellulose, triacetin, talc, titanium dioxide, iron oxide yellow, iron oxide red, and ethylcellulose. Each TRACLEER® 62.5 mg tablet contains 64.541 mg of bosentan, equivalent to 62.5 mg of anhydrous bosentan. Each TRACLEER® 125 mg tablet contains 129.082 mg of bosentan, equivalent to 125 mg of anhydrous bosentan.

CLINICAL PHARMACOLOGY

Mechanism of Action
Endothelin-1 (ET-1) is a neurohormone, the effects of which are mediated by binding to ET_A and ET_B receptors in the endothelium and vascular smooth muscle. ET-1 concentrations are elevated in plasma and lung tissue of patients with pulmonary arterial hypertension, suggesting a pathogenic role for ET-1 in this disease. Bosentan is a specific and competitive antagonist at endothelin receptor types ET_A and ET_B. Bosentan has a slightly higher affinity for ET_A receptors than for ET_B receptors.

Pharmacokinetics
General
After oral administration, maximum plasma concentrations of bosentan are attained within 3–5 hours and the terminal elimination half-life ($t_{1/2}$) is about 5 hours. The exposure to bosentan after intravenous and oral administration is about 2-fold greater in adult patients with pulmonary arterial hypertension than in healthy adult subjects.

Absorption and Distribution
The absolute bioavailability of bosentan in normal volunteers is about 50% and is unaffected by food. The volume of distribution is about 18 L. Bosentan is highly bound (> 98%) to plasma proteins, mainly albumin. Bosentan does not penetrate into erythrocytes.

Metabolism and Elimination
Bosentan has three metabolites, one of which is pharmacologically active and may contribute 10%-20% of the effect of bosentan. Bosentan is an inducer of CYP2C9 and CYP3A4 and possibly also of CYP2C19. Total clearance after a single intravenous dose is about 8 L/hr. Upon multiple dosing, plasma concentrations decrease gradually to 50%-65% of those seen after single dose administration, probably the effect of auto-induction of the metabolizing liver enzymes. Steady-state is reached within 3-5 days. Bosentan is eliminated by biliary excretion following metabolism in the liver. Less than 3% of an administered oral dose is recovered in urine.

Special Populations
It is not known whether bosentan pharmacokinetics is influenced by gender, body weight, race, or age.

Liver Function Impairment
In vitro and *in vivo* evidence showing extensive hepatic metabolism of bosentan suggests that liver impairment could significantly increase exposure of bosentan. In a study comparing 8 patients with mild liver impairment (as indicated by the Child-Pugh method) to 8 controls, the single- and multiple-dose pharmacokinetics of bosentan were not altered in patients with mild hepatic impairment. The influence of moderate or severe liver impairment on the pharmacokinetics of bosentan has not been evaluated. Bosentan should generally be avoided in patients with moderate or severe liver abnormalities and/or elevated aminotransferases > 3 × ULN (See **DOSAGE AND ADMINISTRATION**).

Renal Impairment
In patients with severe renal impairment (creatinine clearance 15–30 ml/min), plasma concentrations of bosentan were essentially unchanged and plasma concentrations of the three metabolites were increased about 2-fold compared to people with normal renal function. These differences do not appear to be clinically important (See **DOSAGE AND ADMINISTRATION**).

Clinical Studies
Pulmonary Arterial Hypertension
Two randomized, double-blind, multi-center, placebo-controlled trials were conducted in 32 and 213 patients. The larger study (BREATHE-1) compared 2 doses (125 mg b.i.d. and 250 mg b.i.d.) of TRACLEER® with placebo. The smaller study (Study 351) compared 125 mg b.i.d. with placebo. Patients had severe (WHO functional Class III–IV) pulmonary arterial hypertension: primary pulmonary hypertension (72%) or pulmonary hypertension secondary to scleroderma or other connective tissue diseases (21%), or to autoimmune diseases (7%). There were no patients with pulmonary hypertension secondary to other conditions such as HIV disease, or recurrent pulmonary emboli.
In both studies, TRACLEER® or placebo was added to patients' current therapy, which could have included a combination of digoxin, anticoagulants, diuretics, and vasodilators (e.g., calcium channel blockers, ACE inhibitors), but not epoprostenol. TRACLEER® was given at a dose of 62.5 mg b.i.d. for 4 weeks and then at 125 mg b.i.d. or 250 mg b.i.d. for either 12 (BREATHE-1) or 8 (Study 351) additional weeks. The primary study endpoint was 6-minute walk distance. In addition, symptoms and functional status were assessed. Hemodynamic measurements were made at 12 weeks in Study 351.
The mean age was about 49 years. About 80% of patients were female, and about 80% were Caucasian. Patients had been diagnosed with pulmonary hypertension for a mean of 2.4 years.

Submaximal Exercise Capacity
Results of the 6-minute walk distance at 3 months (Study 351) or 4 months (BREATHE-1) are shown in Table 1.
[See table 1 above]

Continued on next page

Tracleer—Cont.

In both trials, treatment with TRACLEER® resulted in a significant increase in exercise capacity. The improvement in walk distance was apparent after 1 month of treatment (with 62.5 mg b.i.d.) and fully developed by about 2 months of treatment (Figure 1). It was maintained for up to 7 months of double-blind treatment. Walking distance was somewhat greater with 250 mg b.i.d., but the potential for increased liver injury causes this dose not to be recommended (See **DOSAGE AND ADMINISTRATION**). There were no apparent differences in treatment effects on walk distance among subgroups analyzed by demographic factors, baseline disease severity, or disease etiology, but the studies had little power to detect such differences.

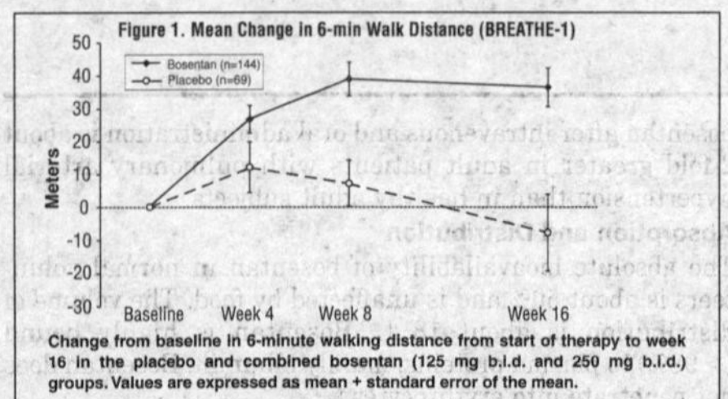

Figure 1. Mean Change in 6-min Walk Distance (BREATHE-1)

Change from baseline in 6-minute walking distance from start of therapy to week 16 in the placebo and combined bosentan (125 mg b.i.d. and 250 mg b.i.d.) groups. Values are expressed as mean + standard error of the mean.

Hemodynamic Changes

Invasive hemodynamic parameters were assessed in Study 351. Treatment with TRACLEER® led to a significant increase in cardiac index (CI) associated with a significant reduction in pulmonary artery pressure (PAP), pulmonary vascular resistance (PVR), and mean right atrial pressure (RAP) (Table 2).

[See table 2 above]

Table 2. Change from Baseline to Week 12: Hemodynamic Parameters

	Bosentan 125 mg b.i.d.		Placebo
Mean CI (L/min/m²)	N=20		N=10
Baseline	2.35±0.73		2.48±1.03
Absolute Change	0.50±0.46		-0.52±0.48
Treatment Effect		1.02[(a)]	
Mean PAP (mmHg)	N=20		N=10
Baseline	53.7±13.4		55.7±10.5
Absolute Change	-1.6±5.1		5.1±8.8
Treatment Effect		-6.7[(b)]	
Mean PVR (dyn•sec•cm⁻⁵)	N=19		N=10
Baseline	896±425		942±430
Absolute Change	-223±245		191±235
Treatment Effect		-415[(a)]	
Mean RAP (mmHg)	N=19		N=10
Baseline	9.7±5.6		9.9±4.1
Absolute Change	-1.3±4.1		4.9±4.6
Treatment Effect		-6.2[(a)]	

Values shown are means ± SD
[(a)] $p \leq 0.001$
[(b)] $p < 0.02$

Symptoms and Functional Status

Symptoms of pulmonary arterial hypertension were assessed by Borg dyspnea score, WHO functional class, and rate of "clinical worsening." Clinical worsening was assessed as the sum of death, hospitalizations for PAH, discontinuation of therapy because of PAH, and need for epoprostenol. There was a significant reduction in dyspnea during walk tests (Borg dyspnea score), and significant improvement in WHO functional class in TRACLEER®-treated patients. There was a significant reduction in the rate of clinical worsening (Table 3 and Figure 2). Figure 2 shows the Log-rank test reflecting clinical worsening over 28 weeks.

[See table 3 above]

Table 3. Incidence of Clinical Worsening, Intent To Treat Population

	BREATHE-1		Study 351	
	Bosentan 125/250 mg b.i.d. (N = 144)	Placebo (N = 69)	Bosentan 125 mg b.i.d. (N = 21)	Placebo (N = 11)
Patients with clinical worsening [n (%)]	9 (6%)[(a)]	14 (20%)	0 (0%)[(b)]	3 (27%)
Death	1 (1%)	2 (3%)	0 (0%)	0 (0%)
Hospitalization for PAH	6 (4%)	9 (13%)	0 (0%)	3 (27%)
Discontinuation due to worsening of PAH	5 (3%)	6 (9%)	0 (0%)	3 (27%)
Receipt of epoprostenol[(c)]	4 (3%)	3 (4%)	0 (0%)	3 (27%)

Note: Patients may have had more than one reason for clinical worsening.
[(a)] p=0.0015 vs. placebo by log-rank test. There was no relevant difference between the 125 mg and 250 mg b.i.d. groups.
[(b)] p=0.033 vs. placebo by Fisher's exact test.
[(c)] Receipt of epoprostenol was always a consequence of clinical worsening.

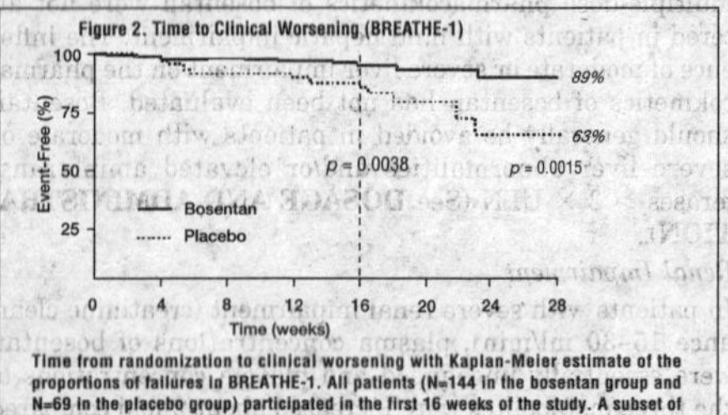

Figure 2. Time to Clinical Worsening (BREATHE-1)

Time from randomization to clinical worsening with Kaplan-Meier estimate of the proportions of failures in BREATHE-1. All patients (N=144 in the bosentan group and N=69 in the placebo group) participated in the first 16 weeks of the study. A subset of this population (N=35 in the bosentan group and 13 in the placebo group) continued double-blind therapy for up to 28 weeks.

Congestive Heart Failure (CHF)

In a pair of studies, 1613 subjects with NYHA Class III-IV heart failure, left ventricular ejection fraction <35%, on diuretics, ACE inhibitor, and other therapies, were randomized to placebo or TRACLEER® (62.5 mg b.i.d. titrated as tolerated to 125 mg b.i.d.) and followed for up to 70 weeks. Use of TRACLEER® was associated with no benefit on patient global assessment (the primary end point) or mortality. However, hospitalizations for heart failure were more common during the first 4 to 8 weeks after bosentan was initiated. Based on these results, bosentan is not effective in the treatment of congestive heart failure with left ventricular dysfunction.

INDICATIONS AND USAGE

TRACLEER® is indicated for the treatment of pulmonary arterial hypertension in patients with WHO Class III or IV symptoms, to improve exercise ability and decrease the rate of clinical worsening (see **Clinical Studies**).

CONTRAINDICATIONS

See **BOX WARNING** for **CONTRAINDICATION** to use in pregnancy.

Pregnancy Category X. TRACLEER® is expected to cause fetal harm if administered to pregnant women. Bosentan was teratogenic in rats given oral doses ≥ 60 mg/kg/day (twice the maximum recommended human oral dose of 125 mg, b.i.d., on a mg/m² basis). In an embryo-fetal toxicity study in rats, bosentan showed dose-dependent teratogenic effects, including malformations of the head, mouth, face and large blood vessels. Bosentan increased stillbirths and pup mortality at oral doses of 60 and 300 mg/kg/day (2 and 10 times, respectively, the maximum recommended human dose on a mg/m² basis). Although birth defects were not observed in rabbits given oral doses of up to 1500 mg/kg/day, plasma concentrations of bosentan in rabbits were lower than those reached in the rat. The similarity of malformations induced by bosentan and those observed in endothelin-1 knockout mice and in animals treated with other endothelin receptor antagonists indicates that teratogenicity is a class effect of these drugs. There are no data on the use of TRACLEER® in pregnant women.

Pregnancy must be excluded before the start of treatment with TRACLEER® and prevented thereafter by use of reliable contraception. Hormonal contraceptives, including oral, injectable, and implantable contraceptives may not be reliable in the presence of TRACLEER® and should not be used as the sole contraceptive method in patients receiving TRACLEER® (see **Drug Interactions**: Hormonal Contraceptives, Including Oral, Injectable, and Implantable Contraceptives). Input from a gynecologist or similar expert on adequate contraception should be sought as needed.

TRACLEER® should be started only in patients known not to be pregnant. For female patients of childbearing potential, a prescription for TRACLEER® should not be issued by the prescriber unless the patient assures the prescriber that she is not sexually active or provides negative results from a urine or serum pregnancy test performed during the first 5 days of a normal menstrual period and at least 11 days after the last unprotected act of sexual intercourse.

Follow-up urine or serum pregnancy tests should be obtained monthly in women of childbearing potential taking TRACLEER®. The patient must be advised that if there is any delay in onset of menses or any other reason to suspect pregnancy, she must notify the physician immediately for pregnancy testing. If the pregnancy test is positive, the physician and patient must discuss the risk to the pregnancy and to the fetus.

Cyclosporine A: Co-administration of cyclosporine A and bosentan resulted in markedly increased plasma concentrations of bosentan. Therefore, concomitant use of TRACLEER® and cyclosporine A is contraindicated.

Glyburide: An increased risk of liver enzyme elevations was observed in patients receiving glyburide concomitantly with bosentan. Therefore co-administration of glyburide and TRACLEER® is contraindicated.

Hypersensitivity: TRACLEER® is also contraindicated in patients who are hypersensitive to bosentan or any component of the medication.

WARNINGS

Potential Liver Injury (see **BOX WARNING**)

Elevations in ALT or AST by more than 3 × ULN were observed in 11% of bosentan-treated patients (N = 658) compared to 2% of placebo-treated patients (N = 280). Three-fold increases were seen in 12% of 95 PAH patients on 125 mg b.i.d. and 14% of 70 PAH patients on 250 mg b.i.d. Eight-fold increases were seen in 2% of PAH patients on 125 mg b.i.d. and 7% of PAH patients on 250 mg b.i.d. Bilirubin increases to ≥ 3 × ULN were associated with aminotransferase increases in 2 of 658 (0.3%) of patients treated with bosentan.

The combination of hepatocellular injury (increases in aminotransferases of > 3 × ULN) and increases in total bilirubin (≥ 3 × ULN) is a marker for potential serious liver injury.[1]

Elevations of AST and/or ALT associated with bosentan are dose-dependent, occur both early and late in treatment, usually progress slowly, are typically asymptomatic, and to date have been reversible after treatment interruption or cessation. These aminotransferase elevations may reverse spontaneously while continuing treatment with TRACLEER®.

Liver aminotransferase levels must be measured prior to initiation of treatment and then monthly. If elevated aminotransferase levels are seen, changes in monitoring and treatment must be initiated (see **DOSAGE AND ADMINISTRATION**). If liver aminotransferase elevations are accompanied by clinical symptoms of liver injury (such as nausea, vomiting, fever, abdominal pain, jaundice, or unusual lethargy or fatigue) or increases in bilirubin ≥ 2 × ULN, treatment should be stopped. There is no experience with the re-introduction of TRACLEER® in these circumstances.

Pre-existing Liver Impairment

Liver aminotransferase levels must be measured prior to initiation of treatment and then monthly. TRACLEER® should generally be avoided in patients with moderate or severe liver impairment (see **Clinical Pharmacology** and **DOSAGE AND ADMINISTRATION**). In addition, TRACLEER® should generally be avoided in patients with elevated aminotransferases (> 3 × ULN) because monitoring liver injury in these patients may be more difficult (see **BOX WARNING**).

PRECAUTIONS

Hematologic Changes

Treatment with TRACLEER® caused a dose-related decrease in hemoglobin and hematocrit. Hemoglobin levels should be monitored after 1 and 3 months of treatment and then every 3 months. The overall mean decrease in hemoglobin concentration for bosentan-treated patients was 0.9 g/dl (change to end of treatment). Most of this decrease of hemoglobin concentration was detected during the first few weeks of bosentan treatment and hemoglobin levels stabilized by 4–12 weeks of bosentan treatment. In placebo-controlled studies of all uses of bosentan, marked decreases in hemoglobin (> 15% decrease from baseline resulting in values < 11 g/dl) were observed in 6% of bosentan-treated patients and 3% of placebo-treated patients. In patients with pulmonary arterial hypertension treated with doses of 125 and 250 mg b.i.d., marked decreases in hemoglobin occurred in 3% compared to 1% in placebo-treated patients. A decrease in hemoglobin concentration by at least 1 g/dl was observed in 57% of bosentan-treated patients as compared to 29% of placebo-treated patients. In 80% of those patients whose hemoglobin decreased by at least 1 g/dl, the decrease occurred during the first 6 weeks of bosentan treatment.

During the course of treatment the hemoglobin concentration remained within normal limits in 68% of bosentan-treated patients compared to 76% of placebo patients. The explanation for the change in hemoglobin is not known, but it does not appear to be hemorrhage or hemolysis.

It is recommended that hemoglobin concentrations be checked after 1 and 3 months, and every 3 months thereafter. If a marked decrease in hemoglobin concentration occurs, further evaluation should be undertaken to determine the cause and need for specific treatment.

Fluid retention

In a placebo-controlled trial of patients with severe chronic heart failure, there was an increased incidence of hospitalization for CHF associated with weight gain and increased leg edema during the first 4-8 weeks of treatment with TRACLEER®. In addition, there have been numerous post-marketing reports of fluid retention in patients with pulmonary hypertension, occurring within weeks after starting TRACLEER®. Patients required intervention with a diuretic, fluid management, or hospitalization for decompensating heart failure (see **CLINICAL STUDIES**; *Congestive Heart Failure*).

Information for Patients

Patients are advised to consult the TRACLEER® Medication Guide on the safe use of TRACLEER®.

The physician should discuss with the patient the importance of monthly monitoring of serum aminotransferases and urine or serum pregnancy testing and of avoidance of pregnancy. The physician should discuss options for effective contraception and measures to prevent pregnancy with their female patients. Input from a gynecologist or similar expert on adequate contraception should be sought as needed.

Drug Interactions

Bosentan is metabolized by CYP2C9 and CYP3A4. Inhibition of these isoenzymes may increase the plasma concentration of bosentan (see ketoconazole). Bosentan is an inducer of CYP3A4 and CYP2C9. Consequently, plasma concentrations of drugs metabolized by these two isoenzymes will be decreased when TRACLEER® is co-administered. Bosentan had no relevant inhibitory effect on any CYP isoenzymes tested (CYP1A2, CYP2C9, CYP2C19, CYP2D6, CYP3A4). Consequently, TRACLEER® is not expected to increase the plasma concentrations of drugs metabolized by these enzymes.

Hormonal Contraceptives, Including Oral, Injectable, and Implantable Contraceptives: Specific interaction studies have not been performed to evaluate the effect of co-administration of bosentan and hormonal contraceptives, including oral, injectable or implantable contraceptives. Since many of these drugs are metabolized by CYP3A4, there is a possibility of failure of contraception when TRACLEER® is co-administered. Women should not rely on hormonal contraception alone when taking TRACLEER®.

Specific interaction studies have demonstrated the following:

Cyclosporine A: During the first day of concomitant administration, trough concentrations of bosentan were increased by about 30-fold. Steady-state bosentan plasma concentrations were 3- to 4-fold higher than in the absence of cyclosporine A. The concomitant administration of bosentan and cyclosporine A is contraindicated (see **CONTRAINDICATIONS**). Co-administration of bosentan decreased the plasma concentrations of cyclosporine A (a CYP3A4 substrate) by approximately 50%.

Tacrolimus: Co-administration of tacrolimus and bosentan has not been studied in man. Co-administration of tacrolimus and bosentan resulted in markedly increased plasma concentrations of bosentan in animals. Caution should be exercised if tacrolimus and bosentan are used together.

Glyburide: An increased risk of elevated liver aminotransferases was observed in patients receiving concomitant therapy with glyburide. Therefore, the concomitant administration of TRACLEER® and glyburide is contraindicated, and alternative hypoglycemic agents should be considered (see **CONTRAINDICATIONS**).

Co-administration of bosentan decreased the plasma concentrations of glyburide by approximately 40%. The plasma concentrations of bosentan were also decreased by approximately 30%. Bosentan is also expected to reduce plasma concentrations of other oral hypoglycemic agents that are predominantly metabolized by CYP2C9 or CYP3A4. The possibility of worsened glucose control in patients using these agents should be considered.

Ketoconazole: Co-administration of bosentan 125 mg b.i.d. and ketoconazole, a potent CYP3A4 inhibitor, increased the plasma concentrations of bosentan by approximately 2-fold. No dose adjustment of bosentan is necessary, but increased effects of bosentan should be considered.

Simvastatin and Other Statins: Co-administration of bosentan decreased the plasma concentrations of simvastatin (a CYP3A4 substrate), and its active β-hydroxy acid metabolite, by approximately 50%. The plasma concentrations of bosentan were not affected. Bosentan is also expected to reduce plasma concentrations of other statins that have significant metabolism by CYP3A4, such as lovastatin and atorvastatin. The possibility of reduced statin efficacy should be considered. Patients using CYP3A4 metabolized statins should have cholesterol levels monitored after TRACLEER® is initiated to see whether the statin dose needs adjustment.

Warfarin: Co-administration of bosentan 500 mg b.i.d. for 6 days decreased the plasma concentrations of both S-warfarin (a CYP2C9 substrate) and R-warfarin (a CYP3A4 substrate) by 29 and 38%, respectively. Clinical experience with concomitant administration of bosentan and warfarin in patients with pulmonary arterial hypertension did not show clinically relevant changes in INR or warfarin dose (baseline vs. end of the clinical studies), and the need to change the warfarin dose during the trials due to changes in INR or due to adverse events was similar among bosentan- and placebo-treated patients.

Digoxin, Nimodipine and Losartan: Bosentan has been shown to have no pharmacokinetic interactions with digoxin and nimodipine, and losartan has no effect on plasma levels of bosentan.

Carcinogenesis, Mutagenesis, Impairment of Fertility

Two years of dietary administration of bosentan to mice produced an increased incidence of hepatocellular adenomas and carcinomas in males at doses as low as 450 mg/kg/day (about 8 times the maximum recommended human dose [MRHD] of 125 mg b.i.d., on a mg/m^2 basis). In the same study, doses greater than 2000 mg/kg/day (about 32 times the MRHD) were associated with an increased incidence of colon adenomas in both males and females. In rats, dietary administration of bosentan for two years was associated with an increased incidence of brain astrocytomas in males at doses as low as 500 mg/kg/day (about 16 times the MRHD). In a comprehensive battery of *in vitro* tests (the microbial mutagenesis assay, the unscheduled DNA synthesis assay, the V-79 mammalian cell mutagenesis assay, and human lymphocyte assay) and an *in vivo* mouse micronucleus assay, there was no evidence for any mutagenic or clastogenic activity of bosentan.

Impairment of Fertility/Testicular Function

Many endothelin receptor antagonists have profound effects on the histology and function of the testes in animals. These drugs have been shown to induce atrophy of the seminiferous tubules of the testes and to reduce sperm counts and male fertility in rats when administered for longer than 10 weeks. Where studied, testicular tubular atrophy and decreases in male fertility observed with endothelin receptor antagonists appear irreversible.

In fertility studies in which male and female rats were treated with bosentan at oral doses of up to 1500 mg/kg/day (50 times the MRHD on a mg/m^2 basis) or intravenous doses up to 40 mg/kg/day, no effects on sperm count, sperm motility, mating performance or fertility were observed. An increased incidence of testicular tubular atrophy was observed in rats given bosentan orally at doses as low as 125 mg/kg/day (about 4 times the MRHD and the lowest doses tested) for two years but not at doses as high as 1500 mg/kg/day (about 50 times the MRHD) for 6 months. Effects on sperm count and motility were evaluated only in the much shorter duration fertility studies in which males had been exposed to the drug for 4-6 weeks. An increased incidence of tubular atrophy was not observed in mice treated for 2 years at doses up to 4500 mg/kg/day (about 75 times the MRHD) or in dogs treated up to 12 months at doses up to 500 mg/kg/day (about 50 times the MRHD).

There are no data on the effects of bosentan or other endothelin receptor antagonists on testicular function in man.

Pregnancy, Teratogenic Effects: Category X (See **CONTRAINDICATIONS**).

Nursing Mothers

It is not known whether this drug is excreted in human milk. Because many drugs are excreted in human milk, breastfeeding while taking TRACLEER® is not recommended.

Pediatric Use

Safety and efficacy in pediatric patients have not been established (see **DOSAGE AND ADMINISTRATION**).

Use in Elderly Patients

Clinical experience with TRACLEER® in subjects aged 65 or older has not included a sufficient number of such subjects to identify a difference in response between elderly and younger patients (see **DOSAGE AND ADMINISTRATION**).

ADVERSE REACTIONS

Adverse Events

See **BOX WARNING** for discussion of liver injury and **PRECAUTIONS** for discussion of hemoglobin and hematocrit abnormalities.

Safety data on bosentan were obtained from 12 clinical studies (8 placebo-controlled and 4 open-label) in 777 patients with pulmonary arterial hypertension, and other diseases. Doses up to 8 times the currently recommended clinical dose (125 mg b.i.d.) were administered for a variety of durations. The exposure to bosentan in these trials ranged from 1 day to 4.1 years (N=89 for 1 year; N=61 for 1.5 years and N=39 for more than 2 years). Exposure of pulmonary arterial hypertension patients (N=235) to bosentan ranged from 1 day to 1.7 years (N=126 more than 6 months and N=28 more than 12 months).

Treatment discontinuations due to adverse events other than those related to pulmonary hypertension during the clinical trials in patients with pulmonary arterial hypertension were more frequent on bosentan (5%; 8/165 patients) than on placebo (3%; 2/80 patients). In this database the only cause of discontinuations > 1%, and occurring more often on bosentan was abnormal liver function.

The adverse drug reactions that occurred in ≥ 3% of the bosentan-treated patients and were more common on bosentan in placebo-controlled trials in pulmonary arterial hypertension at doses of 125 or 250 mg b.i.d. are shown in Table 4:

Table 4. Adverse events* occurring in ≥ 3% of patients treated with bosentan 125-250 mg b.i.d. and more common on bosentanin placebo-controlled studies in pulmonary arterial hypertension

Adverse Event	Bosentan N=165		Placebo N=80	
	No.	%	No.	%
Headache	36	22%	16	20%
Nasopharyngitis	18	11%	6	8%
Flushing	15	9%	4	5%
Hepatic function abnormal	14	8%	2	3%
Edema, lower limb	13	8%	4	5%
Hypotension	11	7%	3	4%
Palpitations	8	5%	1	1%
Dyspepsia	7	4%	0	0%
Edema	7	4%	2	3%
Fatigue	6	4%	1	1%
Pruritus	6	4%	0	0%

***Note: only AEs with onset from start of treatment to 1 calendar day after end of treatment are included. All reported events (at least 3%) are included except those too general to be informative, and those not reasonably associated with the use of the drug because they were associated with the condition being treated or are very common in the treated population.**

In placebo-controlled studies of bosentan in pulmonary arterial hypertension and for other diseases (primarily chronic heart failure), a total of 677 patients were treated with bosentan at daily doses ranging from 100 mg to 2000 mg and 288 patients were treated with placebo. The duration of treatment ranged from 4 weeks to 6 months. For the adverse drug reactions that occurred in ≥ 3% of bosentan-treated patients, the only ones that occurred more frequently on bosentan than on placebo (≥ 2% difference) were headache (16% vs. 13%), flushing (7% vs. 2%), abnormal hepatic function (6% vs. 2%), leg edema (5% vs. 1%), and anemia (3% vs. 1%).

Laboratory Abnormalities

Increased Liver Aminotransferases (see **BOX WARNING** and **WARNINGS**).

Decreased Hemoglobin and Hematocrit (see **PRECAUTIONS**).

Long-term Treatment

The long-term follow-up of the patients who were treated with TRACLEER® in the two pivotal studies and their open-label extensions (N=235) shows that 93% and 84% of patients were still alive at 1 and 2 years, respectively, after the start of treatment with TRACLEER®. These estimates may be influenced by the presence of epoprostenol treatment, which was administered to 43/235 patients. Without a control group, these data must be interpreted cautiously and cannot be interpreted as an improvement in survival.

OVERDOSAGE

Bosentan has been given as a single dose of up to 2400 mg in normal volunteers, or up to 2000 mg/day for 2 months in patients, without any major clinical consequences. The most common side effect was headache of mild to moderate intensity. In the cyclosporine A interaction study, in which doses of 500 and 1000 mg b.i.d. of bosentan were given concomitantly with cyclosporine A, trough plasma concentrations of bosentan increased 30-fold, resulting in severe headache, nausea, and vomiting, but no serious adverse events. Mild decreases in blood pressure and increases in heart rate were observed.

There is no specific experience of overdosage with bosentan beyond the doses described above. Massive overdosage may result in pronounced hypotension requiring active cardiovascular support.

DOSAGE AND ADMINISTRATION

General

TRACLEER® treatment should be initiated at a dose of 62.5 mg b.i.d. for 4 weeks and then increased to the maintenance dose of 125 mg b.i.d. Doses above 125 mg b.i.d. did not appear to confer additional benefit sufficient to offset the increased risk of liver injury.

Tablets should be administered morning and evening with or without food.

Dosage Adjustment and Monitoring in Patients Developing Aminotransferase Abnormalities

ALT/AST levels	Treatment and monitoring recommendations
> 3 and ≤ 5 × ULN	Confirm by another aminotransferase test; if confirmed, reduce the daily dose or interrupt treatment, and monitor aminotransferase levels at least every 2 weeks. If the aminotransferase levels return to pre-treatment values, continue or re-introduce the treatment as appropriate (see below).
> 5 and ≤ 8 × ULN	Confirm by another aminotransferase test; if confirmed, stop treatment and monitor amino-

Continued on next page

Tracleer—Cont.

	transferase levels at least every 2 weeks. Once the aminotransferase levels return to pre-treatment values, consider re-introduction of the treatment (see below).
> 8 × ULN	Treatment should be stopped and re-introduction of TRACLEER® should not be considered. There is no experience with re-introduction of TRACLEER® in these circumstances.

If TRACLEER® is re-introduced it should be at the starting dose; aminotransferase levels should be checked within 3 days and thereafter according to the recommendations above.

If liver aminotransferase elevations are accompanied by clinical symptoms of liver injury (such as nausea, vomiting, fever, abdominal pain, jaundice, or unusual lethargy or fatigue) or increases in bilirubin ≥ 2 × ULN, treatment should be stopped. There is no experience with the re-introduction of TRACLEER® in these circumstances.

Use in Women of Child-bearing Potential

TRACLEER® treatment should only be initiated in women of child-bearing potential following a negative pregnancy test and only in those who practice adequate contraception that does not rely solely upon hormonal contraceptives, including oral, injectable or implantable contraceptives (see **DRUG INTERACTIONS:** Hormonal Contraceptives, Including Oral, Injectable and Implantable Contraceptives). Input from a gynecologist or similar expert on adequate contraception should be sought as needed. Urine or serum pregnancy tests should be obtained monthly in women of child-bearing potential taking TRACLEER®.

Dosage Adjustment in Renally Impaired Patients

The effect of renal impairment on the pharmacokinetics of bosentan is small and does not require dosing adjustment.

Dosage Adjustment in Geriatric Patients

Clinical studies of TRACLEER® did not include sufficient numbers of subjects aged 65 and older to determine whether they respond differently from younger subjects. Clinical experience has not identified differences in responses between elderly and younger patients. In general, caution should be exercised in dose selection for elderly patients given the greater frequency of decreased hepatic, renal, or cardiac function, and of concomitant disease or other drug therapy in this age group.

Dosage Adjustment in Hepatically Impaired Patients

The influence of liver impairment on the pharmacokinetics of TRACLEER® has not been evaluated. Because there is *in vivo* and *in vitro* evidence that the main route of excretion of TRACLEER® is biliary, liver impairment would be expected to increase exposure (Cmax, AUC) to bosentan. There are no specific data to guide dosing in hepatically impaired patients (See **WARNINGS**); caution should be exercised in patients with mildly impaired liver function. TRACLEER® should generally be avoided in patients with moderate or severe liver impairment.

Dosage Adjustment in Children

Safety and efficacy in pediatric patients have not been established.

Dosage Adjustment in Patients with Low Body Weight

In patients with a body weight below 40 kg but who are over 12 years of age the recommended initial and maintenance dose is 62.5 mg b.i.d.

Discontinuation of Treatment

There is limited experience with abrupt discontinuation of TRACLEER®. No evidence for acute rebound has been observed. Nevertheless, to avoid the potential for clinical deterioration, gradual dose reduction (62.5 mg b.i.d. for 3 to 7 days) should be considered.

HOW SUPPLIED

62.5 mg film-coated, round, biconvex, orange-white tablets, embossed with identification marking "62,5" packaged in a white high-density polyethylene bottle and a white polypropylene child-resistant cap.

NDC 66215-101-06: Bottle containing 60 tablets.

125 mg film-coated, oval, biconvex, orange-white tablets, embossed with identification marking "125", packaged in a white high-density polyethylene bottle and a white polypropylene child-resistant cap.

NDC 66215-102-06: Bottle containing 60 tablets.

Rx only.

STORAGE

Store at 20°C – 25°C (68°F – 77°F). Excursions are permitted between 15°C and 30°C (59°F and 86°F). [See USP Controlled Room Temperature].

Manufactured by:

Patheon, Inc.
Mississauga, Ontario, L5N 7K9, CANADA

Distributed by:

ICS
Louisville, KY 40229, USA

Marketed by:

Actelion Pharmaceuticals US, Inc.,
South San Francisco, CA 94080, USA

Reference

1. Zimmerman HJ. Hepatotoxicity - The adverse effects of drugs and other chemicals on the liver. Second ed. Philadelphia: Lippincott, 1999.

October 6, 2003

Medication Guide

Tracleer (tra-KLEER) Tablets

(bosentan)

Read this information carefully before you start taking Tracleer tablets. Read the information you get with Tracleer each time you refill your prescription. There may be new information. This information does not take the place of talking with your doctor.

What is the most important information I should know about Tracleer?

- **Liver damage.**

Tracleer can cause liver damage if liver problems are not found early. Therefore, you must have a blood test to check your liver function before you start Tracleer and each month after that. (See "What are the possible side effects of Tracleer?" for information about the signs of liver problems.)

- **Major birth defects.**

Tracleer can cause major birth defects if taken during pregnancy. Therefore, women must not be pregnant when they start taking Tracleer or during Tracleer treatment. Women who are sexually active must have a negative pregnancy test before beginning treatment. A negative test means you are not pregnant. The test should be during the first five days of a normal menstrual period and at least 11 days after the last unprotected sexual intercourse. **Pregnancy tests must be done each month during Tracleer treatment, if you are sexually active.**

Women who are able to get pregnant must use effective birth control while taking Tracleer. Birth control pills, shots, implants, or other hormone-based birth control may not be enough when Tracleer is used. Talk with your doctor and, if needed, with a gynecologist (a doctor who specializes in female reproduction) or another doctor who knows about birth control, to find out how to avoid pregnancy. **Tell your doctor right away if you miss a period or think you may be pregnant.**

What is Tracleer?

Tracleer is a medicine to treat pulmonary arterial hypertension, which is high blood pressure in the lung arteries. You take it by mouth.

Tracleer can improve your ability to exercise and can slow the worsening of your physical condition and symptoms. Tracleer lowers high blood pressure in your lungs and lets your heart pump blood more effectively.

Who should not take Tracleer?

Do not take Tracleer if:

- **you are pregnant, plan to become pregnant, or become pregnant during Tracleer treatment. Tracleer can cause major birth defects.** All women should read the birth defects section of "What is the most important information I should know about Tracleer?" Severe birth defects from Tracleer happen early in pregnancy. Therefore, you must not be pregnant while taking Tracleer.
- **your blood test shows possible liver injury**
- you are taking cyclosporine-A (used for psoriasis and rheumatoid arthritis, and to prevent rejection of heart or kidney transplants) or glyburide (used for diabetes)
- **you are allergic to any ingredients in Tracleer.** The active ingredient is bosentan. Ask your doctor or pharmacist if you need to know the inactive ingredients.

Tell your doctor if you have moderate or severe liver problems. Tracleer may not be right for you.

Tell your doctor about **all** the medicines you use. They may affect how Tracleer works, or Tracleer may affect how the other medicines work. Be sure to tell your doctor if you take

- ketoconazole (used for fungal infections)
- hormone-based birth control, such as pills, shots, and implants
- cyclosporine A (used for psoriasis and rheumatoid arthritis, and to prevent rejection of heart or kidney transplants)
- tacrolimus (used to prevent rejection of liver or kidney transplants)
- glyburide (used for diabetes)
- cholesterol lowering medicines
- warfarin (used to prevent blood clots).

How should I take Tracleer?

Tracleer will be mailed to you by a central pharmacy. Your doctor will give you complete details:

- In most cases, you will take 1 tablet in the morning and 1 in the evening.
- You can take it with or without food.
- Your doctor will tell you how much to take.
- It will be easier to remember to take Tracleer if you do it at the same time each morning and evening. If you have trouble remembering, ask a family member to remind you, or put written notes where you will be sure to see them.
- If you take more than the prescribed dose of Tracleer, call your doctor right away.
- If you miss a dose, take your tablet as soon as you remember. However, do not take 2 doses to make up for a missed dose. Take your next tablet at the regular time.
- Do not stop taking Tracleer unless your doctor tells you to do so. Suddenly stopping your treatment may cause your symptoms to get worse. If you need to stop taking Tracleer, your doctor may tell you to reduce the dose over a few days before stopping completely.

During treatment, your doctor will test your blood for signs of side effects to your liver and red blood cells.

What should I avoid while taking Tracleer?

- **Do not get pregnant** while taking Tracleer. (See the birth defect section of "What is the most important information I should know about Tracleer?") If you miss a period, call your doctor.
- **Breast feeding is not recommended** while taking Tracleer. It is not known if Tracleer can pass through your milk and harm the baby.
- **Do not use hormone-based birth control (pills, injections, implants) as your only method of birth control.** These may not work when used with Tracleer. Ask your doctor about effective birth control choices.
- **Do not take cyclosporine-A.** This medicine can cause too much Tracleer in your blood and increase your chance of liver damage.
- **Do not take glyburide.** This medicine can increase your chance of liver damage.

What are the possible side effects of Tracleer?

Tracleer can have serious side effects:

- **Liver damage.** Tracleer can cause liver damage if it is not found early. Because this side effect may not cause symptoms at first, only a blood test can show that you have early liver damage. Regular blood tests let your doctor change or stop your therapy before there is permanent damage. **Therefore, it is very important that you have a liver function blood test before you start treatment and every month after that.**

Call your doctor right away if you have any of these symptoms of liver problems:

nausea, vomiting, fever, unusual tiredness, abdominal (stomach area) pain, or yellowing of the skin or the whites of your eyes (jaundice).

- **Major birth defects.** All females should read the birth defects section of "What is the most important information I should know about Tracleer?"
- **Low sperm count.** Drugs like Tracleer lower sperm count in animals. If this happens in men taking Tracleer, they may lose the ability to father children.

Other possible side effects

The most common side effects of Tracleer are:

- low red blood cell levels (anemia)
- headache
- inflamed throat and irritated nose passages
- flushing (hot flashes)
- ankle and leg swelling
- low blood pressure
- irregular heart beats
- upset stomach
- tiredness
- itching

General advice about prescription medicines

Medicines are sometimes prescribed for purposes other than those listed in a Medication Guide. If you have any concerns or questions about Tracleer, ask your doctor or other health-care provider. This Medication Guide is only a summary of some important information about Tracleer. Your doctor can give you information about Tracleer that was written for healthcare professionals. Do not use Tracleer for a condition for which it was not prescribed. Do not share Tracleer with other people.

This Medication Guide has been approved by the US Food and Drug Administration.

October 6, 2003

ACTELION

 ACTU TRA PI 004 1103

Shown in Product Identification Guide, page 304

ZAVESCA® ℞

[ză-vĕs-kă]

(miglustat)

100 mg capsules

DESCRIPTION

ZAVESCA® (miglustat capsules, 100 mg) is an inhibitor of the enzyme glucosylceramide synthase, which is a glucosyl transferase enzyme responsible for the first step in the synthesis of most glycosphingolipids. ZAVESCA® is an N-alkylated imino sugar, a synthetic analogue of D-glucose.

The chemical name for miglustat is 1,5-(butylimino)-1,5-dideoxy-D-glucitol with the chemical formula $C_{10}H_{21}NO_4$ and a molecular weight of 219.28.

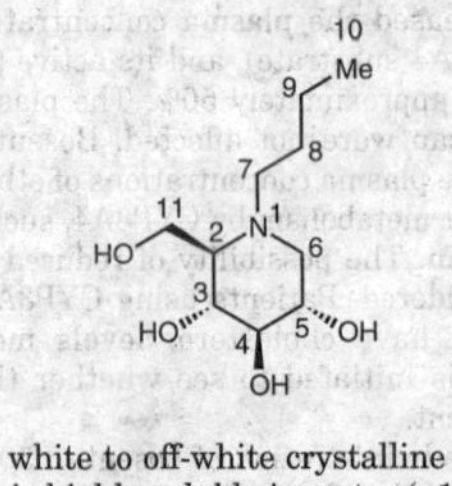

Miglustat is a white to off-white crystalline solid and has a bitter taste. It is highly soluble in water (>1000mg/mL as a free base).

ZAVESCA® is supplied in hard gelatin capsules each containing 100 mg miglustat for oral administration. Each ZAVESCA® 100 mg capsule also contains sodium starch glycollate, povidone (K30), and magnesium stearate. Ingredients in the capsule shell include gelatin and titanium dioxide, and the shells are printed with edible ink consisting of black iron oxide, shellac, soya lecithin, and antifoam.

CLINICAL PHARMACOLOGY

Background

Type 1 Gaucher disease is caused by a functional deficiency of glucocerebrosidase, the enzyme that mediates the degradation of the glycosphingolipid glucosylceramide. The failure to degrade glucosylceramide results in the lysosomal storage of this material within tissue macrophages leading to widespread pathology. Macrophages containing stored glucosylceramide are typically found in the liver, spleen, and bone marrow and occasionally in lung, kidney, and intestine. Secondary hematologic consequences include severe anemia and thrombocytopenia in addition to the characteristic progressive hepatosplenomegaly. Skeletal complications include osteonecrosis and osteopenia with secondary pathological fractures. Enzyme replacement therapy is the standard of care for most patients who require treatment for type 1 Gaucher disease.

Mode of Action

Miglustat functions as a competitive and reversible inhibitor of the enzyme glucosylceramide synthase, the initial enzyme in a series of reactions which results in the synthesis of most glycosphingolipids. The goal of treatment with ZAVESCA® is to reduce the rate of glycosphingolipid biosynthesis so that the amount of glycosphingolipid substrate is reduced to a level which allows the residual activity of the deficient glucocerebrosidase enzyme to be more effective (substrate reduction therapy). *In vitro* and *in vivo* studies have shown that miglustat can reduce the synthesis of glucosylceramide-based glycosphingolipids. In clinical trials, ZAVESCA® improved liver and spleen volume, as well as hemoglobin concentration and platelet count.

Pharmacokinetics

Absorption

After a 100 mg oral dose, the time to maximum observed plasma concentration of miglustat (t_{max}) ranged from 2 to 2.5 hours in Gaucher patients. Plasma concentrations show a biexponential decline, characterized by a short distribution phase and a longer elimination phase. The effective half-life of miglustat is approximately 6 to 7 hours, which predicts that steady-state will be achieved by 1.5 to 2 days following the start of three times daily dosing.

Miglustat, dosed at 50 and 100 mg in Gaucher patients, exhibits dose proportional pharmacokinetics. Miglustat's pharmacokinetics were not altered after repeated dosing three times daily for up to 12 months.

Co-administration of ZAVESCA® with food results in a decrease in the rate of absorption of miglustat (maximum serum concentration [C_{max}] was decreased by 36% and t_{max} delayed 2 h) but has no statistically significant effect on the extent of absorption of miglustat (area-under-the-plasma-concentration curve [AUC] was decreased by 14%). The mean oral bioavailability of a 100 mg miglustat capsule is about 97% relative to an oral solution administered under fasting conditions.

Distribution

Miglustat does not bind to plasma proteins. Mean apparent volume of distribution of miglustat is 83-105 liters in Gaucher patients, indicating that miglustat distributes into extravascular tissues.

Elimination

The major route of excretion of miglustat is renal. Miglustat is excreted unchanged in the urine. Renal impairment has a significant effect on the pharmacokinetics of miglustat resulting in increased systemic exposure of miglustat in such patients. There is no evidence that miglustat is metabolized in humans.

Special Populations

Geriatric Patients

ZAVESCA® has not been evaluated in geriatric patients over 65 years. (See **PRECAUTIONS; Geriatric Use**)

Pediatric Patients

ZAVESCA® has not been evaluated in patients under the age of 18 years. (See **PRECAUTIONS; Pediatric Use**)

Gender

There was no statistically significant gender difference in miglustat pharmacokinetics, based on pooled data analysis.

Race

Ethnic differences in miglustat pharmacokinetics have not been evaluated in Gaucher patients. However, apparent oral clearance of miglustat in patients of Ashkenazi Jewish descent was not statistically different to that in others (1 Asian and 15 Caucasians), based on a cross-study analysis.

Hepatic Insufficiency

No studies have been performed to assess the pharmacokinetics of miglustat in patients with hepatic impairment, since miglustat is not metabolized in the human liver.

Renal Insufficiency

Limited data in patients with Fabry disease and impaired renal function indicate that clearance (CL/F) of miglustat decreases with decreasing renal function. While the number of subjects with mild and moderate renal impairment was very small, the data suggest an approximate decrease in CL/F of 40% and 60%, respectively, in mild and moderate renal impairment, justifying the need to decrease the dosing of miglustat in such patients dependent upon creatinine clearance levels (see **DOSAGE AND ADMINISTRATION**).

Table 1: Liver Volume Changes in 2 Open-Label Uncontrolled Monotherapy Studies of ZAVESCA® with Extension Phases

		Liver Volume	
	n	**Absolute Mean (L) (2-sided 95% CI)**	**Percent Mean (%) (2-sided 95% CI)**
Study 1 (starting dose ZAVESCA® 100 mg three times daily)			
Baseline (Month 0)	21	2.39	
Month 12 Change from baseline		-0.28 (-0.38, -0.18)	-12.1% (-16.4, 7.9)
Study 1 Extension Phase			
Baseline (Month 0)	12	2.54	
Month 24 Change from baseline		-0.36 (-0.48, -0.24)	-14.5% (-19.3, 9.7)
Study 2 (ZAVESCA® 50 mg three times daily)			
Baseline (Month 0)	17	2.45	
Month 6 Change from baseline		-0.14 (-0.25, -0.03)	-5.9% (-9.9, -1.9)
Study 2 Extension Phase			
Baseline (Month 0)	13	2.35	
Month 12 Change from baseline		-0.17 (-0.3, 0.0)	-6.2% (-12.0, -0.5)

Table 2: Spleen Volume Changes in 2 Open-Label Uncontrolled Monotherapy Studies of ZAVESCA® with Extension Phases

		Spleen Volume	
	n	**Absolute Mean (L) (2-sided 95% CI)**	**Percent Mean (%) (2-sided 95% CI)**
Study 1 (starting dose ZAVESCA® 100 mg three times daily)			
Baseline (Month 0)	18	1.64	
Month 12 Change from baseline		-0.32 (-0.42, -0.22)	-19.0% (-23.7, -14.3)
Study 1 Extension Phase			
Baseline (Month 0)	10	1.56	
Month 24 Change from baseline		-0.42 (-0.53, -0.30)	-26.4% (-30.4, -22.4)
Study 2 (ZAVESCA® 50 mg three times daily)			
Baseline (Month 0)	11	1.98	
Month 6 Change from baseline		-0.09 (-0.18, -0.01)	-4.5% (-8.2, -0.7)
Study 2 Extension Phase			
Baseline (Month 0)	9	1.98	
Month 12 Change from baseline		-0.23 (-0.46, 0.00)	-10.1% (-20.1, -0.1)

Data in severe renal impairment are limited to two patients with creatinine clearances in the range 18-29 mL/min and cannot be extrapolated below this range. These data suggest a decrease in CL/F by at least 70% in patients with severe renal impairment. Treatment with miglustat in patients with severe renal impairment is therefore not recommended (see sections on **PRECAUTIONS** and **DOSAGE AND ADMINISTRATION**).

Drug Interactions (See also **PRECAUTIONS**, **Drug Interactions**)

Miglustat does not inhibit or induce various substrates of cytochrome P450 enzymes; consequently significant interactions are unlikely with drugs that are substrates of cytochrome P450 enzymes.

Drug interaction between ZAVESCA® (miglustat 100 mg orally three times daily) and Cerezyme® (imiglucerase; 7.5 or 15 U/kg/day) was assessed in Cerezyme stabilized patients after one month of co-administration. There was no significant effect of Cerezyme on pharmacokinetics of miglustat, with the co-administration of Cerezyme and miglustat resulting in a 22% reduction in C_{max} and a 14% reduction in the AUC for miglustat. While ZAVESCA® appeared to increase the clearance of imiglucerase by 70%, these results are not conclusive because of the small number of subjects studied and because patients took variable doses of Cerezyme (see **PRECAUTIONS**, **Drug Interactions**).

Concomitant therapy with loperamide during clinical trials did not appear to significantly alter the pharmacokinetics of miglustat.

Clinical Studies

The efficacy of ZAVESCA® in type 1 Gaucher disease has been investigated in two open-label, uncontrolled studies and one randomized, open-label, active-controlled study with enzyme replacement given as Cerezyme. Patients who received ZAVESCA® were treated with doses ranging from 100 to 600 mg a day, although the majority of patients were maintained on doses between 200 to 300 mg a day. Efficacy parameters included the evaluation of liver and spleen organ volume, hemoglobin concentration, and platelet count. A total of 80 patients were exposed to ZAVESCA® during the three studies and their extensions.

Open-Label Uncontrolled Monotherapy Studies

In Study 1, ZAVESCA® was administered at a starting dose of 100 mg three times daily for 12 months (dose range of 100 once-daily -200 mg three times daily) to 28 adult patients with type 1 Gaucher disease, who were unable or unwilling to take enzyme replacement therapy, and who had not taken enzyme replacement therapy in the preceding 6 months. Twenty-two patients completed the study. After 12 months of treatment, the results showed significant mean percent reductions from baseline in liver volume of 12% and spleen volume of 19%, a non-significant increase from baseline in mean absolute hemoglobin concentration of 0.26 g/dL and a mean absolute increase from baseline in platelet counts of 8×10^9/L (See Tables 1-4).

In Study 2, ZAVESCA® was administered at a dose of 50 mg three times daily for 6 months to 18 adult patients with type 1 Gaucher disease who were unable or unwilling to take enzyme replacement therapy and who had not in the preceding 6 months. Seventeen patients completed the study. After 6 months of treatment, the results showed significant mean percent reductions from baseline in liver volume of 6% and spleen volume of 5%. There was a non-significant mean absolute decrease from baseline in hemoglobin concentration of 0.13 g/dL and a non-significant mean absolute increase from baseline in platelet counts of 5×10^9/L (See Tables 1-4).

Extension period

Eighteen patients were enrolled in a 12-month extension to Study 1. A subset of patients continuing in the extension had somewhat larger mean baseline liver volumes, and lower mean baseline platelet counts and hemoglobin concentrations than the original study population. After a total of 24 months of treatment, there were significant mean decreases from baseline in liver and spleen organ volume of 15% and 27%, respectively, and significant mean absolute increases from baseline in hemoglobin concentration and platelet counts of 0.9 g/dL and 14×10^9/L, respectively (See Tables 1-4).

Sixteen patients were enrolled in a 6-month extension to Study 2. After a total of 12 months of treatment, there was a mean decrease from baseline in spleen organ volume of 10%, whereas the mean percent decrease in liver organ volume remained at 6%. There were no significant changes in hemoglobin concentrations or platelet counts (See Tables 1-4).

Liver volume results from Studies 1 and 2 and their extensions are summarized in Table 1:

[See table 1 above]

Spleen volume results from Studies 1 and 2 and their extensions are summarized in Table 2:

[See table 2 above]

Hemoglobin concentration results from Studies 1 and 2 and their extensions are summarized in Table 3:

[See table 3 at top of next page]

A more pronounced improvement in hemoglobin concentrations was seen at 18 and 24 months in patients with baseline (Month 0) hemoglobin concentrations <11.5 g/dL.

Platelet count results from Studies 1 and 2 and their extensions are summarized in Table 4:

Continued on next page

Zavesca—Cont.

[See table 4 at right]

Open-Label Active-Controlled Study

Study 3 was an open-label, randomized, active-controlled study of 36 adult patients with type 1 Gaucher disease, who had been receiving enzyme replacement therapy with Cerezyme for a minimum of 2 years prior to study entry. Patients were randomized 1:1:1 to one of three treatment groups, as follows:

- ZAVESCA® 100 mg three times daily alone
- Cerezyme (patient's usual dose) alone
- ZAVESCA® 100 mg three times daily + Cerezyme (usual dose)

Patients were treated for 6 months, and 33 patients completed the study. At Month 6, the results showed a significant decrease in mean percent change in liver volume in the combination treatment group compared to the Cerezyme alone group. There were no significant differences between the groups for mean absolute changes in liver and spleen volume and hemoglobin concentration. However, there was a significant difference between the ZAVESCA® alone and Cerezyme alone groups in platelet counts at Month 6, with the ZAVESCA® alone group having a mean absolute decrease in platelet count of 21.6×10^9/L and the Cerezyme alone group having a mean absolute increase in platelet count of 10.1×10^9/L (see Tables 5-8).

Extension period

Twenty-nine patients were enrolled in a 6-month extension to Study 3. In the extension phase, all 29 patients had withdrawn from Cerezyme and received open-label ZAVESCA® 100 mg three times daily monotherapy. At Month 12, the results showed non-significant decreases in platelet counts from baseline in all three treatment groups (by original randomization). There were significant decreases in platelet counts from Month 6 to Month 12 in the 2 groups originally randomized to treatment with Cerezyme and to combination therapy, and a continued decrease in platelet counts in the group originally randomized to ZAVESCA® alone. There were no significant changes in any treatment group for liver volume, spleen volume, or hemoglobin concentration (see Tables 5-8).

Liver volume results from Study 3 and extension are summarized in Table 5:

[See table 5 at right]

Spleen volume results from Study 3 and extension are summarized in Table 6:

[See table 6 at top of next page]

Hemoglobin concentrations results from Study 3 and extension are summarized in Table 7:

[See table 7 on next page]

Platelet count results from Study 3 and extension are summarized in Table 8:

[See table 8 on next page]

In patients with platelet counts above 150×10^9/L at baseline, there were significant decreases in platelet counts at Month 12 in patients randomized to ZAVESCA® treatment.

Summary of clinical studies

Treatment with ZAVESCA® as monotherapy at a starting dose of 100 mg three times daily (dosage range 100 mg once daily to 200 mg three times daily) in adult type 1 Gaucher disease patients who were either treatment naive or who had not taken enzyme replacement therapy in the previous 6 months resulted in decreases in liver and spleen volume after 12 months of treatment, and increases in platelet counts and hemoglobin concentration after 24 months of treatment. However, in adult type 1 Gaucher disease patients who had been treated with enzyme replacement therapy for at least 2 years, switching to ZAVESCA® as monotherapy was associated with decreases in platelet counts after discontinuation of enzyme replacement therapy. Platelet counts also declined after discontinuation of enzyme replacement therapy in patients treated with combination therapy.

The efficacy and safety of ZAVESCA® has not been evaluated in patients with severe type 1 Gaucher disease, defined as a hemoglobin concentration below 9 g/dL or a platelet count below 50×10^9/L or active bone disease.

INDICATIONS AND USAGE

ZAVESCA® is indicated for the treatment of adult patients with mild to moderate type 1 Gaucher disease for whom enzyme replacement therapy is not a therapeutic option (e.g. due to constraints such as allergy, hypersensitivity, or poor venous access).

CONTRAINDICATIONS

ZAVESCA® is contraindicated in patients who have demonstrated hypersensitivity to the active substance or any of the excipients.

Pregnancy Category X.

Miglustat may cause fetal harm when administered to a pregnant woman. In female rats given miglustat by oral gavage at doses of 20, 60, 180 mg/kg/day beginning 14 days before mating and continuing through gestation day 17 (organogenesis), decreased live births including complete litter loss and decreased fetal weight was observed in the mid- and high-dose groups (systemic exposures ≥2 times the human therapeutic systemic exposure based on body surface area comparison). In pregnant rats given miglustat by oral gavage at doses of 20, 60, 180 mg/kg/day from gestation day 6 through lactation (postpartum day 20), dystocia and delayed parturition were observed in the mid- and high-dose

Table 3: Hemoglobin Concentration Changes in 2 Open-Label Uncontrolled Monotherapy Studies of ZAVESCA® with Extension Phases

		Hemoglobin Concentration	
	n	Absolute Mean (g/dL) (2-sided 95% CI)	Percent Mean (%) (2-sided 95% CI)
Study 1 (starting dose ZAVESCA® 100 mg three times daily)			
Baseline (Month 0)	22	11.94	
Month 12 Change from baseline		0.26 (-0.05, 0.57)	2.6% (-0.5, 5.7)
Study 1 Extension Phase			
Baseline (Month 0)	13	11.03	
Month 24 Change from baseline		0.91 (0.30, 1.53)	9.1% (2.9, 15.2)
Study 2 (ZAVESCA® 50 mg three times daily)			
Baseline (Month 0)	17	11.60	
Month 6 Change from baseline		-0.13 (-0.51, 0.24)	-1.3% (-4.4, 1.8)
Study 2 Extension Phase			
Baseline (Month 0)	13	11.94	
Month 12 Change from baseline		0.06 (-0.73, 0.85)	1.2% (-5.2, 7.7)

Table 4: Platelet Count Changes in 2 Open-Label Uncontrolled Monotherapy Studies of ZAVESCA® with Extension Phases

		Platelet Count	
	n	Absolute Mean (10^9/L) (2-sided 95% CI)	Percent Mean (%) (2-sided 95% CI)
Study 1 (starting dose ZAVESCA® 100 mg three times daily)			
Baseline (Month 0)	22	76.58	
Month 12 Change from baseline		8.28 (1.88, 14.69)	16.0% (-0.8, 32.8)
Study 1 Extension Phase			
Baseline (Month 0)	13	72.35	
Month 24 Change from baseline		13.58 (7.72, 19.43)	26.1% (14.7, 37.5)
Study 2 (ZAVESCA® 50 mg three times daily)			
Baseline (Month 0)	17	116.47	
Month 6 Change from baseline		5.35 (-6.31, 17.02)	2.0% (-6.9, 10.8)
Study 2 Extension Phase			
Baseline (Month 0)	13	122.15	
Month 12 Change from baseline		14.0 (-3.4, 31.4)	14.7% (-1.4, 30.7)

Table 5: Liver Volume Changes from Study 3 and Extension Phase

	Cerezyme alone	ZAVESCA® alone	Combination
Study 3	n=11	n=10	n=9
Month 0	1.81	1.58	2.01
Month 6 Change (L)	0.04	-0.05	-0.09
Month 6% Change	3.6%	-2.9%	-4.9%
Adjusted mean Difference from Cerezyme (95% CI)		-4.5% (-13.2, 4.2)	-8.4% (-16.6, -0.1)
Extension Phase*	n=10	n=8	n=8
Month 0	1.94	1.60	2.04
Month 12 Change (L)	-0.05	-0.01	-0.08
Month 12% Change	-0.7%	-0.8%	-4.0%

*All patients received ZAVESCA® 100 mg three times daily monotherapy from Month 6 to Month 12

groups (systemic exposures ≥2 times the human therapeutic systemic exposure, based on body surface area comparison), in addition decreased live births and pup body weights were observed at >20 mg/kg/day (systemic exposures less than the human therapeutic systemic exposure, based on body surface area comparison).

In pregnant rabbits given miglustat by oral gavage at doses of 15, 30, 45 mg/kg/day during gestation days 6 -18 (organogenesis), maternal death and decreased body weight gain were observed at 15 mg/kg/day (systemic exposures less than the human therapeutic systemic exposure, based on body surface area comparisons).

ZAVESCA® is contraindicated in women who are or may become pregnant. If this drug is administered to a woman with reproductive potential, the patient should be apprised of the potential hazard to a fetus.

WARNINGS

Cases of peripheral neuropathy have been reported in patients treated with ZAVESCA®. All patients undergoing ZAVESCA® treatment should undergo baseline and repeat neurological evaluations at approximately 6-month intervals. Patients who develop symptoms such as numbness and tingling should have a careful reassessment of the risk/benefit of ZAVESCA® therapy and cessation of treatment may be considered.

PRECAUTIONS

General

Therapy should be directed by physicians knowledgeable in the management of patients with Gaucher disease.

Tremor

Approximately 30% of patients have reported tremor or exacerbation of existing tremor on treatment. These tremors were described as an exaggerated physiological tremor of the hands. Tremor usually began within the first month of therapy and in many cases resolved between 1 to 3 months during treatment. Dose reduction may ameliorate the tremor usually within days but discontinuation with treatment may sometimes be required.

Diarrhea and Weight Loss

Diarrhea and weight loss were common in clinical studies of patients treated with ZAVESCA®, approximately 85% and up to 65% of treated patients, respectively, reporting these conditions. Diarrhea appears to be the result of the disaccharidase inhibitory activity of ZAVESCA®, with a resultant osmotic diarrhea. It is unclear if weight loss results from the diarrhea and associated gastrointestinal complaints, a decrease in food intake, or a combination of these or other factors. The incidence of diarrhea was noted to decrease over time with continued ZAVESCA® treatment, and was noted to result in an increase in the use of anti-diarrheal medications, most commonly loperamide. Patients may be instructed to avoid high carbohydrate content foods during treatment with ZAVESCA® if they present with diarrhea. The incidence of weight loss was most evident in the first 12 months of treatment.

Male Fertility

Male patients should maintain reliable contraceptive methods while taking ZAVESCA®. Studies in the rat have shown that miglustat adversely affects spermatogenesis and sperm parameters, thereby reducing fertility. Until further information is available, it is advised that before seeking to conceive, male patients should cease ZAVESCA® and maintain reliable contraceptive methods for 3 months thereafter (see **Carcinogenesis, Mutagenesis, and Impairment of Fertility**).

Information for Patients

Patients should be informed of the potential risks and benefits of ZAVESCA® and of alternative modes of therapy. Patients should be advised that diarrhea, gastrointestinal complaints, and weight loss are common side effects of ZAVESCA® therapy, and to adhere to dietary instructions. Patients should also be advised to promptly report any numbness, pain, or burning in the hands and feet, and the development of tremor or worsening in an existing tremor.

Drug Interactions

While co-administration of ZAVESCA® appeared to increase the clearance of Cerezyme by 70%, these results are not conclusive because of the small number of subjects studied and because patients took variable doses of Cerezyme. Combination therapy with Cerezyme (imiglucerase) and ZAVESCA® is not indicated (see **CLINICAL PHARMACOLOGY, Drug Interactions**).

Animal Toxicology

Histopathology findings in the absence of clinical signs in the central nervous system of the monkey (brain, spine) that included vascular mineralization, in addition to mineralization and necrosis of white matter were observed at >750 mg/kg/day (4 times the human therapeutic systemic exposure based on area-under-the-plasma-concentration curve [AUC] comparisons) in a 52-week oral toxicity study using doses of 750 and 2000 mg/kg/d. Vacuolization of white matter was observed in rats dosed orally by gavage at ≥ 180 mg/kg/d (6 times the human therapeutic exposure based on surface area comparisons, mg/m^2) in a 4-week study using doses of 180, 840, and 4200 mg/kg/d. Vacuolization can sometimes occur as an artifact of tissue processing. Findings in dogs included tremor and absent corneal reflexes at 105 mg/kg/day (10 times the human therapeutic systemic exposure, based on body surface area comparisons mg/m^2) after a 4-week oral gavage toxicity study using doses of 35, 70, 105 , and 140 mg/kg/d. Ataxia, diminished/absent pupillary, palpebral, or patellar reflexes were observed in a dog at ≥495 mg/kg/day (50 times the human therapeutic systemic exposure based on body surface area comparisons, mg/m^2), in a 2-week oral gavage toxicity study using doses of 85, 165, 495, and 825 mg/kg/d.

Cataracts were observed in rats at ≥ 180 mg/kg/day (4 times the human therapeutic systemic exposure, based on AUC) in a 52-week oral gavage toxicity study using doses of 180, 420, 840, and 1680 mg/kg/d.

Gastrointestinal necrosis, inflammation, and hemorrhage were observed in dogs at ≥ 85 mg/kg/day (9 times the human therapeutic systemic exposure based on body surface area comparisons, mg/m^2) after a 2-week oral (capsule) toxicity study using doses of 85, 165, 495, and 825 mg/kg/d. Similar GI toxicity occurred in rats at 1200 mg/kg/day (7 times the human therapeutic systemic exposure, based on AUC) in a 26-week oral gavage toxicity study using doses of 300, 600, and 1200 mg/kg/d. In monkeys, similar GI toxicity occurred at ≥750 mg/kg/day (6x times the human therapeutic systemic exposure based on AUC) following a 52-week oral gavage toxicity study using doses of 750 and 2000 mg/kg/d.

Carcinogenesis, Mutagenesis, and Impairment of Fertility

Long-term studies in animals to evaluate the carcinogenic potential of miglustat have not been conducted. Miglustat was not mutagenic or clastogenic in a battery of *in vitro* and *in vivo* assays including the bacterial reverse mutation (Ames), chromosomal aberration (in human lymphocytes), gene mutation in mammalian cells (Chinese hamster ovary), and mouse micronucleus assays.

Male rats, given 20 mg/kg/day miglustat by (systemic exposure less than the human therapeutic systemic exposure based on body surface area comparisons, mg/m^2) oral gavage 14 days prior to mating, had decreased spermatogenesis with altered sperm morphology and motility and decreased fertility. Decreased spermatogenesis was reversible following 6 weeks of drug withdrawal. A higher doses of 60 mg/kg/day (2 times the human therapeutic systemic exposure based on body surface area comparison, mg/m^2) resulted in seminiferous tubule and testicular atrophy/degeneration.

Female rats were given oral gavage doses of 20, 60, 180 mg/kg/day beginning 14 days before mating and continuing through gestation. Effects observed at 20 mg/kg/day (systemic exposure less than the human therapeutic systemic exposure, based on body surface area comparisons) included decreased corpora lutea, increased postimplantation loss, and decreased live births.

Pregnancy Category X. See **CONTRAINDICATIONS** section.

There are no adequate and well-controlled studies of miglustat in pregnant women. ZAVESCA® should not be used during pregnancy.

Table 6: Spleen Volume Changes from Study 3 and Extension Phase

	Cerezyme alone	ZAVESCA® alone	Combination
Study 3	n=8	n=7	n=7
Month 0	0.61	0.69	0.76
Month 6 Change (L)	-0.02	-0.03	-0.08
Month 6% Change	-2.1%	-4.8%	-8.5%
Adjusted % Difference from Cerezyme (95% CI)		-5.8% (-22.1, 10.5)	-6.4% (-21.0, 8.2)
Extension Phase*	n=7	n=6	n=6
Month 0	0.83	0.57	0.84
Month 12 Change (L)	0.04	-0.05	-0.05
Month 12% Change	1.5%	-6.1%	-4.8%

*All patients received ZAVESCA® 100 mg three times daily monotherapy from Month 6 to Month 12

Table 7: Hemoglobin Concentration Changes from Study 3 and Extension Phase

	Cerezyme alone	ZAVESCA® alone	Combination
Study 3	n=12	n=10	n=11
Month 0	13.18	12.44	12.38
Month 6 Change (g/dL)	-0.15	-0.31	-0.10
Month 6% Change	-1.2%	-2.4%	-0.5%
Adjusted % Difference from Cerezyme (95% Cl)		-1.9% (-6.4, 2.6)	-0.6% (-4.8, 3.5)
Extension Phase*	n=10	n=9	n=9
Month 0	13.39	12.46	12.20
Month 12 Change (g/dL)	-0.48	-0.13	-0.13
Month 12% Change	-3.1%	-1.1%	-0.8%

*All patients received ZAVESCA® 100 mg three times daily monotherapy from Month 6 to Month 12

Table 8: Platelet Count Changes from Study 3 and Extension Phase

	Cerezyme alone	ZAVESCA® alone	Combination
Study 3	n=12	n=10	n=11
Month 0	165.75	170.55	152.14
Month 6 Change (10^9/L)	15.29	-21.60	2.73
Month 6% Change	10.1%	-9.6%	3.2%
Adjusted % Difference from Cerezyme (95% Cl)		-17.1% (-32.9, -1.3)	-4.6% (-19.9, 10.7)
Extension Phase*	n=10	n=9	n=9
Month 0	170.05	184.83	136.33
Month 12 Change (10^9/L)	-3.75	-27.39	-12.22
Month 12% Change	-3.2%	-10.4%	-8.3%

*All patients received ZAVESCA® 100 mg three times daily monotherapy from Month 6 to Month 12

Labor and Delivery

Studies in pregnant rats exposed to ZAVESCA® during gestation through lactation are associated with dystocia and delayed parturition at systemic exposure 2 times the human therapeutic systemic exposure, based on body surface area comparisons.

Nursing Mothers

It is not known whether miglustat is excreted in human milk. Because many drugs are excreted in human milk and because of the potential for serious adverse reactions in nursing infants from miglustat, ZAVESCA® should not be used in nursing mothers unless the potential benefit justifies the potential risk to the infant. A decision should be made whether to discontinue nursing or discontinue the drug, taking into account the importance of the drug to the lactating woman.

Pediatric Use

The safety and effectiveness of ZAVESCA® have not been evaluated in patients under the age of 18. Treatment with ZAVESCA® is associated with diarrhea and weight loss in approximately 85% and up to 65%, respectively, of adult patients. The effects of ZAVESCA® on growth and development in children have not been evaluated.

Geriatric Use

Clinical studies of ZAVESCA® did not include sufficient numbers of patients aged 65 and over to determine whether they respond differently than younger patients. Other reported clinical experience has not identified differences in responses between elderly and younger patients. In general, dose selection for an elderly patient should be cautious, usually starting at the low end of the dosing range, reflecting the greater frequency of decreased hepatic, renal, and cardiac function and of concomitant disease or other drug therapy.

Renal Impairment

Miglustat is known to be substantially excreted by the kidney, and the risk of adverse reactions to this drug may be greater in patients with impaired renal function. The clearance of miglustat is decreased by 40 to 60% in patients with mild to moderate renal impairment, and up to 70% in patients with severe renal impairment. As a result of this, dose reductions are recommended for those patients with mild to moderate renal impairment, the reduction being dependent upon the level of their creatinine clearance adjustment. For those patients with severe renal impairment, treatment with miglustat is not recommended. Since elderly patients are more likely to have decreased renal function, care should be taken in dose selection, and it may be useful to monitor renal function.

ADVERSE REACTIONS

Overview

The safety and tolerability of ZAVESCA® have been evaluated in 80 adult type 1 Gaucher disease patients in two open-label uncontrolled and one open-label active controlled trials. All 80 patients in the combined dataset from the clinical studies reported at least one adverse event during their treatment period.

Adverse Reaction Information

Open-Label Uncontrolled Monotherapy Trials

In two open-label, uncontrolled monotherapy trials in adult type 1 Gaucher disease patients treated with ZAVESCA® at

Continued on next page

Zavesca—Cont.

a starting dose of 100 mg three times daily (dose range 100 – 200 mg three times daily) for 12 months in 28 patients [Study 1], or at a dose of 50 mg three times daily for 6 months in 18 patients [Study 2], gastrointestinal events were observed in more than 80 % of patients either at the outset of treatment, or intermittently during treatment. Diarrhea was observed in approximately 85% of patients. Weight loss has been observed in up to 65% of patients. (see **PRECAUTIONS**, **General**, *Diarrhea and Weight Loss*).
In the two open-label, uncontrolled monotherapy trials, the Adverse Reactions by WHO body system and preferred term occurring with an incidence of ≥5%, are presented in Table 9 below.

Table 9: Adverse Reactions in ≥5% of Patients in Two Open-Label, Uncontrolled Monotherapy Trials of ZAVESCA®

	Incidence of adverse reaction	
	Study 1 (starting dose 100 mg three times daily)	**Study 2 (50 mg three times daily)**
Patients entered in Study (n)	28	18
Body System - Preferred Term	% of patients reporting	% of patients reporting
Gastrointestinal System		
Diarrhea	89	89
Flatulence	29	44
Abdominal Pain	18	50
Nausea	14	22
Vomiting	4	11
Bloating	0	6
Anorexia	7	0
Dyspepsia	7	0
Epigastric pain not food-related	0	6
Metabolic and Nutritional Disorders		
Weight Decrease	39	67
Central and Peripheral Nervous System		
Headache	21	22
Tremor	11	11
Dizziness	0	11
Cramps legs	4	11
Paresthesia	7	0
Migraine	0	6
Vision Disorders		
Visual Disturbance	0	17
Musculoskeletal Disorders		
Cramps	0	11
Platelet, Bleeding, and Clotting Disorders		
Thrombocytopenia	7	6
Reproductive disorders, female		
Menstrual disorder	0	6

Open-Label Active-Controlled Study
In an open-label, active-controlled study, 36 adult type 1 Gaucher disease patients were treated with ZAVESCA®, Cerezyme, or ZAVESCA® + Cerezyme (Study 3). Gastrointestinal adverse events and weight loss were commonly seen in patients exposed to ZAVESCA®. The Adverse Reactions by WHO body system and preferred term occurring with an incidence of ≥5%, are presented in Table 10 below. [See table 10 above]

Table 10: Adverse Reactions in ≥5% of Patients in Open-Label Active Controlled Study

	Incidence of adverse reaction		
	ZAVESCA® alone	**Cerezyme alone**	**ZAVESCA® + Cerezyme**
Patients entered in Study (n)	12	12	12
Body System - Preferred Term	% of patients reporting	% of patients reporting	% of patients reporting
Gastrointestinal System			
Diarrhea	100	0	83
Abdominal Pain	67	0	58
Flatulence	50	0	42
Constipation	8	0	25
Nausea	8	0	8
Mouth dry	8	0	0
Body as a Whole			
Influenza-Like Symptoms	0	0	8
Pain	0	8	8
Pain legs	0	0	8
Weakness generalized	17	0	8
Abdominal distension	8	0	8
Back pain	8	0	0
Abdominal distension gaseous	8	0	0
Chills	0	0	8
Heaviness in limbs	8	0	0
Metabolic and Nutritional Disorders			
Weight Decrease	67	0	42
Central and Peripheral Nervous System			
Tremor	17	0	33
Dizziness	8	0	25
Cramps legs	8	0	0
Gait unsteady	8	0	0
Numbness localized	0	0	8
Shaking	0	0	8
Psychiatric disorders			
Appetite absent	0	0	8
Jitteriness	0	0	8
Memory loss	8	0	0
Vision Disorders			
Eye abnormality	0	0	8
Visual disturbance	0	0	8
Reproductive disorders, female			
Menstrual irregularity	0	0	8

OVERDOSAGE

In the clinical development program for ZAVESCA®, no patient experienced an overdose of study drug. However, ZAVESCA® has been administered at doses of up to 3000 mg/day (approximately 10 times the recommended starting dose administered to Gaucher patients) for up to six months in Human Immunodeficiency Virus (HIV)-positive patients. Adverse events observed in the HIV studies included granulocytopenia, dizziness, and paresthesia. Leukopenia and neutropenia have also been observed in a similar group of patients receiving 800 mg/day or above.

DOSAGE AND ADMINISTRATION

Instructions for Administration
Therapy should be directed by physicians who are knowledgeable in the management of Gaucher disease.
The recommended dose for the treatment of adult patients with type 1 Gaucher disease is one 100 mg capsule administered orally three times a day at regular intervals.
It may be necessary to reduce the dose to one 100 mg capsule once or twice a day in some patients for adverse effects, such as diarrhea or tremor.

Patients with Renal Insufficiency
In patients with mild renal impairment (adjusted creatinine clearance 50-70 mL/min/1.73 m^2), ZAVESCA® administration should commence at a dose of 100 mg twice per day. In patients with moderate renal impairment (adjusted creatinine clearance of 30-50 mL/min/1.73 m^2), ZAVESCA® administration should commence at a dose of one 100 mg capsule per day. Use of ZAVESCA® in patients with severe renal impairment (creatinine clearance of <30 mL/min/ 1.73 m^2) is not recommended.

STORAGE
Store at 20°C to 25°C (68°F to 77°F). Brief exposure to 15°C to 30°C (59°F to 86°F) permitted (see USP Controlled Room Temperature).

HOW SUPPLIED

ZAVESCA® is supplied in hard gelatin capsules containing 100 mg miglustat. ZAVESCA® 100 mg capsules are white opaque with "OGT 918" printed in black on the cap and "100" printed in black on the body.
ZAVESCA® 100 mg capsules are packed in blister cards. Five blister cards of 18 capsules are supplied in each carton.
NDC 66215-201-90: carton containing 90 capsules.
NDC 66215-201-18: blister card containing 18 capsules
Rx only
Manufactured by:
Galen Limited,
Craigavon, Co. Armagh, BT63 5UA, UK
Marketed and Distributed by:
Actelion Pharmaceuticals US Inc
South San Francisco, CA 94080, US.
(650) 624 6900
Package Insert Preparation: July 31, 2003

Patient Information

ZAVESCA® (zah-VEHS-kah) (miglustat) 100 mg Capsules
Read the Patient Information that comes with ZAVESCA® before you start using it and each time you get a refill. There may be new information. This leaflet does not take the place of talking with your healthcare provider about your condition or your treatment.
What is ZAVESCA®?
ZAVESCA® is a prescription medicine taken by mouth for adults with mild to moderate type 1 Gaucher disease. ZAVESCA® is used only in patients who cannot be treated with enzyme replacement therapy.
ZAVESCA® has not been studied in children under 18 years of age.
What is type 1 Gaucher disease?
Type 1 Gaucher disease is an inherited disease that you get from both your parents. People with type 1 Gaucher disease are missing an enzyme that breaks down a chemical in the body called glucosylceramide. Too much glycosylceramide causes liver and spleen enlargement, changes in the blood, and bone disease. ZAVESCA® may stop glucosylceramide from forming.
Who should not take ZAVESCA®?
Do not take ZAVESCA® if you are allergic to any of its ingredients. The active ingredient is miglustat. See the end of this leaflet for a complete list of ingredients. Tell your doctor before taking ZAVESCA®:
- **If you are pregnant or planning to become pregnant.** ZAVESCA® may harm your baby. You should use effective birth control while taking ZAVESCA®. **ZAVESCA® may also harm a man's sperm.** All men should use effective birth control during treatment with ZAVESCA® and for 3 months after stopping ZAVESCA®. Do not use ZAVESCA® if you plan to become pregnant, or if your partner can become pregnant.
- **If you are breast-feeding.** It is not known if ZAVESCA® passes into your milk and if it can harm your baby. You should decide either to breast feed or take ZAVESCA®, but not both.
- **If you have kidney problems**
- **About all of your medical conditions**
- **About all the medicines you take including prescription and non-prescription medicines, vitamins and other dietary supplements.** Some medicines may affect ZAVESCA®. ZAVESCA® may affect other medicines.

How should I take ZAVESCA®?
- Take ZAVESCA® exactly as your doctor has prescribed. Check with your doctor or your pharmacist if you are not sure.
- Take ZAVESCA® at the same time or times each day. Your doctor will prescribe the dose that is right for you.
- Swallow ZAVESCA® capsules whole with water. ZAVESCA® may be taken with or without food
- If you miss a dose of ZAVESCA®, skip that dose. Take the next ZAVESCA® capsule at the usual time.
- If you take too much ZAVESCA® or overdose, call your doctor or local poison control center right away.

What should I avoid while taking ZAVESCA®?
Do not get pregnant while taking ZAVESCA®. Men and women should use effective birth control during treatment with ZAVESCA®. Men should keep using effective birth control for 3 months after treatment with ZAVESCA® stops.
What are the possible side effects of ZAVESCA®?
ZAVESCA® can cause problems affecting your nerves (neurologic problems):
- **Hand tremors (shaky movements) or worsen a hand tremor that you already have.** Tremors may begin within

the first month of starting treatment. Sometimes the tremors may go away between 1 to 3 months with continued treatment. Sometimes a lower dose or stopping ZAVESCA® is needed to help the tremors go away. Call your doctor if you get hand tremors while taking ZAVESCA® or the hand tremors you already have get worse.

- **Numbness and tingling in your hands, arms, legs, or feet (peripheral neuropathy).** Call your doctor right away if you get numbness or tingling in your arms or legs.

Your doctor may test your nerves (neurological exam) before you start ZAVESCA® and may repeat this procedure at a later time.

Diarrhea is the most common side effect for people taking ZAVESCA®. Your doctor may give you another medicine (anti-diarrheal) to treat diarrhea if it is a problem for you, and may recommend changes to your diet. You may also lose weight when you start treatment with ZAVESCA®.

Some of the other side effects with ZAVESCA® are:
- Gas
- Stomach pain
- Headache
- Dizziness
- Nausea
- Constipation
- Muscle cramps
- Weakness
- Cramps
- Do not feel like eating
- Vision problems
- Low platelet count

Call your doctor if you get any side effect that bothers you. Sometimes the side effects will go away. Sometimes a lower dose of ZAVESCA® will help side effects go away.

These are not all the side effects with ZAVESCA®. For more information, ask your doctor or your pharmacist.

How do I store ZAVESCA®?
- Store ZAVESCA® between 20°C to 25°C (68°F to 77°F)
- Do not use ZAVESCA® that has expired.
- **Keep ZAVESCA® and all medicines out of the reach of children.**

General information about ZAVESCA®

Medicines are sometimes prescribed for conditions that are not mentioned in Patient Information leaflets. Do not use ZAVESCA® for a condition for which it was not prescribed. Do not give ZAVESCA® to other people, even if they have the same symptoms you have. It may harm them.

This leaflet summarizes the most important information about ZAVESCA®. If you would like more information, talk with your doctor. You can ask your doctor or pharmacist for information about ZAVESCA® that is written for health professionals. For more information about ZAVESCA® contact:

Medical Information Department
Actelion Pharmaceuticals US Inc.,
601 Gateway Boulevard, Suite 100
South San Francisco, CA 94080 US.
Tel: toll-free (866) 228 3546

What are the ingredients of ZAVESCA®?

Active Ingredient: miglustat

Inactive Ingredients: sodium starch glycollate, povidone (K30) and magnesium stearate in the capsule; the capsule shell contains gelatin and titanium dioxide; the edible printing ink contains, black iron oxide, shellac, soya lecithin and antifoam.

RX Only

Leaflet preparation: July 31, 2003

ACTELION

Shown in Product Identification Guide, page 304

Agouron Pharmaceuticals, A Pfizer Company

(See Pfizer, Inc.)

Alamo Pharmaceuticals, LLC

9 CAMPUS DRIVE
PARSIPPANY, NJ 07054

Direct Inquiries to:
Tel: 973-538-7100
Fax: 973-538-7117

FAZACLO™ ℞

[faz-a-klo]
(clozapine, USP)
Orally Disintegrating Tablets
Rx only

Prescribing Information

Before prescribing FAZACLO™ (clozapine, USP), the physician should be thoroughly familiar with the details of this prescribing information.

WARNING

1. AGRANULOCYTOSIS

BECAUSE OF A SIGNIFICANT RISK OF AGRANULOCYTOSIS, A POTENTIALLY LIFE-THREATENING ADVERSE EVENT, CLOZAPINE SHOULD BE RESERVED FOR USE IN THE TREATMENT OF SEVERELY ILL SCHIZOPHRENIC PATIENTS WHO FAIL TO SHOW AN ACCEPTABLE RESPONSE TO ADEQUATE COURSES OF STANDARD ANTIPSYCHOTIC DRUG TREATMENT.

PATIENTS BEING TREATED WITH CLOZAPINE MUST HAVE A BASELINE WHITE BLOOD CELL (WBC) AND DIFFERENTIAL COUNT BEFORE INITIATION OF TREATMENT AS WELL AS REGULAR WBC COUNTS DURING TREATMENT AND FOR 4 WEEKS AFTER DISCONTINUATION OF TREATMENT.

CLOZAPINE IS AVAILABLE ONLY THROUGH A DISTRIBUTION SYSTEM THAT ENSURES MONITORING OF WBC COUNTS ACCORDING TO THE SCHEDULE DESCRIBED BELOW PRIOR TO DELIVERY OF THE NEXT SUPPLY OF MEDICATION. (SEE WARNINGS.)

2. SEIZURES

SEIZURES HAVE BEEN ASSOCIATED WITH THE USE OF CLOZAPINE. DOSE APPEARS TO BE AN IMPORTANT PREDICTOR OF SEIZURE, WITH A GREATER LIKELIHOOD AT HIGHER CLOZAPINE DOSES. CAUTION SHOULD BE USED WHEN ADMINISTERING CLOZAPINE TO PATIENTS HAVING A HISTORY OF SEIZURES OR OTHER PREDISPOSING FACTORS. PATIENTS SHOULD BE ADVISED NOT TO ENGAGE IN ANY ACTIVITY WHERE SUDDEN LOSS OF CONSCIOUSNESS COULD CAUSE SERIOUS RISK TO THEMSELVES OR OTHERS. (SEE WARNINGS.)

3. MYOCARDITIS

ANALYSES OF POSTMARKETING SAFETY DATABASES SUGGEST THAT CLOZAPINE IS ASSOCIATED WITH AN INCREASED RISK OF FATAL MYOCARDITIS, ESPECIALLY DURING, BUT NOT LIMITED TO, THE FIRST MONTH OF THERAPY. IN PATIENTS IN WHOM MYOCARDITIS IS SUSPECTED, CLOZAPINE TREATMENT SHOULD BE PROMPTLY DISCONTINUED. (SEE WARNINGS.)

4. OTHER ADVERSE CARDIOVASCULAR AND RESPIRATORY EFFECTS

ORTHOSTATIC HYPOTENSION, WITH OR WITHOUT SYNCOPE, CAN OCCUR WITH CLOZAPINE TREATMENT. RARELY, COLLAPSE CAN BE PROFOUND AND BE ACCOMPANIED BY RESPIRATORY AND/OR CARDIAC ARREST. ORTHOSTATIC HYPOTENSION IS MORE LIKELY TO OCCUR DURING INITIAL TITRATION IN ASSOCIATION WITH RAPID DOSE ESCALATION. IN PATIENTS WHO HAVE HAD EVEN A BRIEF INTERVAL OFF CLOZAPINE (i.e., 2 OR MORE DAYS SINCE THE LAST DOSE) TREATMENT SHOULD BE STARTED WITH 12.5 mg ONCE OR TWICE DAILY. (SEE WARNINGS, DOSAGE, AND ADMINISTRATION.)

SINCE COLLAPSE, RESPIRATORY ARREST, AND CARDIAC ARREST DURING INITIAL TREATMENT HAS OCCURRED IN PATIENTS WHO WERE BEING ADMINISTERED BENZODIAZEPINES OR OTHER PSYCHOTROPIC DRUGS, CAUTION IS ADVISED WHEN CLOZAPINE IS INITIATED IN PATIENTS TAKING A BENZODIAZEPINE OR ANY OTHER PSYCHOTROPIC DRUG. (SEE WARNINGS.)

DESCRIPTION

FAZACLO™ (clozapine, USP), an atypical antipsychotic drug, is a tricyclic dibenzodiazepine derivative, 8-chloro-11-(4-methyl-1-piperazinyl)-5*H*-dibenzo[*b,e*][1,4]diazepine.

The structural formula is:

[See chemical structure at top of next column]

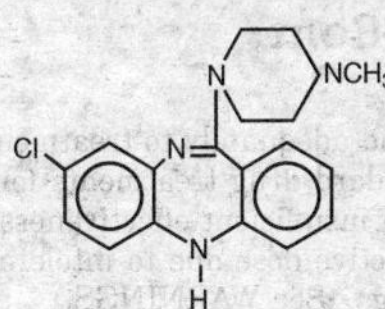

$C_{18}H_{19}ClN_4$ Mol. wt. 326.83

FAZACLO™ (clozapine, USP) is available as scored, yellow, orally disintegrating tablets of 25 and 100 mg for oral administration without water.

Each orally disintegrating tablet contains clozapine equivalent to 25 or 100 mg.

25- and 100-mg Orally Disintegrating Tablets

Active Ingredient: clozapine is a yellow, crystalline powder, very slightly soluble in water

Inactive Ingredients: aminoalkyl methacrylate copolymer E, mannitol, aspartame, microcrystalline cellulose, crospovidone, natural and artificial mint flavor, sodium bicarbonate, citric acid, ferric oxide (yellow), and magnesium stearate

THIS PRODUCT CONTAINS ASPARTAME AND IS NOT INTENDED FOR USE BY INFANTS. PHENYLKETONURICS: CONTAINS PHENYLALANINE. Phenylalanine is a component of aspartame. Each 25-mg, orally disintegrating tablet contains 3.1 mg aspartame, thus, 1.74 mg phenylalanine. Each 100-mg, orally disintegrating tablet contains 12.4 mg aspartame, thus, 6.96 mg phenylalanine. The allowable daily intake of aspartame is 50 mg per kilogram of body weight per day. (See PRECAUTIONS, Phenylketonurics.)

CLINICAL PHARMACOLOGY

Pharmacodynamics

FAZACLO™ (clozapine, USP) is classified as an "atypical" antipsychotic drug because its profile of binding to dopamine receptors and its effects on various dopamine mediated behaviors differ from those exhibited by more typical antipsychotic drug products. In particular, although FAZACLO™ (clozapine, USP) does interfere with the binding of dopamine at D_1, D_2, D_3, and D_5 receptors, and has a high affinity for the D_4 receptor, it does not induce catalepsy nor inhibit apomorphine-induced stereotypy. This evidence, consistent with the view that FAZACLO™ (clozapine, USP) is preferentially more active at limbic than at striatal dopamine receptors, may explain the relative freedom of FAZACLO™ (clozapine, USP) from extrapyramidal side effects.

FAZACLO™ (clozapine, USP) also acts as an antagonist at adrenergic, cholinergic, histaminergic, and serotonergic receptors.

Absorption, Distribution, Metabolism, and Excretion

In man, clozapine tablets (25 and 100 mg) are equally bioavailable relative to a clozapine solution. FAZACLO™ (clozapine, USP) orally disintegrating tablets are bioequivalent to Clozaril (clozapine) tablets. Following a dosage of 100 mg b.i.d., the average steady-state peak plasma concentration was 413 ng/mL (range: 132–854 ng/mL), occurring at the average of 2.3 hours (range: 1–6 hours) after dosing. The average minimum concentration at steady state was 168 ng/mL (range: 45–574 ng/mL), after 100 mg b.i.d. dosing. Food does not appear to affect the systemic bioavailability of clozapine. Thus, FAZACLO™ (clozapine, USP) may be administered with or without food.

Clozapine is approximately 97% bound to serum proteins. The interaction between clozapine and other highly protein-bound drugs has not been fully evaluated but may be important. (See PRECAUTIONS.)

Clozapine is almost completely metabolized prior to excretion and only trace amounts of unchanged drug are detected in the urine and feces. Approximately 50% of the administered dose is excreted in the urine and 30% in the feces. The demethylated, hydroxylated, and *N*-oxide derivatives are components in both urine and feces. Pharmacological testing has shown the desmethyl metabolite (norclozapine) to have only limited activity, while the hydroxylated and *N*-oxide derivatives were inactive.

The mean elimination half-life of clozapine after a single 75-mg dose was 8 hours (range: 4–12 hours), compared to a mean elimination half-life, after achieving steady state with 100 mg b.i.d. dosing, of 12 hours (range: 4–66 hours). A comparison of single-dose and multiple-dose administration of clozapine showed that the elimination half-life increased significantly after multiple dosing relative to that after single-dose administration, suggesting the possibility of concentration-dependent pharmacokinetics. However, at steady state, linearly dose-proportional changes with respect to AUC (area under the curve), peak, and minimum clozapine plasma concentrations were observed after administration of 37.5, 75, and 150 mg b.i.d.

Human Pharmacology

In contrast to more typical antipsychotic drugs, clozapine therapy produces little or no prolactin elevation.

As is true of more typical antipsychotic drugs, clinical electroencephalogram (EEG) studies have shown that clozapine increases delta and theta activity and slows dominant alpha frequencies. Enhanced synchronization occurs; sharp wave activity and spike and wave complexes may also develop. Patients, on rare occasions, may report an intensification of dream activity during clozapine therapy. REM sleep was found to be increased to 85% of the total sleep time. In these patients, the onset of REM sleep occurred almost immediately after falling asleep.

INDICATIONS AND USAGE

FAZACLO™ (clozapine, USP) is indicated for the management of severely ill schizophrenic patients who fail to respond adequately to standard drug treatment for schizophrenia. Because of the significant risk of agranulocytosis and seizure associated with its use, FAZACLO™ (clozapine, USP) should be used only in patients who have

Continued on next page

Fazaclo—Cont.

failed to respond adequately to treatment with appropriate courses of standard drug treatments for schizophrenia, either because of insufficient effectiveness or the inability to achieve an effective dose due to intolerable adverse effects from those drugs. (See WARNINGS.)

The effectiveness of clozapine in a treatment-resistant schizophrenic population was demonstrated in a 6-week study comparing clozapine and chlorpromazine. Patients meeting DSM-III criteria for schizophrenia and having a mean Brief Psychiatric Rating Scale (BPRS) total score of 61 were demonstrated to be treatment-resistant by history and by open, prospective treatment with haloperidol before entering into the double-blind phase of the study. The superiority of clozapine to chlorpromazine was documented in statistical analyses employing both categorical and continuous measures of treatment effect.

Because of the significant risk of agranulocytosis and seizures, events which both present a continuing risk over time, the extended treatment of patients failing to show an acceptable level of clinical response should ordinarily be avoided. In addition, the need for continuing treatment in patients exhibiting beneficial clinical responses should be periodically reevaluated.

CONTRAINDICATIONS

FAZACLO™ (clozapine, USP) is contraindicated in patients with a previous hypersensitivity to clozapine or any other component of this drug, in patients with myeloproliferative disorders, uncontrolled epilepsy, or a history of clozapine-induced agranulocytosis or severe granulocytopenia. As with more typical antipsychotic drugs, FAZACLO™ (clozapine, USP) is contraindicated in severe central nervous system (CNS) depression or comatose states from any cause.

FAZACLO™ (clozapine, USP) should not be used simultaneously with other agents having a well-known potential to cause agranulocytosis or otherwise suppress bone marrow function. The mechanism of clozapine-induced agranulocytosis is unknown; nonetheless, it is possible that causative factors may interact synergistically to increase the risk and/or severity of bone marrow suppression.

WARNINGS

General

BECAUSE OF THE SIGNIFICANT RISK OF AGRANULOCYTOSIS, A POTENTIALLY LIFE-THREATENING ADVERSE EVENT (SEE FOLLOWING), FAZACLO™ (clozapine, USP) SHOULD BE RESERVED FOR USE IN THE TREATMENT OF SEVERELY ILL SCHIZOPHRENIC PATIENTS WHO FAIL TO SHOW AN ACCEPTABLE RESPONSE TO ADEQUATE COURSES OF STANDARD DRUG TREATMENT FOR SCHIZOPHRENIA, EITHER BECAUSE OF INSUFFICIENT EFFECTIVENESS OR THE INABILITY TO ACHIEVE AN EFFECTIVE DOSE DUE TO INTOLERABLE ADVERSE EFFECTS FROM THOSE DRUGS. CONSEQUENTLY, BEFORE INITIATING TREATMENT WITH FAZACLO™ (clozapine, USP), IT IS STRONGLY RECOMMENDED THAT A PATIENT BE GIVEN AT LEAST 2 TRIALS, EACH WITH A DIFFERENT STANDARD DRUG PRODUCT FOR SCHIZOPHRENIA, AT AN ADEQUATE DOSE AND FOR AN ADEQUATE DURATION.

PATIENTS WHO ARE BEING TREATED WITH FAZACLO™ (clozapine, USP) MUST HAVE A BASELINE WBC AND DIFFERENTIAL COUNT BEFORE INITIATION OF TREATMENT, AND A WBC COUNT EVERY WEEK FOR THE FIRST 6 MONTHS. THEREAFTER, IF ACCEPTABLE WBC COUNTS (WBC ≥3,000/mm^3, ABSOLUTE NEUTROPHIL COUNT [ANC] ≥1500/mm^3) HAVE BEEN MAINTAINED DURING THE FIRST 6 MONTHS OF CONTINUOUS THERAPY, WBC COUNTS CAN BE MONITORED EVERY OTHER WEEK. WBC COUNTS MUST BE MONITORED WEEKLY FOR AT LEAST 4 WEEKS AFTER THE DISCONTINUATION OF FAZACLO™ (clozapine, USP).

FAZACLO™ (clozapine, USP) IS AVAILABLE ONLY THROUGH A DISTRIBUTION SYSTEM THAT ENSURES MONITORING OF WBC COUNTS ACCORDING TO THE SCHEDULE DESCRIBED BELOW PRIOR TO DELIVERY OF THE NEXT SUPPLY OF MEDICATION.

Agranulocytosis

Agranulocytosis, defined as an ANC of less than 500/mm^3, has been estimated to occur in association with clozapine use at a cumulative incidence at 1 year of approximately 1.3%, based on the occurrence of 15 U.S. cases out of 1,743 patients exposed to clozapine during its clinical testing prior to domestic marketing. All of these cases occurred at a time when the need for close monitoring of WBC counts was already recognized. This reaction could prove fatal if not detected early and therapy interrupted. Of the 149 cases of agranulocytosis reported worldwide in association with clozapine use as of December 31, 1989, 32% were fatal. However, few of these deaths occurred since 1977, at which time, the knowledge of clozapine-induced agranulocytosis became more widespread and close monitoring of WBC counts more widely practiced. Nevertheless, it is unknown at present what the case fatality rate will be for FAZACLO™ (clozapine, USP) induced agranulocytosis, despite strict adherence to the required frequency of monitoring. In the United States, under a weekly WBC monitoring system with clozapine, there have been 585 cases of agranulocytosis as of August 21, 1997; 19 were fatal. During this period, 150,409 patients received clozapine. A hematologic risk analysis was conducted based upon the available information in the *Clozapine National Registry (CNR)* for U.S. patients. Based upon a cut-off date of April 30, 1995, the incidence rates of agranulocytosis based upon a weekly monitoring schedule rose steeply during the first two months of therapy, peaking in the third month. Among clozapine patients who continued the drug beyond the third month, the weekly incidence of agranulocytosis fell a substantial degree, so that by the sixth month, the weekly incidence of agranulocytosis was reduced to 3 per 1,000 person-years. After 6 months, the weekly incidence of agranulocytosis declines still further, however, never reaching zero. It should be noted that any type of reduction in the frequency of monitoring WBC counts may result in an increased incidence of agranulocytosis.

Because of the substantial risk for developing agranulocytosis in association with FAZACLO™ (clozapine, USP) use, which may persist over an extended period of time, patients must have a blood sample drawn for a WBC count before initiation of treatment with FAZACLO™ (clozapine, USP) and must have subsequent WBC counts done at least weekly for the first 6 months of continuous treatment. If WBC counts remain acceptable (WBC ≥3000/mm^3, ANC ≥1500/mm^3) during this period, WBC counts may be monitored every other week thereafter. After the discontinuation of FAZACLO™ (clozapine, USP), weekly WBC counts should be continued for an additional 4 weeks.

If a patient is on FAZACLO™ (clozapine, USP) therapy for less than 6 months with no abnormal blood events and there is a break in therapy which is less than or equal to 1 month, patients can continue where they left off with weekly WBC testing for 6 months. When this 6-month period has been completed, the frequency of WBC count monitoring can be reduced to every other week. If a patient is on FAZACLO™ (clozapine, USP) therapy for less than 6 months with no abnormal blood events and there is a break in therapy which is greater than 1 month, patients should be tested weekly for an additional 6-month period before biweekly testing is initiated. If a patient is on FAZACLO™ (clozapine, USP) therapy for less than 6 months and experiences an abnormal blood event as described below but remains a rechallengeable patient (patients cannot be reinitiated on FAZACLO™ (clozapine, USP) therapy if WBC counts fall below 2000/mm^3 or the ANC falls below 1000/mm^3 during FAZACLO™ (clozapine, USP) therapy), the patient must restart the 6-month period of weekly WBC monitoring at Day 0.

If a patient is on FAZACLO™ (clozapine, USP) therapy for 6 months or longer with no abnormal blood events and there is a break in therapy which is 1 year or less, the patient can continue WBC count monitoring every other week if FAZACLO™ (clozapine, USP) therapy is reinitiated. If a patient is on FAZACLO™ (clozapine, USP) therapy for 6 months or longer with no abnormal blood events and there is a break in therapy which is greater than 1 year, if FAZACLO™ (clozapine, USP) therapy is reinitiated, the patient must have WBC counts monitored weekly for an additional 6 months. If a patient is on FAZACLO™ (clozapine, USP) therapy for 6 months or longer and subsequently has an abnormal blood event but remains a rechallengeable patient, the patient must restart weekly WBC count monitoring until an additional 6 months of FAZACLO™ (clozapine, USP) therapy has been received. The distribution of FAZACLO™ (clozapine, USP) is contingent upon performance of the required blood tests.

Treatment should not be initiated if the WBC count is less than 3500/mm^3 or if the patient has a history of a myeloproliferative disorder, previous clozapine-induced agranulocytosis, or granulocytopenia. Patients should be advised to immediately report the appearance of lethargy, weakness, fever, sore throat, or any other signs of infection. If, after the initial treatment, the total WBC count has dropped below 3500/mm^3 or it has dropped by a substantial amount from baseline, even if the count is above 3500/mm^3, or if immature forms are present, a repeat WBC count and a differential count should be done. A substantial drop is defined as a single drop of 3000 or more in the WBC count or a cumulative drop of 3000 or more within 3 weeks. If subsequent WBC counts and the differential count reveal a total WBC count between 3000 and 3500/mm^3 and an ANC above 1500/mm^3, twice-weekly WBC counts and differential counts should be performed. If the total WBC count falls below 3000/mm^3 or the ANC below 1500/mm^3, FAZACLO™ (clozapine, USP) therapy should be interrupted, WBC count and differential should be performed daily, and patients should be carefully monitored for flu-like symptoms or other symptoms suggestive of infection. FAZACLO™ (clozapine, USP) therapy may be resumed if no symptoms of infection develop and if the total WBC count returns to levels above 3000/mm^3 and the ANC returns to levels above 1500/mm^3. However, in this event, twice-weekly WBC counts and differential counts should continue until total WBC counts return to levels above 3500/mm^3.

If the total WBC count falls below 2000/mm^3 or the ANC falls below 1000/mm^3, bone-marrow aspiration should be considered to ascertain granulopoietic status. Protective isolation with close observation may be indicated if granulopoiesis is determined to be deficient. Should evidence of infection develop, the patient should have appropriate cultures performed and an appropriate antibiotic regimen instituted.

Patients whose total WBC counts fall below 2000/mm^3 or ANCs below 1000/mm^3 during FAZACLO™ (clozapine, USP) therapy should have daily WBC count and differential. These patients should not be rechallenged with FAZACLO™ (clozapine, USP). Patients discontinued from clozapine therapy due to significant WBC suppression have been found to develop agranulocytosis upon rechallenge, often with a shorter latency on reexposure. To reduce the chances of rechallenge occurring in patients who have experienced significant bone-marrow suppression during FAZACLO™ (clozapine, USP) therapy, a single, national master file will be confidentially maintained.

Except for evidence of significant bone-marrow suppression during initial clozapine therapy, there are no established risk factors based on worldwide experience for the development of agranulocytosis in association with clozapine use. However, a disproportionate number of the U.S. cases of agranulocytosis occurred in patients of Jewish background compared to the overall proportion of such patients exposed during domestic development of clozapine. Most of the U.S. cases occurred within 4–10 weeks of exposure, but neither dose nor duration is a reliable predictor of this problem. No patient characteristics have been clearly linked to the development of agranulocytosis in association with clozapine use, but agranulocytosis associated with other antipsychotic drugs has been reported to occur with a greater frequency in women, the elderly, and in patients who are cachectic or have serious underlying medical illness; such patients may also be at particular risk with FAZACLO™ (clozapine, USP).

To reduce the risk of agranulocytosis developing undetected, FAZACLO™ (clozapine, USP) is available only through a distribution system that ensures monitoring of WBC counts according to the schedule described above prior to delivery of the next supply of medication.

[See graphic at left]

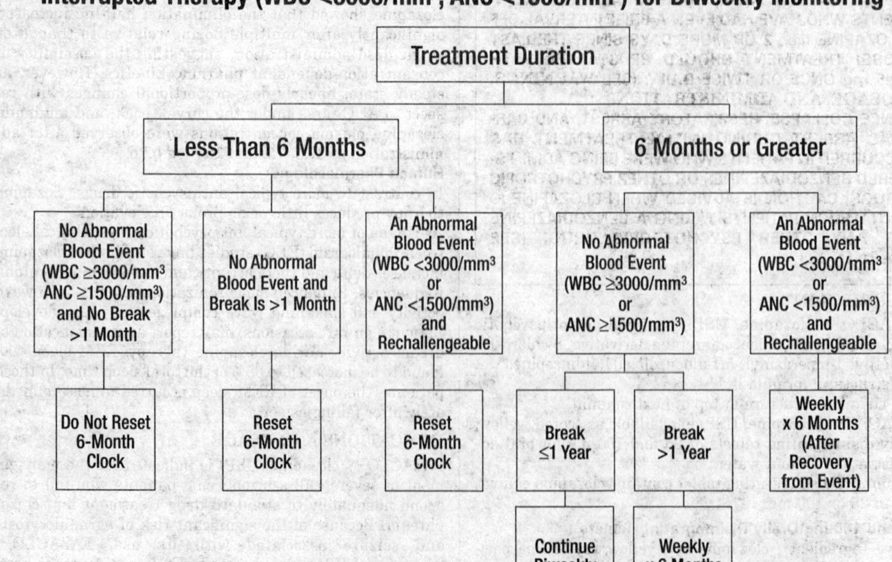

Eosinophilia

In clinical trials, 1% of patients developed eosinophilia, which, in rare cases, can be substantial. If a differential count reveals a total eosinophil count above 4000/mm^3, FAZACLO™ (clozapine, USP) therapy should be interrupted until the eosinophil count falls below 3000/mm^3.

Seizures

Seizure has been estimated to occur in association with clozapine use at a cumulative incidence at one year of approximately 5%, based on the occurrence of one or more seizures in 61 of 1,743 patients exposed to clozapine during its clinical testing prior to domestic marketing (i.e., a crude rate of 3.5%). Dose appears to be an important predictor of seizure, with a greater likelihood of seizure at the higher clozapine doses used.

Caution should be used in administering FAZACLO™ (clozapine, USP) to patients having a history of seizures or other predisposing factors. Because of the substantial risk of seizure associated with clozapine use, patients should be advised not to engage in any activity where sudden loss of consciousness could cause serious risk to themselves or others (e.g., the operation of complex machinery, driving an automobile, swimming, climbing, etc.).

Myocarditis

Postmarketing surveillance data from four countries that employ hematological monitoring of clozapine-treated patients revealed: 30 reports of myocarditis with 17 fatalities in 205,493 U.S. patients (August 2001); 7 reports of myocarditis with 1 fatality in 15,600 Canadian patients (April 2001); 30 reports of myocarditis with 8 fatalities in 24,108 U.K. patients (August 2001); 15 reports of myocarditis with 5 fatalities in 8,000 Australian patients (March 1999). These reports represent an incidence of 5.0, 16.3, 43.2, and 96.6 cases/100,000 patient years, respectively. The number of fatalities represent an incidence of 2.8, 2.3, 11.5, and 32.2 cases/100,000 patient years, respectively.

The overall incidence rate of myocarditis in patients with schizophrenia treated with antipsychotic agents is unknown. However, for the established market economies, World Health Organization (WHO), the incidence of myocarditis is 0.3 cases/100,000 patient years and the fatality rate is 0.2 cases/100,000 patient years. Therefore, the rate of myocarditis in clozapine-treated patients appears to be 17–322 times greater than the general population and is associated with an increased risk of fatal myocarditis that is 14–161 times greater than the general population.

The total reports of myocarditis for these four countries were 82, of which 51 (62%) occurred within the first month of clozapine treatment, 25 (31%) occurred after the first month of therapy, and 6 (7%) were unknown. The median duration of treatment was 3 weeks. Of 5 patients rechallenged with clozapine, 3 had a recurrence of myocarditis. Of the 82 reports, 31 (38%) were fatal, and 25 patients who died had evidence of myocarditis at autopsy. These data also suggest that the incidence of fatal myocarditis may be highest during the first month of therapy.

Therefore, the possibility of myocarditis should be considered in patients receiving FAZACLO™ (clozapine, USP) who present with unexplained fatigue, dyspnea, tachypnea, fever, chest pain, palpitations, other signs or symptoms of heart failure, or electrocardiographic findings such as ST-T wave abnormalities or arrhythmias. It is not known whether eosinophilia is a reliable predictor of myocarditis. Tachycardia, which has been associated with clozapine treatment, has also been noted as a presenting sign in patients with myocarditis. Therefore, tachycardia during the first month of therapy warrants close monitoring for other signs of myocarditis.

Prompt discontinuation of FAZACLO™ (clozapine, USP) treatment is warranted upon suspicion of myocarditis. Patients with clozapine-related myocarditis should not be rechallenged with FAZACLO™ (clozapine, USP).

Other Adverse Cardiovascular and Respiratory Effects

Orthostatic hypotension with or without syncope can occur with FAZACLO™ (clozapine, USP) treatment and may represent a continuing risk in some patients. Rarely (approximately 1 case per 3000 patients), collapse can be profound and accompanied by respiratory and/or cardiac arrest. Orthostatic hypotension is more likely to occur during initial titration in association with rapid-dose escalation and may even occur on first dose. In one report, initial doses as low as 12.5 mg were associated with collapse and respiratory arrest. When restarting patients who have had even a brief interval off FAZACLO™ (clozapine, USP) (i.e., 2 days or more since the last dose), it is recommended that treatment be reinitiated with one-half of a 25-mg, orally-disintegrating tablet (12.5 mg) once or twice daily. (See DOSAGE AND ADMINISTRATION.)

Some of the cases of collapse/respiratory arrest/cardiac arrest during initial treatment occurred in patients who were being administered benzodiazepines; similar events have been reported in patients taking other psychotropic drugs or even clozapine by itself. Although it has not been established that there is an interaction between FAZACLO™ (clozapine, USP) and benzodiazepines or other psychotropics, caution is advised when clozapine is initiated in patients taking a benzodiazepine or any other psychotropic drug.

Tachycardia, which may be sustained, has also been observed in approximately 25% of patients taking clozapine, with patients having an average increase in pulse rate of 10–15 bpm. The sustained tachycardia is not simply a reflex response to hypotension and is present in all positions monitored. Either tachycardia or hypotension may pose a serious risk for an individual with compromised cardiovascular function.

A minority of clozapine-treated patients experience ECG repolarization changes similar to those seen with other antipsychotic drugs, including S-T segment depression and flattening or inversion of T waves, which all normalize after discontinuation of clozapine. The clinical significance of these changes is unclear. However, in clinical trials with clozapine, several patients experienced significant cardiac events, including ischemic changes, myocardial infarction, arrhythmias, and sudden death. In addition, there have been postmarketing reports of congestive heart failure. Causality assessment was difficult in many of these cases because of serious preexisting cardiac disease and plausible alternative causes. Rare instances of sudden death have been reported in psychiatric patients, with or without associated antipsychotic drug treatment, and the relationship of these events to antipsychotic drug use is unknown.

FAZACLO™ (clozapine, USP) should be used with caution in patients with known cardiovascular and/or pulmonary disease, and the recommendation for gradual titration of dose should be carefully observed.

Neuroleptic Malignant Syndrome

A potentially fatal symptom complex sometimes referred to as Neuroleptic Malignant Syndrome (NMS) has been reported in association with antipsychotic drugs. Clinical manifestations of NMS are hyperpyrexia, muscle rigidity, altered mental status, and evidence of autonomic instability (irregular pulse or blood pressure, tachycardia, diaphoresis, and cardiac dysrhythmias).

The diagnostic evaluation of patients with this syndrome is complicated. In arriving at a diagnosis, it is important to identify cases where the clinical presentation includes both serious medical illness (e.g., pneumonia, systemic infection, etc.) and untreated or inadequately treated extrapyramidal signs and symptoms (EPS). Other important considerations in the differential diagnosis include central anticholinergic toxicity, heat stroke, drug fever, and primary CNS pathology.

The management of NMS should include (1) immediate discontinuation of antipsychotic drugs and other drugs not essential to concurrent therapy, (2) intensive symptomatic treatment and medical monitoring, and (3) treatment of any concomitant serious medical problems for which specific treatments are available. There is no general agreement about specific pharmacological treatment regimens for uncomplicated NMS.

If a patient requires antipsychotic drug treatment after recovery from NMS, the potential reintroduction of drug therapy should be carefully considered. The patient should be carefully monitored, since recurrences of NMS have been reported.

There have been several reported cases of NMS in patients receiving clozapine alone or in combination with lithium or other CNS-active agents.

Tardive Dyskinesia

A syndrome consisting of potentially irreversible, involuntary, dyskinetic movements may develop in patients treated with antipsychotic drugs. Although the prevalence of the syndrome appears to be highest among the elderly, especially elderly women, it is impossible to rely upon prevalence estimates to predict at the inception of treatment which patients are likely to develop the syndrome.

There are several reasons for predicting that clozapine may be different from other antipsychotic drugs in its potential for inducing tardive dyskinesia, including the preclinical finding that it has a relatively weak dopamine-blocking effect and the clinical finding of a virtual absence of certain acute extrapyramidal symptoms (e.g., dystonia). A few cases of tardive dyskinesia have been reported in patients on clozapine who had been previously treated with other antipsychotic agents, so that a causal relationship cannot be established. There have been no reports of tardive dyskinesia directly attributable to clozapine alone. Nevertheless, it cannot be concluded without more extended experience that FAZACLO™ (clozapine, USP) is incapable of inducing this syndrome.

Both the risk of developing the syndrome and the likelihood that it will become irreversible are believed to increase as the duration of treatment and the total cumulative dose of antipsychotic drugs administered to the patient increase. However, the syndrome can develop, although much less commonly, after relatively brief treatment periods at low doses. There is no known treatment for established cases of tardive dyskinesia, although the syndrome may remit partially or completely if antipsychotic drug treatment is withdrawn. Antipsychotic drug treatment itself, however, may suppress (or partially suppress) the signs and symptoms of the syndrome and, thereby, may possibly mask the underlying process. The effect that symptom suppression has upon the long-term course of the syndrome is unknown.

Given these considerations, FAZACLO™ (clozapine, USP) should be prescribed in a manner that is most likely to minimize the occurrence of tardive dyskinesia. As with any antipsychotic drug, chronic FAZACLO™ (clozapine, USP) use should be reserved for patients who appear to be obtaining substantial benefit from the drug. In such patients, the smallest dose and the shortest duration of treatment should be sought. The need for continued treatment should be reassessed periodically.

If signs and symptoms of tardive dyskinesia appear in a patient on FAZACLO™ (clozapine, USP), drug discontinuation should be considered. However, some patients may require treatment with FAZACLO™ (clozapine, USP) despite the presence of the syndrome.

Hyperglycemia and Diabetes Mellitus

Hyperglycemia, in some cases extreme and associated with ketoacidosis or hyperosmolar coma or death, has been reported in patients treated with atypical antipsychotics including clozapine. Assessment of the relationship between atypical antipsychotic use and glucose abnormalities is complicated by the possibility of an increased background risk of diabetes mellitus in patients with schizophrenia and the increasing incidence of diabetes mellitus in the general population. Given these confounders, the relationship between atypical antipsychotic use and hyperglycemia-related adverse events is not completely understood. However, epidemiological studies suggest an increased risk of treatment-emergent, hyperglycemia-related adverse events in patients treated with the atypical antipsychotics. Precise risk estimates for hyperglycemia-related adverse events in patients treated with atypical antipsychotics are not available.

Patients with an established diagnosis of diabetes mellitus who are started on atypical antipsychotics should be monitored regularly for worsening of glucose control. Patients with risk factors for diabetes mellitus (e.g., obesity, family history of diabetes) who are starting treatment with atypical antipsychotics should undergo fasting blood glucose testing at the beginning of treatment and periodically during treatment. Any patient treated with atypical antipsychotics should be monitored for symptoms of hyperglycemia including polydipsia, polyuria, polyphagia, and weakness. Patients who develop symptoms of hyperglycemia during treatment with atypical antipsychotics should undergo fasting blood glucose testing. In some cases, hyperglycemia has resolved when the atypical antipsychotic was discontinued; however, some patients required continuation of anti-diabetic treatment despite discontinuation of the suspect drug.

PRECAUTIONS

General

Because of the significant risk of agranulocytosis and seizure, both of which present a continuing risk over time, the extended treatment of patients failing to show an acceptable level of clinical response should ordinarily be avoided. In addition, the need for continuing treatment in patients exhibiting beneficial clinical responses should be periodically reevaluated. Although it is not known whether the risk would be increased, it is prudent to either avoid FAZACLO™ (clozapine, USP) or use it cautiously in patients with a previous history of agranulocytosis induced by other drugs.

Cardiomyopathy

Cases of cardiomyopathy have been reported in patients treated with clozapine. The reporting rate for cardiomyopathy in clozapine-treated patients in the United States (8.9 per 100,000 person-years) was similar to an estimate of the cardiomyopathy incidence in the U.S. general population derived from the 1999 National Hospital Discharge Survey data (9.7 per 100,000 person-years). Approximately 80% of clozapine-treated patients in whom cardiomyopathy was reported were less than 50 years of age; the duration of treatment with clozapine prior to cardiomyopathy diagnosis varied, but was >6 months in 65% of the reports. Dilated cardiomyopathy was most frequently reported, although a large percentage of reports did not specify the type of cardiomyopathy. Signs and symptoms suggestive of cardiomyopathy, particularly exertional dyspnea, fatigue, orthopnea, paroxysmal nocturnal dyspnea, and peripheral edema should alert the clinician to perform further investigations. If the diagnosis of cardiomyopathy is confirmed, the prescriber should discontinue clozapine unless the benefit to the patient clearly outweighs the risk.

Fever

During FAZACLO™ (clozapine, USP) therapy, patients may experience transient temperature elevations above 100.4 °F (38 °C), with the peak incidence within the first 3 weeks of treatment. While this fever is generally benign and self-limiting, it may necessitate discontinuing patients from treatment. On occasion, there may be an associated increase or decrease in WBC count. Patients with fever should be carefully evaluated to rule out the possibility of an underlying infectious process or the development of agranulocytosis. In the presence of high fever, the possibility of NMS must be considered. There have been several reports of NMS in patients receiving clozapine, usually in combination with lithium or other CNS-active drugs. (See Neuroleptic Malignant Syndrome under WARNINGS.)

Pulmonary Embolism

The possibility of pulmonary embolism should be considered in patients receiving FAZACLO™ (clozapine, USP) who present with deep-vein thrombosis, acute dyspnea, chest pain, or with other respiratory signs and symptoms. As of December 31, 1993, there were 18 cases of fatal pulmonary embolism in association with clozapine therapy in users 10–54 years of age. Based upon the extent of use observed in the *Clozapine National Registry*, the mortality rate associated with pulmonary embolus was 1 death per 3,450 person-years of use. This rate was about 27.5 times higher than that in the general population of a similar age and gender (95% confidence interval; 17.1, 42.2). Deep-vein thrombosis has also been observed in association with clozapine therapy. Whether pulmonary embolus can be attributed to clozapine or some characteristic(s) of its users is not clear, but the occurrence of deep-vein thrombosis or respiratory symptomatology should suggest its presence.

Continued on next page

Fazaclo—Cont.

Phenylketonurics
Phenylketonuric patients should be informed that FAZACLO™ (clozapine, USP) contains phenylalanine (a component of aspartame). Each 25-mg, orally disintegrating tablet contains 1.74 mg phenylalanine. Each 100-mg, orally disintegrating tablet contains 6.96 mg phenylalanine.

Hepatitis
Caution is advised in patients using FAZACLO™ (clozapine, USP) who have concurrent hepatic disease. Hepatitis has been reported in both patients with normal and preexisting liver function abnormalities. In patients who develop nausea, vomiting, and/or anorexia during FAZACLO™ (clozapine, USP) treatment, liver function tests should be performed immediately. If the elevation of these values is clinically relevant or if symptoms of jaundice occur, treatment with FAZACLO™ (clozapine, USP) should be discontinued.

Anticholinergic Toxicity
Eye: Clozapine has potent anticholinergic effects and care should be exercised in using this drug in the presence of narrow-angle glaucoma.
Gastrointestinal: Clozapine use has been associated with varying degrees of impairment of intestinal peristalsis, ranging from constipation to intestinal obstruction, fecal impaction, and paralytic ileus. (See ADVERSE REACTIONS.) On rare occasions, these cases have been fatal. Constipation should be initially treated by ensuring adequate hydration and use of ancillary therapy such as bulk laxatives. Consultation with a gastroenterologist is advisable in more serious cases.
Prostate: Clozapine has potent anticholinergic effects and care should be exercised in using this drug in the presence of prostatic enlargement.

Interference with Cognitive and Motor Performance
Because of initial sedation, FAZACLO™ (clozapine, USP) may impair mental and/or physical abilities, especially during the first few days of therapy. The recommendations for gradual-dose escalation should be carefully adhered to and patients cautioned about activities requiring alertness.

Use in Patients with Concomitant Illness
Clinical experience with clozapine in patients with concomitant systemic diseases is limited. Nevertheless, caution is advisable in using FAZACLO™ (clozapine, USP) in patients with renal or cardiac disease.

Use in Patients Undergoing General Anesthesia
Caution is advised in patients being administered general anesthesia because of the CNS effects of clozapine. Check with the anesthesiologist regarding continuation of FAZACLO™ (clozapine, USP) therapy in a patient scheduled for surgery.

Information for Patients
Physicians are advised to discuss the following issues with patients for whom they prescribe FAZACLO™ (clozapine, USP):

— Patients who are to receive FAZACLO™ (clozapine, USP) should be warned about the significant risk of developing agranulocytosis. They should be informed that weekly blood tests are required for the first 6 months;
if acceptable WBC counts (WBC ≥ 3000/mm^3, ANC ≥ 1500/mm^3) have been maintained during the first 6 months of continuous therapy, WBC counts can be evaluated every other week in order to monitor for the occurrence of agranulocytosis; and that FAZACLO™ (clozapine, USP) Orally Disintegrating Tablets will be made available only through a special program designed to ensure the required blood monitoring. Patients should be advised to report immediately the appearance of lethargy, weakness, fever, sore throat, malaise, mucous-membrane ulceration, or other possible signs of infection. Particular attention should be paid to any flu-like complaints or other symptoms that might suggest infection.
— Patients should be informed of the significant risk of seizure during FAZACLO™ (clozapine, USP) treatment, and they should be advised to avoid driving and any other potentially hazardous activity while taking FAZACLO™ (clozapine, USP).
— Patients with phenylketonuria should be aware that FAZACLO™ (clozapine, USP) contains phenylalanine (a component of aspartame). (See PRECAUTIONS, Phenylketonurics.)
— Patients should be advised of the risk of orthostatic hypotension, especially during the period of initial dose titration.
— Patients should be informed that if they stop taking FAZACLO™ (clozapine, USP) for more than 2 days, they should not restart their medication at the same dosage but should contact their physician for dosing instructions.
— Patients should notify their physician if they are taking or plan to take any prescription or over-the-counter drugs or alcohol.
— Patients should notify their physician if they become pregnant or intend to become pregnant during therapy.
— Patients should not breast feed an infant if they are taking FAZACLO™ (clozapine, USP).
— Patients should be advised that FAZACLO™ (clozapine, USP) tablets should remain in the unopened blister until immediately before use.
— Patients should be advised that if FAZACLO™ (clozapine, USP) tablets are split, the half-tablet that is not taken should be destroyed.

Drug Interactions
The risks of using FAZACLO™ (clozapine, USP) in combination with other drugs have not been systematically evaluated. Concurrent psychopharmaceuticals may affect plasma clozapine levels, thus, plasma concentrations of clozapine may fluctuate, and dosage adjustment may be required to avoid adverse effects or clinical failure.

Pharmacodynamic-Related Interactions
Although the exact mechanism of clozapine-induced agranulocytosis is unknown, the possibility that causative factors may interact synergistically with clozapine to increase the risk and/or severity of bone-marrow suppression warrants consideration. Therefore, FAZACLO™ (clozapine, USP) should not be used with other agents having a well-known potential to suppress bone-marrow function.
Given the primary CNS effects of clozapine, caution is advised in using it concomitantly with other CNS-active drugs or alcohol.
Orthostatic hypotension in patients taking clozapine can, in rare cases (approximately 1 case per 3000 patients), be accompanied by profound collapse and respiratory and/or cardiac arrest. Some of the cases of collapse/respiratory arrest/cardiac arrest during initial treatment occurred in patients who were being administered benzodiazepines; similar events have been reported in patients taking other psychotropic drugs or even clozapine by itself. Although it has not been established that there is an interaction between clozapine and benzodiazepines or other psychotropics, caution is advised when clozapine is initiated in patients taking a benzodiazepine or any other psychotropic drug.
FAZACLO™ (clozapine, USP) may potentiate the hypotensive effects of antihypertensive drugs and the anticholinergic effects of atropine-type drugs. The administration of epinephrine should be avoided in the treatment of drug-induced hypotension because of a possible reverse epinephrine effect.

Pharmacokinetic-Related Interactions
Clozapine is a substrate for many cytochrome P450 isozymes, in particular CYP1A2, CYP2D6, and CYP3A4. The risk of metabolic interactions caused by an effect on an individual isoform is, therefore, minimized. Nevertheless, caution should be used in patients receiving concomitant treatment of FAZACLO™ (clozapine, USP) with other drugs which are either inhibitors or inducers of these enzymes.
Concomitant administration of drugs known to induce cytochrome P450 enzymes may decrease the plasma levels of clozapine. Phenytoin, nicotine, carbamazepine, and rifampin may decrease FAZACLO™ (clozapine, USP) plasma levels resulting in a decrease in effectiveness of a previously effective FAZACLO™ (clozapine, USP) dose.
Concomitant administration of drugs known to inhibit the activity of cytochrome P450 isozymes may increase the plasma levels of clozapine. Cimetidine, caffeine, fluvoxamine, and erythromycin may increase plasma levels of FAZACLO™ (clozapine, USP), potentially resulting in adverse effects. Although concomitant use of FAZACLO™ (clozapine, USP) and carbamazepine is not recommended, it should be noted that discontinuation of concomitant carbamazepine administration may result in an increase in FAZACLO™ (clozapine, USP) plasma levels.
In a study of schizophrenic patients who received clozapine under steady-state conditions, fluvoxamine or paroxetine was added in 16 and 14 patients, respectively. After 14 days of coadministration, mean trough concentrations of clozapine and its metabolites, *N*-desmethylclozapine and clozapine *N*-oxide, were elevated with fluvoxamine by about three-fold compared to baseline concentrations. Paroxetine produced only minor changes in the levels of clozapine and its metabolites. However, other published reports describe modest elevations (less than two-fold) of clozapine and metabolite concentrations when clozapine was taken with paroxetine, fluoxetine, and sertraline. Therefore, such combined treatment should be approached with caution and patients should be monitored closely when FAZACLO™ (clozapine, USP) is combined with these drugs, particularly with fluvoxamine. A reduced FAZACLO™ (clozapine, USP) dose should be considered.
A subset (3–10%) of the population has reduced activity of certain drug metabolizing enzymes such as the cytochrome P450 isozyme CYP2D6. Such individuals are referred to as "poor metabolizers" of drugs such as debrisoquin, dextromethorphan, tricyclic antidepressants, and clozapine. These individuals may develop higher than expected plasma concentrations of clozapine when given usual doses. In addition, certain drugs that are metabolized by this isozyme, including many antidepressants (clozapine, selective serotonin reuptake inhibitors, and others), may inhibit the activity of this isozyme and, thus, may make normal metabolizers resemble poor metabolizers with regard to concomitant therapy with other drugs metabolized by this enzyme system, leading to drug interaction.
Concomitant use of clozapine with other drugs metabolized by P450 CYP2D6 may require lower doses than usually prescribed for either FAZACLO™ (clozapine, USP) or the other drug. Therefore, coadministration of FAZACLO™ (clozapine, USP) with other drugs that are metabolized by this isozyme, including antidepressants, phenothiazines, carbamazepine, and Type 1C antiarrhythmics (e.g., propafenone, flecainide, ecainide, and encainide), or that inhibit this enzyme (e.g., quinidine) should be approached with caution.

Carcinogenesis, Mutagenesis, Impairment of Fertility
No carcinogenic potential was demonstrated in long-term studies in mice and rats at doses approximately 7 times the typical human dose on a mg/kg basis. Fertility in male and female rats was not adversely affected by clozapine. Clozapine did not produce genotoxic or mutagenic effects when assayed in appropriate bacterial and mammalian tests.

Pregnancy Category B
Reproduction studies have been performed in rats and rabbits at doses of approximately 2–4 times the human dose and have revealed no evidence of impaired fertility or harm to the fetus due to clozapine. There are, however, no adequate and well-controlled studies in pregnant women. Because animal reproduction studies are not always predictive of human response and in view of the desirability of keeping the administration of all drugs to a minimum during pregnancy, this drug should be used only if clearly needed.

Nursing Mothers
Animal studies suggest that clozapine may be excreted in breast milk and have an effect on the nursing infant. Therefore, women receiving FAZACLO™ (clozapine, USP) should not breast feed.

Pediatric Use
Safety and effectiveness in pediatric patients have not been established.

Geriatric Use
Clinical studies of clozapine did not include sufficient numbers of subjects age 65 and over to determine whether they respond differently than younger subjects.
Orthostatic hypotension can occur with clozapine treatment, and tachycardia, which may be sustained, has been observed in about 25% of patients taking clozapine. (See WARNINGS, Other Adverse Cardiovascular and Respiratory Effects.) Elderly patients, particularly those with compromised cardiovascular functioning, may be more susceptible to these effects.
Also, elderly patients may be particularly susceptible to the anticholinergic effects of clozapine, such as urinary retention and constipation. (See PRECAUTIONS, Anticholinergic Toxicity.)
Dose selection for an elderly patient should be cautious, reflecting the greater frequency of decreased hepatic, renal, or cardiac function, and concomitant disease or other drug therapy. Other reported clinical experience does suggest that the prevalence of tardive dyskinesia appears to be highest among the elderly, especially elderly women. (See WARNINGS, Tardive Dyskinesia.)

ADVERSE REACTIONS

Associated with Discontinuation of Treatment
Sixteen percent of 1,080 patients who received clozapine in premarketing clinical trials discontinued treatment due to an adverse event, including both those that could reasonably be attributed to clozapine treatment and those that might more appropriately be considered intercurrent illness. The more common events considered to be causes of discontinuation included: CNS, primarily drowsiness/sedation, seizures, dizziness/syncope; cardiovascular, primarily tachycardia, hypotension, and ECG changes; gastrointestinal, primarily nausea/vomiting; hematologic, primarily leukopenia/granulocytopenia/agranulocytosis; and fever. None of the events enumerated accounts for more than 1.7% of all discontinuations attributed to adverse clinical events.

Commonly Observed
Adverse events observed in association with the use of clozapine in clinical trials at an incidence of greater than 5% were: CNS complaints, including drowsiness/sedation, dizziness/vertigo, headache, and tremor; autonomic nervous system complaints, including salivation, sweating, dry mouth, and visual disturbances; cardiovascular findings, including tachycardia, hypotension, and syncope; and gastrointestinal complaints, including constipation and nausea; and fever. Complaints of drowsiness/sedation tend to subside with continued therapy or dose reduction. Salivation may be profuse, especially during sleep, but may be diminished with dose reduction.

Incidence in Clinical Trials
The following table enumerates adverse events that occurred at a frequency of 1% or greater among clozapine patients who participated in clinical trials. These rates are not adjusted for duration of exposure.

Treatment-Emergent Adverse Experience Incidence Among Patients Taking Clozapine in Clinical Trials (N = 842) (percentage of patients reporting)

Body System Adverse Event[a]	Percent
Central Nervous System	
Drowsiness/Sedation	39
Dizziness/Vertigo	19
Headache	7
Tremor	6
Syncope	6
Disturbed Sleep/Nightmares	4
Restlessness	4
Hypokinesia/Akinesia	4
Agitation	4
Seizures (convulsions)	3[b]
Rigidity	3
Akathisia	3

Confusion	3
Fatigue	2
Insomnia	2
Hyperkinesia	1
Weakness	1
Lethargy	1
Ataxia	1
Slurred Speech	1
Depression	1
Epileptiform Movements/Myoclonic Jerks	1
Anxiety	1
Cardiovascular	
Tachycardia	25[b]
Hypotension	9
Hypertension	4
Chest Pain/Angina	1
ECG Change/Cardiac Abnormality	1
Gastrointestinal	
Constipation	14
Nausea	5
Abdominal Discomfort/Heartburn	4
Nausea/Vomiting	3
Vomiting	3
Diarrhea	2
Liver Test Abnormality	1
Anorexia	1
Urogenital	
Urinary Abnormalities	2
Incontinence	1
Abnormal Ejaculation	1
Urinary Urgency/Frequency	1
Urinary Retention	1
Autonomic Nervous System	
Salivation	31
Sweating	6
Dry Mouth	6
Visual Disturbances	5
Integumentary (skin)	
Rash	2
Musculoskeletal	
Muscle Weakness	1
Pain (back, neck, legs)	1
Muscle Spasm	1
Muscle Pain, Ache	1
Respiratory	
Throat Discomfort	1
Dyspnea, Shortness of Breath	1
Nasal Congestion	1
Hemic/Lymphatic	
Leukopenia/Decreased WBC/Neutropenia	3
Agranulocytosis	1[b]
Eosinophilia	1
Miscellaneous	
Fever	5
Weight Gain	4
Tongue Numb/Sore	1

[a] Events reported by at least 1% of clozapine patients are included.

[b] Rate based on population of approximately 1700 exposed during premarket clinical evaluation of clozapine.

Other Events Observed During the Premarketing Evaluation of Clozapine

This section reports additional, less frequent adverse events which occurred among the patients taking clozapine in clinical trials. Various adverse events were reported as part of the total experience in these clinical studies; a causal relationship to clozapine treatment cannot be determined in the absence of appropriate controls in some of the studies. The table above enumerates adverse events that occurred at a frequency of at least 1% of patients treated with clozapine. The list below includes all additional adverse experiences reported as being temporally associated with the use of the drug which occurred at a frequency less than 1%, enumerated by organ system.

Central Nervous System: loss of speech, amentia, tics, poor coordination, delusions/hallucinations, involuntary movement, stuttering, dysarthria, amnesia/memory loss, histrionic movements, libido increase or decrease, paranoia, shakiness, Parkinsonism, and irritability

Cardiovascular System: edema, palpitations, phlebitis/thrombophlebitis, cyanosis, premature ventricular contraction, bradycardia, and nose bleed

Gastrointestinal System: abdominal distention, gastroenteritis, rectal bleeding, nervous stomach, abnormal stools, hematemesis, gastric ulcer, bitter taste, and eructation

Urogenital System: dysmenorrhea, impotence, breast pain/discomfort, and vaginal itch/infection

Autonomic Nervous System: numbness, polydypsia, hot flashes, dry throat, and mydriasis

Integumentary (skin): pruritus, pallor, eczema, erythema, bruise, dermatitis, petechiae, and urticaria

Musculoskeletal System: twitching and joint pain

Respiratory System: coughing, pneumonia/pneumonia-like symptoms, rhinorrhea, hyperventilation, wheezing, bronchitis, laryngitis, and sneezing

Hemic and Lymphatic System: anemia and leukocytosis

Miscellaneous: chills/chills with fever, malaise, appetite increase, ear disorder, hypothermia, eyelid disorder, bloodshot eyes, and nystagmus

Postmarketing Clinical Experience

Postmarketing experience has shown an adverse experience profile similar to that presented above. Voluntary reports of adverse events temporally associated with clozapine not mentioned above that have been received since market introduction and that may have no causal relationship with the drug include the following:

Central Nervous System: delirium, EEG abnormal, exacerbation of psychosis, myoclonus, overdose, paresthesia, possible mild cataplexy, and status epilepticus

Cardiovascular System: atrial or ventricular fibrillation and periorbital edema

Gastrointestinal System: acute pancreatitis, dysphagia, fecal impaction, intestinal obstruction/paralytic ileus, and salivary gland swelling

Hepatobiliary System: cholestasis, hepatitis, jaundice

Hepatic System: cholestasis

Urogenital System: acute interstitial nephritis and priapism

Integumentary (skin): hypersensitivity reactions: photosensitivity, vasculitis, erythema multiforme, and Stevens-Johnson Syndrome

Musculoskeletal System: myasthenic syndrome and rhabdomyolysis

Respiratory System: aspiration and pleural effusion

Hemic and Lymphatic System: deep-vein thrombosis, elevated hemoglobin/hematocrit, ESR increased, pulmonary embolism, sepsis, thrombocytosis, and thrombocytopenia

Vision Disorders: narrow-angle glaucoma

Miscellaneous: creatine phosphokinase elevation, hyperglycemia, hyperuricemia, hyponatremia, and weight loss

DRUG ABUSE AND DEPENDENCE

Physical and psychological dependence have not been reported or observed in patients taking clozapine.

OVERDOSAGE

Human Experience

The most commonly reported signs and symptoms associated with clozapine overdose are: altered states of consciousness, including drowsiness, delirium, and coma; tachycardia; hypotension; respiratory depression or failure; and hypersalivation. Aspiration pneumonia and cardiac arrhythmias have also been reported. Seizures have occurred in a minority of reported cases. Fatal overdoses have been reported with clozapine, generally at doses above 2500 mg. There have also been reports of patients recovering from overdoses well in excess of 4 g.

Management of Overdose

Establish and maintain an airway; ensure adequate oxygenation and ventilation. Activated charcoal, which may be used with sorbitol, may be as or more effective than emesis or lavage and should be considered in treating overdosage. Cardiac and vital signs monitoring are recommended along with general symptomatic and supportive measures. Additional surveillance should be continued for several days because of the risk of delayed effects. Avoid epinephrine and derivatives when treating hypotension and quinidine and procainamide when treating cardiac arrhythmia.

There are no specific antidotes for FAZACLO™ (clozapine, USP). Forced diuresis, dialysis, hemoperfusion, and exchange transfusion are unlikely to be of benefit.

In managing overdosage, the physician should consider the possibility of multiple-drug involvement.

Up-to-date information about the treatment of overdose can often be obtained from a certified Regional Poison Control Center. Telephone numbers of certified Poison Control Centers are listed in the *Physicians' Desk Reference*®, a trademark of Medical Economics Company, Inc.

DOSAGE AND ADMINISTRATION

Administration

FAZACLO™ (clozapine, USP) rapidly disintegrates after placement in the mouth. The FAZACLO™ (clozapine, USP) Orally Disintegrating Tablet should be left in the unopened blister until time of use. The orally disintegrating tablet should not be pushed through the foil. Just prior to use, peel the foil from the blister and gently remove the orally disintegrating tablet. Immediately place the tablet in the mouth and allow to disintegrate and swallow with saliva. No water is needed to take FAZACLO™ (clozapine, USP).

Upon initiation of FAZACLO™ (clozapine, USP) therapy, up to a 1-week supply of additional FAZACLO™ (clozapine, USP) orally disintegrating tablets may be provided to the patient to be held for emergencies (e.g., weather, holidays).

Initial Treatment

It is recommended that treatment with FAZACLO™ (clozapine, USP) begin with one-half of a 25-mg, orally disintegrating tablet (12.5 mg) once or twice daily. The remaining one-half tablet should be destroyed. The dosing should be continued with daily dosage increments of 25–50 mg/day, if well-tolerated, to achieve a target dose of 300–450 mg/day by the end of 2 weeks. Subsequent dosage increments should be made no more than once or twice weekly, in increments not to exceed 100 mg. Cautious titration and a divided dosage schedule are necessary to minimize the risks of hypotension, seizure, and sedation.

In the multicenter study that provides primary support for the effectiveness of clozapine in patients resistant to standard drug treatment for schizophrenia, patient's doses were titrated during the first 2 weeks up to a maximum dose of 500 mg/day on a t.i.d. basis. Subsequent dosage increments were then dosed in a total daily dose range of 100–900 mg/day on a t.i.d. basis, with clinical response and adverse effects as guides to correct dosing.

Therapeutic Dose Adjustment

Daily dosing should continue on a divided basis as an effective and tolerable dose level is sought. While many patients may respond adequately at doses between 300–600 mg/day, it may be necessary to raise the dose to the 600–900 mg/day range to obtain an acceptable response. (Note: In the multicenter study providing the primary support for the superiority of clozapine in treatment-resistant patients, the mean and median clozapine doses were both approximately 600 mg/day.)

Because of the possibility of increased adverse reactions at higher doses, particularly seizures, patients should ordinarily be given adequate time to respond to a given dose level before escalation to a higher dose is contemplated. Clozapine can cause EEG changes, including the occurrence of spike and wave complexes. It lowers the seizures threshold in a dose-dependent manner and may induce myoclonic jerks or generalized seizures. These symptoms may be likely to occur with rapid-dose increase and in patients with preexisting epilepsy. In this case, the dose should be reduced and, if necessary, anticonvulsant treatment initiated. Dosing should not exceed 900 mg/day.

Because of the significant risk of agranulocytosis and seizure, events which both present a continuing risk over time, the extended treatment of patients failing to show an acceptable level of clinical response should ordinarily be avoided.

Maintenance Treatment

While the maintenance effectiveness of clozapine in schizophrenia is still under study, the effectiveness of maintenance treatment is well established for many other drugs used to treat schizophrenia. It is recommended that responding patients be continued on FAZACLO™ (clozapine, USP), but at the lowest level needed to maintain remission. Because of the significant risk associated with the use of FAZACLO™ (clozapine, USP), patients should be periodically reassessed to determine the need for maintenance treatment.

Discontinuation of Treatment

In the event of planned termination of FAZACLO™ (clozapine, USP) therapy, gradual reduction in dose is recommended over a 1–2 week period. However, should a patient's medical condition require abrupt discontinuation (e.g., leukopenia), the patient should be carefully observed for the recurrence of psychotic symptoms and symptoms related to cholinergic rebound such as headache, nausea, vomiting, and diarrhea.

Reinitiation of Treatment in Patients Previously Discontinued

When restarting patients who have had even a brief interval off FAZACLO™ (clozapine, USP) (i.e., 2 days or more since the last dose), it is recommended that treatment be reinitiated with one-half of a 25-mg, orally disintegrating tablet (12.5 mg) once or twice daily. The remaining one-half tablet should be destroyed. (See WARNINGS.) If that dose is well tolerated, it may be feasible to titrate patients back to a therapeutic dose more quickly than is recommended for initial treatment. However, any patient who has previously experienced respiratory or cardiac arrest with initial dosing but was then able to be successfully titrated to a therapeutic dose should be retitrated with extreme caution after even 24 hours of discontinuation.

Certain additional precautions seem prudent when reinitiating treatment. The mechanisms underlying clozapine-induced adverse reactions are unknown. It is conceivable, however, that reexposure of a patient might enhance the risk of an untoward event's occurrence and increase its severity. Such phenomena, for example, occur when immune-mediated mechanisms are responsible. Consequently, during the reinitiation of treatment, additional caution is advised. Patients discontinued for WBC counts below 2000/mm^3 or an ANC below 1000/mm^3 must *not* be restarted on FAZACLO™ (clozapine, USP). (See WARNINGS.)

HOW SUPPLIED

FAZACLO™ (clozapine, USP) is available as 25- and 100-mg round, yellow, orally disintegrating tablets with a score on one side.

FAZACLO™ (clozapine, USP) Orally Disintegrating Tablets

25 mg

5/16-inch diameter tablet debossed with "A01" once on the periphery of one side and with a score on the opposite side.

Packages of 48: 8 cards,
6 blisters per card .... NDC 68322-001-01

Packages of 100 unit dose blisters ...... NDC 68322-001-04

100 mg

1/2-inch diameter tablet debossed with "A02" once on the periphery of one side and with a score on the opposite side.

Packages of 48: 8 cards,
6 blisters per card .... NDC 68322-002-01

Packages of 100 unit dose blisters ...... NDC 68322-002-04

Store and Dispense

Store FAZACLO™ (clozapine, USP) at 25 °C (77 °F); excursions permitted to 15–30 °C (59–86 °F). (See *USP* Controlled Room Temperature.) Protect from moisture. The patient should be instructed not to remove the orally disintegrating tablet from the blister until the patient is ready to consume the tablet.

FAZACLO™ (clozapine, USP) must remain in the sealed blister until used by the patient. For out-patient use, dispense sealed blister in a child-resistant container. Drug dispensing should not ordinarily exceed a weekly supply. If a patient is eligible for WBC testing every other week, then a

Continued on next page

Fazaclo—Cont.

two-week supply of FAZACLO™ (clozapine, USP) can be dispensed. Dispensing should be contingent upon the results of a WBC count.
Manufactured for
Alamo Pharmaceuticals, LLC
8501 Wilshire Boulevard, Suite 318
Beverly Hills, California 90211-3119
by
CIMA LABS INC.®
Eden Prairie, Minnesota 55344
CIMA LABS INC.®; U.S. Patent Nos. 5,178,878; 6,155,423
FAZACLO™ is a trademark of Alamo Pharmaceuticals, LLC.
Revised May 2004
Printed in U.S.A.
Shown in Product Identification Guide, page 304

Alcon Laboratories, Inc.

AND ITS AFFILIATES
CORPORATE HEADQUARTERS
6201 SOUTH FREEWAY
FORT WORTH, TX 76134

Direct Inquiries to:
Pharmaceutical/Consumer: (800) 451-3937
(Therapeutic Drugs/Lens Care)
Surgical: (800) 862-5266
(Instrumentation/Surgical Meds)
6201 South Freeway
Fort Worth, TX 76134
(817) 293-0450 (Main Switchboard)

OPHTHALMIC PRODUCTS

For information on Alcon ophthalmic products, consult the PDR For Ophthalmic Medicines. See a complete listing of products in the Manufacturers' Index section of this book. For information, literature, samples or service items contact Alcon at the phone numbers listed above.

AZOPT® ℞
(brinzolamide ophthalmic suspension) 1%

DESCRIPTION

AZOPT® (brinzolamide ophthalmic suspension) 1% contains a carbonic anhydrase inhibitor formulated for multi-dose topical ophthalmic use. Brinzolamide is described chemically as: (R)-(+)-4-Ethylamino-2-(3-methoxypropyl)-3,4-dihydro-2H-thieno [3,2-e]-1,2-thiazine-6-sulfonamide-1,1-dioxide. Its empirical formula is $C_{12}H_{21}N_3O_5S_3$.
Brinzolamide has a molecular weight of 383.5 and a melting point of about 131°C. It is a white powder, which is insoluble in water, very soluble in methanol and soluble in ethanol.
AZOPT® (brinzolamide ophthalmic suspension) 1% is supplied as a sterile, aqueous suspension of brinzolamide which has been formulated to be readily suspended and slow settling, following shaking. It has a pH of approximately 7.5 and an osmolality of 300 mOsm/kg. Each mL of AZOPT® (brinzolamide ophthalmic suspension) 1% contains 10 mg brinzolamide. Inactive ingredients are mannitol, carbomer 974P, tyloxapol, edetate disodium, sodium chloride, hydrochloric acid and/or sodium hydroxide (to adjust pH), and purified water. Benzalkonium chloride 0.01% is added as a preservative.

CLINICAL PHARMACOLOGY

Carbonic anhydrase (CA) is an enzyme found in many tissues of the body including the eye. It catalyzes the reversible reaction involving the hydration of carbon dioxide and the dehydration of carbonic acid. In humans, carbonic anhydrase exists as a number of isoenzymes, the most active being carbonic anhydrase II (CA-II), found primarily in red blood cells (RBCs), but also in other tissues. Inhibition of carbonic anhydrase in the ciliary processes of the eye decreases aqueous humor secretion, presumably by slowing the formation of bicarbonate ions with subsequent reduction in sodium and fluid transport.
The result is a reduction in intraocular pressure (IOP).
AZOPT® (brinzolamide ophthalmic suspension) 1% contains brinzolamide, an inhibitor of carbonic anhydrase II (CA-II). Following topical ocular administration, brinzolamide inhibits aqueous humor formation and reduces elevated intraocular pressure. Elevated intraocular pressure is a major risk factor in the pathogenesis of optic nerve damage and glaucomatous visual field loss.
Following topical ocular administration, brinzolamide is absorbed into the systemic circulation. Due to its affinity for CA-II, brinzolamide distributes extensively into the RBCs and exhibits a long half-life in whole blood (approximately 111 days). In humans, the metabolite N-desethyl brinzolamide is formed, which also binds to CA and accumulates in RBCs. This metabolite binds mainly to CA-I in the presence of brinzolamide. In plasma, both parent brinzolamide and N-desethyl brinzolamide concentrations are low and generally below assay quantitation limits (<10 ng/mL). Binding to plasma proteins is approximately 60%. Brinzolamide is eliminated predominantly in the urine as unchanged drug. N-Desethyl brinzolamide is also found in the urine along with lower concentrations of the N-desmethoxypropyl and O-desmethyl metabolites.
An oral pharmacokinetic study was conducted in which healthy volunteers received 1 mg capsules of brinzolamide twice per day for up to 32 weeks. This regimen approximates the amount of drug delivered by topical ocular administration of AZOPT® (brinzolamide ophthalmic suspension) 1% dosed to both eyes three times per day and simulates systemic drug and metabolite concentrations similar to those achieved with long-term topical dosing. RBC CA activity was measured to assess the degree of systemic CA inhibition. Brinzolamide saturation of RBC CA-II was achieved within 4 weeks (RBC concentrations of approximately 20 μM). N-Desethyl brinzolamide accumulated in RBCs to steady-state within 20–28 weeks reaching concentrations ranging from 6–30 μM. The inhibition of CA-II activity at steady-state was approximately 70–75%, which is below the degree of inhibition expected to have a pharmacological effect on renal function or respiration in healthy subjects.
In two, three-month clinical studies, AZOPT® (brinzolamide ophthalmic suspension) 1% dosed three times per day (TID) in patients with elevated intraocular pressure (IOP), produced significant reductions in IOPs (4–5 mmHg). These IOP reductions are equivalent to the reductions observed with TRUSOPT* (dorzolamide hydrochloride ophthalmic solution) 2% dosed TID in the same studies.
In two clinical studies in patients with elevated intraocular pressure, AZOPT® (brinzolamide ophthalmic suspension) 1% was associated with less stinging and burning upon instillation than TRUSOPT* 2%.

INDICATIONS AND USAGE

AZOPT® (brinzolamide ophthalmic suspension) 1% is indicated in the treatment of elevated intraocular pressure in patients with ocular hypertension or open-angle glaucoma.

CONTRAINDICATIONS

AZOPT® (brinzolamide ophthalmic suspension) 1% is contraindicated in patients who are hypersensitive to any component of this product.

WARNINGS

AZOPT® (brinzolamide ophthalmic suspension) 1% is a sulfonamide and although administered topically it is absorbed systemically. Therefore, the same types of adverse reactions that are attributable to sulfonamides may occur with topical administration of AZOPT® (brinzolamide ophthalmic suspension) 1%. Fatalities have occurred, although rarely, due to severe reactions to sulfonamides including Stevens-Johnson syndrome, toxic epidermal necrolysis, fulminant hepatic necrosis, agranulocytosis, aplastic anemia, and other blood dyscrasias. Sensitization may recur when a sulfonamide is re-administered irrespective of the route of administration. If signs of serious reactions or hypersensitivity occur, discontinue the use of this preparation.

PRECAUTIONS

General:
Carbonic anhydrase activity has been observed in both the cytoplasm and around the plasma membranes of the corneal endothelium. The effect of continued administration of AZOPT® (brinzolamide ophthalmic suspension) 1% on the corneal endothelium has not been fully evaluated. The management of patients with acute angle-closure glaucoma requires therapeutic interventions in addition to ocular hypotensive agents. AZOPT® (brinzolamide ophthalmic suspension) 1% has not been studied in patients with acute angle-closure glaucoma.
AZOPT® (brinzolamide ophthalmic suspension) 1% has not been studied in patients with severe renal impairment (CrCl <30 mL/min). Because AZOPT® (brinzolamide ophthalmic suspension) 1% and its metabolite are excreted predominantly by the kidney, AZOPT® (brinzolamide ophthalmic suspension) 1% is not recommended in such patients.
AZOPT® (brinzolamide ophthalmic suspension) 1% has not been studied in patients with hepatic impairment and should be used with caution in such patients.
There is a potential for an additive effect on the known systemic effects of carbonic anhydrase inhibition in patients receiving an oral carbonic anhydrase inhibitor and AZOPT® (brinzolamide ophthalmic suspension) 1%. The concomitant administration of AZOPT® (brinzolamide ophthalmic suspension) 1% and oral carbonic anhydrase inhibitors is not recommended.
Information For Patients:
AZOPT® (brinzolamide ophthalmic suspension) 1% is a sulfonamide and although administered topically, it is absorbed systemically; therefore, the same types of adverse reactions attributable to sulfonamides may occur with topical administration. Patients should be advised that if serious or unusual ocular or systemic reactions or signs of hypersensitivity occur, they should discontinue the use of the product and consult their physician (see **Warnings**).
Vision may be temporarily blurred following dosing with AZOPT® (brinzolamide ophthalmic suspension) 1%. Care should be exercised in operating machinery or driving a motor vehicle.
Patients should be instructed to avoid allowing the tip of the dispensing container to contact the eye or surrounding structures or other surfaces, since the product can become contaminated by common bacteria known to cause ocular infections. Serious damage to the eye and subsequent loss of vision may result from using contaminated solutions.
Patients should also be advised that if they have ocular surgery or develop an intercurrent ocular condition (e.g., trauma or infection), they should immediately seek their physician's advice concerning the continued use of the present multidose container.
If more than one topical ophthalmic drug is being used, the drugs should be administered at least ten minutes apart.
The preservative in AZOPT® (brinzolamide ophthalmic suspension) 1%, benzalkonium chloride, may be absorbed by soft contact lenses. Contact lenses should be removed during instillation of AZOPT® (brinzolamide ophthalmic suspension) 1%, but may be reinserted 15 minutes after instillation.
Drug Interactions:
AZOPT® (brinzolamide ophthalmic suspension) 1% contains a carbonic anhydrase inhibitor. Acid-base and electrolyte alterations were not reported in the clinical trials with brinzolamide. However, in patients treated with oral carbonic anhydrase inhibitors, rare instances of drug interactions have occurred with high-dose salicylate therapy. Therefore, the potential for such drug interactions should be considered in patients receiving AZOPT® (brinzolamide ophthalmic suspension) 1%.
Carcinogenesis, Mutagenesis, Impairment of Fertility:
Carcinogenicity data on brinzolamide are not available. The following tests for mutagenic potential were negative: (1) *in vivo* mouse micronucleus assay; (2) *in vivo* sister chromatid exchange assay; and (3) Ames *E. coli* test. The *in vitro* mouse lymphoma forward mutation assay was negative in the absence of activation, but positive in the presence of microsomal activation.
In reproduction studies of brinzolamide in rats, there were no adverse effects on the fertility or reproductive capacity of males or females at doses up to 18 mg/kg/day (375 times the recommended human ophthalmic dose).
Pregnancy:
Teratogenic Effects: Pregnancy Category C. Developmental toxicity studies with brinzolamide in rabbits at oral doses of 1, 3, and 6 mg/kg/day (20, 62, and 125 times the recommended human ophthalmic dose) produced maternal toxicity at 6 mg/kg/day and a significant increase in the number of fetal variations, such as accessory skull bones, which was only slightly higher than the historic value at 1 and 6 mg/kg. In rats, statistically decreased body weights of fetuses from dams receiving oral doses of 18 mg/kg/day (375 times the recommended human ophthalmic dose) during gestation were proportional to the reduced maternal weight gain, with no statistically significant effects on organ or tissue development. Increases in unossified sternebrae, reduced ossification of the skull, and unossified hyoid that occurred at 6 and 18 mg/kg were not statistically significant. No treatment-related malformations were seen. Following oral administration of ^{14}C-brinzolamide to pregnant rats, radioactivity was found to cross the placenta and was present in the fetal tissues and blood.
There are no adequate and well-controlled studies in pregnant women. AZOPT® (brinzolamide ophthalmic suspension) 1% should be used during pregnancy only if the potential benefit justifies the potential risk to the fetus.
Nursing Mothers:
In a study of brinzolamide in lactating rats, decreases in body weight gain in offspring at an oral dose of 15 mg/kg/day (312 times the recommended human ophthalmic dose) were seen during lactation. No other effects were observed. However, following oral administration of ^{14}C-brinzolamide to lactating rats, radioactivity was found in milk at concentrations below those in the blood and plasma.
It is not known whether this drug is excreted in human milk. Because many drugs are excreted in human milk and because of the potential for serious adverse reactions in nursing infants from AZOPT® (brinzolamide ophthalmic suspension) 1%, a decision should be made whether to discontinue nursing or to discontinue the drug, taking into account the importance of the drug to the mother.
Pediatric Use:
Safety and effectiveness in pediatric patients have not been established.
Geriatric Use: No overall differences in safety or effectiveness have been observed between elderly and younger patients.

ADVERSE REACTIONS

In clinical studies of AZOPT® (brinzolamide ophthalmic suspension) 1%, the most frequently reported adverse events associated with AZOPT® (brinzolamide ophthalmic suspension) 1% were blurred vision and bitter, sour or unusual taste. These events occurred in approximately 5–10% of patients. Blepharitis, dermatitis, dry eye, foreign body sensation, headache, hyperemia, ocular discharge, ocular discomfort, ocular keratitis, ocular pain, ocular pruritus and rhinitis were reported at an incidence of 1–5%.
The following adverse reactions were reported at an incidence below 1%: allergic reactions, alopecia, chest pain, conjunctivitis, diarrhea, diplopia, dizziness, dry mouth, dyspnea, dyspepsia, eye fatigue, hypertonia, keratoconjunctivitis, keratopathy, kidney pain, lid margin crusting or sticky sensation, nausea, pharyngitis, tearing and urticaria.

OVERDOSAGE

Although no human data are available, electrolyte imbalance, development of an acidotic state, and possible nervous system effects may occur following oral administration of an overdose. Serum electrolyte levels (particularly potassium) and blood pH levels should be monitored.

DOSAGE AND ADMINISTRATION

Shake well before use. The recommended dose is 1 drop of AZOPT® (brinzolamide ophthalmic suspension) 1% in the affected eye(s) three times daily.

AZOPT® (brinzolamide ophthalmic suspension) 1% may be used concomitantly with other topical ophthalmic drug products to lower intraocular pressure.

If more than one topical ophthalmic drug is being used, the drugs should be administered at least ten minutes apart.

HOW SUPPLIED

AZOPT® (brinzolamide ophthalmic suspension) 1% is supplied in plastic DROP-TAINER® dispensers with a controlled dispensing-tip as follows:

NDC 0065-0275-24	2.5 mL
NDC 0065-0275-05	5 mL
NDC 0065-0275-10	10 mL
NDC 0065-0275-15	15 mL

Storage: Store AZOPT® (brinzolamide ophthalmic suspension) 1% at 4–30°C (39–86°F).

℞ **Only**

U.S. Patent Numbers: 5,240,923; 5,378,703; 5,461,081; 6,071,904.

*TRUSOPT is a registered trademark of Merck & Co., Inc.

BETOPTIC S® ℞

(betaxolol HCl)
0.25% as base
Sterile Ophthalmic Suspension

DESCRIPTION

BETOPTIC S® Ophthalmic Suspension 0.25% contains betaxolol hydrochloride, a cardioselective beta-adrenergic receptor blocking agent, in a sterile resin suspension formulation. Betaxolol hydrochloride is a white, crystalline powder, with a molecular weight of 343.89.

Empirical Formula:

$C_{18}H_{29}NO_3 \cdot HCl$

Chemical Name:

(±)-1-[p-[2-(cyclopropylmethoxy)ethyl] phenoxy]-3-(isopropylamino)-2-propanol hydrochloride.

Each mL of BETOPTIC S Ophthalmic Suspension contains: **Active:** betaxolol HCl 2.8 mg equivalent to 2.5 mg of betaxolol base. **Preservative:** benzalkonium chloride 0.01%. **Inactive:** Mannitol, Poly(Styrene-Divinyl Benzene) sulfonic acid, Carbomer 934P, edetate disodium, hydrochloric acid or sodium hydroxide (to adjust pH) and purified water. DM-00

CLINICAL PHARMACOLOGY

Betaxolol HCl, a cardioselective (beta-1-adrenergic) receptor blocking agent, does not have significant membrane-stabilizing (local anesthetic) activity and is devoid of intrinsic sympathomimetic action. Orally administered beta-adrenergic blocking agents reduce cardiac output in healthy subjects and patients with heart disease. In patients with severe impairment of myocardial function, beta-adrenergic receptor antagonists may inhibit the sympathetic stimulatory effect necessary to maintain adequate cardiac function.

When instilled in the eye, BETOPTIC S Ophthalmic Suspension 0.25% has the action of reducing elevated intraocular pressure, whether or not accompanied by glaucoma. Ophthalmic betaxolol has minimal effect on pulmonary and cardiovascular parameters.

Elevated IOP presents a major risk factor in glaucomatous field loss. The higher the level of IOP, the greater the likelihood of optic nerve damage and visual field loss. Betaxolol has the action of reducing elevated as well as normal intraocular pressure and the mechanism of ocular hypotensive action appears to be a reduction of aqueous production as demonstrated by tonography and aqueous fluorophotometry. The onset of action with betaxolol can generally be noted within 30 minutes and the maximal effect can usually be detected 2 hours after topical administration. A single dose provides a 12-hour reduction in intraocular pressure.

In controlled, double-masked studies, the magnitude and duration of the ocular hypotensive effect of BETOPTIC S Ophthalmic Suspension 0.25% and BETOPTIC Ophthalmic Solution 0.5% were clinically equivalent. BETOPTIC S Suspension was significantly more comfortable than BETOPTIC Solution.

Ophthalmic betaxolol solution at 1% (one drop in each eye) was compared to placebo in a crossover study challenging nine patients with reactive airway disease. Betaxolol HCl had no significant effect on pulmonary function as measured by FEV_1, Forced Vital Capacity (FVC), FEV_1/FVC and was not significantly different from placebo. The action of isoproterenol, a beta stimulant, administered at the end of the study was not inhibited by ophthalmic betaxolol.

No evidence of cardiovascular beta adrenergic-blockade during exercise was observed with betaxolol in a double-masked, crossover study in 24 normal subjects comparing ophthalmic betaxolol and placebo for effects on blood pressure and heart rate.

INDICATIONS AND USAGE

BETOPTIC S® Ophthalmic Suspension 0.25% has been shown to be effective in lowering intraocular pressure and may be used in patients with chronic open-angle glaucoma and ocular hypertension. It may be used alone or in combination with other intraocular pressure lowering medications.

CONTRAINDICATIONS

Hypersensitivity to any component of this product. BETOPTIC S Ophthalmic Suspension 0.25% is contraindicated in patients with sinus bradycardia, greater than a first degree atrioventricular block, cardiogenic shock, or patients with overt cardiac failure.

WARNING

FOR TOPICAL OPHTHALMIC USE ONLY.

Topically applied beta-adrenergic blocking agents may be absorbed systemically. The same adverse reactions found with systemic administration of beta-adrenergic blocking agents may occur with topical administration. For example, severe respiratory reactions and cardiac reactions, including death due to bronchospasm in patients with asthma, and rarely death in association with cardiac failure, have been reported with topical application of beta-adrenergic blocking agents.

BETOPTIC S® Ophthalmic Suspension 0.25% has been shown to have a minor effect on heart rate and blood pressure in clinical studies. Caution should be used in treating patients with a history of cardiac failure or heart block. Treatment with BETOPTIC S® Ophthalmic Suspension 0.25% should be discontinued at the first signs of cardiac failure.

PRECAUTIONS

General:

Diabetes Mellitus. Beta-adrenergic blocking agents should be administered with caution in patients subject to spontaneous hypoglycemia or to diabetic patients (especially those with labile diabetes) who are receiving insulin or oral hypoglycemic agents. Beta-adrenergic receptor blocking agents may mask the signs and symptoms of acute hypoglycemia.

Thyrotoxicosis. Beta-adrenergic blocking agents may mask certain clinical signs (e.g., tachycardia) of hyperthyroidism. Patients suspected of developing thyrotoxicosis should be managed carefully to avoid abrupt withdrawal of beta-adrenergic blocking agents, which might precipitate a thyroid storm.

Muscle Weakness. Beta-adrenergic blockade has been reported to potentiate muscle weakness consistent with certain myasthenic symptoms (e.g., diplopia, ptosis and generalized weakness).

Major Surgery. Consideration should be given to the gradual withdrawal of beta-adrenergic blocking agents prior to general anesthesia because of the reduced ability of the heart to respond to beta-adrenergically mediated sympathetic reflex stimuli.

Pulmonary. Caution should be exercised in the treatment of glaucoma patients with excessive restriction of pulmonary function. There have been reports of asthmatic attacks and pulmonary distress during betaxolol treatment. Although rechallenges of some such patients with ophthalmic betaxolol has not adversely affected pulmonary function test results, the possibility of adverse pulmonary effects in patients sensitive to beta blockers cannot be ruled out.

Information for Patients: Do not touch dropper tip to any surface, as this may contaminate the contents. Do not use with contact lenses in eyes.

Drug Interactions: Patients who are receiving a beta-adrenergic blocking agent orally and BETOPTIC S® Ophthalmic Suspension 0.25% should be observed for a potential additive effect either on the intraocular pressure or on the known systemic effects of beta blockade.

Close observation of the patient is recommended when a beta blocker is administered to patients receiving catecholamine-depleting drugs such as reserpine, because of possible additive effects and the production of hypotension and/or bradycardia.

Betaxolol is an adrenergic blocking agent; therefore, caution should be exercised in patients using concomitant adrenergic psychotropic drugs.

Risk from anaphylactic reaction: While taking beta-blockers, patients with a history of atopy or a history of severe anaphylactic reaction to a variety of allergens may be more reactive to repeated accidental, diagnostic, or therapeutic challenge with such allergens. Such patients may be unresponsive to the usual doses of epinephrine used to treat anaphylactic reactions.

Ocular: In patients with angle-closure glaucoma, the immediate treatment objective is to reopen the angle by constriction of the pupil with a miotic agent. Betaxolol has little or no effect on the pupil. When BETOPTIC S Ophthalmic Suspension 0.25% is used to reduce elevated intraocular pressure in angle-closure glaucoma, it should be used with a miotic and not alone.

Carcinogenesis, Mutagenesis, Impairment of Fertility: Lifetime studies with betaxolol HCl have been completed in mice at oral doses of 6, 20 or 60 mg/kg/day and in rats at 3, 12 or 48 mg/kg/day; betaxolol HCl demonstrated no carcinogenic effect. Higher dose levels were not tested.

In a variety of *in vitro* and *in vivo* bacterial and mammalian cell assays, betaxolol HCl was nonmutagenic.

Pregnancy: Pregnancy Category C. Reproduction, teratology, and peri- and postnatal studies have been conducted with orally administered betaxolol HCl in rats and rabbits. There was evidence of drug related postimplantation loss in rabbits and rats at dose levels above 12 mg/kg and 128 mg/kg, respectively. Betaxolol HCl was not shown to be teratogenic, however, and there were no other adverse effects on reproduction at subtoxic dose levels. There are no adequate and well-controlled studies in pregnant women. BETOPTIC S should be used during pregnancy only if the potential benefit justifies the potential risk to the fetus.

Nursing Mothers: It is not known whether betaxolol HCl is excreted in human milk. Because many drugs are excreted in human milk, caution should be exercised when BETOPTIC S® Ophthalmic Suspension 0.25% is administered to nursing women.

Pediatric Use: Safety and effectiveness in pediatric patients have not been established.

Geriatric Use: No overall differences in safety and effectiveness have been observed between elderly and younger patients.

ADVERSE REACTIONS

Ocular: In clinical trials, the most frequent event associated with the use of BETOPTIC S Ophthalmic Suspension 0.25% has been transient ocular discomfort. The following other conditions have been reported in small numbers of patients: blurred vision, corneal punctate keratitis, foreign body sensation, photophobia, tearing, itching, dryness of eyes, erythema, inflammation, discharge, ocular pain, decreased visual acuity and crusty lashes.

Additional medical events reported with other formulations of betaxolol include allergic reactions, decreased corneal sensitivity, corneal punctate staining which may appear in dendritic formations, edema and anisocoria.

Systemic: Systemic reactions following administration of BETOPTIC S Ophthalmic Suspension 0.25% or BETOPTIC Ophthalmic Solution 0.5% have been rarely reported. These include:

Cardiovascular: Bradycardia, heart block and congestive failure.

Pulmonary: Pulmonary distress characterized by dyspnea, bronchospasm, thickened bronchial secretions, asthma and respiratory failure.

Central Nervous System: Insomnia, dizziness, vertigo, headaches, depression, lethargy, and increase in signs and symptoms of myasthenia gravis.

Other: Hives, toxic epidermal necrolysis, hair loss, and glossitis. Perversions of taste and smell have been reported.

OVERDOSAGE

No information is available on overdosage of humans. The oral LD50 of the drug ranged from 350–920 mg/kg in mice and 860–1050 mg/kg in rats. The symptoms which might be expected with an overdose of a systemically administered beta-1-adrenergic receptor blocking agent are bradycardia, hypotension and acute cardiac failure.

A topical overdose of BETOPTIC S® Ophthalmic Suspension 0.25% may be flushed from the eye(s) with warm tap water.

DOSAGE AND ADMINISTRATION

The recommended dose is one to two drops of BETOPTIC S Ophthalmic Suspension 0.25% in the affected eye(s) twice daily. In some patients, the intraocular pressure lowering responses to BETOPTIC S may require a few weeks to stabilize. As with any new medication, careful monitoring of patients is advised.

If the intraocular pressure of the patient is not adequately controlled on this regimen, concomitant therapy with pilocarpine and other miotics, and/or epinephrine and/or carbonic anhydrase inhibitors can be instituted.

HOW SUPPLIED

BETOPTIC S® Ophthalmic Suspension 0.25% is supplied as follows: 2.5, 5, 10 and 15 mL in plastic ophthalmic DROP-TAINER® dispensers.

2.5 mL:	**NDC** 0065-0246-20
5 mL:	**NDC** 0065-0246-05
10 mL:	**NDC** 0065-0246-10
15 mL:	**NDC** 0065-0246-15

STORAGE

Store upright at room temperature. Shake well before using.

℞ **Only.**

U.S. Patents No. 4,911,920

BION® TEARS OTC

Lubricant Eye Drops

DESCRIPTION

BION® TEARS are specially designed to be physiologically compatible with the surface of the eye and to treat dry eye symptoms by replacing needed tear components. BION® TEARS advanced formula contains:

The unique DUASORB® polymeric system which combines with natural tears to soothe and lubricate sensitive dry spots.

A special lubricating vehicle designed to match the electrolyte balance of sodium, potassium, calcium, magnesium, zinc and bicarbonate found in natural tears.

No preservatives or decongestants that may cause irritation or limit use. BION® TEARS may be used as often as necessary to provide relief.

Continued on next page

Bion—Cont.

BION® TEARS special formula requires special packaging. Airtight foil pouches are used to maintain the delicate balance of ingredients until the product is ready for use in the eye. **To ensure optimal effectiveness once the pouch is opened, the containers inside the pouch must be used within four days (96 hours).**

Active Ingredients:
DUASORB® water soluble polymeric system containing Dextran 70 0.1% and Hypromellose 2910 0.3%.

Inactive Ingredients:
Calcium chloride, magnesium chloride, potassium chloride, purified water, sodium bicarbonate, sodium chloride, zinc chloride, hydrochloric acid and/or sodium hydroxide and/or carbon dioxide to adjust pH.

WARNINGS

If you experience eye pain, changes in vision, continued redness or irritation of the eye, or if the condition worsens or persists for more than 72 hours, discontinue use and consult a doctor.
If solution changes color or becomes cloudy, do not use. To avoid contamination, do not touch tip of container to any surface. Do not reuse. Once opened, discard. Keep this and all drugs out of the reach of children. In case of accidental ingestion, seek professional assistance or contact a Poison Control Center immediately.

HOW SUPPLIED

BION® TEARS Lubricant Eye Drops are supplied in boxes of 28 0.015 fl. oz. single-use containers.
Product Code 0065-0419-18

CILOXAN® ℞

(ciprofloxacin hydrochloride ophthalmic ointment)
0.3% as Base
Sterile Ophthalmic Ointment

DESCRIPTION

CILOXAN® (ciprofloxacin hydrochloride ophthalmic ointment) Ophthalmic Ointment is a synthetic, sterile, multiple dose, antimicrobial for topical use. Ciprofloxacin is a fluoroquinolone antibacterial. It is available as the monohydrate monohydrate salt of 1-cyclopropyl-6-fluoro-1,4-dihydro-4-oxo-7-(1-piperazinyl)-3-quinolinecarboxylic acid. Ciprofloxacin is a faint to light yellow crystalline powder with a molecular weight of 385.82. Its empirical formula is $C_{17}H_{18}FN_3O_3 \cdot HCl \cdot H_2O$ and its chemical structure is as follows:

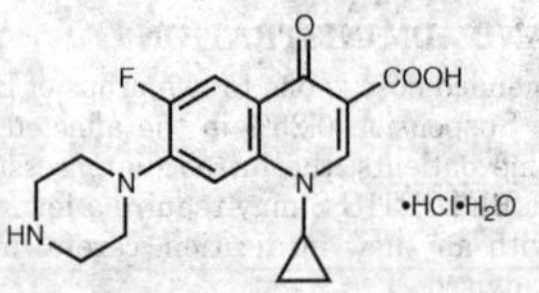

Ciprofloxacin differs from other quinolones in that it has a fluorine atom at the 6-position, a piperazine moiety at the 7-position, and a cyclopropyl ring at the 1-position.

Each gram of CILOXAN (ciprofloxacin hydrochloride ophthalmic ointment) contains: Active: Ciprofloxacin HCl 3.33 mg equivalent to 3 mg base. **Inactives:** Mineral Oil, White Petrolatum.

CLINICAL PHARMACOLOGY

Systemic Absorption: Absorption studies in humans with the ciprofloxacin ointment have not been conducted, however, based on studies with ciprofloxacin solution, 0.3%, mean maximal concentrations are expected to be less than 2.5 ng/mL.

Microbiology: Ciprofloxacin has *in vitro* activity against a wide range of gram-negative and gram-positive organisms. The bactericidal action of ciprofloxacin results from interference with the enzyme DNA gyrase which is needed for the synthesis of bacterial DNA.
Ciprofloxacin has been shown to be active against most strains of the following microorganisms both *in vitro* and in clinical infections (**SEE INDICATIONS AND USAGE** section).

Aerobic gram-positive microorganisms:
Staphylococcus aureus (methicillin-susceptible strains)
Staphylococcus epidermidis (methicillin-susceptible strains)
Streptococcus pneumoniae
Streptococcus Viridans Group

Aerobic gram-negative microorganisms:
Haemophilus influenzae

The following *in vitro* data are available; **but their clinical significance in ophthalmologic infections is unknown.** The safety and effectiveness of ciprofloxacin in treating conjunctivitis due to these microorganisms have not been established in adequate and well controlled trials.
The following organisms are considered susceptible when evaluated using systemic breakpoints. However, a correlation between the *in vitro* systemic breakpoint and ophthalmological efficacy has not been established.
Ciprofloxacin exhibits *in vitro* minimal inhibitory concentrations (MIC's) of 1μg/mL or less (systemic susceptible breakpoint) against most (≥90%) strains of the following ocular pathogens.

Aerobic gram-positive microorganisms:
Bacillus species
Corynebacterium species
Staphylococcus haemolyticus
Staphylococcus hominis

Aerobic gram-negative microorganisms:
Acinetobacter calcoaceticus
Enterobacter aerogenes
Escherichia coli
Haemophilus parainfluenzae
Klebsielle pneumoniae
Moraxella catarrhalis
Neisseria gonorrhoeae
Proteus mirabilis
Pseudomonas aeruginosa
Serratia marcesens

Most strains of *Burkholderia cepacia* and some strains of *Stenotrophomonas maltophilia* are resistant to ciprofloxacin as are most anaerobic bacteria, including *Bacteroides fragilis* and *Clostridium difficile.*
The minimal bactericidal concentration (MBC) generally does not exceed the minimal inhibitory concentration (MIC) by more than a factor of 2. Resistance to ciprofloxacin *in vitro* usually develops slowly (multiple-step mutation).
Ciprofloxacin does not cross-react with other antimicrobial agents such as beta-lactams or aminoglycosides; therefore, organisms resistant to these drugs may be susceptible to ciprofloxacin. Organisms resistant to ciprofloxacin may be susceptible to beta-lactams or aminoglycosides.

Clinical Studies: In multicenter clinical trials, approximately 75% of the patients with signs and symptoms of bacterial conjunctivitis and positive conjunctival cultures were clinically cured and approximately 80% had presumed pathogens eradicated by the end of treatment (day 7).

INDICATIONS AND USAGE

CILOXAN® (ciprofloxacin hydrochloride ophthalmic ointment) is indicated for the treatment of bacterial conjunctivitis caused by susceptible strains of the microorganisms listed below:

Gram-Positive:
Staphylococcus aureus
Staphylococcus epidermidis
Streptococcus pneumoniae
Streptococcus Viridans Group

Gram-Negative:
Haemophilus influenzae

CONTRAINDICATIONS

A history of hypersensitivity to ciprofloxacin or any other component of the medication is a contraindication to its use. A history of hypersensitivity to other quinolones may also contraindicate the use of ciprofloxacin.

WARNINGS

FOR TOPICAL OPHTHALMIC USE ONLY.
NOT FOR INJECTION INTO THE EYE.
Serious and occasionally fatal hypersensitivity (anaphylactic) reactions, some following the first dose, have been reported in patients receiving systemic quinolone therapy. Some reactions were accompanied by cardiovascular collapse, loss of consciousness, tingling, pharyngeal or facial edema, dyspnea, urticaria, and itching. Only a few patients had a history of hypersensitivity reactions. Serious anaphylactic reactions require immediate emergency treatment with epinephrine and other resuscitation measures, including oxygen, intravenous fluids, intravenous antihistamines, corticosteroids, pressor amines and airway management, as clinically indicated.

PRECAUTIONS

General: As with other antibacterial preparations, prolonged use of ciprofloxacin may result in overgrowth of nonsusceptible organisms, including fungi. If superinfection occurs, appropriate therapy should be initiated. Whenever clinical judgment dictates, the patient should be examined with the aid of magnification, such as slit lamp biomicroscopy and, where appropriate, fluorescein staining.
Ciprofloxacin should be discontinued at the first appearance of a skin rash or any other sign of hypersensitivity reaction.
Ophthalmic ointments may retard corneal healing and cause visual blurring.
Patients should be advised not to wear contact lenses if they have signs and symptoms of bacterial conjunctivitis.

Information For Patients: Do not touch tip to any surface as this may contaminate the ointment.
Do not use the product if the imprinted carton seals have been damaged, or removed.

Drug Interactions: Specific drug interaction studies have not been conducted with ophthalmic ciprofloxacin. However, the systemic administration of some quinolones has been shown to elevate plasma concentrations of theophylline, interfere with the metabolism of caffeine, enhance the effects of the oral anticoagulant, warfarin, and its derivatives, and has been associated with transient elevations in serum creatinine in patients receiving cyclosporine concomitantly.

Carcinogenesis, Mutagenesis, Impairment of Fertility: Eight *in vitro* mutagenicity tests have been conducted with ciprofloxacin and the test results are listed below:
Salmonella/Microsome Test (Negative)
E. coli DNA Repair Assay (Negative)
Mouse Lymphoma Cell Forward Mutation Assay (Positive)
Chinese Hamster V79 Cell HGPRT Test (Negative)
Syrian Hamster Embryo Cell Transformation Assay (Negative)
Saccharomyces cerevisiae Point Mutation Assay (Negative)
Saccharomyces cerevisiae Mitotic Crossover and Gene Conversion Assay (Negative)
Rat Hepatocyte DNA Repair Assay (Positive)
Thus, two of the eight tests were positive, but the results of the following three *in vivo* test systems gave negative results:
Rat Hepatocyte DNA Repair Assay
Micronucleus Test (Mice)
Dominant Lethal Test (Mice)
Long-term carcinogenicity studies in mice and rats have been completed. After daily oral dosing for up to two years, there is no evidence that ciprofloxacin had any carcinogenic or tumorigenic effects in these species.

Pregnancy: Pregnancy Category C. Reproduction studies have been performed in rats and mice at doses up to six times the usual daily human oral dose and have revealed no evidence of impaired fertility or harm to the fetus due to ciprofloxacin. In rabbits, as with most antimicrobial agents, ciprofloxacin (30 and 100 mg/kg orally) produced gastrointestinal disturbances resulting in maternal weight loss and an increased incidence of abortion. No teratogenicity was observed at either dose. After intravenous administration, at doses up to 20 mg/kg, no maternal toxicity was produced and no embryotoxicity or teratogenicity was observed. There are no adequate and well controlled studies in pregnant women. CILOXAN® (ciprofloxacin hydrochloride ophthalmic ointment) should be used during pregnancy only if the potential benefit justifies the potential risk to the fetus.

Nursing Mothers: It is not known whether topically applied ciprofloxacin is excreted in human milk. However, it is known that orally administered ciprofloxacin is excreted in the milk of lactating rats and oral ciprofloxacin has been reported in human breast milk after a single 500 mg dose. Caution should be exercised when CILOXAN® (ciprofloxacin hydrochloride ophthalmic ointment) is administered to a nursing mother.

Pediatric Use: Safety and effectiveness of CILOXAN (ciprofloxacin hydrochloride ophthalmic ointment) 0.3% in pediatric patients below the age of two years have not been established. Although ciprofloxacin and other quinolones may cause arthropathy in immature Beagle dogs after oral administration, topical ocular administration of ciprofloxacin to immature animals did not cause any arthropathy and there is no evidence that the ophthalmic dosage form has any effect on the weight bearing joints.

Geriatric Use: No overall clinical differences in safety or effectiveness have been observed between the elderly and other adult patients.

ADVERSE REACTIONS

The following adverse reactions (incidences) were reported in 2% of the patients in clinical studies for CILOXAN (ciprofloxacin hydrochloride ophthalmic ointment): discomfort, keratopathy. Other reactions associated with ciprofloxacin therapy occurring in less than 1% of patients included allergic reactions, blurred vision, corneal staining, decreased visual acuity, dry eye, edema, epitheliopathy, eye pain, foreign body sensation, hyperemia, irritation, keratoconjunctivitis, lid erythema, lid margin hyperemia, photophobia, pruritus, and tearing.
Systemic adverse reactions related to ciprofloxacin therapy occurred at an incidence below 1% and included dermatitis, nausea and taste perversion.

DOSAGE AND ADMINISTRATION

Apply a 1/2″ ribbon into the conjunctival sac three times a day on the first two days, then apply a 1/2″ ribbon two times a day for the next five days.

HOW SUPPLIED

3.5 g sterile ointment supplied in an aluminum tube with a white polyethylene tip and white polyethylene cap. 3.5 g - **NDC** 0065-0654-35
Storage: Store at 36°F to 77°F (2°C to 25°C).

ANIMAL PHARMACOLOGY

Ciprofloxacin and related drugs have been shown to cause arthropathy in immature animals of most species tested following oral administration. However, a one month topical ocular study using immature Beagle dogs did not demonstrate any articular lesions.
Rx Only

CILOXAN® ℞

(ciprofloxacin HCl ophthalmic solution)
0.3% as base
Sterile

DESCRIPTION

CILOXAN® (ciprofloxacin HCl ophthalmic solution) is a synthetic, sterile, multiple dose, antimicrobial for topical ophthalmic use. Ciprofloxacin is a fluoroquinolone antibacterial active against a broad spectrum of gram-positive and gram-negative ocular pathogens. It is available as the monohydrochloride monohydrate salt of 1-cyclopropyl-6-fluoro-1,4-dihydro-4-oxo-7-(1-piperazinyl)-3-quinoline-carboxylic acid. It is a faint to light yellow crystalline powder with a molecular weight of 385.8. Its empirical formula is

$C_{17}H_{18}FN_3O_3 \bullet HCl \bullet H_2O$ and its chemical structure is as follows:

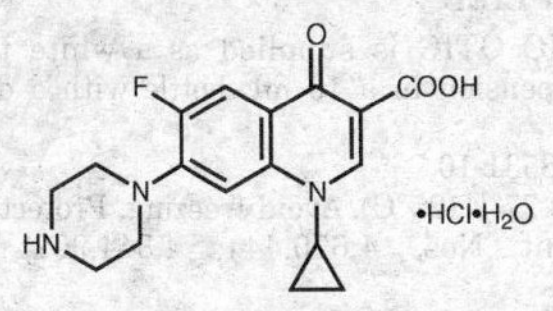

Ciprofloxacin differs from other quinolones in that it has a fluorine atom at the 6-position, a piperazine moiety at the 7-position, and a cyclopropyl ring at the 1-position.

Each mL of CILOXAN Ophthalmic Solution contains: **Active:** Ciprofloxacin HCl 3.5 mg equivalent to 3 mg base. **Preservative:** Benzalkonium Chloride 0.006%. **Inactive:** Sodium Acetate, Acetic Acid, Mannitol 4.6%, Edetate Disodium 0.05%, Hydrochloric Acid and/or Sodium Hydroxide (to adjust pH) and Purified Water. The pH is approximately 4.5 and the osmolality is approximately 300 mOsm. DM-00

CLINICAL PHARMACOLOGY

Systemic Absorption: A systemic absorption study was performed in which CILOXAN Ophthalmic Solution was administered in each eye every two hours while awake for two days followed by every four hours while awake for an additional 5 days. The maximum reported plasma concentration of ciprofloxacin was less than 5 ng/mL. The mean concentration was usually less than 2.5 ng/mL.

Microbiology: Ciprofloxacin has *in vitro* activity against a wide range of gram-negative and gram-positive organisms. The bactericidal action of ciprofloxacin results from interference with the enzyme DNA gyrase which is needed for the synthesis of bacterial DNA.

Ciprofloxacin has been shown to be active against most strains of the following organisms both *in vitro* and in clinical infections. (See INDICATIONS AND USAGE section).

Gram-Positive:

Staphylococcus aureus (including methicillin-susceptible and methicillin-resistant strains)
Staphylococcus epidermidis
Streptococcus pneumoniae
Streptococcus (Viridans Group)

Gram-Negative:

Haemophilus influenzae
Pseudomonas aeruginosa
Serratia marcescens

Ciprofloxacin has been shown to be active *in vitro* against most strains of the following organisms, however, *the clinical significance of these data is unknown:*

Gram-Positive:

Enterococcus faecalis (Many strains are only moderately susceptible)
Staphylococcus haemolyticus
Staphylococcus hominis
Staphylococcus saprophyticus
Streptococcus pyogenes
[See table above]

Other Organisms: *Chlamydia trachomatis* (only moderately susceptible) and *Mycobacterium tuberculosis* (only moderately susceptible).

Most strains of *Pseudomonas cepacia* and some strains of *Pseudomonas maltophilia* are resistant to ciprofloxacin as are most anaerobic bacteria, including *Bacteroides fragilis* and *Clostridium difficile*.

The minimal bactericidal concentration (MBC) generally does not exceed the minimal inhibitory concentration (MIC) by more than a factor of 2. Resistance to ciprofloxacin *in vitro* usually develops slowly (multiple-step mutation).

Ciprofloxacin does not cross-react with other antimicrobial agents such as beta-lactams or aminoglycosides; therefore, organisms resistant to these drugs may be susceptible to ciprofloxacin.

CLINICAL STUDIES

Following therapy with CILOXAN® Ophthalmic Solution, 76% of the patients with corneal ulcers and positive bacterial cultures were clinically cured and complete re-epithelialization occurred in about 92% of the ulcers.

In 3 and 7 day multicenter clinical trials, 52% of the patients with conjunctivitis and positive conjunctival cultures were clinically cured and 70-80% had all causative pathogens eradicated by the end of treatment.

INDICATIONS AND USAGE

CILOXAN Ophthalmic Solution is indicated for the treatment of infections caused by susceptible strains of the designated microorganisms in the conditions listed below:

Corneal Ulcers: *Pseudomonas aeruginosa*
*Serratia marcescens**
Staphylococcus aureus
Staphylococcus epidermidis
Streptococcus pneumoniae
Streptococcus (Viridans Group)*

Conjunctivitis: *Haemophilus influenzae*
Staphylococcus aureus
Staphylococcus epidermidis
Streptococcus pneumoniae

Gram-Negative:

Acinetobacter calcoaceticus subsp. anitratus
Aeromonas caviae
Aeromonas hydrophila
Brucella melitensis
Campylobacter coli
Campylobacter jejuni
Citrobacter diversus
Citrobacter freundii
Edwardsiella tarda
Enterobacter aerogenes
Enterobacter cloacae
Escherichia coli
Haemophilus ducreyi
Haemophilus parainfluenzae
Klebsiella pneumoniae
Klebsiella oxytoca
Legionella pneumophila
Moraxella (Branhamella) catarrhalis
Morganella morganii
Neisseria gonorrhoeae
Neisseria meningitidis
Pasteurella multocida
Proteus mirabilis
Proteus vulgaris
Providencia rettgeri
Providencia stuartii
Salmonella enteritidis
Salmonella typhi
Shigella sonneii
Shigella flexneri
Vibrio cholerae
Vibrio parahaemolyticus
Vibrio vulnificus
Yersinia enterocolitica

*Efficacy for this organism was studied in fewer than 10 infections.

CONTRAINDICATIONS

A history of hypersensitivity to ciprofloxacin or any other component of the medication is a contraindication to its use. A history of hypersensitivity to other quinolones may also contraindicate the use of ciprofloxacin.

WARNINGS

NOT FOR INJECTION INTO THE EYE.

Serious and occasionally fatal hypersensitivity (anaphylactic) reactions, some following the first dose, have been reported in patients receiving systemic quinolone therapy. Some reactions were accompanied by cardiovascular collapse, loss of consciousness, tingling, pharyngeal or facial edema, dyspnea, urticaria, and itching. Only a few patients had a history of hypersensitivity reactions. Serious anaphylactic reactions require immediate emergency treatment with epinephrine and other resuscitation measures, including oxygen, intravenous fluids, intravenous antihistamines, corticosteroids, pressor amines and airway management, as clinically indicated.

Remove contact lenses before using.

PRECAUTIONS

General: As with other antibacterial preparations, prolonged use of ciprofloxacin may result in overgrowth of nonsusceptible organisms, including fungi. If superinfection occurs, appropriate therapy should be initiated. Whenever clinical judgment dictates, the patient should be examined with the aid of magnification, such as slit lamp biomicroscopy and, where appropriate, fluorescein staining.

Ciprofloxacin should be discontinued at the first appearance of a skin rash or any other sign of hypersensitivity reaction.

In clinical studies of patients with bacterial corneal ulcer, a white crystalline precipitate located in the superficial portion of the corneal defect was observed in 35 (16.6%) of 210 patients. The onset of the precipitate was within 24 hours to 7 days after starting therapy. In one patient, the precipitate was immediately irrigated out upon its appearance. In 17 patients, resolution of the precipitate was seen in 1 to 8 days (seven within the first 24-72 hours), in five patients, resolution was noted in 10-13 days. In nine patients, exact resolution days were unavailable; however, at follow-up examinations, 18-44 days after onset of the event, complete resolution of the precipitate was noted. In three patients, outcome information was unavailable. The precipitate did not preclude continued use of ciprofloxacin, nor did it adversely affect the clinical course of the ulcer or visual outcome. (SEE ADVERSE REACTIONS).

Information for patients: Do not touch dropper tip to any surface, as this may contaminate the solution.

Drug Interactions: Specific drug interaction studies have not been conducted with ophthalmic ciprofloxacin. However, the systemic administration of some quinolones has been shown to elevate plasma concentrations of theophylline, interfere with the metabolism of caffeine, enhance the effects of the oral anticoagulant, warfarin, and its derivatives and has been associated with transient elevations in serum creatinine in patients receiving cyclosporine concomitantly.

Carcinogenesis, Mutagenesis, Impairment of Fertility: Eight *in vitro* mutagenicity tests have been conducted with ciprofloxacin and the test results are listed below:

Salmonella/Microsome Test (Negative)
E. coli DNA Repair Assay (Negative)
Mouse Lymphoma Cell Forward Mutation Assay (Positive)
Chinese Hamster V_{79} Cell HGPRT Test (Negative)
Syrian Hamster Embryo Cell Transformation Assay (Negative)
Saccharomyces cerevisiae Point Mutation Assay (Negative)
Saccharomyces cerevisiae Mitotic Crossover and Gene Conversion Assay (Negative)
Rat Hepatocyte DNA Repair Assay (Positive)

Thus, two of the eight tests were positive, but the results of the following three *in vivo* test systems gave negative results:

Rat Hepatocyte DNA Repair Assay
Micronucleus Test (Mice)
Dominant Lethal Test (Mice)

Long term carcinogenicity studies in mice and rats have been completed. After daily oral dosing for up to two years, there is no evidence that ciprofloxacin had any carcinogenic or tumorigenic effects in these species.

Pregnancy — Pregnancy Category C: Reproduction studies have been performed in rats and mice at doses up to six times the usual daily human oral dose and have revealed no evidence of impaired fertility or harm to the fetus due to ciprofloxacin. In rabbits, as with most antimicrobial agents, ciprofloxacin (30 and 100 mg/kg orally) produced gastrointestinal disturbances resulting in maternal weight loss and an increased incidence of abortion. No teratogenicity was observed at either dose. After intravenous administration, at doses up to 20 mg/kg, no maternal toxicity was produced and no embryotoxicity or teratogenicity was observed. There are no adequate and well controlled studies in pregnant women. CILOXAN® Ophthalmic Solution should be used during pregnancy only if the potential benefit justifies the potential risk to the fetus.

Nursing Mothers: It is not known whether topically applied ciprofloxacin is excreted in human milk; however, it is known that orally administered ciprofloxacin is excreted in the milk of lactating rats and oral ciprofloxacin has been reported in human breast milk after a single 500 mg dose. Caution should be exercised when CILOXAN Ophthalmic Solution is administered to a nursing mother.

Pediatric Use: Safety and effectiveness in pediatric patients below the age of 1 year have not been established. Although ciprofloxacin and other quinolones cause arthropathy in immature animals after oral administration, topical ocular administration of ciprofloxacin to immature animals did not cause any arthropathy and there is no evidence that the ophthalmic dosage form has any effect on the weight bearing joints.

ADVERSE REACTIONS

The most frequently reported drug related adverse reaction was local burning or discomfort. In corneal ulcer studies with frequent administration of the drug, white crystalline precipitates were seen in approximately 17% of patients (SEE PRECAUTIONS). Other reactions occurring in less than 10% of patients included lid margin crusting, crystals/scales, foreign body sensation, itching, conjunctival hyperemia and a bad taste following instillation. Additional events occurring in less than 1% of patients included corneal staining, keratopathy/keratitis, allergic reactions, lid edema, tearing, photophobia, corneal infiltrates, nausea and decreased vision.

OVERDOSAGE

A topical overdose of CILOXAN® Ophthalmic Solution may be flushed from the eye(s) with warm tap water.

DOSAGE AND ADMINISTRATION

Corneal Ulcers: The recommended dosage regimen for the treatment of **corneal ulcers** is two drops into the affected eye every 15 minutes for the first six hours and then two drops into the affected eye every 30 minutes for the remainder of the first day. On the second day, instill two drops in the affected eye hourly. On the third through the fourteenth day, place two drops in the affected eye every four hours. Treatment may be continued after 14 days if corneal re-epithelialization has not occurred.

Bacterial Conjunctivitis: The recommended dosage regimen for the treatment of **bacterial conjunctivitis** is one or two drops instilled into the conjunctival sac(s) every two hours while awake for two days and one or two drops every four hours while awake for the next five days.

HOW SUPPLIED

As a sterile ophthalmic solution: 2.5 mL, 5 mL and 10 mL in plastic DROP-TAINER® dispensers.

2.5 mL – **NDC** 0065-0656-25
5 mL – **NDC** 0065-0656-05
10 mL – **NDC** 0065-0656-10

STORAGE: Store at 2° to 25°C (36° to 77°F). Protect from light.

ANIMAL PHARMACOLOGY

Ciprofloxacin and related drugs have been shown to cause arthropathy in immature animals of most species tested following oral administration. However, a one-month topical ocular study using immature Beagle dogs did not demonstrate any articular lesions.

℞ Only

U.S. Patent No. 4,670,444

CIPRO® HC OTIC ℞

(ciprofloxacin hydrochloride and hydrocortisone otic suspension)

DESCRIPTION

CIPRO® HC OTIC (ciprofloxacin hydrochloride and hydrocortisone otic suspension) contains the synthetic broad spectrum antibacterial agent, ciprofloxacin hydro-

Continued on next page

Cipro HC—Cont.

chloride, combined with the anti-inflammatory corticosteroid, hydrocortisone, in a preserved, nonsterile suspension for otic use. Each mL of CIPRO® HC OTIC contains ciprofloxacin hydrochloride (equivalent to 2 mg ciprofloxacin), 10 mg hydrocortisone, and 9 mg benzyl alcohol as a preservative. The inactive ingredients are polyvinyl alcohol, sodium chloride, sodium acetate, glacial acetic acid, phospholipon 90H (modified lecithin), polysorbate, and purified water. Sodium hydroxide or hydrochloric acid may be added for adjustment of pH.

Ciprofloxacin, a fluoroquinolone, is available as the monohydrochloride monohydrate salt of 1-cyclopropyl-6-fluoro-1,4-dihydro-4-oxo-7-(1-piperazinyl)-3-quinolinecarboxylic acid. Its empirical formula is $C_{17}H_{18}FN_3O_3 \bullet HCl \bullet H_2O$ and its chemical structure is as follows:

Hydrocortisone, pregn-4-ene-3, 20-dione, 11, 17, 21-trihydroxy-(11β)-, is an anti-inflammatory corticosteroid. Its empirical formula is $C_{21}H_{30}O_5$ and its chemical structure is:

CLINICAL PHARMACOLOGY

The plasma concentrations of ciprofloxacin were not measured following three drops of otic suspension administration because the systemic exposure to ciprofloxacin is expected to be below the limit of quantitation of the assay (0.05 µg/mL).

Similarly, the predicted C_{max} of hydrocortisone is within the range of endogenous hydrocortisone concentration (0–150 ng/mL), and therefore can not be differentiated from the endogenous cortisol.

Preclinical studies have shown that CIPRO® HC OTIC was not toxic to the guinea pig cochlea when administered intratympanically twice daily for 30 days and was only weakly irritating to rabbit skin upon repeated exposure.

Hydrocortisone has been added to aid in the resolution of the inflammatory response accompanying bacterial infection.

Microbiology

Ciprofloxacin has *in vitro* activity against a wide range of gram-positive and gram-negative microorganisms. The bactericidal action of ciprofloxacin results from interference with the enzyme, DNA gyrase, which is needed for the synthesis of bacterial DNA. Cross-resistance has been observed between ciprofloxacin and other fluoroquinolones. There is generally no cross-resistance between ciprofloxacin and other classes of antibacterial agents such as beta-lactams or aminoglycosides.

Ciprofloxacin has been shown to be active against most strains of the following microorganisms, both *in vitro* and in clinical infections of acute otitis externa as described in the **INDICATIONS AND USAGE** section:

Aerobic gram-positive microorganism
Staphylococcus aureus
Aerobic gram-negative microorganisms
Proteus mirabilis
Pseudomonas aeruginosa

INDICATIONS AND USAGE

CIPRO® HC OTIC is indicated for the treatment of acute otitis externa in adult and pediatric patients, one year and older, due to susceptible strains of *Pseudomonas aeruginosa, Staphylococcus aureus*, and *Proteus mirabilis.*

CONTRAINDICATIONS

CIPRO® HC OTIC is contraindicated in persons with a history of hypersensitivity to hydrocortisone, ciprofloxacin or any member of the quinolone class of antimicrobial agents. This nonsterile product should not be used if the tympanic membrane is perforated. Use of this product is contraindicated in viral infections of the external canal including varicella and herpes simplex infections.

WARNINGS

NOT FOR OPHTHALMIC USE. NOT FOR INJECTION.

CIPRO® HC OTIC should be discontinued at the first appearance of a skin rash or any other sign of hypersensitivity. Serious and occasionally fatal hypersensitivity (anaphylactic) reactions, some following the first dose, have been reported in patients receiving systemic quinolones. Serious acute hypersensitivity reactions may require immediate emergency treatment.

PRECAUTIONS

GENERAL: As with other antibiotic preparations, use of this product may result in overgrowth of nonsusceptible organisms, including fungi. If the infection is not improved after one week of therapy, cultures should be obtained to guide further treatment.

Information for Patients:

If rash or allergic reaction occurs, discontinue use immediately and contact your physician.
Do not use in the eyes.
Avoid contaminating the dropper with material from the ear, fingers, or other sources.
Protect from light.
Shake well immediately before using.
Discard unused portion after therapy is completed.

Carcinogenesis, Mutagenesis, Impairment of Fertility: Eight *in vitro* mutagenicity tests have been conducted with ciprofloxacin, and the test results are listed below:

Salmonella/Microsome Test (Negative)
E. coli DNA Repair Assay (Negative)
Mouse Lymphoma Cell Forward Mutation Assay (Positive)
Chinese Hamster V_{79} Cell HGPRT Test (Negative)
Syrian Hamster Embryo Cell Transformation Assay (Negative)
Saccharomyces cerevisiae Point Mutation Assay (Negative)
Saccharomyces cerevisiae Mitotic Crossover and Gene Conversion Assay (Negative)
Rat Hepatocyte DNA Repair Assay (Positive)

Thus, 2 of the 8 tests were positive, but results of the following 3 *in vivo* test systems gave negative results:

Rat Hepatocyte DNA Repair Assay
Micronucleus Test (Mice)
Dominant Lethal Test (Mice)

Long-term carcinogenicity studies in mice and rats have been completed for ciprofloxacin. After daily oral doses of 750 mg/kg (mice) and 250 mg/kg (rats) were administered for up to 2 years, there was no evidence that ciprofloxacin had any carcinogenic or tumorigenic effects in these species. No long term studies of CIPRO® HC OTIC suspension have been performed to evaluate carcinogenic potential.

Fertility studies performed in rats at oral doses of ciprofloxacin up to 100 mg/kg/day revealed no evidence of impairment. This would be over 1000 times the maximum recommended clinical dose of ototopical ciprofloxacin based upon body surface area, assuming total absorption of ciprofloxacin from the ear of a patient treated with CIPRO® HC OTIC twice per day.

Long term studies have not been performed to evaluate the carcinogenic potential or the effect on fertility of topical hydrocortisone. Mutagenicity studies with hydrocortisone were negative.

Pregnancy: Teratogenic Effects. Pregnancy Category C:
Reproduction studies have been performed in rats and mice using oral doses of up to 100 mg/kg and IV doses up to 30 mg/kg and have revealed no evidence of harm to the fetus as a result of ciprofloxacin. In rabbits, ciprofloxacin (30 and 100 mg/kg orally) produced gastrointestinal disturbances resulting in maternal weight loss and an increased incidence of abortion, but no teratogenicity was observed at either dose. After intravenous administration of doses up to 20 mg/kg, no maternal toxicity was produced in the rabbit, and no embryotoxicity or teratogenicity was observed.

Corticosteroids are generally teratogenic in laboratory animals when administered systemically at relatively low dosage levels. The more potent corticosteroids have been shown to be teratogenic after dermal application in laboratory animals.

Animal reproduction studies have not been conducted with CIPRO® HC OTIC. No adequate and well controlled studies have been performed in pregnant women. Caution should be exercised when CIPRO® HC OTIC is used by a pregnant woman.

Nursing Mothers: Ciprofloxacin is excreted in human milk with systemic use. It is not known whether ciprofloxacin is excreted in human milk following topical otic administration. Because of the potential for serious adverse reactions in nursing infants, a decision should be made whether to discontinue nursing or to discontinue the drug, taking into account the importance of the drug to the mother.

Pediatric use: The safety and efficacy of CIPRO® HC OTIC have been established in pediatric patients 2 years and older (131 patients) in adequate and well-controlled clinical trials. Although no data are available on patients less than age 2 years, there are no known safety concerns or differences in the disease process in this population which would preclude use of this product in patients one year and older. See **DOSAGE AND ADMINISTRATION.**

ADVERSE REACTIONS

In Phase 3 clinical trials, a total of 564 patients were treated with CIPRO® HC OTIC. Adverse events with at least remote relationship to treatment included headache (1.2%) and pruritus (0.4%). The following treatment-related adverse events were each reported in a single patient: migraine, hypesthesia, paresthesia, fungal dermatitis, cough, rash, urticaria, and alopecia.

DOSAGE AND ADMINISTRATION

SHAKE WELL IMMEDIATELY BEFORE USING.

For children (age 1 year and older) and adults, 3 drops of the suspension should be instilled into the affected ear twice daily for seven days. The suspension should be warmed by holding the bottle in the hand for 1–2 minutes to avoid the dizziness which may result from the instillation of a cold solution into the ear canal. The patient should lie with the affected ear upward and then the drops should be instilled. This position should be maintained for 30–60 seconds to facilitate penetration of the drops into the ear. Repeat, if necessary, for the opposite ear. Discard unused portion after therapy is completed.

HOW SUPPLIED

CIPRO® HC OTIC is supplied as a white to off-white opaque suspension in a 10 mL bottle with a dropper dispenser.
NDC 0065-8531-10
Store below 77°F (25°C). Avoid freezing. Protect from light.
U.S. Patent Nos. 4,670,444; 4,844,902; 5,843,930; 5,965,549.
CIPRO is a registered trademark of Bayer AG.
Licensed by Bayer AG
Rx Only

CIPRODEX® ℞

[*sī-prō-dĕks*]
(ciprofloxacin 0.3% and dexamethasone 0.1%)
Sterile Otic Suspension

DESCRIPTION

CIPRODEX® (ciprofloxacin 0.3% and dexamethasone 0.1%) Sterile Otic Suspension contains the synthetic broad-spectrum antibacterial agent, ciprofloxacin hydrochloride, combined with the anti-inflammatory corticosteroid, dexamethasone, in a sterile, preserved suspension for otic use. Each mL of CIPRODEX® Otic contains ciprofloxacin hydrochloride (equivalent to 3 mg ciprofloxacin base), 1 mg dexamethasone, and 0.1 mg benzalkonium chloride as a preservative. The inactive ingredients are boric acid, sodium chloride, hydroxyethyl cellulose, tyloxapol, acetic acid, sodium acetate, edetate disodium, and purified water. Sodium hydroxide or hydrochloric acid may be added for adjustment of pH.

Ciprofloxacin, a fluoroquinolone is available as the monohydrochloride monohydrate salt of 1-cyclopropyl-6-fluoro-1,4-dihydro-4-oxo-7-(1-piperazinyl)-3-quinolinecarboxylic acid. The empirical formula is $C_{17}H_{18}FN_3O_3 \cdot HCl \cdot H_2O$ and the structural formula is:

Dexamethasone, 9-fluoro-11(beta),17,21-trihydroxy-16(alpha)-methylpregna-1,4-diene-3,20-dione, is an anti-inflammatory corticosteroid. The empirical formula is $C_{22}H_{29}FO_5$ and the structural formula is:

CLINICAL PHARMACOLOGY

Pharmacokinetics: Following a single bilateral 4-drop (total dose = 0.28 mL, 0.84 mg ciprofloxacin, 0.28 mg dexamethasone) topical otic dose of CIPRODEX® Otic to pediatric patients after tympanostomy tube insertion, measurable plasma concentrations of ciprofloxacin and dexamethasone were observed at 6 hours following administration in 2 of 9 patients and 5 of 9 patients, respectively.

Mean ± SD peak plasma concentrations of ciprofloxacin were 1.39 ± 0.880 ng/mL (n=9). Peak plasma concentrations ranged from 0.543 ng/mL to 3.45 ng/mL and were on average approximately 0.1% of peak plasma concentrations achieved with an oral dose of 250-mg [1]. Peak plasma concentrations of ciprofloxacin were observed within 15 minutes to 2 hours post dose application.

Mean ± SD peak plasma concentrations of dexamethasone were 1.14 ± 1.54 ng/mL (n=9). Peak plasma concentrations ranged from 0.135 ng/mL to 5.10 ng/mL and were on average approximately 14% of peak concentrations reported in the literature following an oral 0.5-mg tablet dose[2]. Peak plasma concentrations of dexamethasone were observed within 15 minutes to 2 hours post dose application.

Dexamethasone has been added to aid in the resolution of the inflammatory response accompanying bacterial infection (such as otorrhea in pediatric patients with AOM with tympanostomy tubes).

Microbiology: Ciprofloxacin has *in vitro* activity against a wide range of gram-positive and gram-negative microorganisms. The bactericidal action of ciprofloxacin results from interference with the enzyme, DNA gyrase, which is needed for the synthesis of bacterial DNA. Cross-resistance has been observed between ciprofloxacin and other fluoroquinolones. There is generally no cross-resistance between ciprofloxacin and other classes of antibacterial agents such as beta-lactams or aminoglycosides.

Ciprofloxacin has been shown to be active against most isolates of the following microorganisms, both *in vitro* and clinically in otic infections as described in the **INDICATIONS AND USAGE** section.

Aerobic and facultative gram-positive microorganisms
Staphylococcus aureus
Streptococcus pneumoniae
Aerobic and facultative gram-negative microorganisms
Haemophilus influenzae
Moraxella catarrhalis
Pseudomonas aeruginosa

INDICATIONS AND USAGE

CIPRODEX® Otic is indicated for the treatment of infections caused by susceptible isolates of the designated microorganisms in the specific conditions listed below:
Acute Otitis Media in pediatric patients (age 6 months and older) with tympanostomy tubes due to *Staphylococcus aureus, Streptococcus pneumoniae, Haemophilus influenzae, Moraxella catarrhalis,* and *Pseudomonas aeruginosa*.
Acute Otitis Externa in pediatric (age 6 months and older), adult and elderly patients due to *Staphylococcus aureus* and *Pseudomonas aeruginosa*.

CONTRAINDICATIONS

CIPRODEX® Otic is contraindicated in patients with a history of hypersensitivity to ciprofloxacin, to other quinolones, or to any of the components in this medication. Use of this product is contraindicated in viral infections of the external canal including herpes simplex infections.

WARNINGS

FOR OTIC USE ONLY
(This product is not approved for ophthalmic use.)
NOT FOR INJECTION
CIPRODEX® Otic should be discontinued at the first appearance of a skin rash or any other sign of hypersensitivity. Serious and occasionally fatal hypersensitivity (anaphylactic) reactions, some following the first dose, have been reported in patients receiving systemic quinolones. Serious acute hypersensitivity reactions may require immediate emergency treatment.

PRECAUTIONS

General: As with other antibacterial preparations, use of this product may result in overgrowth of nonsusceptible organisms, including yeast and fungi. If the infection is not improved after one week of treatment, cultures should be obtained to guide further treatment. If otorrhea persists after a full course of therapy, or if two or more episodes of otorrhea occur within six months, further evaluation is recommended to exclude an underlying condition such as cholesteatoma, foreign body, or a tumor.
The systemic administration of quinolones, including ciprofloxacin at doses much higher than given or absorbed by the otic route, has led to lesions or erosions of the cartilage in weight-bearing joints and other signs of arthropathy in immature animals of various species.
Guinea pigs dosed in the middle ear with CIPRODEX® Otic for one month exhibited no drug-related structural or functional changes of the cochlear hair cells and no lesions in the ossicles. CIPRODEX® Otic was also shown to lack dermal sensitizing potential in the guinea pig when tested according to the method of Buehler.
No signs of local irritation were found when CIPRODEX® Otic was applied topically in the rabbit eye.

Information for Patients
For otic use only. (This product is not approved for use in the eye.) Warm the bottle in your hand for one to two minutes prior to use and shake well immediately before using.
Avoid contaminating the tip with material from the ear, fingers, or other sources.
Protect from light.
If rash or allergic reaction occurs, discontinue use immediately and contact your physician.
It is very important to use the ear drops for as long as the doctor has instructed, **even if the symptoms improve**.
Discard unused portion after therapy is completed.

Acute Otitis Media in pediatric patients with tympanostomy tubes
Prior to administration of CIPRODEX® Otic in patients (6 months and older) with acute otitis media through tympanostomy tubes, the solution should be warmed by holding the bottle in the hand for one or two minutes to avoid dizziness which may result from the instillation of a cold solution. The patient should lie with the affected ear upward, and then the drops should be instilled. The tragus should then be pumped 5 times by pushing inward to facilitate penetration of the drops into the middle ear. This position should be maintained for 60 seconds. Repeat, if necessary, for the opposite ear (see **DOSAGE AND ADMINISTRATION**).

Acute Otitis Externa
Prior to administration of CIPRODEX® Otic in patients with acute otitis externa, the solution should be warmed by holding the bottle in the hand for one or two minutes to avoid dizziness which may result from the instillation of a cold solution. The patient should lie with the affected ear upward, and then the drops should be instilled. This position should be maintained for 60 seconds to facilitate penetration of the drops into the ear canal. Repeat, if necessary, for the opposite ear (see **DOSAGE AND ADMINISTRATION**).

Drug Interactions
Specific drug interaction studies have not been conducted with CIPRODEX® Otic.

Carcinogenesis, Mutagenesis, Impairment of Fertility
Long-term carcinogenicity studies in mice and rats have been completed for ciprofloxacin. After daily oral doses of 750 mg/kg (mice) and 250 mg/kg (rats) were administered for up to 2 years, there was no evidence that ciprofloxacin had any carcinogenic or tumorigenic effects in these species. No long term studies of CIPRODEX® Otic have been performed to evaluate carcinogenic potential.
Eight *in vitro* mutagenicity tests have been conducted with ciprofloxacin, and the test results are listed below:
Salmonella/Microsome Test (Negative)
E. coli DNA Repair Assay (Negative)
Mouse Lymphoma Cell Forward Mutation Assay (Positive)
Chinese Hamster V_{79} Cell HGPRT Test (Negative)
Syrian Hamster Embryo Cell Transformation Assay (Negative)
Saccharomyces cerevisiae Point Mutation Assay (Negative)
Saccharomyces cerevisiae Mitotic Crossover and Gene Conversion Assay (Negative)
Rat Hepatocyte DNA Repair Assay (Positive)
Thus, 2 of the 8 tests were positive, but results of the following 3 *in vivo* test systems gave negative results:
Rat Hepatocyte DNA Repair Assay
Micronucleus Test (Mice)
Dominant Lethal Test (Mice)
Fertility studies performed in rats at oral doses of ciprofloxacin up to 100 mg/kg/day revealed no evidence of impairment. This would be over 100 times the maximum recommended clinical dose of ototopical ciprofloxacin based upon body surface area, assuming total absorption of ciprofloxacin from the ear of a patient treated with CIPRODEX® Otic twice per day according to label directions.
Long term studies have not been performed to evaluate the carcinogenic potential of topical otic dexamethasone. Dexamethasone has been tested for *in vitro* and *in vivo* genotoxic potential and shown to be positive in the following assays; chromosomal aberrations, sister-chromatid exchange in human lymphocytes and micronuclei and sister-chromatid exchanges in mouse bone marrow. However, the Ames/Salmonella assay, both with and without S9 mix, did not show any increase in His+ revertants.
The effect of dexamethasone on fertility has not been investigated following topical otic application. However, the lowest toxic dose of dexamethasone identified following topical dermal application was 1.802 mg/kg in a 26-week study in male rats and resulted in changes to the testes, epididymis, sperm duct, prostate, seminal vessicle, Cowper's gland and accessory glands. The relevance of this study for short term topical otic use is unknown.

Pregnancy
Teratogenic Effects. Pregnancy Category C:
Reproduction studies have been performed in rats and mice using oral doses of up to 100 mg/kg and IV doses up to 30 mg/kg and have revealed no evidence of harm to the fetus as a result of ciprofloxacin. In rabbits, ciprofloxacin (30 and 100 mg/kg orally) produced gastrointestinal disturbances resulting in maternal weight loss and an increased incidence of abortion, but no teratogenicity was observed at either dose. After intravenous administration of doses up to 20 mg/kg, no maternal toxicity was produced in the rabbit, and no embryotoxicity or teratogenicity was observed.
Corticosteroids are generally teratogenic in laboratory animals when administered systemically at relatively low dosage levels. The more potent corticosteroids have been shown to be teratogenic after dermal application in laboratory animals.
Animal reproduction studies have not been conducted with CIPRODEX® Otic. No adequate and well controlled studies have been performed in pregnant women. Caution should be exercised when CIPRODEX® Otic is used by a pregnant woman.

Nursing Mothers:
Ciprofloxacin and corticosteroids, as a class, appear in milk following oral administration. Dexamethasone in breast milk could suppress growth, interfere with endogenous corticosteroid production, or cause other untoward effects. It is not known whether topical otic administration of ciprofloxacin or dexamethasone could result in sufficient systemic absorption to produce detectable quantities in human milk. Because of the potential for unwanted effects in nursing infants, a decision should be made whether to discontinue nursing or to discontinue the drug, taking into account the importance of the drug to the mother.

Pediatric Use:
The safety and efficacy of CIPRODEX® Otic have been established in pediatric patients 6 months and older (937 patients) in adequate and well-controlled clinical trials. Although no data are available on patients less than age 6 months, there are no known safety concerns or differences in the disease process in this population that would preclude use of this product. (See **DOSAGE AND ADMINISTRATION**.)
No clinically relevant changes in hearing function were observed in 69 pediatric patients (age 4 to 12 years) treated with CIPRODEX® Otic and tested for audiometric parameters.

ADVERSE REACTIONS

In Phases II and III clinical trials, a total of 937 patients were treated with CIPRODEX® Otic. This included 400 patients with acute otitis media with tympanostomy tubes and 537 patients with acute otitis externa. The reported treatment-related adverse events are listed below:

Acute Otitis Media in pediatric patients with tympanostomy tubes
The following treatment-related adverse events occurred in 0.5% or more of the patients with non-intact tympanic membranes.

Adverse Event	Incidence (N=400)
Ear discomfort	3.0%
Ear pain	2.3%
Ear precipitate (residue)	0.5%
Irritability	0.5%
Taste perversion	0.5%

The following treatment-related adverse events were each reported in a single patient: tympanostomy tube blockage; ear pruritus; tinnitus; oral moniliasis; crying; dizziness; and erythema.

Acute Otitis Externa
The following treatment-related adverse events occurred in 0.4% or more of the patients with intact tympanic membranes.

Adverse Event	Incidence (N=537)
Ear pruritus	1.5%
Ear debris	0.6%
Superimposed ear infection	0.6%
Ear congestion	0.4%
Ear pain	0.4%
Erythema	0.4%

The following treatment-related adverse events were each reported in a single patient: ear discomfort; decreased hearing; and ear disorder (tingling).

DOSAGE AND ADMINISTRATION

CIPRODEX® OTIC SHOULD BE SHAKEN WELL IMMEDIATELY BEFORE USE
CIPRODEX® Otic contains 3 mg/mL (3000 μg/mL) ciprofloxacin and 1 mg/mL dexamethasone.
Acute Otitis Media in pediatric patients with tympanostomy tubes: The recommended dosage regimen for the treatment of acute otitis media in pediatric patients (age 6 months and older) through tympanostomy tubes is:
Four drops (0.14 mL, 0.42 mg ciprofloxacin, 0.14 mg dexamethasone) instilled into the affected ear twice daily for seven days. The solution should be warmed by holding the bottle in the hand for one or two minutes to avoid dizziness, which may result from the instillation of a cold solution. The patient should lie with the affected ear upward, and then the drops should be instilled. The tragus should then be pumped 5 times by pushing inward to facilitate penetration of the drops into the middle ear. This position should be maintained for 60 seconds. Repeat, if necessary, for the opposite ear. Discard unused portion after therapy is completed.
Acute Otitis Externa: The recommended dosage regimen for the treatment of acute otitis externa is: For patients (age 6 months and older): Four drops (0.14 mL, 0.42 mg ciprofloxacin, 0.14 mg dexamethasone) instilled into the affected ear twice daily for seven days. The solution should be warmed by holding the bottle in the hand for one or two minutes to avoid dizziness, which may result from the instillation of a cold solution. The patient should lie with the affected ear upward, and then the drops should be instilled. This position should be maintained for 60 seconds to facilitate penetration of the drops into the ear canal. Repeat, if necessary, for the opposite ear. Discard unused portion after therapy is completed.

HOW SUPPLIED

CIPRODEX® (ciprofloxacin 0.3% and dexamethasone 0.1%) Sterile Otic Suspension is supplied as follows: 5 mL fill and 7.5 mL fill in a DROP-TAINER® system. The DROP-TAINER® system consists of a natural polyethylene bottle and natural plug, with a white polypropylene closure. Tamper evidence is provided with a shrink band around the closure and neck area of the package.
NDC 0065-8533-01, 5 mL fill
NDC 0065-8533-02, 7.5 mL fill

Storage:
Store at controlled room temperature, 15°C to 30°C (59°F to 86°F). Avoid freezing. Protect from light.

Clinical Studies:
In a randomized, multicenter, controlled clinical trial, CIPRODEX® Otic dosed 2 times per day for 7 days demonstrated clinical cures in the per protocol analysis in 86% of AOMT patients compared to 79% for ofloxacin solution, 0.3%, dosed 2 times per day for 10 days. Among culture positive patients, clinical cures were 90% for CIPRODEX® Otic compared to 79% for ofloxacin solution, 0.3%. Microbiological eradication rates for these patients in the same clinical trial were 91% for CIPRODEX® Otic compared to 82% for ofloxacin solution, 0.3%. In 2 randomized multicenter, controlled clinical trials, CIPRODEX® Otic dosed 2 times per day for 7 days demonstrated clinical cures in 87% and 94%

Continued on next page

Ciprodex—Cont.

of per protocol evaluable AOE patients, respectively, compared to 84% and 89%, respectively, for otic suspension containing neomycin 0.35%, polymyxin B 10,000 IU/mL, and hydrocortisone 1.0% (neo/poly/HC). Among culture positive patients clinical cures were 86% and 92% for CIPRODEX® Otic compared to 84% and 89%, respectively, for neo/poly/HC. Microbiological eradication rates for these patients in the same clinical trials were 86% and 92% for CIPRODEX® Otic compared to 85% and 85%, respectively, for neo/poly/HC.

References:

1. Campoli-Richards DM, Monk JP, Price A, Benfield P, Todd PA, Ward A. Ciprofloxacin: A review of its antibacterial activity, pharmacokinetic properties and therapeutic use. Drugs 1988;35:373–447.
2. Loew D, Schuster O, and Graul E. Dose-dependent pharmacokinetics of dexamethasone. Eur J Clin Pharmacol 1986;30:225–230.

U.S. Patent Nos. 4,844,902; 6,284,804; 6,359,016
Licensed to Alcon by Bayer AG, CIPRODEX® is a registered trademark of Bayer AG.
Manufactured by Alcon Laboratories, Inc.
Rx Only

PATIENT INFORMATION

CIPRODEX® (CI-PRO-DEX)
(ciprofloxacin 0.3% and dexamethasone 0.1%)
Sterile Otic Suspension

IMPORTANT PATIENT INFORMATION AND INSTRUCTIONS. READ BEFORE USE.

What is CIPRODEX® Otic?

CIPRODEX® Otic is an antibiotic/steroid combination product in a sterile suspension used to treat:

- **Middle Ear Infection with Drainage Through a Tube in Children 6 months and older:** A middle ear infection is a bacterial infection behind the eardrum. People with a tube in the eardrum may notice drainage from the ear canal.
- **Outer Ear Canal Infection in Patients 6 months and older:** An outer ear canal infection, also known as "Swimmer's Ear", is a bacterial infection of the outer ear canal. The ear canal and the outer part of the ear may swell, turn red, and be painful. Also, a fluid discharge may appear in the ear canal.

Who should NOT use CIPRODEX® Otic?

- Do not use this product if allergic to ciprofloxacin or to other quinolone antibiotics.
- Do not use this product if allergic to dexamethasone or to other steroids.
- Do not give this product to pediatric patients who are less than 6 months old.

How should CIPRODEX® Otic be given?

1. Wash hands

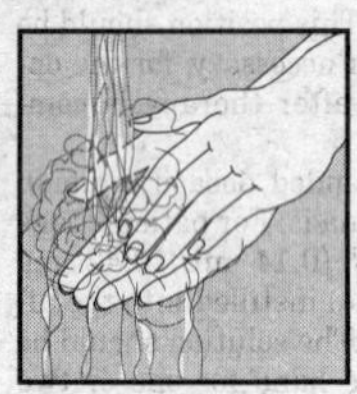

The person giving CIPRODEX® Otic should wash his/her hands with soap and water.

2. Warm & shake bottle

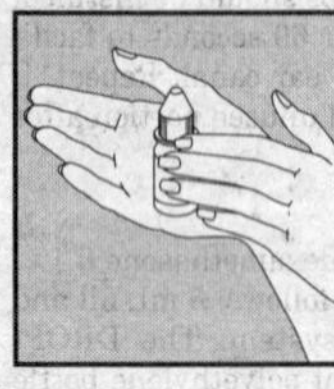

Hold the bottle of CIPRODEX® Otic in the hand for one or two minutes to warm the solution, then shake well.

3. Add drops

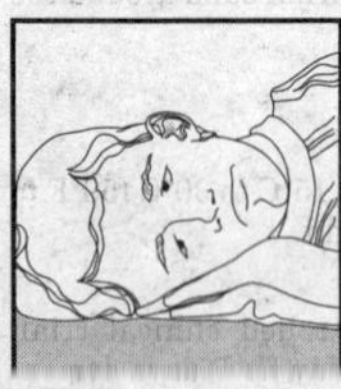

The person receiving CIPRODEX® Otic should lie on his/her side with the infected ear up.

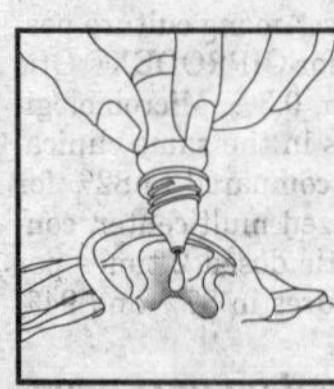

Patients should have 4 drops of CIPRODEX® Otic put into the infected ear. The tip of the bottle should not touch the fingers or the ear or any other surfaces.

BE SURE TO FOLLOW INSTRUCTIONS BELOW FOR THE PATIENT'S SPECIFIC EAR INFECTION.

4. For Patients with Middle Ear Infection with Tubes: While the person receiving CIPRODEX® Otic lies on his/her side, the person giving the drops should gently press the tragus (see diagram) 5 times in a pumping motion. This will allow the drops to pass through the tube in the eardrum and into the middle ear.

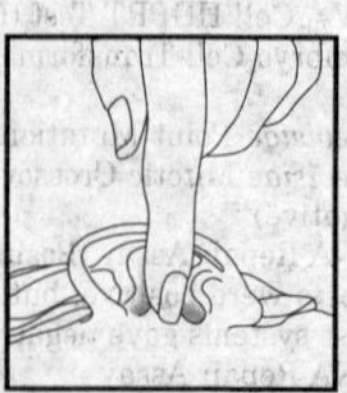

5. For Patients with Outer Ear Infection ("Swimmer's Ear"): While the person receiving the drops lies on his/her side, the person giving the drops should gently pull the outer ear lobe upward and backward. This will allow the ear drops to flow down into the ear canal.

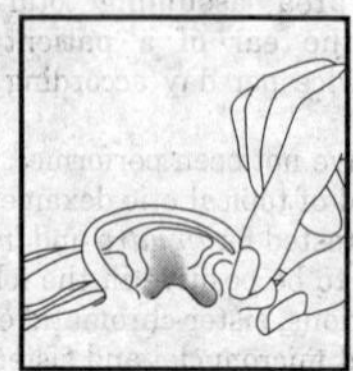

6. Stay on side

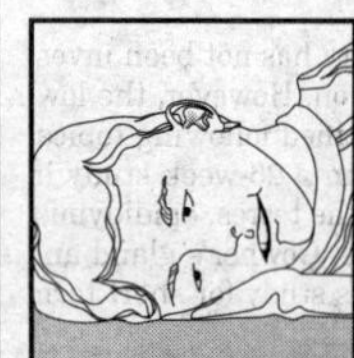

The person who received the ear drops should remain on his/her side for at least 60 seconds.
Repeat Steps 2–5 for the other ear if both ears are infected.

How often should CIPRODEX® Otic be given?

CIPRODEX® Otic ear drops should be given 2 times each day (about 12 hours apart, for example, 8 AM and 8 PM) in each infected ear unless the doctor has instructed otherwise. The best times to use the ear drops are in the morning and at night. It is very important to use the ear drops for as long as the doctor has instructed, **even if the symptoms improve**. If CIPRODEX® Otic ear drops are not used for as long as the doctor has instructed, the infection may return.

What if a dose is missed?

If a dose of CIPRODEX® Otic is missed, it should be given as soon as possible. If it is almost time for the next dose, skip the missed dose and go back to the regular dosing schedule. Do not use a double dose unless the doctor has instructed you to do so. If the infection is not improved after one week, you should consult your doctor. If you have two or more episodes of drainage within six months, it is recommended you see your doctor for further evaluation.

What activities should be avoided while using CIPRODEX® Otic?

It is important that the infected ear(s) remain clean and dry. When bathing, avoid getting the infected ear(s) wet. Avoid swimming unless the doctor has instructed otherwise.

What are the possible side effects of CIPRODEX® Otic?

During the testing of CIPRODEX® Otic for middle ear infections, the most common side effect related to CIPRODEX® Otic was ear discomfort that occurred in up to 3 out of 100 patients. Other common side effects were: ear pain; ear precipitate (residue); irritability; and abnormal taste. During the testing of CIPRODEX® Otic for ear canal infections, the most common side effect related to CIPRODEX® Otic was itching of the ear that occurred in 1 to 2 out of 100 patients. Other common side effects were: ear debris; ear infection in the treated ear; ear congestion; ear pain; and rash.
If any of these side effects persist, call the doctor.
If an allergic reaction to CIPRODEX® Otic occurs, stop using the product and contact your doctor.

DO NOT TAKE BY MOUTH

If CIPRODEX® Otic is accidentally swallowed or overdose occurs, call the doctor immediately. This medicine is available only with a doctor's prescription. Use only as directed. Do not use this medicine if outdated. If you wish to learn more about CIPRODEX® Otic, call your doctor or pharmacist.

HOW SUPPLIED

CIPRODEX® Otic is supplied as follows: 5 mL fill and 7.5 mL fill in a DROP-TAINER® system. The DROP-TAINER® system consists of a natural polyethylene bottle and natural plug, with a white polypropylene closure. Tamper evidence is provided with a shrink band around the closure and neck area of the package.
NDC 0065-8533-01, 5 mL fill
NDC 0065-8533-02, 7.5 mL fill

Storage:
Store at controlled room temperature, 15°C to 30°C (59°F to 86°F). Avoid freezing. Protect from light.

U.S. Patent Nos. 4,844,902; 6,284,804; 6,359,016
CIPRODEX® is a registered trademark of Bayer AG. Licensed to Alcon, Inc. by Bayer AG.
Manufactured by Alcon Laboratories, Inc.
Rx Only

Revision date: 17 July 2003

Shown in Product Identification Guide, page 304

NAPHCON A® OTC

Eye Drops
Relieves Itching & Redness
EYE ALLERGY RELIEF

For the temporary relief of the minor eye symptoms of itching and redness caused by ragweed, pollen, grass, animal dander and hair.

DESCRIPTION

Actives: Naphazoline Hydrochloride 0.025%, Pheniramine Maleate 0.3%. **Preservative:** Benzalkonium Chloride 0.01%. **Inactives:** Boric Acid, Edetate Disodium 0.01%, Purified Water, Sodium Borate, Sodium Chloride, Sodium Hydroxide and/or Hydrochloric Acid (to adjust pH). The sterile ophthalmic solution has a pH of about 6 and a tonicity of about 270 mOsm/Kg.

DIRECTIONS

Put 1 or 2 drops in the affected eye(s) up to 4 times every day.

WARNINGS

To avoid contamination, do not touch tip of container to any surface. Replace cap after using.
If solution changes color or becomes cloudy, do not use.
Stop use and ask a doctor if you feel eye pain, changes in vision occur, redness or irritation of the eye(s) gets worse or lasts more than 72 hours.
Overuse may cause more redness of the eye(s). When using this product, pupils may become enlarged temporarily.
If you are sensitive to any ingredient in this product, do not use. Do not use this product if you have heart disease, high blood pressure, narrow angle glaucoma or trouble urinating unless directed by a physician.
Accidental swallowing by infants and children may lead to coma and marked reduction in body temperature. Before using in children under 6 years of age, consult your physician.
Keep this and all drugs out of the reach of children. If swallowed, get medical help or contact a Poison Control Center right away.
Remove contact lenses before using.
Store at 20°–25°C (68°–77°F).
Protect from light.
Use before the expiration date marked on the carton or bottle.

PATANOL® ℞

[pă'tə-nōl]
(olopatadine hydrochloride ophthalmic solution 0.1%)

DESCRIPTION

PATANOL® (olopatadine hydrochloride ophthalmic solution) 0.1% is a sterile ophthalmic solution containing olopatadine, a relatively selective H_1- receptor antagonist and inhibitor of histamine release from the mast cell for topical administration to the eyes. Olopatadine hydrochloride is a white, crystalline, water-soluble powder with a molecular weight of 373.88. The chemical structure is presented below:

HCl

Chemical Name: 11-[(Z)-3-(Dimethylamino)propylidene]-6-11-dihydrodibenz[b,e] oxepin-2-acetic acid hydrochloride

Each mL of PATANOL contains: **Active:** 1.11 mg olopatadine hydrochloride equivalent to 1 mg olopatadine. **Preservative:** benzalkonium chloride 0.01%. **Inactives:** dibasic sodium phosphate; sodium chloride; hydrochloric acid/sodium hydroxide (adjust pH); and purified water. It has a pH of approximately 7 and an osmolality of approximately 300 mOsm/kg.

CLINICAL PHARMACOLOGY

Olopatadine is an inhibitor of the release of histamine from the mast cell and a relatively selective histamine H_1 –antagonist that inhibits the *in vivo* and *in vitro* type 1 immediate hypersensitivity reaction including inhibition of histamine induced effects on human conjunctival epithelial cells. Olopatadine is devoid of effects on alpha-adrenergic, dopamine and muscarinic type 1 and 2 receptors. Following topical ocular administration in man, olopatadine was shown to have low systemic exposure. Two studies in normal volunteers (totaling 24 subjects) dosed bilaterally with olopatadine 0.15% ophthalmic solution once every 12 hours for 2 weeks demonstrated plasma concentrations to be generally below the quantitation limit of the assay (<0.5 ng/mL). Samples in which olopatadine was quantifiable were typically found within 2 hours of dosing and ranged from 0.5 to 1.3 ng/mL. The half-life in plasma was approximately 3 hours, and elimination was predominantly through renal excretion. Approximately 60–70% of the dose was recovered in the urine as parent drug. Two metabolites, the mono-desmethyl and the N-oxide, were detected at low concentrations in the urine.

Results from an environmental study demonstrated that PATANOL was effective in the treatment of the signs and symptoms of allergic conjunctivitis when dosed twice daily for up to 6 weeks. Results from conjunctival antigen challenge studies demonstrated that PATANOL®, when subjects were challenged with antigen both initially and up to 8 hours after dosing, was significantly more effective than its vehicle in preventing ocular itching associated with allergic conjunctivitis.

INDICATIONS AND USAGE

PATANOL (olopatadine hydrochloride ophthalmic solution) 0.1% is indicated for the treatment of the signs and symptoms of allergic conjunctivitis.

CONTRAINDICATIONS

PATANOL (olopatadine hydrochloride ophthalmic solution) 0.1% is contraindicated in persons with a known hypersensitivity to olopatadine hydrochloride or any components of PATANOL.

WARNINGS

PATANOL (olopatadine hydrochloride ophthalmic solution) 0.1% is for topical use only and not for injection or oral use.

PRECAUTIONS

Information for Patients: To prevent contaminating the dropper tip and solution, care should be taken not to touch the eyelids or surrounding areas with the dropper tip of the bottle. Keep bottle tightly closed when not in use.

Patients should be advised not to wear a contact lens if their eye is red. PATANOL® (olopatadine hydrochloride ophthalmic solution) 0.1% should not be used to treat contact lens related irritation. The preservative in PATANOL, benzalkonium chloride, may be absorbed by soft contact lenses. Patients who wear soft contact lenses and **whose eyes are not red** should be instructed to wait at least ten minutes after instilling PATANOL (olopatadine hydrochloride ophthalmic solution) 0.1% before they insert their contact lenses.

Carcinogenesis, Mutagenesis, Impairment of Fertility: Olopatadine administered orally was not carcinogenic in mice and rats in doses up to 500 mg/kg/day and 200 mg/kg/day, respectively. Based on a 40 µL drop size, these doses were 78,125 and 31,250 times higher than the maximum recommended ocular human dose (MROHD). No mutagenic potential was observed when olopatadine was tested in an *in vitro* bacterial reverse mutation (Ames) test, an *in vitro* mammalian chromosome aberration assay or an *in vivo* mouse micronucleus test. Olopatadine administered to male and female rats at oral doses of 62,500 times MROHD level resulted in a slight decrease in the fertility index and reduced implantation rate; no effects on reproductive function were observed at doses of 7,800 times the maximum recommended ocular human use level.

Pregnancy: Pregnancy Category C. Olopatadine was found not to be teratogenic in rats and rabbits. However, rats treated at 600 mg/kg/day, or 93,750 times the MROHD and rabbits treated at 400 mg/kg/day, or 62,500 times the MROHD, during organogenesis showed a decrease in live fetuses. There are, however, no adequate and well controlled studies in pregnant women. Because animal studies are not always predictive of human responses, this drug should be used in pregnant women only if the potential benefit to the mother justifies the potential risk to the embryo or fetus.

Nursing Mothers: Olopatadine has been identified in the milk of nursing rats following oral administration. It is not known whether topical ocular administration could result in sufficient systemic absorption to produce detectable quantities in the human breast milk. Nevertheless, caution should be exercised when PATANOL® (olopatadine hydrochloride ophthalmic solution) 0.1% is administered to a nursing mother.

Pediatric Use: Safety and effectiveness in pediatric patients below the age of 3 years have not been established.

Geriatric Use: No overall differences in safety or effectiveness have been observed between elderly and younger patients.

ADVERSE REACTIONS

Headaches have been reported at an incidence of 7%. The following adverse experiences have been reported in less than 5% of patients: asthenia, blurred vision, burning or stinging, cold syndrome, dry eye, foreign body sensation, hyperemia, hypersensitivity, keratitis, lid edema, nausea, pharyngitis, pruritus, rhinitis, sinusitis, and taste perversion. Some of these events were similar to the underlying disease being studied.

DOSAGE AND ADMINISTRATION

The recommended dose is one drop in each affected eye two times per day at an interval of 6 to 8 hours.

HOW SUPPLIED

PATANOL (olopatadine hydrochloride ophthalmic solution) 0.1% is supplied as follows: 5 mL in plastic DROP-TAINER® dispenser.

5 mL: **NDC** 0065-0271-05

Storage: Store at 39°F–77°F (4°C–25°C)

Rx Only

U.S. Patents Nos. 4,871,865; 4,923,892; 5,116,863; 5,641,805.

340337-0104 **Revised: December 2003**

ALCON LABORATORIES, INC.
Fort Worth, Texas 76134 USA
Printed in USA

TEARS NATURALE® FORTE OTC
Lubricant Eye Drops
TEARS NATURALE FREE®
Lubricant Eye Drops

DESCRIPTION

Tears Naturale® Forte contains TriSorb™ Triple Demulcent Technology. This unique combination of ingredients works together to retain moisture on the eye and slow evaporation of the tear film. **Tears Naturale® Forte** is preserved with POLYQUAD®, gentle enough for the most sensitive eyes. *In vitro* studies have shown that POLYQUAD substantially avoids the damaging effects of epithelial cell toxicity possible with other tear substitute preservatives and allows epithelial cell growth. POLYQUAD has been shown to be 99% reaction-free in normal subjects and 97% reaction-free in subjects known to be preservative sensitive. **Tears Naturale® Forte** is designed to more closely mimic your natural tears. The unique formulation of **Tears Naturale® Forte** Lubricant Eye Drops protects against the recurrence of dry eye symptoms.

Tears Naturale Free® Lubricant Eye Drops provide lasting relief and are the most convenient preservative-free artificial tears.

- Tears Naturale Free® is the only preservative-free lubricant eye drop with reclosable vials.
- Each vial of Tears Naturale Free® contains up to 3 times as much volume as other products.

With their unique mucin like polymeric formulation, and with their natural pH, low viscosity, and isotonicity, TEARS NATURALE FORTE and TEARS NATURALE FREE provide dry eye patients with comfort and prompt relief of dry eye symptoms.

Sterile-For Topical Eye Use Only

INGREDIENTS

TEARS NATURALE FORTE: Each mL contains:

Active Ingredients: TRISORB™ lubricating and moisturizing demulcents containing: Dextran 70 0.1%, Glycerin 0.2% and Hypromellose 0.3%.

Preservative: POLYQUAD® (Polyquaternium-1) 0.001%.

Inactive Ingredients: boric acid, calcium chloride, glycine, hydrochloric acid and/or sodium hydroxide (to adjust pH), magnesium chloride, polysorbate 80, potassium chloride, purified water, sodium chloride, zinc chloride.

TEARS NATURALE FREE: **Actives:** DUASORB® water soluble polymeric system containing Dextran 70 0.1% and Hypromellose 2910 0.3%. **Inactives:** Sodium Borate, Potassium Chloride, Sodium Chloride, Purified Water. May contain Hydrochloric Acid and/or Sodium Hydroxide to adjust pH.

INDICATIONS

For the temporary relief of burning and irritation due to dryness of the eye and for use as a protectant against further irritation. For the temporary relief of discomfort due to minor irritations of the eye, or to exposure to wind or sun.

WARNINGS

If you experience eye pain, changes in vision, continued redness or irritation of the eye, or if the condition worsens or persists for more than 72 hours, discontinue use and consult a doctor.

If solution changes color or becomes cloudy, do not use.

To avoid contamination, do not touch tip of container to any surface. Replace cap after using. Keep this and all drugs out of the reach of children. In case of accidental ingestion, seek professional assistance or contact a Poison Control Center immediately.

DIRECTIONS

TEARS NATURALE® FORTE: Instill 1 or 2 drops in the affected eye(s) as needed. TEARS NATURALE FREE®: Make sure container is intact before use. To open, completely TWIST off tab and set aside for reclosure. DO NOT pull off. Instill 1 or 2 drops in the affected eye(s) as needed. To close, press tab down over container tip and twist. Reclosed vial may leak under pressure. **DISCARD CONTAINER 12 HOURS AFTER OPENING.**

HOW SUPPLIED

TEARS NATURALE FORTE Lubricant Eye Drops are supplied in 15 mL and 30 mL plastic DROP-TAINER® bottles.

15 mL NDC 0065-0426-15
30 mL NDC 0065-0426-30

TEARS NATURALE FREE Lubricant Eye Drops are supplied in boxes of 36 and 60 0.03 fl. oz. reclosable vials.

36's NDC 0065-0416-25
60's NDC 0065-0416-22

STORAGE: Store at room temperature.

TOBRADEX® ℞
(tobramycin and dexamethasone ophthalmic ointment)
Sterile

DESCRIPTION

TOBRADEX® (tobramycin and dexamethasone ophthalmic ointment) is a sterile, multiple dose antibiotic and steroid combination for topical ophthalmic use.

Each gram of TOBRADEX® Ointment contains: Actives: Tobramycin 0.3% (3mg) and Dexamethasone 0.1% (1mg). **Preservative:** Chlorobutanol 0.5%. **Inactives:** Mineral Oil and White Petrolatum. DM-00

CLINICAL PHARMACOLOGY

Corticoids suppress the inflammatory response to a variety of agents and they probably delay or slow healing. Since corticoids may inhibit the body's defense mechanism against infection, a concomitant antimicrobial drug may be used when this inhibition is considered to be clinically signficant. Dexamethasone is a potent corticoid.

The antibiotic component in the combination (tobramycin) is included to provide action against susceptible organisms. *In vitro* studies have demonstrated that tobramycin is active against susceptible strains of the following microorganisms:

Staphylococci, including *S. aureus* and *S. epidermidis* (coagulase-positive and coagulase-negative), including penicillin-resistant strains.

Streptococci, including some of the Group A-beta-hemolytic species, some nonhemolytic species, and some *Streptococcus pneumoniae.*

Pseudomonas aeruginosa, Escherichia coli, Klebsiella pneumoniae, Enterobacter aerogenes, Proteus mirabilis, Morganella morganii, most *Proteus vulgaris* strains, *Haemophilus influenzae* and *H. aegyptius, Moraxella lacunata, Acinetobacter calcoaceticus* and some *Neisseria* species.

Bacterial susceptibility studies demonstrate that in some cases microorganisms resistant to gentamicin remain susceptible to tobramycin.

No data are available on the extent of systemic absorption from TOBRADEX Ophthalmic Ointment; however, it is known that some systemic absorption can occur with ocularly applied drugs. The usual physiologic replacement dose is 0.75 mg daily. The administered dose for TOBRADEX Ophthalmic Ointment in both eyes four times daily would be 0.4 mg of dexamethasone daily.

INDICATIONS AND USAGE

TOBRADEX Ophthalmic Ointment is indicated for steroid-responsive inflammatory ocular conditions for which a corticosteroid is indicated and where superficial bacterial ocular infection or a risk of bacterial ocular infection exists.

Ocular steroids are indicated in inflammatory conditions of the palpebral and bulbar conjunctiva, cornea and anterior segment of the globe where the inherent risk of steroid use in certain infective conjunctivitides is accepted to obtain a diminution in edema and inflammation. They are also indicated in chronic anterior uveitis and corneal injury from chemical, radiation or thermal burns, or penetration of foreign bodies.

The use of a combination drug with an anti-infective component is indicated where the risk of superficial ocular infection is high or where there is an expectation that potentially dangerous numbers of bacteria will be present in the eye.

The particular anti-infective drug in this product is active against the following common bacterial eye pathogens:

Staphylococci, including *S. aureus* and *S. epidermidis* (coagulase-positive and coagulase-negative), including penicillin-resistant strains.

Streptococci, including some of the Group A-beta-hemolytic species, some nonhemolytic species, and some *Streptococcus pneumoniae.*

Pseudomonas aeruginosa, Escherichia coli, Klebsiella pneumoniae, Enterobacter aerogenes, Proteus mirabilis, Morganella morganii, most *Proteus vulgaris* strains, *Haemophilus influenzae* and *H. aegyptius, Moraxella lacunata, Acinetobacter calcoaceticus* and some *Neisseria* species.

CONTRAINDICATIONS

Epithelial herpes simplex keratitis (dendritic keratitis), vaccinia, varicella, and many other viral diseases of the cornea and conjunctiva. Mycobacterial infection of the eye. Fungal diseases of ocular structures. Hypersensitivity to a component of the medication.

WARNINGS

NOT FOR INJECTION INTO THE EYE. Sensitivity to topically applied aminoglycosides may occur in some patients. If a sensitivity reaction does occur, discontinue use.

Prolonged use of steroids may result in glaucoma, with damage to the optic nerve, defects in visual acuity and fields of vision, and posterior subcapsular cataract formation. In-

Continued on next page

TobraDex Ointment—Cont.

traocular pressure should be routinely monitored even though it may be difficult in pediatric patients and uncooperative patients. Prolonged use may suppress the host response and thus increase the hazard of secondary ocular infections. In those diseases causing thinning of the cornea or sclera, perforations have been known to occur with the use of topical steroids. In acute purulent conditions of the eye, steroids may mask infection or enhance existing infection.

PRECAUTIONS

General. The possibility of fungal infections of the cornea should be considered after long-term steroid dosing. As with other antibiotic preparations, prolonged use may result in overgrowth of nonsusceptible organisms, including fungi. If superinfection occurs, appropriate therapy should be initiated. When multiple prescriptions are required, or whenever clinical judgement dictates, the patient should be examined with the aid of magnification, such as slit lamp biomicroscopy and, where appropriate, fluorescein staining. Cross-sensitivity to other aminoglycoside antibiotics may occur; if hypersensitivity develops with this product, discontinue use and institute appropriate therapy.

Ophthalmic ointment may retard corneal wound healing.

Information for Patients: Do not touch tube tip to any surface, as this may contaminate the contents. Contact lenses should not be worn during the use of this product.

Carcinogenesis, Mutagenesis, Impairment of Fertility. No studies have been conducted to evaluate the carcinogenic or mutagenic potential. No impairment of fertility was noted in studies of subcutaneous tobramycin in rats at doses of 50 and 100 mg/kg/day.

Pregnancy Category C. Corticosteroids have been found to be teratogenic in animal studies. Ocular administration of 0.1% dexamethasone resulted in 15.6% and 32.3% incidence of fetal anomalies in two groups of pregnant rabbits. Fetal growth retardation and increased mortality rates have been observed in rats with chronic dexamethasone therapy. Reproduction studies have been performed in rats and rabbits with tobramycin at doses up to 100 mg/kg/day parenterally and have revealed no evidence of impaired fertility or harm to the fetus. There are no adequate and well controlled studies in pregnant women. TOBRADEX® Ophthalmic Ointment should be used during pregnancy only if the potential benefit justifies the potential risk to the fetus.

Nursing Mothers. Systemically administered corticosteroids appear in human milk and could suppress growth, interfere with endogenous corticosteroid production, or cause other untoward effects. It is not known whether topical administration of corticosteroids could result in sufficient systemic absorption to produce detectable quantities in human milk. Because many drugs are excreted in human milk, caution should be exercised when TOBRADEX® Ophthalmic Ointment is administered to a nursing woman.

Pediatric Use. Safety and effectiveness in pediatric patients below the age of 2 years have not been established.

ADVERSE REACTIONS

Adverse reactions have occurred with steroid/anti-infective combination drugs which can be attributed to the steroid component, the anti-infective component, or the combination. Exact incidence figures are not available. The most frequent adverse reactions to topical ocular tobramycin (TOBREX®) are hypersensitivity and localized ocular toxicity, including lid itching and swelling, and conjunctival erythema. These reactions occur in less than 4% of patients. Similar reactions may occur with the topical use of other aminoglycoside antibiotics. Other adverse reactions have not been reported; however, if topical ocular tobramycin is administered concomitantly with systemic aminoglycoside antibiotics, care should be taken to monitor the total serum concentration. The reactions due to the steroid component are: elevation of intraocular pressure (IOP) with possible development of glaucoma, and infrequent optic nerve damage; posterior subcapsular cataract formation; and delayed wound healing.

Secondary Infection. The development of secondary infection has occurred after use of combinations containing steroids and antimicrobials. Fungal infections of the cornea are particularly prone to develop coincidentally with long-term applications of steroids. The possibility of fungal invasion must be considered in any persistent corneal ulceration where steroid treatment has been used. Secondary bacterial ocular infection following suppression of host responses also occurs.

OVERDOSAGE

Clinically apparent signs and symptoms of an overdose of TOBRADEX® Ophthalmic Ointment (punctate keratitis, erythema, increased lacrimation, edema and lid itching) may be similar to adverse reaction effects seen in some patients.

DOSAGE AND ADMINISTRATION

Apply a small amount (approximately 1/2 inch ribbon) into the conjunctival sac(s) up to three or four times daily.

How to apply TOBRADEX Ophthalmic Ointment:

1. Tilt your head back.
2. Place a finger on your cheek just under your eye and gently pull down until a "V" pocket is formed between your eyeball and your lower lid.
3. Place a small amount (about 1/2 inch) of TOBRADEX Ophthalmic Ointment in the "V" pocket. Do not let the tip of the tube touch your eye.
4. Look downward before closing your eye.

Not more than 8 g should be prescribed initially and the prescription should not be refilled without further evaluation as outlined in the PRECAUTIONS above.

HOW SUPPLIED

Sterile ophthalmic ointment in 3.5 g ophthalmic tube (NDC 0065-0648-35).

STORAGE: Store at 8° to 27°C (46° to 80°F).

Rx Only

U.S. Patent No. 5,149,694

TOBRADEX® ℞

(tobramycin and dexamethasone ophthalmic suspension)
Sterile

DESCRIPTION

TOBRADEX® (tobramycin and dexamethasone ophthalmic suspension) is a sterile, multiple dose antibiotic and steroid combination for topical ophthalmic use.

Each mL of TOBRADEX® Suspension contains: Actives: Tobramycin 0.3% (3 mg) and Dexamethasone 0.1% (1 mg). **Preservative:** Benzalkonium Chloride 0.01%. **Inactives:** Tyloxapol, Edetate Disodium, Sodium Chloride, Hydroxyethyl Cellulose, Sodium Sulfate, Sulfuric Acid and/or Sodium Hydroxide (to adjust pH) and Purified Water. DM-00

CLINICAL PHARMACOLOGY

Corticoids suppress the inflammatory response to a variety of agents and they probably delay or slow healing. Since corticoids may inhibit the body's defense mechanism against infection, a concomitant antimicrobial drug may be used when this inhibition is considered to be clinically significant. Dexamethasone is a potent corticoid.

The antibiotic component in the combination (tobramycin) is included to provide action against susceptible organisms. *In vitro* studies have demonstrated that tobramycin is active against susceptible strains of the following microorganisms:

Staphylococci, including *S. aureus* and *S. epidermidis* (coagulase-positive and coagulase-negative), including penicillin-resistant strains.

Streptococci, including some of the Group A-beta-hemolytic species, some nonhemolytic species, and some *Streptococcus pneumoniae*.

Pseudomonas aeruginosa, Escherichia coli, Klebsiella pneumoniae, Enterobacter aerogenes, Proteus mirabilis, Morganella morganii, most *Proteus vulgaris* strains, *Haemophilus influenzae* and *H. aegyptius, Moraxella lacunata, Acinetobacter calcoaceticus* and some *Neisseria* species.

Bacterial susceptibility studies demonstrate that in some cases microorganisms resistant to gentamicin remain susceptible to tobramycin.

No data are available on the extent of systemic absorption from TOBRADEX Ophthalmic Suspension; however, it is known that some systemic absorption can occur with ocularly applied drugs. If the maximum dose of TOBRADEX Ophthalmic Suspension is given for the first 48 hours (two drops in each eye every 2 hours) and complete systemic absorption occurs, which is highly unlikely, the daily dose of dexamethasone would be 2.4 mg. The usual physiologic replacement dose is 0.75 mg daily. If TOBRADEX Ophthalmic Suspension is given after the first 48 hours as two drops in each eye every 4 hours, the administered dose of dexamethasone would be 1.2 mg daily.

INDICATIONS AND USAGE

TOBRADEX Ophthalmic Suspension is indicated for steroid-responsive inflammatory ocular conditions for which a corticosteroid is indicated and where superficial bacterial ocular infection or a risk of bacterial ocular infection exists.

Ocular steroids are indicated in inflammatory conditions of the palpebral and bulbar conjunctiva, cornea and anterior segment of the globe where the inherent risk of steroid use in certain infective conjunctivitides is accepted to obtain a diminution in edema and inflammation. They are also indicated in chronic anterior uveitis and corneal injury from chemical, radiation or thermal burns, or penetration of foreign bodies.

The use of a combination drug with an anti-infective component is indicated where the risk of superficial ocular infection is high or where there is an expectation that potentially dangerous numbers of bacteria will be present in the eye.

The particular anti-infective drug in this product is active against the following common bacterial eye pathogens:

Staphylococci, including *S. aureus* and *S. epidermidis* (coagulase-positive and coagulase-negative), including penicillin-resistant strains.

Streptococci, including some of the Group A-beta-hemolytic species, some nonhemolytic species, and some *Streptococcus pneumoniae*.

Pseudomonas aeruginosa, Escherichia coli, Klebsiella pneumoniae, Enterobacter aerogenes, Proteus mirabilis, Morganella morganii, most *Proteus vulgaris* strains, *Haemophilus influenzae* and *H. aegyptius, Moraxella lacunata, Acinetobacter calcoaceticus* and some *Neisseria* species.

CONTRAINDICATIONS

Epithelial herpes simplex keratitis (dendritic keratitis), vaccinia, varicella, and many other viral diseases of the cornea and conjunctiva. Mycobacterial infection of the eye. Fungal diseases of ocular structures. Hypersensitivity to a component of the medication.

WARNINGS

NOT FOR INJECTION INTO THE EYE. Sensitivity to topically applied aminoglycosides may occur in some patients. If a sensitivity reaction does occur, discontinue use.

Prolonged use of steroids may result in glaucoma, with damage to the optic nerve, defects in visual acuity and fields of vision, and posterior subcapsular cataract formation. Intraocular pressure should be routinely monitored even though it may be difficult in pediatric patients and uncooperative patients. Prolonged use may suppress the host response and thus increase the hazard of secondary ocular infections. In those diseases causing thinning of the cornea or sclera, perforations have been known to occur with the use of topical steroids. In acute purulent conditions of the eye, steroids may mask infection or enhance existing infection.

PRECAUTIONS

General. The possibility of fungal infections of the cornea should be considered after long-term steroid dosing. As with other antibiotic preparations, prolonged use may result in overgrowth of nonsusceptible organisms, including fungi. If superinfection occurs, appropriate therapy should be initiated. When multiple prescriptions are required, or whenever clinical judgement dictates, the patient should be examined with the aid of magnification, such as slit lamp biomicroscopy and, where appropriate, fluorescein staining. Cross-sensitivity to other aminoglycoside antibiotics may occur; if hypersensitivity develops with this product, discontinue use and institute appropriate therapy.

Information for Patients: Do not touch dropper tip to any surface, as this may contaminate the contents. Contact lenses should not be worn during the use of this product.

Carcinogenesis, Mutagenesis, Impairment of Fertility: No studies have been conducted to evaluate the carcinogenic or mutagenic potential. No impairment of fertility was noted in studies of subcutaneous tobramycin in rats at doses of 50 and 100 mg/kg/day.

Pregnancy Category C. Corticosteroids have been found to be teratogenic in animal studies. Ocular administration of 0.1% dexamethasone resulted in 15.6% and 32.3% incidence of fetal anomalies in two groups of pregnant rabbits. Fetal growth retardation and increased mortality rates have been observed in rats with chronic dexamethasone therapy. Reproduction studies have been performed in rats and rabbits with tobramycin at doses up to 100 mg/kg/day parenterally and have revealed no evidence of impaired fertility or harm to the fetus. There are no adequate and well controlled studies in pregnant women. TOBRADEX® Ophthalmic Suspension should be used during pregnancy only if the potential benefit justifies the potential risk to the fetus.

Nursing Mothers. Systemically administered corticosteroids appear in human milk and could suppress growth, interfere with endogenous corticosteroid production, or cause other untoward effects. It is not known whether topical administration of corticosteroids could result in sufficient systemic absorption to produce detectable quantities in human milk. Because many drugs are excreted in human milk, caution should be exercised when TOBRADEX® Ophthalmic Suspension is administered to a nursing woman.

Pediatric Use. Safety and effectiveness in pediatric patients below the age of 2 years have not been established.

ADVERSE REACTIONS

Adverse reactions have occurred with steroid/anti-infective combination drugs which can be attributed to the steroid component, the anti-infective component, or the combination. Exact incidence figures are not available. The most frequent adverse reactions to topical ocular tobramycin (TOBREX®) are hypersensitivity and localized ocular toxicity, including lid itching and swelling, and conjunctival erythema. These reactions occur in less than 4% of patients. Similar reactions may occur with the topical use of other aminoglycoside antibiotics. Other adverse reactions have not been reported; however, if topical ocular tobramycin is administered concomitantly with systemic aminoglycoside antibiotics, care should be taken to monitor the total serum concentration. The reactions due to the steroid component are: elevation of intraocular pressure (IOP) with possible development of glaucoma, and infrequent optic nerve damage; posterior subcapsular cataract formation; and delayed wound healing.

Secondary Infection. The development of secondary infection has occurred after use of combinations containing steroids and antimicrobials. Fungal infections of the cornea are particularly prone to develop coincidentally with long-term applications of steroids. The possibility of fungal invasion must be considered in any persistent corneal ulceration where steroid treatment has been used. Secondary bacterial ocular infection following suppression of host responses also occurs.

OVERDOSAGE

Clinically apparent signs and symptoms of an overdose of TOBRADEX® Ophthalmic Suspension (punctate keratitis, erythema, increased lacrimation, edema and lid itching) may be similar to adverse reaction effects seen in some patients.

DOSAGE AND ADMINISTRATION

One or two drops instilled into the conjuctival sac(s) every four to six hours. During the initial 24 to 48 hours, the dosage may be increased to one or two drops every two (2) hours. Frequency should be decreased gradually as warranted by improvement in clinical signs. Care should be taken not to discontinue therapy prematurely.

Not more than 20 mL should be prescribed initially and the prescription should not be refilled without further evaluation as outlined in PRECAUTIONS above.

HOW SUPPLIED

Sterile ophthalmic suspension in 2.5 mL (**NDC** 0065-0647-25), 5 mL (**NDC** 0065-0647-05) and 10 mL (**NDC** 0065-0647-10) DROP-TAINER® dispensers.

STORAGE: Store at 8° to 27°C (46° to 80°F).

Store suspension upright and shake well before using.

Rx Only

U.S. Patent No. 5,149,694

TRAVATAN® ℞

[*tra-va-tan*]

(travoprost ophthalmic solution) 0.004%

Sterile

DESCRIPTION

Travoprost is a synthetic prostaglandin $F_{2\alpha}$ analogue. Its chemical name is isopropyl (Z)-7-[(1R,2R,3R,5S)-3,5-dihydroxy-2-[(1*E*,3R)-3-hydroxy-4-[(α,α,α-trifluoro-m-tolyl)oxy]-1-butenyl]cyclopentyl]-5-heptenoate. It has a molecular formula of $C_{26}H_{35}F_3O_6$ and a molecular weight of 500.56. The chemical structure of travoprost is:

Travoprost is a clear, colorless to slightly yellow oil that is very soluble in acetonitrile, methanol, octanol, and chloroform. It is practically insoluble in water.

TRAVATAN® Ophthalmic Solution 0.004% is supplied as sterile, buffered aqueous solution of travoprost with a pH of approximately 6.0 and an osmolality of approximately 290 mOsmol/kg.

Each mL of TRAVATAN® 0.004% contains 40 µg travoprost. Benzalkonium chloride 0.015% is added as a preservative. Inactive ingredients are: polyoxyl 40 hydrogenated castor oil, tromethamine, boric acid, mannitol, edetate disodium, sodium hydroxide and/or hydrochloric acid (to adjust pH) and purified water.

CLINICAL PHARMACOLOGY

Mechanism of Action

Travoprost free acid is a selective FP prostanoid receptor agonist which is believed to reduce intraocular pressure by increasing uveoscleral outflow. The exact mechanism of action is unknown at this time.

Pharmacokinetics/Pharmacodynamics

Absorption: Travoprost is absorbed through the cornea and is hydrolyzed to the active free acid. Data from four multiple dose pharmacokinetic studies (totaling 107 subjects) have shown that plasma concentrations of the free acid are below 0.01 ng/mL (the quantitation limit of the assay) in two-thirds of the subjects. In those individuals with quantifiable plasma concentrations (N=38), the mean plasma C_{max} was 0.018 ± 007 ng/mL (ranged 0.01 to 0.052 ng/mL) and was reached within 30 minutes. From these studies, travoprost is estimated to have a plasma half-life of 45 minutes. There was no difference in plasma concentrations between Days 1 and 7, indicating steady-state was reached early and that there was no significant accumulation.

Metabolism: Travoprost, an isopropyl ester prodrug, is hydrolyzed by esterases in the cornea to its biologically active free acid. Systemically, travoprost free acid is metabolized to inactive metabolites via beta-oxidation of the α(carboxylic acid) chain to give the 1,2-dinor and 1,2,3,4-tetranor analogs, via oxidation of the 15-hydroxyl moiety, as well as via reduction of the 13,14 double bond.

Elimination: The elimination of travoprost free acid from plasma was rapid and levels were generally below the limit of quantification within one hour after dosing. The terminal elimination half-life of travoprost free acid was estimated from fourteen subjects and ranged from 17 minutes to 86 minutes with the mean half-life of 45 minutes. Less than 2% of the topical ocular dose of travoprost was excreted in the urine within 4 hours as the travoprost free acid.

Clinical Studies

In clinical studies, patients with open-angle glaucoma or ocular hypertension and baseline pressure of 25–27 mm Hg who were treated with TRAVATAN® Ophthalmic Solution 0.004% dosed once-daily in the evening demonstrated 7–8 mm Hg reductions in intraocular pressure. In subgroup analyses of these studies, mean IOP reduction in black patients was up to 1.8 mm Hg greater than in non-black patients. It is not known at this time whether this difference is attributed to race or to heavily pigmented irides.

In a multi-center, randomized, controlled trial, patients with mean baseline intraocular pressure of 24–26 mm Hg on TIMOPTIC* 0.5% BID who were treated with TRAVATAN® 0.004% dosed QD adjunctively to TIMOPTIC* 0.5% BID demonstrated 6–7 mm Hg reductions in intraocular pressure.

TRAVATAN® has been studied in patients with hepatic impairment and also in patients with renal impairment. No clinically relevant changes in hematology, blood chemistry, or urinalysis laboratory data were observed in these patients.

INDICATIONS AND USAGE

TRAVATAN® Ophthalmic Solution is indicated for the reduction of elevated intraocular pressure in patients with open-angle glaucoma or ocular hypertension who are intolerant of other intraocular pressure lowering medications or insufficiently responsive (failed to achieve target IOP determined after multiple measurements over time) to another intraocular pressure lowering medication.

CONTRAINDICATIONS

Known hypersensitivity to travoprost, benzalkonium chloride or any other ingredients in this product.

WARNINGS

TRAVATAN® has been reported to cause changes to pigmented tissues. The most frequently reported changes have been increased pigmentation of the iris and periorbital tissue (eyelid) and increased pigmentation and growth of eyelashes. These changes may be permanent.

TRAVATAN® may gradually change eye color, increasing the amount of brown pigmentation in the iris by increasing the number of melanosomes (pigment granules) in melanocytes. The long term effects on the melanocytes and the consequences of potential injury to the melanocytes and/or deposition of pigment granules to other areas of the eye are currently unknown. The change in iris color occurs slowly and may not be noticeable for months to years. Patients should be informed of the possibility of iris color change.

Eyelid skin darkening has been reported in association with the use of TRAVATAN®.

TRAVATAN® Ophthalmic Solution may gradually change eyelashes in the treated eye; these changes include increased length, thickness, pigmentation, and/or number of lashes.

Patients who are expected to receive treatment in only one eye should be informed about the potential for increased brown pigmentation of the iris, periorbital and/or eyelid tissue, and eyelashes in the treated eye and thus heterochromia between the eyes. They should also be advised of the potential for a disparity between the eyes in length, thickness, and/or number of eyelashes.

PRECAUTIONS

General

There have been reports of bacterial keratitis associated with the use of multiple-dose containers of topical ophthalmic products. These containers had been inadvertently contaminated by patients who, in most cases, had a concurrent corneal disease or a disruption of the epithelial surface (see Information for Patients).

Patients may slowly develop increased brown pigmentation of the iris. This change may not be noticeable for months to years (see Warnings). Iris pigmentation changes may be more noticeable in patients with mixed colored irides, i.e., blue-brown, grey-brown, yellow-brown, and green-brown; however, it has also been observed in patients with brown eyes. The color change is believed to be due to increased melanin content in the stromal melanocytes of the iris. The exact mechanism of action is unknown at this time. Typically the brown pigmentation around the pupil spreads concentrically towards the periphery in affected eyes, but the entire iris or parts of it may become more brownish. Until more information about increased brown pigmentation is available, patients should be examined regularly and, depending on the situation, treatment may be stopped if increased pigmentation ensues.

TRAVATAN® should be used with caution in patients with a history of intraocular inflammation (iritis/uveitis) and should generally not be used in patients with active intraocular inflammation.

Macular edema, including cystoid macular edema, has been reported during treatment with prostaglandin $F_{2\alpha}$ analogues. These reports have mainly occurred in aphakic patients, pseudophakic patients with a torn posterior lens capsule, or in patients with known risk factors for macular edema. TRAVATAN® Ophthalmic Solution should be used with caution in these patients.

TRAVATAN® has not been evaluated for the treatment of angle closure, inflammatory or neovascular glaucoma.

TRAVATAN® Ophthalmic Solution should not be administered while wearing contact lenses.

Patients should be advised that TRAVATAN® contains benzalkonium chloride which may be absorbed by contact lenses. Contact lenses should be removed prior to the administration of the solution. Lenses may be reinserted 15 minutes following administration of TRAVATAN®.

Information for Patients

Patients should be advised concerning all the information contained in the Warnings and Precautions sections.

Patients should also be instructed to avoid allowing the tip of the dispensing container to contact the eye or surrounding structures because this could cause the tip to become contaminated by common bacteria known to cause ocular infections. Serious damage to the eye and subsequent loss of vision may result from using contaminated solutions.

Patients also should be advised that if they develop an intercurrent ocular condition (e.g., trauma, or infection) or have ocular surgery, they should immediately seek their physician's advice concerning the continued use of the multi-dose container.

Patients should be advised that if they develop any ocular reactions, particularly conjunctivitis and lid reactions, they should immediately seek their physician's advice.

If more than one topical ophthalmic drug is being used, the drugs should be administered at least five (5) minutes apart.

Carcinogenesis, Mutagenesis, Impairment of Fertility

Two-year carcinogenicity studies in mice and rats at subcutaneous doses of 10, 30, or 100 µg/kg/day did not show any evidence of carcinogenic potential. However, at 100 µg/kg/day, male rats were only treated for 82 weeks, and the maximum tolerated dose (MTD) was not reached in the mouse study. The high dose (100 µg/kg) corresponds to exposure levels over 400 times the human exposure at the maximum recommended human ocular dose (MRHOD) of 0.04 µg/kg, based on plasma active drug levels.

Travoprost was not mutagenic in the Ames test, mouse micronucleus test or rat chromosome aberration assay. A slight increase in the mutant frequency was observed in one of two mouse lymphoma assays in the presence of rat S-9 activation enzymes.

Travoprost did not affect mating or fertility indices in male or female rats at subcutaneous doses up to 10 µg/kg/day [250 times the maximum recommended human ocular dose of 0.04 µg/kg/day on a µg/kg basis (MRHOD)]. At 10 µg/kg/day, the mean number of corpora lutea was reduced, and the post-implantation losses were increased. These effects were not observed at 3 µg/kg/day (75 times the MRHOD).

Pregnancy: Teratogenic Effects

Pregnancy Category: C

Travoprost was teratogenic in rats, at an intravenous (IV) dose up to 10 µg/kg/day (250 times the MRHOD), evidenced by an increase in the incidence of skeletal malformations as well as external and visceral malformations, such as fused sternebrae, domed head and hydrocephaly. Travoprost was not teratogenic in rats at IV doses up to 3 µg/kg/day (75 times the MRHOD), or in mice at subcutaneous doses up to 1.0 µg/kg/day (25 times the MRHOD). Travoprost produced an increase in post-implantation losses and a decrease in fetal viability in rats at IV doses > 3 µg/kg/day (75 times the MRHOD) and in mice at subcutaneous doses > 0.3 µg/kg/day (7.5 times the MRHOD).

In the offspring of female rats that received travoprost subcutaneously from Day 7 of pregnancy to lactation Day 21 at the doses of ≥ 0.12 µg/kg/day (3 times the MRHOD), the incidence of postnatal mortality was increased, and neonatal body weight gain was decreased. Neonatal development was also affected, evidenced by delayed eye opening, pinna detachment and preputial separation, and by decreased motor activity.

There are no adequate and well-controlled studies in pregnant women. TRAVATAN® should be used during pregnancy only if the potential benefit justifies the potential risk to the fetus.

Nursing Mothers

A study in lactating rats demonstrated that radiolabeled travoprost and/or its metabolites were excreted in milk. It is not known whether this drug or its metabolites are excreted in human milk. Because many drugs are excreted in human milk, caution should be exercised when TRAVATAN® is administered to a nursing woman.

Pediatric Use

Safety and effectiveness in pediatric patients have not been established.

Geriatric Use

No overall differences in safety or effectiveness have been observed between elderly and other adult patients.

ADVERSE REACTIONS

The most common ocular adverse event observed in controlled clinical studies with TRAVATAN® 0.004% was ocular hyperemia which was reported in 35 to 50% of patients. Approximately 3% of patients discontinued therapy due to conjunctival hyperemia.

Ocular adverse events reported at an incidence of 5 to 10% included decreased visual acuity, eye discomfort, foreign body sensation, pain, and pruritus.

Ocular adverse events reported at an incidence of 1 to 4% included abnormal vision, blepharitis, blurred vision, cataract, cells, conjunctivitis, dry eye, eye disorder, flare, iris discoloration, keratitis, lid margin crusting, photophobia, subconjunctival hemorrhage, and tearing.

Nonocular adverse events reported at a rate of 1 to 5% were accidental injury, angina pectoris, anxiety, arthritis, back pain, bradycardia, bronchitis, chest pain, cold syndrome, depression, dyspepsia, gastrointestinal disorder, headache, hypercholesterolemia, hypertension, hypotension, infection, pain, prostate disorder, sinusitis, urinary incontinence, and urinary tract infection.

DOSAGE AND ADMINISTRATION

The recommended dosage is one drop in the affected eye(s) once-daily in the evening. The dosage of TRAVATAN® should not exceed once-daily since it has been shown that more frequent administration may decrease the intraocular pressure lowering effect.

Continued on next page

Travatan—Cont.

Reduction of intraocular pressure starts approximately 2 hours after administration and the maximum effect is reached after 12 hours.
TRAVATAN® may be used concomitantly with other topical ophthalmic drug products to lower intraocular pressure. If more than one topical ophthalmic drug is being used, the drugs should be administered at least five (5) minutes apart.

HOW SUPPLIED

TRAVATAN® (travoprost ophthalmic solution) 0.004% is a sterile, isotonic, buffered, preserved, aqueous solution of travoprost (0.04 mg/mL) supplied in Alcon's oval DROP-TAINER® package system.
TRAVATAN® is supplied as a 2.5 mL solution in a 4 mL and a 5 mL solution in a 7.5 mL natural polypropylene dispenser bottle with a natural polypropylene dropper tip and a turquoise polypropylene overcap. Tamper evidence is provided with a shrink band around the closure and neck area of the package.
NDC 0065-0266-25, 2.5 mL fill
NDC 0065-0266-17, 2 units, 2.5 mL fill each
NDC 0065-0266-34, 5 mL fill
Storage
Store at 2°-25°C (36°-77°F).
Rx Only
U.S. Patent Nos. 5,631,287; 5,849,792; 5,889,052; 6,011,062 and 6,235,781.

*TIMOPTIC is a registered trademark of Merck & Co., Inc.
Alcon®
ALCON LABORATORIES, INC.
Fort Worth, Texas 76134 USA
© 2004 Alcon, Inc.

VIGAMOX™ ℞

[*Vi-ga-mox*]
(moxifloxacin hydrochloride ophthalmic solution)
0.5% as base

DESCRIPTION

VIGAMOX™ (moxifloxacin HCl ophthalmic solution) 0.5% is a sterile ophthalmic solution. It is an 8-methoxy fluoroquinolone anti-infective for topical ophthalmic use.

[Chemical structure of moxifloxacin hydrochloride]

$C_{21}H_{24}FN_3O_4 \cdot HCl$ Mol. Wt 437.9

Chemical Name: 1-Cyclopropyl-6-fluoro-1,4-dihydro-8-methoxy-7-[(4aS,7aS)-octahydro-6H-pyrrolol[3,4-b]pyridin-6-yl]-4-oxo-3-quinolinecarboxylic acid, monohydrochloride.
Moxifloxacin hydrochloride is a slightly yellow to yellow crystalline powder. Each mL of VIGAMOX™ contains 5.45 mg moxifloxacin hydrochloride equivalent to 5 mg moxifloxacin base.
Contains:
Active: Moxifloxacin 0.5% (5 mg/mL); **Inactives:** Boric acid, sodium chloride, and purified water. May also contain hydrochloric acid/sodium hydroxide to adjust pH to approximately 6.8.
VIGAMOX™ is an isotonic solution with an osmolality of approximately 290 mOsm/kg.

CLINICAL PHARMACOLOGY

Pharmacokinetics: Plasma concentrations of moxifloxacin were measured in healthy adult male and female subjects who received bilateral topical ocular doses of VIGAMOX™ 3 times a day. The mean steady-state C_{max} (2.7 ng/mL) and estimated daily exposure AUC (45 ng·hr/mL) values were 1,600 and 1,000 times lower than the mean C_{max} and AUC reported after therapeutic 400 mg oral doses of moxifloxacin. The plasma half-life of moxifloxacin was estimated to be 13 hours.
Microbiology
Moxifloxacin is an 8-methoxy fluoroquinolone with a diazabicyclononyl ring at the C7 position. The antibacterial action of moxifloxacin results from inhibition of the topoisomerase II (DNA gyrase) and topoisomerase IV. DNA gyrase is an essential enzyme that is involved in the replication, transcription and repair of bacterial DNA. Topoisomerase IV is an enzyme known to play a key role in the partitioning of the chromosomal DNA during bacterial cell division.
The mechanism of action for quinolones, including moxifloxacin, is different from that of macrolides, aminoglycosides, or tetracyclines. Therefore, moxifloxacin may be active against pathogens that are resistant to these antibiotics and these antibiotics may be active against pathogens that are resistant to moxifloxacin. There is no cross-resistance between moxifloxacin and the aforementioned classes of antibiotics. Cross resistance has been observed between systemic moxifloxacin and some other quinolones.
In vitro resistance to moxifloxacin develops via multiple-step mutations. Resistance to moxifloxacin occurs *in vitro* at a general frequency of between 1.8×10^{-9} to $< 1 \times 10^{-11}$ for Gram-positive bacteria.
Moxifloxacin has been shown to be active against most strains of the following microorganisms, both *in vitro* and in clinical infections as described in the INDICATIONS AND USAGE section:
Aerobic Gram-positive microorganisms:
Corynebacterium species*
*Micrococcus luteus**
Staphylococcus aureus
Staphylococcus epidermidis
Staphylococcus haemolyticus
Staphylococcus hominis
*Staphylococcus warneri**
Streptococcus pneumoniae
Streptococcus viridans group
Aerobic Gram-negative microorganisms:
*Acinetobacter lwoffii**
Haemophilus influenzae
*Haemophilus parainfluenzae**
Other microorganisms:
Chlamydia trachomatis

*Efficacy for this organism was studied in fewer than 10 infections.
The following *in vitro* data are also available, **but their clinical significance in ophthalmic infections is unknown**. The safety and effectiveness of VIGAMOX™ in treating ophthalmological infections due to these microorganisms have not been established in adequate and well-controlled trials.
The following organisms are considered susceptible when evaluated using systemic breakpoints. However, a correlation between the *in vitro* systemic breakpoint and ophthalmological efficacy has not been established. The list of organisms is provided as guidance only in assessing the potential treatment of conjunctival infections. Moxifloxacin exhibits *in vitro* minimal inhibitory concentrations (MICs) of 2 µg/ml or less (systemic susceptible breakpoint) against most (≥ 90%) of strains of the following ocular pathogens.
Aerobic Gram-positive microorganisms:
Streptococcus pyogenes
Aerobic Gram-negative microorganisms:
Escherichia coli
Klebsiella oxytoca
Klebsiella pneumoniae
Moraxella catarrhalis
Proteus mirabilis
Anaerobic microorganisms:
Fusobacterium species
Prevotella species
Clinical Studies:
In two randomized, double-masked, multicenter, controlled clinical trials in which patients were dosed 3 times a day for 4 days, VIGAMOX™ solution produced clinical cures on day 5–6 in 66% to 69% of patients treated for bacterial conjunctivitis. Microbiological success rates for the eradication of the baseline pathogens ranged from 84% to 94%. Please note that microbiologic eradication does not always correlate with clinical outcome in anti-infective trials.

INDICATIONS AND USAGE

VIGAMOX™ solution is indicated for the treatment of bacterial conjunctivitis caused by susceptible strains of the following organisms:
Aerobic Gram-positive microorganisms:
Corynebacterium species*
*Micrococcus luteus**
Staphylococcus aureus
Staphylococcus epidermidis
Staphylococcus haemolyticus
Staphylococcus hominis
*Staphylococcus warneri**
Streptococcus pneumoniae
Streptococcus viridans group
Aerobic Gram-negative microorganisms:
*Acinetobacter lwoffii**
Haemophilus influenzae
*Haemophilus parainfluenzae**
Other microorganisms:
Chlamydia trachomatis

*Efficacy for this organism was studied in fewer than 10 infections.

CONTRAINDICATIONS

VIGAMOX™ (moxifloxacin HCl ophthalmic solution) is contraindicated in patients with a history of hypersensitivity to moxifloxacin, to other quinolones, or to any of the components in this medication.

WARNINGS

NOT FOR INJECTION.
VIGAMOX™ solution should not be injected subconjunctivally, nor should it be introduced directly into the anterior chamber of the eye.
In patients receiving systemically administered quinolones, including moxifloxacin, serious and occasionally fatal hypersensitivity (anaphylactic) reactions have been reported, some following the first dose. Some reactions were accompanied by cardiovascular collapse, loss of consciousness, angioedema (including laryngeal, pharyngeal or facial edema), airway obstruction, dyspnea, urticaria, and itching. If an allergic reaction to moxifloxacin occurs, discontinue use of the drug. Serious acute hypersensitivity reactions may require immediate emergency treatment. Oxygen and airway management should be administered as clinically indicated.

PRECAUTIONS

General: As with other anti-infectives, prolonged use may result in overgrowth of non-susceptible organisms, including fungi. If superinfection occurs, discontinue use and institute alternative therapy. Whenever clinical judgment dictates, the patient should be examined with the aid of magnification, such as slit-lamp biomicroscopy, and, where appropriate, fluorescein staining. Patients should be advised not to wear contact lenses if they have signs and symptoms of bacterial conjunctivitis.
Information for Patients: Avoid contaminating the applicator tip with material from the eye, fingers or other source. Systemically administered quinolones including moxifloxacin have been associated with hypersensitivity reactions, even following a single dose. Discontinue use immediately and contact your physician at the first sign of a rash or allergic reaction.
Drug Interactions: Drug-drug interaction studies have not been conducted with VIGAMOX™ solution. *In vitro* studies indicate that moxifloxacin does not inhibit CYP3A4, CYP2D6, CYP2C9, CYP2C19, or CYP1A2 indicating that moxifloxacin is unlikely to alter the pharmacokinetics of drugs metabolized by these cytochrome P450 isozymes.
Carcinogenesis, Mutagenesis, Impairment of Fertility: Long-term studies in animals to determine the carcinogenic potential of moxifloxacin have not been performed. However, in an accelerated study with initiators and promoters, moxifloxacin was not carcinogenic in rats following up to 38 weeks of oral dosing at 500 mg/kg/day (approximately 21,700 times the highest recommended total daily human ophthalmic dose for a 50 kg person, on a mg/kg basis).
Moxifloxacin was not mutagenic in four bacterial strains used in the Ames *Salmonella* reversion assay. As with other quinolones, the positive response observed with moxifloxacin in strain TA 102 using the same assay may be due to the inhibition of DNA gyrase. Moxifloxacin was not mutagenic in the CHO/HGPRT mammalian cell gene mutation assay. An equivocal result was obtained in the same assay when v79 cells were used. Moxifloxacin was clastogenic in the v79 chromosome aberration assay, but it did not induce unscheduled DNA synthesis in cultured rat hepatocytes. There was no evidence of genotoxicity *in vivo* in a micronucleus test or a dominant lethal test in mice.
Moxifloxacin had no effect on fertility in male and female rats at oral doses as high as 500 mg/kg/day, approximately 21,700 times the highest recommended total daily human ophthalmic dose. At 500 mg/kg orally there were slight effects on sperm morphology (head-tail separation) in male rats and on the estrous cycle in female rats.
Pregnancy: Teratogenic Effects.
Pregnancy Category C: Moxifloxacin was not teratogenic when administered to pregnant rats during organogenesis at oral doses as high as 500 mg/kg/day (approximately 21,700 times the highest recommended total daily human ophthalmic dose); however, decreased fetal body weights and slightly delayed fetal skeletal development were observed. There was no evidence of teratogenicity when pregnant Cynomolgus monkeys were given oral doses as high as 100 mg/kg/day (approximately 4,300 times the highest recommended total daily human ophthalmic dose). An increased incidence of smaller fetuses was observed at 100 mg/kg/day.
Since there are no adequate and well-controlled studies in pregnant women, VIGAMOX™ solution should be used during pregnancy only if the potential benefit justifies the potential risk to the fetus.
Nursing Mothers: Moxifloxacin has not been measured in human milk, although it can be presumed to be excreted in human milk. Caution should be exercised when VIGAMOX™ solution is administered to a nursing mother.
Pediatric Use: The safety and effectiveness of VIGAMOX™ solution in infants below 1 year of age have not been established. There is no evidence that the ophthalmic administration of VIGAMOX™ has any effect on weight bearing joints, even though oral administration of some quinolones has been shown to cause arthropathy in immature animals.
Geriatric Use: No overall differences in safety and effectiveness have been observed between elderly and younger patients.

ADVERSE REACTIONS

The most frequently reported ocular adverse events were conjunctivitis, decreased visual acuity, dry eye, keratitis, ocular discomfort, ocular hyperemia, ocular pain, ocular pruritus, subconjunctival hemorrhage, and tearing. These events occurred in approximately 1-6% of patients.
Nonocular adverse events reported at a rate of 1-4% were fever, increased cough, infection, otitis media, pharyngitis, rash, and rhinitis.

DOSAGE AND ADMINISTRATION

Instill one drop in the affected eye 3 times a day for 7 days.

HOW SUPPLIED

VIGAMOX™ (moxifloxacin hydrochloride ophthalmic solution) 0.5% is supplied as a sterile ophthalmic solution in Alcon's DROP-TAINER® dispensing system consisting of a natural low density polyethylene bottle and dispensing plug

and tan polypropylene closure. Tamper evidence is provided with a shrink band around the closure and neck area of the package.
3 mL in 6 mL bottle - **NDC** 0065-4013-03
Storage: Store at 2°C-25°C (36°F-77°F).
Rx Only
Manufactured by
Alcon Laboratories, Inc.
Fort Worth, Texas 76134 USA
Licensed from Bayer AG to Alcon, Inc.
U.S. PAT. NO. 4,990,517; 5,607,942; 5,849,752

Allergan, Inc.

2525 DUPONT DRIVE
P.O. BOX 19534
IRVINE, CA 92623-9534

Direct Inquiries to:
(714) 246-4500

OPHTHALMIC PRODUCTS

For information on Allergan, Inc., prescription, OTC, and ophthalmic products, consult the Physicians' Desk Reference for Ophthalmology. For literature, service items, or sample material, contact Allergan directly. See a complete listing of products in the Manufacturers' Index section of this book.

ACULAR® ℞

(ketorolac tromethamine ophthalmic solution) 0.5%
Sterile

DESCRIPTION

ACULAR® (ketorolac tromethamine ophthalmic solution) is a member of the pyrrolo-pyrrole group of nonsteroidal anti-inflammatory drugs (NSAIDs) for ophthalmic use. Its chemical name is (±)-5-Benzoyl-2,3-dihydro-1H-pyrrolizine-1-carboxylic acid, compound with 2-amino-2-(hydroxymethyl)-1,3-propanediol (1:1)
ACULAR® ophthalmic solution is supplied as a sterile isotonic aqueous 0.5% solution, with a pH of 7.4. ACULAR® ophthalmic solution is a racemic mixture of R-(+)- and S-(-)-ketorolac tromethamine. Ketorolac tromethamine may exist in three crystal forms. All forms are equally soluble in water. The pKa of ketorolac is 3.5. This white to off-white crystalline substance discolors on prolonged exposure to light. The molecular weight of ketorolac tromethamine is 376.41. The osmolality of ACULAR® ophthalmic solution is 290 mOsm/kg. Each mL of ACULAR® ophthalmic solution contains:
Active: ketorolac tromethamine 0.5%. **Preservative:** benzalkonium chloride 0.01%. **Inactives:** edetate disodium 0.1%; octoxynol 40; purified water; sodium chloride; and hydrochloric acid and/or sodium hydroxide to adjust the pH.

CLINICAL PHARMACOLOGY

Ketorolac tromethamine is nonsteroidal anti-inflammatory drug which, when administered systemically, has demonstrated analgesic, anti-inflammatory, and anti-pyretic activity. The mechanism of its action is thought to be due to its ability to inhibit prostaglandin biosynthesis. Ketorolac tromethamine given systemically does not cause pupil constriction.
Prostaglandins have been shown in many animal models to be mediators of certain kinds of intraocular inflammation. In studies performed in animal eyes, prostaglandins have been shown to produce disruption of the blood-aqueous humor barrier, vasodilation, increased vascular permeability, leukocytosis, and increased intraocular pressure. Prostaglandins also appear to play a role in the miotic response produced during ocular surgery by constricting the iris sphincter independently of cholinergic mechanisms.
Two drops (0.1 mL) of 0.5% ACULAR® ophthalmic solution instilled into the eyes of patients 12 hours and 1 hour prior to cataract extraction achieved measurable levels in 8 of 9 patients' eyes (mean ketorolac concentration 95 ng/mL aqueous humor, range 40 to 170 ng/mL). Ocular administration of ketorolac tromethamine reduces prostaglandin E_2 (PGE_2) levels in aqueous humor. The mean concentration of PGE_2 was 80 pg/mL in the aqueous humor of eyes receiving vehicle and 28 pg/mL in the eyes receiving ACULAR® 0.5% ophthalmic solution.
One drop (0.05 mL) of 0.5% ACULAR® ophthalmic solution was instilled into one eye and one drop of vehicle into the other eye TID in 26 normal subjects. Only 5 of 26 subjects had a detectable amount of ketorolac in their plasma (range 10.7 to 22.5 ng/mL) at Day 10 during topical ocular treatment. When ketorolac tromethamine 10 mg is administered systemically every 6 hours, peak plasma levels at steady state are around 960 ng/mL.
Two controlled clinical studies showed that ACULAR® ophthalmic solution was significantly more effective than its vehicle in relieving ocular itching caused by seasonal allergic conjunctivitis.
Two controlled clinical studies showed that patients treated for two weeks with ACULAR® ophthalmic solution were less likely to have measurable signs of inflammation (cell and flare) than patients treated with its vehicle.
Results from clinical studies indicate that ketorolac tromethamine has no significant effect upon intraocular pressure; however, changes in intraocular pressure may occur following cataract surgery.

INDICATIONS AND USAGE

ACULAR® ophthalmic solution is indicated for the temporary relief of ocular itching due to seasonal allergic conjunctivitis. ACULAR® ophthalmic solution is also indicated for the treatment of postoperative inflammation in patients who have undergone cataract extraction.

CONTRAINDICATIONS

ACULAR® ophthalmic solution is contraindicated in patients with previously demonstrated hypersensitivity to any of the ingredients in the formulation.

WARNINGS

There is the potential for cross-sensitivity to acetylsalicylic acid, phenylacetic acid derivatives, and other nonsteroidal anti-inflammatory agents. Therefore, caution should be used when treating individuals who have previously exhibited sensitivities to these drugs.
With some nonsteroidal anti-inflammatory drugs, there exists the potential for increased bleeding time due to interference with thrombocyte aggregation. There have been reports that ocularly applied nonsteroidal anti-inflammatory drugs may cause increased bleeding of ocular tissues (including hyphemas) in conjunction with ocular surgery.

PRECAUTIONS

General: All topical nonsteroidal anti-inflammatory drugs (NSAIDs) may slow or delay healing. Topical corticosteroids are also known to slow or delay healing. Concomitant use of topical NSAIDs and topical steroids may increase the potential for healing problems.
Use of topical NSAIDs may result in keratitis. In some susceptible patients, continued use of topical NSAIDs may result in epithelial breakdown, corneal thinning, corneal erosion, corneal ulceration or corneal perforation. These events may be sight threatening. Patients with evidence of corneal epithelial breakdown should immediately discontinue use of topical NSAIDs and should be closely monitored for corneal health.
Postmarketing experience with topical NSAIDs suggests that patients with complicated ocular surgeries, corneal denervation, corneal epithelial defects, diabetes mellitus, ocular surface diseases (e.g., dry eye syndrome), rheumatoid arthritis, or repeat ocular surgeries within a short period of time may be at increased risk for corneal adverse events which may become sight threatening. Topical NSAIDs should be used with caution in these patients.
Postmarketing experience with topical NSAIDs also suggests that use more than 24 hours prior to surgery or use beyond 14 days post-surgery may increase patient risk for the occurrence and severity of corneal adverse events.
It is recommended that ACULAR® ophthalmic solution be used with caution in patients with known bleeding tendencies or who are receiving medications which may prolong bleeding time.
Information for Patients: ACULAR® ophthalmic solution should not be administered while wearing contact lenses.
Carcinogenesis, Mutagenesis, and Impairment of Fertility: Ketorolac tromethamine was not carcinogenic in rats given up to 5 mg/kg/day orally for 24 months (151 times the maximum recommended human topical ophthalmic dose, on a mg/kg basis, assuming 100% absorption in humans and animals) nor in mice given 2 mg/kg/day orally for 18 months (60 times the maximum recommended human topical ophthalmic dose, on a mg/kg basis, assuming 100% absorption in human and animals).
Ketorolac tromethamine was not mutagenic *in vitro* in the Ames assay or in forward mutation assays. Similarly, it did not result in an *in vitro* increase in unscheduled DNA synthesis or an *in vivo* increase in chromosome breakage in mice. However, ketorolac tromethamine did result in an increased incidence in chromosomal aberrations in Chinese hamster ovary cells.
Ketorolac tromethamine did not impair fertility when administered orally to male and female rats at doses up to 272 and 484 times the maximum recommended human topical ophthalmic dose, respectively, on a mg/kg basis, assuming 100% absorption in humans and animals.
Pregnancy:
Teratogenic Effects: Pregnancy Category C. Ketorolac tromethamine, administered during organogenesis, was not teratogenic in rabbits or rats at oral doses up to 109 times and 303 times the maximum recommended human topical ophthalmic dose, respectively, on a mg/kg basis assuming 100% absorption in humans and animals. When administered to rats after Day 17 of gestation at oral doses up to 45 times the maximum recommended human topical ophthalmic dose, respectively, on a mg/kg basis, assuming 100% absorption in humans and animals, ketorolac tromethamine resulted in dystocia and increased pup mortality. There are no adequate and well-controlled studies in pregnant women. ACULAR® ophthalmic solution should be used during pregnancy only if the potential benefit justifies the potential risk to the fetus.
Nonteratogenic Effects: Because of the known effects of prostaglandin-inhibiting drugs on the fetal cardiovascular system (closure of the ductus arteriosus), the use of ACULAR® ophthalmic solution during late pregnancy should be avoided.
Nursing Mothers: Caution should be exercised when ACULAR® ophthalmic solution is administered to a nursing woman.
Pediatric Use: Safety and efficacy in pediatric patients below the age of 3 have not been established.
Geriatric Use: No overall differences in safety or effectiveness have been observed between elderly and younger patients.

ADVERSE REACTIONS

The most frequent adverse events reported with the use of ketorolac tromethamine ophthalmic solutions have been transient stinging and burning on instillation. These events were reported by up to 40% of patients participating in clinical trials.
Other adverse events occurring approximately 1 to 10% of the time during treatment with ketorolac tromethamine ophthalmic solutions included allergic reactions, corneal edema, iritis, ocular inflammation, superficial keratitis and superficial ocular infections.
Other adverse events reported rarely with the use of ketorolac tromethamine ophthalmic solutions included: corneal infiltrates, corneal ulcer, eye dryness, headaches, and visual disturbance (blurry vision).
Clinical Practice: The following events have been identified during postmarketing use of ketorolac tromethamine ophthalmic solution 0.5% in clinical practice. Because they are reported voluntarily from a population of unknown size, estimates of frequency cannot be made. The events, which have been chosen for inclusion due to either their seriousness, frequency of reporting, possible causal connection to topical ketorolac tromethamine ophthalmic solution 0.5%, or a combination of these factors, include corneal erosion, corneal perforation, corneal thinning and epithelial breakdown (see **PRECAUTIONS, General**).

DOSAGE AND ADMINISTRATION

The recommended dose of ACULAR® ophthalmic solution is one drop (0.25 mg) four times a day for relief of ocular itching due to seasonal allergic conjunctivitis.
For the treatment of postoperative inflammation in patients who have undergone cataract extraction, one drop of ACULAR® ophthalmic solution should be applied to the affected eye(s) four times daily beginning 24 hours after cataract surgery and continuing through the first 2 weeks of the postoperative period.
ACULAR® ophthalmic solution has been safely administered in conjunction with other ophthalmic medications such as antibiotics, beta blockers, carbonic anhydrase inhibitors, cycloplegics, and mydriatics.

HOW SUPPLIED

ACULAR® (ketorolac tromethamine ophthalmic solution) is supplied sterile in opaque white LDPE plastic bottles with droppers with gray high impact polystyrene (HIPS) caps as follows:

3 mL in 6 mL bottle **NDC** 0023-2181-03
5 mL in 10 mL bottle **NDC** 0023-2181-05
10 ml in 10 mL bottle **NDC** 0023-2181-10

Store at room temperature 15–25°C (59–77°F) with protection from light.
℞ only
This product is covered under one or more of the following U.S. Pat.: 5,110,493. Additional patents may be pending.
ACULAR®, a registered trademark of Roche Palo Alto LLC is manufactured and distributed by Allergan, Inc. under license from its developer, Roche Palo Alto LLC, Palo Alto, California, U.S.A.

Revised February 2002

ALLERGAN

Irvine, CA 92612
Shown in Product Identification Guide, page 304

ACULAR LS™ ℞

[ă-kew-lər]
(ketorolac tromethamine ophthalmic solution) 0.4%
Sterile

DESCRIPTION

ACULAR LS™ (ketorolac tromethamine ophthalmic solution) 0.4% is a member of the pyrrolo-pyrrole group of nonsteroidal anti-inflammatory drugs (NSAIDs) for ophthalmic use.
Structural and Molecular Formula:

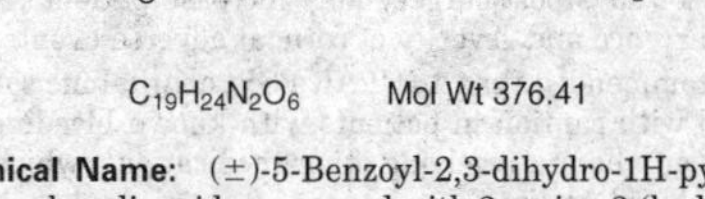

$C_{19}H_{24}N_2O_6$ Mol Wt 376.41

Chemical Name: (±)-5-Benzoyl-2,3-dihydro-1H-pyrrolizine-1-carboxylic acid, compound with 2-amino-2-(hydroxymethyl)-1,3-propanediol (1:1)

Continued on next page

Acular LS—Cont.

Contains: Active: ketorolac tromethamine 0.4%. **Preservative:** benzalkonium chloride 0.006%. Inactives: sodium chloride; edetate disodium 0.015%; octoxynol 40; purified water; and hydrochloric acid and/or sodium hydroxide to adjust the pH.
ACULAR LS™ ophthalmic solution is supplied as a sterile isotonic aqueous 0.4% solution, with a pH of approximately 7.4. ACULAR LS™ ophthalmic solution is a racemic mixture of R-(+) and S-(-)- ketorolac tromethamine. Ketorolac tromethamine may exist in three crystal forms. All forms are equally soluble in water. The pKa of ketorolac is 3.5. This white to off-white crystalline substance discolors on prolonged exposure to light. The osmolality of ACULAR LS™ ophthalmic solution is approximately 290 mOsml/kg.

CLINICAL PHARMACOLOGY

Mechanism of Action

Ketorolac tromethamine is a nonsteroidal anti-inflammatory drug which, when administered systemically, has demonstrated analgesic, anti-inflammatory, and anti-pyretic activity. The mechanism of its action is thought to be due to its ability to inhibit prostaglandin biosynthesis. Ketorolac tromethamine given systemically does not cause pupil constriction.

Pharmacokinetics

One drop (0.05 mL) of 0.5% ketorolac tromethamine ophthalmic solution was instilled into one eye and one drop of vehicle into the other eye TID in 26 normal subjects. Only 5 of 26 subjects had a detectable amount of ketorolac in their plasma (range 10.7 to 22.5 ng/mL) at day 10 during topical ocular treatment. When ketorolac tromethamine 10 mg is administered systemically every 6 hours, peak plasma levels at steady state are around 960 ng/mL.

Clinical Studies

In two double-masked, multi-centered, parallel-group studies, 313 patients who had undergone photorefractive keratectomy received ACULAR LS™ 0.4% or its vehicle QID for up to 4 days. Significant differences favored ACULAR LS™ for the reduction of ocular pain and burning/stinging following photorefractive keratectomy surgery.
Results from clinical studies indicate that ketorolac tromethamine has no significant effect upon intraocular pressure.

INDICATIONS AND USAGE

ACULAR LS™ ophthalmic solution is indicated for the reduction of ocular pain and burning/stinging following corneal refractive surgery.

CONTRAINDICATIONS

ACULAR LS™ ophthalmic solution is contraindicated in patients with previously demonstrated hypersensitivity to any of the ingredients in the formulation.

WARNINGS

There is the potential for cross-sensitivity to acetylsalicylic acid, phenylacetic acid derivatives, and other nonsteroidal anti-inflammatory agents. Therefore, caution should be used when treating individuals who have previously exhibited sensitivities to these drugs.
With some nonsteroidal anti-inflammatory drugs there exists the potential for increased bleeding time due to interference with thrombocyte aggregation. There have been reports that ocularly applied nonsteroidal anti-inflammatory drugs may cause increased bleeding of ocular tissues (including hyphemas) in conjunction with ocular surgery.

PRECAUTIONS

General: All topical nonsteroidal anti-inflammatory drugs (NSAIDs), including ketorolac tromethamine ophthalmic solution, may slow or delay healing. Topical corticosteroids are also known to slow or delay healing. Concomitant use of topical NSAIDS and topical steroids may increase the potential for healing problems.
Use of topical NSAIDs may result in keratitis. In some susceptible patients, continued use of topical NSAIDs may result in epithelial breakdown, corneal thinning, corneal erosion, corneal ulceration or corneal perforation. These events may be sight threatening. Patients with evidence of corneal epithelial breakdown should immediately discontinue use of topical NSAIDs and should be closely monitored for corneal health.
Postmarketing experience with topical NSAIDs suggests that patients with complicated ocular surgeries, corneal denervation, corneal epithelial defects, diabetes mellitus, ocular surface diseases (e.g., dry eye syndrome), rheumatoid arthritis, or repeat ocular surgeries within a short period of time may be at increased risk for corneal adverse events which may become sight threatening. Topical NSAIDs should be used with caution in these patients.
Postmarketing experience with topical NSAIDs also suggests that use more than 24 hours prior to surgery or use beyond 14 days post-surgery may increase patient risk for the occurrence and severity of corneal adverse events.
It is recommended that ACULAR LS™ ophthalmic solution be used with caution in patients with known bleeding tendencies or who are receiving other medications, which may prolong bleeding time.
Information for Patients: ACULAR LS™ ophthalmic solution should not be administered while wearing contact lenses.
Carcinogenesis, Mutagenesis, Impairment of Fertility: Ketorolac tromethamine was neither carcinogenic in rats given up to 5 mg/kg/day orally for 24 months (156 times the maximum recommended human topical ophthalmic dose, on a mg/kg basis, assuming 100% absorption in humans and animals) nor in mice given 2 mg/kg/day orally for 18 months (62.5 times the maximum recommended human topical ophthalmic dose, on a mg/kg basis, assuming 100% absorption in humans and animals).
Ketorolac tromethamine was not mutagenic *in vitro* in the Ames assay or in forward mutation assays. Similarly, it did not result in an *in vitro* increase in unscheduled DNA synthesis or an *in vivo* increase in chromosome breakage in mice. However, ketorolac tromethamine did result in an increased incidence in chromosomal aberrations in Chinese hamster ovary cells.
Ketorolac tromethamine did not impair fertility when administered orally to male and female rats at doses up to 280 and 499 times the maximum recommended human topical ophthalmic dose, respectively, on a mg/kg basis, assuming 100% absorption in humans and animals.
Pregnancy:
Teratogenic Effects: Pregnancy Category C:
Ketorolac tromethamine, administered during organogenesis, was not teratogenic in rabbits or rats at oral doses up to 112 times and 312 times the maximum recommended human topical ophthalmic dose, respectively, on a mg/kg basis assuming 100% absorption in humans and animals. When administered to rats after Day 17 of gestation at oral doses up to 46 times the maximum recommended human topical ophthalmic dose on a mg/kg basis, assuming 100% absorption in humans and animals, ketorolac tromethamine resulted in dystocia and increased pup mortality. There are no adequate and well-controlled studies in pregnant women. ACULAR LS™ ophthalmic solution should be used during pregnancy only if the potential benefit justifies the potential risk to the fetus.
Nonteratogenic Effects:
Because of the known effects of prostaglandin-inhibiting drugs on the fetal cardiovascular system (closure of the ductus arteriosus), the use of ACULAR LS™ ophthalmic solution during late pregnancy should be avoided.
Nursing Mothers: Caution should be exercised when ACULAR LS™ ophthalmic solution is administered to a nursing woman.
Pediatric Use: Safety and effectiveness of ketorolac tromethamine in pediatric patients below the age of 3 have not been established.
Geriatric use: No overall differences in safety or effectiveness have been observed between elderly and younger patients.

ADVERSE REACTIONS

The most frequently reported adverse reactions for ACULAR LS™ ophthalmic solution occurring in approximately 1 to 5% of the overall study population were conjunctival hyperemia, corneal infiltrates, headache, ocular edema and ocular pain.
The most frequent adverse events reported with the use of ketorolac tromethamine ophthalmic solutions have been transient stinging and burning on instillation. These events were reported by 20%-40% of patients participating in these other clinical trials.
Other adverse events occurring approximately 1%-10% of the time during treatment with ketorolac tromethamine ophthalmic solutions included allergic reactions, corneal edema, iritis, ocular inflammation, ocular irritation, ocular pain, superficial keratitis, and superficial ocular infections.
Clinical Practice:
The following events have been identified during postmarketing use of ketorolac tromethamine ophthalmic solutions in clinical practice. Because they are reported voluntarily from a population of unknown size, estimates of frequency cannot be made. The events, which have been chosen for inclusion due to either their seriousness, frequency of reporting, possible causal connection to topical ketorolac tromethamine ophthalmic solutions, or a combination of these factors, include corneal erosion, corneal perforation, corneal thinning and epithelial breakdown (see **PRECAUTIONS, General).**

DOSAGE AND ADMINISTRATION

The recommended dose of ACULAR LS™ ophthalmic solution is one drop four times a day in the operated eye as needed for pain and burning/stinging for up to 4 days following corneal refractive surgery.
Ketorolac tromethamine ophthalmic solution has been safely administered in conjunction with other ophthalmic medications such as antibiotics, beta blockers, carbonic anhydrase inhibitors, cycloplegics, and mydriatics.

HOW SUPPLIED

ACULAR LS™ (ketorolac tromethamine ophthalmic solution) 0.4% is supplied sterile in an opaque white LDPE plastic bottle with a white dropper with a gray high impact polystyrene (HIPS) cap as follows:
5 mL in 10 mL bottle- NDC 0023-9277-05
Note: Store at 15°C-25°C (59°F-77°F).
Rx only
U.S. Pat. 5,110,493

This product is manufactured and distributed by Allergan, Inc. under license from its developer, Roche Palo Alto LLC, Palo Alto, California, U.S.A.
May 2003
9437X
Shown in Product Identification Guide, page 304

ACULAR® PF ℞

(ketorolac tromethamine ophthalmic solution) 0.5%
Preservative-Free

DESCRIPTION

ACULAR® PF (ketorolac tromethamine ophthalmic solution) Preservative-Free is a member of the pyrrolo-pyrrole group of nonsteroidal anti-inflammatory drugs (NSAIDs) for ophthalmic use. Its chemical name is (±)-5-Benzoyl-2,3-dihydro-1H-pyrrolizine-1-carboxylic acid, compound with 2-amino-2-(hydroxymethyl)-1,3-propanediol (1:1)
ACULAR® PF is a racemic mixture of R-(+) and S-(-)-ketorolac tromethamine. Ketorolac tromethamine may exist in three crystal forms. All forms are equally soluble in water. The pKa of ketorolac is 3.5. This white to off-white crystalline substance discolors on prolonged exposure to light. The molecular weight of ketorolac tromethamine is 376.41. The osmolality of ACULAR® PF is 290 mOsmol/kg.
Each ml of ACULAR® PF contains: **Active:** ketorolac tromethamine 0.5%. **Inactives:** purified water; sodium chloride; and hydrochloric acid and/or sodium hydroxide to adjust the pH to 7.4.

CLINICAL PHARMACOLOGY

Ketorolac tromethamine is a nonsteroidal anti-inflammatory drug which, when administered systemically, has demonstrated analgesic, anti-inflammatory, and anti-pyretic activity. The mechanism of its action is thought to be due to its ability to inhibit prostaglandin biosynthesis. Ketorolac tromethamine given systemically does not cause pupil constriction.
One drop (0.05 mL) of ketorolac tromethamine (preserved) was instilled into one eye and one drop of vehicle into the other eye TID in 26 normal subjects. Only 5 of 26 subjects had a detectable amount of ketorolac in their plasma (range 10.7 to 22.5 ng/mL) at day 10 during topical ocular treatment. When ketorolac tromethamine 10 mg is administered systemically every 6 hours, peak plasma levels at steady state are around 960 ng/mL.
In two double-masked, multi-centered, parallel-group studies, 340 patients who had undergone incisional refractive surgery received ACULAR® PF or its vehicle QID for up to 3 days. Significant differences favored ACULAR® PF for the treatment of ocular pain and photophobia.
Results from clinical studies indicate that ketorolac tromethamine has no significant effect upon intraocular pressure.

INDICATIONS AND USAGE

ACULAR® PF ophthalmic solution is indicated for the reduction of ocular pain and photophobia following incisional refractive surgery.

CONTRAINDICATIONS

ACULAR® PF ophthalmic solution is contraindicated in patients with previously demonstrated hypersensitivity to any of the ingredients in the formulation.

WARNINGS

There is the potential for cross-sensitivity to acetylsalicylic acid, phenylacetic acid derivatives, and other nonsteroidal anti-inflammatory agents. Therefore, caution should be used when treating individuals who have previously exhibited sensitivities to these drugs.
With some nonsteroidal anti-inflammatory drugs, there exists the potential for increased bleeding time due to interference with thrombocyte aggregation. There have been reports that ocularly applied nonsteroidal anti-inflammatory drugs may cause increased bleeding of ocular tissues (including hyphemas) in conjunction with ocular surgery.

PRECAUTIONS

General: All topical nonsteroidal anti-inflammatory drugs (NSAIDs) may slow or delay healing. Topical corticosteroids are also known to slow or delay healing. Concomitant use of topical NSAIDs and topical steroids may increase the potential for healing problems.
Use of topical NSAIDs may result in keratitis. In some susceptible patients, continued use of topical NSAIDs may result in epithelial breakdown, corneal thinning, corneal erosion, corneal ulceration or corneal perforation. These events may be sight threatening. Patients with evidence of corneal epithelial breakdown should immediately discontinue use of topical NSAIDs and should be closely monitored for corneal health.
Postmarketing experience with topical NSAIDs suggests that patients with complicated ocular surgeries, corneal denervation, corneal epithelial defects, diabetes mellitus, ocular surface diseases (e.g., dry eye syndrome), rheumatoid arthritis, or repeat ocular surgeries within a short period of time may be at increased risk for corneal adverse events which may become sight threatening. Topical NSAIDs should be used with caution in these patients.
Postmarketing experience with topical NSAIDs also suggests that use more than 24 hours prior to surgery or use beyond 14 days post-surgery may increase patient risk for the occurrence and severity of corneal adverse events.
It is recommended that ACULAR® PF ophthalmic solution be used with caution in patients with known bleeding tendencies or who are receiving other medications which may prolong bleeding time.

Information for Patients: ACULAR® PF should not be administered while wearing contact lenses.
The solution from one individual single-use vial is to be used immediately after opening for administration to one or both eyes, and the remaining contents should be discarded immediately after administration. To avoid contamination, do not touch tip of unit-dose vial to eye or any other surface.
Carcinogenesis, Mutagenesis, and Impairment of Fertility: Ketorolac tromethamine was not carcinogenic in rats given up to 5 mg/kg/day orally for 24 months (151 times the maximum recommended human topical ophthalmic dose, on a mg/kg basis, assuming 100% absorption in humans and animals) nor in mice given 2 mg/kg/day orally for 18 months (60 times the maximum recommended human topical ophthalmic dose, on a mg/kg basis, assuming 100% absorption in humans and animals).
Ketorolac tromethamine was not mutagenic *in vitro* in the Ames assay or in forward mutation assays. Similarly, it did not result in an *in vitro* increase in unscheduled DNA synthesis or an *in vivo* increase in chromosome breakage in mice. However, ketorolac tromethamine did result in an increased incidence in chromosomal aberrations in Chinese hamster ovary cells.
Ketorolac tromethamine did not impair fertility when administered orally to male and female rats at doses up to 272 and 484 times the maximum recommended human topical ophthalmic dose, respectively, on a mg/kg basis, assuming 100% absorption in humans and animals.
Pregnancy:
Teratogenic Effects: Pregnancy Category C. Ketorolac tromethamine, administered during organogenesis, was not teratogenic in rabbits or rats at oral doses up to 109 times and 303 times the maximum recommended human topical ophthalmic dose, respectively, on a mg/kg basis assuming 100% absorption in humans and animals. When administered to rats after Day 17 of gestation at oral doses up to 45 times the maximum recommended human topical ophthalmic dose, respectively, on a mg/kg basis, assuming 100% absorption in humans and animals, ketorolac tromethamine resulted in dystocia and increased pup mortality. There are no adequate and well-controlled studies in pregnant women. ACULAR® PF ophthalmic solution should be used during pregnancy only if the potential benefit justifies the potential risk to the fetus.
Nonteratogenic Effects: Because of the known effects of prostaglandin-inhibiting drugs on the fetal cardiovascular system (closure of the ductus arteriosus), the use of ACULAR® PF during late pregnancy should be avoided.
Nursing Mothers: Caution should be exercised when ACULAR® PF is administered to a nursing woman.
Pediatric Use: Safety and efficacy in pediatric patients below the age of 3 years have not been established.
Geriatric Use: No overall differences in safety or effectiveness have been observed between elderly and younger patients.

ADVERSE REACTIONS

The most frequent adverse events reported with the use of ketorolac tromethamine ophthalmic solutions have been transient stinging and burning on instillation. These events were reported by approximately 20% of patients participating in clinical trials.
Other adverse events occurring approximately 1%–10% of the time during treatment with ketorolac tromethamine ophthalmic solutions included allergic reactions, corneal edema, iritis, ocular inflammation, ocular irritation, superficial keratitis, and superficial ocular infections.
Other adverse events reported rarely with the use of ketorolac tromethamine ophthalmic solutions include: corneal infiltrates, corneal ulcer, eye dryness, headaches, and visual disturbance (blurry vision).
Clinical Practice: The following events have been identified during postmarketing use of ketorolac tromethamine ophthalmic solution 0.5% in clinical practice. Because they are reported voluntarily from a population of unknown size, estimates of frequency cannot be made. The events, which have been chosen for inclusion due to either their seriousness, frequency of reporting, possible causal connection to topical ketorolac tromethamine ophthalmic solution 0.5%, or a combination of these factors, include corneal erosion, corneal perforation, corneal thinning and epithelial breakdown (see **PRECAUTIONS, General**).

DOSAGE AND ADMINISTRATION

The recommended dose of ACULAR® PF is one drop (0.25 mg) four times a day in the operated eye as needed for pain and photophobia for up to 3 days after incisional refractive surgery.

HOW SUPPLIED

ACULAR® PF (ketorolac tromethamine ophthalmic solution) 0.5% Preservative-Free is available as a sterile solution supplied in clear, LDPE single-use vials as follows: ACULAR® PF 12 Single-Use Vials 0.4 mL each - NDC 0023-9055-04. Store ACULAR® PF at 15°C–30°C (59°F–86°F) with protection from light.
℞ only
U.S. Pat.: 5,110,493
ALLERGAN ©2002 Allergan, Irvine, CA 92612, U.S.A.
ACULAR® is a registered trademark of Roche Palo Alto LLC. ACULAR® PF is manufactured and distributed by ALLERGAN under license from its developer, Roche Palo Alto LLC, Palo Alto, California, U.S.A. Revised February 2002

Shown in Product Identification Guide, page 304

ALPHAGAN® P ℞

(brimonidine tartrate ophthalmic solution) 0.15%
STERILE

DESCRIPTION

ALPHAGAN® P (brimonidine tartrate ophthalmic solution) 0.15% is a relatively selective alpha-2 adrenergic agonist for ophthalmic use. The chemical name of brimonidine tartrate is 5-bromo-6- (2-imidazolidinylideneamino) quinoxaline L-tartrate. It is an off-white to pale yellow powder. It has a molecular weight of 442.24 as the tartrate salt, and is both soluble in water (1.5 mg/mL) and in the product vehicle (3.0 mg/mL) at pH 7.2. The structural formula is:

Formula: $C_{11}H_{10}BrN_5 \bullet C_4H_6O_6$
CAS Number: 70359-46-5
In solution, ALPHAGAN® P (brimonidine tartrate ophthalmic solution) 0.15% has a clear, greenish-yellow color. It has an osmolality of 250–350 mOsmol/kg and a pH of 6.6–7.4.
Each mL of ALPHAGAN® P contains:
Active Ingredient: brimonidine tartrate 0.15% (1.5 mg/mL)
Preservative: *Purite*® 0.005% (0.05 mg/mL)
Inactives: boric acid; calcium chloride; magnesium chloride; potassium chloride; purified water; sodium borate; sodium carboxymethylcellulose; sodium chloride; with hydrochloric acid and/or sodium hydroxide to adjust pH.

CLINICAL PHARMACOLOGY

Mechanism of Action: ALPHAGAN® P ophthalmic solution is an alpha adrenergic receptor agonist. It has a peak ocular hypotensive effect occurring at two hours post-dosing. Fluorophotometric studies in animals and humans suggest that brimonidine tartrate has a dual mechanism of action by reducing aqueous humor production and increasing uveoscleral outflow.
Pharmacokinetics: After ocular administration of either a 0.1% or 0.2% solution, plasma concentrations peaked within 0.5 to 2.5 hours and declined with a systemic half-life of approximately 2 hours. In humans, systemic metabolism of brimonidine is extensive. It is metabolized primarily by the liver. Urinary excretion is the major route of elimination of the drug and its metabolites. Approximately 87% of an orally-administered radioactive dose was eliminated within 120 hours, with 74% found in the urine.
Clinical Evaluations: Elevated IOP presents a major risk factor in glaucomatous field loss. The higher the level of IOP, the greater the likelihood of optic nerve damage and visual field loss. Brimonidine tartrate has the action of lowering intraocular pressure with minimal effect on cardiovascular and pulmonary parameters.
Two clinical studies were conducted to evaluate the safety, efficacy, and acceptability of ALPHAGAN® P (brimonidine tartrate ophthalmic solution) 0.15% compared with ALPHAGAN®, administered three-times-daily in patients with open-angle glaucoma or ocular hypertension. Those results indicated that ALPHAGAN® P (brimonidine tartrate ophthalmic solution) 0.15% is comparable in IOP lowering effect to ALPHAGAN® (brimonidine tartrate ophthalmic solution) 0.2%, and effectively lowers IOP in patients with open-angle glaucoma or ocular hypertension by approximately 2–5 mmHg.

INDICATIONS AND USAGE

ALPHAGAN® P is indicated for the lowering of intraocular pressure in patients with open-angle glaucoma or ocular hypertension.

CONTRAINDICATIONS

ALPHAGAN® P is contraindicated in patients with hypersensitivity to brimonidine tartrate or any component of this medication. It is also contraindicated in patients receiving monoamine oxidase (MAO) inhibitor therapy.

PRECAUTIONS

General: Although ALPHAGAN® P ophthalmic solution had minimal effect on the blood pressure of patients in clinical studies, caution should be exercised in treating patients with severe cardiovascular disease.
ALPHAGAN® P has not been studied in patients with hepatic or renal impairment; caution should be used in treating such patients. ALPHAGAN® P should be used with caution in patients with depression, cerebral or coronary insufficiency, Raynaud's phenomenon, orthostatic hypotension, or thromboangiitis obliterans. Patients prescribed IOP-lowering medication should be routinely monitored for IOP.
Information for Patients: As with other drugs in this class, ALPHAGAN® P ophthalmic solution may cause fatigue and/or drowsiness in some patients. Patients who engage in hazardous activities should be cautioned of the potential for a decrease in mental alertness.
Drug Interactions: Although specific drug interaction studies have not been conducted with ALPHAGAN® P, the possibility of an additive or potentiating effect with CNS depressants (alcohol, barbiturates, opiates, sedatives, or anesthetics) should be considered. Alpha-agonists, as a class, may reduce pulse and blood pressure. Caution in using concomitant drugs such as beta-blockers (ophthalmic and systemic), anti-hypertensives and/or cardiac glycosides is advised.
Tricyclic antidepressants have been reported to blunt the hypotensive effect of systemic clonidine. It is not known whether the concurrent use of these agents with ALPHAGAN® P ophthalmic solution in humans can lead to resulting interference with the IOP lowering effect. No data on the level of circulating catecholamines after ALPHAGAN® P administration are available. Caution, however, is advised in patients taking tricyclic antidepressants which can affect the metabolism and uptake of circulating amines.
Carcinogenesis, Mutagenesis, and Impairment of Fertility: No compound-related carcinogenic effects were observed in either mice or rats following a 21-month and 24-month study, respectively. In these studies, dietary administration of brimonidine tartrate at doses up to 2.5 mg/kg/day in mice and 1.0 mg/kg/day in rats achieved 86 and 55 times, respectively, the plasma drug concentration estimated in humans treated with one drop of ALPHAGAN® P ophthalmic solution into both eyes 3 times per day.
Brimonidine tartrate was not mutagenic or cytogenic in a series of *in vitro* and *in vivo* studies including the Ames test, chromosomal aberration assay in Chinese Hamster Ovary (CHO) cells, a host-mediated assay and cytogenic studies in mice, and dominant lethal assay.
Reproductive studies performed in rats with oral doses of 0.66 mg base/kg revealed no evidence of impaired fertility due to ALPHAGAN® P.
Pregnancy: Teratogenic Effects: Pregnancy Category B. Reproductive studies performed in rats with oral doses of 0.66 mg base/kg revealed no evidence of harm to the fetus due to ALPHAGAN® P ophthalmic solution. Dosing at this level produced an exposure that is 189 times higher than the exposure seen in humans following multiple ophthalmic doses.
There are no adequate and well-controlled studies in pregnant women. In animal studies, brimonidine crossed the placenta and entered into the fetal circulation to a limited extent. ALPHAGAN® P should be used during pregnancy only if the potential benefit to the mother justifies the potential risk to the fetus.
Nursing Mothers: It is not known whether this drug is excreted in human milk; in animal studies brimonidine tartrate was excreted in breast milk. A decision should be made whether to discontinue nursing or to discontinue the drug, taking into account the importance of the drug to the mother.
Pediatric Use: In a well-controlled clinical study conducted in pediatric glaucoma patients (ages 2 to 7 years) the most commonly observed adverse events with brimonidine tartrate ophthalmic solution 0.2% dosed three times daily were somnolence (50%–83% in patients ages 2 to 6 years) and decreased alertness. In pediatric patients 7 years of age or older (>20kg), somnolence appears to occur less frequently (25%). Approximately 16% of patients on brimonidine tartrate ophthalmic solution discontinued from the study due to somnolence.
The safety and effectiveness of brimonidine tartrate ophthalmic solution have not been studied in pediatric patients below the age of 2 years. Brimonidine tartrate ophthalmic solution is not recommended for use in pediatric patients under the age of 2 years. (Also refer to Adverse Reactions section.)
Geriatric Use: No overall differences in safety or effectiveness have been observed between elderly and other adult patients.

ADVERSE REACTIONS

Adverse events occurring in approximately 10–20% of the subjects included: allergic conjunctivitis, conjunctival hyperemia, and eye pruritus.
Adverse events occurring in approximately 5–9% of the subjects included: burning sensation, conjunctival folliculosis, hypertension, oral dryness, and visual disturbance.
Events occurring in approximately 1–4% of subjects included: allergic reaction, asthenia, blepharitis, bronchitis, conjunctival edema, conjunctival hemorrhage, conjunctivitis, cough, dizziness, dyspepsia, dyspnea, epiphora, eye discharge, eye dryness, eye irritation, eye pain, eyelid edema, eyelid erythema, flu syndrome, follicular conjunctivitis, foreign body sensation, headache, pharyngitis, photophobia, rash, rhinitis, sinus infection, sinusitis, stinging, superficial punctate keratopathy, visual field defect, vitreous floaters, and worsened visual acuity.
The following events were reported in less than 1% of subjects: corneal erosion, insomnia, nasal dryness, somnolence, and taste perversion.
The following events have been identified during post-marketing use of ALPHAGAN® ophthalmic solution in clinical practice. Because they are reported voluntarily from a population of unknown size, estimates of frequency cannot be made. The events, which have been chosen for inclusion due to either their seriousness, frequency of reporting, possible causal connection to ALPHAGAN®, or a combination of these factors, include: bradycardia; hypotension; iritis; miosis; skin reactions (including erythema, eyelid pruritus, rash, and vasodilation) and tachycardia. Apnea, bradycardia, hypotension, hypothermia, hypotonia, and somnolence have been reported in infants receiving ALPHAGAN® ophthalmic solution.

Continued on next page

Alphagan P—Cont.

OVERDOSAGE

No information is available on overdosage in humans. Treatment of an oral overdose includes supportive and symptomatic therapy; a patent airway should be maintained.

DOSAGE AND ADMINISTRATION

The recommended dose is one drop of ALPHAGAN® P in the affected eye(s) three times daily, approximately 8 hours apart.

ALPHAGAN® P ophthalmic solution may be used concomitantly with other topical ophthalmic drug products to lower intraocular pressure. If more than one topical ophthalmic product is being used, the products should be administered at least 5 minutes apart.

HOW SUPPLIED

ALPHAGAN® P (brimonidine tartrate ophthalmic solution) 0.15% is supplied sterile in opaque teal LDPE plastic bottles and tips with purple high impact polystyrene (HIPS) caps as follows:

5 mL in 10 mL bottle	NDC 0023-9177-05
10 mL in 10 mL bottle	NDC 0023-9177-10
15 mL in 15 mL bottle	NDC 0023-9177-15

NOTE: Store at 15°–25°C (59°–77°F).

Rx Only

® Marks owned by Allergan, Inc.

U.S. Pat. 5,424,078; 5,736,165; 6,194,415; 6,248,741; 6,465,464; 6,562,873; 6,627,210; 6,641,834; 6,673,337

ALLERGAN

Irvine, CA 92612, U.S.A.

Shown in Product Identification Guide, page 304

BLEPHAMIDE® ℞

(sulfacetamide sodium and prednisolone acetate ophthalmic ointment, USP)
10%/0.2% sterile

DESCRIPTION

BLEPHAMIDE® (sulfacetamide sodium and prednisolone acetate ophthalmic ointment, USP) is a sterile topical ophthalmic ointment combining an antibacterial and a corticosteroid.

Chemical Names: Sulfacetamide sodium: N-sulfanilylacetamide monosodium salt monohydrate.

Prednisolone acetate: 11β, 17, 21-trihydroxypregna-1,4-diene-3, 20-dione, 21-acetate.

Contains: Actives: sulfacetamide sodium 10% and prednisolone acetate 0.2%. Preservative: phenylmercuric acetate (0.0008%); Inactives: mineral oil; white petrolatum; and petrolatum (and) lanolin alcohol.

CLINICAL PHARMACOLOGY

Corticosteroids suppress the inflammatory response to a variety of agents and they probably delay or slow healing. Since corticosteroids may inhibit the body's defense mechanism against infection, a concomitant antibacterial drug may be used when this inhibition is considered to be clinically significant in a particular case.

When a decision to administer both a corticosteroid and an antibacterial is made, the administration of such drugs in combination has the advantage of greater patient compliance and convenience, with the added assurance that the appropriate dosage of both drugs is administered, plus assured compatibility of ingredients when both types of drugs are in the same formulation and, particularly, that the correct volume of drug is delivered and retained.

The relative potency of corticosteroids depends on the molecular structure, concentration and release from the vehicle.

Microbiology: Sulfacetamide exerts a bacteriostatic effect against susceptible bacteria by restricting the synthesis of folic acid required for growth through competition with p-amino benzoic acid.

Some strains of these bacteria may be resistant to sulfacetamide or resistant strains may emerge *in vivo.*

The anti-infective component in BLEPHAMIDE® ointment is included to provide action against specific organisms susceptible to it. Sulfacetamide sodium is active *in vitro* against susceptible strains of the following microorganisms: *Escherichia coli, Staphylococcus aureus, Streptococcus pneumoniae, Streptococcus* (*viridans* group), *Haemophilus influenzae, Klebsiella* species, and *Enterobacter* species. This product does not provide adequate coverage against: *Neisseria* species, *Pseudomonas* species, and *Serratia marcescens* (see **INDICATIONS AND USAGE**).

INDICATIONS AND USAGE

BLEPHAMIDE® ophthalmic ointment is indicated for steroid-responsive inflammatory ocular conditions for which a corticosteroid is indicated and where superficial bacterial ocular infection or a risk of bacterial ocular infection exists. Ocular corticosteroids are indicated in inflammatory conditions of the palpebral and bulbar conjunctiva, cornea, and anterior segment of the globe where the inherent risk of corticosteroid use in certain infective conjunctivitides is accepted to obtain diminution in edema and inflammation. They are also indicated in chronic anterior uveitis and corneal injury from chemical, radiation or thermal burns or penetration of foreign bodies.

The use of a combination drug with an anti-infective component is indicated where the risk of superficial ocular infection is high or where there is an expectation that potentially dangerous numbers of bacteria will be present in the eye.

The particular antibacterial drug in this product is active against the following common bacterial eye pathogens: *Escherichia coli, Staphylococcus aureus, Streptococcus pneumoniae, Streptococcus* (*viridans* group), *Haemophilus influenzae, Klebsiella* species, and *Enterobacter* species.

The product does not provide adequate coverage against: *Neisseria* species, *Pseudomonas* species, and *Serratia marcescens.*

A significant percentage of staphylococcal isolates are completely resistant to sulfa drugs.

CONTRAINDICATIONS

BLEPHAMIDE® ophthalmic ointment is contraindicated in most viral diseases of the cornea and conjunctiva including epithelial herpes simplex keratitis (dendritic keratitis), vaccinia, and varicella, and also in mycobacterial infection of the eye and fungal diseases of ocular structures.

This product is also contraindicated in individuals with known or suspected hypersensitivity to any of the ingredients of this preparation, to other sulfonamides and to other corticosteroids. See **WARNINGS**. (Hypersensitivity to the antimicrobial component occurs at a higher rate than for other components).

WARNINGS

NOT FOR INJECTION INTO THE EYE.

Prolonged use of corticosteroids may result in ocular hypertension/glaucoma with damage to the optic nerve, defects in visual acuity and fields of vision, and in posterior subcapsular cataract formation.

Acute anterior uveitis may occur in susceptible individuals, primarily Blacks.

Prolonged use of BLEPHAMIDE® ophthalmic ointment may suppress the host response and thus increase the hazard of secondary ocular infections. In those diseases causing thinning of the cornea or sclera, perforation has been known to occur with the use of topical corticosteroids. In acute purulent conditions of the eye, corticosteroids may mask infection or enhance existing infection.

If the product is used for 10 days or longer, intraocular pressure should be routinely monitored even though it may be difficult in children and uncooperative patients. Corticosteroids should be used with caution in the presence of glaucoma. Intraocular pressure should be checked frequently.

A significant percentage of staphylococcal isolates are completely resistant to sulfonamides.

The use of steroids after cataract surgery may delay healing and increase the incidence of filtering blebs.

The use of ocular corticosteroids may prolong the course and may exacerbate the severity of many viral infections of the eye (including herpes simplex). Employment of corticosteroid medication in the treatment of herpes simplex requires great caution.

Topical steroids are not effective in mustard gas keratitis and Sjögren's keratoconjunctivitis.

Fatalities have occurred, although rarely, due to severe reactions to sulfonamides including Stevens-Johnson syndrome, toxic epidermal necrolysis, fulminant hepatic necrosis, agranulocytosis, aplastic anemia and other blood dyscrasias. Sensitization may recur when a sulfonamide is readministered, irrespective of the route of administration. If signs of hypersensitivity or other serious reactions occur, discontinue use of this preparation. Cross-sensitivity among corticosteroids has been demonstrated (see **ADVERSE REACTIONS**).

PRECAUTIONS

General: The initial prescription and renewal of the medication order beyond 8 g of ointment should be made by a physician only after examination of the patient with the aid of magnification, such as slit lamp biomicroscopy and, where appropriate, fluorescein staining. If signs and symptoms fail to improve after two days, the patient should be re-evaluated. The possibility of fungal infections of the cornea should be considered after prolonged corticosteroid dosing. Use with caution in patients with severe dry eye. Fungal cultures should be taken when appropriate.

The p-amino benzoic acid present in purulent exudates competes with sulfonamides and can reduce their effectiveness. Ophthalmic ointments may retard corneal healing.

Information for Patients: If inflammation or pain persists longer than 48 hours or becomes aggravated, the patient should be advised to discontinue use of the medication and consult a physician (see **WARNINGS**).

This product is sterile when packaged. To prevent contamination, care should be taken to avoid touching the tube tip to eyelids or to any other surface. The use of this tube by more than one person may spread infection. Keep tube tightly closed when not in use. Keep out of the reach of children.

Laboratory Tests: Eyelid cultures and tests to determine the susceptibility of organisms to sulfacetamide may be indicated if signs and symptoms persist or recur in spite of the recommended course of treatment with BLEPHAMIDE® ophthalmic ointment.

Drug Interactions: BLEPHAMIDE® ophthalmic ointment is incompatible with silver preparations. Local anesthetics related to p-amino benzoic acid may antagonize the action of the sulfonamides.

Carcinogenesis, Mutagenesis, Impairment of Fertility: Prednisolone has been reported to be noncarcinogenic. Long-term animal studies for carcinogenic potential have not been performed with sulfacetamide.

One author detected chromosomal nondisjunction in the yeast *Saccharomyces cerevisiae* following application of sulfacetamide sodium. The significance of this finding to topical ophthalmic use of sulfacetamide sodium in the human is unknown.

Mutagenic studies with prednisolone have been negative. Studies on reproduction and fertility have not been performed with sulfacetamide. A long-term chronic toxicity study in dogs showed that high oral doses of prednisolone prevented estrus. A decrease in fertility was seen in male and female rats that were mated following oral dosing with another glucocorticosteroid.

Pregnancy: Teratogenic Effects: Pregnancy Category C. Animal reproduction studies have not been conducted with sulfacetamide sodium. Prednisolone has been shown to be teratogenic in rabbits, hamsters, and mice. In mice, prednisolone has been shown to be teratogenic when given in doses 1 to 10 times the human ocular dose. Dexamethasone, hydrocortisone and prednisolone were ocularly applied to both eyes of pregnant mice five times per day on days 10 through 13 of gestation. A significant increase in the incidence of cleft palate was observed in the fetuses of the treated mice. There are no adequate well-controlled studies in pregnant women dosed with corticosteroids.

Kernicterus may be precipitated in infants by sulfonamides being given systemically during the third trimester of pregnancy. It is not known whether sulfacetamide sodium can cause fetal harm when administered to a pregnant woman or whether it can affect reproductive capacity.

BLEPHAMIDE® ophthalmic ointment should be used during pregnancy only if the potential benefit justifies the potential risk to the fetus.

Nursing Mothers: It is not known whether topical administration of corticosteroids could result in sufficient systemic absorption to produce detectable quantities in human milk. Systemically administered corticosteroids appear in human milk and could suppress growth, interfere with endogenous corticosteroid production, or cause other untoward effects. Systemically administered sulfonamides are capable of producing kernicterus in infants of lactating women. Because of the potential for serious adverse reactions in nursing infants from sulfacetamide sodium and prednisolone acetate ophthalmic ointments, a decision should be made whether to discontinue nursing or to discontinue the medication.

Pediatric Use: Safety and effectiveness in children below the age of six have not been established.

ADVERSE REACTIONS

Adverse reactions have occurred with corticosteroid/antibacterial combination drugs which can be attributed to the corticosteroid component, the antibacterial component, or the combination. Exact incidence figures are not available since no denominator of treated patients is available.

Reactions occurring most often from the presence of the antibacterial ingredient are allergic sensitizations. Fatalities have occurred, although rarely, due to severe reactions to sulfonamides including Stevens-Johnson syndrome, toxic epidermal necrolysis, fulminant hepatic necrosis, agranulocytosis, aplastic anemia, and other blood dyscrasias (See **WARNINGS**).

Sulfacetamide sodium may cause local irritation.

The reactions due to the corticosteroid component in decreasing order of frequency are: elevation of intraocular pressure (IOP) with possible development of glaucoma and infrequent optic nerve damage, posterior subcapsular cataract formation, and delayed wound healing.

Although systemic effects are extremely uncommon, there have been rare occurrences of systemic hypercorticoidism after use of topical steroids.

Corticosteroid-containing preparations can also cause acute anterior uveitis or perforation of the globe. Mydriasis, loss of accommodation and ptosis have occasionally been reported following local use of corticosteroids.

Secondary Infection: The development of secondary infection has occurred after use of combinations containing corticosteroids and antibacterials. Fungal and viral infections of the cornea are particularly prone to develop coincidentally with long-term applications of corticosteroid. The possibility of fungal invasion must be considered in any persistent corneal ulceration where corticosteroid treatment has been used.

Secondary bacterial ocular infection following suppression of host responses also occurs.

DOSAGE AND ADMINISTRATION

A small amount, approximately $^1/_2$ inch ribbon of ointment, should be applied in the conjunctival sac three or four times daily and once or twice at night.

Not more than 8 g should be prescribed initially.

The dosing of BLEPHAMIDE® ophthalmic ointment may be reduced, but care should be taken not to discontinue therapy prematurely. In chronic conditions, withdrawal of treatment should be carried out by gradually decreasing the frequency of application.

If signs and symptoms fail to improve after two days, the patient should be re-evaluated (see **PRECAUTIONS**).

HOW SUPPLIED

BLEPHAMIDE® (sulfacetamide sodium and prednisolone acetate ophthalmic ointment, USP) 10%/0.2% is supplied sterile in 3.5 gram ointment tubes:

NDC 0023-0313-04.

Note: Store between 15–25°C (59–77°F).

℞ **only**

Shown in Product Identification Guide, page 304

BLEPHAMIDE® ℞

(sulfacetamide sodium-prednisolone acetate ophthalmic suspension)

DESCRIPTION

BLEPHAMIDE® ophthalmic suspension is a topical anti-inflammatory/anti-infective combination product for ophthalmic use.

Chemical Names:

Sulfacetamide sodium: N-Sulfanilylacetamide monosodium salt monohydrate.

Prednisolone acetate: 11β, 17, 21-Trihydroxypregna-1, 4-diene-3, 20-dione 21-acetate.

Contains:

Actives: sulfacetamide sodium 10%, prednisolone acetate (microfine suspension) 0.2%: Preservative: benzalkonium chloride (0.004%): Inactives: polyvinyl alcohol 1.4%; polysorbate 80; edetate disodium; sodium phosphate, dibasic; potassium phosphate, monobasic; sodium thiosulfate; hydrochloric acid and/or sodium hydroxide to adjust the pH; and purified water.

CLINICAL PHARMACOLOGY

Corticosteroids suppress the inflammatory response to a variety of agents and they probably delay or slow healing. Since corticosteroids may inhibit the body's defense mechanism against infection, a concomitant antibacterial drug may be used when this inhibition is considered to be clinically significant in a particular case.

When a decision to administer both a corticosteroid and an antibacterial is made, the administration of such drugs in combination has the advantage of greater patient compliance and convenience, with the added assurance that the appropriate dosage of both drugs is administered. When both types of drugs are in the same formulation, compatibility of ingredients is assured and the correct volume of drug is delivered and retained. The relative potency of corticosteroids depends on the molecular structure, concentration, and release from the vehicle.

Microbiology: Sulfacetamide sodium exerts a bacteriostatic effect against susceptible bacteria by restricting the synthesis of folic acid required for growth through competition with p-aminobenzoic acid.

Some strains of these bacteria may be resistant to sulfacetamide or resistant strains may emerge *in vivo.*

The anti-infective component in these products is included to provide action against specific organisms susceptible to it. Sulfacetamide sodium is active *in vitro* against susceptible strains of the following microorganisms: *Escherichia coli, Staphylococcus aureus, Streptococcus pneumoniae, Streptococcus (viridans* group), *Haemophilus influenzae, Klebsiella* species, and *Enterobacter* species. This product does not provide adequate coverage against: *Neisseria* species, *Pseudomonas* species, and *Serratia marcescens* (see **INDICATIONS AND USAGE**).

INDICATIONS AND USAGE

A steroid/anti-infective combination is indicated for steroid-responsive inflammatory ocular conditions for which a corticosteroid is indicated and where superficial bacterial ocular infection or a risk of bacterial ocular infection exists.

Ocular corticosteroids are indicated in inflammatory conditions of the palpebral and bulbar conjunctiva, cornea, and anterior segment of the globe where the inherent risk of corticosteroid use in certain infective conjunctivitides is accepted to obtain a diminution in edema and inflammation. They are also indicated in chronic anterior uveitis and corneal injury from chemical, radiation, or thermal burns or penetration of foreign bodies.

The use of a combination drug with an anti-infective component is indicated where the risk of superficial ocular infection is high or where there is an expectation that potentially dangerous numbers of bacteria will be present in the eye.

The particular antibacterial drug in this product is active against the following common bacterial eye pathogens: *Escherichia coli, Staphylococcus aureus, Streptococcus pneumoniae, Streptococcus (viridans* group), *Haemophilus influenzae, Klebsiella* species, and *Enterobacter* species. This product does not provide adequate coverage against *Neisseria* species, *Pseudomonas* species, and *Serratia marcescens.*

A significant percentage of staphlococcal isolates are completely resistant to sulfa drugs.

CONTRAINDICATIONS

BLEPHAMIDE® ophthalmic suspension is contraindicated in most viral diseases of the cornea and conjunctiva including epithelial herpes simplex keratitis (dendritic keratitis), vaccinia, and varicella, and also in mycobacterial infection of the eye and fungal diseases of ocular structures.

This product is also contraindicated in individuals with known or suspected hypersensitivity to any of the ingredients of this preparation, to other sulfonamides and to other corticosteroids. See **WARNINGS.** (Hypersensitivity to the antimicrobial component occurs at a higher rate than for other components.)

WARNINGS

NOT FOR INJECTION INTO THE EYE.

Prolonged use of corticosteroids may result in ocular hypertension/glaucoma with damage to the optic nerve, defects in visual acuity and fields of vision, and in posterior subcapsular cataract formation.

Acute anterior uveitis may occur in susceptible individuals, primarily Blacks.

Prolonged use of BLEPHAMIDE® ophthalmic suspension may suppress the host response and thus increase the hazard of secondary ocular infections. In those diseases causing thinning of the cornea or sclera, perforation has been known to occur with the use of topical corticosteroids. In acute purulent conditions of the eye, corticosteroids may mask infection or enhance existing infection.

If the product is used for 10 days or longer, intraocular pressure should be routinely monitored even though it may be difficult in children and uncooperative patients. Corticosteroids should be used with caution in the presence of glaucoma. Intraocular pressure should be checked frequently.

A significant percentage of staphylococcal isolates are completely resistant to sulfonamides.

The use of steroids after cataract surgery may delay healing and increase the incidence of filtering blebs.

The use of ocular corticosteroids may prolong the course and may exacerbate the severity of many viral infections of the eye (including herpes simplex). Employment of corticosteroid medication in the treatment of herpes simplex requires great caution.

Topical steroids are not effective in mustard gas keratitis and Sjögren's keratoconjunctivitis.

Fatalities have occurred, although rarely, due to severe reactions to sulfonamides including Stevens-Johnson syndrome, toxic epidermal necrolysis, fulminant hepatic necrosis, agranulocytosis, aplastic anemia and other blood dyscrasias. Sensitization may recur when a sulfonamide is readministered, irrespective of the route of administration. If signs of hypersensitivity or other serious reactions occur, discontinue use of this preparation. Cross-sensitivity among corticosteroids has been demonstrated (see **ADVERSE REACTIONS**).

PRECAUTIONS

General: The initial prescription and renewal of the medication order beyond 20 milliliters of the suspension should be made by a physician only after examination of the patient with the aid of magnification, such as slit lamp biomicroscopy and, where appropriate, fluorescein staining. If signs and symptoms fail to improve after two days, the patient should be re-evaluated.

The possibility of fungal infections of the cornea should be considered after prolonged corticosteroid dosing. Use with caution in patients with severe dry eye. Fungal cultures should be taken when appropriate.

The p-amino benzoic acid present in purulent exudates competes with sulfonamides and can reduce their effectiveness.

Information for Patients: If inflammation or pain persists longer than 48 hours or becomes aggravated, the patient should be advised to discontinue use of the medication and consult a physician (see **WARNINGS**). Contact lenses should not be worn during the use of this product.

This product is sterile when packaged. To prevent contamination, care should be taken to avoid touching the applicator tip to eyelids or to any other surface. The use of this bottle by more than one person may spread infection. Keep bottle tightly closed when not in use. Protect from light. Sulfonamide solutions darken on prolonged standing and exposure to heat and light. Do not use if solution has darkened. Yellowing does not affect activity. Keep out of the reach of children.

Laboratory Tests: Eyelid cultures and tests to determine the susceptibility of organisms to sulfacetamide may be indicated if signs and symptoms persist or recur in spite of the recommended course of treatment with BLEPHAMIDE® ophthalmic suspension.

Drug Interactions: BLEPHAMIDE® ophthalmic suspension is incompatible with silver preparations. Local anesthetics related to p-amino benzoic acid may antagonize the action of the sulfonamides.

Carcinogenesis, Mutagenesis, Impairment of Fertility: Prednisolone has been reported to be noncarcinogenic. Long-term animal studies for carcinogenic potential have not been performed with sulfacetamide.

One author detected chromosomal nondisjunction in the yeast *Saccharomyces cerevisiae* following application of sulfacetamide sodium. The significance of this finding to topical ophthalmic use of sulfacetamide sodium in the human is unknown.

Mutagenic studies with prednisolone have been negative. Studies on reproduction and fertility have not been performed with sulfacetamide. A long-term chronic toxicity study in dogs showed that high oral doses of prednisolone prevented estrus. A decrease in fertility was seen in male and female rats that were mated following oral dosing with another glucocorticosteroid.

Pregnancy: Teratogenic Effects: Pregnancy Category C. Animal reproduction studies have not been conducted with sulfacetamide sodium. Prednisolone has been shown to be teratogenic in rabbits, hamsters, and mice. In mice, prednisolone has been shown to be teratogenic when given in doses 1 to 10 times the human ocular dose. Dexamethasone, hydrocortisone and prednisolone were ocularly applied to both eyes of pregnant mice five times per day on days 10 through 13 of gestation. A significant increase in the incidence of cleft palate was observed in the fetuses of the treated mice. There are no adequate well-controlled studies in pregnant women dosed with corticosteroids.

Kernicterus may be precipitated in infants by sulfonamides being given systemically during the third trimester of pregnancy. It is not known whether sulfacetamide sodium can cause fetal harm when administered to a pregnant woman or whether it can affect reproductive capacity.

BLEPHAMIDE® ophthalmic suspension should be used during pregnancy only if the potential benefit justifies the potential risk to the fetus.

Nursing Mothers: It is not known whether topical administration of corticosteroids could result in sufficient systemic absorption to produce detectable quantities in human milk. Systemically administered corticosteroids appear in human milk and could suppress growth, interfere with endogenous corticosteroid production, or cause other untoward effects. Systemically administered sulfonamides are capable of producing kernicterus in infants of lactating women. Because of the potential for serious adverse reactions in nursing infants from sulfacetamide sodium and prednisolone acetate ophthalmic suspensions, a decision should be made whether to discontinue nursing or to discontinue the medication.

Pediatric Use: Safety and effectiveness in pediatric patients below the age of six have not been established.

ADVERSE REACTIONS

Adverse reactions have occurred with corticosteroid/antibacterial combination drugs which can be attributed to the corticosteroid component, the antibacterial component, or the combination. Exact incidence figures are not available since no denominator of treated patients is available.

Reactions occurring most often from the presence of the anti-bacterial ingredient are allergic sensitizations. Fatalities have occurred, although rarely, due to severe reactions to sulfonamides including Stevens-Johnson syndrome, toxic epidermal necrolysis, fulminant hepatic necrosis, agranulocytosis, aplastic anemia, and other blood dyscrasias (See **WARNINGS**).

Sulfacetamide sodium may cause local irritation.

The reactions due to the corticosteroid component in decreasing order of frequency are: elevation of intraocular pressure (IOP) with possible development of glaucoma and infrequent optic nerve damage, posterior subcapsular cataract formation, and delayed wound healing.

Although systemic effects are extremely uncommon, there have been rare occurrences of systemic hypercorticoidism after use of topical corticosteroids.

Corticosteroid-containing preparations can also cause acute anterior uveitis or perforation of the globe. Mydriasis, loss of accommodation and ptosis have occasionally been reported following local use of corticosteroids.

Secondary Infection: The development of secondary infection has occurred after use of combinations containing corticosteroids and antibacterials. Fungal and viral infections of the cornea are particularly prone to develop coincidentally with long-term applications of corticosteroid. The possibility of fungal invasion must be considered in any persistent corneal ulceration where corticosteroid treatment has been used.

Secondary bacterial ocular infection following suppression of host responses also occurs.

DOSAGE AND ADMINISTRATION

SHAKE WELL BEFORE USING. Two drops should be instilled into the conjunctival sac every four hours during the day and at bedtime.

Not more than 20 milliliters should be prescribed initially, and the prescription should not be refilled without further evaluation as outlined in **PRECAUTIONS** above.

BLEPHAMIDE® dosage may be reduced, but care should be taken not to discontinue therapy prematurely. In chronic conditions, withdrawal of treatment should be carried out by gradually decreasing the frequency of application.

If signs and symptoms fail to improve after two days, the patient should be re-evaluated (see **PRECAUTIONS**).

HOW SUPPLIED

BLEPHAMIDE® ophthalmic suspension is supplied in plastic dropper bottles in the following sizes:

5 mL—NDC 11980-022-05 10 mL—NDC 11980-022-10

Note: Protect from freezing. **Shake well before using.**

Storage: Store BLEPHAMIDE® at 8°–24°C (46°–75°F) in an upright position.

PROTECT FROM LIGHT

Sulfonamide solutions darken on prolonged standing and exposure to heat and light. Do not use if solution has darkened. Yellowing does not affect activity.

KEEP OUT OF REACH OF CHILDREN

℞ **only.**

®Marks owned by Allergan, Inc.

Shown in Product Identification Guide, page 304

Continued on next page

BOTOX® ℞
[bō-tŏks]
(Botulinum Toxin Type A)
botulinum toxin type a
Purified Neurotoxin Complex

DESCRIPTION

BOTOX® (Botulinum Toxin Type A) Purified Neurotoxin Complex is a sterile, vacuum-dried purified botulinum toxin type A, produced from fermentation of Hall strain *Clostridium botulinum* type A grown in a medium containing casein hydrolysate, glucose and yeast extract. It is purified from the culture solution by dialysis and a series of acid precipitations to a complex consisting of the neurotoxin, and several accessory proteins. The complex is dissolved in sterile sodium chloride solution containing Albumin (Human) and is sterile filtered (0.2 microns) prior to filling and vacuum-drying.
One Unit of **BOTOX®** corresponds to the calculated median intraperitoneal lethal dose (LD_{50}) in mice. The method utilized for performing the assay is specific to Allergan's product, **BOTOX®**. Due to specific details of this assay such as the vehicle, dilution scheme and laboratory protocols for the various mouse LD_{50} assays, Units of biological activity of **BOTOX®** cannot be compared to nor converted into Units of any other botulinum toxin or any toxin assessed with any other specific assay method. Therefore, differences in species sensitivities to different botulinum neurotoxin serotypes precludes extrapolation of animal-dose activity relationships to human dose estimates. The specific activity of **BOTOX®** is approximately 20 Units/nanogram of neurotoxin protein complex.
Each vial of **BOTOX®** contains 100 Units (U) of *Clostridium botulinum* type A neurotoxin complex, 0.5 milligrams of Albumin (Human), and 0.9 milligrams of sodium chloride in a sterile, vacuum-dried form without a preservative.

CLINICAL PHARMACOLOGY

BOTOX® blocks neuromuscular transmission by binding to acceptor sites on motor or sympathetic nerve terminals, entering the nerve terminals, and inhibiting the release of acetylcholine. This inhibition occurs as the neurotoxin cleaves SNAP-25, a protein integral to the successful docking and release of acetylcholine from vesicles situated within nerve endings.
When injected intramuscularly at therapeutic doses, **BOTOX®** produces partial chemical denervation of the muscle resulting in a localized reduction in muscle activity. In addition, the muscle may atrophy, axonal sprouting may occur, and extrajunctional acetylcholine receptors may develop. There is evidence that reinnervation of the muscle may occur, thus slowly reversing muscle denervation produced by **BOTOX®**.
When injected intradermally, **BOTOX®** produces temporary chemical denervation of the sweat gland resulting in local reduction in sweating.

Pharmacokinetics
Botulinum Toxin Type A is not expected to be present in the peripheral blood at measurable levels following IM or intradermal injection at the recommended doses. The recommended quantities of neurotoxin administered at each treatment session are not expected to result in systemic, overt distant clinical effects, i.e. muscle weakness, in patients without other neuromuscular dysfunction. However, sub-clinical systemic effects have been shown by single-fiber electromyography after IM doses of botulinum toxins appropriate to produce clinically observable local muscle weakness.

Clinical Studies:
Cervical Dystonia:
A phase 3 randomized, multi-center, double blind, placebo-controlled study of the treatment of cervical dystonia was conducted.[1] This study enrolled adult patients with cervical dystonia and a history of having received **BOTOX®** in an open label manner with perceived good response and tolerable side effects. Patients were excluded if they had previously received surgical or other denervation treatment for their symptoms or had a known history of neuromuscular disorder. Subjects participated in an open label enrichment period where they received their previously employed dose of **BOTOX®**. Only patients who were again perceived as showing a response were advanced to the randomized evaluation period. The muscles in which the blinded study agent injections were to be administered were determined on an individual patient basis.
There were 214 subjects evaluated for the open label period, of which 170 progressed into the randomized, blinded treatment period (88 in the **BOTOX®** group, 82 in the placebo group). Patient evaluations continued for at least 10 weeks post-injection. The primary outcome for the study was a dual endpoint, requiring evidence of both a change in the Cervical Dystonia Severity Scale (CDSS) and an increase in the percentage of patients showing any improvement on the Physicians Global Assessment Scale at 6 weeks after the injection session. The CDSS quantifies the severity of abnormal head positioning and was newly devised for this study. CDSS allots 1 point for each 5 degrees (or part thereof) of head deviation in each of the three planes of head movement (range of scores up to theoretical maximum of 54). The Physician Global Assessment Scale is a 9 category scale scoring the physician's evaluation of the patients' status compared to baseline, ranging from −4 to +4 (very marked worsening to complete improvement), with 0 indicating no change from baseline and +1 slight improvement.

Table 1: Efficacy Outcomes of The Phase 3 Cervical Dystonia Study (Group Means)

	Placebo N=82	BOTOX® N=88	95% CI on Difference
Baseline CDSS	9.3	9.2	
Change in CDSS at Week 6	-0.3	-1.3	(-2.3, 0.3)[a,b]
Percentage Patients with Any Improvement on Physicians Global Assessment	31%	51%	(5%, 34%)[a]
Pain Intensity Baseline	1.8	1.8	
Change in Pain Intensity at Week 6	-0.1	-0.4	(-0.7, -0.2)[c]
Pain Frequency Baseline Change in Pain Frequency at Week 6	1.9 -0.0	1.8 -0.3	(-0.5, -0.0)[c]

[a] Confidence intervals are constructed from the analysis of covariance table with treatment and investigational site as main effects, and baseline CDSS as a covariate.
[b] These values represent the prospectively planned method for missing data imputation and statistical test. Sensitivity analyses indicated that the 95% confidence interval excluded the value of no difference between groups and the p-value was less than 0.05. These analyses included several alternative missing data imputation methods and non-parametric statistical tests.
[c] Confidence intervals are based on the t-distribution

Table 2: Number of Patients Treated Per Muscle And Fraction Of Total Dose Injected Into Involved Muscles

Muscle*	Number of Patients Treated in this Muscle (N=88)	Mean % Dose per Muscle	Mid-Range of % Dose per Muscle*
Splenius capitis/cervicis	83	38	25-50
Sternocleidomastoid	77	25	17-31
Levator scapulae	52	20	16-25
Trapezius	49	29	18-33
Semispinalis	16	21	13-25
Scalene	15	15	6-21
Longissimus	8	29	17-41

*The mid-range of dose is calculated as the 25th to 75th percentiles.
NOTE: There were 16 patients who had additional muscles injected.

Table 3: Study 1. Study Outcomes

Treatment Response	BOTOX® 50 Units N= 104	BOTOX® 75 Units N=110	Placebo N= 108	BOTOX® 50-placebo (95% CI)	BOTOX® 75-placebo (95% CI)
HDSS Score change ≥2 % (n)[a]	55% (57)	49% (54)	6% (6)	49.3% (38.8, 59.7)	43% (33.2, 53.8)
>50% decrease in axillary sweat production % (n)	81% (84)	86% (94)	41% (44)	40% (28.1, 52.0)	45% (33.3, 56.1)

[a] Patients who showed at least a 2-grade improvement from baseline value on the HDSS 4 weeks after both of the first two treatment sessions or had a sustained response after their first treatment session and did not receive re-treatment during the study

Pain is also an important symptom of cervical dystonia and was evaluated by separate assessments of pain frequency and severity on scales of 0 (no pain) to 4 (constant in frequency or extremely severe in intensity). Study results on the primary endpoints and the pain-related secondary endpoints are shown in Table 1.
[See table 1 above]
Exploratory analyses of this study suggested that the majority of patients who had shown a beneficial response by week 6 had returned to their baseline status by 3 months after treatment. Exploratory analyses of subsets by patient sex and age suggest that both sexes receive benefit, although female patients may receive somewhat greater amounts than male patients. There is a consistent treatment-associated effect between subsets greater than and less than age 65 (see also **PRECAUTIONS: Geriatrics**). There were too few non-Caucasian patients enrolled to draw any conclusions regarding relative efficacy in racial subsets.
There were several randomized studies conducted prior to the phase 3 study which were supportive but not adequately designed to assess or quantitatively estimate the efficacy of **BOTOX®**.
In the phase 3 study the median total **BOTOX®** dose in patients randomized to receive **BOTOX®** (n=88) was 236 Units, with 25th to 75th percentile ranges of 198 to 300 Units. Of these 88 patients, most received injections to 3 or 4 muscles; 38 received injections to 3 muscles, 28 to 4 muscles, 5 to 5 muscles and 5 to 2 muscles. The dose was divided amongst the affected muscles in quantities shown in Table 2. The total dose and muscles selected were tailored to meet individual patient needs.
[See table 2 above]
Primary Axillary Hyperhidrosis:
The efficacy and safety of **BOTOX®** for the treatment of primary axillary hyperhidrosis were evaluated in two randomized, multi-center, double-blind, placebo-controlled studies. Study 1 included adult patients with persistent primary axillary hyperhidrosis who scored 3 or 4 on a Hyperhidrosis Disease Severity Scale (HDSS) and who produced at least 50mg of sweat in each axilla at rest over 5 minutes. HDSS is a 4-point scale with 1= "underarm sweating is never noticeable and never interferes with my daily activities"; to 4 = "underarm sweating is intolerable and always interferes with my daily activities". A total of 322 patients were randomized in a 1:1:1 ratio to treatment in both axillae with either 50 Units of **BOTOX®**, 75 Units of **BOTOX®**, or placebo. Patients were evaluated at 4-week intervals. Patients who responded to the first injection were re-injected when they reported a re-increase in HDSS score to 3 or 4 and produced at least 50mg sweat in each axilla by gravimetric measurement, but no sooner than 8 weeks after the initial injection.
Study responders were defined as patients who showed at least a 2-grade improvement from baseline value on the HDSS 4 weeks after both of the first two treatment sessions or had a sustained response after their first treatment session and did not receive re-treatment during the study. Spontaneous resting axillary sweat production was assessed by weighing a filter paper held in the axilla over a period of 5 minutes (gravimetric measurement). Sweat production responders were those patients who demonstrated a reduction in axillary sweating from baseline of at least 50% at week 4.
In the three study groups the percentage of patients with baseline HDSS score of 3 ranged from 50% to 54% and from 46 % to 50% for a score of 4. The median amount of sweat production (averaged for each axilla) was 102 mg, 123 mg, and 114 mg for the placebo, 50 Units and 75 Units groups respectively.
The percentage of responders based on at least a 2-grade decrease from baseline in HDSS or based on a >50% decrease from baseline in axillary sweat production was greater in both **BOTOX®** groups than in the placebo group ($p < 0.001$), but was not significantly different between the 2 **BOTOX®** doses (See Table 3).
[See table 3 above]
Duration of response was calculated as the number of days between injection and the date of the first visit at which patients returned to 3 or 4 on the HDSS scale. The median duration of response following the first treatment in **BOTOX®**-treated patients with either dose was 201 days. Among those who received a second **BOTOX®** injection, the median duration of response was similar to that observed after the first treatment.

In study 2, 320 adults with bilateral axillary primary hyperhidrosis were randomized to receive either 50 Units of **BOTOX®** (n=242) or placebo (n=78). Treatment responders were defined as subjects showing at least a 50% reduction from baseline in axillary sweating measured by gravimetric measurement at 4 weeks. At week 4 post-injection, the percentages of responders were 91% (219/242) in the **BOTOX®** group and 36% (28/78) in the placebo group, $p < 0.001$. The difference in percentage of responders between **BOTOX®** and placebo was 55% (95% CI = 43.3, 65.9).

Blepharospasm:

Botulinum toxin has been investigated for use in patients with blepharospasm in several studies. In an open label uncontrolled study, 27 patients with essential blepharospasm were injected with 2.0 Units of **BOTOX®** at each of six sites on each side. One patient had not received any prior treatment. Twenty-six of the patients had not responded to therapy with benztropine mesylate, clonazepam and/or baclofen. Three of the 26 patients continued to experience spasms following muscle stripping surgery. Twenty-five of the 27 patients treated with botulinum toxin reported improvement within 48 hours. One patient was controlled with a higher dosage at 13 weeks post initial injection and one patient reported mild improvement but remained functionally impaired.[2]

In another study, 12 patients with blepharospasm were evaluated in a double-blind, placebo-controlled study. Patients receiving botulinum toxin (n=8) improved compared with the placebo group (n=4). The mean dystonia score improved by 72%, the self-assessment score rating improved by 61%, and a videotape evaluation rating improved by 39%. The effects of the treatment lasted a mean of 12.5 weeks.[3]

One thousand six hundred eighty-four patients with blepharospasm who were evaluated in an open label trial showed clinical improvement as evaluated by measured eyelid force and clinically observed intensity of lid spasm, lasting an average of 12.5 weeks prior to the need for re-treatment.[4]

Strabismus:

It is postulated that when used for the treatment of strabismus, the administration of **BOTOX®** affects muscle pairs by inducing an atrophic lengthening of the injected muscle and a corresponding shortening of the muscle's antagonist; it was on the basis of this hypothesis that clinical studies were conducted. Six hundred seventy-seven patients with strabismus treated with one or more injections of **BOTOX®** were evaluated in an open label trial. Fifty-five percent of these patients improved to an alignment of 10 prism diopters or less when evaluated six months or more following injection.[5] These results are consistent with results from additional open label trials which were conducted for this indication.[4]

INDICATIONS AND USAGE

BOTOX® is indicated for the treatment of cervical dystonia in adults to decrease the severity of abnormal head position and neck pain associated with cervical dystonia.

BOTOX® is indicated for the treatment of severe primary axillary hyperhidrosis that is inadequately managed with topical agents.

BOTOX® is indicated for the treatment of strabismus and blepharospasm associated with dystonia, including benign essential blepharospasm or VII nerve disorders in patients 12 years of age and above.

The efficacy of **BOTOX®** treatment in deviations over 50 prism diopters, in restrictive strabismus, in Duane's syndrome with lateral rectus weakness, and in secondary strabismus caused by prior surgical over-recession of the antagonist has not been established. **BOTOX®** is ineffective in chronic paralytic strabismus except when used in conjunction with surgical repair to reduce antagonist contracture.

CONTRAINDICATIONS

BOTOX® is contraindicated in the presence of infection at the proposed injection site(s) and in individuals with known hypersensitivity to any ingredient in the formulation.

WARNINGS

The recommended dosage and frequency of administration for **BOTOX®** should not be exceeded. Risks resulting from administration at higher dosages are not known.

Hypersensitivity Reactions

Serious and/or immediate hypersensitivity reactions have been rarely reported. These reactions include anaphylaxis, urticaria, soft tissue edema, and dyspnea. One fatal case of anaphylaxis has been reported in which lidocaine was used as the diluent, and consequently the causal agent cannot be reliably determined. If such a reaction occurs further injection of **BOTOX®** should be discontinued and appropriate medical therapy immediately instituted.

Pre-Existing Neuromuscular Disorders

Individuals with peripheral motor neuropathic diseases (e.g., amyotrophic lateral sclerosis, or motor neuropathy) or neuromuscular junctional disorders (e.g., myasthenia gravis or Lambert-Eaton syndrome) should only receive **BOTOX®** with caution. Patients with neuromuscular disorders may be at increased risk of clinically significant systemic effects including severe dysphagia and respiratory compromise from typical doses of **BOTOX®**. Published medical literature has reported rare cases of administration of a botulinum toxin to patients with known or unrecognized neuromuscular disorders where the patients have shown extreme sensitivity to the systemic effects of typical clinical doses. In some of these cases, dysphagia has lasted several months and required placement of a gastric feeding tube.

Dysphagia

Dysphagia is a commonly reported adverse event following treatment of cervical dystonia patients with all botulinum toxins. In these patients, there are reports of rare cases of dysphagia severe enough to warrant the insertion of a gastric feeding tube. There are also rare case reports where subsequent to the finding of dysphagia a patient developed aspiration pneumonia and died.

Human Albumin

This product contains albumin, a derivative of human blood. Based on effective donor screening and product manufacturing processes, it carries an extremely remote risk for transmission of viral diseases. A theoretical risk for transmission of Creutzfeldt-Jakob disease (CJD) also is considered extremely remote. No cases of transmission of viral diseases or CJD have ever been identified for albumin.

PRECAUTIONS

The safe and effective use of **BOTOX®** depends upon proper storage of the product, selection of the correct dose, and proper reconstitution and administration techniques. Physicians administering **BOTOX®** must understand the relevant neuromuscular and/or orbital anatomy of the area involved and any alterations to the anatomy due to prior surgical procedures. An understanding of standard electromyographic techniques is also required for treatment of strabismus and may be useful for the treatment of cervical dystonia.

Caution should be used when **BOTOX®** treatment is used in the presence of inflammation at the proposed injection site(s) or when excessive weakness or atrophy is present in the target muscle(s).

Cervical Dystonia:

Patients with smaller neck muscle mass and patients who require bilateral injections into the sternocleidomastoid muscle have been reported to be at greater risk for dysphagia. Limiting the dose injected into the sternocleidomastoid muscle may reduce the occurrence of dysphagia. Injections into the levator scapulae may be associated with an increased risk of upper respiratory infection and dysphagia.

Primary Axillary Hyperhidrosis:

Patients should be evaluated for potential causes of secondary hyperhidrosis (e.g. hyperthyroidism) to avoid symptomatic treatment of hyperhidrosis without the diagnosis and/or treatment of the underlying disease. The safety and effectiveness of **BOTOX®** for hyperhidrosis in other body areas have not been established. Weakness of hand muscles and blepharoptosis may occur in patients who receive **BOTOX®** for palmar hyperhidrosis and facial hyperhidrosis, respectively.

Blepharospasm:

Reduced blinking from **BOTOX®** injection of the orbicularis muscle can lead to corneal exposure, persistent epithelial defect and corneal ulceration, especially in patients with VII nerve disorders. One case of corneal perforation in an aphakic eye requiring corneal grafting has occurred because of this effect. Careful testing of corneal sensation in eyes previously operated upon, avoidance of injection into the lower lid area to avoid ectropion, and vigorous treatment of any epithelial defect should be employed. This may require protective drops, ointment, therapeutic soft contact lenses, or closure of the eye by patching or other means.

Strabismus:

During the administration of **BOTOX®** for the treatment of strabismus, retrobulbar hemorrhages sufficient to compromise retinal circulation have occurred from needle penetrations into the orbit. It is recommended that appropriate instruments to decompress the orbit be accessible. Ocular (globe) penetrations by needles have also occurred. An ophthalmoscope to diagnose this condition should be available. Inducing paralysis in one or more extraocular muscles may produce spatial disorientation, double vision or past pointing. Covering the affected eye may alleviate these symptoms.

Information for Patients:

Patients or caregivers should be advised to seek immediate medical attention if swallowing, speech or respiratory disorders arise.

Patients with cervical dystonia should be informed of the possibility of experiencing dysphagia, which is typically mild to moderate, but could be severe. Rare consequences of severe dysphagia include aspiration, dyspnea, pneumonia, and the need to reestablish an airway.

As with any treatment with the potential to allow previously sedentary patients to resume activities, the sedentary patient should be cautioned to resume activity gradually following the administration of **BOTOX®**.

Drug Interactions:

Co-administration of **BOTOX®** and aminoglycosides or other agents interfering with neuromuscular transmission (e.g., curare-like compounds) should only be performed with caution as the effect of the toxin may be potentiated.

The effect of administering different botulinum neurotoxin serotypes at the same time or within several months of each other is unknown. Excessive neuromuscular weakness may be exacerbated by administration of another botulinum toxin prior to the resolution of the effects of a previously administered botulinum toxin.

Pregnancy: Pregnancy Category C

When pregnant mice and rats were injected intramuscularly during the period of organogenesis, the developmental NOEL of **BOTOX®** was 4 U/kg. Higher doses (8 or 16 U/kg) were associated with reductions in fetal body weights and/or delayed ossification which may be reversible.

In a range finding study in rabbits, daily injection of 0.125 U/kg/day (days 6 to 18 of gestation) and 2 U/kg (days 6 and 13 of gestation) produced severe maternal toxicity, abortions and/or fetal malformations. Higher doses resulted in death of the dams. The rabbit appears to be a very sensitive species to **BOTOX®**.

There are no adequate and well-controlled studies of **BOTOX®** in pregnant women. Because animal reproductive studies are not always predictive of human response, **BOTOX®** should be administered during pregnancy only if the potential benefit justifies the potential risk to the fetus. If this drug is used during pregnancy, or if the patient becomes pregnant while taking this drug, the patient should be apprised of the potential risks, including abortion or fetal malformations which have been observed in rabbits.

Carcinogenesis, Mutagenesis, Impairment of Fertility:

Long term studies in animals have not been performed to evaluate carcinogenic potential of **BOTOX®**.

The reproductive NOEL following intramuscular injection of 0, 4, 8, and 16 U/kg was 4 U/kg in male rats and 8 U/kg in female rats. Higher doses were associated with dose-dependent reductions in fertility in male rats (where limb weakness resulted in the inability to mate), and an altered estrous cycle in female rats. There were no adverse effects on the viability of the embryos.

Nursing Mothers: It is not known whether this drug is excreted in human milk. Because many drugs are excreted in human milk, caution should be exercised when **BOTOX®** is administered to a nursing woman.

Pediatric Use: Safety and effectiveness in children below the age of 12 have not been established for blepharospasm or strabismus, or below the age of 16 for cervical dystonia or 18 for hyperhidrosis.

Geriatric Use: Clinical studies of **BOTOX®** did not include sufficient numbers of subjects aged 65 and over to determine whether they respond differently from younger subjects. Other reported clinical experience has not identified differences in responses between the elderly and younger patients. There were too few patients over the age of 75 to enable any comparisons. In general, dose selection for an elderly patient should be cautious, usually starting at the low end of the dosing range, reflecting the greater frequency of decreased hepatic, renal, or cardiac function, and of concomitant disease or other drug therapy.

ADVERSE REACTIONS

General:

There have been rare spontaneous reports of death, sometimes associated with dysphagia, pneumonia, and/or other significant debility or anaphylaxis, after treatment with botulinum toxin.

There have also been rare reports of adverse events involving the cardiovascular system, including arrhythmia and myocardial infarction, some with fatal outcomes. Some of these patients had risk factors including cardiovascular disease. The exact relationship of these events to the botulinum toxin injection has not been established.

The following events have been reported since the drug has been marketed and a causal relationship to the botulinum toxin injected is unknown: skin rash (including erythema multiforme, urticaria and psoriasiform eruption), pruritus, and allergic reaction.

In general, adverse events occur within the first week following injection of **BOTOX®** and while generally transient may have a duration of several months. Localized pain, tenderness and/or bruising may be associated with the injection. Local weakness of the injected muscle(s) represents the expected pharmacological action of botulinum toxin. However, weakness of adjacent muscles may also occur due to spread of toxin.

Cervical Dystonia:

In cervical dystonia patients evaluated for safety in double-blind and open-label studies following injection of **BOTOX®**, the most frequently reported adverse reactions were dysphagia (19%), upper respiratory infection (12%), neck pain (11%), and headache (11%).[7]

Other events reported in 2-10% of patients in any one study in decreasing order of incidence include: increased cough, flu syndrome, back pain, rhinitis, dizziness, hypertonia, soreness at injection site, asthenia, oral dryness, speech disorder, fever, nausea, and drowsiness. Stiffness, numbness, diplopia, ptosis, and dyspnea have been reported rarely.

Dysphagia and symptomatic general weakness may be attributable to an extension of the pharmacology of **BOTOX®** resulting from the spread of the toxin outside the injected muscles.

The most common severe adverse event associated with the use of **BOTOX®** injection in patients with cervical dystonia is dysphagia with about 20% of these cases also reporting dyspnea. (See **Warnings**). Most dysphagia is reported as mild or moderate in severity. However, it may rarely be associated with more severe signs and symptoms (See **Warnings**).

Additionally, reports in the literature include a case of a female patient who developed brachial plexopathy two days after injection of 120 Units of **BOTOX®** for the treatment of cervical dystonia, and reports of dysphonia in patients who have been treated for cervical dystonia.

Primary Axillary Hyperhidrosis:

The most frequently reported adverse events (3-10% of patients) following injection of **BOTOX®** in double-blind studies included injection site pain and hemorrhage, non-

Continued on next page

Botox—Cont.

axillary sweating, infection, pharyngitis, flu syndrome, headache, fever, neck or back pain, pruritus, and anxiety. The data reflect 346 patients exposed to **BOTOX®** 50 Units and 110 patients exposed to **BOTOX®** 75 Units in each axilla.

Because clinical trials are conducted under widely varying conditions, adverse events observed in the clinical trials of a drug cannot be directly compared to rates in the clinical trials of another drug and may not be predictive of rates observed in practice.

Blepharospasm:

In a study of blepharospasm patients who received an average dose per eye of 33 Units (injected at 3 to 5 sites) of the currently manufactured **BOTOX®**, the most frequently reported treatment-related adverse reactions were ptosis (20.8%), superficial punctate keratitis (6.3%) and eye dryness (6.3%).[8]

In this study, the rate for ptosis in the current **BOTOX®** treated group (20.8% of patients) was significantly higher than the original **BOTOX®** treated group (4.0% of patients) (p=0.014%). All of these events were mild or moderate except for one case of ptosis which was rated severe.

Other events reported in prior clinical studies in decreasing order of incidence include: irritation, tearing, lagophthalmos, photophobia, ectropion, keratitis, diplopia and entropion, diffuse skin rash and local swelling of the eyelid skin lasting for several days following eyelid injection.

In two cases of VII nerve disorder (one case of an aphakic eye), reduced blinking from **BOTOX®** injection of the orbicularis muscle led to serious corneal exposure, persistent epithelial defect, and corneal ulceration. Perforation occurred in the aphakic eye and required corneal grafting.

A report of acute angle closure glaucoma one day after receiving an injection of botulinum toxin for blepharospasm was received, with recovery four months later after laser iridotomy and trabeculectomy. Focal facial paralysis, syncope and exacerbation of myasthenia gravis have also been reported after treatment of blepharospasm.

Strabismus:

Extraocular muscles adjacent to the injection site can be affected, causing ptosis or vertical deviation, especially with higher doses of **BOTOX®**. The incidence rates of these adverse effects in 2058 adults who received a total of 3650 injections for horizontal strabismus are 15.7% and 16.9%, respectively.[4]

Inducing paralysis in one or more extraocular muscles may produce spatial disorientation, double vision, or pastpointing. Covering the affected eye may alleviate these symptoms.

The incidence of ptosis was 0.9% after inferior rectus injection and 37.7% after superior rectus injection.

Ptosis (0.3%) and vertical deviation greater than two prism diopters (2.1%) were reported to persist for over six months in a larger series of 5587 injections of horizontal muscles in 3104 patients.

In these patients, the injection procedure itself caused nine scleral perforations. A vitreous hemorrhage occurred in one case and later cleared. No retinal detachment or visual loss occurred in any case. Sixteen retrobulbar hemorrhages occurred without visual loss. Decompression of the orbit after five minutes was done to restore retinal circulation in one case. Five eyes had pupillary change consistent with ciliary ganglion damage (Adie's pupil).

One patient developed anterior segment ischemia after receiving **BOTOX®** injection into the medial rectus muscle under direct visualization for esotropia.

Immunogenicity:

Formation of neutralizing antibodies to botulinum toxin type A may reduce the effectiveness of **BOTOX®** treatment by inactivating the biological activity of the toxin. The rate of formation of neutralizing antibodies in patients receiving **BOTOX®** has not been well studied.

In the phase 3 cervical dystonia study[1] that enrolled only patients with a history of receiving **BOTOX®** for multiple treatment sessions, at study entry there were 192 patients with antibody assay results, of whom 33 (17%) had a positive assay for neutralizing activity. There were 96 patients in the randomized period of the phase 3 study with valid assays at both study entry and end and who were neutralizing activity negative at entry. Of these 96, 2 patients (2%) converted to positive for neutralizing activity. Both of these converting patients were among the 52 who had received two **BOTOX®** treatments between the two assays; none were in the group randomized to placebo in the controlled comparison period of the study.

In the randomized period of the cervical dystonia study, patients in the **BOTOX®** group whose baseline assays were neutralizing antibody negative showed improvements on CDSS (n=64, mean CDSS change -2.1) while patients whose baseline assays were neutralizing antibody positive did not (n=14, mean CDSS change +1.1).

However, in uncontrolled studies there are also individual patients who are perceived as continuing to respond to treatments despite the presence of neutralizing activity. Not all patients who become non-responsive to **BOTOX®** after an initial period of clinical response have demonstrable levels of neutralizing activity.

One patient among the 445 hyperhidrosis patients with analyzed specimens showed the presence of neutralizing antibodies.

The data reflect the patients whose test results were considered positive or negative for neutralizing activity to **BOTOX®** in a mouse protection assay. The results of these tests are highly dependent on the sensitivity and specificity of the assay. Additionally, the observed incidence of neutralizing activity in an assay may be influenced by several factors including sample handling, concomitant medications and underlying disease. For these reasons, comparison of the incidence of neutralizing activity to **BOTOX®** with the incidence reported to other products may be misleading.

The critical factors for neutralizing antibody formation have not been well characterized. The results from some studies suggest that **BOTOX®** injections at more frequent intervals or at higher doses may lead to greater incidence of antibody formation. The potential for antibody formation may be minimized by injecting with the lowest effective dose given at the longest feasible intervals between injections.

OVERDOSAGE

Signs and symptoms of overdose are not apparent immediately post-injection. Should accidental injection or oral ingestion occur, the person should be medically supervised for up to several weeks for signs or symptoms of systemic weakness or muscle paralysis.

An antitoxin is available in the event of immediate knowledge of an overdose or misinjection. In the event of an overdose or injection into the wrong muscle, immediately contact Allergan for additional information at (800) 433-8871 from 8:00 a.m. to 4:00 p.m. Pacific Time, or at (714) 246-5954 for a recorded message at other times. The antitoxin will not reverse any botulinum toxin induced muscle weakness effects already apparent by the time of antitoxin administration.

DOSAGE AND ADMINISTRATION

BOTOX® is supplied in a single use vial. Because the product and diluent do not contain a preservative, once opened and reconstituted, store in a refrigerator and use within four hours. Discard any remaining solution. Do not freeze reconstituted **BOTOX®**.

BOTOX® is to be reconstituted with sterile, non-preserved saline prior to intramuscular injection.

General:

An injection of **BOTOX®** is prepared by drawing into an appropriately sized sterile syringe an amount of the properly reconstituted toxin (see Dilution Table) slightly greater than the intended dose. Air bubbles in the syringe barrel are expelled and the syringe is attached to an appropriate injection needle. Patency of the needle should be confirmed. A new, sterile, needle and syringe should be used to enter the vial on each occasion for removal of **BOTOX®**.

The method utilized for performing the potency assay is specific to Allergan's Botulinum Toxin Type A. Due to specific details of this assay such as the vehicle, dilution scheme and laboratory protocols for the various potency assays, Units of biological activity of Botulinum Toxin Type A cannot be compared to nor converted into Units of any other botulinum toxin or any toxin assessed with any other specific assay method. Therefore, differences in species sensitivities to different botulinum neurotoxin serotypes precludes extrapolation of animal dose-activity relationships to human dose relationships.

Cervical Dystonia:

The phase 3 study enrolled patients who had extended histories of receiving and tolerating **BOTOX®** injections, with prior individualized adjustment of dose. The mean **BOTOX®** dose administered to patients in the phase 3 study was 236 Units (25th to 75th percentile range 198 Units to 300 Units). The **BOTOX®** dose was divided among the affected muscles (see Clinical Studies: Cervical Dystonia). Dosing in initial and sequential treatment sessions should be tailored to the individual patient based on the patient's head and neck position, localization of pain, muscle hypertrophy, patient response and adverse event history.

The initial dose for a patient without prior use of **BOTOX®** should be at a lower dose, with subsequent dosing adjusted based on individual response. Limiting the total dose injected into the sternocleido-mastoid muscles to 100 Units or less may decrease the occurrence of dysphagia (see Precautions: Cervical Dystonia).

A 25, 27 or 30 gauge needle may be used for superficial muscles, and a longer 22 gauge needle may be used for deeper musculature. Localization of the involved muscles with electromyographic guidance may be useful.

Clinical improvement generally begins within the first two weeks after injection with maximum clinical benefit at approximately six weeks post-injection. In the phase 3 study most subjects were observed to have returned to pretreatment status by 3 months post-treatment.

Primary Axillary Hyperhidrosis

The recommended dose is 50 Units per axilla. The hyperhidrotic area to be injected should be defined using standard staining techniques, e.g., Minor's Iodine-Starch Test. **BOTOX®** is reconstituted with 0.9% non-preserved sterile saline (100 Units/4 mL). Using a 30 gauge needle, 50 Units of **BOTOX®** (2mL) is injected intradermally in 0.1 to 0.2 mL aliquots to each axilla evenly distributed in multiple sites (10-15) approximately 1-2 cm apart.

Repeat injections for hyperhidrosis should be administered when the clinical effect of a previous injection diminishes.

Instructions for the Minor's Iodine Starch Test Procedure

Patients should shave underarms and abstain from use of over-the-counter deodorants or antiperspirants for 24 hours prior to the test. Patient should be resting comfortably without exercise, hot drinks, etc. for approximately 30 minutes prior to the test. Dry the underarm area and then immediately paint it with iodine solution. Allow the area to dry, then lightly sprinkle the area with starch powder. Gently blow off any excess starch powder. The hyperhidrotic area will develop a deep blue-black color over approximately 10 minutes.

Each injection site has a ring of effect of up to approximately 2 cm in diameter. To minimize the area of no effect, the injection sites should be evenly spaced as shown in Figure 1:

Figure 1:

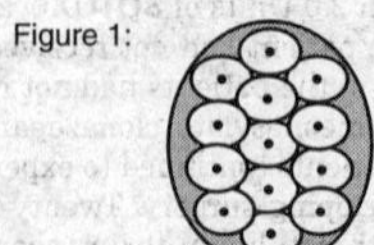

Each dose is injected to a depth of approximately 2mm and at a 45° angle to the skin surface with the bevel side up to minimize leakage and to ensure the injections remain intradermal.

If injection sites are marked in ink do not inject **BOTOX®** directly through the ink mark to avoid a permanent tattoo effect.

Blepharospasm:

For blepharospasm, reconstituted **BOTOX®** (see Dilution Table) is injected using a sterile, 27-30 gauge needle without electromyographic guidance. The initial recommended dose is 1.25-2.5 Units (0.05 mL to 0.1 mL volume at each site) injected into the medial and lateral pre-tarsal orbicularis oculi of the upper lid and into the lateral pre-tarsal orbicularis oculi of the lower lid. Avoiding injection near the levator palpebrae superioris may reduce the complication of ptosis. Avoiding medial lower lid injections, and thereby reducing diffusion into the inferior oblique, may reduce the complication of diplopia. Ecchymosis occurs easily in the soft eyelid tissues. This can be prevented by applying pressure at the injection site immediately after the injection.

In general, the initial effect of the injections is seen within three days and reaches a peak at one to two weeks post-treatment. Each treatment lasts approximately three months, following which the procedure can be repeated. At repeat treatment sessions, the dose may be increased up to two-fold if the response from the initial treatment is considered insufficient-usually defined as an effect that does not last longer than two months. However there appears to be little benefit obtainable from injecting more than 5.0 Units per site. Some tolerance may be found when **BOTOX®** is used in treating blepharospasm if treatments are given any more frequently than every three months, and is rare to have the effect be permanent.

The cumulative dose of **BOTOX®** treatment in a 30-day period should not exceed 200 Units.

Strabismus:

BOTOX® is intended for injection into extraocular muscles utilizing the electrical activity recorded from the tip of the injection needle as a guide to placement within the target muscle. Injection without surgical exposure or electromyographic guidance should not be attempted. Physicians should be familiar with electromyographic technique.

To prepare the eye for **BOTOX®** injection, it is recommended that several drops of a local anesthetic and an ocular decongestant be given several minutes prior to injection.

Note: The volume of **BOTOX®** injected for treatment of strabismus should be between 0.05-0.15 mL per muscle.

The initial listed doses of the reconstituted **BOTOX®** (see Dilution Table below) typically create paralysis of injected muscles beginning one to two days after injection and increasing in intensity during the first week. The paralysis lasts for 2-6 weeks and gradually resolves over a similar time period. Overcorrections lasting over six months have been rare. About one half of patients will require subsequent doses because of inadequate paralytic response of the muscle to the initial dose, or because of mechanical factors such as large deviations or restrictions, or because of the lack of binocular motor fusion to stabilize the alignment.

I. Initial doses in Units. Use the lower listed doses for treatment of small deviations. Use the larger doses only for large deviations.
   A. For vertical muscles, and for horizontal strabismus of less than 20 prism diopters: 1.25-2.5 Units in any one muscle.
   B. For horizontal strabismus of 20 prism diopters to 50 prism diopters: 2.5-5.0 Units in any one muscle.
   C. For persistent VI nerve palsy of one month or longer duration: 1.25-2.5 Units in the medial rectus muscle.

II. Subsequent doses for residual or recurrent strabismus.
   A. It is recommended that patients be re-examined 7-14 days after each injection to assess the effect of that dose.
   B. Patients experiencing adequate paralysis of the target muscle that require subsequent injections should receive a dose comparable to the initial dose.

C. Subsequent doses for patients experiencing incomplete paralysis of the target muscle may be increased up to two-fold compared to the previously administered dose.
D. Subsequent injections should not be administered until the effects of the previous dose have dissipated as evidenced by substantial function in the injected and adjacent muscles.
E. The maximum recommended dose as a single injection for any one muscle is 25 Units.

Dilution Technique:
Prior to injection, reconstitute vacuum-dried **BOTOX®**, with sterile normal saline **without** a preservative; 0.9% Sodium Chloride Injection is the only recommended diluent. Draw up the proper amount of diluent in the appropriate size syringe, and slowly inject the diluent into the vial. Discard the vial if a vacuum does not pull the diluent into the vial. Gently mix **BOTOX®** with the saline by rotating the vial. Record the date and time of reconstitution on the space on the label. **BOTOX®** should be administered within four hours after reconstitution.
During this time period, reconstituted **BOTOX®** should be stored in a refrigerator (2° to 8°C). Reconstituted **BOTOX®** should be clear, colorless and free of particulate matter. Parenteral drug products should be inspected visually for particulate matter and discoloration prior to administration and whenever the solution and the container permit.

Dilution Table

Diluent Added (0.9% Sodium Chloride Injection)	Resulting dose Units per 0.1 mL
1.0 mL	10.0 Units
2.0 mL	5.0 Units
4.0 mL	2.5 Units
8.0 mL	1.25 Units

Note: These dilutions are calculated for an injection volume of 0.1 mL. A decrease or increase in the **BOTOX®** dose is also possible by administering a smaller or larger injection volume—from 0.05 mL (50% decrease in dose) to 0.15 mL (50% increase in dose.)

HOW SUPPLIED

BOTOX® is supplied in a single use vial. Each vial contains 100 Units of vacuum-dried *Clostridium botulinum* type A neurotoxin complex. NDC 0023-1145-01.
Vials of **BOTOX®** have a holographic film on the vial label that contains the name "Allergan" within horizontal lines of rainbow color. In order to see the hologram, rotate the vial back and forth between your fingers under a desk lamp or fluorescent light source. (Note: the holographic film on the label is absent in the date/batch area.) If you do not see the lines of rainbow color or the name "Allergan", do not use the product and contact Allergan for additional information at (800) 890-4345 from 8:00 a.m. to 4:00 p.m. Pacific time.

Rx Only
Single use vial.
Storage:
Unopened vials of **BOTOX®** should be stored in a refrigerator (2° to 8°C) for up to 24 months. Do not use after the expiration date on the vial. Administer **BOTOX®** within 4 hours of reconstitution; during this period reconstituted **BOTOX®** should be stored in a refrigerator (2° to 8°C). Reconstituted **BOTOX®** should be clear, colorless and free of particulate matter.
All vials, including expired vials, or equipment used with the drug should be disposed of carefully as is done with all medical waste.
® Marks owned by Allergan, Inc.
Revised: July 2004
Manufactured by: Allergan Pharmaceuticals Ireland
a subsidiary of: Allergan, Inc., 2525 Dupont Dr., Irvine, CA 92612

REFERENCES

1. Data on file, Allergan, Inc. A randomized, multicenter, double-blind, placebo-controlled study of intramuscular **BOTOX®** (botulinum toxin type A) purified neurotoxin complex (original 79-11 **BOTOX®**[5]) for the treatment of cervical dystonia. 1998.
2. Arthurs B, Flanders M, Codere F, Gauthier S, Dresner S, Stone L. Treatment of blepharospasm with medication, surgery and type A botulinum toxin. Can J Ophthalmol 1987;22:24-28.
3. Jankovic J, Orman J. Botulinum A toxin for cranial-cervical dystonia: A double-blind, placebo-controlled study. Neurology 1987;37:616-623.
4. Data on file, Allergan, Inc.
5. Scott AB. Botulinum toxin treatment of strabismus. American Academy of Ophthalmology, Focal Points 1989: Clinical Modules for Ophthalmologists Vol VII Module 12.
6. Wang YC, Burr DH, Korthals GJ, Sugiyama H. Acute toxicity of aminoglycoside antibiotics as an aid in detecting botulism. Appl Environ Microbiol 1984;48:951-955.
7. Data on file, Allergan, Inc. 1999.
8. Data on file, Allergan, Inc. A randomized, multicenter, double-blind, parallel clinical trial to compare the safety and efficacy of **BOTOX®** (botulinum toxin type A) purified neurotoxin complex manufactured from neurotoxin complex batch BCB2024 to that manufactured from neurotoxin complex batch 79-11 in blepharospasm patients. 1997.

ELESTAT™ ℞

[*ĕl-ĕ-stăt*]
(epinastine HCl ophthalmic solution) 0.05%
Sterile

DESCRIPTION

ELESTAT™ (epinastine HCl ophthalmic solution) 0.05% is a clear, colorless, sterile isotonic solution containing epinastine HCl, an antihistamine and an inhibitor of histamine release from the mast cell for topical administration to the eyes.
Epinastine HCl is represented by the following structural formula:

x HCl

$C_{16}H_{15}N_3$ • HCl Mol. Wt. 285.78

Chemical Name: 3-Amino-9, 13b-dihydro-1H-dibenz[c, f]imidazo[1,5-a]azepine hydrochloride
Each mL contains: Active: Epinastine HCl 0.05% (0.5mg/mL) equivalent to epinastine 0.044% (0.44mg/mL); **Preservative:** Benzalkonium chloride 0.01%; **Inactives:** Edetate disodium; purified water; sodium chloride; sodium phosphate, monobasic; and sodium hydroxide and/or hydrochloric acid (to adjust the pH). ELESTAT™ has a pH of approximately 7 and an osmolality range of 250 to 310 mOsm/kg.

CLINICAL PHARMACOLOGY

Epinastine is a topically active, direct H_1-receptor antagonist and an inhibitor of the release of histamine from the mast cell. Epinastine is selective for the histamine H_1-receptor and has affinity for the histamine H_2-receptor. Epinastine also possesses affinity for the α_1-, α_2-, and 5-HT_2-receptors. Epinastine does not penetrate the blood/brain barrier and, therefore, is not expected to induce side effects of the central nervous system.
Fourteen subjects, with allergic conjunctivitis, received one drop of ELESTAT™ ophthalmic solution in each eye twice daily for seven days. On day seven average maximum epinastine plasma concentrations of 0.04 ± 0.014 ng/ml were reached after about two hours indicating low systemic exposure. While these concentrations represented an increase over those seen following a single dose, the day 1 and day 7 Area Under the Curve (AUC) values were unchanged indicating that there is no increase in systemic absorption with multiple dosing. Epinastine is 64% bound to plasma proteins. The total systemic clearance is approximately 56 L/hr and the terminal plasma elimination half-life is about 12 hours. Epinastine is mainly excreted unchanged. About 55% of an intravenous dose is recovered unchanged in the urine with about 30% in feces. Less than 10% is metabolized. The renal elimination is mainly via active tubular secretion.
Clinical studies: Epinastine HCl 0.05% has been shown to be significantly superior to vehicle for improving ocular itching in patients with allergic conjunctivitis in clinical studies using two different models: (1) conjunctival antigen challenge (CAC) where patients were dosed and then received antigen instilled into the inferior conjunctival fornix; and (2) environmental field studies where patients were dosed and evaluated during allergy season in their natural habitat. Results demonstrated a rapid onset of action for epinastine HCl 0.05% within 3 to 5 minutes after conjunctival antigen challenge. Duration of effect was shown to be 8 hours, making a twice daily regimen suitable. This dosing regimen was shown to be safe and effective for up to 8 weeks, without evidence of tachyphylaxis.

INDICATIONS AND USAGE

ELESTAT™ ophthalmic solution is indicated for the prevention of itching associated with allergic conjunctivitis.

CONTRAINDICATIONS

ELESTAT™ ophthalmic solution is contraindicated in those patients who have shown hypersensitivity to epinastine or to any of the other ingredients.

WARNINGS

ELESTAT™ is for topical ophthalmic use only and not for injection or oral use.

PRECAUTIONS

Information for Patients: Patients should be advised not to wear a contact lens if their eye is red. ELESTAT™ ophthalmic solution should not be used to treat contact lens related irritation. The preservative in ELESTAT™, benzalkonium chloride, may be absorbed by soft contact lenses. Contact lenses should be removed prior to instillation of ELESTAT™ ophthalmic solution and may be reinserted after 10 minutes following its administration.
Patients should be instructed to avoid allowing the tip of the dispensing container to contact the eye, surrounding structures, fingers, or any other surface in order to avoid contamination of the solution by common bacteria known to cause ocular infections. Serious damage to the eye and subsequent loss of vision may result from using contaminated solutions. Bottle should be kept tightly closed when not in use.
Carcinogenesis, Mutagenesis, Impairment of Fertility: In 18-month or 2-year dietary carcinogenicity studies in mice or rats, respectively, epinastine was not carcinogenic at doses up to 40 mg/kg [approximately 30,000 times higher than the maximum recommended ocular human dose of 0.0014 mg/kg/day (MROHD) on a mg/kg basis, assuming 100% absorption in humans and animals].
Epinastine in newly synthesized batches was negative for mutagenicity in the Ames/*Salmonella* assay and *in vitro* chromosome aberration assay using human lymphocytes. Positive results were seen with early batches of epinastine in two *in vitro* chromosomal aberration studies conducted in 1980s with human peripheral lymphocytes and with V79 cells, respectively. Epinastine was negative in the *in vivo* clastogenicity studies, including the mouse micronucleus assay and chromosome aberration assay in Chinese hamsters. Epinastine was also negative in the cell transformation assay using Syrian hamster embryo cells, V79/HGPRT mammalian cell point mutation assay, and *in vivo/in vitro* unscheduled DNA synthesis assay using rat primary hepatocytes.
Epinastine had no effect on fertility of male rats. Decreased fertility in female rats was observed at an oral dose up to approximately 90,000 times the MROHD.
Pregnancy: Teratogenic Effects: Pregnancy Category C In an embryofetal developmental study in pregnant rats, maternal toxicity with no embryofetal effects was observed at an oral dose that was approximately 150,000 times the MROHD. Total resorptions and abortion were observed in an embryofetal study in pregnant rabbits at an oral dose that was approximately 55,000 times the MROHD. In both studies, no drug-induced teratogenic effects were noted.
Epinastine reduced pup body weight gain following an oral dose to pregnant rats that was approximately 90,000 times the MROHD.
There are, however, no adequate and well-controlled studies in pregnant women. Because animal reproduction studies are not always predictive of human response, ELESTAT™ ophthalmic solution should be used during pregnancy only if the potential benefit justifies the potential risk to the fetus.
Nursing Mothers: A study in lactating rats revealed excretion of epinastine in the breast milk. It is not known whether this drug is excreted in human milk. Because many drugs are excreted in human milk, caution should be exercised when ELESTAT™ ophthalmic solution is administered to a nursing woman.
Pediatric Use: Safety and effectiveness in pediatric patients below the age of 3 years have not been established.
Geriatric Use: No overall differences in safety or effectiveness have been observed between elderly and younger patients.

ADVERSE REACTIONS

The most frequently reported ocular adverse events occurring in approximately 1–10% of patients were burning sensation in the eye, folliculosis, hyperemia, and pruritus.
The most frequently reported non-ocular adverse events were infection (cold symptoms and upper respiratory infections) seen in approximately 10% of patients, and headache, rhinitis, sinusitis, increased cough, and pharyngitis seen in approximately 1–3% of patients.
Some of these events were similar to the underlying disease being studied.

DOSAGE AND ADMINISTRATION

The recommended dosage is one drop in each eye twice a day.
Treatment should be continued throughout the period of exposure (i.e., until the pollen season is over or until exposure to the offending allergen is terminated), even when symptoms are absent.

HOW SUPPLIED

ELESTAT™ (epinastine HCl ophthalmic solution) 0.05% is supplied sterile in opaque white LDPE plastic bottles with dropper tips and white high impact polystyrene (HIPS) caps as follows:
5 mL in 8 mL bottle NDC 0023-9201-05
Storage: Store at 15–25°C (59–77°F). Keep bottle tightly closed and out of the reach of children.
Rx Only October 2003

Irvine, CA 92612 U.S.A.
® and ™ Marks owned by Allergan, Inc. 9343X
Licensed from Boehringer Ingelheim Int. GmbH
71634US10M
Inspire and the Inspire logo are registered trademarks of Inspire Pharmaceuticals Inc.

LUMIGAN® ℞

(bimatoprost ophthalmic solution) 0.03%

DESCRIPTION

LUMIGAN® (bimatoprost ophthalmic solution) 0.03% is a synthetic prostamide analog with ocular hypotensive activity. Its chemical name is (Z)-7-[(1R,2R,3R,5S)-3,5-Dihydroxy-2-[1E,3S)-3-hydroxy-5-phenyl-1-pentenyl]cyclopentyl]-5-N-ethylheptenamide, and its molecular weight is

Continued on next page

Lumigan—Cont.

415.58. Its molecular formula is $C_{25}H_{37}NO_4$. Its chemical structure is:

Bimatoprost is a powder, which is very soluble in ethyl alcohol and methyl alcohol and slightly soluble in water. LUMIGAN® is a clear, isotonic, colorless, sterile ophthalmic solution with an osmolality of approximately 290 mOsmol/kg.

Each mL **contains**: **Active:** bimatoprost 0.3 mg; **Preservative:** Benzalkonium chloride 0.05 mg; **Inactives:** Sodium chloride; sodium phosphate, dibasic; citric acid; and purified water. Sodium hydroxide and/or hydrochloric acid may be added to adjust pH. The pH during its shelf life ranges from 6.8–7.8.

CLINICAL PHARMACOLOGY

Mechanism of Action

Bimatoprost is a prostamide, a synthetic structural analog of prostaglandin with ocular hypotensive activity. It selectively mimics the effects of naturally occurring substances, prostamides. Bimatoprost is believed to lower intraocular pressure (IOP) in humans by increasing outflow of aqueous humor through both the trabecular meshwork and uveoscleral routes. Elevated IOP presents a major risk factor for glaucomatous field loss. The higher the level of IOP, the greater the likelihood of optic nerve damage and visual field loss.

Pharmacokinetics

Absorption: After one drop of bimatoprost ophthalmic solution 0.03% was administered once daily to both eyes of 15 healthy subjects for two weeks, blood concentrations peaked within 10 minutes after dosing and were below the lower limit of detection (0.025 ng/mL) in most subjects within 1.5 hours after dosing. Mean C_{max} and AUC_{0-24hr} values were similar on days 7 and 14 at approximately 0.08 ng/mL and 0.09 ng•hr/mL, respectively, indicating that steady state was reached during the first week of ocular dosing. There was no significant systemic drug accumulation over time.

Distribution

Bimatoprost is moderately distributed into body tissues with a steady-state volume of distribution of 0.67 L/kg. In human blood, bimatoprost resides mainly in the plasma. Approximately 12% of bimatoprost remains unbound in human plasma.

Metabolism

Bimatoprost is the major circulating species in the blood once it reaches the systemic circulation following ocular dosing. Bimatoprost then undergoes oxidation, N-deethylation and glucuronidation to form a diverse variety of metabolites.

Elimination

Following an intravenous dose of radiolabeled bimatoprost (3.12 µg/kg) to six healthy subjects, the maximum blood concentration of unchanged drug was 12.2 ng/mL and decreased rapidly with an elimination half-life of approximately 45 minutes. The total blood clearance of bimatoprost was 1.5 L/hr/kg. Up to 67% of the administered dose was excreted in the urine while 25% of the dose was recovered in the feces.

Clinical Studies:

In clinical studies of patients with open angle glaucoma or ocular hypertension with a mean baseline IOP of 26 mm Hg, the IOP-lowering effect of LUMIGAN® (bimatoprost ophthalmic solution) 0.03% once daily (in the evening) was 7–8 mm Hg.

In patients with a history of liver disease or abnormal ALT, AST and/or bilirubin at baseline, LUMIGAN® had no adverse effect on liver function over 24 months.

INDICATIONS AND USAGE

LUMIGAN® (bimatoprost ophthalmic solution) 0.03% is indicated for the reduction of elevated intraocular pressure in patients with open angle glaucoma or ocular hypertension who are intolerant of other intraocular pressure lowering medications or insufficiently responsive (failed to achieve target IOP determined after multiple measurements over time) to another intraocular pressure lowering medication.

CONTRAINDICATIONS

LUMIGAN® (bimatoprost ophthalmic solution) 0.03% is contraindicated in patients with hypersensitivity to bimatoprost or any other ingredient in this product.

WARNINGS

LUMIGAN® (bimatoprost ophthalmic solution) 0.03% has been reported to cause changes to pigmented tissues. These reports include increased pigmentation and growth of eyelashes and increased pigmentation of the iris and periorbital tissue (eyelid). These changes may be permanent.

LUMIGAN® (bimatoprost ophthalmic solution) may gradually change eye color, increasing the amount of brown pigment in the iris by increasing the number of melanosomes (pigment granules) in melanocytes. The long-term effects on the melanocytes and the consequences of potential injury to the melanocytes and/or deposition of pigment granules to other areas of the eye are currently unknown. The change in iris color occurs slowly and may not be noticeable for several months to years. Patients should be informed of the possibility of iris color change.

Eyelid skin darkening has also been reported in association with the use of LUMIGAN®.

LUMIGAN® (bimatoprost ophthalmic solution) may gradually change eyelashes; these changes include increased length, thickness, pigmentation, and number of lashes.

Patients who are expected to receive treatment in only one eye should be informed about the potential for increased brown pigmentation of the iris, periorbital tissue, and eyelashes in the treated eye and thus, heterochromia between the eyes. They should also be advised of the potential for a disparity between the eyes in length, thickness, and/or number of eyelashes.

PRECAUTIONS

General:

There have been reports of bacterial keratitis associated with the use of multiple-dose containers of topical ophthalmic products. These containers had been inadvertently contaminated by patients who, in most cases, had a concurrent corneal disease or a disruption of the ocular epithelial surface (see Information for Patients).

Patients may slowly develop increased brown pigmentation of the iris. This change may not be noticeable for several months to years (see Warnings). Typically the brown pigmentation around the pupil is expected to spread concentrically towards the periphery in affected eyes, but the entire iris or parts of it may also become more brownish. Until more information about increased brown pigmentation is available, patients should be examined regularly and, depending on the clinical situation, treatment may be stopped if increased pigmentation ensues. The increase in brown iris pigment is not expected to progress further upon discontinuation of treatment, but the resultant color change may be permanent. Neither nevi nor freckles of the iris are expected to be affected by treatment.

LUMIGAN® (bimatoprost ophthalmic solution) 0.03% should be used with caution in patients with active intraocular inflammation (e.g., uveitis).

Macular edema, including cystoid macular edema, has been reported during treatment with bimatoprost ophthalmic solution. LUMIGAN® should be used with caution in aphakic patients, in pseudophakic patients with a torn posterior lens capsule, or in patients with known risk factors for macular edema. LUMIGAN® (bimatoprost ophthalmic solution) has not been evaluated for the treatment of angle closure, inflammatory or neovascular glaucoma.

LUMIGAN® should not be administered while wearing contact lenses.

Information for Patients:

Patients should be informed that LUMIGAN® (bimatoprost ophthalmic solution) has been reported to cause increased growth and darkening of eyelashes and darkening of the skin around the eye in some patients. These changes may be permanent.

Some patients may slowly develop darkening of the iris, which may be permanent.

When only one eye is treated, patients should be informed of the potential for a cosmetic difference between the eyes in eyelash length, darkness or thickness, and/or color changes of the eyelid skin or iris.

Patients should be instructed to avoid allowing the tip of the dispensing container to contact the eye, surrounding structures, fingers, or any other surface in order to avoid contamination of the solution by common bacteria known to cause ocular infections. Serious damage to the eye and subsequent loss of vision may result from using contaminated solutions.

Patients should also be advised that if they develop an intercurrent ocular condition (e.g., trauma or infection) or have ocular surgery, they should immediately seek their physician's advice concerning the continued use of the multidose container.

Patients should be advised that if they develop any ocular reactions, particularly conjunctivitis and eyelid reactions, they should immediately seek their physician's advice.

Contact lenses should be removed prior to instillation of LUMIGAN® and may be reinserted 15 minutes following its administration. Patients should be advised that LUMIGAN® (bimatoprost ophthalmic solution) contains benzalkonium chloride, which may be absorbed by soft contact lenses.

If more than one topical ophthalmic drug is being used, the drugs should be administered at least five (5) minutes between applications.

Carcinogenesis, Mutagenesis, Impairment of Fertility:

Carcinogenicity studies were not performed with bimatoprost.

Bimatoprost was not mutagenic or clastogenic in the Ames test, in the mouse lymphoma test, or in the *in vivo* mouse micronucleus tests.

Bimatoprost did not impair fertility in male or female rats up to doses of 0.6 mg/kg/day (approximately 103 times the recommended human exposure based on blood AUC levels).

Pregnancy: *Teratogenic Effects:* ***Pregnancy Category C.***

In embryo/fetal developmental studies in pregnant mice and rats, abortion was observed at oral doses of bimatoprost which achieved at least 33 or 97 times, respectively, the intended human exposure based on blood AUC levels.

At doses 41 times the intended human exposure based on blood AUC levels, the gestation length was reduced in the dams, the incidence of dead fetuses, late resorptions, peri- and postnatal pup mortality was increased, and pup body weights were reduced.

There are no adequate and well-controlled studies of LUMIGAN® administration in pregnant women. Because animal reproductive studies are not always predictive of human response, LUMIGAN® (bimatoprost ophthalmic solution) should be administered during pregnancy only if the potential benefit justifies the potential risk to the fetus.

Nursing Mothers:

It is not known whether LUMIGAN® is excreted in human milk, although in animal studies, bimatoprost has been shown to be excreted in breast milk. Because many drugs are excreted in human milk, caution should be exercised when LUMIGAN® (bimatoprost ophthalmic solution) is administered to a nursing woman.

Pediatric Use:

Safety and effectiveness in pediatric patients have not been established.

Geriatric Use:

No overall clinical differences in safety or effectiveness have been observed between elderly and other adult patients.

ADVERSE REACTIONS

In clinical trials, the most frequent events associated with the use of LUMIGAN® (bimatoprost ophthalmic solution) 0.03% occurring in approximately 15% to 45% of patients, in descending order of incidence, included conjunctival hyperemia, growth of eyelashes, and ocular pruritus. Approximately 3% of patients discontinued therapy due to conjunctival hyperemia.

Ocular adverse events occurring in approximately 3 to 10% of patients, in descending order of incidence, included ocular dryness, visual disturbance, ocular burning, foreign body sensation, eye pain, pigmentation of the periocular skin, blepharitis, cataract, superficial punctate keratitis, eyelid erythema, ocular irritation, and eyelash darkening. The following ocular adverse events reported in approximately 1 to 3% of patients, in descending order of incidence, included: eye discharge, tearing, photophobia, allergic conjunctivitis, asthenopia, increases in iris pigmentation, and conjunctival edema. In less than 1% of patients, intraocular inflammation was reported as iritis.

Systemic adverse events reported in approximately 10% of patients were infections (primarily colds and upper respiratory tract infections). The following systemic adverse events reported in approximately 1 to 5% of patients, in descending order of incidence, included headaches, abnormal liver function tests, asthenia and hirsutism.

OVERDOSAGE

No information is available on overdosage in humans. If overdose with LUMIGAN® (bimatoprost ophthalmic solution) 0.03% occurs, treatment should be symptomatic.

In oral (by gavage) mouse and rat studies, doses up to 100 mg/kg/day did not produce any toxicity. This dose expressed as mg/m^2 is at least 70 times higher than the accidental dose of one bottle of LUMIGAN® for a 10 kg child.

DOSAGE AND ADMINISTRATION

The recommended dosage is one drop in the affected eye(s) once daily in the evening. The dosage of LUMIGAN® (bimatoprost ophthalmic solution) 0.03% should not exceed once daily since it has been shown that more frequent administration may decrease the intraocular pressure lowering effect.

Reduction of the intraocular pressure starts approximately 4 hours after the first administration with maximum effect reached within approximately 8 to 12 hours.

LUMIGAN® may be used concomitantly with other topical ophthalmic drug products to lower intraocular pressure. If more than one topical ophthalmic drug is being used, the drugs should be administered at least five (5) minutes apart.

HOW SUPPLIED

LUMIGAN® (bimatoprost ophthalmic solution) 0.03% is supplied sterile in opaque white low density polyethylene ophthalmic dispenser bottles and tips with turquoise polystyrene caps in the following sizes: 2.5 mL fill in 5 mL container — NDC 0023-9187-03; 5 mL fill in 8 mL container — NDC 0023-9187-05; or 7.5 mL fill in 8 mL container — NDC 0023-9187-07.

℞ only

Storage: LUMIGAN® should be stored in the original container at 2° to 25°C (36° to 77°F).

ALLERGAN

® Marks owned by Allergan, Inc.

US Pat. 5,688,819 and 6,403,649

July 2003

Shown in Product Identification Guide, page 304

RESTASIS® ℞

[*rĕ´stā-sĭs*]

(cyclosporine ophthalmic emulsion) 0.05%

Sterile, Preservative-Free

DESCRIPTION

RESTASIS® (cyclosporine ophthalmic emulsion) 0.05% contains a topical immunomodulator with anti-inflammatory effects. Cyclosporine's chemical name is Cyclo[[(E)-(2S,3R,4R)-3-hydroxy-4-methyl-2-(methylamino)-6-octenoyl]-L-2-aminobutyryl-N-methylglycyl-N-methyl-L-leucyl-L-valyl-N-methyl-L-leucyl-L-alanyl-D-alanyl-N-methyl-L-leucyl-N-methyl-L-leucyl-N-methyl-L-valyl] and it has the following structure:

Cyclosporine is a fine white powder. RESTASIS® appears as a white opaque to slightly translucent homogeneous emulsion. It has an osmolality of 230 to 320 mOsmol/kg and a pH of 6.5-8.0.

Each mL of RESTASIS® ophthalmic emulsion contains: **Active:** cyclosporine 0.05%. **Inactives:** glycerin; castor oil; polysorbate 80; carbomer 1342; purified water and sodium hydroxide to adjust the pH.

CLINICAL PHARMACOLOGY

Mechanism of action:

Cyclosporine is an immunosuppressive agent when administered systemically.

In patients whose tear production is presumed to be suppressed due to ocular inflammation associated with keratoconjunctivitis sicca, cyclosporine emulsion is thought to act as a partial immunomodulator. The exact mechanism of action is not known.

Pharmacokinetics:

Blood cyclosporin A concentrations were measured using a specific high pressure liquid chromatography-mass spectrometry assay.

Blood concentrations of cyclosporine, in all the samples collected, after topical administration of RESTASIS® 0.05%, BID, in humans for up to 12 months, were below the quantitation limit of 0.1 ng/mL. There was no detectable drug accumulation in blood during 12 months of treatment with RESTASIS® ophthalmic emulsion.

Clinical Evaluations:

Four multicenter, randomized, adequate and well-controlled clinical studies were performed in approximately 1200 patients with moderate to severe keratoconjunctivitis sicca. RESTASIS® demonstrated statistically significant increases in Schirmer wetting of 10 mm versus vehicle at six months in patients whose tear production was presumed to be suppressed due to ocular inflammation. This effect was seen in approximately 15% of RESTASIS® ophthalmic emulsion treated patients versus approximately 5% of vehicle treated patients.

Increased tear production was not seen in patients currently taking topical anti-inflammatory drugs or using punctal plugs. No increase in bacterial or fungal ocular infections was reported following administration of RESTASIS®.

INDICATIONS AND USAGE

RESTASIS® ophthalmic emulsion is indicated to increase tear production in patients whose tear production is presumed to be suppressed due to ocular inflammation associated with keratoconjunctivitis sicca. Increased tear production was not seen in patients currently taking topical anti-inflammatory drugs or using punctal plugs.

CONTRAINDICATIONS

RESTASIS® is contraindicated in patients with active ocular infections and in patients with known or suspected hypersensitivity to any of the ingredients in the formulation.

WARNING

RESTASIS® ophthalmic emulsion has not been studied in patients with a history of herpes keratitis.

PRECAUTIONS

General: For ophthalmic use only.

Information for Patients:

The emulsion from one individual single-use vial is to be used immediately after opening for administration to one or both eyes, and the remaining contents should be discarded immediately after administration.

Do not allow the tip of the vial to touch the eye or any surface, as this may contaminate the emulsion.

RESTASIS® should not be administered while wearing contact lenses. Patients with decreased tear production typically should not wear contact lenses. If contact lenses are worn, they should be removed prior to the administration of the emulsion. Lenses may be reinserted 15 minutes following administration of RESTASIS® ophthalmic emulsion.

Carcinogenesis, Mutagenesis, and Impairment of Fertility:

Systemic carcinogenicity studies were carried out in male and female mice and rats. In the 78-week oral (diet) mouse study, at doses of 1, 4, and 16 mg/kg/day, evidence of a statistically significant trend was found for lymphocytic lymphomas in females, and the incidence of hepatocellular carcinomas in mid-dose males significantly exceeded the control value.

In the 24-month oral (diet) rat study, conducted at 0.5, 2, and 8 mg/kg/day, pancreatic islet cell adenomas significantly exceeded the control rate in the low dose level. The hepatocellular carcinomas and pancreatic islet cell adenomas were not dose related. The low doses in mice and rats are approximately 1000 and 500 times greater, respectively, than the daily human dose of one drop (28 µL) of 0.05% RESTASIS® BID into each eye of a 60 kg person (0.001 mg/kg/day), assuming that the entire dose is absorbed.

Cyclosporine has not been found mutagenic/genotoxic in the Ames Test, the V79-HGPRT Test, the micronucleus test in mice and Chinese hamsters, the chromosome-aberration tests in Chinese hamster bone-marrow, the mouse dominant lethal assay, and the DNA-repair test in sperm from treated mice. A study analyzing sister chromatid exchange (SCE) induction by cyclosporine using human lymphocytes in vitro gave indication of a positive effect (i.e., induction of SCE).

No impairment in fertility was demonstrated in studies in male and female rats receiving oral doses of cyclosporine up to 15 mg/kg/day (approximately 15,000 times the human daily dose of 0.001 mg/kg/day) for 9 weeks (male) and 2 weeks (female) prior to mating.

Pregnancy-Teratogenic effects:

Pregnancy category C.

Teratogenic effects: No evidence of teratogenicity was observed in rats or rabbits receiving oral doses of cyclosporine up to 300 mg/kg/day during organogenesis. These doses in rats and rabbits are aproximately 300,000 times greater than the daily human dose of one drop (28 µL) 0.05% RESTASIS® BID into each eye of a 60 kg person (0.001mg/kg/day), assuming that the entire dose is absorbed.

Non-Teratogenic effects: Adverse effects were seen in reproduction studies in rats and rabbits only at dose levels toxic to dams. At toxic doses (rats at 30 mg/kg/day and rabbits at 100 mg/kg/day), cyclosporine oral solution, USP, was embryo- and fetotoxic as indicated by increased pre- and postnatal mortality and reduced fetal weight together with related skeletal retardations. These doses are 30,000 and 100,000 times greater, respectively than the daily human dose of one-drop (28 µL) of 0.05% RESTASIS® BID into each eye of a 60 kg person (0.001 mg/kg/day), assuming that the entire dose is absorbed. No evidence of embryofetal toxicity was observed in rats or rabbits receiving cyclosporine at oral doses up to 17 mg/kg/day or 30 mg/kg/day, respectively, during organogenesis. These doses in rats and rabbits are approximately 17,000 and 30,000 times greater, respectively, than the daily human dose.

Offspring of rats receiving a 45 mg/kg/day oral dose of cyclosporine from Day 15 of pregnancy until Day 21 post partum, a maternally toxic level, exhibited an increase in postnatal mortality; this dose is 45,000 times greater than the daily human topical dose, 0.001 mg/kg/day, assuming that the entire dose is absorbed. No adverse events were observed at oral doses up to 15 mg/kg/day (15,000 times greater than the daily human dose).

There are no adequate and well-controlled studies of RESTASIS® in pregnant women. RESTASIS® should be administered to a pregnant woman only if clearly needed.

Nursing Mothers:

Cyclosporine is known to be excreted in human milk following systemic administration but excretion in human milk after topical treatment has not been investigated. Although blood concentrations are undetectable after topical administration of RESTASIS® ophthalmic emulsion, caution should be exercised when RESTASIS® is administered to a nursing woman.

Pediatric Use:

The safety and efficacy of RESTASIS® ophthalmic emulsion have not been established in pediatric patients below the age of 16.

Geriatric Use:

No overall difference in safety or effectiveness has been observed between elderly and younger patients.

ADVERSE REACTIONS

The most common adverse event following the use of RESTASIS® was ocular burning (17%).

Other events reported in 1% to 5% of patients included conjunctival hyperemia, discharge, epiphora, eye pain, foreign body sensation, pruritus, stinging, and visual disturbance (most often blurring).

DOSAGE AND ADMINISTRATION

Invert the unit dose vial a few times to obtain a uniform, white, opaque emulsion before using. Instill one drop of RESTASIS® ophthalmic emulsion twice a day in each eye approximately 12 hours apart. RESTASIS® can be used concomitantly with artificial tears, allowing a 15 minute interval between products. Discard vial immediately after use.

HOW SUPPLIED

RESTASIS® ophthalmic emulsion is packaged in single use vials. Each vial contains 0.4 mL fill in a 0.9 mL LDPE vial; 32 vials are packaged in a polypropylene tray with an aluminum peelable lid.

RESTASIS® 32 Vials 0.4 mL each - NDC 0023-9163-32

Storage: Store RESTASIS® ophthalmic emulsion at 15° to 25° C (59°-77° F).

KEEP OUT OF THE REACH OF CHILDREN.

Rx Only

U.S. Pat. 4,649,047; 4,839,342; 5,474,979.

INSPIRE PHARMACEUTICALS, INC.

Inspire and the Inspire logo are registered trademarks of Inspire Pharmaceuticals, Inc.

Shown in Product Identification Guide, page 304

POLYTRIM® ℞

(trimethoprim sulfate and polymyxin b sulfate ophthalmic solution) Sterile

DESCRIPTION

POLYTRIM® (trimethoprim sulfate and polymyxin B sulfate ophthalmic solution) is a sterile antimicrobial solution for topical ophthalmic use. It has pH of 4.0 to 6.2 and osmolality of 270 to 310 mOsm/kg.

Chemical Names: Trimethoprim sulfate, 2,4-Diamino-5-(3,4,5-trimethoxybenzyl)pyrimidine sulfate is a white, odorless, crystalline powder with a molecular weight of 678.72.

Polymyxin B sulfate is the sulfate salt of polymyxin B_1 and B_2 which are produced by the growth of *Bacillus polymyxa* (Prazmowski) Migula (Fam. Bacillaceae). It has a potency of not less than 6,000 polymyxin B units per mg, calculated on an anhydrous basis.

Contains: Actives: trimethoprim sulfate equivalent to 1 mg/mL; polymyxin B sulfate 10,000 units/mL. Preservative: benzalkonium chloride 0.04 mg/mL. Inactives: sodium chloride; sulfuric acid and purified water. May also contain sodium hydroxide for pH adjustment.

CLINICAL PHARMACOLOGY

Trimethoprim is a synthetic antibacterial drug active against a wide variety of aerobic gram-positive and gram-negative ophthalmic pathogens. Trimethoprim blocks the production of tetrahydrofolic acid from dihydrofolic acid by binding to and reversibly inhibiting the enzyme dihydrofolate reductase. This binding is stronger for the bacterial enzyme than for the corresponding mammalian enzyme and therefore selectively interferes with bacterial biosynthesis of nucleic acids and proteins.

Polymyxin B, a cyclic lipopeptide antibiotic, is bactericidal for a variety of gram-negative organisms, especially *Pseudomonas aeruginosa*. It increases the permeability of the bacterial cell membrane by interacting with the phospholipid components of the membrane.

Blood samples were obtained from 11 human volunteers at 20 minutes, 1 hour and 3 hours following instillation in the eye of 2 drops of ophthalmic solution containing 1 mg trimethoprim and 10,000 units polymyxin B per mL. Peak serum concentrations were approximately 0.03 µg/mL trimethoprim and 1 unit/mL polymyxin B.

Microbiology: *In vitro* studies have demonstrated that the anti-infective components of POLYTRIM® are active against the following bacterial pathogens that are capable of causing external infections of the eye:

Trimethoprim: *Staphylococcus aureus* and *Staphylococcus epidermidis, Streptococcus pyogenes, Streptococcus faecalis, Streptococcus pneumoniae, Haemophilus influenzae, Haemophilus aegyptius, Escherichia coli, Klebsiella pneumoniae, Proteus mirabilis* (indole-negative), *Proteus vulgaris* (indole-positive), *Enterobacter aerogenes*, and *Serratia marcescens*.

Polymyxin B: *Pseudomonas aeruginosa, Escherichia coli, Klebsiella pneumoniae, Enterobacter aerogenes* and *Haemophilus influenzae*.

INDICATIONS AND USAGE

POLYTRIM® Ophthalmic Solution is indicated in the treatment of surface ocular bacterial infections, including acute bacterial conjunctivitis, and blepharoconjunctivitis, caused by susceptible strains of the following microorganisms: *Staphylococcus aureus, Staphylococcus epidermidis, Streptococcus pneumoniae, Streptococcus viridans, Haemophilus influenzae* and *Pseudomonas aeruginosa.**

*Efficacy for this organism in this organ system was studied in fewer than 10 infections.

CONTRAINDICATIONS

POLYTRIM® Ophthalmic Solution is contraindicated in patients with known hypersensitivity to any of its components.

WARNINGS

NOT FOR INJECTION INTO THE EYE. If a sensitivity reaction to POLYTRIM® occurs, discontinue use. POLYTRIM® Ophthalmic Solution is not indicated for the prophylaxis or treatment of ophthalmia neonatorum.

PRECAUTIONS

General: As with other antimicrobial preparations, prolonged use may result in overgrowth of nonsusceptible organisms, including fungi. If superinfection occurs, appropriate therapy should be initiated.

Information for Patients: Avoid contaminating the applicator tip with material from the eye, fingers, or other source. This precaution is necessary if the sterility of the drops is to be maintained.

If redness, irritation, swelling or pain persists or increases, discontinue use immediately and contact your physician. Patients should be advised not to wear contact lenses if they have signs and symptoms of ocular bacterial infections.

Continued on next page

Polytrim—Cont.

Carcinogenesis, Mutagenesis, Impairment of Fertility:
Carcinogenesis: Long-term studies in animals to evaluate carcinogenic potential have not been conducted with polymyxin B sulfate or trimethoprim.
Mutagenesis: Trimethoprim was demonstrated to be non-mutagenic in the Ames assay. In studies at two laboratories no chromosomal damage was detected in cultured Chinese hamster ovary cells at concentrations approximately 500 times human plasma levels after oral administration; at concentrations approximately 1000 times human plasma levels after oral administration in these same cells, a low level of chromosomal damage was induced at one of the laboratories. Studies to evaluate mutagenic potential have not been conducted with polymyxin B sulfate.
Impairment of Fertility: Polymyxin B sulfate has been reported to impair the motility of equine sperm, but its effects on male or female fertility are unknown.
No adverse effects on fertility or general reproductive performance were observed in rats given trimethoprim in oral dosages as high as 70 mg/kg/day for males and 14 mg/kg/day for females.
Pregnancy: ***Teratogenic Effects:*** Pregnancy Category C. Animal reproduction studies have not been conducted with polymyxin B sulfate. It is not known whether polymyxin B sulfate can cause fetal harm when administered to a pregnant woman or can affect reproduction capacity.
Trimethoprim has been shown to be teratogenic in the rat when given in oral doses 40 times the human dose. In some rabbit studies, the overall increase in fetal loss (dead and resorbed and malformed conceptuses) was associated with oral doses 6 times the human therapeutic dose.
While there are no large well-controlled studies on the use of trimethoprim in pregnant women, Brumfitt and Pursell, in a retrospective study, reported the outcome of 186 pregnancies during which the mother received either placebo or oral trimethoprim in combination with sulfamethoxazole. The incidence of congenital abnormalities was 4.5% (3 of 66) in those who received placebo and 3.3% (4 of 120) in those receiving trimethoprim and sulfamethoxazole. There were no abnormalities in the 10 children whose mothers received the drug during the first trimester. In a separate survey, Brumfitt and Pursell also found no congenital abnormalities in 35 children whose mothers had received oral trimethoprim and sulfamethoxazole at the time of conception or shortly thereafter.
Because trimethoprim may interfere with folic acid metabolism, trimethoprim should be used during pregnancy only if the potential benefit justifies the potential risk to the fetus.
Nonteratogenic Effects: The oral administration of trimethoprim to rats at a dose of 70 mg/kg/day commencing with the last third of gestation and continuing through parturition and lactation caused no deleterious effects on gestation or pup growth and survival.
Nursing mothers: It is not known whether this drug is excreted in human milk. Because many drugs are excreted in human milk, caution should be exercised when POLYTRIM® Ophthalmic Solution is administered to a nursing woman.
Pediatric Use: Safety and effectiveness in children below the age of 2 months have not been established (see WARNINGS).
Geriatric Use: No overall differences in safety or effectiveness have been observed between elderly and other adult patients.

ADVERSE REACTIONS

The most frequent adverse reaction to POLYTRIM® Ophthalmic Solution is local irritation consisting of increased redness, burning, stinging, and/or itching. This may occur on instillation, within 48 hours, or at any time with extended use. There are also multiple reports of hypersensitivity reactions consisting of lid edema, itching, increased redness, tearing, and/or circumocular rash. Photosensitivity has been reported in patients taking oral trimethoprim.

DOSAGE AND ADMINISTRATION

In mild to moderate infections, instill one drop in the affected eye(s) every three hours (maximum of 6 doses per day) for a period of 7 to 10 days.

HOW SUPPLIED

Polytrim® (trimethoprim sulfate and polymyxin B sulfate ophthalmic solution) is supplied sterile in opaque white low density polyethylene ophthalmic dispenser bottles and tips with white high impact polystyrene (HIPS) caps as follows: 10 mL in 10 mL bottle—NDC 0023-7824-10).
Note: Store at 15°–25°C (59°–77°F) and protect from light.
℞ only

Irvine, CA 92612

ZYMAR™ ℞

[zī-mar]
(gatifloxacin ophthalmic solution) 0.3%
Sterile

DESCRIPTION

ZYMAR™ (gatifloxacin ophthalmic solution) 0.3% is a sterile ophthalmic solution. It is an 8-methoxy fluoroquinolone anti-infective for topical ophthalmic use.

Structure and Empirical Formula:

$C_{19}H_{22}FN_3O_4 \cdot 1.5\ H_2O$ Mol Wt 402.42

Chemical Name: (±)-1-cyclopropyl-6-fluoro-1,4-dihydro-8-methoxy-7-(3-methyl-1-piperazinyl)-4-oxo-3-quinolinecarboxylic acid sesquihydrate
Contains: Active: gatifloxacin 0.3% (3 mg/mL).
Preservative: benzalkonium chloride 0.005%.
Inactives: edetate disodium; purified water and sodium chloride. May contain hydrochloric acid and/or sodium hydroxide to adjust pH to approximately 6.
ZYMAR™ is a sterile, clear, pale yellow colored isotonic unbuffered solution. It has an osmolality of 260-330 mOsm/kg.

CLINICAL PHARMACOLOGY

Pharmacokinetics: Gatifloxacin ophthalmic solution 0.3% or 0.5% was administered to one eye of 6 healthy male subjects each in an escalated dosing regimen starting with a single 2 drop dose, then 2 drops 4 times daily for 7 days and finally 2 drops 8 times daily for 3 days.
At all time points, serum gatifloxacin levels were below the lower limit of quantification (5 ng/mL) in all subjects.
Microbiology: Gatifloxacin is an 8-methoxy fluoroquinolone with a 3-methylpiperazinyl substituent at C7. The antibacterial action of gatifloxacin results from inhibition of DNA gyrase and topoisomerase IV. DNA gyrase is an essential enzyme that is involved in the replication, transcription and repair of bacterial DNA. Topoisomerase IV is an enzyme known to play a key role in the partitioning of the chromosomal DNA during bacterial cell division.
The mechanism of action of fluoroquinolones including gatifloxacin is different from that of aminoglycoside, macrolide, and tetracycline antibiotics. Therefore, gatifloxacin may be active against pathogens that are resistant to these antibiotics and these antibiotics may be active against pathogens that are resistant to gatifloxacin. There is no cross-resistance between gatifloxacin and the aforementioned classes of antibiotics. Cross resistance has been observed between systemic gatifloxacin and some other fluoroquinolones.
Resistance to gatifloxacin *in vitro* develops via multiple step mutations. Resistance to gatifloxacin *in vitro* occurs at a general frequency of between 1×10^{-7} to 10^{-10}.
Gatifloxacin has been shown to be active against most strains of the following organisms both *in vitro* and clinically, in conjunctival infections as described in the INDICATIONS AND USAGE section.
Aerobes, Gram-Positive:
*Corynebacterium propinquum**
Staphylococcus aureus
Staphylococcus epidermidis
*Streptococcus mitis**
Streptococcus pneumoniae
Aerobes, Gram-Negative:
Haemophilus influenzae

* Efficacy for this organism was studied in fewer than 10 infections.

The following *in vitro* data are available, **but their clinical significance in ophthalmic infections is unknown.** The safety and effectiveness of ZYMAR™ in treating ophthalmic infections due to the following organisms have not been established in adequate and well-controlled clinical trials.
The following organisms are considered susceptible when evaluated using systemic breakpoints. However, a correlation between the *in vitro* systemic breakpoint and ophthalmological efficacy has not been established. The following list of organisms is provided as guidance only in assessing the potential treatment of conjunctival infections.
Gatifloxacin exhibits *in vitro* minimal inhibitory concentrations (MICs) of 2µg/mL or less (systemic susceptible breakpoint) against most (≥ 90%) strains of the following ocular pathogens.
Aerobes, Gram-Positive:
Listeria monocytogenes
Staphylococcus saprophyticus
Streptococcus agalactiae
Streptococcus pyogenes
Streptococcus viridans Group
Streptococcus Groups C, F, G
Aerobes, Gram-Negative:
Acinetobacter lwoffii
Enterobacter aerogenes
Enterobacter cloacae
Escherichia coli
Citrobacter freundii
Citrobacter koseri
Haemophilus parainfluenzae
Klebsiella oxytoca
Klebsiella pneumoniae
Moraxella catarrhalis
Morganella morganii
Neisseria gonorrhoeae
Neisseria meningitidis
Proteus mirabilis
Proteus vulgaris
Serratia marcescens
Vibrio cholerae
Yersinia enterocolitica
Other Microorganisms:
Chlamydia pneumoniae
Legionella pneumophila
Mycobacterium marinum
Mycobacterium fortuitum
Mycoplasma pneumoniae
Anaerobic Microorganisms:
Bacteroides fragilis
Clostridium perfringens

Clinical Studies:

In a randomized, double-masked, multicenter clinical trial, where patients were dosed for 5 days, ZYMAR™ solution was superior to its vehicle on day 5-7 in patients with conjunctivitis and positive conjunctival cultures. Clinical outcomes for the trial demonstrated clinical cure of 77% (40/52) for the gatifloxacin treated group versus 58% (28/48) for the placebo treated group. Microbiological outcomes for the same clinical trial demonstrated a statistically superior eradication rate for causative pathogens of 92% (48/52) for gatifloxacin vs. 72% (34/48) for placebo. Please note that microbiologic eradication does not always correlate with clinical outcome in anti-infective trials.

INDICATIONS AND USAGE

ZYMAR™ solution is indicated for the treatment of bacterial conjunctivitis caused by susceptible strains of the following organisms:
Aerobic Gram-Positive Bacteria:
*Corynebacterium propinquum**
Staphylococcus aureus
Staphylococcus epidermidis
*Streptococcus mitis**
Streptococcus pneumoniae
Aerobic Gram-Negative Bacteria:
Haemophilus influenzae

* Efficacy for this organism was studied in fewer than 10 infections.

CONTRAINDICATIONS

ZYMAR™ solution is contraindicated in patients with a history of hypersensitivity to gatifloxacin, to other quinolones, or to any of the components in this medication.

WARNINGS

NOT FOR INJECTION.
ZYMAR™ solution should not be injected subconjunctivally, nor should it be introduced directly into the anterior chamber of the eye.
In patients receiving systemic quinolones, including gatifloxacin, serious and occasionally fatal hypersensitivity (anaphylactic) reactions, some following the first dose, have been reported. Some reactions were accompanied by cardiovascular collapse, loss of consciousness, angioedema (including laryngeal, pharyngeal or facial edema), airway obstruction, dyspnea, urticaria, and itching. If an allergic reaction to gatifloxacin occurs, discontinue the drug. Serious acute hypersensitivity reactions may require immediate emergency treatment. Oxygen and airway management should be administered as clinically indicated.

PRECAUTIONS

General: As with other anti-infectives, prolonged use may result in overgrowth of nonsusceptible organisms, including fungi. If superinfection occurs discontinue use and institute alternative therapy. Whenever clinical judgment dictates, the patient should be examined with the aid of magnification, such as slit lamp biomicroscopy and, where appropriate, fluorescein staining.
Patients should be advised not to wear contact lenses if they have signs and symptoms of bacterial conjunctivitis.
Information for Patients: Avoid contaminating the applicator tip with material from the eye, fingers or other source. Systemic quinolones, including gatifloxacin, have been associated with hypersensitivity reactions, even following a single dose. Discontinue use immediately and contact your physician at the first sign of a rash or allergic reaction.
Drug Interactions: Specific drug interaction studies have not been conducted with ZYMAR™ ophthalmic solution. However, the systemic administration of some quinolones has been shown to elevate plasma concentrations of theophylline, interfere with the metabolism of caffeine, and enhance the effects of the oral anticoagulant warfarin and its derivatives, and has been associated with transient elevations in serum creatinine in patients receiving systemic cyclosporine concomitantly.
Carcinogenesis, Mutagenesis, Impairment of Fertility
There was no increase in neoplasms among B6C3F1 mice given gatifloxacin in the diet for 18 months at doses averaging 81 mg/kg/day in males and 90 mg/kg/day in females. These doses are approximately 2000-fold higher than the maximum recommended ophthalmic dose of 0.04 mg/kg/day in a 50 kg human.
There was no increase in neoplasms among Fischer 344 rats given gatifloxacin in the diet for 2 years at doses averaging 47 mg/kg/day in males and 139 mg/kg/day in females (1000 and 3000-fold higher, respectively, than the maximum recommended ophthalmic dose). A statistically significant increase in the incidence of large granular lymphocyte (LGL) leukemia was seen in males treated with a high dose of approximately 2000-fold higher than the maximum recom-

mended ophthalmic dose. Fischer 344 rats have a high spontaneous background rate of LGL leukemia and the incidence in high-dose males only slightly exceeded the historical control range established for this strain.
In genetic toxicity tests, gatifloxacin was positive in 1 of 5 strains used in bacterial reverse mutation assays; Salmonella strain TA102. Gatifloxacin was positive in *in vitro* mammalian cell mutation and chromosome aberration assays. Gatifloxacin was positive in *in vitro* unscheduled DNA synthesis in rat hepatocytes but not human leukocytes. Gatifloxacin was negative in *in vivo* micronucleus tests in mice, cytogenetics test in rats, and DNA repair test in rats. The findings may be due to the inhibitory effects of high concentrations on eukaryotic type II DNA topoisomerase.
There were no adverse effects on fertility or reproduction in rats given gatifloxacin orally at doses up to 200 mg/kg/day (approximately 4500-fold higher than the maximum recommended ophthalmic dose for ZYMAR™).
Pregnancy: Teratogenic Effects. Pregnancy Category C: There were no teratogenic effects observed in rats or rabbits following oral gatifloxacin doses up to 50 mg/kg/day (approximately 1000-fold higher than the maximum recommended ophthalmic dose). However, skeletal/craniofacial malformations or delayed ossification, atrial enlargement, and reduced fetal weight were observed in fetuses from rats given ≥150 mg/kg/day (approximately 3000-fold higher than the maximum recommended ophthalmic dose). In a perinatal/postnatal study, increased late post-implantation loss and neonatal/perinatal mortalities were observed at 200 mg/kg/day (approximately 4500 times the maximum recommended ophthalmic dose).
Because there are no adequate and well-controlled studies in pregnant women, ZYMAR™ solution should be used during pregnancy only if the potential benefit justifies the potential risk to the fetus.
Nursing Mothers: Gatifloxacin is excreted in the breast milk of rats. It is not known whether this drug is excreted in human milk. Because many drugs are excreted in human milk, caution should be exercised when gatifloxacin is administered to a nursing woman.
Pediatric Use: Safety and effectiveness in infants below the age of one year have not been established.
Geriatric use: No overall differences in safety or effectiveness have been observed between elderly and younger patients.

ADVERSE REACTIONS
Ophthalmic Use: The most frequently reported adverse events in the overall study population were conjunctival irritation, increased lacrimation, keratitis, and papillary conjunctivitis. These events occurred in approximately 5-10% of patients. Other reported reactions occurring in 1-4% of patients were chemosis, conjunctival hemorrhage, dry eye, eye discharge, eye irritation, eye pain, eyelid edema, headache, red eye, reduced visual acuity and taste disturbance.

DOSAGE AND ADMINISTRATION
The recommended dosage regimen for the treatment of bacterial conjunctivitis is:
Days 1 and 2: Instill one drop every two hours in the affected eye(s) while awake, up to 8 times daily.
Days 3 through 7: Instill one drop up to four times daily while awake.

HOW SUPPLIED
ZYMAR™ (gatifloxacin ophthalmic solution) 0.3% is supplied sterile in a white, low density polyethylene (LDPE) bottle with a controlled dropper tip and a tan, high impact polystyrene (HIPS) cap in the following sizes:
5 mL in an 8 mL bottle-NDC 0023-9218-05
Note: Store at 15°–25°C (59°–77°F). Protect from freezing.

ANIMAL PHARMACOLOGY
Quinolone antibacterials have been shown to cause bone or cartilage changes in immature animals. There was no evidence of bone cartilage changes following ocular administration of gatifloxacin in rabbits or dogs.
Rx only
October 2003

Licensed from: Kyorin Pharmaceuticals Co., Ltd.
U.S. PAT. 4,980,470; 5,880,283
9415X 71706US11M
Shown in Product Identification Guide, page 304

NOTICE
Before prescribing or administering any product described in PHYSICIANS' DESK REFERENCE check the **PDR Supplements** for revised information.

Alpha Therapeutic Corporation

Please see Grifols Biologicals Inc. for further product information

Alpharma Branded Products Division

ONE NEW ENGLAND AVENUE
PISCATAWAY, NJ 08854

Direct Inquiries to:
Medical Affairs
(877) 4 - KADIAN

KADIAN® Ⓒ℞
Morphine Sulfate Sustained Release Capsules
KADIAN® 20 mg Capsules
KADIAN® 30 mg Capsules
KADIAN® 50 mg Capsules
KADIAN® 60 mg Capsules
KADIAN® 100 mg Capsules

DESCRIPTION
KADIAN® capsules 20, 30, 50, 60 and 100 mg contain identical polymer coated sustained release pellets of morphine sulfate for oral administration.
Chemically, morphine sulfate is 7,8-didehydro-4,5 α- epoxy-17-methyl-morphinan-3,6 α- diol sulfate (2:1) (salt) pentahydrate and has the following structural formula:

$\cdot H_2SO_4 \cdot 5H_2O$

Morphine sulfate is an odorless, white, crystalline powder with a bitter taste and a molecular weight of 758 (as the sulfate). It has a solubility of 1 in 21 parts of water and 1 in 1000 parts of alcohol, but is practically insoluble in chloroform or ether. The octanol: water partition coefficient of morphine is 1.42 at physiologic pH and the pK_b is 7.9 for the tertiary nitrogen (mostly ionized at pH 7.4).
Each KADIAN® sustained release capsule contains either 20, 30, 50, 60, or 100 mg of Morphine Sulfate USP and the following inactive ingredients common to all strengths: hypromellose, ethylcellulose, methacrylic acid copolymer, polyethylene glycol, diethyl phthalate, talc, corn starch, and sucrose. The 20 mg capsule shell contains gelatin, silicon dioxide, sodium lauryl sulfate, D&C yellow #10, titanium dioxide, and black ink SW-9009. The 30 mg capsule shell contains gelatin, silicon dioxide, sodium lauryl sulfate, FD&C red #3, FD&C blue #1, titanium dioxide and black ink S-1-8114 or S-1-8115. The 50 mg capsule shell contains gelatin, silicon dioxide, sodium lauryl sulfate, D&C red #28, FD&C red #40, FD&C blue #1, titanium dioxide, and black ink SW-9009. The 60 mg capsule shell contains gelatin, silicon dioxide, sodium lauryl sulfate, D&C red #28, FD&C red #40, FD&C blue #1, titanium dioxide and black ink S-1-8114 or S-1-8115. The 100 mg capsule shell contains gelatin, silicon dioxide, sodium lauryl sulfate, D&C yellow #10, FD&C blue #1, titanium dioxide, and black ink SW-9009.

CLINICAL PHARMACOLOGY
Morphine is a natural product that is the prototype for the class of natural and synthetic opioid analgesics. Opioids produce a wide spectrum of pharmacologic effects including analgesia, dysphoria, euphoria, somnolence, respiratory depression, diminished gastrointestinal motility, altered circulatory dynamics, histamine release and physical dependence.
Morphine produces both its therapeutic and its adverse effects by interaction with one or more classes of specific opioid receptors located throughout the body. Morphine acts as a pure agonist, binding with and activating opioid receptors at sites in the peri-aqueductal and peri-ventricular grey matter, the ventro-medial medulla and the spinal cord to produce analgesia.
Effects on the Central Nervous System
The principal therapeutic actions of morphine are analgesia, sedation and alterations of mood. Opioids of this class do not usually eliminate pain, but they do reduce the perception of pain by the central nervous system.
Morphine produces respiratory depression by reducing the responsiveness of the brain stem respiratory centers to increases in carbon dioxide tension (or to direct electrical stimulation).
Morphine depresses the cough reflex by direct effect on the cough center in the medulla. Antitussive effects may occur with doses lower than those usually required for analgesia. Morphine causes miosis, even in total darkness, and little tolerance develops to this effect. Pinpoint pupils are a sign of opioid overdose but are not pathognomonic (e.g. pontine lesions of hemorrhagic or ischemic origins may produce similar findings). Marked mydriasis rather than miosis may be seen due to severe hypoxia in overdose situations.
Effects on the Gastrointestinal Tract
Gastric, biliary and pancreatic secretions are decreased by morphine. Morphine causes a reduction in motility associated with an increase in tone in the antrum of the stomach and duodenum. Digestion of food in the small intestine is delayed and propulsive contractions are decreased. Propulsive peristaltic waves in the colon are decreased, while tone is increased to the point of spasm. The end result is constipation. Morphine can cause a marked increase in biliary tract pressure as a result of spasm of the sphincter of Oddi.
Effects on the Cardiovascular System
Morphine produces peripheral vasodilation which may result in orthostatic hypotension or syncope. Release of histamine may be induced by morphine and can contribute to opioid-induced hypotension. Manifestations of histamine release and/or peripheral vasodilation may include pruritus, flushing, red eyes and sweating.
Pharmacodynamics
The relationship between the blood level of morphine and the analgesic response will depend on the patient's age, state of health, medical condition, and the extent of previous opioid treatment.
A minimum effective concentration (MEC) of morphine for pain relief has been reported as 27.2 ± 14.5 ng/mL (mean ± SD) in cancer patients treated with morphine solution. These results compare with the MEC for plasma morphine reported as 14.7 ± 4.8 ng/mL (mean ± SD) in patients with postoperative pain. The high degree of variation is of clinical significance as it may result in either under-dosing or over-dosing if the dosage is not adjusted to the patient's clinical status and analgesic response (see **PRECAUTIONS** and **DOSAGE AND ADMINISTRATION**).
For opioid-tolerant patients the situation is much more complex. Some patients will become rapidly tolerant to the analgesic effects of morphine, and will require high daily oral morphine doses for adequate pain control. Since the development of tolerance to both the therapeutic and adverse effects of opioids is highly individualized, the dose of morphine should be individualized to the patient's condition and should not be based on an arbitrary choice of a dose or blood level to be achieved.
Pharmacokinetics
KADIAN® capsules contain polymer coated sustained release pellets of morphine sulfate that release morphine significantly more slowly than from morphine sulfate tablets and shorter-acting controlled-release oral morphine sulfate preparations. KADIAN® activity is primarily due to morphine. One metabolite, morphine-6-glucuronide, has been shown to have analgesic activity, but poorly crosses the blood-brain barrier.
Following oral administration, the extent of absorption is essentially the same for immediate or sustained release formulations, although the time to peak blood level (T_{max}) will be longer and the C_{max} will be lower for formulations that delay the release of morphine in the gastrointestinal tract.
Elimination of morphine is primarily via hepatic metabolism to glucuronide metabolites (55 to 65%) which are then renally excreted. The terminal half-life of morphine is 2 to 4 hours, however, a longer term half-life of about 15 hours has been reported in studies where blood has been sampled up to 48 hours.
The single-dose pharmacokinetics of KADIAN® are linear over the dosage range of 30 to 100 mg. The single dose and multiple dose pharmacokinetic parameters of KADIAN® in normal volunteers are summarized in Table 1.
[See table 1 at top of next page]
Absorption
Following the administration of oral morphine solution, approximately 50% of the morphine absorbed reaches the systemic circulation within 30 minutes. However, following the administration of an equal amount of KADIAN® to healthy volunteers, this occurs, on average, after 8 hours. As with most forms of oral morphine, because of pre-systemic elimination, only about 20 to 40% of the administered dose reaches the systemic circulation.
Food Effects: While concurrent administration of food slows the rate of absorption of KADIAN®, the extent of absorption is not affected and KADIAN® can be administered without regard to meals.
Steady State: When KADIAN® is given on a fixed dosing regimen to patients with chronic pain due to malignancy, steady state is achieved in about two days. At steady state, KADIAN® will have a significantly lower C_{max} and a higher C_{min} than equivalent doses of oral morphine solution and some other controlled-release preparations (see Graph 1).

Graph 1 (Study # MOB-1/98):
Mean steady state plasma morphine concentrations for KADIAN® (twice a day), controlled-release morphine tablet (twice a day) and oral morphine solution (every 4 hours); plasma concentrations are normalized to 100 mg every 24 hours, (n=24).

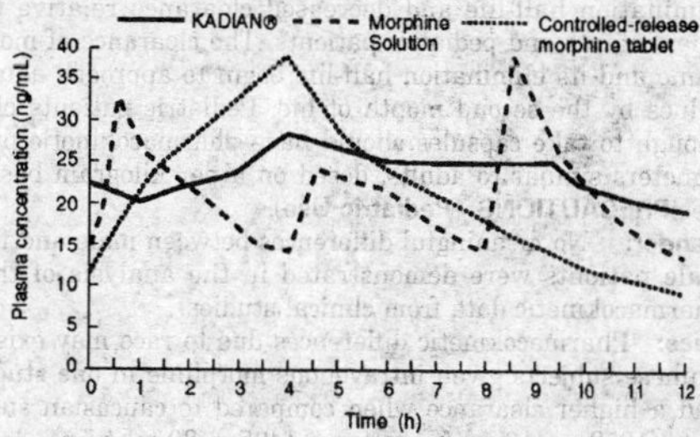

Continued on next page

Kadian—Cont.

Table 1: Mean pharmacokinetic parameters (% coefficient variation) resulting from a fasting single dose study in normal volunteers and a multiple dose study in patients with cancer pain.

Regimen/ Dosage Form	AUC#,+ (ng.h/mL)	C_{max}+ (ng/mL)	T_{max} (h)	C_{min}+ (ng/mL)	Fluctuation*
Single Dose (n=24)					
KADIAN® Capsule	271.0 (19.4)	15.6 (24.4)	8.6 (41.1)	na^	na
Controlled-Release Tablet	304.3 (19.1)	30.5 (32.1)	2.5 (52.6)	na	na
Morphine Solution	362.4 (42.6)	64.4 (38.2)	0.9 (55.8)	na	na
Multiple Dose (n=24)					
KADIAN® Capsule q24h	500.9 (38.6)	37.3 (37.7)	10.3 (32.2)	9.9 (52.3)	3.0 (45.5)
Controlled-Release Tablet q12h	457.3 (40.2)	36.9 (42.0)	4.4 (53.0)	7.6 (60.3)	4.1 (51.5)

\# For single dose AUC = $AUC_{0\text{-}48h}$, for multiple dose AUC = $AUC_{0\text{-}24h}$ at steady state
\+ For single dose parameter normalized to 100 mg, for multiple dose parameter normalized to 100 mg per 24 hours
* Steady-state fluctuation in plasma concentrations = C_{max}–C_{min}/C_{min}
^ Not applicable

When given once-daily (every 24 hours) to 24 patients with malignancy, KADIAN® had a similar C_{max} and higher C_{min} at steady state in clinical usage, when compared to twice-daily (every 12 hours) controlled-release morphine tablets (MS Contin®), given at an equivalent total daily dosage (see Graph 2 and Table 1). Drug-disease interactions are frequently seen in the older and more gravely ill patients, and may result in both altered absorption and reduced clearance as compared to normal volunteers (see **Geriatric, Hepatic Failure,** and **Renal Insufficiency** sections).

Graph 2 (Study # MOR-9/92):

Dose normalized mean steady state plasma morphine concentrations for KADIAN® (once a day), and an equivalent dose of a 12-hour, controlled-release morphine tablet given twice a day. Plasma concentrations are normalized to 100 mg every 24 hours, (n=24).

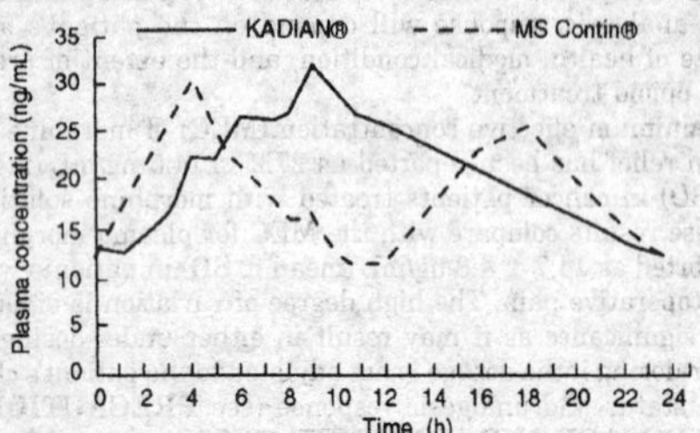

Distribution

Once absorbed, morphine is distributed to skeletal muscle, kidneys, liver, intestinal tract, lungs, spleen and brain.
The volume of distribution of morphine is approximately 3 to 4 L/kg. Morphine is 30 to 35% reversibly bound to plasma proteins.
Although the primary site of action of morphine is in the CNS, only small quantities pass the blood-brain barrier. Morphine also crosses the placental membranes (see **PRECAUTIONS - Pregnancy**) and has been found in breast milk (see **PRECAUTIONS - Nursing Mothers**).

Metabolism

The major pathway of the detoxification of morphine is conjugation, either with D-glucuronic acid in the liver to produce glucuronides or with sulfuric acid to give morphine-3-etheral sulfate. Although a small fraction (less than 5%) of morphine is demethylated, for all practical purposes, virtually all morphine is converted to glucuronide metabolites including morphine-3-glucuronide, M3G (about 50%) and morphine-6-glucuronide, M6G (about 5 to 15%). Studies in healthy subjects and cancer patients have shown that the glucuronide metabolite to morphine mean molar ratios (based on AUC) are similar after both single doses and at steady state for KADIAN®, 12-hour controlled-release morphine sulfate tablets and morphine sulfate solution.
M3G has no significant analgesic activity. M6G has been shown to have opioid agonist and analgesic activity in humans.

Excretion

Approximately 10% of morphine dose is excreted unchanged in the urine. Most of the dose is excreted in the urine as M3G and M6G. A small amount of the glucuronide metabolites is excreted in the bile and there is some minor enterohepatic cycling. Seven to 10% of administered morphine is excreted in the feces.
The mean adult plasma clearance is about 20-30 mL/minute/kg. The effective terminal half-life of morphine after IV administration is reported to be approximately 2.0 hours. Longer plasma sampling in some studies suggests a longer terminal half-life of morphine of about 15 hours.

Special Populations

Geriatric: The elderly may have increased sensitivity to morphine and may achieve higher and more variable serum levels than younger patients. In adults, the duration of analgesia increases progressively with age, though the degree of analgesia remains unchanged. KADIAN® pharmacokinetics have not been investigated in elderly patients (>65 years) although such patients were included in the clinical studies.

Nursing Mothers: Morphine is excreted in the maternal milk, and the milk to plasma morphine AUC ratio is about 2.5:1. The amount of morphine received by the infant depends on the maternal plasma concentration, amount of milk ingested by the infant, and the extent of first pass metabolism.

Pediatric: Infants under 1 month of age have a prolonged elimination half-life and decreased clearance relative to older infants and pediatric patients. The clearance of morphine and its elimination half-life begin to approach adult values by the second month of life. Pediatric patients old enough to take capsules should have pharmacokinetic parameters similar to adults, dosed on a per kilogram basis (see **PRECAUTIONS - Pediatric Use**).

Gender: No meaningful differences between male and female patients were demonstrated in the analysis of the pharmacokinetic data from clinical studies.

Race: Pharmacokinetic differences due to race may exist. Chinese subjects given intravenous morphine in one study had a higher clearance when compared to caucasian subjects (1852 ± 116 mL/min versus 1495 ± 80 mL/min).

Hepatic Failure: The pharmacokinetics of morphine were found to be significantly altered in individuals with alcoholic cirrhosis. The clearance was found to decrease with a corresponding increase in half-life. The M3G and M6G to morphine plasma AUC ratios also decreased in these patients indicating a decrease in metabolic activity.

Renal Insufficiency: The pharmacokinetics of morphine are altered in renal failure patients. AUC is increased and clearance is decreased. The metabolites, M3G and M6G accumulate several fold in renal failure patients compared with healthy subjects.

Drug-Drug Interactions: The known drug interactions involving morphine are pharmacodynamic, not pharmacokinetic (see **PRECAUTIONS - Drug Interactions**).

Clinical Studies

A total of 177 healthy subjects and 337 patients with cancer pain participated in a total of 15 studies (10 pharmacokinetic and 6 clinical; one study reported both pharmacokinetic and clinical data). Of these individuals, 158 healthy subjects and 268 patients received KADIAN®. In the controlled clinical studies patients were followed for a median duration of 7 days and in the open label studies patients were followed for up to 12-24 months. KADIAN® was compared to oral morphine solution and to either MS Contin® or to a 12-hour controlled-release morphine tablet bioequivalent to MS Contin® using trial designs that followed the clinical and pharmacokinetic performance of each treatment in cancer patients receiving chronic opioid therapy.
In two controlled studies, patients with moderate to severe cancer pain were titrated with immediate-release morphine (IRM) solution or tablets to a stable total daily dose of morphine for at least three consecutive days, then randomized to KADIAN® or 12-hour controlled-release morphine for seven days of observation. KADIAN® given once a day proved similar to the same total dose of morphine given in divided doses in a 12-hour dosage form, with respect to pain relief, use of rescue medication, patient and investigator global assessment, and quality of sleep. Individual patient differences in the pattern of pain control emphasize the need to individualize both dose and dosing interval (see **DOSAGE AND ADMINISTRATION**).

INDICATIONS AND USAGE

KADIAN® is indicated for the management of moderate to severe pain where treatment with an opioid analgesic is indicated for more than a few days (see **CLINICAL PHARMACOLOGY; Clinical Studies**).
KADIAN® was developed for use in patients with chronic pain who require repeated dosing with a potent opioid analgesic, and has been tested in patients with pain due to malignant conditions. KADIAN® has not been tested as an analgesic for the treatment of acute pain or in the postoperative setting and is not recommended for such use.

CONTRAINDICATIONS

KADIAN® is contraindicated in patients with a known hypersensitivity to morphine, morphine salts or any of the capsule components.
KADIAN® is contraindicated in patients with respiratory depression in the absence of resuscitative equipment, and in patients with acute or severe bronchial asthma.
KADIAN® is contraindicated in any patient who has or is suspected of having paralytic ileus.

WARNINGS (See also CLINICAL PHARMACOLOGY)

Impaired Respiration

Respiratory depression is the chief hazard of all morphine preparations. Respiratory depression occurs more frequently in elderly and debilitated patients, and those suffering from conditions accompanied by hypoxia, hypercapnia, or upper airway obstruction (when even moderate therapeutic doses may significantly decrease pulmonary ventilation).
Morphine should be used with extreme caution in patients with chronic obstructive pulmonary disease or cor pulmonale, and in patients having a substantially decreased respiratory reserve (e.g. severe kyphoscoliosis), hypoxia, hypercapnia, or pre-existing respiratory depression. In such patients, even usual therapeutic doses of morphine may increase airway resistance and decrease respiratory drive to the point of apnea.

Head Injury and Increased Intracranial Pressure

The respiratory depressant effects of morphine with carbon dioxide retention and secondary elevation of cerebrospinal fluid pressure may be markedly exaggerated in the presence of head injury, other intracranial lesions, or a pre-existing increase in intracranial pressure. Morphine produces effects which may obscure neurologic signs of further increases in pressure in patients with head injuries. Morphine should only be administered under such circumstances when considered essential and then with extreme care.

Hypotensive Effect

KADIAN®, like all opioid analgesics, may cause severe hypotension in an individual whose ability to maintain blood pressure has already been compromised by a reduced blood volume, or a concurrent administration of drugs such as phenothiazines or general anesthetics. (see also **PRECAUTIONS - Drug Interactions**). KADIAN® may produce orthostatic hypotension and syncope in ambulatory patients.
KADIAN®, like all opioid analgesics, should be administered with caution to patients in circulatory shock, as vasodilation produced by the drug may further reduce cardiac output and blood pressure.

Gastrointestinal Obstruction

KADIAN® should not be given to patients with gastrointestinal obstruction, particularly paralytic ileus, as there is a risk of the product remaining in the stomach for an extended period and the subsequent release of a bolus of morphine when normal gut motility is restored. As with other solid morphine formulations diarrhea may reduce morphine absorption.

PRECAUTIONS (See also CLINICAL PHARMACOLOGY)

General

KADIAN® is intended for use in patients who require continuous treatment with a potent opioid analgesic. As with any potent opioid, it is critical to adjust the dosing regimen for KADIAN® for each patient, taking into account the patient's prior analgesic treatment experience. Although it is clearly impossible to enumerate every consideration that is important to the selection of the initial dose of KADIAN®, attention should be given to the points under **DOSAGE AND ADMINISTRATION.**

Cordotomy

Patients taking KADIAN® who are scheduled for cordotomy or other interruption of pain transmission pathways should have KADIAN® ceased 24 hours prior to the procedure and the pain controlled by parenteral short-acting opioids. In addition, the post-procedure titration of analgesics for such patients should be individualized to avoid either oversedation or withdrawal syndromes.

Use in Pancreatic/Biliary Tract Disease

KADIAN® may cause spasm of the sphincter of Oddi and should be used with caution in patients with biliary tract disease, including acute pancreatitis. Opioids may cause increases in the serum amylase level.

Special risk groups

KADIAN® should be administered with caution, and in reduced dosages in elderly or debilitated patients; patients with severe renal or hepatic insufficiency; patients with Addison's disease; myxedema; hypothyroidism; prostatic hypertrophy or urethral stricture.
Caution should also be exercised in the administration of KADIAN® to patients with CNS depression, toxic psychosis, acute alcoholism and delirium tremens, and convulsive disorders.

Driving and operating machinery

Morphine may impair the mental and/or physical abilities needed to perform potentially hazardous activities such as driving a car or operating machinery. Patients must be cautioned accordingly. Patients should also be warned about the potential combined effects of morphine with other CNS depressants, including other opioids, phenothiazines, sedative/hypnotics and alcohol (see **Drug Interactions**).

Information for Patients

If clinically advisable, patients receiving KADIAN® should be given the following instructions by the physician:

1. KADIAN® capsules should be swallowed whole (not chewed, crushed, or dissolved). Alternatively, KADIAN® capsules may be opened and the entire contents sprinkled on a small amount of applesauce immediately prior to ingestion. The pellets should NOT be chewed, crushed, or dissolved due to risk of overdose. When prescribing KADIAN® by the sprinkle method, details of proper technique should be explained to the patient. KADIAN® cap-

sules may also be opened and the entire contents sprinkled over about 10 mL of water in a beaker then flushed with swirling through a pre-wetted 16-French gastrostomy tube fitted with a plastic funnel at the port end. The beaker is rinsed with additional aliquots of water as necessary to transfer all of the pellets to flush the tube. **NASOGASTRIC TUBES SHOULD NOT BE USED.** (also see **DOSAGE AND ADMINISTRATION**)

2. The dose of KADIAN® should not be adjusted without consulting the physician.
3. Morphine may impair mental and/or physical ability required for the performance of potentially hazardous tasks (e.g. driving, operating machinery). Patients started on KADIAN® or whose dose has been changed should refrain from dangerous activity until it is established that they are not adversely affected.
4. Morphine should not be taken with alcohol or other CNS depressants (sleeping medication, tranquilizers) because additive effects including CNS depression may occur. A physician should be consulted if other medications are currently being used or are prescribed for future use.
5. Women of childbearing potential who become or are planning to become pregnant, should consult a physician.
6. Upon completion of therapy, it may be appropriate to taper the morphine dose, rather than abruptly discontinuing it.
7. While psychological dependence ("addiction") to morphine used in the treatment of pain is very rare, morphine is one of a class of drugs known to be abused and should be handled accordingly.
8. As with other opioids, patients taking KADIAN® should be advised that severe constipation could occur and appropriate laxatives, stool softeners and other appropriate treatments should be initiated from the beginning of opioid therapy.

Drug Interactions

CNS Depressants: Morphine should be used with great caution and in reduced dosage in patients who are concurrently receiving other central nervous system (CNS) depressants including sedatives, hypnotics, general anesthetics, antiemetics, phenothiazines, other tranquilizers and alcohol because of the risk of respiratory depression, hypotension and profound sedation or coma. When such combined therapy is contemplated, the initial dose of one or both agents should be reduced by at least 50%.

Muscle Relaxants: Morphine may enhance the neuromuscular blocking action of skeletal relaxants and produce an increased degree of respiratory depression.

Mixed Agonist/Antagonist Opioid Analgesics: From a theoretical perspective, mixed agonist/antagonist analgesics (i.e. pentazocine, nalbuphine and butorphanol) should NOT be administered to patients who have received or are receiving a course of therapy with a pure opioid agonist analgesic. In these patients, mixed agonist/antagonist analgesics may reduce the analgesic effect and/or may precipitate withdrawal symptoms.

Monoamine Oxidase Inhibitors (MAOIs): MAOIs have been reported to intensify the effects of at least one opioid drug causing anxiety, confusion and significant depression of respiration or coma. We do not recommend the use of KADIAN® in patients taking MAOIs or within 14 days of stopping such treatment.

Cimetidine: There is an isolated report of confusion and severe respiratory depression when a hemodialysis patient was concurrently administered morphine and cimetidine.

Diuretics: Morphine can reduce the efficacy of diuretics by inducing the release of antidiuretic hormone. Morphine may also lead to acute retention of urine by causing spasm of the sphincter of the bladder, particularly in men with prostatism.

Food: KADIAN® capsules should be swallowed whole (not chewed, crushed, or dissolved). Alternatively, KADIAN® capsules may be opened and the entire contents sprinkled on a small amount of applesauce immediately prior to ingestion. The pellets in KADIAN® should NOT be chewed, crushed, or dissolved due to risk of overdose. (see **DOSAGE AND ADMINISTRATION,** and **INFORMATION FOR PATIENTS**)

Carcinogenicity/Mutagenicity/Impairment of Fertility

Long-term studies in animals to evaluate the carcinogenic potential of morphine have not been conducted. There are no reports of carcinogenic effects in humans.

In vitro studies have reported that morphine is non-mutagenic in the Ames test with *Salmonella*, and induces chromosomal aberrations in human leukocytes and lethal mutation induction in *Drosophila*. Morphine was found to be mutagenic *in vitro* in human T-cells, increasing the DNA fragmentation. *In vivo*, morphine was mutagenic in the mouse micronucleus test and induced chromosomal aberrations in spermatids and murine lymphocytes.

Chronic opioid abusers (e.g., heroin abusers) and their offspring display higher rates of chromosomal damage. However, the rates of chromosomal abnormalities were similar in nonexposed individuals and in heroin users enrolled in long term opioid maintenance programs.

Pregnancy

Teratogenic effects (Pregnancy Category C)

Teratogenic effects of morphine have been reported in the animal literature. High parental doses during the second trimester were teratogenic in neurological, soft and skeletal tissue. The abnormalities included encephalopathy and axial skeletal fusions. These doses were often maternally toxic and were 0.3 to 3-fold the maximum recommended human dose (MRHD) on a mg/m^2 basis. The relative contribution of morphine-induced maternal hypoxia and malnutrition, each of which can be teratogenic, has not been clearly defined. Treatment of male rats with approximately 3-fold the MRHD for 10 days prior to mating decreased litter size and viability.

Nonteratogenic effects

Morphine given subcutaneously, at non-maternally toxic doses, to rats during the third trimester with approximately 0.15-fold the MRHD caused reversible reductions in brain and spinal cord volume, and testes size and body weight in the offspring, and decreased fertility in female offspring. The offspring of rats and hamsters treated orally or intraperitoneally throughout pregnancy with 0.04- to 0.3-fold the MRHD of morphine have demonstrated delayed growth, motor and sexual maturation and decreased male fertility. Chronic morphine exposure of fetal animals resulted in mild withdrawal, altered reflex and motor skill development, and altered responsiveness to morphine that persisted into adulthood.

There are no well-controlled studies of chronic *in utero* exposure to morphine sulfate in human subjects. However, uncontrolled retrospective studies of human neonates chronically exposed to other opioids *in utero*, demonstrated reduced brain volume which normalized over the first month of life. Infants born to opioid-abusing mothers are more often small for gestational age, have a decreased ventilatory response to CO_2 and increased risk of sudden infant death syndrome.

Morphine should only be used during pregnancy if the need for strong opioid analgesia justifies the potential risk to the fetus.

Labor and Delivery

KADIAN® is not recommended for use in women during and immediately prior to labor, where shorter acting analgesics or other analgesic techniques are more appropriate. Occasionally, opioid analgesics may prolong labor through actions which temporarily reduce the strength, duration and frequency of uterine contractions. However, this effect is not consistent and may be offset by an increased rate of cervical dilatation which tends to shorten labor.

Neonates whose mothers received opioid analgesics during labor should be observed closely for signs of respiratory depression. A specific opioid antagonist, such as naloxone or nalmefene, should be available for reversal of opioid-induced respiratory depression in the neonate.

Neonatal Withdrawal Syndrome

Chronic maternal use of opiates or opioids during pregnancy coexposes the fetus. The newborn may experience subsequent neonatal withdrawal syndrome (NWS). Manifestations of NWS include irritability, hyperactivity, abnormal sleep pattern, high-pitched cry, tremor, vomiting, diarrhea, weight loss, and failure to gain weight. The onset, duration, and severity of the disorder differ based on such factors as the addictive drug used, time and amount of mother's last dose, and rate of elimination of the drug from the newborn. Approaches to the treatment of this syndrome have included supportive care and, when indicated, drugs such as paragoric or phenobarbital.

Nursing Mothers

Low levels of morphine sulfate have been detected in human milk. Withdrawal symptoms can occur in breast-feeding infants when maternal administration of morphine sulfate is stopped. Because of the potential for adverse reactions in nursing infants from KADIAN®, a decision should be made whether to discontinue nursing or discontinue the drug, taking into account the importance of the drug to the mother.

Pediatric Use

There are studies from the literature reporting the safe and effective use of both immediate and sustained release oral morphine preparations for analgesia in pediatric patients who were dosed on a per kilogram basis. However, the safety of KADIAN®, both the entire capsule and the pellets sprinkled on applesauce, have not been directly investigated in pediatric patients below the age of 18 years. The range of doses available is not suitable for the treatment of very young pediatric patients or those who are not old enough to take capsules safely. The applesauce sprinkling method is not an appropriate alternative for these patients.

ADVERSE REACTIONS

Serious adverse reactions that may be associated with KADIAN® therapy in clinical use are those observed with other opioid analgesics and include: respiratory depression, respiratory arrest, circulatory depression, cardiac arrest, hypotension, and/or shock (see **OVERDOSAGE, WARNINGS**).

The less severe adverse events seen on initiation of therapy with KADIAN® are also typical opioid side effects. These events are dose dependent, and their frequency depends on the clinical setting, the patient's level of opioid tolerance, and host factors specific to the individual. They should be expected and managed as a part of opioid analgesia. The most frequent of these include drowsiness, dizziness, constipation and nausea. In many cases, the frequency of these events during initiation of therapy may be minimized by careful individualization of starting dosage, slow titration, and the avoidance of large rapid swings in plasma concentrations of the opioid. Many of these adverse events, will cease or decrease as KADIAN® therapy is continued and some degree of tolerance is developed, but others may be expected to remain troublesome throughout therapy.

Management of Excessive Drowsiness

Most patients receiving morphine will experience initial drowsiness. This usually disappears within 3–5 days and is not a cause of concern unless it is excessive, or accompanied by unsteadiness or confusion. Dizziness and unsteadiness may be associated with postural hypotension, particularly in elderly or debilitated patients, and has been associated with syncope and falls in non-tolerant patients started on opioids.

Excessive or persistent sedation should be investigated. Factors to be considered should include: concurrent sedative medications, the presence of hepatic or renal insufficiency, hypoxia or hypercapnia due to exacerbated respiratory failure, intolerance to the dose used (especially in older patients), disease severity and the patient's general condition. The dosage should be adjusted according to individual needs, but additional care should be used in the selection of initial doses for the elderly patient, the cachectic or gravely ill patient, or in patients not already familiar with opioid analgesic medications to prevent excessive sedation at the onset of treatment.

Management of Nausea and Vomiting

Nausea and vomiting are common after single doses of morphine or as an early undesirable effect of chronic opioid therapy. The prescription of a suitable antiemetic should be considered, with the awareness that sedation may result (see **Drug Interactions**). The frequency of nausea and vomiting usually decreases within a week or so but may persist due to opioid-induced gastric stasis. Metoclopramide is often useful in such patients.

Management of Constipation

Virtually all patients suffer from constipation while taking opioids on a chronic basis. Some patients, particularly elderly, debilitated or bedridden patients may become impacted. Tolerance does not usually develop for the constipating effects of opioids. Patients must be cautioned accordingly and laxatives, softeners and other appropriate treatments should be used prophylactically from the beginning of opioid therapy.

Adverse Events Probably Related to KADIAN® Administration

In controlled clinical trials in patients with chronic cancer pain the most common adverse events reported by patients at least once during therapy were drowsiness (9%), constipation (9%), nausea (7%), dizziness (6%), and anxiety (6%). Other less common side effects expected from morphine or seen in less than 3% of patients in the clinical trials were:

Body as a Whole: Asthenia, accidental injury, fever, pain, chest pain, headache, diaphoresis, chills, flu syndrome, back pain, malaise, withdrawal syndrome

Cardiovascular: Tachycardia, atrial fibrillation, hypotension, hypertension, pallor, facial flushing, palpitations, bradycardia, syncope

Central Nervous System: Confusion, dry mouth, anxiety, abnormal thinking, abnormal dreams, lethargy, depression, tremor, loss of concentration, insomnia, amnesia, paresthesia, agitation, vertigo, foot drop, ataxia, hypesthesia, slurred speech, hallucinations, vasodilation, euphoria, apathy, seizures, myoclonus

Endocrine: Hyponatremia due to inappropriate ADH secretion, gynecomastia

Gastrointestinal: Vomiting, anorexia, dysphagia, dyspepsia, diarrhea, abdominal pain, stomach atony disorder, gastro-esophageal reflux, delayed gastric emptying, biliary colic

Hemic & Lymphatic: Anemia, leukopenia, thrombocytopenia

Metabolic & Nutritional: Peripheral edema, hyponatremia, edema

Musculoskeletal: Back pain, bone pain, arthralgia

Respiratory: Hiccup, rhinitis, atelectasis, asthma, hypoxia, dyspnea, respiratory insufficiency, voice alteration, depressed cough reflex, non-cardiogenic pulmonary edema

Skin and Appendages: Rash, decubitus ulcer, pruritus, skin flush

Special Senses: Amblyopia, conjunctivitis, miosis, blurred vision, nystagmus, diplopia

Urogenital: Urinary abnormality, amenorrhea, urinary retention, urinary hesitancy, reduced libido, reduced potency, prolonged labor

DRUG ABUSE AND DEPENDENCE

Morphine is the prototype of opioid agonist drugs, and may be subject to misuse, abuse and addiction. Addiction to opioids prescribed for pain management is rare, but requests for opioids from patients addicted to opioids are common and physicians should take appropriate care in prescribing this controlled substance.

Opioid analgesics may cause physical dependence. Physical dependence results in withdrawal symptoms in patients who abruptly discontinue the drug. Withdrawal also may be precipitated through the administration of drugs with opioid antagonist activity, e.g. naloxone, nalmefene, or mixed agonist/antagonist analgesics (pentazocine, butorphanol, nalbuphine), (see also **OVERDOSAGE**).

Physical dependence usually does not occur to a clinically significant degree until after several weeks of continued opioid usage. Tolerance, in which increasingly large doses are required in order to produce the same degree of analgesia, is initially manifested by a shortened duration of analgesic effect, and subsequently, by decreases in the intensity of analgesia.

Continued on next page

Kadian—Cont.

In chronic pain patients, and in opioid-tolerant cancer patients, the administration of KADIAN® should be guided by the degree of tolerance manifested. Physical dependence, per se, is not ordinarily a concern when one is dealing with a patient in pain, and fear of tolerance should not deter using adequate doses to adequately relieve pain.
If morphine is abruptly discontinued an abstinence syndrome may occur. This is usually mild and is characterized by rhinitis, myalgia, abdominal cramping and occasional diarrhea. Most observable symptoms disappear in 5–14 days without treatment; however, there may be a phase of secondary or chronic abstinence which may last for 2–6 months characterized by insomnia, irritability and muscular aches.
If treatment of physical dependence of patients taking morphine is necessary, the patient may be detoxified by gradual reduction of the dose. Gastrointestinal disturbances or dehydration should be treated with supportive care.
KADIAN® has no role in the management of opioid addiction.

OVERDOSAGE

Symptoms

Acute overdosage with morphine is manifested by respiratory depression, somnolence progressing to stupor or coma, skeletal muscle flaccidity, cold and clammy skin, constricted pupils, and, sometimes, pulmonary edema, bradycardia, hypotension and death. Marked mydriasis rather than miosis may be seen due to severe hypoxia in overdose situations.

Treatment

Primary attention should be given to the re-establishment of a patent airway and institution of assisted or controlled ventilation. Gastric contents may need to be emptied to remove unabsorbed drug when a sustained release formulation such as KADIAN® has been taken. Care should be taken to secure the airway before attempting treatment by gastric emptying or activated charcoal.
The pure opioid antagonists, naloxone or nalmefene, are specific antidotes to respiratory depression which results from opioid overdose. Since the duration of reversal would be expected to be less than the duration of action of KADIAN®, the patient must be carefully monitored until spontaneous respiration is reliably re-established. KADIAN® will continue to release and add to the morphine load for up to 24 hours after administration and the management of an overdose should be monitored accordingly. If the response to opioid antagonists is suboptimal or not sustained, additional antagonist should be given as directed by the manufacturer of the product.
Opioid antagonists should not be administered in the absence of clinically significant respiratory or circulatory depression secondary to morphine overdose. Such agents should be administered cautiously to persons who are known, or suspected to be physically dependent on KADIAN®. In such cases, an abrupt or complete reversal of opioid effects may precipitate an acute abstinence syndrome.
Opioid Tolerant Individuals: In an individual physically dependent on opioids, administration of the usual dose of the antagonist will precipitate an acute withdrawal. The severity of the withdrawal produced will depend on the degree of physical dependence and the dose of the antagonist administered. Use of an opioid antagonist should be reserved for cases where such treatment is clearly needed. If it is necessary to treat serious respiratory depression in the physically dependent patient, administration of the antagonist should be begun with care and by titration with smaller than usual doses.
Supportive measures (including oxygen, vasopressors) should be employed in the management of circulatory shock and pulmonary edema as indicated. Cardiac arrest or arrhythmias may require cardiac massage or defibrillation.

DOSAGE AND ADMINISTRATION

KADIAN® CAPSULES SHOULD BE SWALLOWED WHOLE (NOT CHEWED, CRUSHED, OR DISSOLVED).
ALTERNATIVELY, KADIAN® CAPSULES MAY BE OPENED AND THE ENTIRE CONTENTS SPRINKLED ON A SMALL AMOUNT OF APPLESAUCE IMMEDIATELY PRIOR TO INGESTION. THE PELLETS IN KADIAN® CAPSULES SHOULD NOT BE CHEWED, CRUSHED, OR DISSOLVED DUE TO RISK OF OVERDOSE.
TAKING CHEWED OR CRUSHED KADIAN® CAPSULES OR PELLETS WILL LEAD TO THE RAPID RELEASE AND ABSORPTION OF A POTENTIALLY TOXIC DOSE OF MORPHINE.
KADIAN® CAPSULES MAY BE OPENED AND THE ENTIRE CONTENTS SPRINKLED OVER ABOUT 10 ML OF WATER AND FLUSHED WITH SWIRLING THROUGH A PRE-WETTED 16 FRENCH GASTROSTOMY TUBE FITTED WITH FUNNEL AT THE PORT END. ADDITIONAL ALIQUOTS OF WATER ARE USED TO TRANSFER ALL PELLETS AND TO FLUSH THE TUBE. THE ADMINISTRATION OF KADIAN® PELLETS THROUGH A NASOGASTRIC TUBE SHOULD NOT BE ATTEMPTED.
The sustained release nature of KADIAN® allows it to be administered on **either** a once-a-day or twice-a-day schedule. KADIAN® produces analgesia similar to that produced by conventional immediate-release and controlled-release formulations for the same total daily dose of morphine. However, peak and trough blood levels depend on the release characteristics of each specific formulation, and other oral morphines may not be therapeutically equivalent to KADIAN® for an individual patient.
KADIAN® capsules have the same extent of absorption (AUC) as immediate-release oral formulations and controlled-release oral formulations of morphine sulfate. However, key pharmacokinetic parameters (e.g. C_{max}, T_{max}) for KADIAN® are significantly different from other controlled-release oral formulations.
As with any potent opioid drug product, it is critical to adjust the dosing regimen for each patient individually, taking into account the patient's prior analgesic treatment experience. In the selection of the initial dose of KADIAN®, attention should be given to:

1) the total daily dose, potency and kind of opioid the patient has been taking previously;
2) the reliability of the relative potency estimate used to calculate the equivalent dose of morphine needed;
3) the patient's degree of opioid tolerance;
4) the general condition and medical status of the patient;
5) concurrent medication;
6) the type and severity of the patient's pain.

The following dosing recommendations, therefore, can only be considered suggested approaches to what is actually a series of clinical decisions over time in the management of the pain of an individual patient.

Conversion from Other Oral Morphine Formulations to KADIAN®

Patients on other oral morphine formulations may be converted to KADIAN® by administering one-half of the patient's total daily oral morphine dose as KADIAN® capsules every 12 hours (twice-a-day) or by administering the total daily oral morphine dose as KADIAN® capsules every 24 hours (once-a-day). KADIAN® should not be given more frequently than every 12 hours.

Conversion from Parenteral Morphine or Other Parenteral or Oral Opioids to KADIAN®

KADIAN® can be administered to patients previously receiving treatment with parenteral morphine or other opioids. While there are useful tables of oral and parenteral equivalents in cancer analgesia, there is substantial inter-patient variation in the relative potency of different opioid drugs and formulations. For these reasons, it is better to underestimate the patient's 24 hour oral morphine requirement and provide rescue medication, than to overestimate and manage an adverse event. The following general points should be considered:
Parenteral to oral morphine ratio: It may take anywhere from 2–6 mg of oral morphine to provide analgesia equivalent to 1 mg of parenteral morphine. A dose of oral morphine three times the daily parenteral morphine requirement may be sufficient in chronic use settings.
Other parenteral or oral opioids to oral morphine sulfate: Physicians are advised to refer to published relative potency data, keeping in mind that such ratios are only approximate. In general, it is safest to give half of the estimated daily morphine demand as the initial dose, and to manage inadequate analgesia by supplementation with immediate-release morphine. (See discussion which follows.)
The first dose of KADIAN® may be taken with the last dose of any immediate-release (short-acting) opioid medication due to the long delay until the peak effect after administration of KADIAN®.

Use of KADIAN® as the First Opioid Analgesic

There has been no evaluation of KADIAN® as an initial opioid analgesic in the management of pain. Because it may be more difficult to titrate a patient to adequate analgesia using a sustained release morphine, it is ordinarily advisable to begin treatment using an immediate-release morphine formulation.

Individualization of Dosage

The best use of opioid analgesics in the management of chronic malignant and non-malignant pain is challenging, and is well described in materials published by the World Health Organization and the Agency for Health Care Policy and Research which are available from Alpharma upon request. KADIAN® is a third step drug which is most useful when the patient requires a constant level of opioid analgesia as a "floor" or "platform" from which to manage breakthrough pain. When a patient has reached the point where comfort cannot be provided with a combination of non-opioid medications (NSAIDs and acetaminophen) and intermittent use of moderate or strong opioids, the patient's total opioid therapy should be converted into a 24 hour oral morphine equivalent.
KADIAN® should be started by administering one-half of the estimated total daily oral morphine dose every 12 hours (twice-a-day) **or** by administering the total daily oral morphine dose every 24 hours (once-a-day). The dose should be titrated no more frequently than every-other-day to allow the patients to stabilize before escalating the dose. If breakthrough pain occurs, the dose may be supplemented with a small dose (less than 20% of the total daily dose) of a short-acting analgesic. Patients who are excessively sedated after a once-a-day dose or who regularly experience inadequate analgesia before the next dose should be switched to twice-a-day dosing.
Patients who do not have a proven tolerance to opioids should be started only on the 20 mg strength, and usually should be increased at a rate not greater than 20 mg every-other-day. Most patients will rapidly develop some degree of tolerance, requiring dosage adjustment until they have achieved their individual best balance between baseline analgesia and opioid side effects such as confusion, sedation and constipation. No guidance can be given as to the recommended maximal dose, especially in patients with chronic pain of malignancy. In such cases the total dose of KADIAN® should be advanced until the desired therapeutic endpoint is reached or clinically significant opioid-related adverse reactions intervene.

Alternative Methods of Administration

In a study of healthy volunteers, KADIAN® pellets sprinkled over applesauce were found to be bioequivalent to KADIAN® capsules swallowed whole with applesauce under fasting conditions. Other foods have not been tested. Patients who have difficulty swallowing whole capsules or tablets may benefit from this alternative method of administration.

1) Sprinkle the pellets onto a small amount of applesauce. Applesauce should be room temperature or cooler.
2) Use immediately.
3) Rinse mouth to ensure all pellets have been swallowed.
4) Patients should consume entire portion and should not divide applesauce into separate doses.

The entire capsule contents may be administered through a 16 French gastrostomy tube.

1) Flush the gastrostomy tube with water to ensure that it is wet.
2) Sprinkle the KADIAN® Pellets into 10 mL of water.
3) Use a swirling motion to pour the pellets and water into the gastrostomy tube through a funnel.
4) Rinse the beaker with a further 10 mL of water and pour this into the funnel.
5) Repeat rinsing until no pellets remain in the beaker.

THE ADMINISTRATION OF KADIAN® PELLETS THROUGH A NASOGASTRIC TUBE SHOULD NOT BE ATTEMPTED.

Considerations in the Adjustment of Dosing Regimens

If signs of excessive opioid effects are observed early in the dosing interval, the next dose should be reduced. If this adjustment leads to inadequate analgesia, that is, if breakthrough pain occurs when KADIAN® is administered on an every 24 hours dosing regimen, consideration should be given to dosing every 12 hours. If breakthough pain occurs on a 12 hour dosing regimen a supplemental dose of short-acting analgesic may be given. As experience is gained, adjustments in both dose and dosing interval can be made to obtain an appropriate balance between pain relief and opioid side effects. To avoid accumulation the dosing interval of KADIAN® should not be reduced below 12 hours.

Conversion from KADIAN® to Other Controlled-Release Oral Morphine Formulations

KADIAN® is not bioequivalent to other controlled-release morphine preparations. Although for a given dose the same total amount of morphine is available from KADIAN® as from morphine solution or controlled-release morphine tablets, the slower release of morphine from KADIAN® results in reduced maximum and increased minimum plasma morphine concentrations than with shorter acting morphine products. Conversion from KADIAN® to the same total daily dose of controlled-release morphine preparations may lead to either excessive sedation at peak or inadequate analgesia at trough and close observation and appropriate dosage adjustments are recommended.

Conversion from KADIAN® to Parenteral Opioids

When converting a patient from KADIAN® to parenteral opioids, it is best to calculate an equivalent parenteral dose, and then initiate treatment at half of this calculated value. For example, to estimate the required 24 hour dose of parenteral morphine for a patient taking KADIAN®, one would take the 24 hour KADIAN® dose, divide by an oral to parenteral conversion ratio of 3, divide the estimated 24 hour parenteral dose into six divided doses (for a four hour dosing interval), then halve this dose as an initial trial.
For example, to estimate the required parenteral morphine dose for a patient taking 360 mg of KADIAN® a day, divide the 360 mg daily oral morphine dose by a conversion ratio of 1 mg of parenteral morphine for every 3 mg of oral morphine. The estimated 120 mg daily parenteral requirement is then divided into six 20 mg doses, and half of this, or 10 mg, is then given every 4 hours as an initial trial dose. This approach is likely to require a dosage increase in the first 24 hours for many patients, but is recommended because it is less likely to cause overdose than trying to establish an equivalent dose without titration.
Opioid analgesic agents may not effectively relieve dysesthetic pain, post-herpetic neuralgia, stabbing pains, activity-related pain, and some forms of headache. This does not mean that patients suffering from these types of pain should not be given an adequate trial of opioid analgesics. However, such patients may need to be promptly evaluated for other types of pain therapy.

Safety and Handling

KADIAN® consists of closed hard gelatin capsules containing polymer coated morphine sulfate pellets that pose no known handling risk to health care workers. Oral morphine products are not known to be associated with a high risk of diversion, but all strong opioids are liable to diversion and misuse both by the general public and health care workers, and should be handled accordingly.

HOW SUPPLIED

KADIAN® capsules contain white to off-white or tan colored polymer coated sustained release pellets of morphine sulfate and are available in five dose strengths:

20 mg size 4 capsule, yellow opaque cap imprinted KADIAN and yellow opaque body imprinted with 20 mg. Capsules are supplied in bottles of 30 (NDC 63857-322-03), 60 (NDC 63857-322-06), and 100 (NDC 63857-322-11).
30 mg size 4 capsule, blue violet opaque cap imprinted KADIAN and blue violet opaque body imprinted with 30 mg. Capsules are supplied in bottles of 30 (NDC 63857-325-03), 60 (NDC 63857-325-06), and 100 (NDC 63857-325-11).
50 mg size 2 capsule, blue opaque cap imprinted KADIAN and blue opaque body imprinted with 50 mg. Capsules are supplied in bottles of 30 (NDC 63857-323-03), 60 (NDC 63857-323-06), and 100 (NDC 63857-323-11).
60 mg size 1 capsule, pink opaque cap imprinted KADIAN and pink opaque body imprinted with 60 mg. Capsules are supplied in bottles of 30 (NDC 63857-326-03), 60 (NDC 63857-326-06), and 100 (NDC 63857-326-11).
100 mg size 0 capsule, green opaque cap imprinted KADIAN and green opaque body imprinted with 100 mg. Capsules are supplied in bottles of 30 (NDC 63857-324-03), 60 (NDC 63857-324-06), and 100 (NDC 63857-324-11).
Store at 25°C (77°F); excursions permitted to 15°–30°C (59°–86°F). Protect from light and moisture.
Dispense in a sealed, tamper-evident, childproof, light-resistant container.

CAUTION

DEA Order Form Required.

℞ only

KADIAN® is a registered trademark of US Oral Pharmaceuticals Pty Ltd.
MS Contin® is a registered trademark of The Purdue Frederick Company
Manufactured for: **Alpharma Branded Products Division**
One New England Avenue
Piscataway, NJ 08854
by: Purepac Pharmaceutical Co.
Elizabeth, NJ 07207 USA
40-8984 Revised—June 2004

Shown in Product Identification Guide, page 304

Alto Pharmaceuticals, Inc.

P.O. BOX 271150
TAMPA, FL 33688-1150
12506 CLENDENNING DR.
TAMPA, FL 33618

Direct Inquiries to:
John J. Cullaro
Customer Service
www.altopharm.com
Tel (800) 330-2891
Fax (813) 968-0527

ZINC-220® CAPSULES OTC

[*zĭnk*]

(zinc sulfate 220 mg.)

COMPOSITION

Each opaque blue and pink capsule contains zinc sulfate 220 mg. delivering 78.5 mg. of elemental zinc. Zinc-220 Capsules do not contain dextrose or glucose. Inactive Ingredients dicalcium phosphate, cellulose, magnesium stearate, magnesium trisilicate and gelatin (capsule shell).

ACTION AND USES

Zinc-220 Capsules are indicated as a dietary supplement. Normal growth and tissue repair are directly dependent upon an adequate supply of zinc in the diet. Zinc functions as an integral part of a number of enzymes important to protein and carbohydrate metabolism. Zinc-220 Capsules are recommended for deficiencies or the prevention of deficiencies of zinc.

WARNINGS

Zinc-220 if administered in stat dosages of 2 grams (9 capsules) will cause an emetic effect. This product should not be used by pregnant or lactating women.

PRECAUTION

It is recommended that Zinc-220 Capsules be taken with meals or milk to avoid gastric distress.

DOSAGE

One capsule daily with milk or meals. One capsule daily provides approximately 523% times the recommended adult requirement for zinc.

HOW SUPPLIED

Product	NDC	SIZE
Zinc-220® Capsules	0731-0401-06	Unit Dose Boxes 100 (10×10)
Zinc-220® Capsules	0731-0401-01	Bottles 100

ALTO® Pharmaceuticals, Inc.

Shown in Product Identification Guide, page 304

Amarin Pharmaceuticals Inc.

For product information see Valeant Pharmaceuticals International

American Red Cross

NATIONAL HEADQUARTERS
BIOMEDICAL SERVICES
2025 E STREET, NW
WASHINGTON, DC 20006-5009

Direct Inquiries to:
Medical Affairs Department
800-293-5023
Customer Service Department
800-261-5772
Please see the American Red Cross Plasma Services Website for Full Prescribing Information:
http://plasmaservices.redcross.org

ALBUMARC® 5% ℞
ALBUMIN (HUMAN), USP, 5% SOLUTION

6 bottles per case	NDC #
250mL bottle	52769-450-25
500mL bottle	52769-450-50

ALBUMARC® 25% ℞
ALBUMIN (HUMAN), USP, 25% SOLUTION

10 bottles per case	NDC #
50mL bottle	52769-451-05
100mL bottle	52769-451-10

ALBUMIN (HUMAN), USP, 25% SOLUTION ℞

Albumin (Human) 25% is supplied in 50mL and 100mL vials, with circular and latex-free, disposable sterile intravenous administration set.

10 bottles per case	NDC #
50mL bottle	52769-251-05
100mL bottle	52769-251-10

ALBUMIN (HUMAN), USP, 5% SOLUTION

Albumin (Human) 5% is supplied in 250 mL and 500 mL vials, with circular and latex-free, disposable sterile intravenous administration set.

10 bottles per case	NDC #
250 mL bottle	52769-250-25
500 mL bottle	52769-250-50

CROSSEAL® ℞
Fibrin Sealant, (Human)

HOW SUPPLIED

Crosseal® is supplied as a kit consisting of two separate packages: (1) a package containing one vial each of Biological Active Component (BAC) (40–60 mg/mL fibrinogen) and Thrombin (800–1200 10/mL human thrombin, 5.6–6.2 mg/mL calcium chloride) frozen solutions and (2) a spray application device. The kit is supplied as 1 mL, 2 mL or 5 mL dosages.
The application device package contains a pre-assembled applicator and an air tube with a 0.2 um filter. The application devices are sterile and for single use only.

NDC #	
1 mL	52769-880-11
2 mL	52769-880-22
5 mL	52769-880-55
5 mL with 45 cm device	52769-880-56

GENARC™ ℞
[*jĕn-ărk*]

Antihemophilic Factor (recombinant)

GENARC™ is available in single-dose bottles which contain nominally 250, 500 and 1,000 International Units per bottle. GENARC™ is packaged with 10 mL of Sterile Water for Injection, USP, a double-ended needle, and a filter needle.

NDC #	
Low range assay	52769-464-02
Mid range assay	52769-464-05
High range assay	52769-464-10

MONARC-M™ ℞
ANTIHEMOPHILIC FACTOR (HUMAN)
Method M
Monoclonal Purified

HOW SUPPLIED

MONARC–M™ is available as single dose bottles. Each bottle is labeled with the potency in International Units, and is packaged together with 10 mL of Sterile Water for Injection, USP, a double-ended needle, and a filter needle.
NDC 52769-460-01

PANGLOBULIN® ℞
IMMUNE GLOBULIN INTRAVENOUS (HUMAN)

CAUTION: US Federal law prohibits dispensing without prescription.

HOW SUPPLIED

Immune Globulin Intravenous (Human), Panglobulin®, is available as a white lyophilized powder in 6 and 12 g size vials. The only diluents which may be used to reconstitute the product are sterile (0.9%) Sodium Chloride Injection USP, 5% Dextrose, or Sterile Water.
Panglobulin® (IgIV) is available in individual vial packages, and each bottle is supplied with a transfer device for use when reconstituting the product.
6 g Individual vial package NDC 52769-268-66
12 g Individual vial package NDC 52769-269-72

PANGLOBULIN® NF ℞
[*păn'glŏb-ew-lĭn*]

Immune Globulin Intravenous (Human) Nanofiltered

Immune Globulin Intravenous (Human), Panglobulin® NF Nanofiltered is available as a white lyophilized powder in 6 and 12 g size vials. The only diluents which may be used to reconstitute the product are sterile (0.9%) Sodium Chloride Injection USP, 5% Dextrose, or Sterile Water.
Panglobulin® NF (IgIV) is available in individual vial packages, and each bottle is supplied with a transfer device for use when reconstituting the product.
6 g Individual vial package NDC 52769-417-06
12 g Individual vial package NDC 52769-418-12

POLYGAM® S/D
IMMUNE GLOBULIN INTRAVENOUS ℞
SOLVENT/DETERGENT TREATED (HUMAN)

HOW SUPPLIED

Immune Globulin Intravenous (Human), Polygam® S/D, is supplied in 5 g or 10 g single use bottles. Each bottle of Immune Globulin Intravenous (Human), Polygam® S/D, is furnished with a suitable volume of Sterile Water for Injection, USP, a transfer device and an administration set which contains an integral airway and a 15 micron filter.
5g NDC 52769-471-75
10g NDC 52769-471-80

Amgen

AMGEN INC.
ONE AMGEN CENTER DRIVE
THOUSAND OAKS, CA 91320-1799

For Medical Information Contact:
Global Medical Affairs
(800) 772-6436
FAX: (805) 480-1299
In Emergencies:
(800) 772-6436
After Hours and Weekends:
(800) 772-6436

Sales and Ordering:
Customer Service Department
(800) 282-6436
FAX: (800) 292-6436

ARANESP® ℞
[*ără-nĕsp*]

(darbepoetin alfa)
For Injection

DESCRIPTION

Aranesp® is an erythropoiesis stimulating protein, closely related to erythropoietin, that is produced in Chinese hamster ovary (CHO) cells by recombinant DNA technology. Aranesp® is a 165-amino acid protein that differs from recombinant human erythropoietin in containing 5 N-linked oligosaccharide chains, whereas recombinant human erythropoietin contains 3 chains[1]. The two additional N-glycosylation sites result from amino acid substitutions in the erythropoietin peptide backbone. The additional carbohydrate chains increase the approximate molecular weight of the glycoprotein from 30,000 to 37,000 daltons. Aranesp® is formulated as a sterile, colorless, preservative-free protein solution for intravenous (IV) or subcutaneous (SC) administration.
Single-dose vials are available containing 25, 40, 60, 100, 150, 200, 300, or 500 mcg of Aranesp®.

Continued on next page

Aranesp—Cont.

Single-dose prefilled syringes are available containing 25, 40, 60, 100, 150, 200, 300, or 500 mcg of Aranesp. To reduce the risk of accidental needlesticks to users, each prefilled syringe is equipped with a needle guard that covers the needle during disposal.

Single-dose vials and prefilled syringes are available in two formulations that contain excipients as follows:

Polysorbate solution Each 1 mL contains 0.05 mg polysorbate 80, and is formulated at pH 6.2 ± 0.2 with 2.12 mg sodium phosphate monobasic monohydrate, 0.66 mg sodium phosphate dibasic anhydrous, and 8.18 mg sodium chloride in Water for Injection, USP (to 1 mL).

Albumin solution Each 1 mL contains 2.5 mg albumin (human), and is formulated at pH 6.0 ± 0.3 with 2.23 mg sodium phosphate monobasic monohydrate, 0.53 mg sodium phosphate dibasic anhydrous, and 8.18 mg sodium chloride in Water for Injection, USP (to 1 mL).

CLINICAL PHARMACOLOGY

Mechanism of Action

Aranesp® stimulates erythropoiesis by the same mechanism as endogenous erythropoietin. A primary growth factor for erythroid development, erythropoietin is produced in the kidney and released into the bloodstream in response to hypoxia. In responding to hypoxia, erythropoietin interacts with progenitor stem cells to increase red blood cell (RBC) production. Production of endogenous erythropoietin is impaired in patients with chronic renal failure (CRF), and erythropoietin deficiency is the primary cause of their anemia. Increased hemoglobin levels are not generally observed until 2 to 6 weeks after initiating treatment with Aranesp® (see **DOSAGE AND ADMINISTRATION: Dose Adjustment**). In patients with cancer receiving concomitant chemotherapy, the etiology of anemia is multifactorial.

Pharmacokinetics

The pharmacokinetics of Aranesp® were studied in patients with CRF and cancer patients receiving chemotherapy.

Over the therapeutic range of 0.45 to 4.5 mcg/kg, pharmacokinetic measures (Cmax, half-life, AUC) were linear with respect to dose, and no evidence of accumulation was observed beyond an expected < 2-fold increase in blood levels when compared to the initial dose.

Following SC administration, absorption is slow and rate limiting. The observed half-life in CRF patients, which reflected the rate of absorption, was 49 hours (range: 27 to 89 hours). Following IV administration to these patients, Aranesp® serum concentration-time profiles are biphasic, with a distribution half-life of approximately 1.4 hours and the mean terminal half-life of 21 hours. Post SC administration in CRF patients' peak concentrations occur at 34 hours (range: 24 to 72 hours), whereas cancer patients' peak concentrations are at 90 hours (range: 71 to 123 hours).

When administered by IV administration, the terminal half-life of Aranesp® is approximately 3-fold longer than Epoetin alfa. The bioavailability of Aranesp® as measured in CRF patients after SC administration is 37% (range: 30% to 50%).

CLINICAL STUDIES

Throughout this section of the package insert, the Aranesp® study numbers associated with the nephrology and cancer clinical programs are designated with the letters "N" and "C", respectively.

Chronic Renal Failure Patients

The safety and effectiveness of Aranesp® have been assessed in multicenter studies. Two studies evaluated the safety and efficacy of Aranesp® for the correction of anemia in adult patients with CRF, and two studies assessed the ability of Aranesp® to maintain hemoglobin concentrations in adult patients with CRF who had been receiving other recombinant erythropoietins.

De Novo Use of Aranesp®

In two open-label studies, Aranesp® or Epoetin alfa were administered for the correction of anemia in CRF patients who had not been receiving prior treatment with exogenous erythropoietin. Study N1 evaluated CRF patients receiving dialysis; Study N2 evaluated patients not requiring dialysis (predialysis patients). In both studies, the starting dose of Aranesp® was 0.45 mcg/kg administered once weekly. The starting dose of Epoetin alfa was 50 U/kg 3 times weekly in Study N1 and 50 U/kg twice weekly in Study N2. When necessary, dosage adjustments were instituted to maintain hemoglobin in the study target range of 11 to 13 g/dL. (Note: The recommended hemoglobin target is lower than the target range of these studies. See **DOSAGE AND ADMINISTRATION: General** for recommended clinical hemoglobin target.) The primary efficacy endpoint was the proportion of patients who experienced at least a 1.0 g/dL increase in hemoglobin concentration to a level of at least 11.0 g/dL by 20 weeks (Study N1) or 24 weeks (Study N2). The studies were designed to assess the safety and effectiveness of Aranesp® but not to support conclusions regarding comparisons between the two products.

In Study N1, the hemoglobin target was achieved by 72% (95% CI: 62%, 81%) of the 90 patients treated with Aranesp® and 84% (95% CI: 66%, 95%) of the 31 patients treated with Epoetin alfa. The mean increase in hemoglobin over the initial 4 weeks of Aranesp® treatment was 1.10 g/dL (95% CI: 0.82 g/dL, 1.37 g/dL).

In Study N2, the primary efficacy endpoint was achieved by 93% (95% CI: 87%, 97%) of the 129 patients treated with Aranesp® and 92% (95% CI: 78%, 98%) of the 37 patients treated with Epoetin alfa. The mean increase in hemoglobin from baseline through the initial 4 weeks of Aranesp® treatment was 1.38 g/dL (95% CI: 1.21 g/dL, 1.55 g/dL).

Conversion From Other Recombinant Erythropoietins

Two studies (N3 and N4) were conducted in adult patients with CRF who had been receiving other recombinant erythropoietins and compared the abilities of Aranesp® and other erythropoietins to maintain hemoglobin concentrations within a study target range of 9 to 13 g/dL. (Note: The recommended hemoglobin target is lower than the target range of these studies. See **DOSAGE AND ADMINISTRATION: General** for recommended clinical hemoglobin target.) CRF patients who had been receiving stable doses of other recombinant erythropoietins were randomized to Aranesp®, or to continue with their prior erythropoietin at the previous dose and schedule. For patients randomized to Aranesp®, the initial weekly dose was determined on the basis of the previous total weekly dose of recombinant erythropoietin. Study N3 was a double-blind study conducted in North America, in which 169 hemodialysis patients were randomized to treatment with Aranesp® and 338 patients continued on Epoetin alfa. Study N4 was an open-label study conducted in Europe and Australia in which 347 patients were randomized to treatment with Aranesp® and 175 patients were randomized to continue on Epoetin alfa or Epoetin beta. Of the 347 patients randomized to Aranesp®, 92% were receiving hemodialysis and 8% were receiving peritoneal dialysis.

In Study N3, a median weekly dose of 0.53 mcg/kg Aranesp® (25th, 75th percentiles: 0.30, 0.93 mcg/kg) was required to maintain hemoglobin in the study target range. In Study N4, a median weekly dose of 0.41 mcg/kg Aranesp® (25th 75th percentiles: 0.26, 0.65 mcg/kg) was required to maintain hemoglobin in the study target range.

Cancer Patients Receiving Chemotherapy

The safety and effectiveness of Aranesp® in reducing the requirement for RBC transfusions in patients undergoing chemotherapy was assessed in a randomized, placebo-controlled, double-blind, multinational study (C1). This study was conducted in anemic (Hgb ≤ 11 g/dL) patients with advanced, small cell or non-small cell lung cancer, who received a platinum-containing chemotherapy regimen. Patients were randomized to receive Aranesp® 2.25 mcg/kg (n = 156) or placebo (n = 158) administered as a single weekly SC injection for up to 12 weeks. The dose was escalated to 4.5 mcg/kg/week at week six, in subjects with an inadequate response to treatment, defined as less than 1 g/dL hemoglobin increase. There were 67 patients in the Aranesp® arm who had their dose increased from 2.25 to 4.5 mcg/kg/week, at any time during the treatment period.

Efficacy was determined by a reduction in the proportion of patients who were transfused over the 12 week treatment period. A significantly lower proportion of patients in the Aranesp® arm, 26% (95% CI: 20%, 33%) required transfusion compared to 60% (95% CI: 52%, 68%) in the placebo arm (Kaplan-Meier estimate of proportion; $p < 0.001$ by Cochran - Mantel - Haenszel test). Of the 67 patients who received a dose increase, 28% had a 2 g/dL increase in hemoglobin over baseline, generally occurring between weeks 8 to 13. Of the 89 patients who did not receive a dose increase, 69% had a 2 g/dL increase in hemoglobin over baseline, generally occurring between weeks 6 to 13.

Studies were conducted that evaluated doses of Aranesp® ranging from 0.5 mcg/kg to 8.0 mcg/kg administered weekly. Data from these studies indicate that there is a dose response relationship with respect to hemoglobin response. The minimally effective starting dose with respect to reducing transfusion requirements was 1.5 mcg/kg/week, with a plateau observed at 4.5 mcg/kg/week.

INDICATIONS AND USAGE

Aranesp® is indicated for the treatment of anemia associated with chronic renal failure, including patients on dialysis and patients not on dialysis, and for the treatment of anemia in patients with non-myeloid malignancies where anemia is due to the effect of concomitantly administered chemotherapy.

CONTRAINDICATIONS

Aranesp® is contraindicated in patients with:

- uncontrolled hypertension
- known hypersensitivity to the active substance or any of the excipients

WARNINGS

Cardiovascular Events, Hemoglobin, and Rate of Rise of Hemoglobin

Aranesp® and other erythropoietic therapies may increase the risk of cardiovascular events, including death. The higher risk of cardiovascular events may be associated with higher hemoglobin and/or higher rates of rise of hemoglobin. The hemoglobin level should be managed carefully to avoid exceeding a target level of 12 g/dL.

In a clinical trial of Epoetin alfa (rHuEPO) treatment in hemodialysis patients with clinically evident cardiac disease, patients were randomized to a target hemoglobin of either 14 ± 1 g/dL or 10 ± 1 g/dL[2]. Higher mortality (35% versus 29%) was observed in the 634 patients randomized to a target hemoglobin of 14 g/dL than in the 631 patients assigned a target hemoglobin of 10 g/dL. The reason for the increased mortality observed in this study is unknown; however, the incidence of nonfatal myocardial infarction, vascular access thrombosis, and other thrombotic events was also higher in the group randomized to a target hemoglobin of 14 g/dL.

In patients treated with Aranesp® or other recombinant erythropoietins in Aranesp® clinical trials, increases in hemoglobin greater than approximately 1.0 g/dL during any 2-week period were associated with increased incidence of cardiac arrest, neurologic events (including seizures and stroke), exacerbations of hypertension, congestive heart failure, vascular thrombosis/ischemia/infarction, acute myocardial infarction, and fluid overload/edema. It is recommended that the dose of Aranesp® be decreased if the hemoglobin increase exceeds 1.0 g/dL in any 2-week period, because of the association of excessive rate of rise of hemoglobin with these events.

Hypertension

Patients with uncontrolled hypertension should not be treated with Aranesp®; blood pressure should be controlled adequately before initiation of therapy. Blood pressure may rise during treatment of anemia with Aranesp® or Epoetin alfa. In Aranesp® clinical trials, approximately 40% of patients with CRF required initiation or intensification of antihypertensive therapy during the early phase of treatment when the hemoglobin was increasing. Hypertensive encephalopathy and seizures have been observed in patients with CRF treated with Aranesp® or Epoetin alfa.

Special care should be taken to closely monitor and control blood pressure in patients treated with Aranesp®. During Aranesp® therapy, patients should be advised of the importance of compliance with antihypertensive therapy and dietary restrictions. If blood pressure is difficult to control by pharmacologic or dietary measures, the dose of Aranesp® should be reduced or withheld (see **DOSAGE AND ADMINISTRATION: Dose Adjustment**). A clinically significant decrease in hemoglobin may not be observed for several weeks.

Seizures

Seizures have occurred in patients with CRF participating in clinical trials of Aranesp® and Epoetin alfa. During the first several months of therapy, blood pressure and the presence of premonitory neurologic symptoms should be monitored closely. While the relationship between seizures and the rate of rise of hemoglobin is uncertain, it is recommended that the dose of Aranesp® be decreased if the hemoglobin increase exceeds 1.0 g/dL in any 2-week period.

Thrombotic Events

An increased incidence of thrombotic events has been observed in patients treated with erythropoietic agents. In patients with cancer who received Aranesp®, pulmonary emboli, thrombophlebitis and thrombosis occurred more frequently than in placebo controls (see **ADVERSE REACTIONS: *Cancer Patients Receiving Chemotherapy*, Table 4**).

Pure Red Cell Aplasia

Pure red cell aplasia (PRCA), in association with neutralizing antibodies to native erythropoietin has been observed in patients treated with recombinant erythropoietins. This has been reported predominantly in patients with CRF. PRCA has been reported in a limited number of subjects exposed to other recombinant erythropoietin products prior to exposure to Aranesp®; therefore, the contribution of Aranesp® to the development of PRCA is unclear. Any patient with loss of response to Aranesp® should be evaluated for the etiology of loss of effect (see **PRECAUTIONS: General**). Aranesp® should be discontinued in any patient with evidence of PRCA and the patient evaluated for the presence of binding and neutralizing antibodies to Aranesp®, native erythropoietin, and any other recombinant erythropoietin administered to the patient. Amgen may be contacted to assist in this evaluation. In patients with PRCA secondary to neutralizing antibodies to erythropoietin, Aranesp® should not be administered.

Albumin (Human)

Aranesp® is supplied in two formulations with different excipients, one containing polysorbate 80 and another containing albumin (human), a derivative of human blood (see **DESCRIPTION**). Based on effective donor screening and product manufacturing processes, Aranesp® formulated with albumin carries an extremely remote risk for transmission of viral diseases. A theoretical risk for transmission of Creutzfeldt-Jakob disease (CJD) also is considered extremely remote. No cases of transmission of viral diseases or CJD have ever been identified for albumin.

PRECAUTIONS

General

The safety and efficacy of Aranesp® therapy have not been established in patients with underlying hematologic diseases (e.g., hemolytic anemia, sickle cell anemia, thalassemia, porphyria).

Lack or Loss of Response to Aranesp®

A lack of response or failure to maintain a hemoglobin response with Aranesp® doses within the recommended dosing range should prompt a search for causative factors. Deficiencies of folic acid or vitamin B_{12} should be excluded or corrected. Depending on the clinical setting, intercurrent infections, inflammatory or malignant processes, osteofibrosis cystica, occult blood loss, hemolysis, severe aluminum toxicity, and bone marrow fibrosis may compromise an erythropoietic response. In the absence of another etiology, the patient should be evaluated for evidence of PRCA and sera should be tested for the presence of antibody to recombinant erythropoietins.

Hematology

Sufficient time should be allowed to determine a patient's responsiveness to a dosage of Aranesp® before adjusting the dose. Because of the time required for erythropoiesis and the RBC half-life, an interval of 2 to 6 weeks may occur between the time of a dose adjustment (initiation, increase, decrease, or discontinuation) and a significant change in hemoglobin.

In order to prevent the hemoglobin from exceeding the recommended target (12 g/dL) or rising too rapidly (greater than 1.0 g/dL in 2 weeks), the guidelines for dose and frequency of dose adjustments should be followed (see **WARNINGS** and **DOSAGE AND ADMINISTRATION: Dose Adjustment**).

Allergic Reactions

There have been rare reports of potentially serious allergic reactions, including skin rash and urticaria, associated with Aranesp®. Symptoms have recurred with rechallenge, suggesting a causal relationship exists in some instances. If a serious allergic or anaphylactic reaction occurs, Aranesp® should be immediately and permanently discontinued and appropriate therapy should be administered.

Patients With CRF Not Requiring Dialysis

Patients with CRF not yet requiring dialysis may require lower maintenance doses of Aranesp® than patients receiving dialysis. Though predialysis patients generally receive less frequent monitoring of blood pressure and laboratory parameters than dialysis patients, predialysis patients may be more responsive to the effects of Aranesp®, and require judicious monitoring of blood pressure and hemoglobin. Renal function and fluid and electrolyte balance should also be closely monitored.

Dialysis Management

Therapy with Aranesp® results in an increase in RBCs and a decrease in plasma volume, which could reduce dialysis efficiency; patients who are marginally dialyzed may require adjustments in their dialysis prescription.

Growth Factor Potential

Aranesp® is a growth factor that primarily stimulates RBC production. The possibility that Aranesp® can act as a growth factor for any tumor type, particularly myeloid malignancies, has not been evaluated. In the randomized, placebo-controlled study in 314 subjects with advanced lung cancer, there were no statistically significant differences in time-to-progression (TTP) or overall survival (OS) observed; however, the study was not designed to detect or exclude clinically meaningful differences in either TTP or OS.

Laboratory Tests

After initiation of Aranesp® therapy, the hemoglobin should be determined weekly until it has stabilized and the maintenance dose has been established (see **DOSAGE AND ADMINISTRATION**). After a dose adjustment, the hemoglobin should be determined weekly for at least 4 weeks, until it has been determined that the hemoglobin has stabilized in response to the dose change. The hemoglobin should then be monitored at regular intervals.

In order to ensure effective erythropoiesis, iron status should be evaluated for all patients before and during treatment, as the majority of patients will eventually require supplemental iron therapy. Supplemental iron therapy is recommended for all patients whose serum ferritin is below 100 mcg/L or whose serum transferrin saturation is below 20%.

Information for Patients

Patients should be informed of the possible side effects of Aranesp® and be instructed to report them to the prescribing physician. Patients should be informed of the signs and symptoms of allergic drug reactions and be advised of appropriate actions. Patients should be counseled on the importance of compliance with their Aranesp® treatment, dietary and dialysis prescriptions, and the importance of judicious monitoring of blood pressure and hemoglobin concentration should be stressed.

It is recommended that Aranesp® should be administered by a healthcare professional. In those rare cases where it is determined that a patient can safely and effectively administer Aranesp® at home, appropriate instruction on the proper use of Aranesp® should be provided for patients and their caregivers, including careful review of the accompanying "Information for Patients" insert. Patients and caregivers should also be cautioned against the reuse of needles, syringes, or drug product, and be thoroughly instructed in their proper disposal. A puncture-resistant container for the disposal of used syringes and needles should be made available to the patient.

Drug Interactions

No formal drug interaction studies of Aranesp® have been performed.

Carcinogenesis, Mutagenesis, and Impairment of Fertility

Carcinogenicity: The carcinogenic potential of Aranesp® has not been evaluated in long-term animal studies. Aranesp® did not alter the proliferative response of non-hematological cells in vitro or in vivo. In toxicity studies of approximately 6 months duration in rats and dogs, no tumorigenic or unexpected mitogenic responses were observed in any tissue type. Using a panel of human tissues, the in vitro tissue binding profile of Aranesp® was identical to Epoetin alfa. Neither molecule bound to human tissues other than those expressing the erythropoietin receptor.

Mutagenicity: Aranesp® was negative in the in vitro bacterial and CHO cell assays to detect mutagenicity and in the in vivo mouse micronucleus assay to detect clastogenicity.

Impairment of Fertility: When administered intravenously to male and female rats prior to and during mating, reproductive performance, fertility, and sperm assessment parameters were not affected at any doses evaluated (up to 10 mcg/kg/dose, administered 3 times weekly). An increase in post implantation fetal loss was seen at doses equal to or greater than 0.5 mcg/kg/dose, administered 3 times weekly.

Pregnancy Category C

When Aranesp® was administered intravenously to rats and rabbits during gestation, no evidence of a direct embryotoxic, fetotoxic, or teratogenic outcome was observed at doses up to 20 mcg/kg/day. The only adverse effect observed was a slight reduction in fetal weight, which occurred at doses causing exaggerated pharmacological effects in the dams (1 mcg/kg/day and higher). No deleterious effects on uterine implantation were seen in either species. No significant placental transfer of Aranesp® was observed in rats. An increase in post implantation fetal loss was observed in studies assessing fertility (see **PRECAUTIONS: Carcinogenesis, Mutagenesis, and Impairment of Fertility: Impairment of Fertility**).

Intravenous injection of Aranesp® to female rats every other day from day 6 of gestation through day 23 of lactation at doses of 2.5 mcg/kg/dose and higher resulted in offspring (F1 generation) with decreased body weights, which correlated with a low incidence of deaths, as well as delayed eye opening and delayed preputial separation. No adverse effects were seen in the F2 offspring.

There are no adequate and well-controlled studies in pregnant women. Aranesp® should be used during pregnancy only if the potential benefit justifies the potential risk to the fetus.

Nursing Mothers

It is not known whether Aranesp® is excreted in human milk. Because many drugs are excreted in human milk, caution should be exercised when Aranesp® is administered to a nursing woman.

Pediatric Use

The safety and efficacy of Aranesp® in pediatric patients have not been established.

Geriatric Use

Of the 1598 CRF patients in clinical studies of Aranesp®, 42% were age 65 and over, while 15% were 75 and over. Of the 873 cancer patients in clinical studies receiving Aranesp® and concomitant chemotherapy, 45% were age 65 and over, while 14% were 75 and over. No overall differences in safety or efficacy were observed between older and younger patients.

ADVERSE REACTIONS

General

Because clinical trials are conducted under widely varying conditions, adverse reaction rates observed in the clinical trials of Aranesp® cannot be directly compared to rates in the clinical trials of other drugs and may not reflect the rates observed in practice.

Chronic Renal Failure Patients

In all studies, the most frequently reported serious adverse reactions with Aranesp® were vascular access thrombosis, congestive heart failure, sepsis, and cardiac arrhythmia. The most commonly reported adverse reactions were infection, hypertension, hypotension, myalgia, headache, and diarrhea, (see **WARNINGS: Cardiovascular Events, Hemoglobin, and Rate of Rise of Hemoglobin,** and **Hypertension**).

The most frequently reported adverse reactions resulting in clinical intervention (e.g., discontinuation of Aranesp®, adjustment in dosage, or the need for concomitant medication to treat an adverse reaction symptom) were hypotension, hypertension, fever, myalgia, nausea, and chest pain.

The data described below reflect exposure to Aranesp® in 1598 CRF patients, including 675 exposed for at least 6 months, of whom 185 were exposed for greater than 1 year. Aranesp® was evaluated in active-controlled (n = 823) and uncontrolled studies (n = 775).

The rates of adverse events and association with Aranesp® are best assessed in the results from studies in which Aranesp® was used to stimulate erythropoiesis in patients anemic at study baseline (n = 348), and, in particular, the subset of these patients in randomized controlled trials (n = 276). Because there were no substantive differences in the rates of adverse reactions between these subpopulations, or between these subpopulations and the entire population of patients treated with Aranesp®, data from all 1598 patients were pooled.

The population encompassed an age range from 18 to 91 years. Fifty-seven percent of the patients were male. The percentages of Caucasian, Black, Asian, and Hispanic patients were 83%, 11%, 3%, and 1%, respectively. The median weekly dose of Aranesp® was 0.45 mcg/kg (25th, 75th percentiles: 0.29, 0.66 mcg/kg).

Some of the adverse events reported are typically associated with CRF, or recognized complications of dialysis, and may not necessarily be attributable to Aranesp® therapy. No important differences in adverse event rates between treatment groups were observed in controlled studies in which patients received Aranesp® or other recombinant erythropoietins.

The data in Table 1 reflect those adverse events occurring in at least 5% of patients treated with Aranesp®.

Table 1. Adverse Events Occurring in ≥ 5% of CRF Patients

Event	Patients Treated With Aranesp® (n = 1598)
APPLICATION SITE	
Injection-site Pain	7%
BODY AS A WHOLE	
Peripheral Edema	11%
Fatigue	9%
Fever	9%
Death	7%
Chest Pain, Unspecified	6%
Fluid Overload	6%
Access Infection	6%
Influenza-like Symptoms	6%
Access Hemorrhage	6%
Asthenia	5%
CARDIOVASCULAR	
Hypertension	23%
Hypotension	22%
Cardiac Arrhythmias/Cardiac Arrest	10%
Angina Pectoris/Cardiac Chest Pain	8%
Thrombosis Vascular Access	8%
Congestive Heart Failure	6%
CNS/PNS	
Headache	16%
Dizziness	8%
GASTROINTESTINAL	
Diarrhea	16%
Vomiting	15%
Nausea	14%
Abdominal Pain	12%
Constipation	5%
MUSCULO-SKELETAL	
Myalgia	21%
Arthralgia	11%
Limb Pain	10%
Back Pain	8%
RESISTANCE MECHANISM	
Infection[a]	27%
RESPIRATORY	
Upper Respiratory Infection	14%
Dyspnea	12%
Cough	10%
Bronchitis	6%
SKIN AND APPENDAGES	
Pruritus	8%

[a] Infection includes sepsis, bacteremia, pneumonia, peritonitis, and abscess.

The incidence rates for other clinically significant events are shown in Table 2

Table 2. Percent Incidence of Other Clinically Significant Events in CRF Patients

Event	Patients Treated With Aranesp® (n = 1598)
Acute Myocardial Infarction	2%
Seizure	1%
Stroke	1%
Transient Ischemic Attack	1%

Thrombotic Events

Vascular access thrombosis in hemodialysis patients occurred in clinical trials at an annualized rate of 0.22 events per patient year of Aranesp® therapy. Rates of thrombotic events (e.g., vascular access thrombosis, venous thrombosis, and pulmonary emboli) with Aranesp® therapy were similar to those observed with other recombinant erythropoietins in these trials; the median duration of exposure was 12 weeks.

Cancer Patients Receiving Chemotherapy

The data described below reflect the exposure to Aranesp® in 873 cancer patients. Aranesp® was evaluated in seven studies that were active-controlled and/or placebo-controlled studies of up to 6 months duration. The Aranesp®-treated patient demographics were as follows: median age of 63 years (range of 20 to 91 years); 40% male; 88% Caucasian, 5% Hispanic, 4% Black, and 3% Asian. Over 90% of patients had locally advanced or metastatic cancer, with the remainder having early stage disease. Patients with solid tumors (e.g., lung, breast, colon, ovarian cancers), and lymphoproliferative malignancies (e.g., lymphoma, multiple myeloma) were enrolled in the clinical studies. All of the 873 Aranesp®-treated subjects also received concomitant cyclic chemotherapy.

The most frequently reported serious adverse events included death (10%), fever (4%), pneumonia (3%), dehydration (3%), vomiting (2%), and dyspnea (2%). The most commonly reported adverse events were fatigue, edema, nausea, vomiting, diarrhea, fever and dyspnea (see **Table 3**). Except for those events listed in Tables 3 and 4, the incidence of adverse events in clinical studies occurred at a similar rate compared with patients who received placebo and were generally consistent with the underlying disease and its treatment with chemotherapy. The most frequently reported reasons for discontinuation of Aranesp® were progressive disease, death, discontinuation of the chemotherapy, asthenia, dyspnea, pneumonia, and gastrointestinal hemorrhage. No important differences in adverse event rates between treatment groups were observed in controlled studies in which patients received Aranesp® or other recombinant erythropoietins.

Continued on next page

Aranesp—Cont.

Table 3. Adverse Events Occurring in ≥ 5% of Patients Receiving Chemotherapy

Event	Aranesp® (n = 873)	Placebo (n = 221)
BODY AS A WHOLE		
Fatigue	33%	30%
Edema	21%	10%
Fever	19%	16%
CNS/PNS		
Dizziness	14%	8%
Headache	12%	9%
GASTROINTESTINAL		
Diarrhea	22%	12%
Constipation	18%	17%
METABOLIC/NUTRITION		
Dehydration	5%	3%
MUSCULO-SKELETAL		
Arthralgia	13%	6%
Myalgia	8%	5%
SKIN AND APPENDAGES		
Rash	7%	3%

Table 4. Incidence of Other Clinically Significant Adverse Events in Patients Receiving Chemotherapy

Event	All Aranesp® (n = 873)	Placebo (n = 221)
Hypertension	3.7%	3.2%
Seizures/Convulsions[a]	0.6%	0.5%
Thrombotic Events	6.2%	4.1%
Pulmonary Embolism	1.3%	0.0%
Thrombosis[b]	5.6%	4.1%

[a] Seizures/Convulsions include the preferred terms: Convulsions, Convulsions Grand Mal, and Convulsions Local.

[b] Thrombosis includes: Thrombophlebitis, Thrombophlebitis Deep, Thrombosis Venous, Thrombosis Venous Deep, Thromboembolism, and Thrombosis

Thrombotic and Cardiovascular Events

Overall, the incidence of thrombotic events was 6.2% for Aranesp® and 4.1% for placebo. However, the following events were reported more frequently in Aranesp®-treated patients than in placebo controls: pulmonary embolism, thromboembolism, thrombosis, and thrombophlebitis (deep and/or superficial). In addition, edema of any type was more frequently reported in Aranesp®-treated (21%) patients than in patients who received placebo (10%).

Immunogenicity

As with all therapeutic proteins, there is a potential for immunogenicity. The incidence of antibody development in patients receiving Aranesp® has not been adequately determined. Radioimmunoprecipitation assays were performed on sera from 1534 CRF and 833 cancer patients treated with Aranesp® in clinical studies. High-titer antibodies were not detected in patients with CRF, but assay sensitivity may be inadequate to reliably detect lower titers. Antibodies were detected by radioimmunoprecipitation in sera from three cancer patients; neutralizing activity, possibly related to antibodies, was detected in one of these three patients. There was no evidence of PRCA in that patient (see **WARNINGS: Pure Red Cell Aplasia**).

The incidence of antibody formation is highly dependent on the sensitivity and specificity of the assay. Additionally, the observed incidence of antibody positivity in an assay may be influenced by several factors including sample handling, timing of sample collection, concomitant medications, and underlying disease. For these reasons, comparison of the incidence of antibodies to Aranesp®, with the incidence of antibodies to other products may be misleading.

OVERDOSAGE

The maximum amount of Aranesp® that can be safely administered in single or multiple doses has not been determined. Doses over 3.0 mcg/kg/week for up to 28 weeks have been administered to CRF patients. Doses up to 8.0 mcg/kg every week and 15.0 mcg/kg every 3 weeks have been administered to cancer patients for up to 12-16 weeks. Excessive rise and rate of rise in hemoglobin concentration, however, have been associated with adverse events (see **WARNINGS** and **DOSAGE AND ADMINISTRATION: Dose Adjustment**). In the event of polycythemia, Aranesp® should be temporarily withheld (see **DOSAGE AND ADMINISTRATION: Dose Adjustment**). If clinically indicated, phlebotomy may be performed.

DOSAGE AND ADMINISTRATION

General

IMPORTANT: Aranesp® dosing regimens are different for each of the indications described in this section of the package insert. Due to the longer serum half-life, Aranesp® should be administered less frequently than Epoetin alfa (for example, where Epoetin alfa is administered three times a week, Aranesp® should be administered weekly). Aranesp® should be administered under the supervision of a healthcare professional.

Single-dose Vial, Polysorbate Solution

1 Vial/Pack, 4 Packs/Case	4 Vials/Pack, 4 Packs/Case	4 Vials/Pack, 10 Packs/Case
200 mcg/1 mL (NDC 55513-006-01)	200 mcg/1 mL (NDC 55513-006-04)	25 mcg/1 mL (NDC 55513-002-04)
300 mcg/1 mL (NDC 55513-110-01)	300 mcg/1 mL (NDC 55513-110-04)	40 mcg/1 mL (NDC 55513-003-04)
500 mcg/1 mL (NDC 55513-008-01)		60 mcg/1 mL (NDC 55513-004-04)
		100 mcg/1 mL (NDC 55513-005-04)
		150 mcg/0.75 mL (NDC 55513-053-04)

Single-dose Vial, Albumin Solution

1 Vial/Pack, 4 Packs/Case	4 Vials/Pack, 4 Packs/Case	4 Vials/Pack, 10 Packs/Case
200 mcg/1 mL (NDC 55513-014-01)	200 mcg/1 mL (NDC 55513-014-04)	25 mcg/1 mL (NDC 55513-010-04)
300 mcg/1 mL (NDC 55513-015-01)	300 mcg/1 mL (NDC 55513-015-04)	40 mcg/1 mL (NDC 55513-011-04)
500 mcg/1 mL (NDC 55513-016-01)		60 mcg/1 mL (NDC 55513-012-04)
		100 mcg/1 mL (NDC 55513-013-04)
		150 mcg/0.75 mL (NDC 55513-054-04)

Single-dose Prefilled Syringe (SingleJect®) With a 27 gauge, ½ inch Needle With an UltraSafe® Needle Guard, Polysorbate Solution

1 Syringe/Pack, 4 Packs/Case	4 Syringes/Pack, 4 Packs/Case	4 Syringes/Pack, 10 Packs/Case
200 mcg/0.4 mL (NDC 55513-028-01)	200 mcg/0.4 mL (NDC 55513-028-04)	25 mcg/0.42 mL (NDC 55513-057-04)
300 mcg/0.6 mL (NDC 55513-111-01)	300 mcg/0.6 mL (NDC 55513-111-04)	40 mcg/0.4 mL (NDC 55513-021-04)
500 mcg/1 mL (NDC 55513-032-01)		60 mcg/0.3 mL (NDC 55513-023-04)
		100 mcg/0.5 mL (NDC 55513-025-04)
		150 mcg/0.3 mL (NDC 55513-027-04)

Single-dose Prefilled Syringe (SingleJect®) With a 27 gauge, ½ inch Needle With an UltraSafe® Needle Guard, Albumin Solution

1 Syringe/Pack, 4 Packs/Case	4 Syringes/Pack, 4 Packs/Case	4 Syringes/Pack, 10 Packs/Case
200 mcg/0.4 mL (NDC 55513-044-01)	200 mcg/0.4 mL (NDC 55513-044-04)	25 mcg/0.42 mL (NDC 55513-058-04)
300 mcg/0.6 mL (NDC 55513-046-01)	300 mcg/0.6 mL (NDC 55513-046-04)	40 mcg/0.4 mL (NDC 55513-037-04)
500 mcg/1 mL (NDC 55513-048-01)		60 mcg/0.3 mL (NDC 55513-039-04)
		100 mcg/0.5 mL (NDC 55513-041-04)
		150 mcg/0.3 mL (NDC 55513-043-04)

Aranesp® is supplied in either vials or in prefilled syringes with UltraSafe® Needle Guards*. Following administration of Aranesp® from the prefilled syringe, the UltraSafe® Needle Guard should be activated to prevent accidental needle sticks.

Chronic Renal Failure Patients

Aranesp® is administered either IV or SC as a single weekly injection. The dose should be started and slowly adjusted as described below based on hemoglobin levels. If a patient fails to respond or maintain a response, other etiologies should be considered and evaluated (see **PRECAUTIONS: General** and **Laboratory Tests**). When Aranesp® therapy is initiated or adjusted, the hemoglobin should be followed weekly until stabilized and monitored at least monthly thereafter.

For patients who respond to Aranesp® with a rapid increase in hemoglobin (e.g., more than 1.0 g/dL in any 2-week period), the dose of Aranesp® should be reduced (see **DOSAGE AND ADMINISTRATION: Dose Adjustment**) because of the association of excessive rate of rise of hemoglobin with adverse events (see **WARNINGS: Cardiovascular Events, Hemoglobin, and Rate of Rise of Hemoglobin**).

The dose should be adjusted for each patient to achieve and maintain a target hemoglobin level not to exceed 12 g/dL.

Starting Dose

Correction of Anemia

The recommended starting dose of Aranesp® for the correction of anemia in CRF patients is 0.45 mcg/kg body weight, administered as a single IV or SC injection once weekly. Because of individual variability, doses should be titrated to not exceed a target hemoglobin concentration of 12 g/dL (see **DOSAGE AND ADMINISTRATION: Dose Adjustment**). For many patients, the appropriate maintenance dose will be lower than this starting dose. Predialysis patients, in particular, may require lower maintenance doses. Also, some patients have been treated successfully with a SC dose of Aranesp® administered once every 2 weeks.

Conversion From Epoetin alfa to Aranesp®

The starting weekly dose of Aranesp® should be estimated on the basis of the weekly Epoetin alfa dose at the time of substitution (see **Table 5**). Because of individual variability, doses should then be titrated to maintain the target hemoglobin. Due to the longer serum half-life, Aranesp® should be administered less frequently than Epoetin alfa. Aranesp® should be administered once a week if a patient was receiving Epoetin alfa 2 to 3 times weekly. Aranesp® should be administered once every 2 weeks if a patient was receiving Epoetin alfa once per week. The route of administration (IV or SC) should be maintained.

Table 5. Estimated Aranesp® Starting Doses (mcg/week) Based on Previous Epoetin alfa Dose (Units/week)

Previous Weekly Epoetin alfa Dose (Units/week)	Weekly Aranesp® Dose (mcg/week)
< 2,500	6.25
2,500 to 4,999	12.5
5,000 to 10,999	25
11,000 to 17,999	40
18,000 to 33,999	60
34,000 to 89,999	100
≥ 90,000	200

Dose Adjustment

The dose should be adjusted for each patient to achieve and maintain a target hemoglobin not to exceed 12 g/dL. Increases in dose should not be made more frequently than once a month. If the hemoglobin is increasing and approaching 12 g/dL, the dose should be reduced by approximately 25%. If the hemoglobin continues to increase, doses should be temporarily withheld until the hemoglobin begins to decrease, at which point therapy should be reinitiated at a dose approximately 25% below the previous dose. If the hemoglobin increases by more than 1.0 g/dL in a 2 week period, the dose should be decreased by approximately 25%. If the increase in hemoglobin is less than 1.0 g/dL over 4 weeks and iron stores are adequate (see **PRECAUTIONS: Laboratory Tests**), the dose of Aranesp® may be increased by approximately 25% of the previous dose. Further increases may be made at 4-week intervals until the specified hemoglobin is obtained.

Maintenance Dose

Aranesp® dosage should be adjusted to maintain a target hemoglobin not to exceed 12 g/dL. If the hemoglobin exceeds 12 g/dL, the dose may be adjusted as described above. Doses must be individualized to ensure that hemoglobin is maintained at an appropriate level for each patient.

Cancer Patients Receiving Chemotherapy

The recommended starting dose for Aranesp® is 2.25 mcg/kg administered as a weekly SC injection.

The dose should be adjusted for each patient to achieve and maintain a target hemoglobin. If there is less than a 1.0 g/dL increase in hemoglobin after 6 weeks of therapy, the dose of Aranesp® should be increased up to 4.5 mcg/kg. If hemoglobin increases by more than 1.0 g/dL in a 2-week period or if the hemoglobin exceeds 12 g/dL, the dose should be reduced by approximately 25%. If the hemoglobin exceeds 13 g/dL, doses should be temporarily withheld until the hemoglobin falls to 12 g/dL. At this point, therapy should be reinitiated at a dose approximately 25% below the previous dose.

Preparation and Administration of Aranesp®

Do not shake Aranesp® or leave vials or syringes exposed to bright light. After removing the vials or prefilled syringes from the cartons, keep them covered to protect from room light until administration. Vigorous shaking or exposure to light may denature Aranesp® causing it to become biologically inactive. Always store vials or prefilled syringes of Aranesp® in their carton until use.

Parenteral drug products should be inspected visually for particulate matter and discoloration prior to administration. Do not use any vials or prefilled syringes exhibiting particulate matter or discoloration.

Do not dilute Aranesp®.

Do not administer Aranesp® in conjunction with other drug solutions.

Aranesp® is packaged in single-dose vials and prefilled syringes and contains no preservative. Discard any unused portion. **Do not pool unused portions from the vials or prefilled syringes. Do not use the vial or prefilled syringe more than one time.**

Following administration of Aranesp® from the prefilled syringe, activate the UltraSafe® Needle Guard. Place your hands behind the needle, grasp the guard with one hand, and slide the guard forward until the needle is completely covered and the guard clicks into place. NOTE: If an audible click is not heard, the needle guard may not be completely activated. The prefilled syringe should be disposed of by placing the entire prefilled syringe with guard activated into an approved puncture-proof container.

See the accompanying "Information for Patients" leaflet for complete instructions on the preparation and administration of Aranesp® for patients.

HOW SUPPLIED

Aranesp® is available in single-dose vials in two solutions, an albumin solution and a polysorbate solution. The words "Albumin Free" appear on the polysorbate container labels and the package main panels as well as other panels as space permits. Aranesp® albumin solution is also available in single-dose prefilled syringes supplied with a 27 gauge, ½ inch needle. To reduce the risk of accidental needlesticks to users, each prefilled syringe is equipped with an UltraSafe® Needle Guard that covers the needle during disposal. Aranesp® is available in the following packages:

[See first table at top of previous page]

[See second table at top of previous page]

Storage

Store at 2° to 8°C (36° to 46°F). Do not freeze or shake. Protect from light.

REFERENCES

1. Egrie JC, Browne JK. Development and characterization of novel erythropoiesis stimulating protein (NESP). *Br J Cancer.* 2001;84(suppl 1):3-10.
2. Besarab A, Bolton WK, Browne JK, et al. The effects of normal as compared with low hematocrit values in patients with cardiac disease who are receiving hemodialysis and epoetin. *N Engl J Med.* 1998;339:584-90.

℞ only

This product, or its use, may be covered by one or more US Patents, including US Patent No. 5,618,698, in addition to others including patents pending.

Manufactured by:

Amgen Manufacturing, Limited, a subsidiary of Amgen Inc.
One Amgen Center Drive
Thousand Oaks, CA 91320-1799

* UltraSafe® is a registered trademark of Safety Syringes, Inc.

Issue Date: 12/12/2003
3240603 – v4

Shown in Product Identification Guide, pages 304, 305

ENBREL® ℞

[ən-brĕl]
(etanercept)

DESCRIPTION

ENBREL® (etanercept) is a dimeric fusion protein consisting of the extracellular ligand-binding portion of the human 75 kilodalton (p75) tumor necrosis factor receptor (TNFR) linked to the Fc portion of human IgG1. The Fc component of etanercept contains the C_H2 domain, the C_H3 domain and hinge region, but not the C_H1 domain of IgG1. Etanercept is produced by recombinant DNA technology in a Chinese hamster ovary (CHO) mammalian cell expression system. It consists of 934 amino acids and has an apparent molecular weight of approximately 150 kilodaltons.

Table 1:
ACR Responses in Placebo- and Active-Controlled Trials
(Percent of Patients)

	Placebo Controlled				Active Controlled	
	Study I		Study II		Study III	
	Placebo	ENBREL®[a]	MTX/ Placebo	MTX/ ENBREL®[a]	MTX	ENBREL®[a]
Response	N = 80	N = 78	N = 30	N = 59	N = 217	N = 207
ACR 20						
Month 3	23%	62%[b]	33%	66%[b]	56%	62%
Month 6	11%	59%[b]	27%	71%[b]	58%	65%
Month 12	NA	NA	NA	NA	65%	72%
ACR 50						
Month 3	8%	41%[b]	0%	42%[b]	24%	29%
Month 6	5%	40%[b]	3%	39%[b]	32%	40%
Month 12	NA	NA	NA	NA	43%	49%
ACR 70						
Month 3	4%	15%[b]	0%	15%[b]	7%	13%[c]
Month 6	1%	15%[b]	0%	15%[b]	14%	21%[c]
Month 12	NA	NA	NA	NA	22%	25%

[a] 25 mg ENBREL® SC twice weekly.
[b] $p < 0.01$, ENBREL® vs. placebo.
[c] $p < 0.05$, ENBREL® vs. MTX.

ENBREL® is supplied as a sterile, white, preservative-free, lyophilized powder for parenteral administration after reconstitution with 1 mL of the supplied Sterile Bacteriostatic Water for Injection (BWFI), USP (containing 0.9% benzyl alcohol). Reconstitution with the supplied BWFI yields a multiple-use, clear, and colorless solution of ENBREL® with a pH of 7.4 ± 0.3. Each vial of ENBREL® contains 25 mg etanercept, 40 mg mannitol, 10 mg sucrose, and 1.2 mg tromethamine.

CLINICAL PHARMACOLOGY

General

Etanercept binds specifically to tumor necrosis factor (TNF) and blocks its interaction with cell surface TNF receptors. TNF is a naturally occurring cytokine that is involved in normal inflammatory and immune responses. It plays an important role in the inflammatory processes of rheumatoid arthritis (RA), polyarticular-course juvenile rheumatoid arthritis (JRA), and ankylosing spondylitis and the resulting joint pathology. In addition, TNF plays a role in the inflammatory process of plaque psoriasis. Elevated levels of TNF are found in involved tissues and fluids of patients with RA, psoriatic arthritis, ankylosing spondylitis (AS), and plaque psoriasis.

Two distinct receptors for TNF (TNFRs), a 55 kilodalton protein (p55) and a 75 kilodalton protein (p75), exist naturally as monomeric molecules on cell surfaces and in soluble forms. Biological activity of TNF is dependent upon binding to either cell surface TNFR.

Etanercept is a dimeric soluble form of the p75 TNF receptor that can bind to two TNF molecules. It inhibits the activity of TNF in vitro and has been shown to affect several animal models of inflammation, including murine collagen-induced arthritis. Etanercept inhibits binding of both TNFα and TNFβ (lymphotoxin alpha [LTα]) to cell surface TNFRs, rendering TNF biologically inactive. Cells expressing transmembrane TNF that bind ENBREL® are not lysed in vitro in the presence or absence of complement.

Etanercept can also modulate biological responses that are induced or regulated by TNF, including expression of adhesion molecules responsible for leukocyte migration (i.e., E-selectin and to a lesser extent intercellular adhesion molecule-1 [ICAM-1]), serum levels of cytokines (e.g., IL-6), and serum levels of matrix metalloproteinase-3 (MMP-3 or stromelysin).

Pharmacokinetics

After administration of 25 mg of ENBREL® by a single subcutaneous (SC) injection to 25 patients with RA, a mean ± standard deviation half-life of 102 ± 30 hours was observed with a clearance of 160 ± 80 mL/hr. A maximum serum concentration (Cmax) of 1.1 ± 0.6 mcg/mL and time to Cmax of 69 ± 34 hours was observed in these patients following a single 25 mg dose. After 6 months of twice weekly 25 mg doses in these same RA patients, the mean Cmax was 2.4 ± 1.0 mcg/mL (N = 23). Patients exhibited a two- to seven-fold increase in peak serum concentrations and approximately four-fold increase in $AUC_{0\text{-}72hr}$ (range 1 to 17 fold) with repeated dosing. Serum concentrations in patients with RA have not been measured for periods of dosing that exceed 6 months. The pharmacokinetic parameters in patients with plaque psoriasis were similar to those seen in patients with RA.

In another study, serum concentration profiles at steady state were comparable among patients with RA treated with 50 mg ENBREL® once weekly and those treated with 25 mg ENBREL® twice weekly. The mean (± standard deviation) Cmax, Cmin, and partial AUC were 2.4 ± 1.5 mg/L, 1.2 ± 0.7 mg/L, and 297 ± 166 mg•h/L, respectively, for patients treated with 50 mg ENBREL® once weekly (N = 21); and 2.6 ± 1.2 mg/L, 1.4 ± 0.7 mg/L, and 316 ± 135 mg•h/L for patients treated with 25 mg ENBREL® twice weekly (N = 16).

Pharmacokinetic parameters were not different between men and women and did not vary with age in adult patients.

No formal pharmacokinetic studies have been conducted to examine the effects of renal or hepatic impairment on ENBREL® disposition.

Patients with JRA (ages 4 to 17 years) were administered 0.4 mg/kg of ENBREL® twice weekly for up to 18 weeks. The mean serum concentration after repeated SC dosing was 2.1 mcg/mL, with a range of 0.7 to 4.3 mcg/mL. Limited data suggests that the clearance of ENBREL® is reduced slightly in children ages 4 to 8 years. Population pharmacokinetic analyses predict that administration of 0.8 mg/kg of ENBREL® once weekly will result in Cmax 11% higher, and Cmin 20% lower at steady state as compared to administration of 0.4 mg/kg of ENBREL® twice weekly. The predicted pharmacokinetic differences between the regimens in JRA patients are of the same magnitude as the differences observed between twice weekly and weekly regimens in adult RA patients. The pharmacokinetics of ENBREL® in children < 4 years of age have not been studied.

CLINICAL STUDIES

Adult Rheumatoid Arthritis

The safety and efficacy of ENBREL® were assessed in three randomized, double-blind, controlled studies. Study I evaluated 234 patients with active RA who were ≥ 18 years old, had failed therapy with at least one but no more than four disease-modifying antirheumatic drugs (DMARDs; e.g., hydroxychloroquine, oral or injectable gold, methotrexate [MTX], azathioprine, D-penicillamine, sulfasalazine), and had ≥ 12 tender joints, ≥ 10 swollen joints, and either ESR ≥ 28 mm/hr, CRP > 2.0 mg/dL, or morning stiffness for ≥ 45 minutes. Doses of 10 mg or 25 mg ENBREL® or placebo were administered SC twice a week for 6 consecutive months. Results from patients receiving 25 mg are presented in Table 1.

Study II evaluated 89 patients and had similar inclusion criteria to Study I except that subjects in Study II had additionally received MTX for at least 6 months with a stable dose (12.5 to 25 mg/week) for at least 4 weeks and they had at least 6 tender or painful joints. Subjects in Study II received a dose of 25 mg ENBREL® or placebo SC twice a week for 6 months in addition to their stable MTX dose.

Study III compared the efficacy of ENBREL® to MTX in patients with active RA. This study evaluated 632 patients who were ≥ 18 years old with early (≤ 3 years disease duration) active RA; had never received treatment with MTX; and had ≥ 12 tender joints, ≥ 10 swollen joints, and either ESR ≥ 28 mm/hr, CRP > 2.0 mg/dL, or morning stiffness for ≥ 45 minutes. Doses of 10 mg or 25 mg ENBREL® were administered SC twice a week for 12 consecutive months. The study was unblinded after all patients had completed at least 12 months (and a median of 17.3 months) of therapy. The majority of patients remained in the study on the treatment to which they were randomized through 2 years, after which they entered an extension study and received open-label 25 mg ENBREL®. Results from patients receiving 25 mg are presented in Table 1. MTX tablets (escalated from 7.5 mg/week to a maximum of 20 mg/week over the first 8 weeks of the trial) or placebo tablets were given once a week on the same day as the injection of placebo or ENBREL® doses, respectively.

The results of all three trials were expressed in percentage of patients with improvement in RA using American College of Rheumatology (ACR) response criteria.

Clinical Response

The percent of ENBREL®-treated patients achieving ACR 20, 50, and 70 responses was consistent across all three trials. The results of the three trials are summarized in Table 1.

[See table 1 above]

The time course for ACR 20 response rates for patients receiving placebo or 25 mg ENBREL® in Studies I and II is

Continued on next page

Enbrel—Cont.

summarized in Figure 1. The time course of responses to ENBREL® in Study III was similar.

Figure 1
Time Course of ACR 20 Responses

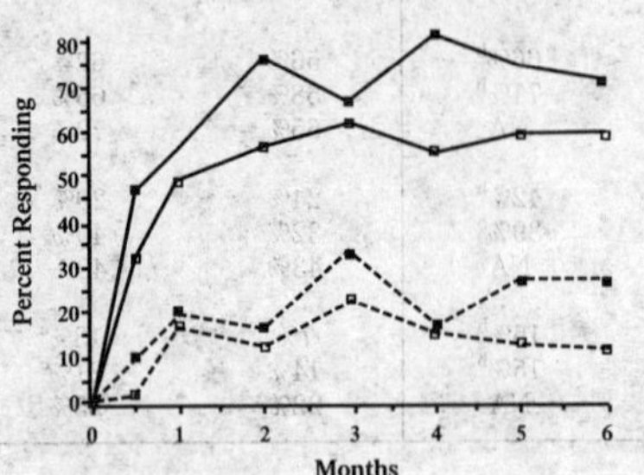

Among patients receiving ENBREL®, the clinical responses generally appeared within 1 to 2 weeks after initiation of therapy and nearly always occurred by 3 months. A dose response was seen in Studies I and III: 25 mg ENBREL® was more effective than 10 mg (10 mg was not evaluated in Study II). ENBREL® was significantly better than placebo in all components of the ACR criteria as well as other measures of RA disease activity not included in the ACR response criteria, such as morning stiffness.

In Study III, ACR response rates and improvement in all the individual ACR response criteria were maintained through 24 months of ENBREL® therapy. Over the 2-year study, 23% of ENBREL® patients achieved a major clinical response, defined as maintenance of an ACR 70 response over a 6-month period.

The results of the components of the ACR response criteria for Study I are shown in Table 2. Similar results were observed for ENBREL®-treated patients in Studies II and III.

[See table 2 at right]

Table 2:
Components of ACR Response in Study I

Parameter (median)	Placebo N = 80 Baseline	3 Months	ENBREL®[a] N = 78 Baseline	3 Months*
Number of tender joints[b]	34.0	29.5	31.2	10.0[f]
Number of swollen joints[c]	24.0	22.0	23.5	12.6[f]
Physician global assessment[d]	7.0	6.5	7.0	3.0[f]
Patient global assessment[d]	7.0	7.0	7.0	3.0[f]
Pain[d]	6.9	6.6	6.9	2.4[f]
Disability index[e]	1.7	1.8	1.6	1.0[f]
ESR (mm/hr)	31.0	32.0	28.0	15.5[f]
CRP (mg/dL)	2.8	3.9	3.5	0.9[f]

* Results at 6 months showed similar improvement.
[a] 25 mg ENBREL® SC twice weekly.
[b] Scale 0-71.
[c] Scale 0-68.
[d] Visual analog scale; 0 = best, 10 = worst.
[e] Health Assessment Questionnaire[1]; 0 = best, 3 = worst; includes eight categories: dressing and grooming, arising, eating, walking, hygiene, reach, grip, and activities.
[f] $p < 0.01$, ENBREL® vs. placebo, based on mean percent change from baseline.

After discontinuation of ENBREL®, symptoms of arthritis generally returned within a month. Reintroduction of treatment with ENBREL® after discontinuations of up to 18 months resulted in the same magnitudes of response as patients who received ENBREL® without interruption of therapy based on results of open-label studies.

Continued durable responses have been seen for up to 36 months in open-label extension treatment trials when patients received ENBREL® without interruption. Some patients receiving ENBREL® for up to 3 years have been able to dose reduce and even discontinue concomitant steroids and/or methotrexate while maintaining a clinical response.

A Health Assessment Questionnaire (HAQ),[1] which included disability, vitality, mental health, general health status, and arthritis-associated health status subdomains, was administered every 3 months during Studies I and III. All subdomains of the HAQ were improved in patients treated with ENBREL®.

In Study III, health outcome measures were assessed by the SF-36 questionnaire. The eight subscales of the SF-36 were combined into two summary scales, the physical component summary (PCS) and the mental component summary (MCS).[2] At 12 months, patients treated with 25 mg ENBREL® showed significantly more improvement in the PCS compared to the 10 mg ENBREL® group, but not in the MCS. Improvement in the PCS was maintained over the 24 months of ENBREL® therapy.

A 24-week study was conducted in 242 patients with active RA on background methotrexate who were randomized to receive either ENBREL® alone or the combination of ENBREL® and anakinra. The ACR_{50} response rate was 31% for patients treated with the combination of ENBREL® and anakinra and 41% for patients treated with ENBREL® alone, indicating no added clinical benefit of the combination over ENBREL® alone. Serious infections were increased with the combination compared to ENBREL® alone (see **WARNINGS**).

Physical Function Response

In Studies I, II, and III, physical function and disability were assessed using the HAQ.[1] Additionally, in Study III, patients were administered the SF-36[2] Health Survey. In Studies I and II, patients treated with 25 mg ENBREL® twice weekly showed greater improvement from baseline in the HAQ score beginning in month 1 through month 6 in comparison to placebo ($p < 0.001$) for the HAQ disability domain (where 0 = none and 3 = severe). In Study I, the mean improvement in the HAQ score from baseline to month 6 was 0.6 (from 1.6 to 1.0) for the 25 mg ENBREL® group and 0 (from 1.7 to 1.7) for the placebo group. In Study II, the mean improvement from baseline to month 6 was 0.6 (from 1.5 to 0.9) for the ENBREL®/MTX group and 0.2 (from 1.3 to 1.2) for the placebo/MTX group. In Study III, the mean improvement in the HAQ score from baseline to month 6 was 0.7 (from 1.5 to 0.7) for 25 mg ENBREL® twice weekly.

In Study III, patients treated with 25 mg ENBREL® twice weekly showed greater improvement from baseline in SF-36 physical component summary score compared to ENBREL® 10 mg twice weekly and no worsening in the SF-36 mental component summary score. In open-label ENBREL® studies, improvements in physical function and disability measures have been maintained for up to 4 years.

Table 3:
Mean Radiographic Change Over 6 and 12 Months In Study III

		MTX	25 mg ENBREL®	MTX-ENBREL® (95% Confidence Interval*)	P-value
12 Months	Total Sharp score	1.59	1.00	0.59 (-0.12, 1.30)	0.110
	Erosion score	1.03	0.47	0.56 (0.11, 1.00)	0.002
	JSN score	0.56	0.52	0.04 (-0.39, 0.46)	0.529
6 Months	Total Sharp score	1.06	0.57	0.49 (0.06, 0.91)	0.001
	Erosion score	0.68	0.30	0.38 (0.09, 0.66)	0.001
	JSN score	0.38	0.27	0.11 (-0.14, 0.35)	0.585

*95% confidence intervals for the differences in change scores between MTX and ENBREL®

Radiographic Response

In Study III, structural joint damage was assessed radiographically and expressed as change in total Sharp score (TSS) and its components, the erosion score and joint space narrowing (JSN) score. Radiographs of hands/wrists and forefeet were obtained at baseline, 6 months, 12 months, and 24 months and scored by readers who were unaware of treatment group. The results are shown in Table 3. A significant difference for change in erosion score was observed at 6 months and maintained at 12 months.

[See table 3 above]

Patients continued on the therapy to which they were randomized for the second year of Study III. Seventy-two percent of patients had x-rays obtained at 24 months. Compared to the patients in the MTX group, greater inhibition of progression in TSS and erosion score was seen in the 25 mg ENBREL® group, and in addition, less progression was noted in the JSN score.

In the open-label extension of Study III, 55% of the original patients treated with 25 mg ENBREL® have been evaluated radiographically at 4 years. Patients had continued inhibition of structural damage, as measured by the TSS, and 65% of them had no progression of structural damage. Patients originally treated with MTX had further reduction in radiographic progression once they began treatment with ENBREL®.

Once Weekly Dosing

The safety and efficacy of 50 mg ENBREL® (two 25 mg SC injections) administered once weekly were evaluated in a double-blind, placebo-controlled study of 420 patients with active RA. Fifty-three patients received placebo, 214 patients received 50 mg ENBREL® once weekly, 153 patients received 25 mg ENBREL® twice weekly. The safety and efficacy profiles of the two ENBREL® treatment groups were similar.

Polyarticular-Course Juvenile Rheumatoid Arthritis (JRA)

The safety and efficacy of ENBREL® were assessed in a two-part study in 69 children with polyarticular-course JRA who had a variety of JRA onset types. Patients ages 4 to 17 years with moderately to severely active polyarticular-course JRA refractory to or intolerant of methotrexate were enrolled; patients remained on a stable dose of a single nonsteroidal anti-inflammatory drug and/or prednisone (≤ 0.2 mg/kg/day or 10 mg maximum). In part 1, all patients received 0.4 mg/kg (maximum 25 mg per dose) ENBREL® SC twice weekly. In part 2, patients with a clinical response at day 90 were randomized to remain on ENBREL® or receive placebo for four months and assessed for disease flare. Responses were measured using the JRA Definition of Improvement (DOI),[3] defined as ≥ 30% improvement in at least three of six and ≥ 30% worsening in no more than one of the six JRA core set criteria, including active joint count, limitation of motion, physician and patient/parent global assessments, functional assessment, and ESR. Disease flare was defined as a ≥ 30% worsening in three of the six JRA core set criteria and ≥ 30% improvement in not more than one of the six JRA core set criteria and a minimum of two active joints.

In part 1 of the study, 51 of 69 (74%) patients demonstrated a clinical response and entered part 2. In part 2, 6 of 25 (24%) patients remaining on ENBREL® experienced a disease flare compared to 20 of 26 (77%) patients receiving placebo ($p = 0.007$). From the start of part 2, the median time to flare was ≥ 116 days for patients who received ENBREL® and 28 days for patients who received placebo. Each component of the JRA core set criteria worsened in the arm that received placebo and remained stable or improved in the arm that continued on ENBREL®. The data suggested the possibility of a higher flare rate among those patients with a higher baseline ESR. Of patients who demonstrated a clinical response at 90 days and entered part 2 of the study, some of the patients remaining on ENBREL® continued to improve from month 3 through month 7, while those who received placebo did not improve.

The majority of JRA patients who developed a disease flare in part 2 and reintroduced ENBREL® treatment up to 4 months after discontinuation re-responded to ENBREL® therapy in open-label studies. Most of the responding patients who continued ENBREL® therapy without interruption have maintained responses for up to 18 months.

Studies have not been done in patients with polyarticular-course JRA to assess the effects of continued ENBREL® therapy in patients who do not respond within 3 months of initiating ENBREL® therapy, or to assess the combination of ENBREL® with methotrexate.

Psoriatic Arthritis

The safety and efficacy of ENBREL® were assessed in a randomized, double-blind, placebo-controlled study in 205 patients with psoriatic arthritis. Patients were between 18 and 70 years of age and had active psoriatic arthritis (≥ 3 swollen joints and ≥ 3 tender joints) in one or more of the following forms: (1) distal interphalangeal (DIP) involvement (N = 104); (2) polyarticular arthritis (absence of rheumatoid nodules and presence of psoriasis; N = 173); (3) arthritis mutilans (N = 3); (4) asymmetric psoriatic arthritis (N = 81); or (5) ankylosing spondylitis-like (N = 7). Patients also had plaque psoriasis with a qualifying target lesion ≥ 2 cm in diameter. Patients currently on MTX therapy (stable for ≥ 2 months) could continue at a stable dose of ≤ 25 mg/week MTX. Doses of 25 mg ENBREL® or placebo were administered SC twice a week for 6 months.

Compared to placebo, treatment with ENBREL® resulted in significant improvements in measures of disease activity (Table 4).

[See table 4 at top of next page]

Among patients with psoriatic arthritis who received ENBREL®, the clinical responses were apparent at the time of the first visit (4 weeks) and were maintained through 6 months of therapy. Responses were similar in patients who were or were not receiving concomitant methotrexate therapy at baseline. At 6 months, the ACR 20/50/70 responses were achieved by 50%, 37%, and 9%, respectively, of patients receiving ENBREL®, compared to 13%, 4%, and 1%, respectively, of patients receiving placebo. Similar responses were seen in patients with each of the subtypes of psoriatic arthritis, although few patients were enrolled with the arthritis mutilans and ankylosing spondylitis-like subtypes. The results of this study were similar to those seen in an earlier single-center, randomized, placebo-controlled study of 60 patients with psoriatic arthritis.

The skin lesions of psoriasis were also improved with ENBREL® , relative to placebo, as measured by percentages of patients achieving improvements in the Psoriasis Area and Severity Index (PASI).[4] Responses increased over time, and at 6 months, the proportions of patients achieving a 50% or 75% improvement in the PASI were 47% and 23%, respectively, in the ENBREL® group (N = 66), compared to 18% and 3%, respectively, in the placebo group (N = 62). Responses were similar in patients who were or were not receiving concomitant methotrexate therapy at baseline.

Radiographic Response

Radiographic changes were also assessed in the psoriatic arthritis study. Radiographs of hands and wrists were obtained at baseline and months 6 and 12. A modified Total Sharp Score (TSS), which included distal interphalangeal joints (i.e., not identical to the modified TSS used for rheumatoid arthritis) was used by readers blinded to treatment group to assess the radiographs. Some radiographic features specific to psoriatic arthritis (e.g., pencil-and-cup deformity, joint space widening, gross osteolysis and ankylosis) were included in the scoring system, but others (e.g., phalangeal tuft resorption, juxta-articular and shaft periostitis) were not.

Most patients showed little or no change in the modified TSS during this 12-month study (median change of 0 in both treatment and placebo groups). However, there was a difference between groups in the distribution of scores (p = 0.0001, van Elteren test). More placebo-treated patients experienced larger magnitudes of radiographic worsening (increased TSS) compared to ENBREL® treatment. In an exploratory analysis, 12 of 104 placebo patients compared to 0 of 101 ENBREL®-treated patients had increases of points or more in TSS.

Ankylosing Spondylitis

The safety and efficacy of ENBREL® were assessed in a randomized, double-blind, placebo-controlled study in 277 patients with active ankylosing spondylitis. Patients were between 18 and 70 years of age and had ankylosing spondylitis as defined by the modified New York Criteria for Ankylosing Spondylitis.[5] Patients were to have evidence of active disease based on values of ≥ 30 on a 0-100 unit Visual Analog Scale (VAS) for the average of morning stiffness duration and intensity, and 2 of the following 3 other parameters: a) patient global assessment, b) average of nocturnal and total back pain, and c) the average score on the Bath Ankylosing Spondylitis Functional Index (BASFI). Patients with complete ankylosis of the spine were excluded from study participation. Patients taking hydroxychloroquine, sulfasalazine, methotrexate or prednisone (≤ 10 mg/day) could continue these drugs at stable doses for the duration of the study. Doses of 25 mg ENBREL® or placebo were administered SC twice a week for 6 months.

The primary measure of efficacy was a 20% improvement in the Assessment in Ankylosing Spondylitis (ASAS) response criteria.[6] Compared to placebo, treatment with ENBREL® resulted in improvements in the ASAS and other measures of disease activity (Figure 2 and Table 5).

Figure 2: ASAS 20 Responses in Ankylosing Spondylitis

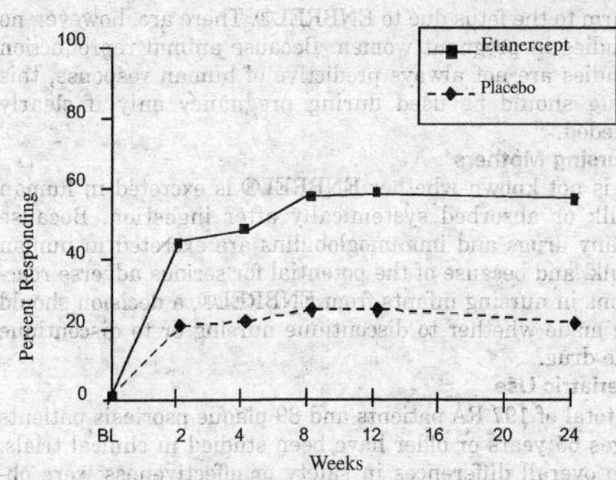

At 12 weeks, the ASAS 20/50/70 responses were achieved by 60%, 45%, and 29%, respectively, of patients receiving ENBREL®, compared to 27%, 13%, and 7%, respectively, of patients receiving placebo (p ≤ 0.0001, ENBREL® vs. placebo). Similar responses were seen at week 24. Responses were similar between those patients receiving concomitant therapies at baseline and those who were not. The results of this study were similar to those seen in a single-center, randomized, placebo-controlled study of 40 patients and a multi-center, randomized, placebo-controlled study of 84 patients with ankylosing spondylitis.

[See table 5 above]

Plaque Psoriasis

The safety and efficacy of ENBREL® were assessed in two randomized, double-blind, placebo-controlled studies in adults with chronic stable plaque psoriasis involving ≥ 10% of the body surface area, a minimum PASI of 10 and who had received or were candidates for systemic anti-psoriatic therapy or phototherapy. Patients with guttate, erythrodermic, or pustular psoriasis and patients with severe infections within 4 weeks of screening were excluded from study. No concomitant major anti-psoriatic therapies were allowed during the study.

Study I evaluated 672 patients who received placebo or ENBREL® SC at doses of 25 mg once a week, 25 mg twice a week or 50 mg twice a week for 3 months. After 3 months, patients continued on blinded treatments for an additional 3 months during which time, patients originally randomized to placebo began treatment with blinded ENBREL® at 25 mg twice weekly (designated as placebo/ENBREL® in

Table 4:
Components of Disease Activity in Psoriatic Arthritis

Parameter (median)	Placebo N = 104 Baseline	6 Months	ENBREL®[a] N = 101 Baseline	6 Months
Number of tender joints[b]	17.0	13.0	18.0	5.0
Number of swollen joints[c]	12.5	9.5	13.0	5.0
Physician global assessment[d]	3.0	3.0	3.0	1.0
Patient global assessment[d]	3.0	3.0	3.0	1.0
Morning stiffness (minutes)	60	60	60	15
Pain[d]	3.0	3.0	3.0	1.0
Disability index[e]	1.0	0.9	1.1	0.3
CRP (mg/dL)[f]	1.1	1.1	1.6	0.2

[a] $p < 0.001$ for all comparisons between ENBREL® and placebo at 6 months.
[b] Scale 0-78.
[c] Scale 0-76.
[d] Likert scale; 0 = best, 5 = worst.
[e] Health Assessment Questionnaire[1]; 0 = best, 3 = worst; includes eight categories: dressing and grooming, arising, eating, walking, hygiene, reach, grip, and activities.
[f] Normal range: 0 -0.79 mg/dL

Table 5:
Components of Ankylosing Spondylitis Disease Activity

Mean values at time points	Placebo N = 139 Baseline	6 Months	ENBREL®[a] N = 138 Baseline	6 Months
ASAS response criteria				
Patient global assessment[b]	63	56	63	36
Back pain[c]	62	56	60	34
BASFI[d]	56	55	52	36
Inflammation[e]	64	57	61	33
Acute phase reactants				
CRP (mg/dL)[f]	2.0	1.9	1.9	0.6
Spinal mobility (cm):				
Modified Schober's test	3.0	2.9	3.1	3.3
Chest expansion	3.2	3.0	3.3	3.9
Occiput-to-wall measurement	5.3	6.0	5.6	4.5

[a] $p < 0.0015$ for all comparisons between ENBREL® and placebo at 6 months. P-values for continuous endpoints were based on percent change from baseline.
[b] Measured on a Visual Analog Scale (VAS) scale with 0 = "none" and 100 = "severe."
[c] Average of total nocturnal and back pain scores, measured on a VAS scale with 0 = "no pain" and 100 = "most severe pain."
[d] Bath Ankylosing Spondylitis Functional Index (BASFI), average of 10 questions.
[e] Inflammation represented by the average of the last 2 questions on the 6-question Bath Ankylosing Spondylitis Disease Activity Index (BASDAI).
[f] C-reactive protein (CRP) normal range: 0 - 1.0 mg/dL.

Table 6: Study I Outcomes at 3 and 6 Months

	Placebo/ENBREL® 25 mg BIW (N = 168)	ENBREL®/ENBREL® 25 mg QW (N = 169)	25 mg BIW (N = 167)	50 mg BIW (N = 168)
3 Months				
PASI 75 n (%)	6 (4%)	23 (14%)[a]	53 (32%)[b]	79 (47%)[b]
Difference (95% CI)		10% (4, 16)	28% (21, 36)	43% (35, 52)
sPGA, "clear" or "minimal" n (%)	8 (5%)	36 (21%)[b]	53 (32%)[b]	79 (47%)[b]
Difference (95% CI)		17% (10, 24)	27% (19, 35)	42% (34, 50)
PASI 50 n (%)	24 (14%)	62 (37%)[b]	90 (54%)[b]	119 (71%)[b]
Difference (95% CI)		22% (13, 31)	40% (30, 49)	57% (48, 65)
6 Months				
PASI 75 n (%)	55 (33%)	36 (21%)	68 (41%)	90 (54%)

[a] $p = 0.001$ compared with placebo
[b] $p < 0.0001$ compared with placebo

Table 6); patients originally randomized to ENBREL® continued on the originally randomized dose (designated as ENBREL®/ENBREL® groups in Table 6).

Study II evaluated 611 patients who received placebo or ENBREL® SC at doses of 25 mg or 50 mg twice a week for 3 months. After 3 months of randomized blinded treatment, patients in all three arms began receiving open-label ENBREL® at 25 mg twice weekly for 9 additional months.

Response to treatment in both studies was assessed after 3 months of therapy and was defined as the proportion of patients who achieved a reduction in score of at least 75% from baseline by the Psoriasis Area and Severity Index (PASI). The PASI is a composite score that takes into consideration both the fraction of body surface area affected and the nature and severity of psoriatic changes within the affected regions (induration, erythema, and scaling).

Other evaluated outcomes included the proportion of patients who achieved a score of "clear" or "minimal" by the Static Physician Global Assessment (sPGA) and the proportion of patients with a reduction of PASI of at least 50% from baseline. The sPGA is a 6 category scale ranging from "5 = severe" to "0 = none" indicating the physician's overall assessment of the psoriasis severity focusing on induration, erythema, and scaling. Treatment success of "clear" or "minimal" consisted of none or minimal elevation in plaque, up to faint red coloration in erythema, and none or minimal fine scale over < 5% of the plaque.

Patients in all treatment groups and in both studies had a median baseline PASI score ranging from 15 to 17; and the percentage of patients with baseline sPGA classifications ranged from 54% to 66% for moderate, 17% to 26% for marked, and 1% to 5% for severe. Across all treatment groups, the percentage of patients who previously received systemic therapy for psoriasis ranged from 61% to 65% in Study I, and 71% to 75% in Study II; and those who previously received phototherapy ranged from 44% to 50% in Study I, and 72% to 73% in Study II.

More patients randomized to ENBREL® than placebo achieved at least a 75% reduction from baseline PASI score (PASI 75) with a dose response relationship across doses of 25 mg once a week, 25 mg twice a week and 50 mg twice a week (Tables 6 and 7). The individual components of the PASI (induration, erythema, and scaling) contributed comparably to the overall treatment-associated improvement in PASI.

[See table 6 above]
[See table 7 at top of next page]

Among PASI 75 achievers in both studies, the median time to PASI 50 and PASI 75 was approximately 1 and approximately 2 months, respectively, after the start of therapy with either 25 or 50 mg twice a week.

In Study I patients who achieved PASI 75 at month 6 were entered into a study drug withdrawal and retreatment period. Following withdrawal of study drug, these patients had a median duration of PASI 75 of between 1 and 2 months.

In Study I, in patients who were PASI 75 responders at 3 months, retreatment with open-label ENBREL® after discontinuation of up to 5 months resulted in a similar proportion of responders as was seen during the initial double-blind portion of the study.

In Study II, most patients initially randomized to 50 mg twice a week continued in the study after month 3 and had

Continued on next page

Enbrel—Cont.

their ENBREL® dose decreased to 25 mg twice a week. Of the 91 patients who were PASI 75 responders at month 3, 70 (77%) maintained their PASI 75 response at month 6.

Efficacy and safety of ENBREL® treatment beyond 12 months has not been adequately evaluated in patients with psoriasis.

INDICATIONS AND USAGE

ENBREL® is indicated for reducing signs and symptoms, inhibiting the progression of structural damage, and improving physical function in patients with moderately to severely active rheumatoid arthritis. ENBREL® can be used in combination with methotrexate in patients who do not respond adequately to methotrexate alone.

ENBREL® is indicated for reducing signs and symptoms of moderately to severely active polyarticular-course juvenile rheumatoid arthritis in patients who have had an inadequate response to one or more DMARDs.

ENBREL® is indicated for reducing signs and symptoms and inhibiting the progression of structural damage of active arthritis in patients with psoriatic arthritis. ENBREL® can be used in combination with methotrexate in patients who do not respond adequately to methotrexate alone.

ENBREL® is indicated for reducing signs and symptoms in patients with active ankylosing spondylitis.

ENBREL® is indicated for the treatment of adult patients (18 years or older) with chronic moderate to severe plaque psoriasis who are candidates for systemic therapy or phototherapy.

CONTRAINDICATIONS

ENBREL® should not be administered to patients with sepsis or with known hypersensitivity to ENBREL® or any of its components.

WARNINGS

INFECTIONS

IN POST-MARKETING REPORTS, SERIOUS INFECTIONS AND SEPSIS, INCLUDING FATALITIES, HAVE BEEN REPORTED WITH THE USE OF ENBREL®. MANY OF THE SERIOUS INFECTIONS HAVE OCCURRED IN PATIENTS ON CONCOMITANT IMMUNOSUPPRESSIVE THERAPY THAT, IN ADDITION TO THEIR UNDERLYING DISEASE, COULD PREDISPOSE THEM TO INFECTIONS. RARE CASES OF TUBERCULOSIS (TB) HAVE BEEN OBSERVED IN PATIENTS TREATED WITH TNF ANTAGONISTS, INCLUDING ENBREL®. PATIENTS WHO DEVELOP A NEW INFECTION WHILE UNDERGOING TREATMENT WITH ENBREL® SHOULD BE MONITORED CLOSELY. ADMINISTRATION OF ENBREL® SHOULD BE DISCONTINUED IF A PATIENT DEVELOPS A SERIOUS INFECTION OR SEPSIS. TREATMENT WITH ENBREL® SHOULD NOT BE INITIATED IN PATIENTS WITH ACTIVE INFECTIONS INCLUDING CHRONIC OR LOCALIZED INFECTIONS. PHYSICIANS SHOULD EXERCISE CAUTION WHEN CONSIDERING THE USE OF ENBREL® IN PATIENTS WITH A HISTORY OF RECURRING INFECTIONS OR WITH UNDERLYING CONDITIONS WHICH MAY PREDISPOSE PATIENTS TO INFECTIONS, SUCH AS ADVANCED OR POORLY CONTROLLED DIABETES (see PRECAUTIONS and ADVERSE REACTIONS: Infections).

IN A 24-WEEK STUDY OF CONCURRENT ENBREL® AND ANAKINRA THERAPY, THE RATE OF SERIOUS INFECTIONS IN THE COMBINATION ARM (7%) WAS HIGHER THAN WITH ENBREL® ALONE (0%). THE COMBINATION OF ENBREL® AND ANAKINRA DID NOT RESULT IN HIGHER ACR RESPONSE RATES COMPARED TO ENBREL® ALONE (see CLINICAL STUDIES: Clinical Response and ADVERSE REACTIONS: Infections).

Neurologic Events

Treatment with ENBREL® and other agents that inhibit TNF have been associated with rare cases of new onset or exacerbation of central nervous system demyelinating disorders, some presenting with mental status changes and some associated with permanent disability. Cases of transverse myelitis, optic neuritis, multiple sclerosis, and new onset or exacerbation of seizure disorders have been observed in association with ENBREL® therapy. The causal relationship to ENBREL® therapy remains unclear. While no clinical trials have been performed evaluating ENBREL® therapy in patients with multiple sclerosis, other TNF antagonists administered to patients with multiple sclerosis have been associated with increases in disease activity.[7, 8] Prescribers should exercise caution in considering the use of ENBREL® in patients with preexisting or recent-onset central nervous system demyelinating disorders (see **ADVERSE REACTIONS**).

Hematologic Events

Rare reports of pancytopenia including aplastic anemia, some with a fatal outcome, have been reported in patients treated with ENBREL®. The causal relationship to ENBREL® therapy remains unclear. Although no high risk group has been identified, caution should be exercised in patients being treated with ENBREL® who have a previous history of significant hematologic abnormalities. All patients should be advised to seek immediate medical attention if they develop signs and symptoms suggestive of blood dyscrasias or infection (e.g., persistent fever, bruising, bleeding, pallor) while on ENBREL®. Discontinuation of ENBREL® therapy should be considered in patients with confirmed significant hematologic abnormalities.

Table 7: Study II Outcomes at 3 Months

	Placebo (N = 204)	ENBREL® 25 mg BIW (N = 204)	ENBREL® 50 mg BIW (N = 203)
PASI 75 n (%)	6 (3%)	66 (32%)[a]	94 (46%)[a]
Difference (95% CI)		29% (23, 36)	43% (36, 51)
sPGA, "clear" or "minimal" n (%)	7 (3%)	75 (37%)[a]	109 (54%)[a]
Difference (95% CI)		34% (26, 41)	50% (43, 58)
PASI 50 n (%)	18 (9%)	124 (61%)[a]	147 (72%)[a]
Difference (95% CI)		52% (44, 60)	64% (56, 71)

[a] $p < 0.0001$ compared with placebo

Two percent of patients treated concurrently with ENBREL® and anakinra developed neutropenia (ANC $< 1 \times 10^9$/L). While neutropenic, one patient developed cellulitis which recovered with antibiotic therapy.

Malignancies

In the controlled portions of clinical trials of all the TNF-blocking agents, more cases of lymphoma have been observed among patients receiving the TNF blocker compared to control patients. During the controlled portions of ENBREL® trials, 2 lymphomas were observed among 3435 ENBREL®-treated patients versus 0 among 1335 control patients (duration of controlled treatment ranged from 3 to 6 months). In the controlled and open-label portions of clinical trials of ENBREL®, 7 lymphomas were observed in 4650 patients over approximately 9062 patient-years of therapy. This is 2-fold higher than that expected in the general population. While patients with rheumatoid arthritis or psoriasis, particularly those with highly active disease, may be at a higher risk (up to several fold) for the development of lymphoma, the potential role of TNF-blocking therapy in the development of malignancies is not known (see **ADVERSE REACTIONS: Malignancies**).[11, 12]

PRECAUTIONS

General

Allergic reactions associated with administration of ENBREL® during clinical trials have been reported in < 2% of patients. If an anaphylactic reaction or other serious allergic reaction occurs, administration of ENBREL® should be discontinued immediately and appropriate therapy initiated.

Information for Patients

If a patient or caregiver is to administer ENBREL®, the patient or caregiver should be instructed in injection techniques and how to measure and administer the correct dose (see the ENBREL® (etanercept) "Patient Information" insert). The first injection should be performed under the supervision of a qualified health care professional. The patient's or caregiver's ability to inject subcutaneously should be assessed. Patients and caregivers should be instructed in the technique as well as proper syringe and needle disposal, and be cautioned against reuse of needles and syringes. A puncture-resistant container for disposal of needles and syringes should be used. If the product is intended for multiple use, additional syringes, needles, and alcohol swabs will be required.

Patients with Heart Failure

Two large clinical trials evaluating the use of ENBREL® in the treatment of heart failure were terminated early due to lack of efficacy. Results of one study suggested higher mortality in patients treated with ENBREL® compared to placebo. Results of the second study did not corroborate these observations. Analyses did not identify specific factors associated with increased risk of adverse outcomes in heart failure patients treated with ENBREL® (see **ADVERSE REACTIONS: Patients with Heart Failure**). There have been post-marketing reports of worsening of congestive heart failure (CHF), with and without identifiable precipitating factors, in patients taking ENBREL®. There have also been rare reports of new onset CHF, including CHF in patients without known pre-existing cardiovascular disease. Some of these patients have been under 50 years of age. Physicians should exercise caution when using ENBREL® in patients who also have heart failure, and monitor patients carefully.

Immunosuppression

Anti-TNF therapies, including ENBREL®, affect host defenses against infections and malignancies since TNF mediates inflammation and modulates cellular immune responses. In a study of 49 patients with RA treated with ENBREL®, there was no evidence of depression of delayed-type hypersensitivity, depression of immunoglobulin levels, or change in enumeration of effector cell populations. The impact of treatment with ENBREL® on the development and course of malignancies, as well as active and/or chronic infections, is not fully understood (see **WARNINGS: Malignancies, ADVERSE REACTIONS: Infections,** and **Malignancies**). The safety and efficacy of ENBREL® in patients with immunosuppression or chronic infections have not been evaluated.

Immunizations

Most psoriatic arthritis patients receiving ENBREL® were able to mount effective B-cell immune responses to pneumococcal polysaccharide vaccine, but titers in aggregate were moderately lower and fewer patients had two-fold rises in titers compared to patients not receiving ENBREL®. The clinical significance of this is unknown. Patients receiving ENBREL® may receive concurrent vaccinations, except for live vaccines. No data are available on the secondary transmission of infection by live vaccines in patients receiving ENBREL® (see **PRECAUTIONS: Immunosuppression**).

It is recommended that JRA patients, if possible, be brought up to date with all immunizations in agreement with current immunization guidelines prior to initiating ENBREL® therapy. Patients with a significant exposure to varicella virus should temporarily discontinue ENBREL® therapy and be considered for prophylactic treatment with Varicella Zoster Immune Globulin.

Autoimmunity

Treatment with ENBREL® may result in the formation of autoantibodies (see **ADVERSE REACTIONS: Autoantibodies**) and, rarely, in the development of a lupus-like syndrome (see **ADVERSE REACTIONS: Adverse Reaction Information from Spontaneous Reports**) which may resolve following withdrawal of ENBREL®. If a patient develops symptoms and findings suggestive of a lupus-like syndrome following treatment with ENBREL®, treatment should be discontinued and the patient should be carefully evaluated.

Drug Interactions

Specific drug interaction studies have not been conducted with ENBREL®. However, it was observed that the pharmacokinetics of ENBREL® was unaltered by concomitant methotrexate in rheumatoid arthritis patients.

In a study in which patients with active RA were treated for up to 24 weeks with concurrent ENBREL® and anakinra therapy, a 7% rate of serious infections was observed, which was higher than that observed with ENBREL® alone (0%) (see also **WARNINGS**). Two percent of patients treated concurrently with ENBREL® and anakinra developed neutropenia (ANC $< 1 \times 10^9$/L).

Carcinogenesis, Mutagenesis, and Impairment of Fertility

Long-term animal studies have not been conducted to evaluate the carcinogenic potential of ENBREL® or its effect on fertility. Mutagenesis studies were conducted in vitro and in vivo, and no evidence of mutagenic activity was observed.

Pregnancy (Category B)

Developmental toxicity studies have been performed in rats and rabbits at doses ranging from 60- to 100-fold higher than the human dose and have revealed no evidence of harm to the fetus due to ENBREL®. There are, however, no studies in pregnant women. Because animal reproduction studies are not always predictive of human response, this drug should be used during pregnancy only if clearly needed.

Nursing Mothers

It is not known whether ENBREL® is excreted in human milk or absorbed systemically after ingestion. Because many drugs and immunoglobulins are excreted in human milk, and because of the potential for serious adverse reactions in nursing infants from ENBREL®, a decision should be made whether to discontinue nursing or to discontinue the drug.

Geriatric Use

A total of 197 RA patients and 89 plaque psoriasis patients ages 65 years or older have been studied in clinical trials. No overall differences in safety or effectiveness were observed between these patients and younger patients. Because there is a higher incidence of infections in the elderly population in general, caution should be used in treating the elderly.

Pediatric Use

ENBREL® is indicated for treatment of polyarticular-course juvenile rheumatoid arthritis in patients who have had an inadequate response to one or more DMARDs. For issues relevant to pediatric patients, in addition to other sections of the label, see also **WARNINGS; PRECAUTIONS: Immunizations;** and **ADVERSE REACTIONS: Adverse Reactions in Patients with JRA**. ENBREL® has not been studied in children < 4 years of age.

The safety and efficacy of ENBREL® in pediatric patients with plaque psoriasis have not been studied.

ADVERSE REACTIONS

Adverse Reactions in Adult Patients with RA, Psoriatic Arthritis, Ankylosing Spondylitis, or Plaque Psoriasis

ENBREL® has been studied in 1440 patients with RA, followed for up to 57 months, in 157 patients with psoriatic arthritis for 6 months, in 222 patients with ankylosing spondylitis for up to 10 months, and 1261 patients with plaque psoriasis for up to 15 months. In controlled trials, the proportion of ENBREL®-treated patients who discontinued treatment due to adverse events was approximately 4% in the indications studied. The vast majority of these patients were treated with 25 mg SC twice weekly. In plaque psoriasis studies, ENBREL® doses studied were 25 mg SC once a week, 25 mg SC twice a week, and 50 mg SC twice a week.

Table 8:
Percent of RA Patients Reporting Adverse Events in Controlled Clinical Trials*

	Placebo Controlled		Active Controlled (Study III)	
	Percent of patients		Percent of patients	
Event	Placebo† (N = 152)	ENBREL® (N = 349)	MTX (N = 217)	ENBREL® (N = 415)
Injection site reaction	10	37	7	34
Infection (total)**	32	35	72	64
Non-upper respiratory infection (non-URI)**	32	38	60	51
Upper respiratory infection (URI)**	16	29	39	31
Headache	13	17	27	24
Nausea	10	9	29	15
Rhinitis	8	12	14	16
Dizziness	5	7	11	8
Pharyngitis	5	7	9	6
Cough	3	6	6	5
Asthenia	3	5	12	11
Abdominal pain	3	5	10	10
Rash	3	5	23	14
Peripheral edema	3	2	4	8
Respiratory disorder	1	5	NA	NA
Dyspepsia	1	4	10	11
Sinusitis	2	3	3	5
Vomiting	–	3	8	5
Mouth ulcer	1	2	14	6
Alopecia	1	1	12	6
Pneumonitis ("MTX lung")	–	–	2	0

* Includes data from the 6-month study in which patients received concurrent MTX therapy.
† The duration of exposure for patients receiving placebo was less than the ENBREL®-treated patients
** Infection (total) includes data from all three placebo-controlled trials. Non-URI and URI include data only from the two placebo-controlled trials where infections were collected separately from adverse events (placebo N = 110, ENBREL® N = 213).

Injection Site Reactions
In controlled trials in rheumatologic indications, approximately 37% of patients treated with ENBREL® developed injection site reactions. In controlled trials in patients with plaque psoriasis, 14% of patients treated with ENBREL® developed injection site reactions during the first 3 months of treatment. All injection site reactions were described as mild to moderate (erythema and/or itching, pain, or swelling) and generally did not necessitate drug discontinuation. Injection site reactions generally occurred in the first month and subsequently decreased in frequency. The mean duration of injection site reactions was 3 to 5 days. Seven percent of patients experienced redness at a previous injection site when subsequent injections were given. In post-marketing experience, injection site bleeding and bruising have also been observed in conjunction with ENBREL® therapy.
Infections
In controlled trials, there were no differences in rates of infection among RA, psoriatic arthritis, ankylosing spondylitis, and plaque psoriasis patients treated with ENBREL® and those treated with placebo (or MTX for RA and psoriatic arthritis patients). The most common type of infection was upper respiratory infection, which occurred at a rate of approximately 20% among both ENBREL®- and placebo-treated patients in RA, psoriatic arthritis, and AS trials, and at a rate of approximately 12% among both ENBREL®- and placebo-treated patients in plaque psoriasis trials in the first 3 months of treatment.
In placebo-controlled trials in RA, psoriatic arthritis, ankylosing spondylitis, and plaque psoriasis no increase in the incidence of serious infections was observed (approximately 1% in both placebo- and ENBREL®-treated groups). In all clinical trials in RA, serious infections experienced by patients have included: pyelonephritis, bronchitis, septic arthritis, abdominal abscess, cellulitis, osteomyelitis, wound infection, pneumonia, foot abscess, leg ulcer, diarrhea, sinusitis, and sepsis. The rate of serious infections has not increased in open-label extension trials and is similar to that observed in ENBREL®- and placebo-treated patients from controlled trials. Serious infections, including sepsis and death, have also been reported during post-marketing use of ENBREL®. Some have occurred within a few weeks after initiating treatment with ENBREL®. Many of the patients had underlying conditions (e.g., diabetes, congestive heart failure, history of active or chronic infections) in addition to their rheumatoid arthritis (see **WARNINGS**). Data from a sepsis clinical trial not specifically in patients with RA suggest that ENBREL® treatment may increase mortality in patients with established sepsis.[9]
In patients who received both ENBREL® and anakinra for up to 24 weeks, the incidence of serious infections was 7%. The most common infections consisted of bacterial pneumonia (4 cases) and cellulitis (4 cases). One patient with pulmonary fibrosis and pneumonia died due to respiratory failure.
In post-marketing experience in rheumatologic indications, infections have been observed with various pathogens including viral, bacterial, fungal, and protozoal organisms. Infections have been noted in all organ systems and have been reported in patients receiving ENBREL® alone or in combination with immunosuppressive agents.
In clinical trials in plaque psoriasis, serious infections experienced by ENBREL®-treated patients have included: cellulitis, gastroenteritis, pneumonia, abscess, and osteomyelitis.
Malignancies
Among 3389 rheumatoid arthritis patients treated with ENBREL® in clinical trials for a mean of 28 months (approximately 8000 patient-years of therapy), 6 lymphomas were observed for a rate of 0.07 cases per 100 patient-years. This is 2-fold higher than the rate of lymphomas expected in the general population based on the Surveillance, Epidemiology, and End Results Database.[10] An increased rate of lymphoma up to several fold has been reported in the rheumatoid arthritis patient population, and may be further increased in patients with more severe disease activity[11, 12] (see **WARNINGS: Malignancies**). Fifty-five malignancies, other than lymphoma, were observed. Of these, the most common malignancies were colon, breast, lung and prostate, which were similar in type and number to what would be expected in the general population.[10] Analysis of the cancer rates at 6 month intervals suggest constant rates over three years of observation.
In the placebo-controlled portions of the psoriasis studies, 8 of 933 patients who received ENBREL® at any dose were diagnosed with a malignancy compared to 1 of 414 patients who received placebo. Among the 1261 patients with psoriasis who received ENBREL® at any dose in the controlled and uncontrolled portions of the psoriasis studies (1062 patient-years), a total of 22 patients were diagnosed with 23 malignancies; 9 patients with non-cutaneous solid tumors, 12 patients with 13 non-melanoma skin cancers (8 basal, 5 squamous), and 1 patient with non-Hodgkin's lymphoma. Among the placebo treated patients (90 patient-years of observation) 1 patient was diagnosed with 2 squamous cell cancers. The size of the placebo group and limited duration of the controlled portions of studies precludes the ability to draw firm conclusions.
Immunogenicity
Patients with RA, psoriatic arthritis, ankylosing spondylitis, or plaque psoriasis were tested at multiple timepoints for antibodies to ENBREL®. Antibodies to the TNF receptor portion or other protein components of the ENBREL® drug product were detected at least once in sera of approximately 6% of adult patients with RA, psoriatic arthritis, ankylosing spondylitis or plaque psoriasis. These antibodies were all non-neutralizing. No apparent correlation of antibody development to clinical response or adverse events was observed. Results from JRA patients were similar to those seen in adult RA patients treated with ENBREL®. The long-term immunogenicity of ENBREL® is unknown.
The data reflect the percentage of patients whose test results were considered positive for antibodies to ENBREL® in an ELISA assay, and are highly dependent on the sensitivity and specificity of the assay. Additionally, the observed incidence of antibody positivity in an assay may be influenced by several factors including sample handling, concomitant medications, and underlying disease. For these reasons, comparison of the incidence of antibodies to ENBREL® with the incidence of antibodies to other products may be misleading.
Autoantibodies
Patients with RA had serum samples tested for autoantibodies at multiple timepoints. In RA Studies I and II, the percentage of patients evaluated for antinuclear antibodies (ANA) who developed new positive ANA (titer ≥ 1:40) was higher in patients treated with ENBREL® (11%) than in placebo-treated patients (5%). The percentage of patients who developed new positive anti-double-stranded DNA antibodies was also higher by radioimmunoassay (15% of patients treated with ENBREL® compared to 4% of placebo-treated patients) and by *Crithidia luciliae* assay (3% of patients treated with ENBREL® compared to none of placebo-treated patients). The proportion of patients treated with ENBREL® who developed anticardiolipin antibodies was similarly increased compared to placebo-treated patients. In Study III, no pattern of increased autoantibody development was seen in ENBREL® patients compared to MTX patients.
The impact of long-term treatment with ENBREL® on the development of autoimmune diseases is unknown. Rare adverse event reports have described patients with rheumatoid factor positive and/or erosive RA who have developed additional autoantibodies in conjunction with rash and other features suggesting a lupus-like syndrome.
Other Adverse Reactions
Table 8 summarizes events reported in at least 3% of all patients with higher incidence in patients treated with ENBREL® compared to controls in placebo-controlled RA trials (including the combination methotrexate trial) and relevant events from Study III. In placebo-controlled plaque psoriasis trials, the percentages of patients reporting injection site reactions were lower in the placebo dose group (6.4%) than in the ENBREL® dose groups (15.5%) in Studies I and II. Otherwise, the percentages of patients reporting adverse events in the 50 mg twice a week dose group were similar to those observed in the 25 mg twice a week dose group or placebo group. In psoriasis Study I, there were no serious adverse events of worsening psoriasis following withdrawal of study drug. However, adverse events of worsening psoriasis including three serious adverse events were observed during the course of the clinical trials. Urticaria and non-infectious hepatitis were observed in a small number of patients and angioedema was observed in one patient in clinical studies. Urticaria and angioedema have also been reported in spontaneous post-marketing reports. Adverse events in psoriatic arthritis, ankylosing spondylitis, and plaque psoriasis trials were similar to those reported in RA clinical trials.
[See table 8 above]
In controlled trials of RA and psoriatic arthritis, rates of serious adverse events were seen at a frequency of approximately 5% among ENBREL®- and control-treated patients. In controlled trials of plaque psoriasis, rates of serious adverse events were seen at a frequency of < 1.5% among ENBREL®- and placebo-treated patients in the first 3 months of treatment. Among patients with RA in placebo-controlled, active-controlled, and open-label trials of ENBREL®, malignancies (see **WARNINGS: Malignancies, ADVERSE REACTIONS: Malignancies**) and infections (see **ADVERSE REACTIONS: Infections**) were the most common serious adverse events observed. Other infrequent serious adverse events observed in RA, psoriatic arthritis, ankylosing spondylitis, or plaque psoriasis clinical trials are listed by body system below:

Cardiovascular:	heart failure, myocardial infarction, myocardial ischemia, hypertension, hypotension, deep vein thrombosis, thrombophlebitis
Digestive:	cholecystitis, pancreatitis, gastrointestinal hemorrhage, appendicitis
Hematologic/ Lymphatic:	lymphadenopathy
Musculoskeletal:	bursitis, polymyositis
Nervous:	cerebral ischemia, depression, multiple sclerosis (see **WARNINGS: Neurologic Events**)
Respiratory:	dyspnea, pulmonary embolism, sarcoidosis
Skin:	worsening psoriasis
Urogenital:	membranous glomerulonephropathy, kidney calculus

In a randomized controlled trial in which 51 patients with RA received ENBREL® 50 mg twice weekly and 25 patients received ENBREL® 25 mg twice weekly, the following serious adverse events were observed in the 50 mg twice weekly arm: gastrointestinal bleeding, normal pressure hydrocephalus, seizure, and stroke. No serious adverse events were observed in the 25 mg arm.
Adverse Reactions in Patients with JRA
In general, the adverse events in pediatric patients were similar in frequency and type as those seen in adult patients (see **WARNINGS** and other sections under **ADVERSE REACTIONS**). Differences from adults and other special considerations are discussed in the following paragraphs.
Severe adverse reactions reported in 69 JRA patients ages 4 to 17 years included varicella (see also **PRECAUTIONS: Immunizations**), gastroenteritis, depression/personality disorder, cutaneous ulcer, esophagitis/gastritis, group A streptococcal septic shock, Type 1 diabetes mellitus, and soft tissue and post-operative wound infection.
Forty-three of 69 (62%) children with JRA experienced an infection while receiving ENBREL® during three months of study (part 1 open-label), and the frequency and severity of infections was similar in 58 patients completing 12 months of open-label extension therapy. The types of infections reported in JRA patients were generally mild and consistent with those commonly seen in outpatient pediatric populations. Two JRA patients developed varicella infection and signs and symptoms of aseptic meningitis which resolved without sequelae.

Continued on next page

Enbrel—Cont.

The following adverse events were reported more commonly in 69 JRA patients receiving 3 months of ENBREL® compared to the 349 adult RA patients in placebo-controlled trials. These included headache (19% of patients, 1.7 events per patient-year), nausea (9%, 1.0 events per patient-year), abdominal pain (19%, 0.74 events per patient-year), and vomiting (13%, 0.74 events per patient-year).

In post-marketing experience, the following additional serious adverse events have been reported in pediatric patients: abscess with bacteremia, optic neuritis, pancytopenia, seizures, tuberculous arthritis, urinary tract infection (see **WARNINGS**), coagulopathy, cutaneous vasculitis, and transaminase elevations. The frequency of these events and their causal relationship to ENBREL® therapy are unknown.

Patients with Heart Failure

Two randomized placebo-controlled studies have been performed in patients with CHF. In one study, patients received either ENBREL® 25 mg twice weekly, 25 mg three times weekly, or placebo. In a second study, patients received either ENBREL® 25 mg once weekly, 25 mg twice weekly, or placebo. Results of the first study suggested higher mortality in patients treated with ENBREL® at either schedule compared to placebo. Results of the second study did not corroborate these observations. Analyses did not identify specific factors associated with increased risk of adverse outcomes in heart failure patients treated with ENBREL® (see **PRECAUTIONS: Patients with Heart Failure**).

Adverse Reaction Information from Spontaneous Reports

Adverse events have been reported during post-approval use of ENBREL®. Because these events are reported voluntarily from a population of uncertain size, it is not always possible to reliably estimate their frequency or establish a causal relationship to ENBREL® exposure.

Additional adverse events are listed by body system below:

Body as a whole:	angioedema, fatigue, fever, flu syndrome, generalized pain, weight gain
Cardiovascular:	chest pain, vasodilation (flushing), new-onset congestive heart failure (see **PRECAUTIONS: Patients with Heart Failure**)
Digestive:	altered sense of taste, anorexia, diarrhea, dry mouth, intestinal perforation
Hematologic/ Lymphatic:	adenopathy, anemia, aplastic anemia, leukopenia, neutropenia, pancytopenia, thrombocytopenia (see **WARNINGS**)
Musculoskeletal:	joint pain, lupus-like syndrome with manifestations including rash consistent with subacute or discoid lupus
Nervous:	paresthesias, stroke, seizures and central nervous system events suggestive of multiple sclerosis or isolated demyelinating conditions such as transverse myelitis or optic neuritis (see **WARNINGS**)
Ocular:	dry eyes, ocular inflammation
Respiratory:	dyspnea, interstitial lung disease, pulmonary disease, worsening of prior lung disorder
Skin:	cutaneous vasculitis, pruritis, subcutaneous nodules, urticaria

OVERDOSAGE

The maximum tolerated dose of ENBREL® has not been established in humans. Toxicology studies have been performed in monkeys at doses up to 30 times the human dose with no evidence of dose-limiting toxicities. No dose-limiting toxicities have been observed during clinical trials of ENBREL®. Single IV doses up to 60 mg/m^2 have been administered to healthy volunteers in an endotoxemia study without evidence of dose-limiting toxicities.

DOSAGE AND ADMINISTRATION

Adult RA, AS, and Psoriatic Arthritis Patients

The recommended dose of ENBREL® for adult patients with rheumatoid arthritis, psoriatic arthritis, or ankylosing spondylitis is 50 mg per week given as two 25 mg subcutaneous (SC) injections at separate sites. The dose should be administered as two 25 mg injections given either on the same day or 3 or 4 days apart (see **CLINICAL STUDIES**). Methotrexate, glucocorticoids, salicylates, nonsteroidal anti-inflammatory drugs (NSAIDs), or analgesics may be continued during treatment with ENBREL®. Based on a study of 50 mg ENBREL® twice weekly in patients with RA that suggested higher incidence of adverse reactions but similar ACR response rates, doses higher than 50 mg per week are not recommended (see **ADVERSE REACTIONS**).

Adult Plaque Psoriasis Patients

The recommended starting dose of ENBREL® for adult patients is a 50 mg dose given twice weekly (administered 3 to 4 days apart) for 3 months followed by a reduction to a maintenance dose of 50 mg per week (see **CLINICAL STUDIES**).

Starting doses of ENBREL® of 25 mg or 50 mg per week were also shown to be efficacious. The proportion of responders were related to ENBREL® dosage (see **CLINICAL STUDIES**).

JRA Patients

The recommended dose of ENBREL® for pediatric patients ages 4 to 17 years with active polyarticular-course JRA is 0.8 mg/kg per week (up to a maximum of 50 mg per week). The maximum dose that should be administered at a single injection site is 25 mg (1.0 mL). Therefore, for pediatric patients weighing more than 31 kg (68 pounds), the total weekly dose should be administered as two subcutaneous (SC) injections, either on the same day or 3 or 4 days apart. The dose for pediatric patients weighing 31 kg (68 pounds) or less should be administered as a single SC injection once weekly. Glucocorticoids, nonsteroidal anti-inflammatory drugs (NSAIDs), or analgesics may be continued during treatment with ENBREL®. Concurrent use with methotrexate and higher doses of ENBREL® have not been studied in pediatric patients.

Preparation of ENBREL®

ENBREL® is intended for use under the guidance and supervision of a physician. Patients may self-inject when deemed appropriate and if they receive medical follow-up, as necessary. Patients should not self-administer until they receive proper training in how to prepare and administer the correct dose.

ENBREL® should be reconstituted aseptically with 1 mL of the supplied Sterile Bacteriostatic Water for Injection, USP (0.9% benzyl alcohol) giving a solution of 1.0 mL containing 25 mg of ENBREL®.

A vial adapter is supplied for use when reconstituting the lyophilized powder. However, the vial adapter should not be used if multiple doses are going to be withdrawn from the vial. If the vial will be used for multiple doses, a 25-gauge needle should be used for reconstituting and withdrawing ENBREL®, and the supplied "Mixing Date:" sticker should be attached to the vial and the date of reconstitution entered. Reconstitution with the supplied BWFI, using a 25-gauge needle, yields a preserved, multiple-use solution that must be used within 14 days.

If using the vial adapter, twist the vial adapter onto the diluent syringe. Then, place the vial adapter over the ENBREL® vial and insert the vial adapter into the vial stopper. Push down on the plunger to inject the diluent into the ENBREL® vial. Keeping the diluent syringe in place, gently swirl the contents of the ENBREL® vial during dissolution. To avoid excessive foaming, do not shake or vigorously agitate.

If using a 25-gauge needle to reconstitute and withdraw ENBREL®, the diluent should be injected very slowly into the ENBREL® vial. It is normal for some foaming to occur. The contents should be swirled gently during dissolution. To avoid excessive foaming, do not shake or vigorously agitate. Generally, dissolution of ENBREL® takes less than 10 minutes. Visually inspect the solution for particulate matter and discoloration prior to administration. The solution should not be used if discolored or cloudy, or if particulate matter remains.

Withdraw the correct dose of reconstituted solution into the syringe. Some foam or bubbles may remain in the vial. Remove the syringe from the vial adapter or remove the 25-gauge needle from the syringe. Attach a 27-gauge needle to inject ENBREL®.

The contents of one vial of ENBREL® solution should not be mixed with, or transferred into, the contents of another vial of ENBREL®. No other medications should be added to solutions containing ENBREL®, and do not reconstitute ENBREL® with other diluents. Do not filter reconstituted solution during preparation or administration.

The ENBREL® (etanercept) "Patient Information" insert contains more detailed instructions on the preparation of ENBREL®. Reconstitution with the supplied BWFI, using a 25-gauge needle, yields a preserved, multiple-use solution that must be used within 14 days. Discard reconstituted solution after 14 days. PRODUCT STABILITY AND STERILITY CANNOT BE ASSURED AFTER 14 DAYS.

Administration of ENBREL®

A 50 mg dose should be given as two 25 mg SC injections. Rotate sites for injection (thigh, abdomen, or upper arm). Never inject into areas where the skin is tender, bruised, red, or hard. See the ENBREL® (etanercept) "Patient Information" insert for detailed information on injection site selection and dose administration.

Storage and Stability

Do not use a dose tray beyond the expiration date stamped on the carton, dose tray label, vial label, or diluent syringe label. The dose tray containing ENBREL® (sterile powder) must be refrigerated at 2°-8°C (36°-46°F). DO NOT FREEZE.

Reconstituted solutions of ENBREL® prepared with the supplied Bacteriostatic Water for Injection, USP (0.9% benzyl alcohol), using a 25-gauge needle, may be stored for up to 14 days if refrigerated at 2°-8°C (36°-46°F). Discard reconstituted solution after 14 days. **PRODUCT STABILITY AND STERILITY CANNOT BE ASSURED AFTER 14 DAYS.**

HOW SUPPLIED

ENBREL® is supplied in a carton containing four dose trays (NDC 58406-425-34). Each dose tray contains one 25 mg vial of etanercept, one diluent syringe (1 mL Sterile Bacteriostatic Water for Injection, USP, containing 0.9% benzyl alcohol), one 27-gauge ½ inch needle, one vial adapter, one plunger, and two alcohol swabs. Each carton contains four "Mixing Date:" stickers.

Rx Only

REFERENCES

1. Ramey DR, Fries JF, Singh G. The Health Assessment Questionnaire 1995 - Status and Review. In: Spilker B, ed. "Quality of Life and Pharmacoeconomics in Clinical Trials." 2nd ed. Philadelphia, PA. Lippincott-Raven 1996;227.
2. Ware JE Jr, Gandek B. Overview of the SF-36 Health Survey and the International Quality of Life Assessment (IQOLA) Project. J. Clin Epidemiol 1998;51(11): 903.
3. Giannini EH, Ruperto N, Ravelli A, et al. Preliminary definition of improvement of juvenile arthritis. Arthritis Rheum 1997;40(7):1202.
4. Fredriksson T, Petersson U. Severe psoriasis-oral therapy with a new retinoid. Dermatologica 1978;157:238.
5. van der Linden S, Valkenburg HA, Cats A. Evaluation of diagnostic criteria for ankylosing spondylitis: a proposal for modification of the New York criteria. Arthritis Rheum 1984;27(4):361-8.
6. Anderson JJ, Baron G, van der Heijde D, Felson DT, Dougados M. Ankylosing spondylitis assessment group preliminary definition of short-term improvement in ankylosing spondylitis. Arthritis Rheum 2001;44(8):1876-86.
7. Van Oosten BW, Barkhof F, Truyen L, et al. Increased MRI activity and immune activation in two multiple sclerosis patients treated with the monoclonal anti-tumor necrosis factor antibody cA2. Neurology 1996;47: 1531.
8. Arnason BGW, et al. (Lenercept Multiple Sclerosis Study Group). TNF neutralization in MS: Results of a randomized, placebo-controlled multicenter study. Neurology 1999;53:457.
9. Fisher CJ Jr, Agosti JM, Opal SM, et al. Treatment of septic shock with the tumor necrosis factor receptor: Fc fusion protein. The Soluble TNF Receptor Sepsis Study Group. N Engl J Med 1996;334(26):1697.
10. National Cancer Institute. Surveillance, Epidemiology, and End Results Database (SEER) Program. SEER Incidence Crude Rates, 11 Registries, 1992-1999.
11. Mellemkjaer L, Linet MS, Gridley G, et al. Rheumatoid Arthritis and Cancer Risk. European Journal of Cancer 1996;32A(10):1753-1757.
12. Baecklund E, Ekbom A, Sparen P, et al. Disease Activity and Risk of Lymphoma in Patients With Rheumatoid Arthritis: Nested Case-Control Study. BMJ 1998;317: 180-181.

AMGEN®
Wyeth®

Manufactured by:
Immunex Corporation
Thousand Oaks, CA 91320-1799
U.S. License Number 1132
Marketed by Amgen and Wyeth Pharmaceuticals

3XXXXXX-v20
Issue Date: 4/30/2004
Immunex U.S. Patent Numbers:
5,395,760; 5,605,690; 5,945,397; 6,201,105; 6,572,852; Re. 36,755

Shown in Product Identification Guide, page 305

EPOGEN® ℞

[ē' pə-gĕn]
(Epoetin alfa)
FOR INJECTION

DESCRIPTION

Erythropoietin is a glycoprotein which stimulates red blood cell production. It is produced in the kidney and stimulates the division and differentiation of committed erythroid progenitors in the bone marrow. EPOGEN® (Epoetin alfa), a 165 amino acid glycoprotein manufactured by recombinant DNA technology, has the same biological effects as endogenous erythropoietin.[1] It has a molecular weight of 30,400 daltons and is produced by mammalian cells into which the human erythropoietin gene has been introduced. The product contains the identical amino acid sequence of isolated natural erythropoietin.

EPOGEN® is formulated as a sterile, colorless liquid in an isotonic sodium chloride/sodium citrate buffered solution or a sodium chloride/sodium phosphate buffered solution for intravenous (IV) or subcutaneous (SC) administration.

Single-dose, Preservative-free Vial: Each 1 mL of solution contains 2000, 3000, 4000 or 10,000 Units of Epoetin alfa, 2.5 mg Albumin (Human), 5.8 mg sodium citrate, 5.8 mg sodium chloride, and 0.06 mg citric acid in Water for Injection, USP (pH 6.9 ± 0.3). This formulation contains no preservative.

Single-dose, Preservative-free Vial: 1 mL (40,000 Units/mL). Each 1 mL of solution contains 40,000 Units of Epoetin alfa, 2.5 mg Albumin (Human), 1.2 mg sodium phosphate monobasic monohydrate, 1.8 mg sodium phosphate dibasic anhydrate, 0.7 mg sodium citrate, 5.8 mg sodium chloride, and 6.8 mcg citric acid in Water for Injection, USP (pH 6.9 ± 0.3). This formulation contains no preservative.

Multidose, Preserved Vial: 2 mL (20,000 Units, 10,000 Units/mL). Each 1 mL of solution contains 10,000 Units of Epoetin alfa, 2.5 mg Albumin (Human), 1.3 mg sodium citrate, 8.2 mg sodium chloride, 0.11 mg citric acid, and 1% benzyl alcohol as preservative in Water for Injection, USP (pH 6.1 ± 0.3).

Multidose, Preserved Vial: 1 mL (20,000 Units/mL). Each 1 mL of solution contains 20,000 Units of Epoetin alfa,

2.5 mg Albumin (Human), 1.3 mg sodium citrate, 8.2 mg sodium chloride, 0.11 mg citric acid, and 1% benzyl alcohol as preservative in Water for Injection, USP (pH 6.1 ± 0.3).

CLINICAL PHARMACOLOGY

Chronic Renal Failure Patients

Endogenous production of erythropoietin is normally regulated by the level of tissue oxygenation. Hypoxia and anemia generally increase the production of erythropoietin, which in turn stimulates erythropoiesis.[2] In normal subjects, plasma erythropoietin levels range from 0.01 to 0.03 Units/mL and increase up to 100- to 1000-fold during hypoxia or anemia.[2] In contrast, in patients with chronic renal failure (CRF), production of erythropoietin is impaired, and this erythropoietin deficiency is the primary cause of their anemia.[3,4]

Chronic renal failure is the clinical situation in which there is a progressive and usually irreversible decline in kidney function. Such patients may manifest the sequelae of renal dysfunction, including anemia, but do not necessarily require regular dialysis. Patients with end-stage renal disease (ESRD) are those patients with CRF who require regular dialysis or kidney transplantation for survival.

EPOGEN® has been shown to stimulate erythropoiesis in anemic patients with CRF, including both patients on dialysis and those who do not require regular dialysis.[4-13] The first evidence of a response to the three times weekly (TIW) administration of EPOGEN® is an increase in the reticulocyte count within 10 days, followed by increases in the red cell count, hemoglobin, and hematocrit, usually within 2 to 6 weeks.[4,5] Because of the length of time required for erythropoiesis — several days for erythroid progenitors to mature and be released into the circulation — a clinically significant increase in hematocrit is usually not observed in less than 2 weeks and may require up to 6 weeks in some patients. Once the hematocrit reaches the suggested target range (30% to 36%), that level can be sustained by EPOGEN® therapy in the absence of iron deficiency and concurrent illnesses.

The rate of hematocrit increase varies between patients and is dependent upon the dose of EPOGEN®, within a therapeutic range of approximately 50 to 300 Units/kg TIW.[4] A greater biologic response is not observed at doses exceeding 300 Units/kg TIW.[6] Other factors affecting the rate and extent of response include availability of iron stores, the baseline hematocrit, and the presence of concurrent medical problems.

Zidovudine-treated HIV-infected Patients

Responsiveness to EPOGEN® in HIV-infected patients is dependent upon the endogenous serum erythropoietin level prior to treatment. Patients with endogenous serum erythropoietin levels ≤ 500 mUnits/mL, and who are receiving a dose of zidovudine ≤ 4200 mg/week, may respond to EPOGEN® therapy. Patients with endogenous serum erythropoietin levels > 500 mUnits/mL do not appear to respond to EPOGEN® therapy. In a series of four clinical trials involving 255 patients, 60% to 80% of HIV-infected patients treated with zidovudine had endogenous serum erythropoietin levels ≤ 500 mUnits/mL.

Response to EPOGEN® in zidovudine-treated HIV-infected patients is manifested by reduced transfusion requirements and increased hematocrit.

Cancer Patients on Chemotherapy

Anemia in cancer patients may be related to the disease itself or the effect of concomitantly administered chemotherapeutic agents. EPOGEN® has been shown to increase hematocrit and decrease transfusion requirements after the first month of therapy (months 2 and 3), in anemic cancer patients undergoing chemotherapy.

A series of clinical trials enrolled 131 anemic cancer patients who were receiving cyclic cisplatin- or non cisplatin-containing chemotherapy. Endogenous baseline serum erythropoietin levels varied among patients in these trials with approximately 75% (n = 83/110) having endogenous serum erythropoietin levels ≤ 132 mUnits/mL, and approximately 4% (n = 4/110) of patients having endogenous serum erythropoietin levels > 500 mUnits/mL. In general, patients with lower baseline serum erythropoietin levels responded more vigorously to EPOGEN® than patients with higher baseline erythropoietin levels. Although no specific serum erythropoietin level can be stipulated above which patients would be unlikely to respond to EPOGEN® therapy, treatment of patients with grossly elevated serum erythropoietin levels (eg, > 200 mUnits/mL) is not recommended.

Pharmacokinetics

Intravenously administered EPOGEN® is eliminated at a rate consistent with first order kinetics with a circulating half-life ranging from approximately 4 to 13 hours in adult and pediatric patients with CRF.[14-16] Within the therapeutic dose range, detectable levels of plasma erythropoietin are maintained for at least 24 hours. After SC administration of EPOGEN® to patients with CRF, peak serum levels are achieved within 5 to 24 hours after administration and decline slowly thereafter. There is no apparent difference in half-life between adult patients not on dialysis whose serum creatinine levels were greater than 3, and adult patients maintained on dialysis.

In normal volunteers, the half-life of IV administered EPOGEN® is approximately 20% shorter than the half-life in CRF patients. The pharmacokinetics of EPOGEN® have not been studied in HIV-infected patients.

The pharmacokinetic profile of EPOGEN® in children and adolescents appears to be similar to that of adults. Limited data are available in neonates.[17]

It has been demonstrated in normal volunteers that the 10,000 Units/mL citrate-buffered Epoetin alfa formulation and the 40,000 Units/mL phosphate-buffered Epoetin alfa formulation are bioequivalent after SC administration of single 750 Units/kg doses. The C_{max} and $t_{1/2}$ after administration of the phosphate buffered Epoetin alfa formulation were 1.8 ± 0.7 Units/mL and 19.0 ± 5.9 hours (mean ± SD), respectively. The corresponding mean ± SD values for the citrate-buffered Epoetin alfa formulation were 2 ± 0.9 Units/mL and 16.3 ± 3.0 hours. There was no notable accumulation in serum after two weekly 750 Units/kg SC doses of Epoetin alfa.

INDICATIONS AND USAGE

Treatment of Anemia of Chronic Renal Failure Patients

EPOGEN® is indicated for the treatment of anemia associated with CRF, including patients on dialysis (ESRD) and patients not on dialysis. EPOGEN® is indicated to elevate or maintain the red blood cell level (as manifested by the hematocrit or hemoglobin determinations) and to decrease the need for transfusions in these patients.

Non-dialysis patients with symptomatic anemia considered for therapy should have a hemoglobin less than 10 g/dL.

EPOGEN® is not intended for patients who require immediate correction of severe anemia. EPOGEN® may obviate the need for maintenance transfusions but is not a substitute for emergency transfusion.

Prior to initiation of therapy, the patient's iron stores should be evaluated. Transferrin saturation should be at least 20% and ferritin at least 100 ng/mL. Blood pressure should be adequately controlled prior to initiation of EPOGEN® therapy, and must be closely monitored and controlled during therapy.

EPOGEN® should be administered under the guidance of a qualified physician (see DOSAGE AND ADMINISTRATION).

Treatment of Anemia in Zidovudine-treated HIV-infected Patients

EPOGEN® is indicated for the treatment of anemia related to therapy with zidovudine in HIV-infected patients. EPOGEN® is indicated to elevate or maintain the red blood cell level (as manifested by the hematocrit or hemoglobin determinations) and to decrease the need for transfusions in these patients. EPOGEN® is not indicated for the treatment of anemia in HIV-infected patients due to other factors such as iron or folate deficiencies, hemolysis, or gastrointestinal bleeding, which should be managed appropriately.

EPOGEN®, at a dose of 100 Units/kg TIW, is effective in decreasing the transfusion requirement and increasing the red blood cell level of anemic, HIV-infected patients treated with zidovudine, when the endogenous serum erythropoietin level is ≤ 500 mUnits/mL and when patients are receiving a dose of zidovudine ≤ 4200 mg/week.

Treatment of Anemia in Cancer Patients on Chemotherapy

EPOGEN® is indicated for the treatment of anemia in patients with non-myeloid malignancies where anemia is due to the effect of concomitantly administered chemotherapy. EPOGEN® is indicated to decrease the need for transfusions in patients who will be receiving concomitant chemotherapy for a minimum of 2 months. EPOGEN® is not indicated for the treatment of anemia in cancer patients due to other factors such as iron or folate deficiencies, hemolysis, or gastrointestinal bleeding, which should be managed appropriately.

Reduction of Allogeneic Blood Transfusion in Surgery Patients

EPOGEN® is indicated for the treatment of anemic patients (hemoglobin >10 to ≤ 13 g/dL) scheduled to undergo elective, noncardiac, nonvascular surgery to reduce the need for allogeneic blood transfusions.[18-20] EPOGEN® is indicated for patients at high risk for perioperative transfusions with significant, anticipated blood loss. EPOGEN® is not indicated for anemic patients who are willing to donate autologous blood. The safety of the perioperative use of EPOGEN® has been studied only in patients who are receiving anticoagulant prophylaxis.

CLINICAL EXPERIENCE: RESPONSE TO EPOGEN®

Chronic Renal Failure Patients

Response to EPOGEN® was consistent across all studies. In the presence of adequate iron stores (see IRON EVALUATION), the time to reach the target hematocrit is a function of the baseline hematocrit and the rate of hematocrit rise. The rate of increase in hematocrit is dependent upon the dose of EPOGEN® administered and individual patient variation. In clinical trials at starting doses of 50 to 150 Units/kg TIW, adult patients responded with an average rate of hematocrit rise of:

Starting Dose (TIW IV)	Hematocrit Increase Points/Day	Hematocrit Increase Points/2 Weeks
50 Units/kg	0.11	1.5
100 Units/kg	0.18	2.5
150 Units/kg	0.25	3.5

Over this dose range, approximately 95% of all patients responded with a clinically significant increase in hematocrit, and by the end of approximately 2 months of therapy virtually all patients were transfusion-independent. Changes in the quality of life of adult patients treated with EPOGEN® were assessed as part of a phase 3 clinical trial.[5,8] Once the target hematocrit (32% to 38%) was achieved, statistically significant improvements were demonstrated for most quality of life parameters measured, including energy and activity level, functional ability, sleep and eating behavior, health status, satisfaction with health, sex life, well-being, psychological effect, life satisfaction, and happiness. Patients also reported improvement in their disease symptoms. They showed a statistically significant increase in exercise capacity (VO_2 max), energy, and strength with a significant reduction in aching, dizziness, anxiety, shortness of breath, muscle weakness, and leg cramps.[8,21]

Adult Patients on Dialysis: Thirteen clinical studies were conducted, involving IV administration to a total of 1010 anemic patients on dialysis for 986 patient-years of EPOGEN® therapy. In the three largest of these clinical trials, the median maintenance dose necessary to maintain the hematocrit between 30% to 36% was approximately 75 Units/kg TIW. In the US multicenter phase 3 study, approximately 65% of the patients required doses of 100 Units/kg TIW, or less, to maintain their hematocrit at approximately 35%. Almost 10% of patients required a dose of 25 Units/kg, or less, and approximately 10% required a dose of more than 200 Units/kg TIW to maintain their hematocrit at this level.

A multicenter unit dose study was also conducted in 119 patients receiving peritoneal dialysis who self-administered EPOGEN® subcutaneously for approximately 109 patient-years of experience. Patients responded to EPOGEN® administered SC in a manner similar to patients receiving IV administration.[22]

Pediatric Patients on Dialysis: One hundred twenty-eight children from 2 months to 19 years of age with CRF requiring dialysis were enrolled in 4 clinical studies of EPOGEN®. The largest study was a placebo-controlled, randomized trial in 113 children with anemia (hematocrit ≤ 27%) undergoing peritoneal dialysis or hemodialysis. The initial dose of EPOGEN® was 50 Units/kg IV or SC TIW. The dose of study drug was titrated to achieve either a hematocrit of 30% to 36% or an absolute increase in hematocrit of 6 percentage points over baseline.

At the end of the initial 12 weeks, a statistically significant rise in mean hematocrit (9.4% vs 0.9%) was observed only in the EPOGEN® arm. The proportion of children achieving a hematocrit of 30%, or an increase in hematocrit of 6 percentage points over baseline, at any time during the first 12 weeks was higher in the EPOGEN® arm (96% vs 58%). Within 12 weeks of initiating EPOGEN® therapy, 92.3% of the pediatric patients were transfusion-independent as compared to 65.4% who received placebo. Among patients who received 36 weeks of EPOGEN®, hemodialysis patients required a higher median maintenance dose (167 Units/kg/week [n = 28] vs 76 Units/kg/week [n = 36]) and took longer to achieve a hematocrit of 30% to 36% (median time to response 69 days vs 32 days) than patients undergoing peritoneal dialysis.

Patients With CRF Not Requiring Dialysis

Four clinical trials were conducted in patients with CRF not on dialysis involving 181 patients treated with EPOGEN® for approximately 67 patient-years of experience. These patients responded to EPOGEN® therapy in a manner similar to that observed in patients on dialysis. Patients with CRF not on dialysis demonstrated a dose-dependent and sustained increase in hematocrit when EPOGEN® was administered by either an IV or SC route, with similar rates of rise of hematocrit when EPOGEN® was administered by either route. Moreover, EPOGEN® doses of 75 to 150 Units/kg per week have been shown to maintain hematocrits of 36% to 38% for up to 6 months. Correcting the anemia of progressive renal failure will allow patients to remain active even though their renal function continues to decrease.[23-24]

Zidovudine-treated HIV-infected Patients

EPOGEN® has been studied in four placebo-controlled trials enrolling 297 anemic (hematocrit < 30%) HIV-infected (AIDS) patients receiving concomitant therapy with zidovudine (all patients were treated with Epoetin alfa manufactured by Amgen Inc). In the subgroup of patients (89/125 EPOGEN® and 88/130 placebo) with prestudy endogenous serum erythropoietin levels ≤ 500 mUnits/mL, EPOGEN® reduced the mean cumulative number of units of blood transfused per patient by approximately 40% as compared to the placebo group.[25] Among those patients who required transfusions at baseline, 43% of patients treated with EPOGEN® versus 18% of placebo-treated patients were transfusion-independent during the second and third months of therapy. EPOGEN® therapy also resulted in significant increases in hematocrit in comparison to placebo. When examining the results according to the weekly dose of zidovudine received during month 3 of therapy, there was a statistically significant ($p < 0.003$) reduction in transfusion requirements in patients treated with EPOGEN® (n = 51) compared to placebo treated patients (n = 54) whose mean weekly zidovudine dose was ≤ 4200 mg/week.[25]

Approximately 17% of the patients with endogenous serum erythropoietin levels ≤ 500 mUnits/mL receiving EPOGEN® in doses from 100 to 200 Units/kg TIW achieved a hematocrit of 38% without administration of transfusions or significant reduction in zidovudine dose. In the subgroup of patients whose prestudy endogenous serum erythropoietin levels were > 500 mUnits/mL, EPOGEN® therapy did not reduce transfusion requirements or increase hematocrit, compared to the corresponding responses in placebo-treated patients.

In a 6 month open-label EPOGEN® study, patients responded with decreased transfusion requirements and sustained increases in hematocrit and hemoglobin with doses of EPOGEN® up to 300 Units/kg TIW.[25-27]

Continued on next page

Epogen—Cont.

Responsiveness to EPOGEN® therapy may be blunted by intercurrent infectious/inflammatory episodes and by an increase in zidovudine dosage. Consequently, the dose of EPOGEN® must be titrated based on these factors to maintain the desired erythropoietic response.

Cancer Patients on Chemotherapy

EPOGEN® has been studied in a series of six placebo-controlled, double-blind trials that enrolled 131 anemic cancer patients receiving EPOGEN® or matching placebo. Across all studies, 72 patients were treated with concomitant non cisplatin-containing chemotherapy regimens and 59 patients were treated with concomitant cisplatin-containing chemotherapy regimens. Patients were randomized to EPOGEN® 150 Units/kg or placebo subcutaneously TIW for 12 weeks in each study.

The results of the pooled data from these six studies are shown in the table below. Because of the length of time required for erythropoiesis and red cell maturation, the efficacy of EPOGEN® (reduction in proportion of patients requiring transfusions) is not manifested until 2 to 6 weeks after initiation of EPOGEN®.

[See table below]

Intensity of chemotherapy in the above trials was not directly assessed, however the degree and timing of neutropenia was comparable across all trials. Available evidence suggests that patients with lymphoid and solid cancers respond similarly to EPOGEN® therapy, and that patients with or without tumor infiltration of the bone marrow respond similarly to EPOGEN® therapy.

Surgery Patients

EPOGEN® has been studied in a placebo-controlled, double-blind trial enrolling 316 patients scheduled for major, elective orthopedic hip or knee surgery who were expected to require ≥ 2 units of blood and who were not able or willing to participate in an autologous blood donation program. Based on previous studies which demonstrated that pretreatment hemoglobin is a predictor of risk of receiving transfusion,[20,28] patients were stratified into one of three groups based on their pretreatment hemoglobin [≤ 10 (n = 2), > 10 to ≤ 13 (n = 96), and > 13 to ≤ 15 g/dL (n = 218)] and then randomly assigned to receive 300 Units/kg EPOGEN®, 100 Units/kg EPOGEN® or placebo by SC injection for 10 days before surgery, on the day of surgery, and for 4 days after surgery.[18] All patients received oral iron and a low-dose post-operative warfarin regimen.[18]

Treatment with EPOGEN® 300 Units/kg significantly (p = 0.024) reduced the risk of allogeneic transfusion in patients with a pretreatment hemoglobin of > 10 to ≤ 13; 5/31 (16%) of EPOGEN® 300 Units/kg, 6/26 (23%) of EPOGEN® 100 Units/kg, and 13/29 (45%) of placebo-treated patients were transfused.[18] There was no significant difference in the number of patients transfused between EPOGEN® (9% 300 Units/kg, 6% 100 Units/kg) and placebo (13%) in the > 13 to ≤ 15 g/dL hemoglobin stratum. There were too few patients in the ≤ 10 g/dL group to determine if EPOGEN® is useful in this hemoglobin strata. In the > 10 to ≤ 13 g/dL pretreatment stratum, the mean number of units transfused per EPOGEN®-treated patient (0.45 units blood for 300 Units/kg, 0.42 units blood for 100 Units/kg) was less than the mean transfused per placebo-treated patient (1.14 units) (overall p = 0.028). In addition, mean hemoglobin, hematocrit, and reticulocyte counts increased significantly during the presurgery period in patients treated with EPOGEN®.[18]

EPOGEN® was also studied in an open-label, parallel-group trial enrolling 145 subjects with a pretreatment hemoglobin level of ≥ 10 to ≤ 13 g/dL who were scheduled for major orthopedic hip or knee surgery and who were not participating in an autologous program.[19] Subjects were randomly assigned to receive one of two SC dosing regimens of EPOGEN® (600 Units/kg once weekly for 3 weeks prior to surgery and on the day of surgery, or 300 Units/kg once daily for 10 days prior to surgery, on the day of surgery and for 4 days after surgery). All subjects received oral iron and appropriate pharmacologic anticoagulation therapy.

From pretreatment to presurgery, the mean increase in hemoglobin in the 600 Units/kg weekly group (1.44 g/dL) was greater than observed in the 300 Units/kg daily group.[19] The mean increase in absolute reticulocyte count was smaller in the weekly group ($0.11 \times 10^6/mm^3$) compared to the daily group ($0.17 \times 10^6/mm^3$). Mean hemoglobin levels were similar for the two treatment groups throughout the postsurgical period.

The erythropoietic response observed in both treatment groups resulted in similar transfusion rates [11/69 (16%) in the 600 Units/kg weekly group and 14/71 (20%) in the 300 Units/kg daily group].[19] The mean number of units transfused per subject was approximately 0.3 units in both treatment groups.

Proportion of Patients Transfused During Chemotherapy (Efficacy Population[a])

Chemotherapy Regimen	On Study[b]		During Months 2 and 3[c]	
	EPOGEN®	Placebo	EPOGEN®	Placebo
Regimens without cisplatin	44% (15/34)	44% (16/36)	21% (6/29)	33% (11/33)
Regimens containing cisplatin	50% (14/28)	63% (19/30)	23% (5/22)[d]	56% (14/25)
Combined	47% (29/62)	53% (35/66)	22% (11/51)[d]	43% (25/58)

[a] Limited to patients remaining on study at least 15 days (1 patient excluded from EPOGEN®, 2 patients excluded from placebo).
[b] Includes all transfusions from day 1 through the end of study.
[c] Limited to patients remaining on study beyond week 6 and includes only transfusions during weeks 5-12.
[d] Unadjusted 2-sided $p < 0.05$

CONTRAINDICATIONS

EPOGEN® is contraindicated in patients with:

1. Uncontrolled hypertension.
2. Known hypersensitivity to mammalian cell-derived products.
3. Known hypersensitivity to Albumin (Human).

WARNINGS

Pediatric Use

The multidose preserved formulation contains benzyl alcohol. Benzyl alcohol has been reported to be associated with an increased incidence of neurological and other complications in premature infants which are sometimes fatal.

Thrombotic Events and Increased Mortality

A randomized, prospective trial of 1265 hemodialysis patients with clinically evident cardiac disease (ischemic heart disease or congestive heart failure) was conducted in which patients were assigned to EPOGEN® treatment targeted to a maintenance hematocrit of either 42 ± 3% or 30 ± 3%.[42] Increased mortality was observed in 634 patients randomized to a target hematocrit of 42% [221 deaths (35% mortality)] compared to 631 patients targeted to remain at a hematocrit of 30% [185 deaths (29% mortality)]. The reason for the increased mortality observed in these studies is unknown, however, the incidence of non-fatal myocardial infarctions (3.1% vs 2.3%), vascular access thromboses (39% vs 29%), and all other thrombotic events (22% vs 18%) were also higher in the group randomized to achieve a hematocrit of 42%.

Increased mortality was also observed in a randomized placebo-controlled study of EPOGEN® in adult patients who did not have CRF who were undergoing coronary artery bypass surgery (7 deaths in 126 patients randomized to EPOGEN® versus no deaths among 56 patients receiving placebo). Four of these deaths occurred during the period of study drug administration and all four deaths were associated with thrombotic events. While the extent of the population affected is unknown, in patients at risk for thrombosis, the anticipated benefits of EPOGEN® treatment should be weighed against the potential for increased risks associated with therapy.

In a randomized, prospective trial conducted with another Epoetin alfa product, in 939 women with metastatic carcinoma of the breast who were receiving chemotherapy, patients were assigned to receive either Epoetin alfa or placebo for up to a year, in a weekly schedule, with the primary goal of showing improved survival and improved quality of life in the Epoetin alfa treatment arm.[25] This study utilized a treatment strategy designed to maintain hemoglobin levels of 12 to14 g/dL (hematocrit 36 to 42%). Increased mortality in the first 4 months after randomization was observed among 469 patients who received the erythropoietin product [41 deaths (8.7% mortality)] compared to 470 patients who received placebo [16 deaths (3.4% mortality)]. In the first four months of the study, the incidence of fatal thrombotic vascular events (1.1% vs 0.2%) and death attributed to disease progression (6.0% vs 2.8%) were both higher in the group randomized to receive Epoetin alfa as compared to placebo. Based on Kaplan-Meier estimates, the proportion of subjects surviving at 12 months after randomization was lower in the Epoetin alfa group than in the placebo group (70% vs 76%), p = 0.012, log rank. However, due to insufficient monitoring and data collection, reliable comparisons cannot be made concerning the effect of Epoetin alfa on overall time to disease progression, progression-free survival, and overall survival.

Pure Red Cell Aplasia

Pure red cell aplasia (PRCA), in association with neutralizing antibodies to native erythropoietin, has been observed in patients treated with recombinant erythropoietins. PRCA has been reported in a limited number of patients exposed to EPOGEN®. This has been reported predominantly in patients with CRF. Any patient with loss of response to EPOGEN® should be evaluated for the etiology of loss of effect (see PRECAUTIONS: LACK OR LOSS OF RESPONSE). EPOGEN® should be discontinued in any patient with evidence of PRCA and the patient evaluated for the presence of binding and neutralizing antibodies to EPOGEN® native erythropoietin, and any other recombinant erythropoietin administered to the patient. Amgen should be contacted to assist in this evaluation. In patients with PRCA secondary to neutralizing antibodies to erythropoietin, EPOGEN® should not be administered and such patients should not be switched to another product as anti-erythropoietin antibodies cross-react with other erythropoietins (see ADVERSE REACTIONS).

Albumin (Human)

EPOGEN® contains albumin, a derivative of human blood. Based on effective donor screening and product manufacturing processes, it carries an extremely remote risk for transmission of viral diseases. A theoretical risk for transmission of Creutzfeldt-Jakob disease (CJD) also is considered extremely remote. No cases of transmission of viral diseases or CJD have ever been identified for albumin.

Chronic Renal Failure Patients

Hypertension: Patients with uncontrolled hypertension should not be treated with EPOGEN®; blood pressure should be controlled adequately before initiation of therapy. Up to 80% of patients with CRF have a history of hypertension.[29] Although there does not appear to be any direct pressor effects of EPOGEN®, blood pressure may rise during EPOGEN® therapy. During the early phase of treatment when the hematocrit is increasing, approximately 25% of patients on dialysis may require initiation of, or increases in, antihypertensive therapy. Hypertensive encephalopathy and seizures have been observed in patients with CRF treated with EPOGEN®.

Special care should be taken to closely monitor and aggressively control blood pressure in patients treated with EPOGEN®. Patients should be advised as to the importance of compliance with antihypertensive therapy and dietary restrictions. If blood pressure is difficult to control by initiation of appropriate measures, the hemoglobin may be reduced by decreasing or withholding the dose of EPOGEN®. A clinically significant decrease in hemoglobin may not be observed for several weeks.

It is recommended that the dose of EPOGEN® be decreased if the hemoglobin increase exceeds 1 g/dL in any 2-week period, because of the possible association of excessive rate of rise of hemoglobin with an exacerbation of hypertension. In CRF patients on hemodialysis with clinically evident ischemic heart disease or congestive heart failure, the hemoglobin should be managed carefully, not to exceed 12 g/dL (see THROMBOTIC EVENTS).

Seizures: Seizures have occurred in patients with CRF participating in EPOGEN® clinical trials.

In adult patients on dialysis, there was a higher incidence of seizures during the first 90 days of therapy (occurring in approximately 2.5% of patients) as compared with later timepoints.

Given the potential for an increased risk of seizures during the first 90 days of therapy, blood pressure and the presence of premonitory neurologic symptoms should be monitored closely. Patients should be cautioned to avoid potentially hazardous activities such as driving or operating heavy machinery during this period.

While the relationship between seizures and the rate of rise of hemoglobin is uncertain, it is recommended that the dose of EPOGEN® be decreased if the hemoglobin increase exceeds 1 g/dL in any 2-week period.

Thrombotic Events: During hemodialysis, patients treated with EPOGEN® may require increased anticoagulation with heparin to prevent clotting of the artificial kidney (see ADVERSE REACTIONS for more information about thrombotic events).

Other thrombotic events (eg, myocardial infarction, cerebrovascular accident, transient ischemic attack) have occurred in clinical trials at an annualized rate of less than 0.04 events per patient year of EPOGEN® therapy. These trials were conducted in adult patients with CRF (whether on dialysis or not) in whom the target hematocrit was 32% to 40%. However, the risk of thrombotic events, including vascular access thrombosis, was significantly increased in adult patients with ischemic heart disease or congestive heart failure receiving EPOGEN® therapy with the goal of reaching a normal hematocrit (42%) as compared to a target hematocrit of 30%. Patients with pre-existing cardiovascular disease should be monitored closely.

Zidovudine-treated HIV-infected Patients

In contrast to CRF patients, EPOGEN® therapy has not been linked to exacerbation of hypertension, seizures, and thrombotic events in HIV-infected patients.

PRECAUTIONS

The parenteral administration of any biologic product should be attended by appropriate precautions in case allergic or other untoward reactions occur (see CONTRAINDICATIONS). In clinical trials, while transient rashes were occasionally observed concurrently with EPOGEN® therapy, no serious allergic or anaphylactic reactions were reported (see ADVERSE REACTIONS for more information regarding allergic reactions).

The safety and efficacy of EPOGEN® therapy have not been established in patients with a known history of a seizure disorder or underlying hematologic disease (eg, sickle cell anemia, myelodysplastic syndromes, or hypercoagulable disorders).

In some female patients, menses have resumed following EPOGEN® therapy; the possibility of pregnancy should be discussed and the need for contraception evaluated.

Hematology

Exacerbation of porphyria has been observed rarely in patients with CRF treated with EPOGEN®. However, EPOGEN® has not caused increased urinary excretion of porphyrin metabolites in normal volunteers, even in the presence of a rapid erythropoietic response. Nevertheless, EPOGEN® should be used with caution in patients with known porphyria.

In preclinical studies in dogs and rats, but not in monkeys, EPOGEN® therapy was associated with subclinical bone marrow fibrosis. Bone marrow fibrosis is a known complication of CRF in humans and may be related to secondary hyperparathyroidism or unknown factors. The incidence of bone marrow fibrosis was not increased in a study of adult patients on dialysis who were treated with EPOGEN® for 12 to 19 months, compared to the incidence of bone marrow fibrosis in a matched group of patients who had not been treated with EPOGEN®.

Hemoglobin in CRF patients should be measured twice a week; zidovudine-treated HIV-infected and cancer patients should have hemoglobin measured once a week until hemoglobin has been stabilized, and measured periodically thereafter.

Lack or Loss of Response

If the patient fails to respond or to maintain a response to doses within the recommended dosing range, the following etiologies should be considered and evaluated:

1. Iron deficiency: Virtually all patients will eventually require supplemental iron therapy (see IRON EVALUATION).
2. Underlying infectious, inflammatory, or malignant processes.
3. Occult blood loss.
4. Underlying hematologic diseases (ie, thalassemia, refractory anemia, or other myelodysplastic disorders).
5. Vitamin deficiencies: Folic acid or vitamin B12.
6. Hemolysis.
7. Aluminum intoxication.
8. Osteitis fibrosa cystica.
9. Pure Red Cell Aplasia (PRCA): In the absence of another etiology, the patient should be evaluated for evidence of PRCA and sera should be tested for the presence of antibodies to recombinant erythropoietins.

Iron Evaluation

During EPOGEN® therapy, absolute or functional iron deficiency may develop. Functional iron deficiency, with normal ferritin levels but low transferrin saturation, is presumably due to the inability to mobilize iron stores rapidly enough to support increased erythropoiesis. Transferrin saturation should be at least 20% and ferritin should be at least 100 ng/mL.

Prior to and during EPOGEN® therapy, the patient's iron status, including transferrin saturation (serum iron divided by iron binding capacity) and serum ferritin, should be evaluated. Virtually all patients will eventually require supplemental iron to increase or maintain transferrin saturation to levels which will adequately support erythropoiesis stimulated by EPOGEN®. All surgery patients being treated with EPOGEN® should receive adequate iron supplementation throughout the course of therapy in order to support erythropoiesis and avoid depletion of iron stores.

Drug Interaction

No evidence of interaction of EPOGEN® with other drugs was observed in the course of clinical trials.

Carcinogenesis, Mutagenesis, and Impairment of Fertility

Carcinogenic potential of EPOGEN® has not been evaluated. EPOGEN® does not induce bacterial gene mutation (Ames Test), chromosomal aberrations in mammalian cells, micronuclei in mice, or gene mutation at the HGPRT locus. In female rats treated IV with EPOGEN®, there was a trend for slightly increased fetal wastage at doses of 100 and 500 Units/kg.

Pregnancy Category C

EPOGEN® has been shown to have adverse effects in rats when given in doses 5 times the human dose. There are no adequate and well-controlled studies in pregnant women. EPOGEN® should be used during pregnancy only if potential benefit justifies the potential risk to the fetus.

In studies in female rats, there were decreases in body weight gain, delays in appearance of abdominal hair, delayed eyelid opening, delayed ossification, and decreases in the number of caudal vertebrae in the F1 fetuses of the 500 Units/kg group. In female rats treated IV, there was a trend for slightly increased fetal wastage at doses of 100 and 500 Units/kg. EPOGEN® has not shown any adverse effect at doses as high as 500 Units/kg in pregnant rabbits (from day 6 to 18 of gestation).

Nursing Mothers

Postnatal observations of the live offspring (F1 generation) of female rats treated with EPOGEN® during gestation and lactation revealed no effect of EPOGEN® at doses of up to 500 Units/kg. There were, however, decreases in body weight gain, delays in appearance of abdominal hair, eyelid opening, and decreases in the number of caudal vertebrae in the F1 fetuses of the 500 Units/kg group. There were no EPOGEN®-related effects on the F2 generation fetuses.

It is not known whether EPOGEN® is excreted in human milk. Because many drugs are excreted in human milk, caution should be exercised when EPOGEN® is administered to a nursing woman.

Pediatric Use

See WARNINGS: PEDIATRIC USE.

Pediatric Patients on Dialysis: EPOGEN® is indicated in infants (1 month to 2 years), children (2 years to 12 years), and adolescents (12 years to 16 years) for the treatment of anemia associated with CRF requiring dialysis. Safety and effectiveness in pediatric patients less than 1 month old have not been established (see CLINICAL EXPERIENCE: CHRONIC RENAL FAILURE, PEDIATRIC PATIENTS ON DIALYSIS). The safety data from these studies show that there is no increased risk to pediatric CRF patients on dialysis when compared to the safety profile of EPOGEN® in adult CRF patients (see ADVERSE REACTIONS and WARNINGS). Published literature[30-33] provides supportive evidence of the safety and effectiveness of EPOGEN® in pediatric CRF patients on dialysis.

Pediatric Patients Not Requiring Dialysis: Published literature[33,34] has reported the use of EPOGEN® in 133 pediatric patients with anemia associated with CRF not requiring dialysis, ages 3 months to 20 years, treated with 50 to 250 Units/kg SC or IV, QW to TIW. Dose-dependent increases in hemoglobin and hematocrit were observed with reductions in transfusion requirements.

Pediatric HIV-infected Patients: Published literature [35,36] has reported the use of EPOGEN® in 20 zidovudine-treated anemic HIV-infected pediatric patients ages 8 months to 17 years, treated with 50 to 400 Units/kg SC or IV, 2 to 3 times per week. Increases in hemoglobin levels and in reticulocyte counts, and decreases in or elimination of blood transfusions were observed.

Pediatric Cancer Patients on Chemotherapy: Published literature[37,38] has reported the use of EPOGEN® in approximately 64 anemic pediatric cancer patients ages 6 months to 18 years, treated with 25 to 300 Units/kg SC or IV, 3 to 7 times per week. Increases in hemoglobin and decreases in transfusion requirements were noted.

Chronic Renal Failure Patients

Patients with CRF Not Requiring Dialysis

Blood pressure and hemoglobin should be monitored no less frequently than for patients maintained on dialysis. Renal function and fluid and electrolyte balance should be closely monitored, as an improved sense of well-being may obscure the need to initiate dialysis in some patients.

Hematology

Sufficient time should be allowed to determine a patient's responsiveness to a dosage of EPOGEN® before adjusting the dose. Because of the time required for erythropoiesis and the red cell half-life, an interval of 2 to 6 weeks may occur between the time of a dose adjustment (initiation, increase, decrease, or discontinuation) and a significant change in hemoglobin.

In order to avoid reaching the suggested target hemoglobin too rapidly, or exceeding the suggested target range (hemoglobin of 10 g/dL to 12 g/dL), the guidelines for dose and frequency of dose adjustments (see DOSAGE AND ADMINISTRATION) should be followed.

For patients who respond to EPOGEN® with a rapid increase in hemoglobin (eg, more than 1 g/dL in any 2-week period), the dose of EPOGEN® should be reduced because of the possible association of excessive rate of rise of hemoglobin with an exacerbation of hypertension.

The elevated bleeding time characteristic of CRF decreases toward normal after correction of anemia in adult patients treated with EPOGEN®. Reduction of bleeding time also occurs after correction of anemia by transfusion.

Laboratory Monitoring

The hemoglobin should be determined twice a week until it has stabilized in the suggested target range and the maintenance dose has been established. After any dose adjustment, the hemoglobin should also be determined twice weekly for at least 2 to 6 weeks until it has been determined that the hemoglobin has stabilized in response to the dose change. The hematocrit should then be monitored at regular intervals.

A complete blood count with differential and platelet count should be performed regularly. During clinical trials, modest increases were seen in platelets and white blood cell counts. While these changes were statistically significant, they were not clinically significant and the values remained within normal ranges.

In patients with CRF, serum chemistry values (including blood urea nitrogen [BUN], uric acid, creatinine, phosphorus, and potassium) should be monitored regularly. During clinical trials in adult patients on dialysis, modest increases were seen in BUN, creatinine, phosphorus, and potassium. In some adult patients with CRF not on dialysis treated with EPOGEN®, modest increases in serum uric acid and phosphorus were observed. While changes were statistically significant, the values remained within the ranges normally seen in patients with CRF.

Diet

As the hemoglobin increases and patients experience an improved sense of well-being and quality of life, the importance of compliance with dietary and dialysis prescriptions should be reinforced. In particular, hyperkalemia is not uncommon in patients with CRF. In US studies in patients on dialysis, hyperkalemia has occurred at an annualized rate of approximately 0.11 episodes per patient-year of EPOGEN® therapy, often in association with poor compliance to medication, diet, and/or dialysis.

Dialysis Management

Therapy with EPOGEN® results in an increase in hematocrit and a decrease in plasma volume which could affect dialysis efficiency. In studies to date, the resulting increase in hematocrit did not appear to adversely affect dialyzer function[9,10] or the efficiency of high flux hemodialysis.[11] During hemodialysis, patients treated with EPOGEN® may require increased anticoagulation with heparin to prevent clotting of the artificial kidney.

Patients who are marginally dialyzed may require adjustments in their dialysis prescription. As with all patients on dialysis, the serum chemistry values (including BUN, creatinine, phosphorus, and potassium) in patients treated with EPOGEN® should be monitored regularly to assure the adequacy of the dialysis prescription.

Information for Patients

In those situations in which the physician determines that a home dialysis patient can safely and effectively self-administer EPOGEN®, the patient should be instructed as to the proper dosage and administration. Home dialysis patients should be referred to the full "Information for Home Dialysis Patients" insert; it is not a disclosure of all possible effects. Patients should be informed of the signs and symptoms of allergic drug reaction and advised of appropriate actions. If home use is prescribed for a home dialysis patient, the patient should be thoroughly instructed in the importance of proper disposal and cautioned against the reuse of needles, syringes, or drug product. A puncture-resistant container for the disposal of used syringes and needles should be available to the patient. The full container should be disposed of according to the directions provided by the physician.

Renal Function

In adult patients with CRF not on dialysis, renal function and fluid and electrolyte balance should be closely monitored, as an improved sense of well-being may obscure the need to initiate dialysis in some patients. In patients with CRF not on dialysis, placebo-controlled studies of progression of renal dysfunction over periods of greater than 1 year have not been completed. In shorter term trials in adult patients with CRF not on dialysis, changes in creatinine and creatinine clearance were not significantly different in patients treated with EPOGEN® compared with placebo-treated patients. Analysis of the slope of 1/serum creatinine versus time plots in these patients indicates no significant change in the slope after the initiation of EPOGEN® therapy.

Zidovudine-treated HIV-infected Patients

Hypertension

Exacerbation of hypertension has not been observed in zidovudine-treated HIV-infected patients treated with EPOGEN®. However, EPOGEN® should be withheld in these patients if pre-existing hypertension is uncontrolled, and should not be started until blood pressure is controlled. In double-blind studies, a single seizure has been experienced by a patient treated with EPOGEN®.[25]

Cancer Patients on Chemotherapy

Hypertension

Hypertension, associated with a significant increase in hemoglobin, has been noted rarely in patients treated with EPOGEN®. Nevertheless, blood pressure in patients treated with EPOGEN® should be monitored carefully, particularly in patients with an underlying history of hypertension or cardiovascular disease.

Seizures

In double-blind, placebo-controlled trials, 3.2% (n = 2/63) of patients treated with EPOGEN® and 2.9% (n = 2/68) of placebo-treated patients had seizures. Seizures in 1.6% (n = 1/63) of patients treated with EPOGEN® occurred in the context of a significant increase in blood pressure and hematocrit from baseline values. However, both patients treated with EPOGEN® also had underlying CNS pathology which may have been related to seizure activity.

Thrombotic Events

In double-blind, placebo-controlled trials, 3.2% (n = 2/63) of patients treated with EPOGEN® and 11.8% (n = 8/68) of placebo-treated patients had thrombotic events (eg, pulmonary embolism, cerebrovascular accident), (See WARNINGS; Thrombotic Events and Increased Mortality).

Tumor Growth Factor Potential

EPOGEN® is a growth factor that primarily stimulates red cell production. Erythropoietin receptors are also found to be present on the surface of some malignant cell lines and tumor biopsy specimens. However, it is not known if these receptors are functional. A randomized, placebo-controlled trial was conducted in 224 chemotherapy-naïve, non-anemic patients with small cell lung cancer receiving cisplatin-based combination chemotherapy, to investigate whether the concurrent use of EPOGEN® stimulated tumor growth as assessed by impact on overall response rate. Patients were randomized to receive EPOGEN® 150 Units/kg or placebo subcutaneously TIW during chemotherapy. The overall response rates, after 3 cycles of treatment, were 72% and 67%, in the EPOGEN® and placebo arms, respectively. Complete response rates (17% vs. 14%) and median overall survival (10.5 mos vs. 10.4 mos) were similar in the EPOGEN® and placebo arms[25].

An additional study explored effect on survival and/or progression of administrations of other exogenous erythropoietin with higher hemoglobin targets.

In a randomized, placebo-controlled study using another Epoetin alfa product, conducted in 939 women with metastatic breast cancer, study drug dosing was titrated to attempt to maintain hemoglobin levels between 12 and 14 g/dL. At four months, death attributed to disease pro-

Continued on next page

Epogen—Cont.

gression was higher (6% vs 3%) in women receiving Epoetin alfa. Overall mortality was significantly higher at 12 months in the Epoetin alfa arm (See WARNINGS; Thrombotic Events and Increased Mortality).

In a randomized, placebo-controlled study using Epoetin beta, conducted in 351 patients with head and neck cancer, study drug was administered with the aim of achieving a hemoglobin level of 14 g/dL in women and 15 g/dL in men. Locoregional progression-free survival was significantly shorter (median PFS: 406 days Epoetin beta vs 745 days placebo, p = 0.04) in patients receiving Epoetin beta.[43]

There is insufficient information to establish whether use of Epoetin products, including EPOGEN®, have an adverse effect on time to tumor progression or progression-free survival.

These trials permitted or required dosing to achieve hemoglobin of greater than 12 g/dL. Until further information is available, the recommended target hemoglobin should not exceed 12 g/dL in men or women.

Surgery Patients

Thrombotic/Vascular Events

In perioperative clinical trials with orthopedic patients, the overall incidence of thrombotic/vascular events was similar in Epoetin alfa and placebo-treated patients who had a pretreatment hemoglobin of > 10 g/dL to ≤ 13 g/dL. In patients with a hemoglobin of > 13 g/dL treated with 300 Units/kg of Epoetin alfa, the possibility that EPOGEN® treatment may be associated with an increased risk of postoperative thrombotic/vascular events cannot be excluded.[18-20,28]

In one study in which Epoetin alfa was administered in the perioperative period to patients undergoing coronary artery bypass graft surgery, there were 7 deaths in the group treated with Epoetin alfa (n = 126) and no deaths in the placebo-treated group (n = 56). Among the 7 deaths in the patients treated with Epoetin alfa, 4 were at the time of therapy (between study day 2 and 8). The 4 deaths at the time of therapy (3%) were associated with thrombotic/vascular events. A causative role of Epoetin alfa cannot be excluded (see WARNINGS).

Hypertension

Blood pressure may rise in the perioperative period in patients being treated with EPOGEN®. Therefore, blood pressure should be monitored carefully.

ADVERSE REACTIONS

Immunogenicity

As with all therapeutic proteins, there is the potential for immunogenicity. The observed incidence of antibody positivity in an assay may be influenced by several factors including assay methodology, sample handling, timing of sample collection, concomitant medications, and underlying disease. For these reasons, comparison of the incidence of antibodies to EPOGEN® with the incidence of antibodies to other products may be misleading.

A few cases of PRCA associated with antibodies with neutralizing activity have been reported in patients receiving EPOGEN® (see WARNINGS: PURE RED CELL APLASIA). These cases were observed in patients treated by either SC or IV routes of administration and occurred predominantly in CRF patients.

Chronic Renal Failure Patients

EPOGEN® is generally well-tolerated. The adverse events reported are frequent sequelae of CRF and are not necessarily attributable to EPOGEN® therapy. In double-blind, placebo-controlled studies involving over 300 patients with CRF, the events reported in greater than 5% of patients treated with EPOGEN® during the blinded phase were:

	Percent of Patients Reporting Event	
Event	Patients Treated With EPOGEN® (n = 200)	Placebo-treated Patients (n = 135)
Hypertension	24%	19%
Headache	16%	12%
Arthralgias	11%	6%
Nausea	11%	9%
Edema	9%	10%
Fatigue	9%	14%
Diarrhea	9%	6%
Vomiting	8%	5%
Chest Pain	7%	9%
Skin Reaction (Administration Site)	7%	12%
Asthenia	7%	12%
Dizziness	7%	13%
Clotted Access	7%	2%

Significant adverse events of concern in patients with CRF treated in double-blind, placebo-controlled trials occurred in the following percent of patients during the blinded phase of the studies:

Seizure	1.1%	1.1%
CVA/TIA	0.4%	0.6%
MI	0.4%	1.1%
Death	0%	1.7%

In the US EPOGEN® studies in adult patients on dialysis (over 567 patients), the incidence (number of events per patient-year) of the most frequently reported adverse events were: hypertension (0.75), headache (0.40), tachycardia (0.31), nausea/vomiting (0.26), clotted vascular access (0.25), shortness of breath (0.14), hyperkalemia (0.11), and diarrhea (0.11). Other reported events occurred at a rate of less than 0.10 events per patient per year.

Events reported to have occurred within several hours of administration of EPOGEN® were rare, mild, and transient, and included injection site stinging in dialysis patients and flu-like symptoms such as arthralgias and myalgias.

In all studies analyzed to date, EPOGEN® administration was generally well-tolerated, irrespective of the route of administration.

Pediatric CRF Patients: In pediatric patients with CRF on dialysis, the pattern of most adverse events was similar to that found in adults. Additional adverse events reported during the double-blind phase in >10% of pediatric patients in either treatment group were: abdominal pain, dialysis access complications including access infections and peritonitis in those receiving peritoneal dialysis, fever, upper respiratory infection, cough, pharyngitis, and constipation. The rates are similar between the treatment groups for each event.

Hypertension: Increases in blood pressure have been reported in clinical trials, often during the first 90 days of therapy. On occasion, hypertensive encephalopathy and seizures have been observed in patients with CRF treated with EPOGEN®. When data from all patients in the US phase 3 multicenter trial were analyzed, there was an apparent trend of more reports of hypertensive adverse events in patients on dialysis with a faster rate of rise of hematocrit (greater than 4 hematocrit points in any 2-week period). However, in a double-blind, placebo-controlled trial, hypertensive adverse events were not reported at an increased rate in the group treated with EPOGEN® (150 Units/kg TIW) relative to the placebo group.

Seizures: There have been 47 seizures in 1010 patients on dialysis treated with EPOGEN® in clinical trials, with an exposure of 986 patient-years for a rate of approximately 0.048 events per patient-year. However, there appeared to be a higher rate of seizures during the first 90 days of therapy (occurring in approximately 2.5% of patients) when compared to subsequent 90-day periods. The baseline incidence of seizures in the untreated dialysis population is difficult to determine; it appears to be in the range of 5% to 10% per patient-year.[39-41]

Thrombotic Events: In clinical trials where the maintenance hematocrit was 35 ± 3% on EPOGEN®, clotting of the vascular access (A-V shunt) has occurred at an annualized rate of about 0.25 events per patient-year, and other thrombotic events (eg, myocardial infarction, cerebral vascular accident, transient ischemic attack, and pulmonary embolism) occurred at a rate of 0.04 events per patient-year. In a separate study of 1111 untreated dialysis patients, clotting of the vascular access occurred at a rate of 0.50 events per patient-year. However, in CRF patients on hemodialysis who also had clinically evident ischemic heart disease or congestive heart failure, the risk of A-V shunt thrombosis was higher (39% vs 29%, $p < 0.001$), and myocardial infarctions, vascular ischemic events, and venous thrombosis were increased, in patients targeted to a hematocrit of 42 ± 3% compared to those maintained at 30 ± 3% (see WARNINGS).

In patients treated with commercial EPOGEN®, there have been rare reports of serious or unusual thrombo-embolic events including migratory thrombophlebitis, microvascular thrombosis, pulmonary embolus, and thrombosis of the retinal artery, and temporal and renal veins. A causal relationship has not been established.

Allergic Reactions: There have been no reports of serious allergic reactions or anaphylaxis associated with EPOGEN® administration during clinical trials. Skin rashes and urticaria have been observed rarely and when reported have generally been mild and transient in nature. There have been rare reports of potentially serious allergic reactions including urticaria with associated respiratory symptoms or circumoral edema, or urticaria alone. Most reactions occurred in situations where a causal relationship could not be established. Symptoms recurred with rechallenge in a few instances, suggesting that allergic reactivity may occasionally be associated with EPOGEN® therapy. If an anaphylactoid reaction occurs, EPOGEN® should be immediately discontinued and appropriate therapy initiated.

Zidovudine-treated HIV-infected Patients

Adverse events reported in clinical trials with EPOGEN® in zidovudine-treated HIV-infected patients were consistent with the progression of HIV infection. In double-blind, placebo-controlled studies of 3 months duration involving approximately 300 zidovudine-treated HIV-infected patients, adverse events with an incidence of ≥ 10% in either patients treated with EPOGEN® or placebo-treated patients were:

	Percent of Patients Reporting Event	
Event	Patients Treated With EPOGEN® (n = 144)	Placebo-treated Patients (n = 153)
Pyrexia	38%	29%
Fatigue	25%	31%
Headache	19%	14%
Cough	18%	14%
Diarrhea	16%	18%
Rash	16%	8%
Congestion, Respiratory	15%	10%
Nausea	15%	12%
Shortness of Breath	14%	13%
Asthenia	11%	14%
Skin Reaction, Medication Site	10%	7%
Dizziness	9%	10%

In the 297 patients studied, EPOGEN® was not associated with significant increases in opportunistic infections or mortality.[25] In 71 patients from this group treated with EPOGEN® at 150 Units/kg TIW, serum p24 antigen levels did not appear to increase.[27] Preliminary data showed no enhancement of HIV replication in infected cell lines in vitro.[25]

Peripheral white blood cell and platelet counts are unchanged following EPOGEN® therapy.

Allergic Reactions: Two zidovudine-treated HIV-infected patients had urticarial reactions within 48 hours of their first exposure to study medication. One patient was treated with EPOGEN® and one was treated with placebo (EPOGEN® vehicle alone). Both patients had positive immediate skin tests against their study medication with a negative saline control. The basis for this apparent pre-existing hypersensitivity to components of the EPOGEN® formulation is unknown, but may be related to HIV-induced immunosuppression or prior exposure to blood products.

Seizures: In double-blind and open-label trials of EPOGEN® in zidovudine-treated HIV-infected patients, 10 patients have experienced seizures.[25] In general, these seizures appear to be related to underlying pathology such as meningitis or cerebral neoplasms, not EPOGEN® therapy.

Cancer Patients on Chemotherapy

Adverse experiences reported in clinical trials with EPOGEN® in cancer patients were consistent with the underlying disease state. In double-blind, placebo-controlled studies of up to 3 months duration involving 131 cancer patients, adverse events with an incidence > 10% in either patients treated with EPOGEN® or placebo-treated patients were as indicated below:

	Percent of Patients Reporting Event	
Event	Patients Treated With EPOGEN® (n = 63)	Placebo-treated Patients (n = 68)
Pyrexia	29%	19%
Diarrhea	21%*	7%
Nausea	17%*	32%
Vomiting	17%	15%
Edema	17%*	1%
Asthenia	13%	16%
Fatigue	13%	15%
Shortness of Breath	13%	9%
Parasthesia	11%	6%
Upper Respiratory Infection	11%	4%
Dizziness	5%	12%
Trunk Pain	3%*	16%

* Statistically significant

Although some statistically significant differences between patients being treated with EPOGEN® and placebo-treated patients were noted, the overall safety profile of EPOGEN® appeared to be consistent with the disease process of advanced cancer. During double-blind and subsequent open-label therapy in which patients (n = 72 for total exposure to EPOGEN®) were treated for up to 32 weeks with doses as high as 927 Units/kg, the adverse experience profile of EPOGEN® was consistent with the progression of advanced cancer.

Surgery Patients

Adverse events with an incidence of ≥ 10% are shown in the following table:

[See first table at top of next page]

Thrombotic/Vascular Events: In three double-blind, placebo-controlled orthopedic surgery studies, the rate of deep venous thrombosis (DVT) was similar among Epoetin alfa and placebo-treated patients in the recommended population of patients with a pretreatment hemoglobin of > 10 g/dL to ≤ 13 g/dL.[18,20,28] However, in 2 of 3 orthopedic surgery studies the overall rate (all pretreatment hemoglobin groups combined) of DVTs detected by postoperative ultrasonography and/or surveillance venography was higher in the group treated with Epoetin alfa than in the placebo-treated group (11% vs 6%). This finding was attributable to the difference in DVT rates observed in the subgroup of patients with pretreatment hemoglobin > 13 g/dL. However, the incidence of DVTs was within the range of that reported in the literature for orthopedic surgery patients.

In the orthopedic surgery study of patients with pretreatment hemoglobin of > 10 g/dL to ≤ 13 g/dL which compared two dosing regimens (600 Units/kg weekly × 4 and 300 Units/kg daily × 15), 4 subjects in the 600 Units/kg weekly EPOGEN® group (5%) and no subjects in the 300 Units/kg daily group had a thrombotic vascular event during the study period.[19]

In a study examining the use of Epoetin alfa in 182 patients scheduled for coronary artery bypass graft surgery, 23% of patients treated with Epoetin alfa and 29% treated with placebo experienced thrombotic/vascular events. There were

4 deaths among the Epoetin alfa-treated patients that were associated with a thrombotic/vascular event. A causative role of Epoetin alfa cannot be excluded (see WARNINGS).

OVERDOSAGE

The maximum amount of EPOGEN® that can be safely administered in single or multiple doses has not been determined. Doses of up to 1500 Units/kg TIW for 3 to 4 weeks have been administered to adults without any direct toxic effects of EPOGEN® itself.[6] Therapy with EPOGEN® can result in polycythemia if the hemoglobin is not carefully monitored and the dose appropriately adjusted. If the suggested target range is exceeded, EPOGEN® may be temporarily withheld until the hemoglobin returns to the suggested target range; EPOGEN® therapy may then be resumed using a lower dose (see DOSAGE AND ADMINISTRATION). If polycythemia is of concern, phlebotomy may be indicated to decrease the hemoglobin.

DOSAGE AND ADMINISTRATION

Chronic Renal Failure Patients

The recommended range for the starting dose of EPOGEN® is 50 to 100 Units/kg TIW for adult patients. The recommended starting dose for pediatric CRF patients on dialysis is 50 Units/kg TIW. The dose of EPOGEN® should be reduced as the hemoglobin approaches 12 g/dL or increases by more than 1 g/dL in any 2-week period. The dosage of EPOGEN® must be individualized to maintain the hemoglobin within the suggested target range. At the physician's discretion, the suggested target hemoglobin range may be expanded to achieve maximal patient benefit.

EPOGEN® may be given either as an IV or SC injection. In patients on hemodialysis, EPOGEN® usually has been administered as an IV bolus TIW. While the administration of EPOGEN® is independent of the dialysis procedure, EPOGEN® may be administered into the venous line at the end of the dialysis procedure to obviate the need for additional venous access. In adult patients with CRF not on dialysis, EPOGEN® may be given either as an IV or SC injection.

Patients who have been judged competent by their physicians to self-administer EPOGEN® without medical or other supervision may give themselves either an IV or SC injection.

[See second table at right]

During therapy, hematological parameters should be monitored regularly (see LABORATORY MONITORING).

Pretherapy Iron Evaluation: Prior to and during EPOGEN® therapy, the patient's iron stores, including transferrin saturation (serum iron divided by iron binding capacity) and serum ferritin, should be evaluated. Transferrin saturation should be at least 20%, and ferritin should be at least 100 ng/mL. Virtually all patients will eventually require supplemental iron to increase or maintain transferrin saturation to levels that will adequately support erythropoiesis stimulated by EPOGEN®.

Dose Adjustment: The dose should be adjusted for each patient to achieve and maintain a target hemoglobin not to exceed 12 g/dL.

Increases in dose should not be made more frequently than once a month. If the hemoglobin is increasing and approaching 12 g/dL, the dose should be reduced by approximately 25%. If the hemoglobin continues to increase, dose should be temporarily withheld until the hemoglobin begins to decrease, at which point therapy should be reinitiated at a dose approximately 25% below the previous dose. If the hemoglobin increases by more than 1 g/dL in a 2-week period, the dose should be decreased by approximately 25%.

If the increase in the hemoglobin is less than 1 g/dL over 4 weeks and iron stores are adequate (see *PRECAUTIONS: Laboratory Tests*), the dose of EPOGEN® may be increased by approximately 25% of the previous dose. Further increases may be made at 4-week intervals until the specified hemoglobin is obtained.

Maintenance Dose: The maintenance dose must be individualized for each patient on dialysis. In the US phase 3 multicenter trial in patients on hemodialysis, the median maintenance dose was 75 Units/kg TIW, with a range from 12.5 to 525 Units/kg TIW. Almost 10% of the patients required a dose of 25 Units/kg, or less, and approximately 10% of the patients required more than 200 Units/kg TIW to maintain their hematocrit in the suggested target range. In pediatric hemodialysis and peritoneal dialysis patients, the median maintenance dose was 167 Units/kg/week (49 to 447 Units/kg per week) and 76 Units/kg per week (24 to 323 Units/kg/week) administered in divided doses (TIW or BIW), respectively to achieve the target range of 30% to 36%.

If the hemoglobin remains below, or falls below, the suggested target range, iron stores should be re-evaluated. If the transferrin saturation is less than 20%, supplemental iron should be administered. If the transferrin saturation is greater than 20%, the dose of EPOGEN® may be increased. Such dose increases should not be made more frequently than once a month, unless clinically indicated, as the response time of the hemoglobin to a dose increase can be 2 to 6 weeks. Hemoglobin should be measured twice weekly for 2 to 6 weeks following dose increases. In adult patients with CRF not on dialysis, the maintenance dose must also be individualized. EPOGEN® doses of 75 to 150 Units/kg/week have been shown to maintain hematocrits of 36% to 38% for up to 6 months.

Lack or Loss of Response: Over 95% of patients with CRF responded with clinically significant increases in hematocrit, and virtually all patients were transfusion-

Percent of Patients Reporting Event

Event	Patients Treated With EPOGEN® 300 U/kg (n = 112)[a]	Patients Treated With EPOGEN® 100 U/kg (n = 101)[a]	Placebo-treated Patients (n = 103)[a]	Patients Treated With EPOGEN® 600 U/kg (n = 73)[b]	Patients Treated With EPOGEN® 300 U/kg (n = 72)[b]
Pyrexia	51%	50%	60%	47%	42%
Nausea	48%	43%	45%	45%	58%
Constipation	43%	42%	43%	51%	53%
Skin reaction, Medication Site	25%	19%	22%	26%	29%
Vomiting	22%	12%	14%	21%	29%
Skin Pain	18%	18%	17%	5%	4%
Pruritus	16%	16%	14%	14%	22%
Insomnia	13%	16%	13%	21%	18%
Headache	13%	11%	9%	10%	19%
Dizziness	12%	9%	12%	11%	21%
Urinary Tract Infection	12%	3%	11%	11%	8%
Hypertension	10%	11%	10%	5%	10%
Diarrhea	10%	7%	12%	10%	6%
Deep Venous Thrombosis	10%	3%	5%	0%[c]	0%[c]
Dyspepsia	9%	11%	6%	7%	8%
Anxiety	7%	2%	11%	11%	4%
Edema	6%	11%	8%	11%	7%

[a] Study including patients undergoing orthopedic surgery treated with EPOGEN® or placebo for 15 days
[b] Study including patients undergoing orthopedic surgery treated with EPOGEN® 600 Units/kg weekly × 4 or 300 Units/kg daily × 15
[c] Determined by clinical symptoms

Starting Dose:	
Adults	50 to 100 Units/kg TIW; IV or SC
Pediatric Patients	50 Units/kg TIW; IV or SC
Reduce Dose When	1. Hgb. approaches 12 g/dL or, 2. Hgb. increases > 1 g/dL in any 2-week period
Increase Dose If:	Hgb. does not increase by 2 g/dL after 8 weeks of therapy, and hgb. is below suggested target range
Maintenance Dose:	Individually titrate
Suggested Target Hgb. Range:	10 g/dL to 12 g/dL

Starting Dose:	
Adults	150 Units/kg SC TIW
Pediatric Patients	See PRECAUTIONS: Pediatric Use.
Reduce Dose by 25% when:	1. Hgb approaches 12 g/dL or, 2. Hgb increases > 1 g/dL in any 2-week period
Withhold Dose if:	Hgb exceeds 13 g/dL, until the hemoglobin fall to 12 g/dL, and restart dose at 25% below the previous dose.
Increase Dose to 300 Units/kg TIW if:	response is not satisfactory [no reduction in transfusion requirements or rise in hemoglobin] after 8 weeks
Suggested Target Hgb. Range:	10 g/dL to 12 g/dL

independent within approximately 2 months of initiation of EPOGEN® therapy.

If a patient fails to respond or maintain a response, other etiologies should be considered and evaluated as clinically indicated (see PRECAUTIONS: LACK OR LOSS OF RESPONSE).

Zidovudine-treated HIV-infected Patients

Prior to beginning EPOGEN®, it is recommended that the endogenous serum erythropoietin level be determined (prior to transfusion). Available evidence suggests that patients receiving zidovudine with endogenous serum erythropoietin levels > 500 mUnits/mL are unlikely to respond to therapy with EPOGEN®.

Starting Dose: For adult patients with serum erythropoietin levels ≤ 500 mUnits/mL who are receiving a dose of zidovudine ≤ 4200 mg/week, the recommended starting dose of EPOGEN® is 100 Units/kg as an IV or SC injection TIW for 8 weeks. For pediatric patients, see PRECAUTIONS: PEDIATRIC USE.

Increase Dose: During the dose adjustment phase of therapy, the hemoglobin should be monitored weekly. If the response is not satisfactory in terms of reducing transfusion requirements or increasing hemoglobin after 8 weeks of therapy, the dose of EPOGEN® can be increased by 50 to 100 Units/kg TIW. Response should be evaluated every 4 to 8 weeks thereafter and the dose adjusted accordingly by 50 to 100 Units/kg increments TIW. If patients have not responded satisfactorily to an EPOGEN® dose of 300 Units/kg TIW, it is unlikely that they will respond to higher doses of EPOGEN®.

Maintenance Dose: After attainment of the desired response (ie, reduced transfusion requirements or increased hemoglobin), the dose of EPOGEN® should be titrated to maintain the response based on factors such as variations in zidovudine dose and the presence of intercurrent infectious or inflammatory episodes. If the hemoglobin exceeds 13 g/dL, the dose should be discontinued until the hemoglobin drops to 12 g/dL. The dose should be reduced by 25% when treatment is resumed and then titrated to maintain the desired hemoglobin.

Cancer Patients on Chemotherapy

Although no specific serum erythropoietin level can be stipulated above which patients would be unlikely to respond to EPOGEN® therapy, treatment of patients with grossly elevated serum erythropoietin levels (eg, > 200 mUnits/mL) is not recommended. The hemoglobin should be monitored on a weekly basis in patients receiving EPOGEN® therapy until hemoglobin becomes stable. The dose of EPOGEN® should be titrated to maintain the desired hemoglobin.

[See third table above]

During therapy, hematological parameters should be monitored regularly (see PRECAUTIONS: Laboratory Monitoring).

Surgery Patients

Prior to initiating treatment with EPOGEN® a hemoglobin should be obtained to establish that it is > 10 to ≤ 13 g/dL.[18] The recommended dose of EPOGEN® is 300 Units/kg/day subcutaneously for 10 days before surgery, on the day of surgery, and for 4 days after surgery.

An alternate dose schedule is 600 Units/kg EPOGEN® subcutaneously in once weekly doses (21, 14, and 7 days before surgery) plus a fourth dose on the day of surgery.[19]

All patients should receive adequate iron supplementation. Iron supplementation should be initiated no later than the beginning of treatment with EPOGEN® and should continue throughout the course of therapy.

PREPARATION AND ADMINISTRATION OF EPOGEN®

1. Do not shake. It is not necessary to shake EPOGEN®. Prolonged vigorous shaking may denature any glycoprotein, rendering it biologically inactive.

Continued on next page

Epogen—Cont.

2. Parenteral drug products should be inspected visually for particulate matter and discoloration prior to administration. Do not use any vials exhibiting particulate matter or discoloration.
3. Using aseptic techniques, attach a sterile needle to a sterile syringe. Remove the flip top from the vial containing EPOGEN®, and wipe the septum with a disinfectant. Insert the needle into the vial, and withdraw into the syringe an appropriate volume of solution.
4. **Single-dose:** 1 mL vial contains no preservative. Use one dose per vial; do not re-enter the vial. Discard unused portions.
   Multidose: 1 mL and 2 mL vials contain preservative. Store at 2° to 8° C after initial entry and between doses. Discard 21 days after initial entry.
5. Do not dilute or administer in conjunction with other drug solutions. However, at the time of SC administration, preservative-free EPOGEN® from single-use vials may be admixed in a syringe with bacteriostatic 0.9% sodium chloride injection, USP, with benzyl alcohol 0.9% (bacteriostatic saline) at a 1:1 ratio using aseptic technique. The benzyl alcohol in the bacteriostatic saline acts as a local anesthetic which may ameliorate SC injection site discomfort. Admixing is not necessary when using the multidose vials of EPOGEN® containing benzyl alcohol.

HOW SUPPLIED

EPOGEN®, containing Epoetin alfa, is available in the following packages:

1 mL **Single-dose, Preservative-free** Solution
2000 Units/mL (NDC 55513-126-10)
3000 Units/mL (NDC 55513-267-10)
4000 Units/mL (NDC 55513-148-10)
10,000 Units/mL (NDC 55513-144-10)
40,000 Units/mL (NDC 55513-823-10)

Supplied in dispensing packs containing 10 single-dose vials.

2 mL **Multidose, Preserved** Solution
10,000 Units/mL (NDC 55513-283-10)

1 mL **Multidose, Preserved** Solution
20,000 Units/mL (NDC 55513-478-10)

Supplied in dispensing packs containing 10 multidose vials.

STORAGE

Store at 2° to 8° C (36° to 46° F). Do not freeze or shake.

REFERENCES

1. Egrie JC, Strickland TW, Lane J, et al. Characterization and Biological Effects of Recombinant Human Erythropoietin. *Immunobiol.* 1986;72:213-224.
2. Graber SE, Krantz SB. Erythropoietin and the Control of Red Cell Production. *Ann Rev Med.* 1978;29:51-66.
3. Eschbach JW, Adamson JW. Anemia of End-Stage Renal Disease (ESRD). *Kidney Intl.* 1985;28:1-5.
4. Eschbach JW, Egrie JC, Downing MR, et al. Correction of the Anemia of End-Stage Renal Disease with Recombinant Human Erythropoietin. *NEJM.* 1987;316:73-78.
5. Eschbach JW, Abdulhadi MH, Browne JK, et al. Recombinant Human Erythropoietin in Anemic Patients with End-Stage Renal Disease. *Ann Intern Med.* 1989;111:992-1000.
6. Eschbach JW, Egrie JC, Downing MR, et al. The Use of Recombinant Human Erythropoietin (r-HuEPO): Effect in End-Stage Renal Disease (ESRD). In: Friedman, Beyer, DeSanto, Giordano, eds. *Prevention of Chronic Uremia.* Philadelphia, PA: Field and Wood Inc; 1989:148-155.
7. Egrie JC, Eschbach JW, McGuire T, Adamson JW. Pharmacokinetics of Recombinant Human Erythropoietin (r-HuEPO) Administered to Hemodialysis (HD) Patients. *Kidney Intl.* 1988;33:262.
8. Evans RW, Rader B, Manninen DL, et al. The Quality of Life of Hemodialysis Recipients Treated with Recombinant Human Erythropoietin. *JAMA.* 1990;263:825-830.
9. Paganini E, Garcia J, Ellis P, et al. Clinical Sequelae of Correction of Anemia with Recombinant Human Erythropoietin (r-HuEPO); Urea Kinetics, Dialyzer Function and Reuse. *Am J Kid Dis.* 1988;11:16.
10. Delano BG, Lundin AP, Golansky R, et al. Dialyzer Urea and Creatinine Clearances Not Significantly Changed in r-HuEPO Treated Maintenance Hemodialysis (MD) Patients. *Kidney Intl.* 1988;33:219.
11. Stivelman J, Van Wyck D, Ogden D. Use of Recombinant Erythropoietin (r-HuEPO) with High Flux Dialysis (HFD) Does Not Worsen Azotemia or Shorten Access Survival. *Kidney Intl.* 1988;33:239.
12. Lim VS, DeGowin RL, Zavala D, et al. Recombinant Human Erythropoietin Treatment in Pre-Dialysis Patients: A Double-Blind Placebo Controlled Trial. *Ann Int Med.* 1989;110:108-114.
13. Stone WJ, Graber SE, Krantz SB, et al. Treatment of the Anemia of Pre-Dialysis Patients with Recombinant Human Erythropoietin: A Randomized, Placebo-Controlled Trial. *Am J Med Sci.* 1988;296:171-179.
14. Braun A, Ding R, Seidel C, Fies T, Kurtz A, Scharer K. Pharmacokinetics of recombinant human erythropoietin applied subcutaneously to children with chronic renal failure. *Pediatr Nephrol.* 1993;7:61-64.
15. Geva P, Sherwood JB. Pharmacokinetics of recombinant human erythropoietin (rHuEPO) in pediatric patients on chronic cycling peritoneal dialysis (CCPD). *Blood.* 1991;78 (Suppl 1):91a.
16. Jabs K, Grant JR, Harmon W, *et al.* Pharmacokinetics of Epoetin alfa (rHuEPO) in pediatric hemodialysis (HD) patients. *J Am Soc Nephrol.* 1991;2:380.
17. Kling PJ, Widness JA, Guillery EN, Veng-Pedersen P, Peters C, DeAlarcon PA. Pharmacokinetics and pharmacodynamics of erythropoietin during therapy in an infant with renal failure. *J Pediatr.* 1992;121:822-825.
18. deAndrade JR and Jove M. Baseline Hemoglobin as a Predictor of Risk of Transfusion and Response to Epoetin alfa in Orthopedic Surgery Patients. *Am. J. of Orthoped.* 1996;25 (8):533-542.
19. Goldberg MA and McCutchen JW. A Safety and Efficacy Comparison Study of Two Dosing Regimens of Epoetin alfa in Patients Undergoing Major Orthopedic Surgery. *Am. J. of Orthoped.* 1996;25 (8):544-552.
20. Faris PM and Ritter MA. The Effects of Recombinant Human Erythropoietin on Perioperative Transfusion Requirements in Patients Having a Major Orthopedic Operation. *J. Bone and Joint surgery.* 1996;78-A:62-72.
21. Lundin AP, Akerman MJH, Chesler RM, et al. Exercise in Hemodialysis Patients after Treatment with Recombinant Human Erythropoietin. *Nephron.* 1991;58:315-319.
22. Amgen Inc., data on file.
23. Eschbach JW, Kelly MR, Haley NR, et al. Treatment of the Anemia of Progressive Renal Failure with Recombinant Human Erythropoietin. *NEJM.* 1989;321:158-163.
24. The US Recombinant Human Erythropoietin Predialysis Study Group. Double-Blind, Placebo-Controlled Study of the Therapeutic Use of Recombinant Human Erythropoietin for Anemia Associated with Chronic Renal Failure in Predialysis Patients. *Am J Kid Dis.* 1991;18:50-59.
25. Ortho Biologics, Inc., data on file.
26. Danna RP, Rudnick SA, Abels RI. Erythropoietin Therapy for the Anemia Associated with AIDS and AIDS Therapy and Cancer. In: MB Garnick, ed. *Erythropoietin in Clinical Applications - An International Perspective.* New York, NY: Marcel Dekker; 1990:301-324.
27. Fischl M, Galpin JE, Levine JD, et al. Recombinant Human Erythropoietin for Patients with AIDS Treated with Zidovudine. *NEJM.* 1990;322:1488-1493.
28. Laupacis A. Effectiveness of Perioperative Recombinant Human Eyrthropoietin in Elective Hip Replacement. *Lancet.* 1993;341:1228-1232.
29. Kerr DN. Chronic Renal Failure. In: Beeson PB, McDermott W, Wyngaarden JB, eds. *Cecil Textbook of Medicine.* Philadelphia, PA: W.B. Saunders; 1979:1351-1367.
30. Campos A, Garin EH. Therapy of renal anemia in children and adolescents with recombinant human erythropoietin (rHuEPO). *Clin Pediatr* (Phila). 1992;31:94-99.
31. Montini G, Zacchello G, Baraldi E, et al. Benefits and risks of anemia correction with recombinant human erythropoietin in children maintained by hemodialysis. *J Pediatr.* 1990;117:556-560.
32. Offner G, Hoyer PF, Latta K, Winkler L, Brodehl J, Scigalla P. One year's experience with recombinant erythropoietin in children undergoing continuous ambulatory or cycling peritoneal dialysis. *Pediatr Nephrol.* 1990;4:498-500.
33. Muller-Wiefel DE, Scigalla P. Specific problems of renal anemia in childhood. *Contrib Nephrol.* 1988;66:71-84.
34. Scharer K, Klare B, Dressel P, Gretz N. Treatment of renal anemia by subcutaneous erythropoietin in children with preterminal chronic renal failure. *Acta Paediatr.* 1993;82:953-958.
35. Mueller BU, Jacobsen RN, Jarosinski P, et al. Erythropoietin for zidovudine-associated anemia in children with HIV infection. *Pediatr AIDS and HIV Infect: Fetus to Adolesc.* 1994;5:169-173.
36. Zuccotti GV, Plebani A, Biasucci G, et al. Granulocyte-colony stimulating factor and erythropoietin therapy in children with human immunodeficiency virus infection. *J Int Med Res.* 1996;24:115-121.
37. Beck MN, Beck D. Recombinant erythropoietin in acute chemotherapy-induced anemia of children with cancer. *Med Pediatr Oncol.* 1995;25:17-21.
38. Bennetts G, Bertolone S, Bray G, Dinndorf P, Feusner J, Cairo M. Erythropoietin reduces volumes of red cell transfusions required in some subsets of children with acute lymphocytic leukemia. *Blood.* 1995;86:853a.
39. Raskin NH, Fishman RA. Neurologic Disorders in Renal Failure (First of Two Parts). *NEJM.* 1976;294:143-148.
40. Raskin NH and Fishman RA. Neurologic Disorders in Renal Failure (Second of Two Parts). *NEJM.* 1976;294:204-210.
41. Messing RO, Simon RP. Seizures as a Manifestation of Systemic Disease. *Neurologic Clinics.* 1986;4:563-584.
42. Besarab A, Bolton WK, Browne JK, et al. The effects of normal as compared with low hematocrit values in patients with cardiac disease who are receiving hemodialysis and epoetin. *NEJM.* 1998;339:584-90.

Manufactured by:
Amgen Manufacturing, Limited,
a subsidiary of Amgen Inc.
One Amgen Center Drive
Thousand Oaks, CA 91320-1799
3XXXXXX – V10
Issue Date: 05/21/2004

Shown in Product Identification Guide, page 305

KINERET® ℞

[*kĭn' ĕ-rĕt*]
(anakinra)

DESCRIPTION

Kineret® (anakinra) is a recombinant, nonglycosylated form of the human interleukin-1 receptor antagonist (IL-1Ra). Kineret® differs from native human IL-1Ra in that it has the addition of a single methionine residue at its amino terminus. Kineret® consists of 153 amino acids and has a molecular weight of 17.3 kilodaltons. It is produced by recombinant DNA technology using an *E coli* bacterial expression system.

Kineret® is supplied in single use prefilled glass syringes with 27 gauge needles as a sterile, clear, colorless-to-white, preservative-free solution for daily subcutaneous (SC) administration. Each prefilled glass syringe contains: 0.67 mL (100 mg) of anakinra in a solution (pH 6.5) containing sodium citrate (1.29 mg), sodium chloride (5.48 mg), disodium EDTA (0.12 mg), and polysorbate 80 (0.70 mg) in Water for Injection, USP.

CLINICAL PHARMACOLOGY

Kineret® blocks the biologic activity of IL-1 by competitively inhibiting IL-1 binding to the interleukin-1 type I receptor (IL-1RI), which is expressed in a wide variety of tissues and organs.[1]

IL-1 production is induced in response to inflammatory stimuli and mediates various physiologic responses including inflammatory and immunological responses. IL-1 has a broad range of activities including cartilage degradation by its induction of the rapid loss of proteoglycans, as well as stimulation of bone resorption.[2] The levels of the naturally occurring IL-1Ra in synovium and synovial fluid from rheumatoid arthritis (RA) patients are not sufficient to compete with the elevated amount of locally produced IL-1.[3,4,5]

Pharmacokinetics

The absolute bioavailability of Kineret® after a 70 mg SC bolus injection in healthy subjects (n = 11) is 95%. In subjects with RA, maximum plasma concentrations of Kineret® occurred 3 to 7 hours after SC administration of Kineret® at clinically relevant doses (1 to 2 mg/kg; n = 18); the terminal half-life ranged from 4 to 6 hours. In RA patients, no unexpected accumulation of Kineret® was observed after daily SC doses for up to 24 weeks.

The influence of demographic covariates on the pharmacokinetics of Kineret® was studied using population pharmacokinetic analysis encompassing 341 patients receiving daily SC injection of Kineret® at doses of 30, 75, and 150 mg for up to 24 weeks. The estimated Kineret® clearance increased with increasing creatinine clearance and body weight. After adjusting for creatinine clearance and body weight, gender and age were not significant factors for mean plasma clearance.

Patients With Renal Impairment: The mean plasma clearance of Kineret® in subjects with mild (creatinine clearance 50-80 mL/min) and moderate (creatinine clearance 30-49 mL/min) renal insufficiency was reduced by 16% and 50%, respectively. In severe renal insufficiency and end stage renal disease (creatinine clearance < 30 mL/min[6]), mean plasma clearance declined by 70% and 75%, respectively. Less than 2.5% of the administered dose of Kineret® was removed by hemodialysis or continuous ambulatory peritoneal dialysis. Based on these observations, a dose schedule change should be considered for subjects with severe renal insufficiency or end stage renal disease (see **DOSAGE AND ADMINISTRATION**).

Patients With Hepatic Dysfunction: No formal studies have been conducted examining the pharmacokinetics of Kineret® administered subcutaneously in rheumatoid arthritis patients with hepatic impairment.

CLINICAL STUDIES

The safety and efficacy of Kineret® have been evaluated in three randomized, double-blind, placebo-controlled trials of 1790 patients ≥ 18 years of age with active rheumatoid arthritis (RA). An additional fourth study was conducted to assess safety. In the efficacy trials, Kineret® was studied in combination with other disease-modifying antirheumatic drugs (DMARDs) other than Tumor Necrosis Factor (TNF) blocking agents (studies 1 and 2) or as a monotherapy (study 3).

Study 1 involved 899 patients with active RA who had been on a stable dose of methotrexate (MTX) (10 to 25 mg/week) for at least 8 weeks. All patients had at least 6 swollen/painful and 9 tender joints and either a C-reactive protein (CRP) of ≥ 1.5 mg/dL or an erythrocyte sedimentation rate (ESR) of ≥ 28 mm/hr. Patients were randomized to Kineret® or placebo in addition to their stable doses of MTX. The first 501 patients were evaluated for signs and symptoms of active RA. The total 899 patients were evaluated for progression of structural damage.

Study 2 evaluated 419 patients with active RA who had received MTX for at least 6 months including a stable dose (15 to 25 mg/week) for at least 3 consecutive months prior to enrollment. Patients were randomized to receive placebo or one of five doses of Kineret® SC daily for 12 to 24 weeks in addition to their stable doses of MTX.

Study 3 evaluated 472 patients with active RA and had similar inclusion criteria to study 1 except that these patients had received no DMARD for the previous 6 weeks or during the study.[7] Patients were randomized to receive either Kineret® or placebo. Patients were DMARD-naïve or had failed no more than 3 DMARDs.

Study 4 was a placebo-controlled, randomized trial designed to assess the safety of Kineret® in 1414 patients receiving a variety of concurrent medications for their RA including some DMARD therapies, as well as patients who were DMARD-free. The TNF blocking agents etanercept and infliximab were specifically excluded. Concurrent DMARDs included MTX, sulfasalazine, hydroxychloroquine, gold, penicillamine, leflunomide, and azathioprine. Unlike studies 1, 2 and 3, patients predisposed to infection due to a history of underlying disease such as pneumonia, asthma, controlled diabetes, and chronic obstructive pulmonary disease (COPD) were also enrolled (see **ADVERSE REACTIONS: Infections**).

In studies 1, 2 and 3, the improvement in signs and symptoms of RA was assessed using the American College of Rheumatology (ACR) response criteria (ACR_{20}, ACR_{50}, ACR_{70}). In these studies, patients treated with Kineret® were more likely to achieve an ACR_{20} or higher magnitude of response (ACR_{50} and ACR_{70}) than patients treated with placebo (Table 1). The treatment response rates did not differ based on gender or ethnic group. The results of the ACR component scores in study 1 are shown in Table 2.

Most clinical responses, both in patients receiving placebo and patients receiving Kineret®, occurred within 12 weeks of enrollment.

[See table 1 at right]

[See table 2 at right]

A 24-week study was conducted in 242 patients with active RA on background methotrexate who were randomized to receive either etanercept alone or the combination of Kineret® and etanercept. The ACR_{50} response rate was 31% for patients treated with the combination of Kineret® and etanercept and 41% for patients treated with etanercept alone, indicating no added clinical benefit of the combination over etanercept alone. Serious infections were increased with the combination compared to etanercept alone (see **WARNINGS**).

In study 1, the effect of Kineret® on the progression of structural damage was assessed by measuring the change from baseline at month 12 in the Total Modified Sharp Score (TSS) and its subcomponents, erosion score, and joint space narrowing (JSN) score.[8] Radiographs of hands/wrists and forefeet were obtained at baseline, 6 months and 12 months and scored by readers who were unaware of treatment group. A difference between placebo and Kineret® for change in TSS, erosion score (ES) and JSN score was observed at 6 months and at 12 months (Table 3).

[See table 3 at right]

The disability index of the Health Assessment Questionnaire (HAQ) was administered monthly for the first six months and quarterly thereafter during study 1. Health outcomes were assessed by the Short Form-36 (SF-36) questionnaire. The 1-year data on HAQ in study 1 showed more improvement with Kineret® than placebo. The physical component summary (PCS) score of the SF-36 also showed more improvement with Kineret® than placebo but not the mental component summary (MCS).

INDICATIONS AND USAGE

Kineret® is indicated for the reduction in signs and symptoms and slowing the progression of structural damage in moderately to severely active rheumatoid arthritis, in patients 18 years of age or older who have failed 1 or more disease modifying antirheumatic drugs (DMARDs). Kineret® can be used alone or in combination with DMARDs other than Tumor Necrosis Factor (TNF) blocking agents (see **WARNINGS**).

CONTRAINDICATIONS

Kineret® is contraindicated in patients with known hypersensitivity to *E coli*-derived proteins, Kineret®, or any components of the product.

WARNINGS

KINERET® HAS BEEN ASSOCIATED WITH AN INCREASED INCIDENCE OF SERIOUS INFECTIONS (2%) VS. PLACEBO (< 1%). ADMINISTRATION OF KINERET® SHOULD BE DISCONTINUED IF A PATIENT DEVELOPS A SERIOUS INFECTION. TREATMENT WITH KINERET® SHOULD NOT BE INITIATED IN PATIENTS WITH ACTIVE INFECTIONS. THE SAFETY AND EFFICACY OF KINERET® IN IMMUNOSUPPRESSED PATIENTS OR IN PATIENTS WITH CHRONIC INFECTIONS HAVE NOT BEEN EVALUATED.

IN A 24-WEEK STUDY OF CONCURRENT KINERET® AND ETANERCEPT THERAPY, THE RATE OF SERIOUS INFECTIONS IN THE COMBINATION ARM (7%) WAS HIGHER THAN WITH ETANERCEPT ALONE (0%). THE COMBINATION OF KINERET® AND ETANERCEPT DID NOT RESULT IN HIGHER ACR RESPONSE RATES COMPARED TO ETANERCEPT ALONE. (see CLINICAL STUDIES). CONCURRENT THERAPY WITH KINERET® AND ETANERCEPT IS NOT RECOMMENDED.

PRECAUTIONS

General

Hypersensitivity reactions associated with Kineret® administration are rare. If a severe hypersensitivity reaction occurs, administration of Kineret® should be discontinued and appropriate therapy initiated.

Immunosuppression

The impact of treatment with Kineret® on active and/or chronic infections and the development of malignancies is not known (see **WARNINGS** and **ADVERSE REACTIONS: Infections and Malignancies**).

Table 1: Percent of Patients with ACR Responses in Studies 1 and 3

Response	Study 1 (Patients on MTX) Placebo (n = 251)	Study 1 Kineret® 100 mg/day (n = 250)	Study 3 (No DMARDs) Placebo (n = 119)	Study 3 Kineret® 75 mg/day (n = 115)	Study 3 Kineret® 150 mg/day (n = 115)
ACR_{20}					
Month 3	24%	34%[a]	23%	33%	33%
Month 6	22%	38%[c]	27%	34%	43%[a]
ACR_{50}					
Month 3	6%	13%[b]	5%	10%	8%
Month 6	8%	17%[b]	8%	11%	19%[a]
ACR_{70}					
Month 3	0%	3%[a]	0%	0%	0%
Month 6	2%	6%[a]	1%	1%	1%

[a] $p < 0.05$, Kineret® versus placebo
[b] $p < 0.01$, Kineret® versus placebo
[c] $p < 0.001$, Kineret® versus placebo

Table 2: Median ACR Component Scores in Study 1

Parameter (median)	Placebo/MTX (n = 251) Baseline	Placebo/MTX Month 6	Kineret®/MTX 100 mg/day (n = 250) Baseline	Kineret®/MTX Month 6
Patient Reported Outcomes				
Disability index[a]	1.38	1.13	1.38	1.00
Patient global assessment[b]	51.0	41.0	51.0	29.0
Pain[b]	56.0	44.0	63.0	34.0
Objective Measures				
ESR (mm/hr)	35.0	32.0	36.0	19.0
CRP (mg/dL)	2.2	1.6	2.2	0.5
Physician's Assessments				
Tender/painful joints[c]	20.0	11.0	23.0	9.0
Physician global assessment[b]	59.0	31.0	59.0	26.0
Swollen joints[d]	18.0	10.5	17.0	9.0

[a] Health assessment questionnaire; 0 = best, 3 = worst; includes eight categories: dressing and grooming, arising, eating, walking, hygiene, reach, grip, and activities.
[b] Visual analog scale; 0 = best, 100 = worst
[c] Scale 0 to 68
[d] Scale 0 to 66

Table 3: Mean Radiographic Changes Over 12 Months in Study 1

	Placebo/MTX (N = 450) Baseline	Placebo/MTX Change at Month 12	Kineret® 100 mg/day/MTX (N = 449) Baseline	Kineret® Change at Month 12	Placebo/MTX vs. Kineret®/MTX 95% Confidence Interval*	p-value**
TSS	52	2.6	50	1.7	0.9 [0.3, 1.6]	<0.001
Erosion	28	1.6	25	1.1	0.5 [0.1, 1.0]	0.024
JSN	24	1.1	25	0.7	0.4 [0.1, 0.7]	<0.001

* Differences and 95% confidence intervals for the differences in change scores between Placebo/MTX and Kineret®/MTX
** Based on Wilcoxon rank-sum test

Immunizations

No data are available on the effects of vaccination in patients receiving Kineret®. Live vaccines should not be given concurrently with Kineret®. No data are available on the secondary transmission of infection by live vaccines in patients receiving Kineret® (see **PRECAUTIONS: Immunosuppression**). Since Kineret® interferes with normal immune response mechanisms to new antigens such as vaccines, vaccination may not be effective in patients receiving Kineret®.

Information for Patients

If a physician has determined that a patient can safely and effectively receive Kineret® at home, patients and their caregivers should be instructed on the proper dosage and administration of Kineret®. All patients should be provided with the "Information for Patients" insert. While this "Information for Patients" insert provides information about the product and its use, it is not intended to take the place of regular discussions between the patient and healthcare provider.

Patients should be informed of the signs and symptoms of allergic and other adverse drug reactions and advised of appropriate actions. Patients and their caregivers should be thoroughly instructed in the importance of proper disposal and cautioned against the reuse of needles, syringes, and drug product. A puncture-resistant container for the disposal of used syringes should be available to the patient. The full container should be disposed of according to the directions provided by the healthcare provider.

Laboratory Tests

Patients receiving Kineret® may experience a decrease in neutrophil counts. In the placebo-controlled studies, 8% of patients receiving Kineret® had decreases in neutrophil counts of at least 1 World Health Organization (WHO) toxicity grade compared with 2% in the placebo control group. Nine Kineret®-treated patients (0.4%) experienced neutropenia (ANC $< 1 \times 10^9$/L). This is discussed in more detail in the **ADVERSE REACTIONS: Hematologic Events** section. Neutrophil counts should be assessed prior to initiating Kineret® treatment, and while receiving Kineret®, monthly for 3 months, and thereafter quarterly for a period up to 1 year.

Drug Interactions

No drug-drug interaction studies in human subjects have been conducted. Toxicologic and toxicokinetic studies in rats did not demonstrate any alterations in the clearance or toxicologic profile of either methotrexate or Kineret® when the two agents were administered together. In a study in which patients with active RA were treated for up to 24 weeks with concurrent Kineret® and etanercept therapy, a 7% rate of serious infections was observed, which was higher than that observed with etanercept alone (0%) (see also **WARNINGS**). Two percent of patients treated concurrently with Kineret® and etanercept developed neutropenia (ANC $< 1 \times 10^9$/L).

Carcinogenesis, Mutagenesis, and Impairment of Fertility

Kineret® has not been evaluated for its carcinogenic potential in animals. Using a standard in vivo and in vitro battery of mutagenesis assays, Kineret® did not induce gene mutations in either bacteria or mammalian cells. In rats and rabbits, Kineret® at doses of up to 100-fold greater than the human dose had no adverse effects on male or female fertility.

Pregnancy Category B

Reproductive studies have been conducted with Kineret® on rats and rabbits at doses up to 100 times the human dose and have revealed no evidence of impaired fertility or harm to the fetus. There are, however, no adequate and well-controlled studies in pregnant women. Because animal reproduction studies are not always predictive of human response, Kineret® should be used during pregnancy only if clearly needed.

Nursing Mothers

It is not known whether Kineret® is secreted in human milk. Because many drugs are secreted in human milk, caution should be exercised if Kineret® is administered to nursing women.

Continued on next page

Kineret—Cont.

Pediatric Use

The safety and efficacy of Kineret® in patients with juvenile rheumatoid arthritis (JRA) have not been established.

Geriatric Use

A total of 752 patients ≥ 65 years of age, including 163 patients ≥ 75 years of age, were studied in clinical trials. No differences in safety or effectiveness were observed between these patients and younger patients, but greater sensitivity of some older individuals cannot be ruled out. Because there is a higher incidence of infections in the elderly population in general, caution should be used in treating the elderly.

This drug is known to be substantially excreted by the kidney, and the risk of toxic reactions to this drug may be greater in patients with impaired renal function.

ADVERSE REACTIONS

The most serious adverse reactions were:

- Serious Infections - see **WARNINGS**
- Neutropenia, particularly when used in combination with TNF blocking agents

The most common adverse reaction with Kineret® is injection-site reactions. These reactions were the most common reason for withdrawing from studies.

Because clinical trials are conducted under widely varying and controlled conditions, adverse reaction rates observed in clinical trials of a drug cannot be directly compared to rates in the clinical trials of another drug and may not predict the rates observed in a broader patient population in clinical practice.

The data described herein reflect exposure to Kineret® in 3025 patients, including 2124 exposed for at least 6 months and 884 exposed for at least one year. Studies 1 and 4 used the recommended dose of 100 mg per day. The patients studied were representative of the general population of patients with rheumatoid arthritis.

Injection-site Reactions

The most common and consistently reported treatment-related adverse event associated with Kineret® is injection-site reaction (ISR). The majority of ISRs were reported as mild. These typically lasted for 14 to 28 days and were characterized by 1 or more of the following: erythema, ecchymosis, inflammation, and pain. In studies 1 and 4, 71% of patients developed an ISR, which was typically reported within the first 4 weeks of therapy. The development of ISRs in patients who had not previously experienced ISRs was uncommon after the first month of therapy.

Infections

In studies 1 and 4 combined, the incidence of infection was 39% in the Kineret®-treated patients and 37% in placebo-treated patients during the first 6 months of blinded treatment. The incidence of serious infections in studies 1 and 4 was 2% in Kineret®-treated patients and 1% in patients receiving placebo over 6 months. The incidence of serious infection over 1 year was 3% in Kineret®-treated patients and 2% in patients receiving placebo. These infections consisted primarily of bacterial events such as cellulitis, pneumonia, and bone and joint infections, rather than unusual, opportunistic, fungal, or viral infections. Patients with asthma appeared to be at higher risk of developing serious infections; Kineret® 4% vs. placebo 0%. Most patients continued on study drug after the infection resolved.

In open-label extension studies, the overall rate of serious infections was stable over time and comparable to that observed in controlled trials. In clinical studies and postmarketing experience, rare cases of opportunistic infections have been observed and included fungal, mycobacterial and bacterial pathogens. Infections have been noted in all organ systems and have been reported in patients receiving Kineret® alone or in combination with immunosuppressive agents.

In patients who received both Kineret® and etanercept for up to 24 weeks, the incidence of serious infections was 7%. The most common infections consisted of bacterial pneumonia (4 cases) and cellulitis (4 cases). One patient with pulmonary fibrosis and pneumonia died due to respiratory failure.

Malignancies

Among 5300 RA patients treated with Kineret® in clinical trials for a mean of 15 months (approximately 6400 patient years of treatment), 8 lymphomas were observed for a rate of 0.12 cases/100 patient years. This is 3.6 fold higher than the rate of lymphomas expected in the general population, based on the National Cancer Institute's Surveillance, Epidemiology and End Results (SEER) database.[9] An increased rate of lymphoma, up to several fold, has been reported in the RA population, and may be further increased in patients with more severe disease activity. Thirty-seven malignancies other than lymphoma were observed. Of these, the most common were breast, respiratory system, and digestive system. There were 3 melanomas observed in study 4 and its long-term open-label extension, greater than the 1 expected case. The significance of this finding is not known. While patients with RA, particularly those with highly active disease, may be at a higher risk (up to several fold) for the development of lymphoma, the role of IL-1 blockers in the development of malignancy is not known.

Hematologic Events

In placebo-controlled studies with Kineret®, treatment was associated with small reductions in the mean values for total white blood count, platelets, and absolute neutrophil count (ANC), and a small increase in the mean eosinophil differential percentage.

In all placebo-controlled studies, 8% of patients receiving Kineret® had decreases in ANC of at least 1 WHO toxicity grade, compared with 2% of placebo patients. Nine Kineret®-treated patients (0.4%) developed neutropenia (ANC $< 1 \times 10^9$/L). Two percent of patients treated concurrently with Kineret® and etanercept developed neutropenia (ANC $< 1 \times 10^9$/L. While neutropenic, one patient developed cellulitis which recovered with antibiotic therapy.

Immunogenicity

In studies 1 and 4, from which data is available for up to 36 months, 49% of patients tested positively at one or more timepoints for anti-anakinra antibodies in a highly sensitive, anakinra-binding biosensor assay. Of the 1615 patients with available data at Week 12 or later, 30 (2%) were seropositive in a cell-based bioassay for antibodies capable of neutralizing the biologic effects of Kineret®. Of the 13 patients with available follow-up data, 5 patients remained positive for neutralizing antibodies at the end of the studies. No correlation between antibody development and adverse events was observed.

Antibody assay results are highly dependent on the sensitivity and specificity of the assays. Additionally, the observed incidence of antibody positivity in an assay may be influenced by several factors, including sample handling, concomitant medications, and underlying disease. For these reasons, comparison of the incidence of antibodies to Kineret® with the incidence of antibodies to other products may be misleading.

Other Adverse Events

Table 4 reflects adverse events in studies 1 and 4, that occurred with a frequency of ≥ 5% in Kineret®-treated patients over a 6-month period.

Table 4. Percent of RA Patients Reporting Adverse Events (Studies 1 and 4)

Preferred term	Placebo (n = 733)	Kineret® 100 mg/day (n = 1565)
Injection Site Reaction	29%	71%
Worsening of RA	29%	19%
URI	17%	14%
Headache	9%	12%
Nausea	7%	8%
Diarrhea	5%	7%
Sinusitis	7%	7%
Arthralgia	6%	6%
Flu Like Symptoms	6%	6%
Abdominal Pain	5%	5%

OVERDOSAGE

There have been no cases of overdose reported with Kineret® in clinical trials of RA. In sepsis trials no serious toxicities attributed to Kineret® were seen when administered at mean calculated doses of up to 35 times those given patients with RA over a 72-hour treatment period.

DOSAGE AND ADMINISTRATION

The recommended dose of Kineret® for the treatment of patients with rheumatoid arthritis is 100 mg/day administered daily by subcutaneous injection. Higher doses did not result in a higher response. The dose should be administered at approximately the same time every day.

Physicians should consider a dose of 100 mg of Kineret® administered every other day for RA patients who have severe renal insufficiency or end stage renal disease (defined as creatinine clearance < 30 mL/min, as estimated from serum creatinine levels). See **CLINICAL PHARMACOLOGY, Pharmacokinetics: Patients with Renal Impairment.**

Kineret® is provided in single-use prefilled glass syringes. The needle cover contains dry natural rubber (latex), which should not be handled by persons sensitive to this substance. Instructions on appropriate use should be given by the healthcare provider to the patient or caregiver. Patients or caregivers should not be allowed to administer Kineret® until the patient or caregiver has demonstrated a thorough understanding of procedures and an ability to inject the product. After administration of Kineret®, it is essential to follow the proper procedure for disposal of syringes and needles. See the "Information for Patients" insert for detailed instructions on the handling and injection of Kineret®.

Do not use Kineret® beyond the expiration date shown on the carton.Visually inspect the solution for particulate matter and discoloration before administration. If particulates or discoloration are observed, the prefilled syringe should not be used.

Administer only one dose (the entire contents of one prefilled glass syringe) per day. Discard any unused portions.

HOW SUPPLIED

Kineret® is supplied in single-use preservative free, prefilled glass syringes with 27 gauge needles. Each prefilled glass syringe contains 0.67 mL (100 mg) of anakinra. Kineret® is dispensed in a 4 x 7 syringe dispensing pack containing 28 syringes (NDC 55513-177-28).

Storage

Kineret® should be stored in the refrigerator at 2° to 8°C (36° to 46°F). **DO NOT FREEZE OR SHAKE.** Protect from light.

Rx only

REFERENCES

1. Hannum CH, Wilcox CJ, Arend WP, et al. Interleukin-1 receptor antagonist activity of a human interleukin-1 inhibitor. *Nature.* 1990; 343:336-40.
2. Van Lent PLEM, Fons AJ, Van De Loo AEM, et al, Major role for interleukin 1 but not for tumor necrosis factor in early cartilage damage in immune complex in mice. *J Rheumatol.* 1995; 22:2250-2258.
3. Deleuran BW, Shu CQ, Field M, et al. Localization of interleukin-1 alpha, type 1 interleukin-1 receptor and interleukin-1 receptor antagonist in the synovial membrane and cartilage/pannus junction in rheumatoid arthritis. *Br J Rheumatol.* 1992; 31:801-809.
4. Chomarat P, Vannier E, Dechanet J, et al. Balance of IL-1 receptor antagonist/IL-1*B* in rheumatoid synovium and its regulation by IL-4 and IL-10. *J Immunol.* 1995; 1432-1439.
5. Firestein GS, Boyle DL, Yu C, et al. Synovial interleukin-1 receptor antagonist and interleukin-1 balance in rheumatoid arthritis. *Arthritis Rheum.* 1994; 37: 644-652.
6. Cockcroft DW and Gault HM. Prediction of creatinine clearance from serum creatinine. *Nephron* 1976; 16:31-41.
7. Bresnihan B, Alvaro-Gracia JM, Cobby M, et al. Treatment of rheumatoid arthritis with recombinant human interleukin-1 receptor antagonist. *Arthritis Rheum.* 1998; 41:2196-2204.
8. Sharp JT, Young DY, Bluhm GB, et al. How many joints in the hands and wrists should be included in a score of radiologic abnormalities used to assess rheumatoid arthritis? *Arthritis Rheum.* 1985; 28:1326-1335.
9. National Cancer Institute. Surveillance, Epidemiology, and End Results Database (SEER) Program. SEER Incidence Crude Rates, 11 Registries, 1992-1999.

This product, its production, and/or its use may be covered by one or more U.S. Patents, including U.S. Patent Nos. 6,599,873 and 5,075,222 as well as other patents or patents pending.

AMGEN®

Manufactured by:
Amgen Manufacturing, Limited,
a subsidiary of Amgen Inc
One Amgen Center Drive
Thousand Oaks, CA 91320-1799

3XXXXXX – v9.0
Issue Date: 04/23/2004

Shown in Product Identification Guide, page 305

NEULASTA™ ℞

[*nū' läs-tă*]
(pegfilgrastim)

DESCRIPTION

Neulasta™ (pegfilgrastim) is a covalent conjugate of recombinant methionyl human G-CSF (Filgrastim) and monomethoxypolyethylene glycol. Filgrastim is a water-soluble 175 amino acid protein with a molecular weight of approximately 19 kilodaltons (kD). Filgrastim is obtained from the bacterial fermentation of a strain of *Escherichia coli* transformed with a genetically engineered plasmid containing the human G-CSF gene. To produce pegfilgrastim, a 20 kD monomethoxypolyethylene glycol molecule is covalently bound to the N-terminal methionyl residue of Filgrastim. The average molecular weight of pegfilgrastim is approximately 39 kD.

Neulasta™ is supplied in 0.6 mL prefilled syringes for subcutaneous (SC) injection. Each syringe contains 6 mg pegfilgrastim (based on protein weight), in a sterile, clear, colorless, preservative-free solution (pH 4.0) containing acetate (0.35 mg), sorbitol (30.0 mg), polysorbate 20 (0.02 mg), and sodium (0.02 mg) in water for injection, USP.

CLINICAL PHARMACOLOGY

Both Filgrastim and pegfilgrastim are Colony Stimulating Factors that act on hematopoietic cells by binding to specific cell surface receptors thereby stimulating proliferation, differentiation, commitment, and end cell functional activation.[1,2] Studies on cellular proliferation, receptor binding, and neutrophil function demonstrate that Filgrastim and pegfilgrastim have the same mechanism of action. Pegfilgrastim has reduced renal clearance and prolonged persistence in vivo as compared to Filgrastim.

Pharmacokinetics

The pharmacokinetics and pharmacodynamics of Neulasta™ were studied in 379 patients with cancer. The pharmacokinetics of Neulasta™ were nonlinear in cancer patients and clearance decreased with increases in dose. Neutrophil receptor binding is an important component of the clearance of Neulasta™, and serum clearance is directly related to the number of neutrophils. For example, the concentration of Neulasta™ declined rapidly at the onset of neutrophil recovery that followed myelosuppressive chemotherapy. In addition to numbers of neutrophils, body weight appeared to be a factor. Patients with higher body weights experienced higher systemic exposure to Neulasta™ after receiving a dose normalized for body weight. A large variability in the pharmacokinetics of Neulasta™ was observed in cancer patients. The half-life of Neulasta™ ranged from 15 to 80 hours after SC injection.

Special Populations

No gender-related differences were observed in the pharmacokinetics of Neulasta™, and no differences were observed in the pharmacokinetics of geriatric patients (≥65 years of age) compared to younger patients (< 65 years of age) (see PRECAUTIONS, Geriatric Use). The pharmacokinetic profile in pediatric populations or in patients with hepatic or renal insufficiency has not been assessed.

CLINICAL STUDIES

Neulasta™ was evaluated in two randomized, double-blind, active control studies, employing doxorubicin 60 mg/m² and docetaxel 75 mg/m² administered every 21 days for up to 4 cycles for the treatment of metastatic breast cancer. Study 1 investigated the utility of a fixed dose of Neulasta™. Study 2 employed a weight-adjusted dose. In the absence of growth factor support, similar chemotherapy regimens have been reported to result in a 100% incidence of severe neutropenia (absolute neutrophil count [ANC] $<0.5 \times 10^9$/L) with a mean duration of 5-7 days, and a 30%-40% incidence of febrile neutropenia. Based on the correlation between the duration of severe neutropenia and the incidence of febrile neutropenia found in studies with Filgrastim, duration of severe neutropenia was chosen as the primary endpoint in both studies, and the efficacy of Neulasta™ was demonstrated by establishing comparability to Filgrastim (NEUPOGEN®)-treated subjects in the mean days of severe neutropenia.

In study 1, 157 subjects were randomized to receive a single SC dose of 6 mg of Neulasta™ on day 2 of each chemotherapy cycle or Filgrastim at 5 mcg/kg/day SC beginning on day 2 of each cycle. In study 2, 310 subjects were randomized to receive a single SC injection of Neulasta™ at 100 mcg/kg on day 2 or Filgrastim at 5 mcg/kg/day SC beginning on day 2 of each cycle of chemotherapy.

Both studies met the primary objective of demonstrating that the mean days of severe neutropenia of Neulasta™-treated patients did not exceed that of Filgrastim-treated patients by more than one day in cycle 1 of chemotherapy (see Table 1). The rates of febrile neutropenia in the two studies were comparable for Neulasta™ and Filgrastim (in the range of 10% to 20%). Other secondary endpoints included days of severe neutropenia in cycles 2-4, the depth of ANC nadir in cycles 1-4, and the time to ANC recovery after nadir. In both studies, the results for the secondary endpoints were similar between the two treatment groups.

Table 1. Mean Days of Severe Neutropenia (in Cycle 1)

Study	Mean days of severe neutropenia		Difference in means (95% CI)
	Neulasta™[a]	NEUPOGEN® (5 mcg/kg/day)	
Study 1 n = 157	1.8	1.6	0.2 (-0.2, 0.6)
Study 2 n = 310	1.7	1.6	0.1 (-0.2, 0.4)

[a]Study 1 dose = 6 mg × 1; study 2 dose = 100 mcg/kg × 1

INDICATIONS AND USAGE

Neulasta™ is indicated to decrease the incidence of infection, as manifested by febrile neutropenia, in patients with non-myeloid malignancies receiving myelosuppressive anticancer drugs associated with a clinically significant incidence of febrile neutropenia.

CONTRAINDICATIONS

Neulasta™ is contraindicated in patients with known hypersensitivity to *E coli*-derived proteins, pegfilgrastim, Filgrastim, or any other component of the product.

WARNINGS

Splenic Rupture

RARE CASES OF SPLENIC RUPTURE HAVE BEEN REPORTED FOLLOWING THE ADMINISTRATION OF THE PARENT COMPOUND OF NEULASTA™, FILGRASTIM, FOR PBPC MOBILIZATION IN BOTH HEALTHY DONORS AND PATIENTS WITH CANCER. SOME OF THESE CASES WERE FATAL. NEULASTA™ HAS NOT BEEN EVALUATED IN THIS SETTING, THEREFORE, NEULASTA™ SHOULD NOT BE USED FOR PBPC MOBILIZATION. PATIENTS RECEIVING NEULASTA™ WHO REPORT LEFT UPPER ABDOMINAL OR SHOULDER TIP PAIN SHOULD BE EVALUATED FOR AN ENLARGED SPLEEN OR SPLENIC RUPTURE.

Adult Respiratory Distress Syndrome (ARDS)

Adult respiratory distress syndrome (ARDS) has been reported in neutropenic patients with sepsis receiving Filgrastim, the parent compound of Neulasta™ and is postulated to be secondary to an influx of neutrophils to sites of inflammation in the lungs. Neutropenic patients receiving Neulasta™ who develop fever, lung infiltrates, or respiratory distress should be evaluated for the possibility of ARDS. In the event that ARDS occurs, Neulasta™ should be discontinued and/or withheld until resolution of ARDS and patients should receive appropriate medical management for this condition.

Allergic Reactions

Allergic-type reactions, including anaphylaxis, skin rash, and urticaria, occurring on initial or subsequent treatment have been reported with the parent compound of Neulasta™ Filgrastim. In some cases, symptoms have recurred with rechallenge, suggesting a causal relationship. Allergic-type reactions to Neulasta™ have not been observed in clinical trials. If a serious allergic reaction or an anaphylactic reaction occurs, appropriate therapy should be administered and further use of Neulasta™ should be discontinued.

Sickle Cell Disease

Severe sickle cell crises have been reported in patients with sickle cell disease (specifically homozygous sickle cell anemia, sickle/hemoglobin C disease, and sickle/β+ thalassemia) who received Filgrastim, the parent compound of pegfilgrastim, for PBPC mobilization or following chemotherapy. One of these cases was fatal. Pegfilgrastim should be used with caution in patients with sickle cell disease, and only after careful consideration of the potential risks and benefits. Patients with sickle cell disease who receive Neulasta™ should be kept well hydrated and monitored for the occurrence of sickle cell crises. In the event of severe sickle cell crisis supportive care should be administered, and interventions to ameliorate the underlying event, such as therapeutic red blood cell exchange transfusion, should be considered.

PRECAUTIONS

General

Use With Chemotherapy and/or Radiation Therapy

Neulasta™ should not be administered in the period between 14 days before and 24 hours after administration of cytotoxic chemotherapy (see DOSAGE AND ADMINISTRATION) because of the potential for an increase in sensitivity of rapidly dividing myeloid cells to cytotoxic chemotherapy.

The use of Neulasta™ has not been studied in patients receiving chemotherapy associated with delayed myelosuppression (eg, nitrosoureas, mitomycin C).

The administration of Neulasta™ concomitantly with 5-fluorouracil or other antimetabolites has not been evaluated in patients. Administration of pegfilgrastim at 0, 1, and 3 days before 5-fluorouracil resulted in increased mortality in mice; administration of pegfilgrastim 24 hours after 5-fluorouracil did not adversely affect survival.

The use of Neulasta™ has not been studied in patients receiving radiation therapy.

Potential Effect on Malignant Cells

Pegfilgrastim is a growth factor that primarily stimulates neutrophils and neutrophil precursors; however, the G-CSF receptor through which pegfilgrastim and Filgrastim act has been found on tumor cell lines, including some myeloid, T-lymphoid, lung, head and neck, and bladder tumor cell lines. The possibility that pegfilgrastim can act as a growth factor for any tumor type cannot be excluded. Use of Neulasta™ in myeloid malignancies and myelodysplasia (MDS) has not been studied. In a randomized study comparing the effects of the parent compound of Neulasta™, Filgrastim, to placebo in patients undergoing remission induction and consolidation chemotherapy for acute myeloid leukemia, important differences in remission rate between the two arms were excluded. Disease-free survival and overall survival were comparable; however, the study was not designed to detect important differences in these endpoints.[3]

Information for Patients

Patients should be informed of the possible side effects of Neulasta™ and be instructed to report them to the prescribing physician. Patients should be informed of the signs and symptoms of allergic drug reactions and be advised of appropriate actions. Patients should be counseled on the importance of compliance with their Neulasta™ treatment, including regular monitoring of blood counts.

If it is determined that a patient or caregiver can safely and effectively administer Neulasta™ (pegfilgrastim) at home, appropriate instruction on the proper use of Neulasta™ (pegfilgrastim) should be provided for patients and their caregivers, including careful review of the "Information for Patients and Caregivers" insert. Patients and caregivers should be cautioned against the reuse of needles, syringes, or drug product, and be thoroughly instructed in their proper disposal. A puncture-resistant container for the disposal of used syringes and needles should be available.

Laboratory Monitoring

To assess a patient's hematologic status and ability to tolerate myelosuppressive chemotherapy, a complete blood count and platelet count should be obtained before chemotherapy is administered. Regular monitoring of hematocrit value and platelet count is recommended.

Drug Interaction

No formal drug interaction studies between Neulasta™ and other drugs have been performed. Drugs such as lithium may potentiate the release of neutrophils; patients receiving lithium and Neulasta™ should have more frequent monitoring of neutrophil counts.

Carcinogenesis, Mutagenesis, Impairment of Fertility

No mutagenesis studies were conducted with pegfilgrastim. The carcinogenic potential of pegfilgrastim has not been evaluated in long-term animal studies. In a toxicity study of 6 months duration in rats given once weekly subcutaneous injections of up to 1000 mcg/kg of pegfilgrastim (approximately 23-fold higher than the recommended human dose), no precancerous or cancerous lesions were noted.

When administered once weekly via subcutaneous injections to male and female rats at doses up to 1000 mcg/kg prior to, and during mating, reproductive performance, fertility, and sperm assessment parameters were not affected.

Pregnancy Category C

Pegfilgrastim has been shown to have adverse effects in pregnant rabbits when administered SC every other day during gestation at doses as low as 50 mcg/kg/dose (approximately 4-fold higher than the recommended human dose). Decreased maternal food consumption, accompanied by a decreased maternal body weight gain and decreased fetal body weights were observed at 50 to 1000 mcg/kg/dose. Pegfilgrastim doses of 200 and 250 mcg/kg/dose resulted in an increased incidence of abortions. Increased post-implantation loss due to early resorptions was observed at doses of 200 to 1000 mcg/kg/dose, and decreased numbers of live rabbit fetuses were observed at pegfilgrastim doses of 200 to 1000 mcg/kg/dose, given every other day.

Subcutaneous injections of pegfilgrastim of up to 1000 mcg/kg/dose every other day during the period of organogenesis in rats were not associated with an embryotoxic or fetotoxic outcome. However, an increased incidence (compared to historical controls) of wavy ribs was observed in rat fetuses at 1000 mcg/kg/dose every other day. Very low levels (< 0.5%) of pegfilgrastim crossed the placenta when administered subcutaneously to pregnant rats every other day during gestation.

Once weekly subcutaneous injections of pegfilgrastim to female rats from day 6 of gestation through day 18 of lactation at doses up to 1000 mcg/kg/dose did not result in any adverse maternal effects.

There were no deleterious effects on the growth and development of the offspring and no adverse effects were found upon assessment of fertility indices.

There are no adequate and well-controlled studies in pregnant women. Neulasta™ should be used during pregnancy only if the potential benefit to the mother justifies the potential risk to the fetus.

Nursing Mothers

It is not known whether pegfilgrastim is excreted in human milk. Because many drugs are excreted in human milk, caution should be exercised when Neulasta™ is administered to a nursing woman.

Pediatric Use

The safety and effectiveness of Neulasta™ in pediatric patients have not been established. The 6 mg fixed dose single-use syringe formulation should not be used in infants, children, and smaller adolescents weighing less than 45 kg.

Geriatric Use

Of the 465 subjects with cancer who received Neulasta™ in clinical studies, 85 (18%) were age 65 and over, and 14 (3%) were age 75 and over. No overall differences in safety or effectiveness were observed between these patients and younger patients; however, due to the small number of elderly subjects, small but clinically relevant differences cannot be excluded.

ADVERSE REACTIONS

See WARNINGS sections regarding Splenic Rupture ARDS, Allergic Reactions and Sickle Cell Disease.

Safety data are based upon 465 subjects with lymphoma and solid tumors (breast, lung, and thoracic tumors) enrolled in six randomized clinical studies. Subjects received Neulasta™ after nonmyeloablative cytotoxic chemotherapy. Most adverse experiences were attributed by the investigators to the underlying malignancy or cytotoxic chemotherapy and occurred at similar rates in subjects who received Neulasta™ (n = 465) or Filgrastim (n = 331). These adverse experiences occurred at rates between 72% and 15% and included: nausea, fatigue, alopecia, diarrhea, vomiting, constipation, fever, anorexia, skeletal pain, headache, taste perversion, dyspepsia, myalgia, insomnia, abdominal pain, arthralgia, generalized weakness, peripheral edema, dizziness, granulocytopenia, stomatitis, mucositis, and neutropenic fever.

The most common adverse event attributed to Neulasta™ in clinical trials was medullary bone pain, reported in 26% of subjects, which was comparable to the incidence of Filgrastim-treated patients. This bone pain was generally reported to be of mild-to-moderate severity. Approximately 12% of all subjects utilized non-narcotic analgesics and less than 6% utilized narcotic analgesics in association with bone pain. No patient withdrew from study due to bone pain.

In clinical studies, leukocytosis (WBC counts $> 100 \times 10^9$/L) was observed in less than 1% of 465 subjects with non-myeloid malignancies receiving Neulasta™. Leukocytosis was not associated with any adverse effects.

In subjects receiving Neulasta™ in clinical trials, the only serious event that was not deemed attributable to underlying or concurrent disease, or to concurrent therapy was a case of hypoxia.

Reversible elevations in LDH, alkaline phosphatase, and uric acid, which did not require treatment intervention, were observed. The incidences of these changes, presented for Neulasta™ relative to Filgrastim, were: LDH (19% vs 29%), alkaline phosphatase (9% vs 16%), and uric acid (8% vs 9% [1% of reported cases for both treatment groups were classified as severe]).

Immunogenicity

As with all therapeutic proteins, there is a potential for immunogenicity. The incidence of antibody development in patients receiving Neulasta™ has not been adequately determined. While available data suggest that a small proportion of patients developed binding antibodies to Filgrastim or pegfilgrastim, the nature and specificity of these antibodies has not been adequately studied. No neutralizing antibodies have been detected using a cell-based bioassay in 46 patients who apparently developed binding antibodies. The detection of antibody formation is highly dependent on the

Continued on next page

Neulasta—Cont.

sensitivity and specificity of the assay, and the observed incidence of antibody positivity in an assay may be influenced by several factors including sample handling, concomitant medications, and underlying disease. Therefore, comparison of the incidence of antibodies to Neulasta™ with the incidence of antibodies to other products may be misleading.
Cytopenias resulting from an antibody response to exogenous growth factors have been reported on rare occasions in patients treated with other recombinant growth factors. There is a theoretical possibility that an antibody directed against pegfilgrastim may cross-react with endogenous G-CSF, resulting in immune-mediated neutropenia, but this has not been observed in clinical studies.

OVERDOSAGE

The maximum amount of Neulasta™ that can be safely administered in single or multiple doses has not been determined. Single doses of 300 mcg/kg have been administered SC to 8 normal volunteers and 3 patients with non-small cell lung cancer without serious adverse effects. These subjects experienced a mean maximum ANC of 55 × 10^9/L, with a corresponding mean maximum WBC of 67 × 10^9/L. The absolute maximum ANC observed was 96 × 10^9/L with a corresponding absolute maximum WBC observed of 120 × 10^9/L. The duration of leukocytosis ranged from 6 to 13 days. Leukapheresis should be considered in the management of symptomatic individuals.

DOSAGE AND ADMINISTRATION

The recommended dosage of Neulasta™ is a single subcutaneous (SC) injection of 6 mg administered once per chemotherapy cycle. Neulasta™ should not be administered in the period between 14 days before and 24 hours after administration of cytotoxic chemotherapy (see PRECAUTIONS).
The 6 mg fixed-dose formulation should not be used in infants, children, and smaller adolescents weighing less than 45 kg.
Neulasta™ should be visually inspected for discoloration and particulate matter before administration. Neulasta™ should not be administered if discoloration or particulates are observed.
Neulasta™ is supplied in prefilled syringes with UltraSafe® Needle Guards. Following administration of Neulasta™ from the prefilled syringe, the UltraSafe® Needle Guard should be activated to prevent accidental needle sticks. To activate the UltraSafe® Needle Guard, place your hands behind the needle, grasp the guard with one hand, and slide the guard forward until the needle is completely covered and the guard clicks into place. NOTE: If an audible click is not heard, the needle guard may not be completely activated. The prefilled syringe should be disposed of by placing the entire prefilled syringe with guard activated into an approved puncture-proof container.

Storage

Neulasta™ should be stored refrigerated at 2° to 8°C (36° to 46°F); syringes should be kept in their carton to protect from light until time of use. Shaking should be avoided. Before injection, Neulasta™ may be allowed to reach room temperature for a maximum of 48 hours but should be protected from light. Neulasta™ left at room temperature for more than 48 hours should be discarded. Freezing should be avoided; however, if accidentally frozen, Neulasta™ should be allowed to thaw in the refrigerator before administration. If frozen a second time, Neulasta™ should be discarded.

HOW SUPPLIED

Neulasta™ is supplied as a preservative-free solution containing 6 mg (0.6 mL) of pegfilgrastim (10 mg/mL) in a single-dose syringe with a 27 gauge, 1/2 inch needle with an UltraSafe® Needle Guard.
Neulasta™ is provided in a dispensing pack containing one syringe (NDC 55513-190-01).

REFERENCES

1. Morstyn G, Dexter T, Foote M. *Filgrastim (r-metHuG-CSF) in clinical practice* 2nd Edition. 1998;3:51-71.
2. Valerius T, Elsasser D, Repp R, et al. HLA Class-II antibodies recruit G-CSF activated neutrophils for treatment of B-cell malignancies. *Leukemia and Lymphoma*. 1997;26, 261-269.
3. Heil G, Hoelzer D, Sanz MA, et al. A randomized, double-blind, placebo-controlled, phase III study of Filgrastim in remission induction and consolidation therapy for adults with de novo Acute Myeloid Leukemia. *Blood*. 1997;90:4710-4718.

Manufactured by:
Amgen Inc.
One Amgen Center Drive
Thousand Oaks, California 91320-1799

Issue Date: 01/31/02
Shown in Product Identification Guide, page 305

NEUPOGEN® ℞

[nūe'pō-jĕn]
(Filgrastim)

DESCRIPTION

Filgrastim is a human granulocyte colony-stimulating factor (G-CSF), produced by recombinant DNA technology. NEUPOGEN® is the Amgen Inc. trademark for Filgrastim, which has been selected as the name for recombinant methionyl human granulocyte colony-stimulating factor (r-metHuG-CSF).
NEUPOGEN® is a 175 amino acid protein manufactured by recombinant DNA technology.[1] NEUPOGEN® is produced by *Escherichia coli* (*E coli*) bacteria into which has been inserted the human granulocyte colony-stimulating factor gene. NEUPOGEN® has a molecular weight of 18,800 daltons. The protein has an amino acid sequence that is identical to the natural sequence predicted from human DNA sequence analysis, except for the addition of an N-terminal methionine necessary for expression in *E coli*. Because NEUPOGEN® is produced in *E coli*, the product is nonglycosylated and thus differs from G-CSF isolated from a human cell.
NEUPOGEN® is a sterile, clear, colorless, preservative-free liquid for parenteral administration containing Filgrastim at a specific activity of 1.0 ± 0.6 × 10^8 U/mg (as measured by a cell mitogenesis assay). The product is available in single use vials and prefilled syringes. The single use vials contain either 300 mcg or 480 mcg Filgrastim at a fill volume of 1.0 mL or 1.6 mL, respectively. The single use prefilled syringes contain either 300 mcg or 480 mcg Filgrastim at a fill volume of 0.5 mL or 0.8 mL, respectively. See table below for product composition of each single use vial or prefilled syringe.
[See table below]

CLINICAL PHARMACOLOGY

Colony-stimulating Factors

Colony-stimulating factors are glycoproteins which act on hematopoietic cells by binding to specific cell surface receptors and stimulating proliferation, differentiation commitment, and some end-cell functional activation.
Endogenous G-CSF is a lineage specific colony-stimulating factor which is produced by monocytes, fibroblasts, and endothelial cells. G-CSF regulates the production of neutrophils within the bone marrow and affects neutrophil progenitor proliferation,[2,3] differentiation,[2,4] and selected end-cell functional activation (including enhanced phagocytic ability,[5] priming of the cellular metabolism associated with respiratory burst,[6] antibody dependent killing,[7] and the increased expression of some functions associated with cell surface antigens[8]). G-CSF is not species specific and has been shown to have minimal direct in vivo or in vitro effects on the production of hematopoietic cell types other than the neutrophil lineage.

Preclinical Experience

Filgrastim was administered to monkeys, dogs, hamsters, rats, and mice as part of a preclinical toxicology program which included single-dose acute, repeated-dose subacute, subchronic, and chronic studies. Single-dose administration of Filgrastim by the oral, intravenous (IV), subcutaneous (SC), or intraperitoneal (IP) routes resulted in no significant toxicity in mice, rats, hamsters, or monkeys. Although no deaths were observed in mice, rats, or monkeys at dose levels up to 3450 mcg/kg or in hamsters using single doses up to approximately 860 mcg/kg, deaths were observed in a subchronic (13-week) study in monkeys. In this study, evidence of neurological symptoms was seen in monkeys treated with doses of Filgrastim greater than 1150 mcg/kg/day for up to 18 days. Deaths were seen in 5 of the 8 treated animals and were associated with 15- to 28-fold increases in peripheral leukocyte counts, and neutrophil-infiltrated hemorrhagic foci were seen in both the cerebrum and cerebellum. In contrast, no monkeys died following 13 weeks of daily IV administration of Filgrastim at a dose level of 115 mcg/kg. In an ensuing 52-week study, one 115 mcg/kg dosed female monkey died after 18 weeks of daily IV administration of Filgrastim. Death was attributed to cardiopulmonary insufficiency.
In subacute, repeated-dose studies, changes observed were attributable to the expected pharmacological actions of Filgrastim (ie, dose-dependent increases in white cell counts, increased circulating segmented neutrophils, and increased myeloid:erythroid ratio in bone marrow). In all species, histopathologic examination of the liver and spleen revealed evidence of ongoing extramedullary granulopoiesis; increased spleen weights were seen in all species and appeared to be dose-related. A dose-dependent increase in serum alkaline phosphatase was observed in rats, and may reflect increased activity of osteoblasts and osteoclasts. Changes in serum chemistry values were reversible following discontinuation of treatment.
In rats treated at doses of 1150 mcg/kg/day for 4 weeks (5 of 32 animals) and for 13 weeks at doses of 100 mcg/kg/day (4 of 32 animals) and 500 mcg/kg/day (6 of 32 animals), articular swelling of the hind legs was observed. Some degree of hind leg dysfunction was also observed; however, symptoms reversed following cessation of dosing. In rats, osteoclasis and osteoanagenesis were found in the femur, humerus, coccyx, and hind legs (where they were accompanied by synovitis) after IV treatment for 4 weeks (115 to 1150 mcg/kg/day), and in the sternum after IV treatment for 13 weeks (115 to 575 mcg/kg/day). These effects reversed to normal within 4 to 5 weeks following cessation of treatment.
In the 52-week chronic, repeated-dose studies performed in rats (IP injection up to 57.5 mcg/kg/day), and cynomolgus monkeys (IV injection of up to 115 mcg/kg/day), changes observed were similar to those noted in the subacute studies. Expected pharmacological actions of Filgrastim included dose-dependent increases in white cell counts, increased circulating segmented neutrophils and alkaline phosphatase levels, and increased myeloid:erythroid ratios in the bone marrow. Decreases in platelet counts were also noted in primates. In no animals tested were hemorrhagic complications observed. Rats displayed dose-related swelling of the hind limb, accompanied by some degree of hind limb dysfunction; osteopathy was noted microscopically. Enlarged spleens (both species) and livers (monkeys), reflective of ongoing extramedullary granulopoiesis, as well as myeloid hyperplasia of the bone marrow, were observed in a dose-dependent manner.

Pharmacologic Effects of NEUPOGEN®

In phase 1 studies involving 96 patients with various nonmyeloid malignancies, NEUPOGEN® administration resulted in a dose-dependent increase in circulating neutrophil counts over the dose range of 1 to 70 mcg/kg/day.[9-11] This increase in neutrophil counts was observed whether NEUPOGEN® was administered IV (1 to 70 mcg/kg twice daily),[9] SC (1 to 3 mcg/kg once daily),[11] or by continuous SC infusion (3 to 11 mcg/kg/day).[10] With discontinuation of NEUPOGEN® therapy, neutrophil counts returned to baseline, in most cases within 4 days. Isolated neutrophils displayed normal phagocytic (measured by zymosan-stimulated chemoluminescence) and chemotactic (measured by migration under agarose using N-formyl-methionyl-leucyl-phenylalanine [fMLP] as the chemotaxin) activity in vitro.
The absolute monocyte count was reported to increase in a dose-dependent manner in most patients receiving NEUPOGEN®; however, the percentage of monocytes in the differential count remained within the normal range. In all studies to date, absolute counts of both eosinophils and basophils did not change and were within the normal range following administration of NEUPOGEN®. Increases in lymphocyte counts following NEUPOGEN® administration have been reported in some normal subjects and cancer patients.
White blood cell (WBC) differentials obtained during clinical trials have demonstrated a shift towards earlier granulocyte progenitor cells (left shift), including the appearance of promyelocytes and myeloblasts, usually during neutrophil recovery following the chemotherapy-induced nadir. In addition, Dohle bodies, increased granulocyte granulation, as well as hypersegmented neutrophils have been observed. Such changes were transient, and were not associated with clinical sequelae nor were they necessarily associated with infection.

Pharmacokinetics

Absorption and clearance of NEUPOGEN® follows first-order pharmacokinetic modeling without apparent concentration dependence. A positive linear correlation occurred between the parenteral dose and both the serum concentration and area under the concentration-time curves. Continuous IV infusion of 20 mcg/kg of NEUPOGEN® over 24 hours resulted in mean and median serum concentrations of approximately 48 and 56 ng/mL, respectively. Subcutaneous administration of 3.45 mcg/kg and 11.5 mcg/kg resulted in maximum serum concentrations of 4 and 49 ng/mL, respectively, within 2 to 8 hours. The volume of distribution averaged 150 mL/kg in both normal subjects and cancer patients. The elimination half-life, in both normal subjects and cancer patients, was approximately 3.5 hours. Clearance rates of NEUPOGEN® were approximately 0.5 to 0.7 mL/minute/kg. Single parenteral doses or daily IV doses, over a 14-day period, resulted in comparable half-lives. The half-lives were similar for IV administration (231 minutes, following doses of 34.5 mcg/kg) and for SC administration (210 minutes, following NEUPOGEN® doses of 3.45 mcg/kg). Continuous 24-hour IV infusions of 20 mcg/kg over an 11- to 20-day period produced steady-state serum concentrations of NEUPOGEN® with no evidence of drug accumulation over the time period investigated.
Pharmacokinetic data in geriatric patients (≥ 65 years) are not available.

	300 mcg/ 1.0 mL Vial	480 mcg/ 1.6 mL Vial	300 mcg/ 0.5 mL Syringe	480 mcg/ 0.8 mL Syringe
Filgrastim	300 mcg	480 mcg	300 mcg	480 mcg
Acetate	0.59 mg	0.94 mg	0.295 mg	0.472 mg
Sorbitol	50.0 mg	80.0 mg	25.0 mg	40.0 mg
Tween® 80	0.004%	0.004%	0.004%	0.004%
Sodium	0.035 mg	0.056 mg	0.0175 mg	0.028 mg
Water for Injection USP q.s. ad	1.0 mL	1.6 mL	0.5 mL	0.8 mL

CLINICAL EXPERIENCE

Cancer Patients Receiving Myelosuppressive Chemotherapy

NEUPOGEN® has been shown to be safe and effective in accelerating the recovery of neutrophil counts following a variety of chemotherapy regimens. In a phase 3 clinical trial in small cell lung cancer, patients received SC administration of NEUPOGEN® (4 to 8 mcg/kg/day, days 4 to 17) or placebo. In this study, the benefits of NEUPOGEN® therapy were shown to be prevention of infection as manifested by febrile neutropenia, decreased hospitalization, and decreased IV antibiotic usage. No difference in survival or disease progression was demonstrated.

In the phase 3, randomized, double-blind, placebo-controlled trial conducted in patients with small cell lung cancer, patients were randomized to receive NEUPOGEN® (n = 99) or placebo (n = 111) starting on day 4, after receiving standard dose chemotherapy with cyclophosphamide, doxorubicin, and etoposide. A total of 210 patients were evaluated for efficacy and 207 evaluated for safety. Treatment with NEUPOGEN® resulted in a clinically and statistically significant reduction in the incidence of infection, as manifested by febrile neutropenia; the incidence of at least one infection over all cycles of chemotherapy was 76% (84/111) for placebo-treated patients, versus 40% (40/99) for NEUPOGEN®-treated patients ($p < 0.001$). The following secondary analyses were also performed. The requirements for in-patient hospitalization and antibiotic use were also significantly decreased during the first cycle of chemotherapy; incidence of hospitalization was 69% (77/111) for placebo-treated patients in cycle 1, versus 52% (51/99) for NEUPOGEN®-treated patients ($p = 0.032$). The incidence of IV antibiotic usage was 60% (67/111) for placebo-treated patients in cycle 1, versus 38% (38/99) for NEUPOGEN®-treated patients ($p = 0.003$). The incidence, severity, and duration of severe neutropenia (absolute neutrophil count [ANC] < 500/mm^3) following chemotherapy were all significantly reduced. The incidence of severe neutropenia in cycle 1 was 84% (83/99) for patients receiving NEUPOGEN® versus 96% (106/110) for patients receiving placebo ($p = 0.004$). Over all cycles, patients randomized to NEUPOGEN® had a 57% (286/500 cycles) rate of severe neutropenia versus 77% (416/543 cycles) for patients randomized to placebo. The median duration of severe neutropenia in cycle 1 was reduced from 6 days (range 0 to 10 days) for patients receiving placebo to 2 days (range 0 to 9 days) for patients receiving NEUPOGEN® ($p < 0.001$). The mean duration of neutropenia in cycle 1 was 5.64 ± 2.27 days for patients receiving placebo versus 2.44 ± 1.90 days for patients receiving NEUPOGEN®. Over all cycles, the median duration of neutropenia was 3 days for patients randomized to placebo versus 1 day for patients randomized to NEUPOGEN®. The median severity of neutropenia (as measured by ANC nadir) was 72/mm^3 (range 0/mm^3 to 7912/mm^3) in cycle 1 for patients receiving NEUPOGEN® versus 38/mm^3 (range 0/mm^3 to 9520/mm^3) for patients receiving placebo ($p = 0.012$). The mean severity of neutropenia in cycle 1 was 496/mm^3 ± 1382/mm^3 for patients receiving NEUPOGEN® versus 204/mm^3 ± 953/mm^3 for patients receiving placebo. Over all cycles, the ANC nadir for patients randomized to NEUPOGEN® was 403/mm^3, versus 161/mm^3 for patients randomized to placebo. Administration of NEUPOGEN® resulted in an earlier ANC nadir following chemotherapy than was experienced by patients receiving placebo (day 10 vs day 12). NEUPOGEN® was well-tolerated when given SC daily at doses of 4 to 8 mcg/kg for up to 14 consecutive days following each cycle of chemotherapy (see ADVERSE REACTIONS).

Several other phase 1/2 studies, which did not directly measure the incidence of infection, but which did measure increases in neutrophils, support the efficacy of NEUPOGEN®. The regimens are presented to provide some background on the clinical experience with NEUPOGEN®. No claim regarding the safety or efficacy of the chemotherapy regimens is made. The effects of NEUPOGEN® on tumor growth or on the anti-tumor activity of the chemotherapy were not assessed. The doses of NEUPOGEN® used in these studies are considerably greater than those found to be effective in the phase 3 study described above. Such phase 1/2 studies are summarized in the following table.

[See table above]

Type of Malignancy	Regimen	Chemotherapy Dose	No. Pts.	Trial Phase	NEUPOGEN® Daily Dosage[a]
Small Cell Lung Cancer	Cyclophosphamide Doxorubicin Etoposide	1 g/m^2/day 50 mg/m^2/day 120 mg/m^2/day × 3 q 21 days	210	3	4-8 mcg/kg SC days 4-17
Small Cell Lung Cancer[11]	Ifosfamide Doxorubicin Etoposide Mesna	5 g/m^2/day 50 mg/m^2/day 120 mg/m^2/day × 3 8 g/m^2/day q 21 days	12	1/2	5.75-46 mcg/kg IV days 4-17
Urothelial Cancer[12]	Methotrexate Vinblastine Doxorubicin Cisplatin	30 mg/m^2/day × 2 3 mg/m^2/day × 2 30 mg/m^2/day 70 mg/m^2/day q 28 days	40	1/2	3.45-69 mcg/kg IV days 4-11
Various Nonmyeloid Malignancies[13]	Cyclophosphamide Etoposide Cisplatin	2.5 g/m^2/day × 2 500 mg/m^2/day × 3 50 mg/m^2/day × 3 q 28 days	18	1/2	23-69 mcg/kg[b] IV days 8-28
Breast/Ovarian Cancer[14]	Doxorubicin[c]	75 mg/m^2 100 mg/m^2 125 mg/m^2 150 mg/m^2 q 14 days	21	2	11.5 mcg/kg IV days 2-9 5.75 mcg/kg IV days 10-12
Neuroblastoma	Cyclophosphamide Doxorubicin Cisplatin	150 mg/m^2 × 7 35 mg/m^2 90 mg/m^2 q 28 days (cycles 1,3,5)[d]	12	2	5.45–17.25 mcg/kg SC days 6-19

[a] NEUPOGEN® doses were those that accelerated neutrophil production. Doses which provided no additional acceleration beyond that achieved at the next lower dose are not reported.
[b] Lowest dose(s) tested in the study.
[c] Patients received doxorubicin at either 75, 100, 125, or 150 mg/m^2.
[d] Cycles 2,6 = cyclophosphamide 150 mg/m^2 × 7 and etoposide 280 mg/m^2 × 3.
Cycle 4 = cisplatin 90 mg/m^2 × 1 and etoposide 280 mg/m^2 × 3.

Patients With Acute Myeloid Leukemia Receiving Induction or Consolidation Chemotherapy

In a randomized, double-blind, placebo-controlled, multicenter, phase 3 clinical trial, 521 patients (median age 54, range 16 to 89 years) were treated for de novo acute myeloid leukemia (AML). Following a standard induction chemotherapy regimen comprising daunorubicin, cytosine arabinoside, and etoposide[15] (DAV 3+7+5), patients received either NEUPOGEN® at 5 mcg/kg/day or placebo, SC, from 24 hours after the last dose of chemotherapy until neutrophil recovery (ANC 1000/mm^3 for 3 consecutive days or 10,000/mm^3 for 1 day) or for a maximum of 35 days.

Treatment with NEUPOGEN® significantly reduced the median time to ANC recovery and the median duration of fever, antibiotic use, and hospitalization following induction chemotherapy. In the NEUPOGEN®-treated group, the median time from initiation of chemotherapy to ANC recovery (ANC ≥ 500/mm^3) was 20 days (vs 25 days in the control group, $p = 0.0001$), the median duration of fever was reduced by 1.5 days ($p = 0.009$), and there were statistically significant reductions in the durations of IV antibiotic use and hospitalization. During consolidation therapy (DAV 2+5+5), patients treated with NEUPOGEN® also experienced significant reductions in the incidence of severe neutropenia, time to neutrophil recovery, the incidence and duration of fever, and in the durations of IV antibiotic use and hospitalization. Patients treated with a further course of standard (DAV 2+5+5) or high-dose cytosine arabinoside consolidation also experienced significant reductions in the duration of neutropenia.

There were no statistically significant differences between NEUPOGEN® and placebo groups in complete remission rate (69% NEUPOGEN® vs 68% placebo, $p = 0.77$), disease-free survival (median 342 days NEUPOGEN® [n = 178], 322 days placebo [n = 177], $p = 0.99$), time to progression of all randomized patients (median 165 days NEUPOGEN®, 186 days placebo, $p = 0.87$), or overall survival (median 380 days NEUPOGEN®, 425 days placebo, $p = 0.83$).

Cancer Patients Receiving Bone Marrow Transplant

In two separate randomized, controlled trials, patients with Hodgkin's disease (HD) and non-Hodgkin's lymphoma (NHL) were treated with myeloablative chemotherapy and autologous bone marrow transplantation (ABMT). In one study (n = 54), NEUPOGEN® was administered at doses of 10 or 30 mcg/kg/day; a third treatment group in this study received no NEUPOGEN®. A statistically significant reduction in the median number of days of severe neutropenia (ANC < 500/mm^3) occurred in the NEUPOGEN®-treated group versus the control group (23 days in the control group, 11 days in the 10 mcg/kg/day group, and 14 days in the 30 mcg/kg/day group, [11 days in the combined treatment groups, $p = 0.004$]). In the second study (n = 44, 43 patients evaluable), NEUPOGEN® was administered at doses of 10 or 20 mcg/kg/day; a third treatment group in this study received no NEUPOGEN®. A statistically significant reduction in the median number of days of severe neutropenia occurred in the NEUPOGEN®-treated group versus the control group (21.5 days in the control group and 10 days in both treatment groups, $p < 0.001$). The number of days of febrile neutropenia was also reduced significantly in this study (13.5 days in the control group, 5 days in the 10 mcg/kg/day group, and 5.5 days in the 20 mcg/kg/day group, [5 days in the combined treatment groups, $p < 0.0001$]). Reductions in the number of days of hospitalization and antibiotic use were also seen, although these reductions were not statistically significant. There were no effects on red blood cell or platelet levels.

In a randomized, placebo-controlled trial, 70 patients with myeloid and nonmyeloid malignancies were treated with myeloablative therapy and allogeneic bone marrow transplant followed by 300 mcg/m^2/day of a Filgrastim product. A statistically significant reduction in the median number of days of severe neutropenia occurred in the treated group versus the control group (19 days in the control group and 15 days in the treatment group, $p < 0.001$) and time to recovery of ANC to ≥ 500/mm^3 (21 days in the control group and 16 days in the treatment group, $p < 0.001$).

In three nonrandomized studies (n = 119), patients received ABMT and treatment with NEUPOGEN®. One study (n = 45) involved patients with breast cancer and malignant melanoma. A second study (n = 39) involved patients with HD. The third study (n = 35) involved patients with NHL, acute lymphoblastic leukemia (ALL), and germ cell tumor. In these studies, the recovery of the ANC to ≥ 500/mm^3 ranged from a median of 11.5 to 13 days.

None of the conditioning regimens used in the ABMT studies included radiation therapy.

While these studies were not designed to compare survival, this information was collected and evaluated. The overall survival and disease progression of patients receiving NEUPOGEN® in these studies were similar to those observed in the respective control groups and to historical data.

Peripheral Blood Progenitor Cell Collection and Therapy in Cancer Patients

All patients in the Amgen-sponsored trials received a similar mobilization/collection regimen: NEUPOGEN® was administered for 6 to 7 days, with an apheresis procedure on days 5, 6, and 7 (except for a limited number of patients receiving apheresis on days 4, 6, and 8). In a non-Amgen-sponsored study, patients underwent mobilization to a target number of mononuclear cells (MNC), with apheresis starting on day 5. There are no data on the mobilization of peripheral blood progenitor cells (PBPC) after days 4 to 5 that are not confounded by leukapheresis.

Mobilization: Mobilization of PBPC was studied in 50 heavily pretreated patients (median number of prior cycles = 9.5) with NHL, HD, or ALL (Amgen study 1). CFU-GM was used as the marker for engraftable PBPC. The median CFU-GM level on each day of mobilization was determined from the data available (CFU-GM assays were not obtained on all patients on each day of mobilization). These data are presented below.

The data from Amgen study 1 were supported by data from Amgen study 2 in which 22 pretreated breast cancer patients (median number of prior cycles = 3) were studied. Both the CFU-GM and CD34$^+$ cells reached a maximum on day 5 at > 10-fold over baseline and then remained elevated with leukapheresis.

[See first table at top of next page]

In three studies of patients with prior exposure to chemotherapy, the median CFU-GM yield in the leukapheresis product ranged from 20.9 to 32.7 × 10^4/kg body weight (n = 105). In two of these studies where CD34$^+$ yields in the leukapheresis product were also determined, the median CD34$^+$ yields were 3.11 and 2.80 × 10^6/kg, respectively (n = 56). In an additional study of 18 chemotherapy-naive patients, the median CFU-GM yield was 123.4 × 10^4/kg.

Continued on next page

Neupogen—Cont.

Engraftment: Engraftment following NEUPOGEN®-mobilized PBPC is summarized for 101 patients in the table below. In all studies, a Cox regression model showed that the total number of CFU-GM and/or CD34⁺ cells collected was a significant predictor of time to platelet recovery.

In a randomized, unblinded study of patients with HD or NHL undergoing myeloablative chemotherapy (Amgen study 3), 27 patients received NEUPOGEN®-mobilized PBPC followed by NEUPOGEN® and 31 patients received ABMT followed by NEUPOGEN®. Patients randomized to the NEUPOGEN®-mobilized PBPC group compared to the ABMT group had significantly fewer days of platelet transfusions (median 6 vs 10 days), a significantly shorter time to a sustained platelet count > 20,000/mm^3 (median 16 vs 23 days), a significantly shorter time to recovery of a sustained ANC ≥ 500/mm^3 (median 11 vs 14 days), significantly fewer days of red blood cell transfusions (median 2 vs 3 days) and a significantly shorter duration of posttransplant hospitalization.

[See second table at right]

Three of the 101 patients (3%) did not achieve the criteria for engraftment as defined by a platelet count ≥ 20,000/mm^3 by day 28. In clinical trials of NEUPOGEN® for the mobilization of PBPC, NEUPOGEN® was administered to patients at 5 to 24 mcg/kg/day after reinfusion of the collected cells until a sustainable ANC (≥ 500/mm^3) was reached. The rate of engraftment of these cells in the absence of NEUPOGEN® posttransplantation has not been studied.

Patients With Severe Chronic Neutropenia

Severe chronic neutropenia (SCN) (idiopathic, cyclic, and congenital) is characterized by a selective decrease in the number of circulating neutrophils and an enhanced susceptibility to bacterial infections.

The daily administration of NEUPOGEN® has been shown to be safe and effective in causing a sustained increase in the neutrophil count and a decrease in infectious morbidity in children and adults with the clinical syndrome of SCN.[16]

In the phase 3 trial, summarized in the following table, daily treatment with NEUPOGEN® resulted in significant beneficial changes in the incidence and duration of infection, fever, antibiotic use, and oropharyngeal ulcers. In this trial, 120 patients with a median age of 12 years (range 1 to 76 years) were treated.

[See third table at right]

The incidence for each of these 5 clinical parameters was lower in the NEUPOGEN® arm compared to the control arm for cohorts in each of the 3 major diagnostic categories. All 3 diagnostic groups showed favorable trends in favor of treatment. An analysis of variance showed no significant interaction between treatment and diagnosis, suggesting that efficacy did not differ substantially in the different diseases. Although NEUPOGEN® substantially reduced neutropenia in all patient groups, in patients with cyclic neutropenia, cycling persisted but the period of neutropenia was shortened to 1 day.

As a result of the lower incidence and duration of infections, there was also a lower number of episodes of hospitalization (28 hospitalizations in 62 patients in the treated group vs 44 hospitalizations in 60 patients in the control group over a 4-month period [p = 0.0034]). Patients treated with NEUPOGEN® also reported a lower number of episodes of diarrhea, nausea, fatigue, and sore throat.

In the phase 3 trial, untreated patients had a median ANC of 210/mm^3 (range 0 to 1550/mm^3). NEUPOGEN® therapy was adjusted to maintain the median ANC between 1500 and 10,000/mm^3. Overall, the response to NEUPOGEN® was observed in 1 to 2 weeks. The median ANC after 5 months of NEUPOGEN® therapy for all patients was 7460/mm^3 (range 30 to 30,880/mm^3). NEUPOGEN® dosing requirements were generally higher for patients with congenital neutropenia (2.3 to 40 mcg/kg/day) than for patients with idiopathic (0.6 to 11.5 mcg/kg/day) or cyclic (0.5 to 6 mcg/kg/day) neutropenia.

Progenitor Cell Levels in Peripheral Blood by Mobilization Day

	Overall Study 1 CFU-GM/mL		Study 2 CFU-GM/mL		Study 2 CD34⁺ (× 10⁴/mL)	
	No. Samples	Median (25%–75%)	No. Samples	Median (25%–75%)	No. Samples	Median (25%–75%)
Day 1	11	18 (13-62)	20	42 (15-151)	20	0.13 (0.02-0.66)
Day 2	7	22 (3-61)	n/a	n/a	n/a	n/a
Day 3	10	138 (39-364)	n/a	n/a	n/a	n/a
Day 4	18	365 (158-864)	18	576 (108-1819)	17	2.11 (0.58-3.93)
Day 5	36	781 (391-1608)	21	960 (72-1677)	22	3.16 (1.08-6.11)
Day 6	46	505 (199-1397)	22	756 (70-3486)	22	2.67 (1.09-4.40)
Day 7	37	333 (111-938)	22	597 (118-2009)	21	2.64 (0.78-4.22)
Day 8	15	383 (94-815)	12	51 (10-746)	12	1.61 (0.38-4.31)

n/a = not available

		Amgen-sponsored Study 1 N = 13	Amgen-sponsored Study 2 N = 22	Amgen-sponsored Study 3 N = 27	Non-Amgen-sponsored Study N = 39
Median PBPC/kg Collected					
	MNC	9.5 × 10⁸	9.5 × 10⁸	8.1 × 10⁸	10.3 × 10⁸
	CD34⁺	n/a	3.1 × 10⁶	2.8 × 10⁶	6.2 × 10⁶
	CFU-GM	63.9 × 10⁴	25.3 × 10⁴	32.6 × 10⁴	n/a
Days to ANC ≥ 500/mm³	Median	9	10	11	10
	Range	8-10	8-15	9-38	7-40
Days to Plt. ≥ 20,000/mm³	Median	10	12.5	16	15.5
	Range	7-16	10-30	8-52	7-63

n/a = not available

Overall Significant Changes in Clinical Endpoints
Median Incidence[a] (events) or Duration (days) per 28-day Period

	Control Patients[b]	NEUPOGEN®-treated Patients	p-value
Incidence of Infection	0.50	0.20	< 0.001
Incidence of Fever	0.25	0.20	< 0.001
Duration of Fever	0.63	0.20	0.005
Incidence of Oropharyngeal Ulcers	0.26	0.00	< 0.001
Incidence of Antibiotic Use	0.49	0.20	< 0.001

[a] Incidence values were calculated for each patient, and are defined as the total number of events experienced divided by the number of 28-day periods of exposure (on-study). Median incidence values were then reported for each patient group.
[b] Control patients were observed for a 4-month period.

INDICATIONS AND USAGE

Cancer Patients Receiving Myelosuppressive Chemotherapy

NEUPOGEN® is indicated to decrease the incidence of infection, as manifested by febrile neutropenia, in patients with nonmyeloid malignancies receiving myelosuppressive anti-cancer drugs associated with a significant incidence of severe neutropenia with fever (see CLINICAL EXPERIENCE). A complete blood count (CBC) and platelet count should be obtained prior to chemotherapy, and twice per week (see LABORATORY MONITORING) during NEUPOGEN® therapy to avoid leukocytosis and to monitor the neutrophil count. In phase 3 clinical studies, NEUPOGEN® therapy was discontinued when the ANC was ≥ 10,000/mm^3 after the expected chemotherapy-induced nadir.

Patients With Acute Myeloid Leukemia Receiving Induction or Consolidation Chemotherapy

NEUPOGEN® is indicated for reducing the time to neutrophil recovery and the duration of fever, following induction or consolidation chemotherapy treatment of adults with AML.

Cancer Patients Receiving Bone Marrow Transplant

NEUPOGEN® is indicated to reduce the duration of neutropenia and neutropenia-related clinical sequelae, eg, febrile neutropenia, in patients with nonmyeloid malignancies undergoing myeloablative chemotherapy followed by marrow transplantation (see CLINICAL EXPERIENCE). It is recommended that CBCs and platelet counts be obtained at a minimum of 3 times per week (see LABORATORY MONITORING) following marrow infusion to monitor the recovery of marrow reconstitution.

Patients Undergoing Peripheral Blood Progenitor Cell Collection and Therapy

NEUPOGEN® is indicated for the mobilization of hematopoietic progenitor cells into the peripheral blood for collection by leukapheresis. Mobilization allows for the collection of increased numbers of progenitor cells capable of engraftment compared with collection by leukapheresis without mobilization or bone marrow harvest. After myeloablative chemotherapy, the transplantation of an increased number of progenitor cells can lead to more rapid engraftment, which may result in a decreased need for supportive care (see CLINICAL EXPERIENCE).

Patients With Severe Chronic Neutropenia

NEUPOGEN® is indicated for chronic administration to reduce the incidence and duration of sequelae of neutropenia (eg, fever, infections, oropharyngeal ulcers) in symptomatic patients with congenital neutropenia, cyclic neutropenia, or idiopathic neutropenia (see CLINICAL EXPERIENCE). It is essential that serial CBCs with differential and platelet counts, and an evaluation of bone marrow morphology and karyotype be performed prior to initiation of NEUPOGEN® therapy (see WARNINGS). The use of NEUPOGEN® prior to confirmation of SCN may impair diagnostic efforts and may thus impair or delay evaluation and treatment of an underlying condition, other than SCN, causing the neutropenia.

CONTRAINDICATIONS

NEUPOGEN® is contraindicated in patients with known hypersensitivity to *E coli*-derived proteins, Filgrastim, or any component of the product.

WARNINGS

Allergic Reactions

Allergic-type reactions occurring on initial or subsequent treatment have been reported in < 1 in 4000 patients treated with NEUPOGEN®. These have generally been characterized by systemic symptoms involving at least 2 body systems, most often skin (rash, urticaria, facial edema), respiratory (wheezing, dyspnea), and cardiovascular (hypotension, tachycardia). Some reactions occurred on initial exposure. Reactions tended to occur within the first 30 minutes after administration and appeared to occur more frequently in patients receiving NEUPOGEN® IV. Rapid resolution of symptoms occurred in most cases after administration of antihistamines, steroids, bronchodilators, and/or epinephrine. Symptoms recurred in more than half the patients who were rechallenged.

SPLENIC RUPTURE

RARE CASES OF SPLENIC RUPTURE HAVE BEEN REPORTED FOLLOWING THE ADMINISTRATION OF COLONY-STIMULATING FACTORS, INCLUDING NEUPOGEN®, FOR PERIPHERAL BLOOD PROGENITOR CELL (PBPC) MOBILI-

ZATION IN BOTH HEALTHY DONORS AND PATIENTS WITH CANCER. SOME OF THESE CASES WERE FATAL. INDIVIDUALS RECEIVING NEUPOGEN® WHO REPORT ABDOMINAL OR SHOULDER TIP PAIN, PARTICULARLY HEALTHY DONORS RECEIVING NEUPOGEN® FOR PBPC MOBILIZATION, SHOULD BE EVALUATED FOR AN ENLARGED SPLEEN OR SPLENIC RUPTURE.

Adult Respiratory Distress Syndrome (ARDS)

Adult respiratory distress syndrome (ARDS) has been reported in neutropenic patients with sepsis receiving NEUPOGEN®, and is postulated to be secondary to an influx of neutrophils to sites of inflammation in the lungs. Neutropenic patients receiving NEUPOGEN® who develop fever, lung infiltrates, or respiratory distress should be evaluated for the possibility of ARDS. In the event that ARDS occurs, NEUPOGEN® should be discontinued until resolution of ARDS and patients should receive appropriate medical management for this condition.

Sickle Cell Disease

Severe sickle cell crises have been reported in patients with sickle cell disease (specifically homozygous sickle cell anemia, sickle/hemoglobin C disease, and sickle/β+ thalassemia) who received NEUPOGEN® for PBPC mobilization or following chemotherapy. One of these cases was fatal. NEUPOGEN® should be used with caution in patients with sickle cell disease, and only after careful consideration of the potential risks and benefits. Patients with sickle cell disease who receive NEUPOGEN® should be kept well hydrated and monitored for the occurrence of sickle cell crises. In the event of severe sickle cell crisis, supportive care should be administered, and interventions to ameliorate the underlying event, such as therapeutic red blood cell exchange transfusion, should be considered.

Patients With Severe Chronic Neutropenia

The safety and efficacy of NEUPOGEN® in the treatment of neutropenia due to other hematopoietic disorders (eg, myelodysplastic syndrome [MDS]) have not been established. Care should be taken to confirm the diagnosis of SCN before initiating NEUPOGEN® therapy.

MDS and AML have been reported to occur in the natural history of congenital neutropenia without cytokine therapy.[17] Cytogenetic abnormalities, transformation to MDS, and AML have also been observed in patients treated with NEUPOGEN® for SCN. Based on available data including a postmarketing surveillance study, the risk of developing MDS and AML appears to be confined to the subset of patients with congenital neutropenia (see ADVERSE REACTIONS). Abnormal cytogenetics and MDS have been associated with the eventual development of myeloid leukemia. The effect of NEUPOGEN® on the development of abnormal cytogenetics and the effect of continued NEUPOGEN® administration in patients with abnormal cytogenetics or MDS are unknown. If a patient with SCN develops abnormal cytogenetics or myelodysplasia, the risks and benefits of continuing NEUPOGEN® should be carefully considered.

PRECAUTIONS

General

Simultaneous Use With Chemotherapy and Radiation Therapy

The safety and efficacy of NEUPOGEN® given simultaneously with cytotoxic chemotherapy have not been established. Because of the potential sensitivity of rapidly dividing myeloid cells to cytotoxic chemotherapy, do not use NEUPOGEN® in the period 24 hours before through 24 hours after the administration of cytotoxic chemotherapy (see DOSAGE AND ADMINISTRATION).

The efficacy of NEUPOGEN® has not been evaluated in patients receiving chemotherapy associated with delayed myelosuppression (eg, nitrosoureas) or with mitomycin C or with myelosuppressive doses of antimetabolites such as 5-fluorouracil.

The safety and efficacy of NEUPOGEN® have not been evaluated in patients receiving concurrent radiation therapy. Simultaneous use of NEUPOGEN® with chemotherapy and radiation therapy should be avoided.

Potential Effect on Malignant Cells

NEUPOGEN® is a growth factor that primarily stimulates neutrophils. However, the possibility that NEUPOGEN® can act as a growth factor for any tumor type cannot be excluded. In a randomized study evaluating the effects of NEUPOGEN® versus placebo in patients undergoing remission induction for AML, there was no significant difference in remission rate, disease-free, or overall survival (see CLINICAL EXPERIENCE).

The safety of NEUPOGEN® in chronic myeloid leukemia (CML) and myelodysplasia has not been established.

When NEUPOGEN® is used to mobilize PBPC, tumor cells may be released from the marrow and subsequently collected in the leukapheresis product. The effect of reinfusion of tumor cells has not been well-studied, and the limited data available are inconclusive.

Leukocytosis

Cancer Patients Receiving Myelosuppressive Chemotherapy

White blood cell counts of 100,000/mm^3 or greater were observed in approximately 2% of patients receiving NEUPOGEN® at doses above 5 mcg/kg/day. There were no reports of adverse events associated with this degree of leukocytosis. In order to avoid the potential complications of excessive leukocytosis, a CBC is recommended twice per week during NEUPOGEN® therapy (see LABORATORY MONITORING).

Premature Discontinuation of NEUPOGEN® Therapy

Cancer Patients Receiving Myelosuppressive Chemotherapy

A transient increase in neutrophil counts is typically seen 1 to 2 days after initiation of NEUPOGEN® therapy. However, for a sustained therapeutic response, NEUPOGEN® therapy should be continued following chemotherapy until the post nadir ANC reaches 10,000/mm^3. Therefore, the premature discontinuation of NEUPOGEN® therapy, prior to the time of recovery from the expected neutrophil nadir, is generally not recommended (see DOSAGE AND ADMINISTRATION).

Immunogenicity

As with all therapeutic proteins, there is a potential for immunogenicity. The incidence of antibody development in patients receiving NEUPOGEN® has not been adequately determined. While available data suggest that a small proportion of patients developed binding antibodies to Filgrastim, the nature and specificity of these antibodies has not been adequately studied. In clinical studies comparing NEUPOGEN® and Neulasta™, the incidence of antibodies binding to NEUPOGEN® was 3% (11/333). In these 11 patients, no evidence of a neutralizing response was observed using a cell-based bioassay. The detection of antibody formation is highly dependent on the sensitivity and specificity of the assay, and the observed incidence of antibody positivity in an assay may be influenced by several factors including timing of sampling, sample handling, concomitant medications, and underlying disease. Therefore, comparison of the incidence of antibodies to NEUPOGEN® with the incidence of antibodies to other products may be misleading. Cytopenias resulting from an antibody response to exogenous growth factors have been reported on rare occasions in patients treated with other recombinant growth factors. There is a theoretical possibility that an antibody directed against Filgrastim may cross-react with endogenous G-CSF, resulting in immune-mediated neutropenia; however, this has not been reported in clinical studies or in post-marketing experience. Patients who develop hypersensitivity to Filgrastim (NEUPOGEN ®) may have allergic or hypersensitivity reactions to other *E coli*-derived proteins.

Other

In studies of NEUPOGEN® administration following chemotherapy, most reported side effects were consistent with those usually seen as a result of cytotoxic chemotherapy (see ADVERSE REACTIONS). Because of the potential of receiving higher doses of chemotherapy (ie, full doses on the prescribed schedule), the patient may be at greater risk of thrombocytopenia, anemia, and nonhematologic consequences of increased chemotherapy doses (please refer to the prescribing information of the specific chemotherapy agents used). Regular monitoring of the hematocrit and platelet count is recommended. Furthermore, care should be exercised in the administration of NEUPOGEN® in conjunction with other drugs known to lower the platelet count. There have been rare reports (< 1 in 7000 patients) of cutaneous vasculitis in patients treated with NEUPOGEN®. In most cases, the severity of cutaneous vasculitis was moderate or severe. Most of the reports involved patients with SCN receiving long-term NEUPOGEN® therapy. Symptoms of vasculitis generally developed simultaneously with an increase in the ANC and abated when the ANC decreased. Many patients were able to continue NEUPOGEN® at a reduced dose.

Information for Patients and Caregivers

Patients should be referred to the "Information for Patients and Caregivers" labeling included with the package insert in each dispensing pack of NEUPOGEN® vials or NEUPOGEN® prefilled syringes. The "Information for Patients and Caregivers" labeling provides information about neutrophils and neutropenia and the safety and efficacy of NEUPOGEN®. It is not intended to be a disclosure of all known or possible effects.

Laboratory Monitoring

Cancer Patients Receiving Myelosuppressive Chemotherapy

A CBC and platelet count should be obtained prior to chemotherapy, and at regular intervals (twice per week) during NEUPOGEN® therapy. Following cytotoxic chemotherapy, the neutrophil nadir occurred earlier during cycles when NEUPOGEN® was administered, and WBC differentials demonstrated a left shift, including the appearance of promyelocytes and myeloblasts. In addition, the duration of severe neutropenia was reduced, and was followed by an accelerated recovery in the neutrophil counts. Therefore, regular monitoring of WBC counts, particularly at the time of the recovery from the post chemotherapy nadir, is recommended in order to avoid excessive leukocytosis.

Cancer Patients Receiving Bone Marrow Transplant

Frequent CBCs and platelet counts are recommended (at least 3 times per week) following marrow transplantation.

Patients With Severe Chronic Neutropenia

During the initial 4 weeks of NEUPOGEN® therapy and during the 2 weeks following any dose adjustment, a CBC with differential and platelet count should be performed twice weekly. Once a patient is clinically stable, a CBC with differential and platelet count should be performed monthly during the first year of treatment. Thereafter, if clinically stable, routine monitoring with regular CBCs (ie, as clinically indicated but at least quarterly) is recommended. Additionally, for those patients with congenital neutropenia, annual bone marrow and cytogenetic evaluations should be performed throughout the duration of treatment (see WARNINGS, ADVERSE REACTIONS).

In clinical trials, the following laboratory results were observed:

- Cyclic fluctuations in the neutrophil counts were frequently observed in patients with congenital or idiopathic neutropenia after initiation of NEUPOGEN® therapy.
- Platelet counts were generally at the upper limits of normal prior to NEUPOGEN® therapy. With NEUPOGEN® therapy, platelet counts decreased but usually remained within normal limits (see ADVERSE REACTIONS).
- Early myeloid forms were noted in peripheral blood in most patients, including the appearance of metamyelocytes and myelocytes. Promyelocytes and myeloblasts were noted in some patients.
- Relative increases were occasionally noted in the number of circulating eosinophils and basophils. No consistent increases were observed with NEUPOGEN® therapy.
- As in other trials, increases were observed in serum uric acid, lactic dehydrogenase, and serum alkaline phosphatase.

Drug Interaction

Drug interactions between NEUPOGEN® and other drugs have not been fully evaluated. Drugs which may potentiate the release of neutrophils, such as lithium, should be used with caution.

Carcinogenesis, Mutagenesis, Impairment of Fertility

The carcinogenic potential of NEUPOGEN® has not been studied. NEUPOGEN® failed to induce bacterial gene mutations in either the presence or absence of a drug metabolizing enzyme system. NEUPOGEN® had no observed effect on the fertility of male or female rats, or on gestation at doses up to 500 mcg/kg.

Pregnancy Category C

NEUPOGEN® has been shown to have adverse effects in pregnant rabbits when given in doses 2 to 10 times the human dose. Since there are no adequate and well-controlled studies in pregnant women, the effect, if any, of NEUPOGEN® the developing fetus or the reproductive capacity of the mother is unknown. However, the scientific literature describes transplacental passage of NEUPOGEN® when administered to pregnant rats during the latter part of gestation[18] and apparent transplacental passage of NEUPOGEN® when administered to pregnant humans by ≤ 30 hours prior to preterm delivery (≤ 30 weeks gestation).[19] NEUPOGEN® should be used during pregnancy only if the potential benefit justifies the potential risk to the fetus.

In rabbits, increased abortion and embryolethality were observed in animals treated with NEUPOGEN® at 80 mcg/kg/day. NEUPOGEN® administered to pregnant rabbits at doses of 80 mcg/kg/day during the period of organogenesis was associated with increased fetal resorption, genitourinary bleeding, developmental abnormalities, decreased body weight, live births, and food consumption. External abnormalities were not observed in the fetuses of dams treated at 80 mcg/kg/day. Reproductive studies in pregnant rats have shown that NEUPOGEN® was not associated with lethal, teratogenic, or behavioral effects on fetuses when administered by daily IV injection during the period of organogenesis at dose levels up to 575 mcg/kg/day.

In Segment III studies in rats, offspring of dams treated at > 20 mcg/kg/day exhibited a delay in external differentiation (detachment of auricles and descent of testes) and slight growth retardation, possibly due to lower body weight of females during rearing and nursing. Offspring of dams treated at 100 mcg/kg/day exhibited decreased body weights at birth, and a slightly reduced 4-day survival rate.

Nursing Mothers

It is not known whether NEUPOGEN® is excreted in human milk. Because many drugs are excreted in human milk, caution should be exercised if NEUPOGEN® is administered to a nursing woman.

Pediatric Use

In a phase 3 study to assess the safety and efficacy of NEUPOGEN® in the treatment of SCN, 120 patients with a median age of 12 years were studied. Of the 120 patients, 12 were infants (1 month to 2 years of age), 47 were children (2 to 12 years of age), and 9 were adolescents (12 to 16 years of age). Additional information is available from a SCN postmarketing surveillance study, which includes long-term follow-up of patients in the clinical studies and information from additional patients who entered directly into the postmarketing surveillance study. Of the 531 patients in the surveillance study as of 31 December 1997, 32 were infants, 200 were children, and 68 were adolescents (see CLINICAL EXPERIENCE, INDICATIONS AND USAGE, LABORATORY MONITORING, DOSAGE AND ADMINISTRATION).

Pediatric patients with congenital types of neutropenia (Kostmann's syndrome, congenital agranulocytosis, or Schwachman-Diamond syndrome) have developed cytogenetic abnormalities and have undergone transformation to MDS and AML while receiving chronic NEUPOGEN® treatment. The relationship of these events to NEUPOGEN® administration is unknown (see WARNINGS, ADVERSE REACTIONS).

Long-term follow-up data from the postmarketing surveillance study suggest that height and weight are not adversely affected in patients who received up to 5 years of

Continued on next page

Neupogen—Cont.

NEUPOGEN® treatment. Limited data from patients who were followed in the phase 3 study for 1.5 years did not suggest alterations in sexual maturation or endocrine function.
The safety and efficacy in neonates and patients with autoimmune neutropenia of infancy have not been established.
In the cancer setting, 12 pediatric patients with neuroblastoma have received up to 6 cycles of cyclophosphamide, cisplatin, doxorubicin, and etoposide chemotherapy concurrently with NEUPOGEN®; in this population, NEUPOGEN® was well-tolerated. There was one report of palpable splenomegaly associated with NEUPOGEN® therapy; however, the only consistently reported adverse event was musculoskeletal pain, which is no different from the experience in the adult population.

Geriatric Use

Among 855 subjects enrolled in 3 randomized, placebo controlled trials of NEUPOGEN® use following myelosuppressive chemotherapy, there were 232 subjects age 65 or older, and 22 subjects age 75 or older. No overall differences in safety or effectiveness were observed between these subjects and younger subjects, and other clinical experience has not identified differences in the responses between elderly and younger patients.
Clinical studies of NEUPOGEN® in other approved indications (ie, bone marrow transplant recipients, PBPC mobilization, and SCN) did not include sufficient numbers of subjects aged 65 and older to determine whether elderly subjects respond differently from younger subjects.

ADVERSE REACTIONS

Cancer Patients Receiving Myelosuppressive Chemotherapy

In clinical trials involving over 350 patients receiving NEUPOGEN® following nonmyeloablative cytotoxic chemotherapy, most adverse experiences were the sequelae of the underlying malignancy or cytotoxic chemotherapy. In all phase 2 and 3 trials, medullary bone pain, reported in 24% of patients, was the only consistently observed adverse reaction attributed to NEUPOGEN® therapy. This bone pain was generally reported to be of mild-to-moderate severity, and could be controlled in most patients with non-narcotic analgesics; infrequently, bone pain was severe enough to require narcotic analgesics. Bone pain was reported more frequently in patients treated with higher doses (20 to 100 mcg/kg/day) administered IV, and less frequently in patients treated with lower SC doses of NEUPOGEN® (3 to 10 mcg/kg/day).
In the randomized, double-blind, placebo-controlled trial of NEUPOGEN® therapy following combination chemotherapy in patients (n = 207) with small cell lung cancer, the following adverse events were reported during blinded cycles of study medication (placebo or NEUPOGEN® at 4 to 8 mcg/kg/day). Events are reported as exposure-adjusted since patients remained on double-blind NEUPOGEN® a median of 3 cycles versus 1 cycle for placebo.

	% of Blinded Cycles With Events	
Event	NEUPOGEN® N = 384 Patient Cycles	Placebo N = 257 Patient Cycles
Nausea/Vomiting	57	64
Skeletal Pain	22	11
Alopecia	18	27
Diarrhea	14	23
Neutropenic Fever	13	35
Mucositis	12	20
Fever	12	11
Fatigue	11	16
Anorexia	9	11
Dyspnea	9	11
Headache	7	9
Cough	6	8
Skin Rash	6	9
Chest Pain	5	6
Generalized Weakness	4	7
Sore Throat	4	9
Stomatitis	5	10
Constipation	5	10
Pain (Unspecified)	2	7

In this study, there were no serious, life-threatening, or fatal adverse reactions attributed to NEUPOGEN® therapy. Specifically, there were no reports of flu-like symptoms, pleuritis, pericarditis, or other major systemic reactions to NEUPOGEN®.
Spontaneously reversible elevations in uric acid, lactate dehydrogenase, and alkaline phosphatase occurred in 27% to 58% of 98 patients receiving blinded NEUPOGEN® therapy following cytotoxic chemotherapy; increases were generally mild-to-moderate. Transient decreases in blood pressure (< 90/60 mmHg), which did not require clinical treatment, were reported in 7 of 176 patients in phase 3 clinical studies following administration of NEUPOGEN®. Cardiac events (myocardial infarctions, arrhythmias) have been reported in 11 of 375 cancer patients receiving NEUPOGEN® in clinical studies; the relationship to NEUPOGEN® therapy is unknown. No evidence of interaction of NEUPOGEN® with other drugs was observed in the course of clinical trials (see PRECAUTIONS).
There has been no evidence for the development of antibodies or of a blunted or diminished response to NEUPOGEN® in treated patients, including those receiving NEUPOGEN® daily for almost 2 years.

Patients With Acute Myeloid Leukemia

In a randomized phase 3 clinical trial, 259 patients received NEUPOGEN® and 262 patients received placebo postchemotherapy. Overall, the frequency of all reported adverse events was similar in both the NEUPOGEN® and placebo groups (83% vs 82% in Induction 1; 61% vs 64% in Consolidation 1). Adverse events reported more frequently in the NEUPOGEN®-treated group included: petechiae (17% vs 14%), epistaxis (9% vs 5%), and transfusion reactions (10% vs 5%). There were no significant differences in the frequency of these events.
There were a similar number of deaths in each treatment group during induction (25 NEUPOGEN® vs 27 placebo). The primary causes of death included infection (9 vs 18), persistent leukemia (7 vs 5), and hemorrhage (6 vs 3). Of the hemorrhagic deaths, 5 cerebral hemorrhages were reported in the NEUPOGEN® group and one in the placebo group. Other serious nonfatal hemorrhagic events were reported in the respiratory tract (4 vs 1), skin (4 vs 4), gastrointestinal tract (2 vs 2), urinary tract (1 vs 1), ocular (1 vs 0), and other nonspecific sites (2 vs 1). While 19 (7%) patients in the NEUPOGEN® group and 5 (2%) patients in the placebo group experienced severe or fatal hemorrhagic events, overall, hemorrhagic adverse events were reported at a similar frequency in both groups (40% vs 38%). The time to transfusion-independent platelet recovery and the number of days of platelet transfusions were similar in both groups.

Cancer Patients Receiving Bone Marrow Transplant

In clinical trials, the reported adverse effects were those typically seen in patients receiving intensive chemotherapy followed by bone marrow transplant (BMT). The most common events reported in both control and treatment groups included stomatitis, nausea, and vomiting, generally of mild-to-moderate severity and were considered unrelated to NEUPOGEN®. In the randomized studies of BMT involving 167 patients who received study drug, the following events occurred more frequently in patients treated with Filgrastim than in controls: nausea (10% vs 4%), vomiting (7% vs 3%), hypertension (4% vs 0%), rash (12% vs 10%), and peritonitis (2% vs 0%). None of these events were reported by the Investigator to be related to NEUPOGEN®. One event of erythema nodosum was reported moderate in severity and possibly related to NEUPOGEN®.
Generally, adverse events observed in nonrandomized studies were similar to those seen in randomized studies, occurred in a minority of patients, and were of mild-to-moderate severity. In one study (n = 45), 3 serious adverse events reported by the investigator were considered possibly related to NEUPOGEN®. These included 2 events of renal insufficiency and one event of capillary leak syndrome. The relationship of these events to NEUPOGEN® remains unclear since they occurred in patients with culture-proven infection with clinical sepsis who were receiving potentially nephrotoxic antibacterial and antifungal therapy.

Cancer Patients Undergoing Peripheral Blood Progenitor Cell Collection and Therapy

In clinical trials, 126 patients received NEUPOGEN® for PBPC mobilization. In this setting, NEUPOGEN® was generally well-tolerated. Adverse events related to NEUPOGEN® consisted primarily of mild-to-moderate musculoskeletal symptoms, reported in 44% of patients. These symptoms were predominantly events of medullary bone pain (33%). Headache was reported related to NEUPOGEN® in 7% of patients. Transient increases in alkaline phosphatase related to NEUPOGEN® were reported in 21% of the patients who had serum chemistries measured; most were mild-to-moderate.
All patients had increases in neutrophil counts during mobilization, consistent with the biological effects of NEUPOGEN®. Two patients had a WBC count > 100,000/mm^3. No sequelae were associated with any grade of leukocytosis.
Sixty-five percent of patients had mild-to-moderate anemia and 97% of patients had decreases in platelet counts; 5 patients (out of 126) had decreased platelet counts to < 50,000/mm^3. Anemia and thrombocytopenia have been reported to be related to leukapheresis; however, the possibility that NEUPOGEN® mobilization may contribute to anemia or thrombocytopenia has not been ruled out.

Patients With Severe Chronic Neutropenia

Mild-to-moderate bone pain was reported in approximately 33% of patients in clinical trials. This symptom was readily controlled with non-narcotic analgesics. Generalized musculoskeletal pain was also noted in higher frequency in patients treated with NEUPOGEN®. Palpable splenomegaly was observed in approximately 30% of patients. Abdominal or flank pain was seen infrequently, and thrombocytopenia (< 50,000/mm^3) was noted in 12% of patients with palpable spleens. Fewer than 3% of all patients underwent splenectomy, and most of these had a prestudy history of splenomegaly. Fewer than 6% of patients had thrombocytopenia (< 50,000/mm^3) during NEUPOGEN® therapy, most of whom had a pre-existing history of thrombocytopenia. In most cases, thrombocytopenia was managed by NEUPOGEN® dose reduction or interruption. An additional 5% of patients had platelet counts between 50,000 to 100,000/mm^3. There were no associated serious hemorrhagic sequelae in these patients. Epistaxis was noted in 15% of patients treated with NEUPOGEN®, but was associated with thrombocytopenia in 2% of patients. Anemia was reported in approximately 10% of patients, but in most cases appeared to be related to frequent diagnostic phlebotomy, chronic illness, or concomitant medications. Other adverse events infrequently observed and possibly related to NEUPOGEN® therapy were: injection site reaction, rash, hepatomegaly, arthralgia, osteoporosis, cutaneous vasculitis, hematuria/proteinuria, alopecia, and exacerbation of some pre-existing skin disorders (eg, psoriasis).
Cytogenetic abnormalities, transformation to MDS, and AML have been observed in patients treated with NEUPOGEN® for SCN (see WARNINGS, PRECAUTIONS: Pediatric Use). As of 31 December 1997, data were available from a postmarketing surveillance study of 531 SCN patients with an average follow-up of 4.0 years. Based on analysis of these data, the risk of developing MDS and AML appears to be confined to the subset of patients with congenital neutropenia. A life-table analysis of these data revealed that the cumulative risk of developing leukemia or MDS by the end of the 8th year of NEUPOGEN® treatment in a patient with congenital neutropenia was 16.5 % (95% C.I. = 9.8%, 23.3%); this represents an annual rate of approximately 2%. Cytogenetic abnormalities, most commonly involving chromosome 7, have been reported in patients treated with NEUPOGEN® who had previously documented normal cytogenetics. It is unknown whether the development of cytogenetic abnormalities, MDS, or AML is related to chronic daily NEUPOGEN® administration or to the natural history of congenital neutropenia. It is also unknown if the rate of conversion in patients who have not received NEUPOGEN® is different from that of patients who have received NEUPOGEN®. Routine monitoring through regular CBCs is recommended for all SCN patients. Additionally, annual bone marrow and cytogenetic evaluations are recommended in all patients with congenital neutropenia (see LABORATORY MONITORING).

OVERDOSAGE

In cancer patients receiving NEUPOGEN® as an adjunct to myelosuppressive chemotherapy, it is recommended, to avoid the potential risks of excessive leukocytosis, that NEUPOGEN® therapy be discontinued if the ANC surpasses 10,000/mm^3 after the chemotherapy-induced ANC nadir has occurred. Doses of NEUPOGEN® that increase the ANC beyond 10,000/mm^3 may not result in any additional clinical benefit.
The maximum tolerated dose of NEUPOGEN® has not been determined. Efficacy was demonstrated at doses of 4 to 8 mcg/kg/day in the phase 3 study of nonmyeloablative chemotherapy. Patients in the BMT studies received up to 138 mcg/kg/day without toxic effects, although there was a flattening of the dose response curve above daily doses of greater than 10 mcg/kg/day.
In NEUPOGEN® clinical trials of cancer patients receiving myelosuppressive chemotherapy, WBC counts > 100,000/mm^3 have been reported in less than 5% of patients, but were not associated with any reported adverse clinical effects.
In cancer patients receiving myelosuppressive chemotherapy, discontinuation of NEUPOGEN® therapy usually results in a 50% decrease in circulating neutrophils within 1 to 2 days, with a return to pretreatment levels in 1 to 7 days.

DOSAGE AND ADMINISTRATION

NEUPOGEN® is supplied in either vials or in prefilled syringes with UltraSafe® Needle Guards. Following administration of NEUPOGEN® from the prefilled syringe, the UltraSafe® Needle Guard should be activated to prevent accidental needle sticks. To activate the UltraSafe® Needle Guard, place your hands behind the needle, grasp the guard with one hand, and slide the guard forward until the needle is completely covered and the guard clicks into place. **NOTE: If an audible click is not heard, the needle guard may not be completely activated.** The prefilled syringe should be disposed of by placing the entire prefilled syringe with guard activated into an approved puncture-proof container.

Cancer Patients Receiving Myelosuppressive Chemotherapy

The recommended starting dose of NEUPOGEN® is 5 mcg/kg/day, administered as a single daily injection by SC bolus injection, by short IV infusion (15 to 30 minutes), or by continuous SC or continuous IV infusion. A CBC and platelet count should be obtained before instituting NEUPOGEN® therapy, and monitored twice weekly during therapy. Doses may be increased in increments of 5 mcg/kg for each chemotherapy cycle, according to the duration and severity of the ANC nadir.

NEUPOGEN® should be administered no earlier than 24 hours after the administration of cytotoxic chemotherapy. NEUPOGEN® should not be administered in the period 24 hours before the administration of chemotherapy (see PRECAUTIONS). NEUPOGEN® should be administered daily for up to 2 weeks, until the ANC has reached 10,000/mm^3 following the expected chemotherapy-induced neutrophil nadir. The duration of NEUPOGEN® therapy needed to attenuate chemotherapy-induced neutropenia may be dependent on the myelosuppressive potential of the chemotherapy regimen employed. NEUPOGEN® therapy should be discontinued if the ANC surpasses 10,000/mm^3 after the expected chemotherapy-induced neutrophil nadir (see PRECAUTIONS). In phase 3 trials, efficacy was observed at doses of 4 to 8 mcg/kg/day.

Cancer Patients Receiving Bone Marrow Transplant

The recommended dose of NEUPOGEN® following BMT is 10 mcg/kg/day given as an IV infusion of 4 or 24 hours, or as a continuous 24-hour SC infusion. For patients receiving BMT, the first dose of NEUPOGEN® should be administered at least 24 hours after cytotoxic chemotherapy and at least 24 hours after bone marrow infusion.

During the period of neutrophil recovery, the daily dose of NEUPOGEN® should be titrated against the neutrophil response as follows:

Absolute Neutrophil Count	NEUPOGEN® Dose Adjustment
When ANC > 1000/mm^3 for 3 consecutive days	Reduce to 5 mcg/kg/day[a]
then: If ANC remains > 1000/mm^3 for 3 more consecutive days	Discontinue NEUPOGEN®
then: If ANC decreases to < 1000/mm^3	Resume at 5 mcg/kg/day

[a] If ANC decreases to < 1000/mm^3 at any time during the 5 mcg/kg/day administration, NEUPOGEN® should be increased to 10 mcg/kg/day, and the above steps should then be followed.

Peripheral Blood Progenitor Cell Collection and Therapy in Cancer Patients

The recommended dose of NEUPOGEN® for the mobilization of PBPC is 10 mcg/kg/day SC, either as a bolus or a continuous infusion. It is recommended that NEUPOGEN® be given for at least 4 days before the first leukapheresis procedure and continued until the last leukapheresis. Although the optimal duration of NEUPOGEN® administration and leukapheresis schedule have not been established, administration of NEUPOGEN® for 6 to 7 days with leukaphereses on days 5, 6, and 7 was found to be safe and effective (see CLINICAL EXPERIENCE for schedules used in clinical trials). Neutrophil counts should be monitored after 4 days of NEUPOGEN®, and NEUPOGEN® dose modification should be considered for those patients who develop a WBC count > 100,000/mm^3.

In all clinical trials of NEUPOGEN® for the mobilization of PBPC, NEUPOGEN® was also administered after reinfusion of the collected cells (see CLINICAL EXPERIENCE).

Patients With Severe Chronic Neutropenia

NEUPOGEN® should be administered to those patients in whom a diagnosis of congenital, cyclic, or idiopathic neutropenia has been definitively confirmed. Other diseases associated with neutropenia should be ruled out.

Starting Dose:

Congenital Neutropenia: The recommended daily starting dose is 6 mcg/kg BID SC every day.

Idiopathic or Cyclic Neutropenia: The recommended daily starting dose is 5 mcg/kg as a single injection SC every day.

Dose Adjustments:

Chronic daily administration is required to maintain clinical benefit. Absolute neutrophil count should not be used as the sole indication of efficacy. The dose should be individually adjusted based on the patients' clinical course as well as ANC. In the SCN postmarketing surveillance study, the reported median daily doses of NEUPOGEN® were: 6.0 mcg/kg (congenital neutropenia), 2.1 mcg/kg (cyclic neutropenia), and 1.2 mcg/kg (idiopathic neutropenia). In rare instances, patients with congenital neutropenia have required doses of NEUPOGEN® ≥ 100 mcg/kg/day.

Dilution

If required, NEUPOGEN® may be diluted in 5% dextrose. NEUPOGEN® diluted to concentrations between 5 and 15 mcg/mL should be protected from adsorption to plastic materials by the addition of Albumin (Human) to a final concentration of 2 mg/mL. When diluted in 5% dextrose or 5% dextrose plus Albumin (Human), NEUPOGEN® is compatible with glass bottles, PVC and polyolefin IV bags, and polypropylene syringes.

Dilution of NEUPOGEN® to a final concentration of less than 5 mcg/mL is not recommended at any time. **Do not dilute with saline at any time; product may precipitate.**

Storage

NEUPOGEN® should be stored in the refrigerator at 2° to 8°C (36° to 46°F). Avoid shaking. Prior to injection, NEUPOGEN® may be allowed to reach room temperature for a maximum of 24 hours. Any vial or prefilled syringe left at room temperature for greater than 24 hours should be discarded. Parenteral drug products should be inspected visually for particulate matter and discoloration prior to administration, whenever solution and container permit; if particulates or discoloration are observed, the container should not be used.

HOW SUPPLIED

NEUPOGEN®: Use Use only one dose per vial; do not reenter the vial. Discard unused portions. Do not save unused drug for later administration.

Use only one dose per prefilled syringe. Discard unused portions. Do not save unused drug for later administration.

Vials

Single-dose, preservative-free vials containing 300 mcg (1 mL) of Filgrastim (300 mcg/mL). Dispensing packs of 10 (NDC 55513-530-10).

Single-dose, preservative-free vials containing 480 mcg (1.6 mL) of Filgrastim (300 mcg/mL). Dispensing packs of 10 (NDC 55513-546-10).

Prefilled Syringes (SingleJect®)

Single-dose, preservative-free, prefilled syringes with 27 gauge, ½ inch needles with an UltraSafe® Needle Guard, containing 300 mcg (0.5 mL) of Filgrastim (600 mcg/mL). Dispensing packs of 10 (NDC 55513-924-10).

Single-dose, preservative-free, prefilled syringes with 27 gauge, ½ inch needles with an UltraSafe® Needle Guard, containing 480 mcg (0.8 mL) of Filgrastim (600 mcg/mL). Dispensing packs of 10 (NDC 55513-209-10).

NEUPOGEN® should be stored at 2° to 8°C (36° to 46°F). Avoid shaking.

REFERENCES

1. Zsebo KM, Cohen AM, Murdock DC, et al. Recombinant human granulocyte colony-stimulating factor: Molecular and biological characterization. *Immunobiol.* 1986;172:175-184.
2. Welte K, Bonilla MA, Gillio AP, et al. Recombinant human G-CSF: Effects on hematopoiesis in normal and cyclophosphamide treated primates. *J Exp Med.* 1987;165:941-948.
3. Duhrsen U, Villeval JL, Boyd J, et al. Effects of recombinant human granulocyte colony-stimulating factor on hematopoietic progenitor cells in cancer patients. *Blood.* 1988;72:2074-2081.
4. Souza LM, Boone TC, Gabrilove J, et al. Recombinant human granulocyte colony-stimulating factor: Effects on normal and leukemic myeloid cells. *Science.* 1986;232:61-65.
5. Weisbart RH, Kacena A, Schuh A, Golde DW. GM-CSF induces human neutrophil IgA-mediated phagocytosis by an IgA Fc receptor activation mechanism. *Nature.* 1988;332:647-648.
6. Kitagawa S, Yuo A, Souza LM, Saito M, Miura Y, Takaku F. Recombinant human granulocyte colony-stimulating factor enhances superoxide release in human granulocytes stimulated by chemotactic peptide. *Biochem Biophys Res Commun.* 1987;1443:1146.
7. Glaspy JA, Baldwin GC, Robertson PA, et al. Therapy for neutropenia in hairy cell leukemia with recombinant human granulocyte colony-stimulating factor. *Ann Int Med.* 1988;109:789-795.
8. Yuo A, Kitagawa S, Ohsaka A, et al. Recombinant human granulocyte colony-stimulating factor as an activator of human granulocytes: Potentiation of responses triggered by receptor-mediated agonists and stimulation of C3bi receptor expression and adherance. *Blood.* 1989;74:2144-2149.
9. Gabrilove JL, Jakubowski A, Fain K, et al. Phase I study of granulocyte colony-stimulating factor in patients with transitional cell carcinoma of the urothelium. *J Clin Invest.* 1988;82:1454-1461.
10. Morstyn G, Souza L, Keech J, et al. Effect of granulocyte colony-stimulating factor on neutropenia induced by cytotoxic chemotherapy. *Lancet.* 1988;1:667-672.
11. Bronchud MH, Scarffe JH, Thatcher N, et al. Phase I/II study of recombinant human granulocyte colony-stimulating factor in patients receiving intensive chemotherapy for small cell lung cancer. *Br J Cancer.* 1987;56:809-813.
12. Gabrilove JL, Jakubowski A, Scher H, et al. Effect of granulocyte colony-stimulating factor on neutropenia and associated morbidity due to chemotherapy for transitional cell carcinoma of the urothelium. *N Engl J Med.* 1988;318:1414-1422.
13. Neidhart J, Mangalik A, Kohler W, et al. Granulocyte colony-stimulating factor stimulates recovery of granulocytes in patients receiving dose-intensive chemotherapy without bone-marrow transplantation. *J Clin Oncol.* 1989;7:1685-1691.
14. Bronchud MH, Howell A, Crowther D, et al. The use of granulocyte colony-stimulating factor to increase the intensity of treatment with doxorubicin in patients with advanced breast and ovarian cancer. *Br J Cancer.* 1989;60:121-128.
15. Heil G, Hoelzer D, Sanz MA, et al. A randomized, double-blind, placebo-controlled, phase III study of Filgrastim in remission induction and consolidation therapy for adults with de novo Acute Myeloid Leukemia. *Blood.* 1997;90:4710-4718.
16. Dale DC, Bonilla MA, Davis MW, et al. A randomized controlled phase III trial of recombinant human granulocyte colony-stimulating factor (Filgrastim) for treatment of severe chronic neutropenia. *Blood.* 1993;81:2496-2502.
17. Schroeder TM and Kurth R. Spontaneous chromosomal breakage and high incidence of leukemia in inherited disease. *Blood.* 1971;37:96-112.
18. Medlock ES, Kaplan DL, Cecchini M, Ulich TR, del Castillo J, Andresen J. Granulocyte colony-stimulating factor crosses the placenta and stimulates fetal rat granulopoiesis. *Blood.* 1993;81:916-922.
19. Calhoun DA, Rosa C, Christensen RD. Transplacental passage of recombinant human granulocyte colony-stimulating factor in women with an imminent preterm delivery. *Am J Obstet Gynecol.* 1996;174:1306-1311.

This product and its use are covered by the following US Patent Nos.: 4,810,643; 4,999,291; 5,582,823; 5,580,755.

Manufactured by:
Amgen Inc.
One Amgen Center Drive
Thousand Oaks, California 91320-1799

Issue Date: 05/29/02

Shown in Product Identification Guide, page 305

SENSIPAR™ TABLETS ℞

[*sĕn-sĭ-par*]

(cinacalcet HCl)

DESCRIPTION

Sensipar™ (cinacalcet hydrochloride) is a calcimimetic agent that increases the sensitivity of the calcium-sensing receptor to activation by extracellular calcium. Its empirical formula is $C_{22}H_{22}F_3N \cdot HCl$ with a molecular weight of 393.9 g/mol (hydrochloride salt) and 357.4 g/mol (free base). It has one chiral center having an R-absolute configuration. The R-enantiomer is the more potent enantiomer and has been shown to be responsible for pharmacodynamic activity.

Cinacalcet HCl is a white to off-white, crystalline solid that is soluble in methanol or 95% ethanol and slightly soluble in water.

Sensipar™ tablets are formulated as light-green, film-coated, oval-shaped tablets for oral administration in strengths of 30 mg, 60 mg, and 90 mg of cinacalcet HCl as the free base equivalent (33 mg, 66 mg, and 99 mg as the hydrochloride salt, respectively).

Cinacalcet HCl is described chemically as N-[1-(R)-(-)-(1-naphthyl)ethyl]-3-[3-(trifluoromethyl)phenyl]-1-aminopropane hydrochloride and has the following structural formula:

F_3C H N •HCl CH_3

Inactive Ingredients: Sensipar™ tablets are comprised of the active ingredient, and the following inactive ingredients: pre-gelatinized starch, microcrystalline cellulose, povidone, crospovidone, colloidal silicon dioxide, and magnesium stearate. Tablets are coated with color (Opadry® II green) and clear film-coat (Opadry® clear), carnauba wax, and Opacode® black ink.

CLINICAL PHARMACOLOGY

Mechanism of Action

Secondary hyperparathyroidism (HPT) in patients with chronic kidney disease (CKD) is a progressive disease, associated with increases in parathyroid hormone (PTH) levels and derangements in calcium and phosphorus metabolism. Increased PTH stimulates osteoclastic activity resulting in cortical bone resorption and marrow fibrosis. The goals of treatment of secondary hyperparathyroidism are to lower levels of PTH, calcium, and phosphorus in the blood, in order to prevent progressive bone disease and the systemic consequences of disordered mineral metabolism. In CKD patients on dialysis with uncontrolled secondary HPT, reductions in PTH are associated with a favorable impact on bone-specific alkaline phosphatase (BALP), bone turnover and bone fibrosis.

The calcium-sensing receptor on the surface of the chief cell of the parathyroid gland is the principal regulator of PTH secretion. Sensipar™ directly lowers PTH levels by increasing the sensitivity of the calcium-sensing receptor to extracellular calcium. The reduction in PTH is associated with a concomitant decrease in serum calcium levels.

Pharmacokinetics

Absorption and Distribution: After oral administration of cinacalcet, maximum plasma concentration (C_{max}) is achieved in approximately 2 to 6 hours. A food-effect study in healthy volunteers indicated that the C_{max} and area under the curve ($AUC_{(0-inf)}$) were increased 82% and 68%, respectively, when cinacalcet was administered with a high-fat meal compared to fasting. C_{max} and $AUC_{(0-inf)}$ of cinacalcet were increased 65% and 50%, respectively, when cinacalcet was administered with a low-fat meal compared to fasting.

After absorption, cinacalcet concentrations decline in a biphasic fashion with a terminal half-life of 30 to 40 hours. Steady-state drug levels are achieved within 7 days. The mean accumulation ratio is approximately 2 with once-daily oral administration. The median accumulation ratio is approximately 2 to 5 with twice-daily oral administration. The

Continued on next page

Sensipar—Cont.

AUC and C_{max} of cinacalcet increase proportionally over the dose range of 30 to 180 mg once daily. The pharmacokinetic profile of cinacalcet does not change over time with once-daily dosing of 30 to 180 mg. The volume of distribution is high (approximately 1000 L), indicating extensive distribution. Cinacalcet is approximately 93 to 97% bound to plasma protein(s). The ratio of blood cinacalcet concentration to plasma cinacalcet concentration is 0.80 at a blood cinacalcet concentration of 10 ng/mL.

Metabolism and Excretion: Cinacalcet is metabolized by multiple enzymes, primarily CYP3A4, CYP2D6 and CYP1A2. After administration of a 75 mg radiolabeled dose to healthy volunteers, cinacalcet was rapidly and extensively metabolized via: 1) oxidative N-dealkylation to hydrocinnamic acid and hydroxy-hydrocinnamic acid, which are further metabolized via β-oxidation and glycine conjugation; the oxidative N-dealkylation process also generates metabolites that contain the naphthalene ring; and 2) oxidation of the naphthalene ring on the parent drug to form dihydrodiols, which are further conjugated with glucuronic acid. The plasma concentrations of the major circulating metabolites including the cinnamic acid derivatives and glucuronidated dihydrodiols markedly exceed parent drug concentrations. The hydrocinnamic acid metabolite was shown to be inactive at concentrations up to 10 μM in a cell-based assay measuring calcium-receptor activation. The glucuronide conjugates formed after cinacalcet oxidation were shown to have a potency approximately 0.003 times that of cinacalcet in a cell-based assay measuring a calcimimetic response. Renal excretion of metabolites was the primary route of elimination of radioactivity. Approximately 80% of the dose was recovered in the urine and 15% in the feces.

Special Populations

Hepatic Insufficiency: The disposition of a 50 mg cinacalcet single dose was compared in patients with hepatic impairment and subjects with normal hepatic function. Cinacalcet exposure, $AUC_{(0\text{-inf})}$, was comparable between healthy volunteers and patients with mild hepatic impairment. However, in patients with moderate and severe hepatic impairment (as indicated by the Child-Pugh method), cinacalcet exposures as defined by the $AUC_{(0\text{-inf})}$ were 2.4 and 4.2 times higher, respectively, than that in normals. The mean half-life of cinacalcet is prolonged by 33% and 70% in patients with moderate and severe hepatic impairment, respectively. Protein binding of cinacalcet is not affected by impaired hepatic function. See PRECAUTIONS and DOSAGE AND ADMINISTRATION.

Renal Insufficiency: The pharmacokinetic profile of a 75 mg Sensipar™ single dose in patients with mild, moderate, and severe renal insufficiency, and those on hemodialysis or peritoneal dialysis is comparable to that in healthy volunteers.

Geriatric Patients: The pharmacokinetic profile of Sensipar™ in geriatric patients (age ≥ 65, n = 12) is similar to that for patients who are < 65 years of age (n = 268).

Pediatric Patients: The pharmacokinetics of Sensipar™ have not been studied in patients < 18 years of age.

Drug Interactions

An in vitro study indicates that cinacalcet is a strong inhibitor of CYP2D6, but not of CYP1A2, CYP2C9, CYP2C19, and CYP3A4.

Ketoconazole: Cinacalcet $AUC_{(0\text{-inf})}$ and C_{max} increased 2.3 and 2.2 times, respectively, when a single 90 mg cinacalcet dose on Day 5 was administered to subjects treated with 200 mg ketoconazole twice daily for 7 days compared to 90 mg cinacalcet given alone (see DOSAGE AND ADMINISTRATION).

Calcium Carbonate: No significant pharmacokinetic interaction was observed when 1500 mg calcium carbonate was coadministered with 100 mg cinacalcet.

Pantoprazole: No significant pharmacokinetic interaction was observed when cinacalcet 90 mg was administered to subjects treated with 80 mg pantoprazole daily for 3 days.

Sevelamer HCl: No significant pharmacokinetic interaction was observed when 2400 mg sevelamer HCl was coadministered with 90 mg cinacalcet tablet (subjects subsequently received 2400 mg sevelamer HCl two more times on Day 1 and three more times on Day 2).

Amitriptyline: Concurrent administration of 25 mg or 100 mg cinacalcet with 50 mg amitriptyline increased amitriptyline exposure and nortriptyline (active metabolite) exposure by approximately 20% in CYP2D6 extensive metabolizers.

Warfarin: R-and S-warfarin pharmacokinetics and warfarin pharmacodynamics were not affected in subjects treated with warfarin 25 mg who received cinacalcet 30 mg twice daily. The lack of effect of cinacalcet on the pharmacokinetics of R- and S-warfarin and the absence of auto-induction upon multiple dosing in patients indicates that cinacalcet is not an inducer of CYP2C9 in humans.

Pharmacodynamics

Reduction in intact PTH (iPTH) levels correlated with cinacalcet concentrations in CKD patients. The nadir in iPTH level occurs approximately 2 to 6 hours post dose, corresponding with the C_{max} of cinacalcet. After steady state is reached, serum calcium concentrations remain constant over the dosing interval in CKD patients.

CLINICAL STUDIES

Secondary Hyperparathyroidism in Patients with Chronic Kidney Disease on Dialysis

Three 6-month, multicenter, randomized, double-blind, placebo-controlled clinical studies of similar design were conducted in CKD patients on dialysis. A total of 665 patients were randomized to Sensipar™ and 471 patients to placebo. The mean age of the patients was 54 years, 62% were male, and 52% Caucasian. The average baseline iPTH level by the Nichols intact immunoradiometric assay (IRMA) was 712 pg/mL, with 26% of the patients having a baseline iPTH level > 800 pg/mL. The mean baseline Ca x P ion product was 61 mg^2/dL^2. The average duration of dialysis prior to study enrollment was 67 months. Ninety-six percent of patients were on hemodialysis and 4% peritoneal dialysis. At study entry, 66% of the patients were receiving vitamin D sterols and 93% were receiving phosphate binders. Sensipar™ (or placebo) was initiated at a dose of 30 mg once daily and titrated every 3 or 4 weeks to a maximum dose of 180 mg once daily to achieve an iPTH of ≤ 250 pg/mL. The dose was not increased if a patient had any of the following: iPTH ≤ 200 pg/mL, serum calcium < 7.8 mg/dL, or any symptoms of hypocalcemia. If a patient experienced symptoms of hypocalcemia or had a serum calcium < 8.4 mg/dL, calcium supplements and/or calcium-based phosphate binders could be increased. If these measures were insufficient, the vitamin D dose could be increased. Approximately 70% of the Sensipar™ patients and 80% of the placebo patients completed the 6-month studies. In the primary efficacy analysis, 40% of Sensipar™ patients and 5% of placebo patients achieved an iPTH ≤ 250 pg/mL (p<0.001) (Table 1, Figure 1). Secondary efficacy parameters also improved in patients treated with Sensipar™. These studies showed that Sensipar™ reduced PTH while lowering Ca x P, calcium and phosphorus levels (Table 1, Figure 2). The median dose of Sensipar™ at the completion of the studies was 90 mg. Patients with milder disease typically required lower doses.

[See table 1 below]

Figure 1. Mean (SE) iPTH Values (Pooled Phase 3 Studies)

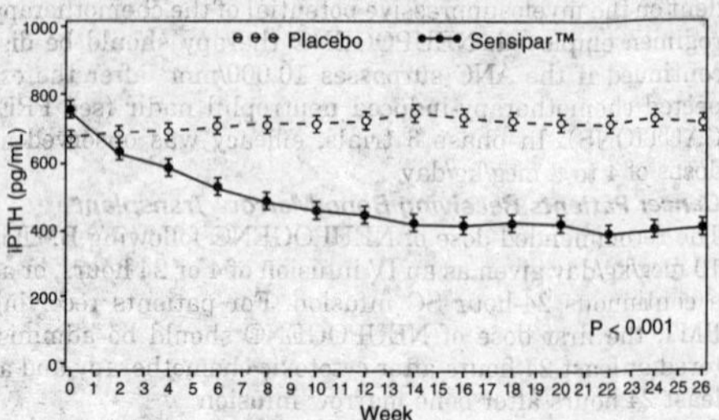

Data are presented for patients who completed the studies; Placebo (N = 342), Sensipar™ (N = 439).

Figure 2. Mean (SE) Ca x P Values (Pooled Phase 3 Studies)

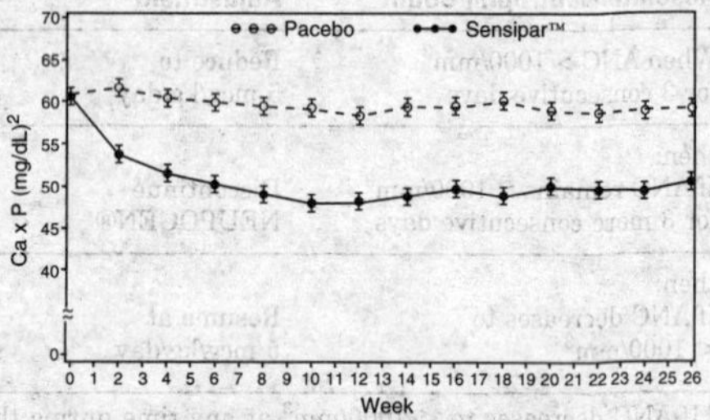

Data are presented for patients who completed the studies; Placebo (N = 342), Sensipar™ (N = 439).

Reductions in iPTH and Ca x P were maintained for up to 12 months of treatment.

Sensipar™ decreased iPTH and Ca x P levels regardless of disease severity (i.e., baseline iPTH value), duration of dialysis, and whether or not vitamin D sterols were administered. Approximately 60% of patients with mild (iPTH ≥ 300 to ≤ 500 pg/mL), 41% with moderate (iPTH > 500 to 800 pg/mL), and 11% with severe (iPTH > 800 pg/mL) secondary HPT achieved a mean iPTH value of 250 pg/mL. Plasma iPTH levels were measured using the Nichols IRMA.

In CKD patients with secondary HPT not on dialysis, the long-term safety and efficacy of Sensipar™ have not been established. Exploratory investigation indicates that CKD patients not on dialysis have an increased risk for hypocalcemia compared to CKD patients on dialysis, which may be due to lower baseline calcium levels. In a small, short-term study, in which the median dose of cinacalcet was 30 mg at the completion of the study, 74% of cinacalcet-treated patients experienced at least one serum calcium value < 8.4 mg/dL (see PRECAUTIONS Hypocalcemia).

Parathyroid Carcinoma

Ten patients with parathyroid carcinoma were enrolled in an open-label study. The study consisted of 2 phases, a dose-titration phase and a maintenance phase.

The range of exposure was 2 to 16 weeks in the titration phase (n = 10) and 16 to 48 weeks (n = 3) for the maintenance phase. Baseline mean (SD) serum calcium was 14.7 (1.8) mg/dL. The range of change from baseline to last measurement was −7.5 to 2.7 mg/dL during the titration phase and −7.4 to 0.9 mg/dL during the maintenance phase (Figure 3). No patients maintained a serum calcium level within the normal range. The doses ranged from 70 mg twice daily to 90 mg four times daily for patients in the maintenance phase.

Figure 3. Serum Calcium Values in Parathyroid Carcinoma Patients Receiving Sensipar™ at Baseline, Titration and Maintenance Phase

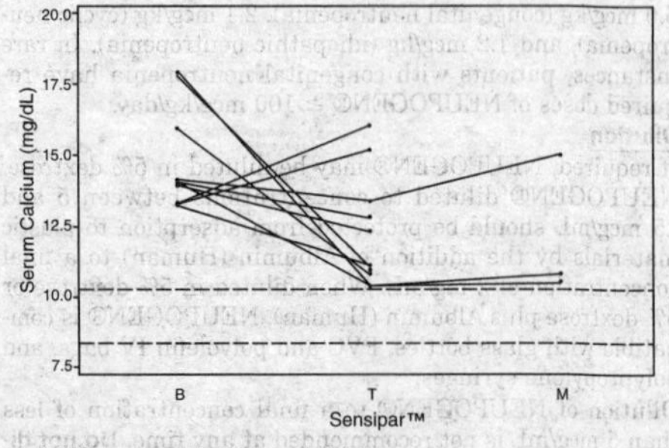

Solid lines represent individual patient data
B = baseline; T = last value in titration phase; M = last value in maintenance phase
Reference lines (dashed) show the normal range for serum calcium values

INDICATIONS AND USAGE

Sensipar™ is indicated for the treatment of secondary hyperparathyroidism in patients with Chronic Kidney Disease on dialysis.

Table 1. Effects of Sensipar™ on iPTH, Ca x P, Serum Calcium, and Serum Phosphorus in 6-month Phase 3 Studies (Patients on Dialysis)

	Study 1		Study 2		Study 3	
	Placebo (N = 205)	Sensipar™ (N = 205)	Placebo (N = 165)	Sensipar™ (N = 166)	Placebo (N = 101)	Sensipar™ (N = 294)
iPTH						
Baseline (pg/mL: Median	535	537	556	547	670	703
Median (SD)	651 (398)	636 (341)	630 (317)	652 (372)	832 (486)	848 (685)
Evaluation Phase (pg/mL)	563	275	592	238	737	339
Median Percent Change	+3.8	-48.3	+8.4	-54.1	+2.3	-48.2
Patients Achieving Primary Endpoint (iPTH) ≤ 250 pg/mL) (%)[a]	4%	41%**	7%	46%**	6%	35%**
Patients Achieving ≥ 30% Reduction in iPTH (%)[a]	11%	61%	12%	68%	10%	59%
Patients Achieving iPTH ≤ 250 pg/mL and Ca x P < 55 mg^2/dL^2(%)	1%	32%	5%	35%	5%	28%
Ca x P						
Baseline (mg^2/dL^2)	62	61	61	61	61	59
Evaluation Phase (mg^2/dL^2)	59	52	59	47	57	48
Median Percent Change	-2.0	-14.9	-3.1	-19.7	-4.8	-15.7
Calcium						
Baseline (mg/dL)	9.8	9.8	9.9	10.0	9.9	9.8
Evaluation Phase (mg/dL)	9.9	9.1	9.9	9.1	10.0	9.1
Median Percent Change	+0.5	-5.5	+0.1	-7.4	+0.3	-6.0
Phosphorus						
Baseline (mg/dL)	6.3	6.1	6.1	6.0	6.1	6.0
Evaluation Phase (mg/dL)	6.0	5.6	5.9	5.1	5.6	5.3
Median Percent Change	-1.0	-9.0	-2.4	-12.4	-5.6	-8.6

** p < 0.001 compared to placebo; p-values presented for primary endpoint only

[a] iPTH value based on averaging over the evaluation phase (defined as weeks 13 to 26 in studies 1 and 2 and weeks 17 to 26 in study 3)

Values shown are medians unless indicated otherwise

Sensipar™ is indicated for the treatment of hypercalcemia in patients with parathyroid carcinoma.

CONTRAINDICATIONS

Sensipar™ is contraindicated in patients with hypersensitivity to any component(s) of this product.

WARNINGS

Seizures

In three clinical studies of CKD patients on dialysis, 5% of the patients in both the Sensipar™ and placebo groups reported a history of seizure disorder at baseline. During the trials, seizures (primarily generalized or tonic-clonic) were observed in 1.4% (9/656) of Sensipar™-treated patients and 0.4% (2/470) of placebo-treated patients. Five of the nine Sensipar™-treated patients had a history of a seizure disorder and two were receiving anti-seizure medication at the time of their seizure. Both placebo-treated patients had a history of seizure disorder and were receiving anti-seizure medication at the time of their seizure. While the basis for the reported difference in seizure rate is not clear, the threshold for seizures is lowered by significant reductions in serum calcium levels. Therefore, serum calcium levels should be closely monitored in patients receiving Sensipar™, particularly in patients with a history of a seizure disorder (see PRECAUTIONS, Hypocalcemia).

PRECAUTIONS

General

Hypocalcemia

Sensipar™ lowers serum calcium, and therefore patients should be carefully monitored for the occurrence of hypocalcemia. Potential manifestations of hypocalcemia include paresthesias, myalgias, cramping, tetany, and convulsions.
Sensipar™ treatment should not be initiated if serum calcium is less than the lower limit of the normal range (8.4 mg/dL). Serum calcium should be measured within 1 week after initiation or dose adjustment of Sensipar™. Once the maintenance dose has been established, serum calcium should be measured approximately monthly (see DOSAGE AND ADMINISTRATION).

If serum calcium falls below 8.4 mg/dL but remains above 7.5 mg/dL, or if symptoms of hypocalcemia occur, calcium-containing phosphate binders and/or vitamin D sterols can be used to raise serum calcium. If serum calcium falls below 7.5 mg/dL, or if symptoms of hypocalcemia persist and the dose of vitamin D cannot be increased, withhold administration of Sensipar™ until serum calcium levels reach 8.0 mg/dL, and/or symptoms of hypocalcemia have resolved. Treatment should be re-initiated using the next lowest dose of Sensipar™ (see DOSAGE AND ADMINISTRATION).

In the 26-week studies of patients with CKD on dialysis, 66% of patients receiving Sensipar™ compared with 25% of patients receiving placebo developed at least one serum calcium value < 8.4 mg/dL. Less than 1% of patients in each group permanently discontinued study drug due to hypocalcemia.

In CKD patients with secondary HPT not on dialysis, the long-term safety and efficacy of Sensipar™ have not been established. Exploratory investigation indicates that CKD patients not on dialysis have an increased risk for hypocalcemia compared to CKD patients on dialysis, which may be due to lower baseline calcium levels. In a small, short-term study, in which the median dose of cinacalcet was 30 mg at the completion of the study, 74% of cinacalcet-treated patients experienced at least one serum calcium value < 8.4 mg/dL.

Adynamic Bone Disease

Adynamic bone disease may develop if iPTH levels are suppressed below 100 pg/mL when assessed using the standard Nichols IRMA. One clinical study evaluated bone histomorphometry in patients treated with Sensipar™ for one year. Three patients with mild hyperparathyroid bone disease at the beginning of the study developed adynamic bone disease during treatment with Sensipar™. Two of these patients had iPTH levels below 100 pg/mL at multiple time points during the study. In the three 6-month, phase 3 studies conducted in CKD patients on dialysis, 11% of patients treated with Sensipar™ had mean iPTH values below 100 pg/mL during the efficacy-assessment phase. If iPTH levels decrease below the NKF-K/DOQI recommended target range (150-300 pg/mL)[1] in patients treated with Sensipar™, the dose of Sensipar™ and/or vitamin D sterols should be reduced or therapy discontinued.

Hepatic Insufficiency

Cinacalcet exposure as assessed by $AUC_{(0\text{-inf})}$ in patients with moderate and severe hepatic impairment (as indicated by the Child-Pugh method) were 2.4 and 4.2 times higher, respectively, than that in normals. Patients with moderate and severe hepatic impairment should be monitored throughout treatment with Sensipar™ (see CLINICAL PHARMACOLOGY, Pharmacokinetics and DOSAGE AND ADMINISTRATION).

Information for Patients

It is recommended that Sensipar™ be taken with food or shortly after a meal. Tablets should be taken whole and should not be divided.

Laboratory Tests

Patients with CKD on Dialysis with Secondary Hyperparathyroidism

Serum calcium and serum phosphorus should be measured within 1 week and iPTH should be measured 1 to 4 weeks after initiation or dose adjustment of Sensipar™. Once the maintenance dose has been established, serum calcium and serum phosphorus should be measured approximately monthly, and PTH every 1 to 3 months (see DOSAGE AND ADMINISTRATION). All iPTH measurements during the Sensipar™ trials were obtained using the Nichols IRMA.

In patients with end-stage renal disease, testosterone levels are often below the normal range. In a placebo-controlled trial in patients with CKD on dialysis, there were reductions in total and free testosterone in male patients following six months of treatment with Sensipar™. Levels of total testosterone decreased by a median of 15.8% in the Sensipar™-treated patients and by 0.6% in the placebo-treated patients. Levels of free testosterone decreased by a median of 31.3% in the Sensipar™-treated patients and by 16.3% in the placebo-treated patients. The clinical significance of these reductions in serum testosterone is unknown.

Patients with Parathyroid Carcinoma

Serum calcium should be measured within 1 week after initiation or dose adjustment of Sensipar™. Once maintenance dose levels have been established, serum calcium should be measured every 2 months (see DOSAGE AND ADMINISTRATION).

Drug Interactions and/or Drug/Laboratory Test Interactions

See CLINICAL PHARMACOLOGY, Pharmacokinetics and Drug Interactions.

Effect of Sensipar™ on other drugs:

Drugs metabolized by cytochrome P450 2D6 (CYP2D6): Sensipar™ is a strong in vitro inhibitor of CYP2D6. Therefore, dose adjustments of concomitant medications that are predominantly metabolized by CYP2D6 and have a narrow therapeutic index (e.g., flecainide, vinblastine, thioridazine and most tricyclic antidepressants) may be required.

Amitriptyline: Concurrent administration of 25 mg or 100 mg cinacalcet with 50 mg amitriptyline increased amitriptyline exposure and nortriptyline (active metabolite) exposure by approximately 20% in CYP2D6 extensive metabolizers.

Effect of other drugs on Sensipar™:

Sensipar™ is metabolized by multiple cytochrome P450 enzymes, primarily CYP3A4, CYP2D6, and CYP1A2.

Ketoconazole: Sensipar™ is metabolized in part by CYP3A4. Co-administration of ketoconazole, a strong inhibitor of CYP3A4, increased cinacalcet exposure following a single 90 mg dose of Sensipar™ by 2.3 fold. Dose adjustment of Sensipar™ may be required and PTH and serum calcium concentrations should be closely monitored if a patient initiates or discontinues therapy with a strong CYP3A4 inhibitor (e.g., ketoconazole, erythromycin, itraconazole; see DOSAGE AND ADMINISTRATION).

Carcinogenesis, Mutagenesis, and Impairment of Fertility

Carcinogenicity: Standard lifetime dietary carcinogenicity bioassays were conducted in mice and rats. Mice were given dietary doses of 15, 50, 125 mg/kg/day in males and 30, 70, 200 mg/kg/day in females (exposures up to 2 times those resulting with a human oral dose of 180 mg/day based on AUC comparison). Rats were given dietary doses of 5, 15, 35 mg/kg/day in males and 5, 20, 35 mg/kg/day in females (exposures up to 2 times those resulting with a human oral dose of 180 mg/day based on AUC comparison). No increased incidence of tumors was observed following treatment with cinacalcet.

Mutagenicity: Cinacalcet was not genotoxic in the Ames bacterial mutagenicity assay or in the Chinese Hamster Ovary (CHO) cell HGPRT forward mutation assay and CHO cell chromosomal aberration assay, with and without metabolic activation or in the in vivo mouse micronucleus assay.

Impairment of fertility: Female rats were given oral gavage doses of 5, 25, 75 mg/kg/day beginning 2 weeks before mating and continuing through gestation day 7. Male rats were given oral doses 4 weeks prior to mating, during mating (3 weeks) and 2 weeks post-mating. No effects were observed in male or female fertility at 5 and 25 mg/kg/day (exposures up to 3 times those resulting with a human oral dose of 180 mg/day based on AUC comparison). At 75 mg/kg/day, there were slight adverse effects (slight decreases in body weight and food consumption) in males and females.

Pregnancy Category C

In pregnant female rats given oral gavage doses of 2, 25, 50 mg/kg/day during gestation no teratogenicity was observed at doses up to 50 mg/kg/day (exposure 4 times those resulting with a human oral dose of 180 mg/day based on AUC comparison). Decreased fetal body weights were observed at all doses (less than 1 to 4 times a human oral dose of 180 mg/day based on AUC comparison) in conjunction with maternal toxicity (decreased food consumption and body weight gain).

In pregnant female rabbits given oral gavage doses of 2, 12, 25 mg/kg/day during gestation no adverse fetal effects were observed (exposures less than with a human oral dose of 180 mg/day based on AUC comparisons). Reductions in maternal food consumption and body weight gain were seen at doses of 12 and 25 mg/kg/day.

In pregnant rats given oral gavage doses of 5, 15, 25 mg/kg/day during gestation through lactation no adverse fetal or pup (post-weaning) effects were observed at 5 mg/kg/day (exposures less than with a human therapeutic dose of 180 mg/day based on AUC comparisons). Higher doses of 15 and 25 mg/kg/day (exposures 2-3 times a human oral dose of 180 mg/day based on AUC comparisons) were accompanied by maternal signs of hypocalcemia (periparturient mortality and early postnatal pup loss), and reductions in postnatal maternal and pup body-weight gain. Sensipar™ has been shown to cross the placental barrier in rabbits.

There are no adequate and well-controlled studies in pregnant women. Sensipar™ should be used during pregnancy only if the potential benefit justifies the potential risk to the fetus.

Lactating Women

Studies in rats have shown that Sensipar™ is excreted in the milk with a high milk-to-plasma ratio. It is not known whether this drug is excreted in human milk. Considering these data in rats and because many drugs are excreted in human milk and because of the potential for clinically significant adverse reactions in infants from Sensipar™, a decision should be made whether to discontinue nursing or to discontinue the drug, taking into account the importance of the drug to the lactating woman.

Pediatric Use

The safety and efficacy of Sensipar™ in pediatric patients have not been established.

Geriatric Use

Of the 1136 patients enrolled in the Sensipar™ phase 3 clinical program, 26% were ≥ 65 years old, and 9% were ≥ 75 years old. No differences in the safety and efficacy of Sensipar™ were observed in patients greater or less than 65 years of age (see DOSAGE AND ADMINISTRATION, Geriatric Patients).

ADVERSE EVENTS

Secondary Hyperparathyroidism in Patients with Chronic Kidney Disease on Dialysis

In 3 double-blind placebo-controlled clinical trials, 1126 CKD patients on dialysis received study drug (656 Sensipar™, 470 placebo) for up to 6 months. The most frequently reported adverse events (incidence of at least 5% in the Sensipar™ group and greater than placebo) are provided in Table 2. The most frequently reported events in the Sensipar™ group were nausea and vomiting.

Table 2. Adverse Event Incidence (≥ 5%) in Patients on Dialysis

Event*:	Placebo (n = 470) (%)	Sensipar™ (n = 656) (%)
Nausea	19	31
Vomiting	15	27
Diarrhea	20	21
Myalgia	14	15
Dizziness	8	10
Hypertension	5	7
Asthenia	4	7
Anorexia	4	6
Pain Chest, Non-Cardiac	4	6
Access Infection	4	5

* Included are events that were reported at a greater incidence in the Sensipar™ group than in the placebo group.

The incidence of serious adverse events (29% vs. 31%) was similar in the Sensipar™ and placebo groups, respectively.

12-Month Experience with Sensipar™: Two hundred and sixty-six patients from 2 phase 3 studies continued to receive Sensipar™ or placebo treatment in a 6-month double-blind extension study (12-month total treatment duration). The incidence and nature of adverse events in this study were similar in the two treatment groups, and comparable to those observed in the phase 3 studies.

Parathyroid Carcinoma

The most frequent adverse events in this patient group were nausea and vomiting.

Laboratory values: Serum calcium levels should be closely monitored in patients receiving Sensipar™ (see PRECAUTIONS and DOSAGE AND ADMINISTRATION).

OVERDOSAGE

Doses titrated up to 300 mg once daily have been safely administered to patients on dialysis. Overdosage of Sensipar™ may lead to hypocalcemia. In the event of overdosage, patients should be monitored for signs and symptoms of hypocalcemia and appropriate measures taken to correct serum calcium levels (see PRECAUTIONS).

Since Sensipar™ is highly protein bound, hemodialysis is not an effective treatment for overdosage of Sensipar™.

DOSAGE AND ADMINISTRATION

Sensipar™ tablets should be taken whole and should not be divided. Sensipar™ should be taken with food or shortly after a meal.

Dosage must be individualized.

Secondary Hyperparathyroidism in Patients with Chronic Kidney Disease on Dialysis

The recommended starting oral dose of Sensipar™ is 30 mg once daily. Serum calcium and serum phosphorus should be measured within 1 week and iPTH should be measured 1 to 4 weeks after initiation or dose adjustment of Sensipar™. Sensipar™ should be titrated no more frequently than every 2 to 4 weeks through sequential doses of 60, 90, 120, and 180 mg once daily to target iPTH consistent with the NKF-K/DOQI recommendation for CKD patients on dialysis of 150-300 pg/mL.

Sensipar™ can be used alone or in combination with vitamin D sterols and/or phosphate binders.

During dose titration, serum calcium levels should be monitored frequently and if levels decrease below the normal range, appropriate steps should be taken to increase serum calcium levels, such as by providing supplemental calcium, initiating or increasing the dose of calcium-based phosphate

Continued on next page

Sensipar—Cont.

binder, initiating or increasing the dose of vitamin D sterols, or temporarily withholding treatment with Sensipar™ (see PRECAUTIONS).

Parathyroid Carcinoma

The recommended starting oral dose of Sensipar™ is 30 mg twice daily.

The dosage of Sensipar™ should be titrated every 2 to 4 weeks through sequential doses of 30 mg twice daily, 60 mg twice daily, 90 mg twice daily, and 90 mg three or four times daily as necessary to normalize serum calcium levels.

Special Populations

Geriatric patients: Age does not alter the pharmacokinetics of Sensipar™; no dosage adjustment is required for geriatric patients.

Patients with renal impairment: Renal impairment does not alter the pharmacokinetics of Sensipar™; no dosage adjustment is necessary for renal impairment.

Patients with hepatic impairment: Cinacalcet exposures, as assessed by $AUC_{(0\text{-}inf)}$, in patients with moderate and severe hepatic impairment (as indicated by the Child-Pugh method) were 2.4 and 4.2 times higher, respectively, than in normals. In patients with moderate and severe hepatic impairment, PTH and serum calcium concentrations should be closely monitored throughout treatment with Sensipar™ (see CLINICAL PHARMACOLOGY, Pharmacokinetics and PRECAUTIONS).

Drug Interactions

Sensipar™ is metabolized in part by the enzyme CYP3A4. Co-administration of ketoconazole, a strong inhibitor of CYP3A4, caused an approximate 2-fold increase in cinacalcet exposure. Dose adjustment of Sensipar™ may be required and PTH and serum calcium concentrations should be closely monitored if a patient initiates or discontinues therapy with a strong CYP3A4 inhibitor (e.g., ketoconazole, erythromycin, itraconazole; see CLINICAL PHARMACOLOGY, Pharmacokinetics and PRECAUTIONS).

HOW SUPPLIED

Sensipar™ 30 mg tablets are formulated as light-green, film-coated, oval-shaped tablets printed with "AMGEN" on one side and "30" on the opposite side, packaged in bottles of 30 tablets. (NDC 55513-073-30)

Sensipar™ 60 mg tablets are formulated as light-green, film-coated, oval-shaped tablets printed with "AMGEN" on one side and "60" on the opposite side, packaged in bottles of 30 tablets. (NDC 55513-074-30)

Sensipar™ 90 mg tablets are formulated as light-green, film-coated, oval-shaped tablets printed with "AMGEN" on one side and "90" on the opposite side, packaged in bottles of 30 tablets. (NDC 55513-075-30)

Storage

Store at 25°C (77°F); excursions permitted to 15-30°C (59-86°F). [See USP controlled room temperature].

Rx Only

This product, or its use, may be covered by one or more US Patents including US Patent Nos. 6313146, 6211244, 6031003 and 6011068, in addition to others, including patents pending.

REFERENCES

1. National Kidney Foundation: K/DOQI clinical practice guidelines: bone metabolism and disease in chronic kidney disease. American Journal of Kidney Disease 4 2:S1-S201, 2003

AMGEN®

Manufactured for: Amgen
Amgen Inc.
One Amgen Center Drive
Thousand Oaks, CA 91320-1799

Issue Date 03/08/2004

3289800-v1

Shown in Product Identification Guide, page 305

Andrx Laboratories, Inc.

411 HACKENSACK AVENUE, 3RD FLOOR
HACKENSACK, NJ 07601

Direct Inquiries to:
phone (800) 595-1883

ALTOPREV™ EXTENDED-RELEASE TABLETS ℞
(Lovastatin)

DESCRIPTION

ALTOPREV™ (Lovastatin) Extended-Release Tablets contain a cholesterol-lowering agent isolated from a strain of *Aspergillus terreus*. After oral ingestion, lovastatin, which is an inactive lactone, is hydrolyzed to the corresponding β-hydroxyacid form. This is a principal metabolite and inhibitor of 3-hydroxy-3-methylglutaryl-coenzyme A (HMG-CoA) reductase. This enzyme catalyzes the conversion of HMG-CoA to mevalonate, which is an early and rate limiting step in the biosynthesis of cholesterol.

Table I
ALTOPREV™ vs Lovastatin Immediate-Release (IR)
(Steady-State Pharmacokinetic Parameters at Day 28)

Drug	C_{max} (ng/mL)				C_{min}(ng/mL)				T_{max} (h)		AUC_{0-24hr} (ng•hr/mL)			
	L	LA	TI	AI	L	LA	TI	AI	L	LA	L	LA	TI	AI
ALTOPREV™ 40 mg*	5.5	5.8	17.3	13.4	2.6	3.1	9.1	4.3	14.2	11.8	77	87	263	171
Lovastatin IR 40 mg**	7.8	11.9	36.2	26.6	0.4	0.7	2.4	2.1	3.3	5.3	45	83	252	186

L=lovastatin, LA=lovastatin acid, TI=total inhibitors of HMG-CoA reductase, AI-active inhibitors of HMG-CoA reductase, C_{max}=highest observed plasma concentration, C_{min}=trough concentration at t=24 hours after dosing, T_{max}=time at which the C_{max} occurred, AUC_{0-24hr}-area under the plasma concentration-time curve from time 0 to 24 hr after dosing, calculated by the linear trapezoidal rule.
* Administered at bedtime
** Administered with the evening meal.

Lovastatin is [1 *S* -[1α(*R**),3α,7β,8β(2 *S**,4 *S**),8aβ]]-1,2,3,7,8,8a-hexahydro-3,7-dimethyl-8-[2-(tetrahydro-4-hydroxy-6-oxo-2 *H*-pyran-2-yl)ethyl]-1-naphthalenyl 2-methylbutanoate. The empirical formula of lovastatin is $C_{24}H_{36}O_5$ and its molecular weight is 404.55. Its structural formula is:

Lovastatin is a white, nonhygroscopic crystalline powder that is insoluble in water and sparingly soluble in ethanol, methanol, and acetonitrile.

ALTOPREV™ Extended-Release Tablets are designed for once-a-day oral administration and deliver 10 mg, 20 mg, 40 mg, or 60 mg of lovastatin. In addition to the active ingredient lovastatin, each tablet contains the following inactive ingredients: acetyltributyl citrate; butylated hydroxyanisole; candelilla wax; cellulose acetate; confectioner's sugar (contains corn starch); F D & C yellow # 6; glyceryl monostearate; hypromellose; hypromellose phthalate; lactose; methacrylic acid copolymer, type B; polyethylene glycols (PEG 400, PEG 8000); polyethylene oxides; polysorbate 80; propylene glycol; silicon dioxide; sodium chloride; sodium lauryl sulfate; synthetic black iron oxide; red iron oxide; talc; titanium dioxide and triacetin.

CLINICAL PHARMACOLOGY

Mechanism of Action

Lovastatin is a lactone that is readily hydrolyzed *in vivo* to the corresponding β-hydroxyacid, a potent inhibitor of HMG-CoA reductase, the enzyme that catalyzes the conversion of HMG-CoA to mevalonate. The conversion of HMG-CoA to mevalonate is an early step in the biosynthetic pathway for cholesterol

The involvement of low-density lipoprotein cholesterol (LDL-C) in atherogenesis has been well documented in clinical and pathological studies, as well as in many animal experiments. Epidemiological and clinical studies have established that high LDL-C and low high-density lipoprotein cholesterol (HDL-C) levels are both associated with coronary heart disease. However, the risk of developing coronary heart disease is continuous and graded over the range of cholesterol levels and many coronary events do occur in patients with total cholesterol (Total-C) and LDL-C levels in the lower end of this range.

ALTOPREV™ has been shown to reduce LDL-C, and Total-C. Across all doses studied, treatment with ALTOPREV™ has been shown to result in variable reductions in triglycerides (TG), and variable increases in HDL-C (see Table III under *Clinical Studies*).

Lovastatin immediate-release tablets have been shown to reduce both normal and elevated LDL-C concentrations. LDL is formed from very low-density lipoprotein (VLDL) and is catabolized predominantly by the high-affinity LDL receptor. The mechanism of the LDL-lowering effect of lovastatin immediate-release may involve both reduction of VLDL-C concentration, and induction of the LDL receptor, leading to reduced production and/or increased catabolism of LDL-C. Apolipoprotein B (Apo B) also falls substantially during treatment with lovastatin immediate-release. Since each LDL particle contains one molecule of Apo B, and since little Apo B is found in other lipoproteins, this strongly suggests that lovastatin immediate-release does not merely cause cholesterol to be lost from LDL, but also reduces the concentration of circulating LDL particles. In addition, lovastatin immediate-release can produce increases of variable magnitude in HDL-C, and modestly reduces VLDL-C and plasma TG (see Table IV under *Clinical Studies*). The independent effect of raising HDL or lowering TG on the risk of coronary and cardiovascular morbidity and mortality has not been determined. The effects of lovastatin immediate-release on lipoprotein (a) [Lp(a)], fibrinogen, and certain other independent biochemical risk markers for coronary heart disease are unknown.

Lovastatin, as well as some of its metabolites, are pharmacologically active in humans. The liver is the primary site of action and the principal site of cholesterol synthesis and LDL clearance (see DOSAGE AND ADMINISTRATION).

Pharmacokinetics and Drug Metabolism

Absorption

ALTOPREV™

The appearance of lovastatin in plasma from an ALTOPREV™ Extended-Release Tablet is slower and more prolonged compared to the lovastatin immediate-release formulation.

A pharmacokinetic study carried out with ALTOPREV™ involved measurement of the systemic concentrations of lovastatin (pro-drug), lovastatin acid (active-drug) and total and active inhibitors of HMG-CoA reductase. The pharmacokinetic parameters in 12 hypercholesterolemic subjects at steady state, after 28 days of treatment, comparing ALTOPREV™ 40 mg to lovastatin immediate-release 40 mg, are summarized in Table I.

[See table I above]

The mean plasma concentration-time profiles of lovastatin and lovastatin acid in patients after multiple doses of ALTOPREV™ or lovastatin immediate-release at day 28 are shown in Figure 1.

Figure 1
Mean (SD) plasma concentration-time profiles of lovastatin and lovastatin acid in hypercholesterolemic patients (n=12) after 28 days of administration of ALTOPREV™ or lovastatin immediate release.

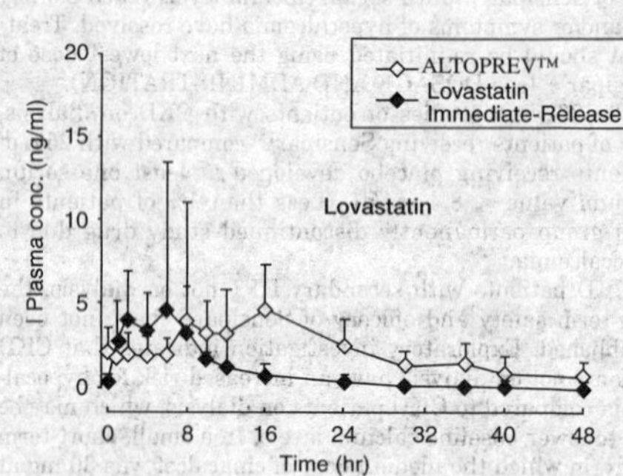

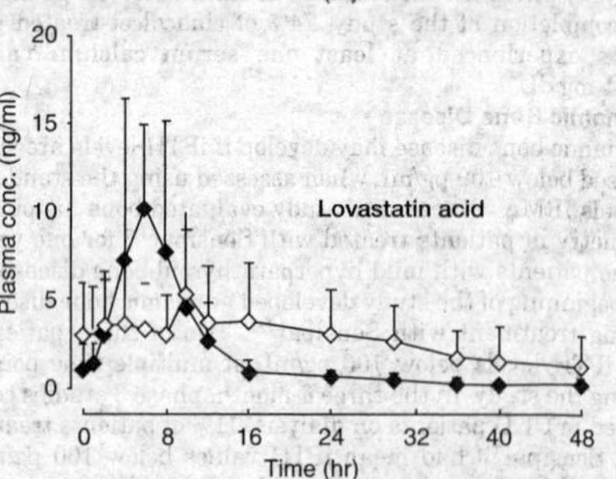

The extended-release properties of ALTOPREV™ are characterized by a prolonged absorptive phase, which results in a longer T_{max} and lower C_{max} for lovastatin (prodrug) and its major metabolite, lovastatin acid, compared to lovastatin immediate-release.

The bioavailability of lovastatin (pro-drug) as measured by the AUC_{0-24hr} was greater for ALTOPREV™ compared to lovastatin immediate-release (as measured by a chemical assay), while the bioavailability of total and active inhibitors of HMG-CoA reductase were equivalent to lovastatin immediate-release (as measured by an enzymatic assay).

With once-a-day dosing, mean values of AUCs of active and total inhibitors at steady state were about 1.8–1.9 times those following a single dose. Accumulation ratio of lovastatin exposure was 1.5 after multiple daily doses of ALTOPREV™ compared to that of a single dose measured using a chemical assay.

ALTOPREV™ appears to have dose linearity for doses from 10 mg up to 60 mg per day.

When ALTOPREV™ was given after a meal, plasma concentrations of lovastatin and lovastatin acid were about 0.5–0.6 times those found when ALTOPREV™ was administered in the fasting state, indicating that food decreases the bioavailability of ALTOPREV™. There was an association between the bioavailability of ALTOPREV™ and dosing after mealtimes. Bioavailability was lowered under the following conditions, (from higher bioavailability to lower bioavailability) in the following order: under overnight fasting conditions, before bedtime, with dinner, and with a high fat breakfast. In a multicenter, randomized, parallel group study, patients were administered 40 mg of ALTOPREV™ at three different times; before breakfast, after dinner and at bedtime. Although there was no statistical difference in the extent of lipid change between the three groups, there was a numerically greater reduction in LDL-C and TG and an increase in HDL-C when ALTOPREV™ was administered at bedtime. Results of this study are displayed in Table II.

Table II
ALTOPREV™ 40 mg
(Least Squares Mean Percent Changes from Baseline to Endpoint at 4 weeks of treatment*)

	LDL-C	HDL-C	TOTAL-C	TG
Before Breakfast	−32.0%	8.4%	−22.2%	−10.2%
After Dinner	−34.1%	7.4%	−23.6%	−11.2%
Before Bedtime	−36.9%	11.1%	−25.5%	−19.7%

N=22 for the Before Breakfast group, N=23 for the After Dinner group, and N=23 for the Before Bedtime group.

* All changes from baseline are statistically significant.

At steady state in humans, the bioavailability of lovastatin, following the administration of ALTOPREV™, was 190% compared to lovastatin immediate-release.

Lovastatin Immediate-Release

Absorption of lovastatin, estimated relative to an intravenous reference dose in each of four animal species tested, averaged about 30% of an oral dose. Following an oral dose of ^{14}C-labeled lovastatin in man, 10% of the dose was excreted in urine and 83% in feces. The latter represents absorbed drug equivalents excreted in bile, as well as any unabsorbed drug. In a single dose study in four hypercholesterolemic patients, it was estimated that less than 5% of an oral dose of lovastatin reaches the general circulation as active inhibitors.

Distribution

Lovastatin

Both lovastatin and its β-hydroxyacid metabolite are highly bound (>95%) to human plasma proteins. Animal studies demonstrated that lovastatin crosses the blood-brain and placental barriers.

In animal studies, after oral dosing, lovastatin had high selectivity for the liver, where it achieved substantially higher concentrations than in non-target tissues.

Lovastatin undergoes extensive first-pass extraction in the liver, its primary site of action, with subsequent excretion of drug equivalents in the bile. As a consequence of extensive hepatic extraction of lovastatin, the availability of drug to the general circulation is low and variable.

Metabolism

Metabolism studies with ALTOPREV™ have not been conducted.

Lovastatin

Lovastatin is a lactone that is readily hydrolyzed *in vivo* to the corresponding β-hydroxyacid, a potent inhibitor of HMG-CoA reductase. Inhibition of HMG-CoA reductase is the basis for an assay in pharmacokinetic studies of the β-hydroxyacid metabolites (active inhibitors) and, following base hydrolysis, active plus latent inhibitors (total inhibitors) in plasma following administration of lovastatin.

The major active metabolites present in human plasma are the β-hydroxyacid of lovastatin, its 6′-hydroxy derivative, and two additional metabolites. The risk of myopathy is increased by high levels of HMG-CoA reductase inhibitory activity in plasma. Potent inhibitors of CYP3A4 can raise the plasma levels of HMG-CoA reductase inhibitory activity and increase the risk of myopathy (see **WARNINGS**, *Myopathy/Rhabdomyolysis* and **PRECAUTIONS**, *Drug Interactions*).

Lovastatin is a substrate for CYP3A4 (see PRECAUTIONS, *Drug Interactions*). Grapefruit juice contains one or more components that inhibit CYP3A4 and can increase the plasma concentrations of drugs metabolized by CYP3A4. In one study,[1] 10 subjects consumed 200 mL of double-strength grapefruit juice (one can of frozen concentrate diluted with one rather than 3 cans of water) three times daily for 2 days and an additional 200 mL double-strength grapefruit juice together with and 30 and 90 minutes following a single dose of 80 mg lovastatin on the third day. This regimen of grapefruit juice resulted in mean increases in the concentration of lovastatin and its beta-hydroxyacid metabolite (as measured by the area under the concentration-time curve) of 15-fold and 5-fold respectively (as measured using a chemical assay—liquid chromatography/tandem mass spectrometry). In a second study, 15 subjects consumed one 8 oz glass of single-strength grapefruit juice (one can of frozen concentrate diluted with 3 cans of water) with breakfast for 3 consecutive days and a single dose of 40 mg lovastatin in the evening of the third day. This regimen of grapefruit juice resulted in a mean increase in the plasma concentration (as measured by the area under the concentration-time curve) of active and total HMG-CoA reductase inhibitory activity [using a validated enzyme inhibition assay different from that used in the first study, both before (for active inhibitors) and after (for total inhibitors) base hydrolysis] of 1.34-fold and 1.36-fold, respectively, and of lovastatin and its β-hydroxyacid metabolite (measured using a chemical assay—liquid chromatography/tandem mass spectrometry) of 1.94-fold and 1.57-fold, respectively. The effect of amounts of grapefruit juice between those used in these two studies on lovastatin pharmacokinetics has not been studied.

Excretion

ALTOPREV™

In a single-dose study with ALTOPREV™, the amounts of lovastatin and lovastatin acid excreted in the urine were below the lower limit of quantitation of the assay (1.0 ng/mL), indicating that negligible excretion of ALTOPREV™ occurs through the kidney.

Lovastatin

Lovastatin undergoes extensive first-pass extraction in the liver, its primary site of action, with subsequent excretion of drug equivalents in the bile.

Special Populations

Geriatric

Lovastatin Immediate-Release

In a study with lovastatin immediate-release which included 16 elderly patients between 70–78 years of age who received lovastatin immediate-release 80 mg/day, the mean plasma level of HMG-CoA reductase inhibitory activity was increased approximately 45% compared with 18 patients between 18–30 years of age (see PRECAUTIONS, *Geriatric Use*)

Pediatric

Pharmacokinetic data in the pediatric population are not available.

Gender

In a single dose pharmacokinetic study with ALTOPREV™, there were no statistically significant differences in pharmacokinetic parameters between men (n=12) and women (n=10), although exposure tended to be higher in men than women.

In clinical studies with ALTOPREV™, there was no clinically significant difference in LDL-C reduction between men and women.

Renal Insufficiency

In a study of patients with severe renal insufficiency (creatinine clearance 10–30 mL/min), the plasma concentrations of total inhibitors after a single dose of lovastatin were approximately two-fold higher than those in healthy volunteers.

Hemodialysis

The effect of hemodialysis on plasma levels of lovastatin and its metabolites have not been studied.

Hepatic Insufficiency

No pharmacokinetic studies with ALTOPREV™ have been conducted in patients with hepatic insufficiency.

Clinical Studies

ALTOPREV™

ALTOPREV™ has been shown to reduce Total-C, LDL-C, and TG and increase HDL-C in patients with hypercholesterolemia. Near maximal response was observed after four weeks of treatment and the response was maintained with continuation of therapy for up to 6 months.

In a 12-week, multicenter, placebo-controlled, double-blind, dose-response study in adult men and women 21 to 70 years of age with primary hypercholesterolemia, once daily administration of ALTOPREV™ 10 to 60 mg in the evening was compared to placebo. ALTOPREV™ produced dose related reductions in LDL-C and Total-C. ALTOPREV™ produced mean reductions in TG across all doses that varied from approximately 10% to 25%. ALTOPREV™ produced mean increases in HDL-C across all doses that varied from approximately 9% to 13%.

The lipid changes with ALTOPREV™ treatment in this study, from baseline to endpoint, are displayed in Table III.

[See table III above]

Table III
ALTOPREV™ vs. Placebo
(Mean Percent Change from Baseline After 12 Weeks)*

Treatment	N	LDL-C	HDL-C	TOTAL-C	TG
Placebo	34	1.3	5.6	3.4	8.7
ALTOPREV™ 10 mg	33	−23.8	9.4	−17.9	−17.3
ALTOPREV™ 20 mg	34**	−29.6	12.0	−20.9	−13.0
ALTOPREV™ 40 mg	33	−35.8	13.1	−25.4	−9.9
ALTOPREV™ 60 mg	35	−40.8	11.6	−29.2	−25.1

N=the number of patients with values at both baseline and endpoint.
*Except for the HDL-C elevation with ALTOPREV™ 10 mg, all lipid changes with ALTOPREV™ were statistically significant compared to placebo.
**For LDL-C, 33 patients had values at baseline and endpoint.

The range of LDL-C responses is represented graphically in the following figure (Figure 2):

[See figure 2 at top of next column]

Figure 2
ALTOPREV™ vs. Placebo
LDL-C Percent Change from Baseline After 12 Weeks

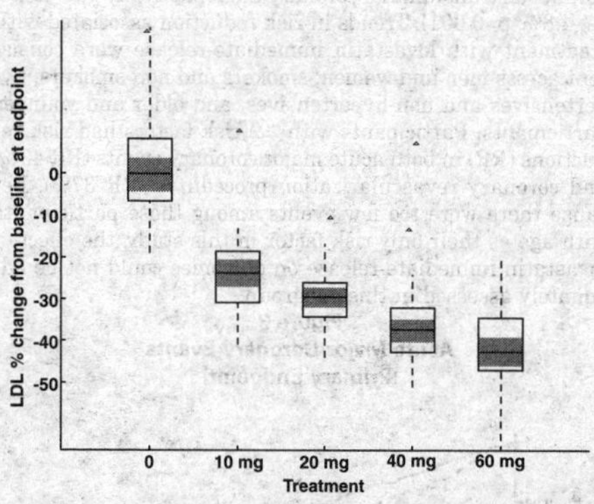

The distribution of LDL-C responses is represented graphically by the boxplots in Figure 2. The bottom line of the box represents the 25th percentile and the top line, the 75th percentile. The horizontal line in the box represents the median and the gray area is the 95% confidence interval for the median. The range of responses is depicted by the tails and outliers.

ALTOPREV™ Long-Term Study

A total of 365 patients were enrolled in an extension study in which all patients were administered ALTOPREV™ 40 mg or 60 mg once daily for up to 6 months of treatment. The lipid-altering effects of ALTOPREV™ were comparable to what was observed in the dose-response study, and were maintained for up to 6 months of treatment.

Special Populations

In clinical studies with ALTOPREV™, there were no statistically significant differences in LDL-C reduction in an older population (≥65 years old), compared to a younger population (<65 years old). There were also no statistically significant differences in LDL-C reduction between male and female patients.

Lovastatin Immediate-Release

Lovastatin immediate-release has been shown to be effective in reducing Total-C and LDL-C in heterozygous familial and non-familial forms of primary hypercholesterolemia and in mixed hyperlipidemia. A marked response was seen within 2 weeks, and the maximum therapeutic response occurred within 4–6 weeks. The response was maintained during continuation of therapy. Single daily doses given in the evening were more effective than the same dose given in the morning, perhaps because cholesterol is synthesized mainly at night.

Lovastatin immediate-release was studied in controlled trials in hypercholesterolemic patients with well-controlled non-insulin dependent diabetes mellitus with normal renal function. The effect of lovastatin immediate-release on lipids and lipoproteins and the safety profile of lovastatin immediate-release were similar to that demonstrated in studies in nondiabetics. Lovastatin immediate-release had no clinically important effect on glycemic control or on the dose requirement of oral hypoglycemic agents.

Expanded Clinical Evaluation of Lovastatin (EXCEL) Study

Lovastatin immediate-release was compared to placebo in 8,245 patients with hypercholesterolemia [Total-C 240–300 mg/dL (6.2 mmol/L–7.6 mmol/L), LDL-C >160 mg/dL (4.1 mmol/L)] in the randomized, double-blind, parallel, 48-week EXCEL study. All changes in the lipid measurements (see Table IV) observed in lovastatin immediate-release-treated patients were dose-related and significantly different from placebo (p≤0.001). These results were sustained throughout the study.

[See table IV at top of next page]

Lovastatin Immediate-Release

Air Force/Texas Coronary Atherosclerosis Prevention Study (AFCAPS/TexCAPS)

The Air Force/Texas Coronary Atherosclerosis Prevention Study (AFCAPS/TexCAPS), a double-blind, randomized, placebo-controlled, primary prevention study, demonstrated that treatment with lovastatin immediate-release decreased the rate of acute major coronary events (composite endpoint of myocardial infarction, unstable angina, and sudden cardiac death) compared with placebo during a median of 5.1 years of follow-up. Participants were middle-aged and elderly men (ages 45–73) and women (ages 55–73) without symptomatic cardiovascular disease with average to moderately elevated Total-C and LDL-C, below average HDL-C, and who were at high risk based on elevated Total-C/HDL-C. In addition to age, 63% of the participants had at least one other risk factor (baseline HDL-C <35 mg/dL, hypertension, family history, smoking and diabetes).

AFCAPS/TexCAPS enrolled 6,605 participants (5,608 men, 997 women) based on the following lipid entry criteria: Total-C range of 180–264 mg/dL, LDL-C range of 130–190 mg/dL, HDL-C of ≤45 mg/dL for men and ≤47 mg/dL for women, and TG of ≤400 mg/dL. Participants were treated

Continued on next page

Altoprev—Cont.

with standard care, including diet, and either lovastatin immediate-release 20 mg - 40 mg daily (n=3,304) or placebo (n=3,301). Approximately 50% of the participants treated with lovastatin immediate-release were titrated to 40 mg daily when their LDL-C remained >110 mg/dL at the 20-mg starting dose.

Lovastatin immediate-release reduced the risk of a first acute major coronary event, the primary efficacy endpoint, by 37% (lovastatin immediate-release 3.5%, placebo 5.5%; p<0.001; Figure 3). A first acute major coronary event was defined as myocardial infarction (54 participants on lovastatin immediate-release, 94 on placebo) or unstable angina (54 vs. 80) or sudden cardiac death (8 vs. 9). Furthermore, among the secondary endpoints, lovastatin immediate-release reduced the risk of unstable angina by 32% (1.8% vs. 2.6%; p=0.023), of myocardial infarction by 40% (1.7% vs. 2.9%; p=0.002), and of undergoing coronary revascularization procedures (e.g., coronary artery bypass grafting or percutaneous transluminal coronary angioplasty) by 33% (3.2% vs. 4.8%; p=0.001). Trends in risk reduction associated with treatment with lovastatin immediate-release were consistent across men and women, smokers and non-smokers, hypertensives and non-hypertensives, and older and younger participants. Participants with ≥2 risk factors had risk reductions (RR) in both acute major coronary events (RR 43%) and coronary revascularization procedures (RR 37%). Because there were too few events among those participants with age as their only risk factor in this study, the effect of lovastatin immediate-release on outcomes could not be adequately assessed in this subgroup.

Figure 3
Acute Major Coronary Events (Primary Endpoint)

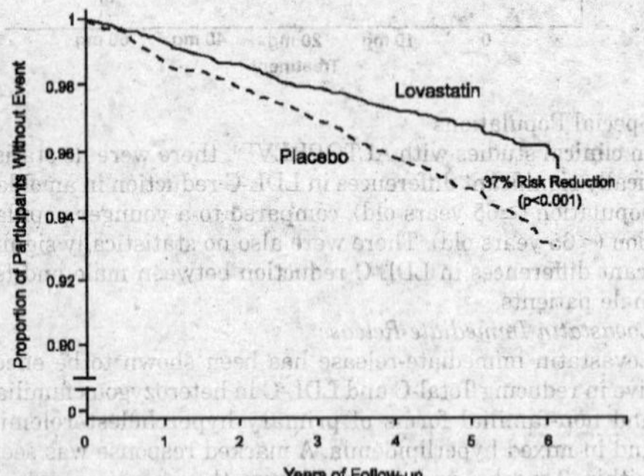

Atherosclerosis

In the Canadian Coronary Atherosclerosis Intervention Trial (CCAIT), the effect of therapy with lovastatin on coronary atherosclerosis was assessed by coronary angiography in hyperlipidemic patients. In this randomized, double-blind, controlled clinical trial, patients were treated with conventional measures (usually diet and 325 mg of aspirin every other day) and either lovastatin 20 mg–80 mg daily or placebo. Angiograms were evaluated at baseline and at two years by computerized quantitative coronary angiography (QCA). Lovastatin significantly slowed the progression of lesions as measured by the mean change per-patient in minimum lumen diameter (the primary endpoint) and percent diameter stenosis, and decreased the proportions of patients categorized with disease progression (33% vs. 50%) and with new lesions (16% vs. 32%).

In a similarly designed trial, the Monitored Atherosclerosis Regression Study (MARS), patients were treated with diet and either lovastatin 80 mg daily or placebo. No statistically significant difference between lovastatin and placebo was seen for the primary endpoint (mean change per patient in percent diameter stenosis of all lesions), or for most secondary QCA endpoints. Visual assessment by angiographers who formed a consensus opinion of overall angiographic change (Global Change Score) was also a secondary endpoint. By this endpoint, significant slowing of disease was seen, with regression in 23% of patients treated with lovastatin compared to 11% of placebo patients.

The effect of lovastatin on the progression of atherosclerosis in the coronary arteries has been corroborated by similar findings in another vasculature. In the Asymptomatic Carotid Artery Progression Study (ACAPS), the effect of therapy with lovastatin on carotid atherosclerosis was assessed by B-mode ultrasonography in hyperlipidemic patients with early carotid lesions and without known coronary heart disease at baseline. In this double-blind, controlled clinical trial, 919 patients were randomized in a 2 × 2 factorial design to placebo, lovastatin 10–40 mg daily and/or warfarin. Ultrasonograms of the carotid walls were used to determine the change per patient from baseline to three years in mean maximum intimal-medial thickness (IMT) of 12 measured segments. There was a significant regression of carotid lesions in patients receiving lovastatin alone compared to those receiving placebo alone (p=0.001). The predictive value of changes in IMT for stroke has not yet been established. In the lovastatin group there was a significant reduction in the number of patients with major cardiovascular events relative to the placebo group (5 vs. 14) and a significant reduction in all-cause mortality (1 vs. 8).

TABLE IV
Lovastatin Immediate-Release (IR) vs. Placebo
(Percent Change from Baseline - Average Values Between Weeks 12 and 48)

DOSAGE	N**	TOTAL-C (mean)	LDL-C (mean)	HDL-C (mean)	LDL-C/ HDL-C (mean)	TOTAL-C/ HDL-C (mean)	TG (median)
Placebo	1663	+0.7	+0.4	+2.0	+0.2	+0.6	+4
Lovastatin IR							
20 mg q.p.m.	1642	−17	−24	+6.6	−27	−21	−10
40 mg q.p.m.	1645	−22	−30	+7.2	−34	−26	−14
20 mg b.i.d.	1646	−24	−34	+8.6	−38	−29	−16
40 mg b.i.d.	1649	−29	−40	+9.5	−44	−34	−19

**Patients enrolled

Table V
NCEP Treatment Guidelines: LDL-C Goals and Cutpoints for Therapeutic Lifestyle Changes and Drug Therapy in Different Risk Categories

Risk Category	LDL Goal (mg/dL)	LDL Level at Which to Initiate Therapeutic Lifestyle Changes (mg/dL)	LDL Level at Which to Consider Drug Therapy (mg/dL)
CHD† or CHD risk equivalents (10-year risk >20%)	<100	≥100	≥130 (100–129: drug optional)††
2+ Risk factors (10-year risk ≤20%)	<130	≥130	10-year risk 10%–20%: ≥130; 10-year risk <10%: ≥160
0–1 Risk factor†††	<160	≥160	≥190 (160–189: LDL-lowering drug optional)

† CHD, coronary heart disease

†† Some authorities recommend use of LDL-lowering drugs in this category if an LDL-C level of <100 mg/dL cannot be achieved by therapeutic lifestyle changes. Others prefer use of drugs that primarily modify triglycerides and HDL-C, e.g., nicotinic acid or fibrate. Clinical judgement also may call for deferring drug therapy in this subcategory.

††† Almost all people with 0–1 risk factor have 10-year risk <10%; thus, 10-year risk assessment in people with 0–1 risk factor is not necessary.

Eye

There was a high prevalence of baseline lenticular opacities in the patients population included in the early clinical trials with lovastatin immediate-release. During these trials the appearance of new opacities was noted in both the lovastatin immediate-release and placebo groups. There was no clinically significant change in visual acuity in the patients who had new opacities reported nor was any patient, including those with opacities noted at baseline, discontinued from therapy because of a decrease in visual acuity.

A three-year, double-blind, placebo-controlled study in hypercholesterolemic patients to assess the effect of lovastatin immediate-release on the human lens demonstrated that there were no clinically or statistically significant differences between the lovastatin immediate-release and placebo groups in the incidence, type or progression of lenticular opacities. There are no controlled clinical data assessing the lens available for treatment beyond three years.

INDICATIONS AND USAGE

Therapy with ALTOPREV™ (Lovastatin) Extended-Release Tablets should be a component of multiple risk factor intervention in those individuals with dyslipidemia who are at risk for atherosclerotic vascular disease. ALTOPREV™ should be used in addition to a diet restricted in saturated fat and cholesterol as part of a treatment strategy to lower Total-C and LDL-C to target levels when the response to diet and other nonpharmacological measures alone has been inadequate to reduce risk.

ALTOPREV™

Primary Prevention of Coronary Heart Disease

In individuals without symptomatic cardiovascular disease, average to moderately elevated Total-C and LDL-C, and below average HDL-C, ALTOPREV™ is indicated to reduce the risk of:

- Myocardial infarction
- Unstable angina
- Coronary revascularization procedures

(See CLINICAL PHARMACOLOGY, *Clinical Studies*.)

Coronary Heart Disease

ALTOPREV™ is indicated to slow the progression of coronary atherosclerosis in patients with coronary heart disease as part of a treatment strategy to lower Total-C and LDL-C to target levels.

Hyperlipidemia

Therapy with lipid-altering agents should be a component of multiple risk factor intervention in those individuals at significantly increased risk for arthérosclerotic vascular disease due to hypercholesterolemia

ALTOPREV™ is indicated as an adjunct to diet for the reduction of elevated Total-C, LDL-C, Apo B, and TG, and to increase HDL-C in patients with primary hypercholesterolemia (heterozygous familial and non-familial) and mixed dyslipidemia (Fredrickson types IIa and IIb, see Table VI) when the response to diet restricted in saturated fat and cholesterol and to other non-pharmacological measures alone has been inadequate.

General Recommendations

Prior to initiating therapy with ALTOPREV™, secondary causes for hypercholesterolemia (e.g., poorly controlled diabetes mellitus, hypothyroidism, nephrotic syndrome, dysproteinemias, obstructive liver disease, other drug therapy, alcoholism) should be excluded, and a lipid profile performed to measure Total-C, HDL-C, and TG. For patients with TG less than 400 mg/dL (<4.5 mmol/L), LDL-C can be estimated using the following equation:

LDL-C = Total-C - [0.2 × (TG) + HDL-C]

For TG levels >400 mg/dL (>4.5 mmol/L), this equation is less accurate and LDL-C concentrations should be determined by ultracentrifugation. In hypertriglyceridemic patients, LDL-C may be low or normal despite elevated Total-C. In such cases, ALTOPREV™ is not indicated.

The National Cholesterol Education Program (NCEP) Treatment Guidelines are summarized below:

[See table V above]

After the LDL-C goal has been achieved, if the TG is still ≥200 mg/dL, non-HDL-C (total-C minus HDL-C) becomes a secondary target of therapy. Non-HDL-C goals are set 30 mg/dL higher than LDL-C goals for each risk category.

At the time of hospitalization for an acute coronary event, consideration can be given to initiating drug therapy at discharge if the LDL-C is ≥130 mg/dL (see NCEP Guidelines above).

Since the goal of treatment is to lower LDL-C, the NCEP recommends that LDL-C levels be used to initiate and assess treatment response. Only if LDL-C levels are not available, should the Total-C be used to monitor therapy.

Although ALTOPREV™ may be useful to reduce elevated LDL-C levels in patients with combined hypercholesterolemia and hypertriglyceridemia where hypercholesterolemia is the major abnormality (Type IIb hyperlipoproteinemia), it has not been studied in conditions where the major abnormality is elevation of chylomicrons, VLDL or IDL (i.e., hyperlipoproteinemia types I, III, IV, or V). [See Table VI]

Table VI
Classification of Hyperlipoproteinemias

Type	Lipoproteins Elevated	Lipid Elevations Major	Lipid Elevations Minor
I (rare)	Chylomicrons	TG	↑→TC
IIa	LDL	TC	-
IIb	LDL, VLDL	TC	TG
III (rare)	IDL	TC/TG	
IV	VLDL	TG	↑→TC
V (rare)	Chylomicrons, VLDL	TG	↑→TC

TC = total cholesterol; TG = triglycerides; LDL = low-density lipoprotein; VLDL = very low-density lipoprotein; IDL = intermediate-density lipoprotein

↑→ = increased or no change

CONTRAINDICATIONS

Hypersensitivity to any component of this medication. Active liver disease or unexplained persistent elevations of serum transaminases (see WARNINGS).

Pregnancy and Lactation

Atherosclerosis is a chronic process and the discontinuation of lipid-lowering drugs during pregnancy should have little impact on the outcome of long-term therapy of primary hypercholesterolemia. Moreover, cholesterol and other products of the cholesterol biosynthesis pathway are essential components for fetal development, including synthesis of steroids and cell membranes. Because of the ability of inhibitors of HMG-CoA reductase such as ALTOPREV™ to decrease the synthesis of cholesterol and possibly other products of the cholesterol biosynthesis pathway, ALTOPREV™ is contraindicated during pregnancy and in nursing mothers. **ALTOPREV™ should be administered to women of childbearing age only when such patients are highly unlikely to conceive.** If the patient becomes pregnant while taking this drug, ALTOPREV™ should be discontinued immediately and the patient should be apprised of the potential hazard to the fetus (see PRECAUTIONS, *Pregnancy*).

WARNINGS

Skeletal Muscle

Lovastatin and other inhibitors of HMG-CoA reductase occasionally cause myopathy, which is manifested as muscle pain or weakness associated with grossly elevated creatine kinase [>10 × the upper limit of normal (ULN)]. Myopathy sometimes takes the form of rhabdomyolysis with or without acute renal failure secondary to myoglobinuria, and rare fatalities have occurred. The risk of myopathy is increased by high levels of HMG-CoA reductase inhibitory activity in plasma.

The risk of myopathy/rhabdomyolysis is increased by concomitant use of lovastatin with the following:

Potent inhibitors of CYP3A4:

Cyclosporine, itraconazole, ketoconazole, erythromycin, clarithromycin, HIV protease inhibitors, nefazodone, or large quantities of grapefruit juice (>1 quart daily), particularly with higher doses of lovastatin (see below: CLINICAL PHARMACOLOGY, *Pharmacokinetics*; PRECAUTIONS, *Drug Interactions, CYP3A4 Interactions*).

Lipid-lowering drugs that can cause myopathy when given alone:

Gemfibrozil, other fibrates, or lipid-lowering doses (≥1 g/day) of niacin, particularly with higher doses of lovastatin (see below; CLINICAL PHARMACOLOGY, *Pharmacokinetics*; PRECAUTIONS, *Drug Interactions, Interactions with lipid-lowering drugs that can cause myopathy when given alone*).

Other drugs: The risk of myopathy/rhabdomyolysis is increased when either amiodarone or verapamil is used concomitantly with higher doses of a closely related member of the HMG-CoA reductase inhibitor class (see PRECAUTIONS, *Drug Interactions, Other drug interactions*).

- **The risk of myopathy/rhabdomyolysis is dose related.** In a clinical study (EXCEL) in which patients were carefully monitored and some interacting drugs were excluded, there was one case of myopathy among 4933 patients randomized to lovastatin 20–40 mg daily for 48 weeks, and 4 among 1649 patients randomized to 80 mg daily.

CONSEQUENTLY:

1. **Use of lovastatin concomitantly with itraconazole, ketoconazole, erythromycin, clarithromycin, HIV protease inhibitors, nefazodone, or large quantities of grapefruit juice (>1 quart daily) should be avoided.** If treatment with itraconazole, ketoconazole, erythromycin, or clarithromycin is unavoidable, therapy with lovastatin should be suspended during the course of treatment. Concomitant use with other medicines labeled as having a potent inhibitory effect on CYP3A4 at therapeutic doses should be avoided unless the benefits of combined therapy outweigh the increased risk.
2. **The dose of lovastatin should not exceed 20 mg daily in patients receiving concomitant medication with cyclosporine, gemfibrozil, other fibrates or lipid-lowering doses (≥1 g/day) of niacin. The combined use of lovastatin with fibrates or niacin should be avoided unless the benefit of further alteration in lipid levels is likely to outweigh the increased risk of this drug combination.** Addition of these drugs to lovastatin typically provides little additional reduction in LDL-C, but further reductions of TG and further increases in HDL-C may be obtained.
3. **The dose of lovastatin should not exceed 20 mg daily in patients receiving concomitant medication with amiodarone or verapamil. The combined use of lovastatin at doses higher than 40 mg daily with amiodarone or verapamil should be avoided unless the clinical benefit is likely to outweigh the increased risk of myopathy.**
4. **All patients starting therapy with lovastatin, or whose dose of lovastatin is being increased, should be advised of the risk of myopathy and told to report promptly any unexplained muscle pain, tenderness or weakness. Lovastatin therapy should be discontinued immediately if myopathy is diagnosed or suspected.** The presence of these symptoms, and/or a CK level >10 times the ULN indicates myopathy. In most cases, when patients were promptly discontinued from treatment, muscle symptoms and CK increases resolved. Periodic CK determinations may be considered in patients starting therapy with lovastatin or whose dose is being increased, but there is no assurance that such monitoring will prevent myopathy.
5. Many of the patients who have developed rhabdomyolysis on therapy with lovastatin have had complicated medical histories, including renal insufficiency usually as a consequence of long-standing diabetes mellitus. Such patients merit closer monitoring. Therapy with lovastatin should be temporarily stopped a few days prior to elective major surgery and when any major medical or surgical condition supervenes.
6. From post-marketing reports with ALTOPREV™, myopathy and rhabdomyolysis have been reported, especially in elderly patients initiating therapy with ALTOPREV™ at a dose of 60 mg per day. Thus, lower starting doses of ALTOPREV™ are recommended for elderly patients, particular those with complicated medical conditions (See **DOSAGE AND ADMINISTRATION**, *Elderly Patients*).

Liver Dysfunction

Persistent increases (to more than 3 times the upper limit of normal) in serum transaminases occurred in 1.9% of adult patients who received lovastatin for at least one year in early clinical trials (see ADVERSE REACTIONS). When the drug was interrupted or discontinued in these patients, the transaminase levels usually fell slowly to pretreatment levels. The increases usually appeared 3 to 12 months after the start of therapy with lovastatin, and were not associated with jaundice or other clinical signs or symptoms. There was no evidence of hypersensitivity.

ALTOPREV™

In controlled clinical trials (467 patients treated with ALTOPREV™ and 329 patients treated with lovastatin immediate-release) no meaningful differences in transaminase elevations between the two treatments were observed.

Lovastatin Immediate-Release

In the EXCEL study (see CLINICAL PHARMACOLOGY, *Clinical Studies*), the incidence of persistent increases in serum transaminases over 48 weeks was 0.1% for placebo, 0.1% at 20 mg/day, 0.9% at 40 mg/day, and 1.5% at 80 mg/day in patients on lovastatin. However, in post-marketing experience with lovastatin immediate-release, symptomatic liver disease has been reported rarely at all dosages (see ADVERSE REACTIONS).

In AFCAPS/TexCAPS, the number of participants with consecutive elevations of either alanine aminotransferase (ALT) or aspartate aminotransferase (AST) (>3 times the upper limit of normal), over a median of 5.1 years of follow-up, was not significantly different between the lovastatin immediate-release and placebo groups [18 (0.6%) vs. 11 (0.3%)]. The starting dose of lovastatin immediate-release was 20 mg/day; 50% of the lovastatin immediate-release treated participants were titrated to 40 mg/day at Week 18. Of the 18 participants on lovastatin immediate-release with consecutive elevations of either ALT or AST, 11 (0.7%) elevations occurred in participants taking 20 mg/day, while 7 (0.4%) elevations occurred in participants titrated to 40 mg/day. Elevated transaminases resulted in discontinuation of 6 (0.2%) participants from therapy in the lovastatin immediate-release group (n=3,304) and 4 (0.1%) in the placebo group (n=3,301).

It is recommended that liver function tests be performed before the initiation of treatment, at 6 and 12 weeks after initiation of therapy or elevation of dose, and periodically thereafter (e.g., semiannually).

Patients who develop increased transaminase levels should be monitored with a second liver function evaluation to confirm the finding and be followed thereafter with frequent liver function tests until the abnormality(ies) return to normal. Should an increase in AST or ALT of three times the upper limit of normal or greater persist, withdrawal of therapy with ALTOPREV™ is recommended.

The drug should be used with caution in patients who consume substantial quantities of alcohol and/or have a past history of liver disease. Active liver disease or unexplained transaminase elevations are contraindications to the use of ALTOPREV™.

As with other lipid-lowering agents, moderate (less than three times the upper limit of normal) elevations of serum transaminases have been reported following therapy with lovastatin (see ADVERSE REACTIONS). These changes appeared soon after initiation of therapy with lovastatin, were often transient, were not accompanied by any symptoms and interruption of treatment was not required.

PRECAUTIONS

General

ALTOPREV™ may elevate creatine phosphokinase and transaminase levels (see WARNINGS and ADVERSE REACTIONS). This should be considered in the differential diagnosis of chest pain in a patient on therapy with ALTOPREV™.

Homozygous Familial Hypercholesterolemia

Lovastatin immediate-release was found to be less effective in patients with the rare homozygous familial hypercholesterolemia, possibly because these patients have no functional LDL receptors. Lovastatin immediate-release appears to be more likely to raise serum transaminases (see ADVERSE REACTIONS) in these homozygous patients.

Information for Patients

The ALTOPREV™ Extended-Release Tablets should be swallowed whole and not chewed or crushed.

Patients should be advised to report promptly unexplained muscle pain, tenderness or weakness (see WARNINGS, *Myopathy/Rhabdomyolsis*).

Drug Interactions

Drug interaction studies have not been performed with ALTOPREV™. The types, frequencies and magnitude of drug interactions that may be encountered when ALTOPREV™ is administered with other drugs may differ from the drug interactions encountered with the lovastatin immediate-release formulation. In addition, as the drug exposure with ALTOPREV™ 60 mg is greater than that with lovastatin immediate-release 80 mg (maximum recommended dose), the severity and magnitude of drug interactions that may be encountered with ALTOPREV™ 60 mg are not known. It is therefore recommended that the following precautions and recommendations for the concomitant administration of lovastatin immediate-release with other drugs be interpreted with caution, and that the monitoring of the pharmacologic effects of ALTOPREV™ and/or other concomitantly administered drugs be undertaken where appropriate.

CYP3A4 Interactions

Lovastatin is metabolized by CYP3A4 but has no CYP3A4 inhibitory activity; therefore it is not expected to affect the plasma concentrations of other drugs metabolized by CYP3A4. Potent inhibitors of CYP3A4 (below) increase the risk of myopathy by reducing the elimination of lovastatin. **See WARNINGS, *Myopathy/Rhabdomyolysis*, and CLINICAL PHARMACOLOGY, *Pharmacokinetics*.**

Itraconazole
Ketoconazole
Erythromycin
Clarithromycin
HIV protease inhibitors
Nefazodone
Cyclosporine
Large quantities of grapefruit juice (>1 quart daily)

Interactions With Lipid-Lowering Drugs That Can Cause Myopathy When Given Alone

The risk of myopathy is also increased by the following lipid-lowering drugs that are not potent CYP3A4 inhibitors, but which can cause myopathy when given alone.

See WARNINGS, Myopathy/Rhabdomyolysis.

Gemfibrozil
Other fibrates
Niacin (nicotinic acid) (≥1 g/day)

Other Drug Interactions Amiodarone or Verapamil: The risk of myopathy/rhabdomyolysis is increased when either amiodarone or verapamil is used concomitantly with a closely related member of the HMG-CoA reductase inhibitor class (see **WARNINGS**, *Myopathy/Rhabdomyolysis*).

Coumarin Anticoagulants: In a small clinical trial in which lovastatin was administered to warfarin treated patients, no effect on prothrombin time was detected. However, another HMG-CoA reductase inhibitor has been found to produce a less than two seconds increase in prothrombin time in healthy volunteers receiving low doses of warfarin. Also, bleeding and/or increased prothrombin time has been reported in a few patients taking coumarin anticoagulants concomitantly with lovastatin. It is recommended that in patients taking anticoagulants, prothrombin time be determined before starting lovastatin and frequently enough during early therapy to ensure that no significant alteration of prothrombin time occurs. Once a stable prothrombin time has been documented, prothrombin times can be monitored at the intervals usually recommended for patients on coumarin anticoagulants. If the dose of lovastatin is changed, the same procedure should be repeated. Lovastatin therapy has not been associated with bleeding or with changes in prothrombin time in patients not taking anticoagulants.

Antipyrine: Lovastatin had no effect on the pharmacokinetics of antipyrine or its metabolites. However, since lovastatin is metabolized by the cytochrome P450 isoform 3A4, this does not preclude an interaction with other drugs metabolized by the same isoform (see WARNINGS, *Myopathy/Rhabdomyolysis*).

Propranolol: In normal volunteers, there was no clinically significant pharmacokinetic or pharmacodynamic interaction with concomitant administration of single doses of lovastatin and propranolol.

Digoxin: In patients with hypercholesterolemia, concomitant administration of lovastatin and digoxin resulted in no effect on digoxin plasma concentrations.

Oral Hypoglycemic Agents: In pharmacokinetic studies of lovastatin immediate-release in hypercholesterolemic non-insulin dependent diabetic patients, there was no drug interaction with glipizide or with chlorpropamide (see CLINICAL PHARMACOLOGY, *Clinical Studies*).

Endocrine Function

HMG-CoA reductase inhibitors interfere with cholesterol synthesis and as such might theoretically blunt adrenal and/or gonadal steroid production. Results of clinical trials with drugs in this class have been inconsistent with regard to drug effects on basal and reserve steroid levels. However, clinical studies have shown that lovastatin does not reduce basal plasma cortisol concentration or impair adrenal reserve, and does not reduce basal plasma testosterone concentration. Another HMG-CoA reductase inhibitor has been shown to reduce the plasma testosterone response to HCG. In the same study, the mean testosterone response to HCG was slightly but not significantly reduced after treatment with lovastatin 40 mg daily for 16 weeks in 21 men. The effects of HMG-CoA reductase inhibitors on male fertility have not been studied in adequate numbers of male patients. The effects, if any, on the pituitary-gonadal axis in premenopausal women are unknown. Patients treated with lovastatin who develop clinical evidence of endocrine dysfunction should be evaluated appropriately. Caution should also be exercised if an HMG-CoA reductase inhibitor or other agent used to lower cholesterol levels is administered to patients also receiving other drugs (e.g., ketoconazole, spironolactone, cimetidine) that may decrease the levels or activity of endogenous steroid hormones.

Continued on next page

Altoprev—Cont.

CNS Toxicity

Lovastatin produced optic nerve degeneration (Wallerian degeneration of retinogeniculate fibers) in clinically normal dogs in a dose-dependent fashion starting at 60 mg/kg/day, a dose that produced mean plasma drug levels about 30 times higher than the mean drug level in humans taking the highest recommended dose (as measured by total enzyme inhibitory activity). Vestibulocochlear Wallerian-like degeneration and retinal ganglion cell chromatolysis were also seen in dogs treated for 14 weeks at 180 mg/kg/day, a dose which resulted in a mean plasma drug level (C_{max}) similar to that seen with the 60 mg/kg/day dose.

CNS vascular lesions, characterized by perivascular hemorrhage and edema, mononuclear cell infiltration of perivascular spaces, perivascular fibrin deposits and necrosis of small vessels, were seen in dogs treated with lovastatin at a dose of 180 mg/kg/day, a dose which produced plasma drug levels (C_{max}) which were about 30 times higher than the mean values in humans taking 80 mg/day.

Similar optic nerve and CNS vascular lesions have been observed with other drugs of this class. Cataracts were seen in dogs treated for 11 and 28 weeks at 180 mg/kg/day and 1 year at 60 mg/kg/day.

Carcinogenesis, Mutagenesis, Impairment of Fertility

In a 21-month carcinogenic study in mice with lovastatin immediate-release, there was a statistically significant increase in the incidence of hepatocellular carcinomas and adenomas in both males and females at 500 mg/kg/day. This dose produced a total plasma drug exposure 3 to 4 times that of humans given the highest recommended dose of lovastatin (drug exposure was measured as total HMG-CoA reductase inhibitory activity in extracted plasma). Tumor increases were not seen at 20 and 100 mg/kg/day, doses that produced drug exposures of 0.3 to 2 times that of humans at the 80 mg/day lovastatin immediate-release dose. A statistically significant increase in pulmonary adenomas was seen in female mice at approximately 4 times the human drug exposure. [Although mice were given 300 times the human dose (HD) on a mg/kg body weight basis, plasma levels of total inhibitory activity were only 4 times higher in mice than in humans given 80 mg of lovastatin immediate-release].

There was an increase in incidence of papilloma in the nonglandular mucosa of the stomach of mice beginning at exposures of 1 to 2 times that of humans given lovastatin immediate-release. The glandular mucosa was not affected. The human stomach contains only glandular mucosa.

In a 24-month carcinogenicity study in rats, there was a positive dose response relationship for hepatocellular carcinogenicity in males at drug exposures between 2–7 times that of human exposure at 80 mg/day lovastatin immediate-release (doses in rats were 5, 30 and 180 mg/kg/day).

An increased incidence of thyroid neoplasms in rats appears to be a response that has been seen with other HMG-CoA reductase inhibitors.

A chemically similar drug in this class was administered to mice for 72 weeks at 25, 100, and 400 mg/kg body weight, which resulted in mean serum drug levels approximately 3, 15, and 33 times higher than the mean human serum drug concentration (as total inhibitory activity) after a 40 mg oral dose of lovastatin immediate-release. Liver carcinomas were significantly increased in high-dose females and mid- and high-dose males, with a maximum incidence of 90 percent in males. The incidence of adenomas of the liver was significantly increased in mid- and high-dose females. Drug treatment also significantly increased the incidence of lung adenomas in mid- and high-dose males and females. Adenomas of the Harderian gland (a gland of the eye of rodents) were significantly higher in high dose mice than in controls.

No evidence of mutagenicity was observed with lovastatin immediate-release in a microbial mutagen test using mutant strains of *Salmonella typhimurium* with or without rat or mouse liver metabolic activation. In addition, no evidence of damage to genetic material was noted in an *in vitro* alkaline elution assay using rat or mouse hepatocytes, a V-79 mammalian cell forward mutation study, an *in vitro* chromosome aberration study in CHO cells, or an *in vivo* chromosomal aberration assay in mouse bone marrow.

Drug-related testicular atrophy, decreased spermatogenesis, spermatocytic degeneration and giant cell formation were seen in dogs starting at 20 mg/kg/day with lovastatin immediate-release. Similar findings were seen with another drug in this class. No drug-related effects on fertility were found in studies with lovastatin in rats. However, in studies with a similar drug in this class, there was decreased fertility in male rats treated for 34 weeks at 25 mg/kg body weight, although this effect was not observed in a subsequent fertility study when this same dose was administered for 11 weeks (the entire cycle of spermatogenesis, including epididymal maturation). In rats treated with this same reductase inhibitor at 180 mg/kg/day, seminiferous tubule degeneration (necrosis and loss of spermatogenic epithelium) was observed. No microscopic changes were observed in the testes from rats of either study. The clinical significance of these findings is unclear.

Pregnancy

Pregnancy Category X

See CONTRAINDICATIONS.

Safety in pregnant women has not been established. Lovastatin immediate-release has been shown to produce skeletal malformations at plasma levels 40 times the human exposure (for mouse fetus) and 80 times the human exposure (for rat fetus) based on mg/m^2 surface area (doses were 800 mg/kg/day). No drug-induced changes were seen in either species at multiples of 8 times (rat) or 4 times (mouse) based on surface area. No evidence of malformations was noted in rabbits at exposures up to 3 times the human exposure (dose of 15 mg/kg/day, highest tolerated dose of lovastatin immediate-release).

Rare reports of congenital anomalies have been received following intrauterine exposure to HMG-CoA reductase inhibitors. In a review[2] of approximately 100 prospectively followed pregnancies in women exposed to lovastatin immediate-release or another structurally related HMG-CoA reductase inhibitor, the incidences of congenital anomalies, spontaneous abortions and fetal deaths/stillbirths did not exceed what would be expected in the general population. The number of cases is adequate only to exclude a 3 to 4-fold increase in congenital anomalies over the background incidence. In 89% of the prospectively followed pregnancies, drug treatment was initiated prior to pregnancy and was discontinued at some point in the first trimester when pregnancy was identified. As safety in pregnant women has not been established and there is no apparent benefit to therapy with ALTOPREV™ during pregnancy (see CONTRAINDICATIONS), treatment should be immediately discontinued as soon as pregnancy is recognized. ALTOPREV™ should be administered to women of child-bearing potential only when such patients are highly unlikely to conceive and have been informed of the potential hazard.

Nursing Mothers

It is not known whether lovastatin is excreted in human milk. Because a small amount of another drug in this class is excreted in human breast milk and because of the potential for serious adverse reactions in nursing infants, women taking ALTOPREV™ should not nurse their infants (see CONTRAINDICATIONS).

Pediatric Use

Safety and effectiveness in pediatric patients have not been established. Because pediatric patients are not likely to benefit from cholesterol lowering for at least a decade and because experience with this drug is limited (no studies in subjects below the age of 20 years), treatment of pediatric patients with ALTOPREV™ is not recommended at this time.

Geriatric Use

ALTOPREV™

Of the 467 patients who received ALTOPREV™ in controlled clinical studies, 18% were 65 years and older. Of the 297 patients who received ALTOPREV™ in uncontrolled clinical studies, 22% were 65 years and older. No overall differences in effectiveness or safety were observed between these patients and other reported clinical experience has not identified differences in response between the elderly and younger patients, but greater sensitivity of some older individuals cannot be ruled out. Thus, lower starting doses of ALTOPREV™ are recommended for elderly patients, particularly those with complicated medical conditions. (See **DOSAGE AND ADMINISTRATION**, *Elderly Patients*).

Lovastatin Immediate-Release

In pharmacokinetic studies with lovastatin immediate-release, the mean plasma level of HMG-CoA reductase inhibitory activity was shown to be approximately 45% higher in elderly patients between 70–78 years of age compared with patients between 18–30 years of age; however, clinical study experience in the elderly indicates that dosage adjustment based on this age-related pharmacokinetic difference is not needed. In the two large clinical studies conducted with lovastatin immediate-release (EXCEL and AFCAPS/TexCAPS), 21% (3094/14850) of patients were ≥65 years of age. Lipid-lowering efficacy with lovastatin was at least as great in elderly patients compared with younger patients, and there were no overall differences in safety over the 20 to 80 mg dosage range (see CLINICAL PHARMACOLOGY).

ADVERSE REACTIONS

ALTOPREV™

ALTOPREV™ Clinical Studies

In clinical studies with ALTOPREV™, adverse reactions have generally been mild and transient. In controlled studies with 467 patients who received ALTOPREV™, <3% of patients were discontinued due to adverse experiences attributable to ALTOPREV™. This was similar to the discontinuation rate in the placebo and lovastatin immediate-release treatment groups. Pooled results from clinical studies with ALTOPREV™ show that the most frequently reported adverse reactions in the ALTOPREV™ group were infection, headache and accidental injury. Similar incidences of these adverse reactions were seen in the lovastatin and placebo groups. The most frequent adverse events thought to be related to ALTOPREV™ were nausea, abdominal pain, insomnia, dyspepsia, headache, asthenia, and myalgia. In controlled trials (e.g., vs. placebo and vs. lovastatin immediate-release), clinical adverse experiences reported as in ≥5% in any treatment group are shown in Table VII below.

[See table VII below]

Lovastatin Immediate-Release

Lovastatin Immediate-Release Phase III Clinical Studies

In Phase III controlled clinical studies involving 613 patients treated with lovastatin immediate-release, the adverse experience profile was similar to that shown below for the 8,245-patient EXCEL study [see *Expanded Clinical Evaluation of Lovastatin (EXCEL) Study*]. Persistent increases of serum transaminases have been noted (see WARNINGS, *Liver Dysfunction*). About 11% of patients had elevations of CK levels of at least twice the normal value on one or more occasions. The corresponding values for the control agent cholestyramine was 9%. This was attributable to the noncardiac fraction of CK. Large increases in CK have sometimes been reported (see WARNINGS, *Skeletal Muscle*).

Expanded Clinical Evaluation of Lovastatin (EXCEL) Study

Lovastatin immediate-release was compared to placebo in 8,245 patients with hypercholesterolemia [Total-C 240-300 mg/dL (6.2–7.8 mmol/L)] in the randomized, double-blind, parallel, 48-week EXCEL study. Clinical adverse experiences reported as possibly, probably or definitely drug-related in ≥1% in any treatment group are shown in the table below. For no event was the incidence on drug and placebo statistically different.

[See table VIII at bottom of next page]

Other clinical adverse experiences reported as possibly, probably or definitely drug-related in 0.5% to 1.0% of patients in any drug-treated group are listed below. In all these cases the incidence on drug and placebo was not statistically different. *Body as a Whole:* chest pain; *Gastrointestinal:* acid regurgitation, dry mouth, vomiting; *Musculoskeletal:* leg pain, shoulder pain, arthralgia; *Nervous System/Psychiatric:* insomnia, paresthesia; *Skin:* alopecia, pruritus; *Special Senses:* eye irritation.

In the EXCEL study (see CLINICAL PHARMACOLOGY, *Clinical Studies*), 4.6% of the patients treated up to 48 weeks were discontinued due to clinical or laboratory adverse experiences which were rated by the investigator as possibly, probably or definitely related to therapy with lovastatin immediate-release. The value for the placebo group was 2.5%.

Air Force/Texas Coronary Atherosclerosis Prevention Study (AFCAPS/TexCAPS)

In AFCAPS/TexCAPS (see CLINICAL PHARMACOLOGY, *Clinical Studies*) involving 6,605 participants treated with 20–40 mg/day of lovastatin immediate-release (n=3,304) or placebo (n=3,301), the safety and tolerability profile of the group treated with lovastatin immediate-release was comparable to that of the group treated with placebo during a

Table VII
Pooled Controlled Studies TESS by Body System and COSTART Term, Most Common (≥5% in Any Group)

		Treatment		
		Placebo	ALTOPREV™	MEVACOR™
Randomized Patients, n =		34	467	329
Body System	**COSTART Term**			
Body as a Whole	Infection	3 (9)	52 (11)	52 (16)
	Accidental Injury	3 (9)	26 (6)	12 (4)
	Asthenia	2 (6)	12 (3)	6 (2)
	Headache	2 (6)	34 (7)	26 (8)
	Back Pain	1 (3)	23 (5)	18 (5)
	Flu Syndrome	1 (3)	24 (5)	18 (5)
	Pain	0	14 (3)	17 (5)
Digestive	Diarrhea	2 (6)	15 (3)	8 (2)
Musculoskeletal	Arthralgia	2 (6)	24 (5)	20 (6)
	Myalgia	5 (15)	14 (3)	11 (3)
Nervous	Dizziness	2 (6)	10 (2)	5 (2)
Respiratory	Sinusitis	1 (3)	17 (4)	20 (6)
Urogenital	Urinary Tract Infection	2 (6)	8 (2)	9 (3)

median of 5.1 years of follow-up. The adverse experiences reported in AFCAPS/TexCAPS were similar to those reported in EXCEL [see ADVERSE REACTIONS, *Expanded Clinical Evaluation of Lovastatin (EXCEL) Study].*

Concomitant Therapy

In controlled clinical studies in which lovastatin immediate-release was administered concomitantly with cholestyramine, no adverse reactions peculiar to this concomitant treatment were observed. The adverse reactions that occurred were limited to those reported previously with lovastatin or cholestyramine. Other lipid-lowering agents were not administered concomitantly with lovastatin during controlled clinical studies. Preliminary data suggests that the addition of gemfibrozil to therapy with lovastatin is not associated with greater reduction in LDL-C than that achieved with lovastatin alone. In uncontrolled clinical studies, most of the patients who have developed myopathy were receiving concomitant therapy with cyclosporine, gemfibrozil or niacin (nicotinic acid) (see WARNINGS, *Myopathy/Rhabdomyolysis*)

The following effects have been reported with drugs in this class. Not all the effects listed below have necessarily been associated with lovastatin therapy.

Skeletal: muscle cramps, myalgia, myopathy, rhabdomyolysis, arthralgias.

Neurological: dysfunction of certain cranial nerves (including alteration of taste, impairment of extra-ocular movement, facial paresis), tremor, dizziness, vertigo, memory loss, paresthesia, peripheral neuropathy, peripheral nerve palsy, psychic disturbances, anxiety, insomnia, depression.

Hypersensitivity Reactions: An apparent hypersensitivity syndrome has been reported rarely which has included one or more of the following features: anaphylaxis, angioedema, lupus erythematous-like syndrome, polymyalgia rheumatica, vasculitis, purpura, thrombocytopenia, leukopenia, hemolytic anemia, positive ANA, ESR increase, eosinophilia, arthritis, arthralgia, urticaria, asthenia, photosensitivity, fever, chills, flushing, malaise, dyspnea, toxic epidermal necrolysis, erythema multiforme, including Stevens-Johnson syndrome.

Gastrointestinal: pancreatitis, hepatitis, including chronic active hepatitis, cholestatic jaundice, fatty change in liver; and rarely, cirrhosis, fulminant hepatic necrosis, and hepatoma; anorexia, vomiting.

Skin: alopecia, pruritus. A variety of skin changes (e.g., nodules, discoloration, dryness of skin/mucous membranes, changes to hair/nails) have been reported.

Reproductive: gynecomastia, loss of libido, erectile dysfunction.

Eye: progression of cataracts (lens opacities), ophthalmoplegia.

Laboratory Abnormalities: elevated transaminases, alkaline phosphatase, γ-glutamyl transpeptidase, and bilirubin; thyroid function abnormalities.

OVERDOSAGE

After oral administration of lovastatin immediate-release to mice the median lethal dose observed was >15 g/m^2.

Five healthy human volunteers have received up to 200 mg of lovastatin as a single dose without clinically significant adverse experiences. A few cases of accidental overdosage with lovastatin immediate-release have been reported; no patients had any specific symptoms, and all patients recovered without sequelae. The maximum dose taken was 5 g–6 g.

Until further experience is obtained, no specific treatment of overdosage with ALTOPREV™ can be recommended.

The dialyzability of lovastatin and its metabolites in man is not known at present.

DOSAGE AND ADMINISTRATION

The patient should be placed on a standard cholesterol-lowering diet before receiving ALTOPREV™ and should continue on this diet during treatment with ALTOPREV™ (see NCEP Treatment Guidelines for details on dietary therapy).

The usual recommended starting dose is 20, 40, or 60 mg once a day given in the evening at bedtime. The recommended dosing range is 10–60 mg/day, in single doses. Doses should be individualized according to the recommended goal of therapy (see NCEP Guidelines and CLINICAL PHARMACOLOGY). A starting dose of 10 mg may be considered for patients requiring smaller reductions. Adjustments should be made at intervals of 4 weeks or more. See below for dosage recommendations in special populations (i.e., elderly patients, or patients with complicated medical conditions or renal insufficiency) or for patients receiving concomitant therapy (i.e., cyclosporine, amiodarone, verapamil, fibrates or niacin).

In patients taking cyclosporine concomitantly with ALTOPREV™ (see WARNINGS, *Skeletal Muscle*), therapy should begin with 10 mg of ALTOPREV™ and should not exceed 20 mg/day.

Cholesterol levels should be monitored periodically and consideration should be given to reducing the dosage of ALTOPREV™ if cholesterol levels fall significantly below the targeted range.

Elderly Patients or Patients with Complicated Medical Conditions

The usual recommended starting dose in elderly patients (age ≥65 years) or patients with complicated medical conditions (renal insufficiency, diabetes) is 20 once a day given in the evening at bedtime. Higher doses should be used only after careful consideration of the potential risks and benefits (See NCEP Guidelines and **WARNINGS, *Myopathy/Rhabdomyolysis***). A starting dose of 10 mg may be considered for patients requiring smaller reductions.

Dosage in Patients Taking Cyclosporine

In patients taking cyclosporine concomitantly with ALTOPREV™ (see **WARNINGS**, *Myopathy/Rhabdomyolysis*), therapy should begin with 10 mg of ALTOPREV™ and should not exceed 20 mg/day.

Dosage in Patients Taking Amiodarone or Verapamil

In patients taking amiodarone or verapamil concomitantly with ALTOPREV™, the dose should not exceed 20 mg/day (see **WARNINGS**, *Myopathy/Rhabdomyolysis and* PRECAUTIONS, *Drug Interactions, Other Drug Interactions*).

Concomitant Lipid-Lowering Therapy

Use of ALTOPREV™ with fibrates or niacin should generally be avoided. However, if ALTOPREV™ is used in combination with fibrates or niacin, the dose of ALTOPREV™ should generally not exceed 20 mg (see WARNINGS, *Myopathy/Rhabdomyolysis* and PRECAUTIONS, *Drug Interactions*).

Dosage in Patients with Renal Insufficiency

In patients with severe renal insufficiency (creatinine clearance <30 mL/min), dosage increases above 20 mg/day should be carefully considered and, if deemed necessary, implemented cautiously (see CLINICAL PHARMACOLOGY and WARNINGS, *Myopathy/Rhabdomyolysis*).

HOW SUPPLIED

ALTOPREV™ (Lovastatin) are supplied as round, convex shaped extended-release tablets containing 10 mg, 20 mg, 40 mg and 60 mg of lovastatin.

NDC 62022-627-30—10 mg extended-release dark orange-colored tablets: imprinted with Andrx logo and 10 on one side, bottles of 30.

NDC 62022-628-30—20 mg extended-release orange-colored tablets: imprinted with Andrx logo and 20 on one side, bottles of 30.

NDC 62022-629-30—40 mg extended-release peach-colored tablets: imprinted with Andrx logo and 40 on one side, bottles of 30.

NDC 62022-630-30—60 mg extended-release light peach-colored tablets: imprinted with Andrx logo and 60 on one side, bottles of 30.

Storage

Store at controlled room temperature 20°–25° C (68°–77°F). Avoid excessive heat and humidity.

Rx only

Distributed by
Andrx Laboratories, Inc.
Weston, Florida 33331

Manufactured by
Andrx Pharmaceuticals, Inc.
Fort Lauderdale, FL 33314

Package Insert #7467
Rev Date: 07/04

References:

1. Kantola, T, et al. Clin Pharmacol Ther 1998; 63(4):397–402.
2. Manson, J.M., Freyssinges, C., Ducrocq, M.B., Stephenson, W.P., Postmarketing Surveillance of Lovastatin and Simvastatin Exposure During Pregnancy. Reproductive Toxicology. 19(6):439–446. 1996.

Shown in Product Identification Guide, page 305

Table VIII
Clinical Adverse Events Reported as Possibly, Probably or Definitely Drug-Related in ≥1% in Any Treatment Group in the EXCEL Study

	Placebo (N=1663) %	Lovastatin IR 20 mg q.p.m. (N=1642) %	Lovastatin IR 40 mg q.p.m. (N=1645) %	Lovastatin IR 20 mg b.i.d. (N=1646) %	Lovastatin IR 40 mg b.i.d. (N=1649) %
Body As a Whole					
Asthenia	1.4	1.7	1.4	1.5	1.2
Gastrointestinal					
Abdominal pain	1.6	2.0	2.0	2.2	2.5
Constipation	1.9	2.0	3.2	3.2	3.5
Diarrhea	2.3	2.6	2.4	2.2	2.6
Dyspepsia	1.9	1.3	1.3	1.0	1.6
Flatulence	4.2	3.7	4.3	3.9	4.5
Nausea	2.5	1.9	2.5	2.2	2.2
Musculoskeletal					
Muscle cramps	0.5	0.6	0.8	1.1	1.0
Myalgia	1.7	2.6	1.8	2.2	3.0
Nervous System/Psychiatric					
Dizziness	0.7	0.7	1.2	0.5	0.5
Headache	2.7	2.6	2.8	2.1	3.2
Skin					
Rash	0.7	0.8	1.0	1.2	1.3
Special Senses					
Blurred vision	0.8	1.1	0.9	0.9	1.2

FORTAMET™ ℞

[fōr-tä mĕt]

(metformin hydrochloride) Extended-Release Tablets
℞ only

DESCRIPTION

FORTAMET™ (metformin hydrochloride) Extended-Release Tablets contain an oral antihyperglycemic drug used in the management of type 2 diabetes. Metformin hydrochloride (N, N-dimethylimidodicarbonimidic diamide hydrochloride) is a member of the biguanide class of oral antihyperglycemics and is not chemically or pharmacologically related to any other class of oral antihyperglycemic agents. The empirical formula of metformin hydrochloride is $C_4H_{11}N_5 \cdot HCl$ and its molecular weight is 165.63. Its structural formula is:

Metformin hydrochloride is a white to off-white crystalline powder that is freely soluble in water and is practically insoluble in acetone, ether, and chloroform. The pKa of metformin is 12.4. The pH of a 1% aqueous solution of metformin hydrochloride is 6.68.

FORTAMET™ Extended-Release Tablets are designed for once-a-day oral administration and deliver 500 mg or 1000 mg of metformin hydrochloride. In addition to the active ingredient metformin hydrochloride, each tablet contains the following inactive ingredients: candellila wax, cellulose acetate, hypromellose, magnesium stearate, polyethylene glycols (PEG 400, PEG 8000), polysorbate 80, povidone, sodium lauryl sulfate, synthetic black iron oxides, titanium dioxide, and triacetin.

SYSTEM COMPONENTS AND PERFORMANCE

FORTAMET™ was developed as an extended-release formulation of metformin hydrochloride and designed for once-a-day oral administration using the patented single-composition osmotic technology (SCOT™). The tablet is similar in appearance to other film-coated oral administered tablets but it consists of an osmotically active core formulation that is surrounded by a semipermeable membrane. Two laser drilled exit ports exist in the membrane, one on either side of the tablet. The core formulation is composed primarily of drug with small concentrations of excipients. The semipermeable membrane is permeable to water but not to higher molecular weight components of biological fluids. Upon ingestion, water is taken up through the membrane, which in turn dissolves the drug and excipients in the core formulation. The dissolved drug and excipients exit through the laser drilled ports in the membrane. The rate of drug delivery is constant and dependent upon the maintenance of a constant osmotic gradient across the membrane. This situation exists so long as there is undissolved drug present in the core tablet. Following the dissolution of the core materials, the rate of drug delivery slowly decreases until the osmotic gradient across the membrane falls to zero at which time delivery ceases. The membrane coating remains intact during the transit of the dosage form through the gastrointestinal tract and is excreted in the feces.

CLINICAL PHARMACOLOGY

Mechanism of Action

Metformin is an antihyperglycemic agent which improves glucose tolerance in patients with type 2 diabetes, lowering both basal and postprandial plasma glucose. Its pharmacologic mechanisms of action are different from other classes

Continued on next page

Fortamet—Cont.

of oral antihyperglycemic agents. Metformin decreases hepatic glucose production, decreases intestinal absorption of glucose, and improves insulin sensitivity by increasing peripheral glucose uptake and utilization. Unlike sulfonylureas, metformin does not produce hypoglycemia in either patients with type 2 diabetes or normal subjects (except in special circumstances, see **PRECAUTIONS**) and does not cause hyperinsulinemia. With metformin therapy, insulin secretion remains unchanged while fasting plasma insulin levels and day-long plasma insulin response may actually decrease.

PHARMACOKINETICS AND DRUG METABOLISM

Absorption and Bioavailability

The appearance of metformin in plasma from a FORTAMET™ Extended-Release Tablet is slower and more prolonged compared to immediate-release metformin.

In a multiple-dose crossover study, 23 patients with type 2 diabetes mellitus were administered either FORTAMET™ 2000 mg once a day (after dinner) or immediate-release (IR) metformin hydrochloride 1000 mg twice a day (after breakfast and after dinner). After 4 weeks of treatment, steady-state pharmacokinetic parameters, area under the concentration-time curve (AUC), time to peak plasma concentration (Tmax), and maximum concentration (Cmax) were evaluated. Results are presented in Table 1.

Table 1
FORTAMET™ vs. Immediate-Release Metformin Steady-State Pharmacokinetic Parameters at 4 Weeks

Pharmacokinetic Parameters (mean ± SD)	FORTAMET™ 2000 mg (administered q.d. after dinner)	Immediate-Release Metformin 2000 mg (1000 mg b.i.d.)
$AUC_{0\text{-}24\ hr}$ (ng•hr/mL)	26,811 ± 7055	27,371 ± 5,781
T_{max} (hr)	6 (3-10)	3 (1-8)
C_{max} (ng/mL)	2849 ± 797	1820 ± 370

In four single-dose studies and one multiple-dose study, the bioavailability of FORTAMET™ 2000 mg given once daily, in the evening, under fed conditions [as measured by the area under the plasma concentration versus time curve (AUC)] was similar to the same total daily dose administered as immediate-release metformin 1000 mg given twice daily. The geometric mean ratios (FORTAMET™/immediate-release metformin) of $AUC_{0\text{-}24hr}$, $AUC_{0\text{-}72hr}$, and $AUC_{0\text{-}inf}$ for these five studies ranged from 0.96 to 1.08.

In a single-dose, four-period replicate crossover design study, comparing two 500 mg FORTAMET™ tablets to one 1000 mg FORTAMET™ tablet administered in the evening with food to 29 healthy male subjects, two 500 mg FORTAMET™ tablets were found to be equivalent to one 1000 mg FORTAMET™ tablet.

In a study carried out with FORTAMET™, there was a dose-associated increase in metformin exposure over 24 hours following oral administration of 1000, 1500, 2000, and 2500 mg.

In three studies with FORTAMET™ using different treatment regimens (2000 mg after dinner; 1000 mg after breakfast and after dinner; and 2500 mg after dinner), the pharmacokinetics of metformin as measured by AUC appeared linear following multiple-dose administration.

The extent of metformin absorption (as measured by AUC) from FORTAMET™ increased by approximately 60% when given with food. When FORTAMET™ was administered with food, Cmax was increased by approximately 30% and Tmax was more prolonged compared with the fasting state (6.1 versus 4.0 hours).

Distribution

Distribution studies with FORTAMET™ have not been conducted. However, the apparent volume of distribution (V/F) of metformin following single oral doses of immediate-release metformin 850 mg averaged 654 ± 358 L. Metformin is negligibly bound to plasma proteins, in contrast to sulfonylureas, which are more than 90% protein bound. Metformin partitions into erythrocytes, most likely as a function of time. At usual clinical doses and dosing schedules of immediate-release metformin, steady state plasma concentrations of metformin are reached within 24-48 hours and are generally <1 µg/mL. During controlled clinical trials of immediate-release metformin, maximum metformin plasma levels did not exceed 5 µg/mL, even at maximum doses.

Metabolism and Excretion

Metabolism studies with FORTAMET™ have not been conducted.

Intravenous single-dose studies in normal subjects demonstrate that metformin is excreted unchanged in the urine and does not undergo hepatic metabolism (no metabolites have been identified in humans) nor biliary excretion.

Table 2
Select Mean (±SD) Metformin Pharmacokinetic Parameters Following Single or Multiple Oral Doses of Immediate-Release Metformin

Subject Groups: Immediate-Release Metformin dose[a] (number of subjects)	C_{max}[b] (µg/mL)	T_{max}[c] (hrs)	Renal Clearance (mL/min)
Healthy, nondiabetic adults:			
500 mg single dose (24)	1.03 (±0.33)	2.75 (±0.81)	600 (±132)
850 mg single dose (74)[d]	1.60 (±0.38)	2.64 (±0.82)	552 (±139)
850 mg three times daily for 19 doses[e] (9)	2.01 (±0.42)	1.79 (±0.94)	642 (±173)
Adults with type 2 diabetes:			
850 mg single dose (23)	1.48 (±0.5)	3.32 (±1.08)	491 (±138)
850 mg three times daily for 19 doses[e] (9)	1.90 (±0.62)	2.01 (±1.22)	550 (±160)
Elderly[f], healthy nondiabetic adults:			
850 mg single dose (12)	2.45 (±0.70)	2.71 (±1.05)	412 (±98)
Renal-impaired adults:			
850 mg single dose			
Mild (CL_{cr}[g] 61-90 mL/min) (5)	1.86 (±0.52)	3.20 (±0.45)	384 (±122)
Moderate (CL_{cr} 31-60 mL/min) (4)	4.12 (±1.83)	3.75 (±0.50)	108 (±57)
Severe (CL_{cr} 10-30 mL/min) (6)	3.93 (±0.92)	4.01 (±1.10)	130 (±90)

[a] All doses given fasting except the first 18 doses of the multiple dose studies
[b] Peak plasma concentration
[c] Time to peak plasma concentration
[d] Combined results (average means) of five studies: mean age 32 years (range 23-59 years)
[e] Kinetic study done following dose 19, given fasting
[f] Elderly subjects, mean age 71 years (range 65-81 years)
[g] CL_{cr} = creatinine clearance normalized to body surface area of 1.73 m^2

Table 3
FORTAMET™ vs. Immediate-Release Metformin Switch Study: Summary of Mean Changes in HbA_{1c}, Fasting Plasma Glucose, Body Weight, Body Mass Index, and Plasma Insulin

	FORTAMET™	Immediate-Release Metformin	Treatment difference for change from baseline (FORTAMET™ minus Immediate-Release Metformin) LS mean (2-sided 95% CI[a])
HbA_{1c} (%)			
N	327	332	0.25
Baseline (mean ± SD)	7.04 ± 0.88	7.07 ± 0.76	(0.14, 0.37) [b]
Change from baseline (mean ± SD)	0.40 ± 0.75	0.14 ± 0.75	
Fasting Plasma Glucose (mg/dL)			
N	329	333	6.43
Baseline (mean ± SD)	146.8 ± 32.1	145.6 ± 29.5	(0.57, 12.29)
Change from baseline (mean ± SD)	10.0 ± 40.8	4.2 ± 35.9	
Plasma Insulin (µu/mL)			
N	304	316	0.02
Baseline (mean ± SD)	17.9 ± 15.1	17.3 ± 10.5	(-1.47, 1.50)
Change from baseline (mean ± SD)	-3.6 ± 13.8	-3.2 ± 8.6	
Body Weight (kg)			
N	313	320	0.30
Baseline (mean ± SD)	94.1 ± 17.8	93.3 ± 17.4	(-0.22, 0.81)
Change from baseline (mean ± SD)	0.3 ± 2.9	0.0 ± 3.7	
Body Mass Index (kg/m^2)			
N	313	320	0.08
Baseline (mean ± SD)	31.1 ± 4.7	31.4 ± 4.5	(-0.11, 0.26)
Change from baseline (mean ± SD)	0.1 ± 1.1	0.0 ± 1.3	

[a] CI = Confidence Interval
[b] FORTAMET was clinically similar to immediate-release metformin based on the pre-defined criterion to establish efficacy. While demonstrating clinical similarity, the response to FORTAMET compared to immediate-release metformin was also shown to be statistically smaller as seen by the 95% CI for the treatment difference which did not include zero.

In healthy nondiabetic adults (N=18) receiving 2500 mg q.d. FORTAMET™, the percent of the metformin dose excreted in urine over 24 hours was 40.9% and the renal clearance was 542 ± 310 mL/min. After repeated administration of FORTAMET™, there is little or no accumulation of metformin in plasma, with most of the drug being eliminated via renal excretion over a 24-hour dosing interval. The $t_{1/2}$ was 5.4 hours for FORTAMET™.

Renal clearance of metformin (Table 2) is approximately 3.5 times greater than creatinine clearance, which indicates that tubular secretion is the major route of metformin elimination. Following oral administration, approximately 90% of the absorbed drug is eliminated via the renal route within the first 24 hours, with a plasma elimination half-life of approximately 6.2 hours. In blood, the elimination half-life is approximately 17.6 hours, suggesting that the erythrocyte mass may be a compartment of distribution.

Special Populations

Geriatrics

Limited data from controlled pharmacokinetic studies of immediate-release metformin in healthy elderly subjects suggest that total plasma clearance of metformin is decreased, the half-life is prolonged, and C_{max} is increased, compared to healthy young subjects. From these data, it appears that the change in metformin pharmacokinetics with aging is primarily accounted for by a change in renal function (Table 2). FORTAMET™ treatment should not be initiated in patients ≥ 80 years of age unless measurement of creatinine clearance demonstrates that renal function is not reduced. (See **WARNINGS, PRECAUTIONS** and **DOSAGE AND ADMINISTRATION.**)

Pediatrics

No pharmacokinetic data from studies of pediatric patients are currently available. (See **PRECAUTIONS**.)

Gender

Five studies indicated that with FORTAMET™ treatment, the pharmacokinetic results for males and females were comparable.

[See table 2 above]

Renal Insufficiency

In patients with decreased renal function (based on measured creatinine clearance), the plasma and blood half-life of metformin is prolonged and the renal clearance is decreased in proportion to the decrease in creatinine clearance (Table 2; also see **WARNINGS**).

Hepatic Insufficiency
No pharmacokinetic studies of metformin have been conducted in patients with hepatic insufficiency.

Race
No studies of metformin pharmacokinetic parameters according to race have been performed. In controlled clinical studies of immediate-release metformin in patients with type 2 diabetes, the antihyperglycemic effect was comparable in whites (n=249), blacks (n=51), and Hispanics (n=24).

Clinical Studies
In a double-blind, randomized, active-controlled, multicenter U.S. clinical study, which compared FORTAMET™ q.d. to immediate-release metformin b.i.d., 680 patients with type 2 diabetes who had been taking metformin-containing medication at study entry were randomly assigned in equal numbers to double-blind treatment with either FORTAMET™ or immediate-release metformin. Doses were adjusted during the first six weeks of treatment with study medication based on patients' FPG levels and were then held constant over a period of 20 weeks. The primary efficacy endpoint was the change in HbA_{1c} from baseline to endpoint. The primary objective was to demonstrate the clinical non-inferiority of FORTAMET™ compared to immediate-release metformin on the primary endpoint.
FORTAMET™ and metformin patients had mean HbA_{1c} changes from baseline to endpoint equal to +0.40 and +0.14, respectively (Table 3). The least-square (LS) mean treatment difference was 0.25 (95% CI = 0.14, 0.37) demonstrating that FORTAMET™ was clinically similar to metformin according to the pre-defined criterion to establish efficacy.
[See table 3 on previous page]
Footnote: Patients were taking metformin-containing medications at baseline that were prescribed by their personal physician.
The mean changes for FPG (Table 3) and plasma insulin (Table 3) were small for both FORTAMET™ and immediate-release metformin, and were not clinically meaningful. Seventy-six (22%) and 49 (14%) of the FORTAMET™ and immediate-release patients, respectively, discontinued prematurely from the trial. Eighteen (5%) patients on FORTAMET™ withdrew because of a stated lack of efficacy, as compared with 8 patients (2%) on immediate-release metformin (p=0.047).
Results from this study also indicated that neither FORTAMET™ nor immediate-release metformin were associated with weight gain or increases in body mass index.
A 24-week, double blind, placebo-controlled study of immediate-release metformin plus insulin, versus insulin plus placebo, was conducted in patients with type 2 diabetes who failed to achieve adequate glycemic control on insulin alone (Table 4). Patients randomized to receive immediate-release metformin plus insulin achieved a reduction in HbA_{1c} of 2.10%, compared to a 1.56% reduction in HbA_{1c} achieved by insulin plus placebo. The improvement in glycemic control was achieved at the final study visit with 16% less insulin, 93.0 U/day versus 110.6 U/day, immediate-release metformin plus insulin versus insulin plus placebo, respectively, p=0.04.

Table 4
Combined Immediate-Release Metformin/Insulin vs. Placebo/Insulin: Summary of Mean Changes from Baseline in HbA_{1c} and Daily Insulin Dose

	Immediate-Release Metformin/Insulin (n = 26)	Placebo/Insulin (n = 28)	Treatment difference Mean ± SE
HbA_{1c} (%)			
Baseline	8.95	9.32	
Change at FINAL VISIT	-2.10	-1.56	-0.54 ± 0.43[a]
Insulin Dose (U/day)			
Baseline	93.12	94.64	
Change at FINAL VISIT	-0.15	15.93	-16.08 ± 7.77[b]

[a] Statistically significant using analysis of covariance with baseline as covariate (p=0.04).
Not significant using analysis of variance (values shown in table)
[b] Statistically significant for insulin (p=0.04)

A second double-blind, placebo-controlled study (n=51), with 16 weeks of randomized treatment, demonstrated that in patients with type 2 diabetes controlled on insulin for 8 weeks with an average HbA_{1c} of 7.46 ± 0.97%, the addition of immediate-release metformin maintained similar glycemic control (HbA_{1c} 7.15 ± 0.61 versus 6.97 ± 0.62 for immediate-release metformin plus insulin and placebo plus insulin, respectively) with 19% less insulin versus baseline (reduction of 23.68 ± 30.22 versus an increase of 0.43 ± 25.20 units for immediate-release metformin plus insulin and placebo plus insulin, p<0.01). In addition, this study demonstrated that the combination of immediate-release metformin plus insulin resulted in reduction in body weight of 3.11 ± 4.30 lbs, compared to an increase of 1.30 ± 6.08 lbs for placebo plus insulin, p=0.01.

Pediatric Clinical Studies
No pediatric clinical studies have been conducted with FORTAMET™. In a double-blind, placebo-controlled study in pediatric patients aged 10 to 16 years with type 2 diabetes (mean FPG 182.2 mg/dL), treatment with immediate-release metformin (up to 2000 mg/day) for up to 16 weeks (mean duration of treatment 11 weeks) resulted in a significant mean net reduction in FPG of 64.3 mg/dL compared with placebo (Table 5).

Table 5
Immediate-Release Metformin vs. Placebo (Pediatrics[a]): Summary of Mean Changes from Baseline* in Plasma Glucose and Body Weight at Final Visit

	Immediate-Release Metformin	Placebo	p-Value
FPG (mg/dL)	(n = 37)	(n = 36)	
Baseline	162.4	192.3	
Change at FINAL VISIT	-42.9	21.4	<0.001
Body Weight (lbs)	(n = 39)	(n = 38)	
Baseline	205.3	189.0	
Change at FINAL VISIT	-3.3	-2.0	NS**

[a] Pediatric patients mean age 13.8 years (range 10-16 years)
* All patients on diet therapy at Baseline
**Not statistically significant

INDICATIONS AND USAGE

FORTAMET™ (metformin hydrochloride) Extended-Release Tablets, used as a once per day monotherapy, are indicated as an adjunct to diet and exercise to lower blood glucose. FORTAMET™ can be used concomitantly with a sulfonylurea or insulin to improve glycemic control in adults. FORTAMET™ is indicated in patients 17 years of age and older as either monotherapy or in combination therapy.

CONTRAINDICATIONS

FORTAMET™ is contraindicated in patients with:
1. Renal disease or renal dysfunction (e.g., as suggested by serum creatinine levels ≥1.5 mg/dL [males], ≥1.4 mg/dL [females] or abnormal creatinine clearance) which may also result from conditions such as cardiovascular collapse (shock), acute myocardial infarction, and septicemia (see **WARNINGS** and **PRECAUTIONS**).
2. Congestive heart failure requiring pharmacologic treatment.
3. Known hypersensitivity to metformin.
4. Acute or chronic metabolic acidosis, including diabetic ketoacidosis, with or without coma. Diabetic ketoacidosis should be treated with insulin.

FORTAMET™ should be temporarily discontinued in patients undergoing radiologic studies involving intravascular administration of iodinated contrast materials, because use of such products may result in acute alteration of renal function. (See also **PRECAUTIONS**.)

WARNINGS

Lactic Acidosis:
Lactic acidosis is a rare, but serious, metabolic complication that can occur due to metformin accumulation during treatment with FORTAMET™ (metformin hydrochloride) Extended-Release Tablets; when it occurs, it is fatal in approximately 50% of cases. Lactic acidosis may also occur in association with a number of pathophysiologic conditions, including diabetes mellitus, and whenever there is significant tissue hypoperfusion and hypoxemia. Lactic acidosis is characterized by elevated blood lactate levels (>5 mmol/L), decreased blood pH, electrolyte disturbances with an increased anion gap, and an increased lactate/pyruvate ratio. When metformin is implicated as the cause of lactic acidosis, metformin plasma levels >5 µg/mL are generally found.
The reported incidence of lactic acidosis in patients receiving metformin hydrochloride is very low (approximately 0.03 cases/1000 patient-years, with approximately 0.015 fatal cases/1000 patient-years). Reported cases have occurred primarily in diabetic patients with significant renal insufficiency, including both intrinsic renal disease and renal hypoperfusion, often in the setting of multiple concomitant medical/surgical problems and multiple concomitant medications. Patients with congestive heart failure requiring pharmacologic management, in particular those with unstable or acute congestive heart failure who are at risk of hypoperfusion and hypoxemia, are at increased risk of lactic acidosis. The risk of lactic acidosis increases with the degree of renal dysfunction and the patient's age. The risk of lactic acidosis may, therefore, be significantly decreased by regular monitoring of renal function in patients taking FORTAMET™ (metformin hydrochloride) Extended-Release Tablets and by use of the minimum effective dose of FORTAMET™. In particular, treatment of the elderly should be accompanied by careful monitoring of renal function. FORTAMET™ treatment should not be initiated in patients ≥80 years of age unless measurement of creatinine clearance demonstrates that renal function is not reduced, as these patients are more susceptible to developing lactic acidosis. In addition, FORTAMET™ should be promptly withheld in the presence of any condition associated with hypoxemia, dehydration, or sepsis. Because impaired hepatic function may significantly limit the ability to clear lactate, FORTAMET™ should generally be avoided in patients with clinical or laboratory evidence of hepatic disease. Patients should be cautioned against excessive alcohol intake, either acute or chronic, when taking FORTAMET™, since alcohol potentiates the effects of metformin hydrochloride on lactate metabolism. In addition, FORTAMET™ should be temporarily discontinued prior to any intravascular radiocontrast study and for any surgical procedure (see also PRECAUTIONS).
The onset of lactic acidosis often is subtle, and accompanied only by nonspecific symptoms such as malaise, myalgias, respiratory distress, increasing somnolence, and nonspecific abdominal distress. There may be associated hypothermia, hypotension, and resistant bradyarrhythmias with more marked acidosis. The patient and the patient's physician must be aware of the possible importance of such symptoms and the patient should be instructed to notify the physician immediately if they occur (see also PRECAUTIONS). FORTAMET™ should be withdrawn until the situation is clarified. Serum electrolytes, ketones, blood glucose and, if indicated, blood pH, lactate levels, and even blood metformin levels may be useful. Once a patient is stabilized on any dose level of FORTAMET™, gastrointestinal symptoms, which are common during initiation of therapy, are unlikely to be drug related. Later occurrence of gastrointestinal symptoms could be due to lactic acidosis or other serious disease.
Levels of fasting venous plasma lactate above the upper limit of normal but less than 5 mmol/L in patients taking FORTAMET™ do not necessarily indicate impending lactic acidosis and may be explainable by other mechanisms, such as poorly controlled diabetes or obesity, vigorous physical activity, or technical problems in sample handling. (See alsoPRECAUTIONS.)
Lactic acidosis should be suspected in any diabetic patient with metabolic acidosis lacking evidence of ketoacidosis (ketonuria and ketonemia).
Lactic acidosis is a medical emergency that must be treated in a hospital setting. In a patient with lactic acidosis who is taking FORTAMET™, the drug should be discontinued immediately and general supportive measures promptly instituted. Because metformin hydrochloride is dialyzable (with a clearance of up to 170 mL/min under good hemodynamic conditions), prompt hemodialysis is recommended to correct the acidosis and remove the accumulated metformin. Such management often results in prompt reversal of symptoms and recovery. (See also CONTRAINDICATIONS and PRECAUTIONS.)

PRECAUTIONS

General
Monitoring of renal function – Metformin is known to be substantially excreted by the kidney, and the risk of metformin accumulation and lactic acidosis increases with the degree of impairment of renal function. Thus, patients with serum creatinine levels above the upper limit of normal for their age should not receive FORTAMET™. In patients with advanced age, FORTAMET™ should be carefully titrated to establish the minimum dose for adequate glycemic effect, because aging is associated with reduced renal function. In elderly patients, particularly those ≥80 years of age, renal function should be monitored regularly and, generally, FORTAMET™ should not be titrated to the maximum dose (see **WARNINGS** and **DOSAGE AND ADMINISTRATION**).
Before initiation of FORTAMET™ therapy and at least annually thereafter, renal function should be assessed and verified as normal. In patients in whom development of renal dysfunction is anticipated, renal function should be assessed more frequently and FORTAMET™ discontinued if evidence of renal impairment is present.
Use of concomitant medications that may affect renal function or metformin disposition – Concomitant medication(s) that may affect renal function or result in significant hemodynamic change or may interfere with the disposition of metformin, such as cationic drugs that are eliminated by renal tubular secretion (see **PRECAUTIONS: Drug Interactions**), should be used with caution.
Radiologic studies involving the use of intravascular iodinated contrast materials (for example, intravenous urogram, intravenous cholangiography, angiography, and computed tomography (CT) scans with intravascular contrast materials) – Intravascular contrast studies with iodinated materials can lead to acute alteration of renal function and have been associated with lactic acidosis in patients receiving metformin (see **CONTRAINDICATIONS**). Therefore, in patients in whom any such study is planned, FORTAMET™ should be temporarily discontinued at the time of or prior to the procedure, and withheld for 48 hours subsequent to the procedure and reinstituted only after renal function has been re-evaluated and found to be normal.
Hypoxic states – Cardiovascular collapse (shock) from whatever cause, acute congestive heart failure, acute myocardial infarction and other conditions characterized by

Continued on next page

Fortamet—Cont.

hypoxemia have been associated with lactic acidosis and may also cause prerenal azotemia. When such events occur in patients on FORTAMET™ therapy, the drug should be promptly discontinued.

Surgical procedures – FORTAMET™ therapy should be temporarily suspended for any surgical procedure (except minor procedures not associated with restricted intake of food and fluids) and should not be restarted until the patient's oral intake has resumed and renal function has been evaluated as normal.

Alcohol intake – Alcohol is known to potentiate the effect of metformin on lactate metabolism. Patients, therefore, should be warned against excessive alcohol intake, acute or chronic, while receiving FORTAMET™.

Impaired hepatic function – Since impaired hepatic function has been associated with some cases of lactic acidosis, FORTAMET™ should generally be avoided in patients with clinical or laboratory evidence of hepatic disease.

Vitamin B_{12} levels – In controlled clinical trials of immediate-release metformin of 29 weeks duration, a decrease to subnormal levels of previously normal serum Vitamin B_{12} levels, without clinical manifestations, was observed in approximately 7% of patients. Such decrease, possibly due to interference with B_{12} absorption from the B_{12}-intrinsic factor complex, is, however, very rarely associated with anemia and appears to be rapidly reversible with discontinuation of immediate-release metformin or Vitamin B_{12} supplementation. Measurement of hematologic parameters on an annual basis is advised in patients on FORTAMET™ and any apparent abnormalities should be appropriately investigated and managed (see **PRECAUTIONS: Laboratory Tests**). Certain individuals (those with inadequate Vitamin B_{12} or calcium intake or absorption) appear to be predisposed to developing subnormal Vitamin B_{12} levels. In these patients, routine serum Vitamin B_{12} measurements at two- to three-year intervals may be useful.

Change in clinical status of patients with previously controlled type 2 diabetes – A patient with type 2 diabetes previously well controlled on FORTAMET™ who develops laboratory abnormalities or clinical illness (especially vague and poorly defined illness) should be evaluated promptly for evidence of ketoacidosis or lactic acidosis. Evaluation should include serum electrolytes and ketones, blood glucose and, if indicated, blood pH, lactate, pyruvate, and metformin levels. If acidosis of either form occurs, FORTAMET™ must be stopped immediately and other appropriate corrective measures initiated (see also **WARNINGS**).

Hypoglycemia – Hypoglycemia does not occur in patients receiving FORTAMET™ alone under usual circumstances of use, but could occur when caloric intake is deficient, when strenuous exercise is not compensated by caloric supplementation, or during concomitant use with other glucose-lowering agents (such as sulfonylureas and insulin) or ethanol. Elderly, debilitated, or malnourished patients, and those with adrenal or pituitary insufficiency or alcohol intoxication are particularly susceptible to hypoglycemic effects. Hypoglycemia may be difficult to recognize in the elderly, and in people who are taking beta-adrenergic blocking drugs.

Loss of control of blood glucose – When a patient stabilized on any diabetic regimen is exposed to stress such as fever, trauma, infection , or surgery, a temporary loss of glycemic control may occur. At such times, it may be necessary to withhold FORTAMET™ and temporarily administer insulin. FORTAMET™ may be reinstituted after the acute episode is resolved.

The effectiveness of oral antidiabetic drugs in lowering blood glucose to a targeted level decreases in many patients over a period of time. This phenomenon, which may be due to progression of the underlying disease or to diminished responsiveness to the drug, is known as secondary failure, to distinguish it from primary failure in which the drug is ineffective during initial therapy. Should secondary failure occur with FORTAMET™ or sulfonylurea monotherapy, combined therapy with FORTAMET™ and sulfonylurea may result in a response. Should secondary failure occur with combined FORTAMET™/sulfonylurea therapy, it may be necessary to consider therapeutic alternatives including initiation of insulin therapy.

Information for Patients

Patients should be informed of the potential risks and benefits of FORTAMET™ and of alternative modes of therapy. They should also be informed about the importance of adherence to dietary instructions, of a regular exercise program, and of regular testing of blood glucose, glycosylated hemoglobin, renal function, and hematologic parameters.

The risks of lactic acidosis, its symptoms, and conditions that predispose to its development, as noted in the **WARNINGS** and **PRECAUTIONS** sections, should be explained to patients. Patients should be advised to discontinue FORTAMET™ immediately and to promptly notify their health practitioner if unexplained hyperventilation, myalgia, malaise, unusual somnolence, or other nonspecific symptoms occur. Once a patient is stabilized on any dose level of FORTAMET™, gastrointestinal symptoms, which are common during initiation of metformin therapy, are unlikely to be drug related. Later occurrence of gastrointestinal symptoms could be due to lactic acidosis or other serious disease.

Patients should be counseled against excessive alcohol intake, either acute or chronic, while receiving FORTAMET™.

FORTAMET™ alone does not usually cause hypoglycemia, although it may occur when FORTAMET™ is used in conjunction with oral sulfonylureas and insulin. When initiating combination therapy, the risks of hypoglycemia, its symptoms and treatment, and conditions that predispose to its development should be explained to patients and responsible family members. (See **Patient Information** Printed Below.)

Patients should be informed that FORTAMET™ must be swallowed whole and not chewed, cut, or crushed, and that the inactive ingredients may occasionally be eliminated in the feces as a soft mass that may resemble the original tablet. (See **Patient Information**.)

Laboratory Tests

Response to all diabetic therapies should be monitored by periodic measurements of fasting blood glucose and glycosylated hemoglobin levels, with a goal of decreasing these levels toward the normal range. During initial dose titration, fasting glucose can be used to determine the therapeutic response. Thereafter, both glucose and glycosylated hemoglobin should be monitored. Measurements of glycosylated hemoglobin may be especially useful for evaluating long-term control (see also **DOSAGE AND ADMINISTRATION**).

Initial and periodic monitoring of hematologic parameters (e.g., hemoglobin/hematocrit and red blood cell indices) and renal function (serum creatinine) should be performed, at least on an annual basis. While megaloblastic anemia has rarely been seen with immediate-release metformin therapy, if this is suspected, Vitamin B_{12} deficiency should be excluded.

Drug Interactions (Clinical Evaluation of Drug Interactions Conducted with Immediate-Release Metformin)

Glyburide – In a single-dose interaction study in type 2 diabetes patients, co-administration of metformin and glyburide did not result in any changes in either metformin pharmacokinetics or pharmacodynamics. Decreases in glyburide AUC and C_{max} were observed, but were highly variable. The single-dose nature of this study and the lack of correlation between glyburide blood levels and pharmacodynamic effects, makes the clinical significance of this interaction uncertain. (See **DOSAGE AND ADMINISTRATION: Concomitant FORTAMET™ and Oral Sulfonylurea Therapy in Adult Patients.**)

Furosemide – A single-dose, metformin-furosemide drug interaction study in healthy subjects demonstrated that pharmacokinetic parameters of both compounds were affected by co-administration. Furosemide increased the metformin plasma and blood C_{max} by 22% and blood AUC by 15%, without any significant change in metformin renal clearance. When administered with metformin, the C_{max} and AUC of furosemide were 31% and 12% smaller, respectively, than when administered alone, and the terminal half-life was decreased by 32%, without any significant change in furosemide renal clearance. No information is available about the interaction of metformin and furosemide when co-administered chronically.

Nifedipine – A single-dose, metformin-nifedipine drug interaction study in normal healthy volunteers demonstrated that co-administration of nifedipine increased plasma metformin C_{max} and AUC by 20% and 9%, respectively, and increased the amount excreted in the urine. T_{max} and half-life were unaffected. Nifedipine appears to enhance the absorption of metformin. Metformin had minimal effects on nifedipine.

Cationic drugs – Cationic drugs (e.g., amiloride, digoxin, morphine, procainamide, quinidine, quinine, ranitidine, triamterene, trimethoprim, or vancomycin) that are eliminated by renal tubular secretion theoretically have the potential for interaction with metformin by competing for common renal tubular transport systems. Such interaction between metformin and oral cimetidine has been observed in normal healthy volunteers in both single- and multiple-dose, metformin-cimetidine drug interaction studies, with a 60% increase in peak metformin plasma and whole blood concentrations and a 40% increase in plasma and whole blood metformin AUC. There was no change in elimination half-life in the single-dose study. Metformin had no effect on cimetidine pharmacokinetics. Although such interactions remain theoretical (except for cimetidine), careful patient monitoring and dose adjustment of FORTAMET™ and/or the interfering drug is recommended in patients who are taking cationic medications that are excreted via the proximal renal tubular secretory system.

Other – Certain drugs tend to produce hyperglycemia and may lead to loss of glycemic control. These drugs include the thiazides and other diuretics, corticosteroids, phenothiazines, thyroid products, estrogens, oral contraceptives, phenytoin, nicotinic acid, sympathomimetics, calcium channel blocking drugs, and isoniazid. When such drugs are administered to a patient receiving FORTAMET™, the patient should be closely observed for loss of blood glucose control. When such drugs are withdrawn from a patient receiving FORTAMET™, the patient should be observed closely for hypoglycemia.

In healthy volunteers, the pharmacokinetics of metformin and propranolol, and metformin and ibuprofen were not affected when co-administered in single-dose interaction studies.

Metformin is negligibly bound to plasma proteins and is, therefore, less likely to interact with highly protein-bound drugs such as salicylates, sulfonamides, chloramphenicol, and probenecid, as compared to the sulfonylureas, which are extensively bound to serum proteins.

Carcinogenesis, Mutagenesis, Impairment of Fertility

Long-term carcinogenicity studies with metformin have been performed in rats (dosing duration of 104 weeks) and mice (dosing duration of 91 weeks) at doses up to and including 900 mg/kg/day and 1500 mg/kg/day, respectively. These doses are both approximately four times the maximum recommended human daily dose of 2000 mg based on body surface area comparisons. No evidence of carcinogenicity with metformin was found in either male or female mice. Similarly, there was no tumorigenic potential observed with metformin in male rats. There was, however, an increased incidence of benign stromal uterine polyps in female rats treated with 900 mg/kg/day.

There was no evidence of mutagenic potential of metformin in the following *in vitro* tests: Ames test (*S. typhimurium*), gene mutation test (mouse lymphoma cells), or chromosomal aberrations test (human lymphocytes). Results in the *in vivo* mouse micronucleus test were also negative.

Fertility of male or female rats was unaffected by metformin when administered at doses as high as 600 mg/kg/day, which is approximately three times the maximum recommended human daily dose based on body surface area comparisons.

Pregnancy

Teratogenic Effects: Pregnancy Category B

Recent information strongly suggests that abnormal blood glucose levels during pregnancy are associated with a higher incidence of congenital abnormalities. Most experts recommend that insulin be used during pregnancy to maintain blood glucose levels as close to normal as possible. Because animal reproduction studies are not always predictive of human response, FORTAMET™ should not be used during pregnancy unless clearly needed.

There are no adequate and well-controlled studies in pregnant women with immediate-release metformin or FORTAMET™. Metformin was not teratogenic in rats and rabbits at doses up to 600 mg/kg/day. This represents an exposure of about two and six times the maximum recommended human daily dose of 2000 mg based on body surface area comparisons for rats and rabbits, respectively. Determination of fetal concentrations demonstrated a partial placental barrier to metformin.

Nursing Mothers

Studies in lactating rats show that metformin is excreted into milk and reaches levels comparable to those in plasma. Similar studies have not been conducted in nursing mothers. Because the potential for hypoglycemia in nursing infants may exist, a decision should be made whether to discontinue nursing or to discontinue the drug, taking into account the importance of the drug to the mother. If FORTAMET™ is discontinued, and if diet alone is inadequate for controlling blood glucose, insulin therapy should be considered.

Pediatric Use

No pediatric clinical studies have been conducted with FORTAMET™. The safety and effectiveness of immediate-release metformin for the treatment of type 2 diabetes have been established in pediatric patients ages 10 to 16 years (studies have not been conducted in pediatric patients below the age of 10 years). Use of immediate-release metformin in this age group is supported by evidence from adequate and well-controlled studies of immediate-release metformin in adults with additional data from a controlled clinical study in pediatric patients ages 10-16 years with type 2 diabetes, which demonstrated a similar response in glycemic control to that seen in adults. (See **CLINICAL PHARMACOLOGY: Pediatric Clinical Studies.**) In this study, adverse effects were similar to those described in adults. (See **ADVERSE REACTIONS: Pediatric Patients.**) A maximum daily dose of 2000 mg of immediate-release metformin is recommended.

The safety and efficacy of FORTAMET™ has not been evaluated in pediatric patients.

Geriatric Use

Of the 389 patients who received FORTAMET™ in controlled Phase III clinical studies, 26.5% [103/389] were 65 years and older. No overall differences in effectiveness or safety were observed between these patients and younger patients.

Controlled clinical studies of immediate-release metformin did not include sufficient numbers of elderly patients to determine whether they respond differently from younger patients, although other reported clinical experience has not identified differences in responses between the elderly and younger patients. Metformin is known to be substantially excreted by the kidney and because of the risk of serious adverse reactions to the drug is greater in patients with impaired renal function, immediate-release metformin should only be used in patients with normal renal function (see **CONTRAINDICATIONS, WARNINGS**, and **CLINICAL PHARMACOLOGY: Pharmacokinetics**). Because aging is associated with reduced renal function, immediate-release metformin should be used with caution as age increases. Care should be taken in dose selection and should be based on careful and regular monitoring of renal function. Generally, elderly patients should not be titrated to the maximum dose of immediate-release metformin (see also **WARNINGS** and **DOSAGE AND ADMINISTRATION**).

ADVERSE REACTIONS

FORTAMET™ Clinical Studies

In the controlled clinical studies of FORTAMET™ in patients with type 2 diabetes, a total of 424 patients received

FORTAMET™ therapy (up to 2500 mg/day) and 430 patients received immediate-release metformin. Adverse reactions reported in ≥5% of the FORTAMET™ or immediate-release metformin patients are listed in Table 6. These pooled results show that the most frequently reported adverse reactions in the FORTAMET™ group were infection, diarrhea, and nausea. Similar incidences of these adverse reactions were seen in the immediate-release metformin group.

Table 6
Number and Percentage of Patients With the Most Common (Incidence ≥5%) Treatment-Emergent Signs or Symptoms by Body System and Preferred Term – Pooled Phase II and III Studies

Body System Preferred Term	FORTAMET™ (N=424) n	(%)	Immediate-Release Metformin (N=430) n	(%)
Body as a Whole				
Accidental Injury	31	(7.3)	24	(5.6)
Headache	20	(4.7)	22	(5.1)
Infection	87	(20.5)	90	(20.9)
Digestive System				
Diarrhea	71	(16.7)	51	(11.9)
Dyspepsia	18	(4.2)	22	(5.1)
Nausea	36	(8.5)	32	(7.4)
Respiratory System				
Rhinitis	18	(4.2)	24	(5.6)

The most frequent adverse events thought to be related to FORTAMET™ were diarrhea, nausea, dyspepsia, flatulence, and abdominal pain. The frequency of dyspepsia was 4.2% in the FORTAMET™ group compared to 5.1% in the immediate-release group, the frequency of flatulence was 3.5% in the FORTAMET™ group compared to 3.7% in the immediate-release group, and the frequency of abdominal pain was 3.3% in the FORTAMET™ group compared to 4.4% in the immediate-release group.
In the controlled studies, 4.7% of patients treated with FORTAMET™ and 4.9% of patients treated with immediate-release metformin were discontinued due to adverse events.

Immediate-Release Metformin

Immediate-Release Metformin Phase III Clinical Studies

In a U.S. double-blind clinical study of immediate-release metformin in patients with type 2 diabetes, a total of 141 patients received immediate-release metformin therapy (up to 2550 mg per day) and 145 patients received placebo. Adverse reactions reported in greater than 5% of the immediate-release metformin patients, and that were more common in immediate-release metformin- than placebo-treated patients, are listed in Table 7.

Table 7
Most Common Adverse Reactions (>5.0%) in a Placebo-Controlled Clinical Study of Immediate-Release Metformin Monotherapy*

Adverse Reaction	Immediate-Release Metformin Monotherapy (n = 141) % of Patients	Placebo (n = 145)
Diarrhea	53.2	11.7
Nausea/Vomiting	25.5	8.3
Flatulence	12.1	5.5
Asthenia	9.2	5.5
Indigestion	7.1	4.1
Abdominal Discomfort	6.4	4.8
Headache	5.7	4.8

* Reactions that were more common in immediate-release metformin than placebo-treated patients

Diarrhea led to discontinuation of study medication in 6% of patients treated with immediate-release metformin. Additionally, the following adverse reactions were reported in ≥1.0 - ≤5.0% of immediate-release metformin patients and were more commonly reported with immediate-release metformin than placebo: abnormal stools, hypoglycemia, myalgia, lightheaded, dyspnea, nail disorder, rash, sweating increased, taste disorder, chest discomfort, chills, flu syndrome, flushing, palpitation.

Pediatric Patients

No pediatric clinical studies have been conducted with FORTAMET™. In clinical trials with immediate-release metformin in pediatric patients with type 2 diabetes, the profile of adverse reactions was similar to that observed in adults.

OVERDOSAGE

Hypoglycemia has not been seen even with ingestion of up to 85 grams of immediate-release metformin, although lactic acidosis has occurred in such circumstances (see **WARNINGS**). Metformin is dialyzable with a clearance of up to 170 mL/min under good hemodynamic conditions. Therefore, hemodialysis may be useful for removal of accumulated drug from patients in whom metformin overdosage is suspected.

DOSAGE AND ADMINISTRATION

There is no fixed dosage regimen for the management of hyperglycemia in patients with type 2 diabetes with FORTAMET™ or any other pharmacologic agent. Dosage of FORTAMET™ must be individualized on the basis of both effectiveness and tolerance, while not exceeding the maximum recommended daily dose. The maximum recommended daily dose of FORTAMET™ Extended-Release Tablets in adults is 2500 mg.
FORTAMET™ should generally be given once daily with the evening meal. FORTAMET™ should be started at a low dose, with gradual dose escalation, both to reduce gastrointestinal side effects and to permit identification of the minimum dose required for adequate glycemic control of the patient.
During treatment initiation and dose titration (see **Recommended Dosing Schedule**), fasting plasma glucose should be used to determine the therapeutic response to FORTAMET™ and identify the minimum effective dose for the patient. Thereafter, glycosylated hemoglobin should be measured at intervals of approximately three months. The therapeutic goal should be to decrease both fasting plasma glucose and glycosylated hemoglobin levels to normal or near normal by using the lowest effective dose of FORTAMET™, either when used as monotherapy or in combination with sulfonylurea or insulin.
Monitoring of blood glucose and glycosylated hemoglobin will also permit detection of primary failure, i.e., inadequate lowering of blood glucose at the maximum recommended dose of medication, and secondary failure, i.e., loss of an adequate blood glucose lowering response after an initial period of effectiveness.
Short-term administration of FORTAMET™ may be sufficient during periods of transient loss of control in patients usually well-controlled on diet alone.

Recommended Dosing Schedule

The usual starting dose of FORTAMET™ (metformin hydrochloride) Extended-Release Tablets is 1000 mg once daily with the evening meal, although 500 mg may be utilized when clinically appropriate. Dosage increases should be made in increments of 500 mg weekly, up to a maximum of 2500 mg once daily with the evening meal. (See **CLINICAL PHARMACOLOGY, Clinical Studies.**)
In randomized trials, patients currently treated with immediate-release metformin were switched to FORTAMET™. Results of this trial suggest that patients receiving immediate-release metformin treatment may be safely switched to FORTAMET™ once daily at the same total daily dose, up to 2500 mg once daily. Following a switch from immediate-release metformin to FORTAMET™, glycemic control should be closely monitored and dosage adjustments made accordingly (see **CLINICAL PHARMACOLOGY, Clinical Studies.**)

Pediatrics – There is no pediatric information available for FORTAMET™.

Transfer From Other Antidiabetic Therapy

When transferring patients from standard oral hypoglycemic agents other than chlorpropamide to FORTAMET™, no transition period generally is necessary. When transferring patients from chlorpropamide, care should be exercised during the first two weeks because of the prolonged retention of chlorpropamide in the body, leading to overlapping drug effects and possible hypoglycemia.

Concomitant FORTAMET™ and Oral Sulfonylurea Therapy in Adult Patients

If patients have not responded to four weeks of the maximum dose of FORTAMET™ monotherapy, consideration should be given to gradual addition of an oral sulfonylurea while continuing FORTAMET™ at the maximum dose, even if prior primary or secondary failure to a sulfonylurea has occurred. Clinical and pharmacokinetic drug-drug interaction data are currently available only for metformin plus glyburide (also known as glibenclamide). With concomitant FORTAMET and sulfonylurea therapy, the desired control of blood glucose may be obtained by adjusting the dose of each drug. However, attempts should be made to identify the minimum effective dose of each drug to achieve this goal. With concomitant FORTAMET™ and sulfonylurea therapy, the risk of hypoglycemia associated with sulfonylurea therapy continues and may be increased. Appropriate precautions should be taken. (See Package Insert of the respective sulfonylurea.)
If patients have not satisfactorily responded to one to three months of concomitant therapy with the maximum dose of FORTAMET™ and the maximum dose of an oral sulfonylurea, consider therapeutic alternatives including switching to insulin with or without FORTAMET™.

Concomitant FORTAMET™ and Insulin Therapy in Adult Patients

The current insulin dose should be continued upon initiation of FORTAMET™ therapy. FORTAMET™ therapy should be initiated at 500 mg once daily in patients on insulin therapy. For patients not responding adequately, the dose of FORTAMET™ should be increased by 500 mg after approximately 1 week and by 500 mg every week thereafter until adequate glycemic control is achieved. The maximum recommended daily dose for FORTAMET™ Extended-Release Tablets is 2500 mg. It is recommended that the insulin dose be decreased by 10% to 25% when fasting plasma glucose concentrations decrease to less than 120 mg/dL in patients receiving concomitant insulin and FORTAMET™. Further adjustment should be individualized based on glucose-lowering response.

Specific Patient Populations

FORTAMET™ is not recommended for use in pregnancy, and is not recommended in patients below the age of 17 years.
The initial and maintenance dosing of FORTAMET™ should be conservative in patients with advanced age, due to the potential for decreased renal function in this population. Any dosage adjustment should be based on a careful assessment of renal function. Generally, elderly, debilitated, and malnourished patients should not be titrated to the maximum dose of FORTAMET™.
Monitoring of renal function is necessary to aid in prevention of lactic acidosis, particularly in the elderly. (See **WARNINGS.**)

HOW SUPPLIED

FORTAMET™ (metformin hydrochloride) Extended-Release Tablets are supplied as biconvex-shaped, film-coated extended-release tablets containing 500 mg or 1000 mg of metformin hydrochloride.
NDC 62022 574 60: 500 mg extended-release white-colored tablets imprinted with Andrx logo and 574 on one side, bottles of 60.
NDC 62022 575 60: 1000 mg extended-release white-colored tablets imprinted Andrx logo and 575 on one side, bottles of 60.

STORAGE

Store at 25°C (77°F); excursions permitted to 15°-30°C (59°-86°F) [see USP Controlled Room Temperature]. Keep tightly closed (protect from moisture). Protect from light. Avoid excessive heat and humidity.

Distributed by:
Andrx Laboratories, Inc.
Weston, Florida 33331
Manufactured by:
Andrx Pharmaceuticals, Inc.
Ft. Lauderdale, Florida 33314

7420
Rev. 04/04

PATIENT INFORMATION ABOUT FORTAMET™

(metformin hydrochloride) extended-release tablets

Q1. Why do I need to take FORTAMET™?

Your doctor has prescribed FORTAMET™ to treat your type 2 diabetes, a condition in which blood sugar (blood glucose) is elevated. There are two types of diabetes. FORTAMET™ is indicated for the most common type, known as type 2 diabetes.

Q2. Why is it important to control type 2 diabetes?

Type 2 diabetes has multiple possible complications, including blindness, kidney failure, and circulatory and heart problems. Lowering your blood sugar to a normal level may prevent or delay these complications.

Q3. How is type 2 diabetes usually controlled?

High blood sugar can be lowered by diet and exercise, by a number of oral medications and by insulin injections. Your doctor may recommend that you try lifestyle modifications such as improved diet and exercise before initiating drug treatment for type 2 diabetes. Each patient will be treated individually by his or her physician, and should follow all treatment recommendations.

Q4. Does FORTAMET™ work differently from other glucose-control medications?

Yes. FORTAMET™, as well as other formulations of metformin, lowers the amount of sugar in your blood by controlling how much sugar is released by the liver. FORTAMET™ (metformin hydrochloride) does not cause your body to produce more insulin. FORTAMET™ rarely causes hypoglycemia (low blood sugar) and it does not usually cause weight gain when taken alone. However, if you do not eat enough, if you take other medications to lower blood sugar, or if you drink alcohol, you can develop hypoglycemia. Specifically, when FORTAMET™ is taken together with a sulfonylurea or with insulin, hypoglycemia and weight gain are more likely to occur.

Q5. What happens if my blood sugar is still too high?

If your blood sugar is high, consult your physician. When blood sugar cannot be lowered enough by either FORTAMET™ (metformin hydrochloride) Extended-Release Tablets or a sulfonylurea, the two medications can be effective when taken together. Other alternatives involve switching to other oral antidiabetic drugs (e.g., alpha glucoside inhibitors or glitazones). FORTAMET™ may be stopped and replaced with other drugs and/or insulin. If you are unable to maintain your blood sugar with diet, exercise and glucose-control medications taken orally, then your doctor may prescribe injectable insulin to control your diabetes.

Continued on next page

Fortamet—Cont.

Q6. Why should I take FORTAMET in addition to insulin if I am already on insulin alone?

Adding FORTAMET™ to insulin can help you better control your blood sugar while reducing the insulin dose and possibly reducing your weight.

Q7. Can FORTAMET™ cause side effects?

FORTAMET™, like all blood sugar-lowering medications, can cause side effects in some patients. Most of these side effects are minor and will go away after you've taken FORTAMET™ for a while. However, there are also serious but rare side effects related to FORTAMET™ (see below).

Q8. What kind of side effects can FORTAMET™ cause?

If side effects occur, they usually occur during the first few weeks of therapy. They are normally minor ones such as diarrhea, nausea, abdominal pain and upset stomach. FORTAMET™ is generally taken with meals, which reduce these side effects.

Although these side effects are likely to go away, call your doctor if you have severe discomfort or if these effects last for more than a few weeks. Some patients may need to have their doses lowered or stop taking FORTAMET™, either temporarily or permanently. You should tell your doctor if the problems come back or start later on during the therapy.

WARNING: A rare number of people who have taken metformin have developed a serious condition called lactic acidosis. Properly functioning kidneys are needed to help prevent lactic acidosis. You should not take FORTAMET™ if you have impaired kidney function, as measured by a blood test (see Q9-13).

Q9. Are there any serious side effects that FORTAMET™ can cause?

FORTAMET™ rarely causes serious side effects. The most serious side effect that FORTAMET™ can cause is called lactic acidosis.

Q10. What is lactic acidosis and can it happen to me?

Lactic acidosis is caused by a build-up of lactic acid in the blood. Lactic acidosis associated with metformin is rare and has occurred mostly in people whose kidneys were not working normally. Lactic acidosis has been reported in about one in 33,000 patients taking metformin over the course of a year. Although rare, if lactic acidosis does occur, it can be fatal in up to half the cases.

It is also important for your liver to be working normally when you take FORTAMET™. Your liver helps to remove lactic acid from your bloodstream. Your doctor will monitor your diabetes and may perform blood tests on you from time to time to make sure your kidneys and your liver are functioning normally. There is no evidence that FORTAMET™ causes harm to the kidneys or liver.

Q11. Are there other risk factors for lactic acidosis?

Your risk of developing lactic acidosis from taking FORTAMET™ is very low as long as your kidneys and liver are healthy. However, some factors can increase your risk because they can affect kidney and liver function. You should discuss your risk with your physician. You should not take FORTAMET™ if:

- You have some forms of kidney or liver problems
- You have congestive heart failure which is treated with medications, e.g., digoxin (Lanoxin®) or furosemide (Lasix®)
- You drink alcohol excessively (all the time or short-term "binge" drinking)
- You are seriously dehydrated (have lost a large amount of body fluids)
- You are going to have, within a few days, certain x-ray tests with injectable contrast agents
- You are going to have surgery
- You develop a serious condition such as a heart attack, severe infection, or a stroke
- You are 80 years of age or older and have NOT had your kidney function tested

Q12. What are the symptoms of lactic acidosis?

Some of the symptoms include feeling very weak, tired or uncomfortable, unusual muscle pain, trouble breathing, unusual or unexpected stomach discomfort, feeling cold, feeling dizzy or lightheaded, or suddenly developing a slow or irregular heartbeat. If you notice these symptoms, or if your medical condition has suddenly changed, stop taking FORTAMET™ and call your doctor right away. Lactic acidosis is a medical emergency that must be treated in a hospital.

Q13. What does my doctor need to know to decrease my risk of lactic acidosis?

Tell your doctor if you have an illness that results in severe vomiting, diarrhea and/or fever, or if your intake of fluids is generally reduced. These situations can lead to severe dehydration, and it may be necessary to stop taking FORTAMET™ temporarily. You should let your doctor know if you are going to have any surgery or specialized x-ray procedures that require injection of contrast agents. FORTAMET™ therapy will need to be stopped temporarily in such instances.

Q14. Can I take FORTAMET™ with other medications?

Remind your doctor and/or pharmacist that you are taking FORTAMET™ when any new drug is prescribed or a change is made in how you take a drug already prescribed. FORTAMET™ may interfere with the way some drugs work and some drugs may interfere with the action of FORTAMET™.

Q15. What if I become pregnant while taking FORTAMET™?

Tell your doctor if you plan to become pregnant or have become pregnant. As with other oral glucose-control medications, you should not take FORTAMET™ during pregnancy. Usually your doctor will prescribe insulin while you are pregnant.

Q16. How do I take FORTAMET™?

FORTAMET™ tablets should be swallowed whole. FORTAMET™ should not be cut, crushed, or chewed. FORTAMET™ should be taken once a day with food. You will be started on a low dose of FORTAMET™ and your dosage will be increased gradually until your blood sugar is controlled.

Q17. Where can I get more information about FORTAMET™?

This leaflet is a summary of the most important information about FORTAMET™. If you have any questions or problems, you should talk to your doctor or other healthcare provider about type 2 diabetes as well as FORTAMET™ and its side effects.

Distributed by:
Andrx Laboratories, Inc.
Weston, Florida 33331
Manufactured by:
Andrx Pharmaceuticals, Inc.
Ft. Lauderdale, Florida 33314
www.Fortamet.com

7446
Rev. 02/04

Arco Pharmaceuticals, Inc.
105 ORVILLE DRIVE
BOHEMIA, NY 11716

Direct Inquiries to:
Customer Service Department
1-800-645-5412

MEGA-B® OTC
(super potency vitamin B complex, sugar & starch free)

COMPOSITION

Each Mega-B Tablet contains the following Mega Vitamins:

B_1 (Thiamine Mononitrate)	100 mg.
B_2 (Riboflavin)	100 mg.
B_6 (Pyridoxine Hydrochloride)	100 mg.
B_{12} (Cyanocobalamin)	100 mcg.
Choline Bitartrate	100 mg.
Inositol	100 mg.
Niacinamide	100 mg.
Folic Acid	100 mcg.
Pantothenic Acid	100 mg.
d-Biotin	100 mcg.
Para-Aminobenzoic Acid (PABA)	100 mg.

In a base of yeast to provide the identified and unidentified B-Complex Factors.

ADVANTAGES

Each Mega-B capsule-shaped tablet provides the highest vitamin B complex available in a single dose.

Mega-B was designed for those patients who require truly Mega vitamin potencies with the convenience of minimum dosage.

INDICATIONS

Mega-B is indicated in conditions characterized by depletions or increased demand of the water-soluble B-complex vitamins. It may be useful in the nutritional management of patients during prolonged convalescence associated with major surgery. It is also indicated for stress conditions, as an adjunct to antibiotics and diuretic therapy, pre and post operative cases, liver conditions, gastrointestinal disorders interferring with intake or absorption of water-soluble vitamins, prolonged or wasting diseases, diabetes, burns, fractures, severe infections, and some psychological disorders.

WARNING

NOT INTENDED FOR TREATMENT OF PERNICIOUS ANEMIA, OR OTHER PRIMARY OR SECONDARY ANEMIAS.

DOSAGE

Usual dosage is one Mega-B tablet daily, or varied, depending on clinical needs.

SUPPLIED

Yellow capsule shaped tablets in bottles of 30, 100 and 500.

AstraZeneca LP
WILMINGTON, DE 19850-5437

For Product Full Prescribing Information, Business Information, Medical Information, Adverse Drug Experiences, and Customer Service:
Information Center
1-800-236-9933

For Product Ordering:
Trade Customer Service
1-800-842-9920

For Product Full Prescribing Information:
Internet: www.astrazeneca-us.com

ASTRAMORPH/PF™ ℞
[ăs'-tră-mŏrf']
(morphine sulfate injection, USP)
Preservative-Free
Rx only

ATACAND® ℞
[ăt'-ă-kănd]
(candesartan cilexetil)
TABLETS

> USE IN PREGNANCY
> **When used in pregnancy during the second and third trimesters, drugs that act directly on the renin-angiotensin system can cause injury and even death to the developing fetus. When pregnancy is detected,** ATACAND should be discontinued as soon as possible. See WARNINGS, Fetal/Neonatal Morbidity and Mortality.

DESCRIPTION

ATACAND (candesartan cilexetil), a prodrug, is hydrolyzed to candesartan during absorption from the gastrointestinal tract. Candesartan is a selective AT_1 subtype angiotensin II receptor antagonist.

Candesartan cilexetil, a nonpeptide, is chemically described as (±)-1-Hydroxyethyl 2-ethoxy-1-[*p*-(*o*-1*H*-tetrazol-5-ylphenyl)benzyl]-7-benzimidazolecarboxylate, cyclohexyl carbonate (ester).

Its empirical formula is $C_{33}H_{34}N_6O_6$, and its structural formula is

site of ester hydrolysis.

Candesartan cilexetil is a white to off-white powder with a molecular weight of 610.67. It is practically insoluble in water and sparingly soluble in methanol. Candesartan cilexetil is a racemic mixture containing one chiral center at the cyclohexyloxycarbonyloxy ethyl ester group. Following oral administration, candesartan cilexetil undergoes hydrolysis at the ester link to form the active drug, candesartan, which is achiral.

ATACAND is available for oral use as tablets containing either 4 mg, 8 mg, 16 mg, or 32 mg of candesartan cilexetil and the following inactive ingredients: hydroxypropyl cellulose, polyethylene glycol, lactose, corn starch, carboxymethylcellulose calcium, and magnesium stearate. Ferric oxide (reddish brown) is added to the 8-mg, 16-mg, and 32-mg tablets as a colorant.

CLINICAL PHARMACOLOGY

Mechanism of Action

Angiotensin II is formed from angiotensin I in a reaction catalyzed by angiotensin-converting enzyme (ACE, kininase II). Angiotensin II is the principal pressor agent of the renin-angiotensin system, with effects that include vasoconstriction, stimulation of synthesis and release of aldosterone, cardiac stimulation, and renal reabsorption of sodium. Candesartan blocks the vasoconstrictor and aldosterone-secreting effects of angiotensin II by selectively blocking the binding of angiotensin II to the AT_1 receptor in many tissues, such as vascular smooth muscle and the adrenal gland. Its action is, therefore, independent of the pathways for angiotensin II synthesis.

There is also an AT_2 receptor found in many tissues, but AT_2 is not known to be associated with cardiovascular homeostasis. Candesartan has much greater affinity (>10,000-fold) for the AT_1 receptor than for the AT_2 receptor.

Blockade of the renin-angiotensin system with ACE inhibitors, which inhibit the biosynthesis of angiotensin II from angiotensin I, is widely used in the treatment of hypertension. ACE inhibitors also inhibit the degradation of bradykinin, a reaction also catalyzed by ACE. Because candesartan does not inhibit ACE (kininase II), it does not affect the response to bradykinin. Whether this difference has clinical relevance is not yet known. Candesartan does not bind to or block other hormone receptors or ion channels known to be important in cardiovascular regulation.

Blockade of the angiotensin II receptor inhibits the negative regulatory feedback of angiotensin II on renin secretion, but the resulting increased plasma renin activity and angiotensin II circulating levels do not overcome the effect of candesartan on blood pressure.

Pharmacokinetics

General

Candesartan cilexetil is rapidly and completely bioactivated by ester hydrolysis during absorption from the gastrointestinal tract to candesartan, a selective AT_1 subtype angiotensin II receptor antagonist. Candesartan is mainly excreted unchanged in urine and feces (via bile). It undergoes minor hepatic metabolism by O-deethylation to an inactive metabolite. The elimination half-life of candesartan is approximately 9 hours. After single and repeated administration, the pharmacokinetics of candesartan are linear for oral doses up to 32 mg of candesartan cilexetil. Candesartan and its inactive metabolite do not accumulate in serum upon repeated once-daily dosing.

Following administration of candesartan cilexetil, the absolute bioavailability of candesartan was estimated to be 15%. After tablet ingestion, the peak serum concentration (C_{max}) is reached after 3 to 4 hours. Food with a high fat content does not affect the bioavailability of candesartan after candesartan cilexetil administration.

Metabolism and Excretion

Total plasma clearance of candesartan is 0.37 mL/min/kg, with a renal clearance of 0.19 mL/min/kg. When candesartan is administered orally, about 26% of the dose is excreted unchanged in urine. Following an oral dose of ^{14}C-labeled candesartan cilexetil, approximately 33% of radioactivity is recovered in urine and approximately 67% in feces. Following an intravenous dose of ^{14}C-labeled candesartan, approximately 59% of radioactivity is recovered in urine and approximately 36% in feces. Biliary excretion contributes to the elimination of candesartan.

Distribution

The volume of distribution of candesartan is 0.13 L/kg. Candesartan is highly bound to plasma proteins (>99%) and does not penetrate red blood cells. The protein binding is constant at candesartan plasma concentrations well above the range achieved with recommended doses. In rats, it has been demonstrated that candesartan crosses the blood-brain barrier poorly, if at all. It has also been demonstrated in rats that candesartan passes across the placental barrier and is distributed in the fetus.

Special Populations

Pediatric—The pharmacokinetics of candesartan cilexetil have not been investigated in patients <18 years of age.

Geriatric and Gender—The pharmacokinetics of candesartan have been studied in the elderly (≥65 years) and in both sexes. The plasma concentration of candesartan was higher in the elderly (C_{max} was approximately 50% higher, and AUC was approximately 80% higher) compared to younger subjects administered the same dose. The pharmacokinetics of candesartan were linear in the elderly, and candesartan and its inactive metabolite did not accumulate in the serum of these subjects upon repeated, once-daily administration. No initial dosage adjustment is necessary. (See DOSAGE AND ADMINISTRATION.) There is no difference in the pharmacokinetics of candesartan between male and female subjects.

Renal Insufficiency—In hypertensive patients with renal insufficiency, serum concentrations of candesartan were elevated. After repeated dosing, the AUC and C_{max} were approximately doubled in patients with severe renal impairment (creatinine clearance <30 mL/min/1.73m^2) compared to patients with normal kidney function. The pharmacokinetics of candesartan in hypertensive patients undergoing hemodialysis are similar to those in hypertensive patients with severe renal impairment. Candesartan cannot be removed by hemodialysis. No initial dosage adjustment is necessary in patients with renal insufficiency. (See DOSAGE AND ADMINISTRATION.)

Hepatic Insufficiency—The pharmacokinetics of candesartan were compared in patients with mild and moderate hepatic impairment to matched healthy volunteers following a single oral dose of 16 mg candesartan cilexetil. The increase in AUC for candesartan was 30% in patients with mild hepatic impairment (Child-Pugh A) and 145% in patients with moderate hepatic impairment (Child-Pugh B). The increase in C_{max} for candesartan was 56% in patients with mild hepatic impairment and 73% in patients with moderate hepatic impairment. The pharmacokinetics after candesartan cilexetil administration have not been investigated in patients with severe hepatic impairment. No initial dosage adjustment is necessary in patients with mild hepatic impairment. In patients with moderate hepatic impairment, consideration should be given to initiation of ATACAND at a lower dose. (See DOSAGE AND ADMINISTRATION.)

Drug Interactions

See PRECAUTIONS, Drug Interactions.

Pharmacodynamics

Candesartan inhibits the pressor effects of angiotensin II infusion in a dose-dependent manner. After 1 week of once-daily dosing with 8 mg of candesartan cilexetil, the pressor effect was inhibited by approximately 90% at peak with approximately 50% inhibition persisting for 24 hours.

Plasma concentrations of angiotensin I and angiotensin II, and plasma renin activity (PRA), increased in a dose-dependent manner after single and repeated administration of candesartan cilexetil to healthy subjects and hypertensive patients. ACE activity was not altered in healthy subjects after repeated candesartan cilexetil administration. The once-daily administration of up to 16 mg of candesartan cilexetil to healthy subjects did not influence plasma aldosterone concentrations, but a decrease in the plasma concentration of aldosterone was observed when 32 mg of candesartan cilexetil was administered to hypertensive patients. In spite of the effect of candesartan cilexetil on aldosterone secretion, very little effect on serum potassium was observed.

In multiple-dose studies with hypertensive patients, there were no clinically significant changes in metabolic function, including serum levels of total cholesterol, triglycerides, glucose, or uric acid. In a 12-week study of 161 patients with non-insulin-dependent (type 2) diabetes mellitus and hypertension, there was no change in the level of HbA_{1c}.

Clinical Trials

The antihypertensive effects of ATACAND were examined in 14 placebo-controlled trials of 4- to 12-weeks duration, primarily at daily doses of 2 to 32 mg per day in patients with baseline diastolic blood pressures of 95 to 114 mm Hg. Most of the trials were of candesartan cilexetil as a single agent, but it was also studied as add-on to hydrochlorothiazide and amlodipine. These studies included a total of 2350 patients randomized to one of several doses of candesartan cilexetil and 1027 to placebo. Except for a study in diabetics, all studies showed significant effects, generally dose related, of 2 to 32 mg on trough (24 hour) systolic and diastolic pressures compared to placebo, with doses of 8 to 32 mg giving effects of about 8–12/4–8 mm Hg. There were no exaggerated first-dose effects in these patients. Most of the antihypertensive effect was seen within 2 weeks of initial dosing and the full effect in 4 weeks. With once-daily dosing, blood pressure effect was maintained over 24 hours, with trough to peak ratios of blood pressure effect generally over 80%. Candesartan cilexetil had an additional blood pressure lowering effect when added to hydrochlorothiazide.

The antihypertensive effects of candesartan cilexetil and losartan potassium at their highest recommended doses administered once-daily were compared in two randomized, double-blind trials. In a total of 1268 patients with mild to moderate hypertension who were not receiving other antihypertensive therapy, candesartan cilexetil 32 mg lowered systolic and diastolic blood pressure by 2 to 3 mm Hg on average more than losartan potassium 100 mg, when measured at the time of either peak or trough effect. The antihypertensive effects of twice daily dosing of either candesartan cilexetil or losartan potassium were not studied.

The antihypertensive effect was similar in men and women and in patients older and younger than 65. Candesartan was effective in reducing blood pressure regardless of race, although the effect was somewhat less in blacks (usually a low-renin population). This has been generally true for angiotensin II antagonists and ACE inhibitors.

In long-term studies of up to 1 year, the antihypertensive effectiveness of candesartan cilexetil was maintained, and there was no rebound after abrupt withdrawal.

There were no changes in the heart rate of patients treated with candesartan cilexetil in controlled trials.

INDICATIONS AND USAGE

ATACAND is indicated for the treatment of hypertension. It may be used alone or in combination with other antihypertensive agents.

CONTRAINDICATIONS

ATACAND is contraindicated in patients who are hypersensitive to any component of this product.

WARNINGS

Fetal/Neonatal Morbidity and Mortality

Drugs that act directly on the renin-angiotensin system can cause fetal and neonatal morbidity and death when administered to pregnant women. Several dozen cases have been reported in the world literature in patients who were taking angiotensin-converting enzyme inhibitors. Post-marketing experience has identified reports of fetal and neonatal toxicity in babies born to women treated with ATACAND during pregnancy. When pregnancy is detected, ATACAND should be discontinued as soon as possible.

The use of drugs that act directly on the renin-angiotensin system during the second and third trimesters of pregnancy has been associated with fetal and neonatal injury, including hypotension, neonatal skull hypoplasia, anuria, reversible or irreversible renal failure, and death. Oligohydramnios has also been reported, presumably resulting from decreased fetal renal function; oligohydramnios in this setting has been associated with fetal limb contractures, craniofacial deformation, and hypoplastic lung development. Prematurity, intrauterine growth retardation, and patent ductus arteriosus have also been reported, although it is not clear whether these occurrences were due to exposure to the drug.

These adverse effects do not appear to have resulted from intrauterine drug exposure that has been limited to the first trimester. Mothers whose embryos and fetuses are exposed to an angiotensin II receptor antagonist only during the first trimester should be so informed. Nonetheless, when patients become pregnant, physicians should have the patient discontinue the use of ATACAND as soon as possible.

Rarely (probably less often than once in every thousand pregnancies), no alternative to a drug acting on the renin-angiotensin system will be found. In these rare cases, the mothers should be apprised of the potential hazards to their fetuses, and serial ultrasound examinations should be performed to assess the intra-amniotic environment.

If oligohydramnios is observed, ATACAND should be discontinued unless it is considered life saving for the mother. Contraction stress testing (CST), a nonstress test (NST), or biophysical profiling (BPP) may be appropriate, depending upon the week of pregnancy. Patients and physicians should be aware, however, that oligohydramnios may not appear until after the fetus has sustained irreversible injury.

Infants with histories of *in utero* exposure to an angiotensin II receptor antagonist should be closely observed for hypotension, oliguria, and hyperkalemia. If oliguria occurs, attention should be directed toward support of blood pressure and renal perfusion. Exchange transfusion or dialysis may be required as means of reversing hypotension and/or substituting for disordered renal function.

Oral doses ≥ 10 mg of candesartan cilexetil/kg/day administered to pregnant rats during late gestation and continued through lactation were associated with reduced survival and an increased incidence of hydronephrosis in the offspring. The 10-mg/kg/day dose in rats is approximately 2.8 times the maximum recommended daily human dose (MRHD) of 32 mg on a mg/m^2 basis (comparison assumes human body weight of 50 kg). Candesartan cilexetil given to pregnant rabbits at an oral dose of 3 mg/kg/day (approximately 1.7 times the MRHD on a mg/m^2 basis) caused maternal toxicity (decreased body weight and death) but, in surviving dams, had no adverse effects on fetal survival, fetal weight, or external, visceral, or skeletal development. No maternal toxicity or adverse effects on fetal development were observed when oral doses up to 1000 mg of candesartan cilexetil/kg/day (approximately 138 times the MRHD on a mg/m^2 basis) were administered to pregnant mice.

Hypotension in Volume- and Salt-Depleted Patients

In patients with an activated renin-angiotensin system, such as volume- and/or salt-depleted patients (eg, those being treated with diuretics), symptomatic hypotension may occur. These conditions should be corrected prior to administration of ATACAND, or the treatment should start under close medical supervision (see DOSAGE AND ADMINISTRATION).

If hypotension occurs, the patients should be placed in the supine position and, if necessary, given an intravenous infusion of normal saline. A transient hypotensive response is not a contraindication to further treatment which usually can be continued without difficulty once the blood pressure has stabilized.

PRECAUTIONS

General

Impaired Hepatic Function—Based on pharmacokinetic data which demonstrate significant increases in candesartan AUC and C_{max} in patients with moderate hepatic impairment, a lower initiating dose should be considered for patients with moderate hepatic impairment. (See DOSAGE AND ADMINISTRATION, and CLINICAL PHARMACOLOGY, Special Populations.)

Impaired Renal Function—As a consequence of inhibiting the renin-angiotensin-aldosterone system, changes in renal function may be anticipated in susceptible individuals treated with ATACAND. In patients whose renal function may depend upon the activity of the renin-angiotensin-aldosterone system (eg, patients with severe congestive heart failure), treatment with angiotensin-converting enzyme inhibitors and angiotensin receptor antagonists has been associated with oliguria and/or progressive azotemia and (rarely) with acute renal failure and/or death. Similar results may be anticipated in patients treated with ATACAND. (See CLINICAL PHARMACOLOGY, Special Populations.)

In studies of ACE inhibitors in patients with unilateral or bilateral renal artery stenosis, increases in serum creatinine or blood urea nitrogen (BUN) have been reported. There has been no long-term use of ATACAND in patients with unilateral or bilateral renal artery stenosis, but similar results may be expected.

Information for Patients

Pregnancy—Female patients of childbearing age should be told about the consequences of second- and third-trimester exposure to drugs that act on the renin-angiotensin system, and they should also be told that these consequences do not appear to have resulted from intrauterine drug exposure that has been limited to the first trimester. These patients should be asked to report pregnancies to their physicians as soon as possible.

Drug Interactions

No significant drug interactions have been reported in studies of candesartan cilexetil given with other drugs such as glyburide, nifedipine, digoxin, warfarin, hydrochlorothiazide, and oral contraceptives in healthy volunteers. Because candesartan is not significantly metabolized by the cytochrome P450 system and at therapeutic concentrations has no effects on P450 enzymes, interactions with drugs that inhibit or are metabolized by those enzymes would not be expected.

Lithium—Reversible increases in serum lithium concentrations and toxicity have been reported during concomitant administration of lithium with ACE inhibitors, and with some angiotensin II receptor antagonists. An increase in serum lithium concentration has been reported during concomitant administration of lithium with ATACAND, so careful monitoring of serum lithium levels is recommended during concomitant use.

Carcinogenesis, Mutagenesis, Impairment of Fertility

There was no evidence of carcinogenicity when candesartan cilexetil was orally administered to mice and rats for up to

Continued on next page

Atacand—Cont.

104 weeks at doses up to 100 and 1000 mg/kg/day, respectively. Rats received the drug by gavage, whereas mice received the drug by dietary administration. These (maximally-tolerated) doses of candesartan cilexetil provided systemic exposures to candesartan (AUCs) that were, in mice, approximately 7 times and, in rats, more than 70 times the exposure in man at the maximum recommended daily human dose (32 mg).

Candesartan and its O-deethyl metabolite tested positive for genotoxicity in the *in vitro* Chinese hamster lung (CHL) chromosomal aberration assay. Neither compound tested positive in the Ames microbial mutagenesis assay or the *in vitro* mouse lymphoma cell assay. Candesartan (but not its O-deethyl metabolite) was also evaluated *in vivo* in the mouse micronucleus test and *in vitro* in the Chinese hamster ovary (CHO) gene mutation assay, in both cases with negative results. Candesartan cilexetil was evaluated in the Ames test, the *in vitro* mouse lymphoma cell and rat hepatocyte unscheduled DNA synthesis assays and the *in vivo* mouse micronucleus test, in each case with negative results. Candesartan cilexetil was not evaluated in the CHL chromosomal aberration or CHO gene mutation assay.

Fertility and reproductive performance were not affected in studies with male and female rats given oral doses of up to 300 mg/kg/day (83 times the maximum daily human dose of 32 mg on a body surface area basis).

Pregnancy

Pregnancy Categories C (first trimester) *and D* (second and third trimesters). See WARNINGS, Fetal/Neonatal Morbidity and Mortality.

Nursing Mothers

It is not known whether candesartan is excreted in human milk, but candesartan has been shown to be present in rat milk. Because of the potential for adverse effects on the nursing infant, a decision should be made whether to discontinue nursing or discontinue the drug, taking into account the importance of the drug to the mother.

Pediatric Use

Safety and effectiveness in pediatric patients have not been established.

Geriatric Use

Of the total number of subjects in clinical studies of ATACAND, 21% (683/3260) were 65 and over, while 3% (87/3260) were 75 and over. No overall differences in safety or effectiveness were observed between these subjects and younger subjects, and other reported clinical experience has not identified differences in responses between the elderly and younger patients, but greater sensitivity of some older individuals cannot be ruled out. In a placebo-controlled trial of about 200 elderly hypertensive patients (ages 65 to 87 years), administration of candesartan cilexetil was well tolerated and lowered blood pressure by about 12/6 mm Hg more than placebo.

ADVERSE REACTIONS

ATACAND has been evaluated for safety in more than 3600 patients/subjects, including more than 3200 patients treated for hypertension. About 600 of these patients were studied for at least 6 months and about 200 for at least 1 year. In general, treatment with ATACAND was well tolerated. The overall incidence of adverse events reported with ATACAND was similar to placebo.

The rate of withdrawals due to adverse events in all trials in patients (7510 total) was 3.3% (ie, 108 of 3260) of patients treated with candesartan cilexetil as monotherapy and 3.5% (ie, 39 of 1106) of patients treated with placebo. In placebo-controlled trials, discontinuation of therapy due to clinical adverse events occurred in 2.4% (ie, 57 of 2350) of patients treated with ATACAND and 3.4% (ie, 35 of 1027) of patients treated with placebo.

The most common reasons for discontinuation of therapy with ATACAND were headache (0.6%) and dizziness (0.3%).

The adverse events that occurred in placebo-controlled clinical trials in at least 1% of patients treated with ATACAND and at a higher incidence in candesartan cilexetil (n = 2350) than placebo (n = 1027) patients included back pain (3% vs 2%), dizziness (4% vs 3%), upper respiratory tract infection (6% vs 4%), pharyngitis (2% vs 1%), and rhinitis (2% vs 1%).

The following adverse events occurred in placebo-controlled clinical trials at a more than 1% rate but at about the same or greater incidence in patients receiving placebo compared to candesartan cilexetil: fatigue, peripheral edema, chest pain, headache, bronchitis, coughing, sinusitis, nausea, abdominal pain, diarrhea, vomiting, arthralgia, albuminuria.

Other potentially important adverse events that have been reported, whether or not attributed to treatment, with an incidence of 0.5% or greater from the 3260 patients worldwide treated in clinical trials with ATACAND are listed below. It cannot be determined whether these events were causally related to ATACAND. **Body as a Whole**: asthenia, fever; **Central and Peripheral Nervous System**: paresthesia, vertigo; **Gastrointestinal System Disorder**: dyspepsia, gastroenteritis; **Heart Rate and Rhythm Disorders**: tachycardia, palpitation; **Metabolic and Nutritional Disorders**: creatine phosphokinase increased, hyperglycemia, hypertriglyceridemia, hyperuricemia; **Musculoskeletal System Disorders**: myalgia; **Platelet/Bleeding-Clotting Disorders**: epistaxis; **Psychiatric Disorders**: anxiety, depression, somnolence; **Respiratory System Disorders**: dyspnea; **Skin and Appendages Disorders**: rash, sweating increased; **Urinary System Disorders**: hematuria.

Other reported events seen less frequently included angina pectoris, myocardial infarction, and angioedema.

Adverse events occurred at about the same rates in men and women, older and younger patients, and black and nonblack patients.

Post-Marketing Experience

The following have been very rarely reported in post-marketing experience:

Digestive: Abnormal hepatic function and hepatitis.

Hematologic: Neutropenia, leukopenia, and agranulocytosis.

Metabolic and Nutritional Disorders: hyperkalemia, hyponatremia.

Renal: renal impairment, renal failure.

Skin and Appendages Disorders: Pruritus and urticaria.

Laboratory Test Findings

In controlled clinical trials, clinically important changes in standard laboratory parameters were rarely associated with the administration of ATACAND.

Creatinine, Blood Urea Nitrogen—Minor increases in blood urea nitrogen (BUN) and serum creatinine were observed infrequently.

Hyperuricemia—Hyperuricemia was rarely found (19 or 0.6% of 3260 patients treated with candesartan cilexetil and 5 or 0.5% of 1106 patients treated with placebo).

Hemoglobin and Hematocrit—Small decreases in hemoglobin and hematocrit (mean decreases of approximately 0.2 grams/dL and 0.5 volume percent, respectively) were observed in patients treated with ATACAND alone but were rarely of clinical importance. Anemia, leukopenia, and thrombocytopenia were associated with withdrawal of one patient each from clinical trials.

Potassium—A small increase (mean increase of 0.1 mEq/L) was observed in patients treated with ATACAND alone but was rarely of clinical importance. One patient from a congestive heart failure trial was withdrawn for hyperkalemia (serum potassium = 7.5 mEq/L). This patient was also receiving spironolactone.

Liver Function Tests—Elevations of liver enzymes and/or serum bilirubin were observed infrequently. Five patients assigned to candesartan cilexetil in clinical trials were withdrawn because of abnormal liver chemistries. All had elevated transaminases. Two had mildly elevated total bilirubin, but one of these patients was diagnosed with Hepatitis A.

OVERDOSAGE

No lethality was observed in acute toxicity studies in mice, rats, and dogs given single oral doses of up to 2000 mg/kg of candesartan cilexetil. In mice given single oral doses of the primary metabolite, candesartan, the minimum lethal dose was greater than 1000 mg/kg but less than 2000 mg/kg.

The most likely manifestation of overdosage with ATACAND would be hypotension, dizziness, and tachycardia; bradycardia could occur from parasympathetic (vagal) stimulation. If symptomatic hypotension should occur, supportive treatment should be instituted.

Candesartan cannot be removed by hemodialysis.

Treatment: To obtain up-to-date information about the treatment of overdose, consult your Regional Poison Control Center. Telephone numbers of certified poison control centers are listed in the *Physicians' Desk Reference (PDR)*. In managing overdose, consider the possibilities of multiple-drug overdoses, drug-drug interactions, and altered pharmacokinetics in your patient.

DOSAGE AND ADMINISTRATION

Dosage must be individualized. Blood pressure response is dose related over the range of 2 to 32 mg. The usual recommended starting dose of ATACAND is 16 mg once daily when it is used as monotherapy in patients who are not volume depleted. ATACAND can be administered once or twice daily with total daily doses ranging from 8 mg to 32 mg. Larger doses do not appear to have a greater effect, and there is relatively little experience with such doses. Most of the antihypertensive effect is present within 2 weeks, and maximal blood pressure reduction is generally obtained within 4 to 6 weeks of treatment with ATACAND.

No initial dosage adjustment is necessary for elderly patients, for patients with mildly impaired renal function, or for patients with mildly impaired hepatic function (see CLINICAL PHARMACOLOGY, Special Populations). In patients with moderate hepatic impairment, consideration should be given to initiation of ATACAND at a lower dose (See CLINICAL PHARMACOLOGY, Special Populations). For patients with possible depletion of intravascular volume (eg, patients treated with diuretics, particularly those with impaired renal function), ATACAND should be initiated under close medical supervision and consideration should be given to administration of a lower dose (see WARNINGS, Hypotension in Volume- and Salt-Depleted Patients).

ATACAND may be administered with or without food.

If blood pressure is not controlled by ATACAND alone, a diuretic may be added. ATACAND may be administered with other antihypertensive agents.

HOW SUPPLIED

No. 3782—Tablets ATACAND, 4 mg, are white to off-white, circular/biconvex-shaped, non-film-coated tablets, coded ACF on one side and 004 on the other. They are supplied as follows:

NDC 0186-0004-31 unit of use bottles of 30.

No. 3780—Tablets ATACAND, 8 mg, are light pink, circular/biconvex-shaped, non-film-coated tablets, coded ACG on one side and 008 on the other. They are supplied as follows:

NDC 0186-0008-31 unit of use bottles of 30.

No. 3781—Tablets ATACAND, 16 mg, are pink, circular/biconvex-shaped, non-film-coated tablets, coded ACH on one side and 016 on the other. They are supplied as follows:

NDC 0186-0016-31 unit of use bottles of 30

NDC 0186-0016-54 unit of use bottles of 90

NDC 0186-0016-28 unit dose packages of 100.

No. 3791—Tablets ATACAND, 32 mg, are pink, circular/biconvex-shaped, non-film-coated tablets, coded ACL on one side and 032 on the other. They are supplied as follows:

NDC 0186-0032-31 unit of use bottles of 30

NDC 0186-0032-54 unit of use bottles of 90

NDC 0186-0032-28 unit dose packages of 100.

Storage

Store at 25°C (77°F); excursions permitted to 15-30°C (59-86°F) [see USP Controlled Room Temperature]. Keep container tightly closed.

ATACAND is a trademark of the AstraZeneca group of companies ©AstraZeneca 2003

Rev. 02/03

Takeda Manufactured under the license from Takeda Chemical Industries, Ltd.

by: AstraZeneca AB, S-151 85 Södertälje, Sweden

for: AstraZeneca LP, Wilmington, DE 19850

9174309

610002-09

AstraZeneca

Shown in Product Identification Guide, page 305

ATACAND HCT® 16-12.5 ℞

[*ăt ă-kănd*]

(candesartan cilexetil – hydrochlorothiazide)

ATACAND HCT® 32-12.5 ℞

(candesartan cilexetil – hydrochlorothiazide)

TABLETS

USE IN PREGNANCY

When used in pregnancy during the second and third trimesters, drugs that act directly on the renin-angiotensin system can cause injury and even death to the developing fetus. When pregnancy is detected, ATACAND HCT should be discontinued as soon as possible. See WARNINGS, Fetal/Neonatal Morbidity and Mortality.

DESCRIPTION

ATACAND HCT (candesartan cilexetil-hydrochlorothiazide) combines an angiotensin II receptor (type AT_1) antagonist and a diuretic, hydrochlorothiazide.

Candesartan cilexetil, a nonpeptide, is chemically described as, (±)-1-Hydroxyethyl 2-ethoxy-1-[*p*-(*o*-1*H*-tetrazol-5-ylphenyl)benzyl]-7-benzimidazolecarboxylate, cyclohexyl carbonate (ester).

Its empirical formula is $C_{33}H_{34}N_6O_6$, and its structural formula is

⬇ site of ester hydrolysis.

Candesartan cilexetil is a white to off-white powder with a molecular weight of 610.67. It is practically insoluble in water and sparingly soluble in methanol. Candesartan cilexetil is a racemic mixture containing one chiral center at the cyclohexyloxycarbonyloxy ethyl ester group. Following oral administration, candesartan cilexetil undergoes hydrolysis at the ester link to form the active drug, candesartan, which is achiral.

Hydrochlorothiazide is 6-chloro-3,4-dihydro-2*H*-1,2,4-benzothiadiazine-7-sulfonamide 1,1-dioxide. Its empirical formula is $C_7H_8ClN_3O_4S_2$ and its structural formula is

Hydrochlorothiazide is a white, or practically white, crystalline powder with a molecular weight of 297.72, which is slightly soluble in water, but freely soluble in sodium hydroxide solution.

ATACAND HCT is available for oral administration in two tablet strengths of candesartan cilexetil and hydrochlorothiazide.

ATACAND HCT 16-12.5 contains 16 mg of candesartan cilexetil and 12.5 mg of hydrochlorothiazide. ATACAND HCT 32-12.5 contains 32 mg of candesartan cilexetil and 12.5 mg of hydrochlorothiazide. The inactive ingredients of the tablets are calcium carboxymethylcellulose, hydroxypropyl cellulose, lactose monohydrate, magnesium stearate, corn starch, polyethylene glycol 8000, and ferric oxide (yellow). Ferric oxide (reddish brown) is also added to the 16-12.5 mg tablet as colorant.

CLINICAL PHARMACOLOGY

Mechanism of Action

Angiotensin II is formed from angiotensin I in a reaction catalyzed by angiotensin-converting enzyme (ACE, kininase II). Angiotensin II is the principal pressor agent of the renin-angiotensin system, with effects that include vasoconstriction, stimulation of synthesis and release of aldosterone, cardiac stimulation, and renal reabsorption of sodium. Candesartan blocks the vasoconstrictor and aldosterone-secreting effects of angiotensin II by selectively blocking the binding of angiotensin II to the AT_1 receptor in many tissues, such as vascular smooth muscle and the adrenal gland. Its action is, therefore, independent of the pathways for angiotensin II synthesis.

There is also an AT_2 receptor found in many tissues, but AT_2 is not known to be associated with cardiovascular homeostasis. Candesartan has much greater affinity (>10,000-fold) for the AT_1 receptor than for the AT_2 receptor.

Blockade of the renin-angiotensin system with ACE inhibitors, which inhibit the biosynthesis of angiotensin II from angiotensin I, is widely used in the treatment of hypertension. ACE inhibitors also inhibit the degradation of bradykinin, a reaction also catalyzed by ACE. Because candesartan does not inhibit ACE (kininase II), it does not affect the response to bradykinin. Whether this difference has clinical relevance is not yet known. Candesartan does not bind to or block other hormone receptors or ion channels known to be important in cardiovascular regulation.

Blockade of the angiotensin II receptor inhibits the negative regulatory feedback of angiotensin II on renin secretion, but the resulting increased plasma renin activity and angiotensin II circulating levels do not overcome the effect of candesartan on blood pressure.

Hydrochlorothiazide is a thiazide diuretic. Thiazides affect the renal tubular mechanisms of electrolyte reabsorption, directly increasing excretion of sodium and chloride in approximately equivalent amounts. Indirectly, the diuretic action of hydrochlorothiazide reduces plasma volume, with consequent increases in plasma renin activity, increases in aldosterone secretion, increases in urinary potassium loss, and decreases in serum potassium. The renin-aldosterone link is mediated by angiotensin II, so coadministration of an angiotensin II receptor antagonist tends to reverse the potassium loss associated with these diuretics.

The mechanism of the antihypertensive effect of thiazides is unknown.

Pharmacokinetics

General

Candesartan Cilexetil

Candesartan cilexetil is rapidly and completely bioactivated by ester hydrolysis during absorption from the gastrointestinal tract to candesartan, a selective AT_1 subtype angiotensin II receptor antagonist. Candesartan is mainly excreted unchanged in urine and feces (via bile). It undergoes minor hepatic metabolism by O-deethylation to an inactive metabolite. The elimination half-life of candesartan is approximately 9 hours. After single and repeated administration, the pharmacokinetics of candesartan are linear for oral doses up to 32 mg of candesartan cilexetil. Candesartan and its inactive metabolite do not accumulate in serum upon repeated once-daily dosing.

Following administration of candesartan cilexetil, the absolute bioavailability of candesartan was estimated to be 15%. After tablet ingestion, the peak serum concentration (C_{max}) is reached after 3 to 4 hours. Food with a high fat content does not affect the bioavailability of candesartan after candesartan cilexetil administration.

Hydrochlorothiazide

When plasma levels have been followed for at least 24 hours, the plasma half-life has been observed to vary between 5.6 and 14.8 hours.

Metabolism and Excretion

Candesartan Cilexetil

Total plasma clearance of candesartan is 0.37 mL/min/kg, with a renal clearance of 0.19 mL/min/kg. When candesartan is administered orally, about 26% of the dose is excreted unchanged in urine. Following an oral dose of ^{14}C-labeled candesartan cilexetil, approximately 33% of radioactivity is recovered in urine and approximately 67% in feces. Following an intravenous dose of ^{14}C-labeled candesartan, approximately 59% of radioactivity is recovered in urine and approximately 36% in feces. Biliary excretion contributes to the elimination of candesartan.

Hydrochlorothiazide

Hydrochlorothiazide is not metabolized but is eliminated rapidly by the kidney. At least 61% of the oral dose is eliminated unchanged within 24 hours.

Distribution

Candesartan Cilexetil

The volume of distribution of candesartan is 0.13 L/kg. Candesartan is highly bound to plasma proteins (>99%) and does not penetrate red blood cells. The protein binding is constant at candesartan plasma concentrations well above the range achieved with recommended doses. In rats, it has been demonstrated that candesartan crosses the blood-brain barrier poorly, if at all. It has also been demonstrated in rats that candesartan passes across the placental barrier and is distributed in the fetus.

Hydrochlorothiazide

Hydrochlorothiazide crosses the placental but not the blood-brain barrier and is excreted in breast milk.

Special Populations

Pediatric

The pharmacokinetics of candesartan cilexetil have not been investigated in patients <18 years of age.

Geriatric

The pharmacokinetics of candesartan have been studied in the elderly (≥65 years). The plasma concentration of candesartan was higher in the elderly (C_{max} was approximately 50% higher, and AUC was approximately 80% higher) compared to younger subjects administered the same dose. The pharmacokinetics of candesartan were linear in the elderly, and candesartan and its inactive metabolite did not accumulate in the serum of these subjects upon repeated, once-daily administration. No initial dosage adjustment is necessary. (See DOSAGE AND ADMINISTRATION.)

Gender

There is no difference in the pharmacokinetics of candesartan between male and female subjects.

Renal Insufficiency

In hypertensive patients with renal insufficiency, serum concentrations of candesartan were elevated. After repeated dosing, the AUC and C_{max} were approximately doubled in patients with severe renal impairment (creatinine clearance <30 mL/min/1.73m^2) compared to patients with normal kidney function. The pharmacokinetics of candesartan in hypertensive patients undergoing hemodialysis are similar to those in hypertensive patients with severe renal impairment. Candesartan cannot be removed by hemodialysis. No initial dosage adjustment is necessary in patients with renal insufficiency.

Thiazide diuretics are eliminated by the kidney, with a terminal half-life of 5-15 hours. In a study of patients with impaired renal function (mean creatinine clearance of 19 mL/min), the half-life of hydrochlorothiazide elimination was lengthened to 21 hours. (See DOSAGE AND ADMINISTRATION.)

Hepatic Insufficiency

The pharmacokinetics of candesartan were compared in patients with mild and moderate hepatic impairment to matched healthy volunteers following a single oral dose of 16 mg candesartan cilexetil. The increase in AUC for candesartan was 30% in patients with mild hepatic impairment (Child-Pugh A) and 145% in patients with moderate hepatic impairment (Child-Pugh B). The increase in C_{max} for candesartan was 56% in patients with mild hepatic impairment and 73% in patients with moderate hepatic impairment. The pharmacokinetics after candesartan cilexetil administration have not been investigated in patients with severe hepatic impairment. No initial dosage adjustment is necessary in patients with mild hepatic impairment. In patients with moderate hepatic impairment, a lower dose of candesartan is recommended.

Thiazide diuretics should be used with caution in patients with hepatic impairment. (See DOSAGE AND ADMINISTRATION.)

Pharmacodynamics

Candesartan Cilexetil

Candesartan inhibits the pressor effects of angiotensin II infusion in a dose-dependent manner. After 1 week of once-daily dosing with 8 mg of candesartan cilexetil, the pressor effect was inhibited by approximately 90% at peak with approximately 50% inhibition persisting for 24 hours.

Plasma concentrations of angiotensin I and angiotensin II, and plasma renin activity (PRA), increased in a dose-dependent manner after single and repeated administration of candesartan cilexetil to healthy subjects and hypertensive patients. ACE activity was not altered in healthy subjects after repeated candesartan cilexetil administration. The once-daily administration of up to 16 mg of candesartan cilexetil to healthy subjects did not influence plasma aldosterone concentrations, but a decrease in the plasma concentration of aldosterone was observed when 32 mg of candesartan cilexetil was administered to hypertensive patients. In spite of the effect of candesartan cilexetil on aldosterone secretion, very little effect on serum potassium was observed.

In multiple-dose studies with hypertensive patients, there were no clinically significant changes in metabolic function including serum levels of total cholesterol, triglycerides, glucose, or uric acid. In a 12-week study of 161 patients with non-insulin-dependent (type 2) diabetes mellitus and hypertension, there was no change in the level of HbA_{1c}.

Hydrochlorothiazide

After oral administration of hydrochlorothiazide, diuresis begins within 2 hours, peaks in about 4 hours and lasts about 6 to 12 hours.

Clinical Trials

Candesartan Cilexetil–Hydrochlorothiazide

Of 12 controlled clinical trials involving 4588 patients, 5 were double-blind, placebo controlled and evaluated the antihypertensive effects of single entities vs the combination. These 5 trials, of 8 to 12 weeks duration, randomized 3037 hypertensive patients. Doses ranged from 2 to 32 mg candesartan cilexetil and from 6.25 to 25 mg hydrochlorothiazide administered once daily in various combinations.

The combination of candesartan cilexetil-hydrochlorothiazide resulted in placebo-adjusted decreases in sitting systolic and diastolic blood pressures of 14-18/8-11 mm Hg at doses of 16-12.5 mg and 32-12.5 mg. The combination of candesartan cilexetil and hydrochlorothiazide 32-25 mg resulted in placebo-adjusted decreases in sitting systolic and diastolic blood pressures of 16-19/9-11 mm Hg. The placebo corrected trough to peak ratio was evaluated in a study of candesartan cilexetil-hydrochlorothiazide 32-12.5 mg and was 88%.

Most of the antihypertensive effect of the combination of candesartan cilexetil and hydrochlorothiazide was seen in 1 to 2 weeks with the full effect observed within 4 weeks. In long- term studies of up to 1 year, the blood pressure lowering effect of the combination was maintained. The antihypertensive effect was similar regardless of age or gender, and overall response to the combination was similar in black and non-black patients. No appreciable changes in heart rate were observed with combination therapy in controlled trials.

INDICATIONS AND USAGE

ATACAND HCT is indicated for the treatment of hypertension. This fixed dose combination is not indicated for initial therapy (see DOSAGE AND ADMINISTRATION).

CONTRAINDICATIONS

ATACAND HCT is contraindicated in patients who are hypersensitive to any component of this product.

Because of the hydrochlorothiazide component, this product is contraindicated in patients with anuria or hypersensitivity to other sulfonamide-derived drugs.

WARNINGS

Fetal/Neonatal Morbidity and Mortality

Drugs that act directly on the renin-angiotensin system can cause fetal and neonatal morbidity and death when administered to pregnant women. Several dozen cases have been reported in the world literature in patients who were taking angiotensin-converting enzyme inhibitors. Post-marketing experience has identified reports of fetal and neonatal toxicity in babies born to women treated with candesartan cilexetil during pregnancy. Because candesartan cilexetil is a component of ATACAND HCT, when pregnancy is detected, ATACAND HCT should be discontinued as soon as possible.

The use of drugs that act directly on the renin-angiotensin system during the second and third trimesters of pregnancy has been associated with fetal and neonatal injury, including hypotension, neonatal skull hypoplasia, anuria, reversible or irreversible renal failure, and death. Oligohydramnios has also been reported, presumably resulting from decreased fetal renal function; oligohydramnios in this setting has been associated with fetal limb contractures, craniofacial deformation, and hypoplastic lung development. Prematurity, intrauterine growth retardation, and patent ductus arteriosus have also been reported, although it is not clear whether these occurrences were due to exposure to the drug.

These adverse effects do not appear to have resulted from intrauterine drug exposure that has been limited to the first trimester. Mothers whose embryos and fetuses are exposed to an angiotensin II receptor antagonist only during the first trimester should be so informed. Nonetheless, when patients become pregnant, physicians should have the patient discontinue the use of ATACAND HCT as soon as possible.

Rarely (probably less often than once in every thousand pregnancies), no alternative to a drug acting on the renin-angiotensin system will be found. In these rare cases, the mothers should be apprised of the potential hazards to their fetuses, and serial ultrasound examinations should be performed to assess the intra-amniotic environment.

If oligohydramnios is observed, ATACAND HCT should be discontinued unless it is considered life saving for the mother. Contraction stress testing (CST), a nonstress test (NST), or biophysical profiling (BPP) may be appropriate, depending upon the week of pregnancy. Patients and physicians should be aware, however, that oligohydramnios may not appear until after the fetus has sustained irreversible injury.

Infants with histories of *in utero* exposure to an angiotensin II receptor antagonist should be closely observed for hypotension, oliguria, and hyperkalemia. If oliguria occurs, attention should be directed toward support of blood pressure and renal perfusion. Exchange transfusion or dialysis may be required as means of reversing hypotension and/or substituting for disordered renal function.

Candesartan Cilexetil-Hydrochlorothiazide

There was no evidence of teratogenicity or other adverse effects on embryo-fetal development when pregnant mice, rats or rabbits were treated orally with candesartan cilexetil alone or in combination with hydrochlorothiazide. For mice, the maximum dose of candesartan cilexetil was 1000 mg/kg/day (about 150 times the maximum recommended daily human dose [MRHD]*). For rats, the maximum dose of candesartan cilexetil was 100 mg/kg/day (about 31 times the MRHD*). For rabbits, the maximum dose of candesartan cilexetil was 1 mg/kg/day (a maternally toxic dose that is about half the MRHD*). In each of these studies, hydrochlorothiazide was tested at the same dose level (10 mg/kg/day, about 4, 8, and 15 times the MRHD* in mouse, rats, and rabbit, respectively). There was no evidence of harm to the rat or mouse fetus or embryo in studies in which hydrochlorothiazide was administered alone to the pregnant rat or mouse at doses of up to 1000 and 3000 mg/kg/day, respectively.

* Doses compared on the basis of body surface area. MRHD considered to be 32 mg for candesartan cilexetil and 12.5 mg for hydrochlorothiazide.

Thiazides cross the placental barrier and appear in cord blood. There is a risk of fetal or neonatal jaundice, thrombocytopenia, and possibly other adverse reactions that have occurred in adults.

Continued on next page

Atacand HCT—Cont.

Hypotension in Volume- and Salt-Depleted Patients
Based on adverse events reported from all clinical trials of ATACAND HCT, excessive reduction of blood pressure was rarely seen in patients with uncomplicated hypertension treated with candesartan cilexetil and hydrochlorothiazide (0.4%). Initiation of antihypertensive therapy may cause symptomatic hypotension in patients with intravascular volume- or sodium-depletion, eg, in patients treated vigorously with diuretics or in patients on dialysis. These conditions should be corrected prior to administration of ATACAND HCT, or the treatment should start under close medical supervision (see DOSAGE AND ADMINISTRATION).
If hypotension occurs, the patients should be placed in the supine position and, if necessary, given an intravenous infusion of normal saline. A transient hypotensive response is not a contraindication to further treatment which usually can be continued without difficulty once the blood pressure has stabilized.

Hydrochlorothiazide
Impaired Hepatic Function
Thiazide diuretics should be used with caution in patients with impaired hepatic function or progressive liver disease, since minor alterations of fluid and electrolyte balance may precipitate hepatic coma.
Hypersensitivity Reaction
Hypersensitivity reactions to hydrochlorothiazide may occur in patients with or without a history of allergy or bronchial asthma, but are more likely in patients with such a history.
Systemic Lupus Erythematosus
Thiazide diuretics have been reported to cause exacerbation or activation of systemic lupus erythematosus.
Lithium Interaction
Lithium generally should not be given with thiazides (see PRECAUTIONS, Drug Interactions, Hydrochlorothiazide, Lithium).

PRECAUTIONS

General
Candesartan Cilexetil–Hydrochlorothiazide
In clinical trials of various doses of candesartan cilexetil and hydrochlorothiazide, the incidence of hypertensive patients who developed hypokalemia (serum potassium <3.5 mEq/L) was 2.5% versus 2.1% for placebo; the incidence of hyperkalemia (serum potassium >5.7 mEq/L) was 0.4% versus 1.0% for placebo. No patient receiving ATACAND HCT 16-12.5 mg or 32-12.5 mg was discontinued due to increases or decreases in serum potassium. Overall, the combination of candesartan cilexetil and hydrochlorothiazide had no clinically significant effect on serum potassium.
Hydrochlorothiazide
Periodic determination of serum electrolytes to detect possible electrolyte imbalance should be performed at appropriate intervals.
All patients receiving thiazide therapy should be observed for clinical signs of fluid or electrolyte imbalance: namely, hyponatremia, hypochloremic alkalosis, and hypokalemia. Serum and urine electrolyte determinations are particularly important when the patient is vomiting excessively or receiving parenteral fluids. Warning signs or symptoms of fluid and electrolyte imbalance, irrespective of cause, include dryness of mouth, thirst, weakness, lethargy, drowsiness, restlessness, confusion, seizures, muscle pains or cramps, muscular fatigue, hypotension, oliguria, tachycardia, and gastrointestinal disturbances such as nausea and vomiting.
Hypokalemia may develop, especially with brisk diuresis, when severe cirrhosis is present, or after prolonged therapy. Interference with adequate oral electrolyte intake will also contribute to hypokalemia. Hypokalemia may cause cardiac arrhythmia and may also sensitize or exaggerate the response of the heart to the toxic effects of digitalis (eg, increased ventricular irritability).
Although any chloride deficit is generally mild and usually does not require specific treatment, except under extraordinary circumstances (as in liver disease or renal disease), chloride replacement may be required in the treatment of metabolic alkalosis.
Dilutional hyponatremia may occur in edematous patients in hot weather; appropriate therapy is water restriction, rather than administration of salt, except in rare instances when the hyponatremia is life-threatening. In actual salt depletion, appropriate replacement is the therapy of choice.
Hyperuricemia may occur or acute gout may be precipitated in certain patients receiving thiazide therapy.
In diabetic patients dosage adjustments of insulin or oral hypoglycemic agents may be required. Hyperglycemia may occur with thiazide diuretics. Thus latent diabetes mellitus may become manifest during thiazide therapy.
The antihypertensive effects of the drug may be enhanced in the post-sympathectomy patient.
If progressive renal impairment becomes evident consider withholding or discontinuing diuretic therapy.
Thiazides have been shown to increase the urinary excretion of magnesium; this may result in hypomagnesemia.
Thiazides may decrease urinary calcium excretion. Thiazides may cause intermittent and slight elevation of serum calcium in the absence of known disorders of calcium metabolism. Marked hypercalcemia may be evidence of hidden hyperparathyroidism. Thiazides should be discontinued before carrying out tests for parathyroid function.
Increases in cholesterol and triglyceride levels may be associated with thiazide diuretic therapy.

Impaired Renal Function
Candesartan cilexetil
As a consequence of inhibiting the renin-angiotensin-aldosterone system, changes in renal function may be anticipated in susceptible individuals treated with candesartan cilexetil. In patients whose renal function may depend upon the activity of the renin- angiotensin-aldosterone system (eg, patients with severe congestive heart failure), treatment with angiotensin-converting enzyme inhibitors and angiotensin receptor antagonists has been associated with oliguria and/or progressive azotemia and (rarely) with acute renal failure and/or death. Similar results may be anticipated in patients treated with candesartan cilexetil. (See CLINICAL PHARMACOLOGY, Special Populations.)
In studies of ACE inhibitors in patients with unilateral or bilateral renal artery stenosis, increases in serum creatinine or blood urea nitrogen (BUN) have been reported. There has been no long-term use of candesartan cilexetil in patients with unilateral or bilateral renal artery stenosis, but similar results may be expected.
Hydrochlorothiazide
Thiazides should be used with caution in severe renal disease. In patients with renal disease, thiazides may precipitate azotemia. Cumulative effects of the drug may develop in patients with impaired renal function.

Impaired Hepatic Function
Candesartan cilexetil
Based on pharmacokinetic data significant increases in candesartan AUC and C_{max} in patients with moderate hepatic impairment have been demonstrated. (See CLINICAL PHARMACOLOGY, Special Populations.)

Information for Patients
Pregnancy
Female patients of childbearing age should be told about the consequences of second- and third-trimester exposure to drugs that act on the renin-angiotensin system, and they should also be told that these consequences do not appear to have resulted from intrauterine drug exposure that has been limited to the first trimester. These patients should be asked to report pregnancies to their physicians as soon as possible.
Symptomatic Hypotension
A patient receiving ATACAND HCT should be cautioned that lightheadedness can occur, especially during the first days of therapy, and that it should be reported to the prescribing physician. The patients should be told that if syncope occurs, ATACAND HCT should be discontinued until the physician has been consulted.
All patients should be cautioned that inadequate fluid intake, excessive perspiration, diarrhea, or vomiting can lead to an excessive fall in blood pressure, with the same consequences of lightheadedness and possible syncope.
Potassium Supplements
A patient receiving ATACAND HCT should be told not to use potassium supplements or salt substitutes containing potassium without consulting the prescribing physician.

Drug Interactions
Candesartan Cilexetil
No significant drug interactions have been reported in studies of candesartan cilexetil given with other drugs such as glyburide, nifedipine, digoxin, warfarin, hydrochlorothiazide, and oral contraceptives in healthy volunteers. Because candesartan is not significantly metabolized by the cytochrome P450 system and at therapeutic concentrations has no effects on P450 enzymes, interactions with drugs that inhibit or are metabolized by those enzymes would not be expected.
Lithium—Reversible increases in serum lithium concentrations and toxicity have been reported during concomitant administration of lithium with ACE inhibitors, and with some angiotensin II receptor antagonists. An increase in serum lithium concentration has been reported during concomitant administration of lithium with candesartan cilexetil, so careful monitoring of serum lithium levels is recommended during concomitant use.
Hydrochlorothiazide
When administered concurrently the following drugs may interact with thiazide diuretics:
Alcohol, barbiturates, or narcotics—Potentiation of orthostatic hypotension may occur.
Antidiabetic drugs (oral agents and insulin)—Dosage adjustment of the antidiabetic drug may be required.
Other antihypertensive drugs—Additive effect or potentiation.
Cholestyramine and colestipol resins—Absorption of hydrochlorothiazide is impaired in the presence of anionic exchange resins. Single doses of either cholestyramine or colestipol resins bind the hydrochlorothiazide and reduce its absorption from the gastrointestinal tract by up to 85 and 43 percent, respectively.
Corticosteroids, ACTH—Intensified electrolyte depletion, particularly hypokalemia.
Pressor amines (eg, norepinephrine)—Possible decreased response to pressor amines but not sufficient to preclude their use.
Skeletal muscle relaxants, nondepolarizing (eg, tubocurarine)—Possible increased responsiveness to the muscle relaxant.
Lithium—Generally should not be given with diuretics. Diuretic agents reduce the renal clearance of lithium and add a high risk of lithium toxicity. Refer to the package insert for lithium preparations before use of such preparations with ATACAND HCT.
Non-steroidal Anti-inflammatory Drugs—In some patients, the administration of a non-steroidal anti-inflammatory agent can reduce the diuretic, natriuretic, and antihypertensive effects of loop, potassium-sparing and thiazide diuretics. Therefore, when ATACAND HCT and non-steroidal anti-inflammatory agents are used concomitantly, the patient should be observed closely to determine if the desired effect of the diuretic is obtained.

Carcinogenesis, Mutagenesis, Impairment of Fertility
Candesartan Cilexetil–Hydrochlorothiazide
No carcinogenicity studies have been conducted with the combination of candesartan cilexetil and hydrochlorothiazide. There was no evidence of carcinogenicity when candesartan cilexetil was orally administered to mice and rats for up to 104 weeks at doses up to 100 and 1000 mg/kg/day, respectively. Rats received the drug by gavage whereas mice received the drug by dietary administration. These (maximally-tolerated) doses of candesartan cilexetil provided systemic exposures to candesartan (AUCs) that were, in mice, approximately 7 times and, in rats, more than 70 times the exposure in man at the maximum recommended daily human dose (32 mg). Two-year feeding studies in mice and rats conducted under the auspices of the National Toxicology Program (NTP) uncovered no evidence of a carcinogenic potential of hydrochlorothiazide in female mice (at doses of up to approximately 600 mg/kg/day) or in male and female rats (at doses of up to approximately 100 mg/kg/day). The NTP, however, found equivocal evidence for hepatocarcinogenicity in male mice.
Candesartan and its O-deethyl metabolite tested positive for genotoxicity in the *in vitro* Chinese hamster lung (CHL) chromosomal aberration assay. Neither compound tested positive in the Ames microbial mutagenesis assay or the *in vitro* mouse lymphoma cell assay. Candesartan (but not its O-deethyl metabolite) was also evaluated *in vivo* in the mouse micronucleus test and *in vitro* in the Chinese hamster ovary (CHO) gene mutation assay, in both cases with negative results. Candesartan cilexetil was evaluated in the Ames test, the *in vitro* mouse lymphoma cell and rat hepatocyte unscheduled DNA synthesis assays and the *in vivo* mouse micronucleus test, in each case with negative results. Candesartan cilexetil was not evaluated in the CHL chromosomal aberration or CHO gene mutation assay. In the *in vitro* CHL chromosomal aberration and mouse lymphoma assays, mutagenic effects were detected when hydrochlorothiazide was tested alone and in the presence of candesartan.
Hydrochlorothiazide alone and in the presence of candesartan cilexetil was negative for mutagenicity in bacteria (Ames test). Under the auspices of the NTP, positive test results were obtained for hydrochlorothiazide in the *in vitro* CHO Sister Chromatid Exchange (clastogenicity) and in the Mouse Lymphoma Cell (mutagenicity) assays and in the *Aspergillus nidulans* non-disjunction assay. In addition, hydrochlorothiazide was not genotoxic *in vitro* in the Ames test for point mutations and the Chinese Hamster Ovary (CHO) test for chromosomal aberrations, or *in vivo* in assays using mouse germinal cell chromosomes, Chinese hamster bone marrow chromosomes, and the Drosophila sex-linked recessive lethal trait gene.
No fertility studies have been conducted with the combination of candesartan cilexetil and hydrochlorothiazide. Fertility and reproductive performance were not affected in studies with male and female rats given oral doses of up to 300 mg candesartan cilexetil/kg/day (83 times the maximum daily human dose of 32 mg on a body surface area basis). Hydrochlorothiazide had no adverse effects on the fertility of mice and rats of either sex in studies wherein these species were exposed, via their diet, to doses of up to 100 and 4 mg/kg, respectively, prior to conception and throughout gestation.

Pregnancy
Pregnancy Categories C (first trimester) *and D* (second and third trimesters). See WARNINGS, Fetal/Neonatal Morbidity and Mortality.

Nursing Mothers
It is not known whether candesartan is excreted in human milk, but candesartan has been shown to be present in rat milk. Thiazides appear in human milk. Because of the potential for adverse effects on the nursing infant, a decision should be made whether to discontinue nursing or discontinue the drug, taking into account the importance of the drug to the mother.

Pediatric Use
Safety and effectiveness in pediatric patients have not been established.

Geriatric Use
Of the total number of subjects in all clinical studies of ATACAND HCT (2831), 611 (22%) were 65 and over, while 94 (3%) were 75 and over. No overall differences in safety or effectiveness were observed between these subjects and younger subjects. Other reported clinical experience has not identified differences in responses between the elderly and younger patients, but greater sensitivity of some older individuals cannot be ruled out.

ADVERSE REACTIONS

Candesartan Cilexetil-Hydrochlorothiazide

ATACAND HCT has been evaluated for safety in more than 2800 patients treated for hypertension. More than 750 of these patients were studied for at least six months and more than 500 patients were treated for at least one year. Adverse experiences have generally been mild and transient in nature and have only infrequently required discontinuation of therapy. The overall incidence of adverse events reported with ATACAND HCT was comparable to placebo. The overall frequency of adverse experiences was not related to dose, age, gender, or race.

In placebo-controlled trials that included 1089 patients treated with various combinations of candesartan cilexetil (doses of 2-32 mg) and hydrochlorothiazide (doses of 6.25-25 mg) and 592 patients treated with placebo, adverse events, whether or not attributed to treatment, occurring in greater than 2% of patients treated with ATACAND HCT and that were more frequent for ATACAND HCT than placebo were: ***Respiratory System Disorder:*** upper respiratory tract infection (3.6% vs 3.0%); ***Body as a Whole:*** back pain (3.3% vs 2.4%); influenza-like symptoms (2.5% vs 1.9%); ***Central/Peripheral Nervous System:*** dizziness (2.9% vs 1.2%).

The frequency of headache was greater than 2% (2.9%) in patients treated with ATACAND HCT but was less frequent than the rate in patients treated with placebo (5.2%).

Other adverse events that have been reported, whether or not attributed to treatment, with an incidence of 0.5% or greater from the more than 2800 patients worldwide treated with ATACAND HCT included: ***Body as a Whole:*** inflicted injury, fatigue, pain, chest pain, peripheral edema, asthenia; ***Central and Peripheral Nervous System:*** vertigo, paresthesia, hypesthesia; ***Respiratory System Disorders:*** bronchitis, sinusitis, pharyngitis, coughing, rhinitis, dyspnea; ***Musculoskeletal System Disorders:*** arthralgia, myalgia, arthrosis, arthritis, leg cramps, sciatica; ***Gastrointestinal System Disorders:*** nausea, abdominal pain, diarrhea, dyspepsia, gastritis, gastroenteritis, vomiting; ***Metabolic and Nutritional Disorders:*** hyperuricemia, hyperglycemia, hypokalemia, increased BUN, creatine phosphokinase increased; ***Urinary System Disorders:*** urinary tract infection, hematuria, cystitis; ***Liver/Biliary System Disorders:*** hepatic function abnormal, increased transaminase levels; ***Heart Rate and Rhythm Disorders:*** tachycardia, palpitation, extrasystoles, bradycardia; ***Psychiatric Disorders:*** depression, insomnia, anxiety; ***Cardiovascular Disorders:*** ECG abnormal; ***Skin and Appendages Disorders:*** eczema, sweating increased, pruritus, dermatitis, rash; ***Platelet/Bleeding-Clotting Disorders:*** epistaxis; ***Resistance Mechanism Disorders:*** infection, viral infection; ***Vision Disorders:*** conjunctivitis; ***Hearing and Vestibular Disorders:*** tinnitus.

Reported events seen less frequently than 0.5% included angina pectoris, myocardial infarction and angioedema.

Candesartan Cilexetil

Other adverse experiences that have been reported with candesartan cilexetil, without regard to causality, were: ***Body as a Whole:*** fever; ***Metabolic and Nutritional Disorders:*** hypertriglyceridemia; ***Psychiatric Disorders:*** somnolence; ***Urinary System Disorders:*** albuminuria.

Post-Marketing Experience

The following have been very rarely reported in post-marketing experience with candesartan cilexetil:

Digestive: Abnormal hepatic function and hepatitis.

Hematologic: Neutropenia, leukopenia, and agranulocytosis.

Metabolic and Nutritional Disorders: hyperkalemia, hyponatremia.

Renal: renal impairment, renal failure.

Skin and Appendages Disorders: Pruritus and urticaria.

Hydrochlorothiazide

Other adverse experiences that have been reported with hydrochlorothiazide, without regard to causality, are listed below:

Body As A Whole: weakness; ***Cardiovascular:*** hypotension including orthostatic hypotension (may be aggravated by alcohol, barbiturates, narcotics or antihypertensive drugs); ***Digestive:*** pancreatitis, jaundice (intrahepatic cholestatic jaundice), sialadenitis, cramping, constipation, gastric irritation, anorexia; ***Hematologic:*** aplastic anemia, agranulocytosis, leukopenia, hemolytic anemia, thrombocytopenia; ***Hypersensitivity:*** anaphylactic reactions, necrotizing angiitis (vasculitis and cutaneous vasculitis), respiratory distress including pneumonitis and pulmonary edema, photosensitivity, urticaria, purpura; ***Metabolic:*** electrolyte imbalance, glycosuria; ***Musculoskeletal:*** muscle spasm; ***Nervous System/Psychiatric:*** restlessness; ***Renal:*** renal failure, renal dysfunction, interstitial nephritis; ***Skin:*** erythema multiforme including Stevens-Johnson syndrome, exfoliative dermatitis including toxic epidermal necrolysis, alopecia; ***Special Senses:*** transient blurred vision, xanthopsia; ***Urogenital:*** impotence.

Laboratory Test Findings

In controlled clinical trials, clinically important changes in standard laboratory parameters were rarely associated with the administration of ATACAND HCT.

Creatinine, Blood Urea Nitrogen—Minor increases in blood urea nitrogen (BUN) and serum creatinine were observed infrequently. One patient was discontinued from ATACAND HCT due to increased BUN. No patient was discontinued due to an increase in serum creatinine.

Hemoglobin and Hematocrit—Small decreases in hemoglobin and hematocrit (mean decreases of approximately 0.2 g/dL and 0.4 volume percent, respectively) were observed in patients treated with ATACAND HCT, but were rarely of clinical importance.

Potassium—A small decrease (mean decrease of 0.1 mEq/L) was observed in patients treated with ATACAND HCT. In placebo-controlled trials, hypokalemia was reported in 0.4% of patients treated with ATACAND HCT as compared to 1.0% of patients treated with hydrochlorothiazide or 0.2% of patients treated with placebo.

Liver Function Tests—Occasional elevations of liver enzymes and/or serum bilirubin have occurred.

OVERDOSAGE

Candesartan Cilexetil–Hydrochlorothiazide

No lethality was observed in acute toxicity studies in mice, rats and dogs given single oral doses of up to 2000 mg/kg of candesartan cilexetil or in rats given single oral doses of up to 2000 mg/kg of candesartan cilexetil in combination with 1000 mg/kg of hydrochlorothiazide. In mice given single oral doses of the primary metabolite, candesartan, the minimum lethal dose was greater than 1000 mg/kg but less than 2000 mg/kg.

Limited data are available in regard to overdosage with candesartan cilexetil in humans. The most likely manifestations of overdosage with candesartan cilexetil would be hypotension, dizziness, and tachycardia; bradycardia could occur from parasympathetic (vagal) stimulation. If symptomatic hypotension should occur, supportive treatment should be initiated. For hydrochlorothiazide, the most common signs and symptoms observed are those caused by electrolyte depletion (hypokalemia, hypochloremia, hyponatremia) and dehydration resulting from excessive diuresis. If digitalis has also been administered, hypokalemia may accentuate cardiac arrhythmias.

Candesartan cannot be removed by hemodialysis. The degree to which hydrochlorothiazide is removed by hemodialysis has not been established.

Treatment

To obtain up-to-date information about the treatment of overdose, consult your Regional Poison Control Center. Telephone numbers of certified poison control centers are listed in the *Physicians' Desk Reference (PDR)*. In managing overdose, consider the possibilities of multiple-drug overdoses, drug-drug interactions, and altered pharmacokinetics in your patient.

DOSAGE AND ADMINISTRATION

The usual recommended starting dose of candesartan cilexetil is 16 mg once daily when it is used as monotherapy in patients who are not volume depleted. ATACAND can be administered once or twice daily with total daily doses ranging from 8 mg to 32 mg. Patients requiring further reduction in blood pressure should be titrated to 32 mg. Doses larger than 32 mg do not appear to have a greater blood pressure lowering effect.

Hydrochlorothiazide is effective in doses of 12.5 to 50 mg once daily.

To minimize dose-independent side effects, it is usually appropriate to begin combination therapy only after a patient has failed to achieve the desired effect with monotherapy.

The side effects (See WARNINGS) of candesartan cilexetil are generally rare and apparently independent of dose; those of hydrochlorothiazide are a mixture of dose-dependent phenomena (primarily hypokalemia) and dose-independent phenomena (eg, pancreatitis), the former much more common than the latter. Therapy with any combination of candesartan cilexetil and hydrochlorothiazide will be associated with both sets of dose-independent side effects.

Replacement Therapy: The combination may be substituted for the titrated components.

Dose Titration by Clinical Effect: A patient whose blood pressure is not controlled on 25 mg of hydrochlorothiazide once daily can expect an incremental effect from ATACAND HCT 16-12.5 mg. A patient whose blood pressure is controlled on 25 mg of hydrochlorothiazide but is experiencing decreases in serum potassium can expect the same or incremental blood pressure effects from ATACAND HCT 16-12.5 mg and serum potassium may improve.

A patient whose blood pressure is not controlled on 32 mg of ATACAND can expect incremental blood pressure effects from ATACAND HCT 32-12.5 mg and then 32-25 mg. The maximal antihypertensive effect of any dose of ATACAND HCT can be expected within 4 weeks of initiating that dose.

Patients with Renal Impairment: The usual regimens of therapy with ATACAND HCT may be followed as long as the patient's creatinine clearance is > 30 mL/min. In patients with more severe renal impairment, loop diuretics are preferred to thiazides, so ATACAND HCT is not recommended.

Patients with Hepatic Impairment: Thiazide diuretics should be used with caution in patients with hepatic impairment; therefore, care should be exercised with dosing of ATACAND HCT.

ATACAND HCT may be administered with other antihypertensive agents.

ATACAND HCT may be administered with or without food.

HOW SUPPLIED

No. 3825—Tablets ATACAND HCT 16-12.5, are peach, oval, biconvex, non-film-coated tablets, coded ACS on one side and 162 on the other. They are supplied as follows:

NDC 0186-0162-28 unit dose packages of 100.

NDC 0186-0162-54 unit of use bottles of 90.

No. 3826—Tablets ATACAND HCT 32-12.5, are yellow, oval, biconvex, non-film-coated tablets, coded ACJ on one side and 322 on the other. They are supplied as follows:

NDC 0186-0322-28 unit dose packages of 100.

NDC 0186-0322-54 unit of use bottles of 90.

Storage

Store at 25°C (77°F); excursions permitted to 15-30°C (59-86°F) [see USP Controlled Room Temperature]. Keep container tightly closed.

ATACAND HCT is a trademark of the AstraZeneca group of companies

Rev 04/03

Manufactured under the license from Takeda Chemical Industries, Ltd.

by: AstraZeneca AB, S-151 85 Södertälje, Sweden

for: AstraZeneca LP, Wilmington, DE 19850

Made in Sweden

9329102

610517-02

AstraZeneca

Shown in Product Identification Guide, page 305

EMLA® CREAM ℞

(lidocaine 2.5% and prilocaine 2.5%)

EMLA® ANESTHETIC DISC

(lidocaine 2.5% and prilocaine 2.5% cream)

Topical Adhesive System

Shown in Product Identification Guide, page 305

ENTOCORT EC CAPSULES ℞

[*ĕn'tō-kōrt*]

(budesonide)

℞ only

DESCRIPTION

Budesonide, the active ingredient of ENTOCORT™ EC capsules, is a synthetic corticosteroid. It is designated chemically as (RS)-11β, 16α, 17,21-tetrahydroxypregna-1,4-diene-3,20-dione cyclic 16,17-acetal with butyraldehyde. Budesonide is provided as a mixture of two epimers (22R and 22S). The empirical formula of budesonide is $C_{25}H_{34}O_6$ and its molecular weight is 430.5. Its structural formula is:

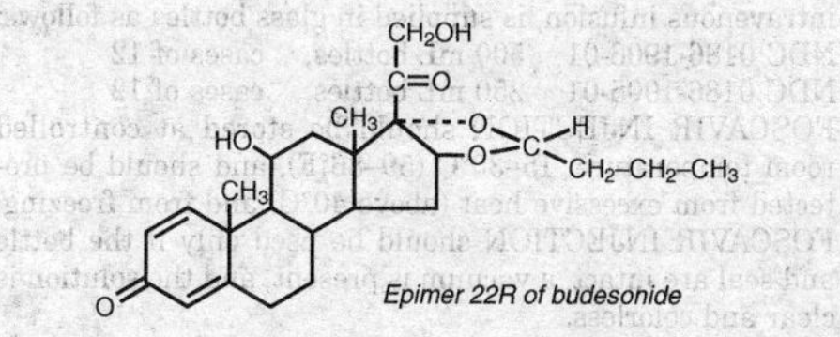

Epimer 22R of budesonide

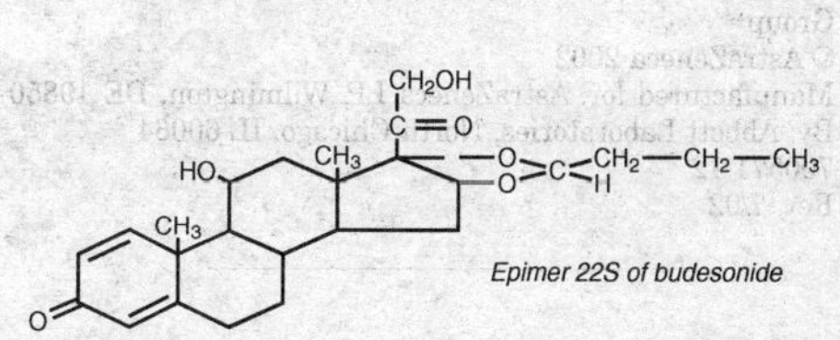

Epimer 22S of budesonide

Budesonide is a white to off-white, tasteless, odorless powder that is practically insoluble in water and heptane, sparingly soluble in ethanol, and freely soluble in chloroform. Its partition coefficient between octanol and water at pH 5 is 1.6×10^3 ionic strength 0.01.

Each capsule contains 3 mg of micronized budesonide with the following inactive ingredients: ethylcellulose, acetyltributyl citrate, methacrylic acid copolymer type C, triethyl citrate, antifoam M, polysorbate 80, talc, and sugar spheres. The capsule shells have the following inactive ingredients: gelatin, iron oxide, and titanium dioxide.

HOW SUPPLIED

ENTOCORT EC 3 mg capsules are hard gelatin capsules with an opaque light grey body and an opaque pink cap, coded with Entocort EC 3 mg on the capsule.

They are supplied as follows:

NDC 0186-0702-10 Bottles of 100

Storage

Store at 25°C (77°F); excursions permitted to 15-30°C (59-86°F) [See USP Controlled Room Temperature].

Keep container tightly closed.

All trademarks are the property of the AstraZeneca group

Manufactured for:

AstraZeneca LP, Wilmington, DE 19850

By: AstraZeneca AB, S-151 85 Södertälje, Sweden

65006–00 Rev 10/02

AstraZeneca

Shown in Product Identification Guide, page 305

Continued on next page

FOSCAVIR® ℞
(foscarnet sodium) Injection
℞ only

WARNING
RENAL IMPAIRMENT IS THE MAJOR TOXICITY OF FOSCAVIR. FREQUENT MONITORING OF SERUM CREATININE, WITH DOSE ADJUSTMENT FOR CHANGES IN RENAL FUNCTION, AND ADEQUATE HYDRATION WITH ADMINISTRATION OF FOSCAVIR, IS IMPERATIVE. (See ADMINISTRATION section; Hydration.)
SEIZURES, RELATED TO ALTERATIONS IN PLASMA MINERALS AND ELECTROLYTES, HAVE BEEN ASSOCIATED WITH FOSCAVIR TREATMENT. THEREFORE, PATIENTS MUST BE CAREFULLY MONITORED FOR SUCH CHANGES AND THEIR POTENTIAL SEQUELAE. MINERAL AND ELECTROLYTE SUPPLEMENTATION MAY BE REQUIRED.
FOSCAVIR IS INDICATED FOR USE ONLY IN IMMUNOCOMPROMISED PATIENTS WITH CMV RETINITIS AND MUCOCUTANEOUS ACYCLOVIR-RESISTANT HSV INFECTIONS. (See INDICATIONS section.)

DESCRIPTION
FOSCAVIR is the brand name for foscarnet sodium. The chemical name of foscarnet sodium is phosphonoformic acid, trisodium salt. Foscarnet sodium is a white, crystalline powder containing 6 equivalents of water of hydration with an empirical formula of $Na_3CO_5P \bullet 6\ H_2O$ and a molecular weight of 300.1. The structural formula is:

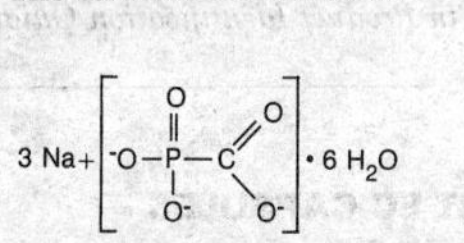

3 Na+ [-O-P(=O)(O-)-C(=O)O-] • 6 H₂O

FOSCAVIR has the potential to chelate divalent metal ions, such as calcium and magnesium, to form stable coordination compounds. FOSCAVIR INJECTION is a sterile, isotonic aqueous solution for intravenous administration only. The solution is clear and colorless. Each milliliter of FOSCAVIR contains 24 mg of foscarnet sodium hexahydrate in Water for Injection, USP. Hydrochloric acid and/or sodium hydroxide may have been added to adjust the pH of the solution to 7.4. FOSCAVIR INJECTION contains no preservatives.

HOW SUPPLIED
FOSCAVIR (foscarnet sodium) INJECTION, 24 mg/mL for intravenous infusion, is supplied in glass bottles as follows:
NDC 0186-1906-01 500 mL bottles, cases of 12
NDC 0186-1905-01 250 mL bottles, cases of 12
FOSCAVIR INJECTION should be stored at controlled room temperature, 15–30°C (59–86°F), and should be protected from excessive heat (above 40°C) and from freezing. FOSCAVIR INJECTION should be used only if the bottle and seal are intact, a vacuum is present, and the solution is clear and colorless.
Trademarks herein are the property of the AstraZeneca Group

Manufactured for: AstraZeneca LP, Wilmington, DE 19850
By: Abbott Laboratories, North Chicago, IL 60064
700571-12
Rev. 7/02

LEXXEL® ℞
(enalapril maleate-felodipine ER)
TABLETS

USE IN PREGNANCY
When used in pregnancy during the second and third trimesters, ACE inhibitors can cause injury and even death to the developing fetus. When pregnancy is detected, LEXXEL should be discontinued as soon as possible. See WARNINGS, Fetal/Neonatal Morbidity and Mortality.

DESCRIPTION
LEXXEL (enalapril maleate-felodipine ER) is a combination product, consisting of an outer layer of enalapril maleate surrounding a core tablet of an extended-release felodipine formulation.
Enalapril maleate is the maleate salt of enalapril, the ethyl ester of a long-acting angiotensin converting enzyme inhibitor, enalaprilat. Enalapril maleate is chemically described as (S)-1-[N-[1-(ethoxycarbonyl)-3-phenylpropyl]-L-alanyl]-L-proline, (Z)-2-butenedioate salt (1:1). Its empirical formula is $C_{20}H_{28}N_2O_5 \bullet C_4H_4O_4$, and its structural formula is:
[See chemical structure at top of next column] 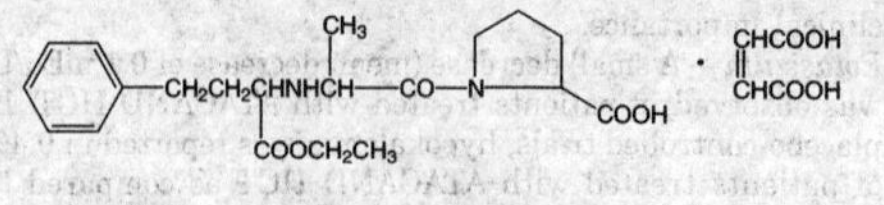
Enalapril maleate is a white to off-white, crystalline powder with a molecular weight of 492.53. It is sparingly soluble in water, soluble in ethanol, and freely soluble in methanol.
Felodipine, a calcium channel blocker, is a dihydropyridine derivative that is chemically described as ± ethyl methyl 4-(2,3-dichlorophenyl)-1,4-dihydro-2,6-dimethyl-3,5-pyridinedicarboxylate. Its empirical formula is $C_{18}H_{19}Cl_2NO_4$ and its structural formula is:

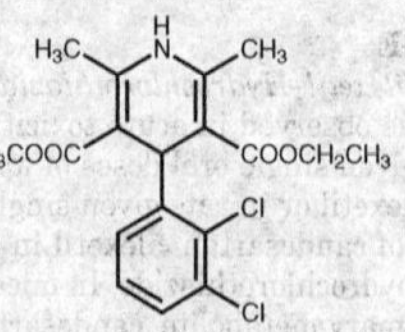

Felodipine is a slightly yellowish, crystalline powder with a molecular weight of 384.26. It is insoluble in water and is freely soluble in dichloromethane and ethanol. Felodipine is a racemic mixture; however, S-felodipine is the more biologically active enantiomer.
LEXXEL is available for oral use in two tablet combinations of enalapril maleate with felodipine as an extended-release formulation: LEXXEL 5-2.5, containing 5 mg of enalapril maleate and 2.5 mg of felodipine ER and LEXXEL 5-5, containing 5 mg of enalapril maleate and 5 mg of felodipine ER. Inactive ingredients include: propyl gallate, polyoxyl 40 hydrogenated castor oil, cellulose compounds, lactose, aluminum silicate, sodium stearyl fumarate, carnauba wax, and iron oxides. The tablets are imprinted with an ink of synthetic red iron oxide (LEXXEL 5-2.5) or synthetic black iron oxide (LEXXEL 5-5) which contains pharmaceutical glaze in SD-45, n-butyl alcohol, propylene glycol, isopropyl alcohol, ammonium hydroxide, and simethicone (LEXXEL 5-2.5) and methyl alcohol (LEXXEL 5-5).

HOW SUPPLIED
No. 3771—Tablets LEXXEL, 5-2.5 are white, round/biconvex-shaped, film-coated tablets, coded LEXXEL 2, 5-2.5 on one side and no markings on the other. Each tablet contains 5 mg of enalapril maleate and 2.5 mg of felodipine as an extended-release formulation. They are supplied as follows:
NDC 0186-0002-31 unit of use bottles of 30 (with desiccants)
No. 3661—Tablets LEXXEL, 5-5 are white, round/biconvex-shaped, film-coated tablets, coded LEXXEL 1, 5-5 on one side and no markings on the other. Each tablet contains 5 mg of enalapril maleate and 5 mg of felodipine as an extended-release formulation. They are supplied as follows:
NDC 0186-0001-31 unit of use bottles of 30 (with desiccants)
NDC 0186-0001-68 bottles of 100 (with desiccants)

Storage
Store at 25°C (77°F); excursions permitted between 15°C and 30°C (59°F and 86°F) [See USP Controlled Room Temperature]. Keep container tightly closed. Protect from moisture and light. Dispense in a tight container, if product package is subdivided.
Rev. 11/03
LEXXEL is a trademark of the AstraZeneca group

Manufactured for: AstraZeneca LP
Wilmington, DE 19850
By: Merck & Co., Inc., Whitehouse Station, NJ 08889, USA
9176508
620008-08
Rev. 11/03
Shown in Product Identification Guide, page 305

NAROPIN® ℞
[nă'rō-pĭn]
(ropivacaine HCl) Injection
℞ only

DESCRIPTION
Naropin® Injection contains ropivacaine HCl which is a member of the amino amide class of local anesthetics. Naropin Injection is a sterile, isotonic solution that contains the enantiomerically pure drug substance, sodium chloride for isotonicity and Water for Injection. Sodium hydroxide and/or hydrochloric acid may be used for pH adjustment. It is administered parenterally.
Ropivacaine HCl is chemically described as S-(-)-1-propyl-2',6'-pipecoloxylidide hydrochloride monohydrate. The drug substance is a white crystalline powder, with a molecular formula of $C_{17}H_{26}N_2O \bullet HCl \bullet H_2O$, molecular weight of 328.89 and the following structural formula:
[See chemical structure at top of next column] 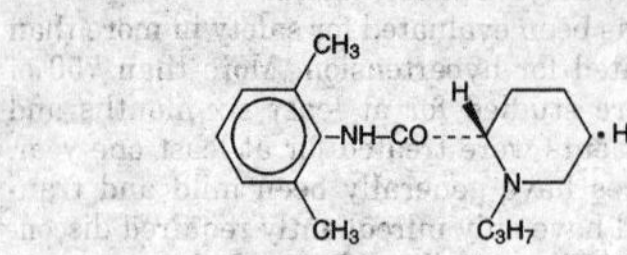
At 25°C ropivacaine HCl has a solubility of 53.8 mg/mL in water, a distribution ratio between n-octanol and phosphate buffer at pH 7.4 of 14:1 and a pKa of 8.07 in 0.1 M KCl solution. The pKa of ropivacaine is approximately the same as bupivacaine (8.1) and is similar to that of mepivacaine (7.7). However, ropivacaine has an intermediate degree of lipid solubility compared to bupivacaine and mepivacaine.
Naropin Injection is preservative-free and is available in single dose containers in 2.0 (0.2%), 5.0 (0.5%), 7.5 (0.75%) and 10.0 mg/mL(1.0%) concentrations. The specific gravity of Naropin solutions range from 1.002 to 1.005 at 25°C.

CLINICAL PHARMACOLOGY
Mechanism of Action
Ropivacaine is a member of the amino amide class of local anesthetics and is supplied as the pure S-(-)-enantiomer. Local anesthetics block the generation and the conduction of nerve impulses, presumably by increasing the threshold for electrical excitation in the nerve, by slowing the propagation of the nerve impulse, and by reducing the rate of rise of the action potential. In general, the progression of anesthesia is related to the diameter, myelination and conduction velocity of affected nerve fibers. Clinically, the order of loss of nerve function is as follows: (1) pain, (2) temperature, (3) touch, (4) proprioception, and (5) skeletal muscle tone.
PHARMACOKINETICS
Absorption
The systemic concentration of ropivacaine is dependent on the total dose and concentration of drug administered, the route of administration, the patient's hemodynamic/circulatory condition, and the vascularity of the administration site.
From the epidural space, ropivacaine shows complete and biphasic absorption. The half-lives of the 2 phases, (mean ± SD) are 14 ± 7 minutes and 4.2 ± 0.9 h, respectively. The slow absorption is the rate limiting factor in the elimination of ropivacaine which explains why the terminal half-life is longer after epidural than after intravenous administration.
Ropivacaine shows dose-proportionality up to the highest intravenous dose studied, 80 mg, corresponding to a mean ± SD peak plasma concentration of 1.9 ± 0.3 µg/mL.
[See table 1 at top of next page]
In some patients after a 300 mg dose for brachial plexus block, free plasma concentrations of ropivacaine may approach the threshold for CNS toxicity. (See PRECAUTIONS.) At a dose of greater than 300 mg, for local infiltration, the terminal half-life may be longer (>30 hours).
Distribution
After intravascular infusion, ropivacaine has a steady state volume of distribution of 41 ± 7 liters. Ropivacaine is 94% protein bound, mainly to α-acid glycoprotein. An increase in total plasma concentrations during continuous epidural infusion has been observed, related to a postoperative increase of α_1-acid glycoprotein. Variations in unbound, ie, pharmacologically active, concentrations have been less than in total plasma concentration. Ropivacaine readily crosses the placenta and equilibrium in regard to unbound concentration will be rapidly reached. (See PRECAUTIONS, Labor and Delivery.)
Metabolism
Ropivacaine is extensively metabolized in the liver, predominantly by aromatic hydroxylation mediated by cytochrome P4501A to 3-hydroxy ropivacaine. After a single IV dose approximately 37% of the total dose is excreted in the urine as both free and conjugated 3-hydroxy ropivacaine. Low concentrations of 3-hydroxy ropivacaine have been found in the plasma. Urinary excretion of the 4-hydroxy ropivacaine, and both the 3-hydroxy N-de-alkylated (3-OH-PPX) and 4-hydroxy N-de-alkylated (4-OH-PPX) metabolites account for less than 3% of the dose. An additional metabolite, 2-hydroxy-methyl-ropivacaine, has been identified but not quantified in the urine. The N-de-alkylated metabolite of ropivacaine (PPX) and 3-OH-ropivacaine are the major metabolites excreted in the urine during epidural infusion. Total PPX concentration in the plasma was about half as that of total ropivacaine; however, mean unbound concentrations of PPX was about 7 to 9 times higher than that of unbound ropivacaine following continuous epidural infusion up to 72 hours. Unbound PPX, 3-hydroxy and 4-hydroxy ropivacaine, have a pharmacological activity in animal models less than that of ropivacaine. There is no evidence of *in vivo* racemization in urine of ropivacaine.
Elimination
The kidney is the main excretory organ for most local anesthetic metabolites. In total, 86% of the ropivacaine dose is excreted in the urine after intravenous administration of which only 1% relates to unchanged drug. Ropivacaine has a mean ± SD total plasma clearance of 387 ± 107 mL/min, an unbound plasma clearance of 7.2 ± 1.6 L/min, and a renal clearance of 1 mL/min. The mean ± SD terminal half-life is 1.8 ± 0.7 h after intravascular administration and 4.2 ± 1.0 h after epidural administration (see Absorption).
Pharmacodynamics
Studies in humans have demonstrated that, unlike most other local anesthetics, the presence of epinephrine has no major effect on either the time of onset or the duration of action of ropivacaine. Likewise, addition of epinephrine to ropivacaine has no effect on limiting systemic absorption of ropivacaine.
Systemic absorption of local anesthetics can produce effects on the central nervous and cardiovascular systems. At blood concentrations achieved with therapeutic doses, changes in cardiac conduction, excitability, refractoriness, contractility, and peripheral vascular resistance have been reported. Toxic blood concentrations depress cardiac conduction and

Table 1:
Pharmacokinetic (plasma concentration-time) data from clinical trials

Route	Epidural Infusion[a]		Epidural Infusion[a]	Epidural Block[b]	Epidural Block[b]	Plexus Block[c]	IV Infusion[d]
Dose (mg)	1493±10	2075±206	1217±277	150	187.5	300	40
N	12	12	11	8	8	10	12
C_{max} (mg/L)	2.4±1[e]	2.8±0.5[e]	2.3±1.1[e]	1.1±0.2	1.6±0.6	2.3±0.8	1.2±0.2[f]
T_{max} (min)	n/a[h]	n/a	n/a	43±14	34±9	54±22	n/a
AUC_0-(mg.h/L)	135.5±50	145±34	161±90	7.2±2	11.3±4	13±3.3	1.8±0.6
CL (L/h)	11.03	13.7	n/a	5.5±2	5±2.6	n/a	21.2±7
$t_{1/2}$ (hr)[g]	5±2.5	5.7±3	6.0±3	5.7±2	7.1±3	6.8±3.2	1.9±0.5

[a] Continuous 72 hour epidural infusion after an epidural block with 5 or 10 mg/mL.
[b] Epidural anesthesia with 7.5 mg/mL (0.75%) for cesarean delivery.
[c] Brachial plexus block with 7.5 mg/mL (0.75%) ropivacaine.
[d] 20 minute IV infusion to volunteers (40 mg).
[e] C_{max} measured at the end of infusion (ie, at 72 hr).
[f] C_{max} measured at the end of infusion (ie, at 20 minutes).
[g] $t_{1/2}$ is the true terminal elimination half-life. On the other hand, $t_{1/2}$ follows absorption-dependent elimination (flip-flop) after non-intravenous administration.
[h] n/a=not applicable

excitability, which may lead to atrioventricular block, ventricular arrhythmias and to cardiac arrest, sometimes resulting in fatalities. In addition, myocardial contractility is depressed and peripheral vasodilation occurs, leading to decreased cardiac output and arterial blood pressure.
Following systemic absorption, local anesthetics can produce central nervous system stimulation, depression or both. Apparent central stimulation is usually manifested as restlessness, tremors and shivering, progressing to convulsions, followed by depression and coma, progressing ultimately to respiratory arrest. However, the local anesthetics have a primary depressant effect on the medulla and on higher centers. The depressed stage may occur without a prior excited stage.
In 2 clinical pharmacology studies (total n=24) ropivacaine and bupivacaine were infused (10 mg/min) in human volunteers until the appearance of CNS symptoms, eg, visual or hearing disturbances, perioral numbness, tingling and others. Similar symptoms were seen with both drugs. In 1 study, the mean ± SD maximum tolerated intravenous dose of ropivacaine infused (124 ± 38 mg) was significantly higher than that of bupivacaine (99 ± 30 mg) while in the other study the doses were not different (115 ± 29 mg of ropivacaine and 103 ± 30 mg of bupivacaine). In the latter study, the number of subjects reporting each symptom was similar for both drugs with the exception of muscle twitching which was reported by more subjects with bupivacaine than ropivacaine at comparable intravenous doses. At the end of the infusion, ropivacaine in both studies caused significantly less depression of cardiac conductivity (less QRS widening) than bupivacaine. Ropivacaine and bupivacaine caused evidence of depression of cardiac contractility, but there were no changes in cardiac output.
Clinical data in one published article indicate that differences in various pharmacodynamic measures were observed with increasing age. In one study, the upper level of analgesia increased with age, the maximum decrease of mean arterial pressure (MAP) declined with age during the first hour after epidural administration, and the intensity of motor blockade increased with age. However, no pharmacokinetic differences were observed between elderly and younger patients.
In non-clinical pharmacology studies comparing ropivacaine and bupivacaine in several animal species, the cardiac toxicity of ropivacaine was less than that of bupivacaine, although both were considerably more toxic than lidocaine. Arrhythmogenic and cardio-depressant effects were seen in animals at significantly higher doses of ropivacaine than bupivacaine. The incidence of successful resuscitation was not significantly different between the ropivacaine and bupivacaine groups.

Clinical Trials

Ropivacaine was studied as a local anesthetic both for surgical anesthesia and for acute pain management. (See DOSAGE AND ADMINISTRATION.)
The onset, depth and duration of sensory block are, in general, similar to bupivacaine. However, the depth and duration of motor block, in general, are less than that with bupivacaine.

Epidural Administration In Surgery

There were 25 clinical studies performed in 900 patients to evaluate Naropin epidural injection for general surgery. Naropin was used in doses ranging from 75 to 250 mg. In doses of 100-200 mg, the median (1st-3rd quartile) onset time to achieve a T10 sensory block was 10 (5-13) minutes and the median (1st-3rd quartile) duration at the T10 level was 4 (3-5) hours. (See DOSAGE AND ADMINISTRATION.) Higher doses produced a more profound block with a greater duration of effect.

Epidural Administration In Cesarean Section

A total of 12 studies were performed with epidural administration of Naropin for cesarean section. Eight of these studies involved 218 patients using the concentration of 5 mg/mL (0.5%) in doses up to 150 mg. Median onset measured at T6 ranged from 11 to 26 minutes. Median duration of sensory block at T6 ranged from 1.7 to 3.2 h, and duration of motor block ranged from 1.4 to 2.9 h. Naropin provided adequate muscle relaxation for surgery in all cases.
In addition, 4 active controlled studies for cesarean section were performed in 264 patients at a concentration of 7.5 mg/mL (0.75%) in doses up to 187.5 mg. Median onset measured at T6 ranged from 4 to 15 minutes. Seventy-seven to 96% of Naropin-exposed patients reported no pain at delivery. Some patients received other anesthetic, analgesic, or sedative modalities during the course of the operative procedure.

Epidural Administration In Labor And Delivery

A total of 9 double-blind clinical studies, involving 240 patients were performed to evaluate Naropin for epidural block for management of labor pain. When administered in doses up to 278 mg as intermittent injections or as a continuous infusion, Naropin produced adequate pain relief.
A prospective meta-analysis on 6 of these studies provided detailed evaluation of the delivered newborns and showed no difference in clinical outcomes compared to bupivacaine. There were significantly fewer instrumental deliveries in mothers receiving ropivacaine as compared to bupivacaine.

Table 2:
LABOR AND DELIVERY META-ANALYSIS: MODE OF DELIVERY

Delivery Mode	Naropin n=199		Bupivacaine n=188	
	n	%	n	%
Spontaneous Vertex	116	58	92	49
Vacuum Extractor	26		33	
		}27*		}40
Forceps	28		42	
Cesarean Section	29	15	21	11

*p=0.004 versus bupivacaine

Epidural Administration In Postoperative Pain Management

There were 8 clinical studies performed in 382 patients to evaluate Naropin 2 mg/mL (0.2%) for postoperative pain management after upper and lower abdominal surgery and after orthopedic surgery. The studies utilized intravascular morphine via PCA as a rescue medication and quantified as an efficacy variable.
Epidural anesthesia with Naropin 5 mg/mL, (0.5%) was used intraoperatively for each of these procedures prior to initiation of postoperative Naropin. The incidence and intensity of the motor block were dependent on the dose rate of Naropin and the site of injection. Cumulative doses of up to 770 mg of ropivacaine were administered over 24 hours (intraoperative block plus postoperative continuous infusion). The overall quality of pain relief, as judged by the patients, in the ropivacaine groups was rated as good or excellent (73% to 100%). The frequency of motor block was greatest at 4 hours and decreased during the infusion period in all groups. At least 80% of patients in the upper and lower abdominal studies and 42% in the orthopedic studies had no motor block at the end of the 21-hour infusion period. Sensory block was also dose rate-dependent and a decrease in spread was observed during the infusion period.
A double blind, randomized, clinical trial compared lumbar epidural infusion of Naropin (n=26) and bupivacaine (n=26) at 2 mg/mL (8 mL/h), for 24 hours after knee replacement. In this study, the pain scores were higher in the Naropin group, but the incidence and the intensity of motor block were lower.
Continuous epidural infusion of Naropin 2 mg/mL (0.2%) during up to 72 hours for postoperative pain management after major abdominal surgery was studied in 2 multicenter, double-blind studies. A total of 391 patients received a low thoracic epidural catheter, and Naropin 7.5 mg/mL (0.75%) was given for surgery, in combination with GA. Postoperatively, Naropin 2 mg/mL (0.2%), 4-14 mL/h, alone or with fentanyl 1, 2, or 4 μg/mL was infused through the epidural catheter and adjusted according to the patient's needs. These studies support the use of Naropin 2 mg/mL (0.2%) for epidural infusion at 6-14 mL/h (12-28 mg) for up to 72 hours and demonstrated adequate analgesia with only slight and nonprogressive motor block in cases of moderate to severe postoperative pain.
Clinical studies with 2 mg/mL (0.2%) Naropin have demonstrated that infusion rates of 6-14 mL (12-28 mg) per hour provide adequate analgesia with nonprogressive motor block in cases of moderate to severe postoperative pain. In these studies, this technique resulted in a significant reduction in patients' morphine rescue dose requirement. Clinical experience supports the use of Naropin epidural infusions for up to 72 hours.

Peripheral Nerve Block

Naropin, 5 mg/mL (0.5%), was evaluated for its ability to provide anesthesia for surgery using the techniques of Peripheral Nerve Block. There were 13 studies performed including a series of 4 pharmacodynamic and pharmacokinetic studies performed on minor nerve blocks. From these, 235 Naropin treated patients were evaluable for efficacy. Naropin was used in doses up to 275 mg. When used for brachial plexus block, onset depended on technique used. Supraclavicular blocks were consistently more successful than axillary blocks. The median onset of sensory block (anesthesia) produced by ropivacaine 0.5% via axillary block ranged from 10 minutes (medial brachial cutaneous nerve) to 45 minutes (musculocutaneous nerve). Median duration ranged from 3.7 hours (medial brachial cutaneous nerve) to 8.7 hours (ulnar nerve). The 5 mg/mL (0.5%) Naropin solution gave success rates from 56% to 86% for axillary blocks, compared with 92% for supraclavicular blocks.
In addition, Naropin, 7.5 mg/mL (0.75%), was evaluated in 99 Naropin treated patients, in 2 double-blind studies, performed to provide anesthesia for surgery using the techniques of Brachial Plexus Block. Naropin 7.5 mg/mL was compared to bupivacaine 5 mg/mL. In 1 study, patients underwent axillary brachial plexus block using injections of 40 mL (300 mg) of Naropin, 7.5 mg/mL (0.75%) or 40 mL injections of bupivacaine, 5 mg/mL (200 mg). In a second study, patients underwent subclavian perivascular brachial plexus block using 30 mL (225 mg) of Naropin, 7.5 mg/mL (0.75%) or 30 mL of bupivacaine 5 mg/mL (150 mg). There was no significant difference between the Naropin and bupivacaine groups in either study with regard to onset of anesthesia, duration of sensory blockade, or duration of anesthesia.
The median duration of anesthesia varied between 11.4 and 14.4 hours with both techniques. In one study, using the axillary technique, the quality of analgesia and muscle relaxation in the Naropin group was judged to be significantly superior to bupivacaine by both investigator and surgeon. However, using the subclavian perivascular technique, no statistically significant difference was found in the quality of analgesia and muscle relaxation as judged by both the investigator and surgeon. The use of Naropin 7.5 mg/mL for block of the brachial plexus via either the subclavian perivascular approach using 30 mL (225 mg) or via the axillary approach using 40 mL (300 mg) both provided effective and reliable anesthesia.

Local Infiltration

A total of 7 clinical studies were performed to evaluate the local infiltration of Naropin to produce anesthesia for surgery and analgesia in postoperative pain management. In these studies 297 patients who received Naropin in doses up to 200 mg (concentrations up to 5 mg/mL, 0.5%) were evaluable for efficacy. With infiltration of 100-200 mg Naropin, the time to first request for analgesic was 2-6 hours. When compared to placebo, Naropin produced lower pain scores and a reduction of analgesic consumption.

INDICATIONS AND USAGE

Naropin is indicated for the production of local or regional anesthesia for surgery and for acute pain management.

Surgical Anesthesia:	epidural block for surgery including cesarean section; major nerve block; local infiltration
Acute Pain Management:	epidural continuous infusion or intermittent bolus, eg, postoperative or labor; local infiltration

CONTRAINDICATIONS

Naropin is contraindicated in patients with a known hypersensitivity to ropivacaine or to any local anesthetic agent of the amide type.

WARNINGS

IN PERFORMING NAROPIN BLOCKS, UNINTENDED INTRAVENOUS INJECTION IS POSSIBLE AND MAY RESULT IN CARDIAC ARRHYTHMIA OR CARDIAC ARREST. THE POTENTIAL FOR SUCCESSFUL RESUSCITATION HAS NOT BEEN STUDIED IN HUMANS. NAROPIN SHOULD BE ADMINISTERED IN INCREMENTAL DOSES. IT IS NOT RECOMMENDED FOR EMERGENCY SITUATIONS, WHERE A FAST ONSET OF SURGICAL ANESTHESIA IS NECESSARY. HISTORICALLY, PREGNANT PATIENTS WERE REPORTED TO HAVE A HIGH RISK FOR CARDIAC ARRHYTHMIAS, CARDIAC/CIRCULATORY ARREST AND DEATH WHEN 0.75% BUPIVACAINE (ANOTHER MEMBER OF THE

Continued on next page

Naropin—Cont.

AMINO AMIDE CLASS OF LOCAL ANESTHETICS) WAS INADVERTENTLY RAPIDLY INJECTED INTRAVENOUSLY.

LOCAL ANESTHETICS SHOULD ONLY BE ADMINISTERED BY CLINICIANS WHO ARE WELL VERSED IN THE DIAGNOSIS AND MANAGEMENT OF DOSE-RELATED TOXICITY AND OTHER ACUTE EMERGENCIES WHICH MIGHT ARISE FROM THE BLOCK TO BE EMPLOYED, AND THEN ONLY AFTER INSURING THE **IMMEDIATE (WITHOUT DELAY)** AVAILABILITY OF OXYGEN, OTHER RESUSCITATIVE DRUGS, CARDIOPULMONARY RESUSCITATIVE EQUIPMENT, AND THE PERSONNEL RESOURCES NEEDED FOR PROPER MANAGEMENT OF TOXIC REACTIONS AND RELATED EMERGENCIES (See also ADVERSE REACTIONS and PRECAUTIONS). DELAY IN PROPER MANAGEMENT OF DOSE-RELATED TOXICITY, UNDERVENTILATION FROM ANY CAUSE, AND/OR ALTERED SENSITIVITY MAY LEAD TO THE DEVELOPMENT OF ACIDOSIS, CARDIAC ARREST AND, POSSIBLY, DEATH. SOLUTIONS OF NAROPIN SHOULD NOT BE USED FOR THE PRODUCTION OF OBSTETRICAL PARACERVICAL BLOCK ANESTHESIA, RETROBULBAR BLOCK, OR SPINAL ANESTHESIA (SUBARACHNOID BLOCK) DUE TO INSUFFICIENT DATA TO SUPPORT SUCH USE. INTRAVENOUS REGIONAL ANESTHESIA (BIER BLOCK) SHOULD NOT BE PERFORMED DUE TO A LACK OF CLINICAL EXPERIENCE AND THE RISK OF ATTAINING TOXIC BLOOD LEVELS OF ROPIVACAINE.

It is essential that aspiration for blood, or cerebrospinal fluid (where applicable), be done prior to injecting any local anesthetic, both the original dose and all subsequent doses, to avoid intravascular or subarachnoid injection. However, a negative aspiration does *not* ensure against an intravascular or subarachnoid injection.

A well-known risk of epidural anesthesia may be an unintentional subarachnoid injection of local anesthetic. Two clinical studies have been performed to verify the safety of Naropin at a volume of 3 mL injected into the subarachnoid space since this dose represents an incremental epidural volume that could be unintentionally injected. The 15 and 22.5 mg doses injected resulted in sensory levels as high as T5 and T4, respectively. Anesthesia to pinprick started in the sacral dermatomes in 2-3 minutes, extended to the T10 level in 10-13 minutes and lasted for approximately 2 hours. The results of these 2 clinical studies showed that a 3 mL dose did not produce any serious adverse events when spinal anesthesia blockade was achieved.

Naropin should be used with caution in patients receiving other local anesthetics or agents structurally related to amide-type local anesthetics, since the toxic effects of these drugs are additive.

PRECAUTIONS

General

The safe and effective use of local anesthetics depends on proper dosage, correct technique, adequate precautions and readiness for emergencies.

Resuscitative equipment, oxygen and other resuscitative drugs should be available for immediate use. (See WARNINGS and ADVERSE REACTIONS.) The lowest dosage that results in effective anesthesia should be used to avoid high plasma levels and serious adverse events. Injections should be made slowly and incrementally, with frequent aspirations before and during the injection to avoid intravascular injection. When a continuous catheter technique is used, syringe aspirations should also be performed before and during each supplemental injection. During the administration of epidural anesthesia, it is recommended that a test dose of a local anesthetic with a fast onset be administered initially and that the patient be monitored for central nervous system and cardiovascular toxicity, as well as for signs of unintended intrathecal administration before proceeding. When clinical conditions permit, consideration should be given to employing local anesthetic solutions, which contain epinephrine for the test dose because circulatory changes compatible with epinephrine may also serve as a warning sign of unintended intravascular injection. An intravascular injection is still possible even if aspirations for blood are negative. Administration of higher than recommended doses of Naropin to achieve greater motor blockade or increased duration of sensory blockade may result in cardiovascular depression, particularly in the event of inadvertent intravascular injection. Tolerance to elevated blood levels varies with the physical condition of the patient. Debilitated, elderly patients and acutely ill patients should be given reduced doses commensurate with their age and physical condition. Local anesthetics should also be used with caution in patients with hypotension, hypovolemia or heart block.

Careful and constant monitoring of cardiovascular and respiratory vital signs (adequacy of ventilation) and the patient's state of consciousness should be performed after each local anesthetic injection. It should be kept in mind at such times that restlessness, anxiety, incoherent speech, lightheadedness, numbness and tingling of the mouth and lips, metallic taste, tinnitus, dizziness, blurred vision, tremors, twitching, depression, or drowsiness may be early warning signs of central nervous system toxicity. Because amide-type local anesthetics such as ropivacaine are metabolized by the liver, these drugs, especially repeat doses, should be used cautiously in patients with hepatic disease. Patients with severe hepatic disease, because of their inability to metabolize local anesthetics normally, are at a greater risk of developing toxic plasma concentrations. Local anesthetics should also be used with caution in patients with impaired cardiovascular function because they may be less able to compensate for functional changes associated with the prolongation of A-V conduction produced by these drugs.

Many drugs used during the conduct of anesthesia are considered potential triggering agents for malignant hyperthermia (MH). Amide-type local anesthetics are not known to trigger this reaction. However, since the need for supplemental general anesthesia cannot be predicted in advance, it is suggested that a standard protocol for MH management should be available.

Epidural Anesthesia

During epidural administration, Naropin should be administered in incremental doses of 3 to 5 mL with sufficient time between doses to detect toxic manifestations of unintentional intravascular or intrathecal injection. Syringe aspirations should also be performed before and during each supplemental injection in continuous (intermittent) catheter techniques. An intravascular injection is still possible even if aspirations for blood are negative. During the administration of epidural anesthesia, it is recommended that a test dose be administered initially and the effects monitored before the full dose is given. When clinical conditions permit, the test dose should contain an appropriate dose of epinephrine to serve as a warning of unintentional intravascular injection. If injected into a blood vessel, this amount of epinephrine is likely to produce a transient "epinephrine response" within 45 seconds, consisting of an increase in heart rate and systolic blood pressure, circumoral pallor, palpitations and nervousness in the unsedated patient. The sedated patient may exhibit only a pulse rate increase of 20 or more beats per minute for 15 or more seconds. Therefore, following the test dose, the heart should be continuously monitored for a heart rate increase. Patients on beta-blockers may not manifest changes in heart rate, but blood pressure monitoring can detect a rise in systolic blood pressure. A test dose of a short-acting amide anesthetic such as lidocaine is recommended to detect an unintentional intrathecal administration. This will be manifested within a few minutes by signs of spinal block (eg, decreased sensation of the buttocks, paresis of the legs, or, in the sedated patient, absent knee jerk). An intravascular or subarachnoid injection is still possible even if results of the test dose are negative. The test dose itself may produce a systemic toxic reaction, high spinal or epinephrine-induced cardiovascular effects.

Use in Brachial Plexus Block

Ropivacaine plasma concentrations may approach the threshold for central nervous system toxicity after the administration of 300 mg of ropivacaine for brachial plexus block. Caution should be exercised when using the 300 mg dose. (See OVERDOSAGE.)

Use in Head and Neck Area

Small doses of local anesthetics injected into the head and neck area may produce adverse reactions similar to systemic toxicity seen with unintentional intravascular injections of larger doses. The injection procedures require the utmost care. Confusion, convulsions, respiratory depression, and/or respiratory arrest, and cardiovascular stimulation or depression have been reported. These reactions may be due to intra-arterial injection of the local anesthetic with retrograde flow to the cerebral circulation. Patients receiving these blocks should have their circulation and respiration monitored and be constantly observed. Resuscitative equipment and personnel for treating adverse reactions should be immediately available. Dosage recommendations should not be exceeded. (See DOSAGE AND ADMINISTRATION.)

Use in Ophthalmic Surgery

The use of Naropin in retrobulbar blocks for ophthalmic surgery has not been studied. Until appropriate experience is gained, the use of Naropin for such surgery is not recommended.

Information for Patients

When appropriate, patients should be informed in advance that they may experience temporary loss of sensation and motor activity in the anesthetized part of the body following proper administration of lumbar epidural anesthesia. Also, when appropriate, the physician should discuss other information including adverse reactions in the Naropin package insert.

Drug Interactions

Naropin should be used with caution in patients receiving other local anesthetics or agents structurally related to amide-type local anesthetics, since the toxic effects of these drugs are additive. Cytochrome P4501A2 is involved in the formation of 3-hydroxy ropivacaine, the major metabolite. *In vivo*, the plasma clearance of ropivacaine was reduced by 70% during coadministration of fluvoxamine (25 mg bid for 2 days), a selective and potent CYP1A2 inhibitor. Thus strong inhibitors of cytochrome P4501A2, such as fluvoxamine, given concomitantly during administration of Naropin, can interact with Naropin leading to increased ropivacaine plasma levels. Caution should be exercised when CYP1A2 inhibitors are coadministered. Possible interactions with drugs known to be metabolized by CYP1A2 via competitive inhibition such as theophylline and imipramine may also occur. Coadministration of a selective and potent inhibitor of CYP3A4, ketoconazole (100 mg bid for 2 days with ropivacaine infusion administered 1 hour after ketoconazole) caused a 15% reduction in *in-vivo* plasma clearance of ropivacaine.

Table 3A
Adverse Events Reported in ≥1 % of Adult Patients Receiving Regional or Local Anesthesia (Surgery, Labor, Cesarean Section, Post-Operative Pain Management, Peripheral Nerve Block and Local Infiltration)

Adverse Reaction	Naropin total N=1661 N	(%)	Bupivacaine total N=1433 N	(%)
Hypotension	536	(32.3)	408	(28.5)
Nausea	283	(17.0)	207	(14.4)
Vomiting	117	(7.0)	88	(6.1)
Bradycardia	96	(5.8)	73	(5.1)
Headache	84	(5.1)	68	(4.7)
Paresthesia	82	(4.9)	57	(4.0)
Back pain	73	(4.4)	75	(5.2)
Pain	71	(4.3)	71	(5.0)
Pruritus	63	(3.8)	40	(2.8)
Fever	61	(3.7)	37	(2.6)
Dizziness	42	(2.5)	23	(1.6)
Rigors (Chills)	42	(2.5)	24	(1.7)
Postoperative complications	41	(2.5)	44	(3.1)
Hypoesthesia	27	(1.6)	24	(1.7)
Urinary retention	23	(1.4)	20	(1.4)
Progression of labor poor/failed	23	(1.4)	22	(1.5)
Anxiety	21	(1.3)	11	(0.8)
Breast disorder, breast-feeding	21	(1.3)	12	(0.8)
Rhinitis	18	(1.1)	13	(0.9)

Table 3B
Adverse Events Reported in ≥1 % of Fetuses or Neonates of Mothers Who Received Regional Anesthesia (Cesarean Section and Labor Studies)

Adverse Reaction	Naropin total N = 639 N	(%)	Bupivacaine total N = 573 N	(%)
Fetal bradycardia	77	(12.1)	68	(11.9)
Neonatal jaundice	49	(7.7)	47	(8.2)
Neonatal complication-NOS	42	(6.6)	38	(6.6)
Apgar score low	18	(2.8)	14	(2.4)
Neonatal respiratory disorder	17	(2.7)	18	(3.1)
Neonatal tachypnea	14	(2.2)	15	(2.6)
Neonatal fever	13	(2.0)	14	(2.4)
Fetal tachycardia	13	(2.0)	12	(2.1)
Fetal distress	11	(1.7)	10	(1.7)
Neonatal infection	10	(1.6)	8	(1.4)
Neonatal hypoglycemia	8	(1.3)	16	(2.8)

Carcinogenesis, Mutagenesis, Impairment of Fertility

Long term studies in animals of most local anesthetics, including ropivacaine, to evaluate the carcinogenic potential have not been conducted.

Weak mutagenic activity was seen in the mouse lymphoma test. Mutagenicity was not noted in the other assays, demonstrating that the weak signs of *in vitro* activity in the mouse lymphoma test were not manifest under diverse *in vivo* conditions.

Studies performed with ropivacaine in rats did not demonstrate an effect on fertility or general reproductive performance over 2 generations.

Pregnancy Category B

Reproduction toxicity studies have been performed in pregnant New Zealand white rabbits and Sprague-Dawley rats. During gestation days 6-18, rabbits received 1.3, 4.2, or 13 mg/kg/day subcutaneously. In rats, subcutaneous doses of 5.3, 11 and 26 mg/kg/day were administered during gestation days 6-15. No teratogenic effects were observed in rats and rabbits at the highest doses tested. The highest doses of 13 mg/kg/day (rabbits) and 26 mg/kg/day (rats) are approximately 1/3 of the maximum recommended human dose (epidural, 770 mg/24 hours) based on a mg/m^2 basis. In 2 prenatal and postnatal studies, the female rats were dosed daily from day 15 of gestation to day 20 postpartum. The doses were 5.3, 11 and 26 mg/kg/day subcutaneously. There were no treatment-related effects on late fetal development, parturition, lactation, neonatal viability, or growth of the offspring.

In another study with rats, the males were dosed daily for 9 weeks before mating and during mating. The females were dosed daily for 2 weeks before mating and then during the mating, pregnancy, and lactation, up to day 42 post coitus. At 23 mg/kg/day, an increased loss of pups was observed during the first 3 days postpartum. The effect was considered secondary to impaired maternal care due to maternal toxicity.

There are no adequate or well-controlled studies in pregnant women of the effects of Naropin on the developing fetus. Naropin should only be used during pregnancy if the benefits outweigh the risk.

Teratogenicity studies in rats and rabbits did not show evidence of any adverse effects on organogenesis or early fetal development in rats (26 mg/kg sc) or rabbits (13 mg/kg). The doses used were approximately equal to total daily dose based on body surface area. There were no treatment-related effects on late fetal development, parturition, lactation, neonatal viability, or growth of the offspring in 2 perinatal and postnatal studies in rats, at dose levels equivalent to the maximum recommended human dose based on body surface area. In another study at 23 mg/kg, an increased pup loss was seen during the first 3 days postpartum, which was considered secondary to impaired maternal care due to maternal toxicity.

Labor and Delivery

Local anesthetics, including ropivacaine, rapidly cross the placenta, and when used for epidural block can cause varying degrees of maternal, fetal and neonatal toxicity (see CLINICAL PHARMACOLOGY and PHARMACOKINETICS.) The incidence and degree of toxicity depend upon the procedure performed, the type and amount of drug used, and the technique of drug administration. Adverse reactions in the parturient, fetus and neonate involve alterations of the central nervous system, peripheral vascular tone and cardiac function.

Maternal hypotension has resulted from regional anesthesia with Naropin for obstetrical pain relief. Local anesthetics produce vasodilation by blocking sympathetic nerves. Elevating the patient's legs and positioning her on her left side will help prevent decreases in blood pressure. The fetal heart rate also should be monitored continuously, and electronic fetal monitoring is highly advisable. Epidural anesthesia has been reported to prolong the second stage of labor by removing the patient's reflex urge to bear down or by interfering with motor function. Spontaneous vertex delivery occurred more frequently in patients receiving Naropin than in those receiving bupivacaine.

Nursing Mothers

Some local anesthetic drugs are excreted in human milk and caution should be exercised when they are administered to a nursing woman. The excretion of ropivacaine or its metabolites in human milk has not been studied. Based on the milk/plasma concentration ratio in rats, the estimated daily dose to a pup will be about 4% of the dose given to the mother. Assuming that the milk/plasma concentration in humans is of the same order, the total Naropin dose to which the baby is exposed by breast-feeding is far lower than by exposure *in utero* in pregnant women at term (see PRECAUTIONS.)

Pediatric Use

The safety and efficacy of Naropin in pediatric patients have not been established.

Geriatric Use

Of the 2,978 subjects that were administered Naropin Injection in 71 controlled and uncontrolled clinical studies, 803 patients (27%) were 65 years of age or older which includes 127 patients (4%) 75 years of age and over. Naropin Injection was found to be safe and effective in the patients in these studies. Clinical data in one published article indicate that differences in various pharmacodynamic measures were observed with increasing age. In one study, the upper level of analgesia increased with age, the maximum de-

Table 4
Common Events (Epidural Administration)

Adverse Reaction	Naropin						Bupivacaine			
	5 mg/mL total N=256		7.5 mg/mL total N=297		10 mg/mL total N=207		5 mg/mL total N=236		7.5 mg/mL total N=174	
	N	(%)	N	(%)	N	(%)	N	(%)	N	(%)
hypotension	99	(38.7)	146	(49.2)	113	(54.6)	91	(38.6)	89	(51.1)
nausea	34	(13.3)	68	(22.9)			41	(17.4)	36	(20.7)
bradycardia	29	(11.3)	58	(19.5)	40	(19.3)	32	(13.6)	25	(14.4)
back pain	18	(7.0)	23	(7.7)	34	(16.4)	21	(8.9)	23	(13.2)
vomiting	18	(7.0)	33	(11.1)	23	(11.1)	19	(8.1)	14	(8.0)
headache	12	(4.7)	20	(6.7)	16	(7.7)	13	(5.5)	9	(5.2)
fever	8	(3.1)	5	(1.7)	18	(8.7)	11	(4.7)		
chills	6	(2.3)	7	(2.4)	6	(2.9)	4	(1.7)	3	(1.7)
urinary retention	5	(2.0)	8	(2.7)	10	(4.8)	10	(4.2)		
paresthesia	5	(2.0)	10	(3.4)	5	(2.4)	7	(3.0)		
pruritus			14	(4.7)	3	(1.4)			7	(4.0)

Table 5
Effects of Age on Hypotension (Epidural Administration)
Total N: Naropin = 760, bupivacaine = 410

	Naropin						Bupivacaine			
Age	5 mg/mL		7.5 mg/mL		10 mg/mL		5 mg/mL		7.5 mg/mL	
	N	(%)	N	(%)	N	(%)	N	(%)	N	(%)
<65	68	(32.2)	99	(43.2)	87	(51.5)	64	(33.5)	73	(48.3)
≥65	31	(68.9)	47	(69.1)	26	(68.4)	27	(60.0)	16	(69.6)

crease of mean arterial pressure (MAP) declined with age during the first hour after epidural administration, and the intensity of motor blockade increased with age.

This drug and its metabolites are known to be excreted by the kidney, and the risk of toxic reactions to this drug may be greater in patients with impaired renal function. Elderly patients are more likely to have decreased hepatic, renal, or cardiac function, as well as concomitant disease. Therefore, care should be taken in dose selection, starting at the low end of the dosage range, and it may be useful to monitor renal function. (See PHARMACOKINETICS, Elimination.)

ADVERSE REACTIONS

Reactions to ropivacaine are characteristic of those associated with other amide-type local anesthetics. A major cause of adverse reactions to this group of drugs may be associated with excessive plasma levels, which may be due to overdosage, unintentional intravascular injection or slow metabolic degradation.

The reported adverse events are derived from clinical studies conducted in the US and other countries. The reference drug was usually bupivacaine. The studies used a variety of premedications, sedatives, and surgical procedures of varying length. A total of 3988 patients have been exposed to Naropin at concentrations up to 1.0% in clinical trials. Each patient was counted once for each type of adverse event.

Incidence ≥5%

For the indications of epidural administration in surgery, cesarean section, postoperative pain management, peripheral nerve block, and local infiltration, the following treatment-emergent adverse events were reported with an incidence of ≥5% in all clinical studies (N=3988): hypotension (37.0%), nausea (24.8%), vomiting (11.6%), bradycardia (9.3%), fever (9.2%), pain (8.0%) postoperative complications (7.1%), anemia (6.1%), paraesthesia (5.6%), headache (5.1%), pruritus (5.1%), and back pain (5.0%).

Incidence 1–5%

Urinary retention, dizziness, rigors, hypertension, tachycardia, anxiety, oliguria, hypoesthesia, chest pain, hypokalemia, dyspnea, cramps, and urinary tract infection.

Incidence in Controlled Clinical Trials

The reported adverse events are derived from controlled clinical studies with Naropin (concentrations ranged from 0.125% to 1.0% for Naropin and 0.25 % to 0.75% for bupivacaine) in the US and other countries involving 3094 patients. Table 3A and 3B list adverse events (number and percentage) that occurred in at least 1% of Naropin-treated patients in these studies. The majority of patients receiving concentrations higher than 5.0 mg/mL (0.5%) were treated with Naropin.

[See table 3A at top of previous page]
[See table 3B at top of previous page]

Incidence < 1%

The following adverse events were reported during the Naropin clinical program in more than one patient (N=3988), occurred at an overall incidence of <1%, and were considered relevant:

Application Site Reactions—injection site pain
Cardiovascular System—vasovagal reaction, syncope, postural hypotension, non-specific ECG abnormalities
Female Reproductive—poor progression of labor, uterine atony
Gastrointestinal System—fecal incontinence, tenesmus, neonatal vomiting
General and Other Disorders—hypothermia, malaise, asthenia, accident and/or injury
Hearing and Vestibular—tinnitus, hearing abnormalities
Heart Rate and Rhythm—extrasystoles, non-specific arrhythmias, atrial fibrillation
Liver and Biliary System—jaundice
Metabolic Disorders—hypomagnesemia
Musculoskeletal System—myalgia
Myo/Endo/Pericardium—ST segment changes, myocardial infarction
Nervous System—tremor, Horner's syndrome, paresis, dyskinesia, neuropathy, vertigo, coma, convulsion, hypokinesia, hypotonia, ptosis, stupor
Psychiatric Disorders—agitation, confusion, somnolence, nervousness, amnesia, hallucination, emotional lability, insomnia, nightmares
Respiratory System—bronchospasm, coughing
Skin Disorders—rash, urticaria
Urinary System Disorders—urinary incontinence, micturition disorder
Vascular—deep vein thrombosis, phlebitis, pulmonary embolism
Vision—vision abnormalities

For the indication epidural anesthesia for surgery, the 15 most common adverse events were compared between different concentrations of Naropin and bupivacaine. Table 4 is based on data from trials in the U.S. and other countries where Naropin was administered as an epidural anesthetic for surgery.

[See table 4 above]

Using data from the same studies, the number (%) of patients experiencing hypotension is displayed by patient age, drug and concentration in Table 5. In Table 6, the adverse events for Naropin are broken down by gender.

[See table 5 above]

Table 6
Most Common Adverse Events by Gender (Epidural Administration) Total N: Females = 405, Males = 355

Adverse Reaction	Female		Male	
	N	(%)	N	(%)
hypotension	220	(54.3)	138	(38.9)
nausea	119	(29.4)	23	(6.5)
bradycardia	65	(16.0)	56	(15.8)
vomiting	59	(14.6)	8	(2.3)
back pain	41	(10.1)	23	(6.5)
headache	33	(8.1)	17	(4.8)
chills	18	(4.4)	5	(1.4)
fever	16	(4.0)	3	(0.8)
pruritus	16	(4.0)	1	(0.3)
pain	12	(3.0)	4	(1.1)
urinary retention	11	(2.7)	7	(2.0)

Continued on next page

Naropin—Cont.

dizziness	9	(2.2)	4	(1.1)
hypoesthesia	8	(2.0)	2	(0.6)
paresthesia	8	(2.0)	10	(2.8)

Systemic Reactions

The most commonly encountered acute adverse experiences that demand immediate countermeasures are related to the central nervous system and the cardiovascular system. These adverse experiences are generally dose-related and due to high plasma levels which may result from overdosage, rapid absorption from the injection site, diminished tolerance or from unintentional intravascular injection of the local anesthetic solution. In addition to systemic dose-related toxicity, unintentional subarachnoid injection of drug during the intended performance of lumbar epidural block or nerve blocks near the vertebral column (especially in the head and neck region) may result in underventilation or apnea ("Total or High Spinal"). Also, hypotension due to loss of sympathetic tone and respiratory paralysis or underventilation due to cephalad extension of the motor level of anesthesia may occur. This may lead to secondary cardiac arrest if untreated. Factors influencing plasma protein binding, such as acidosis, systemic diseases that alter protein production or competition with other drugs for protein binding sites, may diminish individual tolerance.

Epidural administration of Naropin has, in some cases, as with other local anesthetics, been associated with transient increases in temperature to >38.5°C. This occurred more frequently at doses of Naropin >16 mg/h.

Neurologic Reactions

These are characterized by excitation and/or depression. Restlessness, anxiety, dizziness, tinnitus, blurred vision or tremors may occur, possibly proceeding to convulsions. However, excitement may be transient or absent, with depression being the first manifestation of an adverse reaction. This may quickly be followed by drowsiness merging into unconsciousness and respiratory arrest. Other central nervous system effects may be nausea, vomiting, chills, and constriction of the pupils.

The incidence of convulsions associated with the use of local anesthetics varies with the route of administration and the total dose administered. In a survey of studies of epidural anesthesia, overt toxicity progressing to convulsions occurred in approximately 0.1% of local anesthetic administrations.

The incidence of adverse neurological reactions associated with the use of local anesthetics may be related to the total dose and concentration of local anesthetic administered and are also dependent upon the particular drug used, the route of administration, and the physical status of the patient. Many of these observations may be related to local anesthetic techniques, with or without a contribution from the drug. During lumbar epidural block, occasional unintentional penetration of the subarachnoid space by the catheter or needle may occur. Subsequent adverse effects may depend partially on the amount of drug administered intrathecally as well as the physiological and physical effects of a dural puncture. These observations may include spinal block of varying magnitude (including high or total spinal block), hypotension secondary to spinal block, urinary retention, loss of bladder and bowel control (fecal and urinary incontinence), and loss of perineal sensation and sexual function. Signs and symptoms of subarachnoid block typically start within 2-3 minutes of injection. Doses of 15 and 22.5 mg of Naropin resulted in sensory levels as high as T5 and T4, respectively. Analgesia started in the sacral dermatomes in 2-3 minutes and extended to the T10 level in 10-13 minutes and lasted for approximately 2 hours. Other neurological effects following unintentional subarachnoid administration during epidural anesthesia may include persistent anesthesia, paresthesia, weakness, paralysis of the lower extremities, and loss of sphincter control; all of which may have slow, incomplete or no recovery. Headache, septic meningitis, meningismus, slowing of labor, increased incidence of forceps delivery, or cranial nerve palsies due to traction on nerves from loss of cerebrospinal fluid have been reported (see DOSAGE AND ADMINISTRATION discussion of Lumbar Epidural Block.) A high spinal is characterized by paralysis of the arms, loss of consciousness, respiratory paralysis and bradycardia.

Cardiovascular System Reactions

High doses or unintentional intravascular injection may lead to high plasma levels and related depression of the myocardium, decreased cardiac output, heart block, hypotension, bradycardia, ventricular arrhythmias, including ventricular tachycardia and ventricular fibrillation, and possibly cardiac arrest. (See WARNINGS, PRECAUTIONS and OVERDOSAGE sections.)

Allergic Reactions

Allergic type reactions are rare and may occur as a result of sensitivity to the local anesthetic (see WARNINGS). These reactions are characterized by signs such as urticaria, pruritus, erythema, angioneurotic edema (including laryngeal edema), tachycardia, sneezing, nausea, vomiting, dizziness, syncope, excessive sweating, elevated temperature, and possibly, anaphylactoid symptomatology (including severe hypotension). Cross sensitivity among members of the amide-type local anesthetic group has been reported. The usefulness of screening for sensitivity has not been definitively established.

OVERDOSAGE

Acute emergencies from local anesthetics are generally related to high plasma levels encountered, or large doses administered, during therapeutic use of local anesthetics or to unintended subarachnoid or intravascular injection of local anesthetic solution. (See ADVERSE REACTIONS, WARNINGS and PRECAUTIONS.)

MANAGEMENT OF LOCAL ANESTHETIC EMERGENCIES

Therapy with Naropin should be discontinued at the first sign of toxicity. No specific information is available for the treatment of toxicity with Naropin; therefore, treatment should be symptomatic and supportive. The first consideration is prevention, best accomplished by incremental injection of Naropin, careful and constant monitoring of cardiovascular and respiratory vital signs and the patient's state of consciousness after each local anesthetic and during continuous infusion. At the first sign of change in mental status, oxygen should be administered.

The first step in the management of systemic toxic reactions, as well as underventilation or apnea due to unintentional subarachnoid injection of drug solution, consists of immediate attention to the establishment and maintenance of a patent airway and effective assisted or controlled ventilation with 100% oxygen with a delivery system capable of permitting immediate positive airway pressure by mask. Circulation should be assisted as necessary. This may prevent convulsions if they have not already occurred.

If necessary, use drugs to control convulsions. Intravenous barbiturates, anticonvulsant agents, or muscle relaxants should only be administered by those familiar with their use. Immediately after the institution of these ventilatory measures, the adequacy of the circulation should be evaluated. Supportive treatment of circulatory depression may require administration of intravenous fluids, and, when appropriate, a vasopressor dictated by the clinical situation (such as ephedrine or epinephrine to enhance myocardial contractile force).

The mean dosages of ropivacaine producing seizures, after intravenous infusion in dogs, nonpregnant and pregnant sheep were 4.9, 6.1 and 5.9 mg/kg, respectively. These doses were associated with peak arterial total plasma concentrations of 11.4, 4.3 and 5.0 µg/mL, respectively.

In human volunteers given intravenous Naropin, the mean maximum tolerated total and free arterial plasma concentrations were 4.3 and 0.6 µg/mL respectively, at which time moderate CNS symptoms (muscle twitching) were noted.

Clinical data from patients experiencing local anesthetic induced convulsions demonstrated rapid development of hypoxia, hypercarbia and acidosis within a minute of the onset of convulsions. These observations suggest that oxygen consumption and carbon dioxide production are greatly increased during local anesthetic convulsions and emphasize the importance of immediate and effective ventilation with oxygen which may avoid cardiac arrest.

If difficulty is encountered in the maintenance of a patent airway or if prolonged ventilatory support (assisted or controlled) is indicated, endotracheal intubation, employing drugs and techniques familiar to the clinician, may be indicated after initial administration of oxygen by mask.

The supine position is dangerous in pregnant women at term because of aortocaval compression by the gravid uterus. Therefore, during treatment of systemic toxicity, maternal hypotension or fetal bradycardia following regional block, the parturient should be maintained in the left lateral decubitus position if possible, or manual displacement of the uterus off the great vessels should be accomplished. Resuscitation of obstetrical patients may take longer than resuscitation of non-pregnant patients and closed-chest cardiac compression may be ineffective. Rapid delivery of the fetus may improve the response to resuscitative efforts.

DOSAGE AND ADMINISTRATION

The rapid injection of a large volume of local anesthetic solution should be avoided and fractional (incremental) doses should always be used. The smallest dose and concentration required to produce the desired result should be administered.

The dose of any local anesthetic administered varies with the anesthetic procedure, the area to be anesthetized, the vascularity of the tissues, the number of neuronal segments to be blocked, the depth of anesthesia and degree of muscle relaxation required, the duration of anesthesia desired, individual tolerance, and the physical condition of the patient. Patients in poor general condition due to aging or other compromising factors such as partial or complete heart conduction block, advanced liver disease or severe renal dysfunction require special attention although regional anesthesia is frequently indicated in these patients. To reduce the risk of potentially serious adverse reactions, attempts should be made to optimize the patient's condition before major blocks are performed, and the dosage should be adjusted accordingly.

Use an adequate test dose (3-5 mL of a short acting local anesthetic solution containing epinephrine) prior to induction of complete block. This test dose should be repeated if the patient is moved in such a fashion as to have displaced the epidural catheter. Allow adequate time for onset of anesthesia following administration of each test dose.

Parenteral drug products should be inspected visually for particular matter and discoloration prior to administration, whenever solution and container permit. Solutions which are discolored or which contain particulate matter should not be administered.

[See table 7 at left]

The doses in the table are those considered to be necessary to produce a successful block and should be regarded as

Table 7
DOSAGE RECOMMENDATIONS

	Conc. mg/mL	(%)	Volume mL	Dose mg	Onset min	Duration hours
SURGICAL ANESTHESIA						
Lumbar Epidural	5.0	(0.5%)	15-30	75-150	15-30	2-4
Administration	7.5	(0.75%)	15-25	113-188	10-20	3-5
Surgery	10.0	(1.0%)	15-20	150-200	10-20	4-6
Lumbar Epidural	5.0	(0.5%)	20-30	100-150	15-25	2-4
Administration	7.5	(0.75%)	15-20	113-150	10-20	3-5
Cesarean Section						
Thoracic Epidural	5.0	(0.5%)	5-15	25-75	10-20	n/a[1]
Administration	7.5	(0.75%)	5-15	38-113	10-20	n/a[1]
Surgery						
Major Nerve Block	5.0	(0.5%)	35-50	175-250	15-30	5-8
(eg, brachial plexus block)	7.5	(0.75%)	10-40	75-300	10-25	6-10
Field Block	5.0	(0.5%)	1-40	5-200	1-15	2-6
(eg, minor nerve blocks and infiltration)						
LABOR PAIN MANAGEMENT						
Lumbar Epidural Administration						
Initial Dose	2.0	(0.2%)	10-20	20-40	10-15	0.5-1.5
Continuous infusion[2]	2.0	(0.2%)	6-14 mL/h	12-28 mg/h	n/a[1]	n/a[1]
Incremental injections (top-up)[2]	2.0	(0.2%)	10-15 mL/h	20-30 mg/h	n/a[1]	n/a[1]
POSTOPERATIVE PAIN MANAGEMENT						
Lumbar Epidural Administration						
Continuous infusion[3]	2.0	(0.2%)	6-14 mL/h	12-28 mg/h	n/a[1]	n/a[1]
Thoracic Epidural Administration Continuous infusion[3]	2.0	(0.2%)	6-14 mL/h	12-28 mg/h	n/a[1]	n/a[1]
Infiltration	2.0	(0.2%)	1-100	2-200	1-5	2-6
(eg, minor nerve block)	5.0	(0.5%)	1-40	5-200	1-5	2-6

1 = Not Applicable

2 = Median dose of 21 mg per hour was administered by continuous infusion or by incremental injections (top-ups) over a median delivery time of 5.5 hours.

3 = Cumulative doses up to 770 mg of Naropin over 24 hours (intraoperative block plus postoperative infusion); Continuous epidural infusion at rates up to 28 mg per hour for 72 hours have been well tolerated in adults, ie, 2016 mg plus surgical dose of approximately 100-150 mg as top-up.

guidelines for use in adults. Individual variations in onset and duration occur. The figures reflect the expected average dose range needed. For other local anesthetic techniques standard current textbooks should be consulted.

When prolonged blocks are used, either through continuous infusion or through repeated bolus administration, the risks of reaching a toxic plasma concentration or inducing local neural injury must be considered. Experience to date indicates that a cumulative dose of up to 770 mg Naropin administered over 24 hours is well tolerated in adults when used for postoperative pain management: ie, 2016 mg. Caution should be exercised when administering Naropin for prolonged periods of time, eg, > 70 hours in debilitated patients.

For treatment of postoperative pain, the following technique can be recommended: If regional anesthesia was not used intraoperatively, then an initial epidural block with 5-7 mL Naropin is induced via an epidural catheter. Analgesia is maintained with an infusion of Naropin, 2 mg/mL (0.2%). Clinical studies have demonstrated that infusion rates of 6-14 mL (12-28 mg) per hour provide adequate analgesia with nonprogressive motor block. With this technique a significant reduction in the need for opioids was demonstrated. Clinical experience supports the use of Naropin epidural infusions for up to 72 hours.

HOW SUPPLIED

Naropin® Polyamp DuoFit™ Sterile Pak:
Boxes of 5
polypropylene ampules fitting both Luer-lock and Luer-slip (tapered) syringes

2.0 mg/mL (0.2%)	10 mL	NDC 0186-0859-47 Product No. 0186-0859-44
2.0 mg/mL (0.2%)	20 mL	NDC 0186-0859-57 Product No. 0186-0859-54
5.0 mg/mL (0.5%)	20 mL	NDC 0186-0863-57 Product No. 0186-0863-54
7.5 mg/mL (0.75%)	20 mL	NDC 0186-0867-57 Product No. 0186-0867-54
10.0 mg/mL (1.0%)	10 mL	NDC 0186-0868-47 Product No. 0186-0868-44
10.0 mg/mL (1.0%)	20 mL	NDC 0186-0868-57 Product No. 0186-0868-54

Naropin® Single Dose Vials:

5.0 mg/mL (0.5%)	30 mL	NDC 0186-0863-61

Naropin® Single Dose Infusion Bottles:

2.0 mg/mL (0.2%)	100 mL	NDC 0186-0859-81
2.0 mg/mL (0.2%)	200 mL	NDC 0186-0859-91

Naropin® Sterile-Pak® Single Dose Vials:
Boxes of 5

5.0 mg/mL (0.5%)	30 mL	NDC 0186-0863-61 Product No: 0186-0863-69

The solubility of ropivacaine is limited at pH above 6. Thus care must be taken as precipitation may occur if Naropin is mixed with alkaline solutions.

Disinfecting agents containing heavy metals, which cause release of respective ions (mercury, zinc, copper, etc.) should not be used for skin or mucous membrane disinfection since they have been related to incidents of swelling and edema. When chemical disinfection of the container surface is desired, either isopropyl alcohol (91%) or ethyl alcohol (70%) is recommended. It is recommended that chemical disinfection be accomplished by wiping the ampule or vial stopper thoroughly with cotton or gauze that has been moistened with the recommended alcohol just prior to use. When a container is required to have a sterile outside, a Sterile-Pak should be chosen. Glass containers may, as an alternative, be autoclaved once. Stability has been demonstrated using a targeted F_0 of 7 minutes at 121°C.

Solutions should be stored at controlled room temperature 20-25°C (68-77°F) [see USP].

These products are intended for single use and are free from preservatives. Any solution remaining from an opened container should be discarded promptly. In addition, continuous infusion bottles should not be left in place for more than 24 hours.

AstraZeneca LP Wilmington, DE 19850
AstraZeneca
721683-04
721683-05
721697-06
808407-01 Rev. 06/03

Shown in Product Identification Guide, page 305

NESACAINE® ℞
(chloroprocaine HCl Injection, USP)
[nes' a-caine]
NESACAINE®-MPF
(chloroprocaine HCl Injection, USP)
For Infiltration and Nerve Block.

NEXIUM® ℞
(esomeprazole magnesium)
DELAYED-RELEASE CAPSULES
℞ only

DESCRIPTION

The active ingredient in NEXIUM® (esomeprazole magnesium) Delayed-Release Capsules is bis(5-methoxy-2-[(S)-[(4-methoxy-3,5-dimethyl-2-pyridinyl)methyl]sulfinyl]-1*H*-benzimidazole-1-yl) magnesium trihydrate, a compound that inhibits gastric acid secretion. Esomeprazole is the S-isomer of omeprazole, which is a mixture of the S- and R-isomers. Its empirical formula is $(C_{17}H_{18}N_3O_3S)_2Mg \times 3\ H_2O$ with molecular weight of 767.2 as a trihydrate and 713.1 on an anhydrous basis. The structural formula is:

The magnesium salt is a white to slightly colored crystalline powder. It contains 3 moles of water of solvation and is slightly soluble in water.

The stability of esomeprazole magnesium is a function of pH; it rapidly degrades in acidic media, but it has acceptable stability under alkaline conditions. At pH 6.8 (buffer), the half-life of the magnesium salt is about 19 hours at 25°C and about 8 hours at 37°C.

NEXIUM is supplied as Delayed-Release Capsules for oral administration. Each delayed-release capsule contains 20 mg or 40 mg of esomeprazole (present as 22.3 mg or 44.5 mg esomeprazole magnesium trihydrate) in the form of enteric-coated pellets with the following inactive ingredients: glyceryl monostearate 40–50, hydroxypropyl cellulose, hypromellose, magnesium stearate, methacrylic acid copolymer type C, polysorbate 80, sugar spheres, talc, and triethyl citrate. The capsule shells have the following inactive ingredients: gelatin, FD&C Blue #1, FD&C Red #40, D&C Red #28, titanium dioxide, shellac, ethyl alcohol, isopropyl alcohol, n-butyl alcohol, propylene glycol, sodium hydroxide, polyvinyl pyrrolidone, and D&C Yellow #10.

CLINICAL PHARMACOLOGY

Pharmacokinetics

Absorption

NEXIUM Delayed-Release Capsules contain an enteric-coated pellet formulation of esomeprazole magnesium. After oral administration peak plasma levels (C_{max}) occur at approximately 1.5 hours (T_{max}). The C_{max} increases proportionally when the dose is increased, and there is a three-fold increase in the area under the plasma concentration-time curve (AUC) from 20 to 40 mg. At repeated once-daily dosing with 40 mg, the systemic bioavailability is approximately 90% compared to 64% after a single dose of 40 mg. The mean exposure (AUC) to esomeprazole increases from 4.32 μmol*hr/L on day 1 to 11.2 μmol*hr/L on day 5 after 40 mg once daily dosing.

The AUC after administration of a single 40 mg dose of esomeprazole is decreased by 43–53% after food intake compared to fasting conditions. Esomeprazole should be taken at least one hour before meals.

The pharmacokinetic profile of esomeprazole was determined in 36 patients with symptomatic gastroesophageal reflux disease following repeated once daily administration of 20 mg and 40 mg capsules of NEXIUM over a period of five days. The results are shown in the following table:

Pharmacokinetic Parameters of NEXIUM Following Oral Dosing for 5 days

Parameter	NEXIUM 40 mg	NEXIUM 20 mg
AUC (μmol*h/L)	12.6	4.2
Coefficient of variation	42%	59%
C_{max} (μmol/L)	4.7	2.1
T_{max} (h)	1.6	1.6
$t_{1/2}$ (h)	1.5	1.2

Values represent the geometric mean, except the T_{max}, which is the arithmetic mean.

Distribution

Esomeprazole is 97% bound to plasma proteins. Plasma protein binding is constant over the concentration range of 2–20 μmol/L. The apparent volume of distribution at steady state in healthy volunteers is approximately 16 L.

Metabolism

Esomeprazole is extensively metabolized in the liver by the cytochrome P450 (CYP) enzyme system. The metabolites of esomeprazole lack antisecretory activity. The major part of esomeprazole's metabolism is dependent upon the CYP2C19 isoenzyme, which forms the hydroxy and desmethyl metabolites. The remaining amount is dependent on CYP3A4 which forms the sulphone metabolite. CYP2C19 isoenzyme exhibits polymorphism in the metabolism of esomeprazole, since some 3% of Caucasians and 15–20% of Asians lack CYP2C19 and are termed Poor metabolizers. At steady state, the ratio of AUC in Poor metabolizers to AUC in the rest of the population (Extensive metabolizers) is approximately 2.

Following administration of equimolar doses, the S- and R-isomers are metabolized differently by the liver, resulting in higher plasma levels of the S- than of the R-isomer.

Excretion

The plasma elimination half-life of esomeprazole is approximately 1–1.5 hours. Less than 1% of parent drug is excreted in the urine. Approximately 80% of an oral dose of esomeprazole is excreted as inactive metabolites in the urine, and the remainder is found as inactive metabolites in the feces.

Special Populations

Geriatric

The AUC and C_{max} values were slightly higher (25% and 18%, respectively) in the elderly as compared to younger subjects at steady state. Dosage adjustment based on age is not necessary.

Pediatric

The pharmacokinetics of esomeprazole have not been studied in patients < 18 years of age.

Gender

The AUC and C_{max} values were slightly higher (13%) in females than in males at steady state. Dosage adjustment based on gender is not necessary.

Hepatic Insufficiency

The steady state pharmacokinetics of esomeprazole obtained after administration of 40 mg once daily to 4 patients each with mild (Child Pugh A), moderate (Child Pugh Class B), and severe (Child Pugh Class C) liver insufficiency were compared to those obtained in 36 male and female GERD patients with normal liver function. In patients with mild and moderate hepatic insufficiency, the AUCs were within the range that could be expected in patients with normal liver function. In patients with severe hepatic insufficiency the AUCs were 2 to 3 times higher than in the patients with normal liver function. No dosage adjustment is recommended for patients with mild to moderate hepatic insufficiency (Child Pugh Classes A and B). However, in patients with severe hepatic insufficiency (Child Pugh Class C) a dose of 20 mg once daily should not be exceeded (See **DOSAGE AND ADMINISTRATION**).

Renal Insufficiency

The pharmacokinetics of esomeprazole in patients with renal impairment are not expected to be altered relative to healthy volunteers as less than 1% of esomeprazole is excreted unchanged in urine.

Pharmacokinetics: Combination Therapy with Antimicrobials

Esomeprazole magnesium 40 mg once daily was given in combination with clarithromycin 500 mg twice daily and amoxicillin 1000 mg twice daily for 7 days to 17 healthy male and female subjects. The mean steady state AUC and C_{max} of esomeprazole increased by 70% and 18%, respectively during triple combination therapy compared to treatment with esomeprazole alone. The observed increase in esomeprazole exposure during co-administration with clarithromycin and amoxicillin is not expected to produce significant safety concerns.

The pharmacokinetic parameters for clarithromycin and amoxicillin were similar during triple combination therapy and administration of each drug alone. However, the mean AUC and C_{max} for 14-hydroxyclarithromycin increased by 19% and 22%, respectively, during triple combination therapy compared to treatment with clarithromycin alone. This increase in exposure to 14-hydroxyclarithromycin is not considered to be clinically significant.

Pharmacodynamics

Mechanism of Action

Esomeprazole is a proton pump inhibitor that suppresses gastric acid secretion by specific inhibition of the H^+/K^+-ATPase in the gastric parietal cell. The S- and R-isomers of omeprazole are protonated and converted in the acidic compartment of the parietal cell forming the active inhibitor, the achiral sulphenamide. By acting specifically on the proton pump, esomeprazole blocks the final step in acid production, thus reducing gastric acidity. This effect is dose-related up to a daily dose of 20 to 40 mg and leads to inhibition of gastric acid secretion.

Antisecretory Activity

The effect of esomeprazole on intragastric pH was determined in patients with symptomatic gastroesophageal reflux disease in two separate studies. In the first study of 36 patients, NEXIUM 40 mg and 20 mg capsules were administered over 5 days. The results are shown in the following table:

Effect on Intragastric pH on Day 5 (N=36)

Parameter	NEXIUM 40 mg	NEXIUM 20 mg
% Time Gastric pH >4† (Hours)	70%* (16.8 h)	53% (12.7 h)
Coefficient of variation	26%	37%

Continued on next page

Nexium—Cont.

Median 24 Hour pH	4.9*	4.1
Coefficient of variation	16%	27%

† Gastric pH was measured over a 24-hour period
* p< 0.01 NEXIUM 40 mg vs NEXIUM 20 mg

In a second study, the effect on intragastric pH of NEXIUM 40 mg administered once daily over a five day period was similar to the first study. (% time with pH>4 was 68% or 16.3 hours).

Serum Gastrin Effects

The effect of NEXIUM on serum gastrin concentrations was evaluated in approximately 2,700 patients in clinical trials up to 8 weeks and in over 1,300 patients for up to 6–12 months. The mean fasting gastrin level increased in a dose-related manner. This increase reached a plateau within two to three months of therapy and returned to baseline levels within four weeks after discontinuation of therapy.

Enterochromaffin-like (ECL) Cell Effects

In 24-month carcinogenicity studies of omeprazole in rats, a dose-related significant occurrence of gastric ECL cell carcinoid tumors and ECL cell hyperplasia was observed in both male and female animals (see **PRECAUTIONS**, Carcinogenesis, Mutagenesis, Impairment of Fertility). Carcinoid tumors have also been observed in rats subjected to fundectomy or long-term treatment with other proton pump inhibitors or high doses of H_2-receptor antagonists.

Human gastric biopsy specimens have been obtained from more than 3,000 patients treated with omeprazole in long-term clinical trials. The incidence of ECL cell hyperplasia in these studies increased with time; however, no case of ECL cell carcinoids, dysplasia, or neoplasia has been found in these patients.

In over 1,000 patients treated with NEXIUM (10, 20 or 40 mg/day) up to 6–12 months, the prevalence of ECL cell hyperplasia increased with time and dose. No patient developed ECL cell carcinoids, dysplasia, or neoplasia in the gastric mucosa.

Endocrine Effects

NEXIUM had no effect on thyroid function when given in oral doses of 20 or 40 mg for 4 weeks. Other effects of NEXIUM on the endocrine system were assessed using omeprazole studies. Omeprazole given in oral doses of 30 or 40 mg for 2 to 4 weeks had no effect on carbohydrate metabolism, circulating levels of parathyroid hormone, cortisol, estradiol, testosterone, prolactin, cholecystokinin or secretin.

Microbiology

Esomeprazole magnesium, amoxicillin and clarithromycin triple therapy has been shown to be active against most strains of *Helicobacter pylori (H. pylori) in vitro* and in clinical infections as described in the **Clinical Studies** and **INDICATIONS AND USAGE** sections.

Helicobacter

Helicobacter pylori: Susceptibility testing of *H. pylori* isolates was performed for amoxicillin and clarithromycin using agar dilution methodology, and minimum inhibitory concentrations (MICs) were determined.

Pretreatment Resistance: Clarithromycin pretreatment resistance rate (MIC ≥ 1 μg/mL) to *H. pylori* was 15% (66/445) at baseline in all treatment groups combined. A total of > 99% (394/395) of patients had *H. pylori* isolates which were considered to be susceptible (MIC ≤ 0.25 μg/mL) to amoxicillin at baseline. One patient had a baseline *H. pylori* isolate with an amoxicillin MIC = 0.5 μg/mL.

Clarithromycin Susceptibility Test Results and Clinical/Bacteriologic Outcomes: The baseline *H. pylori* clarithromycin susceptibility results and the *H. pylori* eradication results at the Day 38 visit are shown in the table below:

Clarithromycin Susceptibility Test Results and Clinical/Bacteriological Outcomes[a] for Triple Therapy - (Esomeprazole magnesium 40 mg once daily/amoxicillin 1000 mg twice daily/clarithromycin 500 mg twice daily for 10 days)

Clarithromycin Pretreatment Results		*H. pylori* negative (Eradicated)	*H. pylori* positive (Not Eradicated) Post-treatment susceptibility results			
			S[b]	I[b]	R[b]	No MIC
Susceptible[b]	182	162	4	0	2	14
Intermediate[b]	1	1	0	0	0	0
Resistant[b]	29	13	1	0	13	2

[a] Includes only patients with pretreatment and post-treatment clarithromycin susceptibility test results
[b] Susceptible (S) MIC ≤ 0.25 μg/mL, Intermediate (I) MIC =0.5 μg/mL, Resistant (R) MIC ≥ 1.0 μg/mL

Patients not eradicated of *H. pylori* following esomeprazole magnesium/amoxicillin/clarithromycin triple therapy will likely have clarithromycin resistant *H. pylori* isolates. Therefore, clarithromycin susceptibility testing should be done, when possible. Patients with clarithromycin resistant *H. pylori* should not be re-treated with a clarithromycin-containing regimen.

Amoxicillin Susceptibility Test Results and Clinical/Bacteriological Outcomes: In the esomeprazole magnesium/amoxicillin/clarithromycin clinical trials, 83% (176/212) of the patients in the esomeprazole magnesium/amoxicillin/clarithromycin treatment group who had pretreatment amoxicillin susceptible MICs (≤ 0.25 μg/mL) were eradicated of *H. pylori*, and 17% (36/212) were not eradicated of *H. pylori*. Of the 36 patients who were not eradicated of *H. pylori* on triple therapy, 16 had no post-treatment susceptibility test results and 20 had post-treatment *H. pylori* isolates with amoxicillin susceptible MICs. Fifteen of the patients who were not eradicated of *H. pylori* on triple therapy also had post-treatment *H. pylori* isolates with clarithromycin resistant MICs. There were no patients with *H. pylori* isolates who developed treatment emergent resistance to amoxicillin.

Susceptibility Test for Helicobacter pylori: The reference methodology for susceptibility testing of *H. pylori* is agar dilution MICs. One to three microliters of an inoculum equivalent to a No.2 McFarland standard ($1 \times 10^7 - 1 \times 10^8$ CFU/mL for *H. pylori*) are inoculated directly onto freshly prepared antimicrobial containing Mueller-Hinton agar plates with 5% aged defibrinated sheep blood (≥ 2 weeks old). The agar dilution plates are incubated at 35°C in a microaerobic environment produced by a gas generating system suitable for *Campylobacter*. After 3 days of incubation, the MICs are recorded as the lowest concentration of antimicrobial agent required to inhibit growth of the organism. The clarithromycin and amoxicillin MIC values should be interpreted according to the following criteria:

Clarithromycin MIC (μg/mL)[a]	Interpretation
≤ 0.25	Susceptible (S)
0.5	Intermediate (I)
≥ 1.0	Resistant (R)
Amoxicillin MIC (μg/mL)[a,b]	**Interpretation**
≤ 0.25	Susceptible (S)

[a] These are breakpoints for the agar dilution methodology and they should not be used to interpret results obtained using alternative methods.
[b] There were not enough organisms with MICs > 0.25 μg/mL to determine a resistance breakpoint.

Standardized susceptibility test procedures require the use of laboratory control microorganisms to control the technical aspects of the laboratory procedures. Standard clarithromycin and amoxicillin powders should provide the following MIC values:

Erosive Esophagitis Healing Rate (Life-Table Analysis)

Study	No. of Patients	Treatment Groups	Week 4	Week 8	Significance Level*
1	588	NEXIUM 20 mg	68.7%	90.6%	N.S.
	588	Omeprazole 20 mg	69.5%	88.3%	
2	654	NEXIUM 40 mg	75.9%	94.1%	p < 0.001
	656	NEXIUM 20 mg	70.5%	89.9%	p < 0.05
	650	Omeprazole 20 mg	64.7%	86.9%	
3	576	NEXIUM 40 mg	71.5%	92.2%	N.S.
	572	Omeprazole 20 mg	68.6%	89.8%	
4	1216	NEXIUM 40 mg	81.7%	93.7%	p < 0.001
	1209	Omeprazole 20 mg	68.7%	84.2%	

*log-rank test vs omeprazole 20 mg
N.S. = not significant (p > 0.05).

Sustained Resolution[‡] of Heartburn (Erosive Esophagitis Patients)

Study	No. of Patients	Treatment Groups	Cumulative Percent[#] with Sustained Resolution: Day 14	Day 28	Significance Level*
1	573	NEXIUM 20 mg	64.3%	72.7%	N.S.
	555	Omeprazole 20 mg	64.1%	70.9%	
2	621	NEXIUM 40 mg	64.8%	74.2%	p < 0.001
	620	NEXIUM 20 mg	62.9%	70.1%	N.S.
	626	Omeprazole 20 mg	56.5%	66.6%	
3	568	NEXIUM 40 mg	65.4%	73.9%	N.S.
	551	Omeprazole 20 mg	65.5%	73.1%	
4	1187	NEXIUM 40 mg	67.6%	75.1%	p < 0.001
	1188	Omeprazole 20 mg	62.5%	70.8%	

[‡]Defined as 7 consecutive days with no heartburn reported in daily patient diary.
[#]Defined as the cumulative proportion of patients who have reached the start of sustained resolution
*log-rank test vs omeprazole 20 mg
N.S. = not significant (p > 0.05).

Microorganism	Antimicrobial Agent	MIC (μg/mL)[a]
H. pylori ATCC 43504	Clarithromycin	0.016–0.12 (μg/mL)
H. pylori ATCC 43504	Amoxicillin	0.016–0.12 (μg/mL)

[a]These are quality control ranges for the agar dilution methodology and they should not be used to control test results obtained using alternative methods.

Clinical Studies

Healing of Erosive Esophagitis

The healing rates of NEXIUM 40 mg, NEXIUM 20 mg, and omeprazole 20 mg (the approved dose for this indication) were evaluated in patients with endoscopically diagnosed erosive esophagitis in four multicenter, double-blind, randomized studies. The healing rates at weeks 4 and 8 were evaluated and are shown in the table below:

[See first table above]

In these same studies of patients with erosive esophagitis, sustained heartburn resolution and time to sustained heartburn resolution were evaluated and are shown in the table below:

[See second table above]

In these four studies, the range of median days to the start of sustained resolution (defined as 7 consecutive days with no heartburn) was 5 days for NEXIUM 40 mg, 7–8 days for NEXIUM 20 mg and 7–9 days for omeprazole 20 mg.

There are no comparisons of 40 mg of NEXIUM with 40 mg of omeprazole in clinical trials assessing either healing or symptomatic relief of erosive esophagitis.

Long-Term Maintenance of Healing of Erosive Esophagitis

Two multicenter, randomized, double-blind placebo-controlled 4-arm trials were conducted in patients with endoscopically confirmed, healed erosive esophagitis to evaluate NEXIUM 40 mg (n=174), 20 mg (n=180), 10 mg (n=168) or placebo (n=171) once daily over six months of treatment.

No additional clinical benefit was seen with NEXIUM 40 mg over NEXIUM 20 mg.

The percentage of patients that maintained healing of erosive esophagitis at the various time points are shown in the figure below.

[See first figure at top of next column]
[See second figure at top of next column]

Patients remained in remission significantly longer and the number of recurrences of erosive esophagitis was significantly less in patients treated with NEXIUM compared to placebo. In both studies, the proportion of patients on NEXIUM who remained in remission and were free of heartburn and other GERD symptoms was well differentiated from placebo.

In a third multicenter open label study of 808 patients treated for 12 months with NEXIUM 40 mg, the percentage of patients that maintained healing of erosive esophagitis was 93.7% for six months and 89.4% for one year.

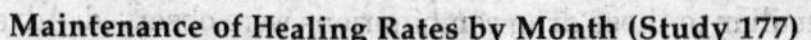
Maintenance of Healing Rates by Month (Study 177)

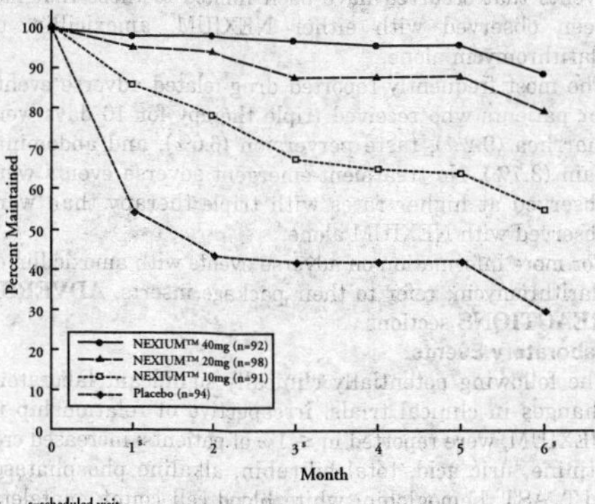

Maintenance of Healing Rates by Month (Study178)

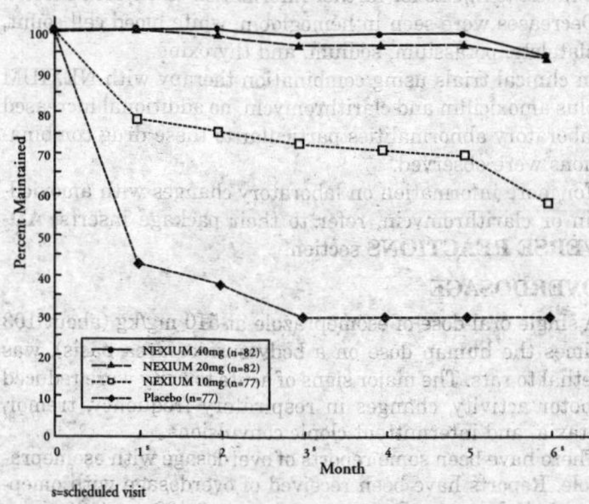

Symptomatic Gastroesophageal Reflux Disease (GERD)

Two multicenter, randomized, double-blind, placebo-controlled studies were conducted in a total of 717 patients comparing four weeks of treatment with NEXIUM 20 mg or 40 mg once daily versus placebo for resolution of GERD symptoms. Patients had ≥ 6-month history of heartburn episodes, no erosive esophagitis by endoscopy, and heartburn on at least four of the seven days immediately preceding randomization.

The percentage of patients that were symptom-free of heartburn was significantly higher in the NEXIUM groups compared to placebo at all follow-up visits (Weeks 1, 2, and 4). No additional clinical benefit was seen with NEXIUM 40 mg over NEXIUM 20 mg.

The percent of patients symptom-free of heartburn by day are shown in the figures below:

Percent of Patients Symptom-Free of Heartburn by Day (Study 225)

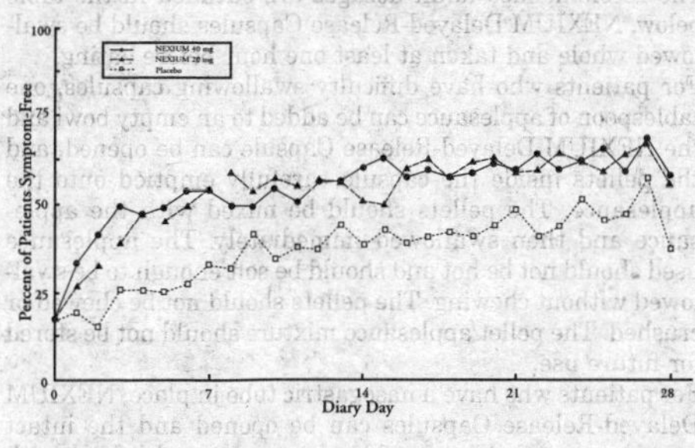

Percent of Patients Symptom-Free of Heartburn by Day (Study 226)

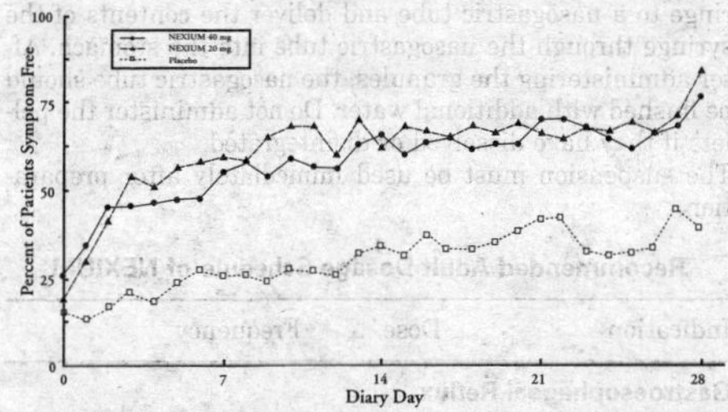

In three European symptomatic GERD trials, NEXIUM 20 mg and 40 mg and omeprazole 20 mg were evaluated. No significant treatment related differences were seen.

Helicobacter pylori *(H. pylori) Eradication in Patients with Duodenal Ulcer Disease*

Triple Therapy (NEXIUM/amoxicillin/clarithromycin): Two multicenter, randomized, double-blind studies were conducted using a 10 day treatment regimen. The first study (191) compared NEXIUM 40 mg once daily in combination with amoxicillin 1000 mg twice daily and clarithromycin 500 mg twice daily to NEXIUM 40 mg once daily plus clarithromycin 500 mg twice daily. The second study (193) compared NEXIUM 40 mg once daily in combination with amoxicillin 1000 mg twice daily and clarithromycin 500 mg twice daily to NEXIUM 40 mg once daily. *H. pylori* eradication rates, defined as at least two negative tests and no positive tests from CLOtest®, histology and/or culture, at 4 weeks post-therapy were significantly higher in the NEXIUM plus amoxicillin and clarithromycin group than in the NEXIUM plus clarithromycin or NEXIUM alone group. The results are shown in the following table *(see next page)*:

***H. pylori* Eradication Rates at 4 Weeks after 10 Day Treatment Regimen**
% of Patients Cured
[95% Confidence Interval]
(Number of patients)

Study	Treatment Group	Per-Protocol†	Intent-to-Treat‡
191	NEXIUM plus amoxicillin and clarithromycin	84%* [78, 89] (n=196)	77%* [71, 82] (n=233)
	NEXIUM plus clarithromycin	55% [48, 62] (n=187)	52% [45, 59] (n=215)
193	NEXIUM plus amoxicillin and clarithromycin	85%** [74, 93] (n=67)	78%** [67, 87] (n=74)
	NEXIUM	5% [0, 23] (n=22)	4% [0, 21] (n=24)

†Patients were included in the analysis if they had *H. pylori* infection documented at baseline, had at least one endoscopically verified duodenal ulcer ≥ 0.5 cm in diameter at baseline or had a documented history of duodenal ulcer disease within the past 5 years, and were not protocol violators. Patients who dropped out of the study due to an adverse event related to the study drug were included in the analysis as not *H. pylori* eradicated.

‡Patients were included in the analysis if they had documented *H. pylori* infection at baseline, had at least one documented duodenal ulcer at baseline, or had a documented history of duodenal ulcer disease, and took at least one dose of study medication. All dropouts were included as not *H. pylori* eradicated.

*$p < 0.05$ compared to NEXIUM plus clarithromycin

**$p < 0.05$ compared to NEXIUM alone

The percentage of patients with a healed baseline duodenal ulcer by 4 weeks after the 10 day treatment regimen in the NEXIUM plus amoxicillin and clarithromycin group was 75% (n=156) and 57% (n=60) respectively, in the 191 and 193 studies (per-protocol analysis).

INDICATIONS AND USAGE

Treatment of Gastroesophageal Reflux Disease (GERD)

Healing of Erosive Esophagitis

NEXIUM is indicated for the short-term treatment (4 to 8 weeks) in the healing and symptomatic resolution of diagnostically confirmed erosive esophagitis. For those patients who have not healed after 4–8 weeks of treatment, an additional 4–8 week course of NEXIUM may be considered.

Maintenance of Healing of Erosive Esophagitis

NEXIUM is indicated to maintain symptom resolution and healing of erosive esophagitis. Controlled studies do not extend beyond 6 months.

Symptomatic Gastroesophageal Reflux Disease

NEXIUM is indicated for treatment of heartburn and other symptoms associated with GERD.

***H. pylori* Eradication to Reduce the Risk of Duodenal Ulcer Recurrence**

Triple Therapy (NEXIUM plus amoxicillin and clarithromycin): NEXIUM, in combination with amoxicillin and clarithromycin, is indicated for the treatment of patients with *H. pylori* infection and duodenal ulcer disease (active or history of within the past 5 years) to eradicate *H. pylori*. Eradication of *H. pylori* has been shown to reduce the risk of duodenal ulcer recurrence. (See **Clinical Studies** and **DOSAGE AND ADMINISTRATION.**)

In patients who fail therapy, susceptibility testing should be done. If resistance to clarithromycin is demonstrated or susceptibility testing is not possible, alternative antimicrobial therapy should be instituted. (See **CLINICAL PHARMACOLOGY, Microbiology** and the clarithromycin package insert, **CLINICAL PHARMACOLOGY, Microbiology.**)

CONTRAINDICATIONS

NEXIUM is contraindicated in patients with known hypersensitivity to any component of the formulation or to substituted benzimidazoles.

Clarithromycin is contraindicated in patients with a known hypersensitivity to any macrolide antibiotic.

Concomitant administration of clarithromycin with pimozide is contraindicated. There have been post-marketing reports of drug interactions when clarithromycin and/or erythromycin are co-administered with pimozide resulting in cardiac arrhythmias (QT prolongation, ventricular tachycardia, ventricular fibrillation, and torsade de pointes) most likely due to inhibition of hepatic metabolism of pimozide by erythromycin and clarithromycin. Fatalities have been reported. (Please refer to full prescribing information for clarithromycin.)

Amoxicillin is contraindicated in patients with a known hypersensitivity to any penicillin. (Please refer to full prescribing information for amoxicillin.)

WARNINGS

CLARITHROMYCIN SHOULD NOT BE USED IN PREGNANT WOMEN EXCEPT IN CLINICAL CIRCUMSTANCES WHERE NO ALTERNATIVE THERAPY IS APPROPRIATE. IF PREGNANCY OCCURS WHILE TAKING CLARITHROMYCIN, THE PATIENT SHOULD BE APPRISED OF THE POTENTIAL HAZARD TO THE FETUS. (See WARNINGS in prescribing information for clarithromycin.)

Amoxicillin: Serious and occasionally fatal hypersensitivity (anaphylactic) reactions have been reported in patients on penicillin therapy. These reactions are more apt to occur in individuals with a history of penicillin hypersensitivity and/or a history of sensitivity to multiple allergens.

There have been well documented reports of individuals with a history of penicillin hypersensitivity reactions who have experienced severe hypersensitivity reactions when treated with a cephalosporin. Before initiating therapy with any penicillin, careful inquiry should be made concerning previous hypersensitivity reactions to penicillins, cephalosporins, and other allergens. If an allergic reaction occurs, amoxicillin should be discontinued and the appropriate therapy instituted.

SERIOUS ANAPHYLACTIC REACTIONS REQUIRE IMMEDIATE EMERGENCY TREATMENT WITH EPINEPHRINE, OXYGEN, INTRAVENOUS STEROIDS, AND AIRWAY MANAGEMENT, INCLUDING INTUBATION, SHOULD ALSO BE ADMINISTERED AS INDICATED.

Pseudomembranous colitis has been reported with nearly all antibacterial agents, including clarithromycin and amoxicillin, and may range in severity from mild to life threatening. Therefore, it is important to consider this diagnosis in patients who present with diarrhea subsequent to the administration of antibacterial agents.

Treatment with antibacterial agents alters the normal flora of the colon and may permit overgrowth of clostridia. Studies indicate that a toxin produced by *Clostridium difficile* is a primary cause of "antibiotic-associated colitis".

After the diagnosis of pseudomembranous colitis has been established, therapeutic measures should be initiated. Mild cases of pseudomembranous colitis usually respond to discontinuation of the drug alone. In moderate to severe cases, consideration should be given to management with fluids and electrolytes, protein supplementation, and treatment with an antibacterial drug clinically effective against *Clostridium difficile colitis*.

PRECAUTIONS

General

Symptomatic response to therapy with NEXIUM does not preclude the presence of gastric malignancy.

Atrophic gastritis has been noted occasionally in gastric corpus biopsies from patients treated long-term with omeprazole, of which NEXIUM is an enantiomer.

Information for Patients

Patients should be informed of the following:

NEXIUM Delayed-Release Capsules should be taken at least one hour before meals.

For patients who have difficulty swallowing capsules, one tablespoon of applesauce can be added to an empty bowl and the NEXIUM Delayed-Release Capsule can be opened, and the pellets inside the capsule carefully emptied onto the applesauce. The pellets should be mixed with the applesauce and then swallowed immediately. The applesauce used should not be hot and should be soft enough to be swallowed without chewing. The pellets should not be chewed or crushed. The pellet/applesauce mixture should not be stored for future use.

Antacids may be used while taking NEXIUM.

Drug Interactions

Esomeprazole is extensively metabolized in the liver by CYP2C19 and CYP3A4.

In vitro and *in vivo* studies have shown that esomeprazole is not likely to inhibit CYPs 1A2, 2A6, 2C9, 2D6, 2E1 and 3A4. No clinically relevant interactions with drugs metabolized by these CYP enzymes would be expected. Drug interaction studies have shown that esomeprazole does not have any clinically significant interactions with phenytoin, warfarin, quinidine, clarithromycin or amoxicillin. Post-marketing reports of changes in prothrombin measures have been received among patients on concomitant warfarin and esomeprazole therapy. Increases in INR and prothrombin time may lead to abnormal bleeding and even death. Patients treated with proton pump inhibitors and warfarin concomitantly may need to be monitored for increases in INR and prothrombin time.

Esomeprazole may potentially interfere with CYP2C19, the major esomeprazole metabolizing enzyme. Coadministration of esomeprazole 30 mg and diazepam, a CYP2C19 substrate, resulted in a 45% decrease in clearance of diazepam. Increased plasma levels of diazepam were observed 12 hours after dosing and onwards. However, at that time, the plasma levels of diazepam were below the therapeutic interval, and thus this interaction is unlikely to be of clinical relevance.

Continued on next page

Nexium—Cont.

Esomeprazole inhibits gastric acid secretion. Therefore, esomeprazole may interfere with the absorption of drugs where gastric pH is an important determinant of bioavailability (e.g., ketoconazole, iron salts and digoxin).
Coadministration of oral contraceptives, diazepam, phenytoin, or quinidine did not seem to change the pharmacokinetic profile of esomeprazole.
Combination Therapy with Clarithromycin
Co-administration of esomeprazole, clarithromycin, and amoxicillin has resulted in increases in the plasma levels of esomeprazole and 14-hydroxyclarithromycin. (See **CLINICAL PHARMACOLOGY, Pharmacokinetics: Combination Therapy with Antimicrobials.**)
Concomitant administration of clarithromycin with pimozide is contraindicated. (See clarithromycin package insert.)

Carcinogenesis, Mutagenesis, Impairment of Fertility
The carcinogenic potential of esomeprazole was assessed using omeprazole studies. In two 24-month oral carcinogenicity studies in rats, omeprazole at daily doses of 1.7, 3.4, 13.8, 44.0 and 140.8 mg/kg/day (about 0.7 to 57 times the human dose of 20 mg/day expressed on a body surface area basis) produced gastric ECL cell carcinoids in a dose-related manner in both male and female rats; the incidence of this effect was markedly higher in female rats, which had higher blood levels of omeprazole. Gastric carcinoids seldom occur in the untreated rat. In addition, ECL cell hyperplasia was present in all treated groups of both sexes. In one of these studies, female rats were treated with 13.8 mg omeprazole/kg/day (about 5.6 times the human dose on a body surface area basis) for 1 year, then followed for an additional year without the drug. No carcinoids were seen in these rats. An increased incidence of treatment-related ECL cell hyperplasia was observed at the end of 1 year (94% treated vs 10% controls). By the second year the difference between treated and control rats was much smaller (46% vs 26%) but still showed more hyperplasia in the treated group. Gastric adenocarcinoma was seen in one rat (2%). No similar tumor was seen in male or female rats treated for 2 years. For this strain of rat no similar tumor has been noted historically, but a finding involving only one tumor is difficult to interpret. A 78-week mouse carcinogenicity study of omeprazole did not show increased tumor occurrence, but the study was not conclusive.
Esomeprazole was negative in the Ames mutation test, in the *in vivo* rat bone marrow cell chromosome aberration test, and the *in vivo* mouse micronucleus test. Esomeprazole, however, was positive in the *in vitro* human lymphocyte chromosome aberration test. Omeprazole was positive in the *in vitro* human lymphocyte chromosome aberration test, the *in vivo* mouse bone marrow cell chromosome aberration test, and the *in vivo* mouse micronucleus test.
The potential effects of esomeprazole on fertility and reproductive performance were assessed using omeprazole studies. Omeprazole at oral doses up to 138 mg/kg/day in rats (about 56 times the human dose on a body surface area basis) was found to have no effect on reproductive performance of parental animals.

Pregnancy
Teratogenic Effects. Pregnancy Category B
Teratology studies have been performed in rats at oral doses up to 280 mg/kg/day (about 57 times the human dose on a body surface area basis) and in rabbits at oral doses up to 86 mg/kg/day (about 35 times the human dose on a body surface area basis) and have revealed no evidence of impaired fertility or harm to the fetus due to esomeprazole. There are, however, no adequate and well-controlled studies in pregnant women. Because animal reproduction studies are not always predictive of human response, this drug should be used during pregnancy only if clearly needed.
Teratology studies conducted with omeprazole in rats at oral doses up to 138 mg/kg/day (about 56 times the human dose on a body surface area basis) and in rabbits at doses up to 69 mg/kg/day (about 56 times the human dose on a body surface area basis) did not disclose any evidence for a teratogenic potential of omeprazole. In rabbits, omeprazole in a dose range of 6.9 to 69.1 mg/kg/day (about 5.5 to 56 times the human dose on a body surface area basis) produced dose-related increases in embryo-lethality, fetal resorptions, and pregnancy disruptions. In rats, dose-related embryo/fetal toxicity and postnatal developmental toxicity were observed in offspring resulting from parents treated with omeprazole at 13.8 to 138.0 mg/kg/day (about 5.6 to 56 times the human doses on a body surface area basis). There are no adequate and well-controlled studies in pregnant women. Sporadic reports have been received of congenital abnormalities occurring in infants born to women who have received omeprazole during pregnancy.
Amoxicillin
Pregnancy Category B. See full prescribing information for amoxicillin before using in pregnant women.
Clarithromycin
Pregnancy Category C. See **WARNINGS** (above) and full prescribing information for clarithromycin before using in pregnant women.

Nursing Mothers
The excretion of esomeprazole in milk has not been studied. However, omeprazole concentrations have been measured in breast milk of a woman following oral administration of 20 mg. Because esomeprazole is likely to be excreted in human milk, because of the potential for serious adverse reactions in nursing infants from esomeprazole, and because of the potential for tumorigenicity shown for omeprazole in rat carcinogenicity studies, a decision should be made whether to discontinue nursing or to discontinue the drug, taking into account the importance of the drug to the mother.

Pediatric Use
Safety and effectiveness in pediatric patients have not been established.

Geriatric Use
Of the total number of patients who received NEXIUM in clinical trials, 778 were 65 to 74 years of age and 124 patients were ≥ 75 years of age.
No overall differences in safety and efficacy were observed between the elderly and younger individuals, and other reported clinical experience has not identified differences in responses between the elderly and younger patients, but greater sensitivity of some older individuals cannot be ruled out.

ADVERSE REACTIONS

The safety of NEXIUM was evaluated in over 10,000 patients (aged 18–84 years) in clinical trials worldwide including over 7,400 patients in the United States and over 2,600 patients in Europe and Canada. Over 2,900 patients were treated in long-term studies for up to 6–12 months. In general, NEXIUM was well tolerated in both short and long-term clinical trials.
The safety in the treatment of healing of erosive esophagitis was assessed in four randomized comparative clinical trials, which included 1,240 patients on NEXIUM 20 mg, 2,434 patients on NEXIUM 40 mg, and 3,008 patients on omeprazole 20 mg daily. The most frequently occurring adverse events (≥1%) in all three groups was headache (5.5, 5.0, and 3.8, respectively) and diarrhea (no difference among the three groups). Nausea, flatulence, abdominal pain, constipation, and dry mouth occurred at similar rates among patients taking NEXIUM or omeprazole.
Additional adverse events that were reported as possibly or probably related to NEXIUM with an incidence < 1% are listed below by body system:
Body as a Whole: abdomen enlarged, allergic reaction, asthenia, back pain, chest pain, chest pain substernal, facial edema, peripheral edema, hot flushes, fatigue, fever, flu-like disorder, generalized edema, leg edema, malaise, pain, rigors; ***Cardiovascular:*** flushing, hypertension, tachycardia; ***Endocrine:*** goiter; ***Gastrointestinal:*** bowel irregularity, constipation aggravated, dyspepsia, dysphagia, dysplasia GI, epigastric pain, eructation, esophageal disorder, frequent stools, gastroenteritis, GI hemorrhage, GI symptoms not otherwise specified, hiccup, melena, mouth disorder, pharynx disorder, rectal disorder, serum gastrin increased, tongue disorder, tongue edema, ulcerative stomatitis, vomiting; ***Hearing:*** earache, tinnitus; ***Hematologic:*** anemia, anemia hypochromic, cervical lymphoadenopathy, epistaxis, leukocytosis, leukopenia, thrombocytopenia; ***Hepatic:*** bilirubinemia, hepatic function abnormal, SGOT increased, SGPT increased; ***Metabolic/Nutritional:*** glycosuria, hyperuricemia, hyponatremia, increased alkaline phosphatase, thirst, vitamin B12 deficiency, weight increase, weight decrease; ***Musculoskeletal:*** arthralgia, arthritis aggravated, arthropathy, cramps, fibromyalgia syndrome, hernia, polymyalgia rheumatica; ***Nervous System/Psychiatric:*** anorexia, apathy, appetite increased, confusion, depression aggravated, dizziness, hypertonia, nervousness, hypoesthesia, impotence, insomnia, migraine, migraine aggravated, paresthesia, sleep disorder, somnolence, tremor, vertigo, visual field defect; ***Reproductive:*** dysmenorrhea, menstrual disorder, vaginitis; ***Respiratory:*** asthma aggravated, coughing, dyspnea, larynx edema, pharyngitis, rhinitis, sinusitis; ***Skin and Appendages:*** acne, angioedema, dermatitis, pruritus, pruritus ani, rash, rash erythematous, rash maculo-papular, skin inflammation, sweating increased, urticaria; ***Special Senses:*** otitis media, parosmia, taste loss, taste perversion; ***Urogenital:*** abnormal urine, albuminuria, cystitis, dysuria, fungal infection, hematuria, micturition frequency, moniliasis, genital moniliasis, polyuria; ***Visual:*** conjunctivitis, vision abnormal.
Endoscopic findings that were reported as adverse events include: duodenitis, esophagitis, esophageal stricture, esophageal ulceration, esophageal varices, gastric ulcer, gastritis, hernia, benign polyps or nodules, Barrett's esophagus, and mucosal discoloration.
The incidence of treatment-related adverse events during 6-month maintenance treatment was similar to placebo. There were no differences in types of related adverse events seen during maintenance treatment up to 12 months compared to short-term treatment.
Two placebo-controlled studies were conducted in 710 patients for the treatment of symptomatic gastroesophageal reflux disease. The most common adverse events that were reported as possibly or probably related to NEXIUM were diarrhea (4.3%), headache (3.8%), and abdominal pain (3.8%).
Postmarketing Reports—There have been spontaneous reports of adverse events with postmarketing use of esomeprazole. These reports have included rare cases of anaphylactic reaction.
Other adverse events not observed with NEXIUM, but occurring with omeprazole can be found in the omeprazole package insert, **ADVERSE REACTIONS** section.

Combination Treatment with Amoxicillin and Clarithromycin
In clinical trials using combination therapy with NEXIUM plus amoxicillin and clarithromycin, no adverse events peculiar to these drug combinations were observed. Adverse events that occurred have been limited to those that had been observed with either NEXIUM, amoxicillin, or clarithromycin alone.
The most frequently reported drug-related adverse events for patients who received triple therapy for 10 days were diarrhea (9.2%), taste perversion (6.6%), and abdominal pain (3.7%). No treatment-emergent adverse events were observed at higher rates with triple therapy than were observed with NEXIUM alone.
For more information on adverse events with amoxicillin or clarithromycin, refer to their package inserts, **ADVERSE REACTIONS** sections.

Laboratory Events
The following potentially clinically significant laboratory changes in clinical trials, irrespective of relationship to NEXIUM, were reported in ≤ 1% of patients: increased creatinine, uric acid, total bilirubin, alkaline phosphatase, ALT, AST, hemoglobin, white blood cell count, platelets, serum gastrin, potassium, sodium, thyroxine and thyroid stimulating hormone (see **CLINICAL PHARMACOLOGY,** *Endocrine Effects* for further information on thyroid effects). Decreases were seen in hemoglobin, white blood cell count, platelets, potassium, sodium, and thyroxine.
In clinical trials using combination therapy with NEXIUM plus amoxicillin and clarithromycin, no additional increased laboratory abnormalities particular to these drug combinations were observed.
For more information on laboratory changes with amoxicillin or clarithromycin, refer to their package inserts, **ADVERSE REACTIONS** section.

OVERDOSAGE

A single oral dose of esomeprazole at 510 mg/kg (about 103 times the human dose on a body surface area basis), was lethal to rats. The major signs of acute toxicity were reduced motor activity, changes in respiratory frequency, tremor, ataxia, and intermittent clonic convulsions.
There have been some reports of overdosage with esomeprazole. Reports have been received of overdosage with omeprazole in humans. Doses ranged up to 2,400 mg (120 times the usual recommended clinical dose). Manifestations were variable, but included confusion, drowsiness, blurred vision, tachycardia, nausea, diaphoresis, flushing, headache, dry mouth, and other adverse reactions similar to those seen in normal clinical experience (see omeprazole package insert—**ADVERSE REACTIONS**). No specific antidote for esomeprazole is known. Since esomeprazole is extensively protein bound, it is not expected to be removed by dialysis. In the event of overdosage, treatment should be symptomatic and supportive.
As with the management of any overdose, the possibility of multiple drug ingestion should be considered. For current information on treatment of any drug overdose, a certified Regional Poison Control Center should be contacted. Telephone numbers are listed in the Physicians' Desk Reference (PDR) or local telephone book.

DOSAGE AND ADMINISTRATION

The recommended adult dosages are outlined in the table below. NEXIUM Delayed-Release Capsules should be swallowed whole and taken at least one hour before eating.
For patients who have difficulty swallowing capsules, one tablespoon of applesauce can be added to an empty bowl and the NEXIUM Delayed-Release Capsule can be opened, and the pellets inside the capsule carefully emptied onto the applesauce. The pellets should be mixed with the applesauce and then swallowed immediately. The applesauce used should not be hot and should be soft enough to be swallowed without chewing. The pellets should not be chewed or crushed. The pellet/applesauce mixture should not be stored for future use.
For patients who have a nasogastric tube in place, NEXIUM Delayed-Release Capsules can be opened and the intact granules emptied into a 60 mL syringe and mixed with 50 mL of water. Replace the plunger and shake the syringe vigorously for 15 seconds. Hold the syringe with the tip up and check for granules remaining in the tip. Attach the syringe to a nasogastric tube and deliver the contents of the syringe through the nasogastric tube into the stomach. After administering the granules, the nasogastric tube should be flushed with additional water. Do not administer the pellets if they have dissolved or disintegrated.
The suspension must be used immediately after preparation.

Recommended Adult Dosage Schedule of NEXIUM

Indication	Dose	Frequency
Gastroesophageal Reflux Disease (GERD)		
Healing of Erosive Esophagitis	20 mg or 40 mg	Once Daily for 4 to 8 Weeks*
Maintenance of Healing of Erosive Esophagitis	20 mg	Once Daily**
Symptomatic Gastroesophageal Reflux Disease	20 mg	Once Daily for 4 Weeks***

***H. pylori* Eradication to Reduce the Risk of Duodenal Ulcer Recurrence**

Triple Therapy:

NEXIUM	40 mg	Once Daily for 10 Days
Amoxicillin	1000 mg	Twice Daily for 10 Days
Clarithromycin	500 mg	Twice Daily for 10 Days

* (see **CLINICAL STUDIES**). The majority of patients are healed within 4 to 8 weeks. For patients who do not heal after 4–8 weeks, an additional 4–8 weeks of treatment may be considered.

** Controlled studies did not extend beyond six months.

*** If symptoms do not resolve completely after 4 weeks, an additional 4 weeks of treatment may be considered.

Please refer to amoxicillin and clarithromycin full prescribing information for **CONTRAINDICATIONS**, **WARNINGS** and dosing in elderly and renally-impaired patients.

Special Populations

Geriatric

No dosage adjustment is necessary. (See **CLINICAL PHARMACOLOGY, Pharmacokinetics**.)

Renal Insufficiency

No dosage adjustment is necessary. (See **CLINICAL PHARMACOLOGY, Pharmacokinetics**.)

Hepatic Insufficiency

No dosage adjustment is necessary in patients with mild to moderate liver impairment (Child Pugh Classes A and B). For patients with severe liver impairment (Child Pugh Class C), a dose of 20 mg of NEXIUM should not be exceeded (See **CLINICAL PHARMACOLOGY, Pharmacokinetics**.)

Gender

No dosage adjustment is necessary. (See **CLINICAL PHARMACOLOGY, Pharmacokinetics**.)

HOW SUPPLIED

NEXIUM Delayed-Release Capsules, 20 mg, are opaque, hard gelatin, amethyst colored capsules with two radial bars in yellow on the cap and NEXIUM 20 mg in yellow on the body. They are supplied as follows:

NDC 0186-5020-31 unit of use bottles of 30
NDC 0186-5022-28 unit dose packages of 100
NDC 0186-5020-54 bottles of 90
NDC 0186-5020-82 bottles of 1000

NEXIUM Delayed-Release Capsules, 40 mg, are opaque, hard gelatin, amethyst colored capsules with three radial bars in yellow on the cap and NEXIUM 40 mg in yellow on the body. They are supplied as follows:

NDC 0186-5040-31 unit of use bottles of 30
NDC 0186-5042-28 unit dose packages of 100
NDC 0186-5040-54 bottles of 90
NDC 0186-5040-82 bottles of 1000

Storage

Store at 25°C (77°F); excursions permitted to 15–30°C (59–86°F). [See USP Controlled Room Temperature]. Keep container tightly closed. Dispense in a tight container if the product package is subdivided.

REFERENCES

1. National Committee for Clinical Laboratory Standards. Methods for Dilution Antimicrobial Susceptibility Tests for Bacteria That Grow Aerobically. Fifth Edition: Approved Standard NCCLS Document M7-A5, Vol. 20, no. 2, NCCLS, Wayne, PA, January 2000.

NEXIUM and the color purple as applied to the capsule are registered trademarks of the AstraZeneca group of companies

Distributed by:
AstraZeneca LP
Wilmington, DE 19850
Product of France
9346607
620514-07
Rev. 04/04

Shown in Product Identification Guide, page 305

PLENDIL® ℞

(felodipine)

EXTENDED-RELEASE TABLETS

DESCRIPTION

PLENDIL® (felodipine) is a calcium antagonist (calcium channel blocker). Felodipine is a dihydropyridine derivative that is chemically described as ± ethyl methyl 4-(2,3-dichlorophenyl)-1,4-dihydro-2,6-dimethyl-3,5-pyridinedicarboxylate. Its empirical formula is $C_{18}H_{19}Cl_2NO_4$ and its structural formula is:

Felodipine is a slightly yellowish, crystalline powder with a molecular weight of 384.26. It is insoluble in water and is freely soluble in dichloromethane and ethanol. Felodipine is a racemic mixture.

Tablets PLENDIL provide extended release of felodipine. They are available as tablets containing 2.5 mg, 5 mg, or 10 mg of felodipine for oral administration. In addition to the active ingredient felodipine, the tablets contain the following inactive ingredients: Tablets PLENDIL 2.5 mg—hydroxypropyl cellulose, lactose, FD&C Blue 2, sodium stearyl fumarate, titanium dioxide, yellow iron oxide, and other ingredients. Tablets PLENDIL 5 mg and 10 mg—cellulose, red and yellow oxide, lactose, polyethylene glycol, sodium stearyl fumarate, titanium dioxide, and other ingredients.

*Trademark of the AstraZeneca Group

HOW SUPPLIED

No. 3584—Tablets PLENDIL, 2.5 mg, are sage green, round convex tablets, with code 450 on one side and PLENDIL on the other. They are supplied as follows:

NDC 0186-0450-28 unit dose packages of 100
NDC 0186-0450-58 unit of use bottles of 100

No. 3585—Tablets PLENDIL, 5 mg, are light red-brown, round convex tablets, with code 451 on one side and PLENDIL on the other. They are supplied as follows:

NDC 0186-0451-28 unit dose packages of 100
NDC 0186-0451-58 unit of use bottles of 100

No. 3586—Tablets PLENDIL, 10 mg, are red-brown, round convex tablets, with code 452 on one side and PLENDIL on the other. They are supplied as follows:

NDC 0186-0452-28 unit dose packages of 100
NDC 0186-0452-58 unit of use bottles of 100

Storage

Store below 30°C (86°F). Keep container tightly closed. Protect from light.

Plendil is a trademark of the AstraZeneca group of companies

Manufactured for: AstraZeneca LP
Wilmington, DE 19850
By: Merck & Co., Inc., Whitehouse Station, NJ, 08889 USA
9179716
630002-16
Rev. 11/03

Shown in Product Identification Guide, page 305

POLOCAINE® ℞

[pō '-lō-caine"]

(Mepivacaine Hydrochloride Injection, USP)

POLOCAINE®-MPF

(Mepivacaine Hydrochloride Injection, USP)

THESE SOLUTIONS ARE NOT INTENDED FOR SPINAL ANESTHESIA OR DENTAL USE

℞ only

PRILOSEC® ℞

[prī-lō-sĕk]

(OMEPRAZOLE)

DELAYED-RELEASE CAPSULES

DESCRIPTION

The active ingredient in PRILOSEC (omeprazole) Delayed-Release Capsules is a substituted benzimidazole, 5-methoxy-2-[[(4-methoxy-3, 5-dimethyl-2-pyridinyl) methyl] sulfinyl]-1*H*-benzimidazole, a compound that inhibits gastric acid secretion. Its empirical formula is $C_{17}H_{19}N_3O_3S$, with a molecular weight of 345.42. The structural formula is:

Omeprazole is a white to off-white crystalline powder which melts with decomposition at about 155°C. It is a weak base, freely soluble in ethanol and methanol, and slightly soluble in acetone and isopropanol and very slightly soluble in water. The stability of omeprazole is a function of pH; it is rapidly degraded in acid media, but has acceptable stability under alkaline conditions.

PRILOSEC is supplied as delayed-release capsules for oral administration. Each delayed-release capsule contains either 10 mg, 20 mg or 40 mg of omeprazole in the form of enteric-coated granules with the following inactive ingredients: cellulose, disodium hydrogen phosphate, hydroxypropyl cellulose, hypromellose, lactose, mannitol, sodium lauryl sulfate and other ingredients. The capsule shells have the following inactive ingredients: gelatin-NF, FD&C Blue #1, FD&C Red #40, D&C Red #28, titanium dioxide, synthetic black iron oxide, isopropanol, butyl alcohol, FD&C Blue #2, D&C Red #7 Calcium Lake, and, in addition, the 10 mg and 40 mg capsule shells also contain D&C Yellow #10.

HOW SUPPLIED

No. 3426 — PRILOSEC Delayed-Release Capsules, 10 mg, are opaque, hard gelatin, apricot and amethyst colored capsules, coded 606 on cap and PRILOSEC 10 on the body. They are supplied as follows:

NDC 0186-0606-31 unit of use bottles of 30
NDC 0186-0606-82 bottles of 1000.

No. 3440 — PRILOSEC Delayed-Release Capsules, 20 mg, are opaque, hard gelatin, amethyst colored capsules, coded 742 on cap and PRILOSEC 20 on body. They are supplied as follows:

NDC 0186-0742-31 unit of use bottles of 30
NDC 0186-0742-82 bottles of 1000.

No. 3428 — PRILOSEC Delayed-Release Capsules, 40 mg, are opaque, hard gelatin, apricot and amethyst colored capsules, coded 743 on cap and PRILOSEC 40 on the body. They are supplied as follows:

NDC 0186-0743-31 unit of use bottles of 30
NDC 0186-0743-68 bottles of 100
NDC 0186-0743-82 bottles of 1000.

Storage

Store PRILOSEC Delayed-Release Capsules in a tight container protected from light and moisture. Store between 15°C and 30°C (59°F and 86°F).

REFERENCES

1. National Committee for Clinical Laboratory Standards. Methods for Dilution Antimicrobial Susceptibility Tests for Bacteria That Grow Aerobically—Fifth Edition. Approved Standard NCCLS Document M7-A5, Vol, 20, No. 2, NCCLS, Wayne, PA, January 2000.

PRILOSEC is a trademark of the AstraZeneca group of companies.

Manufactured for: AstraZeneca LP, Wilmington, DE 19850
By: Merck & Co., Inc., Whitehouse Station, NJ 08889, USA
9194139
640004-39
Rev. 10/03

Shown in Product Identification Guide, page 305

PULMICORT RESPULES® ℞

[pŭl-mĭ-cōrt]

(budesonide inhalation suspension)

0.25 mg and 0.5 mg

℞ only

For inhalation use via compressed air driven jet nebulizers only (not for use with ultrasonic devices). Not for injection. Read patient instructions before using.

DESCRIPTION

Budesonide, the active component of PULMICORT RESPULES®, is a corticosteroid designated chemically as (RS)-11β, 16α, 17, 21-tetrahydroxypregna-1, 4-diene-3, 20-dione cyclic 16, 17-acetal with butyraldehyde. Budesonide is provided as a mixture of two epimers (22R and 22S). The empirical formula of budesonide is $C_{25}H_{34}O_6$ and its molecular weight is 430.5. Its structural formula is:

Budesonide is a white to off-white, tasteless, odorless powder that is practically insoluble in water and in heptane, sparingly soluble in ethanol, and freely soluble in chloroform. Its partition coefficient between octanol and water at pH 7.4 is 1.6×10^3.

PULMICORT RESPULES is a sterile suspension for inhalation via jet nebulizer and contains the active ingredient budesonide (micronized), and the inactive ingredients disodium edetate, sodium chloride, sodium citrate, citric acid, polysorbate 80, and Water for Injection. Two dose strengths are available in single-dose ampules (Respules™ ampules): 0.25 mg and 0.5 mg per 2 mL RESPULE ampule. For PULMICORT RESPULES, like all other nebulized treatments, the amount delivered to the lungs will depend on patient factors, the jet nebulizer utilized, and compressor performance. Using the Pari-LC-Jet Plus Nebulizer/Pari Master compressor system, under *in vitro* conditions, the mean delivered dose at the mouthpiece (% nominal dose) was approximately 17% at a mean flow rate of 5.5 L/min. The mean nebulization time was 5 minutes or less. PULMICORT RESPULES should be administered from jet nebulizers at adequate flow rates, via face masks or mouthpieces (see DOSAGE AND ADMINISTRATION).

CLINICAL PHARMACOLOGY

Mechanism of Action

Budesonide is an anti-inflammatory corticosteroid that exhibits potent glucocorticoid activity and weak mineralocorticoid activity. In standard *in vitro* and animal models, budesonide has approximately a 200-fold higher affinity for

Continued on next page

Pulmicort—Cont.

the glucocorticoid receptor and a 1000-fold higher topical anti-inflammatory potency than cortisol (rat croton oil ear edema assay). As a measure of systemic activity, budesonide is 40 times more potent than cortisol when administered subcutaneously and 25 times more potent when administered orally in the rat thymus involution assay.
The precise mechanism of corticosteroid actions on inflammation in asthma is not well known. Corticosteroids have been shown to have a wide range of inhibitory activities against multiple cell types (eg, mast cells, eosinophils, neutrophils, macrophages, and lymphocytes) and mediators (eg, histamine, eicosanoids, leukotrienes, and cytokines) involved in allergic- and non-allergic-mediated inflammation. The anti-inflammatory actions of corticosteroids may contribute to their efficacy in asthma.
Studies in asthmatic patients have shown a favorable ratio between topical anti-inflammatory activities and systemic corticosteroid effects over a wide dose range of inhaled budesonide in a variety of formulations and delivery systems including Pulmicort Turbuhaler® (an inhalation-driven, multi-dose dry powder inhaler) and the inhalation suspension for nebulization. This is explained by a combination of a relatively high local anti-inflammatory effect, extensive first pass hepatic degradation of orally absorbed drug (85–95%) and the low potency of metabolites (see below).

Pharmacokinetics

The activity of PULMICORT RESPULES is due to the parent drug, budesonide. In glucocorticoid receptor affinity studies, the 22R form was two times as active as the 22S epimer. *In vitro* studies indicated that the two forms of budesonide do not interconvert.
Budesonide is primarily cleared by the liver. In asthmatic children 4–6 years of age, the terminal half-life of budesonide after nebulization is 2.3 hours, and the systemic clearance is 0.5 L/min, which is approximately 50% greater than in healthy adults after adjustment for differences in weight.
After a single dose of 1 mg budesonide, a peak plasma concentration of 2.6 nmol/L was obtained approximately 20 minutes after nebulization in asthmatic children 4–6 years of age. The exposure (AUC) of budesonide following administration of a single 1 mg dose of budesonide by nebulization to asthmatic children 4–6 years of age is comparable to healthy adults given a single 2 mg dose by nebulization.
Absorption: In asthmatic children 4–6 years of age, the total absolute bioavailability (ie, lung + oral) following administration of PULMICORT RESPULES via jet nebulizer was approximately 6% of the labeled dose.
The peak plasma concentration of budesonide occurred 10–30 minutes after start of nebulization.
Distribution: In asthmatic children 4–6 years of age, the volume of distribution at steady-state of budesonide was 3 L/kg, approximately the same as in healthy adults. Budesonide is 85–90% bound to plasma proteins, the degree of binding being constant over the concentration range (1–100 nmol/L) achieved with, and exceeding, recommended doses. Budesonide showed little or no binding to corticosteroid-binding globulin. Budesonide rapidly equilibrated with red blood cells in a concentration independent manner with a blood/plasma ratio of about 0.8.
Metabolism: *In vitro* studies with human liver homogenates have shown that budesonide is rapidly and extensively metabolized. Two major metabolites formed via cytochrome P450 (CYP) isoenzyme 3A4 (CYP3A4) catalyzed biotransformation have been isolated and identified as 16α-hydroxyprednisolone and 6β-hydroxybudesonide. The corticosteroid activity of each of these two metabolites is less than 1% of that of the parent compound. No qualitative difference between the *in vitro* and *in vivo* metabolic patterns has been detected. Negligible metabolic inactivation was observed in human lung and serum preparations.
Excretion: Budesonide is excreted in urine and feces in the form of metabolites. In adults, approximately 60% of an intravenous radiolabeled dose was recovered in the urine. No unchanged budesonide was detected in the urine.
Special Populations: No differences in pharmacokinetics due to race, gender, or age have been identified.
Hepatic Insufficiency: Reduced liver function may affect the elimination of corticosteroids. The pharmacokinetics of budesonide were affected by compromised liver function as evidenced by a doubled systemic availability after oral ingestion. The intravenous pharmacokinetics of budesonide were, however, similar in cirrhotic patients and in healthy adults.

Pharmacodynamics

The therapeutic effects of conventional doses of orally inhaled budesonide are largely explained by its direct local action on the respiratory tract. To confirm that systemic absorption is not a significant factor in the clinical efficacy of inhaled budesonide, a clinical study in adult patients with asthma was performed comparing 400 mcg budesonide administered via a pressurized metered dose inhaler with a tube spacer to 1400 mcg of oral budesonide and placebo. The study demonstrated the efficacy of inhaled budesonide but not orally ingested budesonide despite comparable systemic levels.
Improvement in the control of asthma symptoms following inhalation of PULMICORT RESPULES can occur within 2–8 days of beginning treatment, although maximum benefit may not be achieved for 4–6 weeks.
Budesonide administered via Turbuhaler® has been shown in various challenge models (including histamine, methacholine, sodium metabisulfite, and adenosine monophosphate) to decrease bronchial hyperresponsiveness in asthmatic patients. The clinical relevance of these models is not certain.
Pre-treatment with budesonide administered via TURBUHALER 1600 mcg daily (800 mcg twice daily) for 2 weeks reduced the acute (early-phase reaction) and delayed (late-phase reaction) decrease in FEV_1 following inhaled allergen challenge.
The effects of PULMICORT RESPULES on the hypothalamic-pituitary-adrenal (HPA) axis were studied in three, 12-week, double-blind, placebo-controlled studies in 293 pediatric patients, 6 months to 8 years of age, with persistent asthma. For most patients, the ability to increase cortisol production in response to stress, as assessed by the short cosyntropin (ACTH) stimulation test, remained intact with PULMICORT RESPULES treatment at recommended doses. In the subgroup of children age 6 months to 2 years (n=21) receiving a total daily dose of PULMICORT RESPULES equivalent to 0.25 mg (n=5), 0.5 mg (n=5), 1 mg (n=8), or placebo (n=3), the mean change from baseline in ACTH-stimulated cortisol levels showed a decline in peak stimulated cortisol at 12 weeks compared to an increase in the placebo group. These mean differences were not statistically significant compared to placebo. Another 12-week study in 141 pediatric patients 6 to 12 months of age with mild to moderate asthma or recurrent/persistent wheezing was conducted. All patients were randomized to receive either 0.5 mg or 1 mg of PULMICORT RESPULES or placebo once daily. A total of 28, 17, and 31 patients in the PULMICORT RESPULES 0.5 mg, 1 mg, and placebo arms respectively, had an evaluation of serum cortisol levels post-ACTH stimulation both at baseline and at the end of the study. The mean change from baseline to Week 12 ACTH-stimulated minus basal plasma cortisol levels did not indicate adrenal suppression in patients treated with PULMICORT RESPULES versus placebo. However, 7 patients in this study (4 of whom received PULMICORT RESPULES 0.5 mg, 2 of whom received PULMICORT RESPULES 1 mg and 1 of whom received placebo) showed a shift from normal baseline stimulated cortisol level (≥500 nmol/L) to a subnormal level (<500 nmol/L) at Week 12. In 4 of these patients receiving PULMICORT RESPULES, the cortisol values were near the cutoff value of 500 nmol/L.
The effects of PULMICORT RESPULES at doses of 0.5 mg twice daily, and 1 mg and 2 mg twice daily (2 times and 4 times the highest recommended total daily dose, respectively) on 24-hour urinary cortisol excretion were studied in 18 patients between 6 to 15 years of age with persistent asthma in a cross-over study design (4 weeks of treatment per dose level). There was a dose-related decrease in urinary cortisol excretion at 2 and 4 times the recommended daily dose. The two higher doses of PULMICORT RESPULES (1 and 2 mg twice daily) showed statistically significantly reduced (43–52%) urinary cortisol excretion compared to the run-in period. The highest recommended dose of PULMICORT RESPULES, 1 mg total daily dose, did not show statistically significantly reduced urinary cortisol excretion compared to the run-in period.
PULMICORT RESPULES, like other inhaled corticosteroid products, may impact the HPA axis, especially in susceptible individuals, in younger children, and in patients given high doses for prolonged periods.

CLINICAL TRIALS

Three double-blind, placebo-controlled, parallel group, randomized U.S. clinical trials of 12-weeks duration each were conducted in 1018 pediatric patients, 6 months to 8 years of age, with persistent asthma of varying disease duration (2 to 107 months) and severity. Doses of 0.25 mg, 0.5 mg, and 1 mg administered either once or twice daily were compared to placebo to provide information about appropriate dosing to cover a range of asthma severity. A Pari-LC-Jet Plus Nebulizer (with a face mask or mouthpiece) connected to a Pari Master compressor was used to deliver PULMICORT RESPULES to patients in the 3 U.S. controlled clinical trials. The co-primary endpoints were nighttime and daytime asthma symptom scores (0–3 scale). Each of the five doses discussed below were studied in one or two, but not all three of the U.S. studies.
Results of the 3 controlled clinical trials for recommended dosages of budesonide inhalation suspension (0.25 mg to 0.5 mg once or twice daily, or 1 mg once daily, up to a total daily dose of 1 mg) in 946 patients, 12 months to 8 years of age, are presented below. Compared to placebo, PULMICORT RESPULES significantly decreased both nighttime and daytime symptom scores of asthma at doses of 0.25 mg once daily (one study), 0.25 mg twice daily, and 0.5 mg twice daily. PULMICORT RESPULES significantly decreased either nighttime or daytime symptom scores, but not both, at doses of 1 mg once daily, and 0.5 mg once daily (one study). Symptom reduction in response to PULMICORT RESPULES occurred across gender and age. PULMICORT RESPULES significantly reduced the need for bronchodilator therapy at all the doses studied.
Improvements in lung function were associated with PULMICORT RESPULES in the subgroup of patients capable of performing lung function testing. Significant improvements were seen in FEV_1 [PULMICORT RESPULES 0.5 mg once daily and 1 mg once daily (one study); 0.5 mg twice daily] and morning PEF [PULMICORT RESPULES 1 mg once daily (one study); 0.25 mg twice daily; 0.5 mg twice daily] compared to placebo.
A numerical reduction in nighttime and daytime symptom scores (0–3 scale) of asthma was observed within 2–8 days, although maximum benefit was not achieved for 4–6 weeks after starting treatment. The reduction in nighttime and daytime asthma symptom scores was maintained throughout the 12 weeks of the double-blind trials.

Patients Not Receiving Inhaled Corticosteroid Therapy

The efficacy of PULMICORT RESPULES at doses of 0.25 mg, 0.5 mg, and 1 mg once daily was evaluated in 344 pediatric patients, 12 months to 8 years of age, with mild to moderate persistent asthma (mean baseline nighttime asthma symptom scores of the treatment groups ranged from 1.07 to 1.34) who were not well controlled by bronchodilators alone. The changes from baseline to Weeks 0–12 in nighttime asthma symptom scores are shown in Figure 1. Nighttime asthma symptom scores improved significantly in the patients treated with PULMICORT RESPULES compared to placebo. Similar improvements were also observed for daytime asthma symptom scores.
[See figure 1 below]

Patients Previously Maintained on Inhaled Corticosteroids

The efficacy of PULMICORT RESPULES at doses of 0.25 mg and 0.5 mg twice daily was evaluated in 133 pediatric asthma patients, 4 to 8 years of age, previously maintained on inhaled corticosteroids (mean FEV_1 79.5% predicted; mean baseline nighttime asthma symptom scores of the treatment groups ranged from 1.04 to 1.18; mean baseline dose of beclomethasone dipropionate of 265 mcg/day, ranging between 42 to 1008 mcg/day; mean baseline dose of triamcinolone acetonide of 572 mcg/day, ranging between 200 to 1200 mcg/day). The changes from baseline to Weeks 0–12 in nighttime asthma symptom scores are shown in Figure 2. Nighttime asthma symptom scores were significantly improved in patients treated with PULMICORT RESPULES compared to placebo. Similar improvements were also observed for daytime asthma symptom scores.
PULMICORT RESPULES at a dose of 0.5 mg twice daily significantly improved FEV_1, and both doses (0.25 mg and 0.5 mg twice daily) significantly increased morning PEF, compared to placebo.
[See figure 2 at top of next page]

Patients Receiving Once-Daily or Twice-Daily Dosing

The efficacy of PULMICORT RESPULES at doses of 0.25 mg once daily, 0.25 mg twice daily, 0.5 mg twice daily, and 1 mg once daily, was evaluated in 469 pediatric patients 12 months to 8 years of age (mean baseline nighttime asthma symptom scores of the treatment groups ranged from 1.13 to 1.31). Approximately 70% were not previously receiving inhaled corticosteroids. The changes from baseline to Weeks 0–12 in nighttime asthma symptom scores are shown in Figure 3. PULMICORT RESPULES at doses of 0.25 mg and 0.5 mg twice daily, and 1 mg once daily, significantly improved nighttime asthma symptom scores compared to placebo. Similar improvements were also observed for daytime asthma symptom scores.
PULMICORT RESPULES at a dose of 0.5 mg twice daily significantly improved FEV_1, and at doses of 0.25 mg and 0.5 mg twice daily and 1 mg once daily significantly improved morning PEF, compared to placebo.

Figure 1: A 12-Week Trial in Pediatric Patients Not on Inhaled Corticosteroid Therapy Prior to Study Entry.

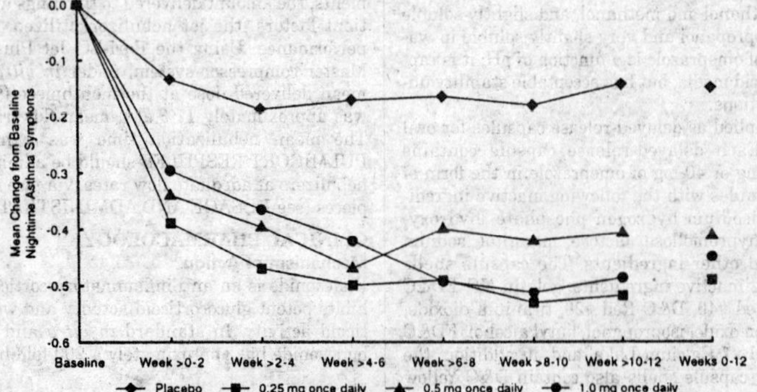

The evidence supports the efficacy of the same nominal dose of PULMICORT RESPULES administered on either a once-daily or twice-daily schedule. However, when all measures are considered together, the evidence is stronger for twice-daily dosing (see DOSAGE AND ADMINISTRATION).
[See figure 3 at right]

INDICATIONS

PULMICORT RESPULES is indicated for the maintenance treatment of asthma and as prophylactic therapy in children 12 months to 8 years of age.
PULMICORT RESPULES is NOT indicated for the relief of acute bronchospasm.

CONTRAINDICATIONS

PULMICORT RESPULES is contraindicated as the primary treatment of status asthmaticus or other acute episodes of asthma where intensive measures are required.
Hypersensitivity to budesonide or any of the ingredients of this preparation contraindicates the use of PULMICORT RESPULES.

WARNINGS

Particular care is needed for patients who are transferred from systemically active corticosteroids to inhaled corticosteroids because deaths due to adrenal insufficiency have occurred in asthmatic patients during and after transfer from systemic corticosteroids to less systemically available inhaled corticosteroids. After withdrawal from systemic corticosteroids, a number of months are required for recovery of HPA-axis function.
Patients who have been previously maintained on 20 mg or more per day of prednisone (or its equivalent) may be most susceptible, particularly when their systemic corticosteroids have been almost completely withdrawn.
During this period of HPA-axis suppression, patients may exhibit signs and symptoms of adrenal insufficiency when exposed to trauma, surgery, infection (particularly gastroenteritis) or other conditions associated with severe electrolyte loss. Although PULMICORT RESPULES may provide control of asthma symptoms during these episodes, in recommended doses it supplies less than normal physiological amounts of corticosteroid systemically and does NOT provide the mineralocorticoid activity that is necessary for coping with these emergencies.
During periods of stress or a severe asthma attack, patients who have been withdrawn from systemic corticosteroids should be instructed to resume oral corticosteroids (in large doses) immediately and to contact their physicians for further instructions. These patients should also be instructed to carry a warning card indicating that they may need supplementary systemic corticosteroids during periods of stress or a severe asthma attack.
Transfer of patients from systemic corticosteroid therapy to PULMICORT RESPULES may unmask allergic conditions previously suppressed by the systemic corticosteroid therapy, eg, rhinitis, conjunctivitis, and eczema (see DOSAGE AND ADMINISTRATION).
Patients who are on drugs which suppress the immune system are more susceptible to infection than healthy individuals. Chicken pox and measles, for example, can have a more serious or even fatal course in susceptible pediatric patients or adults on immunosuppressant doses of corticosteroids. In pediatric or adult patients who have not had these diseases, or who have not been properly vaccinated, particular care should be taken to avoid exposure. How the dose, route, and duration of corticosteroid administration affects the risk of developing a disseminated infection is not known. The contribution of the underlying disease and/or prior corticosteroid treatment to the risk is also not known. If exposed, therapy with varicella zoster immune globulin (VZIG) or pooled intravenous immunoglobulin (IVIG), as appropriate, may be indicated. If exposed to measles, prophylaxis with pooled intramuscular immunoglobulin (IG) may be indicated. (See the respective package inserts for complete VZIG and IG prescribing information.) If chicken pox develops, treatment with antiviral agents may be considered.
PULMICORT RESPULES is not a bronchodilator and is not indicated for the rapid relief of acute bronchospasm or other acute episodes of asthma.
As with other inhaled asthma medications, bronchospasm, with an immediate increase in wheezing, may occur after dosing. If acute bronchospasm occurs following dosing with PULMICORT RESPULES, it should be treated immediately with a fast-acting inhaled bronchodilator. Treatment with PULMICORT RESPULES should be discontinued and alternate therapy instituted.
Patients should be instructed to contact their physician immediately when episodes of asthma not responsive to their usual doses of bronchodilators occur during treatment with PULMICORT RESPULES.

PRECAUTIONS

General

Inhaled corticosteroids may cause a reduction in growth velocity when administered to pediatric patients (see PRECAUTIONS, Pediatric Use).
During withdrawal from oral corticosteroids, some patients may experience symptoms of systemically active corticosteroid withdrawal, eg, joint and/or muscular pain, lassitude, and depression, despite maintenance or even improvement of respiratory function.
Because budesonide is absorbed into the circulation and may be systemically active, particularly at higher doses, suppression of HPA function may be associated when PULMICORT RESPULES is administered at doses exceeding those recommended (see DOSAGE AND ADMINISTRATION), or when the dose is not titrated to the lowest effective dose. Since individual sensitivity to effects on cortisol production exists, physicians should consider this information when prescribing PULMICORT RESPULES.

Figure 2: A 12-Week Trial in Pediatric Patients Previously Maintained on Inhaled Corticosteroid Therapy Prior to Study Entry.

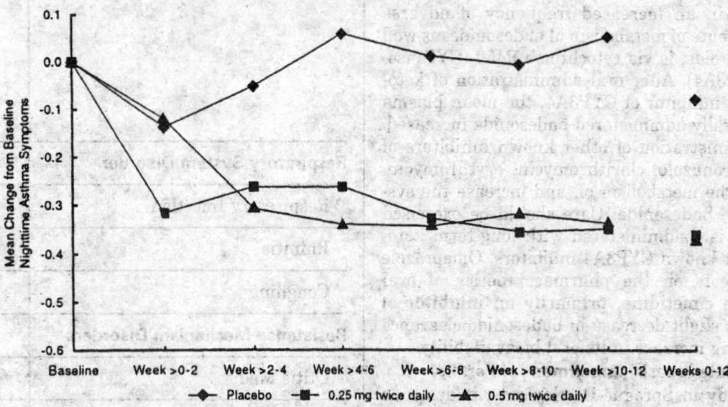

Figure 3: A 12-Week Trial in Pediatric Patients Either Maintained on Bronchodilators Alone or Inhaled Corticosteroid Therapy Prior to Study Entry.

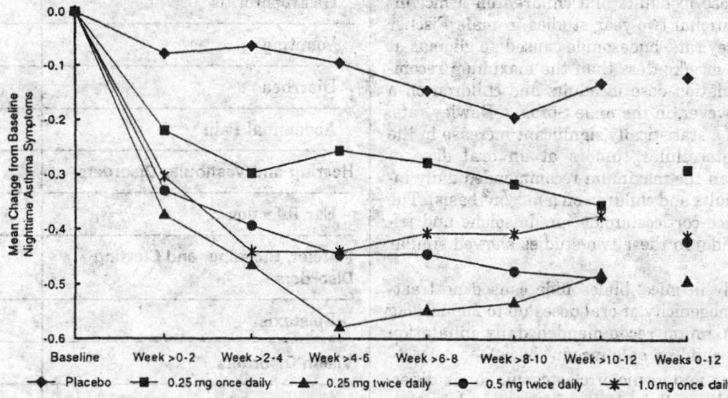

Because of the possibility of systemic absorption of inhaled corticosteroids, patients treated with these drugs should be observed carefully for any evidence of systemic corticosteroid effects. Particular care should be taken in observing patients post-operatively or during periods of stress for evidence of inadequate adrenal response.
It is possible that systemic corticosteroid effects such as hypercorticism and adrenal suppression may appear in a small number of patients, particularly at higher doses. If such changes occur, PULMICORT RESPULES should be reduced slowly, consistent with accepted procedures for management of asthma symptoms and for tapering of systemic corticosteroids.
Although patients in clinical trials have received PULMICORT RESPULES on a continuous basis for periods of up to 1 year, the long-term local and systemic effects of PULMICORT RESPULES in human subjects are not completely known. In particular, the effects resulting from chronic use of PULMICORT RESPULES on developmental or immunological processes in the mouth, pharynx, trachea, and lung are unknown.
In clinical trials with PULMICORT RESPULES, localized infections with *Candida albicans* occurred in the mouth and pharynx in some patients. The incidences of localized infections of *Candida albicans* were similar between the placebo and PULMICORT RESPULES treatment groups. If symptomatic oropharyngeal candidiasis develops, it should be treated with appropriate local or systemic (ie, oral) antifungal therapy while still continuing with PULMICORT RESPULES therapy, but at times therapy with PULMICORT RESPULES may need to be interrupted under close medical supervision.
Inhaled corticosteroids should be used with caution, if at all, in patients with active or quiescent tuberculosis infection of the respiratory tract, untreated systemic fungal, bacterial, viral, or parasitic infections; or ocular herpes simplex.
Rare instances of glaucoma, increased intraocular pressure, and cataracts have been reported following the inhaled administration of corticosteroids.

Information for Patients

For instructions on the proper use of PULMICORT RESPULES and to attain the maximum improvement in asthma symptoms, the patient or the parent/guardian of the patient should receive, read, and follow the accompanying patient information and instructions carefully. In addition, patients being treated with PULMICORT RESPULES should receive the following information and instructions. This information is intended to aid the patient in the safe and effective use of the medication. It is not a disclosure of all possible adverse or intended effects.

- Patients should take PULMICORT RESPULES at regular intervals once or twice a day as directed, since its effectiveness depends on regular use. The patient should not alter the prescribed dosage unless advised to do so by the physician.
- The effects of mixing PULMICORT RESPULES with other nebulizable medications have not been adequately assessed. PULMICORT RESPULES should be administered separately in the nebulizer.
- PULMICORT RESPULES is not a bronchodilator, and its use is not intended to treat acute life-threatening episodes of asthma.
- PULMICORT RESPULES should be administered with a jet nebulizer connected to a compressor with an adequate air flow, equipped with a mouthpiece or suitable face mask. The face mask should be properly adjusted to optimize delivery and to avoid exposing the eyes to the nebulized medication (see DOSAGE AND ADMINISTRATION).
- Ultrasonic nebulizers are not suitable for the adequate administration of PULMICORT RESPULES and, therefore, are not recommended (see DOSAGE AND ADMINISTRATION).
- Rinsing the mouth with water after each treatment may decrease the risk of development of local candidiasis. Corticosteroid effects on the skin can be avoided if the face is washed after the use of a face mask.
- Improvement in asthma control following treatment with PULMICORT RESPULES can occur within 2–8 days of beginning treatment, although maximum benefit may not be achieved for 4–6 weeks after starting treatment. If the asthma symptoms do not improve in that time frame, or if the condition worsens, the patient or the patient's parent/guardian should be instructed to contact the physician.
- Care should be taken to avoid exposure to chicken pox and measles. If exposure occurs, and the child has not had chicken pox or been properly vaccinated, a physician should be consulted without delay.
- PULMICORT RESPULES should be stored upright at controlled room temperature 20–25°C (68–77°F) and protected from light. PULMICORT RESPULES should not be refrigerated or frozen.
- When an aluminum foil envelope has been opened, the shelf life of the unused RESPULES ampules is two weeks when protected from light. The date the envelope was opened should be recorded on the back of the envelope in the space provided.
- After opening the aluminum foil envelope, the unused RESPULES ampules should be returned to the envelope to protect them from light. Any individually opened RESPULES ampules must be used promptly.
- For proper usage of PULMICORT RESPULES and to attain maximum improvement, the accompanying Patient's Instructions for Use should be read and followed.

Drug Interactions

In clinical studies, concurrent administration of budesonide and other drugs commonly used in the treatment of asthma

Continued on next page

Pulmicort—Cont.

has not resulted in an increased frequency of adverse events. The main route of metabolism of budesonide, as well as other corticosteroids, is via cytochrome P450 (CYP) isoenzyme 3A4 (CYP3A4). After oral administration of ketoconazole, a potent inhibitor of CYP3A4, the mean plasma concentration of orally administered budesonide increased. Concomitant administration of other known inhibitors of CYP3A4 (eg, itraconazole, clarithromycin, erythromycin, etc.) may inhibit the metabolism of, and increase the systemic exposure to, budesonide. Care should be exercised when budesonide is coadministered with long-term ketoconazole and other known CYP3A4 inhibitors. Omeprazole did not have effects on the pharmacokinetics of oral budesonide, while cimetidine, primarily an inhibitor of CYP1A2, caused a slight decrease in budesonide clearance and a corresponding increase in its oral bioavailability.

Carcinogenesis, Mutagenesis, Impairment of Fertility

In a two-year study in Sprague-Dawley rats, budesonide caused a statistically significant increase in the incidence of gliomas in male rats at an oral dose of 50 mcg/kg (less than the maximum recommended daily inhalation dose in adults and children on a mcg/m^2 basis). No tumorigenicity was seen in male and female rats at respective oral doses up to 25 and 50 mcg/kg (less than the maximum recommended daily inhalation dose in adults and children on a mcg/m^2 basis). In two additional two-year studies in male Fischer and Sprague-Dawley rats, budesonide caused no gliomas at an oral dose of 50 mcg/kg (less than the maximum recommended daily inhalation dose in adults and children on a mcg/m^2 basis). However, in the male Sprague-Dawley rats, budesonide caused a statistically significant increase in the incidence of hepatocellular tumors at an oral dose of 50 mcg/kg (less than the maximum recommended daily inhalation dose in adults and children on a mcg/m^2 basis). The concurrent reference corticosteroids (prednisolone and triamcinolone acetonide) in these two studies showed similar findings.

In a 91-week study in mice, budesonide caused no treatment-related carcinogenicity at oral doses up to 200 mcg/kg (less than the maximum recommended daily inhalation dose in adults and children on a mcg/m^2 basis).

Budesonide was not mutagenic or clastogenic in six different test systems: Ames *Salmonella*/microsome plate test, mouse micronucleus test, mouse lymphoma test, chromosome aberration test in human lymphocytes, sex-linked recessive lethal test in *Drosophila melanogaster*, and DNA repair analysis in rat hepatocyte culture.

In rats, budesonide had no effect on fertility at subcutaneous doses up to 80 mcg/kg (less than the maximum recommended daily inhalation dose in adults on a mcg/m^2 basis). However, it caused a decrease in prenatal viability and viability in the pups at birth and during lactation, along with a decrease in maternal body-weight gain, at subcutaneous doses of 20 mcg/kg and above (less than the maximum recommended daily inhalation dose in adults on a mcg/m^2 basis). No such effects were noted at 5 mcg/kg (less than the maximum recommended daily inhalation dose in adults on a mcg/m^2 basis).

Pregnancy

Teratogenic Effects: Pregnancy Category B—As with other corticosteroids, budesonide was teratogenic and embryocidal in rabbits and rats. Budesonide produced fetal loss, decreased pup weights, and skeletal abnormalities at subcutaneous doses of 25 mcg/kg in rabbits (less than the maximum recommended daily inhalation dose in adults on a mcg/m^2 basis) and 500 mcg/kg in rats (approximately 4 times the maximum recommended daily inhalation dose in adults on a mcg/m^2 basis). In another study in rats, no teratogenic or embryocidal effects were seen at inhalation doses up to 250 mcg/kg (approximately 2 times the maximum recommended daily inhalation dose in adults on a mcg/m^2 basis).

Experience with oral corticosteroids since their introduction in pharmacologic, as opposed to physiologic, doses suggests that rodents are more prone to teratogenic effects from corticosteroids than humans. In addition, because there is a natural increase in corticosteroid production during pregnancy, most women will require a lower exogenous corticosteroid dose and many will not need corticosteroid treatment during pregnancy.

Studies of pregnant women, however, have not shown that inhaled budesonide increases the risk of abnormalities when administered during pregnancy. The results from a large population-based prospective cohort epidemiological study reviewing data from three Swedish registries covering approximately 99% of the pregnancies from 1995–1997 (ie, Swedish Medical Birth Registry; Registry of Congenital Malformations; Child Cardiology Registry) indicate no increased risk for congenital malformations from the use of inhaled budesonide during early pregnancy. Congenital malformations were studied in 2014 infants born to mothers reporting the use of inhaled budesonide for asthma in early pregnancy (usually 10–12 weeks after the last menstrual period), the period when most major organ malformations occur. The rate of recorded congenital malformations was similar compared to the general population rate (3.8% vs. 3.5%, respectively). In addition, after exposure to inhaled budesonide, the number of infants born with orofacial clefts was similar to the expected number in the normal population (4 children vs. 3.3, respectively).

Adverse Events with ≥ 3% Incidence Reported by Patients on PULMICORT RESPULES

Adverse Events	Vehicle Placebo (n=227) %	PULMICORT RESPULES Total Daily Dose		
		0.25 mg (n=178) %	0.5 mg (n=223) %	1 mg (n=317) %
Respiratory System Disorder				
Respiratory Infection	36	34	35	38
Rhinitis	9	7	11	12
Coughing	5	5	9	8
Resistance Mechanism Disorders				
Otitis Media	11	12	11	9
Viral Infection	3	4	5	3
Moniliasis	2	4	3	4
Gastrointestinal System Disorders				
Gastroenteritis	4	5	5	5
Vomiting	3	2	4	4
Diarrhea	2	4	4	2
Abdominal Pain	2	3	2	3
Hearing and Vestibular Disorders				
Ear Infection	4	2	4	5
Platelet, Bleeding, and Clotting Disorders				
Epistaxis	1	2	4	3
Vision Disorders				
Conjunctivitis	2	<1	4	2
Skin and Appendages Disorders				
Rash	3	<1	4	2

These same data were utilized in a second study bringing the total to 2534 infants whose mothers were exposed to inhaled budesonide. In this study, the rate of congenital malformations among infants whose mothers were exposed to inhaled budesonide during early pregnancy was not different from the rate for all newborn babies during the same period (3.6%).

Despite the animal findings, it would appear that the possibility of fetal harm is remote if the drug is used during pregnancy. Nevertheless, because the studies in humans cannot rule out the possibility of harm, PULMICORT RESPULES should be used during pregnancy only if clearly needed.

Non-teratogenic Effects: Hypoadrenalism may occur in infants born of mothers receiving corticosteroids during pregnancy. Such infants should be carefully observed.

Nursing Mothers

It is not known whether budesonide is excreted in human milk. Because other corticosteroids are excreted in human milk, caution should be exercised if budesonide is administered to nursing women.

Pediatric Use

Safety in children six months to 12 months of age has been evaluated. Safety and effectiveness in children 12 months to 8 years of age have been established (see CLINICAL PHARMACOLOGY, Pharmacodynamics, CLINICAL TRIALS and ADVERSE REACTIONS).

A 12-week study in 141 pediatric patients 6 to 12 months of age with mild to moderate asthma or recurrent/persistent wheezing was conducted. All patients were randomized to receive either 0.5 mg or 1 mg of PULMICORT RESPULES or placebo once daily. Adrenal axis function was assessed with an ACTH stimulation test at the beginning and end of the study, and mean changes from baseline in this variable did not indicate adrenal suppression in patients who received PULMICORT RESPULES versus placebo. However, on an individual basis, 7 patients in this study (6 in the PULMICORT RESPULES treatment arms and 1 in the placebo arm) experienced a shift from having a normal baseline stimulated cortisol level to having a subnormal level at Week 12 (see CLINICAL PHARMACOLOGY, Pharmacodynamics). Pneumonia was observed more frequently in patients treated with PULMICORT RESPULES than in patients treated with placebo, (N = 2, 1, and 0) in the PULMICORT RESPULES 0.5 mg, 1 mg, and placebo groups, respectively.

A dose dependent effect on growth was also noted in this 12-week trial. Infants in the placebo arm experienced an average growth of 3.7 cm over 12 weeks compared with 3.5 cm and 3.1 cm in the PULMICORT RESPULES 0.5 mg and 1 mg arms respectively. This corresponds to estimated mean (95% CI) reductions in 12-week growth velocity between placebo and PULMICORT RESPULES 0.5 mg of 0.2 cm (−0.6 to 1.0) and between placebo and PULMICORT RESPULES 1 mg of 0.6 cm (−0.2 to 1.4). These findings support that the use of PULMICORT RESPULES in infants 6 to 12 months of age may result in systemic effects and are consistent with findings of growth suppression in other studies with inhaled corticosteroids.

Controlled clinical studies have shown that inhaled corticosteroids may cause a reduction in growth velocity in pediatric patients. In these studies, the mean reduction in growth velocity was approximately one centimeter per year (range 0.3 to 1.8 cm per year) and appears to be related to dose and duration of exposure. This effect has been observed in the absence of laboratory evidence of hypothalamic-pituitary-adrenal (HPA)-axis suppression, suggesting that growth velocity is a more sensitive indicator of systemic corticosteroid exposure in pediatric patients than some commonly used tests of HPA-axis function. The long-term effects of this reduction in growth velocity associated with inhaled corticosteroids, including the impact on final adult height, are unknown. The potential for "catch up" growth following discontinuation of treatment with inhaled corticosteroids has not been adequately studied. The growth of pediatric patients receiving inhaled corticosteroids, including PULMICORT RESPULES, should be monitored routinely (eg, via stadiometry). The potential growth effects of prolonged treatment should be weighed against clinical benefits obtained and the risks associated with alternative therapies. To minimize the systemic effects of inhaled corticosteroids, including PULMICORT RESPULES, each patient should be titrated to his/her lowest effective dose.

Geriatric Use

Of the 215 patients in 3 clinical trials of PULMICORT RESPULES in adult patients, 65 (30%) were 65 years of age or older, while 22 (10%) were 75 years of age or older. No overall differences in safety were observed between these patients and younger patients, and other reported clinical or medical surveillance experience has not identified differences in responses between the elderly and younger patients.

ADVERSE REACTIONS

The following adverse reactions were reported in pediatric patients treated with PULMICORT RESPULES.

The incidence of common adverse reactions is based on three double-blind, placebo-controlled, U.S. clinical trials in which 945 patients, 12 months to 8 years of age, (98 patients ≥12 months and <2 years of age; 225 patients ≥2 and <4 years of age; and 622 patients ≥4 and ≤8 years of age) were treated with PULMICORT RESPULES (0.25 to 1 mg total daily dose for 12 weeks) or vehicle placebo. The incidence and nature of adverse events reported for

Previous Therapy	Recommended Starting Dose	Highest Recommended Dose
Bronchodilators alone	0.5 mg total daily dose administered either once daily or twice daily in divided doses	0.5 mg total daily dose
Inhaled Corticosteroids	0.5 mg total daily dose administered either once daily or twice daily in divided doses	1 mg total daily dose
Oral Corticosteroids	1 mg total daily dose administered either as 0.5 mg twice daily or 1 mg once daily	1 mg total daily dose

PULMICORT RESPULES was comparable to that reported for placebo. The following table shows the incidence of adverse events in U.S. controlled clinical trials, regardless of relationship to treatment, in patients previously receiving bronchodilators and/or inhaled corticosteroids. This population included a total of 605 male and 340 female patients.
[See table at top of previous page]
The table above shows all adverse events with an incidence of 3% or more in at least one active treatment group where the incidence was higher with PULMICORT RESPULES than with placebo.
The following adverse events occurred with an incidence of 3% or more in at least one PULMICORT RESPULES group where the incidence was equal to or less than that of the placebo group: fever, sinusitis, pain, pharyngitis, bronchospasm, bronchitis, and headache.

Incidence 1% to ≤3% (by body system)

The information below includes all adverse events with an incidence of 1 to ≤3%, in at least one PULMICORT RESPULES treatment group where the incidence was higher with PULMICORT RESPULES than with placebo, regardless of relationship to treatment.

Body as a whole: allergic reaction, chest pain, fatigue, flu-like disorder
Respiratory system: stridor
Resistance mechanisms: herpes simplex, external ear infection, infection
Central & peripheral nervous system: dysphonia, hyperkinesia
Skin & appendages: eczema, pustular rash, pruritus
Hearing & vestibular: earache
Vision: eye infection
Psychiatric: anorexia, emotional lability
Musculoskeletal system: fracture, myalgia
Application site: contact dermatitis
Platelet, bleeding & clotting: purpura
White cell and resistance: cervical lymphadenopathy

The incidence of reported adverse events was similar between the 447 PULMICORT RESPULES-treated (mean total daily dose 0.5 to 1 mg) and 223 conventional therapy-treated pediatric asthma patients followed for one year in three open-label studies.
Cases of growth suppression have been reported for inhaled corticosteroids including post-marketing reports for PULMICORT RESPULES (see PRECAUTIONS, Pediatric Use).
Less frequent adverse events (<1%) reported in the published literature, long-term, open-label clinical trials, or from marketing experience for inhaled budesonide include: immediate and delayed hypersensitivity reactions including rash, contact dermatitis, angioedema, and bronchospasm; symptoms of hypocorticism and hypercorticism; psychiatric symptoms including depression, aggressive reactions, irritability, anxiety, and psychosis; and bone disorders including avascular necrosis of the femoral head and osteoporosis.

OVERDOSAGE

The potential for acute toxic effects following overdose of PULMICORT RESPULES is low. If inhaled corticosteroids are used at excessive doses for prolonged periods, systemic corticosteroid effects such as hypercorticism or growth suppression may occur (see PRECAUTIONS).
In mice the minimal lethal inhalation dose was 100 mg/kg (approximately 410 or 120 times, respectively, the maximum recommended daily inhalation dose in adults or children on a mg/m^2 basis). In rats there were no deaths at an inhalation dose of 68 mg/kg (approximately 550 or 160 times, respectively, the maximum recommended daily inhalation dose in adults or children on a mg/m^2 basis). In mice the minimal oral lethal dose was 200 mg/kg (approximately 810 or 240 times, respectively, the maximum recommended daily inhalation dose in adults or children on a mg/m^2 basis). In rats, the minimal oral lethal dose was less than 100 mg/kg (approximately 810 or 240 times, respectively, the maximum recommended daily inhalation dose in adults or children on a mg/m^2 basis).

DOSAGE AND ADMINISTRATION

PULMICORT RESPULES is indicated for use in asthmatic patients 12 months to 8 years of age. PULMICORT RESPULES should be administered by the inhaled route via jet nebulizer connected to an air compressor. Individual patients will experience a variable onset and degree of symptom relief. Improvement in asthma control following inhaled administration of PULMICORT RESPULES can occur within 2–8 days of initiation of treatment, although maximum benefit may not be achieved for 4–6 weeks. The safety and efficacy of PULMICORT RESPULES when administered in excess of recommended doses have not been established. In all patients, it is desirable to downward-titrate to the lowest effective dose once asthma stability is achieved. The recommended starting dose and highest recommended dose of PULMICORT RESPULES, based on prior asthma therapy, are listed in the following table.
[See table above]
In symptomatic children not responding to non-steroidal therapy, a starting dose of 0.25 mg once daily of PULMICORT RESPULES may also be considered.
If once-daily treatment with PULMICORT RESPULES does not provide adequate control of asthma symptoms, the total daily dose should be increased and/or administered as a divided dose.

Patients Not Receiving Systemic (Oral) Corticosteroids

Patients who require maintenance therapy of their asthma may benefit from treatment with PULMICORT RESPULES at the doses recommended above. Once the desired clinical effect is achieved, consideration should be given to tapering to the lowest effective dose. For the patients who do not respond adequately to the starting dose, consideration should be given to administering the total daily dose as a divided dose, if a once-daily dosing schedule was followed. If necessary, higher doses, up to the maximum recommended doses, may provide additional asthma control.

Patients Maintained on Chronic Oral Corticosteroids

Initially, PULMICORT RESPULES should be used concurrently with the patient's usual maintenance dose of systemic corticosteroid. After approximately one week, gradual withdrawal of the systemic corticosteroid may be initiated by reducing the daily or alternate daily dose. Further incremental reductions may be made after an interval of one or two weeks, depending on the response of the patient. Generally, these decrements should not exceed 25% of the prednisone dose or its equivalent. A slow rate of withdrawal is strongly recommended. During reduction of oral corticosteroids, patients should be carefully monitored for asthma instability, including objective measures of airway function, and for adrenal insufficiency (see WARNINGS). During withdrawal, some patients may experience symptoms of systemic corticosteroid withdrawal, eg, joint and/or muscular pain, lassitude, and depression, despite maintenance or even improvement in pulmonary function. Such patients should be encouraged to continue with PULMICORT RESPULES but should be monitored for objective signs of adrenal insufficiency. If evidence of adrenal insufficiency occurs, the systemic corticosteroid doses should be increased temporarily and thereafter withdrawal should continue more slowly. During periods of stress or a severe asthma attack, transfer patients may require supplementary treatment with systemic corticosteroids.
A Pari-LC-Jet Plus Nebulizer (with face mask or mouthpiece) connected to a Pari Master compressor was used to deliver PULMICORT RESPULES to each patient in 3 U.S. controlled clinical studies. The safety and efficacy of PULMICORT RESPULES delivered by other nebulizers and compressors have not been established.
PULMICORT RESPULES should be administered via jet nebulizer connected to an air compressor with an adequate air flow, equipped with a mouthpiece or suitable face mask. Ultrasonic nebulizers are not suitable for the adequate administration of PULMICORT RESPULES and, therefore, are NOT recommended.
The effects of mixing PULMICORT RESPULES with other nebulizable medications have not been adequately assessed. PULMICORT RESPULES should be administered separately in the nebulizer (see PRECAUTIONS, Information for Patients).

Directions for Use

Illustrated *Patient's Instructions for Use* accompany each package of PULMICORT RESPULES.

HOW SUPPLIED

PULMICORT RESPULES is supplied in sealed aluminum foil envelopes containing one plastic strip of five single-dose RESPULES ampules together with patient instructions for use. There are 30 RESPULES ampules in a carton. Each single-dose RESPULE ampule contains 2 mL of sterile liquid suspension.
PULMICORT RESPULES is available in two strengths, each containing 2 mL:

NDC 0186-1988-04	0.25 mg/2 mL
NDC 0186-1989-04	0.5 mg/2 mL

Storage

PULMICORT RESPULES should be stored upright at controlled room temperature 20–25°C (68–77°F) [see USP], and protected from light. When an envelope has been opened, the shelf life of the unused RESPULES ampules is 2 weeks when protected. After opening the aluminum foil envelope, the unused RESPULES ampules should be returned to the aluminum foil envelope to protect them from light. Any opened RESPULE ampule must be used promptly. Gently shake the RESPULE ampule using a circular motion before use. Keep out of reach of children. Do not freeze.
All trademarks are the property of the AstraZeneca group

AstraZeneca LP, Wilmington, DE 19850
721851-04
Rev. 03/04

Shown in Product Identification Guide, page 305

PULMICORT TURBUHALER 200 mcg ℞

[pull-mĭ-kŏrt]
(budesonide inhalation powder)
For Oral Inhalation Only.
℞ only

DESCRIPTION

Budesonide, the active component of PULMICORT TURBUHALER 200 mcg, is a corticosteroid designated chemically as (RS)-11β,16α,17,21-Tetrahydroxypregna-1,4-diene-3,20-dione cyclic 16,17-acetal with butyraldehyde. Budesonide is provided as a mixture of two epimers (22R and 22S). The empirical formula of budesonide is $C_{25}H_{34}O_6$ and its molecular weight is 430.5. Its structural formula is:

Budesonide is a white to off-white, tasteless, odorless powder that is practically insoluble in water and in heptane, sparingly soluble in ethanol, and freely soluble in chloroform. Its partition coefficient between octanol and water at pH 7.4 is 1.6×10^3.
PULMICORT TURBUHALER is an inhalation-driven multi-dose dry powder inhaler which contains only micronized budesonide. Each actuation of PULMICORT TURBUHALER provides 200 mcg budesonide per metered dose, which delivers approximately 160 mcg budesonide from the mouthpiece (based on *in vitro* testing at 60 L/min for 2 sec).
In vitro testing has shown that the dose delivery for PULMICORT TURBUHALER is substantially dependent on airflow through the device. Patient factors such as inspiratory flow rates will also affect the dose delivered to the lungs of patients in actual use (see *Patient's Instructions for Use*). In adult patients with asthma (mean FEV_1 2.9 L [0.8–5.1 L]) mean peak inspiratory flow (PIF) through PULMICORT TURBUHALER was 78 (40–111) L/min. Similar results (mean PIF 82 [43–125] L/min) were obtained in asthmatic children (6 to 15 years, mean FEV_1 2.1 L [0.9–5.4 L]). Patients should be carefully instructed on the use of this drug product to assure optimal dose delivery.

HOW SUPPLIED

PULMICORT TURBUHALER consists of a number of assembled plastic details, the main parts being the dosing mechanism, the storage unit for drug substance and the mouthpiece. The inhaler is protected by a white outer tubular cover screwed onto the inhaler. The body of the inhaler is white and the turning grip is brown. The following wording is printed on the grip in raised lettering, "Pulmicort™ 200 mcg". The TURBUHALER inhaler cannot be refilled and should be discarded when empty.
PULMICORT TURBUHALER is available as 200 mcg/dose, 200 doses (NDC 0186-0915-42) and has a target fill weight of 104 mg.
When there are 20 doses remaining in PULMICORT TURBUHALER, a red mark will appear in the indicator window. If the unit is used beyond the point at which the red mark appears at the bottom of the window, the correct amount of medication may not be obtained. The unit should be discarded.
Store with the cover tightened in a dry place at controlled room temperature 20-25°C (68-77°F) [see USP]. Keep out of the reach of children.
All trademarks are the property of the AstraZeneca group

Manufactured for: AstraZeneca LP, Wilmington, DE 19850
By: AstraZeneca AB, Södertälje, Sweden
808179-03 Rev. 12/03

Shown in Product Identification Guide, page 305

Continued on next page

RHINOCORT AQUA® ℞

[rī-nə-kort äquă]
(budesonide)
Nasal Spray 32 mcg
For Intranasal Use Only.
℞ only

DESCRIPTION

Budesonide, the active ingredient of RHINOCORT AQUA® Nasal Spray, is an anti-inflammatory synthetic corticosteroid.
It is designated chemically as (RS)-11-beta, 16-alpha, 17, 21-tetrahydroxypregna-1,4-diene-3,20-dione cyclic 16, 17-acetal with butyraldehyde.
Budesonide is provided as the mixture of two epimers (22R and 22S).
The empirical formula of budesonide is $C_{25}H_{34}O_6$ and its molecular weight is 430.5.
Its structural formula is:

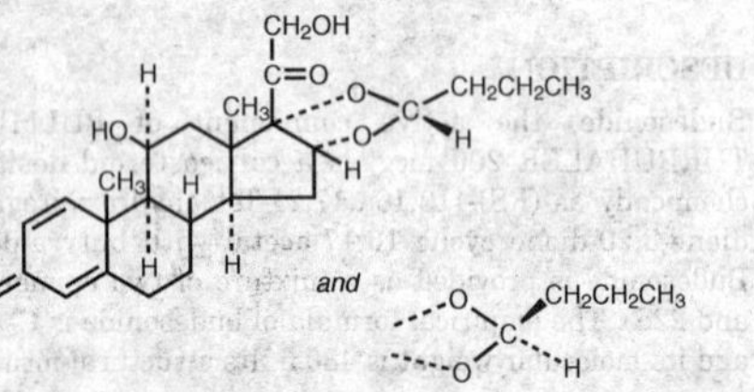

Budesonide is a white to off-white, odorless powder that is practically insoluble in water and in heptane, sparingly soluble in ethanol, and freely soluble in chloroform.
Its partition coefficient between octanol and water at pH 5 is 1.6×10^3.
RHINOCORT AQUA is an unscented, metered-dose, manual-pump spray formulation containing a micronized suspension of budesonide in an aqueous medium. Microcrystalline cellulose and carboxymethyl cellulose sodium, dextrose anhydrous, polysorbate 80, disodium edetate, potassium sorbate, and purified water are contained in this medium; hydrochloric acid is added to adjust the pH to a target of 4.5.
RHINOCORT AQUA Nasal Spray delivers 32 mcg of budesonide per spray.
Each bottle of RHINOCORT AQUA Nasal Spray 32 mcg contains 120 metered sprays after initial priming.
Prior to initial use, the container must be shaken gently and the pump must be primed by actuating eight times. If used daily, the pump does not need to be reprimed. If not used for two consecutive days, reprime with one spray or until a fine spray appears. If not used for more than 14 days, rinse the applicator and reprime with two sprays or until a fine spray appears.

CLINICAL PHARMACOLOGY

Budesonide is a synthetic corticosteroid having potent glucocorticoid activity and weak mineralocorticoid activity. In standard *in vitro* and animal models, budesonide has approximately a 200-fold higher affinity for the glucocorticoid receptor and a 1000-fold higher topical anti-inflammatory potency than cortisol (rat croton oil ear edema assay). As a measure of systemic activity, budesonide is 40 times more potent than cortisol when administered subcutaneously and 25 times more potent when administered orally in the rat thymus involution assay. In glucocorticoid receptor affinity studies, the 22R form was twice as active as the 22S epimer.
The precise mechanism of corticosteroid actions in seasonal and perennial allergic rhinitis is not known. Corticosteroids have been shown to have a wide range of inhibitory activities against multiple cell types (eg, mast cells, eosinophils, neutrophils, macrophages, and lymphocytes) and mediators (eg, histamine, eicosanoids, leukotrienes, and cytokines) involved in allergic mediated inflammation.
Corticosteroids affect the delayed (6 hour) response to an allergen challenge more than the histamine-associated immediate response (20 minute). The clinical significance of these findings is unknown.

Pharmacokinetics

The pharmacokinetics of budesonide have been studied following nasal, oral, and intravenous administration. Budesonide is relatively well absorbed after both inhalation and oral administration, and is rapidly metabolized into metabolites with low corticosteroid potency. The clinical activity of RHINOCORT AQUA Nasal Spray is therefore believed to be due to the parent drug, budesonide. *In vitro* studies indicate that the two epimeric forms of budesonide do not interconvert.

Absorption

Following intranasal administration of RHINOCORT AQUA, the mean peak plasma concentration occurs at approximately 0.7 hours. Compared to an intravenous dose, approximately 34% of the delivered intranasal dose reaches the systemic circulation, most of which is absorbed through the nasal mucosa. While budesonide is well absorbed from the GI tract, the oral bioavailability of budesonide is low (~10%) primarily due to extensive first pass metabolism in the liver.

Distribution

Budesonide has a volume of distribution of approximately 2–3 L/kg. The volume of distribution for the 22R epimer is almost twice that of the 22S epimer. Protein binding of budesonide *in vitro* is constant (85–90%) over a concentration range (1–100 nmol/L) which exceeded that achieved after administration of recommended doses. Budesonide shows little to no binding to glucocorticosteroid binding globulin. It rapidly equilibrates with red blood cells in a concentration independent manner with a blood/plasma ratio of about 0.8.

Metabolism

Budesonide is rapidly and extensively metabolized in humans by the liver. Two major metabolites (16α-hydroxyprednisolone and 6β-hydroxybudesonide) are formed via cytochrome P450 (CYP) isoenzyme 3A4 (CYP3A4)-catalyzed biotransformation. Known metabolic inhibitors of CYP3A4 (eg, ketoconazole), or significant hepatic impairment, may increase the systemic exposure of unmetabolized budesonide (see WARNINGS and PRECAUTIONS). *In vitro* studies on the binding of the two primary metabolites to the glucocorticoid receptor indicate that they have less than 1% of the affinity for the receptor as the parent compound budesonide. *In vitro* studies have evaluated sites of metabolism and showed negligible metabolism in skin, lung, and serum. No qualitative difference between the *in vitro* and *in vivo* metabolic patterns could be detected.

Elimination

Budesonide is excreted in the urine and feces in the form of metabolites. After intranasal administration of a radiolabeled dose, 2/3 of the radioactivity was found in the urine and the remainder in the feces. The main metabolites of budesonide in the 0–24 hour urine sample following IV administration are 16α-hydroxyprednisolone (24%) and 6β-hydroxybudesonide (5%). An additional 34% of the radioactivity recovered in the urine was identified as conjugates.
The 22R form was preferentially cleared with clearance value of 1.4 L/min vs. 1.0 L/min for the 22S form. The terminal half-life, 2 to 3 hours, was similar for both epimers and it appeared to be independent of dose.

Special Populations

Geriatric: No specific pharmacokinetic study has been undertaken in subjects >65 years of age.
Pediatric: After administration of RHINOCORT AQUA Nasal Spray, the time to reach peak drug concentrations and plasma half-life were similar in children and in adults. Children had plasma concentrations approximately twice those observed in adults due primarily to differences in weight between children and adults.
Gender: No specific pharmacokinetic study has been conducted to evaluate the effect of gender on budesonide pharmacokinetics. However, following administration of 400 mcg of RHINOCORT AQUA Nasal Spray to 7 male and 8 female volunteers in a pharmacokinetic study, no major gender differences in the pharmacokinetic parameters were found.
Race: No specific study has been undertaken to evaluate the effect of race on budesonide pharmacokinetics.
Renal Insufficiency: The pharmacokinetics of budesonide have not been investigated in patients with renal insufficiency.
Hepatic Insufficiency: Reduced liver function may affect the elimination of corticosteroids. The pharmacokinetics of orally administered budesonide were affected by compromised liver function as evidenced by a doubled systemic availability. The relevance of this finding to intranasally administered budesonide has not been established.

Pharmacodynamics

A 3-week clinical study in seasonal rhinitis, comparing RHINOCORT Nasal Inhaler, orally ingested budesonide, and placebo in 98 patients with allergic rhinitis due to birch pollen, demonstrated that the therapeutic effect of RHINOCORT Nasal Inhaler can be attributed to the topical effects of budesonide.
The effects of RHINOCORT AQUA Nasal Spray on adrenal function have been evaluated in several clinical trials. In a four-week clinical trial, 61 adult patients who received 256 mcg daily of RHINOCORT AQUA Nasal Spray demonstrated no significant differences from patients receiving placebo in plasma cortisol levels measured before and 60 minutes after 0.25 mg intramuscular cosyntropin. There were no consistent differences in 24-hour urinary cortisol measurements in patients receiving up to 400 mcg daily. Similar results were seen in a study of 150 children and adolescents aged 6 to 17 with perennial rhinitis who were treated with 256 mcg daily for up to 12 months.
After treatment with the recommended maximal daily dose of RHINOCORT AQUA (256 mcg) for seven days, there was a small, but statistically significant decrease in the area under the plasma cortisol-time curve over 24 hours (AUC_{0-24h}) in healthy adult volunteers.
A dose-related suppression of 24-hour urinary cortisol excretion was observed after administration of RHINOCORT AQUA doses ranging from 100–800 mcg daily for up to four days in 78 healthy adult volunteers. The clinical relevance of these results is unknown.

Clinical Trials

The therapeutic efficacy of RHINOCORT AQUA Nasal Spray has been evaluated in placebo-controlled clinical trials of seasonal and perennial allergic rhinitis of 3–6 weeks duration.
The number of patients treated with budesonide in these studies was 90 males and 51 females aged 6–12 years and 691 males and 694 females 12 years and above. The patients were predominantly Caucasian.
Overall, the results of these clinical trials showed that RHINOCORT AQUA Nasal Spray administered once daily provides statistically significant reduction in the severity of nasal symptoms of seasonal and perennial allergic rhinitis including runny nose, sneezing, and nasal congestion.
An improvement in nasal symptoms may be noted in patients within 10 hours of first using RHINOCORT AQUA Nasal Spray. This time to onset is supported by an environmental exposure unit study in seasonal allergic rhinitis patients which demonstrated that RHINOCORT AQUA Nasal Spray led to a statistically significant improvement in nasal symptoms compared to placebo by 10 hours. Further support comes from a clinical study of patients with perennial allergic rhinitis which demonstrated a statistically significant improvement in nasal symptoms for both RHINOCORT AQUA Nasal Spray and for the active comparator (mometasone furoate) compared to placebo by 8 hours. Onset was also assessed in this study with peak nasal inspiratory flow rate and this endpoint failed to show efficacy for either active treatment. Although statistically significant improvements in nasal symptoms compared to placebo were noted within 8–10 hours in these studies, about one half to two thirds of the ultimate clinical improvement with RHINOCORT AQUA Nasal Spray occurs over the first 1–2 days, and maximum benefit may not be achieved until approximately 2 weeks after initiation of treatment.

INDICATIONS AND USAGE

RHINOCORT AQUA Nasal Spray is indicated for the management of nasal symptoms of seasonal or perennial allergic rhinitis in adults and children six years of age and older.

CONTRAINDICATIONS

Hypersensitivity to any of the ingredients in this preparation contraindicates the use of RHINOCORT AQUA Nasal Spray.

WARNINGS

The replacement of a systemic corticosteroid with a topical corticosteroid can be accompanied by signs of adrenal insufficiency, and in addition some patients may experience symptoms of corticosteroid withdrawal, eg, joint and/or muscular pain, lassitude, and depression. Patients previously treated for prolonged periods with systemic corticosteroids and transferred to topical corticosteroids should be carefully monitored for acute adrenal insufficiency in response to stress. In those patients who have asthma or other clinical conditions requiring long-term systemic corticosteroid treatment, too rapid a decrease in systemic corticosteroids may cause a severe exacerbation of their symptoms.
Patients who are on drugs which suppress the immune system are more susceptible to infections than healthy individuals. Chicken pox and measles, for example, can have a more serious or even fatal course in non-immune children or adults on immunosuppressant doses of corticosteroids. In such children or adults who have not had these diseases, particular care should be taken to avoid exposure. How the dose, route, and duration of corticosteroid administration affects the risk of developing a disseminated infection is not known. The contribution of the underlying disease and/or prior corticosteroid treatment to the risk is also not known. If exposed to chicken pox, prophylaxis with varicella zoster immune globulin (VZIG) may be indicated. If exposed to measles, prophylaxis with pooled intramuscular immunoglobulin (IG) may be indicated. (See the respective package inserts for complete VZIG and IG prescribing information). If chicken pox develops, treatment with antiviral agents may be considered.

PRECAUTIONS

General

Intranasal corticosteroids may cause a reduction in growth velocity when administered to pediatric patients (see PRECAUTIONS, Pediatric Use).
Rarely, immediate and/or delayed hypersensitivity reactions may occur after the intranasal administration of budesonide. Rare instances of wheezing, nasal septum perforation, and increased intraocular pressure have been reported following the intranasal application of corticosteroids, including budesonide.
Although systemic effects have been minimal with recommended doses of RHINOCORT AQUA Nasal Spray, any such effect is dose dependent. Therefore, larger than recommended doses of RHINOCORT AQUA Nasal Spray should be avoided and the minimal effective dose for the patient should be used (see DOSAGE AND ADMINISTRATION).
When used at larger doses, systemic corticosteroid effects such as hypercorticism and adrenal suppression may appear. If such changes occur, the dosage of RHINOCORT AQUA Nasal Spray should be discontinued slowly, consistent with accepted procedures for discontinuing oral corticosteroid therapy.
In clinical studies with budesonide administered intranasally, the development of localized infections of the nose and pharynx with *Candida albicans* has occurred only rarely. When such an infection develops, it may require treatment with appropriate local or systemic therapy and discontinuation of treatment with RHINOCORT AQUA Nasal Spray. Patients using RHINOCORT AQUA Nasal Spray over several months or longer should be examined periodically for evidence of *Candida* infection or other signs of adverse effects on the nasal mucosa.
RHINOCORT AQUA Nasal Spray should be used with caution, if at all, in patients with active or quiescent tuberculous infection, untreated fungal, bacterial, or systemic viral infections, or ocular herpes simplex.
Because of the inhibitory effect of corticosteroids on wound healing, patients who have experienced recent nasal septal ulcers, nasal surgery, or nasal trauma should not use a nasal corticosteroid until healing has occurred.

Hepatic dysfunction influences the pharmacokinetics of budesonide, similar to the effect on other corticosteroids, with a reduced elimination rate and increased systemic availability (see CLINICAL PHARMACOLOGY, Special Populations).

Information for Patients

Patients being treated with RHINOCORT AQUA Nasal Spray should receive the following information and instructions. Patients who are on immunosuppressant doses of corticosteroids should be warned to avoid exposure to chicken pox or measles and, if exposed, to obtain medical advice.

Patients should use RHINOCORT AQUA Nasal Spray at regular intervals since its effectiveness depends on its regular use (see DOSAGE AND ADMINISTRATION).

An improvement in nasal symptoms may be noted in patients within 10 hours of first using RHINOCORT AQUA Nasal Spray. This time to onset is supported by an environmental exposure unit study in seasonal allergic rhinitis patients which demonstrated that RHINOCORT AQUA Nasal Spray led to a statistically significant improvement in nasal symptoms compared to placebo by 10 hours. Further support comes from a clinical study of patients with perennial allergic rhinitis which demonstrated a statistically significant improvement in nasal symptoms for both RHINOCORT AQUA Nasal Spray and for the active comparator (mometasone furoate) compared to placebo by 8 hours. Onset was also assessed in this study with peak nasal inspiratory flow rate and this endpoint failed to show efficacy for either active treatment. Although statistically significant improvements in nasal symptoms compared to placebo were noted within 8–10 hours in these studies, about one half to two thirds of the ultimate clinical improvement with RHINOCORT AQUA Nasal Spray occurs over the first 1–2 days, and maximum benefit may not be achieved until approximately 2 weeks after initiation of treatment. Initial assessment for response should be made during this time frame and periodically until the patient's symptoms are stabilized.

The patient should take the medication as directed and should not exceed the prescribed dosage. The patient should contact the physician if symptoms do not improve after two weeks, or if the condition worsens. Patients who experience recurrent episodes of epistaxis (nosebleeds) or nasal septum discomfort while taking this medication should contact their physician. For proper use of this unit and to attain maximum improvement, the patient should read and follow the accompanying patient instructions carefully.

It is important to shake the bottle well before each use. The RHINOCORT AQUA Nasal Spray 32 mcg bottle has been filled with an excess to accommodate the priming activity. The bottle should be discarded after 120 sprays following initial priming, since the amount of budesonide delivered per spray thereafter may be substantially less than the labeled dose. Do not transfer any remaining suspension to another bottle.

Drug Interactions

The main route of metabolism of budesonide, as well as other corticosteroids, is via cytochrome P450 (CYP) isoenzyme 3A4 (CYP3A4). After oral administration of ketoconazole, a potent inhibitor of CYP3A4, the mean plasma concentration of orally administered budesonide increased by more than seven-fold. Concomitant administration of other known inhibitors of CYP3A4 (eg, itraconazole, clarithromycin, erythromycin, etc.) may inhibit the metabolism of, and increase the systemic exposure to, budesonide (see WARNINGS and PRECAUTIONS, General). Care should be exercised when budesonide is coadministered with long-term ketoconazole and other known CYP3A4 inhibitors.

Omeprazole, an inhibitor of CYP2C19, did not have effects on the pharmacokinetics of oral budesonide, while cimetidine, primarily an inhibitor of CYP1A2, caused a slight decrease in budesonide clearance and corresponding increase in its oral bioavailability.

Carcinogenesis, Mutagenesis, Impairment of Fertility

In a two-year study in Sprague-Dawley rats, budesonide caused a statistically significant increase in the incidence of gliomas in the male rats receiving an oral dose of 50 mcg/kg (approximately twice the maximum recommended daily intranasal dose in adults and children on a mcg/m^2 basis). No tumorigenicity was seen in male and female rats at respective oral doses up to 25 and 50 mcg/kg (approximately equal to and two times the maximum recommended daily intranasal dose in adults and children on a mcg/m^2 basis, respectively). In two additional two-year studies in male Fischer and Sprague-Dawley rats, budesonide caused no gliomas at an oral dose of 50 mcg/kg (approximately twice the maximum recommended daily intranasal dose in adults and children on a mcg/m^2 basis). However, in male Sprague-Dawley rats, budesonide caused a statistically significant increase in the incidence of hepatocellular tumors at an oral dose of 50 mcg/kg (approximately twice the maximum recommended daily intranasal dose in adults and children on a mcg/m^2 basis). The concurrent reference corticosteroids (prednisolone and triamcinolone acetonide) in these two studies showed similar findings.

In a 91-week study in mice, budesonide caused no treatment-related carcinogenicity at oral doses up to 200 mcg/kg (approximately 3 times the maximum recommended daily intranasal dose in adults and children on a mcg/m^2 basis).

Budesonide was not mutagenic or clastogenic in six different test systems: Ames *Salmonella*/microsome plate test, mouse micronucleus test, mouse lymphoma test, chromosome aberration test in human lymphocytes, sex-linked recessive lethal test in *Drosophila melanogaster*, and DNA repair analysis in rat hematocyte culture.

In rats, budesonide caused a decrease in prenatal viability and viability of the pups at birth and during lactation, along with a decrease in maternal body-weight gain, at subcutaneous doses of 20 mcg/kg and above (less than the maximum recommended daily intranasal dose in adults on a mcg/m^2 basis). No such effects were noted at 5 mcg/kg (less than the maximum recommended daily intranasal dose in adults on a mcg/m^2 basis).

Pregnancy

Teratogenic Effects: Pregnancy Category C: Budesonide was teratogenic and embryocidal in rabbits and rats. Budesonide produced fetal loss, decreased pup weights, and skeletal abnormalities at subcutaneous doses of 25 mcg/kg in rabbits and 500 mcg/kg in rats (approximately 2 and 16 times the maximum recommended daily intranasal dose in adults on a mcg/m^2 basis). In another study in rats, no teratogenic or embryocidal effects were seen at inhalation doses up to 250 mcg/kg (approximately 8 times the maximum recommended daily intranasal dose in adults on a mcg/m^2 basis).

There are no adequate and well-controlled studies in pregnant women. RHINOCORT AQUA Nasal Spray should be used during pregnancy only if the potential benefit justifies the potential risk to the fetus.

Experience with oral corticosteroids since their introduction in pharmacologic, as opposed to physiologic, doses suggests that rodents are more prone to teratogenic effects from corticosteroids than humans. In addition, because there is a natural increase in corticosteroid production during pregnancy, most women will require a lower exogenous corticosteroid dose and many will not need corticosteroid treatment during pregnancy.

Nonteratogenic Effects: Hypoadrenalism may occur in infants born of mothers receiving corticosteroids during pregnancy. Such infants should be carefully observed.

Nursing Mothers

It is not known whether budesonide is excreted in human milk. Because other corticosteroids are excreted in human milk, caution should be exercised when RHINOCORT AQUA Nasal Spray is administered to nursing women.

Pediatric Use

Safety and effectiveness in pediatric patients below 6 years of age have not been established.

Controlled clinical studies have shown that intranasal corticosteroids may cause a reduction in growth velocity in pediatric patients. This effect has been observed in the absence of laboratory evidence of hypothalamic-pituitary-adrenal (HPA)-axis suppression, suggesting that growth velocity is a more sensitive indicator of systemic corticosteroid exposure in pediatric patients than some commonly used tests of HPA-axis function. The long-term effects of this reduction in growth velocity associated with intranasal corticosteroids, including the impact on final adult height, are unknown. The potential for "catch-up" growth following discontinuation of treatment with intranasal corticosteroids has not been adequately studied. The growth of pediatric patients receiving intranasal corticosteroids, including RHINOCORT AQUA Nasal Spray, should be monitored routinely (eg, via stadiometry). The potential growth effects of prolonged treatment should be weighed against clinical benefits obtained and the availability of safe and effective noncorticosteroid treatment alternatives. To minimize the systemic effects of intranasal corticosteroids, including RHINOCORT AQUA Nasal Spray, each patient should be titrated to the lowest dose that effectively controls his/her symptoms.

Geriatric Use

Of the 2,461 patients in clinical studies of RHINOCORT AQUA Nasal Spray, 5% were 60 years of age and over. No overall differences in safety or effectiveness were observed between these subjects and younger subjects, except for an adverse event reporting frequency of epistaxis which increased with age. Further, other reported clinical experience has not identified any other differences in responses between elderly and younger patients, but greater sensitivity of some older individuals cannot be ruled out.

ADVERSE REACTIONS

The incidence of common adverse reactions is based upon two U.S. and five non-U.S. controlled clinical trials in 1,526 patients [110 females and 239 males less than 18 years of age, and 635 females and 542 males 18 years of age and older] treated with RHINOCORT AQUA Nasal Spray at doses up to 400 mcg once daily for 3–6 weeks. The table below describes adverse events occurring at an incidence of 2% or greater and more common among RHINOCORT AQUA Nasal Spray-treated patients than in placebo-treated patients in controlled clinical trials. The overall incidence of adverse events was similar between RHINOCORT AQUA and placebo.

Adverse Event	RHINOCORT AQUA	Placebo Vehicle
Epistaxis	8%	5%
Pharyngitis	4%	3%
Bronchospasm	2%	1%
Coughing	2%	<1%
Nasal Irritation	2%	<1%

A similar adverse event profile was observed in the subgroup of pediatric patients 6 to 12 years of age.

Two to three percent (2–3%) of patients in clinical trials discontinued because of adverse events. Systemic corticosteroid side effects were not reported during controlled clinical studies with RHINOCORT AQUA Nasal Spray.

If recommended doses are exceeded, however, or if individuals are particularly sensitive, symptoms of hypercorticism, ie, Cushing's Syndrome, could occur.

Rare adverse events reported from post-marketing experience include: nasal septum perforation, pharynx disorders (throat irritation, throat pain, swollen throat, burning throat, and itchy throat), angioedema, anosmia, and palpitations.

Cases of growth suppression have been reported for intranasal corticosteroids including RHINOCORT AQUA Nasal Spray (see PRECAUTIONS, Pediatric Use).

OVERDOSAGE

Acute overdosage with this dosage form is unlikely since one 120 spray bottle of RHINOCORT AQUA Nasal Spray 32 mcg only contains approximately 5.4 mg of budesonide. Chronic overdosage may result in signs/symptoms of hypercorticism (see WARNINGS and PRECAUTIONS).

DOSAGE AND ADMINISTRATION

The recommended starting dose for adults and children 6 years of age and older is 64 mcg per day administered as one spray per nostril of RHINOCORT AQUA Nasal Spray 32 mcg once daily. The maximum recommended dose for adults (12 years of age and older) is 256 mcg per day administered as four sprays per nostril once daily of RHINOCORT AQUA Nasal Spray 32 mcg and the maximum recommended dose for pediatric patients (<12 years of age) is 128 mcg per day administered as two sprays per nostril once daily of RHINOCORT AQUA Nasal Spray 32 mcg (see HOW SUPPLIED).

Prior to initial use, the container must be shaken gently and the pump must be primed by actuating eight times. If used daily, the pump does not need to be reprimed. If not used for two consecutive days, reprime with one spray or until a fine spray appears. If not used for more than 14 days, rinse the applicator and reprime with two sprays or until a fine spray appears.

Individualization of Dosage

It is always desirable to titrate an individual patient to the minimum effective dose to reduce the possibility of side effects. In adults and children 6 years of age and older, the recommended starting dose is 64 mcg daily administered as one spray per nostril of RHINOCORT AQUA Nasal Spray 32 mcg, once daily. Some patients who do not achieve symptom control at the recommended starting dose may benefit from an increased dose. The maximum daily dose is 256 mcg for adults and 128 mcg for pediatric patients (<12 years of age). When the maximum benefit has been achieved and symptoms have been controlled, reducing the dose may be effective in maintaining control of the allergic rhinitis symptoms in patients who were initially controlled on higher doses.

An improvement in nasal symptoms may be noted in patients within 10 hours of first using RHINOCORT AQUA Nasal Spray. This time to onset is supported by an environmental exposure unit study in seasonal allergic rhinitis patients which demonstrated that RHINOCORT AQUA Nasal Spray led to a statistically significant improvement in nasal symptoms compared to placebo by 10 hours. Further support comes from a clinical study of patients with perennial allergic rhinitis which demonstrated a statistically significant improvement in nasal symptoms for both RHINOCORT AQUA Nasal Spray and for the active comparator (mometasone furoate) compared to placebo by 8 hours. Onset was also assessed in this study with peak nasal inspiratory flow rate and this endpoint failed to show efficacy for either active treatment. Although statistically significant improvements in nasal symptoms compared to placebo were noted within 8–10 hours in these studies, about one half to two thirds of the ultimate clinical improvement with RHINOCORT AQUA Nasal Spray occurs over the first 1–2 days, and maximum benefit may not be achieved until approximately 2 weeks after initiation of treatment. Initial assessment for response should be made during this time frame and periodically until the patient's symptoms are stabilized.

Directions for Use

Illustrated *Patient's Instructions for Use* accompany each package of RHINOCORT AQUA Nasal Spray 32 mcg.

HOW SUPPLIED

RHINOCORT AQUA Nasal Spray 32 mcg is available in a green coated glass bottle with a metered-dose pump spray and a green protection cap. RHINOCORT AQUA Nasal Spray 32 mcg provides 120 metered sprays after initial priming; net fill weight 8.6 g. The RHINOCORT AQUA Nasal Spray 32 mcg bottle has been filled with an excess to accommodate the priming activity. The bottle should be discarded after 120 sprays following initial priming, since the amount of budesonide delivered per spray thereafter may be substantially less than the labeled dose. Each spray delivers 32 mcg of budesonide to the patient.

NDC 0186-1070-08

RHINOCORT AQUA Nasal Spray

32 mcg, 120 metered sprays; net fill weight 8.6 g

Continued on next page

Rhinocort Aqua—Cont.

RHINOCORT AQUA Nasal Spray should be stored at controlled room temperature, 20 to 25°C (68 to 77°F) with the valve up. Do not freeze. Protect from light. **Shake gently before use.** Do not spray in eyes.

Distributed by:
AstraZeneca LP, Wilmington, DE 19850
Rev. 03/03 808201-05

Shown in Product Identification Guide, page 306

TOPROL-XL® ℞
[tō'prōl]
(metoprolol succinate)
EXTENDED-RELEASE TABLETS
Tablets: 25 MG, 50 MG, 100 MG, AND 200 MG

DESCRIPTION

TOPROL-XL, metoprolol succinate, is a $beta_1$-selective (cardioselective) adrenoceptor blocking agent, for oral administration, available as extended release tablets. TOPROL-XL has been formulated to provide a controlled and predictable release of metoprolol for once-daily administration. The tablets comprise a multiple unit system containing metoprolol succinate in a multitude of controlled release pellets. Each pellet acts as a separate drug delivery unit and is designed to deliver metoprolol continuously over the dosage interval. The tablets contain 23.75, 47.5, 95 and 190 mg of metoprolol succinate equivalent to 25, 50, 100 and 200 mg of metoprolol tartrate, USP, respectively. Its chemical name is (±)1-(isopropylamino)-3-[p-(2-methoxyethyl) phenoxy]-2-propanol succinate (2:1) (salt). Its structural formula is:

Metoprolol succinate is a white crystalline powder with a molecular weight of 652.8. It is freely soluble in water; soluble in methanol; sparingly soluble in ethanol; slightly soluble in dichloromethane and 2-propanol; practically insoluble in ethylacetate, acetone, diethylether and heptane. Inactive ingredients: silicon dioxide, cellulose compounds, sodium stearyl fumarate, polyethylene glycol, titanium dioxide, paraffin.

CLINICAL PHARMACOLOGY

General

Metoprolol is a $beta_1$-selective (cardioselective) adrenergic receptor blocking agent. This preferential effect is not absolute, however, and at higher plasma concentrations, metoprolol also inhibits $beta_2$-adrenoreceptors, chiefly located in the bronchial and vascular musculature. Metoprolol has no intrinsic sympathomimetic activity, and membrane-stabilizing activity is detectable only at plasma concentrations much greater than required for beta-blockade. Animal and human experiments indicate that metoprolol slows the sinus rate and decreases AV nodal conduction.

Clinical pharmacology studies have confirmed the beta-blocking activity of metoprolol in man, as shown by (1) reduction in heart rate and cardiac output at rest and upon exercise, (2) reduction of systolic blood pressure upon exercise, (3) inhibition of isoproterenol-induced tachycardia, and (4) reduction of reflex orthostatic tachycardia.

The relative $beta_1$-selectivity of metoprolol has been confirmed by the following: (1) In normal subjects, metoprolol is unable to reverse the $beta_2$-mediated vasodilating effects of epinephrine. This contrasts with the effect of nonselective beta-blockers, which completely reverse the vasodilating effects of epinephrine. (2) In asthmatic patients, metoprolol reduces FEV_1 and FVC significantly less than a nonselective beta-blocker, propranolol, at equivalent $beta_1$-receptor blocking doses.

In five controlled studies in normal healthy subjects, the same daily doses of TOPROL-XL and immediate release metoprolol were compared in terms of the extent and duration of $beta_1$-blockade produced. Both formulations were given in a dose range equivalent to 100–400 mg of immediate release metoprolol per day. In these studies, TOPROL-XL was administered once a day and immediate release metoprolol was administered once to four times a day. A sixth controlled study compared the $beta_1$-blocking effects of a 50 mg daily dose of the two formulations. In each study, $beta_1$-blockade was expressed as the percent change from baseline in exercise heart rate following standardized submaximal exercise tolerance tests at steady state. TOPROL-XL administered once a day, and immediate release metoprolol administered once to four times a day, provided comparable total $beta_1$-blockade over 24 hours (area under the $beta_1$-blockade versus time curve) in the dose range 100–400 mg. At a dosage of 50 mg once daily, TOPROL-XL produced significantly higher total $beta_1$-blockade over 24 hours than immediate release metoprolol. For TOPROL-XL, the percent reduction in exercise heart rate was relatively stable throughout the entire dosage interval and the level of $beta_1$-blockade increased with increasing doses from 50 to 300 mg daily. The effects at peak/trough (ie, at 24-hours post-dosing) were: 14/9, 16/10, 24/14, 27/22 and 27/20% reduction in exercise heart rate for doses of 50, 100, 200, 300 and 400 mg TOPROL-XL once a day, respectively. In contrast to TOPROL-XL, immediate release metoprolol given at a dose of 50–100 mg once a day produced a significantly larger peak effect on exercise tachycardia, but the effect was not evident at 24 hours. To match the peak to trough ratio obtained with TOPROL-XL over the dosing range of 200 to 400 mg, a t.i.d. to q.i.d. divided dosing regimen was required for immediate release metoprolol. A controlled cross-over study in heart failure patients compared the plasma concentrations and $beta_1$-blocking effects of 50 mg immediate release metoprolol administered t.i.d., 100 mg and 200 mg TOPROL-XL once daily. A 50 mg dose of immediate release metoprolol t.i.d. produced a peak plasma level of metoprolol similar to the peak level observed with 200 mg of TOPROL-XL. A 200 mg dose of TOPROL-XL produced a larger effect on suppression of exercise-induced and Holter-monitored heart rate over 24 hours compared to 50 mg t.i.d. of immediate release metoprolol.

The relationship between plasma metoprolol levels and reduction in exercise heart rate is independent of the pharmaceutical formulation. Using the E_{max} model, the maximal $beta_1$-blocking effect has been estimated to produce a 30% reduction in exercise heart rate. $Beta_1$-blocking effects in the range of 30–80% of the maximal effect (corresponding to approximately 8–23% reduction in exercise heart rate) are expected to occur at metoprolol plasma concentrations ranging from 30–540 nmol/L. The concentration-effect curve begins reaching a plateau between 200–300 nmol/L, and higher plasma levels produce little additional $beta_1$-blocking effect. The relative $beta_1$-selectivity of metoprolol diminishes and blockade of $beta_2$-adrenoceptors increases at higher plasma concentrations.

Although beta-adrenergic receptor blockade is useful in the treatment of angina, hypertension, and heart failure there are situations in which sympathetic stimulation is vital. In patients with severely damaged hearts, adequate ventricular function may depend on sympathetic drive. In the presence of AV block, beta-blockade may prevent the necessary facilitating effect of sympathetic activity on conduction. $Beta_2$-adrenergic blockade results in passive bronchial constriction by interfering with endogenous adrenergic bronchodilator activity in patients subject to bronchospasm and may also interfere with exogenous bronchodilators in such patients.

In other studies, treatment with TOPROL-XL produced an improvement in left ventricular ejection fraction. TOPROL-XL was also shown to delay the increase in left ventricular end-systolic and end-diastolic volumes after 6 months of treatment.

Hypertension

The mechanism of the antihypertensive effects of beta-blocking agents has not been elucidated. However, several possible mechanisms have been proposed: (1) competitive antagonism of catecholamines at peripheral (especially cardiac) adrenergic neuron sites, leading to decreased cardiac output; (2) a central effect leading to reduced sympathetic outflow to the periphery; and (3) suppression of renin activity.

Clinical Trials

In controlled clinical studies, an immediate release dosage form of metoprolol has been shown to be an effective antihypertensive agent when used alone or as concomitant therapy with thiazide-type diuretics at dosages of 100–450 mg daily. TOPROL-XL, in dosages of 100 to 400 mg once daily, has been shown to possess comparable β_1-blockade as conventional metoprolol tablets administered two to four times daily. In addition, TOPROL-XL administered at a dose of 50 mg once daily has been shown to lower blood pressure 24-hours post-dosing in placebo-controlled studies. In controlled, comparative, clinical studies, immediate release metoprolol appeared comparable as an antihypertensive agent to propranolol, methyldopa, and thiazide-type diuretics, and affected both supine and standing blood pressure. Because of variable plasma levels attained with a given dose and lack of a consistent relationship of antihypertensive activity to drug plasma concentration, selection of proper dosage requires individual titration.

Angina Pectoris

By blocking catecholamine-induced increases in heart rate, in velocity and extent of myocardial contraction, and in blood pressure, metoprolol reduces the oxygen requirements of the heart at any given level of effort, thus making it useful in the long-term management of angina pectoris.

Clinical Trials

In controlled clinical trials, an immediate release formulation of metoprolol has been shown to be an effective antianginal agent, reducing the number of angina attacks and increasing exercise tolerance. The dosage used in these studies ranged from 100 to 400 mg daily. TOPROL-XL, in dosages of 100 to 400 mg once daily, has been shown to possess beta-blockade similar to conventional metoprolol tablets administered two to four times daily.

Heart Failure

The precise mechanism for the beneficial effects of beta-blockers in heart failure has not been elucidated.

Clinical Trials

MERIT-HF was a double-blind, placebo-controlled study of TOPROL-XL conducted in 14 countries including the US. It randomized 3991 patients (1990 to TOPROL-XL) with ejection fraction ≤ 0.40 and NYHA Class II-IV heart failure attributable to ischemia, hypertension, or cardiomyopathy. The protocol excluded patients with contraindications to beta-blocker use, those expected to undergo heart surgery, and those within 28 days of myocardial infarction or unstable angina. The primary endpoints of the trial were (1) all-cause mortality plus all-cause hospitalization (time to first event) and (2) all-cause mortality. Patients were stabilized on optimal concomitant therapy for heart failure, including diuretics, ACE inhibitors, cardiac glycosides, and nitrates. At randomization, 41% of patients were NYHA Class II, 55% NYHA Class III; 65% of patients had heart failure attributed to ischemic heart disease; 44% had a history of hypertension; 25% had diabetes mellitus; 48% had a history of myocardial infarction. Among patients in the trial, 90% were on diuretics, 89% were on ACE inhibitors, 64% were on digitalis, 27% were on a lipid-lowering agent, 37% were on an oral anticoagulant, and the mean ejection fraction was 0.28. The mean duration of follow-up was one year. At the end of the study, the mean daily dose of TOPROL-XL was 159 mg.

Clinical Endpoints in the MERIT-HF Study

Clinical Endpoint	Number of Patients: Placebo n=2001	Number of Patients: TOPROL-XL n=1990	Relative Risk (95% CI)	Risk Reduction with TOPROL-XL	Nominal P-value
All-cause mortality plus all-cause hospitalization†	767	641	0.81 (0.73–0.90)	19%	0.00012
All-cause mortality	217	145	0.66 (0.53–0.81)	34%	0.00009
All-cause mortality plus heart failure hospitalization†	439	311	0.69 (0.60–0.80)	31%	0.0000008
Cardiovascular mortality	203	128	0.62 (0.50–0.78)	38%	0.000022
Sudden death	132	79	0.59 (0.45–0.78)	41%	0.0002
Death due to worsening heart failure	58	30	0.51 (0.33–0.79)	49%	0.0023
Hospitalizations due to worsening heart failure‡	451	317	N/A	N/A	0.0000076
Cardiovascular hospitalization‡	773	649	N/A	N/A	0.00028

† Time to first event
‡ Comparison of treatment groups examines the number of hospitalizations (Wilcoxon test); relative risk and risk reduction are not applicable.

The trial was terminated early for a statistically significant reduction in all-cause mortality (34%, nominal p=0.00009). The risk of all-cause mortality plus all-cause hospitalization was reduced by 19% (p=0.00012). The trial also showed improvements in heart failure-related mortality and heart failure-related hospitalizations, and NYHA functional class. The table below shows the principal results for the overall study population. The figure below illustrates principal results for a wide variety of subgroup comparisons, including US vs. non-US populations (the latter of which was not prespecified). The combined endpoints of all-cause mortality plus all-cause hospitalization and of mortality plus heart failure hospitalization showed consistent effects in the overall study population and the subgroups, including women and the US population. However, in the US subgroup (n=1071) and women (n=898), overall mortality and cardiovascular mortality appeared less affected. Analyses of female and US patients were carried out because they each represented about 25% of the overall population. Nonetheless, subgroup analyses can be difficult to interpret and it is not known whether these represent true differences or chance effects.

[See table at top of previous page]

[See figure above]

Pharmacokinetics

In man, absorption of metoprolol is rapid and complete. Plasma levels following oral administration of conventional metoprolol tablets, however, approximate 50% of levels following intravenous administration, indicating about 50% first-pass metabolism. Metoprolol crosses the blood-brain barrier and has been reported in the CSF in a concentration 78% of the simultaneous plasma concentration.

Plasma levels achieved are highly variable after oral administration. Only a small fraction of the drug (about 12%) is bound to human serum albumin. Metoprolol is a racemic mixture of R- and S-enantiomers, and is primarily metabolized by CYP2D6. When administered orally, it exhibits stereoselective metabolism that is dependent on oxidation phenotype. Elimination is mainly by biotransformation in the liver, and the plasma half-life ranges from approximately 3 to 7 hours. Less than 5% of an oral dose of metoprolol is recovered unchanged in the urine; the rest is excreted by the kidneys as metabolites that appear to have no beta-blocking activity. Following intravenous administration of metoprolol, the urinary recovery of unchanged drug is approximately 10%. The systemic availability and half-life of metoprolol in patients with renal failure do not differ to a clinically significant degree from those in normal subjects. Consequently, no reduction in dosage is usually needed in patients with chronic renal failure.

Metoprolol is metabolized predominantly by CYP2D6, an enzyme that is absent in about 8% of Caucasians (poor metabolizers) and about 2% of most other populations. CYP2D6 can be inhibited by a number of drugs. Concomitant use of inhibiting drugs in poor metabolizers will increase blood levels of metoprolol several-fold, decreasing metoprolol's cardioselectivity (see PRECAUTIONS, Drug Interactions).

In comparison to conventional metoprolol, the plasma metoprolol levels following administration of TOPROL-XL are characterized by lower peaks, longer time to peak and significantly lower peak to trough variation. The peak plasma levels following once-daily administration of TOPROL-XL average one-fourth to one-half the peak plasma levels obtained following a corresponding dose of conventional metoprolol, administered once daily or in divided doses. At steady state the average bioavailability of metoprolol following administration of TOPROL-XL, across the dosage range of 50 to 400 mg once daily, was 77% relative to the corresponding single or divided doses of conventional metoprolol. Nevertheless, over the 24-hour dosing interval, β_1-blockade is comparable and dose-related (see CLINICAL PHARMACOLOGY). The bioavailability of metoprolol shows a dose-related, although not directly proportional, increase with dose and is not significantly affected by food following TOPROL-XL administration.

INDICATIONS AND USAGE

Hypertension

TOPROL-XL is indicated for the treatment of hypertension. It may be used alone or in combination with other antihypertensive agents.

Angina Pectoris

TOPROL-XL is indicated in the long-term treatment of angina pectoris.

Heart Failure

TOPROL-XL is indicated for the treatment of stable, symptomatic (NYHA Class II or III) heart failure of ischemic, hypertensive, or cardiomyopathic origin. It was studied in patients already receiving ACE inhibitors, diuretics, and, in the majority of cases, digitalis. In this population,

TOPROL-XL decreased the rate of mortality plus hospitalization, largely through a reduction in cardiovascular mortality and hospitalizations for heart failure.

CONTRAINDICATIONS

TOPROL-XL is contraindicated in severe bradycardia, heart block greater than first degree, cardiogenic shock, decompensated cardiac failure, sick sinus syndrome (unless a permanent pacemaker is in place) (see WARNINGS) and in patients who are hypersensitive to any component of this product.

Results for Subgroups in MERIT-HF

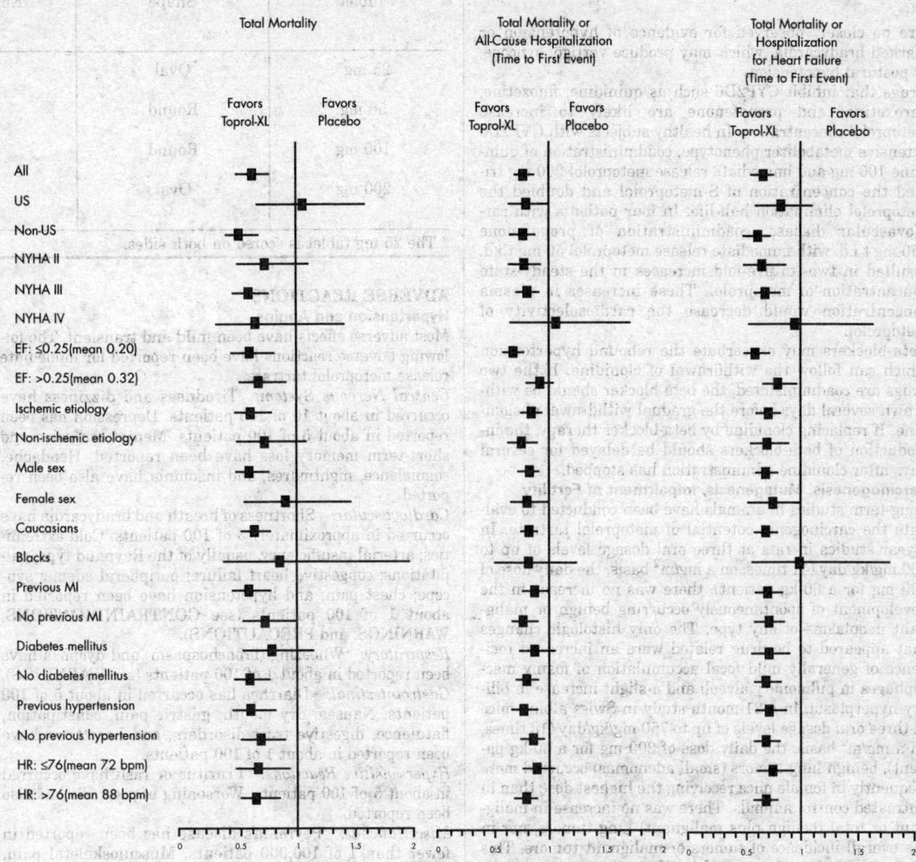

US = United States; NYHA = New York Heart Association; EF = ejection fraction; MI = myocardial infarction; HR = heart rate.

WARNINGS

Ischemic Heart Disease: Following abrupt cessation of therapy with certain beta-blocking agents, exacerbations of angina pectoris and, in some cases, myocardial infarction have occurred. When discontinuing chronically administered TOPROL-XL, particularly in patients with ischemic heart disease, the dosage should be gradually reduced over a period of 1–2 weeks and the patient should be carefully monitored. If angina markedly worsens or acute coronary insufficiency develops, TOPROL-XL administration should be reinstated promptly, at least temporarily, and other measures appropriate for the management of unstable angina should be taken. Patients should be warned against interruption or discontinuation of therapy without the physician's advice. Because coronary artery disease is common and may be unrecognized, it may be prudent not to discontinue TOPROL-XL therapy abruptly even in patients treated only for hypertension.

Bronchospastic Diseases: PATIENTS WITH BRONCHOSPASTIC DISEASES SHOULD, IN GENERAL, NOT RECEIVE BETA-BLOCKERS. Because of its relative $beta_1$-selectivity, however, TOPROL-XL may be used with caution in patients with bronchospastic disease who do not respond to, or cannot tolerate, other antihypertensive treatment. Since $beta_1$-selectivity is not absolute, a $beta_2$-stimulating agent should be administered concomitantly, and the lowest possible dose of TOPROL-XL should be used (see DOSAGE AND ADMINISTRATION).

Major Surgery: The necessity or desirability of withdrawing beta-blocking therapy prior to major surgery is controversial; the impaired ability of the heart to respond to reflex adrenergic stimuli may augment the risks of general anesthesia and surgical procedures.

TOPROL-XL, like other beta-blockers, is a competitive inhibitor of beta-receptor agonists, and its effects can be reversed by administration of such agents, eg, dobutamine or isoproterenol. However, such patients may be subject to protracted severe hypotension. Difficulty in restarting and maintaining the heart beat has also been reported with beta-blockers.

Diabetes and Hypoglycemia: TOPROL-XL should be used with caution in diabetic patients if a beta-blocking agent is required. Beta-blockers may mask tachycardia occurring with hypoglycemia, but other manifestations such as dizziness and sweating may not be significantly affected.

Thyrotoxicosis: Beta-adrenergic blockade may mask certain clinical signs (eg, tachycardia) of hyperthyroidism. Patients suspected of developing thyrotoxicosis should be managed carefully to avoid abrupt withdrawal of beta-blockade, which might precipitate a thyroid storm.

Peripheral Vascular Disease: Beta-blockers can precipitate or aggravate symptoms of arterial insufficiency in patients with peripheral vascular disease. Caution should be exercised in such individuals.

Calcium Channel Blockers: Because of significant inotropic and chronotropic effects in patients treated with beta-blockers and calcium channel blockers of the verapamil and diltiazem type, caution should be exercised in patients treated with these agents concomitantly.

PRECAUTIONS

General

TOPROL-XL should be used with caution in patients with impaired hepatic function. In patients with pheochromocytoma, an alpha-blocking agent should be initiated prior to the use of any beta-blocking agent.

Worsening cardiac failure may occur during up-titration of TOPROL-XL. If such symptoms occur, diuretics should be increased and the dose of TOPROL-XL should not be advanced until clinical stability is restored (see DOSAGE AND ADMINISTRATION). It may be necessary to lower the dose of TOPROL-XL or temporarily discontinue it. Such episodes do not preclude subsequent successful titration of TOPROL-XL.

Information for Patients

Patients should be advised to take TOPROL-XL regularly and continuously, as directed, preferably with or immediately following meals. If a dose should be missed, the patient should take only the next scheduled dose (without doubling it). Patients should not interrupt or discontinue TOPROL-XL without consulting the physician.

Patients should be advised (1) to avoid operating automobiles and machinery or engaging in other tasks requiring alertness until the patient's response to therapy with TOPROL-XL has been determined; (2) to contact the physician if any difficulty in breathing occurs; (3) to inform the physician or dentist before any type of surgery that he or she is taking TOPROL-XL.

Heart failure patients should be advised to consult their physician if they experience signs or symptoms of worsening heart failure such as weight gain or increasing shortness of breath.

Laboratory Tests

Clinical laboratory findings may include elevated levels of serum transaminase, alkaline phosphatase, and lactate dehydrogenase.

Drug Interactions

Catecholamine-depleting drugs (eg, reserpine, mono amine oxidase (MAO) inhibitors) may have an additive effect when given with beta-blocking agents. Patients treated with TOPROL-XL plus a catecholamine depletor should there-

Continued on next page

Toprol-XL—Cont.

fore be closely observed for evidence of hypotension or marked bradycardia, which may produce vertigo, syncope, or postural hypotension.

Drugs that inhibit CYP2D6 such as quinidine, fluoxetine, paroxetine, and propafenone are likely to increase metoprolol concentration. In healthy subjects with CYP2D6 extensive metabolizer phenotype, coadministration of quinidine 100 mg and immediate release metoprolol 200 mg tripled the concentration of S-metoprolol and doubled the metoprolol elimination half-life. In four patients with cardiovascular disease, coadministration of propafenone 150 mg t.i.d. with immediate release metoprolol 50 mg t.i.d. resulted in two- to five-fold increases in the steady-state concentration of metoprolol. These increases in plasma concentration would decrease the cardioselectivity of metoprolol.

Beta-blockers may exacerbate the rebound hypertension which can follow the withdrawal of clonidine. If the two drugs are coadministered, the beta blocker should be withdrawn several days before the gradual withdrawal of clonidine. If replacing clonidine by beta-blocker therapy, the introduction of beta-blockers should be delayed for several days after clonidine administration has stopped.

Carcinogenesis, Mutagenesis, Impairment of Fertility

Long-term studies in animals have been conducted to evaluate the carcinogenic potential of metoprolol tartrate. In 2-year studies in rats at three oral dosage levels of up to 800 mg/kg/day (41 times, on a mg/m^2 basis, the daily dose of 200 mg for a 60-kg patient), there was no increase in the development of spontaneously occurring benign or malignant neoplasms of any type. The only histologic changes that appeared to be drug related were an increased incidence of generally mild focal accumulation of foamy macrophages in pulmonary alveoli and a slight increase in biliary hyperplasia. In a 21-month study in Swiss albino mice at three oral dosage levels of up to 750 mg/kg/day (18 times, on a mg/m^2 basis, the daily dose of 200 mg for a 60-kg patient), benign lung tumors (small adenomas) occurred more frequently in female mice receiving the highest dose than in untreated control animals. There was no increase in malignant or total (benign plus malignant) lung tumors, nor in the overall incidence of tumors or malignant tumors. This 21-month study was repeated in CD-1 mice, and no statistically or biologically significant differences were observed between treated and control mice of either sex for any type of tumor.

All genotoxicity tests performed on metoprolol tartrate (a dominant lethal study in mice, chromosome studies in somatic cells, a *Salmonella*/mammalian-microsome mutagenicity test, and a nucleus anomaly test in somatic interphase nuclei) and metoprolol succinate (a *Salmonella*/mammalian-microsome mutagenicity test) were negative.

No evidence of impaired fertility due to metoprolol tartrate was observed in a study performed in rats at doses up to 22 times, on a mg/m^2 basis, the daily dose of 200 mg in a 60-kg patient.

Pregnancy Category C

Metoprolol tartrate has been shown to increase post-implantation loss and decrease neonatal survival in rats at doses up to 22 times, on a mg/m^2 basis, the daily dose of 200 mg in a 60-kg patient. Distribution studies in mice confirm exposure of the fetus when metoprolol tartrate is administered to the pregnant animal. These studies have revealed no evidence of impaired fertility or teratogenicity. There are no adequate and well-controlled studies in pregnant women. Because animal reproduction studies are not always predictive of human response, this drug should be used during pregnancy only if clearly needed.

Nursing Mothers

Metoprolol is excreted in breast milk in very small quantities. An infant consuming 1 liter of breast milk daily would receive a dose of less than 1 mg of the drug. Caution should be exercised when TOPROL-XL is administered to a nursing woman.

Pediatric Use

Safety and effectiveness in pediatric patients have not been established.

Geriatric Use

Clinical studies of TOPROL-XL in hypertension did not include sufficient numbers of subjects aged 65 and over to determine whether they respond differently from younger subjects. Other reported clinical experience in hypertensive patients has not identified differences in responses between elderly and younger patients.

Of the 1,990 patients with heart failure randomized to TOPROL-XL in the MERIT-HF trial, 50% (990) were 65 years of age and older and 12% (238) were 75 years of age and older. There were no notable differences in efficacy or the rate of adverse events between older and younger patients.

In general, dose selection for an elderly patient should be cautious, usually starting at the low end of the dosing range, reflecting greater frequency of decreased hepatic, renal, or cardiac function, and of concomitant disease or other drug therapy.

Risk of Anaphylactic Reactions

While taking beta-blockers, patients with a history of severe anaphylactic reactions to a variety of allergens may be more reactive to repeated challenge, either accidental, diagnostic, or therapeutic. Such patients may be unresponsive to the usual doses of epinephrine used to treat allergic reaction.

Tablet	Shape	Engraving	Bottle of 100 NDC 0186-	Unit Dose Packages of 100 NDC 0186-
25 mg*	Oval	A β	1088-05	1088-39
50 mg	Round	A mo	1090-05	1090-39
100 mg	Round	A ms	1092-05	1092-39
200 mg	Oval	A my	1094-05	N/A

* The 25 mg tablet is scored on both sides.

ADVERSE REACTIONS

Hypertension and Angina

Most adverse effects have been mild and transient. The following adverse reactions have been reported for immediate release metoprolol tartrate.

Central Nervous System: Tiredness and dizziness have occurred in about 10 of 100 patients. Depression has been reported in about 5 of 100 patients. Mental confusion and short-term memory loss have been reported. Headache, somnolence, nightmares, and insomnia have also been reported.

Cardiovascular: Shortness of breath and bradycardia have occurred in approximately 3 of 100 patients. Cold extremities; arterial insufficiency, usually of the Raynaud type; palpitations; congestive heart failure; peripheral edema; syncope; chest pain; and hypotension have been reported in about 1 of 100 patients (see CONTRAINDICATIONS, WARNINGS, and PRECAUTIONS).

Respiratory: Wheezing (bronchospasm) and dyspnea have been reported in about 1 of 100 patients (see WARNINGS).

Gastrointestinal: Diarrhea has occurred in about 5 of 100 patients. Nausea, dry mouth, gastric pain, constipation, flatulence, digestive tract disorders, and heartburn have been reported in about 1 of 100 patients.

Hypersensitive Reactions: Pruritus or rash have occurred in about 5 of 100 patients. Worsening of psoriasis has also been reported.

Miscellaneous: Peyronie's disease has been reported in fewer than 1 of 100,000 patients. Musculoskeletal pain, blurred vision, decreased libido, and tinnitus have also been reported.

There have been rare reports of reversible alopecia, agranulocytosis, and dry eyes. Discontinuation of the drug should be considered if any such reaction is not otherwise explicable. The oculomucocutaneous syndrome associated with the beta-blocker practolol has not been reported with metoprolol.

Potential Adverse Reactions

A variety of adverse reactions not listed above have been reported with other beta-adrenergic blocking agents and should be considered potential adverse reactions to TOPROL-XL.

Central Nervous System: Reversible mental depression progressing to catatonia; an acute reversible syndrome characterized by disorientation for time and place, short-term memory loss, emotional lability, slightly clouded sensorium, and decreased performance on neuropsychometrics.

Cardiovascular: Intensification of AV block (see CONTRAINDICATIONS).

Hematologic: Agranulocytosis, nonthrombocytopenic purpura, thrombocytopenic purpura.

Hypersensitive Reactions: Fever combined with aching and sore throat, laryngospasm, and respiratory distress.

Heart Failure

In the MERIT-HF study, serious adverse events and adverse events leading to discontinuation of study medication were systematically collected. In the MERIT-HF study comparing TOPROL-XL in daily doses up to 200 mg (mean dose 159 mg once-daily) (n=1990) to placebo (n=2001), 10.3% of TOPROL-XL patients discontinued for adverse events vs. 12.2% of placebo patients.

The table below lists adverse events in the MERIT-HF study that occurred at an incidence of equal to or greater than 1% in the TOPROL-XL group and greater than placebo by more than 0.5%, regardless of the assessment of causality.

Adverse Events Occurring in the MERIT-HF Study at an Incidence ≥ 1% in the TOPROL-XL Group and Greater Than Placebo by More Than 0.5%

	TOPROL-XL N=1990 % of patients	Placebo N=2001 % of patients
Dizziness/vertigo	1.8	1.0
Bradycardia	1.5	0.4
Accident and/or injury	1.4	0.8

Other adverse events with an incidence of > 1% on TOPROL-XL and as common on placebo (within 0.5%) included myocardial infarction, pneumonia, cerebrovascular disorder, chest pain, dyspnea/dyspnea aggravated, syncope, coronary artery disorder, ventricular tachycardia/arrhythmia aggravated, hypotension, diabetes mellitus/diabetes mellitus aggravated, abdominal pain, and fatigue.

Post-Marketing Experience

The following adverse reactions have been reported with TOPROL-XL in worldwide post-marketing use, regardless of causality:

Cardiovascular: 2nd and 3rd degree heart block.

Gastrointestinal: hepatitis, vomiting.

Hematologic: thrombocytopenia.

Musculoskeletal: arthralgia.

Nervous System/Psychiatric: anxiety/nervousness, hallucinations, paresthesia.

Reproductive, male: impotence.

Skin: increased sweating, photosensitivity.

Special Sense Organs: taste disturbances.

OVERDOSAGE

Acute Toxicity

There have been a few reports of overdosage with TOPROL-XL and no specific overdosage information was obtained with this drug, with the exception of animal toxicology data. However, since TOPROL-XL (metoprolol succinate salt) contains the same active moiety, metoprolol, as conventional metoprolol tablets (metoprolol tartrate salt), the recommendations on overdosage for metoprolol conventional tablets are applicable to TOPROL-XL.

Signs and Symptoms

Overdosage of TOPROL-XL may lead to severe hypotension, sinus bradycardia, atrioventricular block, heart failure, cardiogenic shock, cardiac arrest, bronchospasm, impairment of consciousness/coma, nausea, vomiting, and cyanosis.

Treatment

In general, patients with acute or recent myocardial infarction or congestive heart failure may be more hemodynamically unstable than other patients and should be treated accordingly. When possible the patient should be treated under intensive care conditions. On the basis of the pharmacologic actions of metoprolol, the following general measures should be employed:

Elimination of the Drug: Gastric lavage should be performed.

Bradycardia: Atropine should be administered. If there is no response to vagal blockade, isoproterenol should be administered cautiously.

Hypotension: A vasopressor should be administered, eg, levarterenol or dopamine.

Bronchospasm: A beta$_2$-stimulating agent and/or a theophylline derivative should be administered.

Cardiac Failure: A digitalis glycoside and diuretics should be administered. In shock resulting from inadequate cardiac contractility, administration of dobutamine, isoproterenol, or glucagon may be considered.

DOSAGE AND ADMINISTRATION

TOPROL-XL is an extended release tablet intended for once-a-day administration. When switching from immediate release metoprolol tablet to TOPROL-XL, the same total daily dose of TOPROL-XL should be used.

As with immediate release metoprolol, dosages of TOPROL-XL should be individualized and titration may be needed in some patients.

TOPROL-XL tablets are scored and can be divided; however, the whole or half tablet should be swallowed whole and not chewed or crushed.

Hypertension

The usual initial dosage is 50 to 100 mg daily in a single dose, whether used alone or added to a diuretic. The dosage may be increased at weekly (or longer) intervals until optimum blood pressure reduction is achieved. In general, the maximum effect of any given dosage level will be apparent after 1 week of therapy. Dosages above 400 mg per day have not been studied.

Angina Pectoris

The dosage of TOPROL-XL should be individualized. The usual initial dosage is 100 mg daily, given in a single dose. The dosage may be gradually increased at weekly intervals until optimum clinical response has been obtained or there is a pronounced slowing of the heart rate. Dosages above 400 mg per day have not been studied. If treatment is to be discontinued, the dosage should be reduced gradually over a period of 1–2 weeks (see WARNINGS).

Heart Failure

Dosage must be individualized and closely monitored during up-titration. Prior to initiation of TOPROL-XL, the dosing of diuretics, ACE inhibitors, and digitalis (if used) should be stabilized. The recommended starting dose of TOPROL-XL is 25 mg once daily for two weeks in patients with NYHA Class II heart failure and 12.5 mg once daily in patients with more severe heart failure. The dose should then be doubled every two weeks to the highest dosage level tolerated by the patient or up to 200 mg of TOPROL-XL. If transient worsening of heart failure occurs, it may be treated with increased doses of diuretics, and it may also be necessary to lower the dose of TOPROL-XL or temporarily discontinue it. The dose of TOPROL-XL should not be increased until symptoms of worsening heart failure have been stabilized. Initial difficulty with titration should not preclude later attempts to introduce TOPROL-XL. If heart failure patients experience symptomatic bradycardia, the dose of TOPROL-XL should be reduced.

HOW SUPPLIED

Tablets containing metoprolol succinate equivalent to the indicated weight of metoprolol tartrate, USP, are white, biconvex, film-coated, and scored.

[See table at top of previous page]

Store at 25°C (77°F). Excursions permitted to 15–30°C (59–86°F). (See USP Controlled Room Temperature.)

Manufactured for: AstraZeneca LP
Wilmington, DE 19850
By: AstraZeneca AB
S-151 85 Södertälje, Sweden
Made in Sweden
64200-00
Rev. 11/02

Shown in Product Identification Guide, page 306

XYLOCAINE® 2% JELLY ℞
[*zī'lō-kān*]
(lidocaine hydrochloride)

AstraZeneca Pharmaceuticals LP

1800 CONCORD PIKE
WILMINGTON, DE 19850-5437 USA

For Product Full Prescribing Information, Business Information, Medical Information, Adverse Drug Experiences, and Customer Service:

Information Center
1-800-236-9933

For Product Ordering:

Trade Customer Service
1-800-842-9920

For Product Full Prescribing Information:

Internet: www.astrazeneca-us.com

ACCOLATE® ℞
(zafirlukast)
Tablets
[*ac-cō 'late*]

DESCRIPTION

Zafirlukast is a synthetic, selective peptide leukotriene receptor antagonist (LTRA), with the chemical name 4-(5-cyclopentyloxy-carbonylamino-1-methyl-indol-3-ylmethyl)-3-methoxy-N-o-tolylsulfonylbenzamide. The molecular weight of zafirlukast is 575.7 and the structural formula is:

The empirical formula is: $C_{31}H_{33}N_3O_6S$

Zafirlukast, a fine white to pale yellow amorphous powder, is practically insoluble in water. It is slightly soluble in methanol and freely soluble in tetrahydrofuran, dimethylsulfoxide, and acetone.

ACCOLATE is supplied as 10 and 20 mg tablets for oral administration.

Inactive Ingredients: Film-coated tablets containing croscarmellose sodium, lactose, magnesium stearate, microcrystalline cellulose, povidone, hypromellose, and titanium dioxide.

CLINICAL PHARMACOLOGY

Mechanism of Action

Zafirlukast is a selective and competitive receptor antagonist of leukotriene D_4 and E_4 (LTD_4 and LTE_4), components of slow-reacting substance of anaphylaxis (SRSA). Cysteinyl leukotriene production and receptor occupation have been correlated with the pathophysiology of asthma, including airway edema, smooth muscle constriction, and altered cellular activity associated with the inflammatory process, which contribute to the signs and symptoms of asthma. Patients with asthma were found in one study to be 25–100 times more sensitive to the bronchoconstricting activity of inhaled LTD_4 than nonasthmatic subjects.

In vitro studies demonstrated that zafirlukast antagonized the contractile activity of three leukotrienes (LTC_4, LTD_4 and LTE_4) in conducting airway smooth muscle from laboratory animals and humans. Zafirlukast prevented intradermal LTD_4-induced increases in cutaneous vascular permeability and inhibited inhaled LTD_4-induced influx of eosinophils into animal lungs. Inhalational challenge studies in sensitized sheep showed that zafirlukast suppressed the airway responses to antigen; this included both the early- and late-phase response and the nonspecific hyperresponsiveness.

In humans, zafirlukast inhibited bronchoconstriction caused by several kinds of inhalational challenges. Pretreatment with single oral doses of zafirlukast inhibited the bronchoconstriction caused by sulfur dioxide and cold air in patients with asthma. Pretreatment with single doses of zafirlukast attenuated the early- and late-phase reaction caused by inhalation of various antigens such as grass, cat dander, ragweed, and mixed antigens in patients with asthma. Zafirlukast also attenuated the increase in bronchial hyperresponsiveness to inhaled histamine that followed inhaled allergen challenge.

Clinical Pharmacokinetics and Bioavailability:

Absorption

Zafirlukast is rapidly absorbed following oral administration. Peak plasma concentrations are generally achieved 3 hours after oral administration. The absolute bioavailability of zafirlukast is unknown. In two separate studies, one using a high fat and the other a high protein meal, administration of zafirlukast with food reduced the mean bioavailability by approximately 40%.

Distribution

Zafirlukast is more than 99% bound to plasma proteins, predominantly albumin. The degree of binding was independent of concentration in the clinically relevant range. The apparent steady-state volume of distribution (V_{SS}/F) is approximately 70 L, suggesting moderate distribution into tissues. Studies in rats using radiolabeled zafirlukast indicate minimal distribution across the blood-brain barrier.

Metabolism

Zafirlukast is extensively metabolized. The most common metabolic products are hydroxylated metabolites which are excreted in the feces. The metabolites of zafirlukast identified in plasma are at least 90 times less potent as LTD_4 receptor antagonists than zafirlukast in a standard *in vitro* test of activity. *In vitro* studies using human liver microsomes showed that the hydroxylated metabolites of zafirlukast excreted in the feces are formed through the cytochrome P450 2C9 (CYP2C9) pathway. Additional *in vitro* studies utilizing human liver microsomes show that zafirlukast inhibits the cytochrome P450 CYP3A4 and CYP2C9 isoenzymes at concentrations close to the clinically achieved total plasma concentrations (see Drug Interactions).

Excretion

The apparent oral clearance (CL/f) of zafirlukast is approximately 20 L/h. Studies in the rat and dog suggest that biliary excretion is the primary route of excretion. Following oral administration of radiolabeled zafirlukast to volunteers, urinary excretion accounts for approximately 10% of the dose and the remainder is excreted in feces. Zafirlukast is not detected in urine.

In the pivotal bioequivalence study, the mean terminal half-life of zafirlukast is approximately 10 hours in both normal adult subjects and patients with asthma. In other studies, the mean plasma half-life of zafirlukast ranged from approximately 8 to 16 hours in both normal subjects and patients with asthma. The pharmacokinetics of zafirlukast are approximately linear over the range from 5 mg to 80 mg. Steady-state plasma concentrations of zafirlukast are proportional to the dose and predictable from single-dose pharmacokinetic data. Accumulation of zafirlukast in the plasma following twice-daily dosing is approximately 45%.

The pharmacokinetic parameters of zafirlukast 20 mg administered as a single dose to 36 male volunteers are shown with the table below.

Mean (% Coefficient of Variation) pharmacokinetic parameters of zafirlukast following single 20 mg oral dose administration to male volunteers (n=36)

C_{max} ng/mL	t_{max} h	AUC ng·h/mL	$t_{1/2}$ h	CL/f L/h
326 (31.0)	2 (0.5–5.0)	1137 (34)	13.3 (75.6)	19.4 (32)

[1]Median and range

Special Populations

Gender: The pharmacokinetics of zafirlukast are similar in males and females. Weight-adjusted apparent oral clearance does not differ due to gender.

Race: No differences in the pharmacokinetics of zafirlukast due to race have been observed.

Elderly: The apparent oral clearance of zafirlukast decreases with age. In patients above 65 years of age, there is an approximately 2–3 fold greater C_{max} and AUC compared to young adult patients.

Children: Following administration of a single 20 mg dose of zafirlukast to 20 boys and girls between 7 and 11 years of age, and in a second study, to 29 boys and girls between 5 and 6 years of age, the following pharmacokinetic parameters were obtained:

Parameter	Children age 5–6 years Mean (% Coefficient of Variation)	Children age 7–11 years Mean (% Coefficient of Variation)
C_{max} (ng/mL)	756 (39%)	601 (45%)
AUC (ng•h/mL)	2458 (34%)	2027 (38%)
t_{max} (h)	2.1 (61%)	2.5 (55%)
CL/f (L/h)	9.2 (37%)	11.4 (42%)

Weight unadjusted apparent clearance was 11.4 L/h (42%) in the 7–11 year old children and 9.2 L/h (37%) in the 5–6 year old children, which resulted in greater systemic drug exposures than that obtained in adults for an identical dose. To maintain similar exposure levels in children compared to adults, a dose of 10 mg twice daily is recommended in children 5–11 years of age (see DOSAGE AND ADMINISTRATION).

Zafirlukast disposition was unchanged after multiple dosing (20 mg twice daily) in children and the degree of accumulation in plasma was similar to that observed in adults.

Hepatic Insufficiency: In a study of patients with hepatic impairment (biopsy-proven cirrhosis), there was a reduced clearance of zafirlukast resulting in a 50–60% greater C_{max} and AUC compared to normal subjects.

Renal Insufficiency: Based on a cross-study comparison, there are no apparent differences in the pharmacokinetics of zafirlukast between renally-impaired patients and normal subjects.

Drug-Drug Interactions

The following drug interaction studies have been conducted with zafirlukast (see PRECAUTIONS, Drug Interactions).

- Coadministration of multiple doses of zafirlukast (160 mg/day) to steady-state with a single 25 mg dose of warfarin (a substrate of CYP2C9) resulted in a significant increase in the mean AUC (+63%) and half-life (+36%) of S-warfarin. The mean prothrombin time increased by approximately 35%. The pharmacokinetics of zafirlukast were unaffected by coadministration with warfarin.
- Coadministration of zafirlukast (80 mg/day) at steady-state with a single dose of a liquid theophylline preparation (6 mg/kg) in 13 asthmatic patients, 18 to 44 years of age, resulted in decreased mean plasma concentrations of zafirlukast by approximately 30%, but no effect on plasma theophylline concentrations was observed.
- Coadministration of zafirlukast (20 mg/day) or placebo at steady-state with a single dose of sustained release theophylline preparation (16 mg/kg) in 16 healthy boys and girls (6 through 11 years of age) resulted in no significant differences in the pharmacokinetic parameters of theophylline.
- Coadministration of zafirlukast dosed at 40 mg twice daily in a single-blind, parallel-group, 3-week study in 39 healthy female subjects taking oral contraceptives, resulted in no significant effect on ethinyl estradiol plasma concentrations or contraceptive efficacy.
- Coadministration of zafirlukast (40 mg/day) with aspirin (650 mg four times daily) resulted in mean increased plasma concentrations of zafirlukast by approximately 45%.
- Coadministration of a single dose of zafirlukast (40 mg) with erythromycin (500 mg three times daily for 5 days) to steady-state in 11 asthmatic patients resulted in decreased mean plasma concentrations of zafirlukast by approximately 40% due to a decrease in zafirlukast bioavailability.

Clinical Studies

Three U.S. double-blind, randomized, placebo-controlled, 13-week clinical trials in 1380 adults and children 12 years of age and older with mild-to-moderate asthma demonstrated that ACCOLATE improved daytime asthma symptoms, nighttime awakenings, mornings with asthma symptoms, rescue beta$_2$-agonist use, FEV_1, and morning peak expiratory flow rate. In these studies, the patients had a mean baseline FEV_1 of approximately 75% of predicted normal and a mean baseline beta$_2$-agonist requirement of approximately 4–5 puffs of albuterol per day. The results of the largest of the trials are shown in the table below.

Mean Change from Baseline at Study End Point

	ACCOLATE 20 mg twice daily N=514	Placebo N=248
Daytime Asthma symptom score (0–3 scale)	−0.44*	−0.25
Nighttime Awakenings (number per week)	−1.27*	−0.43
Mornings with Asthma Symptoms (days per week)	1.32*	0.75
Rescue β_2-agonist use (puffs per day)	−1.15*	−0.24
FEV_1 (L)	+0.15*	+0.05
Morning PEFR (L/min)	+22.06*	+7.63
Evening PEFR (L/min)	+13.12	+10.14

*p<0.05, compared to placebo

In a second and smaller study, the effect of ACCOLATE on most efficacy parameters was comparable to the active control (inhaled cromolyn sodium 1600 mcg four times per day)

Continued on next page

Accolate—Cont.

and superior to placebo at end point for decreasing rescue beta$_2$-agonist use (figure below).

Mean ß2-agonist use (puffs/day)

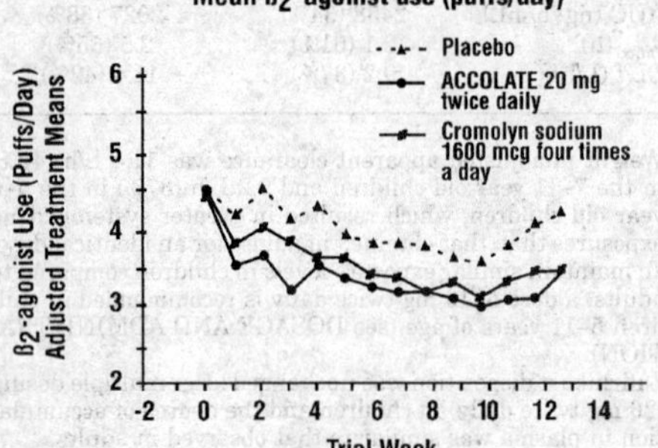

In these trials, improvement in asthma symptoms occurred within one week of initiating treatment with ACCOLATE. The role of ACCOLATE in the management of patients with more severe asthma, patients receiving antiasthma therapy other than as-needed, inhaled beta$_2$-agonists, or as an oral or inhaled corticosteroid-sparing agent remains to be fully characterized.

INDICATIONS AND USAGE

ACCOLATE is indicated for the prophylaxis and chronic treatment of asthma in adults and children 5 years of age and older.

CONTRAINDICATIONS

ACCOLATE is contraindicated in patients who are hypersensitive to zafirlukast or any of its inactive ingredients.

WARNINGS

Hepatotoxicity:

Cases of life-threatening hepatic failure have been reported in patients treated with ACCOLATE. Cases of liver injury without other attributable cause have been reported from post-marketing adverse event surveillance of patients who have received the recommended dose of ACCOLATE (40 mg/day). In most, but not all post-marketing reports, the patient's symptoms abated and the liver enzymes returned to normal or near normal after stopping ACCOLATE. In rare cases, patients have either presented with fulminant hepatitis or progressed to hepatic failure, liver transplantation and death.

Physicians may consider the value of liver function testing. Periodic serum transaminase testing has not proven to prevent serious injury but it is generally believed that early detection of drug-induced hepatic injury along with immediate withdrawal of the suspect drug enhances the likelihood for recovery.

Patients should be advised to be alert for signs and symptoms of liver dysfunction (eg, right upper quadrant abdominal pain, nausea, fatigue, lethargy, pruritus, jaundice, flu-like symptoms, and anorexia)) and to contact their physician immediately if they occur. Ongoing clinical assessment of patients should govern physician interventions, including diagnostic evaluations and treatment.

If liver dysfunction is suspected based upon clinical signs or symptoms (eg, right upper quadrant abdominal pain, nausea, fatigue, lethargy, pruritus, jaundice, flu-like symptoms, anorexia, and enlarged liver), ACCOLATE should be discontinued. Liver function tests, in particular serum ALT, should be measured immediately and the patient managed accordingly. If liver function tests are consistent with hepatic dysfunction. ACCOLATE therapy should not be resumed. Patients in whom ACCOLATE was withdrawn because of hepatic dysfunction where no other attributable cause is identified should not be re-exposed to ACCOLATE (see PRECAUTIONS, Information for Patients and ADVERSE REACTIONS).

Bronchospasm:

ACCOLATE is not indicated for use in the reversal of bronchospasm in acute asthma attacks, including status asthmaticus. Therapy with ACCOLATE can be continued during acute exacerbations of asthma.

Concomitant Warfarin Administration:

Coadministration of zafirlukast with warfarin results in a clinically significant increase in prothrombin time (PT). Patients on oral warfarin anticoagulant therapy and ACCOLATE should have their prothrombin times monitored closely and anticoagulant dose adjusted accordingly (see PRECAUTIONS, Drug Interactions).

PRECAUTIONS

Information for Patients

Patients should be told that a rare side effect of ACCOLATE is hepatic dysfunction, and to contact their physician immediately if they experience symptoms of hepatic dysfunction (eg, right upper quadrant abdominal pain, nausea, fatigue, lethargy, pruritus, jaundice, flu-like symptoms, and anorexia).

ACCOLATE is indicated for the chronic treatment of asthma and should be taken regularly as prescribed, even during symptom-free periods. ACCOLATE is not a bronchodilator and should not be used to treat acute episodes of asthma. Patients receiving ACCOLATE should be instructed not to decrease the dose or stop taking any other antiasthma medications unless instructed by a physician. Women who are breast-feeding should be instructed not to take ACCOLATE (see PRECAUTIONS, Nursing Mothers). Alternative antiasthma medication should be considered in such patients.

The bioavailability of ACCOLATE may be decreased when taken with food. Patients should be instructed to take ACCOLATE at least 1 hour before or 2 hours after meals.

Eosinophilic Conditions

In rare cases, patients on ACCOLATE therapy may present with systemic eosinophilia, eosinophilic pneumonia, or clinical features of vasculitis consistent with Churg-Strauss syndrome, a condition which is often treated with systemic steroid therapy. These events usually, but not always, have been associated with the reduction of oral steroid therapy. Physicians should be alert to eosinophilia, vasculitic rash, worsening pulmonary symptoms, cardiac complications, and/or neuropathy presenting in their patients. A causal association between ACCOLATE and these underlying conditions has not been established (see ADVERSE REACTIONS).

Drug Interactions

In a drug interaction study in 16 healthy male volunteers, coadministration of multiple doses of zafirlukast (160 mg/day) to steady-state with a single 25 mg dose of warfarin resulted in a significant increase in the mean AUC (+63%) and half-life (+36%) of S-warfarin. The mean prothrombin time (PT) increased by approximately 35%. This interaction is probably due to an inhibition by zafirlukast of the cytochrome P450 2C9 isoenzyme system. Patients on oral warfarin anticoagulant therapy and ACCOLATE should have their prothrombin times monitored closely and anticoagulant dose adjusted accordingly (see WARNINGS, Concomitant Warfarin Administration). No formal drug-drug interaction studies with ACCOLATE and other drugs known to be metabolized by the cytochrome P450 2C9 isoenzyme (eg, tolbutamide, phenytoin, carbamazepine) have been conducted; however, care should be exercised when ACCOLATE is coadministered with these drugs.

In a drug interaction study in 11 asthmatic patients, coadministration of a single dose of zafirlukast (40 mg) with erythromycin (500 mg three times daily for 5 days) to steady-state resulted in decreased mean plasma levels of zafirlukast by approximately 40% due to a decrease in zafirlukast bioavailability.

Coadministration of zafirlukast (20 mg/day) or placebo at steady-state with a single dose of sustained release theophylline preparation (16 mg/kg) in 16 healthy boys and girls (6 through 11 years of age) resulted in no significant differences in the pharmacokinetic parameters of theophylline.

Coadministration of zafirlukast (80 mg/day) at steady-state with a single dose of a liquid theophylline preparation (6 mg/kg) in 13 asthmatic patients, 18 to 44 years of age, resulted in decreased mean plasma levels of zafirlukast by approximately 30%, but no effect on plasma theophylline levels was observed.

Rare cases of patients experiencing increased theophylline levels with or without clinical signs or symptoms of theophylline toxicity after the addition of ACCOLATE to an existing theophylline regimen have been reported. The mechanism of the interaction between ACCOLATE and theophylline in these patients is unknown (see ADVERSE REACTIONS).

Coadministration of zafirlukast (40 mg/day) with aspirin (650 mg four times daily) resulted in mean increased plasma levels of zafirlukast by approximately 45%.

In a single-blind, parallel-group, 3-week study in 39 healthy female subjects taking oral contraceptives, 40 mg twice daily of zafirlukast had no significant effect on ethinyl estradiol plasma concentrations or contraceptive efficacy.

No formal drug-drug interaction studies between ACCOLATE and marketed drugs known to be metabolized by the P450 3A4 (CYP3A4) isoenzyme (eg, dihydropyridine calcium-channel blockers, cyclosporin, cisapride) have been conducted. As ACCOLATE is known to be an inhibitor of CYP3A4 *in vitro*, it is reasonable to employ appropriate clinical monitoring when these drugs are coadministered with ACCOLATE.

Carcinogenesis, Mutagenesis, Impairment of Fertility

In two-year carcinogenicity studies, zafirlukast was administered at dietary doses of 10, 100, and 300 mg/kg to mice and 40, 400, and 2000 mg/kg to rats. Male mice at an oral dose of 300 mg/kg/day (approximately 30 times the maximum recommended daily oral dose in adults and in children on a mg/m^2 basis) showed an increased incidence of hepatocellular adenomas; female mice at this dose showed a greater incidence of whole body histocytic sarcomas. Male and female rats at an oral dose of 2000 mg/kg/day (resulting in approximately 160 times the exposure to drug plus metabolites from the maximum recommended daily oral dose in adults and in children based on a comparison of the plasma area-under the curve [AUC] values) of zafirlukast showed an increased incidence of urinary bladder transitional cell papillomas. Zafirlukast was not tumorigenic at oral doses up to 100 mg/kg (approximately 10 times the maximum recommended daily oral dose in adults and in children on a mg/m^2 basis) in mice and at oral doses up to 400 mg/kg (resulting in approximately 140 times the exposure to drug plus metabolites from the maximum recommended daily oral dose in adults and in children based on a comparison of the plasma AUC values) in rats. The clinical significance of these findings for the long-term use of ACCOLATE is unknown.

Zafirlukast showed no evidence of mutagenic potential in the reverse microbial assay, in 2 forward point mutation (CHO-HGPRT and mouse lymphoma) assays or in two assays for chromosomal aberrations (the *in vitro* human peripheral blood lymphocyte clastogenic assay and the *in vivo* rat bone marrow micronucleus assay).

No evidence of impairment of fertility and reproduction was seen in male and female rats treated with zafirlukast at oral doses up to 2000 mg/kg (approximately 410 times the maximum recommended daily oral dose in adults on a mg/m^2 basis).

Pregnancy Category B

No teratogenicity was observed at oral doses up to 1600 mg/kg/day in mice (approximately 160 times the maximum recommended daily oral dose in adults on a mg/m^2 basis), up to 2000 mg/kg/day in rats (approximately 410 times the maximum recommended daily oral dose in adults on a mg/m^2 basis) and up to 2000 mg/kg/day in cynomolgus monkeys (which resulted in approximately 20 times the exposure to drug plus metabolites compared to that from the maximum recommended daily oral dose in adults based on comparison of the AUC values). At an oral dose of 2000 mg/kg/day in rats, maternal toxicity and deaths were seen with increased incidence of early fetal resorption. Spontaneous abortions occurred in cynomolgus monkeys at the maternally toxic oral dose of 2000 mg/kg/day. There are no adequate and well-controlled trials in pregnant women. Because animal reproductive studies are not always predictive of human response, ACCOLATE should be used during pregnancy only if clearly needed.

Nursing Mothers

Zafirlukast is excreted in breast milk. Following repeated 40 mg twice-a-day dosing in healthy women, average steady-state concentrations of zafirlukast in breast milk were 50 ng/mL compared to 255 ng/mL in plasma. Because of the potential for tumorigenicity shown for zafirlukast in mouse and rat studies and the enhanced sensitivity of neonatal rats and dogs to the adverse effects of zafirlukast, ACCOLATE should not be administered to mothers who are breast-feeding.

Pediatric Use

The safety of ACCOLATE at doses of 10 mg twice daily has been demonstrated in 205 pediatric patients 5 through 11 years of age in placebo-controlled trials lasting up to six weeks and with 179 patients in this age range participating in 52 weeks of treatment in an open label extension.

The effectiveness of ACCOLATE for the prophylaxis and chronic treatment of asthma in pediatric patients 5 through 11 years of age is based on an extrapolation of the demonstrated efficacy of ACCOLATE in adults with asthma and the likelihood that the disease course, and pathophysiology and the drug's effect are substantially similar between the two populations. The recommended dose for the patients 5 through 11 years of age is based upon a cross-study comparison of the pharmacokinetics of zafirlukast in adults and pediatric subjects, and on the safety profile of zafirlukast in both adult and pediatric patients at doses equal to or higher than the recommended dose.

The safety and effectiveness of zafirlukast for pediatric patients less than 5 years of age has not been established. The effect of ACCOLATE on growth in children has not been determined.

Geriatric Use

Based on cross-study comparison, the clearance of zafirlukast is reduced in patients 65 years of age and older such that C_{max} and AUC are approximately 2- to 3-fold greater than those of younger patients (see DOSAGE AND ADMINISTRATION and CLINICAL PHARMACOLOGY).

A total of 8094 patients were exposed to zafirlukast in North American and European short-term placebo-controlled clinical trials. Of these, 243 patients were elderly (age 65 years and older). No overall difference in adverse events was seen in the elderly patients, except for an increase in the frequency of infections among zafirlukast-treated elderly patients compared to placebo-treated elderly patients (7.0% vs. 2.9%). The infections were not severe, occurred mostly in the lower respiratory tract, and did not necessitate withdrawal of therapy.

An open-label, uncontrolled, 4-week trial of 3759 asthma patients compared the safety and efficacy of ACCOLATE 20 mg given twice daily in three patient age groups, adolescents (12–17 years), adults (18–65 years), and elderly (greater than 65 years). A higher percentage of elderly patients (n=384) reported adverse events when compared to adults and adolescents. These elderly patients showed less improvement in efficacy measures. In the elderly patients, adverse events occurring in greater than 1% of the population included headache (4.7%), diarrhea and nausea (1.8%), and pharyngitis (1.3%). The elderly reported the lowest percentage of infections of all three age groups in this study.

ADVERSE REACTIONS

Adults and Children 12 years of age and older

The safety database for ACCOLATE consists of more than 4000 healthy volunteers and patients who received ACCOLATE, of which 1723 were asthmatics enrolled in trials of 13 weeks duration or longer. A total of 671 patients received ACCOLATE for 1 year or longer. The majority of the patients were 18 years of age or older; however, 222 patients between the age of 12 and 18 years received ACCOLATE.

A comparison of adverse events reported by =1% of zafirlukast-treated patients, and at rates numerically greater than in placebo-treated patients, is shown for all trials in the table below.

Adverse Event	ACCOLATE N=4058	PLACEBO N=2032
Headache	12.9%	11.7%
Infection	3.5%	3.4%
Nausea	3.1%	2.0%
Diarrhea	2.8%	2.1%
Pain (generalized)	1.9%	1.7%
Asthenia	1.8%	1.6%
Abdominal Pain	1.8%	1.1%
Accidental Injury	1.6%	1.5%
Dizziness	1.6%	1.5%
Myalgia	1.6%	1.5%
Fever	1.6%	1.1%
Back Pain	1.5%	1.2%
Vomiting	1.5%	1.1%
SGPT Elevation	1.5%	1.1%
Dyspepsia	1.3%	1.2%

The frequency of less common adverse events was comparable between ACCOLATE and placebo.

Rarely, elevations of one or more liver enzymes have occurred in patients receiving ACCOLATE in controlled clinical trials. In clinical trials, most of these have been observed at doses four times higher than the recommended dose. The following hepatic events (which have occurred predominantly in females) have been reported from post-marketing adverse event surveillance of patients who have received the recommended dose of ACCOLATE (40 mg/day): cases of symptomatic hepatitis (with or without hyperbilirubinemia) without other attributable cause; and rarely, hyperbilirubinemia without other elevated liver function tests. In most, but not all postmarketing reports, the patient's symptoms abated and the liver enzymes returned to normal or near normal after stopping ACCOLATE. In rare cases, patients have presented with fulminant hepatitis or progressed to hepatic failure, liver transplantation and death (see WARNINGS, Hepatotoxicity and PRECAUTIONS, Information for Patients.)

In clinical trials, an increased proportion of zafirlukast patients over the age of 55 years reported infections as compared to placebo-treated patients. A similar finding was not observed in other age groups studied. These infections were mostly mild or moderate in intensity and predominantly affected the respiratory tract. Infections occurred equally in both sexes, were dose-proportional to total milligrams of zafirlukast exposure, and were associated with coadministration of inhaled corticosteroids. The clinical significance of this finding is unknown.

In rare cases, patients on ACCOLATE therapy may present with systemic eosinophilia, eosinophilic pneumonia, or clinical features of vasculitis consistent with Churg-Strauss syndrome, a condition which is often treated with systemic steroid therapy. These events usually, but not always, have been associated with the reduction of oral steroid therapy. Physicians should be alert to eosinophilia, vasculitic rash, worsening pulmonary symptoms, cardiac complications, and/or neuropathy presenting in their patients. A causal association between ACCOLATE and these underlying conditions has not been established (see PRECAUTIONS, Eosinophilic Conditions).

Hypersensitivity reactions, including urticaria, angioedema and rashes, with or without blistering, have been reported in association with ACCOLATE therapy. Additionally, there have been reports of patients experiencing agranulocytosis, bleeding, bruising, or edema, arthralgia, and myalgia in association with ACCOLATE therapy.

Rare cases of patients experiencing increased theophylline levels with or without clinical signs or symptoms of theophylline toxicity after the addition of ACCOLATE to an existing theophylline regimen have been reported. The mechanism of the interaction between ACCOLATE and theophylline in these patients is unknown and not predicted by available *in vitro* metabolism data and the results of two clinical drug interaction studies (see CLINICAL PHARMACOLOGY and PRECAUTIONS, Drug Interactions).

Pediatric Patients 5 through 11 years of age

ACCOLATE has been evaluated for safety in 788 pediatric patients 5 through 11 years of age. Cumulatively, 313 pediatric patients were treated with ACCOLATE 10 mg twice daily or higher for at least 6 months, and 113 of them were treated for one year or longer in clinical trials. The safety profile of ACCOLATE 10 mg twice daily-versus placebo in the 4- and 6-week double-blind trials was generally similar to that observed in the adult clinical trials with ACCOLATE 20 mg twice daily.

In pediatric patients receiving ACCOLATE in multi-dose clinical trials, the following events occurred with a frequency of ≥2% and more frequently than in pediatric patients who received placebo, regardless of causality assessment: headache (4.5 vs. 4.2%) and abdominal pain (2.8 vs. 2.3%).

The post-marketing experience in this age group is similar to that seen in adults, including hepatic dysfunction, which may lead to liver failure.

OVERDOSAGE

No deaths occurred at oral zafirlukast doses of 2000 mg/kg in mice (approximately 210 times the maximum recommended daily oral dose in adults and children on a mg/m^2 basis), 2000 mg/kg in rats (approximately 420 times the maximum recommended daily oral dose in adults and children on a mg/m^2 basis), and 500 mg/kg in dogs (approximately 350 times the maximum recommended daily oral dose in adults and children on a mg/m^2 basis).

Overdosage with ACCOLATE has been reported in four patients surviving reported doses as high as 200 mg. The predominant symptoms reported following ACCOLATE overdose were rash and upset stomach. There were no acute toxic effects in humans that could be consistently ascribed to the administration of ACCOLATE. It is reasonable to employ the usual supportive measures in the event of an overdose; eg, remove unabsorbed material from the gastrointestinal tract, employ clinical monitoring, and institute supportive therapy, if required.

DOSAGE AND ADMINISTRATION

Because food can reduce the bioavailability of zafirlukast, ACCOLATE should be taken at least 1 hour before or 2 hours after meals.

Adults and Children 12 years of age and older

The recommended dose of ACCOLATE in adults and children 12 years and older is 20 mg twice daily.

Pediatric Patients 5 through 11 years of age

The recommended dose of ACCOLATE in children 5 through 11 years of age is 10 mg twice daily.

Elderly Patients: Based on cross-study comparisons, the clearance of zafirlukast is reduced in elderly patients (65 years of age and older), such that C_{max} and AUC are approximately twice those of younger adults. In clinical trials, a dose of 20 mg twice daily was not associated with an increase in the overall incidence of adverse events or withdrawals because of adverse events in elderly patients.

Patients with Hepatic Impairment: The clearance of zafirlukast is reduced in patients with stable alcoholic cirrhosis such that the C_{max} and AUC are approximately 50–60% greater than those of normal adults. ACCOLATE has not been evaluated in patients with hepatitis or in long-term studies of patients with cirrhosis.

Patients with Renal Impairment: Dosage adjustment is not required for patients with renal impairment.

HOW SUPPLIED

ACCOLATE 10 mg Tablets, (NDC 0310-0401) white, unflavored, round, biconvex, film-coated, mini-tablets identified with "ACCOLATE 10" debossed on one side are supplied in opaque HDPE bottles of 60 tablets and Hospital Unit Dose blister packages of 100 tablets.

ACCOLATE 20 mg Tablets, (NDC 0310-0402) white, round, biconvex, coated tablets identified with "ACCOLATE 20" debossed on one side are supplied in opaque HDPE bottles of 60 tablets and Hospital Unit Dose blister packages of 100 tablets.

Store at controlled room temperature, 20–25°C (68–77°F) [see USP]. Protect from light and moisture. Dispense in the original air-tight container.

ACCOLATE is a trademark of the AstraZeneca group of companies

Manufactured for:
AstraZeneca Pharmaceuticals LP
Wilmington, DE 19850
By: IPR Pharmaceuticals, Inc.
Carolina, PR 00984
64198-02 Rev 3/04

Shown in Product Identification Guide, page 306

ARIMIDEX® ℞

[ă-rĭ-mĭ-dĕx]

(Anastrozole) TABLETS

DESCRIPTION

ARIMIDEX® (anastrozole) tablets for oral administration contain 1 mg of anastrozole, a non-steroidal aromatase inhibitor. It is chemically described as 1,3-Benzenediacetonitrile, α, α, α', α'-tetramethyl-5-(1H-1,2,4-triazol-1-ylmethyl). Its molecular formula is $C_{17}H_{19}N_5$ and its structural formula is:

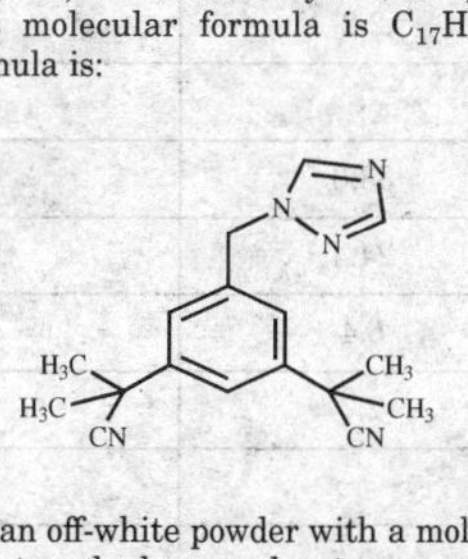

Anastrozole is an off-white powder with a molecular weight of 293.4. Anastrozole has moderate aqueous solubility (0.5 mg/mL at 25°C); solubility is independent of pH in the physiological range. Anastrozole is freely soluble in methanol, acetone, ethanol, and tetrahydrofuran, and very soluble in acetonitrile.

Each tablet contains as inactive ingredients: lactose, magnesium stearate, hydroxypropylmethylcellulose, polyethylene glycol, povidone, sodium starch glycolate, and titanium dioxide.

CLINICAL PHARMACOLOGY

Mechanism of Action

Many breast cancers have estrogen receptors and growth of these tumors can be stimulated by estrogen. In postmenopausal women, the principal source of circulating estrogen (primarily estradiol) is conversion of adrenally-generated androstenedione to estrone by aromatase in peripheral tissues, such as adipose tissue, with further conversion of estrone to estradiol. Many breast cancers also contain aromatase; the importance of tumor-generated estrogens is uncertain.

Treatment of breast cancer has included efforts to decrease estrogen levels, by ovariectomy premenopausally and by use of anti-estrogens and progestational agents both pre- and post-menopausally; and these interventions lead to decreased tumor mass or delayed progression of tumor growth in some women.

Anastrozole is a potent and selective non-steroidal aromatase inhibitor. It significantly lowers serum estradiol concentrations and has no detectable effect on formation of adrenal corticosteroids or aldosterone.

Pharmacokinetics

Inhibition of aromatase activity is primarily due to anastrozole, the parent drug. Studies with radiolabeled drug have demonstrated that orally administered anastrozole is well absorbed into the systemic circulation with 83 to 85% of the radiolabel recovered in urine and feces. Food does not affect the extent of absorption. Elimination of anastrozole is primarily via hepatic metabolism (approximately 85%) and to a lesser extent, renal excretion (approximately 11%), and anastrozole has a mean terminal elimination half-life of approximately 50 hours in postmenopausal women. The major circulating metabolite of anastrozole, triazole, lacks pharmacologic activity. The pharmacokinetic parameters are similar in patients and in healthy postmenopausal volunteers. The pharmacokinetics of anastrozole are linear over the dose range of 1 to 20 mg and do not change with repeated dosing. Consistent with the approximately 2-day terminal elimination half-life, plasma concentrations approach steady-state levels at about 7 days of once daily dosing and steady-state levels are approximately three- to four-fold higher than levels observed after a single dose of ARIMIDEX. Anastrozole is 40% bound to plasma proteins in the therapeutic range.

Metabolism and Excretion

Studies in postmenopausal women demonstrated that anastrozole is extensively metabolized with about 10% of the dose excreted in the urine as unchanged drug within 72 hours of dosing, and the remainder (about 60% of the dose) is excreted in urine as metabolites. Metabolism of anastrozole occurs by N-dealkylation, hydroxylation and glucuronidation. Three metabolites of anastrozole have been identified in human plasma and urine. The known metabolites are triazole, a glucuronide conjugate of hydroxy-anastrozole, and a glucuronide of anastrozole itself. Several minor (less than 5% of the radioactive dose) metabolites have not been identified.

Because renal elimination is not a significant pathway of elimination, total body clearance of anastrozole is unchanged even in severe (creatinine clearance less than 30 mL/min/1.73m^2) renal impairment, dosing adjustment in patients with renal dysfunction is not necessary (see Special Populations and DOSAGE AND ADMINISTRATION sections). Dosage adjustment is also unnecessary in patients with stable hepatic cirrhosis (see Special Populations and DOSAGE AND ADMINISTRATION sections).

Special Populations

Geriatric

Anastrozole pharmacokinetics have been investigated in postmenopausal female volunteers and patients with breast cancer. No age related effects were seen over the range <50 to >80 years.

Race

Estradiol and estrone sulfate levels were similar between Japanese and Caucasian postmenopausal women who received 1 mg of anastrozole daily for 16 days. Anastrozole mean steady-state minimum plasma concentrations in Caucasian and Japanese postmenopausal women were 25.7 and 30.4 ng/mL, respectively.

Renal Insufficiency

Anastrozole pharmacokinetics have been investigated in subjects with renal insufficiency. Anastrozole renal clearance decreased proportionally with creatinine clearance and was approximately 50% lower in volunteers with severe renal impairment (creatinine clearance <30 mL/min/1.73m^2) compared to controls. Since only about 10% of anastrozole is excreted unchanged in the urine, the reduction in renal clearance did not influence the total body clearance (see DOSAGE AND ADMINISTRATION).

Hepatic Insufficiency

Hepatic metabolism accounts for approximately 85% of anastrozole elimination. Anastrozole pharmacokinetics have been investigated in subjects with hepatic cirrhosis related to alcohol abuse. The apparent oral clearance (CL/F) of anastrozole was approximately 30% lower in subjects with stable hepatic cirrhosis than in control subjects with normal liver function. However, plasma anastrozole concentrations in the subjects with hepatic cirrhosis were within the range of concentrations seen in normal subjects across all clinical trials (see DOSAGE AND ADMINISTRATION), so that no dosage adjustment is needed.

Drug-Drug Interactions

Anastrozole inhibited reactions catalyzed by cytochrome P450 1A2, 2C8/9, and 3A4 *in vitro* with Ki values which were approximately 30 times higher than the mean steady-

Continued on next page

Arimidex—Cont.

state C_{max} values observed following a 1 mg daily dose. Anastrozole had no inhibitory effect on reactions catalyzed by cytochrome P450 2A6 or 2D6 *in vitro*. Administration of a single 30 mg/kg or multiple 10 mg/kg doses of anastrozole to healthy subjects had no effect on the clearance of antipyrine or urinary recovery of antipyrine metabolites. Based on these *in vitro* and *in vivo* results, it is unlikely that co-administration of ARIMIDEX 1 mg with other drugs will result in clinically significant inhibition of cytochrome P450 mediated metabolism.

In a study conducted in 16 male volunteers, anastrozole did not alter the pharmacokinetics as measured by C_{max} and AUC, and anticoagulant activity as measured by prothrombin time, activated partial thromboplastine time, and thrombin time of both R- and S-warfarin.

Co-administration of anastrozole and tamoxifen in breast cancer patients reduced anastrozole plasma concentration by 27% compared to those achieved with anastrozole alone; however, the co-administration did not affect the pharmacokinetics of tamoxifen or N-desmethyltamoxifen (see **PRECAUTIONS—Drug Interactions**).

Pharmacodynamics

Effect on Estradiol: Mean serum concentrations of estradiol were evaluated in multiple daily dosing trials with 0.5, 1, 3, 5, and 10 mg of ARIMIDEX in postmenopausal women with advanced breast cancer. Clinically significant suppression of serum estradiol was seen with all doses. Doses of 1 mg and higher resulted in suppression of mean serum concentrations of estradiol to the lower limit of detection (3.7 pmol/L). The recommended daily dose, ARIMIDEX 1 mg, reduced estradiol by approximately 70% within 24 hours and by approximately 80% after 14 days of daily dosing. Suppression of serum estradiol was maintained for up to 6 days after cessation of daily dosing with ARIMIDEX 1 mg.

Effect on Corticosteroids: In multiple daily dosing trials with 3, 5, and 10 mg, the selectivity of anastrozole was assessed by examining effects on corticosteroid synthesis. For all doses, anastrozole did not affect cortisol or aldosterone secretion at baseline or in response to ACTH. No glucocorticoid or mineralocorticoid replacement therapy is necessary with anastrozole.

Other Endocrine Effects: In multiple daily dosing trials with 5 and 10 mg, thyroid stimulating hormone (TSH) was measured; there was no increase in TSH during the administration of ARIMIDEX. ARIMIDEX does not possess direct progestogenic, androgenic, or estrogenic activity in animals, but does perturb the circulating levels of progesterone, androgens, and estrogens.

Table 1 - Demographic and Baseline Characteristics for ATAC Trial

Demographic Characteristic	ARIMIDEX 1 mg (*N=3125)	Tamoxifen 20 mg (*N=3116)	ARIMIDEX 1 mg plus Tamoxifen 20 mg (*N=3125)
Mean Age (yrs.)	64.1	64.1	64.3
Age Range (yrs.)	38.1–92.8	32.8–94.9	37.0–92.2
Age Distribution (%)			
<45 yrs.	0.7	0.4	0.5
45-60 yrs.	34.6	35.0	34.5
>60 <70 yrs.	38.0	37.1	37.7
>70 yrs.	26.7	27.4	27.3
Mean Weight (kg)	70.8	71.1	71.3
Receptor Status (%)			
Positive[1]	83.5	83.1	83.8
Negative[2]	7.4	8.0	7.0
Other[3]	8.8	8.6	9.1
Other Treatment (%) prior to Randomization			
Mastectomy	47.8	47.3	48.1
Breast conservation[4]	52.3	52.8	52
Axillary surgery	95.5	95.7	95.2
Radiotherapy	63.3	62.5	62.0
Chemotherapy	22.3	20.8	20.8
Neoadjuvant Tamoxifen	1.6	1.6	1.7
Primary Tumor Size (%)			
T1 (≤2 cm)	63.9	62.9	64.1
T2 (>2 cm and ≤5 cm)	32.6	34.2	32.9
T3 (>5 cm)	2.7	2.2	2.3
Nodal Status (%)			
Node positive	34.9	33.6	33.5
1-3 (# of nodes)	24.4	24.4	24.3
4-9	7.5	6.4	6.8
>9	2.9	2.7	2.3
Tumor Grade (%)			
Well differentiated	20.8	20.5	21.2
Moderately differentiated	46.8	47.8	46.6
Poorly/undifferentiated	23.7	23.3	23.7
Not assessed/recorded	8.7	8.4	8.5

[1] Includes patients who were estrogen receptor (ER) positive or progesterone receptor (PgR) positive, or both positive

[2] Includes patients with both ER negative and PgR negative receptor status

[3] Includes all other combinations of ER and PgR receptor status unknown

[4] Among the patients who had breast conservation, radiotherapy was administered to 95.0% of patients in the ARIMIDEX arm, 94.1% in the tamoxifen arm and 94.5% in the ARIMIDEX plus tamoxifen arm.

*N=Number of patients randomized to the treatment

Clinical Studies

Adjuvant Treatment of Breast Cancer in Postmenopausal Women: A multicenter, double-blind trial (ATAC) randomized 9,366 postmenopausal women with operable breast cancer to adjuvant treatment with ARIMIDEX 1 mg daily, tamoxifen 20 mg daily, or a combination of the two treatments for five years or until recurrence of the disease. At the time of the efficacy analysis, women had received a median of 31 months of treatment and had been followed for recurrence-free survival for a median of 33 months.

The primary endpoint of the trial is recurrence-free survival, ie, time to occurrence of a distant or local recurrence, or contralateral breast primary or death from any cause. Time to distant recurrence and the incidence of contralateral breast primaries were analyzed.

Demographic and other baseline characteristics were similar among the three treatment groups (see Table 1).

[See table 1 at left]

The recommended duration of tamoxifen therapy is five years; continued benefit of tamoxifen after 3 years has been documented. The results of the ATAC trial in a patient population treated for a median 31 months, thus allow only a preliminary comparison of ARIMIDEX and tamoxifen therapy. At this time, recurrence-free survival was improved in the ARIMIDEX arm compared to the tamoxifen arm: Hazard Ratio (HR) = 0.83, 95% CI 0.71-0.96, p=0.0144. Results were essentially the same in the hormone receptor positive patients (about 84% of the patients): HR = 0.78, 95% CI 0.65-0.93.

Recurrence-free survival in the combination treatment arm was similar to that in the tamoxifen group.

Duration of follow-up in this ongoing trial is too short to permit a mature survival analysis. The duration of therapy on the study arms and frequency of individual events comprising recurrence are described in Table 2.

[See table 2 at top of next page]

First Line Therapy in Postmenopausal Women with Advanced Breast Cancer: Two double-blind, well-controlled clinical studies of similar design (0030, a North American study and 0027, a predominately European study) were conducted to assess the efficacy of ARIMIDEX compared with tamoxifen as first-line therapy for hormone receptor positive or hormone receptor unknown locally advanced or metastatic breast cancer in postmenopausal women. A total of 1021 patients between the ages of 30 and 92 years old were randomized to receive trial treatment. Patients were randomized to receive 1 mg of ARIMIDEX once daily or 20 mg of tamoxifen once daily. The primary end points for both trials were time to tumor progression, objective tumor response rate, and safety.

Demographics and other baseline characteristics, including patients who had measurable and no measurable disease, patients who were given previous adjuvant therapy, the site of metastatic disease and ethnic origin were similar for the two treatment groups for both trials. The following table summarizes the hormone receptor status at entry for all randomized patients in trials 0030 and 0027.

[See table 3 on next page]

For the primary endpoints, trial 0030 showed ARIMIDEX was at least as effective as tamoxifen for objective tumor response rate. ARIMIDEX had a statistically significant advantage over tamoxifen (p=0.006) for time to tumor progression (see Table 4 and Figure 1). Trial 0027 showed ARIMIDEX was at least as effective as tamoxifen for objective tumor response rate and time to tumor progression (see Table 4 and Figure 2).

Table 4 below summarizes the results of trial 0030 and trial 0027 for the primary efficacy endpoints.

[See table 4 on next page]

Figure 1 - Kaplan-Meier probability of time to disease progression for all randomized patients (intent-to-treat) in Trial 0030

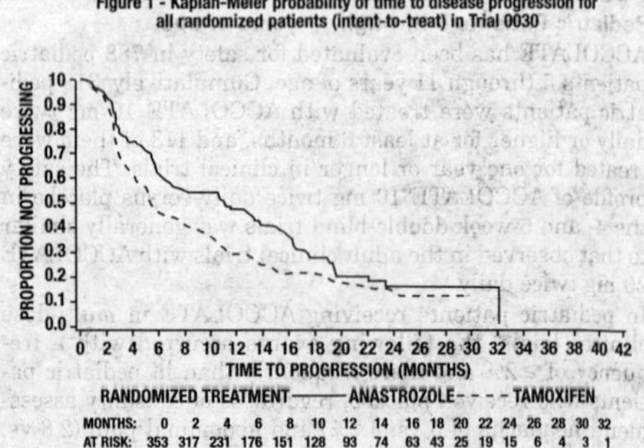

[See figure 2 at top of next column]

Results from the secondary endpoints of time to treatment failure, duration of tumor response, and duration of clinical benefit were supportive of the results of the primary efficacy endpoints. There were too few deaths occurring across treatment groups of both trials to draw conclusions on overall survival differences.

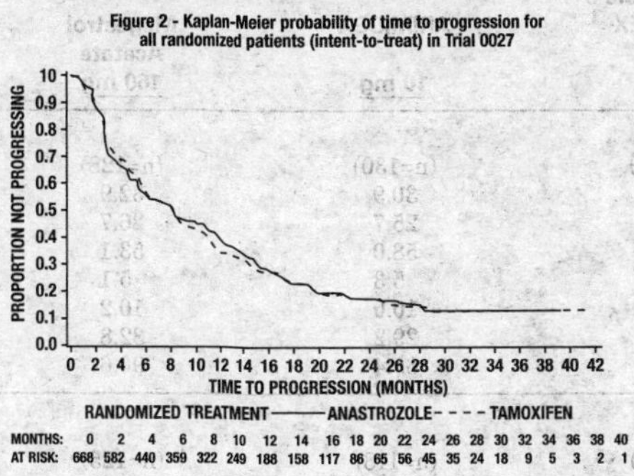

Second Line Therapy in Postmenopausal Women with Advanced Breast Cancer who had Disease Progression following Tamoxifen Therapy: Anastrozole was studied in two well-controlled clinical trials (0004, a North American study; 0005, a predominately European study) in postmenopausal women with advanced breast cancer who had disease progression following tamoxifen therapy for either advanced or early breast cancer. Some of the patients had also received previous cytotoxic treatment. Most patients were ER-positive; a smaller fraction were ER-unknown or ER-negative; the ER-negative patients were eligible only if they had had a positive response to tamoxifen. Eligible patients with measurable and non-measurable disease were randomized to receive either a single daily dose of 1 mg or 10 mg of ARIMIDEX or megestrol acetate 40 mg four times a day. The studies were double-blinded with respect to ARIMIDEX. Time to progression and objective response (only patients with measurable disease could be considered partial responders) rates were the primary efficacy variables. Objective response rates were calculated based on the Union Internationale Contre le Cancer (UICC) criteria. The rate of prolonged (more than 24 weeks) stable disease, the rate of progression, and survival were also calculated.

Both trials included over 375 patients; demographics and other baseline characteristics were similar for the three treatment groups in each trial. Patients in the 0005 trial had responded better to prior tamoxifen treatment. Of the patients entered who had prior tamoxifen therapy for advanced disease (58% in Trial 0004; 57% in Trial 0005), 18% of these patients in Trial 0004 and 42% in Trial 0005 were reported by the primary investigator to have responded. In Trial 0004, 81% of patients were ER-positive, 13% were ER-unknown, and 6% were ER-negative. In Trial 0005, 58% of patients were ER-positive, 37% were ER-unknown, and 5% were ER-negative. In Trial 0004, 62% of patients had measurable disease compared to 79% in Trial 0005. The sites of metastatic disease were similar among treatment groups for each trial. On average, 40% of the patients had soft tissue metastases; 60% had bone metastases; and 40% had visceral (15% liver) metastases.

As shown in the table below, similar results were observed among treatment groups and between the two trials. None of the within-trial differences were statistically significant.

[See table 5 at top of next page]

More than 1/3 of the patients in each treatment group in both studies had either an objective response or stabilization of their disease for greater than 24 weeks. Among the 263 patients who received ARIMIDEX 1 mg, there were 11 complete responders and 22 partial responders. In patients who had an objective response, more than 80% were still responding at 6 months from randomization and more than 45% were still responding at 12 months from randomization.

When data from the two controlled trials are pooled, the objective response rates and median times to progression and death were similar for patients randomized to ARIMIDEX 1 mg and megestrol acetate. There is, in this data, no indication that ARIMIDEX 10 mg is superior to ARIMIDEX 1 mg.

[See table 6 on next page]

Objective response rates and median times to progression and death for ARIMIDEX 1 mg were similar to megestrol acetate for women over or under 65. There were too few non-white patients studied to draw conclusions about racial differences in response.

INDICATIONS AND USAGE

ARIMIDEX is indicated for adjuvant treatment of postmenopausal women with hormone receptor positive early breast cancer.

The effectiveness of ARIMIDEX in early breast cancer is based on an analysis of recurrence-free survival in patients treated for a median of 31 months (see **CLINICAL PHARMACOLOGY—Clinical Studies** subsection). Further follow-up of study patients will be required to determine long-term outcomes.

ARIMIDEX is indicated for the first-line treatment of postmenopausal women with hormone receptor positive or hormone receptor unknown locally advanced or metastatic breast cancer.

ARIMIDEX is indicated for the treatment of advanced breast cancer in postmenopausal women with disease progression following tamoxifen therapy. Patients with ER-negative disease and patients who did not respond to previous tamoxifen therapy rarely responded to ARIMIDEX.

Table 2—ATAC Endpoint Summary

	ARIMIDEX 1 mg (N=3125)	Tamoxifen 20 mg (N=3116)	ARIMIDEX 1 mg plus Tamoxifen 20 mg (N=3125)
Median Duration of Therapy (mo.)[1]	30.9	30.7	30.4
Range Duration of Therapy (mo.)	<1 to 55.3	<1 to 55.7	<1 to 54.5
Median Efficacy Follow-Up (mo.)	33.6	33.2	32.9
Range Follow-Up (mo.)	<1 to 55.2	<1 to 55.7	<1 to 54.4
Recurrence-Free Survival			
First Event (n,%)	318 (10.2)	379 (12.2)	383 (12.3)
Locoregional[2]	67 (2.1)	83 (2.7)	81 (2.6)
Distant	157 (5.0)	181 (5.8)	202 (6.5)
New Contralateral Primaries	14 (0.4)	33 (1.1)	28 (0.9)
Invasive	9 (0.3)	30 (1.0)	23 (0.7)
Ductal carcinoma in situ	5 (0.2)	3 (<0.1)	5 (0.2)
Deaths[3]			
Death — breast cancer	4 (0.12)	1 (0.03)	0 (0.00)
Death — other reason	76 (2.4)	81 (2.6)	72 (2.3)

[1]Based on treatment received
[2]Includes new primary ipsilateral breast cancer (including DCIS), and recurrences at the chest wall, axillary and other regional lymph nodes
[3]Includes only deaths that were first events

Table 3

Number (%) of subjects

Receptor status	Trial 0030 ARIMIDEX 1 mg (n=171)	Trial 0030 Tamoxifen 20 mg (n=182)	Trial 0027 ARIMIDEX 1 mg (n=340)	Trial 0027 Tamoxifen 20 mg (n=328)
ER+ and/or PgR+	151 (88.3)	162 (89.0)	154 (45.3)	144 (43.9)
ER unknown, PgR unknown	19 (11.1)	20 (11.0)	185 (54.4)	183 (55.8)

ER = Estrogen receptor
PgR = Progesterone receptor

Table 4

End point	Trial 0030 ARIMIDEX 1 mg (n=171)	Trial 0030 Tamoxifen 20 mg (n=182)	Trial 0027 ARIMIDEX 1 mg (n=340)	Trial 0027 Tamoxifen 20 mg (n=328)
Time to progression (TTP)				
Median TTP (months)	11.1	5.6	8.2	8.3
Number (%) of subjects who progressed	114 (67%)	138 (76%)	249 (73%)	247 (75%)
Hazard ratio (LCL)[1]	1.42 (1.15)		1.01 (0.87)	
2-sided 95% CI	(1.11, 1.82)		(0.85, 1.20)	
p-value[2]	0.006		0.920	
Best objective response rate				
Number (%) of subjects with CR + PR	36 (21.1%)	31 (17.0%)	112 (32.9%)	107 (32.6%)
Odds Ratio (LCL)[3]	1.30 (0.83)		1.01 (0.77)	

CR = Complete Response
PR = Partial Response
CI = Confidence Interval
LCL = Lower Confidence Limit
[1] Tamoxifen:ARIMIDEX
[2] Two-sided Log Rank
[3] ARIMIDEX:Tamoxifen

CONTRAINDICATIONS

ARIMIDEX is contraindicated in any patient who has shown a hypersensitivity reaction to the drug or to any of the excipients.

WARNINGS

ARIMIDEX can cause fetal harm when administered to a pregnant woman. Anastrozole has been found to cross the placenta following oral administration of 0.1 mg/kg in rats and rabbits (about 1 and 1.9 times the recommended human dose, respectively, on a mg/m² basis). Studies in both rats and rabbits at doses equal to or greater than 0.1 and 0.02 mg/kg/day, respectively (about 1 and 1/3, respectively, the recommended human dose on a mg/m² basis), administered during the period of organogenesis showed that anastrozole increased pregnancy loss (increased pre- and/or post-implantation loss, increased resorption, and decreased numbers of live fetuses); effects were dose related in rats. Placental weights were significantly increased in rats at doses of 0.1 mg/kg/day or more.

Evidence of fetotoxicity, including delayed fetal development (i.e., incomplete ossification and depressed fetal body weights), was observed in rats administered doses of 1 mg/kg/day (which produced plasma anastrozole C_{ssmax} and $AUC_{0-24\ hr}$ that were 19 times and 9 times higher than the respective values found in postmenopausal volunteers at the recommended dose). There was no evidence of teratogenicity in rats administered doses up to 1.0 mg/kg/day. In rabbits, anastrozole caused pregnancy failure at doses equal to or greater than 1.0 mg/kg/day (about 16 times the recommended human dose on a mg/m² basis); there was no evidence of teratogenicity in rabbits administered 0.2 mg/kg/day (about 3 times the recommended human dose on a mg/m² basis).

There are no adequate and well-controlled studies in pregnant women using ARIMIDEX. If ARIMIDEX is used during pregnancy, or if the patient becomes pregnant while receiving this drug, the patient should be apprised of the

Continued on next page

Arimidex—Cont.

potential hazard to the fetus or potential risk for loss of the pregnancy.

PRECAUTIONS

General

Before starting treatment with ARIMIDEX, pregnancy must be excluded (see WARNINGS). ARIMIDEX should be administered under the supervision of a qualified physician experienced in the use of anticancer agents.

Laboratory Tests

During the ATAC trial, more patients receiving ARIMIDEX were reported to have an elevated serum cholesterol compared to patients receiving tamoxifen (7% versus 3%, respectively).

Drug Interactions

(See **CLINICAL PHARMACOLOGY**) Anastrozole inhibited *in vitro* metabolic reactions catalyzed by cytochromes P450 1A2, 2C8/9, and 3A4 but only at relatively high concentrations. Anastrozole did not inhibit P450 2A6 or the polymorphic P450 2D6 in human liver microsomes. Anastrozole did not alter the pharmacokinetics of antipyrine. Although there have been no formal interaction studies other than with antipyrine, based on these *in vivo* and *in vitro* studies, it is unlikely that co-administration of a 1 mg dose of ARIMIDEX with other drugs will result in clinically significant drug inhibition of cytochrome P450-mediated metabolism of the other drugs.

An interaction study with warfarin showed no clinically significant effect of anastrozole on warfarin pharmacokinetics or anticoagulant activity.

Clinical and pharmacokinetic results from the ATAC trial suggest that tamoxifen should not be administered with anastrozole (see **CLINICAL PHARMACOLOGY — Drug Interactions and Clinical Studies** subsections). Co-administration of anastrozole and tamoxifen resulted in a reduction of anastrozole plasma levels by 27% compared with those achieved with anastrozole alone.

Estrogen-containing therapies should not be used with ARIMIDEX as they may diminish its pharmacologic action.

Drug/Laboratory Test Interactions

No clinically significant changes in the results of clinical laboratory tests have been observed.

Carcinogenesis

A conventional carcinogenesis study in rats at doses of 1.0 to 25 mg/kg/day (about 10 to 243 times the daily maximum recommended human dose on a mg/m^2 basis) administered by oral gavage for up to 2 years revealed an increase in the incidence of hepatocellular adenoma and carcinoma and uterine stromal polyps in females and thyroid adenoma in males at the high dose. A dose related increase was observed in the incidence of ovarian and uterine hyperplasia in females. At 25 mg/kg/day, plasma AUC_{0-24hr} levels in rats were 110 to 125 times higher than the level exhibited in postmenopausal volunteers at the recommended dose. A separate carcinogenicity study in mice at oral doses of 5 to 50 mg/kg/day (about 24 to 243 times the daily maximum recommended human dose on a mg/m^2 basis) for up to 2 years produced an increase in the incidence of benign ovarian stromal, epithelial and granulosa cell tumors at all dose levels. A dose related increase in the incidence of ovarian hyperplasia was also observed in female mice. These ovarian changes are considered to be rodent-specific effects of aromatase inhibition and are of questionable significance to humans. The incidence of lymphosarcoma was increased in males and females at the high dose. At 50 mg/kg/day, plasma AUC levels in mice were 35 to 40 times higher than the level exhibited in postmenopausal volunteers at the recommended dose.

Mutagenesis

ARIMIDEX has not been shown to be mutagenic in *in vitro* tests (Ames and E. coli bacterial tests, CHO-K1 gene mutation assay) or clastogenic either *in vitro* (chromosome aberrations in human lymphocytes) or *in vivo* (micronucleus test in rats).

Impairment of Fertility

Oral administration of anastrozole to female rats (from 2 weeks before mating to pregnancy day 7) produced significant incidence of infertility and reduced numbers of viable pregnancies at 1 mg/kg/day (about 10 times the recommended human dose on a mg/m^2 basis and 9 times higher than the AUC $_{0-24hr}$ found in postmenopausal volunteers at the recommended dose). Pre-implantation loss of ova or fetus was increased at doses equal to or greater than 0.02 mg/kg/day (about one-fifth the recommended human dose on a mg/m^2 basis). Recovery of fertility was observed following a 5-week non-dosing period which followed 3 weeks of dosing. It is not known whether these effects observed in female rats are indicative of impaired fertility in humans.

Multiple-dose studies in rats administered anastrozole for 6 months at doses equal to or greater than 1 mg/kg/day (which produced plasma anastrozole C_{ssmax} and AUC_{0-24hr} that were 19 and 9 times higher than the respective values found in postmenopausal volunteers at the recommended dose) resulted in hypertrophy of the ovaries and the presence of follicular cysts. In addition, hyperplastic uteri were observed in 6-month studies in female dogs administered doses equal to or greater than 1 mg/kg/day (which produced plasma anastrozole C_{ssmax} and AUC_{0-24hr} that were 22 times and 16 times higher than the respective values found in postmenopausal women at the recommended dose). It is not

Table 5

	ARIMIDEX 1 mg	ARIMIDEX 10 mg	Megestrol Acetate 160 mg
Trial 0004 (N. America)	(n=128)	(n=130)	(n=128)
Median Follow-up (months)*	31.3	30.9	32.9
Median Time to Death (months)	29.6	25.7	26.7
2 Year Survival Probability (%)	62.0	58.0	53.1
Median Time to Progression (months)	5.7	5.3	5.1
Objective Response (all patients) (%)	12.5	10.0	10.2
Stable Disease for >24 weeks (%)	35.2	29.2	32.8
Progression (%)	86.7	85.4	90.6
Trial 0005 (Europe, Australia, S. Africa)	(n=135)	(n=118)	(n=125)
Median Follow-up (months)*	31.0	30.9	31.5
Median Time to Death (months)	24.3	24.8	19.8
2 Year Survival Probability (%)	50.5	50.9	39.1
Median Time to Progression (months)	4.4	5.3	3.9
Objective Response (all patients) (%)	12.6	15.3	14.4
Stable Disease for >24 weeks (%)	24.4	25.4	23.2
Progression (%)	91.9	89.8	92.0

*Surviving Patients

Table 6

Trials 0004 & 0005 (Pooled Data)	ARIMIDEX 1 mg N=263	ARIMIDEX 10 mg N=248	Megestrol Acetate 160 mg N=253
Median Time to Death (months)	26.7	25.5	22.5
2 Year Survival Probability (%)	56.1	54.6	46.3
Median Time to Progression (months)	4.8	5.3	4.6
Objective Response (all patients) (%)	12.5	12.5	12.3

Table 7 — Adverse events occurring with an incidence of at least 5% in any treatment group during treatment, or within 14 days of the end of treatment

Body system and adverse event by COSTART-preferred term*	ARIMIDEX 1 mg (N = 3092)	Tamoxifen 20 mg (N = 3093)	ARIMIDEX 1 mg plus Tamoxifen 20 mg (N = 3098)
	Number (%) of patients		
Body as a whole			
Asthenia	512 (17)	491 (16)	468 (15)
Pain	461 (15)	435 (14)	407 (13)
Back pain	256 (8)	255 (8)	258 (8)
Headache	277 (9)	216 (7)	214 (7)
Abdominal pain	227 (7)	228 (7)	219 (7)
Infection	223 (7)	225 (7)	211 (7)
Accidental injury	221 (7)	221 (7)	226 (7)
Flu syndrome	154 (5)	170 (5)	170 (5)
Chest pain	164 (5)	122 (4)	152 (5)
Cardiovascular			
Vasodilatation	1082 (35)	1246 (40)	1261 (41)
Hypertension	292 (9)	252 (8)	270 (9)
Digestive			
Nausea	307 (10)	298 (10)	324 (10)
Constipation	201 (7)	214 (7)	232 (7)
Diarrhea	227 (7)	186 (6)	193 (6)
Dyspepsia	166 (5)	137 (4)	156 (5)
Gastrointestinal disorder	155 (5)	122 (4)	127 (4)
Hemic and lymphatic			
Lymphoedema	267 (9)	299 (10)	296 (10)
Metabolic and nutritional			
Peripheral edema	255 (8)	275 (9)	281 (9)
Weight gain	253 (8)	250 (8)	264 (9)
Hypercholesteremia	210 (7)	79 (3)	72 (2)
Musculoskeletal			
Arthritis	431 (14)	344 (11)	364 (12)
Arthralgia	390 (13)	251 (8)	265 (9)
Osteoporosis	229 (7)	161 (5)	174 (6)
Fracture	219 (7)	137 (4)	178 (6)
Bone pain	165 (5)	149 (5)	143 (5)
Arthrosis	179 (6)	136 (4)	119 (4)
Nervous system			
Depression	348 (11)	341 (11)	342 (11)
Insomnia	266 (9)	245 (8)	227 (7)
Dizziness	198 (6)	207 (7)	190 (6)
Anxiety	168 (5)	157 (5)	140 (5)
Paraesthesia	195 (6)	116 (4)	120 (4)
Respiratory			
Pharyngitis	376 (12)	359 (12)	350 (11)
Cough increased	212 (7)	237 (8)	203 (7)
Dyspnea	186 (6)	185 (6)	175 (6)
Skin and appendages			
Rash	300 (10)	331 (11)	326 (11)
Sweating	121 (4)	165 (5)	142 (5)
Urogenital			
Leukorrhea	75 (2)	265 (9)	277 (9)
Urinary tract infection	192 (6)	252 (8)	228 (7)
Breast pain	205 (7)	136 (4)	182 (6)
Vulvovaginitis	180 (6)	134 (4)	134 (4)

COSTART Coding Symbols for Thesaurus of Adverse Reaction Terms.
N = Number of patients receiving the treatment.
*A patient may have had more than 1 adverse event, including more than 1 adverse event in the same body system.

Table 8 — Number (%) of patients with Pre-specified Adverse Event in ATAC Trial

	ARIMIDEX N=3092 (%)	Tamoxifen N=3093 (%)	Odds-ratio	95% CI
All Fractures	224 (7)	145 (5)	1.59	1.28 – 1.97
Fractures of Spine, Hip, Wrist	89 (3)	62 (2)	1.45	1.04 – 2.04
Musculo-skeletal disorders[1]	940 (30)	737 (24)	1.41	1.28 – 1.55
Ischemic Cardiovascular Disease	92 (3)	74 (2)	1.25	0.91 – 1.72
Asthenia	513 (17)	491 (16)	1.05	0.93 – 1.20
Nausea and Vomiting	348 (11)	342 (11)	1.02	0.88 – 1.19
Mood Disturbances	521 (17)	511 (17)	1.02	0.90 – 1.16
Cataracts	128 (4)	140 (5)	0.91	0.71 – 1.17
Hot Flashes	1082 (35)	1246 (40)	0.80	0.73 – 0.87
Venous Thromboembolic events	73 (2)	120 (4)	0.60	0.44 – 0.81
Deep Venous Thromboembolic Events	40 (1)	60 (2)	0.66	0.43 – 1.00
Ischemic Cerebrovascular Event	40 (1)	74 (2)	0.53	0.35 – 0.80
Vaginal Bleeding	147 (5)	270 (9)	0.52	0.42 – 0.64
Vaginal Discharge	94 (3)	378 (12)	0.23	0.18 – 0.28
Endometrial Cancer	3 (0.1)	15 (0.5)	0.20	0.04 – 0.70

[1]Refers to joint symptoms, including arthritis, arthrosis and arthralgia.

known whether these effects on the reproductive organs of animals are associated with impaired fertility in premenopausal women.

Pregnancy

Pregnancy Category D (See **WARNINGS**)

Nursing Mothers

It is not known if anastrozole is excreted in human milk. Because many drugs are excreted in human milk, caution should be exercised when ARIMIDEX is administered to a nursing woman (see WARNINGS and PRECAUTIONS).

Pediatric Use

The safety and efficacy of ARIMIDEX in pediatric patients have not been established.

Geriatric Use

In studies 0030 and 0027 about 50% of patients were 65 or older. Patients ≥ 65 years of age had moderately better tumor response and time to tumor progression than patients < 65 years of age regardless of randomized treatment. In studies 0004 and 0005 50% of patients were 65 or older. Response rates and time to progression were similar for the over 65 and younger patients. In the ATAC adjuvant study, 35% of patients were < 60 years of age; 38% were ≥ 60 to ≤ 70 years of age; and 27% were > 70 years of age. The number of events by age group was insufficient to perform a subset efficacy analysis.

ADVERSE REACTIONS

Adjuvant Therapy

The median duration of adjuvant treatment for safety evaluation was 37.3 months, 36.9 months, and 36.5 months for patients receiving ARIMIDEX 1 mg, tamoxifen 20 mg, and the combination of ARIMIDEX 1 mg plus tamoxifen 20 mg, respectively.

Adverse events occurring with an incidence of at least 5% in any treatment group during treatment or within 14 days of the end of treatment are presented in Table 7.

[See table 7 on previous page]

Non-pathologic fractures were reported more frequently in the ARIMIDEX-treated patients (219 [7%]) than in the tamoxifen-treated patients (137 [4%]).

Certain adverse events and combinations of adverse events were prospectively specified for analysis, based on the known pharmacologic properties and side effect profiles of the two drugs (see Table 8). Patients receiving ARIMIDEX had an increase in musculoskeletal events and fractures (including fractures of spine, hip and wrist) compared with patients receiving tamoxifen. Patients receiving ARIMIDEX had a decrease in hot flashes, vaginal bleeding, vaginal discharge, endometrial cancer, venous thromboembolic events (including deep venous thrombosis) and ischemic cerebrovascular events compared with patients receiving tamoxifen.

[See table 8 above]

Angina pectoris was reported more frequently in the ARIMIDEX-treated patients (52 [1.7%]) than in the tamoxifen-treated patients (30 [1.0%]); the incidence of myocardial infarction was comparable (ARIMIDEX 24 patients [0.8%]; tamoxifen 25 patients [0.8%]).

Preliminary results from the ATAC trial bone substudy demonstrated that patients receiving ARIMIDEX had a mean decrease in both lumbar spine and total hip bone mineral density (BMD) compared to baseline. Patients receiving tamoxifen had a mean increase in both lumbar spine and total hip BMD compared to baseline.

First Line Therapy

ARIMIDEX was generally well tolerated in two well-controlled clinical trials (ie, Trials 0030 and 0027). Adverse events occurring with an incidence of at least 5% in either treatment group of trials 0030 and 0027 during or within 2 weeks of the end of treatment are shown in Table 9.

Table 9

Body system Adverse event[a]	Number (%) of subjects ARIMIDEX (n=506)	Tamoxifen (n=511)
Whole body		
Asthenia	83 (16)	81 (16)
Pain	70 (14)	73 (14)
Back pain	60 (12)	68 (13)
Headache	47 (9)	40 (8)
Abdominal pain	40 (8)	38 (7)
Chest pain	37 (7)	37 (7)
Flu syndrome	35 (7)	30 (6)
Pelvic pain	23 (5)	30 (6)
Cardiovascular		
Vasodilation	128 (25)	106 (21)
Hypertension	25 (5)	36 (7)
Digestive		
Nausea	94 (19)	106 (21)
Constipation	47 (9)	66 (13)
Diarrhea	40 (8)	33 (6)
Vomiting	38 (8)	36 (7)
Anorexia	26 (5)	46 (9)
Metabolic and nutritional		
Peripheral edema	51 (10)	41 (8)
Musculoskeletal		
Bone pain	54 (11)	52 (10)
Nervous		
Dizziness	30 (6)	22 (4)
Insomnia	30 (6)	38 (7)
Depression	23 (5)	32 (6)
Hypertonia	16 (3)	26 (5)
Respiratory		
Cough increased	55 (11)	52 (10)
Dyspnea	51 (10)	47 (9)
Pharyngitis	49 (10)	68 (13)
Skin and appendages		
Rash	38 (8)	34 (8)
Urogenital		
Leukorrhea	9 (2)	31 (6)

[a]A patient may have had more than 1 adverse event.

Less frequent adverse experiences reported in patients receiving ARIMIDEX 1 mg in either Trial 0030 or Trial 0027 were similar to those reported for second-line therapy.

Based on results from second-line therapy and the established safety profile of tamoxifen, the incidences of 9 prespecified adverse event categories potentially causally related to one or both of the therapies because of their pharmacology were statistically analyzed. No significant differences were seen between treatment groups.

Table 10
Number (n) and Percentage of Patients

Adverse Event Group[a]	ARIMIDEX 1 mg (n = 506) n	(%)	NOLVADEX 20 mg (n = 511) n	(%)
Depression	23	(5)	32	(6)
Tumor Flare	15	(3)	18	(4)
Thromboembolic Disease[a]	18	(4)	33	(6)
Venous[b]	5		15	
Coronary and Cerebral[c]	13		19	
Gastrointestinal Disturbance	170	(34)	196	(38)
Hot Flushes	134	(26)	118	(23)
Vaginal Dryness	9	(2)	3	(1)
Lethargy	6	(1)	15	(3)
Vaginal Bleeding	5	(1)	11	(2)
Weight Gain	11	(2)	8	(2)

[a] A patient may have had more than 1 adverse event

[b] Includes pulmonary embolus, thrombophlebitis, retinal vein thrombosis

[c] Includes myocardial infarction, myocardial ischemia, angina pectoris, cerebrovascular accident, cerebral ischemia and cerebral infarct

Despite the lack of estrogenic activity for ARIMIDEX, there was no increase in myocardial infarction or fracture when compared with tamoxifen.

Second Line Therapy

ARIMIDEX was generally well tolerated in two well-controlled clinical trials (ie, Trials 0004 and 0005), with less than 3.3% of the ARIMIDEX-treated patients and 4.0% of the megestrol acetate-treated patients withdrawing due to an adverse event.

The principal adverse event more common with ARIMIDEX than megestrol acetate was diarrhea. Adverse events reported in greater than 5% of the patients in any of the treatment groups in these two well-controlled clinical trials, regardless of causality, are presented below:

Table 11
Number (n) and Percentage of Patients with Adverse Event[†]

Adverse Event	ARIMIDEX 1 mg (n = 262) n	%	ARIMIDEX 10 mg (n = 246) n	%	Megestrol Acetate 160 mg (n = 253) n	%
Asthenia	42	(16)	33	(13)	47	(19)
Nausea	41	(16)	48	(20)	28	(11)
Headache	34	(13)	44	(18)	24	(9)
Hot Flashes	32	(12)	29	(11)	21	(8)
Pain	28	(11)	38	(15)	29	(11)
Back Pain	28	(11)	26	(11)	19	(8)
Dyspnea	24	(9)	27	(11)	53	(21)
Vomiting	24	(9)	26	(11)	16	(6)
Cough Increased	22	(8)	18	(7)	19	(8)
Diarrhea	22	(8)	18	(7)	7	(3)
Constipation	18	(7)	18	(7)	21	(8)
Abdominal Pain	18	(7)	14	(6)	18	(7)
Anorexia	18	(7)	19	(8)	11	(4)
Bone Pain	17	(6)	26	(12)	19	(8)
Pharyngitis	16	(6)	23	(9)	15	(6)
Dizziness	16	(6)	12	(5)	15	(6)
Rash	15	(6)	15	(6)	19	(8)
Dry Mouth	15	(6)	11	(4)	13	(5)
Peripheral Edema	14	(5)	21	(9)	28	(11)
Pelvic Pain	14	(5)	17	(7)	13	(5)
Depression	14	(5)	6	(2)	5	(2)
Chest Pain	13	(5)	18	(7)	13	(5)
Paresthesia	12	(5)	15	(6)	9	(4)
Vaginal Hemorrhage	6	(2)	4	(2)	13	(5)
Weight Gain	4	(2)	9	(4)	30	(12)
Sweating	4	(2)	3	(1)	16	(6)
Increased Appetite	0	(0)	1	(0)	13	(5)

[†]A patient may have more than one adverse event.

Other less frequent (2% to 5%) adverse experiences reported in patients receiving ARIMIDEX 1 mg in either Trial 0004 or Trial 0005 are listed below. These adverse experiences are listed by body system and are in order of decreasing frequency within each body system regardless of assessed causality.

Body as a Whole: Flu syndrome; fever; neck pain; malaise; accidental injury; infection

Cardiovascular: Hypertension; thrombophlebitis

Hepatic: Gamma GT increased; SGOT increased; SGPT increased

Continued on next page

Arimidex—Cont.

Hematologic: Anemia; leukopenia
Metabolic and Nutritional: Alkaline phosphatase increased; weight loss
Mean serum total cholesterol levels increased by 0.5 mmol/L among patients receiving ARIMIDEX. Increases in LDL cholesterol have been shown to contribute to these changes.
Musculoskeletal: Myalgia; arthralgia; pathological fracture
Nervous: Somnolence; confusion; insomnia; anxiety; nervousness
Respiratory: Sinusitis; bronchitis; rhinitis
Skin and Appendages: Hair thinning; pruritus
Urogenital: Urinary tract infection; breast pain

The incidences of the following adverse event groups potentially causally related to one or both of the therapies because of their pharmacology, were statistically analyzed: weight gain, edema, thromboembolic disease, gastrointestinal disturbance, hot flushes, and vaginal dryness. These six groups, and the adverse events captured in the groups, were prospectively defined. The results are shown in the table below.

Table 12
Number (n) and Percentage of Patients

Adverse Event Group	ARIMIDEX 1 mg (n = 262) n	(%)	ARIMIDEX 10 mg (n = 246) n	(%)	Megestrol Acetate 160 mg (n = 253) n	(%)
Gastrointestinal Disturbance	77	(29)	81	(33)	54	(21)
Hot Flushes	33	(13)	29	(12)	35	(14)
Edema	19	(7)	28	(11)	35	(14)
Thromboembolic Disease	9	(3)	4	(2)	12	(5)
Vaginal Dryness	5	(2)	3	(1)	2	(1)
Weight Gain	4	(2)	10	(4)	30	(12)

More patients treated with megestrol acetate reported weight gain as an adverse event compared to patients treated with ARIMIDEX 1 mg ($p<0.0001$). Other differences were not statistically significant.

An examination of the magnitude of change in weight in all patients was also conducted. Thirty-four percent (87/253) of the patients treated with megestrol acetate experienced weight gain of 5% or more and 11% (27/253) of the patients treated with megestrol acetate experienced weight gain of 10% or more. Among patients treated with ARIMIDEX 1 mg, 13% [33/262] experienced weight gain of 5% or more and 3% [6/262] experienced weight gain of 10% or more. On average, this 5 to 10% weight gain represented between 6 and 12 pounds.

No patients receiving ARIMIDEX or megestrol acetate discontinued treatment due to drug-related weight gain.

Vaginal bleeding has been reported infrequently, mainly in patients during the first few weeks after changing from existing hormonal therapy to treatment with ARIMIDEX. If bleeding persists, further evaluation should be considered.

During clinical trials and postmarketing experience joint pain/stiffness has been reported in association with the use of ARIMIDEX.

ARIMIDEX may also be associated with rash including very rare cases of mucocutaneous disorders such as erythema multiforme and Stevens-Johnson syndrome.

OVERDOSAGE

Clinical trials have been conducted with ARIMIDEX, up to 60 mg in a single dose given to healthy male volunteers and up to 10 mg daily given to postmenopausal women with advanced breast cancer; these dosages were well tolerated. A single dose of ARIMIDEX that results in life-threatening symptoms has not been established. In rats, lethality was observed after single oral doses that were greater than 100 mg/kg (about 800 times the recommended human dose on a mg/m^2 basis) and was associated with severe irritation to the stomach (necrosis, gastritis, ulceration, and hemorrhage).

In an oral acute toxicity study in the dog the median lethal dose was greater than 45 mg/kg/day.

There is no specific antidote to overdosage and treatment must be symptomatic. In the management of an overdose, consider that multiple agents may have been taken. Vomiting may be induced if the patient is alert. Dialysis may be helpful because ARIMIDEX is not highly protein bound. General supportive care, including frequent monitoring of vital signs and close observation of the patient, is indicated.

DOSAGE AND ADMINISTRATION

The dose of ARIMIDEX is one 1 mg tablet taken once a day. For patients with advanced breast cancer, ARIMIDEX should be continued until tumor progression.

For adjuvant treatment of early breast cancer in postmenopausal women, the optimal duration of therapy is unknown. The median duration of therapy at the time of data analysis was 31 months; the ongoing ATAC trial is planned for five years of treatment.

Patients with Hepatic Impairment
(See **CLINICAL PHARMACOLOGY**) Hepatic metabolism accounts for approximately 85% of anastrozole elimination. Although clearance of anastrozole was decreased in patients with cirrhosis due to alcohol abuse, plasma anastrozole concentrations stayed in the usual range seen in patients without liver disease. Therefore, no changes in dose are recommended for patients with mild-to-moderate hepatic impairment, although patients should be monitored for side effects. ARIMIDEX has not been studied in patients with severe hepatic impairment.

Patients with Renal Impairment
No changes in dose are necessary for patients with renal impairment.

Use in the Elderly
No dosage adjustment is necessary.

HOW SUPPLIED

White, biconvex, film-coated tablets containing 1 mg of anastrozole. The tablets are impressed on one side with a logo consisting of a letter "A" (upper case) with an arrowhead attached to the foot of the extended right leg of the "A" and on the reverse with the tablet strength marking "Adx 1". These tablets are supplied in bottles of 30 tablets (NDC 0310-0201-30).

Storage
Store at controlled room temperature, 20–25°C (68–77°F) [see USP].

AstraZeneca Pharmaceuticals LP
Wilmington, DE 19850
Made in USA
All trademarks are the property of the AstraZeneca group

Rev 09-02 SIC No. 64206-00
Shown in Product Identification Guide, page 306

CASODEX® ℞
[kăs'ō-dĕks]
(bicalutamide) Tablets

DESCRIPTION

CASODEX® (bicalutamide) Tablets for oral administration contain 50 mg of bicalutamide, a non-steroidal antiandrogen with no other known endocrine activity. The chemical name is propanamide, N-[4-cyano-3-(trifluoromethyl)phenyl]-3-[(4-fluorophenyl)sulfonyl]-2-hydroxy-2-methyl-,(+-). The structural and empirical formulas are:

$C_{18}H_{14}N_2O_4F_4S$

Bicalutamide has a molecular weight of 430.37. The pKa' is approximately 12. Bicalutamide is a fine white to off-white powder which is practically insoluble in water at 37°C (5 mg per 1000 mL), slightly soluble in chloroform and absolute ethanol, sparingly soluble in methanol, and soluble in acetone and tetrahydrofuran.

CASODEX is a racemate with its antiandrogenic activity being almost exclusively exhibited by the R-enantiomer of bicalutamide; the S-enantiomer is essentially inactive.

The inactive ingredients of CASODEX Tablets are lactose, magnesium stearate, methylhydroxypropylcellulose, polyethylene glycol, polyvidone, sodium starch glycollate, and titanium dioxide.

CLINICAL PHARMACOLOGY

Mechanism of Action: CASODEX is a non-steroidal antiandrogen. It competitively inhibits the action of androgens by binding to cytosol androgen receptors in the target tissue. Prostatic carcinoma is known to be androgen sensitive and responds to treatment that counteracts the effect of androgen and/or removes the source of androgen.

When CASODEX is combined with luteinizing hormone-releasing hormone (LHRH) analogue therapy, the suppression of serum testosterone induced by the LHRH analogue is not affected. However, in clinical trials with CASODEX as a single agent for prostate cancer, rises in serum testosterone and estradiol have been noted.

Pharmacokinetics
Absorption: Bicalutamide is well-absorbed following oral administration, although the absolute bioavailability is unknown. Co-administration of bicalutamide with food has no clinically significant effect on rate or extent of absorption.
Distribution: Bicalutamide is highly protein-bound (96%). See Drug-Drug Interactions below.
Metabolism/Elimination: Bicalutamide undergoes stereospecific metabolism. The S (inactive) isomer is metabolized primarily by glucuronidation. The R (active) isomer also undergoes glucuronidation but is predominantly oxidized to an inactive metabolite followed by glucuronidation. Both the parent and metabolite glucuronides are eliminated in the urine and feces. The S-enantiomer is rapidly cleared relative to the R-enantiomer, with the R-enantiomer accounting for about 99% of total steady-state plasma levels.

Special Populations
Geriatric: In two studies in patients given 50 or 150 mg daily, no significant relationship between age and steady-state levels of total bicalutamide or the active R-enantiomer has been shown.
Hepatic Insufficiency: No clinically significant difference in the pharmacokinetics of either enantiomer of bicalutamide was noted in patients with mild-to-moderate hepatic disease as compared to healthy controls. However, the half-life of the R-enantiomer was increased approximately 76% (5.9 and 10.4 days for normal and impaired patients, respectively) in patients with severe liver disease (n=4).
Renal Insufficiency: Renal impairment (as measured by creatinine clearance) had no significant effect on the elimination of total bicalutamide or the active R-enantiomer.
Women, Pediatrics: Bicalutamide has not been studied in women or pediatric subjects.
Drug-Drug Interactions: Clinical studies have not shown any drug interactions between bicalutamide and LHRH analogues (goserelin or leuprolide). There is no evidence that bicalutamide induces hepatic enzymes. *In vitro* protein-binding studies have shown that bicalutamide can displace coumarin anticoagulants from binding sites. Prothrombin times should be closely monitored in patients already receiving coumarin anticoagulants who are started on CASODEX.

Pharmacokinetics of the active enantiomer of CASODEX in normal males and patients with prostate cancer are presented in Table 1.

Table 1

Parameter	Mean	Standard Deviation
Normal Males (n=30)		
Apparent Oral Clearance (L/hr)	0.320	0.103
Single Dose Peak Concentration (μg/mL)	0.768	0.178
Single Dose Time to Peak Concentration (hours)	31.3	14.6
Half-Life (days)	5.8	2.29
Patients with Prostate Cancer (n=40)		
C_{SS} (μg/mL)	8.939	3.504

C_{SS} = Mean Steady-State Concentration

Clinical Studies
In a multicenter, double-blind, controlled clinical trial, 813 patients with previously untreated advanced prostate cancer were randomized to receive CASODEX 50 mg once daily (404 patients) or flutamide 250 mg (409 patients) three times a day, each in combination with LHRH analogues (either goserelin acetate implant or leuprolide acetate depot). In an analysis conducted after a median follow-up of 160 weeks was reached, 213 (52.7%) patients treated with CASODEX-LHRH analogue therapy and 235 (57.5%) patients treated with flutamide-LHRH analogue therapy had died. There was no significant difference in survival between treatment groups (see Figure 1). The hazard ratio for time to death (survival) was 0.87 (95% confidence interval 0.72 to 1.05).

Figure 1 - The Kaplan-Meier probability of death for both antiandrogen treatment groups.

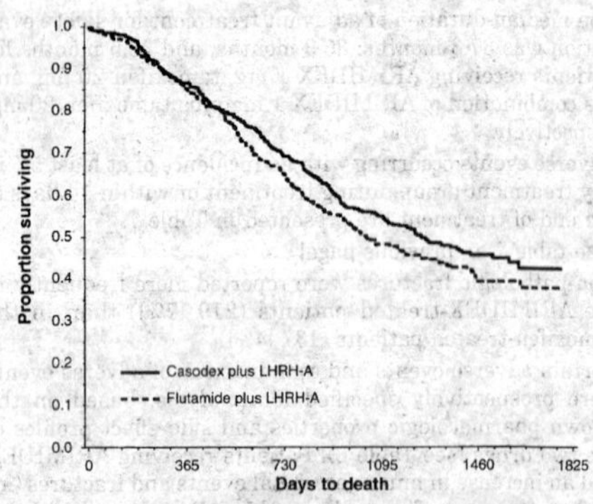

There was no significant difference in time to objective tumor progression between treatment groups (see Figure 2). Objective tumor progression was defined as the appearance of any bone metastases or the worsening of any existing bone metastases on bone scan attributable to metastatic disease, or an increase by 25% or more of any existing measurable extraskeletal metastases. The hazard ratio for time to progression of CASODEX plus LHRH analogue to that of flutamide plus LHRH analogue was 0.93 (95% confidence interval, 0.79 to 1.10).

[See figure 2 at top of next column]

Quality of life was assessed with self-administered patient questionnaires on pain, social functioning, emotional well-being, vitality, activity limitation, bed disability, overall health, physical capacity, general symptoms, and treatment related symptoms. Assessment of the Quality of Life questionnaires did not indicate consistent significant differences between the two treatment groups.

Figure 2 - Kaplan-Meier curve for time to progression for both antiandrogen treatment groups

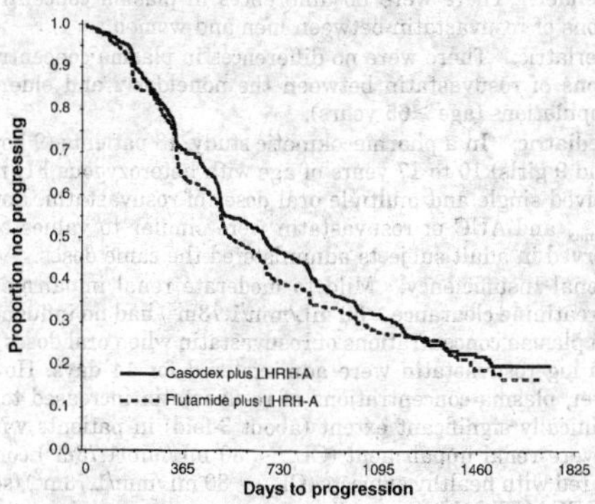

INDICATIONS AND USAGE

CASODEX is indicated for use in combination therapy with a luteinizing hormone-releasing hormone (LHRH) analogue for the treatment of Stage D_2 metastatic carcinoma of the prostate.

CONTRAINDICATIONS

CASODEX is contraindicated in any patient who has shown a hypersensitivity reaction to the drug or any of the tablet's components.

CASODEX has no indication for women, and should not be used in this population, particularly for non-serious or non-life threatening conditions. Further, CASODEX should not be used by women who are or may become pregnant. If this drug is used during pregnancy, or if the patient becomes pregnant while taking this drug, the patient should be apprised of the potential hazard to the fetus. CASODEX may cause fetal harm when administered to pregnant women. The male offspring of rats receiving doses of 10 mg/kg/day (plasma drug concentrations in rats equal to approximately 2/3 human therapeutic concentrations*) and above were observed to have reduced anogenital distance and hypospadias in reproductive toxicology studies. These pharmacological effects have been observed with other antiandrogens. No other teratogenic effects were observed in rabbits receiving doses up to 200 mg/kg/day (approximately 1/3 human therapeutic concentrations*) or rats receiving doses up to 250 mg/kg/day (approximately 2 times human therapeutic concentrations*).

*Based on a maximum dose of 50 mg/day of bicalutamide for an average 70 kg patient.

WARNINGS

Hepatitis: Rare cases of death or hospitalization due to severe liver injury have been reported post-marketing in association with the use of CASODEX. Hepatotoxicity in these reports generally occurred within the first three to four months of treatment. Hepatitis or marked increases in liver enzymes leading to drug discontinuation occurred in approximately 1% of CASODEX patients in controlled clinical trials.

Serum transaminase levels should be measured prior to starting treatment with CASODEX, at regular intervals for the first four months of treatment, and periodically thereafter. If clinical symptoms or signs suggestive of liver dysfunction occur (e.g., nausea, vomiting, abdominal pain, fatigue, anorexia, "flu-like" symptoms, dark urine, jaundice, or right upper quadrant tenderness), the serum transaminases, in particular the serum ALT, should be measured immediately. If at any time a patient has jaundice, or their ALT rises above two times the upper limit of normal, CASODEX should be immediately discontinued with close follow-up of liver function.

PRECAUTIONS

General:

1. CASODEX should be used with caution in patients with moderate-to-severe hepatic impairment. CASODEX is extensively metabolized by the liver. Limited data in subjects with severe hepatic impairment suggest that excretion of CASODEX may be delayed and could lead to further accumulation. Periodic liver function tests should be considered for hepatic-impaired patients on long-term therapy (See WARNINGS).
2. In clinical trials with CASODEX as a single agent for prostate cancer, gynecomastia and breast pain have been reported in up to 38% and 39% of patients, respectively.
3. Regular assessments of serum Prostate Specific Antigen (PSA) may be helpful in monitoring the patient's response. If PSA levels rise during CASODEX therapy, the patient should be evaluated for clinical progression. For patients who have objective progression of disease together with an elevated PSA, a treatment-free period of antiandrogen, while continuing the LHRH analogue, may be considered.

Information for Patients: Patients should be informed that therapy with CASODEX and the LHRH analogue should be initiated concomitantly, and that they should not interrupt or stop taking these medications without consulting their physician. Treatment with CASODEX should be started at the same time as treatment with an LHRH analogue.

Drug Interactions: *In vitro* studies have shown CASODEX can displace coumarin anticoagulants, such as warfarin, from their protein-binding sites. It is recommended that if CASODEX is started in patients already receiving coumarin anticoagulants, prothrombin times should be closely monitored and adjustment of the anticoagulant dose may be necessary (see CLINICAL PHARMACOLOGY, Drug-Drug Interactions).

Carcinogenesis, Mutagenesis, Impairment of Fertility: Two-year oral carcinogenicity studies were conducted in both male and female rats and mice at doses of 5, 15 or 75 mg/kg/day of bicalutamide. A variety of tumor target organ effects were identified and were attributed to the antiandrogenicity of bicalutamide, namely, testicular benign interstitial (Leydig) cell tumors in male rats at all dose levels (the steady-state plasma concentration with the 5 mg/kg/day dose is approximately 2/3 human therapeutic concentrations*) and uterine adenocarcinoma in female rats at 75 mg/kg/day (approximately 1 1/2 times the human therapeutic concentrations*). There is no evidence of Leydig cell hyperplasia in patients; uterine tumors are not relevant to the indicated patient population.

A small increase in the incidence of hepatocellular carcinoma in male mice given 75 mg/kg/day of bicalutamide (approximately 4 times human therapeutic concentrations*) and an increased incidence of benign thyroid follicular cell adenomas in rats given 5 mg/kg/day (approximately 2/3 human therapeutic concentrations*) and above were recorded. These neoplastic changes were progressions of non-neoplastic changes related to hepatic enzyme induction observed in animal toxicity studies. Enzyme induction has not been observed following bicalutamide administration in man. There were no tumorigenic effects suggestive of genotoxic carcinogenesis.

A comprehensive battery of both *in vitro* and *in vivo* genotoxicity tests (yeast gene conversion, Ames, *E. coli*, CHO/HGPRT, human lymphocyte cytogenetic, mouse micronucleus, and rat bone marrow cytogenetic tests) has demonstrated that CASODEX does not have genotoxic activity.

Administration of CASODEX may lead to inhibition of spermatogenesis. The long-term effects of CASODEX on male fertility have not been studied.

In male rats dosed at 250 mg/kg/day (approximately 2 times human therapeutic concentrations*), the precoital interval and time to successful mating were increased in the first pairing but no effects on fertility following successful mating were seen. These effects were reversed by 7 weeks after the end of an 11-week period of dosing.

No effects on female rats dosed at 10, 50 and 250 mg/kg/day (approximately 2/3, 1 and 2 times human therapeutic concentrations, respectively*) or their female offspring were observed. Administration of bicalutamide to pregnant females resulted in feminization of the male offspring leading to hypospadias at all dose levels. Affected male offspring were also impotent.

*Based on a maximum dose of 50 mg/day of bicalutamide for an average 70 kg patient.

Pregnancy: Pregnancy Category X (see CONTRAINDICATIONS).

Nursing Mothers: CASODEX is not indicated for use in women. It is not known whether this drug is excreted in human milk. Because many drugs are excreted in human milk, caution should be exercised when CASODEX is administered to a nursing woman.

Pediatric Use: Safety and effectiveness of CASODEX in pediatric patients have not been established.

ADVERSE REACTIONS

In patients with advanced prostate cancer treated with CASODEX in combination with an LHRH analogue, the most frequent adverse experience was hot flashes (53%).

In the multicenter, double-blind, controlled clinical trial comparing CASODEX 50 mg once daily with flutamide 250 mg three times a day, each in combination with an LHRH analogue, the following adverse experiences with an incidence of 5% or greater, regardless of causality, have been reported.

Table 2
Incidence of Adverse Events
(≥ 5% in Either Treatment Group)
Regardless of Causality

Body System Adverse Event	Treatment Group Number of Patients (%)	
	CASODEX Plus LHRH Analogue (n = 401)	Flutamide Plus LHRH Analogue (n = 407)
Body as a Whole		
Pain (General)	142 (35)	127 (31)
Back Pain	102 (25)	105 (26)
Asthenia	89 (22)	87 (21)
Pelvic Pain	85 (21)	70 (17)
Infection	71 (18)	57 (14)
Abdominal Pain	46 (11)	46 (11)
Chest Pain	34 (8)	34 (8)
Headache	29 (7)	27 (7)
Flu Syndrome	28 (7)	30 (7)
Cardiovascular		
Hot Flashes	211 (53)	217 (53)
Hypertension	34 (8)	29 (7)
Digestive		
Constipation	87 (22)	69 (17)
Nausea	62 (15)	58 (14)
Diarrhea	49 (12)	107 (26)
Increased Liver Enzyme Test†	30 (7)	46 (11)
Dyspepsia	30 (7)	23 (6)
Flatulence	26 (6)	22 (5)
Anorexia	25 (6)	29 (7)
Vomiting	24 (6)	32 (8)
Hemic and Lymphatic		
Anemia††	45 (11)	53 (13)
Metabolic and Nutritional		
Peripheral Edema	53 (13)	42 (10)
Weight Loss	30 (7)	39 (10)
Hyperglycemia	26 (6)	27 (7)
Alkaline Phosphatase Increased	22 (5)	24 (6)
Weight Gain	22 (5)	18 (4)
Musculoskeletal		
Bone Pain	37 (9)	43 (11)
Myasthenia	27 (7)	19 (5)
Arthritis	21 (5)	29 (7)
Pathological Fracture	17 (4)	32 (8)
Nervous System		
Dizziness	41 (10)	35 (9)
Paresthesia	31 (8)	40 (10)
Insomnia	27 (7)	39 (10)
Anxiety	20 (5)	9 (2)
Depression	16 (4)	33 (8)
Respiratory System		
Dyspnea	51 (13)	32 (8)
Cough Increased	33 (8)	24 (6)
Pharyngitis	32 (8)	23 (6)
Bronchitis	24 (6)	22 (3)
Pneumonia	18 (4)	19 (5)
Rhinitis	15 (4)	22 (5)
Skin and Appendages		
Rash	35 (9)	30 (7)
Sweating	25 (6)	20 (5)
Urogenital		
Nocturia	49 (12)	55 (14)
Hematuria	48 (12)	26 (6)
Urinary Tract Infection	35 (9)	36 (9)
Gynecomastia	36 (9)	30 (7)
Impotence	27 (7)	35 (9)
Breast Pain	23 (6)	15 (4)
Urinary Frequency	23 (6)	29 (7)
Urinary Retention	20 (5)	14 (3)
Urination Impaired	19 (5)	15 (4)
Urinary Incontinence	15 (4)	32 (8)

†Increased liver enzyme test includes increases in AST, ALT or both.

††Anemia includes anemia, hypochromic- and iron deficiency anemia.

Other adverse experiences (greater than or equal to 2%, but less than 5%) reported in the CASODEX-LHRH analogue treatment group are listed below by body system and are in order of decreasing frequency within each body system regardless of causality.

Body as a Whole: Neoplasm; Neck pain; Fever; Chills; Sepsis; Hernia; Cyst

Cardiovascular: Angina pectoris; Congestive heart failure; Myocardial infarct; Heart arrest; Coronary artery disorder; Syncope

Digestive: Melena; Rectal hemorrhage; Dry mouth; Dysphagia; Gastrointestinal disorder; Periodontal abscess; Gastrointestinal carcinoma

Metabolic and Nutritional: Edema; Bun increased; Creatinine increased; Dehydration; Gout; Hypercholesteremia

Musculoskeletal: Myalgia; Leg cramps

Nervous: Hypertonia; Confusion; Somnolence; Libido decreased; Neuropathy; Nervousness

Respiratory: Lung disorder; Asthma; Epistaxis; Sinusitis

Skin and Appendages: Dry skin; Alopecia; Pruritus; Herpes zoster; Skin carcinoma; Skin disorder

Special Senses: Cataract specified

Urogenital: Dysuria; Urinary urgency; Hydronephrosis; Urinary tract disorder

Abnormal Laboratory Test Values: Laboratory abnormalities including elevated AST, ALT, bilirubin, BUN, and creatinine and decreased hemoglobin and white cell count have been reported in both CASODEX-LHRH analogue treated and flutamide-LHRH analogue treated patients.

Postmarketing Experience: Rare cases of interstitial pneumonitis and pulmonary fibrosis have been reported with CASODEX.

OVERDOSAGE

Long-term clinical trials have been conducted with dosages up to 200 mg of CASODEX daily and these dosages have been well tolerated. A single dose of CASODEX that results in symptoms of an overdose considered to be life-threatening has not been established.

There is no specific antidote; treatment of an overdose should be symptomatic.

In the management of an overdose with CASODEX, vomiting may be induced if the patient is alert. It should be remembered that, in this patient population, multiple drugs may have been taken. Dialysis is not likely to be helpful since CASODEX is highly protein bound and is extensively

Continued on next page

Casodex—Cont.

metabolized. General supportive care, including frequent monitoring of vital signs and close observation of the patient, is indicated.

DOSAGE AND ADMINISTRATION

The recommended dose for CASODEX therapy in combination with an LHRH analogue is one 50 mg tablet once daily (morning or evening), with or without food. It is recommended that CASODEX be taken at the same time each day. Treatment with CASODEX should be started at the same time as treatment with an LHRH analogue.

Dosage Adjustment in Renal Impairment: No dosage adjustment is necessary for patients with renal impairment (see CLINICAL PHARMACOLOGY, Special Populations, Renal Insufficiency).

Dosage Adjustment in Hepatic Impairment: No dosage adjustment is necessary for patients with mild to moderate hepatic impairment. Although there is a 76% (5.9 and 10.4 days for normal and impaired patients, respectively) increase in the half-life of the active enantiomer of bicalutamide in patients with severe liver impairment (n=4), no dosage adjustment is necessary (see CLINICAL PHARMACOLOGY, Special Populations, Hepatic Impairment, PRECAUTIONS and WARNINGS sections).

HOW SUPPLIED

50 mg Tablets. (NDC 0310-0705) White, film-coated tablets (identified on one side with "CDX50" and on the reverse with the "CASODEX logo") are supplied in unit dose blisters of 30 tablets per carton (0310-0705-39), bottles of 30 tablets (0310-0705-30) and bottles of 100 tablets (0310-0705-10).

Store at controlled room temperature, 20-25°C (68-77°F).

AstraZeneca

Manufactured for
AstraZeneca Pharmaceuticals LP
Wilmington, DE 19850
by AstraZeneca GmbH, Plankstadt, Germany
Made in Germany
O:\CAS NEWARK 09-02 Rev. 09/02

Shown in Product Identification Guide, page 306

CEFOTAN® ℞

[cef 'o-tan]

cefotetan disodium for injection

For Intravenous or Intramuscular Use

CEFOTAN® ℞

cefotetan injection

In GALAXY® Plastic Container (PL 2040)

For Intravenous Use Only

Shown in Product Identification Guide, page 306

CRESTOR® ℞

[krĕs-tōr]

(rosuvastatin calcium)

DESCRIPTION

CRESTOR® (rosuvastatin calcium) is a synthetic lipid-lowering agent. Rosuvastatin is an inhibitor of 3-hydroxy-3-methylglutaryl-coenzyme A (HMG-CoA) reductase. This enzyme catalyzes the conversion of HMG-CoA to mevalonate, an early and rate-limiting step in cholesterol biosynthesis.

Rosuvastatin calcium is bis[(E)-7-[4-(4-fluorophenyl)-6-isopropyl-2-[methyl(methylsulfonyl)amino] pyrimidin-5-yl](3R,5S)-3,5-dihydroxyhept-6-enoic acid] calcium salt. The empirical formula for rosuvastatin calcium is $(C_{22}H_{27}FN_3O_6S)_2Ca$. Its molecular weight is 1001.14. Its structural formula is:

Rosuvastatin calcium is a white amorphous powder that is sparingly soluble in water and methanol, and slightly soluble in ethanol. Rosuvastatin is a hydrophilic compound with a partition coefficient (octanol/water) of 0.13 at pH of 7.0.

CRESTOR Tablets for oral administration contain 5, 10, 20, or 40 mg of rosuvastatin and the following inactive ingredients: microcrystalline cellulose NF, lactose monohydrate NF, tribasic calcium phosphate NF, crospovidone NF, magnesium stearate NF, hypromellose NF, triacetin NF, titanium dioxide USP, yellow ferric oxide, and red ferric oxide NF.

CLINICAL PHARMACOLOGY

General: In the bloodstream, cholesterol and triglycerides (TG) circulate as part of lipoprotein complexes. With ultracentrifugation, these complexes separate into very-low-density lipoprotein (VLDL), intermediate-density lipoprotein (IDL), and low-density lipoprotein (LDL) fractions that contain apolipoprotein B-100 (ApoB-100) and high-density lipoprotein (HDL) fractions.

Cholesterol and TG synthesized in the liver are incorporated into VLDL and secreted into the circulation for delivery to peripheral tissues. TG are removed by the action of lipases, and in a series of steps, the modified VLDL is transformed first into IDL and then into cholesterol-rich LDL. IDL and LDL are removed from the circulation mainly by high affinity ApoB/E receptors, which are expressed to the greatest extent on liver cells. HDL is hypothesized to participate in the reverse transport of cholesterol from tissues back to the liver.

Epidemiologic, experimental, and clinical studies have established that high LDL cholesterol (LDL-C), low HDL cholesterol (HDL-C), and high plasma TG promote human atherosclerosis and are risk factors for developing cardiovascular disease. In contrast, higher levels of HDL-C are associated with decreased cardiovascular risk.

Like LDL, cholesterol-enriched triglyceride-rich lipoproteins, including VLDL, IDL, and remnants, can also promote atherosclerosis. Elevated plasma triglycerides are frequently found with low HDL-C levels and small LDL particles, as well as in association with non-lipid metabolic risk factors for coronary heart disease (CHD). As such, total plasma TG has not consistently been shown to be an independent risk factor for CHD. Furthermore, the independent effect of raising HDL or lowering TG on the risk of coronary and cardiovascular morbidity and mortality has not been determined.

Mechanism of Action: Rosuvastatin is a selective and competitive inhibitor of HMG-CoA reductase, the rate-limiting enzyme that converts 3-hydroxy-3-methylglutaryl coenzyme A to mevalonate, a precursor of cholesterol. *In vivo* studies in animals, and *in vitro* studies in cultured animal and human cells have shown rosuvastatin to have a high uptake into, and selectivity for, action in the liver, the target organ for cholesterol lowering. In *in vivo* and *in vitro* studies, rosuvastatin produces its lipid-modifying effects in two ways. First, it increases the number of hepatic LDL receptors on the cell-surface to enhance uptake and catabolism of LDL. Second, rosuvastatin inhibits hepatic synthesis of VLDL, which reduces the total number of VLDL and LDL particles.

Rosuvastatin reduces total cholesterol (total-C), LDL-C, ApoB, and nonHDL-C (total cholesterol minus HDL-C) in patients with homozygous and heterozygous familial hypercholesterolemia (FH), nonfamilial forms of hypercholesterolemia, and mixed dyslipidemia. Rosuvastatin also reduces TG and produces increases in HDL-C. Rosuvastatin reduces total-C, LDL-C, VLDL-cholesterol (VLDL-C), ApoB, nonHDL-C, and TG, and increases HDL-C in patients with isolated hypertriglyceridemia. The effect of rosuvastatin on cardiovascular morbidity and mortality has not been determined.

Pharmacokinetics and Drug Metabolism

Absorption: In clinical pharmacology studies in man, peak plasma concentrations of rosuvastatin were reached 3 to 5 hours following oral dosing. Both peak concentration (C_{max}) and area under the plasma concentration-time curve (AUC) increased in approximate proportion to rosuvastatin dose. The absolute bioavailability of rosuvastatin is approximately 20%.

Administration of rosuvastatin with food decreased the rate of drug absorption by 20% as assessed by C_{max}, but there was no effect on the extent of absorption as assessed by AUC.

Plasma concentrations of rosuvastatin do not differ following evening or morning drug administration.

Significant LDL-C reductions are seen when rosuvastatin is given with or without food, and regardless of the time of day of drug administration.

Distribution: Mean volume of distribution at steady-state of rosuvastatin is approximately 134 liters. Rosuvastatin is 88% bound to plasma proteins, mostly albumin. This binding is reversible and independent of plasma concentrations.

Metabolism: Rosuvastatin is not extensively metabolized; approximately 10% of a radiolabeled dose is recovered as metabolite. The major metabolite is N-desmethyl rosuvastatin, which is formed principally by cytochrome P450 2C9, and *in vitro* studies have demonstrated that N-desmethyl rosuvastatin has approximately one-sixth to one-half the HMG-CoA reductase inhibitory activity of rosuvastatin. Overall, greater than 90% of active plasma HMG-CoA reductase inhibitory activity is accounted for by rosuvastatin.

Excretion: Following oral administration, rosuvastatin and its metabolites are primarily excreted in the feces (90%). The elimination half-life ($t_{1/2}$) of rosuvastatin is approximately 19 hours.

After an intravenous dose, approximately 28% of total body clearance was via the renal route, and 72% by the hepatic route.

Special Populations

Race: A population pharmacokinetic analysis revealed no clinically relevant differences in pharmacokinetics among Caucasian, Hispanic, and Black or Afro-Caribbean groups. However, pharmacokinetic studies show an approximate 2-fold elevation in median exposure (AUC) in Japanese subjects residing in Japan and in Chinese subjects residing in Singapore when compared with Caucasians residing in North America and Europe. No studies directly examining Asian ethnic populations residing in the U.S. are available, so the contribution of environmental and genetic factors to the observed increases in rosuvastatin drug levels have not been determined. (See WARNINGS, Myopathy/Rhabdomyolysis, and PRECAUTIONS, General.)

Gender: There were no differences in plasma concentrations of rosuvastatin between men and women.

Geriatric: There were no differences in plasma concentrations of rosuvastatin between the nonelderly and elderly populations (age ≥65 years).

Pediatric: In a pharmacokinetic study, 18 patients (9 boys and 9 girls) 10 to 17 years of age with heterozygous FH received single and multiple oral doses of rosuvastatin. Both C_{max} and AUC of rosuvastatin were similar to values observed in adult subjects administered the same doses.

Renal Insufficiency: Mild to moderate renal impairment (creatinine clearance ≥30 mL/min/1.73m²) had no influence on plasma concentrations of rosuvastatin when oral doses of 20 mg rosuvastatin were administered for 14 days. However, plasma concentrations of rosuvastatin increased to a clinically significant extent (about 3-fold) in patients with severe renal impairment (CL_{cr} < 30 mL/min/1.73m²) compared with healthy subjects (CL_{cr} > 80 mL/min/1.73m²) (see PRECAUTIONS, General).

Hemodialysis: Steady-state plasma concentrations of rosuvastatin in patients on chronic hemodialysis were approximately 50% greater compared with healthy volunteer subjects with normal renal function.

Hepatic Insufficiency: In patients with chronic alcohol liver disease, plasma concentrations of rosuvastatin were modestly increased. In patients with Child-Pugh A disease, C_{max} and AUC were increased by 60% and 5%, respectively, as compared with patients with normal liver function. In patients with Child-Pugh B disease, C_{max} and AUC were increased 100% and 21%, respectively, compared with patients with normal liver function (see CONTRAINDICATIONS and WARNINGS, Liver Enzymes).

Drug-Drug Interactions

Cytochrome P450 3A4: *In vitro* and *in vivo* data indicate that rosuvastatin clearance is not dependent on metabolism by cytochrome P450 3A4 to a clinically significant extent. This has been confirmed in studies with known cytochrome P450 3A4 inhibitors (ketoconazole, erythromycin, itraconazole).

Ketoconazole: Coadministration of ketoconazole (200 mg twice daily for 7 days) with rosuvastatin (80 mg) resulted in no change in plasma concentrations of rosuvastatin.

Erythromycin: Coadministration of erythromycin (500 mg four times daily for 7 days) with rosuvastatin (80 mg) decreased AUC and C_{max} of rosuvastatin by 20% and 31%, respectively. These reductions are not considered clinically significant.

Itraconazole: Itraconazole (200 mg once daily for 5 days) resulted in a 39% and 28% increase in AUC of rosuvastatin after 10 mg and 80 mg dosing, respectively. These increases are not considered clinically significant.

Fluconazole: Coadministration of fluconazole (200 mg once daily for 11 days) with rosuvastatin (80 mg) resulted in a 14% increase in AUC of rosuvastatin. This increase is not considered clinically significant.

Cyclosporine: Coadministration of cyclosporine with rosuvastatin resulted in no significant changes in cyclosporine plasma concentrations. However, C_{max} and AUC of rosuvastatin increased 11- and 7-fold, respectively, compared with historical data in healthy subjects. These increases are considered to be clinically significant (see PRECAUTIONS, Drug Interactions, WARNINGS, Myopathy/Rhabdomyolysis, and DOSAGE AND ADMINISTRATION).

Warfarin: Coadministration of warfarin (20 mg) with rosuvastatin (40 mg) did not change warfarin plasma concentrations but increased the International Normalized Ratio (INR) (see PRECAUTIONS, Drug Interactions).

Digoxin: Coadministration of digoxin (0.5 mg) with rosuvastatin (40 mg) resulted in no change to digoxin plasma concentrations.

Fenofibrate: Coadministration of fenofibrate (67 mg three times daily) with rosuvastatin (10 mg) resulted in no significant changes in plasma concentrations of rosuvastatin or fenofibrate (see PRECAUTIONS, Drug Interactions and WARNINGS, Myopathy/Rhabdomyolysis).

Gemfibrozil: Coadministration of gemfibrozil (600 mg twice daily for 7 days) with rosuvastatin (80 mg) resulted in a 90% and 120% increase for AUC and C_{max} of rosuvastatin, respectively. This increase is considered to be clinically significant (see PRECAUTIONS, Drug Interactions, WARNINGS, Myopathy/Rhabdomyolysis, DOSAGE AND ADMINISTRATION).

Antacid: Coadministration of an antacid (aluminum and magnesium hydroxide combination) with rosuvastatin (40 mg) resulted in a decrease in plasma concentrations of rosuvastatin by 54%. However, when the antacid was given 2 hours after rosuvastatin, there were no clinically significant changes in plasma concentrations of rosuvastatin (see PRECAUTIONS, Information for Patients).

Oral contraceptives: Coadministration of oral contraceptives (ethinyl estradiol and norgestrel) with rosuvastatin resulted in an increase in plasma concentrations of ethinyl estradiol and norgestrel by 26% and 34%, respectively.

Clinical Studies

Hypercholesterolemia (Heterozygous Familial and Nonfamilial) and Mixed Dyslipidemia (Fredrickson Type IIa and IIb)

CRESTOR reduces total-C, LDL-C, ApoB, nonHDL-C, and TG, and increases HDL-C, in patients with hypercholesterolemia and mixed dyslipidemia. Therapeutic response is seen within 1 week, and maximum response is usually achieved within 4 weeks and maintained during long-term therapy.

CRESTOR is effective in a wide variety of adult patient populations with hypercholesterolemia, with and without hypertriglyceridemia, regardless of race, gender, or age and in special populations such as diabetics or patients with heterozygous FH. Experience in pediatric patients has been limited to patients with homozygous FH.

Dose-Ranging Study: In a multicenter, double-blind, placebo-controlled, dose-ranging study in patients with hypercholesterolemia, CRESTOR given as a single daily dose for 6 weeks significantly reduced total-C, LDL-C, nonHDL-C, and ApoB, across the dose range (Table 1).

Table 1.
Dose-Response in Patients With Primary Hypercholesterolemia (Adjusted Mean % Change From Baseline at Week 6)

Dose	N	Total-C	LDL-C	Non HDL-C	ApoB	TG	HDL-C
Placebo	13	-5	-7	-7	-3	-3	3
5	17	-33	-45	-44	-38	-35	13
10	17	-36	-52	-48	-42	-10	14
20	17	-40	-55	-51	-46	-23	8
40	18	-46	-63	-60	-54	-28	10

Active-Controlled Study: CRESTOR was compared with the HMG-CoA reductase inhibitors atorvastatin, simvastatin, and pravastatin in a multicenter, open-label, dose-ranging study of 2,240 patients with Type IIa and IIb hypercholesterolemia. After randomization, patients were treated for 6 weeks with a single daily dose of either CRESTOR, atorvastatin, simvastatin, or pravastatin (Figure 1 and Table 2).

Figure 1.
Percent LDL-C Change by Dose of CRESTOR, Atorvastatin, Simvastatin, and Pravastatin at Week 6 in Patients With Type IIa/IIb Dyslipidemia

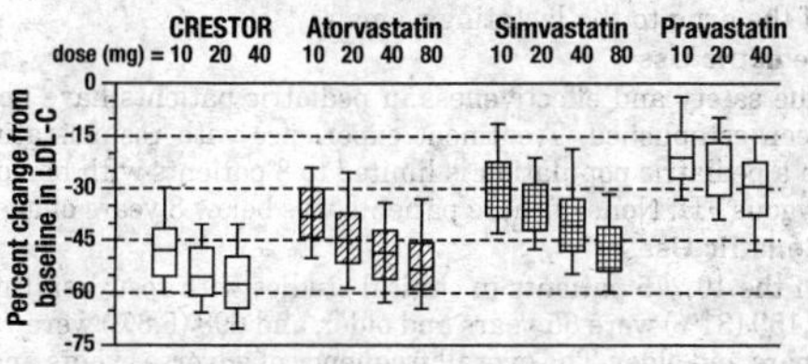

Box plots are a representation of the 25th, 50th, and 75th percentile values, with whiskers representing the 10th and 90th percentile values. Mean baseline LDL-C: 189 mg/dL.

Table 2.
Percent Change in LDL-C From Baseline to Week 6 (LS means§) by Treatment Group (sample sizes ranging from 156-157 patients per group)

Treatment	Treatment Daily Dose 10 mg	20 mg	40 mg	80 mg
CRESTOR	-46*	-52†	-55‡	—
Atorvastatin	-37	-43	-48	-51
Pravastatin	-20	-24	-30	—
Simvastatin	-28	-35	-39	-46

* CRESTOR 10 mg reduced LDL-C significantly more than atorvastatin 10 mg; pravastatin 10 mg, 20 mg, and 40 mg; simvastatin 10 mg, 20 mg, and 40 mg. ($p<0.002$)

† CRESTOR 20 mg reduced LDL-C significantly more than atorvastatin 20 mg and 40 mg; pravastatin 20 mg, and 40 mg; simvastatin 20 mg, 40 mg, and 80 mg. ($p<0.002$)

‡ CRESTOR 40 mg reduced LDL-C significantly more than atorvastatin 40 mg; pravastatin 40 mg; simvastatin 40 mg and 80 mg. ($p<0.002$)

§ Corresponding standard errors are approximately 1.00

Heterozygous Familial Hypercholesterolemia

In a study of patients with heterozygous FH (baseline mean LDL of 291), patients were randomized to CRESTOR 20 mg or atorvastatin 20 mg. The dose was increased by 6-week intervals. Significant LDL-C reductions from baseline were seen at each dose in both treatment groups (Table 3).

Table 3.
Mean LDL-C Percentage Change from Baseline

		CRESTOR (n=435) LS Mean* (95% CI)	Atorvastatin (n=187) LS Mean (95% CI)
Week 6	20 mg	-47% (-49%, -46%)	-38% (-40%, -36%)
Week 12	40 mg	-55% (-57%, -54%)	-47% (-49%, -45%)
Week 18	80 mg	NA	-52% (-54%, -50%)

*LS Means are least square means adjusted for baseline LDL.

Table 4.
Dose-Response in Patients With Primary Hypertriglyceridemia Over 6 Weeks Dosing Median (Min, Max) Percent Change From Baseline

Dose	Placebo N=26	CRESTOR 5 mg N=25	CRESTOR 10 mg N=23	CRESTOR 20 mg N=27	CRESTOR 40 mg N=25
Triglycerides	1 (-40, 72)	-21 (-58, 38)	-37 (-65, 5)	-37 (-72, 11)	-43 (-80, -7)
NonHDL-C	2 (-13, 19)	-29 (-43, -8)	-49 (-59, -20)	-43 (-74, 12)	-51 (-62, -6)
VLDL-C	2 (-36, 53)	-25 (-62, 49)	-48 (-72, 14)	-49 (-83, 20)	-56 (-83, 10)
Total-C	1 (-13, 17)	-24 (-40, -4)	-40 (-51, -14)	-34 (-61, -11)	-40 (-51, -4)
LDL-C	5 (-30, 52)	-28 (-71, 2)	-45 (-59, 7)	-31 (-66, 34)	-43 (-61, -3)
HDL-C	-3 (-25, 18)	3 (-38, 33)	8 (-8, 24)	22 (-5, 50)	17 (-14, 63)

Table 5.
NCEP Treatment Guidelines: LDL-C Goals and Cutpoints for Therapeutic Lifestyle Changes and Drug Therapy in Different Risk Categories

Risk Category	LDL Goal	LDL level at which to initiate TLC	LDL level at which to consider drug therapy
CHD[a] or CHD Risk Equivalent (10-year risk > 20%)	<100 mg/dL	≥100 mg/dL	≥130 mg/dL (100-129 mg/dL: drug optional)[c]
2+ Risk Factors (10-year risk ≤ 20%)	<130 mg/dL	≥ 130 mg/dL	≥130 mg/dL 10-year risk 10-20%
			≥160 mg/dL 10-year risk <10%
0-1 Risk Factor[b]	<160 mg/dL	≥160 mg/dL	≥190 mg/dL (160-189 mg/dL LDL-lowering drug optional)

[a] CHD = coronary heart disease.

[b] Some authorities recommend use of LDL-lowering drugs in this category if an LDL-C <100 mg/dL cannot be achieved by TLC. Others prefer use of drugs that primarily modify triglycerides and HDL-C, e.g., nicotinic acid or fibrate. Clinical judgment also may call for deferring drug therapy in this subcategory.

[c] Almost all people with 0-1 risk factor have 10-year risk <10%; thus, 10-year risk assessment in people with 0-1 risk factor is not necessary.

Hypertriglyceridemia (Fredrickson Type IIb & IV)

In a double-blind, placebo-controlled dose-response study in patients with baseline TG levels from 273 to 817 mg/dL, CRESTOR given as a single daily dose (5 to 40 mg) over 6 weeks significantly reduced serum TG levels (Table 4).

[See table 4 above]

Homozygous Familial Hypercholesterolemia

In an open-label, forced-titration study, homozygous FH patients (n=40, 8-63 years) were evaluated for their response to CRESTOR 20 to 40 mg titrated at a 6-week interval. In the overall population, the mean LDL-C reduction from baseline was 22%. About one-third of the patients benefited from increasing their dose from 20 mg to 40 mg with further LDL lowering of greater than 6%. In the 27 patients with at least a 15% reduction in LDL-C, the mean LDL-C reduction was 30% (median 28% reduction). Among 13 patients with an LDL-C reduction of <15%, 3 had no change or an increase in LDL-C. Reductions in LDL-C of 15% or greater were observed in 3 of 5 patients with known receptor negative status.

INDICATIONS AND USAGE

CRESTOR is indicated:

1. as an adjunct to diet to reduce elevated total-C, LDL-C, ApoB, nonHDL-C, and TG levels and to increase HDL-C in patients with primary hypercholesterolemia (heterozygous familial and nonfamilial) and mixed dyslipidemia (Fredrickson Type IIa and IIb);
2. as an adjunct to diet for the treatment of patients with elevated serum TG levels (Fredrickson Type IV);
3. to reduce LDL-C, total-C, and ApoB in patients with homozygous familial hypercholesterolemia as an adjunct to other lipid-lowering treatments (e.g., LDL apheresis) or if such treatments are unavailable.

According to NCEP-ATPIII guidelines, therapy with lipid-altering agents should be a component of multiple-risk-factor intervention in individuals at increased risk for coronary heart disease due to hypercholesterolemia. The two major modalities of LDL-lowering therapy are therapeutic lifestyle changes (TLC) and drug therapy. The TLC Diet stresses reductions in saturated fat and cholesterol intake. Table 5 defines LDL-C goals and cutpoints for initiation of TLC and for drug consideration.

[See table 5 above]

After the LDL-C goal has been achieved, if the TG is still ≥ 200 mg/dL, nonHDL-C (total-C minus HDL-C) becomes a secondary target of therapy. NonHDL-C goals are set 30 mg/dL higher than LDL-C goals for each risk category.

At the time of hospitalization for a coronary event, consideration can be given to initiating drug therapy at discharge if the LDL-C is ≥ 130 mg/dL (see NCEP Treatment Guidelines, above).

Patients >20 years of age should be screened for elevated cholesterol levels every 5 years.

Prior to initiating therapy with CRESTOR, secondary causes for hypercholesterolemia (e.g., poorly-controlled diabetes mellitus, hypothyroidism, nephrotic syndrome, dyslipoproteinemias, obstructive liver disease, other drug therapy, and alcoholism) should be excluded, and a lipid profile performed to measure total-C, LDL-C, HDL-C, and TG. For patients with TG <400 mg/dL (<4.5 mmol/L), LDL-C can be estimated using the following equation: $\text{LDL-C} = \text{total-C} - (0.20 \times [\text{TG}] + \text{HDL-C})$. For TG levels >400 mg/dL (>4.5 mmol/L), this equation is less accurate and LDL-C concentrations should be determined by ultracentrifugation.

CRESTOR has not been studied in Fredrickson Type I, III, and V dyslipidemias.

CONTRAINDICATIONS

CRESTOR is contraindicated in patients with a known hypersensitivity to any component of this product.

Rosuvastatin is contraindicated in patients with active liver disease or with unexplained persistent elevations of serum transaminases (see WARNINGS, Liver Enzymes).

Pregnancy and Lactation

Atherosclerosis is a chronic process and discontinuation of lipid-lowering drugs during pregnancy should have little impact on the outcome of long-term therapy of primary hypercholesterolemia. Cholesterol and other products of cholesterol biosynthesis are essential components for fetal development (including synthesis of steroids and cell membranes). Since HMG-CoA reductase inhibitors decrease cholesterol synthesis and possibly the synthesis of other biologically active substances derived from cholesterol, they may cause fetal harm when administered to pregnant women. Therefore, HMG-CoA reductase inhibitors are contraindicated during pregnancy and in nursing mothers. ROSUVASTATIN SHOULD BE ADMINISTERED TO WOMEN OF CHILDBEARING AGE ONLY WHEN SUCH PATIENTS ARE HIGHLY UNLIKELY TO CONCEIVE AND HAVE BEEN INFORMED OF THE POTENTIAL HAZARDS. If the patient becomes pregnant while taking this drug, therapy should be discontinued immediately and the patient apprised of the potential hazard to the fetus.

WARNINGS

Liver Enzymes

HMG-CoA reductase inhibitors, like some other lipid-lowering therapies, have been associated with biochemical abnormalities of liver function. The incidence of persistent elevations (>3 times the upper limit of normal [ULN] occurring on 2 or more consecutive occasions) in serum transaminases in fixed dose studies was 0.4, 0, 0, and 0.1% in patients who received rosuvastatin 5, 10, 20, and 40 mg, respectively. In most cases, the elevations were transient and resolved or improved on continued therapy or after a brief interruption in therapy. There were two cases of jaundice, for which a relationship to rosuvastatin therapy could not be determined, which resolved after discontinuation of therapy. There were no cases of liver failure or irreversible liver disease in these trials.

It is recommended that liver function tests be performed before and at 12 weeks following both the initiation of therapy and any elevation of dose, and periodically (e.g., semiannually) thereafter. Liver enzyme changes generally occur in the first 3 months of treatment with rosuvastatin. Patients who develop increased transaminase levels should be monitored until the abnormalities have resolved. Should an increase in ALT or AST of >3 times ULN persist, reduction of dose or withdrawal of rosuvastatin is recommended.

Rosuvastatin should be used with caution in patients who consume substantial quantities of alcohol and/or have a history of liver disease (see CLINICAL PHARMACOLOGY, Special Populations, Hepatic Insufficiency). Active liver

Continued on next page

Crestor—Cont.

disease or unexplained persistent transaminase elevations are contraindications to the use of rosuvastatin (see CONTRAINDICATIONS).

Myopathy/Rhabdomyolysis

Rare cases of rhabdomyolysis with acute renal failure secondary to myoglobinuria have been reported with rosuvastatin and with other drugs in this class.

Uncomplicated myalgia has been reported in rosuvastatin-treated patients (see ADVERSE REACTIONS). Creatine kinase (CK) elevations (>10 times upper limit of normal) occurred in 0.2% to 0.4% of patients taking rosuvastatin at doses up to 40 mg in clinical studies. Treatment-related myopathy, defined as muscle aches or muscle weakness in conjunction with increases in CK values >10 times upper limit of normal, was reported in up to 0.1% of patients taking rosuvastatin doses of up to 40 mg in clinical studies. Rare cases of rhabdomyolysis were seen with higher than recommended doses (80 mg) of rosuvastatin in clinical trials. Factors that may predispose patients to myopathy with HMG-CoA reductase inhibitors include advanced age (≥65 years), hypothyroidism, and renal insufficiency. The incidence of myopathy increased at doses of rosuvastatin above the recommended dosage range.

Consequently:

1. Rosuvastatin should be prescribed with caution in patients with predisposing factors for myopathy, such as, renal impairment (see DOSAGE AND ADMINISTRATION), advanced age, and hypothyroidism.
2. Patients should be advised to promptly report unexplained muscle pain, tenderness, or weakness, particularly if accompanied by malaise or fever. Rosuvastatin therapy should be discontinued if markedly elevated CK levels occur or myopathy is diagnosed or suspected.
3. The risk of myopathy during treatment with rosuvastatin may be increased with concurrent administration of other lipid-lowering therapies or cyclosporine, (see CLINICAL PHARMACOLOGY, Drug Interactions, PRECAUTIONS, Drug Interactions, and DOSAGE AND ADMINISTRATION). **The benefit of further alterations in lipid levels by the combined use of rosuvastatin with fibrates or niacin should be carefully weighed against the potential risks of this combination. Combination therapy with rosuvastatin and gemfibrozil should generally be avoided. (See DOSAGE AND ADMINISTRATION and PRECAUTIONS, Drug Interactions).**
4. **The risk of myopathy during treatment with rosuvastatin may be increased in circumstances which increase rosuvastatin drug levels (see CLINICAL PHARMACOLOGY, Special Populations, Race and Renal Insufficiency, and PRECAUTIONS, General).**
5. **Rosuvastatin therapy should also be temporarily withheld in any patient with an acute, serious condition suggestive of myopathy or predisposing to the development of renal failure secondary to rhabdomyolysis (e.g., sepsis, hypotension, major surgery, trauma, severe metabolic, endocrine, and electrolyte disorders, or uncontrolled seizures).**

PRECAUTIONS

General

Before instituting therapy with rosuvastatin, an attempt should be made to control hypercholesterolemia with appropriate diet and exercise, weight reduction in obese patients, and treatment of underlying medical problems (see INDICATIONS AND USAGE).

Administration of rosuvastatin 20 mg to patients with severe renal impairment (CL_{cr} <30 mL/min/1.73 m^2) resulted in a 3-fold increase in plasma concentrations of rosuvastatin compared with healthy volunteers (see WARNINGS, Myopathy/Rhabdomyolysis and DOSAGE AND ADMINISTRATION).

Pharmacokinetic studies show an approximate 2-fold elevation in median exposure in Japanese subjects residing in Japan and in Chinese subjects residing in Singapore compared with Caucasians residing in North America and Europe. The contribution of environmental and genetic factors to the difference observed has not been determined. However, these increases should be considered when making rosuvastatin dosing decisions for patients of Japanese and Chinese ancestry. (See WARNINGS Myopathy/Rhabdomyolysis; CLINICAL PHARMACOLOGY, Special Populations, Race.)

Information for Patients

Patients should be advised to report promptly unexplained muscle pain, tenderness, or weakness, particularly if accompanied by malaise or fever.

When taking rosuvastatin with an aluminum and magnesium hydroxide combination antacid, the antacid should be taken at least 2 hours after rosuvastatin administration (see CLINICAL PHARMACOLOGY, Drug Interactions).

Laboratory Tests

In the rosuvastatin clinical trial program, dipstick-positive proteinuria and microscopic hematuria were observed among rosuvastatin treated patients, predominantly in patients dosed above the recommended dose range (i.e., 80 mg). However, this finding was more frequent in patients taking rosuvastatin 40 mg, when compared to lower doses of rosuvastatin or comparator statins, though it was generally transient and was not associated with worsening renal function. Although the clinical significance of this finding is unknown, a dose reduction should be considered for patients on rosuvastatin 40 mg therapy with unexplained persistent proteinuria during routine urinalysis testing.

Drug Interactions

Cyclosporine: When rosuvastatin 10 mg was coadministered with cyclosporine in cardiac transplant patients, rosuvastatin mean C_{max} and mean AUC were increased 11-fold and 7-fold, respectively, compared with healthy volunteers. These increases are considered to be clinically significant and require special consideration in the dosing of rosuvastatin to patients taking concomitant cyclosporine (see WARNINGS, Myopathy/Rhabdomyolysis, and DOSAGE AND ADMINISTRATION).

Warfarin: Coadministration of rosuvastatin to patients on stable warfarin therapy resulted in clinically significant rises in INR (>4, baseline 2-3). In patients taking coumarin anticoagulants and rosuvastatin concomitantly, INR should be determined before starting rosuvastatin and frequently enough during early therapy to ensure that no significant alteration of INR occurs. Once a stable INR time has been documented, INR can be monitored at the intervals usually recommended for patients on coumarin anticoagulants. If the dose of rosuvastatin is changed, the same procedure should be repeated. Rosuvastatin therapy has not been associated with bleeding or with changes in INR in patients not taking anticoagulants.

Gemfibrozil: Coadministration of a single rosuvastatin dose to healthy volunteers on gemfibrozil (600 mg twice daily) resulted in 2.2- and 1.9-fold, respectively, increase in mean C_{max} and mean AUC of rosuvastatin (see DOSAGE AND ADMINISTRATION).

Endocrine Function

Although clinical studies have shown that rosuvastatin alone does not reduce basal plasma cortisol concentration or impair adrenal reserve, caution should be exercised if any HMG-CoA reductase inhibitor or other agent used to lower cholesterol levels is administered concomitantly with drugs that may decrease the levels or activity of endogenous steroid hormones such as ketoconazole, spironolactone, and cimetidine.

CNS Toxicity

CNS vascular lesions, characterized by perivascular hemorrhages, edema, and mononuclear cell infiltration of perivascular spaces, have been observed in dogs treated with several other members of this drug class. A chemically similar drug in this class produced dose-dependent optic nerve degeneration (Wallerian degeneration of retinogeniculate fibers) in dogs, at a dose that produced plasma drug levels about 30 times higher than the mean drug level in humans taking the highest recommended dose. Edema, hemorrhage, and partial necrosis in the interstitium of the choroid plexus was observed in a female dog sacrificed moribund at day 24 at 90 mg/kg/day by oral gavage (systemic exposures 100 times the human exposure at 40 mg/day based on AUC comparisons). Corneal opacity was seen in dogs treated for 52 weeks at 6 mg/kg/day by oral gavage (systemic exposures 20 times the human exposure at 40 mg/day based on AUC comparisons). Cataracts were seen in dogs treated for 12 weeks by oral gavage at 30 mg/kg/day (systemic exposures 60 times the human exposure at 40 mg/day based on AUC comparisons). Retinal dysplasia and retinal loss were seen in dogs treated for 4 weeks by oral gavage at 90 mg/kg/day (systemic exposures 100 times the human exposure at 40 mg/day based on AUC). Doses ≤30 mg/kg/day (systemic exposures ≤60 times the human exposure at 40 mg/day based on AUC comparisons) following treatment up to one year, did not reveal retinal findings.

Carcinogenesis, Mutagenesis, Impairment of Fertility

In a 104-week carcinogenicity study in rats at dose levels of 2, 20, 60, or 80 mg/kg/day by oral gavage, the incidence of uterine stromal polyps was significantly increased in females at 80 mg/kg/day at systemic exposure 20 times the human exposure at 40 mg/day based on AUC. Increased incidence of polyps was not seen at lower doses.

In a 107-week carcinogenicity study in mice given 10, 60, 200 mg/kg/day by oral gavage, an increased incidence of hepatocellular adenoma/carcinoma was observed at 200 mg/kg/day at systemic exposures 20 times human exposure at 40 mg/day based on AUC. An increased incidence of hepatocellular tumors was not seen at lower doses.

Rosuvastatin was not mutagenic or clastogenic with or without metabolic activation in the Ames test with *Salmonella typhimurium* and *Escherichia coli*, the mouse lymphoma assay, and the chromosomal aberration assay in Chinese hamster lung cells. Rosuvastatin was negative in the *in vivo* mouse micronucleus test.

In rat fertility studies with oral gavage doses of 5, 15, 50 mg/kg/day, males were treated for 9 weeks prior to and throughout mating and females were treated 2 weeks prior to mating and throughout mating until gestation day 7. No adverse effect on fertility was observed at 50 mg/kg/day (systemic exposures up to 10 times human exposure at 40 mg/day based on AUC comparisons). In testicles of dogs treated with rosuvastatin at 30 mg/kg/day for one month, spermatidic giant cells were seen. Spermatidic giant cells were observed in monkeys after 6-month treatment at 30 mg/kg/day in addition to vacuolation of seminiferous tubular epithelium. Exposures in the dog were 20 times and in the monkey 10 times human exposure at 40 mg/day based on body surface area comparisons. Similar findings have been seen with other drugs in this class.

Pregnancy

Pregnancy Category X

See CONTRAINDICATIONS.

Rosuvastatin may cause fetal harm when administered to a pregnant woman. Rosuvastatin is contraindicated in women who are or may become pregnant. Safety in pregnant women has not been established. There are no adequate and well-controlled studies of rosuvastatin in pregnant women. Rosuvastatin crosses the placenta and is found in fetal tissue and amniotic fluid at 3% and 20%, respectively, of the maternal plasma concentration following a single 25 mg/kg oral gavage dose on gestation day 16 in rats. A higher fetal tissue distribution (25% maternal plasma concentration) was observed in rabbits after a single oral gavage dose of 1 mg/kg on gestation day 18. If this drug is administered to a woman with reproductive potential, the patient should be apprised of the potential hazard to a fetus.

In female rats given oral gavage doses of 5, 15, 50 mg/kg/day rosuvastatin before mating and continuing through day 7 postcoitus results in decreased fetal body weight (female pups) and delayed ossification at the high dose (systemic exposures 10 times human exposure at 40 mg/day based on AUC comparisons).

In pregnant rats given oral gavage doses of 2, 20, 50 mg/kg/day from gestation day 7 through lactation day 21 (weaning), decreased pup survival occurred in groups given 50 mg/kg/day, systemic exposures ≥12 times human exposure at 40 mg/day based on body surface area comparisons.

In pregnant rabbits given oral gavage doses of 0.3, 1, 3 mg/kg/day from gestation day 6 to lactation day 18 (weaning), exposures equivalent to human exposure at 40 mg/day based on body surface area comparisons, decreased fetal viability and maternal mortality was observed.

Rosuvastatin was not teratogenic in rats at ≤25 mg/kg/day or in rabbits ≤3 mg/kg/day (systemic exposures equivalent to human exposure at 40 mg/day based on AUC or body surface comparison, respectively).

Nursing Mothers

It is not known whether rosuvastatin is excreted in human milk. Studies in lactating rats have demonstrated that rosuvastatin is secreted into breast milk at levels 3 times higher than that obtained in the plasma following oral gavage dosing. Because many drugs are excreted in human milk and because of the potential for serious adverse reactions in nursing infants from rosuvastatin, a decision should be made whether to discontinue nursing or administration of rosuvastatin taking into account the importance of the drug to the lactating woman.

Pediatric Use

The safety and effectiveness in pediatric patients have not been established. Treatment experience with rosuvastatin in a pediatric population is limited to 8 patients with homozygous FH. None of these patients was below 8 years of age.

Geriatric Use

Of the 10,275 patients in clinical studies with rosuvastatin, 3,159 (31%) were 65 years and older, and 698 (6.8%) were 75 years and older. The overall frequency of adverse events and types of adverse events were similar in patients above and below 65 years of age. (See WARNINGS, Myopathy/Rhabdomyolysis.)

The efficacy of rosuvastatin in the geriatric population (≥65 years of age) was comparable to the efficacy observed in the non-elderly.

ADVERSE REACTIONS

Rosuvastatin is generally well tolerated. Adverse reactions have usually been mild and transient. In clinical studies of 10,275 patients, 3.7% were discontinued due to adverse experiences attributable to rosuvastatin.

The most frequent adverse events thought to be related to rosuvastatin were myalgia, constipation, asthenia, abdominal pain, and nausea.

Clinical Adverse Experiences

Adverse experiences, regardless of causality assessment, reported in ≥2% of patients in placebo-controlled clinical studies of rosuvastatin are shown in Table 6; discontinuations due to adverse events in these studies of up to 12 weeks duration occurred in 3% of patients on rosuvastatin and 5% on placebo.

Table 6. Adverse Events in Placebo-Controlled Studies

Adverse Event	Rosuvastatin N=744	Placebo N=382
Pharyngitis	9.0	7.6
Headache	5.5	5.0
Diarrhea	3.4	2.9
Dyspepsia	3.4	3.1
Nausea	3.4	3.1
Myalgia	2.8	1.3
Asthenia	2.7	2.6
Back Pain	2.6	2.4
Flu syndrome	2.3	1.8
Urinary tract infection	2.3	1.6
Rhinitis	2.2	2.1
Sinusitis	2.0	1.8

In addition, the following adverse events were reported, regardless of causality assessment, in ≥1% of 10,275 patients treated with rosuvastatin in clinical studies. The events in *italics* occurred in ≥2% of these patients.

Body as a Whole: *Abdominal pain, accidental injury, chest pain, infection, pain,* pelvic pain, and neck pain.

Cardiovascular System: *Hypertension*, angina pectoris, vasodilatation, and palpitation.

Digestive System: *Constipation, gastroenteritis*, vomiting, flatulence, periodontal abscess, and gastritis.

Endocrine: Diabetes mellitus.

Hemic and Lymphatic System: Anemia and ecchymosis.
Metabolic and Nutritional Disorders: *Peripheral edema.*
Musculoskeletal System: *Arthritis, arthralgia*, and pathological fracture.
Nervous System: *Dizziness, insomnia, hypertonia, paresthesia, depression*, anxiety, vertigo and neuralgia.
Respiratory System: *Bronchitis, cough increased*, dyspnea, pneumonia, and asthma.
Skin and Appendages: *Rash* and pruritus.
Laboratory Abnormalities: In the rosuvastatin clinical trial program, dipstick-positive proteinuria and microscopic hematuria were observed among rosuvastatin-treated patients, predominantly in patients dosed above the recommended dose range (i.e., 80 mg). However, this finding was more frequent in patients taking rosuvastatin 40 mg, when compared to lower doses of rosuvastatin or comparator statins, though it was generally transient and was not associated with worsening renal function. (See PRECAUTIONS, Laboratory Tests.)
Other abnormal laboratory values reported were elevated creatinine phosphokinase, transaminases, hyperglycemia, glutamyl transpeptidase, alkaline phosphatase, bilirubin, and thyroid function abnormalities.
Other adverse events reported less frequently than 1% in the rosuvastatin clinical study program, regardless of causality assessment, included arrhythmia, hepatitis, hypersensitivity reactions (i.e., face edema, thrombocytopenia, leukopenia, vesiculobullous rash, urticaria, and angioedema), kidney failure, syncope, myasthenia, myositis, pancreatitis, photosensitivity reaction, myopathy, and rhabdomyolysis.

OVERDOSAGE

There is no specific treatment in the event of overdose. In the event of overdose, the patient should be treated symptomatically and supportive measures instituted as required. Hemodialysis does not significantly enhance clearance of rosuvastatin.

DOSAGE AND ADMINISTRATION

The patient should be placed on a standard cholesterol-lowering diet before receiving CRESTOR and should continue on this diet during treatment. CRESTOR can be administered as a single dose at any time of day, with or without food.

Hypercholesterolemia (Heterozygous Familial and Nonfamilial) and Mixed Dyslipidemia (Fredrickson Type IIa and IIb)

The dose range for CRESTOR is 5 to 40 mg once daily. Therapy with CRESTOR should be individualized according to goal of therapy and response. The usual recommended starting dose of CRESTOR is 10 mg once daily. Initiation of therapy with 5 mg once daily may be considered for patients requiring less aggressive LDL-C reductions or who have predisposing factors for myopathy (see WARNINGS, Myopathy/Rhabdomyolysis). For patients with marked hypercholesterolemia (LDL-C > 190 mg/dL) and aggressive lipid targets, a 20-mg starting dose may be considered. The 40-mg dose of CRESTOR should be reserved for those patients who have not achieved goal LDL-C at 20 mg (see WARNINGS, Myopathy/Rhabdomyolysis). After initiation and/or upon titration of CRESTOR, lipid levels should be analyzed within 2 to 4 weeks and dosage adjusted accordingly.

Homozygous Familial Hypercholesterolemia

The recommended starting dose of CRESTOR is 20 mg once daily in patients with homozygous FH. The maximum recommended daily dose is 40 mg. CRESTOR should be used in these patients as an adjunct to other lipid-lowering treatments (e.g., LDL apheresis) or if such treatments are unavailable. Response to therapy should be estimated from pre-apheresis LDL-C levels.

Dosage in Patients Taking Cyclosporine

In patients taking cyclosporine, therapy should be limited to CRESTOR 5 mg once daily (see WARNINGS, Myopathy/Rhabdomyolysis, and PRECAUTIONS, Drug Interactions).

Concomitant Lipid-Lowering Therapy

The effect of CRESTOR on LDL-C and total-C may be enhanced when used in combination with a bile acid binding resin. If CRESTOR is used in combination with gemfibrozil, the dose of CRESTOR should be limited to 10 mg once daily (see WARNINGS, Myopathy/Rhabdomyolysis, and PRECAUTIONS, Drug Interactions).

Dosage in Patients With Renal Insufficiency

No modification of dosage is necessary for patients with mild to moderate renal insufficiency. For patients with severe renal impairment (CL_{cr} <30 mL/min/1.73 m^2) not on hemodialysis, dosing of CRESTOR should be started at 5 mg once daily and not to exceed 10 mg once daily (see PRECAUTIONS, General, and CLINICAL PHARMACOLOGY, Special Populations, Renal Insufficiency).

HOW SUPPLIED

CRESTOR® (rosuvastatin calcium) Tablets are supplied as:
5 mg tablets: Yellow, round, biconvex, coated tablets identified as "ZD4522" and "5" debossed on one side and plain on the other side of the tablet.
(NDC 0310-0755-90) bottles of 90
10 mg tablets: Pink, round, biconvex, coated tablets identified as "ZD4522" and "10" debossed on one side and plain on the other side of the tablet.
(NDC 0310-0751-90) bottles of 90
(NDC 0310-0751-39) unit dose packages of 100
20 mg tablets: Pink, round, biconvex, coated tablets identified as "ZD4522" and "20" debossed on one side and plain on the other side of the tablet.
(NDC 0310-0752-90) bottles of 90
(NDC 0310-0752-39) unit dose packages of 100
40 mg tablets: Pink, oval, biconvex, coated tablets identified as "ZD4522" debossed on one side and "40" debossed on the other side of the tablet.
(NDC 0310-0754-30) bottles of 30
(NDC 0310-0754-39) unit dose packages of 100

Storage

Store at controlled room temperature, 20-25°C (68-77°F) [see USP]. Protect from moisture.

Rx only

CRESTOR is a trademark of the AstraZeneca group of companies.

Licensed from SHIONOGI & CO., LTD., Osaka, Japan
Manufactured for:
AstraZeneca Pharmaceuticals LP
Wilmington, DE 19850
By: IPR Pharmaceuticals, Inc.
Carolina, PR 00984
IPR (trade) 630100
IPR (sample) 630200
API (sample) 23073-00
Rev. 08/03
AstraZeneca

Shown in Product Identification Guide, page 306

DIPRIVAN® ℞

[dĭ′prĭ-văn]

(propofol) Injectable Emulsion
FOR IV ADMINISTRATION

DESCRIPTION

DIPRIVAN® (propofol) Injectable Emulsion is a sterile, nonpyrogenic emulsion containing 10 mg/mL of propofol suitable for intravenous administration. Propofol is chemically described as 2,6-diisopropylphenol and has a molecular weight of 178.27. The structural and molecular formulas are:

OH
$(CH_3)_2CH$ — $CH(CH_3)_2$
$C_{12}H_{18}O$

Propofol is very slightly soluble in water and, thus, is formulated in a white, oil-in-water emulsion. The pKa is 11. The octanol/water partition coefficient for propofol is 6761:1 at a pH of 6-8.5. In addition to the active component, propofol, the formulation also contains soybean oil (100 mg/mL), glycerol (22.5 mg/mL), egg lecithin (12 mg/mL); and disodium edetate (0.005%); with sodium hydroxide to adjust pH. The DIPRIVAN Injectable Emulsion is isotonic and has a pH of 7-8.5.

STRICT ASEPTIC TECHNIQUE MUST ALWAYS BE MAINTAINED DURING HANDLING. DIPRIVAN INJECTABLE EMULSION IS A SINGLE-USE PARENTERAL PRODUCT WHICH CONTAINS 0.005% DISODIUM EDETATE TO RETARD THE RATE OF GROWTH OF MICROORGANISMS IN THE EVENT OF ACCIDENTAL EXTRINSIC CONTAMINATION. HOWEVER, DIPRIVAN INJECTABLE EMULSION CAN STILL SUPPORT THE GROWTH OF MICROORGANISMS AS IT IS NOT AN ANTIMICROBIALLY PRESERVED PRODUCT UNDER USP STANDARDS. ACCORDINGLY, STRICT ASEPTIC TECHNIQUE MUST STILL BE ADHERED TO. DO NOT USE IF CONTAMINATION IS SUSPECTED. DISCARD UNUSED PORTIONS AS DIRECTED WITHIN THE REQUIRED TIME LIMITS (SEE DOSAGE AND ADMINISTRATION, HANDLING PROCEDURES). THERE HAVE BEEN REPORTS IN WHICH FAILURE TO USE ASEPTIC TECHNIQUE WHEN HANDLING DIPRIVAN INJECTABLE EMULSION WAS ASSOCIATED WITH MICROBIAL CONTAMINATION OF THE PRODUCT AND WITH FEVER, INFECTION/SEPSIS, OTHER LIFE-THREATENING ILLNESS, AND/OR DEATH.

CLINICAL PHARMACOLOGY

General

DIPRIVAN Injectable Emulsion is an intravenous sedative-hypnotic agent for use in the induction and maintenance of anesthesia or sedation. Intravenous injection of a therapeutic dose of propofol produces hypnosis rapidly with minimal excitation, usually within 40 seconds from the start of an injection (the time for one arm-brain circulation). As with other rapidly acting intravenous anesthetic agents, the half-time of the blood-brain equilibration is approximately 1 to 3 minutes, and this accounts for the rapid induction of anesthesia.

Pharmacodynamics

Pharmacodynamic properties of propofol are dependent upon the therapeutic blood propofol concentrations. Steady state propofol blood concentrations are generally proportional to infusion rates, especially within an individual patient. Undesirable side effects such as cardiorespiratory depression are likely to occur at higher blood concentrations which result from bolus dosing or rapid increase in infusion rate. An adequate interval (3 to 5 minutes) must be allowed between clinical dosage adjustments in order to assess drug effects.

The hemodynamic effects of DIPRIVAN Injectable Emulsion during induction of anesthesia vary. If spontaneous ventilation is maintained, the major cardiovascular effects are arterial hypotension (sometimes greater than a 30% decrease) with little or no change in heart rate and no appreciable decrease in cardiac output. If ventilation is assisted or controlled (positive pressure ventilation), the degree and incidence of decrease in cardiac output are accentuated. Addition of a potent opioid (e.g., fentanyl) when used as a premedicant further decreases cardiac output and respiratory drive.

If anesthesia is continued by infusion of DIPRIVAN Injectable Emulsion, the stimulation of endotracheal intubation and surgery may return arterial pressure towards normal. However, cardiac output may remain depressed. Comparative clinical studies have shown that the hemodynamic effects of DIPRIVAN Injectable Emulsion during induction of anesthesia are generally more pronounced than with other IV induction agents traditionally used for this purpose.

Clinical and preclinical studies suggest that DIPRIVAN Injectable Emulsion is rarely associated with elevation of plasma histamine levels.

Induction of anesthesia with DIPRIVAN Injectable Emulsion is frequently associated with apnea in both adults and pediatric patients. In 1573 adult patients who received DIPRIVAN Injectable Emulsion (2 to 2.5 mg/kg), apnea lasted less than 30 seconds in 7% of patients, 30-60 seconds in 24% of patients, and more than 60 seconds in 12% of patients. In 218 pediatric patients from birth through 16 years of age assessable for apnea who received bolus doses of DIPRIVAN Injectable Emulsion (1 to 3.6 mg/kg), apnea lasted less than 30 seconds in 12% of patients, 30-60 seconds in 10% of patients, and more than 60 seconds in 5% of patients.

During maintenance, DIPRIVAN Injectable Emulsion causes a decrease in ventilation usually associated with an increase in carbon dioxide tension which may be marked depending upon the rate of administration and other concurrent medications (e.g., opioids, sedatives, etc.).

During monitored anesthesia care (MAC) sedation, attention must be given to the cardiorespiratory effects of DIPRIVAN Injectable Emulsion. Hypotension, oxyhemoglobin desaturation, apnea, airway obstruction, and/or oxygen desaturation can occur, especially following a rapid bolus of DIPRIVAN Injectable Emulsion. During initiation of MAC sedation, slow infusion or slow injection techniques are preferable over rapid bolus administration, and during maintenance of MAC sedation, a variable rate infusion is preferable over intermittent bolus administration in order to minimize undesirable cardiorespiratory effects. In the elderly, debilitated, or ASA III/IV patients, rapid (single or repeated) bolus dose administration should not be used for MAC sedation. (See WARNINGS.)

Clinical studies in humans and studies in animals show that DIPRIVAN Injectable Emulsion does not suppress the adrenal response to ACTH.

Preliminary findings in patients with normal intraocular pressure indicate that DIPRIVAN Injectable Emulsion anesthesia produces a decrease in intraocular pressure which may be associated with a concomitant decrease in systemic vascular resistance.

Animal studies and limited experience in susceptible patients have not indicated any propensity of DIPRIVAN Injectable Emulsion to induce malignant hyperthermia.

Studies to date indicate that DIPRIVAN Injectable Emulsion when used in combination with hypocarbia increases cerebrovascular resistance and decreases cerebral blood flow, cerebral metabolic oxygen consumption, and intracranial pressure. DIPRIVAN Injectable Emulsion does not affect cerebrovascular reactivity to changes in arterial carbon dioxide tension (see Clinical Trials - Neuroanesthesia).

Hemosiderin deposits have been observed in the livers of dogs receiving DIPRIVAN Injectable Emulsion containing 0.005% disodium edetate over a four-week period; the clinical significance is unknown.

Pharmacokinetics

The proper use of DIPRIVAN Injectable Emulsion requires an understanding of the disposition and elimination characteristics of propofol.

The pharmacokinetics of propofol are well described by a three compartment linear model with compartments representing the plasma, rapidly equilibrating tissues, and slowly equilibrating tissues.

Following an IV bolus dose, there is rapid equilibration between the plasma and the highly perfused tissue of the brain, thus accounting for the rapid onset of anesthesia. Plasma levels initially decline rapidly as a result of both rapid distribution and high metabolic clearance. Distribution accounts for about half of this decline following a bolus of propofol.

However, distribution is not constant over time, but decreases as body tissues equilibrate with plasma and become saturated. The rate at which equilibration occurs is a function of the rate and duration of the infusion. When equilibration occurs there is no longer a net transfer of propofol between tissues and plasma.

Discontinuation of the recommended doses of DIPRIVAN Injectable Emulsion after the maintenance of anesthesia for approximately one-hour, or for sedation in the ICU for one-day, results in a prompt decrease in blood propofol concentrations and rapid awakening. Longer infusions (10 days of ICU sedation) result in accumulation of significant tissue stores of propofol, such that the reduction in circulating propofol is slowed and the time to awakening is increased.

Continued on next page

Diprivan—Cont.

By daily titration of DIPRIVAN Injectable Emulsion dosage to achieve only the minimum effective therapeutic concentration, rapid awakening within 10 to 15 minutes will occur even after long-term administration. If, however, higher than necessary infusion levels have been maintained for a long time, propofol will be redistributed from fat and muscle to the plasma, and this return of propofol from peripheral tissues will slow recovery.

The figure below illustrates the fall of plasma propofol levels following ICU sedation infusions of various durations.

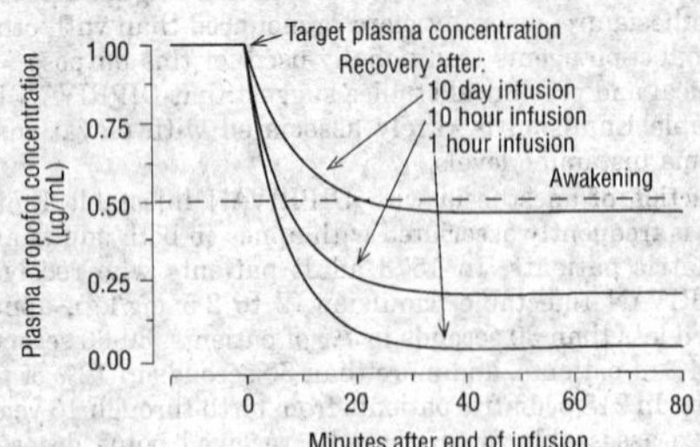

The large contribution of distribution (about 50%) to the fall of propofol plasma levels following brief infusions means that after very long infusions (at steady state), about half the initial rate will maintain the same plasma levels. Failure to reduce the infusion rate in patients receiving DIPRIVAN Injectable Emulsion for extended periods may result in excessively high blood concentrations of the drug. Thus, titration to clinical response and daily evaluation of sedation levels are important during use of DIPRIVAN Injectable Emulsion infusion for ICU sedation, especially of long duration.

Adults: Propofol clearance ranges from 23-50 mL/kg/min (1.6 to 3.4 L/min in 70 kg adults). It is chiefly eliminated by hepatic conjugation to inactive metabolites which are excreted by the kidney. A glucuronide conjugate accounts for about 50% of the administered dose. Propofol has a steady state volume of distribution (10-day infusion) approaching 60 L/kg in healthy adults. A difference in pharmacokinetics due to gender has not been observed. The terminal half-life of propofol after a 10-day infusion is 1 to 3 days.

Geriatrics: With increasing patient age, the dose of propofol needed to achieve a defined anesthetic end point (dose-requirement) decreases. This does not appear to be an age-related change of pharmacodynamics or brain sensitivity, as measured by EEG burst suppression. With increasing patient age pharmacokinetic changes are such that for a given IV bolus dose, higher peak plasma concentrations occur, which can explain the decreased dose requirement. These higher peak plasma concentrations in the elderly can predispose patients to cardiorespiratory effects including hypotension, apnea, airway obstruction, and/or oxygen desaturation. The higher plasma levels reflect an age-related decrease in volume of distribution and reduced intercompartmental clearance. Lower doses are thus recommended for initiation and maintenance of sedation/anesthesia in elderly patients. (See CLINICAL PHARMACOLOGY - Individualization of Dosage.)

Pediatrics: The pharmacokinetics of propofol were studied in 53 children between the ages of 3 and 12 years who received DIPRIVAN Injectable Emulsion for periods of approximately 1-2 hours. The observed distribution and clearance of propofol in these children were similar to adults.

Organ Failure: The pharmacokinetics of propofol do not appear to be different in people with chronic hepatic cirrhosis or chronic renal impairment compared to adults with normal hepatic and renal function. The effects of acute hepatic or renal failure on the pharmacokinetics of propofol have not been studied.

Clinical Trials

Anesthesia and Monitored Anesthesia Care (MAC) Sedation

DIPRIVAN Injectable Emulsion was compared to intravenous and inhalational anesthetic or sedative agents in 91 trials involving a total of 5,135 patients. Of these, 3,354 received DIPRIVAN Injectable Emulsion and comprised the overall safety database for anesthesia and MAC sedation. Fifty-five of these trials, 20 for anesthesia induction and 35 for induction and maintenance of anesthesia or MAC sedation, were carried out in the US or Canada and provided the basis for dosage recommendations and the adverse event profile during anesthesia or MAC sedation.

Pediatric Anesthesia

DIPRIVAN Injectable Emulsion was studied in 14 clinical trials involving 691 pediatric patients, including 42 cardiac surgical patients. Of the total 691 patients, 90 were less than 3 years of age and 601 were 3 years of age or older. Of these, 506 were from US/Canadian clinical trials and comprised the overall safety and efficacy database for Pediatric Anesthesia. The majority of the remaining patients were healthy ASA I/II patients. (See Table 1)

[See table 1 above]

[See table 2 above]

Also includes all time following induction dose.

TABLE 1. PEDIATRIC INDUCTION OF ANESTHESIA
Patients Receiving DIPRIVAN Injectable Emulsion Median and (Range)

Age Range	No. of Patients	Induction Dose	Injection Duration
Birth through 16 years	353	2.5 mg/kg (1-3.6)	20 sec. (6-45)

TABLE 2. PEDIATRIC MAINTENANCE OF ANESTHESIA
Patients Receiving DIPRIVAN Injectable Emulsion Median and (Range)

Age Range	No. of Patients	Maintenance Dosage µg/kg/min	Duration Minutes
2 months to 2 years	68	199 (82 - 394)	65 (12 - 282)
2 to 12 years	165	188 (12 - 1041)	69 (23 - 374)
>12 through 16 years	27	161 (84 - 359)	69 (26 - 251)

Neuroanesthesia

DIPRIVAN Injectable Emulsion was studied in 50 patients undergoing craniotomy for supratentorial tumors in two clinical trials. The mean lesion size (anterior/posterior and lateral) was 31 mm and 32 mm in one trial and 55 mm and 42 mm in the other trial respectively.

[See table 3 above]

TABLE 3. NEUROANESTHESIA CLINICAL TRIALS
Patients Receiving DIPRIVAN Injectable Emulsion Median and (Range)

Patient Type	No. of Patients	Induction Bolus Dosages (mg/kg)	Maintenance Dosage (µg/kg/min)	Maintenance Duration (min)
Craniotomy patients	50	1.36 (0.9-6.9)	146 (68-425)	285 (48-622)

In ten of these patients, DIPRIVAN Injectable Emulsion was administered by infusion in a controlled clinical trial to evaluate the effect of DIPRIVAN Injectable Emulsion on cerebrospinal fluid pressure (CSFP). The mean arterial pressure was maintained relatively constant over 25 minutes with a change from baseline of -4% ± 17% (mean ± SD), whereas the percent change in cerebrospinal fluid pressure (CSFP) was -46% ± 14%. As CSFP is an indirect measure of intracranial pressure (ICP), when given by infusion or slow bolus, DIPRIVAN Injectable Emulsion, in combination with hypocarbia, is capable of decreasing ICP independent of changes in arterial pressure.

Intensive Care Unit (ICU) Sedation

Adult Patients:

DIPRIVAN Injectable Emulsion was compared to benzodiazepines and/or opioids in 14 clinical trials involving a total of 550 ICU patients. Of these, 302 received DIPRIVAN Injectable Emulsion and comprise the overall safety database for ICU sedation. Six of these studies were carried out in the US or Canada and provide the basis for dosage recommendations and the adverse event profile.

Information from 193 literature reports of DIPRIVAN Injectable Emulsion used for ICU sedation in over 950 patients and information from the clinical trials are summarized below:

[See table 4 above]

TABLE 4. ADULT ICU SEDATION CLINICAL TRIALS AND LITERATURE
Patients receiving DIPRIVAN Injectable Emulsion Median and (Range)

ICU Patient Type	Number of Trials	Patient Literature	Sedation Dose (µg/kg/min)	Sedation Dose mg/kg/h	Sedation Duration Hours
Post-CABG	41	—	11 (0.1-30)	0.66 (0.006-1.8)	10 (2-14)
	—	334	(5-100)	(0.3-6)	(4-24)
Post-Surgical	60	—	20 (6-53)	1.2 (0.4-3.2)	18 (0.3-187)
	—	142	(23-82)	(1.4-4.9)	(6-96)
Neuro/Head Trauma	7	—	25 (13-37)	1.5 (0.8-2.2)	168 (112-282)
	—	184	(8.3-87)	(0.5-5.2)	(8 hr-5 days)
Medical	49	—	41 (9-131)	2.5 (0.5-7.9)	72 (0.4-337)
		76	(3.3-62)	(0.2-3.7)	(4-96)
Special Patients					
ARDS/Resp. Failure	—	56	(10-142)	(0.6-8.5)	(1 hr-8 days)
COPD/Asthma	—	49	(17-75)	(1-4.5)	(1-8 days)
Status Epilepticus	—	15	(25-167)	(1.5-10)	(1-21 days)
Tetanus	—	11	(5-100)	(0.3-6)	(1-25 days)

Trials (Individual patients from clinical studies)
Literature (Individual patients from published reports)
CABG (Coronary Artery Bypass Graft)
ARDS (Adult Respiratory Distress Syndrome)

Cardiac Anesthesia

DIPRIVAN Injectable Emulsion was evaluated in 5 clinical trials conducted in the US and Canada, involving a total of 569 patients undergoing coronary artery bypass graft (CABG). Of these, 301 patients received DIPRIVAN Injectable Emulsion. They comprise the safety database for cardiac anesthesia and provide the basis for dosage recommendations in this patient population, in conjunction with reports in the published literature.

Individualization of Dosage

General: STRICT ASEPTIC TECHNIQUE MUST ALWAYS BE MAINTAINED DURING HANDLING. DIPRIVAN INJECTABLE EMULSION IS A SINGLE-USE PARENTERAL PRODUCT WHICH CONTAINS 0.005% DISODIUM EDETATE TO RETARD THE RATE OF GROWTH OF MICROORGANISMS IN THE EVENT OF ACCIDENTAL EXTRINSIC CONTAMINATION. HOWEVER, DIPRIVAN INJECTABLE EMULSION CAN STILL SUPPORT THE GROWTH OF MICROORGANISMS AS IT IS NOT AN ANTIMICROBIALLY PRESERVED PRODUCT UNDER USP STANDARDS. ACCORDINGLY, STRICT ASEPTIC TECHNIQUE MUST STILL BE ADHERED TO. DO NOT USE IF CONTAMINATION IS SUSPECTED. DISCARD UNUSED PORTIONS AS DIRECTED WITHIN THE REQUIRED TIME LIMITS (SEE DOSAGE AND ADMINISTRATION, HANDLING PROCEDURES). THERE HAVE BEEN REPORTS IN WHICH FAILURE TO USE ASEPTIC TECHNIQUE WHEN HANDLING DIPRIVAN INJECTABLE EMULSION WAS ASSOCIATED WITH MICROBIAL CONTAMINATION OF THE PRODUCT AND WITH FEVER, INFECTION/SEPSIS, OTHER LIFE-THREATENING ILLNESS, AND/OR DEATH.

Propofol blood concentrations at steady state are generally proportional to infusion rates, especially in individual patients. Undesirable effects such as cardiorespiratory depression are likely to occur at higher blood concentrations which result from bolus dosing or rapid increases in the infusion rate. An adequate interval (3 to 5 minutes) must be allowed between clinical dosage adjustments in order to assess drug effects.

When administering DIPRIVAN Injectable Emulsion by infusion, syringe pumps or volumetric pumps are recommended to provide controlled infusion rates. When infusing DIPRIVAN Injectable Emulsion to patients undergoing magnetic resonance imaging, metered control devices may be utilized if mechanical pumps are impractical.

Changes in vital signs (increases in pulse rate, blood pressure, sweating, and/or tearing) that indicate a response to surgical stimulation or lightening of anesthesia may be controlled by the administration of DIPRIVAN Injectable Emulsion 25 mg (2.5 mL) to 50 mg (5 mL) incremental boluses and/or by increasing the infusion rate.

For minor surgical procedures (e.g., body surface) nitrous oxide (60%-70%) can be combined with a variable rate DIPRIVAN Injectable Emulsion infusion to provide satisfactory anesthesia. With more stimulating surgical procedures (e.g., intra-abdominal), or if supplementation with nitrous oxide is not provided, administration rate(s) of DIPRIVAN Injectable Emulsion and/or opioids should be increased in order to provide adequate anesthesia.

Infusion rates should always be titrated downward in the absence of clinical signs of light anesthesia until a mild response to surgical stimulation is obtained in order to avoid administration of DIPRIVAN Injectable Emulsion at rates higher than are clinically necessary. Generally, rates of 50 to 100 µg/kg/min in adults should be achieved during maintenance in order to optimize recovery times.

Other drugs that cause CNS depression (hypnotics/sedatives, inhalational anesthetics, and opioids) can increase

CNS depression induced by propofol. Morphine premedication (0.15 mg/kg) with nitrous oxide 67% in oxygen has been shown to decrease the necessary propofol injection maintenance infusion rate and therapeutic blood concentrations when compared to non-narcotic (lorazepam) premedication.

Induction of General Anesthesia

Adult Patients: Most adult patients under 55 years of age and classified ASA I/II require 2 to 2.5 mg/kg of DIPRIVAN Injectable Emulsion for induction when unpremedicated or when premedicated with oral benzodiazepines or intramuscular opioids. For induction, DIPRIVAN Injectable Emulsion should be titrated (approximately 40 mg every 10 seconds) against the response of the patient until the clinical signs show the onset of anesthesia. As with other sedative-hypnotic agents, the amount of intravenous opioid and/or benzodiazepine premedication will influence the response of the patient to an induction dose of DIPRIVAN Injectable Emulsion.

Elderly, Debilitated, or ASA III/IV Patients: It is important to be familiar and experienced with the intravenous use of DIPRIVAN Injectable Emulsion before treating elderly, debilitated, or ASA III/IV patients. Due to the reduced clearance and higher blood concentrations, most of these patients require approximately 1 to 1.5 mg/kg (approximately 20 mg every 10 seconds) of DIPRIVAN Injectable Emulsion for induction of anesthesia according to their condition and responses. A rapid bolus should not be used, as this will increase the likelihood of undesirable cardiorespiratory depression including hypotension, apnea, airway obstruction, and/or oxygen desaturation. (See DOSAGE AND ADMINISTRATION.)

Pediatric Patients: Most patients aged 3 years through 16 years and classified ASA I or II require 2.5 to 3.5 mg/kg of DIPRIVAN Injectable Emulsion for induction when unpremedicated or when lightly premedicated with oral benzodiazepines or intramuscular opioids. Within this dosage range, younger pediatric patients may require higher induction doses than older pediatric patients. As with other sedative-hypnotic agents, the amount of intravenous opioid and/or benzodiazepine premedication will influence the response of the patient to an induction dose of DIPRIVAN Injectable Emulsion. A lower dosage is recommended for pediatric patients classified as ASA III or IV. Attention should be paid to minimize pain on injection when administering DIPRIVAN Injectable Emulsion to pediatric patients. Boluses of DIPRIVAN Injectable Emulsion may be administered via small veins if pretreated with lidocaine or via antecubital or larger veins (See PRECAUTIONS - General).

Neurosurgical Patients: Slower induction is recommended using boluses of 20 mg every 10 seconds. Slower boluses or infusions of DIPRIVAN Injectable Emulsion for induction of anesthesia, titrated to clinical responses, will generally result in reduced induction dosage requirements (1 to 2 mg/kg). (See PRECAUTIONS and DOSAGE AND ADMINISTRATION.)

Cardiac Anesthesia: DIPRIVAN Injectable Emulsion has been well-studied in patients with coronary artery disease, but experience in patients with hemodynamically significant valvular or congenital heart disease is limited. As with other anesthetic and sedative-hypnotic agents, DIPRIVAN Injectable Emulsion in healthy patients causes a decrease in blood pressure that is secondary to decreases in preload (ventricular filling volume at the end of the diastole) and afterload (arterial resistance at the beginning of the systole). The magnitude of these changes is proportional to the blood and effect site concentrations achieved. These concentrations depend upon the dose and speed of the induction and maintenance infusion rates.

In addition, lower heart rates are observed during maintenance with DIPRIVAN Injectable Emulsion, possibly due to reduction of the sympathetic activity and/or resetting of the baroreceptor reflexes. Therefore, anticholinergic agents should be administered when increases in vagal tone are anticipated.

As with other anesthetic agents, DIPRIVAN Injectable Emulsion reduces myocardial oxygen consumption. Further studies are needed to confirm and delineate the extent of these effects on the myocardium and the coronary vascular system.

Morphine premedication (0.15 mg/kg) with nitrous oxide 67% in oxygen has been shown to decrease the necessary DIPRIVAN Injectable Emulsion maintenance infusion rates and therapeutic blood concentrations when compared to non-narcotic (lorazepam) premedication. The rate of DIPRIVAN Injectable Emulsion administration should be determined based on the patient's premedication and adjusted according to clinical responses.

A rapid bolus induction should be avoided. A slow rate of approximately 20 mg every 10 seconds until induction onset (0.5 to 1.5 mg/kg) should be used. In order to assure adequate anesthesia, when DIPRIVAN Injectable Emulsion is used as the primary agent, maintenance infusion rates should not be less than 100 µg/kg/min and should be supplemented with analgesic levels of continuous opioid administration. When an opioid is used as the primary agent, DIPRIVAN Injectable Emulsion maintenance rates should not be less than 50 µg/kg/min, and care should be taken to ensure amnesia with concomitant benzodiazepines. Higher doses of DIPRIVAN Injectable Emulsion will reduce the opioid requirements (see Table 5). When DIPRIVAN Injectable Emulsion is used as the primary anesthetic, it should not be administered with the high-dose opioid technique as this may increase the likelihood of hypotension (see PRECAUTIONS - Cardiac Anesthesia).

Table 5. Cardiac Anesthesia Techniques

Primary Agent	Rate	Secondary Agent/Rate (Following Induction with Primary Agent)
DIPRIVAN Injectable Emulsion		OPIOID[a]/0.05-0.075 g/kg/min (no bolus)
Preinduction anxiolysis	25 µg/kg/min	
Induction	0.5-1.5 mg/kg over 60 sec	
Maintenance (Titrated to Clinical Response)	100-150 µg/kg/min	
OPIOID[b]		DIPRIVAN Injectable Emulsion/50-100 µg/kg/min (no bolus)
Induction	25-50 µg/kg	
Maintenance	0.2-0.3 µg/kg/min	

[a]OPIOID is defined in terms of fentanyl equivalents, i.e.,
1 µg of fentanyl = 5 µg of alfentanil (for bolus)
= 10 µg of alfentanil (for maintenance)
or
= 0.1 µg of sufentanil

[b]Care should be taken to ensure amnesia with concomitant benzodiazepine therapy

[See table 5 above]

Maintenance of General Anesthesia

Adult Patients:

In adults, anesthesia can be maintained by administering DIPRIVAN Injectable Emulsion by infusion or intermittent IV bolus injection. The patient's clinical response will determine the infusion rate or the amount and frequency of incremental injections.

Continuous Infusion: DIPRIVAN Injectable Emulsion 100 to 200 µg/kg/min administered in a variable rate infusion with 60%-70% nitrous oxide and oxygen provides anesthesia for patients undergoing general surgery. Maintenance by infusion of DIPRIVAN Injectable Emulsion should immediately follow the induction dose in order to provide satisfactory or continuous anesthesia during the induction phase. During this initial period following the induction dose, higher rates of infusion are generally required (150 to 200 µg/kg/min) for the first 10 to 15 minutes. Infusion rates should subsequently be decreased 30%-50% during the first half-hour of maintenance. Generally, rates of 50-100 µg/kg/min in adults should be achieved during maintenance in order to optimize recovery times.

Other drugs that cause CNS depression (hypnotics/sedatives, inhalational anesthetics, and opioids) can increase the CNS depression induced by propofol.

Intermittent Bolus: Increments of DIPRIVAN Injectable Emulsion 25 mg (2.5 mL) to 50 mg (5 mL) may be administered with nitrous oxide in adult patients undergoing general surgery. The incremental boluses should be administered when changes in vital signs indicate a response to surgical stimulation or light anesthesia.

Pediatric Patients: DIPRIVAN Injectable Emulsion administered as a variable rate infusion supplemented with nitrous oxide 60%-70% provides satisfactory anesthesia for most children 2 months of age or older, ASA class I or II, undergoing general anesthesia.

In general, for the pediatric population, maintenance by infusion of DIPRIVAN Injectable Emulsion at a rate of 200-300 µg/kg/min should immediately follow the induction dose. Following the first half-hour of maintenance, infusion rates of 125-150 µg/kg/min are typically needed. DIPRIVAN Injectable Emulsion SHOULD BE TITRATED TO ACHIEVE THE DESIRED CLINICAL EFFECT. Younger pediatric patients may require higher maintenance infusion rates than older pediatric patients. (See Table 2 Clinical Trials.)

DIPRIVAN Injectable Emulsion has been used with a variety of agents commonly used in anesthesia such as atropine, scopolamine, glycopyrrolate, diazepam, depolarizing and nondepolarizing muscle relaxants, and opioid analgesics, as well as with inhalational and regional anesthetic agents.

In the elderly, debilitated, or ASA III/IV patients, rapid bolus doses should not be used, as this will increase cardiorespiratory effects including hypotension, apnea, airway obstruction, and/or oxygen desaturation.

Monitored Anesthesia Care (MAC) Sedation

Adult Patients:

When DIPRIVAN Injectable Emulsion is administered for MAC sedation, rates of administration should be individualized and titrated to clinical response. In most patients, the rates of DIPRIVAN Injectable Emulsion administration will be in the range of 25–75 µg/kg/min.

During initiation of MAC sedation, slow infusion or slow injection techniques are preferable over rapid bolus administration. During maintenance of MAC sedation, a variable rate infusion is preferable over intermittent bolus dose administration. In the elderly, debilitated, or ASA III/IV patients, rapid (single or repeated) bolus dose administration should not be used for MAC sedation. (See WARNINGS.) **A rapid bolus injection can result in undesirable cardiorespiratory depression including hypotension, apnea, airway obstruction, and/or oxygen desaturation.**

Initiation of MAC Sedation: For initiation of MAC sedation, either an infusion or a slow injection method may be utilized while closely monitoring cardiorespiratory function. With the infusion method, sedation may be initiated by infusing DIPRIVAN Injectable Emulsion at 100 to 150 µg/kg/min (6 to 9 mg/kg/h) for a period of 3 to 5 minutes and titrating to the desired clinical effect while closely monitoring respiratory function. With the slow injection method for initiation, patients will require approximately 0.5 mg/kg administered over 3 to 5 minutes and titrated to clinical responses. When DIPRIVAN Injectable Emulsion is administered slowly over 3 to 5 minutes, most patients will be adequately sedated, and the peak drug effect can be achieved while minimizing undesirable cardiorespiratory effects occurring at high plasma levels.

In the elderly, debilitated, or ASA III/IV patients, rapid (single or repeated) bolus dose administration should not be used for MAC sedation. (See WARNINGS.) The rate of administration should be over 3-5 minutes and the dosage of DIPRIVAN Injectable Emulsion should be reduced to approximately 80% of the usual adult dosage in these patients according to their condition, responses, and changes in vital signs. (See DOSAGE AND ADMINISTRATION.)

Maintenance of MAC Sedation: For maintenance of sedation, a variable rate infusion method is preferable over an intermittent bolus dose method. With the variable rate infusion method, patients will generally require maintenance rates of 25 to 75 µg/kg/min (1.5 to 4.5 mg/kg/h) during the first 10 to 15 minutes of sedation maintenance. Infusion rates should subsequently be decreased over time to 25 to 50 µg/kg/min and adjusted to clinical responses. In titrating to clinical effect, allow approximately 2 minutes for onset of peak drug effect.

Infusion rates should always be titrated downward in the absence of clinical signs of light sedation until mild responses to stimulation are obtained in order to avoid sedative administration of DIPRIVAN Injectable Emulsion at rates higher than are clinically necessary.

If the intermittent bolus dose method is used, increments of DIPRIVAN Injectable Emulsion 10 mg (1 mL) or 20 mg (2 mL) can be administered and titrated to desired clinical effect. With the intermittent bolus method of sedation maintenance, there is the potential for respiratory depression, transient increases in sedation depth, and/or prolongation of recovery.

In the elderly, debilitated, or ASA III/IV patients, rapid (single or repeated) bolus dose administration should not be used for MAC sedation. (See WARNINGS.) The rate of administration and the dosage of DIPRIVAN Injectable Emulsion should be reduced to approximately 80% of the usual adult dosage in these patients according to their condition, responses, and changes in vital signs. (See DOSAGE AND ADMINISTRATION.)

DIPRIVAN Injectable Emulsion can be administered as the sole agent for maintenance of MAC sedation during surgical/diagnostic procedures. When DIPRIVAN Injectable Emulsion sedation is supplemented with opioid and/or benzodiazepine medications, these agents increase the sedative and respiratory effects of DIPRIVAN Injectable Emulsion and may also result in a slower recovery profile. (See PRECAUTIONS, Drug Interactions.)

ICU Sedation: (See WARNINGS and DOSAGE AND ADMINISTRATION, Handling Procedures.)

Adult Patients: For intubated, mechanically ventilated adult patients, Intensive Care Unit (ICU) sedation should be initiated slowly with a continuous infusion in order to titrate to desired clinical effect and minimize hypotension. (See DOSAGE AND ADMINISTRATION.)

Across all 6 US/Canadian clinical studies, the mean infusion maintenance rate for all DIPRIVAN Injectable Emulsion patients was 27 ± 21 µg/kg/min. The maintenance infusion rates required to maintain adequate sedation ranged from 2.8 µg/kg/min to 130 µg/kg/min. The infusion rate was lower in patients over 55 years of age (approximately 20 µg/kg/min) compared to patients under 55 years of age (approximately 38 µg/kg/min). In these studies, morphine or fentanyl was used as needed for analgesia.

Most adult ICU patients recovering from the effects of general anesthesia or deep sedation will require maintenance rates of 5 to 50 µg/kg/min (0.3 to 3 mg/kg/h) individualized and titrated to clinical response. (See DOSAGE AND ADMINISTRATION.) With medical ICU patients or patients who have recovered from the effects of general anesthesia or deep sedation, the rate of administration of 50 µg/kg/min or higher may be required to achieve adequate sedation. These higher rates of administration may increase the likelihood of patients developing hypotension.

Although there are reports of reduced analgesic requirements, most patients received opioids for analgesia during maintenance of ICU sedation. Some patients also received benzodiazepines and/or neuromuscular blocking agents.

Continued on next page

Diprivan—Cont.

During long-term maintenance of sedation, some ICU patients were awakened once or twice every 24 hours for assessment of neurologic or respiratory function. (See Clinical Trials, Table 4.)

In post-CABG (coronary artery bypass graft) patients, the maintenance rate of propofol administration was usually low (median 11 μg/kg/min) due to the intraoperative administration of high opioid doses. Patients receiving DIPRIVAN Injectable Emulsion required 35% less nitroprusside than midazolam patients; this difference was statistically significant ($P<0.05$). During initiation of sedation in post-CABG patients, a 15% to 20% decrease in blood pressure was seen in the first 60 minutes. It was not possible to determine cardiovascular effects in patients with severely compromised ventricular function (See Clinical Trials, Table 4).

In Medical or Postsurgical ICU studies comparing DIPRIVAN Injectable Emulsion to benzodiazepine infusion or bolus, there were no apparent differences in maintenance of adequate sedation, mean arterial pressure, or laboratory findings. Like the comparators, DIPRIVAN Injectable Emulsion reduced blood cortisol during sedation while maintaining responsivity to challenges with adrenocorticotropic hormone (ACTH). Case reports from the published literature generally reflect that DIPRIVAN Injectable Emulsion has been used safely in patients with a history of porphyria or malignant hyperthermia.

In hemodynamically stable head trauma patients ranging in age from 19-43 years, adequate sedation was maintained with DIPRIVAN Injectable Emulsion or morphine (N=7 in each group). There were no apparent differences in adequacy of sedation, intracranial pressure, cerebral perfusion pressure, or neurologic recovery between the treatment groups. In literature reports from Neurosurgical ICU and severely head-injured patients DIPRIVAN Injectable Emulsion infusion with or without diuretics and hyperventilation controlled intracranial pressure while maintaining cerebral perfusion pressure. In some patients, bolus doses resulted in decreased blood pressure and compromised cerebral perfusion pressure. (See Clinical Trials, Table 4.)

DIPRIVAN Injectable Emulsion was found to be effective in status epilepticus which was refractory to the standard anticonvulsant therapies. For these patients, as well as for ARDS/respiratory failure and tetanus patients, sedation maintenance dosages were generally higher than those for other critically ill patient populations. (See Clinical Trials, Table 4.)

Abrupt discontinuation of DIPRIVAN Injectable Emulsion prior to weaning or for daily evaluation of sedation levels should be avoided. This may result in rapid awakening with associated anxiety, agitation, and resistance to mechanical ventilation. Infusions of DIPRIVAN Injectable Emulsion should be adjusted to maintain a light level of sedation through the weaning process or evaluation of sedation level. (See PRECAUTIONS.)

INDICATIONS AND USAGE

DIPRIVAN Injectable Emulsion is an IV sedative-hypnotic agent that can be used for both induction and/or maintenance of anesthesia as part of a balanced anesthetic technique for inpatient and outpatient surgery in adult patients and pediatric patients greater than 3 years of age. DIPRIVAN Injectable Emulsion can also be used for maintenance of anesthesia as part of a balanced anesthetic technique for inpatient and outpatient surgery in adult patients and in pediatric patients greater than 2 months of age. DIPRIVAN Injectable Emulsion is not recommended for induction of anesthesia below the age of 3 years or for maintenance of anesthesia below the age of 2 months because its safety and effectiveness have not been established in those populations.

In adult patients, DIPRIVAN Injectable Emulsion, when administered intravenously as directed, can be used to initiate and maintain monitored anesthesia care (MAC) sedation during diagnostic procedures. DIPRIVAN Injectable Emulsion may also be used for MAC sedation in conjunction with local/regional anesthesia in patients undergoing surgical procedures. (See PRECAUTIONS.)

Safety, effectiveness and dosing guidelines for DIPRIVAN Injectable Emulsion have not been established for MAC Sedation/light general anesthesia in the pediatric population undergoing diagnostic or nonsurgical procedures and therefore it is not recommended for this use. (See PRECAUTIONS, Pediatric Use).

DIPRIVAN Injectable Emulsion should only be administered to intubated, mechanically ventilated adult patients in the Intensive Care Unit (ICU) to provide continuous sedation and control of stress responses. In this setting, DIPRIVAN Injectable Emulsion should be administered only by persons skilled in the medical management of critically ill patients and trained in cardiovascular resuscitation and airway management.

DIPRIVAN Injectable Emulsion is not indicated for use in Pediatric ICU sedation since the safety of this regimen has not been established. (See PRECAUTIONS, Pediatric Use).

DIPRIVAN Injectable Emulsion is not recommended for obstetrics, including cesarean section deliveries. DIPRIVAN Injectable Emulsion crosses the placenta, and as with other general anesthetic agents, the administration of DIPRIVAN Injectable Emulsion may be associated with neonatal depression. (See PRECAUTIONS.)

DIPRIVAN Injectable Emulsion is not recommended for use in nursing mothers because DIPRIVAN Injectable Emulsion has been reported to be excreted in human milk, and the effects of oral absorption of small amounts of propofol are not known. (See PRECAUTIONS.)

CONTRAINDICATIONS

DIPRIVAN Injectable Emulsion is contraindicated in patients with a known hypersensitivity to DIPRIVAN Injectable Emulsion or its components, or when general anesthesia or sedation are contraindicated.

WARNINGS

For general anesthesia or monitored anesthesia care (MAC) sedation, DIPRIVAN Injectable Emulsion should be administered only by persons trained in the administration of general anesthesia and not involved in the conduct of the surgical/diagnostic procedure. Patients should be continuously monitored, and facilities for maintenance of a patent airway, artificial ventilation, and oxygen enrichment and circulatory resuscitation must be immediately available.

For sedation of intubated, mechanically ventilated adult patients in the Intensive Care Unit (ICU), DIPRIVAN Injectable Emulsion should be administered only by persons skilled in the management of critically ill patients and trained in cardiovascular resuscitation and airway management.

In the elderly, debilitated, or ASA III/IV patients, rapid (single or repeated) bolus administration should not be used during general anesthesia or MAC sedation in order to minimize undesirable cardiorespiratory depression, including hypotension, apnea, airway obstruction, and/or oxygen desaturation.

MAC sedation patients should be continuously monitored by persons not involved in the conduct of the surgical or diagnostic procedure; oxygen supplementation should be immediately available and provided where clinically indicated; and oxygen saturation should be monitored in all patients. Patients should be continuously monitored for early signs of hypotension, apnea, airway obstruction, and/or oxygen desaturation. These cardiorespiratory effects are more likely to occur following rapid initiation (loading) boluses or during supplemental maintenance boluses, especially in the elderly, debilitated, or ASA III/IV patients.

DIPRIVAN Injectable Emulsion should not be coadministered through the same IV catheter with blood or plasma because compatibility has not been established. *In vitro* tests have shown that aggregates of the globular component of the emulsion vehicle have occurred with blood/plasma/serum from humans and animals. The clinical significance is not known.

STRICT ASEPTIC TECHNIQUE MUST ALWAYS BE MAINTAINED DURING HANDLING. DIPRIVAN INJECTABLE EMULSION IS A SINGLE-USE PARENTERAL PRODUCT WHICH CONTAINS 0.005% DISODIUM EDETATE TO RETARD THE RATE OF GROWTH OF MICROORGANISMS IN THE EVENT OF ACCIDENTAL EXTRINSIC CONTAMINATION. HOWEVER, DIPRIVAN INJECTABLE EMULSION CAN STILL SUPPORT THE GROWTH OF MICROORGANISMS AS IT IS NOT AN ANTIMICROBIALLY PRESERVED PRODUCT UNDER USP STANDARDS. ACCORDINGLY, STRICT ASEPTIC TECHNIQUE MUST STILL BE ADHERED TO. DO NOT USE IF CONTAMINATION IS SUSPECTED. DISCARD UNUSED PORTIONS AS DIRECTED WITHIN THE REQUIRED TIME LIMITS (SEE DOSAGE AND ADMINISTRATION, HANDLING PROCEDURES). THERE HAVE BEEN REPORTS IN WHICH FAILURE TO USE ASEPTIC TECHNIQUE WHEN HANDLING DIPRIVAN INJECTABLE EMULSION WAS ASSOCIATED WITH MICROBIAL CONTAMINATION OF THE PRODUCT AND WITH FEVER, INFECTION/SEPSIS, OTHER LIFE-THREATENING ILLNESS, AND/OR DEATH.

PRECAUTIONS

General

Adult and Pediatric Patients: A lower induction dose and a slower maintenance rate of administration should be used in elderly, debilitated, or ASA III/IV patients. (See CLINICAL PHARMACOLOGY - Individualization of Dosage.) Patients should be continuously monitored for early signs of significant hypotension and/or bradycardia. Treatment may include increasing the rate of intravenous fluid, elevation of lower extremities, use of pressor agents, or administration of atropine. Apnea often occurs during induction and may persist for more than 60 seconds. Ventilatory support may be required. Because DIPRIVAN Injectable Emulsion is an emulsion, caution should be exercised in patients with disorders of lipid metabolism such as primary hyperlipoproteinemia, diabetic hyperlipemia, and pancreatitis.

Very rarely the use of DIPRIVAN Injectable Emulsion may be associated with the development of a period of postoperative unconsciousness which may be accompanied by an increase in muscle tone. This may or may not be preceded by a brief period of wakefulness. Recovery is spontaneous. The clinical criteria for discharge from the recovery/day surgery area established for each institution should be satisfied before discharge of the patient from the care of the anesthesiologist.

When DIPRIVAN Injectable Emulsion is administered to an epileptic patient, there may be a risk of seizure during the recovery phase.

Attention should be paid to minimize pain on administration of DIPRIVAN Injectable Emulsion. Transient local pain can be minimized if the larger veins of the forearm or antecubital fossa are used. Pain during intravenous injection may also be reduced by prior injection of IV lidocaine (1 mL of a 1% solution). Pain on injection occurred frequently in pediatric patients (45%) when a small vein of the hand was utilized without lidocaine pretreatment. With lidocaine pretreatment or when antecubital veins were utilized, pain was minimal (incidence less than 10%) and well-tolerated.

Venous sequelae (phlebitis or thrombosis) have been reported rarely (<1%). In two well-controlled clinical studies using dedicated intravenous catheters, no instances of venous sequelae were observed up to 14 days following induction.

Intra-arterial injection in animals did not induce local tissue effects. Accidental intra-arterial injection has been reported in patients, and, other than pain, there were no major sequelae.

Intentional injection into subcutaneous or perivascular tissues of animals caused minimal tissue reaction. During the post-marketing period, there have been rare reports of local pain, swelling, blisters, and/or tissue necrosis following accidental extravasation of DIPRIVAN Injectable Emulsion.

Perioperative myoclonia, rarely including convulsions and opisthotonos, has occurred in temporal relationship in cases in which DIPRIVAN Injectable Emulsion has been administered.

Clinical features of anaphylaxis, which may include angioedema, bronchospasm, erythema, and hypotension, occur rarely following DIPRIVAN Injectable Emulsion administration, although use of other drugs in most instances makes the relationship to DIPRIVAN Injectable Emulsion unclear.

There have been rare reports of pulmonary edema in temporal relationship to the administration of DIPRIVAN Injectable Emulsion, although a causal relationship is unknown.

Very rarely, cases of unexplained postoperative pancreatitis (requiring hospital admission) have been reported after anesthesia in which DIPRIVAN Injectable Emulsion was one of the induction agents used. Due to a variety of confounding factors in these cases, including concomitant medications, a causal relationship to DIPRIVAN Injectable Emulsion is unclear.

DIPRIVAN Injectable Emulsion has no vagolytic activity. Reports of bradycardia, asystole, and rarely, cardiac arrest have been associated with DIPRIVAN Injectable Emulsion. Pediatric patients are susceptible to this effect, particularly when fentanyl is given concomitantly. The intravenous administration of anticholinergic agents (e.g., atropine or glycopyrrolate) should be considered to modify potential increases in vagal tone due to concomitant agents (e.g., succinylcholine) or surgical stimuli.

Intensive Care Unit Sedation

Adult Patients (See WARNINGS and DOSAGE AND ADMINISTRATION, Handling Procedures.) The administration of DIPRIVAN Injectable Emulsion should be initiated as a continuous infusion and changes in the rate of administration made slowly (>5 min) in order to minimize hypotension and avoid acute overdosage. (See CLINICAL PHARMACOLOGY - Individualization of Dosage.)

Patients should be monitored for early signs of significant hypotension and/or cardiovascular depression, which may be profound. These effects are responsive to discontinuation of DIPRIVAN Injectable Emulsion, IV fluid administration, and/or vasopressor therapy.

As with other sedative medications, there is wide interpatient variability in DIPRIVAN Injectable Emulsion dosage requirements, and these requirements may change with time.

Failure to reduce the infusion rate in patients receiving DIPRIVAN Injectable Emulsion for extended periods may result in excessively high blood concentrations of the drug. Thus, titration to clinical response and daily evaluation of sedation levels are important during use of DIPRIVAN Injectable Emulsion infusion for ICU sedation, especially of long duration.

Opioids and paralytic agents should be discontinued and respiratory function optimized prior to weaning patients from mechanical ventilation. Infusions of DIPRIVAN Injectable Emulsion should be adjusted to maintain a light level of sedation prior to weaning patients from mechanical ventilatory support. Throughout the weaning process, this level of sedation may be maintained in the absence of respiratory depression. Because of the rapid clearance of DIPRIVAN Injectable Emulsion, abrupt discontinuation of a patient's infusion may result in rapid awakening of the patient with associated anxiety, agitation, and resistance to mechanical ventilation, making weaning from mechanical ventilation difficult. It is therefore recommended that administration of DIPRIVAN Injectable Emulsion be continued in order to maintain a light level of sedation throughout the weaning process until 10-15 minutes prior to extubation, at which time the infusion can be discontinued.

There have been very rare reports of rhabdomyolysis associated with the administration of DIPRIVAN Injectable Emulsion for ICU sedation.

Since DIPRIVAN Injectable Emulsion is formulated in an oil-in-water emulsion, elevations in serum triglycerides may occur when DIPRIVAN Injectable Emulsion is administered for extended periods of time. Patients at risk of hyperlipidemia should be monitored for increases in serum triglycerides or serum turbidity. Administration of DIPRIVAN Injectable Emulsion should be adjusted if fat is being inadequately cleared from the body. A reduction in the quantity of concurrently administered lipids is indicated to compensate for the amount of lipid infused as part of the

DIPRIVAN Injectable Emulsion formulation; 1 mL of DIPRIVAN Injectable Emulsion contains approximately 0.1 g of fat (1.1 kcal).

EDTA is a strong chelator of trace metals — including zinc. Although with DIPRIVAN Injectable Emulsion there are no reports of decreased zinc levels or zinc deficiency-related adverse events, DIPRIVAN Injectable Emulsion should not be infused for longer than 5 days without providing a drug holiday to safely replace estimated or measured urine zinc losses.

In clinical trials mean urinary zinc loss was approximately 2.5 to 3.0 mg/day in adult patients and 1.5 to 2.0 mg/day in pediatric patients.

In patients who are predisposed to zinc deficiency, such as those with burns, diarrhea, and/or major sepsis, the need for supplemental zinc should be considered during prolonged therapy with DIPRIVAN Injectable Emulsion.

At high doses (2-3 grams per day), EDTA has been reported, on rare occasions, to be toxic to the renal tubules. Studies to-date, in patients with normal or impaired renal function have not shown any alteration in renal function with DIPRIVAN Injectable Emulsion containing 0.005% disodium edetate. In patients at risk for renal impairment, urinalysis and urine sediment should be checked before initiation of sedation and then be monitored on alternate days during sedation.

The long-term administration of DIPRIVAN Injectable Emulsion to patients with renal failure and/or hepatic insufficiency has not been evaluated.

Neurosurgical Anesthesia: When DIPRIVAN Injectable Emulsion is used in patients with increased intracranial pressure or impaired cerebral circulation, significant decreases in mean arterial pressure should be avoided because of the resultant decreases in cerebral perfusion pressure. To avoid significant hypotension and decreases in cerebral perfusion pressure, an infusion or slow bolus of approximately 20 mg every 10 seconds should be utilized instead of rapid, more frequent, and/or larger boluses of DIPRIVAN Injectable Emulsion. Slower induction titrated to clinical responses, will generally result in reduced induction dosage requirements (1 to 2 mg/kg). When increased ICP is suspected, hyperventilation and hypocarbia should accompany the administration of DIPRIVAN Injectable Emulsion. (See DOSAGE AND ADMINISTRATION.)

Cardiac Anesthesia: Slower rates of administration should be utilized in premedicated patients, geriatric patients, patients with recent fluid shifts, or patients who are hemodynamically unstable. Any fluid deficits should be corrected prior to administration of DIPRIVAN Injectable Emulsion. In those patients where additional fluid therapy may be contraindicated, other measures, e.g., elevation of lower extremities, or use of pressor agents, may be useful to offset the hypotension which is associated with the induction of anesthesia with DIPRIVAN Injectable Emulsion.

Information for Patients: Patients should be advised that performance of activities requiring mental alertness, such as operating a motor vehicle, or hazardous machinery or signing legal documents may be impaired for some time after general anesthesia or sedation.

Drug Interactions: The induction dose requirements of DIPRIVAN Injectable Emulsion may be reduced in patients with intramuscular or intravenous premedication, particularly with narcotics (e.g., morphine, meperidine, and fentanyl, etc.) and combinations of opioids and sedatives (e.g., benzodiazepines, barbiturates, chloral hydrate, droperidol, etc.). These agents may increase the anesthetic or sedative effects of DIPRIVAN Injectable Emulsion and may also result in more pronounced decreases in systolic, diastolic, and mean arterial pressures and cardiac output.

During maintenance of anesthesia or sedation, the rate of DIPRIVAN Injectable Emulsion administration should be adjusted according to the desired level of anesthesia or sedation and may be reduced in the presence of supplemental analgesic agents (e.g., nitrous oxide or opioids). The concurrent administration of potent inhalational agents (e.g., isoflurane, enflurane, and halothane) during maintenance with DIPRIVAN Injectable Emulsion has not been extensively evaluated. These inhalational agents can also be expected to increase the anesthetic or sedative and cardiorespiratory effects of DIPRIVAN Injectable Emulsion.

DIPRIVAN Injectable Emulsion does not cause a clinically significant change in onset, intensity or duration of action of the commonly used neuromuscular blocking agents (e.g., succinylcholine and nondepolarizing muscle relaxants).

No significant adverse interactions with commonly used premedications or drugs used during anesthesia or sedation (including a range of muscle relaxants, inhalational agents, analgesic agents, and local anesthetic agents) have been observed in adults. In pediatric patients, administration of fentanyl concomitantly with DIPRIVAN Injectable Emulsion may result in serious bradycardia.

Carcinogenesis, Mutagenesis, Impairment of Fertility: Animal carcinogenicity studies have not been performed with propofol.

In vitro and *in vivo* animal tests failed to show any potential for mutagenicity by propofol. Tests for mutagenicity included the Ames (using *Salmonella* sp) mutation test, gene mutation/gene conversion using *Saccharomyces cerevisiae*, *in vitro* cytogenetic studies in Chinese hamsters, and a mouse micronucleus test.

Studies in female rats at intravenous doses up to 15 mg/kg/day (approximately equivalent to the recommended human induction dose on a mg/m^2 basis) for 2 weeks before pregnancy to day 7 of gestation did not show impaired fertility.

Incidence greater than 1% - Probably Causally Related

	Anesthesia/MAC Sedation	ICU Sedation
Cardiovascular:	Bradycardia Arrhythmia [Peds: 1.2%] Tachycardia Nodal [Peds: 1.6%] Hypotension* [Peds: 17%] (see also CLINICAL PHARMACOLOGY) [Hypertension Peds: 8%]	Bradycardia Decreased Cardiac Output Hypotension 26%
Central Nervous System:	Movement* [Peds: 17%]	
Injection Site:	Burning/Stinging or Pain, 17.6% [Peds: 10%]	
Metabolic/Nutritional:		Hyperlipemia*
Respiratory:	Apnea (see also CLINICAL PHARMACOLOGY)	Respiratory Acidosis During Weaning*
Skin and Appendages:	Rash [Peds: 5%] Pruritus [Peds: 2%]	

Events without an * or % had an incidence of 1%–3%

*Incidence of events 3% to 10%

Incidence less than 1% - Probably Causally Related

	Anesthesia/MAC Sedation	ICU Sedation
Body as a Whole:	Anaphylaxis/Anaphylactoid Reaction Perinatal Disorder [Tachycardia] [Bigeminy] [Bradycardia] [Premature Ventricular Contractions] [Hemorrhage] [ECG Abnormal] [Arrhythmia Atrial] [Fever] [Extremities Pain] [Anticholinergic Syndrome]	
Cardiovascular:	Premature Atrial Contractions Syncope	
Central Nervous System:	Hypertonia/Dystonia, Paresthesia	Agitation
Digestive:	[Hypersalivation] [Nausea]	
Hemic/Lymphatic:	[Leukocytosis]	
Injection Site:	[Phlebitis] [Pruritus]	
Metabolic:	[Hypomagnesemia]	
Musculoskeletal:	Myalgia	
Nervous:	[Dizziness] [Agitation] [Chills] [Somnolence] [Delirium]	
Respiratory:	Wheezing [Cough] [Laryngospasm] [Hypoxia]	Decreased Lung Function
Skin and Appendages:	Flushing, Pruritus	
Special Senses:	Amblyopia [Vision Abnormal]	
Urogenital:	Cloudy Urine	Green Urine

Incidence less than 1% - Causal Relationship Unknown

	Anesthesia/MAC Sedation	ICU Sedation
Body as a Whole:	Asthenia, Awareness, Chest Pain, Extremities Pain, Fever, Increased Drug Effect, Neck Rigidity/Stiffness, Trunk Pain	Fever, Sepsis, Trunk Pain, Whole Body Weakness
Cardiovascular:	Arrhythmia, Atrial Fibrillation, Atrioventricular Heart Block, Bigeminy, Bleeding, Bundle Branch Block, Cardiac Arrest, ECG Abnormal, Edema, Extrasystole, Heart Block, Hypertension, Myocardial Infarction, Myocardial Ischemia, Premature Ventricular Contractions, ST Segment Depression, Supraventricular Tachycardia, Tachycardia, Ventricular Fibrillation	Arrhythmia, Atrial Fibrillation, Bigeminy, Cardiac Arrest, Extrasystole, Right Heart Failure, ventricular Tachycardia
Central Nervous System:	Abnormal Dreams, Agitation, Amorous Behavior, Anxiety, Bucking/Jerking/Thrashing, Chills/Shivering/Clonic/Myoclonic Movement, Combativeness, Confusion, Delirium, Depression, Dizziness, Emotional Lability, Euphoria, Fatigue, Hallucinations, Headache, Hypotonia, Hysteria, Insomnia, Moaning, Neuropathy, Opisthotonos, Rigidity, Seizures, Somnolence, Tremor, Twitching	Chills/Shivering, Intracranial Hypertension, Seizures, Somnolence, Thinking Abnormal
Digestive:	Cramping, Diarrhea, Dry Mouth, Enlarged Parotid, Nausea, Swallowing, Vomiting	Ileus, Liver Function Abnormal
Hematologic/Lymphatic:	Coagulation Disorder, Leukocytosis	
Injection Site:	Hives/Itching, Phlebitis, Redness/Discoloration	
Metabolic/Nutritional:	Hyperkalemia, Hyperlipemia	BUN Increased, Creatinine Increased, Dehydration, Hyperglycemia, Metabolic Acidosis, Osmolality Increased
Respiratory:	Bronchospasm, Burning in Throat, Cough, Dyspnea, Hiccough, Hyperventilation, Hypoventilation, Hypoxia, Laryngospasm, Pharyngitis, Sneezing, Tachypnea, Upper Airway Obstruction	Hypoxia
Skin and Appendages:	Conjunctival Hyperemia, Diaphoresis, Urticaria	Rash
Special Senses:	Diplopia, Ear Pain, Eye Pain, Nystagmus, Taste Perversion, Tinnitus	
Urogenital:	Oliguria, Urine Retention	Kidney Failure

Male fertility in rats was not affected in a dominant lethal study at intravenous doses up to 15 mg/kg/day for 5 days.

Pregnancy Category B: Reproduction studies have been performed in rats and rabbits at intravenous doses of 15 mg/kg/day (approximately equivalent to the recommended human induction dose on a mg/m^2 basis) and have revealed no evidence of impaired fertility or harm to the fetus due to propofol. Propofol, however, has been shown to cause maternal deaths in rats and rabbits and decreased pup survival during the lactating period in dams treated with 15 mg/kg/day (approximately equivalent to the recommended human induction dose on a mg/m^2 basis). The pharmacological activity (anesthesia) of the drug on the mother is probably responsible for the adverse effects seen in the offspring. There are, however, no adequate and well-controlled studies in pregnant women. Because animal reproduction studies are not always predictive of human responses, this drug should be used during pregnancy only if clearly needed.

Labor and Delivery: DIPRIVAN Injectable Emulsion is not recommended for obstetrics, including cesarean section deliveries. DIPRIVAN Injectable Emulsion crosses the placenta, and as with other general anesthetic agents, the administration of DIPRIVAN Injectable Emulsion may be associated with neonatal depression.

Continued on next page

Diprivan—Cont.

Nursing Mothers: DIPRIVAN Injectable Emulsion is not recommended for use in nursing mothers because DIPRIVAN Injectable Emulsion has been reported to be excreted in human milk and the effects of oral absorption of small amounts of propofol are not known.

Pediatric Use: The safety and effectiveness of DIPRIVAN Injectable Emulsion have been established for induction of anesthesia in pediatric patients aged 3 years and older and for the maintenance of anesthesia aged 2 months and older. DIPRIVAN Injectable Emulsion is not recommended for the induction of anesthesia in patients younger than 3 years of age and for the maintenance of anesthesia in patients younger than 2 months of age as safety and effectiveness have not been established.

In pediatric patients, administration of fentanyl concomitantly with DIPRIVAN Injectable Emulsion may result in serious bradycardia (see PRECAUTIONS – General).

DIPRIVAN Injectable Emulsion is not indicated for use in pediatric patients for ICU sedation or for MAC sedation for surgical, nonsurgical or diagnostic procedures as safety and effectiveness have not been established.

There have been anecdotal reports of serious adverse events and death in pediatric patients with upper respiratory tract infections receiving DIPRIVAN Injectable Emulsion for ICU sedation.

In one multicenter clinical trial of ICU sedation in critically ill pediatric patients that excluded patients with upper respiratory tract infections, the incidence of mortality observed in patients who received DIPRIVAN Injectable Emulsion (n=222) was 9%, while that for patients who received standard sedative agents (n=105) was 4%. While causality has not been established, DIPRIVAN Injectable Emulsion is not indicated for sedation in pediatric patients until further studies have been performed to document its safety in that population. (See CLINICAL PHARMACOLOGY – Pediatric Patients: and Dosage and Administration).

In pediatric patients, abrupt discontinuation following prolonged infusion may result in flushing of the hands and feet, agitation, tremulousness and hyperirritability. Increased incidences of bradycardia (5%), agitation (4%), and jitteriness (9%) have also been observed.

Geriatric Use: The effect of age on induction dose requirements for propofol was assessed in an open study involving 211 unpremedicated patients with approximately 30 patients in each decade between the ages of 16 and 80. The average dose to induce anesthesia was calculated for patients up to 54 years of age and for patients 55 years of age or older. The average dose to induce anesthesia in patients up to 54 years of age was 1.99 mg/kg and in patients above 54 it was 1.66 mg/kg. Subsequent clinical studies have demonstrated lower dosing requirements for subjects greater than 60 years of age.

A lower induction dose and a slower maintenance rate of administration of DIPRIVAN Injectable Emulsion should be used in elderly patients. In this group of patients, rapid (single or repeated) bolus administration should not be used in order to minimize undesirable cardiorespiratory depression including hypotension, apnea, airway obstruction, and/or oxygen desaturation. All dosing should be titrated according to patient condition and response. (See DOSAGE AND ADMINISTRATION – Elderly, debilitated or ASA III/IV patients and CLINICAL PHARMACOLOGY – Geriatrics.)

ADVERSE REACTIONS

General

Adverse event information is derived from controlled clinical trials and worldwide marketing experience. In the description below, rates of the more common events represent US/Canadian clinical study results. Less frequent events are also derived from publications and marketing experience in over 8 million patients; there are insufficient data to support an accurate estimate of their incidence rates. These studies were conducted using a variety of premedicants, varying lengths of surgical/diagnostic procedures, and various other anesthetic/sedative agents. Most adverse events were mild and transient.

Anesthesia and MAC Sedation in Adults

The following estimates of adverse events for DIPRIVAN Injectable Emulsion include data from clinical trials in general anesthesia/MAC sedation (N=2889 adult patients). The adverse events listed below as probably causally related are those events in which the actual incidence rate in patients treated with DIPRIVAN Injectable Emulsion was greater than the comparator incidence rate in these trials. Therefore, incidence rates for anesthesia and MAC sedation in adults generally represent estimates of the percentage of clinical trial patients which appeared to have probable causal relationship.

The adverse experience profile from reports of 150 patients in the MAC sedation clinical trials is similar to the profile established with DIPRIVAN Injectable Emulsion during anesthesia (see below). During MAC sedation clinical trials, significant respiratory events included cough, upper airway obstruction, apnea, hypoventilation, and dyspnea.

Anesthesia in Pediatric Patients

Generally the adverse experience profile from reports of 506 DIPRIVAN Injectable Emulsion pediatric patients from 6 days through 16 years of age in the US/Canadian anesthesia clinical trials is similar to the profile established with DIPRIVAN Injectable Emulsion during anesthesia in adults (see Pediatric percentages [Peds %] below). Although not reported as an adverse event in clinical trials, apnea is frequently observed in pediatric patients.

ICU Sedation in Adults

The following estimates of adverse events include data from clinical trials in ICU sedation (N=159 adult patients). Probably related incidence rates for ICU sedation were determined by individual case report form review. Probable causality was based upon an apparent dose response relationship and/or positive responses to rechallenge. In many instances the presence of concomitant disease and concomitant therapy made the causal relationship unknown. Therefore, incidence rates for ICU sedation generally represent estimates of the percentage of clinical trial patients which appeared to have a probable causal relationship.

[See table at top of previous page]

DRUG ABUSE AND DEPENDENCE

Rare cases of self-administration of DIPRIVAN Injectable Emulsion by health care professionals have been reported, including some fatalities. DIPRIVAN Injectable Emulsion should be managed to prevent the risk of diversion, including restriction of access and accounting procedures as appropriate to the clinical setting.

OVERDOSAGE

If overdosage occurs, DIPRIVAN Injectable Emulsion administration should be discontinued immediately. Overdosage is likely to cause cardiorespiratory depression. Respiratory depression should be treated by artificial ventilation with oxygen. Cardiovascular depression may require repositioning of the patient by raising the patient's legs, increasing the flow rate of intravenous fluids, and administering pressor agents and/or anticholinergic agents.

DOSAGE AND ADMINISTRATION

Dosage and rate of administration should be individualized and titrated to the desired effect, according to clinically relevant factors, including preinduction and concomitant medications, age, ASA physical classification, and level of debilitation of the patient.

The following is abbreviated dosage and administration information which is only intended as a general guide in the use of DIPRIVAN Injectable Emulsion. Prior to administering DIPRIVAN Injectable Emulsion, it is imperative that the physician review and be completely familiar with the specific dosage and administration information detailed in the CLINICAL PHARMACOLOGY - Individualization of Dosage section.

In the elderly, debilitated, or ASA III/IV patients, rapid bolus doses should not be the method of administration. (See WARNINGS.)

Intensive Care Unit Sedation:

STRICT ASEPTIC TECHNIQUE MUST ALWAYS BE MAINTAINED DURING HANDLING. DIPRIVAN INJECTABLE EMULSION IS A SINGLE-USE PARENTERAL PRODUCT WHICH CONTAINS 0.005% DISODIUM EDETATE TO RETARD THE RATE OF GROWTH OF MICROORGANISMS IN THE EVENT OF ACCIDENTAL EXTRINSIC CONTAMINATION. HOWEVER, DIPRIVAN INJECTABLE EMULSION CAN

INDICATION	DOSAGE AND ADMINISTRATION
Induction of General Anesthesia	**Healthy Adults Less Than 55 Years of Age:** 40 mg every 10 seconds until induction onset (2 to 2.5 mg/kg). **Elderly, Debilitated, or ASA III/IV Patients:** 20 mg every 10 seconds until induction onset (1 to 1.5 mg/kg). **Cardiac Anesthesia:** 20 mg every 10 seconds until induction onset (0.5 to 1.5 mg/kg). **Neurosurgical Patients:** 20 mg every 10 seconds until induction onset (1 to 2 mg/kg) **Pediatric Patients - healthy, from 3 years to 16 years of age:** 2.5 to 3.5 mg/kg administered over 20-30 seconds. See PRECAUTIONS—Pediatric Use: and CLINICAL PHARMACOLOGY—Pediatric patients)
Maintenance of General Anesthesia:	**Infusion** **Healthy Adults Less Than 55 Years of Age:** 100 to 200 µg/kg/min (6 to 12 mg/kg/h). **Elderly, Debilitated, ASA III/IV Patients:** 50 to 100 µg/kg/min (3 to 6 mg/kg/h). **Cardiac Anesthesia:** Most patients require: Primary DIPRIVAN Injectable Emulsion with Secondary Opioid-100-150 µg/kg/min Low-Dose DIPRIVAN Injectable Emulsion with Primary Opioid-50-100 µg/kg/min (See CLINICAL PHARMACOLOGY, Table 5) **Neurosurgical Patients:** 100 to 200 µg/kg/min (6 to 12 mg/kg/h). **Pediatric Patients—healthy, from 2 months of age to 16 years of age:** 125 to 300 µg/kg/min (7.5 to 18 mg/kg/h) Following the first half hour of maintenance, if clinical signs of light anesthesia are not present, the infusion rate should be decreased. (See PRECAUTIONS—Pediatric Use: and CLINICAL PHARMACOLOGY—Pediatric patients)
Maintenance of General Anesthesia:	**Intermittent Bolus** **Healthy Adults Less Than 55 Years of Age:** Increments of 20 to 50 mg as needed.
Initiation of MAC Sedation:	**Healthy Adults Less Than 55 Years of Age:** Slow infusion or slow injection techniques are recommended to avoid apnea or hypotension. Most patients require an infusion of 100 to 150 µg/kg/min (6 to 9 mg/kg/h) for 3 to 5 minutes or a slow injection of 0.5 mg/kg over 3 to 5 minutes followed immediately by a maintenance infusion. **Elderly, Debilitated, Neurosurgical, or ASA III/IV Patients:** Most patients require dosages similar to healthy adults. Rapid boluses are to be avoided. (See WARNINGS.)
Maintenance of MAC Sedation	**Healthy Adults Less Than 55 Years of Age:** A variable rate infusion technique is preferable over an intermittent bolus technique. Most patients require an infusion of 25 to 75 µg/kg/min (1.5 to 4.5 mg/kg/h) or incremental bolus doses of 10 mg or 20 mg. **In Elderly, Debilitated, Neurosurgical, or ASA III/IV Patients:** Most patients require 80% of the usual adult dose. A rapid (single or repeated) bolus dose should not be used. (See WARNINGS.)
Initiation and Maintenance of ICU Sedation in Intubated, Mechanically Ventilated	**Adult Patients**—Because of the residual effects of previous anesthetic or sedative agents, in most patients the initial infusion should be 5 µg/kg/min (0.3 mg/kg/h) for at least 5 minutes. Subsequent increments of 5 to 10 µg/kg/min (0.3 to 0.6 mg/kg/h) over 5 to 10 minutes may be used until desired clinical effect is achieved. Maintenance rates of 5 to 50 µg/kg/min (0.3 to 3 mg/kg/h) or higher may be required. **Evaluation of clinical effect and assessment of CNS function should be carried out daily throughout maintenance to determine the minimum dose of DIPRIVAN Injectable Emulsion required for sedation.** **The tubing and any unused portions of DIPRIVAN Injectable Emulsion should be discarded after 12 hours because DIPRIVAN Injectable Emulsion contains no preservatives and is capable of supporting rapid growth of microorganisms. (See WARNINGS, and DOSAGE AND ADMINISTRATION.)**

STILL SUPPORT THE GROWTH OF MICROORGANISMS AS IT IS NOT AN ANTIMICROBIALLY PRESERVED PRODUCT UNDER USP STANDARDS. ACCORDINGLY, STRICT ASEPTIC TECHNIQUE MUST STILL BE ADHERED TO. DO NOT USE IF CONTAMINATION IS SUSPECTED. (See DOSAGE AND ADMINISTRATION, Handling Procedures.)

DIPRIVAN Injectable Emulsion should be individualized according to the patient's condition and response, blood lipid profile, and vital signs. (See PRECAUTIONS - ICU Sedation.) For intubated, mechanically ventilated adult patients, Intensive Care Unit (ICU) sedation should be initiated slowly with a continuous infusion in order to titrate to desired clinical effect and minimize hypotension. When indicated, initiation of sedation should begin at 5 µg/kg/min (0.3 mg/kg/h). The infusion rate should be increased by increments of 5 to 10 µg/kg/min (0.3 to 0.6 mg/kg/h) until the desired level of sedation is achieved. A minimum period of 5 minutes between adjustments should be allowed for onset of peak drug effect. Most adult patients require maintenance rates of 5 to 50 µg/kg/min (0.3 to 3 mg/kg/h) or higher. Dosages of DIPRIVAN Injectable Emulsion should be reduced in patients who have received large dosages of narcotics. Conversely, the DIPRIVAN Injectable Emulsion dosage requirement may be reduced by adequate management of pain with analgesic agents. As with other sedative medications, there is interpatient variability in dosage requirements, and these requirements may change with time. (See dosage guide.) **EVALUATION OF LEVEL OF SEDATION AND ASSESSMENT OF CNS FUNCTION SHOULD BE CARRIED OUT DAILY THROUGHOUT MAINTENANCE TO DETERMINE THE MINIMUM DOSE OF DIPRIVAN INJECTABLE EMULSION REQUIRED FOR SEDATION (SEE CLINICAL TRIALS, ICU SEDATION).** Bolus administration of 10 or 20 mg should only be used to rapidly increase depth of sedation in patients where hypotension is not likely to occur. Patients with compromised myocardial function, intravascular volume depletion, or abnormally low vascular tone (e.g., sepsis) may be more susceptible to hypotension. (See PRECAUTIONS).

EDTA is a strong chelator of trace metals – including zinc. Although with DIPRIVAN Injectable Emulsion there are no reports of decreased zinc levels or zinc deficiency-related adverse events, DIPRIVAN Injectable Emulsion should not be infused for longer than 5 days without providing a drug holiday to safely replace estimated or measured urine zinc losses.

At high doses (2-3 grams per day), EDTA has been reported, on rare occasions, to be toxic to the renal tubules. Studies to-date, in patients with normal or impaired renal function have not shown any alteration in renal function with DIPRIVAN Injectable Emulsion containing 0.005% disodium edetate. In patients at risk for renal impairment, urinalysis and urine sediment should be checked before initiation of sedation and then be monitored on alternate days during sedation.

SUMMARY OF DOSAGE GUIDELINES -

Dosages and rates of administration in the following table should be individualized and titrated to clinical response. Safety and dosing requirements for induction of anesthesia in pediatric patients have only been established for children 3 years of age or older. Safety and dosing requirements for the maintenance of anesthesia have only been established for children 2 months of age and older.

For complete dosage information, see CLINICAL PHARMACOLOGY - Individualization of Dosage.

[See table at top of previous page]

Compatibility and Stability: DIPRIVAN Injectable Emulsion should not be mixed with other therapeutic agents prior to administration.

Dilution Prior to Administration: DIPRIVAN Injectable Emulsion is provided as a ready to use formulation. However, should dilution be necessary, it should only be diluted with 5% Dextrose Injection, USP, and it should not be diluted to a concentration less than 2 mg/mL because it is an emulsion. In diluted form it has been shown to be more stable when in contact with glass than with plastic (95% potency after 2 hours of running infusion in plastic).

Administration with Other Fluids: Compatibility of DIPRIVAN Injectable Emulsion with the coadministration of blood/serum/plasma has not been established. (See WARNINGS.) When administered using a y-type infusion set, DIPRIVAN Injectable Emulsion has been shown to be compatible with the following intravenous fluids.

— 5% Dextrose Injection, USP
— Lactated Ringers Injection, USP
— Lactated Ringers and 5% Dextrose Injection
— 5% Dextrose and 0.45% Sodium Chloride Injection, USP
— 5% Dextrose and 0.2% Sodium Chloride Injection, USP

Assembly Instructions for Pre-Filled Syringe

1. Remove the Luer connector from packaging.
2. Remove glass syringe barrel from tray and check for cracks or leaks. Shake. Remove the plastic cover. Applying moderate pressure, disinfect the surface of the rubber stopper using the alcohol swab provided in the package prior to attachment of the Luer connector.
3. Pull off needle cover from Luer connector. The bevel of the needle spike is slightly bent (c-tip) to prevent potential coring.

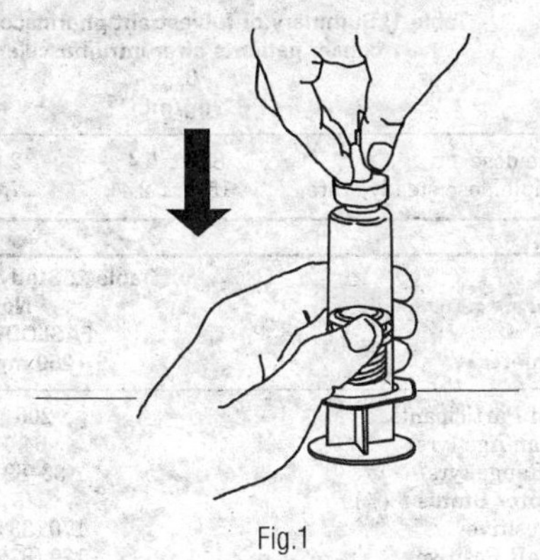

Fig.1

4. Stand the syringe barrel vertically on a hard surface and push Luer connector on to syringe barrel so needle penetrates rubber seal and connector slides over the aluminum seal until firmly seated. (Fig. 1)

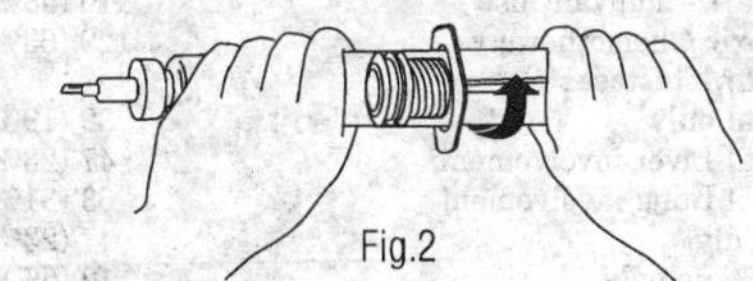

Fig.2

5. Add plunger rod by screwing clockwise. CAUTION: the rod must be fully screwed on, otherwise it may detach which could result in siphoning of the syringe contents. (Fig. 2)
6. Unscrew Luer cover and remove excess nitrogen gas from the syringe (a small nitrogen gas bubble may remain). Assemble administration line and connect syringe.

Handling Procedures

General

Parenteral drug products should be inspected visually for particulate matter and discoloration prior to administration whenever solution and container permit.

Clinical experience with the use of in-line filters and DIPRIVAN Injectable Emulsion during anesthesia or ICU/MAC sedation is limited. DIPRIVAN Injectable Emulsion should only be administered through a filter with a pore size of 5 µm or greater unless it has been demonstrated that the filter does not restrict the flow of DIPRIVAN Injectable Emulsion and/or cause the breakdown of the emulsion. Filters should be used with caution and where clinically appropriate. Continuous monitoring is necessary due to the potential for restricted flow and/or breakdown of the emulsion. Do not use if there is evidence of separation of the phases of the emulsion.

Rare cases of self-administration of DIPRIVAN Injectable Emulsion by health care professionals have been reported, including some fatalities (See DRUG ABUSE AND DEPENDENCE).

STRICT ASEPTIC TECHNIQUE MUST ALWAYS BE MAINTAINED DURING HANDLING. DIPRIVAN INJECTABLE EMULSION IS A SINGLE-USE PARENTERAL PRODUCT WHICH CONTAINS 0.005% DISODIUM EDETATE TO RETARD THE RATE OF GROWTH OF MICROORGANISMS IN THE EVENT OF ACCIDENTAL EXTRINSIC CONTAMINATION. HOWEVER, DIPRIVAN INJECTABLE EMULSION CAN STILL SUPPORT THE GROWTH OF MICROORGANISMS AS IT IS NOT AN ANTIMICROBIALLY PRESERVED PRODUCT UNDER USP STANDARDS. ACCORDINGLY, STRICT ASEPTIC TECHNIQUE MUST STILL BE ADHERED TO. DO NOT USE IF CONTAMINATION IS SUSPECTED. DISCARD UNUSED PORTIONS AS DIRECTED WITHIN THE REQUIRED TIME LIMITS (SEE DOSAGE AND ADMINISTRATION, HANDLING PROCEDURES). THERE HAVE BEEN REPORTS IN WHICH FAILURE TO USE ASEPTIC TECHNIQUE WHEN HANDLING DIPRIVAN INJECTABLE EMULSION WAS ASSOCIATED WITH MICROBIAL CONTAMINATION OF THE PRODUCT AND WITH FEVER, INFECTION/SEPSIS, OTHER LIFE-THREATENING ILLNESS, AND/OR DEATH.

Guidelines for Aseptic Technique for General Anesthesia/MAC Sedation

DIPRIVAN Injectable Emulsion should be prepared for use just prior to initiation of each individual anesthetic/sedative procedure. The vial/pre-filled syringe rubber stopper should be disinfected using 70% isopropyl alcohol. DIPRIVAN Injectable Emulsion should be drawn into sterile syringes immediately after vials are opened. When withdrawing DIPRIVAN Injectable Emulsion from vials, a sterile vent spike should be used. The syringe(s) should be labeled with appropriate information including the date and time the vial was opened. Administration should commence promptly and be completed within 6 hours after the vials or pre-filled syringes have been opened.

DIPRIVAN Injectable Emulsion should be prepared for single-patient use only. Any unused portions of DIPRIVAN Injectable Emulsion, reservoirs, dedicated administration tubing and/or solutions containing DIPRIVAN Injectable Emulsion must be discarded at the end of the anesthetic procedure or at 6 hours, whichever occurs sooner. The IV line should be flushed every 6 hours and at the end of the anesthetic procedure to remove residual DIPRIVAN Injectable Emulsion.

Guidelines for Aseptic Technique for ICU Sedation

DIPRIVAN Injectable Emulsion should be prepared for single-patient use only. When DIPRIVAN Injectable Emulsion is administered directly from the vial/pre-filled syringe, strict aseptic techniques must be followed. The vial/pre-filled syringe rubber stopper should be disinfected using 70% isopropyl alcohol. A sterile vent spike and sterile tubing must be used for administration of DIPRIVAN Injectable Emulsion. As with other lipid emulsions, the number of IV line manipulations should be minimized. Administration should commence promptly and must be completed within 12 hours after the vial has been spiked. The tubing and any unused portions of DIPRIVAN Injectable Emulsion must be discarded after 12 hours.

If DIPRIVAN Injectable Emulsion is transferred to a syringe or other container prior to administration, the handling procedures for General anesthesia/MAC sedation should be followed, and the product should be discarded and administration lines changed after 6 hours.

HOW SUPPLIED

DIPRIVAN Injectable Emulsion is available in ready to use 20 mL infusion vials, 50 mL infusion vials, 100 mL infusion vials, and 50 mL pre-filled syringes containing 10 mg/mL of propofol.

20 mL infusion vials (NDC 0310-0300-22)
50 mL infusion vials (NDC 0310-0300-50)
100 mL infusion vials (NDC 0310-0300-11)
50 mL pre-filled syringes (NDC 0310-0300-54)

Propofol undergoes oxidative degradation, in the presence of oxygen, and is therefore packaged under nitrogen to eliminate this degradation path.

Store between 4-22°C (40-72°F). Do not freeze. Shake well before use.

All trademarks are the property of the AstraZeneca group

Manufactured for:
AstraZeneca Pharmaceuticals, LP
Wilmington, DE 19850
By: AstraZeneca S.p.A., Caponago, Italy
Made in Italy
Rev 2/01 SIC 64180-02

Shown in Product Identification Guide, page 306

FASLODEX® ℞

[făs'lō-dĕks]

fulvestrant injection

DESCRIPTION

FASLODEX® (fulvestrant) Injection for intramuscular administration is an estrogen receptor antagonist without known agonist effects. The chemical name is 7-alpha-[9-(4,4,5,5,5-penta fluoropentylsulphinyl) nonyl]estra-1,3,5-(10)- triene-3,17-beta-diol. The molecular formula is $C_{32}H_{47}F_5O_3S$ and its structural formula is:

OH
HO
$(CH_2)_9SO(CH_2)_3CF_2CF_3$

Fulvestrant is a white powder with a molecular weight of 606.77. The solution for injection is a clear, colorless to yellow, viscous liquid.

Each injection contains as inactive ingredients: Alcohol, USP, Benzyl Alcohol, NF, and Benzyl Benzoate, USP, as co-solvents, and Castor Oil, USP as a co-solvent and release rate modifier.

FASLODEX is supplied in sterile single patient pre-filled syringes containing 50-mg/mL fulvestrant either as a single 5 mL or two concurrent 2.5 mL injections to deliver the required monthly dose. FASLODEX is administered as an intramuscular injection of 250 mg once monthly.

CLINICAL PHARMACOLOGY

Mechanism of Action

Many breast cancers have estrogen receptors (ER), and the growth of these tumors can be stimulated by estrogen. Fulvestrant is an estrogen receptor antagonist that binds to the estrogen receptor in a competitive manner with affinity comparable to that of estradiol. Fulvestrant down regulates the ER protein in human breast cancer cells.

In a clinical study in postmenopausal women with primary breast cancer treated with single doses of FASLODEX 15–22 days prior to surgery, there was evidence of increasing down regulation of ER with increasing dose. This was associated with a dose-related decrease in the expression of the progesterone receptor, an estrogen-regulated protein. These effects on the ER pathway were also associated with a decrease in Ki67 labeling index, a marker of cell proliferation.

In vitro studies demonstrated that fulvestrant is a reversible inhibitor of the growth of tamoxifen-resistant, as well as estrogen-sensitive human breast cancer (MCF-7) cell lines. In *in vivo* tumor studies, fulvestrant delayed the establishment of tumors from xenografts of human breast cancer MCF-7 cells in nude mice. Fulvestrant inhibited the growth of established MCF-7 xenografts and of tamoxifen-

Continued on next page

Faslodex—Cont.

resistant breast tumor xenografts. Fulvestrant resistant breast tumor xenografts may also be cross-resistant to tamoxifen.

Fulvestrant showed no agonist-type effects in *in vivo* uterotropic assays in immature or ovariectomized mice and rats. In *in vivo* studies in immature rats and ovariectomized monkeys, fulvestrant blocked the uterotrophic action of estradiol. In postmenopausal women, the absence of changes in plasma concentrations of FSH and LH in response to fulvestrant treatment (250 mg monthly) suggests no peripheral steroidal effects.

Pharmacokinetics

Following intravenous administration, fulvestrant is rapidly cleared at a rate approximating hepatic blood flow (about 10.5 mL plasma/min/Kg). After an intramuscular injection plasma concentrations are maximal at about 7 days and are maintained over a period of at least one month, with trough concentration about one-third of C_{max}. The apparent half-life was about 40 days. After administration of 250 mg of fulvestrant intramuscularly every month, plasma levels approach steady-state after 3 to 6 doses, with an average 2.5 fold increase in plasma AUC, compared to single dose AUC and trough levels about equal to the single dose C_{max} (see **Table 1**).

[See table 1 at right]

Fulvestrant was subject to extensive and rapid distribution. The apparent volume of distribution at steady state was approximately 3 to 5 L/kg. This suggests that distribution is largely extravascular. Fulvestrant was highly (99%) bound to plasma proteins; VLDL, LDL and HDL lipoprotein fractions appear to be the major binding components. The role of sex hormone-binding globulin, if any, could not be determined.

Metabolism and Excretion

Biotransformation and disposition of fulvestrant in humans have been determined following intramuscular and intravenous administration of ^{14}C-labeled fulvestrant. Metabolism of fulvestrant appears to involve combinations of a number of possible biotransformation pathways analogous to those of endogenous steroids, including oxidation, aromatic hydroxylation, conjugation with glucuronic acid and/or sulphate at the 2, 3 and 17 positions of the steroid nucleus, and oxidation of the side chain sulphoxide. Identified metabolites are either less active or exhibit similar activity to fulvestrant in antiestrogen models. Studies using human liver preparations and recombinant human enzymes indicate that cytochrome P-450 3A4 (CYP 3A4) is the only P-450 isoenzyme involved in the oxidation of fulvestrant; however, the relative contribution of P-450 and non-P-450 routes *in vivo* is unknown.

Fulvestrant was rapidly cleared by the hepatobiliary route, with excretion primarily via the feces (approximately 90%). Renal elimination was negligible (less than 1%).

Special Populations

Geriatric: In patients with breast cancer, there was no difference in fulvestrant pharmacokinetic profile related to age (range 33 to 89 years).

Gender: Following administration of a single intravenous dose, there were no pharmacokinetic differences between men and women or between premenopausal and postmenopausal women. Similarly, there were no differences between men and postmenopausal women after intramuscular administration.

Race: In the advanced breast cancer treatment trials, the potential for pharmacokinetic differences due to race have been evaluated in 294 women including 87.4% Caucasian, 7.8% Black, and 4.4% Hispanic. No differences in fulvestrant plasma pharmacokinetics were observed among these groups. In a separate trial, pharmacokinetic data from postmenopausal ethnic Japanese women were similar to those obtained in non-Japanese patients.

Renal Impairment: Negligible amounts of fulvestrant are eliminated in urine; therefore, a study in patients with renal impairment was not conducted. In the advanced breast cancer trials, fulvestrant concentrations in women with estimated creatinine clearance as low as 30 mL/min were similar to women with normal creatinine.

Hepatic Impairment: Fulvestrant is metabolized primarily in the liver. In clinical trials in patients with locally advanced or metastatic breast cancer, pharmacokinetic data were obtained following administration of a 250 mg dose of FASLODEX to 261 patients classified as having normal liver function and to 24 patients with mild impairment. Mild impairment was defined as an alanine aminotransferase concentration (at any visit) greater than the upper limit of the normal (ULN) reference range, but less than 2 times the ULN; or if any 2 of the following 3 parameters were between 1- and 2-times the ULN: aspartate aminotransferase, alkaline phosphatase, or total bilirubin.

There was no clear relationship between fulvestrant clearance and hepatic impairment and the safety profile in patients with mild hepatic impairment was similar to that seen in patients with no hepatic impairment. Safety and efficacy have not been evaluated in patients with moderate to severe hepatic impairment (see **PRECAUTIONS-Hepatic Impairment** and **DOSAGE AND ADMINISTRATION-Hepatic Impairment** sections).

Pediatric: The pharmacokinetics of fulvestrant have not been evaluated in pediatric patients.

Table 1: Summary of fulvestrant pharmacokinetic parameters in postmenopausal advanced breast cancer patients after intramuscular administration of a 250 mg dose (Mean ± SD)

	C_{max} ng/mL	C_{min} ng/mL	AUC ng.d/mL	t½ days	CL mL/min
Single dose	8.5 ± 5.4	2.6 ± 1.1	131 ± 62	40 ± 11	690 ± 226
Multiple dose steady state	15.8 ± 2.4	7.4 ± 1.7	328 ± 48		

Table 2: Study Population Demographics

	North American Trial		European Trial	
Parameter	**FASLODEX 250 mg**	**Anastrozole 1 mg**	**FASLODEX 250 mg**	**Anastrozole 1 mg**
No. of Participants	206	194	222	229
Median Age (yrs)	64	61	64	65
Age Range (yrs)	33–89	36–94	35–86	33–89
Receptor Status # (%)				
ER Positive	170 (83%)	156 (80%)	156 (70%)	173 (76%)
ER/PgR Positive	179 (87%)	169 (87%)	163 (73%)	183 (80%)
ER/PgR Unknown	13 (6%)	15 (8%)	51 (23%)	37 (16%)
Previous Therapy				
Tamoxifen	196 (95%)	187 (96%)	215 (97%)	225 (98%)
Adjuvant antiestrogen only	94 (46%)	94 (48%)	95 (43%)	100 (44%)
Antiestrogen for advanced disease +/- adjuvant use	110 (53%)	97 (50%)	126 (57%)	129 (56%)
Cytotoxic Chemotherapy	129 (63%)	122 (63%)	94 (42%)	98 (43%)
Site of Metastases				
Visceral only*	39 (19%)	45 (23%)	30 (14%)	41 (18%)
Visceral Liver involvement	47 (23%)	45 (23%)	48 (22%)	56 (24%)
Visceral Lung involvement	63 (31%)	60 (31%)	56 (25%)	60 (26%)
Bone only	47 (23%)	43 (22%)	38 (17%)	40 (17%)
Soft Tissue only	12 (6%)	13 (7%)	11 (5%)	8 (3%)
Skin and soft tissue	43 (21%)	41 (21%)	40 (18%)	35 (15%)

*Defined as liver or lung metastatic, or recurrent, disease
ER/PgR Positive defined as ER positive or PgR positive
ER/PgR Unknown defined as ER unknown and PgR unknown

Table 3: Efficacy Results

	North American Trial		European Trial	
Endpoint	**FASLODEX 250 mg (n=206)**	**Anastrozole 1 mg (n=194)**	**FASLODEX 250 mg (n=222)**	**Anastrozole 1 mg (n=229)**
Objective tumor response				
Number (%) of subjects with CR + PR	35 (17.0)	33 (17.0)	45 (20.3)	34 (14.9)
% Difference in Tumor Response Rate (FAS-ANA)	0.0		5.4	
2-sided 95.4% CI	(−6.3, 8.9)		(−1.4, 14.8)	
Time to progression (TTP)				
Median TTP (days)	165	103	166	156
Hazard ratio (FAS/ANA)	0.9		1.0	
2-sided 95.4% CI	(0.7, 1.1)		(0.8, 1.2)	
Stable Disease for ≥24 weeks (%)	26.7	19.1	24.3	30.1
Survival Time				
Died n (%)	109 (52.9%)	92 (47.4%)	125 (56.3%)	130 (56.8%)
Median Survival (days)	837	901	803	742
Hazard ratio	1.1		1.0	
2-sided 95% CI	(0.8, 1.5)		(0.8, 1.3)	

CR = Complete Response; PR = Partial Response; CI = Confidence Interval; FAS = FASLODEX; ANA = anastrazole

Drug-Drug Interactions

There are no known drug-drug interactions. Fulvestrant does not significantly inhibit any of the major CYP isoenzymes, including CYP 1A2, 2C9, 2C19, 2D6, and 3A4 *in vitro*, and studies of co-administration of fulvestrant with midazolam indicate that therapeutic doses of fulvestrant have no inhibitory effects on CYP 3A4 or alter blood levels of drug metabolized by that enzyme. Also, although fulvestrant is partly metabolized by CYP 3A4, a clinical study with rifampin, an inducer of CYP 3A4, showed no effect on the pharmacokinetics of fulvestrant. Clinical studies of the effect of strong CYP 3A4 inhibitors on the pharmacokinetics of fulvestrant have not been performed.

Clinical Studies

Efficacy of FASLODEX was established by comparison to the selective aromatase inhibitor anastrozole in two randomized, controlled clinical trials (one conducted in North America, the other in predominately Europe) in postmenopausal women with locally advanced or metastatic breast cancer. All patients had progressed after previous therapy with an antiestrogen or progestin for breast cancer in the adjuvant or advanced disease setting. The majority of patients in these trials had ER+ and/or PgR+ tumors. Patients who had ER-/PgR- or unknown disease must have shown prior response to endocrine therapy.

In both trials, eligible patients with measurable and/or evaluable disease were randomized to receive either FASLODEX 250 mg intramuscularly once a month (28 days ± 3 days) or anastrozole 1 mg orally once a day. All patients were assessed monthly for the first three months and every three months thereafter. The North American trial was a double-blind, randomized trial in 400 postmenopausal women. The European trial was an open, randomized trial conducted in 451 patients. Patients on the FASLODEX arm of the North American trial received two separate injections (2 x 2.5 mL), whereas FASLODEX patients received a single injection (1 x 5 mL) in the European trial. In both trials, patients were initially randomized to a 125 mg per month dose as well, but interim analysis showed a very low response rate and low dose groups were dropped.

The effectiveness endpoints were response rates (RR), based on the Union Internationale Contre le Cancer (UICC) criteria, and time to progression (TTP). Survival time was also determined. Confidence intervals (95.4%) were calculated for the difference in RR between the FASLODEX and anastrozole groups. The hazard ratio for an unfavorable event, (such as disease progression or death) between FASLODEX and anastrozole groups was also determined.

Table 2 provides the demographics and baseline characteristics of the postmenopausal women randomized to FASLODEX 250 mg or anastrozole 1 mg.

[See table 2 above]

Results of the trials, after a minimum follow-up duration of 14.6 months, are summarized in Table 3. The effectiveness of FASLODEX 250 mg was determined by comparing RR and TTP results to anastrozole 1 mg, the active control. With respect to response rate, the two studies ruled out (by one-sided 97.7% confidence limit) inferiority of FASLODEX to anastrozole of 6.3% and 1.4%.

[See table 3 above]

There are no efficacy data for the use of FASLODEX in premenopausal women with advanced breast cancer (women with functioning ovaries as evidenced by menstruation and/or premenopausal LH, FSH and estradiol levels).

INDICATIONS AND USAGE

FASLODEX is indicated for the treatment of hormone receptor positive metastatic breast cancer in postmenopausal women with disease progression following antiestrogen therapy.

CONTRAINDICATIONS

FASLODEX is contraindicated in pregnant women, and in patients with a known hypersensitivity to the drug or to any of its components.

WARNINGS

Women of childbearing potential should be advised not to become pregnant while receiving FASLODEX. FASLODEX can cause fetal harm when administered to a pregnant woman and has been shown to cross the placenta following single intramuscular doses in rats and in rabbits. In studies in the pregnant rat, intramuscular doses of fulvestrant 100 times lower than the maximum recommended human dose (based on body surface area [BSA]), caused an increased incidence of fetal abnormalities and death. Similarly, rabbits failed to maintain pregnancy and the fetuses showed an increased incidence of skeletal variations when fulvestrant was administered at one-half the recommended human dose (based on BSA).

There are no studies in pregnant women using FASLODEX. If FASLODEX is used during pregnancy or if the patient becomes pregnant while receiving this drug, the patient should be apprised of the potential hazard to the fetus, or potential risk for loss of the pregnancy. See **Pregnancy** section of **PRECAUTIONS**.

Because FASLODEX is administered intramuscularly, it should not be used in patients with bleeding diatheses, thrombocytopenia or in patients on anticoagulants.

PRECAUTIONS

General

Before starting treatment with FASLODEX, pregnancy must be excluded (see **WARNINGS**).

Hepatic Impairment

Safety and efficacy have not been evaluated in patients with moderate to severe hepatic impairment (see **CLINICAL PHARMACOLOGY-Hepatic Impairment** and **DOSAGE AND ADMINISTRATION-Hepatic Impairment** sections).

Drug Interactions

There are no known drug-drug interactions. Although, fulvestrant is metabolized by CYP 3A4 in vitro, drug interactions studies with ketoconazole or rifampin did not alter fulvestrant pharmacokinetics. Dose adjustment is not needed in patients co-prescribed CYP3A4 inhibitors or inducers (see **CLINICAL PHARMACOLOGY-Drug-Drug Interactions**).

Carcinogenesis, Mutagenesis and Impairment of Fertility

A two-year carcinogenesis study was conducted in female and male rats, at intramuscular doses of 15 mg/kg/30 days, 10 mg/rat/30 days and 10 mg/rat/15 days. These doses correspond to approximately 1-, 3-, and 5-fold (in females) and 1.3-, 1.3-, and 1.6-fold (in males) the systemic exposure [$AUC_{0-30\ days}$] achieved in women receiving the recommended dose of 250 mg/month. An increased incidence of benign ovarian granulosa cell tumors and testicular Leydig cell tumors was evident, in females dosed at 10 mg/rat/15 days and males dosed at 15 mg/rat/30 days, respectively. Induction of such tumors is consistent with the pharmacology-related endocrine feedback alterations in gonadotropin levels caused by an antiestrogen.

Fulvestrant was not mutagenic or clastogenic in multiple *in vitro* tests with and without the addition of a mammalian liver metabolic activation factor (bacterial mutation assay in strains of Salmonella typhimurium and Escherichia coli, in vitro cytogenetics study in human lymphocytes, mammalian cell mutation assay in mouse lymphoma cells and *in vivo* micronucleus test in rat.

In female rats, fulvestrant administered at doses ≥ 0.01 mg/kg/day (approximately one-hundredth of the human recommended dose based on body surface area [BSA], for 2 weeks prior to and for 1 week following mating, caused a reduction in fertility and embryonic survival). No adverse effects on female fertility and embryonic survival were evident in female animals dosed at 0.001 mg/kg/day (approximately one-thousandth of the human dose based on BSA). Restoration of female fertility to values similar to controls was evident following a 29-day withdrawal period after dosing at 2 mg/kg/day (twice the human dose based on BSA). The effects of fulvestrant on the fertility of female rats appear to be consistent with its antiestrogenic activity. The potential effects of fulvestrant on the fertility of male animals were not studied but, in a 6-month toxicology study, male rats treated with intramuscular doses of 15 mg/kg/30 days, 10 mg/rat/30 days, or 10 mg/rat/15 days fulvestrant showed a loss of spermatozoa from the seminiferous tubules, seminiferous tubular atrophy, and degenerative changes in the epididymides. Changes in the testes and epididymides had not recovered 20 weeks after cessation of dosing. These fulvestrant doses correspond to approximately 2-, 3-, and 3-fold the systemic exposure [$AUC_{0-30\ days}$] achieved in women.

Pregnancy

Pregnancy Category D: (See **WARNINGS**).

In studies in female rats at doses ≥ 0.01 mg/kg/day (IM; approximately one-hundredth of the human recommended dose based on body surface area [BSA]), fulvestrant caused a reversible reduction in female fertility, as well as effects on embryo/fetal development consistent with its antiestrogenic activity. Fulvestrant caused an increased incidence of fetal abnormalities in rats (tarsal flexure of the hind paw at 2 mg/kg/day IM; twice the human dose on BSA) and non-ossification of the odontoid and ventral tubercle of the first cervical vertebra at doses ≥ 0.1 mg/kg/day IM (approximately one-tenth of the human dose on BSA) when administered during the period of organogenesis. Rabbits failed to maintain pregnancy when dosed with 1 mg/kg/day fulvestrant IM (twice the human dose on BSA) during the period of organogenesis. Further, in rabbits dosed at 0.25 mg/kg/day (about one-half the human dose on BSA), increases in placental weight and post-implantation loss were observed but, there were no observed effects on fetal development. Fulvestrant was associated with an increased incidence of fetal variations in rabbits (backwards displacement of the pelvic girdle, and 27 pre-sacral vertebrae at 0.25 mg/kg/day IM; one-half the human dose on BSA) when administered during the period of organogenesis. Because pregnancy could not be maintained in the rabbit following doses of fulvestrant of 1 mg/kg/day and above, this study was inadequate to fully define the possible adverse effects on fetal development at clinically relevant exposures.

Nursing Mothers

Fulvestrant is found in rat milk at levels significantly higher (approximately 12-fold) than plasma after administration of 2 mg/kg. Drug exposure in rodent pups from fulvestrant-treated lactating dams was estimated as 10% of the administered dose. It is not known if fulvestrant is excreted in human milk. Because many drugs are excreted in human milk, and because of the potential for serious adverse reactions from FASLODEX in nursing infants, a decision should be made whether to discontinue nursing or to discontinue the drug taking into account the importance of the drug to the mother.

Pediatric Use

The safety and efficacy of FASLODEX in pediatric patients have not been established.

Geriatric Use

When tumor response was considered by age, objective responses were seen in 24% and 22% of patients under 65 years of age and in 16% and 11% of patients 65 years of age and older, who were treated with FASLODEX in the European and North American trials, respectively.

ADVERSE REACTIONS

The most commonly reported adverse experiences in the FASLODEX and anastrozole treatment groups, regardless of the investigator's assessment of causality, were gastrointestinal symptoms (including nausea, vomiting, constipation, diarrhea and abdominal pain), headache, back pain, vasodilatation (hot flushes), and pharyngitis.

Injection site reactions with mild transient pain and inflammation were seen with FASLODEX and occurred in 7% of patients (1% of treatments) given the single 5 mL injection (predominately European Trial) and in 27% of patients (4.6% of treatments) given the 2 x 2.5 mL injections (North American Trial).

Table 4 lists adverse experiences reported with an incidence of 5% or greater, regardless of assessed causality, from the two controlled clinical trials comparing the administration of FASLODEX 250 mg intramuscularly once a month with anastrozole 1 mg orally once a day.

Table 4: Combined Trials Adverse Events ≥ 5%

Body system and adverse event[a]	FASLODEX 250 mg N=423 (%)	Anastrozole 1 mg N=423 (%)
Body as a whole	68.3	67.6
Asthenia	22.7	27.0
Pain	18.9	20.3
Headache	15.4	16.8
Back pain	14.4	13.2
Abdominal pain	11.8	11.6
Injection site pain*	10.9	6.6
Pelvic pain	9.9	9.0
Chest pain	7.1	5.0
Flu syndrome	7.1	6.4
Fever	6.4	6.4
Accidental injury	4.5	5.7
Cardiovascular system	30.3	27.9
Vasodilatation	17.7	17.3
Digestive system	51.5	48.0
Nausea	26.0	25.3
Vomiting	13.0	11.8
Constipation	12.5	10.6
Diarrhea	12.3	12.8
Anorexia	9.0	10.9
Hemic and lymphatic systems	13.7	13.5
Anemia	4.5	5.0
Metabolic and Nutritional disorders	18.2	17.7
Peripheral edema	9.0	10.2
Musculoskeletal system	25.5	27.9
Bone pain	15.8	13.7
Arthritis	2.8	6.1
Nervous system	34.3	33.8
Dizziness	6.9	6.6
Insomnia	6.9	8.5
Paresthesia	6.4	7.6
Depression	5.7	6.9
Anxiety	5.0	3.8
Respiratory system	38.5	33.6
Pharyngitis	16.1	11.6
Dyspnea	14.9	12.3
Cough increased	10.4	10.4
Skin and appendages	22.2	23.4
Rash	7.3	8.0
Sweating	5.0	5.2
Urogenital system	18.2	14.9
Urinary tract infection	6.1	3.5

[a] A patient may have more than one adverse event.

*All patients on FASLODEX received injections, but only those anastrozole patients who were in the North American study received placebo injections.

Other adverse events reported as drug-related and seen infrequently (<1%) include thromboembolic phenomena, myalgia, vertigo, and leukopenia.

Vaginal bleeding has been reported infrequently (<1%), mainly in patients during the first 6 weeks after changing from existing hormonal therapy to treatment with FASLODEX. If bleeding persists, further evaluation should be considered.

OVERDOSAGE

Animal studies have shown no effects other than those related directly or indirectly to antiestrogen activity with intramuscular doses of fulvestrant higher than the recommended human dose. There is no clinical experience with overdosage in humans. No adverse effects were seen in healthy male and female volunteers who received intravenous fulvestrant, which resulted in peak plasma concentrations at the end of the infusion, that were approximately 10 to 15 times those seen after intramuscular injection.

DOSAGE AND ADMINISTRATION

Adults (including the elderly): The recommended dose is 250 mg to be administered intramuscularly into the buttock at intervals of one month as either a single 5 mL injection or two concurrent 2.5 mL injections (see **HOW SUPPLIED**). The injection should be administered slowly.

Patients with Hepatic Impairment

FASLODEX has not been studied in patients with moderate or severe hepatic compromise. No dosage adjustment is recommended in patients with mild hepatic impairment (see **CLINICAL PHARMACOLOGY-Hepatic Impairment** and **PRECAUTIONS-Hepatic Impairment** sections).

Instructions for Intramuscular use, handling and disposal

1. Remove glass syringe barrel from tray and check that it is not damaged.
2. Remove perforated patient record label from syringe.
3. Peel open the safety needle (SafetyGlide™) outer packaging. For complete SafetyGlide™ instructions refer below to the "Directions for Use of SafetyGlide™."
4. Break the seal of the white plastic cover on the syringe luer connector to remove the cover with the attached rubber tip cap (see Figure 1).
5. Twist to lock the needle to the luer connector.
6. Remove needle sheath.
7. Remove excess gas from the syringe (a small gas bubble may remain).
8. Administer intramuscularly slowly in the buttock.
9. Immediately activate needle protection device upon withdrawal from patient by pushing lever arm completely forward until needle tip is fully covered (see Figure 2).
10. Visually confirm that the lever arm has fully advanced and the needle tip is covered. If unable to activate, discard immediately into an approved sharps collector.
11. Repeat steps 1 through 10 for second syringe.

For the 2 x 2.5 mL syringe package only, both syringes must be administered to receive the 250 mg recommended monthly dose.

SAFETYGLIDE™ INSTRUCTIONS FROM BECTON DICKINSON

SafetyGlide™ is a trademark of Becton Dickinson and Company

Reorder number 305917

CAUTION CONCERNING SAFETYGLIDE™

Federal (USA) law restricts this device to sale by or on the order of a physician. To help avoid HIV (AIDS), HBV (Hepatitis), and other infectious diseases due to accidental needlesticks, contaminated needles should not be recapped or removed, unless there is no alternative or that such action is required by a specific medical procedure.

WARNING CONCERNING SAFETYGLIDE™

Do not autoclave SafetyGlide™ Needle before use. Hands must remain behind the needle at all times during use and disposal.

DIRECTIONS FOR USE OF SAFETYGLIDE™

Peel apart packaging of the SafetyGlide™, break the seal of the white plastic cover on the syringe Luer connector and attach the SafetyGlide™ needle to the Luer Lock of the syringe by twisting.

Transport filled syringe to point of administration.

Pull shield straight off needle to avoid damaging needle point.

Administer injection following package instruction.

For user convenience, the needle 'bevel up' position is orientated to the lever arm, as shown in Figure 3.

Immediately activate needle protection device upon withdrawal from patient by pushing lever arm completely forward until needle tip is fully covered (Figure 2).

Visually confirm that the lever arm has fully advanced and the needle tip is covered. If unable to activate, discard immediately into an approved sharps collector.

Activation of the protective mechanism may cause minimal splatter of fluid that may remain on the needle after injection.

For greatest safety, use a one-handed technique and activate away from self and others.

After single use, discard in an approved sharps collector in accordance with applicable regulations and institutional policy.

Continued on next page

Faslodex—Cont.

Becton Dickinson guarantees the contents of their unopened or undamaged packages to be sterile, nontoxic and nonpyrogenic.

Figure 1

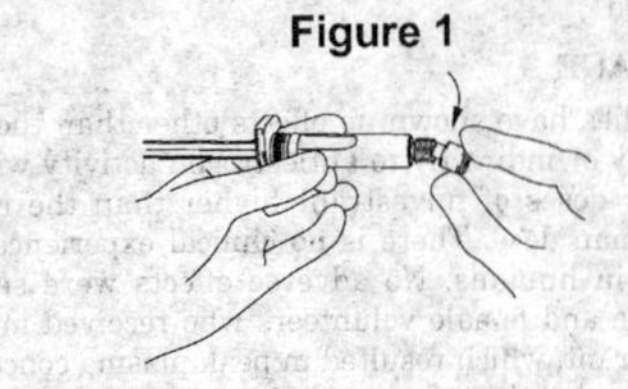

Figure 2

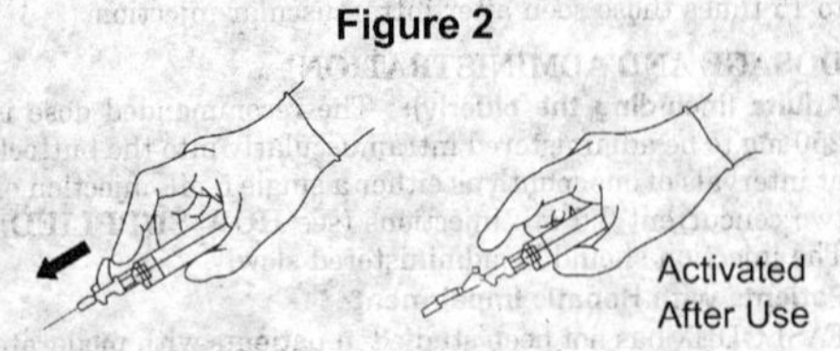

Figure 3

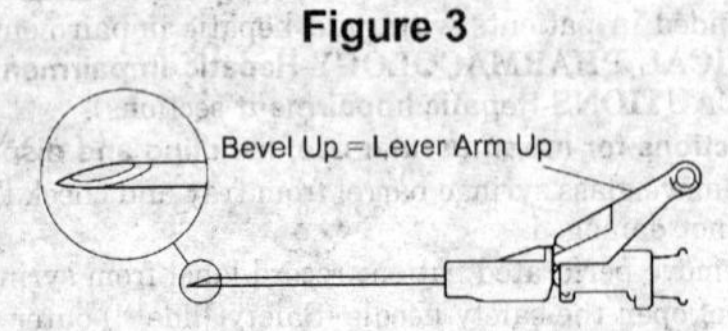

HOW SUPPLIED

FASLODEX is supplied in two different packaging configurations:

1. FASLODEX is supplied as one clear neutral glass (Type 1) barrel containing 250 mg/5mL (50 mg/mL) FASLODEX Injection for intramuscular injection and fitted with a tamper evident closure.
NDC 0310-0720-50

2. FASLODEX is also supplied as two clear neutral glass (Type 1) barrels each containing 125 mg/2.5 mL (50 mg/mL) FASLODEX Injection for intramuscular injection and fitted with a tamper-evident closure. **PLEASE NOTE: THE SYRINGES ARE SUPPLIED HALF FULL. BOTH SYRINGES MUST BE ADMINISTERED TO RECEIVE THE 250 MG RECOMMENDED MONTHLY DOSE.**
NDC 0310-0720-25

The syringes are presented in a tray with polystyrene plunger rod and safety needles (SafetyGlide™) for connection to the barrel.

Storage

REFRIGERATE, 2°–8°C (36°–46°F). TO PROTECT FROM LIGHT, STORE IN THE ORIGINAL CARTON UNTIL TIME OF USE.

SafetyGlide™ is a trademark of Becton Dickinson and Company

All other trademarks are the property of the AstraZeneca group of companies.

Distributed by:
AstraZeneca Pharmaceuticals LP
Wilmington, DE 19850
Manufactured for:
AstraZeneca UK Ltd.
Macclesfield, England
By: Vetter Pharma-Fertigung GmbH & Co. KG
Ravensburg, Germany
22073-00
Rev 12/03

Shown in Product Identification Guide, page 306

IRESSA® ℞

[ēr′ əs-sə]
(gefitinib tablets)
250 mg
FOR ONCOLOGY USE ONLY

DESCRIPTION

IRESSA® (gefitinib tablets) contain 250 mg of gefitinib and are available as brown film-coated tablets for daily oral administration.

Gefitinib is an anilinoquinazoline with the chemical name 4-Quinazolinamine, *N*-(3-chloro-4-fluorophenyl)-7-methoxy-6-[3-4-morpholin) propoxy] and the following structural formula:

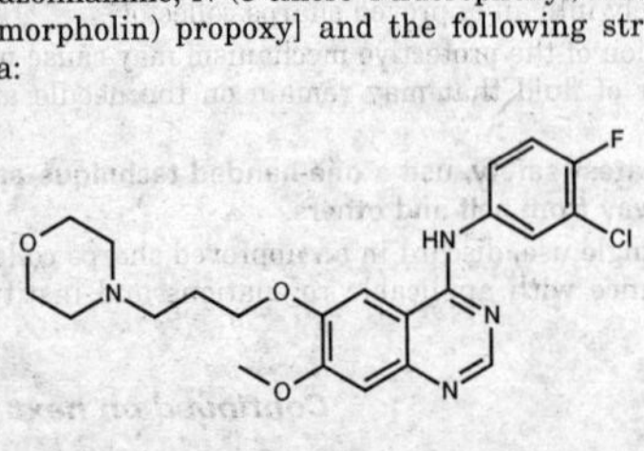

It has the molecular formula $C_{22}H_{24}ClFN_4O_3$, a relative molecular mass of 446.9 and is a white-colored powder. Gefitinib is a free base. The molecule has pK_as of 5.4 and 7.2 and therefore ionizes progressively in solution as the pH falls. Gefitinib can be defined as sparingly soluble at pH 1, but is practically insoluble above pH 7, with the solubility dropping sharply between pH 4 and pH 6. In non-aqueous solvents, gefitinib is freely soluble in glacial acetic acid and dimethylsulphoxide, soluble in pyridine, sparingly soluble in tetrahydrofuran, and slightly soluble in methanol, ethanol (99.5%), ethyl acetate, propan-2-ol and acetonitrile.

The inactive ingredients of IRESSA tablets are: **Tablet core:** Lactose monohydrate, microcrystalline cellulose, croscarmellose sodium, povidone, sodium lauryl sulfate and magnesium stearate. **Coating:** Hydroxypropyl methylcellulose, polyethylene glycol 300, titanium dioxide, red ferric oxide and yellow ferric oxide.

CLINICAL PHARMACOLOGY

Mechanism of Action

The mechanism of the clinical antitumor action of gefitinib is not fully characterized. Gefitinib inhibits the intracellular phosphorylation of numerous tyrosine kinases associated with transmembrane cell surface receptors, including the tyrosine kinases associated with the epidermal growth factor receptor (EGFR-TK). EGFR is expressed on the cell surface of many normal cells and cancer cells. No clinical studies have been performed that demonstrate a correlation between EGFR receptor expression and response to gefitinib.

Pharmacokinetics

Gefitinib is absorbed slowly after oral administration with mean bioavailability of 60%. Elimination is by metabolism (primarily CYP3A4) and excretion in feces. The elimination half-life is about 48 hours. Daily oral administration of gefitinib to cancer patients resulted in a 2-fold accumulation compared to single dose administration. Steady state plasma concentrations are achieved within 10 days.

Absorption and Distribution:

Gefitinib is slowly absorbed, with peak plasma levels occurring 3-7 hours after dosing and mean oral bioavailability of 60%. Bioavailability is not significantly altered by food. Gefitinib is extensively distributed throughout the body with a mean steady state volume of distribution of 1400 L following intravenous administration. *In vitro* binding of gefitinib to human plasma proteins (serum albumin and α1-acid glycoprotein) is 90% and is independent of drug concentrations.

Metabolism and Elimination:

Gefitinib undergoes extensive hepatic metabolism in humans, predominantly by CYP3A4. Three sites of biotransformation have been identified: metabolism of the N-propoxymorpholino-group, demethylation of the methoxy-substituent on the quinazoline, and oxidative defluorination of the halogenated phenyl group.

Five metabolites were identified in human plasma. Only O-desmethyl gefitinib has exposure comparable to gefitinib. Although this metabolite has similar EGFR-TK activity to gefitinib in the isolated enzyme assay, it had only 1/14 of the potency of gefitinib in one of the cell-based assays.

Gefitinib is cleared primarily by the liver, with total plasma clearance and elimination half-life values of 595 mL/min and 48 hours, respectively, after intravenous administration. Excretion is predominantly via the feces (86%), with renal elimination of drug and metabolites accounting for less than 4% of the administered dose.

Special Populations:

In population based data analyses, no relationships were identified between predicted steady state trough concentration and patient age, body weight, gender, ethnicity or creatinine clearance.

Pediatric:

There are no pharmacokinetic data in pediatric patients.

Hepatic Impairment:

The influence of hepatic metastases with elevation of serum aspartate aminotransferase (AST/SGOT), alkaline phosphatase, and bilirubin has been evaluated in patients with normal (14 patients), moderately elevated (13 patients) and severely elevated (4 patients) levels of one or more of these biochemical parameters. Patients with moderately and severely elevated biochemical liver abnormalities had gefitinib pharmacokinetics similar to individuals without liver abnormalities (see **PRECAUTIONS** section).

Renal Impairment:

No clinical studies were conducted with IRESSA in patients with severely compromised renal function (see **PRECAUTIONS** section). Gefitinib and its metabolites are not significantly excreted via the kidney (<4%).

Drug-Drug Interactions:

In human liver microsome studies, gefitinib had no inhibitory effect on CYP1A2, CYP2C9, and CYP3A4 activities at concentrations ranging from 2–5000 ng/mL. At the highest concentration studied (5000 ng/mL), gefitinib inhibited CYP2C19 by 24% and CYP2D6 by 43%. Exposure to metoprolol, a substrate of CYP2D6, was increased by 30% when it was given in combination with gefitinib (500 mg daily for 28 days) in patients with solid tumors.

Rifampicin, an inducer of CYP3A4, reduced mean AUC of gefitinib by 85% in healthy male volunteers (see **PRECAUTIONS—Drug Interactions** and **DOSAGE AND ADMINISTRATION—Dosage Adjustment** sections).

Concomitant administration of itraconazole (200 mg QD for 12 days), an inhibitor of CYP3A4, with gefitinib (250 mg single dose) to healthy male volunteers, increased mean gefitinib AUC by 88% (see **PRECAUTIONS—Drug Interactions** section).

Co-administration of high doses of ranitidine with sodium bicarbonate (to maintain the gastric pH above pH 5.0) reduced mean gefitinib AUC by 44% (See **PRECAUTIONS—Drug Interactions** section).

International Normalized Ratio (INR) elevations and/or bleeding events have been reported in some patients taking warfarin while on IRESSA therapy. Patients taking warfarin should be monitored regularly for changes in prothrombin time or INR (see **PRECAUTIONS—Drug Interactions** and **ADVERSE REACTIONS** sections).

Clinical Studies

Non-Small Cell Lung Cancer (NSCLC)—A multicenter clinical trial in the United States evaluated the tumor response rate of IRESSA 250 and 500 mg/day in patients with advanced non-small cell lung cancer whose disease had progressed after at least two prior chemotherapy regimens including a platinum drug and docetaxel. IRESSA was taken once daily at approximately the same time each day.

Two hundred and sixteen patients received IRESSA, 102 (47%) and 114 (53%) receiving 250 mg and 500 mg daily doses, respectively. Study patient demographics and disease characteristics are summarized in Table 1. Forty-one percent of the patients had received two prior treatment regimens, 33% three prior treatment regimens, and 25% four or more prior treatment regimens. Effectiveness of IRESSA as

Table 1: Demographic and Disease Characteristics

Characteristic	IRESSA Dose 250 mg/day N = 66 (%)	500 mg/day N = (76%)
Age Group		
18–64 years	43 (65)	43 (57)
64–74 years	19 (29)	30 (39)
75 years and above	4 (6)	3 (4)
Sex		
Male	38 (58)	41 (54)
Female	28 (42)	35 (46)
Race		
White	61 (92)	68 (89)
Black	1 (2)	2 (3)
Asian/Oriental	1 (2)	2 (3)
Hispanic	0 (0)	3 (4)
Other	3 (5)	1 (1)
Smoking History		
Yes (Previous or current smoker)	45 (68)	62 (82)
No (Never smoked)	21 (32)	14 (18)
Baseline WHO Performance Status		
0	14 (21)	9 (12)
1	36 (55)	53 (70)
2	15 (23)	14 (18)
Not recorded	1 (2)	0 (0)
Tumor Histology		
Squamous	9 (14)	11 (14)
Adenocarcinoma	47 (71)	50 (66)
Undifferentiated	6 (9)	4 (5)
Large Cell	1 (2)	2 (3)
Squamous & Adenocarcinoma	3 (5)	7 (9)
Not Recorded	0 (0)	2 (3)
Current Disease Status		
Locally advanced	11 (17)	5 (7)
Metastatic	55 (83)	71 (93)

third line therapy was determined in the 142 evaluable patients with documented disease progression on platinum and docetaxel therapies or who had had unacceptable toxicity on these agents.
[See table 1 at top of previous page]
Table 2 shows tumor response rates and response duration. The overall response rate for the 250 and 500 mg doses combined was 10.6% (95% CI: 6%, 16.8%). Response rates appeared to be highly variable in subgroups of the treated population: 5.1% (4/79) in males, 17.5% (11/63) in females, 4.6% (5/108) in previous or current smokers, 29.4% (10/34) in nonsmokers, 12.4% (12/97) with adenocarcinoma histology, and 6.7% (3/45) with other NSCLC histologies. Similar differences were seen in a multinational study in patients who had received 1 or 2 prior chemotherapy regimens, at least 1 of which was platinum-based. In responders, the median time from diagnosis to study randomization was 16.7 months (range 8 to 34 months).
[See table 2 at right]

Non-Small Cell Lung Cancer (NSCLC); Studies of First-line Treatment in Combination with Chemotherapy—Two large trials were conducted in chemotherapy-naïve patients with stage III and IV non-small cell lung cancer. Two thousand one hundred thirty patients were randomized to receive IRESSA 250 mg daily, IRESSA 500 mg daily, or placebo in combination with platinum-based chemotherapy regimens. The chemotherapies given in these first-line trials were gemcitabine and cis-platinum (N=1093) or carboplatin and paclitaxel (N=1037). The addition of IRESSA did not demonstrate any increase, or trend toward such an increase, in tumor response rates, time to progression, or overall survival.

INDICATIONS AND USAGE

IRESSA is indicated as monotherapy for the treatment of patients with locally advanced or metastatic non-small cell lung cancer after failure of both platinum-based and docetaxel chemotherapies.
The effectiveness of IRESSA is based on objective response rates (see **CLINICAL PHARMACOLOGY—Clinical Studies** section). There are no controlled trials demonstrating a clinical benefit, such as improvement in disease-related symptoms or increased survival.
Results from two large, controlled, randomized trials in first-line treatment of non-small cell lung cancer showed no benefit from adding IRESSA to doublet, platinum-based chemotherapy. Therefore, IRESSA is not indicated for use in this setting.

CONTRAINDICATIONS

IRESSA is contraindicated in patients with severe hypersensitivity to gefitinib or to any other component of IRESSA.

WARNINGS

Pulmonary Toxicity
Cases of interstitial lung disease (ILD) have been observed in patients receiving IRESSA at an overall incidence of about 1%. Approximately 1/3 of the cases have been fatal. The reported incidence of ILD was about 2% in the Japanese post-marketing experience, about 0.3% in approximately 23,000 patients treated with IRESSA in a US expanded access program and about 1% in the studies of first-line use in NSCLC (but with similar rates in both treatment and placebo groups). Reports have described the adverse event as interstitial pneumonia, pneumonitis and alveolitis. Patients often present with the acute onset of dyspnea, sometimes associated with cough or low-grade fever, often becoming severe within a short time and requiring hospitalization. ILD has occurred in patients who have received prior radiation therapy (31% of reported cases), prior chemotherapy (57% of reported patients), and no previous therapy (12% of reported cases). Patients with concurrent idiopathic pulmonary fibrosis whose condition worsens while receiving IRESSA have been observed to have an increased mortality compared to those without concurrent idiopathic pulmonary fibrosis.
In the event of acute onset or worsening of pulmonary symptoms (dyspnea, cough, fever), IRESSA therapy should be interrupted and a prompt investigation of these symptoms should occur. If interstitial lung disease is confirmed, IRESSA should be discontinued and the patient treated appropriately (see **PRECAUTIONS—Information for Patients, ADVERSE REACTIONS** and **DOSAGE AND ADMINISTRATION—Dosage Adjustment** sections).

Pregnancy Category D
IRESSA may cause fetal harm when administered to a pregnant woman. A single dose study in rats showed that gefitinib crosses the placenta after an oral dose of 5 mg/kg (30 mg/m^2, about 1/5 the recommended human dose on a mg/m^2 basis). When pregnant rats were treated with 5 mg/kg from the beginning of organogenesis to the end of weaning gave birth, there was a reduction in the number of offspring born alive. This effect was more severe at 20 mg/kg and was accompanied by high neonatal mortality soon after parturition. In this study a dose of 1 mg/kg caused no adverse effects.
In rabbits, a dose of 20 mg/kg/day (240 mg/m^2, about twice the recommended dose in humans on a mg/m^2 basis) caused reduced fetal weight.
There are no adequate and well-controlled studies in pregnant women using IRESSA. If IRESSA is used during pregnancy or if the patient becomes pregnant while receiving this drug, she should be apprised of the potential hazard to the fetus or potential risk for loss of the pregnancy.

PRECAUTIONS

Hepatotoxicity
Asymptomatic increases in liver transaminases have been observed in IRESSA treated patients; therefore, periodic liver function (transaminases, bilirubin, and alkaline phosphatase) testing should be considered. Discontinuation of IRESSA should be considered if changes are severe.

Table 2: Efficacy Results

	Evaluable Patients		
	250 mg (N=66)	500 mg (N=76)	Combined (N=142)
Objective Tumor Response Rate (%)	13.6	7.9	10.6
95% CI (%)	6.4-24.3	3.0-16.4	6.0-16.8
Median Duration of Objective Response (months)	8.9	4.5	7.0
Range (months)	4.6-18.6+	4.4-7.6	4.4-18.6+

+=data are ongoing

Patients with Hepatic Impairment
In vitro and *in vivo* evidence suggest that gefitinib is cleared primarily by the liver. Therefore, gefitinib exposure may be increased in patients with hepatic dysfunction. In patients with liver metastases and moderately to severely elevated biochemical liver abnormalities, however, gefitinib pharmacokinetics were similar to the pharmacokinetics of individuals without liver abnormalities (see **CLINICAL PHARMACOLOGY—Pharmacokinetics—Special Populations** section). The influence of non-cancer related hepatic impairment on the pharmacokinetics of gefitinib has not been evaluated.

Information for Patients
Patients should be advised to seek medical advice promptly if they develop 1) severe or persistent diarrhea, nausea, anorexia, or vomiting, as these have sometimes been associated with dehydration; 2) an onset or worsening of pulmonary symptoms, ie, shortness of breath or cough; 3) an eye irritation; or, 4) any other new symptom (see **WARNINGS—Pulmonary Toxicity, ADVERSE REACTIONS** and **DOSAGE AND ADMINISTRATION—Dosage Adjustment** sections).
Women of childbearing potential must be advised to avoid becoming pregnant (see **WARNINGS—Pregnancy Category D**).

Drug Interactions
Substances that are inducers of CYP3A4 activity increase the metabolism of gefitinib and decrease its plasma concentrations. In patients receiving a potent CYP3A4 inducer such as rifampicin or phenytoin, a dose increase to 500 mg daily should be considered in the absence of severe adverse drug reaction, and clinical response and adverse events should be carefully monitored (see **CLINICAL PHARMACOLOGY—Pharmacokinetics—Drug-Drug Interactions** and **DOSAGE AND ADMINISTRATION—Dosage Adjustment** sections).
International Normalized Ratio (INR) elevations and/or bleeding events have been reported in some patients taking warfarin while on IRESSA therapy. Patients taking warfarin should be monitored regularly for changes in prothrombin time or INR (see **CLINICAL PHARMACOLOGY—Pharmacokinetics—Drug-Drug Interactions** and **ADVERSE REACTIONS** sections).
Substances that are potent inhibitors of CYP3A4 activity (eg, ketoconazole and itraconazole) decrease gefitinib metabolism and increase gefitinib plasma concentrations. This increase may be clinically relevant as adverse experiences are related to dose and exposure; therefore, caution should be used when administering CYP3A4 inhibitors with IRESSA (see **CLINICAL PHARMACOLOGY—Pharmacokinetics—Drug-Drug Interactions** and **ADVERSE REACTIONS** sections).
Drugs that cause significant sustained elevation in gastric pH (histamine H_2-receptor antagonists such as ranitidine or cimetidine) may reduce plasma concentrations of IRESSA and therefore potentially may reduce efficacy (see **CLINICAL PHARMACOLOGY—Drug-Drug Interactions** section).

Carcinogenesis, Mutagenesis, Impairment of Fertility
Gefitinib has been tested for genotoxicity in a series of *in vitro* (bacterial mutation, mouse lymphoma, and human lymphocyte) assays and an *in vivo* rat micronucleus test. Under the conditions of these assays, gefitinib did not cause genetic damage.
Carcinogenicity studies have not been conducted with gefitinib.

Pregnancy
Pregnancy Category D (see **WARNINGS** and **PRECAUTIONS—Information for Patients** sections).

Nursing Mothers
It is not known whether IRESSA is excreted in human milk. Following oral administration of carbon-14 labeled gefitinib to rats 14 days postpartum, concentrations of radioactivity in milk were higher than in blood. Levels of gefitinib and its metabolites were 11-to-19-fold higher in milk than in blood, after oral exposure of lactating rats to a dose of 5 mg/kg. Because many drugs are excreted in human milk and because of the potential for serious adverse reactions in nursing infants, women should be advised against breastfeeding while receiving IRESSA therapy.

Pediatric Use
Safety and effectiveness of IRESSA in pediatric patients have not been studied.

Geriatric Use
Of the total number of patients participating in trials of second- and third-line IRESSA treatment of NSCLC, 65% were aged 64 years or less, 30.5 % were aged 65 to 74 years, and 5% of patients were aged 75 years or older. No differences in safety or efficacy were observed between younger and older patients.

Patients with Severe Renal Impairment
The effect of severe renal impairment on the pharmacokinetics of gefitinib is not known. Patients with severe renal impairment should be treated with caution when given IRESSA.

ADVERSE REACTIONS

The safety database includes 941 patients from clinical trials and approximately 23,000 patients in the Expanded Access Program.
Table 3 includes drug-related adverse events with an incidence of ≥5% for the 216 patients who received either 250 mg or 500 mg of IRESSA monotherapy for treatment of NSCLC. The most common adverse events reported at the recommended 250 mg daily dose were diarrhea, rash, acne, dry skin, nausea, and vomiting (see **PRECAUTIONS—Information for Patients** and **DOSAGE AND ADMINISTRATION—Dosage Adjustment** sections). The 500 mg dose showed a higher rate for most of these adverse events.
Table 4 provides drug-related adverse events with an incidence of ≥5% by CTC grade for the patients who received the 250 mg/day dose of IRESSA monotherapy for treatment of NSCLC. Only 2% of patients stopped therapy due to an adverse drug reaction (ADR). The onset of these ADRs occurred within the first month of therapy.

Table 3: Drug-Related Adverse Events with an Incidence of ≥5% in either 250 mg or 500 mg Dose Group

	Number (%) of Patients	
Drug-related adverse event[a]	250 mg/day (N=102) %	500 mg/day (N=114) %
Diarrhea	49 (48)	76 (67)
Rash	44 (43)	61 (54)
Acne	25 (25)	37 (33)
Dry skin	13 (13)	30 (26)
Nausea	13 (13)	20 (18)
Vomiting	12 (12)	10 (9)
Pruritus	8 (8)	10 (9)
Anorexia	7 (7)	11 (10)
Asthenia	6 (6)	5 (4)
Weight loss	3 (3)	6 (5)

[a]A patient may have had more than 1 drug-related adverse event.

Table 4: Drug Related Adverse Events ≥5% at 250 mg dose by Worst CTC Grade (n=102)

	% of Patients				
Adverse event	All Grades	CTC Grade 1	CTC Grade 2	CTC Grade 3	CTC Grade 4
Diarrhea	48	41	6	1	0
Rash	43	39	4	0	0
Acne	25	19	6	0	0
Dry Skin	13	12	1	0	0
Nausea	13	7	5	1	0
Vomiting	12	9	2	1	0
Pruritus	8	7	1	0	0
Anorexia	7	3	4	0	0
Asthenia	6	2	2	1	1

Other adverse events reported at an incidence of <5% in patients who received either 250 mg or 500 mg as monotherapy for treatment of NSCLC (along with their frequency at the 250 mg recommended dose) include the following: peripheral edema (2%), amblyopia (2%), dyspnea (2%), conjunctivitis (1%), vesiculobullous rash (1%), and mouth ulceration (1%).

Interstitial Lung Disease
Cases of interstitial lung disease (ILD) have been observed in patients receiving IRESSA at an overall incidence of about 1%. Approximately 1/3 of the cases have been fatal. The reported incidence of ILD was about 2% in the Japanese post-marketing experience, about 0.3% in approximately 23,000 patients treated with IRESSA in a US expanded access program and about 1% in the studies of first-line use in NSCLC (but with similar rates in both treatment and placebo groups). Reports have described the adverse event as interstitial pneumonia, pneumonitis and alveolitis. Patients often present with the acute onset of dyspnea, sometimes associated with cough or low-grade fever, often becoming severe within a short time and requir-

Continued on next page

Iressa—Cont.

ing hospitalization. ILD has occurred in patients who have received prior radiation therapy (31% of reported cases), prior chemotherapy (57% of reported patients), and no previous therapy (12% of reported cases). Patients with concurrent idiopathic pulmonary fibrosis whose condition worsens while receiving IRESSA have been observed to have an increased mortality compared to those without concurrent idiopathic pulmonary fibrosis.

In the event of acute onset or worsening of pulmonary symptoms (dyspnea, cough, fever), IRESSA therapy should be interrupted and a prompt investigation of these symptoms should occur. If interstitial lung disease is confirmed, IRESSA should be discontinued and the patient treated appropriately (see **WARNINGS—Pulmonary Toxicity, PRECAUTIONS—Information for Patients** and **DOSAGE AND ADMINISTRATION—Dosage Adjustment** sections).

In patients receiving IRESSA therapy, there were reports of eye pain and corneal erosion/ulcer, sometimes in association with aberrant eyelash growth (see **PRECAUTIONS—Information for Patients** section). There were also rare reports of pancreatitis and very rare reports of corneal membrane sloughing, ocular ischemia/hemorrhage, toxic epidermal necrolysis, erythema multiforme, and allergic reactions, including angioedema and urticaria.

International Normalized Ratio (INR) elevations and/or bleeding events have been reported in some patients taking warfarin while on IRESSA therapy. Patients taking warfarin should be monitored regularly for changes in prothrombin time or INR (see **CLINICAL PHARMACOLOGY—Drug-Drug Interactions** and **PRECAUTIONS—Drug Interactions** sections).

Data from non-clinical (*in vitro and in vivo*) studies indicate that gefitinib has the potential to inhibit the cardiac action potential repolarization process (eg, QT interval). The clinical relevance of these findings is unknown.

OVERDOSAGE

The acute toxicity of gefitinib up to 500 mg in clinical studies has been low. In non-clinical studies, a single dose of 12,000 mg/m^2 (about 80 times the recommended clinical dose on a mg/m^2 basis) was lethal to rats. Half this dose caused no mortality in mice.

There is no specific treatment for an IRESSA overdose and possible symptoms of overdose are not established. However, in Phase 1 clinical trials, a limited number of patients were treated with daily doses of up to 1000 mg. An increase in frequency and severity of some adverse reactions was observed, mainly diarrhea and skin rash. Adverse reactions associated with overdose should be treated symptomatically; in particular, severe diarrhea should be managed appropriately.

DOSAGE AND ADMINISTRATION

The recommended daily dose of IRESSA is one 250 mg tablet with or without food. Higher doses do not give a better response and cause increased toxicity.

Dosage Adjustment

Patients with poorly tolerated diarrhea (sometimes associated with dehydration) or skin adverse drug reactions may be successfully managed by providing a brief (up to 14 days) therapy interruption followed by reinstatement of the 250 mg daily dose.

In the event of acute onset or worsening of pulmonary symptoms (dyspnea, cough, fever), IRESSA therapy should be interrupted and a prompt investigation of these symptoms should occur and appropriate treatment initiated. If interstitial lung disease is confirmed, IRESSA should be discontinued and the patient treated appropriately (see **WARNINGS—Pulmonary Toxicity, PRECAUTIONS—Information for Patients** and **ADVERSE REACTIONS** sections).

Patients who develop onset of new eye symptoms such as pain should be medically evaluated and managed appropriately, including IRESSA therapy interruption and removal of an aberrant eyelash if present. After symptoms and eye changes have resolved, the decision should be made concerning reinstatement of the 250 mg daily dose (see **PRECAUTIONS—Information for Patients** and **ADVERSE REACTIONS** sections).

In patients receiving a potent CYP3A4 inducer such as rifampicin or phenytoin, a dose increase to 500 mg daily should be considered in the absence of severe adverse drug reaction, and clinical response and adverse events should be carefully monitored (see **CLINICAL PHARMACOLOGY—Pharmacokinetics—Drug-Drug Interactions** and **PRECAUTIONS—Drug Interactions** sections).

No dosage adjustment is required on the basis of patient age, body weight, gender, ethnicity, or renal function; or in patients with moderate to severe hepatic impairment due to liver metastases (see **CLINICAL PHARMACOLOGY—Pharmacokinetics—Special Populations** section).

HOW SUPPLIED

IRESSA tablets are supplied as round, biconvex, brown film-coated tablets intagliated with "IRESSA 250" on one side and plain on the other side, each containing 250 mg of gefitinib.

Bottles of 30 Tablets (NDC 0310-0482-30)

Storage

Store at controlled room temperature 20-25°C (68-77°F) [see USP].

Manufactured for:
AstraZeneca Pharmaceuticals LP
Wilmington, DE 19850
By: AstraZeneca UK Limited
Macclesfield, Cheshire, England
Made in the United Kingdom
64218-00
Rev 02/04

Shown in Product Identification Guide, page 306

MERREM® I.V. ℞

(meropenem for injection)
For Intravenous Use Only

To reduce the development of drug-resistant bacteria and maintain the effectiveness of MERREM® I.V. (meropenem for injection) and other antibacterial drugs, MERREM I.V. should be used only to treat or prevent infections that are proven or strongly suspected to be caused by bacteria.

DESCRIPTION

MERREM® I.V. (meropenem for injection) is a sterile, pyrogen-free, synthetic, broad-spectrum, carbapenem antibiotic for intravenous administration. It is (4R,5S,6S)-3-[[(3S, 5S)-5-(Dimethylcarbamoyl)-3-pyrrolidinyl]thio]-6-[(1R)-1-hydroxyethyl]-4-methyl-7-oxo-1-azabicyclo[3.2.0]hept-2-ene-2-carboxylic acid trihydrate. Its empirical formula is $C_{17}H_{25}N_3O_5S \cdot 3H_2O$ with a molecular weight of 437.52. Its structural formula is:

MERREM I.V. is a white to pale yellow crystalline powder. The solution varies from colorless to yellow depending on the concentration. The pH of freshly constituted solutions is between 7.3 and 8.3. Meropenem is soluble in 5% monobasic potassium phosphate solution, sparingly soluble in water, very slightly soluble in hydrated ethanol, and practically insoluble in acetone or ether.

When constituted as instructed (see **DOSAGE AND ADMINISTRATION; PREPARATION OF SOLUTION**), each 1 g MERREM I.V. vial will deliver 1 g of meropenem and 90.2 mg of sodium as sodium carbonate (3.92 mEq). Each 500 mg MERREM I.V. vial will deliver 500 mg meropenem and 45.1 mg of sodium as sodium carbonate (1.96 mEq).

MERREM I.V. in the ADD-Vantage† vial is intended for intravenous use only after dilution with the appropriate volume of diluent solution in the Abbott ADD-Vantage® diluent container. (See **DOSAGE AND ADMINISTRATION; PREPARATION OF SOLUTION.**) MERREM I.V. in the ADD-Vantage vial is available in two strengths. Each 1 g ADD-Vantage vial of MERREM I.V. will deliver 90.2 mg of sodium as sodium carbonate (3.92 mEq), and each 500 mg ADD-Vantage vial will deliver 45.1 mg of sodium as sodium carbonate (1.96 mEq).

CLINICAL PHARMACOLOGY

At the end of a 30-minute intravenous infusion of a single dose of MERREM I.V. in normal volunteers, mean peak plasma concentrations are approximately 23 µg/mL (range 14-26) for the 500 mg dose and 49 µg/mL (range 39-58) for the 1 g dose. A 5-minute intravenous bolus injection of MERREM I.V. in normal volunteers results in mean peak plasma concentrations of approximately 45 µg/mL (range 18-65) for the 500 mg dose and 112 µg/mL (range 83-140) for the 1 g dose.

Following intravenous doses of 500 mg, mean plasma concentrations of meropenem usually decline to approximately 1 µg/mL at 6 hours after administration.

In subjects with normal renal function, the elimination half-life of MERREM I.V. is approximately 1 hour. Approximately 70% of the intravenously administered dose is recovered as unchanged meropenem in the urine over 12 hours, after which little further urinary excretion is detectable. Urinary concentrations of meropenem in excess of 10 µg/mL are maintained for up to 5 hours after a 500 mg dose. No accumulation of meropenem in plasma or urine was observed with regimens using 500 mg administered every 8 hours or 1 g administered every 6 hours in volunteers with normal renal function.

Plasma protein binding of meropenem is approximately 2%. There is one metabolite which is microbiologically inactive.

Meropenem penetrates well into most body fluids and tissues including cerebrospinal fluid, achieving concentrations matching or exceeding those required to inhibit most susceptible bacteria. After a single intravenous dose of MERREM I.V., the highest mean concentrations of meropenem were found in tissues and fluids at 1 hour (0.5 to 1.5 hours) after the start of infusion, except where indicated in the tissues and fluids listed in the table below.

[See table below]

The pharmacokinetics of MERREM I.V. in pediatric patients 2 years of age or older are essentially similar to those in adults. The elimination half-life for meropenem was approximately 1.5 hours in pediatric patients of age 3 months to 2 years. The pharmacokinetics are linear over the dose range from 10 to 40 mg/kg.

Pharmacokinetic studies with MERREM I.V. in patients with renal insufficiency have shown that the plasma clearance of meropenem correlates with creatinine clearance. Dosage adjustments are necessary in subjects with renal impairment. (See **DOSAGE AND ADMINISTRATION-Use in Adults with Renal Impairment.**) A pharmacokinetic study with MERREM I.V. in elderly patients with renal insufficiency has shown a reduction in plasma clearance of meropenem that correlates with age-associated reduction in creatinine clearance.

Meropenem I.V. is hemodialyzable. However, there is no information on the usefulness of hemodialysis to treat overdosage. (See **OVERDOSAGE.**)

A pharmacokinetic study with MERREM I.V. in patients with hepatic impairment has shown no effects of liver disease on the pharmacokinetics of meropenem.

Microbiology

The bactericidal activity of meropenem results from the inhibition of cell wall synthesis. Meropenem readily penetrates the cell wall of most gram-positive and gram-negative bacteria to reach penicillin-binding-protein (PBP) targets. Its strongest affinities are toward PBPs 2, 3 and 4 of *Escherichia coli* and *Pseudomonas aeruginosa;* and PBPs 1, 2, and 4 of *Staphylococcus aureus.* Bactericidal concentrations (defined as a 3 $\log_{10}$ reduction in cell counts within 12 to 24 hours) are typically 1-2 times the bacteriostatic concentrations of meropenem, with the exception of *Listeria monocytogenes,* against which lethal activity is not observed.

Meropenem has significant stability to hydrolysis by β-lactamases of most categories, both penicillinases and cephalosporinases produced by gram-positive and gram-

Meropenem Concentrations in Selected Tissues (Highest Concentrations Reported)

Tissue	I.V. Dose (g)	Number of Samples	Mean [µg/mL or µg/(g)]***	Range [µg/mL or µg/(g)]
Endometrium	0.5	7	4.2	1.7-10.2
Myometrium	0.5	15	3.8	0.4-8.1
Ovary	0.5	8	2.8	0.8-4.8
Cervix	0.5	2	7.0	5.4-8.5
Fallopian tube	0.5	9	1.7	0.3-3.4
Skin	0.5	22	3.3	0.5-12.6
Skin	1.0	10	5.3	1.3-16.7
Colon	1.0	2	2.6	2.5-2.7
Bile	1.0	7	14.6 (3 h)	4.0-25.7
Gall bladder	1.0	1	—	3.9
Interstitial fluid	1.0	5	26.3	20.9-37.4
Peritoneal fluid	1.0	9	30.2	7.4-54.6
Lung	1.0	2	4.8 (2 h)	1.4-8.2
Bronchial mucosa	1.0	7	4.5	1.3-11.1
Muscle	1.0	2	6.1 (2 h)	5.3-6.9
Fascia	1.0	9	8.8	1.5-20
Heart valves	1.0	7	9.7	6.4-12.1
Myocardium	1.0	10	15.5	5.2-25.5
CSF (inflamed)	20 mg/kg*	8	1.1 (2 h)	0.2-2.8
	40 mg/kg**	5	3.3 (3 h)	0.9-6.5
CSF (uninflamed)	1.0	4	0.2 (2 h)	0.1-0.3

* in pediatric patients of age 5 months to 8 years
** in pediatric patients of age 1 month to 15 years
***at 1 hour unless otherwise noted

negative bacteria, with the exception of metallo-β-lactamases. Meropenem should not be used to treat methicillin-resistant staphylococci. Cross resistance is sometimes observed with strains resistant to other carbapenems.

In vitro tests show meropenem to act synergistically with aminoglycoside antibiotics against some isolates of *Pseudomonas aeruginosa*.

Meropenem has been shown to be active against most strains of the following microorganisms, both *in vitro* and in clinical infections as described in the **INDICATIONS AND USAGE** section.

Gram-Positive Aerobes

Streptococcus pneumoniae (excluding penicillin-resistant strains)

Viridans group streptococci

NOTE: Penicillin-resistant strains had meropenem MIC_{90} values of 1 or 2 µg/mL, which is above the 0.12 µg/mL susceptible breakpoint for this species.

Gram-Negative Aerobes

Escherichia coli

Haemophilus influenzae (β-lactamase and non-β-lactamase producing)

Klebsiella pneumoniae

Neisseria meningitidis

Pseudomonas aeruginosa

Anaerobes

Bacteroides fragilis

Bacteroides thetaiotaomicron

Peptostreptococcus species

The following in vitro data are available, **but their clinical significance is unknown.**

Meropenem exhibits *in vitro* minimum inhibitory concentrations (MIC's) of 0.12 µg/mL against most (≥ 90%) strains of *Streptococcus pneumoniae*, 0.5 µg/mL or less against most (≥ 90%) strains of *Haemophilus influenzae*, and 4 µg/mL or less against most (≥ 90%) strains of the other microorganisms in the following list; however, the safety and effectiveness of meropenem in treating clinical infections due to these microorganisms have not been established in adequate and well-controlled clinical trials.

Gram-Positive Aerobes

Staphylococcus aureus (β-lactamase and non-β-lactamase producing)

Staphylococcus epidermidis (β-lactamase and non-β-lactamase-producing)

NOTE: Staphylococci which are resistant to methicillin/oxacillin must be considered resistant to meropenem.

Gram-Negative Aerobes

Acinetobacter species

Aeromonas hydrophila

Campylobacter jejuni

Citrobacter diversus

Citrobacter freundii

Enterobacter cloacae

Haemophilus influenzae (ampicillin-resistant, non-β-lactamase-producing strains [BLNAR strains])

Hafnia alvei

Klebsiella oxytoca

Moraxella catarrhalis (β-lactamase and non-β-lactamase-producing strains)

Morganella morganii

Pasteurella multocida

Proteus mirabilis

Proteus vulgaris

Salmonella species

Serratia marcescens

Shigella species

Yersinia enterocolitica

Anaerobes

Bacteroides distasonis

Bacteroides ovatus

Bacteroides uniformis

Bacteroides ureolyticus

Bacteroides vulgatus

Clostridium difficile

Clostridium perfringens

Eubacterium lentum

Fusobacterium species

Prevotella bivia

Prevotella intermedia

Prevotella melaninogenica

Porphyromonas asaccharolytica

Propionibacterium acnes

Susceptibility Tests

Dilution Techniques:

Quantitative methods are used to determine antimicrobial minimum inhibitory concentrations (MIC's). These MIC's provide estimates of the susceptibility of bacteria to antimicrobial compounds. The MIC's should be determined using a standardized procedure. Standardized procedures are based on a dilution method[1] (broth or agar) or equivalent with standardized inoculum concentrations and standardized concentrations of meropenem powder. The MIC values should be interpreted according to the following criteria for indicated aerobic organisms other than *Haemophilus* species and streptococci:

MIC (µg/mL)	Interpretation
≤ 4	(S) Susceptible
8	(I) Intermediate
≥ 16	(R) Resistant

Haemophilus Test Media (HTM) and the following interpretive criteria should be used when testing *Haemophilus* species:

MIC (µg/mL)	Interpretation
≤ 0.5	(S) Susceptible

The current absence of resistant strains precludes defining any categories other than "Susceptible". Strains yielding results suggestive of a "Nonsusceptible" category should be submitted to a reference laboratory for further testing.

The following criteria should be used when testing streptococci including *Streptococcus pneumoniae*:

When testing *S. pneumoniae*:

MIC (µg/mL)	Interpretation
≤ 0.12	(S) Susceptible

When testing viridans group streptococci:

MIC (µg/mL)	Interpretation
≤ 0.5	(S) Susceptible

The current absence of resistant strains precludes defining any categories other than "Susceptible". Strains yielding results suggestive of a "Nonsusceptible" category should be submitted to a reference laboratory for further testing.

A report of 'Susceptible' indicates that the pathogen is likely to be inhibited if the antimicrobial compound in the blood reaches the concentrations usually achievable. A report of 'Intermediate' indicates that the result should be considered equivocal, and, if the microorganism is not fully susceptible to alternative, clinically feasible drugs, the test should be repeated. This category implies possible clinical applicability in body sites where the drug is physiologically concentrated or in situations where high dosage of drug can be used. This category also provides a buffer zone which prevents small uncontrolled technical factors from causing major discrepancies in interpretation. A report of 'Resistant' indicates that the pathogen is not likely to be inhibited if the antimicrobial compound in the blood reaches the concentrations usually achievable; other therapy should be selected.

Standardized susceptibility test procedures require the use of laboratory control microorganisms to control the technical aspects of the laboratory procedures. Standard meropenem powder should provide the following MIC values:

Microorganism	ATCC	MIC (µg/mL)
Enterococcus faecalis	29212	2.0-8.0
Escherichia coli	25922	0.008-0.06
Haemophilus influenzae	49766	0.03-0.12
Pseudomonas aeruginosa	27853	0.25-1.0
Streptococcus pneumoniae	49619	0.06-0.25

Diffusion Techniques:

Quantitative methods that require measurement of zone diameters also provide reproducible estimates of the susceptibility of bacteria to antimicrobial compounds. One such standardized procedure[2] requires the use of standardized inoculum concentrations. This procedure uses paper disks impregnated with 10-µg of meropenem to test the susceptibility of microorganisms to meropenem.

Reports from the laboratory providing results of the standard single-disk susceptibility test with a 10-µg disk should be interpreted according to the following criteria for indicated aerobic organisms other than *Haemophilus* species and streptococci:

Zone Diameter (mm)	Interpretation
≥ 16	(S) Susceptible
14-15	(I) Intermediate
≤ 13	(R) Resistant

Haemophilus Test Media and the following criteria should be used when testing *Haemophilus* species:

Zone Diameter (mm)	Interpretation
≥ 20	(S) Susceptible

The current absence of resistant strains precludes defining any categories other than "Susceptible". Strains yielding results suggestive of a "Nonsusceptible" category should be submitted to a reference laboratory for further testing.

Streptococcus pneumoniae isolates should be tested using 1-µg/mL oxacillin disk. Isolates with oxacillin zone sizes of ≥ 20 mm are susceptible (MIC ≤ 0.06 µg/mL) to penicillin and can be considered susceptible to meropenem for approved indications, and meropenem need not be tested. A meropenem MIC should be determined on isolates of *S. pneumoniae* with oxacillin zone sizes of ≤ 19 mm. The disk test does not distinguish penicillin intermediate strains (i.e., MIC's = 0.12-1.0 µg/mL) from strains that are penicillin resistant (i.e., MIC's ≥ 2 µg/mL). Viridans group streptococci should be tested for meropenem susceptibility using an MIC method. Reliable disk diffusion tests for meropenem do not yet exist for testing streptococci.

Interpretation should be as stated above for results using dilution techniques. Interpretation involves correlation of the diameter obtained in the disk test with the MIC for meropenem.

As with standardized dilution techniques, diffusion methods require the use of laboratory control microorganisms that are used to control the technical aspects of the laboratory procedures. For the diffusion technique, the 10-µg meropenem disk should provide the following zone diameters in these laboratory test quality control strains:

Microorganism	ATCC	Zone Diameter (mm)
Escherichia coli	25922	28-34
Haemophilus influenzae	49247	20-28
Pseudomonas aeruginosa	27853	27-33

Anaerobic Techniques:

For anaerobic bacteria, susceptibility to meropenem as MIC's can be determined by standardized test methods.[3] The MIC values obtained should be interpreted according to the following criteria:

MIC (µg/mL)	Interpretation
≤ 4	(S) Susceptible
8	(I) Intermediate
≥ 16	(R) Resistant

Interpretation is identical to that stated above for results using dilution techniques.

As with other susceptibility techniques, the use of laboratory control microorganisms is required to control the technical aspects of the laboratory standardized procedures. Standardized meropenem powder should provide the following MIC values:

Microorganism	ATCC	MIC (µg/mL)
Bacteroides fragilis	25285	0.06-0.25
Bacteroides thetaiotaomicron	29741	0.125-0.5

INDICATIONS AND USAGE

To reduce the development of drug-resistant bacteria and maintain the effectiveness of MERREM I.V. and other antibacterial drugs, MERREM I.V. should only be used to treat or prevent infections that are proven or strongly suspected to be caused by susceptible bacteria. When culture and susceptibility information are available, they should be considered in selecting or modifying antibacterial therapy. In the absence of such data, local epidemiology and susceptibility patterns may contribute to the empiric selection of therapy.

MERREM I.V. is indicated as single agent therapy for the treatment of the following infections when caused by susceptible strains of the designated microorganisms:

Intra-abdominal Infections

Complicated appendicitis and peritonitis caused by viridans group streptococci, *Escherichia coli, Klebsiella pneumoniae, Pseudomonas aeruginosa, Bacteroides fragilis, B. thetaiotaomicron,* and *Peptostreptococcus* species.

Bacterial Meningitis (Pediatric patients ≥ 3 months only)

Bacterial meningitis caused by *Streptococcus pneumoniae*‡, *Haemophilus influenzae* (β-lactamase and non-β-lactamase-producing strains), and *Neisseria meningitidis*.

‡The efficacy of meropenem as monotherapy in the treatment of meningitis caused by penicillin nonsusceptible strains of *Streptococcus pneumoniae* has not been established.

MERREM I.V. has been found to be effective in eliminating concurrent bacteremia in association with bacterial meningitis.

For information regarding use in pediatric patients (3 months of age and older) see **PRECAUTIONS-Pediatrics, ADVERSE REACTIONS**, and **DOSAGE AND ADMINISTRATION** sections.

Appropriate cultures should usually be performed before initiating antimicrobial treatment in order to isolate and identify the organisms causing infection and determine their susceptibility to MERREM I.V.

MERREM I.V. is useful as presumptive therapy in the indicated condition (i.e., intra-abdominal infections) prior to the identification of the causative organisms because of its broad spectrum of bactericidal activity.

Antimicrobial therapy should be adjusted, if appropriate, once the results of culture(s) and antimicrobial susceptibility testing are known.

CONTRAINDICATIONS

MERREM I.V. is contraindicated in patients with known hypersensitivity to any component of this product or to other drugs in the same class or in patients who have demonstrated anaphylactic reactions to β-lactams.

WARNINGS

SERIOUS AND OCCASIONALLY FATAL HYPERSENSITIVITY (ANAPHYLACTIC) REACTIONS HAVE BEEN REPORTED IN PATIENTS RECEIVING THERAPY WITH β-LACTAMS. THESE REACTIONS ARE MORE LIKELY TO OCCUR IN INDIVIDUALS WITH A HISTORY OF SENSITIVITY TO MULTIPLE ALLERGENS.

THERE HAVE BEEN REPORTS OF INDIVIDUALS WITH A HISTORY OF PENICILLIN HYPERSENSITIVITY WHO HAVE EXPERIENCED SEVERE HYPERSENSITIVITY REACTIONS WHEN TREATED WITH ANOTHER β-LACTAM. BEFORE INITIATING THERAPY WITH MERREM I.V., CAREFUL INQUIRY SHOULD BE MADE CONCERNING PREVIOUS HYPERSENSITIVITY REACTIONS TO PENICILLINS, CEPHALOSPORINS, OTHER β-LACTAMS, AND OTHER ALLERGENS. IF AN ALLERGIC REACTION TO MERREM I.V. OCCURS, DISCONTINUE THE DRUG IMMEDIATELY. **SERIOUS ANAPHYLACTIC REACTIONS REQUIRE IMMEDIATE EMERGENCY TREATMENT WITH EPINEPHRINE, OXYGEN, INTRAVE-**

Continued on next page

Merrem I.V.—Cont.

NOUS STEROIDS, AND AIRWAY MANAGEMENT, INCLUDING INTUBATION. OTHER THERAPY MAY ALSO BE ADMINISTERED AS INDICATED.

Seizures and other CNS adverse experiences have been reported during treatment with MERREM I.V. (See **PRECAUTIONS** and **ADVERSE REACTIONS**.)

Pseudomembranous colitis has been reported with nearly all antibacterial agents, including meropenem, and may range in severity from mild to life-threatening. Therefore, it is important to consider this diagnosis in patients who present with diarrhea subsequent to the administration of antibacterial agents.

Treatment with antibacterial agents alters the normal flora of the colon and may permit overgrowth of clostridia. Studies indicate that a toxin produced by *Clostridium difficile* is a primary cause of "antibiotic-associated colitis".

After the diagnosis of pseudomembranous colitis has been established, therapeutic measures should be initiated. Mild cases of pseudomembranous colitis usually respond to drug discontinuation alone. In moderate-to-severe cases, consideration should be given to management with fluids and electrolytes, protein supplementation, and treatment with an antibacterial drug clinically effective against *Clostridium difficile* colitis.

PRECAUTIONS

General: Prescribing MERREM I.V. in the absence of a proven or strongly suspected bacterial infection or a prophylactic indication is unlikely to provide benefit to the patient and increases the risk of the development of drug-resistant bacteria.

Seizures and other adverse CNS experiences have been reported during treatment with MERREM I.V. These experiences have occurred most commonly in patients with CNS disorders (e.g., brain lesions or history of seizures) or with bacterial meningitis and/or compromised renal function.

During the initial clinical investigations, 2904 immunocompetent adult patients were treated for infections outside the CNS, with the overall seizure rate being 0.7% (based on 20 patients with this adverse event). All meropenem-treated patients with seizures had pre-existing contributing factors. Among these are included prior history of seizures or CNS abnormality and concomitant medications with seizure potential. Dosage adjustment is recommended in patients with advanced age and/or reduced renal function. (See **DOSAGE AND ADMINISTRATION - Use in Adults with Renal Impairment**.)

Close adherence to the recommended dosage regimens is urged, especially in patients with known factors that predispose to convulsive activity. Anticonvulsant therapy should be continued in patients with known seizure disorders. If focal tremors, myoclonus, or seizures occur, patients should be evaluated neurologically, placed on anticonvulsant therapy if not already instituted, and the dosage of MERREM I.V. re-examined to determine whether it should be decreased or the antibiotic discontinued.

In patients with renal dysfunction, thrombocytopenia has been observed but no clinical bleeding reported. (See **DOSAGE AND ADMINISTRATION - Use in Adults with Renal Impairment**.)

There is inadequate information regarding the use of MERREM I.V. in patients on hemodialysis.

As with other broad-spectrum antibiotics, prolonged use of meropenem may result in overgrowth of nonsusceptible organisms. Repeated evaluation of the patient is essential. If superinfection does occur during therapy, appropriate measures should be taken.

Laboratory Tests: While MERREM I.V. possesses the characteristic low toxicity of the beta-lactam group of antibiotics, periodic assessment of organ system functions, including renal, hepatic, and hematopoietic, is advisable during prolonged therapy.

Drug Interactions: Probenecid competes with meropenem for active tubular secretion and thus inhibits the renal excretion of meropenem. This led to statistically significant increases in the elimination half-life (38%) and in the extent of systemic exposure (56%). Therefore, the coadministration of probenecid with meropenem is not recommended.

There is evidence that meropenem may reduce serum levels of valproic acid to subtherapeutic levels (therapeutic range considered to be 50 to 100 µg/mL total valproate).

Carcinogenesis, Mutagenesis, Impairment of Fertility:

Carcinogenesis: Carcinogenesis studies have not been performed.

Mutagenesis: Genetic toxicity studies were performed with meropenem using the bacterial reverse mutation test, the Chinese hamster ovary HGPRT assay, cultured human lymphocytes cytogenic assay, and the mouse micronucleus test. There was no evidence of mutagenic potential found in any of these tests.

Impairment of fertility: Reproductive studies were performed with meropenem in rats at doses up to 1000 mg/kg/day, and cynomolgus monkeys at doses up to 360 mg/kg/day (on the basis of AUC comparisons, approximately 1.8 times and 3.7 times, respectively, to the human exposure at the usual dose of 1 g every 8 hours). There was no reproductive toxicity seen.

Pregnancy Category B: Reproductive studies have been performed with meropenem in rats at doses of up to 1000 mg/kg/day, and cynomolgus monkeys at doses of up to 360 mg/kg/day (on the basis of AUC comparisons, approximately 1.8 times and 3.7 times, respectively, to the human exposure at the usual dose of 1 g every 8 hours). These studies revealed no evidence of impaired fertility or harm to the fetus due to meropenem, although there were slight changes in fetal body weight at doses of 250 mg/kg/day (on the basis of AUC comparisons, 0.4 times the human exposure at a dose of 1 g every 8 hours) and above in rats. There are, however, no adequate and well-controlled studies in pregnant women. Because animal reproduction studies are not always predictive of human response, this drug should be used during pregnancy only if clearly needed.

Pediatric Use: The safety and effectiveness of MERREM I.V. have been established for pediatric patients ≥ 3 months of age. Use of MERREM I.V. in pediatric patients with bacterial meningitis is supported by evidence from adequate and well-controlled studies in the pediatric population. Use of MERREM I.V. in pediatric patients with intra-abdominal infections is supported by evidence from adequate and well-controlled studies with adults with additional data from pediatric pharmacokinetics studies and controlled clinical trials in pediatric patients. (See **CLINICAL PHARMACOLOGY, INDICATIONS AND USAGE, ADVERSE REACTIONS, DOSAGE AND ADMINISTRATION**, and **CLINICAL STUDIES** sections.)

Nursing Mothers: It is not known whether this drug is excreted in human milk. Because many drugs are excreted in human milk, caution should be exercised when MERREM I.V. is administered to a nursing woman.

Geriatric Use: Of the total number of subjects in clinical studies of MERREM I.V., approximately 1100 (30%) were 65 years of age and older, while 400 (11%) were 75 years and older. No overall differences in safety or effectiveness were observed between these subjects and younger subjects; spontaneous reports and other reported clinical experience have not identified differences in responses between the elderly and younger patients, but greater sensitivity of some older individuals cannot be ruled out.

A pharmacokinetic study with MERREM I.V. in elderly patients with renal insufficiency has shown a reduction in plasma clearance of meropenem that correlates with age-associated reduction in creatinine clearance. (See **DOSAGE AND ADMINISTRATION; Use in Adults with Renal Impairment.**)

MERREM I.V. is known to be substantially excreted by the kidney, and the risk of toxic reactions to this drug may be greater in patients with impaired renal function. Because elderly patients are more likely to have decreased renal function, care should be taken in dose selection, and it may be useful to monitor renal function.

Information For Patients: Patients should be counseled that antibacterial drugs including MERREM I.V. should only be used to treat bacterial infections. They do not treat viral infections (eg, the common cold). When MERREM I.V. is prescribed to treat a bacterial infection, patients should be told that although it is common to feel better early in the course of therapy, the medication should be taken exactly as directed. Skipping doses or not completing the full course of therapy may (1) decrease the effectiveness of the immediate treatment and (2) increase the likelihood that bacteria will develop resistance and will not be treatable by MERREM I.V. or other antibacterial drugs in the future.

ADVERSE REACTIONS

Adult Patients:

During clinical investigations, 2904 immunocompetent adult patients were treated for infections outside the CNS with MERREM I.V. (500 mg or 1000 mg q 8 hours). Deaths in 5 patients were assessed as possibly related to meropenem; 36 (1.2%) patients had meropenem discontinued because of adverse events. Many patients in these trials were severely ill and had multiple background diseases, physiological impairments and were receiving multiple other drug therapies. In the seriously ill patient population, it was not possible to determine the relationship between observed adverse events and therapy with MERREM I.V.

The following adverse reaction frequencies were derived from the clinical trials in the 2904 patients treated with MERREM I.V.

Local Adverse Reactions

Local adverse reactions that were reported irrespective of the relationship to therapy with MERREM I.V. were as follows:

Inflammation at the injection site	2.4%
Injection site reaction	0.9%
Phlebitis/thrombophlebitis	0.8%
Pain at the injection site	0.4%
Edema at the injection site	0.2%

Systemic Adverse Reactions

Systemic adverse clinical reactions that were reported irrespective of the relationship to therapy with MERREM I.V. occurring in greater than 1.0% of the patients were diarrhea (4.8%), nausea/vomiting (3.6%), headache (2.3%), rash (1.9%), sepsis (1.6%), constipation (1.4%), apnea (1.3%), shock (1.2%), and pruritus (1.2%).

Additional adverse systemic clinical reactions that were reported irrespective of relationship to therapy with MERREM I.V. and occurring in less than or equal to 1.0% but greater than 0.1% of the patients are listed below within each body system in order of decreasing frequency:

Bleeding events were seen as follows: gastrointestinal hemorrhage (0.5%), melena (0.3%), epistaxis (0.2%), hemoperitoneum (0.2%), summing to 1.2%.

Body as a Whole: pain, abdominal pain, chest pain, fever, back pain, abdominal enlargement, chills, pelvic pain

Cardiovascular: heart failure, heart arrest, tachycardia, hypertension, myocardial infarction, pulmonary embolus, bradycardia, hypotension, syncope

Digestive System: oral moniliasis, anorexia, cholestatic jaundice/jaundice, flatulence, ileus, hepatic failure, dyspepsia, intestinal obstruction

Hemic/Lymphatic: anemia, hypochromic anemia, hypervolemia

Metabolic/Nutritional: peripheral edema, hypoxia

Nervous System: insomnia, agitation/delirium, confusion, dizziness, seizure (see **PRECAUTIONS**), nervousness, paresthesia, hallucinations, somnolence, anxiety, depression, asthenia

Respiratory: respiratory disorder, dyspnea, pleural effusion, asthma, cough increased, lung edema

Skin and Appendages: urticaria, sweating, skin ulcer

Urogenital System: dysuria, kidney failure, vaginal moniliasis, urinary incontinence

Adverse Laboratory Changes

Adverse laboratory changes that were reported irrespective of relationship to MERREM I.V. and occurring in greater than 0.2% of the patients were as follows:

Hepatic: increased SGPT (ALT), SGOT (AST), alkaline phosphatase, LDH, and bilirubin

Hematologic: increased platelets, increased eosinophils, decreased platelets, decreased hemoglobin, decreased hematocrit, decreased WBC, shortened prothrombin time and shortened partial thromboplastin time, leukocytosis, hypokalemia

Renal: increased creatinine and increased BUN

NOTE: For patients with varying degrees of renal impairment, the incidence of heart failure, kidney failure, seizure and shock reported irrespective of relationship to MERREM I.V., increased in patients with moderately severe renal impairment (creatinine clearance >10 to 26 mL/min).

Urinalysis: presence of urine red blood cells

Pediatric Patients:

Clinical Adverse Reactions

MERREM I.V. was studied in 515 pediatric patients (≥ 3 months to < 13 years of age) with serious bacterial infections (excluding meningitis. See next section.) at dosages of 10 to 20 mg/kg every 8 hours. The types of clinical adverse events seen in these patients are similar to the adults, with the most common adverse events reported as possibly, probably, or definitely related to MERREM I.V. and their rates of occurrence as follows:

Diarrhea	3.5%
Rash	1.6%
Nausea and Vomiting	0.8%

MERREM I.V. was studied in 321 pediatric patients (≥ 3 months to < 17 years of age) with meningitis at a dosage of 40 mg/kg every 8 hours. The types of clinical adverse events seen in these patients are similar to the adults, with the most common adverse events reported as possibly, probably, or definitely related to MERREM I.V. and their rates of occurrence as follows:

Diarrhea	4.7%
Rash (mostly diaper area moniliasis)	3.1%
Oral Moniliasis	1.9%
Glossitis	1.0%

In the meningitis studies the rates of seizure activity during therapy were comparable between patients with no CNS abnormalities who received meropenem and those who received comparator agents (either cefotaxime or ceftriaxone). In the MERREM I.V. treated group, 12/15 patients with seizures had late onset seizures (defined as occurring on day 3 or later) versus 7/20 in the comparator arm.

Adverse Laboratory Changes:

Laboratory abnormalities seen in the pediatric-aged patients in both the pediatric and the meningitis studies are similar to those reported in adult patients.

There is no experience in pediatric patients with renal impairment.

Post-marketing Experience:

Worldwide post-marketing adverse events not previously listed in the product label and reported as possibly, probably, or definitely drug related are listed within each body system in order of decreasing severity. Hematologic - agranulocytosis, neutropenia, and leukopenia. Skin - toxic epidermal necrolysis, Stevens-Johnson Syndrome, angioedema, and erythema multiform.

OVERDOSAGE

In mice and rats, large intravenous doses of meropenem (2200-4000 mg/kg) have been associated with ataxia, dyspnea, convulsions, and mortalities.

Intentional overdosing of MERREM I.V. is unlikely, although accidental overdosing might occur if large doses are given to patients with reduced renal function. The largest dose of meropenem administered in clinical trials has been 2 g given intravenously every 8 hours. At this dosage, no adverse pharmacological effects or increased safety risks have been observed.

No specific information is available for the treatment of MERREM I.V. overdosage. In the event of an overdose, MERREM I.V. should be discontinued and general supportive treatment given until renal elimination takes place. Meropenem and its metabolite are readily dialyzable and ef-

Treatment Arm	No. evaluable/ No. enrolled (%)	Microbiologic Eradication Rate	Clinical Cure Rate	Outcome
meropenem	146/516 (28%)	98/146 (67%)	101/146 (69%)	
imipenem	65/220 (30%)	40/65 (62%)	42/65 (65%)	Meropenem equivalent to control
cefotaxime/ metronidazole	26/85 (30%)	22/26 (85%)	22/26 (85%)	Meropenem not equivalent to control
clindamycin/ tobramycin	50/212 (24%)	38/50 (76%)	38/50 (76%)	Meropenem equivalent to control

MICROORGANISM	MERREM I.V.	COMPARATOR
S. pneumoniae	17/24 (71)	19/30 (63)
H. influenzae (+)	8/10 (80)	6/6 (100)
H. influenzae (−/NT)	44/59 (75)	44/60 (73)
N. meningitidis	30/35 (86)	35/39 (90)
TOTAL (including others)	102/131 (78)	108/140 (77)

(+) β-lactamase-producing; (−/NT) non-β-lactamase-producing or not tested

Recommended MERREM I.V. Dosage Schedule for Adults With Impaired Renal Function

Creatinine Clearance (mL/min)	Dose (dependent on type of infection)	Dosing Interval
26-50	recommended dose (1000 mg)	every 12 hours
10-25	one-half recommended dose	every 12 hours
<10	one-half recommended dose	every 24 hours

$$\text{Males: Creatinine Clearance (mL/min)} = \frac{\text{Weight (kg)} \times (140 - \text{age})}{72 \times \text{serum creatinine (mg/dL)}}$$

Females: 0.85 × above value

fectively removed by hemodialysis; however, no information is available on the use of hemodialysis to treat overdosage.

CLINICAL STUDIES

Intra-abdominal:

One controlled clinical study of complicated intra-abdominal infection was performed in the United States where meropenem was compared to clindamycin/tobramycin. Three controlled clinical studies of complicated intra-abdominal infections were performed in Europe; meropenem was compared to imipenem (two trials) and cefotaxime/metronidazole (one trial).

Using strict evaluability criteria and microbiologic eradication and clinical cures at follow-up which occurred 7 or more days after completion of therapy, the following presumptive microbiologic eradication/clinical cure rates and statistical findings were obtained:

[See first table above]

The finding that meropenem was not statistically equivalent to cefotaxime/metronidazole may have been due to uneven assignment of more seriously ill patients to the meropenem arm. Currently there is no additional information available to further interpret this observation.

Bacterial Meningitis:

Four hundred forty-six patients (397 pediatric patients ≥ 3 months to < 17 years of age) were enrolled in 4 separate clinical trials and randomized to treatment with meropenem (n=225) at a dose of 40 mg/kg q 8 hours or a comparator drug, i.e., cefotaxime (n=187) or ceftriaxone (n=34), at the approved dosing regimens. A comparable number of patients were found to be clinically evaluable (ranging from 61-68%) and with a similar distribution of pathogens isolated on initial CSF culture.

Patients were defined as clinically not cured if any one of the following three criteria were met:

1. At the 5-7 week post-completion of therapy visit, the patient had any one of the following: moderate to severe motor, behavior or development deficits, hearing loss of >60 decibels in one or both ears, or blindness.
2. During therapy the patient's clinical status necessitated the addition of other antibiotics.
3. Either during or post-therapy, the patient developed a large subdural effusion needing surgical drainage, or a cerebral abscess, or a bacteriologic relapse.

Using the definition, the following efficacy rates were obtained, per organism. The values represent the number of patients clinically cured/number of clinically evaluable patients, with the percent cure in parentheses.

[See second table above]

Sequelae were the most common reason patients were assessed as clinically not cured.

Five patients were found to be bacteriologically not cured, 3 in the comparator group (1 relapse and 2 patients with cerebral abscesses) and 2 in the meropenem group (1 relapse and 1 with continued growth of *Pseudomonas aeruginosa*).

The adverse events seen were comparable between the two treatment groups both in type and frequency. The meropenem group did have a statistically higher number of patients with transient elevation of liver enzymes. (See **ADVERSE REACTIONS**.) Rates of seizure activity during therapy were comparable between patients with no CNS abnormalities who received meropenem and those who received comparator agents. In the MERREM I.V. treated group, 12/15 patients with seizures had late onset seizures (defined as occurring on day 3 or later) versus 7/20 in the comparator arm.

With respect to hearing loss, 263 of the 271 evaluable patients had at least one hearing test performed post-therapy. The following table shows the degree of hearing loss between the meropenem-treated patients and the comparator-treated patients.

Degree of Hearing Loss (in one or both ears)	Meropenem n = 128	Comparator n = 135
No loss	61%	56%
20-40 decibels	20%	24%
>40-60 decibels	8%	7%
>60 decibels	9%	10%

DOSAGE AND ADMINISTRATION

Adults: One gram (1 g) by intravenous administration every 8 hours. MERREM I.V. should be given by intravenous infusion, over approximately 15 to 30 minutes or as an intravenous bolus injection (5 to 20 mL) over approximately 3-5 minutes.

Use in Adults with Renal Impairment: Dosage should be reduced in patients with creatinine clearance less than 51 mL/min. (see dosing table below.)

[See third table above]

When only serum creatinine is available, the following formula (Cockcroft and Gault equation)[4] may be used to estimate creatinine clearance.

[See fourth table above]

There is inadequate information regarding the use of MERREM I.V. in patients on hemodialysis.

There is no experience with peritoneal dialysis.

Use in Adults With Hepatic Insufficiency: No dosage adjustment is necessary in patients with impaired hepatic function.

Use in Elderly Patients: No dosage adjustment is required for elderly patients with creatinine clearance values above 50 mL/min.

Use in Pediatric Patients: For pediatric patients from 3 months of age and older, the MERREM I.V. dose is 20 or 40 mg/kg every 8 hours (maximum dose is 2 g every 8 hours), depending on the type of infection (intra-abdominal or meningitis). (See dosing table below.) Pediatric patients weighing over 50 kg should be administered MERREM I.V. at a dose of 1 g every 8 hours for intra-abdominal infections and 2 g every 8 hours for meningitis. MERREM I.V. should be given as intravenous infusion over approximately 15 to 30 minutes or as an intravenous bolus injection (5 to 20 mL) over approximately 3-5 minutes.

Recommended MERREM I.V. Dosage Schedule for Pediatrics With Normal Renal Function

Type of Infection	Dose(mg/kg)	Dosing Interval
Intra-abdominal	20	every 8 hours
Meningitis	40	every 8 hours

There is no experience in pediatric patients with renal impairment.

PREPARATION OF SOLUTION

For Intravenous Bolus Administration

Constitute injection vials (500 mg and 1 g) with sterile Water for Injection. (See table below.) Shake to dissolve and let stand until clear.

Vial Size	Amount of Diluent Added (mL)	Approximate Withdrawable Volume (mL)	Approximate Average Concentration (mg/mL)
500 mg	10	10	50
1 g	20	20	50

For Infusion

Infusion vials (500 mg and 1 g) may be directly constituted with a compatible infusion fluid. (See **COMPATIBILITY AND STABILITY.**) Alternatively, an injection vial may be constituted, then the resulting solution added to an I.V. container and further diluted with an appropriate infusion fluid. (See **COMPATIBILITY AND STABILITY.**)

NOTE: ADD-VANTAGE VIALS ARE NOT TO BE USED IN THIS MANNER.

For ADD-Vantage Vials

ADD-Vantage vials of MERREM I.V. are to be constituted only with Sodium Chloride Injection 0.45%, Sodium Chloride Injection 0.9% or Dextrose Injection 5% in the 50, 100, and 250 mL Abbott ADD-Vantage® flexible diluent containers. MERREM I.V. supplied in single-use ADD-Vantage vials should be prepared as directed.

DIRECTIONS FOR USE OF MERREM I.V. (meropenem for injection) IN ADD-VANTAGE VIALS:

To Open Diluent Container: Peel overwrap from the corner and remove container. Some opacity of the plastic due to moisture absorption during the sterilization process may be observed. This is normal and does not affect the solution quality or safety. The opacity will diminish gradually.

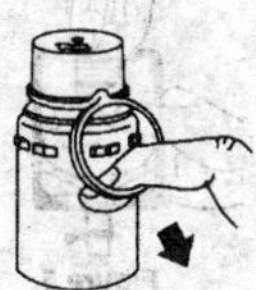

Figure 1

To Assemble ADD-Vantage Vial and Flexible Diluent Container: (Use Aseptic Technique)

1. Remove the protective covers from the top of the vial and the vial port on the diluent container as follows:

a. To remove the breakaway vial cap, swing the pull ring over the top of the vial and pull down far enough to start the opening (see Figure 1), then pull straight up to remove the cap. (See Figure 2.)

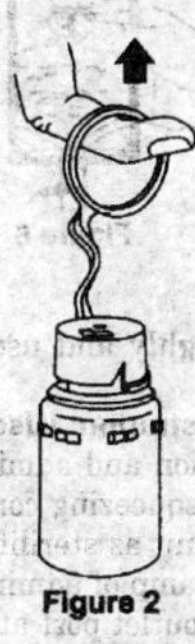

Figure 2

NOTE: Once the breakaway cap has been removed, do not access vial with syringe.

b. To remove the vial port cover, grasp the tab on the pull ring, pull up to break the three tie strings, then pull back to remove the cover. (See Figure 3.)

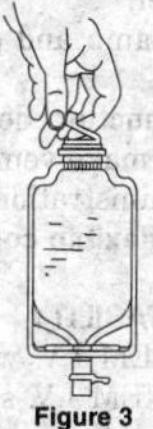

Figure 3

2. Screw the vial into the vial port until it will go no further. THE VIAL MUST BE SCREWED IN TIGHTLY TO ASSURE A SEAL. This occurs approximately 1/2 turn (180°) after the first audible click. (See Figure 4.) The clicking sound does not assure a seal; the vial must be turned as far as it will go.

Continued on next page

Merrem I.V.—Cont.

NOTE: ONCE VIAL IS SEATED, DO NOT ATTEMPT TO REMOVE.

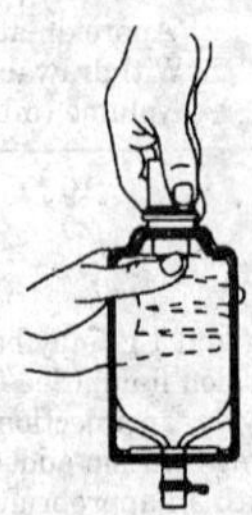

Figure 4

3. Recheck the vial to assure that it is tight by trying to turn it further in the direction of assembly.
4. Label appropriately.

To Prepare Admixture:

1. Squeeze the bottom of the diluent container gently to inflate the portion of the container surrounding the end of the drug vial.
2. With the other hand, push the drug vial down into the container telescoping the walls of the container. Grasp the inner cap of the vial through the walls of the container. (See Figure 5.)

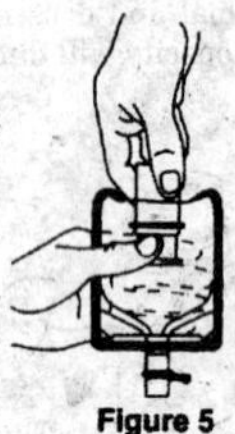

Figure 5

3. Pull the inner cap from the drug vial. (See Figure 6.) Verify that the rubber stopper has been pulled out and invert the system several times, allowing the drug and diluent to mix.

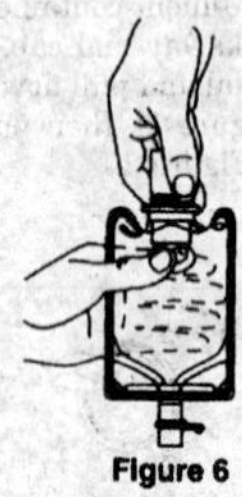

Figure 6

4. Mix contents thoroughly and use within the specified time.

Preparation For Administration: (Use Aseptic Technique)

1. Confirm the activation and admixture of vial contents.
2. Check for leaks by squeezing container firmly. If leaks are found, discard unit as sterility may be impaired.
3. Close flow control clamp of administration set.
4. Remove cover from outlet port at bottom of container.
5. Insert piercing pin of administration set into port with a twisting motion until the pin is firmly seated.
   NOTE: See full directions on administration set carton.
6. Lift the free end of the hanger loop on the bottom of the vial, breaking the two tie strings. Bend the loop outward to lock it in the upright position, then suspend container from hanger.
7. Squeeze and release drip chamber to establish proper fluid level in chamber.
8. Open flow control clamp and clear air from set. Close clamp.
9. Attach set to venipuncture device. If device is not indwelling, prime and make venipuncture.
10. Regulate rate of administration with flow control clamp.

WARNING: Do not use flexible container in series connections.

COMPATIBILITY AND STABILITY

Compatibility of MERREM I.V. with other drugs has not been established. MERREM I.V. should not be mixed with or physically added to solutions containing other drugs.

Freshly prepared solutions of MERREM I.V. should be used whenever possible. However, constituted solutions of MERREM I.V. maintain satisfactory potency at controlled room temperature 15-25°C (59-77°F) or under refrigeration at 4°C (39°F) as described below. Solutions of intravenous MERREM I.V. should not be frozen.

Intravenous Bolus Administration

MERREM I.V. injection vials constituted with sterile Water for Injection for bolus administration (up to 50 mg/mL of MERREM I.V.) may be stored for up to 2 hours at controlled room temperature 15-25°C (59-77°F) or for up to 12 hours at 4°C (39°F).

	Number of Hours Stable at Controlled Room Temperature 15-25°C (59-77°F)	Number of Hours Stable at 4°C (39°F)
Sodium Chloride Injection 0.9%	4	24
Dextrose Injection 5.0%	1	4
Dextrose Injection 10.0%	1	2
Dextrose and Sodium Chloride Injection 5.0%/0.9%	1	2
Dextrose and Sodium Chloride Injection 5.0%/0.2%	1	4
Potassium Chloride in Dextrose Injection 0.15%/5.0%	1	6
Sodium Bicarbonate in Dextrose Injection 0.02%/5.0%	1	6
Dextrose Injection 5.0% in Normosol®-M	1	8
Dextrose Injection 5.0% in Ringers Lactate Injection	1	4
Dextrose and Sodium Chloride Injection 2.5%/0.45%	3	12
Mannitol Injection 2.5%	2	16
Ringers Injection	4	24
Ringers Lactate Injection	4	12
Sodium Lactate Injection 1/6 N	2	24
Sodium Bicarbonate Injection 5.0%	1	4

Intravenous Infusion Administration

Stability in Infusion Vials: MERREM I.V. infusion vials constituted with Sodium Chloride Injection 0.9% (MERREM I.V. concentrations ranging from 2.5 to 50 mg/mL) are stable for up to 2 hours at controlled room temperature 15-25°C (55-77°F) or for up to 18 hours at 4°C (39°F). Infusion vials of MERREM I.V. constituted with Dextrose Injection 5% (MERREM I.V. concentrations ranging from 2.5 to 50 mg/mL) are stable for up to 1 hour at controlled room temperature 15-25°C (59-77°F) or for up to 8 hours at 4°C (39°F).

Stability in Plastic I.V. Bags: Solutions prepared for infusion (MERREM I.V. concentrations ranging from 1 to 20 mg/mL) may be stored in plastic intravenous bags with diluents as shown below:
[See table above]

Stability in Baxter Minibag Plus: Solutions of MERREM I.V. (MERREM I.V. concentrations ranging from 2.5 to 20 mg/mL) in Baxter Minibag Plus bags with Sodium Chloride Injection 0.9% may be stored for up to 4 hours at controlled room temperatures 15-25°C (59-77°F) or for up to 24 hours at 4°C (39°F). Solutions of MERREM I.V. (MERREM I.V. concentrations ranging from 2.5 to 20 mg/mL) in Baxter Minibag Plus bags with Dextrose Injection 5.0% may be stored up to 1 hour at controlled room temperatures 15-25°C (59-77°F) or for up to 6 hours at 4°C (39°F).

Stability in Plastic Syringes, Tubing and Intravenous Infusion Sets: Solutions of MERREM I.V. (MERREM I.V. concentrations ranging from 1 to 20 mg/mL) in Water for Injection or Sodium Chloride Injection 0.9% (for up to 4 hours) or in Dextrose Injection 5.0% (for up to 2 hours) at controlled room temperatures 15-25°C (59-77°F) are stable in plastic tubing and volume control devices of common intravenous infusion sets.

Solutions of MERREM I.V. (MERREM I.V. concentrations ranging from 1 to 20 mg/mL) in Water for Injection or Sodium Chloride Injection 0.9% (for up to 48 hours) or in Dextrose Injection 5% (for up to 6 hours) are stable at 4°C (39°F) in plastic syringes.

ADD-Vantage Vials: ADD-Vantage vials diluted in Sodium Chloride Injection 0.45% (MERREM I.V. concentrations ranging from 5 to 20 mg/mL) may be stored for up to 6 hours at controlled room temperature 15-25°C (59-77°F) or for 24 hours at 4°C (39°F). ADD-Vantage vials diluted in Sodium Chloride Injection 0.9% (MERREM I.V. concentrations ranging from 1-20 mg/mL) may be stored for up to 4 hours at controlled room temperature 15-25°C (59-77°F) or for 24 hours at 4°C (39°F). ADD-Vantage vials diluted with Dextrose Injection 5.0% (MERREM I.V. concentrations ranging from 1-20 mg/mL) may be stored for up to 1 hour at controlled room temperature 15-25°C (59-77°F) or for 8 hours at 4°C (39°F).

NOTE: Parenteral drug products should be inspected visually for particulate matter and discoloration prior to administration, whenever solution and container permit.

HOW SUPPLIED

MERREM I.V. is supplied in 20 mL and 30 mL injection vials containing sufficient meropenem to deliver 500 mg or 1 g for intravenous administration, respectively. MERREM I.V. is supplied in 100 mL infusion vials containing sufficient meropenem to deliver 500 mg or 1 g for intravenous administration. The dry powder should be stored at controlled room temperature 20-25°C (68-77°F) [see USP].

MERREM I.V. is also supplied as ADD-Vantage Vials containing sufficient meropenem to deliver 500 mg or 1 g for intravenous administration.

500 mg Injection Vial	(NDC 0310-0325-20)
1 g Injection Vial	(NDC 0310-0321-30)
500 mg ADD-Vantage	(NDC 0310-0325-15)
1 g ADD-Vantage	(NDC 0310-0321-15)

REFERENCES

1. National Committee for Clinical Laboratory Standards. Methods for Dilution Antimicrobial Susceptibility Tests for Bacteria that Grow Aerobically—Third Edition. Approved Standard NCCLS Document M7-A3, Vol. 13, No. 25, NCCLS, Villanova, PA; December, 1993.
2. National Committee for Clinical Laboratory Standards. Performance Standards for Antimicrobial Disk Susceptibility Tests—Fifth Edition. Approved Standard NCCLS Document M2-A5, Vol. 13, No. 24, NCCLS, Villanova, PA; December 1993.
3. National Committee for Clinical Laboratory Standards. Methods for Antimicrobial Susceptibility Testing of Anaerobic Bacteria—Third Edition. Approved Standard NCCLS Document M11-A3, Vol. 13, No. 26, NCCLS, Villanova, PA; December 1993.
4. Cockcroft DW, Gault MH. Prediction of creatinine clearance from serum creatinine. Nephron. 1976; 16:31-41.

† ADD-Vantage is a registered trademark of Abbott Laboratories Inc.

All other trademarks are the property of the AstraZeneca group of companies.

Manufactured for:
AstraZeneca Pharmaceuticals LP
Wilmington, DE 19850
By: ACS Dobfar SpA
Viale Addetta, 4/12
20067 Tribiano, Milano, Italy
Made in Italy
64213-01
Rev 01/04

Shown in Product Identification Guide, page 306

NOLVADEX® ℞

[*nōl-vă-dĕks*]
(tamoxifen citrate)

Please visit www.NOLVADEX.com or call the AstraZeneca Information Center at 1-800-236-9933 for the most current full prescribing information.

Shown in Product Identification Guide, page 306

SEROQUEL® ℞

(quetiapine fumarate)

DESCRIPTION

SEROQUEL (quetiapine fumarate) is a psychotropic agent belonging to a new chemical class, the dibenzothiazepine derivatives. The chemical designation is 2-[2-(4-dibenzo [*b,f*] [1,4]thiazepin-11-yl-1-piperazinyl)ethoxy]-ethanol fumarate (2:1) (salt). It is present in tablets as the fumarate salt. All doses and tablet strengths are expressed as milligrams of base, not as fumarate salt. Its molecular formula is $C_{42}H_{50}N_6O_4S_2 \bullet C_4H_4O_4$ and it has a molecular weight of 883.11 (fumarate salt). The structural formula is:

Quetiapine fumarate is a white to off-white crystalline powder which is moderately soluble in water.

SEROQUEL is supplied for oral administration as 25 mg (round, peach), 100 mg (round, yellow), 200 mg (round, white), and 300 mg (capsule-shaped, white) tablets.

Inactive ingredients are povidone, dibasic dicalcium phosphate dihydrate, microcrystalline cellulose, sodium starch glycolate, lactose monohydrate, magnesium stearate, hypromellose, polyethylene glycol and titanium dioxide.

The 25 mg tablets contain red ferric oxide and yellow ferric oxide and the 100 mg tablets contain only yellow ferric oxide.

CLINICAL PHARMACOLOGY

Pharmacodynamics

SEROQUEL is an antagonist at multiple neurotransmitter receptors in the brain: serotonin $5HT_{1A}$ and $5HT_2$ (IC_{50s}=717 & 148nM respectively), dopamine D_1 and D_2

(IC_{50s}=1268 & 329nM respectively), histamine H_1 (IC_{50}=30nM), and adrenergic α_1 and α_2 receptors (IC_{50s}=94 & 271nM, respectively). SEROQUEL has no appreciable affinity at cholinergic muscarinic and benzodiazepine receptors (IC_{50s}>5000 nM).

The mechanism of action of SEROQUEL, as with other drugs having efficacy in the treatment of schizophrenia and acute manic episodes associated with bipolar disorder, is unknown. However, it has been proposed that this drug's efficacy in schizophrenia is mediated through a combination of dopamine type 2 (D_2) and serotonin type 2 ($5HT_2$) antagonism. Antagonism at receptors other than dopamine and $5HT_2$ with similar receptor affinities may explain some of the other effects of SEROQUEL.

SEROQUEL's antagonism of histamine H_1 receptors may explain the somnolence observed with this drug.

SEROQUEL's antagonism of adrenergic α_1 receptors may explain the orthostatic hypotension observed with this drug.

Pharmacokinetics

Quetiapine fumarate activity is primarily due to the parent drug. The multiple-dose pharmacokinetics of quetiapine are dose-proportional within the proposed clinical dose range, and quetiapine accumulation is predictable upon multiple dosing. Elimination of quetiapine is mainly via hepatic metabolism with a mean terminal half-life of about 6 hours within the proposed clinical dose range. Steady-state concentrations are expected to be achieved within two days of dosing. Quetiapine is unlikely to interfere with the metabolism of drugs metabolized by cytochrome P450 enzymes.

Absorption: Quetiapine fumarate is rapidly absorbed after oral administration, reaching peak plasma concentrations in 1.5 hours. The tablet formulation is 100% bioavailable relative to solution. The bioavailability of quetiapine is marginally affected by administration with food, with C_{max} and AUC values increased by 25% and 15%, respectively.

Distribution: Quetiapine is widely distributed throughout the body with an apparent volume of distribution of 10±4 L/kg. It is 83% bound to plasma proteins at therapeutic concentrations. *In vitro*, quetiapine did not affect the binding of warfarin or diazepam to human serum albumin. In turn, neither warfarin nor diazepam altered the binding of quetiapine.

Metabolism and Elimination: Following a single oral dose of ^{14}C-quetiapine, less than 1% of the administered dose was excreted as unchanged drug, indicating that quetiapine is highly metabolized. Approximately 73% and 20% of the dose was recovered in the urine and feces, respectively.

Quetiapine is extensively metabolized by the liver. The major metabolic pathways are sulfoxidation to the sulfoxide metabolite and oxidation to the parent acid metabolite; both metabolites are pharmacologically inactive. *In vitro* studies using human liver microsomes revealed that the cytochrome P450 3A4 isoenzyme is involved in the metabolism of quetiapine to its major, but inactive, sulfoxide metabolite.

Population Subgroups

Age: Oral clearance of quetiapine was reduced by 40% in elderly patients (≥ 65 years, n=9) compared to young patients (n=12), and dosing adjustment may be necessary (See **DOSAGE AND ADMINISTRATION**).

Gender: There is no gender effect on the pharmacokinetics of quetiapine.

Race: There is no race effect on the pharmacokinetics of quetiapine.

Smoking: Smoking has no effect on the oral clearance of quetiapine.

Renal Insufficiency: Patients with severe renal impairment (Clcr=10–30 mL/min/1.73 m^2, n=8) had a 25% lower mean oral clearance than normal subjects (Clcr > 80 mL/min/1.73 m^2, n=8), but plasma quetiapine concentrations in the subjects with renal insufficiency were within the range of concentrations seen in normal subjects receiving the same dose. Dosage adjustment is therefore not needed in these patients.

Hepatic Insufficiency: Hepatically impaired patients (n=8) had a 30% lower mean oral clearance of quetiapine than normal subjects. In two of the 8 hepatically impaired patients, AUC and C_{max} were 3-times higher than those observed typically in healthy subjects. Since quetiapine is extensively metabolized by the liver, higher plasma levels are expected in the hepatically impaired population, and dosage adjustment may be needed (See **DOSAGE AND ADMINISTRATION**).

Drug-Drug Interactions: *In vitro* enzyme inhibition data suggest that quetiapine and 9 of its metabolites would have little inhibitory effect on *in vivo* metabolism mediated by cytochromes P450 1A2, 2C9, 2C19, 2D6 and 3A4.

Quetiapine oral clearance is increased by the prototype cytochrome P450 3A4 inducer, phenytoin, and decreased by the prototype cytochrome P450 3A4 inhibitor, ketoconazole. Dose adjustment of quetiapine will be necessary if it is coadministered with phenytoin or ketoconazole (See **Drug Interactions** under **PRECAUTIONS** and **DOSAGE AND ADMINISTRATION**).

Quetiapine oral clearance is not inhibited by the nonspecific enzyme inhibitor, cimetidine.

Quetiapine at doses of 750 mg/day did not affect the single dose pharmacokinetics of antipyrine, lithium or lorazepam (See **Drug Interactions** under **PRECAUTIONS**).

Clinical Efficacy Data

Bipolar Mania

The efficacy of SEROQUEL in the treatment of acute manic episodes was established in 3 short-term (3-week) placebo-controlled trials in patients who met DSM-IV criteria for Bipolar I disorder with manic episodes. These trials included patients with or without psychotic features and excluded patients with rapid cycling and mixed episodes. Of these trials, 2 were monotherapy and 1 was adjunct therapy to either lithium or divalproex. Adjunct therapy is defined as the simultaneous initiation or subsequent administration of SEROQUEL with lithium or divalproex.

The primary rating instrument used for assessing manic symptoms in these trials was the Young Mania Rating Scale (YMRS), an 11-item clinician-rated scale traditionally used to assess the degree of manic symptomatology (irritability, disruptive/aggressive behavior, sleep, elevated mood, speech, increased activity, sexual interest, language/thought disorder, thought content, appearance, and insight) in a range from 0 (no manic features) to 60 (maximum score). The primary outcome in these trials was change from baseline in the YMRS total score at Day 21.

The results of the trials follow:

Monotherapy

In two 3-week trials (n=300, n=299) comparing SEROQUEL to placebo, SEROQUEL was superior to placebo in the reduction of the YMRS total score. The majority of patients in these trials taking SEROQUEL were dosed in a range of 400 and 800 mg per day.

Adjunct Therapy

In this 3-week placebo-controlled trial, 170 patients with acute bipolar mania (YMRS ≥ 20) were randomized to receive SEROQUEL or placebo as adjunct treatment to lithium or divalproex. Patients may or may not have received an adequate treatment course of lithium or divalproex prior to randomization. SEROQUEL was superior to placebo when added to lithium or divalproex alone in the reduction of YMRS total score.

The majority of patients in this trial taking SEROQUEL were dosed in a range between 400 and 800 mg per day. In a similarly designed trial (n=200), SEROQUEL was associated with an improvement in YMRS scores but did not demonstrate superiority to placebo, possibly due to a higher placebo effect.

Schizophrenia

The efficacy of SEROQUEL in the treatment of schizophrenia was established in 3 short-term (6-week) controlled trials of inpatients with schizophrenia who met DSM III-R criteria for schizophrenia. Although a single fixed dose haloperidol arm was included as a comparative treatment in one of the three trials, this single haloperidol dose group was inadequate to provide a reliable and valid comparison of SEROQUEL and haloperidol.

Several instruments were used for assessing psychiatric signs and symptoms in these studies, among them the Brief Psychiatric Rating Scale (BPRS), a multi-item inventory of general psychopathology traditionally used to evaluate the effects of drug treatment in schizophrenia. The BPRS psychosis cluster (conceptual disorganization, hallucinatory behavior, suspiciousness, and unusual thought content) is considered a particularly useful subset for assessing actively psychotic schizophrenic patients. A second traditional assessment, the Clinical Global Impression (CGI), reflects the impression of a skilled observer, fully familiar with the manifestations of schizophrenia, about the overall clinical state of the patient. In addition, the Scale for Assessing Negative Symptoms (SANS), a more recently developed but less well evaluated scale, was employed for assessing negative symptoms.

The results of the trials follow:

(1) In a 6-week, placebo-controlled trial (n=361) involving 5 fixed doses of SEROQUEL (75, 150, 300, 600 and 750 mg/day on a tid schedule), the 4 highest doses of SEROQUEL were generally superior to placebo on the BPRS total score, the BPRS psychosis cluster and the CGI severity score, with the maximal effect seen at 300 mg/day, and the effects of doses of 150 to 750 were generally indistinguishable. SEROQUEL, at a dose of 300 mg/day, was superior to placebo on the SANS.

(2) In a 6-week, placebo-controlled trial (n=286) involving titration of SEROQUEL in high (up to 750 mg/day on a tid schedule) and low (up to 250 mg/day on a tid schedule) doses, only the high dose SEROQUEL group (mean dose, 500 mg/day) was generally superior to placebo on the BPRS total score, the BPRS psychosis cluster, the CGI severity score, and the SANS.

(3) In a 6-week dose and dose regimen comparison trial (n=618) involving two fixed doses of SEROQUEL (450 mg/day on both bid and tid schedules and 50 mg/day on a bid schedule), only the 450 mg/day (225 mg bid schedule) dose group was generally superior to the 50 mg/day (25 mg bid) SEROQUEL dose group on the BPRS total score, the BPRS psychosis cluster, the CGI severity score, and on the SANS.

Examination of population subsets (race, gender, and age) did not reveal any differential responsiveness on the basis of race or gender, with an apparently greater effect in patients under the age of 40 compared to those older than 40. The clinical significance of this finding is unknown.

INDICATIONS AND USAGE

Bipolar Mania

SEROQUEL is indicated for the short-term treatment of acute manic episodes associated with bipolar I disorder, as either monotherapy or adjunct therapy to lithium or divalproex.

The efficacy of SEROQUEL in acute bipolar mania was established in two 3-week monotherapy trials and one 3-week adjunct therapy trial of bipolar I patients initially hospitalized for up to 7 days for acute mania (See **CLINICAL PHARMACOLOGY**). Effectiveness for more than 3 weeks has not been systematically evaluated in clinical trials. Therefore, the physician who elects to use SEROQUEL for extended periods should periodically re-evaluate the long-term risks and benefits of the drug for the individual patient (See **DOSAGE AND ADMINISTRATION**).

Schizophrenia

SEROQUEL is indicated for the treatment of schizophrenia. The efficacy of SEROQUEL in schizophrenia was established in short-term (6-week) controlled trials of schizophrenic inpatients (See **CLINICAL PHARMACOLOGY**).

The effectiveness of SEROQUEL in long-term use, that is, for more than 6 weeks, has not been systematically evaluated in controlled trials. Therefore, the physician who elects to use SEROQUEL for extended periods should periodically re-evaluate the long-term usefulness of the drug for the individual patient (See **DOSAGE AND ADMINISTRATION**).

CONTRAINDICATIONS

SEROQUEL is contraindicated in individuals with a known hypersensitivity to this medication or any of its ingredients.

WARNINGS

Neuroleptic Malignant Syndrome (NMS)

A potentially fatal symptom complex sometimes referred to as Neuroleptic Malignant Syndrome (NMS) has been reported in association with administration of antipsychotic drugs, including SEROQUEL. Rare cases of NMS have been reported with SEROQUEL. Clinical manifestations of NMS are hyperpyrexia, muscle rigidity, altered mental status, and evidence of autonomic instability (irregular pulse or blood pressure, tachycardia, diaphoresis, and cardiac dysrhythmia). Additional signs may include elevated creatine phosphokinase, myoglobinuria (rhabdomyolysis) and acute renal failure.

The diagnostic evaluation of patients with this syndrome is complicated. In arriving at a diagnosis, it is important to exclude cases where the clinical presentation includes both serious medical illness (e.g., pneumonia, systemic infection, etc.) and untreated or inadequately treated extrapyramidal signs and symptoms (EPS). Other important considerations in the differential diagnosis include central anticholinergic toxicity, heat stroke, drug fever and primary central nervous system (CNS) pathology.

The management of NMS should include: 1) immediate discontinuation of antipsychotic drugs and other drugs not essential to concurrent therapy; 2) intensive symptomatic treatment and medical monitoring; and 3) treatment of any concomitant serious medical problems for which specific treatments are available. There is no general agreement about specific pharmacological treatment regimens for NMS.

If a patient requires antipsychotic drug treatment after recovery from NMS, the potential reintroduction of drug therapy should be carefully considered. The patient should be carefully monitored since recurrences of NMS have been reported.

Tardive Dyskinesia

A syndrome of potentially irreversible, involuntary, dyskinetic movements may develop in patients treated with antipsychotic drugs. Although the prevalence of the syndrome appears to be highest among the elderly, especially elderly women, it is impossible to rely upon prevalence estimates to predict, at the inception of antipsychotic treatment, which patients are likely to develop the syndrome. Whether antipsychotic drug products differ in their potential to cause tardive dyskinesia is unknown.

The risk of developing tardive dyskinesia and the likelihood that it will become irreversible are believed to increase as the duration of treatment and the total cumulative dose of antipsychotic drugs administered to the patient increase. However, the syndrome can develop, although much less commonly, after relatively brief treatment periods at low doses.

There is no known treatment for established cases of tardive dyskinesia, although the syndrome may remit, partially or completely, if antipsychotic treatment is withdrawn. Antipsychotic treatment, itself, however, may suppress (or partially suppress) the signs and symptoms of the syndrome and thereby may possibly mask the underlying process. The effect that symptomatic suppression has upon the long-term course of the syndrome is unknown.

Given these considerations, SEROQUEL should be prescribed in a manner that is most likely to minimize the occurrence of tardive dyskinesia. Chronic antipsychotic treatment should generally be reserved for patients who appear to suffer from a chronic illness that (1) is known to respond to antipsychotic drugs, and (2) for whom alternative, equally effective, but potentially less harmful treatments are not available or appropriate. In patients who do require chronic treatment, the smallest dose and the shortest duration of treatment producing a satisfactory clinical response should be sought. The need for continued treatment should be reassessed periodically.

If signs and symptoms of tardive dyskinesia appear in a patient on SEROQUEL, drug discontinuation should be considered. However, some patients may require treatment with SEROQUEL despite the presence of the syndrome.

Hyperglycemia and Diabetes Mellitus

Hyperglycemia, in some cases extreme and associated with ketoacidosis or hyperosmolar coma or death, has been reported in patients treated with atypical antipsychotics, including Seroquel. Assessment of the relationship between

Continued on next page

Seroquel—Cont.

atypical antipsychotic use and glucose abnormalities is complicated by the possibility of an increased background risk of diabetes mellitus in patients with schizophrenia and the increasing incidence of diabetes mellitus in the general population. Given these confounders, the relationship between atypical antipsychotic use and hyperglycemia-related adverse events is not completely understood. However, epidemiological studies suggest an increased risk of treatment-emergent hyperglycemia-related adverse events in patients treated with the atypical antipsychotics. Precise risk estimates for hyperglycemia-related adverse events in patients treated with atypical antipsychotics are not available.

Patients with an established diagnosis of diabetes mellitus who are started on atypical antipsychotics should be monitored regularly for worsening of glucose control. Patients with risk factors for diabetes mellitus (eg, obesity, family history of diabetes) who are starting treatment with atypical antipsychotics should undergo fasting blood glucose testing at the beginning of treatment and periodically during treatment. Any patient treated with atypical antipsychotics should be monitored for symptoms of hyperglycemia including polydipsia, polyuria, polyphagia, and weakness. Patients who develop symptoms of hyperglycemia during treatment with atypical antipsychotics should undergo fasting blood glucose testing. In some cases, hyperglycemia has resolved when the atypical antipsychotic was discontinued; however, some patients required continuation of anti-diabetic treatment despite discontinuation of the suspect drug.

PRECAUTIONS

General

Orthostatic Hypotension: SEROQUEL may induce orthostatic hypotension associated with dizziness, tachycardia and, in some patients, syncope, especially during the initial dose-titration period, probably reflecting its α_1-adrenergic antagonist properties. Syncope was reported in 1% (23/2567) of the patients treated with SEROQUEL, compared with 0% (0/607) on placebo and about 0.4% (2/527) on active control drugs.

SEROQUEL should be used with particular caution in patients with known cardiovascular disease (history of myocardial infarction or ischemic heart disease, heart failure or conduction abnormalities), cerebrovascular disease or conditions which would predispose patients to hypotension (dehydration, hypovolemia and treatment with antihypertensive medications). The risk of orthostatic hypotension and syncope may be minimized by limiting the initial dose to 25 mg bid (See **DOSAGE AND ADMINISTRATION**). If hypotension occurs during titration to the target dose, a return to the previous dose in the titration schedule is appropriate.

Cataracts: The development of cataracts was observed in association with quetiapine treatment in chronic dog studies (see Animal Toxicology). Lens changes have also been observed in patients during long-term SEROQUEL treatment, but a causal relationship to SEROQUEL use has not been established. Nevertheless, the possibility of lenticular changes cannot be excluded at this time. Therefore, examination of the lens by methods adequate to detect cataract formation, such as slit lamp exam or other appropriately sensitive methods, is recommended at initiation of treatment or shortly thereafter, and at 6 month intervals during chronic treatment.

Seizures: During clinical trials, seizures occurred in 0.6% (18/2792) of patients treated with SEROQUEL compared to 0.2% (1/607) on placebo and 0.7% (4/527) on active control drugs. As with other antipsychotics SEROQUEL should be used cautiously in patients with a history of seizures or with conditions that potentially lower the seizure threshold, e.g., Alzheimer's dementia. Conditions that lower the seizure threshold may be more prevalent in a population of 65 years or older.

Hypothyroidism: Clinical trials with SEROQUEL demonstrated a dose-related decrease in total and free thyroxine (T4) of approximately 20% at the higher end of the therapeutic dose range and was maximal in the first two to four weeks of treatment and maintained without adaptation or progression during more chronic therapy. Generally, these changes were of no clinical significance and TSH was unchanged in most patients, and levels of TBG were unchanged. In nearly all cases, cessation of SEROQUEL treatment was associated with a reversal of the effects on total and free T4, irrespective of the duration of treatment. About 0.4% (12/2791) of SEROQUEL patients did experience TSH increases in monotherapy studies. Six of the patients with TSH increases needed replacement thyroid treatment. In the mania adjunct studies, where SEROQUEL was added to lithium or divalproate, 12% (24/196) of SEROQUEL treated patients compared to 7% (15/203) of placebo treated patients had elevated TSH levels. Of the SEROQUEL treated patients with elevated TSH levels, 3 had simultaneous low free T4 levels.

Cholesterol and Triglyceride Elevations: In schizophrenia trials, SEROQUEL-treated patients had increases from baseline in cholesterol and triglyceride of 11% and 17%, respectively, compared to slight decreases for placebo patients. These changes were only weakly related to the increases in weight observed in SEROQUEL-treated patients.

Hyperprolactinemia: Although an elevation of prolactin levels was not demonstrated in clinical trials with SEROQUEL, increased prolactin levels were observed in rat studies with this compound, and were associated with an increase in mammary gland neoplasia in rats (see **Carcinogenesis**). Tissue culture experiments indicate that approximately one-third of human breast cancers are prolactin dependent *in vitro*, a factor of potential importance if the prescription of these drugs is contemplated in a patient with previously detected breast cancer. Although disturbances such as galactorrhea, amenorrhea, gynecomastia, and impotence have been reported with prolactin-elevating compounds, the clinical significance of elevated serum prolactin levels is unknown for most patients. Neither clinical studies nor epidemiologic studies conducted to date have shown an association between chronic administration of this class of drugs and tumorigenesis in humans; the available evidence is considered too limited to be conclusive at this time.

Transaminase Elevations: Asymptomatic, transient and reversible elevations in serum transaminases (primarily ALT) have been reported. In schizophrenia trials, the proportions of patients with transaminase elevations of > 3 times the upper limits of the normal reference range in a pool of 3- to 6-week placebo-controlled trials were approximately 6% for SEROQUEL compared to 1% for placebo. In acute bipolar mania trials, the proportions of patients with transaminase elevations of > 3 times the upper limits of the normal reference range in a pool of 3- to 12-week placebo-controlled trials were approximately 1% for both SEROQUEL and placebo. These hepatic enzyme elevations usually occurred within the first 3 weeks of drug treatment and promptly returned to pre-study levels with ongoing treatment with SEROQUEL.

Potential for Cognitive and Motor Impairment: Somnolence was a commonly reported adverse event reported in patients treated with SEROQUEL especially during the 3–5 day period of initial dose-titration. In schizophrenia trials, somnolence was reported in 18% of patients on SEROQUEL compared to 11% of placebo patients. In acute bipolar mania trials using SEROQUEL as monotherapy, somnolence was reported in 16% of patients on SEROQUEL compared to 4% of placebo patients. In acute bipolar mania trials using SEROQUEL as adjunct therapy, somnolence was reported in 34% of patients on SEROQUEL compared to 9% of placebo patients. Since SEROQUEL has the potential to impair judgment, thinking, or motor skills, patients should be cautioned about performing activities requiring mental alertness, such as operating a motor vehicle (including automobiles) or operating hazardous machinery until they are reasonably certain that SEROQUEL therapy does not affect them adversely.

Priapism: One case of priapism in a patient receiving SEROQUEL has been reported prior to market introduction. While a causal relationship to use of SEROQUEL has not been established, other drugs with alpha-adrenergic blocking effects have been reported to induce priapism, and it is possible that SEROQUEL may share this capacity. Severe priapism may require surgical intervention.

Body Temperature Regulation: Although not reported with SEROQUEL, disruption of the body's ability to reduce core body temperature has been attributed to antipsychotic agents. Appropriate care is advised when prescribing SEROQUEL for patients who will be experiencing conditions which may contribute to an elevation in core body temperature, e.g., exercising strenuously, exposure to extreme heat, receiving concomitant medication with anticholinergic activity, or being subject to dehydration.

Dysphagia: Esophageal dysmotility and aspiration have been associated with antipsychotic drug use. Aspiration pneumonia is a common cause of morbidity and mortality in elderly patients, in particular those with advanced Alzheimer's dementia. SEROQUEL and other antipsychotic drugs should be used cautiously in patients at risk for aspiration pneumonia.

Suicide: The possibility of a suicide attempt is inherent in bipolar disorder and schizophrenia: close supervision of high risk patients should accompany drug therapy. Prescriptions for SEROQUEL should be written for the smallest quantity of tablets consistent with good patient management in order to reduce the risk of overdose.

Use in Patients with Concomitant Illness: Clinical experience with SEROQUEL in patients with certain concomitant systemic illnesses (see Renal Impairment and Hepatic Impairment under **CLINICAL PHARMACOLOGY**, Special Populations) is limited. SEROQUEL has not been evaluated or used to any appreciable extent in patients with a recent history of myocardial infarction or unstable heart disease. Patients with these diagnoses were excluded from premarketing clinical studies. Because of the risk of orthostatic hypotension with SEROQUEL, caution should be observed in cardiac patients (see **Orthostatic Hypotension**).

Information for Patients

Physicians are advised to discuss the following issues with patients for whom they prescribe SEROQUEL.

Orthostatic Hypotension: Patients should be advised of the risk of orthostatic hypotension, especially during the 3–5 day period of initial dose titration, and also at times of re-initiating treatment or increases in dose.

Interference with Cognitive and Motor Performance: Since somnolence was a commonly reported adverse event associated with SEROQUEL treatment, patients should be advised of the risk of somnolence, especially during the 3–5 day period of initial dose titration. Patients should be cautioned about performing any activity requiring mental alertness, such as operating a motor vehicle (including automobiles) or operating hazardous machinery, until they are reasonably certain that SEROQUEL therapy does not affect them adversely.

Pregnancy: Patients should be advised to notify their physician if they become pregnant or intend to become pregnant during therapy.

Nursing: Patients should be advised not to breast feed if they are taking SEROQUEL.

Concomitant Medication: As with other medications, patients should be advised to notify their physicians if they are taking, or plan to take, any prescription or over-the-counter drugs.

Alcohol: Patients should be advised to avoid consuming alcoholic beverages while taking SEROQUEL.

Heat Exposure and Dehydration: Patients should be advised regarding appropriate care in avoiding overheating and dehydration.

Laboratory Tests

No specific laboratory tests are recommended.

Drug Interactions

The risks of using SEROQUEL in combination with other drugs have not been extensively evaluated in systematic studies. Given the primary CNS effects of SEROQUEL, caution should be used when it is taken in combination with other centrally acting drugs. SEROQUEL potentiated the cognitive and motor effects of alcohol in a clinical trial in subjects with selected psychotic disorders, and alcoholic beverages should be avoided while taking SEROQUEL.

Because of its potential for inducing hypotension, SEROQUEL may enhance the effects of certain antihypertensive agents.

SEROQUEL may antagonize the effects of levodopa and dopamine agonists.

The Effect of Other Drugs on Quetiapine

Phenytoin: Coadministration of quetiapine (250 mg tid) and phenytoin (100 mg tid) increased the mean oral clearance of quetiapine by 5-fold. Increased doses of SEROQUEL may be required to maintain control of symptoms of schizophrenia in patients receiving quetiapine and phenytoin, or other hepatic enzyme inducers (e.g., carbamazepine, barbiturates, rifampin, glucocorticoids). Caution should be taken if phenytoin is withdrawn and replaced with a non-inducer (e.g., valproate) (see **DOSAGE AND ADMINISTRATION**).

Divalproex: Coadministration of quetiapine (150 mg bid) and divalproex (500 mg bid) increased the mean maximum plasma concentration of quetiapine at steady state by 17% without affecting the extent of absorption or mean oral clearance.

Thioridazine: Thioridazine (200 mg bid) increased the oral clearance of quetiapine (300 mg bid) by 65%.

Cimetidine: Administration of multiple daily doses of cimetidine (400 mg tid for 4 days) resulted in a 20% decrease in the mean oral clearance of quetiapine (150 mg tid). Dosage adjustment for quetiapine is not required when it is given with cimetidine.

P450 3A Inhibitors: Coadministration of ketoconazole (200 mg once daily for 4 days), a potent inhibitor of cytochrome P450 3A, reduced oral clearance of quetiapine by 84%, resulting in a 335% increase in maximum plasma concentration of quetiapine. Caution is indicated when SEROQUEL is administered with ketoconazole and other inhibitors of cytochrome P450 3A (e.g., itraconazole, fluconazole, and erythromycin).

Fluoxetine, Imipramine, Haloperidol, and Risperidone: Coadministration of fluoxetine (60 mg once daily); imipramine (75 mg bid), haloperidol (7.5 mg bid), or risperidone (3 mg bid) with quetiapine (300 mg bid) did not alter the steady-state pharmacokinetics of quetiapine.

Effect of Quetiapine on Other Drugs

Lorazepam: The mean oral clearance of lorazepam (2 mg, single dose) was reduced by 20% in the presence of quetiapine administered as 250 mg tid dosing.

Divalproex: The mean maximum concentration and extent of absorption of total and free valproic acid at steady state were decreased by 10 to 12% when divalproex (500 mg bid) was administered with quetiapine (150 mg bid). The mean oral clearance of total valproic acid (administered as divalproex 500 mg bid) was increased by 11% in the presence of quetiapine (150 mg bid). The changes were not significant

Lithium: Concomitant administration of quetiapine (250 mg tid) with lithium had no effect on any of the steady-state pharmacokinetic parameters of lithium.

Antipyrine: Administration of multiple daily doses up to 750 mg/day (on a tid schedule) of quetiapine to subjects with selected psychotic disorders had no clinically relevant effect on the clearance of antipyrine or urinary recovery of antipyrine metabolites. These results indicate that quetiapine does not significantly induce hepatic enzymes responsible for cytochrome P450 mediated metabolism of antipyrine.

Carcinogenesis, Mutagenesis, Impairment of Fertility

Carcinogenesis: Carcinogenicity studies were conducted in C57BL mice and Wistar rats. Quetiapine was administered in the diet to mice at doses of 20, 75, 250, and 750 mg/kg and to rats by gavage at doses of 25, 75, and 250 mg/kg for two years. These doses are equivalent to 0.1, 0.5, 1.5, and 4.5 times the maximum human dose (800 mg/day) on a mg/m^2 basis (mice) or 0.3, 0.9, and 3.0 times the maximum human dose on a mg/m^2 basis (rats). There were statistically significant increases in thyroid gland follicular adenomas in male mice at doses of 250 and 750 mg/kg or 1.5 and 4.5 times the maximum human dose on a mg/m^2 basis and in male rats at a dose of 250 mg/kg or 3.0 times the maximum human dose on a mg/m^2 basis. Mammary gland adenocarcinomas were statistically significantly increased in female rats at all doses tested (25, 75, and 250 mg/kg or

0.3, 0.9, and 3.0 times the maximum recommended human dose on a mg/m^2 basis).

Thyroid follicular cell adenomas may have resulted from chronic stimulation of the thyroid gland by thyroid stimulating hormone (TSH) resulting from enhanced metabolism and clearance of thyroxine by rodent liver. Changes in TSH, thyroxine, and thyroxine clearance consistent with this mechanism were observed in subchronic toxicity studies in rat and mouse and in a 1-year toxicity study in rat; however, the results of these studies were not definitive. The relevance of the increases in thyroid follicular cell adenomas to human risk, through whatever mechanism, is unknown.

Antipsychotic drugs have been shown to chronically elevate prolactin levels in rodents. Serum measurements in a 1-yr toxicity study showed that quetiapine increased median serum prolactin levels a maximum of 32- and 13-fold in male and female rats, respectively. Increases in mammary neoplasms have been found in rodents after chronic administration of other antipsychotic drugs and are considered to be prolactin-mediated. The relevance of this increased incidence of prolactin-mediated mammary gland tumors in rats to human risk is unknown (see Hyperprolactinemia in **PRECAUTIONS, General**).

Mutagenesis: The mutagenic potential of quetiapine was tested in six *in vitro* bacterial gene mutation assays and in an *in vitro* mammalian gene mutation assay in Chinese Hamster Ovary cells. However, sufficiently high concentrations of quetiapine may not have been used for all tester strains. Quetiapine did produce a reproducible increase in mutations in one *Salmonella typhimurium* tester strain in the presence of metabolic activation. No evidence of clastogenic potential was obtained in an *in vitro* chromosomal aberration assay in cultured human lymphocytes or in the *in vivo* micronucleus assay in rats.

Impairment of Fertility: Quetiapine decreased mating and fertility in male Sprague-Dawley rats at oral doses of 50 and 150 mg/kg or 0.6 and 1.8 times the maximum human dose on a mg/m^2 basis. Drug-related effects included increases in interval to mate and in the number of matings required for successful impregnation. These effects continued to be observed at 150 mg/kg even after a two-week period without treatment. The no-effect dose for impaired mating and fertility in male rats was 25 mg/kg, or 0.3 times the maximum human dose on a mg/m^2 basis. Quetiapine adversely affected mating and fertility in female Sprague-Dawley rats at an oral dose of 50 mg/kg, or 0.6 times the maximum human dose on a mg/m^2 basis. Drug-related effects included decreases in matings and in matings resulting in pregnancy, and an increase in the interval to mate. An increase in irregular estrus cycles was observed at doses of 10 and 50 mg/kg, or 0.1 and 0.6 times the maximum human dose on a mg/m^2 basis. The no-effect dose in female rats was 1 mg/kg, or 0.01 times the maximum human dose on a mg/m^2 basis.

Pregnancy

Pregnancy Category C

The teratogenic potential of quetiapine was studied in Wistar rats and Dutch Belted rabbits dosed during the period of organogenesis. No evidence of a teratogenic effect was detected in rats at doses of 25 to 200 mg/kg or 0.3 to 2.4 times the maximum human dose on a mg/m^2 basis or in rabbits at 25 to 100 mg/kg or 0.6 to 2.4 times the maximum human dose on a mg/m^2 basis. There was, however, evidence of embryo/fetal toxicity. Delays in skeletal ossification were detected in rat fetuses at doses of 50 and 200 mg/kg (0.6 and 2.4 times the maximum human dose on a mg/m^2 basis) and in rabbits at 50 and 100 mg/kg (1.2 and 2.4 times the maximum human dose on a mg/m^2 basis). Fetal body weight was reduced in rat fetuses at 200 mg/kg and rabbit fetuses at 100 mg/kg (2.4 times the maximum human dose on a mg/m^2 basis for both species). There was an increased incidence of a minor soft tissue anomaly (carpal/tarsal flexure) in rabbit fetuses at a dose of 100 mg/kg (2.4 times the maximum human dose on a mg/m^2 basis). Evidence of maternal toxicity (i.e., decreases in body weight gain and/or death) was observed at the high dose in the rat study and at all doses in the rabbit study. In a peri/postnatal reproductive study in rats, no drug-related effects were observed at doses of 1, 10, and 20 mg/kg or 0.01, 0.12, and 0.24 times the maximum human dose on a mg/m^2 basis. However, in a preliminary peri/postnatal study, there were increases in fetal and pup death, and decreases in mean litter weight at 150 mg/kg, or 3.0 times the maximum human dose on a mg/m^2 basis.

There are no adequate and well-controlled studies in pregnant women and quetiapine should be used during pregnancy only if the potential benefit justifies the potential risk to the fetus.

Labor and Delivery: The effect of SEROQUEL on labor and delivery in humans is unknown.

Nursing Mothers: SEROQUEL was excreted in milk of treated animals during lactation. It is not known if SEROQUEL is excreted in human milk. It is recommended that women receiving SEROQUEL should not breast feed.

Pediatric Use: The safety and effectiveness of SEROQUEL in pediatric patients have not been established.

Geriatric Use: Of the approximately 3400 patients in clinical studies with SEROQUEL, 7% (232) were 65 years of age or over. In general, there was no indication of any different tolerability of SEROQUEL in the elderly compared to younger adults. Nevertheless, the presence of factors that might decrease pharmacokinetic clearance, increase the pharmacodynamic response to SEROQUEL, or cause poorer tolerance or orthostasis, should lead to consideration of a lower starting dose, slower titration, and careful monitoring during the initial dosing period in the elderly. The mean plasma clearance of SEROQUEL was reduced by 30% to 50% in elderly patients when compared to younger patients (see Pharmacokinetics under **CLINICAL PHARMACOLOGY** and **DOSAGE AND ADMINISTRATION**).

ADVERSE REACTIONS

The information below is derived from a clinical trial database for SEROQUEL consisting of over 3000 patients. This database includes 405 patients exposed to SEROQUEL for the treatment of acute bipolar mania (monotherapy and adjunct therapy) and approximately 2600 patients and/or normal subjects exposed to 1 or more doses of SEROQUEL for the treatment of schizophrenia.

Of these approximately 3000 subjects, approximately 2700 (2300 in schizophrenia and 405 in acute bipolar mania) were patients who participated in multiple dose effectiveness trials, and their experience corresponded to approximately 914.3 patient-years. The conditions and duration of treatment with SEROQUEL varied greatly and included (in overlapping categories) open-label and double-blind phases of studies, inpatients and outpatients, fixed-dose and dose-titration studies, and short-term or longer-term exposure.

Adverse reactions were assessed by collecting adverse events, results of physical examinations, vital signs, weights, laboratory analyses, ECGs, and results of ophthalmologic examinations.

Adverse events during exposure were obtained by general inquiry and recorded by clinical investigators using terminology of their own choosing. Consequently, it is not possible to provide a meaningful estimate of the proportion of individuals experiencing adverse events without first grouping similar types of events into a smaller number of standardized event categories. In the tables and tabulations that follow, standard COSTART terminology has been used to classify reported adverse events.

The stated frequencies of adverse events represent the proportion of individuals who experienced, at least once, a treatment-emergent adverse event of the type listed. An event was considered treatment emergent if it occurred for the first time or worsened while receiving therapy following baseline evaluation.

Adverse Findings Observed in Short-Term, Controlled Trials

Adverse Events Associated with Discontinuation of Treatment in Short-Term, Placebo-Controlled Trials

Acute Bipolar Mania: Overall, discontinuations due to adverse events were 5.7 % for SEROQUEL vs. 5.1% for placebo in monotherapy and 3.6% for SEROQUEL vs. 5.9% for placebo in adjunct therapy.

Schizophrenia: Overall, there was little difference in the incidence of discontinuation due to adverse events (4% for SEROQUEL vs. 3% for placebo) in a pool of controlled trials. However, discontinuations due to somnolence and hypotension were considered to be drug related (see **PRECAUTIONS**):

Adverse Event	SEROQUEL	Placebo
Somnolence	0.8%	0%
Hypotension	0.4%	0%

Adverse Events Occurring at an Incidence of 1% or More Among SEROQUEL Treated Patients in Short-Term, Placebo-Controlled Trials: The prescriber should be aware that the figures in the tables and tabulations cannot be used to predict the incidence of side effects in the course of usual medical practice where patient characteristics and other factors differ from those that prevailed in the clinical trials. Similarly, the cited frequencies cannot be compared with figures obtained from other clinical investigations involving different treatments, uses, and investigators. The cited figures, however, do provide the prescribing physician with some basis for estimating the relative contribution of drug and nondrug factors to the side effect incidence in the population studied.

Table 1 enumerates the incidence, rounded to the nearest percent, of treatment-emergent adverse events that occurred during acute therapy of schizophrenia (up to 6 weeks) and bipolar mania (up to 12 weeks) in 1% or more of patients treated with SEROQUEL (doses ranging from 75 to 800 mg/day) where the incidence in patients treated with SEROQUEL was greater than the incidence in placebo-treated patients.

Table 1. Treatment-Emergent Adverse Experience Incidence in 3- to 12-Week Placebo-Controlled Clinical Trials[1] for the Treatment of Schizophrenia and Acute Bipolar Mania (monotherapy)

Body System/ Preferred Term	SEROQUEL (n=719)	Placebo (n=404)
Body as a Whole		
Headache	21%	14%
Pain	7%	5%
Asthenia	5%	3%
Abdominal pain	4%	1%
Back pain	3%	1%
Fever	2%	1%
Cardiovascular		
Tachycardia	6%	4%
Postural Hypotension	4%	1%
Digestive		
Dry Mouth	9%	3%
Constipation	8%	3%
Vomiting	6%	5%
Dyspepsia	5%	1%
Gastroenteritis	2%	0%
Gamma Glutamyl Transpeptidase Increased	1%	0%
Metabolic and Nutritional		
Weight Gain	5%	1%
SGPT Increased	5%	1%
SGOT Increased	3%	1%
Nervous		
Agitation	20%	17%
Somnolence	18%	8%
Dizziness	11%	5%
Anxiety	4%	3%
Respiratory System		
Pharyngitis	4%	3%
Rhinitis	3%	1%
Skin and Appendages		
Rash	4%	2%
Special Senses		
Amblyopia	2%	1%

[1] Events for which the SEROQUEL incidence was equal to or less than placebo are not listed in the table, but included the following: accidental injury, akathisia, chest pain, cough increased, depression, diarrhea, extrapyramidal syndrome, hostility, hypertension, hypertonia, hypotension, increased appetite, infection, insomnia, leukopenia, malaise, nausea, nervousness, paresthesia, peripheral edema, sweating, tremor, and weight loss.

In these studies, the most commonly observed adverse events associated with the use of SEROQUEL (incidence of 5% or greater) and observed at a rate on SEROQUEL at least twice that of placebo were somnolence (18%), dizziness (11%), dry mouth (9%), constipation (8%), SGPT increased (5%), weight gain (5%), and dyspepsia (5%).

Table 2 enumerates the incidence, rounded to the nearest percent, of treatment-emergent adverse events that occurred during therapy (up to 3-weeks) of acute mania in 5% or more of patients treated with SEROQUEL (doses ranging from 100 to 800 mg/day) used as adjunct therapy to lithium and divalproex where the incidence in patients treated with SEROQUEL was greater than the incidence in placebo-treated patients.

Table 2. Treatment-Emergent Adverse Experience Incidence in 3-Week Placebo-Controlled Clinical Trials[1] for the Treatment of Acute Bipolar Mania (Adjunct Therapy)

Body System/ Preferred Term	SEROQUEL (n=196)	Placebo (n=203)
Body as a Whole		
Headache	17%	13%
Asthenia	10%	4%
Abdominal pain	7%	3%
Back pain	5%	3%
Cardiovascular		
Postural Hypotension	7%	2%
Digestive		
Dry Mouth	19%	3%
Constipation	10%	5%
Metabolic and Nutritional		
Weight gain	6%	3%
Nervous		
Somnolence	34%	9%
Dizziness	9%	6%
Tremor	8%	7%
Agitation	6%	4%
Respiratory		
Pharyngitis	6%	3%

[1] Events for which the SEROQUEL incidence was equal to or less than placebo are not listed in the table, but included the following: akathisia, diarrhea, insomnia, and nausea.

In these studies, the most commonly observed adverse events associated with the use of SEROQUEL (incidence of 5% or greater) and observed at a rate on SEROQUEL at least twice that of placebo were somnolence (34%), dry mouth (19%), asthenia (10%), constipation (10%), abdominal pain (7%), postural hypotension (7%), pharyngitis (6%), and weight gain (6%).

Explorations for interactions on the basis of gender, age, and race did not reveal any clinically meaningful differences in the adverse event occurrence on the basis of these demographic factors.

Dose Dependency of Adverse Events in Short-Term, Placebo-Controlled Trials

Dose-related Adverse Events: Spontaneously elicited adverse event data from a study of schizophrenia comparing five fixed doses of SEROQUEL (75 mg, 150 mg, 300 mg, 600 mg, and 750 mg/day) to placebo were explored for dose-relatedness of adverse events. Logistic regression analyses revealed a positive dose response ($p<0.05$) for the following adverse events: dyspepsia, abdominal pain, and weight gain.

Extrapyramidal Symptoms: Data from one 6-week clinical trial of schizophrenia comparing five fixed doses of

Continued on next page

Seroquel—Cont.

SEROQUEL (75, 150, 300, 600, 750 mg/day) provided evidence for the lack of treatment-emergent extrapyramidal symptoms (EPS) and dose-relatedness for EPS associated with SEROQUEL treatment. Three methods were used to measure EPS: (1) Simpson-Angus total score (mean change from baseline) which evaluates parkinsonism and akathisia, (2) incidence of spontaneous complaints of EPS (akathisia, akinesia, cogwheel rigidity, extrapyramidal syndrome, hypertonia, hypokinesia, neck rigidity, and tremor), and (3) use of anticholinergic medications to treat emergent EPS.

Dose Groups	Placebo	SEROQUEL 75mg	150mg	300mg	600mg	750mg
Parkinsonism	0.6	-1.0	-1.2	-1.6	-1.8	-1.8
EPS incidence	16%	6%	6%	4%	8%	6%
Anticholinergic Medications	14%	11%	10%	8%	12%	11%

In six additional placebo-controlled clinical trials (3 in acute mania and 3 in schizophrenia) using variable doses of SEROQUEL, there were no differences between the SEROQUEL and placebo treatment groups in the incidence of EPS, as assessed by Simpson-Angus total scores, spontaneous complaints of EPS and the use of concomitant anticholinergic medications to treat EPS.

Vital Signs and Laboratory Studies

Vital Sign Changes: SEROQUEL is associated with orthostatic hypotension (see **PRECAUTIONS**).

Weight Gain: In schizophrenia trials the proportions of patients meeting a weight gain criterion of ≥7% of body weight were compared in a pool of four 3- to 6-week placebo-controlled clinical trials, revealing a statistically significantly greater incidence of weight gain for SEROQUEL (23%) compared to placebo (6%). In mania monotherapy trials the proportions of patients meeting the same weight gain criterion were 21% compared to 7% for placebo and in mania adjunct therapy trials the proportion of patients meeting the same weight criterion were 13% compared to 4% for placebo.

Laboratory Changes: An assessment of the premarketing experience for SEROQUEL suggested that it is associated with asymptomatic increases in SGPT and increases in both total cholesterol and triglycerides (see **PRECAUTIONS**).

An assessment of hematological parameters in short-term, placebo-controlled trials revealed no clinically important differences between SEROQUEL and placebo.

ECG Changes: Between group comparisons for pooled placebo-controlled trials revealed no statistically significant SEROQUEL/placebo differences in the proportions of patients experiencing potentially important changes in ECG parameters, including QT, QTc, and PR intervals. However, the proportions of patients meeting the criteria for tachycardia were compared in four 3- to 6-week placebo-controlled clinical trials for the treatment of schizophrenia revealing a 1% (4/399) incidence for SEROQUEL compared to 0.6% (1/156) incidence for placebo. In acute (monotherapy) bipolar mania trials the proportions of patients meeting the criteria for tachycardia was 0.5% (1/192) for SEROQUEL compared to 0% (0/178) incidence for placebo. In acute bipolar mania (adjunct) trials the proportions of patients meeting the same criteria was 0.6% (1/166) for SEROQUEL compared to 0% (0/171) incidence for placebo. SEROQUEL use was associated with a mean increase in heart rate, assessed by ECG, of 7 beats per minute compared to a mean increase of 1 beat per minute among placebo patients. This slight tendency to tachycardia may be related to SEROQUEL's potential for inducing orthostatic changes (see **PRECAUTIONS**).

Other Adverse Events Observed During the Pre-Marketing Evaluation of SEROQUEL

Following is a list of COSTART terms that reflect treatment-emergent adverse events as defined in the introduction to the ADVERSE REACTIONS section reported by patients treated with SEROQUEL at multiple doses ≥ 75 mg/day during any phase of a trial within the premarketing database of approximately 2200 patients treated for schizophrenia. All reported events are included except those already listed in Table 1 or elsewhere in labeling, those events for which a drug cause was remote, and those event terms which were so general as to be uninformative. It is important to emphasize that, although the events reported occurred during treatment with SEROQUEL, they were not necessarily caused by it.

Events are further categorized by body system and listed in order of decreasing frequency according to the following definitions: frequent adverse events are those occurring in at least 1/100 patients (only those not already listed in the tabulated results from placebo-controlled trials appear in this listing); infrequent adverse events are those occurring in 1/100 to 1/1000 patients; rare events are those occurring in fewer than 1/1000 patients.

Nervous System: ***Frequent:*** hypertonia, dysarthria; ***Infrequent:*** abnormal dreams, dyskinesia, thinking abnormal, tardive dyskinesia, vertigo, involuntary movements, confusion, amnesia, psychosis, hallucinations, hyperkinesia, libido increased*, urinary retention, incoordination, paranoid reaction, abnormal gait, myoclonus, delusions, manic reaction, apathy, ataxia, depersonalization, stupor, bruxism, catatonic reaction, hemiplegia; ***Rare:*** aphasia, buccoglossal syndrome, choreoathetosis, delirium, emotional lability, euphoria, libido decreased*, neuralgia, stuttering, subdural hematoma.

Body as a Whole: ***Frequent:*** flu syndrome; ***Infrequent:*** neck pain, pelvic pain*, suicide attempt, malaise, photosensitivity reaction, chills, face edema, moniliasis; ***Rare:*** abdomen enlarged.

Digestive System: ***Frequent:*** anorexia; ***Infrequent:*** increased salivation, increased appetite, gamma glutamyl transpeptidase increased, gingivitis, dysphagia, flatulence, gastroenteritis, gastritis, hemorrhoids, stomatitis, thirst, tooth caries, fecal incontinence, gastroesophageal reflux, gum hemorrhage, mouth ulceration, rectal hemorrhage, tongue edema; ***Rare:*** glossitis, hematemesis, intestinal obstruction, melena, pancreatitis.

Cardiovascular System: ***Frequent:*** palpitation; ***Infrequent:*** vasodilatation, QT interval prolonged, migraine, bradycardia, cerebral ischemia, irregular pulse, T wave abnormality, bundle branch block, cerebrovascular accident, deep thrombophlebitis, T wave inversion; ***Rare:*** angina pectoris, atrial fibrillation, AV block first degree, congestive heart failure, ST elevated, thrombophlebitis, T wave flattening, ST abnormality, increased QRS duration.

Respiratory System: ***Frequent:*** pharyngitis, rhinitis, cough increased, dyspnea; ***Infrequent:*** pneumonia, epistaxis, asthma; ***Rare:*** hiccup, hyperventilation.

Metabolic and Nutritional System: ***Frequent:*** peripheral edema; ***Infrequent:*** weight loss, alkaline phosphatase increased, hyperlipemia, alcohol intolerance, dehydration, hyperglycemia, creatinine increased, hypoglycemia; ***Rare:*** glycosuria, gout, hand edema, hypokalemia, water intoxication.

Skin and Appendages System: ***Frequent:*** sweating; ***Infrequent:*** pruritis, acne, eczema, contact dermatitis, maculopapular rash, seborrhea, skin ulcer; ***Rare:*** exfoliative dermatitis, psoriasis, skin discoloration.

Urogenital System: ***Infrequent:*** dysmenorrhea*, vaginitis*, urinary incontinence, metrorrhagia*, impotence*, dysuria, vaginal moniliasis*, abnormal ejaculation*, cystitis, urinary frequency, amenorrhea*, female lactation*, leukorrhea*, vaginal hemorrhage*, vulvo-vaginitis* orchitis*; ***Rare:*** gynecomastia*, nocturia, polyuria, acute kidney failure.

Special Senses: ***Infrequent:*** conjunctivitis, abnormal vision, dry eyes, tinnitus, taste perversion, blepharitis, eye pain; ***Rare:*** abnormality of accommodation, deafness, glaucoma.

Musculoskeletal System: ***Infrequent:*** pathological fracture, myasthenia, twitching, arthralgia, arthritis, leg cramps, bone pain.

Hemic and Lymphatic System: ***Frequent:*** leukopenia; ***Infrequent:*** leukocytosis, anemia, ecchymosis, eosinophilia, hypochromic anemia; lymphadenopathy, cyanosis; ***Rare:*** hemolysis, thrombocytopenia.

Endocrine System: ***Infrequent:*** hypothyroidism, diabetes mellitus; ***Rare:*** hyperthyroidism.

*adjusted for gender

Post Marketing Experience: Adverse events reported since market introduction which were temporally related to SEROQUEL therapy include: leukopenia/neutropenia. If a patient develops a low white cell count consider discontinuation of therapy. Possible risk factors for leukopenia/neutropenia include pre-existing low white cell count and history of drug induced leukopenia/neutropenia.

Other adverse events reported since market introduction, which were temporally related to SEROQUEL therapy, but not necessarily causally related, include the following: agranulocytosis, anaphylaxis, hyponatremia, rhabdomyolysis, syndrome of inappropriate antidiuretic hormone secretion (SIADH), and Steven Johnson syndrome (SJS).

DRUG ABUSE AND DEPENDENCE

Controlled Substance Class: SEROQUEL is not a controlled substance.

Physical and Psychologic dependence: SEROQUEL has not been systematically studied, in animals or humans, for its potential for abuse, tolerance or physical dependence. While the clinical trials did not reveal any tendency for any drug-seeking behavior, these observations were not systematic and it is not possible to predict on the basis of this limited experience the extent to which a CNS-active drug will be misused, diverted, and/or abused once marketed. Consequently, patients should be evaluated carefully for a history of drug abuse, and such patients should be observed closely for signs of misuse or abuse of SEROQUEL, e.g., development of tolerance, increases in dose, drug-seeking behavior.

OVERDOSAGE

Human experience: Experience with SEROQUEL (quetiapine fumarate) in acute overdosage was limited in the clinical trial database (6 reports) with estimated doses ranging from 1200 mg to 9600 mg and no fatalities. In general, reported signs and symptoms were those resulting from an exaggeration of the drug's known pharmacological effects, i.e., drowsiness and sedation, tachycardia and hypotension. One case, involving an estimated overdose of 9600 mg, was associated with hypokalemia and first degree heart block. In post-marketing experience, there have been very rare reports of overdose of SEROQUEL alone resulting in death, coma or QTc prolongation.

Management of Overdosage: In case of acute overdosage, establish and maintain an airway and ensure adequate oxygenation and ventilation. Gastric lavage (after intubation, if patient is unconscious) and administration of activated charcoal together with a laxative should be considered. The possibility of obtundation, seizure or dystonic reaction of the head and neck following overdose may create a risk of aspiration with induced emesis. Cardiovascular monitoring should commence immediately and should include continuous electro-cardiographic monitoring to detect possible arrhythmias. If antiarrhythmic therapy is administered, disopyramide, procainamide and quinidine carry a theoretical hazard of additive QT-prolonging effects when administered in patients with acute overdosage of SEROQUEL. Similarly it is reasonable to expect that the alpha-adrenergic-blocking properties of bretylium might be additive to those of quetiapine, resulting in problematic hypotension.

There is no specific antidote to SEROQUEL. Therefore appropriate supportive measures should be instituted. The possibility of multiple drug involvement should be considered. Hypotension and circulatory collapse should be treated with appropriate measures such as intravenous fluids and/or sympathomimetic agents (epinephrine and dopamine should not be used, since beta stimulation may worsen hypotension in the setting of quetiapine-induced alpha blockade). In cases of severe extrapyramidal symptoms, anticholinergic medication should be administered. Close medical supervision and monitoring should continue until the patient recovers.

DOSAGE AND ADMINISTRATION

Acute Bipolar Mania

Usual Dose: When used as monotherapy or adjunct therapy (with lithium or divalproex), SEROQUEL should be initiated in BID doses totaling 100 mg/day on Day 1, increased to 400 mg/day on Day 4 in increments of up to 100 mg/day in BID divided doses. Further dosage adjustments up to 800 mg/day by Day 6 should be in increments of no greater than 200 mg/day. Data indicates that the majority of patients responded between 400 to 800 mg/day. The safety of doses above 800 mg/day has not been evaluated in clinical trials.

Schizophrenia

Usual Dose: SEROQUEL should generally be administered with an initial dose of 25 mg bid, with increases in increments of 25–50 mg bid or tid on the second and third day, as tolerated, to a target dose range of 300 to 400 mg daily by the fourth day, given bid or tid. Further dosage adjustments, if indicated, should generally occur at intervals of not less than 2 days, as steady state for SEROQUEL would not be achieved for approximately 1–2 days in the typical patient. When dosage adjustments are necessary, dose increments/decrements of 25–50 mg bid are recommended. Most efficacy data with SEROQUEL were obtained using tid regimens, but in one controlled trial 225 mg bid was also effective.

Efficacy in schizophrenia was demonstrated in a dose range of 150 to 750 mg/day in the clinical trials supporting the effectiveness of SEROQUEL. In a dose response study, doses above 300 mg/day were not demonstrated to be more efficacious than the 300 mg/day dose. In other studies, however, doses in the range of 400–500 mg/day appeared to be needed. The safety of doses above 800 mg/day has not been evaluated in clinical trials.

Dosing in Special Populations

Consideration should be given to a slower rate of dose titration and a lower target dose in the elderly, and in patients who are debilitated or who have a predisposition to hypotensive reactions (see **CLINICAL PHARMACOLOGY**). When indicated, dose escalation should be performed with caution in these patients.

Patients with hepatic impairment should be started on 25 mg/day. The dose should be increased daily in increments of 25–50 mg/day to an effective dose, depending on the clinical response and tolerability of the patient.

The elimination of quetiapine was enhanced in the presence of phenytoin. Higher maintenance doses of quetiapine may be required when it is coadministered with phenytoin and other enzyme inducers such as carbamazepine and phenobarbital (See Drug Interactions under **PRECAUTIONS**).

Maintenance Treatment: While there is no body of evidence available to answer the question of how long the patient treated with SEROQUEL should remain on it, the effectiveness of maintenance treatment is well established for many other drugs used to treat schizophrenia. It is recommended that responding patients be continued on SEROQUEL, but at the lowest dose needed to maintain remission. Patients should be periodically reassessed to determine the need for maintenance treatment.

Reinitiation of Treatment in Patients Previously Discontinued: Although there are no data to specifically address reinitiation of treatment, it is recommended that when restarting patients who have had an interval of less than one week off SEROQUEL, titration of SEROQUEL is not required and the maintenance dose may be reinitiated. When restarting therapy of patients who have been off SEROQUEL for more than one week, the initial titration schedule should be followed.

Switching from Antipsychotics: There are no systematically collected data to specifically address switching patients with schizophrenia from antipsychotics to SEROQUEL, or concerning concomitant administration with antipsychotics. While immediate discontinuation of the previous antipsychotic treatment may be acceptable for some patients with schizophrenia, more gradual discontinuation may be most appropriate for others. In all cases, the period of overlapping antipsychotic administration should be minimized. When switching patients with schizophrenia from depot antipsychotics, if medically appropriate, initiate SEROQUEL therapy in place of the next scheduled injection. The need for continuing existing EPS medication should be reevaluated periodically.

HOW SUPPLIED

25 mg Tablets (NDC 0310-0275) peach, round, biconvex, film coated tablets, identified with 'SEROQUEL' and '25' on one side and plain on the other side, are supplied in bottles of 100 tablets and 1000 tablets, and hospital unit dose packages of 100 tablets.

100 mg Tablets (NDC 0310-0271) yellow, round, biconvex film coated tablets, identified with 'SEROQUEL' and '100' on one side and plain on the other side, are supplied in bottles of 100 tablets and hospital unit dose packages of 100 tablets.

200 mg Tablets (NDC 0310-0272) white, round, biconvex, film coated tablets, identified with 'SEROQUEL' and '200' on one side and plain on the other side, are supplied in bottles of 100 tablets and hospital unit dose packages of 100 tablets.

300 mg Tablets (NDC 0310-0274) white, capsule-shaped, biconvex, film coated tablets, intagliated with 'SEROQUEL' on one side and '300' on the other side, are supplied in bottles of 60 tablets and hospital unit dose packages of 100 tablets.

Store at 25°C (77°F); excursions permitted to 15–30°C (59–86°F) [See USP].

ANIMAL TOXICOLOGY

Quetiapine caused a dose-related increase in pigment deposition in thyroid gland in rat toxicity studies which were 4 weeks in duration or longer and in a mouse 2 year carcinogenicity study. Doses were 10–250 mg/kg in rats, 75–750 mg/kg in mice; these doses are 0.1–3.0, and 0.1–4.5 times the maximum recommended human dose (on a mg/m^2 basis), respectively. Pigment deposition was shown to be irreversible in rats. The identity of the pigment could not be determined, but was found to be co-localized with quetiapine in thyroid gland follicular epithelial cells. The functional effects and the relevance of this finding to human risk are unknown.

In dogs receiving quetiapine for 6 or 12 months, but not for 1 month, focal triangular cataracts occurred at the junction of posterior sutures in the outer cortex of the lens at a dose of 100 mg/kg, or 4 times the maximum recommended human dose on a mg/m^2 basis. This finding may be due to inhibition of cholesterol biosynthesis by quetiapine. Quetiapine caused a dose related reduction in plasma cholesterol levels in repeat-dose dog and monkey studies; however, there was no correlation between plasma cholesterol and the presence of cataracts in individual dogs. The appearance of delta-8-cholestanol in plasma is consistent with inhibition of a late stage in cholesterol biosynthesis in these species. There also was a 25% reduction in cholesterol content of the outer cortex of the lens observed in a special study in quetiapine treated female dogs. Drug-related cataracts have not been seen in any other species; however, in a 1-year study in monkeys, a striated appearance of the anterior lens surface was detected in 2/7 females at a dose of 225 mg/kg or 5.5 times the maximum recommended human dose on a mg/m^2 basis.

SEROQUEL is a trademark of the AstraZeneca group of companies.

AstraZeneca Pharmaceuticals LP
Wilmington, DE 19850
Made in USA
64245-01
Rev 01/04
AstraZeneca

Shown in Product Identification Guide, page 306

TENORMIN® ℞

[tən or' min]
(atenolol)
ONE TABLET A DAY

DESCRIPTION

TENORMIN® (atenolol), a synthetic, beta$_1$-selective (cardioselective) adrenoreceptor blocking agent, may be chemically described as benzeneacetamide, 4-[2'-hydroxy-3'-[(1-methylethyl) amino] propoxy]-. The molecular and structural formulas are:

OH
$OCH_2CHCH_2NHCH(CH_3)_2$
$C_{14}H_{22}N_2O_3$
CH_2CONH_2

Atenolol (free base) has a molecular weight of 266. It is a relatively polar hydrophilic compound with a water solubility of 26.5 mg/mL at 37°C and a log partition coefficient (octanol/water) of 0.23. It is freely soluble in 1N HCl (300 mg/mL at 25°C) and less soluble in chloroform (3 mg/mL at 25°C).

TENORMIN is available as 25, 50 and 100 mg tablets for oral administration.

Inactive Ingredients: Magnesium stearate, microcrystalline cellulose, povidone, sodium starch glycolate.

HOW SUPPLIED

TENORMIN Tablets: Tablets of 25 mg atenolol, NDC 0310-0107, (round, flat, uncoated white tablets identified with "T" debossed on one side and 107 debossed on the other side) are supplied in bottles of 100 tablets.

Tablets of 50 mg atenolol, NDC 0310-0105, (round, flat, uncoated white tablets identified with "TENORMIN" debossed on one side and 105 debossed on the other side, bisected) are supplied in bottles of 100 tablets.

Tablets of 100 mg atenolol, NDC 0310-0101, (round, flat, uncoated white tablets identified with "TENORMIN" debossed on one side and 101 debossed on the other side) are supplied in bottles of 100 tablets.

Store at controlled room temperature, 20-25°C (68-77°F) [see USP]. Dispense in well-closed, light-resistant containers.

All trademarks are the property of the AstraZeneca group

Manufactured for:
AstraZeneca Pharmaceuticals LP
Wilmington, DE 19850
By: IPR Pharmaceuticals, Inc.
Carolina, PR 00984
610200
Rev 04/03
AstraZeneca

Shown in Product Identification Guide, page 306

TENORMIN® I.V. Injection ℞

[tən or' min]
(atenolol)

DESCRIPTION

TENORMIN® (atenolol), a synthetic, beta$_1$-selective (cardioselective) adrenoreceptor blocking agent, may be chemically described as benzeneacetamide, 4-[2'-hydroxy-3'-[(1-methylethyl)amino]propoxy]-. The molecular and structural formulas are:

OH
$O\text{-}CH_2\text{-}CH\text{-}CH_2\text{-}NHCH(CH_3)_2$
$C_{14}H_{22}N_2O_3$
CH_2CONH_2

Atenolol (free base) has a molecular weight of 266. It is a relatively polar hydrophilic compound with a water solubility of 26.5 mg/mL at 37°C and a log partition coefficient (octanol/water) of 0.23. It is freely soluble in 1N HCl (300 mg/mL at 25°C) and less soluble in chloroform (3 mg/mL at 25°C).

TENORMIN for parenteral administration is available as TENORMIN I.V. Injection containing 5 mg atenolol in 10 mL sterile, isotonic, citrate-buffered, aqueous solution. The pH of the solution is 5.5-6.5.

Inactive Ingredients: Sodium chloride for isotonicity and citric acid and sodium hydroxide to adjust pH.

HOW SUPPLIED

TENORMIN I.V. Injection TENORMIN I.V. Injection, NDC 0310-0108, is supplied as 5 mg atenolol in 10 mL ampules of isotonic citrate-buffered aqueous solution.

Protect from light. Keep ampules in outer packaging until time of use. Store at controlled room temperature, 20-25°C (68-77°F) [see USP].

All trademarks are the property of the AstraZeneca group

Manufactured for: AstraZeneca Pharmaceuticals LP, Wilmington, DE 19850
By: AstraZeneca LP, Wilmington, DE 19850
808348-01 Rev. 05/03
AstraZeneca

Shown in Product Identification Guide, page 306

ZESTORETIC® ℞

(lisinopril/hydrochlorothiazide)

USE IN PREGNANCY

When used in pregnancy during the second and third trimesters, ACE inhibitors can cause injury and even death to the developing fetus. When pregnancy is detected, ZESTORETIC should be discontinued as soon as possible. See WARNINGS, Pregnancy, Lisinopril, Fetal/Neonatal Morbidity and Mortality.

DESCRIPTION

ZESTORETIC® (Lisinopril and Hydrochlorothiazide) combines an angiotensin converting enzyme inhibitor, lisinopril, and a diuretic, hydrochlorothiazide.

Lisinopril, a synthetic peptide derivative, is an oral long-acting angiotensin converting enzyme inhibitor. It is chemically described as (S)-1-[N^2-(1-carboxy-3-phenylpropyl)-L-lysyl]-L-proline dihydrate. Its empirical formula is $C_{21}H_{31}N_3O_5 \bullet 2H_2O$ and its structural formula is:

$CH_2CH_2 \cdots C \cdots N \cdots C \cdots C-N$ • $2H_2O$
COOH $(CH_2)_4$ COOH
NH_2

Lisinopril is a white to off-white, crystalline powder, with a molecular weight of 441.53. It is soluble in water, sparingly soluble in methanol, and practically insoluble in ethanol.

Hydrochlorothiazide is 6-chloro-3,4-dihydro-2H-1,2,4-benzothiadiazine-7-sulfonamide 1,1-dioxide. Its empirical formula is $C_7H_8ClN_3O_4S_2$ and its structural formula is:

H_2N O_2S SO_2 NH Cl N H

Hydrochlorothiazide is a white, or practically white, crystalline powder with a molecular weight of 297.72, which is slightly soluble in water, but freely soluble in sodium hydroxide solution.

ZESTORETIC is available for oral use in three tablet combinations of lisinopril with hydrochlorothiazide: ZESTORETIC 10-12.5 containing 10 mg lisinopril and 12.5 mg hydrochlorothiazide; ZESTORETIC 20-12.5 containing 20 mg lisinopril and 12.5 mg hydrochlorothiazide; and, ZESTORETIC 20-25 containing 20 mg lisinopril and 25 mg hydrochlorothiazide.

Inactive Ingredients:

10-12.5 Tablets - calcium phosphate, magnesium stearate, mannitol, red ferric oxide, starch, yellow ferric oxide.

20-12.5 Tablets - calcium phosphate, magnesium stearate, mannitol, starch.

20-25 Tablets - calcium phosphate, magnesium stearate, mannitol, red ferric oxide, starch, yellow ferric oxide.

HOW SUPPLIED

ZESTORETIC 10-12.5 Tablets (NDC 0310-0141) Peach, round, biconvex, uncoated tablets identified with "141" debossed on one side and "ZESTORETIC" on the other side are supplied in bottles of 100 tablets.

ZESTORETIC 20-12.5 Tablets (NDC 0310-0142) White, round, biconvex, uncoated tablets identified with "142" debossed on one side and "ZESTORETIC" on the other side are supplied in bottles of 100 tablets.

ZESTORETIC 20-25 Tablets (NDC 0310-0145) Peach, round, biconvex, uncoated tablets identified with "145" debossed on one side and "ZESTORETIC" on the other side are supplied in bottles of 100 tablets.

Store at controlled room temperature, 20-25°C (68-77°F) [see USP]. Protect from excessive light and humidity.

¶Registered trademark of Hospal Ltd.

All other trademarks are the property of the AstraZeneca group

Manufactured for:
AstraZeneca Pharmaceuticals LP
Wilmington, DE 19850
By: IPR Pharmaceuticals, Inc.
Carolina, PR 00984
AstraZeneca
660007
Rev 05/03

Shown in Product Identification Guide, page 306

ZESTRIL® ℞

[zĕs-trĭl]
(lisinopril)

USE IN PREGNANCY

When used in pregnancy during the second and third trimesters, ACE inhibitors can cause injury and even death to the developing fetus. When pregnancy is detected, ZESTRIL should be discontinued as soon as possible. See WARNINGS, Fetal/Neonatal Morbidity and Mortality.

DESCRIPTION

Lisinopril is an oral long-acting angiotensin converting enzyme inhibitor. Lisinopril, a synthetic peptide derivative, is chemically described as (S)-1-[N^2-(1-carboxy-3-phenylpropyl)-L-lysyl]-L-proline dihydrate. Its empirical formula is $C_{21}H_{31}N_3O_5 \bullet 2H_2O$ and its structural formula is:

$CH_2CH_2 \cdots C \cdots N \cdots C \cdots C-N$ • $2H_2O$
COOH $(CH_2)_4$ COOH
NH_2

Lisinopril is a white to off-white, crystalline powder, with a molecular weight of 441.53. It is soluble in water and sparingly soluble in methanol and practically insoluble in ethanol.

ZESTRIL is supplied as 2.5 mg, 5 mg, 10 mg, 20 mg, 30 mg and 40 mg tablets for oral administration.

Inactive Ingredients:

Continued on next page

Zestril—Cont.

2.5 mg tablets—calcium phosphate, magnesium stearate, mannitol, starch.
5, 10, 20 and 30 mg tablets—calcium phosphate, magnesium stearate, mannitol, red ferric oxide, starch.
40 mg tablets—calcium phosphate, magnesium stearate, mannitol, starch, yellow ferric oxide.

HOW SUPPLIED

2.5 mg Tablets (NDC 0310-0135) white, round, biconvex, uncoated tablets identified as "ZESTRIL 2 1/2" on one side and "135" on the other side are supplied in bottles of 100 tablets.
5 mg Tablets (NDC 0310-0130) pink, capsule-shaped, biconvex, bisected, uncoated tablets, identified "ZESTRIL" on one side and "130" on the other side are supplied in bottles of 100 tablets and unit dose packages of 100 tablets.
10 mg Tablets (NDC 0310-0131) pink, round, biconvex, uncoated tablets identified "ZESTRIL 10" debossed on one side, and "131" debossed on the other side are supplied in bottles of 100 tablets and unit dose packages of 100 tablets.
20 mg Tablets (NDC 0310-0132) red, round, biconvex, uncoated tablets identified "ZESTRIL 20" debossed on one side, and "132" debossed on the other side are supplied in bottles of 100 tablets and unit dose packages of 100 tablets.
30 mg Tablets (NDC 0310-0133) red, round, biconvex, uncoated tablets identified "ZESTRIL 30" debossed on one side, and "133" debossed on the other side are supplied in bottles of 100 tablets.
40 mg Tablets (NDC 0310-0134) yellow, round, biconvex, uncoated tablets identified "ZESTRIL 40" debossed on one side, and "134" debossed on the other side are supplied in bottles of 100 tablets.

Storage
Store at controlled room temperature, 20–25°C (68–77°F) [see USP]. Protect from moisture, freezing and excessive heat. Dispense in a tight container.

Manufactured for:
AstraZeneca Pharmaceuticals LP
Wilmington, DE 19850
By: IPR Pharmaceuticals, Inc.
Carolina, PR 00984
Rev 07/03 PCC 650305
AstraZeneca
Shown in Product Identification Guide, page 306

ZOLADEX® 3.6 MG ℞
[*zōl'-ă-dĕx*]
(goserelin acetate implant)
Equivalent to 3.6 mg goserelin

DESCRIPTION

ZOLADEX® (goserelin acetate implant), contains a potent synthetic decapeptide analogue of luteinizing hormone-releasing hormone (LHRH), also known as a gonadotropin releasing hormone (GnRH) agonist analogue. Goserelin acetate is chemically described as an acetate salt of [D-Ser(Bu^t)^6,Azgly^{10}]LHRH. Its chemical structure is pyro-Glu-His-Trp-Ser-Tyr-D-Ser(Bu^t)-Leu-Arg-Pro-Azgly-NH_2 acetate [$C_{59}H_{84}N_{18}O_{14} \cdot (C_2H_4O_2)_x$ where x = 1 to 2.4]. Goserelin acetate is an off-white powder with a molecular weight of 1269 Daltons (free base). It is freely soluble in glacial acetic acid. It is soluble in water, 0.1M hydrochloric acid, 0.1M sodium hydroxide, dimethylformamide and dimethyl sulfoxide. Goserelin acetate is practically insoluble in acetone, chloroform and ether.

ZOLADEX is supplied as a sterile, biodegradable product containing goserelin acetate equivalent to 3.6 mg of goserelin. ZOLADEX is designed for subcutaneous injection with continuous release over a 28-day period. Goserelin acetate is dispersed in a matrix of D,L-lactic and glycolic acids copolymer (13.3-14.3 mg/dose) containing less than 2.5% acetic acid and up to 12% goserelin-related substances and presented as a sterile, white to cream colored 1-mm diameter cylinder, preloaded in a special single use syringe with a 16-gauge needle x 0.5 mm needle and protective needle sleeve (SafeSystem™ Syringe) in a sealed, light and moisture proof, aluminum foil laminate pouch containing a desiccant capsule. Studies of the D,L-lactic and glycolic acids copolymer have indicated that it is completely biodegradable and has no demonstrable antigenic potential.

CLINICAL PHARMACOLOGY

Mechanism of Action: ZOLADEX is a synthetic decapeptide analogue of LHRH. ZOLADEX acts as a potent inhibitor of pituitary gonadotropin secretion when administered in the biodegradable formulation.

Following initial administration in males, ZOLADEX causes an initial increase in serum luteinizing hormone (LH) and follicle stimulating hormone (FSH) levels with subsequent increases in serum levels of testosterone. Chronic administration of ZOLADEX leads to sustained suppression of pituitary gonadotropins, and serum levels of testosterone consequently fall into the range normally seen in surgically castrated men approximately 2-4 weeks after initiation of therapy. This leads to accessory sex organ regression. In animal and in vitro studies, administration of goserelin resulted in the regression or inhibition of growth of the hormonally sensitive dimethylbenzanthracene (DMBA)-induced rat mammary tumor and Dunning R3327 prostate tumor. In clinical trials with follow-up of more than 2 years, suppression of serum testosterone to castrate levels has been maintained for the duration of therapy.

In females, a similar down-regulation of the pituitary gland by chronic exposure to ZOLADEX leads to suppression of gonadotropin secretion, a decrease in serum estradiol to levels consistent with the postmenopausal state, and would be expected to lead to a reduction of ovarian size and function, reduction in the size of the uterus and mammary gland, as well as a regression of sex hormone-responsive tumors, if present. Serum estradiol is suppressed to levels similar to those observed in postmenopausal women within 3 weeks following initial administration; however, after suppression was attained, isolated elevations of estradiol were seen in 10% of the patients enrolled in clinical trials. Serum LH and FSH are suppressed to follicular phase levels within four weeks after initial administration of drug and are usually maintained at that range with continued use of ZOLADEX. In 5% or less of women treated with ZOLADEX, FSH and LH levels may not be suppressed to follicular phase levels on day 28 post treatment with use of a single 3.6 mg depot injection. In certain individuals, suppression of any of these hormones to such levels may not be achieved with ZOLADEX. Estradiol, LH and FSH levels return to pretreatment values within 12 weeks following the last implant administration in all but rare cases.

Pharmacokinetics: The pharmacokinetics of ZOLADEX have been determined in both male and female healthy volunteers and patients. In these studies, ZOLADEX was administered as a single 250 µg (aqueous solution) dose and as a single or multiple 3.6 mg depot dose by subcutaneous route.

Absorption: The absorption of radiolabeled drug was rapid, and the peak blood radioactivity levels occurred between 0.5 and 1.0 hour after dosing. The mean (± standard deviation) pharmacokinetic parameter estimates of ZOLADEX after administration of 3.6 mg depot for 2 months in males and females are presented in the following table.

[See table below]

Parameters (Units)	Males n=7	Females n=9
Peak Plasma Concentration (ng/mL)	2.84 ± 1.81	1.46 ± 0.82
Time to Peak Concentration (days)	12-15	8-22
Area Under the Curve (0–28 days) (ng.h/mL)	27.8 ± 15.3	18.5 ± 10.3
Systemic Clearance (mL/min)	110.5 ± 47.5	163.9 ± 71.0
*Apparent Volume of Distribution (L)	44.1 ± 13.6	20.3 ± 4.1
*Elimination Half-life (h)	4.2 ± 1.1	2.3 ± 0.6

* The apparent volume of distribution and the elimination half-life were determined after subcutaneous administration of 250 µg aqueous solution of goserelin.

Pharmacokinetic data were obtained using a nonspecific RIA method.

Goserelin is released from the depot at a much slower rate initially for the first 8 days, and then there is more rapid and continuous release for the remainder of the 28-day dosing period. Despite the change in the releasing rate of goserelin, administration of ZOLADEX every 28 days resulted in testosterone levels that were suppressed to and maintained in the range normally seen in surgically castrated men.

When ZOLADEX 3.6 mg depot was used for treating male and female patients with normal renal and hepatic function, there was no significant evidence of drug accumulation. However, in clinical trials the minimum serum levels of a few patients were increased. These levels can be attributed to interpatient variation.

Distribution: The apparent volumes of distribution determined after subcutaneous administration of 250 µg aqueous solution of goserelin were 44.1 and 20.3 liters for males and females, respectively. The plasma protein binding of goserelin obtained from one sample was found to be 27.3%.

Metabolism: Metabolism of goserelin, by hydrolysis of the C-terminal amino acids, is the major clearance mechanism. The major circulating component in serum appeared to be 1–7 fragment, and the major component presented in urine of one healthy male volunteer was 5-10 fragment. The metabolism of goserelin in humans yields a similar but narrow profile of metabolites to that found in other species. All metabolites found in humans have also been found in toxicology species.

Excretion: Clearance of goserelin following subcutaneous administration of the solution formulation of goserelin is very rapid and occurs via a combination of hepatic metabolism and urinary excretion. More than 90% of a subcutaneous radiolabeled solution formulation dose of goserelin is excreted in urine. Approximately 20% of the dose in urine is accounted for by unchanged goserelin. The total body clearance of goserelin (administered subcutaneously as a 3.6 mg depot) was significantly ($p<0.05$) greater (163.9 versus 110.5 L/min) in females compared to males.

Special Populations
Renal Insufficiency: In clinical trials with the solution formulation of goserelin, male patients with impaired renal function (creatinine clearance < 20 mL/min) had a total body clearance and serum elimination half-life of 31.5 mL/min and 12.1 hours, respectively, compared to 133 mL/min and 4.2 hours for subjects with normal renal function (creatinine clearance > 70 mL/min). In females, the effects of reduced goserelin clearance due to impaired renal function on drug efficacy and toxicity are unknown. Pharmacokinetic studies using the aqueous formulation of goserelin in patients with renal impairment do not indicate a need for dose adjustment with the use of the depot formulation.

Hepatic Insufficiency: The total body clearances and serum elimination half-lives were similar between normal and hepatic impaired patients receiving 250 µg solution formulation of goserelin. Pharmacokinetic studies using the aqueous formulation of goserelin in patients with hepatic impairment do not indicate a need for dose adjustment with the use of the depot formulation.

Drug-Drug Interactions: No formal drug-drug interaction studies have been performed.

Clinical Studies-Prostatic Carcinoma: In controlled studies of patients with advanced prostatic cancer comparing ZOLADEX to orchiectomy, the long-term endocrine responses and objective responses were similar between the two treatment arms. Additionally, duration of survival was similar between the two treatment arms in a comparative trial.

Clinical Studies-Stage B2-C Prostatic Carcinoma: The effects of hormonal treatment combined with radiation were studied in 466 patients (231 ZOLADEX + flutamide + radiation, 235 radiation alone) with bulky primary tumors confined to the prostate (stage B2) or extending beyond the capsule (stage C), with or without pelvic node involvement.

In this multicentered, controlled trial, administration of ZOLADEX (3.6 mg depot) and flutamide capsules (250 mg t.i.d.) prior to and during radiation was associated with a significantly lower rate of local failure compared to radiation alone (16% vs 33% at 4 years, $P<0.001$). The combination therapy also resulted in a trend toward reduction in the incidence of distant metastases (27% vs 36% at 4 years, $P=0.058$). Median disease-free survival was significantly increased in patients who received complete hormonal therapy combined with radiation as compared to those patients who received radiation alone (4.4 vs 2.6 years, $P<0.001$). Inclusion of normal PSA level as a criterion for disease-free survival also resulted in significantly increased median disease-free survival in patients receiving the combination therapy (2.7 vs 1.5 years, $P<0.001$).

Clinical Studies-Endometriosis: In controlled clinical studies using the 3.6 mg formulation every 28 days for 6 months, ZOLADEX was shown to be as effective as danazol therapy in relieving clinical symptoms (dysmenorrhea, dyspareunia and pelvic pain) and signs (pelvic tenderness, pelvic induration) of endometriosis and decreasing the size of endometrial lesions as determined by laparoscopy. In one study comparing ZOLADEX with danazol (800 mg/day), 63% of ZOLADEX-treated patients and 42% of danazol-treated patients had a greater than or equal to 50% reduction in the extent of endometrial lesions. In the second study comparing ZOLADEX with danazol (600 mg/day), 62% of ZOLADEX-treated and 51% of danazol-treated patients had a greater than or equal to 50% reduction in the extent of endometrial lesions. The clinical significance of a decrease in endometriotic lesions is not known at this time; and in addition, laparoscopic staging of endometriosis does not necessarily correlate with severity of symptoms.

In these two studies, ZOLADEX led to amenorrhea in 92% and 80%, respectively, of all treated women within 8 weeks after initial administration. Menses usually resumed within 8 weeks following completion of therapy.

Within 4 weeks following initial administration, clinical symptoms were significantly reduced, and at the end of treatment were, on average, reduced by approximately 84%.

During the first two months of ZOLADEX use, some women experience vaginal bleeding of variable duration and intensity. In all likelihood, this bleeding represents estrogen withdrawal bleeding, and is expected to stop spontaneously. There is insufficient evidence to determine whether pregnancy rates are enhanced or adversely affected by the use of ZOLADEX.

Clinical Studies-Breast Cancer: The Southwest Oncology Group conducted a prospective, randomized clinical trial (SWOG-8692 [INT-0075]) in premenopausal women with advanced estrogen receptor positive or progesterone receptor positive breast cancer which compared ZOLADEX with oophorectomy. On the basis of interim data from 124 women, the best objective response (CR+PR) for the ZOLADEX group is 22% versus 12% for the oophorectomy group. The median time to treatment failure is 6.7 months for patients treated with ZOLADEX and 5.5 months for patients treated with oophorectomy. The median survival time for the ZOLADEX arm is 33.2 months and for the oophorectomy arm is 33.6 months.

Subjective responses based on measures of pain control and performance status were observed with both treatments; 48% of the women in the ZOLADEX treatment group and 50% in the oophorectomy group had subjective responses. In the clinical trial (SWOG-8692 [INT 0075]), the mean post treatment estradiol level was reported as 17.8 pg/mL. (The mean estradiol level in post-menopausal women as reported

in the literature is 13 pg/mL). During the conduct of the clinical trial, women whose estradiol levels were not reduced to the postmenopausal range, received two ZOLADEX depots, thus, increasing the dose of ZOLADEX from 3.6 mg to 7.2 mg.
Findings were similar in uncontrolled clinical trials involving patients with hormone receptor positive and negative breast cancer. Premenopausal women with estrogen receptor (ER) status of positive, negative, or unknown participated in the uncontrolled (Phase II and Trial 2302) clinical trials. Objective tumor responses were seen regardless of ER status, as shown in the following table.

OBJECTIVE RESPONSE BY ER STATUS

ER status	CR + PR/Total No. (%) Phase II (N = 228)	Trial 2302 (N = 159)
Positive	43/119 (36)	31/86 (36)
Negative	6/33 (18)	3/26 (10)
Unknown	20/76 (26)	18/44 (41)

Clinical Studies-Endometrial Thinning: Two trials were conducted with ZOLADEX prior to endometrial ablation for dysfunctional uterine bleeding.
Trial 0022, was a double-blind, prospective, randomized, parallel-group multicenter trial conducted in 358 premenopausal women with dysfunctional uterine bleeding. Eligible patients were randomized to receive either two depots of ZOLADEX 3.6 mg (n=180) or two placebo injections (n=178) administered four weeks apart. 175 patients in each group underwent endometrial ablation using either diathermy loop alone or in combination with rollerball approximately 2 weeks after the second injection. Endometrial thickness was assessed immediately before surgery using a transvaginal ultrasonic probe. The incidence of amenorrhea was compared between the ZOLADEX and placebo groups at 24 weeks after endometrial ablation.
The median endometrial thickness before surgery was significantly less in the ZOLADEX treatment group (1.50 mm) compared to the placebo group (3.55 mm). Six months after surgery, 40% of patients (70/175) treated with ZOLADEX in Trial 0022 reported amenorrhea as compared with 26% who had received placebo injections (44/171), a difference that was statistically significant.
Trial 0003, was a single center, open-label, randomized trial in premenopausal women with dysfunctional uterine bleeding. The trial allowed for a comparison of 1 depot of ZOLADEX and 2 depots of ZOLADEX administered 4 weeks apart with ablation using Nd: YAG laser occurring 4 weeks after ZOLADEX administration. Forty patients were randomized into each of the ZOLADEX treatment groups.
The median endometrial thickness before surgery was significantly less in the group treated with two depots (0.5 mm) compared to the group treated with one depot (1 mm). No difference in the incidence of amenorrhea was found at 24 weeks (24% in both groups). Of the 74 patients that completed the trial, 53 % reported hypomenorrhea and 20% reported normal menses six months after surgery.

INDICATIONS AND USAGE

Prostatic Carcinoma: ZOLADEX is indicated in the palliative treatment of advanced carcinoma of the prostate.
Stage B2-C Prostatic Carcinoma: ZOLADEX is indicated for use in combination with flutamide for the management of locally confined Stage T2b–T4 (Stage B2-C) carcinoma of the prostate. Treatment with ZOLADEX and flutamide should start 8 weeks prior to initiating radiation therapy and continue during radiation therapy.
Endometriosis: ZOLADEX is indicated for the management of endometriosis, including pain relief and reduction of endometriotic lesions for the duration of therapy. Experience with ZOLADEX for the management of endometriosis has been limited to women 18 years of age and older treated for 6 months.
Advanced Breast Cancer: ZOLADEX is indicated for use in the palliative treatment of advanced breast cancer in pre- and perimenopausal women.
The estrogen and progesterone receptor values may help to predict whether ZOLADEX therapy is likely to be beneficial. (See CLINICAL PHARMACOLOGY.)
Endometrial Thinning: ZOLADEX is indicated for use as an endometrial-thinning agent prior to endometrial ablation for dysfunctional uterine bleeding.
The automatic safety feature of the syringe aids in the prevention of needlestick injury.

CONTRAINDICATIONS

A report of an anaphylactic reaction to synthetic GnRH (Factrel) has been reported in the medical literature. ZOLADEX is contraindicated in those patients who have a known hypersensitivity to LHRH, LHRH agonist analogues or any of the components in ZOLADEX.
ZOLADEX is contraindicated in women being treated for endometriosis or endometrial thinning who are or may become pregnant while receiving the drug. ZOLADEX can cause fetal harm when administered to a pregnant woman. Effects on reproductive function, as a result of antigonadotrophic properties of the drug, are expected to occur on chronic administration.
Effective nonhormonal contraception must be used by all premenopausal women during ZOLADEX therapy and for 12 weeks following discontinuation of therapy. There are no adequate and well-controlled studies in pregnant women using ZOLADEX. If this drug is used during pregnancy, or the patient being treated for endometriosis or endometrial thinning becomes pregnant while taking this drug, the patient should be apprised of the potential hazard to the fetus or potential risk for loss of the pregnancy. Women of childbearing potential should be advised to avoid becoming pregnant.
For a description of findings in animal reproductive toxicity studies, see **WARNINGS**.
ZOLADEX is contraindicated in women who are breast feeding (see Nursing Mothers Section).

WARNINGS

Before starting treatment with ZOLADEX, pregnancy must be excluded. Safe use of ZOLADEX in pregnancy has not been established. ZOLADEX can cause fetal harm when administered to a pregnant woman. ZOLADEX has been found to cross the placenta following subcutaneous administration of 50 and 1000 µg/kg in rats and rabbits, respectively. Studies in both rats and rabbits at doses equal to or greater than 2 and 20 µg/kg/day, respectively (about 1/10 and 2 times the daily maximum recommended human dose, respectively, on a mg/m^2 basis), administered during the period of organogenesis, have confirmed that ZOLADEX will increase pregnancy loss, and is embryotoxic/fetotoxic (characterized by increased preimplantation loss, increased resorption and an increase in umbilical hernia in rats at a dose of ≥ 10 µg/kg/day [about 1/2 the recommended human dose on a mg/m^2 basis]); effects were dose-related. In additional reproduction studies in rats, ZOLADEX was found to decrease fetus and pup survival.
There are no adequate and well-controlled studies in pregnant women using ZOLADEX. Women of childbearing potential should be advised to avoid becoming pregnant.
When used every 28 days, ZOLADEX usually inhibits ovulation and stops menstruation. Contraception is not ensured, however, by taking ZOLADEX. During treatment, pregnancy must be avoided by the use of nonhormonal methods of contraception. If ZOLADEX is used during pregnancy (in a patient with advanced breast cancer) or the patient becomes pregnant while receiving this drug, the patient must be apprised of the potential risk for loss of the pregnancy due to possible hormonal imbalance as a result of the expected pharmacologic action of ZOLADEX treatment. Following the last ZOLADEX injection, nonhormonal methods of contraception must be continued until the return of menses or for at least 12 weeks. (See **CONTRAINDICATIONS**.)
Prostate and Breast Cancer: Initially, ZOLADEX, like other LHRH agonists, causes transient increases in serum levels of testosterone in men with prostate cancer, and estrogen in women with breast cancer. Transient worsening of symptoms, or the occurrence of additional signs and symptoms of prostate or breast cancer, may occasionally develop during the first few weeks of ZOLADEX treatment. A small number of patients may experience a temporary increase in bone pain, which can be managed symptomatically. As with other LHRH agonists, isolated cases of ureteral obstruction and spinal cord compression have been observed in patients with prostate cancer. If spinal cord compression or renal impairment develops, standard treatment of these complications should be instituted. For extreme cases in prostate cancer patients, an immediate orchiectomy should be considered.
As with other LHRH agonists or hormonal therapies (antiestrogens, estrogens, etc.), hypercalcemia has been reported in some prostate and breast cancer patients with bone metastases after starting treatment with ZOLADEX. If hypercalcemia does occur, appropriate treatment measures should be initiated.

PRECAUTIONS

General: Hypersensitivity, antibody formation and acute anaphylactic reactions have been reported with LHRH agonist analogues.
Of 115 women worldwide treated with ZOLADEX and tested for development of binding to goserelin following treatment with ZOLADEX, one patient showed low-titer binding to goserelin. On further testing of this patient's plasma obtained following treatment, her goserelin binding component was found not to be precipitated with rabbit antihuman immunoglobulin polyvalent sera. These findings suggest the possibility of antibody formation.
The pharmacologic action of ZOLADEX on the uterus and cervix may cause an increase in cervical resistance. Therefore, care should be taken when dilating the cervix for endometrial ablation.

Information for Patients

Males: The use of ZOLADEX in patients at particular risk of developing ureteral obstruction or spinal cord compression should be considered carefully and the patients monitored closely during the first month of therapy. Patients with ureteral obstruction or spinal cord compression should have appropriate treatment prior to initiation of ZOLADEX therapy.

Females: Patients must be made aware of the following information:

1. Since menstruation should stop with effective doses of ZOLADEX the patient should notify her physician if regular menstruation persists. Patients missing one or more successive doses of ZOLADEX may experience breakthrough menstrual bleeding.
2. ZOLADEX should not be prescribed if the patient is pregnant, breast feeding, lactating, has nondiagnosed abnormal vaginal bleeding, or is allergic to any of the components of ZOLADEX.
3. Use of ZOLADEX in pregnancy is contraindicated in women being treated for endometriosis or endometrial thinning. Therefore, a nonhormonal method of contraception should be used during treatment. Patients should be advised that if they miss one or more successive doses of ZOLADEX, breakthrough menstrual bleeding or ovulation may occur with the potential for conception. If a patient becomes pregnant during treatment for endometriosis or endometrial thinning, ZOLADEX treatment should be discontinued and the patient should be advised of the possible risks to the pregnancy and fetus. (See **CONTRAINDICATIONS**.)
   For patients being treated for advanced breast cancer, see **WARNINGS**.
4. Those adverse events occurring most frequently in clinical studies with ZOLADEX are associated with hypoestrogenism; of these, the most frequently reported are hot flashes (flushes), headaches, vaginal dryness, emotional lability, change in libido, depression, sweating and change in breast size. Clinical studies in endometriosis suggest the addition of Hormone Replacement Therapy (estrogens and/or progestins) to ZOLADEX may decrease the occurrence of vasomotor symptoms and vaginal dryness associated with hypoestrogenism without compromising the efficacy of ZOLADEX in relieving pelvic symptoms. The optimal drugs, dose and duration of treatment has not been established.
5. As with other LHRH agonist analogues, treatment with ZOLADEX induces a hypoestrogenic state which results in a loss of bone mineral density (BMD) over the course of treatment, some of which may not be reversible. In patients with a history of prior treatment that may have resulted in bone mineral density loss and/or in patients with major risk factors for decreased bone mineral density such as chronic alcohol abuse and/or tobacco abuse, significant family history of osteoporosis, or chronic use of drugs that can reduce bone density such as anticonvulsants or corticosteroids, ZOLADEX therapy may pose an additional risk. In these patients the risks and benefits must be weighed carefully before therapy with ZOLADEX is instituted. Clinical studies suggest the addition of Hormone Replacement Therapy (estrogens and/or progestins) to ZOLADEX is effective in reducing the bone mineral loss which occurs with ZOLADEX alone. The optimal drugs, dose and duration of treatment has not been established.
6. Currently, there are no clinical data on the effects of retreatment or treatment of benign gynecological conditions with ZOLADEX for periods in excess of 6 months.
7. As with other hormonal interventions that disrupt the pituitary-gonadal axis, some patients may have delayed return to menses. The rare patient, however, may experience persistent amenorrhea.

Drug Interactions: No formal drug-drug interaction studies have been performed. No confirmed interactions have been reported between ZOLADEX and other drugs.
Drug/Laboratory Test Interactions: Administration of ZOLADEX in therapeutic doses results in suppression of the pituitary-gonadal system. Because of this suppression, diagnostic tests of pituitary-gonadotropic and gonadal functions conducted during treatment and until the resumption of menses may show results which are misleading. Normal function is usually restored within 12 weeks after treatment is discontinued.
Carcinogenesis, Mutagenesis, Impairment of Fertility: Subcutaneous implant of ZOLADEX in male and female rats once every 4 weeks for 1 year and recovery for 23 weeks at doses of about 80 and 150 µg/kg (males) and 50 and 100 µg/kg (females) daily (about 3 to 9 times the recommended human dose on a mg/m^2 basis) resulted in an increased incidence of pituitary adenomas. An increased incidence of pituitary adenomas was also observed following subcutaneous implant of ZOLADEX in rats at similar dose levels for a period of 72 weeks in males and 101 weeks in females. The relevance of the rat pituitary adenomas to humans has not been established. Subcutaneous implants of ZOLADEX every 3 weeks for 2 years delivered to mice at doses of up to 2400 µg/kg/day (about 70 times the recommended human dose on a mg/m^2 basis) resulted in an increased incidence of histiocytic sarcoma of the vertebral column and femur.
Mutagenicity tests using bacterial and mammalian systems for point mutations and cytogenetic effects have provided no evidence for mutagenic potential.
Administration of goserelin led to changes that were consistent with gonadal suppression in both male and female rats as a result of its endocrine action. In male rats administered 500-1000 µg/kg/day (about 30-60 times the recommended human dose on a mg/m^2 basis), a decrease in weight and atrophic histological changes were observed in the testes, epididymis, seminal vesicle and prostate gland with complete suppression of spermatogenesis. In female rats administered 50-1000 µg/kg/day (about 3-60 times the recommended daily human dose on a mg/m^2 basis), suppression of ovarian function led to decreased size and weight of ovaries and secondary sex organs; follicular development was arrested at the antral stage and the corpora lutea were reduced in size and number. Except for the testes, almost com-

Continued on next page

Zoladex—Cont.

plete histologic reversal of these effects in males and females was observed several weeks after dosing was stopped; however, fertility and general reproductive performance were reduced in those that became pregnant after goserelin was discontinued. Fertile matings occurred within 2 weeks after cessation of dosing, even though total recovery of reproductive function may not have occurred before mating took place; and, the ovulation rate, the corresponding implantation rate, and number of live fetuses were reduced. Based on histological examination, drug effects on reproductive organs were reversible in male and female dogs administered 107-214 µg/kg/day ZOLADEX (about 20-40 times the recommended daily human dose on a mg/m^2 basis) when drug treatment was stopped after continuous administration for 1 year.

Pregnancy: Pregnancy Category X for treatment of endometriosis and endometrial thinning. See **CONTRAINDICATIONS** and **WARNINGS** sections. **Pregnancy Category D** for treatment of advanced breast cancer in pre- and perimenopausal women. See **WARNINGS** section.

Nursing Mothers: ZOLADEX has been shown to be excreted in the milk of lactating rats. It is not known if this drug is excreted in human milk. Because many drugs are excreted in human milk, and because of the potential for serious adverse reactions from ZOLADEX in nursing infants, mothers should discontinue nursing prior to taking the drug.

Pediatric Use: The safety and efficacy of ZOLADEX in pediatric patients have not been established.

ADVERSE REACTIONS

General: Rarely, hypersensitivity reactions (including urticaria and anaphylaxis) have been reported in patients receiving ZOLADEX.

Changes in blood pressure, manifest as hypotension or hypertension, have been occasionally observed in patients administered ZOLADEX. The changes are usually transient, resolving either during continued therapy or after cessation of therapy with ZOLADEX. Rarely, such changes have been sufficient to require medical intervention including withdrawal of treatment from ZOLADEX.

As with other agents in this class, very rare cases of pituitary apoplexy have been reported following initial administration in patients with a functional pituitary adenoma.

Males-Prostatic Carcinoma: ZOLADEX has been found to be generally well tolerated in clinical trials. Adverse reactions reported in these trials were rarely severe enough to result in the patients' withdrawal from ZOLADEX treatment. As seen with other hormonal therapies, the most commonly observed adverse events during ZOLADEX therapy were due to the expected physiological effects from decreased testosterone levels. These included hot flashes, sexual dysfunction and decreased erections.

Initially, ZOLADEX, like other LHRH agonists, causes transient increases in serum levels of testosterone. A small percentage of patients experienced a temporary worsening of signs and symptoms (see **WARNINGS** section), usually manifested by an increase in cancer-related pain which was managed symptomatically. Isolated cases of exacerbation of disease symptoms, either ureteral obstruction or spinal cord compression, occurred at similar rates in controlled clinical trials with both ZOLADEX and orchiectomy. The relationship of these events to therapy is uncertain.

There have been post-marketing reports of osteoporosis, decreased bone mineral density and bony fracture in men treated with ZOLADEX for prostate cancer.

In the controlled clinical trials of ZOLADEX versus orchiectomy, the following events were reported as adverse reactions in greater than 5% of the patients.

	TREATMENT RECEIVED	
	ZOLADEX (n=242)	ORCHIECTOMY (n=254)
ADVERSE EVENT	%	%
Hot Flashes	62	53
Sexual Dysfunction	21	15
Decreased Erections	18	16
Lower Urinary Tract Symptoms	13	8
Lethargy	8	4
Pain (worsened in the first 30 days)	8	3
Edema	7	8
Upper Respiratory Infection	7	2
Rash	6	1
Sweating	6	4
Anorexia	5	2
Chronic Obstructive Pulmonary Disease	5	3
Congestive Heart Failure	5	1
Dizziness	5	4
Insomnia	5	1
Nausea	5	2
Complications of Surgery	0	18†

†Complications related to surgery were reported in 18% of the orchiectomy patients, while only 3% of ZOLADEX patients reported adverse reactions at the injection site. The surgical complications included scrotal infection (5.9%), groin pain (4.7%), wound seepage (3.1%), scrotal hematoma (2.8%), incisional discomfort (1.6%) and skin necrosis (1.2%).

The following additional adverse reactions were reported in greater than 1% but less than 5% of the patients treated with ZOLADEX: CARDIOVASCULAR - arrhythmia, cerebrovascular accident, hypertension, myocardial infarction, peripheral vascular disorder, chest pain; CENTRAL NERVOUS SYSTEM - anxiety, depression, headache; GASTROINTESTINAL - constipation, diarrhea, ulcer, vomiting; HEMATOLOGIC - anemia; METABOLIC/NUTRITIONAL - gout, hyperglycemia, weight increase; MISCELLANEOUS - chills, fever; UROGENITAL - renal insufficiency, urinary obstruction, urinary tract infection, breast swelling and tenderness.

Stage B2-C Prostatic Carcinoma: Treatment with ZOLADEX and flutamide did not add substantially to the toxicity of radiation treatment alone. The following adverse experiences were reported during a multicenter clinical trial comparing ZOLADEX + flutamide + radiation versus radiation alone. The most frequently reported (greater than 5%) adverse experiences are listed below:

ADVERSE EVENTS DURING ACUTE RADIATION THERAPY (within first 90 days of radiation therapy)

	(n=231) flutamide + ZOLADEX + Radiation % All	(n=235) Radiation Only % All
Rectum/Large Bowel	80	76
Bladder	58	60
Skin	37	37

ADVERSE EVENTS DURING LATE RADIATION PHASE (after 90 days of radiation therapy)

	(n=231) flutamide + ZOLADEX + Radiation % All	(n=235) Radiation Only % All
Diarrhea	36	40
Cystitis	16	16
Rectal Bleeding	14	20
Proctitis	8	8
Hematuria	7	12

Additional adverse event data was collected for the combination therapy with radiation group over both the hormonal treatment and hormonal treatment plus radiation phases of the study. Adverse experiences occurring in more than 5% of patients in this group, over both parts of the study, were hot flashes (46%), diarrhea (40%), nausea (9%), and skin rash (8%).

Females: As would be expected with a drug that results in hypoestrogenism, the most frequently reported adverse reactions were those related to this effect.

As with other LHRH agonists, there have been reports of ovarian cyst formation and, when ZOLADEX 3.6 mg is used in combination with gonadotropins, of ovarian hyperstimulation syndrome (OHSS).

Endometriosis: In controlled clinical trials comparing ZOLADEX every 28 days and danazol daily for the treatment of endometriosis, the following events were reported at a frequency of 5% or greater:

	TREATMENT RECEIVED	
	ZOLADEX (n=411)	DANAZOL (n=207)
ADVERSE EVENT	%	%
Hot Flushes	96	67
Vaginitis	75	43
Headache	75	63
Emotional Lability	60	56
Libido Decreased	61	44
Sweating	45	30
Depression	54	48
Acne	42	55
Breast Atrophy	33	42
Seborrhea	26	52
Peripheral Edema	21	34
Breast Enlargement	18	15
Pelvic Symptoms	18	23
Pain	17	16
Dyspareunia	14	5
Libido Increased	12	19
Infection	13	11
Asthenia	11	13
Nausea	8	14
Hirsutism	7	15
Insomnia	11	4
Breast Pain	7	4
Abdominal Pain	7	7
Back Pain	7	13
Flu Syndrome	5	5
Dizziness	6	4
Application Site Reaction	6	-
Voice Alterations	3	8
Pharyngitis	5	2
Hair Disorders	4	11
Myalgia	3	11
Nervousness	3	5
Weight Gain	3	23
Leg Cramps	2	6
Increased Appetite	2	5
Pruritus	2	6
Hypertonia	1	10

The following adverse events not already listed above were reported at a frequency of 1% or greater, regardless of causality, in ZOLADEX-treated women from all clinical trials: WHOLE BODY - allergic reaction, chest pain, fever, malaise; CARDIOVASCULAR - hemorrhage, hypertension, migraine, palpitations, tachycardia; DIGESTIVE - anorexia, constipation, diarrhea, dry mouth, dyspepsia, flatulence; HEMATOLOGIC - ecchymosis; METABOLIC AND NUTRITIONAL - edema; MUSCULOSKELETAL - arthralgia, joint disorder; CNS - anxiety, paresthesia, somnolence, thinking abnormal; RESPIRATORY - bronchitis, cough increased, epistaxis, rhinitis, sinusitis; SKIN - alopecia, dry skin, rash, skin discoloration; SPECIAL SENSES - amblyopia, dry eyes; UROGENITAL - dysmenorrhea, urinary frequency, urinary tract infection, vaginal hemorrhage.

Hormone Replacement Therapy: Clinical studies suggest the addition of Hormone Replacement Therapy (estrogens and/or progestins) to ZOLADEX may decrease the occurrence of vasomotor symptoms and vaginal dryness associated with hypoestrogenism without compromising the efficacy of ZOLADEX in relieving pelvic symptoms. The optimal drugs, dose and duration of treatment has not been established.

Changes in Bone Mineral Density: After 6 months of ZOLADEX treatment, 109 female patients treated with ZOLADEX showed an average 4.3% decrease of vertebral trabecular bone mineral density (BMD) as compared to pretreatment values. BMD was measured by dual-photon absorptiometry or dual energy x-ray absorptiometry. Sixty-six of these patients were assessed for BMD loss 6 months after the completion (posttherapy) of the 6-month therapy period. Data from these patients showed an average 2.4% BMD loss compared to pretreatment values. Twenty-eight of the 109 patients were assessed for BMD at 12 months posttherapy. Data from these patients showed an average decrease of 2.5% in BMD compared to pretreatment values. These data suggest a possibility of partial reversibility. Clinical studies suggest the addition of Hormone Replacement Therapy (estrogens and/or progestins) to ZOLADEX is effective in reducing the bone mineral loss which occurs with ZOLADEX alone without compromising the efficacy of ZOLADEX in relieving the symptoms of endometriosis. The optimal drugs, dose and duration of treatment has not been established.

Changes in Laboratory Values During Treatment

Plasma Enzymes. Elevation of liver enzymes (AST, ALT) have been reported in female patients exposed to ZOLADEX (representing less than 1% of all patients).

Lipids. In a controlled trial, ZOLADEX therapy resulted in a minor, but statistically significant effect on serum lipids. In patients treated for endometriosis at 6 months following initiation of therapy, danazol treatment resulted in a mean increase in LDL cholesterol of 33.3 mg/dL and a decrease in HDL cholesterol of 21.3 mg/dL compared to increases of 21.3 and 2.7 mg/dL in LDL cholesterol and HDL cholesterol, respectively, for ZOLADEX-treated patients. Triglycerides increased by 8.0 mg/dL in ZOLADEX-treated patients compared to a decrease of 8.9 mg/dL in danazol-treated patients.

In patients treated for endometriosis, ZOLADEX increased total cholesterol and LDL cholesterol during 6 months of treatment. However, ZOLADEX therapy resulted in HDL cholesterol levels which were significantly higher relative to danazol therapy. At the end of 6 months of treatment, HDL cholesterol fractions (HDL_2 and HDL_3) were decreased by 13.5 and 7.7 mg/dL, respectively, for danazol-treated patients compared to treatment increases of 1.9 and 0.8 mg/dL, respectively, for ZOLADEX treated patients.

Breast Cancer: The adverse event profile for women with advanced breast cancer treated with ZOLADEX is consistent with the profile described above for women treated with ZOLADEX for endometriosis. In a controlled clinical trial (SWOG-8692) comparing ZOLADEX with oophorectomy in premenopausal and perimenopausal women with advanced breast cancer, the following events were reported at a frequency of 5% or greater in either treatment group regardless of causality.

	TREATMENT RECEIVED	
	ZOLADEX (n=57)	OOPHORECTOMY (n=55)
ADVERSE EVENT	% of Pts.	% of Pts.
Hot Flashes	70	47
Tumor Flare	23	4
Nausea	11	7
Edema	5	0
Malaise/Fatigue/ Lethargy	5	2
Vomiting	4	7

In the Phase II clinical trial program in 333 pre- and perimenopausal women with advanced breast cancer, hot flashes were reported in 75.9% of patients and decreased libido was noted in 47.7% of patients. These two adverse events reflect the pharmacological actions of ZOLADEX. Injection site reactions were reported in less than 1% of patients.

Endometrial Thinning: The following adverse events were reported at a frequency of 5% or greater in premenopausal women presenting with dysfunctional uterine bleeding in Trial 0022 for endometrial thinning. These results indicate that headache, hot flushes and sweating were more common in the ZOLADEX group than in the placebo group.

ADVERSE EVENTS REPORTED AT A FREQUENCY OF 5% OR GREATER IN ZOLADEX AND PLACEBO TREATMENT GROUPS OF TRIAL 0022

ADVERSE EVENT	ZOLADEX 3.6 mg (n=180) %	Placebo (n=177) %
Whole body		
Headache	32	22
Abdominal Pain	11	10
Pelvic Pain	9	6
Back Pain	4	7
Cardiovascular		
Vasodilatation	57	18
Migraine	7	4
Hypertension	6	2
Digestive		
Nausea	5	6
Nervous		
Nervousness	5	3
Depression	3	7
Respiratory		
Pharyngitis	6	9
Sinusitis	3	6
Skin and appendages		
Sweating	16	5
Urogenital		
Dysmenorrhea	7	9
Uterine Hemorrhage	6	4
Vulvovaginitis	5	1
Menorrhagia	4	5
Vaginitis	1	6

OVERDOSAGE

The pharmacologic properties of ZOLADEX and its mode of administration make accidental or intentional overdosage unlikely. There is no experience of overdosage from clinical trials. Animal studies indicate that no increased pharmacologic effect occurred at higher doses or more frequent administration. Subcutaneous doses of the drug as high as 1 mg/kg/day in rats and dogs did not produce any nonendocrine related sequelae; this dose is greater than 400 times that proposed for human use. If overdosage occurs, it should be managed symptomatically.

DOSAGE AND ADMINISTRATION

ZOLADEX, at a dose of 3.6 mg, should be administered subcutaneously every 28 days into the anterior abdominal wall below the navel line using an aseptic technique under the supervision of a physician.

While a delay of a few days is permissible, every effort should be made to adhere to the 28-day schedule.

Prostate Cancer: For the management of advanced prostate cancer, ZOLADEX is intended for long-term administration unless clinically inappropriate.

Stage B2-C Prostatic Carcinoma: When ZOLADEX is given in combination with radiotherapy and flutamide for patients with Stage T2b-T4 (Stage B2-C) prostatic carcinoma, treatment should be started 8 weeks prior to initiating radiotherapy and should continue during radiation therapy. A treatment regimen using a ZOLADEX 3.6 mg depot 8 weeks before radiotherapy, followed in 28 days by the ZOLADEX 10.8 mg depot, can be administered. Alternatively, four injections of 3.6 mg depot can be administered at 28 day intervals, two depots preceding and two during radiotherapy.

Endometriosis: For the management of endometriosis, the recommended duration of administration is 6 months.

Currently, there are no clinical data on the effect of treatment of benign gynecological conditions with ZOLADEX for periods in excess of 6 months.

Retreatment cannot be recommended for the management of endometriosis since safety data for retreatment are not available. If the symptoms of endometriosis recur after a course of therapy, and further treatment with ZOLADEX is contemplated, consideration should be given to monitoring bone mineral density. Clinical studies suggest the addition of Hormone Replacement Therapy (estrogens and/or progestins) to ZOLADEX is effective in reducing the bone mineral loss which occurs with ZOLADEX alone without compromising the efficacy of ZOLADEX in relieving the symptoms of endometriosis. The addition of Hormone Replacement Therapy may also reduce the occurrence of vasomotor symptoms and vaginal dryness associated with hypoestrogenism. The optimal drugs, dose and duration of treatment has not been established.

Breast Cancer: For the management of advanced breast cancer, ZOLADEX is intended for long-term administration unless clinically inappropriate.

Endometrial Thinning: For use as an endometrial-thinning agent prior to endometrial ablation, the dosing recommendation is one or two depots (with each depot given four weeks apart). When one depot is administered, surgery should be performed at four weeks. When two depots are administered, surgery should be performed within two to four weeks following administration of the second depot.

Renal or Hepatic Impairment: No dosage adjustment is necessary for patients with renal or hepatic impairment.

Administration Technique: The proper method of administration of ZOLADEX is described in the instructions that follow.

1. Put the patient in a comfortable position with the upper part of the body slightly raised. Prepare an area of the anterior abdominal wall below the navel line with an alcohol swab.
2. Examine the foil pouch and syringe for damage. Remove the syringe from the opened foil pouch and hold the syringe at a slight angle to the light. Check that at least part of the ZOLADEX implant is visible.
3. Grasp the red plastic safety tab and pull away from the syringe, and discard. Remove needle cover. **Unlike liquid injections, there is no need to remove air bubbles as attempts to do so may displace the ZOLADEX implant.**
4. Holding the syringe around the protective sleeve, using an aseptic technique, pinch the skin of the patient's anterior abdominal wall below the navel line. With the bevel of the needle facing up, insert the needle at a 30 to 45 degree angle to the skin in one continuous deliberate motion until the protective sleeve touches the patient's skin (Figure 3).
   NOTE: The ZOLADEX syringe cannot be used for aspiration. If the hypodermic needle penetrates a large vessel, blood will be seen instantly in the syringe chamber. If a vessel is penetrated, withdraw the needle and inject with a new syringe elsewhere.
5. Do not penetrate into muscle or peritoneum.
6. To administer the ZOLADEX implant and to activate the protective sleeve, grasp the barrel at the finger grip and depress the plunger until you cannot depress it any further. If the plunger is not depressed **fully** the protective sleeve will **NOT** activate. When the protective sleeve 'clicks', the protective sleeve will automatically begin to slide to cover the needle.
   NOTE: The needle does not retract.
7. Withdraw the needle and allow protective sleeve to slide and cover needle. Dispose of the syringe in an approved sharps collector.

NOTE: In the unlikely event of the need to surgically remove ZOLADEX, it may be localized by ultrasound.

HOW SUPPLIED

ZOLADEX is supplied as a sterile and totally biodegradable D,L-lactic and glycolic acids copolymer (13.3-14.3 mg/dose) impregnated with goserelin acetate equivalent to 3.6 mg of goserelin in a disposable syringe device fitted with a 16 gauge x 0.5 mm hypodermic needle with protective needle sleeve [SafeSystem™ Syringe] (NDC 0310-0950-36). The unit is sterile and comes in a sealed, light and moisture proof, aluminum foil laminate pouch containing a desiccant capsule. Store at room temperature (do not exceed 25°C [77°F]).

Zoladex is a trademark of the AstraZeneca group of companies.

Manufactured for:
AstraZeneca Pharmaceuticals LP
Wilmington, DE 19850
by: AstraZeneca UK Limited
Macclesfield, England
Made in United Kingdom
64216-00
Rev. 12/03

Shown in Product Identification Guide, page 306

ZOLADEX® 10.8 mg 3-MONTH ℞

[zōl′-ă-dĕx]

goserelin acetate implant
Equivalent to 10.8 mg goserelin
FOR USE IN MEN WITH PROSTATE CANCER

DESCRIPTION

ZOLADEX® (goserelin acetate implant), contains a potent synthetic decapeptide analogue of luteinizing hormone-releasing hormone (LHRH), also known as a gonadotropin releasing hormone (GnRH) agonist analogue. Goserelin acetate is chemically described as an acetate salt of [D-Ser(Bu^t)^6,Azgly^{10}]LHRH. Its chemical structure is pyro-Glu-His-Trp-Ser-Tyr-D-Ser(Bu^t)-Leu-Arg-Pro-Azgly-NH_2 acetate [$C_{59}H_{84}N_{18}O_{14} \cdot (C_2H_4O_2)_x$ where x = 1 to 2.4].

Goserelin acetate is an off-white powder with a molecular weight of 1269 Daltons (free base). It is freely soluble in glacial acetic acid. It is soluble in water, 0.1M hydrochloric acid, 0.1M sodium hydroxide, dimethylformamide and dimethyl sulfoxide. Goserelin acetate is practically insoluble in acetone, chloroform and ether.

ZOLADEX 10.8 mg implant is supplied as a sterile, biodegradable product containing goserelin acetate equivalent to 10.8 mg of goserelin. ZOLADEX is designed for subcutaneous implantation with continuous release over a 12-week period. Goserelin acetate is dispersed in a matrix of D,L-lactic and glycolic acids copolymer (12.82-14.76 mg/dose) containing less than 2% acetic acid and up to 10% goserelin-related substances and presented as a sterile, white to cream colored 1.5 mm diameter cylinder, preloaded in a special single-use syringe with a 14-gauge x 0.5 mm needle and protective needle sleeve (SafeSystem™ Syringe) in a sealed, light- and moisture-proof, aluminum foil laminate pouch containing a desiccant capsule.

Studies of the D,L-lactic and glycolic acids copolymer have indicated that it is completely biodegradable and has no demonstrable antigenic potential.

ZOLADEX is also supplied as a sterile, biodegradable product containing goserelin acetate equivalent to 3.6 mg of goserelin designed for administration every 28 days.

CLINICAL PHARMACOLOGY

Mechanism of Action: ZOLADEX is a synthetic decapeptide analogue of LHRH. ZOLADEX acts as a potent inhibitor of pituitary gonadotropin secretion when administered in the biodegradable formulation.

Following initial administration, ZOLADEX causes an initial increase in serum-luteinizing hormone (LH) and follicle-stimulating hormone (FSH) levels with subsequent increases in serum levels of testosterone. Chronic administration of ZOLADEX leads to sustained suppression of pituitary gonadotropins, and serum levels of testosterone consequently fall into the range normally seen in surgically castrated men approximately 21 days after initiation of therapy. This leads to accessory sex organ regression.

In animal and in *in vitro* studies, administration of goserelin resulted in the regression or inhibition of growth of the hormonally sensitive dimethylbenzanthracene (DMBA)-induced rat mammary tumor and Dunning R3327 prostate tumor.

In clinical trials using ZOLADEX 3.6 mg with follow-up of more than 2 years, suppression of serum testosterone to castrate levels has been maintained for the duration of therapy.

Pharmacokinetics:

Absorption: The pharmacokinetics of goserelin have been determined in healthy male volunteers and patients. In healthy males, radiolabeled goserelin was administered as a single 250 µg (aqueous solution) dose by the subcutaneous route. The absorption of radiolabeled drug was rapid, and the peak blood radioactivity levels occurred between 0.5 and 1.0 hour after dosing.

The overall pharmacokinetic profile of goserelin following administration of a ZOLADEX 10.8 mg depot to patients with prostate cancer was determined. The initial release of goserelin from the depot was relatively rapid resulting in a peak concentration at 2 hours after dosing. From Day 4 until the end of the 12-week dosing interval, the sustained release of goserelin from the depot produced reasonably stable systemic exposure. Mean (Standard Deviation) pharmacokinetic data are presented in Table 1. There is no clinically significant accumulation of goserelin following administration of four depots administered at 12-week intervals. Pharmacokinetic data were obtained using an RIA method, which has been shown to be specific for goserelin in the presence of its metabolites.

[See table 1 at top of next page]

Serum goserelin concentrations in prostate cancer patients administered three 3.6 mg depots followed by one 10.8 mg depot are displayed in Figure 1. The profiles for both formulations are primarily dependent upon the rate of drug release from the depots. For the 3.6 mg depot, mean concentrations gradually rise to reach a peak of about 3 ng/mL at around 15 days after administration and then decline to approximately 0.5 ng/mL by the end of the treatment period. For the 10.8 mg depot, mean concentrations increase to reach a peak of about 8 ng/mL within the first 24 hours and then decline rapidly up to Day 4. Thereafter, mean concentrations remain relatively stable in the range of about 0.3 to 1 ng/mL up to the end of the treatment period.

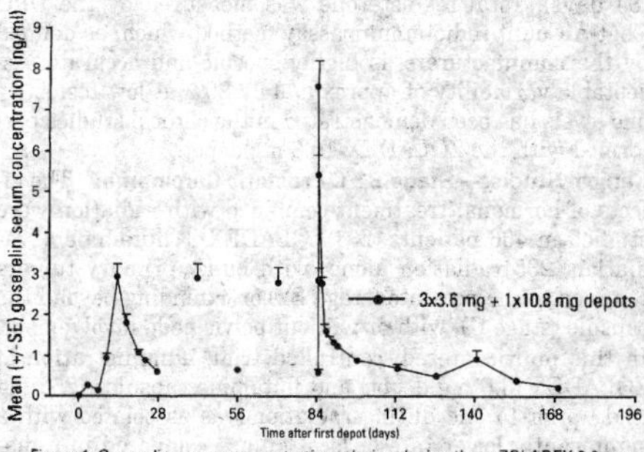

Figure 1: Goserelin serum concentrations during dosing three ZOLADEX 3.6 mg depots (0, 28, 56 days) then one ZOLADEX 10.8 mg depot (84 days) to prostate cancer patients.

Administration of four ZOLADEX 10.8 mg depots to patients with prostate cancer resulted in testosterone levels that were suppressed to and maintained within the range normally observed in surgically castrated men (0-1.73 nmol/L or 0-50 ng/dL), over the dosing interval in approximately 91% (145/160) of patients studied. In 6 of 15 patients that escaped from castrate range, serum testosterone levels were maintained below 2.0 nmol/L (58 ng/dL) and in only one of the 15 patients did the depot completely fail to maintain serum testosterone levels to within the castrate range over a 336-day period (4 depot injections). In the 8 additional patients, a transient escape was followed 14 days later by a level within the castrate range.

Continued on next page

Zoladex 3 Month—Cont.

Distribution: The apparent volume of distribution determined after subcutaneous administration of 250 µg aqueous solution of goserelin was 44.1 ± 13.6 liters for healthy males. The plasma protein binding of goserelin was found to be 27%.
Metabolism: Metabolism of goserelin, by hydrolysis of the C-terminal amino acids, is the major clearance mechanism. The major circulating component in serum appeared to be 1-7 fragment, and the major component present in urine of one healthy male volunteer was 5-10 fragment. The metabolism of goserelin in humans yields a similar but narrow profile of metabolites to that found in other species. All metabolites found in humans have also been found in toxicology species.
Excretion: Clearance of goserelin following subcutaneous administration of a radiolabeled solution of goserelin was very rapid and occurred via a combination of hepatic and urinary excretion. More than 90% of a subcutaneous radiolabeled solution formulation dose of goserelin was excreted in urine. Approximately 20% of the dose recovered in urine was accounted for by unchanged goserelin.
Special Populations
Renal Insufficiency: In clinical trials with the solution formulation of goserelin, subjects with impaired renal function (creatinine clearance less than 20 mL/min) had a serum elimination half-life of 12.1 hours compared to 4.2 hours for subjects with normal renal function (creatinine clearance greater than 70 mL/min). However, there was no evidence for any accumulation of goserelin on multiple dosing of the ZOLADEX 10.8 mg depot to subjects with impaired renal function. There was no evidence for any increase in incidence of adverse events in renally impaired patients administered the 10.8 mg depot. These data indicate that there is no need for any dosage adjustment when administering ZOLADEX 10.8 mg to subjects with impaired renal function.
Hepatic Insufficiency: The clearance and half-life of goserelin administered as an aqueous solution are not affected by hepatic impairment. These data indicate that there is no need for any dosage adjustment when administering ZOLADEX 10.8 mg to subjects with impaired hepatic function.
Geriatric: There is no need for any dosage adjustment when administering ZOLADEX 10.8 mg to geriatric patients.
Body Weight: A decline of approximately 1 to 2.5% in the AUC after administration of a 10.8 mg depot was observed with a kilogram increase in body weight. In obese patients who have not responded clinically, testosterone levels should be monitored closely.
Drug-Drug Interactions: No formal drug-drug interaction studies have been performed.
Clinical Studies—Prostatic Carcinoma: In two controlled clinical trials, 160 patients with advanced prostate cancer were randomized to receive either one 3.6 mg ZOLADEX implant every four weeks or a single 10.8 mg ZOLADEX implant every 12 weeks. Mean serum testosterone suppression was similar between the two arms. PSA falls at three months were 94% in patients who received the 10.8 mg implant and 92.5% in patients that received three 3.6 mg implants.
Periodic monitoring of serum testosterone levels should be considered if the anticipated clinical or biochemical response to treatment has not been achieved. A clinical outcome similar to that produced with the use of the 3.6 mg implant administered every 28 days is predicted with ZOLADEX 10.8 mg implant administered every 12 weeks (84 days). Total testosterone was measured by the DPC Coat-A-Count radioimmunoassay method which, as defined by the manufacturers, is highly specific and accurate. Acceptable variability of approximately 20% at low testosterone levels has been demonstrated in the clinical studies performed with the ZOLADEX 10.8 mg depot.
Clinical Studies—Stage B2-C Prostatic Carcinoma: The effects of hormonal treatment combined with radiation were studied in 466 patients (231 ZOLADEX + flutamide + radiation, 235 radiation alone) with bulky primary tumors confined to the prostate (stage B2) or extending beyond the capsule (stage C), with or without pelvic node involvement. In this multicentered, controlled trial, administration of ZOLADEX (3.6 mg depot) and flutamide capsules (250 mg t.i.d.) prior to and during radiation was associated with a significantly lower rate of local failure compared to radiation alone (16% vs 33% at 4 years, $P<0.001$). The combination therapy also resulted in a trend toward reduction in the incidence of distant metastases (27% vs 36% at 4 years, $P=0.058$). Median disease-free survival was significantly increased in patients who received complete hormonal therapy combined with radiation as compared to those patients who received radiation alone (4.4 vs 2.6 years, $P<0.001$). Inclusion of normal PSA level as a criterion for disease-free survival also resulted in significantly increased median disease-free survival in patients receiving the combination therapy (2.7 vs 1.5 years, $P<0.001$).

INDICATIONS AND USAGE

Prostatic Carcinoma: ZOLADEX is indicated in the palliative treatment of advanced carcinoma of the prostate.
In controlled studies of patients with advanced prostatic cancer comparing ZOLADEX 3.6 mg to orchiectomy, the long-term endocrine responses and objective responses were similar between the two treatment arms. Additionally, duration of survival was similar between the two treatment arms in a major comparative trial.
In controlled studies of patients with advanced prostatic cancer, ZOLADEX 10.8 mg implant produced pharmacodynamically similar effect in terms of suppression of serum testosterone to that achieved with ZOLADEX 3.6 mg implant. Clinical outcome similar to that produced with the use of the ZOLADEX 3.6 mg implant administered every 28 days is predicted with the ZOLADEX 10.8 mg implant administered every 12 weeks.
Stage B2-C Prostatic Carcinoma: ZOLADEX is indicated for use in combination with flutamide for the management of locally confined Stage T2b-T4 (Stage B2-C) carcinoma of the prostate. Treatment with ZOLADEX and flutamide should start 8 weeks prior to initiating radiation therapy and continue during radiation therapy.
The automatic safety feature of the syringe aids in the prevention of needlestick injury.

Table 1
Goserelin pharmacokinetic parameters for the 10.8 mg depot

Parameter	n	Mean	(SD)	95% CI Lower	95% CI Upper
Systemic clearance (mL/min)	41	121	(42.4)	108	134
C_{max} (ng/mL)	41	8.85	(2.83)	7.96	9.74
T_{max} (h)	41	1.80	(0.34)	1.70	1.92
C_{min} (ng/mL)	44	0.37	(0.21)	0.30	0.43
Elimination Half-life (h) ¶	7	4.16	(1.12)	3.12	5.20

¶ = determined after subcutaneous administration of 250 µg aqueous solution of goserelin.
SD = standard deviation
95% CI = 95% confidence interval

CONTRAINDICATIONS

A report of an anaphylactic reaction to synthetic GnRH (Factrel) has been reported in the medical literature.
ZOLADEX is contraindicated in those patients who have a known hypersensitivity to LHRH, LHRH agonist analogues or any of the components in ZOLADEX.
ZOLADEX 10.8 mg implant is not indicated in women as the data are insufficient to support reliable suppression of serum estradiol. For female patients requiring treatment with goserelin, refer to the prescribing information for ZOLADEX 3.6 mg implant.
ZOLADEX is contraindicated in women who are or may become pregnant while receiving the drug. In studies in rats and rabbits, ZOLADEX increased preimplantation loss, resorptions, and abortions (see Pregnancy section). In rats and dogs, ZOLADEX suppressed ovarian function, decreased ovarian weight and size, and led to atrophic changes in secondary sex organs. Further evidence suggests that fertility was reduced in female rats that became pregnant after ZOLADEX was stopped. These effects are an expected consequence of the hormonal alterations produced by ZOLADEX in humans. If a patient becomes pregnant during treatment, the drug must be discontinued and the patient must be apprised of the potential risk for loss of the pregnancy due to possible hormonal imbalance as a result of the expected pharmacologic action of ZOLADEX treatment. In animal studies, there was no evidence that ZOLADEX possessed the potential to cause teratogenicity in rabbits; however, in rats the incidence of umbilical hernia was significantly increased with treatment. (See Pregnancy, Teratogenic Effects.)

WARNINGS

Initially, ZOLADEX, like other LHRH agonists, causes transient increases in serum levels of testosterone. Transient worsening of symptoms, or the occurrence of additional signs and symptoms of prostatic cancer, may occasionally develop during the first few weeks of ZOLADEX treatment. A small number of patients may experience a temporary increase in bone pain, which can be managed symptomatically. As with other LHRH agonists, isolated cases of ureteral obstruction and spinal cord compression have been observed. If spinal cord compression or renal impairment develops, standard treatment of these complications should be instituted, and in extreme cases an immediate orchiectomy considered.

PRECAUTIONS

General: Hypersensitivity, antibody formation and acute anaphylactic reactions have been reported with LHRH agonist analogues.
Of 115 women worldwide treated with ZOLADEX 3.6 mg and tested for development of binding to goserelin following treatment with ZOLADEX, one patient showed low-titer binding to goserelin. On further testing of this patient's plasma obtained following treatment, her goserelin binding component was found not to be precipitated with rabbit antihuman immunoglobulin polyvalent sera. These findings suggest the possibility of antibody formation.
Information for Patients: The use of ZOLADEX in patients at particular risk of developing ureteral obstruction or spinal cord compression should be considered carefully and the patients monitored closely during the first month of therapy. Patients with ureteral obstruction or spinal cord compression should have appropriate treatment prior to initiation of ZOLADEX therapy.
Drug Interactions: No No drug interaction studies with other drugs have been conducted with ZOLADEX. No confirmed interactions have been reported between ZOLADEX and other drugs.
Drug/Laboratory Test Interactions: Administration of ZOLADEX in therapeutic doses results in suppression of the pituitary-gonadal system. Because of this suppression, diagnostic tests of pituitary-gonadotropic and gonadal functions conducted during treatment may show results which are misleading.
Carcinogenesis, Mutagenesis, Impairment of Fertility: Subcutaneous implant of ZOLADEX in male and female rats once every 4 weeks for 1 year and recovery for 23 weeks at doses of about 80 and 150 µg/kg (males) and 50 and 100 µg/kg (females) daily (about 3 to 9 times the recommended human dose on a mg/m^2 basis) resulted in an increased incidence of pituitary adenomas. An increased incidence of pituitary adenomas was also observed following subcutaneous implant of ZOLADEX in rats at similar dose levels for a period of 72 weeks in males and 101 weeks in females. The relevance of the rat pituitary adenomas to humans has not been established. Subcutaneous implants of ZOLADEX every 3 weeks for 2 years delivered to mice at doses of up to 2400 µg/kg/day (about 70 times the recommended human dose on a mg/m^2 basis) resulted in an increased incidence of histiocytic sarcoma of the vertebral column and femur.
Mutagenicity tests using bacterial and mammalian systems for point mutations and cytogenetic effects have provided no evidence for mutagenic potential.
Administration of goserelin led to changes that were consistent with gonadal suppression in both male and female rats as a result of its endocrine action. In male rats administered 500-1000 µg/kg/day (about 30-60 times the recommended human dose on a mg/m^2 basis), a decrease in weight and atrophic histological changes were observed in the testes, epididymis, seminal vesicle and prostate gland with complete suppression of spermatogenesis. In female rats administered 50-1000 µg/kg/day (about 3-60 times the recommended daily human dose on a mg/m^2 basis), suppression of ovarian function led to decreased size and weight of ovaries and secondary sex organs; follicular development was arrested at the antral stage and the corpora lutea were reduced in size and number. Except for the testes, almost complete histologic reversal of these effects in males and females was observed several weeks after dosing was stopped; however, fertility and general reproductive performance were reduced in those that became pregnant after goserelin was discontinued. Fertile matings occurred within 2 weeks after cessation of dosing, even though total recovery of reproductive function may not have occurred before mating took place; and, the ovulation rate, the corresponding implantation rate, and number of live fetuses were reduced. Based on histological examination, drug effects on reproductive organs seem to be completely reversible in male and female dogs when drug treatment was stopped after continuous administration for 1 year at 100 times the recommended monthly dose.
Pregnancy, Teratogenic Effects: Pregnancy Category X. See CONTRAINDICATIONS section. ZOLADEX 10.8 mg is not indicated in women as the data are insufficient to support reliable suppression of serum estradiol. Studies in both rats and rabbits at doses of 2, 10, 20, and 50 µg/kg/day and 20, 250, and 1,000 µg/kg/day, respectively (about 1/10 to 3 times and 2 to 100 times the daily maximum recommended human dose, respectively, on a mg/m^2 basis) administered during the period of organogenesis, have confirmed that ZOLADEX will increase pregnancy loss in a dose-related manner. While there was no evidence that ZOLADEX possessed the potential to cause teratogenicity in rabbits, in rats the incidence of umbilical hernia was significantly increased at doses greater than 10 mg/kg/day (about 1/2 the recommended dose on a mg/m^2 basis).
Nursing Mothers: It is not known if this drug is excreted in human milk. Many drugs are excreted in human milk and there is a potential for serious adverse reactions in nursing infants of mothers receiving ZOLADEX (See CONTRAINDICATIONS).
Pediatric Use: Safety and efficacy of ZOLADEX in pediatric patients have not been established.

ADVERSE REACTIONS

General: Rarely, hypersensitivity reactions (including urticaria and anaphylaxis) have been reported in patients receiving ZOLADEX.
As with other endocrine therapies, hypercalcemia (increased calcium) has rarely been reported in cancer patients with bone metastases following initiation of treatment with ZOLADEX or other LHRH agonists.
ZOLADEX has been found to be generally well tolerated in clinical trials. Adverse reactions reported in these trials were rarely severe enough to result in the patients' withdrawal from ZOLADEX treatment. As seen with other hormonal therapies, the most commonly observed adverse

events during ZOLADEX therapy were due to the expected physiological effects from decreased testosterone levels. These included hot flashes, sexual dysfunction and decreased erections.

As with other agents in this class, very rare cases of pituitary apoplexy have been reported following initial administration in patients with a functional pituitary adenoma.

Initially, ZOLADEX, like other LHRH agonists, causes transient increases in serum levels of testosterone. A small percentage of patients experienced a temporary worsening of signs and symptoms (see WARNINGS section), usually manifested by an increase in cancer-related pain which was managed symptomatically. Isolated cases of exacerbation of disease symptoms, either ureteral obstruction or spinal cord compression, occurred at similar rates in controlled clinical trials with both ZOLADEX and orchiectomy. The relationship of these events to therapy is uncertain.

There have been post-marketing reports of osteoporosis, decreased bone mineral density and bony fracture in men treated with ZOLADEX for prostate cancer.

Changes in blood pressure, manifest as hypotension or hypertension, have been occasionally observed in patients administered ZOLADEX. The changes are usually transient, resolving either during continued therapy or after cessation of therapy with ZOLADEX. Rarely, such changes have been sufficient to require medical intervention including withdrawal of treatment from ZOLADEX.

Prostatic Carcinoma: Two controlled clinical trials using ZOLADEX 10.8 mg versus ZOLADEX 3.6 mg were conducted. During a comparative phase, patients were randomized to receive either a single 10.8 mg implant or three consecutive 3.6 mg implants every 4 weeks over weeks 0-12. During this phase, the only adverse event reported in greater than 5% of patients was hot flashes, with an incidence of 47% in the ZOLADEX 10.8 mg group and 48% in the ZOLADEX 3.6 mg group.

From weeks 12-48 all patients were treated with a 10.8 mg implant every 12 weeks. During this noncomparative phase, the following adverse events were reported in greater than 5% of patients:

Adverse Event	ZOLADEX 10.8 mg (n = 157) %
Hot Flashes	64
Pain (General)	14
Gynecomastia	8
Pelvic Pain	6
Bone Pain	6
Asthenia	5

The following adverse events were reported in greater than 1%, but less than 5% of patients treated with ZOLADEX 10.8 mg implant every 12 weeks. Some of these are commonly reported in elderly patients.

WHOLE BODY—Abdominal pain, Back pain, Flu syndrome, Headache, Sepsis, Aggravation reaction

CARDIOVASCULAR—Angina pectoris, Cerebral ischemia, Cerebrovascular accident, Heart failure, Pulmonary embolus, Varicose veins

DIGESTIVE—Diarrhea, Hematemesis

ENDOCRINE—Diabetes mellitus

HEMATOLOGIC—Anemia

METABOLIC—Peripheral edema

NERVOUS SYSTEM—Dizziness, Paresthesia, Urinary retention

RESPIRATORY—Cough increased, Dyspnea, Pneumonia

SKIN—Herpes simplex, Pruritus

UROGENITAL—Bladder neoplasm, Breast pain, Hematuria, Impotence, Urinary frequency, Urinary incontinence, Urinary tract disorder, Urinary tract infection, Urination impaired.

The following adverse events not already listed above were reported in patients receiving ZOLADEX 3.6 mg in other clinical trials. Inclusion does not necessarily represent a causal relationship to ZOLADEX 10.8 mg.

WHOLE BODY: Allergic reaction, Chills, Fever, Infection, Injection site reaction, Lethargy, Malaise

CARDIOVASCULAR: Arrhythmia, Chest pain, Hemorrhage, Hypertension, Migraine, Myocardial infarction, Palpitations, Peripheral vascular disorder, Tachycardia

DIGESTIVE: Anorexia, Constipation, Dry mouth, Dyspepsia, Flatulence, Increased appetite, Nausea, Ulcer, Vomiting

HEMATOLOGIC: Ecchymosis

METABOLIC: Edema, Gout, Hyperglycemia, Weight increase

MUSCULOSKELETAL: Arthralgia, Hypertonia, Joint disorder, Leg cramps, Myalgia, Osteoporosis

NERVOUS SYSTEM: Anxiety, Depression, Emotional lability, Headache, Insomnia, Nervousness, Somnolence, Thinking abnormal

RESPIRATORY: Bronchitis, Chronic obstructive pulmonary disease, Epistaxis, Rhinitis, Sinusitis, Upper respiratory infection, Voice alterations

SKIN: Acne, Alopecia, Dry skin, Hair disorders, Rash, Seborrhea, Skin discoloration, Sweating

SPECIAL SENSES: Amblyopia, Dry eyes

UROGENITAL: Breast tenderness, Decreased erections, Renal insufficiency, Sexual dysfunction, Urinary obstruction

Stage B2-C Prostatic Carcinoma: Treatment with ZOLADEX and flutamide did not add substantially to the toxicity of radiation treatment alone. The following adverse experiences were reported during a multicenter clinical trial comparing ZOLADEX + flutamide + radiation versus radiation alone. The most frequently reported (greater than 5%) adverse experiences are listed below:

ADVERSE EVENTS DURING ACUTE RADIATION THERAPY
(within first 90 days of radiation therapy)

	(n=231) flutamide + ZOLADEX + Radiation % All	(n=235) Radiation Only % All
Rectum/Large Bowel	80	76
Bladder	58	60
Skin	37	37

ADVERSE EVENTS DURING LATE RADIATION PHASE
(after 90 days of radiation therapy)

	(n=231) flutamide + ZOLADEX + Radiation % All	(n=235) Radiation Only % All
Diarrhea	36	40
Cystitis	16	16
Rectal Bleeding	14	20
Proctitis	8	8
Hematuria	7	12

Additional adverse event data was collected for the combination therapy with radiation group over both the hormonal treatment and hormonal treatment plus radiation phases of the study. Adverse experiences occurring in more than 5% of patients in this group, over both parts of the study, were hot flashes (46%), diarrhea (40%), nausea (9%), and skin rash (8%).

Changes in Laboratory Values During Treatment

Plasma Enzymes: Elevation of liver enzymes (AST, ALT) have been reported in female patients exposed to ZOLADEX 3.6 mg (representing less than 1% of all patients). There was no other evidence of abnormal liver function. Causality between these changes and ZOLADEX have not been established.

Lipids: In a controlled trial in females, ZOLADEX 3.6 mg implant therapy resulted in a minor, but statistically significant effect on serum lipids (i.e., increases in LDL cholesterol of 21.3 mg/dL; increases in HDL cholesterol of 2.7 mg/dL; and triglycerides increased by 8.0 mg/dL).

OVERDOSAGE

The pharmacologic properties of ZOLADEX and its mode of administration make accidental or intentional overdosage unlikely. There is no experience of overdosage from clinical trials. Animal studies indicate that no increased pharmacologic effect occurred at higher doses or more frequent administration. Subcutaneous doses of the drug as high as 1 mg/kg/day in rats and dogs did not produce any nonendocrine related sequelae; this dose is greater than 400 times that proposed for human use. If overdosage occurs, it should be managed symptomatically.

DOSAGE AND ADMINISTRATION

ZOLADEX, at a dose of 10.8 mg, should be administered subcutaneously every 12 weeks into the anterior abdominal wall below the navel line using an aseptic technique under the supervision of a physician.

While a delay of a few days is permissible, every effort should be made to adhere to the 12-week schedule.

Prostatic Carcinoma: For the management of advanced prostate cancer, ZOLADEX is intended for long-term administration unless clinically inappropriate.

Stage B2-C Prostatic Carcinoma: When ZOLADEX is given in combination with radiotherapy and flutamide for patients with Stage T2b-T4 (Stage B2-C) prostatic carcinoma, treatment should be started 8 weeks prior to initiating radiotherapy and should continue during radiation therapy. A treatment regimen using one ZOLADEX 3.6 mg depot, followed in 28 days by one ZOLADEX 10.8 mg depot, should be administered.

Renal or Hepatic Impairment: No dosage adjustment is necessary for patients with renal or hepatic impairment.

Females: ZOLADEX 10.8 mg implant is not indicated in women as the data are insufficient to support reliable suppression of serum estradiol. For female patients requiring treatment with goserelin, refer to the prescribing information for ZOLADEX 3.6 mg implant.

Administration Technique: The proper method of administration of ZOLADEX is described in the instructions that follow.

1. Put the patient in a comfortable position with the upper part of the body slightly raised. Prepare an area of the anterior abdominal wall below the navel line with an alcohol swab.
2. Examine the foil pouch and syringe for damage. Remove the syringe from the opened foil pouch and hold the syringe at a slight angle to the light. Check that at least part of the ZOLADEX implant is visible.
3. Grasp the blue plastic safety tab and pull away from the syringe, and discard. Remove needle cover. **Unlike liquid injections, there is no need to remove air bubbles as attempts to do so may displace the ZOLADEX implant.**
4. Holding the syringe around the protective sleeve, using an aseptic technique, pinch the skin of the patient's anterior abdominal wall below the navel line. With the bevel of the needle facing up, insert the needle at a 30 to 45 degree angle to the skin in one continuous deliberate motion until the protective sleeve touches the patient's skin (Figure 3).
   NOTE: The ZOLADEX syringe cannot be used for aspiration. If the hypodermic needle penetrates a large vessel, blood will be seen instantly in the syringe chamber. If a vessel is penetrated, withdraw the needle and inject with a new syringe elsewhere.
5. Do not penetrate into muscle or peritoneum.
6. To administer the ZOLADEX implant and to activate the protective sleeve, grasp the barrel at the finger grip and depress the plunger until you cannot depress it any further. If the plunger is not depressed **fully** the protective sleeve will **NOT** activate. When the protective sleeve 'clicks', the protective sleeve will automatically begin to slide to cover the needle.
   NOTE: The needle does not retract.
7. Withdraw the needle and allow protective sleeve to slide and cover needle. Dispose of the syringe in an approved sharps collector.
   NOTE: In the unlikely event of the need to surgically remove ZOLADEX, it may be localized by ultrasound.

HOW SUPPLIED

ZOLADEX 10.8 mg implant is supplied as a sterile and totally biodegradable D,L-lactic and glycolic acids copolymer (12.82-14.76 mg/dose) impregnated with goserelin acetate equivalent to 10.8 mg of goserelin in a disposable syringe device fitted with a 14-gauge x 0.5 mm hypodermic needle with protective needle sleeve [SafeSystem™ Syringe] (NDC 0310-0951-30). The unit is sterile and comes in a sealed, light- and moisture-proof, aluminum foil laminate pouch containing a desiccant capsule. Store at room temperature (do not exceed 25°C [77°F]).

Zoladex is a trademark of the AstraZeneca group of companies.

Manufactured for:
AstraZeneca Pharmaceuticals LP
Wilmington, DE 19850
by AstraZeneca UK Limited
Macclesfield, England
Made in the United Kingdom
64225-00
Rev 12/03

Auxilium Pharmaceuticals, Inc.

160 WEST GERMANTOWN PIKE
NORRISTOWN, PA 19401

Direct Inquiries to:
610-239-1499

TESTIM® 1% Ⓒ℞

[*tĕs-tĭm*]
(testosterone gel)
Rx only

DESCRIPTION

Testim® (testosterone gel) is a clear to translucent hydroalcoholic topical gel containing 1% testosterone. Testim® provides continuous transdermal delivery of testosterone for 24 hours, following a single application to intact, clean, dry skin of the shoulders and upper arms.

One 5 g or two 5 g tubes of Testim® contains 50 mg or 100 mg of testosterone, respectively, to be applied daily to the skin's surface. Approximately 10% of the applied testosterone dose is absorbed across skin of average permeability during a 24-hour period.

The active pharmacological ingredient in Testim® is testosterone.

Testosterone ($C_{19}H_{28}O_2$) MW: 288.42

Testosterone

Testosterone USP is a white to practically white crystalline powder chemically described as 17-β hydroxyandrost-4-en-3-one. Inactive ingredients in Testim® are purified water, pentadecalactone, carbopol, acrylates, propylene glycol, glycerin, polyethylene glycol, ethanol (74%), and tromethamine.

Continued on next page

Testim—Cont.

CLINICAL PHARMACOLOGY

Testim® 1% (testosterone gel) delivers physiologic amounts of testosterone, producing circulating testosterone levels that approximate normal levels (e.g., 300 – 1000 ng/dL) seen in healthy men.

Testosterone – General Androgen Effects:

Testosterone and dihydrotestosterone (DHT), endogenous androgens, are responsible for normal growth and development of the male sex organs and for maintenance of secondary sex characteristics. These effects include the growth and maturation of the prostate, seminal vesicles, penis, and scrotum; the development of male hair distribution, such as facial, pubic, chest, and axillary hair; laryngeal enlargement; vocal cord thickening; alterations in body musculature; and fat distribution.

Male hypogonadism results from insufficient secretion of testosterone and is characterized by low serum testosterone concentrations. Symptoms associated with male hypogonadism include decreased sexual desire with or without impotence, fatigue and loss of energy, mood depression, regression of secondary sexual characteristics, and osteoporosis. Hypogonadism is a risk factor for osteoporosis in men.

Drugs in the androgen class also promote retention of nitrogen, sodium, potassium, phosphorus, and decreased urinary excretion of calcium.

Androgens have been reported to increase protein anabolism and decrease protein catabolism. Nitrogen balance is improved only when there is sufficient intake of calories and protein. Androgens have been reported to stimulate the production of red blood cells by enhancing erythropoietin production.

Androgens are responsible for the growth spurt of adolescence and for the eventual termination of linear growth brought about by fusion of the epiphyseal growth centers. In children, exogenous androgens accelerate linear growth rates but may cause a disproportionate advancement in bone maturation. Use over long periods may result in fusion of the epiphyseal growth centers and termination of the growth process.

During exogenous administration of androgens, endogenous testosterone release may be inhibited through feedback inhibition of pituitary luteinizing hormone (LH). At large doses of exogenous androgens, spermatogenesis may also be suppressed through feedback inhibition of pituitary follicle-stimulating hormone (FSH).

There is a lack of substantial evidence that androgens are effective in accelerating fracture healing or in shortening post-surgical convalescence.

Pharmacokinetics

The pharmacokinetics of Testim® have been evaluated with administration of doses containing 50 mg and 100 mg of testosterone to adult males with morning testosterone levels ≤300 ng/dL.

Absorption

Testim® is a topical formulation that dries quickly when applied to the skin surface. The skin serves as a reservoir for the sustained release of testosterone into the systemic circulation. Approximately 10% of the testosterone applied on the skin surface is absorbed into the systemic circulation during a 24-hour period.

Single Dose

In single dose studies, when either Testim® 50 mg or 100 mg was administered, absorption of testosterone into the blood continued for the entire 24 hour dosing period. Also, mean peak and average serum concentrations within the normal range were achieved within 24 hours.

Multiple Dose

With single daily applications of Testim® 50 mg and 100 mg, follow-up measurements at 30 and 90 days after starting treatment have confirmed that serum testosterone and DHT concentrations are generally maintained within the normal range.

Figure 1 summarizes the 24-hour pharmacokinetic profile of testosterone for patients maintained on Testim® 50 mg or Testim® 100 mg for 30 days.

Figure 1
Mean Steady-Stae Serum Testosterone (±SD) (ng/mL)
Concentrations on Day 30 in Patients Applying Testim™ Once Daily

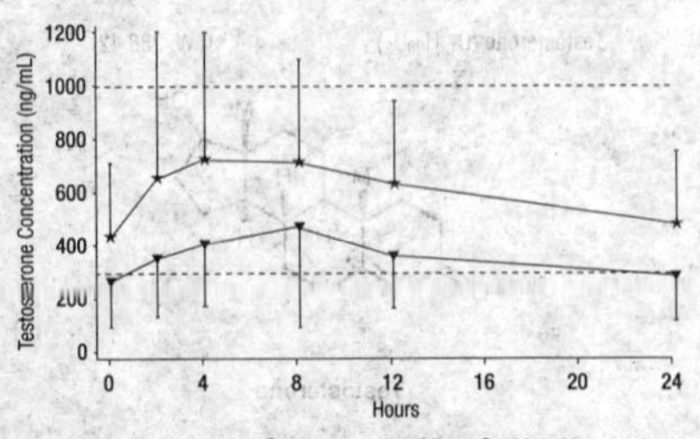

The average daily testosterone concentration produced by Testim® 100 mg at Day 30 was 612 (± 286) ng/dL and by Testim® 50 mg at Day 30 was 365 (± 187) ng/dL.

Figure 2 summarizes the 24-hour pharmacokinetic profile of DHT for patients maintained on Testim® 50 mg or Testim® 100 mg for 30 days.

Figure 2
Mean Steady-Stae Serum Dihydrotestosterone (±SD) (pg/mL)
Concentrations on Day 30 in Patients Applying Testim™ Once Daily

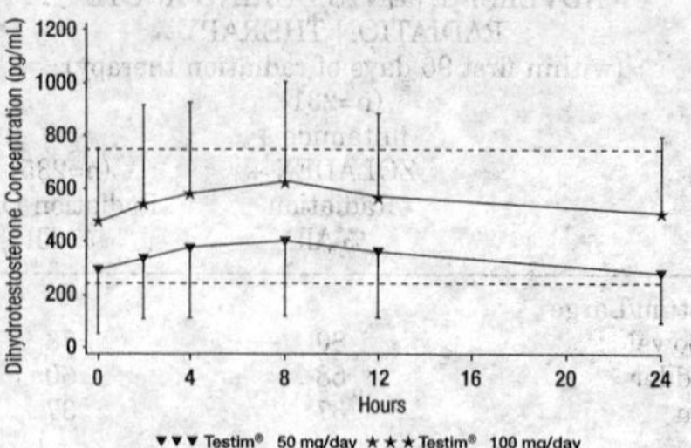

The average daily DHT concentration produced by Testim® 100 mg at Day 30 was 555 (± 293) pg/mL and by Testim® 50 mg at Day 30 was 346 (± 212) pg/mL.

Washing

The effect of showering (with mild soap) at 1, 2 and 6 hours post application of Testim® 100 mg was evaluated in a clinical trial in 12 men. The study demonstrated that the overall effect of washing was to lessen testosterone levels; however, when washing occurred two or more hours post drug application, serum testosterone levels remained within the normal range.

Distribution

Circulating testosterone is chiefly bound in the serum to sex hormone-binding globulin (SHBG) and albumin. The albumin-bound fraction of testosterone easily dissociates from albumin and is presumed to be bioactive. The portion of testosterone bound to SHBG is not considered biologically active. Approximately 40% of testosterone in plasma is bound to SHBG, 2% remains unbound (free) and the rest is bound to albumin and other proteins. The amount of SHBG in the serum and the total testosterone level will determine the distribution of bioactive and nonbioactive androgen.

Metabolism

There is considerable variation in the half-life of testosterone as reported in the literature, ranging from ten to 100 minutes.

Testosterone is metabolized to various 17-keto steroids through two different pathways. The major active metabolites of testosterone are estradiol and DHT. Testosterone is metabolized to DHT by steroid 5α-reductase located in the skin, liver, and the urogenital tract of the male. DHT binds with greater affinity to SHBG than does testosterone. In many tissues, the activity of testosterone depends on its reduction to DHT, which binds to cytosol receptor proteins. The steroid-receptor complex is transported to the nucleus where it initiates transcription and cellular changes related to androgen action. In reproductive tissues, DHT is further metabolized to 3α and 3ß androstanediol. Inactivation of testosterone occurs primarily in the liver.

DHT concentrations increased in parallel with testosterone concentrations during Testim® treatment. After 90 days of treatment, mean DHT concentrations remained generally within the normal range for Testim®-treated subjects.

Excretion

About 90% of a testosterone dose given intramuscularly is excreted in the urine as glucuronic and sulfuric acid conjugates of testosterone and metabolites; about 6% of a dose is excreted in the feces, mostly in the unconjugated form.

Special Population

In patients treated with Testim® there are no observed differences in the average daily serum testosterone concentration at steady-state based on age or cause of hypogonadism. No formal studies were conducted in a pediatric age population or in patients with renal or hepatic insufficiencies.

Clinical Studies

Testim® was evaluated in a randomized multicenter, multidose, active and placebo controlled 90-day study in 406 adult males with morning testosterone levels ≤300 ng/dL. The study was double-blind for the doses of Testim® and placebo, but open label for the non-scrotal testosterone transdermal system. During the first 60 days, patients were evenly randomized to Testim® 50 mg, Testim® 100 mg, placebo gel, or testosterone transdermal system. At Day 60, patients receiving Testim® were maintained at the same dose, or were titrated up or down within their treatment group, based on 24-hour averaged serum testosterone concentration levels obtained on Day 30.

Of 192 hypogonadal men who were appropriately titrated with Testim® and who had sufficient data for analysis, 74% achieved an average serum testosterone level within the normal range on treatment Day 90.

Table 1 summarizes the mean testosterone concentrations on Day 30 for patients receiving Testim® 50 mg or 100 mg.

Table 1: Mean (± SD) Steady-State Serum Testosterone Concentrations on Day 30

	Testim® 50 mg n=94	Testim® 100 mg n=95	Placebo n=93
C_{avg} (ng/dL)	365 ± 187	612 ± 286	216 ± 79
C_{max} (ng/dL)	538 ± 371	897 ± 565	271 ± 110
C_{min} (ng/dL)	223 ± 126	394 ± 189	164 ± 64

At Day 30, patients receiving Testim® 100 mg daily showed significant improvement from baseline in multiple sexual function parameters as measured by patient questionnaires when compared to placebo. These parameters included sexual motivation, sexual desire, sexual activity and spontaneous erections. For Testim® 100 mg, improvements in sexual motivation, spontaneous erections, and sexual desire were maintained through Day 90. Sexual enjoyment and satisfaction with erection duration were improved compared to baseline but these improvements were not significant compared to the placebo group.

In Testim®-treated patients, the number of days in which sexual activity was reported to occur increased by 123% from baseline at Day 30 and was still increased from baseline by 59% at Day 90. The number of days with spontaneous erections increased by 137% at Day 30 and was maintained at 78% at Day 90 for Testim®-treated patients compared to baseline.

Table 2 summarizes the changes in body composition at Day 90 for patients receiving Testim® 50 mg or 100 mg as measured by standardized whole body DEXA (Dual Energy X-ray Absorptiometry) scanning.

[See table 2 at top of next page]

At Day 90, mean increases from baseline in lean body mass and mean decreases from baseline in total fat mass and percent body fat in Testim®-treated patients were significant when compared to placebo-treated patients.

Potential for Testosterone Transfer

The potential for dermal testosterone transfer following Testim® use was evaluated in two clinical trials with males dosed with Testim® and their untreated female partners.

In the first trial (AUX-TG-206), 30 couples were evenly randomized to five groups. In the first four groups, 100 mg of Testim® was applied to the male abdomen and the couples were then asked to rub abdomen-to-abdomen for 15 minutes at 1 hour, 4 hours, 8 hours or 12 hours after dose application, respectively. In these couples, serum testosterone concentrations in female partners increased from baseline by at least 4 times and potential for transfer was seen at all timepoints.

When 6 males used a shirt to cover the abdomen at 15 minutes post-application and partners again rubbed abdomens for 15 minutes at the 1 hour timepoint, the potential for transfer was markedly reduced.

In the second trial (AUX-TG-209), 24 couples were evenly randomized to four groups. Testim® 100 mg was applied to the male arms and shoulders. In one group, 15 minutes of direct skin-to-skin rubbing began at 4 hours after application. In these six women, all of whom showered immediately after the rubbing activity, mean maximum serum testosterone concentrations increased from baseline by approximately 4 times. When males wore a long-sleeved T-shirt and rubbing was started at 1 and at 4 hours after application, the transfer of testosterone from male to female partners was prevented.

INDICATIONS AND USAGE

Testim® is indicated for testosterone replacement therapy in adult males for conditions associated with a deficiency or absence of endogenous testosterone:

1. Primary hypogonadism (congenital or acquired): testicular failure due to cryptorchidism, bilateral torsion, orchitis, vanishing testis syndrome, orchiectomy, Klinefelter's syndrome, chemotherapy, or toxic damage from alcohol or heavy metals. These men usually have low serum testosterone levels and gonadotropins (FSH, LH) above the normal range.
2. Hypogonadotropic hypogonadism (congenital or acquired): idiopathic gonadotropin or luteinizing hormone-releasing hormone (LHRH) deficiency or pituitary-hypothalamic injury from tumors, trauma, or radiation. These men have low testosterone serum levels but have gonadotropins in the normal or low range.

Testim® has not been clinically evaluated in males under 18 years of age.

CONTRAINDICATIONS

Androgens are contraindicated in men with carcinoma of the breast or known or suspected carcinoma of the prostate.

Testim® is not indicated for use in women, has not been evaluated for use in women, and must not be used in women.

Pregnant and nursing women should avoid skin contact with Testim® application sites on men. Testosterone may cause fetal harm. Testosterone exposure during pregnancy has been reported to be associated with fetal abnormalities. In the event that unwashed or unclothed skin to which Testim® has been applied comes in direct contact with the skin of a pregnant or nursing woman, the general area of contact on the woman should be immediately washed with soap and water.

Testim® should not be used in patients with known hypersensitivity to any of its ingredients, including testosterone USP that is chemically synthesized from soy.

WARNINGS

1. Testim® should not be applied to the abdomen.
2. Prolonged use of high doses of orally active 17-alpha-alkyl androgens (e.g., methyltestosterone) has been associated with serious hepatic adverse effects (peliosis hepatitis, hepatic neoplasms, cholestatic hepatitis, and

jaundice). Peliosis hepatitis can be a life-threatening or fatal complication. Long-term therapy with testosterone enanthate, which elevates blood levels for prolonged periods has produced multiple hepatic adenomas. Transdermal testosterone is not known to produce these adverse effects.
3. Geriatric patients treated with androgens may be at an increased risk for the development of prostatic hyperplasia and prostatic carcinoma.
4. Geriatric patients and other patients with clinical or demographic characteristics that are recognized to be associated with an increased risk of prostate cancer should be evaluated for the presence of prostate cancer prior to initiation of testosterone replacement therapy. In men receiving testosterone replacement therapy, surveillance for prostate cancer should be consistent with current practices for eugonadal men (see PRECAUTIONS: Carcinogenesis, Mutagenesis, Impairment of Fertility and Laboratory Tests).
5. Edema, with or without congestive heart failure, may be a serious complication in patients with preexisting cardiac, renal, or hepatic disease. In addition to discontinuation of the drug, diuretic therapy may be required.
6. Gynecomastia occasionally develops and occasionally persists in patients being treated for hypogonadism.
7. The treatment of hypogonadal men with testosterone may potentiate sleep apnea in some patients, especially those with risk factors such as obesity or chronic lung diseases.

PRECAUTIONS

Transfer of testosterone to another person can occur when vigorous skin-to-skin contact is made with the application site (See Clinical Studies).

The following precautions are recommended to minimize potential transfer of testosterone from Testim®-treated skin to another person:

- Patients should wash their hands thoroughly and immediately with soap and water after application of Testim®. Studies of hand-washing show that Testim® is effectively removed from the skin surface by thorough washing with soap and water.
- Patients should cover the application site(s) with clothing after the gel has dried (e.g. a shirt).
- Prior to any situation in which direct skin-to-skin contact is anticipated, patients should wash the application sites thoroughly with soap and water so as to remove drug residue.
- In the event that unwashed or unclothed skin to which Testim® has been applied does come in direct contact with the skin of another person, the general area of contact on the other person should be washed thoroughly with soap and water as soon as possible.

Changes in body hair distribution, significant increase in acne, or other signs of virilization of the female partner should be brought to the attention of a physician.

General

The physician should instruct patients to report any of the following:

- Too frequent or persistent erections of the penis.
- Any changes in skin color, ankle swelling or unexplained nausea and vomiting.
- Breathing disturbances, including those associated with sleep.

Information for Patients

Advise patients to carefully read the information brochure that accompanies each carton of 30 Testim® single-use tubes.

Advise patients of the following:

- Testim® should not be applied to the scrotum, penis, or abdomen.
- Testim® should be applied once daily at approximately the same time each day to clean dry skin of the shoulders and/or upper arms.
- Washing or swimming may lessen testosterone levels; however, when washing occurs two or more hours post drug application, serum testosterone levels remain within the normal range.
- Testim® may be transferred to another person by vigorous contact with the application site. Potential for transfer may be reduced by washing hands thoroughly after application, by wearing clothing to cover the sites, and by washing the application sites thoroughly with soap and water prior to any direct skin-to-skin contact.

Laboratory Tests

1. Hemoglobin and hematocrit levels should be checked periodically (to detect polycythemia) in patients on long-term androgen therapy.
2. Liver function, prostate specific antigen (PSA), cholesterol, and high-density lipoprotein (HDL) should be checked periodically.
3. To ensure proper dosing, serum testosterone concentrations should be measured (see DOSAGE AND ADMINISTRATION).

Drug Interactions

Oxyphenbutazone: Concurrent administration of oxyphenbutazone and androgens may result in elevated serum levels of oxyphenbutazone.

Insulin: In diabetic patients, the metabolic effects of androgens may decrease blood glucose and, therefore, insulin requirements.

Propranolol: In a published pharmacokinetic study of an injectable testosterone product, administration of testosterone cypionate led to an increased clearance of propranolol in the majority of men tested. It is unknown if this would apply to Testim®.

Table 2: Effect of Testim® on Lean Body Mass, Total Fat Mass and % Body Fat

Days of Treatment	Lean Body Mass (Muscle) (kg)	Total Fat Mass (kg)	% Body Fat
Baseline	61.6	29.4	30.9
Day 90	63.3	28.6	29.8
Change from Baseline	↑1.6	↓0.8	↓1.1

Table 3: Incidence of Adverse Events Judged Possibly, Probably or Definitely Related to Use of Testim® in the Controlled Clinical Trial

Event	Testim® 50 mg	Testim® 100 mg	Placebo
Application Site Reactions	2%	4%	3%
Benign Prostatic Hyperplasia	0%	1%	1%
Blood Pressure Diastolic Decreased	1%	0%	0%
Blood Pressure Increased	1%	1%	0%
Gynecomastia	1%	0%	0%
Headache	1%	1%	0%
Hematocrit/hemoglobin Increased	1%	2%	0%
Hot Flushes	1%	0%	0%
Insomnia	1%	0%	0%
Lacrimation Increased	1%	0%	0%
Mood Swings	1%	0%	0%
Smell Disorder	1%	0%	0%
Spontaneous Penile Erection	1%	0%	0%
Taste Disorder	1%	1%	0%

Corticosteroids: The concurrent administration of testosterone with ACTH or corticosteroids may enhance edema formation; thus these drugs should be administered cautiously, particularly in patients with cardiac or hepatic disease.

Drug/Laboratory Test Interactions

Androgens may decrease levels of thyroxin-binding globulin, resulting in decreased total T4 serum levels and increased resin uptake of T3 and T4. Free thyroid hormone levels remain unchanged, however, and there is no clinical evidence of thyroid dysfunction.

Carcinogenesis, Mutagenesis, Impairment of Fertility

Animal Data: Testosterone has been tested by subcutaneous injection and implantation in mice and rats. In mice, the implant induced cervical-uterine tumors, which metastasized in some cases. There is suggestive evidence that injection of testosterone into some strains of female mice increases their susceptibility to hepatoma. Testosterone is also known to increase the number of tumors and decrease the degree of differentiation of chemically induced carcinomas of the liver in rats.

Human Data: There are rare reports of hepatocellular carcinoma in patients receiving long-term oral therapy with androgens in high doses. Withdrawal of the drugs did not lead to regression of the tumors in all cases.

Geriatric patients treated with androgens may be at an increased risk for the development of prostatic hyperplasia and prostatic carcinoma. Geriatric patients and other patients with clinical or demographic characteristics that are recognized to be associated with an increased risk of prostate cancer should be evaluated for the presence of prostate cancer prior to initiation of testosterone replacement therapy.

In men receiving testosterone replacement therapy, surveillance for prostate cancer should be consistent with current practices for eugonadal men.

Pregnancy Category X (see Contraindications) – Teratogenic Effects: Testim® is not indicated for women and must not be used in women. Testosterone may cause fetal harm.

Nursing Mothers: Testim® is not indicated for women and must not be used in nursing mothers.

Pediatric Use: Safety and efficacy of Testim® in patients <18 years old has not been established.

ADVERSE REACTIONS

In a controlled clinical study, 304 patients were treated with Testim® 50 mg or 100 mg or placebo gel for up to 90 days. Two hundred-five (205) patients received Testim® 50 mg or 100 mg daily and 99 patients received placebo. Patients with adverse events that were possibly or probably related to study drug and reported by ≥1% of the Testim® patients and greater than placebo are listed in Table 3.

[See table 3 above]

The following adverse events possibly or probably related to Testim® occurred in fewer than 1% of patients but were greater in Testim® groups compared to the placebo group: activated partial thromboplastin time prolonged, blood creatinine increased, prothrombin time prolonged, appetite increased, sensitive nipples, and acne.

In this clinical trial of Testim®, six patients had adverse events that led to their discontinuation. These events included: vertigo, coronary artery disease, depression with suicidal ideation, urinary tract infection/pneumonia (none of which were considered related to Testim® administration), mood swings and hypertension. No Testim® patients discontinued due to skin reaction.

In one foreign Phase 3 trial, one subject discontinued due to a skin-related adverse event. In the pivotal U.S. and European Phase 3 trials combined, at the 50 mg dosage strength, the percentage of subjects reporting clinically notable increases in hematocrit or hemoglobin were similar to placebo. However, in the 100 mg dose group, 2.3% and 2.8% of patients had a clinically notable increase in hemoglobin (≥ 19 gm/dL) or hematocrit (≥ 58%), respectively.

In the combined ongoing U.S. and European open label extension studies, approximately 140 patients received Testim® for at least 6 months. The preliminary results from these studies are consistent with those reported for the U.S. controlled clinical trial.

DRUG ABUSE AND DEPENDENCE

Testim® contains testosterone, a Schedule III controlled substance as defined by the Anabolic Steroids Control Act. Oral ingestion of Testim® will not result in clinically significant serum testosterone concentrations due to extensive first-pass metabolism.

OVERDOSAGE

There were no reports of overdose in the Testim® clinical trials. There is one report of acute overdosage by injection of testosterone enanthate: testosterone levels of up to 11,400 ng/dL were implicated in a cerebrovascular accident.

DOSAGE AND ADMINISTRATION

The recommended starting dose of Testim® is 5 g of gel (one tube) containing 50 mg of testosterone applied once daily (preferably in the morning) to clean, dry intact skin of the shoulders and/or upper arms. Morning serum testosterone levels should then be measured approximately 14 days after initiation of therapy to ensure proper serum testosterone levels are achieved. If the serum testosterone concentration is below the normal range, or if the desired clinical response is not achieved, the daily Testim® dose may be increased from 5 g (one tube) to 10 g (two tubes) as instructed by the physician.

Upon opening the tube the entire contents should be squeezed into the palm of the hand and immediately applied to the shoulders and/or upper arms. Application sites

Continued on next page

Testim—Cont.

should be allowed to dry for a few minutes prior to dressing. Hands should be washed thoroughly with soap and water after Testim® has been applied.
In order to prevent transfer to another person, clothing should be worn to cover the application sites. If direct skin-to-skin contact with another person is anticipated, the application sites must be washed thoroughly with soap and water.
In order to maintain serum testosterone levels in the normal range, the sites of application should not be washed for at least two hours after application of Testim®.
Do not apply Testim® to the genitals or to the abdomen.

HOW SUPPLIED

Testim® contains testosterone, a Schedule III controlled substance as defined by the Anabolic Steroids Control Act. Testim® is supplied in unit-dose tubes in cartons of 30. Each tube contains 50 mg testosterone in 5 g of gel, and is supplied as follows:

NDC Number	Strength	Package Size
66887-001-05	1% (50 mg)	30 tubes: 5 g per tube

Storage
Store at room temperature 25°C (77°F); Excursions permitted to 15°-30°C (59°-86°F) [See USP Controlled Room Temperature].
Disposal
Used Testim® tubes should be discarded in household trash in a manner that prevents accidental application or ingestion by children or pets; contents flammable.
Manufactured for:
Auxilium Pharmaceuticals, Inc.
Norristown, PA, 19401 USA
By: DPT Laboratories, Ltd.
San Antonio, TX 78215
Labeling Code: AA2500.08
Issued: September 2003
0904-05
127997

Aventis Pharmaceuticals Inc.
300 SOMERSET CORPORATE BOULEVARD
BRIDGEWATER, NJ 08807-0977

Direct Inquiries to:
Customer Service
300 Somerset Corporate Boulevard
Bridgewater, NJ 08807-0977
(800) 207-8049

For Medical Information Contact:
Generally:
Medical Information Services
300 Somerset Corporate Boulevard
Bridgewater, NJ 08807-0977
(800) 633-1610
For Oncology Medical Information
call (866) 662-6411

PRODUCT IDENTIFICATION
NUMERICAL SUMMARY
SOLID ORAL DOSAGE FORMS

Aventis Pharmaceuticals
Bridgewater, NJ 08807-0977
To provide quick and positive identification of Aventis Pharmaceuticals prescription drug products, we have imprinted an identifying number and the name MARION on the following tablets.
ALLEGRA® 60-mg capsules are imprinted in black ink, with "ALLEGRA" on the cap and "60 mg" on the body.
ALLEGRA® 30-mg tablets have 03 on one side and either 0088 or scripted E on the other.
ALLEGRA® 60-mg tablets have 06 on one side and either 0088 or scripted E on the other.
ALLEGRA® 180-mg tablets have 018 on one side and either 0088 or scripted E on the other.
ALLEGRA-D® Extended-Release Tablets are engraved with "Allegra-D".
AMARYL® (glimepiride) Tablets 1 mg, 2 mg, and 4 mg are either imprinted with "AMA RYL" on one side, or imprinted with "AMA RYL" on one side and the Hoechst logo on both sides of the bisect on the other side.
ANZEMET® 50 mg tablets are imprinted with "A" on one side and "50" on the other.
ANZEMET® 100 mg tablets are imprinted with "100" on one side and "ANZEMET" on the other.
ARAVA™ (leflunomide) Tablets, 10 mg, are embossed with "ZBN" on one side.
ARAVA™ Tablets, 20 mg, are embossed with "ZBO" on one side.
ARAVA™ Tablets, 100 mg, are embossed with "ZBP" on one side.
CANTIL® Tablets, 25 mg (mepenzolate bromide USP) is debossed MERRELL 37.
CLOMID® Tablets, 50 mg (clomiphene citrate) is debossed CLOMID 50.
DDAVP® (desmopressin acetate) 0.1 mg Tablets are coded with "DDAVP" on one side of the bisect and "0.1" on the other side of the bisect. "RPR" is coded on the reverse.
DDAVP® (desmopressin acetate) 0.2 mg Tablets are coded with "DDAVP" on one side of the bisect and "0.2" on the other side of the bisect. "RPR" is coded on the reverse.
DIAβETA® (glyburide) Tablets 1.25 mg, 2.5 mg, and 5 mg are either imprinted with "DiaB" on one side, or with "Hoechst" on one side and "Diaβ" on the other side.
HIPREX® Tablets, 1 g (methenamine hippurate) is debossed MERRELL 277.
KETEK™ (telithromycin) Tablets are imprinted with "H3647" on one side and "400" on the other side.
LASIX® (furosemide) Tablets 20 mg are imprinted with "Lasix® " on one side and "HOECHST" on the other.
LASIX® (furosemide) Tablets 40 mg are imprinted with "Lasix® 40" on one side and the Hoechst logo on the other.
LASIX® (furosemide) Tablets 80 mg are imprinted with "Lasix® 80" on one side and the Hoechst logo on the other.
NILANDRON® Tablets have a triangular logo on one side and an internal reference number (168 D) on the other.
NORPRAMIN® Tablets, 10 mg (desipramine hydrochloride USP) is imprinted 68-7.
NORPRAMIN® Tablets, 25 mg (desipramine hydrochloride USP) is imprinted NORPRAMIN 25.
NORPRAMIN® Tablets, 50 mg (desipramine hydrochloride USP) is imprinted NORPRAMIN 50.
NORPRAMIN® Tablets, 75 mg (desipramine hydrochloride USP) is imprinted NORPRAMIN 75.
NORPRAMIN® Tablets, 100 mg (desipramine hydrochloride USP) is imprinted NORPRAMIN 100.
NORPRAMIN® Tablets, 150 mg (desipramine hydrochloride USP) is imprinted NORPRAMIN 150.
RIFADIN® Capsules, 150 mg (rifampin) is imprinted "RIFADIN 150".
RIFADIN® Capsules, 300 mg (rifampin) is imprinted "RIFADIN 300".
RIFAMATE® Capsules, 300 mg rifampin and 150 mg isoniazid is imprinted "RIFAMATE" on both ends of the capsule.
RIFATER® Tablets, 120 mg rifampin, 50 mg isoniazid, and 300 mg pyrazinamide is imprinted with "RIFATER".
RILUTEK® (riluzole) 50 mg Tablets are engraved with "RPR 202" on one side.
TENUATE® Tablets, 25 mg (diethylpropion hydrochloride USP) is debossed TENUATE 25 or MERRELL 697.
TENUATE® DOSPAN® Controlled-Release Tablets, 75 mg (diethylpropion hydrochloride USP) is debossed TENUATE 75 or MERRELL 698.
TRENTAL® (pentoxifylline) Tablets 400 mg are imprinted "TRENTAL".
UAS-AM-10497-1

ALLEGRA® ℞
[ə- 'lĕgrə]
(fexofenadine hydrochloride)
Capsules and Tablets

Rev. May 2003a

DESCRIPTION

Fexofenadine hydrochloride, the active ingredient of ALLEGRA, is a histamine H_1-receptor antagonist with the chemical name (±)-4-[1-hydroxy-4-[4-(hydroxydiphenylmethyl)-1-piperidinyl]-butyl]-α, α-dimethyl benzeneacetic acid hydrochloride. It has the following chemical structure

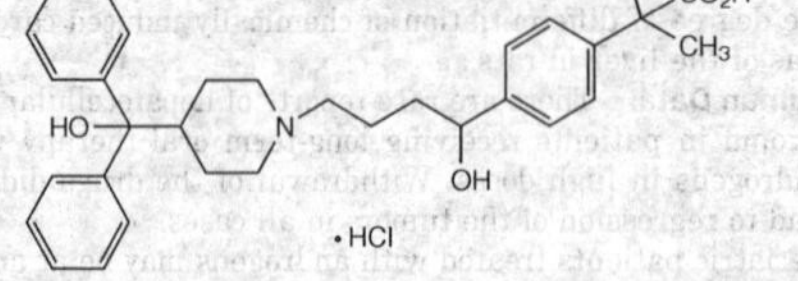

The molecular weight is 538.13 and the empirical formula is $C_{32}H_{39}NO_4 \cdot HCl$.
Fexofenadine hydrochloride is a white to off-white crystalline powder. It is freely soluble in methanol and ethanol, slightly soluble in chloroform and water, and insoluble in hexane. Fexofenadine hydrochloride is a racemate and exists as a zwitterion in aqueous media at physiological pH.
ALLEGRA is formulated as a capsule or tablet for oral administration. Each capsule contains 60 mg fexofenadine hydrochloride and the following excipients: croscarmellose sodium, gelatin, lactose, microcrystalline cellulose, and pregelatinized starch. The printed capsule shell is made from gelatin, iron oxide, silicon dioxide, sodium lauryl sulfate, titanium dioxide, and other ingredients.
Each tablet contains 30, 60, or 180 mg fexofenadine hydrochloride (depending on the dosage strength) and the following excipients: croscarmellose sodium, magnesium stearate, microcrystalline cellulose, and pregelatinized starch. The aqueous tablet film coating is made from hypromellose, iron oxide blends, polyethylene glycol, povidone, silicone dioxide, and titanium dioxide.

CLINICAL PHARMACOLOGY

Mechanism of Action

Fexofenadine hydrochloride is an antihistamine with selective peripheral H_1-receptor antagonist activity. Both enantiomers of fexofenadine hydrochloride displayed approximately equipotent antihistaminic effects. Fexofenadine inhibited histamine release from peritoneal mast cells in rats. In laboratory animals, no anticholinergic, $alpha_1$-adrenergic or beta-adrenergic-receptor blocking effects were observed. No sedative or other central nervous system effects were observed. Radiolabeled tissue distribution studies in rats indicated that fexofenadine does not cross the blood-brain barrier.

Pharmacokinetics

Absorption:
Fexofenadine hydrochloride was rapidly absorbed following oral administration of a single dose of two 60 mg capsules to healthy male volunteers with a mean time to maximum plasma concentration occurring at 2.6 hours post-dose. After administration of a single 60 mg capsule to healthy subjects, the mean maximum plasma concentration was 131 ng/mL. Following single dose oral administrations of either the 60 and 180 mg tablet to healthy, adult male volunteers, mean maximum plasma concentrations were 142 and 494 ng/mL, respectively. The tablet formulations are bioequivalent to the capsule when administered at equal doses. Fexofenadine hydrochloride pharmacokinetics are linear for oral doses up to a total daily dose of 240 mg (120 mg twice daily). The administration of the 60 mg capsule contents mixed with applesauce did not have a significant effect on the pharmacokinetics of fexofenadine in adults.

Distribution:
Fexofenadine hydrochloride is 60% to 70% bound to plasma proteins, primarily albumin and α_1-acid glycoprotein.

Elimination:
The mean elimination half-life of fexofenadine was 14.4 hours following administration of 60 mg, twice daily, in normal volunteers.
Human mass balance studies documented a recovery of approximately 80% and 11% of the [^{14}C] fexofenadine hydrochloride dose in the feces and urine, respectively. Because the absolute bioavailability of fexofenadine hydrochloride has not been established, it is unknown if the fecal component represents unabsorbed drug or the result of biliary excretion.

Metabolism:
Approximately 5% of the total oral dose was metabolized.

Special Populations:
Special population pharmacokinetics (for geriatric subjects, renal and hepatic impairment), obtained after a single dose of 80 mg fexofenadine hydrochloride, were compared to those for normal subjects from a separate study of similar design. While subject weights were relatively uniform between studies, these adult special population patients were substantially older than the healthy, young volunteers. Thus, an age effect may be confounding the pharmacokinetic differences observed in some of the special populations.

Seasonal allergic rhinitis (SAR) and chronic idiopathic urticaria (CIU) patients. The pharmacokinetics of fexofenadine hydrochloride in seasonal allergic rhinitis and chronic idiopathic urticaria patients were similar to those in healthy subjects.

Geriatric Subjects. In older subjects (≥65 years old), peak plasma levels of fexofenadine were 99% greater than those observed in normal volunteers (<65 years old). Mean elimination half-lives were similar to those observed in normal volunteers.

Pediatric Patients. Cross study comparisons indicated that fexofenadine hydrochloride area under the curve (AUC) following oral administration of a 60 mg dose to 7–12 year old pediatric allergic rhinitis patients was 56% greater compared to healthy adult subjects given the same dose. Plasma exposure in pediatric patients given 30 mg fexofenadine hydrochloride is comparable to adults given 60 mg.

Renal Impairment. In patients with mild to moderate (creatinine clearance 41–80 mL/min) and severe (creatinine clearance 11–40 mL/min) renal impairment, peak plasma levels of fexofenadine were 87% and 111% greater, respectively, and mean elimination half-lives were 59% and 72% longer, respectively, than observed in normal volunteers. Peak plasma levels in patients on dialysis (creatinine clearance ≤10 mL/min) were 82% greater and half-life was 31% longer than observed in normal volunteers. Based on increases in bioavailability and half-life, a dose of 60 mg once daily is recommended as the starting dose in patients with decreased renal function. (See DOSAGE AND ADMINISTRATION).

Hepatic Impairment. The pharmacokinetics of fexofenadine hydrochloride in patients with hepatic disease did not differ substantially from that observed in healthy patients.

Effect of Gender. Across several trials, no clinically significant gender-related differences were observed in the pharmacokinetics of fexofenadine hydrochloride.

Pharmacodynamics

Wheal and Flare. Human histamine skin wheal and flare studies following single and twice daily doses of 20 and 40 mg fexofenadine hydrochloride demonstrated that the drug exhibits an antihistamine effect by 1 hour, achieves maximum effect at 2 to 3 hours, and an effect is still seen at 12 hours. There was no evidence of tolerance to these effects after 28 days of dosing.
Histamine skin wheal and flare studies in 7 to 12 year old patients showed that following a single dose of 30 or 60 mg, antihistamine effect was observed at 1 hour and reached a maximum by 3 hours. Greater than 49% inhibition of wheal area, and 74% inhibition of flare area were maintained for 8 hours following the 30 and 60 mg dose.

Effects on QT_c. In dogs (30 mg/kg/orally twice a day), and in rabbits (10 mg/kg, infused intravenously over 1 hour) fexofenadine hydrochloride did not prolong QT_c. In dogs, the plasma fexofenadine concentration was approximately 9 times the therapeutic plasma concentrations in adults receiving the maximum recommended daily oral dose. In rabbits, the plasma fexofenadine concentration was approximately 20 times the therapeutic plasma concentration in adults receiving the maximum recommended daily oral dose. No effect was observed on calcium channel current, delayed potassium channel current, or action potential duration in guinea pig myocytes, sodium current in rat neonatal myocytes, or on several delayed rectifier potassium channels cloned from human heart at concentrations up to 1 x 10^{-5} M of fexofenadine hydrochloride.

No statistically significant increase in mean QT_c interval compared to placebo was observed in 714 seasonal allergic rhinitis patients given fexofenadine hydrochloride capsules in doses of 60 to 240 mg twice daily for two weeks. Pediatric patients from two placebo controlled trials (n=855) treated with up to 60 mg fexofenadine hydrochloride twice daily demonstrated no significant treatment or dose-related increases in QT_c. In addition, no statistically significant increase in mean QT_c interval compared to placebo was observed in 40 healthy volunteers given fexofenadine hydrochloride as an oral solution at doses up to 400 mg twice daily for 6 days, or in 231 healthy volunteers given fexofenadine hydrochloride 240 mg once daily for 1 year.

Clinical Studies

Seasonal Allergic Rhinitis:

Adults. In three, 2-week, multicenter, randomized, double-blind, placebo-controlled trials in patients 12 to 68 years of age with seasonal allergic rhinitis (n=1634), fexofenadine hydrochloride 60 mg twice daily significantly reduced total symptom scores (the sum of the individual scores for sneezing, rhinorrhea, itchy nose/palate/throat, itchy/watery/red eyes) compared to placebo. Statistically significant reductions in symptom scores were observed following the first 60 mg dose, with the effect maintained throughout the 12-hour interval. In these studies, there was no additional reduction in total symptom scores with higher doses of fexofenadine hydrochloride up to 240 mg twice daily.

In one 2-week, multicenter, randomized, double-blind clinical trial in patients 12 to 65 years of age with seasonal allergic rhinitis (n=863), fexofenadine hydrochloride 180 mg once daily significantly reduced total symptom scores (the sum of the individual scores for sneezing, rhinorrhea, itchy nose/palate/throat, itchy/watery/red eyes) compared to placebo. Although the number of patients in some of the subgroups was small, there were no significant differences in the effect of fexofenadine hydrochloride across subgroups of patients defined by gender, age, and race. Onset of action for reduction in total symptom scores, excluding nasal congestion, was observed at 60 minutes compared to placebo following a single 60 mg fexofenadine hydrochloride dose administered to patients with seasonal allergic rhinitis who were exposed to ragweed pollen in an environmental exposure unit. In one clinical trial conducted with ALLEGRA 60 mg capsules, and in one clinical trial conducted with ALLEGRA-D extended release tablets, onset of action was seen within 1 to 3 hours.

Pediatrics. Two 2-week multicenter, randomized, placebo-controlled, double-blind trials in 877 pediatric patients 6 to 11 years of age with seasonal allergic rhinitis were conducted at doses of 15, 30, and 60 mg twice daily. In one of these two studies, conducted in 411 pediatric patients, all three doses of fexofenadine hydrochloride significantly reduced total symptom scores (the sum of the individual scores for sneezing, rhinorrhea, itchy nose/palate/throat, itchy/watery/red eyes) compared to placebo, however a dose response relationship was not seen. The 60 mg twice daily dose did not provide any additional benefit over the 30 mg twice daily dose. Furthermore, exposure in pediatric patients given 30 mg fexofenadine hydrochloride is comparable to adults given 60 mg (see CLINICAL PHARMACOLOGY).

Three clinical safety studies in 845 children aged 6 months to 5 years with allergic rhinitis comparing 15 mg BID (n=85) and 30 mg BID (n=330) of an experimental formulation of fexofenadine to placebo (n=430) have been conducted. In general, fexofenadine hydrochloride was well tolerated in these studies. No unexpected adverse events were seen given the known safety profile of fexofenadine and likely adverse reactions for this patient population. (See PRECAUTIONS Pediatric Use and ADVERSE REACTIONS.)

Chronic Idiopathic Urticaria:

Two 4-week multicenter, randomized, double-blind, placebo-controlled clinical trials compared four different doses of fexofenadine hydrochloride tablet (20, 60, 120, and 240 mg twice daily) to placebo in patients aged 12 to 70 years with chronic idiopathic urticaria (n=726). Efficacy was demonstrated by a significant reduction in mean pruritus scores (MPS), mean number of wheals (MNW), and mean total symptom scores (MTSS, the sum of the MPS and MNW score). Although all four doses were significantly superior to placebo, symptom reduction was greater and efficacy was maintained over the entire 4-week treatment period with fexofenadine hydrochloride doses of ≥60 mg twice daily. However, no additional benefit of the 120 or 240 mg fexofenadine hydrochloride twice daily dose was seen over the 60 mg twice daily dose in reducing symptom scores. There were no significant differences in the effect of fexofenadine hydrochloride across subgroups of patients defined by gender, age, weight, and race.

Effects on steady-state fexofenadine hydrochloride pharmacokinetics after 7 days of co-administration with fexofenadine hydrochloride 120 mg every 12 hours (two times the recommended twice daily dose) in normal volunteers (n=24)

Concomitant Drug	C_{maxSS} *(Peak plasma concentration)*	$AUC_{SS(0-12h)}$ *(Extent of systemic exposure)*
Erythromycin (500 mg every 8 hrs)	+82%	+109%
Ketoconazole (400 mg once daily)	+135%	+164%

INDICATIONS AND USAGE

Seasonal Allergic Rhinitis

ALLEGRA is indicated for the relief of symptoms associated with seasonal allergic rhinitis in adults and children 6 years of age and older. Symptoms treated effectively were sneezing, rhinorrhea, itchy nose/palate/throat, itchy/watery/red eyes.

Chronic Idiopathic Urticaria

ALLEGRA is indicated for treatment of uncomplicated skin manifestations of chronic idiopathic urticaria in adults and children 6 years of age and older. It significantly reduces pruritus and the number of wheals.

CONTRAINDICATIONS

ALLEGRA is contraindicated in patients with known hypersensitivity to any of its ingredients.

PRECAUTIONS

Drug Interaction with Erythromycin and Ketoconazole

Fexofenadine hydrochloride has been shown to exhibit minimal (ca. 5%) metabolism. However, co-administration of fexofenadine hydrochloride with ketoconazole and erythromycin led to increased plasma levels of fexofenadine hydrochloride. Fexofenadine hydrochloride had no effect on the pharmacokinetics of erythromycin and ketoconazole. In two separate studies, fexofenadine hydrochloride 120 mg twice daily (two times the recommended twice daily dose) was co-administered with erythromycin 500 mg every 8 hours or ketoconazole 400 mg once daily under steady-state conditions to normal, healthy volunteers (n=24, each study). No differences in adverse events or QT_c interval were observed when patients were administered fexofenadine hydrochloride alone or in combination with erythromycin or ketoconazole. The findings of these studies are summarized in the following table:

[See table above]

The changes in plasma levels were within the range of plasma levels achieved in adequate and well-controlled clinical trials.

The mechanism of these interactions has been evaluated in *in vitro, in situ,* and *in vivo* animal models. These studies indicate that ketoconazole or erythromycin co-administration enhances fexofenadine gastrointestinal absorption. *In vivo* animal studies also suggest that in addition to increasing absorption, ketoconazole decreases fexofenadine hydrochloride gastrointestinal secretion, while erythromycin may also decrease biliary excretion.

Drug Interactions with Antacids

Administration of 120 mg of fexofenadine hydrochloride (2 x 60 mg capsule) within 15 minutes of an aluminum and magnesium containing antacid (Maalox®) decreased fexofenadine AUC by 41% and C_{max} by 43%. ALLEGRA should not be taken closely in time with aluminum and magnesium containing antacids.

Carcinogenesis, Mutagenesis, Impairment of Fertility

The carcinogenic potential and reproductive toxicity of fexofenadine hydrochloride were assessed using terfenadine studies with adequate fexofenadine hydrochloride exposure (based on plasma area-under-the-concentration vs. time [AUC] values). No evidence of carcinogenicity was observed in an 18-month study in mice and in a 24-month study in rats at oral doses up to 150 mg/kg of terfenadine (which led to fexofenadine exposures that were respectively approximately 3 and 5 times the exposure from the maximum recommended daily oral dose of fexofenadine hydrochloride in adults and children).

In *in vitro* (Bacterial Reverse Mutation, CHO/HGPRT Forward Mutation, and Rat Lymphocyte Chromosomal Aberration assays) and *in vivo* (Mouse Bone Marrow Micronucleus assay) tests, fexofenadine hydrochloride revealed no evidence of mutagenicity.

In rat fertility studies, dose-related reductions in implants and increases in postimplantation losses were observed at an oral dose of 150 mg/kg of terfenadine (which led to fexofenadine hydrochloride exposures that were approximately 3 times the exposure of the maximum recommended daily oral dose of fexofenadine hydrochloride in adults).

Pregnancy

Teratogenic Effects: Category C. There was no evidence of teratogenicity in rats or rabbits at oral doses of terfenadine up to 300 mg/kg (which led to fexofenadine exposures that were approximately 4 and 31 times, respectively, the exposure from the maximum recommended daily oral dose of fexofenadine in adults).

There are no adequate and well controlled studies in pregnant women. Fexofenadine should be used during pregnancy only if the potential benefit justifies the potential risk to the fetus.

Nonteratogenic Effects. Dose-related decreases in pup weight gain and survival were observed in rats exposed to an oral dose of 150 mg/kg of terfenadine (approximately 3 times the maximum recommended daily oral dose of fexofenadine hydrochloride in adults based on comparison of fexofenadine hydrochloride AUCs).

Nursing Mothers

There are no adequate and well-controlled studies in women during lactation. Because many drugs are excreted in human milk, caution should be exercised when fexofenadine hydrochloride is administered to a nursing woman.

Pediatric Use

The recommended dose in patients 6 to 11 years of age is based on cross-study comparison of the pharmacokinetics of ALLEGRA in adults and pediatric patients and on the safety profile of fexofenadine hydrochloride in both adult and pediatric patients at doses equal to or higher than the recommended doses.

The safety of ALLEGRA tablets at a dose of 30 mg twice daily has been demonstrated in 438 pediatric patients 6 to 11 years of age in two placebo-controlled 2-week seasonal allergic rhinitis trials. The safety of ALLEGRA for the treatment of chronic idiopathic urticaria in patients 6 to 11 years of age is based on cross-study comparison of the pharmacokinetics of ALLEGRA in adult and pediatric patients and on the safety profile of fexofenadine in both adult and pediatric patients at doses equal to or higher than the recommended dose.

The effectiveness of ALLEGRA for the treatment of seasonal allergic rhinitis in patients 6 to 11 years of age was demonstrated in one trial (n=411) in which ALLEGRA tablets 30 mg twice daily significantly reduced total symptom scores compared to placebo, along with extrapolation of demonstrated efficacy in patients ages 12 years and above, and the pharmacokinetic comparisons in adults and children. The effectiveness of ALLEGRA for the treatment of chronic idiopathic urticaria in patients 6 to 11 years of age is based on an extrapolation of the demonstrated efficacy of ALLEGRA in adults with this condition and the likelihood that the disease course, pathophysiology and the drug's effect are substantially similar in children to that of adult patients.

Three clinical safety studies comparing 15 mg BID (n=85) and 30 mg BID (n=330) of an experimental formulation of fexofenadine to placebo (n=430) have been conducted in pediatric patients aged 6 months to 5 years. In general, fexofenadine hydrochloride was well tolerated in these studies. No unexpected adverse events were seen given the known safety profile of fexofenadine and likely adverse reactions for this patient population. (See ADVERSE REACTIONS and CLINICAL PHARMACOLOGY.)

The safety and effectiveness of fexofenadine hydrochloride in pediatric patients under 6 years of age have not been established.

Geriatric Use

Clinical studies of ALLEGRA tablets and capsules did not include sufficient numbers of subjects aged 65 years and over to determine whether this population responds differently from younger patients. Other reported clinical experience has not identified differences in responses between the geriatric and younger patients. This drug is known to be substantially excreted by the kidney, and the risk of toxic reactions to this drug may be greater in patients with impaired renal function. Because elderly patients are more likely to have decreased renal function, care should be taken in dose selection, and may be useful to monitor renal function. (See CLINICAL PHARMACOLOGY).

ADVERSE REACTIONS

Seasonal Allergic Rhinitis

Adults. In placebo-controlled seasonal allergic rhinitis clinical trials in patients 12 years of age and older, which included 2461 patients receiving fexofenadine hydrochloride capsules at doses of 20 mg to 240 mg twice daily, adverse events were similar in fexofenadine hydrochloride and placebo-treated patients. All adverse events that were reported by greater than 1% of patients who received the recommended daily dose of fexofenadine hydrochloride (60 mg capsules twice daily), and that were more common with fexofenadine hydrochloride than placebo, are listed in Table 1.

In a placebo-controlled clinical study in the United States, which included 570 patients aged 12 years and older receiving fexofenadine hydrochloride tablets at doses of 120 or 180 mg once daily, adverse events were similar in fexofenadine hydrochloride and placebo-treated patients. Table 1 also lists adverse experiences that were reported by greater than 2% of patients treated with fexofenadine hydrochloride tablets at doses of 180 mg once daily and that were more common with fexofenadine hydrochloride than placebo.

Continued on next page

Allegra—Cont.

The incidence of adverse events, including drowsiness, was not dose-related and was similar across subgroups defined by age, gender, and race.
[See table 1 below]
The frequency and magnitude of laboratory abnormalities were similar in fexofenadine hydrochloride and placebo-treated patients.
Pediatric. Table 2 lists adverse experiences in patients aged 6 to 11 years of age which were reported by greater than 2% of patients treated with fexofenadine hydrochloride tablets at a dose of 30 mg twice daily in placebo-controlled seasonal allergic rhinitis studies in the United States and Canada that were more common with fexofenadine hydrochloride than placebo.
[See table 2 below]
Three clinical safety studies in 845 children aged 6 months to 5 years comparing 15 mg BID (n=85) and 30 mg BID (n=330) of an experimental formulation of fexofenadine to placebo (n=430) have been conducted. In general, fexofenadine hydrochloride was well tolerated in these studies. No unexpected adverse events were seen given the known safety profile of fexofenadine and likely adverse reactions for this patient population. (See PRECAUTIONS Pediatric Use.)

Chronic Idiopathic Urticaria
Adverse events reported by patients 12 years of age and older in placebo-controlled chronic idiopathic urticaria studies were similar to those reported in placebo-controlled seasonal allergic rhinitis studies. In placebo-controlled chronic idiopathic urticaria clinical trials, which included 726 patients 12 years of age and older receiving fexofenadine hydrochloride tablets at doses of 20 to 240 mg twice daily, adverse events were similar in fexofenadine hydrochloride and placebo-treated patients. Table 3 lists adverse experiences in patients aged 12 years and older which were reported by greater than 2% of patients treated with fexofenadine hydrochloride 60 mg tablets twice daily in controlled clinical studies in the United States and Canada and that were more common with fexofenadine hydrochloride than placebo. The safety of fexofenadine hydrochloride in the treatment of chronic idiopathic urticaria in pediatric patients 6 to 11 years of age is based on the safety profile of fexofenadine hydrochloride in adults and adolescent patients at doses equal to or higher than the recommended dose (see Pediatric Use).
[See table 3 below]
Events that have been reported during controlled clinical trials involving seasonal allergic rhinitis and chronic idiopathic urticaria patients with incidences less than 1% and similar to placebo and have been rarely reported during postmarketing surveillance include: insomnia, nervousness, and sleep disorders or paroniria. In rare cases, rash, urticaria, pruritus and hypersensitivity reactions with manifestations such as angioedema, chest tightness, dyspnea, flushing and systemic anaphylaxis have been reported.

OVERDOSAGE

Reports of fexofenadine hydrochloride overdose have been infrequent and contain limited information. However, dizziness, drowsiness, and dry mouth have been reported. Single doses of fexofenadine hydrochloride up to 800 mg (six normal volunteers at this dose level), and doses up to 690 mg twice daily for 1 month (three normal volunteers at this dose level) or 240 mg once daily for 1 year (234 normal volunteers at this dose level) were administered without the development of clinically significant adverse events as compared to placebo.
In the event of overdose, consider standard measures to remove any unabsorbed drug. Symptomatic and supportive treatment is recommended.
Hemodialysis did not effectively remove fexofenadine hydrochloride from blood (1.7% removed) following terfenadine administration.
No deaths occurred at oral doses of fexofenadine hydrochloride up to 5000 mg/kg in mice (110 times the maximum recommended daily oral dose in adults and 200 times the maximum recommended daily oral dose in children based on mg/m^2) and up to 5000 mg/kg in rats (230 times the maximum recommended daily oral dose in adults and 400 times the maximum recommended daily oral dose in children based on mg/m^2). Additionally, no clinical signs of toxicity or gross pathological findings were observed. In dogs, no evidence of toxicity was observed at oral doses up to 2000 mg/kg (300 times the maximum recommended daily oral dose in adults and 530 times the maximum recommended daily oral dose in children based on mg/m^2).

Table 1
Adverse experiences in patients ages 12 years and older reported in placebo-controlled seasonal allergic rhinitis clinical trials in the United States

Twice daily dosing with fexofenadine capsules at rates of greater than 1%

Adverse experience	*Fexofenadine 60 mg Twice Daily (n=679)*	*Placebo Twice Daily (n=671)*
Viral Infection (cold, flu)	2.5%	1.5%
Nausea	1.6%	1.5%
Dysmenorrhea	1.5%	0.3%
Drowsiness	1.3%	0.9%
Dyspepsia	1.3%	0.6%
Fatigue	1.3%	0.9%

Once daily dosing with fexofenadine hydrochloride tablets at rates of greater than 2%

Adverse experience	*Fexofenadine 180 mg once daily (n=283)*	*Placebo (n=293)*
Headache	10.6%	7.5%
Upper Respiratory Tract Infection	3.2%	3.1%
Back Pain	2.8%	1.4%

Table 2
Adverse experiences reported in placebo-controlled seasonal allergic rhinitis studies in pediatric patients ages 6 to 11 in the United States and Canada at rates of greater than 2%

Adverse experience	*Fexofenadine 30 mg twice daily (n=209)*	*Placebo (n=229)*
Headache	7.2%	6.6%
Accidental Injury	2.9%	1.3%
Coughing	3.8%	1.3%
Fever	2.4%	0.9%
Pain	2.4%	0.4%
Otitis Media	2.4%	0.0%
Upper Respiratory Tract Infection	4.3%	1.7%

Table 3
Adverse experiences reported in patients 12 years and older in placebo-controlled chronic idiopathic urticaria studies in the United States and Canada at rates of greater than 2%

Adverse experience	*Fexofenadine 60 mg twice daily (n=186)*	*Placebo (n=178)*
Back Pain	2.2%	1.1%
Sinusitis	2.2%	1.1%
Dizziness	2.2%	0.6%
Drowsiness	2.2%	0.0%

DOSAGE AND ADMINISTRATION

Seasonal Allergic Rhinitis
Adults and Children 12 Years and Older. The recommended dose of ALLEGRA is 60 mg twice daily, or 180 mg once daily. A dose of 60 mg once daily is recommended as the starting dose in patients with decreased renal function (see CLINICAL PHARMACOLOGY).
Children 6 to 11 Years. The recommended dose of ALLEGRA is 30 mg twice daily. A dose of 30 mg once daily is recommended as the starting dose in pediatric patients with decreased renal function (see CLINICAL PHARMACOLOGY).
Chronic Idiopathic Urticaria
Adults and Children 12 Years and Older. The recommended dose of ALLEGRA is 60 mg twice daily. A dose of 60 mg once daily is recommended as the starting dose in patients with decreased renal function (see CLINICAL PHARMACOLOGY).
Children 6 to 11 Years. The recommended dose of ALLEGRA is 30 mg twice daily. A dose of 30 mg once daily is recommended as the starting dose in pediatric patients with decreased renal function (see CLINICAL PHARMACOLOGY).

HOW SUPPLIED

ALLEGRA 60 mg capsules are available in: high-density polyethylene (HDPE) bottles of 60 (NDC 0088-1102-41); HDPE bottles of 100 (NDC 0088-1102-47); HDPE bottles of 500 (NDC 0088-1102-55); and aluminum-foil blister packs of 100 (NDC 0088-1102-49).
ALLEGRA capsules have a white opaque cap and a pink opaque body. The capsules are imprinted in black ink, with "ALLEGRA" on the cap and "60 mg" on the body.
ALLEGRA 30 mg tablets are available in: high-density polyethylene (HDPE) bottles of 100 (NDC 0088-1106-47) with a polypropylene screw cap containing a pulp/wax liner with heat-sealed foil inner seal and HDPE bottles of 500 (NDC 0088-1106-55) with a polypropylene screw cap containing a pulp/wax liner with heat-sealed foil inner seal.
ALLEGRA 60 mg tablets are available in: HDPE bottles of 100 (NDC 0088-1107-47) with a polypropylene screw cap containing a pulp/wax liner with heat-sealed foil inner seal; HDPE bottles of 500 (NDC 0088-1107-55) with a polypropylene screw cap containing a pulp/wax liner with heat-sealed foil inner seal; and aluminum foil-backed clear blister packs of 100 (NDC 0088-1107-49).
ALLEGRA 180 mg tablets are available in: HDPE bottles of 100 (NDC 0088-1109-47) with a polypropylene screw cap containing a pulp/wax liner with heat-sealed foil inner seal; and HDPE bottles of 500 (NDC 0088-1109-55) with a polypropylene screw cap containing a pulp/wax liner with heat-sealed foil inner seal.
ALLEGRA tablets are coated with a peach colored film coating. Tablets have the following unique identifiers: 30 mg tablets have 03 on one side and either 0088 or scripted E on the other; 60 mg tablets have 06 on one side and either 0088 or scripted E on the other; and 180 mg tablets have 018 on one side and either 0088 or scripted E on the other.
Store ALLEGRA capsules and tablets at controlled room temperature 20–25°C (68–77°F). (See USP Controlled Room Temperature). Foil-backed blister packs containing ALLEGRA capsules and all tablet packaging should be protected from excessive moisture.
Rx only
Rev. May 2003a
Aventis Pharmaceuticals Inc.
Kansas City, MO 64137 USA
US Patents 4,254,129; 5,375,693; 5,578,610

www.allegra.com
Shown in Product Identification Guide, page 306

ALLEGRA-D® ℞

[ə-'lĕgra-D]
(fexofenadine HCl 60 mg and pseudoephedrine HCl 120 mg)
Extended-Release Tablets

Prescribing Information as of January 2003

DESCRIPTION

ALLEGRA-D® (fexofenadine hydrochloride and pseudoephedrine hydrochloride) Extended-Release Tablets for oral administration contain 60 mg fexofenadine hydrochloride for immediate-release and 120 mg pseudoephedrine hydrochloride for extended-release. Tablets also contain as excipients: microcrystalline cellulose, pregelatinized starch, croscarmellose sodium, magnesium stearate, carnauba wax, stearic acid, silicon dioxide, hypromellose and polyethylene glycol.
Fexofenadine hydrochloride, one of the active ingredients of ALLEGRA-D, is a histamine H_1-receptor antagonist with the chemical name (±)-4-[1-hydroxy-4-[4-(hydroxydiphenylmethyl)-1-piperidinyl]-butyl]-α, α-dimethyl benzeneacetic acid hydrochloride and the following chemical structure:
[See chemical structure at top of next column]
The molecular weight is 538.13 and the empirical formula is $C_{32}H_{39}NO_4{\cdot}HCl$. Fexofenadine hydrochloride is a white to off-white crystalline powder. It is freely soluble in methanol and ethanol, slightly soluble in chloroform and water, and insoluble in hexane. Fexofenadine hydrochloride is a racemate and exists as a zwitterion in aqueous media at physiological pH.
Pseudoephedrine hydrochloride, the other active ingredient of ALLEGRA-D, is an adrenergic (vasoconstrictor) agent

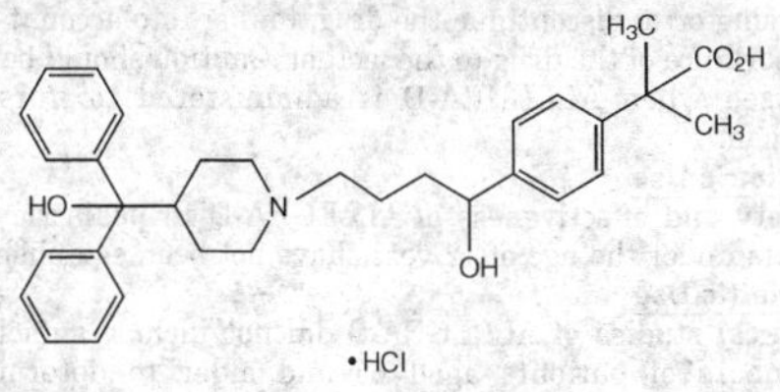

with the chemical name [S-(R*,R*)]-α-[1-(methylamino) ethyl]-benzenemethanol hydrochloride and the following chemical structure:

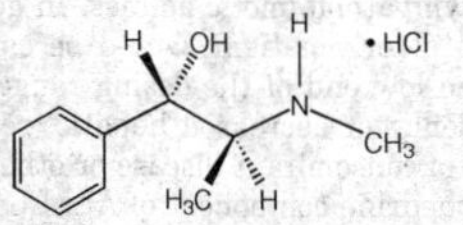

The molecular weight is 201.70. The molecular formula is $C_{10}H_{15}NO \cdot HCl$. Pseudoephedrine hydrochloride occurs as fine, white to off-white crystals or powder, having a faint characteristic odor. It is very soluble in water, freely soluble in alcohol, and sparingly soluble in chloroform.

CLINICAL PHARMACOLOGY

Mechanism of Action

Fexofenadine hydrochloride, the major active metabolite of terfenadine, is an antihistamine with selective peripheral H_1-receptor antagonist activity. Fexofenadine hydrochloride inhibited antigen-induced bronchospasm in sensitized guinea pigs and histamine release from peritoneal mast cells in rats. In laboratory animals, no anticholinergic or alpha$_1$-adrenergic-receptor blocking effects were observed. Moreover, no sedative or other central nervous system effects were observed. Radiolabeled tissue distribution studies in rats indicated that fexofenadine does not cross the blood-brain barrier.

Pseudoephedrine hydrochloride is an orally active sympathomimetic amine and exerts a decongestant action on the nasal mucosa. Pseudoephedrine hydrochloride is recognized as an effective agent for the relief of nasal congestion due to allergic rhinitis. Pseudoephedrine produces peripheral effects similar to those of ephedrine and central effects similar to, but less intense than, amphetamines. It has the potential for excitatory side effects. At the recommended oral dose, it has little or no pressor effect in normotensive adults.

Pharmacokinetics

The pharmacokinetics of fexofenadine hydrochloride and pseudoephedrine hydrochloride when administered separately have been well characterized. Fexofenadine pharmacokinetics were linear for oral doses of fexofenadine hydrochloride up to 120 mg twice daily. The mean elimination half-life of fexofenadine was 14.4 hours following administration of 60 mg fexofenadine hydrochloride, twice daily, to steady-state in normal volunteers. Human mass balance studies documented a recovery of approximately 80% and 11% of the [^{14}C] fexofenadine hydrochloride dose in the feces and urine, respectively. Approximately 5% of the total dose was metabolized. Because the absolute bioavailability of fexofenadine hydrochloride has not been established, it is unknown if the fecal component is unabsorbed drug or the result of biliary excretion. The pharmacokinetics of fexofenadine hydrochloride in seasonal allergic rhinitis patients were similar to those in healthy subjects. Peak fexofenadine plasma concentrations were similar between adolescent (12–16 years of age) and adult patients. Fexofenadine is 60% to 70% bound to plasma proteins, primarily albumin and α_1-acid glycoprotein.

Pseudoephedrine has been shown to have a mean elimination half-life of 4–6 hours which is dependent on urine pH. The elimination half-life is decreased at urine pH lower than 6 and may be increased at urine pH higher than 8.

The bioavailability of fexofenadine hydrochloride and pseudoephedrine hydrochloride from ALLEGRA-D Extended-Release Tablets is similar to that achieved with separate administration of the components. Coadministration of fexofenadine and pseudoephedrine does not significantly affect the bioavailability of either component.

Fexofenadine hydrochloride was rapidly absorbed following single-dose administration of the 60 mg fexofenadine hydrochloride/120 mg pseudoephedrine hydrochloride tablet with median time to mean maximum fexofenadine plasma concentration of 191 ng/mL occurring 2 hours postdose. Pseudoephedrine hydrochloride produced a mean single-dose pseudoephedrine peak plasma concentration of 206 ng/mL which occurred 6 hours postdose. Following multiple dosing to steady-state, a fexofenadine peak concentration of 255 ng/mL was observed 2 hours postdose. Following multiple dosing to steady-state, a pseudoephedrine peak concentration of 411 ng/mL was observed 5 hours postdose. Co-administration of ALLEGRA-D with a high-fat meal decreased fexofenadine plasma concentrations C_{max} (−46%) and AUC (−42%). Time to maximum concentration (T_{max}) was delayed by 50%. The rate or extent of pseudoephedrine absorption was not affected by food. It is recommended that the administration of ALLEGRA-D with food should be avoided. (See DOSAGE AND ADMINISTRATION).

Special Populations

Special population pharmacokinetics (for renal and hepatic impairment and age), obtained after a single dose of 80 mg fexofenadine hydrochloride, were compared to those from normal subjects in a separate study of similar design. While subject weights were relatively uniform between studies, these special population patients were substantially older than the healthy, young volunteers. Thus, an age effect may be confounding the pharmacokinetic differences observed in some of the special populations.

Effect of Age. In older subjects (≥65 years old), peak plasma levels of fexofenadine were 99% greater than those observed in younger subjects (<65 years old). Mean elimination half-lives were similar to those observed in younger subjects.

Renally Impaired. In patients with mild (creatinine clearance 41–80 mL/min) to severe (creatinine clearance 11–40 mL/min) renal impairment, peak plasma levels of fexofenadine were 87% and 111% greater, respectively, and mean elimination half-lives were 59% and 72% longer, respectively, than observed in normal volunteers. Peak plasma levels in patients on dialysis (creatinine clearance ≤10 mL/min) were 82% greater and half-life was 31% longer than observed in normal volunteers.

About 55–75% of an administered dose of pseudoephedrine hydrochloride is excreted unchanged in the urine; the remainder is apparently metabolized in the liver. Therefore, pseudoephedrine may accumulate in patients with renal insufficiency.

Based on increases in bioavailability and half-life of fexofenadine hydrochloride and pseudoephedrine hydrochloride, a dose of one tablet once daily is recommended as the starting dose in patients with decreased renal function (See DOSAGE AND ADMINISTRATION).

Hepatically Impaired. The pharmacokinetics of fexofenadine hydrochloride in patients with hepatic disease did not differ substantially from that observed in healthy subjects. The effect on pseudoephedrine pharmacokinetics is unknown.

Effect of Gender. Across several trials, no clinically significant gender-related differences were observed in the pharmacokinetics of fexofenadine hydrochloride.

Pharmacodynamics

Wheal and Flare. Human histamine skin wheal and flare studies following single and twice daily doses of 20 mg and 40 mg fexofenadine hydrochloride demonstrated that the drug exhibits an antihistamine effect by 1 hour, achieves maximum effect at 2–3 hours, and an effect is still seen at 12 hours. There was no evidence of tolerance to these effects after 28 days of dosing. The clinical significance of these observations is not known.

Effects on QT_c. In dogs, (10 mg/kg/day, orally for 5 days) and rabbits (10 mg/kg, intravenously over one hour) fexofenadine hydrochloride did not prolong QT_c at plasma concentrations that were at least 28 and 63 times, respectively, the therapeutic plasma concentrations in man (based on a 60 mg twice daily fexofenadine hydrochloride dose). No effect was observed on calcium channel current, delayed K^+ channel current, or action potential duration in guinea pig myocytes, Na^+ current in rat neonatal myocytes, or on the delayed rectifier K^+ channel cloned from human heart at concentrations up to 1×10^{-5} M of fexofenadine. This concentration was at least 32 times the therapeutic plasma concentration in man (based on a 60 mg twice daily fexofenadine hydrochloride dose).

No statistically significant increase in mean QT_c interval compared to placebo was observed in 714 seasonal allergic rhinitis patients given fexofenadine hydrochloride capsules in doses of 60 mg to 240 mg twice daily for two weeks or in 40 healthy volunteers given fexofenadine hydrochloride as an oral solution at doses up to 400 mg twice daily for 6 days.

A one year study designed to evaluate safety and tolerability of 240 mg of fexofenadine hydrochloride (n=240) compared to placebo (n=237) in healthy subjects, did not reveal a statistically significant increase in the mean QT_c interval for the fexofenadine hydrochloride treated group when evaluated pretreatment and after 1, 2, 3, 6, 9, and 12 months of treatment.

Administration of the 60 mg fexofenadine hydrochloride/120 mg pseudoephedrine hydrochloride combination tablet for approximately 2 weeks to 213 patients with seasonal allergic rhinitis demonstrated no statistically significant increase in the mean QT_c interval compared to fexofenadine hydrochloride administered alone (60 mg twice daily, n=215), or compared to pseudoephedrine hydrochloride (120 mg twice daily, n=215) administered alone.

Clinical Studies

In a 2-week, multicenter, randomized, double-blind, active-controlled trial in patients 12–65 years of age with seasonal allergic rhinitis due to ragweed allergy (n=651), the 60 mg fexofenadine hydrochloride/120 mg pseudoephedrine hydrochloride combination tablet administered twice daily significantly reduced the intensity of sneezing, rhinorrhea, itchy nose/palate/throat, itchy/watery/red eyes, and nasal congestion.

In three, 2-week, multicenter, randomized, double-blind, placebo-controlled trials in patients 12–68 years of age with seasonal allergic rhinitis (n=1634), fexofenadine hydrochloride 60 mg twice daily significantly reduced total symptom scores (the sum of the individual scores for sneezing, rhinorrhea, itchy nose/palate/throat, itchy/watery/red eyes) compared to placebo. Statistically significant reductions in symptom scores were observed following the first 60 mg dose, with the effect maintained throughout the 12-hour interval. In general, there was no additional reduction in total symptom scores with higher doses of fexofenadine hydrochloride up to 240 mg twice daily. Although the number of subjects in some of the subgroups was small, there were no significant differences in the effect of fexofenadine hydrochloride across subgroups of patients defined by gender, age, and race. Onset of action for reduction in total symptom scores, excluding nasal congestion, was observed at 60 minutes compared to placebo following a single 60 mg fexofenadine hydrochloride dose administered to patients with seasonal allergic rhinitis who were exposed to ragweed pollen in an environmental exposure unit.

INDICATIONS AND USAGE

ALLEGRA-D is indicated for the relief of symptoms associated with seasonal allergic rhinitis in adults and children 12 years of age and older. Symptoms treated effectively include sneezing, rhinorrhea, itchy nose/palate/ and/or throat, itchy/watery/red eyes, and nasal congestion.

ALLEGRA-D should be administered when both the antihistaminic properties of fexofenadine hydrochloride and the nasal decongestant properties of pseudoephedrine hydrochloride are desired (see CLINICAL PHARMACOLOGY).

CONTRAINDICATIONS

ALLEGRA-D is contraindicated in patients with known hypersensitivity to any of its ingredients.

Due to its pseudoephedrine component, ALLEGRA-D is contraindicated in patients with narrow-angle glaucoma or urinary retention, and in patients receiving monoamine oxidase (MAO) inhibitor therapy or within fourteen (14) days of stopping such treatment (see Drug Interactions section). It is also contraindicated in patients with severe hypertension, or severe coronary artery disease, and in those who have shown hypersensitivity or idiosyncrasy to its components, to adrenergic agents, or to other drugs of similar chemical structures. Manifestations of patient idiosyncrasy to adrenergic agents include: insomnia, dizziness, weakness, tremor, or arrhythmias.

WARNINGS

Sympathomimetic amines should be used judiciously and sparingly in patients with hypertension, diabetes mellitus, ischemic heart disease, increased intraocular pressure, hyperthyroidism, renal impairment, or prostatic hypertrophy (see CONTRAINDICATIONS). Sympathomimetic amines may produce central nervous system stimulation with convulsions or cardiovascular collapse with accompanying hypotension.

PRECAUTIONS

General

Due to its pseudoephedrine component, ALLEGRA-D should be used with caution in patients with hypertension, diabetes mellitus, ischemic heart disease, increased intraocular pressure, hyperthyroidism, renal impairment, or prostatic hypertrophy (see WARNINGS and CONTRAINDICATIONS). Patients with decreased renal function should be given a lower initial dose (one tablet per day) because they have reduced elimination of fexofenadine and pseudoephedrine (See CLINICAL PHARMACOLOGY and DOSAGE AND ADMINISTRATION).

Information for Patients

Patients taking ALLEGRA-D tablets should receive the following information: ALLEGRA-D tablets are prescribed for the relief of symptoms of seasonal allergic rhinitis. Patients should be instructed to take ALLEGRA-D tablets only as prescribed. **Do not exceed the recommended dose.** If nervousness, dizziness, or sleeplessness occur, discontinue use and consult the doctor. Patients should also be advised against the concurrent use of ALLEGRA-D tablets with over-the-counter antihistamines and decongestants.

The product should not be used by patients who are hypersensitive to it or to any of its ingredients. Due to its pseudoephedrine component, this product should not be used by patients with narrow-angle glaucoma, urinary retention, or by patients receiving a monoamine oxidase (MAO) inhibitor or within 14 days of stopping use of MAO inhibitor. It also should not be used by patients with severe hypertension or severe coronary artery disease.

Patients should be told that this product should be used in pregnancy or lactation only if the potential benefit justifies the potential risk to the fetus or nursing infant. Patients should be cautioned not to break or chew the tablet. Patients should be directed to swallow the tablet whole. Patients should be instructed not to take the tablet with food. Patients should also be instructed to store the medication in a tightly closed container in a cool, dry place, away from children.

Drug Interactions

Fexofenadine hydrochloride and pseudoephedrine hydrochloride do not influence the pharmacokinetics of each other when administered concomitantly.

Fexofenadine has been shown to exhibit minimal (ca. 5%) metabolism. However, co-administration of fexofenadine with ketoconazole and erythromycin led to increased plasma levels of fexofenadine. Fexofenadine had no effect on the pharmacokinetics of erythromycin and ketoconazole. In two separate studies, fexofenadine HCl 120 mg BID (twice the recommended dose) was co-administered with erythromycin 500 mg every 8 hours or ketoconazole 400 mg once daily under steady-state conditions to normal, healthy volunteers (n=24, each study). No differences in adverse events or QT_c interval were observed when subjects were administered fexofenadine HCl alone or in combination with erythromycin or ketoconazole. The findings of these studies are summarized in the following table:

Continued on next page

Allegra-D—Cont.

Effects on Steady-State Fexofenadine Pharmacokinetics After 7 Days of Co-Administration with Fexofenadine Hydrochloride 120 mg Every 12 Hours (twice recommended dose) in Normal Volunteers (n=24)

Concomitant Drug	$C_{max,SS}$ (Peak plasma concentration)	AUC_{SS} (0–12h) (Extent of systemic exposure)
Erythromycin (500 mg every 8 hrs)	+82%	+109%
Ketoconazole (400 mg once daily)	+135%	+164%

The changes in plasma levels were within the range of plasma levels achieved in adequate and well-controlled clinical trials.
The mechanism of these interactions has been evaluated in *in vitro*, *in situ* and *in vivo* animal models. These studies indicate that ketoconazole or erythromycin co-administration enhances fexofenadine gastrointestinal absorption. *In vivo* animal studies also suggest that in addition to enhancing absorption, ketoconazole decreases fexofenadine gastrointestinal secretion, while erythromycin may also decrease biliary excretion.
ALLEGRA-D tablets (pseudoephedrine component) are contraindicated in patients taking monoamine oxidase inhibitors and for 14 days after stopping use of an MAO inhibitor. Concomitant use with antihypertensive drugs which interfere with sympathetic activity (eg, methyldopa, mecamylamine, and reserpine) may reduce their antihypertensive effects. Increased ectopic pacemaker activity can occur when pseudoephedrine is used concomitantly with digitalis.
Care should be taken in the administration of ALLEGRA-D concomitantly with other sympathomimetic amines because combined effects on the cardiovascular system may be harmful to the patient (see WARNINGS).

Carcinogenesis, Mutagenesis, Impairment of Fertility
There are no animal or in vitro studies on the combination product fexofenadine hydrochloride and pseudoephedrine hydrochloride to evaluate carcinogenesis, mutagenesis, or impairment of fertility.
The carcinogenic potential and reproductive toxicity of fexofenadine hydrochloride were assessed using terfenadine studies with adequate fexofenadine exposure (area-under-the plasma concentration versus time curve [AUC]). No evidence of carcinogenicity was observed when mice and rats were given daily oral doses up to 150 mg/kg of terfenadine for 18 and 24 months, respectively. In both species, 150 mg/kg of terfenadine produced AUC values of fexofenadine that were approximately 3 times the human AUC at the maximum recommended daily oral dose in adults.
Two-year feeding studies in rats and mice conducted under the auspices of the National Toxicology Program (NTP) demonstrated no evidence of carcinogenic potential with ephedrine sulfate, a structurally related drug with pharmacological properties similar to pseudoephedrine, at doses up to 10 and 27 mg/kg, respectively (approximately 1/3 and 1/2, respectively, the maximum recommended daily oral dose of pseudoephedrine hydrochloride in adults on a mg/m^2 basis).
In *in vitro* (Bacterial Reverse Mutation, CHO/HGPRT Forward Mutation, and Rat Lymphocyte Chromosomal Aberration assays) and *in vivo* (Mouse Bone Marrow Micronucleus assay) tests, fexofenadine hydrochloride revealed no evidence of mutagenicity.
Reproduction and fertility studies with terfenadine in rats produced no effect on male or female fertility at oral doses up to 300 mg/kg/day. However, reduced implants and post implantation losses were reported at 300 mg/kg. A reduction in implants was also observed at an oral dose of 150 mg/kg/day. Oral doses of 150 and 300 mg/kg of terfenadine produced AUC values of fexofenadine that were approximately 3 and 4 times, respectively, the human AUC at the maximum recommended daily oral dose in adults.

Pregnancy
Teratogenic Effects: Category C. Terfenadine alone was not teratogenic in rats and rabbits at oral doses up to 300 mg/kg; 300 mg/kg of terfenadine produced fexofenadine AUC values that were approximately 4 and 30 times, respectively, the human AUC at the maximum recommended daily oral dose in adults.
The combination of terfenadine and pseudoephedrine hydrochloride in a ratio of 1:2 by weight was studied in rats and rabbits. In rats, an oral combination dose of 150/300 mg/kg produced reduced fetal weight and delayed ossification with a finding of wavy ribs. The dose of 150 mg/kg of terfenadine in rats produced an AUC value of fexofenadine that was approximately 3 times the human AUC at the maximum recommended daily oral dose in adults. The dose of 300 mg/kg of pseudoephedrine hydrochloride in rats was approximately 10 times the maximum recommended daily oral dose in adults on a mg/m^2 basis. In rabbits, an oral combination dose of 100/200 mg/kg produced decreased fetal weight. By extrapolation, the AUC of fexofenadine for 100 mg/kg orally of terfenadine was approximately 10 times the human AUC at the maximum recommended daily oral dose in adults. The dose of 200 mg/kg of pseudoephedrine hydrochloride was approximately 15 times the maximum recommended daily oral dose in adults on a mg/m^2 basis.
There are no adequate and well-controlled studies in pregnant women. ALLEGRA-D should be used during pregnancy only if the potential benefit justifies the potential risk to the fetus.
Nonteratogenic Effects. Dose-related decreases in pup weight gain and survival were observed in rats exposed to an oral dose of 150 mg/kg of terfenadine; this dose produced an AUC of fexofenadine that was approximately 3 times the human AUC at the maximum recommended daily oral dose in adults.

Nursing Mothers
It is not known if fexofenadine is excreted in human milk. Because many drugs are excreted in human milk, caution should be used when fexofenadine hydrochloride is administered to a nursing woman. Pseudoephedrine hydrochloride administered alone distributes into breast milk of lactating human females. Pseudoephedrine concentrations in milk are consistently higher than those in plasma. The total amount of drug in milk as judged by AUC is 2 to 3 times greater than the plasma AUC. The fraction of a pseudoephedrine dose excreted in milk is estimated to be 0.4% to 0.7%. A decision should be made whether to discontinue nursing or to discontinue the drug, taking into account the importance of the drug to the mother. Caution should be exercised when ALLEGRA-D is administered to nursing women.

Pediatric Use
Safety and effectiveness of ALLEGRA-D in pediatric patients under the age of 12 years have not been established.

Geriatric Use
Clinical studies of ALLEGRA-D did not include sufficient numbers of patients aged 65 and older to determine whether they respond differently from younger patients. Other reported clinical experience has not identified differences in responses between the elderly and younger patients, although the elderly are more likely to have adverse reactions to sympathomimetic amines. In general, dose selection for an elderly patient should be cautious, usually starting at the low end of the dosing range, reflecting the greater frequency of decreased hepatic, renal, or cardiac function, and of concomitant disease or other drug therapy.
The pseudoephedrine component of ALLEGRA-D is known to be substantially excreted by the kidney, and the risk of toxic reactions to this drug may be greater in patients with impaired renal function. Because elderly patients are more likely to have decreased renal function, care should be taken in dose selection, and it may be useful to monitor renal function.

ADVERSE REACTIONS

ALLEGRA-D
In one clinical trial (n=651) in which 215 patients with seasonal allergic rhinitis received the 60 mg fexofenadine hydrochloride/120 mg pseudoephedrine hydrochloride combination tablet twice daily for up to 2 weeks, adverse events were similar to those reported either in patients receiving fexofenadine hydrochloride 60 mg alone (n=218 patients) or in patients receiving pseudoephedrine hydrochloride 120 mg alone (n=218). A placebo group was not included in this study.
The percent of patients who withdrew prematurely because of adverse events was 3.7% for the fexofenadine hydrochloride/pseudoephedrine hydrochloride combination group, 0.5% for the fexofenadine hydrochloride group, and 4.1% for the pseudoephedrine hydrochloride group. All adverse events that were reported by greater than 1% of patients who received the recommended daily dose of the fexofenadine hydrochloride/pseudoephedrine hydrochloride combination are listed in the following table.
[See table below]

Adverse Experiences Reported in One Active-Controlled Seasonal Allergic Rhinitis Clinical Trial at Rates of Greater than 1%

Adverse Experience	60 mg Fexofenadine Hydrochloride/120 mg Pseudoephedrine Hydrochloride Combination Tablet Twice Daily (n=215)	Fexofenadine Hydrochloride 60 mg Twice Daily (n=218)	Pseudoephedrine Hydrochloride 120 mg Twice Daily (n=218)
Headache	13.0%	11.5%	17.4%
Insomnia	12.6%	3.2%	13.3%
Nausea	7.4%	0.5%	5.0%
Dry Mouth	2.8%	0.5%	5.5%
Dyspepsia	2.8%	0.5%	0.9%
Throat Irritation	2.3%	1.8%	0.5%
Dizziness	1.9%	0.0%	3.2%
Agitation	1.9%	0.0%	1.4%
Back Pain	1.9%	0.5%	0.5%
Palpitation	1.9%	0.0%	0.9%
Nervousness	1.4%	0.5%	1.8%
Anxiety	1.4%	0.0%	1.4%
Upper Respiratory Infection	1.4%	0.9%	0.9%
Abdominal Pain	1.4%	0.5%	0.5%

Many of the adverse events occurring in the fexofenadine hydrochloride/pseudoephedrine hydrochloride combination group were adverse events also reported predominately in the pseudoephedrine hydrochloride group, such as insomnia, headache, nausea, dry mouth, dizziness, agitation, nervousness, anxiety, and palpitation.

Fexofenadine Hydrochloride
In placebo-controlled clinical trials, which included 2461 patients receiving fexofenadine hydrochloride at doses of 20 mg to 240 mg twice daily, adverse events were similar in fexofenadine hydrochloride and placebo-treated patients. The incidence of adverse events, including drowsiness, was not dose related and was similar across subgroups defined by age, gender, and race. The percent of patients who withdrew prematurely because of adverse events was 2.2% with fexofenadine hydrochloride vs 3.3% with placebo.
Events that have been reported during controlled clinical trials involving seasonal allergic rhinitis and chronic idiopathic urticaria patients with incidences less than 1% and similar to placebo and have been rarely reported during postmarketing surveillance include: insomnia, nervousness, and sleep disorders or paroniria. In rare cases, rash, urticaria, pruritus and hypersensitivity reactions with manifestations such as angioedema, chest tightness, dyspnea, flushing and systemic anaphylaxis have been reported.

Pseudoephedrine Hydrochloride
Pseudoephedrine hydrochloride may cause mild CNS stimulation in hypersensitive patients. Nervousness, excitability, restlessness, dizziness, weakness, or insomnia may occur. Headache, drowsiness, tachycardia, palpitation, pressor activity, and cardiac arrhythmias have been reported. Sympathomimetic drugs have also been associated with other untoward effects such as fear, anxiety, tenseness, tremor, hallucinations, seizures, pallor, respiratory difficulty, dysuria, and cardiovascular collapse.

OVERDOSAGE

Most reports of fexofenadine hydrochloride overdose contain limited information. However, dizziness, drowsiness, and dry mouth have been reported. For the pseudoephedrine hydrochloride component of ALLEGRA-D, information on acute overdose is limited to the marketing history of pseudoephedrine hydrochloride. Single doses of fexofenadine hydrochloride up to 800 mg (6 normal volunteers at this dose level), and doses up to 690 mg twice daily for one month (3 normal volunteers at this dose level), were administered without the development of clinically significant adverse events.
In large doses, sympathomimetics may give rise to giddiness, headache, nausea, vomiting, sweating, thirst, tachycardia, precordial pain, palpitations, difficulty in micturition, muscular weakness and tenseness, anxiety, restlessness, and insomnia. Many patients can present a toxic psychosis with delusions and hallucinations. Some may develop cardiac arrhythmias, circulatory collapse, convulsions, coma, and respiratory failure.

In the event of overdose, consider standard measures to remove any unabsorbed drug. Symptomatic and supportive treatment is recommended. Hemodialysis did not effectively remove fexofenadine from blood (up to 1.7% removed) following terfenadine administration.
The effect of hemodialysis on the removal of pseudoephedrine is unknown.
No deaths occurred in mature mice and rats at oral doses of fexofenadine hydrochloride up to 5000 mg/kg (approximately 170 and 340 times, respectively, the maximum recommended daily oral dose in adults on a mg/m^2 basis.) The median oral lethal dose in newborn rats was 438 mg/kg (approximately 30 times the maximum recommended daily oral dose in adults on a mg/m^2 basis). In dogs, no evidence of toxicity was observed at oral doses up to 2000 mg/kg (approximately 450 times the maximum recommended human daily oral dose in adults on a mg/m^2 basis). The oral median lethal dose of pseudoephedrine hydrochloride in rats was 1674 mg/kg (approximately 55 times the maximum recommended daily oral dose in adults on a mg/m^2 basis).

DOSAGE AND ADMINISTRATION

The recommended dose of ALLEGRA-D is one tablet twice daily for adults and children 12 years of age and older. It is recommended that the administration of ALLEGRA-D with food should be avoided. A dose of one tablet once daily is recommended as the starting dose in patients with decreased renal function. (See CLINICAL PHARMACOLOGY and PRECAUTIONS.)

HOW SUPPLIED

ALLEGRA-D (fexofenadine hydrochloride and pseudoephedrine hydrochloride) Extended-Release Tablets contain 60 mg fexofenadine hydrochloride for immediate-release and 120 mg pseudoephedrine hydrochloride for extended-release. ALLEGRA-D (fexofenadine hydrochloride and pseudoephedrine hydrochloride) Extended-Release Tablets are available in: high-density polyethylene (HDPE) bottles of 60 (NDC 0088-1090-41) with a polypropylene child-resistant cap containing a pulp/wax liner with heat-sealed foil inner seal; HDPE bottles of 100 (NDC 0088-1090-47) with a polypropylene screw cap containing a pulp/wax liner with heat-sealed foil inner seal; HDPE bottles of 500 (NDC 0088-1090-55) with a polypropylene screw cap containing a pulp/wax liner with heat-sealed foil inner seal; and aluminum foil-backed clear blister packs of 100 (NDC 0088-1090-49).
ALLEGRA-D is a two-layer tablet, one white layer and one tan layer with a clear film coating on the tablet. The tablets are engraved with "Allegra-D" on the white layer.
Store ALLEGRA-D Extended-Release Tablets at 20–25°C (68–77°F). (See USP Controlled Room Temperature.)
Rx only
Prescribing Information as of January 2003
Aventis Pharmaceuticals Inc.
Kansas City, MO 64137 USA
US Patents 4,254,129; 5,375,693; 5,578,610.

www.allegra.com
alldp0103p
Shown in Product Identification Guide, page 306

AMARYL® ℞

[am'ə ril]
(glimepiride tablets)
1, 2, and 4 mg
℞ Only
Prescribing Information as of February 2003

DESCRIPTION

AMARYL® (glimepiride tablets) is an oral blood-glucose-lowering drug of the sulfonylurea class. Glimepiride is a white to yellowish-white, crystalline, odorless to practically odorless powder formulated into tablets of 1-mg, 2-mg, and 4-mg strengths for oral administration. AMARYL tablets contain the active ingredient glimepiride and the following inactive ingredients: lactose (hydrous), sodium starch glycolate, povidone, microcrystalline cellulose, and magnesium stearate. In addition, AMARYL 1-mg tablets contain Ferric Oxide Red, AMARYL 2-mg tablets contain Ferric Oxide Yellow and FD&C Blue #2 Aluminum Lake, and AMARYL 4-mg tablets contain FD&C Blue #2 Aluminum Lake.
Chemically, glimepiride is identified as 1-[[p-[2-(3-ethyl-4-methyl-2-oxo-3-pyrroline-1-carboxamido)ethyl]phenyl]sulfonyl]-3-(trans-4-methylcyclohexyl)urea.
The CAS Registry Number is 93479-97-1
The structural formula is:

Molecular Formula: $C_{24}H_{34}N_4O_5S$
Molecular Weight: 490.62
Glimepiride is practically insoluble in water.

CLINICAL PHARMACOLOGY

Mechanism Of Action

The primary mechanism of action of glimepiride in lowering blood glucose appears to be dependent on stimulating the release of insulin from functioning pancreatic beta cells. In addition, extrapancreatic effects may also play a role in the activity of sulfonylureas such as glimepiride. This is supported by both preclinical and clinical studies demonstrating that glimepiride administration can lead to increased sensitivity of peripheral tissues to insulin. These findings are consistent with the results of a long-term, randomized, placebo-controlled trial in which AMARYL therapy improved postprandial insulin/C-peptide responses and overall glycemic control without producing clinically meaningful increases in fasting insulin/C-peptide levels. However, as with other sulfonylureas, the mechanism by which glimepiride lowers blood glucose during long-term administration has not been clearly established.
AMARYL is effective as initial drug therapy. In patients where monotherapy with AMARYL or metformin has not produced adequate glycemic control, the combination of AMARYL and metformin may have a synergistic effect, since both agents act to improve glucose tolerance by different primary mechanisms of action. This complementary effect has been observed with metformin and other sulfonylureas, in multiple studies.

Pharmacodynamics

A mild glucose-lowering effect first appeared following single oral doses as low as 0.5–0.6 mg in healthy subjects. The time required to reach the maximum effect (i.e., minimum blood glucose level [T_{min}]) was about 2 to 3 hours. In noninsulin-dependent (Type II) diabetes mellitus (NIDDM) patients, both fasting and 2-hour postprandial glucose levels were significantly lower with glimepiride (1, 2, 4, and 8 mg once daily) than with placebo after 14 days of oral dosing. The glucose-lowering effect in all active treatment groups was maintained over 24 hours.
In larger dose-ranging studies, blood glucose and HbA_{1c} were found to respond in a dose-dependent manner over the range of 1 to 4 mg/day of AMARYL. Some patients, particularly those with higher fasting plasma glucose (FPG) levels, may benefit from doses of AMARYL up to 8 mg once daily. No difference in response was found when AMARYL was administered once or twice daily.
In two 14-week, placebo-controlled studies in 720 subjects, the average net reduction in HbA_{1c} for AMARYL (glimepiride tablets) patients treated with 8 mg once daily was 2.0% in absolute units compared with placebo-treated patients. In a long-term, randomized, placebo-controlled study of NIDDM patients unresponsive to dietary management, AMARYL therapy improved postprandial insulin/C-peptide responses, and 75% of patients achieved and maintained control of blood glucose and HbA_{1c}. Efficacy results were not affected by age, gender, weight, or race.
In long-term extension trials with previously-treated patients, no meaningful deterioration in mean fasting blood glucose (FBG) or HbA_{1c} levels was seen after 2 1/2 years of AMARYL therapy.
Combination therapy with AMARYL and insulin (70% NPH/30% regular) was compared to placebo/insulin in secondary failure patients whose body weight was >130% of their ideal body weight. Initially, 5–10 units of insulin were administered with the main evening meal and titrated upward weekly to achieve predefined FPG values. Both groups in this double-blind study achieved similar reductions in FPG levels but the AMARYL/insulin therapy group used approximately 38% less insulin.
AMARYL therapy is effective in controlling blood glucose without deleterious changes in the plasma lipoprotein profiles of patients treated for NIDDM.

Pharmacokinetics

Absorption. After oral administration, glimepiride is completely (100%) absorbed from the GI tract. Studies with single oral doses in normal subjects and with multiple oral doses in patients with NIDDM have shown significant absorption of glimepiride within 1 hour after administration and peak drug levels (C_{max}) at 2 to 3 hours. When glimepiride was given with meals, the mean T_{max} (time to reach C_{max}) was slightly increased (12%) and the mean C_{max} and AUC (area under the curve) were slightly decreased (8% and 9%, respectively).
Distribution. After intravenous (IV) dosing in normal subjects, the volume of distribution (Vd) was 8.8 L (113 mL/kg), and the total body clearance (CL) was 47.8 mL/min. Protein binding was greater than 99.5%.
Metabolism. Glimepiride is completely metabolized by oxidative biotransformation after either an IV or oral dose. The major metabolites are the cyclohexyl hydroxy methyl derivative (M1) and the carboxyl derivative (M2). Cytochrome P450 II C9 has been shown to be involved in the biotransformation of glimepiride to M1. M1 is further metabolized to M2 by one or several cytosolic enzymes. M1, but not M2, possesses about 1/3 of the pharmacological activity as compared to its parent in an animal model; however, whether the glucose-lowering effect of M1 is clinically meaningful is not clear.
Excretion. When ^{14}C-glimepiride was given orally, approximately 60% of the total radioactivity was recovered in the urine in 7 days and M1 (predominant) and M2 accounted for 80–90% of that recovered in the urine. Approximately 40% of the total radioactivity was recovered in feces and M1 and M2 (predominant) accounted for about 70% of that recovered in feces. No parent drug was recovered from urine or feces. After IV dosing in patients, no significant biliary excretion of glimepiride or its M1 metabolite has been observed.
Pharmacokinetic Parameters. The pharmacokinetic parameters of glimepiride obtained from a single-dose, crossover, dose-proportionality (1, 2, 4, and 8 mg) study in normal subjects and from a single- and multiple-dose, parallel, dose-proportionality (4 and 8 mg) study in patients with NIDDM are summarized below:
[See table above]

	Volunteers Single Dose Mean±SD	Patients with NIDDM Single Dose (Day 1) Mean±SD	Multiple Dose (Day 10) Mean±SD
C_{max} (ng/mL)			
1 mg	103 ± 34 (12)	—	—
2 mg	177 ± 44 (12)	—	—
4 mg	308 ± 69 (12)	352 ± 222 (12)	309 ± 134 (12)
8 mg	551 ± 152 (12)	591 ± 232 (14)	578 ± 265 (11)
T_{max} (h)	2.4 ± 0.8 (48)	2.5 ± 1.2 (26)	2.8 ± 2.2 (23)
CL/f (mL/min)	52.1 ± 16.0 (48)	48.5 ± 29.3 (26)	52.7 ± 40.3 (23)
Vd/f (L)	21.8 ± 13.9 (48)	19.8 ± 12.7 (26)	37.1 ± 18.2 (23)
T1/2 (h)	5.3 ± 4.1 (48)	5.0 ± 2.5 (26)	9.2 ± 3.6 (23)

( ) = No. of subjects
CL/f = Total body clearance after oral dosing
Vd/f = Volume of distribution calculated after oral dosing

These data indicate that glimepiride did not accumulate in serum, and the pharmacokinetics of glimepiride were not different in healthy volunteers and in NIDDM patients. Oral clearance of glimepiride did not change over the 1-8-mg dose range, indicating linear pharmacokinetics.
Variability. In normal healthy volunteers, the intra-individual variabilities of C_{max}, AUC, and CL/f for glimepiride were 23%, 17%, and 15%, respectively, and the inter-individual variabilities were 25%, 29%, and 24%, respectively.

Special Populations

Geriatric. Comparison of glimepiride pharmacokinetics in NIDDM patients ≤65 years and those >65 years was performed in a study using a dosing regimen of 6 mg daily. There were no significant differences in glimepiride pharmacokinetics between the two age groups. The mean AUC at steady state for the older patients was about 13% lower than that for the younger patients; the mean weight-adjusted clearance for the older patients was about 11% higher than that for the younger patients.
Pediatric. No studies were performed in pediatric patients.
Gender. There were no differences between males and females in the pharmacokinetics of glimepiride when adjustment was made for differences in body weight.
Race. No pharmacokinetic studies to assess the effects of race have been performed, but in placebo-controlled studies of AMARYL (glimepiride tablets) in patients with NIDDM, the antihyperglycemic effect was comparable in whites (n = 536), blacks (n = 63), and Hispanics (n = 63).
Renal Insufficiency. A single-dose, open-label study was conducted in 15 patients with renal impairment. AMARYL (3 mg) was administered to 3 groups of patients with different levels of mean creatinine clearance (CLcr); (Group I, CLcr = 77.7 mL/min, n = 5), (Group II, CLcr = 27.7 mL/min, n = 3), and (Group III, CLcr = 9.4 mL/min, n = 7). AMARYL was found to be well tolerated in all 3 groups. The results showed that glimepiride serum levels decreased as renal function decreased. However, M1 and M2 serum levels (mean AUC values) increased 2.3 and 8.6 times from Group I to Group III. The apparent terminal half-life ($T_{1/2}$) for glimepiride did not change, while the half-lives for M1 and M2 increased as renal function decreased. Mean urinary excretion of M1 plus M2 as percent of dose, however, decreased (44.4%, 21.9%, and 9.3% for Groups I to III).
A multiple-dose titration study was also conducted in 16 NIDDM patients with renal impairment using doses ranging from 1–8 mg daily for 3 months. The results were consistent with those observed after single doses. All patients with a CLcr less than 22 mL/min had adequate control of their glucose levels with a dosage regimen of only 1 mg daily. The results from this study suggested that a starting dose of 1 mg AMARYL may be given to NIDDM patients with kidney disease, and the dose may be titrated based on fasting blood glucose levels.
Hepatic Insufficiency. No studies were performed in patients with hepatic insufficiency.
Other Populations. There were no important differences in glimepiride metabolism in subjects identified as phenotypically different drug-metabolizers by their metabolism of sparteine.
The pharmacokinetics of glimepiride in morbidly obese patients were similar to those in the normal weight group, except for a lower C_{max} and AUC. However, since neither C_{max} nor AUC values were normalized for body surface area, the lower values of C_{max} and AUC for the obese patients were likely the result of their excess weight and not due to a difference in the kinetics of glimepiride.

Continued on next page

Amaryl—Cont.

Drug Interactions. The hypoglycemic action of sulfonylureas may be potentiated by certain drugs, including nonsteroidal anti-inflammatory drugs and other drugs that are highly protein bound, such as salicylates, sulfonamides, chloramphenicol, coumarins, probenecid, monoamine oxidase inhibitors, and beta adrenergic blocking agents. When these drugs are administered to a patient receiving AMARYL, the patient should be observed closely for hypoglycemia. When these drugs are withdrawn from a patient receiving AMARYL, the patient should be observed closely for loss of glycemic control.

Certain drugs tend to produce hyperglycemia and may lead to loss of control. These drugs include the thiazides and other diuretics, corticosteroids, phenothiazines, thyroid products, estrogens, oral contraceptives, phenytoin, nicotinic acid, sympathomimetics, and isoniazid. When these drugs are administered to a patient receiving AMARYL, the patient should be closely observed for loss of control. When these drugs are withdrawn from a patient receiving AMARYL, the patient should be observed closely for hypoglycemia.

Coadministration of aspirin (1 g tid) and AMARYL led to a 34% decrease in the mean glimepiride AUC and, therefore, a 34% increase in the mean CL/f. The mean C_{max} had a decrease of 4%. Blood glucose and serum C-peptide concentrations were unaffected and no hypoglycemic symptoms were reported. Pooled data from clinical trials showed no evidence of clinically significant adverse interactions with uncontrolled concurrent administration of aspirin and other salicylates.

Coadministration of either cimetidine (800 mg once daily) or ranitidine (150 mg bid) with a single 4-mg oral dose of AMARYL did not significantly alter the absorption and disposition of glimepiride, and no differences were seen in hypoglycemic symptomatology. Pooled data from clinical trials showed no evidence of clinically significant adverse interactions with uncontrolled concurrent administration of H2-receptor antagonists.

Concomitant administration of propranolol (40 mg tid) and AMARYL significantly increased C_{max}, AUC, and $T_{1/2}$ of glimepiride by 23%, 22%, and 15%, respectively, and it decreased CL/f by 18%. The recovery of M1 and M2 from urine, however, did not change. The pharmacodynamic responses to glimepiride were nearly identical in normal subjects receiving propranolol and placebo. Pooled data from clinical trials in patients with NIDDM showed no evidence of clinically significant adverse interactions with uncontrolled concurrent administration of beta-blockers. However, if beta-blockers are used, caution should be exercised and patients should be warned about the potential for hypoglycemia.

Concomitant administration of AMARYL (glimepiride tablets) (4 mg once daily) did not alter the pharmacokinetic characteristics of R- and S-warfarin enantiomers following administration of a single dose (25 mg) of racemic warfarin to healthy subjects. No changes were observed in warfarin plasma protein binding. AMARYL treatment did result in a slight, but statistically significant, decrease in the pharmacodynamic response to warfarin. The reductions in mean area under the prothrombin time (PT) curve and maximum PT values during AMARYL treatment were very small (3.3% and 9.9%, respectively) and are unlikely to be clinically important.

The responses of serum glucose, insulin, C-peptide, and plasma glucagon to 2 mg AMARYL were unaffected by coadministration of ramipril (an ACE inhibitor) 5 mg once daily in normal subjects. No hypoglycemic symptoms were reported. Pooled data from clinical trials in patients with NIDDM showed no evidence of clinically significant adverse interactions with uncontrolled concurrent administration of ACE inhibitors.

A potential interaction between oral miconazole and oral hypoglycemic agents leading to severe hypoglycemia has been reported. Whether this interaction also occurs with the intravenous, topical, or vaginal preparations of miconazole is not known. Potential interactions of glimepiride with other drugs metabolized by cytochrome P450 II C9 also include phenytoin, diclofenac, ibuprofen, naproxen, and mefenamic acid.

Although no specific interaction studies were performed, pooled data from clinical trials showed no evidence of clinically significant adverse interactions with uncontrolled concurrent administration of calcium-channel blockers, estrogens, fibrates, NSAIDS, HMG CoA reductase inhibitors, sulfonamides, or thyroid hormone.

INDICATIONS AND USAGE

AMARYL is indicated as an adjunct to diet and exercise to lower the blood glucose in patients with noninsulin-dependent (Type II) diabetes mellitus (NIDDM) whose hyperglycemia cannot be controlled by diet and exercise alone. AMARYL may be used concomitantly with metformin when diet, exercise, and AMARYL or metformin alone do not result in adequate glycemic control.

AMARYL is also indicated for use in combination with insulin to lower blood glucose in patients whose hyperglycemia cannot be controlled by diet and exercise in conjunction with an oral hypoglycemic agent. Combined use of glimepiride and insulin may increase the potential for hypoglycemia.

In initiating treatment for noninsulin-dependent diabetes, diet and exercise should be emphasized as the primary form of treatment. Caloric restriction, weight loss, and exercise are essential in the obese diabetic patient. Proper dietary management and exercise alone may be effective in controlling the blood glucose and symptoms of hyperglycemia. In addition to regular physical activity, cardiovascular risk factors should be identified and corrective measures taken where possible.

If this treatment program fails to reduce symptoms and/or blood glucose, the use of an oral sulfonylurea or insulin should be considered. Use of AMARYL must be viewed by both the physician and patient as a treatment in addition to diet and exercise and not as a substitute for diet and exercise or as a convenient mechanism for avoiding dietary restraint. Furthermore, loss of blood glucose control on diet and exercise alone may be transient, thus requiring only short-term administration of AMARYL.

During maintenance programs, AMARYL monotherapy should be discontinued if satisfactory lowering of blood glucose is no longer achieved. Judgments should be based on regular clinical and laboratory evaluations. Secondary failures to AMARYL monotherapy can be treated with AMARYL-insulin combination therapy.

In considering the use of AMARYL in asymptomatic patients, it should be recognized that blood glucose control in NIDDM has not definitely been established to be effective in preventing the long-term cardiovascular and neural complications of diabetes. However, the Diabetes Control and Complications Trial (DCCT) demonstrated that control of HbA_{1c} and glucose was associated with a decrease in retinopathy, neuropathy, and nephropathy for insulin-dependent diabetic (IDDM) patients.

CONTRAINDICATIONS

AMARYL is contraindicated in patients with

1. Known hypersensitivity to the drug.
2. Diabetic ketoacidosis, with or without coma. This condition should be treated with insulin.

WARNINGS

SPECIAL WARNING ON INCREASED RISK OF CARDIOVASCULAR MORTALITY

The administration of oral hypoglycemic drugs has been reported to be associated with increased cardiovascular mortality as compared to treatment with diet alone or diet plus insulin. This warning is based on the study conducted by the University Group Diabetes Program (UGDP), a long-term, prospective clinical trial designed to evaluate the effectiveness of glucose-lowering drugs in preventing or delaying vascular complications in patients with non-insulin-dependent diabetes. The study involved 823 patients who were randomly assigned to one of four treatment groups (Diabetes, 19 supp. 2: 747–830, 1970).

UGDP reported that patients treated for 5 to 8 years with diet plus a fixed dose of tolbutamide (1.5 grams per day) had a rate of cardiovascular mortality approximately 2-1/2 times that of patients treated with diet alone. A significant increase in total mortality was not observed, but the use of tolbutamide was discontinued based on the increase in cardiovascular mortality, thus limiting the opportunity for the study to show an increase in overall mortality. Despite controversy regarding the interpretation of these results, the findings of the UGDP study provide an adequate basis for this warning. The patient should be informed of the potential risks and advantages of AMARYL (glimepiride tablets) and of alternative modes of therapy.

Although only one drug in the sulfonylurea class (tolbutamide) was included in this study, it is prudent from a safety standpoint to consider that this warning may also apply to other oral hypoglycemic drugs in this class, in view of their close similarities in mode of action and chemical structure.

PRECAUTIONS

General

Hypoglycemia: All sulfonylurea drugs are capable of producing severe hypoglycemia. Proper patient selection, dosage, and instructions are important to avoid hypoglycemic episodes. Patients with impaired renal function may be more sensitive to the glucose-lowering effect of AMARYL. A starting dose of 1 mg once daily followed by appropriate dose titration is recommended in those patients. Debilitated or malnourished patients, and those with adrenal, pituitary, or hepatic insufficiency are particularly susceptible to the hypoglycemic action of glucose-lowering drugs. Hypoglycemia may be difficult to recognize in the elderly and in people who are taking beta-adrenergic blocking drugs or other sympatholytic agents. Hypoglycemia is more likely to occur when caloric intake is deficient, after severe or prolonged exercise, when alcohol is ingested, or when more than one glucose-lowering drug is used. Combined use of glimepiride with insulin or metformin may increase the potential for hypoglycemia.

Loss of control of blood glucose: When a patient stabilized on any diabetic regimen is exposed to stress such as fever, trauma, infection, or surgery, a loss of control may occur. At such times, it may be necessary to add insulin in combination with AMARYL or even use insulin monotherapy. The effectiveness of any oral hypoglycemic drug, including AMARYL, in lowering blood glucose to a desired level decreases in many patients over a period of time, which may be due to progression of the severity of the diabetes or to diminished responsiveness to the drug. This phenomenon is known as secondary failure, to distinguish it from primary failure in which the drug is ineffective in an individual patient when first given. Should secondary failure occur with AMARYL or metformin monotherapy, combined therapy with AMARYL and metformin or AMARYL and insulin may result in a response. Should secondary failure occur with combined AMARYL/metformin therapy, it may be necessary to initiate insulin therapy.

Information for Patients

Patients should be informed of the potential risks and advantages of AMARYL and of alternative modes of therapy. They should also be informed about the importance of adherence to dietary instructions, of a regular exercise program, and of regular testing of blood glucose.

The risks of hypoglycemia, its symptoms and treatment, and conditions that predispose to its development should be explained to patients and responsible family members. The potential for primary and secondary failure should also be explained.

Laboratory Tests

Fasting blood glucose should be monitored periodically to determine therapeutic response. Glycosylated hemoglobin should also be monitored, usually every 3 to 6 months, to more precisely assess long-term glycemic control.

Drug Interactions

(See CLINICAL PHARMACOLOGY, Drug Interactions.)

Carcinogenesis, Mutagenesis, and Impairment of Fertility

Studies in rats at doses of up to 5000 ppm in complete feed (approximately 340 times the maximum recommended human dose, based on surface area) for 30 months showed no evidence of carcinogenesis. In mice, administration of glimepiride for 24 months resulted in an increase in benign pancreatic adenoma formation which was dose related and is thought to be the result of chronic pancreatic stimulation. The no-effect dose for adenoma formation in mice in this study was 320 ppm in complete feed, or 46–54 mg/kg body weight/day. This is about 35 times the maximum human recommended dose of 8 mg once daily based on surface area.

Glimepiride was non-mutagenic in a battery of *in vitro* and *in vivo* mutagenicity studies (Ames test, somatic cell mutation, chromosomal aberration, unscheduled DNA synthesis, mouse micronucleus test).

There was no effect of glimepiride on male mouse fertility in animals exposed up to 2500 mg/kg body weight (>1,700 times the maximum recommended human dose based on surface area). Glimepiride had no effect on the fertility of male and female rats administered up to 4000 mg/kg body weight (approximately 4,000 times the maximum recommended human dose based on surface area).

Pregnancy

Teratogenic Effects. Pregnancy Category C. Glimepiride did not produce teratogenic effects in rats exposed orally up to 4000 mg/kg body weight (approximately 4,000 times the maximum recommended human dose based on surface area) or in rabbits exposed up to 32 mg/kg body weight (approximately 60 times the maximum recommended human dose based on surface area). Glimepiride has been shown to be associated with intrauterine fetal death in rats when given in doses as low as 50 times the human dose based on surface area and in rabbits when given in doses as low as 0.1 times the human dose based on surface area. This fetotoxicity, observed only at doses inducing maternal hypoglycemia, has been similarly noted with other sulfonylureas, and is believed to be directly related to the pharmacologic (hypoglycemic) action of glimepiride.

There are no adequate and well-controlled studies in pregnant women. On the basis of results from animal studies, AMARYL (glimepiride tablets) should not be used during pregnancy. Because recent information suggests that abnormal blood glucose levels during pregnancy are associated with a higher incidence of congenital abnormalities, many experts recommend that insulin be used during pregnancy to maintain glucose levels as close to normal as possible.

Nonteratogenic Effects. In some studies in rats, offspring of dams exposed to high levels of glimepiride during pregnancy and lactation developed skeletal deformities consisting of shortening, thickening, and bending of the humerus during the postnatal period. Significant concentrations of glimepiride were observed in the serum and breast milk of the dams as well as in the serum of the pups. These skeletal deformations were determined to be the result of nursing from mothers exposed to glimepiride.

Prolonged severe hypoglycemia (4 to 10 days) has been reported in neonates born to mothers who were receiving a sulfonylurea drug at the time of delivery. This has been reported more frequently with the use of agents with prolonged half-lives. Patients who are planning a pregnancy should consult their physician, and it is recommended that they change over to insulin for the entire course of pregnancy and lactation.

Nursing Mothers

In rat reproduction studies, significant concentrations of glimepiride were observed in the serum and breast milk of the dams, as well as in the serum of the pups. Although it is not known whether AMARYL is excreted in human milk, other sulfonylureas are excreted in human milk. Because the potential for hypoglycemia in nursing infants may exist, and because of the effects on nursing animals, AMARYL should be discontinued in nursing mothers. If AMARYL is discontinued, and if diet and exercise alone are inadequate for controlling blood glucose, insulin therapy should be considered. (See above Pregnancy, Nonteratogenic Effects.)

Pediatric Use

Safety and effectiveness in pediatric patients have not been established.

Geriatric Use
In US clinical studies of AMARYL, 608 of 1986 patients were 65 and over. No overall differences in safety or effectiveness were observed between these subjects and younger subjects, but greater sensitivity of some older individuals cannot be ruled out.
Comparison of glimepiride pharmacokinetics in NIDDM patients ≤65 years (n=49) and those >65 years (n=42) was performed in a study using a dosing regimen of 6 mg daily. There were no significant differences in glimepiride pharmacokinetics between the two age groups (see CLINICAL PHARMACOLOGY, Special Populations, Geriatric).
The drug is known to be substantially excreted by the kidney, and the risk of toxic reactions to this drug may be greater in patients with impaired renal function. Because elderly patients are more likely to have decreased renal function, care should be taken in dose selection, and it may be useful to monitor renal function.
Elderly patients are particularly susceptible to hypoglycemic action of glucose-lowering drugs. In elderly, debilitated, or malnourished patients, or in patients with renal and hepatic insufficiency, the initial dosing, dose increments, and maintenance dosage should be conservative based upon blood glucose levels prior to and after initiation of treatment to avoid hypoglycemic reactions. Hypoglycemia may be difficult to recognize in the elderly and in people who are taking beta-adrenergic blocking drugs or other sympatholytic agents (see CLINICAL PHARMACOLOGY, Special Populations, Renal Insufficiency; PRECAUTIONS, General; and DOSING AND ADMINISTRATION, Special Patient Population).

ADVERSE REACTIONS

The incidence of hypoglycemia with AMARYL, as documented by blood glucose values <60 mg/dL, ranged from 0.9–1.7% in two large, well-controlled, 1-year studies. (See WARNINGS and PRECAUTIONS.)
AMARYL has been evaluated for safety in 2,013 patients in US controlled trials, and in 1,551 patients in foreign controlled trials. More than 1,650 of these patients were treated for at least 1 year.
Adverse events, other than hypoglycemia, considered to be possibly or probably related to study drug that occurred in US placebo-controlled trials in more than 1% of patients treated with AMARYL are shown below.

Adverse Events Occurring in ≥1% AMARYL Patients

	AMARYL		Placebo	
	No.	%	No.	%
Total Treated	746	100	294	100
Dizziness	13	1.7	1	0.3
Asthenia	12	1.6	3	1.0
Headache	11	1.5	4	1.4
Nausea	8	1.1	0	0.0

Gastrointestinal Reactions
Vomiting, gastrointestinal pain, and diarrhea have been reported, but the incidence in placebo-controlled trials was less than 1%. In rare cases, there may be an elevation of liver enzyme levels. In isolated instances, impairment of liver function (e.g. with cholestasis and jaundice), as well as hepatitis, which may also lead to liver failure have been reported with sulfonylureas, including AMARYL.
Dermatologic Reactions
Allergic skin reactions, e.g., pruritus, erythema, urticaria, and morbilliform or maculopapular eruptions, occur in less than 1% of treated patients. These may be transient and may disappear despite continued use of AMARYL. If those hypersensitivity reactions persist or worsen, the drug should be discontinued. Porphyria cutanea tarda, photosensitivity reactions, and allergic vasculitis have been reported with sulfonylureas.
Hematologic Reactions
Leukopenia, agranulocytosis, thrombocytopenia, hemolytic anemia, aplastic anemia, and pancytopenia have been reported with sulfonylureas.
Metabolic Reactions
Hepatic porphyria reactions and disulfiram-like reactions have been reported with sulfonylureas; however, no cases have yet been reported with AMARYL (glimepiride tablets). Cases of hyponatremia have been reported with glimepiride and all other sulfonylureas, most often in patients who are on other medications or have medical conditions known to cause hyponatremia or increase release of antidiuretic hormone. The syndrome of inappropriate antidiuretic hormone (SIADH) secretion has been reported with certain other sulfonylureas, and it has been suggested that these sulfonylureas may augment the peripheral (antidiuretic) action of ADH and/or increase release of ADH.
Other Reactions
Changes in accommodation and/or blurred vision may occur with the use of AMARYL. This is thought to be due to changes in blood glucose, and may be more pronounced when treatment is initiated. This condition is also seen in untreated diabetic patients, and may actually be reduced by treatment. In placebo-controlled trials of AMARYL, the incidence of blurred vision was placebo, 0.7%, and AMARYL, 0.4%.

OVERDOSAGE

Overdosage of sulfonylureas, including AMARYL, can produce hypoglycemia. Mild hypoglycemic symptoms without loss of consciousness or neurologic findings should be treated aggressively with oral glucose and adjustments in drug dosage and/or meal patterns. Close monitoring should continue until the physician is assured that the patient is out of danger. Severe hypoglycemic reactions with coma, seizure, or other neurological impairment occur infrequently, but constitute medical emergencies requiring immediate hospitalization. If hypoglycemic coma is diagnosed or suspected, the patient should be given a rapid intravenous injection of concentrated (50%) glucose solution. This should be followed by a continuous infusion of a more dilute (10%) glucose solution at a rate that will maintain the blood glucose at a level above 100 mg/dL. Patients should be closely monitored for a minimum of 24 to 48 hours, because hypoglycemia may recur after apparent clinical recovery.

DOSAGE AND ADMINISTRATION

There is no fixed dosage regimen for the management of diabetes mellitus with AMARYL or any other hypoglycemic agent. The patient's fasting blood glucose and HbA_{1c} must be measured periodically to determine the minimum effective dose for the patient; to detect primary failure, i.e., inadequate lowering of blood glucose at the maximum recommended dose of medication; and to detect secondary failure, i.e., loss of adequate blood glucose lowering response after an initial period of effectiveness. Glycosylated hemoglobin levels should be performed to monitor the patient's response to therapy.
Short-term administration of AMARYL may be sufficient during periods of transient loss of control in patients usually controlled well on diet and exercise.
Usual Starting Dose
The usual starting dose of AMARYL as initial therapy is 1–2 mg once daily, administered with breakfast or the first main meal. Those patients who may be more sensitive to hypoglycemic drugs should be started at 1 mg once daily, and should be titrated carefully. (See PRECAUTIONS Section for patients at increased risk.)
No exact dosage relationship exists between AMARYL and the other oral hypoglycemic agents. The maximum starting dose of AMARYL should be no more than 2 mg.
Failure to follow an appropriate dosage regimen may precipitate hypoglycemia. Patients who do not adhere to their prescribed dietary and drug regimen are more prone to exhibit unsatisfactory response to therapy.
Usual Maintenance Dose
The usual maintenance dose is 1 to 4 mg once daily. The maximum recommended dose is 8 mg once daily. After reaching a dose of 2 mg, dosage increases should be made in increments of no more than 2 mg at 1–2 week intervals based upon the patient's blood glucose response. Long-term efficacy should be monitored by measurement of HbA_{1c} levels, for example, every 3 to 6 months.
AMARYL-Metformin Combination Therapy
If patients do not respond adequately to the maximal dose of AMARYL monotherapy, addition of metformin may be considered. Published clinical information exists for the use of other sulfonylureas including glyburide, glipizide, chlorpropamide, and tolbutamide in combination with metformin.
With concomitant AMARYL and metformin therapy, the desired control of blood glucose may be obtained by adjusting the dose of each drug. However, attempts should be made to identify the minimum effective dose of each drug to achieve this goal. With concomitant AMARYL and metformin therapy, the risk of hypoglycemia associated with AMARYL therapy continues and may be increased. Appropriate precautions should be taken.
AMARYL-Insulin Combination Therapy
Combination therapy with AMARYL and insulin may also be used in secondary failure patients. The fasting glucose level for instituting combination therapy is in the range of >150 mg/dL in plasma or serum depending on the patient. The recommended AMARYL dose is 8 mg once daily administered with the first main meal. After starting with low-dose insulin, upward adjustments of insulin can be done approximately weekly as guided by frequent measurements of fasting blood glucose. Once stable, combination-therapy patients should monitor their capillary blood glucose on an ongoing basis, preferably daily. Periodic adjustments of insulin may also be necessary during maintenance as guided by glucose and HbA_{1c} levels.
Specific Patient Populations
AMARYL (glimepiride tablets) is not recommended for use in pregnancy, nursing mothers, or children. In elderly, debilitated, or malnourished patients, or in patients with renal or hepatic insufficiency, the initial dosing, dose increments, and maintenance dosage should be conservative to avoid hypoglycemic reactions (See CLINICAL PHARMACOLOGY, Special Populations and PRECAUTIONS, General).
Patients Receiving Other Oral Hypoglycemic Agents
As with other sulfonylurea hypoglycemic agents, no transition period is necessary when transferring patients to AMARYL. Patients should be observed carefully (1–2 weeks) for hypoglycemia when being transferred from longer half-life sulfonylureas (e.g., chlorpropamide) to AMARYL due to potential overlapping of drug effect.

HOW SUPPLIED

AMARYL tablets are available in the following strengths and package sizes:
1 mg (pink, flat-faced, oblong with notched sides at double bisect, either imprinted with "AMA RYL" on one side, and the Hoechst logo on both sides of the bisect on the other side)
Bottles of 100 (NDC 0039-0221-10)
2 mg (green, flat-faced, oblong with notched sides at double bisect, either imprinted with "AMA RYL" on one side, or imprinted with "AMA RYL" on one side and the Hoechst logo on both sides of the bisect on the other side)
Bottles of 100 (NDC 0039-0222-10)
Unit Dose Cartons (100) (NDC 0039-0222-11)
4 mg (blue, flat-faced, oblong with notched sides at double bisect, either imprinted with "AMA RYL" on one side, or imprinted with "AMA RYL" on one side and the Hoechst logo on both sides of the bisect on the other side)
Bottles of 100 (NDC 0039-0223-10)
Unit Dose Cartons (100) (NDC 0039-0223-11)
Store between 59 and 86° F (15 and 30° C).
Dispense in well-closed containers with safety closures.

ANIMAL TOXICOLOGY

Reduced serum glucose values and degranulation of the pancreatic beta cells were observed in beagle dogs exposed to 320 mg glimepiride/kg/day for 12 months (approximately 1,000 times the recommended human dose based on surface area). No evidence of tumor formation was observed in any organ. One female and one male dog developed bilateral subcapsular cataracts. Non-GLP studies indicated that glimepiride was unlikely to exacerbate cataract formation. Evaluation of the co-cataractogenic potential of glimepiride in several diabetic and cataract rat models was negative and there was no adverse effect of glimepiride on bovine ocular lens metabolism in organ culture.

HUMAN OPHTHALMOLOGY DATA

Ophthalmic examinations were carried out in over 500 subjects during long-term studies using the methodology of Taylor and West and Laties et al. No significant differences were seen between AMARYL and glyburide in the number of subjects with clinically important changes in visual acuity, intra-ocular tension, or in any of the five lens-related variables examined.
Ophthalmic examinations were carried out during long-term studies using the method of Chylack et al. No significant or clinically meaningful differences were seen between AMARYL and glipizide with respect to cataract progression by subjective LOCS II grading and objective image analysis systems, visual acuity, intraocular pressure, and general ophthalmic examination.
Prescribing Information as of February 2003
Aventis Pharmaceuticals NJ
Bridgewater, NJ 08807 USA
www.aventispharma-us.com
US Patent 4,379,785

amap0203p
Shown in Product Identification Guide, page 307

ANZEMET® Injection ℞

[an-zĕmĕt]
(dolasetron mesylate injection)

Prescribing Information as of October 2003

DESCRIPTION

ANZEMET (dolasetron mesylate) is an antinauseant and antiemetic agent. Chemically, dolasetron mesylate is (2α,6α,8α,9aβ)-octahydro-3-oxo-2,6-methano-*2H*-quinolizin-8-yl-*1H*-indole-3-carboxylate monomethanesulfonate, monohydrate. It is a highly specific and selective serotonin subtype 3 ($5\text{-}HT_3$) receptor antagonist both in vitro and in vivo. Dolasetron mesylate has the following structural formula:

$\cdot CH_3SO_3H \cdot H_2O$

The empirical formula is $C_{19}H_{20}N_2O_3 \cdot CH_3SO_3H \cdot H_2O$, with a molecular weight of 438.50. Approximately 74% of dolasetron mesylate monohydrate is dolasetron base.
Dolasetron mesylate monohydrate is a white to off-white powder that is freely soluble in water and propylene glycol, slightly soluble in ethanol, and slightly soluble in normal saline.
ANZEMET Injection is a clear, colorless, nonpyrogenic, sterile solution for intravenous administration. Each milliliter of ANZEMET Injection contains 20 mg of dolasetron mesylate and 38.2 mg mannitol, USP, with an acetate buffer in water for injection. The pH of the resulting solution is 3.2 to 3.8.
ANZEMET Injection multidose vials contain a clear, colorless, nonpyrogenic, sterile solution for intravenous administration. Each ANZEMET multidose vial contains 25 mL (500 mg) dolasetron mesylate. Each milliliter contains 20 mg dolasetron mesylate, 29 mg mannitol, USP, and 5 mg phenol, USP, with an acetate buffer in water for injection. The pH of the resulting solution is 3.2 to 3.7.

CLINICAL PHARMACOLOGY

Dolasetron mesylate and its active metabolite, hydrodolasetron (MDL 74,156), are selective serotonin $5\text{-}HT_3$ receptor

Continued on next page

Anzemet Injection—Cont.

antagonists not shown to have activity at other known serotonin receptors and with low affinity for dopamine receptors. The serotonin 5-HT_3 receptors are located on the nerve terminals of the vagus in the periphery and centrally in the chemoreceptor trigger zone of the area postrema. It is thought that chemotherapeutic agents produce nausea and vomiting by releasing serotonin from the enterochromaffin cells of the small intestine, and that the released serotonin then activates 5-HT_3 receptors located on vagal efferents to initiate the vomiting reflex.

Acute, usually reversible, ECG changes (PR and QT_c prolongation; QRS widening), caused by dolasetron mesylate, have been observed in healthy volunteers and in controlled clinical trials. The active metabolites of dolasetron may block sodium channels, a property unrelated to its ability to block 5-HT_3 receptors. QT_c prolongation is primarily due to QRS widening. Dolasetron appears to prolong both depolarization and, to a lesser extent, repolarization time. The magnitude and frequency of the ECG changes increased with dose (related to peak plasma concentrations of hydrodolasetron but not the parent compound). These ECG interval prolongations usually returned to baseline within 6 to 8 hours, but in some patients were present at 24 hour follow up. Dolasetron mesylate administration has little or no effect on blood pressure.

In healthy volunteers (N=64), dolasetron mesylate in single intravenous doses up to 5 mg/kg produced no effect on pupil size or meaningful changes in EEG tracings. Results from neuropsychiatric tests revealed that dolasetron mesylate did not alter mood or concentration. Multiple daily doses of dolasetron have had no effect on colonic transit in humans. Dolasetron mesylate has no effect on plasma prolactin concentrations.

Pharmacokinetics in Humans

Intravenous dolasetron mesylate is rapidly eliminated ($t_{1/2}$ <10 min) and completely metabolized to the most clinically relevant species, hydrodolasetron.

The reduction of dolasetron to hydrodolasetron is mediated by a ubiquitous enzyme, carbonyl reductase. Cytochrome P-450 (CYP)IID6 is primarily responsible for the subsequent hydroxylation of hydrodolasetron and both CYPIIIA and flavin monooxygenase are responsible for the N-oxidation of hydrodolasetron.

Hydrodolasetron is excreted in the urine unchanged (53.0% of administered intravenous dose). Other urinary metabolites include hydroxylated glucuronides and N-oxide.

Hydrodolasetron appeared rapidly in plasma, with a maximum concentration occurring approximately 0.6 hour after the end of intravenous treatment, and was eliminated with a mean half-life of 7.3 hours (%CV=24) and an apparent clearance of 9.4 mL/min/kg (%CV=28) in 24 adults. Hydrodolasetron is eliminated by multiple routes, including renal excretion and, after metabolism, mainly glucuronidation, and hydroxylation. Hydrodolasetron exhibits linear pharmacokinetics over the intravenous dose range of 50 to 200 mg and they are independent of infusion rate. Doses lower than 50 mg have not been studied. Two thirds of the administered dose is recovered in the urine and one third in the feces. Hydrodolasetron is widely distributed in the body with a mean apparent volume of distribution of 5.8 L/kg (%CV=25, N=24) in adults.

Sixty-nine to 77% of hydrodolasetron is bound to plasma protein. In a study with ^{14}C labeled dolasetron, the distribution of radioactivity to blood cells was not extensive. The binding of hydrodolasetron to α_1-acid glycoprotein is approximately 50%. The pharmacokinetics of hydrodolasetron are linear and similar in men and women.

The pharmacokinetics of hydrodolasetron, in special and targeted patient populations following intravenous administration of ANZEMET Injection, are summarized in Table 1. The pharmacokinetics of hydrodolasetron are similar in adult healthy volunteers and in adult cancer patients receiving chemotherapeutic agents. The apparent clearance of hydrodolasetron in pediatric and adolescent patients is 1.4 times to twofold higher than in adults. The apparent clearance of hydrodolasetron is not affected by age in adult cancer patients. Following intravenous administration, the apparent clearance of hydrodolasetron remains unchanged with severe hepatic impairment and decreases 47% with severe renal impairment. No dose adjustment is necessary for elderly patients or for patients with hepatic or renal impairment.

In a pharmacokinetic study in pediatric cancer patients (ages 3 to 11, N=25; ages 12 to 17, N=21) given a single 0.6, 1.2, 1.8, or 2.4 mg/kg dose of ANZEMET Injection intravenously, apparent clearance values were highest and half-lives were lowest in the youngest age group. For the 3 to 11 and the 12 to 17 year age groups, all receiving doses between 0.6 to 2.4 mg/kg, mean apparent clearances are 2 and 1.3 times greater, respectively, than for healthy adults receiving the same range of doses.

Thirty-two pediatric cancer patients ages 3 to 11 years (N=19) and 12 to 17 years (N=13), received 0.6, 1.2, or 1.8 mg/kg ANZEMET Injection diluted with either apple or apple-grape juice and administered orally. In this study, the mean apparent clearances were 3 times greater in the younger pediatric group and 1.8 times greater in the older pediatric group than those observed in healthy adult volunteers. Across this spectrum of pediatric patients, maximum plasma concentrations were 0.6 to 0.7 times those observed in healthy adults receiving similar doses.

Table 1. Pharmacokinetic Values for Plasma Hydrodolasetron Following Intravenous Administration of ANZEMET Injection*

	Age (years)	Dose	CL_{app} (mL/min/kg)	$t_{1/2}$ (h)	C_{max} (ng/mL)
Young Healthy Volunteers (N=24)	19–40	100 mg	9.4 (28%)	7.3 (24%)	320 (25%)
Elderly Healthy Volunteers (N=15)	65–75	2.4 mg/kg	8.3 (30%)	6.9 (22%)	620 (31%)
Cancer Patients					
Adults (N=273)	19–87	0.6–3.0 mg/kg	10.2 (34%)†	7.5 (43%)†	505 (26%)‡
Adolescents (N=21)	12–17	0.6–3.0 mg/kg	12.5 (37%)	5.5 (31%)	562 (45%)§
Children (N=25)	3–11	0.6–2.4 mg/kg	19.2 (30%)	4.4 (24%)	505 (100%)‖
Pediatric Surgery Patients (N=18)	2–11	1.2 mg/kg	13.1 (47%)	4.8 (23%)	255 (22%)
Patients with Severe Renal Impairment (N=12) (Creatinine clearance ≤10 mL/min)	28–74	200 mg	5.0 (33%)	10.9 (30%)	867 (31%)
Patients with Severe Hepatic Impairment (N=3)	42–52	150 mg	9.6 (19%)	11.7 (22%)	396 (45%)

CL_{app}: apparent clearance $t_{1/2}$: terminal elimination half-life ( ): coefficient of variation in %
*: mean values
†: results from population kinetic study
‡: results from adult cancer study (dose=1.8 mg/kg, N=8)
§: results from adolescents (dose=1.8 mg/kg, N=7)
‖: results from children (dose=1.8 mg/kg, N=5)

Table 2. Prevention of Chemotherapy-Induced Nausea and Emesis from Cisplatin Chemotherapy*

	ANZEMET Injection 1.8 mg/kg†	Metoclopramide‡	*p*-value
Number of Patients	72	69	
Response Over 24 Hours			
Complete Response§	41 (57%)	24 (35%)	0.0009
Nausea Score‖	4	30	0.0400

*: Dose ≥80 mg/m²
†: Administered intravenously
‡: 3 mg/kg intravenous bolus and 0.5 mg/kg/h intravenously over 8 h.
§: No emetic episodes and no rescue medication.
‖: Median 24-h change from baseline nausea score using visual analog scale (VAS): Score range 0="none" to 100="nausea as bad as it could be."

Table 3. Prevention of Chemotherapy-Induced Nausea and Emesis from Cisplatin Chemotherapy*

	ANZEMET Injection 1.8 mg/kg†	Ondansetron 32 mg‡	*p*-value
Number of Patients	198	206	
Response Over 24 Hours			
Complete Response§	88 (44%)	88 (43%)	NS
Nausea Score‖	10	16	NS

*: Dose ≥70 mg/m²
†: Administered intravenously
‡: Includes 12 patients who received 3 doses 0.15 mg/kg of ondansetron intravenously.
§: No emetic episodes and no rescue medication.
‖: Median 24-h change from baseline nausea score using visual analog scale (VAS): Score range 0="none" to 100="nausea as bad as it could be."

In a pharmacokinetic study in 18 pediatric patients (2 to 11 years of age) undergoing surgery with general anesthesia and administered a single 1.2 mg/kg intravenous dose of ANZEMET Injection, mean apparent clearance was greater (40%) and terminal half-life shorter (36%) for hydrodolasetron than in healthy adults receiving the same dose.

For 12 pediatric patients, ages 2 to 12 years receiving 1.2 mg/kg ANZEMET Injection diluted in apple or apple-grape juice and administered orally, the mean apparent clearance was 34% greater and half-life was 21% shorter than in healthy adults receiving the same dose.

[See table 1 above]

CLINICAL STUDIES

Prevention of Cancer Chemotherapy-Induced Nausea and Vomiting

ANZEMET Injection administered intravenously at a dose of 1.8 mg/kg gave similar results in preventing nausea and vomiting as the other selective serotonin 5-HT_3 receptor antagonists studied as active comparators. It was more effective than metoclopramide. Efficacy was based on complete response rates (0 emetic episodes and no rescue medication).

Cisplatin Based Chemotherapy

A randomized, double-blind trial compared single intravenous doses of ANZEMET Injection with metoclopramide in 226 (160 men and 66 women) adult cancer patients receiving ≥80 mg/m² cisplatin. ANZEMET Injection at a dose of 1.8 mg/kg was significantly more effective than metoclopramide in the prevention of chemotherapy-induced nausea and vomiting in this study (Table 2).

[See table 2 above]

A second randomized, double-blind trial compared single intravenous doses of ANZEMET Injection with intravenous ondansetron in 609 (377 men and 232 women) adult cancer patients receiving ≥70 mg/m² cisplatin. A single intravenous 1.8 mg/kg dose of ANZEMET Injection was shown to be equivalent to a single intravenous 32 mg dose of ondansetron (Table 3).

[See table 3 above]

Another randomized, double-blind trial compared single IV doses of ANZEMET with a single 3-mg IV dose of granisetron in 474 (315 men and 159 women) patients receiving ≥80 mg/m² cisplatin chemotherapy. A single intravenous 1.8-mg/kg dose of ANZEMET gave similar results as those from granisetron.

Cyclophosphamide Based Chemotherapy

In a study of ANZEMET Injection in 309 patients (96 men and 213 women) receiving moderately emetogenic chemotherapy such as cyclophosphamide based regimens, a single intravenous 1.8 mg/kg dose of ANZEMET Injection was equivalent to metoclopramide administered as a 2 mg/kg intravenous bolus followed by 3 mg/kg intravenously over 8 hours. Complete response rates were 63% and 52%, respectively, p=0.12.

Prevention of Postoperative Nausea and Vomiting

ANZEMET Injection administered intravenously at a dose of 12.5 mg approximately 15 minutes before the cessation of general balanced anesthesia (short-acting barbiturate, nitrous oxide, narcotic and analgesic, and skeletal muscle relaxant) was significantly more effective than placebo in preventing postoperative nausea and vomiting. No increased efficacy was seen with higher doses.

One trial compared single intravenous ANZEMET Injection doses of 12.5, 25, 50, and 100 mg with placebo in 635 women surgical patients undergoing laparoscopic procedures. ANZEMET Injection at a dose of 12.5 mg was statistically superior to placebo for complete response (no vomiting, no rescue medication) (p=.0003). Complete response rates were 50% and 31%, respectively.

Another trial compared single intravenous ANZEMET Injection doses of 12.5, 25, 50, and 100 mg with placebo in 1030 (722 women and 308 men) surgical patients. In women, the 12.5 mg dose was statistically superior to placebo for complete response. The complete response rates were 50% and 40%, respectively. However, in men, there was no statistically significant difference in complete response between any ANZEMET dose and placebo.

Treatment of Postoperative Nausea and/or Vomiting

Two randomized, double-blinded trials compared single intravenous ANZEMET Injection doses of 12.5, 25, 50, and 100 mg with placebo in 124 male and 833 female patients who had undergone surgery with general balanced anesthesia and presented with early postoperative nausea or vomiting requiring antiemetic treatment.

In both studies, the 12.5 mg intravenous dose of ANZEMET was statistically superior to placebo for complete response (no vomiting, no escape medication). No significant increased efficacy was seen with higher doses.

INDICATIONS AND USAGE

ANZEMET Injection is indicated for the following:

(1) the prevention of nausea and vomiting associated with initial and repeat courses of emetogenic cancer chemotherapy, including high dose cisplatin;

(2) the prevention of postoperative nausea and vomiting. As with other antiemetics, routine prophylaxis is not recommended for patients in whom there is little expectation that nausea and/or vomiting will occur postoperatively. In patients where nausea and/or vomiting must be avoided postoperatively, ANZEMET Injection is recommended even where the incidence of postoperative nausea and/or vomiting is low;

(3) the treatment of postoperative nausea and/or vomiting.

CONTRAINDICATIONS

ANZEMET Injection is contraindicated in patients known to have hypersensitivity to the drug.

WARNINGS

ANZEMET can cause ECG interval changes (PR, QT_c, JT prolongation and QRS widening). These changes are related in magnitude and frequency to blood levels of the active metabolite. These changes are self-limiting with declining blood levels. Some patients have interval prolongations for 24 hours or longer. Interval prolongation could lead to cardiovascular consequences, including heart block or cardiac arrhythmias. These have rarely been reported.

A cardiac conduction abnormality observed on an intraoperative cardiac rhythm monitor (interpreted as complete heart block) was reported in a 61-year-old woman who received 200 mg ANZEMET for the prevention of postoperative nausea and vomiting. This patient was also taking verapamil. A similar event also interpreted as complete heart block was reported in one patient receiving placebo.

A 66-year-old man with Stage IV non-Hodgkins lymphoma died suddenly 6 hours after receiving 1.8 mg/kg (119 mg) intravenous ANZEMET Injection. This patient had other potential risk factors including substantial exposure to doxorubicin and concomitant cyclophosphamide.

PRECAUTIONS

General

Dolasetron should be administered with caution in patients who have or may develop prolongation of cardiac conduction intervals, particularly QT_c. These include patients with hypokalemia or hypomagnesemia, patients taking diuretics with potential for inducing electrolyte abnormalities, patients with congenital QT syndrome, patients taking anti-arrhythmic drugs or other drugs which lead to QT prolongation, and cumulative high dose anthracycline therapy.

Cross hypersensitivity reactions have been reported in patients who received other selective $5\text{-}HT_3$ receptor antagonists. These reactions have not been seen with dolasetron mesylate.

Drug Interactions

The potential for clinically significant drug-drug interactions posed by dolasetron and hydrodolasetron appears to be low for drugs commonly used in chemotherapy or surgery, because hydrodolasetron is eliminated by multiple routes. See PRECAUTIONS, General for information about potential interaction with other drugs that prolong the QT_c interval. Blood levels of hydrodolasetron increased 24% when dolasetron was coadministered with cimetidine (nonselective inhibitor of cytochrome P 450) for 7 days, and decreased 28% with coadministration of rifampin (potent inducer of cytochrome P-450) for 7 days.

ANZEMET Injection has been safely coadministered with drugs used in chemotherapy and surgery. As with other agents which prolong ECG intervals, caution should be exercised in patients taking drugs which prolong ECG intervals, particularly QT_c.

In patients taking furosemide, nifedipine, diltiazem, ACE inhibitors, verapamil, glyburide, propranolol, and various chemotherapy agents, no effect was shown on the clearance of hydrodolasetron. Clearance of hydrodolasetron decreased by about 27% when dolasetron mesylate was administered intravenously concomitantly with atenolol. ANZEMET did not influence anesthesia recovery time in patients. Dolasetron mesylate did not inhibit the antitumor activity of four chemotherapeutic agents (cisplatin, 5-fluorouracil, doxorubicin, cyclophosphamide) in four murine models.

Table 4. Adverse Events ≥2% from Chemotherapy-Induced Nausea and Vomiting Studies

Event	ANZEMET Injection 1.8 mg/kg (n=695)	Ondansetron/ Granisetron* (n=356)
Headache	169 (24.3%)	73 (20.5%)
Diarrhea	86 (12.4%)	25 (7.0%)
Fever	30 (4.3%)	18 (5.1%)
Fatigue	25 (3.6%)	12 (3.4%)
Hepatic Function Abnormal†	25 (3.6%)	12 (3.4%)
Abdominal Pain	22 (3.2%)	7 (2.0%)
Hypertension	20 (2.9%)	9 (2.5%)
Pain	17 (2.4%)	7 (2.0%)
Dizziness	15 (2.2%)	7 (2.0%)
Chills/Shivering	14 (2.0%)	6 (1.7%)

*: Ondansetron 32 mg intravenous, granisetron 3 mg intravenous.
†: Includes events coded as SGOT- and/or SGPT-increased (see also Liver and Biliary System below)

Table 5. Adverse Events ≥2% from Placebo-Controlled Postoperative Nausea and Vomiting Studies

Event	ANZEMET Injection 12.5 mg (n=615)	Placebo (n=739)
Headache	58 (9.4%)	51 (6.9%)
Dizziness	34 (5.5%)	23 (3.1%)
Drowsiness	15 (2.4%)	18 (2.4%)
Pain	15 (2.4%)	21 (2.8%)
Urinary Retention	12 (2.0%)	16 (2.2%)

Carcinogenesis, Mutagenesis, Impairment of Fertility

In a 24-month carcinogenicity study, there was a statistically significant (P<0.001) increase in the incidence of combined hepatocellular adenomas and carcinomas in male mice treated with 150 mg/kg/day and above. In this study, mice (CD-1) were treated orally with dolasetron mesylate 75, 150 or 300 mg/kg/day (225, 450 or 900 mg/m^2/day). For a 50 kg person of average height (1.46 m^2 body surface area), these doses represent 3.4, 6.8 and 13.5 times the recommended clinical dose (66.6 mg/m^2, intravenous) on a body surface area basis. No increase in liver tumors was observed at a dose of 75 mg/kg/day in male mice and at doses up to 300 mg/kg/day in female mice.

In a 24-month rat (Sprague-Dawley) carcinogenicity study, oral dolasetron mesylate was not tumorigenic at doses up to 150 mg/kg/day (900 mg/m^2/day, 13.5 times the recommended human dose based on body surface area) in male rats and 300 mg/kg/day (1800 mg/m^2/day, 27 times the recommended human dose based on body surface area) in female rats.

Dolasetron mesylate was not genotoxic in the Ames test, the rat lymphocyte chromosomal aberration test, the Chinese hamster ovary (CHO) cell (HGPRT) forward mutation test, the rat hepatocyte unscheduled DNA synthesis (UDS) test or the mouse micronucleus test.

Dolasetron mesylate was found to have no effect on fertility and reproductive performance at oral doses up to 100 mg/kg/day (600 mg/m^2/day, 9 times the recommended human dose based on body surface area) in female rats and up to 400 mg/kg/day (2400 mg/m^2/day, 36 times the recommended human dose based on body surface area) in male rats.

Pregnancy: Teratogenic Effects, Pregnancy Category B.

Teratology studies have not revealed evidence of impaired fertility or harm to the fetus due to dolasetron mesylate. These studies have been performed in pregnant rats at intravenous doses up to 60 mg/kg/day (5.4 times the recommended human dose based on body surface area) and pregnant rabbits at intravenous doses up to 20 mg/kg/day (3.2 times the recommended human dose based on body surface area). There are, however, no adequate and well-controlled studies in pregnant women. Because animal reproduction studies are not always predictive of human response, this drug should be used during pregnancy only if clearly needed.

Nursing Mothers

It is not known whether dolasetron mesylate is excreted in human milk. Because many drugs are excreted in human milk, caution should be exercised when ANZEMET Injection is administered to a nursing woman.

Pediatric Use

Four open-label, noncomparative pharmacokinetic studies have been performed in a total of 108 pediatric patients receiving emetogenic chemotherapy or undergoing surgery with general anesthesia. These patients received ANZEMET Injection either intravenously or orally in juice. Pediatric patients from 2 to 17 years of age participated in these trials, which included intravenous ANZEMET Injection doses of 0.6, 1.2, 1.8, or 2.4 mg/kg, and oral doses of 0.6, 1.2, or 1.8 mg/kg. There is no experience in pediatric patients under 2 years of age. Overall, ANZEMET Injection was well tolerated in these pediatric patients. Efficacy information collected in pediatric patients receiving cancer chemotherapy are consistent with those obtained in adults. No efficacy information was collected in the pediatric postoperative nausea and vomiting studies.

Use in Elderly Patients

Dosage adjustment is not needed in patients over 65. Effectiveness in prevention of nausea and vomiting in elderly patients was no different than in younger age groups.

ADVERSE REACTIONS

Chemotherapy Patients

In controlled clinical trials, 2265 adult patients received ANZEMET Injection. The overall adverse event rates were similar with 1.8 mg/kg ANZEMET Injection and ondansetron or granisetron. Patients were receiving concurrent chemotherapy, predominantly high-dose (≥50 mg/m^2) cisplatin. Following is a combined listing of all adverse events reported in ≥2% of patients in these controlled trials (Table 4).

[See table 4 above]

Postoperative Patients

In controlled clinical trials with 2550 adult patients, headache and dizziness were reported more frequently with 12.5 mg ANZEMET Injection than with placebo. Rates of other adverse events were similar. Following is a listing of all adverse events reported in ≥2% of patients receiving either placebo or 12.5 mg ANZEMET Injection for the prevention or treatment of postoperative nausea and vomiting in controlled clinical trials (Table 5).

[See table 5 above]

In clinical trials, the following infrequently reported adverse events, assessed by investigators as treatment-related or causality unknown, occurred following oral or intravenous administration of ANZEMET to adult patients receiving concomitant cancer chemotherapy or surgery:

Cardiovascular: Hypotension; rarely–edema, peripheral edema. The following events also occurred rarely and with a similar frequency as placebo and/or active comparator: Mobitz I AV block, chest pain, orthostatic hypotension, myocardial ischemia, syncope, severe bradycardia, and palpitations. See PRECAUTIONS section for information on potential effects on ECG.

In addition, the following asymptomatic treatment-emergent ECG changes were seen at rates less than or equal to those for active or placebo controls: bradycardia, tachycardia, T wave change, ST-T wave change, sinus arrhythmia, extrasystole (APCs or VPCs), poor R-wave progression, bundle branch block (left and right), nodal arrhythmia, U wave change, atrial flutter/fibrillation.

Continued on next page

ANZEMET® Injection
(dolasetron mesylate injection)
20 mg/mL

Strength	Description	NDC Number
12.5 mg	0.625mL single-use ampules* (Box of 6)	0088-1208-65
12.5 mg	0.625mL single use vial* (Box of 6)	0088-1208-06
12.5 mg	0.625mL fill in single-use 2mL Carpuject with Luer Lock† (Box of 10)	0088-1208-76
100 mg/5 mL	5mL single-use vial*	0088-1206-32
500 mg/25 mL	25 mL multidose vial††	0088-1209-26

Anzemet Injection—Cont.

Furthermore, severe hypotension, bradycardia and syncope have been reported immediately or closely following IV administration.

Dermatologic: Rash, increased sweating.

Gastrointestinal System: Constipation, dyspepsia, abdominal pain, anorexia; rarely–pancreatitis.

Hearing, Taste and Vision: Taste perversion, abnormal vision; rarely–tinnitus, photophobia.

Hematologic: Rarely–hematuria, epistaxis, prothrombin time prolonged, PTT increased, anemia, purpura/hematoma, thrombocytopenia.

Hypersensitivity: Rarely–anaphylactic reaction, facial edema, urticaria.

Liver and Biliary System: Transient increases in AST (SGOT) and/or ALT (SGPT) values have been reported as adverse events in less than 1% of adult patients receiving ANZEMET in clinical trials. The increases did not appear to be related to dose or duration of therapy and were not associated with symptomatic hepatic disease. Similar increases were seen with patients receiving active comparator. Rarely–hyperbilirubinemia, increased GGT.

Metabolic and Nutritional: Rarely–alkaline phosphatase increased.

Musculoskeletal: Rarely–myalgia, arthralgia.

Nervous System: Flushing, vertigo, paraesthesia, tremor; rarely–ataxia, twitching.

Psychiatric: Agitation, sleep disorder, depersonalization; rarely–confusion, anxiety, abnormal dreaming.

Respiratory System: Rarely–dyspnea, bronchospasm.

Urinary System: Rarely–dysuria, polyuria, acute renal failure.

Vascular (Extracardiac): Local pain or burning on IV administration; rarely–peripheral ischemia, thrombophlebitis/phlebitis.

OVERDOSAGE

A 59-year-old man with metastatic melanoma and no known pre-existing cardiac conditions developed severe hypotension and dizziness 40 minutes after receiving a 15 minute intravenous infusion of 1000 mg (13 mg/kg) of dolasetron mesylate. Treatment for the overdose consisted of infusion of 500 mL of a plasma expander, dopamine, and atropine. The patient had normal sinus rhythm and prolongation of PR, QRS and QT_c intervals on an ECG recorded 2 hours after the infusion. The patient's blood pressure was normal 3 hours after the event and the ECG intervals returned to baseline on follow-up. The patient was released from the hospital 6 hours after the event.

Following a suspected overdose of ANZEMET Injection, a patient found to have second-degree or higher AV conduction block with ECG should undergo cardiac telemetry monitoring.

There is no known specific antidote for dolasetron mesylate, and patients with suspected overdose should be managed with supportive therapy. Individual doses as large as 5 mg/kg intravenously or 400 mg orally have been safely given to healthy volunteers or cancer patients.

It is not known if dolasetron mesylate is removed by hemodialysis or peritoneal dialysis.

A 7-year-old boy received 6 mg/kg dolasetron mesylate orally before surgery. No symptoms occurred and no treatment was required.

Single intravenous doses of dolasetron mesylate at 160 mg/kg in male mice and 140 mg/kg in female mice and rats of both sexes (6.3 to 12.6 times the recommended human dose based on body surface area) were lethal. Symptoms of acute toxicity were tremors, depression and convulsions.

DOSAGE AND ADMINISTRATION

The recommended dose of ANZEMET Injection should not be exceeded.

Prevention of Cancer Chemotherapy-Induced Nausea and Vomiting

Adults: The recommended intravenous dosage of ANZEMET Injection from clinical trial results is 1.8 mg/kg given as a single dose approximately 30 minutes before chemotherapy (see Administration). Alternatively, for most patients, a fixed dose of 100 mg can be administered over 30 seconds.

Pediatric Patients: The recommended intravenous dosage in pediatric patients 2 to 16 years of age is 1.8 mg/kg given as a single dose approximately 30 minutes before chemotherapy, up to a maximum of 100 mg (see Administration). Safety and effectiveness in pediatric patients under 2 years of age have not been established.

ANZEMET Injection mixed in apple or apple-grape juice may be used for oral dosing of pediatric patients. When ANZEMET Injection is administered orally, the recommended dosage in pediatric patients 2 to 16 years of age is 1.8 mg/kg up to a maximum 100 mg dose given within 1 hour before chemotherapy.

The diluted product may be kept up to 2 hours at room temperature before use.

Use in the Elderly, in Renal Failure Patients, or in Hepatically Impaired Patients: No dosage adjustment is recommended.

Prevention or Treatment of Postoperative Nausea and/or Vomiting

Adults: The recommended intravenous dosage of ANZEMET Injection is 12.5 mg given as a single dose approximately 15 minutes before the cessation of anesthesia (prevention) or as soon as nausea or vomiting presents (treatment).

Pediatric Patients: The recommended intravenous dosage in pediatric patients 2 to 16 years of age is 0.35 mg/kg, with a maximum dose of 12.5 mg, given as a single dose approximately 15 minutes before the cessation of anesthesia or as soon as nausea or vomiting presents. Safety and effectiveness in pediatric patients under 2 years of age have not been established.

ANZEMET Injection mixed in apple or apple-grape juice may be used for oral dosing of pediatric patients. When ANZEMET Injection is administered orally, the recommended oral dosage in pediatric patients 2 to 16 years of age is 1.2 mg/kg up to a maximum 100-mg dose given within 2 hours before surgery. The diluted product may be kept up to 2 hours at room temperature before use.

Use in the Elderly, in Renal Failure Patients, or in Hepatically Impaired Patients: No dosage adjustment is recommended.

Administration

ANZEMET Injection can be safely infused intravenously as rapidly as 100 mg/30 seconds or diluted in a compatible intravenous solution (see below) to 50 mL and infused over a period of up to 15 minutes. ANZEMET Injection should not be mixed with other drugs. Flush the infusion line before and after administration of ANZEMET Injection.

Stability

After dilution, ANZEMET Injection is stable under normal lighting conditions at room temperature for 24 hours or under refrigeration for 48 hours with the following compatible intravenous fluids: 0.9% sodium chloride injection, 5% dextrose injection, 5% dextrose and 0.45% sodium chloride injection, 5% dextrose and Lactated Ringer's injection, Lactated Ringer's injection, and 10% mannitol injection. Although ANZEMET Injection is chemically and physically stable when diluted as recommended, sterile precautions should be observed because diluents generally do not contain preservative. After dilution, do not use beyond 24 hours, or 48 hours if refrigerated.

Parenteral drug products should be inspected visually for particulate matter and discoloration before administration whenever solution and container permit.

HOW SUPPLIED

ANZEMET Injection (dolasetron mesylate injection) is supplied as a clear, colorless solution in single-use ampules, single and multidose vials, and Carpuject® sterile cartridges with Luer Lock.

[See table above]

Store at 20–25°C (68–77°F) with excursions permitted to 15–30°C (59–86°F) [See USP Controlled Room Temperature]. Protect from light.

Prescribing information as of October 2003

Mfd for Aventis Pharmaceuticals Inc.
Kansas City, MO 64137 USA

*Mfd by Gruppo Lepetit S.p.A.
20020 Lainate, Italy—Made in Italy
†Mfd by Abbott Laboratories
McPherson, KS 67460 USA
††Mfd by Gruppo Lepetit S.p.A.
20020 Lainate, Italy—Made in Italy

Carpuject is a registered trademark of Abbott Laboratories.
www.aventis-us.com

Shown in Product Identification Guide, page 307

ANZEMET® Tablets ℞

[*an-zĕmĕt*]
(dolasetron mesylate)

Prescribing Information as of October 2003

DESCRIPTION

ANZEMET (dolasetron mesylate) is an antinauseant and antiemetic agent. Chemically, dolasetron mesylate is (2α,6α,8α,9aβ)-octahydro-3-oxo-2,6-methano-2*H*-quinolizin-8-yl-l*H*-indole-3-carboxylate monomethanesulfonate, monohydrate. It is a highly specific and selective serotonin subtype 3 ($5\text{-}HT_3$) receptor antagonist both in vitro and in vivo. Dolasetron mesylate has the following structural formula:

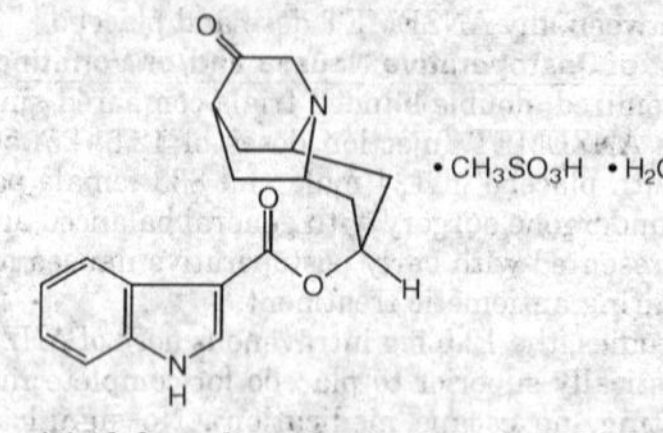

• CH_3SO_3H • H_2O

The empirical formula is $C_{19}H_{20}N_2O_3 \bullet CH_3SO_3H \bullet H_2O$, with a molecular weight of 438.50. Approximately 74% of dolasetron mesylate monohydrate is dolasetron base.

Dolasetron mesylate monohydrate is a white to off-white powder that is freely soluble in water and propylene glycol, slightly soluble in ethanol, and slightly soluble in normal saline.

Each ANZEMET Tablet for oral administration contains dolasetron mesylate (as the monohydrate) and also contains the inactive ingredients: carnauba wax, croscarmellose sodium, hypromellose, lactose, magnesium stearate, polyethylene glycol, polysorbate 80, pregelatinized starch, synthetic red iron oxide, titanium dioxide, and white wax. The tablets are printed with black ink, which contains lecithin, pharmaceutical glaze, propylene glycol, and synthetic black iron oxide.

CLINICAL PHARMACOLOGY

Dolasetron mesylate and its active metabolite, hydrodolasetron (MDL 74,156), are selective serotonin $5\text{-}HT_3$ receptor antagonists not shown to have activity at other known serotonin receptors and with low affinity for dopamine receptors. The serotonin $5\text{-}HT_3$ receptors are located on the nerve terminals of the vagus in the periphery and centrally in the chemoreceptor trigger zone of the area postrema. It is thought that chemotherapeutic agents produce nausea and vomiting by releasing serotonin from the enterochromaffin cells of the small intestine, and that the released serotonin then activates $5\text{-}HT_3$ receptors located on vagal efferents to initiate the vomiting reflex.

Acute, usually reversible, ECG changes (PR and QT_c prolongation; QRS widening), caused by dolasetron mesylate, have been observed in healthy volunteers and in controlled clinical trials. The active metabolites of dolasetron may block sodium channels, a property unrelated to its ability to block $5\text{-}HT_3$ receptors. QT_c prolongation is primarily due to QRS widening. Dolasetron appears to prolong both depolarization and, to a lesser extent, repolarization time. The magnitude and frequency of the ECG changes increased with dose (related to peak plasma concentrations of hydrodolasetron but not the parent compound). These ECG interval prolongations usually returned to baseline within 6 to 8 hours, but in some patients were present at 24 hour follow up. Dolasetron mesylate administration has little or no effect on blood pressure.

In healthy volunteers (N=64), dolasetron mesylate in single intravenous doses up to 5 mg/kg produced no effect on pupil size or meaningful changes in EEG tracings. Results from neuropsychiatric tests revealed that dolasetron mesylate did not alter mood or concentration. Multiple daily doses of dolasetron have had no effect on colonic transit in humans. Dolasetron has no effect on plasma prolactin concentrations.

Pharmacokinetics in Humans

Oral dolasetron is well absorbed, although parent drug is rarely detected in plasma due to rapid and complete metabolism to the most clinically relevant species, hydrodolasetron.

The reduction of dolasetron to hydrodolasetron is mediated by a ubiquitous enzyme, carbonyl reductase. Cytochrome P-450 (CYP)IID6 is primarily responsible for the subsequent hydroxylation of hydrodolasetron and both CYPIIIA and flavin monooxygenase are responsible for the N-oxidation of hydrodolasetron.

Hydrodolasetron is excreted in the urine unchanged (61.0% of administered oral dose). Other urinary metabolites include hydroxylated glucuronides and N-oxide.

Hydrodolasetron appears rapidly in plasma, with a maximum concentration occurring approximately 1 hour after dosing, and is eliminated with a mean half-life of 8.1 hours (%CV=18%) and an apparent clearance of 13.4 mL/min/kg (%CV=29%) in 30 adults. The apparent absolute bioavailability of oral dolasetron, determined by the major active metabolite hydrodolasetron, is approximately 75%. Orally administered dolasetron intravenous solution and tablets are bioequivalent. Food does not affect the bioavailability of dolasetron taken by mouth.

Hydrodolasetron is eliminated by multiple routes, including renal excretion and, after metabolism, mainly, glucuronidation and hydroxylation. Two thirds of the administered dose is recovered in the urine and one third in the feces.

Hydrodolasetron is widely distributed in the body with a mean apparent volume of distribution of 5.8 L/kg (%CV=25%, N=24) in adults.

Sixty-nine to 77% of hydrodolasetron is bound to plasma protein. In a study with ^{14}C labeled dolasetron, the distribution of radioactivity to blood cells was not extensive. Approximately 50% of hydrodolasetron is bound to α_1-acid glycoprotein. The pharmacokinetics of hydrodolasetron are linear and similar in men and women.

The pharmacokinetics of hydrodolasetron, in special and targeted patient populations following oral administration of dolasetron, are summarized in Table 1. The pharmacokinetics of hydrodolasetron are similar in adult healthy volunteers and in adult cancer patients receiving chemotherapeutic agents. The apparent clearance following oral administration of hydrodolasetron is approximately 1.6- to 3.4-fold higher in children and adolescents than in adults. The clearance following oral administration of hydrodolasetron is not affected by age in adult cancer patients. The apparent oral clearance of hydrodolasetron decreases 42% with severe hepatic impairment and 44% with severe renal impairment. No dose adjustment is necessary for elderly patients or for patients with hepatic or renal impairment.

The pharmacokinetics of ANZEMET Tablets have not been studied in the pediatric population. However, the following pharmacokinetic data are available on intravenous ANZEMET Injection administered orally to children.

Thirty-two pediatric cancer patients ages 3 to 11 years (N=19) and 12 to 17 years (N=13), received 0.6, 1.2, or 1.8 mg/kg ANZEMET Injection diluted with either apple or apple-grape juice and administered orally. In this study, the mean apparent clearances of hydrodolasetron were 3 times greater in the younger pediatric group and 1.8 times greater in the older pediatric group than those observed in healthy adult volunteers. Across this spectrum of pediatric patients, maximum plasma concentrations were 0.6 to 0.7 times those observed in healthy adults receiving similar doses.

For 12 pediatric patients, ages 2 to 12 years receiving 1.2 mg/kg ANZEMET Injection diluted in apple or apple-grape juice and administered orally, the mean apparent clearance was 34% greater and half-life was 21% shorter than in healthy adults receiving the same dose.

[See table 1 at right]

CLINICAL STUDIES

Prevention of Cancer Chemotherapy-Induced Nausea and Vomiting

Oral ANZEMET at a dose of 100 mg prevents nausea and vomiting associated with moderately emetogenic cancer therapy as shown by 24 hour efficacy data from two double-blind studies. Efficacy was based on complete response (ie, no vomiting, no rescue medication).

The first randomized, double-blind trial compared single oral ANZEMET doses of 25, 50, 100 and 200 mg in 60 men and 259 women cancer patients receiving cyclophosphamide and/or doxorubicin. There was no statistically significant difference in complete response between the 100 mg and 200 mg dose. Results are summarized in Table 2.

[See table 2 at right]

Another trial also compared single oral ANZEMET doses of 25, 50, 100, and 200 mg in 307 patients receiving moderately emetogenic chemotherapy. In this study, the 100 mg ANZEMET dose gave a 73% complete response rate.

Prevention of Postoperative Nausea and Vomiting

ANZEMET Tablets at a dose of 100 mg administered orally 1–2 hours before surgery and before general balanced anesthesia (short-acting barbiturate, nitrous oxide, narcotic analgesic, and skeletal muscle relaxant) was significantly more effective than placebo in preventing postoperative nausea and vomiting. Efficacy was based on complete response rates (0 emetic episodes and no rescue medication over 24 hours). No increased efficacy was seen with higher doses.

One trial compared single ANZEMET Tablet doses of 25, 50, 100, and 200 mg with placebo in 789 women undergoing gynecological surgery. In this study the 100 mg dose produced a complete response rate statistically superior to placebo. The study results are summarized in Table 3.

[See table 3 at right]

Another trial also compared single oral ANZEMET doses of 25, 50, 100, and 200 mg with placebo in 373 women undergoing gynecological surgery. In this study, the 100 mg ANZEMET dose gave a 54% complete response rate as compared to the 29% rate of placebo.

INDICATIONS AND USAGE

ANZEMET Tablets are indicated for:

1) **the prevention of nausea and vomiting associated with moderately emetogenic cancer chemotherapy, including initial and repeat courses;**
2) **the prevention of postoperative nausea and vomiting.**

CONTRAINDICATIONS

ANZEMET Tablets are contraindicated in patients known to have hypersensitivity to the drug.

WARNINGS

ANZEMET can cause ECG interval changes (PR, QT_C, JT prolongation and QRS widening). These changes are related in magnitude and frequency to blood levels of the active metabolite. These changes are self-limiting with declining blood levels. Some patients have interval prolongations for 24 hours or longer. Interval prolongation could lead to cardiovascular consequences, including heart block or cardiac arrhythmias. These have rarely been reported.

Table 1. Pharmacokinetic Values for Plasma Hydrodolasetron Following Oral Administration of ANZEMET*

	Age (years)	Dose	CL_{app} (mL/min/kg)	$t_{1/2}$ (h)	C_{max} (ng/mL)
Young Healthy Volunteers (N=30)	19–45	200 mg	13.4 (29%)	8.1 (18%)	556 (28%)
Elderly Healthy Volunteers (N=15)	65–75	2.4 mg/kg	9.5 (36%)	7.2 (32%)	662 (28%)
Cancer Patients					
Adults (N=61)†	24–84	25–200 mg	12.9 (49%)	7.9 (43%)	— ‡
Adolescents (N=13)	12–17	0.6–1.8 mg/kg	26.5 (67%)	6.4 (30%)	374§ (32%)
Children (N=19)	3–11	0.6–1.8 mg/kg	44.2 (49%)	5.5 (39%)	217‖ (67%)
Pediatric Surgery Patients (N=11)	2–12	1.2 mg/kg	20.8 (49%)	5.9 (24%)	159 (32%)
Patients with Severe Renal Impairment (N=12) (Creatinine clearance ≤10 mL/min)	28–74	200 mg	7.2 (48%)	10.7 (29%)	701 (21%)
Patients with Severe Hepatic Impairment (N=3)	42–52	150 mg	8.8 (57%)	11.0 (36%)	410 (12%)

CL_{app}: apparent clearance $t_{1/2}$: terminal elimination half-life ( ): coefficient of variation in %
*: mean values
†: analyzed by nonlinear mixed effect modeling with data pooled across dose strengths
‡: sampling times did not allow calculation
§: results from adolescents (dose=1.8 mg/kg, N=3)
‖: results from children (dose=1.8 mg/kg, N=7)

Table 2. Prevention of Chemotherapy-Induced Nausea and Vomiting from Moderately Emetogenic Chemotherapy

	ANZEMET Tablets				
Response Over 24 Hours	25 mg (N=78)	50 mg (N=83)	**100 mg† (N=80)**	200 mg (N=78)	*p*-value for Linear Trend
Complete Response‡	24 (31%)	34 (41%)	**49 (61%)**	46 (59%)	P<.0001
Nausea Score§	49	10	**11**	7	P=.0006

†: The recommended dose
‡: No emetic episodes and no rescue medication.
§: Median 24-h change from baseline nausea score using visual analog scale (VAS): Score range 0="none" to 100="nausea as bad as it could be."

Table 3. Prevention of Postoperative Nausea and Vomiting

	ANZEMET Tablets				
Response Over 24 Hours	25 mg (N=159)	50 mg (N=166)	**100 mg† (N=154)**	200 mg (N=154)	Placebo (N=156)
Complete Response‡	71 (45%)	95 (57%)*	**78 (51%)***	73 (47%)*	55 (35%)
Nausea Score§	5*	4*	**5***	6*	15

*: p<.05 vs placebo
†: The recommended dose
‡: No emetic episodes and no rescue medication.
§: Median 24-h change from baseline nausea score using visual analog scale (VAS): Score range 0="none" to 100="nausea as bad as it could be."

A cardiac conduction abnormality observed on an intraoperative cardiac rhythm monitor (interpreted as complete heart block) was reported in a 61-year-old woman who received 200 mg ANZEMET for the prevention of postoperative nausea and vomiting. This patient was also taking verapamil. A similar event also interpreted as complete heart block was reported in one patient receiving placebo.

A 66-year-old man with Stage IV non-Hodgkins lymphoma died suddenly 6 hours after receiving 1.8 mg/kg (119 mg) intravenous ANZEMET Injection. This patient had other potential risk factors including substantial exposure to doxorubicin and concomitant cyclophosphamide.

PRECAUTIONS

General

Dolasetron should be administered with caution in patients who have or may develop prolongation of cardiac conduction intervals, particularly QT_c. These include patients with hypokalemia or hypomagnesemia, patients taking diuretics with potential for inducing electrolyte abnormalities, patients with congenital QT syndrome, patients taking anti-arrhythmic drugs or other drugs which lead to QT prolongation, and cumulative high dose anthracycline therapy.

Cross hypersensitivity reactions have been reported in patients who received other selective 5-HT_3 receptor antagonists. These reactions have not been seen with dolasetron mesylate.

Drug Interactions

The potential for clinically significant drug-drug interactions posed by dolasetron and hydrodolasetron appears to be low for drugs commonly used in chemotherapy or surgery, because hydrodolasetron is eliminated by multiple routes. See PRECAUTIONS, General for information about potential interaction with other drugs that prolong the QT_c interval. Blood levels of hydrodolasetron increased 24% when dolasetron was coadministered with cimetidine (nonselective inhibitor of cytochrome P-450) for 7 days, and decreased 28% with coadministration of rifampin (potent inducer of cytochrome P-450) for 7 days.

ANZEMET has been safely coadministered with drugs used in chemotherapy and surgery. As with other agents which prolong ECG intervals, caution should be exercised in patients taking drugs which prolong ECG intervals, particularly QT_c.

In patients taking furosemide, nifedipine, diltiazem, ACE inhibitors, verapamil, glyburide, propranolol, and various chemotherapy agents, no effect was shown on the clearance of hydrodolasetron. Clearance of hydrodolasetron decreased by about 27% when dolasetron mesylate was administered intravenously concomitantly with atenolol. ANZEMET did not influence anesthesia recovery time in patients. Dolasetron mesylate did not inhibit the antitumor activity of four chemotherapeutic agents (cisplatin, 5-fluorouracil, doxorubicin, cyclophosphamide) in four murine models.

Carcinogenesis, Mutagenesis, Impairment of Fertility

In a 24-month carcinogenicity study, there was a statistically significant (P<0.001) increase in the incidence of combined hepatocellular adenomas and carcinomas in male mice treated with 150 mg/kg/day and above. In this study, mice (CD-1) were treated orally with dolasetron mesylate 75, 150, or 300 mg/kg/day (225, 450 or 900 mg/m^2/day). For a 50 kg person of average height (1.46 m^2 body surface area), these doses represent 3, 6, and 12 times the recommended clinical dose (74 mg/m^2) on a body surface area basis. No increase in liver tumors was observed at a dose of 75 mg/kg/day in male mice and at doses up to 300 mg/kg/day in female mice.

In a 24-month rat (Sprague-Dawley) carcinogenicity study, oral dolasetron mesylate was not tumorigenic at doses up to 150 mg/kg/day (900 mg/m^2/day, 12 times the recommended

Continued on next page

Anzemet Tablets—Cont.

human dose based on body surface area) in male rats and 300 mg/kg/day (1800 mg/m^2/day, 24 times the recommended human dose based on body surface area) in female rats.
Dolasetron mesylate was not genotoxic in the Ames test, the rat lymphocyte chromosomal aberration test, the Chinese hamster ovary (CHO) cell (HGPRT) forward mutation test, the rat hepatocyte unscheduled DNA synthesis (UDS) test or the mouse micronucleus test.
Dolasetron mesylate was found to have no effect on fertility and reproductive performance at oral doses up to 100 mg/kg/day (600 mg/m^2/day, 8 times the recommended human dose based on body surface area) in female rats and up to 400 mg/kg/day (2400 mg/m^2/day, 32 times the recommended human dose based on body surface area) in male rats.

Pregnancy: Teratogenic Effects, Pregnancy Category B.
Teratology studies have not revealed evidence of impaired fertility or harm to the fetus due to dolasetron mesylate. These studies have been performed in pregnant rats at oral doses up to 100 mg/kg/day (8 times the recommended human dose based on body surface area) and pregnant rabbits at oral doses up to 100 mg/kg/day (16 times the recommended human dose based on body surface area). There are, however, no adequate and well-controlled studies in pregnant women. Because animal reproduction studies are not always predictive of human response, this drug should be used during pregnancy only if clearly needed.

Nursing Mothers
It is not known whether dolasetron mesylate is excreted in human milk. Because many drugs are excreted in human milk, caution should be exercised when ANZEMET Tablets are administered to a nursing woman.

Pediatric Use
ANZEMET Tablets are expected to be as safe and effective as when ANZEMET Injection is given orally to pediatric patients. ANZEMET Tablets are recommended for children old enough to swallow tablets (see CLINICAL PHARMACOLOGY, Pharmacokinetics in Humans).

Elderly
Dosage adjustment is not needed in patients over 65. Effectiveness in prevention of nausea and vomiting in elderly patients was no different than in younger age groups.

ADVERSE REACTIONS

Chemotherapy Patients
In controlled clinical trials, 943 adult cancer patients received ANZEMET Tablets. These patients were receiving concurrent chemotherapy, predominantly cyclophosphamide and doxorubicin regimens. The following adverse events were reported in ≥2% of patients receiving either ANZEMET 25 mg or ANZEMET 100 mg tablets for prevention of cancer chemotherapy induced nausea and vomiting in controlled clinical trials (Table 4).

Table 4. Adverse Events ≥ 2% from Chemotherapy-Induced Nausea and Vomiting Studies

	ANZEMET	
Event	25 mg (N=235)	100 mg (N=227)
Headache	42 (17.9%)	52 (22.9%)
Fatigue	6 (2.6%)	13 (5.7%)
Diarrhea	5 (2.1%)	12 (5.3%)
Bradycardia	12 (5.1%)	9 (4.0%)
Dizziness	3 (1.3%)	7 (3.1%)
Pain	0	7 (3.1%)
Tachycardia	7 (3.0%)	6 (2.6%)
Dyspepsia	7 (3.0%)	5 (2.2%)
Chills/Shivering	3 (1.3%)	5 (2.2%)

Postoperative Patients
In controlled clinical trials, 936 adult female patients have received oral ANZEMET for the prevention of postoperative nausea and vomiting. Following is a listing of all adverse events reported in ≥2% of patients receiving either placebo or ANZEMET for prevention of postoperative nausea and vomiting in controlled clinical trials (Table 5).

Table 5. Adverse Events ≥ 2% from Placebo-Controlled Postoperative Nausea and Vomiting Studies

Event	ANZEMET 100 mg (N=228)	Placebo (N=231)
Headache	16 (7.0%)	11 (4.8%)
Hypotension	12 (5.3%)	15 (6.5%)
Dizziness	10 (4.4%)	0 (0.0%)
Fever	8 (3.5%)	7 (3.0%)
Pruritus	7 (3.1%)	8 (3.5%)
Oliguria	6 (2.6%)	3 (1.3%)
Hypertension	5 (2.2%)	7 (3.0%)
Tachycardia	5 (2.2%)	2 (0.9%)

In clinical trials, the following infrequently reported adverse events, assessed by investigators as treatment-related or causality unknown, occurred following oral or intravenous administration of ANZEMET to adult patients receiving concomitant cancer chemotherapy or surgery:
Cardiovascular: Hypotension; rarely–edema, peripheral edema. The following events also occurred rarely and with a similar frequency as placebo and/or active comparator: Mobitz I AV block, chest pain, orthostatic hypotension, myocardial ischemia, syncope, severe bradycardia, and palpitations. See PRECAUTIONS section for information on potential effects on ECG.
In addition, the following asymptomatic treatment-emergent ECG changes were seen at rates less than or equal to those for active or placebo controls: bradycardia, T wave change, ST-T wave change, sinus arrhythmia, extrasystole (APCs or VPCs), poor R-wave progression, bundle branch block (left and right), nodal arrhythmia, U wave change, atrial flutter/fibrillation.
Furthermore, severe hypotension, bradycardia and syncope have been reported immediately or closely following IV administration.
Dermatologic: Rash, increased sweating.
Gastrointestinal System: Constipation, dyspepsia, abdominal pain, anorexia; rarely—pancreatitis.
Hearing, Taste and Vision: Taste perversion, abnormal vision; rarely—tinnitus, photophobia.
Hematologic: Rarely—hematuria, epistaxis, prothrombin time prolonged, PTT increased, anemia, purpura/hematoma, thrombocytopenia.
Hypersensitivity: Rarely—anaphylactic reaction, facial edema, urticaria.
Liver and Biliary System: Transient increases in AST (SGOT) and/or ALT (SGPT) values have been reported as adverse events in less than 1% of adult patients receiving ANZEMET in clinical trials. The increases did not appear to be related to dose or duration of therapy and were not associated with symptomatic hepatic disease. Similar increases were seen with patients receiving active comparator. Rarely—hyperbilirubinemia, increased GGT.
Metabolic and Nutritional: Rarely—alkaline phosphatase increased.
Musculoskeletal: Rarely—myalgia, arthralgia.
Nervous System: Flushing, vertigo, paresthesia, tremor; rarely—ataxia, twitching.
Psychiatric: Agitation, sleep disorder, depersonalization; rarely—confusion, anxiety, abnormal dreaming.
Respiratory System: Rarely—dyspnea, bronchospasm.
Urinary System: Rarely—dysuria, polyuria, acute renal failure.
Vascular (Extracardiac): Local pain or burning on IV administration; rarely—peripheral ischemia, thrombophlebitis/phlebitis.

OVERDOSAGE

A 59-year-old man with metastatic melanoma and no known pre-existing cardiac conditions developed severe hypotension and dizziness 40 minutes after receiving a 15 minute intravenous infusion of 1000 mg (13 mg/kg) of dolasetron mesylate. Treatment for the overdose consisted of infusion of 500 mL of a plasma expander, dopamine, and atropine. The patient had normal sinus rhythm and prolongation of PR, QRS and QT$_c$ intervals on an ECG recorded 2 hours after the infusion. The patient's blood pressure was normal 3 hours after the event and the ECG intervals returned to baseline on follow-up. The patient was released from the hospital 6 hours after the event.
Following a suspected overdose of ANZEMET Injection, a patient found to have second-degree or higher AV conduction block with ECG should undergo cardiac telemetry monitoring.
There is no known specific antidote for dolasetron mesylate, and patients with suspected overdose should be managed with supportive therapy. Individual doses as large as 5 mg/kg intravenously or 400 mg orally have been safely given to healthy volunteers or cancer patients.
It is not known if dolasetron mesylate is removed by hemodialysis or peritoneal dialysis.
A 7-year-old boy received 6 mg/kg of dolasetron mesylate orally before surgery. No symptoms occurred and no treatment was required.
Single intravenous doses of dolasetron mesylate at 160 mg/kg in male mice and 140 mg/kg in female mice and rats of both sexes (6.3 to 12.6 times the recommended human dose based on body surface area) were lethal. Symptoms of acute toxicity were tremors, depression and convulsions.

DOSAGE AND ADMINISTRATION

The recommended doses of ANZEMET Tablets should not be exceeded.

Prevention of Cancer Chemotherapy-Induced Nausea and Vomiting
Adults: The recommended oral dosage of ANZEMET (dolasetron mesylate) is 100 mg given within one hour before chemotherapy.
Pediatric Patients: The recommended oral dosage in pediatric patients 2 to 16 years of age is 1.8 mg/kg given within one hour before chemotherapy, up to a maximum of 100 mg. Safety and effectiveness in pediatric patients under 2 years of age have not been established.
Use in the Elderly, Renal Failure Patients, or Hepatically Impaired Patients: No dosage adjustment is recommended. (See Pharmacokinetics in Humans.)

Prevention of Postoperative Nausea and Vomiting
Adults: The recommended oral dosage of ANZEMET (dolasetron mesylate) is 100 mg within two hours before surgery.
Pediatric Patients: The recommended oral dosage in pediatric patients 2 to 16 years of age is 1.2 mg/kg given within two hours before surgery, up to a maximum of 100 mg. Safety and effectiveness in pediatric patients under 2 years of age have not been established.
Use in the Elderly, Renal Failure Patients, or Hepatically Impaired Patients: No dosage adjustment is recommended. (See Pharmacokinetics in Humans.)

HOW SUPPLIED

[See table below]
Store at controlled room temperature 20–25°C (68–77°F). Protect from light.

Prescribing Information as of October 2003

Manufactured by: Patheon Pharmaceuticals Inc.
Cincinnati, OH 45215 USA
Manufactured for: Aventis Pharmaceuticals Inc.
Kansas City, MO 64137 USA
www.aventis-us.com
Shown in Product Identification Guide, page 307

ANZEMET® Tablets
(dolasetron mesylate)

Strength	Quantity	NDC Number	Description
50 mg	5 ct Bottle 10 ct Unit Dose 5 ct Blister Pack	0088-1202-05 0088-1202-43 0088-1202-29	Light pink, film coated, round tablet imprinted with "A" on one side and "50" on the other.
100 mg	5 ct Bottle 10 ct Unit Dose 5 ct Blister Pack	0088-1203-05 0088-1203-43 0088-1203-29	Pink, film coated, elongated oval tablet imprinted with "100" on one side and "ANZEMET" on the other.

APIDRA™ ℞

[a'pĭ-dră]
Insulin glulisine (rDNA origin) injection
Rx only
Prescribing Information as of April 2004a

DESCRIPTION

APIDRA™ (insulin glulisine [rDNA origin]) is a human insulin analog that is a rapid-acting, parenteral blood glucose lowering agent. Insulin glulisine is produced by recombinant DNA technology utilizing a non-pathogenic laboratory strain of *Escherichia coli* (K12). Insulin glulisine differs from human insulin in that the amino acid asparagine at position B3 is replaced by lysine and the lysine in position B29 is replaced by glutamic acid. Chemically, it is 3^B-lysine-29^B-glutamic acid-human insulin, has the empirical formula $C_{258}H_{384}N_{64}O_{78}S_6$ and a molecular weight of 5823. It has the following structural formula:

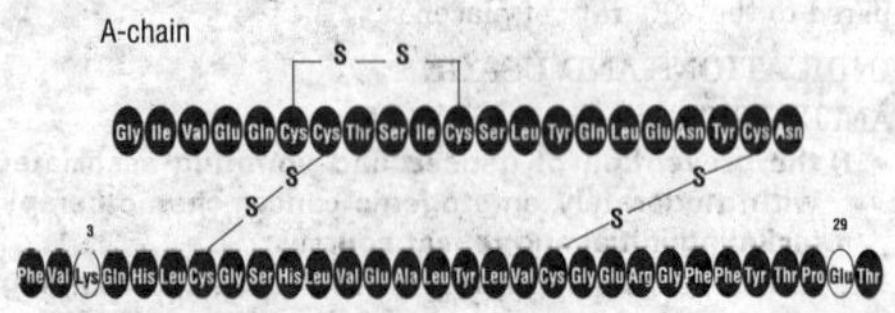

APIDRA is a sterile, aqueous, clear, and colorless solution. Each milliliter of APIDRA (insulin glulisine injection) contains 100 IU (3.49 mg) insulin glulisine, 3.15 mg m-cresol, 6 mg tromethamine, 5 mg sodium chloride, 0.01 mg polysorbate 20, and water for injection. APIDRA has a pH of approximately 7.3. The pH is adjusted by addition of aqueous solutions of hydrochloric acid and/or sodium hydroxide.

CLINICAL PHARMACOLOGY

Mechanism of Action
The primary activity of insulins and insulin analogs, including insulin glulisine, is regulation of glucose metabolism.

Insulins lower blood glucose levels by stimulating peripheral glucose uptake by skeletal muscle and fat, and by inhibiting hepatic glucose production. Insulins inhibit lipolysis in the adipocyte, inhibit proteolysis, and enhance protein synthesis.

The glucose lowering activities of APIDRA and of regular human insulin are equipotent when administered by the intravenous route. After subcutaneous administration, the effect of APIDRA is more rapid in onset and of shorter duration compared to regular human insulin.

Pharmacokinetics

Absorption and Bioavailability

Pharmacokinetic profiles in healthy volunteers and patients with diabetes (type 1 or type 2) demonstrated that absorption of insulin glulisine was faster than regular human insulin.

In a study in patients with type 1 diabetes (n=20) after subcutaneous administration of 0.15 IU/kg, the median time to maximum concentration (T_{max}) was 55 minutes (range 34 to 91 minutes) and the peak concentration (C_{max}) was 82 µIU/mL (range 42 to 134 µIU/mL) for insulin glulisine compared to a median T_{max} of 82 minutes (range 52 to 308 minutes) and a C_{max} of 46 µIU/mL (range 32 to 70 µIU/mL) for regular human insulin. The mean residence time of insulin glulisine was shorter (median: 98 minutes, range 55 to 149 minutes) than for regular human insulin (median: 161 minutes, range 133 to 193 minutes). (See Figure 1.)

Figure 1. Pharmacokinetic profile of insulin glulisine and regular human insulin in patients with type 1 diabetes after a dose of 0.15 IU/kg.

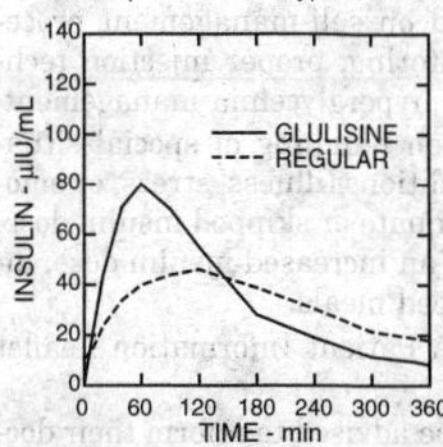

In a euglycemic clamp study in patients with type 2 diabetes (n=24) with a body mass index (BMI) between 20 to 36 kg/m² after subcutaneous administration of 0.2 IU/kg, the median time to maximum concentration (T_{max}) was 89 minutes (range 74 to 103 minutes) and the median peak concentration (C_{max}) was 81µIU/mL (range 75 to 112 µIU/mL) for insulin glulisine compared to a median T_{max} of 94 minutes (range 55 to 140 minutes) and a median C_{max} of 39 µIU/mL (range 30 to 56 µIU/mL) for regular human insulin. The mean residence time of insulin glulisine was shorter (median: 154 minutes, range 122 to 174 minutes) than for regular human insulin (median: 280 minutes, range 227 to 294 minutes).

Figure 2. Pharmacokinetic profile of insulin glulisine and regular human insulin in patients with type 2 diabetes after a dose of 0.2 IU/kg.

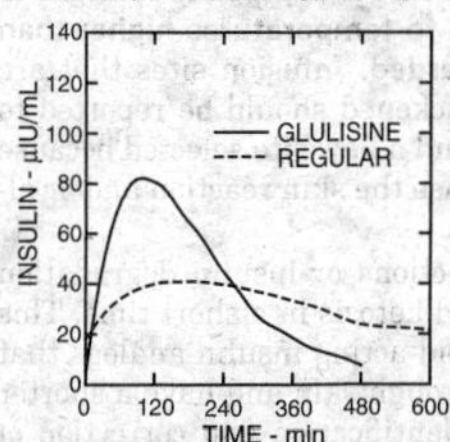

In a euglycemic clamp study in obese, non-diabetic subjects (n=18) with a body mass index (BMI) between 30 to 40 kg/m² after subcutaneous administration of 0.3 IU/kg, the median time to maximum concentration (T_{max}) was 76 minutes (range 51 to 118 minutes) and the median peak concentration (C_{max}) was 199 µIU/mL (range 99 to 387 µIU/mL) for insulin glulisine compared to a median T_{max} of 144 minutes (range 110 to 207 minutes) and a median C_{max} of 79 µIU/mL (range 39 to 166 µIU/mL) for regular human insulin. The mean residence time of insulin glulisine was shorter (median: 141 minutes, range 105 to 210 minutes) than for regular human insulin (median: 226 minutes, range 188 to 293 minutes).

When APIDRA was injected subcutaneously into different areas of the body, the time-concentration profiles were similar. The absolute bioavailability of insulin glulisine after subcutaneous administration is about 70%, regardless of injection area (abdomen 73%, deltoid 71%, thigh 68%).

Distribution and Elimination

The distribution and elimination of insulin glulisine and regular human insulin after intravenous administration are similar with volumes of distribution of 13 L and 21 L and half-lives of 13 and 17 minutes, respectively. After subcutaneous administration, insulin glulisine is eliminated more rapidly than regular human insulin with an apparent half-life of 42 minutes compared to 86 minutes.

Pharmacodynamics

Studies in healthy volunteers and patients with diabetes demonstrated that APIDRA has a more rapid onset of action and a shorter duration of activity than regular human insulin when given subcutaneously.

In a study in patients with type 1 diabetes (n= 20), the glucose-lowering profiles of APIDRA and regular human insulin were assessed at various times in relation to a standard meal at a dose of 0.15 IU/kg. (See Figure 3.)

Figure 3. Serial mean blood glucose collected up to 6 hours following single dose of APIDRA and regular human insulin. APIDRA given 2 minutes (APIDRA - pre) before the start of a meal compared to regular human insulin given 30 minutes (Regular - 30 min) before start of the meal (Figure 3A) and compared to regular human insulin (Regular - pre) given 2 minutes before a meal (Figure 3B). APIDRA given 15 minutes (APIDRA - post) after start of a meal compared to regular human insulin (Regular - pre) given 2 minutes before a meal (Figure 3C). On the x-axis zero (0) is the start of a 15-minute meal.

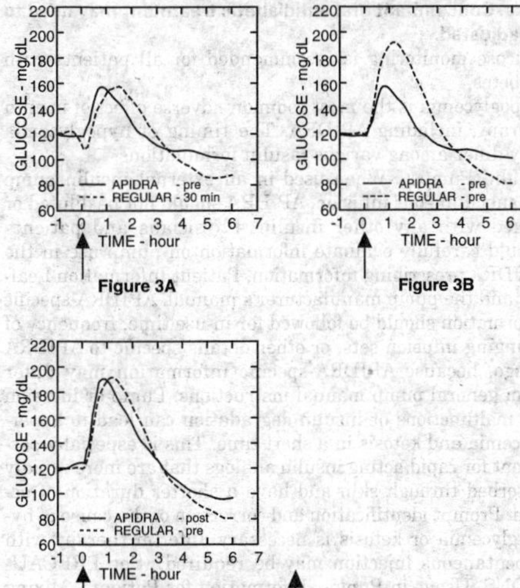

The maximum blood glucose excursion (ΔGLU_{max}; baseline subtracted glucose concentration) for APIDRA injected 2 minutes before meal was 65 mg/dL compared to 64 mg/dL for regular human insulin injected 30 minutes before meal (see Figure 3A), and 84 mg.h/dL for regular human insulin injected 2 minutes before meal (see Figure 3B). The maximum blood glucose excursion for APIDRA injected 15 minutes after the start of a meal was 85 mg/dL compared to 84 mg.h/dL for regular human insulin injected 2 minutes before meal (see Figure 3C).

Special Populations

Pediatric Patients

The pharmacokinetic and pharmacodynamic properties of APIDRA and regular human insulin were assessed in a study conducted in pediatric patients with type 1 diabetes (children [7 to 11 years, n = 10] and adolescents [12 to 16 years, n = 10]). The relative differences in pharmacokinetics and pharmacodynamics between APIDRA and regular human insulin in pediatric patients with type 1 diabetes were similar to those in healthy adult subjects and adults with type 1 diabetes.

Gender

Information on the effect of gender on the pharmacokinetics of APIDRA is not available.

Race

A study was performed in 24 healthy Caucasians and Japanese to compare the pharmacokinetic and pharmacodynamic parameters after subcutaneous injection of insulin glulisine, insulin lispro, and regular human insulin. With subcutaneous injection of insulin glulisine, Japanese subjects had a greater initial exposure (33%) for the ratio of AUC(0-1hr) to AUC (0-clamp end) than that in Caucasians (21%) though the total exposures were similar. Similar findings were observed with insulin lispro and regular human insulin for the racial difference.

Obesity

The more rapid onset of action and shorter duration of activity of APIDRA and insulin lispro compared to regular human insulin were maintained in an obese non-diabetic population (n= 18). (See Figure 4.)

Figure 4. Glucose infusion rates (GIR) in a euglycemic clamp study after subcutaneous injection of 0.3 IU/kg of APIDRA, insulin lispro or regular human insulin in an obese population.

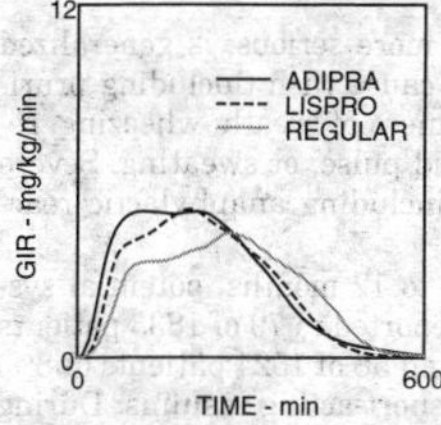

Renal Impairment

Studies with human insulin have shown increased circulating levels of insulin in patients with renal failure. In a study performed in 24 non-diabetic subjects covering a wide range of renal function (Cl_{Cr} >80 mL/min; 30-50 mL/min; <30 mL/min), the subjects with moderate and severe renal impairment showed increased exposure of insulin glulisine by 29% to 40% and reduced clearance of insulin glulisine by 20 to 25% compared to normal subjects. Careful glucose monitoring and dose adjustments of insulin, including APIDRA, may be necessary in patients with renal dysfunction. (See PRECAUTIONS, Renal Impairment.)

Hepatic Impairment

The effect of hepatic impairment on the pharmacokinetics of APIDRA has not been studied. Some studies with human insulin have shown increased circulating levels of insulin in patients with liver failure. Careful glucose monitoring and dose adjustments of insulin, including APIDRA, may be necessary in patients with hepatic dysfunction. (See PRECAUTIONS, Hepatic Impairment.)

Pregnancy

The effect of pregnancy on the pharmacokinetics and pharmacodynamics of APIDRA has not been studied. (See PRECAUTIONS, Pregnancy.)

Smoking

The effect of smoking on the pharmacokinetics and pharmacodynamics of APIDRA has not been studied.

CLINICAL STUDIES

The safety and efficacy of APIDRA was studied in adult patients with type 1 and type 2 diabetes (n=1833). The primary efficacy parameter was glycemic control, as measured by glycated hemoglobin (GHb), and expressed as hemoglobin A1c equivalents (HbA1c).

Type 1 Diabetes:

A 26-week, randomized, open-label, active-control study was conducted in patients with type 1 diabetes to assess the safety and efficacy of APIDRA (n= 339) compared to insulin lispro (n= 333) when administered subcutaneously within 15 minutes before a meal. Lantus® (insulin glargine)† was administered once daily in the evening as the basal insulin. There was a 4-week run-in period combining insulin lispro and Lantus followed by randomization. Most patients were Caucasian (97%). Fifty eight percent of the patients were male. The mean age was 38.5 years (range 18 to 74 years). Glycemic control (see Table 1) and the rates of hypoglycemia requiring intervention from a third party (see Adverse Reactions), were comparable for the two treatment regimens. The number of daily short-acting insulin injections and the total daily doses of APIDRA and insulin lispro were similar. (See Table 1.)

Table 1: Type 1 Diabetes Mellitus–Adult

Treatment duration	26 weeks	
Treatment in combination with:	Lantus®	
	APIDRA	Insulin Lispro
HbA1c (%)		
Number of patients	331	322
Baseline mean	7.60	7.58
Adj. mean change from baseline	-0.14	-0.14
APIDRA – Insulin Lispro	0.00	
95% CI for treatment difference	(-0.09; 0.10)	
Basal insulin dose (IU/day)		
Endstudy mean	24.16	26.43
Adj. mean change from baseline	0.12	1.82
Short-acting insulin dose (IU/day)		
Endstudy mean	29.03	30.12
Adj. mean change from baseline	-1.07	-0.81
Mean number of short-acting insulin injections per day	3.36	3.42

Type 2 Diabetes:

A 26-week, randomized, open-label, active-control study was conducted in insulin-treated patients with type 2 diabetes to assess the safety and efficacy of APIDRA (n= 435) given within 15 minutes before a meal compared to regular human insulin (n=441) administered 30 to 45 minutes prior to a meal. NPH human insulin was given twice a day as the basal insulin. All patients participated in a 4-week run-in period combining regular human insulin and NPH human insulin. Eighty-five percent of patients were Caucasian and 11% were Black. The mean age was 58.3 years (range 26 to 84 years). The average body mass index (BMI) was 34.55 kg/m². At randomization, 58% of the patients were on an oral antidiabetic agent and were instructed to continue use of their oral antidiabetic agent at the same dose. The majority of patients (79%) mixed their short-acting insulin with NPH human insulin immediately prior to injection. The reductions from baseline in HbA1c were similar between treatment groups (see Table 2). The rates of hypoglycemia, requiring intervention from a third party, were comparable for the two treatment regimens (see Adverse Reactions). No differences between APIDRA and regular human insulin groups were seen in the number of daily short-acting insulin injections or basal or short-acting insulin doses. (See Table 2.)

Table 2: Type 2 Diabetes Mellitus–Adult

Treatment duration	26 weeks	
Treatment in combination with:	NPH human insulin	
	APIDRA	Regular Human Insulin
HbA1c (%)		
Number of patients	404	403
Baseline mean	7.57	7.50
Adj. mean change from baseline	-0.46	-0.30
APIDRA – Regular Human Insulin	-0.16	
95% CI for treatment difference	(-0.26; -0.05)	

Continued on next page

Apidra—Cont.

Basal insulin dose (IU/day)		
Endstudy mean	65.34	63.05
Adj. mean change from baseline	5.73	6.03
Short-acting insulin dose (IU/day)		
Endstudy mean	35.99	36.16
Adj. mean change from baseline	3.69	5.00
Mean number of short-acting insulin injections per day	2.27	2.24

Pre- and Post-Meal Administration (Type 1 Diabetes):
A 12-week, randomized, open-label, active-control study was conducted in patients with type 1 diabetes to assess the safety and efficacy of APIDRA administered at different times with respect to a meal. APIDRA was administered subcutaneously either within 15 minutes before a meal (n=286) or immediately after a meal (n=296) and regular human insulin (n= 278) was administered subcutaneously 30 to 45 minutes prior to a meal. Lantus® was administered once daily at bedtime as the basal insulin. There was a 4-week run-in period combining regular human insulin and Lantus followed by randomization. Most patients were Caucasian (94%). The mean age was 40.3 years (range 18 to 73 years). Glycemic control (see Table 3) and the rates of hypoglycemia requiring intervention from a third party (see Adverse Reactions) were comparable for the treatment regimens. No changes from baseline between the treatments were seen in the total daily number of short-acting insulin injections. (See Table 3.)

Table 3: Type 1 Diabetes Mellitus–Adult

Treatment duration Treatment in combination with:	12 weeks Lantus® APIDRA pre meal	12 weeks Lantus® APIDRA post meal	12 weeks Lantus® Regular Human Insulin
HbA1c (%)			
Number of patients	268	276	257
Baseline mean	7.73	7.70	7.64
Adj. mean change from baseline*	-0.26	-0.11	-0.13
Basal insulin dose (IU/day)			
Endstudy mean	29.49	28.77	28.46
Adj. mean change from baseline	0.99	0.24	0.65
Short-acting insulin dose (IU/day)			
Endstudy mean	28.44	28.06	29.23
Adj. mean change from baseline	-0.88	-0.47	1.75
Mean number of short-acting insulin injections per day	3.15	3.13	3.03

*Adj. mean change from baseline treatment difference (98.33% CI for treatment difference): APIDRA pre meal vs. Regular Human Insulin - 0.13 (-0.26; 0.01); APIDRA post meal vs. Regular Human Insulin 0.02 (-0.11; 0.16); APIDRA post meal vs. pre meal 0.15 (0.02; 0.29).

Continuous Subcutaneous Insulin Infusion (CSII) (Type 1 Diabetes):
To evaluate the use of APIDRA for administration using an external pump, a 12-week randomized, active control study (APIDRA versus insulin aspart) was conducted in patients with type 1 diabetes (APIDRA n=29, insulin aspart n=30). All patients were Caucasian. The mean age was 45.8 (range 21-73 years). Glycemic control (mean HbA1c value at endpoint 6.98% with APIDRA and 7.18% with insulin aspart) and the rates of hypoglycemia requiring intervention from a third party were comparable for the two treatment regimens.

INDICATIONS AND USAGE

APIDRA is indicated for the treatment of adult patients with diabetes mellitus for the control of hyperglycemia.
APIDRA has a more rapid onset of action and a shorter duration of action than regular human insulin. APIDRA should normally be used in regimens that include a longer-acting insulin or basal insulin analog. (See WARNINGS and DOSAGE AND ADMINISTRATION.)
APIDRA may also be infused subcutaneously by external insulin infusion pumps. (See WARNINGS, PRECAUTIONS, Usage in Pumps, Information for Patients, Mixing of Insulins, DOSAGE AND ADMINISTRATION, RECOMMENDED STORAGE.)

CONTRAINDICATIONS

APIDRA is contraindicated during episodes of hypoglycemia and in patients hypersensitive to APIDRA or one of its excipients.

WARNINGS

APIDRA differs from regular human insulin by its rapid onset of action and shorter duration of action. When used as a meal time insulin, the dose of APIDRA should be given within 15 minutes before or immediately after a meal. Because of the short duration of action of APIDRA, patients with diabetes also require a longer-acting insulin or insulin infusion pump therapy to maintain adequate glucose control.
Any change of insulin should be made cautiously and only under medical supervision. Changes in insulin strength, manufacturer, type (e.g., regular, NPH, analogs), or species (animal, human) may result in the need for a change in dose. Concomitant oral antidiabetic treatment may need to be adjusted.
Glucose monitoring is recommended for all patients with diabetes.
Hypoglycemia is the most common adverse effect of insulin therapy, including APIDRA. The timing of hypoglycemia may differ among various insulin formulations.
Insulin Pumps: When used in an external insulin pump for subcutaneous infusion, APIDRA should not be diluted or mixed with any other insulin. Physicians and patients should carefully evaluate information on pump use in the APIDRA prescribing information, Patient Information Leaflet, and the pump manufacturer's manual. APIDRA-specific information should be followed for in-use time, frequency of changing infusion sets, or other details specific to APIDRA usage, because APIDRA-specific information may differ from general pump manual instructions. Pump or infusion set malfunctions or insulin degradation can lead to hyperglycemia and ketosis in a short time. This is especially pertinent for rapid-acting insulin analogs that are more rapidly absorbed through skin and have a shorter duration of action. Prompt identification and correction of the cause of hyperglycemia or ketosis is necessary. Interim therapy with subcutaneous injection may be required. (See PRECAUTIONS, Usage in Pumps, Information for Patients, Mixing of Insulins, DOSAGE AND ADMINISTRATION, and RECOMMENDED STORAGE.)

PRECAUTIONS

General
As with all insulin preparations, the time course of APIDRA action may vary in different individuals or at different times in the same individual and is dependent on site of injection, blood supply, temperature, and physical activity.
Adjustment of dosage of any insulin may be necessary if patients change their physical activity or their usual meal plan.
Insulin requirements may be altered during intercurrent conditions such as illness, emotional disturbances, or stress.
Hypoglycemia
As with all insulin preparations, hypoglycemic reactions may be associated with the administration of APIDRA. Rapid changes in serum glucose levels may induce symptoms similar to hypoglycemia in persons with diabetes, regardless of the glucose value. Early warning symptoms of hypoglycemia may be different or less pronounced under certain conditions, such as long duration of diabetes, diabetic nerve disease, use of medications such as beta-blockers, or intensified diabetes control. (See PRECAUTIONS, Drug Interactions.)
Such situations may result in severe hypoglycemia (and, possibly, loss of consciousness) prior to patients' awareness of hypoglycemia.
Renal Impairment
The requirements for APIDRA may be reduced in patients with renal impairment. (See CLINICAL PHARMACOLOGY, Special Populations.)
Hepatic Impairment
Studies have not been performed in patients with hepatic impairment. APIDRA requirements may be diminished due to reduced capacity for gluconeogenesis and reduced insulin metabolism, similar to observations found with other insulins. (See CLINICAL PHARMACOLOGY, Special Populations.)
Allergy
Local Allergy
As with other insulin therapy, patients may experience redness, swelling, or itching at the site of injection. These minor reactions usually resolve in a few days to a few weeks. In some instances, these reactions may be related to factors other than insulin, such as irritants in a skin cleansing agent or poor injection technique.
Systemic Allergy
Less common, but potentially more serious, is generalized allergy to insulin, which may cause rash (including pruritus) over the whole body, shortness of breath, wheezing, reduction in blood pressure, rapid pulse, or sweating. Severe cases of generalized allergy, including anaphylactic reactions, may be life threatening.
In controlled clinical trials up to 12 months, potential systemic allergic reactions were reported in 79 of 1833 patients (4.3%) who received APIDRA and 58 of 1524 patients (3.8%) who received the comparator short-acting insulins. During these trials treatment with APIDRA was permanently discontinued in 1 of 1833 patients due to a potential systemic allergic reaction.
Localized reactions and generalized myalgias have been reported with the use of cresol as an injectable excipient.
As with any insulin therapy, lipodystrophy may occur at the injection site and delay insulin absorption.
Antibody Production
In a study in patients with type 1 diabetes (n=333), the concentrations of insulin antibodies that react with both human insulin and insulin glulisine (cross-reactive insulin antibodies) remained near baseline during the first 6 months of the study in the patients treated with APIDRA. A decrease in antibody concentration was observed during the following 6 months of the study. In a study in patients with type 2 diabetes (n=411), a similar increase in cross-reactive insulin antibody concentration was observed in the patients treated with APIDRA and in the patients treated with human insulin during the first 9 months of the study. Thereafter the concentration of antibodies decreased in the APIDRA patients and remained stable in the human insulin patients. There was no correlation between cross-reactive insulin antibody concentration and changes in HbA1c, insulin doses, or incidences of hypoglycemia.
Usage in Pumps
APIDRA has been studied in the following pumps and infusion sets: Disetronic® H-Tron® plus V100 and D-Tron® with Disetronic catheters (Rapid™, Rapid C™, Rapid D™, and Tender™); MiniMed® Models 506, 507, 507c and 508 with MiniMed catheters (Sof-set Ultimate QR™, and Quick-set™)‡.
Based on *in vitro* studies which have shown loss of m-cresol, and insulin degradation, APIDRA should not be used beyond 48 hours at 98.6°F (37°C) in infusion sets and reservoirs. APIDRA in clinical use should not be exposed to temperatures greater than 98.6°F (37°C). **APIDRA should not be mixed with other insulins or with a diluent when used in the pump.** (See WARNINGS, PRECAUTIONS, Information for Patients, Mixing of Insulins, DOSAGE AND ADMINISTRATION, and RECOMMENDED STORAGE.)
Information for Patients
For all patients
Patients should be instructed on self-management procedures including glucose monitoring, proper injection technique, and hypoglycemia and hyperglycemia management. Patients must be instructed on handling of special situations such as intercurrent conditions (illness, stress, or emotional disturbances), an inadequate or skipped insulin dose, inadvertent administration of an increased insulin dose, inadequate food intake, or skipped meals.
Refer patients to the APIDRA Patient Information Leaflet for additional information.
Women with diabetes should be advised to inform their doctor if they are pregnant or are contemplating pregnancy.
For patients using pumps
Patients using external pump infusion therapy should be trained appropriately. APIDRA has been studied in the following pumps and infusion sets: Disetronic H-Tron plus V100 and D-Tron with Disetronic catheters (Rapid, Rapid C, Rapid D, and Tender); MiniMed Models 506, 507, 507c and 508 with MiniMed catheters (Sof-set Ultimate QR, and Quick-set).
To minimize insulin degradation, infusion set occlusion, and loss of the preservative (m-cresol), the infusion sets (reservoir, tubing, and catheter) and the APIDRA in the reservoir should be replaced every 48 hours or less and a new infusion site should be selected. The temperature of the insulin may exceed ambient temperature when the pump housing, cover, tubing or sport case is exposed to sunlight or radiant heat. **Insulin exposed to temperatures higher than 98.6°F (37°C) should be discarded.** Infusion sites that are erythematous, pruritic, or thickened should be reported to the healthcare professional, and a new site selected because continued infusion may increase the skin reaction and/or alter the absorption of APIDRA.
Pump or infusion set malfunctions or insulin degradation can lead to hyperglycemia and ketosis in a short time. This is especially pertinent for rapid-acting insulin analogs that are more rapidly absorbed through skin and have a shorter duration of action. Prompt identification and correction of the cause of hyperglycemia or ketosis is necessary. Problems include pump malfunction, infusion set occlusion, leakage, disconnection or kinking, and degraded insulin. Less commonly, hypoglycemia from pump malfunction may occur. If these problems cannot be promptly corrected, patients should resume therapy with subcutaneous insulin injection and contact their healthcare professional. (See WARNINGS, PRECAUTIONS, Usage in Pumps, Mixing of Insulins, DOSAGE AND ADMINISTRATION, and RECOMMENDED STORAGE.)
Drug Interactions
A number of substances affect glucose metabolism and may require insulin dose adjustment and particularly close monitoring.
The following are examples of substances that may reduce the blood-glucose-lowering effect of insulin: corticosteroids, danazol, diazoxide, diuretics, sympathomimetic agents (e.g., epinephrine, albuterol, terbutaline), glucagon, isoniazid, phenothiazine derivatives, somatropin, thyroid hormones, estrogens, progestogens (e.g., in oral contraceptives), protease inhibitors, and atypical antipsychotic medications (e.g., olanzepine and clozapine).
The following are examples of substances that may increase the blood-glucose-lowering effect and susceptibility to hypoglycemia: oral antidiabetic products, ACE inhibitors, disopyramide, fibrates, fluoxetine, MAO inhibitors, pentoxifylline, propoxyphene, salicylates, sulfonamide antibiotics.
Beta-blockers, clonidine, lithium salts, and alcohol may either potentiate or weaken the blood-glucose-lowering effect of insulin. Pentamidine may cause hypoglycemia, which may sometimes be followed by hyperglycemia.
In addition, under the influence of sympatholytic medicinal products such as beta-blockers, clonidine, guanethidine, and reserpine, the signs of hypoglycemia may be reduced or absent.

Mixing of Insulins
In a clinical study in healthy volunteers (n=32) the total insulin glulisine bioavailability was similar after subcutaneous injection of insulin glulisine and NPH insulin (premixed in the syringe) and following separate simultaneous subcutaneous injections. There was some attenuation (27%) of the maximum concentration (C_{max}) after premixing, however the time to maximum concentration (T_{max}) was not affected. If APIDRA is mixed with NPH human insulin, APIDRA should be drawn into the syringe first. Injection should be made immediately after mixing. No data are available on mixing APIDRA with insulin preparations other than NPH. (See CLINICAL STUDIES.) APIDRA should not be mixed with insulin preparations other than NPH.
Mixtures should not be administered intravenously.
The effects of mixing APIDRA with diluents or other insulins when used in external subcutaneous infusion pumps for insulin have not been studied. Therefore, APIDRA should not be mixed in these instances.

Carcinogenesis, Mutagenesis, Impairment of Fertility
Standard 2-year carcinogenicity studies in animals have not been performed. In Sprague Dawley rats, a 12-month repeat dose toxicity study was conducted with insulin glulisine at subcutaneous doses of 2.5, 5, 20 or 50 IU/kg twice daily (dose resulting in an exposure 1, 2, 8, and 20 times the average human dose, based on body surface area comparison). There was a non-dose dependent higher incidence of mammary gland tumors in female rats administered insulin glulisine compared to untreated controls. The incidence of mammary tumors for insulin glulisine and regular human insulin was similar. The relevance of these findings to humans is not known.
Insulin glulisine was not mutagenic in the following tests: Ames test, *in vitro* mammalian chromosome aberration test in V79 Chinese hamster cells, and *in vivo* mammalian erythrocyte micronucleus test in rats.
In fertility studies in male and female rats at subcutaneous doses up to 10 IU/kg once daily (dose resulting in an exposure 2 times the average human dose, based on body surface area comparison), no clear adverse effects on male and female fertility, or general reproductive performance of animals were observed.

Pregnancy - Teratogenic Effects - Pregnancy Category C
Reproduction and teratology studies have been performed with insulin glulisine in rats and rabbits using regular human insulin as a comparator.
The drug was given to female rats throughout pregnancy at subcutaneous doses up to 10 IU/kg once daily (dose resulting in an exposure 2 times the average human dose, based on body surface area comparison). Insulin glulisine did not have any remarkable toxic effects on the embryo-fetal development in rats.
The drug was given to female rabbits throughout pregnancy at subcutaneous doses up to 1.5 IU/kg/day (dose resulting in an exposure 0.5 times the average human dose, based on body surface area comparison). Adverse effects on embryo-fetal development were only seen at maternal toxic dose levels inducing hypoglycemia. Increased incidence of post-implantation losses and skeletal defects were observed at a dose level of 1.5 IU/kg once daily (dose resulting in an exposure 0.5 times the average human dose, based on body surface area comparison) that also caused mortality in dams. A slight increased incidence of post-implantation losses was seen at the next lower dose level of 0.5 IU/kg once daily (dose resulting in an exposure 0.2 times the average human dose, based on body surface area comparison) which was also associated with severe hypoglycemia but there were no defects at that dose. No effects were observed in rabbits at a dose of 0.25 IU/kg once daily (dose resulting in an exposure 0.1 times the average human dose, based on body surface area comparison). The effects of insulin glulisine did not differ from those observed with subcutaneous regular human insulin at the same doses and were attributed to secondary effects of maternal hypoglycemia.
There are no well-controlled clinical studies of the use of insulin glulisine in pregnant women. Because animal reproduction studies are not always predictive of human response, this drug should be used during pregnancy only if the potential benefit justifies the potential risk to the fetus.
It is essential for patients with diabetes or a history of gestational diabetes to maintain good metabolic control before conception and throughout pregnancy. Insulin requirements may decrease during the first trimester, generally increase during the second and third trimesters, and rapidly decline after delivery. Careful monitoring of glucose control is essential in such patients.

Nursing Mothers
It is unknown whether insulin glulisine is excreted in human milk. Many drugs, including human insulin, are excreted in human milk. For this reason, caution should be exercised when APIDRA is administered to a nursing woman. Patients with diabetes who are lactating may require adjustments in APIDRA dose, meal plan, or both.

Pediatric Use
Safety and effectiveness of APIDRA in pediatric patients have not been established.

Geriatric Use
In Phase III clinical trials (n=2408), APIDRA was administered to 147 patients ≥65 years of age and 27 patients ≥75 years of age. The majority of these were patients with type 2 diabetes. The change in HbA1c values and hypoglycemia frequencies did not differ by age, but greater sensitivity of some older individuals cannot be ruled out.

Table 4: Severe Symptomatic Hypoglycemia

	Type 1 Diabetes Mellitus – Adult 12 weeks in combination with Lantus®*			Type 1 Diabetes Mellitus– Adult 26 weeks in combination with Lantus®**		Type 2 Diabetes Mellitus– Adult 26 weeks in combination with NPH human insulin**	
	APIDRA Pre-meal	APIDRA Post-meal	Regular Human Insulin	APIDRA	Insulin Lispro	APIDRA	Regular Human Insulin
Severe symptomatic hypoglycemia (events/month/patient)	0.05	0.05	0.13	0.02	0.02	0.00	0.00
Severe symptomatic hypoglycemia Percent of patients (n/total N)	8.4% (24/286)	8.4% (25/296)	10.1% (28/278)	4.8% (16/335)	4.0% (13/326)	1.4% (6/416)	1.2% (5/420)

*Entire treatment phase (3 months) has been included.
**Last three months of treatment have been considered.

ADVERSE REACTIONS

Overall, clinical studies comparing APIDRA with short-acting insulins did not demonstrate a difference in frequency of adverse events.
Adverse events commonly associated with human insulin therapy include the following:
Body as a whole: allergic reactions. (See PRECAUTIONS.)
Skin and appendages: injection site reaction, lipodystrophy, pruritus, rash. (See PRECAUTIONS.)
Other: hypoglycemia. (See WARNINGS and PRECAUTIONS.)
The rates and incidence of severe symptomatic hypoglycemia, defined as hypoglycemia requiring intervention from a third party, were comparable for all treatment regimens (see Table 4).
[See table 4 above]

Continuous Subcutaneous Insulin Infusion (CSII) (Type 1 Diabetes):
The rates of catheter occlusions and infusion site reactions were similar for APIDRA and insulin aspart (see Table 5).

Table 5: Catheter Occlusions and Infusion Site Reactions.

	APIDRA	Insulin aspart
Catheter occlusions/ month	0.08	0.15
Infusion site reactions	10.3% (3/29)	13.3% (4/30)

OVERDOSAGE

Hypoglycemia may occur as a result of an excess of insulin relative to food intake, energy expenditure, or both.
Mild/Moderate episodes of hypoglycemia usually can be treated with oral glucose. Adjustments in drug dosage, meal patterns, or exercise may be needed.
Severe episodes with coma, seizure, or neurologic impairment may be treated with intramuscular/subcutaneous glucagon or concentrated intravenous glucose. Sustained carbohydrate intake and observation may be necessary because hypoglycemia may recur after apparent clinical recovery.

DOSAGE AND ADMINISTRATION

APIDRA is a recombinant insulin analog that has been shown to be equipotent to human insulin. One unit of APIDRA has the same glucose-lowering effect as one unit of regular human insulin. After subcutaneous administration, it has a more rapid onset and shorter duration of action.
APIDRA should be given within 15 minutes before a meal or within 20 minutes after starting a meal.
APIDRA is intended for subcutaneous administration and for use by external infusion pump.
The dosage of APIDRA should be individualized and determined based on the physician's advice in accordance with the needs of the patient. APIDRA should normally be used in regimens that include a longer-acting insulin or basal insulin analog.
APIDRA should be administered by subcutaneous injection in the abdominal wall, the thigh or the deltoid or by continuous subcutaneous infusion in the abdominal wall. As with all insulins, injection sites and infusion sites within an injection area (abdomen, thigh or deltoid) should be rotated from one injection to the next.
As for all insulins, the rate of absorption, and consequently the onset and duration of action, may be affected by injection site, exercise and other variables. Blood glucose monitoring is recommended for all patients with diabetes.

Preparation and Handling
Parenteral drug products should be inspected visually prior to administration whenever the solution and the container permit. APIDRA must only be used if the solution is clear and colorless with no particles visible.
When it is used in a pump, APIDRA should not be mixed with other insulins or with a diluent.

HOW SUPPLIED

APIDRA 100 units per mL (U-100) is available in the following package size:
10 mL vials NDC 0088-2500-33

Storage:
Unopened Vial:
Unopened APIDRA vials should be stored in a refrigerator, 36°F to 46°F (2°C to 8°C). Protect from light. APIDRA should not be stored in the freezer and it should not be allowed to freeze. Discard vial if frozen.
Open (In-Use) Vial:
Opened vials, whether or not refrigerated, must be used within 28 days. They must be discarded if not used within 28 days. If refrigeration is not possible, the open vial in use can be kept unrefrigerated for up to 28 days away from direct heat and light, as long as the temperature is not greater than 77°F (25°C).

	Not in-use (unopened) Refrigerated	Not in-use (unopened) Room Temperature, below 77°F (25°C)	In-use (opened) Room Temperature, below 77°F (25°C)
10 mL Vial	Until expiration date	28 days	28 days, refrigerated/ room temperature

Infusion sets:
Infusion sets (reservoirs, tubing, and catheters) and the APIDRA in the reservoir should be discarded after no more than 48 hours of use or after exposure to temperatures that exceed 98.6°F (37°C).
Rx only
Rev. April 2004a
Manufactured by:
Aventis Pharma Deutschland GmbH
D-65926 Frankfurt am Main
Frankfurt, Germany
Manufactured for:
Aventis Pharmaceuticals Inc.
Kansas City, MO 64137 USA
US Patent Number 6,221,633
www.aventis-us.com

†Lantus® is a registered trademark of Aventis Pharmaceuticals Inc.
‡The brands listed are the registered trademarks of their respective owners and are not trademarks of Aventis Pharmaceuticals Inc.

Patient Information

APIDRA™ 10 mL vial (1000 units per vial) 100 units per mL (U-100) (insulin glulisine [recombinant DNA origin] injection)
Read the Patient Information that comes with APIDRA (uh-PEE-druh) before you start using it and each time you get a refill. There may be new information. This leaflet does not take the place of talking with your healthcare provider about your condition or treatment. If you have questions about APIDRA or about diabetes, talk with your healthcare provider.

What is the most important information I should know about APIDRA?
Do not change the insulin you are using without talking to your healthcare provider. Any change in insulin strength, manufacturer, type (regular, NPH, analogs), or species (animal, human) may need a change in the dose. This dose change may be needed right away or later on during the first several weeks or months on the new insulin. Doses of oral antidiabetic medicines may also need to change, if your insulin is changed.
You must test your blood sugar levels while using an insulin such as APIDRA. Your healthcare provider will tell you how often you should test your blood sugar level, and what to do if it is high or low.
When used in a pump do not mix APIDRA with any other insulin or liquid.
APIDRA comes as U-100 insulin and contains 100 units of APIDRA. One milliliter (mL) of U-100 insulin contains 100 units of insulin. (1 mL = 1 cc).

Continued on next page

Apidra—Cont.

What is APIDRA?
APIDRA is a rapid-acting man-made insulin that is like insulin made by your body. APIDRA is used to treat adults with diabetes for the control of high blood sugar. APIDRA starts working faster than regular insulin and does not work as long. APIDRA is used with a longer-acting insulin or by itself as insulin pump therapy to maintain proper blood sugar control.
Your body needs insulin to turn sugar (glucose) into energy. If your body does not make enough insulin, you need to take more insulin so you will not have too much sugar in your blood.
Insulin injections are important in keeping your diabetes under control. But the way you live, your diet, careful checking of your blood sugar levels, exercise, and planned physical activity, all work with your insulin to help you control your diabetes.
You need a prescription to get APIDRA. Always be sure you receive the right insulin from the pharmacy.
Who should not take APIDRA?
Do not take APIDRA if you are allergic to insulin glulisine or any of the inactive ingredients in APIDRA. See the end of this leaflet for a list of the inactive ingredients.
Before starting APIDRA, tell your healthcare provider
- **about all your medical problems including if you:**
  - **have liver or kidney problems.** Your dose may need to be adjusted.
  - **are pregnant or plan to become pregnant.** It is not known if APIDRA may harm your unborn baby. It is very important to maintain control of your blood sugar levels during pregnancy. Your healthcare provider will decide which insulin is best for you during your pregnancy.
  - **are breast-feeding or plan to breast-feed.** It is not known whether APIDRA passes into your milk. Many medicines, including insulin, pass into human milk, and could affect your baby. Talk to your healthcare provider about the best way to feed your baby.
- **about all the medicines you take including** prescription and non-prescription medicines, vitamins and herbal supplements.

How should I use APIDRA?
See the end of this leaflet for the **"Instructions for Use"** including the sections **"How do I draw the insulin into the syringe?"** and **"How should I infuse APIDRA with an external subcutaneous insulin infusion pump?"**
- Follow the instructions given by your healthcare provider about the type or types of insulin you are using. Do not make any changes with your insulin unless you have talked to your healthcare provider. Your insulin needs may change because of illness, stress, other medicines, or changes in diet or activity level. Talk to your healthcare provider about how to adjust your insulin dose.
- You should take APIDRA within 15 minutes before a meal or within 20 minutes after starting the meal. Only use APIDRA that is clear and colorless. If your APIDRA is cloudy or colored, return it to your pharmacy for a replacement.
- Follow your healthcare provider's instructions for testing your blood sugar.
- Inject APIDRA under your skin (subcutaneously) in your upper arm, abdomen (stomach area), or thigh (upper leg). Never inject it into a vein or muscle. If you use a pump, infuse APIDRA through the skin of your abdomen.
- Change (rotate) injection sites within the same body area.

What kind of syringe should I use?
- Always use a syringe that is marked for U-100 insulin. If you use the wrong syringe, you may get the wrong dose. You could get a blood sugar level that is too low or too high.

Mixing with APIDRA
- If you are mixing APIDRA with NPH human insulin, draw APIDRA into the syringe first. Inject the mixture right away. **Do not mix APIDRA with any other type of insulin than NPH.**
- **Do not mix APIDRA with any other insulin when used in a pump.**

What can affect how much insulin I need?
Illness. Illness may change how much insulin you need. It is a good idea to think ahead and make a "sick day" plan with your healthcare provider in advance so you will be ready when this happens. Be sure to test your blood sugar more often and call your healthcare provider if you are sick.
Medicines. Many medicines can affect your insulin needs. Other medicines, including prescription and non-prescription medicines, vitamins and herbal supplements, can change the way insulin works. You may need a different dose of insulin when you are taking certain other medicines. **Know all the medicines you take,** including prescription and non-prescription medicines, vitamins and herbal supplements. You may want to keep a list of the medicines you take. You can show this list to all your healthcare providers and pharmacists anytime you get a new medicine or refill. They will tell you if your insulin dose needs to be changed.
Meals. The amount of food you eat can affect your insulin needs. If you eat less food, skip meals, or eat more food than usual, you may need a different dose of insulin. Talk to your healthcare provider if you change your diet so that you know how to adjust your APIDRA and other insulin doses.
Alcohol. Alcohol, including beer and wine, may affect the way APIDRA works and affect your blood sugar levels. Talk to your healthcare provider about drinking alcohol.
Exercise or Activity level. Exercise or activity level may change the way your body uses insulin. Check with your healthcare provider before you start an exercise program because your dose may need to be changed.
Travel. If you travel across time zones, talk with your healthcare professional about how to time your injections. When you travel, wear your medical alert identification. Take extra insulin and supplies with you.
What are the possible side effects of APIDRA and other insulins?
Hypoglycemia (low blood glucose):
Hypoglycemia is often called an "insulin reaction" or "low blood sugar". It may happen when you do not have enough sugar in your blood. Common causes of hypoglycemia are illness, emotional or physical stress, too much insulin, too little food or missed meals, and too much exercise or activity. Early warning signs of hypoglycemia may be different, less noticeable or not noticeable at all in some people. That is why it is important to check your blood sugar as you have been advised by your healthcare provider.
Hypoglycemia can happen with:
- **The wrong insulin dose.** This can happen when too much insulin is injected. For pump users it could happen if the pump dose is too high.
- **Not enough carbohydrate (sugar or starch) intake.** This can happen if: a meal or snack is missed or delayed.
- **Vomiting or diarrhea** that decreases the amount of sugar absorbed by your body.
- **Intake of alcohol.**
- **Medicines that affect insulin.** Be sure to discuss all your medicines with your healthcare provider. Do not start any new medicines until you know how they may affect your insulin dose.
- **Medical conditions that can affect your blood sugar levels or insulin.** These conditions include diseases of the adrenal glands, the pituitary, the thyroid gland, the liver, and the kidney.
- **Too much glucose use by the body.** This can happen if you exercise too much or have a fever.
- **Injecting insulin the wrong way or in the wrong injection area.**

Hypoglycemia can be mild to severe. Its onset may be rapid. Some patients have few or no warning symptoms, including:
- patients with diabetes for a long time
- patients with diabetic neuropathy (nerve problems)
- or patients using certain medicines for high blood pressure or heart problems.

Hypoglycemia may reduce your ability to drive a car or use mechanical equipment and you may risk injury to yourself or others.
Severe hypoglycemia can be dangerous and can cause temporary or permanent harm to your heart or brain. **It may cause unconsciousness, seizures, or death.**
Symptoms of hypoglycemia may include:
- anxiety, irritability, restlessness, trouble concentrating, personality changes, mood changes, or other abnormal behavior
- tingling in your hands, feet, lips, or tongue
- dizziness, light-headedness, or drowsiness
- nightmares or trouble sleeping
- headache
- blurred vision
- slurred speech
- palpitations (fast heart beat)
- sweating
- tremor (shaking)
- unsteady gait (walking).

If you have hypoglycemia often or it is hard for you to know if you have the symptoms of hypoglycemia, talk to your healthcare provider.
Mild to moderate hypoglycemia can be treated by eating or drinking carbohydrates such as fruit juice, raisins, sugar candies, milk or glucose tablets. Talk to your healthcare provider about the amount of carbohydrates you should eat to treat mild to moderate hypoglycemia.
Severe hypoglycemia may require the help of another person or emergency medical people. Someone with hypoglycemia who cannot take foods or liquids with sugar by mouth needs medical help fast and will need treatment with a glucagon injection or glucose given intravenously (IV). Without medical help right away, serious reactions or even death could happen.
Hyperglycemia (high blood glucose):
Hyperglycemia occurs when you have too much sugar in your blood. Usually, it means there is not enough insulin to break down the food you eat into energy your body can use. Hyperglycemia can be caused by a fever, an infection, stress, eating more than you should, taking less insulin than prescribed, or it can mean your diabetes is getting worse.
Hyperglycemia can happen with:
- **The wrong insulin dose.** This can happen from:
  — injecting too little or no insulin
  — incorrect storage (freezing, excessive heat)
  — use after the expiration date.

For pump users this can also be caused when the bolus dose of APIDRA infusion or the basal infusion is set too low or the pump is delivering too little insulin.
- **Too much carbohydrate intake.** This can happen if you eat larger meals, eat more often or increase the amount of carbohydrate in your meals.
- **Medicines that affect insulin.** Be sure to discuss all your medicines with your healthcare provider. **Do not start any new medicines until you know how they may affect your insulin dose.**
- **Medical conditions that affect insulin.** These medical conditions include fevers, infections, heart attacks, and stress.
- **Injecting insulin the wrong way or in the wrong injection area.**

Testing your blood or urine often will let you know if you have hyperglycemia. If your tests are often high, tell your healthcare provider so your dose of medicine can be changed.
Hyperglycemia can be mild or severe. It can **progress to diabetic acidosis (DKA) (ketoacidosis) or very high glucose levels (hyperosmolar coma) and result in unconsciousness and death.**
Diabetic ketoacidosis occurs most often in patients with type 1 diabetes. It can also happen in patients with type 2 diabetes who become very sick. Because some patients get few symptoms of hyperglycemia, it is important to check your blood sugar regularly.
Symptoms of hyperglycemia include:
- confusion or drowsiness
- increased thirst
- decreased appetite, nausea, or vomiting
- rapid heart rate
- increased urination and dehydration (too little fluid in your body).

Symptoms of DKA also include:
- fruity smelling breath
- fast, deep breathing
- stomach area (abdominal) pain.

Severe or continuing hyperglycemia or DKA needs evaluation and treatment right away by your healthcare provider.
Other possible side effects of APIDRA include:
Serious allergic reactions:
Some times severe, life-threatening allergic reactions can happen with insulin. If you think you are having a severe allergic reaction, get medical help right away. Signs of insulin allergy include:
- a rash all over your body
- shortness of breath
- wheezing (trouble breathing)
- a fast pulse
- sweating
- low blood pressure.

Reactions at the injection site:
Injecting insulin can cause the following reactions on the skin at the injection site:
- a little depression in the skin (lipoatrophy)
- skin thickening (lipohypertrophy)
- red, swelling, itchy skin (injection site reaction).

You can reduce the chance of getting an injection site reaction if you change (rotate) the injection site each time. An injection site reaction should clear up in a few days or a few weeks. If injection site reactions do not go away or keep happening call your healthcare provider.
Tell your healthcare provider if you have any side effects that bother you.
These are not all the side effects of APIDRA. Ask your healthcare provider or pharmacist for more information.
How should I store APIDRA?
- **Unopened vial:**
  Store new unopened APIDRA vials in the refrigerator (not the freezer) between 36°F to 46°F (2°C to 8°C). Do not freeze APIDRA. Keep APIDRA out of direct heat and light. If a vial freezes or overheats, throw it away.
- **Open (In-Use) vial:**
  Once a vial is opened, you can keep it in the refrigerator or as cool as possible (below 77°F [25°C]), but the opened vial must be used within 28 days. If refrigeration is not possible, the open vial in use can be kept unrefrigerated for up to 28 days away from direct heat and light, as long as the temperature is not greater than 77°F (25°C). For example, do not leave it in a car on a summer day.

	Not in-use (unopened) Refrigerated	**Not in-use (unopened) Room Temperature, below 77°F (25°C)**	**In-use (opened) Room Temperature, below 77°F (25°C)**
10 mL Vial	Until expiration date	28 days	28 days, refrigerated/ room temperature

- **Insulin pump infusion sets:** Infusion sets (reservoirs, tubing, and catheters) and the APIDRA in the reservoir should be thrown away:
  - after no more than 48 hours of use or
  - after exposure to temperatures higher than 98.6°F (37°C).
- Do not use a vial of APIDRA after the expiration date stamped on the label.
- Do not use APIDRA if it is cloudy or if you see particles.

General Information about APIDRA

Use APIDRA only to treat your diabetes. **Do not** give or share APIDRA with another person, even if they have diabetes also. It may harm them.

This leaflet summarizes the most important information about APIDRA. If you would like more information, talk with your healthcare provider. You can ask your healthcare provider or pharmacist for information about APIDRA that is written for health professionals. For more information about APIDRA call 1-800-633-1610 or go to website www.aventis-us.com.

What are the ingredients in APIDRA?

Active Ingredient: insulin glulisine

Inactive Ingredients: m-cresol, tromethamine, sodium chloride, polysorbate 20, and water for injection.

Instructions for Use

How do I draw the insulin into the syringe?

- **The syringe must be new and not contain any other medicine.**
- **Do not mix APIDRA with any other type of insulin than NPH.** If you are mixing APIDRA with NPH human insulin, draw APIDRA into the syringe first. Inject the mixture right away.

Follow these steps:

1. Wash your hands.
2. Check the insulin to make sure it is clear and colorless. Do not use it after the expiration date or if it is cloudy or if you see particles.
3. If you are using a new vial, remove the protective cap. **Do not** remove the stopper.
4. Wipe the top of the vial with an alcohol swab. You do not have to shake the vial of APIDRA before use.
5. Use a new needle and syringe every time you take a dose. Use disposable syringes and needles only once. Throw them away properly. **Never** share needles and syringes.
6. Draw air into the syringe equal to your insulin dose. Put the needle through the rubber top of the vial and push the plunger to inject the air into the vial.
7. Leave the syringe in the vial and turn both upside down. Hold the syringe and vial firmly in one hand.
8. Make sure the tip of the needle is in the insulin. With your free hand, pull the plunger to withdraw the correct dose into the syringe.
9. Before you take the needle out of the vial, check the syringe for air bubbles. If bubbles are in the syringe, hold the syringe straight up and tap the side of the syringe until the bubbles float to the top. Push the bubbles out with the plunger and draw insulin back in until you have the correct dose. If you are mixing APIDRA with NPH insulin check with your healthcare professional on how to mix.
10. Remove the needle from the vial. Do not let the needle touch anything. You are now ready to inject.

How do I inject APIDRA?

Inject APIDRA under your skin. Take APIDRA as prescribed by your healthcare provider.

You should look at the medicine in the vial. If the medicine is cloudy or has particles in it, do not use it. Contact your healthcare provider. Use a new vial.

Follow these steps:

1. Decide on an injection area - either upper arm, thigh or abdomen. Injection sites within an injection area must be different from one injection to the next.
2. Use alcohol or soap and water to clean the skin where you are going to inject. The injection site should be dry before you inject.
3. Pinch the skin. Stick the needle in the way your healthcare provider showed you. Release the skin.
4. Slowly push in the plunger of the syringe all the way, making sure you have injected all the insulin. Leave the needle in the skin for about 10 seconds.
   Pull the needle straight out and gently press on the spot where you injected yourself for several seconds. **Do not rub the area.**
5. Follow your healthcare provider's instructions for throwing away the needle and syringe. Do not recap the syringe. Used needle and syringe should be placed in sharps containers (such as red biohazard containers), hard plastic containers (such as detergent bottles), or metal containers (such as an empty coffee can). Such containers should be sealed and disposed of properly.

How should I infuse APIDRA with an external subcutaneous insulin infusion pump?

Do not mix APIDRA with any other insulin or liquid when used in a pump.

- APIDRA is recommended for use in the following pumps and infusion sets: Disetronic® H-Tron® plus V100 and D-Tron® with Disetronic catheters (Rapid™, Rapid C™, Rapid D™, and Tender™); MiniMed® Models 506, 507, 507c and 508 with MiniMed catheters (Sof-set Ultimate QR™, and Quick-set™)‡. Refer to the instruction manual of your specific pump on proper use of insulin in a pump. Call your healthcare provider if you have questions about using the pump.
- If the pump or infusion set does not work right you may not receive the right dose of insulin. Hypoglycemia, hyperglycemia or ketosis can happen. Problems should be identified and corrected as quickly as possible, see instruction manual for your pump. Because APIDRA starts working faster and does not work as long, you may have less time to identify and correct the problem than with regular insulin.
- If you start using APIDRA by pump infusion, you may need to adjust your insulin doses. Check with your healthcare provider.
- You must use insulin from a new vial of APIDRA if unexplained hyperglycemia happens, or if pump alarms do not respond to all of the following:
  - a repeat dose (injection or bolus) of APIDRA
  - a change in the infusion set, including the reservoir with APIDRA
  - a change in the infusion site.

If these actions do not work, you may need to restart your injections with syringes and you must call your healthcare provider. Continue to check your blood sugar often.

The infusion set, reservoir with insulin, and infusion site should be changed:

- every 48 hours or less
- when unexpected hyperglycemia or ketosis occurs
- when alarms sound, as specified by your pump manual
- if the insulin has been exposed to temperatures over 98.6°F (37°C). If the insulin or pump could have absorbed radiant heat, for example from sunlight, that would heat the insulin to over 98.6°F (37°C). Dark colored pump cases or sport covers can increase this type of heat. The location where the pump is worn may affect the temperature.
- Patients who get skin reactions at the infusion site may need to change infusion sites more often.

ADDITIONAL INFORMATION

DIABETES FORECAST is a national magazine designed especially for patients with diabetes and their families and is available by subscription from the American Diabetes Association, National Service Center, 1701 N. Beauregard Street, Alexandria, Virginia 22311, 1-800-DIABETES (1-800-342-2383). You may also visit the ADA website at www.diabetes.org.

Another publication, **DIABETES COUNTDOWN**, is available from the Juvenile Diabetes Research Foundation International (JDRF), 120 Wall Street, 19th Floor, New York, New York 10005, 1-800-JDF-CURE (1-800-533-2873). You may also visit the JDRF website at www.jdf.org.

To get more information about diabetes, check with your healthcare professional or diabetes educator or visit www.DiabetesWatch.com.

Rev. April 2004a
Aventis Pharmaceuticals Inc.
Kansas City, MO 64137 USA

† Lantus® is a registered trademark of Aventis Pharmaceuticals Inc.
‡ The brands listed are the registered trademarks of their respective owners and are not trademarks of Aventis Pharmaceuticals, Inc.

API-APRIL04a-F-A

ARAVA® Tablets ℞

[ă-ră-vă]
(leflunomide)
10 mg, 20 mg, 100 mg
℞ only
Prescribing Information as of March 2004

> **CONTRAINDICATIONS AND WARNINGS**
> **PREGNANCY MUST BE EXCLUDED BEFORE THE START OF TREATMENT WITH ARAVA. ARAVA IS CONTRAINDICATED IN PREGNANT WOMEN, OR WOMEN OF CHILDBEARING POTENTIAL WHO ARE NOT USING RELIABLE CONTRACEPTION. (SEE CONTRAINDICATIONS AND WARNINGS.) PREGNANCY MUST BE AVOIDED DURING ARAVA TREATMENT OR PRIOR TO THE COMPLETION OF THE DRUG ELIMINATION PROCEDURE AFTER ARAVA TREATMENT.**

DESCRIPTION

ARAVA® (leflunomide) is a pyrimidine synthesis inhibitor. The chemical name for leflunomide is N-(4′-trifluoromethylphenyl)-5-methylisoxazole-4-carboxamide. It has an empirical formula $C_{12}H_9F_3N_2O_2$, a molecular weight of 270.2 and the following structural formula:

CO—NH—⟨phenyl⟩—CF3; N, O, CH3

ARAVA is available for oral administration as tablets containing 10, 20, or 100 mg of active drug. Combined with leflunomide are the following inactive ingredients: colloidal silicon dioxide, crospovidone, hypromellose, lactose monohydrate, magnesium stearate, polyethylene glycol, povidone, starch, talc, titanium dioxide, and yellow ferric oxide (20 mg tablet only).

CLINICAL PHARMACOLOGY

Mechanism of Action

Leflunomide is an isoxazole immunomodulatory agent which inhibits dihydroorotate dehydrogenase (an enzyme involved in de novo pyrimidine synthesis) and has antiproliferative activity. Several *in vivo* and *in vitro* experimental models have demonstrated an anti-inflammatory effect.

Pharmacokinetics

Following oral administration, leflunomide is metabolized to an active metabolite A77 1726 (hereafter referred to as M1) which is responsible for essentially all of its activity *in vivo*. Plasma levels of leflunomide are occasionally seen, at very low levels. Studies of the pharmacokinetics of leflunomide have primarily examined the plasma concentrations of this active metabolite.

F3C, NH—C(=O)—C(=C(CH3)OH)—C≡N

A77 1726 (M1)

Absorption

Following oral administration, peak levels of the active metabolite, M1, occurred between 6-12 hours after dosing. Due to the very long half-life of M1 (~2 weeks), a loading dose of 100 mg for 3 days was used in clinical studies to facilitate the rapid attainment of steady-state levels of M1. Without a loading dose, it is estimated that attainment of steady-state plasma concentrations would require nearly two months of dosing. The resulting plasma concentrations following both loading doses and continued clinical dosing indicate that M1 plasma levels are dose proportional.

[See table 1 below]

Relative to an oral solution, ARAVA tablets are 80% bioavailable. Co-administration of leflunomide tablets with a high fat meal did not have a significant impact on M1 plasma levels.

Distribution

M1 has a low volume of distribution (Vss = 0.13 L/kg) and is extensively bound (>99.3%) to albumin in healthy subjects. Protein binding has been shown to be linear at therapeutic concentrations. The free fraction of M1 is slightly higher in patients with rheumatoid arthritis and approximately doubled in patients with chronic renal failure; the mechanism and significance of these increases are unknown.

Metabolism

Leflunomide is metabolized to one primary (M1) and many minor metabolites. Of these minor metabolites, only 4-trifluoromethylaniline (TFMA) is quantifiable, occurring at low levels in the plasma of some patients. The parent compound is rarely detectable in plasma. At the present time the specific site of leflunomide metabolism is unknown. *In vivo* and *in vitro* studies suggest a role for both the GI wall and the liver in drug metabolism. No specific enzyme has been identified as the primary route of metabolism for leflunomide; however, hepatic cytosolic and microsomal cellular fractions have been identified as sites of drug metabolism.

Elimination

The active metabolite M1 is eliminated by further metabolism and subsequent renal excretion as well as by direct biliary excretion. In a 28 day study of drug elimination (n=3) using a single dose of radiolabeled compound, approximately 43% of the total radioactivity was eliminated in the urine and 48% was eliminated in the feces. Subsequent analysis of the samples revealed the primary urinary metabolites to be leflunomide glucuronides and an oxanilic acid derivative of M1. The primary fecal metabolite was M1. Of these two routes of elimination, renal elimination is more significant over the first 96 hours after which fecal elimination begins to predominate. In a study involving the intravenous administration of M1, the clearance was estimated to be 31 mL/hr.

In small studies using activated charcoal (n=1) or cholestyramine (n=3) to facilitate drug elimination, the *in*

Continued on next page

Table 1. Pharmacokinetic Parameters for M1 after Administration of Leflunomide at Doses of 5, 10, and 25 mg/day for 24 Weeks to Patients (n=54) with Rheumatoid Arthritis (Mean ± SD) (Study YU204)

Maintenance (Loading) Dose			
Parameter	5 mg (50 mg)	10 mg (100 mg)	25 mg (100 mg)
C_{24} (Day 1) (µg/mL)[1]	4.0 ± 0.6	8.4 ± 2.1	8.5 ± 2.2
C_{24} (ss) (µg/mL)[2]	8.8 ± 2.9	18 ± 9.6	63 ± 36
$t_{1/2}$ (DAYS)	15 ± 3	14 ± 5	18 ± 9

[1] Concentration at 24 hours after loading dose
[2] Concentration at 24 hours after maintenance doses at steady state

Arava—Cont.

vivo plasma half-life of M1 was reduced from >1 week to approximately 1 day (see PRECAUTIONS—General—Need for Drug Elimination). Similar reductions in plasma half-life were observed for a series of volunteers (n=96) enrolled in pharmacokinetic trials who were given cholestyramine. This suggests that biliary recycling is a major contributor to the long elimination half-life of M1. Studies with both hemodialysis and CAPD (chronic ambulatory peritoneal dialysis) indicate that M1 is not dialyzable.

Special Populations

Gender. Gender has not been shown to cause a consistent change in the *in vivo* pharmacokinetics M1.

Age. Age has been shown to cause a change in the *in vivo* pharmacokinetics of M1 (see Pediatrics).

Smoking. A population based pharmacokinetic analysis of the phase III data indicates that smokers have a 38% increase in clearance over non-smokers; however, no difference in clinical efficacy was seen between smokers and nonsmokers.

Chronic Renal Insufficiency. In single dose studies in patients (n=6) with chronic renal insufficiency requiring either chronic ambulatory peritoneal dialysis (CAPD) or hemodialysis, neither had a significant impact on circulating levels of M1. The free fraction of M1 was almost doubled, but the mechanism of this increase is not known. In light of the fact that the kidney plays a role in drug elimination, and without adequate studies of leflunomide use in subjects with renal insufficiency, caution should be used when ARAVA is administered to these patients.

Hepatic Insufficiency. Studies of the effect of hepatic insufficiency on M1 pharmacokinetics have not been done. Given the need to metabolize leflunomide into the active species, the role of the liver in drug elimination/recycling, and the possible risk of increased hepatic toxicity, the use of leflunomide in patients with hepatic insufficiency is not recommended.

Pediatrics

The pharmacokinetics of M1 following oral administration of leflunomide have been investigated in 73 pediatric patients with polyarticular course Juvenile Rheumatoid Arthritis (JRA) who ranged in age from 3 to 17 years. The results of a population pharmacokinetic analysis of these trials have demonstrated that pediatric patients with body weights ≤40 kg have a reduced clearance of M1 (see Table 2) relative to adult rheumatoid arthritis patients.

Table 2: Population Pharmacokinetic Estimate of M1 Clearance Following Oral Administration of Leflunomide in Pediatric Patients with Polyarticular Course JRA Mean ± SD [Range]

N	Body Weight (kg)	CL (mL/h)
10	<20	18 ± 9.8 [6.8-37]
30	20-40	18 ± 9.5 [4.2-43]
33	>40	26 ± 16 [9.7-93.6]

Drug Interactions

In vivo drug interaction studies have demonstrated a lack of a significant drug interaction between leflunomide and tri-phasic oral contraceptives, and cimetidine.

In vitro studies of protein binding indicated that warfarin did not affect M1 protein binding. At the same time M1 was shown to cause increases ranging from 13–50% in the free fraction of diclofenac, ibuprofen and tolbutamide at concentrations in the clinical range. *In vitro* studies of drug metabolism indicate that M1 inhibits CYP 450 2C9, which is responsible for the metabolism of phenytoin, tolbutamide, warfarin and many NSAIDs. M1 has been shown to inhibit the formation of 4′-hydroxydiclofenac from diclofenac *in vitro*. The clinical significance of these findings with regard to phenytoin and tolbutamide is unknown, however, there was extensive concomitant use of NSAIDs in the clinical studies and no differential effect was observed. (see **PRECAUTIONS—Drug Interactions**).

Methotrexate. Coadministration, in 30 patients, of ARAVA (100 mg/day × 2 days followed by 10-20 mg/day) with methotrexate (10-25 mg/week, with folate) demonstrated no pharmacokinetic interaction between the two drugs. However, co-administration increased risk of hepatotoxicity (see PRECAUTIONS—Drug Interactions—Hepatotoxic Drugs).

Rifampin. Following concomitant administration of a single dose of ARAVA to subjects receiving multiple doses of rifampin, M1 peak levels were increased (~40%) over those seen when ARAVA was given alone. Because of the potential for ARAVA levels to continue to increase with multiple dosing, caution should be used if patients are to receive both ARAVA and rifampin.

CLINICAL STUDIES

A. ADULTS

The efficacy of ARAVA in the treatment of rheumatoid arthritis (RA) was demonstrated in three controlled trials showing reduction in signs and symptoms, and inhibition of structural damage. In two placebo controlled trials, efficacy was demonstrated for improvement in physical function.

1. Reduction of signs and symptoms

Relief of signs and symptoms was assessed using the American College of Rheumatology (ACR) 20 Responder Index, a composite of clinical, laboratory, and functional measures in rheumatoid arthritis. An "ACR20 Responder" is a patient who had ≥ 20% improvement in both tender and swollen joint counts and in 3 of the following 5 criteria: physician global assessment, patient global assessment, functional ability measure [Modified Health Assessment Questionnaire (MHAQ)], visual analog pain scale, and erythrocyte sedimentation rate or C-reactive protein. An "ACR20 Responder at Endpoint" is a patient who completed the study and was an ACR20 Responder at the completion of the study.

2. Inhibition of structural damage

Inhibition of structural damage compared to control was assessed using the Sharp Score (Sharp, JT. Scoring Radiographic Abnormalities in Rheumatoid Arthritis, Radiologic Clinics of North America, 1996; vol. 34, pp. 233-241), a composite score of X-ray erosions and joint space narrowing in hands/wrists and forefeet.

3. Improvement in physical function

Improvement in physical function was assessed using the Health Assessment Questionnaire (HAQ) and the Medical Outcomes Survey Short Form (SF-36).

In all Arava monotherapy studies, an initial loading dose of 100 mg per day for three days only was used followed by 20 mg per day thereafter.

US301 Clinical Trial in Adults

Study US301, a 2 year study, randomized 482 patients with active RA of at least 6 months duration to leflunomide 20 mg/day (n=182), methotrexate 7.5 mg/week increasing to 15 mg/week (n=182), or placebo (n=118). All patients received folate 1 mg BID. Primary analysis was at 52 weeks with blinded treatment to 104 weeks.

Overall, 235 of the 508 randomized treated patients (482 in primary data analysis and an additional 26 patients), continued into a second 12 months of double-blind treatment (98 leflunomide, 101 methotrexate, 36 placebo). Leflunomide dose continued at 20 mg/day and the methotrexate dose could be increased to a maximum of 20 mg/week. In total 190 patients (83 leflunomide, 80 methotrexate, 27 placebo) completed 2 years of double-blind treatment.

The rate and reason for withdrawal is summarized in table 3.

[See table 3 above]

Table 3: Withdrawals in US301

	n(%) patients		
	Leflunomide 190	Placebo 128	Methotrexate 190
Withdrawals in Year-1			
Lack of efficacy	33 (17.4)	70 (54.7)	50 (26.3)
Safety	44 (23.2)	12 (9.4)	22 (11.6)
Other[1]	15 (7.9)	10 (7.8)	17 (9.0)
Total	92 (48.4)	92 (71.9)	89 (46.8)
Patients entering Year 2	98	36	101
Withdrawals in Year-2			
Lack of efficacy	4 (4.1)	1 (2.8)	4 (4.0)
Safety	8 (8.2)	0 (0.0)	10 (9.9)
Other[1]	3 (3.1)	8 (22.2)	7 (6.9)
Total	15 (15.3)	9 (25.0)	21 (20.8)

[1]Includes: lost to follow up, protocol violation, noncompliance, voluntary withdrawal, investigator discretion.

MN301/303/305 Clinical Trial in Adults

Study MN301 randomized 358 patients with active RA to leflunomide 20 mg/day (n=133), sulfasalazine 2.0 g/day (n=133), or placebo (n=92). Treatment duration was 24 weeks. An extension of the study was an optional 6-month blinded continuation of MN301 without the placebo arm, resulting in a 12-month comparison of leflunomide and sulfasalazine (study MN303).

Of the 168 patients who completed 12 months of treatment in MN301 and MN303, 146 patients (87%) entered a 1-year extension study of double blind active treatment (MN305; 60 leflunomide, 60 sulfasalazine, 26 placebo/sulfasalazine). Patients continued on the same daily dosage of leflunomide or sulfasalazine that they had been taking at the completion

Table 4: Withdrawals in study MN301/303/305

	n(%) patients		
	Leflunomide 133	Placebo 92	Sulfasalazine 133
Withdrawals in MN301 (Mo 0–6)			
Lack of efficacy	10 (7.5)	29 (31.5)	14 (10.5)
Safety	19 (14.3)	6 (6.5)	25 (18.8)
Other[1]	8 (6.0)	6 (6.5)	11 (8.3)
Total	37 (27.8)	41 (44.6)	50 (37.6)
Patients entering MN303	80		76
Withdrawals in MN303 (Mo 7-12)			
Lack of efficacy	4 (5.0)		2 (2.6)
Safety	2 (2.5)		5 (6.6)
Other[1]	3 (3.8)		1 (1.3)
Total	9 (11.3)		8 (10.5)
Patients entering MN305	60		60
Withdrawals in MN305 (Mo 13-24)			
Lack of efficacy	0 (0.0)		3 (5.0)
Safety	6 (10.0)		8 (13.3)
Other[1]	1 (1.7)		2 (3.3)
Total	7 (11.7)		13 (21.7)

[1]Includes: lost to follow up, protocol violation, noncompliance, voluntary withdrawal, investigator discretion.

Table 5: Withdrawals in MN302/304

	n(%) patients	
	Leflunomide 501	Methotrexate 498
Withdrawals in MN302 (Year-1)		
Lack of efficacy	37 (7.4)	15 (3.0)
Safety	98 (19.6)	79 (15.9)
Other[1]	17 (3.4)	17 (3.4)
Total	152 (30.3)	111 (22.3)
Patients entering MN304	292	320
Withdrawals in MN304 (Year-2)		
Lack of efficacy	13 (4.5)	9 (2.8)
Safety	11 (3.8)	22 (6.9)
Other[1]	12 (4.1)	12 (3.8)
Total	36 (12.3)	43 (13.4)

[1] Includes: lost to follow up, protocol violation, noncompliance, voluntary withdrawal, investigator discretion.

of MN301/303. A total of 121 patients (53 leflunomide, 47 sulfasalazine, 21 placebo/sulfasalazine) completed the 2 years of double-blind treatment.

Patient withdrawal data in MN301/303/305 is summarized in table 4.

[See table 4 on previous page]

MN302/304 Clinical Trial in Adults

Study MN302 randomized 999 patients with active RA to leflunomide 20 mg/day (n=501) or methotrexate at 7.5 mg/week increasing to 15 mg/week (n=498). Folate supplementation was used in 10% of patients. Treatment duration was 52 weeks.

Of the 736 patients who completed 52 weeks of treatment in study MN302, 612 (83%) entered the double-blind, 1-year extension study MN304 (292 leflunomide, 320 methotrexate). Patients continued on the same daily dosage of leflunomide or methotrexate that they had been taking at the completion of MN302. There were 533 patients (256 leflunomide, 277 methotrexate) who completed 2 years of double-blind treatment.

Patient withdrawal data in MN302/304 is summarized in table 5.

[See table 5 on previous page]

Clinical Trial Data

1. Signs and symptoms Rheumatoid Arthritis

The ACR20 Responder at Endpoint rates are shown in Figure 1. ARAVA was statistically significantly superior to placebo in reducing the signs and symptoms of RA by the primary efficacy analysis, ACR20 Responder at Endpoint, in study US301 (at the primary 12 months endpoint) and MN301 (at 6 month endpoint). ACR20 Responder at Endpoint rates with ARAVA treatment were consistent across the 6 and 12 month studies (41-49%). No consistent differences were demonstrated between leflunomide and methotrexate or between leflunomide and sulfasalazine. ARAVA treatment effect was evident by 1 month, stabilized by 3-6 months, and continued throughout the course of treatment as shown in Figure 2.

Figure 1

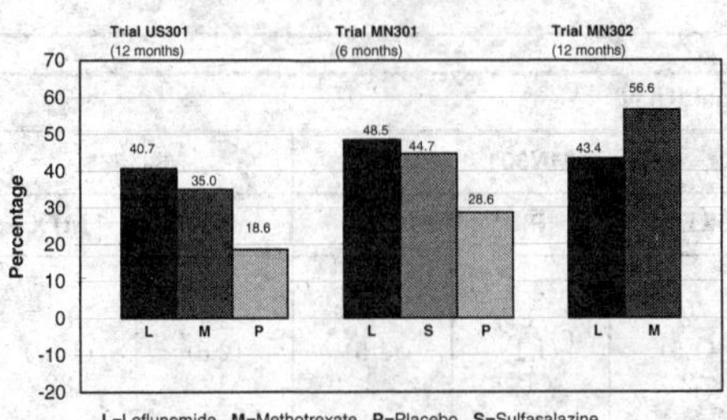

L=Leflunomide, M=Methotrexate, P=Placebo, S=Sulfasalazine

	Comparisons	95% Confidence Interval	p Value
US301	Leflunomide vs. Placebo	(12, 32)	<0.0001
	Methotrexate vs. Placebo	(8, 30)	<0.0001
	Leflunomide vs. Methotrexate	(-4, 16)	NS
MN301	Leflunomide vs. Placebo	(7, 33)	0.0026
	Sulfasalazine vs. Placebo	(4, 29)	0.0121
	Leflunomide vs. Sulfasalazine	(-8, 16)	NS
MN302	Leflunomide vs. Methotrexate	(-19, -7)	<0.000

Figure 2

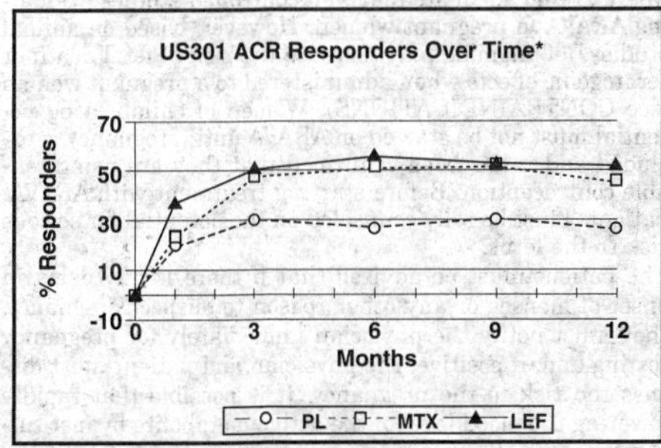

*Last Observation Carried Forward.

ACR50 and ACR70 Responders are defined in an analogous manner to the ACR20 Responder, but use improvements of 50% or 70%, respectively (Table 6). Mean change for the individual components of the ACR Responder Index are shown in Table 7.

[See table 6 above]

Table 7 shows the results of the components of the ACR response criteria for US301, MN301, and MN302. ARAVA was significantly superior to placebo in all components of the ACR Response criteria in study US301 and MN301. In addition Arava was significantly superior to placebo in improving morning stiffness, a measure of RA disease activity, not included in the ACR Response criteria. No consistent differences were demonstrated between ARAVA and the active comparators.

[See table 7 at top of next page]

Table 6. Summary of ACR Response Rates*

Study and Treatment Group	ACR20	ACR50	ACR70
Placebo-Controlled Studies			
US301 (12 months)			
Leflunomide (n=178)†	52.2‡	34.3‡	20.2‡
Placebo (n=118)†	26.3	7.6	4.2
Methotrexate (n=180)†	45.6	22.8	9.4
MN301 (6 months)			
Leflunomide (n=130)†	54.6‡	33.1‡	10.0§
Placebo (n=91)†	28.6	14.3	2.2
Sulfasalazine (n=132)†	56.8	30.3	7.6
Non-Placebo Active-Controlled Studies			
MN302 (12 months)			
Leflunomide (n=495)†	51.1	31.1	9.9
Methotrexate (n=489)†	65.2	43.8	16.4

* Intent to treat (ITT) analysis using last observation carried forward (LOCF) technique for patients who discontinued early.

† N is the number of ITT patients for whom adequate data were available to calculate the indicated rates.

‡ p<0.001 leflunomide vs placebo

§ p<0.02 leflunomide vs placebo

Maintenance of effect

After completing 12 months of treatment, patients continuing on study treatment were evaluated for an additional 12 months of double-blind treatment (total treatment period of 2 years) in studies US301, MN305, and MN304. ACR Responder rates at 12 months were maintained over 2 years in most patients continuing a second year of treatment.

Improvement from baseline in the individual components of the ACR responder criteria was also sustained in most patients during the second year of Arava treatment in all three trials.

2. Inhibition of structural damage

The change from baseline to endpoint in progression of structural disease, as measured by the Sharp X-ray score, is displayed in Figure 3. ARAVA was statistically significantly superior to placebo in inhibiting the progression of disease by the Sharp Score. No consistent differences were demonstrated between leflunomide and methotrexate or between leflunomide and sulfasalazine.

Figure 3

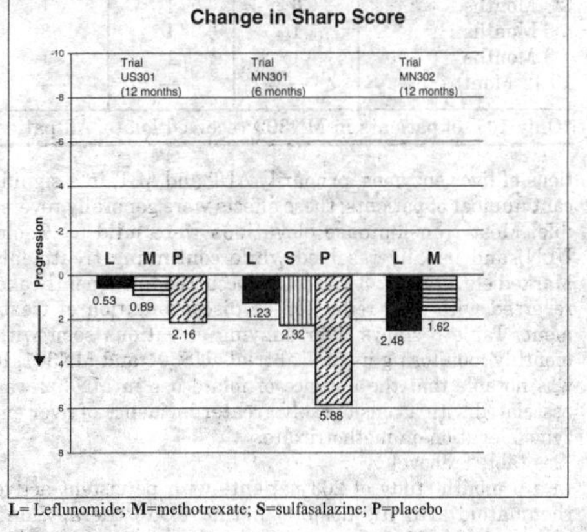

L= Leflunomide; M=methotrexate; S=sulfasalazine; P=placebo

	Comparisons	95% Confidence Interval	p Value
US301	Leflunomide vs. Placebo	(-4.0, -1.1)	0.0007
	Methotrexate vs. Placebo	(-2.6, -0.2)	0.0196
	Leflunomide vs. Methotrexate	(-2.3, 0.0)	0.0499
MN301	Leflunomide vs. Placebo	(-6.2, -1.8)	0.0004
	Sulfasalazine vs. Placebo	(-6.9, 0.0)	0.0484
	Leflunomide vs. Sulfasalazine	(-3.3, 1.2)	NS
MN302	Leflunomide vs. Methotrexate	(-2.2, 7.4)	NS

3. Improvement in physical function

The Health Assessment Questionnaire (HAQ) assesses a patient's physical function and degree of disability. The mean change from baseline in functional ability as measured by the HAQ Disability Index (HAQ DI) in the 6 and 12 month placebo and active controlled trials is shown in Figure 4. ARAVA was statistically significantly superior to placebo in improving physical function. Superiority to placebo was demonstrated consistently across all eight HAQ DI subscales (dressing, arising, eating, walking, hygiene, reach, grip and activities) in both placebo controlled studies.

The Medical Outcomes Survey Short Form 36 (SF-36), a generic health-related quality of life questionnaire, further addresses physical function. In US301, at 12 months, ARAVA provided statistically significant improvements compared to placebo in the Physical Component Summary (PCS) Score.

Figure 4

Change in Functional Ability Measure*

Trial US301 (12 months) — L: -0.45, M: -0.26, P: -0.03
Trial MN301 (6 months) — L: -0.56, S: -0.37, P: -0.08
Trial MN302 (12 months) — L: -0.44, M: -0.54

Improvement

* as measured by HAQ Disability Index

L=Leflunomide, M=Methotrexate, P=Placebo, S=Sulfasalazine

	Comparison	95% Confidence Interval	p Value
US301	Leflunomide vs. Placebo	(-0.58, -0.29)	0.0001
	Leflunomide vs. Methotrexate	(-0.34, -0.07)	0.0026
MN301	Leflunomide vs. Placebo	(-0.67, -0.36)	<0.0001
	Leflunomide vs. Sulfasalazine	(-0.33, -0.03)	0.0163
MN302	Leflunomide vs. Methotrexate	(0.01, 0.16)	0.0221

Maintenance of effect

The improvement in physical function demonstrated at 6 and 12 months was maintained over two years. In those patients continuing therapy for a second year, this improvement in physical function as measured by HAQ and SF-36 (PCS) was maintained.

Clinical Trials in Pediatrics

ARAVA was studied in a single multicenter, double-blind, active-controlled trial in 94 patients (1:1 randomization) with polyarticular course juvenile rheumatoid arthritis (JRA) as defined by the American College of Rheumatology (ACR). Approximately 68% of pediatric patients receiving ARAVA, versus 89% of pediatric patients receiving the active comparator, improved by Week 16 (end-of-study) employing the JRA Definition of Improvement (DOI) ≥ 30 % responder endpoint. In this trial, the loading dose and maintenance dose of ARAVA was based on three weight categories: <20 kg, 20-40kg, and ≥40 kg. The response rate to ARAVA in pediatric patients ≤40 kg was less robust than in pediatric patients >40 kg suggesting suboptimal dosing in smaller weight pediatric patients, as studied, resulting in less than efficacious plasma concentrations, despite reduced clearance of M1. (See PHARMACOKINETICS).

INDICATIONS AND USAGE

ARAVA is indicated in adults for the treatment of active rheumatoid arthritis (RA):

1. to reduce signs and symptoms
2. to inhibit structural damage as evidenced by X-ray erosions and joint space narrowing
3. to improve physical function.

(see CLINICAL STUDIES)

Aspirin, nonsteroidal anti-inflammatory agents and/or low dose corticosteroids may be continued during treatment with ARAVA (see PRECAUTIONS—Drug Interactions—NSAIDs). The combined use of ARAVA with antimalarials, intramuscular or oral gold, D penicillamine, azathioprine, or methotrexate has not been adequately studied (see WARNINGS—Immunosuppression Potential/Bone Marrow Suppression).

Continued on next page

Arava—Cont.

CONTRAINDICATIONS

ARAVA is contraindicated in patients with known hypersensitivity to leflunomide or any of the other components of ARAVA.

ARAVA can cause fetal harm when administered to a pregnant woman. Leflunomide, when administered orally to rats during organogenesis at a dose of 15 mg/kg, was teratogenic (most notably anophthalmia or microphthalmia and internal hydrocephalus). The systemic exposure of rats at this dose was approximately 1/10 the human exposure level based on AUC. Under these exposure conditions, leflunomide also caused a decrease in the maternal body weight and an increase in embryolethality with a decrease in fetal body weight for surviving fetuses. In rabbits, oral treatment with 10 mg/kg of leflunomide during organogenesis resulted in fused, dysplastic sternebrae. The exposure level at this dose was essentially equivalent to the maximum human exposure level based on AUC. At a 1 mg/kg dose, leflunomide was not teratogenic in rats and rabbits.

When female rats were treated with 1.25 mg/kg of leflunomide beginning 14 days before mating and continuing until the end of lactation, the offspring exhibited marked (greater than 90%) decreases in postnatal survival. The systemic exposure level at 1.25 mg/kg was approximately 1/100 the human exposure level based on AUC.

ARAVA is contraindicated in women who are or may become pregnant. If this drug is used during pregnancy, or if the patient becomes pregnant while taking this drug, the patient should be apprised of the potential hazard to the fetus.

WARNINGS

Immunosuppression Potential/Bone Marrow Suppression

ARAVA is not recommended for patients with severe immunodeficiency, bone marrow dysplasia, or severe, uncontrolled infections. In the event that a serious infection occurs, it may be necessary to interrupt therapy with ARAVA and administer cholestyramine or charcoal (see PRECAUTIONS—General—Need for Drug Elimination). Medications like leflunomide that have immunosuppression potential may cause patients to be more susceptible to infections, including opportunistic infections. Rarely, severe infections including sepsis, which may be fatal, have been reported in patients receiving ARAVA. Most of the reports were confounded by concomitant immunosuppressant therapy and/or comorbid illness which, in addition to rheumatoid disease, may predispose patients to infection.

There have been rare reports of pancytopenia, agranulocytosis and thrombocytopenia in patients receiving ARAVA alone. These events have been reported most frequently in patients who received concomitant treatment with methotrexate or other immunosuppressive agents, or who had recently discontinued these therapies; in some cases, patients had a prior history of a significant hematologic abnormality.

Patients taking ARAVA should have platelet, white blood cell count and hemoglobin or hematocrit monitored at baseline and monthly for six months following initiation of therapy and every 6- to 8 weeks thereafter. If used with concomitant methotrexate and/or other potential immunosuppressive agents, chronic monitoring should be monthly. If evidence of bone marrow suppression occurs in a patient taking ARAVA, treatment with ARAVA should be stopped, and cholestyramine or charcoal should be used to reduce the plasma concentration of leflunomide active metabolite (see PRECAUTIONS—General—Need for Drug Elimination).

In any situation in which the decision is made to switch from ARAVA to another anti-rheumatic agent with a known potential for hematologic suppression, it would be prudent to monitor for hematologic toxicity, because there will be overlap of systemic exposure to both compounds. ARAVA washout with cholestyramine or charcoal may decrease this risk, but also may induce disease worsening if the patient had been responding to ARAVA treatment.

Hepatotoxicity

RARE CASES OF SEVERE LIVER INJURY, INCLUDING CASES WITH FATAL OUTCOME, HAVE BEEN REPORTED DURING TREATMENT WITH LEFLUNOMIDE. MOST CASES OF SEVERE LIVER INJURY OCCUR WITHIN 6 MONTHS OF THERAPY AND IN A SETTING OF MULTIPLE RISK FACTORS FOR HEPATOTOXICITY (liver disease, other hepatotoxins). (See PRECAUTIONS).

At minimum, ALT (SGPT) must be performed at baseline and monitored initially at monthly intervals during the first six months then, if stable, every 6 to 8 weeks thereafter. In addition, if ARAVA and methotrexate are given concomitantly, ACR guidelines for monitoring methotrexate liver toxicity must be followed with ALT, AST, and serum albumin testing monthly.

Guidelines for dose adjustment or discontinuation based on the severity and persistence of ALT elevation are recommended as follows: For confirmed ALT elevations between 2- and 3-fold ULN, dose reduction to 10 mg/day may allow continued administration of ARAVA under close monitoring. If elevations between 2- and 3-fold ULN persist despite dose reduction or if ALT elevations of >3-fold ULN are present, ARAVA should be discontinued and cholestyramine or charcoal should be administered (see PRECAUTIONS—General—Need for Drug Elimination) with close monitoring, including retreatment with cholestyramine or charcoal as indicated.

In clinical trials, ARAVA treatment as monotherapy or in combination with methotrexate was associated with elevations of liver enzymes, primarily ALT and AST, in a significant number of patients; these effects were generally reversible. Most transaminase elevations were mild (≤ 2-fold ULN) and usually resolved while continuing treatment. Marked elevations (>3-fold ULN) occurred infrequently and reversed with dose reduction or discontinuation of treatment. Table 8 shows liver enzyme elevations seen with monthly monitoring in clinical trials US301 and MN301. It was notable that the absence of folate use in MN302 was associated with a considerably greater incidence of liver enzyme elevation on methotrexate.

[See table 8 above]

Table 7. Mean Change in the Components of the ACR Responder Index*

Components	Placebo-Controlled Studies						Non-placebo Controlled Study	
	US301 (12 months)			MN301 Non-US (6 months)			MN302 Non-US (12 months)	
	Leflunomide	Methotrexate	Placebo	Leflunomide	Sulfasalazine	Placebo	Leflunomide	Methotrexate
Tender joint count[1]	-7.7	-6.6	-3.0	-9.7	-8.1	-4.3	-8.3	-9.7
Swollen joint count[1]	-5.7	-5.4	-2.9	-7.2	-6.2	-3.4	-6.8	-9.0
Patient global assessment[2]	-2.1	-1.5	0.1	-2.8	-2.6	-0.9	-2.3	-3.0
Physician global assessment[2]	-2.8	-2.4	-1.0	-2.7	-2.5	-0.8	-2.3	-3.1
Physical function/ disability (MHAQ/HAQ)	-0.29	-0.15	0.07	-0.50	-0.29	-0.04	-0.37	-0.44
Pain intensity[2]	-2.2	-1.7	-0.5	-2.7	-2.0	-0.9	-2.1	-2.9
Erythrocyte Sedimentation rate	-6.26	-6.48	2.56	-7.48	-16.56	3.44	-10.12	-22.18
C-reactive protein	-0.62	-0.50	0.47	-2.26	-1.19	0.16	-1.86	-2.45
Not included in the ACR Responder Index								
Morning Stiffness (min)	-101.4	-88.7	14.7	-93.0	-42.4	-6.8	-63.7	-86.6

* Last Observation Carried Forward; Negative Change Indicates Improvement

[1] Based on 28 joint count

[2] Visual Analog Scale - 0=Best; 10=Worst

Table 8. Liver Enzyme Elevations >3-fold Upper Limits of Normal (ULN)

	US301			MN301			MN302*	
	LEF	PL	MTX	LEF	PL	SSZ	LEF	MTX
ALT (SGPT) >3-fold ULN (n %)	8 (4.4)	3 (2.5)	5 (2.7)	2 (1.5)	1 (1.1)	2 (1.5)	13 (2.6)	83 (16.7)
Reversed to ≤2-fold ULN:	8	3	5	2	1	2	12	82
Timing of Elevation								
0-3 Months	6	1	1	2	1	2	7	27
4-6 Months	1	1	3	—	—	—	1	34
7-9 Months	1	1	1	—	—	—	—	16
10-12 Months	—	—	—	—	—	—	5	6

*Only 10% of patients in MN302 received folate. All patients in US301 received folate.

In a 6 month study of 263 patients with persistent active rheumatoid arthritis despite methotrexate therapy, and with normal LFTs, leflunomide was added to a group of 133 patients starting at 10 mg per day and increased to 20 mg as needed. An increase in ALT greater than or equal to three times the ULN was observed in 3.8% of patients compared to 0.8% in 130 patients continued on methotrexate with placebo added.

Pre-existing Hepatic Disease

Given the possible risk of increased hepatotoxicity, and the role of the liver in drug activation, elimination and recycling, the use of ARAVA is not recommended in patients with significant hepatic impairment or evidence of infection with hepatitis B or C viruses. (See Warnings—Hepatotoxicity).

Skin Reactions

Rare cases of Stevens-Johnson syndrome and toxic epidermal necrolysis have been reported in patients receiving ARAVA. If a patient taking ARAVA develops any of these conditions, ARAVA therapy should be stopped, and a drug elimination procedure is recommended (see PRECAUTIONS— General—Need for Drug Elimination).

Malignancy

The risk of malignancy, particularly lymphoproliferative disorders, is increased with the use of some immunosuppression medications. There is a potential for immunosuppression with ARAVA. No apparent increase in the incidence of malignancies and lymphoproliferative disorders was reported in the clinical trials of ARAVA, but larger and longer-term studies would be needed to determine whether there is an increased risk of malignancy or lymphoproliferative disorders with ARAVA.

Use in Women of Childbearing Potential

There are no adequate and well-controlled studies evaluating ARAVA in pregnant women. However, based on animal studies, leflunomide may increase the risk of fetal death or teratogenic effects when administered to a pregnant woman (see CONTRAINDICATIONS). Women of childbearing potential must not be started on ARAVA until pregnancy is excluded and it has been confirmed that they are using reliable contraception. Before starting treatment with ARAVA, patients must be fully counseled on the potential for serious risk to the fetus.

The patient must be advised that if there is any delay in onset of menses or any other reason to suspect pregnancy, they must notify the physician immediately for pregnancy testing and, if positive, the physician and patient must discuss the risk to the pregnancy. It is possible that rapidly lowering the blood level of the active metabolite by instituting the drug elimination procedure described below at the first delay of menses may decrease the risk to the fetus from ARAVA.

Upon discontinuing ARAVA, it is recommended that all women of childbearing potential undergo the drug elimination procedure described below. Women receiving ARAVA treatment who wish to become pregnant must discontinue ARAVA and undergo the drug elimination procedure described below which includes verification of M1 metabolite plasma levels less than 0.02 mg/L (0.02 µg/mL). Human plasma levels of the active metabolite (M1) less than 0.02 mg/L (0.02 µg/mL) are expected to have minimal risk based on available animal data.

Drug Elimination Procedure

The following drug elimination procedure is recommended to achieve non-detectable plasma levels (less than 0.02 mg/L or 0.02 µg/mL) after stopping treatment with ARAVA:

1) Administer cholestyramine 8 grams 3 times daily for 11 days. (The 11 days do not need to be consecutive unless there is a need to lower the plasma level rapidly.)

2) Verify plasma levels less than 0.02 mg/L (0.02 μg/mL) by two separate tests at least 14 days apart. If plasma levels are higher than 0.02 mg/L, additional cholestyramine treatment should be considered.

Without the drug elimination procedure, it may take up to 2 years to reach plasma M1 metabolite levels less than 0.02 mg/L due to individual variation in drug clearance.

PRECAUTIONS

General

Need for Drug Elimination

The active metabolite of leflunomide is eliminated slowly from the plasma. In instances of any serious toxicity from ARAVA, including hypersensitivity, use of a drug elimination procedure as described in this section is highly recommended to reduce the drug concentration more rapidly after stopping ARAVA therapy. If hypersensitivity is the suspected clinical mechanism, more prolonged cholestyramine or charcoal administration may be necessary to achieve rapid and sufficient clearance. The duration may be modified based on the clinical status of the patient.

Cholestyramine given orally at a dose of 8 g three times a day for 24 hours to three healthy volunteers decreased plasma levels of M1 by approximately 40% in 24 hours and by 49 to 65% in 48 hours.

Administration of activated charcoal (powder made into a suspension) orally or via nasogastric tube (50 g every 6 hours for 24 hours) has been shown to reduce plasma concentrations of the active metabolite, M1, by 37% in 24 hours and by 48% in 48 hours.

These drug elimination procedures may be repeated if clinically necessary.

Renal Insufficiency

Single dose studies in dialysis patients show a doubling of the free fraction of M1 in plasma. There is no clinical experience in the use of ARAVA in patients with renal impairment. Caution should be used when administering this drug in this population.

Vaccinations

No clinical data are available on the efficacy and safety of vaccinations during ARAVA treatment. Vaccination with live vaccines is, however, not recommended. The long half-life of ARAVA should be considered when contemplating administration of a live vaccine after stopping ARAVA.

Information for Patients

The potential for increased risk of birth defects should be discussed with female patients of childbearing potential. It is recommended that physicians advise women that they may be at increased risk of having a child with birth defects if they are pregnant when taking ARAVA, become pregnant while taking ARAVA, or do not wait to become pregnant until they have stopped taking ARAVA and followed the drug elimination procedure (as described in WARNINGS—Use In Women of Childbearing Potential—Drug Elimination Procedure).

Patients should be advised of the possibility of rare, serious skin reactions. Patients should be instructed to inform their physicians promptly if they develop a skin rash or mucous membrane lesions.

Patients should be advised of the potential hepatotoxic effects of ARAVA and of the need for monitoring liver enzymes.

Patients should be instructed to notify their physicians if they develop symptoms such as unusual tiredness, abdominal pain or jaundice.

Patients should be advised that they may develop a lowering of their blood counts and should have frequent hematologic monitoring. This is particularly important for patients who are receiving other immunosuppressive therapy concurrently with ARAVA, who have recently discontinued such therapy before starting treatment with ARAVA, or who have had a history of a significant hematologic abnormality. Patients should be instructed to notify their physicians promptly if they notice symptoms of pancytopenia (such as easy bruising or bleeding, recurrent infections, fever, paleness or unusual tiredness).

Laboratory Tests

Hematologic Monitoring

At minimum, patients taking ARAVA should have platelet, white blood cell count and hemoglobin or hematocrit monitored at baseline and monthly for six months following initiation of therapy and every 6 to 8 weeks thereafter.

Bone Marrow Suppression Monitoring

If used with concomitantly with immunosuppressants such as methotrexate, chronic monitoring should be monthly. (see WARNINGS—Immunosuppression Potential/Bone Marrow Suppression).

Liver Enzyme Monitoring

ALT (SGPT) must be performed at baseline and monitored at monthly intervals during the first six months then, if stable, every 6 to 8 weeks thereafter. In addition, if ARAVA and methotrexate are given concomitantly, ACR guidelines for monitoring methotrexate liver toxicity must be followed with ALT, AST, and serum albumin testing every month. (See WARNINGS—Hepatotoxicity.)

Due to a specific effect on the brush border of the renal proximal tubule, ARAVA has a uricosuric effect. A separate effect of hypophosphaturia is seen in some patients. These effects have not been seen together, nor have there been alterations in renal function.

Carcinogenesis, Mutagenesis, and Impairment of Fertility

No evidence of carcinogenicity was observed in a 2-year bioassay in rats at oral doses of leflunomide up to the maximally tolerated dose of 6 mg/kg (approximately 1/40 the maximum human M1 systemic exposure based on AUC). However, male mice in a 2-year bioassay exhibited an increased incidence in lymphoma at an oral dose of 15 mg/kg, the highest dose studied (1.7 times the human M1 exposure based on AUC). Female mice, in the same study, exhibited a dose-related increased incidence of bronchoalveolar adenomas and carcinomas combined beginning at 1.5 mg/kg (approximately 1/10 the human M1 exposure based on AUC). The significance of the findings in mice relative to the clinical use of ARAVA is not known.

Leflunomide was not mutagenic in the Ames Assay, the Unscheduled DNA Synthesis Assay, or in the HGPRT Gene Mutation Assay. In addition, leflunomide was not clastogenic in the *in vivo* Mouse Micronucleus Assay nor in the *in vivo* Cytogenetic Test in Chinese Hamster Bone Marrow Cells. However, 4-trifluoromethylaniline (TFMA), a minor metabolite of leflunomide, was mutagenic in the Ames Assay and in the HGPRT Gene Mutation Assay, and was clastogenic in the *in vitro* Assay for Chromosome Aberrations in the Chinese Hamster Cells. TFMA was not clastogenic in the *in vivo* Mouse Micronucleus Assay nor in the *in vivo* Cytogenetic Test in Chinese Hamster Bone Marrow Cells.

Leflunomide had no effect on fertility in either male or female rats at oral doses up to 4.0 mg/kg (approximately 1/30 the human M1 exposure based on AUC).

Pregnancy

Pregnancy Category X. See CONTRAINDICATIONS section. Pregnancy Registry: To monitor fetal outcomes of pregnant women exposed to leflunomide, health care providers are encouraged to register such patients by calling 1-877-311-8972.

Table 9. Percentage Of Patients With Adverse Events ≥3% In Any Leflunomide Treated Group

	All RA Studies	Placebo-Controlled Trials				Active-Controlled Trials	
		MN 301 and US 301				MN 302*	
	LEF (N=1339)[1]	LEF (N=315)	PBO (N=210)	SSZ (N=133)	MTX (N=182)	LEF (N=501)	MTX (N=498)
BODY AS A WHOLE							
Allergic Reaction	2%	5%	2%	0%	6%	1%	2%
Asthenia	3%	6%	4%	5%	6%	3%	3%
Flu Syndrome	2%	4%	2%	0%	7%	0%	0%
Infection, upper respiratory	4%	0%	0%	0%	0%	0%	0%
Injury Accident	5%	7%	5%	3%	11%	6%	7%
Pain	2%	4%	2%	2%	5%	1%	<1%
Abdominal Pain	6%	5%	4%	4%	8%	6%	4%
Back Pain	5%	6%	3%	4%	9%	8%	7%
CARDIOVASCULAR							
Hypertension[2]	10%	9%	4%	4%	3%	10%	4%
- New onset of hypertension		1%	<1%	0%	2%	2%	<1%
Chest Pain	2%	4%	2%	2%	4%	1%	2%
GASTROINTESTINAL							
Anorexia	3%	3%	2%	5%	2%	3%	3%
Diarrhea	17%	27%	12%	10%	20%	22%	10%
Dyspepsia	5%	10%	10%	9%	13%	6%	7%
Gastroenteritis	3%	1%	1%	0%	6%	3%	3%
Abnormal Liver Enzymes	5%	10%	2%	4%	10%	6%	17%
Nausea	9%	13%	11%	19%	18%	13%	18%
GI/Abdominal Pain	5%	6%	4%	7%	8%	8%	8%
Mouth Ulcer	3%	5%	4%	3%	10%	3%	6%
Vomiting	3%	5%	4%	4%	3%	3%	3%
METABOLIC AND NUTRITIONAL							
Hypokalemia	1%	3%	1%	1%	1%	1%	<1%
Weight Loss[3]	4%	2%	1%	2%	0%	2%	2%
MUSCULO-SKELETAL SYSTEM							
Arthralgia	1%	4%	3%	0%	9%	<1%	1%
Leg Cramps	1%	4%	2%	2%	6%	0%	0%
Joint Disorder	4%	2%	2%	2%	2%	8%	6%
Synovitis	2%	<1%	1%	0%	2%	4%	2%
Tenosynovitis	3%	2%	0%	1%	2%	5%	1%
NERVOUS SYSTEM							
Dizziness	4%	5%	3%	6%	5%	7%	6%
Headache	7%	13%	11%	12%	21%	10%	8%
Paresthesia	2%	3%	1%	1%	2%	4%	3%

(Table continued on next page)

Continued on next page

Arava—Cont.

Nursing Mothers
ARAVA should not be used by nursing mothers. It is not known whether ARAVA is excreted in human milk. Many drugs are excreted in human milk, and there is a potential for serious adverse reactions in nursing infants from ARAVA. Therefore, a decision should be made whether to proceed with nursing or to initiate treatment with ARAVA, taking into account the importance of the drug to the mother.

Use in Males
Available information does not suggest that ARAVA would be associated with an increased risk of male-mediated fetal toxicity. However, animal studies to evaluate this specific risk have not been conducted. To minimize any possible risk, men wishing to father a child should consider discontinuing use of ARAVA and taking cholestyramine 8 grams 3 times daily for 11 days.

Drug Interactions

Cholestyramine and Charcoal
Administration of cholestyramine or activated charcoal in patients (n=13) and volunteers (n=96) resulted in a rapid and significant decrease in plasma M1 (the active metabolite of leflunomide) concentration (see PRECAUTIONS—General—Need for Drug Elimination).

Hepatotoxic Drugs
Increased side effects may occur when leflunomide is given concomitantly with hepatotoxic substances. This is also to be considered when leflunomide treatment is followed by such drugs without a drug elimination procedure. In a small (n=30) combination study of ARAVA with methotrexate, a 2- to 3-fold elevation in liver enzymes was seen in 5 of 30 patients. All elevations resolved, 2 with continuation of both drugs and 3 after discontinuation of leflunomide. A >3-fold increase was seen in another 5 patients. All of these also resolved, 2 with continuation of both drugs and 3 after discontinuation of leflunomide. Three patients met "ACR criteria" for liver biopsy (1: Roegnik Grade I, 2: Roegnik Grade IIIa). No pharmacokinetic interaction was identified (see CLINICAL PHARMACOLOGY).

NSAIDs
In *in vitro* studies, M1 was shown to cause increases ranging from 13-50% in the free fraction of diclofenac and ibuprofen at concentrations in the clinical range. The clinical significance of this finding is unknown, however, there was extensive concomitant use of NSAIDs in clinical studies and no differential effect was observed.

Tolbutamide
In *in vitro* studies, M1 was shown to cause increases ranging from 13-50% in the free fraction of tolbutamide at concentrations in the clinical range. The clinical significance of this finding is unknown.

Rifampin
Following concomitant administration of a single dose of ARAVA to subjects receiving multiple doses of rifampin, M1 peak levels were increased (~40%) over those seen when ARAVA was given alone. Because of the potential for ARAVA levels to continue to increase with multiple dosing, caution should be used if patients are to be receiving both ARAVA and rifampin.

Warfarin
Increased INR (International Normalized Ratio) when ARAVA and warfarin were co-administered has been rarely reported.

Pediatric Use
The safety and effectiveness of ARAVA in pediatric patients with polyarticular course juvenile rheumatoid arthritis (JRA) have not been fully evaluated. (See CLINICAL STUDIES and ADVERSE REACTIONS).

Geriatric Use
No dosage adjustment is needed in patients over 65.

ADVERSE REACTIONS

Adverse reactions associated with the use of leflunomide in RA include diarrhea, elevated liver enzymes (ALT and AST), alopecia and rash. In the controlled studies at one year, the following adverse events were reported, regardless of causality. (See Table 9.)

[See table 9 on previous page and above]

Adverse events during a second year of treatment with leflunomide in clinical trials were consistent with those observed during the first year of treatment and occurred at a similar or lower incidence.

In addition, the following adverse events have been reported in 1% to <3% of the RA patients in the leflunomide treatment group in controlled clinical trials.

Body as a Whole: abscess, cyst, fever, hernia, malaise, pain, neck pain, pelvic pain;
Cardiovascular: angina pectoris, migraine, palpitation, tachycardia, varicose vein, vasculitis, vasodilatation;
Gastrointestinal: cholelithiasis, colitis, constipation, esophagitis, flatulence, gastritis, gingivitis, melena, oral moniliasis, pharyngitis, salivary gland enlarged, stomatitis (or aphthous stomatitis), tooth disorder;
Endocrine: diabetes mellitus, hyperthyroidism;
Hemic and Lymphatic System: anemia (including iron deficiency anemia), ecchymosis;
Metabolic and Nutritional: creatine phosphokinase increased, hyperglycemia, hyperlipidemia, peripheral edema;
Musculo-Skeletal System: arthrosis, bone necrosis, bone pain, bursitis, muscle cramps, myalgia, tendon rupture;

Table 9 *(cont.)*. Percentage Of Patients With Adverse Events ≥3% In Any Leflunomide Treated Group

	All RA Studies	Placebo-Controlled Trials				Active-Controlled Trials	
		MN 301 and US 301				MN 302*	
	LEF (N=1339)[1]	LEF (N=315)	PBO (N=210)	SSZ (N=133)	MTX (N=182)	LEF (N=501)	MTX (N=498)
RESPIRATORY SYSTEM							
Bronchitis	7%	5%	2%	4%	7%	8%	7%
Increased Cough	3%	4%	5%	3%	6%	5%	7%
Respiratory Infection	15%	21%	21%	20%	32%	27%	25%
Pharyngitis	3%	2%	1%	2%	1%	3%	3%
Pneumonia	2%	3%	0%	0%	1%	2%	2%
Rhinitis	2%	5%	2%	4%	3%	2%	2%
Sinusitis	2%	5%	5%	0%	10%	1%	1%
SKIN AND APPENDAGES							
Alopecia	10%	9%	1%	6%	6%	17%	10%
Eczema	2%	1%	1%	1%	1%	3%	2%
Pruritus	4%	5%	2%	3%	2%	6%	2%
Rash	10%	12%	7%	11%	9%	11%	10%
Dry Skin	2%	3%	2%	2%	0%	3%	1%
UROGENITAL SYSTEM							
Urinary Tract Infection	5%	5%	7%	4%	2%	5%	6%

* Only 10% of patients in MN302 received folate. All patients in US301 received folate; none in MN301 received folate.
[1] Includes all controlled and uncontrolled trials with leflunomide (duration up to 12 months).
[2] Hypertension as a preexisting condition was overrepresented in all leflunomide treatment groups in phase III trials.
[3] In a meta-analysis of all phase II and III studies, during the first 6 months in patients receiving leflunomide, 10% lost 10-19 lbs (24 cases per 100 patient years) and 2% lost at least 20 lbs (4 cases/100 patient years). Of patients receiving leflunomide 4% lost 10% of their baseline weight during the first 6 months of treatment.

ARAVA® (leflunomide) Tablets

Strength	Quantity	NDC Number	Description
10 mg	30 count bottle	0088-2160-30	White, round film-coated tablet embossed with "ZBN" on one side.
20 mg	30 count bottle	0088-2161-30	Light yellow, triangular film-coated tablet embossed with "ZBO" on one side.
100 mg	3 count blister pack	0088-2162-03	White, round film-coated tablet embossed with "ZBP" on one side.

Nervous System: anxiety, depression, dry mouth, insomnia, neuralgia, neuritis, sleep disorder, sweating increased, vertigo;
Respiratory System: asthma, dyspnea, epistaxis, lung disorder;
Skin and Appendages: acne, contact dermatitis, fungal dermatitis, hair discoloration, hematoma, herpes simplex, herpes zoster, maculopapular rash, nail disorder, skin discoloration, skin disorder, skin nodule, subcutaneous nodule, ulcer skin;
Special Senses: blurred vision, cataract, conjunctivitis, eye disorder, taste perversion;
Urogenital System: albuminuria, cystitis, dysuria, hematuria, menstrual disorder, prostate disorder, urinary frequency, vaginal moniliasis.

Other less common adverse events seen in clinical trials include: 1 case of anaphylactic reaction occurred in Phase 2 following rechallenge of drug after withdrawal due to rash (rare); urticaria; eosinophilia; transient thrombocytopenia (rare); and leukopenia <2000 WBC/mm^3 (rare).

Adverse events during a second year of treatment with leflunomide in clinical trials were consistent with those observed during the first year of treatment and occurred at a similar or lower incidence.

In post-marketing experience, the following have been reported rarely:

Body as a whole: opportunistic infections, severe infections including sepsis that may be fatal;
Gastrointestinal: pancreatitis;
Hematologic: agranulocytosis, leukopenia, neutropenia, pancytopenia, thrombocytopenia;
Hypersensitivity: angioedema;
Hepatic: hepatitis, jaundice/cholestasis, severe liver injury such as hepatic failure and acute hepatic necrosis that may be fatal;
Respiratory: interstitial lung disease;
Nervous system: peripheral neuropathy
Skin and Appendages: erythema multiforme, Stevens-Johnson syndrome, toxic epidermal necrolysis.

Adverse Reactions (Pediatric Patients)
The safety of ARAVA was studied in 74 patients with polyarticular course juvenile rheumatoid arthritis ranging in age from 3-17 years (47 patients from the active-controlled study and 27 from the open-label safety and pharmacokinetic study). The most common adverse events included abdominal pain, diarrhea, nausea, vomiting, oral ulcers, upper respiratory tract infections, alopecia, rash, headache, and dizziness. Less common adverse events included anemia, hypertension, and weight loss. Fourteen pediatric patients experienced ALT and/or AST elevations, nine between 1.2 and 3-fold the upper limit of normal, five between 3 and 8-fold the upper limit of normal.

DRUG ABUSE AND DEPENDENCE

ARAVA has no known potential for abuse or dependence.

OVERDOSAGE

In mouse and rat acute toxicology studies, the minimally toxic dose for oral leflunomide was 200-500 mg/kg and 100 mg/kg, respectively (approximately >350 times the maximum recommended human dose, respectively).

There have been reports of chronic overdose in patients taking ARAVA at daily dose up to five times the recommended daily dose and reports of acute overdose in adults or children. There were no adverse events reported in the majority of case reports of overdose. Adverse events were consistent with the safety profile for ARAVA (see ADVERSE REACTIONS). The most frequent adverse events observed were diarrhea, abdominal pain, leukopenia, anemia and elevated liver function tests.

In the event of a significant overdose or toxicity, cholestyramine or charcoal administration is recommended to accelerate elimination (see PRECAUTIONS—General—Need for Drug Elimination).

Studies with both hemodialysis and CAPD (chronic ambulatory peritoneal dialysis) indicate that M1, the primary metabolite of leflunomide, is not dialyzable. (see CLINICAL PHARMACOLOGY—Elimination).

DOSAGE AND ADMINISTRATION

Loading Dose

Due to the long half-life in patients with RA and recommended dosing interval (24 hours), a loading dose is needed to provide steady-state concentrations more rapidly. It is recommended that ARAVA therapy be initiated with a loading dose of one 100 mg tablet per day for 3 days. Elimination of the loading dose regimen may decrease the risk of adverse events. This could be especially important for patients at increased risk of hematologic or hepatic toxicity, such as those receiving concomitant treatment with methotrexate or other immunosuppressive agents or on such medications in the recent past. (See WARNINGS—Hepatotoxicity).

Maintenance Therapy

Daily dosing of 20 mg is recommended for treatment of patients with RA. A small cohort of patients (n=104), treated with 25 mg/day, experienced a greater incidence of side effects; alopecia, weight loss, liver enzyme elevations. Doses higher than 20 mg/day are not recommended. If dosing at 20 mg/day is not well tolerated clinically, the dose may be decreased to 10 mg daily. Liver enzymes must be monitored and dose adjustments may be necessary (see WARNINGS—Hepatotoxicity). Due to the prolonged half-life of the active metabolite of leflunomide, patients should be carefully observed after dose reduction, since it may take several weeks for metabolite levels to decline.

HOW SUPPLIED

ARAVA Tablets in 10 and 20 mg strengths are packaged in bottles. ARAVA Tablets 100 mg strength are packaged in blister packs.

[See second table on previous page]

Store at 25°C (77°F); excursions permitted to 15-30°C (59-86°F) [see USP Controlled Room Temperature]. Protect from light.

Rx only.

Rev. March 2004

Manufactured by
Usiphar, 60200 Compiegne, France
for
Aventis Pharmaceuticals Inc.
Kansas City, MO 64137
Made in France

Shown in Product Identification Guide, page 307

CLAFORAN® ℞

[*kla 'fər-an*]

Sterile (cefotaxime for injection, USP)
and Injection (cefotaxime injection, USP)
Rx only
Prescribing Information as of January 2004

To reduce the development of drug-resistant bacteria and maintain the effectiveness of CLAFORAN® (cefotaxime sodium) and other antibacterial drugs, CLAFORAN should be used only to treat or prevent infections that are proven or strongly suspected to be caused by bacteria.

DESCRIPTION

Sterile CLAFORAN® (cefotaxime sodium) is a semisynthetic, broad spectrum cephalosporin antibiotic for parenteral administration. It is the sodium salt of 7-[2-(2-amino-4-thiazolyl) glyoxylamido]-3-(hydroxymethyl)-8-oxo-5-thia-1-azabicyclo [4.2.0] oct-2-ene-2-carboxylate 7^2 (Z)-(o-methyloxime), acetate (ester). CLAFORAN contains approximately 50.5 mg (2.2 mEq) of sodium per gram of cefotaxime activity. Solutions of CLAFORAN range from very pale yellow to light amber depending on the concentration and the diluent used. The pH of the injectable solutions usually ranges from 5.0 to 7.5. The CAS Registry Number is 64485-93-4.

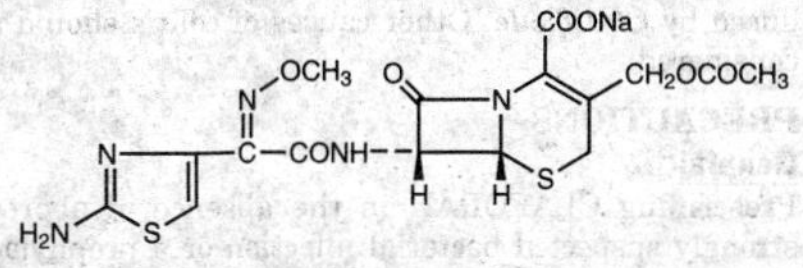

CLAFORAN is supplied as a dry powder in conventional and ADD-Vantage® System compatible vials, infusion bottles, pharmacy bulk package bottles, and as a frozen, premixed, iso-osmotic injection in a buffered diluent solution in plastic containers. CLAFORAN, equivalent to 1 gram and 2 grams cefotaxime, is supplied as frozen, premixed, iso-osmotic injections in plastic containers. Solutions range from very pale yellow to light amber. Dextrose Hydrous, USP has been added to adjust osmolality (approximately 1.7 g and 700 mg to the 1 g and 2 g cefotaxime dosages, respectively). The injections are buffered with sodium citrate hydrous, USP. The pH is adjusted with hydrochloric acid and may be adjusted with sodium hydroxide.

The plastic container is fabricated from a specially designed multilayer plastic (PL 2040). Solutions are in contact with the polyethylene layer of this container and can leach out certain chemical components of the plastic in very small amounts within the expiration period. The suitability of the plastic has been confirmed in tests in animals according to the USP biological tests for plastic containers, as well as by tissue culture toxicity studies.

CLINICAL PHARMACOLOGY

Following IM administration of a single 500 mg or 1 g dose of CLAFORAN to normal volunteers, mean peak serum concentrations of 11.7 and 20.5 mcg/mL respectively were attained within 30 minutes and declined with an elimination half-life of approximately 1 hour. There was a dose-dependent increase in serum levels after the IV administration of 500 mg, 1 g, and 2 g of CLAFORAN (38.9, 101.7, and 214.4 mcg/mL respectively) without alteration in the elimination half-life. There is no evidence of accumulation following repetitive IV infusion of 1 g doses every 6 hours for 14 days as there are no alterations of serum or renal clearance. About 60% of the administered dose was recovered from urine during the first 6 hours following the start of the infusion.

Approximately 20-36% of an intravenously administered dose of ^{14}C-cefotaxime is excreted by the kidney as unchanged cefotaxime and 15–25% as the desacetyl derivative, the major metabolite. The desacetyl metabolite has been shown to contribute to the bactericidal activity. Two other urinary metabolites (M_2 and M_3) account for about 20-25%. They lack bactericidal activity.

A single 50 mg/kg dose of CLAFORAN was administered as an intravenous infusion over a 10- to 15-minute period to 29 newborn infants grouped according to birth weight and age. The mean half-life of cefotaxime in infants with lower birth weights (≤1500 grams), regardless of age, was longer (4.6 hours) than the mean half-life (3.4 hours) in infants whose birth weight was greater than 1500 grams. Mean serum clearance was also smaller in the lower birth weight infants. Although the differences in mean half-life values are statistically significant for weight, they are not clinically important. Therefore, dosage should be based solely on age. (See DOSAGE AND ADMINISTRATION section.)

Additionally, no disulfiram-like reactions were reported in a study conducted in 22 healthy volunteers administered CLAFORAN and ethanol.

Microbiology

The bactericidal activity of cefotaxime sodium results from inhibition of cell wall synthesis. Cefotaxime sodium has *in vitro* activity against a wide range of gram-positive and gram-negative organisms. Cefotaxime sodium has a high degree of stability in the presence of β-lactamases, both penicillinases and cephalosporinases, of gram-negative and gram-positive bacteria. Cefotaxime sodium has been shown to be active against most strains of the following microorganisms both *in vitro* and in clinical infections as described in the INDICATIONS AND USAGE section.

Aerobes, Gram-positive:

Enterococcus spp.
*Staphylococcus aureus**, including β-lactamase-positive and negative strains
Staphylococcus epidermidis
Streptococcus pneumoniae
Streptococcus pyogenes (Group A beta-hemolytic streptococci)
Streptococcus spp.

---

*Staphylococci which are resistant to methicillin/oxacillin must be considered resistant to cefotaxime sodium.

Aerobes, Gram-negative:

Acinetobacter spp.
Citrobacter spp.
Enterobacter spp.
Escherichia coli
Haemophilus influenzae (including ampicillin-resistant strains)
Haemophilus parainfluenzae
Klebsiella spp. (including *Klebsiella pneumoniae*)
Morganella morganii
Neisseria gonorrhoeae (including β-lactamase-positive and negative strains)
Neisseria meningitidis
Proteus mirabilis
Proteus vulgaris
Providencia rettgeri
Providencia stuartii
Serratia marcescens

NOTE: Many strains of the above organisms that are multiply resistant to other antibiotics, e.g. penicillins, cephalosporins, and aminoglycosides, are susceptible to cefotaxime sodium. Cefotaxime sodium is active against some strains of *Pseudomonas aeruginosa*.

Anaerobes:

Bacteroides spp., including some strains of *Bacteroides fragilis*
Clostridium spp. (**Note:** Most strains of *Clostridium difficile* are resistant.)
Fusobacterium spp. (Including *Fusobacterium nucleatum*).
Peptococcus spp.
Peptostreptococcus spp.

Cefotaxime sodium also demonstrates *in vitro* activity against the following microorganisms **but the clinical significance is unknown**. Cefotaxime sodium exhibits *in vitro* minimal inhibitory concentrations (MICs) of 8 mcg/mL or less against most (≥90%) strains of the following microorganisms; however, the safety and effectiveness of cefotaxime sodium in treating clinical infections due to these microorganisms have not been established in adequate and well-controlled clinical trials:

Aerobes, Gram-negative:

Providencia spp.
Salmonella spp. (including *Salmonella typhi*)
Shigella spp.

Cefotaxime sodium is highly stable *in vitro* to four of the five major classes of ß-lactamases described by Richmond et al.[1], including type IIIa (TEM) which is produced by many gram-negative bacteria. The drug is also stable to β-lactamase (penicillinase) produced by staphylococci. In addition, cefotaxime sodium shows high affinity for penicillin-binding proteins in the cell wall, including PBP: Ib and III.

Cefotaxime sodium and aminoglycosides have been shown to be synergistic *in vitro* against some strains of *Pseudomonas aeruginosa* but the clinical significance is unknown.

Susceptibility Tests

Dilution techniques:

Quantitative methods that are used to determine minimum inhibitory concentrations (MICs) provide reproducible estimates of the susceptibility of bacteria to antimicrobial compounds. One such standardized procedure uses a standardized dilution method[1] (broth or agar) or equivalent with cefotaxime sodium powder. The MIC values obtained should be interpreted according to the following criteria:

When testing organisms[a] other than *Haemophilus* spp., *Neisseria gonorrhoeae*, and *Streptococcus* spp.

MIC (mcg/mL)	Interpretation
≤8	Susceptible (S)
16-32	Intermediate (I)
≥64	Resistant (R)

When testing *Haemophilus* spp.[b]

MIC (mcg/mL)	Interpretation[c]
≤2	Susceptible (S)

When testing *Streptococcus*[d]

MIC (mcg/mL)	Interpretation
≤0.5	Susceptible (S)
1	Intermediate (I)
≥2	Resistant (R)

When testing *Neisseria gonorrhoeae*[e]

MIC (mcg/mL)	Interpretation[c]
≤0.5	Susceptible (S)

---

a. Staphylococci exhibiting resistance to methicillin/oxacillin, should be reported as also resistant to cefotaxime despite apparent *in vitro* susceptibility.
b. Interpretive criteria is applicable only to tests performed by broth microdilution method using Haemophilus Test Media.[2]
c. The absence of resistant strains precludes defining any interpretations other than susceptible.
d. *Streptococcus pneumoniae* must be tested using cation-adjusted Mueller-Hinton broth with 2-5% lysed horse blood.
e. Interpretive criteria applicable only to tests performed by agar dilution method using GC agar base with 1% defined growth supplement.[2]

A report of "Susceptible" indicates that the pathogen is likely to be inhibited if the antimicrobial compound in the blood reaches the concentrations usually achievable. A report of "Intermediate" indicates that the result should be considered equivocal and if the microorganism is not fully susceptible to alternative clinically feasible drugs the test should be repeated. This category implies possible clinical applicability in body sites where the drug is physiologically concentrated or in situations where high dosage of drug can be used. This category also provides a buffer zone that prevents small uncontrolled technical factors from causing major discrepancies in interpretation. A report of "Resistant" indicates that the pathogen is not likely to be inhibited if the antimicrobial compound in the blood reaches the concentrations usually achievable, other therapy should be selected.

Standardized susceptibility test procedures require the use of laboratory control microorganisms to control the technical aspects of the laboratory procedure. Standard cefotaxime sodium powder should provide the following MIC values:

Microorganism	MIC (mcg/mL)
Escherichia coli ATCC 25922	0.06-0.25
Staphylococcus aureus ATCC 29213	1-4
Pseudomonas aeruginosa ATCC 27853	4-16
Haemophilus influenzae[a] ATCC 49247	0.12-0.5
Streptococcus pneumoniae[b] ATCC 49619	0.06-0.25
Neisseria gonorrhoeae[c] ATCC 49226	0.015-0.06

---

a. Ranges applicable only to tests performed by broth microdilution method using Haemophilus Test Media.[2]
b. Ranges applicable only to tests performed by broth microdilution method using cation-adjusted Mueller-Hinton broth with 2–5% lysed horse blood.[2]
c. Ranges applicable only to tests performed by agar dilution method using GC agar base with 1% defined growth supplement.[2]

Continued on next page

Claforan—Cont.

Diffusion Techniques:

Quantitative methods that require measurements of zone diameters also provide reproducible estimates of the susceptibility of bacteria to antimicrobial compounds. One such standardized procedure[3] requires the use of standardized inoculum concentrations. This procedure uses paper disks impregnated with 30 mcg cefotaxime sodium to test the susceptibility of microorganisms to cefotaxime sodium. Reports from the laboratory providing results of the standard single-disk susceptibility test using a 30 mcg cefotaxime sodium disk should be interpreted according to the following criteria: When testing organisms[a] other than *Haemophilus* spp., *Neisseria gonorrhoeae*, and *Streptococcus* spp.

MIC (mcg/mL)	Interpretation
≥23	Susceptible (S)
15-22	Intermediate (I)
≤14	Resistant (R)

When testing *Haemophilus* spp.[b]

Zone Diameter (mm)	Interpretation[c]
≥26	Susceptible (S)

When testing *Streptococcus* other than *Streptococcus pneumoniae*

Zone Diameter (mm)	Interpretation[c]
≥28	Susceptible (S)
26-27	Intermediate (I)
≤25	Resistant (R)

When testing *Neisseria gonorrhoeae*[d]

Zone Diameter (mm)	Interpretation[c]
≥31	Susceptible (S)

a. Staphylococci exhibiting resistance to methicillin/oxacillin, should be reported as also resistant to cefotaxime despite apparent *in vitro* susceptibility.
b. Interpretive criteria is applicable only to tests performed by disk diffusion method using Haemophilus Test Media.[3]
c. The absence of resistant strains precludes defining any interpretations other than susceptible.
d. Interpretive criteria applicable only to tests performed by disk diffusion method using GC agar base with 1% defined growth supplement.[3]

Interpretation should be as stated above for results using dilution techniques. Interpretation involves correlation of the diameter obtained in the disk test with the MIC for cefotaxime sodium.

As with standardized dilution techniques, diffusion methods require the use of laboratory control microorganisms that are used to control the technical aspects of the laboratory procedures. For the diffusion technique, the 30 mcg cefotaxime sodium disk should provide the following zone diameters in these laboratory test quality control strains:

Microorganism	Zone Diameter (mm)
Escherichia coli ATCC 25922	29-35
Staphylococcus aureus ATCC 25923	25-31
Pseudomonas aeruginosa ATCC 27853	18-22
Haemophilus influenzae[a] ATCC 49247	31-39
Neisseria gonorrhoeae[b] ATCC 49226	38-48

a. Ranges applicable only to tests performed by disk diffusion method using Haemophilus Test Media.[3]
b. Ranges applicable only to tests performed by disk diffusion method using GC agar base with 1% defined growth supplement.[3]

Anaerobic Techniques:

For anaerobic bacteria, the susceptibility to cefotaxime sodium as MICs can be determined by standardized test methods.[4] The MIC values obtained should be interpreted according to the following criteria:

MIC (mcg/mL)	Interpretation
≤16	Susceptible (S)
32	Intermediate (I)
≥64	Resistant (R)

Interpretation is identical to that stated above for results using dilution techniques.

As with other susceptibility techniques, the use of laboratory control microorganisms is required to control the technical aspects of the laboratory standardized procedures. Standardized cefotaxime sodium powder should provide the following MIC values:

Microorganism	MIC (mcg/mL)
Bacteroides fragilis[a] ATCC 25285	8-32
Bacteroides thetaiotaomicron ATCC 29741	16-64
Eubacterium lantem ATCC 43055	64-256

a. Ranges applicable only to tests performed by agar dilution method.

INDICATIONS AND USAGE

Treatment

CLAFORAN is indicated for the treatment of patients with serious infections caused by susceptible strains of the designated microorganisms in the diseases listed below.

(1) Lower respiratory tract infections, including pneumonia, caused by *Streptococcus pneumoniae* (formerly *Diplococcus pneumoniae*), *Streptococcus pyogenes** (Group A streptococci) and other streptococci (excluding enterococci, e.g., *Enterococcus faecalis*), *Staphylococcus aureus* (penicillinase and non-penicillinase producing), *Escherichia coli, Klebsiella* species, *Haemophilus influenzae* (including ampicillin resistant strains), *Haemophilus parainfluenzae, Proteus mirabilis, Serratia marcescens**, *Enterobacter* species, indole positive *Proteus* and *Pseudomonas* species (including *P. aeruginosa*).

(2) Genitourinary infections. Urinary tract infections caused by *Enterococcus* species, *Staphylococcus epidermidis, Staphylococcus aureus**, (penicillinase and non-penicillinase producing), *Citrobacter* species, *Enterobacter* species, *Escherichia coli, Klebsiella* species, *Proteus mirabilis, Proteus vulgaris**, *Providencia stuartii, Morganella morganii**, *Providencia rettgeri**, *Serratia marcescens* and *Pseudomonas* species (including *P. aeruginosa*). Also, uncomplicated gonorrhea (cervical/urethral and rectal) caused by *Neisseria gonorrhoeae*, including penicillinase producing strains.

(3) Gynecologic infections, including pelvic inflammatory disease, endometritis and pelvic cellulitis caused by *Staphylococcus epidermidis, Streptococcus* species, *Enterococcus* species, *Enterobacter* species*, *Klebsiella* species*, *Escherichia coli, Proteus mirabilis, Bacteroides* species (including *Bacteroides fragilis**), *Clostridium* species, and anaerobic cocci (including *Peptostreptococcus* species and *Peptococcus* species) and *Fusobacterium* species (including *F. nucleatum**).

CLAFORAN, like other cephalosporins, has no activity against *Chlamydia trachomatis*. Therefore, when cephalosporins are used in the treatment of patients with pelvic inflammatory disease and *C. trachomatis* is one of the suspected pathogens, appropriate antichlamydial coverage should be added.

(4) Bacteremia/Septicemia caused by *Escherichia coli, Klebsiella* species, and *Serratia marcescens, Staphylococcus aureus* and *Streptococcus* species (including *S. pneumonia*).

(5) Skin and skin structure infections caused by *Staphylococcus aureus* (penicillinase and non-penicillinase producing), *Staphylococcus epidermidis, Streptococcus pyogenes* (Group A streptococci) and other streptococci, *Enterococcus* species, *Acinetobacter* species*, *Escherichia coli, Citrobacter* species (including *C. freundii**), *Enterobacter* species, *Klebsiella* species, *Proteus mirabilis, Proteus vulgaris**, *Morganella morganii, Providencia rettgeri**, *Pseudomonas* species, *Serratia marcescens, Bacteroides* species, and anaerobic cocci (including *Peptostreptococcus** species and *Peptococcus* species).

(6) Intra-abdominal infections including peritonitis caused by *Streptococcus* species*, *Escherichia coli, Klebsiella* species, *Bacteroides* species, and anaerobic cocci (including *Peptostreptococcus** species and *Peptococcus** species) *Proteus mirabilis**, and *Clostridium* species*.

(7) Bone and/or joint infections caused by *Staphylococcus aureus* (penicillinase and non-penicillinase producing strains), *Streptococcus* species (including *S. pyogenes**), *Pseudomonas* species (including *P. aeruginosa**), and *Proteus mirabilis**.

(8) Central nervous system infections, e.g., meningitis and ventriculitis, caused by *Neisseria meningitidis, Haemophilus influenzae, Streptococcus pneumoniae, Klebsiella pneumoniae** and *Escherichia coli**.

(*) Efficacy for this organism, in this organ system, has been studied in fewer than 10 infections.

Although many strains of enterococci (e.g., *S. faecalis*) and *Pseudomonas* species are resistant to cefotaxime sodium *in vitro*, CLAFORAN has been used successfully in treating patients with infections caused by susceptible organisms.

Specimens for bacteriologic culture should be obtained prior to therapy in order to isolate and identify causative organisms and to determine their susceptibilities to CLAFORAN. Therapy may be instituted before results of susceptibility studies are known; however, once these results become available, the antibiotic treatment should be adjusted accordingly.

In certain cases of confirmed or suspected gram-positive or gram-negative sepsis or in patients with other serious infections in which the causative organism has not been identified, CLAFORAN may be used concomitantly with an aminoglycoside. The dosage recommended in the labeling of both antibiotics may be given and depends on the severity of the infection and the patient's condition. Renal function should be carefully monitored, especially if higher dosages of the aminoglycosides are to be administered or if therapy is prolonged, because of the potential nephrotoxicity and ototoxicity of aminoglycoside antibiotics. It is possible that nephrotoxicity may be potentiated if CLAFORAN is used concomitantly with an aminoglycoside.

Prevention

The administration of CLAFORAN preoperatively reduces the incidence of certain infections in patients undergoing surgical procedures (e.g., abdominal or vaginal hysterectomy, gastrointestinal and genitourinary tract surgery) that may be classified as contaminated or potentially contaminated.

In patients undergoing cesarean section, intraoperative (after clamping the umbilical cord) and postoperative use of CLAFORAN may also reduce the incidence of certain postoperative infections. See **DOSAGE AND ADMINISTRATION** section.

Effective use for elective surgery depends on the time of administration. To achieve effective tissue levels, CLAFORAN should be given 1/2 or 1 1/2 hours before surgery. See **DOSAGE AND ADMINISTRATION** section. For patients undergoing gastrointestinal surgery, preoperative bowel preparation by mechanical cleansing as well as with a non-absorbable antibiotic (e.g., neomycin) is recommended.

If there are signs of infection, specimens for culture should be obtained for identification of the causative organism so that appropriate therapy may be instituted.

To reduce the development of drug-resistant bacteria and maintain the effectiveness of CLAFORAN and other antibacterial drugs, CLAFORAN should be used only to treat or prevent infections that are proven or strongly suspected to be caused by susceptible bacteria. When culture and susceptibility information are available, they should be considered in selecting or modifying antibacterial therapy. In the absence of such data, local epidemiology and susceptibility patterns may contribute to the empiric selection of therapy.

CONTRAINDICATIONS

CLAFORAN is contraindicated in patients who have shown hypersensitivity to cefotaxime sodium or the cephalosporin group of antibiotics.

WARNINGS

BEFORE THERAPY WITH CLAFORAN IS INSTITUTED, CAREFUL INQUIRY SHOULD BE MADE TO DETERMINE WHETHER THE PATIENT HAS HAD PREVIOUS HYPERSENSITIVITY REACTIONS TO CEFOTAXIME SODIUM, CEPHALOSPORINS, PENICILLINS, OR OTHER DRUGS. THIS PRODUCT SHOULD BE GIVEN WITH CAUTION TO PATIENTS WITH TYPE I HYPERSENSITIVITY REACTIONS TO PENICILLIN. ANTIBIOTICS SHOULD BE ADMINISTERED WITH CAUTION TO ANY PATIENT WHO HAS DEMONSTRATED SOME FORM OF ALLERGY, PARTICULARLY TO DRUGS. IF AN ALLERGIC REACTION TO CLAFORAN OCCURS, DISCONTINUE TREATMENT WITH THE DRUG. SERIOUS HYPERSENSITIVITY REACTIONS MAY REQUIRE EPINEPHRINE AND OTHER EMERGENCY MEASURES.

During post-marketing surveillance, a potentially life-threatening arrhythmia was reported in each of six patients who received a rapid (less than 60 seconds) bolus injection of cefotaxime through a central venous catheter. Therefore, cefotaxime should only be administered as instructed in the **DOSAGE AND ADMINISTRATION** section.

Pseudomembranous colitis has been reported with nearly all antibacterial agents, including cefotaxime, and may range from mild to life threatening. Therefore, it is important to consider its diagnosis in patients with diarrhea subsequent to the administration of antibacterial agents.

Treatment with antibacterial agents alters the normal flora of the colon and may permit overgrowth of Clostridia. Studies indicate that a toxin produced by *Clostridium difficile* is one primary cause of antibiotic-associated colitis.

After the diagnosis of pseudomembranous colitis has been established, appropriate therapeutic measures should be initiated. Mild cases of colitis may respond to drug discontinuance alone. In moderate to severe cases, consideration should be given to management with fluids and electrolytes, protein supplementation, and treatment with an antibacterial drug clinically effective against *Clostridium difficile* colitis.

When the colitis is not relieved by drug discontinuance or when it is severe, oral vancomycin is the treatment of choice for antibiotic-associated pseudomembranous colitis produced by *C. difficile*. Other causes of colitis should also be considered.

PRECAUTIONS

General

Prescribing CLAFORAN in the absence of a proven or strongly suspected bacterial infection or a prophylactic indication is unlikely to provide benefit to the patient and increases the risk of the development of drug-resistant bacteria.

CLAFORAN should be prescribed with caution in individuals with a history of gastrointestinal disease, particularly colitis.

Because high and prolonged serum antibiotic concentrations can occur from usual doses in patients with transient or persistent reduction of urinary output because of renal insufficiency, the total daily dosage should be reduced when CLAFORAN is administered to such patients. Continued dosage should be determined by degree of renal impairment, severity of infection, and susceptibility of the causative organism.

Although there is no clinical evidence supporting the necessity of changing the dosage of cefotaxime sodium in patients with even profound renal dysfunction, it is suggested that, until further data are obtained, the dose of cefotaxime sodium be halved in patients with estimated creatinine clearances of less than 20 mL/min/1.73 m^2.

When only serum creatinine is available, the following formula[5] (based on sex, weight, and age of the patient) may be used to convert this value into creatinine clearance. The serum creatinine should represent a steady state of renal function.

	Weight (kg × (140 - age))
Males:	72 × serum creatinine
Females:	0.85 × above value

As with other antibiotics, prolonged use of CLAFORAN may result in overgrowth of nonsusceptible organisms. Repeated evaluation of the patient's condition is essential. If superinfection occurs during therapy, appropriate measures should be taken.

As with other beta-lactam antibiotics, granulocytopenia and, more rarely, agranulocytosis may develop during treatment with CLAFORAN, particularly if given over long periods. For courses of treatment lasting longer than 10 days, blood counts should therefore be monitored.

CLAFORAN, like other parenteral anti-infective drugs, may be locally irritating to tissues. In most cases, perivascular extravasation of CLAFORAN responds to changing of the infusion site. In rare instances, extensive perivascular extravasation of CLAFORAN may result in tissue damage and require surgical treatment. To minimize the potential for tissue inflammation, infusion sites should be monitored regularly and changed when appropriate.

Information for patients

Patients should be counseled that antibacterial drugs including CLAFORAN should only be used to treat bacterial infections. They do not treat viral infections (e.g., the common cold). When CLAFORAN is prescribed to treat a bacterial infection, patients should be told that although it is common to feel better early in the course of therapy, the medication should be taken exactly as directed. Skipping doses or not completing the full course of therapy may (1) decrease the effectiveness of the immediate treatment and (2) increase the likelihood that bacteria will develop resistance and will not be treatable by CLAFORAN or other antibacterial drugs in the future.

Drug Interactions

Increased nephrotoxicity has been reported following concomitant administration of cephalosporins and aminoglycoside antibiotics.

Drug/Laboratory Test Interactions

Cephalosporins, including cefotaxime sodium, are known to occasionally induce a positive direct Coombs' test.

Carcinogenesis, Mutagenesis

Lifetime studies in animals to evaluate carcinogenic potential have not been conducted. CLAFORAN was not mutagenic in the mouse micronucleus test or in the Ames' test. CLAFORAN did not impair fertility to rats when administered subcutaneously at doses up to 250 mg/kg/day (0.2 times the maximum recommended human dose based on mg/m^2) or in mice when administered intravenously at doses up to 2000 mg/kg/day (0.7 times the recommended human dose based on mg/m^2).

Pregnancy: Teratogenic Effects: Pregnancy Category B:

Reproduction studies have been performed in pregnant mice given CLAFORAN intravenously at doses up to 1200 mg/kg/day (0.4 times the recommended human dose based on mg/m^2) or in pregnant rats when administered intravenously at doses up to 1200 mg/kg/day (0.8 times the recommended human dose based on mg/m^2). No evidence of embryotoxicity or teratogenicity was seen in these studies. There are no well-controlled studies in pregnant women. Because animal reproductive studies are not always predictive of human response, this drug should be used during pregnancy only if clearly needed.

Nonteratogenic Effects

Use of the drug in women of child-bearing potential requires that the anticipated benefit be weighed against the possible risks.

In perinatal and postnatal studies with rats, the pups in the group given 1200 mg/kg/day of CLAFORAN were significantly lighter in weight at birth and remained smaller than pups in the control group during the 21 days of nursing.

Nursing Mothers

CLAFORAN is excreted in human milk in low concentrations. Caution should be exercised when CLAFORAN is administered to a nursing woman.

Pediatric Use

See Precautions above regarding perivascular extravasation. The potential for toxic effects in pediatric patients from chemicals that may leach from the plastic in single dose Galaxy® containers (premixed CLAFORAN Injection) has not been determined.

ADVERSE REACTIONS

CLAFORAN is generally well tolerated. The most common adverse reactions have been local reactions following IM or IV injection. Other adverse reactions have been encountered infrequently.

The most frequent adverse reactions (greater than 1%) are:

Local (4.3%)—Injection site inflammation with IV administration. Pain, induration, and tenderness after IM injection.

Hypersensitivity (2.4%)—Rash, pruritus, fever, eosinophilia and less frequently urticaria and anaphylaxis.

Gastrointestinal (1.4%)—Colitis, diarrhea, nausea, and vomiting.

Symptoms of pseudomembranous colitis can appear during or after antibiotic treatment.

Nausea and vomiting have been reported rarely.

Strength	Diluent (mL)	Withdrawable Volume (mL)	Approximate Concentration (mg/mL)
500 mg vial*(IM)	2	2.2	230
1g vial* (IM)	3	3.4	300
2g vial* (IM)	5	6.0	330
500 mg vial* (IV)	10	10.2	50
1g vial* (IV)	10	10.4	95
2g vial* (IV)	10	11.0	180
1g infusion	50-100	50-100	20-10
2g infusion	50-100	50-100	40-20

(*) in conventional vials

Less frequent adverse reactions (less than 1%) are:

Cardiovascular System—Potentially life-threatening arrhythmias following rapid (less than 60 seconds) bolus administration via central venous catheter have been observed.

Hematologic System—Neutropenia, transient leukopenia, eosinophilia, thrombocytopenia and agranulocytosis have been reported. Some individuals have developed positive direct Coombs Tests during treatment with CLAFORAN and other cephalosporin antibiotics. Rare cases of hemolytic anemia have been reported.

Genitourinary System—Moniliasis, vaginitis.

Central Nervous System—Headache.

Liver—Transient elevations in SGOT, SGPT, serum LDH, and serum alkaline phosphatase levels have been reported.

Kidney—As with some other cephalosporins, interstitial nephritis and transient elevations of BUN and creatinine have been occasionally observed with CLAFORAN.

Cutaneous—As with other cephalosporins, isolated cases of erythema multiforme, Stevens-Johnson syndrome, and toxic epidermal necrolysis have been reported.

Cephalosporin Class Labeling

In addition to the adverse reactions listed above which have been observed in patients treated with cefotaxime sodium, the following adverse reactions and altered laboratory tests have been reported for cephalosporin class antibiotics: allergic reactions, hepatic dysfunction including cholestasis, aplastic anemia, hemorrhage, and false-positive test for urinary glucose.

Several cephalosporins have been implicated in triggering seizures, particularly in patients with renal impairment when the dosage was not reduced. See **DOSAGE AND ADMINISTRATION** and **OVERDOSAGE**. If seizures associated with drug therapy occur, the drug should be discontinued. Anticonvulsant therapy can be given if clinically indicated.

OVERDOSAGE

The acute toxicity of CLAFORAN was evaluated in neonatal and adult mice and rats. Significant mortality was seen at parenteral doses in excess of 6000 mg/kg/day in all groups. Common toxic signs in animals that died were a decrease in spontaneous activity, tonic and clonic convulsions, dyspnea, hypothermia, and cyanosis.

Cefotaxime sodium overdosage has occurred in patients. Most cases have shown no overt toxicity. The most frequent reactions were elevations of BUN and creatinine. Patients who receive an acute overdosage should be carefully observed and given supportive treatment.

DOSAGE AND ADMINISTRATION

Adults

Dosage and route of administration should be determined by susceptibility of the causative organisms, severity of the infection, and the condition of the patient (see table for dosage guideline). CLAFORAN may be administered IM or IV after reconstitution. Premixed CLAFORAN Injection is intended for IV administration after thawing. The maximum daily dosage should not exceed 12 grams.

GUIDELINES FOR DOSAGE OF CLAFORAN

Type of Infection	Daily Dose (grams)	Frequency and Route
Gonococcal urethritis/cervicitis in males and females	0.5	0.5 gram IM (single dose)
Rectal gonorrhea in females	0.5	0.5 gram IM (single dose)
Rectal gonorrhea in males	1	1 gram IM (single dose)
Uncomplicated infections	2	1 gram every 12 hours IM or IV dose)
Moderate to severe infections	3–6	1-2 grams every 8 hours IM or IV
Infections commonly needing antibiotics in higher dosage (e.g., septicemia)	6–8	2 grams every 6-8 hours IV
Life-threatening infections	up to 12	2 grams every 4 hours IV

If *C. trachomatis* is a suspected pathogen, appropriate antichlamydial coverage should be added, because cefotaxime sodium has no activity against this organism.

To prevent postoperative infection in contaminated or potentially contaminated surgery, the recommended dose is a single 1 gram IM or IV administered 30 to 90 minutes prior to start of surgery.

Cesarean Section Patients

The first dose of 1 gram is administered intravenously as soon as the umbilical cord is clamped. The second and third doses should be given as 1 gram intravenously or intramuscularly at 6 and 12 hours after the first dose.

Neonates, Infants, and Children

The following dosage schedule is recommended:

Neonates (birth to 1 month):

0-1 week of age	50 mg/kg per dose every 12 hours IV
1-4 weeks of age	50 mg/kg per dose every 8 hours IV

It is not necessary to differentiate between premature and normal-gestational age infants.

Infants and Children (1 month to 12 years):

For body weights less than 50 kg, the recommended daily dose is 50 to 180 mg/kg IM or IV body weight divided into four to six equal doses. The higher dosages should be used for more severe or serious infections, including meningitis. For body weights 50 kg or more, the usual adult dosage should be used; the maximum daily dosage should not exceed 12 grams.

Impaired Renal Function—see **PRECAUTIONS** section.

NOTE: As with antibiotic therapy in general, administration of CLAFORAN should be continued for a minimum of 48 to 72 hours after the patient defervesces or after evidence of bacterial eradication has been obtained; a minimum of 10 days of treatment is recommended for infections caused by Group A beta-hemolytic streptococci in order to guard against the risk of rheumatic fever or glomerulonephritis; frequent bacteriologic and clinical appraisal is necessary during therapy of chronic urinary tract infection and may be required for several months after therapy has been completed; persistent infections may require treatment of several weeks and doses smaller than those indicated above should not be used.

Preparation of CLAFORAN Sterile

CLAFORAN for IM or IV administration should be reconstituted as follows:

[See table above]

Shake to dissolve; inspect for particulate matter and discoloration prior to use. Solutions of CLAFORAN range from very pale yellow to light amber, depending on concentration, diluent used, and length and condition of storage.

For intramuscular use: Reconstitute VIALS with Sterile Water for Injection or Bacteriostatic Water for Injection as described above.

For intravenous use: Reconstitute VIALS with at least 10 mL of Sterile Water for Injection. Reconstitute INFUSION BOTTLES with 50 or 100 mL of 0.9% Sodium Chloride Injection or 5% Dextrose Injection. For other diluents, see **COMPATIBILITY AND STABILITY** section.

NOTE: Solutions of CLAFORAN must not be admixed with aminoglycoside solutions. If CLAFORAN and aminoglycosides are to be administered to the same patient, they must be administered separately and not as mixed injection.

A SOLUTION OF 1 G CLAFORAN IN 14 ML OF STERILE WATER FOR INJECTION IS ISOTONIC.

IM Administration: As with all IM preparations, CLAFORAN should be injected well within the body of a relatively large muscle such as the upper outer quadrant of the buttock (i.e., gluteus maximus); aspiration is necessary to avoid inadvertent injection into a blood vessel. Individual IM doses of 2 grams may be given if the dose is divided and is administered in different intramuscular sites.

IV Administration: The IV route is preferable for patients with bacteremia, bacterial septicemia, peritonitis, meningitis, or other severe or life-threatening infections, or for patients who may be poor risks because of lowered resistance resulting from such debilitating conditions as malnutrition, trauma, surgery, diabetes, heart failure, or malignancy, particularly if shock is present or impending.

For intermittent IV administration, a solution containing 1 gram or 2 grams in 10 mL of Sterile Water for Injection can be injected over a period of three to five minutes. Cefotaxime should not be administered over a period of less than three minutes. (See WARNINGS). With an infusion system, it may also be given over a longer period of time through the tubing system by which the patient may be receiving other

Continued on next page

Claforan—Cont.

IV solutions. However, during infusion of the solution containing CLAFORAN, it is advisable to discontinue temporarily the administration of other solutions at the same site. For the administration of higher doses by continuous IV infusion, a solution of CLAFORAN may be added to IV bottles containing the solutions discussed below.

Directions for use of CLAFORAN Injection in Galaxy Container (PL 2040 Plastic)

CLAFORAN Injection in Galaxy containers (PL 2040 plastic) is for continuous or intermittent infusion using sterile equipment.

Storage

Store in a freezer capable of maintaining a temperature of −20°C/−4°F.

Thawing of Plastic Container

Thaw frozen container at room temperature or under refrigeration (at or below 5°C). [DO NOT FORCE THAW BY IMMERSION IN WATER BATHS OR BY MICROWAVE IRRADIATION.]

Check for minute leaks by squeezing container firmly. If leaks are detected, discard solution as sterility may be impaired.

DO NOT ADD SUPPLEMENTARY MEDICATION.

The container should be visually inspected. Components of the solution may precipitate in the frozen state and will dissolve upon reaching room temperature with little or no agitation. Potency is not affected. Agitate after solution has reached room temperature. If after visual inspection the solution remains cloudy or if an insoluble precipitate is noted or if any seals or outlet ports are not intact, the container should be discarded.

The thawed solution is stable for 10 days under refrigeration (at or below 5°C) or 24 hours at or below 22°C. Do not refreeze thawed antibiotics.

CAUTION: Do not use plastic containers in series connections. Such use could result in air embolism due to residual air being drawn from the primary container before administration of the fluid from the secondary container is complete.

Preparation for Intravenous Administration:

1. Suspend container from eyelet support.
2. Remove protector from outlet port at bottom of container.
3. Attach administration set. Refer to complete directions accompanying set.

Preparation of CLAFORAN Sterile in ADD-Vantage® System

CLAFORAN Sterile 1 g or 2 g may be reconstituted in 50 mL or 100 mL of 5% Dextrose or 0.9% Sodium Chloride in the ADD-Vantage® diluent container. Refer to enclosed, separate INSTRUCTIONS FOR ADD-VANTAGE® SYSTEM.

Compatibility and Stability

Solutions of CLAFORAN Sterile reconstituted as described above (**Preparation of CLAFORAN Sterile**) remain chemically stable (potency remains above 90%) as follows when stored in original containers and disposable plastic syringes:

[See table below]

Reconstituted solutions stored in original containers and plastic syringes remain stable for 13 weeks frozen.

Reconstituted solutions may be further diluted up to 1000 mL with the following solutions and maintain satisfactory potency for 24 hours at or below 22°C, and at least 5 days under refrigeration (at or below 5°C): 0.9% Sodium Chloride Injection; 5 or 10% Dextrose Injection; 5% Dextrose and 0.9% Sodium Chloride Injection, 5% Dextrose and 0.45% Sodium Chloride Injection; 5% Dextrose and 0.2% Sodium Chloride Injection; Lactated Ringer's Solution; Sodium Lactate Injection (M/6); 10% Invert Sugar Injection, 8.5% TRAVASOL® (Amino Acid) Injection without Electrolytes.

Solutions of CLAFORAN Sterile reconstituted in 0.9% Sodium Chloride Injection or 5% Dextrose Injection in Viaflex® plastic containers maintain satisfactory potency for 24 hours at or below 22°C, 5 days under refrigeration (at or below 5°C) and 13 weeks frozen. Solutions of CLAFORAN Sterile reconstituted in 0.9% Sodium Chloride Injection or 5% Dextrose Injection in the ADD-Vantage® flexible containers maintain satisfactory potency for 24 hours at or below 22°C. DO NOT FREEZE.

NOTE: CLAFORAN solutions exhibit maximum stability in the pH 5-7 range. Solutions of CLAFORAN should not be prepared with diluents having a pH above 7.5, such as Sodium Bicarbonate Injection.

Parenteral drug products should be inspected visually for particulate matter and discoloration prior to administration, whenever solution and container permit.

HOW SUPPLIED

Sterile CLAFORAN is a dry off-white to pale yellow crystalline powder supplied in vials and bottles containing cefotaxime sodium as follows:

500 mg cefotaxime (free acid equivalent) in vials in packages of 10 (NDC 0039-0017-10).

1 g cefotaxime (free acid equivalent) in vials in packages of 10 (NDC 0039-0018-10), packages of 25 (NDC 0039-0018-25), packages of 50 (NDC 0039-0018-50); infusion bottles in packages of 10 (NDC 0039-0018-11).

2 g cefotaxime (free acid equivalent) in vials in packages of 10 (NDC 0039-0019-10), packages of 25 (NDC 0039-0019-25), packages of 50 (NDC 0039-0019-50); infusion bottles in packages of 10 (NDC 0039-0019-11).

1 g cefotaxime (free acid equivalent) in ADD-Vantage® System vials in packages of 25 (NDC 0039-0023-25) and 50 (NDC 0039-0023-50).

2 g cefotaxime (free acid equivalent) in ADD-Vantage® System vials in packages of 25 (NDC 0039-0024-25) and 50 (NDC 0039-0024-50).

ADD-Vantage® System diluents (5% Dextrose or 0.9% Sodium Chloride) are available from Abbott Laboratories.

Also available:

Pharmacy Bulk Package:

10g cefotaxime (free acid equivalent) in bottles (NDC 0039-0020-01)

NOTE: CLAFORAN in the dry state should be stored below 30°C. The dry material as well as solutions tend to darken depending on storage conditions and should be protected from elevated temperatures and excessive light.

Premixed CLAFORAN Injection is supplied as a frozen, iso-osmotic, sterile, nonpyrogenic solution in 50 mL single dose Galaxy® containers (PL 2040 plastic) as follows:

1 g cefotaxime (free acid equivalent) in packages of 12 (NDC 0039-0037-05) 2G3518.

2 g cefotaxime (free acid equivalent) in packages of 12 (NDC 0039-0038-05) 2G3519.

NOTE: Store Premixed CLAFORAN Injection at or below −20°C/−4°F. [See DIRECTIONS FOR USE OF CLAFORAN (cefotaxime injection) IN GALAXY® CONTAINERS (PL 2040 PLASTIC)].

Claforan® Injection supplied as a frozen, iso-osmotic, sterile, nonpyrogenic solution in Galaxy® containers (PL 2040 plastic) is manufactured for Aventis Pharmaceuticals by Baxter Healthcare Corporation.

REFERENCES

1) Richmond, M. H. and Sykes R. B.: The β-Lactamases of Gram-Negative Bacteria and their Possible Physiological Role, Advances in Microbial Physiology 9:31-88, 1973.
2) National Committee for Clinical Laboratory Standards. Methods for Dilution Antimicrobial Susceptibility Tests for Bacteria that Grow Aerobically—Third Edition. Approved Standard NCCLS Document M7-A3, Vol. 13, No. 25, NCCLS, Villanova, PA, December, 1993.
3) National Committee for Clinical Laboratory Standards. Performance Standard for Antimicrobial Disk Susceptibility Tests—Fifth Edition. Approved Standard NCCLS Document M2-A5, Vol. 13, No. 24, NCCLS, Villanova, PA, December, 1993.
4) National Committee for Clinical Laboratory Standards. Methods for Antimicrobial Susceptibility Testing of Anaerobic Bacteria—Third Edition. Approved Standard NCCLS Document M11-A3, NCCLS, Villanova, PA, December, 1993.
5) Cockcroft, D.W. and Gault, M.H.: Prediction of Creatinine Clearance from Serum Creatinine, Nephron 16:31-41, 1976.

Sterile cefotaxime sodium US Patents 4,298,606; 5,583,216; 5,159,070; 4,376,203; 5,336,776.

Cefotaxime sodium injection US Patents 4,298,606; 5,583,216; 5,159,070; 4,376,203; 5,336,776.

Galaxy and PL 2040 REG TM Baxter International Inc.

ADD-Vantage REG TM Abbott Laboratories.

US Patents ADD-Vantage System: 4,614,267; 4,614,515; 4,757,911; 4,703,864; 4,784,658; 4,784,259; 4,948,000; 4,936,445; 5,583,216; 5,159,070; 4,376,203; 5,336,776.

Rev. January 2004

Manufactured by:
Patheon UK Limited,
Swindon, Wiltshire SN3 5BZ, England

Manufactured for:
Aventis Pharmaceuticals NJ
Bridgewater, NJ 08807 USA

Made in United Kingdom

Strength	Reconstituted Concentration mg/mL	Stability at or below 22°C	Stability under Refrigeration (at or below 5°C) Original Containers	Plastic Syringes
500 mg vial IM	230	12 hours	7 days	5 days
1g vial IM	300	12 hours	7 days	5 days
2g vial IM	330	12 hours	7 days	5 days
500 mg vial IV	50	24 hours	7 days	5 days
1g vial IV	95	24 hours	7 days	5 days
2g vial IV	180	12 hours	7 days	5 days
1g infusion bottle	10-20	24 hours	10 days	
2g infusion bottle	20-40	24 hours	10 days	

Claforan Injection in Galaxy Containers:

Manufactured by:
Baxter Healthcare Corporation
Deerfield, IL 60015 USA

Manufactured for:
Aventis Pharmaceuticals NJ
Bridgewater, NJ 08807 USA

www.aventis-us.com

CLA-JAN04-F-A

Shown in Product Identification Guide, page 307

CLOMID® ℞

[clo'-mid]

(clomiphene citrate tablets USP)

Prescribing Information as of June 2000

DESCRIPTION

CLOMID (clomiphene citrate tablets USP) is an orally administered, nonsteroidal, ovulatory stimulant designated chemically as 2-[p-(2-chloro-1,2-diphenylvinyl)phenoxy] triethylamine citrate (1:1). It has the molecular formula of $C_{26}H_{28}ClNO \cdot C_6H_8O_7$ and a molecular weight of 598.09. It is represented structurally as:

$(C_2H_5)_2NCH_2CH_2O$–(phenyl)–C(phenyl)=C(Cl)–(phenyl) • $C_6H_8O_7$

Clomiphene citrate is a white to pale yellow, essentially odorless, crystalline powder. It is freely soluble in methanol; soluble in ethanol; slightly soluble in acetone, water, and chloroform; and insoluble in ether.

CLOMID is a mixture of two geometric isomers [cis (zuclomiphene) and trans (enclomiphene)] containing between 30% and 50% of the cis-isomer.

Each white scored tablet contains 50 mg clomiphene citrate USP. The tablet also contains the following inactive ingredients: corn starch, lactose, magnesium stearate, pregelatinized corn starch, and sucrose.

CLINICAL PHARMACOLOGY

Action

CLOMID is a drug of considerable pharmacologic potency. With careful selection and proper management of the patient, CLOMID has been demonstrated to be a useful therapy for the anovulatory patient desiring pregnancy.

Clomiphene citrate is capable of interacting with estrogen-receptor-containing tissues, including the hypothalamus, pituitary, ovary, endometrium, vagina, and cervix. It may compete with estrogen for estrogen-receptor-binding sites and may delay replenishment of intracellular estrogen receptors. Clomiphene citrate initiates a series of endocrine events culminating in a preovulatory gonadotropin surge and subsequent follicular rupture. The first endocrine event in response to a course of clomiphene therapy is an increase in the release of pituitary gonadotropins. This initiates steroidogenesis and folliculogenesis, resulting in growth of the ovarian follicle and an increase in the circulating level of estradiol. Following ovulation, plasma progesterone and estradiol rise and fall as they would in a normal ovulatory cycle.

Available data suggest that both the estrogenic and antiestrogenic properties of clomiphene may participate in the initiation of ovulation. The two clomiphene isomers have been found to have mixed estrogenic and antiestrogenic effects, which may vary from one species to another. Some data suggest that zuclomiphene has greater estrogenic activity than enclomiphene.

Clomiphene citrate has no apparent progestational, androgenic, or antiandrogenic effects and does not appear to interfere with pituitary-adrenal or pituitary-thyroid function. Although there is no evidence of a "carryover effect" of CLOMID, spontaneous ovulatory menses have been noted in some patients after CLOMID therapy.

Pharmacokinetics

Based on early studies with ^{14}C-labeled clomiphene citrate, the drug was shown to be readily absorbed orally in humans and excreted principally in the feces. Cumulative urinary and fecal excretion of the ^{14}C averaged about 50% of the oral dose and 37% of an intravenous dose after 5 days. Mean urinary excretion was approximately 8% with fecal excretion of about 42%.

Some ^{14}C label was still present in the feces 6 weeks after administration. Subsequent single-dose studies in normal volunteers showed that zuclomiphene (cis) has a longer half-life than enclomiphene (trans). Detectable levels of zuclomiphene persisted for longer than a month in these subjects. This may be suggestive of stereo-specific enterohepatic recycling or sequestering of the zuclomiphene. Thus, it is possible that some active drug may remain in the body during early pregnancy in women who conceive in the menstrual cycle during CLOMID therapy.

CLINICAL STUDIES

During clinical investigations, 7578 patients received CLOMID, some of whom had impediments to ovulation other than ovulatory dysfunction (see INDICATIONS AND USAGE). In those clinical trials, successful therapy characterized by pregnancy occurred in approximately 30% of these patients.

There were a total of 2635 pregnancies reported during the clinical trial period. Of those pregnancies, information on outcome was only available for 2369 of the cases. Table 1 summarizes the outcome of these cases.
Of the reported pregnancies, the incidence of multiple pregnancies was 7.98%: 6.9% twin, 0.5% triplet, 0.3% quadruplet, and 0.1% quintuplet. Of the 165 twin pregnancies for which sufficient information was available, the ratio of monozygotic to dizygotic twins was about 1:5. Table 1 reports the survival rate of the live multiple births.
A sextuplet birth was reported after completion of original clinical studies; none of the sextuplets survived (each weighed less than 400 g), although each appeared grossly normal.

Table 1. Outcome of Reported Pregnancies in Clinical Trials (n = 2369)

Outcome	Total Number of Pregnancies	Survival Rate
Pregnancy Wastage		
Spontaneous Abortions	483*	
Stillbirths	24	
Live Births		
Single Births	1697	98.16%†
Multiple Births	165	83.25%†

* Includes 28 ectopic pregnancies, 4 hydatiform moles, and 1 fetus papyraceous.
† Indicates percentage of surviving infants from these pregnancies.

The overall survival of infants from multiple pregnancies including spontaneous abortions, stillbirths, and neonatal deaths is 73%.

INDICATIONS AND USAGE

CLOMID is indicated for the treatment of ovulatory dysfunction in women desiring pregnancy. Impediments to achieving pregnancy must be excluded or adequately treated before beginning CLOMID therapy. Those patients most likely to achieve success with clomiphene therapy include patients with polycystic ovary syndrome (see WARNINGS: Ovarian Hyperstimulation Syndrome), amenorrhea-galactorrhea syndrome, psychogenic amenorrhea, post-oral-contraceptive amenorrhea, and certain cases of secondary amenorrhea of undetermined etiology.
Properly timed coitus in relationship to ovulation is important. A basal body temperature graph or other appropriate tests may help the patient and her physician determine if ovulation occurred. Once ovulation has been established, each course of CLOMID should be started on or about the 5th day of the cycle. Long-term cyclic therapy is not recommended beyond a total of about six cycles (including three ovulatory cycles). (See DOSAGE AND ADMINISTRATION and PRECAUTIONS.)
CLOMID is indicated only in patients with demonstrated ovulatory dysfunction who meet the conditions described below (see CONTRAINDICATIONS):

1. Patients who are not pregnant.
2. Patients without ovarian cysts. CLOMID should not be used in patients with ovarian enlargement except those with polycystic ovary syndrome. Pelvic examination is necessary prior to the first and each subsequent course of CLOMID treatment.
3. Patients without abnormal vaginal bleeding. If abnormal vaginal bleeding is present, the patient should be carefully evaluated to ensure that neoplastic lesions are not present.
4. Patients with normal liver function.

In addition, patients selected for CLOMID therapy should be evaluated in regard to the following:

1. **Estrogen Levels.** Patients should have adequate levels of endogenous estrogen (as estimated from vaginal smears, endometrial biopsy, assay of urinary estrogen, or from bleeding in response to progesterone). Reduced estrogen levels, while less favorable, do not preclude successful therapy.
2. **Primary Pituitary or Ovarian Failure.** CLOMID therapy cannot be expected to substitute for specific treatment of other causes of ovulatory failure.
3. **Endometriosis and Endometrial Carcinoma.** The incidence of endometriosis and endometrial carcinoma increases with age as does the incidence of ovulatory disorders. Endometrial biopsy should always be performed prior to CLOMID therapy in this population.
4. **Other Impediments to Pregnancy.** Impediments to pregnancy can include thyroid disorders, adrenal disorders, hyperprolactinemia, and male factor infertility.
5. **Uterine Fibroids.** Caution should be exercised when using CLOMID in patients with uterine fibroids due to the potential for further enlargement of the fibroids.

There are no adequate or well-controlled studies that demonstrate the effectiveness of CLOMID in the treatment of male infertility. In addition, testicular tumors and gynecomastia have been reported in males using clomiphene. The cause and effect relationship between reports of testicular tumors and the administration of CLOMID is not known.
Although the medical literature suggests various methods, there is no universally accepted standard regimen for combined therapy (ie, CLOMID in conjunction with other ovulation-inducing drugs). Similarly, there is no standard CLOMID regimen for ovulation induction in *in vitro* fertilization programs to produce ova for fertilization and reintroduction. Therefore, CLOMID is not recommended for these uses.

CONTRAINDICATIONS

Hypersensitivity
CLOMID is contraindicated in patients with a known hypersensitivity or allergy to clomiphene citrate or to any of its ingredients.

Pregnancy
CLOMID should not be administered during pregnancy. CLOMID may cause fetal harm in animals (see Animal Fetotoxicity). Although no causative evidence of a deleterious effect of CLOMID therapy on the human fetus has been established, there have been reports of birth anomalies which, during clinical studies, occurred at an incidence within the range reported for the general population (see Fetal/Neonatal Anomalies and Mortality; ADVERSE REACTIONS).
To avoid inadvertent CLOMID administration during early pregnancy, appropriate tests should be utilized during each treatment cycle to determine whether ovulation occurs. The patient should be evaluated carefully to exclude pregnancy, ovarian enlargement, or ovarian cyst formation between each treatment cycle. The next course of CLOMID therapy should be delayed until these conditions have been excluded.
Fetal/Neonatal Anomalies and Mortality. The following fetal abnormalities have been reported subsequent to pregnancies following ovulation induction therapy with CLOMID during clinical trials. Each of the following fetal abnormalities were reported at a rate of <1% (experiences are listed in order of decreasing frequency): Congenital heart lesions, Down syndrome, club foot, congenital gut lesions, hypospadias, microcephaly, harelip and cleft palate, congenital hip, hemangioma, undescended testicles, polydactyly, conjoined twins and teratomatous malformation, patent ductus arteriosus, amaurosis, arteriovenous fistula, inguinal hernia, umbilical hernia, syndactyly, pectus excavatum, myopathy, dermoid cyst of scalp, omphalocele, spina bifida occulta, ichthyosis, and persistent lingual frenulum. Neonatal death and fetal death/stillbirth in infants with birth defects have also been reported at a rate of <1%. The overall incidence of reported birth anomalies from pregnancies associated with maternal CLOMID ingestion during clinical studies was within the range of that reported for the general population.
In addition, reports of birth anomalies have been received during postmarketing surveillance of CLOMID (see ADVERSE REACTIONS).
Animal Fetotoxicity. Oral administration of clomiphene citrate to pregnant rats during organogenesis at doses of 1 to 2 mg/kg/day resulted in hydramnion and weak, edematous fetuses with wavy ribs and other temporary bone changes. Doses of 8 mg/kg/day or more also caused increased resorptions and dead fetuses, dystocia, and delayed parturition, and 40 mg/kg/day resulted in increased maternal mortality. Single doses of 50 mg/kg caused fetal cataracts, while 200 mg/kg caused cleft palate.
Following injection of clomiphene citrate 2 mg/kg to mice and rats during pregnancy, the offspring exhibited metaplastic changes of the reproduction tract. Newborn mice and rats injected during the first few days of life also developed metaplastic changes in uterine and vaginal mucosa, as well as premature vaginal opening and anovulatory ovaries. These findings are similar to the abnormal reproductive behavior and sterility described with other estrogens and antiestrogens.
In rabbits, some temporary bone alterations were seen in fetuses from dams given oral doses of 20 or 40 mg/kg/day during pregnancy, but not following 8 mg/kg/day. No permanent malformations were observed in those studies. Also, rhesus monkeys given oral doses of 1.5 to 4.5 mg/kg/day for various periods during pregnancy did not have any abnormal offspring.
Liver Disease. CLOMID therapy is contraindicated in patients with liver disease or a history of liver dysfunction (see also INDICATIONS AND USAGE and ADVERSE REACTIONS).
Abnormal Uterine Bleeding. CLOMID is contraindicated in patients with abnormal uterine bleeding of undetermined origin (see INDICATIONS AND USAGE).
Ovarian Cysts. CLOMID is contraindicated in patients with ovarian cysts or enlargement not due to polycystic ovarian syndrome (see INDICATIONS AND USAGE and WARNINGS).
Other. CLOMID is contraindicated in patients with uncontrolled thyroid or adrenal dysfunction or in the presence of an organic intracranial lesion such as pituitary tumor (see INDICATIONS AND USAGE).

WARNINGS

Visual Symptoms
Patients should be advised that blurring or other visual symptoms such as spots or flashes (scintillating scotomata) may occasionally occur during therapy with CLOMID. These visual symptoms increase in incidence with increasing total dose or therapy duration and generally disappear within a few days or weeks after CLOMID is discontinued. Patients should be warned that these visual symptoms may render such activities as driving a car or operating machinery more hazardous than usual, particularly under conditions of variable lighting.
These visual symptoms appear to be due to intensification and prolongation of afterimages. Symptoms often first appear or are accentuated with exposure to a brightly lit environment. While measured visual acuity usually has not been affected, a study patient taking 200 mg CLOMID daily developed visual blurring on the 7th day of treatment, which progressed to severe diminution of visual acuity by the 10th day. No other abnormaltiy was found, and the visual acuity returned to normal on the 3rd day after treatment was stopped.
Ophthalmologically definable scotomata and retinal cell function (electroretinographic) changes have also been reported. A patient treated during clinical studies developed phosphenes and scotomata during prolonged CLOMID administration, which disappeared by the 32nd day after stopping therapy.
Postmarketing surveillance of adverse events has also revealed other visual signs and symptoms during CLOMID therapy (see ADVERSE REACTIONS).
While the etiology of these visual symptoms is not yet understood, patients with any visual symptoms should discontinue treatment and have a complete ophthalmological evaluation carried out promptly.

Ovarian Hyperstimulation Syndrome
The ovarian hyperstimulation syndrome (OHSS) has been reported to occur in patients receiving clomiphene citrate therapy for ovulation induction. In some cases, OHSS occurred following cyclic use of clomiphene citrate therapy or when clomiphene citrate was used in combination with gonadotropins. Transient liver function test abnormalities suggestive of hepatic dysfunction, which may be accompanied by morphologic changes on liver biopsy, have been reported in association with ovarian hyperstimulation syndrome (OHSS).
OHSS is a medical event distinct from uncomplicated ovarian enlargement. The clinical signs of this syndrome in severe cases can include gross ovarian enlargement, gastrointestinal symptoms, ascites, dyspnea, oliguria, and pleural effusion. In addition, the following symptoms have been reported in association with this syndrome: pericardial effusion, anasarca, hydrothorax, acute abdomen, hypotension, renal failure, pulmonary edema, intraperitoneal and ovarian hemorrhage, deep venous thrombosis, torsion of the ovary, and acute respiratory distress. The early warning signs of OHSS are abdominal pain and distention, nausea, vomiting, diarrhea, and weight gain. Elevated urinary steroid levels, varying degrees of electrolyte imbalance, hypovolemia, hemoconcentration, and hypoproteinemia may occur. Death due to hypovolemic shock, hemoconcentration, or thromboembolism has occurred. Due to fragility of enlarged ovaries in severe cases, abdominal and pelvic examination should be performed very cautiously. If conception results, rapid progression to the severe form of the syndrome may occur.
To minimize the hazard associated with occasional abnormal ovarian enlargement associated with CLOMID therapy, the lowest dose consistent with expected clinical results should be used. Maximal enlargement of the ovary, whether physiologic or abnormal, may not occur until several days after discontinuation of the recommended dose of CLOMID. Some patients with polycystic ovary syndrome who are unusually sensitive to gonadotropin may have an exaggerated response to usual doses of CLOMID. Therefore, patients with polycystic ovary syndrome should be started on the lowest recommended dose and shortest treatment duration for the first course of therapy (see DOSAGE AND ADMINISTRATION).
If enlargement of the ovary occurs, additional CLOMID therapy should not be given until the ovaries have returned to pretreatment size, and the dosage or duration of the next course should be reduced. Ovarian enlargement and cyst formation associated with CLOMID therapy usually regress spontaneously within a few days or weeks after discontinuing treatment. The potential benefit of subsequent CLOMID therapy in these cases should exceed the risk. Unless surgical indication for laparotomy exists, such cystic enlargement should always be managed conservatively.
A causal relationship between ovarian hyperstimulation and ovarian cancer has not been determined. However, because a correlation between ovarian cancer and nulliparity, infertility, and age has been suggested, if ovarian cysts do not regress spontaneously, a thorough evaluation should be performed to rule out the presence of ovarian neoplasia.

PRECAUTIONS

General
Careful attention should be given to the selection of candidates for CLOMID therapy. Pelvic examination is necessary prior to CLOMID treatment and before each subsequent course (see CONTRAINDICATIONS and WARNINGS).

Information for Patients
The purpose and risks of CLOMID therapy should be presented to the patient before starting treatment. It should be emphasized that the goal of CLOMID therapy is ovulation for subsequent pregnancy. The physician should counsel the patient with special regard to the following potential risks:
Visual Symptoms: Advise that blurring or other visual symptoms occasionally may occur during or shortly after CLOMID therapy. Warn that visual symptoms may render such activities as driving a car or operating machinery more hazardous than usual, particularly under conditions of variable lighting (see WARNINGS).
The patient should be instructed to inform the physician whenever any unusual visual symptoms occur. If the patient has any visual symptoms, treatment should be discontinued and complete ophthalmologic evaluation performed.

Continued on next page

Clomid—Cont.

Abdominal/Pelvic Pain or Distention: Ovarian enlargement may occur during or shortly after therapy with CLOMID. To minimize the risks associated with ovarian enlargement, the patient should be instructed to inform the physician of any abdominal or pelvic pain, weight gain, discomfort, or distention after taking CLOMID (see WARNINGS).

Multiple Pregnancy: Inform the patient that there is an increased chance of multiple pregnancy, including bilateral tubal pregnancy and coexisting tubal and intrauterine pregnancy, when conception occurs in relation to CLOMID therapy. The potential complications and hazards of multiple pregnancy should be explained.

Pregnancy Wastage and Birth Anomalies: The physician should explain the assumed risk of any pregnancy, whether ovulation is induced with the aid of CLOMID or occurs naturally. The patient should be informed of the greater risks associated with certain characteristics or conditions of any pregnant woman, eg, age of female and male partner, history of spontaneous abortions, Rh genotype, abnormal menstrual history, infertility history, organic heart disease, diabetes, exposure to infectious agents such as rubella, familial history of birth anomaly, that may be pertinent to the patient for whom CLOMID is being considered. Based upon the evaluation of the patient, genetic counseling may be indicated.

The overall incidence of reported birth anomalies from pregnancies associated with maternal CLOMID ingestion during the investigational studies was within the range of that reported in published references for the general population. (See CONTRAINDICATIONS: Pregnancy.)

During clinical investigation, the experience from patients with known pregnancy outcome (Table 1) shows a spontaneous abortion rate of 20.4% and stillbirth rate of 1.0%. (See CLINICAL PHARMACOLOGY.)

Drug Interactions

Drug interactions with CLOMID have not been documented.

Carcinogenesis, Mutagenesis, Impairment of Fertility

Long-term toxicity studies in animals have not been performed to evaluate the carcinogenic or mutagenic potential of clomiphene citrate.

Oral administration of CLOMID to male rats at doses of 0.3 or 1 mg/kg/day caused decreased fertility, while higher doses caused temporary infertility. Oral doses of 0.1 mg/kg/day in female rats temporarily interrupted the normal cyclic vaginal smear pattern and prevented conception. Doses of 0.3 mg/kg/day slightly reduced the number of ovulated ova and corpora lutea, while 3 mg/kg/day inhibited ovulation.

Pregnancy

Pregnancy Category X. (See CONTRAINDICATIONS.)

Nursing Mothers

It is not known whether CLOMID is excreted in human milk. Because many drugs are excreted in human milk, caution should be exercised if CLOMID is administered to a nursing woman. In some patients, CLOMID may reduce lactation.

Ovarian Cancer

Prolonged use of clomiphene citrate tablets USP may increase the risk of a borderline or invasive ovarian tumor (see ADVERSE REACTIONS).

ADVERSE REACTIONS

Clinical Trial Adverse Events. CLOMID, at recommended dosages, is generally well tolerated. Adverse reactions usually have been mild and transient and most have disappeared promptly after treatment has been discontinued. Adverse experiences reported in patients treated with clomiphene citrate during clinical studies are shown in Table 2.

Table 2. Incidence of Adverse Events In Clinical Studies (Events Greater than 1%) (n = 8029*)

Adverse Event	%
Ovarian Enlargement	13.6
Vasomotor Flushes	10.4
Abdominal-Pelvic Discomfort/ Distention/Bloating	5.5
Nausea and Vomiting	2.2
Breast Discomfort	2.1
Visual Symptoms	1.5
Blurred vision, lights, floaters, waves, unspecified visual complaints, photophobia, diplopia, scotomata, phosphenes	
Headache	1.3
Abnormal Uterine Bleeding	1.3
Intermenstrual spotting, menorrhagia	

* Includes 498 patients whose reports may have been duplicated in the event totals and could not be distinguished as such. Also, excludes 47 patients who did not report symptom data.

The following adverse events have been reported in fewer than 1% of patients in clinical trials: Acute abdomen, appetite increase, constipation, dermatitis or rash, depression, diarrhea, dizziness, fatigue, hair loss/dry hair, increased urinary frequency/volume, insomnia, light-headedness, nervous tension, vaginal dryness, vertigo, weight gain/loss.

Patients on prolonged CLOMID therapy may show elevated serum levels of desmosterol. This is most likely due to a direct interference with cholesterol synthesis. However, the serum sterols in patients receiving the recommended dose of CLOMID are not significantly altered. Ovarian cancer has been infrequently reported in patients who have received fertility drugs. Infertility is a primary risk factor for ovarian cancer; however, epidemiology data suggest that prolonged use of clomiphene may increase the risk of a borderline or invasive ovarian tumor.

Postmarketing Adverse Events

The following adverse experiences were reported spontaneously with CLOMID. The cause and effect relationship of the listed events to the administration of CLOMID is not known.

Dermatologic: Acne, allergic reaction, erythema, erythema multiforme, erythema nodosum, hypertrichosis, pruritus

Central Nervous System: Migraine headache, paresthesia, seizure, stroke, syncope

Psychiatric: Anxiety, irritability, mood changes, psychosis

Visual Disorders: Abnormal accommodation, cataract, eye pain, macular edema, optic neuritis, photopsia, posterior vitreous detachment, retinal hemorrhage, retinal thrombosis, retinal vascular spasm, temporary loss of vision

Cardiovascular: Arrhythmia, chest pain, edema, hypertension, palpitation, phlebitis, pulmonary embolism, shortness of breath, tachycardia, thrombophlebitis

Musculoskeletal: Arthralgia, back pain, myalgia

Hepatic: Transaminases increased, hepatitis

Neoplasms: Liver (hepatic hemangiosarcoma, liver cell adenoma, hepatocellular carcinoma); breast (fibrocystic disease, breast carcinoma); endometrium (endometrial carcinoma); nervous system (astrocytoma, pituitary tumor, prolactinoma, neurofibromatosis, glioblastoma multiforme, brain abcess); ovary (luteoma of pregnancy, dermoid cyst of the ovary, ovarian carcinoma); trophoblastic (hydatiform mole, choriocarcinoma); miscellaneous (melanoma, myeloma, perianal cysts, renal cell carcinoma, Hodgkin's lymphoma, tongue carcinoma, bladder carcinoma); and neoplasms of offspring (neuroectodermal tumor, thyroid tumor, hepatoblastoma, lymphocytic leukemia)

Genitourinary: Endometriosis, ovarian cyst (ovarian enlargement or cysts could, as such, be complicated by adnexal torsion), ovarian hemorrhage, tubal pregnancy, uterine hemorrhage

Body as a Whole: Fever, tinnitus, weakness

Other: Leukocytosis, thyroid disorder

Fetal/Neonatal anomalies. The following fetal abnormalities have also been reported during postmarketing surveillance: delayed development; abnormal bone development including skeletal malformations of the skull, face, nasal passages, jaw, hand, limb (ectromelia including amelia, hemimelia, and phocomelia), foot, and joints; tissue malformations including imperforate anus, tracheoesophageal fistula, diaphragmatic hernia, renal agenesis and dysgenesis, and malformations of the eye and lens (cataract), ear, lung, heart (ventricular septal defect and tetralogy of Fallot), and genitalia; as well as dwarfism, deafness, mental retardation, chromosomal disorders, and neural tube defects (including anencephaly).

DRUG ABUSE AND DEPENDENCE

Tolerance, abuse, or dependence with CLOMID has not been reported.

OVERDOSAGE

Signs and Symptoms

Toxic effects accompanying acute overdosage of CLOMID have not been reported. Signs and symptoms of overdosage as a result of the use of more than the recommended dose during CLOMID therapy include nausea, vomiting, vasomotor flushes, visual blurring, spots or flashes, scotomata, ovarian enlargement with pelvic or abdominal pain. (See CONTRAINDICATIONS: Ovarian Cyst.)

Oral LD_{50}. The acute oral LD_{50} of CLOMID is 1700 mg/kg in mice and 5750 mg/kg in rats. The toxic dose in humans is not known.

Dialysis: It is not known if CLOMID is dialyzable.

Treatment

In the event of overdose, appropriate supportive measures should be employed in addition to gastrointestinal decontamination.

DOSAGE AND ADMINISTRATION

General Considerations

The workup and treatment of candidates for CLOMID therapy should be supervised by physicians experienced in management of gynecologic or endocrine disorders. Patients should be chosen for therapy with CLOMID only after careful diagnostic evaluation (see INDICATIONS AND USAGE). The plan of therapy should be outlined in advance. Impediments to achieving the goal of therapy must be excluded or adequately treated before beginning CLOMID. The therapeutic objective should be balanced with potential risks and discussed with the patient and others involved in the achievement of a pregnancy.

Ovulation most often occurs from 5 to 10 days after a course of CLOMID. Coitus should be timed to coincide with the expected time of ovulation. Appropriate tests to determine ovulation may be useful during this time.

Recommended Dosage

Treatment of the selected patient should begin with a low dose, 50 mg daily (1 tablet) for 5 days. The dose should be increased only in those patients who do not ovulate in response to cyclic 50 mg CLOMID. A low dosage or duration of treatment course is particularly recommended if unusual sensitivity to pituitary gonadotropin is suspected, such as in patients with polycystic ovary syndrome (see WARNINGS: Ovarian Hyperstimulation Syndrome).

The patient should be evaluated carefully to exclude pregnancy, ovarian enlargement, or ovarian cyst formation between each treatment cycle.

If progestin-induced bleeding is planned, or if spontaneous uterine bleeding occurs prior to therapy, the regimen of 50 mg daily for 5 days should be started on or about the 5th day of the cycle. Therapy may be started at any time in the patient who has had no recent uterine bleeding. When ovulation occurs at this dosage, there is no advantage to increasing the dose in subsequent cycles of treatment.

If ovulation does not appear to occur after the first course of therapy, a second course of 100 mg daily (two 50 mg tablets given as a single daily dose) for 5 days should be given. This course may be started as early as 30 days after the previous one after precautions are taken to exclude the presence of pregnancy. Increasing the dosage or duration of therapy beyond 100 mg/day for 5 days is not recommended.

The majority of patients who are going to ovulate will do so after the first course of therapy. If ovulation does not occur after three courses of therapy, further treatment with CLOMID is not recommended and the patient should be reevaluated. If three ovulatory responses occur, but pregnancy has not been achieved, further treatment is not recommended. If menses does not occur after an ovulatory response, the patient should be reevaluated. Long-term cyclic therapy is not recommended beyond a total of about six cycles (see PRECAUTIONS).

HOW SUPPLIED

NDC 0068-0226-30: 50 mg tablets in cartons of 30

Tablets are round, white, scored, and debossed CLOMID 50.

Store tablets at controlled room temperature 59–86°F (15–30°C). Protect from heat, light, and excessive humidity, and store in closed containers.

Rx only

Prescribing Information as of June 2000

Merrell Pharmaceuticals Inc.
Subsidiary of Aventis Pharmaceuticals Inc.
Kansas City, MO 64137 USA
www.aventispharma-us.com
50058984

Shown in Product Identification Guide, page 307

DDAVP® Injection ℞
(desmopressin acetate)
4 µg/mL

Prescribing Information as of December 2002

DESCRIPTION

DDAVP® Injection (desmopressin acetate) 4 µg/mL is a synthetic analogue of the natural pituitary hormone 8-arginine vasopressin (ADH), an antidiuretic hormone affecting renal water conservation. It is chemically defined as follows:

Mol. Wt. 1183.34

Empirical Formula: $C_{46}H_{64}N_{14}O_{12}S_2 \bullet C_2H_4O_2 \bullet 3H_2O$

$SCH_2CH_2C(=O)$-Tyr-Phe-Gln-Asn-Cys-Pro-D-Arg-Gly-NH_2 • CH_3COOH • $3H_2O$ (positions 1 2 3 4 5 6 7 8 9; S of position 1 bridged to Cys 6)

1-(3-mercaptopropionic acid)-8-D-arginine vasopressin monoacetate (salt) trihydrate.

DDAVP Injection 4 µg/mL is provided as a sterile, aqueous solution for injection.

Each mL provides:

Desmopressin acetate	4.0 µg
Sodium chloride	9.0 mg
Hydrochloric acid to adjust pH to 4	

The 10 mL vial contains chlorobutanol as a preservative (5.0 mg/mL).

CLINICAL PHARMACOLOGY

DDAVP Injection 4 µg/mL contains as active substance, desmopressin acetate, a synthetic analogue of the natural hormone arginine vasopressin. One mL (4 µg) of DDAVP (desmopressin acetate) solution has an antidiuretic activity of about 16 IU; 1 µg of DDAVP is equivalent to 4 IU.

DDAVP has been shown to be more potent than arginine vasopressin in increasing plasma levels of factor VIII activity in patients with hemophilia and von Willebrand's disease Type I.

Dose-response studies were performed in healthy persons, using doses of 0.1 to 0.4 µg/kg body weight, infused over a 10-minute period. Maximal dose response occurred at 0.3 to 0.4 µg/kg. The response to DDAVP of factor VIII activity and plasminogen activator is dose-related, with maximal plasma levels of 300 to 400 percent of initial concentrations obtained after infusion of 0.4 µg/kg body weight. The increase is rapid and evident within 30 minutes, reaching a maximum at a point ranging from 90 minutes to two hours. The factor VIII related antigen and ristocetin cofactor activity were also increased to a smaller degree, but still are dose-dependent.

1. The biphasic half-lives of DDAVP were 7.8 and 75.5 minutes for the fast and slow phases, respectively, compared with 2.5 and 14.5 minutes for lysine vasopressin, another form of the hormone. As a result, DDAVP provides a prompt onset of antidiuretic action with a long duration after each administration.
2. The change in structure of arginine vasopressin to DDAVP has resulted in a decreased vasopressor action and decreased actions on visceral smooth muscle relative to the enhanced antidiuretic activity, so that clinically effective antidiuretic doses are usually below threshold levels for effects on vascular or visceral smooth muscle.
3. When administered by injection, DDAVP has an antidiuretic effect about ten times that of an equivalent dose administered intranasally.
4. The bioavailability of the subcutaneous route of administration was determined qualitatively using urine output data. The exact fraction of drug absorbed by that route of administration has not been quantitatively determined.
5. The percentage increase of factor VIII levels in patients with mild hemophilia A and von Willebrand's disease was not significantly different from that observed in normal healthy individuals when treated with 0.3 µg/kg of DDAVP infused over 10 minutes.
6. Plasminogen activator activity increases rapidly after DDAVP infusion, but there has been no clinically significant fibrinolysis in patients treated with DDAVP.
7. The effect of repeated DDAVP administration when doses were given every 12 to 24 hours has generally shown a gradual diminution of the factor VIII activity increase noted with a single dose. The initial response is reproducible in any particular patient if there are 2 or 3 days between administrations.

INDICATIONS AND USAGE

Hemophilia A: DDAVP Injection 4 µg/mL is indicated for patients with hemophilia A with factor VIII coagulant activity levels greater than 5%.

DDAVP will often maintain hemostasis in patients with hemophilia A during surgical procedures and postoperatively when administered 30 minutes prior to scheduled procedure.

DDAVP will also stop bleeding in hemophilia A patients with episodes of spontaneous or trauma-induced injuries such as hemarthroses, intramuscular hematomas or mucosal bleeding.

DDAVP is not indicated for the treatment of hemophilia A with factor VIII coagulant activity levels equal to or less than 5%, or for the treatment of hemophilia B, or in patients who have factor VIII antibodies.

In certain clinical situations, it may be justified to try DDAVP in patients with factor VIII levels between 2% to 5%; however, these patients should be carefully monitored.

von Willebrand's Disease (Type I): DDAVP Injection 4 µg/mL is indicated for patients with mild to moderate classic von Willebrand's disease (Type I) with factor VIII levels greater than 5%. DDAVP will often maintain hemostasis in patients with mild to moderate von Willebrand's disease during surgical procedures and postoperatively when administered 30 minutes prior to the scheduled procedure.

DDAVP will usually stop bleeding in mild to moderate von Willebrand's patients with episodes of spontaneous or trauma-induced injuries such as hemarthroses, intramuscular hematomas or mucosal bleeding.

Those von Willebrand's disease patients who are least likely to respond are those with severe homozygous von Willebrand's disease with factor VIII coagulant activity and factor VIII von Willebrand factor antigen levels less than 1%. Other patients may respond in a variable fashion depending on the type of molecular defect they have. Bleeding time and factor VIII coagulant activity, ristocetin cofactor activity, and von Willebrand factor antigen should be checked during administration of DDAVP to ensure that adequate levels are being achieved.

DDAVP is not indicated for the treatment of severe classic von Willebrand's disease (Type I) and when there is evidence of an abnormal molecular form of factor VIII antigen. (See **WARNINGS**.)

Diabetes Insipidus: DDAVP Injection 4 µg/mL is indicated as antidiuretic replacement therapy in the management of central (cranial) diabetes insipidus and for the management of the temporary polyuria and polydipsia following head trauma or surgery in the pituitary region. DDAVP is ineffective for the treatment of nephrogenic diabetes insipidus. DDAVP is also available as an intranasal preparation. However, this means of delivery can be compromised by a variety of factors that can make nasal insufflation ineffective or inappropriate. These include poor intranasal absorption, nasal congestion and blockage, nasal discharge, atrophy of nasal mucosa, and severe atrophic rhinitis. Intranasal delivery may be inappropriate where there is an impaired level of consciousness. In addition, cranial surgical procedures, such as transsphenoidal hypophysectomy, create situations where an alternative route of administration is needed as in cases of nasal packing or recovery from surgery.

CONTRAINDICATIONS

DDAVP Injection 4 µg/mL is contraindicated in individuals with known hypersensitivity to desmopressin acetate or to any of the components of **DDAVP Injection** 4 µg/mL.

WARNINGS

When DDAVP Injection is administered to patients who do not have need of antidiuretic hormone for its antidiuretic effect, in particular in pediatric and geriatric patients, fluid intake should be adjusted downward to decrease the potential occurrence of water intoxication and hyponatremia with accompanying signs and symptoms (headache, nausea/vomiting, decreased serum sodium and weight gain).

Particular attention should be paid to the possibility of the rare occurrence of an extreme decrease in plasma osmolality that may result in seizures which could lead to coma.

DDAVP should not be used to treat patients with Type IIB von Willebrand's disease since platelet aggregation may be induced.

PRECAUTIONS

General: For injection use only.

DDAVP® Injection (desmopressin acetate) 4 µg/mL has infrequently produced changes in blood pressure causing either a slight elevation in blood pressure or a transient fall in blood pressure and a compensatory increase in heart rate. The drug should be used with caution in patients with coronary artery insufficiency and/or hypertensive cardiovascular disease.

DDAVP (desmopressin acetate) should be used with caution in patients with conditions associated with fluid and electrolyte imbalance, such as cystic fibrosis, because these patients are prone to hyponatremia.

There have been rare reports of thrombotic events following **DDAVP Injection** 4 µg/mL in patients predisposed to thrombus formation. No causality has been determined, however, the drug should be used with caution in these patients.

Severe allergic reactions have been reported rarely. Anaphylaxis has been reported rarely with intravenous and intranasal DDAVP, including isolated cases of fatal anaphylaxis with intravenous DDAVP. It is not known whether antibodies to **DDAVP Injection** 4 µg/mL are produced after repeated injections.

Hemophilia A: Laboratory tests for assessing patient status include levels of factor VIII coagulant, factor VIII antigen and factor VIII ristocetin cofactor (von Willebrand factor) as well as activated partial thromboplastin time. Factor VIII coagulant activity should be determined before giving DDAVP for hemostasis. If factor VIII coagulant activity is present at less than 5% of normal, DDAVP should not be relied on.

von Willebrand's Disease: Laboratory tests for assessing patient status include levels of factor VIII coagulant activity, factor VIII ristocetin cofactor activity, and factor VIII von Willebrand factor antigen. The skin bleeding time may be helpful in following these patients.

Diabetes Insipidus: Laboratory tests for monitoring the patient include urine volume and osmolality. In some cases, plasma osmolality may be required.

Drug Interactions: Although the pressor activity of DDAVP is very low compared with the antidiuretic activity, use of doses as large as 0.3 µg/kg of DDAVP with other pressor agents should be done only with careful patient monitoring.

DDAVP has been used with epsilon aminocaproic acid without adverse effects.

Carcinogenicity, Mutagenicity, Impairment of Fertility: Studies with DDAVP have not been performed to evaluate carcinogenic potential, mutagenic potential or effects on fertility.

Pregnancy Category B: Fertility studies have not been done. Teratology studies in rats and rabbits at doses from 0.05 to 10 µg/kg/day (approximately 0.1 times the maximum systemic human exposure in rats and up to 38 times the maximum systemic human exposure in rabbits based on surface area, mg/m^2) revealed no harm to the fetus due to DDAVP. There are, however, no adequate and well controlled studies in pregnant women. Because animal reproduction studies are not always predictive of human response, this drug should be used during pregnancy only if clearly needed.

Several publications of desmopressin acetate's use in the management of diabetes insipidus during pregnancy are available; these include a few anecdotal reports of congenital anomalies and low birth weight babies. However, no causal connection between these events and desmopressin acetate has been established. A fifteen year, Swedish epidemiologic study of the use of desmopressin acetate in pregnant women with diabetes insipidus found the rate of birth defects to be no greater than that in the general population; however, the statistical power of this study is low. As opposed to preparations containing natural hormones, desmopressin acetate in antidiuretic doses has no uterotonic action and the physician will have to weigh the therapeutic advantages against the possible risks in each case.

Nursing Mothers: There have been no controlled studies in nursing mothers. A single study in postpartum women demonstrated a marked change in plasma, but little if any change in assayable DDAVP in breast milk following an intranasal dose of 10 µg. It is not known whether this drug is excreted in human milk. Because many drugs are excreted in human milk, caution should be exercised when DDAVP is administered to a nursing woman.

Pediatric Use: Use in infants and pediatric patients will require careful fluid intake restriction to prevent possible hyponatremia and water intoxication. **DDAVP Injection** 4 µg/mL *should not be used in infants less than three months of age* in the treatment of hemophilia A or von Willebrand's disease; safety and effectiveness in pediatric patients under 12 years of age with diabetes insipidus have not been established.

ADVERSE REACTIONS

Infrequently, DDAVP has produced transient headache, nausea, mild abdominal cramps and vulval pain. These symptoms disappeared with reduction in dosage. Occasionally, injection of DDAVP has produced local erythema, swelling or burning pain. Occasional facial flushing has been reported with the administration of DDAVP. **DDAVP Injection** has infrequently produced changes in blood pressure causing either a slight elevation or a transient fall and a compensatory increase in heart rate. Severe allergic reactions including anaphylaxis have been reported rarely with **DDAVP Injection**.

See **WARNINGS** for the possibility of water intoxication and hyponatremia.

There have been rare reports of thrombotic events (acute cerebrovascular thrombosis, acute myocardial infarction) following **DDAVP Injection** in patients predisposed to thrombus formation.

OVERDOSAGE

(See **ADVERSE REACTIONS**.) In case of overdosage, the dosage should be reduced, frequency of administration decreased, or the drug withdrawn according to the severity of the condition.

There is no known specific antidote for desmopressin acetate or **DDAVP Injection** 4 µg/mL.

An oral LD_{50} has not been established. An intravenous dose of 2 mg/kg in mice demonstrated no effect.

DOSAGE AND ADMINISTRATION

Hemophilia A and von Willebrand's Disease (Type I): DDAVP Injection 4 µg/mL is administered as an intravenous infusion at a dose of 0.3 µg DDAVP/kg body weight diluted in sterile physiological saline and infused slowly over 15 to 30 minutes. In adults and children weighing more than 10 kg, 50 mL of diluent is recommended; in children weighing 10 kg or less, 10 mL of diluent is recommended. Blood pressure and pulse should be monitored during infusion. If **DDAVP Injection** 4 µg/mL is used preoperatively, it should be administered 30 minutes prior to the scheduled procedure.

The necessity for repeat administration of DDAVP or use of any blood products for hemostasis should be determined by laboratory response as well as the clinical condition of the patient. The tendency toward tachyphylaxis (lessening of response) with repeated administration given more frequently than every 48 hours should be considered in treating each patient.

Diabetes Insipidus: This formulation is administered subcutaneously or by direct intravenous injection. **DDAVP Injection** 4 µg/mL dosage must be determined for each patient and adjusted according to the pattern of response. Response should be estimated by two parameters: adequate duration of sleep and adequate, not excessive, water turnover.

The usual dosage range in adults is 0.5 mL (2.0 µg) to 1 mL (4.0 µg) daily, administered intravenously or subcutaneously, usually in two divided doses. The morning and evening doses should be separately adjusted for an adequate diurnal rhythm of water turnover. For patients who have been controlled on intranasal DDAVP and who must be switched to the injection form, either because of poor intranasal absorption or because of the need for surgery, the comparable antidiuretic dose of the injection is about one-tenth the intranasal dose.

Parenteral drug products should be inspected visually for particulate matter and discoloration prior to administration whenever solution and container permit.

See directions for use of One Point Cut (OPC) ampules for **DDAVP Injection** on back of carton.

HOW SUPPLIED

DDAVP Injection 4 µg/mL is available as a sterile solution in cartons of ten 1 mL single-dose ampules (NDC 0075-2451-01) and in 10 mL multiple-dose vials (NDC 0075-2451-53), each containing 4.0 µg DDAVP per mL.

Store refrigerated 2 to 8°C (36 to 46°F).

Rx Only.

Keep out of the reach of children.

Manufactured for
Aventis Pharmaceuticals Inc.
Bridgewater, NJ 08807
By Ferring AB, Soldattorpsvägen 5
SE-200 61 Limhamn, Sweden
US Patents 5,500,413; 5,596,078; 5,763,407
Rev. December 2002

Shown in Product Identification Guide, page 307

DDAVP® Nasal Spray ℞
(desmopressin acetate)

Prescribing Information as of December 2002

DESCRIPTION

DDAVP® Nasal Spray (desmopressin acetate) is a synthetic analogue of the natural pituitary hormone 8-arginine vasopressin (ADH), an antidiuretic hormone affecting renal water conservation. It is chemically defined as follows:

Mol. wt. 1183.34

Continued on next page

DDAVP Nasal Spray—Cont.

Empirical formula: $C_{46}H_{64}N_{14}O_{12}S_2 \cdot C_2H_4O_2 \cdot 3H_2O$

```
 ┌─────────────────────────────────┐
 │           O                     │
 │           ‖                     │
SCH2CH2C-Tyr-Phe-Gln-Asn-Cys-Pro-D-Arg-Gly-NH2 • CH3COOH • 3H2O
     1      2   3   4   5   6   7     8   9
```

1-(3-mercaptopropionic acid)-8-D-arginine vasopressin monoacetate (salt) trihydrate.

DDAVP Nasal Spray is provided as an aqueous solution for intranasal use.

Each mL contains:

Desmopressin acetate	0.1 mg
Sodium Chloride	7.5 mg
Citric acid monohydrate	1.7 mg
Disodium phosphate dihydrate	3.0 mg
Benzalkonium chloride solution (50%)	0.2 mg

The **DDAVP Nasal Spray** compression pump delivers 0.1 mL (10 µg) of DDAVP (desmopressin acetate) per spray.

CLINICAL PHARMACOLOGY

DDAVP contains as active substance desmopressin acetate, a synthetic analogue of the natural hormone arginine vasopressin. One mL (0.1 mg) of intranasal DDAVP has an antidiuretic activity of about 400 IU; 10 µg of desmopressin acetate is equivalent to 40 IU.

1. The biphasic half-lives for intranasal DDAVP were 7.8 and 75.5 minutes for the fast and slow phases, compared with 2.5 and 14.5 minutes for lysine vasopressin, another form of the hormone used in this condition. As a result, intranasal DDAVP provides a prompt onset of antidiuretic action with a long duration after each administration.
2. The change in structure of arginine vasopressin to DDAVP has resulted in a decreased vasopressor action and decreased actions on visceral smooth muscle relative to the enhanced antidiuretic activity, so that clinically effective antidiuretic doses are usually below threshold levels for effects on vascular or visceral smooth muscle.
3. DDAVP administered intranasally has an antidiuretic effect about one-tenth that of an equivalent dose administered by injection.

INDICATIONS AND USAGE

Primary Nocturnal Enuresis: DDAVP Nasal Spray is indicated for the management of primary nocturnal enuresis. It may be used alone or adjunctive to behavioral conditioning or other nonpharmacological intervention. It has been shown to be effective in some cases that are refractory to conventional therapies.

Central Cranial Diabetes Insipidus: DDAVP Nasal Spray is indicated as antidiuretic replacement therapy in the management of central cranial diabetes insipidus and for management of the temporary polyuria and polydipsia following head trauma or surgery in the pituitary region. It is ineffective for the treatment of nephrogenic diabetes insipidus.

The use of **DDAVP Nasal Spray** in patients with an established diagnosis will result in a reduction in urinary output with increase in urine osmolality and a decrease in plasma osmolality. This will allow the resumption of a more normal life-style with a decrease in urinary frequency and nocturia.

There are reports of an occasional change in response with time, usually greater than 6 months. Some patients may show a decreased responsiveness, others a shortened duration of effect. There is no evidence this effect is due to the development of binding antibodies but may be due to a local inactivation of the peptide.

Patients are selected for therapy by establishing the diagnosis by means of the water deprivation test, the hypertonic saline infusion test, and/or the response to antidiuretic hormone. Continued response to intranasal DDAVP can be monitored by urine volume and osmolality.

DDAVP is also available as a solution for injection when the intranasal route may be compromised. These situations include nasal congestion and blockage, nasal discharge, atrophy of nasal mucosa, and severe atrophic rhinitis. Intranasal delivery may also be inappropriate where there is an impaired level of consciousness. In addition, cranial surgical procedures, such as transphenoidal hypophysectomy create situations where an alternative route of administration is needed as in cases of nasal packing or recovery from surgery.

CONTRAINDICATIONS

DDAVP Nasal Spray is contraindicated in individuals with known hypersensitivity to desmopressin acetate or to any of the components of **DDAVP Nasal Spray**.

WARNINGS

1. For intranasal use only.
2. When DDAVP Nasal Spray is administered, in particular in pediatric and geriatric patients, fluid intake should be adjusted downward in order to decrease the potential occurrence of water intoxication and hyponatremia with accompanying signs and symptoms (headache, nausea/vomiting, decreased serum sodium and weight gain). Particular attention should be paid to the possibility of the rare occurrence of an extreme decrease in plasma osmolality that may result in seizures which could lead to coma.

PRECAUTIONS

General: Intranasal DDAVP at high dosage has infrequently produced a slight elevation of blood pressure, which disappeared with a reduction in dosage. The drug should be used with caution in patients with coronary artery insufficiency and/or hypertensive cardiovascular disease because of possible rise in blood pressure.

DDAVP should be used with caution in patients with conditions associated with fluid and electrolyte imbalance, such as cystic fibrosis, because these patients are prone to hyponatremia. Rare severe allergic reactions have been reported with DDAVP. Anaphylaxis has been reported rarely with intravenous and intranasal administration of DDAVP.

Central Cranial Diabetes Insipidus: Since DDAVP is used intranasally, changes in the nasal mucosa such as scarring, edema, or other disease may cause erratic, unreliable absorption in which case intranasal DDAVP should not be used. For such situations, DDAVP Injection should be considered.

Primary Nocturnal Enuresis: If changes in the nasal mucosa have occurred, unreliable absorption may result. **DDAVP Nasal Spray** should be discontinued until the nasal problems resolve.

Information for Patients: Patients should be informed that the **DDAVP Nasal Spray** bottle accurately delivers 50 doses of 10 µg each. Any solution remaining after 50 doses should be discarded since the amount delivered thereafter may be substantially less than 10 µg of drug. No attempt should be made to transfer remaining solution to another bottle. Patients should be instructed to read accompanying directions on use of the spray pump carefully before use.

Laboratory Tests: Laboratory tests for following the patient with central cranial diabetes insipidus or post-surgical or head trauma-related polyuria and polydipsia include urine volume and osmolality. In some cases plasma osmolality measurements may be required. For the healthy patient with primary nocturnal enuresis, serum electrolytes should be checked at least once if therapy is continued beyond 7 days.

Drug Interactions: Although the pressor activity of DDAVP is very low compared to the antidiuretic activity, use of large doses of intranasal DDAVP with other pressor agents should only be done with careful patient monitoring.

Carcinogenesis, Mutagenesis, Impairment of Fertility: Studies with DDAVP have not been performed to evaluate carcinogenic potential, mutagenic potential or effects on fertility.

Pregnancy: *Category B:* Fertility studies have not been done. Teratology studies in rats and rabbits at doses from 0.05 to 10 µg/kg/day (approximately 0.1 times the maximum systemic human exposure in rats and up to 38 times the maximum systemic human exposure in rabbits based on surface area, mg/m^2) revealed no harm to the fetus due to DDAVP (desmopressin acetate). There are, however, no adequate and well controlled studies in pregnant women. Because animal reproduction studies are not always predictive of human response, this drug should be used during pregnancy only if clearly needed.

Several publications of desmopressin acetate's use in the management of diabetes insipidus during pregnancy are available; these include a few anecdotal reports of congenital anomalies and low birth weight babies. However, no causal connection between these events and desmopressin acetate has been established. A fifteen year Swedish epidemiologic study of the use of desmopressin acetate in pregnant women with diabetes insipidus found the rate of birth defects to be no greater than that in the general population; however, the statistical power of this study is low. As opposed to preparations containing natural hormones, desmopressin acetate in antidiuretic doses has no uterotonic action and the physician will have to weigh the therapeutic advantages against the possible risks in each case.

Nursing Mothers: There have been no controlled studies in nursing mothers. A single study in a post-partum woman demonstrated a marked change in plasma, but little if any change in assayable DDAVP in breast milk following an intranasal dose of 10 µg. It is not known whether this drug is excreted in human milk. Because many drugs are excreted in human milk, caution should be exercised when DDAVP is administered to a nursing woman.

Pediatric Use: *Primary Nocturnal Enuresis:*

DDAVP Nasal Spray (desmopressin acetate) has been used in childhood nocturnal enuresis. Short-term (4–8 weeks) **DDAVP Nasal Spray** administration has been shown to be safe and modestly effective in pediatric patients aged 6 years or older with severe childhood nocturnal enuresis. Adequately controlled studies with intranasal DDAVP in primary nocturnal enuresis have not been conducted beyond 4–8 weeks. The dose should be individually adjusted to achieve the best results.

Central Cranial Diabetes Insipidus: DDAVP Nasal Spray has been used in children with diabetes insipidus. Use in infants and children will require careful fluid intake restriction to prevent possible hyponatremia and water intoxication. The dose must be individually adjusted to the patient with attention in the very young to the danger of an extreme decrease in plasma osmolality with resulting convulsions. Dose should start at 0.05 mL or less.

Since the spray cannot deliver less than 0.1 mL (10 µg), smaller doses should be administered using the rhinal tube delivery system. Do not use the nasal spray in pediatric patients requiring less than 0.1 mL (10 µg) per dose.

There are reports of an occasional change in response with time, usually greater than 6 months. Some patients may show a decreased responsiveness, others a shortened duration of effect. There is no evidence this effect is due to the development of binding antibodies but may be due to a local inactivation of the peptide.

ADVERSE REACTIONS

Infrequently, high dosages of intranasal DDAVP have produced transient headache and nausea. Nasal congestion, rhinitis and flushing have also been reported occasionally along with mild abdominal cramps. These symptoms disappeared with reduction in dosage. Nosebleed, sore throat, cough and upper respiratory infections have also been reported.

The following table lists the percentage of patients having adverse experiences without regard to relationship to study drug from the pooled pivotal study data for nocturnal enuresis.

ADVERSE REACTION	PLACEBO (N=59) %	DDAVP 20 µg (N=60) %	DDAVP 40 µg (N=61) %
BODY AS A WHOLE			
Abdominal Pain	0	2	2
Asthenia	0	0	2
Chills	0	0	2
Headache	0	2	5
Throat Pain	2	0	0
NERVOUS SYSTEM			
Depression	2	0	0
Dizziness	0	0	3
RESPIRATORY SYSTEM			
Epistaxis	2	3	0
Nostril Pain	0	2	0
Respiratory Infection	2	0	0
Rhinitis	2	8	3
CARDIOVASCULAR SYSTEM			
Vasodilation	2	0	0
DIGESTIVE SYSTEM			
Gastrointestinal Disorder	0	2	0
Nausea	0	0	2
SKIN & APPENDAGES			
Leg Rash	2	0	0
Rash	2	0	0
SPECIAL SENSES			
Conjunctivitis	0	2	0
Edema Eyes	0	2	0
Lachrymation Disorder	0	0	2

See **WARNINGS** for the possibility of water intoxication and hyponatremia.

OVERDOSAGE

(See **ADVERSE REACTIONS**.) In case of overdosage, the dose should be reduced, frequency of administration decreased, or the drug withdrawn according to the severity of the condition. There is no known specific antidote for desmopressin acetate or **DDAVP Nasal Spray**.

An oral LD_{50} has not been established. An intravenous dose of 2 mg/kg in mice demonstrated no effect.

DOSAGE AND ADMINISTRATION

Primary Nocturnal Enuresis: Dosage should be adjusted according to the individual. The recommended initial dose for those 6 years of age and older is 20 µg or 0.2 mL solution intranasally at bedtime. Adjustment up to 40 µg is suggested if the patient does not respond.

Some patients may respond to 10 µg and adjustment to that lower dose may be done if the patient has shown a response to 20 µg. It is recommended that one-half of the dose be administered per nostril. Adequately controlled studies with intranasal DDAVP in primary nocturnal enuresis have not been conducted beyond 4–8 weeks.

Central Cranial Diabetes Insipidus: DDAVP Nasal Spray dosage must be determined for each individual patient and adjusted according to the diurnal pattern of response. Response should be estimated by two parameters: adequate duration of sleep and adequate, not excessive, water turnover. Patients with nasal congestion and blockage have often responded well to intranasal DDAVP. The usual dosage range in adults is 0.1 to 0.4 mL daily, either as a single dose or divided into two or three doses. Most adults require 0.2 mL daily in two divided doses. The morning and evening doses should be separately adjusted for an adequate diurnal rhythm of water turnover. For children aged 3 months to 12 years, the usual dosage range is 0.05 to 0.3 mL daily, either as a single dose or divided into two doses. About $^1/_4$ to $^1/_3$ of patients can be controlled by a single daily dose of DDAVP administered intranasally.

The nasal spray pump can only deliver doses of 0.1 mL (10 µg) or multiples of 0.1 mL. If doses other than these are required, the rhinal tube delivery system may be used.

The spray pump must be primed prior to the first use. To prime pump, press down four times. The bottle will now deliver 10 µg of drug per spray. Discard **DDAVP Nasal Spray** after 50 sprays since the amount delivered thereafter per spray may be substantially less than 10 µg of drug.

HOW SUPPLIED

DDAVP Nasal Spray is available in a 5-mL bottle with spray pump delivering 50 sprays of 10 µg (NDC 0075-2452-01). Desmopressin acetate is also available as DDAVP Rhinal Tube, a refrigerated product with 2.5 mL per vial, packaged with two rhinal tube applicators per carton (NDC 0075-2450-01).

Store at Controlled Room Temperature 20 to 25°C (68 to 77°F) [see USP].
STORE BOTTLE IN UPRIGHT POSITION.
Rx Only.
Keep out of the reach of children.
Manufactured for:
Aventis Pharmaceuticals Inc.
Bridgewater, NJ 08807
By Ferring AB, Soldattorpsvägen 5
SE-200 G1 Limhamn, Sweden
Rev. December 2002

Shown in Product Identification Guide, page 307

DDAVP® Tablets ℞
(desmopressin acetate)

Prescribing Information as of November 2002
Rx only

DESCRIPTION

DDAVP® Tablets (desmopressin acetate) are a synthetic analogue of the natural pituitary hormone 8-arginine vasopressin (ADH), an antidiuretic hormone affecting renal water conservation. It is chemically defined as follows:
Mol. Wt. 1183.34
Empirical Formula:
$C_{46}H_{64}N_{14}O_{12}S_2 \cdot C_2H_4O_2 \cdot 3H_2O$

$SCH_2CH_2C(=O)$-Tyr-Phe-Gln-Asn-Cys-Pro-D-Arg-Gly-$NH_2 \cdot CH_3COOH \cdot 3H_2O$
1 2 3 4 5 6 7 8 9

1-(3-mercaptopropionic acid)-8-D-arginine vasopressin monoacetate (salt) trihydrate.
DDAVP Tablets contain either 0.1 or 0.2 mg desmopressin acetate. Inactive ingredients include: lactose, potato starch, magnesium stearate and povidone.

CLINICAL PHARMACOLOGY

DDAVP Tablets contain as active substance, desmopressin acetate, a synthetic analogue of the natural hormone arginine vasopressin.
Central Diabetes Insipidus: Dose response studies in patients with diabetes insipidus have demonstrated that oral doses of 0.025 mg to 0.4 mg produced clinically significant antidiuretic effects. In most patients, doses of 0.1 mg to 0.2 mg produced optimal antidiuretic effects lasting up to eight hours. With doses of 0.4 mg, antidiuretic effects were observed for up to 12 hours; measurements beyond 12 hours were not recorded. Increasing oral doses produced dose dependent increases in the plasma levels of DDAVP (desmopressin acetate).
The plasma half-life of DDAVP followed a monoexponential time course with $t_{1/2}$ values of 1.5 to 2.5 hours which was independent of dose.
The bioavailability of DDAVP oral tablets is about 5% compared to intranasal DDAVP, and about 0.16% compared to intravenous DDAVP. The time to reach maximum plasma DDAVP levels ranged from 0.9 to 1.5 hours following oral or intranasal administration, respectively. Following administration of **DDAVP Tablets**, the onset of antidiuretic effect occurs at around 1 hour, and it reaches a maximum at about 4 to 7 hours based on the measurement of increased urine osmolality.
The use of **DDAVP Tablets** in patients with an established diagnosis will result in a reduction in urinary output with an accompanying increase in urine osmolality. These effects usually will allow resumption of a more normal life style, with a decrease in urinary frequency and nocturia.
There are reports of an occasional change in response to the intranasal formulations of DDAVP (DDAVP Nasal Spray and DDAVP Rhinal Tube). Usually, the change occurred over a period of time greater than six months. This change may be due to decreased responsiveness, or to shortened duration of effect. There is no evidence that this effect is due to the development of binding antibodies, but may be due to a local inactivation of the peptide. No lessening of effect was observed in the 46 patients who were treated with **DDAVP Tablets** for 12 to 44 months and no serum antibodies to desmopressin were detected.
The change in structure of arginine vasopressin to desmopressin acetate resulted in less vasopressor activity and decreased action on visceral smooth muscle relative to enhanced antidiuretic activity. Consequently, clinically effective antidiuretic doses are usually below the threshold for effects on vascular or visceral smooth muscle. In the four long-term studies of **DDAVP Tablets**, no increases in blood pressure in 46 patients receiving **DDAVP Tablets** for periods of 12 to 44 months were reported.
In one study, the pharmacodynamic characteristics of **DDAVP Tablets** and intranasal formulation were compared during an 8-hour dosing interval at steady state. The doses administered to 36 hydrated (water loaded) healthy male adult volunteers every 8 hours were 0.1, 0.2, 0.4 mg orally and 0.01 mg intranasally by rhinal tube. The results are shown in the following table:

Response to DDAVP and Placebo at Two Weeks of Treatment
Mean (SE) Number of Wet Nights/2 Weeks

	Placebo (n = 85)	0.2 mg/day (n = 79)	0.4 mg/day (n = 82)	0.6 mg/day (n = 83)
Baseline	10 (0.3)	11 (0.3)	10 (0.3)	10 (0.3)
Reduction from Baseline	1 (0.3)	3 (0.4)	3 (0.4)	4 (0.4)
Percent Reduction from Baseline	10%	27%	30%	40%
p-value vs placebo	—	<0.05	<0.05	<0.05

Mean Changes from Baseline (SE) in Pharmacodynamic Parameters in Normal Healthy Adult Volunteers

Treatment	Total Urine Volume in mL	Maximum Urine Osmolality in mOsm/kg
0.1 mg PO q8h	−3689.3 (149.6)	514.8 (21.9)
0.2 mg PO q8h	−4429.9 (149.6)	686.3 (21.9)
0.4 mg PO q8h	−4998.8 (149.6)	769.3 (21.9)
0.01 mg IN q8h	−4844.9 (149.6)	754.1 (21.9)

(SE) = Standard error of the mean

With respect to the mean values of total urine volume decrease and maximum urine osmolality increase from baseline, the 90% confidence limits estimated that the 0.4 mg and 0.2 mg oral dose produced between 95% and 110% and 84% to 99% of pharmacodynamic activity, respectively, when compared to the 0.01 mg intranasal dose.
While both the 0.2 mg and 0.4 mg oral doses are considered pharmacodynamically similar to the 0.01 mg intranasal dose, the pharmacodynamic data on an inter-subject basis was highly variable and, therefore, individual dosing is recommended.
In another study in diabetes insipidus patients, the pharmacodynamic characteristics of **DDAVP Tablets** and intranasal formulations were compared over a 12-hour period. Ten fluid-controlled patients under age 18 were administered tablet doses of 0.2 mg and 0.4 mg, and intranasal doses of 0.01 mg and 0.02 mg.

Mean Peak Pharmacodynamic Parameters (SD) in Pediatric and Adolescent Diabetes Insipidus Patients

Treatment	Urine Volume in mL/min	Maximum Urine Osmolality in mOsm/kg
0.01 mg IN	0.3 (0.15)	717.0 (224.63)
0.02 mg IN	0.3 (0.25)	761.8 (298.82)
0.2 mg PO	0.3 (0.12)	678.3 (147.91)
0.4 mg PO	0.2 (0.15)	787.2 (73.34)

(SD) = Standard Deviation

All four dose formulations (0.01 mg IN, 0.02 mg IN, 0.2 mg PO and 0.4 mg PO) have a similar, pronounced pharmacodynamic effect on urine volume and urine osmolality. At two hours after study drug administration, mean urine volume was 4 mL/min and urine osmolality was >500 mOsm/kg. Mean plasma osmolality remained relatively constant over the time course recorded (0 to 12 hours). A statistical separation from baseline did not occur at any dose or time point. In these patients, the 0.2 mg tablets and the 0.01 mg intranasal spray exhibited similar pharmacodynamic profiles as did the 0.4 mg tablets and the 0.02 mg intranasal spray formulation. In another study of adult diabetes insipidus patients previously controlled on DDAVP intranasal spray, after one week of self-titration from spray to tablets, patients' diuresis was controlled with 0.1 mg **DDAVP Tablets** three times a day.
Primary Nocturnal Enuresis: Two double-blind, randomized, placebo-controlled studies were conducted in 340 patients with primary nocturnal enuresis. Patients were 5–17 years old, and 72% were males. A total of 329 patients were evaluated for efficacy. Patients were evaluated over a two-week baseline period in which the average number of wet nights was 10 (range 4–14). Patients were then randomized to receive 0.2, 0.4, or 0.6 mg of DDAVP or placebo. The pooled results after two weeks are shown in the following table:
[See table above]
Patients treated with **DDAVP Tablets** showed a statistically significant reduction in the number of wet nights compared to placebo-treated patients. A greater response was observed with increasing doses up to 0.6 mg.
In a six month, open-label extension study, patients completing the placebo-controlled studies were started on 0.2 mg/day DDAVP, and the dose was progressively increased until the optimal response was achieved (maximum dose 0.6 mg/day). A total of 230 patients were evaluated for efficacy; the average number of wet nights/2 weeks during the untreated baseline period was 10 (range 4–14), and the average duration (SD) of treatment was 4.2 (1.8) months. Twenty-five (25) patients (11%) achieved a complete or near complete response (≤2 wet nights/2 weeks) and did not require titration to the 0.6 mg/day dose. The majority of patients (198 of 230, 86%) were titrated to the highest dose. When all dose groups were combined, 128 (56%) showed at least a 50% reduction from baseline in the number of wet nights/2 weeks, while 87 (38%) patients achieved a complete or near complete response.

INDICATIONS AND USAGE

Central Diabetes Insipidus: DDAVP Tablets are indicated as antidiuretic replacement therapy in the management of central diabetes insipidus and for the management of the temporary polyuria and polydipsia following head trauma or surgery in the pituitary region. DDAVP is ineffective for the treatment of nephrogenic diabetes insipidus.
Patients were selected for therapy based on the diagnosis by means of the water deprivation test, the hypertonic saline infusion test, and/or response to antidiuretic hormone. Continued response to DDAVP can be monitored by measuring urine volume and osmolality.
Primary Nocturnal Enuresis: DDAVP® Tablets (desmopressin acetate) are indicated for the management of primary nocturnal enuresis. DDAVP may be used alone or as an adjunct to behavioral conditioning or other non-pharmacologic intervention.

CONTRAINDICATIONS

DDAVP Tablets are contraindicated in individuals with known hypersensitivity to desmopressin acetate or to any of the components of **DDAVP Tablets.**

WARNINGS

When DDAVP Tablets are administered, in particular and geriatric patients, fluid intake should be adjusted downward to decrease the potential occurrence of water intoxication and hyponatremia with accompanying signs and symptoms (headache, nausea/vomiting, decreased serum sodium and weight gain). Particular attention should be paid to the possibility of the rare occurrence of an extreme decrease in plasma osmolality that may result in seizures which could lead to coma.

PRECAUTIONS

General: Intranasal formulations of DDAVP at high doses and DDAVP Injection have infrequently produced a slight elevation of blood pressure which disappears with a reduction of dosage. Although this effect has not been observed when single oral doses up to 0.6 mg have been administered, the drug should be used with caution in patients with coronary artery insufficiency and/or hypertensive cardiovascular disease, because of a possible rise in blood pressure.
DDAVP should be used with caution in patients with conditions associated with fluid and electrolyte imbalance, such as cystic fibrosis, since these patients may develop hyponatremia.
Rare severe allergic reactions have been reported with DDAVP. Anaphylaxis has been reported with intravenous and intranasal administration of DDAVP Injection, but not with **DDAVP Tablets.**
Laboratory Tests: *Central Diabetes Insipidus:* Laboratory tests for monitoring the patient with central diabetes insipidus or post-surgical or head trauma-related polyuria and polydipsia include urine volume and osmolality. In some cases, measurements of plasma osmolality may be useful.
Drug Interactions: Although the pressor activity of DDAVP is very low compared to its antidiuretic activity, large doses of **DDAVP Tablets** should be used with other pressor agents only with careful patient monitoring.
Carcinogenicity, Mutagenicity, Impairment of Fertility: Studies with DDAVP have not been performed to evaluate carcinogenic potential, mutagenic potential or effects on fertility.
Pregnancy: *Category B:* Fertility studies have not been done. Teratology studies in rats and rabbits at doses from 0.05 to 10 μg/kg/day (approximately 0.1 times the maximum systemic human exposure in rats and up to 38 times the maximum systemic human exposure in rabbits based on surface area, mg/m^2) revealed no harm to the fetus due to DDAVP (desmopressin acetate). There are, however, no adequate and well-controlled studies in pregnant women. Because animal studies are not always predictive of human response, this drug should be used during pregnancy only if clearly needed.
Several publications where desmopressin acetate was used in the management of diabetes insipidus during pregnancy are available; these include a few anecdotal reports of congenital anomalies and low birth weight babies. However, no causal connection between these events and desmopressin acetate has been established. A fifteen year Swedish epidemiologic study of the use of desmopressin acetate in preg-

Continued on next page

DDAVP Tablets—Cont.

nant women with diabetes insipidus found the rate of birth defects to be no greater than that in the general population; however, the statistical power of this study is low. As opposed to preparations containing natural hormones, desmopressin acetate in antidiuretic doses has no uterotonic action and the physician will have to weigh the possible therapeutic advantages against the possible risks in each case.

Nursing Mothers: There have been no controlled studies in nursing mothers. A single study in postpartum women demonstrated a marked change in plasma, but little if any change in assayable DDAVP in breast milk following an intranasal dose of 0.01 mg.

It is not known whether the drug is excreted in human milk. Because many drugs are excreted in human milk, caution should be exercised when DDAVP is administered to nursing mothers.

Pediatric Use: *Central Diabetes Insipidus:* **DDAVP® Tablets** (desmopressin acetate) have been used safely in pediatric patients, age 4 years and older, with diabetes insipidus for periods up to 44 months. In younger pediatric patients the dose must be individually adjusted in order to prevent an excessive decrease in plasma osmolality leading to hyponatremia and possible convulsions; dosing should start at 0.05 mg (1/2 of the 0.1 mg tablet). Use of **DDAVP Tablets** in pediatric patients requires careful fluid intake restrictions to prevent possible hyponatremia and water intoxication.

Primary Nocturnal Enuresis: **DDAVP Tablets** have been safely used in pediatric patients age 6 years and older with primary nocturnal enuresis for up to 6 months. Some patients respond to a dose of 0.2 mg; however, increasing responses are seen at doses of 0.4 mg and 0.6 mg. No increase in the frequency or severity of adverse reactions or decrease in efficacy was seen with an increased dose or duration. The dose should be individually adjusted to achieve the best results.

ADVERSE REACTIONS

Infrequently, large doses of the intranasal formulations of DDAVP and DDAVP Injection have produced transient headache, nausea, flushing and mild abdominal cramps. These symptoms have disappeared with reduction in dosage.

Central Diabetes Insipidus: In long-term clinical studies in which patients with diabetes insipidus were followed for periods up to 44 months of **DDAVP Tablet** therapy, transient increases in AST (SGOT) no higher than 1.5 times the upper limit of normal were occasionally observed. Elevated AST (SGOT) returned to the normal range despite continued use of **DDAVP Tablets.**

Primary Nocturnal Enuresis: The only adverse event occurring in ≥3% of patients in controlled clinical trials with **DDAVP Tablets** that was probably, possibly, or remotely related to study drug was headache (4% DDAVP, 3% placebo).

Other: The following adverse events have been reported; however their relationship to DDAVP has not been established: abnormal thinking, diarrhea, and edema-weight gain.

See **WARNINGS** for the possibility of water intoxication and hyponatremia.

OVERDOSAGE

(See **ADVERSE REACTIONS.**) In case of overdose, the dose should be reduced, frequency of administration decreased, or the drug withdrawn according to the severity of the condition. There is no known specific antidote for DDAVP. The patient should be observed and treated with appropriate symptomatic therapy.

An oral LD_{50} has not been established. Oral doses up to 0.2 mg/kg/day have been administered to dogs and rats for 6 months without any significant drug-related toxicities reported. An intravenous dose of 2 mg/kg in mice demonstrated no effect.

DOSAGE AND ADMINISTRATION

Central Diabetes Insipidus: The dosage of **DDAVP Tablets** must be determined for each individual patient and adjusted according to the diurnal pattern of response. Response should be estimated by two parameters: adequate duration of sleep and adequate, not excessive, water turnover. Patients previously on intranasal DDAVP therapy should begin tablet therapy twelve hours after the last intranasal dose. During the initial dose titration period, patients should be observed closely and appropriate safety parameters measured to assure adequate response. Patients should be monitored at regular intervals during the course of **DDAVP Tablet** therapy to assure adequate antidiuretic response. Modifications in dosage regimen should be implemented as necessary to assure adequate water turnover.

Adults and Children: It is recommended that patients be started on doses of 0.05 mg (1/2 of the 0.1 mg tablet) two times a day and individually adjusted to their optimum therapeutic dose. Most patients in clinical trials found that the optimal dosage range is 0.1 mg to 0.8 mg daily, administered in divided doses. Each dose should be separately adjusted for an adequate diurnal rhythm of water turnover. Total daily dosage should be increased or decreased in the range of 0.1 mg to 1.2 mg divided into two or three daily doses as needed to obtain adequate antidiuresis. See **Pediatric Use** subsection for special considerations when administering desmopressin acetate to pediatric diabetes insipidus patients.

Primary Nocturnal Enuresis: The dosage of **DDAVP Tablets** must be determined for each individual patient and adjusted according to response. Patients previously on intranasal DDAVP therapy can begin tablet therapy the night following (24 hours after) the last intranasal dose. The recommended initial dose for patients age 6 years and older is 0.2 mg at bedtime. The dose may be titrated up to 0.6 mg to achieve the desired response.

HOW SUPPLIED

Strength	Size	NDC 0075-	Color	Markings
0.1 mg	Bottle of 100	0016-00	White	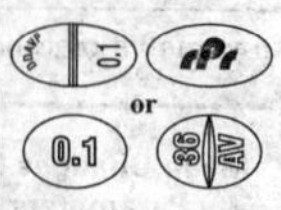 DDAVP 0.1 / rPr or 0.1 / 36 AV
0.2 mg	Bottle of 100	0026-00	White	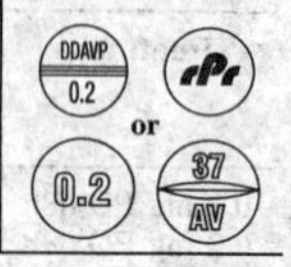 DDAVP 0.2 / rPr or 0.2 / 37 AV

Store at Controlled Room Temperature 20 to 25°C (68 to 77°F) [see USP]. Avoid exposure to excessive heat or light. This product should be dispensed in a container with a child-resistant cap.

Keep out of the reach of children.

U.S. Patent Nos. 5,500,413, 5,596,078, 5,674,850, 5,047,398

Manufactured for
Aventis Pharmaceuticals Inc.
Bridgewater, NJ 08807 USA
By Ferring AB, Soldattorpsvägen 5, SE-200 61 Limhamn, Sweden
Rev. November 2002

Shown in Product Identification Guide, page 307

DIAβETA® ℞

[*dī "ə-bū 'ta*]
(glyburide USP)
Tablets 1.25, 2.5 and 5 mg

Prescribing Information as of April 2004

DESCRIPTION

Diaβeta (glyburide USP) is an oral blood-glucose-lowering drug of the sulfonylurea class. It is a white, crystalline compound, formulated as tablets of 1.25 mg, 2.5 mg, and 5 mg strengths for oral administration. Diaβeta tablets contain the active ingredient glyburide and the following inactive ingredients: dibasic calcium phosphate USP, magnesium stearate NF, microcrystalline cellulose NF, sodium alginate NF, talc USP. Diaβeta 1.25 mg tablets also contain D&C Yellow #10 Aluminum Lake and FD&C Red #40 Aluminum Lake. Diaβeta 2.5 mg tablets also contain FD&C Red #40 Aluminum Lake. Diaβeta 5 mg tablets also contain D&C Yellow #10 Aluminum Lake, and FD&C Blue #1. Chemically, Diaβeta is identified as 1-[[p-[2-(5-Chloro-*o*-anisamido)ethyl]phenyl]sulfonyl]-3-cyclohexylurea.

The CAS Registry Number is 10238-21-8.

The structural formula is:

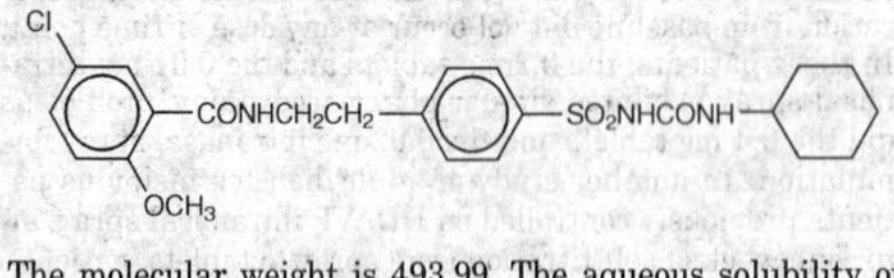

Cl — $CONHCH_2CH_2$ — $SO_2NHCONH$ — ; OCH_3

The molecular weight is 493.99. The aqueous solubility of Diaβeta increases with pH as a result of salt formation.

CLINICAL PHARMACOLOGY

Diaβeta appears to lower the blood glucose acutely by stimulating the release of insulin from the pancreas, an effect dependent upon functioning beta cells in the pancreatic islets. The mechanism by which Diaβeta lowers blood glucose during long-term administration has not been clearly established.

With chronic administration in Type II diabetic patients, the blood glucose lowering effect persists despite a gradual decline in the insulin secretory response to the drug. Extrapancreatic effects may play a part in the mechanism of action of oral sulfonylurea hypoglycemic drugs.

In addition to its blood glucose lowering actions, Diaβeta produces a mild diuresis by enhancement of renal free water clearance. Clinical experience to date indicates an extremely low incidence of disulfiram-like reactions in patients while taking Diaβeta.

Pharmacokinetics

Single-dose studies with Diaβeta in normal subjects demonstrate significant absorption within one hour, peak drug levels at about four hours, and low but detectable levels at twenty-four hours. Mean serum levels of glyburide, as reflected by areas under the serum concentration-time curve, increase in proportion to corresponding increases in dose. Multiple-dose studies with Diaβeta in diabetic patients demonstrate drug level concentration-time curves similar to single-dose studies, indicating no build-up of drug in tissue depots. The decrease of glyburide in the serum of normal healthy individuals is biphasic, the terminal half-life being about 10 hours. In single-dose studies in fasting normal subjects, the degree and duration of blood glucose lowering is proportional to the dose administered and to the area under the drug level concentration-time curve. The blood glucose lowering effect persists for 24 hours following single morning doses in non-fasting diabetic patients. Under conditions of repeated administration in diabetic patients, however, there is no reliable correlation between blood drug levels and fasting blood glucose levels. A one-year study of diabetic patients treated with Diaβeta showed no reliable correlation between administered dose and serum drug level.

The major metabolite of Diaβeta is the 4-trans-hydroxy derivative. A second metabolite, the 3-cis-hydroxy derivative, also occurs. These metabolites contribute no significant hypoglycemic action since they are only weakly active (1/400th and 1/40th, respectively, as glyburide) in rabbits.

Diaβeta is excreted as metabolites in the bile and urine, approximately 50% by each route. This dual excretory pathway is qualitatively different from that of other sulfonylureas, which are excreted primarily in the urine.

Sulfonylurea drugs are extensively bound to serum proteins. Displacement from protein binding sites by other drugs may lead to enhanced hypoglycemic action. In vitro, the protein binding exhibited by Diaβeta is predominantly non-ionic, whereas that of other sulfonylureas (chlorpropamide, tolbutamide, tolazamide) is predominantly ionic. Acidic drugs such as phenylbutazone, warfarin, and salicylates displace the ionic-binding sulfonylureas from serum proteins to a far greater extent than the non-ionic binding Diaβeta. It has not been shown that this difference in protein binding will result in fewer drug-drug interactions with Diaβeta in clinical use.

INDICATIONS AND USAGE

Diaβeta is indicated as an adjunct to diet to lower the blood glucose in patients with non-insulin-dependent diabetes mellitus (Type II) whose hyperglycemia cannot be controlled by diet alone.

In initiating treatment for non-insulin-dependent diabetes, diet should be emphasized as the primary form of treatment. Caloric restriction and weight loss are essential in the obese diabetic patient. Proper dietary management alone may be effective in controlling the blood glucose and symptoms of hyperglycemia. The importance of regular physical activity should also be stressed, and cardiovascular risk factors should be identified and corrective measures taken where possible.

If this treatment program fails to reduce symptoms and/or blood glucose, the use of an oral sulfonylurea or insulin should be considered. Use of Diaβeta must be viewed by both the physician and patient as a treatment in addition to diet, and not as a substitute for diet or as a convenient mechanism for avoiding dietary restraint. Furthermore, loss of blood glucose control on diet alone may be transient, thus requiring only short-term administration of Diaβeta.

During maintenance programs, Diaβeta should be discontinued if satisfactory lowering of blood glucose is no longer achieved. Judgments should be based on regular clinical and laboratory evaluations.

In considering the use of Diaβeta in asymptomatic patients, it should be recognized that controlling the blood glucose in non-insulin dependent diabetes has not been definitely established to be effective in preventing the long-term cardiovascular or neural complications of diabetes.

CONTRAINDICATIONS

Diaβeta is contraindicated in patients with:

1. Known hypersensitivity to the drug.
2. Diabetic ketoacidosis, with or without coma. This condition should be treated with insulin.

WARNINGS

SPECIAL WARNING ON INCREASED RISK OF CARDIOVASCULAR MORTALITY

The administration of oral hypoglycemic drugs has been reported to be associated with increased cardiovascular mortality as compared to treatment with diet alone or diet plus insulin. This warning is based on the study conducted by the University Group Diabetes Program (UGDP), a long-term prospective clinical trial designed to evaluate the effectiveness of glucose-lowering drugs in preventing or delaying vascular complications in patients with non-insulin-dependent diabetes. The study involved 823 patients who were randomly assigned to one of four treatment groups (Diabetes 19 (supp. 2): 747-830, 1970).

UGDP reported that patients treated for 5 to 8 years with diet plus a fixed dose of tolbutamide (1.5 grams per day) had a rate of cardiovascular mortality approximately 2½ times that of patients treated with diet alone. A significant increase in total mortality was not observed, but the use of tolbutamide was discontinued based on the increase in cardiovascular mortality, thus limiting the opportunity for the study to show an increase in overall mortality. Despite controversy regarding the interpretation of these results, the findings of the UGDP study provide an adequate basis for this warning. The patient should be informed of the potential risks and advantages of Diaβeta and of alternative modes of therapy.

Although only one drug in the sulfonylurea class (tolbutamide) was included in this study, it is prudent from a safety standpoint to consider that this warning may also apply to other oral hypoglycemic drugs in this class, in view of their close similarities in mode of action and chemical structure.

PRECAUTIONS

General

Hypoglycemia: All sulfonylurea drugs are capable of producing severe hypoglycemia. Proper patient selection, dosage, and instructions are important to avoid hypoglycemic episodes. Renal or hepatic insufficiency may cause elevated blood levels of Diaβeta and the latter may also diminish gluconeogenic capacity, both of which increase the risk of serious hypoglycemic reactions. Elderly, debilitated or malnourished patients, and those with adrenal or pituitary insufficiency are particularly susceptible to the hypoglycemic action of glucose-lowering drugs. Hypoglycemia may be difficult to recognize in the elderly, and in people who are taking beta-adrenergic blocking drugs or other sympatholytic agents. Hypoglycemia is more likely to occur when caloric intake is deficient, after severe or prolonged exercise, when alcohol is ingested, or when more than one glucose-lowering drug is used. Loss of control of blood glucose: When a patient stabilized on any diabetic regimen is exposed to stress such as fever, trauma, infection, or surgery, a loss of control may occur. At such times, it may be necessary to discontinue Diaβeta and administer insulin.

The effectiveness of any oral hypoglycemic drug, including Diaβeta, in lowering blood glucose to a desired level decreases in many patients over a period of time, which may be due to progression of the severity of the diabetes or to diminished responsiveness to the drug. This phenomenon is known as secondary failure, to distinguish it from primary failure in which the drug is ineffective in an individual patient when first given.

Information for Patients

Patients should be informed of the potential risks and advantages of Diaβeta and of alternative modes of therapy. They should also be informed about the importance of adherence to dietary instructions, of a regular exercise program, and of regular testing of blood glucose.

The risks of hypoglycemia, its symptoms and treatment, and conditions that predispose to its development should be explained to patients and responsible family members. Primary and secondary failure should also be explained.

Laboratory Tests

Periodic fasting blood glucose measurements should be performed to monitor therapeutic response. A glycosylated hemoglobin determination should also be performed periodically.

Drug Interactions

The hypoglycemic action of sulfonylureas may be potentiated by certain drugs including nonsteroidal anti-inflammatory agents and other drugs that are highly protein bound, salicylates, sulfonamides, chloramphenicol, probenecid, monoamine oxidase inhibitors and beta adrenergic blocking agents. When such drugs are administered to a patient receiving Diaβeta, the patient should be observed closely for hypoglycemia. When such drugs are withdrawn from a patient receiving Diaβeta, the patient should be observed closely for loss of control.

A possible interaction between glyburide and fluoroquinolone antibiotics has been reported resulting in a potentiation of the hypoglycemic action of glyburide. The mechanism for this interaction is not known.

Possible interactions between glyburide and coumarin derivatives have been reported that may either potentiate or weaken the effects of coumarin derivatives. The mechanism of these interactions is not known.

Certain drugs tend to produce hyperglycemia and may lead to loss of control. These drugs include the thiazides and other diuretics, corticosteroids, phenothiazines, thyroid products, estrogens, oral contraceptives, phenytoin, nicotinic acid, sympathomimetics, calcium channel blocking drugs, and isoniazid. When such drugs are administered to a patient receiving Diaβeta, the patient should be closely observed for loss of control. When such drugs are withdrawn from a patient receiving Diaβeta, the patient should be observed closely for hypoglycemia. A potential interaction between oral miconazole and oral hypoglycemic agents leading to severe hypoglycemia has been reported. Whether this interaction also occurs with the intravenous, topical or vaginal preparations of miconazole is not known.

Carcinogenesis, Mutagenesis, and Impairment of Fertility

Diaβeta is non-mutagenic when studied in the Salmonella microsome test (Ames test) and in the DNA damage/alkaline elution assay. Studies in rats at doses up to 300 mg/kg/day for 18 months showed no carcinogenic effects.

No drug related effects were noted in any of the criteria evaluated in the two year oncogenicity study of glyburide in mice.

Pregnancy

Teratogenic Effects: Pregnancy Category C

Diaβeta has been shown to affect the maturation of the long bones (humerus and femur) in rat pups when given in doses 6250 times the maximum recommended human dose. These effects, which were seen during the period of lactation and not during organogenesis, are a shortening of the bones with effects to various structures of the long bones, especially in humerus and femur.

There are no adequate and well-controlled studies in pregnant women. Because animal reproduction studies are not always predictive of human response, Diaβeta should be used during pregnancy only if the potential benefit justifies the risk to the fetus. Because recent information suggests that abnormal blood glucose levels during pregnancy are associated with a higher incidence of congenital abnormalities, many experts recommend that insulin be used during pregnancy to maintain blood glucose levels as close to normal as possible.

Nonteratogenic Effects: Prolonged severe hypoglycemia (4 to 10 days) has been reported in neonates born to mothers who were receiving a sulfonylurea drug at the time of delivery. This has been reported more frequently with the use of agents with prolonged half-lives. If Diaβeta is used during pregnancy, it should be discontinued at least two weeks before the expected delivery date.

Nursing Mothers

Although it is not known whether Diaβeta is excreted in human milk, some sulfonylureas are known to be excreted in human milk. Because the potential for hypoglycemia in nursing infants may exist, a decision should be made whether to discontinue nursing or to discontinue administering the drug, taking into account the importance of the drug to the mother. If Diaβeta is discontinued and if diet alone is inadequate for controlling blood glucose, insulin therapy should be considered.

Pediatric Use

Safety and effectiveness in pediatric patients have not been established.

Geriatric Use

In US clinical studies of glyburide, 1406 of 2897 patients were ≥60 years and 515 patients were ≥70 years. Differences in safety and efficacy were not determined between these patients and younger patients, but greater sensitivity of some older individuals cannot be ruled out.

Elderly patients are particularly susceptible to hypoglycemic action of glucose-lowering drugs. Hypoglycemia may be difficult to recognize in the elderly (see PRECAUTIONS). The initial and maintenance dosing should be conservative to avoid hypoglycemic reactions.

In three published studies of 20 to 51 subjects each, mixed results were seen in comparing the pharmacokinetics of glyburide in elderly versus younger subjects. However, observed pharmacodynamic differences indicate the necessity for dosage titration to a specified therapeutic response.

This drug is known to be substantially excreted by the kidney, and the risk of toxic reactions to this drug may be greater in patients with impaired renal function. Because elderly patients are more likely to have decreased renal function, care should be taken in dose selection, and it may be useful to monitor renal function.

In elderly, debilitated, or malnourished patients, or in patients with renal or hepatic insufficiency, the initial dosing, dose increments, and maintenance dosage should be conservative to avoid hypoglycemic reactions. Hypoglycemia may be difficult to recognize in the elderly and in people who are taking beta-adrenergic blocking drugs or other sympatholytic agents. (See PRECAUTIONS, General; and DOSAGE AND ADMINISTRATION.)

ADVERSE REACTIONS

Hypoglycemia: See PRECAUTIONS and OVERDOSAGE Sections.

Gastrointestinal Reactions: Cholestatic jaundice and hepatitis may occur rarely; Diaβeta should be discontinued if this occurs. Liver function abnormalities, including isolated transaminase elevations, have been reported. Gastrointestinal disturbances, e.g., nausea, epigastric fullness, and heartburn, are the most common reactions and occur in 1.8% of treated patients. They tend to be dose-related and may disappear when dosage is reduced.

Dermatologic Reactions: Allergic skin reactions, e.g., pruritus, erythema, urticaria, and morbilliform or maculopapular eruptions, occur in 1.5% of treated patients. These may be transient and may disappear despite continued use of Diaβeta; if skin reactions persist, the drug should be discontinued.

Porphyria cutanea tarda and photosensitivity reactions have been reported with sulfonylureas.

Hematologic Reactions: Leukopenia, agranulocytosis, thrombocytopenia, which occasionally may present as purpura, hemolytic anemia, aplastic anemia, and pancytopenia have been reported with sulfonylureas.

Metabolic Reactions: Hepatic porphyria reactions have been reported with sulfonylureas; however, these have not been reported with Diaβeta. Disulfiram-like reactions have been reported very rarely with Diaβeta. Cases of hyponatremia have been reported with glyburide and all other sulfonylureas, most often in patients who are on other medications or have medical conditions known to cause hyponatremia or increase release of antidiuretic hormone. The syndrome of inappropriate antidiuretic hormone (SIADH) secretion has been reported with certain other sulfonylureas, and it has been suggested that these sulfonylureas may augment the peripheral (antidiuretic) action of ADH and/or increase release of ADH.

Other Reactions: Changes in accommodation and/or blurred vision have been reported with glyburide and other sulfonylureas. These are thought to be related to fluctuation in glucose levels.

In addition to dermatologic reactions, allergic reactions such as angioedema, arthralgia, myalgia and vasculitis have been reported.

OVERDOSAGE

Overdosage of sulfonylureas, including Diaβeta, can produce hypoglycemia. Mild hypoglycemic symptoms without loss of consciousness or neurologic findings should be treated aggressively with oral glucose and adjustments in drug dosage and/or meal patterns. Close monitoring should continue until the physician is assured that the patient is out of danger. Severe hypoglycemic reactions with coma, seizure, or other neurological impairment occur infrequently, but constitute medical emergencies requiring immediate hospitalization. If hypoglycemic coma is diagnosed or suspected, the patient should be given a rapid intravenous injection of concentrated (50%) glucose solution. This should be followed by a continuous infusion of a more dilute (10%) glucose solution at a rate that will maintain the blood glucose at a level above 100 mg/mL. Patients should be closely monitored for a minimum of 24 to 48 hours, since hypoglycemia may recur after apparent clinical recovery.

DOSAGE AND ADMINISTRATION

There is no fixed dosage regimen for the management of diabetes mellitus with Diaβeta or any other hypoglycemic agent. The patient's fasting blood glucose must be measured periodically to determine the minimum effective dose for the patient; to detect primary failure, i.e., inadequate lowering of blood glucose at the maximum recommended dose of medication; and to detect secondary failure, i.e., loss of adequate blood glucose lowering response after an initial period of effectiveness. Periodic glycosylated hemoglobin determinations should be performed.

Short-term administration of Diaβeta may be sufficient during periods of transient loss of control in patients usually controlled well on diet.

1. Usual Starting Dose

The usual starting dose of Diaβeta as initial therapy is 2.5 to 5 mg daily, administered with breakfast or the first main meal. Those patients who may be more sensitive to hypoglycemic drugs should be started at 1.25 mg daily. (See PRECAUTIONS Section for patients at increased risk). Failure to follow an appropriate dosage regimen may precipitate hypoglycemia. Patients who do not adhere to their prescribed dietary and drug regimen are more prone to exhibit unsatisfactory response to therapy.

Transfer of patients from other oral antidiabetic regimens to Diaβeta should be done conservatively and the initial daily dose should be 2.5 to 5 mg. When transferring patients from oral hypoglycemic agents other than chlorpropamide, to Diaβeta, no transition period and no initial priming dose is necessary. When transferring patients from chlorpropamide, particular care should be exercised during the first two weeks because the prolonged retention of chlorpropamide in the body and subsequent overlapping drug effects may provoke hypoglycemia.

Bioavailability studies have demonstrated that Glynase® PresTab® Tablets 3 mg are not bioequivalent to Diaβeta Tablets 5 mg. Therefore, these products are not substitutable and patients should be retitrated if transferred.

Some Type II diabetic patients being treated with insulin may respond satisfactorily to Diaβeta. If the insulin dose is less than 20 units daily, substitution of Diaβeta 2.5 to 5 mg as a single daily dose may be tried. If the insulin dose is between 20 and 40 units daily, the patient may be placed directly on Diaβeta 5 mg daily as a single dose. If the insulin dose is more than 40 units daily, a transition period is required for conversion to Diaβeta. In these patients, insulin dosage is decreased by 50% and Diaβeta 5 mg daily is started. Please refer to Usual Maintenance Dose for further explanation.

2. Usual Maintenance Dose

The usual maintenance dose is in the range of 1.25 to 20 mg daily, which may be given as a single dose or in divided doses (See Dosage Interval Section). Dosage increases should be made in increments of no more than 2.5 mg at weekly intervals based upon the patient's blood glucose response.

No exact dosage relationship exists between Diaβeta and the other oral hypoglycemic agents. Although patients may be transferred from the maximum dose of other sulfonylureas, the maximum starting dose of 5 mg of Diaβeta should be observed. A maintenance dose of 5 mg Diaβeta provides approximately the same degree of blood glucose control as 250 to 375 mg chlorpropamide, 250 to 375 mg tolazamide, 500 to 750 mg acetohexamide, or 1000 to 1500 mg tolbutamide.

When transferring patients receiving more than 40 units of insulin daily, they may be started on a daily dose of Diaβeta 5 mg concomitantly with a 50% reduction in insulin dose. Progressive withdrawal of insulin and increase of Diaβeta in increments of 1.25 to 2.5 mg every 2 to 10 days is then carried out. During this conversion period when both insulin and Diaβeta are being used, hypoglycemia may rarely occur. During insulin withdrawal, patients should self-test their blood for glucose and their urine for acetone at least 3 times daily and report results to their physician. Self-testing of urinary glucose is a less desirable alternative. The appearance of persistent acetonuria with glycosuria indicates that the patient is a Type I diabetic who requires insulin therapy.

3. Maximum Dose

Daily doses of more than 20 mg are not recommended.

4. Dosage Interval

Once-a-day therapy is usually satisfactory, based upon usual meal patterns and a 10 hour half-life of Diaβeta. Some patients, particularly those receiving more than 10 mg daily, may have a more satisfactory response with twice-a-day dosage.

In elderly patients, debilitated or malnourished patients, and patients with impaired renal or hepatic function, the

Continued on next page

Diaβeta—Cont.

initial and maintenance dosing should be conservative to avoid hypoglycemic reactions. (See PRECAUTIONS Section.)

HOW SUPPLIED

Diaβeta (glyburide USP) tablets are available in the following strengths and package sizes:

1.25 mg (peach oblong, scored tablets with beveled edges, either imprinted with "Dia β" on one side, or with "Hoechst" on one side and "Dia β" on the other side).

Bottles of 50 (NDC 0039-0053-05)

2.5 mg (pink oblong, scored tablets with beveled edges, either imprinted with "Dia β" on one side, or with "Hoechst" on one side and "Dia β" on the other side).

Bottles of 100 (NDC 0039-0051-10)
Bottles of 500 (NDC 0039-0051-50)

5 mg (green oblong, scored tablets with beveled edges, either imprinted with "Dia β" on one side, or with "Hoechst" on one side and "Dia β" on the other side).

Bottles of 100 (NDC 0039-0052-10)
Bottles of 500 (NDC 0039-0052-50)
Bottles of 1000 (NDC 0039-0052-70)

Store at 25°C (77°F); excursions permitted to 15–30°C (59–86°F) [See USP Controlled Room Temperature].
Dispense in well-closed containers with safety closures.

Rev. April 2004

Manufactured by:
Patheon Pharmaceuticals Inc.
Cincinnati, OH 45215 USA
Manufactured for:
Aventis Pharmaceuticals NJ
Bridgewater, NJ 08807 USA
www.aventis-us.com

Glynase and PresTab are registered trademarks of The Upjohn Company

Shown in Product Identification Guide, page 307

KETEK™ ℞

[kē-tĕk]

(telithromycin) Tablets

Prescribing Information as of March 2004

To reduce the development of drug-resistant bacteria and maintain the effectiveness of KETEK and other antibacterial drugs, KETEK should be used only to treat infections that are proven or strongly suspected to be caused by bacteria.

DESCRIPTION

KETEK™ tablets contain telithromycin, a semisynthetic antibacterial in the ketolide class for oral administration. Chemically, telithromycin is designated as Erythromycin, 3-de[(2,6-dideoxy-3-C-methyl-3-O-methyl-α-L-ribo-hexopyranosyl)oxy]-11,12-dideoxy-6-O-methyl-3-oxo-12,11-[oxycarbonyl[[4-[4-(3-pyridinyl)-1H-imidazol-1-yl]butyl]imino]]-.

Telithromycin, a ketolide, differs chemically from the macrolide group of antibacterials by the lack of α-L-cladinose at position 3 of the erythronolide A ring, resulting in a 3-keto function. It is further characterized by a C11-12 carbamate substituted by an imidazolyl and pyridyl ring through a butyl chain. Its empirical formula is $C_{43}H_{65}N_5O_{10}$ and its molecular weight is 812.03.

Telithromycin is a white to off-white crystalline powder. The following represents the chemical structure of telithromycin.

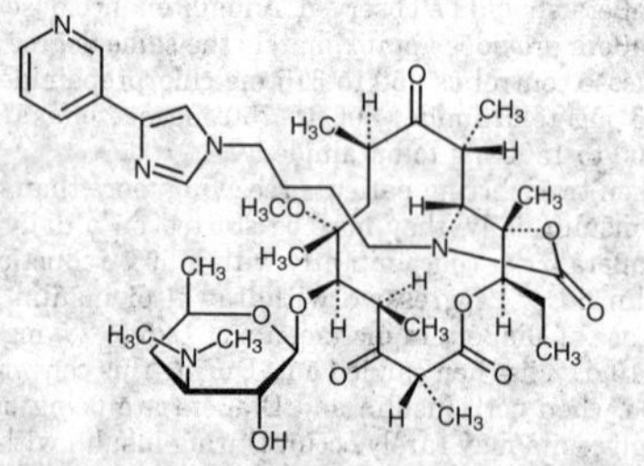

KETEK tablets are light-orange, oval, film-coated tablets, each containing 400 mg telithromycin, plus the following inactive ingredients: cornstarch, croscarmellose sodium, hypromellose, lactose monohydrate, magnesium stearate, microcrystalline cellulose, polyethylene glycol, povidone, red ferric oxide, talc, titanium dioxide, and yellow ferric oxide.

CLINICAL PHARMACOLOGY

Pharmacokinetics

Absorption:

Following oral administration, telithromycin reached maximal concentration at about 1 hour (0.5 - 4 hours). It has an absolute bioavailability of 57% in both young and elderly subjects.

The rate and extent of absorption are unaffected by food intake, thus KETEK tablets can be given without regard to food.

In healthy adult subjects, peak plasma telithromycin concentrations of approximately 2 μg/mL are attained at a median of 1 hour after an 800-mg oral dose.

Steady-state plasma concentrations are reached within 2 to 3 days of once daily dosing with telithromycin 800 mg. Following oral dosing, the mean terminal elimination half-life of telithromycin is 10 hours.

The pharmacokinetics of telithromycin after administration of single and multiple (7 days) once daily 800-mg doses to healthy adult subjects are shown in Table 1.

Table 1

Parameter	Mean (SD) Single dose (n=18)	Mean (SD) Multiple dose (n=18)
C_{max}(μg/mL)	1.9 (0.80)	2.27 (0.71)
T_{max}(h)*	1.0 (0.5-4.0)	1.0 (0.5-3.0)
$AUC_{(0\text{-}24)}$ (μg.h/mL)	8.25 (2.6)	12.5 (5.4)
Terminal $t_{1/2}$ (h)	7.16 (1.3)	9.81 (1.9)
C_{24h}(μg/mL)	0.03 (0.013)	0.07 (0.051)

* Median (min-max) values
SD=Standard deviation
C_{max}=Maximum plasma concentration
T_{max}=Time to C_{max}
AUC=Area under concentration vs. time curve
$t_{1/2}$=Terminal plasma half-life
C_{24h} =Plasma concentration at 24 hours post-dose

In a patient population, mean peak and trough plasma concentrations were 2.9 μg/mL (±1.55), (n=219) and 0.2 μg/mL (±0.22), (n=204), respectively, after 3 to 5 days of KETEK 800 mg once daily.

Distribution: Total *in vitro* protein binding is approximately 60% to 70% and is primarily due to human serum albumin.

Protein binding is not modified in elderly subjects and in patients with hepatic impairment.

The volume of distribution of telithromycin after intravenous infusion is 2.9 L/kg.

Telithromycin concentrations in bronchial mucosa, epithelial lining fluid, and alveolar macrophages after 800 mg once daily dosing for 5 days in patients are displayed in Table 2.

[See table 2 below]

Telithromycin concentration in white blood cells exceeds the concentration in plasma and is eliminated more slowly from white blood cells than from plasma. Mean white blood cell concentrations of telithromycin peaked at 72.1 μg/mL at 6 hours, and remained at 14.1 μg/mL 24 hours after 5 days of repeated dosing of 600 mg once daily. After 10 days, repeated dosing of 600 mg once daily, white blood cell concentrations remained at 8.9 μg/mL 48 hours after the last dose.

Metabolism: In total, metabolism accounts for approximately 70% of the dose. In plasma, the main circulating compound after administration of an 800-mg radiolabeled dose was parent compound, representing 56.7% of the total radioactivity. The main metabolite represented 12.6% of the AUC of telithromycin. Three other plasma metabolites were quantified, each representing 3% or less of the AUC of telithromycin.

It is estimated that approximately 50% of its metabolism is mediated by CYP 450 3A4 and the remaining 50% is CYP 450-independent.

Elimination: The systemically available telithromycin is eliminated by multiple pathways as follows: 7% of the dose is excreted unchanged in feces by biliary and/or intestinal secretion; 13% of the dose is excreted unchanged in urine by renal excretion; and 37% of the dose is metabolized by the liver.

Special populations

Gender: There was no significant difference between males and females in mean AUC, C_{max}, and elimination half-life in two studies; one in 18 healthy young volunteers (18 to 40 years of age) and the other in 14 healthy elderly volunteers (65 to 92 years of age), given single and multiple once daily doses of 800 mg of KETEK.

Hepatic insufficiency: In a single-dose study (800 mg) in 12 patients and a multiple-dose study (800 mg) in 13 patients with mild to severe hepatic insufficiency (Child Pugh Class A, B and C), the C_{max}, AUC and $t_{1/2}$ of telithromycin were similar to those obtained in age- and sex-matched healthy subjects. In both studies, an increase in renal elimination was observed in hepatically impaired patients indicating that this pathway may compensate for some of the decrease in metabolic clearance. No dosage adjustment is recommended due to hepatic impairment. (See **PRECAUTIONS, General** and **DOSAGE AND ADMINISTRATION.**)

Renal insufficiency: In a multiple-dose study, 36 subjects with varying degrees of renal impairment received 400 mg, 600 mg, or 800 mg KETEK once daily for 5 days. There was a 1.4-fold increase in $C_{max,ss}$, and a 1.9-fold increase in AUC $(0\text{-}24)_{ss}$ at 800 mg multiple doses in the severely renally impaired group (CL_{CR} < 30 mL/min) compared to healthy volunteers. Renal excretion may serve as a compensatory elimination pathway for telithromycin in situations where metabolic clearance is impaired. Patients with severe renal impairment are prone to conditions that may impair their metabolic clearance.

In a single-dose study in patients with end-stage renal failure on hemodialysis (n=10), the mean C_{max} and AUC values were similar to normal healthy subjects when KETEK was administered 2 hours post-dialysis. However, the effect of dialysis on removing telithromycin from the body has not been studied.

At present, no dose has been established in severely renal-impaired patients including those who need dialysis. (See **DOSAGE AND ADMINISTRATION.**)

Multiple insufficiency: The effects of co-administration of ketoconazole in 12 subjects (age ≥ 60 years), with impaired renal function were studied (CL_{CR}=24 to 80 mL/min). In this study, when severe renal insufficiency (CL_{CR} < 30 mL/min, n=2) and concomitant impairment of CYP 3A4 metabolism pathway were present, telithromycin exposure (AUC (0-24) was increased by approximately 4- to 5-fold compared with the exposure in healthy subjects with normal renal function receiving telithromycin alone. In the presence of severe renal impairment (CL_{CR} < 30 mL/min), no dose has been established.

Geriatric: Pharmacokinetic data show that there is an increase of 1.4-fold in exposure (AUC) in 20 patients ≥ 65 years of age with community acquired pneumonia in a Phase III study, and a 2.0-fold increase in exposure (AUC) in 14 subjects ≥ 65 years of age as compared with subjects less than 65 years of age in a Phase I study. No dosage adjustment is required based on age alone.

Drug-drug interactions

Studies were performed to evaluate the effect of CYP 3A4 inhibitors on telithromycin and the effect of telithromycin on drugs that are substrates of CYP 3A4 and CYP 2D6. In addition, drug interaction studies were conducted with several other concomitantly prescribed drugs.

CYP 3A4 inhibitors:

Itraconazole: A multiple-dose interaction study with itraconazole showed that C_{max} of telithromycin was increased by 22% and AUC by 54%.

Ketoconazole: A multiple-dose interaction study with ketoconazole showed that C_{max} of telithromycin was increased by 51% and AUC by 95%.

Grapefruit juice: When telithromycin was given with 240 mL of grapefruit juice after an overnight fast to healthy subjects, the pharmacokinetics of telithromycin were not affected.

CYP 3A4 substrates:

Cisapride: Steady-state peak plasma concentrations of cisapride (an agent with the potential to increase QT interval) were increased by 95% when co-administered with repeated doses of telithromycin, resulting in significant increases in QTc. (See **CONTRAINDICATIONS.**)

Simvastatin: When simvastatin was co-administered with telithromycin, there was a 5.3-fold increase in simvastatin C_{max}, an 8.9-fold increase in simvastatin AUC, a 15-fold increase in the simvastatin active metabolite C_{max}, and a 12-fold increase in the simvastatin active metabolite AUC. (See **PRECAUTIONS.**)

In another study, when simvastatin and telithromycin were administered 12 hours apart, there was a 3.4-fold increase in simvastatin C_{max}, a 4.0-fold increase in simvastatin AUC, a 3.2-fold increase in the active metabolite C_{max}, and a 4.3-fold increase in the active metabolite AUC. (See **PRECAUTIONS.**)

Table 2

	Hours post-dose	Mean concentration (μg/mL) Tissue or fluid	Mean concentration (μg/mL) Plasma	Tissue/ Plasma Ratio
Bronchial mucosa	2	3.88*	1.86	2.11
	12	1.41*	0.23	6.33
	24	0.78*	0.08	12.11
Epithelial lining fluid	2	14.89	1.86	8.57
	12	3.27	0.23	13.8
	24	0.84	0.08	14.41
Alveolar macrophages	2	65	1.07	55
	8	100	0.605	180
	24	41	0.073	540

*Units in mg/kg

Table 3. Susceptibility Test Result Interpretive Criteria for Telithromycin

Pathogen	Minimal Inhibitory Concentrations (μg/mL)			Disk Diffusion (zone diameters in mm)		
	S	I	R[a]	S	I	R[a]
Staphylococcus aureus	≤ 0.25			≥ 22		
Streptococcus pneumoniae	≤ 1	2	≥ 4	≥ 19	16–18	≤ 15
Haemophilus influenzae	≤ 4	8	≥ 16	≥ 15	12–14	≤ 11

[a] The current absence of data on resistant isolates precludes defining any category other than "Susceptible". If strains yield MIC results other than susceptible, they should be submitted to a reference laboratory for further testing.

Midazolam: Concomitant administration of telithromycin with intravenous or oral midazolam resulted in 2- and 6-fold increases, respectively, in the AUC of midazolam due to inhibition of CYP 3A4-dependent metabolism of midazolam. (See **PRECAUTIONS**.)

CYP 2D6 substrates:

Paroxetine: There was no pharmacokinetic effect on paroxetine when telithromycin was co-administered.

Metoprolol: When metoprolol was co-administered with telithromycin, there was an increase of approximately 38% on the C_{max} and AUC of metoprolol, however, there was no effect on the elimination half-life of metoprolol. Telithromycin exposure is not modified with concomitant single-dose administration of metoprolol. (See **PRECAUTIONS, Drug interactions.**)

Other drug interactions:

Digoxin: The plasma peak and trough levels of digoxin were increased by 73% and 21%, respectively, in healthy volunteers when co-administered with telithromycin. However, trough plasma concentrations of digoxin (when equilibrium between plasma and tissue concentrations has been achieved) ranged from 0.74 to 2.17 ng/mL. There were no significant changes in ECG parameters and no signs of digoxin toxicity. (See **PRECAUTIONS.**)

Theophylline: When theophylline was co-administered with repeated doses of telithromycin, there was an increase of approximately 16% and 17% on the steady-state C_{max} and AUC of theophylline. Co-administration of theophylline may worsen gastrointestinal side effects such as nausea and vomiting, especially in female patients. It is recommended that telithromycin should be taken with theophylline 1 hour apart to decrease the likelihood of gastrointestinal side effects.

Sotalol: Telithromycin has been shown to decrease the C_{max} and AUC of sotalol by 34% and 20%, respectively, due to decreased absorption.

Warfarin: When co-administered with telithromycin, there were no pharmacodynamic or pharmacokinetic effects on racemic warfarin in healthy subjects.

Oral contraceptives: When oral contraceptives containing ethinyl estradiol and levonorgestrel were co-administered with telithromycin, the steady-state AUC of ethinyl estradiol did not change and the steady-state AUC of levonorgestrel was increased by 50%. The pharmacokinetic/pharmacodynamic study showed that telithromycin did not interfere with the antiovulatory effect of oral contraceptives containing ethinyl estradiol and levonorgestrel.

Ranitidine, antacid: There was no clinically relevant pharmacokinetic interaction of ranitidine or antacids containing aluminum and magnesium hydroxide on telithromycin.

Rifampin: During concomitant administration of rifampin and KETEK in repeated doses, C_{max} and AUC of telithromycin were decreased by 79%, and 86%, respectively. (See **PRECAUTIONS, Drug Interactions.**)

Microbiology

Telithromycin belongs to the ketolide class of antibacterials and is structurally related to the macrolide family of antibiotics. Telithromycin concentrates in phagocytes where it exhibits activity against intracellular respiratory pathogens. *In vitro,* telithromycin has been shown to demonstrate concentration-dependent bactericidal activity against isolates of *Streptococcus pneumoniae* (including multi-drug resistant isolates [MDRSP*]).

*MDRSP=Multi-drug resistant *Streptococcus pneumoniae* includes isolates known as PRSP (penicillin-resistant *Streptococcus pneumoniae*), and are isolates resistant to two or more of the following antimicrobials: penicillin, 2nd generation cephalosporins (e.g., cefuroxime), macrolides, tetracyclines, and trimethoprim/sulfamethoxazole.

Mechanism of action

Telithromycin blocks protein synthesis by binding to domains II and V of 23S rRNA of the 50S ribosomal subunit. By binding at domain II, telithromycin retains activity against gram-positive cocci (e.g., *Streptococcus pneumoniae*) in the presence of resistance mediated by methylases (*erm* genes) that alter the domain V binding site of telithromycin. Telithromycin may also inhibit the assembly of nascent ribosomal units.

Mechanism of resistance

Staphylococcus aureus and *Streptococcus pyogenes* with the constitutive macrolide-lincosamide-streptogramin B ($cMLS_B$) phenotype are resistant to telithromycin.

Mutants of *Streptococcus pneumoniae* derived in the laboratory by serial passage in subinhibitory concentrations of telithromycin have demonstrated resistance based on L22 riboprotein mutations (telithromycin MICs are elevated but still within the susceptible range), one of two reported mutations affecting the L4 riboprotein, and production of K-peptide. The clinical significance of these laboratory mutants is not known.

Cross resistance

Telithromycin does not induce resistance through methylase gene expression in erythromycin-inducibly resistant bacteria, a function of its 3-keto moiety. Telithromycin has not been shown to induce resistance to itself.

List of Microorganisms

Telithromycin has been shown to be active against most strains of the following microorganisms, both *in vitro* and in clinical settings as described in the **INDICATIONS AND USAGE** section.

Aerobic gram-positive microorganisms

Staphylococcus aureus (methicillin and erythromycin susceptible isolates only)

Streptococcus pneumoniae (including multi-drug resistant isolates [MDRSP*])

*MDRSP=Multi-drug resistant *Streptococcus pneumoniae* includes isolates known as PRSP (penicillin-resistant *S. pneumoniae*), and are isolates resistant to two or more of the following antimicrobials: penicillin, 2nd generation cephalosporins (e.g., cefuroxime), macrolides, tetracyclines, and trimethoprim/sulfamethoxazole.

Aerobic gram-negative microorganisms

Haemophilus influenzae

Moraxella catarrhalis

Other microorganisms

Chlamydophila (Chlamydia) pneumoniae

Mycoplasma pneumoniae

The following *in vitro* data are available, **but their clinical significance is unknown.**

At least 90% of the following microorganisms exhibit *in vitro* minimum inhibitory concentrations (MICs) less than or equal to the susceptible breakpoint for telithromycin. However, the safety and efficacy of telithromycin in treating clinical infections due to these microorganisms have not been established in adequate and well-controlled clinical trials.

Aerobic gram-positive microorganisms

Streptococcus pyogenes (erythromycin susceptible isolates only)

Streptococci (Lancefield groups C and G)

Viridans group streptococci

Anaerobic bacteria

Prevotella bivia

Prevotella intermedia

Peptostreptococcus spp.

Other microorganisms

Legionella pneumophila

Susceptibility Test Methods

When available, the clinical microbiology laboratory should provide cumulative results of *in vitro* susceptibility test results for antimicrobial drugs used in local hospitals and practice areas to the physician as periodic reports that describe the susceptibility profile of nosocomial and community-acquired pathogens. These reports should aid the physician in selecting the most effective antimicrobial.

Dilution techniques:

Quantitative methods are used to determine antimicrobial minimum inhibitory concentrations (MICs). These MICs provide estimates of the susceptibility of bacteria to antibacterial compounds. The MICs should be determined using a standardized procedure. Standardized procedures are based on dilution methods (broth or agar dilution)[1,3] or equivalent with standardized inoculum and concentrations of telithromycin powder. The MIC values should be interpreted according to criteria provided in Table 3.

Diffusion techniques:

Quantitative methods that require measurement of zone diameters also provide reproducible estimates of the susceptibility of bacteria to antibiotics. One such standardized procedure[2,3] requires the use of standardized inoculum concentrations. This procedure uses paper disks impregnated with 15 μg telithromycin to test the susceptibility of microorganisms to telithromycin. Disc diffusion zone sizes should be interpreted according to criteria in Table 3.

[See table 3 above]

A report of "Susceptible" indicates that the antimicrobial is likely to inhibit growth of the pathogen if the antibacterial compound in the blood reaches the concentrations usually achievable. A report of "Intermediate" indicates that the result should be considered equivocal, and, if the microorganism is not fully susceptible to alternative, clinically feasible drugs, the test should be repeated. This category implies possible clinical applicability in body sites where the drug is physiologically concentrated or in situations where high dosage of drug can be used. This category also provides a buffer zone that prevents small uncontrolled technical factors from causing major discrepancies in interpretation. A report of "Resistant" indicates that the antimicrobial is not likely to inhibit growth of the pathogen if the antimicrobial compound in the blood reaches the concentrations usually achievable; other therapy should be selected.

Quality control:

Standardized susceptibility test procedures require the use of quality control microorganisms to determine the performance of the test procedures[1,2,3]. Standard telithromycin powder should provide the MIC ranges for the quality control organisms in Table 4. For the disk diffusion technique, the 15-μg telithromycin disk should provide the zone diameter ranges for the quality control organisms in Table 4.

Table 4. Acceptable Quality Control Ranges for Telithromycin

QC Strain	Minimal Inhibitory Concentrations (μg/mL)	Disk Diffusion (Zone diameters in mm)
Staphylococcus aureus ATCC® 29213	0.06-0.25	Not Applicable
Staphylococcus aureus ATCC 25923	Not Applicable	24-30
Streptococcus pneumoniae ATCC 49619	0.004-0.03	27-33
Haemophilus influenzae ATCC 49247	1.0-4.0	17-23

ATCC = American Type Culture Collection

INDICATIONS AND USAGE

KETEK tablets are indicated for the treatment of infections caused by susceptible strains of the designated microorganisms in the conditions listed below for patients 18 years old and above.

Acute bacterial exacerbation of chronic bronchitis due to *Streptococcus pneumoniae, Haemophilus influenzae*, or *Moraxella catarrhalis*.

Acute bacterial sinusitis due to *Streptococcus pneumoniae, Haemophilus influenzae, Moraxella catarrhalis*, or *Staphylococcus aureus*.

Community-acquired pneumonia (of mild to moderate severity) due to *Streptococcus pneumoniae*, (including multi-drug resistant isolates [MDRSP*]), *Haemophilus influenzae, Moraxella catarrhalis, Chlamydophila pneumoniae*, or *Mycoplasma pneumoniae*.

*MDRSP, Multi-drug resistant *Streptococcus pneumoniae* includes isolates known as PRSP (penicillin-resistant *Streptococcus pneumoniae*), and are isolates resistant to two or more of the following antibiotics: penicillin, 2nd generation cephalosporins, e.g., cefuroxime, macrolides, tetracyclines and trimethoprim/sulfamethoxazole.

To reduce the development of drug-resistant bacteria and maintain the effectiveness of KETEK and other antibacterial drugs, KETEK should be used only to treat infections that are proven or strongly suspected to be caused by susceptible bacteria. When culture and susceptibility information are available, they should be considered in selecting or modifying antibacterial therapy. In the absence of such data, local epidemiology and susceptibility patterns may contribute to the empiric selection of therapy.

CONTRAINDICATIONS

KETEK is contraindicated in patients with a history of hypersensitivity to telithromycin and/or any components of KETEK tablets, or any macrolide antibiotic.

Concomitant administration of KETEK with cisapride or pimozide is contraindicated. (See **CLINICAL PHARMACOLOGY, Drug-drug Interactions** and **PRECAUTIONS.**)

WARNINGS

Pseudomembranous colitis has been reported with nearly all antibacterial agents, including telithromycin, and may range in severity from mild to life-threatening. Therefore, it is important to consider this diagnosis in patients who present with diarrhea subsequent to the administration of any antibacterial agents.

Treatment with antibacterial agents alters the flora of the colon and may permit overgrowth of clostridia. Studies indicate that toxin-producing strains of *Clostridium difficile* are the primary cause of "antibiotic-associated colitis".

After the diagnosis of pseudomembranous colitis has been established, therapeutic measures should be initiated. Mild cases of pseudomembranous colitis usually respond to drug discontinuation alone. In moderate to severe cases, consideration should be given to management with fluids and electrolytes, protein supplementation, and treatment with an antibacterial drug clinically effective against *C. difficile* colitis. (See **ADVERSE REACTIONS.**)

Telithromycin has the potential to prolong the QTc interval of the electrocardiogram in some patients. QTc prolongation may lead to an increased risk for ventricular arrhythmias, including torsades de pointes. Thus, telithromycin should be avoided in patients with congenital prolongation of the QTc interval, and in patients with ongoing proarrhythmic conditions such as uncorrected hypokalemia or hypomagnesemia, clinically significant bradycardia, and in patients receiving Class IA (e.g., quinidine and procainamide) or Class III (e.g., dofetilide) antiarrhythmic agents.

Continued on next page

Ketek—Cont.

No cardiovascular morbidity or mortality attributable to QTc prolongation occurred with telithromycin treatment in 4780 patients in clinical efficacy trials, including 204 patients having a prolonged QTc at baseline.
Exacerbations of myasthenia gravis have been reported in patients with myasthenia gravis treated with telithromycin. This has sometimes occurred within a few hours after intake of the first dose of telithromycin. Reports have included life-threatening acute respiratory failure with a rapid onset in patients with myasthenia gravis treated for respiratory tract infections with telithromycin. Telithromycin is not recommended in patients with myasthenia gravis unless no other therapeutic alternatives are available. If other therapeutic alternatives are not available, patients with myasthenia gravis taking telithromycin must be closely monitored. Patients must be advised that if they experience exacerbation of their symptoms, they should discontinue treatment of KETEK and immediately seek medical attention. Supportive measures should be instituted as medically necessary.

PRECAUTIONS

General

Prescribing KETEK in the absence of a proven or strongly suspected bacterial infection or a prophylactic indication is unlikely to provide benefit to the patient and increases the risk of the development of drug-resistant bacteria.
KETEK may cause visual disturbances particularly in slowing the ability to accommodate and the ability to release accommodation. Visual disturbances included blurred vision, difficulty focusing, and diplopia. Most events were mild to moderate; however, severe cases have been reported. Patients should be cautioned about the potential effects of these visual disturbances on driving a vehicle, operating machinery or engaging in other potentially hazardous activities. (See **ADVERSE REACTIONS, CLINICAL STUDIES.**)
Hepatic dysfunction, including increased liver enzymes and hepatitis, with or without jaundice, has been reported with the use of KETEK. These events were generally reversible. Caution should be used in patients with a previous history of hepatitis/jaundice associated with the use of KETEK. (See **ADVERSE REACTIONS, Liver and biliary system.**)
Telithromycin is principally excreted via the liver and kidney. Telithromycin may be administered without dosage adjustment in the presence of hepatic impairment. In the presence of severe renal impairment (CL_{CR} < 30 mL/min), the dose of KETEK has not been established. (See **DOSAGE AND ADMINISTRATION.**)

Information for patients

The following information and instructions should be communicated to the patient.
KETEK may cause problems with vision particularly when looking quickly between objects close by and objects far away. These events include blurred vision, difficulty focusing, and objects looking doubled. Most events were mild to moderate; however, severe cases have been reported. Problems with vision were reported as having occurred after any dose during treatment, but most occurred following the first or second dose. These problems lasted several hours and in some patients came back with the next dose. (See **PRECAUTIONS, General** and **ADVERSE REACTIONS.**)
If visual difficulties occur:

- patients should avoid driving a motor vehicle, operating heavy machinery, or engaging in otherwise hazardous activities.
- avoiding quick changes in viewing between objects in the distance and objects nearby may help to decrease the effects of these visual difficulties.
- patients should contact their physician if these visual difficulties interfere with their daily activities.

Patients should also be advised:

- that antibacterial drugs including KETEK should only be used to treat bacterial infections. They do not treat viral infections (e.g., the common cold). When KETEK is prescribed to treat a bacterial infection, patients should be told that although it is common to feel better early in the course of therapy, the medication should be taken exactly as directed. Skipping doses or not completing the full course of therapy may (1) decrease the effectiveness of the immediate treatment and (2) increase the likelihood that bacteria will develop resistance and will not be treatable by KETEK or other antibacterial drugs in the future.
- that KETEK has the potential to produce changes in the electrocardiogram (QTc interval prolongation) and that they should report any fainting occurring during drug treatment.
- that KETEK should be avoided in patients receiving Class 1A (e.g., quinidine, procainamide) or Class III (e.g., dofetilide) antiarrhythmic agents.
- to inform their physician of any personal or family history of QTc prolongation or proarrhythmic conditions such as uncorrected hypokalemia, or clinically significant bradycardia.
- that telithromycin is not recommended in patients with myasthenia gravis. Patients should inform their physician if they have myasthenia gravis.
- that simvastatin, lovastatin, or atorvastatin should be avoided in patients receiving KETEK. If KETEK is prescribed, therapy with simvastatin, lovastatin, or atorvastatin should be stopped during the course of treatment.
- that KETEK tablets can be taken with or without food.
- to inform their physician of any other medications taken concurrently with KETEK, including over-the-counter medications and dietary supplements.

Drug interactions

Telithromycin is a strong inhibitor of the cytochrome P450 3A4 system. Co-administration of KETEK tablets and a drug primarily metabolized by the cytochrome P450 3A4 enzyme system may result in increased plasma concentration of the drug co-administered with telithromycin that could increase or prolong both the therapeutic and adverse effects. Therefore, appropriate dosage adjustments may be necessary for the drug co-administered with telithromycin.
The use of KETEK is contraindicated with cisapride. (See **CONTRAINDICATIONS** and **CLINICAL PHARMACOLOGY, Drug-drug interactions.**)
The use of KETEK is contraindicated with pimozide. Although there are no studies looking at the interaction between KETEK and pimozide, there is a potential risk of increased pimozide plasma levels by inhibition of CYP 3A4 pathways by KETEK as with macrolides. (See **CONTRAINDICATIONS.**)
In a pharmacokinetic study, simvastatin levels were increased due to CYP 3A4 inhibition by telithromycin. (See **CLINICAL PHARMACOLOGY, Other drug interactions.**)
Similarly, an interaction may occur with lovastatin or atorvastatin, but not with pravastatin or fluvastatin. High levels of HMG-CoA reductase inhibitors increase the risk of myopathy. Use of simvastatin, lovastatin, or atorvastatin concomitantly with KETEK should be avoided. If KETEK is prescribed, therapy with simvastatin, lovastatin, or atorvastatin should be suspended during the course of treatment.
Monitoring of digoxin side effects or serum levels should be considered during concomitant administration of digoxin and KETEK. (See **CLINICAL PHARMACOLOGY, Drug-drug interactions.**)
Patients should be monitored with concomitant administration of midazolam and dosage adjustment of midazolam should be considered if necessary. Precaution should be used with other benzodiazepines, which are metabolized by CYP 3A4 and undergo a high first-pass effect (e.g., triazolam). (See **CLINICAL PHARMACOLOGY, Drug-drug interactions.**)

Table 5

All and Possibly Related Treatment-Emergent Adverse Events Reported in Controlled Phase III Clinical Studies (Percent Incidence)

Adverse Event*	All TEAEs		Possibly-Related TEAEs	
	KETEK	Comparator†	KETEK	Comparator†
	n= 2702	n= 2139	n= 2702	n= 2139
Diarrhea	10.8%	8.6%	10.0%	8.0%
Nausea	7.9%	4.6%	7.0%	4.1%
Headache	5.5%	5.8%	2.0%	2.5%
Dizziness (excl. vertigo)	3.7%	2.7%	2.8%	1.5%
Vomiting	2.9%	2.2%	2.4%	1.4%
Loose Stools	2.3%	1.5%	2.1%	1.4%
Dysgeusia	1.6%	3.6%	1.5%	3.6%

*Based on a frequency of all and possibly related treatment-emergent adverse events of ≥ 2% in KETEK or comparator groups.
†Includes comparators from all controlled Phase III studies.

Concomitant treatment of KETEK with rifampin, a CYP 3A4 inducer, should be avoided. Concomitant administration of other CYP 3A4 inducers such as phenytoin, carbamazepine, or phenobarbital is likely to result in subtherapeutic levels of telithromycin and loss of effect. (See **CLINICAL PHARMACOLOGY, Other drug interactions.**)
In patients treated with metoprolol for heart failure, the increased exposure to metoprolol, a CYP 2D6 substrate, may be of clinical importance. Therefore, co-administration of KETEK and metoprolol in patients with heart failure should be considered with caution. (See **CLINICAL PHARMACOLOGY, Drug-drug interactions.**)
No specific drug interaction studies have been performed to evaluate the following potential drug-drug interactions with KETEK. However, these drug interactions have been observed with macrolide products.

Drugs metabolized by the cytochrome P450 system such as carbamazepine, cyclosporine, tacrolimus, sirolimus, hexobarbital, and phenytoin: elevation of serum levels of these drugs may be observed when co-administered with telithromycin. As a result, increases or prolongation of the therapeutic and/or adverse effects of the concomitant drug may be observed.

Ergot alkaloid derivatives (such as ergotamine or dihydroergotamine): acute ergot toxicity characterized by severe peripheral vasospasm and dysesthesia has been reported when macrolide antibiotics were co-administered. Without further data, the co-administration of KETEK and these drugs is not recommended.

Laboratory test interactions

There are no reported laboratory test interactions.

Carcinogenesis, mutagenesis, impairment of fertility

Long-term studies in animals to determine the carcinogenic potential of KETEK have not been conducted.
Telithromycin showed no evidence of genotoxicity in four tests: gene mutation in bacterial cells, gene mutation in mammalian cells, chromosome aberration in human lymphocytes, and the micronucleus test in the mouse.
No evidence of impaired fertility in the rat was observed at doses estimated to be 0.61 times the human daily dose on a mg/m^2 basis. At doses of 1.8-3.6 times the human daily dose, at which signs of parental toxicity were observed, moderate reductions in fertility indices were noted in male and female animals treated with telithromycin.

Pregnancy

Teratogenic effects: Pregnancy Category C. Telithromycin was not teratogenic in the rat or rabbit. Reproduction studies have been performed in rats and rabbits, with effect on pre-post natal development studied in the rat. At doses estimated to be 1.8 times (900 mg/m^2) and 0.49 times (240 mg/m^2) the daily human dose of 800 mg (492 mg/m^2) in the rat and rabbit, respectively, no evidence of fetal terata was found. At doses higher than the 900 mg/m^2 and 240 mg/m^2 in rats and rabbits, respectively, maternal toxicity may have resulted in delayed fetal maturation. No adverse effects on prenatal and postnatal development of rat pups were observed at 1.5 times (750 $mg/m^2/d$) the daily human dose.
There are no adequate and well-controlled studies in pregnant women. Telithromycin should be used during pregnancy only if the potential benefit justifies the potential risk to the fetus.

Nursing mothers

Telithromycin is excreted in breast milk of rats. Telithromycin may also be excreted in human milk. Because many drugs are excreted in human milk, caution should be exercised when KETEK is administered to a nursing mother.

Pediatric use

The safety and effectiveness of KETEK in pediatric patients has not been established.

Geriatric use

In all Phase III clinical trials (n=4,780), KETEK was administered to 694 patients who were 65 years and older, including 231 patients who were 75 years and older. Efficacy and safety in elderly patients ≥ 65 years were generally similar to that observed in younger patients; however, greater sensitivity of some older individuals cannot be ruled out. No dosage adjustment is required based on age alone. (See **CLINICAL PHARMACOLOGY, Special populations, Geriatric** and **DOSAGE AND ADMINISTRATION.**)

ADVERSE REACTIONS

In Phase III clinical trials, 4,780 patients (n=2702 in controlled trials) received daily oral doses of KETEK 800 mg once daily for 5 days or 7 to 10 days. Most adverse events were mild to moderate in severity. In the combined Phase III studies, discontinuation due to treatment-emergent adverse events occurred in 4.4% of KETEK-treated patients and 4.3% of combined comparator-treated patients. Most discontinuations in the KETEK group were due to treatment-emergent adverse events in the gastrointestinal body system, primarily diarrhea (0.9% for KETEK vs. 0.7% for comparators), nausea (0.7% for KETEK vs. 0.5% for comparators).
All and possibly related treatment-emergent adverse events (TEAEs) occurring in controlled clinical studies in ≥ 2.0% of all patients are included below:
[See table 5 at left]
The following events judged by investigators to be at least possibly drug related were observed infrequently (≥ 0.2% and < 2%), in KETEK-treated patients in the controlled Phase III studies.
Gastrointestinal system: abdominal distension, dyspepsia, gastrointestinal upset, flatulence, constipation, gastroenteritis, gastritis, anorexia, oral candidiasis, glossitis, stomatitis, watery stools.

Table 6

Infection	Daily dose and route of administration	Frequency of administration	Duration of treatment
Acute bacterial exacerbation of chronic bronchitis	800 mg oral (2 tablets of 400 mg)	once daily	5 days
Acute bacterial sinusitis	800 mg oral (2 tablets of 400 mg)	once daily	5 days
Community-acquired pneumonia	800 mg oral (2 tablets of 400 mg)	once daily	7-10 days

Table 7. CAP: Clinical cure rate at post-therapy follow-up (17–24 days)

	Patients (n)		Clinical cure rate	
Controlled Studies	**KETEK**	**Comparator**	**KETEK**	**Comparator**
KETEK vs. clarithromycin 500 mg BID for 10 days	162	156	88.3%	88.5%
KETEK vs. trovafloxacin* 200 mg QD for 7 to 10 days	80	86	90.0%	94.2%
KETEK vs. amoxicillin 1000 mg TID for 10 days	149	152	94.6%	90.1%
KETEK for 7 days vs. clarithromycin 500 mg BID for 10 days	161	146	88.8%	91.8%

*This study was stopped prematurely after trovafloxacin was restricted for use in hospitalized patients with severe infection.

Table 10. Acute Sinusitis: Clinical cure rate at post-therapy follow-up (17–24 days)

	Patients (n)		Clinical cure rate	
Controlled Studies	**KETEK (5 day treatment)**	**Comparator (10 day treatment)**	**KETEK (5 day treatment)**	**Comparator (10 day treatment)**
KETEK vs. amoxicillin/clavulanic acid 500/125 mg TID	146	137	75.3%	74.5%
KETEK vs. cefuroxime axetil 250 mg BID	189	89	85.2%	82.0%

Liver and biliary system: abnormal liver function tests: increased transaminases, increased liver enzymes (e.g., ALT, AST) were usually asymptomatic and reversible. ALT elevations above 3 times the upper limit of normal were observed in 1.6%, and 1.7% of patients treated with KETEK and comparators, respectively. Hepatitis, with or without jaundice, occurred in 0.07% of patients treated with KETEK, and was reversible. (See **PRECAUTIONS, General.**)

Nervous system: dry mouth, somnolence, insomnia, vertigo, increased sweating

Body as a whole: abdominal pain, upper abdominal pain, fatigue

Special senses: Visual adverse events most often included blurred vision, diplopia, or difficulty focusing. Most events were mild to moderate; however, severe cases have been reported. Some patients discontinued therapy due to these adverse events. Visual adverse events were reported as having occurred after any dose during treatment, but most visual adverse events (65%) occurred following the first or second dose. Visual events lasted several hours and recurred upon subsequent dosing in some patients. For patients who continued treatment, some resolved on therapy while others continued to have symptoms until they completed the full course of treatment. (See **PRECAUTIONS, General** and **PRECAUTIONS, Information for patients.**)

Females and patients under 40 years old experienced a higher incidence of telithromycin-associated visual adverse events. (See **CLINICAL STUDIES.**)

Urogenital system: vaginal candidiasis, vaginitis, vaginosis fungal

Skin: rash

Hematologic: increased platelet count

Other possibly related clinically-relevant events occurring in <0.2% of patients treated with KETEK from the controlled Phase III studies included: anxiety, bradycardia, eczema, elevated blood bilirubin, erythema multiforme, flushing, hypotension, increased blood alkaline phosphatase, increased eosinophil count, paresthesia, pruritus, urticaria.

Post-Marketing Adverse Event Reports:

In addition to adverse events reported from clinical trials, the following events have been reported from worldwide post-marketing experience with KETEK.

Allergic: face edema, rare reports of severe allergic reactions, including angioedema and anaphylaxis.

Cardiovascular: atrial arrhythmias

Liver and biliary system: Hepatic dysfunction, including increased liver enzymes, and hepatocellular and/or cholestatic hepatitis, with or without jaundice, has been infrequently reported with telithromycin. This hepatic dysfunction may be severe and is usually reversible.

Musculoskeletal: muscle cramps, rare reports of exacerbation of myasthenia gravis. (See **WARNINGS.**)

OVERDOSAGE

In the event of acute overdosage, the stomach should be emptied by gastric lavage. The patient should be carefully monitored (e.g., ECG, electrolytes) and given symptomatic and supportive treatment. Adequate hydration should be maintained. The effectiveness of hemodialysis in an overdose situation with KETEK is unknown.

DOSAGE AND ADMINISTRATION

The dose of KETEK tablets is 800 mg taken orally once every 24 hours. The duration of therapy depends on the infection type and is described below. KETEK tablets can be administered with or without food.

[See table 6 above]

KETEK may be administered without dosage adjustment in the presence of hepatic impairment.

In the presence of severe renal impairment (CL_{CR} < 30 mL/min), including patients who need dialysis, the dose of KETEK has not been established.

HOW SUPPLIED

KETEK™ 400 mg tablets are supplied as light-orange, oval, film-coated tablets, imprinted "H3647" on one side and "400" on the other side. These are packaged in bottles and blister cards (Ketek Pak™ and unit dose) as follows:

Bottles of 60 (NDC 0088-2225-41)
Ketek Pak™, 10-tablet cards
(2 tablets per blister cavity) (NDC 0088-2225-07)
Unit dose package of 100
(blister pack) (NDC 0088-2225-49)

Store at 25°C (77°F); excursions permitted to 15-30°C (59-86°F) [see USP Controlled Room Temperature].

CLINICAL STUDIES

Community-acquired pneumonia (CAP)

KETEK was studied in four randomized, double-blind, controlled studies and four open-label studies for the treatment of community-acquired pneumonia. Patients with mild to moderate CAP who were considered appropriate for oral outpatient treatment were enrolled in these trials. Patients with severe pneumonia were excluded based on any one of the following: ICU admission, need for parenteral antibiotics, respiratory rate > 30/minute, hypotension, altered mental status, < 90% oxygen saturation by pulse oximetry, or white blood cell count < 4000/mm^3. Total number of clinically evaluable patients in the telithromycin group included 2016 patients.

[See table 7 above]

Clinical cure rates by pathogen from the four CAP controlled clinical trials in microbiologically evaluable patients given KETEK for 7-10 days or a comparator are displayed in Table 8.

Table 8. CAP: Clinical cure rate by pathogen at post-therapy follow-up (17-24 days)

Pathogen	KETEK	Comparator
Streptococcus pneumoniae	73/78 (93.6%)	63/70 (90.0%)
Haemophilus influenzae	39/47 (83.0%)	42/44 (95.5%)
Moraxella catarrhalis	12/14 (85.7%)	7/9 (77.8%)
Chlamydophila (Chlamydia) pneumoniae	23/25 (92.0%)	18/19 (94.7%)
Mycoplasma pneumoniae	22/23 (95.7%)	20/22 (90.9%)

Clinical cure rates for patients with CAP due to *Streptococcus pneumoniae* were determined from patients in controlled and uncontrolled trials. Of 333 evaluable patients with CAP due to *Streptococcus pneumoniae*, 312 (93.7%) achieved clinical success. Only patients considered appropriate for oral outpatient therapy were included in these trials. More severely ill patients were not enrolled. Blood cultures were obtained in all patients participating in the clinical trials of mild to moderate community-acquired pneumonia. In a limited number of outpatients with incidental pneumococcal bacteremia treated with KETEK, a clinical cure rate of 88% (67/76) has been observed. KETEK is not indicated for the treatment of severe community-acquired pneumonia or suspected pneumococcal bacteremia.

Clinical cure rates for patients with CAP due to multi-drug resistant *Streptococcus pneumoniae* (MDRSP*) were determined from patients in controlled and uncontrolled trials. Of 36 evaluable patients with CAP due to MDRSP, 33 (91.7%) achieved clinical success.

*MDRSP: Multi-drug resistant *Streptococcus pneumoniae* includes isolates known as PRSP (penicillin-resistant *Streptococcus pneumoniae*), and are isolates resistant to two or more of the following antibiotics: penicillin, 2nd generation cephalosporins, e.g., cefuroxime, macrolides, tetracyclines and trimethoprim/sulfamethoxazole.

Table 9. Clinical cure rate for 36 evaluable patients with MDRSP treated with KETEK in studies of community-acquired pneumonia

Screening Susceptibility	Clinical Success in Evaluable MDRSP Patients	
	n/N[a]	**%**
Penicillin-resistant	20/23	86.9
2nd generation cephalosporin-resistant	20/22	90.9
Macrolide-resistant	25/28	89.3
Trimethoprim/ sulfamethoxazole-resistant	24/27	88.9
Tetracycline-resistant[b]	11/13	84.6

[a] n = the number of patients successfully treated; N = the number with resistance to the listed drug of the 36 evaluable patients with CAP due to MDRSP.

[b] Includes isolates tested for resistance to either tetracycline or doxycycline.

Acute bacterial sinusitis

KETEK was studied in two randomized, double-blind, comparative studies for the treatment of acute sinusitis. Clinical cure rates with KETEK given for 5 days and comparator drug are shown in Table 10.

[See table 10 above]

A third study compared 5 days with 10 days of KETEK for the treatment of acute bacterial sinusitis, clinical cure rates for the two treatments were similar (91.1% vs. 91.0% respectively).

Clinical cure rates in microbiologically evaluable patients for KETEK against the most common pathogens from the two acute sinusitis controlled clinical trials are displayed in Table 11.

Table 11. Acute Sinusitis: Clinical cure rate by pathogen

Pathogen	KETEK 5 days	Comparator 10-days
Streptococcus pneumoniae	27/31 (87.1%)	14/16 (87.5%)
Haemophilus influenzae	28/34 (82.4%)	13/15 (86.7%)
Moraxella catarrhalis	7/7 (100%)	7/7 (100%)
Staphylococcus aureus	8/8 (100%)	2/3 (66.7%)

Continued on next page

Table 12. AECB: Clinical cure rate at post-therapy follow-up (17–24 days)

Controlled Studies	Patients (n)		Clinical cure rate	
	KETEK	Comparator	KETEK	Comparator
KETEK (5 day therapy) vs. cefuroxime axetil 500mg BID (10 day therapy)	140	142	86.4%	83.1%
KETEK (5 day therapy) vs. amoxicillin/clavulanic acid 500/125 mg TID (10 day therapy)	115	112	86.1%	82.1%
KETEK (5 day therapy) vs. clarithromycin 500mg BID (10 day therapy)	225	231	85.8%	89.2%

Ketek—Cont.

Acute bacterial exacerbation of chronic bronchitis (AECB)
KETEK was studied in three randomized, double-blind, controlled studies for the treatment of acute exacerbation of chronic bronchitis. Clinical cure rates are displayed in Table 12.
[See table 12 above]
Clinical cure rates in microbiologically evaluable patients treated with KETEK against the most common pathogens from the three acute exacerbation of chronic bronchitis clinical trials are displayed in Table 13.

Table 13. AECB: Clinical cure rate by pathogen at post-therapy follow-up (17–24 days)

Pathogen	KETEK	Comparator
Streptococcus pneumoniae	22/27 (81.5%)	15/19 (78.9%)
Haemophilus influenzae	44/60 (73.3%)	45/53 (84.9%)
Moraxella catarrhalis	27/29 (93.1%)	29/34 (85.3%)

Visual Adverse Events
Table 14 provides the incidence of all treatment-emergent visual adverse events in controlled Phase III studies by age and gender. The group with the highest incidence was females under the age of 40, while males over the age of 40 had rates of visual adverse events similar to comparator-treated patients.

Table 14. Incidence of All Treatment-Emergent Visual Adverse Events in Controlled Phase III Studies

Gender/Age	Telithromycin	Comparators*
Female ≤ 40	2.1% (14/682)	0.0% (0/534)
Female > 40	1.0% (7/703)	0.35% (2/574)
Male ≤ 40	1.2% (7/563)	0.48% (2/417)
Male > 40	0.27% (2/754)	0.33% (2/614)
Total	1.1% (30/2702)	0.28% (6/2139)

* Includes all comparators combined

ANIMAL PHARMACOLOGY

Repeated dose toxicity studies of 1, 3, and 6 months' duration with telithromycin conducted in rat, dog and monkey showed that the liver was the principal target for toxicity with elevations of liver enzymes and histological evidence of damage. There was evidence of reversibility after cessation of treatment. Plasma exposures based on free fraction of drug at the no observed adverse effect levels ranged from 1 to 10 times the expected clinical exposure.
Phospholipidosis (intracellular phospholipid accumulation) affecting a number of organs and tissues (e.g., liver, kidney, lung, thymus, spleen, gall bladder, mesenteric lymph nodes, GI-tract) has been observed with the administration of telithromycin in rats at repeated doses of 900 mg/m²/day (1.8× the human dose) or more for 1 month, and 300 mg/m²/day (0.61× the human dose) or more for 3–6 months. Similarly, phospholipidosis has been observed in dogs with telithromycin at repeated doses of 3000 mg/m2/day (6.1× the human dose) or more for 1 month and 1000 mg/ m²/day (2.0× the human dose) or more for 3 months. The significance of these findings for humans is unknown.
Pharmacology/toxicology studies showed an effect both in prolonging QTc interval in dogs *in vivo* and *in vitro* action potential duration (APD) in rabbit Purkinje fibers. These effects were observed at concentrations of free drug at least 8.8 (in dogs) times those circulating in clinical use. *In vitro* electrophysiological studies (hERG assays) suggested an inhibition of the rapid activating component of the delayed rectifier potassium current (I_{Kr}) as an underlying mechanism.

Rev. March 2004
Aventis Pharmaceuticals Inc.
Kansas City, MO 64137

US Patent Nos.: 5,527,780; 5,969,161; and 6,022,965
Rx only
www.aventispharma-us.com

References

1. National Committee for Clinical Laboratory Standards. Methods for Dilution Antimicrobial Susceptibility Tests for Bacteria That Grow Aerobically – Sixth Edition; Approved Standard, NCCLS Document M7-A6, Vol. 23, No. 2, NCCLS, Wayne, PA, January, 2003.
2. National Committee for Clinical Laboratory Standards. Performance Standards for Antimicrobial Disk Susceptibility Tests - Eighth Edition; Approved Standard, NCCLS Document M2-A8, Vol. 23, No. 1, NCCLS, Wayne, PA, January, 2003.
3. National Committee for Clinical Laboratory Standards. Performance Standards for Antimicrobial Susceptibility Testing: Twelfth Informational Supplement; Approved Standard, NCCLS Document M2-A8 and M7-A6, Vol. 23, No. 1, NCCLS, Wayne, PA, January, 2004.

Rx only

Patient Information About:
KETEK™
(telithromycin) Tablets
400mg Tablets

Before beginning your treatment, please read this section to learn important information about KETEK™ (telithromycin). Although the information presented here will be useful during your therapy, not all the benefits and risks of treatment with KETEK are discussed in this document. This section is not intended to take the place of conversations with your doctor or healthcare provider about your treatment or medical condition. The medicine described here can only be prescribed by a licensed healthcare provider. With this in mind, be sure to talk to your healthcare provider if you have any questions. It's important to note that only a doctor or healthcare provider can determine if KETEK is right for you.

What is KETEK?
KETEK (*KEE tek*) is an antibiotic used to treat adults 18 years of age and older with certain respiratory (lung and sinus) infections caused by certain germs called bacteria. KETEK kills many of the types of bacteria that can infect the lungs and sinuses, and has been found to treat these infections safely and effectively in clinical trials.
Not all respiratory infections are caused by bacteria. For example, common colds are caused by viruses. KETEK, like other antibiotics, does not kill viruses.
KETEK Tablets are light orange, oval, film-coated tablets, imprinted with "H3647" on one side and "400" on the other side, and each containing 400 mg of active drug.

How and when should I take KETEK?
The usual dose is two KETEK Tablets taken at the same time once daily for 5 to 10 days.
KETEK tablets should be swallowed whole and may be taken with or without food. Try to take your tablets at the same time every day, unless your healthcare provider tells you otherwise.
Follow the dosing instructions carefully, and do not take more than the prescribed amount. If you miss a dose, take it as soon as you remember. Do not take more than one dose (e.g., two tablets) of KETEK in a 24-hour period. If you have any questions, talk to your healthcare provider.
To make sure that all bacteria are killed, take all of the medicine that was prescribed for you even if you begin to feel better, unless instructed otherwise. You should contact your healthcare provider if your condition is not improving while taking KETEK.

Who should not take KETEK?
You must not take KETEK if:
- You have ever had a severe allergic reaction to KETEK or to any of the group of antibiotics known as "macrolides" such as erythromycin, azithromycin (Zithromax®), clarithromycin (Biaxin®) or dirithromycin (Dynabac®).
- You are currently taking cisapride (Propulsid®) or pimozide (Orap®).

You should be sure to talk to your healthcare provider before taking KETEK if any of the following are true, so he/she can determine if KETEK is right for you:
- If you have, or if a relative has, a rare heart condition known as congenital prolongation of the QT interval.
- If you are being treated for heart rhythm disturbances with certain medicines known as antiarrhythmics (such as quinidine, procainamide, or dofetilide) or if you have low blood potassium (hypokalemia), or low blood magnesium (hypomagnesemia).
- If you have a disease known as myasthenia gravis.
- If you are pregnant, planning to become pregnant, or are nursing.
- If you have ever experienced jaundice (yellow color of the skin and/or eyes) while taking KETEK.
- If you have any other serious medical conditions, including heart, liver, or kidney disease.

What about other medications I am taking?
It is important to let your healthcare provider know about all of the medicines you are taking, including those obtained without a prescription. Also see section **"Who should not take KETEK?"**
It is important to tell your healthcare provider if you are taking:
- Simvastatin, lovastatin, or atorvastatin (used for lowering cholesterol). You should stop treatment with these medications while you are taking KETEK.
- Medicines that correct heart rhythm called "antiarrhythmics" (such as quinidine, procainamide, or dofetilide).
- Any of the following medicines: itraconazole, ketoconazole, midazolam, digoxin, ergot alkaloid derivatives, cyclosporine, carbamazepine, hexobarbital, phenytoin, tacrolimus, sirolimus, metoprolol, theophylline or rifampin.
- Medicines called diuretics (also sometimes called water pills) such as furosemide or hydrochlorothiazide.

What are the possible side effects of KETEK?
KETEK is generally well tolerated. Most side effects are mild to moderate.
The most common side effects are nausea, headache, dizziness, vomiting, and diarrhea. If diarrhea persists call your healthcare provider.
KETEK may cause problems with vision, particularly when looking quickly between objects close by and objects far away. These events include blurred vision, difficulty focusing, and objects looking doubled. Most events were mild to moderate; however, severe cases have been reported. Problems with vision were reported as having occurred after any dose during treatment, but most occurred following the first or second dose. These problems lasted several hours and sometimes came back with the next dose.
If visual difficulties occur:
- You should avoid driving a motor vehicle, operating heavy machinery, or engaging in otherwise hazardous activities.
- Avoiding quickly looking between objects in the distance and objects nearby may help you to decrease these visual difficulties.
- You should contact your physician if these visual difficulties interfere with your daily activities.

There have been reports of side effects on the liver. If you develop jaundice (yellow color of the skin and/or eyes), stop your medication and contact your healthcare provider.
KETEK has the potential to affect the heart, as seen on an electrocardiogram (EKG) test. In very rare cases, this condition may result in a serious abnormal heartbeat. Contact your healthcare provider if you have a fainting spell.
There have been reports of worsening of myasthenia gravis symptoms in patients with myasthenia gravis. If you have myasthenia gravis and experience any worsening of your symptoms (such as muscle weakness, difficulty breathing) during treatment with KETEK, you should stop taking KETEK and seek immediate medical attention.
If you have other side effects not mentioned in this section or have concerns about side effects, be sure to talk to your healthcare provider.

How can I find out more about KETEK?
This is a summary of selected key points about KETEK. If you'd like more information or if you have concerns, talk to your healthcare provider. You can also visit the KETEK website at www.KETEK.com. But remember, neither this Patient Information nor the website can replace discussions with your doctor or healthcare provider.

Other key points to remember:
- Take your prescribed dose of KETEK once a day at the same time each day.
- Complete the course of medication (take all the tablets prescribed), even if you start to feel better, unless instructed otherwise.
- As with all other medications, do not use KETEK for other conditions or give tablets to others.
- Store KETEK tablets at room temperature.
- Keep this medication out of the reach of children.
- Do not take your tablets after the expiration date noted.
- Talk to your healthcare provider if you have questions or concerns.

Patient Information as of March 2004
BIAXIN® (clarithromycin) is a registered trademark of Abbott Laboratories.
ZITHROMAX® (azithromycin) is a registered trademark of Pfizer Inc.
DYNABAC® (dirithromycin) is a registered trademark of Eli Lilly and Company.
PROPULSID® (cisapride) is a registered trademark of Johnson & Johnson.
ORAP® (pimozide) is a registered trademark of Teva Pharmaceuticals USA, Inc.

Aventis Pharmaceuticals Inc.
Kansas City, MO 64137
US Patent Nos.: 5,527,780; 5,969,161; and 6,022,965
Rx only

KET-PI-15249-1
Shown in Product Identification Guide, page 307

LANTUS® ℞

[lăn' tus]
(insulin glargine [rDNA origin] injection)

LANTUS® must NOT be diluted or mixed with any other insulin or solution.
Prescribing Information as of May 2003a

DESCRIPTION

LANTUS® (insulin glargine [rDNA origin] injection) is a sterile solution of insulin glargine for use as an injection. Insulin glargine is a recombinant human insulin analog that is a long-acting (up to 24-hour duration of action), parenteral blood-glucose-lowering agent. (See CLINICAL PHARMACOLOGY). LANTUS is produced by recombinant DNA technology utilizing a non-pathogenic laboratory strain of *Escherichia coli* (K12) as the production organism. Insulin glargine differs from human insulin in that the amino acid asparagine at position A21 is replaced by glycine and two arginines are added to the C-terminus of the B-chain. Chemically, it is 21^A-Gly-30^Ba-L-Arg-30^Bb-L-Arg-human insulin and has the empirical formula $C_{267}H_{404}N_{72}O_{78}S_6$ and a molecular weight of 6063. It has the following structural formula:

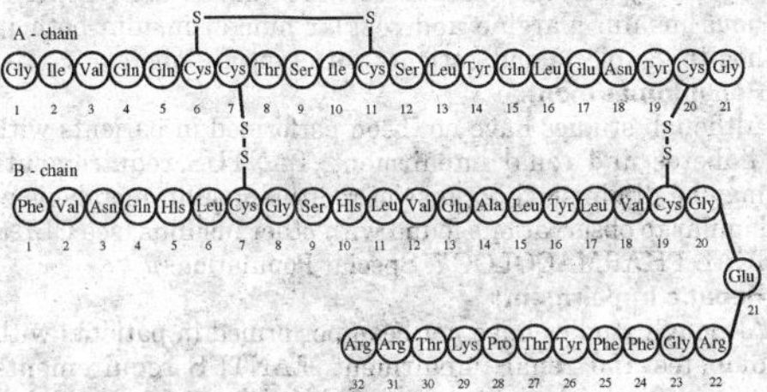

LANTUS consists of insulin glargine dissolved in a clear aqueous fluid. Each milliliter of LANTUS (insulin glargine injection) contains 100 IU (3.6378 mg) insulin glargine, 30 mcg zinc, 2.7 mg m-cresol, 20 mg glycerol 85%, and water for injection. The pH is adjusted by addition of aqueous solutions of hydrochloric acid and sodium hydroxide. LANTUS has a pH of approximately 4.

CLINICAL PHARMACOLOGY

Mechanism of Action:
The primary activity of insulin, including insulin glargine, is regulation of glucose metabolism. Insulin and its analogs lower blood glucose levels by stimulating peripheral glucose uptake, especially by skeletal muscle and fat, and by inhibiting hepatic glucose production. Insulin inhibits lipolysis in the adipocyte, inhibits proteolysis, and enhances protein synthesis.

Pharmacodynamics:
Insulin glargine is a human insulin analog that has been designed to have low aqueous solubility at neutral pH. At pH 4, as in the LANTUS injection solution, it is completely soluble. After injection into the subcutaneous tissue, the acidic solution is neutralized, leading to formation of microprecipitates from which small amounts of insulin glargine are slowly released, resulting in a relatively constant concentration/time profile over 24 hours with no pronounced peak. This profile allows once-daily dosing as a patient's basal insulin.
In clinical studies, the glucose-lowering effect on a molar basis (i.e., when given at the same doses) of intravenous insulin glargine is approximately the same as human insulin. In euglycemic clamp studies in healthy subjects or in patients with type 1 diabetes, the onset of action of subcutaneous insulin glargine was slower than NPH human insulin. The effect profile of insulin glargine was relatively constant with no pronounced peak and the duration of its effect was prolonged compared to NPH human insulin. *Figure 1* shows results from a study in patients with type 1 diabetes conducted for a maximum of 24 hours after the injection. The median time between injection and the end of pharmacological effect was 14.5 hours (range: 9.5 to 19.3 hours) for NPH human insulin, and 24 hours (range: 10.8 to >24.0 hours) (24 hours was the end of the observation period) for insulin glargine.
[See figure at top of next column]
The longer duration of action (up to 24 hours) of LANTUS is directly related to its slower rate of absorption and supports once-daily subcutaneous administration. The time course of action of insulins, including LANTUS, may vary between individuals and/or within the same individual.

Pharmacokinetics:
Absorption and Bioavailability. After subcutaneous injection of insulin glargine in healthy subjects and in patients with diabetes, the insulin serum concentrations indicated a slower, more prolonged absorption and a relatively constant concentration/time profile over 24 hours with no pronounced peak in comparison to NPH human insulin. Serum insulin concentrations were thus consistent with the time profile of the pharmacodynamic activity of insulin glargine.

Table 1: Type 1 Diabetes Mellitus—Adult

	Study A		Study B		Study C	
Treatment duration	28 weeks		28 weeks		16 weeks	
Treatment in combination with	Regular insulin		Regular insulin		Insulin lispro	
	LANTUS	NPH	LANTUS	NPH	LANTUS	NPH
Number of subjects treated	292	293	264	270	310	309
HbA1c						
Endstudy mean	8.13	8.07	7.55	7.49	7.53	7.60
Adj. mean change from baseline	+0.21	+0.10	−0.16	−0.21	−0.07	−0.08
LANTUS—NPH	+0.11		+0.05		+0.01	
95% CI for Treatment difference	(−0.03; +0.24)		(−0.08; +0.19)		(−0.11; +0.13)	
Basal insulin dose						
Endstudy mean	19.2	22.8	24.8	31.3	23.9	29.2
Mean change from baseline	−1.7	−0.3	−4.1	+1.8	−4.5	+0.9
Total insulin dose						
Endstudy mean	46.7	51.7	50.3	54.8	47.4	50.7
Mean change from baseline	−1.1	−0.1	+0.3	+3.7	−2.9	+0.3
Fasting blood glucose (mg/dL)						
Endstudy mean	146.3	150.8	147.8	154.4	144.4	161.3
Adj. mean change from baseline	−21.1	−16.0	−20.2	−16.9	−29.3	−11.9

Table 2: Type 1 Diabetes Mellitus—Pediatric

	Study D	
Treatment duration	28 weeks	
Treatment in combination with	Regular insulin	
	LANTUS	NPH
Number of subjects treated	174	175
HbA1c		
Endstudy mean	8.91	9.18
Adj. mean change from baseline	+0.28	+0.27
LANTUS—NPH	+0.01	
95% CI for Treatment difference	(−0.24; +0.26)	
Basal insulin dose		
Endstudy mean	18.2	21.1
Mean change from baseline	−1.3	+2.4
Total insulin dose		
Endstudy mean	45.0	46.0
Mean change from baseline	+1.9	+3.4
Fasting blood glucose (mg/dL)		
Endstudy mean	171.9	182.7
Adj. mean change from baseline	−23.2	−12.2

Figure 1. Activity Profile in Patients with Type 1 Diabetes†

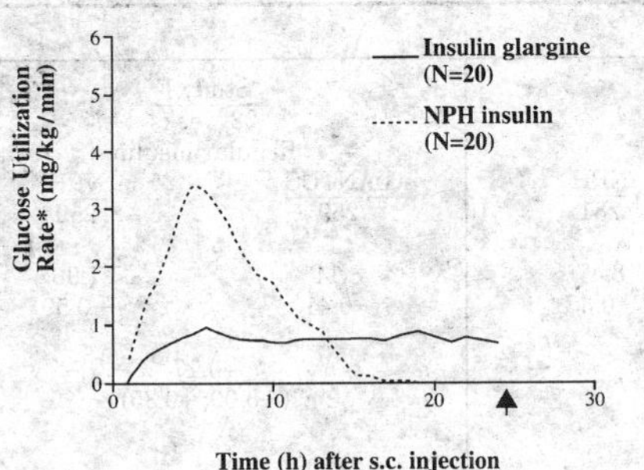

* Determined as amount of glucose infused to maintain constant plasma glucose levels (hourly mean values); indicative of insulin activity.
† Between-patient variability (CV, coefficient of variation); insulin glargine, 84% and NPH, 78%.

After subcutaneous injection of 0.3 IU/kg insulin glargine in patients with type 1 diabetes, a relatively constant concentration/time profile has been demonstrated. The duration of action after abdominal, deltoid, or thigh subcutaneous administration was similar.

Metabolism. A metabolism study in humans indicates that insulin glargine is partly metabolized at the carboxyl terminus of the B chain in the subcutaneous depot to form two active metabolites with in vitro activity similar to that of insulin, M1 (21^A-Gly-insulin) and M2 (21^A-Gly-des-30^B-Thr-insulin). Unchanged drug and these degradation products are also present in the circulation.

Special Populations:
Age, Race, and Gender. Information on the effect of age, race, and gender on the pharmacokinetics of LANTUS is not available. However, in controlled clinical trials in adults (n=3890) and a controlled clinical trial in pediatric patients (n=349), subgroup analyses based on age, race, and gender did not show differences in safety and efficacy between insulin glargine and NPH human insulin.

Smoking. The effect of smoking on the pharmacokinetics/pharmacodynamics of LANTUS has not been studied.

Pregnancy. The effect of pregnancy on the pharmacokinetics and pharmacodynamics of LANTUS has not been studied (see PRECAUTIONS, Pregnancy).

Obesity. In controlled clinical trials, which included patients with Body Mass Index (BMI) up to and including 49.6 kg/m^2, subgroup analyses based on BMI did not show any differences in safety and efficacy between insulin glargine and NPH human insulin.

Renal Impairment. The effect of renal impairment on the pharmacokinetics of LANTUS has not been studied. However, some studies with human insulin have shown increased circulating levels of insulin in patients with renal failure. Careful glucose monitoring and dose adjustments of insulin, including LANTUS, may be necessary in patients with renal dysfunction (see PRECAUTIONS, Renal Impairment).

Hepatic Impairment. The effect of hepatic impairment on the pharmacokinetics of LANTUS has not been studied. However, some studies with human insulin have shown increased circulating levels of insulin in patients with liver failure. Careful glucose monitoring and dose adjustments of insulin, including LANTUS, may be necessary in patients with hepatic dysfunction (see PRECAUTIONS, Hepatic Impairment).

CLINICAL STUDIES

The safety and effectiveness of insulin glargine given once-daily at bedtime was compared to that of once-daily and twice-daily NPH human insulin in open-label, randomized, active-control, parallel studies of 2327 adult patients and 349 pediatric patients with type 1 diabetes mellitus and 1563 adult patients with type 2 diabetes mellitus (see Tables 1–3). In general, the reduction in glycated hemoglobin (HbA1c) with LANTUS was similar to that with NPH human insulin. The overall rates of hypoglycemia did not differ between patients with diabetes treated to LANTUS compared with NPH human insulin.

Type 1 Diabetes—Adult (see Table 1). In two large, randomized, controlled clinical studies (Studies A and B), patients with type 1 diabetes (Study A; n=585, Study B; n=534) were randomized to basal-bolus treatment with LANTUS once daily at bedtime or to NPH human insulin once or twice daily and treated for 28 weeks. Regular human insulin was administered before each meal. LANTUS was administered at bedtime. NPH human insulin was administered once daily at bedtime or in the morning and at bedtime when used twice daily. In one large, randomized, controlled clinical study (Study C), patients with type 1 diabetes (n=619) were treated for 16 weeks with a basal-bolus insulin regimen where insulin lispro was used before each meal. LANTUS was administered once daily at bedtime and NPH human insulin was administered once or twice daily. In these studies, LANTUS and NPH human insulin had a similar effect on glycohemoglobin with a similar overall rate of hypoglycemia.
[See table 1 above]

Type 1 Diabetes—Pediatric (see Table 2). In a randomized, controlled clinical study (Study D), pediatric patients (age range 6 to 15 years) with type 1 diabetes (n=349) were treated for 28 weeks with a basal-bolus insulin regimen where regular human insulin was used before each meal. LANTUS was administered once daily at bedtime and NPH

Continued on next page

Lantus—Cont.

human insulin was administered once or twice daily. Similar effects on glycohemoglobin and the incidence of hypoglycemia were observed in both treatment groups.

[See table 2 at top of previous page]

Type 2 Diabetes—Adult (see Table 3). In a large, randomized, controlled clinical study (Study E) (n=570), LANTUS was evaluated for 52 weeks as part of a regimen of combination therapy with insulin and oral antidiabetes agents (a sulfonylurea, metformin, acarbose, or combinations of these drugs). LANTUS administered once daily at bedtime was as effective as NPH human insulin administered once daily at bedtime in reducing glycohemoglobin and fasting glucose. There was a low rate of hypoglycemia that was similar in LANTUS and NPH human insulin treated patients. In a large, randomized, controlled clinical study (Study F), in patients with type 2 diabetes not using oral antidiabetic agents (n=518), a basal-bolus regimen of LANTUS once daily at bedtime or NPH human insulin administered once or twice daily was evaluated for 28 weeks. Regular human insulin was used before meals as needed. LANTUS had similar effectiveness as either once- or twice-daily NPH human insulin in reducing glycohemoglobin and fasting glucose with a similar incidence of hypoglycemia.

[See table 3 below]

LANTUS Flexible Daily Dosing

The safety and efficacy of LANTUS administered pre-breakfast, pre-dinner, or at bedtime were evaluated in a large, randomized, controlled clinical study, in patients with type 1 diabetes (study G, n=378). Patients were also treated with insulin lispro at mealtime. LANTUS administered at different times of the day resulted in similar reductions in glycated hemoglobin compared to that with bedtime administration (see Table 4). In these patients, data are available from 8-point home glucose monitoring. The maximum mean blood glucose level was observed just prior to injection of LANTUS regardless of time of administration, i.e. pre-breakfast, pre-dinner, or bedtime.

In this study, 5% of patients in the LANTUS-breakfast arm discontinued treatment because of lack of efficacy. No patients in the other two arms discontinued for this reason. Routine monitoring during this trial revealed the following mean changes in systolic blood pressure: pre-breakfast group, 1.9 mm Hg; pre-dinner group, 0.7 mm Hg; pre-bedtime group, −2.0 mm Hg.

The safety and efficacy of LANTUS administered pre-breakfast or at bedtime were also evaluated in a large, randomized, active-controlled clinical study (Study H, n=697) in type 2 diabetes patients no longer adequately controlled on oral agent therapy. All patients in this study also received AMARYL® (glimepiride) 3 mg daily. LANTUS given before breakfast was at least as effective in lowering glycated hemoglobin A1c (HbA1c) as LANTUS given at bedtime or NPH human insulin given at bedtime (see Table 4).

[See table 4 below]

INDICATIONS AND USAGE

LANTUS is indicated for once-daily subcutaneous administration for the treatment of adult and pediatric patients with type 1 diabetes mellitus or adult patients with type 2 diabetes mellitus who require basal (long-acting) insulin for the control of hyperglycemia.

CONTRAINDICATIONS

LANTUS is contraindicated in patients hypersensitive to insulin glargine or the excipients.

WARNINGS

Hypoglycemia is the most common adverse effect of insulin, including LANTUS. As with all insulins, the timing of hypoglycemia may differ among various insulin formulations. Glucose monitoring is recommended for all patients with diabetes.

Any change of insulin should be made cautiously and only under medical supervision. Changes in insulin strength, timing of dosing, manufacturer, type (e.g., regular, NPH, or insulin analogs), species (animal, human), or method of manufacture (recombinant DNA versus animal-source insulin) may result in the need for a change in dosage. Concomitant oral antidiabetes treatment may need to be adjusted.

PRECAUTIONS

General:

LANTUS is not intended for intravenous administration. The prolonged duration of activity of insulin glargine is dependent on injection into subcutaneous tissue. Intravenous administration of the usual subcutaneous dose could result in severe hypoglycemia.

LANTUS must NOT be diluted or mixed with any other insulin or solution. If LANTUS is diluted or mixed, the solution may become cloudy, and the pharmacokinetic/pharmacodynamic profile (e.g., onset of action, time to peak effect) of LANTUS and/or the mixed insulin may be altered in an unpredictable manner. When LANTUS and regular human insulin were mixed immediately before injection in dogs, a delayed onset of action and time to maximum effect for regular human insulin was observed. The total bioavailability of the mixture was also slightly decreased compared to separate injections of LANTUS and regular human insulin. The relevance of these observations in dogs to humans is not known.

As with all insulin preparations, the time course of LANTUS action may vary in different individuals or at different times in the same individual and the rate of absorption is dependent on blood supply, temperature, and physical activity.

Insulin may cause sodium retention and edema, particularly if previously poor metabolic control is improved by intensified insulin therapy.

Hypoglycemia:

As with all insulin preparations, hypoglycemic reactions may be associated with the administration of LANTUS. Hypoglycemia is the most common adverse effect of insulins. Early warning symptoms of hypoglycemia may be different or less pronounced under certain conditions, such as long duration of diabetes, diabetic nerve disease, use of medications such as beta-blockers, or intensified diabetes control (see PRECAUTIONS, Drug Interactions). Such situations may result in severe hypoglycemia (and, possibly, loss of consciousness) prior to patient's awareness of hypoglycemia. The time of occurrence of hypoglycemia depends on the action profile of the insulins used and may, therefore, change when the treatment regimen is changed. Patients being switched from twice daily NPH insulin to once-daily LANTUS should have their initial LANTUS dose reduced by 20% from the previous total daily NPH dose to reduce the risk of hypoglycemia (see DOSAGE AND ADMINISTRATION, Changeover to LANTUS).

The prolonged effect of subcutaneous LANTUS may delay recovery from hypoglycemia.

In a clinical study, symptoms of hypoglycemia or counterregulatory hormone responses were similar after intravenous insulin glargine and regular human insulin both in healthy subjects and patients with type 1 diabetes.

Renal Impairment:

Although studies have not been performed in patients with diabetes and renal impairment, LANTUS requirements may be diminished because of reduced insulin metabolism, similar to observations found with other insulins (see CLINICAL PHARMACOLOGY, Special Populations).

Hepatic Impairment:

Although studies have not been performed in patients with diabetes and renal impairment, LANTUS requirements may be diminished due to reduced insulin metabolism, similar to observations found with other insulins (see CLINICAL PHARMACOLOGY, Special Populations).

Injection Site and Allergic Reactions:

As with any insulin therapy, lipodystrophy may occur at the injection site and delay insulin absorption. Other injection site reactions with insulin therapy include redness, pain, itching, hives, swelling, and inflammation. Continuous rotation of the injection site within a given area may help to reduce or prevent these reactions. Most minor reactions to insulins usually resolve in a few days to a few weeks.

Reports of injection site pain were more frequent with LANTUS than NPH human insulin (2.7% insulin glargine versus 0.7% NPH). The reports of pain at the injection site were usually mild and did not result in discontinuation of therapy.

Immediate-type allergic reactions are rare. Such reactions to insulin (including insulin glargine) or the excipients may, for example, be associated with generalized skin reactions, angioedema, bronchospasm, hypotension, or shock and may be life threatening.

Intercurrent Conditions:

Insulin requirements may be altered during intercurrent conditions such as illness, emotional disturbances, or stress.

Information for Patients:

LANTUS must only be used if the solution is clear and colorless with no particles visible (see DOSAGE AND ADMINISTRATION, Preparation and Handling).

Patients must be advised that LANTUS must NOT be diluted or mixed with any other insulin or solution (see PRECAUTIONS, General).

Patients should be instructed on self-management procedures including glucose monitoring, proper injection technique, and hypoglycemia and hyperglycemia management. Patients must be instructed on handling of special situations such as intercurrent conditions (illness, stress, or emotional disturbances), an inadequate or skipped insulin dose, inadvertent administration of an increased insulin dose, inadequate food intake, or skipped meals. Refer patients to the LANTUS Information for the Patient circular for additional information.

As with all patients who have diabetes, the ability to concentrate and/or react may be impaired as a result of hypoglycemia or hyperglycemia.

Patients with diabetes should be advised to inform their health care practitioner if they are pregnant or are contemplating pregnancy.

Drug Interactions:

A number of substances affect glucose metabolism and may require insulin dose adjustment and particularly close monitoring.

The following are examples of substances that may increase the blood-glucose-lowering effect and susceptibility to hypoglycemia: oral antidiabetic products, ACE inhibitors, disopyramide, fibrates, fluoxetine, MAO inhibitors, propoxyphene, salicylates, somatostatin analog (e.g., octreotide), sulfonamide antibiotics.

The following are examples of substances that may reduce the blood-glucose-lowering effect of insulin: corticosteroids,

Table 3: Type 2 Diabetes Mellitus—Adult

	Study E		Study F	
Treatment duration	52 weeks		28 weeks	
Treatment in combination with	Oral agents		Regular insulin	
	LANTUS	NPH	LANTUS	NPH
Number of subjects treated	289	281	259	259
HbA1c				
Endstudy mean	8.51	8.47	8.14	7.96
Adj. mean change from baseline	−0.46	−0.38	−0.41	−0.59
LANTUS—NPH	−0.08		+0.17	
95% CI for Treatment difference	(−0.28; +0.12)		(−0.00; +0.35)	
Basal insulin dose				
Endstudy mean	25.9	23.6	42.9	52.5
Mean change from baseline	+11.5	+9.0	−1.2	+7.0
Total insulin dose				
Endstudy mean	25.9	23.6	74.3	80.0
Mean change from baseline	+11.5	+9.0	+10.0	+13.1
Fasting blood glucose (mg/dL)				
Endstudy mean	126.9	129.4	141.5	144.5
Adj. mean change from baseline	−49.0	−46.3	−23.8	−21.6

Table 4: Flexible LANTUS Daily Dosing in Type 1 (Study G) and Type 2 (Study H) Diabetes Mellitus

	Study G			Study H		
Treatment duration	**24 weeks**			**24 weeks**		
Treatment in combination with:	**Insulin lispro**			**AMARYL® (glimepiride)**		
	LANTUS Breakfast	**LANTUS Dinner**	**LANTUS Bedtime**	**LANTUS Breakfast**	**LANTUS Bedtime**	**NPH Bedtime**
Number of subjects treated*	112	124	128	234	226	227
HbA1c						
Baseline mean	7.56	7.53	7.61	9.13	9.07	9.09
Endstudy mean	7.39	7.42	7.57	7.87	8.12	8.27
Mean change from baseline	−0.17	−0.11	−0.04	−1.26	−0.95	−0.83
Basal insulin dose (IU)						
Endstudy mean	27.3	24.6	22.8	40.4	38.5	36.8
Mean change from baseline	5.0	1.8	1.5			
Total insulin dose (IU)				NA**	NA	NA
Endstudy mean	53.3	54.7	51.5			
Mean change from baseline	1.6	3.0	2.3			

*Intent to treat

**Not applicable

danazol, diuretics, sympathomimetic agents (e.g., epinephrine, albuterol, terbutaline), isoniazid, phenothiazine derivatives, somatropin, thyroid hormones, estrogens, progestogens (e.g., in oral contraceptives).
Beta-blockers, clonidine, lithium salts, and alcohol may either potentiate or weaken the blood-glucose-lowering effect of insulin. Pentamidine may cause hypoglycemia, which may sometimes be followed by hyperglycemia.
In addition, under the influence of sympatholytic medicinal products such as beta-blockers, clonidine, guanethidine, and reserpine, the signs of hypoglycemia may be reduced or absent.

Carcinogenesis, Mutagenesis, Impairment of Fertility:
In mice and rats, standard two-year carcinogenicity studies with insulin glargine were performed at doses up to 0.455 mg/kg, which is for the rat approximately 10 times and for the mouse approximately 5 times the recommended human subcutaneous starting dose of 10 IU (0.008 mg/kg/day), based on mg/m^2. The findings in female mice were not conclusive due to excessive mortality in all dose groups during the study. Histiocytomas were found at injection sites in male rats (statistically significant) and male mice (not statistically significant) in acid vehicle containing groups. These tumors were not found in female animals, in saline control, or insulin comparator groups using a different vehicle. The relevance of these findings to humans is unknown.
Insulin glargine was not mutagenic in tests for detection of gene mutations in bacteria and mammalian cells (Ames- and HGPRT-test) and in tests for detection of chromosomal aberrations (cytogenetics in vitro in V79 cells and in vivo in Chinese hamsters).
In a combined fertility and prenatal and postnatal study in male and female rats at subcutaneous doses up to 0.36 mg/kg/day, which is approximately 7 times the recommended human subcutaneous starting dose of 10 IU (0.008 mg/kg/day), based on mg/m^2, maternal toxicity due to dose-dependent hypoglycemia, including some deaths, was observed. Consequently, a reduction of the rearing rate occurred in the high-dose group only. Similar effects were observed with NPH human insulin.

Pregnancy:
Teratogenic Effects: Pregnancy Category C. Subcutaneous reproduction and teratology studies have been performed with insulin glargine and regular human insulin in rats and Himalayan rabbits. The drug was given to female rats before mating, during mating, and throughout pregnancy at doses up to 0.36 mg/kg/day, which is approximately 7 times the recommended human subcutaneous starting dose of 10 IU (0.008 mg/kg/day), based on mg/m^2. In rabbits, doses of 0.072 mg/kg/day, which is approximately 2 times the recommended human subcutaneous starting dose of 10 IU (0.008 mg/kg/day), based on mg/m^2, were administered during organogenesis. The effects of insulin glargine did not generally differ from those observed with regular human insulin in rats or rabbits. However, in rabbits, five fetuses from two litters of the high-dose group exhibited dilation of the cerebral ventricles. Fertility and early embryonic development appeared normal.
There are no well-controlled clinical studies of the use of insulin glargine in pregnant women. It is essential for patients with diabetes or a history of gestational diabetes to maintain good metabolic control before conception and throughout pregnancy. Insulin requirements may decrease during the first trimester, generally increase during the second and third trimesters, and rapidly decline after delivery. Careful monitoring of glucose control is essential in such patients. Because animal reproduction studies are not always predictive of human response, this drug should be used during pregnancy only if clearly needed.

Nursing Mothers:
It is unknown whether insulin glargine is excreted in significant amounts in human milk. Many drugs, including human insulin, are excreted in human milk. For this reason, caution should be exercised when LANTUS is administered to a nursing woman. Lactating women may require adjustments in insulin dose and diet.

Pediatric Use:
Safety and effectiveness of LANTUS have been established in the age group 6 to 15 years with type 1 diabetes.

Geriatric Use:
In controlled clinical studies comparing insulin glargine to NPH human insulin, 593 of 3890 patients with type 1 and type 2 diabetes were 65 years and older. The only difference in safety or effectiveness in this subpopulation compared to the entire study population was an expected higher incidence of cardiovascular events in both insulin glargine and NPH human insulin-treated patients.
In elderly patients with diabetes, the initial dosing, dose increments, and maintenance dosage should be conservative to avoid hypoglycemic reactions. Hypoglycemia may be difficult to recognize in the elderly (see PRECAUTIONS, Hypoglycemia).

ADVERSE REACTIONS

The adverse events commonly associated with LANTUS include the following:
Body as a whole: allergic reactions (see PRECAUTIONS).
Skin and appendages: injection site reaction, lipodystrophy, pruritus, rash (see PRECAUTIONS).
Other: hypoglycemia (se WARNINGS and PRECAUTIONS)
In clinical studies in adult patients, there was a higher incidence of treatment-emergent injection site pain in LANTUS-treated patients (2.7%) compared to NPH insulin-treated patients (0.7%). The reports of pain at the injection site were usually mild and did not result in discontinuation of therapy. Other treatment-emergent injection site reactions occurred at similar incidences with both insulin glargine and NPH human insulin.
Retinopathy was evaluated in the clinical studies by means of retinal adverse events reported and fundus photography. The numbers of retinal adverse events reported for LANTUS and NPH treatment groups were similar for patients with type 1 and type 2 diabetes. Progression of retinopathy was investigated by fundus photography using a grading protocol derived from the Early Treatment Diabetic Retinopathy Study (ETDRS). In one clinical study involving patients with type 2 diabetes, a difference in the number of subjects with ≥3-step progression in ETDRS scale over a 6-month period was noted by fundus photography (7.5% in LANTUS group versus 2.7% in NPH treated group). The overall relevance of this isolated finding cannot be determined due to the small number of patients involved, the short follow-up period, and the fact that this finding was not observed in other clinical studies.

OVERDOSAGE

An excess of insulin relative to food intake, energy expenditure, or both may lead to severe and sometimes long-term and life-threatening hypoglycemia. Mild episodes of hypoglycemia can usually be treated with oral carbohydrates. Adjustments in drug dosage, meal patterns, or exercise may be needed.
More severe episodes with coma, seizure, or neurologic impairment may be treated with intramuscular/subcutaneous glucagon or concentrated intravenous glucose. After apparent clinical recovery from hypoglycemia, continued observation and additional carbohydrate intake may be necessary to avoid reoccurrence of hypoglycemia.

DOSAGE AND ADMINISTRATION

LANTUS is a recombinant human insulin analog. Its potency is approximately the same as human insulin. It exhibits a relatively constant glucose-lowering profile over 24 hours that permits once-daily dosing.
LANTUS may be administered at any time during the day. LANTUS should be administered subcutaneously once a day at the same time every day. For patients adjusting timing of dosing with LANTUS, see **WARNINGS** and **PRECAUTIONS, Hypoglycemia**. LANTUS is not intended for intravenous administration (see PRECAUTIONS). Intravenous administration of the usual subcutaneous dose could result in severe hypoglycemia. The desired blood glucose levels as well as the doses and timing of antidiabetic medications must be determined individually. Blood glucose monitoring is recommended for all patients with diabetes. The prolonged duration of activity of LANTUS is dependent on injection into subcutaneous space.
As with all insulins, injection sites within an injection area (abdomen, thigh or deltoid) must be rotated from one injection to the next.
In clinical studies, there was no relevant difference in insulin glargine absorption after abdominal, deltoid, or thigh subcutaneous administration. As for all insulins, the rate of absorption, and consequently the onset and duration of action, may be affected by exercise and other variables.
LANTUS is not the insulin of choice for the treatment of diabetic ketoacidosis. Intravenous short-acting insulin is the preferred treatment.

Pediatric Use:
LANTUS can be safely administrated to pediatric patients ≥6 years of age. Administration to pediatric patients <6 years has not been studied. Based on the results of a study in pediatric patients, the dose recommendation for changeover to LANTUS is the same as described for adults in DOSAGE AND ADMINISTRATION, Changeover to LANTUS.

Initiation of LANTUS Therapy:
In a clinical study with insulin naïve patients with type 2 diabetes already treated with oral antidiabetic drugs, LANTUS was started at an average dose of 10 IU once daily, and subsequently adjusted according to the patient's need to a total daily dose ranging from 2 to 100 IU.

Changeover to LANTUS:
If changing from a treatment regimen with an intermediate- or long-acting insulin to a regimen with LANTUS, the amount and timing of short-acting insulin or fast-acting insulin analog or the dose of any oral antidiabetes drug may need to be adjusted. In clinical studies, when patients were transferred from once-daily NPH human insulin or ultralente human insulin to once-daily LANTUS, the initial dose was usually not changed. However, when patients were transferred from twice-daily NPH human insulin to LANTUS once daily, to reduce the risk of hypoglycemia, the initial dose (IU) was usually reduced by approximately 20% (compared to total daily IU of NPH human insulin) and then adjusted based on patient response (see PRECAUTIONS, Hypoglycemia).
A program of close metabolic monitoring under medical supervision is recommended during transfer and in the initial weeks thereafter. The amount and timing of short-acting insulin or fast-acting insulin analog may need to be adjusted. This is particularly true for patients with acquired antibodies to human insulin needing high-insulin doses and occurs with all insulin analogs. Dose adjustment of LANTUS and other insulins or oral antidiabetes drugs may be required; for example, if the patient's timing of dosing, weight or lifestyle changes, or other circumstances arise that increase susceptibility to hypoglycemia or hyperglycemia (see PRECAUTIONS, Hypoglycemia).
The dose may also have to be adjusted during intercurrent illness (see PRECAUTIONS, Intercurrent Conditions).

Preparation and Handling:
Parenteral drug products should be inspected visually prior to administration whenever the solution and the container permit. LANTUS must only be used if the solution is clear and colorless with no particles visible.
The syringes must not contain any other medicinal product or residue.
Mixing and diluting. LANTUS must NOT be diluted or mixed with any other insulin or solution (see PRECAUTIONS, General).

HOW SUPPLIED

LANTUS 100 units per mL (U-100) is available in the following package sizes:
10 mL vials (NDC 0088-2220-33)

Storage:
Unopened LANTUS vials should be stored in a refrigerator, 36°F–46°F (2°C–8°C). LANTUS should not be stored in the freezer and it should not be allowed to freeze. Discard vial if frozen.

Open (in Use) Vial:
Opened vials, whether or not refrigerated, must be used within 28 days. They must be discarded if not used within 28 days. If refrigeration is not possible, the open vial in use can be kept unrefrigerated for up to 28 days away from direct heat and light, as long as the temperature is not greater than 86°F (30°C).

Rev. May 2003a
Manufactured by:
Aventis Pharma Deutschland GmbH
D-65926 Frankfurt am Main
Frankfurt, Germany
Manufactured for:
Aventis Pharmaceuticals Inc.
Kansas City, MO 64137 USA
US Patents 5,656,722, 5,370,629, and 5,509,905
Made in Germany
www.aventis-us.com

LANTUS®

(insulin glargine [Recombinant DNA origin] injection)

Patient Information for the LANTUS 10 mL vial (1000 units per vial) 100 units per mL (U-100)
This leaflet tells you about LANTUS (LAN-tus) and about how to use LANTUS in a vial. At the end of the leaflet is a list of vocabulary words you may find useful. Read this information carefully before you use LANTUS. Read the information you get when you refill your LANTUS prescriptions because there may be new information. This leaflet does not take the place of complete discussions with your health care professional. If you have questions about LANTUS or about diabetes, talk with your health care professional.

What is the most important information I should know about LANTUS?
Do NOT dilute or mix LANTUS with any other insulin or solution. It will not work as intended, and you may lose blood sugar control, which could be serious.

What is LANTUS?
LANTUS is a long-acting synthetic (man-made) human insulin to treat diabetes. You need a prescription to get LANTUS. Always be sure the pharmacy gives you the right insulin. The carton and vial should look like the ones in this picture.

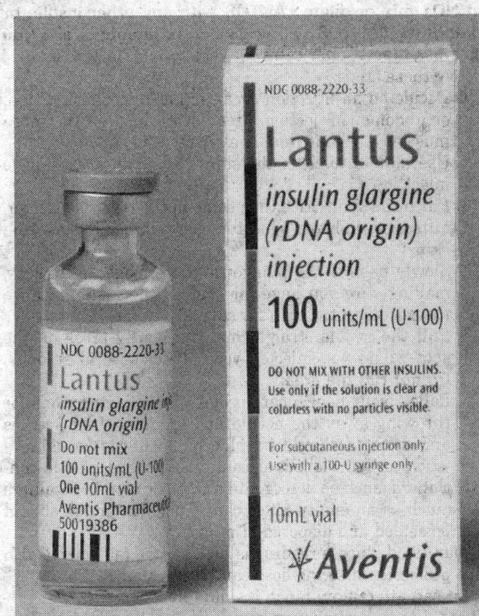

Diabetes is a disease caused when the body cannot produce or use insulin. Insulin is a hormone produced by the pancreas. Your body needs insulin to turn glucose (sugar) from food into energy. If your body does not make enough insulin,

Continued on next page

Lantus—Cont.

you need another source of insulin so you will not have too much sugar in your blood. That is why you must take insulin injections.
LANTUS is similar to the insulin made by your body. It is used once a day to lower blood glucose. Like other insulins, you take LANTUS by injecting it in the fatty layer under the skin (subcutaneously). The dose your health care professional prescribes helps keep the glucose level in your blood close to normal.
You will be able to tell if LANTUS is working by testing your blood and/or urine for glucose.
LANTUS contains active and inactive ingredients. The active ingredient is insulin. It is dissolved in a colorless sterile (germ-free) fluid. The concentration is 100 units/mL (U-100). Inactive ingredients are zinc, glycerol, m-cresol, and water for injection.
Insulin injections play an important role in keeping your diabetes in control. But the way you live—your diet, careful monitoring of your glucose levels, exercise, and planned physical activity—all work with your insulin to help you control your diabetes.

Who should NOT take LANTUS?
You should not take LANTUS if you are allergic to insulin or any of the inactive ingredients in LANTUS.

What sort of syringe should I use?
Always use a syringe that is marked for U-100 insulin preparations. If you use the wrong syringe, you may get the wrong dose and develop a blood glucose level that is too low or too high.
Use disposable syringes and needles only once. Throw them away properly. Use a new needle and syringe every time you dose. **Never** share needles and syringes.

How do I draw the insulin into the syringe?
Do NOT dilute or mix LANTUS with any other insulin or solution. The syringe must not contain any other medicine or residue.
Follow these steps:
1. Wash your hands.
2. Check the insulin to make sure it is clear and colorless. Do not use it if it is cloudy or if you see particles.
3. If you are using a new vial, remove the protective cap. **Do not** remove the stopper.
4. Wipe the top of the vial with an alcohol swab.
5. Draw air into the syringe equal to your insulin dose. Put the needle through the rubber top of the vial and push the plunger to inject the air into the vial.
6. Leave the syringe in the vial and turn both upside down. Hold the syringe and vial firmly in one hand.
7. Make sure the tip of the needle is in the insulin. With your free hand, pull the plunger to withdraw the correct dose into the syringe.
8. Before you take the needle out of the vial, check the syringe for air bubbles. If bubbles are in the syringe, hold the syringe straight up and tap the side of the syringe until the bubbles float to the top. Push the bubbles out with the plunger and draw insulin back in until you have the correct dose.
9. Remove the needle from the vial. Do not let the needle touch anything. You are now ready to inject.

How do I inject LANTUS?
Inject LANTUS under your skin once a day. You may take LANTUS at any time during the day but you must take it at the same time every day. You do not need to shake the vial before use. You should look at the medicine in the vial. If the medicine is cloudy or has particles in it, throw the vial away and get a new one. Check the expiration date.
Do NOT mix or dilute LANTUS with any other insulin or solution or LANTUS will not work as intended, and you may lose blood sugar control, which could be serious.
Follow these steps:
1. Decide on an injection area—either upper arm, thigh, or abdomen. Injection sites within an injection area must be different from one injection to the next.
2. Use alcohol to clean the skin where you are going to inject.
3. Pinch the skin. Stick the needle in the way your doctor, nurse, or diabetes educator showed you. Release the skin.
4. Slowly push in the plunger of the syringe all the way, making sure you have injected all the insulin. Leave the needle in the skin for several seconds.
5. Pull the needle straight out and gently press on the spot where you injected yourself for several seconds. **Do not rub the area.**
6. Follow your health care professional's instructions for throwing away the needle and syringe. Used needles and syringe should be placed in sharps containers (such as red biohazard containers), hard plastic containers (such as detergent bottles), or metal containers (such as an empty coffee can). Such containers should be sealed and disposed of properly.

If your blood glucose reading is high or low, tell your health care professional so the dose can be adjusted.

What can affect how much insulin I need?
Illness. Illness may change how much insulin you need. It is a good idea to think ahead and make a "sick day" plan with your health care professional so you will be ready when this happens. Be sure to test your blood and urine often and call your health care professional if you are sick.
Pregnancy and nursing. The effects of LANTUS on an unborn child or on a nursing baby are unknown, therefore, tell your health care professional if you plan to become pregnant or breast feed, or if you become pregnant. You may need to use another medicine.
Your diabetes may be harder to control when you are pregnant. It is important for you to monitor your glucose closer than usual during this time.
Medicines. Other medicines, including non-prescription medicines, and dietary supplements can change the way insulin works. Therefore, tell your health care professional about all other medicines and supplements you are taking. Do not change your medicine doses yourself.
For example, your body may need more insulin if you take birth control, thyroid, decongestant, or diet pills. Your body may need less insulin if you are taking antidepressants, antidiabetes pills, or ACE inhibitors (used to lower blood pressure, for certain heart conditions and kidney disease).
Exercise. Exercise may change the way your body uses insulin. Be sure to check with your health care professional before you start an exercise program.
Travel. If you travel across time zones, talk with your health care professional about how to time your injections. When you travel, wear your medical alert identification. Take extra insulin and supplies with you.

What if I want to drink alcohol?
Before you drink alcohol, talk to your health care professional about its effect on diabetes.

What are the possible side effects of insulins?

1. Hypoglycemia (low blood sugar):
Hypoglycemia is often called an "insulin reaction" or "low blood sugar." It may occur when you do not have enough glucose in your blood.
Early warning signs of hypoglycemia may be different or less noticeable in some people. That is why it is important to check your glucose as you have been advised by your health care professional.
Hypoglycemia can occur with:
- **The wrong insulin dose.** This can happen when too much insulin is injected.
- **Medicines that directly lower glucose or increase sensitivity to insulin.** This can happen with oral (taken by mouth) antidiabetes drugs, sulfa antibiotics (for infections), ACE inhibitors (used to lower blood pressure, for certain heart conditions and kidney disease), salicylates including aspirin, some antidepressants, and with other medicines.
- **Medical conditions that limit the body's glucose reserve, lengthen the time insulin stays in the body, or that increase sensitivity to insulin.** These conditions include diseases of the adrenal glands, the pituitary, the thyroid gland, the liver, and the kidney.
- **Not enough carbohydrate (sugar or starch) intake.** This can happen if a meal or snack is missed or delayed, you have vomiting or diarrhea that decreases the amount of glucose absorbed by your body or you have consumed alcohol as it interferes with carbohydrate metabolism
- **Too much glucose in the body.** This can happen if you exercise too much or have higher than normal metabolism rates due to fever.
- **Poor injection technique**

Hypoglycemia can be mild or severe. Its onset may be rapid. Patients with very good (tight) glucose control, patients with diabetes neuropathy (nerve problems), or patients using some beta-blockers (used for high blood pressure and heart conditions) may have few warning symptoms before severe hypoglycemia develops.
Hypoglycemia may reduce your ability to drive a car or use mechanical equipment without risk of injury to yourself or others. Severe hypoglycemia can cause temporary or permanent harm to your heart or brain. **It may cause unconsciousness, seizures, or death.**
Symptoms of hypoglycemia include:
- anxiety, irritability, restlessness, trouble concentrating, personality changes, mood changes, or other abnormal behavior
- tingling in your hands, feet, lips, or tongue
- dizziness, light-headedness, or drowsiness
- nightmares or trouble sleeping
- headache
- blurred vision or slurred speech
- palpitations (rapid heart beat)
- sweating
- tremor (shaking) or unsteady gait (walking)

If you have frequent or severe hypoglycemia or if you have trouble recognizing the symptoms of hypoglycemia, talk to your health care professional. Mild to moderate hypoglycemia can be treated by eating or drinking carbohydrates (fruit juice, raisins, sugar candies, milk or glucose tablets). More severe or continuing hypoglycemia may require the help of another person or emergency medical personnel. Someone with hypoglycemia who cannot take sugar by mouth needs medical help fast and will need treatment with a glucagon injection or glucose given intravenously. Without immediate medical help, serious reactions or even death could occur.
Talk with your health care professional about severe, continuing, or frequent hypoglycemia, and hypoglycemia for which you had few warning symptoms.

2. Hyperglycemia (high blood sugar):
Hyperglycemia occurs when you have too much glucose in your blood. Usually, it means there is not enough insulin to break down the food you eat into energy your body can use. Hyperglycemia can be caused by a fever, an infection, stress, eating more than you should, taking less insulin or antidiabetes agents than prescribed, or it can be part of the natural progression of diabetes.
Hyperglycemia can occur with:
- **The wrong insulin dose.** This can happen from injecting too little or no insulin, or the insulin's ability to lower glucose is changed by incorrect storage (freezing, excessive heat), or usage after the expiration date.
- **Too much carbohydrate intake.** This can happen if you eat larger meals, eat more often or increase the proportion of carbohydrate in your meals.
- **Medicines that directly increase glucose or decrease sensitivity to insulin.** This can happen, for example, with thiazides (water pills), corticosteroids, or birth control pills.
- **Medical conditions that increase the body's production of glucose or decrease sensitivity to insulin.** These medical conditions include fevers, infections, heart attacks, and stress.
- **Poor injection technique**

Routine testing of your blood will let you know if you have hyperglycemia. If your tests are often high, tell your health care professional so your dose of medicine can be changed.
Hyperglycemia can be mild or severe. It can **progress to diabetic ketoacidosis (DKA), very high glucose levels or hyperosmolar coma and result in unconsciousness and death.**
Diabetic ketoacidosis occurs most often in patients with type 1 diabetes but it can occur in patients with type 2 diabetes who become seriously ill.
Because some patients experience few symptoms of hyperglycemia and ketosis, it is important to monitor your glucose regularly.
Symptoms of hyperglycemia or DKA include:
- confusion or drowsiness
- fruity smelling breath
- rapid, deep breathing
- increased thirst
- decreased appetite, nausea, or vomiting
- abdominal (stomach area) pain
- rapid heart rate
- increased urination and dehydration (too little fluid in your body)

More severe or continuing hyperglycemia or DKA requires prompt evaluation and treatment by your health care professional.
Do not use LANTUS to treat diabetic ketoacidosis.

3. Allergic reactions:
In rare cases, a patient may be allergic to an insulin product. Severe insulin allergies may be life-threatening. If you think you are having an allergic reaction, get medical help right away. Signs of insulin allergy are:
- a rash all over your body
- shortness of breath
- wheezing (trouble breathing)
- a fast pulse
- sweating
- low blood pressure

4. Possible reactions on the skin at the injection site:
Injecting insulin can cause the following reactions on the skin at the injection site:
- a little depression in the skin (lipoatrophy)
- skin thickening (lipohypertrophy)
- red, swelling, itchy skin (injection site reaction)

An injection site reaction should clear up in a few days or a few weeks. If it does not go away and it continues to occur, tell your health care professional.
You can reduce the chance of getting lipoatrophy and lipohypertrophy if you change the injection site each time. Tell your health care professional if you have these problems. You may need to learn to inject your insulin a different way.

How should I store LANTUS?
Unopened Vials:
Store new unopened LANTUS vials in the refrigerator (not the freezer) between 36°F–46°F (2°C–8°C). Do not freeze LANTUS. If a vial freezes, throw it away. Keep LANTUS out of direct heat and light.
Open (In Use) vial:
Once a vial is opened, you can keep it in the refrigerator or as cool as possible (below 86°F [30°C]), but the opened 10 mL vial must be used within 28 days. If refrigeration is not possible, the open vial in use can be kept unrefrigerated for up to 28 days away from direct heat and light, as long as the temperature is not greater than 86°F (30°C). For example, do not leave it in your car on a summer day.
Do not use a vial of LANTUS after the expiration date stamped on the label.

VOCABULARY

Glucose—A form of sugar that the body uses for fuel. It is made when food is broken down in the digestive system. Blood carries glucose to the cells.
Hyperglycemia—Too much glucose in the blood. Usually testing, not symptoms, reveals a too-high level.
Hypoglycemia—Also called insulin reaction. It means that glucose levels in the blood are too low.
Insulin—A hormone that helps the cells in your body use glucose.
Ketoacidosis (kee-toe-as-ih-DOE-sis)—A dangerous condition caused when the body does not have enough insulin.
LANTUS—A long-acting insulin similar to insulin made by your body. It is used once a day at bedtime to lower blood glucose.
Lipoatrophy (LIP-o-AT-troe-fee)—Loss of fat under the skin. Can be caused by repeated insulin injections in the same place.
Lipohypertrophy (LIP-o-hi-PER-troe-fee)—A lump under the skin caused by an overgrowth of fat cells. Can be caused by repeated insulin injections in the same place.

Pancreas (PAN-kree-as)—A gland near the stomach that produces insulin.
Subcutaneous (sub-ku-TAE-nee-us)—The fatty layer under the skin.

ADDITIONAL INFORMATION

DIABETES FORECAST is a national magazine designed especially for patients with diabetes and their families and is available by subscription from the American Diabetes Association, National Service Center, 1701 N. Beauregard Street, Alexandria, Virginia 22311, 1-800-DIABETES (1-800-342-2383).
Another publication, **DIABETES COUNTDOWN**, is available from the Juvenile Diabetes Foundation International (JDF), 120 Wall Street, 19th Floor, New York, New York 10005, 1-800-JDF-CURE (1-800-533-2873). You may also visit the JDF website at www.jdf.org.
To get more information about diabetes, check with your health care professional or diabetes educator or visit www.DiabetesWatch.com. To get more information about LANTUS, ask your health care professional or call 1-800-633-1610.
Rev. May 2003a
Aventis Pharmaceuticals Inc.
Kansas City, MO 64137 USA

Shown in Product Identification Guide, page 307

LOVENOX® ℞

[lō′və-nŏks]
(enoxaparin sodium injection)
Rx only

Rev. April 2004

SPINAL / EPIDURAL HEMATOMAS

When neuraxial anesthesia (epidural/spinal anesthesia) or spinal puncture is employed, patients anticoagulated or scheduled to be anticoagulated with low molecular weight heparins or heparinoids for prevention of thromboembolic complications are at risk of developing an epidural or spinal hematoma which can result in long-term or permanent paralysis.
The risk of these events is increased by the use of indwelling epidural catheters for administration of analgesia or by the concomitant use of drugs affecting hemostasis such as non steroidal anti-inflammatory drugs (NSAIDs), platelet inhibitors, or other anticoagulants. The risk also appears to be increased by traumatic or repeated epidural or spinal puncture.
Patients should be frequently monitored for signs and symptoms of neurological impairment. If neurologic compromise is noted, urgent treatment is necessary.
The physician should consider the potential benefit versus risk before neuraxial intervention in patients anticoagulated or to be anticoagulated for thromboprophylaxis (see also **WARNINGS, Hemorrhage,** and **PRECAUTIONS, Drug Interactions**).

DESCRIPTION

Lovenox Injection is a sterile aqueous solution containing enoxaparin sodium, a low molecular weight heparin.
Lovenox Injection is available in two concentrations:

1. 100 mg per mL

-Prefilled Syringes	30 mg / 0.3 mL, 40 mg / 0.4 mL
-Graduated Prefilled Syringes	60 mg / 0.6 mL, 80 mg / 0.8 mL, 100 mg / 1 mL
-Multiple-Dose Vials	300 mg / 3.0 mL

Lovenox Injection 100 mg/mL Concentration contains 10 mg enoxaparin sodium (approximate anti-Factor Xa activity of 1000 IU [with reference to the W.H.O. First International Low Molecular Weight Heparin Reference Standard]) per 0.1 mL Water for Injection.

2. 150 mg per mL

-Graduated Prefilled Syringes	120 mg / 0.8 mL, 150 mg / 1 mL

Lovenox Injection 150 mg/mL Concentration contains 15 mg enoxaparin sodium (approximate anti-Factor Xa activity of 1500 IU [with reference to the W.H.O. First International Low Molecular Weight Heparin Reference Standard]) per 0.1 mL Water for Injection.
The Lovenox prefilled syringes and graduated prefilled syringes are preservative-free and intended for use only as a single-dose injection. The multiple-dose vial contains 15 mg/1.0 mL benzyl alcohol as a preservative. (See **DOSAGE AND ADMINISTRATION** and **HOW SUPPLIED** for dosage unit descriptions.) The pH of the injection is 5.5 to 7.5.
Enoxaparin sodium is obtained by alkaline degradation of heparin benzyl ester derived from porcine intestinal mucosa. Its structure is characterized by a 2-O-sulfo-4-enepyranosuronic acid group at the non-reducing end and a 2-N,6-O-disulfo-D-glucosamine at the reducing end of the chain. The drug substance is the sodium salt. The average molecular weight is about 4500 daltons. The molecular weight distribution is:

<2000 daltons	≤20%
2000 to 8000 daltons	≥68%
>8000 daltons	≤18%

Pharmacokinetic Parameters* After 5 Days of 1.5 mg/kg SC Once Daily Doses of Enoxaparin Sodium Using 100 mg/mL *or* 200 mg/mL Concentrations

	Concentration	Anti-Xa	Anti-IIa	Heptest	aPTT
Amax (IU/mL or Δ sec)	100 mg/mL	1.37 (±0.23)	0.23 (±0.05)	104.5 (±16.6)	19.3 (±4.7)
	200 mg/mL	1.45 (±0.22)	0.26 (±0.05)	110.9 (±17.1)	22 (±6.7)
	90% CI	102-110%		102-111%	
tmax** (h)	100 mg/mL	3 (2-6)	4 (2-5)	2.5 (2-4.5)	3 (2-4.5)
	200 mg/mL	3.5 (2-6)	4.5 (2.5-6)	3.3 (2-5)	3 (2-5)
AUC (ss) (h*IU/mL or h*Δ sec)	100 mg/mL	14.26 (±2.93)	1.54 (±0.61)	1321 (±219)	
	200 mg/mL	15.43 (±2.96)	1.77 (±0.67)	1401 (±227)	
	90% CI	105-112%		103-109%	

*Means ± SD at Day 5 and 90% Confidence Interval (CI) of the ratio
**Median (range)

STRUCTURAL FORMULA

R	R′	n
– H or – SO_3Na	– SO_3Na or – C–CH_3 (=O)	3 to 20

CLINICAL PHARMACOLOGY

Enoxaparin is a low molecular weight heparin which has antithrombotic properties. In humans, enoxaparin given at a dose of 1.5 mg/kg subcutaneously (SC) is characterized by a higher ratio of anti-Factor Xa to anti-Factor IIa activity (mean±SD, 14.0±3.1) (based on areas under anti-Factor activity versus time curves) compared to the ratios observed for heparin (mean±SD, 1.22±0.13). Increases of up to 1.8 times the control values were seen in the thrombin time (TT) and the activated partial thromboplastin time (aPTT). Enoxaparin at a 1 mg/kg dose (100 mg / mL concentration), administered SC every 12 hours to patients in a large clinical trial resulted in aPTT values of 45 seconds or less in the majority of patients (n = 1607).

Pharmacokinetics (conducted using 100 mg / mL concentration):

Absorption. Maximum anti-Factor Xa and anti-thrombin (anti-Factor IIa) activities occur 3 to 5 hours after SC injection of enoxaparin. Mean peak anti-Factor Xa activity was 0.16 IU/mL (1.58 µg/mL) and 0.38 IU/mL (3.83 µg/mL) after the 20 mg and the 40 mg clinically tested SC doses, respectively. Mean (n = 46) peak anti-Factor Xa activity was 1.1 IU/mL at steady state in patients with unstable angina receiving 1mg/kg SC every 12 hours for 14 days. Mean absolute bioavailability of enoxaparin, after 1.5 mg/kg given SC, based on anti-Factor Xa activity is approximately 100% in healthy volunteers.
Enoxaparin pharmacokinetics appear to be linear over the recommended dosage ranges (see **Dosage and Administration**). After repeated subcutaneous administration of 40 mg once daily and 1.5 mg/kg once-daily regimens in healthy volunteers, the steady state is reached on day 2 with an average exposure ratio about 15% higher than after a single dose. Steady-state enoxaparin activity levels are well predicted by single-dose pharmacokinetics. After repeated subcutaneous administration of the 1 mg/kg twice daily regimen, the steady state is reached from day 4 with mean exposure about 65% higher than after a single dose and mean peak and trough levels of about 1.2 and 0.52 IU/mL, respectively. Based on enoxaparin sodium pharmacokinetics, this difference in steady state is expected and within the therapeutic range.
Although not studied clinically, the 150 mg/mL concentration of enoxaparin sodium is projected to result in anticoagulant activities similar to those of 100 mg/mL and 200 mg/mL concentrations at the same enoxaparin dose. When a daily 1.5 mg/kg SC injection of enoxaparin sodium was given to 25 healthy male and female subjects using a 100 mg/mL or a 200 mg/mL concentration the following pharmacokinetic profiles were obtained (see table below):
[See table above]

Distribution. The volume of distribution of anti-Factor Xa activity is about 4.3 L.

Elimination. Following intravenous (i.v.) dosing, the total body clearance of enoxaparin is 26 mL/min. After i.v. dosing of enoxaparin labeled with the gamma-emitter, ^{99m}Tc, 40% of radioactivity and 8 to 20% of anti-Factor Xa activity were recovered in urine in 24 hours. Elimination half-life based on anti-Factor Xa activity was 4.5 hours after a single SC dose to about 7 hours after repeated dosing. Following a 40 mg SC once a day dose, significant anti-Factor Xa activity persists in plasma for about 12 hours.
Following SC dosing, the apparent clearance (CL/F) of enoxaparin is approximately 15 mL/min.

Metabolism. Enoxaparin sodium is primarily metabolized in the liver by desulfation and/or depolymerization to lower molecular weight species with much reduced biological potency. Renal clearance of active fragments represents about 10% of the administered dose and total renal excretion of active and non-active fragments 40% of the dose.

Special Populations

Gender: Apparent clearance and A_{max} derived from anti-Factor Xa values following single SC dosing (40 mg and 60 mg) were slightly higher in males than in females. The source of the gender difference in these parameters has not been conclusively identified, however, body weight may be a contributing factor.

Geriatric: Apparent clearance and A_{max} derived from anti-Factor Xa values following single and multiple SC dosing in elderly subjects were close to those observed in young subjects. Following once a day SC dosing of 40 mg enoxaparin, the Day 10 mean area under anti-Factor Xa activity versus time curve (AUC) was approximately 15% greater than the mean Day 1 AUC value. (See **PRECAUTIONS**.)

Renal Impairment: A linear relationship between anti-Factor Xa plasma clearance and creatinine clearance at steady-state has been observed, which indicates decreased clearance of enoxaparin sodium in patients with reduced renal function. Anti-Factor Xa exposure represented by AUC, at steady-state, is marginally increased in mild (creatinine clearance 50–80 mL/min) and moderate (creatinine clearance 30–50 mL/min) renal impairment after repeated subcutaneous 40 mg once daily doses. In patients with severe renal impairment (creatinine clearance <30 mL/ min), the AUC at steady state is significantly increased on average by 65% after repeated subcutaneous 40-mg once-daily doses (see **PRECAUTIONS** and **DOSAGE AND ADMINISTRATION**).

Weight: After repeated subcutaneous 1.5 mg/kg once daily dosing, mean AUC of anti-Factor Xa activity is marginally higher at steady-state in obese healthy volunteers (BMI 30-48 kg/m^2) compared to non-obese control subjects, while Amax is not increased.
When non-weight adjusted dosing was administered, it was found after a single-subcutaneous 40-mg dose, that anti-Factor Xa exposure is 52% higher in low-weight women (<45 kg) and 27% higher in low-weight men (<57 kg) when compared to normal weight control subjects (see **PRECAUTIONS**).

Hemodialysis: In a single study, elimination rate appeared similar but AUC was two-fold higher than control population, after a single 0.25 or 0.50 mg/kg intravenous dose.

CLINICAL TRIALS

Prophylaxis of Deep Vein Thrombosis Following Abdominal Surgery in Patients at Risk for Thromboembolic Complications: Abdominal surgery patients at risk include those who are over 40 years of age, obese, undergoing surgery under general anesthesia lasting longer than 30 minutes or who have additional risk factors such as malignancy or a history of deep vein thrombosis or pulmonary embolism.
In a double-blind, parallel group study of patients undergoing elective cancer surgery of the gastrointestinal, urological, or gynecological tract, a total of 1116 patients were enrolled in the study, and 1115 patients were treated. Patients ranged in age from 32 to 97 years (mean age 67 years) with 52.7% men and 47.3% women. Patients were 98% Caucasian, 1.1% Black, 0.4% Oriental, and 0.4% others. Lovenox Injection 40 mg SC, administered once a day, beginning 2 hours prior to surgery and continuing for a maximum of 12 days after surgery, was comparable to heparin 5000 U every 8 hours SC in reducing the risk of deep vein thrombosis (DVT). The efficacy data are provided below.

Efficacy of Lovenox Injection in the Prophylaxis of Deep Vein Thrombosis Following Abdominal Surgery

	Dosing Regimen	
Indication	**Lovenox Inj.** 40 mg q.d. SC n (%)	**Heparin** 5000 U q8h SC n (%)
All Treated Abdominal Surgery Patients	555 (100)	560 (100)

Continued on next page

Lovenox—Cont.

Treatment Failures		
Total VTE[1] (%)	56 (10.1) (95% CI[2]: 8 to 13)	63 (11.3) (95% CI: 9 to 14)
DVT Only (%)	54 (9.7) (95% CI: 7 to 12)	61 (10.9) (95% CI: 8 to 13)

[1] VTE = Venous thromboembolic events which included DVT, PE, and death considered to be thromboembolic in origin.
[2] CI = Confidence Interval

In a second double-blind, parallel group study, Lovenox Injection 40 mg SC once a day was compared to heparin 5000 U every 8 hours SC in patients undergoing colorectal surgery (one-third with cancer). A total of 1347 patients were randomized in the study and all patients were treated. Patients ranged in age from 18 to 92 years (mean age 50.1 years) with 54.2% men and 45.8% women. Treatment was initiated approximately 2 hours prior to surgery and continued for approximately 7 to 10 days after surgery. The efficacy data are provided below.

Efficacy of Lovenox Injection in the Prophylaxis of Deep Vein Thrombosis Following Colorectal Surgery

	Dosing Regimen	
Indication	**Lovenox Inj.** 40 mg q.d. SC n (%)	**Heparin** 5000 U q8h SC n (%)
All Treated Colorectal Surgery Patients	673 (100)	674 (100)
Treatment Failures		
Total VTE[1] (%)	47 (7.1) (95% CI[2]: 5 to 9)	45 (6.7) (95% CI: 5 to 9)
DVT Only (%)	47 (7.0) (95% CI: 5 to 9)	44 (6.5) (95% CI: 5 to 8)

[1] VTE = Venous thromboembolic events which included DVT, PE, and death considered to be thromboembolic in origin.
[2] CI = Confidence Interval

Prophylaxis of Deep Vein Thrombosis Following Hip or Knee Replacement Surgery: Lovenox Injection has been shown to reduce the risk of post-operative deep vein thrombosis (DVT) following hip or knee replacement surgery.
In a double-blind study, Lovenox Injection 30 mg every 12 hours SC was compared to placebo in patients with hip replacement. A total of 100 patients were randomized in the study and all patients were treated. Patients ranged in age from 41 to 84 years (mean age 67.1 years) with 45% men and 55% women. After hemostasis was established, treatment was initiated 12 to 24 hours after surgery and was continued for 10 to 14 days after surgery. The efficacy data are provided below.

Efficacy of Lovenox Injection in the Prophylaxis of Deep Vein Thrombosis Following Hip Replacement Surgery

	Dosing Regimen	
Indication	**Lovenox Inj.** 30 mg q12h SC n (%)	**Placebo** q12h SC n (%)
All Treated Hip Replacement Patients	50 (100)	50 (100)
Treatment Failures		
Total DVT (%)	5 (10)[1]	23 (46)
Proximal DVT (%)	1 (2)[2]	11 (22)

[1] p value versus placebo = 0.0002
[2] p value versus placebo = 0.0134

A double-blind, multicenter study compared three dosing regimens of Lovenox Injection in patients with hip replacement. A total of 572 patients were randomized in the study and 568 patients were treated. Patients ranged in age from 31 to 88 years (mean age 64.7 years) with 63% men and 37% women. Patients were 93% Caucasian, 6% Black, <1% Oriental, and 1% others. Treatment was initiated within two days after surgery and was continued for 7 to 11 days after surgery. The efficacy data are provided below.
[See first table above]
There was no significant difference between the 30 mg every 12 hours and 40 mg once a day regimens. In a double-blind study, Lovenox Injection 30 mg every 12 hours SC was compared to placebo in patients undergoing knee replacement

Efficacy of Lovenox Injection in the Prophylaxis of Deep Vein Thrombosis Following Hip Replacement Surgery

	Dosing Regimen		
Indication	**10 mg q.d. SC** n (%)	**30 mg q12h SC** n (%)	**40 mg q.d. SC** n (%)
All Treated Hip Replacement Patients	161 (100)	208 (100)	199 (100)
Treatment Failures			
Total DVT (%)	40 (25)	22 (11)[1]	27 (14)
Proximal DVT (%)	17 (11)	8 (4)[2]	9 (5)

[1] p value versus Lovenox 10 mg once a day = 0.0008
[2] p value versus Lovenox 10 mg once a day = 0.0168

Efficacy of Lovenox Injection in the Prophylaxis of Deep Vein Thrombosis in Medical Patients With Severely Restricted Mobility During Acute Illness

	Dosing Regimen		
Indication	**Lovenox Inj.** 20 mg q.d. SC n (%)	**Lovenox Inj.** 40 mg q.d. SC n (%)	**Placebo** n (%)
All Treated Medical Patients During Acute Illness	351 (100)	360 (100)	362 (100)
Treatment Failure[1] Total VTE[2] (%)	43 (12.3)	16 (4.4)	43 (11.9)
Total DVT (%)	43 (12.3) (95% CI[3] 8.8 to 15.7)	16 (4.4) (95% CI[3] 2.3 to 6.6)	41 (11.3) (95% CI[3] 8.1 to 14.6)
Proximal DVT (%)	13 (3.7)	5 (1.4)	14 (3.9)

[1] Treatment failures during therapy, between Days 1 and 14.
[2] VTE = Venous thromboembolic events which included DVT, PE, and death considered to be thromboembolic in origin.
[3] CI = Confidence Interval

surgery. A total of 132 patients were randomized in the study and 131 patients were treated, of which 99 had total knee replacement and 32 had either unicompartmental knee replacement or tibial osteotomy. The 99 patients with total knee replacement ranged in age from 42 to 85 years (mean age 70.2 years) with 36.4% men and 63.6% women. After hemostasis was established, treatment was initiated 12 to 24 hours after surgery and was continued up to 15 days after surgery. The incidence of proximal and total DVT after surgery was significantly lower for Lovenox Injection compared to placebo. The efficacy data are provided below.

Efficacy of Lovenox Injection in the Prophylaxis of Deep Vein Thrombosis Following Total Knee Replacement Surgery

	Dosing Regimen	
Indication	**Lovenox Inj.** 30 mg q12h SC n (%)	**Placebo** q12h SC n (%)
All Treated Total Knee Replacement Patients	47 (100)	52 (100)
Treatment Failures		
Total DVT (%)	5 (11)[1] (95% CI[2]: 1 to 21)	32 (62) (95% CI: 47 to 76)
Proximal DVT (%)	0 (0)[3] (95% Upper CL[4]: 5)	7 (13) (95% CI: 3 to 24)

[1] p value versus placebo = 0.0001
[2] CI = Confidence Interval
[3] p value versus placebo = 0.013
[4] CL = Confidence Limit

Additionally, in an open-label, parallel group, randomized clinical study, Lovenox Injection 30 mg every 12 hours SC in patients undergoing elective knee replacement surgery was compared to heparin 5000 U every 8 hours SC. A total of 453 patients were randomized in the study and all were treated. Patients ranged in age from 38 to 90 years (mean age 68.5 years) with 43.7% men and 56.3% women. Patients were 92.5% Caucasian, 5.3% Black, 0.2% Oriental, and 0.4% others. Treatment was initiated after surgery and continued up to 14 days. The incidence of deep vein thrombosis was significantly lower for Lovenox Injection compared to heparin.
Extended Prophylaxis of Deep Vein Thrombosis Following Hip Replacement Surgery: In a study of extended prophylaxis for patients undergoing hip replacement surgery, patients were treated, while hospitalized, with Lovenox Injection 40 mg SC, initiated up to 12 hours prior to surgery for the prophylaxis of post-operative DVT. At the end of the peri-operative period, all patients underwent bilateral venography. In a double-blind design, those patients with no venous thromboembolic disease were randomized to a post-discharge regimen of either Lovenox Injection 40 mg (n = 90) once a day SC or to placebo (n = 89) for 3 weeks. A total of 179 patients were randomized in the double-blind phase of the study and all patients were treated. Patients ranged in age from 47 to 87 years (mean age 69.4 years) with 57% men and 43% women. In this population of patients, the incidence of DVT during extended prophylaxis was significantly lower for Lovenox Injection compared to placebo. The efficacy data are provided below.

Efficacy of Lovenox Injection in the Extended Prophylaxis of Deep Vein Thrombosis Following Hip Replacement Surgery

	Post-Discharge Dosing Regimen	
Indication (Post-Discharge)	**Lovenox Inj.** 40 mg q.d. SC n (%)	**Placebo** q.d. SC n (%)
All Treated Extended Prophylaxis Patients	90 (100)	89 (100)
Treatment Failures		
Total DVT (%)	6 (7)[1] (95% CI[2]: 3 to 14)	18 (20) (95% CI: 12 to 30)
Proximal DVT (%)	5 (6)[3] (95% CI: 2 to 13)	7 (8) (95% CI: 3 to 16)

[1] p value versus placebo = 0.008
[2] CI= Confidence Interval
[3] p value versus placebo = 0.537

In a second study, patients undergoing hip replacement surgery were treated, while hospitalized, with Lovenox Injection 40 mg SC, initiated up to 12 hours prior to surgery. All patients were examined for clinical signs and symptoms of venous thromboembolic (VTE) disease. In a double-blind design, patients without clinical signs and symptoms of VTE disease were randomized to a post-discharge regimen of either Lovenox Injection 40 mg (n = 131) once a day SC or to placebo (n = 131) for 3 weeks. A total of 262 patients were randomized in the study double-blind phase and all patients were treated. Patients ranged in age from 44 to 87 years (mean age 68.5 years) with 43.1% men and 56.9% women. Similar to the first study the incidence of DVT during extended prophylaxis was significantly lower for Lovenox Injection compared to placebo, with a statistically significant difference in both total DVT (Lovenox Injection 21 [16%] versus placebo 45 [34%]; p = 0.001) and proximal DVT (Lovenox Injection 8 [6%] versus placebo 28 [21%]; p = <0.001).

Prophylaxis of Deep Vein Thrombosis (DVT) In Medical Patients with Severely Restricted Mobility During Acute Illness: In a double blind multicenter, parallel group study, Lovenox Injection 20 mg or 40 mg once a day SC was compared to placebo in the prophylaxis of DVT in medical patients with severely restricted mobility during acute illness (defined as walking distance of <10 meters for ≤ 3 days). This study included patients with heart failure (NYHA Class III or IV); acute respiratory failure or complicated chronic respiratory insufficiency (not requiring ventilatory

Efficacy of Lovenox Injection in the Prophylaxis of Ischemic Complications in Unstable Angina and Non-Q-Wave Myocardial Infarction (Combined Endpoint of Death, Myocardial Infarction, or Recurrent Angina)

Indication	Dosing Regimen[1] Lovenox Inj. 1 mg/kg q12h SC n (%)	Heparin aPTT Adjusted i.v. Therapy n (%)	Reduction (%)	p Value
All Treated Unstable Angina and Non-Q-Wave MI Patients	1578 (100)	1529 (100)		
Timepoint[2]				
48 Hours	96 (6.1)	112 (7.3)	1.2	0.120
14 Days	261 (16.5)	303 (19.8)	3.3	0.017
30 Days	313 (19.8)	358 (23.4)	3.6	0.014

[1] All patients were also treated with aspirin 100 to 325 mg per day.
[2] Evaluation timepoints are after initiation of treatment. Therapy continued for up to 8 days (median duration 2.6 days).

Efficacy of Lovenox Injection in the Prophylaxis of Ischemic Complications in Unstable Angina and Non-Q-Wave Myocardial Infarction (Combined Endpoint of Death or Myocardial Infarction)

Indication	Dosing Regimen[1] Lovenox Inj. 1 mg/kg q12h SC n (%)	Heparin aPTT Adjusted i.v. Therapy n (%)	Reduction (%)	p Value
All Treated Unstable Angina and Non-Q-Wave MI Patients	1578 (100)	1529 (100)		
Timepoint[2]				
48 Hours	16 (1.0)	20 (1.3)	0.3	0.126
14 Days	76 (4.8)	93 (6.1)	1.3	0.115
30 Days	96 (6.1)	118 (7.7)	1.6	0.069

[1] All patients were also treated with aspirin 100 to 325 mg per day.
[2] Evaluation timepoints are after initiation of treatment. Therapy continued for up to 8 days (median duration 2.6 days).

Efficacy of Lovenox Injection in Treatment of Deep Vein Thrombosis With or Without Pulmonary Embolism

Indication	Dosing Regimen[1] Lovenox Inj. 1.5 mg/kg q.d. SC n (%)	Lovenox Inj. 1 mg/kg q12h SC n (%)	Heparin aPTT Adjusted i.v. Therapy n (%)
All Treated DVT Patients with or without PE	298 (100)	312 (100)	290 (100)
Patient Outcome Total VTE[2] (%)	13 (4.4)[3]	9 (2.9)[3]	12 (4.1)
DVT Only (%)	11 (3.7)	7 (2.2)	8 (2.8)
Proximal DVT (%)	9 (3.0)	6 (1.9)	7 (2.4)
PE (%)	2 (0.7)	2 (0.6)	4 (1.4)

[1] All patients were also treated with warfarin sodium commencing within 72 hours of Lovenox Injection or standard heparin therapy.
[2] VTE = venous thromboembolic event (DVT and/or PE).
[3] The 95% Confidence Intervals for the treatment differences for total VTE were:
Lovenox Injection once a day versus heparin (-3.0 to 3.5)
Lovenox Injection every 12 hours versus heparin (-4.2 to 1.7).

support): acute infection (excluding septic shock); or acute rheumatic disorder [acute lumbar or sciatic pain, vertebral compression (due to osteoporosis or tumor), acute arthritic episodes of the lower extremities]. A total of 1102 patients were enrolled in the study, and 1073 patients were treated. Patients ranged in age from 40 to 97 years (mean age 73 years) with equal proportions of men and women. Treatment continued for a maximum of 14 days (median duration 7 days). When given at a dose of 40 mg once a day SC, Lovenox Injection significantly reduced the incidence of DVT as compared to placebo. The efficacy data are provided below.

[See second table at top of previous page]

At approximately 3 months following enrollment, the incidence of venous thromboembolism remained significantly lower in the Lovenox Injection 40 mg treatment group versus the placebo treatment group.

Prophylaxis of Ischemic Complications in Unstable Angina and Non-Q-Wave Myocardial Infarction: In a multicenter, double-blind, parallel group study, patients who recently experienced unstable angina or non-Q-wave myocardial infarction were randomized to either Lovenox Injection 1 mg/kg every 12 hours SC or heparin i.v. bolus (5000 U) followed by a continuous infusion (adjusted to achieve an aPTT of 55 to 85 seconds). A total of 3171 patients were enrolled in the study, and 3107 patients were treated. Patients ranged in age from 25-94 years (median age 64 years), with 33.4% of patients female and 66.6% male. Race was distributed as follows: 89.8% Caucasian, 4.8% Black, 2.0% Oriental, and 3.5% other. **All** patients were also treated with aspirin 100 to 325 mg per day. Treatment was initiated within 24 hours of the event and continued until clinical stabilization, revascularization procedures, or hospital discharge, with a maximal duration of 8 days of therapy. The combined incidence of the triple endpoint of death, myocardial infarction, or recurrent angina was lower for Lovenox Injection compared with heparin therapy at 14 days after initiation of treatment. The lower incidence of the triple endpoint was sustained up to 30 days after initiation of treatment. These results were observed in an analysis of both all-randomized and all-treated patients. The efficacy data are provided below.

[See first table above]

The combined incidence of death or myocardial infarction at all time points was lower for Lovenox Injection compared to standard heparin therapy, but did not achieve statistical significance. The efficacy data are provided below.

[See second table above]

In a survey one year following treatment, with information available for 92% of enrolled patients, the combined incidence of death, myocardial infarction, or recurrent angina remained lower for Lovenox Injection versus heparin (32.0% vs 35.7%).

Urgent revascularization procedures were performed less frequently in the Lovenox Injection group as compared to the heparin group, 6.3% compared to 8.2% at 30 days (p = 0.047).

Treatment of Deep Vein Thrombosis (DVT) with or without Pulmonary Embolism (PE): In a multicenter, parallel group study, 900 patients with acute lower extremity DVT with or without PE were randomized to an inpatient (hospital) treatment of either (i) Lovenox Injection 1.5 mg/kg once a day SC, (ii) Lovenox Injection 1 mg/kg every 12 hours SC, or (iii) heparin i.v. bolus (5000 IU) followed by a continuous infusion (administered to achieve an aPTT of 55 to 85 seconds). A total of 900 patients were randomized in the study and all patients were treated. Patients ranged in age from 18 to 92 years (mean age 60.7 years) with 54.7% men and 45.3% women. All patients also received warfarin sodium (dose adjusted according to PT to achieve an International Normalization Ratio [INR] of 2.0 to 3.0), commencing within 72 hours of initiation of Lovenox Injection or standard heparin therapy, and continuing for 90 days. Lovenox Injection or standard heparin therapy was administered for a minimum of 5 days and until the targeted warfarin sodium INR was achieved. Both Lovenox Injection regimens were equivalent to standard heparin therapy in reducing the risk of recurrent venous thromboembolism (DVT and/or PE). The efficacy data are provided below.

[See third table above]

Similarly, in a multicenter, open-label, parallel group study, patients with acute proximal DVT were randomized to Lovenox Injection or heparin. Patients who could not receive outpatient therapy were excluded from entering the study. Outpatient exclusion criteria included the following: inability to receive outpatient heparin therapy because of associated co-morbid conditions or potential for non-compliance and inability to attend follow-up visits as an outpatient because of geographic inaccessibility. Eligible patients could be treated in the hospital, but ONLY Lovenox Injection patients were permitted to go home on therapy (72%). A total of 501 patients were randomized in the study and all patients were treated. Patients ranged in age from 19 to 96 years (mean age 57.8 years) with 60.5% men and 39.5% women. Patients were randomized to either Lovenox Injection 1 mg/kg every 12 hours SC or heparin i.v. bolus (5000 IU) followed by a continuous infusion administered to achieve an aPTT of 60 to 85 seconds (in-patient treatment). All patients also received warfarin sodium as described in the previous study. Lovenox Injection or standard heparin therapy was administered for a minimum of 5 days. Lovenox Injection was equivalent to standard heparin therapy in reducing the risk of recurrent venous thromboembolism. The efficacy data are provided below.

Efficacy of Lovenox Injection in Treatment of Deep Vein Thrombosis

Indication	Dosing Regimen[1] Lovenox Inj. 1 mg/kg q12h SC n (%)	Heparin aPTT Adjusted i.v. Therapy n (%)
All Treated DVT Patients	247 (100)	254 (100)
Patient Outcome Total VTE[2] (%)	13 (5.3)[3]	17 (6.7)
DVT Only (%)	11 (4.5)	14 (5.5)
Proximal DVT (%)	10 (4.0)	12 (4.7)
PE (%)	2 (0.8)	3 (1.2)

[1] All patients were also treated with warfarin sodium commencing on the evening of the second day of Lovenox Injection or standard heparin therapy.
[2] VTE = venous thromboembolic event (deep vein thrombosis [DVT] and/or pulmonary embolism [PE]).
[3] The 95% Confidence Intervals for the treatment difference for total VTE was: Lovenox Injection versus heparin (-5.6 to 2.7).

INDICATIONS AND USAGE

- Lovenox Injection is indicated for the prophylaxis of deep vein thrombosis, which may lead to pulmonary embolism:
  - in patients undergoing abdominal surgery who are at risk for thromboembolic complications;
  - in patients undergoing hip replacement surgery, during and following hospitalization;
  - in patients undergoing knee replacement surgery;
  - in medical patients who are at risk for thromboembolic complications due to severely restricted mobility during acute illness.
- Lovenox Injection is indicated for the prophylaxis of ischemic complications of unstable angina and non-Q-wave myocardial infarction, when concurrently administered with aspirin.

Continued on next page

Lovenox—Cont.

- Lovenox Injection is indicated for:
- the **inpatient treatment** of acute deep vein thrombosis **with or without pulmonary embolism**, when administered in conjunction with warfarin sodium;
- the **outpatient treatment** of acute deep vein thrombosis **without pulmonary embolism** when administered in conjunction with warfarin sodium.

See **DOSAGE AND ADMINISTRATION: Adult Dosage** for appropriate dosage regimens.

CONTRAINDICATIONS

Lovenox Injection is contraindicated in patients with active major bleeding, in patients with thrombocytopenia associated with a positive *in vitro* test for anti-platelet antibody in the presence of enoxaparin sodium, or in patients with hypersensitivity to enoxaparin sodium. Patients with known hypersensitivity to heparin or pork products should not be treated with Lovenox Injection or any of its constituents.

WARNINGS

Lovenox Injection is not intended for intramuscular administration. Lovenox Injection cannot be used interchangeably (unit for unit) with heparin or other low molecular weight heparins as they differ in manufacturing process, molecular weight distribution, anti-Xa and anti-IIa activities, units, and dosage. Each of these medicines has its own instructions for use.

Lovenox Injection should be used with extreme caution in patients with a history of heparin-induced thrombocytopenia.

Hemorrhage: Lovenox Injection, like other anticoagulants, should be used with extreme caution in conditions with increased risk of hemorrhage, such as bacterial endocarditis, congenital or acquired bleeding disorders, active ulcerative and angiodysplastic gastrointestinal disease, hemorrhagic stroke, or shortly after brain, spinal, or ophthalmological surgery, or in patients treated concomitantly with platelet inhibitors.

Cases of epidural or spinal hematomas have been reported with the associated use of Lovenox Injection and spinal/epidural anesthesia or spinal puncture resulting in long-term or permanent paralysis. The risk of these events is higher with the use of post-operative indwelling epidural catheters or by the concomitant use of additional drugs affecting hemostasis such as NSAIDs (see boxed WARNING; ADVERSE REACTIONS, Ongoing Safety Surveillance; and PRECAUTIONS, Drug Interactions).

Major hemorrhages including retroperitoneal and intracranial bleeding have been reported. Some of these cases have been fatal.

Bleeding can occur at any site during therapy with Lovenox Injection. An unexplained fall in hematocrit or blood pressure should lead to a search for a bleeding site.

Thrombocytopenia: Thrombocytopenia can occur with the administration of Lovenox Injection.

Moderate thrombocytopenia (platelet counts between 100,000/mm^3 and 50,000/mm^3) occurred at a rate of 1.3% in patients given Lovenox Injection, 1.2% in patients given heparin, and 0.7% in patients given placebo in clinical trials.

Platelet counts less than 50,000/mm^3 occurred at a rate of 0.1% in patients given Lovenox Injection, in 0.2% of patients given heparin, and 0.4% of patients given placebo in the same trials.

Thrombocytopenia of any degree should be monitored closely. If the platelet count falls below 100,000/mm^3, Lovenox Injection should be discontinued. Cases of heparin-induced thrombocytopenia with thrombosis have also been observed in clinical practice. Some of these cases were complicated by organ infarction, limb ischemia, or death.

Pregnant Women with Mechanical Prosthetic Heart Valves: The use of Lovenox Injection for thromboprophylaxis in pregnant women with mechanical prosthetic heart valves has not been adequately studied. In a clinical study of pregnant women with mechanical prosthetic heart valves given enoxaparin (1 mg/kg bid) to reduce the risk of thromboembolism, 2 of 8 women developed clots resulting in blockage of the valve and leading to maternal and fetal death. Although a causal relationship has not been established these deaths may have been due to therapeutic failure or inadequate anticoagulation. No patients in the heparin/warfarin group (0 of 4 women) died. There also have been isolated postmarketing reports of valve thrombosis in pregnant women with mechanical prosthetic heart valves while receiving enoxaparin for thromboprophylaxis. Women with mechanical prosthetic heart valves may be at higher risk for thromboembolism during pregnancy, and, when pregnant, have a higher rate of fetal loss from stillbirth, spontaneous abortion and premature delivery. Therefore, frequent monitoring of peak and trough anti-Factor Xa levels, and adjusting of dosage may be needed.

Miscellaneous: Lovenox multiple-dose vials contain benzyl alcohol as a preservative. The administration of medications containing benzyl alcohol as a preservative to premature neonates has been associated with a fatal "Gasping Syndrome". Because benzyl alcohol may cross the placenta, Lovenox multiple-dose vials, preserved with benzyl alcohol, should be used with caution in pregnant women and only if clearly needed (see **PRECAUTIONS, Pregnancy**).

PRECAUTIONS

General: Lovenox Injection should not be mixed with other injections or infusions.

Lovenox Injection should be used with care in patients with a bleeding diathesis, uncontrolled arterial hypertension or a history of recent gastrointestinal ulceration, diabetic retinopathy, and hemorrhage. Lovenox Injection should be used with care in elderly patients who may show delayed elimination of enoxaparin.

If thromboembolic events occur despite Lovenox Injection prophylaxis, appropriate therapy should be initiated.

Mechanical Prosthetic Heart Valves: The use of Lovenox Injection has not been adequately studied for thromboprophylaxis in patients with mechanical prosthetic heart valves and has not been adequately studied for long-term use in this patient population. Isolated cases of prosthetic heart valve thrombosis have been reported in patients with mechanical prosthetic heart valves who have received enoxaparin for thromboprophylaxis. Some of these cases were pregnant women in whom thrombosis led to maternal and fetal deaths. Insufficient data, the underlying disease and the possibility of inadequate anticoagulation complicate the evaluation of these cases. Pregnant women with mechanical prosthetic heart valves may be at higher risk for thromboembolism (see **WARNINGS, Pregnant Women with Mechanical Prosthetic Heart Valves**).

Renal Impairment: In patients with renal impairment, there is an increase in exposure of enoxaparin sodium. All such patients should be observed carefully for signs and symptoms of bleeding. Because exposure of enoxaparin sodium is significantly increased in patients with severe renal impairment (creatinine clearance <30 mL/min), a dosage adjustment is recommended for therapeutic and prophylactic dosage ranges. No dosage adjustment is recommended in patients with moderate (creatinine clearance 30–50 mL/min) and mild (creatinine clearance 50-80 mL/min) renal impairment. (see **DOSAGE AND ADMINISTRATION** and **CLINICAL PHARMACOLOGY, Pharmacokinetics, Special Populations**).

Low-Weight Patients: An increase in exposure of enoxaparin sodium with prophylactic dosages (non-weight adjusted) has been observed in low-weight women (<45 kg) and low-weight men (<57 kg). All such patients should be observed carefully for signs and symptoms of bleeding (see **CLINICAL PHARMACOLOGY, Pharmacokinetics, Special Populations**).

Laboratory Tests: Periodic complete blood counts, including platelet count, and stool occult blood tests are recommended during the course of treatment with Lovenox Injection. When administered at recommended prophylaxis doses, routine coagulation tests such as Prothrombin Time (PT) and Activated Partial Thromboplastin Time (aPTT) are relatively insensitive measures of Lovenox Injection activity and, therefore, unsuitable for monitoring. Anti-Factor Xa may be used to monitor the anticoagulant effect of Lovenox Injection in patients with significant renal impairment. If during Lovenox Injection therapy abnormal coagulation parameters or bleeding should occur, anti-Factor Xa levels may be used to monitor the anticoagulant effects of Lovenox Injection (see **CLINICAL PHARMACOLOGY: Pharmacokinetics**).

Drug Interactions: Unless really needed, agents which may enhance the risk of hemorrhage should be discontinued prior to initiation of Lovenox Injection therapy. These agents include medications such as: anticoagulants, platelet inhibitors including acetylsalicylic acid, salicylates, NSAIDs (including ketorolac tromethamine), dipyridamole, or sulfinpyrazone. If co-administration is essential, conduct close clinical and laboratory monitoring (see **PRECAUTIONS: Laboratory Tests**).

Carcinogenesis, Mutagenesis, Impairment of Fertility: No long-term studies in animals have been performed to evaluate the carcinogenic potential of enoxaparin. Enoxaparin was not mutagenic in *in vitro* tests, including the Ames test, mouse lymphoma cell forward mutation test, and human lymphocyte chromosomal aberration test, and the *in vivo* rat bone marrow chromosomal aberration test. Enoxaparin was found to have no effect on fertility or reproductive performance of male and female rats at SC doses up to 20 mg/kg/day or 141 mg/m^2/day. The maximum human dose in clinical trials was 2.0 mg/kg/day or 78 mg/m^2/day (for an average body weight of 70 kg, height of 170 cm, and body surface area of 1.8 m^2).

Pregnancy: Pregnancy Category B:

All pregnancies have a background risk of birth defects, loss, or other adverse outcome regardless of drug exposure. The fetal risk summary below describes Lovenox's potential to increase the risk of developmental abnormalities above background risk.

Fetal Risk Summary

Lovenox is not predicted to increase the risk of developmental abnormalities. Lovenox does not cross the placenta, based on human and animal studies, and shows no evidence of teratogenic effects or fetotoxicity.

Clinical Considerations

It is not known if dose adjustment or monitoring of anti-Xa activity of enoxaparin are necessary during pregnancy.

Pregnancy alone confers an increased risk for thromboembolism, that is even higher for women with thromboembolic disease and certain high risk pregnancy conditions. While not adequately studied, pregnant women with mechanical prosthetic heart valves may be at even higher risk for thrombosis (See **WARNINGS, Pregnant Women with Mechanical Prosthetic Heart Valves** and **PRECAUTIONS, Mechanical Prosthetic Heart Valves**.) Pregnant women with thromboembolic disease, including those with mechanical prosthetic heart valves, and those with inherited or acquired thrombophilias, also have an increased risk of other maternal complications and fetal loss regardless of the type of anticoagulant used.

All patients receiving anticoagulants such as enoxaparin, including pregnant women, are at risk for bleeding. Pregnant women receiving enoxaparin should be carefully monitored for evidence of bleeding or excessive anticoagulation. Consideration for use of a shorter acting anticoagulant should be specifically addressed as delivery approaches (see **BOXED WARNING, SPINAL/EPIDURAL HEMATOMAS**). Hemorrhage can occur at any site and may lead to death of mother and/or fetus. Pregnant women should be apprised of the potential hazard to the fetus and the mother if enoxaparin is administered during pregnancy.

Data

- Human Data - There are no adequate and well-controlled studies in pregnant women.

  A retrospective study reviewed the records of 604 women who used enoxaparin during pregnancy. A total of 624 pregnancies resulted in 693 live births. There were 72 hemorrhagic events (11 serious) in 63 women. There were 14 cases of neonatal hemorrhage. Major congenital anomalies in live births occurred at rates (2.5%) similar to background rates.[1]

  There have been postmarketing reports of fetal death when pregnant women received Lovenox Injection. Causality for these cases has not been determined. Insufficient data, the underlying disease, and the possibility of inadequate anticoagulation complicate the evaluation of these cases.

  See **WARNINGS: Pregnant Women with Mechanical Prosthetic Heart Valves** for a clinical study of pregnant women with mechanical prosthetic heart valves.
- Animal Data - Teratology studies have been conducted in pregnant rats and rabbits at SC doses of enoxaparin up to 30 mg/kg/day or 211 mg/m^2/day and 410 mg/m^2/day, respectively. There was no evidence of teratogenic effects or fetotoxicity due to enoxaparin. Because animal reproduction studies are not always predictive of human response, this drug should be used during pregnancy only if clearly needed.

Cases of "Gasping Syndrome" have occurred in premature infants when large amounts of benzyl alcohol have been administered (99-405 mg/kg/day). The multiple-dose vial of Lovenox solution contains 15 mg/1.0 mL benzyl alcohol as a preservative (see **WARNINGS, Miscellaneous**).

Nursing Mothers: It is not known whether this drug is excreted in human milk. Because many drugs are excreted in human milk, caution should be exercised when Lovenox Injection is administered to nursing women.

Pediatric Use: Safety and effectiveness of Lovenox Injection in pediatric patients have not been established.

Geriatric Use: Over 2800 patients, 65 years and older, have received Lovenox Injection in pivotal clinical trials. The efficacy of Lovenox Injection in the elderly (≥65 years) was similar to that seen in younger patients (<65 years). The incidence of bleeding complications was similar between elderly and younger patients when 30 mg every 12 hours or 40 mg once a day doses of Lovenox Injection were employed. The incidence of bleeding complications was higher in elderly patients as compared to younger patients when Lovenox Injection was administered at doses of 1.5 mg/kg once a day or 1 mg/kg every 12 hours. The risk of Lovenox Injection-associated bleeding increased with age. Serious adverse events increased with age for patients receiving Lovenox Injection. Other clinical experience (including postmarketing surveillance and literature reports) has not revealed additional differences in the safety of Lovenox Injection between elderly and younger patients. Careful attention to dosing intervals and concomitant medications (especially antiplatelet medications) is advised. Monitoring of geriatric patients with low body weight (<45 kg) and those predisposed to decreased renal function should be considered (see **CLINICAL PHARMACOLOGY** and **General** and **Laboratory Tests** subsections of **PRECAUTIONS**).

ADVERSE REACTIONS

Hemorrhage: The incidence of major hemorrhagic complications during Lovenox Injection treatment has been low. The following rates of major bleeding events have been reported during clinical trials with Lovenox Injection.

Major Bleeding Episodes Following Abdominal and Colorectal Surgery[1]

	Dosing Regimen	
Indications	**Lovenox Inj.** 40 mg q.d. SC	**Heparin** 5000 U q8h SC
Abdominal Surgery	n = 555 23 (4%)	n = 560 16 (3%)
Colorectal Surgery	n = 673 28 (4%)	n = 674 21 (3%)

[1] Bleeding complications were considered major: (1) if the hemorrhage caused a significant clinical event, or (2) if accompanied by a hemoglobin decrease ≥2 g/dL or transfusion of 2 or more units of blood products. Retroperitoneal, intraocular, and intracranial hemorrhages were always considered major.

Major Bleeding Episodes Following Hip or Knee Replacement Surgery[1]

Indications	Dosing Regimen		
	Lovenox Inj. 40 mg q.d. SC	Lovenox Inj. 30 mg q12h SC	Heparin 15,000 U/24h SC
Hip Replacement Surgery Without Extended Prophylaxis[2]		n = 786 31 (4%)	n = 541 32 (6%)
Hip Replacement Surgery With Extended Prophylaxis			
Peri-operative Period[3]	n = 288 4 (2%)		
Extended Prophylaxis Period[4]	n = 221 0 (0%)		
Knee Replacement Surgery Without Extended Prophylaxis[2]		n = 294 3 (1%)	n = 225 3 (1%)

[1] Bleeding complications were considered major: (1) if the hemorrhage caused a significant clinical event, or (2) if accompanied by a hemoglobin decrease ≥ 2 g/dL or transfusion of 2 or more units of blood products. Retroperitoneal and intracranial hemorrhages were always considered major. In the knee replacement surgery trials, intraocular hemorrhages were also considered major hemorrhages.

[2] Lovenox Injection 30 mg every 12 hours SC initiated 12 to 24 hours after surgery and continued for up to 14 days after surgery.

[3] Lovenox Injection 40 mg SC once a day initiated up to 12 hours prior to surgery and continued for up to 7 days after surgery.

[4] Lovenox Injection 40 mg SC once a day for up to 21 days after discharge.

NOTE: At no time point were the 40 mg once a day preoperative and the 30 mg every 12 hours post-operative hip replacement surgery prophylactic regimens compared in clinical trials.

Injection site hematomas during the extended prophylaxis period after hip replacement surgery occurred in 9% of the Lovenox Injection patients versus 1.8% of the placebo patients.

Major Bleeding Episodes in Medical Patients With Severely Restricted Mobility During Acute Illness[1]

Indications	Dosing Regimen		
	Lovenox Inj.[2] 20 mg q.d. SC	Lovenox Inj.[2] 40 mg q.d. SC	Placebo[2]
Medical Patients During Acute Illness	n = 351 1 (<1%)	n = 360 3 (<1%)	n = 362 2 (<1%)

[1] Bleeding complications were considered major: (1) if the hemorrhage caused a significant clinical event, (2) if the hemorrhage caused a decrease in hemoglobin of ≥ 2 g/dL or transfusion of 2 or more units of blood products. Retroperitoneal and intracranial hemorrhages were always considered major although none were reported during the trial.

[2] The rates represent major bleeding on study medication up to 24 hours after last dose.

Major Bleeding Episodes in Unstable Angina and Non-Q-Wave Myocardial Infarction

Indication	Dosing Regimen	
	Lovenox Inj.[1] 1 mg/kg q12h SC	Heparin[1] aPTT Adjusted i.v. Therapy
Unstable Angina and Non-Q-Wave MI[2,3]	n = 1578 17 (1%)	n = 1529 18 (1%)

[1] The rates represent major bleeding on study medication up to 12 hours after dose.

[2] Aspirin therapy was administered concurrently (100 to 325 mg per day).

[3] Bleeding complications were considered major: (1) if the hemorrhage caused a significant clinical event, or (2) if accompanied by a hemoglobin decrease by ≥ 3 g/dL or transfusion of 2 or more units of blood products. Intraocular, retroperitoneal, and intracranial hemorrhages were always considered major.

Adverse Events Occurring at ≥2% Incidence in Lovenox Injection Treated Patients[1] Undergoing Hip or Knee Replacement Surgery

	Dosing Regimen									
	Lovenox Inj. 40 mg q.d. SC				Lovenox Inj. 30 mg q12h SC		Heparin 15,000 U/24h SC		Placebo q12h SC	
	Peri-operative Period n = 288[2]		Extended Prophylaxis Period n = 131[3]		n = 1080		n = 766		n = 115	
Adverse Event	Severe	Total	Severe	Total	Severe	Total	Severe	Total	Severe	Total
Fever	0%	8%	0%	0%	<1%	5%	<1%	4%	0%	3%
Hemorrhage	<1%	13%	0%	5%	<1%	4%	1%	4%	0%	3%
Nausea					<1%	3%	<1%	2%	0%	2%
Anemia	0%	16%	0%	<2%	<1%	2%	2%	5%	<1%	7%
Edema					<1%	2%	<1%	2%	0%	2%
Peripheral edema	0%	6%	0%	0%	<1%	3%	<1%	4%	0%	3%

[1] Excluding unrelated adverse events.

[2] Data represents Lovenox Injection 40 mg SC once a day initiated up to 12 hours prior to surgery in 288 hip replacement surgery patients who received Lovenox Injection peri-operatively in an unblinded fashion in one clinical trial.

[3] Data represents Lovenox Injection 40 mg SC once a day given in a blinded fashion as extended prophylaxis at the end of the peri-operative period in 131 of the original 288 hip replacement surgery patients for up to 21 days in one clinical trial.

Major Bleeding Episodes in Deep Vein Thrombosis With or Without Pulmonary Embolism Treatment[1]

Indication	Dosing Regimen[2]		
	Lovenox Inj. 1.5 mg/kg q.d. SC	Lovenox Inj. 1 mg/kg q12h SC	Heparin aPTT Adjusted i.v. Therapy
Treatment of DVT and PE	n = 298 5 (2%)	n = 559 9 (2%)	n = 554 9 (2%)

[1] Bleeding complications were considered major: (1) if the hemorrhage caused a significant clinical event, or (2) if accompanied by a hemoglobin decrease ≥2 g/dL or transfusion of 2 or more units of blood products. Retroperitoneal, intraocular, and intracranial hemorrhages were always considered major.

[2] All patients also received warfarin sodium (dose-adjusted according to PT to achieve an INR of 2.0 to 3.0) commencing within 72 hours of Lovenox Injection or standard heparin therapy and continuing for up to 90 days.

Thrombocytopenia: see **WARNINGS: Thrombocytopenia.**

Elevations of Serum Aminotransferases: Asymptomatic increases in aspartate (AST [SGOT]) and alanine (ALT [SGPT]) aminotransferase levels greater than three times the upper limit of normal of the laboratory reference range have been reported in up to 6.1% and 5.9% of patients, respectively, during treatment with Lovenox Injection. Similar significant increases in aminotransferase levels have also been observed in patients and healthy volunteers treated with heparin and other low molecular weight heparins. Such elevations are fully reversible and are rarely associated with increases in bilirubin.

Since aminotransferase determinations are important in the differential diagnosis of myocardial infarction, liver disease, and pulmonary emboli, elevations that might be caused by drugs like Lovenox Injection should be interpreted with caution.

Local Reactions: Mild local irritation, pain, hematoma, ecchymosis, and erythema may follow SC injection of Lovenox Injection.

Other: Other adverse effects that were thought to be possibly or probably related to treatment with Lovenox Injection, heparin, or placebo in clinical trials with patients undergoing hip or knee replacement surgery, abdominal or colorectal surgery, or treatment for DVT and that occurred at a rate of at least 2% in the Lovenox Injection group, are provided below.

Adverse Events Occurring at ≥2% Incidence in Lovenox Injection Treated Patients[1] Undergoing Abdominal or Colorectal Surgery

	Dosing Regimen			
	Lovenox Inj. 40 mg q.d. SC n = 1228		Heparin 5000 U q8h SC n = 1234	
Adverse Event	Severe	Total	Severe	Total
Hemorrhage	<1%	7%	<1%	6%
Anemia	<1%	3%	<1%	3%
Ecchymosis	0%	3%	0%	3%

[1] Excluding unrelated adverse events.

[See table above]

Adverse Events Occurring at ≥2% Incidence in Lovenox Injection Treated Medical Patients[1] With Severely Restricted Mobility During Acute Illness

	Dosing Regimen	
Adverse Event	Lovenox Inj. 40 mg q.d. SC n = 360 (%)	Placebo q.d. SC n = 362 (%)
Dyspnea	3.3	5.2
Thrombocytopenia	2.8	2.8
Confusion	2.2	1.1
Diarrhea	2.2	1.7
Nausea	2.5	1.7

[1] Excluding unrelated and unlikely adverse events.

Adverse Events in Lovenox Injection Treated Patients With Unstable Angina or Non-Q-Wave Myocardial Infarction: Non-hemorrhagic clinical events reported to be related to Lovenox Injection therapy occurred at an incidence of ≤ 1%.

Non-major hemorrhagic episodes, primarily injection site ecchymoses and hematomas, were more frequently reported in patients treated with SC Lovenox Injection than in patients treated with i.v. heparin.

Serious adverse events with Lovenox Injection or heparin in a clinical trial in patients with unstable angina or non-Q-wave myocardial infarction that occurred at a rate of at least 0.5% in the Lovenox Injection group, are provided below (irrespective of relationship to drug therapy).

Serious Adverse Events Occurring at ≥0.5% Incidence in Lovenox Injection Treated Patients With Unstable Angina or Non-Q-Wave Myocardial Infarction

	Dosing Regimen	
Adverse Event	Lovenox Inj. 1 mg/kg q12h SC n = 1578 n (%)	Heparin aPTT Adjusted i.v. Therapy n = 1529 n (%)
Atrial fibrillation	11 (0.70)	3 (0.20)
Heart failure	15 (0.95)	11 (0.72)
Lung edema	11 (0.70)	11 (0.72)
Pneumonia	13 (0.82)	9 (0.59)

[See first table at top of next page]

Ongoing Safety Surveillance: Since 1993, there have been over 80 reports of epidural or spinal hematoma formation with concurrent use of Lovenox Injection and spinal/epidural anesthesia or spinal puncture. The majority of patients had a post-operative indwelling epidural catheter placed for analgesia or received additional drugs affecting hemostasis such as NSAIDs. Many of the epidural or spinal hematomas caused neurologic injury, including long-term or permanent paralysis. Because these events were reported voluntarily from a population of unknown size, estimates of frequency cannot be made.

Other Ongoing Safety Surveillance Reports: local reactions at the injection site (i.e., skin necrosis, nodules, in-

Continued on next page

Lovenox—Cont.

flammation, oozing), systemic allergic reactions (i.e., pruritus, urticaria, anaphylactoid reactions), vesiculobullous rash, rare cases of hypersensitivity cutaneous vasculitis, purpura, thrombocytosis, and thrombocytopenia with thrombosis (see **WARNINGS, Thrombocytopenia**). Very rare cases of hyperlipidemia have been reported, with one case of hyperlipidemia, with marked hypertriglyceridemia, reported in a diabetic pregnant woman; causality has not been determined.

OVERDOSAGE

Symptoms/Treatment: Accidental overdosage following administration of Lovenox Injection may lead to hemorrhagic complications. Injected Lovenox Injection may be largely neutralized by the slow i.v. injection of protamine sulfate (1% solution). The dose of protamine sulfate should be equal to the dose of Lovenox Injection injected: 1 mg protamine sulfate should be administered to neutralize 1 mg Lovenox Injection, if enoxaparin sodium was administered in the previous 8 hours. An infusion of 0.5 mg protamine per 1 mg of enoxaparin sodium may be administered if enoxaparin sodium was administered greater than 8 hours previous to the protamine administration, or if it has been determined that a second dose of protamine is required. The second infusion of 0.5 mg protamine sulfate per 1 mg of Lovenox Injection may be administered if the aPTT measured 2 to 4 hours after the first infusion remains prolonged.

After 12 hours of the enoxaparin sodium injection, protamine administration may not be required. However, even with higher doses of protamine, the aPTT may remain more prolonged than under normal conditions found following administration of heparin. In all cases, the anti-Factor Xa activity is never completely neutralized (maximum about 60%). Particular care should be taken to avoid overdosage with protamine sulfate. Administration of protamine sulfate can cause severe hypotensive and anaphylactoid reactions. Because fatal reactions, often resembling anaphylaxis, have been reported with protamine sulfate, it should be given only when resuscitation techniques and treatment of anaphylactic shock are readily available. For additional information consult the labeling of Protamine Sulfate Injection, USP, products.

A single SC dose of 46.4 mg/kg enoxaparin was lethal to rats. The symptoms of acute toxicity were ataxia, decreased motility, dyspnea, cyanosis, and coma.

DOSAGE AND ADMINISTRATION

All patients should be evaluated for a bleeding disorder before administration of Lovenox Injection, unless the medication is needed urgently. Since coagulation parameters are unsuitable for monitoring Lovenox Injection activity, routine monitoring of coagulation parameters is not required (see **PRECAUTIONS, Laboratory Tests**).

Note: Lovenox Injection is available in two concentrations:

1. 100 mg/mL Concentration: 30 mg / 0.3 mL and 40 mg / 0.4 mL prefilled single-dose syringes, 60 mg / 0.6 mL, 80 mg / 0.8 mL, and 100 mg / 1 mL prefilled, graduated, single-dose syringes, 300 mg / 3.0 mL multiple-dose vials.

2. 150 mg/mL Concentration: 120 mg / 0.8 mL and 150 mg / 1 mL prefilled, graduated, single-dose syringes.

Adult Dosage:

Abdominal Surgery: In patients undergoing abdominal surgery who are at risk for thromboembolic complications, the recommended dose of Lovenox Injection is **40 mg once a day** administered by SC injection with the initial dose given 2 hours prior to surgery. The usual duration of administration is 7 to 10 days; up to 12 days administration has been well tolerated in clinical trials.

Hip or Knee Replacement Surgery: In patients undergoing hip or knee replacement surgery, the recommended dose of Lovenox Injection is **30 mg every 12 hours** administered by SC injection. Provided that hemostasis has been established, the initial dose should be given 12 to 24 hours after surgery. For hip replacement surgery, a dose of **40 mg once a day** SC, given initially 12 (±3) hours prior to surgery, may be considered. Following the initial phase of thromboprophylaxis in hip replacement surgery patients, continued prophylaxis with Lovenox Injection 40 mg once a day administered by SC injection for 3 weeks is recommended. The usual duration of administration is 7 to 10 days; up to 14 days administration has been well tolerated in clinical trials.

Medical Patients During Acute Illness: In medical patients at risk for thromboembolic complications due to severely restricted mobility during acute illness, the recommended dose of Lovenox Injection is **40 mg once a day** administered by SC injection. The usual duration of administration is 6 to 11 days; up to 14 days of Lovenox Injection has been well tolerated in the controlled clinical trial.

Unstable Angina and Non-Q-Wave Myocardial Infarction: In patients with unstable angina or non-Q-wave myocardial infarction, the recommended dose of Lovenox Injection is **1 mg/kg** administered SC **every 12 hours** in conjunction with oral aspirin therapy (100 to 325 mg once daily). Treatment with Lovenox Injection should be prescribed for a minimum of 2 days and continued until clinical stabilization. To minimize the risk of bleeding following vascular instrumentation during the treatment of unstable angina, adhere precisely to the intervals recommended between Lovenox Injection doses. The vascular access sheath for instrumentation should remain in place for 6 to 8 hours following a dose of Lovenox Injection. The next scheduled dose should be given no sooner than 6 to 8 hours after sheath removal. The site of the procedure should be observed for signs of bleeding or hematoma formation. The usual duration of treatment is 2 to 8 days; up to 12.5 days of Lovenox Injection has been well tolerated in clinical trials.

Treatment of Deep Vein Thrombosis With or Without Pulmonary Embolism: In **outpatient treatment**, patients with acute deep vein thrombosis without pulmonary embolism who can be treated at home, the recommended dose of Lovenox Injection is **1 mg/kg every 12 hours** administered SC. In **inpatient (hospital) treatment**, patients with acute deep vein thrombosis with pulmonary embolism or patients with acute deep vein thrombosis without pulmonary embolism (who are not candidates for outpatient treatment), the recommended dose of Lovenox Injection is **1 mg/kg every 12 hours** administered SC **or 1.5 mg/kg once a day** administered SC at the same time every day. In both outpatient and inpatient (hospital) treatments, warfarin sodium therapy should be initiated when appropriate (usually within 72 hours of Lovenox Injection). Lovenox Injection should be continued for a minimum of 5 days and until a therapeutic oral anticoagulant effect has been achieved (International Normalization Ratio 2.0 to 3.0). The average duration of administration is 7 days; up to 17 days of Lovenox Injection administration has been well tolerated in controlled clinical trials.

Renal Impairment: Although no dose adjustment is recommended in patients with moderate (creatinine clearance 30–50 mL/min) and mild (creatinine clearance 50–80 mL/min) renal impairment, all such patients should be observed carefully for signs and symptoms of bleeding.

The recommended prophylaxis and treatment dosage regimens for patients with severe renal impairment (creatinine clearance <30 mL/min) are described in the following table (see **CLINICAL PHARMACOLOGY, Pharmacokinetics, Special Populations** and **PRECAUTIONS, Renal Impairment**).

Adverse Events Occurring at ≥2% Incidence in Lovenox Injection Treated Patients[1] Undergoing Treatment of Deep Vein Thrombosis With or Without Pulmonary Embolism

	Dosing Regimen					
	Lovenox Inj. 1.5 mg/kg q.d. SC n = 298		Lovenox Inj. 1 mg/kg q12h SC n = 559		Heparin aPTT Adjusted i.v. Therapy n = 544	
Adverse Event	**Severe**	**Total**	**Severe**	**Total**	**Severe**	**Total**
Injection Site Hemorrhage	0%	5%	0%	3%	<1%	<1%
Injection Site Pain	0%	2%	0%	2%	0%	0%
Hematuria	0%	2%	0%	<1%	<1%	2%

[1] Excluding unrelated adverse events.

100 mg/mL Concentration

Dosage Unit/Strength[1]	Anti-Xa Activity[2]	Package Size (per carton)	Label Color	NDC # 0075-
Prefilled Syringes[3]				
30 mg / 0.3 mL	3000 IU	10 syringes	Medium Blue	0624-30
40 mg / 0.4 mL	4000 IU	10 syringes	Yellow	0620-40
Graduated Prefilled Syringes[3]				
60 mg / 0.6 mL	6000 IU	10 syringes	Orange	0621-60
80 mg / 0.8 mL	8000 IU	10 syringes	Brown	0622-80
100 mg / 1 mL	10,000 IU	10 syringes	Black	0623-00
Multiple-Dose Vial[4]				
300 mg / 3.0 mL	30,000 IU	1 vial	Red	0626-03

[1] Strength represents the number of milligrams of enoxaparin sodium in Water for Injection. **Lovenox Injection** 30 and 40 mg prefilled syringes, and 60, 80, and 100 mg graduated prefilled syringes each contain **10 mg enoxaparin sodium per 0.1 mL Water for Injection.**

[2] Approximate anti-Factor Xa activity based on reference to the W.H.O. First International Low Molecular Weight Heparin Reference Standard.

[3] Each **Lovenox Injection** syringe is affixed with a 27 gauge × 1/2 inch needle.

[4] Each Lovenox multiple-dose vial contains 15 mg / 1.0 mL of benzyl alcohol as a preservative.

150 mg/mL Concentration

Dosage Unit/Strength[1]	Anti-Xa Activity[2]	Package Size (per carton)	Syringe Label Color	NDC # 0075-
Graduated Prefilled Syringes[3]				
120 mg / 0.8 mL	12,000 IU	10 syringes	Purple	2912-01
150 mg / 1 mL	15,000 IU	10 syringes	Navy Blue	2915-01

[1] Strength represents the number of milligrams of enoxaparin sodium in Water for Injection. **Lovenox Injection** 120 and 150 mg graduated prefilled syringes contain **15 mg enoxaparin sodium per 0.1 mL** Water for Injection.

[2] Approximate anti-Factor Xa activity based on reference to the W.H.O. First International Low Molecular Weight Heparin Reference Standard.

[3] Each **Lovenox Injection** graduated prefilled syringe is affixed with a 27 gauge × 1/2 inch needle.

Dosage Regimens for Patients with Severe Renal Impairment (creatinine clearance <30mL/minute)

Indication	Dosage Regimen
Prophylaxis in abdominal surgery	30 mg administered SC once daily
Prophylaxis in hip or knee replacement surgery	30 mg administered SC once daily
Prophylaxis in medical patients during acute illness	30 mg administered SC once daily
Prophylaxis of ischemic complications of unstable angina and non-Q-wave myocardial infarction, when concurrently administered with aspirin	1 mg/kg administered SC once daily
Inpatient treatment of acute deep vein thrombosis with or without pulmonary embolism, when administered in conjunction with warfarin sodium	1 mg/kg administered SC once daily
Outpatient treatment of acute deep vein thrombosis without pulmonary embolism, when administered in conjunction with warfarin sodium	1 mg/kg administered SC once daily

Administration: Lovenox Injection is a clear, colorless to pale yellow sterile solution, and as with other parenteral drug products, should be inspected visually for particulate matter and discoloration prior to administration.

The use of a tuberculin syringe or equivalent is recommended when using Lovenox multiple-dose vials to assure withdrawal of the appropriate volume of drug.

Lovenox Injection is administered by SC injection. It must not be administered by intramuscular injection. Lovenox Injection is intended for use under the guidance of a physician. Patients may self-inject only if their physician determines that it is appropriate and with medical follow-up, as necessary. Proper training in subcutaneous injection technique (with or without the assistance of an injection device) should be provided.

Subcutaneous Injection Technique: Patients should be lying down and Lovenox Injection administered by deep SC injection. To avoid the loss of drug when using the 30 and 40 mg prefilled syringes, do not expel the air bubble from the syringe before the injection. Administration should be alternated between the left and right anterolateral and left and right posterolateral abdominal wall. The whole length of the needle should be introduced into a skin fold held between the thumb and forefinger; the skin fold should be held throughout the injection. To minimize bruising, do not rub the injection site after completion of the injection.

Lovenox Injection prefilled syringes and graduated prefilled syringes are available with a system that shields the needle after injection.

- Remove the needle shield by pulling it straight off the syringe. If adjusting the dose is required, the dose adjustment must be done prior to injecting the prescribed dose to the patient.

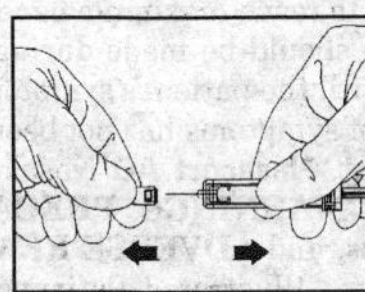

- Inject using standard technique, pushing the plunger to the bottom of the syringe.

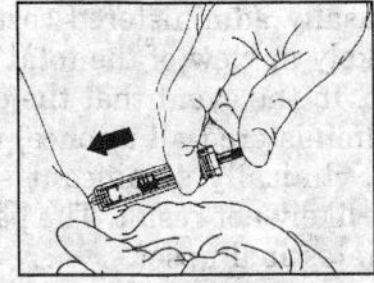

- Remove the syringe from the injection site keeping your finger on the plunger rod.

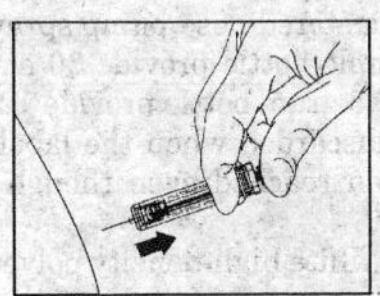

- Orienting the needle away from you and others, activate the safety system by firmly pushing the plunger rod. The protective sleeve will automatically cover the needle and an audible "click" will be heard to confirm shield activation.

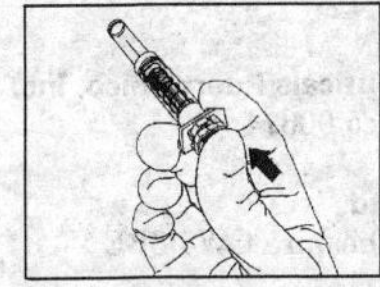

- Immediately dispose of the syringe in the nearest sharps container.

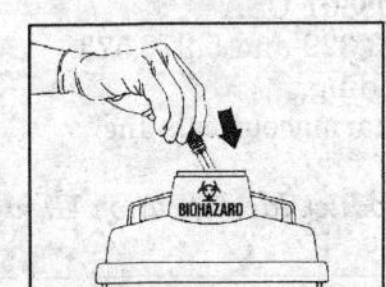

NOTE:

- The safety system can only be activated once the syringe has been emptied.
- Activation of the safety system must be done only after removing the needle from the patient's skin.
- Do not replace the needle shield after injection.
- The safety system should not be sterilized.
- Activation of the safety system may cause minimal splatter of fluid. For optimal safety activate the system while orienting it downwards away from yourself and others.

HOW SUPPLIED

Lovenox® (enoxaparin sodium injection) is available in two concentrations:

[See second table at top of previous page]

[See third table at top of previous page]

Store at 25°C (77°F); excursions permitted to 15–30°C (59–86°F) [see USP Controlled Room Temperature].

Keep out of the reach of children.

[1]Lepercq J, Conard J, Borel-Derlon A, et al. Venous thromboembolism during pregnancy: a retrospective study of enoxaparin safety in 624 pregnancies. *Br J Obstet Gynec* 2001; 108 (11): 1134–40.

Lovenox Injection prefilled and graduated prefilled syringes manufactured by:

Aventis Pharma Specialties
94700 Maisons-Alfort
France
And
Aventis Pharma
Boulevard Industriel
76580 Le Trait
France

Lovenox multiple-dose vials manufactured by:
DSM Pharmaceuticals, Inc.
Greenville, NC 27835

Manufactured for:
Aventis Pharmaceuticals Inc.
Bridgewater, NJ 08807

Rev. April 2004
LOV-April04-F-A

Shown in Product Identification Guide, page 307

NASACORT® AQ ℞

[na 'za · cort]
(triamcinolone acetonide)
Nasal Spray
For intranasal use only.
Shake Well Before Using

Prescribing Information as of March 2004a

DESCRIPTION

Triamcinolone acetonide, USP, the active ingredient in **Nasacort® AQ** Nasal Spray, is a corticosteroid with a molecular weight of 434.51 and with the chemical designation 9-Fluoro-11β,16α,17,21-tetrahydroxypregna-1,4-diene-3,20-dione cyclic 16,17-acetal with acetone ($C_{24}H_{31}FO_6$).

Nasacort AQ Nasal Spray is an unscented, thixotropic, water-based metered-dose pump spray formulation unit containing a microcrystalline suspension of triamcinolone acetonide in an aqueous medium. Microcrystalline cellulose, carboxymethylcellulose sodium, polysorbate 80, dextrose, benzalkonium chloride, and edetate disodium are contained in this aqueous medium; hydrochloric acid or sodium hydroxide may be added to adjust the pH to a target of 5.0 within a range of 4.5 and 6.0.

Each actuation delivers 55 mcg triamcinolone acetonide from the nasal actuator after an initial priming of 5 sprays. It will remain adequately primed for 2 weeks. If the product is not used for more than 2 weeks, then it can be adequately reprimed with one spray. The contents of one 6.5 gram sample bottle provide 30 actuations, and the contents of one 16.5 gram bottle provide 120 actuations. **After either 30 actuations or 120 actuations, the amount of triamcinolone acetonide delivered per actuation may not be consistent and the unit should be discarded.** Each 30 actuation sample bottle contains 3.575 mg of triamcinolone acetonide and each 120 actuation bottle contains 9.075 mg of triamcinolone acetonide.

In the **Information for Patients** tear-off sheet, patients are provided with a check-off form to track usage.

CLINICAL PHARMACOLOGY

Triamcinolone acetonide is a more potent derivative of triamcinolone. Although triamcinolone itself is approximately one to two times as potent as prednisone in animal models of inflammation, triamcinolone acetonide is approximately 8 times more potent than prednisone.

Although the precise mechanism of corticosteroid antiallergic action is unknown, corticosteroids are very effective. However, when allergic symptoms are very severe, local treatment with recommended doses (microgram) of any available topical corticosteroid are not as effective as treatment with larger doses (milligram) of oral or parenteral formulations.

Based upon intravenous dosing of triamcinolone acetonide phosphate ester in adults, the half-life of triamcinolone acetonide was reported to be 88 minutes. The volume of distribution (Vd) reported was 99.5 L (SD ± 27.5) and clearance was 45.2 L/hour (SD ± 9.1) for triamcinolone acetonide. The plasma half-life of corticosteroids does not correlate well with the biologic half-life.

Pharmacokinetic characterization of the **Nasacort AQ** Nasal Spray formulation was determined in both normal adult subjects and patients with allergic rhinitis. Single dose intranasal administration of 220 mcg of **Nasacort AQ** Nasal Spray in normal adult subjects and patients demonstrated minimal absorption of triamcinolone acetonide. The mean peak plasma concentration was approximately 0.5 ng/mL (range: 0.1 to 1.0 ng/mL) and occurred at 1.5 hours post dose. The mean plasma drug concentration was less than 0.06 ng/mL at 12 hours, and below the assay detection limit at 24 hours. The average terminal half-life was 3.1 hours. The range of mean $AUC_{0-\infty}$ values was 1.4 ng•hr/mL to 4.7 ng•hr/mL between doses of 110 mcg to 440 mcg in both patients and healthy volunteers. Dose proportionality was demonstrated in both normal adult subjects and in allergic rhinitis patients following single intranasal doses of 110 mcg or 220 mcg **Nasacort AQ** Nasal Spray. The C_{max} and AUC of the 440 mcg dose increased less than proportionally when compared to 110 and 220 mcg doses. Following multiple doses in pediatric patients receiving 440 mcg/day, plasma drug concentrations, AUC, C_{max} and T_{max} were similar to those values observed in adult patients.

In animal studies using rats and dogs, three metabolites of triamcinolone acetonide have been identified. They are 6β-hydroxytriamcinolone acetonide, 21-carboxytriamcinolone acetonide and 21-carboxy-6β-hydroxytriamcinolone acetonide. All three metabolites are expected to be substantially less active than the parent compound due to (a) the dependence of anti-inflammatory activity on the presence of a 21-hydroxyl group, (b) the decreased activity observed upon 6-hydroxylation, and (c) the markedly increased water solubility favoring rapid elimination. There appeared to be some quantitative differences in the metabolites among species. No differences were detected in metabolic pattern as a function of route of administration.

In order to determine if systemic absorption plays a role in **Nasacort AQ's** treatment of allergic rhinitis symptoms, a two week double-blind, placebo-controlled clinical study was conducted comparing **Nasacort AQ**, orally ingested triamcinolone acetonide, and placebo in 297 adult patients with seasonal allergic rhinitis. The study demonstrated that the therapeutic efficacy of **Nasacort AQ** Nasal Spray can be attributed to the topical effects of triamcinolone acetonide.

In order to evaluate the effects of systemic absorption on the Hypothalamic-Pituitary-Adrenal (HPA) axis, a clinical study was performed in adults comparing 220 mcg or 440 mcg **Nasacort AQ** per day, or 10 mg prednisone per day with placebo for 42 days. Adrenal response to a six-hour cosyntropin stimulation test showed that **Nasacort AQ** administered at doses of 220 mcg and 440 mcg had no statistically significant effect on HPA activity versus placebo. Conversely, oral prednisone at 10 mg/day significantly reduced the response to ACTH.

A study evaluating plasma cortisol response thirty and sixty minutes after cosyntropin stimulation in 80 pediatric patients who received 220 mcg or 440 mcg (twice the maximum recommended daily dose) daily for six weeks was conducted. No abnormal response to cosyntropin infusion (peak serum cortisol <18 mcg/dL) was observed in any pediatric patient after six weeks of dosing with **Nasacort AQ** at 440 mcg per day.

CLINICAL TRIALS

The safety and efficacy of **Nasacort AQ** Nasal Spray have been evaluated in 10 double-blind, placebo-controlled clinical trials of two- to four-weeks duration in adults and children 12 years and older with seasonal or perennial allergic rhinitis. The number of patients treated with **Nasacort AQ** Nasal Spray in these studies was 1266; of these patients, 675 were males and 591 were females.

Overall, the results of these clinical trials in adults and children 12 years and older demonstrated that **Nasacort AQ** Nasal Spray 220 mcg once daily (2 sprays in each nostril), when compared to placebo, provides statistically significant relief of nasal symptoms of seasonal or perennial allergic rhinitis including sneezing, stuffiness, discharge, and itching.

The safety and efficacy of **Nasacort AQ** Nasal Spray, at doses of 110 mcg or 220 mcg once daily, have also been adequately studied in two double-blind, placebo-controlled trials of two- and twelve-weeks duration in children ages 6 through 12 years with seasonal and perennial allergic rhinitis. These trials included 341 males and 177 females. **Nasacort AQ** administered at either dose resulted in statistically significant reductions in the severity of nasal symptoms of allergic rhinitis.

INDICATIONS AND USAGE

Nasacort AQ Nasal Spray is indicated for the treatment of the nasal symptoms of seasonal and perennial allergic rhinitis in adults and children 6 years of age and older.

CONTRAINDICATIONS

Hypersensitivity to any of the ingredients of this preparation contraindicates its use.

WARNINGS

The replacement of a systemic corticosteroid with a topical corticosteroid can be accompanied by signs of adrenal insufficiency and, in addition, some patients may experience symptoms of withdrawal; *e.g.,* joint and/or muscular pain, lassitude and depression. Patients previously treated for prolonged periods with systemic corticosteroids and transferred to topical corticosteroids should be carefully monitored for acute adrenal insufficiency in response to stress. In those patients who have asthma or other clinical conditions requiring long-term systemic corticosteroid treatment, too rapid a decrease in systemic corticosteroids may cause a severe exacerbation of their symptoms.

Children who are on immunosuppressant drugs are more susceptible to infections than healthy children. Chickenpox and measles, for example, can have a more serious or even fatal course in children on immunosuppressant doses of corticosteroids. In such children, or in adults who have not had these diseases, particular care should be taken to avoid exposure. If exposed, therapy with varicella-zoster immune globulin (VZIG) or pooled intravenous immunoglobulin

Continued on next page

Nasacort AQ—Cont.

(IVIG), as appropriate, may be indicated. If chickenpox develops, treatment with antiviral agents may be considered.

PRECAUTIONS

General: In clinical studies with triamcinolone acetonide nasal spray, the development of localized infections of the nose and pharynx with *Candida albicans* has rarely occurred. When such an infection develops it may require treatment with appropriate local or systemic therapy and discontinuance of treatment with **Nasacort AQ** Nasal Spray.

Nasacort AQ Nasal Spray should be used with caution, if at all, in patients with active or quiescent tuberculous infection of the respiratory tract or in patients with untreated fungal, bacterial, or systemic viral infections or ocular herpes simplex.

Because of the inhibitory effect of corticosteroids, in patients who have experienced recent nasal septal ulcers, nasal surgery, or trauma, a corticosteroid should be used with caution until healing has occurred. As with other nasally inhaled corticosteroids, nasal septal perforations have been reported in rare instances.

When used at excessive doses, systemic corticosteroid effects such as hypercorticism and adrenal suppression may appear. If such changes occur, **Nasacort AQ** Nasal Spray should be discontinued slowly, consistent with accepted procedures for discontinuing oral steroid therapy.

Information for Patients: Patients being treated with **Nasacort AQ** Nasal Spray should receive the following information and instructions. Patients who are on immunosuppressant doses of corticosteroids should be warned to avoid exposure to chickenpox or measles and, if exposed, to obtain medical advice.

Patients should use **Nasacort AQ** Nasal Spray at regular intervals since its effectiveness depends on its regular use. (See **DOSAGE AND ADMINISTRATION.**)

An improvement in some patient symptoms may be seen within the first day of treatment, and generally, it takes one week of treatment to reach maximum benefit. Initial assessment for response should be made during this time frame and periodically until the patient's symptoms are stabilized. The patient should take the medication as directed and should not exceed the prescribed dosage. The patient should contact the physician if symptoms do not improve after three weeks, or if the condition worsens. Patients who experience recurrent episodes of epistaxis (nose bleeds) or nasal septum discomfort while taking this medication should contact their physician. For the proper use of this unit and to attain maximum improvement, the patient should read and follow the accompanying patient instructions carefully.

It is important to shake the bottle well before each use. **Also, the bottle should be discarded after either 30 actuations or 120 actuations since the amount of triamcinolone acetonide delivered thereafter per actuation may be substantially less than 55 mcg of drug.** Do not transfer any remaining suspension to another bottle.

Carcinogenesis, Mutagenesis, and Impairment of Fertility: In a two-year study in rats, triamcinolone acetonide caused no treatment-related carcinogenicity at oral doses up to 1.0 mcg/kg (approximately 1/30 and 1/50 of the maximum recommended daily intranasal dose in adults and children on a mcg/m^2 basis, respectively). In a two-year study in mice, triamcinolone acetonide caused no treatment-related carcinogenicity at oral doses up to 3.0 mcg/kg (approximately 1/12 and 1/30 of the maximum recommended daily intranasal dose in adults and children on a mcg/m^2 basis, respectively).

No evidence of mutagenicity was detected from *in vitro* tests (a reverse mutation test in *Salmonella* bacteria and a forward mutation test in Chinese hamster ovary cells) conducted with triamcinolone acetonide.

In male and female rats, triamcinolone acetonide caused no change in pregnancy rate at oral doses up to 15.0 mcg/kg (approximately 1/2 of the maximum recommended daily intranasal dose in adults on a mcg/m^2 basis). Triamcinolone acetonide caused increased fetal resorptions and stillbirths and decreases in pup weight and survival at doses of 5.0 mcg/kg and above (approximately 1/5 of the maximum recommended daily intranasal dose in adults on a mcg/m^2 basis). At 1.0 mcg/kg (approximately 1/30 of the maximum recommended daily intranasal dose in adults on a mcg/m^2 basis), it did not induce the above mentioned effects.

Pregnancy: *Teratogenic Effects: Pregnancy Category C.* Triamcinolone acetonide was teratogenic in rats, rabbits, and monkeys. In rats, triamcinolone acetonide was teratogenic at inhalation doses of 20 mcg/kg and above (approximately 7/10 of the maximum recommended daily intranasal dose in adults on a mcg/m^2 basis). In rabbits, triamcinolone acetonide was teratogenic at inhalation doses of 20 mcg/kg and above (approximately 2 times the maximum recommended daily intranasal dose in adults on a mcg/m^2 basis). In monkeys, triamcinolone acetonide was teratogenic at an inhalation dose of 500 mcg/kg (approximately 37 times the maximum recommended daily intranasal dose in adults on a mcg/m^2 basis). Dose-related teratogenic effects in rats and rabbits included cleft palate and/or internal hydrocephaly and axial skeletal defects, whereas the effects observed in the monkey were cranial malformations.

There are no adequate and well-controlled studies in pregnant women. **Nasacort AQ** Nasal Spray, like other corticosteroids, should be used in pregnancy only if the potential benefit justifies the potential risk to the fetus. Since their introduction, experience with oral corticosteroids in pharmacologic as opposed to physiologic doses suggests that rodents are more prone to teratogenic effects from corticosteroids than humans. In addition, because there is a natural increase in glucocorticoid production during pregnancy, most women will require a lower exogenous corticosteroid dose and many will not need corticosteroid treatment during pregnancy.

Nonteratogenic Effects: Hypoadrenalism may occur in infants born of mothers receiving corticosteroids during pregnancy. Such infants should be carefully observed.

Nursing Mothers: It is not known whether triamcinolone acetonide is excreted in human milk. Because other corticosteroids are excreted in human milk, caution should be exercised when **Nasacort AQ** Nasal Spray is administered to nursing women.

Pediatric Use: Safety and effectiveness in pediatric patients below the age of 6 years have not been established.

Corticosteroids have been shown to cause growth suppression in children and teenagers, particularly with higher doses over extended periods. If a child or teenager on any corticosteroid appears to have growth suppression, the possibility that they are particularly sensitive to this effect of corticosteroids should be considered.

Geriatric Use: Clinical studies of **Nasacort AQ** did not include sufficient numbers of subjects aged 65 and over to determine whether they respond differently from younger subjects. Other reported clinical experience has not identified differences in responses between the elderly and younger patients.

ADVERSE REACTIONS

In placebo-controlled, double-blind, and open-label clinical studies, 1483 adults and children 12 years and older received treatment with triamcinolone acetonide aqueous nasal spray. These patients were treated for an average duration of 51 days. In the controlled trials (2–5 weeks duration) from which the following adverse reaction data are derived, 1394 patients were treated with **Nasacort AQ** Nasal Spray for an average of 19 days. In a long-term, open-label study, 172 patients received treatment for an average duration of 286 days.

Adverse events occurring at an incidence of 2% or greater and more common among **Nasacort AQ**-treated patients than placebo-treated patients in controlled adult clinical trials were:

[See table below]

A total of 602 children 6 to 12 years of age were studied in 3 double-blind, placebo-controlled clinical trials. Of these, 172 received 110 mcg/day and 207 received 220 mcg/day of **Nasacort AQ** Nasal Spray for two, six, or twelve weeks. The longest average durations of treatment for patients receiving 110 mcg/day and 220 mcg/day were 76 days and 80 days, respectively. Only 1% of those patients treated with **Nasacort AQ** were discontinued due to adverse experiences. No patient receiving 110 mcg/day discontinued due to a serious adverse event and one patient receiving 220 mcg/day discontinued due to a serious event that was considered not drug related. Overall, these studies found the adverse experience profile for **Nasacort AQ** to be similar to placebo. A similar adverse event profile was observed in pediatric patients 6–12 years of age as compared to older children and adults with the exception of epistaxis which occurred in less than 2% of the pediatric patients studied.

Adverse events occurring at an incidence of 2% or greater and more common among adult patients treated with placebo than **Nasacort AQ** were: headache, and rhinitis. In children aged 6 to 12 years these events included: asthma, epistaxis, headache, infection, otitis media, sinusitis, and vomiting.

In clinical trials, nasal septum perforation was reported in one adult patient although relationship to **Nasacort AQ** Nasal Spray has not been established.

In the event of accidental overdose, an increased potential for these adverse experiences may be expected, but acute systemic adverse experiences are unlikely. (See **OVERDOSAGE.**)

DOSAGE AND ADMINISTRATION

Recommended Doses: *Adults and children 12 years of age and older:* The recommended starting and maximum dose is 220 mcg per day as two sprays in each nostril once daily. *Children 6 to 12 years of age:* The recommended starting dose is 110 mcg per day given as one spray in each nostril once daily. The maximum recommended dose is 220 mcg per day as two sprays per nostril once daily.

Nasacort AQ Nasal Spray is not recommended for children under 6 years of age since adequate numbers of patients have not been studied in this age group.

Individualization of Dosage: It is always desirable to titrate an individual patient to the minimum effective dose to reduce the possibility of side effects. In adults, when the maximum benefit has been achieved and symptoms have been controlled, reducing the dose to 110 mcg per day (one spray in each nostril once a day) has been shown to be effective in maintaining control of the allergic rhinitis symptoms in patients who were initially controlled at 220 mcg/day.

In children six to twelve years of age, the recommended starting dose is 110 mcg per day given as one spray in each nostril once daily. The maximum recommended daily dose in children 6 to 12 years of age is 220 mcg per day (two sprays in each nostril once daily). Some patients who do not achieve maximum symptom control at a dose of 110 mcg per day may benefit from a dose of 220 mcg given as two sprays in each nostril once daily. The minimum effective dose should be used to ensure continued control of symptoms. Once symptoms are controlled, pediatric patients may be able to be maintained on 110 mcg per day (1 spray in each nostril once daily).

An improvement in some patient symptoms may be seen within the first day of treatment, and generally, it takes one week of treatment to reach maximum benefit. Initial assessment for response should be made during this time frame and periodically until the patient's symptoms are stabilized. If adequate relief of symptoms has not been obtained after 3 weeks of treatment, **Nasacort AQ** Nasal Spray should be discontinued. (See **WARNINGS, PRECAUTIONS, Information for Patients,** and **ADVERSE REACTIONS.**)

Directions For Use: Illustrated Patient's Instructions for use accompany each package of **Nasacort AQ** Nasal Spray.

OVERDOSAGE

Like any other nasally administered corticosteroid, acute overdosing is unlikely in view of the total amount of active ingredient present. In the event that the entire contents of the bottle were administered all at once, via either oral or nasal application, clinically significant systemic adverse events would most likely not result. The patient may experience some gastrointestinal upset.

HOW SUPPLIED

Nasacort AQ Nasal Spray is a nonchlorofluorocarbon (non-CFC) containing metered-dose pump spray. The contents of one 6.5 gram sample bottle provide 30 actuations, and the contents of one 16.5 gram bottle provide 120 actuations. The bottle should be discarded when the labeled number of actuations have been reached even though the bottle is not completely empty.

It is supplied in a white high-density polyethylene container with a metered-dose pump unit, white nasal adapter, and patient instructions.

NDC 0075-1506-16

Keep out of reach of children.

Store at Controlled Room Temperature, 20 to 25°C (68 to 77°F) [see USP].

Rx Only.

Manufactured by:
Aventis Pharmaceuticals Puerto Rico, Inc.
Manati, Puerto Rico 00674
And
Aventis Pharma Ltd.
Holmes Chapel, Cheshire CW4 8BE
United Kingdom
Manufactured for:
Aventis Pharmaceuticals Inc.
Bridgewater, NJ 08807 USA
US Pat. Nos. 6,143,329 and 5,976,573.
Other patents pending.

Rev. March 2004a

Shown in Product Identification Guide, page 307

Adverse Events	Patients treated with 220 mcg triamcinolone acetonide (n=857) %	Vehicle Placebo (n=962) %
Pharyngitis	5.1	3.6
Epistaxis	2.7	0.8
Increase in cough	2.1	1.5

NASACORT® HFA ℞

[na' za-cort]
(triamcinolone acetonide)
Nasal Aerosol
For Intranasal Use Only
Shake Well Before Using
Rev. April 2004c

DESCRIPTION

Triamcinolone acetonide, USP, the active ingredient in **Nasacort® HFA Nasal Aerosol**, is a glucocorticosteroid with a molecular weight of 434.5, the chemical designation 9-Fluoro-11β,16α ,17, 21-tetrahydroxypregna-1, 4-diene-3, 20-dione cyclic 16,17-acetal with acetone ($C_{24}H_{31}FO_6$), and the following chemical structure:

Triamcinolone acetonide is a white to cream-colored crystalline powder, practically insoluble in water, very soluble in dehydrated alcohol, chloroform, and methyl alcohol.
Nasacort HFA Nasal Aerosol is a metered-dose aerosol unit containing a microcrystalline suspension of triamcinolone acetonide in tetrafluoroethane (HFA-134a) and dehydrated alcohol USP 0.7% w/w. Each canister contains 15 mg of triamcinolone acetonide.
The canister must be primed with 3 actuations prior to the first use or after a period of non-use (3 days). After priming, each actuation meters 100 mcg of triamcinolone acetonide in 65 mg of suspension from the valve and delivers 55 mcg of triamcinolone acetonide from the nasal actuator to the patient. If the product is not used for more than 3 days, it should be re-primed with 3 actuations.
Each 9.3 g canister of Nasacort HFA Nasal Aerosol provides 100 metered sprays. After 100 metered sprays, this amount of medication delivered per actuation may not be consistent and the unit should be discarded. Patients are provided with a check-off card to track usage as part of the **PATIENT'S INSTRUCTIONS FOR USE** tear-off sheet.

CLINICAL PHARMACOLOGY

Triamcinolone acetonide, a synthetic glucocorticosteroid, is a more potent derivative of triamcinolone. Although triamcinolone itself is approximately 1 to 2 times as potent as prednisone in animal models of inflammation, triamcinolone acetonide is approximately 8 times more potent than prednisone. The clinical relevance of *in vitro* or animal models of potency comparison is unknown.
The precise mechanism of corticosteroid action on allergic rhinitis is not known. Corticosteroids have been shown to have a wide range of effects on multiple cell types (e.g., mast cells, eosinophils, neutrophils, macrophages, and lymphocytes) and mediators (e.g., histamine, eicosanoids, leukotrienes, and cytokines) involved in inflammation. Nasacort HFA Nasal Aerosol, like other corticosteroids, does not have an immediate effect on allergic rhinitis signs and symptoms. When corticosteroids are discontinued, symptoms may not recur for several days.

Pharmacokinetics:

Absorption: Triamcinolone acetonide is absorbed into the systemic circulation in humans following intranasal administration. In a study involving 24 patients with allergic rhinitis and 24 healthy subjects, absorption of triamcinolone from the nasal mucosa was similar. Following a single intranasal administration of 440 mcg of Nasacort HFA Nasal Aerosol to healthy subjects, the mean maximum triamcinolone acetonide plasma concentration of 0.2 (SD ± 0.1) ng/mL was observed at 3.8 (SD ± 2.4) hours postdosing.
Distribution: Based on an intravenous dose of 2 mg of triamcinolone acetonide phosphate ester in 12 healthy subjects, the mean volume of distribution (Vd) was 103.4 L (SD ± 58.7). The binding of triamcinolone acetonide to plasma proteins is relatively low, and remains consistent over a wide plasma triamcinolone acetonide concentration range (0.03–3.2 ng/mL). Based on an *ex vivo* study, the overall mean percent bound to plasma protein was approximately 68% (SD ± 4.3%).
Metabolism: The metabolism and excretion of triamcinolone acetonide were both rapid and extensive with no parent compound being detected in plasma after 24 hours post oral [^{14}C]-triamcinolone radiolabeled dose.
The disposition and metabolic profile of [^{14}C]-triamcinolone acetonide in human plasma, urine, and feces was evaluated in 6 healthy male subjects. Three major metabolites in plasma were 6β-hydroxytriamcinolone acetonide, triamcinolone acetonide-21-oic acid, and 6β-hydroxytriamcinolone acetonide-21-oic acid. Two major metabolites in the urine were 6β-hydroxytriamcinolone acetonide and its derivative following further oxidation (possibly 6-oxo-triamcinolone acetonide or 11-oxo-triamcinolone acetonide). A trace amount of triamcinolone acetonide-21-oic acid was also found in urine. Primary metabolites in the feces were the same as those in plasma. All three major metabolites in the plasma had no activity as determined by *in vitro* studies.
Elimination: Based on an intravenous dose of 2 mg of triamcinolone acetonide phosphate ester in 12 healthy subjects, the mean half-life of triamcinolone acetonide was 2 hours (SD ± 0.7), and the mean clearance was 37.3 L/hour (SD ± 12.8). Following a single intranasal administration of 440 mcg of triamcinolone acetonide in 24 healthy subjects, the mean half-life was 5.4 hours (SD ± 4.1). However, this value probably reflects lingering absorption of triamcinolone acetonide.
Following a single 800 mcg oral dose of radiolabeled [^{14}C]-triamcinolone acetonide in 6 healthy subjects, urinary and fecal excretion accounted for approximately 90% of the oral [^{14}C]-radiolabeled dose. Of the recovered [^{14}C]-radioactivity, approximately 40% and 60% were found in the urine and feces, respectively. Urinary excretion of [^{14}C]-radioactivity was essentially complete within 24 hours post-dose with most of the fecal elimination completed between 48 and 96 hours post-dose. The plasma half-life of corticosteroids does not correlate well with the duration of the drug's activity.
Special Populations: Formal pharmacokinetic studies using intranasal triamcinolone acetonide were not carried out in any special populations. The effects of renal impairment, hepatic impairment, age, or gender on the pharmacokinetics of triamcinolone acetonide following intranasal administration have not been investigated.
Pharmacodynamics: Several studies were performed to determine if systemic absorption played a role in the response to triamcinolone acetonide in the treatment of allergic rhinitis. An open-label, multiple-dose study was conducted comparing intranasal CFC and depot intramuscular formulations of triamcinolone acetonide in 25 adult patients with seasonal or perennial allergic rhinitis. The doses used were based on bioavailability studies of each formulation. The intranasal CFC formulation was administered at a dose of 440 mcg once daily for 42 days, and the 4 mg depot intramuscular formulation was administered once a week for 42 days. Weekly injection yielded sustained plasma levels throughout the dosing interval while daily intranasal administration resulted in daily peak and trough concentrations, the mean of which was 3.5 times below the mean plasma levels achieved with intramuscular administration. Both intranasal and intramuscular triamcinolone acetonide were clinically effective on allergic rhinitis symptoms. This suggests that triamcinolone acetonide is both systemically and topically active.
The potential systemic effects of triamcinolone acetonide aqueous formulation (Nasacort AQ Nasal Spray) on the hypothalamic-pituitary-adrenal (HPA) axis were studied in 64 patients with allergic rhinitis. Nasacort AQ Nasal Spray administered to adults at doses of 220 or 440 mcg once daily was compared to placebo or 10 mg prednisone administered as oral capsules for 42 days. Plasma cortisol concentrations were not affected in patients treated with either placebo or Nasacort AQ Nasal Spray in response to a 6-hour cosyntropin stimulation test, while oral prednisone significantly reduced the response to cosyntropin.
In another trial, the potential systemic effects of triamcinolone acetonide CFC formulation (Nasacort Nasal Inhaler) on the HPA axis were studied in 64 patients with allergic rhinitis. Nasacort Nasal Inhaler administered to adults at doses of 220 or 440 mcg once daily was compared to placebo or 10 mg prednisone once daily administered as oral capsules for 42 days. Plasma cortisol concentrations, 24-hour urinary 17-OHCS, and 24-hour urinary free cortisol concentrations were not affected in patients treated with either placebo or Nasacort Nasal Inhaler in response to a 6-hour cosyntropin stimulation test, while oral prednisone significantly reduced the response to cosyntropin for plasma cortisol concentrations and 24-hour urinary 17-OHCS concentrations.
A study was conducted evaluating plasma cortisol response 30 and 60 minutes after cosyntropin stimulation in 80 pediatric patients aged 6 to 12 years with allergic rhinitis who received 220 mcg or 440 mcg (twice the maximum recommended daily dose) of Nasacort AQ Nasal Spray daily for 6 weeks. No abnormal response to cosyntropin infusion (peak serum cortisol <18 mcg/dL) was observed after 6 weeks of dosing at 440 mcg per day.

Clinical Trials

The determination of efficacy and safety of Nasacort HFA Nasal Aerosol is based on the clinical program linking Nasacort HFA Nasal Aerosol to Nasacort Nasal Inhaler (triamcinolone acetonide CFC formulation), and by extrapolation from the known efficacy and safety of the Nasacort Nasal Inhaler. The clinical program of Nasacort HFA Nasal Aerosol included 2 studies conducted in the United States involving 1176 patients 12 to 83 years of age with allergic rhinitis, of whom 729 patients were treated with Nasacort HFA Nasal Aerosol. One study was a 2-week, double-blind, parallel-group, placebo-controlled trial comparing Nasacort HFA Nasal Aerosol to Nasacort Nasal Inhaler (triamcinolone acetonide CFC formulation) in 780 patients 18 years of age and older with seasonal allergic rhinitis. The design incorporated 2 doses of Nasacort Nasal Inhaler that were known to be effective (110 mcg and 440 mcg once daily), and 2 doses of Nasacort HFA Nasal Aerosol (110 mcg and 440 mcg once daily). Another study was a 12-month, open-label safety study in 396 patients 12 years of age and older with perennial allergic rhinitis. The dose of Nasacort HFA Nasal Aerosol was 220 mcg once daily for the first 2 weeks and 440 mcg once daily for the remainder of the study.
In the 2-week, double-blind study, Nasacort HFA Nasal Aerosol and Nasacort Nasal Inhaler (triamcinolone acetonide CFC formulation) were comparable, and both formulations showed a significant reduction in symptoms of allergic rhinitis (see table below). There were no significant differences in the effectiveness of Nasacort HFA Nasal Aerosol across subgroups of patients defined by gender, age, or race.

Effect of Nasacort HFA Nasal Aerosol on Total Symptom Score in a 2-Week Clinical Trial in Patients with Seasonal Allergic Rhinitis.

Treatment Group (n)	Baseline Mean Score (SEM)*	Mean Change From Baseline (SEM)**	Placebo Comparison (p-value)
Nasacort HFA 440 mcg Once Daily (111)	6.78 (0.1)	−2.64 (0.18)	< 0.05
Nasacort HFA 110 mcg Once Daily (105)	6.41 (0.1)	−2.29 (0.18)	< 0.05
Placebo (109)	6.75 (0.1)	−1.39 (0.18)	

* Baseline score was an average of the morning and evening scores of 3 symptoms of allergic rhinitis (nasal discharge, nasal stuffiness, and sneezing) for 3 days preceding randomization and the morning of randomization. Each symptom was scored by patients 2 times a day by reflection over the preceding 12 hours on a scale of 0 to 3 where 0=no symptom and 3=severe symptoms.
** Changes were averaged over the 2-week treatment period compared to the baseline. Symptom scoring during treatment period was the same as that for the baseline.

[See table above]

Individualization of Dosage: Individual patients will experience a variable time to onset and degree of symptom relief when using Nasacort HFA Nasal Aerosol. After starting patients on appropriate doses of Nasacort HFA Nasal Aerosol (see **DOSAGE AND ADMINISTRATION**) it is recommended that the effect be assessed in 4 to 7 days. If adequate relief has not been obtained by a reasonable time, alternate forms of treatment should be considered.
The maximum total daily dose should not exceed 440 mcg (4 sprays in each nostril) in patients 12 years of age and older and 220 mcg (2 sprays in each nostril) in patients 6 through 11 years of age. There is no evidence that exceeding the recommended dose is more effective. In general, it is always desirable to titrate an individual patient to the minimum effective dose to reduce the possibility of side effects. (See **WARNINGS, PRECAUTIONS: Information for Patients**, and **ADVERSE REACTIONS**.)

INDICATIONS AND USAGE

Nasacort HFA Nasal Aerosol is indicated for the treatment of the nasal symptoms of allergic rhinitis (seasonal and perennial) in adults and children 6 years of age and older.
Safety and effectiveness of Nasacort HFA Nasal Aerosol in children below 6 years of age have not been adequately established.

CONTRAINDICATIONS

Nasacort HFA Nasal Aerosol is contraindicated in patients with a hypersensitivity to any of the ingredients.

WARNINGS

The replacement of a systemic corticosteroid with a topical corticosteroid can be accompanied by signs of adrenal insufficiency and, in addition, some patients may experience symptoms of withdrawal, e.g., joint and/or muscular pain, lassitude, and depression. Patients previously treated for prolonged periods with systemic corticosteroids and transferred to topical corticosteroids should be carefully monitored for acute adrenal insufficiency in response to stress. In those patients who have asthma or other clinical conditions requiring long-term systemic corticosteroid treatment, too rapid a decrease in systemic corticosteroids may cause a severe exacerbation of their symptoms.
The concomitant use of intranasal corticosteroids with other inhaled corticosteroids could increase the risk of signs or symptoms of hypercorticism and/or suppression of the HPA axis.
Persons who are using drugs that suppress the immune system are more susceptible to infections than healthy individuals. Chickenpox and measles, for example, can have a more serious or even fatal course in susceptible children or adults using corticosteroids. In children or adults who have not had these diseases or been properly immunized, particular care should be taken to avoid exposure. How the dose, route, and duration of corticosteroid administration affect the risk of developing a disseminated infection is not known. The contribution of the underlying disease and/or prior corticosteroid treatment to the risk is also not known. If exposed to chickenpox, prophylaxis with varicella zoster immune globulin (VZIG) may be indicated. If exposed to measles, prophylaxis with pooled intramuscular immunoglobulin (IG) may be indicated. (See the respective package inserts for complete VZIG and IG prescribing information.) If chickenpox develops, treatment with antiviral agents may be considered.
Avoid spraying in eyes.

PRECAUTIONS

General:

Intranasal corticosteroids may cause a reduction in growth velocity when administered to pediatric patients (see **PRECAUTIONS: Pediatric Use**).
Triamcinolone acetonide administered intranasally has been shown to be absorbed into the systemic circulation in humans. Patients with active rhinitis showed absorption similar to that found in normal volunteers.
Rarely, immediate hypersensitivity reactions or contact dermatitis occur after the administration of Nasacort HFA Nasal Aerosol. Rare instances of wheezing, nasal septum perforation, cataracts, glaucoma, and increased intraocular pressure have been reported following the intranasal application of corticosteroids, including triamcinolone acetonide.

Continued on next page

Nasacort HFA—Cont.

Because of the inhibitory effect of corticosteroids on wound healing in patients who have experienced recent nasal septal ulcers, nasal surgery or trauma, a corticosteroid should be used with caution until healing has occurred.

In clinical studies with triamcinolone acetonide administered intranasally, the development of localized infections of the nose and pharynx with *Candida albicans* has rarely occurred. When such an infection develops, it may require treatment with appropriate local or systemic therapy and discontinuance of treatment with Nasacort HFA Nasal Aerosol. As with any long-term topical treatment of the nasal cavity, patients using Nasacort HFA Nasal Aerosol over several months or longer should be examined periodically for evidence of *Candida* infection or other adverse effects on the nasal mucosa.

Intranasal corticosteroids should be used with caution, if at all, in patients with active or quiescent tuberculosis infections of the respiratory tract or in patients with untreated local or systemic fungal or bacterial infections, systemic viral or parasitic infections, or ocular herpes simplex.

When used at higher than recommended doses or in rare individuals at recommended doses, systemic corticosteroid effects such as hypercorticism and adrenal suppression may appear. Therefore, larger than recommended doses of Nasacort HFA Nasal Aerosol should be avoided. If signs or symptoms of hypercorticism and/or suppression of HPA function occur, Nasacort HFA Nasal Aerosol should be discontinued slowly, consistent with accepted procedures for discontinuing oral steroid therapy.

Information for Patients:

Patients being treated with Nasacort HFA Nasal Aerosol should receive the following information and instructions. This information is intended to aid them in the safe and effective use of this medication. It is not a disclosure of all possible adverse or intended effects.

Patients who are on immunosuppressant doses of corticosteroids should be warned to avoid exposure to chickenpox or measles and, if exposed, to obtain medical advice.

Patients should use Nasacort HFA Nasal Aerosol at regular intervals since its effectiveness depends on regular use (see **DOSAGE AND ADMINISTRATION**). Individual patients will experience a variable time to onset and degree of symptom relief, and generally takes 1 week of treatment to reach maximum benefit. The patient should take the medication as directed and should not exceed the prescribed dosage. The patient should contact the physician if symptoms do not improve by a reasonable time, or if the condition worsens. Nasal irritation occurred in 6.2% of adults who used 440 mcg/day, the maximum recommended daily intranasal dose. The patient should contact the physician if nasal irritation occurs. It is advisable for patients who experience nasal septum discomfort to re-evaluate their technique in the application of Nasacort HFA Nasal Aerosol to minimize deposition of drug onto the septum.

For the proper use of this unit and to attain maximum improvement, the patient should read and follow the accompanying patient instructions carefully. Spraying Nasacort HFA Nasal Aerosol directly into the eyes or onto the nasal septum should be avoided. It is important to shake the canister well prior to each actuation to insure that a consistent amount is dispensed per actuation. The canister should be discarded after 100 actuations.

Drug-Drug Interactions:

No drug interaction studies with triamcinolone acetonide have been performed.

Carcinogenesis, Mutagenesis, Impairment of Fertility:

In a 2-year study in rats, triamcinolone acetonide caused no treatment-related carcinogenicity at oral doses up to 1.0 mcg/kg (approximately 1/50 of the maximum recommended daily intranasal dose in adults and children on a mcg/m^2 basis). In a 2-year study in mice, triamcinolone acetonide caused no treatment-related carcinogenicity at oral doses up to 3.0 mcg/kg (approximately 1/30 of the maximum recommended daily intranasal dose in adults and children on a mcg/m^2 basis).

No evidence of mutagenicity was detected from *in vitro* tests (a reverse mutation test in *Salmonella* bacteria and a forward mutation test in Chinese hamster ovary cells) conducted with triamcinolone acetonide.

In male and female rats, triamcinolone acetonide caused no change in pregnancy rate at oral doses up to 15 mcg/kg (approximately 1/3 of the maximum recommended daily intranasal dose in adults on a mcg/m^2 basis). Triamcinolone acetonide caused increased fetal resorptions and stillbirths and decreases in pup weight and survival at doses of 5.0 mcg/kg and above (approximately 1/10 of the maximum recommended daily intranasal dose in adults on a mcg/m^2 basis). At 1.0 mcg/kg (approximately 1/50 of the maximum recommended daily intranasal dose in adults on a mcg/m^2 basis), it did not induce the above mentioned effects.

Pregnancy:

Teratogenic Effects: ***Pregnancy category C.*** Triamcinolone acetonide was teratogenic in rats, rabbits, and monkeys. In rats, triamcinolone acetonide was teratogenic at inhalation doses of 20 mcg/kg and above (approximately 2/5 of the maximum recommended daily intranasal dose in adults on a mcg/m^2 basis). In rabbits, triamcinolone acetonide was also teratogenic at inhalation doses of 20 mcg/kg and above (approximately 4/5 of the maximum recommended daily intranasal dose in adults on a mcg/m^2 basis). In monkeys, triamcinolone acetonide was teratogenic at an inhalation dose of 500 mcg/kg (approximately 20 times the maximum recommended daily intranasal dose in adults on a mcg/m^2 basis). Dose-related teratogenic effects in rats and rabbits included cleft palate and/or internal hydrocephaly and axial skeletal defects, whereas the effects observed in monkeys were cranial malformations.

There are no adequate and well-controlled studies in pregnant women. Therefore, Nasacort HFA Nasal Aerosol should be used during pregnancy only if the potential benefit justifies the potential risk to the fetus. Experience with oral corticosteroids since their introduction in pharmacologic, as opposed to physiologic, doses suggests that rodents are more prone to teratogenic effects from corticosteroids than humans. In addition, because there is an increase in corticosteroid production during pregnancy, most women will require a lower exogenous corticosteroid dose and many will not need corticosteroid treatment during pregnancy.

Nonteratogenic Effects: Hypoadrenalism may occur in infants born of mothers receiving corticosteroids during pregnancy. Such infants should be carefully monitored.

Nursing Mothers:

It is not known whether triamcinolone acetonide is excreted in human milk. Because other corticosteroids are excreted in human milk, caution should be exercised when this product is administered to nursing women.

Pediatric Use:

Safety and effectiveness have not been established in pediatric patients below the age of 6 years.

A placebo-controlled clinical growth study in children has not been conducted with Nasacort HFA Nasal Aerosol. Controlled clinical studies have shown that intranasal corticosteroids may cause a reduction in growth velocity in pediatric patients. This effect has been observed in the absence of laboratory evidence of HPA axis suppression, suggesting that growth velocity is a more sensitive indicator of systemic corticosteroid exposure in pediatric patients than some commonly used tests of HPA axis function. The long-term effects of this reduction in growth velocity associated with intranasal corticosteroids, including the impact on final adult height, are unknown. The potential for "catch-up" growth following discontinuation of treatment with intranasal corticosteroids has not been adequately studied. The growth of pediatric patients receiving intranasal corticosteroids, including Nasacort HFA Nasal Aerosol, should be monitored routinely (e.g., via stadiometry). The potential growth effects of prolonged treatment should be weighed against the clinical benefits obtained and the risks/benefits of treatment alternatives. To minimize the systemic effects of intranasal corticosteroids, including Nasacort HFA Nasal Aerosol, each patient should be titrated to the lowest dose that effectively controls his/her symptoms.

Geriatric Use:

Clinical studies of Nasacort HFA Nasal Aerosol did not include sufficient numbers of subjects aged 65 and over to determine whether they respond differently from younger subjects. Other reported clinical experience has not identified differences in responses between the elderly and younger patients.

ADVERSE REACTIONS

Clinical Trials: A total of 1176 patients with allergic rhinitis were enrolled in placebo-controlled and open-label clinical studies of Nasacort HFA Nasal Aerosol.

In the placebo-controlled trial, 220 patients were treated with Nasacort HFA Nasal Aerosol for an average of 15 days (range 1–19 days). No changes in mucous membranes were noted from physical and visual examinations during this trial.

Adverse events occurring with an incidence of 3% or greater and more commonly with Nasacort HFA Nasal Aerosol arms compared to placebo irrespective of drug relationship are presented in the following table:

Adverse Event	Nasacort HFA Nasal Aerosol 110 mcg (n=107) %	Nasacort HFA Nasal Aerosol 440 mcg (n=113) %	Placebo (n=111) %
Sneezing	14.0	15.9	7.2
Headache	10.3	6.2	8.1
Nasal irritation	7.5	6.2	3.6
Rhinitis	4.7	3.5	1.8

Of the 396 patients enrolled in the 12-month open-label study, 75% received treatment for greater than 6 months. In this study, patients were treated with Nasacort HFA Nasal Aerosol at 220 mcg once daily for the first 2 weeks and 440 mcg once daily for remainder of the study. Adverse events that were considered possibly or probably related to Nasacort HFA Nasal Aerosol and reported at an incidence of 3% or greater included: headache, epistaxis, nasal septum discomfort, rhinitis, nasal burning, and sneezing.

In the open-label study only 2% of patients receiving recommended doses discontinued due to nasal adverse effects. In the rest of the patients the nasal adverse events usually did not interfere with treatment. Seven of the 18 patients who reported nasal septum discomfort had objective evidence of ulceration, abrasion, erosion, or excoriation of the nasal septum, and 22 of the 396 (5.5%) enrolled patients developed nasal septum disorders, of whom 8 had evidence of ulceration, erosion, or excoriation of the septum, and 14 had epistaxis. It is advisable for patients who experience nasal septum discomfort to re-evaluate their technique in the application of Nasacort HFA Nasal Aerosol to minimize deposition of drug onto the septum.

If recommended doses are exceeded, or if individuals taking Nasacort HFA Nasal Aerosol are particularly sensitive or take the drug in conjunction with other corticosteroids, symptoms of hypercorticism, e.g., Cushing syndrome, could occur.

In the event of accidental overdose, an increased potential for these adverse experiences may be expected, but systemic adverse experiences are unlikely (see **OVERDOSAGE**).

Observed During Clinical Practice: In addition to adverse events reported from clinical trials, the following events have been identified during use of Nasacort Nasal Inhaler (triamcinolone acetonide CFC formulation) in clinical practice: nasal septal perforation, infection of the nose and pharynx with *Candida albicans*, cataracts, glaucoma, increased intraocular pressure, wheezing, rash, pruritus, urticaria, dizziness, paresthesia, dry mouth, nausea, coughing, dyspnea, and allergic reaction. Because they were reported voluntarily from a population of unknown size, estimates of frequency cannot be made. These events have been chosen for inclusion due to either their seriousness, frequency of reporting, or possible causal connection to triamcinolone acetonide or a combination of these factors.

DOSAGE AND ADMINISTRATION

Recommended Doses:

Adults and Adolescents 12 years of age and older: The recommended starting dose of Nasacort HFA Nasal Aerosol is 220 mcg per day given as 2 sprays (55 mcg/spray) in each nostril once daily. If needed, the dose may be increased to 440 mcg per day given as 4 sprays (55 mcg/spray) in each nostril once daily. Once the maximal effect has been achieved, it is always desirable to titrate the patient to the minimum effective dose.

Children 6 through 11 years of age: The recommended dose of Nasacort HFA Nasal Aerosol is 220 mcg per day given as 2 sprays (55 mcg/spray) in each nostril once daily. Once the maximal effect has been achieved, it is always desirable to titrate the patient to the minimum effective dose. Safety and effectiveness have not been established in pediatric patients below the age of 6 years (see **PRECAUTIONS, Pediatric Use**).

Directions for Use:

Illustrated **PATIENT'S INSTRUCTIONS FOR USE** accompanies each package.

OVERDOSAGE

Chronic overdosage may result in signs/symptoms of hypercorticism (see **PRECAUTIONS**).

The acute topical application of the entire 15 mg contents of the canister may cause nasal irritation and headache. Acute overdosage with this dosage form is unlikely since one canister of Nasacort HFA Nasal Aerosol contains 15 mg of triamcinolone acetonide.

HOW SUPPLIED

Nasacort HFA Nasal Aerosol is supplied with an aerosol canister which provides 100 metered dose actuations. The correct amount of medication delivered per actuation cannot be assured after 100 actuations have been dispensed, after which the unit should be discarded. Each actuation delivers 55 mcg triamcinolone acetonide through the nasal actuator. The Nasacort HFA Nasal Aerosol canister and accompanying nasal actuator are designed to be used together. The Nasacort HFA Nasal Aerosol canister should not be used with other nasal actuators and the supplied nasal actuator should not be used with other products' canisters. Nasacort HFA Nasal Aerosol is supplied with a molecular sieve sachet as a propellant adsorbent and a white plastic protective cap, and enclosed in a foil laminate overwrap pouch. Patient instructions are also provided. Net weight of the canister contents is 9.3 grams.

NDC 0075-9403-43

CONTENTS UNDER PRESSURE

Avoid spraying in eyes.

Do not puncture. Do not use or store near heat or open flame. Exposure to temperatures above 120°F may cause bursting. Never throw container into fire or incinerator.

Store at controlled room temperature, 20 to 25°C (68 to 77°F) [see USP].

Keep out of reach of children.

Rx only.

Rev. April 2004c

Manufactured for:
Aventis Pharmaceuticals Inc.
Bridgewater, NJ 08807

Manufactured by:
Aventis Pharma Ltd.
Holmes Chapel, Cheshire CW4 8BE
United Kingdom

NASHFA-APRIL04c-F-A
Rev. April 2004c

NASACORT® HFA
[na' za-cort]
(triamcinolone acetonide)
Nasal Aerosol

PATIENT'S INSTRUCTIONS FOR USE

Using your
Nasacort® HFA
(triamcinolone acetonide)
Nasal Aerosol

IMPORTANT:
Please read these instructions carefully before using your **Nasacort® HFA Nasal Aerosol.**

Before each use of Nasacort® HFA Nasal Aerosol, gently blow your nose, making sure your nostrils are clear. Then follow these steps:

Step 1
The Nasacort® HFA Nasal Aerosol device (canister and actuator assembly) is supplied with a protective cap in a pouch. Tear open the pouch and discard it before using the Nasacort HFA Nasal Aerosol device. Remove the white protective cap from the device prior to use. The canister and actuator are designed to be used together. Do not remove the canister from the actuator during regular use of the product.

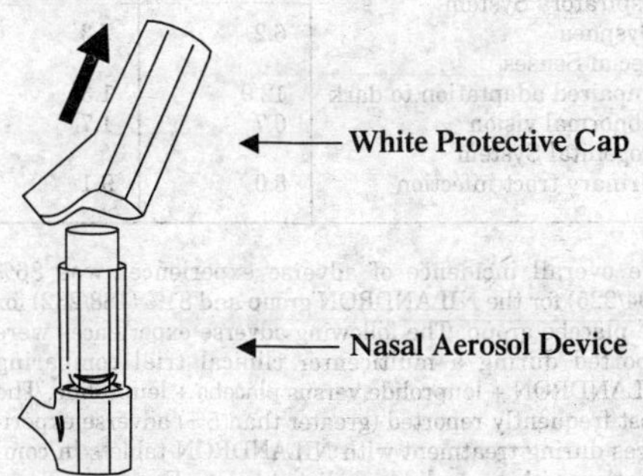

Figure 1: Nasacort HFA Nasal Aerosol device with protective cap

Step 2
Shake the device well.

Step 3
The device must be primed **prior to the first use.** To prime, hold the device between your thumb and forefinger and press down on the canister to release one spray. Repeat this until you have released a total of 3 sprays. Now your device is primed and ready for use.

Re-priming of the device is only necessary when it has not been used for more than 3 days. To re-prime the device, shake it and release 3 sprays (as described in Step 3 above). Now the device is re-primed. There is no need to re-prime the device between more frequent uses.

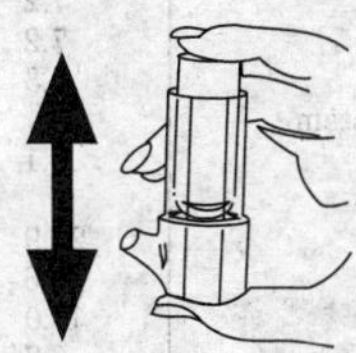

Step 4
To use, hold the device between your thumb and forefinger.

Step 5
Tilt your head back slightly and insert the end of the actuator into one nostril, pointing it slightly toward the outside nostril wall away from the nasal septum, while holding your other nostril closed with one finger. **Avoid spraying in eyes.**

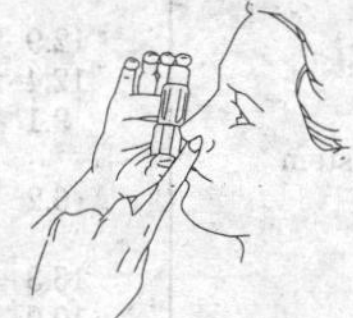

Step 6
Press down on the canister to release one spray and, at the same time, inhale gently through the nostril.

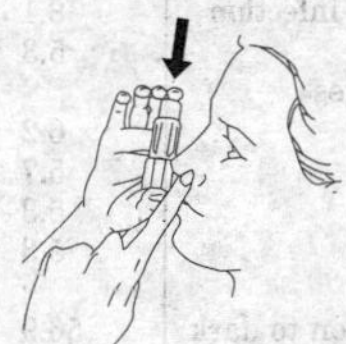

Step 7
Hold your breath for a few seconds, then breathe out slowly through your mouth.

Step 8
Withdraw the device from your nostril.

Step 9
Repeat the process in your other nostril.

NOTE: When the physician prescribes more than one spray per nostril, for each spray repeat steps 5 through 9.

Step 10
Replace the white protective inhaler cap on the device.

NOTE: AVOID BLOWING YOUR NOSE FOR THE NEXT 15 MINUTES.

DOSAGE: Use only as directed by your physician.

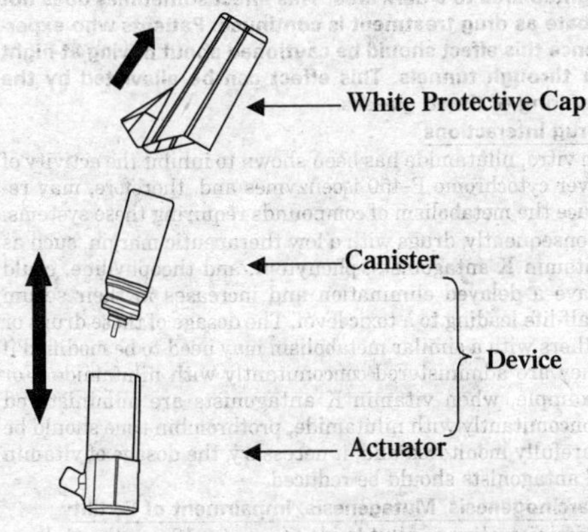

The actuator of your Nasacort® HFA Nasal Aerosol should be cleaned weekly. Remove the white protective cap from the device. Remove the canister from the actuator. Clean the actuator *thoroughly* in lukewarm water. The use of soap, detergent, or disinfectant is not necessary. Allow the actuator to *dry completely*. To replace the canister, gently center and insert the canister with the plastic stem downward into the small hole at the bottom of the actuator. Replace the white protective cap. The correct amount of medication delivered per actuation cannot be assured after 100 actuations have been dispensed (see dose check-off chart below). The Nasacort HFA Nasal Aerosol device should be discarded after 100 actuations. The canister and actuator (the device) are designed to be used together. Never use this canister or actuator with those from any other product.

NOTE: Nasacort® HFA Nasal Aerosol is not intended to give immediate relief of your nasal symptoms. Your particular symptoms may require regular use of this drug for a few days or more before improvement. Therefore, it is important that you use the Nasacort® HFA Nasal Aerosol regularly as recommended by your physician.

CAUTION: Contents under pressure. Do not puncture. Do not use or store near heat or open flame. Exposure to temperatures above 120°F may cause bursting. Never throw canister into fire or incinerator.

Keep out of the reach of children.

Store at Controlled Room Temperature 20 to 25°C (68 to 77°F) [see USP].

Rx Only.

Rev. April 2004c
Manufactured for:
Aventis Pharmaceuticals Inc.
Bridgewater, NJ 08807
Manufactured by:
Aventis Pharma Ltd.
Holmes Chapel, Cheshire CW4 8BE
United Kingdom
NASHFA-APRIL04c-F-A

How to check contents of your Nasacort® HFA Nasal Aerosol

Shaking your canister will NOT give you a good estimate of how much is left. We have included a convenient check-off chart to assist you in keeping track of medication sprays used. This will help assure that you receive the 100 "Full Sprays" of medication present.

Nasacort® HFA 100 Spray Check-Off

1	2	3	4	5	6	7	8
9	10	11	12	13	14	15	16
17	18	19	20	21	22	23	24
25	26	27	28	29	30	31	32
33	34	35	36	37	38	39	40
41	42	43	44	45	46	47	48
49	50	51	52	53	54	55	56
57	58	59	60	61	62	63	64
65	66	67	68	69	70	71	72
73	74	75	76	77	78	79	80
81	82	83	84	85	86	87	88
89	90	91	92	93	94	95	96
97	98	99	100				

— Retain with medication or affix to convenient location.
— Starting with spray #1, check off after each use.
— **DISCARD MEDICATION AFTER 100 SPRAYS.**

Your physician has determined that this product is likely to help your personal health. **USE THIS PRODUCT AS DIRECTED, UNLESS INSTRUCTED TO DO OTHERWISE BY YOUR PHYSICIAN.** If you have any questions about alternatives, consult with your physician.

NILANDRON® ℞
(nilutamide)
Tablets

Prescribing Information as of April 2004

DESCRIPTION

NILANDRON® tablets contain nilutamide, a nonsteroidal, orally active antiandrogen having the chemical name 5,5-dimethyl-3-[4-nitro-3-(trifluoromethyl)phenyl]-2,4-imidazolidinedione with the following structural formula:

Nilutamide is a microcrystalline, white to practically white powder with a molecular weight of 317.25. Its molecular formula is $C_{12}H_{10}F_3N_3O_4$.

It is freely soluble in ethyl acetate, acetone, chloroform, ethyl alcohol, dichloromethane, and methanol. It is slightly soluble in water [< 0.1% W/V at 25°C (77°F)]. It melts between 153°C and 156°C (307.4°F and 312.8°F).

Each NILANDRON tablet contains 150 mg of nilutamide. Other ingredients in NILANDRON tablets are corn starch, lactose, povidone, docusate sodium, magnesium stearate, and talc.

CLINICAL PHARMACOLOGY

Mechanism of Action

Prostate cancer is known to be androgen sensitive and responds to androgen ablation. In animal studies, nilutamide has demonstrated antiandrogenic activity without other hormonal (estrogen, progesterone, mineralocorticoid, and glucocorticoid) effects. In vitro, nilutamide blocks the effects of testosterone at the androgen receptor level. In vivo, nilutamide interacts with the androgen receptor and prevents the normal androgenic response.

Pharmacokinetics

Absorption: Analysis of blood, urine, and feces samples following a single oral 150-mg dose of [^{14}C]-nilutamide in patients with metastatic prostate cancer showed that the drug is rapidly and completely absorbed and that it yields high and persistent plasma concentrations.

Distribution: After absorption of the drug, there is a detectable distribution phase. There is moderate binding of the drug to plasma proteins and low binding to erythrocytes. The binding is nonsaturable except in the case of alpha-1-glycoprotein, which makes a minor contribution to the total concentration of proteins in the plasma. The results of binding studies do not indicate any effects that would cause nonlinear pharmacokinetics.

Metabolism: The results of a human metabolism study using ^{14}C-radiolabelled tablets show that nilutamide is extensively metabolized and less than 2% of the drug is excreted unchanged in urine after 5 days. Five metabolites have been isolated from human urine. Two metabolites display an asymmetric center, due to oxidation of a methyl group, resulting in the formation of D- and L-isomers. One of the metabolites was shown, in vitro, to possess 25 to 50% of the pharmacological activity of the parent drug, and the D-isomer of the active metabolite showed equal or greater potency compared to the L-isomer. However, the pharmacokinetics and the pharmacodynamics of the metabolites have not been fully investigated.

Elimination: The majority (62%) of orally administered [^{14}C]-nilutamide is eliminated in the urine during the first 120 hours after a single 150-mg dose. Fecal elimination is negligible, ranging from 1.4% to 7% of the dose after 4 to 5 days. Excretion of radioactivity in urine likely continues beyond 5 days. The mean elimination half-life of nilutamide determined in studies in which subjects received a single dose of 100–300 mg ranged from 38.0 to 59.1 hours with most values between 41 and 49 hours. The elimination of at least one metabolite is generally longer than that of unchanged nilutamide (59–126 hours). During multiple dosing of 150 mg nilutamide (given as 3 x 50 mg) twice a day, steady state was reached within 2 to 4 weeks for most patients, and mean steady state AUC_{0-12} was 110% higher than the $AUC_{0-\infty}$ obtained from the first 150 mg dose. These data and in vitro metabolism data suggest that, upon multiple dosing, metabolic enzyme inhibition may occur for this drug.

Clinical Studies

Nilutamide through its antiandrogenic activity can complement surgical castration, which suppresses only testicular androgens. The effects of the combined therapy were studied in patients with previously untreated metastatic prostate cancer.

In a double-blind, randomized, multicenter study that enrolled 457 patients (225 treated with orchiectomy and NILANDRON, 232 treated with orchiectomy and placebo), the NILANDRON group showed a statistically significant benefit in time to progression and time to death. The results are summarized below.

Continued on next page

Nilandron—Cont.

	NILANDRON	PLACEBO
Median Survival (months)	27.3	23.6
Progression-Free Survival (months)	21.1	14.9
Complete or Partial Regression	41%	24%
Improvement in Bone Pain	54%	37%

INDICATIONS AND USAGE

Metastatic Prostate Cancer

NILANDRON tablets are indicated for use in combination with surgical castration for the treatment of metastatic prostate cancer (Stage D_2).

For maximum benefit, NILANDRON treatment must begin on the same day as or on the day after surgical castration.

CONTRAINDICATIONS

NILANDRON tablets are contraindicated:

- in patients with severe hepatic impairment (baseline hepatic enzymes should be evaluated prior to treatment)
- in patients with severe respiratory insufficiency
- in patients with hypersensitivity to nilutamide or any component of this preparation.

WARNINGS

Interstitial Pneumonitis

Interstitial pneumonitis has been reported in 2% of patients in controlled clinical trials in patients exposed to nilutamide. A small study in Japanese subjects showed that 8 of 47 patients (17%) developed interstitial pneumonitis. Reports of interstitial changes including pulmonary fibrosis that led to hospitalization and death have been reported rarely post-marketing. Symptoms included exertional dyspnea, cough, chest pain, and fever. X-rays showed interstitial or alveolo-interstitial changes, and pulmonary function tests revealed a restrictive pattern with decreased DLco. Most cases occurred within the first 3 months of treatment with NILANDRON, and most reversed with discontinuation of therapy.

A routine chest X-ray should be performed prior to initiating treatment with NILANDRON. Baseline pulmonary function tests may be considered. Patients should be instructed to report any new or worsening shortness of breath that they experience while on NILANDRON. **If symptoms occur, NILANDRON should be immediately discontinued until it can be determined if the symptoms are drug related.**

Hepatitis

Rare cases of death or hospitalization due to severe liver injury have been reported post-marketing in association with the use of NILANDRON. Hepatotoxicity in these reports generally occurred within the first 3 to 4 months of treatment. Hepatitis or marked increases in liver enzymes leading to drug discontinuation occurred in 1% of NILANDRON patients in controlled clinical trials.

Serum transaminase levels should be measured prior to starting treatment with NILANDRON, at regular intervals for the first 4 months of treatment, and periodically thereafter. Liver function tests should also be obtained at the first sign or symptom suggestive of liver dysfunction, e.g. nausea, vomiting, abdominal pain, fatigue, anorexia, "flu-like" symptoms, dark urine, jaundice, or right upper quadrant tenderness. If at any time, a patient has jaundice, or their ALT rises above 2 times the upper limit of normal, NILANDRON should be immediately discontinued with close followup of liver function tests until resolution.

Use in Women

NILANDRON has no indication for women, and should not be used in this population, particularly for non-serious or non-life threatening conditions.

Other

Foreign postmarketing surveillance has revealed isolated cases of aplastic anemia in which a causal relationship with NILANDRON could not be ascertained.

PRECAUTIONS

Information for Patients

Patients should be informed that NILANDRON tablets should be started on the day of, or on the day after, surgical castration. They should also be informed that they should not interrupt their dosing of NILANDRON or stop taking this medication without consulting their physician.

Because of the possibility of interstitial pneumonitis, patients should also be told to report immediately any dyspnea or aggravation of pre-existing dyspnea.

Because of the possibility of hepatitis, patients should be told to consult with their physician should nausea, vomiting, abdominal pain, or jaundice occur.

Because of the possibility of an intolerance to alcohol (facial flushes, malaise, hypotension) following ingestion of NILANDRON, it is recommended that intake of alcoholic beverages be avoided by patients who experience this reaction. This effect has been reported in about 5% of patients treated with NILANDRON.

In clinical trials, 13% to 57% of patients receiving NILANDRON reported a delay in adaptation to dark, ranging from seconds to a few minutes, when passing from a lighted area to a dark area. This effect sometimes does not abate as drug treatment is continued. Patients who experience this effect should be cautioned about driving at night or through tunnels. This effect can be alleviated by the wearing of tinted glasses.

Drug Interactions

In vitro, nilutamide has been shown to inhibit the activity of liver cytochrome P-450 isoenzymes and, therefore, may reduce the metabolism of compounds requiring these systems. Consequently, drugs with a low therapeutic margin, such as vitamin K antagonists, phenytoin, and theophylline, could have a delayed elimination and increases in their serum half-life leading to a toxic level. The dosage of these drugs or others with a similar metabolism may need to be modified if they are administered concomitantly with nilutamide. For example, when vitamin K antagonists are administered concomitantly with nilutamide, prothrombin time should be carefully monitored and, if necessary, the dosage of vitamin K antagonists should be reduced.

Carcinogenesis, Mutagenesis, Impairment of Fertility

Administration of nilutamide to rats for 18 months at doses of 0, 5, 15, or 45 mg/kg/day produced benign Leydig cell tumors in 35% of the high-dose male rats (AUC exposures in high-dose rats were approximately 1–2 times human AUC exposures with therapeutic doses). The increased incidence of Leydig cell tumors is secondary to elevated luteinizing hormone (LH) concentrations resulting from loss of feedback inhibition at the pituitary. Elevated LH and testosterone concentrations are not observed in castrated men receiving NILANDRON. Nilutamide had no effect on the incidence, size, or time of onset of any spontaneous tumor in rats.

Nilutamide displayed no mutagenic effects in a variety of in vitro and in vivo tests (Ames test, mouse micronucleus test, and two chromosomal aberration tests).

In reproduction studies in rats, nilutamide had no effect on the reproductive function of males and females, and no lethal, teratogenic, or growth-suppressive effects on fetuses were found. The maximal dose at which nilutamide did not affect reproductive function in either sex or have an effect on fetuses was estimated to be 45 mg/kg orally (AUC exposures in rats approximately 1–2 times human therapeutic AUC exposures).

Pregnancy

Pregnancy Category C; Animal reproduction studies have not been conducted with nilutamide. It is also not known whether nilutamide can cause fetal harm when administered to a pregnant woman or can affect reproductive capacity. Nilutamide should be given to a pregnant woman only if clearly needed.

Pediatric Use

Safety and effectiveness in pediatric patients have not been determined.

Animal Pharmacology and Toxicology

Administration of NILANDRON to beagle dogs resulted in drug-related deaths at dose levels that produce AUC exposures in dogs much lower than the AUC exposures of men receiving the therapeutic doses of 150 and 300 mg/day. Nilutamide-induced toxicity in dogs was cumulative with progressively lower doses producing death when given for longer durations. Nilutamide given to dogs at 60 mg/kg/day (1–2 times human AUC exposure) for 1 month produced 100% mortality. Administration of 20 and 30 mg/kg/day nilutamide (1/2–1 times human AUC exposure) for 6 months resulted in 20% and 70% mortality in treated dogs. Administration to dogs of 3, 6, and 12 mg/kg/day nilutamide (1/10–1/2 human AUC exposure) for 1 year resulted in 8%, 33%, and 50% mortality, respectively. **A "no-effect level" for nilutamide-induced mortality in dogs was not identified.** Pathology data from the one-year oral toxicity study suggest that the deaths in dogs were secondary to liver toxicity. Marked-to-massive hepatocellular swelling and vacuolization were observed in affected dogs. Liver toxicity in dogs was not consistently associated with elevations of liver enzymes.

Administration of nilutamide to rats at a dose level of 45 mg/kg/day (AUC exposure in rats 1–2 times human therapeutic AUC exposures) for 18 months increased the incidence of lung pathology (granulomatous inflammation and chronic alveolitis).

The hepatic and pulmonary adverse effects observed in nilutamide-treated animals and men are similar to effects observed with another nitroaromatic compound, nitrofurantoin. Nilutamide and nitrofurantoin are both metabolized in vitro to nitroanion free radicals by microsomal NADPH-cytochrome P450 reductase in the lungs and liver of rats and humans.

ADVERSE REACTIONS

The following adverse experiences were reported during a multicenter clinical trial comparing NILANDRON + surgical castration versus placebo + surgical castration. The most frequently reported (greater than 5%) adverse experiences during treatment with NILANDRON tablets in combination with surgical castration are listed below. For comparison, adverse experiences seen with surgical castration and placebo are also listed.

Adverse Experience	NILANDRON + surgical castration (N=225) % All	Placebo + surgical castration (N=232) % All
Cardiovascular System		
Hypertension	5.3	2.6
Digestive System		
Nausea	9.8	6.0
Constipation	7.1	3.9
Endocrine System		
Hot flushes	28.4	22.4
Metabolic and Nutritional System		
Increased AST	8.0	3.9
Increased ALT	7.6	4.3
Nervous System		
Dizziness	7.1	3.4
Respiratory System		
Dyspnea	6.2	7.3
Special Senses		
Impaired adaptation to dark	12.9	1.3
Abnormal vision	6.7	1.7
Urogenital System		
Urinary tract infection	8.0	9.1

The overall incidence of adverse experiences was 86% (194/225) for the NILANDRON group and 81% (188/232) for the placebo group. The following adverse experiences were reported during a multicenter clinical trial comparing NILANDRON + leuprolide versus placebo + leuprolide. The most frequently reported (greater than 5%) adverse experiences during treatment with NILANDRON tablets in combination with leuprolide are listed below. For comparison, adverse experiences seen with leuprolide and placebo are also listed.

Adverse Experience	NILANDRON + leuprolide (N=209) % All	Placebo + leuprolide (N=202) % All
Body as a Whole		
Pain	26.8	27.7
Headache	13.9	10.4
Asthenia	19.1	20.8
Back pain	11.5	16.8
Abdominal pain	10.0	5.4
Chest pain	7.2	4.5
Flu syndrome	7.2	3.0
Fever	5.3	6.4
Cardiovascular System		
Hypertension	9.1	9.9
Digestive System		
Nausea	23.9	8.4
Constipation	19.6	16.8
Anorexia	11.0	6.4
Dyspepsia	6.7	4.5
Vomiting	5.7	4.0
Endocrine System		
Hot flushes	66.5	59.4
Impotence	11.0	12.9
Libido decreased	11.0	4.5
Hemic and Lymphatic System		
Anemia	7.2	6.4
Metabolic and Nutritional System		
Increased AST	12.9	13.9
Peripheral edema	12.4	17.3
Increased ALT	9.1	8.9
Musculoskeletal System		
Bone Pain	6.2	5.0
Nervous System		
Insomnia	16.3	15.8
Dizziness	10.0	11.4
Depression	8.6	7.4
Hypesthesia	5.3	2.0
Respiratory System		
Dyspnea	10.5	7.4
Upper respiratory infection	8.1	10.9
Pneumonia	5.3	3.5
Skin and Appendages		
Sweating	6.2	3.0
Body hair loss	5.7	0.5
Dry skin	5.3	2.5
Rash	5.3	4.0
Special Senses		
Impaired adaptation to dark	56.9	5.4
Chromatopsia	8.6	0.0
Impaired adaptation to light	7.7	1.0
Abnormal vision	6.2	4.5
Urogenital System		
Testicular atrophy	16.3	12.4
Gynecomastia	10.5	11.9
Urinary tract infection	8.6	21.3
Hematuria	8.1	7.9
Urinary tract disorder	7.2	10.4
Nocturia	6.7	6.4

The overall incidence of adverse experiences is 99.5% (208/209) for the NILANDRON group and 98.5% (199/202) for the placebo group.

Some frequently occurring adverse experiences, for example hot flushes, impotence, and decreased libido, are known to be associated with low serum androgen levels and known to occur with medical or surgical castration alone. Notable was the higher incidence of visual disturbances (variously described as impaired adaptation to darkness, abnormal vision, and colored vision), which led to treatment discontinuation in 1% to 2% of patients.

Interstitial pneumonitis occurred in one (<1%) patient receiving NILANDRON in combination with surgical castration and in seven patients (3%) receiving NILANDRON in combination with leuprolide and one patient receiving placebo in combination with leuprolide. Overall, it has been reported in 2% of patients receiving NILANDRON. This included a report of interstitial pneumonitis in 8 of 47 patients (17%) in a small study performed in Japan.

In addition, the following adverse experiences were reported in 2 to 5% of patients treated with NILANDRON in combination with leuprolide or orchiectomy.

Body as a Whole: Malaise (2%).

Cardiovascular System: Angina (2%), heart failure (3%), syncope (2%).

Digestive System: Diarrhea (2%), gastrointestinal disorder (2%), gastrointestinal hemorrhage (2%), melena (2%).

Metabolic and Nutritional System: Alcohol intolerance (5%), edema (2%), weight loss (2%).

Musculoskeletal System: Arthritis (2%).

Nervous System: Dry mouth (2%), nervousness (2%), paresthesia (3%).

Respiratory System: Cough increased (2%), interstitial lung disease (2%), lung disorder (4%), rhinitis (2%).

Skin and Appendages: Pruritus (2%).

Special Senses: Cataract (2%), photophobia (2%).

Laboratory Values: Haptoglobin increased (2%), leukopenia (3%), alkaline phosphatase increased (3%), BUN increased (2%), creatinine increased (2%), hyperglycemia (4%).

OVERDOSAGE

One case of massive overdosage has been published. A 79-year-old man attempted suicide by ingesting 13 g of nilutamide (i.e., 43 times the maximum recommended dose). Despite immediate gastric lavage and oral administration of activated charcoal, plasma nilutamide levels peaked at 6 times the normal range 2 hours after ingestion. There were no clinical signs or symptoms or changes in parameters such as transaminases or chest X-ray. Maintenance treatment (150 mg/day) was resumed 30 days later.

In repeated-dose tolerance studies, doses of 600 mg/day and 900 mg/day were administered to 9 and 4 patients, respectively. The ingestion of these doses was associated with gastrointestinal disorders, including nausea and vomiting, malaise, headache, and dizziness. In addition, a transient elevation in hepatic enzyme levels was noted in one patient. Since nilutamide is protein bound, dialysis may not be useful as treatment for overdose. As in the management of overdosage with any drug, it should be borne in mind that multiple agents may have been taken. If vomiting does not occur spontaneously, it should be induced if the patient is alert. General supportive care, including frequent monitoring of the vital signs and close observation of the patient, is indicated.

DOSAGE AND ADMINISTRATION

The recommended dosage is 300 mg once a day for 30 days, followed thereafter by 150 mg once a day. NILANDRON tablets can be taken with or without food.

HOW SUPPLIED

NILANDRON 150 mg tablets are supplied in boxes of 30 tablets. Each box contains 3 child-resistant, PVC, aluminum foil-backed blisters of 10 tablets (NDC 0088-1111-14). Each white, biconvex, cylindrical (10 mm in diameter) tablet has a triangular logo on one side and an internal reference number (168D) on the other.

Store at 25°C (77°F); excursions permitted between 15–30°C (59–86°F) [see USP Controlled Room Temperature]. Protect from light.

Prescribing information as of April 2004

Manufactured by
Aventis Pharma Specialites, 60200 Compiegne, France for:
Aventis Pharmaceuticals Inc.
Kansas City, MO 64137
Made in France
www.aventis-us.com

NIL-APRIL04-F-A

Shown in Product Identification Guide, page 307

NORPRAMIN® ℞

[nor-pram' in]

(desipramine hydrochloride tablets USP)

Prescribing Information as of February 2003

DESCRIPTION

NORPRAMIN® (desipramine hydrochloride USP) is an antidepressant drug of the tricyclic type, and is chemically:

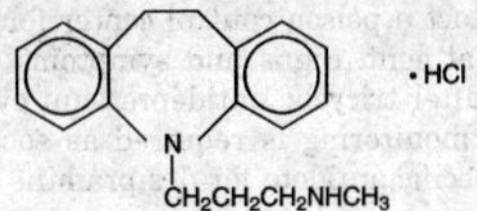

5*H*-Dibenz[*bf*]azepine-5-propanamine, 10,11-dihydro-*N*-methyl-, monohydrochloride.

Inactive Ingredients

The following inactive ingredients are contained in all dosage strengths: acacia, calcium carbonate, corn starch, D&C Red No. 30 and D&C Yellow No. 10 (except 10 mg and 150 mg), FD&C Blue No. 1 (except 50 mg, 75 mg, and 100 mg), hydrogenated soy oil, iron oxide, light mineral oil, magnesium stearate, mannitol, polyethylene glycol 8000, pregelatinized corn starch, sodium benzoate (except 150 mg), sucrose, talc, titanium dioxide, and other ingredients.

CLINICAL PHARMACOLOGY

Mechanism of Action

Available evidence suggests that many depressions have a biochemical basis in the form of a relative deficiency of neurotransmitters such as norepinephrine and serotonin. Norepinephrine deficiency may be associated with relatively low urinary 3-methoxy-4-hydroxyphenyl glycol (MHPG) levels, while serotonin deficiencies may be associated with low spinal fluid levels of 5-hydroxyindoleacetic acid.

While the precise mechanism of action of the tricyclic antidepressants is unknown, a leading theory suggests that they restore normal levels of neurotransmitters by blocking the re-uptake of these substances from the synapse in the central nervous system. Evidence indicates that the secondary amine tricyclic antidepressants, including NORPRAMIN, may have greater activity in blocking the re-uptake of norepinephrine. Tertiary amine tricyclic antidepressants, such as amitriptyline, may have greater effect on serotonin re-uptake.

NORPRAMIN (desipramine hydrochloride) is not a monoamine oxidase (MAO) inhibitor and does not act primarily as a central nervous system stimulant. It has been found in some studies to have a more rapid onset of action than imipramine. Earliest therapeutic effects may occasionally be seen in 2 to 5 days, but full treatment benefit usually requires 2 to 3 weeks to obtain.

Metabolism

Tricyclic antidepressants, such as desipramine hydrochloride, are rapidly absorbed from the gastrointestinal tract. Tricyclic antidepressants or their metabolites are to some extent excreted through the gastric mucosa and reabsorbed from the gastrointestinal tract. Desipramine is metabolized in the liver, and approximately 70% is excreted in the urine.

The rate of metabolism of tricyclic antidepressants varies widely from individual to individual, chiefly on a genetically determined basis. Up to a 36-fold difference in plasma level may be noted among individuals taking the same oral dose of desipramine. The ratio of 2-hydroxydesipramine to desipramine may be increased in the elderly, most likely due to decreased renal elimination with aging.

Certain drugs, particularly the psychostimulants and the phenothiazines, increase plasma levels of concomitantly administered tricyclic antidepressants through competition for the same metabolic enzyme systems. Concurrent administration of cimetidine and tricyclic antidepressants can produce clinically significant increases in the plasma concentrations of the tricyclic antidepressants. Conversely, decreases in plasma levels of the tricyclic antidepressants have been reported upon discontinuation of cimetidine, which may result in the loss of the therapeutic efficacy of the tricyclic antidepressant. Other substances, particularly barbiturates and alcohol, induce liver enzyme activity and thereby reduce tricyclic antidepressant plasma levels. Similar effects have been reported with tobacco smoke.

Research on the relationship of plasma level to therapeutic response with the tricyclic antidepressants has produced conflicting results. While some studies report no correlation, many studies cite therapeutic levels for most tricyclics in the range of 50 to 300 nanograms per milliliter. The therapeutic range is different for each tricyclic antidepressant. For desipramine, an optimal range of therapeutic plasma levels has not been established.

INDICATIONS AND USAGE

NORPRAMIN (desipramine hydrochloride) is indicated for the treatment of depression.

CONTRAINDICATIONS

Desipramine hydrochloride should not be given in conjunction with, or within 2 weeks of, treatment with an MAO inhibitor drug; hyperpyretic crises, severe convulsions, and death have occurred in patients taking MAO inhibitors and tricyclic antidepressants. When NORPRAMIN (desipramie hydrochloride) is substituted for an MAO inhibitor, at least 2 weeks should elapse between treatments. NORPRAMIN should then be started cautiously and should be increased gradually.

The drug is contraindicated in the acute recovery period following myocardial infarction. It should not be used in those who have shown prior hypersensitivity to the drug. Cross-sensitivity between this and other dibenzazepines is a possibility.

WARNINGS

Extreme caution should be used when this drug is given in the following situations:

a. In patients with cardiovascular disease, because of the possibility of conduction defects, arrhythmias, tachycardias, strokes, and acute myocardial infarction.
b. In patients with a history of urinary retention or glaucoma, because of the anticholinergic properties of the drug.
c. In patients with thyroid disease or those taking thyroid medication, because of the possibility of cardiovascular toxicity, including arrhythmias.
d. In patients with a history of seizure disorder, because this drug has been shown to lower the seizure threshold.

This drug is capable of blocking the antihypertensive effect of guanethidine and similarly acting compounds.

The patient should be cautioned that this drug may impair the mental and/or physical abilities required for the performance of potentially hazardous tasks such as driving a car or operating machinery.

In patients who may use alcohol excessively, it should be borne in mind that the potentiation may increase the danger inherent in any suicide attempt or overdosage.

Use in Pregnancy

Safe use of desipramine hydrochloride during pregnancy and lactation has not been established; therefore, if it is to be given to pregnant patients, nursing mothers, or women of childbearing potential, the possible benefits must be weighed against the possible hazards to mother and child. Animal reproductive studies have been inconclusive.

Use in Children

NORPRAMIN (desipramine hydrochloride) is not recommended for use in children since safety and effectiveness in the pediatric age group have not been established. (See ADVERSE REACTIONS, Cardiovascular.)

Geriatric Use

Clinical studies of NORPRAMIN did not include sufficient numbers of subjects aged 65 and over to determine whether they respond differently from younger subjects. Other reported clinical experience has not identified differences in responses between the elderly and younger patients. Lower doses are recommended for elderly patients. (See DOSAGE AND ADMINISTRATION.)

The ratio of 2-hydroxydesipramine to desipramine may be increased in the elderly, most likely due to decreased renal elimination with aging.

This drug is known to be substantially excreted by the kidney, and the risk of toxic reactions to this drug may be greater in patients with impaired renal function. Because elderly patients are more likely to have decreased renal function, care should be taken in dose selection, and it may be useful to monitor renal function.

NORPRAMIN use in the elderly has been associated with a proneness to falling as well as confusional states. (See ADVERSE REACTIONS.)

PRECAUTIONS

General

It is important that this drug be dispensed in the least possible quantities to depressed outpatients, since suicide has been accomplished with this class of drug. Ordinary prudence requires that children not have access to this drug or to potent drugs of any kind; if possible, this drug should be dispensed in containers with child-resistant safety closures. Storage of this drug in the home must be supervised responsibly.

If serious adverse effects occur, dosage should be reduced or treatment should be altered.

NORPRAMIN (desipramine hydrochloride) therapy in patients with manic-depressive illness may induce a hypomanic state after the depressive phase terminates.

The drug may cause exacerbation of psychosis in schizophrenic patients.

Both elevation and lowering of blood sugar levels have been reported.

Leukocyte and differential counts should be performed in any patient who develops fever and sore throat during therapy; the drug should be discontinued if there is evidence of pathologic neutrophil depression.

Clinical experience in the concurrent administration of ECT and antidepressant drugs is limited. Thus, if such treatment is essential, the possibility of increased risk relative to benefits should be considered.

This drug should be discontinued as soon as possible prior to elective surgery because of possible cardiovascular effects. Hypertensive episodes have been observed during surgery in patients taking desipramine hydrochloride.

Drug Interactions

Drugs Metabolized by P450 2D6. The biochemical activity of the drug metabolizing isozyme cytochrome P450 2D6 (debrisoquin hydroxylase) is reduced in a subset of the Caucasian population (about 7% to 10% of Caucasians are so called "poor metabolizers"); reliable estimates of the prevalence of reduced P450 2D6 isozyme activity among Asian, African and other populations are not yet available. Poor metabolizers have higher than expected plasma concentrations of tricyclic antidepressants (TCAs) when given usual doses. Depending on the fraction of drug metabolized by P450 2D6, the increase in plasma concentration may be small, or quite large (8 fold increase in plasma AUC of the TCA).

In addition, certain drugs inhibit the activity of this isozyme and make normal metabolizers resemble poor metabolizers. An individual who is stable on a given dose of TCA may become abruptly toxic when given one of these inhibiting

Continued on next page

Norpramin—Cont.

drugs as concomitant therapy. The drugs that inhibit cytochrome P450 2D6 include some that are not metabolized by the enzyme (quinidine; cimetidine) and many that are substrates for P450 2D6 (many other antidepressants, phenothiazines, and the Type IC antiarrhythmics propafenone and flecainide). While all the selective serotonin reuptake inhibitors (SSRIs), e.g., fluoxetine, sertraline, paroxetine, inhibit P450 2D6, they may vary in the extent of inhibition. The extent to which SSRI TCA interactions may pose clinical problems will depend on the degree of inhibition and the pharmacokinetics of the SSRI involved. Nevertheless, caution is indicated in the co-administration of TCAs with any of the SSRIs and also in switching from one class to the other. Of particular importance, sufficient time must elapse before initiating TCA treatment in a patient being withdrawn from fluoxetine, given the long half-life of the parent and active metabolite (at least 5 weeks may be necessary). Concomitant use of tricyclic antidepressants with drugs that can inhibit cytochrome P450 2D6 may require lower doses than usually prescribed for either the tricyclic antidepressant or the other drug. Furthermore, whenever one of these other drugs is withdrawn from co-therapy, an increased dose of tricyclic antidepressant may be required. It is desirable to monitor TCA plasma levels whenever a TCA is going to be co-administered with another drug known to be an inhibitor of P450 2D6.

Close supervision and careful adjustment of dosage are required when this drug is given concomitantly with anticholinergic or sympathomimetic drugs.

Patients should be warned that while taking this drug their response to alcoholic beverages may be exaggerated.

If NORPRAMIN (desipramine hydrochloride) is to be combined with other psychotropic agents such as tranquilizers or sedative/hypnotics, careful consideration should be given to the pharmacology of the agents employed since the sedative effects of NORPRAMIN and benzodiazepines (e.g., chlordiazepoxide or diazepam) are additive. Both the sedative and anticholinergic effects of the major tranquilizers are also additive to those of NORPRAMIN.

ADVERSE REACTIONS

Included in the following listing are a few adverse reactions that have not been reported with this specific drug. However, the pharmacologic similarities among the tricyclic antidepressant drugs require that each of the reactions be considered when NORPRAMIN (desipramine hydrochloride) is given.

Cardiovascular: hypotension, hypertension, palpitations, heart block, myocardial infarction, stroke, arrhythmias, premature ventricular contractions, tachycardia, ventricular tachycardia, ventricular fibrillation, sudden death

There has been a report of an "acute collapse" and "sudden death" in an 8-year-old (18 kg) male, treated for 2 years for hyperactivity.

There have been additional reports of sudden death in children. (See WARNINGS, Use in Children.)

Psychiatric: confusional states (especially in the elderly) with hallucinations, disorientation, delusions; anxiety, restlessness, agitation; insomnia and nightmares; hypomania; exacerbation of psychosis

Neurologic: numbness, tingling, paresthesias of extremities; incoordination, ataxia, tremors; peripheral neuropathy; extrapyramidal symptoms; seizures; alterations in EEG patterns; tinnitus

Symptoms attributed to Neuroleptic Malignant Syndrome have been reported during desipramine use with and without concomitant neuroleptic therapy.

Anticholinergic: dry mouth, and rarely associated sublingual adenitis; blurred vision, disturbance of accommodation, mydriasis, increased intraocular pressure; constipation, paralytic ileus; urinary retention, delayed micturition, dilation of urinary tract

Allergic: skin rash, petechiae, urticaria, itching, photosensitization (avoid excessive exposure to sunlight), edema (of face and tongue or general), drug fever, cross-sensitivity with other tricyclic drugs

Hematologic: bone marrow depressions including agranulocytosis, eosinophilia, purpura, thrombocytopenia

Gastrointestinal: anorexia, nausea and vomiting, epigastric distress, peculiar taste, abdominal cramps, diarrhea, stomatitis, black tongue, hepatitis, jaundice (simulating obstructive), altered liver function, elevated liver function tests, increased pancreatic enzymes

Endocrine: gynecomastia in the male, breast enlargement and galactorrhea in the female; increased or decreased libido, impotence, painful ejaculation, testicular swelling; elevation or depression of blood sugar levels; syndrome of inappropriate antidiuretic hormone secretion (SIADH)

Other: weight gain or loss; perspiration, flushing; urinary frequency, nocturia; parotid swelling; drowsiness, dizziness, weakness and fatigue, headache; fever; alopecia; elevated alkaline phosphatase

Withdrawal Symptoms: Though not indicative of addiction, abrupt cessation of treatment after prolonged therapy may produce nausea, headache, and malaise.

OVERDOSAGE*

Deaths may occur from overdosage with this class of drugs. Multiple drug ingestion (including alcohol) is common in deliberate tricyclic antidepressant overdose. As the management is complex and changing, it is recommended that the physician contact a poison control center for current information on treatment. Signs and symptoms of toxicity develop rapidly after tricyclic antidepressant overdose; therefore, hospital monitoring is required as soon as possible. There is no specific antidote for desipramine overdosage.

Oral LD_{50}

The oral LD_{50} of desipramine is 290 mg/kg in male mice and 320 mg/kg in female rats.

Manifestations of Overdosage

Critical manifestations of overdose include: cardiac dysrhythmias, severe hypotension, convulsions, and CNS depression, including coma. Changes in the electrocardiogram, particularly in QRS axis or width, are clinically significant indicators of tricyclic antidepressant toxicity.

Other signs of overdose may include: confusion, disturbed concentration, transient visual hallucinations, dilated pupils, agitation, hyperactive reflexes, stupor, drowsiness, muscle rigidity, vomiting, hypothermia, hyperpyrexia, or any of the symptoms listed under ADVERSE REACTIONS.

Management

Aggressive supportive care and serum alkalinization are the mainstays of therapy.

General. Obtain an ECG and immediately initiate cardiac monitoring. Protect the patient's airway, establish an intravenous line, and initiate gastric decontamination. A minimum of 6 hours of observation with cardiac monitoring and observation for signs of CNS or respiratory depression, hypotension, cardiac dysrhythmias and/or conduction blocks, and seizures is necessary. If signs of toxicity occur at any time during this period, extended monitoring is required. Follow ECG, renal function, CPK, and arterial blood gasses as clinically indicated. There are case reports of patients succumbing to fatal dysrhythmias late after overdose; these patients had clinical evidence of significant poisoning prior to death, and most received inadequate gastrointestinal decontamination. Monitoring of plasma drug levels should not guide management of the patient.

Gastrointestinal Decontamination. All patients suspected of tricyclic antidepressant overdose should receive gastrointestinal decontamination. This should include large volume gastric lavage followed by activated charcoal. If consciousness is impaired, the airway should be secured prior to lavage. Emesis is contraindicated.

Cardiovascular. A maximal limb-lead QRS duration of ≥0.10 seconds may be the best indication of the severity of the overdose. Serum alkalinization, to a pH of 7.45 to 7.55, using intravenous sodium bicarbonate and hyperventilation (as needed) should be instituted for patients with dysrhythmias and/or QRS widening. A pH >7.60 or a pCO_2 <20mm Hg is undesirable. Dysrhythmias unresponsive to sodium bicarbonate therapy/hyperventilation may respond to lidocaine, bretylium or phenytoin. Type IA and IC antiarrhythmics are generally contraindicated (eg, quinidine, disopyramide, and procainamide).

In rare instances, hemoperfusion may be beneficial in acute refractory cardiovascular instability in patients with acute toxicity. However, hemodialysis, peritoneal dialysis, exchange transfusions, and forced diuresis generally have been reported as ineffective in tricyclic antidepressant poisoning.

CNS. In patients with CNS depression, early intubation is advised because of the potential for abrupt deterioration. Seizures should be controlled with benzodiazepines. If these are ineffective or seizures recur, other anticonvulsants (eg, phenobarbital, phenytoin) may be used. Physostigmine is not recommended except to treat life-threatening symptoms that have been unresponsive to other therapies, and then only in consultation with a poison control center.

Psychiatric Follow-up. Since overdosage is often deliberate, patients may attempt suicide by other means during the recovery phase. Psychiatric referral may be appropriate.

Pediatric Management. The principles of management of child and adult overdosages are similar. It is strongly recommended that the physician contact the local poison control center for specific pediatric treatment.

* Poisindex®: Toxicologic Management
Topic: Antidepressants, Tricyclic
Micromedex Inc. Vol. 85

DOSAGE AND ADMINISTRATION

Not recommended for use in children (see WARNINGS).

Lower dosages are recommended for elderly patients and adolescents. Lower dosages are also recommended for outpatients compared to hospitalized patients, who are closely supervised. Dosage should be initiated at a low level and increased according to clinical response and any evidence of intolerance. Following remission, maintenance medication may be required for a period of time and should be at the lowest dose that will maintain remission.

Usual Adult Dose

The usual adult dose is 100 to 200 mg per day. In more severely ill patients, dosage may be further increased gradually to 300 mg/day if necessary. Dosages above 300 mg/day are not recommended.

Dosage should be initiated at a lower level and increased according to tolerance and clinical response.

Treatment of patients requiring as much as 300 mg should generally be initiated in hospitals, where regular visits by the physician, skilled nursing care, and frequent electrocardiograms (ECGs) are available.

The best available evidence of impending toxicity from very high doses of NORPRAMIN is prolongation of the QRS or QT intervals on the ECG. Prolongation of the PR interval is also significant, but less closely correlated with plasma levels. Clinical symptoms of intolerance, especially drowsiness, dizziness, and postural hypotension, should also alert the physician to the need for reduction in dosage. Plasma desipramine measurement would constitute the optimal guide to dosage monitoring.

Initial therapy may be administered in divided doses or a single daily dose.

Maintenance therapy may be given on a once-daily schedule for patient convenience and compliance.

Adolescent and Geriatric Dose

The usual adolescent and geriatric dose is 25 to 100 mg daily.

Dosage should be initiated at a lower level and increased according to tolerance and clinical response to a usual maximum of 100 mg daily. In more severely ill patients, dosage may be further increased to 150 mg/day. Doses above 150 mg/day are not recommended in these age groups.

Initial therapy may be administered in divided doses or a single daily dose.

Maintenance therapy may be given on a once-daily schedule for patient convenience and compliance.

HOW SUPPLIED

10 mg blue coated tablets imprinted 68-7
NDC 0068-0007-01: bottles of 100

25 mg yellow coated tablets imprinted NORPRAMIN 25
NDC 0068-0011-01: bottles of 100

50 mg green coated tablets imprinted NORPRAMIN 50
NDC 0068-0015-01: bottles of 100

75 mg orange coated tablets imprinted NORPRAMIN 75
NDC 0068-0019-01: bottles of 100

100 mg peach coated tablets imprinted NORPRAMIN 100
NDC 0068-0020-01: bottles of 100

150 mg white coated tablets imprinted NORPRAMIN 150
NDC 0068-0021-50: bottles of 50

NORPRAMIN tablets should be stored at room temperature, preferably below 86°F (30°C). Protect from excessive heat. Dispense in tight container.

Rx only

Prescribing Information as of February 2003

Mfd by:
Patheon Pharmaceuticals Inc.
Cincinnati, OH 45215 USA
Mfd for:
Merrell Pharmaceuticals Inc.
An Aventis Pharmaceuticals Company
Kansas City, MO 64137 USA
www.aventis-us.com
50058407

Shown in Product Identification Guide, page 307

PRIFTIN® ℞

[*prĭf-tĭn*]
(rifapentine)
150 mg Tablets

Prescribing information as of February 2003

DESCRIPTION

PRIFTIN® (rifapentine) for oral administration contains 150 mg of the active ingredient rifapentine per tablet.

The 150 mg tablets also contain, as inactive ingredients: calcium stearate, disodium EDTA, FD&C Blue No. 2 aluminum lake, hydroxypropyl cellulose, hypromellose USP, microcrystalline cellulose, polyethylene glycol, pregelatinized starch, propylene glycol, sodium ascorbate, sodium lauryl sulfate, sodium starch glycolate, synthetic red iron oxide, and titanium dioxide.

Rifapentine is a rifamycin derivative antibiotic and has a similar profile of microbiological activity to rifampin (rifampicin). The molecular weight is 877.04.

The molecular formula is $C_{47}H_{64}N_4O_{12}$.

The chemical name for rifapentine is rifamycin, 3-[[(4-cyclopentyl-1-piperazinyl)imino]methyl]- or 3-[N-(4-Cyclopentyl-1-piperazinyl)formimidoyl] rifamycin or 5,6,9,17,19,21-hexahydroxy-23-methoxy-2,4,12,16,18,20, 22-heptamethyl-8-[N-(4-cyclopentyl-l-piperazinyl)-formimidoyl]-2,7-(epoxypenta-deca[1,11,13]trienimino)naphtho [2,1-b]furan-1,11-(2H)-dione 21-acetate. It has the following structure:

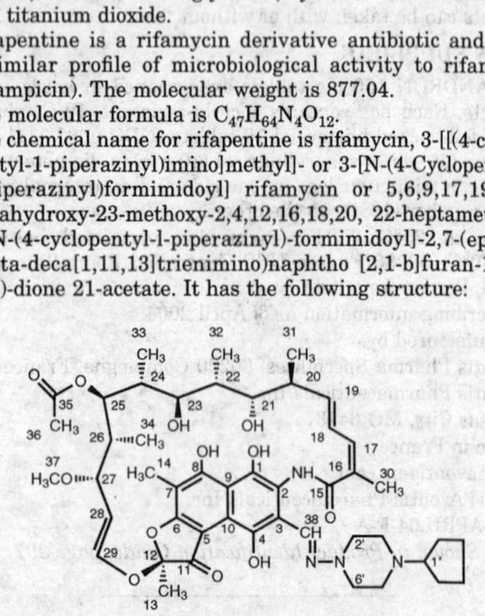

ACTIONS/CLINICAL PHARMACOLOGY

Pharmacokinetics

Absorption

The absolute bioavailability of rifapentine has not been determined. The relative bioavailability (with an oral solution as a reference) of rifapentine after a single 600 mg dose to healthy adult volunteers was 70%. The maximum concentrations were achieved from 5 to 6 hours after administration of the 600 mg rifapentine dose. Food (850 total calories: 33 g protein, 55 g fat and 58 g carbohydrate) increased

AUC(0-∞) and C_{max} by 43% and 44%, respectively over that observed when administered under fasting conditions. When oral doses of rifapentine were administered once daily or once every 72 hours to healthy volunteers for 10 days, single dose AUC(0-∞) value of rifapentine was similar to its steady-state AUC_{ss} (0–24h) or AUC_{ss} (0–72h) values, suggesting no significant auto-induction effect on steady-state pharmacokinetics of rifapentine. Steady-state conditions were achieved by day 10 following daily administration of rifapentine 600 mg. The pharmacokinetic characteristics of rifapentine and 25-desacetyl rifapentine (active metabolite) on day 10 following oral administration of 600 mg rifapentine every 72 hours to healthy volunteers are contained in the following table.

Table 1. Pharmacokinetics and rifapentine and 25-desacetyl rifapentine in healthy volunteers

Parameter	Rifapentine	25-desacetyl Rifapentine
	Mean ± SD (n=12)	
C_{max} (μg/mL)	15.05 ± 4.62	6.26 ± 2.06
AUC (0–72h)(μg*h/mL)	319.54 ± 91.52	215.88 ± 85.96
$T_{½}$(h)	13.19 ± 1.38	13.35 ± 2.67
T_{max} (h)	4.83 ± 1.80	11.25 ± 2.73
Clpo (L/h)	2.03 ± 0.60	–

Distribution

In a population pharmacokinetic analysis in 351 tuberculosis patients who received 600 mg rifapentine in combination with isoniazid, pyrazinamide and ethambutol, the estimated apparent volume of distribution was 70.2 ± 9.1 L. In healthy volunteers, rifapentine and 25-desacetyl rifapentine were 97.7% and 93.2% bound to plasma proteins, respectively. Rifapentine was mainly bound to albumin. Similar extent of protein binding was observed in healthy volunteers, asymptomatic HIV-infected subjects and hepatically impaired subjects.

Metabolism/Excretion

Following a single 600 mg oral dose of radiolabelled rifapentine to healthy volunteers (n=4), 87% of the total ^{14}C rifapentine was recovered in the urine (17%) and feces (70%). Greater than 80% of the total ^{14}C rifapentine dose was excreted from the body within 7 days. Rifapentine was hydrolyzed by an esterase enzyme to form a microbiologically active 25-desacetyl rifapentine. Rifapentine and 25-desacetyl rifapentine accounted for 99% of the total radioactivity in plasma. Plasma AUC (0-∞) and C_{max} values of the 25-desacetyl rifapentine metabolite were one-half and one-third those of the rifapentine, respectively. Based upon relative in vitro activities and AUC(0-∞) values, rifapentine and 25-desacetyl rifapentine potentially contributes 62% and 38% to the clinical activities against *M. tuberculosis*, respectively.

Special Populations

Gender: In a population pharmacokinetics analysis of sparse blood samples obtained from 351 tuberculosis patients who received 600 mg rifapentine in combination with isoniazid, pyrazinamide and ethambutol, the estimated apparent oral clearance of rifapentine for males and females was 2.51 ± 0.14 L/h and 1.69 ± 0.41 L/h, respectively. The clinical significance of the difference in the estimated apparent oral clearance is not known.

Elderly: Following oral administration of a single 600 mg dose of rifapentine to elderly (≥65 years) male healthy volunteers (n=14), the pharmacokinetics of rifapentine and 25-desacetyl metabolite were similar to that observed for young (18 to 45 years) healthy male volunteers (n=20).

Pediatric (Adolescents): In a pharmacokinetics study of rifapentine in healthy adolescents (age 12 to 15), 600 mg rifapentine was administered to those weighing ≥45 kg (n=10) and 450 mg was administered to those weighing <45 kg (n=2). The pharmacokinetics of rifapentine were similar to those observed in healthy adults.

Renal Impaired Patients: The pharmacokinetics of rifapentine have not been evaluated in renal impaired patients. Although only about 17% of an administered dose is excreted via the kidneys, the clinical significance of impaired renal function on the disposition of rifapentine and its 25-desacetyl metabolite is not known.

Hepatic Impaired Patients: Following oral administration of a single 600 mg dose of rifapentine to mild to severe hepatic impaired patients (n=15), the pharmacokinetics of rifapentine and 25-desacetyl metabolite were similar in patients with various degrees of hepatic impairment and to that observed in another study for healthy volunteers (n=12). Since the elimination of these agents are primarily via the liver, the clinical significance of impaired hepatic function on the disposition of rifapentine and its 25-desacetyl metabolite is not known.

Asymptomatic HIV-Infected Volunteers: Following oral administration of a single 600 mg dose of rifapentine to asymptomatic HIV-infected volunteers (n=15) under fasting conditions, mean C_{max} and AUC(0-∞) of rifapentine were lower (20–32%) than that observed in other studies in healthy volunteers (n=55). In a cross-study comparison, mean C_{max} and AUC values of the 25-desacetyl metabolite of rifapentine, when compared to healthy volunteers were higher (6–21%) in one study (n=20), but lower (15–16%) in a different study (n=40). The clinical significance of this observation is not known. Food (850 total calories: 33 g protein, 55 g fat, and 58 g carbohydrate) increases the mean AUC and C_{max} of rifapentine observed under fasting conditions in asymptomatic HIV-infected volunteers by about 51% and 53%, respectively.

Table 2-1. Dose of Rifapentine, Rifampin, Isoniazid, Pyrazinamide, and Ethambutol

Rifapentine Combination Treatment				
Intensive Phase	*Rifapentine (mg)*	*Isoniazid (mg)*	*Pyrazinamide (mg)*	*Ethambutol* (mg)*
	Twice Weekly	*Daily*	*Daily*	*Daily*
Patient Weight				
<50 kg	600	300	1500	800
≥50 kg	600	300	2000	1200
Continuation Phase	*Rifapentine (mg)*	*Isoniazid (mg)*		
	Once Weekly	*Once Weekly*		
Patient Weight				
<50 kg	600	600		
≥50 kg	600	900		
Rifampin Combination Treatment				
Intensive Phase	*Rifampin (mg)*	*Isoniazid (mg)*	*Pyrazinamide (mg)*	*Ethambutol (mg)*
	Daily	*Daily*	*Daily*	*Daily*
Patient Weight				
<50 kg	450	300	1500	800
≥50 kg	600	300	2000	1200
Continuation Phase	*Rifampin (mg)*	*Isoniazid (mg)*		
	Twice Weekly	*Twice Weekly*		
Patient Weight				
<50 kg	450	600		
≥50 kg	600	900		

*Ethambutol was to be discontinued once baseline susceptibility test results were available

Table 2-2. Clinical Outcome in Study 008*

	Rifapentine Combination	Rifampin Combination
Status of End of Treatment		
Converted	87% (248/286)	80% (226/283)
Not Converted	1% (4/286)	3% (8/283)
Lost to Follow-up	12% (34/286)	17% (49/283)
Status Through 24 Month Follow-up:		
Relapsed	12% (29/248)	7% (15/226)
Sputum Negative	57% (142/248)	64% (145/226)
Lost to Follow-up	31% (77/248)	29% (66/226)

*All data for patients with confirmed susceptible MTB (rifapentine combination, n=286; rifampin combination, n=283).

Microbiology

Mechanism of Action

Rifapentine, a cyclopentyl rifamycin, inhibits DNA-dependent RNA polymerase in susceptible strains of *Mycobacterium tuberculosis* but not in mammalian cells. At therapeutic levels, rifapentine exhibits bactericidal activity against both intracellular and extracellular *M. tuberculosis* organisms. Both rifapentine and the 25-desacetyl metabolite accumulate in human monocyte-derived macrophages with intracellular/extracellular ratios of approximately 24:1 and 7:1, respectively.

Resistance Development

In the treatment of tuberculosis (see INDICATIONS AND USAGE), a small number of resistant cells present within large populations of susceptible cells can rapidly become predominant. Rifapentine resistance development in *M. tuberculosis* strains is principally due to one of several single point mutations that occur in the rpoB portion of the gene coding for the beta subunit of the DNA-dependent RNA polymerase. The incidence of rifapentine resistant mutants in an otherwise susceptible population of *M. tuberculosis* strains is approximately one in 10^7 to 10^8 bacilli. Due to the potential for resistance development to rifapentine, appropriate susceptibility tests should be performed in the event of persistently positive cultures.

M. tuberculosis organisms resistant to other rifamycins are likely to be resistant to rifapentine. A high level of cross-resistance between rifampin and rifapentine has been demonstrated with *M. tuberculosis* strains. Cross-resistance does not appear between rifapentine and non-rifamycin antimycobacterial agents such as isoniazid and streptomycin.

In Vitro Activity of Rifapentine against *M. tuberculosis*

Rifapentine and its 25-desacetyl metabolite have demonstrated in vitro activity against rifamycin-susceptible strains of *Mycobacterium tuberculosis* including cidal activity against phagocytized *M. tuberculosis* organisms grown in activated human macrophages.

In vitro results indicate that rifapentine MIC values for *M. tuberculosis* organisms are influenced by study conditions. Rifapentine MIC values were substantially increased employing egg-based medium compared to liquid or agar-based solid media. The addition of Tween 80 in these assays has been shown to lower MIC values for rifamycin compounds.

In mouse infection studies a therapeutic effect, in terms of enhanced survival time or reduction of organ bioburden, has been observed in *M. tuberculosis*-infected animals treated with various intermittent rifapentine-containing regimens. Animal studies have shown that the activity of rifapentine is influenced by dose and frequency of administration.

Susceptibility testing for *Mycobacterium tuberculosis*

Breakpoints to determine whether clinical isolates of *M. tuberculosis* are susceptible or resistant to rifapentine have not been established. The clinical relevance of rifapentine in vitro susceptibility test results for other mycobacterial species has not been determined.

CLINICAL TRIALS

A total of 722 patients were enrolled in Clinical Study 008, an open label, prospective, randomized, parallel group, active controlled trial, for the treatment of pulmonary tuberculosis. This population was mostly comprised of Black (>60%) or Multiracial (>31%) patients and the mean ± standard deviation age was 37 ± 11 years. Treatment groups were comparable with respect to age and race. The percentage of male patients was higher in the rifapentine combination group (80%) than in the rifampin combination group (73%). The study was divided into two phases on the basis of dosing frequency. For the first phase, designated as the Intensive Phase, 361 patients were randomized to receive rifapentine, isoniazid, pyrazinamide, and ethambutol for 60 days and 361 patients were randomized to receive rifampin, isoniazid, pyrazinamide, and ethambutol for 60 days. (Ethambutol was to be discontinued once baseline susceptibility test results were available.) Rifapentine and isoniazid were each administered at a fixed dose regardless of body weight. Rifampin, pyrazinamide, and ethambutol were administered based on body weight according to Table 2-1. **Note:** All drugs were administered ***daily*** in the Intensive Phase **except for rifapentine** which was administered twice weekly. During the second phase, designated as the Continuation Phase, 321 patients who had received rifapentine in the Intensive Phase continued to receive rifapentine and isoniazid once weekly for up to 120 days. Three hundred seven patients who had received rifampin in the Intensive Phase continued to receive rifampin and isoniazid during the Continuation Phase twice weekly for up to 120 days. Rifampin and isoniazid were administered based on body weight according to Table 2-1.

Continued on next page

Priftin—Cont.

Patients in either treatment group were scheduled to receive study drug over a 180-day period with a subsequent 24-month follow-up. Additionally, both treatment groups received pyridoxine (Vitamin B_6) over the 180-day treatment period.

[See table 2-1 at top of previous page]

Table 2-2 presents clinical outcome in Study 008.

[See table 2-2 on previous page]

Risk of relapse was higher in the rifapentine regimen. During the Intensive Phase of treatment the rate of noncompliance with companion medications was somewhat higher for the rifapentine regimen than for the rifampin regimen. Most of the relapses occurred among those with poor compliance with these companion medications and this group also had the largest risk of relapse for the rifapentine regimen relative to the rifampin regimen. This factor appears to explain most, but not all, of the higher relapse rate observed in the rifapentine arm. Failure to convert sputum after two months of treatment (ie, end of Intensive Phase) was associated with a greater risk of relapse for both treatment regimens. Relapse rates were also higher for males in both regimens. Relapse in the rifapentine group was not associated with development of mono-resistance to rifampin.

In vitro susceptibility testing was conducted against *M. tuberculosis* isolates recovered from 620 patients enrolled in the study. Rifapentine and rifampin MIC values were determined employing the radiometric susceptibility testing method utilizing 7H12 broth at pH 6.8 (NCCLS procedure M24-T). Six hundred and twelve patients had *M. tuberculosis* isolates that were susceptible to rifampin (MIC < 0.5 µg/ml). Of these patients, six hundred and ten had *M. tuberculosis* isolates (99.7%) with rifapentine MICs of < 0.125 µg/ml. The other two patients that had rifampin susceptible *M. tuberculosis* isolates had rifapentine MICs of 0.25 µg/ml. The remaining eight patients had *M. tuberculosis* isolates that were resistant to rifampin (MIC > 8.0 µg/ml). These *M. tuberculosis* isolates had rifapentine MICs of > 8.0 µg/ml. In this study high rifampin and rifapentine MICs were associated with multi-drug resistant *M. tuberculosis* (MDRTB) isolates. Rifamycin mono-resistance was not observed in either treatment arm. This information is provided for comparative purposes only as rifapentine breakpoints have not been established.

INDICATIONS AND USAGE

PRIFTIN is indicated for the treatment of pulmonary tuberculosis. PRIFTIN must always be used in conjunction with at least one other antituberculosis drug to which the isolate is susceptible. In the intensive phase of the short-course treatment of pulmonary tuberculosis, **PRIFTIN should be administered twice weekly for two months,** with an interval of no less than 3 days (72 hours) between doses, as part of an appropriate regimen which includes daily companion drugs (Table 2-1). It may also be necessary to add either streptomycin or ethambutol until the results of susceptibility testing are known. ***Compliance with all drugs in the Intensive Phase (ie, PRIFTIN, isoniazid, pyrazinamide, ethambutol or streptomycin) is imperative to assure early sputum conversion and protection against relapse.*** Following the intensive phase, Continuation Phase treatment should be continued with PRIFTIN for 4 months. **During this phase, PRIFTIN should be administered on a once-weekly basis** in combination with an appropriate antituberculous agent for susceptible organisms (Table 2-1) (see DOSAGE AND ADMINISTRATION section).

In the treatment of tuberculosis, the small number of resistant cells present within large populations of susceptible cells can rapidly become the predominant type. Consequently, clinical samples for mycobacterial culture and susceptibility testing should be obtained prior to the initiation of therapy, as well as during treatment to monitor therapeutic response. The susceptibility of *M. tuberculosis* organisms to isoniazid, rifampin, pyrazinamide, ethambutol, rifapentine and other appropriate agents should be measured. If test results show resistance to any of these drugs and the patient is not responding to therapy, the drug regimen should be modified.

CONTRAINDICATIONS

This product is contraindicated in patients with a history of hypersensitivity to any of the rifamycins (eg, rifampin and rifabutin).

WARNINGS

Poor compliance with the dosage regimen, particularly the daily administered non-rifamycin drugs in the Intensive Phase, was associated with late sputum conversion and a high relapse rate in the rifapentine arm of Clinical Study 008. Therefore, compliance with the full course of therapy must be emphasized, and the importance of not missing any doses must be stressed. (See PRECAUTIONS and DOSAGE AND ADMINISTRATION.)

Since antituberculous multidrug treatments, including the rifamycin class, are associated with serious hepatic events, patients with abnormal liver tests and/or liver disease should only be given rifapentine in cases of necessity and then with caution and under strict medical supervision. In these patients, careful monitoring of liver tests (especially serum transaminases) should be carried out prior to therapy and then every 2 to 4 weeks during therapy. If signs of liver disease occur or worsen, rifapentine should be discontinued. Hepatotoxicity of other antituberculosis drugs (eg, isoniazid, pyrazinamide) used in combination with rifapentine should also be taken into account.

Hyperbilirubinemia resulting from competition for excretory pathways between rifapentine and bilirubin cannot be excluded since competition between the related drug rifampin and bilirubin can occur. An isolated report showing a moderate rise in bilirubin and/or transaminase level is not in itself an indication for interrupting treatment; rather, the decision should be made after repeating the tests, noting trends in the levels and considering them in conjunction with the patient's clinical condition.

Pseudomembranous colitis has been reported to occur with various antibiotics, including other rifamycins. Diarrhea, particularly if severe and/or persistent, occurring during treatment or in the initial weeks following treatment may be symptomatic of *Clostridium difficile*-associated disease, the most severe form of which is pseudomembranous colitis. If pseudomembranous colitis is suspected, rifapentine should be stopped immediately and the patient should be treated with supportive and specific treatment without delay (eg, oral vancomycin). Products inhibiting peristalsis are contraindicated in this clinical situation.

Experience in HIV-infected patients is limited. In an ongoing CDC TB trial, five out of 30 HIV-infected patients randomized to once weekly rifapentine (plus INH) in the Continuation Phase who completed treatment, relapsed. Four of these patients developed rifampin mono-resistant (RMR) TB. Each RMR patient had late-stage HIV infection, low CD4 counts and extrapulmonary disease, and documented co-administration of antifungal azoles (See Reference 1). These findings are consistent with the literature in which an emergence of RMR TB in HIV-infected TB patients has been reported in recent years. Further study in this subpopulation is warranted. As with other antituberculous treatments, when rifapentine is used in HIV-infected patients, a more aggressive regimen should be employed (eg, more frequent dosing). Based on results to date of the CDC trial (see above), once weekly dosing during the Continuation Phase of treatment is not recommended at this time.

Because rifapentine has been shown to increase indinavir metabolism (see DRUG INTERACTIONS), it should be used with extreme caution, if at all, in patients who are also taking protease inhibitors.

PRECAUTIONS

General

Rifapentine may produce a predominately red-orange discoloration of body tissues and/or fluids (eg, skin, teeth, tongue, urine, feces, saliva, sputum, tears, sweat, and cerebrospinal fluid).

Contact lenses or dentures may become permanently stained.

Rifapentine should not be used in patients with porphyria. Rifampin has enzyme-inducing properties, including induction of delta amino levulinic acid synthetase. Isolated reports have associated porphyria exacerbation with rifampin administration. Based on these isolated reports with rifampin, it may be assumed that rifapentine has a similar effect.

Information for Patients

The patient should be told that PRIFTIN may produce a reddish coloration of the urine, sweat, sputum, tears, and breast milk and the patient should be forewarned that contact lenses or dentures may be permanently stained. The patient should be advised that the reliability of oral or other systemic hormonal contraceptives may be affected; consideration should be given to using alternative contraceptive measures. For those patients with a propensity to nausea, vomiting, or gastrointestinal upset, administration of PRIFTIN with food may be useful. Patients should be instructed to notify their physician promptly if they experience any of the following: fever, loss of appetite, malaise, nausea and vomiting, darkened urine, yellowish discoloration of the skin and eyes, and pain or swelling of the joints. Compliance with the full course of therapy must be emphasized, and the importance of not missing any doses of the daily administered companion medications in the Intensive Phase must be stressed. (See DOSAGE AND ADMINISTRATION and WARNINGS).

Laboratory Tests

Adults treated for tuberculosis with rifapentine should have baseline measurements of hepatic enzymes, bilirubin, a complete blood count, and a platelet count (or estimate). Patients should be seen at least monthly during therapy and should be specifically questioned concerning symptoms associated with adverse reactions. All patients with abnormalities should have follow-up, including laboratory testing, if necessary. Routine laboratory monitoring for toxicity in people with normal baseline measurements is generally not necessary.

Therapeutic concentrations of rifampin have been shown to inhibit standard microbiological assays for serum folate and Vitamin B_{12}. Similar drug-laboratory interactions should be considered for rifapentine; thus, alternative assay methods should be considered.

Drug Interaction

Rifapentine-Indinavir Interaction: In a study in which 600 mg rifapentine was administered twice weekly for 14 days followed by rifapentine twice weekly plus 800 mg indinavir 3 times a day for an additional 14 days, indinavir C_{max} decreased by 55% while AUC reduced by 70%. Clearance of indinavir increased by 3-fold in the presence of rifapentine while half-life did not change. But when indinavir was administered for 14 days followed by coadministration with rifapentine for an additional 14 days, indinavir did not affect the pharmacokinetics of rifapentine. **Rifapentine should be used with extreme caution, if at all, in patients who are also taking protease inhibitors.** (See WARNINGS and DOSAGE AND ADMINISTRATION.)

Rifapentine is an inducer of cytochromes P4503A4 and P4502C8/9. Therefore, rifapentine may increase the metabolism of other coadministered drugs that are metabolized by these enzymes. Induction of enzyme activities by rifapentine occurred within 4 days after the first dose. Enzyme activities returned to baseline levels 14 days after discontinuing rifapentine. In addition, the magnitude of enzyme induction by rifapentine was dose and dosing frequency dependent; less enzyme induction occurred when 600 mg oral doses of rifapentine were given once every 72 hours versus daily. In vitro and in vivo enzyme induction studies have suggested rifapentine induction potential may be less than rifampin but more potent than rifabutin.

Rifampin has been reported to accelerate the metabolism and may reduce the activity of the following drugs; hence, rifapentine may also increase the metabolism and decrease the activity of these drugs. Dosage adjustments of the following drugs or of drugs metabolized by cytochrome P4503A4 or P4502C8/9 may be necessary if they are given concurrently with rifapentine. Patients using oral or other systemic hormonal contraceptives should be advised to change to nonhormonal methods of birth control.

Anticonvulsants: eg, phenytoin
Antiarrhythmics: eg, disopyramide, mexiletine, quinidine, tocainide
Antibiotics: eg, chloramphenicol, clarithromycin, dapsone, doxycycline, fluoroquinolones (such as ciprofloxacin)
Oral anticoagulants: eg, warfarin
Antifungals: eg, fluconazole, itraconazole, ketoconazole
Barbiturates
Benzodiazepines: eg, diazepam
Beta-blockers, calcium channel blockers: eg, diltiazem, nifedipine, verapamil
Corticosteroids
Cardiac glycoside preparations
Clofibrate
Oral or other systemic hormonal contraceptives
Haloperidol
HIV protease inhibitors: eg, indinavir, ritonavir, nelfinavir, saquinavir (see Rifapentine-Indinavir Interaction above)
Oral hypoglycemic agents: eg, sulfonylureas
Immunosuppressants: eg, cyclosporine, tacrolimus
Levothyroxine
Narcotic analgesics: eg, methadone
Progestins
Quinine
Reverse transcriptase inhibitors: eg, delavirdine, zidovudine
Sildenafil
Theophylline
Tricyclic antidepressants: eg, amitriptyline, nortriptyline

The conversion of rifapentine to 25-desacetyl rifapentine is mediated by an esterase enzyme. There is minimal potential for rifapentine metabolism to be inhibited or induced by another drug, or for rifapentine to inhibit the metabolism of another drug based upon the characteristics of the esterase enzymes. Rifapentine does not induce its own metabolism. Since rifapentine is highly bound to albumin, drug displacement interactions may also occur.

In Clinical Study 008 patients were advised to take rifapentine at least 1 hour before or 2 hours after ingestion of antacids.

Carcinogenesis, Mutagenesis, Impairment of Fertility

Carcinogenicity studies with rifapentine have not been completed. Rifapentine was negative in the following genotoxicity tests: in vitro gene mutation assay in bacteria (Ames test); in vitro point mutation test in *Aspergillus nidulans*; in vitro gene conversion assay in *Saccharomyces cerevisiae*; host-mediated (mouse) gene conversion assay with *Saccharomyces cerevisiae*; in vitro Chinese hamster ovary cell/hypoxanthine-guanine-phosphoribosyl transferase (CHO/HGPRT) forward mutation assay; in vitro chromosomal aberration assay utilizing rat lymphocytes; and in vivo mouse bone marrow micronucleus assay. The 25-desacetyl metabolite of rifapentine was also negative in the in vitro gene mutation assay in bacteria (Ames test), the in vitro Chinese hamster ovary cell/hypoxanthine-guanine-phosphoribosyl transferase (CHO/HGPRT) forward mutation assay, and the in vivo mouse bone marrow micronucleus assay. This metabolite did induce chromosomal aberrations in an in vitro chromosomal aberration assay. Fertility and reproductive performance were not affected by oral administration of rifapentine to male and female rats at doses of up to one-third of the human dose (based on body surface area conversions).

Pregnancy Category C

Teratogenic Effects

Rifapentine has been shown to be teratogenic in rats and rabbits. In rats, when given in doses 0.6 times the human dose (based on body surface area comparisons) during the period of organogenesis, pups showed cleft palates, right aortic arch and increased incidence of delayed ossification and increased number of ribs. Rabbits treated with drug at doses between 0.3 and 1.3 times the human dose (based on body surface area comparison) displayed major malformations including ovarian agenesis, pes varus, arhinia, microphthalmia and irregularities of the ossified facial tissues (4 of 321 examined fetuses).

Nonteratogenic Effects
In rats, rifapentine administration was associated with increased resorption rate and post implantation loss, decreased mean fetus weight, increased number of stillborn pups and slightly increased mortality during lactation. Rabbits given 1.3 times the human dose (based on body surface area comparisons) showed higher post-implantation losses and an increased incidence of stillborn pups.
When rifapentine was administered at 0.3 times the human dose (based on body surface area comparisons) to mated female rats late in gestation (from day 15 of gestation to day 21 postpartum), pup weights and gestational survival (live pups born/pups born) were reduced compared to controls.

Pregnancy–Human Experience
There are no adequate and well-controlled studies in pregnant women. In Clinical Study 008, six patients randomized to rifapentine became pregnant; two had normal deliveries; two had first trimester spontaneous abortions, one had an elective abortion and one patient was lost to follow-up. Of the two patients who spontaneously aborted, co-morbid conditions of ethanol abuse in one and HIV infection in the other were noted.
When administered during the last few weeks of pregnancy, rifampin can cause postnatal hemorrhages in the mother and infant for which treatment with Vitamin K may be indicated. Thus, patients and infants who receive rifapentine during the last few weeks of pregnancy should have appropriate clotting parameters evaluated.
Rifapentine should be used during pregnancy only if the potential benefit justifies the potential risk to the fetus.

Nursing Mothers
It is not known whether rifapentine is excreted in human milk. Because many drugs are excreted in human milk and because of the potential for serious adverse reactions in nursing infants, a decision should be made whether to discontinue nursing or discontinue the drug, taking into account the importance of the drug to the mother. Since rifapentine may produce a red-orange discoloration of body fluids, there is a potential for discoloration of breast milk.

Pediatric Use
The safety and effectiveness of rifapentine in pediatric patients under the age of 12 have not been established. A pharmacokinetic study was conducted in 12- to 15-year-old healthy volunteers. (See ACTIONS/CLINICAL PHARMACOLOGY Special Populations for pharmacokinetic information).

Geriatric Use
Clinical studies of PRIFTIN did not include sufficient numbers of subjects aged 65 and over to determine whether they respond differently from younger subjects. Other reported clinical experience has not identified differences in responses between the elderly and younger patients. In general, dose selection for an elderly patient should be cautious, usually starting at the low end of the dosing range, reflecting the greater frequency of decreased hepatic, renal, or cardiac function and of concomitant disease or other drug therapy. (See ACTIONS/CLINICAL PHARMACOLOGY, Pharmacokinetics, Special Populations-Elderly).

ADVERSE REACTIONS

The investigators in the tuberculosis treatment clinical trial (Study 008) assessed the causality of adverse events as definitely, probably, possibly, unlikely or not related to one of the two drug regimens tested. The following table (Table 2-3) presents treatment-related adverse events deemed by the investigators to be at least possibly related to any of the four drugs in the regimens (rifapentine/rifampin, isoniazid, pyrazinamide, or ethambutol) which occurred in ≥1% of patients. Hyperuricemia was the most frequently reported event that was assessed as treatment related and was most likely related to the pyrazinamide since no cases were reported in the Continuation Phase when this drug was no longer included in the treatment regimen.
[See table 2-3 at right]

Table 2-3. Treatment-Related Adverse Events Occurring in ≥1% of the Patients in Study 008

	Intensive Phase[1]		*Continuation Phase*[2]		*Total*	
Preferred Term	*Rifapentine Combination (N=361) N (%)*	*Rifampin Combination (N=361) N (%)*	*Rifapentine Combination (N=321) N (%)*	*Rifampin Combination (N=307) N (%)*	*Rifapentine Combination (N=361) N (%)*	*Rifampin Combination (N=361) N (%)*
Hyperuricemia	78 (21.6)	55 (15.2)	0	0	78 (21.6)	55 (15.2)
ALT increased	12 (3.3)	17 (4.7)	6 (1.9)	7 (2.3)	18 (5.0)	24 (6.6)
AST increased	11 (3.0)	16 (4.4)	5 (1.6)	7 (2.3)	15 (4.2)	23 (6.4)
Neutropenia	7 (1.9)	9 (2.5)	12 (3.7)	9 (2.9)	18 (5.0)	18 (5.0)
Pyuria	11 (3.0)	10 (2.8)	6 (1.9)	3 (1.0)	14 (3.9)	12 (3.3)
Proteinuria	15 (4.2)	10 (2.8)	2 (0.6)	1 (0.3)	17 (4.7)	11 (3.0)
Hematuria	10 (2.8)	12 (3.3)	4 (1.2)	4 (1.3)	13 (3.6)	15 (4.2)
Lymphopenia	14 (3.9)	13 (3.6)	3 (0.9)	1 (0.3)	16 (4.4)	14 (3.9)
Urinary casts	11 (3.0)	3 (0.8)	4 (1.2)	0	14 (3.9)	3 (0.8)
Rash	9 (2.5)	19 (5.3)	4 (1.2)	3 (1.0)	13 (3.6)	21 (5.8)
Pruritus	8 (2.2)	15 (4.2)	1 (0.3)	1 (0.3)	9 (2.5)	16 (4.4)
Acne	5 (1.4)	3 (0.8)	2 (0.6)	1 (0.3)	7 (1.9)	4 (1.1)
Anorexia	6 (1.7)	8 (2.2)	3 (0.9)	4 (1.3)	8 (2.2)	10 (2.8)
Anemia	7 (1.9)	9 (2.5)	2 (0.6)	1 (0.3)	9 (2.5)	10 (2.8)
Leukopenia	4 (1.1)	4 (1.1)	3 (0.9)	5 (1.6)	7 (1.9)	8 (2.2)
Arthralgia	9 (2.5)	7 (1.9)	0	0	9 (2.5)	7 (1.9)
Pain	7 (1.9)	5 (1.4)	0	1 (0.3)	7 (1.9)	6 (1.7)
Nausea	7 (1.9)	2 (0.6)	0	1 (0.3)	7 (1.9)	3 (0.8)
Vomiting	4 (1.1)	6 (1.7)	1 (0.3)	1 (0.3)	5 (1.4)	7 (1.9)
Headache	3 (0.8)	4 (1.1)	1 (0.3)	3 (1.0)	4 (1.1)	7 (1.9)
Dyspepsia	3 (0.8)	5 (1.4)	2 (0.6)	3 (1.0)	4 (1.1)	8 (2.2)
Hypertension	3 (0.8)	0 (0.0)	1 (0.3)	1 (0.3)	4 (1.1)	1 (0.3)
Dizziness	4 (1.1)	0	0	1 (0.3)	4 (1.1)	1 (0.3)
Thrombocytosis	4 (1.1)	2 (0.6)	0	0	4 (1.1)	2 (0.6)
Diarrhea	4 (1.1)	0	0	0	4 (1.1)	0
Rash maculopapular	4 (1.1)	3 (0.8)	0	0	4 (1.1)	3 (0.8)
Hemoptysis	2 (0.6)	0	2 (0.6)	0	4 (1.1)	0

Note: ≥1% refers to rifapentine in the TOTAL column.

Note: A patient may have experienced the same adverse event more than once during the course of the study, therefore, patient counts across the columns may not equal the patient counts in the TOTAL column.

[1] Intensive Phase consisted of therapy with either rifapentine or rifampin combined with isoniazid, pyrazinamide, and ethambutol administered daily (rifapentine twice weekly) for 60 days.
[2] Continuation Phase consisted of therapy with either rifapentine or rifampin combined with isoniazid for 120 days. Rifapentine patients were dosed once weekly; rifampin patients were dosed twice weekly. Events recorded in this phase includes those reported up to 3 months after Continuation Phase therapy was completed.

Treatment-related adverse events of moderate or severe intensity in <1% of the rifapentine combination therapy patients in Study 008 are presented below by body system.
Hepatic & Biliary: bilirubinemia, hepatitis
Dermatologic: urticaria, skin discoloration
Hematologic: thrombocytopenia, neutrophilia, leukocytosis, purpura, hematoma
Metabolic & Nutritional: hyperkalemia, hypovolemia, alkaline phosphatase increased, LDH increased
Body as a Whole - General: peripheral edema, fatigue
Gastrointestinal: constipation, esophagitis, gastritis, pancreatitis
Musculoskeletal: gout, arthrosis
Psychiatric: aggressive reaction
Three patients (two rifampin combination therapy patients and one rifapentine combination therapy patient) were discontinued in the Intensive Phase as a result of hepatitis with increased liver function tests (ALT, AST, LDH, and bilirubin). Concomitant medications for all three patients included isoniazid, pyrazinamide, ethambutol, and pyridoxine. The two rifampin patients and one rifapentine patient recovered without sequelae.
Twenty-two deaths occurred in Study 008 (eleven in the rifampin combination therapy group and eleven in the rifapentine combination therapy group). None of the deaths were attributed to study medication. In the study, 18/361 (5.0%) rifampin combination therapy patients discontinued the study due to an adverse event compared to 11/361 (3.0%) rifapentine combination therapy patients.
The overall occurrence rate of treatment-related adverse events was higher in males with the rifapentine combination regimen (50%) versus the rifampin combination regimen (43%), while in females the overall rate was greater in the rifampin combination group (68%) compared to the rifapentine combination group (59%). However, there were higher frequencies of treatment-related hematuria and ALT increases for female patients in both treatment groups compared to those for male patients.
Adverse events associated with rifampin may occur with rifapentine: effects of enzyme induction to increase metabolism resulting in decreased concentration of endogenous substrates, including adrenal hormones, thyroid hormones, and vitamin D.

OVERDOSAGE

There is no experience with the treatment of acute overdose with rifapentine at doses exceeding 1200 mg per dose.
In a pharmacokinetic study involving healthy volunteers (n=9), single oral doses up to 1200 mg have been administered without serious adverse events. The only adverse events reported with the 1200 mg dose were heartburn (3/8), headache (2/8) and increased urinary frequency (1/8). In clinical trials, tuberculosis patients ranging in age from 20 to 74 years accidentally received continuous daily doses of rifapentine 600 mg. Some patients received continuous daily dosing for up to 20 days without evidence of serious adverse effects. One patient experienced a transient elevation in SGPT and glucose (the latter attributed to pre-existing diabetes); a second patient experienced slight pruritus. While there is no experience with the treatment of acute overdose with rifapentine, clinical experience with rifamycins suggests that gastric lavage to evacuate gastric contents (within a few hours of overdose), followed by instillation of an activated charcoal slurry into the stomach, may help adsorb any remaining drug from the gastrointestinal tract.
Rifapentine and 25-desacetyl rifapentine are 97.7% and 93.2% plasma protein bound, respectively. Rifapentine and related compounds excreted in urine account for only 17% of the administered dose, therefore, neither hemodialysis nor forced diuresis is expected to enhance the systemic elimination of unchanged rifapentine from the body of a patient with PRIFTIN overdose.

DOSAGE AND ADMINISTRATION

PRIFTIN should not be used alone, in initial treatment or in retreatment of pulmonary tuberculosis. In the intensive phase of short-course therapy which is to continue for 2 months, 600 mg **(four 150 mg tablets)** of PRIFTIN should be given twice weekly with an interval of not less than 3 days (72 hours) between doses. For those patients with propensity to nausea, vomiting or gastrointestinal upset, administration of PRIFTIN with food may be useful. In the Intensive Phase, PRIFTIN must be administered in combination as part of an appropriate regimen which includes daily companion drugs. *Compliance with all drugs in the Intensive Phase (ie, PRIFTIN, isoniazid, pyrazinamide, ethambutol, or streptomycin), especially on days when rifapentine is not administered, is imperative to assure early sputum conversion and protection against relapse.* The Advisory Council for the Elimination of Tuberculosis, the American Thoracic Society and the Centers for Disease Control and Prevention also recommend that either streptomycin or ethambutol be

Continued on next page

Priftin—Cont.

added to the regimen unless the likelihood of isoniazid resistance is very low. The need for streptomycin or ethambutol should be reassessed when the results of susceptibility testing are known. An initial treatment regimen with less than four drugs may be considered if there is little possibility of drug resistance (that is, less than 4% primary resistance to isoniazid in the community, and the patient has had no previous treatment with antituberculosis medications, is not from a country with a high prevalence of drug resistance, and has no known exposure to a drug-resistant case) (see Reference 2).
Following the intensive phase, treatment should be continued with PRIFTIN once weekly for 4 months in combination with isoniazid or an appropriate agent for susceptible organisms. If the patient is still sputum smear or culture positive, if resistant organisms are present, or if the patient is HIV positive, follow the ATS/CDC treatment guidelines (see Reference 2).
Concomitant administration of pyridoxine (Vitamin B_6) is recommended in the malnourished, in those predisposed to neuropathy (eg, alcoholics and diabetics), and in adolescents.
The above recommendations apply to patients with drug-susceptible organisms. Patients with drug-resistant organisms may require longer duration treatment with other drug regimens.

HOW SUPPLIED

PRIFTIN (rifapentine) 150 mg round normal convex dark-pink film-coated tablets debossed "Priftin" on top and "150" on the bottom, are packaged in aluminum formable foil blister strips placed in cartons of 32 tablets (4 strips of 8). Each strip of 8 tablets is inserted into an aluminum foil laminated pouch. (NDC 0088-2100-03).
Store at 25°C (77°F); excursions permitted 15–30°C (59–86°F) (see USP Controlled Room Temperature). Protect from excessive heat and humidity.
Prescribing Information as of February 2003
Manufactured by:
Gruppo Lepetit S.p.A.
20020 Lainate, Italy
Manufactured for:
Aventis Pharmaceuticals Inc.
Kansas City, MO 64137 USA
MADE IN ITALY

REFERENCES

1. Vernon A, et al. Acquired rifamycin monoresistance in patients with HIV-related tuberculosis treated with once-weekly rifapentine and isoniazid. The Lancet 1999; 353: 1843–1847.
2. American Thoracic Society, CDC. Treatment of tuberculosis and tuberculosis infection in adults and children. Am J Respir Crit Care Med. 149:1359–1374, 1994.

RIFADIN® ℞

[rĭf' uh-din]
(rifampin capsules USP)
and

RIFADIN® IV

(rifampin for injection USP)

Prescribing Information as of January 2004

To reduce the development of drug-resistant bacteria and maintain the effectiveness of RIFADIN (rifampin capsules USP) and RIFADIN IV (rifampin for injection USP) and other antibacterial drugs, rifampin should be used only to treat or prevent infections that are proven or strongly suspected to be caused by bacteria.

DESCRIPTION

RIFADIN (rifampin capsules USP) for oral administration contain 150 mg or 300 mg of rifampin per capsule. The 150 mg and 300 mg capsules also contain, as inactive ingredients: corn starch, D&C Red No. 28, FD&C Blue No. 1, FD&C Red No. 40, gelatin, magnesium stearate, and titanium dioxide.
RIFADIN IV (rifampin for injection USP) contains rifampin 600 mg, sodium formaldehyde sulfoxylate 10 mg, and sodium hydroxide to adjust pH.
Rifampin is a semisynthetic antibiotic derivative of rifamycin SV. Rifampin is a red-brown crystalline powder very slightly soluble in water at neutral pH, freely soluble in chloroform, soluble in ethyl acetate and in methanol. Its molecular weight is 822.95 and its chemical formula is $C_{43}H_{58}N_4O_{12}$. The chemical name for rifampin is either:

3-[[(4-Methyl-1-piperazinyl)imino]methyl]rifamycin

or

5,6,9,17,19,21-hexahydroxy-23-methoxy-2,4,12,16,20,22-heptamethyl-8-[N-(4-methyl-1-piperazinyl)formimidoyl]-2,7-(epoxypentadeca[1,11,13]trienimino)naphtho[2,1-*b*]furan-1,11(2H)-dione 21-acetate.
Its structural formula is:
[See chemical structure at top of next column]

CLINICAL PHARMACOLOGY

Oral Administration

Rifampin is readily absorbed from the gastrointestinal tract. Peak serum concentrations in healthy adults and pediatric populations vary widely from individual to individual. Following a single 600 mg oral dose of rifampin in healthy adults, the peak serum concentration averages 7 mcg/mL but may vary from 4 to 32 mcg/mL. Absorption of rifampin is reduced by about 30% when the drug is ingested with food.
Rifampin is widely distributed throughout the body. It is present in effective concentrations in many organs and body fluids, including cerebrospinal fluid. Rifampin is about 80% protein bound. Most of the unbound fraction is not ionized and, therefore, diffuses freely into tissues.
In healthy adults, the mean biological half-life of rifampin in serum averages 3.35 ± 0.66 hours after a 600 mg oral dose, with increases up to 5.08 ± 2.45 hours reported after a 900 mg dose. With repeated administration, the half-life decreases and reaches average values of approximately 2 to 3 hours. The half-life does not differ in patients with renal failure at doses not exceeding 600 mg daily, and consequently, no dosage adjustment is required. Following a single 900 mg oral dose of rifampin in patients with varying degrees of renal insufficiency, the mean half-life increased from 3.6 hours in healthy adults to 5.0, 7.3, and 11.0 hours in patients with glomerular filtration rates of 30 to 50 mL/min, less than 30 mL/min, and in anuric patients, respectively. Refer to the WARNINGS section for information regarding patients with hepatic insufficiency.
Rifampin is rapidly eliminated in the bile, and an enterohepatic circulation ensues. During this process, rifampin undergoes progressive deacetylation so that nearly all the drug in the bile is in this form in about 6 hours. This metabolite is microbiologically active. Intestinal reabsorption is reduced by deacetylation, and elimination is facilitated. Up to 30% of a dose is excreted in the urine, with about half of this being unchanged drug.

Intravenous Administration

After intravenous administration of a 300 or 600 mg dose of rifampin infused over 30 minutes to healthy male volunteers (n=12), mean peak plasma concentrations were 9.0 ± 3.0 and 17.5 ± 5.0 mcg/mL, respectively. Total body clearances after the 300 and 600 mg IV doses were 0.19 ± 0.06 and 0.14 ± 0.03 L/hr/kg, respectively. Volumes of distribution at steady state were 0.66 ± 0.14 and 0.64 ± 0.11 L/kg for the 300 and 600 mg IV doses, respectively. After intravenous administration of 300 or 600 mg doses, rifampin plasma concentrations in these volunteers remained detectable for 8 and 12 hours, respectively (see Table).
[See table above]

Plasma Concentrations (mean ± standard deviation, mcg/mL)

Rifampin Dosage IV	30 min	1 hr	2 hr	4 hr	8 hr	12 hr
300 mg	8.9±2.9	4.9±1.3	4.0±1.3	2.5±1.0	1.1±0.6	<0.4
600 mg	17.4±5.1	11.7±2.8	9.4±2.3	6.4±1.7	3.5±1.4	1.2±0.6

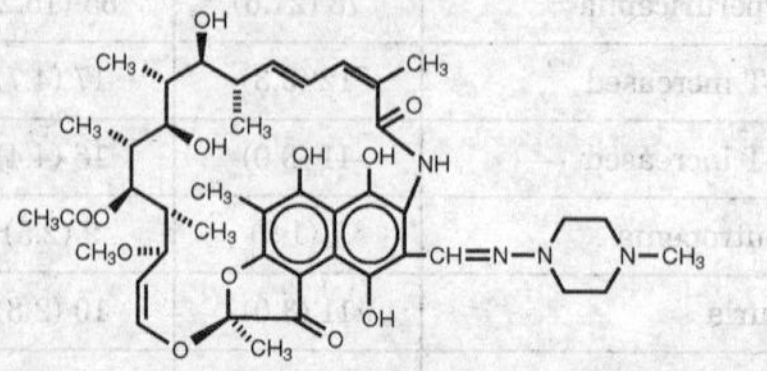

Plasma concentrations after the 600 mg dose, which were disproportionately higher (up to 30% greater than expected) than those found after the 300 mg dose, indicated that the elimination of larger doses was not as rapid.
After repeated once-a-day infusions (3 hr duration) of 600 mg in patients (n=5) for 7 days, concentrations of IV rifampin decreased from 5.81 ± 3.38 mcg/mL 8 hours after the infusion on day 1 to 2.6 ± 1.88 mcg/mL 8 hours after the infusion on day 7.
Rifampin is widely distributed throughout the body. It is present in effective concentrations in many organs and body fluids, including cerebrospinal fluid. Rifampin is about 80% protein bound. Most of the unbound fraction is not ionized and therefore diffuses freely into tissues.
Rifampin is rapidly eliminated in the bile and undergoes progressive enterohepatic circulation and deacetylation to the primary metabolite, 25-desacetyl-rifampin. This metabolite is microbiologically active. Less than 30% of the dose is excreted in the urine as rifampin or metabolites. Serum concentrations do not differ in patients with renal failure at a studied dose of 300 mg and consequently, no dosage adjustment is required.

Pediatrics

Oral Administration. In one study, pediatric patients 6 to 58 months old were given rifampin suspended in simple syrup or as dry powder mixed with applesauce at a dose of 10 mg/kg body weight. Peak serum concentrations of 10.7 ± 0.7 and 11.5 ± 5.1 mcg/mL were obtained 1 hour after preprandial ingestion of the drug suspension and the applesauce mixture, respectively. After the administration of either preparation, the $t_{1/2}$ of rifampin averaged 2.9 hours. It should be noted that in other studies in pediatric populations, at doses of 10 mg/kg body weight, mean peak serum concentrations of 3.5 mcg/mL to 15 mcg/mL have been reported.

Intravenous Administration. In pediatric patients 0.25 to 12.8 years old (n=12), the mean peak serum concentration of rifampin at the end of a 30 minute infusion of approximately 300 mg/m² was 25.9 ± 1.3 mcg/mL; individual peak concentrations 1 to 4 days after initiation of therapy ranged from 11.7 to 41.5 μg/mL; individual peak concentrations 5 to 14 days after initiation of therapy were 13.6 to 37.4 mcg/mL. The individual serum half-life of rifampin changed from 1.04 to 3.81 hours early in therapy to 1.17 to 3.19 hours 5 to 14 days after therapy was initiated.

Microbiology

Rifampin inhibits DNA-dependent RNA polymerase activity in susceptible cells. Specifically, it interacts with bacterial RNA polymerase but does not inhibit the mammalian enzyme. Rifampin at therapeutic levels has demonstrated bactericidal activity against both intracellular and extracellular *Mycobacterium tuberculosis* organisms.
Organisms resistant to rifampin are likely to be resistant to other rifamycins.
Rifampin has bactericidal activity against slow and intermittently growing *M tuberculosis* organisms. It also has significant activity against *Neisseria meningitidis* isolates (see INDICATIONS AND USAGE).
In the treatment of both tuberculosis and the meningococcal carrier state (see INDICATIONS AND USAGE), the small number of resistant cells present within large populations of susceptible cells can rapidly become predominant. In addition, resistance to rifampin has been determined to occur as single-step mutations of the DNA-dependent RNA polymerase. Since resistance can emerge rapidly, appropriate susceptibility tests should be performed in the event of persistent positive cultures.
Rifampin has been shown to be active against most strains of the following microorganisms, both in vitro and in clinical infections as described in the INDICATIONS AND USAGE section.

Aerobic Gram-Negative Microorganisms:
Neisseria meningitidis

"Other" Microorganisms:
Mycobacterium tuberculosis

The following in vitro data are available, but their clinical significance is unknown.
Rifampin exhibits in vitro activity against most strains of the following microorganisms; however, the safety and effectiveness of rifampin in treating clinical infections due to these microorganisms have not been established in adequate and well-controlled trials.

Aerobic Gram-Positive Microorganisms:
Staphylococcus aureus (including Methicillin-Resistant *S. aureus*/MRSA)
Staphylococcus epidermidis

Aerobic Gram-Negative Microorganisms:
Haemophilus influenzae

"Other" Microorganisms:
Mycobacterium leprae

β-lactamase production should have no effect on rifampin activity.

Susceptibility Tests

Prior to initiation of therapy, appropriate specimens should be collected for identification of the infecting organism and in vitro susceptibility tests.
In vitro testing for *Mycobacterium tuberculosis* isolates:
Two standardized in vitro susceptibility methods are available for testing rifampin against *M tuberculosis* organisms. The agar proportion method (CDC or NCCLS[1] M24-P) utilizes Middlebrook 7H10 medium impregnated with rifampin at a final concentration of 1.0 mcg/mL to determine drug resistance. After three weeks of incubation MIC_{99} values are calculated by comparing the quantity of organisms growing in the medium containing drug to the control cultures. Mycobacterial growth in the presence of drug, of at least 1% of the growth in the control culture, indicates resistance.
The radiometric broth method employs the BACTEC 460 machine to compare the growth index from untreated control cultures to cultures grown in the presence of 2.0 mcg/mL of rifampin. Strict adherence to the manufacturer's instructions for sample processing and data interpretation is required for this assay.
Susceptibility test results obtained by the two different methods can only be compared if the appropriate rifampin concentration is used for each test method as indicated above. Both procedures require the use of *M tuberculosis* H37Rv ATCC 27294 as a control organism.
The clinical relevance of in vitro susceptibility test results for mycobacterial species other than *M tuberculosis* using either the radiometric or the proportion method has not been determined.
In vitro testing for *Neisseria meningitidis* isolates:
Dilution Techniques: Quantitative methods that are used to determine minimum inhibitory concentrations provide reproducible estimates of the susceptibility of bacteria to antimicrobial compounds. One such standardized procedure uses a standardized dilution method[2,4] (broth, agar, or microdilution) or equivalent with rifampin powder. The MIC values obtained should be interpreted according to the following criteria for *Neisseria meningitidis:*

MIC (mcg/mL)	Interpretation
≤1	(S) Susceptible
2	(I) Intermediate
≥4	(R) Resistant

A report of "susceptible" indicates that the pathogen is likely to be inhibited by usually achievable concentrations of the antimicrobial compound in the blood. A report of "intermediate" indicates that the result should be considered equivocal, and if the microorganism is not fully susceptible to alternative, clinically feasible drugs, the test should be repeated. This category implies possible clinical applicability in body sites where the drug is physiologically concentrated or in situations where the maximum acceptable dose of drug can be used. This category also provides a buffer zone that prevents small-uncontrolled technical factors from causing major discrepancies in interpretation. A report of "resistant" indicates that usually achievable concentrations of the antimicrobial compound in the blood are unlikely to be inhibitory and that other therapy should be selected.
Measurement of MIC or minimum bactericidal concentrations (MBC) and achieved antimicrobial compound concentrations may be appropriate to guide therapy in some infections. (See CLINICAL PHARMACOLOGY section for further information on drug concentrations achieved in infected body sites and other pharmacokinetic properties of this antimicrobial drug product.)
Standardized susceptibility test procedures require the use of laboratory control microorganisms. The use of these microorganisms does not imply clinical efficacy (see INDICATIONS AND USAGE); they are used to control the technical aspects of the laboratory procedures. Standard rifampin powder should give the following MIC values:

Microorganism		MIC (mcg/mL)
Staphylococcus aureus	ATCC 29213	0.008–0.06
Enterococcus faecalis	ATCC 29212	1–4
Escherichia coli	ATCC 25922	8–32
Pseudomonas aeruginosa	ATCC 27853	32–64
Haemophilus influenzae	ATCC 49247	0.25–1

Diffusion Techniques: Quantitative methods that require measurement of zone diameters provide reproducible estimates of the susceptibility of bacteria to antimicrobial compounds. One such standardized procedure[3,4] that has been recommended for use with disks to test the susceptibility of microorganisms to rifampin uses the 5 mcg rifampin disk. Interpretation involves correlation of the diameter obtained in the disk test with the MIC for rifampin.
Reports from the laboratory providing results of the standard single-disk susceptibility test with a 5 mcg rifampin disk should be interpreted according to the following criteria for *Neisseria meningitidis*:

Zone Diameter (mm)	Interpretation
≥20	(S) Susceptible
17–19	(I) Intermediate
≤16	(R) Resistant

Interpretation should be as stated above for results using dilution techniques.
As with standard dilution techniques, diffusion methods require the use of laboratory control microorganisms. The use of these microorganisms does not imply clinical efficacy (see INDICATIONS AND USAGE); they are used to control the technical aspects of the laboratory procedures. The 5 mcg rifampin disk should provide the following zone diameters in these quality control strains:

Microorganism		Zone Diameter (mm)
S. aureus	ATCC 25923	26–34
E. coli	ATCC 25922	8–10
H. influenzae	ATCC 49247	22–30

INDICATIONS AND USAGE

In the treatment of both tuberculosis and the meningococcal carrier state, the small number of resistant cells present within large populations of susceptible cells can rapidly become the predominant type. Bacteriologic cultures should be obtained before the start of therapy to confirm the susceptibility of the organism to rifampin and they should be repeated throughout therapy to monitor the response to treatment. Since resistance can emerge rapidly, susceptibility tests should be performed in the event of persistent positive cultures during the course of treatment. If test results show resistance to rifampin and the patient is not responding to therapy, the drug regimen should be modified.

Tuberculosis

Rifampin is indicated in the treatment of all forms of tuberculosis.
A three-drug regimen consisting of rifampin, isoniazid, and pyrazinamide (eg, RIFATER®) is recommended in the initial phase of short-course therapy which is usually continued for 2 months. The Advisory Council for the Elimination of Tuberculosis, the American Thoracic Society, and Centers for Disease Control and Prevention recommend that either streptomycin or ethambutol be added as a fourth drug in a regimen containing isoniazid (INH), rifampin, and pyrazinamide for initial treatment of tuberculosis unless the likelihood of INH resistance is very low. The need for a fourth drug should be reassessed when the results of susceptibility testing are known. If community rates of INH resistance are currently less than 4%, an initial treatment regimen with less than four drugs may be considered.
Following the initial phase, treatment should be continued with rifampin and isoniazid (eg, RIFAMATE®) for at least 4 months. Treatment should be continued for longer if the patient is still sputum or culture positive, if resistant organisms are present, or if the patient is HIV positive.
RIFADIN IV is indicated for the initial treatment and retreatment of tuberculosis when the drug cannot be taken by mouth.

Meningococcal Carriers

Rifampin is indicated for the treatment of asymptomatic carriers of *Neisseria meningitidis* to eliminate meningococci from the nasopharynx. **Rifampin is not indicated for the treatment of meningococcal infection because of the possibility of the rapid emergence of resistant organisms.** (See WARNINGS.)
Rifampin should not be used indiscriminately, and therefore, diagnostic laboratory procedures, including serotyping and susceptibility testing, should be performed for establishment of the carrier state and the correct treatment. So that the usefulness of rifampin in the treatment of asymptomatic meningococcal carriers is preserved, the drug should be used only when the risk of meningococcal disease is high.
To reduce the development of drug-resistant bacteria and maintain the effectiveness of rifampin and other antibacterial drugs, rifampin should be used only to treat or prevent infections that are proven or strongly suspected to be caused by susceptible bacteria. When culture and susceptibility information are available, they should be considered in selecting or modifying antibacterial therapy. In the absence of such data, local epidemiology and susceptibility patterns may contribute to the empiric selection of therapy.

CONTRAINDICATIONS

Rifampin is contraindicated in patients with a history of hypersensitivity to any of the rifamycins. (See WARNINGS.)

WARNINGS

Rifampin has been shown to produce liver dysfunction. Fatalities associated with jaundice have occurred in patients with liver disease and in patients taking rifampin with other hepatotoxic agents. Patients with impaired liver function should be given rifampin only in cases of necessity and then with caution and under strict medical supervision. In these patients, careful monitoring of liver function, especially SGPT/ALT and SGOT/AST should be carried out prior to therapy and then every 2 to 4 weeks during therapy. If signs of hepatocellular damage occur, rifampin should be withdrawn.
In some cases, hyperbilirubinemia resulting from competition between rifampin and bilirubin for excretory pathways of the liver at the cell level can occur in the early days of treatment. An isolated report showing a moderate rise in bilirubin and/or transaminase level is not in itself an indication for interrupting treatment; rather, the decision should be made after repeating the tests, noting trends in the levels, and considering them in conjunction with the patient's clinical condition.
Rifampin has enzyme-inducing properties, including induction of delta amino levulinic acid synthetase. Isolated reports have associated porphyria exacerbation with rifampin administration.
The possibility of rapid emergence of resistant meningococci restricts the use of RIFADIN to short-term treatment of the asymptomatic carrier state. **RIFADIN is not to be used for the treatment of meningococcal disease.**

PRECAUTIONS

General

Prescribing rifampin in the absence of a proven or strongly suspected bacterial infection or a prophylactic indication is unlikely to provide benefit to the patient and increases the risk of the development of drug-resistant bacteria.
For the treatment of tuberculosis, rifampin is usually administered on a daily basis. Doses of rifampin greater than 600 mg given once or twice weekly have resulted in a higher incidence of adverse reactions, including the "flu syndrome" (fever, chills and malaise), hematopoietic reactions (leukopenia, thrombocytopenia, or acute hemolytic anemia), cutaneous, gastrointestinal, and hepatic reactions, shortness of breath, shock, anaphylaxis, and renal failure. Recent studies indicate that regimens using twice-weekly doses of rifampin 600 mg plus isoniazid 15 mg/kg are much better tolerated.
Intermittent therapy may be used if the patient cannot (or will not) self-administer drugs on a daily basis. Patients on intermittent therapy should be closely monitored for compliance and cautioned against intentional or accidental interruption of prescribed therapy, because of the increased risk of serious adverse reactions.
Rifampin has enzyme induction properties that can enhance the metabolism of endogenous substrates including adrenal hormones, thyroid hormones, and vitamin D. Rifampin and isoniazid have been reported to alter vitamin D metabolism. In some cases, reduced levels of circulating 25-hydroxy vitamin D and 1,25-dihydroxy vitamin D have been accompanied by reduced serum calcium and phosphate, and elevated parathyroid hormone.

RIFADIN IV

For intravenous infusion only. Must not be administered by intramuscular or subcutaneous route. Avoid extravasation during injection: local irritation and inflammation due to extravascular infiltration of the infusion have been observed. If these occur, the infusion should be discontinued and restarted at another site.

Information for Patients

Patients should be counseled that antibacterial drugs including rifampin should only be used to treat bacterial infections. They do not treat viral infections (e.g., the common cold). When rifampin is prescribed to treat a bacterial infection, patients should be told that although it is common to feel better early in the course of therapy, the medication should be taken exactly as directed. Skipping doses or not completing the full course of therapy may (1) decrease the effectiveness of the immediate treatment and (2) increase the likelihood that bacteria will develop resistance and will not be treatable by rifampin or other antibacterial drugs in the future.
The patient should be told that rifampin may produce a reddish coloration of the urine, sweat, sputum, and tears, and the patient should be forewarned of this. Soft contact lenses may be permanently stained.
The patient should be advised that the reliability of oral or other systemic hormonal contraceptives may be affected; consideration should be given to using alternative contraceptive measures.
Patients should be instructed to take rifampin either 1 hour before or 2 hours after a meal with a full glass of water.
Patients should be instructed to notify their physicians promptly if they experience any of the following: fever, loss of appetite, malaise, nausea and vomiting, darkened urine, yellowish discoloration of the skin and eyes, and pain or swelling of the joints.
Compliance with the full course of therapy must be emphasized, and the importance of not missing any doses must be stressed.

Laboratory Tests

Adults treated for tuberculosis with rifampin should have baseline measurements of hepatic enzymes, bilirubin, serum creatinine, a complete blood count, and a platelet count (or estimate). Baseline tests are unnecessary in pediatric patients unless a complicating condition is known or clinically suspected.
Patients should be seen at least monthly during therapy and should be specifically questioned concerning symptoms associated with adverse reactions. All patients with abnormalities should have follow-up, including laboratory testing, if necessary. Routine laboratory monitoring for toxicity in people with normal baseline measurements is generally not necessary.

Drug Interactions

ENZYME INDUCTION: Rifampin is known to induce certain cytochrome P-450 enzymes. Administration of rifampin with drugs that undergo biotransformation through these metabolic pathways may accelerate elimination of coadministered drugs. To maintain optimum therapeutic blood levels, dosages of drugs metabolized by these enzymes may require adjustment when starting or stopping concomitantly administered rifampin.
Rifampin has been reported to accelerate the metabolism of the following drugs: anticonvulsants (eg, phenytoin), antiarrhythmics (eg, disopyramide, mexiletine, quinidine, tocainide), oral anticoagulants, antifungals (eg, fluconazole, itraconazole, ketoconazole), barbiturates, beta-blockers, calcium channel blockers (eg, diltiazem, nifedipine, verapamil), chloramphenicol, clarithromycin, corticosteroids, cyclosporine, cardiac glycoside preparations, clofibrate, oral or other systemic hormone contraceptives, dapsone, diazepam, doxycycline, fluoroquinolones (eg, ciprofloxacin), haloperidol, oral hypoglycemic agents (sulfonylureas), levothyroxine, methadone, narcotic analgesics, nortriptyline, progestins, quinine, tacrolimus, theophylline tricyclic antidepressants (eg, amitriptyline, nortriptyline), and zidovudine. It may be necessary to adjust the dosages of these drugs if they are given concurrently with rifampin.
Patients using oral or other systemic hormonal contraceptives should be advised to change to nonhormonal methods of birth control during rifampin therapy.
Rifampin has been observed to increase the requirements for anticoagulant drugs of the coumarin type. In patients receiving anticoagulants and rifampin concurrently, it is recommended that the prothrombin time be performed daily or as frequently as necessary to establish and maintain the required dose of anticoagulant.
Diabetes may become more difficult to control.
OTHER INTERACTIONS: When the two drugs were taken concomitantly, decreased concentrations of atovaquone and increased concentrations of rifampin were observed.
Concurrent use of ketoconazole and rifampin has resulted in decreased serum concentrations of both drugs. Concurrent use of rifampin and enalapril has resulted in decreased concentrations of enalaprilat, the active metabolite of enalapril. Dosage adjustments should be made if indicated by the patient's clinical condition.
Concomitant antacid administration may reduce the absorption of rifampin. Daily doses of rifampin should be given at least 1 hour before the ingestion of antacids.
Probenecid and cotrimoxazole have been reported to increase the blood level of rifampin.
When rifampin is given concomitantly with either halothane or isoniazid, the potential for hepatotoxicity is increased. The concomitant use of rifampin and halothane should be avoided. Patients receiving both rifampin and isoniazid should be monitored close for hepatotoxicity.
Plasma concentrations of sulfapyridine may be reduced following the concomitant administration of sulfasalazine and

Continued on next page

Rifadin—Cont.

rifampin. This finding may be the result of alteration in the colonic bacteria responsible for the reduction of sulfasalazine to sulfapyridine and mesalamine.

Drug/Laboratory Interactions

Cross-reactivity and false-positive urine screening tests for opiates have been reported in patients receiving rifampin when using the KIMS (Kinetic Interaction of Microparticles in Solution) method (eg, Abuscreen OnLine opiates assay; Roche Diagnostic Systems). Confirmatory tests, such as gas chromatography/mass spectrometry, will distinguish rifampin from opiates.

Therapeutic levels of rifampin have been shown to inhibit standard microbiological assays for serum folate and vitamin B_{12}. Thus, alternate assay methods should be considered. Transient abnormalities in liver function tests (eg, elevation in serum bilirubin, alkaline phosphatase, and serum transaminases) and reduced biliary excretion of contrast media used for visualization of the gallbladder have also been observed. Therefore, these tests should be performed before the morning dose of rifampin.

Carcinogenesis, Mutagenesis, Impairment of Fertility

There are no known human data on long-term potential for carinogenicity, mutagenicity, or impairment of fertility. A few cases of accelerated growth of lung carcinoma have been reported in man, but a causal relationship with the drug has not been established. An increase in the incidence of hepatomas in female mice (of a strain known to be particularly susceptible to the spontaneous development of hepatomas) was observed when rifampin was administered in doses 2 to 10 times the average daily human dose for 60 weeks, followed by an observation period of 46 weeks. No evidence of carcinogenicity was found in male mice of the same strain, mice of a different strain, or rats under similar experimental conditions.

Rifampin has been reported to possess immunosuppressive potential in rabbits, mice, rats, guinea pigs, human lymphocytes in vitro, and humans. Antitumor activity in vitro has also been shown with rifampin.

There was no evidence of mutagenicity in bacteria, *Drosophila melanogaster*, or mice. An increase in chromotid breaks was noted when whole blood cell cultures were treated with rifampin. Increased frequency of chromosomal aberrations was observed in vitro in lymphocytes obtained from patients treated with combinations of rifampin, isoniazid, and pyrazinamide and combinations of streptomycin, rifampin, isoniazid, and pyrazinamide.

Pregnancy—Teratogenic Effects

Category C. Rifampin has been shown to be teratogenic in rodents given oral doses of rifampin 15 to 25 times the human dose. Although rifampin has been reported to cross the placental barrier and appear in cord blood, the effect of RIFADIN, alone or in combination with other antituberculosis drugs, on the human fetus is not known. Neonates of rifampin-treated mothers should be carefully observed for any evidence of adverse effects. Isolated cases of fetal malformations have been reported; however, there are no adequate and well-controlled studies in pregnant women. Rifampin should be used during pregnancy only if the potential benefit justifies the potential risk to the fetus. Rifampin in oral doses of 150 to 250 mg/kg produced teratogenic effects in mice and rats. Malformations were primarily cleft palate in the mouse and spina bifida in the rat. The incidence of these anomalies was dose-dependent. When rifampin was given to pregnant rabbits in doses up to 20 times the usual daily human dose, imperfect osteogenesis and embryotoxicity were reported.

Pregnancy—Non-Teratogenic Effects

When administered during the last few weeks of pregnancy, rifampin can cause post-natal hemorrhages in the mother and infant for which treatment with vitamin K may be indicated.

Nursing Mothers

Because of the potential for tumorigenicity shown for rifampin in animal studies, a decision should be made whether to discontinue nursing or discontinue the drug, taking into account the importance of the drug to the mother.

Pediatric Use

See CLINICAL PHARMACOLOGY—Pediatrics; see also DOSAGE AND ADMINISTRATION.

Geriatric Use

Clinical studies of RIFADIN did not include sufficient numbers of subjects aged 65 and over to determine whether they respond differently from younger subjects. Other reported clinical experience has not identified differences in responses between the elderly and younger patients. Caution should therefore be observed in using rifampin in elderly patients. (See WARNINGS).

ADVERSE REACTIONS

Gastrointestinal

Heartburn, epigastric distress, anorexia, nausea, vomiting, jaundice, flatulence, cramps, and diarrhea have been noted in some patients. Although *Clostridium difficile* has been shown in vitro to be sensitive to rifampin, pseudomembranous colitis has been reported with the use of rifampin (and other broad spectrum antibiotics). Therefore, it is important to consider this diagnosis in patients who develop diarrhea in association with antibiotic use. Rarely, hepatitis or a shock-like syndrome with hepatic involvement and abnormal liver function tests has been reported.

Hematologic

Thrombocytopenia has occurred primarily with high dose intermittent therapy, but has also been noted after resumption of interrupted treatment. It rarely occurs during well supervised daily therapy. This effect is reversible if the drug is discontinued as soon as purpura occurs. Cerebral hemorrhage and fatalities have been reported when rifampin administration has been continued or resumed after the appearance of purpura.

Rare reports of disseminated intravascular coagulation have been observed.

Leukopenia, hemolytic anemia, and decreased hemoglobin have been observed.

Agranulocytosis has been reported very rarely.

Central Nervous System

Headache, fever, drowsiness, fatigue, ataxia, dizziness, inability to concentrate, mental confusion, behavioral changes, pains in extremities, and generalized numbness have been observed.

Psychoses have been rarely reported.

Ocular

Visual disturbances have been observed.

Endocrine

Menstrual disturbances have been observed.

Rare reports of adrenal insufficiency in patients with compromised adrenal function have been observed.

Renal

Elevations in BUN and serum uric acid have been reported. Rarely, hemolysis, hemoglobinuria, hematuria, interstitial nephritis, acute tubular necrosis, renal insufficiency, and acute renal failure have been noted. These are generally considered to be hypersensitivity reactions. They usually occur during intermittent therapy or when treatment is resumed following intentional or accidental interruption of a daily dosage regimen, and are reversible when rifampin is discontinued and appropriate therapy instituted.

Dermatologic

Cutaneous reactions are mild and self-limiting and do not appear to be hypersensitivity reactions. Typically, they consist of flushing and itching with or without a rash. More serious cutaneous reactions which may be due to hypersensitivity occur but are uncommon.

Hypersensitivity Reactions

Occasionally, pruritus, urticaria, rash, pemphigoid reaction, erythema multiforme including Stevens-Johnson Syndrome, toxic epidermal necrolysis, vasculitis, eosinophilia, sore mouth, sore tongue, and conjunctivitis have been observed.

Anaphylaxis has been reported rarely.

Miscellaneous

Rare reports of myopathy and muscular weakness have also been observed.

Edema of the face and extremities has been reported. Other reactions reported to have occurred with intermittent dosage regimens include "flu syndrome" (such as episodes of fever, chills, headache, dizziness, and bone pain), shortness of breath, wheezing, decrease in blood pressure and shock. The "flu syndrome" may also appear if rifampin is taken irregularly by the patient or if daily administration is resumed after a drug free interval.

OVERDOSAGE

Signs and Symptoms

Nausea, vomiting, abdominal pain, pruritus, headache, and increasing lethargy will probably occur within a short time after ingestion; unconsciousness may occur when there is severe hepatic disease. Transient increases in liver enzymes and/or bilirubin may occur. Brownish-red or orange discoloration of the skin, urine, sweat, saliva, tears, and feces will occur, and its intensity is proportional to the amount ingested.

Facial or periorbital edema has also been reported in pediatric patients. Hypotension, sinus tachycardia, ventricular arrhythmias, seizures and cardiac arrest were reported in some fatal cases.

Acute Toxicity

The LD_{50} of rifampin is approximately 885 mg/kg in the mouse, 1720 mg/kg in the rat, and 2120 mg/kg in the rabbit. The minimum acute lethal or toxic dose is not well established. However, nonfatal acute overdoses in adults have been reported with doses ranging from 9 to 12 gm rifampin. Fatal acute overdoses in adults have been reported with doses ranging from 14 to 60 gm. Alcohol or a history of alcohol abuse was involved in some of the fatal and nonfatal reports. Nonfatal overdoses in pediatric patients ages 1 to 4 years old of 100 mg/kg for one to two doses has been reported.

Treatment

Intensive support measures should be instituted and individual symptoms treated as they arise. Since nausea and vomiting are likely to be present, gastric lavage is probably preferable to induction of emesis. Following evacuation of the gastric contents, the instillation of activated charcoal slurry into the stomach may help absorb any remaining drug from the gastrointestinal tract. Antiemetic medication may be required to control severe nausea and vomiting. Active diuresis (with measured intake and output) will help promote excretion of the drug. Hemodialysis may be of value in some patients.

DOSAGE AND ADMINISTRATION

Rifampin can be administered by the oral route or by IV infusion (see INDICATIONS AND USAGE). IV doses are the same as those for oral.

See CLINICAL PHARMACOLOGY for dosing information in patients with renal failure.

Tuberculosis

Adults: 10 mg/kg, in a single daily administration, not to exceed 600 mg/day, oral or IV

Pediatric Patients: 10–20 mg/kg, not to exceed 600 mg/day, oral or IV

It is recommended that oral rifampin be administered once daily, either 1 hour before or 2 hours after a meal with a full glass of water.

Rifampin is indicated in the treatment of all forms of tuberculosis. A three-drug regimen consisting of rifampin, isoniazid, and pyrazinamide (eg, RIFATER®) is recommended in the initial phase of short-course therapy which is usually continued for 2 months. The Advisory Council for the Elimination of Tuberculosis, the American Thoracic Society, and the Centers for Disease Control and Prevention recommend that either streptomycin or ethambutol be added as a fourth drug in a regimen containing isoniazid (INH), rifampin and pyrazinamide for initial treatment of tuberculosis unless the likelihood of INH resistance is very low. The need for a fourth drug should be reassessed when the results of susceptibility testing are known. If community rates of INH resistance are currently less than 4%, an initial treatment regimen with less than four drugs may be considered.

Following the initial phase, treatment should be continued with rifampin and isoniazid (eg, RIFAMATE®) for at least 4 months. Treatment should be continued for longer if the patient is still sputum or culture positive, if resistant organisms are present, or if the patient is HIV positive.

Preparation of Solution for IV Infusion: Reconstitute the lyophilized powder by transferring 10 mL of sterile water for injection to a vial containing 600 mg of rifampin for injection. Swirl vial gently to completely dissolve the antibiotic. The reconstituted solution contains 60 mg rifampin per mL and is stable at room temperature for 24 hours. Prior to administration, withdraw from the reconstituted solution a volume equivalent to the amount of rifampin calculated to be administered and add to 500 mL of infusion medium. Mix well and infuse at a rate allowing for complete infusion within 3 hours. Alternatively, the amount of rifampin calculated to be administered may be added to 100 mL of infusion medium and infused in 30 minutes.

Dilutions in dextrose 5% for injection (D5W) are stable at room temperature for up to 4 hours and should be prepared and used within this time. Precipitation of rifampin from the infusion solution may occur beyond this time. Dilutions in normal saline are stable at room temperature for up to 24 hours and should be prepared and used within this time. Other infusion solutions are not recommended.

Incompatibilities: Physical incompatibility (precipitate) was observed with undiluted (5 mg/mL) and diluted (1 mg/mL in normal saline) diltiazem hydrochloride and rifampin (6 mg/mL in normal saline) during simulated Y-site administration.

Meningococcal Carriers

Adults: For adults, it is recommended that 600 mg rifampin be administered twice daily for two days.

Pediatric Patients: Pediatric patients 1 month of age or older: 10 mg/kg (not to exceed 600 mg per dose) every 12 hours for two days.

Pediatric patients under 1 month of age: 5 mg/kg every 12 hours for two days.

Preparation of Extemporaneous Oral Suspension

For pediatric and adult patients in whom capsule swallowing is difficult or where lower doses are needed, a liquid suspension may be prepared as follows:

RIFADIN 1% w/v suspension (10 mg/mL) can be compounded using one of four syrups—Simple Syrup (Syrup NF), Simple Syrup (Humco Laboratories), Syrpalta® Syrup (Emerson Laboratories), or Raspberry Syrup (Humco Laboratories).

1. Empty the contents of four RIFADIN 300 mg capsules or eight RIFADIN 150 mg capsules onto a piece of weighing paper.
2. If necessary, gently crush the capsule contents with a spatula to produce a fine powder.
3. Transfer the rifampin powder blend to a 4-ounce amber glass or plastic (high density polyethylene [HDPE], polypropylene, or polycarbonate) prescription bottle.
4. Rinse the paper and spatula with 20 mL of one of the above-mentioned syrups, and add the rinse to the bottle. Shake vigorously.
5. Add 100 mL of syrup to the bottle and shake vigorously.

This compounding procedure results in a 1% w/v suspension containing 10 mg rifampin/mL. Stability studies indicate that the suspension is stable when stored at room temperature (25 ± 3°C) or in a refrigerator (2–8°C) for four weeks. This extemporaneously prepared suspension must be shaken well prior to administration.

HOW SUPPLIED

150 mg maroon and scarlet capsules imprinted "RIFADIN 150."

Bottles of 30 (NDC 0068-0510-30)

300 mg maroon and scarlet capsules imprinted "RIFADIN 300."

Bottles of 30 (NDC 0068-0508-30)
Bottles of 60 (NDC 0068-0508-60)
Bottles of 100 (NDC 0068-0508-61)

Storage: Keep tightly closed. Store in a dry place. Avoid excessive heat.

RIFADIN IV (rifampin for injection USP) is available in glass vials containing 600 mg rifampin (NDC 0068-0597-01).
Storage: Avoid excessive heat (temperatures above 40°C or 104°F). Protect from light.

References:

1. National Committee for Clinical Laboratory Standards, Antimycobacterial Susceptibility Testing. Proposed Standard NCCLS Document M24-P, Vol. 10, No. 10, NNCLS, Villanova, PA, 1990.
2. National Committee for Clinical Laboratory Standards. Methods for Dilution Antimicrobial Susceptibility Tests for Bacteria that Grow Aerobically—Third Edition. Approved Standard NCCLS Document M7-A3, Vol. 13, No. 25, NCCLS, Villanova, PA, December 1993.
3. National Committee for Clinical Laboratory Standards. Performance Standards for Antimicrobial Disk Susceptibility Tests—Fifth Edition. Approved Standard NCCLS Document M2-A5, Vol. 13, No. 24, NCCLS, Villanova, PA, December 1993.
4. National Committee for Clinical Laboratory Standards. Performance Standards for Antimicrobial Susceptibility Testing; Fifth Informational Supplement, NCCLS Document M100-S5, Vol. 14, No. 16, NCCLS, Villanova, PA, December 1994.

Rx Only
Prescribing Information as of January 2004
Rifadin capsules are manufactured by:
Patheon Pharmaceuticals Inc.
Cincinnati, OH 45215 USA
Rifadin IV (rifampin for injection USP) is manufactured by:
GRUPPO LEPETIT S.p.A.
20020 Lainate, Italy
Made in Italy
Manufactured for:
Merrell Pharmaceuticals Inc.
An Aventis Pharmaceuticals Company
Bridgewater, NJ 08807 USA
www.aventis-us.com

RFD-MAR04-F-A
Shown in Product Identification Guide, page 307

RIFAMATE® ℞

[*rĭf 'uh-māt*]
(rifampin and isoniazid capsules USP)

Prescribing Information as of January 2001

WARNING

Severe and sometimes fatal hepatitis associated with isoniazid therapy may occur and may develop even after many months of treatment. The risk of developing hepatitis is age related. Approximate case rates by age are: 0 per 1,000 for persons under 20 years of age, 3 per 1,000 for persons in the 20–34 year age group, 12 per 1,000 for persons in the 35–49 year age group, 23 per 1,000 for persons in the 50–64 year age group, and 8 per 1,000 for persons over 65 years of age. The risk of hepatitis is increased with daily consumption of alcohol. Precise data to provide a fatality rate for isoniazid-related hepatitis is not available; however, in a U.S. Public Health Service Surveillance Study of 13,838 persons taking isoniazid, there were 8 deaths among 174 cases of hepatitis.

Therefore, patients given isoniazid should be carefully monitored and interviewed at monthly intervals. Serum transaminase concentration becomes elevated in about 10–20 percent of patients, usually during the first few months of therapy, but it can occur at any time. Usually enzyme levels return to normal despite continuance of drug, but in some cases progressive liver dysfunction occurs. Patients should be instructed to report immediately any of the prodromal symptoms of hepatitis, such as fatigue, weakness, malaise, anorexia, nausea, or vomiting. If these symptoms appear or if signs suggestive of hepatic damage are detected, isoniazid should be discontinued promptly, since continued use of the drug in these cases has been reported to cause a more severe form of liver damage.

Patients with tuberculosis should be given appropriate treatment with alternative drugs. If isoniazid must be reinstituted, it should be reinstituted only after symptoms and laboratory abnormalities have cleared. The drug should be restarted in very small and gradually increasing doses and should be withdrawn immediately if there is any indication of recurrent liver involvement. Treatment should be deferred in persons with acute hepatic diseases.

DESCRIPTION

RIFAMATE is a combination capsule containing 300 mg rifampin and 150 mg isoniazid. The capsules also contain as inactive ingredients: colloidal silicon dioxide, FD&C Blue No. 1, FD&C Red No. 40, gelatin, magnesium stearate, sodium starch glycolate, and titanium dioxide.

Rifampin is a semisynthetic antibiotic derivative of rifamycin B. The chemical name for rifampin is 3-(4-methyl-1-piperazinyliminomethyl) rifamycin SV.

Isoniazid is the hydrazide of isonicotinic acid. It exists as colorless or white crystals or as a white, crystalline powder that is water soluble, odorless, and slowly affected by exposure to air and light.

CLINICAL PHARMACOLOGY

Rifampin

Rifampin inhibits DNA-dependent RNA polymerase activity in susceptible cells. Specifically, it interacts with bacterial RNA polymerase but does not inhibit the mammalian enzyme. This is the mechanism of action by which rifampin exerts its therapeutic effect. Rifampin cross resistance has only been shown with other rifamycins.

In a study of 14 normal human adult males, peak blood levels of rifampin occured $1^1/_2$ to 3 hours following oral administration of two RIFAMATE capsules. The peaks ranged from 6.9 to 14 mcg/ml with an average of 10 mcg/ml.

In normal subjects the $T^1/_2$ (biological half-life) of rifampin in blood is approximately 3 hours. Elimination occurs mainly through the bile and, to a much lesser extent, the urine.

Isoniazid

Isoniazid acts against actively growing tubercle bacilli.

After oral administration isoniazid produces peak blood levels within 1 to 2 hours which decline to 50% or less within 6 hours. It diffuses readily into all body fluids (cerebrospinal, pleural, and ascitic fluids), tissues, organs, and excreta (saliva, sputum, and feces). The drug also passes through the placental barrier and into milk in concentrations comparable to those in the plasma. From 50 to 70% of a dose of isoniazid is excreted in the urine in 24 hours.

Isoniazid is metabolized primarily by acetylation and dehydrazination. The rate of acetylation is genetically determined. Approximately 50% of Blacks and Caucasians are "slow inactivators"; the majority of Eskimos and Orientals are "rapid inactivators."

The rate of acetylation does not significantly alter the effectiveness of isoniazid. However, slow acetylation may lead to higher blood levels of the drug, and thus an increase in toxic reactions.

Pyridoxine deficiency (B_6) is sometimes observed in adults with high doses of isoniazid and is considered probably due to its competition with pyridoxal phosphate for the enzyme apotryptophanase.

INDICATIONS AND USAGE

For pulmonary tuberculosis in which organisms are susceptible, and when the patient has been titrated on the individual components and it has therefore been established that this fixed dosage is therapeutically effective.

This fixed-dosage combination drug is not recommended for initial therapy of tuberculosis or for preventive therapy.

In the treatment of tuberculosis, small numbers of resistant cells, present within large populations of susceptible cells, can rapidly become the predominating type. Since rapid emergence of resistance can occur, culture and susceptibility tests should be performed in the event of persistent positive cultures.

This drug is not indicated for the treatment of meningococcal infections or asymptomatic carriers of *N. meningitidis* to eliminate meningococci from the nasopharynx.

CONTRAINDICATIONS

Previous isoniazid-associated hepatic injury; severe adverse reactions to isoniazid, such as drug fever, chills, and arthritis; acute liver disease of any etiology. A history of previous hypersensitivity reaction to any of the rifamycins or to isoniazid, including drug-induced hepatitis.

WARNINGS

RIFAMATE (rifampin and isoniazid capsules USP) is a combination of two drugs, each of which has been associated with liver dysfunction. Liver function tests should be performed prior to therapy with RIFAMATE and periodically during treatment.

Rifampin

Rifampin has been shown to produce liver dysfunction. There have been fatalities associated with jaundice in patients with liver disease or receiving rifampin concomitantly with other hepatoxic agents. Since an increased risk may exist for individuals with liver disease, benefits must be weighed carefully against the risk of further liver damage.

Several studies of tumorigenicity potential have been done in rodents. In one strain of mice known to be particularly susceptible to the spontaneous development of hepatomas, rifampin given at a level 2–10 times the maximum dosage used clinically resulted in a significant increase in the occurrence of hepatomas in female mice of this strain after one year of administration.

There was no evidence of tumorigenicity in the males of this strain, in males or females of another mouse strain, or in rats.

Isoniazid

See the boxed warning.

PRECAUTIONS

Rifampin

Rifampin is not recommended for intermittent therapy; the patient should be cautioned against intentional or accidental interruption of the daily dosage regimen since rare renal hypersensitivity reactions have been reported when therapy was resumed in such cases.

Rifampin has been observed to increase the requirements for anticoagulant drugs of the coumarin type. The cause of the phenomenon is unknown. In patients receiving anticoagulants and rifampin concurrently, it is recommended that the prothrombin time be performed daily or as frequently as necessary to establish and maintain the required dose of anticoagulant.

Urine, feces, saliva, sputum, sweat, and tears may be colored red-orange by rifampin and its metabolites. Soft contact lenses may be permanently stained. Individuals to be treated should be made aware of these possibilities.

It has been reported that the reliability of oral contraceptives may be affected in some patients being treated for tuberculosis with rifampin in combination with at least one other antituberculosis drug. In such cases, alternative contraceptive measures may need to be considered.

It has also been reported that rifampin given in combination with other antituberculosis drugs may decrease the pharmacologic activity of methadone, oral hypoglycemics, digitoxin, quinidine, disopyramide, dapsone, and corticosteroids. In these cases, dosage adjustment of the interacting drugs is recommended.

Therapeutic levels of rifampin have been shown to inhibit standard microbiological assays for serum folate and vitamin B_{12}. Alternative methods must be considered when determining folate and vitamin B_{12} concentrations in the presence of rifampin.

Since rifampin has been reported to cross the placental barrier and appear in cord blood and in maternal milk, neonates and newborns of rifampin-treated mothers should be carefully observed for any evidence of untoward effects.

Isoniazid

All drugs should be stopped and an evaluation of the patient should be made at the first sign of a hypersensitivity reaction.

Use of isoniazid should be carefully monitored in the following:

1. Patients who are receiving phenytoin (diphenylhydantoin) concurrently. Isoniazid may decrease the excretion of phenytoin or may enhance its effects. To avoid phenytoin intoxication, appropriate adjustment of the anticonvulsant dose should be made.
2. Daily users of alcohol. Daily ingestion of alcohol may be associated with a higher incidence of isoniazid hepatitis.
3. Patients with current chronic liver disease or severe renal dysfunction.

Periodic ophthalmoscopic examination during isoniazid therapy is recommended when visual symptoms occur.

Usage in Pregnancy and Lactation

Rifampin

Although rifampin has been reported to cross the placental barrier and appear in cord blood, the effect of rifampin, alone or in combination with other antituberculosis drugs, on the human fetus is not known. An increase in congenital malformations, primarily spina bifida and cleft palate, has been reported in the offspring of rodents given oral doses of 150–250 mg/kg/day of rifampin during pregnancy.

The possible teratogenic potential in women capable of bearing children should be carefully weighed against the benefits of therapy.

Isoniazid

It has been reported that in both rats and rabbits, isoniazid may exert an embryocidal effect when administered orally during pregnancy, although no isoniazid-related congenital anomalies have been found in reproduction studies in mammalian species (mice, rats, and rabbits). Isoniazid should be prescribed during pregnancy only when therapeutically necessary. The benefit of preventive therapy should be weighed against a possible risk to the fetus. Preventive treatment generally should be started after delivery because of the increased risk of tuberculosis for new mothers.

Since isoniazid is known to cross the placental barrier and to pass into maternal breast milk, neonates and breast-fed infants of isoniazid treated mothers should be carefully observed for any evidence of adverse effects.

Carcinogenesis: Isoniazid has been reported to induce pulmonary tumors in a number of strains of mice.

ADVERSE REACTIONS

Rifampin

Nervous system reactions: headache, drowsiness, fatigue, ataxia, dizziness, inability to concentrate, mental confusion, visual disturbances, muscular weakness, pain in extremities, and generalized numbness

Gastrointestinal disturbances: in some patients heartburn, epigastric distress, anorexia, nausea, vomiting, gas, cramps, and diarrhea

Hepatic reactions: transient abnormalities in liver function tests (e.g., elevations in serum bilirubin, BSP, alkaline phosphatase, serum transaminases) have been observed. Rarely, hepatitis or a shocklike syndrome with hepatic involvement and abnormal liver function tests.

Renal reactions: elevations in BUN and serum uric acid have been reported. Rarely, hemolysis, hemoglobinuria, hematuria, interstitial nephritis, renal insufficiency, and acute renal failure have been noted. These are generally considered to be hypersensitivity reactions. They usually occur during intermittent therapy or when treatment is resumed following intentional or accidental interruption of a daily dosage regimen, and are reversible when rifampin is discontinued and appropriate therapy instituted.

Hematologic reactions: thrombocytopenia, transient leukopenia, hemolytic anemia, eosinophilia, and decreased hemoglobin have been observed. Thrombocytopenia has

Continued on next page

Rifamate—Cont.

occurred when rifampin and ethambutol were administered concomitantly according to an intermittent dose schedule twice weekly and in high doses.

Allergic and immunological reactions: occasionally pruritus, urticaria, rash, pemphigoid reaction, eosinophilia, sore mouth, sore tongue, and exudative conjunctivitis. Rarely, hemolysis, hemoglobinuria, hematuria, renal insufficiency or acute renal failure have been reported which are generally considered to be hypersensitivity reactions. These have usually occurred during intermittent therapy or when treatment was resumed following intentional or accidental interruption of a daily dosage regimen and were reversible when rifampin was discontinued and appropriate therapy instituted.

Although rifampin has been reported to have an immunosuppressive effect in some animal experiments, available human data indicate that this has no clinical significance.

Metabolic reactions: elevations in BUN and serum uric acid have occurred.

Miscellaneous reactions: fever and menstrual disturbances have been noted.

Isoniazid

The most frequent reactions are those affecting the nervous system and the liver.

Nervous system reactions: peripheral neuropathy is the most common toxic effect. It is dose-related, occurs most often in the malnourished and in those predisposed to neuritis (e.g., alcoholics and diabetics), and is usually preceded by paresthesias of the feet and hands. The incidence is higher in "slow inactivators."

Other neurotoxic effects, which are uncommon with conventional doses, are convulsions, toxic encephalopathy, optic neuritis and atrophy, memory impairment, and toxic psychosis.

Gastrointestinal reactions: nausea, vomiting, and epigastric distress

Hepatic reactions: elevated serum transaminases (SGOT; SGPT), bilirubinemia, bilirubinuria, jaundice, and occasionally severe and sometimes fatal hepatitis. The common prodromal symptoms are anorexia, nausea, vomiting, fatigue, malaise, and weakness. Mild and transient elevations of serum transaminase levels occurs in 10 to 20 percent of persons taking isoniazid. The abnormality usually occurs in the first 4 to 6 months of treatment but can occur at any time during therapy. In most instances, enzyme levels return to normal with no necessity to discontinue medication. In occasional instances, progressive liver damage occurs, with accompanying symptoms. In these cases, the drug should be discontinued immediately. The frequency of progressive liver damage increases with age. It is rare in persons under 20, but occurs in up to 2.3 percent of those over 50 years of age.

Hematologic reactions: agranulocytosis, hemolytic sideroblastic or aplastic anemia, thrombocytopenia, and eosinophilia

Hypersensitivity reactions: fever, skin eruptions (morbilliform, maculopapular, purpuric, or exfoliative), lymphadenopathy, and vasculitis

Metabolic and endocrine reactions: pyridoxine deficiency, pellagra, hyperglycemia, metabolic acidosis, and gynecomastia

Miscellaneous reactions: rheumatic syndrome and systemic lupus erythematosus-like syndrome

OVERDOSAGE

Rifampin

Signs and Symptoms

Nausea, vomiting, and increasing lethargy will probably occur within a short time after ingestion; actual unconsciousness may occur with severe hepatic involvement. Brownish-red or orange discoloration of the skin, urine, sweat, saliva, tears, and feces is proportional to amount ingested.

Liver enlargement, possibly with tenderness, can develop within a few hours after severe overdosage, and jaundice may develop rapidly. Hepatic involvement may be more marked in patients with prior impairment of hepatic function. Other physical findings remain essentially normal.

Direct and total bilirubin levels may increase rapidly with severe overdosage; hepatic enzyme levels may be affected, especially with prior impairment of hepatic function. A direct effect upon hemopoietic system, electrolyte levels, or acid-base balance is unlikely.

Isoniazid

Signs and Symptoms

Isoniazid overdosage produces signs and symptoms within 30 minutes to 3 hours. Nausea, vomiting, dizziness, slurring of speech, blurring of vision, visual hallucinations (including bright colors and strange designs), are among the early manifestations. With marked overdosage, respiratory distress and CNS depression, progressing rapidly from stupor to profound coma, are to be expected, along with severe, intractable seizures. Severe metabolic acidosis, acetonuria, and hyperglycemia are typical laboratory findings.

RIFAMATE (rifampin and isoniazid capsules USP)

Treatment

The airway should be secured and adequate respiratory exchange established. Only then should gastric emptying (lavage-aspiration) be attempted; this may be difficult because of seizures. Since nausea and vomiting are likely to be present, gastric lavage is probably preferable to induction of emesis.

Activated charcoal slurry instilled into the stomach following evacuation of gastric contents can help absorb any remaining drug in the GI tract. Antiemetic medication may be required to control severe nausea and vomiting.

Blood samples should be obtained for immediate determination of gases, electrolytes, BUN, glucose, etc. Blood should be typed and crossmatched in preparation for possible hemodialysis.

Rapid control of metabolic acidosis is fundamental to management. Intravenous sodium bicarbonate should be given at once and repeated as needed, adjusting subsequent dosage on the basis of laboratory findings (i.e., serum sodium, pH, etc.). At the same time, anticonvulsants should be given intravenously (i.e., barbiturates, diphenylhydantoin, diazepam) as required, and large doses of intravenous pyridoxine.

Forced osmotic diuresis must be started early and should be continued for some hours after clinical improvement to hasten renal clearance of drug and help prevent relapse. Fluid intake and output should be monitored.

Bile drainage may be indicated in presence of serious impairment of hepatic function lasting more than 24–48 hours. Under these circumstances and for severe cases, extracorporeal hemodialysis may be required; if this is not available, peritoneal dialysis can be used along with forced diuresis.

Along with measures based on initial and repeated determination of blood gases and other laboratory tests as needed, meticulous respiratory and other intensive care should be utilized to protect against hypoxia, hypotension, aspiration, pneumonitis, etc.

In patients with previously adequate hepatic function, reversal of liver enlargement and impaired hepatic excretory function probably will be noted within 72 hours, with rapid return toward normal thereafter.

Untreated or inadequately treated cases of gross isoniazid overdosage can terminate fatally, but good response has been reported in most patients brought under adequate treatment within the first few hours after drug ingestion.

DOSAGE AND ADMINISTRATION

In general, therapy should be continued until bacterial conversion and maximal improvement have occurred.

Adults: Two RIFAMATE (rifampin and isoniazid capsules USP) capsules (600 mg rifampin, 300 mg isoniazid) once daily, administered one hour before or two hours after a meal.

Concomitant administration of pyridoxine (B_6) is recommended in the malnourished, in those predisposed to neuropathy (e.g., diabetic), and in adolescents.

Susceptibility Testing

Rifampin

Rifampin susceptibility powders are available for both direct and indirect methods of determining the susceptibility of strains of mycobacteria. The MIC's of susceptible clinical isolates when determined in 7H10 or other non-egg-containing media have ranged from 0.1 to 2 mcg/ml.

Quantitative methods that require measurement of zone diameters give the most precise estimates of antibiotic susceptibility. One such procedure has been recommended for use with discs for testing susceptibility to rifampin. Interpretations correlate zone diameters from the disc test with MIC (minimal inhibitory concentration) values for rifampin.

HOW SUPPLIED

Capsules (opaque red), imprinted "RIFAMATE" on both ends of the capsule, containing 300 mg rifampin and 150 mg isoniazid; bottles of 60 (NDC 0068-0509-60).

Prescribing Information as of January 2001

Merrell Pharmaceuticals Inc.
Subsidiary of
Aventis Pharmaceuticals Inc.
Kansas City, MO 64137 USA
rfmp0101p

Shown in Product Identification Guide, page 307

RIFATER® ℞

[*rĭf ' uh-ter*]

(rifampin, isoniazid and pyrazinamide) Tablets

Prescribing Information as of April 2000

WARNING

Severe and sometimes fatal hepatitis associated with isoniazid therapy may occur and may develop even after many months of treatment. The risk of developing hepatitis is age related. Approximate case rates by age are: 0 per 1,000 for persons under 20 years of age, 3 per 1,000 for persons in the 20 to 34 year age group, 12 per 1,000 for persons in the 35 to 49 year age group, 23 per 1,000 for persons in the 50 to 64 year age group, and 8 per 1,000 for persons over 65 years of age. The risk of hepatitis is increased with daily consumption of alcohol. Precise data to provide a fatality rate for isoniazid-related hepatitis is not available; however, in a U.S. Public Health Service Surveillance Study of 13,838 persons taking isoniazid, there were 8 deaths among 174 cases of hepatitis.

Therefore, patients given isoniazid should be carefully monitored and interviewed at monthly intervals. Serum transaminase concentration becomes elevated in about 10% to 20% of patients, usually during the first few months of therapy, but it can occur at any time. Usually enzyme levels return to normal despite continuance of drug, but in some cases progressive liver dysfunction occurs. Patients should be instructed to report immediately any of the prodromal symptoms of hepatitis, such as fatigue, weakness, malaise, anorexia, nausea, or vomiting. If these symptoms appear or if signs suggestive of hepatic damage are detected, isoniazid should be discontinued promptly since continued use of the drug in these cases has been reported to cause a more severe form of liver damage.

Patients with tuberculosis should be given appropriate treatment with alternative drugs. If isoniazid must be reinstituted, it should be reinstituted only after symptoms and laboratory abnormalities have cleared. The drug should be restarted in very small and gradually increasing doses and should be withdrawn immediately if there is any indication of recurrent liver involvement. Treatment should be deferred in persons with acute hepatic diseases.

DESCRIPTION

RIFATER (rifampin/isoniazid/pyrazinamide) tablets are combination tablets containing 120 mg rifampin, 50 mg isoniazid, and 300 mg pyrazinamide for use in antibacterial therapy. The tablets also contain as inactive ingredients: povidone, carboxymethylcellulose sodium, calcium stearate, sodium lauryl sulfate, sucrose, talc, acacia, titanium dioxide, kaolin, magnesium carbonate, colloidal silicon dioxide, dried aluminum hydroxide gel, ferric oxide, black iron oxide, carnauba wax, white beeswax, colophony, hard paraffin, lecithin, shellac, and propylene glycol. The RIFATER triple therapy combination was developed for dosing convenience.

Rifampin is a semisynthetic antibiotic derivative of rifamycin SV. Rifampin is a red-brown crystalline powder very slightly soluble in water at neutral pH, freely soluble in chloroform, soluble in ethyl acetate and methanol. Its molecular weight is 822.95 and its chemical formula is $C_{43}H_{58}N_4O_{12}$. The chemical name for rifampin is either:

3-[[(4-methyl-1-piperazinyl) imino]-methyl]-rifamycin;

or

5,6,9,17,19,21-hexahydroxy-23methoxy-2,4,12,16,18,20,22 heptamethyl-8-[N-(4-methyl-1-piperazinyl)formimidoyl]-2,7-(epoxypentadeca[1,11,13]trienimino)naphtho-[2,1-b]furan-1,11 (2H)-dione 21-acetate.

Its structural formula is:

Isoniazid is the hydroxide of isonicotinic acid. It is a colorless or white crystalline powder or white crystals. It is odorless and slowly affected by exposure to air and light. It is freely soluble in water, sparingly soluble in alcohol and slightly soluble in chloroform and in ether. Its molecular weight is 137.14 and its chemical formula is $C_6H_7N_3O$.

The chemical name for isoniazid is 4-pyridinecarboxylic acid, hydrazide and its structural formula is:

Pyrazinamide, the pyrazine analogue of nicotinamide, is a white, crystalline powder, stable at room temperature, and sparingly soluble in water. The chemical name for pyrazinamide is pyrazinecarboxamide and its molecular weight is 123.11. Its chemical formula is $C_5H_5N_3O$ and its structural formula is:

CLINICAL PHARMACOLOGY

General

Rifampin. Rifampin is readily absorbed from the gastrointestinal tract. Peak serum levels in normal adults and pediatric populations vary widely from individual to individual. Following a single 600 mg oral dose of rifampin in healthy adults, the peak serum level averages 7 µg/mL but may vary from 4 to 32 µg/mL. Absorption of rifampin is reduced when the drug is ingested with food.

In normal subjects, the biological half-life of rifampin in serum averages about 3 hours after a 600 mg oral dose, with increases up to 5.1 hours reported after a 900 mg dose. With repeated administration, the half-life decreases and reaches

average values of approximately 2 to 3 hours. The half-life does not differ in patients with renal failure at doses not exceeding 600 mg daily and, consequently, no dosage adjustment is required. The half-life of rifampin at a dose of 720 mg daily has not been established in patients with renal failure. Following a single 900 mg oral dose of rifampin in patients with varying degrees of renal insufficiency, the half-life increased from 3.6 hours in normal subjects to 5.0, 7.3, and 11.0 hours in patients with glomerular filtration rates of 30–50 mL/min, less than 30 mL/min, and in anuric patients, respectively. Refer to the WARNINGS section for information regarding patients with hepatic insufficiency.
After absorption, rifampin is rapidly eliminated in the bile, and an enterohepatic circulation ensues. During this process, rifampin undergoes progressive deacetylation so that nearly all the drug in the bile is in this form in about 6 hours. This metabolite has antibacterial activity. Intestinal reabsorption is reduced by deacetylation, and elimination is facilitated. Up to 30% of a dose is excreted in the urine, with about half as unchanged drug.
Rifampin is widely distributed throughout the body. It is present in effective concentrations in many organs and body fluids, including cerebrospinal fluid. Rifampin is about 80% protein bound. Most of the unbound fraction is not ionized and therefore is diffused freely in tissues.

Isoniazid. After oral administration, isoniazid is readily absorbed from the GI tract and produces peak blood levels within 1 to 2 hours. It diffuses readily into all body fluids (cerebrospinal, pleural, and ascitic fluids), tissues, organs, and excreta (saliva, sputum, and feces). Isoniazid is not substantially bound to plasma proteins. The drug also passes through the placental barrier and into milk in concentrations comparable to those in the plasma. The plasma half-life of isoniazid in patients with normal renal and hepatic function ranges from 1–4 hours, depending on the rate of metabolism. From 50% to 70% of a dose of isoniazid is excreted in the urine within 24 hours, mostly as metabolites. Isoniazid is metabolized in the liver mainly by acetylation and dehydrazination. The rate of acetylation is genetically determined. Approximately 50% of African Americans and Caucasians are "slow inactivators" and the rest are "rapid inactivators"; the majority of Eskimos and Asians are "rapid inactivators." The rate of acetylation does not significantly alter the effectiveness of isoniazid. However, slow acetylation may lead to higher blood levels of the drug, and thus, an increase in toxic reactions.
Pyridoxin (B_6) deficiency is sometimes observed in adults with high doses of isoniazid and is probably due to its competition with pyridoxal phosphate for the enzyme apotryptophanase.

Pyrazinamide. Pyrazinamide is well absorbed from the gastrointestinal tract and attains peak plasma concentrations within 2 hours. Plasma concentrations generally range from 30 to 50 μg/mL with doses of 20 to 25 mg/kg. It is widely distributed in body tissues and fluids including the liver, lungs, and cerebrospinal fluid (CSF). The CSF concentration is approximately equal to concurrent steady-state plasma concentrations in patients with inflamed meninges. Pyrazinamide is approximately 10% bound to plasma proteins. The plasma half-life of pyrazinamide is 9 to 10 hours in patients with normal renal and hepatic function. The half-life of the drug may be prolonged in patients with impaired renal or hepatic function. Pyrazinamide is hydrolyzed in the liver to its major active metabolite, pyrazinoic acid. Pyrazinoic acid is hydroxylated to the main excretory product, 5-hydroxypyrazinoic acid.
Within 24 hours, approximately 70% of an oral dose of pyrazinamide is excreted in urine, mainly by glomerular filtration. About 4% to 14% of the dose is excreted as unchanged drug; the remainder is excreted as metabolites.

RIFATER

In a single-dose bioavailabilty study of five RIFATER tablets (Treatment A, n=23) versus RIFADIN 600 mg, isoniazid 250 mg, and pyrazinamide 1500 mg (Treatment B, n=24) administered concurrently in normal subjects, there was no difference in extent of absorption, as measured by the area under the plasma concentration versus time curve (AUC), of all three components. However, the mean peak plasma concentration of rifampin was approximately 18% lower following the single-dose administration of RIFATER tablets as compared to RIFADIN administered in combination with pyrazinamide and isoniazid. Mean (±SD) pharmacokinetic parameters are summarized in the following table.
[See first table above]
The effect of food on the pharmacokinetics of RIFATER tablets was not studied.

Microbiology

Rifampin, isoniazid, and pyrazinamide at therapeutic levels have demonstrated bactericidal activity against both intracellular and extracellular *Mycobacterium tuberculosis* organisms.

Mechanism of Action

Rifampin. Rifampin inhibits DNA-dependent RNA polymerase activity in susceptible *Mycobacterium tuberculosis* organisms. Specifically, it interacts with bacterial RNA polymerase, but does not inhibit the mammalian enzyme. Organisms resistant to rifampin are likely to be resistant to other rifamycins.

Isoniazid. Isoniazid kills actively growing tubercle bacilli by inhibiting the biosynthesis of mycolic acids which are major components of the cell wall of *Mycobacterium tuberculosis*.

Pyrazinamide. The exact mechanism of action by which pyrazinamide inhibits the growth of *Mycobacterium tuberculosis* organisms is unknown. *In vitro* and *in vivo* studies have demonstrated that pyrazinamide is only active at a slightly acidic pH (pH 5.5).

Parameter	C_{max} (μg/mL)		Half-life (hr)		Apparent Oral Clearance (L/hr)		Bioavailability (%)
Treatment	A	B	A	B	A	B	A
Isoniazid	3.09 ± 0.88	3.14 ± 0.92	2.80 ± 1.02	2.80 ± 1.11	24.02 ± 15.29	25.72 ± 18.38	100.6 ± 16.6
Rifampin	11.04 ± 3.08	13.61 ± 3.96	3.19 ± 0.63	3.41 ± 0.86	9.62 ± 3.00	8.30 ± 2.50	88.8 ± 16.5
Pyrazinamide	28.02 ± 4.52	29.21 ± 4.35	10.04 ± 1.54	10.08 ± 1.29	3.82 ± 0.65	3.70 ± 0.59	96.8 ± 7.6

Dose of Isoniazid, Rifampin and Pyrazinamide Administered as Separate Drugs

Patient Weight	Isoniazid (mg)	Rifampin (mg)	Pyrazinamide (mg)
<50 kg	300	450	1500
≥50 kg	300	600	2000

Dose of Isoniazid, Rifampin and Pyrazinamide Administered as RIFATER

Patient Weight	Number of Tablets	Isoniazid (mg)	Rifampin (mg)	Pyrazinamide (mg)
≤44 kg	4	200	480	1200
45 to 54 kg	5	250	600	1500
≥55 kg	6	300	720	1800

Negative Sputums/No. of Patients (Percent Negative)

Treatment	2 Months	6 Months	Follow-up Period*
RIFATER	91/96 (95%)	100/104 (96%)	99/101 (98%)
Separate†	99/108 (92%)	95/96 (99%)	105/106 (99%)

* The median follow-up time for all the RIFATER patients was 756 days with a range of 42 to 1325 days and 745 days with a range of 50 to 1427 days for the patients dosed with separate tablets and capsules.
† Isoniazid, rifampin, and pyrazinamide dosed as separate tablets and capsules.

Susceptibility Testing

Prior to initiation of therapy, appropriate specimens should be collected for identification of the infecting organism and *in vitro* susceptibility tests
Two standardized *in vitro* susceptibility methods are available for testing isoniazid, rifampin, and pyrazinamide against *Mycobacterium tuberculosis* organisms. The agar proportion method (CDC or NCCLS M24-P) utilizes Middlebrook 7H10 medium impregnated with isoniazid at 0.2 and 1.0 μg/mL for the final concentrations of drug. The final concentration for pyrazinamide is 25.0 μg/mL at pH 5.5. After 3 weeks of incubation MIC_{99} values are calculated by comparing the quantity of organisms growing in the medium-containing drug to the control cultures. Mycobacterial growth in the presence of drug ≥1% of the control indicates resistance.
The radiometric broth method employs the BACTEC 460 machine to compare the growth index from untreated control cultures to cultures grown in the presence of 0.2 and 1.0 μg/mL of isoniazid and 2.0 μg/mL of rifampin. Strict adherence to the manufacturer's instructions for sample processing and data interpretation is required for this assay. The radiometric broth method has not been approved for the testing of pyrazinamide.
Susceptibility test results obtained by the two different methods can only be compared if the appropriate rifampin or isoniazid concentrations are used for each test method as indicated above. Both test procedures require the use of *Mycobacterium tuberculosis* H37Rv, ATCC 27294, as a control organism.
The clinical relevance of *in vitro* susceptibility test results for mycobacterial species other than *Mycobacterium tuberculosis* using either the radiometric broth method or the proportion method has not been determined.

CLINICAL TRIALS

A total of 250 patients were enrolled in an open label, prospective, randomized, parallel group, active controlled trial, for the treatment of pulmonary tuberculosis. There were 241 patients evaluable for efficacy, 123 patients received isoniazid, rifampin and pyrazinamide as separate tablets and capsules for 56 days, and 118 patients received 4 to 6 RIFATER tablets based on body weight for 56 days. RIFATER tablets and the drugs dosed as separate tablets and capsules were administered based on body weight during the intensive phase of treatment according to the following table.
[See second table above]
During the continuation phase, both treatment groups received 450 mg of rifampin and 300 mg of isoniazid per day for 4 months if the patient weighed <50 kg or 600 mg of rifampin and 300 mg of isoniazid per day for 4 months if the patient weighed ≥50 kg. Patients were followed for occurrence of relapses for up to 30 months after the end of therapy.
There were no significant differences in the negative bacteriological sputum results (available in a subset of patients) between the two treatments at 2 and 6 months during the trial and during the follow-up period. See table below.
[See third table above]
For adverse events, see ADVERSE REACTIONS section.

INDICATIONS AND USAGE

RIFATER is indicated in the initial phase of the short-course treatment of pulmonary tuberculosis. During this phase, which should last 2 months, RIFATER should be administered on a daily, continuous basis (see DOSAGE AND ADMINISTRATION section).
Following the initial phase and treatment with RIFATER, treatment should be continued with rifampin and isoniazid (eg, RIFAMATE) for at least 4 months. Treatment should be continued for a longer period of time if the patient is still sputum or culture positive, if resistant organisms are present, or if the patient is HIV positive.
In the treatment of tuberculosis, the small number of resistant cells present within large populations of susceptible cells can rapidly become the predominant type. Since resistance can emerge rapidly, susceptibility tests should be performed in the event of persistent positive cultures during the course of treatment. Bacteriologic smears or cultures should be obtained before the start of therapy to confirm the susceptibility of the organism to rifampin, isoniazid, and pyrazinamide and they should be repeated throughout therapy to monitor response to the treatment. If test results show resistance to any of the components of RIFATER and the patient is not responding to therapy, the drug regimen should be modified.

CONTRAINDICATIONS

RIFATER is contraindicated in patients with a history of hypersensitivity to rifampin, isoniazid, pyrazinamide, or any of the components. Other contraindications include patients with severe hepatic damage; severe adverse reactions to isoniazid, such as drug fever, chills, and arthritis; patients with acute liver disease of any etiology; and patients with acute gout.

WARNINGS

RIFATER is a combination of the three drugs, rifampin, isoniazid, and pyrazinamide. Each of these individual drugs has been associated with liver dysfunction.

Rifampin. Rifampin has been shown to produce liver dysfunction. Fatalities associated with jaundice have occurred in patients with liver disease and in patients taking rifampin with other hepatoxic agents. Because RIFATER contains both rifampin and isoniazid, it should only be given with caution and under strict medical supervision to patients with impaired liver function. In these patients, careful monitoring of liver function, especially serum glutamic pyruvic transaminase (SGPT) and serum glutamic oxaloacetic transaminase (SGOT) should be carried out prior to ther-

Continued on next page

Rifater—Cont.

apy and then every 2 to 4 weeks during therapy. If signs of hepatocellular damage occur, RIFATER should be withdrawn.

In some cases, hyperbilirubinemia resulting from competition between rifampin and bilirubin for excretory pathways of the liver at the cell level can occur in the early days of treatment. An isolated report showing a moderate rise in bilirubin and/or transminase level is not in itself an indication for interrupting treatment; rather, the decision should be made after repeating the tests, noting trends in the levels, and considering them in conjunction with the patient's clinical condition.

Rifampin has enzyme-inducing properties, including induction of delta amino levulinic acid synthetase. Isolated reports have associated porphyria exacerbation with rifampin administration.

Isoniazid. See the boxed WARNING.

Since RIFATER contains isoniazid, ophthalmologic examinations (including ophthalmoscopy) should be done before treatment is started and periodically thereafter, even without occurrence of visual symptoms.

Pyrazinamide. Since RIFATER contains pyrazinamide, patients started on RIFATER should have baseline serum uric acid and liver function determinations. Patients with preexisting liver disease or those patients at increased risk for drug related hepatitis (eg, alcohol abusers) should be followed closely.

Because it contains pyrazinamide, RIFATER should be discontinued and not be resumed if signs of hepatocellular damage or hyperuricemia accompanied by an acute gouty arthritis appear. If hyperuricemia accompanied by an acute gouty arthritis occurs without liver dysfunction, the patient should be transferred to a regimen not containing pyrazinamide.

PRECAUTIONS

General

RIFATER should be used with caution in patients with a history of diabetes mellitus, as diabetes management may be more difficult.

Rifampin. For treatment of tuberculosis, rifampin is usually administered on a daily basis. Doses of rifampin (>600 mg) given once or twice weekly have resulted in a higher incidence of adverse reactions, including the "flu syndrome" (fever, chills and malaise); hematopoietic reactions (leukopenia, thrombocytopenia, or acute hemolytic anemia); cutaneous, gastrointestinal, and hepatic reactions; shortness of breath; shock and renal failure.

The patient should be advised that the reliability of oral contraceptives may be affected; consideration should be given to using alternative contraceptive measures.

Isoniazid. All drugs should be stopped and an evaluation of the patient should be made at the first sign of a hypersensitivity reaction. Use of RIFATER, because it contains isoniazid, should be carefully monitored in the following:

1. Patients who are receiving phenytoin (diphenylhydantoin) concurrently. Isoniazid may decrease the excretion of phenytoin or may enhance its effects. To avoid phenytoin intoxication, appropriate adjustment of the anticonvulsant dose should be made.
2. Daily users of alcohol. Daily ingestion of alcohol may be associated with a higher incidence of isoniazid hepatitis.
3. Patients with current chronic liver disease or severe renal dysfunction.

Pyrazinamide. Pyrazinamide inhibits renal excretion of urates, frequently resulting in hyperuricemia which is usually asymptomatic. If hyperuricemia is accompanied by acute gouty arthritis, RIFATER, because it contains pyrazinamide, should be discontinued.

Information for Patients

Food Interactions: Because isoniazid has some monoamine oxidase inhibiting activity, an interaction with tyramine-containing foods (cheese, red wine) may occur. Diamine oxidase may also be inhibited, causing exaggerated response (eg, headache, sweating, palpitations, flushing, hypotension) to foods containing histamine (eg, skipjack, tuna, other tropical fish). Tyramine- and histamine-containing foods should be avoided in patients receiving RIFATER.

RIFATER, because it contains rifampin, may produce a reddish coloration of the urine, sweat, sputum, and tears, and the patient should be forewarned of this. Soft contact lenses may be permanently stained.

Patients should be instructed to take RIFATER either 1 hour before or 2 hours after a meal.

Patients should be instructed to notify their physicians promptly if they experience any of the following: fever, loss of appetite, malaise, nausea and vomiting, darkened urine, yellowish discoloration of the skin and eyes, pain or swelling of the joints.

Compliance with the full course of therapy must be emphasized, and the importance of not missing any doses must be stressed.

Laboratory Tests

A complete blood count (CBC), liver function tests, and blood uric acid determinations should be obtained prior to instituting therapy and periodically throughout the course of therapy. Because of a possible transient rise in transaminase and bilirubin values, blood for baseline clinical chemistries should be obtained before RIFATER dosing.

Drug Interactions

Rifampin. Enzyme Induction: Rifampin is known to induce certain cytochrome P-450 enzymes. Coadministration of RIFATER, because it contains rifampin, with drugs that undergo biotransformation through these metabolic pathways may accelerate elimination. To maintain optimum therapeutic blood levels, dosages of drugs metabolized by these enzymes may require adjustment when starting or stopping concomitantly administered rifampin.

Rifampin has been reported to accelerate the metabolism of the following drugs: anticonvulsants (eg, phenytoin), antiarrythmics (eg, disopyramide, mexiletine, quinidine, tocainide), anticoagulants, antifungals (eg, fluconazole, itraconazole, ketoconazole), barbiturates, beta-blockers, calcium channel blockers (eg, diltiazem, nifedipine, verapamil), chloramphenicol, ciprofloxacin, corticosteroids, cyclosporine, cardiac glycoside preparations, clofibrate, oral contraceptives, dapsone, diazepam, haloperidol, oral hypoglycemic agents (sulfonylureas), methadone, narcotic analgesics, nortriptyline, progestins, and theophylline. It may be necessary to adjust dosages of these drugs if they are given concurrently with RIFATER since it contains rifampin.

Rifampin has been observed to increase the requirements for anticoagulant drugs of the coumarin type. In patients receiving anticoagulants and RIFATER concurrently, it is recommended that the prothrombin time be performed daily or as frequently as necessary to establish and maintain the required dose of anticoagulant.

Concurrent use of ketoconazole and rifampin has resulted in decreased serum concentration of both drugs. Concurrent use of rifampin and enalapril has resulted in decreased concentrations of enalaprilat, the active metabolite of enalapril. Since RIFATER contains rifampin, dosage adjustments should be made if RIFATER is concurrently administered with ketoconazole or enalapril if indicated by the patient's clinical condition.

Other Interactions: Concomitant antacid administration may reduce the absorption of rifampin. Daily doses of RIFATER, because it contains rifampin, should be given at least 1 hour before the ingestion of antacids.

Probenecid and cotrimoxazole have been reported to increase the blood level of rifampin.

When rifampin is given concomitantly with either halothane or isoniazid the potential for hepatotoxicity is increased. The concomitant use of RIFATER, because it contains both rifampin and isoniazid, and halothane should be avoided. Patients receiving both rifampin and isoniazid as in RIFATER should be monitored closely for hepatotoxicity. See the boxed WARNING.

Plasma concentrations of sulfapyridine may be reduced following the concomitant administration of sulfasalazine and RIFATER, because it contains rifampin. This finding may be the result of alteration in the colonic bacteria responsible for the reduction of sulfasalazine to sulfapyridine and mesalamine.

Isoniazid. Enzyme Inhibition: Isoniazid is known to inhibit certain cytochrome P-450 enzymes. Coadministration of isoniazid with drugs that undergo biotransformation through these metabolic pathways may decrease elimination. Consequently, dosages of drugs metabolized by these enzymes may require adjustment when starting or stopping concomitantly administered RIFATER, because it contains isoniazid, to maintain optimum therapeutic blood levels.

Isoniazid has been reported to inhibit the metabolism of the following drugs: anticonvulsants (eg, carbamazepine, phenytoin, primidone, valproic acid), benzodiazepines (eg, diazepam), haloperidol, ketoconazole, theophylline, and warfarin. It may be necessary to adjust the dosages of these drugs if they are given concurrently with RIFATER because it contains isoniazid. The impact of the competing effects of rifampin and isoniazid on the metabolism of these drugs is unknown.

Other Interactions: Concomitant antacid administration may reduce the absorption of isoniazid. Ingestion with food may also reduce the absorption of isoniazid. Daily doses of RIFATER, because it contains isoniazid, should be given on an empty stomach at least 1 hour before the ingestion of antacids or food.

Corticosteroids (eg, prednisolone) may decrease the serum concentration of isoniazid by increasing acetylation rate and/or renal clearance. Para-aminosalicylic acid may increase the plasma concentration and elimination half-life of isoniazid by competition of acetylating enzymes.

Pharmacodynamic Interactions: Daily ingestion of alcohol may be associated with a higher incidence of isoniazid hepatitis. Isoniazid, when given concomitantly with rifampin, has been reported to increase the hepatotoxicity of both drugs. Patients receiving both rifampin and isoniazid as in RIFATER should be monitored closely for hepatotoxicity.

The CNS effects of meperidine (drowsiness), cycloserine (dizziness, drowsiness), and disulfiram (acute behavioral and coordination changes) may be exaggerated when concomitant RIFATER, because it contains isoniazid, is given. Concurrent RIFATER, because it contains isoniazid, and levodopa administration may produce symptoms of excess catecholamine stimulation (agitation, flushing, palpitations) or lack of levodopa effect.

Isoniazid may produce hyperglycemia and lead to loss of glucose control in patients on oral hypoglycemics.

Fast acetylation of isoniazid may produce high concentrations of hydrazine that facilitate deflorination of enflurane. Renal function should be monitored in patients receiving both RIFATER and enflurane.

Food Interactions: Because isoniazid has some monoamine oxidase inhibiting activity, an interaction with tyramine-containing foods (cheese, red wine) may occur. Diamine oxidase may also be inhibited, causing exaggerated response (eg, headache, sweating, palpitations, flushing, hypotension) to foods containing histamine (eg, skipjack, tuna, other tropical fish). Tyramine- and histamine-containing foods should be avoided by patients receiving RIFATER.

Drug/Laboratory Tests Interaction

Rifampin. Therapeutic levels of rifampin have been shown to inhibit standard microbiological assays for serum folate and vitamin B_{12}. Therefore, alternative assay methods should be considered. Transient abnormalities in liver function tests (eg, elevation in serum bilirubin, abnormal bromsulphalein [BSP] excretion, alkaline phosphatase and serum transaminases), and reduced biliary excretion of contrast media used for visualization of the gallbladder have also been observed. Therefore, these tests should be performed before the morning dose of RIFATER.

Rifampin and isoniazid have been reported to alter vitamin D metabolism. In some cases, reduced levels of circulating 25-hydroxy vitamin D and 1,25-dihydroxy vitamin D have been accompanied by reduced serum calcium and phosphate, and elevated parathyroid hormone.

Pyrazinamide. Pyrazinamide has been reported to interfere with ACETEST® and KETOSTIX® urine tests to produce a pink-brown color.

Carcinogenesis, Mutagenesis, Impairment of Fertility

Increased frequency of chromosomal aberrations was observed *in vitro* in lymphocytes obtained from patients treated with combinations of rifampin, isoniazid, and pyrazinamide and combinations of streptomycin, rifampin, isoniazid, and pyrazinamide.

Rifampin. There are no known human data on long-term potential for carcinogenicity, mutagenicity, or impairment of fertility. A few cases of accelerated growth of lung carcinoma have been reported in man, but a causal relationship with the drug has not been established. An increase in the incidence of hepatomas in female mice (of a strain known to be particularly susceptible to the spontaneous development of hepatomas) was observed when rifampicin was administered in doses two to ten times the average daily human dose for 60 weeks followed by an observation period of 46 weeks. No evidence of carcinogenicity was found in male mice of the same strain, mice of a different strain, or rats under similar experimental conditions.

Rifampin has been reported to possess immunosuppressive potential in rabbits, mice, rats, guinea pigs, human lymphocytes *in vitro*, and humans. Antitumor activity *in vitro* has also been shown with rifampin.

There was no evidence of mutagenicity in bacteria, *Drosophila melanogaster*, or mice. An increase in chromatid breaks was noted when whole blood cell cultures were treated with rifampin.

Isoniazid. Isoniazid has been reported to induce pulmonary tumors in a number of strains of mice.

Pyrazinamide. In lifetime bioassays in rats and mice, pyrazinamide was administered in the diet at concentrations of up to 10,000 ppm. This resulted in estimated daily doses of 2 g/kg for the mouse, or 40 times the maximum human dose, and 0.5 g/kg for the rat, or 10 times the maximum human dose. Pyrazinamide was not carcinogenic in rats or male mice and no conclusion was possible for female mice.

Pyrazinamide was not mutagenic in the Ames bacterial test, but induced chromosomal aberrations in human lymphocyte cell cultures.

Pregnancy – Teratogenic Effects

Category C. Animal reproduction studies have not been conducted with RIFATER. It is also not known whether RIFATER can cause fetal harm when administered to a pregnant woman. RIFATER should be given to a pregnant woman only if clearly needed.

Rifampin. Although rifampin has been reported to cross the placental barrier and appear in cord blood, the effect of rifampin, alone or in combination with other antituberculosis drugs, on the human fetus is not known. An increase in congenital malformations, primarily spina bifida and cleft palate, has been reported in the offspring of rodents given oral doses of 150 to 250 mg/kg/day of rifampin during pregnancy. The possible teratogenic potential in women capable of bearing children should be carefully weighed against the benefits of RIFATER therapy.

Isoniazid. It has been reported that in both rats and rabbits, isoniazid may exert an embryocidal effect when administered orally during pregnancy, although no isoniazid-related congenital anomalies have been found in reproduction studies in mammalian species (mice, rats, and rabbits). RIFATER, because it contains isoniazid, should be prescribed during pregnancy only when therapeutically necessary. The benefit of preventive therapy should be weighed against a possible risk to the fetus. Preventive treatment generally should be started after delivery because of the increased risk of tuberculosis for new mothers.

Pyrazinamide. Animal reproduction studies have not been conducted with pyrazinamide. It is also not known whether pyrazinamide can cause fetal harm when administered to a pregnant woman. RIFATER, because it contains pyrazinamide, should be given to a pregnant women only if clearly needed.

Pregnancy – Non-Teratogenic Effects

It is not known whether RIFATER can affect reproduction capacity.

Rifampin. When administered during the last few weeks of pregnancy, rifampin can cause postnatal hemorrhages in the mother and infant. In this case, treatment with vitamin K may be indicated for postnatal hemorrhage.

Nursing Mothers

Since rifampin, isoniazid, and pyrazinamide are known to pass into maternal breast milk, a decision should be made whether to discontinue nursing or to discontinue RIFATER, taking into account the importance of the drug to the mother.

Pediatric Use

Safety and effectiveness in pediatric patients under the age of 15 have not been established.

Geriatric Use

Clinical studies of RIFATER did not include sufficient numbers of subjects aged 65 and over to determine whether they respond differently from younger subjects. Other reported clinical experience has not identified differences in responses between the elderly and younger patients. Caution should therefore be observed in using rifampin in elderly patients. (See WARNINGS)

ADVERSE REACTIONS

Adverse Experiences During the Clinical Trial

Adverse event data reported for the RIFATER and the separate drug treatment groups during the first 2 months of the trial are shown in the table below.

Adverse Events Reported During the Clinical Study

Adverse Events by Body Systems During First 2 Months of Trial	Number of Patients With Adverse Events* RIFATER n = 122‡	Separate† n = 123‡
Cutaneous (rash, erythrodema, erythema, exfoliative dermatitis, Lyell syndrome, urticaria, localized skin rash, diffuse skin rash, pruritus, generalized hypersensitivity)	8 (7%)	21 (17%)
Gastrointestinal (nausea, vomiting, digestive pain, diarrhea)	8 (7%)	14 (11%)
Musculoskeletal (arthralgia, long bones pain, phlebitis, localized joint pain, diffuse joint pain, edema of the legs)	5 (4%)	8 (7%)
Hearing and Vestibular (tinnitus, vertigo, vertigo with loss of equilibrium)	3 (2%)	6 (5%)
Liver and Biliary (hepatitis with conjunctival jaundice, hepatitis with deep jaundice)	0 (0%)	2 (2%)
Central and Peripheral Nervous System (sweating, headache, insomnia, diffuse paresthesia of the legs, anxiety, diabetic coma)	5 (4%)	4 (3%)
Total Body (spiking fever, persistent fever)	2 (2%)	4 (3%)
Cardiorespiratory (tightness in chest, coughing, diffuse chest pain, hemoptysis, angina, palpitation, total pneumothorax)	8 (7%)	3 (2%)
Total number of patients with one or more adverse events	29	43

* A given patient may have experienced ≥1 adverse event.

† Isoniazid, rifampin and pyrazinamide dosed as separate tablets and capsules.

‡ A total of 250 patients (124 RIFATER; 126 separate) were originally enrolled in the study. Five patients (2 RIFATER; 3 separate) were excluded due to admission errors.

No serious adverse events were reported in the patients receiving RIFATER tablets. Three serious adverse events were reported in the patients given isoniazid, rifampin, and pyrazinamide as separate tablets and capsules. The three serious adverse events were two general hypersensitivity reactions and one jaundice reaction.

There were no significant differences between the two treatment groups in standard liver function, renal function and hematological laboratory test values measured at baseline and after 8 weeks of treatment. As would be expected for these drugs, there were alterations in liver enzymes (SGOT, SGPT) and serum uric acid levels. The adverse reactions reported during therapy with RIFATER are consistent with those described below for the individual components.

Adverse Reactions Reported for Individual Components

Rifampin, Gastrointestinal: Heartburn, epigastric distress, anorexia, nausea, vomiting, jaundice, flatulence, cramps, and diarrhea have been noted in some patients. Although *Clostridium difficile* has been shown *in vitro* to be sensitive to rifampin, pseudomembranous colitis has been reported with the use of rifampin (and other broad spectrum antibiotics). Therefore, it is important to consider this diagnosis in patients who develop diarrhea in association with antibiotic use. Rarely, hepatitis or a shocklike syndrome with hepatic involvement and abnormal liver function tests has been reported.

Hematologic: Thrombocytopenia has occurred primarily with high dose intermittent therapy, but has also been noted after resumption of interrupted treatment. It rarely occurs during well-supervised daily therapy. This effect is reversible if the drug is discontinued as soon as purpura occurs. Cerebral hemorrhage and fatalities have been reported when rifampin administration has been continued or resumed after the appearance of purpura.

Transient leukopenia, hemolytic anemia, and decreased hemoglobin have been observed.

Central Nervous System: Headache, fever, drowsiness, fatigue, ataxia, dizziness, inability to concentrate, mental confusion, behavioral changes, muscular weakness, pains in extremities, and generalized numbness have been observed.

Rare reports of myopathy have also been observed.

Ocular: Visual disturbances have been observed.

Endocrine: Menstrual disturbances have been observed.

Renal: Elevations in BUN and serum uric acid have been reported. Rarely, hemolysis, hemoglobinuria, hematuria, interstitial nephritis, renal insufficiency, and acute renal failure have been noted. These are generally considered to be hypersensitivity reactions. They usually occur during intermittent therapy or when treatment is resumed following intentional or accidental interruption of a daily dosage regimen, and are reversible when rifampin is discontinued and appropriate therapy instituted.

Dermatologic: Cutaneous reactions are mild and self-limiting and do not appear to be hypersensitivity reactions. Typically, they consist of flushing and itching with or without a rash. More serious cutaneous reactions which may be due to hypersensitivity occur but are uncommon.

Hypersensitivity Reactions: Occasionally pruritus, urticaria, rash, pemphigoid reaction, eosinophilia, sore mouth, sore tongue and conjunctivitis have been observed.

Miscellaneous: Edema of the face and extremities have been reported. Other reactions which have occurred with intermittent dosage regimens include "flu" syndrome (such as episodes of fever, chills, headache, dizziness, and bone pain), shortness of breath, wheezing, decrease in blood pressure and shock. The "flu" syndrome may also appear if rifampin is taken irregularly by the patient or if daily administration is resumed after a drug free interval.

Isoniazid. The most frequent reactions are those affecting the nervous system and the liver. See the boxed WARNING.

Nervous System: Peripheral neuropathy is the most common toxic effect. It is dose-related, occurs most often in the malnourished and in those predisposed to neuritis (eg, alcoholics and diabetics), and is usually preceded by paresthesias of the feet and hands. The incidence is higher in "slow inactivators."

Other neurotoxic effects, which are uncommon with conventional doses, are convulsions, toxic encephalopathy, optic neuritis and atrophy, memory impairment, and toxic psychosis.

Gastrointestinal: Nausea, vomiting, and epigastric distress.

Hepatic: Elevated serum transaminases (SGOT, SGPT), bilirubinemia, bilirubinuria, jaundice, and occasionally severe and sometimes fatal hepatitis. The common prodromal symptoms are anorexia, nausea, vomiting, fatigue, malaise, and weakness. Mild and transient elevation of serum transaminase levels occurs in 10 to 20% of persons taking isoniazid. The abnormality usually occurs in the first 4 to 6 months of treatment but can occur at any time during therapy. In most instances, enzyme levels return to normal with no necessity to discontinue medication. In occasional instances, progressive liver damage occurs, with accompanying symptoms. In these cases, the drug should be discontinued immediately. The frequency of progressive liver damage increases with age. It is rare in persons under 20, but occurs in up to 2.3% of those over 50 years of age.

Hematologic: Agranulocytosis; hemolytic, sideroblastic, or aplastic anemia; thrombocytopenia; and eosinophilia.

Hypersensitivity Reactions: Fever, skin eruptions (morbilliform, maculopapular, purpuric, or exfoliative), lymphadenopathy, and vasculitis.

Metabolic and Endocrine: Pyridoxine deficiency, pellagra, hyperglycemia, metabolic acidosis, and gynecomastia.

Miscellaneous: Rheumatic syndrome and systemic lupus erythematosus-like syndrome.

Pyrazinamide. The principal adverse effect is a hepatic reaction (see WARNINGS). Hepatotoxicity appears to be dose related and may appear at any time during therapy. Pyrazinamide can cause hyperuricemia and gout (see PRECAUTIONS).

Gastrointestinal: GI disturbances including nausea, vomiting, and anorexia have also been reported.

Hematologic and Lymphatic: Thrombocytopenia and sideroblastic anemia with erythroid hyperplasia, vacuolation of erythrocytes and increased serum concentration have occurred rarely with this drug. Adverse effects on blood clotting mechanisms have also been rarely reported.

Other: Mild arthralgia and myalgia have been reported frequently. Hypersensitivity reactions including rashes, urticaria, and pruritus have been reported. Fever, acne, photosensitivity, porphyria, dysuria, and interstitial nephritis have been reported rarely.

OVERDOSAGE

RIFATER. There is no human experience with RIFATER overdosage.

Rifampin. Non-fatal overdoses with as high as 12 g of rifampin have been reported.

One case of fatal overdose is known: A 26-year-old man died after self-administering 60 g of rifampin.

Isoniazid. Untreated or inadequately treated cases of gross isoniazid overdosage can be fatal, but good response has been reported in most patients treated within the first few hours after drug ingestion.

Ingested acutely, as little as 1.5 g isoniazid may cause toxicity in adults. Doses of 35 to 40 mg/kg have resulted in seizures. Ingestion of 80 to 150 mg/kg isoniazid has been associated with severe toxicity and, if untreated, significant mortality.

Pyrazinamide. Overdosage experience with pyrazinamide is limited.

Signs and Symptoms

The following signs and symptoms have been seen with each individual component in an overdosage situation.

Rifampin. Nausea, vomiting, and increasing lethargy will probably occur within a short time after rifampin overdosage; unconsciousness may occur when there is severe hepatic disease. Brownish red or orange discoloration of the skin, urine, sweat, saliva, tears, and feces will occur, and its intensity is proportional to the amount ingested.

Liver enlargement, possibly with tenderness, can develop within a few hours after severe overdosage; bilirubin levels may increase and jaundice may develop rapidly. Hepatic involvement may be more marked in patients with prior impairment of hepatic function. Other physical findings remain essentially normal. A direct effect upon the hematopoietic system, electrolyte levels, or acid-base balance is unlikely.

Isoniazid. Isoniazid overdosage produces signs and symptoms within 30 minutes to 3 hours. Nausea, vomiting, dizziness, slurring of speech, blurring of vision, and visual hallucinations (including bright colors and strange designs) are among the early manifestations. With marked overdosage, respiratory distress and CNS depression progressing rapidly from stupor to profound coma, are to be expected along with severe, intractable seizures. Severe metabolic acidosis, acetonuria, and hyperglycemia are typical laboratory findings.

Pyrazinamide. In one case of pyrazinamide overdosage, abnormal liver function tests developed. These spontaneously reverted to normal when the drug was stopped.

Treatment

The airway should be secured and adequate respiratory exchange should be established in cases of overdosage with RIFATER.

Obtain blood samples for immediate determination of gases, electrolytes, BUN, glucose, etc; type and cross-match blood in preparation for possible hemodialysis.

Gastric lavage within the first 2 to 3 hours after ingestion is advised, but it should not be attempted until convulsions are under control. To treat convulsions, administer IV diazepam or short-acting barbiturates, and IV pyridoxine (usually 1 mg/1 mg isoniazid ingested). Following evacuation of gastric contents, the instillation of activated charcoal slurry into the stomach may help absorb any remaining drug from the gastrointestinal tract. Antiemetic medication may be required to control severe nausea and vomiting.

RAPID CONTROL OF METABOLIC ACIDOSIS IS FUNDAMENTAL TO MANAGEMENT. Give IV sodium bicarbonate at once and repeat as needed, adjusting subsequent dosage on the basis of laboratory findings (ie, serum sodium, pH, etc).

Forced osmotic diuresis must be started early and should be continued for some hours after clinical improvement to hasten renal clearance of drug and help prevent relapse; monitor fluid intake and output.

Hemodialysis is advised for severe cases; if this is not available, peritoneal dialysis can be used along with forced diuresis.

Along with measures based on initial and repeated determination of blood gases and other laboratory tests as needed, utilize meticulous respiratory and other intensive care to protect against hypoxia, hypotension, aspiration pneumonitis, etc.

DOSAGE AND ADMINISTRATION

Adults: Patients should be given the following single daily dose of RIFATER either 1 hour before or 2 hours after a meal with a full glass of water.

Patients weighing ≤44 kg – 4 tablets

Patients weighing between 45–54 kg – 5 tablets

Patients weighing ≥55 kg – 6 tablets

Pediatric Patients: The ratio of the drugs in RIFATER may not be appropriate in pediatric patients under the age of 15 (eg, higher mg/kg doses of isoniazid are usually given in pediatric patients than adults).

RIFATER is recommended in the initial phase of short-course therapy which is usually continued for 2 months. The Advisory Council for the Elimination of Tuberculosis, the American Thoracic Society, and the Centers for Disease Control and Prevention recommend that either streptomycin or ethambutol be added as a fourth drug in a regimen containing isoniazid (INH), rifampin and pyrazinamide for initial treatment of tuberculosis unless the likelihood of INH or rifampin resistance is very low. The need for a fourth drug should be reassessed when the results of sus-

Continued on next page

Rifater—Cont.

ceptibility testing are known. If community rates of INH resistance are currently less than 4%, an initial treatment regimen with less than four drugs may be considered.
Following the initial phase, treatment should be continued with rifampin and isoniazid (eg, RIFAMATE®) for at least 4 months. Treatment should be continued for longer if the patient is still sputum or culture positive, if resistant organisms are present, or if the patient is HIV positive.
Concomitant administration of pyridoxine (B_6) is recommended in the malnourished, in those predisposed to neuropathy (eg, alcoholics and diabetics), and in adolescents.
See CLINICAL PHARMACOLOGY: General for dosing information in patients with renal failure.

HOW SUPPLIED

RIFATER tablets are light beige, smooth, round, and shiny sugar-coated tablets imprinted with "RIFATER" in black ink and contain 120 mg rifampin, 50 mg isoniazid, and 300 mg pyrazinamide, and are supplied as:
Bottles of 60 tablets (NDC 0088-0576-41).
Storage Conditions: Store at controlled room temperature 59–86°F (15–30°C). Protect from excessive humidity.

REFERENCE 1. National Committee for Clinical Laboratory Standards. 1990. Antimycobacterial Susceptibility Testing (Proposed Standard). Document M24-P.

Prescribing Information as of April 2000
Rx only
Merrell Pharmaceuticals Inc.
Subsidiary of Aventis Pharmaceuticals Inc.
Kansas City, MO 64137 USA
www.aventispharma-us.com
Rifater Tablets are manufactured by:
GRUPPO LEPETIT S.p.A.
20020 Lainate, Italy
MADE IN ITALY rftp0400p
Shown in Product Identification Guide, page 307

RILUTEK® ℞
(riluzole) Tablets
[rĭl-ū-tĕk]

Prescribing Information as of May 2003

DESCRIPTION

RILUTEK® (riluzole) is a member of the benzothiazole class. Chemically, riluzole is 2-amino-6-(trifluoromethoxy) benzothiazole. Its molecular formula is $C_8H_5F_3N_2OS$ and its molecular weight is 234.2. Its structural formula is as follows:

[structural formula: F_3C–O–benzothiazole ring with S, N, and NH_2]

Riluzole is a white to slightly yellow powder that is very soluble in dimethylformamide, dimethylsulfoxide and methanol, freely soluble in dichloromethane, sparingly soluble in 0.1 N HCl and very slightly soluble in water and in 0.1 N NaOH. RILUTEK is available as a capsule-shaped, white, film-coated tablet for oral administration containing 50 mg of riluzole. Each tablet is engraved with "RPR 202" on one side.
Inactive Ingredients: Core: anhydrous dibasic calcium phosphate, USP; microcrystalline cellulose, NF; anhydrous colloidal silica, NF; magnesium stearate, NF; croscarmellose sodium, NF. **Film coating:** hypromellose, USP; polyethylene glycol 6000; titanium dioxide, USP.

CLINICAL PHARMACOLOGY

Mechanism of Action

The etiology and pathogenesis of amyotrophic lateral sclerosis (ALS) are not known, although a number of hypotheses have been advanced. One hypothesis is that motor neurons, made vulnerable through either genetic predisposition or environmental factors, are injured by glutamate. In some cases of familial ALS the enzyme superoxide dismutase has been found to be defective.
The mode of action of RILUTEK is unknown. Its pharmacological properties include the following, some of which may be related to its effect: 1) an inhibitory effect on glutamate release, 2) inactivation of voltage-dependent sodium channels, and 3) ability to interfere with intracellular events that follow transmitter binding at excitatory amino acid receptors.
Riluzole has also been shown, in a single study, to delay median time to death in a transgenic mouse model of ALS. These mice express human superoxide dismutase bearing one of the mutations found in one of the familial forms of human ALS.
It is also neuroprotective in various *in vivo* experimental models of neuronal injury involving excitotoxic mechanisms. In *in vitro* tests, riluzole protected cultured rat motor neurons from the excitotoxic effects of glutamic acid and prevented the death of cortical neurons induced by anoxia.
Due to its blockade of glutamatergic neurotransmission, riluzole also exhibits myorelaxant and sedative properties in animal models at doses of 30 mg/kg (about 20 times the recommended human daily dose) and anticonvulsant properties at a dose of 2.5 mg/kg (about 2 times the recommended human daily dose).

Pharmacokinetics

Riluzole is well-absorbed (approximately 90%), with average absolute oral bioavailability of about 60% (CV=30%). Pharmacokinetics are linear over a dose range of 25 to 100 mg given every 12 hours. A high fat meal decreases absorption, reducing AUC by about 20% and peak blood levels by about 45%. The mean elimination half-life of riluzole is 12 hours (CV=35%) after repeated doses. With multiple-dose administration, riluzole accumulates in plasma by about twofold and steady-state is reached in less than 5 days. Riluzole is 96% bound to plasma proteins, mainly to albumin and lipoproteins over the clinical concentration range.
The 50 mg market tablet was equivalent, with respect to AUC, to the tablet used in the dose ranging clinical trials, while the C_{max} was approximately 30% higher. Both tablets have been used in clinical trials. However, if doses greater than those recommended are given, it is likely that higher plasma levels will be achieved, the safety of which has not been established (see DOSAGE AND ADMINISTRATION).

Metabolism and Elimination

Riluzole is extensively metabolized to six major and a number of minor metabolites, not all of which have been identified. Some metabolites appear pharmacologically active in *in vitro* assays. The metabolism of riluzole is mostly hepatic and consists of cytochrome P450-dependent hydroxylation and glucuronidation.
There is marked interindividual variability in the clearance of riluzole, probably attributable to variability of CYP 1A2 activity, the principal isozyme involved in N-hydroxylation.
In vitro studies using liver microsomes show that hydroxylation of the primary amine group producing N-hydroxyriluzole is the main metabolic pathway in human, monkey, dog and rabbit. In humans, cytochrome P450 1A2 is the principal isozyme involved in N-hydroxylation. *In vitro* studies predict that CYP 2D6, CYP 2C19, CYP 3A4 and CYP 2E1 are unlikely to contribute significantly to riluzole metabolism in humans. Whereas direct glucuroconjugation of riluzole (involving the glucurotransferase isoform UGT-HP4) is very slow in human liver microsomes, N-hydroxyriluzole is readily conjugated at the hydroxylamine group resulting in the formation of O- (>90%) and N-glucuronides.
Following a single 150 mg dose of ^{14}C-riluzole to 6 healthy males, 90% and 5% of the radioactivity was recovered in the urine and feces respectively over a period of 7 days. Glucuronides accounted for more than 85% of the metabolites in urine. Only 2% of a riluzole dose was recovered in the urine as unchanged drug.

Special Populations

Hepatic Impairment: The area-under-the-curve (AUC) of riluzole, after a single 50 mg oral dose, increases by about 1.7-fold in patients with mild chronic liver insufficiency (n=6; Child-Pugh's score A) and by about 3-fold in patients with moderate chronic liver insufficiency (n=6; Child-Pugh's score B) compared to healthy volunteers (n=12) (see WARNINGS and PRECAUTIONS). The pharmacokinetics of riluzole have not been studied in patients with severe hepatic impairment.
Renal Impairment: There is no significant difference in pharmacokinetic parameters between patients with moderate (n=5; creatinine clearance 30–50 ml.min^{-1}) and severe (n=7; creatinine clearance <30 ml.min^{-1}) renal insufficiency and healthy volunteers (n=12) after a single oral dose of 50 mg riluzole. The pharmacokinetics of riluzole have not been studied in patients undergoing hemodialysis.
Age: The pharmacokinetic parameters of riluzole after multiple dose administration (4.5 days of treatment at 50 mg riluzole b.i.d.) are not affected in the elderly (≥ 70 years).
Gender: No gender effect on riluzole pharmacokinetics has been found in young or elderly healthy subjects. However, in one placebo-controlled clinical trial with population pharmacokinetics, riluzole mean clearance was found to be 30% lower in female patients (corresponding to an approximate increase in AUC of 45%) as compared to male patients. No favorable or adverse effects of riluzole in relation to gender were seen in controlled trials, however.
Smoking: Patients who smoke cigarettes eliminate riluzole 20% faster than non-smoking patients, based on a population pharmacokinetic analysis on data from 128 ALS patients, of whom 19 were smokers. However, there is no need for dosage adjustment in these patients.
Race: Clearance of riluzole in Japanese subjects native to Japan was found to be 50% lower as compared to Caucasians after normalizing for body weight. Although it is not clear if this difference is due to genetic or environmental factors (*e.g.,* smoking, alcohol, coffee, and dietary preferences), it is possible that Japanese subjects may possess a lower capacity (oxidative and/or conjugative) for metabolizing riluzole. There are no studies, however, of lower doses in Japanese subjects (see PRECAUTIONS).

Clinical Trials

The efficacy of RILUTEK as a treatment of ALS was established in two adequate and well-controlled trials in which the time to tracheostomy or death was longer for patients randomized to RILUTEK than for those randomized to placebo.
These studies admitted patients with either familial or sporadic ALS, a disease duration of less than 5 years, and a baseline forced vital capacity greater than or equal to 60%.
In one study, performed in France and Belgium, 155 ALS patients were followed for at least 13 months (maximum duration 18 months) after being randomized to either 100 mg/day (given 50 mg BID) of RILUTEK or placebo.
Figure 1, which follows, displays the survival curves for time to death or tracheostomy. The vertical axis represents the proportion of individuals alive without tracheostomy at various times following treatment initiation (horizontal axis). Although these survival curves were not statistically significantly different when evaluated by the analysis specified in the study protocol (Logrank test p=0.12), the difference was found to be significant by another appropriate analysis (Wilcoxon test p=0.05). As seen, the study showed an early increase in survival in patients given riluzole. Among the patients in whom treatment failed during the study (tracheostomy or death) there was a difference between the treatment groups in median survival of approximately 90 days. There was no statistically significant difference in mortality at the end of the study.

Figure 1: Kaplan-Meier Survival Curves

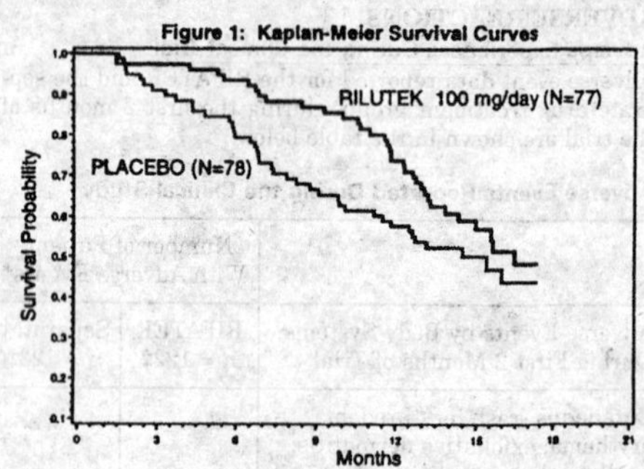

In the second study, performed in both Europe and North America, 959 ALS patients were followed for at least 1 year (North American centers) and up to 18 months (European centers) after being randomized to either 50, 100, 200 mg/day of RILUTEK or placebo.
Figure 2, which follows, displays the survival curves for time to death or tracheostomy for patients randomized to either 100 mg/day of RILUTEK or placebo. Although these survival curves were not statistically significantly different when evaluated by the analysis specified in the study protocol (Logrank test p = 0.076), the difference was found to be significant by another appropriate analysis (Wilcoxon test p = 0.05). Not displayed in Figure 2 are the results of 50 mg/day of RILUTEK which could not be statistically distinguished from placebo and the results of 200 mg/day which are essentially identical to 100 mg/day. As seen, the study showed an early increase in survival in patients given riluzole. Among the patients in whom treatment failed during the study (tracheostomy or death) there was a difference between the treatment groups in median survival of approximately 60 days. There was no statistically significant difference in mortality at the end of the study.

Figure 2: Kaplan-Meier Survival Curves

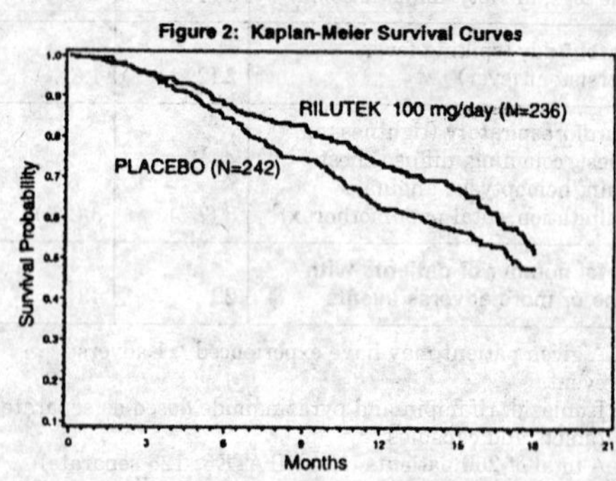

Although riluzole improved early survival in both studies, measures of muscle strength and neurological function did not show a benefit.

INDICATIONS AND USAGE

RILUTEK is indicated for the treatment of patients with amyotrophic lateral sclerosis (ALS). Riluzole extends survival and/or time to tracheostomy.

CONTRAINDICATIONS

RILUTEK is contraindicated in patients who have a history of severe hypersensitivity reactions to riluzole or any of the tablet components.

WARNINGS

Liver Injury/Monitoring Liver Chemistries

RILUTEK should be prescribed with care in patients with current evidence or history of abnormal liver function indicated by significant abnormalities in serum transaminase (ALT/SGPT; AST/SGOT), bilirubin, and/or gamma-glutamate transferase (GGT) levels (see PRECAUTIONS and DOSAGE AND ADMINISTRATION sections). Baseline elevations of several LFTs (especially elevated bilirubin) should preclude the use of RILUTEK.
RILUTEK, even in patients without a prior history of liver disease, causes serum aminotransferase elevations. Experience in almost 800 ALS patients indicates that about 50%

of riluzole-treated patients will experience at least one ALT/SGPT level above the upper limit of normal, about 8% will have elevations > 3 × ULN, and about 2% of patients will have elevations > 5 × ULN. A single non-ALS patient with epilepsy treated with concomitant carbamazepine and phenobarbital experienced marked, rapid elevations of liver enzymes with jaundice (ALT 26 × ULN, AST 17 × ULN, and bilirubin 11 × ULN) four months after starting RILUTEK; these returned to normal 7 weeks after treatment discontinuation.

Maximum increases in serum ALT usually occurred within 3 months after the start of riluzole therapy and were usually transient when < 5 times ULN. In trials, if ALT levels were <5 times ULN, treatment continued and ALT levels usually returned to below 2 times ULN within 2 to 6 months. Treatment in studies was discontinued, however, if ALT levels exceeded 5 × ULN, so that there is no experience with continued treatment of ALS patients once ALT values exceed 5 times ULN (see PRECAUTIONS: Laboratory Tests). There were rare instances of jaundice.

Liver chemistries should be monitored (see PRECAUTIONS).

Neutropenia

Among approximately 4000 patients given riluzole for ALS, there were three cases of marked neutropenia (absolute neutrophil count less than 500/mm^3), all seen within the first 2 months of riluzole treatment. In one case, neutrophil counts rose on continued treatment. In a second case, counts rose after therapy was stopped. A third case was more complex, with marked anemia as well as neutropenia and the etiology of both is uncertain. Patients should be warned to report any febrile illness to their physicians. The report of a febrile illness should prompt treating physicians to check white blood cell counts.

PRECAUTIONS

Use in Patients with Concomitant Disease

RILUTEK should be used with caution in patients with concomitant liver and/or renal insufficiency (see WARNINGS, CLINICAL PHARMACOLOGY). In particular, in cases of RILUTEK-induced hepatic injury manifested by elevated liver enzymes, the effect of the hepatic injury on RILUTEK metabolism is unknown.

Special Populations

Riluzole should be used with caution in elderly patients whose hepatic function may be compromised due to age. Also, females and Japanese patients may possess a lower metabolic capacity to eliminate riluzole compared to males and Caucasian subjects, respectively (see CLINICAL PHARMACOLOGY: Special Populations).

Information for the Patient

Patients should be advised to report any febrile illness to their physicians (see WARNINGS: Neutropenia).

Patients and caregivers should be advised that RILUTEK should be taken on a regular basis and at the same time of the day (*e.g.,* in the morning and evening) each day. If a dose is missed, take the next tablet as originally planned (see DOSAGE AND ADMINISTRATION).

Patients should be warned about the potential for dizziness, vertigo, or somnolence and advised not to drive or operate machinery until they have gained sufficient experience on RILUTEK to gauge whether or not it affects their mental and/or motor performance adversely.

Whether alcohol increases the risk of serious hepatotoxicity with RILUTEK is unknown; therefore, patients being treated with RILUTEK should be discouraged from drinking excessive amounts of alcohol.

Patients should also be made aware that RILUTEK should be stored at temperatures between 20°–25°C (68°–77°F) and protected from bright light.

RILUTEK must be kept out of the reach of children.

Laboratory Tests

It is recommended that serum aminotransferases including ALT levels be measured before and during riluzole therapy. Serum ALT levels should be evaluated every month during the first 3 months of treatment, every 3 months during the remainder of the first year, and periodically thereafter. Serum ALT levels should be evaluated more frequently in patients who develop elevations (see WARNINGS).

As noted in the WARNINGS Section, there is no experience with continued treatment of patients once ALT exceeds 5 × ULN. If a decision is made to continue to treat these patients, frequent monitoring (at least weekly) of complete liver function is recommended. Treatment should be discontinued if ALT exceeds 10 × ULN or if clinical jaundice develops. Because there is no experience with rechallenge of patients who have had RILUTEK discontinued for ALT > 5 × ULN, no recommendations about restarting RILUTEK can be made.

In the two controlled trials in patients with ALS, the frequency with which values for hemoglobin, hematocrit, and erythrocyte counts fell below the lower limit of normal was greater in RILUTEK-treated patients than in placebo-treated patients; however, these changes were mild and transient. The proportions of patients observed with abnormally low values for these parameters showed a dose-response relationship. Only one patient was discontinued from treatment because of severe anemia. The significance of this finding is unknown.

Drug Interactions

There have been no clinical studies designed to evaluate the interaction of riluzole with other drugs.

As with all drugs, the potential for interaction by a variety of mechanisms is a possibility.

Hepatotoxic Drugs: The clinical trials in ALS excluded patients on concomitant medications which were potentially hepatotoxic, (*e.g.,* allopurinol, methyldopa, sulfasalazine). Accordingly, there is no information about the safety of administering RILUTEK in conjunction with such medications. If the practitioner chooses to prescribe such a combination, caution should be exercised.

Drugs Highly Bound To Plasma Proteins: Riluzole is highly bound (96%) to plasma proteins, binding mainly to serum albumin and to lipoproteins. The effect of riluzole (up to 5 mcg/mL) on warfarin (5 mcg/mL) binding did not show any displacement of warfarin. Conversely, riluzole binding was unaffected by the addition of warfarin, digoxin, imipramine and quinine at high therapeutic concentrations.

Effect of Other Drugs On Riluzole Metabolism: *In vitro* studies using human liver microsomal preparations suggest that CYP 1A2 is the principal isozyme involved in the initial oxidative metabolism of riluzole and, therefore, potential interactions may occur when riluzole is given concurrently with agents that affect CYP 1A2 activity. Potential inhibitors of CYP 1A2 (*e.g.,* caffeine, phenacetin, theophylline, amitriptyline, and quinolones) could decrease the rate of riluzole elimination, while inducers of CYP 1A2 (*e.g.,* cigarette smoke, charcoal-broiled food, rifampicin, and omeprazole) could increase the rate of riluzole elimination.

Effect of Riluzole On the Metabolism of Other Drugs: CYP 1A2 is the principal isozyme involved in the initial oxidative metabolism of riluzole; potential interactions may occur when riluzole is given concurrently with other agents which are also metabolized primarily by CYP 1A2 (*e.g.,* theophylline, caffeine, and tacrine). Currently, it is not known whether riluzole has any potential for enzyme induction in humans.

Drug Laboratory Test Interactions: None known

Carcinogenesis, Mutagenesis, Impairment of Fertility

Riluzole was not carcinogenic in mice or rats when administered for 2 years at daily oral doses up to 20 mg/kg and 10 mg/kg, respectively, which are approximately equivalent to the maximum human dose on a mg/m^2 basis.

The genotoxic potential of riluzole was evaluated in the bacterial mutagenicity (Ames) test, the mouse lymphoma mutation assay in L5178Y cells, the *in vitro* chromosomal aberration assay in human lymphocytes and the *in vivo* rat cytogenetic assay and *in vivo* mouse micronucleus assay in bone marrow. There was no evidence of mutagenic or clastogenic potential in the Ames test, the mouse lymphoma assay, or the *in vivo* assays in the mouse and rat. There was an equivocal clastogenic response in the *in vitro* lymphocyte chromosomal aberration assay.

Riluzole impaired fertility when administered to male and female rats prior to and during mating at an oral dose of 15 mg/kg or 1.5 times the maximum daily dose on a mg/m^2 basis (see PRECAUTIONS: "Pregnancy" for effects on fertility).

Pregnancy

Pregnancy category C:

Oral administration of riluzole to pregnant animals during the period of organogenesis caused embryotoxicity in rats and rabbits at doses of 27 mg/kg and 60 mg/kg, respectively, or 2.6 and 11.5 times, respectively, the recommended maximum human daily dose on a mg/m^2 basis. Evidence of maternal toxicity was also observed at these doses.

When administered to rats prior to and during mating (males and females) and throughout gestation and lactation (females), riluzole produced adverse effects on pregnancy (decreased implantations, increased intrauterine death) and offspring viability and growth at an oral dose of 15 mg/kg or 1.5 times the maximum daily dose on a mg/m^2 basis.

There are no adequate and well-controlled studies in pregnant women. Riluzole should be used during pregnancy only if the potential benefit justifies the potential risk to the fetus.

Nursing Women

In rat studies, ^{14}C-riluzole was detected in maternal milk. It is not known whether riluzole is excreted in human breast milk. Because many drugs are excreted in human milk, and because the potential for serious adverse reactions in nursing infants from RILUTEK® is unknown, women should be advised not to breast-feed during treatment with RILUTEK.

Geriatric Use

Age-related compromised renal and hepatic function may cause a decrease in clearance of riluzole (see CLINICAL PHARMACOLOGY: Special Populations). In controlled clinical trials, about 30% of patients were over 65. There were no differences in adverse effects between younger and older patients.

Pediatric Use

The safety and the effectiveness of RILUTEK in pediatric patients have not been established.

ADVERSE REACTIONS

The most commonly observed AEs associated with the use of RILUTEK more frequently than placebo treated patients were: asthenia, nausea, dizziness, decreased lung function, diarrhea, abdominal pain, pneumonia, vomiting, vertigo, circumoral paresthesia, anorexia, and somnolence. Asthenia, nausea, dizziness, diarrhea, anorexia, vertigo, somnolence, and circumoral paresthesia were dose related.

Approximately 14% (n=141) of the 982 individuals with ALS who received RILUTEK in pre-marketing clinical trials discontinued treatment because of an adverse experience. Of those patients who discontinued due to adverse events, the most commonly reported were: nausea, abdominal pain, constipation, and ALT elevations. In a dose response study in ALS patients, the rates of discontinuation of RILUTEK for asthenia, nausea, abdominal pain, and ALT elevation were dose related.

Incidence in Controlled ALS Clinical Studies

Table 1 lists treatment-emergent signs and symptoms that occurred in at least 2% of patients with ALS treated with RILUTEK (n=794) participating in placebo-controlled trials and were numerically greater in the patients treated with RILUTEK 100 mg/day than with placebo or for which a dose response relationship is suggested.

The prescriber should be aware that these figures cannot be used to predict the frequency of adverse experiences in the course of usual medical practice where patient characteristics and other factors may differ from those prevailing during clinical studies. Inspection of these frequencies, however, does provide the prescriber with one basis to estimate the relative contribution of drug and non-drug factors to the AE incidences in the population studied.

Table 1
Adverse Events Occurring in Placebo-Controlled Clinical Trials

†Percentage of patients reporting events

Body System/ Adverse Event†	Riluzole 50 mg/day (N=237)	Riluzole 100 mg/day (N=313)	Riluzole 200 mg/day (N=244)	Placebo (N=320)
Body as a Whole				
Asthenia	14.8	19.2	20.1	12.2
Headache	8.0	7.3	7.0	6.6
Abdominal pain	6.8	5.1	7.8	3.8
Back pain	1.7	3.2	4.1	2.5
Aggravation reaction	0.4	1.3	2.0	0.9
Malaise	0.4	0.6	1.2	0.0
Digestive				
Nausea	12.2	16.3	20.5	10.6
Vomiting	4.2	4.2	4.5	1.6
Dyspepsia	2.5	3.8	6.1	5.0
Anorexia	3.8	3.2	8.6	3.8
Diarrhea	5.5	2.9	9.0	3.1
Flatulence	2.5	2.6	2.0	1.9
Stomatitis	0.8	1.0	1.2	0.0
Tooth disorder	0.0	1.0	1.2	0.3
Oral Moniliasis	0.4	0.6	1.2	0.3
Nervous				
Hypertonia	5.9	6.1	5.3	5.9
Depression	4.2	4.5	6.1	5.0
Dizziness	5.1	3.8	12.7	2.5
Dry mouth	3.0	3.5	2.0	3.4
Insomnia	2.1	3.5	2.9	3.4
Somnolence	0.8	1.9	4.1	1.3
Vertigo	2.5	1.9	4.5	0.9
Circumoral paresthesia	1.3	1.6	3.3	0.0
Skin and Appendages				
Pruritus	3.8	3.8	2.5	3.1
Eczema	0.8	1.6	1.6	0.6
Alopecia	0.0	1.0	1.2	0.6
Exfoliative dermatitis	0.0	0.6	1.2	0.0
Respiratory				
Decreased lung function	13.1	10.2	16.0	9.4
Rhinitis	8.9	6.4	7.8	6.3
Increased cough	2.1	2.6	3.7	1.6
Sinusitis	0.4	1.0	1.6	0.9
Cardiovascular				
Hypertension	6.8	5.1	3.3	4.1
Tachycardia	1.3	2.6	2.0	1.3
Phlebitis	0.4	1.0	0.8	0.3
Palpitation	0.4	0.6	1.2	0.9
Postural hypotension	0.8	0.0	1.6	0.6
Metabolic and Nutritional Disorders				
Weight loss	4.6	4.8	3.7	4.7
Peripheral edema	4.2	2.9	3.3	2.2
Musculoskeletal System				
Arthralgia	5.1	3.5	1.6	3.4
Urogenital System				
Urinary tract infection	2.5	2.6	4.5	2.2
Dysuria	0.0	1.0	1.2	0.3

Other Adverse Events Observed

Other events which occurred in more than 2% of patients treated with RILUTEK 100 mg/day but equally or more frequently in the placebo group included: accidental injury, apnea, bronchitis, constipation, death, dysphagia, dyspnea, flu syndrome, heart arrest, increased sputum, pneumonia, and respiratory disorder.

The overall adverse event profile for RILUTEK was similar between females and males, and was independent of age. Because the largest non-white racial subgroup was only 2% of patients exposed to RILUTEK (18/794) in placebo-controlled trials, there are insufficient data to support a statement regarding the distribution of adverse experience re-

Continued on next page

Rilutek—Cont.

ports by race. In ALS studies, dizziness did occur more commonly in females (11%) than in males (4%). There was not a difference between females and males in the rates of discontinuation of RILUTEK for individual adverse experiences.

Other Adverse Events Observed During All Clinical Trials
RILUTEK has been administered to 1713 individuals during all clinical trials, some of which were placebo-controlled. During these trials, all adverse events were recorded by the clinical investigators using terminology of their own choosing. To provide a meaningful estimate of the proportion of individuals having adverse events, similar types of events were grouped into a smaller number of standardized categories using modified COSTART dictionary terminology. The frequencies presented represent the proportion of the 1713 individuals exposed to RILUTEK who experienced an event of the type cited on at least one occasion while receiving RILUTEK. All reported events are included except those already listed in the previous table, those too general to be informative, and those not reasonably associated with the use of the drug.
Events are further classified within body system categories and enumerated in order of decreasing frequency using the following definitions: *frequent* adverse events are defined as those occurring in at least 1/100 patients; *infrequent* adverse events are those occurring in 1/100 to 1/1000 patients; *rare* adverse events are those occurring in fewer than 1/1000 patients.

***=AE frequency ≤to placebo**

Body as a Whole: *Frequent:* Hostility*. *Infrequent:* Abscess*, sepsis*, photosensitivity reaction*, cellulitis, face edema*, hernia, peritonitis, attempted suicide, injection site reaction, chills*, flu syndrome, intentional injury, enlarged abdomen, neoplasm. *Rare:* Acrodynia, hypothermia, moniliasis*, rheumatoid arthritis.

Digestive System: *Infrequent:* Increased appetite, intestinal obstruction*, fecal impaction, gastrointestinal hemorrhage, gastrointestinal ulceration, gastritis*, fecal incontinence, jaundice, hepatitis, glossitis, gum hemorrhage*, pancreatitis, tenesmus, esophageal stenosis. *Rare:* Cheilitis*, cholecystitis, hematemesis, melena*, biliary pain, proctitis, pseudomembranous enterocolitis, enlarged salivary gland, tongue discoloration, tooth caries.

Nervous System: *Frequent:* Agitation*, tremor. *Infrequent:* Hallucinations, personality disorder*, abnormal thinking*, coma, paranoid reaction*, manic reaction, ataxia, extrapyramidal syndrome, hypokinesia, urinary retention, emotional lability, delusions, apathy, hypesthesia, incoordination, confusion*, convulsion, leg cramps, amnesia, dysarthria, increased libido, stupor, subdural hematoma, abnormal gait, delirium, depersonalization, facial paralysis, hemiplegia, decreased libido, myoclonus. *Rare:* Abnormal dreams, acute brain syndrome, CNS depression, dementia, cerebral embolism, euphoria*, hypotonia, ileus*, peripheral neuritis, psychosis*, psychotic depression, schizophrenic reaction, trismus, wristdrop.

Skin and Appendages: *Infrequent:* Skin ulceration, urticaria, psoriasis, seborrhea*, skin disorder, fungal dermatitis*. *Rare:* Angioedema, contact dermatitis, erythema multiforme, furunculosis*, skin moniliasis, skin granuloma, skin nodule.

Respiratory System: *Infrequent:* Hiccup, pleural disorder*, asthma, epistaxis, hemoptysis, yawn, hyperventilation*, lung edema*, hypoventilation*, lung carcinoma, hypoxia, laryngitis, pleural effusion, pneumothorax*, respiratory moniliasis, stridor.

Cardiovascular System: *Infrequent:* Syncope*, hypotension, heart failure, migraine, peripheral vascular disease, angina pectoris*, myocardial infarction*, ventricular extrasystoles, cerebral hemorrhage, atrial fibrillation*, bundle branch block, congestive heart failure, pericarditis, lower extremity embolus, myocardial ischemia*, shock*. *Rare:* Bradycardia, cerebral ischemia, hemorrhage, mesenteric artery occlusion, subarachnoid hemorrhage, supraventricular tachycardia*, thrombosis, ventricular fibrillation, ventricular tachycardia.

Metabolic and Nutritional Disorders: *Infrequent:* Gout*, respiratory acidosis, edema, thirst*, hypokalemia, hyponatremia, weight gain*. *Rare:* Generalized edema, hypercalcemia, hypercholesteremia.

Endocrine System: *Infrequent:* Diabetes mellitus, thyroid neoplasia. *Rare:* Diabetes insipidus, parathyroid disorder.

Hemic and Lymphatic System: *Infrequent:* Anemia*, leukocytosis, leukopenia, ecchymosis. *Rare:* Neutropenia, aplastic anemia, cyanosis, hypochromic anemia, iron deficiency anemia, lymphadenopathy, petechiae*, purpura.

Musculoskeletal System: *Infrequent:* Arthrosis, myasthenia*, bone neoplasm. *Rare:* Bone necrosis, osteoporosis, tetany.

Special Senses: *Infrequent:* Amblyopia, ophthalmitis. *Rare:* Blepharitis, cataract, deafness, diplopia*, ear pain, glaucoma, hyperacusis, photophobia, taste loss, vestibular disorder.

Urogenital System: *Infrequent:* Urinary urgency, urine abnormality, urinary incontinence, kidney calculus, hematuria, impotence, prostate carcinoma, kidney pain, metrorrhagia, priapism. *Rare:* Amenorrhea, breast abscess, breast pain, nephritis*, nocturia, pyelonephritis, enlarged uterine fibroids, uterine hemorrhage, vaginal moniliasis.

Laboratory Tests: *Infrequent:* Increased gamma glutamyl transferase, abnormal liver function/tests, increased alkaline phosphatase, positive direct Coombs test, increased gamma globulins. *Rare:* increased lactic dehydrogenase.

OVERDOSAGE

No specific antidote or information on treatment of overdosage with RILUTEK is available. In the event of overdose, RILUTEK therapy should be discontinued immediately. Treatment should be supportive and directed toward alleviating symptoms.
Experience with riluzole overdose in humans is limited. Methemoglobinemia of undetermined origin has been reported in association with a riluzole overdose many times the recommended daily dose. This was rapidly reversible after treatment with methylene blue.
The estimated oral median lethal dose is 94 mg/kg and 39 mg/kg for male mice and rats, respectively.

DOSAGE AND ADMINISTRATION

The recommended dose for RILUTEK is 50 mg every 12 hours. No increased benefit can be expected from higher daily doses, but adverse events are increased.
RILUTEK tablets should be taken at least an hour before, or two hours after, a meal to avoid a food-related decrease in bioavailability.

Special Populations
Patients with Impaired Renal or Hepatic Function: see WARNINGS, PRECAUTIONS, CLINICAL PHARMACOLOGY.

HOW SUPPLIED

RILUTEK 50 mg tablets are white, film-coated, capsule-shaped and engraved with "RPR 202" on one side. RILUTEK is supplied in bottles of 60 tablets, NDC 0075-7700-60.

STORE AT CONTROLLED ROOM TEMPERATURE 20°–25°C (68°–77°F) AND PROTECT FROM BRIGHT LIGHT.
KEEP OUT OF THE REACH OF CHILDREN.

Manufactured by:
Usiphar, 60200 Campiegne, France
Manufactured for:
Aventis Pharmaceuticals Inc.
Bridgewater, NJ 08807 USA

Rev. May 2003
US Patent No. 5,527,814

Shown in Product Identification Guide, page 307

TAXOTERE® ℞

[*tax-ō-tĕr*]
(docetaxel)
Injection Concentrate

Prescribing Information as of May 2004
℞ only

WARNING

TAXOTERE® (docetaxel) Injection Concentrate should be administered under the supervision of a qualified physician experienced in the use of antineoplastic agents. Appropriate management of complications is possible only when adequate diagnostic and treatment facilities are readily available.
The incidence of treatment-related mortality associated with TAXOTERE therapy is increased in patients with abnormal liver function, in patients receiving higher doses, and in patients with non-small cell lung carcinoma and a history of prior treatment with platinum-based chemotherapy who receive TAXOTERE as a single agent at a dose of 100 mg/m^2 (see **WARNINGS**).
TAXOTERE should generally not be given to patients with bilirubin > upper limit of normal (ULN), or to patients with SGOT and/or SGPT >1.5 × ULN concomitant with alkaline phosphatase > 2.5 × ULN. Patients with elevations of bilirubin or abnormalities of transaminase concurrent with alkaline phosphatase are at increased risk for the development of grade 4 neutropenia, febrile neutropenia, infections, severe thrombocytopenia, severe stomatitis, severe skin toxicity, and toxic death. Patients with isolated elevations of transaminase > 1.5 × ULN also had a higher rate of febrile neutropenia grade 4 but did not have an increased incidence of toxic death. Bilirubin, SGOT or SGPT, and alkaline phosphatase values should be obtained prior to each cycle of TAXOTERE therapy and reviewed by the treating physician.
TAXOTERE therapy should not be given to patients with neutrophil counts of < 1500 cells/mm^3. In order to monitor the occurrence of neutropenia, which may be severe and result in infection, frequent blood cell counts should be performed on all patients receiving TAXOTERE.
Severe hypersensitivity reactions characterized by hypotension and/or bronchospasm, or generalized rash/erythema occurred in 2.2% (2/92) of patients who received the recommended 3-day dexamethasone premedication. Hypersensitivity reactions requiring discontinuation of the TAXOTERE infusion were reported in five patients who did not receive premedication. These reactions resolved after discontinuation of the infusion and the administration of appropriate therapy. TAXOTERE must not be given to patients who have a history of severe hypersensitivity reactions to TAXOTERE or to other drugs formulated with polysorbate 80 (see **WARNINGS**).
Severe fluid retention occurred in 6.5% (6/92) of patients despite use of a 3-day dexamethasone premedication regimen. It was characterized by one or more of the following events: poorly tolerated peripheral edema, generalized edema, pleural effusion requiring urgent drainage, dyspnea at rest, cardiac tamponade, or pronounced abdominal distention (due to ascites) (see **PRECAUTIONS**).

DESCRIPTION

Docetaxel is an antineoplastic agent belonging to the taxoid family. It is prepared by semisynthesis beginning with a precursor extracted from the renewable needle biomass of yew plants. The chemical name for docetaxel is (2R,3S)-N-carboxy-3-phenylisoserine,N-*tert*-butyl ester, 13-ester with 5β-20-epoxy-1,2α,4,7β,10β,13α-hexahydroxytax-11-en-9-one 4-acetate 2-benzoate, trihydrate. Docetaxel has the following structural formula:

Docetaxel is a white to almost-white powder with an empirical formula of $C_{43}H_{53}NO_{14}{\bullet}3H_2O$, and a molecular weight of 861.9. It is highly lipophilic and practically insoluble in water. TAXOTERE (docetaxel) Injection Concentrate is a clear yellow to brownish-yellow viscous solution. TAXOTERE is sterile, non-pyrogenic, and is available in single-dose vials containing 20 mg (0.5 mL) or 80 mg (2 mL) docetaxel (anhydrous). Each mL contains 40 mg docetaxel (anhydrous) and 1040 mg polysorbate 80.
TAXOTERE Injection Concentrate requires dilution prior to use. A sterile, non-pyrogenic, single-dose diluent is supplied for that purpose. The diluent for TAXOTERE contains 13% ethanol in water for injection, and is supplied in vials.

CLINICAL PHARMACOLOGY

Docetaxel is an antineoplastic agent that acts by disrupting the microtubular network in cells that is essential for mitotic and interphase cellular functions. Docetaxel binds to free tubulin and promotes the assembly of tubulin into stable microtubules while simultaneously inhibiting their disassembly. This leads to the production of microtubule bundles without normal function and to the stabilization of microtubules, which results in the inhibition of mitosis in cells. Docetaxel's binding to microtubules does not alter the number of protofilaments in the bound microtubules, a feature which differs from most spindle poisons currently in clinical use.

HUMAN PHARMACOKINETICS
The pharmacokinetics of docetaxel have been evaluated in cancer patients after administration of 20-115 mg/m^2 in phase I studies. The area under the curve (AUC) was dose proportional following doses of 70-115 mg/m^2 with infusion times of 1 to 2 hours. Docetaxel's pharmacokinetic profile is consistent with a three-compartment pharmacokinetic model, with half-lives for the α, β, and γ phases of 4 min, 36 min, and 11.1 hr, respectively. The initial rapid decline represents distribution to the peripheral compartments and the late (terminal) phase is due, in part, to a relatively slow efflux of docetaxel from the peripheral compartment. Mean values for total body clearance and steady state volume of distribution were 21 L/h/m^2 and 113 L, respectively. Mean total body clearance for Japanese patients dosed at the range of 10-90 mg/m^2 was similar to that of European/American populations dosed at 100 mg/m^2, suggesting no significant difference in the elimination of docetaxel in the two populations.
A study of ^{14}C-docetaxel was conducted in three cancer patients. Docetaxel was eliminated in both the urine and feces following oxidative metabolism of the *tert*-butyl ester group, but fecal excretion was the main elimination route. Within 7 days, urinary and fecal excretion accounted for approximately 6% and 75% of the administered radioactivity, respectively. About 80% of the radioactivity recovered in feces is excreted during the first 48 hours as 1 major and 3 minor metabolites with very small amounts (less than 8%) of unchanged drug.
A population pharmacokinetic analysis was carried out after TAXOTERE treatment of 535 patients dosed at 100 mg/m^2. Pharmacokinetic parameters estimated by this analysis were very close to those estimated from phase I studies. The pharmacokinetics of docetaxel were not influenced by age or gender and docetaxel total body clearance was not modified by pretreatment with dexamethasone. In patients with clinical chemistry data suggestive of mild to moderate liver function impairment (SGOT and/or SGPT >1.5 times the upper limit of normal [ULN] concomitant with alkaline phosphatase >2.5 times ULN), total body clearance was lowered by an average of 27%, resulting in a 38% increase in systemic exposure (AUC). This average, however, includes a substantial range and there is, at present, no measurement

that would allow recommendation for dose adjustment in such patients. Patients with combined abnormalities of transaminase and alkaline phosphatase should, in general, not be treated with TAXOTERE.

Clearance of docetaxel in combination therapy with cisplatin was similar to that previously observed following monotherapy with docetaxel. The pharmacokinetic profile of cisplatin in combination therapy with docetaxel was similar to that observed with cisplatin alone.

A population pharmacokinetic analysis of plasma data from 40 patients with hormone-refractory metastatic prostate cancer indicated that docetaxel systemic clearance in combination with prednisone is similar to that observed following administration of docetaxel alone.

In vitro studies showed that docetaxel is about 94% protein bound, mainly to α_1-acid glycoprotein, albumin, and lipoproteins. In three cancer patients, the *in vitro* binding to plasma proteins was found to be approximately 97%. Dexamethasone does not affect the protein binding of docetaxel. *In vitro* drug interaction studies revealed that docetaxel is metabolized by the CYP3A4 isoenzyme, and its metabolism can be inhibited by CYP3A4 inhibitors, such as ketoconazole, erythromycin, troleandomycin, and nifedipine. Based on *in vitro* findings, it is likely that CYP3A4 inhibitors and/or substrates may lead to substantial increases in docetaxel blood concentrations. No clinical studies have been performed to evaluate this finding (see **PRECAUTIONS**).

CLINICAL STUDIES

Breast Cancer: The efficacy and safety of TAXOTERE have been evaluated in locally advanced or metastatic breast cancer after failure of previous chemotherapy (alkylating agent-containing regimens or anthracycline-containing regimens), primarily at a dose of 100 mg/m^2 given as a 1-hour infusion every 3 weeks, but with some experience at 60 mg/m^2, in two large randomized trials and a number of smaller single arm studies.

Randomized Trials: In one randomized trial, patients with a history of prior treatment with an anthracycline-containing regimen were assigned to treatment with TAXOTERE or the combination of mitomycin (12 mg/m^2 every 6 weeks) and vinblastine (6 mg/m^2 every 3 weeks). 203 patients were randomized to TAXOTERE and 189 to the comparator arm. Most patients had received prior chemotherapy for metastatic disease; only 27 patients on the TAXOTERE arm and 33 patients on the comparator arm entered the study following relapse after adjuvant therapy. Three-quarters of patients had measurable, visceral metastases. The primary endpoint was time to progression. The following table summarizes the study results:

[See first table above]

In a second randomized trial, patients previously treated with an alkylating-containing regimen were assigned to treatment with TAXOTERE or doxorubicin (75 mg/m^2 every 3 weeks). 161 patients were randomized to TAXOTERE and 165 patients to doxorubicin. Approximately one-half of patients had received prior chemotherapy for metastatic disease, and one-half entered the study following relapse after adjuvant therapy. Three-quarters of patients had measurable, visceral metastases. The primary endpoint was time to progression. The study results are summarized below:

[See second table at right]

Single Arm Studies: TAXOTERE at a dose of 100 mg/m^2 was studied in six single arm studies involving a total of 309 patients with metastatic breast cancer in whom previous chemotherapy had failed. Among these, 190 patients had anthracycline-resistant breast cancer, defined as progression during an anthracycline-containing chemotherapy regimen for metastatic disease, or relapse during an anthracycline-containing adjuvant regimen. In anthracycline-resistant patients, the overall response rate was 37.9% (72/190; 95% C.I.: 31.0-44.8) and the complete response rate was 2.1%.

TAXOTERE was also studied in three single arm Japanese studies at a dose of 60 mg/m^2, in 174 patients who had received prior chemotherapy for locally advanced or metastatic breast cancer. Among 26 patients whose best response to an anthracycline had been progression, the response rate was 34.6% (95% C.I.: 17.2-55.7), similar to the response rate in single arm studies of 100 mg/m^2.

Hematologic and Other Toxicity: Relation to dose and baseline liver chemistry abnormalities. Hematologic and other toxicity is increased at higher doses and in patients with elevated baseline liver function tests (LFTs). In the following tables, adverse drug reactions are compared for three populations: 730 patients with normal LFTs given TAXOTERE at 100 mg/m^2 in the randomized and single arm studies of metastatic breast cancer after failure of previous chemotherapy; 18 patients in these studies who had abnormal baseline LFTs (defined as SGOT and/or SGPT > 1.5 times ULN concurrent with alkaline phosphatase > 2.5 times ULN); and 174 patients in Japanese studies given TAXOTERE at 60 mg/m^2 who had normal LFTs.

[See third table at right]
[See first table at top of next page]

Non-Small Cell Lung Cancer (NSCLC): The efficacy and safety of TAXOTERE has been evaluated in patients with unresectable, locally advanced or metastatic non-small cell lung cancer whose disease has failed prior platinum-based chemotherapy or in patients who are chemotherapy-naïve.

Monotherapy with TAXOTERE for NSCLC Previously Treated with Platinum-Based Chemotherapy

Two randomized, controlled trials established that a TAXOTERE dose of 75 mg/m^2 was tolerable and yielded a favorable outcome in patients previously treated with platinum-based chemotherapy (see below). TAXOTERE at a dose of 100 mg/m^2, however, was associated with unacceptable hematologic toxicity, infections, and treatment-related mortality and this dose should not be used (see **BOXED WARNING, WARNINGS,** and **DOSAGE AND ADMINISTRATION** sections).

One trial (TAX317), randomized patients with locally advanced or metastatic non-small cell lung cancer, a history of prior platinum-based chemotherapy, no history of taxane exposure, and an ECOG performance status ≤2 to TAXOTERE or best supportive care. The primary endpoint

Continued on next page

Efficacy of TAXOTERE in the Treatment of Breast Cancer Patients Previously Treated with an Anthracycline-Containing Regimen (Intent-to-Treat Analysis)

Efficacy Parameter	Docetaxel (n=203)	Mitomycin/ Vinblastine (n=189)	p-value
Median Survival	11.4 months	8.7 months	
Risk Ratio*, Mortality (Docetaxel: Control)	0.73		p=0.01 Log Rank
95% CI (Risk Ratio)	0.58-0.93		
Median Time to Progression	4.3 months	2.5 months	
Risk Ratio*, Progression (Docetaxel: Control)	0.75		p=0.01 Log Rank
95% CI (Risk Ratio)	0.61-0.94		
Overall Response Rate Complete Response Rate	28.1% 3.4%	9.5% 1.6%	p<0.0001 Chi Square

*For the risk ratio, a value less than 1.00 favors docetaxel.

Efficacy of TAXOTERE in the Treatment of Breast Cancer Patients Previously Treated with an Alkylating-Containing Regimen (Intent-to-Treat Analysis)

Efficacy Parameter	Docetaxel (n=161)	Doxorubicin (n=165)	p-value
Median Survival	14.7 months	14.3 months	
Risk Ratio*, Mortality (Docetaxel: Control)	0.89		p=0.39 Log Rank
95% CI (Risk Ratio)	0.68-1.16		
Median Time to Progression	6.5 months	5.3 months	
Risk Ratio*, Progression (Docetaxel: Control)	0.93		p=0.45 Log Rank
95% CI (Risk Ratio)	0.71-1.16		
Overall Response Rate Complete Response Rate	45.3% 6.8%	29.7% 4.2%	p=0.004 Chi Square

*For the risk ratio, a value less than 1.00 favors docetaxel.

Hematologic Adverse Events in Breast Cancer Patients Previously Treated with Chemotherapy Treated at TAXOTERE 100 mg/m^2 with Normal or Elevated Liver Function Tests or 60 mg/m^2 with Normal Liver Function Tests

	TAXOTERE 100 mg/m^2		TAXOTERE 60 mg/m^2
Adverse Event	Normal LFTs* n=730 %	Elevated LFTs** n=18 %	Normal LFTs* n=174 %
Neutropenia			
Any <2000 cells/mm^3	98.4	100	95.4
Grade 4 <500 cells/mm^3	84.4	93.8	74.9
Thrombocytopenia			
Any <100,000 cells/mm^3	10.8	44.4	14.4
Grade 4 <20,000 cells/mm^3	0.6	16.7	1.1
Anemia <11 g/dL	94.6	94.4	64.9
Infection* **			
Any	22.5	38.9	1.1
Grade 3 and 4	7.1	33.3	0
Febrile Neutropenia******			
By Patient	11.8	33.3	0
By Course	2.4	8.6	0
Septic Death	1.5	5.6	1.1
Non-Septic Death	1.1	11.1	0

*Normal Baseline LFTs: Transaminases ≤ 1.5 times ULN or alkaline phosphatase ≤ 2.5 times ULN or isolated elevations of transaminases or alkaline phosphatase up to 5 times ULN
**Elevated Baseline LFTs: SGOT and/or SGPT >1.5 times ULN concurrent with alkaline phosphatase >2.5 times ULN
***Incidence of infection requiring hospitalization and/or intravenous antibiotics was 8.5% (n=62) among the 730 patients with normal LFTs at baseline; 7 patients had concurrent grade 3 neutropenia, and 46 patients had grade 4 neutropenia.
****Febrile Neutropenia: For 100 mg/m^2, ANC grade 4 and fever > 38°C with IV antibiotics and/or hospitalization; for 60 mg/m^2, ANC grade 3/4 and fever > 38.1°C

Taxotere—Cont.

of the study was survival. Patients were initially randomized to TAXOTERE 100 mg/m² or best supportive care, but early toxic deaths at this dose led to a dose reduction to TAXOTERE 75 mg/m². A total of 104 patients were randomized in this amended study to either TAXOTERE 75 mg/m² or best supportive care.

In a second randomized trial (TAX320), 373 patients with locally advanced or metastatic non-small cell lung cancer, a history of prior platinum-based chemotherapy, and an ECOG performance status ≤2 were randomized to TAXOTERE 75 mg/m², TAXOTERE 100 mg/m² and a treatment in which the investigator chose either vinorelbine 30 mg/m² days 1, 8, and 15 repeated every 3 weeks or ifosfamide 2 g/m² days 1-3 repeated every 3 weeks. Forty percent of the patients in this study had a history of prior paclitaxel exposure. The primary endpoint was survival in both trials. The efficacy data for the TAXOTERE 75 mg/m² arm and the comparator arms are summarized in the table below and in figures 1 and 2 showing the survival curves for the two studies.

[See second table at right]

Only one of the two trials (TAX317) showed a clear effect on survival, the primary endpoint; that trial also showed an increased rate of survival to one year. In the second study (TAX320) the rate of survival at one year favored TAXOTERE 75 mg/m².

Figure 1: TAX317 Survival K-M Curves - TAXOTERE 75 mg/m² vs. Best Supportive Care

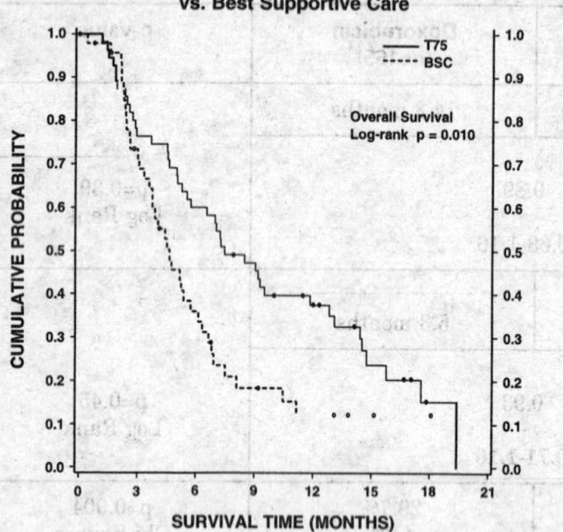

Figure 2: TAX320 Survival K-M Curves - TAXOTERE 75 mg/m² vs. Vinorelbine or Ifosfamide Control

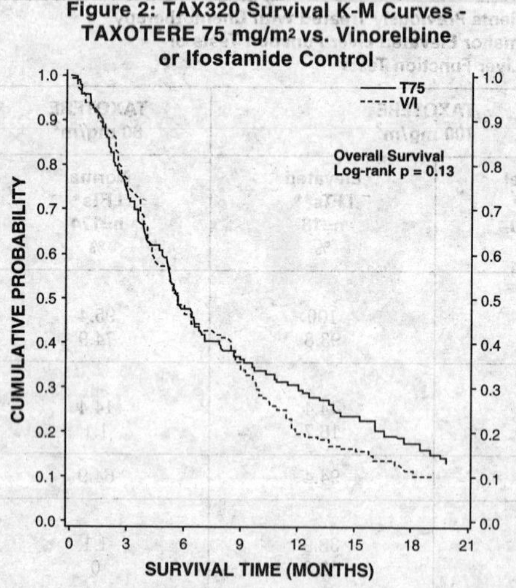

Patients treated with TAXOTERE at a dose of 75 mg/m² experienced no deterioration in performance status and body weight relative to the comparator arms used in these trials.

Combination Therapy with TAXOTERE for Chemotherapy-Naïve NSCLC

In a randomized controlled trial (TAX326), 1218 patients with unresectable stage IIIB or IV NSCLC and no prior chemotherapy were randomized to receive one of three treatments: TAXOTERE 75 mg/m² as a 1 hour infusion immediately followed by cisplatin 75 mg/m² over 30-60 minutes every 3 weeks; vinorelbine 25 mg/m² administered over 6-10 minutes on days 1, 8, 15, 22 followed by cisplatin 100 mg/m² administered on day 1 of cycles repeated every 4 weeks; or a combination of TAXOTERE and carboplatin.

The primary efficacy endpoint was overall survival. Treatment with TAXOTERE+cisplatin did not result in a statistically significantly superior survival compared to vinorelbine+cisplatin (see table below). The 95% confidence interval of the hazard ratio (adjusted for interim analysis and multiple comparisons) shows that the addition of TAXOTERE to cisplatin results in an outcome ranging from a 6% inferior to a 26% superior survival compared to the addition of vinorelbine to cisplatin. The results of a further statistical analysis showed that at least (the lower bound of the 95% confidence interval) 62% of the known survival effect of vinorelbine when added to cisplatin (about a 2-month increase in median survival; Wozniak et al. JCO, 1998) was maintained. The efficacy data for the TAXOTERE+cisplatin arm and the comparator arm are summarized in the table below.

Non-Hematologic Adverse Events in Breast Cancer Patients Previously Treated with Chemotherapy Treated at TAXOTERE 100 mg/m² with Normal or Elevated Liver Function Tests or 60 mg/m² with Normal Liver Function Tests

Adverse Event	TAXOTERE 100 mg/m² Normal LFTs* n=730 %	TAXOTERE 100 mg/m² Elevated LFTs** n=18 %	TAXOTERE 60 mg/m² Normal LFTs* n=174 %
Acute Hypersensitivity Reaction Regardless of Premedication			
Any	13.0	5.6	0.6
Severe	1.2	0	0
Fluid Retention* Regardless of Premedication**			
Any	56.2	61.1	12.6
Severe	7.9	16.7	0
Neurosensory			
Any	56.8	50	19.5
Severe	5.8	0	0
Myalgia	22.7	33.3	3.4
Cutaneous			
Any	44.8	61.1	30.5
Severe	4.8	16.7	0
Asthenia			
Any	65.2	44.4	65.5
Severe	16.6	22.2	0
Diarrhea			
Any	42.2	27.8	NA
Severe	6.3	11.1	
Stomatitis			
Any	53.3	66.7	19.0
Severe	7.8	38.9	0.6

*Normal Baseline LFTs: Transaminases ≤ 1.5 times ULN or alkaline phosphatase ≤ 2.5 times ULN or isolated elevations of transaminases or alkaline phosphatase up to 5 times ULN

**Elevated Baseline Liver Function: SGOT and/or SGPT >1.5 times ULN concurrent with alkaline phosphatase >2.5 times ULN

***Fluid Retention includes (by COSTART): edema (peripheral, localized, generalized, lymphedema, pulmonary edema, and edema otherwise not specified) and effusion (pleural, pericardial, and ascites); no premedication given with the 60 mg/m² dose

NA = not available

Efficacy of TAXOTERE in the Treatment of Non-Small Cell Lung Cancer Patients Previously Treated with a Platinum-Based Chemotherapy Regimen (Intent-to-Treat Analysis)

	TAX317 Docetaxel 75 mg/m² n=55	TAX317 Best Supportive Care/75 n=49	TAX320 Docetaxel 75 mg/m² n=125	TAX320 Control (V/I) n=123
Overall Survival Log-rank Test	p=0.01		p=0.13	
Risk Ratio[††], Mortality (Docetaxel: Control) 95% CI (Risk Ratio)	0.56 (0.35, 0.88)		0.82 (0.63, 1.06)	
Median Survival 95% CI	7.5 months* (5.5, 12.8)	4.6 months (3.7, 6.1)	5.7 months (5.1, 7.1)	5.6 months (4.4, 7.9)
% 1-year Survival 95% CI	37%*† (24, 50)	12% (2, 23)	30%*† (22, 39)	20% (13, 27)
Time to Progression 95% CI	12.3 weeks* (9.0, 18.3)	7.0 weeks (6.0, 9.3)	8.3 weeks (7.0, 11.7)	7.6 weeks (6.7, 10.1)
Response Rate 95% CI	5.5% (1.1, 15.1)	Not Applicable	5.7% (2.3, 11.3)	0.8% (0.0, 4.5)

* p≤0.05; † uncorrected for multiple comparisons; †† a value less than 1.00 favors docetaxel.

Survival Analysis of TAXOTERE in Combination Therapy for Chemotherapy-Naïve NSCLC

Comparison	Taxotere +Cisplatin n=408	Vinorelbine +Cisplatin n=405
Kaplan-Meier Estimate of Median Survival	10.9 months	10.0 months
p-value[a]	0.122	
Estimated Hazard Ratio[b]	0.88	
Adjusted 95% CI[c]	(0.74, 1.06)	

[a]From the superiority test (stratified log rank) comparing TAXOTERE+cisplatin to vinorelbine+cisplatin

[b]Hazard ratio of TAXOTERE+cisplatin vs. vinorelbine+cisplatin. A hazard ratio of less than 1 indicates that TAXOTERE+cisplatin is associated with a longer survival.

[c]Adjusted for interim analysis and multiple comparisons.

The second comparison in the study, vinorelbine+cisplatin versus TAXOTERE+carboplatin, did not demonstrate superior survival associated with the TAXOTERE arm (Kaplan-Meier estimate of median survival was 9.1 months for TAXOTERE+carboplatin compared to 10.0 months on the vinorelbine+cisplatin arm) and the TAXOTERE+carboplatin arm did not demonstrate preservation of at least 50% of the survival effect of vinorelbine added to cisplatin. Secondary endpoints evaluated in the trial included objective response and time to progression. There was no statistically significant difference between TAXOTERE+cisplatin and vinorelbine+cisplatin with respect to objective response and time to progression (see table below).

Response and TTP Analysis of TAXOTERE in Combination Therapy for Chemotherapy-Naïve NSCLC

Endpoint	TAXOTERE +Cisplatin	Vinorelbine +Cisplatin	p-value
Objective Response Rate (95% CI)[a]	31.6% (26.5%, 36.8%)	24.4% (19.8%, 29.2%)	Not Significant
Median Time to Progresion[b] (95% CI)[a]	21.4 weeks (19.3, 24.6)	22.1 weeks (18.1, 25.6)	Not Significant

[a]Adjusted for multiple comparisons.
[b]Kaplan-Meier estimates.

Prostate Cancer
The safety and efficacy of TAXOTERE in combination with prednisone in patients with androgen independent (hormone refractory) metastatic prostate cancer were evaluated in a randomized multicenter active control trial. A total of 1006 patients with Karnofsky Performance Status (KPS) ≥60 were randomized to the following treatment groups:

- TAXOTERE 75 mg/m^2 every 3 weeks for 10 cycles.
- TAXOTERE 30 mg/m^2 administered weekly for the first 5 weeks in a 6-week cycle for 5 cycles.
- Mitoxantrone 12 mg/m^2 every 3 weeks for 10 cycles.

All 3 regimens were administered in combination with prednisone 5 mg twice daily, continuously.
In the TAXOTERE every three week arm, a statistically significant overall survival advantage was demonstrated compared to mitoxantrone. In the TAXOTERE weekly arm, no overall survival advantage was demonstrated compared to the mitoxantrone control arm. Efficacy results for the TAXOTERE every 3 week arm versus the control arm are summarized in the following table and figure 3:

Efficacy of TAXOTERE in the Treatment of Patients with Androgen Independent (Hormone Refractory) Metastatic Prostate Cancer (Intent-to-Treat Analysis)

	TAXOTERE every 3 weeks	Mitoxantrone every 3 weeks
Number of patients	335	337
Median survival (months)	18.9	16.5
95% CI	(17.0-21.2)	(14.4-18.6)
Hazard ratio	0.761	–
95% CI	(0.619-0.936)	–
p-value*	0.0094	–

*Stratified log rank test. Threshold for statistical significance = 0.0175 because of 3 arms.

Figure 3 - TAX327 Survival K-M Curves

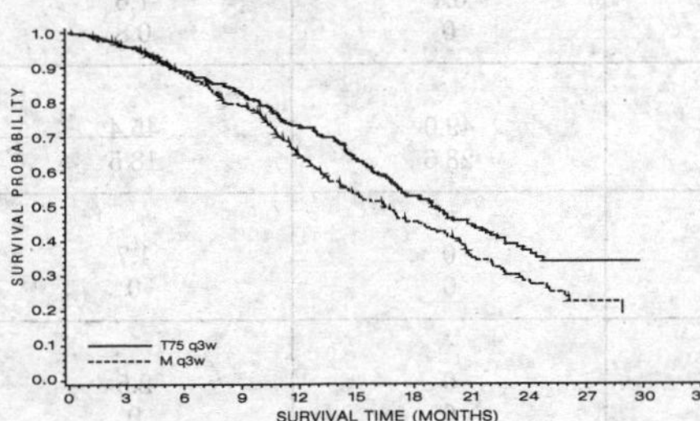

INDICATIONS AND USAGE

Breast Cancer: TAXOTERE is indicated for the treatment of patients with locally advanced or metastatic breast cancer after failure of prior chemotherapy.
Non-Small Cell Lung Cancer: TAXOTERE as a single agent is indicated for the treatment of patients with locally advanced or metastatic non-small cell lung cancer after failure of prior platinum-based chemotherapy.
TAXOTERE in combination with cisplatin is indicated for the treatment of patients with unresectable, locally advanced or metastatic non-small cell lung cancer who have not previously received chemotherapy for this condition.
Prostate Cancer: TAXOTERE in combination with prednisone is indicated for the treatment of patients with androgen independent (hormone refractory) metastatic prostate cancer.

CONTRAINDICATIONS

TAXOTERE is contraindicated in patients who have a history of severe hypersensitivity reactions to docetaxel or to other drugs formulated with polysorbate 80.

Summary of Adverse Events in Patients Receiving TAXOTERE at 100 mg/m^2

Adverse Event	All Tumor Types Normal LFTs* n=2045 %	All Tumor Types Elevated LFTs** n=61 %	Breast Cancer Normal LFTs* n=965 %
Hematologic			
Neutropenia			
<2000 cells/mm^3	95.5	96.4	98.5
<500 cells/mm^3	75.4	87.5	85.9
Leukopenia			
<4000 cells/mm^3	95.6	98.3	98.6
<1000 cells/mm^3	31.6	46.6	43.7
Thrombocytopenia			
<100,000 cells/mm^3	8.0	24.6	9.2
Anemia			
<11 g/dL	90.4	91.8	93.6
<8 g/dL	8.8	31.1	7.7
Febrile Neutropenia***	11.0	26.2	12.3
Septic Death	1.6	4.9	1.4
Non-Septic Death	0.6	6.6	0.6
Infections			
Any	21.6	32.8	22.2
Severe	6.1	16.4	6.4
Fever in Absence of Infection			
Any	31.2	41.0	35.1
Severe	2.1	8.2	2.2
Hypersensitivity Reactions			
Regardless of Premedication			
Any	21.0	19.7	17.6
Severe	4.2	9.8	2.6
With 3-day Premedication	n=92	n=3	n=92
Any	15.2	33.3	15.2
Severe	2.2	0	2.2
Fluid Retention			
Regardless of Premedication			
Any	47.0	39.3	59.7
Severe	6.9	8.2	8.9
With 3-day Premedication	n=92	n=3	n=92
Any	64.1	66.7	64.1
Severe	6.5	33.3	6.5
Neurosensory			
Any	49.3	34.4	58.3
Severe	4.3	0	5.5
Cutaneous			
Any	47.6	54.1	47.0
Severe	4.8	9.8	5.2
Nail Changes			
Any	30.6	23.0	40.5
Severe	2.5	4.9	3.7
Gastrointestinal			
Nausea	38.8	37.7	42.1
Vomiting	22.3	23.0	23.4
Diarrhea	38.7	32.8	42.6
Severe	4.7	4.9	5.5
Stomatitis			
Any	41.7	49.2	51.7
Severe	5.5	13.0	7.4
Alopecia	75.8	62.3	74.2
Asthenia			
Any	61.8	52.5	66.3
Severe	12.8	24.6	14.9
Myalgia			
Any	18.9	16.4	21.1
Severe	1.5	1.6	1.8
Arthralgia	9.2	6.6	8.2
Infusion Site Reactions	4.4	3.3	4.0

***Normal Baseline LFTs: Transaminases ≤ 1.5 times ULN or alkaline phosphatase ≤ 2.5 times ULN or isolated elevations of transaminases or alkaline phosphatase up to 5 times ULN**
****Elevated Baseline LFTs: SGOT and/or SGPT >1.5 times ULN concurrent with alkaline phosphatase >2.5 times ULN**
*****Febrile Neutropenia: ANC grade 4 with fever > 38°C with IV antibiotics and/or hospitalization**

TAXOTERE should not be used in patients with neutrophil counts of <1500 cells/mm^3.

WARNINGS

TAXOTERE should be administered under the supervision of a qualified physician experienced in the use of antineoplastic agents. Appropriate management of complications is possible only when adequate diagnostic and treatment facilities are readily available.

Toxic Deaths
Breast Cancer: TAXOTERE administered at 100 mg/m^2 was associated with deaths considered possibly or probably related to treatment in 2.0% (19/965) of metastatic breast cancer patients, both previously treated and untreated, with normal baseline liver function and in 11.5% (7/61) of patients with various tumor types who had abnormal baseline liver function (SGOT and/or SGPT > 1.5 times ULN together with AP > 2.5 times ULN). Among patients dosed at 60 mg/m2, mortality related to treatment occurred in 0.6% (3/481) of patients with normal liver function, and in 3 of 7 patients with abnormal liver function. Approximately half of these deaths occurred during the first cycle. Sepsis accounted for the majority of the deaths.
Non-Small Cell Lung Cancer: TAXOTERE administered at a dose of 100 mg/m^2 in patients with locally advanced or metastatic non-small cell lung cancer who had a history of prior platinum-based chemotherapy was associated with increased treatment-related mortality (14% and 5% in two randomized, controlled studies). There were 2.8% treatment-related deaths among the 176 patients treated at the 75 mg/m^2 dose in the randomized trials. Among patients who experienced treatment-related mortality at the

Continued on next page

Taxotere—Cont.

75 mg/m^2 dose level, 3 of 5 patients had a PS of 2 at study entry (see **BOXED WARNING, CLINICAL STUDIES**, and **DOSAGE AND ADMINISTRATION** sections).

Premedication Regimen: All patients should be premedicated with oral corticosteroids (see below for prostate cancer) such as dexamethasone 16 mg per day (*e.g.,* 8 mg BID) for 3 days starting 1 day prior to TAXOTERE to reduce the severity of fluid retention and hypersensitivity reactions (see **DOSAGE AND ADMINISTRATION** section). This regimen was evaluated in 92 patients with metastatic breast cancer previously treated with chemotherapy given TAXOTERE at a dose of 100 mg/m^2 every 3 weeks.

The pretreatment regimen for hormone-refractory metastatic prostate cancer is oral dexamethasone 8 mg, at 12 hours, 3 hours and 1 hour before the TAXOTERE infusion (see **DOSAGE AND ADMINISTRATION** section).

Hypersensitivity Reactions: Patients should be observed closely for hypersensitivity reactions, especially during the first and second infusions. Severe hypersensitivity reactions characterized by hypotension and/or bronchospasm, or generalized rash/erythema occurred in 2.2% of the 92 patients premedicated with 3-day corticosteroids. Hypersensitivity reactions requiring discontinuation of the TAXOTERE infusion were reported in 5 out of 1260 patients with various tumor types who did not receive premedication, but in 0/92 patients premedicated with 3-day corticosteroids. Patients with a history of severe hypersensitivity reactions should not be rechallenged with TAXOTERE.

Hematologic Effects: Neutropenia (< 2000 neutrophils/mm^3) occurs in virtually all patients given 60-100 mg/m^2 of TAXOTERE and grade 4 neutropenia (<500 cells/mm^3) occurs in 85% of patients given 100 mg/m^2 and 75% of patients given 60 mg/m^2. Frequent monitoring of blood counts is, therefore, essential so that dose can be adjusted. TAXOTERE should not be administered to patients with neutrophils < 1500 cells/mm^3.

Febrile neutropenia occurred in about 12% of patients given 100 mg/m^2 but was very uncommon in patients given 60 mg/m^2. Hematologic responses, febrile reactions and infections, and rates of septic death for different regimens are dose related and are described in **CLINICAL STUDIES**.

Three breast cancer patients with severe liver impairment (bilirubin > 1.7 times ULN) developed fatal gastrointestinal bleeding associated with severe drug-induced thrombocytopenia.

Hepatic Impairment: (see **BOXED WARNING**).

Fluid Retention: (see **BOXED WARNING**).

Pregnancy: TAXOTERE can cause fetal harm when administered to pregnant women. Studies in both rats and rabbits at doses ≥ 0.3 and 0.03 mg/kg/day, respectively (about 1/50 and 1/300 the daily maximum recommended human dose on a mg/m^2 basis), administered during the period of organogenesis, have shown that TAXOTERE is embryotoxic and fetotoxic (characterized by intrauterine mortality, increased resorption, reduced fetal weight, and fetal ossification delay). The doses indicated above also caused maternal toxicity.

There are no adequate and well-controlled studies in pregnant women using TAXOTERE. If TAXOTERE is used during pregnancy, or if the patient becomes pregnant while receiving this drug, the patient should be apprised of the potential hazard to the fetus or potential risk for loss of the pregnancy. Women of childbearing potential should be advised to avoid becoming pregnant during therapy with TAXOTERE.

PRECAUTIONS

General: Responding patients may not experience an improvement in performance status on therapy and may experience worsening. The relationship between changes in performance status, response to therapy, and treatment-related side effects has not been established.

Hematologic Effects: In order to monitor the occurrence of myelotoxicity, it is recommended that frequent peripheral blood cell counts be performed on all patients receiving TAXOTERE. Patients should not be retreated with subsequent cycles of TAXOTERE until neutrophils recover to a level > 1500 cells/mm^3 and platelets recover to a level > 100,000 cells/mm^3.

A 25% reduction in the dose of TAXOTERE is recommended during subsequent cycles following severe neutropenia (<500 cells/mm^3) lasting 7 days or more, febrile neutropenia, or a grade 4 infection in a TAXOTERE cycle (see **DOSAGE AND ADMINISTRATION** section).

Hypersensitivity Reactions: Hypersensitivity reactions may occur within a few minutes following initiation of a TAXOTERE infusion. If minor reactions such as flushing or localized skin reactions occur, interruption of therapy is not required. More severe reactions, however, require the immediate discontinuation of TAXOTERE and aggressive therapy. All patients should be premedicated with an oral corticosteroid prior to the initiation of the infusion of TAXOTERE (see **BOXED WARNING** and **WARNINGS: Premedication Regimen**).

Cutaneous: Localized erythema of the extremities with edema followed by desquamation has been observed. In case of severe skin toxicity, an adjustment in dosage is recommended (see **DOSAGE AND ADMINISTRATION** section). The discontinuation rate due to skin toxicity was 1.6% (15/965) for metastatic breast cancer patients. Among 92 breast cancer patients premedicated with 3-day corticosteroids, there were no cases of severe skin toxicity reported and no patient discontinued TAXOTERE due to skin toxicity.

Treatment Emergent Adverse Events Regardless of Relationship to Treatment in Patients Receiving TAXOTERE as Monotherapy for Non-Small Cell Lung Cancer Previously Treated with Platinum-Based Chemotherapy*

Adverse Event	TAXOTERE 75 mg/m^2 n=176 %	Best Supportive Care n=49 %	Vinorelbine/ Ifosfamide n=119 %
Neutropenia			
Any	84.1	14.3	83.2
Grade 3/4	65.3	12.2	57.1
Leukopenia			
Any	83.5	6.1	89.1
Grade 3/4	49.4	0	42.9
Thrombocytopenia			
Any	8.0	0	7.6
Grade 3/4	2.8	0	1.7
Anemia			
Any	91.0	55.1	90.8
Grade 3/4	9.1	12.2	14.3
Febrile Neutropenia**	6.3	NA†	0.8
Infection			
Any	33.5	28.6	30.3
Grade 3/4	10.2	6.1	9.2
Treatment Related Mortality	2.8	NA†	3.4
Hypersensitivity Reactions			
Any	5.7	0	0.8
Grade 3/4	2.8	0	0
Fluid Retention			
Any	33.5	ND††	22.7
Severe	2.8		3.4
Neurosensory			
Any	23.3	14.3	28.6
Grade 3/4	1.7	6.1	5.0
Neuromotor			
Any	15.9	8.2	10.1
Grade 3/4	4.5	6.1	3.4
Skin			
Any	19.9	6.1	16.8
Grade 3/4	0.6	2.0	0.8
Gastrointestinal			
Nausea			
Any	33.5	30.6	31.1
Grade 3/4	5.1	4.1	7.6
Vomiting			
Any	21.6	26.5	21.8
Grade 3/4	2.8	2.0	5.9
Diarrhea			
Any	22.7	6.1	11.8
Grade 3/4	2.8	0	4.2
Alopecia	56.3	34.7	49.6
Asthenia			
Any	52.8	57.1	53.8
Severe***	18.2	38.8	22.7
Stomatitis			
Any	26.1	6.1	7.6
Grade 3/4	1.7	0	0.8
Pulmonary			
Any	40.9	49.0	45.4
Grade 3/4	21.0	28.6	18.5
Nail Disorder			
Any	11.4	0	1.7
Severe***	1.1	0	0
Myalgia			
Any	6.3	0	2.5
Severe***	0	0	0
Arthralgia			
Any	3.4	2.0	1.7
Severe***	0	0	0.8
Taste Perversion			
Any	5.7	0	0
Severe***	0.6	0	0

*Normal Baseline LFTs: Transaminases ≤ 1.5 times ULN or alkaline phosphatase ≤ 2.5 times ULN or isolated elevations of transaminases or alkaline phosphatase up to 5 times ULN

** Febrile Neutropenia: ANC grade 4 with fever > 38°C with IV antibiotics and/or hospitalization

*** COSTART term and grading system

† Not Applicable; †† Not Done

Fluid Retention: Severe fluid retention has been reported following TAXOTERE therapy (see **BOXED WARNING** and **WARNINGS: Premedication Regimen**). Patients should be premedicated with oral corticosteroids prior to each TAXOTERE administration to reduce the incidence and severity of fluid retention (see **DOSAGE AND ADMINISTRATION** section). Patients with pre-existing effusions should be closely monitored from the first dose for the possible exacerbation of the effusions.

When fluid retention occurs, peripheral edema usually starts in the lower extremities and may become generalized with a median weight gain of 2 kg.

Among 92 breast cancer patients premedicated with 3-day corticosteroids, moderate fluid retention occurred in 27.2% and severe fluid retention in 6.5%. The median cumulative dose to onset of moderate or severe fluid retention was 819 mg/m^2. 9.8% (9/92) of patients discontinued treatment due to fluid retention: 4 patients discontinued with severe fluid retention; the remaining 5 had mild or moderate fluid retention. The median cumulative dose to treatment discontinuation due to fluid retention was 1021 mg/m^2. Fluid retention was completely, but sometimes slowly, reversible with a median of 16 weeks from the last infusion of TAXOTERE to resolution (range: 0 to 42+ weeks). Patients developing peripheral edema may be treated with standard measures, e.g., salt restriction, oral diuretic(s).

Neurologic: Severe neurosensory symptoms (paresthesia, dysesthesia, pain) were observed in 5.5% (53/965) of metastatic breast cancer patients, and resulted in treatment discontinuation in 6.1%. When these symptoms occur, dosage must be adjusted. If symptoms persist, treatment should be discontinued (see **DOSAGE AND ADMINISTRATION** section). Patients who experienced neurotoxicity in clinical trials and for whom follow-up information on the complete resolution of the event was available had spontaneous reversal of symptoms with a median of 9 weeks from onset (range: 0 to 106 weeks). Severe peripheral motor neuropathy mainly manifested as distal extremity weakness occurred in 4.4% (42/965).

Asthenia: Severe asthenia has been reported in 14.9% (144/965) of metastatic breast cancer patients but has led to treatment discontinuation in only 1.8%. Symptoms of fatigue and weakness may last a few days up to several weeks and may be associated with deterioration of performance status in patients with progressive disease.

Information for Patients: For additional information, see the accompanying Patient Information Leaflet.

Drug Interactions: There have been no formal clinical studies to evaluate the drug interactions of TAXOTERE with other medications. *In vitro* studies have shown that the metabolism of docetaxel may be modified by the concomitant administration of compounds that induce, inhibit, or are metabolized by cytochrome P450 3A4, such as cyclosporine, terfenadine, ketoconazole, erythromycin, and troleandomycin. Caution should be exercised with these drugs when treating patients receiving TAXOTERE as there is a potential for a significant interaction.

Carcinogenicity, Mutagenicity, Impairment of Fertility: No studies have been conducted to assess the carcinogenic potential of TAXOTERE. TAXOTERE has been shown to be clastogenic in the *in vitro* chromosome aberration test in CHO-K$_1$ cells and in the *in vivo* micronucleus test in the mouse, but it did not induce mutagenicity in the Ames test or the CHO/HGPRT gene mutation assays. TAXOTERE produced no impairment of fertility in rats when administered in multiple IV doses of up to 0.3 mg/kg (about 1/50 the recommended human dose on a mg/m^2 basis), but decreased testicular weights were reported. This correlates with findings of a 10-cycle toxicity study (dosing once every 21 days for 6 months) in rats and dogs in which testicular atrophy or degeneration was observed at IV doses of 5 mg/kg in rats and 0.375 mg/kg in dogs (about 1/3 and 1/15 the recommended human dose on a mg/m^2 basis, respectively). An increased frequency of dosing in rats produced similar effects at lower dose levels.

Pregnancy: Pregnancy Category D (see **WARNINGS** section).

Nursing Mothers: It is not known whether TAXOTERE is excreted in human milk. Because many drugs are excreted in human milk, and because of the potential for serious adverse reactions in nursing infants from TAXOTERE, mothers should discontinue nursing prior to taking the drug.

Pediatric Use: The safety and effectiveness of TAXOTERE in pediatric patients have not been established.

Geriatric Use: In a study conducted in chemotherapy-naïve patients with NSCLC (TAX326), 148 patients (36%) in the TAXOTERE+cisplatin group were 65 years of age or greater. There were 128 patients (32%) in the vinorelbine+cisplatin group 65 years of age or greater. In the TAXOTERE+cisplatin group, patients less than 65 years of age had a median survival of 10.3 months (95% CI : 9.1 months, 11.8 months) and patients 65 years or older had a median survival of 12.1 months (95% CI : 9.3 months, 14 months). In patients 65 years of age or greater treated with TAXOTERE+cisplatin, diarrhea (55%), peripheral edema (39%) and stomatitis (28%) were observed more frequently than in the vinorelbine+cisplatin group (diarrhea 24%, peripheral edema 20%, stomatitis 20%). Patients treated with TAXOTERE+cisplatin who were 65 years of age or greater were more likely to experience diarrhea (55%), infections (42%), peripheral edema (39%) and stomatitis (28%) compared to patients less than the age of 65 administered the same treatment (43%, 31%, 31% and 21%, respectively).

When TAXOTERE was combined with carboplatin for the treatment of chemotherapy-naïve, advanced non-small cell lung carcinoma, patients 65 years of age or greater (28%) experienced higher frequency of infection compared to similar patients treated with TAXOTERE+cisplatin, and a higher frequency of diarrhea, infection and peripheral edema than elderly patients treated with vinorelbine+cisplatin.

Of the 333 patients treated with TAXOTERE every three weeks plus prednisone in the prostate cancer study (TAX327), 209 patients were 65 years of age or greater and 68 patients were older than 75 years. In patients treated with TAXOTERE every three weeks, the following TEAEs occurred at rates ≥ 10% higher in patients 65 years of age or greater compared to younger patients: anemia (71% vs. 59%), infection (37% vs. 24%), nail changes (34% vs. 23%), anorexia (21% vs. 10%), weight loss (15% vs. 5%) respectively.

ADVERSE REACTIONS

Adverse reactions are described for TAXOTERE according to indication:

— in the treatment of breast cancer, at the maximum dose of 100 mg/m^2

— in the treatment of advanced non-small cell lung cancer after prior platinum-based chemotherapy, at a dose of 75 mg/m^2

— in the treatment of non-small cell lung cancer in patients who have not previously received chemotherapy for this condition, at a dose of 75 mg/m^2, in combination with cisplatin

— in the treatment of androgen independent (hormone refractory) metastatic prostate cancer, at a dose of 75 mg/m^2 every three weeks in combination with prednisone

Monotherapy with TAXOTERE for Locally Advanced or Metastatic Breast Cancer After Failure of Prior Chemotherapy

TAXOTERE 100 mg/m^2: Adverse drug reactions occurring in at least 5% of patients are compared for three populations who received TAXOTERE administered at 100 mg/m^2 as a 1-hour infusion every 3 weeks: 2045 patients with various tumor types and normal baseline liver function tests; the subset of 965 patients with locally advanced or metastatic breast cancer, both previously treated and untreated with chemotherapy, who had normal baseline liver function tests; and an additional 61 patients with various tumor types who had abnormal liver function tests at baseline. These reactions were described using COSTART terms and were considered possibly or probably related to TAXOTERE. At least 95% of these patients did not receive hematopoietic support. The safety profile is generally similar in patients receiving TAXOTERE for the treatment of breast cancer and in patients with other tumor types.

[See table at top of page 749]

Hematologic: (see **WARNINGS**). Reversible marrow suppression was the major dose-limiting toxicity of TAXOTERE. The median time to nadir was 7 days, while the median duration of severe neutropenia (<500 cells/mm^3) was 7 days. Among 2045 patients with solid tumors and normal baseline LFTs, severe neutropenia occurred in 75.4% and lasted for more than 7 days in 2.9% of cycles.

Febrile neutropenia (<500 cells/mm^3 with fever > 38°C with IV antibiotics and/or hospitalization) occurred in 11% of patients with solid tumors, in 12.3% of patients with metastatic breast cancer, and in 9.8% of 92 breast cancer patients premedicated with 3-day corticosteroids.

Severe infectious episodes occurred in 6.1% of patients with solid tumors, in 6.4% of patients with metastatic breast cancer, and in 5.4% of 92 breast cancer patients premedicated with 3-day corticosteroids.

Thrombocytopenia (<100,000 cells/mm^3) associated with fatal gastrointestinal hemorrhage has been reported.

Hypersensitivity Reactions: Severe hypersensitivity reactions are discussed in the **BOXED WARNING, WARNINGS**, and **PRECAUTIONS** sections. Minor events, including flushing, rash with or without pruritus, chest tightness, back pain, dyspnea, drug fever, or chills, have been reported and resolved after discontinuing the infusion and appropriate therapy.

Fluid Retention: (see **BOXED WARNING, WARNINGS: Premedication Regimen**, and **PRECAUTIONS** sections).

Cutaneous: Severe skin toxicity is discussed in **PRECAUTIONS**. Reversible cutaneous reactions characterized by a rash including localized eruptions, mainly on the feet and/or hands, but also on the arms, face, or thorax, usually associated with pruritus, have been observed. Eruptions generally occurred within 1 week after TAXOTERE infusion, recovered before the next infusion, and were not disabling.

Severe nail disorders were characterized by hypo- or hyperpigmentation, and occasionally by onycholysis (in 0.8% of patients with solid tumors) and pain.

Neurologic: (see **PRECAUTIONS**).

Gastrointestinal: Gastrointestinal reactions (nausea and/or vomiting and/or diarrhea) were generally mild to moderate. Severe reactions occurred in 3-5% of patients with solid tumors and to a similar extent among metastatic breast cancer patients. The incidence of severe reactions was 1% or less for the 92 breast cancer patients premedicated with 3-day corticosteroids.

Severe stomatitis occurred in 5.5% of patients with solid tumors, in 7.4% of patients with metastatic breast cancer, and in 1.1% of the 92 breast cancer patients premedicated with 3-day corticosteroids.

Cardiovascular: Hypotension occurred in 2.8% of patients with solid tumors; 1.2% required treatment. Clinically meaningful events such as heart failure, sinus tachycardia, atrial flutter, dysrhythmia, unstable angina, pulmonary edema, and hypertension occurred rarely. 8.1% (7/86) of metastatic breast cancer patients receiving TAXOTERE 100 mg/m^2 in a randomized trial and who had serial left ventricular ejection fractions assessed developed deterioration of LVEF by ≥ 10% associated with a drop below the institutional lower limit of normal.

Infusion Site Reactions: Infusion site reactions were generally mild and consisted of hyperpigmentation, inflammation, redness or dryness of the skin, phlebitis, extravasation, or swelling of the vein.

Hepatic: In patients with normal LFTs at baseline, bilirubin values greater than the ULN occurred in 8.9% of patients. Increases in SGOT or SGPT > 1.5 times the ULN, or alkaline phosphatase > 2.5 times ULN, were observed in 18.9% and 7.3% of patients, respectively. While on TAXOTERE, increases in SGOT and/or SGPT > 1.5 times ULN concomitant with alkaline phosphatase > 2.5 times ULN occurred in 4.3% of patients with normal LFTs at baseline. (Whether these changes were related to the drug or underlying disease has not been established.)

Monotherapy with TAXOTERE for Unresectable, Locally Advanced or Metastatic NSCLC Previously Treated with Platinum-Based Chemotherapy

TAXOTERE 75 mg/m^2: Treatment emergent adverse drug reactions are shown below. Included in this table are safety data for a total of 176 patients with non-small cell lung carcinoma and a history of prior treatment with platinum-based chemotherapy who were treated in two randomized, controlled trials. These reactions were described using NCI Common Toxicity Criteria regardless of relationship to study treatment, except for the hematologic toxicities or otherwise noted.

[See table at top of previous page]

Combination Therapy with TAXOTERE in Chemotherapy-Naïve Advanced Unresectable or Metastatic NSCLC

The table below presents safety data from two arms of an open label, randomized controlled trial (TAX326) that enrolled patients with unresectable stage IIIB or IV non-small cell lung cancer and no history of prior chemotherapy. Adverse reactions were described using the NCI Common Toxicity Criteria except where otherwise noted.

Adverse Events Regardless of Relationship to Treatment in Chemotherapy-Naïve Advanced Non-Small Cell Lung Cancer Patients Receiving TAXOTERE in Combination with Cisplatin

Adverse Event	TAXOTERE 75 mg/m^2 + Cisplatin 75 mg/m^2 n=406 %	Vinorelbine 25 mg/m^2 + Cisplatin 100 mg/m^2 n=396 %
Neutropenia		
Any	91	90
Grade 3/4	74	78
Febrile Neutropenia	5	5
Thrombocytopenia		
Any	15	15
Grade 3/4	3	4
Anemia		
Any	89	94
Grade 3/4	7	25
Infection		
Any	35	37
Grade 3/4	8	8
Fever in absence of infection		
Any	33	29
Grade 3/4	< 1	1
Hypersensitivity Reaction*		
Any	12	4
Grade 3/4	3	< 1
Fluid Retention**		
Any	54	42
All severe or life-threatening events	2	2
Pleural effusion		
Any	23	22
All severe or life-threatening events	2	2
Peripheral edema		
Any	34	18
All severe or life-threatening events	< 1	< 1
Weight gain		
Any	15	9
All severe or life-threatening events	< 1	< 1
Neurosensory		
Any	47	42
Grade 3/4	4	4
Neuromotor		
Any	19	17
Grade 3/4	3	6

Continued on next page

Taxotere—Cont.

Skin		
Any	16	14
Grade 3/4	< 1	1
Nausea		
Any	72	76
Grade 3/4	10	17
Vomiting		
Any	55	61
Grade 3/4	8	16
Diarrhea		
Any	47	25
Grade 3/4	7	3
Anorexia**		
Any	42	40
All severe or life threatening events	5	5
Stomatitis		
Any	24	21
Grade 3/4	2	1
Alopecia		
Any	75	42
Grade 3/4	< 1	0
Asthenia**		
Any	74	75
All severe or life threatening events	12	14
Nail Disorder**		
Any	14	< 1
All severe events	< 1	0
Myalgia**		
Any	18	12
All severe events	< 1	< 1

*** Replaces NCI term "Allergy"**
**** COSTART term and grading system**

Deaths within 30 days of last study treatment occurred in 31 patients (7.6%) in the docetaxel+cisplatin arm and 37 patients (9.3%) in the vinorelbine+cisplatin arm. Deaths within 30 days of last study treatment attributed to study drug occurred in 9 patients (2.2%) in the docetaxel+cisplatin arm and 8 patients (2.0%) in the vinorelbine+ cisplatin arm. The second comparison in the study, vinorelbine+cisplatin versus TAXOTERE+carboplatin (which did not demonstrate a superior survival associated with TAXOTERE, see **CLINICAL STUDIES** section) demonstrated a higher incidence of thrombocytopenia, diarrhea, fluid retention, hypersensitivity reactions, skin toxicity, alopecia and nail changes on the TAXOTERE+carboplatin arm, while a higher incidence of anemia, neurosensory toxicity, nausea, vomiting, anorexia and asthenia was observed on the vinorelbine+cisplatin arm.

Combination Therapy with TAXOTERE in Patients with Prostate Cancer

The following data are based on the experience of 332 patients, who were treated with TAXOTERE 75 mg/m² every 3 weeks in combination with prednisone 5 mg orally twice daily.

[See table above]

Clinically Important Treatment Emergent Adverse Events (Regardless of Relationship) in Patients with Prostate Cancer who Received TAXOTERE in Combination with Prednisone (TAX 327)

	TAXOTERE 75 mg/m² every 3 weeks + prednisone 5 mg twice daily n=332 %		Mitoxantrone 12 mg/m² every 3 weeks + prednisone 5 mg twice daily n=335 %	
Adverse Event	**Any**	**G 3/4**	**Any**	**G 3/4**
Anemia	66.5	4.9	57.8	1.8
Neutropenia	40.9	32.0	48.2	21.7
Thrombocytopenia	3.4	0.6	7.8	1.2
Febrile neutropenia	2.7	N/A	1.8	N/A
Infection	32.2	5.7	20.3	4.2
Epistaxis	5.7	0.3	1.8	0.0
Allergic Reactions	8.4	0.6	0.6	0.0
Fluid Retention*	24.4	0.6	4.5	0.3
Weight Gain*	7.5	0.3	3.0	0.0
Peripheral Edema*	18.1	0.3	1.5	0.0
Neuropathy Sensory	30.4	1.8	7.2	0.3
Neuropathy Motor	7.2	1.5	3.0	0.9
Rash/Desquamation	6.0	0.3	3.3	0.6
Alopecia	65.1	N/A	12.8	N/A
Nail Changes	29.5	0.0	7.5	0.0
Nausea	41.0	2.7	35.5	1.5
Diarrhea	31.6	2.1	9.6	1.2
Stomatitis/Pharyngitis	19.6	0.9	8.4	0.0
Taste Disturbance	18.4	0.0	6.6	0.0
Vomiting	16.9	1.5	14.0	1.5
Anorexia	16.6	1.2	14.3	0.3
Cough	12.3	0.0	7.8	0.0
Dyspnea	15.1	2.7	8.7	0.9
Cardiac left ventricular function	9.6	0.3	22.1	1.2
Fatigue	53.3	4.5	34.6	5.1
Myalgia	14.5	0.3	12.8	0.9
Tearing	9.9	0.6	1.5	0.0
Arthralgia	8.1	0.6	5.1	1.2

*Related to treatment

Post-marketing Experiences

The following adverse events have been identified from clinical trials and/ or post-marketing surveillance. Because they are reported from a population of unknown size, precise estimates of frequency cannot be made.

Body as a whole: diffuse pain, chest pain, radiation recall phenomenon

Cardiovascular: atrial fibrillation, deep vein thrombosis, ECG abnormalities, thrombophlebitis, pulmonary embolism, syncope, tachycardia, myocardial infarction

Cutaneous: rare cases of bullous eruption such as erythema multiforme or Stevens-Johnson syndrome. Multiple factors may have contributed to the development of these effects.

Gastrointestinal: abdominal pain, anorexia, constipation, duodenal ulcer, esophagitis, gastrointestinal hemorrhage, gastrointestinal perforation, ischemic colitis, colitis, intestinal obstruction, ileus, neutropenic enterocolitis and dehydration as a consequence to gastrointestinal events have been reported.

Hematologic: bleeding episodes

Hepatic: rare cases of hepatitis have been reported.

Neurologic: confusion, rare cases of seizures or transient loss of consciousness have been observed, sometimes appearing during the infusion of the drug.

Ophthalmologic: conjunctivitis, lacrimation or lacrimation with or without conjunctivitis. Excessive tearing which may be attributable to lacrimal duct obstruction has been reported. Rare cases of transient visual disturbances (flashes, flashing lights, scotomata) typically occurring during drug infusion and in association with hypersensitivity reactions have been reported. These were reversible upon discontinuation of the infusion.

Respiratory: dyspnea, acute pulmonary edema, acute respiratory distress syndrome, interstitial pneumonia. Pulmonary fibrosis has been rarely reported.

Urogenital: renal insufficiency

OVERDOSAGE

There is no known antidote for TAXOTERE overdosage. In case of overdosage, the patient should be kept in a specialized unit where vital functions can be closely monitored. Anticipated complications of overdosage include: bone marrow suppression, peripheral neurotoxicity, and mucositis. Patients should receive therapeutic G-CSF as soon as possible after discovery of overdose. Other appropriate symptomatic measures should be taken, as needed.

In two reports of overdose, one patient received 150 mg/m² and the other received 200 mg/m² as 1-hour infusions. Both patients experienced severe neutropenia, mild asthenia, cutaneous reactions, and mild paresthesia, and recovered without incident.

In mice, lethality was observed following single IV doses that were ≥154 mg/kg (about 4.5 times the recommended human dose on a mg/m² basis); neurotoxicity associated with paralysis, non-extension of hind limbs, and myelin degeneration was observed in mice at 48 mg/kg (about 1.5 times the recommended human dose on a mg/m² basis). In male and female rats, lethality was observed at a dose of 20 mg/kg (comparable to the recommended human dose on a mg/m² basis) and was associated with abnormal mitosis and necrosis of multiple organs.

DOSAGE AND ADMINISTRATION

Breast Cancer: The recommended dose of TAXOTERE is 60–100 mg/m² administered intravenously over 1 hour every 3 weeks.

Non-Small Cell Lung Cancer: For treatment after failure of prior platinum-based chemotherapy, TAXOTERE was evaluated as monotherapy, and the recommended dose is 75 mg/m² administered intravenously over 1 hour every 3 weeks. A dose of 100 mg/m² in patients previously treated with chemotherapy was associated with increased hematologic toxicity, infection, and treatment-related mortality in randomized, controlled trials (see **BOXED WARNING, WARNINGS** and **CLINICAL STUDIES** sections).

For chemotherapy-naïve patients, TAXOTERE was evaluated in combination with cisplatin. The recommended dose of TAXOTERE is 75 mg/m² administered intravenously over 1 hour immediately followed by cisplatin 75 mg/m² over 30–60 minutes every 3 weeks.

Prostate cancer: For hormone-refractory metastatic prostate cancer, the recommended dose of TAXOTERE is 75 mg/m² every 3 weeks as a 1 hour infusion. Prednisone 5 mg orally twice daily is administered continuously.

Premedication Regimen: All patients should be premedicated with oral corticosteroids (see below for prostate cancer) such as dexamethasone 16 mg per day (*e.g.,* 8 mg BID) for 3 days starting 1 day prior to TAXOTERE administration in order to reduce the incidence and severity of fluid retention as well as the severity of hypersensitivity reactions (see **BOXED WARNING, WARNINGS,** and **PRECAUTIONS** sections).

For hormone-refractory metastatic prostate cancer, given the concurrent use of prednisone, the recommended premedication regimen is oral dexamethasone 8 mg, at 12 hours, 3 hours and 1 hour before the TAXOTERE infusion (see **WARNINGS,** and **PRECAUTIONS** sections).

Dosage Adjustments During Treatment

Breast Cancer: Patients who are dosed initially at 100 mg/m² and who experience either febrile neutropenia, neutrophils < 500 cells/mm³ for more than 1 week, or severe or cumulative cutaneous reactions during TAXOTERE therapy should have the dosage adjusted from 100 mg/m² to 75 mg/m². If the patient continues to experience these reactions, the dosage should either be decreased from 75 mg/m² to 55 mg/m² or the treatment should be discontinued. Conversely, patients who are dosed initially at 60 mg/m² and who do not experience febrile neutropenia, neutrophils <500 cells/mm³ for more than 1 week, severe or cumulative cutaneous reactions, or severe peripheral neuropathy during TAXOTERE therapy may tolerate higher doses. Patients who develop ≥ grade 3 peripheral neuropathy should have TAXOTERE treatment discontinued entirely.

Non-Small Cell Lung Cancer:

Monotherapy with TAXOTERE for NSCLC Treatment After Failure of Prior Platinum-Based Chemotherapy

Patients who are dosed initially at 75 mg/m² and who experience either febrile neutropenia, neutrophils <500 cells/mm³ for more than one week, severe or cumulative cutaneous reactions, or other grade 3/4 non-hematological toxicities during TAXOTERE treatment should have treatment withheld until resolution of the toxicity and then resumed at 55 mg/m². Patients who develop ≥ grade 3 peripheral neuropathy should have TAXOTERE treatment discontinued entirely.

Combination Therapy with TAXOTERE for Chemotherapy-Naïve NSCLC

For patients who are dosed initially at TAXOTERE 75 mg/m² in combination with cisplatin, and whose nadir of platelet count during the previous course of therapy is <25,000 cells/mm³, in patients who experience febrile neutropenia, and in patients with serious non-hematologic toxicities, the TAXOTERE dosage in subsequent cycles should be reduced to 65 mg/m². In patients who require a further dose reduction, a dose of 50 mg/m² is recommended. For cisplatin dosage adjustments, see manufacturers' prescribing information.

Combination Therapy with TAXOTERE for Hormone-Refractory Metastatic Prostate Cancer

TAXOTERE should be administered when the neutrophil count is ≥ 1,500 cells/mm³. Patients who experience either febrile neutropenia, neutrophils < 500 cells/mm³ for more than one week, severe or cumulative cutaneous reactions or moderate neurosensory signs and/or symptoms during TAXOTERE therapy should have the dosage of TAXOTERE reduced from 75 to 60 mg/m². If the patient continues to experience these reactions at 60 mg/m², the treatment should be discontinued.

Special Populations:

Hepatic Impairment: Patients with bilirubin > ULN should generally not receive TAXOTERE. Also, patients with SGOT and/or SGPT > 1.5 × ULN concomitant with alkaline phosphatase > 2.5 × ULN should generally not receive TAXOTERE.

Children: The safety and effectiveness of docetaxel in pediatric patients below the age of 16 years have not been established.

Elderly: See **Precautions, Geriatric Use.** In general, dose selection for an elderly patient should be cautious, reflecting the greater frequency of decreased hepatic, renal, or cardiac function and of concomitant disease or other drug therapy in elderly patients.

PREPARATION AND ADMINISTRATION

Administration Precautions

TAXOTERE is a cytotoxic anticancer drug and, as with other potentially toxic compounds, caution should be exercised when handling and preparing TAXOTERE solutions. The use of gloves is recommended. Please refer to **Handling and Disposal** section.

If TAXOTERE Injection Concentrate, initial diluted solution, or final dilution for infusion should come into contact with the skin, immediately and thoroughly wash with soap and water.

If TAXOTERE Injection Concentrate, initial diluted solution, or final dilution for infusion should come into contact with mucosa, immediately and thoroughly wash with water.

Contact of the TAXOTERE concentrate with plasticized PVC equipment or devices used to prepare solutions for infusion is not recommended. In order to minimize patient exposure to the plasticizer DEHP (di-2-ethylhexyl phthalate), which may be leached from PVC infusion bags or sets, the final TAXOTERE dilution for infusion should be stored in bottles (glass, polypropylene) or plastic bags (polypropylene, polyolefin) and administered through polyethylene-lined administration sets.

TAXOTERE Injection Concentrate requires two dilutions prior to administration. Please follow the preparation instructions provided below. **Note:** Both the TAXOTERE Injection Concentrate and the diluent vials contain an overfill to compensate for liquid loss during preparation. This overfill ensures that after dilution with the **entire** contents of the accompanying diluent, there is an initial diluted solution containing 10 mg/mL docetaxel.

The table below provides the fill range of the diluent, the approximate extractable volume of diluent when the entire contents of the diluent vial are withdrawn, and the concentration of the initial diluted solution for TAXOTERE 20 mg and TAXOTERE 80 mg.

Product	Diluent 13% (w/w) ethanol in water for injection Fill Range (mL)	Approximate extractable volume of diluent when entire contents are withdrawn (mL)	Concentration of the initial diluted solution (mg/mL docetaxel)
Taxotere® 20 mg/0.5 mL	1.88 – 2.08 mL	1.8 mL	10 mg/mL
Taxotere® 80 mg/2 mL	6.96 – 7.70 mL	7.1 mL	10 mg/mL

Preparation and Administration

A. Initial Diluted Solution

1. TAXOTERE vials should be stored between 2 and 25°C (36 and 77°F). If the vials are stored under refrigeration, allow the appropriate number of vials of TAXOTERE Injection Concentrate and diluent (13% ethanol in water for injection) vials to stand at room temperature for approximately 5 minutes.
2. Aseptically withdraw the **entire** contents of the appropriate diluent vial (approximately 1.8 mL for TAXOTERE 20 mg and approximately 7.1 mL for TAXOTERE 80 mg) into a syringe by partially inverting the vial, and transfer it to the appropriate vial of TAXOTERE Injection Concentrate. **If the procedure is followed as described, an initial diluted solution of 10mg docetaxel/mL will result.**
3. Mix the initial diluted solution by repeated inversions for at least 45 seconds to assure full mixture of the concentrate and diluent. Do not shake.
4. The initial diluted TAXOTERE solution (10 mg docetaxel/mL) should be clear; however, there may be some foam on top of the solution due to the polysorbate 80. Allow the solution to stand for a few minutes to allow any foam to dissipate. It is not required that all foam dissipate prior to continuing the preparation process.
   The initial diluted solution may be used immediately or stored either in the refrigerator or at room temperature for a maximum of 8 hours.

B. Final Dilution for Infusion

1. Aseptically withdraw the required amount of initial diluted TAXOTERE solution (10 mg docetaxel/mL) with a calibrated syringe and injectinto a 250 mL infusion bag or bottle of either 0.9% Sodium Chloride solution or 5% Dextrose solution to produce a final concentration of 0.3 to 0.74 mg/mL.
   If a dose greater than 200 mg of TAXOTERE is required, use a larger volume of the infusion vehicle so that a concentration of 0.74 mg/mL TAXOTERE is not exceeded.
2. Thoroughly mix the infusion by manual rotation.
3. As with all parenteral products, TAXOTERE should be inspected visually for particulate matter or discoloration prior to administration whenever the solution and container permit. If the TAXOTERE initial diluted solution or final dilution for infusion is not clear or appears to have precipitation, these should be discarded.

The final TAXOTERE dilution for infusion should be administered intravenously as a 1-hour infusion under ambient room temperature and lighting conditions.

Stability: TAXOTERE infusion solution, if stored between 2 and 25°C (36 and 77°F) is stable for 4 hours. Fully prepared TAXOTERE infusion solution (in either 0.9% Sodium Chloride solution or 5% Dextrose solution) should be used within 4 hours (including the 1 hour i.v. administration).

HOW SUPPLIED

TAXOTERE Injection Concentrate is supplied in a single-dose vial as a sterile, pyrogen-free, non-aqueous, viscous solution with an accompanying sterile, non-pyrogenic, Diluent (13% ethanol in water for injection) vial. The following strengths are available:

TAXOTERE 80 MG/2 ML (NDC 0075-8001-80)

TAXOTERE (docetaxel) Injection Concentrate 80 mg/2 mL: 80 mg docetaxel in 2 mL polysorbate 80 and Diluent for TAXOTERE 80 mg (13% (w/w) ethanol in water for injection). Both items are in a blister pack in one carton.

TAXOTERE 20 MG/0.5 ML (NDC 0075-8001-20)

TAXOTERE (docetaxel) Injection Concentrate 20 mg/0.5 mL: 20 mg docetaxel in 0.5 mL polysorbate 80 and diluent for TAXOTERE 20 mg (13% (w/w) ethanol in water for injection). Both items are in a blister pack in one carton.

Storage: Store between 2 and 25°C (36 and 77°F). Retain in the original package to protect from bright light. Freezing does not adversely affect the product.

Handling and Disposal: Procedures for proper handling and disposal of anticancer drugs should be considered. Several guidelines on this subject have been published[1–7]. There is no general agreement that all of the procedures recommended in the guidelines are necessary or appropriate.

REFERENCES

1. OSHA Work-Practice Guidelines for Controlling Occupational Exposure to Hazardous Drugs. *Am J Health-Syst Pharm.* 1996; 53: 1669-1685.
2. American Society of Hospital Pharmacists Technical Assistance Bulletin on Handling Cytotoxic and Hazardous Drugs. *Am J Hosp Pharm.* 1990; 47(95): 1033-1049.
3. AMA Council Report. Guidelines for Handling Parenteral Antineoplastics. *JAMA.* 1985; 253(11): 1590-1592.
4. Recommendations for the Safe Handling of Parenteral Antineoplastic Drugs. NIH Publication No. 83-2621. For sale by the Superintendent of Documents, US Government Printing Office, Washington, DC 20402.
5. National Study Commission on Cytotoxic Exposure - Recommendations for Handling Cytotoxic Agents. Available from Louis P. Jeffry, Chairman, National Study Commission on Cytotoxic Exposure. Massachusetts College of Pharmacy and Allied Health Sciences, 179 Longwood Avenue, Boston, MA 02115.
6. Clinical Oncological Society of Australia. Guidelines and Recommendations for Safe Handling of Antineoplastic Agents. *Med J Austr.* 1983; 426-428.
7. Jones, RB, et al. Safe Handling of Chemotherapeutic Agents: A Report from the Mt. Sinai Medical Center. *CA-A Cancer Journal for Clinicians.* 1983; Sept/Oct: 258-263.

Prescribing Information as of May 2004
Manufactured by Aventis Pharma Ltd.
Dagenham, Essex RM10 7XS
United Kingdom
Manufactured for
Aventis Pharmaceuticals Inc.
Bridgewater, NJ 08807 USA
www.aventis-us.com

TAX-MAY04-F-A

Patient Information Leaflet

Questions and Answers About Taxotere® Injection Concentrate

(generic name = docetaxel)
(pronounced as TAX-O-TEER)

What is Taxotere?

Taxotere is a medication to treat breast cancer, non-small cell lung cancer and prostate cancer. It has severe side effects in some patients. This leaflet is designed to help you understand how to use Taxotere and avoid its side effects to the fullest extent possible. The more you understand your treatment, the better you will be able to participate in your care. If you have questions or concerns, be sure to ask your doctor or nurse. They are always your best source of information about your condition and treatment.

What is the most important information about Taxotere?

- Since this drug, like many other cancer drugs, affects your blood cells, your doctor will ask for routine blood tests. These will include regular checks of your white blood cell counts. People with low blood counts can develop life-threatening infections. The earliest sign of infection may be fever, so if you experience a fever, tell your doctor right away.
- Occasionally, serious allergic reactions have occurred with this medicine. If you have any allergies, tell your doctor before receiving this medicine.
- A small number of people who take Taxotere have severe fluid retention, which can be life-threatening. To help avoid this problem, you must take another medication such as dexamethasone (DECKS-A-METH-A-SONE) prior to each Taxotere treatment. You must follow the schedule and take the exact dose of dexamethasone prescribed (see schedule at end of brochure). If you forget to take a dose or do not take it on schedule you must tell the doctor or nurse prior to your Taxotere treatment.
- If you are using any other medicines, tell your doctor before receiving your infusions of Taxotere.

How does Taxotere work?

Taxotere works by attacking cancer cells in your body. Different cancer medications attack cancer cells in different ways.

Here's how Taxotere works: Every cell in your body contains a supporting structure (like a skeleton). Damage to this "skeleton" can stop cell growth or reproduction. Taxotere makes the "skeleton" in some cancer cells very stiff, so that the cells can no longer grow.

How will I receive Taxotere?

Taxotere is given by an infusion directly into your vein. Your treatment will take about 1 hour. Generally, people receive Taxotere every 3 weeks. The amount of Taxotere and the frequency of your infusions will be determined by your doctor.

As part of your treatment, to reduce side effects your doctor will prescribe another medicine called dexamethasone. Your doctor will tell you how and when to take this medicine. It is important that you take the dexamethasone on the schedule set by your doctor. If you forget to take your medication, or do not take it on schedule, make sure to tell your doctor or nurse **BEFORE** you receive your Taxotere treatment. **Included with this information leaflet is a chart to help you remember when to take your dexamethasone.**

What should be avoided while receiving Taxotere?

Taxotere can interact with other medicines. Use only medicines that are prescribed for you by your doctor and **be sure** to tell your doctor all the medicines that you use, including nonprescription drugs.

What are the possible side effects of Taxotere?

Low Blood Cell Count—Many cancer medications, including Taxotere, cause a temporary drop in the number of white blood cells. These cells help protect your body from infection. Your doctor will routinely check your blood count and tell you if it is too low. Although most people receiving Taxotere do not have an infection even if they have a low white blood cell count, the risk of infection is increased.

Fever is often one of the most common and earliest signs of infection. Your doctor will recommend that you take your temperature frequently, especially during the days after treatment with Taxotere. If you have a fever, tell your doctor or nurse immediately.

Allergic Reactions—This type of reaction, which occurs during the infusion of Taxotere, is infrequent. If you feel a warm sensation, a tightness in your chest, or itching during or shortly after your treatment, tell your doctor or nurse immediately.

Continued on next page

Taxotere—Cont.

Fluid Retention—This means that your body is holding extra water. If this fluid retention is in the chest or around the heart it can be life-threatening. If you notice swelling in the feet and legs or a slight weight gain, this may be the first warning sign. Fluid retention usually does not start immediately; but, if it occurs, it may start around your 5th treatment. Generally, fluid retention will go away within weeks or months after your treatments are completed.

Dexamethasone tablets may protect patients from significant fluid retention. It is important that you take this medicine on schedule. If you have not taken dexamethasone on schedule, you must tell your doctor or nurse before receiving your next Taxotere treatment.

Gastrointestinal—Diarrhea has been associated with TAXOTERE use and can be severe in some patients. Nausea and/or vomiting are common in patients receiving TAXOTERE. Severe inflammation of the bowel can also occur in some patients and may be life threatening.

Hair Loss—Loss of hair occurs in most patients taking Taxotere (including the hair on your head, underarm hair, pubic hair, eyebrows, and eyelashes). Hair loss will begin after the first few treatments and varies from patient to patient. Once you have completed all your treatments, hair generally grows back.

Your doctor or nurse can refer you to a store that carries wigs, hairpieces, and turbans for patients with cancer.

Fatigue—A number of patients (about 10%) receiving Taxotere feel very tired following their treatments. If you feel tired or weak, allow yourself extra rest before your next treatment. If it is bothersome or lasts for longer than 1 week, inform your doctor or nurse.

Muscle Pain—This happens about 20% of the time, but is rarely severe. You may feel pain in your muscles or joints. Tell your doctor or nurse if this happens. They may suggest ways to make you more comfortable.

Rash—This side effect occurs commonly but is severe in about 5%. You may develop a rash that looks like a blotchy, hive-like reaction. This usually occurs on the hands and feet but may also appear on the arms, face, or body. Generally, it will appear between treatments and will go away before the next treatment. Inform your doctor or nurse if you experience a rash. They can help you avoid discomfort.

Odd Sensations—About half of patients getting Taxotere will feel numbness, tingling, or burning sensations in their hands and feet. If you do experience this, tell your doctor or nurse. Generally, these go away within a few weeks or months after your treatments are completed. About 14% of patients may also develop weakness in their hands and feet.

Nail Changes—Color changes to your fingernails or toenails may occur while taking Taxotere. In extreme, but rare, cases nails may fall off. After you have finished Taxotere treatments, your nails will generally grow back.

Eye Changes—Excessive tearing, which can be related to conjunctivitis or blockage of the tear ducts, may occur.

If you are interested in learning more about this drug, ask your doctor for a copy of the package insert.

Aventis Pharmaceuticals Inc.
Bridgewater, NJ 08807 USA
www.aventis-us.com
Rev. May 2004
TAX-May04-PIL-A

Every three-week injection of TAXOTERE for breast and non-small cell lung cancers
Take dexamethasone tablets, 8 mg twice daily
Dexamethasone dosing:
Day 1 Date:_____ Time:_____ AM _____ PM
Day 2 Date:_____ Time:_____ AM _____ PM
(Taxotere Treatment Day)
Day 3 Date:_____ Time:_____ AM _____ PM

Every three-week injection of TAXOTERE for prostate cancer
Take dexamethasone 8 mg, at 12 hours, 3 hours and 1 hour before TAXOTERE infusion.
Dexamethasone dosing:
Date:_____ Time:_____
Date:_____ Time:_____
(Taxotere Treatment Day)
Time:_____

Shown in Product Identification Guide, page 307

TRENTAL® ℞

[tren 'tal]
(pentoxifylline)
Tablets, 400 mg

Prescribing Information as of May 2003

DESCRIPTION

TRENTAL® (pentoxifylline) tablets for oral administration contain 400 mg of the active drug and the following inactive ingredients: D&C Red No. 27 Aluminum Lake or FD&C Red No. 3, hypromellose USP, magnesium stearate NF, polyethylene glycol NF, povidone USP, talc USP, titanium dioxide USP, and other ingredients in a controlled-release formulation. TRENTAL is a tri-substituted xanthine derivative designated chemically as 1-(5-oxohexyl)-3,7-dimethylxanthine that, unlike theophylline, is a hemorrheologic agent, i.e. an agent that affects blood viscosity. Pentoxifylline is soluble in water and ethanol, and sparingly soluble in toluene. The CAS Registry Number is 6493-05-6. The chemical structure is:

CLINICAL PHARMACOLOGY

Mode of Action

Pentoxifylline and its metabolites improve the flow properties of blood by decreasing its viscosity. In patients with chronic peripheral arterial disease, this increases blood flow to the affected microcirculation and enhances tissue oxygenation. The precise mode of action of pentoxifylline and the sequence of events leading to clinical improvement are still to be defined. Pentoxifylline administration has been shown to produce dose-related hemorrheologic effects, lowering blood viscosity, and improving erythrocyte flexibility. Leukocyte properties of hemorrheologic importance have been modified in animal and *in vitro* human studies. Pentoxifylline has been shown to increase leukocyte deformability and to inhibit neutrophil adhesion and activation. Tissue oxygen levels have been shown to be significantly increased by therapeutic doses of pentoxifylline in patients with peripheral arterial disease.

Pharmacokinetics and Metabolism

After oral administration in aqueous solution pentoxifylline is almost completely absorbed. It undergoes a first-pass effect and the various metabolites appear in plasma very soon after dosing. Peak plasma levels of the parent compound and its metabolites are reached within 1 hour. The major metabolites are Metabolite I (1-[5-hydroxyhexyl]-3,7-dimethylxanthine) and Metabolite V (1-[3-carboxypropyl]-3,7-dimethylxanthine), and plasma levels of these metabolites are 5 and 8 times greater, respectively, than pentoxifylline.

Following oral administration of aqueous solutions containing 100 to 400 mg of pentoxifylline, the pharmacokinetics of the parent compound and Metabolite I are dose-related and not proportional (non-linear), with half-life and area under the blood-level time curve (AUC) increasing with dose. The elimination kinetics of Metabolite V are not dose-dependent. The apparent plasma half-life of pentoxifylline varies from 0.4 to 0.8 hours and the apparent plasma half-lives of its metabolites vary from 1 to 1.6 hours. There is no evidence of accumulation or enzyme induction (Cytochrome P450) following multiple oral doses.

Excretion is almost totally urinary; the main biotransformation product is Metabolite V. Essentially no parent drug is found in the urine. Despite large variations in plasma levels of parent compound and its metabolites, the urinary recovery of Metabolite V is consistent and shows dose proportionality. Less than 4% of the administered dose is recovered in feces. Food intake shortly before dosing delays absorption of an immediate-release dosage form but does not affect total absorption. The pharmacokinetics and metabolism of TRENTAL have not been studied in patients with renal and/or hepatic dysfunction, but AUC was increased and elimination rate decreased in an older population (60–68 years) compared to younger individuals (22–30 years).

After administration of the 400 mg controlled-release TRENTAL tablet, plasma levels of the parent compound and its metabolites reach their maximum within 2 to 4 hours and remain constant over an extended period of time. Coadministration of TRENTAL tablets with meals resulted in an increase in mean C_{max} and AUC by about 28% and 13% for pentoxifylline, respectively. C_{max} for Metabolite 1 also increased by about 20%. The controlled release of pentoxifylline from the tablet eliminates peaks and troughs in plasma levels for improved gastrointestinal tolerance.

INDICATIONS AND USAGE

TRENTAL is indicated for the treatment of patients with intermittent claudication on the basis of chronic occlusive arterial disease of the limbs. TRENTAL can improve function and symptoms but is not intended to replace more definitive therapy, such as surgical bypass, or removal of arterial obstructions when treating peripheral vascular disease.

CONTRAINDICATIONS

TRENTAL should not be used in patients with recent cerebral and/or retinal hemorrhage or in patients who have previously exhibited intolerance to this product or methylxanthines such as caffeine, theophylline, and theobromine.

PRECAUTIONS

General

Patients with chronic occlusive arterial disease of the limbs frequently show other manifestations of arteriosclerotic disease. TRENTAL has been used safely for treatment of peripheral arterial disease in patients with concurrent coronary artery and cerebrovascular diseases, but there have been occasional reports of angina, hypotension, and arrhythmia. Controlled trials do not show that TRENTAL causes such adverse effects more often than placebo, but, as it is a methylxanthine derivative, it is possible some individuals will experience such responses. Patients on Warfarin should have more frequent monitoring of prothrombin times, while patients with other risk factors complicated by hemorrhage (e.g., recent surgery, peptic ulceration, cerebral and/or retinal bleeding) should have periodic examinations for bleeding including hematocrit and/or hemoglobin.

Drug Interactions

Although a causal relationship has not been established, there have been reports of bleeding and/or prolonged prothrombin time in patients treated with TRENTAL with and without anticoagulants or platelet aggregation inhibitors. Patients on Warfarin should have more frequent monitoring of prothrombin times, while patients with other risk factors complicated by hemorrhage (e.g., recent surgery, peptic ulceration) should have periodic examinations for bleeding including hematocrit and/or hemoglobin. Concomitant administration of TRENTAL and theophylline-containing drugs leads to increased theophylline levels and theophylline toxicity in some individuals. Such patients should be closely monitored for signs of toxicity and have their theophylline dosage adjusted as necessary. TRENTAL has been used concurrently with antihypertensive drugs, beta blockers, digitalis, diuretics, antidiabetic agents, and antiarrhythmics, without observed problems. Small decreases in blood pressure have been observed in some patients treated with TRENTAL; periodic systemic blood pressure monitoring is recommended for patients receiving concomitant antihypertensive therapy. If indicated, dosage of the antihypertensive agents should be reduced.

Carcinogenesis, Mutagenesis and Impairment of Fertility

Long-term studies of the carcinogenic potential of pentoxifylline were conducted in mice and rats by dietary administration of the drug at doses up to 450 mg/kg (approximately 19 times the maximum recommended human daily dose (MRHD) in both species when based on body weight; 1.5 times the MRHD in the mouse and 3.3 times the MRHD in the rat when based on body surface area). In mice, the drug was administered for 18 months, whereas in rats, the drug was administered for 18 months followed by an additional 6 months without drug exposure. In the rat study, there was a statistically significant increase in benign mammary fibroadenomas in females of the 450 mg/kg group. The relevance of this finding to human use is uncertain. Pentoxifyl-

INCIDENCE (%) OF SIDE EFFECTS

	Controlled-Release Tablets		Immediate-Release Capsules	
	Commercially Available		Used only for Controlled Clinical Trials	
	TRENTAL	**Placebo**	**TRENTAL**	**Placebo**
(Numbers of Patients at Risk)	(321)	(128)	(177)	(138)
Discontinued for Side Effect	3.1	0	9.6	7.2
CARDIOVASCULAR SYSTEM				
Angina/Chest pain	0.3	—	1.1	2.2
Arrhythmia/Palpitation	—	—	1.7	0.7
Flushing	—	—	2.3	0.7
DIGESTIVE SYSTEM				
Abdominal Discomfort	—	—	4.0	1.4
Belching/Flatus/Bloating	0.6	—	9.0	3.6
Diarrhea	—	—	3.4	2.9
Dyspepsia	2.8	4.7	9.6	2.9
Nausea	2.2	0.8	28.8	8.7
Vomiting	1.2	—	4.5	0.7
NERVOUS SYSTEM				
Agitation/Nervousness	—	—	1.7	0.7
Dizziness	1.9	3.1	11.9	4.3
Drowsiness	—	—	1.1	5.8
Headache	1.2	1.6	6.2	5.8
Insomnia	—	—	2.3	2.2
Tremor	0.3	0.8	—	—
Blurred Vision	—	—	2.3	1.4

line was devoid of mutagenic activity in various strains of *Salmonella* (Ames test) and in cultured mammalian cells (unscheduled DNA synthesis test) when tested in the presence and absence of metabolic activation. It was also negative in the *in vivo* mouse micronucleus test.

Pregnancy

Category C. Teratogenicity studies have been performed in rats and rabbits using oral doses up to 576 and 264 mg/kg, respectively. On a weight basis, these doses are 24 and 11 times the maximum recommended human daily dose (MRHD); on a body-surface-area basis, they are 4.2 and 3.5 times the MRHD. No evidence of fetal malformation was observed. Increased resorption was seen in rats of the 576 mg/kg group.

There are no adequate and well controlled studies in pregnant women. TRENTAL (pentoxifylline) should be used during pregnancy only if the potential benefit justifies the potential risk to the fetus.

Nursing Mothers

Pentoxifylline and its metabolites are excreted in human milk. Because of the potential for tumorigenicity shown for pentoxifylline in rats, a decision should be made whether to discontinue nursing or discontinue the drug, taking into account the importance of the drug to the mother.

Pediatric Use

Safety and effectiveness in pediatric patients have not been established.

ADVERSE REACTIONS

Clinical trials were conducted using either controlled-release TRENTAL tablets for up to 60 weeks or immediate-release TRENTAL capsules for up to 24 weeks. Dosage ranges in the tablet studies were 400 mg bid to tid and in the capsule studies, 200–400 mg tid. The table summarizes the incidence (in percent) of adverse reactions considered drug related, as well as the numbers of patients who received controlled-release TRENTAL tablets, immediate-release TRENTAL capsules, or the corresponding placebos. The incidence of adverse reactions was higher in the capsule studies (where dose related increases were seen in digestive and nervous system side effects) than in the tablet studies. Studies with the capsule include domestic experience, whereas studies with the controlled-release tablets were conducted outside the U.S.

The table indicates that in the tablet studies few patients discontinued because of adverse effects.

[See table at bottom of previous page]

TRENTAL has been marketed in Europe and elsewhere since 1972. In addition to the above symptoms, the following have been reported spontaneously since marketing or occurred in other clinical trials with an incidence of less than 1%; the causal relationship was uncertain:

Cardiovascular—dyspnea, edema, hypotension.

Digestive—anorexia, cholecystitis, constipation, dry mouth/thirst.

Nervous—anxiety, confusion, depression, seizures.

Respiratory—epistaxis, flu-like symptoms, laryngitis, nasal congestion.

Skin and Appendages—brittle fingernails, pruritus, rash, urticaria, angioedema.

Special Senses—blurred vision, conjunctivitis, earache, scotoma.

Miscellaneous—bad taste, excessive salivation, leukopenia, malaise, sore throat/swollen neck glands, weight change.

A few rare events have been reported spontaneously worldwide since marketing in 1972. Although they occurred under circumstances in which a causal relationship with pentoxifylline could not be established, they are listed to serve as information for physicians: Cardiovascular—angina, arrhythmia, tachycardia, anaphylactoid reactions. Digestive—hepatitis, jaundice, increased liver enzymes; and Hemic and Lymphatic—decreased serum fibrinogen, pancytopenia, aplastic anemia, leukemia, purpura, thrombocytopenia.

OVERDOSAGE

Overdosage with TRENTAL has been reported in pediatric patients and adults. Symptoms appear to be dose related. A report from a poison control center on 44 patients taking overdoses of enteric-coated pentoxifylline tablets noted that symptoms usually occurred 4–5 hours after ingestion and lasted about 12 hours. The highest amount ingested was 80 mg/kg; flushing, hypotension, convulsions, somnolence, loss of consciousness, fever, and agitation occurred. All patients recovered. In addition to symptomatic treatment and gastric lavage, special attention must be given to supporting respiration, maintaining systemic blood pressure, and controlling convulsions. Activated charcoal has been used to absorb pentoxifylline in patients who have overdosed.

DOSAGE AND ADMINISTRATION

The usual dosage of TRENTAL in controlled-release tablet form is one tablet (400 mg) three times a day with meals.

While the effect of TRENTAL may be seen within 2 to 4 weeks, it is recommended that treatment be continued for at least 8 weeks. Efficacy has been demonstrated in double-blind clinical studies of 6 months duration.

Digestive and central nervous system side effects are dose related. If patients develop these side effects it is recommended that the dosage be lowered to one tablet twice a day (800 mg/day). If side effects persist at this lower dosage, the administration of TRENTAL should be discontinued.

HOW SUPPLIED

TRENTAL (pentoxifylline) is available for oral administration as 400 mg pink film-coated oblong tablets imprinted Trental®; supplied in bottles of 100 (NDC 0039-0078-10), and Unit Dose Packs of 100 (NDC 0039-0078-11).

Store between 59 and 86° F (15 and 30° C).

Dispense in well-closed, light-resistant containers.

Protect blisters from light.

Rx only.

Rev. May 2003

US Patents 3,737,433 & 4,189,469

US Patent 3,737,433 patent term has been extended.

Manufactured by:
Patheon Pharmaceuticals Inc.
Cincinnati, OH 45215 USA

Manufactured for:
Aventis Pharmaceuticals NJ
Bridgewater, NJ 08807 USA

©2002 Aventis Pharmaceuticals Inc.

Shown in Product Identification Guide, page 307

Aventis Behring L.L.C.

for product information see ZLB Behring

Aventis Pasteur Inc.

SWIFTWATER PA 18370

Aventis Pasteur Inc.
For Medical Information Contact:
Generally:
Medical Affairs
(800) VACCINE
(800) 822-2463

Adverse Drug Experiences:
Pharmacovigilance Department
(570) 839-7187
(800) 822-2463

Sales and Ordering:
Aventis Pasteur Inc.
Customer Service
(800) VACCINE
(800) 822-2463
(570) 839-7187
www.vaccineshoppe.com

DAPTACEL® ℞

Diphtheria and Tetanus Toxoids and Acellular Pertussis Vaccine Adsorbed
℞ only

DESCRIPTION

DAPTACEL®, Diphtheria and Tetanus Toxoids and Acellular Pertussis Vaccine Adsorbed, for intramuscular use, manufactured by Aventis Pasteur Limited, is a sterile suspension of pertussis antigens and diphtheria and tetanus toxoids adsorbed on aluminum phosphate in a sterile isotonic sodium chloride solution. After shaking, the vaccine is a white homogeneous cloudy suspension. Each dose of DAPTACEL® contains the following active ingredients:

pertussis toxoid	10 µg
filamentous hemagglutinin (FHA)	5 µg
pertactin (PRN)	3 µg
fimbriae types 2 and 3	5 µg
diphtheria toxoid	15 Lf
tetanus toxoid	5 Lf

Other ingredients per dose include 3.3 mg (0.6% v/v) 2-phenoxyethanol as the preservative, 0.33 mg of aluminum as the adjuvant, ≤0.1 mg residual formaldehyde and <50 ng residual glutaraldehyde.

The acellular pertussis vaccine components are produced from *Bordetella pertussis* cultures grown in Stainer-Scholte medium[1] modified by the addition of casamino acids and dimethyl-beta-cyclodextrin. The fimbriae types 2 and 3 are extracted from the bacterial cells and the pertussis toxin, FHA and PRN are prepared from the supernatant. These proteins are purified by sequential filtration, salt-precipitation, ultrafiltration and chromatography. Pertussis toxin is inactivated with glutaraldehyde and FHA is treated with formaldehyde. The individual antigens are adsorbed separately onto aluminum phosphate.

Corynebacterium diphtheriae is grown in modified Mueller's growth medium.[2] After ammonium sulfate fractionation, the diphtheria toxin is detoxified with formalin and diafiltered. *Clostridium tetani* is grown in modified Mueller-Miller casamino acid medium without beef heart infusion.[3] Tetanus toxin is detoxified with formalin and purified by ammonium sulfate fractionation and diafiltration. Diphtheria and tetanus toxoids are individually adsorbed onto aluminum phosphate.

The adsorbed diphtheria, tetanus and acellular pertussis components are combined in a sterile isotonic sodium chloride solution containing 2-phenoxyethanol as preservative. Both diphtheria and tetanus toxoids induce at least 2 units of antitoxin per mL in the guinea pig potency test. The potency of the acellular pertussis vaccine components is evaluated by the antibody response of immunized mice to pertussis toxin, FHA, PRN and fimbriae types 2 and 3 measured by enzyme-linked immunosorbent assay (ELISA).

CLINICAL PHARMACOLOGY

Simultaneous immunization of infants and children against diphtheria, tetanus and pertussis with conventional whole-cell pertussis DTP vaccine (Diphtheria and Tetanus Toxoids and Pertussis Vaccine Adsorbed - For Pediatric Use) has been a routine practice in the US since the late 1940s. This has played a major role in markedly reducing disease and deaths from these infections.[4] DTaP (Diphtheria and Tetanus Toxoids and Acellular Pertussis Vaccine Adsorbed) vaccines were first available for use in infants in the US in 1996 and have been routinely recommended for all doses of the vaccination series for infants and children <7 years of age since 1997.[5]

Diphtheria

Corynebacterium diphtheriae may cause both localized and generalized disease. The systemic intoxication is caused by diphtheria exotoxin, an extracellular protein of toxigenic strains of *C. diphtheriae*. Protection against disease is due to the development of neutralizing antibody to diphtheria toxin.

Both toxigenic and nontoxigenic strains of *C. diphtheriae* can cause disease but only strains that produce diphtheria toxin cause severe manifestations such as myocarditis and neuritis. Diphtheria is a serious disease, with the highest case-fatality rates among infants and the elderly.[4,6]

Prior to the widespread use of diphtheria toxoid in the late 1940s, diphtheria disease was common in the US. More than 200,000 cases, primarily among children, were reported in 1921. Approximately 5%–10% of cases were fatal; the highest case-fatality rates were in the very young and the elderly. More recently, reported cases of diphtheria of all types declined from 306 in 1975 to 59 in 1979; most were cutaneous diphtheria reported from a single state. After 1979, cutaneous diphtheria was no longer reportable.[4] From 1980 through 2000, only 50 cases of diphtheria were reported in the US. During the period 1980–1996, six fatal cases of diphtheria were reported. Only 1 case of diphtheria was reported each year in 1998–2000 with no fatalities.[7] Of 40 reported cases with known age in 1982–1998, 63% were in persons ≥20 years of age. Most cases have occurred in unimmunized or inadequately immunized persons. Although diphtheria disease is rare in the US, it appears that *C. diphtheriae* continues to circulate in areas of the country with previously endemic diphtheria.[8]

Diphtheria continues to occur in other parts of the world. A major epidemic of diphtheria occurred in the newly Independent States of the former Soviet Union beginning in 1990. This epidemic resulted in approximately 150,000 cases and 5,000 deaths during the years 1990–1997.[9] This outbreak is believed to be due to several factors, including a lack of routine immunization of adults in these countries.[10] Complete immunization significantly reduces the risk of developing diphtheria and immunized persons who develop disease have milder illness. Following adequate immunization with diphtheria toxoid, protection is thought to last for at least 10 years. Immunization does not, however, eliminate carriage of *C. diphtheriae* in the pharynx, nose or on the skin.[4]

Tetanus

Tetanus manifests systemic toxicity primarily by neuromuscular dysfunction caused by a potent exotoxin elaborated by *Clostridium tetani*.

Spores of *C. tetani* are ubiquitous. Serological tests indicate that naturally acquired immunity to tetanus toxin does not occur in the US. Thus, universal primary immunization, with subsequent maintenance of adequate antitoxin levels by means of appropriately timed boosters, is necessary to protect all age groups. Tetanus toxoid is a highly effective antigen and a completed primary series generally induces protective levels of serum antitoxin that persist for 10 years or more.[4]

Following routine use of tetanus toxoid in the US, the occurrence of tetanus disease decreased dramatically from 560 reported cases in 1947 to an average of 50–100 cases reported annually from the mid 1970s through the late 1990s to 35 cases in 2000.[7] The case-fatality rate has been relatively constant at approximately 30%. During the years 1982–1998, 52% of reported cases were among persons 60 years of age or older. In the mid to late 1990s, the age distribution of reported cases shifted to a younger age group, in part due to an increased number of cases among injection drug users in California. From 1995–1997, persons 20–59 years of age accounted for 60% of all cases, with persons 60 years of age or older accounting for only 35%. In the US, tetanus occurs almost exclusively among unvaccinated or inadequately vaccinated persons.[8]

Pertussis

Pertussis (whooping cough) is a disease of the respiratory tract caused by *Bordetella pertussis*. This gram-negative coccobacillus produces a variety of biologically active components. The role of the different components produced by *B. pertussis* in either the pathogenesis of, or immunity to, pertussis is not well understood.[6]

Pertussis is highly communicable (attack rates of 90% have been reported for susceptible individuals exposed to a case

Continued on next page

Daptacel—Cont.

in the home)[11] and can cause severe disease, particularly among young infants. Since pertussis became a nationally reportable disease in the US in 1922, the highest number of pertussis cases (approximately 260,000) was reported in 1934. Following the introduction and widespread use of whole-cell pertussis DTP vaccine among infants and children in the mid to late 1940s, pertussis incidence gradually declined, reaching a historical low of 1,010 cases reported in 1976.[12]

During the 1980s and 1990s, the number of reported pertussis cases in the US has gradually increased, particularly among adolescents and adults.[12,13] Improvements in the diagnosis and reporting of pertussis in older age groups is thought to have contributed, at least in part, to the increase in reported cases. The number of cases of pertussis reported among children aged 6 months to 4 years has remained stable throughout the 1990s, suggesting that protection offered by vaccination has continued with the introduction of DTaP vaccines.[12]

During 1997–2000, a total of 29,134 cases were reported, for an estimated average annual incidence rate of 2.7 per 100,000 population.[12] Among 29,048 cases for whom age was known, 29% were aged < 1 year, 12% were aged 1–4 years, 10% were aged 5–9 years, 29% were aged 10–19 years and 20% were ≥20 years of age.[12] Average annual incidence rates during 1997–2000 were highest among infants aged <1 year (55.5 cases per 100,000 population) and lower in children aged 1–4 years (5.5), children aged 5–9 years (3.6), persons aged 10–19 years (5.5) and persons aged ≥20 years (0.8).[12]

The severity of pertussis remains highest in infants. Of 7,203 infants <6 months of age reported as having pertussis during the period 1997–2000, 63% were hospitalized, 12% had pneumonia, 1.4% had one or more seizures, 0.2% had encephalopathy and 0.8% died.[12]

Atypical infection, including nonspecific symptoms of bronchitis or upper respiratory tract infection, may occur at any age but more commonly in older children and adults, including some who were previously immunized. In these cases, pertussis may not be diagnosed because classic signs, particularly the inspiratory whoop, may be absent. Older preschool-aged and school-aged children, as well as adolescents and adults who develop pertussis, may play a role in transmission to young infants.[8]

Concerns about the safety of whole-cell pertussis DTP vaccines prompted the development of less reactogenic DTaP vaccines that contain purified antigens of *B. pertussis*. The pertussis component of DTaP vaccines contains inactivated pertussis toxin and may contain one or more of FHA, PRN and fimbriae types 2 and 3. DTaP vaccines were first available for use in infants in the US in 1996 and have been routinely recommended by the Advisory Committee on Immunization Practices (ACIP) for all doses of the vaccination series for infants and children <7 years of age since 1997.[5]

Since 1991, 7 studies conducted in Europe and Africa have evaluated the efficacy of 8 DTaP vaccines administered to infants. The vaccines, produced by different manufacturers, contained a varying number and quantity of antigens. The derivation and formulation of the individual antigens also varied among different vaccines. The studies differed in study design and 3, including the Sweden I Efficacy Trial (1992–1995), were randomized placebo-controlled clinical trials. Because of these and other differences, comparisons among studies should be made with caution. Within individual studies, however, the efficacy of acellular pertussis vaccines can be compared directly with that of a placebo control or whole-cell pertussis DTP. The efficacy of 3 doses of acellular pertussis vaccines in preventing moderate to severe pertussis disease was within the range expected for most whole-cell pertussis DTP vaccines. Point estimates of the efficacy of DTaP vaccines ranged from 59%–89%.[5]

The effectiveness of pertussis vaccine among US children aged 7–18 months in 1998 and 1999 was calculated using the screening method. During this time, the National Immunization Survey reported 66% of children aged ≤18 months received DTaP rather than whole-cell pertussis DTP.[12] The screening estimate of 88% reflects the effectiveness of the overall vaccination program that used approximately two thirds DTaP and one third whole-cell pertussis DTP in children aged 7–18 months. This estimate is similar to that observed in clinical trials for acellular pertussis vaccines. During 1997–2000, the incidence rates were highest among infants aged <1 year, lower in children aged 1–4 years and remained stable among children aged 5–9 years.[12]

Efficacy of DAPTACEL®

Pertussis

A randomized, double-blinded, placebo-controlled efficacy and safety study was conducted in Sweden from 1992–1995 (Sweden I Efficacy Trial) under the sponsorship of the National Institute of Allergy and Infectious Diseases (NIAID). A total of 9,829 infants received 1 of 4 vaccines: DAPTACEL® (n = 2,587); another investigational acellular pertussis vaccine (n = 2,566); whole-cell pertussis DTP vaccine (n = 2,102); or DT vaccine as placebo (Swedish National Bacteriological Laboratory, n = 2,574). Infants were immunized at 2, 4 and 6 months of age. The mean length of follow-up was 2 years after the third dose of vaccine. The protective efficacy of DAPTACEL® against pertussis after 3 doses of vaccine using the World Health Organization (WHO) case definition (≥21 consecutive days of paroxysmal cough with culture or serologic confirmation or epidemiologic link to a confirmed case) was 84.9% (95% confidence interval [CI] 80.1 to 88.6).[14] The protective efficacy of DAPTACEL® against mild pertussis (≥1 day of cough with laboratory confirmation) was 77.9% (95% CI 72.6 to 82.2).[15] Protection against pertussis by DAPTACEL® was sustained for the 2-year follow-up period.[14,15]

In order to assess the antibody response to the pertussis antigens of DAPTACEL® in the US population, 2 lots of DAPTACEL®, including the lot used in the Sweden I Efficacy Trial, were administered to US infants in the US Bridging Study.[15] In this study, antibody responses following 3 doses of DAPTACEL® given to US children at 2, 4 and 6 months of age were compared to those from a subset of the infants enrolled in the Sweden I Efficacy Trial. Assays were performed in parallel on the available sera from the US and Swedish infants. Antibody responses to all the antigens were similar except for those to the PRN component. For both lots of DAPTACEL®, the geometric mean concentration (GMC) and percent response to PRN in US infants (Lot 006, n = 107; Lot 009, n = 108) were significantly lower after 3 doses of vaccine than in Swedish infants (n = 83). In a separate study performed in Canada (Phase II), in which children received 4 doses of DAPTACEL® at 2, 4, 6 and 17–18 months of age, antibody responses following the fourth dose (n = 275) were equivalent or higher than those seen in the Swedish infants after 3 doses. While a serologic correlate of protection for pertussis has not been established, the antibody response to all antigens in North American infants after 4 doses of DAPTACEL® at 2, 4, 6 and 17–20 months of age was comparable to that achieved in Swedish infants in whom efficacy was demonstrated after 3 doses of DTaP at 2, 4 and 6 months of age.[15]

Diphtheria and Tetanus

In a Canadian clinical study, 324 children were enrolled to receive DAPTACEL® at 2, 4, 6 and 17–18 months of age. The proportion of children with post-dose 3 diphtheria (n = 313) and tetanus (n = 313) antitoxin levels ≥0.01 IU/mL was 100% and ≥0.10 IU/mL was 85% and 100%, respectively.[15] The proportion with post-dose 4 diphtheria (n = 296) and tetanus (n = 296) antitoxin levels ≥0.10 IU/mL was 100%.[15] The efficacy of the diphtheria and tetanus toxoids used in DAPTACEL® was determined on the basis of immunogenicity studies with a comparison to a serological correlate of protection (0.01 antitoxin units/mL) established by the Panel on Review of Bacterial Vaccines and Toxoids.[16]

In the US Bridging Study, for which data are only available following 3 doses, 99.2% (n = 261) achieved diphtheria antitoxin levels of ≥0.01 IU/mL, 80.6% (n = 261) achieved levels of ≥0.10 IU/mL and 100% (n = 260) achieved tetanus antitoxin levels of 0.01 IU/mL and 0.10 IU/mL.[15]

Concurrently Administered Vaccines

In a clinical trial conducted in the US, DAPTACEL® was given simultaneously with *Haemophilus influenzae* type b vaccine and with live oral poliovirus vaccine (OPV) at 2, 4 and 6 months of age according to local practices. Two hundred eighty-one infants received 3 doses of *Haemophilus influenzae* type b vaccine and 305 received 3 doses of OPV. Immune responses to these vaccines were evaluated in a subset of 258 children. One month after the third dose, 96.9% (n = 253) achieved anti-PRP antibody levels of at least 0.15 µg/mL, 82.7% (n = 216) achieved antibody levels of at least 1.0 µg/mL; and 100% (n = 178), had protective neutralizing antibody of ≥1:8 for poliovirus types 1 and 2 and 98.3% (n = 175) for poliovirus type 3.[15]

In the same study, hepatitis B vaccine (supplied by different manufacturers) was also given to children by different schedules. Hepatitis B vaccine was given concurrently with DAPTACEL® at 2 and 6 months of age to a subset of infants who received a birth dose of hepatitis B vaccine. Of infants with adequate serum available for serology testing (n = 82), 97% achieved anti-HBs antibody levels ≥10 mIU/mL post dose 3.[15]

No immunogenicity data are available for concurrent administration of DAPTACEL® with IPV; pneumococcal conjugate vaccine; measles, mumps and rubella vaccine (MMR) or varicella vaccine.

INDICATIONS AND USAGE

DAPTACEL® is indicated for active immunization against diphtheria, tetanus and pertussis in infants and children 6 weeks through 6 years of age (prior to seventh birthday).

Children who have had well-documented pertussis (culture positive for *B. pertussis* or epidemiologic linkage to a culture positive case) should complete the vaccination series with DT; some experts recommend including acellular pertussis vaccine as well. Although well-documented pertussis disease is likely to confer immunity, the duration of protection is unknown.[17]

DAPTACEL® is not to be used for the treatment of *B. pertussis, C. diphtheriae or C. tetani* infections.

When passive protection is required, Tetanus Immune Globulin and/or Diphtheria Antitoxin may also be administered at separate sites with separate needles and syringes.[4] (See DOSAGE AND ADMINISTRATION.)

As with any vaccine, vaccination with DAPTACEL® may not protect 100% of susceptible individuals.

CONTRAINDICATIONS

This vaccine is contraindicated in children and adults seven years of age and older.

Hypersensitivity to any component of the vaccine is a contraindication to further administration.[5]

The following events after receipt of DAPTACEL® are contraindications to further administration of any pertussis-containing vaccine:[5]

- *An immediate anaphylactic reaction.* Because of uncertainty as to which component of the vaccine may be responsible, no further vaccination with diphtheria, tetanus or pertussis components should be carried out. Alternatively, such individuals may be referred to an allergist for evaluation if further immunizations are to be considered.
- *Encephalopathy not attributable to another identifiable cause* (e.g., an acute, severe central nervous system disorder occurring within 7 days after vaccination and consisting of major alterations in consciousness, unresponsiveness or generalized or focal seizures that persist more than a few hours, without recovery within 24 hours). In such cases, DT vaccine should be administered for the remaining doses in the vaccination schedule.

The decision to administer or delay vaccination because of a current or recent febrile illness depends on the severity of symptoms and on the etiology of the disease. According to the ACIP, all vaccines can be administered to persons with mild illness such as diarrhea, mild upper-respiratory infection with or without low-grade fever, or other low-grade febrile illness.[17,18] However, children with moderate or serious illness should not be immunized until recovered.[4]

Elective immunization procedures should be deferred during an outbreak of poliomyelitis because of the risk of provoking paralysis.[19,20,21]

WARNINGS

The stopper to the vial of this product contains dry natural latex rubber that may cause allergic reactions.

If any of the following events occur within the specified period after administration of a whole-cell pertussis DTP or DTaP vaccine, providers and parents should evaluate the risks and benefits of subsequent doses of whole-cell pertussis DTP or DTaP vaccines:[5]

- Temperature of ≥40.5°C (105°F) within 48 hours, not attributable to another identifiable cause.
- Collapse or shock-like state (hypotonic-hyporesponsive episode) within 48 hours.
- Persistent crying lasting ≥3 hours within 48 hours.
- Convulsions with or without fever within 3 days.

When a decision is made to withhold pertussis vaccine, immunization with DT vaccine should be continued.[4]

Because of the risk of hemorrhage, DAPTACEL® should not be given to children with any coagulation disorder, including thrombocytopenia, which would contraindicate intramuscular injection unless the potential benefit clearly outweighs the risk of administration.

Studies suggest that, when given whole-cell pertussis DTP vaccine, infants and children with a history of convulsions in first-degree family members have a 2.4-fold increased risk for neurologic events.[22] However, ACIP has concluded that a history of convulsions or other central nervous system disorders in parents or siblings is not a contraindication to pertussis vaccination and that children with such family histories should receive DTaP vaccines according to the recommended schedule.[4,17,18]

If an infant or young child with a personal or family history of febrile or non-febrile convulsions is to be immunized, acetaminophen or other appropriate antipyretic should be given at the time of DTaP vaccination and for the ensuing 24 hours according to the respective package insert recommended dosage to reduce the possibility of post-vaccination fever.[4,17,18]

A committee of the Institute of Medicine (IOM) has concluded that the evidence is consistent with a causal relationship between whole-cell pertussis DTP vaccine and acute neurologic illness and, under special circumstances, between whole-cell pertussis DTP vaccine and chronic neurologic disease in the context of the National Childhood Encephalopathy Study (NCES) report.[23,24] However, the IOM committee concluded that the evidence was insufficient to determine whether whole-cell pertussis DTP vaccine increased the overall risk of chronic neurologic disease.[24]

Acute encephalopathy (with or without permanent neurological injury) or permanent neurological injury has not been reported following administration of DAPTACEL® but the experience with this vaccine is insufficient to rule this out. (See ADVERSE REACTIONS.)

Infants and children with recognized possible or potential underlying neurologic conditions seem to be at enhanced risk for the appearance of manifestations of the underlying neurologic disorder within 2 or 3 days following whole-cell pertussis DTP vaccine immunization.[4] Whether to administer DAPTACEL® to children with proven or suspected underlying neurologic disorders must be decided on an individual basis after consideration of the risks and benefits. An important consideration includes the current local incidence of pertussis. The ACIP has issued guidelines for such children.[25]

PRECAUTIONS

General

Care is to be taken by the health-care provider for the safe and effective use of this vaccine.

Epinephrine Hydrochloride Solution (1:1,000), other appropriate agents and equipment must be available for immediate use in case an anaphylactic or acute hypersensitivity reaction occurs. Health-care providers must be familiar with current recommendations for the initial management of anaphylaxis in non-hospital settings, including proper airway management.[17,26]

Before an injection of any vaccine, all known precautions should be taken to prevent adverse reactions. This includes a review of the patient's history with respect to possible sensitivity to the vaccine, similar vaccines or to dry natural latex rubber (see WARNINGS), previous immunization history, current health status (see CONTRAINDICATIONS) and a current knowledge of the literature concerning the use of the vaccine under consideration including the nature of adverse events that may follow its use.

The expected immune response to DAPTACEL® may not be obtained in immunosuppressed persons.[4] Pertussis-containing vaccines are not contraindicated in persons with HIV infection.[17]

Special care should be taken to ensure that the injection does not enter a blood vessel.

A separate, sterile syringe and needle or a sterile disposable unit should be used for each patient to prevent transmission of hepatitis or other infectious agents from person to person. Needles should not be recapped but should be disposed of according to biohazard waste guidelines.

Information for Vaccine Recipients and Parents/Guardians

Before administration of this vaccine, health-care personnel should inform the parent, guardian or other responsible adult of the benefits and risks of the vaccine and the importance of completing the immunization series unless a contraindication to further immunization exists. (See ADVERSE REACTIONS and WARNINGS.)

The physician should inform the parent or guardian about the potential for adverse reactions that have been temporally associated with DAPTACEL® and other pertussis-containing vaccines. The health-care provider should provide the Vaccine Information Statements (VIS) which are required by the National Childhood Vaccine Injury Act of 1986 to be given with each immunization. The parent or guardian should be instructed to report any serious adverse reactions to their health-care provider.

IT IS EXTREMELY IMPORTANT WHEN A CHILD RETURNS FOR THE NEXT DOSE IN THE SERIES THAT THE PARENT OR GUARDIAN SHOULD BE QUESTIONED CONCERNING ANY SYMPTOMS AND/OR SIGNS OF AN ADVERSE REACTION AFTER THE PREVIOUS DOSE OF VACCINE. (See CONTRAINDICATIONS and ADVERSE REACTIONS.)

Adverse events following immunization should be reported by health-care providers to the Vaccine Adverse Events Reporting System (VAERS). (See ADVERSE REACTIONS, Reporting of Adverse Events.)

Drug Interactions

As with other intramuscular (I.M.) injections, use with caution in patients on anticoagulant therapy.

Immunosuppressive therapies, including irradiation, antimetabolites, alkylating agents, cytotoxic drugs and corticosteroids (used in greater than physiologic doses), may reduce the immune response to vaccines. Although no specific studies with pertussis vaccine are available, if immunosuppressive therapy is to be soon discontinued, it seems reasonable to defer immunization until the patient has been off therapy for one month; otherwise, the patient should be vaccinated while still on therapy.[4]

If DAPTACEL® is administered to persons with an immunodeficiency disorder, on immunosuppressive therapy or after a recent injection of immune globulin, an adequate immunologic response may not occur.

For information regarding simultaneous administration with other vaccines refer to DOSAGE AND ADMINISTRATION.

If passive immunization is needed for tetanus or diphtheria prophylaxis, Tetanus Immune Globulin (Human) (TIG), or Diphtheria Antitoxin, if used, should be given in a separate site, with a separate needle and syringe.[18]

Carcinogenesis, Mutagenesis, Impairment of Fertility

DAPTACEL® has not been evaluated for its carcinogenic or mutagenic potential or impairment of fertility.

Pregnancy Category C

Animal reproduction studies have not been conducted with DAPTACEL®. It is not known whether DAPTACEL® can cause fetal harm when administered to a pregnant woman or can affect reproductive capacity. DAPTACEL® is NOT recommended for use in a pregnant woman.

Geriatric Use

This product is NOT recommended for use in adult populations.

Pediatric Use

SAFETY AND EFFECTIVENESS OF DAPTACEL® IN INFANTS BELOW 6 WEEKS OF AGE HAVE NOT BEEN ESTABLISHED. (See DOSAGE AND ADMINISTRATION.)

THIS VACCINE IS NOT RECOMMENDED FOR PERSONS 7 YEARS OF AGE OR OLDER. Tetanus and Diphtheria Toxoids Adsorbed For Adult Use (Td) is to be used in individuals 7 years of age or older.

ADVERSE REACTIONS

Over 11,400 doses of DAPTACEL® have been administered to infants and toddlers in 6 clinical studies. In all, 3,694 children received a total of 3 doses and 476 children received 4 doses of DAPTACEL®.[14,15,27,28,29,30,31]

In the Sweden I Efficacy Trial, DAPTACEL® was compared with DT and a whole-cell pertussis DTP vaccine. A standard diary card was kept for 14 days after each dose and follow-up telephone calls were made 1 and 14 days after each injection. Telephone calls were made monthly to monitor the occurrence of severe events and/or hospitalizations for the 2 months after the last injection. There were fewer of the common local and systemic reactions following DAPTACEL® than following the whole-cell pertussis DTP vaccine. As shown in Table 1, the 2,587 infants who enrolled to receive DAPTACEL® at 2, 4 and 6 months of age had similar rates of reactions within 24 hours as recipients of DT and significantly lower rates than infants receiving whole-cell pertussis DTP.[14]

The rates of local reactions reported 1 day after any dose were lower in the DAPTACEL® and DT groups than in the whole-cell pertussis DTP vaccine group.

[See table 1 above]

TABLE 1[14,15] PERCENTAGE OF INFANTS FROM SWEDEN I EFFICACY TRIAL WITH LOCAL OR SYSTEMIC REACTIONS WITHIN 24 HOURS POST-DOSE 1, 2 AND 3 OF DAPTACEL® COMPARED WITH DT AND WHOLE-CELL PERTUSSIS DTP VACCINES

EVENT	Dose 1 (2 MONTHS)			Dose 2 (4 MONTHS)			Dose 3 (6 MONTHS)		
	DAPTACEL® N = 2,587	DT N = 2,574	DTP N = 2,102	DAPTACEL® N = 2,563	DT N = 2,555	DTP N = 2,040	DAPTACEL® N = 2,549	DT N = 2,538	DTP N = 2,001
Local									
Tenderness (Any)	8.0*	8.4	59.5	10.1*	10.3	60.2	10.8*	10.0	50.0
Redness ≥2 cm	0.3*	0.3	6.0	1.0*	0.8	5.1	3.7*	2.4	6.4
Swelling ≥2 cm	0.9*	0.7	10.6	1.6*	2.0	10.0	6.3*§	3.9	10.5
Systemic									
Fever† ≥38°C (100.4°F)	7.8*	7.6	72.3	19.1*	18.4	74.3	23.6*	22.1	65.1
Fretfulness††	32.3	33.0	82.1	39.6	39.8	85.4	35.9	37.7	73.0
Anorexia	11.2*	10.3	39.2	9.1*	8.1	25.6	8.4*	7.7	17.5
Drowsiness	32.7*	32.0	56.9	25.9*	25.6	50.6	18.9*	20.6	37.6
Crying ≥1 hour	1.7*	1.6	11.8	2.5*	2.7	9.3	1.2*	1.0	3.3
Vomiting	6.9*	6.3	9.5	5.2**	5.8	7.4	4.3	5.2	5.5

N = Number of evaluable subjects
* $p<0.001$: DAPTACEL® versus whole-cell pertussis DTP
** $p<0.003$: DAPTACEL® versus whole-cell pertussis DTP
§ $p<0.0001$: DAPTACEL® versus DT
† Rectal temperature
†† Statistical comparisons were not made for this variable
DT: Swedish National Biologics Laboratories
DTP: Aventis Pasteur Inc.

The incidence of serious and less common selected systemic events in this trial are summarized in Table 2.[14,15]

[See table 2 above]

TABLE 2[14,15] SELECTED SYSTEMIC EVENTS: RATES PER 1,000 DOSES AFTER VACCINATION AT 2, 4, AND 6 MONTHS OF AGE IN SWEDEN I EFFICACY TRIAL

EVENT	Dose 1 (2 MONTHS)			Dose 2 (4 MONTHS)			Dose 3 (6 MONTHS)		
	DAPTACEL® N = 2,587	DT N = 2,574	DTP N = 2,102	DAPTACEL® N = 2,565	DT N = 2,556	DTP N = 2,040	DAPTACEL® N = 2,551	DT N = 2,539	DTP N = 2,002
Rectal temperature ≥40°C (104°F) within 48 hours of vaccination.	0.39	0.78	3.33	0	0.78	3.43	0.39	1.18	6.99
Hypotonic-hyporesponsive episode within 24 hours of vaccination.	0	0	1.9	0	0	0.49	0.39	0	0
Persistent crying ≥3 hours within 24 hours of vaccination.	1.16	0	8.09	0.39	0.39	1.96	0	0	1.0
Seizures within 72 hours of vaccination.	0	0.39	0	0	0.39	0.49	0	0.39	0

N = Number of evaluable subjects

One case of whole limb swelling and generalized symptoms, with resolution within 24 hours, was observed following dose 2 of DAPTACEL®. No episodes of anaphylaxis or encephalopathy were observed. No seizures were reported within 3 days of vaccination with DAPTACEL®. Over the entire study period, 6 seizures were reported in the DAPTACEL® group, 9 in the DT group and 3 in the whole-cell pertussis DTP group, for overall rates of 2.3, 3.5 and 1.4 per 1,000 vaccinees, respectively. One case of infantile spasms was reported in the DAPTACEL® group. There were no instances of invasive bacterial infection or death.[14,15]

Rates of serious adverse events that are less common than those reported in the Sweden I Efficacy Trial are not known at this time.

Table 3 summarizes the safety results from the Phase II Study in Canada in children who were immunized at 2, 4, 6 and 17–18 months of age with DAPTACEL®. For adverse events, parents recorded information for 72 hours post-immunization in a diary card. Local reactions of redness and swelling were assessed and measured by the parents using a template with graded size markings. Study staff collected the information from the parents during a structured telephone interview at 2–6, 8–12, 24, 48 and 72 hours and 7 days post-immunization and recorded the information in the case report form.[15,29]

Local and systemic adverse events were consistently less common in DAPTACEL® recipients at 2, 4 and 6 months of age than in those who received whole-cell pertussis DTP vaccine. Following the fourth dose, the same trends were observed, except for rates of severe redness and swelling which did not differ between the 2 vaccine groups. Rates of local reactions of redness and swelling were increased following the fourth dose compared with the first 3 doses as was mild tenderness but there was no increase in severe tenderness.

[See table 3 at top of next page]

The US Bridging Study was designed, in part, to assess the safety of DAPTACEL® in infants at 2, 4 and 6 months of age, with routinely recommended, concurrently given childhood vaccines (*Haemophilus influenzae* type b vaccine, OPV and hepatitis B). For adverse events, parents recorded information for 72 hours post-immunization in a diary card. Local reactions were assessed and measured by the parents. Study staff collected the information from the parents during a structured telephone interview on days 4 and 14 post-immunization and recorded the information in the case report form.[15] The incidence of redness, swelling, pain or tenderness at the injection site and systemic symptoms after each dose is shown as pooled data from 2 lots of DAPTACEL® (Lots 006 and 009) in Table 4. Fever ≥38°C (100.4°F) was observed in 9.9%–11.9% of subjects. The incidence of severe systemic symptoms including irritability, tiredness, anorexia, rash and vomiting ranged from 0.3%–0.6%. One afebrile seizure occurred within 24 hours post dose 2 immunization (n = 321).[15]

In an ongoing study (P3T06) initiated in May 2001 and anticipated to be completed in 2004, which was designed to assess the safety of DAPTACEL® given with routinely recommended vaccines (*Haemophilus influenzae* type b vaccine, IPV, hepatitis B and pneumococcal conjugate vaccine) in the US (in which 777 children have received their first

Continued on next page

Daptacel—Cont.

dose, 350 have received their second dose and 86 their third dose with safety data still being collected from children in this study), one afebrile seizure was reported within 24 hours of receipt of dose 1.

[See table 4 at right]

NIAID sponsored a multicenter Phase I/II clinical trial to compare the safety and immunogenicity of 13 acellular pertussis vaccines with a conventional whole-cell pertussis DTP vaccine in infants in the US. The common local and systemic adverse experiences, after all 3 doses, for DAPTACEL® and the participating acellular vaccines that have subsequently been licensed in the US were generally similar in type and frequency and were reduced in comparison to the whole-cell pertussis DTP vaccine.[28]

Additional adverse reactions evaluated in conjunction with pertussis, diphtheria and tetanus vaccination are as follows:

- As with other aluminum-containing vaccines, a nodule may be palpable at the injection sites for several weeks. Sterile abscess formation at the site of injection has been reported.[4,32]
- Rarely, anaphylactic reactions (i.e., hives, swelling of the mouth, difficulty breathing, hypotension or shock) have been reported after receiving preparations containing diphtheria, tetanus and/or pertussis antigens.[4]

Arthus-type hypersensitivity reactions, characterized by severe local reactions (generally starting 2–8 hours after an injection), may follow receipt of tetanus toxoid. A few cases of peripheral neuropathy have been reported following tetanus toxoid administration, although the evidence is inadequate to accept or reject a causal relation.[33]

A review by the Institute of Medicine (IOM) found a causal relation between tetanus toxoid and brachial neuritis and Guillain-Barré syndrome.[34] The following illnesses have been reported as temporally associated with some vaccines containing tetanus toxoid: neurological complications[35,36] including cochlear lesion, brachial plexus neuropathies,[37] paralysis of the radial nerve,[33] paralysis of the recurrent nerve, accommodation paresis and EEG disturbances with encephalopathy (with or without permanent intellectual or motor function impairment).[38,39] In the differential diagnosis of polyradiculoneuropathies following administration of a vaccine containing tetanus toxoid, tetanus toxoid should be considered as a possible etiology.[39]

Onset of infantile spasms has occurred in infants who have recently received whole-cell pertussis DTP or DT. Analysis of data from the National Childhood Encephalopathy Study (NCES) on children with infantile spasms failed to demonstrate that receipt of DT or whole-cell pertussis DTP vaccines was causally related to infantile spasms.[23,40] The incidence of onset of infantile spasms increases at 3–9 months of age, the time period in which the second and third doses of whole-cell pertussis DTP are generally given. Therefore, some cases of infantile spasms can be expected to be related by chance alone to recent receipt of whole-cell pertussis DTP.[4]

Persistent, inconsolable crying lasting ≥3 hours and high-pitched, unusual screaming, 1% and 0.1% respectively, after 15,752 doses of whole-cell pertussis DTP vaccine have been reported.[38] Convulsions and hypotonic-hyporesponsive episodes (HHE) have each been reported to occur at a frequency of about 1:1,750 injections of whole-cell pertussis DTP.[17,26,38] Most convulsions are brief, generalized and self-limited and are usually associated with fever. Neither febrile nor afebrile convulsions associated with whole-cell pertussis DTP vaccine have been shown to be associated with subsequent seizure disorder.[17] Persistent, inconsolable crying ≥3 hours, convulsions and HHE have also been reported following DTaP vaccines, including DAPTACEL®.[5]

In another large study (Sweden II Efficacy Trial), 3 DTaP vaccines and a whole-cell pertussis DTP vaccine, none of which are licensed in the US, were evaluated to assess relative safety and efficacy.[41] This study included HCPDT, a vaccine made of the same components as DAPTACEL® but containing twice the amount of PT and four times the amount of FHA (20 µg pertussis toxoid and 20 µg FHA). Hypotonic-hyporesponsive episodes (HHE) were observed following 29 (0.047%) of 61,220 doses of HCPDT; 16 (0.026%) of 61,219 doses of an acellular pertussis vaccine made by another manufacturer; and 34 (0.056%) of 60,792 doses of a whole-cell pertussis DTP vaccine. There were 4 additional cases of HHE in other studies using HCPDT vaccine for an overall rate of 33 (0.047%) in 69,525 doses.[15,41] (See CONTRAINDICATIONS and PRECAUTIONS.)

Sudden Infant Death Syndrome (SIDS) has occurred in infants following administration of whole-cell pertussis DTP and DTaP. Large case-control studies of SIDS in the US have shown that receipt of whole-cell pertussis DTP was not causally related to SIDS.[42,43] It should be recognized that the first 3 immunizing doses of whole-cell pertussis DTP and DTaP (including DAPTACEL®) are usually administered to infants 2–6 months of age and that approximately 85% of SIDS cases occur at ages 1–6 months with the peak incidence occurring at 6 weeks to 4 months of age. By chance alone, some cases of SIDS can be expected to follow receipt of whole-cell pertussis DTP[17] and acellular pertussis vaccines. A review by a committee of the IOM concluded that available evidence did not indicate a causal relation between whole-cell pertussis DTP vaccine and SIDS.[23]

TABLE 3[15,29] PERCENTAGE OF CHILDREN FROM PHASE II STUDY IN CANADA WITH LOCAL OR SYSTEMIC REACTIONS WITHIN 72 HOURS OF VACCINATION WITH DAPTACEL® AND WHOLE-CELL PERTUSSIS DTP VACCINE AT 2, 4, 6 AND 17–18 MONTHS OF AGE

EVENT	Dose 1 (2 MONTHS)		Dose 2 (4 MONTHS)		Dose 3 (6 MONTHS)		Dose 4 (18 MONTHS)	
	DAPTACEL® N = 324	DTP# N = 108	DAPTACEL® N = 321	DTP# N = 106	DAPTACEL® N = 320	DTP# N = 104	DAPTACEL® N = 301	DTP# N = 97
Local								
Redness								
Any	12.7*	44.4	20.6*	57.5	22.2*	51.9	36.5*	55.7
≥10 mm	1.2*	13.9	7.8*	22.6	10.0*	17.3	27.9	36.1
≥35 mm	0.3*	3.7	0.3*	5.7	1.6	1.9	21.9	20.6
Swelling								
Any	4.3*	23.1	4.3*	32.1	4.7*	25.0	18.6*	28.9
≥10 mm	1.9*	15.7	2.2*	21.7	3.8*	14.4	15.9*	25.8
≥35 mm	0.3*	6.5	0*	5.7	0.9*	4.8	11.3	15.5
Tenderness†								
Any	10.2*	37.0	7.5*	51.9	8.8*	48.1	23.9*	86.6
Moderate + Severe	0.9*	13.0	1.2*	20.8	1.3*	17.3	3.0*	53.6
Severe	0*	4.6	0.3*	7.5	0*	4.8	0.3*	12.4
Systemic								
Fever†§								
Any ≥37.5°C (99.5°F)	12.0*	43.7	7.7*	50.0	14.8*	53.2	14.5*	67.9
≥38°C (100.4°F)	0.7	1.9	0*	7.8	1.2*	11.7	1.9*	17.9
≥40°C (104°F)	0.3	0	0	1.0	0	1.1	0	0
Irritability$^{\gamma}$								
Any	41.0*	65.7	41.4*	68.9	40.9*	67.3	36.9*	79.4
Moderate + Severe	9.0*	18.5	6.9*	22.6	5.0*	22.1	5.0*	24.7
Severe	0	1.9	0.3	0	0	1.0	0	2.1
Anorexia$^{\Omega}$								
Any	16.0	22.2	9.0*	16.0	11.6*	23.1	17.6*	41.2
Moderate + Severe	1.5	3.7	0.9	2.8	1.3	1.9	2.0*	13.4
Severe	0	0	0.3	0	0	0	0	2.1
Drowsiness$^{\nabla}$								
Any	43.2	52.8	21.8*	33.0	14.4*	32.7	13.3*	29.9
Moderate + Severe	7.7	8.3	2.8*	7.5	1.3	0	1.0*	6.2
Severe	0.3	0	0	0	0	0	0	0
Crying ≥3 Hours	0.6	0.9	0.3	0.9	0	1.0	0	1.0

N = Number of evaluable subjects
\# DTP: whole-cell pertussis DTP vaccine (Aventis Pasteur Limited)
* Significantly less reactogenic than whole-cell DTP vaccine, $p<0.05$
† Moderate = sustained cry with gentle pressure at injection site; Severe = cries when leg is moved
‡ Temperature measurements were axillary
§ Number of evaluable subjects for DAPTACEL®/DTP = 301/103, 298/102, 257/94 and 207/78 at 2, 4, 6 and 18 months, respectively
γ Moderate = more difficulty with settling, even with cuddling; Severe = persistent crying/screaming and inability to console
Ω Moderate = missed one or two feeds; Severe = little or no intake for more than two feeds
∇ Moderate = sleeping much more than normal; Severe = sleeping most of the time with difficulty arousing

TABLE 4[15] PERCENTAGE OF CHILDREN FROM US BRIDGING STUDY WITH ANY LOCAL AND SYSTEMIC REACTIONS WITHIN 72 HOURS OF VACCINATION WITH DAPTACEL® AT 2, 4 AND 6 MONTHS OF AGE (LOTS 006 AND 009 POOLED)

EVENT	Dose 1 (2 MONTHS) N = 321	Dose 2 (4 MONTHS) N = 317	Dose 3 (6 MONTHS) N = 315
Local			
Redness			
Any	12.5	15.8	19.7
<1 inch	11.8	15.1	18.7
≥1 inch	0.6	0.6	1.0
Swelling			
Any	14.3	15.4	17.8
<1 inch	13.7	15.1	16.2
≥1 inch	0.6	0.3	1.6
Tenderness			
Any	30.5	19.6	15.9
Moderate + Severe	8.1	4.4	1.0
Severe	0	0	0
Systemic			
Fever*†			
Any ≥38°C (100.4°F)	11.9	9.9	9.9
≥39°C (102.2°F)	0.3	0.3	0.6
≥40°C (104°F)	0	0	0
Irritability			
Any	72.0	61.2	56.2
Moderate + Severe	33.6	25.2	18.7
Severe	0.3	0.3	0
Anorexia			
Any	26.2	14.8	17.8
Moderate + Severe	5.6	3.8	4.8
Severe	0	0.3	0
Drowsiness			
Any	62.0	44.8	35.6
Moderate + Severe	24.0	8.5	7.3
Severe	0.6	0.3	0
Crying ≥3 Hours	0.3	0	0

N = Number of evaluable subjects
* Rectal temperature
† N = 319, 314 and 313 at 2, 4 and 6 months respectively
Moderate = discomforting enough to interfere with or limit usual daily activity
Severe = disabling, unable to perform daily activities

Whole-cell pertussis DTP vaccine has been associated with acute encephalopathy.[23] A 10-year follow-up to the National Childhood Encephalopathy Study (NCES) of children who experienced acute neurologic disorders in infancy concluded that serious acute neurologic illness increased the risk of chronic neurologic disease or death.[44] A committee of the Institute of Medicine (IOM) has concluded that, because whole-cell pertussis DTP may cause acute neurologic illness, whole-cell pertussis DTP may also cause chronic neurologic disease in the context of the NCES report.[24] However, the IOM committee concluded that the evidence was insufficient to indicate whether or not whole-cell pertussis DTP increased the overall risk of chronic neurologic disease.[24]

A bulging fontanel associated with increased intracranial pressure which occurred within 24 hours following whole-cell pertussis DTP immunization has been reported, although a causal relationship has not been established.[45,46,47]

Reporting of Adverse Events

The National Vaccine Injury Compensation Program, established by the National Childhood Vaccine Injury Act of 1986, requires physicians and other health-care providers who administer vaccines to maintain permanent vaccination records of the manufacturer and lot number of the vaccine administered in the vaccine recipient's permanent medical record along with the date of administration of the vaccine and the name, address and title of the person administering the vaccine. The Act (or statute) further requires the health-care professional to report to the Secretary of the US Department of Health and Human Services the occurrence following immunization of any events set forth in the statute or the Vaccine Injury Table, including anaphylaxis or anaphylactic shock within 7 days; encephalopathy or encephalitis within 7 days, brachial neuritis within 28 days; or an acute complication or sequelae (including death) of an illness, disability, injury, or condition referred to above, or any events that would contraindicate further doses of vaccine, according to this DAPTACEL® package insert.[17,48]

Reporting by parents or guardians of all adverse events after vaccine administration should be encouraged. Adverse events following immunization with vaccine should be reported by health-care providers to VAERS. Reporting forms and information about reporting requirements or completion of the form can be obtained from VAERS through a toll-free number 1-800-822-7967.[48,49]

Health-care providers should also report these events to the Pharmacovigilance Department, Aventis Pasteur Inc., Discovery Drive, Swiftwater, PA 18370 or call 1-800-822-2463.

DOSAGE AND ADMINISTRATION

DAPTACEL® is a sterile white homogenous cloudy suspension of acellular pertussis vaccine components and diphtheria and tetanus toxoids adsorbed on aluminum in a sterile isotonic sodium chloride solution and containing 2-phenoxyethanol as preservative. Inspect the vial visually for extraneous particulate matter and/or discoloration before administration. If these conditions exist, the product should not be administered.

JUST BEFORE USE, SHAKE THE VIAL WELL, until a uniform, cloudy suspension results. WITHDRAW AND INJECT A 0.5 mL DOSE. When administering a dose from a rubber-stoppered vial, do not remove either the rubber stopper or the metal seal holding it in place. Aseptic technique must be used for withdrawal of each dose.

Before injection, the skin over the site to be injected should be cleansed with a suitable germicide. After insertion of the needle into the muscle, aspirate to ensure that the needle has not entered a blood vessel.

Administer the vaccine **intramuscularly** (I.M.). In children younger than 1 year (i.e., infants), the anterolateral aspect of the thigh provides the largest muscle and is the preferred site of injection. In older children, the deltoid muscle is usually large enough for I.M. injection. The vaccine should not be injected into the gluteal area or areas where there may be a major nerve trunk.[17]

Fractional doses (doses <0.5 mL) should not be given. The effect of fractional doses on the frequency of serious adverse events and on efficacy has not been determined.

Do NOT administer this product intravenously or subcutaneously.

Immunization Series

A 0.5 mL dose of DAPTACEL® is approved for administration as a 4 dose series at 2, 4 and 6 months of age, at intervals of 6–8 weeks and at 17–20 months of age. (See CLINICAL PHARMACOLOGY.) The customary age for the first dose is 2 months of age, but it may be given as early as 6 weeks of age and up to the seventh birthday. The interval between the third and fourth dose should be at least 6 months. It is recommended that DAPTACEL® be given for all doses in the series because no data on the interchangeability of DAPTACEL® with other DTaP vaccines exist. At this time, data are insufficient to establish the frequency of adverse events following a fifth dose of DAPTACEL® in children who have previously received 4 doses of DAPTACEL®.[50]

DAPTACEL® may be used to complete the immunization series in infants who have received 1 or more doses of whole-cell pertussis DTP. However, the safety and efficacy of DAPTACEL® in such infants have not been fully demonstrated.[5]

PERSONS 7 YEARS OF AGE AND OLDER SHOULD NOT BE IMMUNIZED WITH DAPTACEL® OR ANY OTHER PERTUSSIS-CONTAINING VACCINES.[18]

DAPTACEL® should not be combined through reconstitution or mixed with any other vaccine.

If any recommended dose of pertussis vaccine cannot be given, DT (For Pediatric Use) should be given as needed to complete the series.

Pre-term infants should be vaccinated according to their chronological age from birth.[17]

Interruption of the recommended schedule with a delay between doses should not interfere with the final immunity achieved with DAPTACEL®. There is no need to start the series over again, regardless of the time between doses.

Simultaneous Vaccine Administration

In clinical trials, DAPTACEL® was routinely administered, at separate sites, concomitantly with one or more of the following vaccines: OPV, hepatitis B vaccine and *Haemophilus influenzae* type b vaccine.[15] No safety and immunogenicity data are currently available on the simultaneous administration of pneumococcal conjugate vaccine, MMR vaccine and varicella vaccine and no immunogenicity data are currently available on the simultaneous administration of IPV. Two afebrile seizures, occurring within 24 hours of immunization, have been reported from 2 US trials where DAPTACEL® was given with other concomitant vaccines. (See ADVERSE REACTIONS.) When concomitant administration of other vaccines is required, they should be given with different syringes and at different injection sites.

ACIP encourages routine simultaneous administration of DTaP, IPV, *Haemophilus influenzae* type b vaccine, pneumococcal conjugate vaccine, MMR, varicella vaccine and hepatitis B vaccine for children who are the recommended age to receive these vaccines and for whom no specific contraindications exist at the time of the visit, unless, in the judgment of the provider, complete vaccination of the child will not be compromised by administering different vaccines at different visits. Simultaneous administration is particularly important if the child might not return for subsequent vaccinations.[18] (See CLINICAL PHARMACOLOGY.)

If passive immunization is needed for tetanus prophylaxis, Tetanus Immune Globulin (Human) (TIG) is the product of choice. It provides longer protection than antitoxin of animal origin and is associated with few adverse reactions. The currently recommended prophylactic dose of TIG for wounds of average severity is 250 units intramuscularly. When tetanus toxoid-containing vaccines and TIG and/or Diphtheria Antitoxin are administered concurrently, separate syringes and separate sites should be used.

HOW SUPPLIED

Vial, 1 × 1 Dose—Product No. 49281-286-01
Vial, 5 × 1 Dose—Product No. 49281-286-05
Vial, 10 × 1 Dose—Product No. 49281-286-10

STORAGE

DAPTACEL® should be stored at 2° to 8°C (35° to 46°F). DO NOT FREEZE. Product which has been exposed to freezing should not be used. Do not use after expiration date.

REFERENCES

1. Stainer DW, Scholte MJ. A simple chemically defined medium for the production of phase I *Bordetella pertussis*. J Gen Microbiol 1970;63:211–220.
2. Stainer DW. Production of diphtheria toxin. In: Manclark CR, ed. Proceeding of an informal consultation on the World Health Organization requirements for diphtheria, tetanus, pertussis and combined vaccines. United States Public Health Service, Bethesda, MD. DHHS Publication No. (FDA) 91-1174. 1991:7–11.
3. Mueller JH, Miller PA. Variable factors influencing the production of tetanus toxin. J Bacteriol 1954;67:271–277.
4. Recommendations of the Advisory Committee on Immunization Practices (ACIP). Diphtheria, Tetanus, and Pertussis: Recommendations for vaccine use and other preventive measures. MMWR 1991;40(RR-10):1–28.
5. Recommendations of the Advisory Committee on Immunization Practices (ACIP). Pertussis vaccination: Use of acellular pertussis vaccines among infants and young children. MMWR 1997;46(RR-7):1–25.
6. Plotkin SA, et al. *Vaccines. 3rd ed.* Philadelphia, W. B. Saunders Company. 1999:140–157,293–344,441–474.
7. Centers for Disease Control and Prevention (CDC). Notice to readers: Final 2000 reports of notifiable diseases. MMWR 2001;50(33):1–10.
8. Atkinson W, et al, editors. *Epidemiology and Prevention of Vaccine-Preventable Diseases. 6th ed.* Centers for Disease Control and Prevention (CDC); Public Health Foundation. 2000:51–72.
9. American Public Health Association (APHA). Control of Communicable Diseases Manual. 2000;(17):166–167.
10. Hardy IRB, et al. Current situation and control strategies for resurgence of diphtheria in newly independent states of the former Soviet Union. Lancet 1996;347:1739–1744.
11. Bedson SP, et al. The prevention of whooping-cough by vaccination. A Medical Research Council Investigation. Br Med J 1951;1:1463–1471.
12. Centers for Disease Control and Prevention (CDC). Pertussis-United States,1997–2000. MMWR 2002;51(4):1–92.
13. Güris D, et al. Changing epidemiology of pertussis in the United States: Increasing reported incidence among adolescents and adults, 1990–1996. Clin Infect Dis 1999;28:1230–1237.
14. Gustafsson L, et al. A controlled trial of a two-component acellular, a five-component acellular, and a whole-cell pertussis vaccine. N Engl J Med 1996;6:349–355.
15. Aventis Pasteur Limited: Data on File.
16. Department of Health and Human Services, Food and Drug Administration. Biological Products; Bacterial Vaccines and Toxoids; Implementation of Efficacy Review; Proposed Rule. Federal Register 1985; 50(240): 51002–51117.
17. American Academy of Pediatrics. In: Pickering LK, ed. *2000 Red Book: Report on the Committee of Infectious Diseases. 25th ed.* Elk Grove Village, IL: American Academy of Pediatrics 2000:17,31–35,51–53,54,65,68,440–445,759–765.
18. Recommendations of the Advisory Committee on Immunization Practices (ACIP). General recommendations on immunization. MMWR 1994;43(RR-1):1–38.
19. Expanded programme on immunization, injection and paralytic poliomyelitis. Wkly Epidem Rec 1980;5:38–40.
20. Sutter RW, et al. Attributable risk of DTP (diphtheria and tetanus toxoids and pertussis vaccine) injection in provoking paralytic poliomyelitis during a large outbreak in Oman. J Infect Dis 1992;165:444–449.
21. Christie AB. *Infectious diseases: Epidemiology and Clinical Practice. 4th ed.* Edinburgh, Churchill Livingstone. 1987;2:817–825.
22. Livengood JR, et al. Family history of convulsion and use of pertussis vaccine. J Pediatr 1989;115(4):527–531.
23. Howson CP, et al. *Adverse Effects of Pertussis and Rubella Vaccines, Pertussis Vaccines and CNS Disorders.* Institute of Medicine (IOM). National Academy Press, Washington, DC, 1991:7–169.
24. Institute of Medicine (IOM). DTP vaccine and chronic nervous system dysfunction: A new analysis. National Academy Press, Washington, DC, 1994;Supplement:1–17.
25. Recommendations of the Advisory Committee on Immunization Practices (ACIP). Update: Vaccine side effects, adverse reactions, contraindications, and precautions. MMWR 1996;45(RR-12):1–35.
26. National Advisory Committee on Immunization (NACI): *Canadian Immunization Guide, 5th ed.* Minister of Public Works and Government Services Canada. 1998:9–13,133–139.
27. Edwards KM, et al. Comparison of 13 acellular pertussis vaccines: Overview and serologic response. American Academy of Pediatrics 1995;Supplement:548–557.
28. Decker MD, et al. Comparison of 13 acellular pertussis vaccines: Adverse reactions. Pediatr 1995;96:557–566.
29. Halperin SA, et al. Adverse reactions and antibody response to four doses of acellular or whole-cell pertussis combined with diphtheria and tetanus toxoids in the first 19 months of life. Vaccine 1996;14(18):767–772.
30. Halperin SA, et al. Safety and immunogenicity of two acellular pertussis vaccines with different pertussis toxoid and filamentous hemagglutinin content in infants 2–6 months old. Scand J Infect Dis 1995;27:279–287.
31. Halperin SA, et al. Acellular pertussis vaccine as a booster dose for seventeen- to nineteen-month-old children immunized with either whole cell acellular pertussis vaccine at two, four and six months of age. Pediatr Infect Dis J 1995;14:792–797.
32. Fawcett HA, Smith NP. Injection-site granuloma due to aluminum. Arch Dermatol 1984;120:1318–1322.
33. Blumstein GI, et al. Peripheral neuropathy following tetanus toxoid administration. JAMA 1966;198(9):1030–1031.
34. Institute of Medicine (U.S.). *Adverse Effects of Pertussis and Rubella Vaccines.* Howson CP, et al, editors. Washington: National Academy Press. 1991:154–157.
35. Rutledge SL, et al. Neurological complications of immunizations. J Pediatr 1986;109:917–924.
36. Walker AM, et al. Neurologic events following diphtheria-tetanus-pertussis immunization. Pediatr 1988;81: 345–349.
37. Tsairis P, et al. Natural history of brachial plexus neuropathy. Arch Neurol 1972;27:109–117.
38. Cody CL, et al. Nature and rates of adverse reactions associated with DTP and DT immunizations in infants and children. Pediatr 1981;68(5):650–660.
39. Schlenska GK. Unusual neurological complications following tetanus toxoid administration. J Neurol 1977;215:299–302.
40. Alderslade R, et al. The National Childhood Encephalopathy Study: a report on 1000 cases of serious neurological disorders in infants and young children from the NCES Research Team. In: Department of Health and Social Security. Whooping cough: reports from the Committee on the Safety of Medicines and the Joint Committee on Vaccination and Immunization. London: Her Majesty's Stationery Office 1981:79–169.
41. Olin P, et al. Randomized controlled trial of two-component, three-component, and five-component acellular pertussis vaccines compared with whole-cell pertussis vaccine. Lancet 1997:1569–1577.
42. Griffin MR, et al. Risk of sudden infant death syndrome after immunization with the diphtheria-tetanus-pertussis vaccine. N Engl J Med 1988:618–623.
43. Hoffman HJ, et al. Diphtheria-tetanus-pertussis immunization and sudden infant death: Results of the National Institute of Child Health and Human Development cooperative epidemiological study of sudden infant death syndrome risk factors. Pediatr 1987;79(4):598–611.
44. Miller D, et al. *Pertussis Immunisation and Serious Acute Neurological Illnesses in Children.* Academic Department of Public Health, St. Mary's Hospital Medical School, University of London, 1993.

Continued on next page

Daptacel—Cont.

45. Jacob J, et al. Increased intracranial pressure after diphtheria, tetanus and pertussis immunization. Am J Dis Child 1979;133:217–218.
46. Mathur R, et al. Bulging fontanel following triple vaccine. Indian Pediatr 1981;18(6):417–418.
47. Shendurnikar N, et al. Bulging fontanel following DTP vaccine. Indian Pediatr 1986;23(11):960.
48. Centers for Disease Control and Prevention (CDC). National Childhood Vaccine Injury Act: Requirements for permanent vaccination records and for reporting of selected events after vaccination. MMWR 1988;37(13): 197–200.
49. Center for Disease Control and Prevention (CDC). Vaccine Adverse Event Reporting System—United States. MMWR 1990;39:730–733.
50. Pichichero MD, et al. Safety and immunogenicity of six acellular pertussis vaccines and one whole-cell pertussis vaccine given as a fifth dose in four six-year-old children. Pediatr 2000;105(1),e11:1–8.

Manufactured by:
Aventis Pasteur Limited
Toronto Ontario Canada
Distributed by:
Aventis Pasteur Inc.
Swiftwater PA 18370 USA
US Patents: 4500639, 4687738, 4784589, 4997915, 5444159, 5667787, 5877298.
Product information
as of January 2003.
R2-0103 USA
4825

MENOMUNE®–A/C/Y/W-135 ℞

Meningococcal Polysaccharide Vaccine Groups A, C, Y and W-135 Combined

DESCRIPTION

Menomune®–A/C/Y/W-135, Meningococcal Polysaccharide Vaccine, Groups A, C, Y and W-135 Combined, for subcutaneous use, is a freeze-dried preparation of the group-specific polysaccharide antigens from *Neisseria meningitidis*, Group A, Group C, Group Y and Group W-135. *N meningitidis* are cultivated with Mueller Hinton agar[1] and Watson Scherp[2] media. The purified polysaccharide is extracted from the *Neisseria meningitidis* cells and separated from the media by procedures which include centrifugation, detergent precipitation, alcohol precipitation, solvent or organic extraction and diafiltration. No preservative is added during manufacture.

The 0.78 mL vial of diluent contains sterile, preservative-free, pyrogen-free distilled water and is used for reconstitution of product supplied in 1 mL vials. The 6 mL vial of diluent contains sterile, pyrogen-free distilled water to which thimerosal (mercury derivative) 1:10,000 is added as a preservative. The 6 mL vial is for reconstitution of product supplied in 10 mL vials. After reconstitution with diluent as indicated on the label, the 0.5 mL dose is formulated to contain 50 µg of "isolated product" from each of Groups A, C, Y and W-135 in an isotonic sodium chloride solution.

Each dose of vaccine is also formulated to contain 2.5 mg to 5 mg of lactose added as a stabilizer.[3] The vaccine when reconstituted is a clear colorless liquid.

Potency is evaluated by measuring the molecular size of each polysaccharide component using a column chromatography method as standardized by the US Food and Drug Administration (FDA) and the World Health Organization (WHO)[4] for Meningococcal Polysaccharide Vaccine.

THIS VACCINE CONFORMS TO THE WORLD HEALTH ORGANIZATION (WHO) REQUIREMENTS.

CLINICAL PHARMACOLOGY

N meningitidis causes both endemic and epidemic disease, principally meningitis and meningococcemia. As a result of the control of *Haemophilus influenzae* type b infections, *N meningitidis* has become the leading cause of bacterial meningitis in children and young adults in the United States (US), with an estimated 2,600 cases each year.[5,6] The case-fatality rate is 13% for meningitis disease (defined as the isolation of *N meningitidis* from cerebrospinal fluid) and 11.5% for persons who have *N meningitidis* isolated from blood,[5,6] despite therapy with antimicrobial agents (eg, penicillin) to which US strains remain clinically sensitive.[5]

The incidence of meningococcal disease peaks in late winter to early spring. Based on multistate surveillance conducted during 1989 to 1991, serogroup B organisms accounted for 46% of all cases and serogroup C for 45%; serogroups W-135 and Y and strains that could not be serotyped accounted for most of the remaining cases.[5,6] Recent data indicate that the proportion of cases caused by serogroup Y strains is increasing.[5] In 1995, among the 30 states reporting supplemental data on culture-confirmed cases of meningococcal disease, serogroup Y accounted for 21% of cases.[7] Because of the success of *H influenzae* type b vaccinations, the median age of persons with bacterial meningitis increased from 15 months in 1986 to 25 years in 1995.[8] The predominate organism causing meningitis in children 2 to 18 years of age is *N meningitidis* based on 1995 surveillance data.[8] Serogroup A, which rarely causes disease in the US, is the most common cause of epidemics in Africa and Asia. A statewide serogroup B epidemic has been reported in the US.[9] Within the US, a vaccine for serogroup B is not yet available.

Outbreaks of serogroup C meningococcal disease (SCMD) have been occurring more frequently in the US since the early 1990s, and the use of vaccine to control these outbreaks has increased.[5] During 1980-1993, 21 outbreaks of SCMD were identified; eight of these occurred during 1992-1993.[10] Each of these 21 outbreaks involved from three to 45 cases of SCMD, and most outbreaks had attack rates exceeding 10 cases per 100,000 population, which is approximately 20 times higher than rates of endemic SCMD.[5] During 1981-1988, only 7,600 doses of meningococcal vaccine were used to control four outbreaks; whereas, from January 1992 through June 1993, 180,000 doses of vaccine were used in response to eight outbreaks.[5]

Several discoveries impacted the future of meningococcal polysaccharide vaccines and demonstrated the significance of anti-capsular antibodies in protection.[11] In the late 1930s, serogroup-specific antigens of meningococcal serogroups A and C were identified as polysaccharides.[9] During the mid 1940s, investigators demonstrated that the protection of mice by anti-serogroup A meningococcal horse serum was directly related to its content of anti-polysaccharide antibodies.[11] Meningococcal polysaccharide vaccines were first demonstrated to be immunogenic in humans by Gotschlich and his co-workers in the 1960s when immunization of US Army recruits with serogroup A and C polysaccharides induced protective antibodies.[11] The investigators recorded a significantly reduced acquisition rate of serogroup C carriage among vaccinated recruits compared with unvaccinated individuals.[11]

Persons who have certain medical conditions are at increased risk for developing meningococcal infection. Meningococcal disease is particularly common among persons who have component deficiencies in the terminal common complement pathway (C3, C5-C9); many of these persons experience multiple episodes of infection.[5] Asplenic persons also may be at increased risk for acquiring meningococcal disease with particularly severe infections.[5] Persons who have other diseases associated with immunosuppression (eg, human immunodeficiency virus [HIV] and *Streptococcus pneumoniae)* may be at higher risk for developing meningococcal disease and for disease caused by some other encapsulated bacteria.[5] Evidence suggests that HIV-infected persons are not at substantially increased risk for epidemic serogroup A meningococcal disease;[5] however, such patients may be at increased risk for sporadic meningococcal disease or disease caused by other meningococcal serogroups.[5] Previously, military recruits had high rates of meningococcal disease, particularly serogroup C disease; however, since the initiation of routine vaccination of recruits with bivalent A/C meningococcal vaccine in 1971, the high rates of meningococcal disease caused by those serogroups have decreased substantially and cases occur infrequently.[5]

A retrospective, epidemiological study was conducted in Maryland to compare the incidence of invasive meningococcal infection in college students with that of the general population of the same age. For the years 1992 to 1997, the incidence of meningococcal infection in Maryland college students was similar to the incidence of the general Maryland population of the same age. However, college students residing on-campus appeared to be at higher risk than those residing off campus.[12]

Vaccine efficacy. The immunogenicity and clinical efficacy of serogroups A and C meningococcal vaccines have been well established.[5] The serogroup A polysaccharide induces antibody in some children as young as 3 months of age, although a response comparable with that among adults is not achieved until 4 or 5 years of age; the serogroup C component is poorly immunogenic in recipients who are less than 18 to 24 months of age.[5] The serogroups A and C vaccines have demonstrated estimated clinical efficacies of 85% to 100% in older children and adults and are useful in controlling epidemics.[5] Serogroups Y and W-135 polysaccharides are safe and immunogenic in adults and in children greater than 2 years of age.[5] Although clinical protection has not been documented, vaccination with these polysaccharides induces bactericidal antibody. The antibody responses to each of the four polysaccharides in the quadrivalent vaccine are serogroup-specific and independent.[5]

Efficacy of serogroup A meningococcal vaccines was demonstrated in the 1970s in Africa and Finland, Egyptian school children aged 6 to 15 years showed 90% or greater protection during the first year after immunization with two different molecular sizes of serogroup A polysaccharide.[11] The higher molecular weight vaccine provided protection for at least three years.[11] In Finland, a randomized controlled mass immunization trial with serogroup A vaccine was conducted in response to a serogroup A epidemic. Results indicated 90 to 100% protection for three years.[11] In Rwanda, vaccination with bivalent A/C polysaccharide vaccine was performed in response to a serogroup A epidemic. A complete cessation of meningococcal disease was observed within two weeks of vaccination, yet the serogroup A carrier rate remained unchanged.[11]

Efficacy of serogroup C meningococcal vaccines was demonstrated in a field trial involving 20,000 troops in the US Army. Results suggested 90% efficacy under epidemic conditions which existed in basic training centers.[13] In Brazil, young children were vaccinated with serogroup C polysaccharide in response to a serogroup C epidemic. Results indicated that the vaccine was not effective in children under 24 months of age and only 52% effective in children aged 24 to 36 months.[11] However, studies suggested that the vaccine used in this trial was less immunogenic than other batches of similar vaccine that were used in US children; also, it was shown that the molecular size of the vaccine was smaller than the serogroup C polysaccharide in the present vaccine.[13] Thus, it is quite probable that the current serogroup C polysaccharide vaccine is more effective.[11]

A study performed using 4 lots of Menomune®–A/C/Y/W-135 in 150 adults showed at least a 4-fold increase in bactericidal antibodies to all groups in greater than 90 percent of the subjects.[14,15]

A study was conducted in 73 children 2 to 12 years of age. Post-immunization sera were not obtained on four children; seroconversion rates were calculated on 69 paired samples. Seroconversion rates as measured by bactericidal antibody were: Group A – 72%, Group C – 58%, Group Y – 90% and Group W-135 – 82%. Seroconversion rates as measured by a 2-fold rise in antibody titers based on Solid Phase Radioimmunoassay were: Group A – 99%, Group C – 99%, Group Y – 97% and Group W-135 – 89%.[16]

Duration of efficacy. Measurable levels of antibodies against the group A and C polysaccharides decrease markedly during the first 3 years following a single dose of vaccine.[5] This decrease in antibody occurs more rapidly in infants and young children than in adults. Similarly, although vaccine-induced clinical protection probably persists in schoolchildren and adults for at least 3 years, the efficacy of the group A vaccine in young children may decrease markedly with the passage of time. In a 3-year study, efficacy declined from greater than 90% to less than 10% among children who were less than 4 years of age at the time of vaccination, whereas among children who were greater than or equal to 4 years of age when vaccinated, efficacy was 67% 3 years later.[5,17] In a New Zealand study, children 2 to 13 years of age received a single dose of monovalent group A vaccine, 26% of children 3 to 23 months of age in this study received two doses of the vaccine, given approximately 3 months apart. After 2-1/2 years of active surveillance (1987 to 1989) there were no cases of invasive group A disease in children vaccinated at 2 years of age and older.[18]

INDICATIONS AND USAGE

Meningococcal Polysaccharide Vaccine, Groups A, C, Y and W-135 Combined, is indicated for active immunization against invasive meningococcal disease caused by these serogroups.[5]

Meningococcal Polysaccharide Vaccine, Groups A, C, Y and W-135 Combined may be used to prevent and control outbreaks of serogroup C meningococcal disease.[5]

For evaluation and management of suspected outbreaks, it is recommended that the health-care workers consult the MMWR for guidance.[5]

Routine vaccination is recommended for the following high-risk groups:[5]

1. Deficiencies in late Complement components (C3, C5-C9).
2. Functional or actual asplenia.
3. Persons with laboratory or industrial exposure to *N meningitidis* aerosols.
4. Travelers to, and residents of, hyperendemic areas such as sub-Saharan Africa. For information concerning geographic areas for which vaccination is recommended, contact CDC at 404-332-4559.

The American College Health Association (ACHA) also recommends that college students consider vaccination to reduce the risk for potentially fatal meningococcal disease.[19]

Vaccinations also should be considered for household or institutional contacts of persons with meningococcal disease and for medical and laboratory personnel at risk of exposure to meningococcal disease.

This vaccine will not stimulate protection against infections caused by organisms other than Groups A, C, Y and W-135 meningococci.

Protective antibody levels may be achieved within 7 to 10 days after vaccination.[5]

Menomune®–A/C/Y/W-135 vaccine is not to be used for treatment of actual infection.

Menomune®–A/C/Y/W-135 vaccine will not protect against other etiologic agents, including *N meningitidis* serogroup B, that cause meningitis.

Menomune®–A/C/Y/W-135 vaccine is not indicated for infants and children younger than 2 years of age except as short-term protection of infants 3 months and older against Group A.[11]

As with any vaccine, vaccination with Menomune®–A/C/Y/W-135 may not protect 100% of susceptible individuals.

For persons remaining at high-risk, especially children who were first vaccinated at < 4 years of age, revaccination may be indicated.[5] (See **DOSAGE AND ADMINISTRATION** section.)

CONTRAINDICATIONS

Immunization should be deferred during the course of any acute illness.

IT IS A CONTRAINDICATION TO ADMINISTER MENOMUNE®–A/C/Y/W-135 TO INDIVIDUALS KNOWN TO BE SENSITIVE TO THIMEROSAL OR ANY OTHER COMPONENT OF THE VACCINE. FOR INDIVIDUALS SENSITIVE TO THIMEROSAL, ADMINISTER THE ONE DOSE PACKAGE SIZE AND RECONSTITUTE WITH THE 0.78 ML VIAL OF DILUENT THAT CONTAINS NO PRESERVATIVE.

WARNING

This product contains dry natural latex rubber as follows: The stopper to the vial contains dry natural latex rubber.

If the vaccine is used in persons receiving immunosuppressive therapy, the expected immune response may not be obtained.

Menomune®–A/C/Y/W-135 should NOT be given at the same time as whole-cell pertussis or whole-cell typhoid vaccines due to combined endotoxin content.[20,21]

PRECAUTIONS

GENERAL

Care is to be taken by the health-care provider for the safe and effective use of Menomune®–A/C/Y/W-135.

EPINEPHRINE INJECTION (1:1000) MUST BE IMMEDIATELY AVAILABLE TO COMBAT UNEXPECTED ANAPHYLACTIC OR OTHER ALLERGIC REACTIONS.

Prior to an injection of any vaccine, all known precautions should be taken to prevent adverse reactions. This includes a review of the patient's history with respect to possible sensitivity to the vaccine or similar vaccines and to possible sensitivity to dry natural latex rubber.

Special care should be taken to avoid injecting the vaccine intradermally, intramuscularly, or intravenously since clinical studies have not been done to establish safety and efficacy of the vaccine using these routes of administration.

Health-care providers should obtain the previous immunization history of the vaccinee, and inquire about the current health status of the vaccinee.

A separate, sterile syringe and needle or a sterile disposable unit should be used for each patient to prevent transmission of hepatitis and other infectious agents from person to person. Needles should not be recapped and should be disposed of according to biohazard waste guidelines.

INFORMATION FOR PATIENT

Patients, parents or guardians should be fully informed of the benefits and risks of immunization with Menomune®–A/C/Y/W-135.

Patients, parents or guardians should be instructed to report any serious adverse reactions to their health-care provider.

As part of the patient's immunization record, the date, lot number and manufacturer of the vaccine administered should be recorded.[22,23,24]

DRUG INTERACTIONS

If Menomune®–A/C/Y/W-135 is administered to immunosuppressed persons or persons receiving immunosuppressive therapy, an adequate immunologic response may not be obtained.

CARCINOGENESIS, MUTAGENESIS, IMPAIRMENT OF FERTILITY

Menomune®–A/C/Y/W-135 has not been evaluated in animals for its carcinogenic, mutagenic potentials or impairment of fertility.

PREGNANCY

REPRODUCTIVE STUDIES–PREGNANCY CATEGORY C

Animal reproduction studies have not been conducted with Meningococcal Polysaccharide Vaccine, Groups A, C, Y and W-135. It is also not known whether Meningococcal Polysaccharide Vaccine, Groups A, C, Y and W-135 can cause fetal harm when administered to a pregnant woman or can affect reproduction capacity. Meningococcal Polysaccharide Vaccine, Groups A, C, Y and W-135 should be given to a pregnant woman only if clearly needed.

Although there is limited data, studies to date have found no evidence of teratogenicity of the polysaccharide quadrivalent meningococcal vaccine when given to pregnant women.[25]

NURSING MOTHERS

It is not known whether this drug is excreted in human milk. Because many drugs are excreted in human milk, caution should be exercised when Menomune®–A/C/Y/W-135 is administered to a nursing woman.

PEDIATRIC USE

SAFETY AND EFFECTIVENESS OF MENOMUNE®–A/C/Y/W-135 IN CHILDREN BELOW THE AGE OF 2 YEARS HAVE NOT BEEN ESTABLISHED.

ADVERSE REACTIONS

Adverse reactions to meningococcal vaccine are mild and consist principally of pain and redness at the injection site for 1 to 2 days. Pain at the site of injection is the most commonly reported adverse reaction, and a transient fever might develop in less than or equal to 2% of young children.[5]

Adverse events reported by 150 adults following vaccination with Menomune®–A/C/Y/W-135 are shown in Table 1.[14] The subjects were observed for three weeks following vaccination. Local reactions resolved within 48 hours and no significant systemic reactions were reported.[14]

[See table above]

In a clinical study involving 73 children 2 to 12 years of age, who received Menomune®–A/C/Y/W-135, local reactions consisting of erythema or tenderness were seen in approximately 40% of the children.[15] In another clinical study involving 53 children 4 to 6 years of age, who received Menomune®–A/C/Y/W-135, erythema was seen in 89% of the children, swelling in 92% and tenderness in 64%. None of these reactions were considered serious or necessitated medical intervention.[26]

On rare occasions, IgA nephropathy has occurred following vaccinations with Menomune®–A/C/Y/W-135. However, a cause and effect relationship has not been established.[16]

Menomune®–A/C/Y/W-135 should NOT be given at the same time as whole-cell pertussis or whole-cell typhoid vaccines due to combined endotoxin content.[20,21]

TABLE 1[14] ADVERSE EVENTS (%) FOLLOWING VACCINATION OF 150 ADULTS WITH MENOMUNE®–A/C/Y/W-135

REACTIONS		MILD	MODERATE
Local			
Pain		2.6	2.0
Tenderness		36.0	9.0
Diameter		< 2 in.	≥ 2 in.
Erythema		3.8	1.2
Induration		4.4	1.2
Systemic			
Headaches		5.2	1.8
Malaise		2.5	0
Chills		2.5	0
Oral Temperature (°F)		2.6 (100–101)	0.6 (> 101)

As with the administration of any vaccine, vaccine components can cause hypersensitivity reactions in some recipients.

Reporting of Adverse Events

The National Vaccine Injury Compensation Program, established by the National Childhood Vaccine Injury Act of 1986, requires physicians and other health-care providers who administer vaccines to maintain permanent vaccination records and to report occurrences of certain adverse events to the US Department of Health and Human Services. Reportable events include those listed in the Act for each vaccine and events specified in the package insert as contraindications to further doses of that vaccine.[22,23,24]

Reporting by patients, parents or guardians of all adverse events occurring after vaccine administration should be encouraged. Adverse events following immunization with vaccine should be reported by the health-care provider to the US Department of Health and Human Services (DHHS) Vaccine Adverse Event Reporting Systems (VAERS). Reporting forms and information about reporting requirements or completion of the form can be obtained from VAERS through a toll-free number 1-800-822-7967.[24]

Health-care providers also should report these events to the Pharmacovigilance Department, Aventis Pasteur Inc., Discovery Drive, Swiftwater, PA 18370 or call 1-800-822-2463.

DOSAGE AND ADMINISTRATION

Parenteral drug products should be inspected visually for extraneous particulate matter and/or discoloration prior to administration whenever solution and container permit. If either of these conditions exist, the vaccine should not be administered.

Reconstitute the vaccine using only the diluent supplied for this purpose. Draw the volume of diluent shown on the diluent label into a suitable size syringe and inject into the vial containing the vaccine. Shake vial until the vaccine is dissolved.

The immunizing dose is a single injection of 0.5 mL administered **subcutaneously.**

Special care should be taken to avoid injecting the vaccine intradermally, intramuscularly, or intravenously since clinical studies have not been done to establish safety and efficacy of the vaccine using these routes of administration.

Primary Immunization

For both adults and children, vaccine is administered subcutaneously as a single 0.5 mL dose. Protective antibody levels may be achieved within 7 to 10 days after vaccination.[5]

REVACCINATION

Revaccination of a single 0.5 mL dose administered subcutaneously may be indicated for individuals at high-risk of infection, particularly children who were first vaccinated when they were less than 4 years of age; such children should be considered for revaccination after 2 or 3 years if they remain at high-risk. Although the need for revaccination in older children and adults has not been determined, antibody levels decline rapidly over 2 to 3 years, and if indications still exist for immunization, revaccination may be considered within 3 to 5 years.[5,18]

Simultaneous administration of Menomune®–A/C/Y/W-135 can be given concurrently with other vaccines at separate sites and separate syringes.[27] However, due to the combined endotoxin content, the vaccine should NOT be administered at the same time as whole-cell pertussis or whole-cell typhoid vaccines.[20,21] (See **WARNINGS** section.)

HOW SUPPLIED

Vial, 1 Dose, with 0.78 mL vial of diluent (contains NO preservative). Product No. 49281-489-01

Vial, 1 Dose (5 per package) with 0.78 mL vial of diluent (5 per package) (contains NO preservative). Product No. 49281-489-05

Vial, 10 Dose, with 6 mL vial of diluent (contains preservative) for administration with needle and syringe (NOT to be used with jet injector). Product No. 49281-489-91

STORAGE

Store freeze-dried vaccine and reconstituted vaccine, when not in use, between 2° – 8°C (35° – 46°F). Discard remainder of multidose vials of vaccine within 35 days after reconstitution. The single dose vial should be used within 30 minutes after reconstitution.

REFERENCES

1. Mueller H, et al. A protein-free medium for primary isolation of the gonococcus and meningococcus. Proc Soc Exp Biol Med 48: 330, 1941
2. Watson RG, et al. The specific hapten of group C (group II *a*) meningococcus. II. Chemical nature. J Immunol. 81: 337, 1958
3. Tiesjema RH, et al. Enhanced stability of meningococcal polysaccharide vaccines by using lactose as a menstruum for lyophilization. Bull WHO 55:43-48, 1977
4. WHO Technical Report Series, No. 658, 1981
5. Recommendation of the Advisory Committee on Immunization Practices (ACIP). Control and prevention of meningococcal disease and control and prevention of serogroup C meningococcal disease: evaluation and management of suspected outbreaks. MMWR 46: No. RR-5, 1997
6. CDC. Laboratory-based surveillance for meningococcal disease in selected areas – United States, 1989-1991. MMWR 42: No. SS-2, 1993
7. CDC. Serogroup Y Meningococcal Disease – Illinois, Connecticut, and Selected Areas, United States, 1989-1996. MMWR 46: Vol. 45, 1010-1013, 1996
8. Schuchat A, et al. Bacterial Meningitis in the United States in 1995. N Engl J Med 337: 970-976, 1997
9. CDC. Serogroup B meningococcal disease – Oregon 1994. MMWR 44: 121-124, 1995
10. Jackson LA, et al. Serogroup C meningococcal outbreaks in the United States: an emerging threat. JAMA 273: 383-389, 1995
11. Frasch CE. Meningococcal vaccines; past, present and future. Ed. K. Cartwright. John Wiley and Sons Ltd, 1995
12. Harrison LH, et al. Risk of meningococcal infection in college students. JAMA 281: 1906-1910, 1999
13. Lepow ML. Meningococcal vaccines, in Vaccines, ed. SA Plotkin and EA Mortimer. WB Saunders Co., 1994
14. Hankins WA, et al. Clinical and serological evaluation of a Meningococcal Polysaccharide Vaccine Groups A, C, Y and W-135. Proc Soc Exper Biol Med 169: 54-57, 1982
15. Lepow ML, et al. Reactogenicity and immunogenicity of a quadrivalent combined meningococcal polysaccharide vaccine in children. J Infect Dis 154: 1033-1036, 1986
16. Unpublished data available from Aventis Pasteur Inc.
17. Reingold AL, et al. Age-specific differences in duration of clinical protection after vaccination with meningococcal polysaccharide A vaccine. Lancet. No. 8447: 114-118, 1985
18. Lennon D, et al. Successful intervention in a Group A meningococcal outbreak in Auckland, New Zealand. Pediatr Infect Dis J 11: 617-623, 1992
19. Collins MJ, et al. Student Health Centers urged to alert students to danger of the disease and provide campus vaccination programs. American College Health Association (ACHA), Baltimore, MD, Press Release 1997
20. Kuronen T, et al. Adverse reactions and endotoxin content of polysaccharide vaccines. Develop Biol Standard, Vol. 34: 117-125, 1977
21. Peltola H, et al. Meningococcus group A vaccine in children three months to five years of age: adverse reactions and immunogenicity related to endotoxin content and molecular weight of the polysaccharide. J Pediatr Vol 92: No 5, 818-822, 1978
22. CDC. National Childhood Vaccine Injury Act: requirements for permanent vaccination records and for reporting of selected events after vaccination. MMWR 37: 197-200, 1988
23. Food and Drug Administration. New reporting requirements for vaccine adverse events. FDA Drug Bull 18 (2), 16-18, 1988
24. CDC. Vaccine Adverse Event Reporting System – United States. MMWR 39: 730-733, 1990
25. Letson GW, et al. Meningococcal vaccine in pregnancy: an assessment of infant risk. Pediatr Infect Dis J 17 (3), 261-263, 1998
26. Scheifele DW, et al. Local adverse effects of meningococcal vaccine. Can Med Assoc J 150: 14-15, 1994
27. American Academy of Pediatrics, Meningococcal infections. In: Peter G, ed. 1997 Red Book: Report of the Committee on Infectious Diseases. 24th ed. Elk Grove Village, IL: American Academy of Pediatrics; 361, 1997

Product information as of January 2003

Manufactured by:
Aventis Pasteur Inc.
Swiftwater PA 18370 USA

Printed in USA

Aventis Pasteur ***Aventis***

4813/4875

Continued on next page

YF-VAX® YELLOW FEVER VACCINE ℞

℞ only

DESCRIPTION

YF-VAX®, Yellow Fever Vaccine, for subcutaneous use, is prepared by culturing the 17D-204 strain of yellow fever virus in living avian leukosis virus-free (ALV-free) chicken embryos. The vaccine contains sorbitol and gelatin as a stabilizer, is lyophilized, and is hermetically sealed under nitrogen. No preservative is added. The vaccine must be reconstituted immediately before use with the sterile diluent provided (Sodium Chloride Injection USP – contains no preservative). YF-VAX® is formulated to contain not less than 4.74 $\log_{10}$ plaque forming units (PFU) per 0.5 mL dose. The vaccine appears slightly opalescent and light orange in color after reconstitution.

CLINICAL PHARMACOLOGY

Yellow fever is an acute viral illness caused by a mosquito-borne flavivirus. The clinical spectrum of yellow fever is highly variable, from subclinical infection to overwhelming pansystemic disease. Yellow fever has an abrupt onset after an incubation period of 3 to 6 days, and usually includes fever, prostration, headache, photophobia, lumbosacral pain, extremity pain (especially the knee joints), epigastric pain, anorexia, and vomiting. The illness may progress to liver and renal failure, and hemorrhagic symptoms and signs caused by thrombocytopenia and abnormal clotting and coagulation may occur. The case-fatality rate of yellow fever varies widely in different studies and may be different for Africa compared to South America, but is typically 20% or higher. Jaundice or other gross evidence of severe liver disease is associated with higher mortality rates.[1]

Two live, attenuated yellow fever vaccines, strains 17D-204 and 17DD, were derived in parallel in the 1930s. Historical data suggest that these "17D vaccines" have identical safety and immunogenicity profiles. Despite a marked reduction in the world-wide incidence of yellow fever in the last five decades due to the extensive use of 17D vaccines and mosquito eradication programs, at least seven tropical South American countries (Bolivia, Brazil, Colombia, Ecuador, French Guiana, Peru, and Venezuela) and much of sub-Saharan Africa[2] currently experience yellow fever epidemics. However, the actual areas of yellow fever virus activity far exceed the infected zones officially reported for epidemics. Approximately 200,000 yellow fever cases have been reported to occur world-wide each year. Six fatalities from yellow fever were reported between 1996 and July 2002, among unimmunized American and European travelers who visited rural areas within the yellow fever endemic zone.[3–8]

Vaccination with 17D strain viruses is predicted to elicit an immune response identical in quality to that induced by wild-type infection. This response is presumed to result from initial infection of cells in the dermis or other subcutaneous tissues near the injection site, with subsequent replication and limited spread of virus leading to the processing and presentation of viral antigens to the immune system, as would occur during infection with wild-type yellow fever virus. The humoral immune response to the viral structural proteins, as opposed to a cell-mediated response, is most important in the protective effect induced by 17D vaccines. Yellow fever antibodies with specificities that prevent or abort infection of cells are detected as neutralizing antibodies in assays that measure the ability of serum to reduce plaque formation in tissue culture cells. The titer of virus neutralizing antibodies in sera of vaccinees is a surrogate for efficacy. A $\log_{10}$ neutralization index (LNI, measured by a plaque reduction assay) of 0.7 or greater was shown to protect 90% of monkeys from lethal intracerebral challenge.[9] This is the definition of seroconversion adopted for clinical trials of yellow fever vaccine. The standard has also been adopted by the World Health Organization (WHO) for efficacy of yellow fever vaccines in humans.[10]

The neutralizing antibody response to 17D vaccines has been evaluated in several uncontrolled studies since the late 1930s. In 24 studies conducted world-wide between 1962 and 1997 using 17D vaccines involving a total of 2,529 adults and 991 infants and children, the seroconversion rate was greater than 91% in all but two studies and never lower than 81%. There were no significant age-related differences in immunogenicity.[1]

Five of these 24 studies were conducted in the US between 1962 and 1993 and included 208 adults who received YF-VAX®. The seroconversion rate was 81% in one study involving 32 subjects and 97% to 100% in the other four studies.[11–15]

In 2001, YF-VAX® was used as a control in a double-blind, randomized comparison trial with another 17D-204 vaccine, conducted at nine centers in the US. YF-VAX® was administered to 725 adults ≥18 years old with a mean age of 38 years. Three hundred twelve of these subjects who received YF-VAX® were evaluated serologically, and 99.3% of them seroconverted with a mean LNI of 2.21. The LNI was slightly higher among males compared to females and slightly lower among Hispanic and African-American subjects compared to others, but these differences were not significant with respect to the protective effect of the vaccine. There was no difference in mean LNI for subjects <40 years old compared to subjects ≥40 years old. Due to the small number of subjects (1.7%) with prior flavivirus immunity, it was not possible to draw conclusions about the role of this factor in the immune response.[16]

Results of one clinical trial involving 33 HIV-positive adults residing in the US indicate that the seroconversion rate to 17D-204 vaccine may be reduced in these patients.[17]

In pregnancy or in immunosuppressed individuals the seroconversion rate after administration of yellow fever vaccine may be significantly reduced.[18]

Existing data suggest that the small percentage of immunologically normal subjects who fail to develop an immune response to an initial vaccination may do so upon revaccination.[19]

In two separate clinical trials of 17D-204 vaccines, 90% of subjects seroconverted within 10 days after vaccination,[20] and 100% of subjects seroconverted within 14 days.[11] Thus, International Health regulations stipulate that the vaccination certificate for yellow fever is valid 10 days after administration of YF-VAX®.[21]

INDICATIONS AND USAGE

YF-VAX® is recommended for active immunization of persons 9 months of age and older in the following categories:

Persons Living In or Traveling To Endemic Areas

While the actual risk for contracting yellow fever during travel is probably low, variability of itineraries and behaviors and the seasonal incidence of disease make it difficult to predict the actual risk for a given individual traveling to a known endemic or epidemic area. Persons greater than or equal to 9 months of age traveling to or living in areas of South America and Africa where yellow fever infection is officially reported at the time of travel should be vaccinated. Vaccination is also recommended for travel outside the urban areas of countries that do not officially report the disease but that lie in a yellow fever endemic zone.

International Travel

Yellow fever vaccination may be required for international travel. Some countries in Africa require evidence of vaccination from all entering travelers and some countries may waive the requirements for travelers staying less than 2 weeks that are coming from areas where there is no current evidence of significant risk for contracting yellow fever. Some countries require an individual, even if only in transit, to have a valid International Certificate of Vaccination if the individual has been in countries either known or thought to harbor yellow fever virus. The certificate becomes valid 10 days after vaccination with YF-VAX®.[2,21]

In no instance should infants less than 9 months of age receive yellow fever vaccine, because of the risk of encephalitis (see **CONTRAINDICATIONS** and **ADVERSE REACTIONS** sections).

Laboratory Personnel

Those laboratory personnel who might be exposed to virulent yellow fever virus or to concentrated preparations of the yellow fever vaccine strain by direct or indirect contact or by aerosols should be vaccinated.[2]

As with any vaccine, vaccination with YF-VAX® may not protect 100% of susceptible individuals (see **CLINICAL PHARMACOLOGY** section).

For simultaneous administration of other vaccines see **PRECAUTIONS** section, **Drug Interactions** subsection.

CONTRAINDICATIONS

Hypersensitivity

Because the yellow fever virus used in the production of this vaccine is propagated in chicken embryos, YF-VAX® should not be administered to anyone with a history of acute hypersensitivity to eggs or egg products; anaphylaxis may occur. *Less severe or localized manifestations of allergy to eggs or to feathers are not contraindications to vaccine administration and do not usually warrant vaccine skin testing (see* ***PRECAUTIONS*** *section,* ***Hypersensitivity Reactions*** *subsection). Generally, persons who are able to eat eggs or egg products may receive the vaccine.*[2,22]

Infants

Vaccination of infants less than 9 months of age IS CONTRAINDICATED because of the risk of encephalitis, and travel of such persons to rural areas in yellow fever endemic zones or to countries experiencing an epidemic should be postponed or avoided, whenever possible.

Immunosuppressed Patients

Exposure to yellow fever vaccine, which is a live virus vaccine, poses a risk of encephalitis or other serious adverse events to patients with illnesses that commonly result in immunosuppression (eg, acquired immunodeficiency syndrome or other manifestations of human immunodeficiency virus (HIV) infection, leukemia, lymphoma, thymoma, generalized malignancy), or patients whose immunologic responses are suppressed by drug therapy (eg, corticosteroids, alkylating drugs, or antimetabolites) or radiation. Therefore, immunosuppressed subjects should not be immunized, and travel to yellow fever endemic areas should be postponed or avoided. If travel to a yellow fever-infected zone is unavoidable, immunosuppressed patients should be advised of the risk, instructed in methods for avoiding vector mosquitoes, and supplied with vaccination waiver letters by their physicians (see **ADVERSE REACTIONS** section).

Family members of immunosuppressed persons, who themselves have no contraindications, may receive yellow fever vaccine.[2,23]

WARNINGS

Anaphylaxis may occur following the use of YF-VAX®, even in individuals with no prior history of hypersensitivity to the vaccine components.

EPINEPHRINE INJECTION (1:1000) SHOULD ALWAYS BE IMMEDIATELY AVAILABLE IN CASE OF AN UNEXPECTED ANAPHYLACTIC OR OTHER SERIOUS ALLERGIC REACTION.

Yellow fever vaccines must be considered as a possible, but rare, cause of vaccine-associated viscerotropic disease[2] (previously described as multiple organ system failure),[2,24] that is similar to fulminant yellow fever caused by wild type yellow fever virus. Available evidence suggests that the occurrence of this syndrome may depend upon the presence of undefined host factors, rather than intrinsic virulence of the yellow fever strain 17D vaccine viruses isolated from subjects with vaccine-associated viscerotropic disease.[24–27] (See **ADVERSE REACTIONS** section).

Vaccine-associated neurotropic disease[2] (previously described as post-vaccinal encephalitis[1]) is a known rare adverse event associated with yellow fever vaccination. Age less than 9 months and immunosuppression are known risk factors for this adverse event. (See **CONTRAINDICATIONS** and **ADVERSE REACTIONS** sections).

PRECAUTIONS

General

Prior to an injection of any vaccine, all known precautions should be taken to prevent adverse events. The patient's previous immunization history, current health status, and medical history should be reviewed for previous hypersensitivity reactions and other adverse events related to this vaccine or similar vaccines and for possible sensitivity to dry natural latex rubber. **The stopper of the vial contains dry natural latex rubber that may cause allergic reactions.** In some instances where symptoms appear soon after a vaccine is administered, differentiation between allergic reaction to the vaccine and reaction to an environmental allergen may not be possible.[22]

EPINEPHRINE INJECTION (1:1000) SHOULD ALWAYS BE IMMEDIATELY AVAILABLE IN CASE OF AN UNEXPECTED ANAPHYLACTIC OR OTHER SERIOUS ALLERGIC REACTION.

A separate, sterile syringe and needle should be used for each patient to prevent transmission of hepatitis or other infectious agents from person to person. Needles should not be recapped and should be properly disposed (eg, sterilized or disposed in red hazardous waste containers).

Hypersensitivity Reactions

YF-VAX® should not be administered to an individual with a history of hypersensitivity to egg or chicken protein (see **CONTRAINDICATIONS** section). However, if a subject is suspect as being an egg-sensitive individual, the following test can be performed before the vaccine is administered:[22]

1. ***Scratch, prick, or puncture test:*** Place a drop of a 1:10 dilution of the vaccine in physiologic saline on a superficial scratch, prick, or puncture on the volar surface of the forearm. Positive (histamine) and negative (physiologic saline) controls should also be used. The test is read after 15 to 20 minutes. A positive test is a wheal 3 mm larger than that of the saline control, usually with surrounding erythema. The histamine control must be positive for valid interpretation. If the result of this test is negative, an intradermal (ID) test should be performed.
2. ***Intradermal test:*** Inject a dose of 0.02 mL of a 1:100 dilution of the vaccine in physiologic saline. Positive and negative control skin tests should be performed concurrently. A wheal 5 mm or larger than the negative control with surrounding erythema is considered a positive reaction.

If vaccination is considered essential, despite a positive skin test, then desensitization can be considered (see **DOSAGE AND ADMINISTRATION** section, **Desensitization** subsection).

Information For Patients

Prior to administration of YF-VAX®, potential vaccinees or their parents or guardians should be asked about their recent health status. All potential vaccinees or their parents or guardians should be fully informed of the benefits and risks of immunization and potential for adverse events that have been temporally associated with YF-VAX® administration. Vaccinees or their parents or guardians should be instructed to report all serious adverse events that occur up to 30 days post-vaccination to their health-care provider.

All travelers should seek information regarding vaccination requirements by consulting local health departments, the Centers for Disease Control and Prevention (CDC), and WHO. Travel agencies, international airlines, and/or shipping lines may also have up-to-date information. Such requirements may be strictly enforced, particularly for persons traveling from Africa or South America to Asia. Travelers should consult the latest published version of Health Information for International Travel to determine requirements and regulations for vaccination.[23]

An International Certificate of Vaccination should be completed, signed, and validated with the center's stamp where the vaccine is administered and provided to all vaccinees. The immunization record should contain the date, lot number and manufacturer of the vaccine administered.[28–30] Subjects should be told that US vaccination certificates are valid for a period of 10 years commencing 10 days after initial vaccination or revaccination.

Drug Interactions

Data are limited in regard to the interaction of YF-VAX® with other vaccines.

- Measles (Schwartz strain) vaccine, diphtheria and tetanus toxoids and pertussis vaccine adsorbed (DTP),[31] Hepatitis A and Hepatitis B vaccines,[2,12,32,33] meningococcal vaccine, Menomune® - A/C/Y/W-135, and typhoid vaccine, Typhim Vi®,[2,12,32] have been administered with yellow fever vaccine at separate injection sites.

- No data exist on possible interference between yellow fever and rabies or Japanese encephalitis vaccines.[2]
- In a prospective study, persons given 5 cc of commercially available immune globulin did not experience alterations in immunologic responses to the yellow fever vaccine.[2,34]
- The anti-malarial drug chloroquine has been administered with yellow fever vaccine.[2,35]

Patients on Corticosteroid Therapy

Oral Prednisone or other systemic corticosteroid therapy may have an immunosuppressive effect on recipients of yellow fever vaccine that potentially decreases immunogenicity and increases the risk of adverse events (see **CONTRAINDICATIONS** section). Intra-articular, bursal, or tendon injections with Prednisone or other corticosteroids should not constitute an increased hazard to recipients of yellow fever vaccine.

Patients With Asymptomatic HIV Infection

Subjects with asymptomatic HIV infection who have had recent laboratory verification of adequate immune system function and who cannot avoid potential exposure to yellow fever virus should be offered the choice of vaccination. Vaccinees should be monitored for possible adverse effects. The seroconversion rate to 17D vaccines is likely to be reduced in these patients.[17] Therefore, documentation of a protective antibody response is recommended before travel. (See **CLINICAL PHARMACOLOGY** section.) For discussion of this subject and for documentation of the immune response to vaccine where it is deemed essential, the CDC may be contacted (970) 221-6400.

Carcinogenesis, Mutagenesis, Impairment of Fertility

YF-VAX® has not been evaluated for its carcinogenic or mutagenic potential or its effect on fertility.

Pregnancy

Reproductive Studies — Pregnancy Category C

Animal reproduction studies have not been conducted with YF-VAX®. It is also not known whether YF-VAX® can cause fetal harm when administered to a pregnant woman or can affect reproductive capacity. Because of the lack of large-scale controlled studies to verify its safety in pregnancy, YF-VAX® should be given to a pregnant woman only if clearly needed. The seroconversion rate to 17D vaccines is markedly reduced in pregnant women. (See **CLINICAL PHARMACOLOGY** section.)[18] For discussion of this subject and for documentation of a protective immune response to vaccine where it is deemed essential, the CDC may be contacted at (970) 221-6400.

Nursing Mothers

It is not known whether this vaccine is excreted in human milk. There have been no reports of adverse events or transmission of 17D vaccine virus from nursing mother to infant. However, vaccination of nursing mothers should be avoided when possible, because of the theoretical risk of the transmission of 17D virus to the breast-fed infant. When travel of nursing mothers to high-risk yellow fever endemic areas cannot be avoided or postponed, such individuals may be immunized.

Pediatric Use

Vaccination of infants less than 9 months of age IS CONTRAINDICATED because of the risk of encephalitis. (See **CONTRAINDICATIONS** and **ADVERSE REACTIONS** sections.)

Geriatric Use

Vaccination of subjects greater than 65 years of age should be limited to individuals who are traveling to or reside in known yellow fever endemic or epidemic areas, because of the increased risk for systemic adverse events in this age group. When vaccination is deemed necessary, the health status of such individuals should be evaluated prior to vaccination. Additionally, if vaccinated, elderly subjects should be carefully monitored for adverse events for 10 days post-vaccination (see **ADVERSE REACTIONS** section).[36,37]

ADVERSE REACTIONS

Adverse reactions to 17D yellow fever vaccine include mild headaches, myalgia, low-grade fevers, or other minor symptoms for 5 to 10 days. Local reactions including edema, hypersensitivity, pain or mass at the injection site have also been reported following yellow fever vaccine administration. Immediate hypersensitivity reactions, characterized by rash, urticaria, and/or asthma, are uncommon and occur principally among persons with histories of egg allergy.[1,2,36]

No placebo-controlled trials to assess the safety of yellow fever 17D vaccines have been performed. However, between 1953 and 1994, reactogenicity of 17D-204 vaccine was monitored in 10 uncontrolled clinical trials. The trials included a total of 3,933 adults and 264 infants greater than 4 months old residing in Europe or in yellow fever endemic areas. Self-limited and mild local reactions consisting of erythema and pain at the injection site and systemic reactions consisting of headache and/or fever occurred in a minority of subjects (typically less than 5%) 5 to 7 days after immunization. In one study involving 115 infants age 4 to 24 months the incidence of fever was as high as 21%. Also in this study, reactogenicity of the vaccine was markedly reduced among a subset of subjects who had serological evidence of previous exposure to yellow fever virus. Only two of the ten studies provided diary cards for daily reporting; this method resulted in a slightly higher incidence of local and systemic complaints.[1]

In 2001, YF-VAX® was used as a control in a double-blind, randomized comparative trial with another 17D-204 vaccine, conducted at nine centers in the US. YF-VAX® was administered to 725 adults ≥18 years old with a mean age of 38 years. Safety data were collected by diary card for days 1 through 10 after vaccination and by interview on days 5, 11, and 31. Among subjects who received YF-VAX®, there were no serious adverse events, and 71.9% experienced non-serious adverse events judged to have been related to vaccination. Most of these were injection site reactions of mild to moderate severity. Four such local reactions were considered severe. Rash occurred in 3.2% and urticaria in two subjects. Systemic reactions (headache, myalgia, malaise, and asthenia) were usually mild and occurred in 10% to 30% of subjects during the first few days after vaccination. The incidence of non-serious adverse reactions, including headache, malaise, injection site edema, and pain, was significantly lower in subjects >60 years compared to younger subjects. Adverse events were less frequent in the 1.7% of vaccinated subjects who had pre-existing immunity to yellow fever virus, compared to those who had not been previously exposed.[16]

A CDC analysis of data submitted to the Vaccine Adverse Events Reporting System (VAERS) between 1990 and 1998 suggests that patients aged 65 or older are at increased risk for systemic adverse events temporally associated with vaccination, compared to the 25- to 44-year-old age group (see **PRECAUTIONS** section, **Geriatric Use** subsection). The rate of systemic adverse events occurring post-vaccination in patients age 65 to 74 was 2.5 times higher than the rate occurring in patients age 25 to 44, based on incidence rates of 6.21 and 2.49 per 100,000 doses of vaccine in the two groups, respectively.[37]

Neurotropic Disease

Vaccine-associated neurotropic disease,[2] (previously described as post-vaccinal encephalitis[1]) is a known rare serious adverse event associated with 17D vaccination. Age less than 9 months and immunosuppression are known risk factors. Twenty-one cases of vaccine-associated neurotropic disease associated with all licensed 17D vaccines have been reported between 1952 and the present, 18 in children or adolescents. Fifteen of these cases occurred prior to 1960, thirteen of which occurred in infants 4 months of age or younger, and two of which occurred in infants six and seven months old. Six cases were reported between 1960 and 1996, world-wide. Three occurred in children, including a one-month-old infant, a three-year-old, and a thirteen-year-old. The three-year-old died of encephalitis, and a genetic variant of the vaccine virus was isolated from the brain in this case.[38] This is the only verified fatality due to yellow fever vaccine-associated neurotropic disease. The three remaining cases of vaccine-associated neurotropic disease since 1960 occurred in adults.[1]

The incidence of vaccine-associated neurotropic disease in infants less than 4 months old is estimated to be between 0.5 and 4 per 1000, based on two historical reports where denominators are available.[39,40] No data are available for calculation of an age-specific incidence rate in the 4- to 9-month-age group. A study in Senegal[41] described two fatal cases of encephalitis possibly associated with 17D-204 vaccination among 67,325 children between the ages of 6 months and 2 years, for an incidence rate of 3 per 100,000. One study conducted in Kenya in 1993 detected four cases of encephalitis temporally associated with vaccination, one in a 2-year-old child and three in adults, for an incidence of 5.3 cases per million vaccinees of all ages.[1]

Viscerotropic Disease

Between 1996 and 1998, four patients, ages 63, 67, 76, and 79, became severely ill 2 to 5 days after vaccination with YF-VAX®. Three of these 4 subjects died. The clinical presentations were characterized by a non-specific febrile syndrome with fatigue, myalgia, and headache, rapidly progressing to a severe illness including respiratory failure, elevated hepatocellular enzymes, lymphocytopenia and thrombocytopenia, hyperbilirubinemia, and renal failure requiring hemodialysis.[24] None of these subjects had vaccine-associated neurotropic disease. This severe adverse event is known as "vaccine-associated viscerotropic disease"[2] (previously described as multiple organ system failure[24]). No cause and effect relationship has been established between vaccination and these subsequent illnesses. In two cases where vaccine virus was recovered from serum, limited nucleotide sequence analysis of the viral genome suggested that the isolates had not undergone a mutation associated with an increase in virulence. The incidence rate for these serious adverse events was estimated at 1 per 400,000 doses of YF-VAX®, based on the total number of doses administered in the US civilian population during the surveillance period.

Vaccine-associated viscerotropic disease temporally associated with yellow fever vaccination has also been reported in Australia and Brazil. One Australian citizen became ill after receiving an immunization with the 17D-204 strain of yellow fever vaccine in his home country,[26] and two Brazilian citizens (age 5 and 22 years) became ill three to four days after receiving 17DD vaccine in Brazil.[27] In the Brazilian and Australian cases, histopathologic changes in the liver included midzonal necrosis, microvesicular fatty change, and Councilman bodies, which are characteristic of wild-type yellow fever. Vaccine-type yellow fever virus was isolated from blood and autopsy material (ie, brain, liver, kidney, spleen, lung, skeletal muscle, or skin) of each of these three persons, all of whom died 8 to 11 days after vaccination. In Brazil, an estimated 23 million vaccine doses were administered during the 15-month period during which the two cases of multiple organ system failure were reported.[27]

In view of the data cited above, both the 17D-204 and 17DD yellow fever vaccines may be considered as a possible, but rare, cause of vaccine-associated viscerotropic disease[2] that is similar to fulminant yellow fever caused by wild-type yellow fever virus. All available evidence from complete nucleotide sequence analysis and testing in experimental animals of vaccine-type yellow fever viruses isolated from the Brazilian subjects suggests that the occurrences are due to undefined host factors, rather than to intrinsic virulence of the 17DD vaccine viruses.[25]

Because of a lack of tissue specimens from most of the US cases of vaccine-associated viscerotropic disease and the qualitative differences between the US cases and those identified in Brazil and Australia, no definitive support for a causal relationship exists between receipt of YF-VAX® and vaccine-associated viscerotropic disease. However, the temporal association with recent receipt of yellow fever vaccine and the similarity of the clinical presentations among all four US cases suggest that the vaccine may play a role in pathogenesis of the cases. Physicians should therefore be cautious to administer yellow fever vaccine only to those persons truly at risk of exposure to wild-type yellow fever virus infection.[2]

Pregnancy

Safety of YF-VAX® was evaluated in a study involving 101 Nigerian women, the majority of whom (88%) were in the third trimester of pregnancy. In this study, it appeared that vaccinating pregnant women with the 17D-204 strain of yellow fever vaccine was not associated with adverse events affecting the mother or fetus. There were no adverse events among 40 infants who were carefully followed up for one year after birth, and none of these infants tested positive for IgM antibodies as a criterion for transplacental infection. However, the percentage of pregnant women who seroconverted was significantly reduced compared to a non-pregnant control group (38.6% vs. 81.5%).[18]

Following a mass immunization campaign in Trinidad, during which 100 to 200 pregnant females were immunized, no adverse events related to pregnancy were reported. In addition, 41 cord blood samples were obtained from infants born to mothers immunized during the first trimester. One of these infants tested positive for IgM antibodies in cord blood. The infant appeared normal at delivery and no subsequent adverse sequelae of infection were reported. However, this result suggests that transplacental infection with 17D vaccine viruses can occur.[42]

A recent case-control study of spontaneous abortion following vaccination of Brazilian women found no significant difference in the odds ratio among vaccinated women compared to a similar unvaccinated group.[43]

Reporting of Adverse Events

The US Department of Health and Human Services has established a Vaccine Adverse Event Reporting System (VAERS) to accept all reports of suspected adverse events after the administration of any vaccine, including but not limited to the reporting of events required by the National Childhood Vaccine Injury Act of 1986.[28,29] Reporting by patients, parents or guardians of all adverse events occurring after vaccine administration is encouraged. Adverse events following immunization with vaccine should be reported by the health-care provider to the US Department of Health and Human Services (DHHS) Vaccine Adverse Event Reporting System. The VAERS toll-free number for forms and information is 1-800-822-7967.[29] Forms may also be available for downloading at the DHHS website www.hhs.gov.

Health-care providers also should report these events to the Pharmacovigilance Department, Aventis Pasteur Inc., Discovery Drive, Swiftwater, PA 18370 or call 1-800-822-2463.

DOSAGE AND ADMINISTRATION

Primary vaccination: For all eligible persons, a single subcutaneous injection of 0.5 mL of reconstituted vaccine (formulated to contain not less than 4.74 $\log_{10}$ PFU) should be administered. Immunity develops by the 10th day after primary vaccination.[11,23,44]

Booster Doses: Re-immunization with 17D vaccine is recommended every 10 years for those at continuing risk of exposure and is required by International Health Regulations.[22] Revaccination boosts antibody titer, although evidence from several studies suggests that yellow fever vaccine immunity persists for at least 30 to 35 years and probably for life,[45] and epidemiologic data suggest that a single infection with wild-type yellow fever virus provides lifelong immunity against illness due to subsequent exposure.

Simultaneous Administration of Other Vaccines

Determination of whether to administer yellow fever vaccine and other immunobiologics simultaneously should be made on the basis of convenience to the traveler in completing the desired vaccinations before travel and on information regarding possible interference. Limited data are available related to administration of YF-VAX® with other vaccines. (See **PRECAUTIONS** section, **Drug Interactions** subsection.) In those specific instances where vaccines may be given concurrently, injections should be administered at separate sites. Where there are no data to support administration of YF-VAX® concurrently with other vaccines, 4 weeks should elapse between sequential vaccinations.[2]

Vaccine Preparation:

- Reconstitute the vaccine using only the diluent supplied (0.6 mL vial of Sodium Chloride Injection USP for single dose vial of vaccine and 3 mL vial of Sodium Chloride Injection USP for 5 dose vial of vaccine). Draw the volume of

Continued on next page

Temperature °C	Test	Number of Lots Tested	Computed Half-Life (Days)
35° – 37°C	Mouse Assay	3	14.0
35° – 37°C	Vero Cell Assay	3	13.9
45° – 47°C	Mouse Assay	3	3.3
45° – 47°C	Vero Cell Assay	3	4.5

YF-Vax—Cont.

the diluent, shown on the diluent label, into a suitable size syringe and slowly inject into the vial containing the vaccine. Allow the reconstituted vaccine to sit for one to two minutes and then carefully swirl mixture until a uniform suspension is achieved. Avoid vigorous shaking as this tends to cause foaming of the suspension. Do not dilute reconstituted vaccine.

- The vaccine should appear slightly opalescent and light orange in color after reconstitution. If the product contains extraneous particulate matter or is discolored, do not administer the vaccine.
- SWIRL VACCINE WELL before withdrawing each dose. Administer the single immunizing dose of 0.5 mL subcutaneously using a 5/8- to 3/4-inch long needle[22] within 60 minutes of reconstituting the vial.

Properly dispose of all reconstituted vaccine and containers that remain unused after one hour (eg, sterilized or disposed in red hazardous waste containers).[2]

Desensitization[22]

If immunization is imperative and the individual has a history of severe egg sensitivity and has a positive skin test to the vaccine, this desensitization procedure may be used to administer the vaccine.

The following successive doses should be administered subcutaneously at 15- to 20-minute intervals:

1.0.05 mL of 1:10 dilution
2.0.05 mL of full strength
3.0.10 mL of full strength
4.0.15 mL of full strength
5.0.20 mL of full strength

Desensitization should only be performed under the direct supervision of a physician experienced in the management of anaphylaxis with necessary emergency equipment immediately available.

HOW SUPPLIED

Vial, 1 Dose (5 per package) with 0.6 mL vial of diluent (5 per package) for administration with needle and syringe. Product No. 49281-915-01

Vial, 5-Dose, with 3 mL vial of diluent, for administration with needle and syringe. Product No. 49281-915-05

YF-VAX® (Yellow Fever Vaccine) in the US is supplied only to designated Yellow Fever Vaccination Centers authorized to issue valid certificates of Yellow Fever Vaccination. Location of the nearest Yellow Fever Vaccination Centers may be obtained from the Centers for Disease Control and Prevention, Atlanta, GA 30333, state or local health departments.

STORAGE

Shipping Conditions and Temperatures

YF-VAX® is shipped frozen in a container with solid carbon dioxide; do not use unless the shipping case contains some dry ice upon arrival.

Upon receipt, lyophilized vaccine must be maintained continuously at 0° – 5°C (32° – 41°F). **DO NOT REFREEZE.**

YF-VAX® does not contain a preservative; therefore, all reconstituted vaccine and containers which remain unused after one hour must be properly disposed (eg, sterilized or disposed in red hazardous waste containers).[2]

The following stability information for YF-VAX® is provided for those countries or areas of the world where an adequate cold chain is a problem and inadvertent exposure to abnormal temperatures has occurred.

[See table above]

YF-VAX® is formulated to satisfy the current US potency requirements of not less than 4.74 $\log_{10}$ PFU per 0.5 mL dose and meets the minimum requirements of WHO.[10]

REFERENCES

1. Monath TP. Vaccines. 3rd Edition, WB Saunders Company. 1999;815–879. **2.** Recommendations of the Advisory Committee on Immunization Practices (ACIP). MMWR 2002;51(RR17):1–10. **3.** Teichmann D, et al. Lancet 354: 1608. **4.** ACIP. MMWR 2000;49:(14);303–305. **5.** McFarland JM, et al. Clin Infect Dis 1997;25:1143–1147. **6.** Centers for Disease Control and Prevention (CDC). MMWR 2002;51(15):324–325. **7.** World Health Organization (WHO). Weekly Epidemiological Record 2001;76:365–372. **8.** Barros MLB, et al. Lancet 1996;348:969–970. **9.** Mason RA, et al. Appl Microbiol 1973;25(4):539–544. **10.** WHO Technical Report Series 594, 1976. **11.** Wisseman CL, et al. Am J Trop Med Hyg 1962;11:550. **12.** American Society for Microbiology. JAMA: HIV/AIDS Resource Center 1996;Sept 15–18. **13.** Meyer HM, et al. Bull World Health Org 1964;30:783. **14.** Bancroft WH, et al. J Infect Dis 1984;149:1005–1010. **15.** Jackson J, et al. Third International Conference on Travel Medicine; Paris 1993;April 25–29. **16.** Monath TP, et al. Am J Trop Med Hyg 2002;533–541. **17.** Goujon C, et al. Fourth International Conference on Travel Medicine; Acapulco, Mexico 1995;April 23–27. **18.** Nasidi A, et al. Transactions of the Royal Society of Tropical Medicine and Hygiene 1993;87:337–339. **19.** Bonnevie-Nielson V, et al. Clin Diag Lab Immunol 1995;2:302–306. **20.** Smithburn KC, et al. Am J Trop Med Hyg 1945;45:217. **21.** WHO. Geneva 1983. **22.** American Academy of Pediatrics. 2000;35–175. **23.** CDC. US Department of Health and Human Services, Public Health Service 2001;3-6,12-21,154-160,207–220. **24.** Martin M, et al. Lancet 2001;358:98–104. **25.** Galler R, et al. Virology 2001;290:309–319. **26.** Chan RC, et al. Lancet 2001;358: 121–122. **27.** Vasconcelos PFC, et al. Lancet 2001;358:91. **28.** CDC. MMWR 1990;39:730–733. **29.** CDC. MMWR 1988;37:197–200. **30.** Food and Drug Administration. FDA Drug Bull 1988;18(2):16–18. **31.** Ruben FL, et al. Bull WHO 1973;48:175–181. **32.** Dumas R, et al. Adv Therapy 1997;14: 160–167. **33.** Coursaget P, et al. Vaccine 1995;13:109–111. **34.** Kaplan JE, et al. Bull WHO 1984;62(4):585–590. **35.** Tsai TF, et al. J Infect Dis 1986;154(4):726–727. **36.** Aventis Pasteur Inc. Data on File – 080601. **37.** Martin M, et al. Emerg Infect Dis 2001;7:945–951. **38.** Jennings AD, et al. J Infect Dis 1994;169:512–518. **39.** Stuart G. WHO 1956;143. **40.** Louis JJ, et al. Pediatr 1981;36:439. **41.** Rey M, et al. Bull Soc Med Afr Noire Lgue Fr 1966;11:617. **42.** Tsai TF, et al. J Infect Dis 1993;168:1520-1523. **43.** Nishioka SA, et al. Trop Med Int Health 1998;3(1):29–33. **44.** ACIP. MMWR 2002;51(RR02):1–36. **45.** Poland JD, et al. Bull WHO 1981;59(6):895–900.

Product information as of April 2003

Manufactured by:
Aventis Pasteur Inc.
Swiftwater PA 18370 USA

4291/4292

Aventis Pasteur ***Aventis***

Axcan Scandipharm Inc.

22 INVERNESS CENTER PARKWAY
BIRMINGHAM, AL 35242

Direct Inquiries to:
Customer Service
(800) 950-8085
Fax: (205) 991-8426

For Medical Information Contact:
Marie-Helene Doyon
(800) 565-3255
Fax: (450) 467-5857

BENTYL® ℞

[bĕn-tĭl]
(dicyclomine hydrochloride USP)

DESCRIPTION

BENTYL is an antispasmodic and anticholinergic (antimuscarinic) agent available in the following forms:

1. BENTYL capsules for oral used contain 10 mg dicyclomine hydrochloride USP. BENTYL 10 mg capsules also contain inactive ingredients: calcium sulfate, corn starch, FD&C Blue No. 1, FD&C Red No. 40, gelatin, lactose, magnesium stearate, pregelatinized corn starch, and titanium dioxide.
2. BENTYL tables for oral use contain 20 mg dicyclomine hydrochloride USP. BENTYL 20 mg tablets also contain inactive ingredients: acacia, dibasic calcium phosphate, corn starch, FD&C Blue No. 1, lactose, magnesium stearate, pregelatinized corn starch, and sucrose.
3. BENTYL syrup for oral use contains 10 mg dicyclomine hydrochloride USP in each 5 mL (1 teaspoonful). BENTYL syrup also contains inactive ingredients: citric acid, D&C Red No. 33, FD&C Blue No. 1, FD&C Red No. 40, FD&C Yellow No. 6, flavors, glucose, methylparaben, propylene glycol, propylparaben, saccharin sodium, and water.
4. BENTYL injection is a sterile, pyrogen-free, aqueous solution for intramuscular injection (NOT FOR INTRAVENOUS USE).

Ampul. 2 mL-Each mL contains 10 mg dicyclomine hydrochloride USP in sterile water for injection, made isotonic with sodium chloride.

Chemically, BENTYL (dicyclomine hydrochloride) is [bicyclohexyl]-1-carboxylic acid, 2-(diethylamino) ethylester, hydrochloride with the following chemical structure:

C(=O)–O–CH₂–CH₂–N(CH₂–CH₃)(CH₂–CH₃) • HCl

Dicyclomine hydrochloride occurs as a fine, white, crystalline, practically odorless powder with a bitter taste. It is soluble in water, freely soluble in alcohol and chloroform, and very slightly soluble in ether.

CLINICAL PHARMACOLOGY

Dicyclomine relieves smooth muscle spasm of the gastrointestinal tract. Animal studies indicate that this action is achieved via a dual mechanism: (1) a specific anticholinergic effect (antimuscarinic) at the acetylcholinereceptor sites with approximately 1/8 the milligram potency of atropine (in vitro, guinea pig ileum); and (2) a direct effect upon smooth muscle (musculotropic) as evidenced by dicyclomine's antagonism of bradykinin- and histamine-induced spasms of the isolated guinea pig ileum. Atropine did not affect responses to these two agonists. In vivo studies in cats and dogs showed dicyclomine to be equally potent against acetyl-choline (ACh)- or barium chloride ($BaCl_2$)-induced intestinal spasm while atropine was at least 200 times more potent against effects of ACh than $BaCl_2$. Tests for mydriatic effects in mice showed that dicyclomine was approximately 1/500 as potent as atropine; antisialagogue tests in rabbits showed dicyclomine to be 1/300 as potent as atropine.

In man, dicyclomine is rapidly absorbed after oral administration, reaching peak values within 60-90 minutes. The principal route of elimination is via the urine (79.5% of the dose). Excretion also occurs in the feces, but to a lesser extent (8.4%). Mean half-life of plasma elimination in one study was determined to be approximately 1.8 hours when plasma concentration were measured for 9 hours after a single dose. In subsequent studies, plasma concentrations were followed for up to 24 hours after a single dose, showing a secondary phase of elimination with a somewhat longer half-life. Mean volume of distribution for a 20 mg oral dose is approximately 3.65 L/kg suggesting extensive distribution in tissues.

In controlled clinical trials involving over 100 patients who received drug, 82% of patients treated for functional bowel/ irritable bowel syndrome with dicyclomine hydrochloride at initial doses of 160 mg daily (40 mg q.i.d.) demonstrated a favorable clinical response compared with 55% treated with placebo. ($P<.05$). In these trials most of the side effects were typically anticholinergic in nature (see table) and were reported by 61% of the patients.

Side Effect	Dicyclomine Hydrochloride (40 mg q.i.d.) %	Placebo %
Dry Mouth	33	5
Dizziness	29	2
Blurred Vision	27	2
Nausea	14	6
Light-Headedness	11	3
Drowsiness	9	1
Weakness	7	1
Nervousness	6	2

Nine percent (9%) of patients were discontinued from the drug because of one or more of these side effects (compared with 2% in the placebo group). In 41% of the patients with side effects, side effects disappeared or were tolerated at the 160 mg daily dose without reduction. A dose reduction from 160 mg daily to an average daily dose of 90 mg was required in 46% of the patients with side effects who then continued to experience a favorable clinical response; their side effects either disappeared or were tolerated (See ADVERSE REACTIONS.)

INDICATIONS AND USAGE

For the treatment of functional bowel/irritable bowel syndrome.

CONTRAINDICATIONS

1. Obstructive uropathy
2. Obstructive disease of the gastrointestinal tract.
3. Severe ulcerative colitis (See PRECAUTIONS)
4. Reflux esophagitis
5. Unstable cardiovascular status in acute hemorrhage
6. Glaucoma
7. Myasthenia gravis
8. Evidence of prior hypersensitivity to dicyclomine hydrochloride or other ingredients of these formulations.
9. Infants less than 6 months of age (See WARNINGS and PRECAUTIONS: Information for Patients.)
10. Nursing Mothers (See WARNINGS and PRECAUTIONS: Information for Patients.)

WARNINGS

In the presence of a high environmental temperature, heat prostration can occur with drug use (fever and heat stroke due to decreased sweating). If symptoms occur, the drug should be discontinued and supportive measures instituted. Diarrhea may be an early symptom of incomplete intestinal obstruction, especially in patients with ileostomy or colostomy. In this instance, treatment with this drug would be inappropriate and possibly harmful.

BENTYL may produce drowsiness or blurred vision. The patient should be warned not to engage in activities requiring mental alertness, such as operating a motor vehicle or other machinery or performing hazardous work while taking this drug.

Psychosis has been reported in sensitive individuals given anticholinergic drugs. CNS signs and symptoms include confusion, disorientation, short-term memory loss, hallucinations, drysarthria, ataxia, coma, euphoria, decreased anxiety, fatigue, insomnia, agitation and mannerisms, and inappropriate affect.

These CNS signs and symptoms usually resolve within 12 to 24 hours after discontinuation of the drug.

There are reports that administration of dicyclomine hydrochloride syrup to infants has been followed by serious respiratory symptoms (dyspnea, shortness of breath, breathlessness, respiratory collapse, apnea, asphyxia), seizures, syncope, pulse rate fluctuations, muscular hypotonia, and coma. Death has been reported. No causal relationship between these effects observed in infants and dicyclomine administration has been established. BENTYL IS CONTRAINDICATID IN INFANTS LESS THAN 6 MONTHS OF AGE AND IN NURSING MOTHERS. (See CONTRAINDICATIONS and PRECAUTIONS: Nursing Mothers and Pediatric Use.)

Safety and efficacy of dicyclomine hydrochloride in pediatric patients have not been established.

PRECAUTIONS

General

Use with caution in patients with:

1. Autonomic neuropathy
2. Hepatic or renal disease
3. Ulcerative colitis-large doses may suppress intestinal motility to the point of producing a paralytic ileus and the use of this drug may precipitate or aggravate the serious complication of toxic megacolon (see CONTRAINDICATIONS)
4. Hyperthyroidism
5. Hypertension
6. Coronary heart disease
7. Congestive heart failure
8. Cardiac tachyarrhythmia
9. Hiatal hernia (see CONTRAINDICATIONS: reflux esophagitis)
10. Known or suspected prostatic hypertrophy.

Investigate any tachycardia before administration of dicyclomine hydrochloride, since it may increase the heart rate. With overdosage, a curare-like action may occur (i.e., neuromuscular blockade leading to muscular weakness and possible paralysis).

Information For Patients

BENTYL may produce drowsiness or blurred vision. The patient should be warned not to engage in activities requiring mental alertness, such as operating a motor vehicle or other machinery or to perform hazardous work while taking this drug.

BENTYL is contraindicated in infants less than 6 months of age and in nursing mothers. (See CONTRAINDICATIONS, WARNINGS, and PRECAUTIONS: Nursing Mothers and Pediatric Use.) In the presence of a high environmental temperature, heat prostration can occur with drug use (fever and heat stroke due to decreased sweating). If symptoms occur, the drug should be discontinued and a physician contacted.

Drug Interactions

The following agents may increase certain actions or side effects of anticholinergic drugs: amantadine, antiarrhythmic agents of Class I (e.g., quinidine), antihistamines, antipsychotic agents (e.g., phenothiazines), MAO inhibitors, narcotic analgesics (e.g., meperidine), nitrates and nitrites, sympathomimetic agents, tricyclic antidepressants, and other drugs having anticholinergic activity.

Anticholinergics antagonize the effects of antiglaucoma agents. Anticholinergic drugs in the presence of increased intraocular pressure may be hazardous when taken concurrently with agents such as corticosteroids. (See also CONTRAINDICATIONS).

Anticholinergic agents may affect gastrointestinal absorption of various drugs, such as slowly dissolving dosage forms of digoxin; increased serum digoxin concentration may result.

Anticholinergic drugs may antagonize the effects of drugs that alter gastrointestinal motility, such as metoclopramide. Because antacids may interfere with the absorption of anticholinergic agents, simultaneous use of these drugs should be avoided. The inhibiting effects of anticholinergic drugs on gastric hydrochloric acid secretion are antagonized by agents used to treat achlorhydria and those used to test gastric secretion.

Carcinogenesis, Mutagenesis, Impairment of Fertility

There are no known human data on long-term potential for carcinogenicity or mutagenicity. Long-term studies in animals to determine carcinogenic potential are not known to have been conducted. In studies in rats at doses of up to 100 mg/kg/day, BENTYL produced no deleterious effects on breeding, conception, or parturition.

Pregnancy

Teratogenic Effects. Pregnancy Category B. Reproduction studies have been performed in rats and rabbits at doses up to 33 times the maximum recommended human dose based on 160 mg/day (3 mg/kg) and have revealed no evidence of impaired fertility or harm to the fetus due to dicyclomine. Epidemiologic studies in pregnant women with products containing dicyclomine hydrochloride (at doses up to 40 mg/day) have not shown that dicyclomine increases the risk of fetal abnormalities if administered during the first trimester of pregnancy. There are, however, no adequate and well-controlled studies in pregnant women at the recommended doses (80–160 mg/day). Because animal reproduction studies are not always predictive of human response. BENTYL as indicated for functional bowel/irritable bowel syndrome should be used during pregnancy only if clearly needed.

Nursing Mothers

Since dicyclomine hydrochloride has been reported to be excreted in human milk, BENTYL IS CONTRAINDICATED IN NURSING MOTHERS (See CONTRAINDICATIONS, WARNINGS, PRECAUTIONS: Pediatric Use and ADVERSE REACTIONS.)

Pediatric Use

(See CONTRAINDICATIONS, WARNINGS, PRECAUTIONS: Nursing Mothers.) BENTYL IS CONTRAINDICATED IN INFANTS LESS THAN 6 MONTHS OF AGE. Safety and effectiveness in pediatric patients have not been established.

ADVERSE REACTIONS

Controlled clinical trials have provided frequency information for reported adverse effects of dicyclomine hydrochloride listed in a decreasing order of frequency. (See CLINICAL PHARMACOLOGY.)

Not all of the following adverse reactions have been reported with dicyclomine hydrochloride. Adverse reactions are included here that have been reported for pharmacologically similar drugs with anticholinergic/antispasmodic action.

Gastrointestinal: dry mouth, nausea, vomiting, constipation, bloated feeling, abdominal pain, taste loss, anorexia.

Central Nervous System: dizziness, light-headedness, tingling, headache, drowsiness, weakness, nervousness, numbness, mental confusion and/or excitement (especially in elderly persons), dyskinesia, lethargy, syncope, speech disturbance, insomnia

Ophthalmologic: blurred vision, diplopia, mydriasis, cycloplegia, increased ocular tension.

Dermatologic/Allergic: rash, urticaria, itching, and other dermal manifestations; severe allergic reaction or drug idiosyncrasies including anaphylaxis.

Genitourinary: urinary hesitancy, urinary retention

Cardiovascular: tachycardia, palpitations.

Respiratory: Dyspnea, apnea, asphyxia (see WARNINGS).

Other: decreased sweating, nasal stuffiness or congestion, sneezing, throat congestion, impotence, suppression of lactation (see PRECAUTIONS: Nursing Mothers)

With the injectable form, there may be temporary sensation of light-headedness. Some local irritation and focal coagulation necrosis may occur following the I.M. injection of the drug.

DRUG ABUSE AND DEPENDENCE

Abuse of and/or dependence on dicyclomine for anticholinergic effects have been rarely reported.

OVERDOSAGE

Signs and Symptoms

The signs and symptoms of overdosage are headache, nausea; vomiting; blurred vision; dilated pupils; hot, dry skin; dizziness; dryness of the mouth; difficulty in swallowing; and CNS stimulation. A curare-like action may occur (i.e., neuromuscular blockade leading to muscular weakness and possible paralysis).

A 37-year-old female reported numbness on the left side, cold fingertips, blurred vision, abdominal and flank pain, decreased appetite, dry mouth, and nervousness following ingestion of 320 mg daily (four 20 mg tablets QID) for four days. These events resolved after discontinuing the dicyclomine.

Oral LD_{50}

The acute oral LD_{50} of the drug is 625 mg/kg in mice.

Minimum Human Lethal Dose/Maximum Human Dose Recorded

The amount of drug in a single dose that is ordinarily associated with symptoms of overdosage or that is likely to be life-threatening, has not been defined. The maximum human oral dose recorded was 600 mg by mouth in a 10-month-old child and approximately 1500 mg in an adult each of whom survived. In three of the infants who died following administration of dicyclomine hydrochloride (see WARNINGS), the blood concentrations of drug were 200, 220, and 505 ng/mL, respectively.

Dialysis

It is not know if BENTYL is dialyzable.

Treatment

Treatment should consist of gastric lavage, emetics, and activated charcoal. Sedatives (e.g., short-acting barbiturates, benzodiazepines) may be used for management of overt signs of excitement. If indicated, an appropriate parenteral cholinergic agent may be used as an antidote.

DOSAGE AND ADMINSTRATION

DOSAGE MUST BE ADJUSTED TO INDIVIDUAL PATIENT NEEDS (See CLINICAL PHARMACOLOGY.)

Adults-Oral. The only oral dose clearly shown to be effective is 160 mg per day (in 4 equally divided doses). Since this dose is associated with a significant incidence of side effects, it is prudent to begin with 80 mg per day (in 4 equally divided doses). Depending upon the patient's response during the first week of therapy, the dose should be increased to 160 mg per day unless side effects limit dosage escalation. If efficacy is not achieved within 2 weeks or side effects require doses below 80 mg per day, the drug should be discontinued. Documented safety data are not available for doses above 80 mg daily for periods longer than 2 weeks.

Adults-Intramuscular Injection. NOT FOR INTRAVENOUS USE.

The intramuscular dosage form is to be used temporarily when the patient cannot take oral medication. Intramuscular injection is about twice as bioavailable as oral dosage forms; consequently the recommended intramuscular dose is 80 mg daily (in 4 equally divided doses). Oral dicyclomine hydrochloride should be started as soon as possible and the intramuscular form should not be used for periods longer than 1 or 2 days.

ASPIRATE THE SYRINGE BEFORE INJECTING TO AVOID INTRAVASUCLAR INJECTION, SINCE THROMBOSIS MAY OCCUR IF THE DRUG IS INADVERTENTLY INJECTED INTRAVEASCUALRLY. Partenteral drug products should be inspected visually for particulate matter and discoloration prior to administration, whenever solution and container permit.

HOW SUPPLIED

10 mg blue capsules, imprinted BENTYL 10 NDC 58914-012-10: bottles of 100. Store at room temperature, preferably below 86°F (30°C).

20 mg compressed, light blue, round tablets, debossed BENTYL 20 NDC 58914-013-10: bottles of 100. To prevent fading, avoid exposure to direct sunlight. Store at room temperature, preferably below 86°F (30°C).

10 mg/5 mL pink syrup NDC 58914-015-16; 16 ounce bottle Store at room temperature, preferably below 86°F (30°C). Protect from excessive heat.

10 mg/mL injection (for intramuscular use only, NOT FOR INTRAVENOUS USE) NDC 58914-080-52: 10 mL multiple dose vials

Store at room temperature, preferably below 86°F (30°C). Protect from freezing.

Rx only

Rev. April 2004

Bentyl Capsules, Bently Tablets and Bentyl Syrup Manufactured by:
Patheon Pharmaceuticals Inc.
Cincinnati, OH 45215
Manufactured for:
Axcan Scandipharm Inc.
22 Inverness Center Parkway
Birmingham, AL 35242
www.axcan.com
Bentyl Injection Manufactured by:
Akorn Inc.
Decatur, IL 62522
Manufactured for:
Axcan Scandipharm Inc.
22 Inverness Center Parkway
Birmingham, AL 35242
www.axcan.com

CANASA® ℞

(Mesalamine)
Rectal Suppositories 500 mg
NDC 58914-500-56
Rx Only

DESCRIPTION

The active ingredient in CANASA®, is mesalamine, also known as 5-aminosalicylic acid (5-ASA). Chemically, mesalamine is 5-amino-2-hydroxybenzoic acid, and is classified as an anti-inflammatory drug.

The empirical formula is $C_7H_7NO_3$, representing a molecular weight of 153.14. The structural formula is:

Each CANASA® Rectal Suppository contains 500 mg of mesalamine in a base of Hard Fat NF.

CLINICAL PHARMACOLOGY

Sulfasalazine has been used in the treatment of ulcerative colitis for over 55 years. It is split by bacterial action in the colon into sulfapyridine (SP) and mesalamine (5-ASA). It is thought that the mesalamine component only is therapeutically active in ulcerative colitis.

Mechanism of Action

The mechanism of action of mesalamine (and sulfasalazine) is unknown, but appears to be topical rather than systemic. Although the pathology of inflammatory bowel disease is uncertain, both prostaglandins and leukotrienes have been implicated as mediators of mucosal injury and inflammation. Recently, however, the role of mesalamine as a free radical scavenger or inhibitor of tumor necrosis factor (TNF) has also been postulated.

Pharmacokinetics

Absorption: Mesalamine (5-ASA) administered as a rectal suppository is variably absorbed. In patients with ulcerative colitis treated with mesalamine 500 mg rectal suppositories, administered once every eight hours for six days, the mean

Continued on next page

Canasa—Cont.

mesalamine peak plasma concentration (C_{max}) was 353 ng/mL (CV=55%) following the initial dose and 361 ng/mL (CV=67%) at steady state. The mean minimum steady state plasma concentration (C_{min}) was 89 ng/mL (CV=89 %). Absorbed mesalamine does not accumulate in the plasma.

Distribution: Mesalamine administered as rectal suppositories distributes in rectal tissue to some extent. In patients with ulcerative proctitis treated with CANASA® 500 mg rectal suppositories, rectal tissue concentrations for 5-ASA and N-acetyl-5-ASA have not been rigorously quantified.

Metabolism: Mesalamine is extensively metabolized, mainly to N-acetyl-5-ASA. The site of metabolism has not been elucidated. In patients with ulcerative colitis treated with one 500 mg mesalamine rectal suppository every eight hours for six days, peak concentration (C_{max}) of N-acetyl-5-ASA ranged from 467 ng/mL to 1399 ng/mL following the initial dose and from 193 ng/mL to 1304 ng/mL at steady state.

Elimination: Mesalamine is eliminated from plasma mainly by urinary excretion, predominantly as N-acetyl-5-ASA. In patients with ulcerative proctitis treated with one mesalamine 500 mg rectal suppository every eight hours for six days, ≤12% of the dose was eliminated in urine as 5-ASA and 8–77% as N-acetyl-5-ASA following the initial dose. At steady state, ≤ 11% of the dose was eliminated as 5-ASA and 3–35% as N-acetyl-5-ASA. The mean elimination half-life was five hours (CV=73%) for 5-ASA and six hours (CV=63%) for N-acetyl-5-ASA following the initial dose. At steady state, the mean elimination half-life was seven hours for both 5-ASA and N-acetyl-5-ASA (CV=102% for 5-ASA and 82% for N-acetyl-5-ASA).

Drug-Drug Interactions: The potential for interactions between mesalamine, administered as 500 mg rectal suppositories, and other drugs has not been studied.

Special Populations (Patients with Renal or Hepatic Impairment): The effect of renal or hepatic impairment on elimination of mesalamine in ulcerative proctitis patients treated with mesalamine 500 mg suppositories has not been studied.

Preclinical Toxicology

Preclinical studies of mesalamine were conducted in rats, mice, rabbits and dogs and kidney was the main target organ of toxicity. In rats, adverse renal effects were observed at a single oral dose of 600 mg/kg (about 3.2 times the recommended human intra-rectal dose, based on body surface area) and at IV doses of >214 mg/kg (about 1.2 times the recommended human intra-rectal dose, based on body surface area). In a 13-week oral gavage toxicity study in rats, papillary necrosis and/or multifocal tubular injury were observed in males receiving 160 mg/kg (about 0.86 times the recommended human intra-rectal dose, based on body surface area) and in both males and females at 640 mg/kg (about 3.5 times the recommended human intra-rectal dose, based on body surface area). In a combined 52-week toxicity and 127-week carcinogenicity study in rats, degeneration of the kidneys and hyalinization of basement membranes and Bowman's capsule were observed at oral doses of 100 mg/kg/day (about 0.54 times the recommended human intra-rectal dose, based on body surface area) and above. In a 14-day rectal toxicity study of mesalamine suppositories in rabbits, intra-rectal doses up to 800 mg/kg (about 8.6 times the recommended human intra-rectal dose, based on body surface area) was not associated with any adverse effects. In a six-month oral toxicity study in dogs, doses of 80 mg/kg (about 1.4 times the recommended human intra-rectal dose, based on body surface area) and higher caused renal pathology similar to that described for the rat. In a rectal toxicity study of mesalamine suppositories in dogs, a dose of 166.6 mg/kg (about 3.0 times the recommended human intra-rectal dose, based on body surface area) produced chronic nephritis and pyelitis. In the 12-month eye toxicity study in dogs, Keratoconjunctivitis sicca (KCS) occurred at oral doses of 40 mg/kg (about 0.72 times the recommended human intra-rectal dose, based on body surface area) and above.

CLINICAL STUDIES

Two double-blind placebo-controlled multicenter studies were conducted in North America in patients with mild to moderate active ulcerative proctitis. The primary measures of efficacy were the same in all trials (clinical disease activity index, sigmoidoscopic and histologic evaluations). The main difference between the studies was dosage regimen: 500 mg three times daily (1.5 g/d) in Study 1; and 500 mg twice daily (1.0 g/d) in Study 2. A total of 173 patients were studied (Study 1, N=79; Study 2, N=94). Eighty-nine (89) patients received mesalamine suppositories and eighty-four (84) patients received placebo suppositories. Patients were evaluated clinically and sigmoidoscopically after three and six weeks of suppository treatment. In Study No. 1 patients were 17 to 73 years of age (mean = 39 yrs), 57% were female, and 97% were white. Patients had an average extent of proctitis (upper disease boundary) of 10.8 cm. Eighty-four percent (84%) of the study patients had multiple prior episodes of proctitis. In Study No. 2, patients were 21 to 72 years of age (mean = 39 yrs), 62% were female, and 96% were white. Patients had an average extent of proctitis (upper disease boundary) of 10.3 cm. Seventy-eight percent (78%) of the study patients had multiple prior episodes of proctitis.

Compared to placebo, mesalamine suppository treatment was statistically (p<0.01) superior to placebo in all trials with respect to improvement in stool frequency, rectal bleeding, mucosal appearance, disease severity, and overall disease activity after three and six weeks of treatment. Daily diary records indicated significant improvement in rectal bleeding in the first week of therapy while tenesmus and diarrhea improved significantly within two weeks. Investigators rated patients receiving mesalamine much improved compared to patients receiving placebo (p<0.001).

The effectiveness of mesalamine suppositories was statistically significant irrespective of sex, extent of proctitis, duration of current episode or duration of disease.

INDICATIONS AND USAGE

CANASA® Suppositories are indicated for the treatment of active ulcerative proctitis.

CONTRAINDICATIONS

CANASA® Suppositories are contraindicated for patients known to have hypersensitivity to mesalamine (5-aminosalicylic acid) or to the suppository vehicle [saturated vegetable fatty acid esters (Hard Fat, NF)].

PRECAUTIONS

Mesalamine has been implicated in the production of an acute intolerance syndrome characterized by cramping, acute abdominal pain and bloody diarrhea, sometimes fever, headache and a rash; in such cases prompt withdrawal is required. The patient's history of sulfasalazine intolerance, if any, should be re-evaluated. If a rechallenge is performed later in order to validate the hypersensitivity it should be carried out under close supervision and only if clearly needed, giving consideration to reduced dosage. In the literature, one patient previously sensitive to sulfasalazine was rechallenged with 400 mg oral mesalamine; within eight hours she experienced headache, fever, intensive abdominal colic, profuse diarrhea and was readmitted as an emergency. She responded poorly to steroid therapy and two weeks later a pancolectomy was required. The possibility of increased absorption of mesalamine and concomitant renal tubular damage as noted in the preclinical studies must be kept in mind. Patients on CANASA®, especially those on concurrent oral products which contain or release mesalamine and those with preexisting renal disease, should be carefully monitored with urinalysis, BUN and creatinine testing.

In a clinical trial most patients who were hypersensitive to sulfasalazine were able to take mesalamine enemas without evidence of any allergic reaction. Nevertheless, caution should be exercised when mesalamine is initially used in patients known to be allergic to sulfasalazine. These patients should be instructed to discontinue therapy if signs of rash or fever become apparent.

A small proportion of patients have developed pancolitis while using mesalamine. However, extension of upper disease boundary and/or flare-ups occurred less often in the mesalamine-treated group than in the placebo-treated group.

Rare instances of pericarditis have been reported with mesalamine containing products including sulfasalazine. Cases of pericarditis have also been reported as manifestations of inflammatory bowel disease. In the cases reported there have been positive rechallenges with mesalamine or mesalamine containing products. In one of these cases, however, a second rechallenge with sulfasalazine was negative throughout a 2 month follow-up. Chest pain or dyspnea in patients treated with mesalamine should be investigated with this information in mind. Discontinuation of CANASA® may be warranted in some cases, but rechallenge with mesalamine can be performed under careful clinical observation should the continued therapeutic need for mesalamine be present.

There have been two reports in the literature of additional serious adverse events: one patient who developed leukopenia and thrombocytopenia after seven months of treatment with one 500 mg suppository nightly, and one patient with rash and fever which was a similar reaction to sulfasalazine.

Information for Patients: See patient information printed at the end of this insert.

Carcinogenesis, Mutagenesis, Impairment of Fertility

Mesalamine caused no increase in the incidence of neoplastic lesions over controls in a two-year study of Wistar rats fed up to 320 mg/kg/day of mesalamine admixed with diet (about 1.7 times the recommended human intra-rectal dose, based on body surface area).

Mesalamine was not mutagenic in the Ames test, the mouse lymphoma cell ($TK^{+/-}$) forward mutation test, or the mouse micronucleus test.

No effects on fertility or reproductive performance of the male and female rats were observed at oral mesalamine doses up to 320 mg/kg/day (about 1.7 times the recommended human intra-rectal dose, based on body surface area). The oligospermia and infertility in men associated with sulfasalazine have not been reported with mesalamine.

Pregnancy, Teratogenic Effects, Pregnancy Category B

Teratology studies have been performed in rats at oral doses up to 320 mg/kg/day (about 1.7 times the recommended human intra-rectal dose, based on body surface area) and in rabbits at oral doses up to 495 mg/kg/day (about 5.4 times the recommended human intra-rectal dose, based on body surface area) and have revealed no evidence of impaired fertility or harm to the fetus due to mesalamine. There are, however, no adequate and well controlled studies in pregnant women. Because animal reproduction studies are not always predictive of human response, this drug should be used in pregnancy only if clearly needed.

Nursing Mothers

It is not known whether mesalamine or its metabolite(s) are excreted in human milk. Because many drugs are excreted in human milk, caution should be exercised when CANASA® is administered to a nursing woman.

Pediatric Use

Safety and effectiveness in pediatric patients have not been established.

Geriatric Use

Clinical studies of CANASA® did not include sufficient numbers of subjects aged 65 and over to determine whether they respond differently from younger subjects. Other reported clinical experience has not identified differences in responses between the elderly and younger patients. In general, dose selection for an elderly patient should be cautious, reflecting the greater frequency of decreased hepatic, renal, or cardiac function, and of concomitant disease or other drug therapy.

Mesalamine is known to be substantially excreted by the kidney, and the risk of toxic reactions to this drug may be greater in patients with impaired renal function. Because elderly patients are more likely to have decreased renal function, it may be useful to monitor renal function.

ADVERSE REACTIONS

Clinical Adverse Experience

ADVERSE REACTIONS OCCURRING IN MORE THAN 1% OF MESALAMINE SUPPOSITORY TREATED PATIENTS (COMPARISON TO PLACEBO)

Symptom	Mesalamine (n=177)		Placebo (n=84)	
	N	%	N	%
Dizziness	5	3.0	2	2.4
Rectal Pain	3	1.8	0	0.0
Fever	2	1.2	0	0.0
Rash	2	1.2	0	0.0
Acne	2	1.2	0	0.0
Colitis	2	1.2	0	0.0

In addition, the following adverse events have been associated with mesalamine containing products: nephrotoxicity, pancreatitis, fibrosing alveolitis and elevated liver enzymes. Cases of pancreatitis and fibrosing alveolitis have been reported as manifestations of inflammatory bowel disease as well.

Hair Loss

Mild hair loss characterized by "more hair in the comb" but no withdrawal from clinical trials has been observed in seven of 815 mesalamine patients but none of the placebo-treated patients. In the literature there are at least six additional patients with mild hair loss who received either mesalamine or sulfasalazine. Retreatment is not always associated with repeated hair loss.

OVERDOSAGE

There have been no documented reports of serious toxicity in man resulting from massive overdosing with mesalamine. Under ordinary circumstances, mesalamine absorption from the colon is limited.

DOSAGE AND ADMINISTRATION

The usual dosage of CANASA® (mesalamine) Suppositories is one 500 mg rectal suppository 2 times daily with possible increase to 3 times daily if inadequate response at two weeks. The suppository should be retained for one to three hours or longer, if possible, to achieve the maximum benefit. While the effect of CANASA® Suppositories may be seen within three to twenty-one days, the usual course of therapy would be from three to six weeks depending on symptoms and sigmoidoscopic findings. Studies have suggested that CANASA® Suppositories will delay relapse after the six-week short-term treatment.

Patient Instructions:

NOTE: CANASA® Suppositories will cause staining of direct contact surfaces, including but not limited to fabrics, flooring, painted surfaces, marble, granite, vinyl, and enamel.

I. Detach one suppository from strip of suppositories.
II. Hold suppository upright and carefully remove the plastic wrapper.
III. Avoid excessive handling of suppository, which is designed to melt at body temperature.
IV. Insert suppository completely into rectum with gentle pressure, pointed end first.
V. A small amount of lubricating gel may be used on the tip of the suppository to assist insertion.

HOW SUPPLIED

CANASA® Suppositories: CANASA® Suppositories for rectal administration are available as bullet shaped, light

tan suppositories containing 500 mg mesalamine supplied in boxes of 30 individually plastic wrapped suppositories (NDC 58914-500-56).
Boxes of 30.
Store below 25°C, do not freeze. Keep away from direct heat, light or humidity.
Rx only
Axcan Scandipharm Inc.
Birmingham, AL 35242
Date: January 4, 2001

Patient Information

CANASA® Rectal Suppositories (mesalamine)

Read this information carefully before you begin treatment. Also, read the information you get whenever you get more medicine. There may be new information. This information does not take the place of talking with your doctor about your medical condition or your treatment. If you have any questions about this medicine, ask your doctor or pharmacist.

What is CANASA®?
CANASA® (can-AH-sah) is a medicine used to treat ulcerative proctitis (ulcerative rectal colitis). CANASA® works inside your rectum (lower intestine) to help reduce bleeding, mucous and bloody diarrhea caused by inflammation (swelling and soreness) of the rectal area. You use CANASA® by inserting it into your rectum.

Who should not use CANASA®?
Do not use CANASA® if you are allergic to the active ingredient mesalamine (also found in drugs such as Rowasa, Asacol, Pentasa, Azulfidine, and Dipentum), if you are allergic to the inactive ingredients, or if you have had any unusual reaction to the ingredients.
Tell your doctor if you

- Have kidney problems. Using CANASA® may make them worse.
- Have had inflamed pancreas (pancreatitis).
- Are pregnant. You and your doctor will decide if you should use CANASA®.
- Have ever had pericarditis (inflamed sac around your heart).
- Are allergic to sulfasalazine. You may need to watch for signs of an allergic reaction to CANASA®.
- Are allergic to aspirin.
- Are allergic to other things, such as foods, preservatives, or dyes.

How should I use CANASA®?
Follow your doctor's instructions about how often to use CANASA® and how long to use it. The usual dose of adults and teenagers is 1 suppository 2 times a day for 3–6 weeks. We do not know if CANASA® will work for children or is safe for them.
Follow these steps to use CANASA®:

1. For best results, empty your rectum (have a bowel movement) just before using CANASA®.
2. Detach one CANASA® suppository from the strip of suppositories.
3. Hold the suppository upright and carefully peel open the plastic at the pre-cut line to take out the suppository.
4. Insert the suppository with the pointed end first completely into your rectum, using gentle pressure.
5. For best results, keep the suppository in your rectum for 3 hours or longer, if possible.

If you have trouble inserting CANASA®, you may put a little bit of lubricating gel on the suppository.
Do not handle the suppository too much, since it may begin to melt from the heat from your hands and body.
If you miss a dose of CANASA®, use it as soon as possible, unless it is almost time for next dose. Do not use 2 suppositories at the same time to make up for a missed dose.
Keep using CANASA® as long as your doctor tells you to use it, even if you feel better.
CANASA® can cause stains on things it touches. Therefore keep it away from clothing and other fabrics, flooring, painted surfaces, marble, granite, plastics, and enamel. Be careful when you use CANASA® to avoid stains.

What should I avoid while taking CANASA®?
Do not breast feed while using CANASA®. We do not know if CANASA® can pass through the milk and harm the baby. Tell your doctor if you become pregnant while using CANASA®.

What are the possible side effects of CANASA®?

- The most common side effects of CANASA® are: headache, gas or flatulence, and diarrhea. These events also occurred when patients were given an inactive suppository.
- Less common, but possibly serious side effects include a reaction to the medicine (acute intolerance syndrome) that includes cramps, sharp abdominal (stomach area) pain, bloody diarrhea, and sometimes fever, headache and rash. Stop use and tell your doctor right away if you get any of these symptoms.
- In rare cases, the sac around the heart may become inflamed (pericarditis). Tell your doctor right away if you develop chest pain or shortness of breath, which are signs of this problem.
- In rare cases, patients using CANASA® develop worsening colitis (pancolitis).
- A very few patients using CANASA® may have mild hair loss.
- Other side effects not listed above may also occur in some patients.

If you notice any other side effects, check with your doctor or pharmacist.

How should I store CANASA®?
Store CANASA® below 25°C, and do not freeze. Keep it away from direct heat, light, or humidity. Keep it out of the reach of children.

General advice about prescription medicines
Medicines are sometimes prescribed for conditions that are not mentioned in patient information leaflets. Do not use CANASA® for a condition for which it was not prescribed. Do not give CANASA® to other people, even if they have the same symptoms you have.
This leaflet summarizes the most important information about CANASA®. If you would like more information, talk with your doctor. You can ask your pharmacist or doctor for information about CANASA® that is written for health professionals.

Shown in Product Identification Guide, page 307

CARAFATE® ℞

[*kăr 'afăt*]
(sucralfate)
Suspension

DESCRIPTION

CARAFATE Suspension contains sucralfate and sucralfate is an α-D-glucopyranoside, β-D-fructofuranosyl-, octakis-(hydrogen sulfate), aluminum complex.

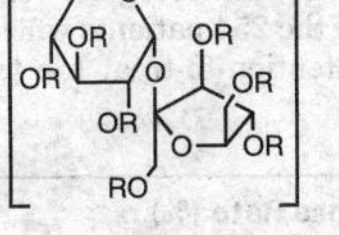

$[Al(OH)_3] \times [H_2O]_y$
(x = 8 to 10 and y = 22 to 31)

$R = SO_3Al(OH)_2$

CARAFATE Suspension for oral administration contains 1 g of sucralfate per 10 mL.
CARAFATE Suspension also contains: colloidal silicon dioxide NF, FD&C Red #40, flavor, glycerin USP, methylcellulose USP, methylparaben NF, microcrystalline cellulose NF, purified water USP, simethicone USP, and sorbitol solution USP. Therapeutic category: antiulcer.

CLINICAL PHARMACOLOGY

Sucralfate is only minimally absorbed from the gastrointestinal tract. The small amounts of the sulfated disaccharide that are absorbed are excreted primarily in the urine.
Although the mechanism of sucralfate's ability to accelerate healing of duodenal ulcers remains to be fully defined, it is known that it exerts its effect through a local, rather than systemic, action.
The following observations also appear pertinent:

1. Studies in human subjects and with animal models of ulcer disease have shown that sucralfate forms an ulcer-adherent complex with proteinaceous exudate at the ulcer site.
2. In vitro, a sucralfate-albumin film provides a barrier to diffusion of hydrogen ions.
3. In human subjects, sucralfate given in doses recommended for ulcer therapy inhibits pepsin activity in gastric juice by 32%.
4. In vitro, sucralfate adsorbs bile salts.

These observations suggest that sucralfate's antiulcer activity is the result of formation of an ulcer-adherent complex that covers the ulcer site and protects it against further attack by acid, pepsin, and bile salts. There are approximately 14 to 16 mEq of acid-neutralizing capacity per 1-g dose of sucralfate.

CLINICAL TRIALS

In a multicenter, double-blind, placebo-controlled study of CARAFATE Suspension, a dosage regiment of 1 g (10 mL) four times daily was demonstrated to be superior to placebo in ulcer healing.

Results From Clinical Trials Healing Rates for Acute Duodenal Ulcer

Treatment	n	Week 2 Healing Rates	Week 4 Healing Rates	Week 8 Healing Rates
CARAFATE Suspension	145	23(16%)*	66(46%)†	95(66%)‡
Placebo	147	10(7%)	39(27%)	58(39%)

*P=0.016
†P=0.001
‡P=0.0001

Equivalence of sucralfate suspension to sucralfate tablets has not been demonstrated.

INDICATIONS AND USAGE

CARAFATE (sucralfate) Suspension is indicated in the short-term (up to 8 weeks) treatment of active duodenal ulcer.

CONTRAINDICATIONS

There are no known contraindications to the use of sucralfate.

PRECAUTIONS

Duodenal ulcer is a chronic, recurrent disease. While short-term treatment with sucralfate can result in complete healing of the ulcer, a successful course of treatment with sucralfate should not be expected to alter the posthealing frequency or severity of duodenal ulceration.

Special Populations: Chronic Renal Failure and Dialysis Patients
When sucralfate is administered orally, small amounts of aluminum are absorbed from the gastrointestinal tract. Concomitant use of sucralfate with other products that contain aluminum, such as aluminum-containing antacids, may increase the total body burden of aluminum. Patients with normal renal function receiving the recommended doses of sucralfate and aluminum-containing products adequately excrete aluminum in the urine. Patients with chronic renal failure or those receiving dialysis have impaired excretion of absorbed aluminum. In addition, aluminum does not cross dialysis membranes because it is bound to albumin and transferrin plasma proteins. Aluminum accumulation and toxicity (aluminum osteodystrophy, osteomalacia, encephalopathy) have been described in patients with renal impairment. Sucralfate should be used with caution in patients with chronic renal failure.

Drug Interactions
Some studies have shown that simultaneous sucralfate administration in healthy volunteers reduced the extent of absorption (bioavailability) of single doses of the following cimetidine, digoxin, fluoroquinolone antibiotics, ketoconazole, I-thyroxine, phenytoin, quinidine, ranitidine, tetracycline, and theophylline. Subtherapeutic prothrombin times with concomitant warfarin and sucralfate therapy have been reported in spontaneous and published case reports. However, two clinical studies have demonstrated no change in either serum warfarin concentration or prothrombin time with the addition of sucralfate to chronic warfarin therapy.
The mechanism of these interactions appears to be nonsystemic in nature, presumably resulting from sucralfate binding to the concomitant agent in the gastrointestinal tract. In all cases studied to date (cimetidine, ciprofloxacin, digoxin, norfloxacin, ofloxacin, and ranitidine), dosing the concomitant medication 2 hours before sucralfate eliminated the interaction. Because of the potential of CARAFATE to alter the absorption of some drugs, CARAFATE should be administered separately from other drugs when alterations in bioavailabity are felt to be critical. In these cases, patients should be monitored appropriately.

Carcinogenesis, Mutagenesis, Impairment of Fertility
Chronic oral toxicity studies of 24 months' duration were conducted in mice and rats at doses up to 1 g/kg (12 times the human dose).
There was no evidence of drug-related tumorigenicity. A reproduction study in rats at doses up to 38 times the human dose did not reveal any indication of fertility impairment. Mutagenicity studies were not conducted.

Pregnancy
Teratogenic effects. Pregnancy Category B.
Teratogenicity studies have been performed in mice, rats, and rabbits at doses up to 50 times the human dose and have revealed no evidence of harm to the fetus due to sucralfate. There are, however, no adequate and well-controlled studies in pregnant women. Because animal reproduction studies are not always predictive of human response, this drug should be used during pregnancy only if clearly needed.

Nursing Mothers
It is not known whether this drug is excreted in human milk. Because many drugs are excreted in human milk, caution should be exercised when sucralfate is administered to a nursing woman.

Pediatric Use
Safety and effectiveness in pediatric patients have not been established.

ADVERSE REACTIONS

Adverse reactions to sucralfate tablets in clinical trials were minor and only rarely led to discontinuation of the drug. In studies involving over 2700 patients treated with sucralfate, adverse effects were reported in 129 (4.7%).
Constipation was the most frequent complaint (2%). Other adverse effects reported in less than 0.5% of the patients are listed below by body system:
Gastrointestinal: diarrhea, dry mouth, flatulence, gastric discomfort, indigestion, nausea, vomiting
Dermatological: pruritus, rash
Nervous System: dizziness, insomnia, sleepiness, vertigo
Other: back pain, headache
Postmarketing reports of hypersensitivity reactions, including urticaria (hives), angioedema, respiratory difficulty, rhinitis, laryngospasm, and facial swelling have been reported in patients receiving sucralfate tablets. Similar events were reported with sucralfate suspension. However, a causal relationship has not been established.
Bezoars have been reported in patients treated with sucralfate. The majority of patients had underlying medical conditions that may predispose to bezoar formation (such as delayed gastric emptying) or were receiving concomitant enteral tube feedings.

Continued on next page

Carafate Suspension—Cont.

Inadvertent injection of insoluble sucralfate and its insoluble excipients has led to fatal complications, including pulmonary and cerebral emboli. Sucralfate is **not** intended for intravenous administration.

OVERDOSAGE

Due to limited experience in humans with overdosage of sucralfate, no specific treatment recommendations can be given. Acute oral studies in animals, however, using doses up to 12 g/kg body weight, could not find a lethal dose. Sucralfate is only minimally absorbed from the gastrointestinal tract. Risks associated with acute overdosage should, therefore, be minimal. In rare reports describing sucralfate overdose, most patients remained asymptomatic. Those few reports where adverse events were described included symptoms of dyspepsia, abdominal pain, nausea, and vomiting.

DOSAGE AND ADMINISTRATION

Active Duodenal Ulcer. The recommended adult oral dosage for duodenal ulcer is 1 g (10 mL/2 teaspoonfuls) four times per day. CARAFATE should be administered on an empty stomach.

Antacids may be prescribed as needed for relief of pain but should not be taken within one-half hour before or after sucralfate.

While healing with sucralfate may occur during the first week or two, treatment should be continued for 4 to 8 weeks unless healing has been demonstrated by x-ray or endoscopic examination.

HOW SUPPLIED

CARAFATE (sucralfate) Suspension 1 g/10 mL is a pink suspension supplied in bottles of 14 fl oz (NDC 58914-170-14).

SHAKE WELL BEFORE USING.

Store at controlled room temperature 20-25°C (68-77°F)[see USP]

Rx Only

Prescribing Information as of April 2004

Axcan Scandipharm Inc.
22 Inverness Center Parkway
Birmingham, AL 35242
www.axcan.com

CARAFATE® Tablets ℞

[kār 'afāt]
(sucralfate)

DESCRIPTION

CARAFATE Tablets contain sucralfate and sucralfate is an α-D-glucopyranoside, β-D-fructofuranosyl-, octakis-(hydrogen sulfate), aluminum complex.

$[Al(OH)_3]\ x\ [H_2O]y$
(x = 8 to 10 and y = 22 to 31)

$R = SO_3Al(OH)_2$

Tablets for oral administration contains 1 g of sucralfate.
Also contain: D & C Red #30 Lake, FD&C Blue #1 Lake, magnesium stearate, microcrystalline cellulose, and starch
Therapeutic category: antiulcer.

CLINICAL PHARMACOLOGY

Sucralfate is only minimally absorbed from the gastrointestinal tract. The small amounts of the sulfated disaccharide that are absorbed are excreted primarily in the urine.

Although the mechanism of sucralfate's ability to accelerate healing of duodenal ulcers remains to be fully defined, it is known that it exerts its effect through a local, rather than systemic, action.

The following observations also appear pertinent:

1. Studies in human subjects and with animal models of ulcer disease have shown that sucralfate forms an ulcer-adherent complex with proteinaceous exudate at the ulcer site.
2. In vitro, a sucralfate-albumin film provides a barrier to diffusion of hydrogen ions.
3. In human subjects, sucralfate given in doses recommended for ulcer therapy inhibits pepsin activity in gastric juice by 32%.
4. In vitro, sucralfate adsorbs bile salts.

These observations suggest that sucralfate's antiulcer activity is the result of formation of an ulcer-adherent complex that covers the ulcer site and protects it against further attack by acid, pepsin, and bile salts. There are approximately 14 to 16 mEq of acid-neutralizing capacity per 1-g dose of sucralfate.

CLINICAL TRIALS

Acute Duodenal Ulcer

Over 600 patients have participated in well-controlled clinical trials worldwide. Multicenter trials conducted in the Untied States, both of them placebo-controlled studies with endoscopic evaluation at 2 and 4 weeks, showed:

STUDY 1

Treatment Groups	Ulcer Healing/ No. Patients	
	2 wk	4 wk (Overall)
Sucralfate	37/105 (35.2%)	82/109 (75.2%)
Placebo	26/106 (24.5%)	68/107 (63.6%)

STUDY 2

Treatment Groups	Ulcer Healing/ No. Patients	
	2 wk	4 wk (Overall)
Sucralfate	8/24 (33%)	22/24 (92%)
Placebo	4/31 (13%)	18/31 (58%)

The sucralfate-placebo differences were statistically significant in both studies at 4 weeks but not at 2 weeks. The poorer result in the first study may have occurred because sucralfate was given 2 hour after meals and at bedtime rather than 1 hour before meals and at bedtime, the regimen used in internation studies and in the second United States study. In addition, in the first study liquid antacid was utilized as needed, whereas in the second study antacid tablets were used.

Maintenance Therapy After Healing of Duodenal Ulcer

Two double-blind randomized placebo-controlled U.S. multicenter trials have demonstrated that sucralfate (1 g bid) is effective as maintenance therapy following healing of duodenal ulcers. In one study, endoscopies were performed monthly for 4 months. Of the 254 patients who enrolled, 239 were analyzed in the intention-to-treat life table analysis presented below.

Duodenal Ulcer Recurrence Rate (%)

	Months of Therapy				
Drug	n	1	2	3	4
CARAFATE	122	20*	30*	38†	42†
Placebo	117	33	46	55	63

*P<0.05, †P<0.01

In this study, prn antacids were not permitted.

In the other study, scheduled endoscopies were performed at 6 and 12 months, but for-cause endoscopies were permitted as symptoms dictated. Median symptom scores between the sucralfate and placebo groups were not significantly different. A life table intention-to-treat analysis for the 94 patients enrolled in the trial had the following results:

Duodenal Ulcer Recurrence Rate (%)

Drug	n	6 months	12 months
CARAFATE	48	19*	27*
Placebo	46	54	65

*P<0.002

In this study, prn antacids were permitted.

Data from placebo-controlled studies longer than 1 year are not available.

INDICATIONS AND USAGE

CARAFATE® (sucralfate) is indicated in:

- Short-term treatment (up to 8 weeks) of active duodenal ulcer. While healing with sucralfate may occur during the first week or two, treatment should be continued for 4 to 8 weeks unless healing has been demonstrated by x-ray or endoscopic examination.
- Maintenance therapy for duodenal ulcer patients at reduced dosage after healing of acute ulcers.

CONTRAINDICATIONS

There are no known contraindications to the use of sucralfate.

PRECAUTIONS

Duodenal ulcer is a chronic, recurrent disease. While short-term treatment with sucralfate can result in complete healing of the ulcer, a successful course of treatment with sucralfate should not be expected to alter the posthealing frequency or severity of duodenal ulceration.

Special Populations: Chronic Renal Failure and Dialysis Patients

When sucralfate is administered orally, small amounts of aluminum are absorbed from the gastrointestinal tract. Concomitant use of sucralfate with other products that contain aluminum, such as aluminum-containing antacids, may increase the total body burden of aluminum. Patients with normal renal function receiving the recommended doses of sucralfate and aluminum-containing products adequately excrete aluminum in the urine. Patients with chronic renal failure or those receiving dialysis have impaired excretion of absorbed aluminum. In addition, aluminum does not cross dialysis membranes because it is bound to albumin and transferrin plasma proteins. Aluminum accumulation and toxicity (aluminum osteodystrophy, osteomalacia, encephalopathy) have been described in patients with renal impairment. Sucralfate should be used with caution in patients with chronic renal failure.

Drug Interactions

Some studies have shown that simultaneous sucralfate administration in healthy volunteers reduced the extent of absorption (bioavailability) of single doses of the following cimetidine, digoxin, fluoroquinolone antibiotics, ketoconazole, I-thyroxine, phenytoin, quinidine, ranitidine, tetracycline, and theophylline. Subtherapeutic prothrombin times with concomitant warfarin and sucralfate therapy have been reported in spontaneous and published case reports. However, two clinical studies have demonstrated no change in either serum warfarin concentration or prothrombin time with the addition of sucralfate to chronic warfarin therapy.

The mechanism of these interactions appears to be nonsystemic in nature, presumably resulting from sucralfate binding to the concomitant agent in the gastrointestinal tract. In all cases studies to date (cimetidine, ciprofloxacin, digoxin, norfloxacin, ofloxacin, and ranitidine), dosing the concomitant medication 2 hours before sucralfate eliminated the interaction. Because of the potential of CARAFATE to alter the absorption of some drugs, CARAFATE should be administered separately from other drugs when alterations in bioavailability are felt to be critical. In these cases, patients should be monitored appropriately.

Carcinogenesis, Mutagenesis, Impairment of Fertility

Chronic oral toxicity studies of 24 months' duration were conducted in mice and rats at doses up to 1 g/kg (12 times the human dose).

There was no evidence of drug-related tumorigenicity. A reproduction study in rats at doses up to 38 times the human dose did not reveal any indication of fertility impairment. Mutagenicity studies were not conducted.

Pregnancy

Teratogenic effects. Pregnancy Category B.

Teratogenicity studies have been performed in mice, rats, and rabbits at doses up to 50 times the human dose and have revealed no evidence of harm to the fetus due to sucralfate. There are, however, no adequate and well-controlled studies in pregnant women. Because animal reproduction studies are not always predictive of human response, this drug should be used during pregnancy only if clearly needed.

Nursing Mothers

It is not known whether this drug is excreted in human milk. Because many drugs are excreted in human milk, caution should be exercised when sucralfate is administered to a nursing woman.

Pediatric Use

Safety and effectiveness in pediatric patients have not been established.

ADVERSE REACTIONS

Adverse reactions to sucralfate in clinical trials were minor and only rarely led to discontinuation of the drug. In studies involving over 2700 patients treated with sucralfate tablets, adverse effects were reported in 129 (4.7%).

Constipation was the most frequent complaint (2%). Other adverse effects reported in less than 0.5% of the patients are listed below by body system:

Gastrointestinal: diarrhea, nausea, vomiting, gastric discomfort, indigestion, flatulence, dry mouth
Dermatological: pruritus, rash
Nervous System: dizziness, insomnia, sleepiness, vertigo
Other: back pain, headache

Postmarketing reports of hypersensitivity reactions, including urticaria (hives), angioedema, respiratory difficulty, rhinitis, laryngospasm, and facial swelling have been reported in patients receiving sucralfate tablets. Similar events were reported with sucralfate suspension. However, a causal relationship has not been established.

Bezoars have been reported in patients treated with sucralfate. The majority of patients had underlying medical conditions that may predispose to bezoar formation (such as delayed gastric emptying) or were receiving concomitant enteral tube feedings.

Inadvertent injection of insoluble sucralfate and its insoluble excipients has led to fatal complications, including pulmonary and cerebral emboli. Sucralfate is **not** intended for intravenous administration.

OVERDOSAGE

Due to limited experience in humans with overdosage of sucralfate, no specific treatment recommendations can be given. Acute oral toxicity studies in animals, however, using doses up to 12 g/kg body weight, could not find a lethal dose. Sucralfate is only minimally absorbed from the gastrointestinal tract. Risks associated with acute overdosage should, therefore, be minimal. In rare reports describing sucralfate overdose, most patients remained asymptomatic. Those few reports where adverse events were described included symptoms of dyspepsia, abdominal pain, nausea, and vomiting.

DOSAGE AND ADMINISTRATION

Active Duodenal Ulcer. The recommended adult oral dosage for duodenal ulcer is 1 g four times per day on an empty stomach.

Antacids may be prescribed as needed for relief of pain but should not be taken within one-half hour before or after sucralfate.

While healing with sucralfate may occur during the first week or two, treatment should be continued for 4 to 8 weeks unless healing has been demonstrated by x-ray or endoscopic examination.

Maintenance Therapy: The recommended adult oral dosage is 1 g twice a day.

HOW SUPPLIED

CARAFATE (sucralfate) 1-g tablets are supplied in bottles of 100 (NDC 58914-171-10), 120 (NDC 58914-171-21), and 500 (NDC 58914-171-50). Light pink, scored, oblong tablets are embossed with CARAFATE on one side and 1712 on the other.

Rx Only

Prescribing Information as of April 2004

Axcan Scandipharm Inc.
22 Inverness Center Parkway
Birmingham, AL 35242
www.axcan.com

R = HO—CH(CH$_3$) and/or —CH=CH$_2$

n = 0 - 6

PHOTOFRIN® ℞

[fō'tō-frĭn]

(porfimer sodium)
for Injection

DESCRIPTION

PHOTOFRIN® (porfimer sodium) for Injection is a photosensitizing agent used in the photodynamic therapy (PDT) of tumors and of high-grade dysplasia (HGD) in Barrett's esophagus (BE). Following reconstitution of the freeze-dried product with 5% Dextrose Injection (USP) or 0.9% Sodium Chloride Injection (USP), it is injected intravenously. This is followed 40–50 hours later by illumination of the tumor or HGD in BE with laser light (630 nm wavelength). PHOTOFRIN® is not a single chemical entity; it is a mixture of oligomers formed by ether and ester linkages of up to eight porphyrin units. It is a dark red to reddish brown cake or powder. Each vial of PHOTOFRIN® contains 75 mg of porfimer sodium as a sterile freeze-dried cake or powder. Hydrochloric Acid and/or Sodium Hydroxide may be added during manufacture to adjust the pH to within 7.2–7.9. There are no preservatives or other additives. The structural formula below is representative of the components present in PHOTOFRIN®.

[See chemical structure above]

CLINICAL PHARMACOLOGY

Pharmacology

The cytotoxic and antitumor actions of PHOTOFRIN® are light and oxygen dependent. Photodynamic therapy with PHOTOFRIN® is a two-stage process. The first stage is the intravenous injection of PHOTOFRIN®. Clearance from a variety of tissues occurs over 40–72 hours, but tumors, skin, and organs of the reticuloendothelial system (including liver and spleen) retain PHOTOFRIN® for a longer period. Illumination with 630 nm wavelength laser light constitutes the second stage of therapy. Tumor selectivity in treatment occurs through a combination of selective retention of PHOTOFRIN® and selective delivery of light. Cellular damage caused by PHOTOFRIN® PDT is a consequence of the propagation of radical reactions. Radical initiation may occur after PHOTOFRIN® absorbs light to form a porphyrin excited state. Spin transfer from PHOTOFRIN® to molecular oxygen may then generate singlet oxygen. Subsequent radical reactions can form superoxide and hydroxyl radicals. Tumor death also occurs through ischemic necrosis secondary to vascular occlusion that appears to be partly mediated by thromboxane A_2 release. The laser treatment induces a photochemical, not a thermal, effect. The necrotic reaction and associated inflammatory responses may evolve over several days.

Pharmacokinetics

Following a 2 mg/kg dose of porfimer sodium to 4 male cancer patients, the average peak plasma concentration was 15 ± 3 mcg/mL, the elimination half-life was 250 ± 285 hours, the steady-state volume of distribution was 0.49 ± 0.28 L/kg, and the total plasma clearance was 0.051 ± 0.035 mL/min/kg. The mean plasma concentration at 48 hours was 2.6 ± 0.4 mcg/mL. The influence of impaired hepatic function on PHOTOFRIN® disposition has not been evaluated.

PHOTOFRIN® was approximately 90% protein bound in human serum, studied *in vitro*. The binding was independent of concentration over the concentration range of 20–100 mcg/mL.

The pharmacokinetics of PHOTOFRIN® was also studied in 24 healthy subjects (12 men and 12 women) who received a single dose of 2 mg/kg PHOTOFRIN® given via the intravenous route. The serum decay was bi-exponential, with a slow distribution phase and a very long elimination phase. The elimination half-life was 415 ± 104 hours (17 ± 4.3 days). C_{max} was determined to be 40 ± 11.6 mcg/mL and AUC_{inf} was 2400 ± 552 mcg•hour/mL. Women had a lower C_{max} and a higher AUC. The clinical significance of these differences is unknown. T_{max} was approximately 1.5 hours in women and 0.17 hours in men. At the time of intended photoactivation 40–50 hours after injection, the pharmacokinetic profiles of PHOTOFRIN® in men and women were similar.

Clinical Studies

Clinical studies of PDT with PHOTOFRIN® were conducted in patients with obstructing esophageal and endobronchial nonsmall cell lung cancers, in patients with early-stage radiologically occult endobronchial cancer, and in patients with high-grade dysplasia (HGD) associated with Barrett's Esophagus (BE). In all clinical studies, the method of PDT administration was essentially identical. A course of therapy consisted of one injection of PHOTOFRIN® (2 mg/kg administered as a slow intravenous injection over 3–5 minutes) followed by up to two non-thermal applications of 630 nm laser light. Doses of 300 Joules/cm (J/cm) of diffuser length were used in esophageal cancer. Doses of 200 J/cm were used in endobronchial cancer for both palliation of obstructing cancer and treatment of superficial lesions. For the ablation of HGD in BE, the light dose administered was 130 J/cm of diffuser length using a centering balloon (for details, see DOSAGE AND ADMINISTRATION). In all cases, the first application of light occurred 40–50 hours after PHOTOFRIN® injection.

For treatment of esophageal and endobronchial cancer, debridement of residua was performed via endoscopy/bronchoscopy 96–120 hours after injection, after which any residual tumor could be retreated with a second laser light application at the same dose used for the initial treatment. Additional courses of PDT with PHOTOFRIN® were allowed after 1 month, up to a maximum of three courses. For ablation of HGD in BE, a second laser light application of 50 J/cm of diffuser length without a centering balloon could be given 96–120 hours after the PHOTOFRIN® injection for untreated areas ("skip" areas). Additional courses of PDT with PHOTOFRIN® were allowed after 3 months, up to a maximum of three courses.

Esophageal Cancer

Photodynamic therapy with PHOTOFRIN® was utilized in a multicenter, single-arm study in 17 patients with completely obstructing esophageal carcinoma. Assessments were made at 1 week and 1 month after the last treatment procedure. As shown in Table 1, after a single course of therapy, 94% of patients obtained an objective tumor response and 76% of patients experienced some palliation of their dysphagia. On average, before treatment these patients had difficulty swallowing liquids, even saliva. After one course of therapy, there was a statistically significant improvement in mean dysphagia grade (1.5 units, $p < 0.05$) and 13 of 17 patients could swallow liquids without difficulty 1 week and/or 1 month after treatment. Based on all courses, three patients achieved a complete tumor response (CR). In two of these patients, the CR was documented only at Week 1 as they had no further assessments. The third patient achieved a CR after a second course of therapy, which was supported by negative histopathology and maintained for the entire follow-up of 6 months.

Of the 17 treated patients, 11 (65%) received clinically important benefit from PDT. Clinically important benefit was defined hierarchically as a complete tumor response (3 patients), achievement of normal swallowing (2 patients went from Grade 5 dysphagia to Grade 1), or achievement of a marked improvement of two or more grades of dysphagia with minimal adverse reactions (6 patients). The median duration of benefit in these patients was 69 days. Duration of benefit was calculated only for the period with documented evidence of improvement. All of these patients were still in response at their last assessment and, therefore, the estimate of 69 days is conservative. The median survival for these 11 patients was 115 days.

TABLE 1. Course 1 Efficacy Results in Patients with Completely Obstructing Esophageal Cancer

EFFICACY PARAMETER	PDT N=17
OBJECTIVE TUMOR RESPONSE[a]	
Week 1	82%
Month 1	35%[b]
Any assessment[c]	94%
IMPROVEMENT[d] IN DYSPHAGIA	
Week 1	71%
Month 1	47%
Any assessment[c]	76%
MEAN DYSPHAGIA GRADE[e] AT BASELINE	4.6
MEAN IMPROVEMENT[e] IN DYSPHAGIA GRADE (units)	
Week 1	1.4
Month 1	1.5
MEAN NUMBER OF LASER APPLICATIONS	1.4

[a] CR+PR, CR = complete response (absence of endoscopically visible tumor), PR = partial response (appearance of a visible lumen)

[b] Eight of the 17 treated patients did not have assessments at Month 1.

[c] Week 1 or Month 1

[d] Patients with at least a one-grade improvement in dysphagia grade

[e] Dysphagia Scale: Grade 1 = normal swallowing, Grade 2 = difficulty swallowing some hard solids; can swallow semi-solids, Grade 3 = unable to swallow any solids; can swallow liquids, Grade 4 = difficulty swallowing liquids, Grade 5 = unable to swallow saliva.

Endobronchial Cancer

Two randomized multicenter Phase 3 studies were conducted to compare the safety and efficacy of PHOTOFRIN® PDT versus Nd:YAG laser therapy for reduction of obstruction and palliation of symptomatic patients with partially or completely obstructing endobronchial nonsmall cell lung cancer. Assessments were made at 1 week and at monthly intervals after treatment. Table 2 shows the results from all randomized patients in the two studies combined. Objective tumor response rates (CR + PR), which demonstrate reduction of obstruction, were 59% for PDT and 58% for Nd:YAG at Week 1. The response rate at 1 month or later was 60% for PDT and 41% for Nd:YAG.

TABLE 2. Efficacy Results from Studies in Late-stage Obstructing Endobronchial Cancer—All Randomized Patients[a]

EFFICACY PARAMETER	PDT N=102 (% of Patients)	Nd:YAG N=109 (% of Patients)
OBJECTIVE TUMOR RESPONSE[b]		
Week 1	59%	58%
Month 1 or later	60%	41%[a]
ATELECTASIS IMPROVEMENT[c]	n=60	n=71
Week 1	35%	18%
Month 1 or later	35%	20%

[a] Statistical comparisons were precluded by the amount of missing data at Month 1 or later (e.g. for tumor response, PDT 28% missing, Nd:YAG 38%).

[b] CR+PR, CR = complete response (absence of bronchoscopically visible tumor), PR = partial response (increase of ≥50% in the smallest luminal diameter); for completely obstructing tumors, any appearance of a lumen).

[c] In patients with atelectasis at baseline

Patient symptoms were evaluated using a 5- or 6-grade pulmonary symptom severity rating scale for dyspnea, cough, and hemoptysis. Patients with moderate to severe symptoms are those most in need of palliation. Improvements of 2 or more grades are considered to be clinically significant. Table 3 shows the percentages of patients with moderate to severe symptoms at baseline who demonstrated a 2-grade improvement at any time during the interval evaluated.

TABLE 3. Efficacy Results from Studies in Late-stage Obstructing Endobronchial Cancer – Clinically Significant Improvements in Patients with Moderate to Severe Symptoms at Baseline[a]

CLINICALLY SIGNIFICANT SYMPTOM IMPROVEMENT[b]	PDT N=102 (% of Patients)	Nd:YAG N=109 (% of Patients)
ANY SYMPTOM	n=89	n=89
Week 1	25%	29%
Month 1 or later	40%	27%[a]
DYSPNEA	n=60	n=68
Week 1	15%	18%
Month 1 or later	23%	13%
COUGH	n=63	n=65
Week 1	6%	9%
Month 1 or later	24%	8%
HEMOPTYSIS	n=24	n=31
Week 1	58%	29%
Month 1 or later	79%	35%

[a] Statistical comparisons were precluded by the amount of missing data at Month 1 or later.

Continued on next page

Photofrin—Cont.

[b] Dyspnea was graded on a 6-point severity rating scale; cough and hemoptysis on 5-point scales. Clinically significant improvement was defined as a change of at least two grades from baseline.

In a separate retrospective analysis, patients were individually evaluated to identify those patients whose benefit to risk ratio was most favorable, i.e., those who obtained clinically important benefit with minimal adverse reactions. Clinically important benefit was defined as one of the following:

1. A substantial improvement in pulmonary symptoms at Month 1 or later (dyspnea ≥2 grades, hemoptysis ≥3 grades, cough ≥3 grades or increase in FEV_1 ≥40%);
2. A moderate improvement in symptoms at Month 2 or later (dyspnea 1 grade, cough 2 grades, hemoptysis 2 grades or increase in FEV_1 ≥20%); or
3. A durable objective tumor response (CR or PR maintained to Month 2 or longer).

Thirty-six (36) of the 99 PDT-treated patients (36%) and 23 of the 99 Nd:YAG-treated patients (23%) received clinically important benefit with only minimal or moderate toxicities of short duration. Thirty-four of 99 PDT-treated patients demonstrated improvements in 2 or more efficacy endpoints (dyspnea, cough, hemoptysis, sputum, atelectasis, pulmonary function tests of FEV_1 or FVC, Karnofsky Performance Score or tumor response) and 29 patients had improvements in 3 or more. The median duration of documented benefit in the 36 patients was 63 days. In these patients with late-stage obstructing lung cancer, median survival was 174 days in PDT-treated patients and 161 days in Nd:YAG-treated patients.

The efficacy of PHOTOFRIN® PDT was also evaluated in the treatment of microinvasive endobronchial tumors in 62 inoperable patients in three noncomparative studies. Microinvasive lung cancer is defined histologically as disease, which invades beyond the basement membrane but not through or into the cartilage. For 11 of the 62 patients, it was clearly documented that surgery and radiotherapy were not indicated. These 11 patients were all inoperable for medical or technical reasons. Radiotherapy was not indicated due to prior high-dose radiotherapy (7 patients), poor pulmonary function (2 patients), multifocal multilobar disease (1 patient), and poor medical condition (1 patient). As shown in Table 4, the complete tumor response rate, biopsy-proven at least 3 months after treatment, was 50%, median time to tumor recurrence was more than 2.7 years, median survival was 2.9 years and disease-specific survival was 4.1 years.

[See table 4 below]

High-Grade Dysplasia in Barrett's Esophagus

The safety and efficacy of PDT with PHOTOFRIN® in ablation of HGD in patients with BE was assessed in one controlled clinical study and two supportive studies.

Controlled Study

A multicenter, partially blinded, randomized, controlled study was conducted in North America and Europe to assess the efficacy of PDT with PHOTOFRIN® for Injection plus omeprazole (PHOTOFRIN® PDT + OM) in producing complete ablation of HGD in patients with BE compared to control patients receiving omeprazole alone (OM Only). A total of 485 patients with the diagnosis of HGD were screened for the study; 208 (43%) were randomized to treatment, 237 (49%) were excluded because the diagnosis of HGD was not confirmed and 40 (8%) did not meet other screening criteria or declined to participate in the study. The high patient exclusion rate re-enforces the recommendation by the American College of Gastroenterology that the diagnosis of HGD in BE should be confirmed by an expert GI pathologist. Patients were centrally randomized in a 2:1 proportion to receive PHOTOFRIN® PDT + OM (138 patients) or OM Only (70 patients). All patients underwent rigorous systematic quarterly endoscopic biopsy surveillance. Four-quadrant jumbo biopsies at every 2 cm of the entire Barrett's mucosa were obtained at each follow-up visit (every three months or six months if four consecutive quarterly follow-up endoscopic biopsy results were negative for HGD). All histological assessments were carried out at a central pathology laboratory and read by pathologists blinded to the treatment administered.

A total of 208 patients who had biopsy-proven HGD in BE were enrolled in the study. Of those, 199 patients were considered evaluable: 130 of 138 (94%) patients randomized to the PHOTOFRIN® PDT + OM group and 69 of 70 (99%) randomized to the OM Only group had no esophageal invasive cancer, suspicion of esophageal invasive cancer, lymph node involvement, or metastases, and had received at least one PHOTOFRIN® PDT course or one week of OM treatment, respectively. The mean age was 66 years (38 to 89 years) in the PHOTOFRIN® PDT + OM group, and 67 (36 to 88) in the OM Only group. The patients in both treatment groups were predominantly male (85%), Caucasian (99%), and former smokers (64%). These characteristics are typical of patients with HGD. Patients randomized to the PHOTOFRIN® PDT + OM treatment received up to three courses of treatment separated by at least 90 days. Each course consisted of intravenous administration of 2.0 mg/kg of PHOTOFRIN® followed 40–50 hours later by a 630 nm laser light dose of 130 J/cm delivered using a centering balloon. A second laser light dose of 50 J/cm could be administered without a centering balloon 96–120 hours after the injection of PHOTOFRIN® for treatment of "skip" areas. Since centering balloons are up to 7 cm in length, patients with more extensive HGD were treated with two or three courses. Both the PHOTOFRIN® PDT treatment group and the control group received 20 mg of omeprazole BID to decrease reflux esophagitis.

The primary efficacy endpoint was the Complete Response rate (CR3 or better) at any one of the endoscopic assessment time points. The CR3 or better response was defined as the complete ablation of HGD and referred to as a composite of the following three response levels.

1. CR1—Complete replacement of all Barrett's metaplasia and dysplasia with normal squamous cell epithelium;
2. CR2—Ablation of all histological grades of dysplasia, including patients with indefinite grade of dysplasia, but some areas of Barrett's epithelium still remain; and
3. CR3—Ablation of all areas of HGD but with some areas of low-grade dysplasia with or without areas which are indefinite for dysplasia, or areas of Barrett's metaplastic epithelium.

TABLE 4. Overall Efficacy Results in Patients with Superficial Endobronchial Tumors

	PDT	
EFFICACY PARAMETER	**n=11**	**n=62**
COMPLETE TUMOR RESPONSE, BIOPSY-PROVEN AT 3 MONTHS		
Number of Patients (%)	3 (27%)	31 (50%)[a]
TIME TO TUMOR RECURRENCE IN PATIENTS WITH COMPLETE RESPONSE		
Number of Patients (%) with Recurrences	1 (33%)	11 (35%)
Median Time to Tumor Recurrence	—	>2.7 years
[95% Confidence Interval]		[1.6,—[b]]
SURVIVAL		
Number of Patients (%) who Died of Any Cause	4 (36%)	32 (52%)
Median Survival	—	2.9 years
[95% Confidence Interval]		[2.1, 5.7]
DISEASE-SPECIFIC SURVIVAL		
Number of Patients (%) who Died of Lung Cancer	3 (27%)	22 (35%)
Median Disease-Specific Survival	—	4.1 years
[95% Confidence Interval]		[2.5,—[b]]

[a] Not included are an additional 18 patients (6 patients not eligible for surgery or radiotherapy) who had complete tumor responses which were documented earlier than 3 months after treatment.

[b] The upper limit of the confidence interval could not be estimated due to an insufficient number of patients whose tumors recurred (Time to Tumor Recurrence) or who died (Survival).

Table 5. Complete Response Rates After a Minimum Follow-Up of 24 Months in the ITT population

		Treatment Groups		
Responders		PHOTOFRIN® PDT + OM	OM Only	p-value[A]
Numbers of patients	N	138	70	
CR3 or better[B]	n	106	27	
	Proportion (%)	0.768 (76.8)	0.386 (38.6)	< 0.0001
	95% CI	(0.689, 0.836)	(0.272, 0.510)	

[A] Fisher's Exact test.

[B] CR3 or better: Ablation of all areas HGD.

NOTE: Six patients in the PHOTOFRIN® PDT + OM group and three patients in the OM Only group without post-baseline biopsy data are considered as non-responders.

There were five secondary efficacy endpoints:

1. Quality of Complete Response, which consisted of two parameters:
   a) CR1 response (complete replacement of all Barrett's metaplasia and dysplasia with normal squamous cell epithelium); and
   b) CR2 or better response (a composite endpoint of complete ablation of all grades of dysplasia and of CR1 response as defined above);
2. Duration of CR;
3. Time to Progression to Cancer;
4. Time to Treatment Failure (a composite endpoint of progression to cancer and other therapeutic intervention for HGD); and
5. Survival time

Table 5 presents the overall clinical response for both treatment groups in the intent-to-treat (ITT) population whose response was CR3 or better at any one of the evaluation time points. Overall, PHOTOFRIN® PDT + OM was effective in eliminating HGD in patients with BE. The proportion of responders was significantly higher in the PHOTOFRIN® PDT + OM group than in the OM Only group (77% versus 39%, respectively; p < 0.0001).

[See table 5 at left]

The quality of response in the PHOTOFRIN® PDT + OM group was significantly better than that measured in the OM Only group at all response levels (p<0.0001). Seventy-two (52%) patients in the PHOTOFRIN® PDT + OM group achieved a CR1 response as compared to only five (7%) patients in the OM Only group. Eighty-one (59%) patients in the PHOTOFRIN® PDT + OM group achieved a CR2 or better response as compared to ten (14%) patients in the OM Only group. The probability of maintaining a complete response (CR3 or better) by the end of the follow-up period was 53% in PHOTOFRIN® PDT + OM group and only 13% in OM Only group.

The time to patients' progression to cancer was significantly longer in the PHOTOFRIN® PDT + OM group than in OM Only group (see Kaplan-Meier plot below).

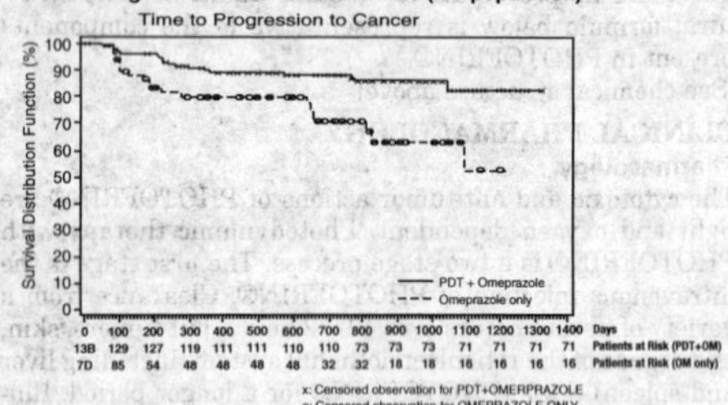

Figure 1. Comparison by Treatment Group of the Time to Progression to Cancer Over Time (ITT population)

At the end of 24 months of follow-up, patients in the PHOTOFRIN® PDT + OM group had an 83% chance of being cancer-free compared to 53% chance among patients in the OM Only group (p=0.0014). Durability of cancer risk reduction beyond two years has not been demonstrated.

At the minimum follow-up of 24 months, the proportion of patients' progression to cancer was statistically lower in the PHOTOFRIN® PDT + OM group than in the OM Only group: 13% (18 of 138 patients) versus 28% (20 of 70 patients), p=0.0060. Progression to cancer was related to complete response status. Patients who did not have a complete response had a greater risk of progression to cancer than patients who achieved a CR3 or better response, both in the PHOTOFRIN® PDT + OM group (38% vs. 6%) and in the OM Only group (44% vs. 4%). Patients who progressed to cancer after a complete response had mostly a CR3 response. No CR1 patients had progressed to cancer during the follow-up period.

Eighteen (13%) patients in the PHOTOFRIN® PDT + OM group and 22 (31%) patients in the OM Only group had another therapeutic intervention for HGD. Patients who experienced a progression of HGD to cancer, or who underwent therapy for HGD other than specified in the treatment arm were discontinued from the study. A disproportionate percentage of patients were discontinued from the OM Only group during the course of the study. By the end of the minimum 24-month follow-up period, 81 (59%) patients in the PHOTOFRIN® PDT + OM group and 28 (40%) patients in the OM Only group remained in their respective treatment arms.

Median survival time could not be estimated for either group, because very few (3) patients died during the follow-up period.

Complete response was influenced by the following factors: treatment with PHOTOFRIN® PDT + OM (vs. OM Only), single focus of HGD (vs. multiple foci), and prior omeprazole intake of at least 3 months (yes vs. no). Complete response was not influenced by the duration of HGD, length of BE, nodular conditions, gender, age, smoking history, and study center's size.

Supportive Studies

Two uncontrolled, supportive studies were conducted that were physician-sponsored, single center Phase II trials. Both studies included patients that had low-grade dysplasia (LGD), HGD and early adenocarcinoma. All HGD in BE patients were treated with PHOTOFRIN® PDT and omeprazole.

The first study enrolled 99 patients (44 with HGD); the purpose of this study was to determine the required light dose to produce effective results. The second study enrolled 86 patients (42 with HGD), who were randomized to receive either PHOTOFRIN® PDT with prednisone or PHOTOFRIN® PDT without prednisone to determine whether steroid treatment would reduce the incidence and severity of esophageal strictures.

A CR3 or better response was demonstrated in 93% of 44 patients with HGD in the first study and in 95% of 42 patients with HGD in the second study after a minimum follow-up of 12 months. A CR2 or better response was achieved in 82% of patients in the first study and in 91% of patients in the second study. A CR1 response occurred in 57% of patients in the first study and in 60% of the second study. Progression to cancer during the above follow-up period occurred in 18% of patients in the first study and in 7% of patients in the second study. No reduction in the incidence or severity of esophageal strictures was found in the prednisone group in the second study.

INDICATIONS AND USAGE

Photodynamic therapy with PHOTOFRIN® is indicated for:

— Palliation of patients with completely obstructing esophageal cancer, or of patients with partially obstructing esophageal cancer who, in the opinion of their physician, cannot be satisfactorily treated with Nd:YAG laser therapy.

— Reduction of obstruction and palliation of symptoms in patients with completely or partially obstructing endobronchial nonsmall cell lung cancer (NSCLC).

— Treatment of microinvasive endobronchial NSCLC in patients for whom surgery and radiotherapy are not indicated.

— Ablation of high-grade dysplasia in Barrett's esophagus patients who do not undergo esophagectomy.

CONTRAINDICATIONS

PHOTOFRIN® is contraindicated in patients with porphyria or in patients with known allergies to porphyrins.

Photodynamic therapy is contraindicated in patients with an existing tracheoesophageal or bronchoesophageal fistula.

Photodynamic therapy is contraindicated in patients with tumors eroding into a major blood vessel.

Photodynamic therapy is not suitable for emergency treatment of patients with severe acute respiratory distress caused by an obstructing endobronchial lesion because 40 to 50 hours are required between injection with PHOTOFRIN® and laser light treatment.

Photodynamic therapy is not suitable for patients with esophageal or gastric varices, or patients with esophageal ulcers >1 cm in diameter.

WARNINGS

Following injection with PHOTOFRIN® precautions must be taken to avoid exposure of skin and eyes to direct sunlight or bright indoor light (see PRECAUTIONS, General Precautions and Information for Patients).

Esophageal Cancer

If the esophageal tumor is eroding into the trachea or bronchial tree, the likelihood of tracheoesophageal or bronchoesophageal fistula resulting from treatment is sufficiently high that PDT is not recommended.

Patients with esophageal varices should be treated with extreme caution. Light should not be given directly to the variceal area because of the high risk of bleeding.

Endobronchial Cancer

Patients should be assessed for the possibility that a tumor may be eroding into a pulmonary blood vessel (see CONTRAINDICATIONS). Patients at high risk for fatal massive hemoptysis (FMH) include those with large, centrally located tumors, those with cavitating tumors or those with extensive tumor extrinsic to the bronchus.

If the endobronchial tumor invades deeply into the bronchial wall, the possibility exists for fistula formation upon resolution of tumor.

Photodynamic therapy should be used with extreme caution for endobronchial tumors in locations where treatment-induced inflammation could obstruct the main airway, e.g., long or circumferential tumors of the trachea, tumors of the carina that involve both mainstem bronchi circumferentially, or circumferential tumors in the mainstem bronchus in patients with prior pneumonectomy.

High-Grade Dysplasia (HGD) in Barrett's Esophagus (BE)

The long-term effect of PDT on HGD in BE is unknown. There is always a risk of leaving cancerous cells behind or leaving residual abnormal epithelium beneath the new squamous cell epithelium; these facts emphasize the risk of overlooking cancer in such patients and the need for rigorous continuing surveillance despite the endoscopic appearance of complete squamous cell reepithelialization. It is recommended that endoscopic biopsy surveillance be conducted every three months, until four consecutive negative evaluations for HGD have been recorded; further follow-up may be scheduled every 6 to 12 months, as per judgment of physicians. The follow-up period of the pivotal study at the time of analysis was a minimum of two years (ranging from 2 to 3.6 years).

PRECAUTIONS

General Precautions and Information for Patients

Photosensitivity

All patients who receive PHOTOFRIN® will be photosensitive and must observe precautions to avoid exposure of skin and eyes to direct sunlight or bright indoor light (from examination lamps, including dental lamps, operating room lamps, unshaded light bulbs at close proximity, etc.) for at least 30 days. Some patients may remain photosensitive for up to 90 days or more. The photosensitivity is due to residual drug, which will be present in all parts of the skin. Exposure of the skin to ambient indoor light is, however, beneficial because the remaining drug will be inactivated gradually and safely through a photobleaching reaction. Therefore, patients should not stay in a darkened room during this period and should be encouraged to expose their skin to ambient indoor light. The level of photosensitivity will vary for different areas of the body, depending on the extent of previous exposure to light. Before exposing any area of skin to direct sunlight or bright indoor light, the patient should test it for residual photosensitivity. A small area of skin should be exposed to sunlight for 10 minutes. If no photosensitivity reaction (erythema, edema, blistering) occurs within 24 hours, the patient can gradually resume normal outdoor activities, initially continuing to exercise caution and gradually allowing increased exposure. If some photosensitivity reaction occurs with the limited skin test, the patient should continue precautions for another 2 weeks before retesting. The tissue around the eyes may be more sensitive, and therefore, it is not recommended that the face be used for testing. If patients travel to a different geographical area with greater sunshine, they should retest their level of photosensitivity. **Conventional UV (ultraviolet) sunscreens are of no value in protecting against photosensitivity reactions because photoactivation is caused by visible light.**

Ocular Sensitivity

Ocular discomfort, commonly described as sensitivity to sun, bright lights, or car headlights, has been reported in patients who received PHOTOFRIN®. For 30 days, when outdoors, patients should wear dark sunglasses which have an average white light transmittance of <4%.

Use Before or After Radiotherapy

If PDT is to be used before or after radiotherapy, sufficient time should be allotted between the two therapies to ensure that the inflammatory response produced by the first treatment has subsided before commencing the second treatment. The inflammatory response from PDT will depend on tumor size and extent of surrounding normal tissue that receives light. It is recommended that 2 to 4 weeks be allowed after PDT before commencing radiotherapy. Similarly, if PDT is to be given after radiotherapy, the acute inflammatory reaction from radiotherapy usually subsides within 4 weeks after completing radiotherapy, after which PDT may be given.

Chest Pain

As a result of PDT treatment, patients may complain of substernal chest pain because of inflammatory responses within the area of treatment. Such pain may be of sufficient intensity to warrant the short-term prescription of opiate analgesics.

Respiratory Distress

Patients with endobronchial lesions must be closely monitored between the laser light therapy and the mandatory debridement bronchoscopy for any evidence of respiratory distress. Inflammation, mucositis, and necrotic debris may cause obstruction of the airway. If respiratory distress occurs, the physician should be prepared to carry out immediate bronchoscopy to remove secretions and debris to open the airway.

Esophageal Strictures

Esophageal strictures as a result of PDT of HGD in BE are common adverse events. An esophageal stricture was defined as a fixed lumen narrowing with solid food dysphagia and requiring dilation.

Regardless of the indication, esophageal strictures were reported in 122 of the 318 (38%) patients enrolled in the three clinical studies. Overall, esophageal strictures occurred within six months following PDT and were manageable through dilations. Multiple dilations of esophageal strictures may be required, as shown in Table 6. Special care should be taken during dilation to avoid perforation of the esophagus.

TABLE 6. Esophageal Dilations in Patients with Treatment-related Strictures

Number of Dilations	Number of Patients with Strictures, N=122	Percentage of Patients with Strictures
1–2 Dilations	38	31%
3–5 Dilations	33	27%
6–10 Dilations	26	21%
> 10 Dilations	25	20%

A high proportion of patients who developed an esophageal stricture received a nodule pre-treatment prior to developing the event (49%) and/or had a mucosal segment treated twice (82%). Therefore, nodule pre-treatment and re-treating the same mucosal segment more than once may influence the risk of developing an esophageal stricture.

Prior to initiating treatment with PHOTOFRIN® PDT, the diagnosis of HGD in BE should be confirmed by an expert GI pathologist. Photodynamic therapy with PHOTOFRIN® should be applied by physicians trained in the endoscopic use of PDT with PHOTOFRIN®, and only in those facilities properly equipped for the procedure.

Avoidance of Pregnancy

Women of childbearing potential should practice an effective method of contraception during therapy (see Pregnancy).

Drug Interactions

There have been no formal interaction studies of PHOTOFRIN® and any other drugs. However, it is possible that concomitant use of other photosensitizing agents (e.g., tetracyclines, sulfonamides, phenothiazines, sulfonylurea hypoglycemic agents, thiazide diuretics, griseofulvin, and fluoroquinolones) could increase the risk of photosensitivity reaction.

PHOTOFRIN® PDT causes direct intracellular damage by initiating radical chain reactions that damage intracellular membranes and mitochondria. Tissue damage also results from ischemia secondary to vasoconstriction, platelet activation and aggregation and clotting. Research in animals and in cell culture has suggested that many drugs could influence the effects of PDT, possible examples of which are described below. There are no human data that support or rebut these possibilities.

Compounds that quench active oxygen species or scavenge radicals, such as dimethyl sulfoxide, b-carotene, ethanol, formate and mannitol would be expected to decrease PDT activity. Preclinical data also suggest that tissue ischemia, allopurinol, calcium channel blockers and some prostaglandin synthesis inhibitors could interfere with PHOTOFRIN® PDT. Drugs that decrease clotting, vasoconstriction or platelet aggregation, e.g., thromboxane A_2 inhibitors, could decrease the efficacy of PDT. Glucocorticoid hormones given before or concomitant with PDT may decrease the efficacy of the treatment.

Carcinogenesis, Mutagenesis, Impairment of Fertility

No long-term studies have been conducted to evaluate the carcinogenic potential of PHOTOFRIN®. *In vitro,* PHOTOFRIN® PDT did not cause mutations in the Ames test, nor did it cause chromosome aberrations or mutations (HGPRT locus) in Chinese hamster ovary (CHO) cells. PHOTOFRIN® caused <2-fold, but significant, increases in sister chromatid exchange in CHO cells irradiated with visible light and a 3-fold increase in Chinese hamster lung fibroblasts irradiated with near UV light. PHOTOFRIN® PDT caused an increase in thymidine kinase mutants and DNA-protein cross-links in mouse L5178Y cells, but not mouse LYR83 cells. PHOTOFRIN® PDT caused a light-dose dependant increase in DNA-strand breaks in malignant human cervical carcinoma cells, but not in normal cells. PHOTOFRIN® was negative in a Chinese hamster ovarian cells (CHO/HGPRT) mutation test. *In vivo,* PHOTOFRIN® did not cause chromosomal aberrations in the mouse micronucleus test.

PHOTOFRIN® given to male and female rats intravenously, at 4 mg/kg/d (0.32 times the clinical dose on a mg/m^2 basis) before conception and through Day 7 of pregnancy caused no impairment of fertility. In this study, long-term dosing with PHOTOFRIN® caused discoloration of testes and ovaries and hypertrophy of the testes. PHOTOFRIN® also caused decreased body weight in the parent rats.

Pregnancy: Pregnancy Category C

There are no adequate and well-controlled studies in pregnant women. PHOTOFRIN® should be used during pregnancy only if the potential benefit justifies the potential risk to the fetus.

PHOTOFRIN® given to rat dams during fetal organogenesis intravenously at 8 mg/kg/d (0.64 times the clinical dose on a mg/m^2 basis) for 10 days caused no major malformations or developmental changes. This dose caused maternal and fetal toxicity resulting in increased resorptions, decreased litter size, delayed ossification, and reduced fetal weight. PHOTOFRIN® caused no major malformations when given to rabbits intravenously during organogenesis at 4 mg/kg/d (0.65 times the clinical dose on a mg/m^2 basis) for 13 days. This dose caused maternal toxicity resulting in increased resorptions, decreased litter size, and reduced fetal body weight.

PHOTOFRIN® given to rats during late pregnancy through lactation intravenously at 4 mg/kg/d (0.32 times the clinical dose on a mg/m^2 basis) for at least 42 days caused a reversible decrease in growth of offspring. Parturition was unaffected.

Nursing Mothers

It is not known whether this drug is excreted in human milk. Because many drugs are excreted in human milk and because of the potential for serious adverse reactions in nursing infants from PHOTOFRIN®, women receiving PHOTOFRIN® must not breast feed.

Pediatric Use

Safety and effectiveness in children have not been established.

Use in Elderly Patients

Approximately 70% of the patients treated with PDT using PHOTOFRIN® in clinical trials were over 60 years of age. There was no apparent difference in effectiveness or safety in these patients compared to younger people. Dose modification based upon age is not required.

ADVERSE REACTIONS

Systemically induced effects associated with PDT with PHOTOFRIN® consist of photosensitivity and mild constipation. All patients who receive PHOTOFRIN® will be photosensitive and must observe precautions to avoid sunlight and bright indoor light (see PRECAUTIONS). Photosensitivity reactions occurred in approximately 20% of cancer patients and in 68% of high-grade dysplasia (HGD) in Barrett's esophagus (BE) patients treated with PHOTOFRIN®. Typically these reactions were mostly mild to moderate er-

Continued on next page

Photofrin—Cont.

ythema but they also included swelling, itching, burning sensation, feeling hot, or blisters. In a single study of 24 healthy subjects, some evidence of photosensitivity reactions occurred in all subjects. Other less common skin manifestations were also reported in areas where photosensitivity reactions had occurred, such as increased hair growth, skin discoloration, skin nodules, increased wrinkles and increased skin fragility. These manifestations may be attributable to a pseudoporphyria state (temporary drug-induced cutaneous porphyria).

Most toxicities associated with this therapy are local effects seen in the region of illumination and occasionally in surrounding tissues. The local adverse reactions are characteristic of an inflammatory response induced by the photodynamic effect.

Esophageal Carcinoma

The following adverse events were reported over the entire follow-up period in at least 5% of patients treated with PHOTOFRIN® PDT, who had completely or partially obstructing esophageal cancer. Table 7 presents data from 88 patients who received the currently marketed formulation. The relationship of many of these adverse events to PDT with PHOTOFRIN® is uncertain.

TABLE 7. Adverse Events Reported in 5% or More of Patients[a] with Obstructing Esophageal Cancer

BODY SYSTEM/ Adverse Event	Number (%) of Patients n=88	
Patients with at Least One Adverse Event	84	(95%)
AUTONOMIC NERVOUS SYSTEM		
Hypertension	5	(6%)
Hypotension	6	(7%)
BODY AS A WHOLE		
Asthenia	5	(6%)
Back pain	10	(11%)
Chest pain	19	(22%)
Chest pain (substernal)	4	(5%)
Edema generalized	4	(5%)
Edema peripheral	6	(7%)
Fever	27	(31%)
Pain	19	(22%)
Surgical complication	4	(5%)
CARDIOVASCULAR		
Cardiac failure	6	(7%)
GASTROINTESTINAL		
Abdominal pain	18	(20%)
Constipation	21	(24%)
Diarrhea	4	(5%)
Dyspepsia	5	(6%)
Dysphagia	9	(10%)
Eructation	4	(5%)
Esophageal edema	7	(8%)
Esophageal tumor bleeding	7	(8%)
Esophageal stricture	5	(6%)
Esophagitis	4	(5%)
Hematemesis	7	(8%)
Melena	4	(5%)
Nausea	21	(24%)
Vomiting	15	(17%)
HEART RATE/RHYTHM		
Atrial fibrillation	9	(10%)
Tachycardia	5	(6%)
METABOLIC & NUTRITIONAL		
Dehydration	6	(7%)
Weight decrease	8	(9%)
PSYCHIATRIC		
Anorexia	7	(8%)
Anxiety	6	(7%)
Confusion	7	(8%)
Insomnia	12	(14%)
RED BLOOD CELL		
Anemia	28	(32%)
RESISTANCE MECHANISM		
Moniliasis	8	(9%)
RESPIRATORY		
Coughing	6	(7%)
Dyspnea	18	(20%)
Pharyngitis	10	(11%)
Pleural effusion	28	(32%)
Pneumonia	16	(18%)
Respiratory insufficiency	9	(10%)
Tracheoesophageal fistula	5	(6%)
SKIN & APPENDAGES		
Photosensitivity reaction	17	(19%)
URINARY		
Urinary tract infection	6	(7%)

[a] Based on adverse events reported at any time druing the entire period of follow-up.

Location of the tumor was a prognostic factor for three adverse events: upper-third of the esophagus (esophageal edema), middle-third (atrial fibrillation), and lower-third, the most vascular region (anemia). Also, patients with large tumors (>10 cm) were more likely to experience anemia. Two of 17 patients with complete esophageal obstruction from tumor experienced esophageal perforations, which were considered to be possibly treatment associated; these perforations occurred during subsequent endoscopies.

TABLE 8. Adverse Events Reported in 5% or More of Patients with Obstructing Endobronchial Cancers Number (%) of Patients

BODY SYSTEM/ Adverse Event	Within 30 Days of Treatment				Entire Follow-up Period[a]			
	PDT n=86		Nd:YAG n=86		PDT n=86		Nd:YAG n=86	
Patients with at Least One Adverse Event	43	(50%)	33	(38%)	62	(72%)	48	(56%)
BODY AS A WHOLE								
Back pain	3	(3%)	1	(1%)	3	(3%)	5	(6%)
Chest pain	6	(7%)	6	(7%)	7	(8%)	8	(9%)
Edema peripheral	3	(3%)	3	(3%)	4	(5%)	3	(3%)
Fever	7	(8%)	7	(8%)	14	(16%)	8	(9%)
Pain	1	(1%)	4	(5%)	4	(5%)	8	(9%)
CENTRAL NERVOUS SYSTEM								
Dysphonia	3	(3%)	2	(2%)	4	(5%)	2	(2%)
GASTROINTESTINAL								
Constipation	4	(5%)	1	(1%)	4	(5%)	2	(2%)
Dyspepsia	1	(1%)	4	(5%)	2	(2%)	5	(6%)
PSYCHIATRIC								
Anxiety	3	(3%)	0	(0%)	5	(6%)	0	(0%)
Insomnia	4	(5%)	2	(2%)	4	(5%)	3	(4%)
RESPIRATORY								
Bronchitis	9	(10%)	2	(2%)	9	(10%)	2	(2%)
Coughing	5	(6%)	8	(9%)	13	(15%)	11	(13%)
Dyspnea	15	(17%)	7	(8%)	26	(30%)	13	(15%)
Hemoptysis	6	(7%)	5	(6%)	14	(16%)	7	(8%)
Pleural effusion	0	(0%)	0	(0%)	4	(5%)	1	(1%)
Pneumonia	5	(6%)	4	(5%)	10	(12%)	5	(6%)
Pneumothorax	0	(0%)	0	(0%)	0	(0%)	4	(5%)
Respiratory insufficiency	0	(0%)	0	(0%)	5	(6%)	1	(1%)
Sputum increased	4	(5%)	5	(6%)	7	(8%)	6	(7%)
SKIN & APPENDAGES								
Photosensitivity reaction	16	(19%)	0	(0%)	18	(21%)	0	(0%)

[a] Follow-up was 33% longer for the PDT group than for the Nd:YAG group, introducing a bias against PDT when adverse events are compared for the entire follow-up period.

Serious and other notable adverse events observed in less than 5% of PDT-treated patients with obstructing esophageal cancer in the clinical studies include the following; their relationship to therapy is uncertain. In the gastrointestinal system, esophageal perforation, gastric ulcer, ileus, jaundice, and peritonitis have occurred. Sepsis has been reported occasionally. Cardiovascular events have included angina pectoris, bradycardia, myocardial infarction, sick sinus syndrome, and supraventricular tachycardia. Respiratory events of bronchitis, bronchospasm, laryngotracheal edema, pneumonitis, pulmonary hemorrhage, pulmonary edema, respiratory failure, and stridor have occurred. The temporal relationship of some gastrointestinal, cardiovascular and respiratory events to the administration of light was suggestive of mediastinal inflammation in some patients. Vision-related events of abnormal vision, diplopia, eye pain and photophobia have been reported.

Obstructing Endobronchial Cancer

Table 8 presents adverse events that were reported over the entire follow-up period in at least 5% of patients with obstructing endobronchial cancer treated with PHOTOFRIN® PDT or Nd:YAG. These data are based on the 86 patients who received the currently marketed formulation. Since it seems likely that most adverse events caused by these acute acting therapies would occur within 30 days of treatment, Table 8 presents those events occurring within 30 days of a treatment procedure, as well as those occurring over the entire follow-up period. It should be noted that follow-up was 33% longer for the PDT group than for the Nd:YAG group, thereby introducing a bias against PDT when adverse event rates are compared for the entire follow-up period. The extent of follow-up in the 30-day period following treatment was comparable between groups (only 9% more for PDT).

[See table 8 above]

Transient inflammatory reactions in PDT-treated patients occur in about 10% of patients and manifest as fever, bronchitis, chest pain, and dyspnea. The incidences of bronchitis and dyspnea were higher with PDT than with Nd:YAG. Most cases of bronchitis occurred within 1 week of treatment and all but one were mild or moderate in intensity. The events usually resolved within 10 days with antibiotic therapy. Treatment-related worsening of dyspnea is generally transient and self-limiting. Debridement of the treated area is mandatory to remove exudate and necrotic tissue. Life-threatening respiratory insufficiency likely due to therapy occurred in 3% of PDT-treated patients and 2% of Nd:YAG-treated patients (see WARNINGS and PRECAUTIONS).

There was a trend toward a higher rate of fatal massive hemoptysis (FMH) occurring on the PDT arm (10%) versus the Nd:YAG arm (5%), however, the rate of FMH occurring within 30 days of treatment was the same for PDT and Nd:YAG (4% total events, 3% treatment-associated events). Patients who have received radiation therapy have a higher incidence of FMH after treatment with PDT and after other forms of local therapy than patients who have not received radiation therapy, but analyses suggest that this increased risk may be due to associated prognostic factors such as having a centrally located tumor. The incidence of FMH in patients previously treated with radiotherapy was 21% (6/29) in the PDT group and 10% (3/29) in the Nd:YAG group. In patients with no prior radiotherapy, the overall incidence of FMH was less than 1%. Characteristics of patients at high risk for FMH are described in WARNINGS and CONTRAINDICATIONS.

Other serious or notable adverse events were observed in less than 5% of PDT-treated patients with endobronchial cancer; their relationship to therapy is uncertain. In the respiratory system, pulmonary thrombosis, pulmonary embolism, and lung abscess have occurred. Cardiac failure, sepsis, and possible cerebrovascular accident have also been reported in one patient each.

Superficial Endobronchial Tumors

The following adverse events were reported over the entire follow-up period in at least 5% of patients with superficial tumors (microinvasive or carcinoma *in situ*) who received the currently marketed formulation.

TABLE 9. Adverse Events Reported in 5% or More of Patients[a] with Superficial Endobronchial Tumors

Adverse Event	Number (%) of Patients n=90	
Patients with at Least One Adverse Event	44	(49%)
Photosensitivity reaction	20	(22%)
Coughing	8	(9%)
Dyspnea	6	(7%)
Edema	16	(18%)
Exudate	20	(22%)
Obstruction	19	(21%)
Stricture	10	(11%)
Ulceration	8	(9%)

[a] Based on adverse events reported at any time during the entire period of follow-up.

In patients with superficial endobronchial tumors, 44 of 90 patients (49%) experienced an adverse event, two-thirds of which were related to the respiratory system. The most common reaction to therapy was a mucositis reaction in one-fifth of the patients, which manifested as edema, exudate, and obstruction. The obstruction (mucus plug) is easily removed with suction or forceps. Mucositis can be minimized by avoiding exposure of normal tissue to excessive light (see PRECAUTIONS). Three patients experienced life-threatening dyspnea: one was given a double dose of light, one was treated concurrently in both mainstem bronchi and the other had had prior pneumonectomy and was treated in the sole remaining main airway (see WARNINGS). Stent placement was required in 3% of the patients due to endobronchial stricture. Fatal massive hemoptysis occurred within 30 days of treatment in one patient with superficial tumors (1%).

High-Grade Dysplasia (HGD) in Barrett's Esophagus (BE)

Table 10 presents adverse events that were reported, regardless of the relationship to treatment, over the follow-up period in at least 5% of patients with HGD in BE in either controlled or uncontrolled clinical trials.

[See table 10 on pages 773 and 774]

In the PHOTOFRIN® PDT + OM group, severe treatment-associated adverse events included chest pain of non-cardiac origin, dysphagia, nausea, vomiting, regurgitation, and heartburn. The severity of these symptoms decreased within 4 to 6 weeks following treatment.

The majority of the photosensitivity reactions occurred within 90 days following PHOTOFRIN® injection and was of mild (69%) or moderate (24%) intensity. Almost all (98%) of the photosensitivity reactions were considered to be associated with treatment. Fourteen (10%) patients reported severe reactions, all of which resolved. The typical reaction was described as skin disorder, sunburn or rash, and affected mostly the face, hands, and neck. Associated symptoms and signs were swelling, pruritis, erythema, blisters, itching, burning sensation, and feeling of heat.

The majority of esophageal stenosis and strictures reported in the PHOTOFRIN® PDT + OM group were of mild (55%) or moderate (37%) intensity, while approximately 8% were of severe intensity. The majority of esophageal strictures were reported during Course 2 of treatment. All esophageal strictures were considered to be associated with treatment. Most esophageal strictures were manageable through dilations (see PRECAUTIONS).

Laboratory Abnormalities

In patients with esophageal cancer, PDT with PHOTOFRIN® may result in anemia due to tumor bleeding. No significant effects were observed for other parameters in patients with endobronchial carcinoma or with HGD in BE.

OVERDOSAGE

PHOTOFRIN® Overdose

There is no information on overdosage situations involving PHOTOFRIN®. Higher than recommended drug doses of two 2 mg/kg doses given two days apart (10 patients) and three 2 mg/kg doses given within two weeks (1 patient), were tolerated without notable adverse reactions. Effects of overdosage on the duration of photosensitivity are unknown. Laser treatment should not be given if an overdose of PHOTOFRIN® is administered. In the event of an overdose, patients should protect their eyes and skin from direct sunlight or bright indoor lights for 30 days. At this time, patients should test for residual photosensitivity (see PRECAUTIONS). PHOTOFRIN® is not dialyzable.

Overdose of Laser Light Following PHOTOFRIN® Injection

Light doses of two to three times the recommended dose have been administered to a few patients with superficial endobronchial tumors. One patient experienced life-threatening dyspnea and the others had no notable complications. Increased symptoms and damage to normal tissue might be expected following an overdose of light. There is no information on overdose of laser light following PHOTOFRIN® injection in patients with esophageal cancer or in patients with high-grade dysplasia in Barrett's esophagus.

DOSAGE AND ADMINISTRATION

Photodynamic therapy with PHOTOFRIN® is a two-stage process requiring administration of both drug and light. The first stage of PDT is the intravenous injection of PHOTOFRIN® at 2 mg/kg. Illumination with laser light 40–50 hours following injection with PHOTOFRIN® constitutes the second stage of therapy. A second laser light application may be given 96–120 hours after injection, preceded by gentle debridement of residual tumor (see Administration of Laser Light). In clinical studies on esophageal and endobronchial cancers, debridement via endoscopy was required 2–3 days after the initial light application. Standard endoscopic techniques are used for light administration and debridement. Practitioners should be fully familiar with the patient's condition and trained in the safe and efficacious treatment of esophageal or endobronchial cancer, or high-grade dysplasia in Barrett's esophagus using photodynamic therapy with PHOTOFRIN® and associated light delivery devices.

For the treatment of esophageal and endobronchial cancer, patients may receive a second course of PDT a minimum of 30 days after the initial therapy; up to three courses of PDT (each separated by a minimum of 30 days) can be given. Before each course of treatment, patients with esophageal cancer should be evaluated for the presence of a tracheoesophageal or bronchoesophageal fistula (see CONTRAINDICATIONS). In patients with endobronchial lesions who have recently undergone radiotherapy, sufficient time (approximately 4 weeks) should be allowed between the therapies to ensure that the acute inflammation produced by radiotherapy has subsided prior to PDT (see PRECAUTIONS, Use Before or After Radiotherapy). All patients should be evaluated for the possibility that the tumor may be eroding into a major blood vessel (see CONTRAINDICATIONS).

For the ablation of high-grade dysplasia in Barrett's esophagus, patients may receive an additional course of PDT at a minimum of 90 days after the initial therapy; up to three courses of PDT (each injection separated by a minimum of 90 days) can be given to a previously treated segment which still shows high-grade dysplasia, low-grade dysplasia, or Barrett's metaplasia, or to a new segment if the initial Barrett's segment was >7 cm in length. Both residual and additional segments may be treated in the same light session(s) provided that the total length of the segments treated with the balloon/diffuser combination is not greater than 7 cm. In the case of a previously treated esophageal segment, if it has not sufficiently healed and/or histological assessment of biopsies is not clear, the subsequent course of PDT may be delayed for an additional 1–2 months.

PHOTOFRIN® Administration

PHOTOFRIN® should be administered as a single slow intravenous injection over 3 to 5 minutes at 2 mg/kg body weight. Reconstitute each vial of PHOTOFRIN® with 31.8 mL of either 5% Dextrose Injection (USP) or 0.9% Sodium Chloride Injection (USP), resulting in a final concentration of 2.5 mg/mL. Shake well until dissolved. Do not mix

Table 10. Treatment Emergent Adverse Events Reported in ≥5% of Patients Treated with PHOTOFRIN® PDT in the Clinical Trials on High-Grade Dysplasia in Barrett's Esophagus[a]

BODY SYSTEM/ Adverse Event	Treatment Groups			
	HGD[A] PHOTOFRIN® PDT + OM N=219 n (%)	HGD[B] OM Only N=69 n (%)	Other[C] PHOTOFRIN® PDT N=99 n (%)	Total PHOTOFRIN® PDT N=318 n (%)
Patients with at Least One Adverse Event	217 (99)	51 (74)	99 (100)	316 (99)
GASTROINTESTINAL	180 (82)	25 (36)	87 (88)	267 (84)
Nausea	61 (28)	5 (7)	63 (64)	124 (39)
Esophageal Stricture[d]	85 (39)	0	37 (37)	122 (38)
Vomiting	72 (33)	4 (6)	35 (35)	107 (34)
Dysphagia	50 (23)	1 (1)	27 (27)	77 (24)
Esophageal Narrowing[e]	60 (27)	4 (6)	16 (16)	76 (24)
Constipation	45 (21)	5 (7)	9 (9)	54 (17)
Abdominal Pain (Upper, lower, NOS)	32 (15)	4 (6)	8 (8)	40 (12)
Diarrhea	22 (10)	7 (10)	6 (6)	28 (9)
Esophageal Pain	15 (7)	0	9 (9)	24 (8)
Hiccup	18 (8)	0	1 (1)	19 (6)
Dyspepsia	12 (5)	3 (4)	6 (6)	18 (6)
Odynophagia	13 (6)	0	4 (4)	17 (5)
Eructation	11 (5)	0	4 (4)	15 (5)
GENERAL and ADMINISTRATION SITE CONDITIONS	135 (62)	17 (25)	66 (67)	201 (63)
Chest Pain	71 (32)	8 (12)	40 (40)	111 (35)
Pyrexia	47 (21)	3 (4)	13 (13)	60 (19)
Chest Discomfort	14 (6)	1 (1)	21 (21)	35 (11)
Pain	17 (8)	2 (3)	7 (7)	24 (8)
Fatigue	13 (6)	2 (3)	0	13 (4)
SKIN and SUBCUTANEOUS TISSUE	120 (55)	8 (12)	29 (29)	149 (47)
Photosensitivity Reaction	101 (46)	0	16 (16)	117 (37)
Rash	14 (6)	3 (4)	7 (7)	21 (7)
Pruritis	13 (6)	1 (1)	1 (1)	14 (4)
RESPIRATORY, THORACIC and MEDIASTINAL	67 (31)	21 (30)	22 (22)	89 (28)
Pleural Effusion	25 (11)	0	15 (15)	40 (13)
Dyspnea	16 (7)	3 (4)	4 (4)	20 (6)
INFECTIONS and INFESTATIONS	58 (26)	22 (32)	8 (8)	66 (21)
Sinusitis	11 (5)	3 (4)	2 (2)	13 (4)
Bronchitis	10 (5)	3 (4)	2 (2)	12 (4)
METABOLISM and NUTRITION	53 (24)	9 (13)	16 (16)	69 (22)
Dehydration	24 (11)	2 (3)	8 (8)	32 (10)
Anorexia	6 (3)	2 (3)	8 (8)	14 (4)
NERVOUS SYSTEM	51 (23)	14 (20)	11 (11)	62 (19)
Headache	17 (8)	6 (9)	2 (2)	19 (6)
INJURY, POISONING and PROCEDURAL	42 (19)	10 (14)	19 (19)	61 (19)
Post Procedural Pain	16 (7)	1 (1)	14 (14)	30 (9)
Sunburn	8 (4)	0	6 (6)	14 (4)

(Table continued on next page)

PHOTOFRIN® with other drugs in the same solution. PHOTOFRIN® , reconstituted with 5% Dextrose Injection (USP) or with 0.9% Sodium Chloride Injection (USP), has a pH in the range of 7 to 8. PHOTOFRIN® has been formulated with an overage to deliver the 75 mg labeled quantity. **The reconstituted product should be protected from bright light and used immediately.** Reconstituted PHOTOFRIN® is an opaque solution, in which detection of particulate matter by visual inspection is extremely difficult. Reconstituted PHOTOFRIN® , however, like all parenteral drug products, should be inspected visually for particulate matter and discoloration prior to administration whenever solution and container permit.

Precautions should be taken to prevent extravasation at the injection site. If extravasation occurs, care must be taken to protect the area from light. There is no known benefit from injecting the extravasation site with another substance.

Administration of Laser Light

Esophageal and Endobronchial Cancer

Initiate 630 nm wavelength laser light delivery to the patient 40–50 hours following injection with PHOTOFRIN® . A second laser light treatment may be given as early as 96 hours or as late as 120 hours after the initial injection with PHOTOFRIN® . No further injection of PHOTOFRIN®

Continued on next page

Photofrin—Cont.

should be given for such retreatment with laser light. Before providing a second laser light treatment, the residual tumor should be debrided. Vigorous debridement may cause tumor bleeding. For endobronchial tumors, debridement of necrotic tissue should be discontinued when the volume of bleeding increases, as this may indicate that debridement has gone beyond the zone of the PDT treatment effect.

The laser system must be approved for delivery of a stable power output at a wavelength of 630 ± 3 nm. Light is delivered to the tumor by cylindrical OPTIGUIDE™ fiber optic diffusers passed through the operating channel of an endoscope/bronchoscope. Instructions for use of the fiber optic and the selected laser system should be read carefully before use. OPTIGUIDE™ cylindrical diffusers are available in several lengths. The choice of diffuser tip length depends on the length of the tumor. Diffuser length should be sized to avoid exposure of nonmalignant tissue to light and to prevent overlapping of previously treated malignant tissue.

Photoactivation of PHOTOFRIN® is controlled by the total light dose delivered:

In the treatment of esophageal cancer, a light dose of 300 J/cm of diffuser length should be delivered. The total power output at the fiber tip is set to deliver the appropriate light dose using exposure times of 12 minutes and 30 seconds.

In the treatment of endobronchial cancer, the light dose should be 200 J/cm of diffuser length. The total power output at the fiber tip is set to deliver the appropriate light dose using exposure times of 8 minutes and 20 seconds. For noncircumferential endobronchial tumors that are soft enough to penetrate, interstitial fiber placement is preferred to intraluminal activation, since this method produces better efficacy and results in less exposure of the normal bronchial mucosa to light. It is important to perform a debridement 2 to 3 days after each light administration to minimize the potential for obstruction caused by necrotic debris (see PRECAUTIONS).

Refer to the OPTIGUIDE™ instructions for use for complete instructions concerning the fiber optic diffuser.

High-Grade Dysplasia (HGD) in Barrett's Esophagus (BE)

Approximately 40–50 hours after PHOTOFRIN® administration light should be delivered by a X-Cell Photodynamic Therapy (PDT) Balloon with Fiber Optic Diffuser. The choice of fiber optic/balloon diffuser combination will depend on the length of Barrett's mucosa to be treated (Table 11).

TABLE 11. Fiber Optic Diffuser/Balloon Combination[a]

Treated Barrett's Mucosa Length (cm)	Fiber Optic Diffuser Size (cm)	Balloon Window Size (cm)
6–7	9	7
4–5	7	5
1–3	5	3

[a] Whenever possible, the BE segment selected for treatment should include normal tissue margins of a few millimeters at the proximal and distal ends.

Light Doses: Photoactivation is controlled by the total light dose delivered. The objective is to expose and treat all areas of HGD and the entire length of BE. The light dose administered will be 130 J/cm of diffuser length using a centering balloon. Based on the pivotal clinical study, acceptable light intensity for the balloon/diffuser combinations range from 200–270 mW/cm of diffuser.

To calculate the light dose, the following specific light dosimetry equation applies for all fiber optic diffusers:

[See second table at right]

Table 12 provides the settings that will be used to deliver the dose within the shortest time (light intensity of 270 mW/cm). A second option (light intensity of 200 mW/cm) has also been included where necessary to accommodate lasers with a total capacity that does not exceed 2.5 W.

[See table 12 at right]

Short fiber diffusers (≤ 2.5 cm) are to be used to pretreat nodules with 50 J/cm diffuser length prior to regular balloon treatment in the first laser light session or for the treatment of "skip" areas (i.e., an area that does not show sufficient mucosal response) after the first light session. For this treatment, the fiber optic diffuser is used without a centering balloon, and a light intensity of 400 mW/cm should be used. For nodule pre-treatment and treatment of skipped areas, care should be taken to minimize exposure to normal tissue as it is also sensitized. Table 13 lists appropriate fiber optic power outputs and treatment times using a light intensity of 400 mW/cm.

TABLE 13. Short Fiber Optic Diffusers to be Used Without a Centering Balloon to Deliver 50 J/cm of Diffuser Length at a Light Intensity of 400 mW/cm

Diffuser Length (cm)	Required Power Output From Diffuser[a] (mW)	Treatment Time (sec)	Treatment Time (min:sec)
1.0	400	125	2:05
1.5	600	125	2:05
2.0	800	125	2:05
2.5	1000	125	2:05

[a] as measured by immersing the diffuser into the cuvet in the power meter and slowly increasing the laser power. Note: No more than 1.5 times the required diffuser power output should be needed from the laser. If more than this is required, the system should be checked.

Table 10 *(cont.)*. Treatment Emergent Adverse Events Reported in ≥5% of Patients Treated with PHOTOFRIN® PDT in the Clinical Trials on High-Grade Dysplasia in Barrett's Esophagus[a]

BODY SYSTEM/ Adverse Event	Treatment Groups			
	HGD[A] PHOTOFRIN® PDT + OM N=219 n (%)	HGD[B] OM Only N=69 n (%)	Other[C] PHOTOFRIN® PDT N=99 n (%)	Total PHOTOFRIN® PDT N=318 n (%)
MUSCULOSKELETAL and CONNECTIVE TISSUE	46 (21)	18 (26)	9 (9)	55 (17)
Back Pain	15 (7)	4 (6)	1 (1)	16 (5)
Arthralgia	10 (5)	6 (9)	1 (1)	11 (3)
INVESTIGATIONS	41 (19)	5 (7)	14 (14)	55 (17)
Weight Decreased	17 (8)	2 (3)	3 (3)	20 (6)
Body Temperature Increased	8 (4)	0	8 (8)	16 (5)
PSYCHIATRIC	37 (17)	8 (12)	4 (4)	41 (13)
Insomnia	11 (5)	3 (4)	1 (1)	12 (4)
Depression	10 (5)	3 (4)	0	10 (3)
Anxiety	10 (5)	1 (1)	0	10 (3)
VASCULAR	25 (11)	6 (9)	4 (4)	29 (9)
Hypertension	10 (5)	1 (1)	0	10 (3)

[A] Includes all HGD patients in the Safety population from PHO BAR 01 (N=133), TCSC 93-07 (N=44), and 96-01 N=42)
[B] Includes all HGD patients in the Safety population from PHO BAR 01 (N=69)
[C] Includes patients with Barrett's metaplasia, indefinite dysplasia, LGD, and adenocarcinoma at baseline in the Safety population from TCSC 93-07 (N=55) and TCSC 96-01 (N=44)
[d] In the controlled clinical trial, an esophageal stricture was defined as a fixed lumen narrowing with solid food dysphagia which required dilations; In the uncontrolled clinical trials, an esophageal stricture was defined as any dilated esophageal narrowing.
[e] An esophageal narrowing was defined as an undilated esophageal stenosis.
NOTE: Adverse events classified using MedDRA 5.0 dictionary, except esophageal strictures/narrowing.

$$\text{Light Dose (J/cm)} = \frac{\text{Power Output From Diffuser (W)} \times \text{Treatment Time (s)}}{\text{Diffuser Length (cm)}}$$

TABLE 12. Fiber Optic Power Outputs and Treatment Times Required to Deliver 130 J/cm of Diffuser Length Using the Centering Balloon

Balloon Window Length (cm)	Diffuser Length (cm)	Light Intensity (mW/cm)	Required Power Output from Diffuser[a] (mW)	Treatment Time (secs)	Treatment Time (min:sec)
3	5	270	1350	480	8:00
5	7	270	1900	480	8:00
7	9	270	2440	480	8:00
		200	1800	650	10:50

[a] as measured by immersing the diffuser into the cuvet in the power meter and slowly increasing the laser power. Note: No more than 1.5 times the required diffuser power output should be needed from the laser. If more than this is required, the system should be checked.

TABLE 14. High-Grade Dysplasia in Barrett's Esophagus of > 7 cm

Procedure	Study Day	Light Delivery Devices	Treatment Intent
PHOTOFRIN® Injection	Day 1	NA	Uptake of photosensitizer
Laser Light Application	Day 3[a]	3, 5 or 7 cm balloon (130 J/cm)	Photoactivation
Laser Light Application *(Optional)*	Day 5	Short (≤ 2.5 cm) fiber optic diffuser (50 J/cm)	Treatment of "skip" areas only

[a] Discrete nodules will receive an initial light application of 50 J/cm (using a short diffuser) before the balloon light application.

A maximum of 7 cm of esophageal mucosa is treated at the first light session using an appropriate size of centering balloon and fiber optic diffuser (Table 11). Whenever possible, the segment selected for the first light application should contain all the areas of HGD. Also, whenever possible, the Barrett's esophagus (BE) segment selected for the first light application should include normal tissue margin of a few millimeters at the proximal and distal ends.

Nodules are to be pretreated at a light dose of 50 J/cm of diffuser length with a short (≤ 2.5 cm) fiber optic diffuser placed directly against the nodule followed by standard balloon application as described above.

Repeat Light Application

A second laser light application may be given to a previously treated segment that shows a "skip" area, using a short, ≤ 2.5 cm fiber optic diffuser at the light dose of 50 J/cm of the diffuser length. Patients with BE >7 cm, should have the remaining untreated length of Barrett's epithelium treated with a second PDT course at least 90 days later.

The treatment regimen is summarized in Table 14.

[See table 14 above]

HOW SUPPLIED

PHOTOFRIN® (porfimer sodium) for Injection is supplied as a freeze-dried cake or powder as follows:

NDC 58914-155-75 — 75 mg vial

PHOTOFRIN® freeze-dried cake or powder should be stored at Controlled Room Temperature 20–25°C (68–77°F) [see USP].

Spills and Disposal

Spills of PHOTOFRIN® should be wiped up with a damp cloth. Skin and eye contact should be avoided due to the potential for photosensitivity reactions upon exposure to light; use of rubber gloves and eye protection is recommended. All contaminated materials should be disposed of in a polyethylene bag in a manner consistent with local regulations.

Accidental Exposure

PHOTOFRIN® is neither a primary ocular irritant nor a primary dermal irritant. However, because of its potential to induce photosensitivity, PHOTOFRIN® might be an eye and/or skin irritant in the presence of bright light. It is important to avoid contact with the eyes and skin during preparation and/or administration. As with therapeutic overdosage, any overexposed person must be protected from bright light.

AXCAN PHARMA
Manufactured by
WYETH-AYERST LEDERLE PARENTERALS, INC.
Carolina, Puerto Rico 00987
for
Axcan Scandipharm Inc.
Birmingham, AL 35242
For inquiries call Axcan Scandipharm Inc. at: 1-800-742-6706
2000072-03
August 2003

Shown in Product Identification Guide, page 307

ULTRASE® ℞

[*ul 'trāce*]
(pancrelipase, USP) Capsules
Enteric-Coated Microspheres

Prescribing Information

DESCRIPTION

ULTRASE® (pancrelipase) Capsules are orally administered capsules containing enteric-coated microspheres of porcine pancreatic enzyme concentrate, predominantly pancreatic lipase, amylase, and protease.

Each ULTRASE ® capsule contains:

Lipase	4,500 U.S.P. Units
Amylase	20,000 U.S.P. Units
Protease	25,000 U.S.P. Units

Inactive ingredients: povidone, talc, sugar, methacrylic acid copolymer (Type C), triethyl citrate, simethicone emulsion.

CLINICAL PHARMACOLOGY

ULTRASE® (pancrelipase) Capsules are designed to prevent inactivation by gastric acid thereby resulting in the delivery of high levels of biologically active enzymes into the duodenum. The enzymes catalyze the hydrolysis of fats into glycerol and fatty acids, starch into dextrins and sugars, and protein into proteoses and derived substances.

INDICATIONS AND USAGE

ULTRASE® (pancrelipase) Capsules are indicated for patients with partial or complete exocrine pancreatic insufficiency caused by:

- Cystic fibrosis (CF)
- Chronic pancreatitis due to alcohol use or other causes
- Surgery (pancreatico-duodenectomy or Whipple's procedure, with or without Wirsung duct injection, total pancreatectomy)
- Obstruction (pancreatic and biliary duct lithiasis, pancreatic and duodenal neoplasms, ductal stenosis)
- Other pancreatic disease (hereditary, post traumatic and allograft pancreatitis, hemochromatosis, Shwachman's Syndrome, lipomatosis, hyperparathyroidism)
- Poor mixing (Billroth II gastrectomy, other types of gastric bypass surgery, gastrinoma)

Pancrelipase capsules are effective in controlling steatorrhea.[1–9]

CONTRAINDICATIONS

Pancrelipase capsules are contraindicated in patients known to be hypersensitive to pork protein. Pancrelipase capsules are contraindicated in patients with acute pancreatitis or with acute exacerbations of chronic pancreatic diseases.

WARNINGS

Should hypersensitivity occur, discontinue medication and treat symptomatically.

PRECAUTIONS

General

TO PROTECT ENTERIC COATING, MICROSPHERES MUST NOT BE CRUSHED OR CHEWED. Where swallowing of capsules is difficult, they may be opened and the microspheres added to a small quantity of a soft food (e.g. applesauce, gelatin, etc.) that does not require chewing, and swallowed immediately. Contact of the microsphere with foods having a pH greater than 5.5 can dissolve the protective enteric shell.

Carcinogenesis, Mutagenesis, Impairment of Fertility

Long-term studies in animals have not been performed to evaluate carcinogenic potential. Methacrylic acid, a minor component of the methacrylic acid copolymer enteric-coating contained in ULTRASE® (pancrelipase) Capsules, has been reported to act as a teratogen in rat embryo cultures. However, the copolymer enteric-coating of ULTRASE® (pancrelipase) Capsules was not mutagenic by the Ames test, and it did not produce chromosome damage in a test for unscheduled DNA synthesis in rat hepatocytes.

Pregnancy: Category C.

Animal reproduction studies have not been conducted with ULTRASE® (pancrelipase) Capsules. It is not known whether ULTRASE® (pancrelipase) Capsules can cause fetal harm when administered to a pregnant woman or can affect reproduction capacity. ULTRASE® (pancrelipase) Capsules should be given to a pregnant woman only if the potential benefit outweighs the potential risk to the fetus.

Nursing Mothers

It is not known whether ULTRASE® (pancrelipase) is excreted in human milk. Because many drugs are excreted in human milk, caution should be exercised when ULTRASE® (pancrelipase) Capsules are administered to a nursing mother.

ADVERSE REACTIONS

The most frequently reported adverse reactions to products containing pancrelipase are gastrointestinal in nature. Less frequently, allergic-type reactions have also been observed. Extremely high doses of exogenous pancreatic enzymes have been associated with hyperuricosuria and hyperuricemia when the preparations given were pancrelipase in powdered or capsule form, or pancreatin in tablet form.

Colonic strictures have been reported in cystic fibrosis patients treated with both high- and lower-strength enzyme supplements.[10] A causal relationship has not been established. The possibility of bowel stricture should be considered if symptoms suggestive of gastrointestinal obstruction occur. Since impaired fluid secretion may be a factor in the development of intestinal obstruction, care should be taken to maintain adequate hydration, particularly in warm weather.[11]

"Fibrosing colonopathy" is a term used to describe a condition seen in patients with CF who have taken high amounts of pancreatic enzyme supplements (>6,000 lipase U/kg/meal). At its most advanced, this condition leads to colonic strictures.

1. In whom should one consider the diagnosis of fibrosing colonopathy?
a. Patients with cystic fibrosis who have evidence of partial or complete obstruction, bloody diarrhea or chylous ascites.
b. Patients who have two of the following three symptoms:
- abdominal pain
- ongoing diarrhea
- poor weight gain

ESPECIALLY if they have:
- taken >6,000 lipase U/kg/meal
- age less than twelve years
- history of meconium ileus
- prior intestinal surgery
- history of recurrent DIOS
- "inflammatory bowel disease"[12]

DOSAGE AND ADMINISTRATION

The enzymatic activity of ULTRASE® (pancrelipase) Capsules is expressed in U.S.P. units. The smallest effective dose should be used. Dosage should be adjusted according to the severity of the exocrine pancreatic insufficiency. Begin therapy with one or two capsules with meals or snacks and adjust dosage according to symptoms.

The number of capsules or capsule strength given with meals and/or snacks should be estimated by assessing which dose minimizes steatorrhea and maintains good nutritional status. Dosages should be adjusted according to the response of the patient. Where swallowing of capsules is difficult, they may be opened and the microspheres added to a small quantity of a soft food (e.g. applesauce, gelatin, etc.) that does not require chewing, and swallowed immediately. It is recommended that the total dose of pancrelipase being ingested for a meal or snack be dispersed equally (with fluids) before, during, and after the meal or snack.

SUGGESTION FOR THE USE OF PANCREATIC ENZYMES IN CYSTIC FIBROSIS [12]

1. Patients should be receiving optimal diet for age and clinical status, recognizing that those with failure to thrive or malnutrition require additional calories and other nutrients for catch-up growth.
2. Nutrition assessment should be a part of routine clinical evaluations.
3. Initial dosing of pancreatic enzyme supplements should begin with 500 lipase U/kg/meal using enteric-coated microsphere products.
4. Patients should be reassessed 2–4 weeks after initiation of therapy. The following items should be assessed:
- Clinical status, e.g. abdominal symptoms and exam;
- Nutritional intake and growth (height, weight, head circumference);
- Character of stools—greasy, oily (for information, not for decision making);
- Quantitative 72-hour fecal fat when indicated but not less than annually (perform on a normal diet for age);
- Fat soluble vitamin measures.
5. Corollaries to dosing suggestions:

a. Dose may be altered in a stepwise fashion according to the response of the patient (see 4. above).

b. Dose approaching 2,000 lipase U/kg/meal would indicate the need for further investigation (see below). Patients presently on higher doses should be reevaluated; either immediately decrease the dose or titrate down to a lower dose range at, or below, 2,000 lipase U/kg/meal. Doses >6,000 lipase U/kg/meal have been associated with colonic strictures.

c. Pancreatic supplements mixed with applesauce or other acidic food substances should be administered immediately, not stored.

d. Enteric-coated microspheres should not be crushed.

e. Enzyme doses (as lipase U/kg/meal) tend to decrease with advancing age.

f. Patients should accept only product brands prescribed by their physician.

g. Adjustment of dosage is the responsibility of the physician. Patients should be advised not to adjust doses without consulting their physician. Changes in product or dosage may require an adjustment period.

h. Complaints transmitted by phone should be investigated thoroughly before dose is adjusted. If indicated, this investigation should include 72-hour fecal fat testing.

i. Pancreatic supplements should be stored in a cool, dry place and checked regularly for expiration date.

HOW SUPPLIED

ULTRASE ® (pancrelipase) Capsules

Gelatin capsules (opaque white and opaque white), imprinted "ULTRASE". Bottles of 100 (NDC 58914-045-10).

Store at controlled room temperature, between 15°C and 25°C (59°F and 77°F), in a dry place. Do not refrigerate.

REFERENCES

1. Delchier JC, Vidon N. *et al.* Fate of orally ingested enzymes in pancreatic insufficiency: comparison of two pancreatic enzyme preparations. *Aliment Pharmacol Therap.* 1991;5:365-378.
2. Duhamel JP, Vidailhet M, *et al.* Étude multicentrique comparative d'une nouvelle présentation de pancréatine en microgranules gastrorésistants dans l'insuffisance pancréatique exocrine de la mucoviscidose chez l'enfant. *Ann Pediatr.* 1988;35:69-74.
3. Dutta SK, Tilley DK. The pH-sensitive enteric-coated pancreatic enzyme preparations: an evaluation of therapeutic efficacy in adult patients with pancreatic insufficiency. *J Clin Gastroenterol.* 1983;5:51-54.
4. Dutta SK, Rubin J, Harvey J. Comparative evaluation of the therapeutic efficacy of a pH-sensitive enteric-coated pancreatic enzyme preparation with conventional pancreatic enzyme therapy in the treatment of exocrine pancreatic insufficiency. *Gastroenterol.* 1983;84:476-482.
5. Gouerou H, Dain MP, *et al.* Alipase versus nonenteric-coated enzymes in pancreatic insufficiency. *Int J Pancreatol.* 1989;5:45-50.
6. Mischler EH, Parrell S, *et al.* Comparison of effectiveness of pancreatic enzyme preparations in cystic fibrosis. *Am J Dis Child.* 1982;136:1060-1063.
7. Salen G, Prakash A. Evaluation of enteric-coated microspheres for enzyme replacement therapy in adults with pancreatic insufficiency. *Cur Ther Res.* 1979;25:650-656.
8. Schneider MU, Knoll-Ruzicka ML, *et al.* Pancreatic enzyme replacement therapy: comparative effects of conventional and enteric-coated microspheric pancreatin and acid-stable fungal enzyme preparations on steatorrhea in chronic pancreatitis. *Hepatogastroenterol.* 1985;32:97-102.
9. Halgreen H, Thorsgaard Pedersen N, Worning H. Symptomatic effect of pancreatic enzyme therapy in patients with chronic pancreatitis. *Scand J Gastroenterol.* 1986;21:104-108.
10. Smyth RL, van Velzen D, *et al.* Strictures of ascending colon in cystic fibrosis and high-strength pancreatic enzymes. *The Lancet.* 1994;343:85-86.
11. Lands L, Zinman R, *et al.* Pancreatic function testing in meconium disease in CF: two case reports. *J Ped Gastroenterol and Nut.* 1988;7:276-279.
12. Cystic Fibrosis Foundation Conference on Pancreatic Enzyme Supplementation in the Context of Fibrosing Colonopathy; Washington, D.C., March 23-24, 1995.

Rx only
REV. 06/03

Marketed as ULTRASE® by: **AXCAN SCANDIPHARM INC.**
22 Inverness Center Parkway
Birmingham, AL 35242 USA
www.axcan.com

ULTRASE® is manufactured by Eurand International, Milan, Italy using its DIFFUCAPS® technology for Axcan Scandipharm Inc. ULTRASE® is a registered trademark of Axcan Scandipharm Inc. Axcan Pharma™ and the Axcan Pharma™ logo are trademarks of Axcan Pharma Inc., the parent corporation of Axcan Scandipharm Inc.

Shown in Product Identification Guide, page 307

ULTRASE® MT ℞

[*ul 'trāce*]
(pancrelipase, USP) Capsules
Enteric-Coated Minitablets

Prescribing Information

DESCRIPTION

ULTRASE® MT (pancrelipase) Capsules are orally administered capsules containing enteric-coated minitablets of porcine pancreatic enzyme concentrate, predominantly pancreatic lipase, amylase, and protease.

Each ULTRASE ® MT12 Capsule contains:

Lipase	12,000 U.S.P. Units
Amylase	39,000 U.S.P. Units
Protease	39,000 U.S.P. Units

Each ULTRASE ® MT18 Capsule contains:

Lipase	18,000 U.S.P. Units
Amylase	58,500 U.S.P. Units
Protease	58,500 U.S.P. Units

Each ULTRASE ® MT20 Capsule contains:

Lipase	20,000 U.S.P. Units
Amylase	65,000 U.S.P. Units
Protease	65,000 U.S.P. Units

Continued on next page

Ultrase MT—Cont.

Inactive ingredients: gelatin, hydrogenated castor oil, silicon dioxide, sodium carboxymethylcellulose, magnesium stearate, croscarmellose sodium, microcrystalline cellulose, hydroxypropyl methycellulose phthalate (HP 55) (as dry substance), talc, triethyl citrate, iron oxides and titanium oxide.

CLINICAL PHARMACOLOGY

ULTRASE® MT (pancrelipase) Capsules are designed to prevent inactivation by gastric acid thereby resulting in the delivery of high levels of biologically active enzymes into the duodenum. The enzymes catalyze the hydrolysis of fats into glycerol and fatty acids, starch into dextrins and sugars, and protein into proteoses and derived substances.

INDICATIONS AND USAGE

ULTRASE® MT (pancrelipase) Capsules are indicated for patients with partial or complete exocrine pancreatic insufficiency caused by:

- Cystic fibrosis (CF)
- Chronic pancreatitis due to alcohol use or other causes
- Surgery (pancreatico-duodenectomy or Whipple's procedure, with or without Wirsung duct injection, total pancreatectomy)
- Obstruction (pancreatic and biliary duct lithiasis, pancreatic and duodenal neoplasms, ductal stenosis)
- Other pancreatic disease (hereditary, post traumatic and allograft pancreatitis, hemochromatosis, Shwachman's Syndrome, lipomatosis, hyperparathyroidism)
- Poor mixing (Billroth II gastrectomy, other types of gastric bypass surgery, gastrinoma)

Pancrelipase capsules are effective in controlling steatorrhea.[1–9]

CONTRAINDICATIONS

Pancrelipase capsules are contraindicated in patients known to be hypersensitive to pork protein. Pancrelipase capsules are contraindicated in patients with acute pancreatitis or with acute exacerbations of chronic pancreatic diseases.

WARNINGS

Should hypersensitivity occur, discontinue medication and treat symptomatically.

PRECAUTIONS

General

TO PROTECT ENTERIC COATING, MINITABLETS MUST NOT BE CRUSHED OR CHEWED. Where swallowing of capsules is difficult, they may be opened and the minitablets added to a small quantity of a soft food (e.g. applesauce, gelatin, etc.) that does not require chewing, and swallowed immediately. Contact of the minitablet with foods having a pH greater than 5.5 can dissolve the protective enteric shell.

Carcinogenesis, Mutagenesis, Impairment of Fertility

Long-term studies in animals have not been performed to evaluate carcinogenic potential.

Pregnancy: Category C.

Animal reproduction studies have not been conducted with ULTRASE® MT (pancrelipase) Capsules. It is not known whether ULTRASE® MT (pancrelipase) Capsules can cause fetal harm when administered to a pregnant woman or can affect reproduction capacity. ULTRASE® MT (pancrelipase) Capsules should be given to a pregnant woman only if the potential benefit outweighs the potential risk to the fetus.

Nursing Mothers

It is not known whether ULTRASE® MT (pancrelipase) is excreted in human milk. Because many drugs are excreted in human milk, caution should be exercised when ULTRASE® MT (pancrelipase) Capsules are administered to a nursing mother.

ADVERSE REACTIONS

The most frequently reported adverse reactions to products containing pancrelipase are gastrointestinal in nature. Less frequently, allergic-type reactions have also been observed. Extremely high doses of exogenous pancreatic enzymes have been associated with hyperuricosuria and hyperuricemia when the preparations given were pancrelipase in powdered or capsule form, or pancreatin in tablet form.

In two clinical studies with ULTRASE® MT in 193 patients with cystic fibrosis, the adverse events described were all gastrointestinal in nature and may actually represent symptoms of the underlying disease, such as abdominal pain/cramps (5.7%), diarrhea (3.6%), and greasy stools and flatulence (1.5% each). In a postmarketing trial with another enteric-coated formulation, 160 adverse events occurred in the 15,711 patients (0.97%) evaluated.[10] The most frequent events reported were diarrhea, skin reaction, and abdominal discomfort (0.2% each).

Colonic strictures have been reported in cystic fibrosis patients treated with both high- and lower-strength enzyme supplements.[11] A causal relationship has not been established. The possibility of bowel stricture should be considered if symptoms suggestive of gastrointestinal obstruction occur. Since impaired fluid secretion may be a factor in the development of intestinal obstruction, care should be taken to maintain adequate hydration, particularly in warm weather.[12]

"Fibrosing colonopathy" is a term used to describe a condition seen in patients with CF who have taken high amounts of pancreatic enzyme supplements (>6,000 lipase U/kg/meal). At its most advanced, this condition leads to colonic strictures.

1. In whom should one consider the diagnosis of fibrosing colonopathy?

a. Patients with cystic fibrosis who have evidence of partial or complete obstruction, bloody diarrhea or chylous ascites.

b. Patients who have two of the following three symptoms:
- abdominal pain
- ongoing diarrhea
- poor weight gain

ESPECIALLY if they have:
- taken >6,000 lipase U/kg/meal
- age less than twelve years
- history of meconium ileus
- prior intestinal surgery
- history of recurrent DIOS
- "inflammatory bowel disease"[13]

DOSAGE AND ADMINISTRATION

The enzymatic activity of ULTRASE® MT (pancrelipase) Capsules is expressed in U.S.P. units.

The smallest effective dose should be used. Dosage should be adjusted according to the severity of the exocrine pancreatic insufficiency. Begin therapy with one or two capsules with meals or snacks and adjust dosage according to symptoms. The number of capsules or capsule strength given with meals and/or snacks should be estimated by assessing which dose minimizes steatorrhea and maintains good nutritional status. Dosages should be adjusted according to the response of the patient. Where swallowing of capsules is difficult, they may be opened and the minitablets added to a small quantity of a soft food (e.g. applesauce, gelatin, etc.) that does not require chewing, and swallowed immediately. It is recommended that the total dose of pancrelipase being ingested for a meal or snack be dispersed equally (with fluids) before, during, and after the meal or snack.

SUGGESTIONS FOR THE USE OF PANCREATIC ENZYMES IN CYSTIC FIBROSIS[13]

1. Patients should be receiving optimal diet for age and clinical status, recognizing that those with failure to thrive or malnutrition require additional calories and other nutrients for catch-up growth.
2. Nutrition assessment should be a part of routine clinical evaluations.
3. Initial dosing of pancreatic enzyme supplements should begin with 500 lipase U/kg/meal using enteric-coated minitablet products.
4. Patients should be reassessed 2–4 weeks after initiation of therapy.
   The following items should be assessed:
   - Clinical status, e.g. abdominal symptoms and exam;
   - Nutritional intake and growth (height, weight, head circumference);
   - Character of stools—greasy, oily (for information, not for decision making);
   - Quantitative 72-hour fecal fat when indicated but not less than annually (perform on a normal diet for age);
   - Fat soluble vitamin measures.
5. Corollaries to dosing suggestions:
   a. Dose may be altered in a stepwise fashion according to the response of the patient (see 4. above).
   b. Dose approaching 2,000 lipase U/kg/meal would indicate the need for further investigation (see below). Patients presently on higher doses should be reevaluated; either immediately decrease the dose or titrate down to a lower dose range at, or below, 2,000 lipase U/kg/meal. Doses >6,000 lipase U/kg/meal have been associated with colonic strictures.
   c. Pancreatic supplements mixed with applesauce or other acidic food substances should be administered immediately, not stored.
   d. Enteric-coated minitablets should not be crushed.
   e. Enzyme doses (as lipase U/kg/meal) tend to decrease with advancing age.
   f. Patient should accept only product brands prescribed by their physician.
   g. Adjustment of dosage is the responsibility of the physician. Patients should be advised not to adjust doses without consulting their physician. Changes in product or dosage may require an adjustment period.
   h. Complaints transmitted by phone should be investigated thoroughly before dose is adjusted. If indicated, this investigation should include 72-hour fecal fat testing.
   i. Pancreatic supplements should be stored in a cool, dry place and checked regularly for expiration date.

HOW SUPPLIED

ULTRASE ® MT12 (pancrelipase) Capsules

Gelatin capsules (white and yellow), imprinted "ULTRASE MT12". Bottles of 100 (NDC 58914-002-10).

ULTRASE ® MT18 (pancrelipase) Capsules

Gelatin capsules (gray and white), imprinted "ULTRASE MT18". Bottles of 100 (NDC 58914-018-10).

ULTRASE ® MT20 (pancrelipase) Capsules

Gelatin capsules (light gray and yellow), imprinted "ULTRASE MT20". Bottles of 100 (NDC 58914-004-10), and bottles of 500 (NDC 58914-004-50).

Store at controlled room temperature, between 15°C and 25°C (59°F and 77°F), in a dry place. Do not refrigerate.

REFERENCES

1. Delchier JC, Vidon N, *et al.* Fate of orally ingested enzymes in pancreatic insufficiency: comparison of two pancreatic enzyme preparations. *Aliment Pharmacol Therap.* 1991;5:365–378.
2. Duhamel JP, Vidailhet M, *et al.* Étude multicentrique comparative d'une nouvelle présentation de pancréatine en microgranules gastrorésistants dans l'insuffisance pancréatique exocrine de la mucoviscidose chez l'enfant. *Ann Pediatr.* 1988;35:69–74.
3. Dutta SK, Tilley DK. The pH-sensitive enteric-coated pancreatic enzyme preparations: an evaluation of therapeutic efficacy in adult patients with pancreatic insufficiency. *J Clin Gastroenterol.* 1983;5:51–54.
4. Dutta SK, Rubin J, Harvey J. Comparative evaluation of the therapeutic efficacy of a pH-sensitive enteric-coated pancreatic enzyme preparation with conventional pancreatic enzyme therapy in the treatment of exocrine pancreatic insufficiency. *Gastroenterol.* 1983;84:476–482.
5. Gouerou H, Dain MP, *et al.* Alipase versus nonenteric-coated enzymes in pancreatic insufficiency. *Int J Pancreatol.* 1989;5:45–50.
6. Mischler EH, Parrell S, *et al.* Comparison of effectiveness of pancreatic enzyme preparations in cystic fibrosis. *Am J Dis Child.* 1982;136:1060–1063.
7. Salen G, Prakash A. Evaluation of enteric-coated microspheres for enzyme replacement therapy in adults with pancreatic insufficiency. *Cur Ther Res.* 1979;25: 650–656.
8. Schneider MU, Knoll-Ruzicka ML, *et al.* Pancreatic enzyme replacement therapy: comparative effects of conventional and enteric-coated microspheric pancreatin and acid-stable fungal enzyme preparations on steatorrhea in chronic pancreatitis. *Hepatogastroenterol.* 1985;32:97–102.
9. Halgreen H, Thorsgaard Pedersen N, Worning H. Symptomatic effect of pancreatic enzyme therapy in patients with chronic pancreatitis. *Scand J Gastroenterol.* 1986;21:104–108.
10. Gretzmacher I, Rüther HG. Maldigestion. *Therapiewoche.* 1983;33:6776–6782.
11. Smyth RL, van Velzen D, *et al.* Strictures of ascending colon in cystic fibrosis and high-strength pancreatic enzymes. *The Lancet.* 1994;343:85–86.
12. Lands L, Zinman R, *et al.* Pancreatic function testing in meconium disease in CF: two case reports. *J Ped Gastroenterol and Nut.* 1988;7:276–279.
13. Cystic Fibrosis Foundation Conference on Pancreatic Enzyme Supplementation in the Context of Fibrosing Colonopathy; Washington, D.C., March 23–24, 1995.

Rx only

REV. 06/03

Marketed as ULTRASE® MT by: **AXCAN SCANDIPHARM INC.**
22 Inverness Center Parkway
Birmingham, AL 35242 USA
www.axcan.com

ULTRASE® MT is manufactured by Eurand International, Milan, Italy using its EURAND MINITABS® technology for Axcan Scandipharm Inc. ULTRASE® is a registered trademark of Axcan Scandipharm Inc. Axcan Pharma™ and the Axcan Pharma™ logo are trademarks of Axcan Pharma Inc., the parent corporation of Axcan Scandipharm Inc.

Shown in Product Identification Guide, page 307

URSO 250™ ℞

[*ūr-so*]

(Ursodiol Tablets, USP) 250 mg

Rx only

DESCRIPTION

URSO 250™ is a bile acid available as 250 mg film-coated tablets for oral administration.

URSO 250™ is ursodiol (ursodeoxycholic acid), a naturally occurring bile acid found in small quantities in normal human bile and in larger quantities in the biles of certain species of bears. It is a bitter-tasting white powder consisting of crystalline particles freely soluble in ethanol and glacial acetic acid, slightly soluble in chloroform, sparingly soluble in ether, and practically insoluble in water. The chemical name of ursodiol is 3α,7β-dihydroxy-5β-cholan-24-oic ($C_{24}H_{40}O_4$). Ursodiol has a molecular weight of 392.56. Its structure is shown below.

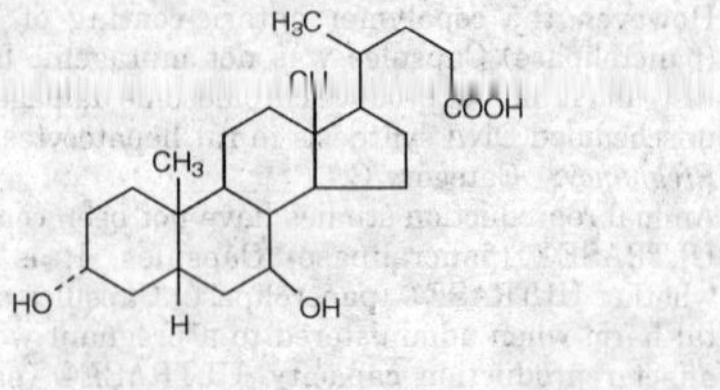

Inactive ingredients: microcrystalline cellulose, povidone, sodium starch glycolate, magnesium stearate, ethylcellulose, dibutyl sebacate, carnauba wax, hydroxypropyl methylcellulose, PEG 3350, PEG 8000, cetyl alcohol, sodium lauryl sulfate and hydrogen peroxide.

CLINICAL PHARMACOLOGY

Ursodiol (UDCA) is normally present as a minor fraction of the total bile acids in humans (about 5%). Following oral administration, the majority of ursodiol is absorbed by passive diffusion and its absorption is incomplete. Once absorbed, ursodiol undergoes hepatic extraction to the extent of about 50% in the absence of liver disease. As the severity of liver disease increases, the extent of extraction decreases. In the liver, ursodiol is conjugated with glycine or taurine, then secreted into bile. These conjugates of ursodiol are absorbed in the small intestine by passive and active mechanisms. The conjugates can also be deconjugated in the ileum by intestinal enzymes, leading to the formation of free ursodiol that can be reabsorbed and reconjugated in the liver. Nonabsorbed ursodiol passes into the colon where it is mostly 7-dehydroxylated to lithocholic acid. Some ursodiol is epimerized to chenodiol (CDCA) via a 7-oxo intermediate. Chenodiol also undergoes 7-dehydroxylation to form lithocholic acid. These metabolites are poorly soluble and excreted in the feces. A small portion of lithocholic acid is reabsorbed, conjugated in the liver with glycine, or taurine and sulfated at the 3 position. The resulting sulfated lithocholic acid conjugates are excreted in bile and then lost in feces.

Lithocholic acid, when administered chronically to animals, causes cholestatic liver injury that may lead to death from liver failure in certain species unable to form sulfate conjugates. Ursodiol is 7-dehydroxylated more slowly than chenodiol. For equimolar doses of ursodiol and chenodiol, steady state levels of lithocholic acid in biliary bile acids are lower during ursodiol administration than with chenodiol administration. Humans and chimpanzees can sulfate lithocholic acid. Although liver injury has not been associated with ursodiol therapy, a reduced capacity to sulfate may exist in some individuals. Nonetheless, such a deficiency has not yet been clearly demonstrated and must be extremely rare, given the several thousand patient-years of clinical experience with ursodiol.

In healthy subjects, at least 70% of ursodiol (unconjugated) is bound to plasma protein. No information is available on the binding of conjugated ursodiol to plasma protein in healthy subjects or primary biliary cirrhosis (PBC) patients. Its volume of distribution has not been determined, but is expected to be small since the drug is mostly distributed in the bile and small intestine. Ursodiol is excreted primarily in the feces. With treatment, urinary excretion increases, but remains less than 1% except in severe cholestatic liver disease.

During chronic administration of ursodiol, it becomes a major biliary and plasma bile acid. At a chronic dose of 13–15 mg/kg/day, ursodiol constitutes 30–50% of biliary and plasma bile acids.

CLINICAL STUDIES

A U.S., multicenter, randomized, double-blind, placebo-controlled study was conducted to evaluate the efficacy of ursodeoxycholic acid at a dose of 13–15 mg/kg/day, administered in 4 divided doses in 180 patients with PBC. Upon completion of the double-blind portion, all patients entered an open-label active treatment extension phase.

Treatment failure, the main efficacy end point measured during this study, was defined as death, need for liver transplantation, histologic progression by two stages or to cirrhosis, development of varices, ascites or encephalopathy, marked worsening of fatigue or pruritus, inability to tolerate the drug, doubling of serum bilirubin and voluntary withdrawal. After two years of double-blind treatment, the incidence of treatment failure was significantly reduced in the URSO 250™ group (n=89) as compared to the placebo group (n=91). Time to treatment failure was also significantly delayed in the URSO 250™ treated group regardless of either histologic stage or baseline bilirubin levels (>1.8 or ≤1.8 mg/dl).

Using a definition of treatment failure which excluded doubling of serum bilirubin and voluntary withdrawal, time to treatment failure was significantly delayed in the URSO 250™ group. In comparison with placebo, treatment with URSO 250™ resulted in a significant improvement in the following serum hepatic biochemistries when compared to baseline: total bilirubin, SGOT, alkaline phosphatase and IgM.

A second study conducted in Canada randomized 222 PBC patients to ursodiol, 14 mg/kg/day or placebo, in a double-blind manner during a two-year period. At two years, a statistically significant difference between the two treatments, in favor of ursodiol, was demonstrated in the following: reduction in the proportion of patients exhibiting a more than 50% increase in serum bilirubin; median percent decrease in bilirubin, transaminases and alkaline phosphatase; incidence of treatment failure; and time to treatment failure. The definition of treatment failure included: discontinuing the study for any reason; a total serum bilirubin level greater than or equal to 1.5 mg/dl or increasing to a level equal to or greater than two times the baseline level; and the development of ascites or encephalopathy.

INDICATIONS AND USAGE

URSO 250™ (ursodiol) tablets are indicated for the treatment of patients with primary biliary cirrhosis.

CONTRAINDICATIONS

Hypersensitivity or intolerance to ursodiol or any of the components of the formulation.

ADVERSE EVENTS (AEs)

ADVERSE EVENTS	*VISIT AT 12 MONTHS*		*VISIT AT 24 MONTHS*	
	UDCA n (%)	Placebo n (%)	UDCA n (%)	Placebo n (%)
Diarrhea	—	—	1 (1.32)	—
Elevated creatinine	—	—	1 (1.32)	—
Elevated blood glucose	1 (1.18)	—	1 (1.32)	—
Leukopenia	—	—	2 (2.63)	—
Peptic ulcer	—	—	1 (1.32)	—
Skin rash	—	—	2 (2.63)	—

PRECAUTIONS

Patients with variceal bleeding, hepatic encephalopathy, ascites or in need of an urgent liver transplant, should receive appropriate specific treatment.

Drug Interactions

Bile acid sequestering agents such as cholestyramine and colestipol may interfere with the action of **URSO 250™** by reducing its absorption. Aluminum-based antacids have been shown to adsorb bile acids *in vitro* and may be expected to interfere with **URSO 250™** in the same manner as the bile acid sequestering agents. Estrogens, oral contraceptives, and clofibrate (and perhaps other lipid-lowering drugs) increase hepatic cholesterol secretion, and encourage cholesterol gallstone formation and hence may counteract the effectiveness of **URSO 250™**.

Carcinogenicity, Mutagenicity and Impairment of Fertility

In two 24-month oral carcinogenicity studies in mice, ursodiol at doses up to 1,000 mg/kg/day (3,000 mg/m^2/day) was not tumorigenic. Based on body surface area, for a 50 kg person of average height (1.46 m^2 body surface area), this dose represents 5.4 times the recommended maximum clinical dose of 15 mg/kg/day (555 mg/m^2/day).

In a two-year oral carcinogenicity study in Fischer 344 rats, ursodiol at doses up to 300 mg/kg/day (1,800 mg/m^2/day, 3.2 times the recommended maximum human dose based on body surface area) was not tumorigenic.

In a life-span (126–138 weeks) oral carcinogenicity study, Sprague-Dawley rats were treated with doses of 33 to 300 mg/kg/day, 0.4 to 3.2 times the recommended maximum human dose based on body surface area. Ursodiol produced a significantly ($p \leq 0.5$, Fisher's exact test) increased incidence of pheochromocytomas of the adrenal medulla in females of the highest dose group.

In 103-week oral carcinogenicity studies of lithocholic acid, a metabolite of ursodiol, doses up to 250 mg/kg/day in mice and 500 mg/kg/day in rats did not produce any tumors. In a 78-week rat study, intrarectal instillation of lithocholic acid (1 mg/kg/day) for 13 months did not produce colorectal tumors. A tumor-promoting effect was observed when it was administered after a single intrarectal dose of a known carcinogen N-methyl-N′-nitro-N-nitroguanidine. On the other hand, in a 32-week rat study, ursodiol at a daily dose of 240 mg/kg (1,440 mg/m^2, 2.6 times the maximum recommended human dose based on body surface area) suppressed the colonic carcinogenic effect of another known carcinogen azoxymethane.

Ursodiol was not genotoxic in the Ames test, the mouse lymphoma cell (L5178Y, TK$^{+/-}$) forward mutation test, the human lymphocyte sister chromatid exchange test, the mouse spermatogenia chromosome aberration test, the Chinese hamster micronucleus test and the Chinese hamster bone marrow cell chromosome aberration test.

Ursodiol at oral doses of up to 2,700 mg/kg/day (16,200 mg/m^2/day, 29 times the recommended maximum human dose based on body surface area) was found to have no effect on fertility and reproductive performance of male and female rats.

Pregnancy, Teratogenic Effects. Pregnancy Category B

Teratology studies have been performed in pregnant rats at oral doses up to 2,000 mg/kg/day (12,000 mg/m^2/day, 22 times the recommended maximum human dose based on body surface area) and in pregnant rabbits at oral doses up to 300 mg/kg/day (3,600 mg/m^2/day, 7 times the recommended maximum human dose based on body surface area) and have revealed no evidence of impaired fertility or harm to the fetus due to ursodiol.

There are no adequate or well-controlled studies in pregnant women. Because animal reproduction studies are not always predictive of human response, this drug should be used during pregnancy only if clearly needed.

Nursing Mothers

It is not known whether ursodiol is excreted in human milk. Because many drugs are excreted in human milk, caution should be exercised when **URSO 250™** is administered to a nursing mother.

Pediatric Use

The safety and effectiveness of **URSO 250™** in pediatric patients have not been established.

[See table above]

Note: Those AEs occurring at the same or higher incidence in the placebo as in the UDCA group have been deleted from this table (this includes diarrhea and thrombocytopenia at 12 months, nausea/vomiting, fever and other toxicity).

UDCA = Ursodeoxycholic acid = Ursodiol

Adverse events are reported regardless of attribution to the test medication.

OVERDOSE

Accidental or intentional overdosage with ursodiol has not been reported. The most severe manifestation of overdosage would likely consist of diarrhea which should be treated symptomatically.

Single oral doses of ursodiol at 10, 5 and 10 g/kg in mice, rats and dogs, respectively were not lethal. A single oral dose of ursodiol at 1.5 g/kg was lethal in hamsters. Symptoms of acute toxicity were salivation and vomiting in dogs, and ataxia, dyspnea, ptosis, agonal convulsions and coma in hamsters.

DOSAGE AND ADMINISTRATION

The recommended adult dosage for **URSO 250™** in the treatment of PBC is 13–15 mg/kg/day administered in four divided doses with food.

HOW SUPPLIED

Each **URSO 250™** film-coated tablet, white, engraved with "URS785", contains 250 mg of ursodiol. Available in bottles of 500 tablets (NDC 58914-785-50) and 100 tablets (NDC 58914-785-10). Store at 20°C to 25°C (68°F to 77°F). Dispense in a tight container.

Manufactured in Canada for:
Axcan Scandipharm Inc.
22 Inverness Center Parkway
Birmingham, AL 35242
USA
URSO 250™ is a trademark of
Axcan Pharma US Inc.
July 2002

Shown in Product Identification Guide, page 307

VIOKASE® ℞

[*vī′ō-kās*]
Pancrelipase, USP
Tablets, Powder
Rx only

For product information please call 1-800-742-6706.

DESCRIPTION

VIOKASE® (pancrelipase, USP) is a pancreatic enzyme concentrate of porcine origin containing standardized lipase, protease, and amylase as well as other pancreatic enzymes. VIOKASE® is available in tablet and powder dosage form for oral administration.

The enzyme potencies of the tablets and powder are:

[See first table at top of next page]

Inactive Ingredients: VIOKASE® 8 and VIOKASE® 16 Tablets: Lactose, croscarmellose sodium, microcrystalline cellulose, silicon dioxide, stearic acid, talc.

VIOKASE® Powder: Lactose, sodium chloride.

CLINICAL PHARMACOLOGY

The natural digestive enzymes in VIOKASE® hydrolyze fats into fatty acids and glycerol, split protein into amino acids, and convert carbohydrates to dextrins and short chain sugars.

Under conditions of the USP test method (in vitro) VIOKASE® has the following total digestive capacity:

[See second table at top of next page]

VIOKASE® 8 and 16 Tablets are immediate release and are not enteric coated.

The digestive capacity of a pancreatic enzyme concentrate depends on the amount that passes through the stomach unchanged and is available at the site of action in the small intestine.

Continued on next page

	VIOKASE® 8 Tablet	VIOKASE® 16 Tablet	VIOKASE® Powder Each 0.7 g (1/4 Teaspoonful)
Lipase, USP units	8,000	16,000	16,800
Protease, USP units	30,000	60,000	70,000
Amylase, USP units	30,000	60,000	70,000

	VIOKASE® 8 Tablet	VIOKASE® 16 Tablet	VIOKASE® Powder Each 0.7 g (1/4 Teaspoonful)
Dietary fat, grams	28	56	59
Dietary protein, grams	30	60	70
Dietary starch, grams	30	60	70

Viokase—Cont.

INDICATIONS

VIOKASE® (pancrelipase, USP) is indicated in the treatment of exocrine pancreatic insufficiency as associated with but not limited to cystic fibrosis, chronic pancreatitis, pancreatectomy, or obstruction of the pancreas ducts.

CONTRAINDICATIONS

Should not be used in patients hypersensitive to pork protein.

PRECAUTIONS

General: Individuals previously sensitized to trypsin, pancreatin or pancrelipase may have allergic manifestations.
Information for Patients: VIOKASE® should not be held in the mouth as the proteolytic action may cause irritation of the mucosa.
Avoid inhalation of the powder when administering VIOKASE®.
Carcinogenesis, Mutagenesis: Long-term studies in animals have not been performed to evaluate the carcinogenic potential.
Pregnancy Category C: Animal reproduction studies have not been conducted with VIOKASE®. It is also not known whether VIOKASE® can cause fetal harm when administered to a pregnant woman or can affect reproduction capacity. VIOKASE® should be given to a pregnant woman only if clearly needed.
Nursing Mothers: It is not known whether this drug is excreted in human milk. Because many drugs are excreted in human milk, caution should be exercised when pancrelipase is administered to a nursing mother.

ADVERSE EFFECTS

The dust or finely powdered pancreatic enzyme concentrate is irritating to the nasal mucosa and the respiratory tract. It has been documented that inhalation of the airborne powder can precipitate an asthma attack. The literature also contains several references to asthma due to inhalation in patients sensitized to pancreatic enzyme concentrates. Extremely high doses of exogenous pancreatic enzymes have been associated with hyperuricemia and hyperuricosuria. Overdosage of pancreatic enzyme concentrate may cause diarrhea or transient intestinal upset.

OVERDOSE

Acute toxicity determinations in animals have not been possible since the maximum dose that could be given orally produced no toxic reaction. In chronic feeding tests rats developed swollen salivary glands. This is believed due to the proteolytic activity and the mucosal irritation caused by tissue digestion.
No acute toxic reactions have been reported.

DOSAGE AND ADMINISTRATION

Powder: Dosage for patients with cystic fibrosis: 1/4 teaspoonful (0.7g) with meals.
Tablets: Dosage range for patients with cystic fibrosis or chronic pancreatitis is from 8,000 to 32,000 Lipase USP Units taken with meals, i.e., one to four VIOKASE® 8 tablets or one to two VIOKASE® 16 tablets with meals or as directed by a physician.
In patients with pancreatectomy or obstruction of pancreatic ducts: one to two VIOKASE® 8 tablets or one VIOKASE® 16 tablet taken at 2-hour intervals or as directed by a physician.

HOW SUPPLIED

VIOKASE® 8 Tablets: Tan, round, compressed tablets engraved VIOKASE® on one side and 9111 on the other side in bottles of 100 (NDC 58914-111-10) and 500 (NDC 58914-111-50).
VIOKASE® 16 Tablets: Tan, oval, biconvex tablets engraved V^{16} on one side and 9116 on the other side in bottles of 100 (NDC 58914-116-10) and 500 (NDC 58914-116-50).
Powder: Tan powder in bottles of 8 oz (227 g) (NDC 58914-115-08).
Store in tightly closed container in a dry place at a temperature not exceeding 25°C (77°F).
Dispense tablets and powder in tight container, preferably with a desiccant.

REFERENCES

1. Regan PT, Malagelada J-R, DiMagno EP, Gianzman SL, Go VLW. Comparative effects of antacids, cimetidine and enteric coating on the therapeutic response to oral enzymes in severe pancreatic insufficiency. N Engl J Med 1977;297:854–8.
2. Graham DY. Enzyme replacement therapy of exocrine pancreatic insufficiency in man. N Eng J Med 1977;296: 1314–7.

VIOKASE® is a registered trademark of Axcan Pharma US Inc.
Rev. February 2003
Manufactured in Canada for:
Axcan Scandipharm Inc.
Birmingham, AL 35242 USA

Shown in Product Identification Guide, page 307

Ballay Pharmaceuticals, Inc.

P.O. BOX 1356
WIMBERLEY, TX 78676

Direct Inquiries to:
Terry Ballay, President
512-847-6458

In addition to the full labeling of the products listed below, the following products are also available from Ballay Pharmaceuticals:
Nortemp®
Baltussin

ALACOL® DM SYRUP ℞

[alə - kōl]
Alcohol Free–Sugar Free

DESCRIPTION

Antihistamine/Nasal Decongestant/Antitussive syrup for oral administration. An alcohol-free, sugar-free, black raspberry flavored syrup. Each teaspoonful (5 mL) contains: Dextromethorphan HBr. 10 mg; Phenylephrine HCl, 5mg; Brompheniramine Maleate, 2 mg.

INACTIVE INGREDIENTS

Propylene Glycol, Sodium Saccharin, Glycerin, Sorbitol, Purified Water, Raspberry Flavor, FD&C Red#40, and FD&C Blue#1

CLINICAL PHARMACOLOGY

Dextromethorphan Hydrobromide acts centrally to elevate the threshold for coughing. It has no analgesic or addictive properties. The onset of antitussive action occurs in 15 to 30 minutes after administration and is of long duration. Phenylephrine HCl is a sympathomimetic drug which is readily absorbed from the gastrointestinal tract and produces nasal vasoconstriction (decongestion). Phenylephrine effects its vasoconstrictor activity by releasing noradrenaline from sympathetic nerve endings and from direct stimulation of α-adreno receptors in blood vessels. Brompheniramine Maleate is a histamine antagonist, specifically an H_1-receptor blocking agent belonging to the alkylamine class of antihistamines. Antihistamines appear to compete with histamine for receptor sites on effector cells. Brompheniramine also has anticholinergic (drying) and sedative effects. Among the antihistaminic effects, it antagonizes the allergic response (vasodilatation, increased vascular permeability, increased mucous secretion) of nasal tissue. Brompheniramine is well absorbed from the gastrointestinal tract, with peak plasma concentration after a single oral dose of 4 mg reached in 5 hours: urinary excretion is the major route of elimination, mostly as products of biodegradation; the liver is assumed to be the main sight of metabolic transformation.

INDICATIONS

ALACOL DM is indicated for the relief of coughs and upper respiratory symptoms, including nasal congestion, associated with allergy or the common cold.

CONTRAINDICATIONS

Hypersensitivity to any of the ingredients. Do not use in newborns, in premature infants, in nursing mothers, in patients with severe hypertension or severe coronary artery disease, or in those receiving MAO inhibitors. Antihistamines should not be used to treat lower respiratory tract conditions including asthma.

WARNINGS

A persistent cough may be a sign of a serious condition. If cough persists for more than one week, tends to recur or is accompanied by fever, rash, or persistent headache, consult a physician. Do not take this product for persistent or chronic cough such as occurs with smoking, asthma, emphysema, or if cough is accompanied by excessive phlegm (mucus) unless directed by a physician. Especially in infants and small children, antihistamines in overdosage may cause hallucinations, convulsions, and death. Antihistamines may diminish mental alertness. In young children they may produce excitation.

PRECAUTIONS

General- Because of its antihistamine component, ALACOL DM should be used with caution in patients with a history of bronchial asthma, narrow-angle glaucoma, gastrointestinal obstruction, urinary bladder neck obstruction. Because of its sympathomimetic component, ALACOL DM should be used with caution in patients with diabetes, hypertension, heart disease, thyroid disease.
Information for Patients- Patients should be warned about engaging in activities requiring mental alertness, such as driving a car or operating dangerous machinery.
Drug Interactions: Antihistamines have additive effects with alcohol and other CNS depressants (hypnotics, sedatives, tranquilizers, antianxiety agents, etc.). MAO inhibitors prolong and intensify the anticholinergic (drying) effects of antihistamines. MAO inhibitors may enhance the effect of phenylephrine. Sympathomimetics may reduce the effects of antihypertensive drugs.
Carcinogenesis, Mutagenesis, Impairment of Fertility- Animal studies of ALACOL DM to assess carcinogenic and mutagenic potential, or the effect on fertility have not been performed.
Usage in Pregnancy-Pregnancy Category C. Teratogenic Effects- Animal reproduction studies have not been conducted with ALACOL DM. It is also not known whether ALACOL DM can cause fetal harm when administered to a pregnant woman or can affect reproduction capacity. ALACOL DM should be used during pregnancy only if the potential benefit justifies the potential risk to the fetus. Reproduction studies of brompheniramine maleate in rats and mice at doses up to 16 times the maximum human dose have revealed no evidence of impaired fertility or harm to the fetus.
Nursing Mothers- Because of the higher risk of intolerance of antihistamines in small infants generally, and in newborns and prematures in particular, ALACOL DM is contraindicated in nursing mothers.

ADVERSE REACTIONS

The most frequent adverse reactions to ALACOL DM include sedation, dryness of mouth, nose and throat, thickening of bronchial secretions, and dizziness. Other adverse reactions may include: ***Dermatologic***- Urticaria, drug rash, photosensitivity, and pruritus. ***Cardiovascular System***- Hypotension, hypertension, cardiac arrhythmias. ***Central Nervous System***- disturbed coordination, tremor, irritability, insomnia, visual disturbance, weakness, nervousness, convulsions, headache, euphoria and dysphoria. ***G.U. System***- Urinary frequency, difficult urination. ***G.I. System***- Epigastric discomfort, anorexia, nausea, vomiting, diarrhea, or constipation. ***Respiratory System***- Tightness of chest and wheezing, shortness of breath. ***Hematologic System***- Hemolytic anemia, thrombocytopenia, agranulocytosis.

OVERDOSAGE

Signs and Symptoms- Dextromethorphan in toxic doses will cause drowsiness, ataxia, nystagmus, opisthotonos, and convulsive seizures. Overdosage of phenylephrine may be associated with tachycardia, hypertension, and cardiac arrhythmias. The effect on the central nervous system of an overdosage of brompheniramine may vary from depression to stimulation, especially in children. Anticholinergic effects may also occur. ***Treatment***- Induce emesis if patient is alert and is seen by a physician prior to 6 hours following ingestion. Precautions against aspiration must be taken, especially in infants and small children. Gastric lavage may be carried out, although in some instances tracheostomy may be necessary prior to lavage. Naloxone HCl 0.005 mg/kg intravenously may be of value in reversing the CNS depression that may occur from an overdose of Dextromethorphan. CNS stimulants may counter CNS depression. Should CNS hyperactivity or convulsive seizures occur, intravenous short-acting barbiturates may be indicated. Hypertensive responses and/or tachycardia should be treated appropriately. Oxygen, intravenous fluids, and other supportive measures should be employed as indicated.

DOSAGE AND ADMINISTRATION

Adults and Children over 12 years- 2 teaspoonsful (10 mL) every 4 hours. ***Children 6 to 12 years***- 1 teaspoonful (5 mL) every 4 hours. ***Children 2 to 6 years***- ½ teaspoonful (2.5 mL) every 4 hours. ***Children under 2 years***- as directed by a physician. Do not exceed 6 doses during a 24 hour period.

HOW SUPPLIED

NDC 63162-507-16 16 oz (473 mL) bottles, and NDC 63162-507-20 20 mL sample bottles.
Store between 59°-86°F (15°-30°C)
Dispense in tight, light resistant containers as defined by the USP.

KEEP THIS AND ALL MEDICATIONS OUT OF THE REACH OF CHILDREN.
Rx Only
Manufactured in USA for
BALLAY PHARMACEUTICALS, INC.
Wimberley, TX 78676
By
Elge, Inc. Rosenberg, TX 77471 REV 11/01

BALAMINE® DM ORAL DROPS ℞
[*bal'-ə' mīn*]
For Infants

BALAMINE® DM SYRUP ℞
[*bal'-ə' mīn*]
For adults and children (18 months and over)

DESCRIPTION

Antihistamine/Decongestant/Antitussive for oral use

ACTIVE INGREDIENTS

BALAMINE DM ORAL DROPS

Each dropperful (1 mL) contains:
Carbinoxamine Maleate .... 2 mg
Pseudoephedrine Hydrochloride .... 25 mg
Dextromethorphan Hydrobromide .... 3.5 mg

BALAMINE DM SYRUP

Each teaspoonful (5 mL) contains:
Carbinoxamine Maleate .... 4 mg
Pseudoephedrine Hydrochloride .... 60 mg
Dextromethorphan Hydrobromide .... 12.5 mg

INACTIVE INGREDIENTS

BALAMINE DM ORAL DROPS

Citric acid, D&C Red No. 33, FD&C Blue No. 1, glycerin, sodium benzoate, sodium citrate, sorbitol, purified water, flavoring and other ingredients.

BALAMINE DM SYRUP

Citric acid, D&C Red No. 33, FD&C Blue No. 1, glycerin, menthol, povidone, purified water, sodium benzoate, sodium citrate, sorbitol, and flavoring.

Carbinoxamine maleate (2-[p-Chloro-α-[2-(dimethylamino) ethoxyl] benzyl]pyridine maleate) is one of the ethanolamine class of H_1 antihistamines. Pseudoephedrine hydrochloride (Benzenemethanol,α-[1-(methylamino) ethyl]-,[S-R*,R*)]-, hydrochloride) is the hydrochloride of pseudoephedrine, a naturally occurring dextrorotatory stereoisomer of ephedrine. Dextromethorphan Hydrobromide (Morphinan, 3-methoxy-17-methyl-, (9α, 13α, 14α)-, hydrobromide, monohydrate) is the hydrobromide of d-form racemethorphan.

CLINICAL PHARMACOLOGY

Antihistaminic, decongestant and antitussive actions.
Carbinoxamine maleate possesses H_1 antihistaminic activity and mild anticholinergic and sedative effects. Serum half-life for carbinoxamine is estimated to be 10 to 20 hours. Virtually no intact drug is excreted in the urine.
Pseudoephedrine hydrochloride is an oral sympathomimetic amine that acts as a decongestant to respiratory tract mucous membranes. While its vasoconstrictor action is similar to that of ephedrine, pseudoephedrine has less pressor effect in normotensive adults. Serum half-life for pseudoephedrine is 6 to 8 hours. Acidic urine is associated with faster elimination of the drug. About one-half of the administered dose is excreted in the urine.
Dextromethorphan hydrobromide is a nonnarcotic antitussive with effectiveness equal to codeine. It acts in the medulla oblongata to elevate the cough threshold. Dextromethorphan does not produce analgesia or induce tolerance, and has no potential for addiction. At usual doses, it will not depress respiration or inhibit ciliary activity. Dextromethorphan is rapidly metabolized with trace amounts of the parent compound in blood and urine. About one-half of the administered dose is excreted in the urine as conjugated metabolites.

INDICATIONS AND USAGE

For relief of coughs and upper respiratory symptoms, including nasal congestion, associated with allergy or the common cold.

CONTRAINDICATIONS

Patients with hypersensitivity or idiosyncrasy to any of its ingredients. Sympathomimetic amines are contraindicated in patients with severe hypertension, severe coronary artery disease and patients on monoamine oxidase (MAO) inhibitor therapy. Antihistamines are contraindicated in patients with narrow-angle glaucoma, urinary retention, peptic ulcer and during an asthma attack. Dextromethorphan should not be used in patients receiving a monoamine oxidase inhibitor (MAOI) or for 2 weeks after stopping the MAOI drug.

WARNINGS

Sympathomimetic amines should be used judiciously and sparingly in patients with hypertension, diabetes, ischemic heart disease, hyperthyroidism, increased intraocular pressure or prostatic hypertrophy. See Contraindications. Sympathomimetic amines may produce CNS stimulation with convulsions or cardiovascular collapse with accompanying

AGE	DOSE*	FREQUENCY*
Balamine DM Oral Drops		
For Oral Use Only		
1-3 months	1/4 dropperful (1/4 mL)	q.i.d.
3-6 months	1/2 dropperful (1/2 mL)	q.i.d.
6-9 months	3/4 dropperful (3/4 mL)	q.i.d.
9-18 months	1 dropperful (1 mL)	q.i.d.
Balamine DM Syrup		
18 months-6 years	1/2 teaspoonful (2.5 mL)	q.i.d.
adults and children 6 years and over	1 teaspoonful (5 mL)	q.i.d.

* In mild cases or in particularly sensitive patients, less frequent or reduced doses may be adequate.

hypotension. The elderly (60 years and older) are more likely to exhibit adverse reactions. Antihistamines may cause excitability, especially in children. At doses higher than the recommended dose, nervousness, dizziness, or sleeplessness may occur. Do not exceed recommended dosage. Administration of dextromethorphan may be accompanied by histamine release and should be used with caution in atopic children.

PRECAUTIONS

General
Before prescribing medication to suppress or modify cough, identify and provide therapy for the underlying cause of cough and take caution that modification of cough does not increase the risk of clinical or physiologic complications. Dextromethorphan should be used with caution in sedated or debilitated patients and in patients confined to supine positions.
Use with caution in patients with hypertension, heart disease, asthma, hyperthyroidism, increased intraocular pressure, diabetes mellitus and prostatic hypertrophy.
Information for Patients: Avoid alcohol and other CNS depressants while taking these products. Patients sensitive to antihistamines may experience moderate to severe drowsiness. Patients sensitive to sympathomimetic amines may note mild CNS stimulation. While taking these products, exercise care in driving or operating appliances, machinery, etc.
Drug Interactions: Antihistamines may enhance the effects of tricyclic antidepressants, barbiturates, alcohol, and other CNS depressants. MAO inhibitors prolong and intensify the anticholinergic effects of antihistamines.
Sympathomimetic amines may reduce the antihypertensive effects of reserpine, veratrum alkaloids, methyldopa and mecamylamine. Effects of sympathomimetics are increased with MAO inhibitors and beta-adrenergic blockers. The cough-suppressant action of dextromethorphan and narcotic antitussives are additive. Dextromethorphan is contraindicated with monoamine oxidase inhibitors (MAOI). See Contraindications section.
Pregnancy Category C: Animal reproduction studies have not been conducted with Balamine DM. It is also not known whether these products can cause fetal harm when administered to a pregnant woman or affect reproduction capacity. Give to pregnant women only if clearly needed.
Nursing Mothers: It is not known whether the drugs in Balamine DM are excreted in human milk. Because many drugs are excreted in human milk and because of the potential for serious adverse reactions in nursing infants, a decision should be made whether to discontinue nursing or discontinue the product, taking into account the importance of the drug to the mother.

ADVERSE REACTIONS

Antihistamines: Sedation, dizziness, diplopia, vomiting, diarrhea, dry mouth, headache, nervousness, nausea, anorexia, heartburn, weakness, polyuria and dysuria and, rarely, excitability in children. Urinary retention may occur in patients with prostatic hypertrophy.
Sympathomimetic Amines: Convulsions, CNS stimulation, cardiac arrhythmias, respiratory difficulty, increased heart rate or blood pressure, hallucinations, tremors, nervousness, insomnia, weakness, pallor and dysuria.
Dextromethorphan: Drowsiness, dizziness, and GI disturbance.

OVERDOSAGE

No information is available as to specific results of an overdose of these products. The signs, symptoms and treatment described below are those of H_1 antihistamine, ephedrine and dextromethorphan overdose.
Symptoms: Should antihistamine effects predominate, central action constitutes the greatest danger. In the small child, predominant symptoms are excitation, hallucination, ataxia, incoordination, tremors, flushed face and fever.
Convulsions, fixed and dilated pupils, coma and death may occur in severe cases. In the adult, fever and flushing are uncommon; excitement leading to convulsions and postictal depression is often preceded by drowsiness and coma. Respiration is usually not seriously depressed; blood pressure is usually stable.
Should sympathomimetic symptoms predominate, central effects include restlessness, dizziness, tremor, hyperactive reflexes, talkativeness, irritability and insomnia. Cardiovascular and renal effects include difficulty in micturition, headache, flushing, palpitation, cardiac arrhythmias, hypertension with subsequent hypotension and circulatory collapse. Gastrointestinal effects include dry mouth, metallic taste, anorexia, nausea, vomiting, diarrhea, and abdominal cramps.
Dextromethorphan may cause respiratory depression with a large overdose.
Treatment: a) Evacuate stomach as condition warrants. Activated charcoal may be useful. b) Maintain a nonstimulating environment. c) Monitor cardiovascular status. d) Do not give stimulants. e) Reduce fever with cool sponging. f) Treat respiratory depression with naloxone if dextromethorphan toxicity is suspected. g) Use sedatives or anticonvulsants to control CNS excitation and convulsions. h) Physostigmine may reverse anticholinergic symptoms. i) Ammonium chloride may acidify the urine to increase urinary excretion of pseudoephedrine. j) Further care is symptomatic and supportive.

DOSAGE AND ADMINISTRATION

[See table above]

HOW SUPPLIED

Balamine DM Oral Drops, grape flavored, in 30 mL bottles, with calibrated droppers, **NDC** 63162-509-30.
Balamine DM Syrup, grape flavored, in 16 fl. oz. (1-pint) bottles, **NDC** 63162-508-16.
Dispense in USP tight, light-resistant container. Avoid exposure to excessive heat.
Rx ONLY
Revised 12/01
BALLAY
Manufactured for: **Ballay Pharmaceuticals, Inc.**
Wimberley, Tx. 78676
Manufactured by: Elge, Inc.
Rosenberg, Tx. 77471

Barr Laboratories, Inc.
2 QUAKER RD. P.O. BOX 2900
POMONA, NY 10970

Direct Inquiries to:
1-800-BARRLAB (227-7522)

PLAN B® ℞
[*plăn b*]
(Levonorgestrel)
Tablets, 0.75 mg

Plan B® is intended to prevent pregnancy after known or suspected contraceptive failure or unprotected intercourse. Emergency contraceptive pills (like all oral contraceptives) do not protect against infection with HIV (the virus that causes AIDS) and other sexually transmitted diseases.

DESCRIPTION

Emergency contraceptive tablet. Each Plan B® tablet contains 0.75 mg of a single active steroid ingredient, levonorgestrel [18,19-Dinorpregn-4-en-20-yn-3-one-13-ethyl-17-hydroxy-, (17α)-(-)-], a totally synthetic progestogen. The inactive ingredients present are colloidal silicon dioxide, potato starch, gelatin, magnesium stearate, talc, corn starch, and lactose monohydrate. Levonorgestrel has a molecular weight of 312.45, and the following structural and molecular formulas:

$C_{21}H_{28}O_2$

CLINICAL PHARMACOLOGY

Emergency contraceptives are not effective if the woman is already pregnant. Plan B® is believed to act as an emergency contraceptive principally by preventing ovulation or fertilization (by altering tubal transport of sperm and/or

Continued on next page

Plan B—Cont.

ova). In addition, it may inhibit implantation (by altering the endometrium). It is not effective once the process of implantation has begun.

Pharmacokinetics

Absorption

No specific investigation of the absolute bioavailability of Plan B® in humans has been conducted. However, literature indicates that levonorgestrel is rapidly and completely absorbed after oral administration (bioavailability about 100%) and is not subject to first pass metabolism.

After a single dose of Plan B® (0.75 mg) administered to 16 women under fasting conditions, maximum serum concentrations of levonorgestrel are 14.1 ± 7.7 ng/mL (mean ± SD) at an average of 1.6 ± 0.7 hours. No formal study of the effect of food on the absorption of levonorgestrel has been undertaken.

Table 1 Pharmacokinetic Parameter Values Following Single Dose Administration of Plan B® (Levonorgestrel) Tablets, 0.75 mg to Healthy Female Volunteers

N	Mean (± S.D.)					
	C_{max} (ng/mL)	T_{max} (h)	CL (L/h)	V_d (L)	$T_{1/2}$ (h)	$AUC_{0-\infty}$ (ng/mL/h)
16	14.1 ± 7.7	1.6 ± 0.7	7.7 ± 2.7	260.0	24.4 ± 5.3	123.1 ± 50.1

Distribution

Levonorgestrel in serum is primarily protein bound. Approximately 50% is bound to albumin and 47.5% is bound to sex hormone binding globulin (SHBG).

Metabolism

Following a single oral dosage, levonorgestrel does not appear to be extensively metabolized by the liver. The primary metabolites are 3α,5β- and 3α,5∝-tetrahydrolevonorgestrel with 16β-hydroxynorgestrel also identified. Together, these account for less than 10% of parent plasma levels. Urinary metabolites hydroxylated at the 2α and 16β positions have also been identified. Small amounts of the metabolites are present in plasma as sulfate and glucuronide conjugates.

Excretion

The elimination half-life of levonorgestrel following single dose administration as Plan B® (0.75 mg) is 24.4 ± 5.3 hours. Excretion following single dose administration as emergency contraception is unknown, but based on chronic, low-dose contraceptive use, levonorgestrel and its metabolites are primarily excreted in the urine, with smaller amounts recovered in the feces.

Special Populations

Geriatric

This product is not intended for use in geriatric (age 65 years or older) populations and pharmacokinetic data are not available for this population.

Pediatric

This product is not intended for use in pediatric (premenarcheal) populations, and pharmacokinetic data are not available for this population.

Race

No formal studies have evaluated the effect of race. However, clinical trials demonstrated a higher pregnancy rate in the Chinese population with both Plan B® and the Yuzpe regimen (another form of emergency contraception consisting of two doses of ethinyl estradiol 0.1 mg + levonorgestrel 0.5 mg). The reason for this apparent increase in the pregnancy rate of emergency contraceptives in Chinese women is unknown.

Hepatic Insufficiency and Renal Insufficiency

No formal studies have evaluated the effect of hepatic insufficiency or renal insufficiency on the disposition of emergency contraceptive tablets.

Drug-Drug Interactions

No formal studies of drug-drug interactions were conducted.

INDICATIONS & USAGE

Indication

Plan B® is an emergency contraceptive that can be used to prevent pregnancy following unprotected intercourse or a known or suspected contraceptive failure. To obtain optimal efficacy, the first tablet should be taken as soon as possible within 72 hours of intercourse. The second tablet must be taken 12 hours later.

Clinical Studies

A double-blind, controlled clinical trial in 1,955 evaluable women compared the efficacy and safety of Plan B® (one 0.75 mg tablet of levonorgestrel taken within 72 hours of intercourse, and one tablet taken 12 hours later) to the Yuzpe regimen (two tablets of 0.25 mg levonorgestrel and 0.05 mg ethinyl estradiol, taken within 72 hours of intercourse, and two tablets taken 12 hours later). Plan B® was at least as effective as the Yuzpe regimen in preventing pregnancy. After a single act of intercourse, the expected pregnancy rate of 8% (with no contraception) was reduced to approximately 1% with Plan B®. Thus, Plan B® reduced the expected number of pregnancies by 89%.

Emergency contraceptives are not as effective as routine contraception since their failure rate, while low based on a single use, would accumulate over time with repeated use (see Warnings). See Table 2 below.

Table 2 Percentage of Women Experiencing an Unintended Pregnancy During the First Year of Typical Use and the First Year of Perfect Use of Contraception, and the Percentage Continuing Use at the End of the first Year – United States

	% of Women Experiencing an Unintended Pregnancy within the First Year of Use		% of Women Continuing Use at One Year
Method (1)	Typical Use[1] (2)	Perfect Use[2] (3)	(4)[3]
Chance[4]	85	85	
Spermicide[5]	26	6	40
Periodic Abstinence	25		63
Calendar		9	
Ovulation Method		3	
Symptom-thermal[6]		2	
Post-ovulation		1	
Withdrawal	19	4	
Cap[7]			
Parous Women	40	26	42
Nulliparous Women	20	9	56
Sponge			
Parous Women	40	20	42
Nulliparous Women	20	9	56
Diaphragm[7]	20	6	56
Condom[8]			
Female (Reality)	21	5	56
Male	14	3	56
Oral Contraceptives	5		71
Progestin Only		0.5	
Combined		0.1	
IUD			
Progestin T	2.0	1.5	81
Copper T 380A	0.8	0.6	78
LNG	0.1	0.1	81
Depo-Provera	0.3	0.3	
Norplant and Norplant-2	0.05	0.05	88
Female Sterilization	0.5	0.5	100
Male Sterilization	0.15	0.10	100

Emergency Contraceptive Pills: Treatment initiated within 72 hours after unprotected intercourse reduces the risk of pregnancy by at least 75%.

Lactational Amenorrhea Method: LAM is a highly effective temporary method of contraception.[9]

1. Among typical couples who initiate use of a method (not necessarily for the first time) who experience an accidental pregnancy during the first year if they do not stop use for any other reason.
2. Among couples who initiate use of a method (not necessarily for the first time) and who use it perfectly (both consistently and correctly) the percentage who experience an accidental pregnancy during the first year if they do not stop use for any other reason.
3. Among couples attempting to avoid pregnancy, the percentage (column 4) who continue to use a method for 1 year.
4. The percent becoming pregnant in columns (2) and (3) are based on data from populations where contraception is not used and from women who cease using contraception in order to become pregnant. Among such populations, about 89% become pregnant within 1 year among women now relying on reversible methods of contraception if they abandoned contraception altogether.
5. Foams, creams, gels, vaginal suppositories, and vaginal film.
6. Cervical mucus (ovulation) method supplemented by calendar in the pre-ovulatory and basal body temperature in the post-ovulatory phase.
7. With spermicidal cream or jelly.
8. Without spermicides.
9. However, to maintain an effective protection against pregnancy, another method of contraception must be used as soon as menstruation resumes, the frequency or duration of breast feeds is reduced, bottle feeds are introduced, or the baby reaches 6 months of age.

Source: Trussell J. Contraceptive efficacy. In Hatcher RA, Trussell J, Stewart F, Cates W, Stewart GK, Guest F, Kowal D. Contraceptive Technology; Seventeenth Revised Edition. New York, NY: Irvington Publishers, 1998.

CONTRAINDICATIONS

Progestin-only contraceptive pills (POPs) are used as a routine method of birth control over longer periods of time, and are contraindicated in some conditions. It is not known whether these same conditions apply to the Plan B® regimen consisting of the emergency use of two progestin pills. POPs however, are not recommended for use in the following conditions:

- Known or suspected pregnancy
- Hypersensitivity to any component of the product
- Undiagnosed abnormal genital bleeding

WARNINGS

Plan B® is not recommended for routine use as a contraceptive.

Plan B® is not effective in terminating an existing pregnancy.

Effects on Menses

Menstrual bleeding patterns are often irregular among women using progestin-only oral contraceptives and in clinical studies of levonorgestrel for postcoital and emergency contraceptive use. Some women may experience spotting a few days after taking Plan B®. At the time of expected menses, approximately 75% of women using Plan B® had vaginal bleeding similar to their normal menses, 12–13% bled more than usual, and 12% bled less than usual. The majority of women (87%) had their next menstrual period at the expected time or within ± 7 days, while 13% had a delay of more than 7 days beyond the anticipated onset of menses. If there is a delay in the onset of menses beyond 1 week, the possibility of pregnancy should be considered.

Ectopic Pregnancy

Ectopic pregnancies account for approximately 2% of reported pregnancies (19.7 per 1,000 reported pregnancies). Up to 10% of pregnancies reported in clinical studies of routine use of progestin-only contraceptives are ectopic. A history of ectopic pregnancy need not be considered a contraindication to use of this emergency contraceptive method. Health providers, however, should be alert to the possibility of an ectopic pregnancy in women who become pregnant or complain of lower abdominal pain after taking Plan B®.

PRECAUTIONS

Pregnancy

Many studies have found no effects on fetal development associated with long-term use of contraceptive doses of oral progestins (POPs). The few studies of infant growth and development that have been conducted with POPs have not demonstrated significant adverse effects.

STD/HIV

Plan B®, like progestin-only contraceptives, does not protect against HIV infection (AIDS) and other sexually transmitted diseases.

Physical Examination and Follow-up

A physical examination is not required prior to prescribing Plan B®. A follow-up physical or pelvic examination, however, is recommended if there is any doubt concerning the general health or pregnancy status of any woman after taking Plan B®.

Carbohydrate Metabolism

The effects of Plan B® on carbohydrate metabolism are unknown. Some users of progestin-only oral contraceptives (POPs) may experience slight deterioration in glucose tolerance, with increases in plasma insulin; however, women with diabetes mellitus who use POPs do not generally experience changes in their insulin requirements. Nonetheless, diabetic women should be monitored while taking Plan B®.

Drug Interactions

Theoretically, the effectiveness of low-dose progestin-only pills is reduced by hepatic enzyme-inducing drugs such as the anticonvulsants phenytoin, carbamazepine, and barbiturates, and the antituberculosis drug rifampin. No significant interaction has been found with broad-spectrum antibiotics. It is not known whether the efficacy of Plan B® would be affected by these or any other medications.

Nursing Mothers

Small amounts of progestin pass into the breast milk in women taking progestin-only pills for long-term contraception resulting in steroid levels in infant plasma of 1–6% of the levels of maternal plasma. However, no adverse effects due to progestin-only pills have been found on breastfeeding performance, either in the quality or quantity of the milk, or on the health, growth or development of the infant.

Pediatric Use

Safety and efficacy of progestin-only pills have been established in women of reproductive age for long-term contraception. Safety and efficacy are expected to be the same for postpubertal adolescents under the age of 16 and for users 16 years and older. Use of Plan B® emergency contraception before menarche is not indicated.

Fertility Following Discontinuation

The limited available data indicate a rapid return of normal ovulation and fertility following discontinuation of progestin-only pills for emergency contraception and long-term contraception.

ADVERSE REACTIONS

The most common adverse events in the clinical trial for women receiving Plan B® included nausea (23%), abdominal pain (18%), fatigue (17%), headache (17%), and menstrual changes. The table below shows those adverse events that occurred in ≥5% of Plan B® users.

Table 3 Adverse Events in ≥5% of Women, by % Frequency

Most Common Adverse Events	Plan B® Levonorgestrel N=977 (%)
Nausea	23.1
Abdominal Pain	17.6
Fatigue	16.9
Headache	16.8
Heavier Menstrual Bleeding	13.8
Lighter Menstrual Bleeding	12.5
Dizziness	11.2
Breast Tenderness	10.7
Other complaints	9.7
Vomiting	5.6
Diarrhea	5.0

Plan B® demonstrated a superior safety profile over the Yuzpe regimen for the following adverse events:

- Nausea: Occurred in 23% of women taking Plan B® (compared to 50% with Yuzpe)
- Vomiting: Occurred in 6% of women taking Plan B® (compared to 19% with Yuzpe)

DRUG ABUSE AND DEPENDENCE

There is no information about dependence associated with the use of Plan B®.

OVERDOSAGE

There are no data on overdosage of Plan B®, although the common adverse event of nausea and its associated vomiting may be anticipated.

DOSAGE AND ADMINISTRATION

One tablet of Plan B® should be taken orally within 72 hours after unprotected intercourse. The second tablet should be taken 12 hours after the first dose. Efficacy is better if Plan B® is taken as directed as soon as possible after unprotected intercourse. Plan B® can be used at any time during the menstrual cycle.

The user should be instructed that if she vomits within one hour of taking either dose of medication she should contact her health care professional to discuss whether to repeat that dose.

HOW SUPPLIED

Plan B® (Levonorgestrel) Tablets, 0.75 mg are available for a single course of treatment in PVC/aluminum foil blister packages of two tablets each. The tablet is white, round and marked: INOR.

Available as:

Unit-of-use NDC 51285-038-93

Store Plan B® tablets at controlled room temperature, 20° to 25°C (68° to 77°F); excursions permitted between 15° to 30°C (59° to 86°F) [See USP].

Mfg. by Gedeon Richter, Ltd., Budapest, Hungary
for Duramed Pharmaceuticals, Inc.
Subsidiary of Barr Pharmaceuticals, Inc.
Pomona, New York 10970
Phone: 1-800-330-1271 Website: www.go2planb.com
Revised FEBRUARY 2004
BR- 038 / 21000382503

Shown in Product Identification Guide, page 311

SEASONALE® ℞

[sĕ-sŏn-ăl]

(levonorgestrel/ethinyl estradiol tablets)

0.15 mg/0.03 mg

Patients should be counseled that this product does not protect against HIV-infection (AIDS) and other sexually transmitted diseases.

DESCRIPTION

Seasonale® (levonorgestrel/ethinyl estradiol tablets) is an extended-cycle oral contraceptive consisting of 84 pink active tablets each containing 0.15 mg of levonorgestrel, a synthetic progestogen and 0.03 mg of ethinyl estradiol, and 7 white inert tablets (without hormones). The chemical formula of levonorgestrel USP is 18,19-Dinorpregn-4-en-20-yn-3-one, 13-ethyl-17-hydroxy-, (17α)-, (-)-, and the chemical formula of ethinyl estradiol USP is 19-Norpregna-1,3,5(10)-trien-20-yne-3,17-diol, (17α)-. The structural formulas are as follows:

Levonorgestrel
$C_{21}H_{28}O_2$ MW: 312.4

Ethinyl Estradiol
$C_{20}H_{24}O_2$ MW: 296.4

Each pink active tablet contains the following inactive ingredients: anhydrous lactose NF, FD&C blue no. 1, FD&C red no. 40, hydroxypropyl methylcellulose USP, microcrystalline cellulose NF, polyethylene glycol NF, magnesium stearate NF, polysorbate 80 NF, and titanium dioxide USP.

Each white inert tablet contains the following inactive ingredients: anhydrous lactose NF, hydroxypropyl methylcellulose USP, microcrystalline cellulose NF, and magnesium stearate NF.

CLINICAL PHARMACOLOGY

Mode of Action

Combination oral contraceptives act by suppression of gonadotropins. Although the primary mechanism of this action is inhibition of ovulation, other alterations include changes in the cervical mucus (which increase the difficulty of sperm entry into the uterus) and changes in the endometrium (which reduce the likelihood of implantation).

Pharmacokinetics

Absorption

No specific investigation of the absolute bioavailability of Seasonale® in humans has been conducted. However, literature indicates that levonorgestrel is rapidly and completely absorbed after oral administration (bioavailability nearly 100%) and is not subject to first-pass metabolism. Ethinyl estradiol is rapidly and almost completely absorbed from the gastrointestinal tract but, due to first-pass metabolism in gut mucosa and liver, the bioavailability of ethinyl estradiol is approximately 43%.

[See table 1 above]

Table 1: Mean ± SD Pharmacokinetic Parameters Following A Single Dose Administration of Two Tablets of Seasonale® in Healthy Female Subjects Under Fasting Conditions

Analyte	AUC_t (mean ± SD)	C_{max} (mean ± SD)	T_{max} (mean ± SD)	$T_{1/2}$ (mean ± SD)
Levonorgestrel	60.8 ± 25.6 ng*hr/mL	5.6 ± 1.5 ng/mL	1.4 ± 0.3 hours	29.8 ± 8.3 hours
Ethinyl estradiol	1307 ± 361 pg*hr/mL	145 ± 45 pg/mL	1.6 ± 0.5 hours	15.4 ± 3.2 hours

The effect of food on the rate and the extent of levonorgestrel and ethinyl estradiol absorption following oral administration of Seasonale® has not been evaluated.

Distribution

The apparent volume of distribution of levonorgestrel and ethinyl estradiol are reported to be approximately 1.8 L/kg and 4.3 L/kg, respectively. Levonorgestrel is about 97.5-99% protein-bound, principally to sex hormone binding globulin (SHBG) and, to a lesser extent, serum albumin. Ethinyl estradiol is about 95–97% bound to serum albumin. Ethinyl estradiol does not bind to SHBG, but induces SHBG synthesis, which leads to decreased levonorgestrel clearance. Following repeated daily dosing of combination levonorgestrel/ethinyl estradiol oral contraceptives, levonorgestrel plasma concentrations accumulate more than predicted based on single-dose kinetics, due in part, to increased SHBG levels that are induced by ethinyl estradiol, and a possible reduction in hepatic metabolic capacity.

Metabolism

Following absorption, levonorgestrel is conjugated at the 17β-OH position to form sulfate and to a lesser extent, glucuronide conjugates in plasma. Significant amounts of conjugated and unconjugated 3α,5β-tetrahydrolevonorgestrel are also present in plasma, along with much smaller amounts of 3α,5α-tetrahydrolevonorgestrel and 16β-hydroxylevonorgestrel. Levonorgestrel and its phase I metabolites are excreted primarily as glucuronide conjugates. Metabolic clearance rates may differ among individuals by several-fold, and this may account in part for the wide variation observed in levonorgestrel concentrations among users.

First-pass metabolism of ethinyl estradiol involves formation of ethinyl estradiol-3-sulfate in the gut wall, followed by 2-hydroxylation of a portion of the remaining untransformed ethinyl estradiol by hepatic cytochrome P-450 3A4 (CYP3A4). Levels of CYP3A4 vary widely among individuals and can explain the variation in rates of ethinyl estradiol hydroxylation. Hydroxylation at the 4-, 6-, and 16- positions may also occur, although to a much lesser extent than 2-hydroxylation. The various hydroxylated metabolites are subject to further methylation and/or conjugation.

Excretion

About 45% of levonorgestrel and its metabolites are excreted in the urine and about 32% are excreted in feces, mostly as glucuronide conjugates. The terminal elimination half-life for levonorgestrel after a single dose of Seasonale® was about 30 hours.

Ethinyl estradiol is excreted in the urine and feces as glucuronide and sulfate conjugates, and it undergoes enterohepatic recirculation. The terminal elimination half-life of ethinyl estradiol after a single dose of Seasonale® was found to be about 15 hours.

SPECIAL POPULATIONS

Race

No formal studies on the effect of race on the pharmacokinetics of Seasonale® were conducted.

Hepatic Insufficiency

No formal studies have been conducted to evaluate the effect of hepatic disease on the pharmacokinetics of Seasonale®. However, steroid hormones may be poorly metabolized in patients with impaired liver function.

Renal Insufficiency

No formal studies have been conducted to evaluate the effect of renal disease on the pharmacokinetics of Seasonale®.

Drug-Drug Interactions

See PRECAUTIONS section – Drug Interactions.

INDICATIONS AND USAGE

Seasonale® tablets are indicated for the prevention of pregnancy in women who elect to use oral contraceptives as a method of contraception.

In a 1-year controlled clinical trial, 4 pregnancies occurred in women 18-35 years of age during 809 completed 91-day cycles of Seasonale® during which no backup contraception was utilized. This represents an overall use-efficacy (typical user efficacy) pregnancy rate of 1.98 per 100 women-years of use.

Oral contraceptives are highly effective for pregnancy prevention. Table 2 lists the typical unintended pregnancy rates for users of combination oral contraceptives and other methods of contraception. The efficacy of these contraceptive methods, except sterilization, the IUD, and Norplant® Implant System, depends upon the reliability with which they are used. Correct and consistent use of methods can result in lower failure rates.

TABLE 2

Percentage of women experiencing an unintended pregnancy during the first year of typical use and the first year of perfect use of contraception and the percentage continuing use at the end of the first year: United States.

Method (1)	% of Women Experiencing an Unintended Pregnancy within the First Year of Use: Typical Use[1] (2)	Perfect Use[2] (3)	% of Women Continuing Use at One Year[3] (4)
Chance[4]	85	85	
Spermicides[5]	26	6	40
Periodic abstinence	25		63
Calendar		9	
Ovulation method		3	
Sympto-thermal[6]		2	
Post-ovulation		1	
Withdrawal	19	4	
Cap[7]			
Parous women	40	26	42
Nulliparous women	20	9	56
Sponge			
Parous women	40	20	42
Nulliparous women	20	9	56
Diaphragm[7]	20	6	56

Continued on next page

Seasonale—Cont.

Condom[8]			
Female (Reality)	21	5	56
Male	14	3	61
Pill	5		71
Progestin only		0.5	
Combined		0.1	
IUD:			
Progesterone T	2.0	1.5	81
Copper T 380A	0.8	0.6	78
LNg 20	0.1	0.1	81
Depo Provera	0.3	0.3	70
Norplant and Norplant-2	0.05	0.05	88
Female sterilization	0.5	0.5	100
Male sterilization	0.15	0.10	100

Emergency Contraceptive Pills: Treatment initiated within 72 hours after unprotected intercourse reduces the risk of pregnancy by at least 75%.[9]

Lactational Amenorrhea Method: LAM is a highly effective, *temporary* method of contraception.[10]

Source: Trussell J, Contraceptive efficacy. In Hatcher RA, Trussell J, Stewart F, Cates W, Stewart GK, Kowal D, Guest F, Contraceptive Technology: Seventeenth Revised Edition. New York NY: Irvington Publishers, 1998.

[1] Among *typical* couples who initiate use of a method (not necessarily for the first time), the percentage who experience an unintended pregnancy during the first year if they do not stop use for any other reason.

[2] Among couples who initiate use of a method (not necessarily for the first time) and who use it *perfectly* (both consistently and correctly), the percentage who experience an unintended pregnancy during the first year if they do not stop use for any other reason.

[3] Among couples attempting to avoid pregnancy, the percentage who continue to use a method for one year.

[4] The percentages of women becoming pregnant in columns (2) and (3) are based on data from populations where contraception is not used and from women who cease using contraception in order to become pregnant. Among such populations, about 89% become pregnant within one year. This estimate was lowered slightly (to 85%) to represent the percentage who would become pregnant within one year among women now relying on reversible methods of contraception if they abandoned contraception altogether.

[5] Foams, creams, gels, vaginal suppositories and vaginal film.

[6] Cervical mucus (ovulation) method supplemented by calendar in the pre-ovulatory and basal body temperature in the post-ovulatory phases.

[7] With spermicidal cream or jelly.

[8] Without spermicides.

[9] The treatment schedule is one dose within 72 hours after unprotected intercourse and a second dose 12 hours after the first dose. The Food and Drug Administration has declared the following brands of oral contraceptives to be safe and effective for emergency contraception: Ovral (1 dose is 2 white pills), Alesse (1 dose is 5 pink pills), Nordette or Levlen (1 dose is 2 light-orange pills), Lo/Ovral (1 dose is 4 white pills), Triphasil or Tri-Levlen (1 dose is 4 yellow pills).

[10] However, to maintain effective protection against pregnancy, another method of contraception must be used as soon as menstruation resumes, the frequency or duration of breastfeeds is reduced, bottle feeds are introduced or the baby reaches six months of age.

CONTRAINDICATIONS

Oral contraceptives should not be used in women who currently have the following conditions:

- Thrombophlebitis or thromboembolic disorders
- A past history of deep vein thrombophlebitis or thromboembolic disorders
- Cerebrovascular or coronary artery disease (current or history)
- Valvular heart disease with thrombogenic complications
- Uncontrolled hypertension
- Diabetes with vascular involvement
- Headaches with focal neurological symptoms
- Major surgery with prolonged immobilization
- Known or suspected carcinoma of the breast or personal history of breast cancer
- Carcinoma of the endometrium or other known or suspected estrogen-dependent neoplasia
- Undiagnosed abnormal genital bleeding
- Cholestatic jaundice of pregnancy or jaundice with prior pill use
- Hepatic adenomas or carcinomas, or active liver disease
- Known or suspected pregnancy
- Hypersensitivity to any component of this product

WARNINGS

Cigarette smoking increases the risk of serious cardiovascular side effects from oral contraceptive use. This risk increases with age and with heavy smoking (15 or more cigarettes per day) and is quite marked in women over 35 years of age. Women who use oral contraceptives should be strongly advised not to smoke.

The use of oral contraceptives is associated with increased risk of several serious conditions including venous and arterial thrombotic and thromboembolic events (such as myocardial infarction, thromboembolism, and stroke), hepatic neoplasia, gallbladder disease, and hypertension. The risk of serious morbidity or mortality is very small in healthy women without underlying risk factors. The risk of morbidity and mortality increases significantly in the presence of other underlying risk factors such as certain inherited thrombophilias, hypertension, hyperlipidemias, obesity and diabetes.

Practitioners prescribing oral contraceptives should be familiar with the following information relating to these risks. The information contained in this package insert is principally based on studies carried out in patients who used oral contraceptives with higher formulations of estrogens and progestogens than those in common use today. The effect of long-term use of the oral contraceptives with lower doses of both estrogens and progestogens remains to be determined.

Throughout this labeling, epidemiological studies reported are of two types: retrospective or case control studies and prospective or cohort studies. Case control studies provide a measure of the relative risk of a disease, namely, a ratio of the incidence of a disease among oral contraceptive users to that among nonusers. The relative risk does not provide information on the actual clinical occurrence of a disease. Cohort studies provide a measure of attributable risk, which is the difference in the incidence of disease between oral contraceptive users and nonusers. The attributable risk does provide information about the actual occurrence of a disease in the population. For further information, the reader is referred to a text on epidemiological methods.

1. Thromboembolic Disorders and Other Vascular Problems

Use of Seasonale® provides women with more hormonal exposure on a yearly basis than conventional monthly oral contraceptives containing similar strength synthetic estrogens and progestins (an additional 9 weeks per year). While this added exposure may pose an additional risk of thrombotic and thromboembolic disease, studies to date with Seasonale have not suggested an increased risk of these disorders.

a. *Myocardial Infarction:* An increased risk of myocardial infarction has been attributed to oral contraceptive use. This risk is primarily in smokers or women with other underlying risk factors for coronary artery disease such as hypertension, hypercholesterolemia, morbid obesity, and diabetes. The relative risk of heart attack for current oral contraceptive users has been estimated to be two to six. The risk is very low under the age of 30. Smoking in combination with oral contraceptive use has been shown to contribute substantially to the incidence of myocardial infarction in women in their mid-thirties or older with smoking accounting for the majority of excess cases. Mortality rates associated with circulatory disease have been shown to increase substantially in smokers over the age of 35 and nonsmokers over the age of 40 (Figure 1) among women who use oral contraceptives. [See figure 1 at top of next column]

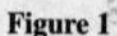
Figure 1

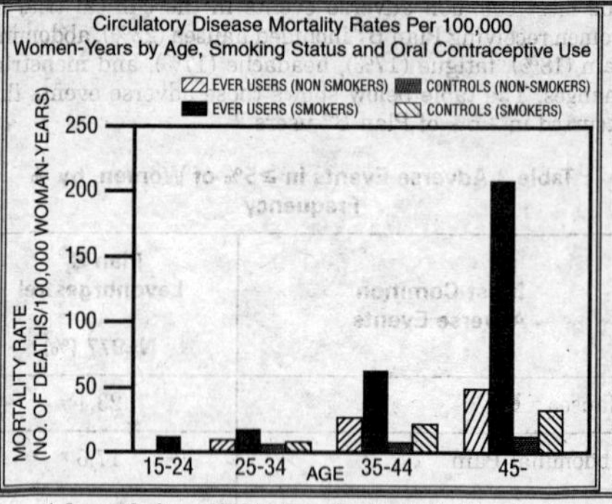

Adapted from P.M. Layde and V. Beral, Lancet, *1*:541–546, 1981

Oral contraceptives may compound the effects of well-known risk factors, such as hypertension, diabetes, hyperlipidemias, age and obesity. In particular, some progestogens are known to decrease HDL cholesterol and cause glucose intolerance, while estrogens may create a state of hyperinsulinism. Oral contraceptives have been shown to increase blood pressure among users (see section 9 in **WARNINGS**). The severity and number of risk factors increase heart disease risk. Oral contraceptives must be used with caution in women with cardiovascular disease risk factors.

b. *Thromboembolism:* An increased risk of thromboembolic and thrombotic disease associated with the use of oral contraceptives is well established. Case control studies have found the relative risk of users compared to non-users to be 3 for the first episode of superficial venous thrombosis, 4 to 11 for deep vein thrombosis or pulmonary embolism, and 1.5 to 6 for women with predisposing conditions for venous thromboembolic disease. Cohort studies have shown the relative risk to be somewhat lower, about 3 for new cases and about 4.5 for new cases requiring hospitalization. The approximate incidence of deep vein thrombosis and pulmonary embolism in users of low dose (<50 µg ethinyl estradiol) combination oral contraceptives is up to 4 per 10,000 woman-years compared to 0.5-3 per 10,000 woman-years for non-users. However, the incidence is less than that associated with pregnancy (6 per 10,000 woman-years). The risk of thromboembolic disease due to oral contraceptives is not related to length of use and disappears after pill use is stopped.

A two- to four-fold increase in relative risk of postoperative thromboembolic complications has been reported with the use of oral contraceptives. The relative risk of venous thrombosis in women who have predisposing conditions is twice that of women without such medical conditions. If feasible, oral contraceptives should be discontinued at least four weeks prior to and for two weeks after elective surgery of a type associated with an increase in risk of thromboembolism and during and following prolonged immobilization. Since the immediate postpartum period is also associated with an increased risk of thromboembolism, oral contraceptives should be started no earlier than four weeks after delivery in women who elect not to breast-feed.

c. *Cerebrovascular Diseases:* Oral contraceptives have been shown to increase both the relative and attributable risks of cerebrovascular events (thrombotic and hemorrhagic strokes), although, in general, the risk is greatest among older (>35 years), hypertensive women who also smoke. Hypertension was found to be a risk factor for both users and nonusers, for both types of strokes, while smoking interacted to increase the risk for hemorrhagic strokes. In a large study, the relative risk of thrombotic strokes has been shown to range from 3 for normotensive users to 14 for users with severe hypertension. The relative risk of hemorrhagic stroke is reported to be 1.2 for nonsmokers who used oral contraceptives, 2.6 for smokers who did not use oral contraceptives, 7.6 for smokers who used oral contraceptives, 1.8 for normotensive users and 25.7 for users with severe hypertension. The attributable risk is also greater in older women. Oral contraceptives also increase the risk for stroke in women with other underlying risk factors such as certain inherited or acquired thrombophilias, hyperlipidemias, and obesity. Women with migraine (particularly migraine with aura) who take combination oral contraceptives may be at an increased risk of stroke.

d. *Dose-Related Risk of Vascular Disease from Oral Contraceptives:* A positive association has been observed between the amount of estrogen and progestogen in oral contraceptives and the risk of vascular disease. A decline in serum high-density lipoproteins (HDL) has been reported with many progestational agents. A decline in serum high-density lipoproteins has been associated with an increased incidence of ischemic heart disease. Because estrogens increase HDL cholesterol, the net effect of an oral contraceptive depends on a balance achieved between doses of estrogen and progestogen and the nature and absolute amount of progestogen used in the contraceptive. The amount of both hormones should be considered in the choice of an oral contraceptive.

Minimizing exposure to estrogen and progestogen is in keeping with good principles of therapeutics. For any particular estrogen/progestogen combination, the dosage regimen prescribed should be one which contains the least amount of estrogen and progestogen that is compatible with a low failure rate and the needs of the individual patient. New acceptors of oral contraceptive agents should be started on preparations containing the lowest estrogen content which is judged appropriate for the individual patient.

e. *Persistence of Risk of Vascular Disease:* There are two studies which have shown persistence of risk of vascular disease for ever-users of oral contraceptives. In a study in the United States, the risk of developing myocardial infarction after discontinuing oral contraceptives persists for at least 9 years for women 40 to 49 years old who had used oral contraceptives for five or more years, but this increased risk was not demonstrated in other age groups. In another study in Great Britain, the risk of developing cerebrovascular disease persisted for at least 6 years after discontinuation of oral contraceptives, although excess risk was very small. However, both studies were performed with oral contraceptive formulations containing 50 micrograms or higher of estrogens.

2. Estimates of Mortality from Contraceptive Use
One study gathered data from a variety of sources which have estimated the mortality rate associated with different methods of contraception at different ages (Table 3). These estimates include the combined risk of death associated with contraceptive methods plus the risk attributable to pregnancy in the event of method failure. Each method of contraception has its specific benefits and risks. The study concluded that with the exception of oral contraceptive users 35 and older who smoke and 40 and older who do not smoke, mortality associated with all methods of birth control is less than that associated with childbirth. The observation of a possible increase in risk of mortality with age for oral contraceptive users is based on data gathered in the 1970's--but not reported until 1983. However, current clinical practice involves the use of lower estrogen dose formulations combined with careful restriction of oral contraceptive use to women who do not have the various risk factors listed in this labeling. Because of these changes in practice and, also, because of some limited new data which suggest that the risk of cardiovascular disease with the use of oral contraceptives may now be less than previously observed, the Fertility and Maternal Health Drugs Advisory Committee was asked to review the topic in 1989. The Committee concluded that although cardiovascular disease risks may be increased with oral contraceptive use after age 40 in healthy nonsmoking women (even with the newer low-dose formulations), there are greater potential health risks associated with pregnancy in older women and with the alternative surgical and medical procedures which may be necessary if such women do not have access to effective and acceptable means of contraception.
Therefore, the Committee recommended that the benefits of oral contraceptive use by healthy nonsmoking women over 40 may outweigh the possible risks. Of course, older women, as all women who take oral contraceptives, should take the lowest possible dose formulation that is effective.

TABLE 3: ANNUAL NUMBER OF BIRTH-RELATED OR METHOD-RELATED DEATHS ASSOCIATED WITH CONTROL OF FERTILITY PER 100,000 NONSTERILE WOMEN, BY FERTILITY-CONTROL METHOD AND ACCORDING TO AGE

Method of control and outcome	AGE 15-19	20-24	25-29	30-34	35-39	40-44
No fertility-control methods*	7.0	7.4	9.1	14.8	25.7	28.2
Oral contraceptives non-smoker**	0.3	0.5	0.9	1.9	13.8	31.6
Oral contraceptives smoker**	2.2	3.4	6.6	13.5	51.1	117.2
IUD**	0.8	0.8	1.0	1.0	1.4	1.4
Condom*	1.1	1.6	0.7	0.2	0.3	0.4
Diaphragm/ spermicide*	1.9	1.2	1.2	1.3	2.2	2.8
Periodic abstinence*	2.5	1.6	1.6	1.7	2.9	3.6

* Deaths are birth related
** Deaths are method related

Adapted from H.W. Ory, Family Planning Perspectives, *15*: 57-63, 1983.

3. Carcinoma of the Reproductive Organs and Breasts
Numerous epidemiological studies have been performed on the incidence of breast, endometrial, ovarian and cervical cancer in women using oral contraceptives. Although the risk of having breast cancer diagnosed may be slightly increased among current and recent users of combined oral contraceptives (RR=1.24), this excess risk decreases over time after combination oral contraceptive discontinuation and by 10 years after cessation the increased risk disappears. The risk does not increase with duration of use and no consistent relationships have been found with dose or type of steroid. The patterns of risk are also similar regardless of a woman's reproductive history or her family breast cancer history. The subgroup for whom risk has been found to be significantly elevated is women who first used oral contraceptives before age 20, but because breast cancer is so rare at these young ages, the number of cases attributable to this early oral contraceptive use is extremely small. Breast cancers diagnosed in current or previous oral contraceptive users tend to be less clinically advanced than in never-users. Women who currently have or have had breast cancer should not use oral contraceptives because breast cancer is a hormone sensitive tumor.
Some studies suggest that oral contraceptive use has been associated with an increase in the risk of cervical intraepithelial neoplasia or invasive cervical cancer in some populations of women. However, there continues to be controversy about the extent to which such findings may be due to differences in sexual behavior and other factors. In spite of many studies of the relationship between oral contraceptive use and breast cancer and cervical cancers, a cause-and-effect relationship has not been established.

4. Hepatic Neoplasia
Benign hepatic adenomas are associated with oral contraceptive use, although their occurrence is rare in the United States. Indirect calculations have estimated the attributable risk to be in the range of 3.3 cases/100,000 for users, a risk that increases after four or more years of use. Rupture of hepatic adenomas may cause death through intra-abdominal hemorrhage.
Studies from Britain have shown an increased risk of developing hepatocellular carcinoma in long-term (>8 years) oral contraceptive users. However, these cancers are extremely rare in the U.S., and the attributable risk (the excess incidence) of liver cancers in oral contraceptive users approaches less than one per million users.

5. Ocular Lesions
There have been clinical case reports of retinal thrombosis associated with the use of oral contraceptives that may lead to partial or complete loss of vision. Oral contraceptives should be discontinued if there is unexplained partial or complete loss of vision; onset of proptosis or diplopia; papilledema; or retinal vascular lesions. Appropriate diagnostic and therapeutic measures should be undertaken immediately.

6. Oral contraceptive Use Before or During Early Pregnancy
Because women using Seasonale® will likely have withdrawal bleeding only 4 times per year, pregnancy should be ruled out at the time of any missed menstrual period (see **DOSAGE AND ADMINISTRATION** section). Oral contraceptive use should be discontinued if pregnancy is confirmed.
Extensive epidemiological studies have revealed no increased risk of birth defects in women who have used oral contraceptives prior to pregnancy. Studies also do not suggest a teratogenic effect, particularly in so far as cardiac anomalies and limb-reduction defects are concerned, when taken inadvertently during early pregnancy (see **CONTRAINDICATIONS** section).
The administration of oral contraceptives to induce withdrawal bleeding should not be used as a test for pregnancy. Oral contraceptives should not be used during pregnancy to treat threatened or habitual abortion.

7. Gallbladder Disease
Earlier studies have reported an increased lifetime relative risk of gallbladder surgery in users of oral contraceptives and estrogens. More recent studies, however, have shown that the relative risk of developing gallbladder disease among oral contraceptive users may be minimal. The recent findings of minimal risk may be related to the use of oral contraceptive formulations containing lower hormonal doses of estrogens and progestogens.

8. Carbohydrate and Lipid Metabolic Effects
Oral contraceptives have been shown to cause glucose intolerance in a significant percentage of users. Oral contraceptives containing greater than 75 micrograms of estrogens cause hyperinsulinism, while lower doses of estrogen cause less glucose intolerance. Progestogens increase insulin secretion and create insulin resistance, this effect varying with different progestational agents. However, in the nondiabetic woman, oral contraceptives appear to have no effect on fasting blood glucose. Because of these demonstrated effects, prediabetic and diabetic women should be carefully observed while taking oral contraceptives.
A small proportion of women will have persistent hypertriglyceridemia while on the pill. As discussed earlier (see **WARNINGS** 1a. and 1d.), changes in serum triglycerides and lipoprotein levels have been reported in oral contraceptive users.

9. Elevated Blood Pressure
Women with significant hypertension should not be started on hormonal contraceptive. An increase in blood pressure has been reported in women taking oral contraceptives and this increase is more likely in older oral contraceptive users and with continued use. Data from the Royal College of General Practitioners and subsequent randomized trials have shown that the incidence of hypertension increases with increasing concentrations of progestogens.
Women with a history of hypertension or hypertension-related diseases, or renal disease should be encouraged to use another method of contraception. If women with hypertension elect to use oral contraceptives, they should be monitored closely, and if significant elevation of blood pressure occurs, oral contraceptives should be discontinued (see **CONTRAINDICATIONS** section). For most women, elevated blood pressure will return to normal after stopping oral contraceptives, and there is no difference in the occurrence of hypertension among ever- and never-users.

10. Headache
The onset or exacerbation of migraine or development of headache with a new pattern that is recurrent, persistent, or severe requires discontinuation of oral contraceptives and evaluation of the cause. (See **WARNINGS**, 1c.)

11. Bleeding Irregularities
When prescribing Seasonale®, the convenience of fewer planned menses (4 per year instead of 13 per year) should be weighed against the inconvenience of increased intermenstrual bleeding and/or spotting.
The clinical trial (SEA 301) that compared the efficacy of Seasonale® (91-day cycles) to an equivalent dosage 28-day cycle regimen also assessed intermenstrual bleeding. The participants in the study were composed primarily of women who had used oral contraceptives previously as opposed to new users. Women with a history of breakthrough bleeding/spotting ≥ 10 consecutive days on oral contraceptives were excluded from the study. More Seasonale® subjects, compared to subjects on the 28-day cycle regimen, discontinued prematurely for unacceptable bleeding (7.7% [Seasonale®] vs. 1.8% [28-day cycle regimen]).
Table 4 shows the percentages of women with ≥ 7 days and ≥ 20 days of intermenstrual spotting and/or bleeding in the Seasonale® and the 28-day cycle treatment groups.

Table 4. Percentage of Subjects with Intermenstrual Bleeding and/or Spotting

Days of intermenstrual bleeding and/or spotting	Percentage of Subjects*	
Seasonale®	Cycle 1 (N=385)	Cycle 4 (N=261)
≥ 7 days	65%	42%
≥ 20 days	35%	15%
28-day regimen	Cycles 1-4 (N=194)	Cycles 10-13 (N=158)
≥ 7 days	38%	39%
≥ 20 days	6%	4%

* Based on spotting and/or bleeding on days 1-84 of a 91 day cycle in the Seasonale subjects and days 1-21 of a 28 day cycle over 4 cycles in the 28-day dosing regimen.

Total days of bleeding and/or spotting (withdrawal plus intermenstrual) were similar over one year of treatment for Seasonale® subjects and subjects on the 28-day cycle regimen.
As in any case of bleeding irregularities, nonhormonal causes should always be considered and adequate diagnostic measures taken to rule out malignancy or pregnancy.
In the event of amenorrhea, pregnancy should be ruled out. Some women may encounter post-pill amenorrhea or oligomenorrhea (possibly with anovulation), especially when such a condition was preexistent.

PRECAUTIONS

1. Sexually Transmitted Diseases
Patients should be counseled that this product does not protect against HIV infection (AIDS) and other sexually transmitted diseases.

2. Physical Examination and Follow-up
A periodic history and physical examination are appropriate for all women, including women using oral contraceptives. The physical examination, however, may be deferred until after initiation of oral contraceptives if requested by the woman and judged appropriate by the clinician. The physical examination should include special reference to blood pressure, breasts, abdomen and pelvic organs, including cervical cytology, and relevant laboratory tests. In case of undiagnosed, persistent or recurrent abnormal vaginal bleeding, appropriate diagnostic measures should be conducted to rule out malignancy. Women with a strong family history of breast cancer or who have breast nodules should be monitored with particular care.

3. Lipid Disorders
Women who are being treated for hyperlipidemias should be followed closely if they elect to use oral contraceptives. Some progestogens may elevate LDL levels and may render the control of hyperlipidemias more difficult. (See **WARNINGS** 1d.)
In patients with familial defects of lipoprotein metabolism receiving estrogen-containing preparations, there have been case reports of significant elevations of plasma triglycerides leading to pancreatitis.

4. Liver Function
If jaundice develops in any woman receiving such drugs, the medication should be discontinued. Steroid hormones may be poorly metabolized in patients with impaired liver function.

5. Fluid Retention
Oral contraceptives may cause some degree of fluid retention. They should be prescribed with caution, and only with careful monitoring, in patients with conditions, which might be aggravated by fluid retention.

6. Emotional Disorders
Women with a history of depression should be carefully observed and the drug discontinued if depression recurs to a serious degree. Patients becoming significantly depressed

Continued on next page

Seasonale—Cont.

while taking oral contraceptives should stop the medication and use an alternate method of contraception in an attempt to determine whether the symptom is drug related.

7. Contact Lenses

Contact-lens wearers who develop visual changes or changes in lens tolerance should be assessed by an ophthalmologist.

8. Drug Interactions

Changes in contraceptive effectiveness associated with co-administration of other products

a. Anti-infective agents and anticonvulsants

Contraceptive effectiveness may be reduced when hormonal contraceptives are co-administered with antibiotics, anticonvulsants, and other drugs that increase the metabolism of contraceptive steroids. This could result in unintended pregnancy or breakthrough bleeding. Examples include rifampin, barbiturates, phenylbutazone, phenytoin, carbamazepine, felbamate, oxcarbazepine, topiramate, and griseofulvin. Several cases of contraceptive failure and breakthrough bleeding have been reported in the literature with concomitant administration of antibiotics such as ampicillin and tetracyclines. However, clinical pharmacology studies investigating drug interaction between combined oral contraceptives and these antibiotics have reported inconsistent results.

b. Anti-HIV protease inhibitors

Several of the anti-HIV protease inhibitors have been studied with co-administration of oral combination hormonal contraceptives; significant changes (increase and decrease) in the plasma levels of the estrogen and progestin have been noted in some cases. The safety and efficacy of combination oral contraceptive products may be affected with co-administration of anti-HIV protease inhibitors. Healthcare providers should refer to the label of the individual anti-HIV protease inhibitors for further drug-drug interaction information.

c. Herbal products

Herbal products containing St. John's Wort (hypericum perforatum) may induce hepatic enzymes (cytochrome P450) and p-glycoprotein transporter and may reduce the effectiveness of contraceptive steroids. This may also result in breakthrough bleeding.

Increase in plasma levels of estradiol associated with co-administered drugs

Co-administration of atorvastatin and certain combination oral contraceptives containing ethinyl estradiol increase AUC values for ethinyl estradiol by approximately 20%. Ascorbic acid and acetaminophen may increase plasma ethinyl estradiol levels, possibly by inhibition of conjugation. CYP 3A4 inhibitors such as itraconazole or ketoconazole may increase plasma hormone levels.

Changes in plasma levels of co-administered drugs

Combination hormonal contraceptives containing some synthetic estrogens (e.g., ethinyl estradiol) may inhibit the metabolism of other compounds. Increased plasma concentrations of cyclosporin, prednisolone, and theophylline have been reported with concomitant administration of combination oral contraceptives. Decreased plasma concentrations of acetaminophen and increased clearance of temazepam, salicylic acid, morphine and clofibric acid, due to induction of conjugation have been noted when these drugs were administered with combination oral contraceptives.

9. Interactions with Laboratory Tests

Certain endocrine and liver function tests and blood components may be affected by oral contraceptives:

a) Increased prothrombin and factors VII, VIII, IX, and X; decreased antithrombin 3; increased norepinephrine-induced platelet aggregability.

b) Increased thyroid-binding globulin (TBG) leading to increased circulating total thyroid hormone, as measured by protein-bound iodine (PBI), T4 by column or by radioimmunoassay. Free T3 resin uptake is decreased, reflecting the elevated TBG, free T4 concentration is unaltered.

c) Other binding proteins may be elevated in serum.

d) Sex hormone binding globulins are increased and result in elevated levels of total circulating sex steroids and corticoids; however, free or biologically active levels remain unchanged.

e) Triglycerides may be increased and levels of various other lipids and lipoproteins may be affected.

f) Glucose tolerance may be decreased.

g) Serum folate levels may be depressed by oral contraceptive therapy. This may be of clinical significance if a woman becomes pregnant shortly after discontinuing oral contraceptives.

10. Carcinogenesis

See **WARNINGS** section.

11. Pregnancy

Pregnancy Category X. See **CONTRAINDICATIONS** and **WARNINGS** sections.

12. Nursing Mothers

Small amounts of oral contraceptive steroids and/or metabolites have been identified in the milk of nursing mothers, and a few adverse effects on the child have been reported, including jaundice and breast enlargement. In addition, oral contraceptives given in the postpartum period may interfere with lactation by decreasing the quantity and quality of breast milk. If possible, the nursing mother should be advised not to use oral contraceptives but to use other forms of contraception until she has completely weaned her child.

13. Pediatric Use:

Safety and efficacy of Seasonale® tablets have been established in women of reproductive age. Safety and efficacy are expected to be the same in postpubertal adolescents under the age of 16 and users 16 and older. Use of Seasonale® before menarche is not indicated.

14. Geriatric Use:

Seasonale® tablets have not been studied in women who have reached menopause.

INFORMATION FOR THE PATIENT

See Patient Labeling Printed Below.

ADVERSE REACTIONS

An increased risk of the following serious adverse reactions has been associated with the use of oral contraceptives (see **WARNINGS** section):

- Thrombophlebitis
- Arterial thromboembolism
- Pulmonary embolism
- Myocardial infarction
- Cerebral hemorrhage
- Cerebral thrombosis
- Hypertension
- Gallbladder disease
- Hepatic adenomas or benign liver tumors

There is evidence of an association between the following conditions and the use of oral contraceptives:

- Mesenteric thrombosis
- Retinal thrombosis

The following adverse reactions have been reported in patients receiving oral contraceptives and are believed to be drug related:

- Nausea
- Vomiting
- Gastrointestinal symptoms (such as abdominal cramps and bloating)
- Breakthrough bleeding
- Spotting
- Change in menstrual flow
- Amenorrhea
- Temporary infertility after discontinuation of treatment
- Edema/fluid retention
- Melasma/chloasma which may persist
- Breast changes: tenderness, enlargement, and secretion
- Change in weight or appetite (increase or decrease)
- Change in cervical ectropion and secretion
- Possible diminution in lactation when given immediately postpartum
- Cholestatic jaundice
- Migraine headache
- Rash (allergic)
- Mood changes, including depression
- Vaginitis, including candidiasis
- Change in corneal curvature (steepening)
- Intolerance to contact lenses
- Decrease in serum folate levels
- Exacerbation of systemic lupus erythematosus
- Exacerbation of porphyria
- Exacerbation of chorea
- Aggravation of varicose veins
- Anaphylactic/anaphylactoid reactions, including urticaria, angioedema, and severe reactions with respiratory and circulatory symptoms

The following adverse reactions have been reported in users of oral contraceptives and the association has been neither confirmed nor refuted:

- Premenstrual syndrome
- Cataracts
- Optic neuritis which may lead to partial or complete loss of vision
- Cystitis-like syndrome
- Headache
- Nervousness
- Dizziness
- Hirsutism
- Loss of scalp hair
- Erythema multiforme
- Erythema nodosum
- Hemorrhagic eruption
- Impaired renal function
- Hemolytic uremic syndrome
- Budd-Chiari syndrome
- Acne
- Changes in libido
- Colitis
- Pancreatitis
- Dysmenorrhea

OVERDOSAGE

Serious ill effects have not been reported following acute ingestion of large doses of oral contraceptives by young children. Overdosage may cause nausea, and withdrawal bleeding may occur in females.

NONCONTRACEPTIVE HEALTH BENEFITS

The following noncontraceptive health benefits related to the use of oral contraceptives are supported by epidemiological studies which largely utilized oral contraceptive formulations containing doses exceeding 0.035 mg of ethinyl estradiol or 0.05 mg of mestranol.

Effects on menses:

- May decrease blood loss and may decrease incidence of iron-deficiency anemia
- May decrease incidence of dysmenorrhea

Effects related to inhibition of ovulation:

- May decrease incidence of functional ovarian cysts
- May decrease incidence of ectopic pregnancies

Effects from long-term use:

- May decrease incidence of fibroadenomas and fibrocystic disease of the breast
- May decrease incidence of acute pelvic inflammatory disease
- May decrease incidence of endometrial cancer
- May decrease incidence of ovarian cancer

DOSAGE AND ADMINISTRATION

Although the occurrence of pregnancy is unlikely if Seasonale® is taken according to directions, if withdrawal bleeding does not occur while taking white (inactive) tablets, the possibility of pregnancy must be considered. Appropriate diagnostic measures to rule out pregnancy should be taken at the time of any missed menstrual period. Seasonale should be discontinued if pregnancy is confirmed. The dosage of Seasonale® is one pink (active) tablet daily for 84 consecutive days, followed by 7 days of white (inert) tablets. To achieve maximum contraceptive effectiveness, Seasonale® must be taken exactly as directed and at intervals not exceeding 24 hours. Ideally, the tablets should be taken at the same time of the day on each day of active treatment. The tablets should not be removed from the protective blister packaging and outer plastic dispenser to avoid damage to the product. The plastic dispenser should be kept in the foil pouch until dispensed to the patient.

During the first cycle of medication, the patient is instructed to begin taking Seasonale® on the first Sunday after the onset of menstruation. If menstruation begins on a Sunday, the first tablet (pink) is taken that day. One pink tablet should be taken daily for 84 consecutive days, followed by 7 days on which a white (inert) tablet is taken. Withdrawal bleeding should occur during the 7 days following discontinuation of pink active tablets. During the first cycle, contraceptive reliance should not be placed on Seasonale® until a pink (active) tablet has been taken daily for 7 consecutive days and a non-hormonal back-up method of birth control (such as condoms or spermicide) should be used during those 7 days. The possibility of ovulation and conception prior to initiation of medication should be considered.

The patient begins her next and all subsequent 91-day courses of tablets without interruption on the same day of the week (Sunday) on which she began her first course, following the same schedule: 84 days on which pink tablets are taken followed by 7 days on which white tablets are taken. If in any cycle the patient starts tablets later than the proper day, she should protect herself against pregnancy by using a non-hormonal back-up method of birth control until she has taken a pink tablet daily for 7 consecutive days.

If spotting or breakthrough bleeding occurs, the patient is instructed to continue on the same regimen. This type of bleeding may be transient and without significance; however, if the bleeding is persistent or prolonged, the patient is advised to consult her healthcare provider.

For patient instructions regarding missed pills, see the **"WHAT TO DO IF YOU MISS PILLS"** section in the **DETAILED PATIENT LABELING**. Any time the patient misses two or more pink tablets, she should also use another method of non-hormonal back-up contraception until she has taken a pink tablet daily for seven consecutive days. If the patient misses one or more white tablets, she is still protected against pregnancy provided she begins taking pink tablets again on the proper day. The possibility of ovulation increases with each successive day that scheduled pink tablets are missed. The risk of pregnancy increases with each active (pink) tablet missed.

In the nonlactating mother, Seasonale® may be initiated no earlier than day 28 postpartum, for contraception due to the increased risk for thromboembolism. When the tablets are administered in the postpartum period, the increased risk of thromboembolic disease associated with the postpartum period must be considered (See **CONTRAINDICATIONS**, **WARNINGS** and **PRECAUTIONS** concerning thromboembolic disease). The patient should be advised to use a nonhormonal back-up method for the first 7 days of tablet-taking. However, if intercourse has already occurred, the possibility of ovulation and conception prior to initiation of medication should be considered. Seasonale® may be initiated immediately after a first-trimester abortion; if the patient starts Seasonale® immediately, additional contraceptive measures are not needed.

HOW SUPPLIED

Seasonale® tablets (levonorgestrel/ethinyl estradiol tablets) 0.15 mg/0.03 mg are available in Extended-Cycle Tablet Dispensers (**NDC 51285-058-66**), each containing a 13-week supply of tablets: 84 pink tablets, each containing 0.15 mg of levonorgestrel and 0.03 mg ethinyl estradiol, and 7 white inert tablets. The active pink tablets are round, film-coated, biconvex, unscored tablets with a debossed ***S*** on one side and **62** on the other side. The inert tablets are white, round, biconvex, unscored tablet debossed with ***S*** on one side and **197** on the other side. Store at controlled room temperature 20°–25° C (68°–77° F) [See USP].

References available upon request.

Brief Summary Patient Package Insert

This product (like all oral contraceptives) is intended to prevent pregnancy. It does not protect against HIV infection (AIDS) and other sexually transmitted diseases such as chlamydia, genital herpes, genital warts, gonorrhea, hepatitis B, and syphilis.

Oral contraceptives, also known as "birth control pills" or "the pill", are taken to prevent pregnancy, and when taken correctly, have a failure rate of approximately 1.0% per year (1 pregnancy per 100 women per year of use). The typical failure rate of pill users is approximately 5% per year when women who miss pills are included.

For the majority of women, oral contraceptives can be taken safely. But for some women oral contraceptive use is associated with certain serious diseases that can be life-threatening or may cause temporary or permanent disability or death. The risks associated with taking oral contraceptives increase significantly if you:

- smoke
- have high blood pressure, diabetes, high cholesterol or are obese
- have or have had clotting disorders, heart attack, stroke, angina pectoris, cancer of the breast or sex organs, jaundice, or malignant or benign liver tumors

You should not take the pill if you are pregnant.

Although cardiovascular disease risks may be increased with oral contraceptive use after age 40 in healthy, nonsmoking women (even with the newer low-dose formulations), there are also greater potential health risks associated with pregnancy in older women.

Cigarette smoking increases the risk of serious cardiovascular side effects from oral contraceptive use. This risk increases with age and with the amount of smoking (15 or more cigarettes per day has been associated with a significantly increased risk) and is quite marked in women over 35 years of age. Women who use oral contraceptives should not smoke.

Most side effects of the pill are not serious. The most common are nausea, vomiting, bleeding or spotting between menstrual periods, weight gain, breast tenderness, and difficulty wearing contact lenses. Some of these side effects, especially nausea and vomiting, may subside within the first 3 months of use.

The serious side effects of the pill occur very infrequently, especially if you are in good health and do not smoke. However, you should know that the following medical conditions have been associated with or made worse by the pill:

1. Blood clots in the legs (thrombophlebitis), lungs (pulmonary embolism), stoppage or rupture of a blood vessel in the brain (stroke), blockage of blood vessels in the heart (heart attack or angina pectoris) or other organs of the body. As mentioned above, smoking increases the risk of heart attacks and strokes and subsequent serious medical consequences. Women with migraine also may be at increased risk of stroke when taking the pill.
2. Liver tumors, which may rupture and cause severe bleeding. A possible but not definite association has been found with the pill and liver cancer. However, liver cancers are extremely rare. The chance of developing liver cancer from using the pill is thus even rarer.
3. High blood pressure, although blood pressure usually returns to normal when the pill is stopped.

The symptoms associated with these serious side effects are discussed in the detailed patient information leaflet. Notify your healthcare provider if you notice any unusual physical disturbances while taking the pill. In addition, drugs such as rifampin, as well as some anticonvulsants and some antibiotics, and herbal preparations containing St. John's Wort (hypericum perforatum) may decrease oral contraceptive effectiveness.

Breast cancer has been diagnosed slightly more often in women who use the pill than in women of the same age who do not use the pill. This very small increase in the number of breast cancer diagnoses gradually disappears during the 10 years after stopping use of the pill. It is not known whether the difference is caused by the pill. It maybe that women taking the pill were examined more often, so that breast cancer was more likely to be detected. You should have regular breast examinations by a healthcare provider and examine your own breasts monthly. Tell your healthcare provider if you have a family history of breast cancer or if you have had breast nodules or an abnormal mammogram. Women who currently have or have had breast cancer should not use hormonal contraceptives because breast cancer is usually a hormone-sensitive tumor.

Some studies have found an increase in the incidence of cancer or precancerous lesions of the cervix in women who use the pill. However, this finding may be related to factors other than the use of the pill.

Be sure to discuss any medical condition you may have with your healthcare provider. Your healthcare provider will take a medical and family history before prescribing oral contraceptives and will examine you. The physical examination may be delayed to another time if you request it and the healthcare provider believes that it is appropriate to postpone it. You should be reexamined at least once a year while taking oral contraceptives. The detailed patient information leaflet gives you further information, which you should read and discuss with your healthcare provider.

What You Should Know About Your Menstrual Cycle When Taking Seasonale®

When you take Seasonale®, which has a 91-day treatment cycle, you should expect to have 4 menstrual periods per year (bleeding when you are taking the 7 white pills). However, you also should expect to have more bleeding or spotting between your menstrual periods than if you were taking an oral contraceptive with a 28-day treatment cycle. During the first Seasonale® treatment cycle, about 1 in 3 women may have 20 or more days of unplanned bleeding or spotting (bleeding when you are taking pink pills). This bleeding or spotting tends to decrease during later cycles. Do not stop Seasonale® because of the bleeding. If the spotting continues for more than 7 consecutive days or if the bleeding is heavy, call your healthcare provider.

If You Miss Your Menstrual Period When Taking Seasonale

You should consider the possibility that you are pregnant if you miss your menstrual period (no bleeding on the days that you are taking white tablets). Since scheduled menstrual periods are less frequent when you are taking Seasonale®, notify your healthcare provider that you have missed your period and are taking Seasonale®. Also notify your healthcare provider if you have symptoms of pregnancy such as morning sickness or unusual breast tenderness. It is important that your healthcare provider evaluates you to determine if you are pregnant. Stop taking Seasonale® if it is determined that you are pregnant.

HOW TO TAKE SEASONALE®

IMPORTANT POINTS TO REMEMBER *BEFORE* YOU START TAKING SEASONALE®

1. BE SURE TO READ THESE DIRECTIONS:
   - Before you start taking your pills.
   - Anytime you are not sure what to do.
2. THE RIGHT WAY TO TAKE SEASONALE® IS TO TAKE ONE PILL EVERY DAY AT THE SAME TIME.
   If you miss pills you could get pregnant. This includes starting the pack late. The more pills you miss, the more likely you are to get pregnant.
3. MANY WOMEN MAY FEEL SICK TO THEIR STOMACH DURING THE FIRST FEW WEEKS OF TAKING PILLS.
   If you feel sick to your stomach, do not stop taking the pill. The problem will usually go away. If it doesn't go away, check with your healthcare provider.
4. MANY WOMEN HAVE SPOTTING OR LIGHT BLEEDING DURING THE FIRST FEW MONTHS OF TAKING SEASONALE®. **Do not stop taking your pills even if you are having irregular bleeding.** If the bleeding lasts for more than 7 consecutive days, talk to your healthcare provider.
5. MISSING PILLS CAN ALSO CAUSE SPOTTING OR LIGHT BLEEDING, even when you make up these missed pills. On the days you take 2 pills to make up for missed pills, you could also feel a little sick to your stomach.
6. IF YOU HAVE VOMITING OR DIARRHEA, or IF YOU TAKE SOME MEDICINES, including some antibiotics and the herbal supplement St. John's Wort, Seasonale may not work as well. Use a back-up method (such as condoms or spermicides) until you check with your healthcare provider.
7. IF YOU HAVE TROUBLE REMEMBERING TO TAKE SEASONALE®, talk to your healthcare provider about how to make pill-taking easier or about using another method of birth control.
8. IF YOU HAVE ANY QUESTIONS OR ARE UNSURE ABOUT THE INFORMATION IN THIS LEAFLET, call your healthcare provider.

***BEFORE* YOU START TAKING SEASONALE®**

1. DECIDE WHAT TIME OF DAY YOU WANT TO TAKE YOUR PILL. It is important to take it at about the same time every day.
2. LOOK AT YOUR EXTENDED-CYCLE TABLET DISPENSER. Your Tablet Dispenser consists of 3 trays with cards that hold 91 individually sealed pills (a 13-week or 91-day cycle). The 91 pills consist of 84 pink pills (active pills with hormones) and 7 white pills (inactive pills without hormone). Trays 1 and 2 each contain 28 pink pills (4 rows of 7 pills). Tray 3 contains 35 pills consisting of 28 pink pills (4 rows of 7 pills) and 7 white pills (1 row of 7 pills).

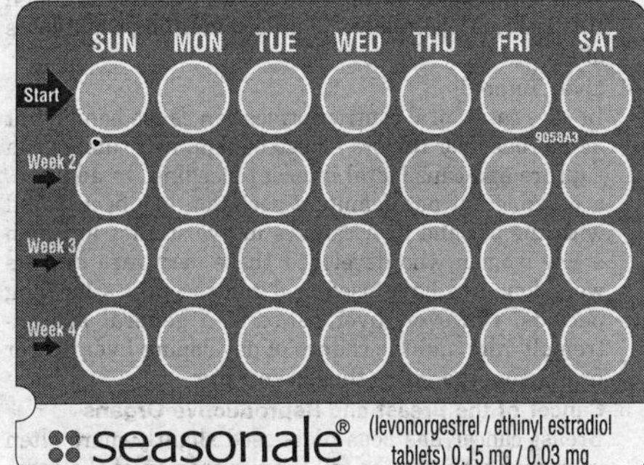

[See first figure at top of next column]
[See second figure at top of next column]

3. ALSO FIND:
   - Where on the first tray in the pack to start taking pills (upper left corner at the start arrow) and
   - In what order to take the pills (follow the weeks and arrow).
4. BE SURE YOU HAVE READY AT ALL TIMES ANOTHER KIND OF BIRTH CONTROL (such as condoms or spermicides), to use as a back-up in case you miss pills.

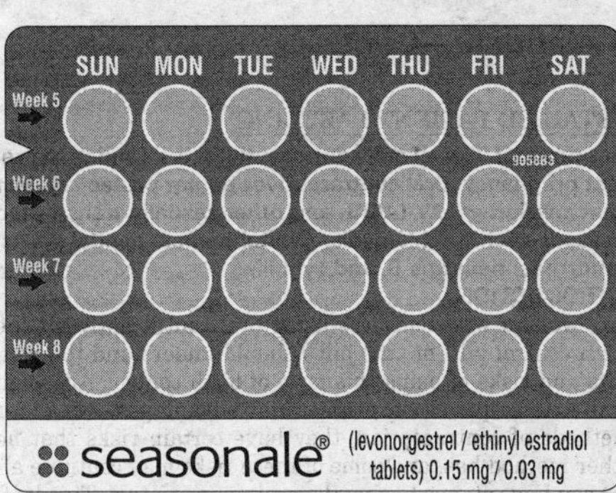

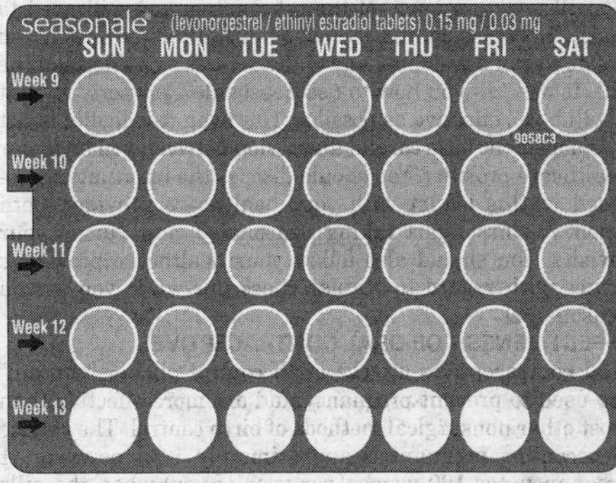

WHEN TO START SEASONALE®

1. Take the first "active" pink pill on the *Sunday after your period starts*, even if you are still bleeding. If your period begins on Sunday, start the first pink pill that same day.
2. *Use another method of birth control (such as condom or spermicide)* as a back-up method if you have sex anytime from the Sunday you start your first pink pill until the next Sunday (first 7 days).

HOW TO TAKE SEASONALE®

1. **Take one pill at the same time every day until you have taken the last pill in the tablet dispenser.**
   Do not skip pills even if you are spotting or bleeding or feel sick to your stomach (nausea).
   Do not skip pills even if you do not have sex very often.
2. **WHEN YOU FINISH A TABLET DISPENSER.**
   After taking the last white pill, start taking the first pink pill from a new Extended-Cycle Tablet Dispenser **the very next day** regardless of when your period started. This should be on a Sunday.
3. **If you miss your period when you are taking the white pills, call your healthcare provider because you may be pregnant.**

WHAT TO DO IF YOU MISS PILLS

If you **MISS 1** pink "active" pill:

1. Take it as soon as you remember. Take the next pill at your regular time. This means you may take 2 pills in 1 day.
2. You do not need to use a back-up birth control method if you have sex.

If you **MISS 2** pink "active" pills in a row:

1. Take 2 pills on the day you remember, and 2 pills the next day.
2. Then take 1 pill a day until you finish the pack.
3. You COULD BECOME PREGNANT if you have sex in the *7 days after* you restart your pills. You MUST use another birth control method (such as condoms or spermicide) as a back-up on the 7 days after you restart your pills.

If you **MISS 3 OR MORE** pink "active" pills in a row:

1. Do not remove the missed pills from the pack as they will not be taken. Keep taking 1 pill every day as indicated on the pack until you have completed all of the remaining pills in the pack. For example: If you resume taking the pill on Thursday, take the pill under "Thursday" and do not take the missed pills. You may experience bleeding during the week following the missed pills.
2. You COULD BECOME PREGNANT if you have sex during the days of missed pills or during the first 7 days after restarting your pills.
3. You **must** use a non-hormonal birth control method (such as condoms or spermicide) as a back-up when you miss pills and for the first 7 days after you restart your pills. **If you miss your period when you are taking the white pills, call your healthcare provider because you may be pregnant.**

If you **MISS ANY** of the 7 white inactive pills.

1. Throw away the missed pills.
2. Keep taking the scheduled pills until the pack is finished.
3. You do not need a back-up method of birth control.

FINALLY, IF YOU ARE STILL NOT SURE WHAT TO DO ABOUT THE PILLS YOU HAVE MISSED

1. Use a BACK-UP METHOD anytime you have sex.
2. KEEP TAKING ONE PILL EACH DAY until you contact your healthcare provider.

Continued on next page

Seasonale—Cont.

DETAILED PATIENT LABELING

This product (like all oral contraceptives) is intended to prevent pregnancy. Oral contraceptives do not protect against transmission of HIV (AIDS) and other sexually transmitted diseases such as chlamydia, genital herpes, genital warts, gonorrhea, hepatitis B, and syphilis.

INTRODUCTION

Any woman who considers using oral contraceptives ("the birth control pill" or "the pill") should understand the benefits and risks of using this form of birth control. Although oral contraceptives have important advantages over other methods of contraception, they have certain risks that no other method has, and some of these risks may continue after you have stopped using the oral contraceptive. This leaflet will give you much of the information you will need to make this decision and will also help you determine if you are at risk of developing any of the serious side effects of the pill. It will tell you how to use Seasonale® properly so that it will be as effective as possible. However, this leaflet is not a replacement for a careful discussion between you and your healthcare provider. You should discuss the information provided in this leaflet with your healthcare provider, both when you first start taking Seasonale® and during your revisits. You should also follow your healthcare provider's advice with regard to regular check-ups while you are on Seasonale®.

EFFECTIVENESS OF ORAL CONTRACEPTIVES

Oral contraceptives or "the birth control pill" or "the pill" are used to prevent pregnancy and are more effective than most other nonsurgical methods of birth control. The chance of becoming pregnant is approximately 1.0% per year (1 pregnancy per 100 women per year of use) when the pills are used correctly, and no pills are missed. Typical failure rates are approximately 5.0% per year when women who miss pills are included. The chance of becoming pregnant increases with each missed pill during the menstrual cycle.

In comparison, typical failure rates for other methods of birth control during the first year of use are as follows:

No methods: 85%
Vaginal sponge: 20 to 40%
Cervical cap: 20 to 40%
Spermicides alone: 26%
Periodic abstinence: 25%
Condom (female): 21%
Diaphragm with spermicides: 20%
Withdrawal: 19%
Condom (male): 14%
Female sterilization: 0.5%
IUD: 0.1 to 2.0%
Injectable progestogen: 0.3%
Male sterilization: 0.15%
Norplant system: 0.05%

WHO SHOULD NOT TAKE ORAL CONTRACEPTIVES

Cigarette smoking increases the risk of serious cardiovascular side effects from oral contraceptive use. This risk increases with age and with the amount of smoking (15 or more cigarettes per day has been associated with a significantly increased risk) and is quite marked in women over 35 years of age. Women who use oral contraceptives should not smoke.

Some women should not use the pill. You should not use the pill if you have any of the following conditions:

- A history of heart attack or stroke
- A history of blood clots in the legs (thrombophlebitis), lungs (pulmonary embolism), or eyes
- A history of blood clots in the deep veins of your legs
- Chest pain (angina pectoris)
- Known or suspected breast cancer or cancer of the lining of the uterus, cervix, vagina, or certain hormonally-sensitive cancers
- Unexplained vaginal bleeding (until a diagnosis is reached by your healthcare provider)
- Yellowing of the whites of the eyes or of the skin (jaundice) during pregnancy or during previous use of the pill
- Liver tumor (benign or cancerous)
- Known or suspected pregnancy
- Heart valve or heart rhythm disorders that may be associated with formation of blood clots
- Diabetes affecting your circulation
- Uncontrolled high blood pressure
- Active liver disease with abnormal liver function tests
- Allergy or hypersensitivity to any of the components of Seasonale®
- A need for surgery with prolonged bedrest

Tell your healthcare provider if you have any of the above conditions. Your healthcare provider can recommend a safer method of birth control.

OTHER CONSIDERATIONS BEFORE TAKING ORAL CONTRACEPTIVES

Tell your healthcare provider if you or any family member has ever had:

- Breast nodules, fibrocystic disease of the breast, an abnormal breast X-ray or mammogram
- Diabetes
- Elevated cholesterol or triglycerides
- High blood pressure
- Migraine or other headaches or epilepsy
- Depression
- Gallbladder, liver, heart or kidney disease
- History of scanty or irregular menstrual periods

Women with any of these conditions should be checked often by their healthcare provider if they choose to use oral contraceptives. Also, be sure to inform your healthcare provider if you smoke or are on any medications.

RISKS OF TAKING ORAL CONTRACEPTIVES

If you use Seasonale® you will receive more exposure to hormones on a yearly basis than if you used a conventional 28-day cycle oral contraceptives containing a similar amount of estrogen and progestin (an additional 9 weeks exposure per year). While this added exposure may pose an additional risk of thrombotic and thromboembolic disease, studies to date with Seasonale have not suggested an increased risk of these disorders.

1. **Risk of Developing Blood Clots**
   Blood clots and blockage of blood vessels are the most serious side effects of taking oral contraceptives and can cause death or serious disability. In particular, a clot in the legs can cause thrombophlebitis and a clot that travels to the lungs can cause a sudden blocking of the vessel carrying blood to the lungs. Rarely, clots occur in the blood vessels of the eye and may cause blindness, double vision, or impaired vision. If you take oral contraceptives and need elective surgery, need to stay in bed for a prolonged illness, or have recently delivered a baby, you may be at risk of developing blood clots. You should consult your healthcare provider about stopping oral contraceptives three to four weeks before surgery and not taking oral contraceptives for two weeks after surgery or during bed rest. You should also not take oral contraceptives soon after delivery of a baby. It is advisable to wait for at least four weeks after delivery if you are not breastfeeding. If you are breastfeeding, you should wait until you have weaned your child before using the pill (See also the section on **Breastfeeding** in **"GENERAL PRECAUTIONS"**.)
   The risk of circulatory disease in oral contraceptive users may be higher in users of high-dose pills (containing 50 micrograms or higher of ethinyl estradiol) and may be greater with longer duration of oral contraceptive use. In addition, some of these increased risks may continue for a number of years after stopping oral contraceptives. The risk of abnormal blood clotting increases with age in both users and nonusers of oral contraceptives, but the increased risk from the oral contraceptive appears to be present at all ages. For women aged 20 to 44, it is estimated that about 1 in 2,000 using oral contraceptives will be hospitalized each year because of abnormal clotting. Among nonusers in the same age group, about 1 in 20,000 would be hospitalized each year. For oral contraceptive users in general, it has been estimated that in women between the ages of 15 and 34 the risk of death due to a circulatory disorder is about 1 in 12,000 per year, whereas for nonusers the rate is about 1 in 50,000 per year. In the age group 35 to 44, the risk is estimated to be about 1 in 2,500 per year for oral contraceptive users and about 1 in 10,000 per year for nonusers.
2. **Heart Attacks and Strokes**
   Oral contraceptives may increase the tendency to develop strokes (stoppage or rupture of blood vessels in the brain) and angina pectoris and heart attacks (blockage of blood vessels in the heart). Any of these conditions can cause death or serious disability. Smoking greatly increases the possibility of suffering heart attacks and strokes. Furthermore, smoking and the use of oral contraceptives greatly increase the chances of developing and dying of heart disease.
   Women with migraine (especially migraine with aura) who take oral contraceptives also may be at higher risk of stroke.
3. **Gallbladder Disease**
   Oral contraceptive users probably have a greater risk than nonusers of having gallbladder disease, although this risk may be related to pills containing high doses of estrogens.
4. **Liver Tumors**
   In rare cases, oral contraceptives can cause benign but dangerous liver tumors. These benign liver tumors can rupture and cause fatal internal bleeding. In addition, a possible but not definite association has been found with the pill and liver cancers in two studies in which a few women who developed these very rare cancers were found to have used oral contraceptives for long periods. However, liver cancers in general are extremely rare and the chance of developing liver cancer from using the pill is thus even rarer.
5. **Cancer of the Breast and Reproductive Organs**
   Breast cancer has been diagnosed slightly more often in women who use the pill than in women of the same age who do not use the pill. This small increase in the number of breast cancer diagnoses gradually disappears during the 10 years after stopping use of the pill. It is not known whether the difference is caused by the pill. It may be that women taking the pill are examined more often, so that breast cancer is more likely to be detected. You should have regular breast examinations by a healthcare provider and examine your own breasts monthly. Tell your healthcare provider if you have a family history of breast cancer or if you have had breast nodules or an abnormal mammogram.
   Women who currently have or have had breast cancer should not use oral contraceptives because breast cancer is usually a hormone-sensitive tumor.
   Some studies have found an increase in the incidence of cancer or precancerous lesions of the cervix in women who use oral contraceptives. However, this finding may be related to factors other than the use of oral contraceptives. There is insufficient evidence to rule out the possibility that the pill may cause such cancers.
6. **Lipid Metabolism and Inflammation of the Pancreas**
   In patients with inherited defects of the lipid metabolism, there have been reports of significant elevations of plasma triglycerides during estrogen therapy. This has led to pancreatitis in some cases.

ESTIMATED RISK OF DEATH FROM A BIRTH CONTROL METHOD OR PREGNANCY

All methods of birth control and pregnancy are associated with a risk of developing certain diseases, which may lead to disability or death. An estimate of the number of deaths associated with different methods of birth control and pregnancy has been calculated and is shown in the following table.

ANNUAL NUMBER OF BIRTH-RELATED OR METHOD-RELATED DEATHS ASSOCIATED WITH CONTROL OF FERTILITY PER 100,000 NONSTERILE WOMEN, BY FERTILITY-CONTROL METHOD AND ACCORDING TO AGE

Method of control and outcome	AGE 15-19	20-24	25-29	30-34	35-39	40-44
No fertility-control methods*	7.0	7.4	9.1	14.8	25.7	28.2
Oral contraceptives non-smoker**	0.3	0.5	0.9	1.9	13.8	31.6
Oral contraceptives smoker**	2.2	3.4	6.6	13.5	51.1	117.2
IUD**	0.8	0.8	1.0	1.0	1.4	1.4
Condom*	1.1	1.6	0.7	0.2	0.3	0.4
Diaphragm/spermicide*	1.9	1.2	1.2	1.3	2.2	2.8
Periodic abstinence*	2.5	1.6	1.6	1.7	2.9	3.6

* Deaths are birth related
** Deaths are method related

In the above table, the risk of death from any birth control method is less than the risk of childbirth, except for oral contraceptive users over the age of 35 who smoke and pill users over the age of 40 even if they do not smoke. It can be seen in the table that for women aged 15 to 39, the risk of death was highest with pregnancy (7 to 26 deaths per 100,000 women, depending on age). Among pill users who do not smoke, the risk of death was always lower than that associated with pregnancy for any age group, although over the age of 40, the risk increases to 32 deaths per 100,000 women, compared to 28 associated with pregnancy at that age. However, for pill users who smoke and are over the age of 35, the estimated number of deaths exceeds those for other methods of birth control. If a woman is over the age of 40 and smokes, her estimated risk of death is four times higher (117/100,000 women) than the estimated risk associated with pregnancy (28/100,000 women) in that age group.

The suggestion that women over 40 who don't smoke should not take oral contraceptives is based on information from older high-dose pills. An Advisory Committee of the FDA discussed this issue in 1989 and recommended that the benefits of oral contraceptive use by healthy, nonsmoking women over 40 years of age may outweigh the possible risks. Older women, as all women who take oral contraceptives, should take an oral contraceptive that contains the least amount of estrogen and progestin that is compatible with the individual patient needs.

WARNING SIGNALS

If any of these adverse effects occur while you are taking oral contraceptives, call your healthcare provider immediately:

- Sharp chest pain, coughing of blood, or sudden shortness of breath (indicating a possible clot in the lung).
- Pain in the calf (indicating a possible clot in the leg).
- Crushing chest pain or heaviness in the chest (indicating a possible heart attack).
- Sudden severe headache or vomiting, dizziness or fainting, disturbances of vision or speech, weakness, or numbness in an arm or leg (indicating a possible stroke).
- Sudden partial or complete loss of vision (indicating a possible clot in the eye).
- Breast lumps (indicating possible breast cancer or fibrocystic disease of the breast; ask your doctor or healthcare provider to show you how to examine your breasts).
- Severe pain or tenderness in the stomach area (indicating a possibly ruptured liver tumor).
- Difficulty in sleeping, weakness, lack of energy, fatigue, or change in mood (possibly indicating severe depression).
- Jaundice or a yellowing of the skin or eyeballs, accompanied frequently by fever, fatigue, loss of appetite, dark-colored urine, or light-colored bowel movements (indicating possible liver problems).

SIDE EFFECTS OF ORAL CONTRACEPTIVES

In addition to the risks and more serious side effects discussed above (see **RISKS OF TAKING ORAL CONTRACEPTIVES, ESTIMATED RISK OF DEATH FROM A BIRTH CONTROL METHOD OR PREGNANCY** and **WARNING SIGNALS** sections), the following may also occur:

1. **Irregular vaginal bleeding**
Irregular vaginal bleeding or spotting (bleeding or spotting between your expected period) is likely to occur while you are taking Seasonale®. Irregular bleeding may vary from slight staining between menstrual periods to breakthrough bleeding which is a flow much like a regular period. Irregular bleeding occurs most often during the first few 91-day cycles of Seasonale® use, tends to decrease during later cycles, but may also occur after you have been taking Seasonale® for some time. Such bleeding usually does not indicate any serious problems. **It is important to continue taking your pills on schedule even if you are having irregular bleeding.** If the bleeding lasts for more than 7 consecutive days, talk to your healthcare provider.
When you take Seasonale®, you need to consider the convenience of fewer expected menstrual periods (4 per year instead of 13) and the inconvenience of more irregular vaginal bleeding or spotting. In a clinical trial comparing Seasonale® (91-day cycles) to a conventional equivalent dosage 28-day cycle oral contraceptive, more women using Seasonale® discontinued treatment because of bleeding problems (7.7% of the Seasonale® users compared to 1.8% of the 28-day cycle users).
The following Table shows the percentages of women with 7 or more and 20 or more days of intermenstrual bleeding and/or spotting in the Seasonale® and the 28-day cycle treatment groups.

Percentages (%) of Women with Intermenstrual Bleeding and/or Spotting

Number of days of intermenstrual bleeding and/or spotting	Percentage of subjects with intermenstrual bleeding or spotting*	
Seasonale®	Cycle 1	Cycle 4
7 or more days	65%	42%
20 or more days	35%	15%
28-day cycle pill	Cycles 1-4	Cycles 10-13
7 or more	38%	39%
20 or more days	6%	4%

* Based on spotting and/or bleeding on days 1-84 of a 91 day cycle in the Seasonale® subjects and days 1-21 of a 28 day cycle over 4 cycles in the 28-day dosing regimen.

Total days of bleeding and/or spotting (withdrawal plus intermenstrual) were similar over one year of treatment for Seasonale® subjects and subjects on the 28-day cycle regimen.

2. **Contact lenses**
If you wear contact lenses and notice a change in vision or an inability to wear your lenses, contact your healthcare provider.
3. **Fluid retention**
Oral contraceptives may cause edema (fluid retention) with swelling of the fingers or ankles and may raise your blood pressure. If you experience fluid retention, contact your healthcare provider.
4. **Melasma**
A spotty darkening of the skin is possible, particularly of the face.
5. **Other side effects**
Other side effects may include nausea and vomiting, change in appetite, breast tenderness, headache, nervousness, depression, dizziness, loss of scalp hair, rash, vaginal infections, and allergic reactions.
If any of these side effects bother you, call your healthcare provider.

GENERAL PRECAUTIONS

1. **Missed Periods and Use of Oral Contraceptives Before or During Early Pregnancy**
If you miss any periods (no bleeding on the days that you take white pills), you must consider the possibility that you may be pregnant. Notify your healthcare provider that you are taking Seasonale® and have missed your period. Also notify your healthcare provider if you have symptoms of pregnancy such as morning sickness or unusual breast tenderness. Because you are taking Seasonale®, it is very important that your healthcare provider evaluates you to determine if you are pregnant. Stop taking Seasonale® if you are pregnant.
There is no conclusive evidence that oral contraceptive use is associated with an increase in birth defects, when taken inadvertently during early pregnancy. Previously, a few studies had reported that oral contraceptives might be associated with birth defects, but these studies have not been confirmed. Nevertheless, oral contraceptives should not be used during pregnancy. You should check with your healthcare provider about risks to your unborn child of any medication taken during pregnancy.
2. **While Breastfeeding**
If you are breastfeeding, consult your healthcare provider before starting oral contraceptives. Some of the drug will be passed on to the child in the milk. A few adverse effects on the child have been reported, including yellowing of the skin (jaundice) and breast enlargement. In addition, oral contraceptives may decrease the amount and quality of your milk. If possible, do not use oral contraceptives while breastfeeding. You should use another method of contraception since breastfeeding provides only partial protection from becoming pregnant and this partial protection decreases significantly as you breast-feed for longer periods of time. You should consider starting oral contraceptives only after you have weaned your child completely.
3. **Laboratory Tests**
If you are scheduled for any laboratory tests, tell your healthcare provider you are taking birth control pills. Certain blood tests may be affected by birth control pills.
4. **Drug Interactions**
Certain drugs may interact with birth control pills to make them less effective in preventing pregnancy or cause an increase in breakthrough bleeding. Such drugs include rifampin, drugs used for epilepsy such as barbiturates (for example, phenobarbital), carbamazepine (Tegretol is one brand of this drug), and phenytoin (Dilantin® is one brand of this drug), primidone (Mysoline®), topiramate (Topamax®), phenylbutazone (Butazolidin® is one brand), some drugs used for HIV such as ritonavir (Norvir®), modafinil (Provigil®) and possibly certain antibiotics (such as ampicillin and other penicillins, and tetracyclines). Pregnancies and breakthrough bleeding have been reported by users of combined hormonal contraceptives who also used some form of the herbal supplement St. John's Wort. You may need to use a non-hormonal method of contraception during any cycle in which you take drugs that can make oral contraceptives less effective. Be sure to tell your healthcare provider if you are taking or start taking any other medications, including nonprescription products or herbal products while taking birth control pills.
You may be at higher risk of a specific type of liver dysfunction if you take troleandomycin and oral contraceptives at the same time.
5. **Sexually transmitted diseases**
This product (like all oral contraceptives) is intended to prevent pregnancy. It does not protect against transmission of HIV (AIDS) and other sexually transmitted diseases such as chlamydia, genital herpes, genital warts, gonorrhea, hepatitis B, and syphilis.

What You Should Know About Your Menstrual Cycle When Taking Seasonale®

When you take Seasonale®, which has a 91-day treatment cycle, you should expect to have 4 menstrual periods per year (bleeding when you are taking the 7 white pills). However, you should expect to have more bleeding or spotting between your menstrual periods than if you were taking an oral contraceptive with a 28-day treatment cycle. During the first Seasonale® treatment cycle, about 1 in 3 women may have 20 or more days of unplanned bleeding or spotting (bleeding when you are taking pink pills). This bleeding or spotting tends to decrease during later cycles. Do not stop Seasonale® because of the bleeding. If the spotting continues for more than 7 consecutive days or if the bleeding is heavy, call your healthcare provider.

HOW TO TAKE SEASONALE®

IMPORTANT POINTS TO REMEMBER *BEFORE* YOU START TAKING SEASONALE®

1. BE SURE TO READ THESE DIRECTIONS:
   - Before you start taking your pills.
   - Anytime you are not sure what to do.
2. THE RIGHT WAY TO TAKE SEASONALE® IS TO TAKE ONE PILL EVERY DAY AT THE SAME TIME.
If you miss pills you could get pregnant. This includes starting the pack late. The more pills you miss, the more likely you are to get pregnant.
3. MANY WOMEN MAY FEEL SICK TO THEIR STOMACH DURING THE FIRST FEW WEEKS OF TAKING PILLS.
If you feel sick to your stomach, do not stop taking the pill. The problem will usually go away. If it doesn't go away, check with your healthcare provider.
4. MANY WOMEN HAVE SPOTTING OR LIGHT BLEEDING DURING THE FIRST FEW MONTHS OF TAKING SEASONALE®. **Do not stop taking your pills even if you are having irregular bleeding.** If the bleeding lasts for more than a few days, talk to your healthcare provider.
5. MISSING PILLS CAN ALSO CAUSE SPOTTING OR LIGHT BLEEDING, even when you make up these missed pills. On the days you take 2 pills to make up for missed pills, you could also feel a little sick to your stomach.
6. IF YOU HAVE VOMITING OR DIARRHEA, or IF YOU TAKE SOME MEDICINES, including some antibiotics and the herbal supplement St. John's Wort, Seasonale may not work as well. Use a back-up method (such as condoms or spermicides) until you check with your healthcare provider.
7. IF YOU HAVE TROUBLE REMEMBERING TO TAKE SEASONALE®, talk to your healthcare provider about how to make pill-taking easier or about using another method of birth control.
8. IF YOU HAVE ANY QUESTIONS OR ARE UNSURE ABOUT THE INFORMATION IN THIS LEAFLET, call your healthcare provider.

***BEFORE* YOU START TAKING SEASONALE®**

1. DECIDE WHAT TIME OF DAY YOU WANT TO TAKE YOUR PILL. It is important to take it at about the same time every day.
2. LOOK AT YOUR EXTENDED-CYCLE TABLET DISPENSER. Your Tablet Dispenser consists of 3 trays with cards that hold 91 individually sealed pills (a 13-week or 91-day cycle). The 91 pills consist of 84 pink pills (active pills with hormones) and 7 white pills (inactive pills without hormone). Trays 1 and 2 each contain 28 pink pills (4 rows of 7 pills). Tray 3 contains 35 pills consisting of 28 pink pills (4 rows of 7 pills) and 7 white pills (1 row of 7 pills).

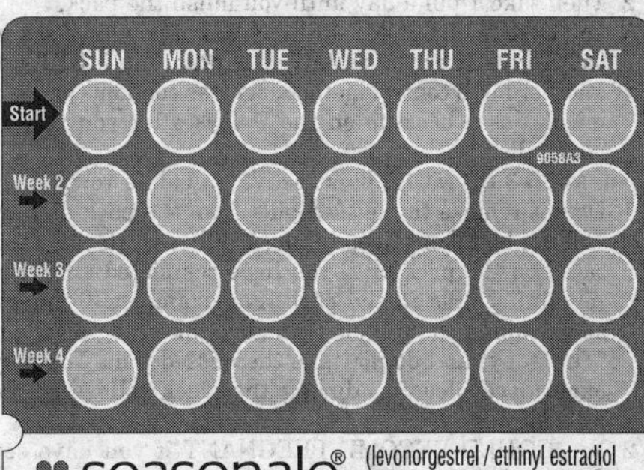

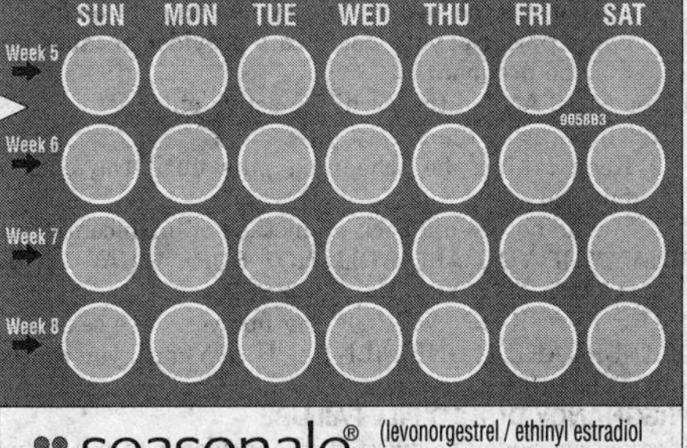

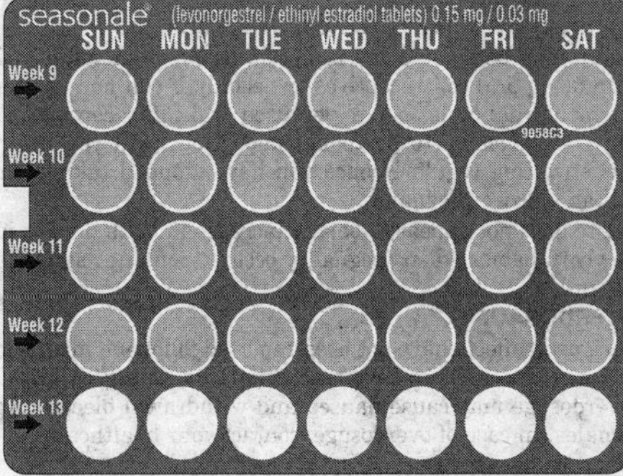

3. ALSO FIND:
   - Where on the first tray in the pack to start taking pills (upper left corner at the start arrow) and
   - In what order to take the pills (follow the weeks and arrow).
4. BE SURE YOU HAVE READY AT ALL TIMES ANOTHER KIND OF BIRTH CONTROL (such as condoms or spermicides), to use as a back-up in case you miss pills.

WHEN TO START SEASONALE®

1. Take the first "active" pink pill on the *Sunday after your period starts*, even if you are still bleeding. If your period begins on Sunday, start the first pink pill that same day.
2. *Use another method of birth control (such as condom or spermicide)* as a back-up method if you have sex anytime from the Sunday you start your first pink pill until the next Sunday (first 7 days).

HOW TO TAKE SEASONALE®

1. **Take one pill at the same time every day until you have taken the last pill in the tablet dispenser. Do not skip pills even if you are spotting or bleeding** or feel sick to your stomach (nausea).
Do not skip pills even if you do not have sex very often.
2. **WHEN YOU FINISH A TABLET DISPENSER.**
After taking the last white pill, start taking the first pink pill from a new Extended-Cycle Tablet Dispenser

Continued on next page

Seasonale—Cont.

the very next day regardless of when your period started. This should be on a Sunday.

3. **If you miss your period when you are taking the white pills, call your healthcare provider because you may be pregnant.**

WHAT TO DO IF YOU MISS PILLS

If you **MISS 1** pink "active" pill:

1. Take it as soon as you remember. Take the next pill at your regular time. This means you may take 2 pills in 1 day.
2. You do not need to use a back-up birth control method if you have sex.

If you **MISS 2** pink "active" pills in a row:

1. Take 2 pills on the day you remember, and 2 pills the next day.
2. Then take 1 pill a day until you finish the pack.
3. You COULD BECOME PREGNANT if you have sex in the *7 days* after you restart your pills. You MUST use another birth control method (such as condoms or spermicide) as a back-up on the 7 days after you restart your pills.

If you **MISS 3 OR MORE** pink "active" pills in a row:

1. Do not remove the missed pills from the pack as they will not be taken. Keep taking 1 pill every day as indicated on the pack until you have completed all of the remaining pills in the pack. For example: If you resume taking the pill on Thursday, take the pill under "Thursday" and do not take the missed pills. You may experience bleeding during the week following the missed pills.
2. You COULD BECOME PREGNANT if you have sex during the days of missed pills or during the first 7 days after restarting your pills.
3. You **must** use a non-hormonal birth control method (such as condoms or spermicide) as a back-up when you miss pills and for the first 7 days after you restart your pills. **If you miss your period when you are taking the white pills, call your healthcare provider because you may be pregnant.**

If you **MISS ANY** of the 7 white inactive pills.

1. Throw away the missed pills.
2. Keep taking the scheduled pills until the pack is finished.
3. You do not need a back-up method of birth control.

FINALLY, IF YOU ARE STILL NOT SURE WHAT TO DO ABOUT THE PILLS YOU HAVE MISSED

1. Use a BACK-UP METHOD anytime you have sex.
2. KEEP TAKING ONE PILL EACH DAY until you contact your healthcare provider.

PREGNANCY DUE TO PILL FAILURE

If taken every day as directed, the incidence of pill failure resulting in pregnancy is approximately 1 % (ie, one pregnancy per 100 women per year), but more typical failure rates are about 5%. If failure does occur, the risk to the fetus is minimal.

PREGNANCY AFTER STOPPING THE PILL

There may be some delay in becoming pregnant after you stop using oral contraceptives, especially if you had irregular menstrual cycles before you used oral contraceptives. It may be advisable to postpone conception until you begin menstruating regularly once you have stopped taking the pill and desire pregnancy.

There does not appear to be any increase in birth defects in newborn babies when pregnancy occurs soon after stopping the pill.

OVERDOSAGE

Serious ill effects have not been reported following ingestion of large doses of oral contraceptives by young children. Overdosage may cause nausea and withdrawal bleeding in females. In case of overdosage, contact your healthcare provider or pharmacist.

OTHER INFORMATION

Your healthcare provider will take a medical and family history before prescribing oral contraceptives and will examine you. The physical examination may be delayed to another time if you request it and the healthcare provider believes that it is appropriate to postpone it. You should be reexamined at least once a year. Be sure to inform your healthcare provider if there is a family history of any of the conditions listed previously in this leaflet. Be sure to keep all appointments with your healthcare provider, because this is a time to determine if there are early signs of side effects of oral contraceptive use.

Do not use the drug for any condition other than the one for which it was prescribed. This drug has been prescribed specifically for you; do not give it to others who may want birth control pills.

NONCONTRACEPTIVE HEALTH BENEFITS

The following noncontraceptive health benefits related to the use of oral contraceptives are supported by epidemiological studies which largely utilized oral contraceptive formulations containing doses exceeding 0.035 mg of ethinyl estradiol or 0.05 mg of mestranol.

Effects on menses:

- May decrease blood loss and may decrease incidence of iron-deficiency anemia
- May decrease incidence of dysmenorrhea

Effects related to inhibition of ovulation:

- May decrease incidence of functional ovarian cysts
- May decrease incidence of ectopic pregnancies

Effects from long-term use:

- May decrease incidence of fibroadenomas and fibrocystic disease of the breast
- May decrease incidence of acute pelvic inflammatory disease
- May decrease incidence of endometrial cancer
- May decrease incidence of ovarian cancer

If you want more information about birth control pills, ask your doctor or pharmacist. They have a more technical leaflet called the Professional Labeling which you may wish to read.

MANUFACTURED BY:
DURAMED PHARMACEUTICALS, INC.
A subsidiary of Barr Laboratories, Inc.
Pomona, NY 10970-0519
Revised September 2003
310905825001
BR 9058

Shown in Product Identification Guide, page 311

Baxter Healthcare Corporation

BIOSCIENCE
ONE BAXTER WAY
WESTLAKE VILLAGE, CA 91362

Direct Inquiries to:
Product Management
(800) 423-2090

For Medical Information Contact:
In Emergencies:
Edward Gomperts, M.D.
Medical Director,
Baxter Healthcare Corporation:
(800) 423-2862

ADVATE ℞

[ăd-vāt]
Antihemophilic Factor (Recombinant)
Plasma/Albumin-Free Method (rAHF-PFM)

DESCRIPTION

ADVATE Antihemophilic Factor (Recombinant), Plasma/Albumin-Free Method (rAHF-PFM) is a purified glycoprotein consisting of 2,332 amino acids that is synthesized by a genetically engineered Chinese hamster ovary (CHO) cell line. In culture, the CHO cell line expresses recombinant antihemophilic factor (rAHF) into the cell culture medium. The rAHF is purified from the culture medium using a series of chromatography columns. The cornerstone of the purification process is an immunoaffinity chromatography step in which a monoclonal antibody directed against Factor VIII is employed to selectively isolate the rAHF from the medium. The cell culture and purification processes used in the manufacture of ADVATE rAHF-PFM employ no additives of human or animal origin. The production process includes a dedicated, viral inactivation solvent-detergent treatment step. The rAHF synthesized by the CHO cells has the same biological effects as Antihemophilic Factor (Human) [AHF (Human)]. Structurally the recombinant protein has a similar combination of heterogeneous heavy and light chains as found in AHF (Human).

ADVATE rAHF-PFM is formulated as a sterile, non-pyrogenic, white to off-white powder for intravenous injection. ADVATE rAHF-PFM is available in single-dose vials that contain nominally 250, 500, 1000 and 1500 International Units (IU) per vial. When reconstituted with the appropriate volume of diluent, the product contains the following stabilizers in maximal amounts: 38 mg/mL mannitol, 10 mg/mL trehalose, 108 mEq/L sodium, 12 mM histidine, 12 mM Tris, 1.9 mM calcium, 0.17 mg/mL polysorbate-80, and 0.10 mg/mL glutathione. Von Willebrand Factor (vWF) is co-expressed with FVIII, and helps to stabilize it in culture. The final product contains no more than 2 ng vWF/IU rAHF, which will not have any clinically relevant effect in patients with von Willebrand's Disease. The product contains no preservative.

Each vial of ADVATE rAHF-PFM is labeled with the AHF activity expressed in IU per vial. Biological potency is determined by an in vitro assay, which employs a Factor VIII concentrate standard that is referenced to a World Health Organization (WHO) International Standard for Factor VIII: C concentrates. The specific activity of ADVATE rAHF-PFM is 4000 to 10,000 IU per milligram of protein.

CLINICAL PHARMACOLOGY

The pharmacokinetics of ADVATE rAHF-PFM were investigated in a Phase 2/3 multicenter pivotal study of previously treated subjects. In addition, an interim analysis comparing the pharmacokinetics of ADVATE rAHF-PFM at the onset of treatment and after a period of at least 75 exposure days was performed in the context of an ongoing continuation study in subjects who completed treatment in the multicenter pivotal Phase 2/3 study. Post-infusion levels and clearance of Factor VIII during the perioperative period were examined in an interim analysis of subjects from the pivotal and continuation studies who were enrolled in an ongoing Phase 2/3 surgical study. Finally, the pharmacokinetics of ADVATE rAHF-PFM were investigated in an interim analysis of an ongoing study of pediatric previously treated subjects < 6 years of age (see Pediatric Use subsection under "PRECAUTIONS").

Pharmacokinetics

A randomized, crossover pharmacokinetic comparison of ADVATE rAHF-PFM produced at a pilot-scale facility in Orth, Austria (the test article) and RECOMBINATE rAHF (the control article) was conducted in the context of the pivotal Phase 2/3 study. Study subjects were initially infused with one of the two preparations at a dose of 50 ± 5 IU/kg body weight while in a non-bleeding state. The second study preparation was infused in a non-bleeding state at 50 ± 5 IU/kg after a washout period of 72 hours to 4 weeks following the first study infusion. The order in which each study preparation was administered was assigned by randomization. Pharmacokinetic parameters (area under the Factor VIII plasma concentration versus time curve [AUC], maximal post-infusion Factor VIII level [C_{max}], in vivo recovery, half-life, clearance [CL], mean residence time [MRT], and volume of distribution in steady-state [V_{ss}]) were calculated from Factor VIII activity measurements in blood samples obtained immediately before and at standardized time intervals up to 48 hours following each infusion.

A total of 56 study subjects were enrolled and randomized. Of these, 50 (modified intent-to-treat population) received both infusions of study medication and had sufficient pharmacokinetic data for the comparison of ADVATE rAHF-PFM and RECOMBINATE rAHF. Thirty subjects (per-protocol population) received both pharmacokinetic infusions of study medication and had data for all pharmacokinetic time points. Pharmacokinetic parameters for each study preparation in the per-protocol analysis are presented in Table 1. [See table 1 below]

For the pharmacokinetic parameters $AUC_{0\text{-}48h}$ and in vivo recovery, the 90% confidence intervals for the ratios of the mean values for the test and control articles were within the pre-established limits of 0.80 and 1.25 for both the per-protocol (n = 30) and intent-to-treat study (n = 50) populations. In addition, in vivo recovery at the onset of treatment and after 75 exposure days was compared for 62 subjects. Results of this analysis indicated no significant change in the in vivo recovery at the onset of treatment and after ≥ 75 exposure days.

Additionally, the pharmacokinetics of ADVATE rAHF-PFM produced at the Orth facility were compared with those of ADVATE rAHF-PFM produced at a commercial-scale facility in Neuchâtel, Switzerland. For the pharmacokinetic parameters $AUC_{0\text{-}48h}$ and in vivo recovery, the 90% confidence intervals for the ratios of the mean values for the test and control articles were within the pre-established limits of 0.80 and 1.25 for both the per-protocol and intent-to-treat study populations.

The Phase 2/3 continuation study provided a means for examining potential changes in all pharmacokinetic parameters of ADVATE rAHF-PFM at the onset of treatment and after a period of at least 75 exposure days. This comparison utilized data for ADVATE rAHF-PFM produced in the Orth facility obtained at the onset of treatment on the pivotal

Table 1.
Pharmacokinetic Parameters for ADVATE rAHF-PFM and RECOMBINATE rAHF (Per-Protocol Analysis)

Parameter	RECOMBINATE rAHF		ADVATE rAHF-PFM	
	N	Mean ± SD	N	Mean[a] ± SD
$AUC_{0\text{-}48h}$ (IU·h/dL)[a]	30	1530 ± 380	30	1534 ±436
In vivo recovery (IU/dL/IU/kg)[b]	30	2.59 ± 0.52	30	2.41 ± 0.50
Half-life (h)	30	11.24 ± 2.53	30	11.98 ± 4.28
C_{max} (IU/dL)	30	129 ± 27	30	120 ± 26
MRT (h)	30	20.03 ± 7.80	30	22.82 ± 13.94
V_{ss} (dL/kg)	30	0.58 ± 0.15	30	0.60 ± 0.15
CL (dL/kg/hr)	30	0.03 ± 0.01	30	0.03 ± 0.01

[a] Area under the plasma Factor VIII concentration × time curve from 0 to 48 hours post-infusion
[b] Calculated as (C_{max} - baseline Factor VIII) divided by the dose in IU/kg, where C_{max} is the maximal post-infusion Factor VIII measurement

Phase 2/3 study with data for ADVATE rAHF-PFM produced in the Neuchâtel facility obtained in the continuation study. A total of 13 of 34 eligible subjects were included in an interim per-protocol analysis (Table 2). Ninety-five percent (95%) confidence intervals calculated for the ratios of the mean values for AUC_{0-48h} and in vivo recovery before and after at least 75 exposure days indicated no evidence of a difference in the pharmacokinetics of ADVATE rAHF-PFM at the two time points.

[See table 2 at right]

In an interim analysis of data from 10 of 25 planned subjects in the Phase 2/3 surgery study, the target Factor VIII level was met or exceeded in all cases following a single loading dose ranging from 48.0 to 69.8 IU/kg.

Hemostatic Efficacy

In the Phase 2/3 pivotal study, a global assessment of efficacy was rendered by the subject (for home treatment) or study site investigator (for treatment under medical supervision) using an ordinal scale of excellent, good, fair, or none, based on the quality of hemostasis achieved with ADVATE rAHF-PFM produced in the Orth facility for the treatment of each new bleeding episode. A total of 510 bleeding episodes were reported, with a mean (± SD) of 6.1 ± 8.2 bleeding episodes per subject. Of the 510 new bleeding episodes treated with ADVATE rAHF-PFM, 439 (86%) were rated excellent or good in their response to treatment, 61 (12%) were rated fair, 1 (0.2%) was rated as having no response, and for 9 (2%), the response to treatment was unknown. A total of 411 (81%) new bleeding episodes were managed with a single infusion, 62 (12%) required 2 infusions, 15 (3%) required 3 infusions, and 22 (4%) required 4 or more infusions of ADVATE rAHF-PFM for satisfactory resolution. A total of 162 (32%) new bleeding episodes occurred spontaneously, 228 (45%) were the result of antecedent trauma, and for 120 (24%) bleeding episodes, the etiology was unknown.

The rate of new bleeding episodes during the protocol-mandated 75 exposure day prophylactic regimen (≥ 25 IU/kg body weight 3–4 times per week) was calculated as a function of the etiology of bleeding episodes for 107 evaluable subjects (n = 274 new bleeding episodes). These rates are presented in Table 3.

Table 3.
Rate of New Bleeding Episodes During Prophylaxis

Bleeding Episode Etiology	Mean (± SD) New Bleeding Episodes/Subject/Month
Spontaneous	0.34 ± 0.49
Post-traumatic	0.39 ± 0.46
Unknown[a]	0.33± 0.34
Overall	0.52 ± 0.71

[a] Etiology was indeterminate

In a post-hoc analysis, the overall rate of bleeding was correlated inversely with the degree of compliance with the prescribed prophylactic regimen. Subjects who infused less than 25 IU ADVATE rAHF-PFM per kg per dose for more than 20% of prophylactic infusions or administered less than 3 infusions per week for more than 20% of study weeks (n = 37) experienced a 2.3-fold higher rate of bleeding in comparison with subjects who complied with the prescribed prophylactic regimen at least 80% of the time and for ≥ 80% of doses (n = 70).

The Phase 2/3 continuation study involved subjects previously treated on the pivotal Phase 2/3 study and provided additional efficacy data on ADVATE rAHF-PFM. An interim analysis of efficacy was conducted for 27 of 82 enrolled subjects who self-administered ADVATE rAHF-PFM produced in Neuchâtel on a routine prophylactic regimen during a minimum period of 50 exposure days to ADVATE rAHF-PFM. As in the pivotal Phase 2/3 study, new bleeding episodes were treated with ADVATE rAHF-PFM and the outcome of treatment was rated as excellent, good, fair, or none, based on the quality of hemostasis achieved. A total of 51 new bleeding episodes occurred in 13 of the 27 subjects being treated with ADVATE rAHF-PFM. By etiology, 53% of these bleeding events resulted from trauma and 27% occurred spontaneously; the other 20% had an undetermined etiology. The response to treatment with ADVATE rAHF-PFM for the majority (63%) of all new bleeding episodes was rated as excellent or good. In addition, 86% of the bleeding episodes resolved with only 1 infusion and an additional 6% were resolved by a second infusion. Thus, 92% of all bleeding episodes required 1 or 2 infusions of study product.

An interim analysis of the hemostatic efficacy of ADVATE rAHF-PFM during the perioperative management of subjects undergoing surgical procedures was conducted for 10 of 25 planned subjects. Ten subjects underwent 10 surgical procedures while receiving ADVATE rAHF-PFM. Eight subjects received the test product by intermittent bolus infusion and 2 subjects received a combination of continuous and intermittent bolus infusion. Nine of the 10 subjects completed the study. Six of the surgical procedures were classified as major, and 4 were minor. Of the 6 major surgeries, 5 were for orthopedic complications of hemophilia. A brief description of each surgical procedure, along with study duration and study medication exposure, are presented in Table 4.

Table 2.
Pharmacokinetic Parameters for ADVATE rAHF-PFM Before and After at Least 75 Exposure Days

Parameter	Parameters at the Onset of Treatment[a]					Parameters after ≥ 75 Exposure Days[b]				
	N	Mean	SD	Min	Max	N	Mean	SD	Min	Max
AUC_{0-48h} (IU·h/dL)	13	1315	405	876	2314	13	1262	497	831	2731
C_{max} (IU/dL)	13	111	23	77	151	13	111	25	73	151
Adjusted Recovery (IU/dL/IU/kg)	13	2.24	0.47	1.54	3.02	13	2.20	0.51	1.46	3.06
Total AUMC (IU·h^2/dL)	13	32995	31768	10527	129569	13	28231	23573	10065	100710
Half-life (h)	13	11.10	2.72	8.38	17.96	13	10.89	1.37	9.24	13.92
Clearance (dL/(kg·h)	13	0.04	0.01	0.02	0.06	13	0.04	0.01	0.01	0.06
Mean residence time (h)	13	19.15	8.40	9.80	40.56	13	18.14	5.32	9.39	29.82
V_{ss} (dL/kg)	13	0.64	0.13	0.42	0.90	13	0.68	0.16	0.43	0.94

[a] Data from the Phase 2/3 pivotal study for ADVATE rAHF-PFM produced in Orth
[b] Data from the Phase 2/3 continuation study for ADVATE rAHF-PFM produced in Neuchâtel

Table 4.
Surgical Procedures, Study Duration, and Study Medication Exposure

Surgery Type	Days of Study	ADVATE rAHF-PFM Exposure Days	Cumulative ADVATE rAHF-PFM Exposure (IU)
Total hip replacement	16	15	61,600
Knee joint replacement	22	18	76,060
Knee arthrodesis	24	22	66,080
Transposition of the left ulnar nerve	5	3	14,560
Insertion of Mediport	28	8[a]	46,893
Dental extraction	18	6	16,599
Left elbow synovectomy	43	32	102,180
Teeth extraction	2	2	10,350
Right knee arthroscopy, chondroplasty and synovectomy	13	10[a]	32,334
Wisdom teeth extraction	14	5	15,357

[a] ADVATE rAHF-PFM was administered by continuous infusion for the first 48 hours post-operatively, followed by bolus infusions for the remainder of study treatment.

For each of the 10 subjects, intra- and post-operative quality of hemostasis achieved with ADVATE rAHF-PFM was assessed by the operating surgeon and study site investigator, respectively, using an ordinal scale of excellent, good, fair, or none. The same rating scale was used to evaluate control of hemorrhage from a surgical drain placed at the incision site in one subject. The quality of hemostasis achieved with ADVATE rAHF-PFM was rated as excellent or good for all assessments.

INDICATIONS AND USAGE

ADVATE rAHF-PFM is indicated in hemophilia A (classical hemophilia) for the prevention and control of bleeding episodes. ADVATE rAHF-PFM is also indicated in the perioperative management of patients with hemophilia A. ADVATE rAHF-PFM can be of therapeutic value in patients with Factor VIII inhibitors not exceeding 10 Bethesda Units (BU) per mL.[1, 2] However, in patients with a known or suspected inhibitor to Factor VIII, the plasma Factor VIII level should be monitored frequently and the dose of ADVATE rAHF-PFM should be adjusted accordingly.

ADVATE rAHF-PFM is not indicated for the treatment of von Willebrand's disease.

CONTRAINDICATIONS

Known hypersensitivity to mouse or hamster proteins may be a contraindication to the use of ADVATE rAHF-PFM (see PRECAUTIONS). Known intolerance or allergic reaction to any of the constituents in the formulation may be a contraindication to the use of ADVATE rAHF-PFM. ADVATE rAHF-PFM is contraindicated in patients who have manifested life-threatening immediate hypersensitivity reactions, including anaphylaxis, to the product.

WARNINGS

None.

PRECAUTIONS

General

Identification of the clotting defect as Factor VIII deficiency is essential before the administration of ADVATE rAHF-PFM. No benefit may be expected from this product in treating other coagulation factor deficiencies.

Formation of Inhibitors to Factor VIII

The formation of neutralizing antibodies to Factor VIII (Factor VIII inhibitors) is a known complication in the management of individuals with hemophilia A. The reported prevalence of these antibodies in previously-untreated patients who were administered rAHF products over several years is 20.7 to 31.7%.[3, 4, 5, 6, 7, 8] These inhibitors are invariably of the immunoglobulin G (IgG) isotype, and the Factor VIII inhibitory activity is expressed as BU per mL of plasma. Patients treated with AHF products should be carefully monitored for the development of Factor VIII inhibitors by appropriate clinical observations and laboratory tests.

Factor VIII inhibitor testing was performed throughout all studies in the rAHF-PFM clinical program. Among 136 treated subjects ≥ 10 years of age, all of whom had ≥ 150 exposure days to Factor VIII products at study entry, 102 had at least 75 exposure days to ADVATE rAHF-PFM. None of these subjects developed an inhibitor. One subject who had < 50 exposure days to ADVATE rAHF-PFM while on study developed an inhibitor. This subject manifested a low titer inhibitor (2.0 BU by the Bethesda assay) after 26 ADVATE rAHF-PFM exposure days. Eight weeks later, the inhibitor was no longer detectable, and in vivo recovery was normal at 1 and 3 hours after infusion of RECOMBINATE rAHF. For the group comprising all subjects with at least 75 exposure days to ADVATE rAHF-PFM and the single subject who developed an inhibitor, the 95% confidence interval (Poisson distribution) for the risk of developing an inhibitor to Factor VIII was 0.02 to 5.4 %.

An interim analysis of inhibitor development in 15 of 50 planned pediatric subjects < 6 years of age who had at least 50 prior exposure days to factor VIII at study entry was conducted. No subject completed 50 exposure days to ADVATE rAHF-PFM. Ten of the 15 enrolled subjects completed at least 10 exposure days to ADVATE rAHF-PFM or 120 total days on study; among this subset, there were no inhibitors.

Formation of Antibodies to Mouse or Hamster Protein

ADVATE rAHF-PFM contains trace amounts of mouse immunoglobulin G (MuIgG; maximum of 0.1 ng/IU ADVATE rAHF-PFM) and hamster (CHO) proteins (maximum of 1.5 ng/IU ADVATE rAHF-PFM). As such, there exists a remote possibility that patients treated with this product may develop hypersensitivity to these non-human mammalian proteins.

In the Phase 2/3 pivotal study of ADVATE rAHF-PFM, serum samples were tested by enzyme immunoassays at baseline and after every 15 ± 2 exposure days, for the presence of antibodies to CHO protein and MuIgG. Regression analysis of assay results was conducted to evaluate trends in levels of antibodies to heterologous proteins as a function of time on study. Four study subjects showed a statistically significant increasing trend in the levels of anti-CHO (n = 1) or anti-MuIgG (n = 3) antibody levels over the course of the study. A fifth study subject showed a marked increase in anti-MuIgG antibodies coincident with the 60 and 75 exposure day interval study visits. None of these subjects exhibited adverse experiences (AEs) or other study findings consistent with an allergic or hypersensitivity response.

Information For Patients

Although allergic type hypersensitivity reactions were not observed in any study subjects receiving ADVATE rAHF-PFM, such reactions are theoretically possible. Patients should be informed of the early signs of hypersensitivity reactions including hives, generalized urticaria, tightness of the chest, wheezing, hypotension, and anaphylaxis. Patients should be advised to discontinue use of the product and contact their physician immediately if these symptoms occur.

Laboratory Tests

Although the dose can be estimated by the calculations that follow, it is highly recommended that, whenever possible, appropriate laboratory tests be performed on the patient's plasma at suitable intervals to assure that adequate Factor VIII levels have been reached and are maintained.

If the patient's plasma Factor VIII level fails to increase as expected or if bleeding is not controlled after adequate dos-

Continued on next page

Advate—Cont.

ing, the presence of an inhibitor should be suspected. By performing the appropriate laboratory procedures, the presence of an inhibitor can be demonstrated and quantified in terms of the number of BU per mL (i.e. the amount of Factor VIII activity neutralized by one mL of patient plasma). If the inhibitor is present at levels less than 10 BU per mL, the administration of additional AHF concentrate may neutralize the inhibitor, and may permit an appropriate hemostatic response. The close monitoring of plasma Factor VIII levels by laboratory assays is necessary in this situation. Inhibitor titers above 10 BU per mL are likely to make the control of hemostasis with AHF concentrates either impossible or impractical because of the very large dose required. In addition, the inhibitor titer may rise following AHF infusion as a result of an anamnestic response to Factor VIII. The treatment or prevention of bleeding in such patients requires the use of alternative therapeutic approaches and agents.

Carcinogenesis, Mutagenesis, Impairment of Fertility

No studies were conducted with the active ingredient in ADVATE rAHF-PFM to assess its mutagenic or carcinogenic potential. The CHO cell line employed in the production of ADVATE rAHF-PFM is derived from that used in the biosynthesis of RECOMBINATE rAHF. ADVATE rAHF-PFM has been shown to be comparable to RECOMBINATE rAHF with respect to its biochemical and physicochemical properties, as well as its non-clinical in vivo pharmacology and toxicology.[9] By inference, RECOMBINATE rAHF and ADVATE rAHF-PFM would be expected to have equivalent mutagenic and carcinogenic potential.

RECOMBINATE rAHF was tested for mutagenicity at doses considerably exceeding plasma concentrations in vitro, and at doses up to ten times the expected maximal clinical dose in vivo. At that concentration, it did not cause reverse mutations, chromosomal aberrations, or an increase in micronuclei formation in bone marrow polychromatic erythrocytes. Studies in animals have not been performed to evaluate carcinogenic potential.

Pediatric Use

Use of ADVATE rAHF-PFM is being examined in the context of an ongoing study of previously treated subjects under 6 years of age and in a planned study of previously untreated subjects with severe or moderately severe hemophilia A. In addition, pediatric subjects between 10 and 16 years of age were treated on the Phase 2/3 pivotal study, and those over 5 years of age were eligible for treatment on the ongoing Phase 2/3 surgery study.

A total of 54 subjects ≤ 16 years of age have been treated across all studies of ADVATE rAHF-PFM to date. Interim pharmacokinetic data for 34 subjects (per-protcol analysis population) ≤ 16 years of age were obtained from a combined dataset comprising subjects 10 to 16 years of age treated on the Phase 2/3 pivotal study and subjects enrolled and treated on the ongoing study of pediatric previously treated subjects < 6 years of age. Among these, 0 were neonates (birth to < 1 month of age), 2 were infants (1 month to < 2 years of age), 15 were children (2 to 12 years of age), and 17 were adolescents (12 to ≤ 16 years of age).

Pharmacokinetic parameters were not significantly different for the different age categories. A summary of the pharmacokinetic parameters for the 34 subjects ≤ 16 years of age in the per-protocol analysis population are shown in Table 5. The mean (± SD) plasma half-life was 11.21 ± 2.92 hours (range: 8.31–24.7 hours). The mean AUC_{0-48h} was 1363 ± 440 IU•h/dL. The mean values for C_{max} and adjusted recovery were 109 ± 23 IU/dL and 2.17 ± 0.44 IU/dL / IU/kg, respectively.

[See table 5 below]

Pregnancy

Pregnancy Category C. Animal reproduction studies have not been conducted with ADVATE rAHF-PFM. It is not known whether ADVATE rAHF-PFM can cause fetal harm when administered to a pregnant woman, or whether it can affect reproductive capacity. ADVATE rAHF-PFM should be given to a pregnant woman only if clearly needed.

ADVERSE REACTIONS

Adverse reactions were examined among a total of 96 subjects > 16 years of age and 54 subjects ≤ 16 years of age who received at least one infusion of ADVATE rAHF-PFM. For subjects > 16 years of age, the mean ± SD and median (range) values for time on study per subject were 319 ± 213 days and 403 days (1 to 654); the mean ± SD and median (range) exposure days to ADVATE rAHF-PFM per subject were 130 ± 84 days and 140 days (1 to 289); and the mean ± SD and median (interquartile range) IU/kg per infusion were 32.0 ± 8.27 IU/kg and 30.7 IU/kg (27.8 to 33.8).

For subjects ≤ 16 years of age, the mean ± SD and median (range) values for time on study per subject were 321 ± 210 days and 428 days (1 to 651); the mean ± SD and median (range) exposure days to ADVATE rAHF-PFM per subject were 138 ± 93 days and 181 days (1 to 284); and the mean ± SD and median (interquartile range) IU/kg per infusion were 36.5 ± 11.7 IU/kg and 33.4 IU/kg (29.7 to 40.4).

Across all clinical studies, a total of 1304 adverse events were reported among 128 of the 150 subjects who received at least 1 infusion of ADVATE rAHF-PFM. Of the 1304 adverse events, 696 were reported among 85 subjects > 16 years of age and 608 were reported among 43 subjects ≤ 16 years of age. All adverse events (product-related and unrelated) reported by at least 10% of subjects are shown in Table 6.

[See table 6 below]

Eighteen of the 1304 adverse events were deemed serious; none were related to the study medication. There were no deaths. Among the 1286 non-serious adverse events, only 28 in 12 subjects were judged by the investigator to be related to the study drug. Severity ratings among the 28 events were mild in 8 cases, moderate in 16 cases, and severe in 4 cases (Table 7).

Table 5.
Pharmacokinetic Parameters with ADVATE rAHF-PFM in Pediatric Previously Treated Subjects (Per-protocol Analysis)

	N	Mean	SD	Min	Max
AUC_{0-48h}(IU·h/dL)	34	1363	440	792	2398
C_{max} (IU/dL)	34	109	23	51	181
Adjusted Recovery (IU/dL/IU/kg)	34	2.17	0.44	1.23	3.39
Total AUMC (IU·h²/dL)	34	36823	47250	9749	283097
Half-life (h)	34	11.21	2.92	8.31	24.7
Clearance (dL/(kg·h))	34	0.04	0/01	0.01	0.06
Mean residence time (h)	34	19.79	9.92	10.70	66.66
Vss(dL/kg)	34	0.64	0.12	0.32	0.86

Table 6.
Summary of All Adverse Experiences (Product-Related and Unrelated) that Occurred in Greater than or Equal to 10% of Study Subjects

MedDRA System Organ Class	MedDRA Preferred Term	Number of Events	Number of Subjects	Percent of Evaluable Subjects[a]
Gastrointestinal disorders	Pharyngolaryngeal pain	22	17	11.3
General disorders and administration site conditions	Fall	25	19	12.7
	Pyrexia	37	25	16.7
Infections and infestations	Nasopharyngitis	32	22	14.7
Injury, poisoning and procedural complications	Accident nos	62	26	17.3
	Limb injury nos	195	52	34.7
Musculoskeletal and connective tissue disorders	Arthralgia	74	35	23.3
Nervous system disorders	Headache nos	138	44	29.3
Respiratory, thoracic and mediastinal disorders	Cough	37	23	15.3

[a] Percent relative to 150, the total number of subjects across all studies who received at least one infusion of ADVATE rAHF-PFM

Table 7.
Summary of Non-Serious, Study-Drug Related Adverse Events

Severity	MedDRA Preferred Term	Number of Events
Mild	Dysgeusia	3
	Pruritis	1
	Dizziness	1
	Catheter-related infection	1
	Rigors	1
	Headache nos	1
	Total	8
Moderate	Dysgeusia	1
	Dizziness	2
	Headache nos	1
	Hot flushes	2
	Diarrhoea nos	1
	Oedema lower limb	1
	Sweating increased	1
	Nausea	1
	Dyspnoea nos	1
	Abdominal pain upper	1
	Chest pain	1
	Bleeding tendency[a]	1
	Haematocrit decreased	1
	Joint Swelling	1
	Total	16
Severe	Headache nos	1
	Pyrexia	1
	Haematoma nos	1
	Coagulation factor VIII decreased	1
	Total	4

[a] Recorded as prolonged bleeding after postoperative drain removal on the case report form

The unexpected decreased coagulation factor VIII levels occurred in one subject during continuous infusion of ADVATE rAHF-PFM following surgery (postoperative Days 10–14). Hemostasis was maintained at all times during this period and both plasma Factor VIII levels and clearance rates returned to appropriate levels by postoperative Day 15. Factor VIII inhibitor assays performed after completion of continuous infusion and at study termination were negative.

Factor VIII inhibitor testing was performed throughout all studies in the rAHF-PFM clinical program. Among 136 treated subjects ≥10 years of age, all of whom had ≥150 exposure days to Factor VIII products at study entry, 102 had at least 75 exposure days to ADVATE rAHF-PFM. None of these subjects developed an inhibitor. One subject who had < 50 exposure days to ADVATE rAHF-PFM while on study developed an inhibitor. This subject manifested a low titer inhibitor (2.0 BU by the Bethesda assay) after 26 ADVATE rAHF-PFM exposure days. Eight weeks later, the inhibitor was no longer detectable, and in vivo recovery was normal at 1 and 3 hours after infusion of RECOMBINATE rAHF. For the group comprising all subjects with at least 75 exposure days to ADVATE rAHF-PFM and the single subject who developed an inhibitor, the 95% confidence interval (Poisson distribution) for the risk of developing an inhibitor to Factor VIII was 0.02 to 5.4%.

DOSAGE AND ADMINISTRATION

Each vial of ADVATE rAHF-PFM is labeled with the rAHF activity expressed in IU per vial. This potency assignment employs a Factor VIII concentrate standard that is referenced to a WHO International Standard for Factor VIII:C Concentrates, and is evaluated by appropriate methodology to ensure accuracy of the results.

The expected in vivo peak increase in Factor VIII level expressed as IU/dL of plasma or percent of normal can be estimated by multiplying the dose administered per kg body weight (IU/kg) by 2. This calculation is based on the findings of several pharmacokinetic studies of rAHF concentrates,[10, 11, 12, 13] and is supported by the data generated by 223 pharmacokinetic studies with ADVATE rAHF-PFM in

Table 8.
Guide to ADVATE rAHF-PFM Dosing for Treatment of Hemorrhages

Degree of Hemorrhage	Required Peak Post infusion Factor VIII Activity in the Blood (as % of normal or IU/dL)	Frequency of Infusion
Early hemarthrosis, muscle bleeding episode, or mild oral bleeding episode	20–40	Begin infusions every 12 to 24 hours for one to three days until the bleeding episode is resolved (as indicated by relief of pain) or healing is achieved.
More extensive hemarthrosis, muscle bleeding episode, or hematoma	30–60	Repeat infusions every 12 to 24 hours for (usually) three days or more until pain and disability are resolved.
Life-threatening bleeding episodes such as head injury, throat bleeding episode, or severe abdominal pain	60–100	Repeat infusions every 8 to 24 hours until resolution of the bleeding episode has occurred.

Table 9.
Guide to ADVATE rAHF-PFM Dosing for Surgical Procedures

Type of Procedure	Required Peak Post infusion Factor VIII Activity in the Blood (as % of Normal or IU/dL)	Frequency of Infusion
Minor surgery, including tooth extraction	60-100	Give a single bolus infusion beginning within one hour of the operation, with optional additional dosing every 12–24 hours as needed to control bleeding. For dental procedures, adjunctive therapy may be considered.
Major surgery	80-120 (pre- and post-operative)	For bolus infusion replacement, repeat infusions every 8 to 24 hours, depending on the desired level of Factor VIII and state of wound healing.

107 Phase 2/3 pivotal study subjects. These pharmacokinetic data demonstrated a peak post-infusion recovery of approximately 1.5–2.5 IU/dL per IU/kg above the pre-infusion baseline.

Examples (assuming patient's baseline Factor VIII level is < 1% of normal):

1. A dose of 1,750 IU ADVATE rAHF-PFM administered to a 70 kg patient should be expected to result in a peak post-infusion Factor VIII increase of 1750 IU × {[2IU/dL]/[IU/kg]}/[70 kg]= 50 IU/dL (50% of normal).
2. A peak level of 70% is required in a 40 kg child. In this situation, the appropriate dose would be 70 IU/dL/{[2IU/dL]/[IU/kg]} × 40 kg = 1400 IU.

Recommended Dose Schedule

Physician supervision of the treatment regimen is required. A guide for dosing in the treatment of hemorrhages is provided in Table 8. A guide for dosing in perioperative management is provided in Table 9. The careful control of replacement therapy is especially important in cases of major surgery or life-threatening hemorrhages.

[See table 8 above]
[See table 9 above]

Although dose can be estimated by the calculations above, it is highly recommended that, whenever possible, appropriate laboratory tests including serial Factor VIII activity assays be performed on the patient's plasma at suitable intervals to assure that adequate Factor VIII levels have been reached and are maintained.

Reconstitution: Use Aseptic Technique

1. Bring the ADVATE rAHF-PFM (dry concentrate) and Sterile Water for Injection (diluent) to room temperature.
2. Remove caps from the concentrate and diluent vials.
3. Cleanse stoppers with germicidal solution, and allow to dry prior to use.
4. Remove protective covering from one end of the double-ended needle and insert exposed needle through the center of the stopper.
5. Remove protective covering from the other end of the double-ended needle. Invert diluent bottle over the upright ADVATE rAHF-PFM bottle, then rapidly insert the free end of the needle through the ADVATE rAHF-PFM bottle stopper at its center. The vacuum in the bottle will draw in the diluent.
6. Disconnect the two bottles by removing the needle from the diluent bottle stopper, then remove the needle from the ADVATE rAHF-PFM bottle. Swirl gently until all material is dissolved. Be sure that ADVATE rAHF-PFM is completely dissolved, otherwise active materials will be removed by the filter needle.

NOTE: Do not refrigerate after reconstitution.

Administration: Use Aseptic Technique

Parenteral drug products should be inspected for particulate matter and discoloration prior to administration, whenever solution and container permit. A colorless appearance is acceptable for ADVATE rAHF-PFM. ADVATE rAHF-PFM should be administered at room temperature not more than 3 hours after reconstitution. Plastic syringes must be used with this product, since proteins such as ADVATE rAHF-PFM tend to stick to the surface of glass syringes.

1. Attach filter needle to a disposable syringe and draw back plunger to admit air into the syringe.
2. Insert needle into reconstituted ADVATE rAHF-PFM.
3. Inject air into bottle and then withdraw the reconstituted material into the syringe.
4. Remove and discard the filter needle from the syringe; attach a suitable needle and inject intravenously as instructed under **Administration by bolus infusion**.
5. If a patient is to receive more than one bottle of ADVATE rAHF-PFM, the contents of the multiple bottles may be drawn into the same syringe by drawing up each bottle through a separate unused filter needle. Filter needles are intended to filter the contents of a single bottle of ADVATE rAHF-PFM only.

Administration by bolus infusion

A dose of ADVATE rAHF-PFM should be administered over a period of ≤ 5 minutes (maximum infusion rate, 10 mL/min). The pulse rate should be determined before and during administration of ADVATE rAHF-PFM. Should a significant increase in pulse rate occur, reducing the rate of administration or temporarily halting the injection usually allows the symptoms to disappear promptly.

HOW SUPPLIED

ADVATE rAHF-PFM is available in single-dose vials that contain nominally 250, 500, 1000, and 1500 IU per vial. ADVATE rAHF-PFM is packaged with 5 mL of Sterile Water for Injection, a double-ended needle, a filter needle, infusion set/blood collection set*, 10 mL sterile syringe, alcohol swabs, bandages, one full prescribing physician insert, and one patient insert.

STORAGE

ADVATE rAHF-PFM should be refrigerated (2°–8°C [36°–46°F]). Avoid freezing to prevent damage to the diluent vial. ADVATE rAHF-PFM may be stored at room temperature (22°–28°C [72°–82°F]) for a period of up to 6 months until the expiration date. Do not use beyond the expiration date printed on the vial.

* Approved for both indications under 510(k).

REFERENCES

1. Aledort L: Inhibitors in hemophilia patients: Current status and management. Am J Hematol 47:208–217, 1994.
2. Kessler CM: An introduction to factor VIII inhibitors: The detection and quantitation. Am J Med 91 (Suppl 5A):1S–5S, 1991.
3. Lusher J, Arkin S, Hurst D: Recombinant FVIII (Kogenate) treatment of previously untreated patients (PUPs) with hemophilia A. Update of safety, efficacy and inhibitor development after seven study years. Abstract no. PD-664, ISTH, Florence. Thromb Haemost (suppl.):162, 1997.
4. Gruppo R, Chen H, Schroth P, Bray GL: Safety and immunogenicity of recombinant factor VIII (Recombinate) in previously untreated patients (PUPs): A 7.3 year update. Abstract no. 291, XXIII Congress of the World Federation of Haemophilia, The Hague. Haemophilia 4:228, 1998.
5. Rothschild C, Laurian Y, Satre EP, et al: French previously untreated patients with severe hemophilia A after exposure to recombinant factor VIII: Incidence of inhibitor and evaluation of immune tolerance. Thromb Haemost 80:779–783, 1998.
6. Gringeri A, Kreuz W, Escuriola-Ettinghausen C, et al: Anti-FVIII inhibitor incidence in previously untreated patients (PUPs) with hemophilia exposed to Kogenate (G.I.P.S.I.—German-Italian PUP Study on Inhibitor). Abstract no. 2642, ISTH, Florence. Thromb Haemost (suppl.):648, 1997.
7. Courter SG, Bedrosian CL: Clinical evaluation of B-domain deleted recombinant factor VIII in previously untreated patients. Semin Hematol 38:52–59, 2001.
8. Scharrer I, Bray GL, Neutzling O: Incidence of inhibitors in haemophilia A patients—A review of studies of recombinant and plasma-derived factor VIII concentrates. Haemophilia 5:45–54, 1999.
9. Baxter Healthcare Corporation, Glendale, CA. U.S.A. Data on file, 2002.
10. White II GC, Courter S, Bray GL, et al: A multicenter study of recombinant factor VIII (Recombinate™) in previously treated patients with hemophilia A. Thromb Haemost 77:660–667, 1997.
11. Abshire TC, Brackmann H-H, Scharrer I, et al: Sucrose formulated recombinant human antihemophilic factor VIII is safe and efficacious for treatment of hemophilia A in home therapy. Thromb Haemost 83:811–816, 2000.
12. Lee CA, Owens D, Bray G, et al: Pharmacokinetics of recombinant factor VIII (Recombinate) using one-stage clotting and chromogenic factor VIII assay. Thromb Haemost 82:1644–1647, 1999.
13. Fijnvandraat K, Berntorp E, ten Cate JW, et al: Recombinant, B-domain deleted factor VIII (r-VIII SQ): Pharmacokinetics and initial safety aspects in hemophilia A patients. Thromb Haemost 77:298–302, 1997.

To enroll in the confidential, industry-wide Patient Notification System, call 1-888-UPDATE U (1-888-873-2838).

Baxter, ADVATE, and RECOMBINATE are trademarks of Baxter International, Inc.

Baxter is registered in the U.S. Patent and Trademark office.

Baxter Healthcare Corporation
Westlake Village, CA 91362 USA
U.S. License No. 140
NDC 0944-2940-01/02/03/04
Issued July 2003 LE-07-00036

ARALAST™

[*ă-ră-lăst*]

Alpha$_1$–Proteinase Inhibitor (Human)
Solvent Detergent Treated Nanofiltered
FOR INTRAVENOUS USE ONLY
Product Information

DESCRIPTION

Alpha$_1$–Proteinase Inhibitor (Human), Aralast™, is a sterile, stable, lyophilized preparation of purified human alpha$_1$–proteinase inhibitor (α_1–PI), also known as alpha$_1$–antitrypsin.[1]

Aralast™ is prepared from large pools of human plasma by using the Cohn–Oncley cold alcohol fractionation process, followed by purification steps including polyethylene glycol and zinc chloride precipitations and ion exchange chromatography. To reduce the risk of viral transmission, the manufacturing process includes treatment with a solvent detergent (SD) mixture [tri–n–butyl phosphate and polysorbate 80] to inactivate enveloped viral agents such as HIV and Hepatitis B and C. In addition, a nanofiltration step is incorporated prior to final sterile filtration to reduce the risk of transmission of non–enveloped viral agents. Based on *in vitro* studies, the process used to produce Aralast™ has been shown to inactivate and/or partition various viruses as shown in the table below.[2]

Processing Step	Elimination of Deliberately Added Virus (Number of logs inactivated/removed)				
	HIV–1*	BVD†	PRV†	HAV‡	PPV‡
Alcohol Fractionation	≥ 4.8	N/A	N/A	N/A	N/A
Solvent Detergent Treatment	≥ 7.2	≥ 4.8	≥ 5.1	N/A	N/A
Nanofiltration	N/A	≥ 6.0	≥ 5.5	8.6	≥ 5.8
Accumulated Reduction	≥ 12.0	≥ 10.8	≥ 10.6	8.6	≥ 5.8

* HIV–1: Fractionation units $\log_{10}$ SFU SD Treatment units $\log_{10}$ $TCID_{50}$/mL
† BVD (Bovine Viral Diarrhea), PRV (Pseudorables Virus): SD Treatment units $\log_{10}$ PFU/mL, Nanofiltration units $\log_{10}$ PFU
‡ HAV (Hepatitis A), PPV (Porcine Parvovirus) Nanofiltration units $\log_{10}$ PFU
N/A Not Applicable

When reconstituted as directed, the concentration of α_1–PI is not less than 16 mg/mL and the specific activity is not less than 0.55 mg active α_1–PI/mg total protein. The composition of the reconstituted product is as follows:

Continued on next page

Aralast—Cont.

Component	Quantity/mL
Elastase Inhibitory Activity	NLT 400 mg Active α_1–PI/0.5 g vial*
	NLT 800 mg Active α_1–PI/1.0 g vial**
Albumin	NMT 5 mg/mL
Polyethylene Glycol	NMT 112 µg/mL
Polysorbate 80	NMT 50 µg/mL
Sodium	NMT 230 mEq/L
Tri–n–butyl Phosphate	NMT 1.0 µg/mL
Zinc	NMT 3 ppm

NLT: Not Less Than
NMT: Not More Than
* Reconstitution volume: 25 mL/0.5 g vial
** Reconstitution volume: 50 mL/1.0 g vial

Each vial of Aralast™ is labeled with the amount of functionally active α_1–PI expressed in mg/vial. The formulation contains no preservative. The pH of the solution ranges from 7.2 to 7.8. Product must only be administered intravenously.

CLINICAL PHARMACOLOGY

Alpha$_1$–Proteinase Inhibitor (Human), Aralast™, functions in the lungs to inhibit serine proteases such as neutrophil elastase (NE), which is capable of degrading protein components of the alveolar walls and which is chronically present in the lung. In the normal lung, α_1–PI is thought to provide more than 90% of the anti–NE protection in the lower respiratory tract.[3,4]

α_1–PI deficiency is an autosomal, co-dominant, hereditary disorder characterized by low serum and lung levels of α_1–PI.[1,3,5,6] Severe forms of the deficiency are frequently associated with slowly progressive, moderate-to-severe panacinar emphysema that most often manifests in the third to fourth decades of life, resulting in a significantly lower life expectancy.[1,3,4,6–8] Individuals with α_1–PI deficiency have little protection against NE released by a chronic, low–level of neutrophils in their lower respiratory tract, resulting in a protease:protease inhibitor imbalance in the lung.[7] The emphysema associated with α_1–PI deficiency is typically worse in the lower lung zones[5]. It is believed to develop because there are insufficient amounts of α_1–PI in the lower respiratory tract to inhibit NE. This imbalance allows unopposed destruction of the connective tissue framework of the lung parenchyma.[7,8]

There are a large number of phenotypic variants of this disorder.[1,3,4] Individuals with the PiZZ variant typically have serum α_1–PI levels less than 35% of the average normal level.[1,5] Individuals with the Pi(null)(null) variant have undetectable α_1–PI protein in their serum.[1,3] Individuals with these low serum α_1-PI levels, i.e., less than 11 µmolar (80 mg/dL), have an unknown risk of developing emphysema over their lifetimes. Two Registry studies have shown risks of 54.2 and 57.0%.[1,3,9] The risk of accelerated development and progression of emphysema in individuals with severe α_1–PI deficiency is higher in smokers than in ex-smokers or non-smokers.[3] The deficiency in α_1–PI represents one of the most common, potentially lethal hereditary disorders.[4]

A clinical study was conducted to compare Aralast™ (test drug) to a commercially available preparation of α_1–PI (Prolastin®), manufactured by Bayer Corporation. All subjects were to have been diagnosed as having congenital α_1–PI deficiency and emphysema but no α_1–PI augmentation therapy within the preceding six months.

Twenty–eight subjects were randomized to receive either test drug or control drug, 60 mg/kg intravenously per week, for 10 consecutive weeks. Two subjects withdrew from the study prematurely: 1 subject receiving Aralast™ withdrew consent after 6 infusions; 1 subject receiving Prolastin® withdrew after 1 infusion due to pneumonia following unscheduled bronchoscopy to remove a foreign body. Trough levels of serum α_1–PI (antigenic determination) and anti–NE capacity (functional determination) were measured prior to treatment at Weeks 8 through 11. Following their first 10 weekly infusions, the subjects who were receiving control drug were switched to Aralast™ while those who already were receiving Aralast™ continued to receive it. Maintenance of mean serum α_1–PI trough levels was assessed prior to treatments at Weeks 12 through 24. Bronchoalveolar lavages (BALs) were performed on subjects at baseline and prior to treatment at Week 7. The ELF from each BAL meeting acceptance criteria was analyzed for the α_1–PI level and anti–NE capacity.

With weekly augmentation therapy, a gradual increase in peak and trough serum α_1–PI levels was noted, with stabilization after several weeks. The metabolic half–life of Alpha$_1$–Proteinase Inhibitor (Human), Aralast™, was 5.9 days. Serum anti–NE capacity trough levels rose substantially in all subjects by Week 2, and by Week 3, serum anti–NE capacity trough levels exceeded 11 µM in the majority of subjects. With few exceptions, levels remained above this recommended threshold level in individual subjects for the duration of the period Weeks 3 through 24 on study. Although only five of fourteen subjects (35.7%) receiving Aralast™ had BALs meeting acceptance criteria for analysis at both baseline and Week 7, a statistically significant increase in the antigenic level of α_1–PI in the ELF was observed. No statistically significant increase in the anti-NE capacity in the ELF was detected.

Viral serology of all subjects was determined periodically throughout the study, including testing for antibodies to hepatitis A (HAV) and C (HCV), presence of circulating HBsAg, and presence of antibodies to HIV–1, HIV–2, and Parvovirus B–19. Subjects who were seronegative to parvovirus B–19 at enrollment were retested by PCR at Week 2. There were no seroconversions in subjects treated with Aralast™ through Week 24. None of the subjects became HBsAg positive during the study, although five of 13 (38%) evaluable subjects in the test group and eight of 13 (62%) in the control group had not been vaccinated to hepatitis B. No patient developed antibodies against α_1–PI.

It was concluded that at a dose of 60 mg/kg administered intravenously once weekly, Aralast™ and the control α_1–PI preparation had similar effects in maintaining target serum α_1–PI trough levels and increasing antigenic levels of α_1–PI in epithelial lining fluid (ELF) with maintenance augmentation therapy.

INDICATIONS AND USAGE

Congenital Alpha$_1$–Proteinase Inhibitor deficiency

Alpha$_1$–Proteinase Inhibitor (Human), Aralast™, is indicated for chronic augmentation therapy in patients having congenital deficiency of α_1–PI with clinically evident emphysema. Clinical and biochemical studies have demonstrated that with such therapy, Aralast™ is effective in maintaining target serum α_1–PI trough levels and increasing α_1–PI levels in epithelial lining fluid (ELF). Clinical data demonstrating the long–term effects of chronic augmentation or replacement therapy of individuals with Aralast™ are not available.

Safety and effectiveness in pediatric patients have not been established. Aralast™ is not indicated as therapy for lung disease patients in whom congenital α_1–PI deficiency has not been established.

CONTRAINDICATIONS

Aralast™ is contraindicated in individuals with selective IgA deficiencies (IgA level less than 15 mg/dL) who have known antibody against IgA, since they may experience severe reactions, including anaphylaxis, to IgA which may be present.

WARNINGS

Because Alpha$_1$–Proteinase Inhibitor (Human), Aralast™, is derived from pooled human plasma, it may carry a risk of transmitting infectious agents, e.g., viruses and theoretically, the Creutzfeldt–Jakob disease (CJD) agent. Stringent procedures designed to reduce the risk of adventitious agent transmission have been employed in the manufacture of this product, from the screening of plasma donors and the collection and testing of plasma through the application of viral elimination/reduction steps such as alcohol fractionation, PEG precipitation, solvent detergent treatment, and nanofiltration. Despite these measures, such products can still potentially transmit disease; therefore, the risk of infectious agents can not be totally eliminated. ALL infections thought by a physician possibly to have been transmitted by this product should be reported to the manufacturer at 1–888–675–2762 (US) or 1–323–225–9735 (International). The physician should weigh the risks and benefits of the use of this product and should discuss these with the patient.

The rate of administration specified in DOSAGE AND ADMINISTRATION should be closely followed, at least until the physician has had sufficient experience with a given patient. Vital signs should be monitored continuously and the patient should be carefully observed throughout the infusion. **IF ANAPHYLACTIC OR SEVERE ANAPHYLACTOID REACTIONS OCCUR, THE INFUSION SHOULD BE DISCONTINUED IMMEDIATELY.** Epinephrine and other appropriate supportive therapy should be available for the treatment of any acute anaphylactic or anaphylactoid reaction.

PRECAUTIONS

General

Alpha$_1$–Proteinase Inhibitor (Human), Aralast™, should be administered within three (3) hours after the reconstituted product is warmed to room temperature. Partially used vials should be discarded and not saved for future use. The solution contains no preservative.

Aralast™ should be administered alone, without mixing with other agents or diluting solutions.

Pregnancy Category C

Animal reproduction studies have not been conducted with Aralast™. It is also not known whether Aralast™ can cause fetal harm when administered to pregnant women or can affect reproductive capacity.

Nursing Mothers

It is not known whether alpha$_1$–proteinase inhibitor is excreted in human milk. Because many drugs are excreted in human milk, caution should be exercised when Aralast™ is administered to a nursing woman.

Pediatric Use

Safety and effectiveness in pediatric patients have not been established.

ADVERSE REACTIONS

Aralast™ was evaluated for up to 96 weeks in 27 subjects with a congenital deficiency of α_1–PI and clinically evident emphysema. The number of subjects with an adverse event, regardless of causality, was 22 of 27 (81.5%). The number of subjects with an adverse event deemed possibly, probably, or definitely related to study drug was 7 of 27 (25.9%).

The frequency of infusions associated with an adverse event, regardless of causality, was 108 of 1127 (9.6%) infusions administered per protocol. The most common symptoms were pharyngitis (1.6%), headache (0.7%), and increased cough (0.6%). Symptoms of bronchitis, sinusitis, pain, rash, back pain, viral infection, peripheral edema, bloating, dizziness, somnolence, asthma, and rhinitis were each associated with ≥ 0.2% of infusions. All symptoms were mild to moderate in severity.

The overall frequency of adverse events deemed to be possibly, probably, or definitely related to study drug was 15 of 1127 (1.3%) infusions. The most common symptoms included headache (0.3%) and somnolence (0.3%). Symptoms of chills and fever, vasodilation, dizziness, pruritus, rash, abnormal vision, chest pain, increased cough, and dyspnea were each associated with one (0.1%) infusion. Five (5) of 27 (18.5%) subjects experienced eight (8) serious adverse reactions during the study. None of these were considered to be causally related to the administration of Aralast™.

Twenty-six (26) of 27 (96.3%) subjects experienced a total of 94 upper and lower respiratory-tract infections during the 96-week study (median: 3.0; range: 1 – 8; mean ± SD: 3.6 ± 2.3 infections). Twenty-eight (29.8%) of the respiratory infections occurred in 19 (70.4%) subjects during the first 24 weeks of the 96-week study suggesting that the risk of infection did not change with time on Aralast™. In a post-hoc analysis, subjects experienced a range of 0 to 8 exacerbations of COPD over the 96-week study with a median of less than one exacerbation per year (median: 0.61; mean ± SD: 0.83 ± 0.87 exacerbations per year).

Treatment-emergent elevations (> two times the upper limit of normal) in aminotransferases (ALT or AST), up to 3.7 times the upper limit of normal, were noted in 3 of 27 (11.1%) subjects. Elevations were transient lasting three months or less. No subject developed any evidence of viral hepatitis or hepatitis serocon-version while being treated with Aralast™, including 13 evaluable subjects who were not vaccinated against hepatitis B.

No clinically relevant alterations in blood pressure, heart rate, respiratory rate, or body temperature occurred during infusion of Aralast™. Mean hematology and laboratory parameters were little changed over the duration of the study, with individual variations not clinically meaningful.

During the initial 10 weeks of the study, subjects were randomized to receive either Aralast™ or a commercially available preparation of α_1-PI (Prolastin®). Both products were well tolerated with the frequency, severity, and symptomatology of adverse reactions similar in both groups. There were no serious adverse events in the group receiving Aralast™. There were two serious adverse events in the control group, one of which was considered to be possibly related to the control drug and included chest pain, dyspnea, and bilateral pulmonary infiltrates. In addition, one subject in the control group became seropositive to Parvovirus B-19. No seroconversions were observed during the entire 96 week study that were attributable to Aralast™. No subject developed an antibody to α_1–PI.

DOSAGE AND ADMINISTRATION

Chronic Augmentation Therapy

FOR INTRAVENOUS USE ONLY. The recommended dosage of Aralast™ is 60 mg/kg body weight administered once weekly by intravenous infusion. Each vial of Aralast™ has the functional activity, as determined by inhibition of porcine pancreatic elastase, stated on the label. Administration of Aralast™ within three hours after reconstitution is recommended to avoid the potential ill effect of any inadvertent microbial contamination occurring during reconstitution. Discard any unused contents.

Infusion Rate

Aralast™ should be administered at a rate not exceeding 0.08 mL/kg body weight/minute. If adverse events occur, the rate should be reduced or the infusion interrupted until the symptoms subside. The infusion may then be resumed at a rate tolerated by the subject.

RECONSTITUTION

Use Aseptic Technique

1. Aralast™ and diluent should be at room temperature before reconstitution.
2. Remove caps from the diluent and product vials.
3. Swab the exposed stopper surfaces with alcohol.
4. Remove cover from one end of the double–ended transfer needle. Insert the exposed end of the needle through the center of the stopper in the DILUENT vial.
5. Remove plastic cap from the other end of the double–ended transfer needle now seated in the stopper of the diluent vial. To reduce any foaming, invert the vial of diluent and insert the exposed end of the needle through the center of the stopper in the PRODUCT vial at an angle, making certain that the diluent vial is always above the product vial. The angle of insertion directs the flow of diluent against the side of the product vial. Refer to Figure below. The vacuum in the vial is sufficient to allow transfer of all of the diluent.

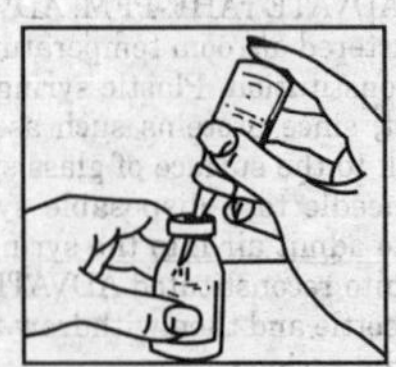

6. Disconnect the two vials by removing the transfer needle from the diluent vial stopper. Remove the double-ended transfer needle from the product vial and discard the needle into the appropriate safety container.
7. Let the vial stand until most of the contents is in solution, then GENTLY swirl until the powder is completely dissolved. Reconstitution requires no more than five minutes for a 0.5 gram vial and no more than 10 minutes for a 1.0 gram vial.
8. DO NOT SHAKE THE CONTENTS OF THE VIAL. DO NOT INVERT THE VIAL UNTIL READY TO WITHDRAW CONTENTS.
9. Use within three hours of reconstitution.
10. After reconstitution, inspect product visually for particulate matter and discoloration prior to administration. When reconstitution procedure is strictly followed, a few small particles may occasionally remain. These will be removed by the microaggregate filter.
11. Reconstituted product from several vials may be pooled into an empty, sterile IV solution container by using aseptic technique. A sterile, 20 micron filter spike is provided for this purpose.

HOW SUPPLIED

Alpha$_1$–Proteinase Inhibitor (Human), Aralast™, is supplied as a sterile, nonpyrogenic, lyophilized powder in single-dose vials. A suitable volume of Sterile Water for Injection, USP diluent is provided (25 mL/0.5 g vial; 50 mL/1.0 g vial). Each vial is labeled with the total α_1–PI functional activity in mg. Aralast™ is packaged with a sterile double-ended transfer needle and a sterile 20 micron filter.

STORAGE

Aralast™ should be stored at 2-8 °C (35-46 °F). Aralast™ may be removed from refrigeration and stored at temperatures not to exceed 25 °C (77 °F). Product removed from refrigeration must be used within one month. Do not freeze. Do not use after the expiration date printed on the label.

Rx only

REFERENCES

1. Brantly M, Nukiwa T, Crystal RG. Molecular basis of alpha–1–antitrypsin deficiency. Am J Med 1988 (Suppl 6A);84:13–31.
2. Data on file at Alpha Therapeutic Corporation.
3. Crystal RG, Brantly ML, Hubbard RC, Curiel DT, et al. The alpha1–antitrypsin gene and its mutations: Clinical consequences and strategies for therapy. Chest 1989;95: 196–208.
4. Crystal RG. α_1–Antitrypsin deficiency: pathogenesis and treatment. Hospital Practice 1991; Feb.15:81–94.
5. Hutchison DCS. Natural history of alpha–1–protease inhibitor deficiency. Am J Med 1988;84(Suppl 6A):3–12.
6. Hubbard RC, Crystal RG. Alpha–1–antitrypsin augmentation therapy for alpha–1–antitrypsin deficiency. Am J Med 1988;84(Suppl 6A):52–62.
7. Ogushi F, Fells GA, Hubbard RC, et al. Z–Type α_1–antitrypsin as an inhibitor of neutrophil elastase. J Clin Investigation 1987;80:1366–1374.
8. Buist SA, Burrows B, Cohen A, et al. Guidelines for the approach to the patient with severe hereditary alpha–1–antitrypsin deficiency. Am Rev Respir Dis 1989;140:1494–1497.
9. Stoller JK, Brantly M, Fleming LE, et al. Formation and current results of a patient-organized registry for α_1–antitrypsin deficiency. Chest 2000; 118(3):843-848.

DATE OF REVISION: January 2003

Manufactured by:
alpha®
THERAPEUTIC CORPORATION
LOS ANGELES, CA 90032 USA
U.S. LICENSE NO. 744
Distributed by:
Baxter
Baxter Healthcare Corporation
One Baxter Way
Westlake Village, CA 91362 USA

Printed In USA
08-8127-01

BUMINATE® 5%

℞

[*bew-mĭ-nāt*]

Albumin (Human), USP, 5% Solution

DESCRIPTION

BUMINATE 5%, Albumin (Human), 5% Solution, is a sterile, nonpyrogenic preparation of albumin in a single dosage form for intravenous administration. Each 100 mL contains 5 g of albumin and was prepared from human venous plasma using the Cohn cold ethanol fractionation process. Source material for fractionation may be obtained from another U.S. licensed manufacturer. It has been adjusted to physiological pH with sodium bicarbonate and/or sodium hydroxide and has been stabilized with sodium acetyltryptophanate and sodium caprylate. The sodium content is 145 ± 15 mEq/L. The solution contains no preservative and none of the coagulation factors found in fresh whole blood or plasma. BUMINATE 5%, Albumin (Human), 5% Solution, is a transparent or slightly opalescent solution which may have a greenish tint or may vary from a pale straw to an amber color.

Table 1
Summary of Viral Reduction Factor for Each Virus and Processing Step

Process Step	Viral Reduction Factor ($\log_{10}$)				
	Lipid Enveloped			Non-lipid Enveloped	
	BVD	HIV-1	PRV	HAV	PPV
Step 1: Processing of cryo-poor plasma to Fraction I+II+III centrifugate	1.2±0.0	5.8±0.0	4.6±0.05	1.9±0.8	1.4±0.1
Step 2: Processing of Fraction I+II+III centrifugate to Fraction IV_1 centrifugate	2.8±0.5	NCM	3.4±0.4	1.9±0.7	(1.2±0.3)*
Step 3: Processing of Fraction IV_1 centrifugate to Fraction IV_4 centrifugate/filter press filtrate†	>2.4±0.1/ >2.4±0.1	≥4.4±0.5/ ≥4.5±0.5	>4.8±0.1/ >4.8±0.1	3.8±0.1/ 2.9±0.2	2.2±0.3/ 2.0±0.3
Step 4: Processing of Fraction IV_4 centrifugate/filter press filtrate to Fraction IV_4 Cuno 70C filtrate††	>1.6±0.2/ >1.7±0.1	NCM	>4.1±0.5/ >4.4±0.1	4.7±0.1/ 4.6±0.1	2.3±0.3/ 3.0±0.8
Step 5: Processing of Fraction V suspension to Cuno 90LP filtrate	(0.2±0.2)*	≥5.0±0.5	>4.6±0.0	4.2±0.4	3.4±0.5
Step 6: Pasteurization	>4.9±0.1	>5.1±0.3	>5.3±0.1	5.3±0.4	NT
Cumulative Reduction Factor, $\log_{10}$**	**>12.9/13.0**	**>20.3/20.4**	**>26.8/27.1**	**21.8/20.8**	**9.3/9.8**

NT Not tested.
NCM No virus reduction claim made at this step.
* Since the reduction factor of =1.0 is within the variability limit of the assay, these values are not included in the computation of the cumulative reduction factor.
† Two reduction factors indicate the two liquid-solid separation options available at this step.
†† Two reduction factors indicate the two starting materials at this step.
** Two cumulative reduction factors derived from the use of the two liquid-solid separation options available at Step 3.

The likelihood of the presence of viable hepatitis viruses has been reduced by heating the product for 10 hours at 60°C. This procedure has been shown to be an effective method of inactivating hepatitis virus in albumin solutions even when those solutions were prepared from plasma known to be infective.[1–3]

BUMINATE 5%, Albumin (Human), 5% Solution, contains no blood group isoagglutinins thereby permitting its administration without regard to the recipient's blood group.

CLINICAL PHARMACOLOGY

Albumin is responsible for 70–80% of the colloid osmotic pressure of normal plasma, thus making it useful in regulating and increasing blood volume.[4,5,6] It is also a transport protein and binds naturally occurring, therapeutic and toxic materials in the circulation.[5,6] BUMINATE 5%, Albumin (Human), 5% Solution, is osmotically equivalent to an equal volume of normal human plasma and will increase circulating plasma volume by an amount approximately equal to the volume infused. The degree and duration of volume expansion depends upon the initial blood volume. With patients treated for diminished blood volume, the effect of infused albumin may last for many hours. In patients with normal blood volumes, the hemodilution lasts for a shorter period.[7,8]

Total body albumin is estimated to be 350 g for a 70 kg man and is distributed throughout the extracellular compartments. The half-life of albumin is 15 to 20 days with a turnover of approximately 15 g per day.[5]

The minimum plasma albumin level necessary to prevent or reverse peripheral edema is unknown. Some investigators recommend that plasma albumin levels be maintained at approximately 2.5 g/dL. This concentration provides a plasma oncotic pressure value of 20 mm Hg.[4]

BUMINATE 5%, Albumin (Human), 5% Solution, is manufactured by the modified Cohn-Oncley cold ethanol fractionation process which includes a series of cold-ethanol precipitation, centrifugation and/or filtration of human plasma followed by pasteurization of the final product at 60 ± 0.5°C for 10–11 hours. This process accomplishes both purification of albumin and the reduction of viruses.

In vitro studies demonstrate that the manufacturing process for BUMINATE 5%, Albumin (Human), 5% Solution, provides for significant viral reduction. These viral reduction studies, summarized in Table 1, demonstrate viral clearance during the manufacturing process for BUMINATE 5%, Albumin (Human), 5% Solution, using human immunodeficiency virus, type 1 (HIV-1) both as a relevant and model virus for HIV-2 and other enveloped RNA viruses; bovine viral diarrheal virus (BVD), a model for lipid enveloped RNA viruses, such as hepatitis C virus (HCV); porcine parvovirus (PPV), a model for non-lipid enveloped DNA viruses such as human parvovirus B19; hepatitis A virus (HAV), a relevant virus and a model for non-lipid enveloped RNA viruses.

These studies indicate that specific manufacturing steps for BUMINATE 5%, Albumin (Human), 5% Solution, are capable of eliminating/inactivating a wide range of relevant and model viruses. Since the mechanism of virus elimination/inactivation at each step is different, the overall manufacturing process of BUMINATE 5%, Albumin (Human), 5% Solution, is robust in reducing viral load.

[See table 1 above]

INDICATIONS AND USAGE

1. Hypovolemia

Hypovolemia is a possible indication for use of BUMINATE 5%, Albumin (Human), 5% Solution. Its effectiveness in reversing hypovolemia depends largely upon its colloid osmotic pressure. Although crystalloid solutions and colloid-containing plasma substitutes can be used in emergency treatment of shock, Albumin (Human) has a longer intravascular half-life than crystalloid solutions.[9]

When the hypovolemia is long-standing and hypoalbuminemia exists accompanied by adequate hydration or edema, treatment with BUMINATE 25%, Albumin (Human), 25% Solution, is preferable.[4,6]

When blood volume deficit is the result of hemorrhage, compatible red blood cells or whole blood should be administered as quickly as possible.

2. Hypoalbuminemia

A. General

Hypoalbuminemia is another possible indication for use of BUMINATE 5%, Albumin (Human), 5% Solution. Hypoalbuminemia can result from one or more of the following:[5]

(1) Inadequate production (malnutrition, burns, major injury, infections, etc.)
(2) Excessive catabolism (burns, major injury, pancreatitis, etc.)
(3) Loss from the body (hemorrhage, excessive renal excretion, burn exudates, etc.)
(4) Redistribution within the body (major surgery, various inflammatory conditions, etc.)

When albumin deficit is the result of excessive protein loss, the effect of administration of albumin will be temporary unless the underlying disorder is reversed. In most cases, increased nutritional replacement of amino acids and/or protein with concurrent treatment of the underlying disorder will restore normal plasma albumin levels more effectively than administration of albumin solutions. Occasionally hypoalbuminemia accompanying severe injuries, infections or severe pancreatitis cannot be quickly reversed and nutritional supplements may fail to restore adequate plasma albumin levels. In these cases, BUMINATE 5%, Albumin (Human), 5% Solution, may be useful.

B. Burns

In conjunction with appropriate crystalloid therapy, BUMINATE 5%, Albumin (Human), 5% Solution, may be useful for treatment of protein deficits after the initial 24-hour period following extensive burns.[4]

3. Miscellaneous Indications

BUMINATE 5%, Albumin (Human), 5% Solution, may be indicated prior to or during cardiopulmonary bypass surgery, though the data do not indicate a clear-cut advantage over crystalloid solutions.[4,6,10]

There is no valid reason for use of albumin as an intravenous nutrient.

CONTRAINDICATIONS

A history of allergic reactions to albumin is a specific contraindication to the use of this product.

BUMINATE 5%, Albumin (Human), 5% Solution, is also contraindicated in severely anemic patients and in patients with cardiac failure.

WARNINGS

Do not use if turbid. Do not begin administration more than 4 hours after the container has been entered.

BUMINATE 5%, Albumin (Human), 5% Solution, is made from human plasma. Products made from human plasma may contain infectious agents, such as viruses, that can cause disease. The risk that such products will transmit an infectious agent has been reduced by screening plasma donors for prior exposure to certain viruses, by testing for the presence of certain current virus infections, and by

Continued on next page

Buminate 5%—Cont.

inactivating and/or removing certain viruses (See DESCRIPTION). Despite these measures, such products can still potentially transmit disease. Based on effective donor screening and product manufacturing processes, albumin carries an extremely remote risk for transmission of viral diseases. A theoretical risk for transmission of Creutzfeldt-Jakob disease (CJD) also is considered extremely remote. No cases of transmission of viral diseases or CJD have ever been identified for albumin. ALL infections thought by a physician possibly to have been transmitted by this product should be reported by the physician or other healthcare provider to Baxter Healthcare Corporation at 1-800-423-2862. The physician should discuss the risks and benefits of this product with the patient.

PRECAUTIONS

Certain components used in the packaging of this product contain natural rubber latex.

BUMINATE 5%, Albumin (Human), 5% Solution, may be given rapidly to individuals with reduced plasma volume with the following exception: if a patient has a history of cardiac or circulatory disease, BUMINATE 5%, Albumin (Human), 5% Solution, should be administered slowly (5 to 10 mL per minute) to avoid too rapid a rise in the blood pressure.

Patients should always be carefully monitored in order to guard against the possibility of circulatory overload.

When BUMINATE 5%, Albumin (Human), 5% Solution, is used following injuries or surgery, the quick rise in blood pressure which follows administration makes it necessary to monitor the patient to detect and treat severed blood vessels that may not have bled at a lower blood pressure.

Pregnancy - Category C

Animal reproduction studies have not been conducted with BUMINATE 5%, Albumin (Human), 5% Solution. It is not known whether BUMINATE 5%, Albumin (Human), 5% Solution, can cause fetal harm when administered to a pregnant woman or can affect reproductive capacity. BUMINATE 5%, Albumin (Human), 5% Solution, should be given to a pregnant woman only if clearly needed.

Pediatric Use

The use of BUMINATE 5%, Albumin (Human), 5% Solution, in children has not been associated with any special or specific hazard, if the dose is appropriate for the child's body weight.

ADVERSE REACTIONS

Untoward reactions to BUMINATE 5%, Albumin (Human), 5% Solution, are extremely rare, although nausea, fever, chills or urticaria may occasionally occur. Such symptoms usually disappear when the infusion is slowed or stopped for a short period of time.

DOSAGE AND ADMINISTRATION

BUMINATE 5%, Albumin (Human), 5% Solution, must be administered intravenously. It may be administered either in conjunction with or combined with other parenterals such as whole blood, plasma, saline, glucose or sodium lactate. The volume of the total dose and the rate of infusion depends on the patient's condition and response.

Recommended Dosages

1. Hypovolemia
   Although the volume of BUMINATE 5%, Albumin (Human), 5% Solution, administered must be individualized, the initial dose should be 250 to 500 mL for older children and adults and 12 to 20 mL per kilogram of body weight for infants and young children. It may be repeated after 30 minutes intervals if the response is not adequate.
2. Hypoalbuminemia
   Hypoalbuminemia is usually accompanied by a hidden extravascular albumin deficiency of equal magnitude. This total body albumin deficit must be considered when determining the amount of albumin necessary to reverse the hypoalbuminemia. When using the patient's serum albumin concentration to estimate the deficit, the body albumin compartment should be calculated to be 80 to 100 mL per kilogram of body weight.[5,6] Daily dose should not exceed 2 g of albumin per kilogram of body weight.
3. Burns
   When BUMINATE 5%, Albumin (Human), 5% Solution, is administered after the first 24 hours following burns, an initial dose of 500 mL is recommended.

Preparation for Administration

Parenteral drug products should be inspected visually for particulate matter and discoloration prior to administration, whenever solution and container permit.

1. Remove cap from bottle to expose center portion of rubber stopper.
2. Clean stopper with germicidal solution.

Administration

Follow directions for use printed on the administration set container. Make certain that the administration set contains an adequate filter.

HOW SUPPLIED

BUMINATE 5%, Albumin (Human), 5% Solution, is supplied in 250 mL and 500 mL bottles.

Storage

Store BUMINATE 5%, Albumin (Human), 5% Solution, at room temperature, not to exceed 30°C (86°F). Avoid freezing to prevent damage to the bottle.

REFERENCES

1. Gellis SS, Neefe JR, Stokes J Jr, *et al:* Chemical, clinical and immunological studies on the products of human plasma fractionation. XXXVI. Inactivation of the virus of homologous serum hepatitis in solutions of normal human serum albumin by means of heat. **J Clin Invest 27**:239-244,1948.
2. Gerety RJ, Aronson DL: Plasma derivatives and viral hepatitis. **Transfusion 22**: 347-351, 1982
3. Murray R, Diefenbach WCL, Geller H, *et al:* Problem of reducing danger of serum hepatitis from blood and blood products. **NY State J Med 55**:1145-1150, 1955
4. Tullis JL: Albumin, 1. Background and use, and 2. Guidelines for clinical use. **JAMA 237**:355-360, 460-463, 1977
5. Peters T Jr: Serum albumin, in **The Plasma Proteins, 2nd ed, Vol 1.** Putnam FW (ed). New York, Academic Press, 1975, pp 133-181
6. Finlayson JS: Albumin products. **Sem Thromb Hemostas 6**:85-120, 1980
7. Janeway CA, Berenberg W, Hutchins G: Indications and uses of blood, blood derivatives and blood substitutes. **Med Clin N Amer 29**:1069-1094, 1945
8. Janeway CA, Gibson ST, Woodruff LM, *et al:* Chemical, clinical, and immunological studies on the products of human plasma fractionation. VII. Concentrated human serum albumin. **J Clin Invest 23**:465-490, 1944
9. Shoemaker WC, Schlichter M, Hopkins JA, *et al:* Comparison of the relative effectiveness of colloids and crystalloids in emergency resuscitation. **Am J Surg 142**: 73-83, 1981
10. Lowenstein E, Hallowell P, Bland JHL: Use of colloid and crystalloid solutions in open heart surgery: Physiological basis and clinical results, in **Proceedings of the Workshop on Albumin.** Sgouris JT, Rene A (eds.) DHEW Publication No. (NIH) 76-925, Washington DC, U.S. Government Printing Office, 1976, pp 195-210

Baxter and BUMINATE are trademarks of Baxter International, Inc., and are registered in the U.S. Patent and Trademark office.

Baxter Healthcare Corporation
Glendale, CA 91203 USA
U.S. License No. 140
Revised September 2002

BUMINATE® 25% ℞

[*bew-mĭ-nāt*]

Albumin (Human), USP, 25% Solution

DESCRIPTION

BUMINATE 25%, Albumin (Human), 25% Solution is a sterile, nonpyrogenic preparation of albumin in a single dosage form for intravenous administration. Each 100 mL contains 25 g of albumin and is prepared from human venous plasma using the Cohn cold ethanol fractionation process. Source material for fractionation may be obtained from another U.S. licensed manufacturer. It has been adjusted to physiological pH with sodium bicarbonate and/or sodium hydroxide and stabilized with sodium acetyltryptophanate and sodium caprylate. The sodium content is 145 ± 15 mEq/L. This solution contains no preservative and none of the coagulation factors found in fresh whole blood or plasma. BUMINATE 25%, Albumin (Human), 25% Solution is a transparent or slightly opalescent solution which may have a greenish tint or may vary from a pale straw to an amber color.

The likelihood of the presence of viable hepatitis viruses has been minimized by heating the product for 10 hours at 60°C. This procedure has been shown to be an effective method of inactivating hepatitis virus in albumin solutions even when those solutions were prepared from plasma known to be infective.[1–3]

CLINICAL PHARMACOLOGY

Albumin is responsible for 70–80% of the colloid osmotic pressure of normal plasma, thus making it useful in regulating the volume of circulating blood.[4–6] Albumin is also a transport protein and binds naturally occurring, therapeutic and toxic materials in the circulation.[5,6]

BUMINATE 25%, Albumin (Human), 25% Solution is osmotically equivalent to approximately five times its volume of human plasma. When injected intravenously, 25% albumin will draw about 3.5 times its volume of additional fluid into the circulation within 15 minutes, except when the patient is markedly dehydrated. This extra fluid reduces hemoconcentration and blood viscosity. The degree and duration of volume expansion depends upon the initial blood volume. With patients treated for diminished blood volume, the effect of infused albumin may persist for many hours; however, in patients with normal volume, the duration will be shorter.[7,8]

Total body albumin is estimated to be 350 g for a 70 kg man and is distributed throughout the extracellular compartments; more than 60% is located in the extravascular fluid compartment. The half-life of albumin is 15 to 20 days with a turnover of approximately 15 g per day.[5]

The minimum plasma albumin level necessary to prevent or reverse peripheral edema is unknown. Some investigators recommend that plasma albumin levels be maintained at approximately 2.5 g/dL. This concentration provides a plasma oncotic value of 20 mm Hg.[4]

BUMINATE 25%, Albumin (Human), 25% Solution is manufactured from human plasma by the modified Cohn-Oncley cold ethanol fractionation process, which includes a series of cold-ethanol precipitation, centrifugation and/or filtration steps followed by pasteurization of the final product at 60 ± 0.5°C for 10–11 hours. This process accomplishes both purification of albumin and reduction of viruses.

In vitro studies, demonstrate that the manufacturing process for BUMINATE 25%, Albumin (Human), 25% Solution provides for significant viral reduction. These viral reduction studies, summarized in Table 1, demonstrate viral clearance during the manufacturing process for BUMINATE 25%, Albumin (Human), 25% Solution using human immunodeficiency virus, type 1 (HIV-1) both as a relevant virus in its own right and as model virus for HIV-2 and other enveloped RNA viruses; bovine viral diarrheal virus (BVD), a model for lipid enveloped RNA viruses, such as hepatitis C virus (HCV); porcine parvovirus (PPV), a model for non-lipid enveloped DNA viruses such as human parvovirus B19; hepatitis A virus (HAV), a relevant virus in its own right and a model for other non-lipid enveloped RNA viruses.

These studies indicate that specific steps in the manufacture of BUMINATE 25%, Albumin (Human), 25% Solution are capable of eliminating/inactivating a wide range of relevant and model viruses. Since the mechanism of virus elimination/inactivation at each step is different, the overall manufacturing process of BUMINATE 25%, Albumin (Human), 25% Solution is robust in reducing viral load.

[See table 1 at top of next page]

INDICATIONS AND USAGE

1. Hypovolemia

Hypovolemia is a possible indication for BUMINATE 25%, Albumin (Human), 25% Solution. Its effectiveness in reversing hypovolemia depends largely upon its ability to draw interstitial fluid into the circulation. It is most effective with patients who are well hydrated.

When hypovolemia is long standing and hypoalbuminemia exists accompanied by adequate hydration or edema, 25% albumin is preferable to 5% protein solutions.[4,6] However, in the absence of adequate or excessive hydration, 5% protein solutions should be used or 25% albumin should be diluted with crystalloid.

Although crystalloid solutions and colloid-containing plasma substitutes can be used in emergency treatment of shock, Albumin (Human) has a prolonged intravascular half-life.[9] When blood volume deficit is the result of hemorrhage, compatible red blood cells or whole blood should be administered as quickly as possible.

2. Hypoalbuminemia

A. General

Hypoalbuminemia is another possible indication for use of BUMINATE 25%, Albumin (Human), 25% Solution. Hypoalbuminemia can result from one or more of the following:[5]

(1) Inadequate production (malnutrition, burns, major injury, infections, etc.)
(2) Excessive catabolism (burns, major injury, pancreatitis, etc.)
(3) Loss from the body (hemorrhage, excessive renal excretion, burn exudates, etc.)
(4) Redistribution within the body (major surgery, various inflammatory conditions, etc.)

When albumin deficit is the result of excessive protein loss, the effect of administration of albumin will be temporary unless the underlying disorder is reversed. In most cases, increased nutritional replacement of amino acids and/or protein with concurrent treatment of the underlying disorder will restore normal plasma albumin levels more effectively than albumin solutions. Occasionally hypoalbuminemia accompanying severe injuries, infections or pancreatitis cannot be quickly reversed and nutritional supplements may fail to restore serum albumin levels. In these cases, BUMINATE 25%, Albumin (Human), 25% Solution might be a useful therapeutic adjunct.

B. Burns

An optimum regimen for the use of albumin, electrolytes and fluid in the early treatment of burns has not been established, however, in conjunction with appropriate crystalloid therapy, BUMINATE 25%, Albumin (Human), 25% Solution may be indicated for treatment of oncotic deficits after the initial 24 hour period following extensive burns and to replace the protein loss which accompanies any severe burn.[4,6]

C. Adult Respiratory Distress Syndrome (ARDS)

A characteristic of ARDS is a hypoproteinemic state which may be causally related to the interstitial pulmonary edema. Although uncertainty exists concerning the precise indication of albumin infusion in these patients, if there is a pulmonary overload accompanied by hypoalbuminemia, 25% albumin solution may have a therapeutic effect when used with a diuretic.[4]

D. Nephrosis

BUMINATE 25%, Albumin (Human), 25% Solution may be a useful aid in treating edema in patients with severe nephrosis who are receiving steroids and/or diuretics.

3. Cardiopulmonary Bypass Surgery

BUMINATE 25%, Albumin (Human), 25% Solution has been recommended prior to or during cardiopulmonary bypass surgery, although no clear data exist indicating its advantage over crystalloid solutions.[4,6,10]

4. **Hemolytic Disease of the Newborn (HDN)**
BUMINATE 25%, Albumin (Human), 25% Solution may be administered in an attempt to bind and detoxify unconjugated bilirubin in infants with severe HDN.

There is no valid reason for use of albumin as an intravenous nutrient.

CONTRAINDICATIONS

A history of allergic reactions to albumin is a specific contraindication to the use of this product. BUMINATE 25%, Albumin (Human), 25% Solution is also contraindicated in severely anemic patients and in patients with cardiac failure.

WARNINGS

Do not use if turbid. Do not begin administration more than 4 hours after the container has been entered. Discard unused portion.

There exists a risk of potentially fatal hemolysis and acute renal failure from the inappropriate use of Sterile Water for Injection as a diluent for BUMINATE 25%, Albumin (Human), 25% Solution. Acceptable diluents include 0.9% Sodium Chloride or 5% Dextrose in Water.

BUMINATE 25%, Albumin (Human), 25% Solution is made from human plasma. Products made from human plasma may contain infectious agents, such as viruses, that can cause disease. The risk that such products will transmit an infectious agent has been reduced by screening plasma donors for prior exposure to certain viruses, by testing for the presence of certain current virus infections, and by inactivating and/or removing certain viruses (See Description). Despite these measures, such products can still potentially transmit disease. Based on effective donor screening and product manufacturing processes, albumin carries an extremely remote risk for transmission of viral diseases. A theoretical risk for transmission of Creutzfeldt-Jakob disease (CJD) also is considered extremely remote. No cases of transmission of viral diseases or CJD have ever been identified for albumin. ALL infections thought by a physician possibly to have been transmitted by this product should be reported by the physician or other healthcare provider to Baxter Healthcare Corporation at 1-800-423-2862. The physician should discuss the risks and benefits of this product with the patient.

PRECAUTIONS

Certain components used in the packaging of this product contain natural rubber latex.

BUMINATE 25%, Albumin (Human), 25% Solution must be administered intravenously at a rate not to exceed 1mL/min to patients with normal blood volume. More rapid administration might cause circulatory overload and pulmonary edema.

A rise in blood pressure after 25% albumin infusion necessitates careful observation of the injured or post-operative patient in order to detect and treat severed blood vessels that may not have bled at a lower blood pressure.

Pregnancy—Category C
Animal reproduction studies have not been conducted with BUMINATE 25%, Albumin (Human), 25% Solution. It is not known whether BUMINATE 25%, Albumin (Human), 25% Solution can cause fetal harm when administered to a pregnant woman or can affect reproductive capacity. BUMINATE 25%, Albumin (Human), 25% Solution should be given to a pregnant woman only if clearly needed.

Pediatric Use
The use of BUMINATE 25%, Albumin (Human), 25% Solution in children has not been associated with any special or specific hazard, if the dose is appropriate for the child's body weight.

ADVERSE REACTIONS

Untoward reactions to BUMINATE 25%, Albumin (Human), 25% Solution are extremely rare, although nausea, fever, chills or urticaria may occasionally occur. Such symptoms usually disappear when the infusion is slowed or stopped for a short period of time.

DOSAGE AND ADMINISTRATION

BUMINATE 25%, Albumin (Human), 25% Solution must be administered intravenously. This solution may be administered in conjunction with or combined with other parenterals such as whole blood, plasma, saline, glucose or sodium lactate. The addition of four volumes of normal saline or 5% glucose to 1 volume of BUMINATE 25%, Albumin (Human), 25% Solution gives a solution which is approximately isotonic and isosmotic with citrated plasma.

Albumin solutions should not be mixed with protein hydrolysates or solutions containing alcohol.

Recommended Dosages

1. Hypovolemic Shock
The dosage of BUMINATE 25%, Albumin (Human), 25% Solution must be individualized. As a guideline, the initial treatment should be in the range of 100 to 200 mL for adults and 2.5 to 5 mL per kilogram body weight for children. This may be repeated after 15 to 30 minutes, if the response is not adequate. For patients with significant plasma volume deficits, albumin replacement is best administered in the form of 5% Albumin (Human).
Upon administration of additional albumin or if hemorrhage has occurred, hemodilution and a relative anemia will follow. This condition should be controlled by the supplemental administration of compatible red blood cells or compatible whole blood.

Table 1
Summary of Viral Reduction Factor for Each Virus and Processing Step

Process Step	Viral Reduction Factor (log_{10})				
	Lipid Enveloped			Non-lipid Enveloped	
	BVD	HIV-1	PRV	HAV	PPV
Step 1: Processing of cryo-poor plasma to Fraction I+II+III centrifugate	1.2±0.0	5.8±0.0	4.6±0.5	1.9±0.8	1.4±0.1
Step 2: Processing of Fraction I+II+III centrifugate to Fraction IV_1 centrifugate	2.8±0.5	NCM	3.4±0.4	1.9±0.7	(1.2±0.3)*
Step 3: Processing of Fraction IV_1 centrifugate to Fraction IV_4 centrifugate/filter press filtrate†	>2.4±0.1/ >2.4±0.1	≥4.4±0.5/ ≥4.5±0.5	>4.8±0.1/ >4.8±0.1	3.8±0.1/ 2.9±0.2	2.2±0.3/ 2.0±0.3
Step 4: Processing of Fraction IV_4 centrifugate/filter press filtrate to Fraction IV_4 Cuno 70C filtrate††	>1.6±0.2/ >1.7±0.1	NCM	>4.1±0.5/ >4.4±0.1	4.7±0.1/ 4.6±0.1	2.3±0.3/ 3.0±0.8
Step 5: Processing of Fraction V suspension to Cuno 90LP filtrate	(0.2±0.2)*	≥5.0±0.5	>4.6±0.0	4.2±0.4	3.4±0.5
Step 6: Pasteurization	>4.9±0.1	>5.1±0.3	>5.3±0.1	5.3±0.4	NT
Cumulative Reduction Factor, log_{10}**	**>12.9/13.0**	**>20.3/20.4**	**>26.8/27.1**	**21.8/20.8**	**9.3/9.8**

NT Not tested.
NCM No virus reduction claim made at this step.
* Since the reduction factor of =1.0 is within the variability limit of the assay, these values are not included in the computation of the cumulative reduction factor.
† Two reduction factors indicate the two liquid-solid separation options available at this step.
†† Two reduction factors indicate the two starting materials at this step.
** Two cumulative reduction factors derived from the use of the two liquid-solid separation options available at Step 3.

2. Burns
The optimal therapeutic regimen for administration of crystalloid and colloid solutions after extensive burns has not been established. When BUMINATE 25%, Albumin (Human), 25% Solution is administered after the first 24 hours following burns, the dose should be determined according to the patient's condition and response to treatment.
3. Hypoalbuminemia
Hypoalbuminemia is usually accompanied by a hidden extravascular albumin deficiency of equal magnitude. This total body albumin deficit must be considered when determining the amount of albumin necessary to reverse the hypoalbuminemia. When using patient's serum albumin concentration to estimate the deficit, the body albumin compartment should be calculated to be 80 to 100 mL per kg of body weight.[5,6] Daily dose should not exceed 2 g of albumin per kilogram of body weight.
4. Hemolytic Disease of the Newborn
BUMINATE 25%, Albumin (Human), 25% Solution may be administered prior to or during exchange transfusion in a dose of 1 g per kilogram body weight.[11]

Preparation for Administration
Parenteral drug products should be inspected visually for particulate matter and discoloration prior to administration, whenever solution and container permit.
1. Remove cap from bottle to expose center portion of rubber stopper.
2. Clean stopper with germicidal solution.

Administration
Follow directions for use printed on the administration set container. Make certain that the administration set contains an adequate filter.

HOW SUPPLIED

BUMINATE 25%, Albumin (Human), 25% Solution is supplied in 20 mL, 50 mL and 100 mL bottles.

Storage
Store BUMINATE 25%, Albumin (Human), 25% Solution at room temperature, not to exceed 30°C (86°F). Avoid freezing to prevent damage to the bottle.

REFERENCES

1. Gellis SS, Neefe JR, Stokes J Jr, *et al*: Chemical, clinical and immunological studies on the products of human plasma fractionation. XXXVI. Inactivation of the virus of homologous serum hepatitis in solutions of normal human serum albumin by means of heat. **J Clin Invest 27**:239–244, 1948
2. Gerety RJ, Aronson DL: Plasma derivatives and viral hepatitis. **Transfusion 22**:347–351, 1982
3. Murray R, Diefenbach WCL, Geller H, *et al*: Problem of reducing danger of serum hepatitis from blood and blood products. **NY State J Med 55**:1145–1150, 1955
4. Tullis JL: Albumin, 1. Background and use, and 2. Guidelines for clinical use. **JAMA 237**:355–360, 460–463, 1977
5. Peters T Jr: Serum albumin, in **The Plasma Proteins, 2nd ed, Vol 1**. Putnam FW (ed). New York, Academic Press, 1975, pp 133–181
6. Finlayson JS: Albumin products. **Semin Thromb Hemostas 6**:85–120, 1980
7. Janeway CA, Berenberg W, Hutchins G: Indications and uses of blood, blood derivatives and blood substitutes. **Med Clin N Amer 29**:1069–1094, 1945
8. Janeway CA, Gibson ST, Woodruff LM, *et al*: Chemical, clinical and immunological studies on the products of human plasma fractionation. VII. Concentrated human serum albumin. **J Clin Invest 23**:465–490, 1944
9. Shoemaker WC, Schluchter M, Hopkins JA, *et al*: Comparison of the relative effectiveness of colloids and crystalloids in emergency resuscitation. **Am J Surg 142**:73–83, 1981
10. Lowenstein E, Hallowell P, Bland JHL: Use of colloid and crystalloid solutions in open heart surgery: Physiological basis and clinical results in, **Proceedings of the Workshop on Albumin.** Sgouris JT, Rene A (eds). DHEW Publication No. (NIH) 76-925, Washington, DC, US Government Printing Office, 1976, pp 195–210
11. Tsao YC, Yu VYH: Albumin in management of neonatal hyperbilirubinaemia. **Arch Dis Childhood 47**:250–256, 1972

Baxter and Buminate are trademarks of Baxter International, and are registered in the U.S. Patent and Trademark office.

Baxter Healthcare Corporation
Glendale, CA 91203 USA
U.S. License No. 140
Revised September 2002

FEIBA VH ℞

[*fī-băh*]
Anti-Inhibitor, Coagulant Complex, Vapor Heated

DESCRIPTION

FEIBA VH Anti-Inhibitor Coagulant Complex, Vapor Heated (AICC) is a freeze-dried sterile human plasma fraction with Factor VIII inhibitor bypassing activity. In vitro, **FEIBA** VH AICC shortens the activated partial thromboplastin time (APTT) of plasma containing Factor VIII inhibitor. Factor VIII inhibitor bypassing activity is expressed in arbitrary units. One IMMUNO Unit of activity is defined as that amount of **FEIBA** VH AICC that shortens the APTT of a high titer Factor VIII inhibitor reference plasma to 50% of the blank value. The product is intended for intravenous administration.

FEIBA VH AICC contains Factors II, IX, and X, mainly non-activated, and Factor VII[1–3] mainly in the activated form. The product contains approximately equal unitages of Factor VIII inhibitor bypassing activity and Prothrombin Complex Factors. In addition, 1 – 6 units of Factor VIII coagulant antigen (FVIII C:Ag) per mL are present. The preparation contains only traces of factors of the kinin generating system. It contains no heparin.

Reconstituted **FEIBA** VH AICC contains 4 mg of trisodium citrate and 8 mg of sodium chloride per mL.

FEIBA VH Anti-Inhibitor Coagulant Complex, Vapor Heated has been prepared from Source Plasma and/or Plasma.

The product has been subjected to in-process virus inactivation where vapor is first applied for 10 hours at 60° ± 0.5°C and an excess pressure of 190 ± 20 mbar followed by 1 hour at 80°± 0.5°C and an excess pressure of 370 ± 30 mbar. (Refer to Clinical Pharmacology and Warnings sections).

Continued on next page

Feiba VH—Cont.

CLINICAL PHARMACOLOGY

In a preclinical study to determine the virus inactivating efficacy of vapor heating, samples of bulk **FEIBA** IMMUNO Anti-Inhibitor Coagulant Complex were spiked with 2 × 10^6/mL infectious units of HIV and subjected to vapor heat treatment. The residual virus titer was found to be less than 1 infectious unit/0.5 mL. A clinical study[4] testing Antihemophilic Factor treated by a similar vapor heating procedure has shown none of 4 lots used in the study to produce non A, non B hepatitis in intensively followed patients naive to blood product administration.

The safety and efficacy of **FEIBA** IMMUNO AICC has been demonstrated by two prospective clinical trials[5–7]. The first, conducted by Sixma and collaborators during 1979 and early 1980, was a randomized double-blind study comparing the effect of **FEIBA** IMMUNO AICC and PROTHROMPLEX IMMUNO (a non-activated prothrombin complex concentrate) in 15 patients with hemophilia A and inhibitors to Factor VIII. A total of 150 bleeding episodes (primarily joint and musculoskeletal plus a few mucocutaneous) were treated. A single dose of 88 Units per kg of body weight was used uniformly for treatments with **FEIBA** IMMUNO AICC. The study showed that, based on subjective patient evaluation, **FEIBA** IMMUNO AICC was fully effective in 41.0% and partly effective in 24.6% of episodes (i.e. combined effectiveness of 65.6%), while PROTHROMPLEX IMMUNO was rated fully effective in 25.0% and partly effective in 21.4% of episodes (i.e. combined effectiveness of 46.4%).

The second study with **FEIBA** IMMUNO AICC was a multiclinic study conducted by Hilgartner et al. It was designed to evaluate the efficacy of **FEIBA** IMMUNO AICC in the treatment of joint, mucous membrane, musculocutaneous and emergency bleeding episodes such as central nervous system hemorrhages and surgical bleedings. In 49 patients with inhibitor titers of greater than 5 Bethesda Units (from nine co-operating hemophilia centers), 489 single doses were given for the treatment of 165 bleeding episodes. The usual dosage was 50 Units per kg of body weight, repeated at 12-hour intervals (6-hour intervals in mucous membrane bleedings), if necessary. Bleeding was controlled in 153 episodes (93%). In 130 (78%) of the episodes, hemostasis was achieved with one or more infusions within 36 hours. Of these, 36% were controlled with one infusion within 12 hours. An additional 14% of episodes responded after more than 36 hours.

Of the 489 single doses, only 18 (3.7%) caused minor transient reactions in recipients. 10 out of 49 patients (20%) showed a rise in their inhibitor titers. In 5 of these patients (10%), the rise was tenfold or more. However, of these 10 patients, 3 had received Factor VIII or Factor IX concentrates within 2 weeks prior to treatment with **FEIBA** IMMUNO AICC. These anamnestic rises have not been observed to interfere with the efficacy of **FEIBA** IMMUNO Anti-Inhibitor Coagulant Complex.

INDICATIONS AND USAGE

FEIBA VH AICC is indicated for the control of spontaneous bleeding episodes or to cover surgical interventions in hemophilia A and hemophilia B patients with inhibitors.

In addition, the use of **FEIBA** IMMUNO AICC has been described in a few non-hemophiliacs with acquired inhibitors to Factors VIII, XI, and XII[8–12]. One case has been reported where **FEIBA** IMMUNO AICC was effective in a patient with von Willebrand's disease with an inhibitor[16].

Clinical experience suggests that patients with a Factor VIII inhibitor titer of less than 5 B.U. may be successfully treated with Antihemophilic Factor. Patients with titers ranging between 5 and 10 B.U. may either be treated with Antihemophilic Factor or **FEIBA** VH AICC. Cases with Factor VIII inhibitor titers greater than 10 B.U. have generally been refractory to treatment with Antihemophilic Factor.

Guidelines to First and Second Choice Treatment:

AICC = **FEIBA** VH Anti-Inhibitor Coagulant Complex, Vapor Heated

AHF = Antihemophilic Factor

Patient's Inhibitor	Clinical Situation		
Titer	Minor Bleeding	Major Bleeding	Surgery (Emergency)
less than 5 B.U.	AHF	AHF	AHF
5 to 10 B.U.	AHF	AHF	AHF
	AICC	AICC	AICC
more than 10 B.U.	AICC	AICC	AICC

Inadequate response to treatment may result from an abnormal platelet count or impaired platelet function[13–15] which were present before treatment with **FEIBA** VH Anti-Inhibitor Coagulant Complex, Vapor Heated.

CONTRAINDICATIONS

The use of **FEIBA** VH AICC is contraindicated in patients who are known to have a normal coagulation mechanism.

WARNINGS

FEIBA VH Anti-Inhibitor Coagulant Complex, Vapor Heated, is made from human plasma. Products made from plasma may contain infectious agents, such as viruses, that can cause disease. The risk that such products will transmit an infectious agent has been reduced by effective donor screening, testing for the presence of certain current virus infections, by inactivating and/or removing certain viruses. Despite these measures, such products can still potentially transmit disease. Because this product is made from human blood, it may carry a risk of transmitting infectious agents, e.g. viruses, and theoretically the Creutzfeldt-Jacob disease (CJD) agent. ALL infections thought by a physician possibly to have been transmitted by this product should be reported by the physician or other health care provider to Baxter Healthcare Corporation, at 1-800-423-2862 (in the U.S.). The physician should discuss the risks and benefits of this product with the patient.

FEIBA VH Anti-Inhibitor Coagulant Complex, Vapor Heated must be used only in patients with circulating inhibitors to one or more coagulation factors and should not be used for the treatment of bleeding episodes resulting from coagulation factor deficiencies. It should not be given to patients with significant signs of disseminated intravascular coagulation (DIC) or fibrinolysis.

Thromboembolic events may occur in the course of treatment with preparations containing the prothrombin complex, particularly following the administration of high doses and/or in patients with thrombotic risk factors.

Infusion of **FEIBA** VH AICC should not exceed single dosage of 100 units per kg of body weight and daily doses of 200 units per kg of body weight. Patients receiving more than 100 units per kg of body weight of **FEIBA** VH AICC must be monitored for the development of DIC and/or symptoms of acute coronary ischemia (see Adverse Reactions section).

High doses of **FEIBA** VH AICC should be given only as long as absolutely necessary to stop bleeding.

It has been reported that **FEIBA** VH AICC and antifibrinolytics have been given simultaneously without complications. It is, however, recommended not to use antifibrinolytics until 12 hours after the administration of **FEIBA** VH AICC.

Anamnestic responses with rise in Factor VIII inhibitor titer have been observed in 20% of the cases (see Clinical Pharmacology section).

Individuals who receive infusions of blood or plasma products may develop signs and/or symptoms of some viral infections, particularly non A, non B hepatitis.

PRECAUTIONS

Monitoring of Therapy

If clinical signs of intravascular coagulation occur, which include changes in blood pressure, pulse rate, respiratory distress, chest pain and cough, the infusion should be stopped promptly and appropriate diagnostic and therapeutic measures are to be initiated.

Laboratory indications of DIC are decreased fibrinogen, decreased platelet count, and/or presence of fibrin-fibrinogen degradation products (FDP). Other indications of DIC include significantly prolonged thrombin time, prothrombin time, or partial thromboplastin time.

Information for Patients

Some viruses, such as parvovirus B19 or hepatitis A, are particularly difficult to remove or inactivate at this time. Parvovirus B19 most seriously affects pregnant women or immune-compromised individuals. Symptoms of parvovirus B19 infection include fever, drowsiness, chills, and runny nose followed about two weeks later by a rash, and joint pain. Evidence of hepatitis A may include several days to weeks of poor appetite, tiredness, and low-grade fever followed by nausea, vomiting, and pain in the belly. Dark urine and a yellowed complexion are also common symptoms. Patients should be encouraged to consult their physician if such symptoms appear.

Non-Hemophilic Patients

Non-hemophilic patients with acquired inhibitors against Factors VIII, IX or XII may have both a bleeding tendency and an increased risk of thrombosis at the same time.

Laboratory Tests and Clinical Efficacy

Tests used to control efficacy such as APTT, WBCT, and TEG do not correlate with clinical improvement. For this reason, attempts at normalizing these values by increasing the dose of **FEIBA** VH Anti-Inhibitor Coagulant Complex,Vapor Heated may not be successful and are strongly discouraged because of the potential hazard of producing DIC by overdose.

Pregnancy Category C

Animal reproduction studies have not been conducted with **FEIBA** VH AICC. It is also not known whether **FEIBA** VH AICC can cause fetal harm when administered to a pregnant woman or can affect reproductive capacity. **FEIBA** VH AICC should be given to a pregnant woman only if clearly needed.

Pediatric Use

No data are available regarding the use of **FEIBA** VH AICC in newborns.

ADVERSE REACTIONS

In the course of treatment with preparations containing the prothrombin complex, thromboembolic events may occur particularly after high doses and/or in patients with thrombotic risk factors.

After application of high doses (single infusion of 100 units per kg of body weight, and daily doses of 200 units per kg of body weight) of **FEIBA** VH AICC, laboratory and/or clinical signs of DIC have occasionally been observed.

In individual instances myocardial infarction was found to occur after high doses and/or prolonged administration and/or in the presence of risk factors predisposing to myocardial infarction.

As with all human plasma products, any kind of allergic reaction may be seen ranging from mild, short-term urticarial rashes to severe anaphylactoid reactions. Administration of **FEIBA** VH Anti-Inhibitor Coagulant Complex, Vapor Heated should be discontinued immediately, if such signs appear. Allergic reactions should be treated with antihistamines and glucocorticoids. Shock should be treated in the usual way.

DOSAGE AND ADMINISTRATION

(See under intravenous Injection/Infusion).

Clinical trials[5–7] have demonstrated that the response to treatment with **FEIBA** IMMUNO AICC may differ from patient to patient with no correlation to the patient's inhibitor titer. Response may also vary between different types of hemorrhage (e.g. joint hemorrhage vs. CNS hemorrhage).

As a general guideline, a dosage range of 50 to 100 Units of **FEIBA** VH AICC per kg of body weight is recommended. However, care should be taken to distinguish between the following four indications, all of which have undergone careful clinical evaluation:

Joint Hemorrhage

In joint hemorrhage, a dose of 50 units per kg of body weight is recommended at 12-hour intervals, which may be increased to doses of 100 units per kg of body weight at 12-hour intervals.

Treatment should be continued until clear signs of clinical improvement appear, such as relief of pain, reduction of swelling or mobilization of the joint.

Mucous Membrane Bleeding

A dose of 50 units per kg of body weight is recommended to be given at 6-hour intervals under careful monitoring (visible bleeding site, repeated measurements of the patient's hematocrit). Again, if hemorrhage does not stop, the dose may be increased to 100 units per kg of body weight at 6-hour intervals. However, 2 such administrations or 200 units per kg of body weight a day should not be exceeded.

Soft Tissue Hemorrhage

For serious soft tissue bleeding such as retroperitoneal bleeding, doses of 100 units per kg of body weight at 12-hour intervals are recommended. A daily dosage of 200 units per kg of body weight should not be exceeded.

Other Severe Hemorrhages

Severe hemorrhages, such as CNS bleedings have been effectively treated with doses of 100 units per kg of body weight at 12-hour intervals. Sometimes, **FEIBA** VH Anti-Inhibitor Coagulant Complex, Vapor Heated may be indicated at 6-hour intervals until clear clinical improvement is achieved.

Reconstitution

1. Warm the unopened vial containing Sterile Water for Injection (diluent) to room temperature (not above 37°C, 98°F).
2. Remove caps from the concentrate and diluent vials to expose central portions of the rubber stoppers.
3. Cleanse exposed surface of the rubber stoppers with germicidal solution and allow to dry.
4. Open the package of BAXJECT device by peeling away the lid without touching the inside (Fig a).

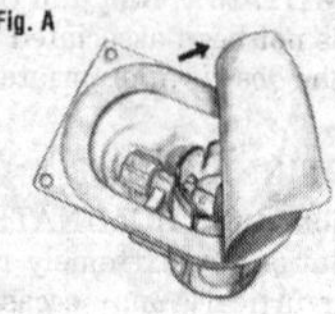

5. **Do not remove the device from the package.** Turn the package over and insert the plastic spike through diluent stopper (Fig. b).

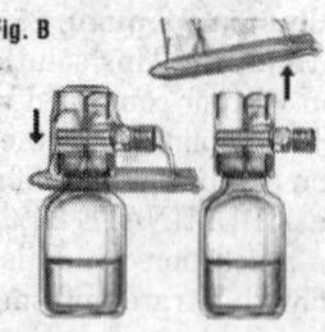

6. Grip the package at its edge and pull the package off the device (Fig.b).
7. Turn the system over,so that the bottle is on top. Quickly insert the other plastic spike into the **FEIBA** VH AICC stopper (Fig.c). The vacuum will draw the diluent into the **FEIBA** VH AICC vial.
[See figure C at top of next column]
8. Swirl gently until **FEIBA** VH AICC is completely dissolved.

Do not refrigerate after reconstitution!

After complete reconstitution of **FEIBA** VH AICC, its injection or infusion should be commenced as promptly as practicable, but must be completed within three hours following reconstitution.

The solution must be given by intravenous injection or intravenous drip infusion and the maximum injection or infu-

Fig. C

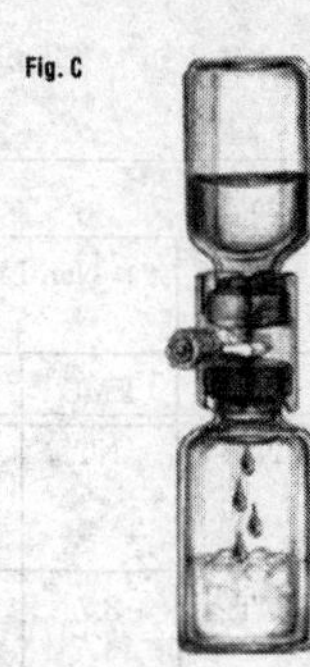

sion rate must not exceed 2 units per kg of body weight per minute. In a patient with a body weight of 75 kg, this corresponds to an infusion rate of 2.5 – 7.5 mL per minute depending on the number of units per vial (see label on vial).

For Intravenous Injection or Infusion

1. After reconstituting the concentrate as described under Reconstitution, parenteral drug products should be inspected for particulate matter and discoloration prior to administration, whenever solution and container permit. Plastic luer lock syringes are recommended for use with this product since protein such as **FEIBA** VH AICC tends to stick to the surface of all-glass syringes.
2. Turn the BAXJECT device handle down towards the **FEIBA** VH AICC concentrate vial and remove the cap attached to the syringe connection of the BAXJECT device (Fig. d).

Fig. D

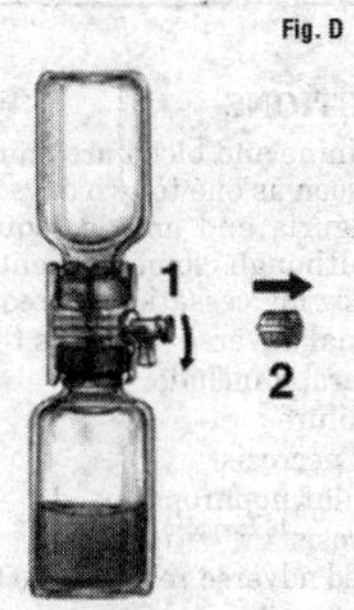

3. Draw air into the syringe, connect the syringe to the BAXJECT device, inject air into the concentrate vial (Fig e).

Fig. E

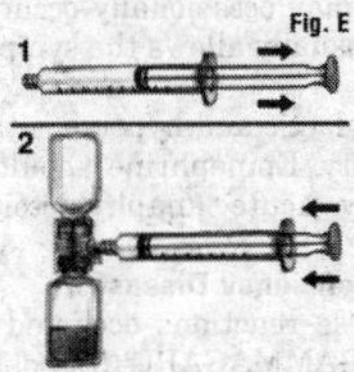

4. While keeping the syringe plunger in place, turn the system upside down (concentrate vial now on top). Draw the concentrate into the syringe by pulling the plunger back slowly (Fig. f).

Fig. F

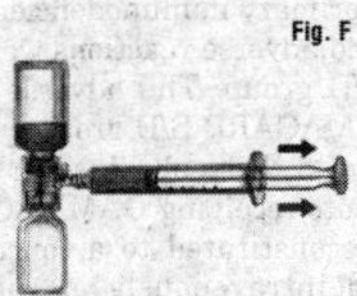

5. Turn the BAXJECT handle to its original position (facing sideways).
6. Disconnect the syringe, attach a suitable needle and inject or infuse intravenously as instructed under **Rate of Administration.**

HOW SUPPLIED

FEIBA VH Anti-Inhibitor Coagulant Complex, Vapor Heated is supplied as freeze-dried powder accompanied by a suitable volume of Sterile Water for Injection U.S.P., one BAXJECT Needleless Transfer device, Package insert.

The number of Units of Factor VIII inhibitor bypassing activity is stated on the label of each vial.

STORAGE

Store at refrigerated temperature (2° to 8°C, 35° to 46°F). **Avoid freezing, which may damage the diluent vial.**

REFERENCES

1. Elsinger F.: Aktivierter Faktor VII in Prothrombinkomplex-Konzentraten. 23rd Annual Meeting of "Deutsche Arbeitsgemeinschaft für Blutgerinnungsforschung" (DAB), Heidelberg, 1979. F. K. Schattauer Verlag, Stuttgart-New York, 367, 1980.
2. Seligsohn U., Østerud B., Rapaport S. I.: Coupled Amidolytic Assay for Factor VII: Its Use With a Clotting Assay to Determine the Activity State of Factor VII. Blood 52: 978, 1978.
3. Seligsohn U., Kasper C. K., Østerud B., Rapaport S. I.: Activated Factor VII: Presence in Factor IX Concentrates and Persistence in the Circulation After Infusion. Blood 53: 828, 1979.
4. Mannucci P. M.: Personal communication
5. Sjamsoedin L. J. M., Heijnen L., Mauser-Bunschoten E. P., van Geijlswijk J. L., van Houwelingen H., van Asten P., Sixma J. J.: The Effect of Activated Prothrombin-Complex Concentrate (**FEIBA**) on Joint and Muscle Bleeding in Patients with Hemophilia A and Antibodies to Factor VIII. The New Engl. J. of Med. 305: 717, 1981.
6. Roberts H. R.: Hemophiliacs with Inhibitors: Therapeutic Options. The New Engl. J. of Med. 305:757, 1981.
7. Hilgartner M. W., Knatterud G. AND THE **FEIBA** STUDY GROUP: The Use of Factor-Eight-Inhibitor-By-Passing-Activity (**FEIBA** IMMUNO) Product for Treatment of Bleeding Episodes in Hemophiliacs with Inhibitors. Blood 61: 36, 1983.
8. Thomas T., William. H., Williams Y., Hunt J.: **FEIBA** in Haemophiliacs with Factor VIII Inhibitor. Brit. Med. J. 1: 52, 1977.
9. Rolovic Z., Elezovic I., Oobrrenovic B.: Life-Threatening Bleeding Due to an Acquired Inhibitor to Factor XII– XI Successfully Treated with **Feiba**. Proceedings of Joint Meeting of the 18th Congress of the International Society of Hematology and 16th Congress of the International Society of Blood Transfusion, Montreal. Abstract 703, 1980.
10. Dormandy K.: Unpublished data.
11. Vinazzer H.: Personal communication.
12. Preston F. E.: A Review of Cases Treated with **FEIBA** in 1977/78. Presentation at the Second Workshop on Factor VIII Inhibitor Patients, Vienna, 1979.
13. Vermylen J., Sschetz J., Semeraro N., Mertens F., Verstraete M.: Evidence that 'Activated' Prothrombin Concentrates Enhance Platelet Coagulant Activity. Brit. J. Haematol. 38: 235, 1978.
14. Semeraro N., Vermylen J.: Evidence that Washed Human Platelets Possess Factor-X Activator Activity. Brit. J. Haematol. 36: 107, 1977.
15. Wensley R. T.: General Summary of the Use of **FEIBA** in Haemophiliacs with Inhibitors to FVIII. Presentation at the Second Workshop on Factor VIII Inhibitor Patients, Vienna, 1979.
16. Hilgartner M. W.: Personal communication.

To enroll in the confidential, Industry-wide Patient Notification System, call 1-888-UPDATE U (1-888-873-2838)

Baxter, **FEIBA VH, FEIBA** IMMUNO, PROTHROMPLEX IMMUNO and BAXJECT are trademarks of Baxter AG, Vienna, Austria; Baxter is a trademark of Baxter International, Inc., registered in the U.S. Patent and Trademark Office.

Baxter Healthcare Corporation
Westlake Village, CA 91362 USA

U.S. License No. 140

Revised 02/2003

U.S. Pat. Nos. 4,395,396 and 4,640,834

6205820EH18

GAMMAGARD S/D ℞

[găm-măh-gărd]

Immune Globulin Intravenous (Human)

SOLVENT DETERGENT TREATED

DESCRIPTION

GAMMAGARD S/D,* Immune Globulin Intravenous (Human) [IGIV] is a solvent/detergent treated, sterile, freeze-dried preparation of highly purified immunoglobulin G (IgG) derived from large pools of human plasma. The product is manufactured by the Cohn-Oncley cold ethanol fractionation process followed by ultrafiltration and ion exchange chromatography. Source material for fractionation may be obtained from another U.S. licensed manufacturer. The manufacturing process includes treatment with an organic solvent/detergent mixture,[1,2] composed of tri-n-butyl phosphate, octoxynol 9 and polysorbate 80.[3] The GAMMAGARD S/D manufacturing process provides a significant viral reduction in *in vitro* studies.[3] These studies, summarized in Table 1, demonstrate virus clearance during GAMMAGARD S/D manufacturing using infectious human immunodeficiency virus, Types 1 and 2 (HIV-1, HIV-2); bovine viral diarrhea virus (BVD), a model virus for hepatitis C virus; sindbis virus (SIN), a model virus for lipid-enveloped viruses; pseudorabies virus (PRV), a model virus for lipid-enveloped DNA viruses such as herpes; vesicular stomatitis virus (VSV), a model virus for lipid-enveloped RNA viruses; hepatitis A virus (HAV) and encephalomyocarditis virus (EMC), a model virus for non-lipid enveloped RNA viruses; and porcine parvovirus (PPV), a model virus for non-lipid enveloped DNA viruses.[3] These reductions are achieved through a combination of process chemistry, partitioning and/or inactivation during cold ethanol fractionation and the solvent/detergent treatment.[3]

***Manufactured under U.S. Patent No. 4,439,421**

[See table 1 at top of next page]

When reconstituted with the total volume of diluent (Sterile Water for Injection, USP) supplied, this preparation contains approximately 50 mg of protein per mL (5%), of which at least 90% is gamma globulin. The product, reconstituted to 5%, contains a physiological concentration of sodium chloride (approximately 8.5 mg/mL) and has a pH of 6.8 ± 0.4. Stabilizing agents and additional components are present in the following maximum amounts for a 5% solution: 3 mg/mL Albumin (Human), 22.5 mg/mL glycine, 20 mg/mL glucose, 2 mg/mL polyethylene glycol (PEG), 1 µg/mL tri-n-butyl phosphate, 1 µg/mL octoxynol 9, and 100 µg/mL polysorbate 80. If it is necessary to prepare a 10% (100 mg/mL) solution for infusion, half the volume of diluent should be added, as described in the **DOSAGE AND ADMINISTRATION** section. In this case, the stabilizing agents and other components will be present at double the concentrations given for the 5% solution. The manufacturing process for GAMMAGARD S/D, isolates IgG without additional chemical or enzymatic modification, and the Fc portion is maintained intact. GAMMAGARD S/D contains all of the IgG antibody activities which are present in the donor population. On the average, the distribution of IgG subclasses present in this product is similar to that in normal plasma.[3] GAMMAGARD S/D contains only trace amounts of IgA (≤ 2.2µg/mL in a 5% solution). IgM is also present in trace amounts.

GAMMAGARD S/D, Immune Globulin Intravenous (Human) contains no preservative.

CLINICAL PHARMACOLOGY

GAMMAGARD S/D, Immune Globulin Intravenous (Human), contains a broad spectrum of IgG antibodies against bacterial and viral agents that are capable of opsonization and neutralization of microbes and toxins.

Peak levels of IgG are reached immediately after infusion of GAMMAGARD S/D. It has been shown that, after infusion, exogenous IgG is distributed relatively rapidly between plasma and extravascular fluid until approximately half is partitioned in the extravascular space. Therefore, a rapid initial drop in serum IgG levels is to be expected.[4] As a class, IgG survives longer *in vivo* than other serum proteins.[4,5] Studies show that the half-life of GAMMAGARD S/D is approximately 37.7 ± 15 days.[3] Previous studies reported IgG half-life values of 21 to 25 days.[4,5,6] The half-life of IgG can vary considerably from person to person, however. In particular, high concentrations of IgG and hypermetabolism associated with fever and infection have been seen to coincide with a shortened half-life of IgG.[4–7]

INDICATIONS AND USAGE

GAMMAGARD S/D is not indicated in patients with selective IgA deficiency where the IgA deficiency is the only abnormality of concern (see **WARNINGS** section).

Primary Immunodeficiency Diseases

GAMMAGARD S/D is indicated for the treatment of primary immunodeficient states, such as: congenital agammaglobulinemia, common variable immunodeficiency, Wiskott-Aldrich syndrome, and severe combined immunodeficiencies.[6,7] This indication was supported by a clinical trial of 17 patients with primary immunodeficiency who received a total of 341 infusions. GAMMAGARD S/D is especially useful when high levels or rapid elevation of circulating IgG are desired or when intramuscular injections are contraindicated (e.g., small muscle mass).

B-cell Chronic Lymphocytic Leukemia (CLL)

GAMMAGARD S/D is indicated for prevention of bacterial infections in patients with hypogammaglobulinemia and/or recurrent bacterial infections associated with B-cell Chronic Lymphocytic Leukemia (CLL). In a study of 81 patients, 41 of whom were treated with GAMMAGARD, Immune Globulin Intravenous (Human), bacterial infections were significantly reduced in the treatment group.[8,9] In this study, the placebo group had approximately twice as many bacterial infections as the IGIV group. The median time to first bacterial infection for the IGIV group was greater than 365 days. By contrast, the time to first bacterial infection in the placebo group was 192 days. The number of viral and fungal infections, which were for the most part minor, was not statistically different between the two groups.

Idiopathic Thrombocytopenic Purpura (ITP)

When a rapid rise in platelet count is needed to prevent and/or to control bleeding in a patient with Idiopathic Thrombocytopenic Purpura, the administration of GAMMAGARD S/D, should be considered.

The efficacy of GAMMAGARD has been demonstrated in a clinical study involving 16 patients. Of these 16 patients, 13 had chronic ITP (11 adults, 2 children), and 3 patients had acute ITP (one adult, 2 children). All 16 patients (100%) demonstrated a clinically significant rise in platelet count to a level greater than $40,000/mm^3$ following the administration of GAMMAGARD. Ten of the 16 patients (62.5%) exhibited a significant rise to greater than $80,000$ platelets/mm^3. Of these 10 patients, 7 had chronic ITP (5 adults, 2 children), and 3 patients had acute ITP (one adult, 2 children). The rise in platelet count to greater than $40,000/mm^3$ occurred after a single 1 g/kg infusion of GAMMAGARD in 8 patients with chronic ITP (6 adults, 2 children), and in 2 patients with acute ITP (one adult, one child). A similar response was observed after two 1 g/kg infusions in 3 adult patients with chronic ITP, and one child with acute ITP. The remaining 2 adult patients with chronic ITP received more than two 1 g/kg infusions before achieving a platelet count

Continued on next page

Gammagard S/D—Cont.

greater than 40,000/mm^3. The rise in platelet count was generally rapid, occurring within 5 days. However, this rise was transient and not considered curative. Platelet count rises lasted 2 to 3 weeks, with a range of 12 days to 6 months. It should be noted that childhood ITP may resolve spontaneously without treatment.

Kawasaki Syndrome

GAMMAGARD S/D, is indicated for the prevention of coronary artery aneurysms associated with Kawasaki syndrome. The percentage incidence of coronary artery aneurysm in patients with Kawasaki syndrome receiving GAMMAGARD either at a single dose of 1 g/kg (n=22) or at a dose of 400 mg/kg for four consecutive days (n=22), beginning within seven days of onset of fever, was 3/44 (6.8%). This was significantly different (p=0.008) from a comparable group of patients that received aspirin only in previous trials and of whom 42/185 (22.7%) experienced coronary artery aneurysms.[10,11,12] All patients in the GAMMAGARD trial received concomitant aspirin therapy and none experienced hypersensitivity-type reactions (urticaria, bronchospasm or generalized anaphylaxis).[13]

Several studies have documented the efficacy of intravenous gammaglobulin in reducing the incidence of coronary artery abnormalities resulting from Kawasaki syndrome.[10–12, 14–17]

CONTRAINDICATIONS

Patients may experience severe hypersensitivity reactions or anaphylaxis in the setting of detectable IgA levels following infusion of GAMMAGARD S/D. The occurrence of severe hypersensitivity reactions or anaphylaxis under such conditions should prompt consideration of an alternative therapy.

GAMMAGARD S/D is contraindicated in patients with selective IgA deficiency where the IgA deficiency is the only abnormality of concern (see **INDICATIONS AND USAGE** and **WARNINGS** sections).

WARNINGS

Warning

Immune Globulin Intravenous (Human) products have been reported to be associated with renal dysfunction, acute renal failure, osmotic nephrosis, and death.[16,18] Patients predisposed to acute renal failure include patients with any degree of pre-existing renal insufficiency, diabetes mellitus, age greater than 65, volume depletion, sepsis, paraproteinemia, or patients receiving known nephrotoxic drugs. Especially in such patients, IGIV products should be administered at the minimum concentration available and the minimum rate of infusion practicable. While these reports of renal dysfunction and acute renal failure have been associated with the use of many of the licensed IGIV products, those containing sucrose as a stabilizer accounted for a disproportionate share of the total number.* See PRECAUTIONS and DOSAGE AND ADMINISTRATION sections for important information intended to reduce the risk of acute renal failure.

***GAMMAGARD S/D does not contain sucrose.**

GAMMAGARD S/D, Immune Globulin Intravenous (Human) is made from human plasma. Products made from human plasma may contain infectious agents, such as viruses, that can cause disease. The risk that such products will transmit an infectious agent has been reduced by screening plasma donors for prior exposure to certain viruses, by testing for the presence of certain current virus infections, and by inactivating and/or removing certain viruses. (See DESCRIPTION section). Despite these measures, such products can still potentially transmit disease. Because this product is made from human blood, it may carry a risk of transmitting infectious agents, e.g., viruses and theoretically, the Creutzfeldt-Jakob disease (CJD) agent. ALL infections thought by a physician possibly to have been transmitted by this product should be reported by the physician or other healthcare provider to Baxter Healthcare Corporation at 1-800-423-2862 (in the U.S.). The physician should discuss the risks and benefits of this product with the patient.

GAMMAGARD S/D, Immune Globulin Intravenous (Human), should only be administered intravenously. Other routes of administration have not been evaluated.

Immediate anaphylactic and hypersensitivity reactions are a remote possibility. Epinephrine should be available for treatment of any acute anaphylactoid reactions.

GAMMAGARD S/D contains only trace amounts of IgA (≤ 2.2 μg/mL in a 5% solution). GAMMAGARD S/D is not indicated in patients with selective IgA deficiency where the IgA deficiency is the only abnormality of concern and it should be given with caution to patients with antibodies to IgA or IgA deficiencies, that are a component of an underlying primary immunodeficiency disease for which IGIV therapy is indicated.[7,19] In such instances, a risk of anaphylaxis may exist despite the fact that GAMMAGARD S/D contains only trace amounts of IgA.

PRECAUTIONS

General

Some viruses, such as parvovirus B19 or hepatitis A, are particularly difficult to remove or inactivate at this time. Parvovirus B19 most seriously affects pregnant women, or immune-compromised individuals. Symptoms of parvovirus B19 infection include fever, drowsiness, chills, and runny nose followed about two weeks later by a rash and joint pain. Evidence of hepatitis A may include several days to weeks of poor appetite, tiredness, and low-grade fever followed by nausea, vomiting, and abdominal pain. Dark urine and a yellowed complexion are also common symptoms. Patients should be encouraged to consult their physician if such symptoms appear.

There is clinical evidence of a possible association between Immune Globulin Intravenous (Human) [IGIV] administration and the potential for the development of thrombotic events. The exact cause of this is unknown; therefore, caution should be exercised in the prescribing and infusion of IGIV in patients with a history of and predisposing factors towards cardiovascular disease or thrombotic episodes.[20–25; 33–38] Analysis of adverse event reports[13,37] has indicated that a rapid rate of infusion may be a risk factor for vascular occlusive events.

An aseptic meningitis syndrome (AMS) has been reported to occur infrequently in association with Immune Globulin Intravenous (Human) [IGIV] treatment. Discontinuation of IGIV treatment has resulted in remission of AMS within several days without sequelae. The syndrome usually begins within several hours to two days following IGIV treatment. It is characterized by symptoms and signs including severe headache, nuchal rigidity, drowsiness, fever, photophobia, painful eye movements, and nausea and vomiting. Cerebrospinal fluid (CSF) studies are frequently positive with pleocytosis up to several thousand cells per cu.mm., predominantly from the granulocytic series, and elevated protein levels up to several hundred mg/dL. Patients exhibiting such symptoms and signs should receive a thorough neurological examination, including CSF studies, to rule out other causes of meningitis. AMS may occur more frequently in association with high dose (2 g/kg) IGIV treatment.

Assure that patients are not volume depleted prior to the initiation of the infusion of IGIV.

Periodic monitoring of renal function tests and urine output is particularly important in patients judged to have a potential increased risk for developing acute renal failure. Renal function, including measurement of blood urea nitrogen (BUN)/serum creatinine, should be assessed prior to the initial infusion of GAMMAGARD S/D and again at appropriate intervals thereafter. If renal function deteriorates, discontinuation of the product should be considered.

For patients judged to be at risk for developing renal dysfunction, it may be prudent to reduce the amount of product infused per unit time by infusing GAMMAGARD S/D at a rate less than 4 mL/kg/Hr (<3.3 mg IG/kg/min) for a 5% solution or at a rate less than 2 mL/kg/Hr (< 3.3 mg IG/kg/min) for a 10 % solution.

Certain components used in the packaging of this product contain natural rubber latex.

Information For Patients

Patients should be instructed to immediately report symptoms of decreased urine output, sudden weight gain, fluid retention/edema, and/or shortness of breath (which may suggest kidney damage) to their physician.

Drug Interactions

See **DOSAGE AND ADMINISTRATION** section.

Pregnancy Category C

Animal reproduction studies have not been conducted with GAMMAGARD S/D, Immune Globulin Intravenous (Human). It is also not known whether GAMMAGARD S/D can cause fetal harm when administered to a pregnant woman or can affect reproduction capacity. GAMMAGARD S/D should be given to a pregnant woman only if clearly needed.

TABLE 1
***In Vitro* Virus Clearance During GAMMAGARD S/D Manufacturing**

Process Step Evaluated	Virus Clearance ($\log_{10}$)								
	Lipid Enveloped Viruses						Non-Lipid Enveloped Viruses		
	BVD	HIV-1	HIV-2	PRV	SIN	VSV	EMC	HAV	PPV
Step 1: Processing of Cryo-Poor Plasma to Fraction I+II+III Precipitate	0.6*	5.7	NT	1.0*	NT	NT	NT	0.5*	0.2*
Step 2: Processing of Resuspended Suspension A Precipitate to Suspension B Filter Press Filtrate	1.3	4.9	NT	3.7	NT	NT	3.7	4.1	3.5
Step 3: Processing of Suspension B Filter Press to Suspension B Cuno 70 Filtrate	0.7*	4.0	NT	4.5	NT	NT	3.0	3.9	3.9
Step 4: Solvent/Detergent Treatment	>4.9	>3.7	5.7	>4.1	5.1	6.0	NA	NA	NA
Cumulative Reduction of Virus ($\log_{10}$)	6.2	18.3	5.7	12.3	5.1	6.0	6.7	8.0	7.4

* These values are not included in the computation of the cumulative reduction of virus since the virus clearance is within the variability limit of the assay (≤1.0).

NA Not Applicable. Solvent/detergent treatment does not effect non-lipid enveloped viruses.

NT Not Tested.

ADVERSE REACTIONS

Increases in creatinine and blood urea nitrogen (BUN) have been observed as soon as one to two days following infusion. Progression to oliguria and anuria requiring dialysis has been observed, although some patients have improved spontaneously following cessation of treatment.[26]

Types of severe renal adverse reactions that have been seen following IGIV therapy include:

- acute renal failure
- acute tubular necrosis[27]
- proximal tubular nephropathy
- osmotic nephrosis[18 (see also 28–30)]

In general, reported adverse reactions to GAMMAGARD, in patients with either congenital or acquired immunodeficiencies are similar in kind and frequency. Various minor reactions, such as mild to moderate hypotension, headache, fatigue, chills, backache, leg cramps, lightheadedness, fever, urticaria, flushing, slight elevation of blood pressure, nausea and vomiting may occasionally occur. Slowing or stopping the infusion usually allows the symptoms to disappear promptly.

Immediate anaphylactic and hypersensitivity reactions are a remote possibility. Epinephrine should be available for treatment of any acute anaphylactoid reaction. (See **WARNINGS**).

Primary Immunodeficiency Diseases

Twenty-one adverse reactions occurred in 341 infusions (6%), when using GAMMAGARD (5% solution), in a clinical trial of 17 patients with primary immunodeficiency.[31] Of the 17 patients, 12 (71%) were adults, and 5 (29%) were children (16 years or younger).

In a cross-over study comparing GAMMAGARD and GAMMAGARD S/D (5% solutions) conducted in a small number (n=10) of primary immunodeficient patients, no unusual or unexpected adverse reactions were observed in the GAMMAGARD S/D group. The adverse reactions experienced in the GAMMAGARD S/D group were similar in frequency and nature to those observed in the control group consisting of patients receiving GAMMAGARD.

GAMMAGARD, reconstituted to a concentration of 10%, was administered intravenously at rates varying from 2-11 mL/kg/Hr. Systemic reactions occurred in 23 (10.5%) of 219 infusions. This compares with an adverse reaction incidence of 6% (only systemic reactions reported) for primary immunodeficient patients previously treated with a 5% solution at infusion rates varying between 2 and 8 mL/kg/Hr, as described above (also, see reference 31). Local pain or irritation was experienced during 35 (16%) of 219 infusions. Application of a warm compress to the infusion site alleviated local symptoms. These local reactions tended to be associated with hand vein infusions and their incidence may be reduced by infusions via the antecubital vein.

B-cell Chronic Lymphocytic Leukemia (CLL)

In the study of patients with B-cell Chronic Lymphocytic Leukemia, the incidence of adverse reactions associated with GAMMAGARD infusions was approximately 1.3% while that associated with placebo (normal saline) infusions was 0.6%.[9]

Idiopathic Thrombocytopenic Purpura (ITP)

During the clinical study of GAMMAGARD for the treatment of Idiopathic Thrombocytopenic Purpura, the only adverse reaction reported was headache which occurred in 12 of 16 patients (75%). Of these 12 patients, 11 had chronic ITP (9 adults, 2 children), and one child had acute ITP. Oral antihistamines and analgesics alleviated the symptoms and were used as pretreatment for those patients requiring additional IGIV therapy. The remaining 4 patients did not report any side effects and did not require pretreatment.

Kawasaki Syndrome

In a study of patients (n=51) with Kawasaki syndrome, no hypersensitivity-type reactions (urticaria, bronchospasm or generalized anaphylaxis) were reported in patients receiving either a single 1g/kg dose of IGIV, GAMMAGARD, or 400 mg/kg of IGIV, GAMMAGARD, for four consecutive days.[20] Mild adverse reactions, including chills, flushing, cramping, headache, hypotension, nausea, rash and wheezing, were reported with both dose regimens. These adverse reactions occurred in 7/51 (13.7%) patients and in association with 7/129 (5.4%) infusions. Of the 25 patients who received a single 1 g/kg dose, 4 patients experienced adverse reactions for an incidence of 16%. Of the 26 patients who received 400 mg/kg/day over 4 days, 3 experienced a single adverse reaction for an incidence of 11.5%.[3]

DOSAGE AND ADMINISTRATION

Primary Immunodeficiency Diseases

For patients with primary immunodeficiencies, monthly doses of at least 100 mg/kg are recommended. Initially, patients may receive 200–400 mg/kg. As there are significant differences in the half-life of IgG among patients with primary immunodeficiencies, the frequency and amount of immunoglobulin therapy may vary from patient to patient. The proper amount can be determined by monitoring clinical response. The minimum serum concentration of IgG necessary for protection has not been established.

B-cell Chronic Lymphocytic Leukemia (CLL)

For patients with hypogammaglobulinemia and/or recurrent bacterial infections due to B-cell Chronic Lymphocytic Leukemia, a dose of 400 mg/kg every 3 to 4 weeks is recommended.

Kawasaki Syndrome

For patients with Kawasaki syndrome, either a single 1 g/kg dose or a dose of 400 mg/kg for four consecutive days beginning within seven days of the onset of fever, administered concomitantly with appropriate aspirin therapy (80–100 mg/kg/day in four divided doses) is recommended.

Idiopathic Thrombocytopenic Purpura (ITP)

For patients with acute or chronic Idiopathic Thrombocytopenic Purpura, a dose of 1 g/kg is recommended. The need for additional doses can be determined by clinical response and platelet count. Up to three separate doses may be given on alternate days if required.

No prospective data are presently available to identify a maximum safe dose, concentration, and rate of infusion in patients determined to be at increased risk of acute renal failure. In the absence of prospective data, the recommended doses should not be exceeded and the concentration and infusion rate selected should be the minimum level practicable. Reduction in dose, concentration, and/or rate of administration in patients at risk of acute renal failure has been proposed in the literature in order to reduce the risk of acute renal failure.[32]

Reconstitution: Use Aseptic Technique

When reconstitution is performed aseptically outside of a sterile laminar air flow hood, administration should begin as soon as possible, but not more than 2 hours after reconstitution.

When reconstitution is performed aseptically in a sterile laminar air flow hood, the reconstituted product may be either maintained in the original glass container or pooled into VIAFLEX bags and stored under constant refrigeration (2–8°C), for up to 24 hours. (The date and time of reconstitution/pooling should be recorded). If these conditions are not met, sterility of the reconstituted product cannot be maintained. Partially used vials should be discarded.

A. 5% Solution

1. **Note: Reconstitute immediately before use.**
2. If refrigerated, warm the Sterile Water for Injection, USP (diluent) and GAMMAGARD S/D, Immune Globulin Intravenous (Human) (dried concentrate), to room temperature.
3. Remove caps from concentrate and diluent bottles to expose central portion of rubber stoppers.
4. Cleanse stoppers with germicidal solution.
5. Remove protective covering from the spike at one end of the transfer device (Fig. 1)

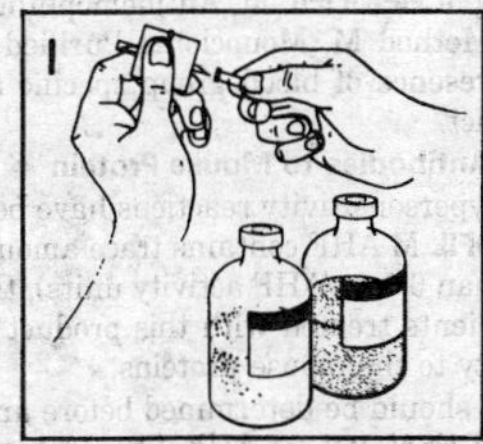

6. Place the diluent bottle on a flat surface and, while holding the bottle to prevent slipping, insert the spike of the transfer device **perpendicularly through the center** of the bottle stopper.
7. Press down firmly so that the transfer device fits snugly against the diluent bottle (Fig. 2). **Caution: Failure to use center of stopper may result in dislodging the stopper.**
   [See figure 2 at top of next column]
8. Remove the protective covering from the other end of the transfer device. Hold diluent bottle to prevent slipping.

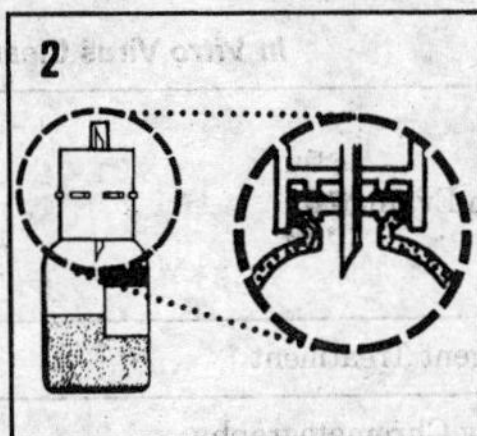

9. Hold concentrate bottle firmly and at an angle of approximately 45 degrees. Invert the diluent bottle with the transfer device at an angle complementary to the concentrate bottle (approximately 45 degrees) and firmly insert the transfer device into the concentrate bottle through the center of the rubber stopper (Fig. 3).

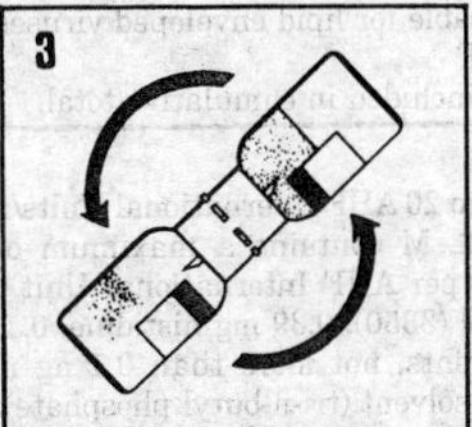

Note: Invert the diluent bottle with attached transfer device rapidly into the concentrate bottle in order to avoid loss of diluent.

Caution: Failure to use center of stopper may result in dislodging the stopper and loss of vacuum.

10. The diluent will flow into the concentrate bottle quickly. When diluent transfer is complete, remove empty diluent bottle and transfer device from concentrate bottle. Discard transfer device after single use.
11. Thoroughly wet the dried material by tilting or inverting and gently rotating the bottle (Fig. 4). **Do not shake. Avoid foaming.**

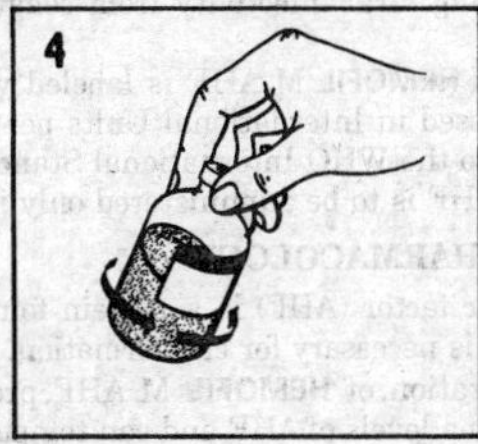

12. Repeat gentle rotation as long as undissolved product is observed.

B. 10% Solution

Follow steps 1–4 as previously described in **A.**

5. To prepare a 10% solution, reconstitute with the appropriate volume of diluent as indicated in Table 2, which indicates the volume of diluent required for a 5% or 10% concentration. Using aseptic technique, draw the required volume of diluent into a sterile hypodermic syringe and needle. Discard the filled syringe.
6. Using the residual diluent in the diluent vial, follow steps 5–12 as previously described in **A.**

TABLE 2
Required Diluent Volume

Concentration	2.5 g bottle	5 g bottle	10 g bottle
5%	50 mL	96 mL	192 mL
10%	25 mL	48 mL	96 mL

Rate of Administration

It is recommended that initially a 5% solution be infused at a rate of 0.5 mL/kg/Hr. If infusion at this rate and concentration causes the patient no distress, the administration rate may be gradually increased to a maximum rate of 4 mL/kg/Hr. Patients who tolerate the 5% concentration at 4 mL/kg/Hr can be infused with the 10% concentration starting at 0.5 mL/kg/Hr. If no adverse effects occur, the rate can be increased gradually up to a maximum of 8 mL/kg/Hr. For patients judged to be at risk for developing renal dysfunction, it may be prudent to reduce the amount of product infused per unit time by infusing GAMMAGARD S/D, at a rate less than 4 mL/kg/Hr (<3.3 mg IG/kg/min) for a 5% solution or at a rate less than 2 mL/kg/Hr (< 3.3 mg IG/kg/min) for a 10 % solution.

It is recommended that antecubital veins be used especially for 10% solutions, if possible. This may reduce the likelihood of the patient experiencing discomfort at the infusion site (see **ADVERSE REACTIONS**).

A rate of administration which is too rapid may cause flushing and changes in pulse rate and blood pressure. Slowing or stopping the infusion usually allows the symptoms to disappear promptly.

Drug Interactions

Admixtures of GAMMAGARD S/D, Immune Globulin Intravenous (Human), with other drugs and intravenous solutions have not been evaluated. It is recommended that GAMMAGARD S/D be administered separately from other drugs or medications which the patient may be receiving. The product should not be mixed with Immune Globulin Intravenous (Human) from other manufacturers.

Antibodies in immune globulin preparations may interfere with patient responses to live vaccines, such as those for measles, mumps, and rubella. The immunizing physician should be informed of recent therapy with Immune Globulin Intravenous (Human) so that appropriate precautions can be taken.

Administration

GAMMAGARD S/D should be administered as soon after reconstitution as possible, or as described in the **DOSAGE AND ADMINISTRATION** section.

The reconstituted material should be at room temperature during administration.

Parenteral drug products should be inspected visually for particulate matter and discoloration prior to administration, whenever solution and container permit.

Reconstituted material should be a clear to slightly opalescent and colorless to pale yellow solution. Do not use if particulate matter and/or discoloration is observed.

Follow directions for use which accompany the administration set provided. If another administration set is used, ensure that the set contains a similar filter.

HOW SUPPLIED

GAMMAGARD S/D is supplied in 2.5 g, 5 g, or 10 g single use bottles. Each bottle of GAMMAGARD S/D is furnished with a suitable volume of Sterile Water for Injection, USP, a transfer device and an administration set which contains an integral airway and a 15 micron filter.

Storage

GAMMAGARD S/D is to be stored at a temperature not to exceed 25°C (77°F). Freezing should be avoided to prevent the diluent bottle from breaking.

REFERENCES

1. Prince AM, Horowitz B, Brotman B: Sterilisation of hepatitis and HTLV-III viruses by exposure to tri-n-butyl phosphate and sodium cholate. **Lancet 1**: 706-710, 1986
2. Horowitz B, Wiebe ME, Lippin A, et al: Inactivation of viruses in labile blood derivatives: I. Disruption of lipid enveloped viruses by tri-n-butyl phosphate detergent combinations. **Transfusion 25**:516-522, 1985
3. Unpublished data in the files of Baxter Healthcare Corporation
4. Waldmann TA, Storber W: Metabolism of immunoglobulins. **Prog Allergy 13**:1-110, 1969
5. Morell A, Riesen W: Structure, function and catabolism of immuno-globulins in **Immunohemotherapy.** Nydegger UE (ed), London, Academic Press, 1981, pp 17-26
6. Stiehm ER: Standard and special human immune serum globulins as therapeutic agents. **Pediatrics 63**: 301-319, 1979
7. Buckley RH: Immunoglobulin replacement therapy: Indications and contraindications for use and variable IgG levels achieved in **Immunoglobulins: Characteristics and Use of Intravenous Preparations.** Alving BM, Finlayson JS (eds), Washington, DC, U.S. Department of Health and Human Services, 1979, pp 3-8
8. Bunch C, Chapel HM, Rai K, *et al*: Intravenous Immune Globulin reduces bacterial infections in Chronic Lymphocytic Leukemia: A controlled randomized clinical trial. **Blood 70 Suppl 1**:753, 1987
9. Cooperative Group for the Study of Immunoglobulin in Chronic Lymphocytic Leukemia: Intravenous immunoglobulin for the prevention of infection in Chronic Lymphocytic Leukemia: A randomized, controlled clinical trial. **N Eng J Med 319**:902-907, 1988
10. Newburger J, Takahashi M, Burns JG, *et al*: The Treatment of Kawasaki Syndrome with Intravenous Gamma Globulin. **New England Journal of Medicine 315**:341-347, 1986
11. Furusho K, Sato K, Soeda T, *et al*: High Dose Intravenous Gammaglobulin for Kawasaki Disease [letter]. **Lancet 2**:1359, 1983
12. Nagashima M, Matsushima M, Matsucka H, Ogawa A, Okumura N: High Dose Gammaglobulin Therapy for Kawasaki Disease. **Journal of Pediatrics 110**:710-712, 1987.
13. Data in the files of Baxter Healthcare Corporation
14. Furusho K, Hroyuki N, Shinomiya K, *et al*: High Dose Intravenous Gammaglobulin for Kawasaki Disease. **Lancet 2**:1055-1058, 1984
15. Engle MA, Fatica NS, Bussel JB, O'Laughlin JE, Snyder MS, Lesser ML: Clinical Trial of Single-Dose Intravenous Gammaglobulin in Acute Kawasaki Disease. **AJDC143**:1300-1304, 1989
16. Isawa M, Sugiyama K, Kawase A, *et al*: Prevention of Coronary Artery Involvement in Kawasaki Disease by Early Intravenous High Dose Gammaglobulin. In: Doyle EF, Engle MA, Gersony WM, Rashkind EJ, Talner NS, eds **Pediatric Cardiology.** New York: Springer-Verlag, 1986:1083-1085
17. Okuri M, Harada K, Yamaguchi H, *et al*: Intravenous Gammaglobulin Therapy in Kawasaki Disease: Trial of Low-Dose Gammaglobulin. In: Shulman ST, ed. **Kawasaki Disease.** New York: Alan R. Liss, 1987:433-439
18. Cayco AV, Perazella MA, Hayslett JP: Renal insufficiency after intravenous immune globulin therapy: A Report of Two Cases and an Analysis of the Literature. 1997; **J Amer Soc Nephrology 8**:1788-1793

Continued on next page

Gammagard S/D—Cont.

19. Burks AW, Sampson HA, Buckley RH: Anaphylactic reactions after gammaglobulin administration in patients with hypogammaglobulinemia: Detection of IgE antibodies to IgA. **N Eng J Med 314**:560-564, 1986
20. Reinhart WH, Berchtold PE: Effect of high-dose intravenous immunoglobulin therapy on blood rheology. **Lancet 339 (8794)**:662-664, 1992
21. Dalakas MC: High-dose intravenous immunoglobulin and serum viscosity: Risk of precipitating thromboembolic events. **Neurology 44 (2)**:223-226, 1994
22. Harkness K, Howell SJL, Davies-Jones GAB: Encephalopathy associated with intravenous immunoglobulin treatment for Guillain-Barre syndrome. **Journal of Neurology Neurosurgery, Psychiatry 60 (5)**:586-598, 1996
23. Woodruff RK, Grigg AP, Firkin FC, Smith IL: Fatal thrombotic events during treatment of autoimmune thrombocytopenia with intravenous immunoglobulin in elderly patients. **Lancet ii (8500)**:217-218, 1986
24. Silbert PL, Knezevic WV, Bridge DT: Cerebral infarction complicating intravenous immunoglobulin therapy for polyneuritis cranialis.**Neurology 42 (1)**:257-258, 1992
25. Duhem C, Dicato MA, Ries F: Side effects of intravenous immune globulins. **Clin Exp Immunol 97: (Suppl 1)** 79-83, 1994
26. Winward DB, Brophy MT: Acute renal failure after administration of intravenous immunoglobulin: review of the literature and case report. 1995; **Pharmacotherapy 15**:765-772
27. Phillips AO: Renal failure and intravenous immunoglobulin [letter, comment]. 1992; **Clin Nephrol 36**:83-86
28. Anderson W, Bethea W: Renal lesions following administration of hypertonic solutions of sucrose. 1940; **JAMA 114**:1983-1987
29. Lindberg H, Wald A: Renal changes following the administration of hypertonic solutions. 1939; **Arch Intern Med 63**:907-918
30. Rigdon RH, Cardwell ES: Renal lesions following the intravenous injection of hypertonic solution of sucrose: A clinical and experimental study. 1942; **Arch Intern Med 69**:670-690
31. Ochs HD, Lee ML, Fischer SH, *et al*: Efficacy of a New Intravenous Immunoglobulin Preparation in Primary Immunodeficient Patients. **Clinical Therapeutics 9**:512-522, 1987
32. Tan E, Hajinazarian M, Bay, *et al*: Acute renal failure resulting from intravenous immunoglobulin therapy. 1993; **Arch Neurology 50**:137-139
33. Brannagan TH 3rd, Nagle KJ, Lange DJ, Rowland LP: Complications of intravenous immune globulin treatment in neurologic disease. **Neurology 47 (3)**:674-677, 1996
34. Haplea SS, Farrar JT, Gibson GA, Laskin M, Pizzi LT, Ashbury AK: Thromboembolic Events Associated with Intravenous Immunoglobulin Therapy: **Neurology 48**: A54, 1997
35. Kwan T, and Keith P: Stroke Following Intravenous Immunoglobulin Infusion in a 28-Year-Old Male with Common Variable Immune Deficiency: A Case Report and Literature Review. **Canadian Journal of Allergy & Clinical Immunology 4**: 250-253, 1999
36. Elkayam O, Paran D, Milo R, Davidovitz Y, Almoznino-Sarafian D, Zelster D, Yaron M, Caspi D: Acute Myocardial Infarction Associated with High Dose Intravenous Immunoglobulin Infusion for Autoimmune Disorders. A study of four cases. **Ann Rheum Dis 59 (1)**: 77-80, 2000
37. Grillo JA, Gorson KC, Ropper AH, Lewis J, Weinstein R: Rapid infusion of intravenous immune globulin in patients with neuromuscular disorders. **Neurology 57(9)**: 1699-1701, 2001
38. Gomperts ED, Darr F: Letter to the Editor: Reference article – Rapid infusion of intravenous immune globulin in patients with neuromuscular disorders. **Neurology**, 2002. In Press

BIBLIOGRAPHY

Bussel JB, Kimberly RP, Inman RD, *et al*: Intravenous gammaglobulin treatment of chronic idiopathic thrombocytopenic purpura. **Blood 62**:480-486, 1983

To enroll in the confidential, industry-wide Patient Notification System, call 1-888-UPDATE U (1-888-873-2838)

Baxter, Gammagard and Viaflex are trademarks of Baxter International, Inc., and are registered in the U.S. Patent and Trademark Office.

Baxter Healthcare Corporation
Westlake Village, CA 91362 USA
U.S. License No. 140
Revised (August) 2002
30-5K-03-240

HEMOFIL M ℞

[*hē-mō-fīl*]

Antihemophilic Factor (Human)
Method M, Monoclonal Purified

DESCRIPTION

HEMOFIL M, Antihemophilic Factor (Human) (AHF), Method M, Monoclonal Purified, is a sterile, nonpyrogenic, dried preparation of antihemophilic factor (Factor VIII, Factor VIII:C, AHF) in concentrated form with a specific activity range of 2 to 20 AHF International Units/mg of total protein. **HEMOFIL** M contains a maximum of 12.5 mg/mL Albumin, and per AHF International Unit, 0.07 mg polyethylene glycol (3350), 0.39 mg histidine, 0.1 mg glycine as stabilizing agents, not more than 0.1 ng mouse protein, 18 ng organic solvent (tri-n-butyl phosphate) and 50 ng detergent (octoxynol 9). In the absence of the added Albumin (Human), the specific activity is approximately 2,000 AHF International Units/mg of protein. See **CLINICAL PHARMACOLOGY**.

HEMOFIL M AHF is prepared by the Method M process from pooled human plasma by immunoaffinity chromatography utilizing a murine monoclonal antibody to Factor VIII:C, followed by an ion exchange chromatography step for further purification. Source material may be provided by other US licensed manufacturers. **HEMOFIL** M AHF also includes an organic solvent (tri-n-butyl phosphate) and detergent (octoxynol 9) virus inactivation step designed to reduce the risk of transmission of hepatitis and other viral diseases. However, no procedure has been shown to be totally effective in removing viral infectivity from coagulation factor products.

Each bottle of **HEMOFIL** M AHF is labeled with the AHF activity expressed in International Units per bottle, which is referenced to the WHO International Standard.

HEMOFIL M AHF is to be administered only intravenously.

CLINICAL PHARMACOLOGY

Antihemophilic factor (AHF) is a protein found in normal plasma which is necessary for clot formation.

The administration of **HEMOFIL** M AHF provides an increase in plasma levels of AHF and can temporarily correct the coagulation defect of patients with hemophilia A (classical hemophilia). The administration of **HEMOFIL** M AHF will also correct deficiencies caused by circulating inhibitors when the inhibitor level does not exceed 10 Bethesda Units per mL.

The half-life of **HEMOFIL** M, Antihemophilic Factor (Human) (AHF), Method M, Monoclonal Purified, administered to Factor VIII deficient patients has been shown to be 14.8 ± 3.0 hours.

Use of an organic solvent (tri-n-butyl phosphate; TNBP) in the manufacture of Antihemophilic Factor (Human) has little or no effect on AHF activity, while lipid enveloped viruses, such as hepatitis B and human immunodeficiency virus (HIV) are inactivated.[1] Prince, *et al*, report inactivation of at least 10,000 Chimpanzee Infectious Doses (CID-50) of hepatitis B virus, 10,000 CID-50 of hepatitis non A, non B virus, and 30,000 Tissue Culture Infectious Doses of HIV with TNBP/detergent treatment during manufacture of an Antihemophilic Factor (Human) concentrate.[2]

In vitro studies demonstrate that the **HEMOFIL** M AHF, manufacturing process provides for significant viral reduction. These studies, summarized in Table 1, demonstrate virus clearance during the **HEMOFIL** M AHF manufacturing process using human immunodeficiency virus, Type 1 (HIV-1); bovine viral diarrhea virus (BVD), a model for lipid enveloped RNA viruses, such as hepatitis C virus (HCV); pseudorabies virus (PRV), a model for lipid enveloped DNA viruses, such as herpes; porcine parvovirus (PPV), a model for non-lipid enveloped DNA viruses, such as human parvovirus B19; and hepatitis A virus (HAV), a model for non-lipid enveloped RNA viruses. These reductions are achieved through a combination of process chemistry, partitioning and/or inactivation during solvent/detergent treatment, immunoaffinity chromatography, Q-Sepharose column chromatography and lyophilization.

[See table 1 above]

Table 1
***In Vitro* Virus Clearance During the Manufacture of HEMOFIL M AHF**

Process Step Evaluated	Virus Clearance, $\log_{10}$				
	Lipid-enveloped			Non-Lipid enveloped	
	HIV-1	BVD	PRV	PPV	HAV
Solvent/Detergent Treatment	10.3	3.8	4.3	*	*
Immunoaffinity Chromatography	N.A.**	N.A.**	N.A.**	4.2	5.3
Q-Sepharose Column Chromatography	N.T.†	2.3	1.1	1.4	<0.9‡
Lyophilization	N.T.†	N.T.†	N.T.†	N.T.†	1.9
Cumulative Total, $\log_{10}$	**10.3**	**6.1**	**5.4**	**5.6**	**7.3**

* Solvent/Detergent treatment inactivates only lipid enveloped viruses. PPV and HAV are non-lipid enveloped viruses.
** Not Applicable for lipid enveloped viruses due to the presence of solvent/detergent in the starting material.
† Not Tested.
‡ Value not included in cumulative total.

HEMOFIL M AHF was administered to 11 patients previously untreated with Antihemophilic Factor (Human). They have shown no signs of hepatitis or HIV infection following three to nine months of evaluation.

A study of 25 patients treated with **HEMOFIL** M AHF, and monitored for three to six months has demonstrated no evidence of antibody response to mouse protein. More than 1,000 infusions of **HEMOFIL** M AHF have been administered during the clinical trials with no significant reactions. Reported events included a single episode each of chest tightness, fuzziness and dizziness, and one patient reported an unusual taste after each infusion.

INDICATIONS AND USAGE

The use of **HEMOFIL** M, Antihemophilic Factor (Human) (AHF), Method M, Monoclonal Purified, is indicated in hemophilia A (classical hemophilia) for the prevention and control of hemorrhagic episodes.

HEMOFIL M AHF can be of significant therapeutic value in patients with acquired Factor VIII inhibitors not exceeding 10 Bethesda Units per mL.[3] However, in such uses, the dosage should be controlled by frequent laboratory determinations of circulating AHF.

HEMOFIL M AHF is not indicated in von Willebrand's disease.

CONTRAINDICATIONS

Known hypersensitivity to mouse protein is a contraindication to the use of **HEMOFIL** M AHF.

WARNINGS

HEMOFIL M, Antihemophilic Factor (Human) (AHF), Method M, Monoclonal Purified, is made from human plasma. Products made from human plasma may contain infectious agents, such as viruses, that can cause disease. The risk that such products will transmit an infectious agent has been reduced by screening plasma donors for prior exposure to certain viruses, by testing for the presence of certain current virus infections, and by inactivating and/or removing certain viruses. Despite these measures, such products can still potentially transmit disease. Because this product is made from human blood, it may carry a risk of transmitting infectious agents, e.g., viruses and theoretically, the Creutzfeldt-Jakob disease (CJD) agent. ALL infections thought by a physician possibly to have been transmitted by this product should be reported by the physician or other healthcare provider to Baxter Healthcare Corporation, at 1-800-423-2862 (in the U.S.). The physician should discuss the risks and benefits of this product with the patient.

Individuals who receive infusions of blood or plasma products may develop signs and/or symptoms of some viral infections, particularly non A, non B hepatitis. As indicated under **CLINICAL PHARMACOLOGY**, however, a group of such patients treated with **HEMOFIL** M AHF did not demonstrate signs or symptoms of non A, non B hepatitis over observation periods ranging from three to nine months.

PRECAUTIONS

General

Certain components used in the packaging of this product contain natural rubber latex.

Identification of the clotting defect as a Factor VIII deficiency is essential before the administration of HEMOFIL M, Antihemophilic Factor (Human) (AHF), Method M, Monoclonal Purified, is initiated.

No benefit may be expected from this product in treating other deficiencies.

The processing of **HEMOFIL** M, Antihemophilic Factor (Human) (AHF), Method M, Monoclonal Purified significantly reduces the presence of blood group specific antibodies in the final product.

Formation of Antibodies to Mouse Protein

Although no hypersensitivity reactions have been observed, because **HEMOFIL** M AHF contains trace amounts of mouse protein (less than 0.1 ng/AHF activity units), the possibility exists that patients treated with this product may develop hypersensitivity to the mouse proteins.

The pulse rate should be determined before and during administration of **HEMOFIL** M AHF. Should a significant increase occur, reducing the rate of administration or temporarily halting the injection usually allows the symptoms to disappear promptly.

Information for Patients

Some viruses, such as parvovirus B19 or hepatitis A, are particularly difficult to remove or inactivate at this time. Parvovirus B19 most seriously affects pregnant women, or immune-compromised individuals. Symptoms of parvovirus B19 infection include fever, drowsiness, chills, and runny nose followed about two weeks later by a rash, and joint pain. Evidence of hepatitis A may include several days to weeks of poor appetite, tiredness, and low-grade fever followed by nausea, vomiting, and pain in the belly. Dark urine and a yellowed complexion are also common symptoms. Patients should be encouraged to consult their physician if such symptoms appear.

Patients should be informed of the early signs of hypersensitivity reactions including hives, generalized urticaria, tightness of the chest, wheezing, hypotension, and anaphylaxis, and should be advised to discontinue use of the product and contact their physician if these symptoms occur.

Laboratory Tests

Although dosage can be estimated by the calculations which follow, it is strongly recommended that whenever possible, appropriate laboratory tests be performed on the patient's plasma at suitable intervals to assure that adequate AHF levels have been reached and are maintained.

If the AHF content of the patient's plasma fails to reach expected levels or if bleeding is not controlled after apparently adequate dosage, the presence of inhibitor should be suspected. By appropriate laboratory procedures, the presence of inhibitor can be demonstrated and quantified in terms of AHF units neutralized by each mL of plasma or by the total estimated plasma volume.

If the inhibitor is at low levels (i.e., <10 Bethesda Units/mL), after administration of sufficient AHF units to neutralize the inhibitor, additional AHF units will elicit the predicted response.

Pregnancy

Pregnancy Category C. Animal reproduction studies have not been conducted with **HEMOFIL** M, Antihemophilic Factor (Human) (AHF), Method M, Monoclonal Purified. It is not known whether **HEMOFIL** M AHF can cause fetal harm when administered to a pregnant woman or can affect reproduction capacity. **HEMOFIL** M AHF should be given to a pregnant woman only if clearly needed.

ADVERSE REACTIONS

Allergic reactions may be encountered from the use of Antihemophilic Factor (Human) preparations. See **Information for Patients.**

The protein in greatest concentration in **HEMOFIL** M AHF is Albumin (Human). Reactions associated with albumin are extremely rare, although nausea, fever, chills or urticaria have been reported.

DOSAGE AND ADMINISTRATION

Each bottle of **HEMOFIL** M AHF is labeled with the AHF activity expressed in IU per bottle. This potency assignment is referenced to the World Health Organization International Standard.

The high purity of **HEMOFIL** M AHF has been thought to influence the difficulty of producing an accurate potency measurement. Experiments have shown that to achieve accurate activity levels, such a potency assay should be conducted using plastic test tubes and pipets as well as substrate containing normal levels of von Willebrand's Factor.

The expected *in vivo* peak AHF level, expressed as IU/dL of plasma or % (percent) of normal, can be calculated by multiplying the dose administered per kg body weight (IU/kg) by two. This calculation is based on the clinical finding by Abildgaard, *et al*,[4] which is supported by data from the collaborative study of *in vivo* recovery and survival with 15 different lots of **HEMOFIL** M AHF on 56 hemophiliacs that demonstrated a mean peak recovery point above the mean pre-infusion baseline of about 2.0 IU/dL per infused IU/kg body weight.[5]

Example:

(1) A dose of 1750 IU AHF administered to a 70 kg patient, i.e. 25 IU/kg (1750/70), should be expected to cause a peak post-infusion AHF increase of 25 × 2 = 50 IU/dL (50% of normal).

(2) A peak level of 70% is required in a 40 kg child. In this situation the dose would be 70/2 × 40 = 1400 IU.

Recommended Dosage Schedule

Physician supervision of the dosage is required. The following dosage schedule may be used as a guide.

[See table above]

HEMORRHAGE		
Degree of hemorrhage	**Required peak post-infusion AHF activity in the blood (as % of normal or IU/dL plasma)**	**Frequency of Infusion**
Early hemarthrosis or muscle or oral bleed	20-40	Begin infusion every 12 to 24 hours for one-three days until the bleeding episode as indicated by pain is resolved or healing is achieved.
More extensive hemarthrosis, muscle bleed, or hematoma	30-60	Repeat infusion every 12 to 24 hours for usually three days or more until pain and disability are resolved.
Life threatening bleeds such as head injury, throat bleed, severe abdominal pain	60-100	Repeat infusion every 18 to 24 hours until threat is resolved.
SURGERY		
Type of operation		
Minor surgery, including tooth extraction	60-80	A single infusion plus oral antifibrinolytic therapy within one hour is sufficient in approximately 70% of cases.
Major surgery	80-100 (pre- and post-operative)	Repeat infusion every 8 to 24 hours depending on state of healing.

The careful control of the substitution therapy is especially important in cases of major surgery or life threatening hemorrhages.

Although dosage can be estimated by the calculations above, it is strongly recommended that whenever possible, appropriate laboratory tests including serial AHF assays be performed on the patient's plasma at suitable intervals to assure that adequate AHF levels have bee reached and are maintained.

Other dosage regimens have been proposed such as that of Schimpf, *et al*, which describes continuous maintenance therapy.[6]

Reconstitution: Use Aseptic Technique

1. Bring **HEMOFIL** M AHF (dry concentrate) and Sterile Water for Injection, USP, (diluent) to room temperature.
2. Remove caps from concentrate and diluent bottles to expose central portion of rubber stoppers.
3. Cleanse stoppers with germicidal solution.
4. Remove protective covering from one end of double-ended needle and insert exposed needle through diluent stopper.
5. Remove protective covering from other end of double-ended needle. Invert diluent bottle over upright **HEMOFIL** M AHF bottle, then rapidly insert free end of the needle through the **HEMOFIL** M AHF bottle stopper at its center. The vacuum in the **HEMOFIL** M AHF bottle will draw in the diluent.
6. Disconnect the two bottles by removing needle from diluent bottle stopper, then remove needle from **HEMOFIL** M AHF bottle. Swirl gently until all material is dissolved. Be sure that **HEMOFIL** M AHF is completely dissolved, otherwise active material will be removed by the filter.

Note: Do not refrigerate after reconstitution.

Administration: Use Aseptic Technique

Administer at room temperature.

HEMOFIL M, Antihemophilic Factor (Human) (AHF), Method M, Monoclonal Purified, should be administered not more than three hours after reconstitution.

Intravenous Syringe Injection

Parenteral drug products should be inspected for particulate matter and discoloration prior to administration, whenever solution and container permit.

Plastic syringes are recommended for use with this product. The ground glass surface of all-glass syringes tend to stick with solutions of this type.

1. Attach filter needle to a disposable syringe and draw back plunger to admit air into syringe.
2. Insert needle into reconstituted **HEMOFIL** M AHF.
3. Inject air into bottle and then withdraw the reconstituted material into the syringe.
4. Remove and discard the filter needle from the syringe; attach a suitable needle and inject intravenously as instructed under **Rate of Administration.**
5. If a patient is to receive more than one bottle of **HEMOFIL** M AHF, the contents of two bottles may be drawn into the same syringe by drawing up each bottle through a separate unused filter needle. This practice lessens the loss of **HEMOFIL** M AHF. Please note, filter needles are intended to filter the contents of a single bottle of **HEMOFIL** M AHF only.

Rate of Administration

Preparations of **HEMOFIL** M AHF can be administered at a rate of up to 10 mL per minute with no significant reactions. The pulse rate should be determined before and during administration of **HEMOFIL** M AHF. Should a significant increase occur, reducing the rate of administration or temporarily halting the injection usually allows the symptoms to disappear promptly.

HOW SUPPLIED

HEMOFIL M AHF is available as single dose bottles. Each bottle is labeled with the potency in International Units, and is packaged together with 10 mL of Sterile Water for Injection, USP, a double-ended needle, and a filter needle.

Storage

HEMOFIL M AHF can be stored under refrigeration [2°-8°C (36°-46°F)] or at room temperature, not to exceed 30°C (86°F), until expiration date noted on the package. Avoid freezing to prevent damage to the diluent bottle.

REFERENCES

1. Horowitz B, Wiebe ME, Lippin A, *et al:* Inactivation of viruses in labile blood derivatives: 1. Disruption of lipid enveloped viruses by tri(n-butyl)phosphate detergent combinations. **Transfusion 25**:516-522, 1985
2. Prince AM, Horowitz B, Brotman B: Sterilisation of hepatitis and HTLV-III viruses by exposure to tri(n-butyl)phosphate and sodium cholate. **Lancet 1**:706-710, 1986
3. Kessler CM: An Introduction to Factor VIII Inhibitors: The Detection and Quantitation. **Am J Med 91 (Suppl 5A)**:1S-5S, 1991
4. Abildgaard CF, Simone JV, Corrigan JJ, *et al:* Treatment of hemophilia with glycine-precipitated Factor VIII. **New Eng J Med 275**:471-475, 1966
5. Addiego, Jr. JE, Gomperts E, Liu S. *et al:* Treatment of hemophilia A with a highly purified Factor VIII concentrate prepared by Anti-FVIIIc immunoaffinity chromatography. **Thrombosis and Haemostasis 67**:19-27, 1992
6. Schimpf K, Rothmann P, Zimmermann K: Factor VIII dosis in prophylaxis of hemophilia A; A further controlled study, in **Proc XIth Cong W.F.H.** Kyoto, Japan, Academic Press, 1976, pp 363-366

To enroll in the confidential, industry-wide Patient Notification System, call 1-888-UPDATE U (1-888-873-2838).

Baxter and Hemofil are trademarks of Baxter International, Inc., and are registered in the U.S. Patent and Trademark office.

Baxter Healthcare Corporation
Glendale, CA 91203 USA
U.S. License No. 140
Revised June 2002

RECOMBINATE ℞

[*rē-kŏm-bĭnāt*]
Antihemophilic Factor (Recombinant)

DESCRIPTION

RECOMBINATE, Antihemophilic Factor (Recombinant) (rAHF) is a glycoprotein synthesized by a genetically engineered Chinese Hamster Ovary (CHO) cell line. In culture, the CHO cell line secretes recombinant antihemophilic factor (rAHF) into the cell culture medium. The rAHF is purified from the culture medium utilizing a series of chromatography columns. A key step in the purification process is an immunoaffinity chromatography methodology in which a purification matrix, prepared by immobilization of a monoclonal antibody directed to factor VIII, is utilized to selectively isolate the rAHF in the medium. The synthesized rAHF produced by the CHO cells has the same biological effects as Antihemophilic Factor (Human) [AHF (Human)]. Structurally the protein has a similar combination of heterogenous heavy and light chains as found in AHF (Human).

RECOMBINATE rAHF is formulated as a sterile, nonpyrogenic, off-white to faint yellow, lyophilized powder preparation of concentrated recombinant AHF for intravenous injection. RECOMBINATE rAHF is available in single-dose bottles which contain nominally 250, 500 and 1000 International Units per bottle. When reconstituted with the appropriate volume of diluent, the product contains the following stabilizers in maximum amounts: 12.5 mg/mL Albumin (Human), 0.20 mg/mL calcium, 1.5 mg/mL polyethylene glycol (3350), 180 mEq/L sodium, 55 mM histidine, 1.5 μg/AHF International Unit (IU) polysorbate-80. Von Willebrand Factor (vWF) is coexpressed with the Antihemophilic Factor (Recombinant) and helps to stabilize it. The final product contains not more than 2 ng vWF/IU rAHF which will not have any clinically relevant effect in patients with von Willebrand's disease. The product contains no preservative.

Manufacturing of RECOMBINATE rAHF is shared by Baxter Healthcare Corporation and Genetics Institute, Inc. The recombinant Antihemophilic Factor Concentrate (For Further Manufacturing Use), is produced by Baxter Healthcare Corporation and Genetics Institute (For Further Manufacturing Use) and subsequently formulated and packaged at Baxter Healthcare Corporation.

Each bottle of RECOMBINATE rAHF is labeled with the AHF activity expressed in IU per bottle. Biological potency is determined by an *in vitro* assay which is referenced to the World Health Organization (WHO) International Standard for Factor VIII:C Concentrate.

CLINICAL PHARMACOLOGY

AHF is the specific clotting factor deficient in patients with hemophilia A (classical hemophilia). Hemophilia A is a genetic bleeding disorder characterized by hemorrhages which may occur spontaneously or after minor trauma. The administration of RECOMBINATE rAHF provides an increase in plasma levels of AHF and can temporarily correct the co-

Continued on next page

Recombinate—Cont.

agulation defect in these patients. Pharmacokinetic studies on sixty-nine (69) patients revealed the circulating mean half-life for rAHF to be 14.6 ± 4.9 hours (n=67), which was not statistically significantly different from plasma-derived **HEMOFIL** M, Antihemophilic Factor (Human) (AHF) (pdAHF). The mean half-life of **HEMOFIL** M AHF was 14.7 ± 5.1 hours (n=61). The actual baseline recovery observed with rAHF was 123.9 ± 47.7 IU/dl (n=23) which is significantly higher than the actual **HEMOFIL** M AHF baseline recovery of 101.7 ± 31.6 IU/dl (n=61). However, the calculated ratio of actual to expected recovery with rAHF (121.2 ± 48.9%) is not different on average from **HEMOFIL** M AHF (123.4 ± 16.4%). The clinical study of rAHF in previously treated patients (individuals with hemophilia A who had been treated with plasma derived AHF) was based on observations made on a study group of 69 patients. These individuals received cumulative amounts of Factor VIII ranging from 20,914 to 1,383,063 IU over the 48 month study. Patients were given a total of 17,700 infusions totaling 28,090,769 IU rAHF.

These patients were successfully treated for bleeding episodes on a demand basis and also for the prevention of bleeds (prophylaxis). Spontaneous bleeding episodes successfully managed include hemarthroses, soft tissue and muscle bleeds. Management of hemostasis was also evaluated in surgeries. A total of 24 procedures on 13 patients were performed during this study. These included minor (e.g. tooth extraction) and major (e.g. bilateral osteotomies, thoracotomy and liver transplant) procedures. Hemostasis was maintained perioperatively and postoperatively with individualized AHF replacement.

A study of rAHF in previously untreated patients was also performed as part of an ongoing study. The study group was comprised of seventy-nine (79) patients, of whom seventy-six (76) had received at least one infusion of rAHF. To date, this cohort has been given 12,209 infusions totaling over 11,277,043 IU rAHF. Hemostasis was appropriately managed in spontaneous bleeding episodes, intracranial hemorrhage and surgical procedures.

INDICATIONS AND USAGE

The use of RECOMBINATE rAHF is indicated in hemophilia A (classical hemophilia) for the prevention and control of hemorrhagic episodes.1 RECOMBINATE rAHF is also indicated in the perioperative management of patients with hemophilia A (classical hemophilia).

RECOMBINATE rAHF can be of therapeutic value in patients with acquired AHF inhibitors not exceeding 10 Bethesda Units per mL[2]. In clinical studies with RECOMBINATE rAHF, patients with inhibitors who were entered into the previously treated patient trial and those previously untreated children who have developed inhibitor activity on study, showed clinical hemostatic response when the titer of inhibitor was less than 10 Bethesda Units per mL. However, in such uses, the dosage of RECOMBINATE rAHF should be controlled by frequent laboratory determinations of circulating AHF levels.

RECOMBINATE rAHF is not indicated in von Willebrand's disease.

CONTRAINDICATIONS

Known hypersensitivity to mouse, hamster or bovine protein may be a contraindication to the use of Antihemophilic Factor (Recombinant) (see **Precautions**).

WARNINGS

None.

PRECAUTIONS

General

Certain components used in the packaging of this product contain natural rubber latex.

Identification of the clotting defect as a Factor VIII deficiency is essential before the administration of RECOMBINATE, Antihemophilic Factor (Recombinant) (rAHF) is initiated. No benefit may be expected from this product in treating other deficiencies.

The formation of neutralizing antibodies, inhibitors to factor VIII, is a known complication in the management of individuals with hemophilia A. The reported prevalence of these antibodies in patients receiving plasma derived AHF is 10-20%[3-7, 10-12]. These inhibitors are invariably IgG immunoglobulins, the factor VIII procoagulant inhibitory activity of which is expressed as Bethesda Units (B.U.) per mL of plasma or serum[3-7]. Over the investigational period, none of the 69 previously treated individuals, without an inhibitor at entry into the study, developed an inhibitor. In the previously untreated patient group there were 73 eligible patients with factor VIII levels less than or equal to 2% who received at least one rAHF treatment (median days 100, range 3-8[21]) and who were tested for inhibitor after treatment with RECOMBINATE rAHF. Of this group, 23 individuals developed detectable inhibitor (median days 10, range 3-69) and of these, 8 patients showed a titer greater than 10 B.U. Patients treated with rAHF should be carefully monitored for the development of antibodies to rAHF by appropriate clinical observations and laboratory tests.

Formation of Antibodies to Mouse, Hamster or Bovine Protein

As RECOMBINATE rAHF contains trace amounts of mouse protein (maximum of 0.1 ng/IU rAHF), hamster protein (maximum of 1.5 ng CHO protein/IU rAHF), and bovine protein (maximum of 1 ng BSA/IU rAHF), the remote possibility exists that patients treated with this product may develop hypersensitivity to these non-human mammalian proteins.

Information for Patients

The patient and physician should discuss the risks and benefits of this product.

Although allergic type hypersensitivity reactions were not observed in any patient receiving RECOMBINATE rAHF on study, such reactions are theoretically possible. Patients should be informed of the early signs of hypersensitivity reactions including hives, generalized urticaria, tightness of the chest, wheezing, hypotension, and anaphylaxis. Patients should be advised to discontinue use of the product and contact their physician if these symptoms occur.

Laboratory Tests

Although dosage can be estimated by the calculations which follow, it is strongly recommended that whenever possible, appropriate laboratory tests be performed on the patient's plasma at suitable intervals to assure that adequate AHF levels have been reached and are maintained.

If the patient's plasma AHF fails to reach expected levels or if bleeding is not controlled after adequate dosage, the presence of inhibitor should be suspected. By performing appropriate laboratory procedures, the presence of an inhibitor can be demonstrated and quantified in terms of AHF International Units neutralized by each mL of plasma or by the total estimated plasma volume. If the inhibitor is present at levels less than 10 Bethesda Units per mL, administration of additional AHF may neutralize the inhibitor. Thereafter, the administration of additional AHF International Units should elicit the predicted response. The control of AHF levels by laboratory assay is necessary in this situation.

Inhibitor titers above 10 Bethesda Units per mL may make hemostasis control with AHF either impossible or impractical because of the very large dose required. In addition, the inhibitor titer may rise following AHF infusion because of an anamnestic response to the AHF antigen.

Carcinogenesis, Mutagenesis, Impairment of Fertility

RECOMBINATE rAHF was tested for mutagenicity at doses considerably exceeding plasma concentrations of rAHF *in vitro* and at doses up to ten times the expected maximum clinical dose *in vivo*, and did not cause reverse mutations, chromosomal aberrations, or an increase in micronuclei in bone marrow polychromatic erythrocytes. Long term studies in animals have not been performed to evaluate carcinogenic potential.

Pediatric Use

RECOMBINATE, Antihemophilic Factor (Recombinant) (rAHF) is appropriate for use in children of all ages, including the newborn. Safety and efficacy studies have been performed in both previously treated (n=23) and previously untreated (n=75) children. (See Clinical Pharmacology and Precautions).

Pregnancy

Pregnancy Category C. Animal reproduction studies have not been conducted with Antihemophilic Factor (Recombinant). It is not known whether Antihemophilic Factor (Recombinant) can cause fetal harm when administered to a pregnant woman or can affect reproductive capacity. Antihemophilic Factor (Recombinant) should be given to a pregnant woman only if clearly needed.

ADVERSE REACTIONS

During the clinical studies conducted in the previously treated patient group, there were 13 infusion related minor adverse reactions reported out of 10,446 infusions (0.12%). One patient experienced flushing and nausea during his first infusion which abated on decreasing the infusion rate. A second patient experienced mild fatigue during and following one infusion and a third patient had a series of eleven nose bleeds with a periodicity associated with the infusions.

The protein in greatest concentration in RECOMBINATE rAHF is Albumin (Human). Reactions associated with intravenous administration of albumin are extremely rare, although nausea, fever, chills or urticaria have been reported. Other allergic reactions could theoretically be encountered in the use of this Antihemophilic Factor preparation. See Information for Patients.

DOSAGE AND ADMINISTRATION

Each bottle of RECOMBINATE rAHF is labeled with the AHF activity expressed in IU per bottle. This potency assignment is referenced to the World Health Organization International Standard for Factor VIII:C Concentrate and is evaluated by appropriate methodology to ensure accuracy of the results. The expected *in vivo* peak increase in AHF level expressed as IU/dL of plasma or % (percent) of normal can be estimated by multiplying the dose administered per kg body weight (IU/kg) by two. This calculation is based on the clinical findings of Abildgaard *et al*[8] and is supported by the data generated by 419 clinical pharmacokinetic studies with rAHF in 67 patients over time. This pharmacokinetic data demonstrated a peak recovery point above the pre-infusion baseline of approximately 2.0 IU/dL per IU/kg body weight.

Example (Assuming patient's baseline AHF level is at <1%):

(1) A dose of 1750 IU AHF administered to a 70 kg patient, i.e. 25 IU/kg (1750/70), should be expected to cause a peak post-infusion AHF increase of 25 × 2 = 50 IU/dL (50% of normal).

(2) A peak level of 70% is required in a 40 kg child. In this situation the dose would be 70/2 × 40 = 1400 IU.

Recommended Dosage Schedule

Physician supervision of the dosage is required. The following dosage schedule may be used as a guide.

[See table below]

Hemorrhage		
Degree of hemorrhage	**Required peak post-infuson AHF activity in the blood (as % of normal or IU/dL plasma)**	**Frequency of infusion**
Early hemarthrosis or muscle bleed or oral bleed	20-40	Begin infusion every 12 to 24 hours for one-three days until the bleeding episode as indicated by pain is resolved or healing is achieved.
More extensive hemarthrosis, muscle bleed, or hematoma	30-60	Repeat infusion every 12 to 24 hours for usually three days or more until pain and disability are resolved.
Life threatening bleeds such as head injury, throat bleed, severe abdominal pain	60-100	Repeat infusion every 8 to 24 hours until threat is resolved.
Surgery		
Type of Operation		
Minor surgery, including tooth extraction	60-80	A single infusion plus oral antifibrinolytic therapy within one hour is sufficient in approximately 70% of cases.
Major surgery	80-100 (pre- and post-operative)	Repeat infusion every 8 to 24 hours depending on state of healing.

The careful control of the substitution therapy is especially important in cases of major surgery or life threatening hemorrhages.

Although dosage can be estimated by the calculations above, it is strongly recommended that whenever possible, appropriate laboratory tests including serial AHF assays be performed on the patient's plasma at suitable intervals to assure that adequate AHF levels have been reached and are maintained.

Other dosage regimens have been proposed such as that of Schimpf, *et al*, which describes continuous maintenance therapy.[9]

Reconstitution: Use Aseptic Technique

1. Bring RECOMBINATE, Antihemophilic Factor (Recombinant) (rAHF) (dry concentrate) and Sterile Water for Injection, USP, (diluent) to room temperature.
2. Remove caps from concentrate and diluent bottles.
3. Cleanse stoppers with germicidal solution and allow to dry prior to use.
4. Remove protective covering from one end of double-ended needle and insert exposed needle through the center of the stopper.
5. Remove protective covering from other end of double-ended needle. Invert diluent bottle over the upright RECOMBINATE rAHF bottle, then rapidly insert free end of the needle through the RECOMBINATE rAHF bottle stopper at its center. The vacuum in the bottle will draw in the diluent.
6. Disconnect the two bottles by removing needle from diluent bottle stopper, then remove needle from RECOMBINATE rAHF bottle. Swirl gently until all material is dissolved. Be sure that RECOMBINATE rAHF is completely dissolved, otherwise active material will be removed by the filter needle.

NOTE: Do not refrigerate after reconstitution. See **Administration.**

Administration: Use Aseptic Technique

Administer at room temperature.

RECOMBINATE rAHF should be administered not more than 3 hours after reconstitution.

Intravenous Syringe Injection

Parenteral drug products should be inspected for particulate matter and discoloration prior to administration, whenever solution and container permit. A colorless to faint yellow appearance is acceptable for RECOMBINATE rAHF.

Plastic syringes are recommended for use with this product since proteins such as AHF tend to stick to the surface of all-glass syringes.

1. Attach filter needle to a disposable syringe and draw back plunger to admit air into the syringe.
2. Insert needle into reconstituted RECOMBINATE rAHF.
3. Inject air into bottle and then withdraw the reconstituted material into the syringe.
4. Remove and discard the filter needle from the syringe; attach a suitable needle and inject intravenously as instructed under Rate of Administration.
5. If a patient is to receive more than one bottle of RECOMBINATE rAHF, the contents of multiple bottles may be drawn into the same syringe by drawing up each bottle through a separate unused filter needle. Filter needles are intended to filter the contents of a single bottle of RECOMBINATE rAHF only.

Rate of Administration

Preparations of RECOMBINATE, Antihemophilic Factor (Recombinant) (rAHF) can be administered at a rate of up to 10 mL per minute with no significant reactions.

The pulse rate should be determined before and during administration of RECOMBINATE rAHF. Should a significant increase in pulse rate occur, reducing the rate of administration or temporarily halting the injection usually allows the symptoms to disappear promptly.

HOW SUPPLIED

RECOMBINATE rAHF is available in single-dose bottles which contain nominally 250, 500 and 1000 International Units per bottle. RECOMBINATE rAHF is packaged with 10 mL of Sterile Water for Injection, USP, a double-ended needle, a filter needle, one physician insert and one patient insert.

Storage

RECOMBINATE rAHF can be stored under refrigeration [2°-8°C (36°-46°F)] or at room temperature, not to exceed 30°C (86°F). Avoid freezing to prevent damage to the diluent bottle. Do not use beyond the expiration date printed on the bottle.

REFERENCES

1. White GC, McMillan CW, Kingdon HS, *et al*: Use of recombinant antihemophilic factor in the treatment of two patients with classic hemophilia. **New Eng J Med 320**: 166-170, 1989
2. Kessler CM: An Introduction to Factor VIII Inhibitors: The Detection and Quantitation. **Am J Med 91 (Suppl 5A)**:1S-5S, 1991
3. Schwarzinger I, Pabinger I, Korninger C, Haschke F, Kundi M, Niessner H, Lechner K: Incidence of inhibitors in patients with severe and moderate hemophilia A treated with factor VIII concentrates. **Am J Hematology 24**:241-245, 1987
4. Penner JA, Kelly PE: Management of patients with factor VIII or IX inhibitors. **Sem Thromb Hemostasis 1**:386-399, 1975
5. Ehrenforth S, Kreuz W, Scharrer I, *et al*: Incidence of development of factor VIII and factor IX inhibitors in haemophiliacs. **Lancet 339**:594-598, 1992
6. McMillan CW, Shapiro SS, Whitehurst D, *et al*: The natural history of factor VIII inhibitors in patients with hemophilia A: a national cooperative study. II. Observations on the initial development of factor VIII:C inhibitors. **Blood 71**:344-348, 1988
7. Addiego JE Jr., Gomperts E, Liu S, *et al*: Treatment of hemophilia A with a highly purified Factor VIII concentrate prepared by Anti-FVIIIc immunoaffinity chromatography. **Thrombosis and Haemostasis 67**:19-27, 1992
8. Abildgaard CF, Simone JV, Corrigan JJ, *et al*: Treatment of hemophilia with glycine-precipitated Factor VIII. **New Eng J Med 275**:471-475, 1966
9. Schimpf K, Rothman P, Zimmermann K: Factor VIII dosis in prophylaxis of hemophilia A; A further controlled study in **Proc XIth Cong W.F.H.** Kyoto, Japan, Academic Press, 1976, pp 363-366
10. Gill FM: The Natural History of Factor VIII Inhibitors in Patients with Hemophilia A. Hoyer LW (ed), Factor VIII Inhibitors, **N.Y. AR Liss**, 1984, pp 19-29
11. Rasi V, Ikkala E: Haemophiliacs with factor VIII inhibitors in Finland: prevalence, incidence and outcome. **Br J Haematol** 76:369-371, 1990
12. Lusher JM, Salzman PM: Viral Safety and Inhibitor Development Associated with Factor VIIIC Ultra-Purified From Plasma in Hemophiliacs Previously Unexposed to Factor VIIIC Concentrates. **Seminars in Hematology 27**:1-7, 1990

To enroll in the confidential, industry-wide Patient Notification System, call 1-888-UPDATE U (1-888-873-2838).

Baxter, Recombinate, and Hemofil are trademarks of Baxter International, Inc.

Baxter and Hemofil are registered in the U.S. Patent and Trademark office.

Manufactured by:	Imported in Canada by:
Baxter Healthcare Corporation	**Baxter Corporation**
Westlake Village, CA 91362 USA	Toronto, Ontario
U.S. License No. 140	

Revised January 2003

7965

RECOMBINATE
Antihemophilic Factor
(Recombinant)
Information for Patients
Recombinate
Antihemophilic Factor (Recombinant)

Pronounced: ant-eye-hee-mo-fee-lick factor

Please read this leaflet carefully before using RECOMBINATE, Antihemophilic Factor Recombinant) (rAHF). This leaflet is a summary of the important information you need to know about your medicine for your factor deficiency. This summary is based on the information provided to your doctor and does not contain all of the information available about RECOMBINATE rAHF. This summary should be used only after you have received instructions from your doctor. If you have any questions after reading this leaflet, ask your doctor or pharmacist.

1. What is RECOMBINATE rAHF?

RECOMBINATE rAHF is a coagulation factor VIII protein that is made in a laboratory by inserting the human gene (DNA piece) that codes for Factor VIII into animal cells which then produce the human coagulation factor protein. In the manufacture of RECOMBINATE rAHF, the human Factor VIII is purified and separated from animal cell components. Albumin, a protein purified from human plasma, is included in RECOMBINATE rAHF to make the Factor VIII protein more stable. Factor VIII (also called antihemophilic factor), is the clotting factor that people with hemophilia A are missing. Hemophilia A is a hereditary bleeding disorder that prevents blood from clotting well. RECOMBINATE rAHF has the same effects as factor VIII protein made from human plasma.

2. What is RECOMBINATE rAHF used for?

RECOMBINATE rAHF can temporarily correct your body's blood clotting process so it helps prevent and control bleeding in people with hemophilia A (classical hemophilia). But you must follow your doctor or other health care provider's instructions and schedule for infusing RECOMBINATE rAHF carefully in order for your RECOMBINATE rAHF treatment to work effectively. Adults and children of all ages, including newborns, may use RECOMBINATE rAHF. Hemophilia A is a disorder that requires ongoing care. RECOMBINATE rAHF will not work in treating other clotting disorders.

3. How does RECOMBINATE rAHF work?

RECOMBINATE rAHF temporarily raises the level of factor VIII in the blood to a more normal level, allowing your body's blood clotting process to function temporarily. Because of this, you must follow your doctor or other health care provider's instructions and schedule for infusing RECOMBINATE rAHF.

4. Who should not use RECOMBINATE rAHF?

You should not use RECOMBINATE rAHF unless your doctor confirms that your clotting disorder is a factor VIII deficiency. Pregnant women should use this product only if clearly needed, since it is not known whether RECOMBINATE rAHF can harm your unborn child. It is also not known if RECOMBINATE rAHF affects a woman's ability to have children. If you are considering becoming pregnant you should talk to your doctor.

5. What is the most important information I need to know about RECOMBINATE rAHF?

You will need to check your pulse rate before and during your administration with RECOMBINATE rAHF. Your doctor or someone at your local hemophilia treatment center can show you how to check your pulse rate. If your pulse rate is much higher than usual you should slow the rate of infusion or temporarily stop the infusion. This should allow for your pulse to return to its normal rate. Ask your doctor how fast your pulse should be for you to slow or temporarily stop the rate of rAHF infusion.

Your body may form inhibitors to factor VIII. An inhibitor is an antibody (part of your body's normal defense system) that forms against factor VIII and prevents the factor VIII from working properly. These inhibitors can cause you to fail to respond to factor VIII therapy. This is not an uncommon complication in the treatment of people with hemophilia A. Work with your doctor to make sure you are carefully monitored for the development of inhibitors to factor VIII.

There is a possibility that you could have an allergic reaction to RECOMBINATE rAHF. You should be aware of early signs of allergic reactions. They are: rash, hives, itching, tightness of the chest, difficulty breathing, throat tightness, weak pulse (due to low blood pressure), feeling lightheaded or feeling dizzy when you stand, and shortness of breath. If you experience any of these symptoms, stop the infusion immediately and contact your doctor. Severe symptoms, including difficulty breathing and (near) fainting require prompt emergency treatment.

6. What are the possible side effects of RECOMBINATE rAHF?

The most common side effects are flushing, nausea, fever, chills, mild fatigue, nose bleeds, and hives.

7. How do I use RECOMBINATE rAHF?

RECOMBINATE, Antihemophilic Factor (Recombinant) (rAHF) is injected directly into the blood stream. When you are first starting treatment you may need or want to go to a Hemophilia Treatment Center or hospital to receive your infusions. Many people with hemophilia learn to infuse their factor by themselves or with the help of a family member. Your doctor or other health care provider can teach you the proper technique for self-infusion. Once you learn how to self-infuse, you can follow the instructions on the back of this leaflet.

8. How do I know what dose to take of RECOMBINATE rAHF?

Your doctor will provide you with a dose that is based on your body weight, the severity of your hemophilia, and the location and severity of bleeding.

Your doctor may periodically need to check laboratory blood test results following infusion of RECOMBINATE rAHF to be sure that the blood level of active Factor VIII is high enough to allow satisfactory blood clotting. If your bleeding is not controlled after infusing RECOMBINATE rAHF, contact your doctor.

RECOMBINATE rAHF comes in three different strengths. The boxes and bottles are color coded. The color bar on the box and bottle show you which one you have. A light blue color bar is for the low potency (220–400 IU). A light pink color bar is for the medium potency (401–800 IU). A light green color bar is for high potency (801–1240 IU). Always check the potency printed on the label to make sure you are using the potency prescribed by your doctor. Always check the expiration date printed on the bottle or box. You should not use the product after the expiration date printed on the bottle or box.

Each bottle of RECOMBINATE rAHF is for single use only. After you add the diluent to the RECOMBINATE rAHF it should be used within 3 hours. Any RECOMBINATE rAHF left in the bottle at the end of your infusion should be discarded. You should not refrigerate RECOMBINATE rAHF after you add the diluent.

9. How do I store RECOMBINATE rAHF?

You may store RECOMBINATE rAHF without the diluent added to it either in the refrigerator or at normal room temperature (not to exceed 86°F). DO NOT FREEZE.

10. How can I find out more about Baxter's patient assistance programs?

You can call Baxter to receive more information on patient assistance programs available to you:

Reimbursement Support 1-800-548-4448
Factor Assist (insurance gap program) 1-800-888-4502
Factor Plus (indigent care program) 1-800-548-4448
Patient Notification System 1-888-873-2838
Baxter Customer Service 1-800-423-2090
Hemophilia Galaxy (www.hemophiliagalaxy.com)

Baxter, Recombinate, Hemophilia Galaxy and Factor Assist, are trademarks of Baxter International, Inc. Baxter and Factor Assist are registered in the U.S. Patent and Trademark office. Factor Plus is a service mark of Baxter International, Inc.

Manufactured by:	Imported in Canada by:
Baxter Healthcare Corporation	**Baxter Corporation**
Westlake Village, CA 91362 USA	Toronto, Ontario
U.S. License No. 14	

Revised January 2003

RECOMBINATE
Antihemophilic Factor (Recombinant)
(For intravenous use only)

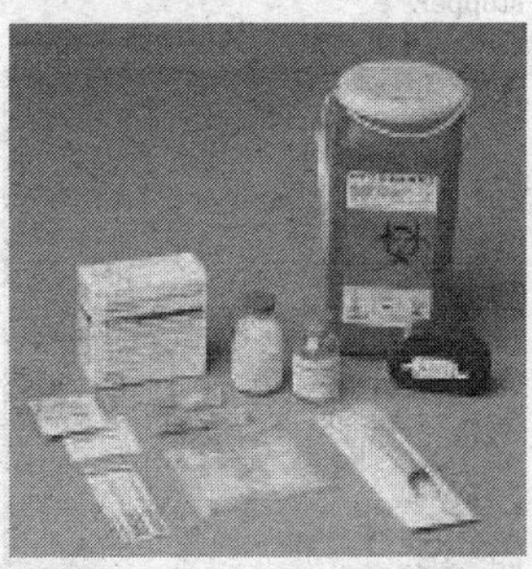

1. In a quiet place, prepare a clean surface. Let the bottle with the FVIII concentrate and the Sterile Water for Injection (diluent) warm up to room temperature.

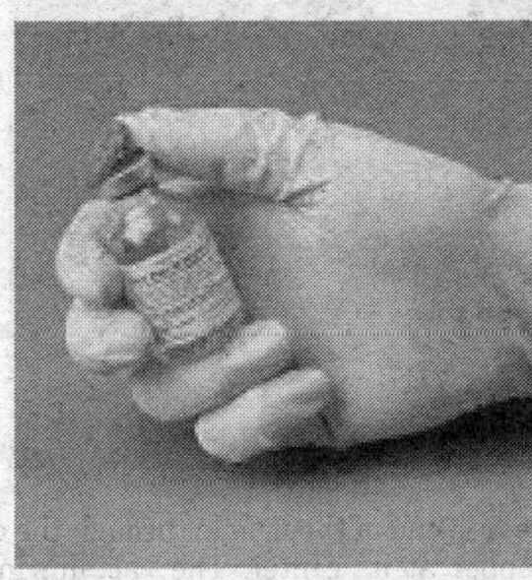

2. After washing your hands and putting on sterile gloves, remove caps from the concentrate and diluent bottles to expose the centers of the rubber stoppers.

Continued on next page

Recombinate—Cont.

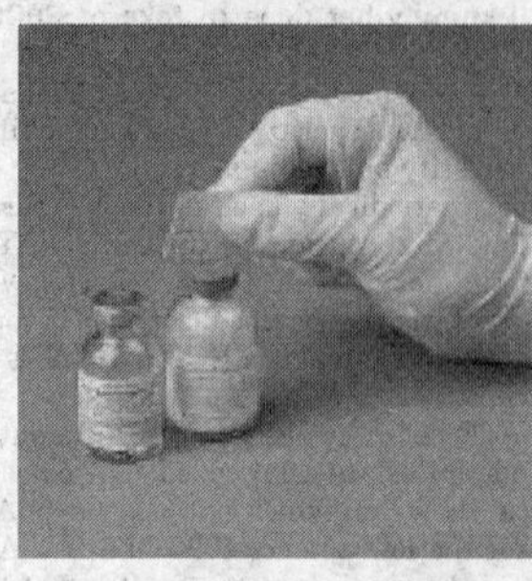

3. Disinfect the stoppers with an alcohol swab or other suitable solution suggested by your doctor or hemophilia center.

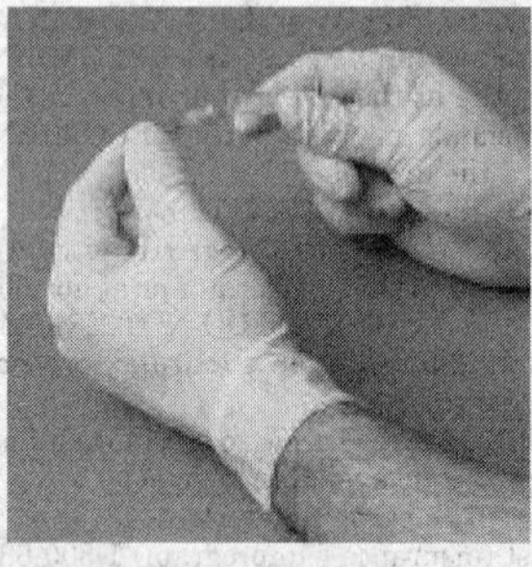

4. Remove the protective covering from one end of the double-ended transfer needle.

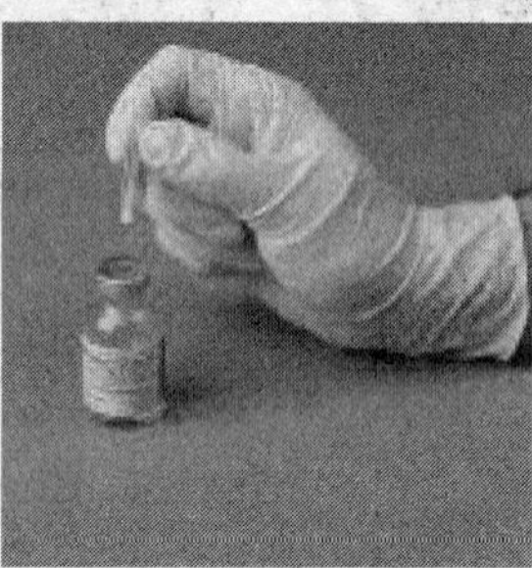

5. Insert the exposed short part of the needle through the diluent stopper.

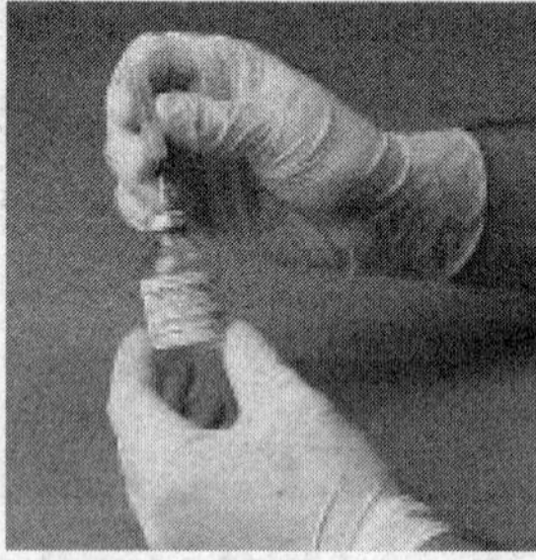

6. Remove the protective covering from the other end of the double-ended transfer needle.

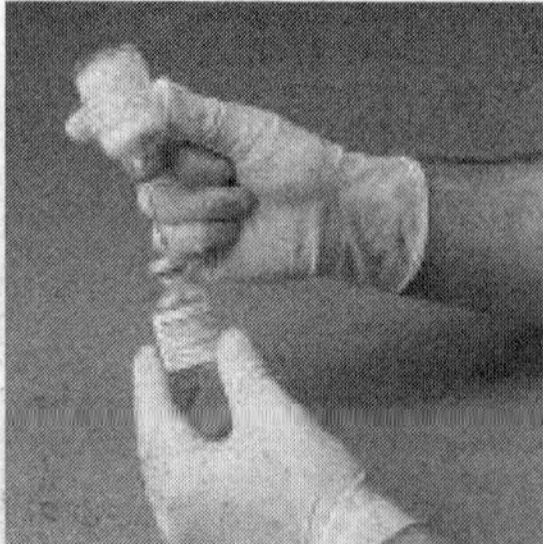

7. Insert the free end of the needle through the concentrate bottle stopper at its center. The vacuum in the bottle will draw in the diluent. Invert the diluent bottle over the upright concentrate bottle.
[See figure at top of next column]
8. Disconnect the two bottles by removing the needle from the diluent bottle stopper, then remove the needle from the concentrate bottle. Do not recap the needle! Place

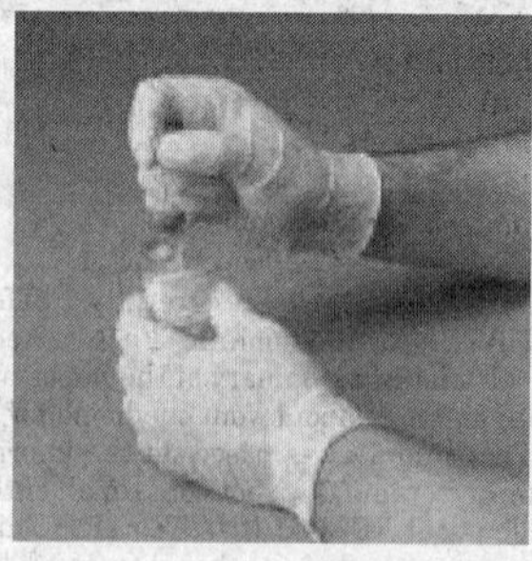

the needle in a hard-walled Sharps container for proper disposal.

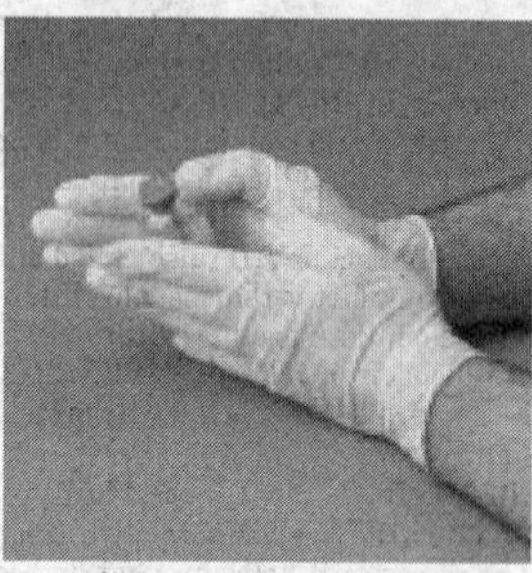

9. Gently roll the vial between palms until all material is dissolved. Do not shake. Check to make sure the product is completely dissolved.

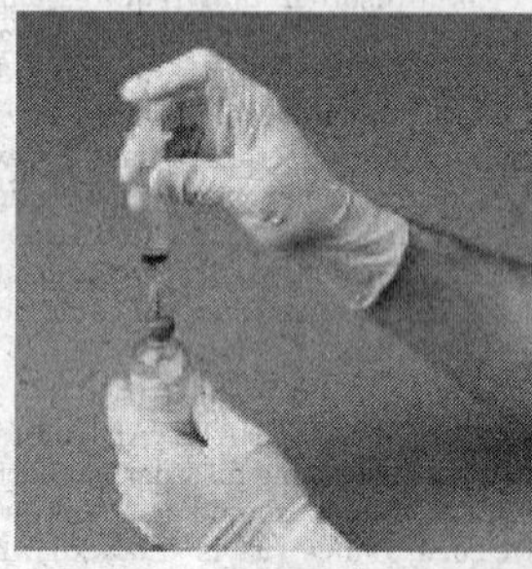

10. Attach filter needle to a disposable syringe and draw back the plunger to allow air into the syringe. Insert the needle into the reconstituted FVIII concentrate. Inject air into the bottle.

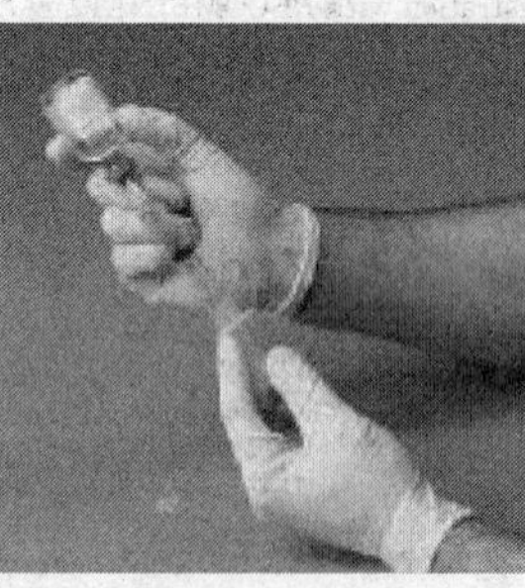

11. Withdraw the solution into the syringe.

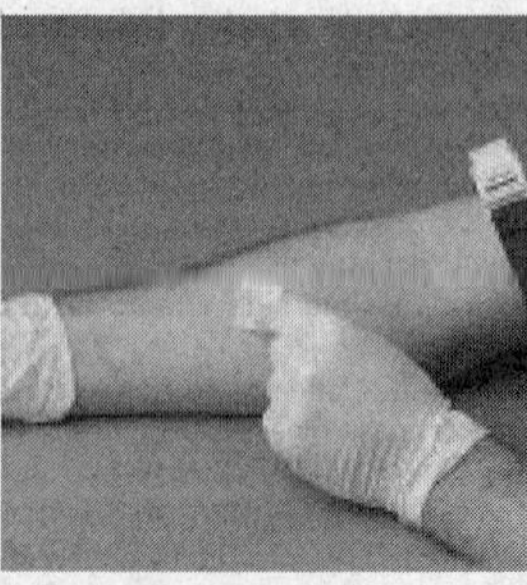

12. Prepare the injection site by wiping with an alcohol swab or other suitable solution suggested by your doctor or hemophilia center.

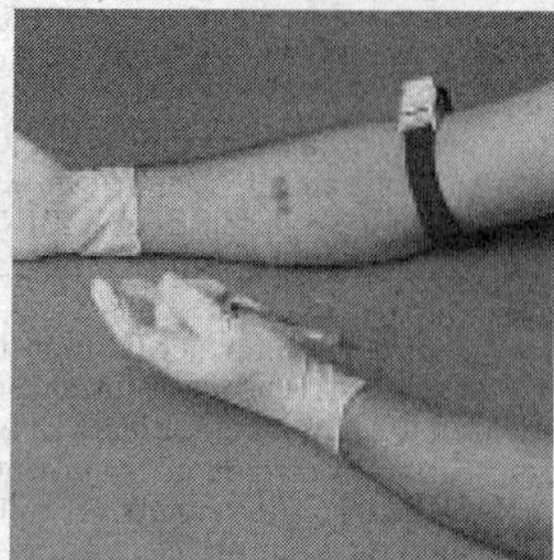

13. Do not infuse the product any faster than 10 mL per minute. Use a winged infusion set if available. After infusion, apply pressure with sterile gauze to the infusion site for 3 minutes. Do not recap the needle after infusion. Place it with the used syringe in a hard-walled Sharps container for proper disposal.

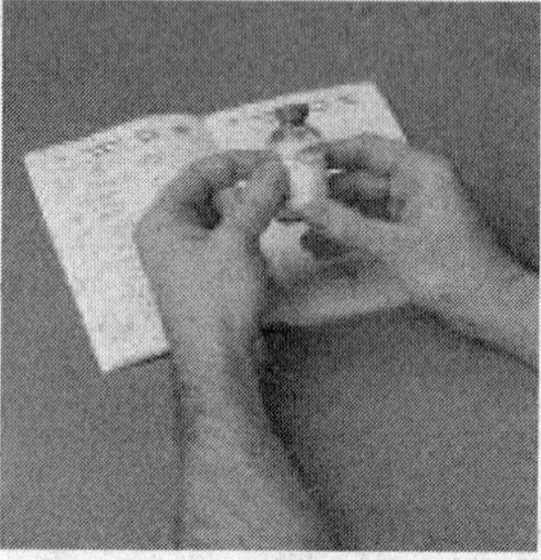

14. After infusion, remove peel-off label from the concentrate bottle and place it in your factor log. Clean up any spilled blood with freshly prepared 10% bleach solution or soap and water.

IMPORTANT: Contact your doctor or local Hemophilia Treatment Center if you experience any problems. These instructions are intended as a visual aid only for those patients who have been instructed by their doctor or hemophilia center on the proper way to self-infuse the product. If you have not been taught by your doctor, do not attempt to self-infuse.

Baxter Healthcare Corporation
Anesthesia & Critical Care

95 SPRING ST
NEW PROVIDENCE, NJ 07974

Direct Inquiries to:
Professional Services Department
(800) ANA DRUG
(800) 262-3784

For Medical Information Contact:
In Emergencies:
Paula Dimopoulos PharmD
Director Medical Affairs
(800) ANA-DRUG
(800) 262-3784

Sales and Ordering:
To place an order, call or fax:
(800) 667-0959
Fax 877-702-3580

BREVIBLOC PREMIXED INJECTION ℞

[brĕv-ĭ-blŏk]
(Esmolol Hydrochloride)
2,500 mg/250 mL (10 mg/mL) Ready-to-use Bags
250 mL Bags
Iso-Osmotic Solution of Esmolol Hydrochloride in Sodium Chloride
For Intravenous Use
Can be used for direct intravenous use.
Esmolol Hydrochloride concentration = 10 milligrams/mL (10,000 micrograms/mL)
Single Patient Use Only
No Preservatives Added

BREVIBLOC DOUBLE STRENGTH PREMIXED INJECTION

(Esmolol Hydrochloride)
2,000 mg/100 mL (20 mg/mL) Ready-to-use Bags
100 mL Bags
Iso-Osmotic Solution of Esmolol Hydrochloride in Sodium Chloride
For Intravenous Use
Can be used for direct intravenous use.
Esmolol Hydrochloride concentration = 20 milligrams/mL (20,000 micrograms/mL)
Single Patient Use Only
No Preservatives Added

BREVIBLOC INJECTION
(Esmolol Hydrochloride)
100 mg/10 mL (10 mg/mL) Ready-to-use Vials
10 mL Vials
Iso-Osmotic Solution of Esmolol Hydrochloride in Sodium Chloride
For Intravenous Use
Can be used for direct intravenous use.
Esmolol Hydrochloride concentration = 10 milligrams/ mL (10,000 micrograms/mL)
Single Patient Use Only
No Preservatives Added

BREVIBLOC DOUBLE STRENGTH INJECTION
(Esmolol Hydrochloride)
100 mg/5 mL (20 mg/mL) Ready-to-use Vials
5 mL Vials
Iso-Osmotic Solution of Esmolol Hydrochloride in Sodium Chloride
For Intravenous Use
Can be used for direct intravenous use.
Esmolol Hydrochloride concentration = 20 milligrams/ mL (20,000 micrograms/mL)
Single Patient Use Only
No Preservatives Added

BREVIBLOC CONCENTRATE
(Esmolol Hydrochloride)
2,500 mg/10 mL (250 mg/mL) Ampuls for Dilution
10 mL Ampuls
NOT FOR DIRECT INTRAVENOUS INJECTION.
Esmolol Hydrochloride concentration = 250 milligrams/ mL (250,000 micrograms/mL)
AMPULS MUST BE DILUTED PRIOR TO INFUSION—SEE DOSAGE AND ADMINISTRATION, Directions for Use of the Brevibloc Concentrate 10 mL Ampul (250 milligrams/mL).

DESCRIPTION

BREVIBLOC (Esmolol Hydrochloride) is a beta$_1$-selective (cardioselective) adrenergic receptor blocking agent with a very short duration of action (elimination half-life is approximately 9 minutes). Esmolol Hydrochloride is:
(±)-Methyl p-[2-hydroxy-3-(isopropylamino) propoxy] hydrocinnamate hydrochloride and has the following structure:

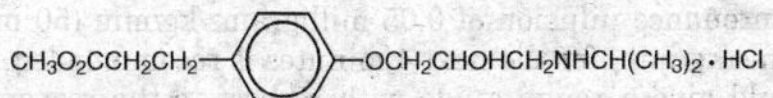

Esmolol Hydrochloride has the empirical formula $C_{16}H_{26}NO_4Cl$ and a molecular weight of 331.8. It has one asymmetric center and exists as an enantiomeric pair.
Esmolol Hydrochloride is a white to off-white crystalline powder. It is a relatively hydrophilic compound which is very soluble in water and freely soluble in alcohol. Its partition coefficient (octanol/water) at pH 7.0 is 0.42 compared to 17.0 for propranolol.

Brevibloc Premixed Injection
BREVIBLOC PREMIXED INJECTION is a clear, colorless to light yellow, sterile, nonpyrogenic, iso-osmotic solution of esmolol hydrochloride in sodium chloride.

2500 mg, 250 mL Single Use Premixed Bag—Each mL contains 10 mg Esmolol Hydrochloride, 5.9 mg Sodium Chloride, USP and Water for Injection, USP; buffered with 2.8 mg Sodium Acetate Trihydrate, USP and 0.546 mg Glacial Acetic Acid, USP. Sodium Hydroxide and/or Hydrochloric Acid added, as necessary, to adjust pH to 5.0 (4.5-5.5). The calculated osmolarity is 312 mOsmol/L. The 250 mL bag is a non-latex, non-PVC IntraVia bag with dual PVC ports. The IntraVia bag is manufactured from a specially designed multilayer plastic (PL 2408). Solutions in contact with the plastic container leach out certain chemical compounds from the plastic in very small amounts; however, biological testing was supportive of the safety of the plastic container materials. See **DOSAGE AND ADMINISTRATION, Directions for Use of the Premixed Bag** for additional information.

2000 mg, 100 mL Single Use Premixed Bag DOUBLE STRENGTH—Each mL contains 20 mg Esmolol Hydrochloride, 4.1 mg Sodium Chloride, USP and Water for Injection, USP; buffered with 2.8 mg Sodium Acetate Trihydrate, USP and 0.546 mg Glacial Acetic Acid, USP. Sodium Hydroxide and/or Hydrochloric Acid added, as necessary, to adjust pH to 5.0 (4.5-5.5). The calculated osmolarity is 312 mOsmol/L. The 100 mL bag is a non-latex, non-PVC IntraVia bag with dual PVC ports. The IntraVia bag is manufactured from a specially designed multilayer plastic (PL 2408). Solutions in contact with the plastic container leach out certain chemical compounds from the plastic in very small amounts; however, biological testing was supportive of the safety of the plastic container materials. See **DOSAGE AND ADMINISTRATION, Directions for Use of the Premixed Bag** for additional information.

Brevibloc Injection
BREVIBLOC INJECTION is a clear, colorless to light yellow, sterile, nonpyrogenic, iso-osmotic solution of esmolol hydrochloride in sodium chloride.

100 mg, 10 mL Single Dose Vial—Each mL contains 10 mg Esmolol Hydrochloride, 5.9 mg Sodium Chloride, USP and Water for Injection, USP; buffered with 2.8 mg Sodium Acetate Trihydrate, USP and 0.546 mg Glacial Acetic Acid, USP. Sodium Hydroxide and/or Hydrochloric Acid added, as necessary to adjust pH to 5.0 (4.5-5.5).

100 mg, 5 mL DOUBLE STRENGTH Single Dose Vial—Each mL contains 20 mg Esmolol Hydrochloride, 4.1 mg Sodium Chloride, USP and Water for Injection, USP; buffered with 2.8 mg Sodium Acetate Trihydrate, USP and 0.546 mg Glacial Acetic Acid, USP. Sodium Hydroxide and/or Hydrochloric Acid added, as necessary to adjust pH to 5.0 (4.5-5.5).

Brevibloc Concentrate
BREVIBLOC CONCENTRATE is a clear, colorless to light yellow, sterile, nonpyrogenic concentrate.

2500 mg, 10 mL Ampul—Each mL contains 250 mg Esmolol Hydrochloride in 25% Propylene Glycol, USP, 25% Alcohol, USP and Water for Injection, USP; buffered with 17.0 mg Sodium Acetate Trihydrate, USP, and 0.00715 mL Glacial Acetic Acid, USP. Sodium Hydroxide and/or Hydrochloric Acid added, as necessary, to adjust pH to 3.5-5.5. NOT FOR DIRECT INTRAVENOUS USE - AMPUL MUST BE DILUTED PRIOR TO INFUSION. See **DOSAGE AND ADMINISTRATION, Directions for Use of the Brevibloc Concentrate 10 mL Ampul (250 milligrams/mL).**

CLINICAL PHARMACOLOGY

BREVIBLOC (Esmolol Hydrochloride) is a beta$_1$-selective (cardioselective) adrenergic receptor blocking agent with rapid onset, a very short duration of action, and no significant intrinsic sympathomimetic or membrane stabilizing activity at therapeutic dosages. Its elimination half-life after intravenous infusion is approximately 9 minutes. BREVIBLOC inhibits the beta$_1$ receptors located chiefly in cardiac muscle, but this preferential effect is not absolute and at higher doses it begins to inhibit beta$_2$ receptors located chiefly in the bronchial and vascular musculature.

Pharmacokinetics and Metabolism
BREVIBLOC (Esmolol Hydrochloride) is rapidly metabolized by hydrolysis of the ester linkage, chiefly by the esterases in the cytosol of red blood cells and not by plasma cholinesterases or red cell membrane acetylcholinesterase. Total body clearance in man was found to be about 20 L/kg/hr, which is greater than cardiac output; thus the metabolism of BREVIBLOC is not limited by the rate of blood flow to metabolizing tissues such as the liver or affected by hepatic or renal blood flow. BREVIBLOC has a rapid distribution half-life of about 2 minutes and an elimination half-life of about 9 minutes.
Using an appropriate loading dose, steady-state blood levels of BREVIBLOC for dosages from 50-300 mcg/kg/min (0.05-0.3 mg/kg/min) are obtained within five minutes. (Steady-state is reached in about 30 minutes without the loading dose.) Steady-state blood levels of BREVIBLOC increase linearly over this dosage range and elimination kinetics are dose-independent over this range. Steady-state blood levels are maintained during infusion but decrease rapidly after termination of the infusion. Because of its short half-life, blood levels of BREVIBLOC can be rapidly altered by increasing or decreasing the infusion rate and rapidly eliminated by discontinuing the infusion.
Consistent with the high rate of blood-based metabolism of BREVIBLOC, less than 2% of the drug is excreted unchanged in the urine. Within 24 hours of the end of infusion, approximately 73-88% of the dosage has been accounted for in the urine as the acid metabolite of BREVIBLOC.
Metabolism of BREVIBLOC results in the formation of the corresponding free acid and methanol. The acid metabolite has been shown in animals to have about 1/1500th the activity of esmolol and in normal volunteers its blood levels do not correspond to the level of beta blockade. The acid metabolite has an elimination half-life of about 3.7 hours and is excreted in the urine with a clearance approximately equivalent to the glomerular filtration rate. Excretion of the acid metabolite is significantly decreased in patients with renal disease, with the elimination half-life increased to about ten-fold that of normals, and plasma levels considerably elevated.
Methanol blood levels, monitored in subjects receiving BREVIBLOC for up to 6 hours at 300 mcg/kg/min (0.3 mg/kg/min) and 24 hours at 150 mcg/kg/min (0.15 mg/kg/min), approximated endogenous levels and were less than 2% of levels usually associated with methanol toxicity.
BREVIBLOC has been shown to be 55% bound to human plasma protein, while the acid metabolite is only 10% bound.

Pharmacodynamics
Clinical pharmacology studies in normal volunteers have confirmed the beta blocking activity of BREVIBLOC (Esmolol Hydrochloride), showing reduction in heart rate at rest and during exercise, and attenuation of isoproterenol-induced increases in heart rate. Blood levels of BREVIBLOC have been shown to correlate with extent of beta blockade. After termination of infusion, substantial recovery from beta blockade is observed in 10-20 minutes.
In human electrophysiology studies, BREVIBLOC produced effects typical of a beta blocker; a decrease in the heart rate, increase in sinus cycle length, prolongation of the sinus node recovery time, prolongation of the AH interval during normal sinus rhythm and during atrial pacing, and an increase in antegrade Wenckebach cycle length.
In patients undergoing radionuclide angiography, BREVIBLOC, at dosages of 200 mcg/kg/min (0.2 mg/kg/min), produced reductions in heart rate, systolic blood pressure, rate pressure product, left and right ventricular ejection fraction and cardiac index at rest, which were similar in magnitude to those produced by intravenous propranolol (4 mg). During exercise, BREVIBLOC produced reductions in heart rate, rate pressure product and cardiac index which were also similar to those produced by propranolol, but produced a significantly larger fall in systolic blood pressure. In patients undergoing cardiac catheterization, the maximum therapeutic dose of 300 mcg/kg/min (0.3 mg/kg/min) of BREVIBLOC produced similar effects and, in addition, there were small, clinically insignificant increases in the left ventricular end diastolic pressure and pulmonary capillary wedge pressure. At thirty minutes after the discontinuation of BREVIBLOC infusion, all of the hemodynamic parameters had returned to pretreatment levels.
The relative cardioselectivity of BREVIBLOC was demonstrated in 10 mildly asthmatic patients. Infusions of BREVIBLOC [100, 200 and 300 mcg/kg/min (0.1, 0.2 and 0.3 mg/kg/min)] produced no significant increases in specific airway resistance compared to placebo. At 300 mcg/kg/min (0.3 mg/kg/min), BREVIBLOC produced slightly enhanced bronchomotor sensitivity to dry air stimulus. These effects were not clinically significant, and BREVIBLOC was well tolerated by all patients. Six of the patients also received intravenous propranolol, and at a dosage of 1 mg, two experienced significant, symptomatic bronchospasm requiring bronchodilator treatment. One other propranolol-treated patient also experienced dry air-induced bronchospasm. No adverse pulmonary effects were observed in patients with COPD who received therapeutic dosages of BREVIBLOC for treatment of supraventricular tachycardia (51 patients) or in perioperative settings (32 patients).

Supraventricular Tachycardia
In two multicenter, randomized, double-blind, controlled comparisons of BREVIBLOC (Esmolol Hydrochloride) with placebo and propranolol, maintenance doses of 50 to 300 mcg/kg/min (0.05 to 0.3 mg/kg/min) of BREVIBLOC were found to be more effective than placebo and about as effective as propranolol, 3-6 mg given by bolus injections, in the treatment of supraventricular tachycardia, principally atrial fibrillation and atrial flutter. The majority of these patients developed their arrhythmias postoperatively. About 60-70% of the patients treated with BREVIBLOC had a desired therapeutic effect (either a 20% reduction in heart rate, a decrease in heart rate to less than 100 bpm, or, rarely, conversion to NSR) and about 95% of those who responded did so at a dosage of 200 mcg/kg/min (0.2 mg/kg/min) or less. The average effective dosage of BREVIBLOC was approximately 100-115 mcg/kg/min (0.1-0.115 mg/kg/min) in the two studies. Other multicenter baseline-controlled studies gave essentially similar results. In the comparison with propranolol, about 50% of patients in both the BREVIBLOC and propranolol groups were on concomitant digoxin. Response rates were slightly higher with both beta blockers in the digoxin-treated patients.
In all studies significant decreases of blood pressure occurred in 20-50% of patients, identified either as adverse reaction reports by investigators, or by observation of systolic pressure less than 90 mmHg or diastolic pressure less than 50 mmHg. The hypotension was symptomatic (mainly diaphoresis or dizziness) in about 12% of patients, and therapy was discontinued in about 11% of patients, about half of whom were symptomatic. In comparison to propranolol, hypotension was about three times as frequent with BREVIBLOC, 53% vs. 17%. The hypotension was rapidly reversible with decreased infusion rate or after discontinuation of therapy with BREVIBLOC. For both BREVIBLOC and propranolol, hypotension was reported less frequently in patients receiving concomitant digoxin.

INDICATIONS AND USAGE

Supraventricular Tachycardia
BREVIBLOC (Esmolol Hydrochloride) is indicated for the rapid control of ventricular rate in patients with atrial fibrillation or atrial flutter in perioperative, postoperative, or other emergent circumstances where short term control of ventricular rate with a short-acting agent is desirable. BREVIBLOC is also indicated in noncompensatory sinus tachycardia where, in the physician's judgment, the rapid heart rate requires specific intervention. BREVIBLOC is not intended for use in chronic settings where transfer to another agent is anticipated.

Intraoperative and Postoperative Tachycardia and/or Hypertension
BREVIBLOC (Esmolol Hydrochloride) is indicated for the treatment of tachycardia and hypertension that occur during induction and tracheal intubation, during surgery, on emergence from anesthesia, and in the postoperative period, when in the physician's judgment such specific intervention is considered indicated.
Use of BREVIBLOC to prevent such events is not recommended.

CONTRAINDICATIONS

BREVIBLOC (Esmolol Hydrochloride) is contraindicated in patients with sinus bradycardia, heart block greater than first degree, cardiogenic shock or overt heart failure (see **WARNINGS**).

WARNINGS

Hypotension: In clinical trials 20-50% of patients treated with BREVIBLOC (Esmolol Hydrochloride) have experienced hypotension, generally defined as systolic pressure less than 90 mmHg and/or diastolic pressure less than 50 mmHg. About 12% of the patients have been symptomatic (mainly diaphoresis or dizziness). Hypotension can occur at any dose but is dose-related so that doses beyond

Continued on next page

Brevibloc—Cont.

200 mcg/kg/min (0.2 mg/kg/min) are not recommended. Patients should be closely monitored, especially if pretreatment blood pressure is low. Decrease of dose or termination of infusion reverses hypotension, usually within 30 minutes.

Cardiac Failure: Sympathetic stimulation is necessary in supporting circulatory function in congestive heart failure, and beta blockade carries the potential hazard of further depressing myocardial contractility and precipitating more severe failure. Continued depression of the myocardium with beta blocking agents over a period of time can, in some cases, lead to cardiac failure. At the first sign or symptom of impending cardiac failure, BREVIBLOC (Esmolol Hydrochloride) should be withdrawn. Although withdrawal may be sufficient because of the short elimination half-life of BREVIBLOC, specific treatment may also be considered (see **OVERDOSAGE**). The use of BREVIBLOC for control of ventricular response in patients with supraventricular arrhythmias should be undertaken with caution when the patient is compromised hemodynamically or is taking other drugs that decrease any or all of the following: peripheral resistance, myocardial filling, myocardial contractility, or electrical impulse propagation in the myocardium. Despite the rapid onset and offset of the effects of BREVIBLOC, several cases of death have been reported in complex clinical states where BREVIBLOC was presumably being used to control ventricular rate.

Intraoperative and Postoperative Tachycardia and/or Hypertension: BREVIBLOC (Esmolol Hydrochloride) should not be used as the treatment for hypertension in patients in whom the increased blood pressure is primarily due to the vasoconstriction associated with hypothermia.

Bronchospastic Diseases: PATIENTS WITH BRONCHOSPASTIC DISEASES SHOULD, IN GENERAL, NOT RECEIVE BETA BLOCKERS. Because of its relative $beta_1$ selectivity and titratability, BREVIBLOC (Esmolol Hydrochloride) may be used with caution in patients with bronchospastic diseases. However, since $beta_1$ selectivity is not absolute, BREVIBLOC should be carefully titrated to obtain the lowest possible effective dose. In the event of bronchospasm, the infusion should be terminated immediately; a $beta_2$ stimulating agent may be administered if conditions warrant but should be used with particular caution as patients already have rapid ventricular rates.

Diabetes Mellitus and Hypoglycemia: BREVIBLOC (Esmolol Hydrochloride) should be used with caution in diabetic patients requiring a beta blocking agent. Beta blockers may mask tachycardia occurring with hypoglycemia, but other manifestations such as dizziness and sweating may not be significantly affected.

PRECAUTIONS

General

Infusion concentrations of 20 mg/mL were associated with more serious venous irritation, including thrombophlebitis, than concentrations of 10 mg/mL with BREVIBLOC CONCENTRATE, extravasation of 20 mg/mL or higher may lead to a serious local reaction and possible skin necrosis. Concentrations greater than 10 mg/mL or infusion into small veins or through a butterfly catheter should be avoided.

Because the acid metabolite of BREVIBLOC is primarily excreted unchanged by the kidney, BREVIBLOC (Esmolol Hydrochloride) should be administered with caution to patients with impaired renal function. The elimination half-life of the acid metabolite was prolonged ten-fold and the plasma level was considerably elevated in patients with end-stage renal disease.

Care should be taken in the intravenous administration of BREVIBLOC CONCENTRATE as sloughing of the skin and necrosis have been reported in association with infiltration and extravasation of intravenous infusions.

Drug Interactions

Catecholamine-depleting drugs, e.g., reserpine, may have an additive effect when given with beta blocking agents. Patients treated concurrently with BREVIBLOC (Esmolol Hydrochloride) and a catecholamine depletor should therefore be closely observed for evidence of hypotension or marked bradycardia, which may result in vertigo, syncope, or postural hypotension.

A study of interaction between BREVIBLOC and warfarin showed that concomitant administration of BREVIBLOC and warfarin does not alter warfarin plasma levels. BREVIBLOC concentrations were equivocally higher when given with warfarin, but this is not likely to be clinically important.

When digoxin and BREVIBLOC were concomitantly administered intravenously to normal volunteers, there was a 10-20% increase in digoxin blood levels at some time points. Digoxin did not affect BREVIBLOC pharmacokinetics. When intravenous morphine and BREVIBLOC were concomitantly administered in normal subjects, no effect on morphine blood levels was seen, but BREVIBLOC steady-state blood levels were increased by 46% in the presence of morphine. No other pharmacokinetic parameters were changed.

The effect of BREVIBLOC on the duration of succinylcholine-induced neuromuscular blockade was studied in patients undergoing surgery. The onset of neuromuscular blockade by succinylcholine was unaffected by BREVIBLOC, but the duration of neuromuscular blockade was prolonged from 5 minutes to 8 minutes.

Although the interactions observed in these studies do not appear to be of major clinical importance, BREVIBLOC should be titrated with caution in patients being treated concurrently with digoxin, morphine, succinylcholine or warfarin.

While taking beta blockers, patients with a history of severe anaphylactic reaction to a variety of allergens may be more reactive to repeated challenge, either accidental, diagnostic, or therapeutic. Such patients may be unresponsive to the usual doses of epinephrine used to treat allergic reaction.

Caution should be exercised when considering the use of BREVIBLOC and verapamil in patients with depressed myocardial function. Fatal cardiac arrests have occurred in patients receiving both drugs. Additionally, BREVIBLOC should not be used to control supraventricular tachycardia in the presence of agents which are vasoconstrictive and inotropic such as dopamine, epinephrine, and norepinephrine because of the danger of blocking cardiac contractility when systemic vascular resistance is high.

Carcinogenesis, Mutagenesis, Impairment of Fertility

Because of its short term usage no carcinogenicity, mutagenicity or reproductive performance studies have been conducted with BREVIBLOC (Esmolol Hydrochloride).

Pregnancy Category C

Teratogenicity studies in rats at intravenous dosages of BREVIBLOC (Esmolol Hydrochloride) up to 3000 mcg/kg/min (3 mg/kg/min) (ten times the maximum human maintenance dosage) for 30 minutes daily produced no evidence of maternal toxicity, embryotoxicity or teratogenicity, while a dosage of 10,000 mcg/kg/min (10 mg/kg/min) produced maternal toxicity and lethality. In rabbits, intravenous dosages up to 1000 mcg/kg/min (1 mg/kg/min) for 30 minutes daily produced no evidence of maternal toxicity, embryotoxicity or teratogenicity, while 2500 mcg/kg/min (2.5 mg/kg/min) produced minimal maternal toxicity and increased fetal resorptions.

Although there are no adequate and well-controlled studies in pregnant women, use of esmolol in the last trimester of pregnancy or during labor or delivery has been reported to cause fetal bradycardia, which continued after termination of drug infusion. BREVIBLOC should be used during pregnancy only if the potential benefit justifies the potential risk to the fetus.

Nursing Mothers

It is not known whether BREVIBLOC (Esmolol Hydrochloride) is excreted in human milk; however, caution should be exercised when BREVIBLOC is administered to a nursing woman.

Pediatric Use

The safety and effectiveness of BREVIBLOC (Esmolol Hydrochloride) in pediatric patients have not been established.

ADVERSE REACTIONS

The following adverse reaction rates are based on use of BREVIBLOC (Esmolol Hydrochloride) in clinical trials involving 369 patients with supraventricular tachycardia and over 600 intraoperative and postoperative patients enrolled in clinical trials. Most adverse effects observed in controlled clinical trial settings have been mild and transient. The most important adverse effect has been hypotension (see **WARNINGS**). Deaths have been reported in post-marketing experience occurring during complex clinical states where BREVIBLOC was presumably being used simply to control ventricular rate (see **WARNINGS**, **Cardiac Failure**).

Cardiovascular—Symptomatic hypotension (diaphoresis, dizziness) occurred in 12% of patients, and therapy was discontinued in about 11%, about half of whom were symptomatic. Asymptomatic hypotension occurred in about 25% of patients. Hypotension resolved during BREVIBLOC (Esmolol Hydrochloride) infusion in 63% of these patients and within 30 minutes after discontinuation of infusion in 80% of the remaining patients. Diaphoresis accompanied hypotension in 10% of patients. Peripheral ischemia occurred in approximately 1% of patients. Pallor, flushing, bradycardia (heart rate less than 50 beats per minute), chest pain, syncope, pulmonary edema and heart block have each been reported in less than 1% of patients. In two patients without supraventricular tachycardia but with serious coronary artery disease (post inferior myocardial infarction or unstable angina), severe bradycardia/sinus pause/asystole has developed, reversible in both cases with discontinuation of treatment.

Central Nervous System—Dizziness has occurred in 3% of patients; somnolence in 3%; confusion, headache, and agitation in about 2%; and fatigue in about 1% of patients. Paresthesia, asthenia, depression, abnormal thinking, anxiety, anorexia, and lightheadedness were reported in less than 1% of patients. Seizures were also reported in less than 1% of patients, with one death.

Respiratory—Bronchospasm, wheezing, dyspnea, nasal congestion, rhonchi, and rales have each been reported in less than 1% of patients.

Gastrointestinal—Nausea was reported in 7% of patients. Vomiting has occurred in about 1% of patients. Dyspepsia, constipation, dry mouth, and abdominal discomfort have each occurred in less than 1% of patients. Taste perversion has also been reported.

Skin (Infusion Site)—Infusion site reactions including inflammation and induration were reported in about 8% of patients. Edema, erythema, skin discoloration, burning at the infusion site, thrombophlebitis, and local skin necrosis from extravasation have each occurred in less than 1% of patients.

Miscellaneous—Each of the following has been reported in less than 1% of patients: Urinary retention, speech disorder, abnormal vision, midscapular pain, rigors, and fever.

OVERDOSAGE

Acute Toxicity

Overdoses of BREVIBLOC (Esmolol Hydrochloride) can cause cardiac arrest. In addition, overdoses can produce bradycardia, hypotension, electromechanical dissociation and loss of consciousness. Cases of massive accidental overdoses of BREVIBLOC have occurred due to dilution errors. Use of BREVIBLOC PREMIXED INJECTION and BREVIBLOC DOUBLE STRENGTH PREMIXED INJECTION may reduce the potential for dilution errors. Some of these overdoses have been fatal while others resulted in permanent disability. Bolus doses in the range of 625 mg to 2.5 g (12.5-50 mg/kg) have been fatal. Patients have recovered completely from overdoses as high as 1.75 g given over one minute or doses of 7.5 g given over one hour for cardiovascular surgery. The patients who survived appear to be those whose circulation could be supported until the effects of BREVIBLOC resolved.

Because of its approximately 9-minute elimination half-life, the first step in the management of toxicity should be to discontinue the BREVIBLOC infusion. Then, based on the observed clinical effects, the following general measures should also be considered.

Bradycardia: Intravenous administration of atropine or another anticholinergic drug.

Bronchospasm: Intravenous administration of a $beta_2$ stimulating agent and/or a theophylline derivative.

Cardiac Failure: Intravenous administration of a diuretic and/or digitalis glycoside. In shock resulting from inadequate cardiac contractility, intravenous administration of dopamine, dobutamine, isoproterenol, or amrinone may be considered.

Symptomatic Hypotension: Intravenous administration of fluids and/or pressor agents.

DOSAGE AND ADMINISTRATION

Dosing Information:

SUPRAVENTRICULAR TACHYCARDIA

Dosage needs to be titrated, using ventricular rate as the guide.

An initial loading dose of 0.5 milligrams/kg (500 micrograms/kg) infused over a minute duration followed by a maintenance infusion of 0.05 milligrams/kg/min (50 micrograms/kg/min) for the next 4 minutes is recommended. This should give a rough guide with respect to the responsiveness of ventricular rate.

After the 4 minutes of initial maintenance infusion (total treatment duration being 5 minutes), depending upon the desired ventricular response, the maintenance infusion may be continued at 0.05 mg/kg/min or increased step-wise (e.g. 0.1 mg/kg/min, 0.15 mg/kg/min to a maximum of 0.2 mg/kg/min) with each step being maintained for 4 or more minutes.

If more rapid slowing of ventricular response is imperative, the 0.5 mg/kg loading dose infused over a 1 minute period may be repeated, followed by a maintenance infusion of 0.1 mg/kg/min for 4 minutes. Then, depending upon ventricular rate, another (and final) loading dose of 0.5 mg/kg/min infused over a 1 minute period may be administered followed by a maintenance infusion of 0.15 mg/kg/min. If needed, after 4 minutes of the 0.15 mg/kg/min maintenance infusion, the maintenance infusion may be increased to a maximum of 0.2 mg/kg/min.

In the absence of loading doses, constant infusion of a single concentration of esmolol reaches pharmacokinetic and pharmacodynamic steady-state in about 30 minutes. Maintenance infusions (with or without loading doses) may be continued for as long as 24 hours.

The following table summarizes the above and assumes that 3 loading doses (the maximum recommended) are infused over 1 minute and incremental maintenance doses are required after each loading dose. There should be no 4th loading dose, but the maintenance dose may be incremented one more time.

[See table at bottom of next page]

In the treatment of supraventricular tachycardia, responses to BREVIBLOC (Esmolol Hydrochloride) usually (over 95%) occur within the range of 50 to 200 micrograms/kg/min (0.05 to 0.2 milligrams/kg/min). The average effective dosage is approximately 100 micrograms/kg/min (0.1 milligrams/kg/min) although dosages as low as 25 micrograms/kg/min (0.025 milligrams/ kg/min) have been adequate in some patients. Dosages as high as 300 micrograms/kg/min (0.3 milligrams/kg/min) have been used, but these provide little added effect and increase the rate of adverse effects, so doses greater than 200 micrograms/kg/min are not recommended. Dosage of BREVIBLOC in supraventricular tachycardia must be individualized by titration in which each step consists of a loading dosage followed by a maintenance dosage.

This specific dosage regimen has not been studied intraoperatively and, because of the time required for titration, may not be optimal for intraoperative use.

The safety of dosages above 300 mcg/kg/min (0.3 mg/kg/min) has not been studied.

In the event of an adverse reaction, the dosage of BREVIBLOC may be reduced or discontinued. If a local infusion site reaction develops, an alternate infusion site should be used and caution should be taken to prevent extravasation. The use of butterfly needles should be avoided.

Abrupt cessation of BREVIBLOC in patients has not been reported to produce the withdrawal effects which may occur with abrupt withdrawal of beta blockers following chronic use in coronary artery disease (CAD) patients. However, caution should still be used in abruptly discontinuing infusions of BREVIBLOC in CAD patients.

After achieving an adequate control of the heart rate and a stable clinical status in patients with supraventricular tachycardia, transition to alternative antiarrhythmic agents such as propranolol, digoxin, or verapamil, may be accomplished.

A recommended guideline for such a transition is given below but the physician should carefully consider the labeling instructions for the alternative agent selected.

Alternative Agent	Dosage
Propranolol hydrochloride	10-20 mg q 4-6 hrs
Digoxin	0.125-0.5 mg q 6 hrs (p.o. or i.v.)
Verapamil	80 mg q 6 hrs

The dosage of BREVIBLOC (Esmolol Hydrochloride) should be reduced as follows:

1. Thirty minutes following the first dose of the alternative agent, reduce the infusion rate of BREVIBLOC by one-half (50%).
2. Following the second dose of the alternative agent, monitor the patient's response and if satisfactory control is maintained for the first hour, discontinue BREVIBLOC.

The use of infusions of BREVIBLOC up to 24 hours has been well documented; in addition, limited data from 24-48 hrs (N=48) indicate that BREVIBLOC is well tolerated up to 48 hours.

INTRAOPERATIVE AND POSTOPERATIVE TACHYCARDIA AND/OR HYPERTENSION

In the intraoperative and postoperative settings it is not always advisable to slowly titrate the dose of BREVIBLOC (Esmolol Hydrochloride) to a therapeutic effect. Therefore, two dosing options are presented: immediate control dosing and a gradual control when the physician has time to titrate.

1. Immediate Control
   For intraoperative treatment of tachycardia and/or hypertension give an 80 mg (approximately 1 mg/kg) bolus dose over 30 seconds followed by a 150 mcg/kg/min infusion, if necessary. Adjust the infusion rate as required up to 300 mcg/kg/min to maintain desired heart rate and/or blood pressure.
2. Gradual Control
   For postoperative tachycardia and hypertension, the dosing schedule is the same as that used in supraventricular tachycardia. To initiate treatment, administer a loading dosage infusion of 500 mcg/kg/min of BREVIBLOC for one minute followed by a four-minute maintenance infusion of 50 mcg/kg/min. If an adequate therapeutic effect is not observed within five minutes, repeat the same loading dosage and follow with a maintenance infusion increased to 100 mcg/kg/min (see above SUPRAVENTRICULAR TACHYCARDIA).

Notes:

1. Higher dosages (250-300 mcg/kg/min) may be required for adequate control of blood pressure than those required for the treatment of atrial fibrillation, flutter and sinus tachycardia. One third of the postoperative hypertensive patients required these higher doses.
2. Parenteral drug products should be inspected visually for particulate matter and discoloration prior to administration, whenever solution and container permit.

Directions for Use of Brevibloc Premixed Injection (10 mg/mL) and Brevibloc DOUBLE STRENGTH Premixed Injection (20 mg/mL)

This dosage form is prediluted to 100 or 250 mL to provide a ready-to-use, iso-osmotic solution of either 20 or 10 mg/mL esmolol hydrochloride in sodium chloride. It is important not to introduce additives to BREVIBLOC PREMIXED INJECTION or BREVIBLOC DOUBLE STRENGTH PREMIXED INJECTION. See **Directions for Use of the Premixed Bag** for additional information.

Directions for Use of the Premixed Bag

Brevibloc Premixed Injection (10 mg/mL) 250 mL IntraVia Bag

Brevibloc DOUBLE STRENGTH Premixed Injection (20 mg/mL) 100 mL IntraVia Bag

BREVIBLOC PREMIXED INJECTION (10 mg/mL) and BREVIBLOC DOUBLE STRENGTH PREMIXED INJECTION (20 mg/mL) are provided in ready-to-use, non-latex, non-PVC bags with two PVC ports, a medication port and a delivery port. **The medication port is to be used solely for withdrawing an initial bolus from the bag; the medication withdrawal port is not intended for repeat bolus administration. The sterility of the premixed bag cannot be assured after repeat withdrawals from the bag. The use of aseptic technique is required when withdrawing the bolus dose. Do not add any additional medications to BREVIBLOC PREMIXED INJECTION.** Each bag is for single-patient use only and contains no preservative. It is advised that once drug has been withdrawn from BREVIBLOC PREMIXED INJECTION, the bag should be used within 24 hours, with any unused portion discarded.

The Brevibloc Premixed Injection contains Esmolol Hydrochloride at a concentration of 10 milligrams/mL. When using a 10 milligrams/mL concentration, a loading dose of 0.5 milligrams/kg infused over 1 minute period of time, for a 70 kg patient, is 3.5 mL. The loading dose can be removed from the medication port of the premixed bag.

The Brevibloc DOUBLE STRENGTH Premixed Injection contains Esmolol Hydrochloride at a concentration of 20 milligrams/mL. When using a 20 milligrams/mL concentration, a loading dose of 0.5 milligrams/kg infused over 1 minute period of time, for a 70 kg patient, is 1.75 mL. The loading dose can be removed from the medication port of the premixed bag.

Figure 1. Two-Port IntraVia Bag

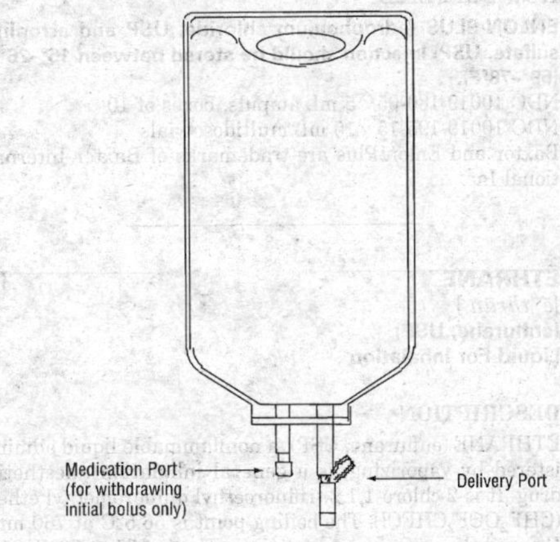

CAUTION

Do not use plastic containers in series connections. Such use could result in an embolism due to residual air being drawn from the primary container before administration of the fluid from the secondary container is completed.

TO OPEN

Do not remove unit from overwrap until ready to use. Do not use if overwrap has been previously opened or damaged. The overwrap is a moisture barrier. The inner bag maintains sterility of the solution.

Tear overwrap at notch and remove premixed bag. Some opacity of the plastic due to moisture absorption during the sterilization process may be observed. This is normal and does not affect the solution quality or safety. The opacity will diminish gradually.

Check for minute leaks by squeezing the inner bag firmly. If leaks are found, discard solution as sterility may be impaired. Do not use unless the solution is clear, colorless to light yellow, and the seal is intact.

Fill out the patient information label supplied and apply to the inner bag.

Elapsed Time (minutes)	Loading Dose (over 1 minute) micrograms/kg/min	Loading Dose (over 1 minute) milligrams/kg/min	Maintenance Dose (over 4 minutes) micrograms/kg/min	Maintenance Dose (over 4 minutes) milligrams/kg/min
0-1	500	0.5		
1-5			50	0.05
5-6	500	0.5		
6-10			100	0.1
10-11	500	0.5		
11-15			150	0.15
15-16	•	•		
16-20			*200	*0.2
>20			Maintenance dose titrated to heart rate or other clinical endpoint.	

*As the desired heart rate or endpoint is approached, the loading infusion may be omitted and the maintenance infusion titrated to 300 mcg/kg/min (0.3 mg/kg/min) or downward as appropriate. Maintenance dosages above 200 mcg/kg/min (0.2 mg/kg/min) have not been shown to have significantly increased benefits. The interval between titration steps may be increased.

Do not introduce additives to BREVIBLOC PREMIXED INJECTION or BREVIBLOC DOUBLE STRENGTH PREMIXED INJECTION.

PREPARATION FOR INTRAVENOUS ADMINISTRATION (use aseptic technique)

1. Suspend premixed bag from eyelet support.
2. Remove plastic protector from delivery port at bottom of bag.
3. Attach administration set. Refer to complete directions accompanying set.

Directions for Use of the Ready-to-use Vials

Brevibloc Injection (10 mg/mL) 10 mL Ready-to-use Vial

Brevibloc DOUBLE STRENGTH Injection (20 mg/mL) 5 mL Ready-to-use Vial

This dosage form is prediluted to provide a ready-to-use, iso-osmotic solution of either 10 or 20 mg/mL esmolol hydrochloride in sodium chloride recommended for BREVIBLOC intravenous administration. It may be used to administer the appropriate BREVIBLOC (Esmolol Hydrochloride) loading dosage infusions by hand-held syringe while the maintenance infusion is being prepared.

The 10 mL Ready-to-use Vial contains Esmolol Hydrochloride at a concentration of 10 milligrams/mL. When using a 10 milligrams/mL concentration, a loading dose of 0.5 mg/kg infused over 1 minute period of time, for a 70 kg patient is 3.5 mL.

The 5 mL DOUBLE STRENGTH Ready-to-use Vial contains Esmolol Hydrochloride at a concentration of 20 milligrams/mL. When using a 20 milligrams/mL concentration, a loading dose of 0.5 mg/kg infused over 1 minute period of time, for a 70 kg patient is 1.75 mL.

Directions for Use of the Brevibloc Concentrate 10 mL Ampul (250 milligrams/mL)

THE 2500 mg AMPUL IS NOT FOR DIRECT INTRAVENOUS INJECTION. THIS DOSAGE FORM IS A CONCENTRATED, POTENT DRUG WHICH MUST BE DILUTED PRIOR TO ITS INFUSION. BREVIBLOC SHOULD NOT BE ADMIXED WITH SODIUM BICARBONATE. BREVIBLOC SHOULD NOT BE MIXED WITH OTHER DRUGS PRIOR TO DILUTION IN A SUITABLE INTRAVENOUS FLUID. (See Compatibility Section below.)

Dilution: Aseptically prepare a 10 mg/mL infusion by adding two 2500 mg ampuls to a 500 mL container or one 2500 mg ampul to a 250 mL container of a compatible intravenous solution listed below. (Remove overage prior to dilution as appropriate.) This yields a final concentration of 10 mg/mL. The diluted solution is stable for at least 24 hours at room temperature. Note: The use of esmolol with propylene glycol has been associated with a higher incidence of venous irritation at concentrations greater than 10 mg/mL on continued infusion. Mixed from the ampul at concentrations of greater than 10 mg/mL BREVIBLOC has, however, been well tolerated when administered *via* a central vein.

Compatibility with Commonly Used Intravenous Fluids

BREVIBLOC was tested for compatibility with ten commonly used intravenous fluids at a final concentration of 10 mg Esmolol Hydrochloride per mL. BREVIBLOC was found to be compatible with the following solutions and was stable for at least 24 hours at controlled room temperature or under refrigeration:

Dextrose (5%) Injection, USP
Dextrose (5%) in Lactated Ringer's Injection
Dextrose (5%) in Ringer's Injection
Dextrose (5%) and Sodium Chloride (0.45%) Injection, USP
Dextrose (5%) and Sodium Chloride (0.9%) Injection, USP
Lactated Ringer's Injection, USP
Potassium Chloride (40 mEq/liter) in Dextrose (5%) Injection, USP
Sodium Chloride (0.45%) Injection, USP
Sodium Chloride (0.9%) Injection, USP

BREVIBLOC is NOT compatible with Sodium Bicarbonate (5%) Injection, USP.

HOW SUPPLIED

BREVIBLOC PREMIXED INJECTION
NDC 10019-055-61, 2500 mg - 250 mL in Ready-to-use 250 mL IntraVia Bags
BREVIBLOC DOUBLE STRENGTH PREMIXED INJECTION
NDC 10019-075-87, 2000 mg - 100 mL in Ready-to-use 100 mL IntraVia Bags
BREVIBLOC INJECTION
NDC 10019-115-01, 100 mg - 10 mL Ready-to-use Vials, Package of 25
BREVIBLOC DOUBLE STRENGTH INJECTION
NDC 10019-085-01, 100 mg - 5 mL Ready-to-use Vials, Package of 10
BREVIBLOC CONCENTRATE
NDC 10019-025-18, 2500 mg - 10 mL Ampuls for Dilution, Package of 10

Store at 25° C (77°F). Excursions permitted to 15°-30°C (59°-86°F). [See USP Controlled Room Temperature.] PROTECT FROM FREEZING. Avoid excessive heat.

Baxter
Manufactured for
Baxter Healthcare Corporation
Deerfield, IL 60015 USA
BREVIBLOC INJECTION, BREVIBLOC DOUBLE STRENGTH INJECTION, and BREVIBLOC CONCENTRATE manufactured by Faulding Puerto Rico, Inc.
P.O. Box 471 Aguadilla, PR 00604 USA

Continued on next page

Brevibloc—Cont.

BREVIBLOC PREMIXED INJECTION and BREVIBLOC DOUBLE STRENGTH PREMIXED INJECTION manufactured by Baxter Healthcare Corporation
Deerfield, IL 60015 USA
Baxter, Brevibloc, Brevibloc Premixed and IntraVia are trademarks of Baxter International Inc. Brevibloc (esmolol hydrochloride) and its packaging are protected by one or more of the following: U.S. Pat. Nos. 5,017,609; 5,849,843; 5,998,019; 6,310,094; 6,528,540; Pat. Pending.
For Product Inquiry 1 800 ANA DRUG
(1-800-262-3784)
Revised: June 2003 460-278-03

DOPRAM INJECTION ℞

[dō 'prăm]
(Doxapram Hydrochloride Injection, USP)
NOT FOR USE IN NEONATES
CONTAINS BENZYL ALCOHOL

DESCRIPTION

DOPRAM Injection (Doxapram Hydrochloride Injection, USP) is a clear, colorless, sterile, non-pyrogenic, aqueous solution with pH 3.5 to 5.0, for intravenous administration.
Each 1 mL contains:

Doxapram Hydrochloride, USP	20 mg
Benzyl Alcohol, NF (as preservative)	0.9%
Water for Injection, USP	q.s.

Doxapram Injection is a respiratory stimulant.
Doxapram hydrochloride is a white to off-white, crystalline powder, sparingly soluble in water, alcohol and chloroform. Chemically, doxapram hydrochloride is 1-ethyl-4-[2-(4-morpholinyl)ethyl]-3,3-diphenyl-2-pyrrolidinone monohydrochloride, monohydrate.

HOW SUPPLIED

DOPRAM Injection (Doxapram Hydrochloride Injection, USP) containing 20 mg of doxapram hydrochloride per mL with benzyl alcohol 0.9% as the preservative is available in: 20 mL multiple dose vials in packages of 6 (NDC 60977-144-02).
CONTAINS BENZYL ALCOHOL.
The vial stopper in this product contains dry natural rubber (latex).
Store at 20°–25°C (68°–77°F), excursions permitted to 15°–30°C (59°–86°F) [see USP Controlled Room Temperature].
DOPRAM is a trademark of Baxter International Inc., or its subsidiaries.
Baxter Healthcare Corporation
Deerfield, IL 60015 USA

ENLON ℞

[ĕn 'lon]
(edrophonium chloride injection, USP)

DESCRIPTION

ENLON is a short and rapid-acting cholinergic drug. Chemically, edrophonium chloride is ethyl(m-hydroxyphenyl) dimethylammonium chloride and its structural formula is:

Each mL contains, in a sterile solution, 10 mg edrophonium chloride compounded with 0.45% phenol as a preservative, and 0.2% sodium sulfite as an antioxidant, buffered with sodium citrate and citric acid, and pH adjusted to approximately 5.4.
ENLON is intended for IV and IM use.

HOW SUPPLIED

ENLON (edrophonium chloride injection, USP):
NDC 10019-873-15 15 mL vials
ENLON (edrophonium chloride injection, USP) should be stored at controlled room temperature 15°–30°C (59°–86°F).
Baxter and Enlon are trademarks of Baxter International Inc.

ENLON-PLUS ℞

[ĕn '-lon ' plus]
(edrophonium chloride, USP and atropine sulfate, USP) Injection

DESCRIPTION

ENLON-PLUS (edrophonium chloride, USP and atropine sulfate, USP) Injection, for intravenous use, is a sterile, nonpyrogenic, nondepolarizing neuromuscular relaxant antagonist. ENLON-PLUS is a combination drug containing a rapid acting acetylcholinesterase inhibitor, edrophonium chloride, and an anticholinergic, atropine sulfate. Chemically, edrophonium chloride is ethyl (m-hydroxyphenyl) dimethylammonium chloride; its structural formula is:

Molecular Formula: $C_{10}H_{16}ClNO$
Molecular Weight: 201.70
Chemically, atropine sulfate is:
endo-(±)-alpha-(hydroxymethyl)-8-methyl-8-azabicyclo [3.2.1]oct-3-yl benzeneacetate sulfate (2:1) monohydrate. Its structural formula is:

Molecular Formula: $(C_{17}H_{23}NO_3)_2.H_2SO_4.H_2O$
Molecular Weight: 694.84
ENLON-PLUS contains in each mL of sterile solution:
5 mL Ampuls: 10 mg edrophonium chloride and 0.14 mg atropine sulfate compounded with 2.0 mg sodium sulfite as a preservative and buffered with sodium citrate and citric acid. The pH range is 4.0–5.0.
15 mL Multidose Vials: 10 mg edrophonium chloride and 0.14 mg atropine sulfate compounded with 2.0 mg sodium sulfite and 4.5 mg phenol as a preservative and buffered with sodium citrate and citric acid. The pH range is 4.0–5.0.

HOW SUPPLIED

ENLON-PLUS (edrophonium chloride, USP and atropine sulfate, USP) Injection should be stored between 15°–26°C (59°–78°F).
NDC 10019-180-05 5 mL ampuls, boxes of 10
NDC 10019-195-15 15 mL multidose vials
Baxter and Enlon-Plus are trademarks of Baxter International Inc.

ĒTHRANE ℞

[ē 'thrān]
(enflurane, USP)
Liquid For Inhalation

DESCRIPTION

ĒTHRANE (enflurane, USP), a nonflammable liquid administered by vaporizing, is a general inhalation anesthetic drug. It is 2-chloro-1,1,2-trifluoroethyl difluoromethyl ether (CHF_2OCF_2CHFCl). The boiling point is 56.5°C at 760 mm Hg, and the vapor pressure (in mm Hg) is 175 at 20°C, 218 at 25°C, and 345 at 36°C. Vapor pressures can be calculated using the equation:

$$\log_{10}P_{vap} = A + \frac{B}{T} \qquad A = 7.967,\ B = -1678.4,\ T = °C + 273.16\ (\text{Kelvin})$$

The specific gravity (25°/25°C) is 1.517. The refractive index at 20°C is 1.3026–1.3030. The blood/gas coefficient is 1.91 at 37°C and the oil/gas coefficient is 98.5 at 37°C.
Enflurane is a clear, colorless, stable liquid whose purity exceeds 99.9% (area percent by gas chromatography). No stabilizers are added as these have been found, through controlled laboratory tests, to be unnecessary even in the presence of ultraviolet light. Enflurane is stable to strong base, does not decompose in contact with soda lime (at normal operating temperatures), and does not react with aluminum, tin, brass, iron or copper. The partition coefficients of enflurane at 25°C are 74 in conductive rubber and 120 in polyvinyl chloride.

HOW SUPPLIED

ĒTHRANE (enflurane, USP) is packaged in 125 and 250 mL amber-colored bottles.
125 mL—NDC 10019-350-50
250 mL—NDC 10019-350-60
Storage: Store at room temperature 15°–30°C (59°–86°F).
Enflurane contains no additives and has been demonstrated to be stable at room temperature for periods in excess of five years.
Baxter and ĒTHRANE (enflurane, USP) are trademarks of Baxter International Inc. registered in the United States Patent and Trademark Office.

FORANE® ℞

[for 'ān]
(isoflurane, USP)
Liquid For Inhalation

DESCRIPTION

FORANE® (isoflurane, USP), a nonflammable liquid administered by vaporizing, is a general inhalation anesthetic drug. It is 1-chloro-2,2,2-trifluoroethyl difluoromethyl ether, and its structural formula is:

Some physical constants are:

Molecular weight		184.5
Boiling point at 760 mm Hg		48.5 °C (uncorr.)
Refractive index n_D^{20}		1.2990–1.3005
Specific gravity 25°/25°C		1.496
Vapor pressure in mm Hg**	20°C	238
	25°C	295
	30°C	367
	35°C	450

**Equation for vapor pressure calculation:

$$\log_{10}P_{vap} = A + \frac{B}{T} \quad \text{where:} \quad A = 8.056,\ B = -1664.58,\ T = °C + 273.16\ (\text{Kelvin})$$

Partition coefficients at 37°C	
Water/gas	0.61
Blood/gas	1.43
Oil/gas	90.8
Partition coefficients at 25°C—rubber and plastic	
Conductive rubber/gas	62.0
Butyl rubber/gas	75.0
Polyvinyl chloride/gas	110.0
Polyethylene/gas	~2.0
Polyurethane/gas	~1.4
Polyolefin/gas	~1.1
Butyl acetate/gas	~2.5
Purity by gas chromatography	>99.9%
Lower limit of flammability in oxygen or nitrous oxide at 9 joules/sec. and 23°C	None
Lower limit of flammability in oxygen or nitrous oxide at 900 joules/sec. and 23°C	Greater than useful concentration in anesthesia.

Isoflurane is a clear, colorless, stable liquid containing no additives or chemical stabilizers. Isoflurane has a mildly pungent, musty, ethereal odor. Samples stored in indirect sunlight in clear, colorless glass for five years, as well as samples directly exposed for 30 hours to a 2 amp, 115 volt, 60 cycle long wave U.V. light were unchanged in composition as determined by gas chromatography. Isoflurane in one normal sodium methoxide-methanol solution, a strong base, for over six months consumed essentially no alkali, indicative of strong base stability. Isoflurane does not decompose in the presence of soda lime (at normal operating temperatures), and does not attack aluminum, tin, brass, iron or copper.

HOW SUPPLIED

FORANE® (isoflurane, USP) is packaged in 100 mL and 250 mL amber-colored bottles.
100 mL – NDC 10019-360-40
250 mL – NDC 10019-360-60
Storage: Store at room temperature 15°–30° C (59°–86° F).
Isoflurane contains no additives and has been demonstrated to be stable at room temperature for periods in excess of five years.

PHENERGAN ℞

[fĕn 'ĕr-găn]
(promethazine HCl)
INJECTION

DESCRIPTION

PHENERGAN (promethazine HCl) Injection, is a sterile, pyrogen-free solution for deep intramuscular or intravenous administration. Promethazine HCl (10*H*-phenothiazine-10-ethanamine, *N,N*,α-trimethyl-, monohydrochloride, (±)-) is a racemic compound and has the following structural formula:

$C_{17}H_{21}ClN_2S$ MW=320.88

Each mL of ampul contains either 25 mg or 50 mg promethazine HCl with 0.1 mg edetate disodium, 0.04 mg calcium chloride, 0.25 mg sodium metabisulfite, and 5 mg phenol in Water for Injection. The pH range is 4.0 to 5.5, buffered with acetic acid-sodium acetate, and it is sealed under nitrogen. PHENERGAN (promethazine HCl) Injection is a clear, colorless solution. The product is light sensitive. It should be inspected before use and discarded if either color or particulate is observed.

HOW SUPPLIED

PHENERGAN (promethazine HCl) Injection is available in 1 mL ampuls, in packages of 25 ampuls, as follows:
25 mg per mL, NDC 60977-001-01
50 mg per mL, NDC 60977-002-02

Store at 20°–25°C (68°–77°F), excursions permitted to 15°–30°C (59°–86°F) [see USP Controlled Room Temperature].
Protect from light. Keep covered in carton until time of use.
Do not use if solution has developed color or contains a precipitate.
PHENERGAN is a registered trademark of Wyeth and used under license.
Baxter Healthcare Corporation
Deerfield, IL 60015 USA

PROPOFOL ℞
Injectable Emulsion 1%
10 mg/mL propofol
Contains a Sulfite
For IV Administration

DESCRIPTION
Propofol injectable emulsion is a sterile, nonpyrogenic emulsion containing 10 mg/mL of propofol suitable for intravenous administration. Propofol is chemically described as 2, 6-diisopropylphenol and has a molecular weight of 178.27. The structural and molecular formulas are:

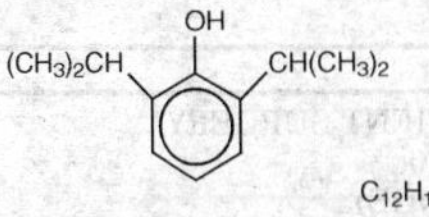

OH (CH3)2CH CH(CH3)2

$C_{12}H_{18}O$

Propofol is very slightly soluble in water and, thus, is formulated in a white, oil-in-water emulsion. The pK_a is 11. The octanol/water partition coefficient for propofol is 6761:1 at a pH of 6-8.5. In addition to the active component, propofol, the formulation also contains soybean oil (100 mg/mL), glycerol (22.5 mg/mL), egg yolk phospholipid (12 mg/mL), and sodium metabisulfite (0.25 mg/mL); with sodium hydroxide to adjust pH. The propofol injectable emulsion is isotonic and has a pH of 4.5-6.4.

STRICT ASEPTIC TECHNIQUE MUST ALWAYS BE MAINTAINED DURING HANDLING. PROPOFOL INJECTABLE EMULSION IS A SINGLE-USE PARENTERAL PRODUCT WHICH CONTAINS SODIUM METABISULFITE (0.25 MG/ML) TO RETARD THE RATE OF GROWTH OF MICROORGANISMS IN THE EVENT OF ACCIDENTAL EXTRINSIC CONTAMINATION. HOWEVER, PROPOFOL INJECTABLE EMULSION CAN STILL SUPPORT THE GROWTH OF MICROORGANISMS AS IT IS NOT AN ANTIMICROBIALLY PRESERVED PRODUCT UNDER USP STANDARDS. ACCORDINGLY, STRICT ASEPTIC TECHNIQUE MUST STILL BE ADHERED TO. DO NOT USE IF CONTAMINATION IS SUSPECTED. DISCARD UNUSED PORTIONS AS DIRECTED WITHIN THE REQUIRED TIME LIMITS (SEE DOSAGE AND ADMINISTRATION, HANDLING PROCEDURES IN FULL PRESCRIBING INFORMATION). THERE HAVE BEEN REPORTS IN WHICH FAILURE TO USE ASEPTIC TECHNIQUE WHEN HANDLING PROPOFOL INJECTABLE EMULSION WAS ASSOCIATED WITH MICROBIAL CONTAMINATION OF THE PRODUCT AND WITH FEVER, INFECTION/SEPSIS, OTHER LIFE-THREATENING ILLNESS, AND/OR DEATH.

HOW SUPPLIED
Propofol injectable emulsion is available in ready-to-use 10 mL vials, 20 mL vials, 50 mL infusion vials, and 100 mL infusion vials containing 10 mg/mL of propofol.

NDC Number	Propofol	Available Packaging
10019-013-06	10 mL vial	10 vials/shelf tray
10019-013-01	20 mL vial	25 vials/shelf tray
10019-013-02	50 mL infusion vial	20 vials/shelf tray
10019-013-03	100 mL infusion vial	10 vials/shelf tray

Propofol undergoes oxidative degradation in the presence of oxygen, and is, therefore, packaged under nitrogen to eliminate this degradation path.
Store between 4°–22°C (40°–72°F). Do not freeze. Shake well before use.

PROTOPAM CHLORIDE ℞
(pralidoxime chloride) for Injection

DESCRIPTION
Chemical name: 2-formyl-1-methylpyridinium chloride oxime. Available in the United States as PROTOPAM Chloride, pralidoxime chloride is frequently referred to as 2-PAM Chloride.
Structural formula:

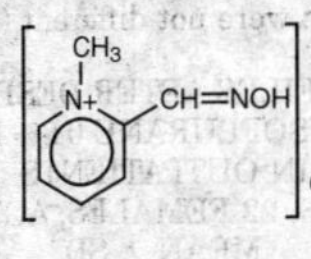

$C_7H_9ClN_2O$ CH3 N+ CH=NOH Cl⁻ M.W. 172.61

Pralidoxime chloride occurs as an odorless, white, nonhygroscopic, crystalline powder which is soluble in water. Stable in air, it melts between 215° and 225°C, with decomposition.
The specific activity of the drug resides in the 2-formyl-1-methylpyridinium ion and is independent of the particular salt employed. The chloride is preferred because of physiologic compatibility, excellent water solubility at all temperatures, and high potency per gram, due to its low (173) molecular weight.
Pralidoxime chloride is a cholinesterase reactivator.
PROTOPAM Chloride for intravenous injection or infusion is prepared by cryodesiccation. Each vial contains 1 g of sterile pralidoxime chloride, and NaOH to adjust pH, to be reconstituted with 20 mL of Sterile Water for Injection, USP. The pH of the reconstituted solution is 3.5 to 4.5. Intramuscular or subcutaneous injection may be used when intravenous injection is not feasible.

HOW SUPPLIED
NDC 60977-141-01—*Hospital Package:* This contains six 20 mL vials of 1 g each of sterile PROTOPAM Chloride (pralidoxime chloride) white to off-white porous cake*, without diluent or syringe. Solution may be prepared by adding 20 mL of Sterile Water for Injection, USP. These are single-dose vials for intravenous injection or for intravenous infusion after further dilution with physiologic saline. Intramuscular or subcutaneous injection may be used when intravenous injection is not feasible.

*When necessary, sodium hydroxide is added during processing to adjust the pH.

Store at 20°–25°C (68°–77°F), excursions permitted to 15°–30°C (59°–86°F) [see USP Controlled Room Temperature].
Baxter and Protopam are trademarks of Baxter International Inc., or it subsidiaries.
Baxter Healthcare Corporation
Deerfield, IL 60015 USA

REVEX ℞
[*Rē-vĕx*]
(nalmefene hydrochloride injection)

DESCRIPTION
REVEX (nalmefene hydrochloride injection), an opioid antagonist, is a 6-methylene analogue of naltrexone. The chemical structure is shown below:

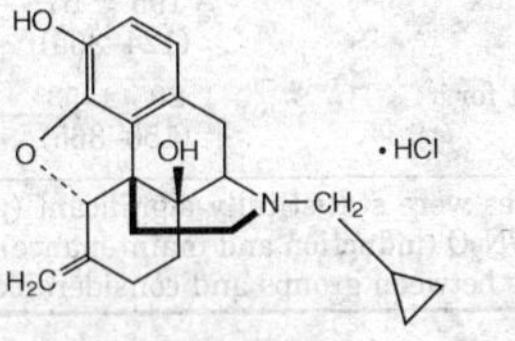

HO O OH N–CH2 H2C • HCl

Molecular Formula: $C_{21}H_{25}NO_3$•HCl
Molecular Weight: 375.9, CAS # 58895-64-0
Chemical Name: 17-(Cyclopropylmethyl)-4,5α-epoxy-6-methylenemorphinan-3,14-diol, hydrochloride salt.
Nalmefene hydrochloride is a white to off-white crystalline powder which is freely soluble in water up to 130 mg/mL and slightly soluble in chloroform up to 0.13 mg/mL, with a pK_a of 7.6.
REVEX is available as a sterile solution for intravenous, intramuscular, and subcutaneous administration in two concentrations, containing 100 µg or 1.0 mg of nalmefene free base per mL. The 100 µg/mL concentration contains 110.8 µg of nalmefene hydrochloride and the 1.0 mg/mL concentration contains 1.108 mg of nalmefene hydrochloride per mL. Both concentrations contain 9.0 mg of sodium chloride per mL and the pH is adjusted to 3.9 with hydrochloric acid.
Concentrations and dosages of REVEX are expressed as the free base equivalent of nalmefene.

HOW SUPPLIED
REVEX (nalmefene hydrochloride injection) is available in the following presentations:
An ampul containing 1 mL of 100 µg/mL nalmefene base (Blue Label) Box of 10 (NDC 10019-315-21)
An ampul containing 2 mL of 1 mg/mL nalmefene base (Green Label) Box of 10 (NDC 10019-311-22)
Store at controlled room temperature.
REVEX is a registered trademark of Ivax Laboratories, Inc.

ROBAXIN INJECTABLE ℞
[*rō 'băks-ĭn*]
(methocarbamol injection, USP)

DESCRIPTION
Robaxin (methocarbamol injection, USP) Injectable, a carbamate derivative of guaifenesin, is a central nervous system (CNS) depressant with sedative and musculoskeletal relaxant properties. It is a sterile, pyrogen-free solution intended for intramuscular or intravenous administration.
Each mL contains: methocarbamol, USP 100 mg, polyethylene glycol 300, NF 0.5 mL, Water for Injection, USP q.s. The pH is adjusted, when necessary, with hydrochloric acid and/or sodium hydroxide. The chemical name of methocarbamol is 3-(2-methoxyphenoxy)-1,2-propanediol 1-carbamate and has the empirical formula of $C_{11}H_{15}NO_5$. Its molecular weight is 241.24. The structural formula is shown below:

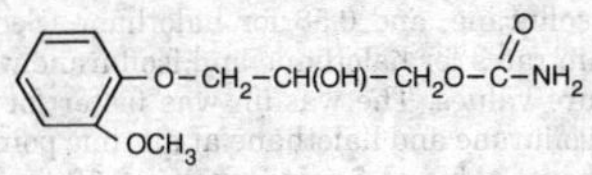

O–CH2–CH(OH)–CH2O–C(=O)–NH2 OCH3

Methocarbamol is a white powder, sparingly soluble in water and chloroform, soluble in alcohol (only with heating) and propylene glycol, and insoluble in benzene and *n*-hexane.
ROBAXIN Injectable has a pH between 3.5 and 6.0.
AFTER MIXING WITH I.V. INFUSION FLUIDS, **DO NOT REFRIGERATE.**

HOW SUPPLIED
ROBAXIN Injectable (100 mg/mL) supplied in – 10 mL single dose vials in packages of 25 (NDC 60977-150-01). Each 10 mL vial contains a total of 1 gram methocarbamol.
Store at 20°-25°C (68°-77°F), excursions permitted to 15°-30°C (59°-86°F) [see USP Controlled Room Temperature].
ROBAXIN is a registered trademark of Wyeth and used under license.
Baxter Healthcare Corporation
Deerfield, IL 60015 USA

SUPRANE® ℞
[*sū 'prān*]
(desflurane, USP)
Volatile Liquid for Inhalation

DESCRIPTION
SUPRANE® (desflurane, USP), a nonflammable liquid administered via vaporizer, is a general inhalation anesthetic. It is (±)1,2,2,2-tetrafluoroethyl difluoromethyl ether:

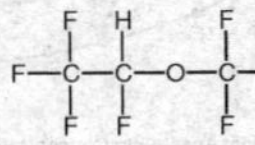

F–C(F)(F)–C(H)(F)–O–C(F)(F)–H

Some physical constants are:

Molecular weight	168.04
Specific gravity (at 20°C/4°C)	1.465
Vapor pressure in mm Hg	669 mm Hg @ 20°C
	731 mm Hg @ 22°C
	757 mm Hg @ 22.8°C (boiling point; 1atm)
	764 mm Hg @ 23°C
	798 mm Hg @ 24°C
	869 mm Hg @ 26°C

Partition coefficients at 37°C:

Blood/Gas	0.424
Olive Oil/Gas	18.7
Brain/Gas	0.54

Mean Component/Gas Partition Coefficients:

Polypropylene (Y piece)	6.7
Polyethylene (circuit tube)	16.2
Latex rubber (bag)	19.3
Latex rubber (bellows)	10.4
Polyvinylchloride (endotracheal tube)	34.7

Desflurane is nonflammable as defined by the requirements of International Electrotechnical Commission 601-2-13.
Desflurane is a colorless, volatile liquid below 22.8°C. Data indicate that desflurane is stable when stored under normal room lighting conditions according to instructions.
Desflurane is chemically stable. The only known degradation reaction is through prolonged direct contact with soda lime producing low levels of fluoroform (CHF_3). The amount of CHF_3 obtained is similar to that produced with MAC-equivalent doses of isoflurane. No discernible degradation occurs in the presence of strong acids.
Desflurane does not corrode stainless steel, brass, aluminum, anodized aluminum, nickel plated brass, copper, or beryllium.

CLINICAL PHARMACOLOGY
SUPRANE® (desflurane, USP) is a volatile liquid inhalation anesthetic minimally biotransformed in the liver in humans. Less than 0.02% of the SUPRANE® absorbed can be recovered as urinary metabolites (compared to 0.2% for isoflurane).
Minimum alveolar concentration (MAC) of desflurane in oxygen for a 25 year-old adult is 7.3%. The MAC of SUPRANE® (desflurane, USP) decreases with increasing age and with addition of depressants such as opioids or benzodiazepines. (See **DOSAGE AND ADMINISTRATION** for details).

Pharmacokinetics
Due to the volatile nature of desflurane in plasma samples, the washin-washout profile of desflurane was used as a surrogate of plasma pharmacokinetics. Eight healthy male volunteers first breathed 70% N_2O/30% O_2 for 30 minutes and then a mixture of SUPRANE® (desflurane, USP) 2.0%, isoflurane 0.4%, and halothane 0.2% for another 30 minutes. During this time, inspired and end-tidal concentrations (F_I and F_A) were measured. The F_A/F_I (washin) value at 30 minutes for desflurane was 0.91, compared to 1.00 for N_2O,

Continued on next page

Suprane—Cont.

0.74 for isoflurane, and 0.58 for halothane (See **Figure 1**). The washin rates for halothane and isoflurane were similar to literature values. The washin was faster for desflurane than for isoflurane and halothane at all time points. The F_A/F_{AO} (washout) value at 5 minutes was 0.12 for desflurane, 0.22 for isoflurane, and 0.25 for halothane (See **Figure 2**). The washout for SUPRANE® was more rapid than that for isoflurane and halothane at all elimination time points. By 5 days, the F_A/F_{AO} for desflurane is 1/20th of that for halothane or isoflurane.

Figure 1.
Desflurane Washin

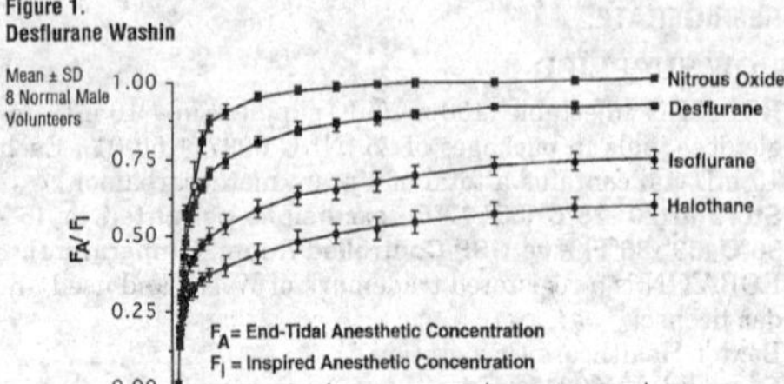

Figure 2.
Desflurane Washout

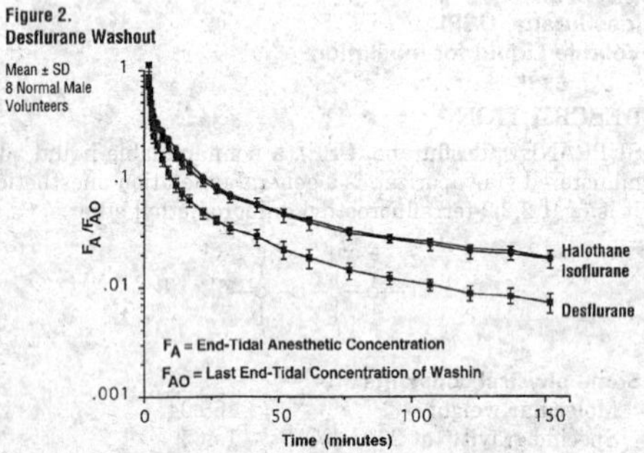

Pharmacodynamics

Changes in the clinical effects of SUPRANE® (desflurane, USP) rapidly follow changes in the inspired concentration. The duration of anesthesia and selected recovery measures for SUPRANE® are given in the following tables:

In 178 female outpatients undergoing laparoscopy, premedicated with fentanyl (1.5–2.0 µg/kg), anesthesia was initiated with propofol 2.5 mg/kg, desflurane/N_2O 60% in O_2 or desflurane/O_2 alone. Anesthesia was maintained with either propofol 1.5–9.0 mg/kg/hr, desflurane 2.6–8.4% in N_2O 60% in O_2, or desflurane 3.1–8.9% in O_2.

[See first table above]

In 88 unpremedicated outpatients, anesthesia was initiated with thiopental 3–9 mg/kg or desflurane in O_2. Anesthesia was maintained with isoflurane 0.7–1.4% in N_2O 60%, desflurane 1.8–7.7% in N_2O 60%, or desflurane 4.4–11.9% in O_2.

[See second table at right]

Recovery from anesthesia was assessed at 30, 60, and 90 minutes following 0.5 MAC desflurane (3%) or isoflurane (0.6%) in N_2O 60% using subjective and objective tests. At 30 minutes after anesthesia, only 43% of the isoflurane group were able to perform the psychometric tests compared to 76% in the desflurane group ($p < 0.05$).

[See third table at right]

SUPRANE® (desflurane, USP) was studied in twelve volunteers receiving no other drugs. Hemodynamic effects during controlled ventilation ($PaCO_2$ 38mm Hg) were:

[See first table at top of next page]

When the same volunteers breathed spontaneously during desflurane anesthesia, systemic vascular resistance and mean arterial blood pressure decreased; cardiac index, heart rate, stroke volume, and central venous pressure (CVP) increased compared to values when the volunteers were conscious. Cardiac index, stroke volume, and CVP were greater during spontaneous ventilation than during controlled ventilation.

During spontaneous ventilation in the same volunteers, increasing the concentration of SUPRANE® (desflurane, USP) from 3% to 12% decreased tidal volume and increased arterial carbon dioxide tension and respiratory rate. The combination of N_2O 60% with a given concentration of desflurane gave results similar to those with desflurane alone. Respiratory depression produced by desflurane is similar to that produced by other potent inhalation agents.

The use of desflurane concentrations higher than 1.5 MAC may produce apnea.

[See figure 3 at right]

CLINICAL TRIALS

SUPRANE® (desflurane, USP) was evaluated in 1,843 patients including ambulatory (N=1,061), cardiovascular (N=277), geriatric (N=103), neurosurgical (N=40), and pediatric (N=235) patients. Clinical experience with these patients and with 1,087 control patients in these studies not receiving desflurane are described below. Although desflurane can be used in adults for the inhalation induction of anesthesia via mask, it produces a high incidence of respiratory irritation (coughing, breathholding, apnea, increased secretions, laryngospasm). For incidence, see **ADVERSE REACTIONS**. Oxyhemoglobin saturation below 90% occurred in 6% of patients (from pooled data, N = 370 adults).

Ambulatory Surgery

SUPRANE® (desflurane, USP) plus N_2O was compared to isoflurane plus N_2O in multicenter studies (21 sites) of 792 ASA physical status I, II, or III patients aged 18–76 years (median 32).

EMERGENCE AND RECOVERY AFTER OUTPATIENT LAPAROSCOPY
178 FEMALES, AGES 20-47
TIMES IN MINUTES: MEAN ± SD (RANGE)

Induction:	Propofol	Propofol	Desflurane/N_2O	Desflurane/O_2
Maintenance:	Propofol/N_2O	Desflurane/N_2O	Desflurane/N_2O	Desflurane/O_2
Number of Pts:	N = 48	N = 44	N = 43	N = 43
Median age	30 (20–43)	26 (21–47)	29 (21–42)	30 (20–40)
Anesthetic Time	49 ± 53 (8–336)	45 ± 35 (11–178)	44 ± 29 (14–149)	41 ± 26 (19–126)
Time to open eyes	7 ± 3 (2–19)	5 ± 2* (2–10)	5 ± 2* (2–12)	4 ± 2* (1–11)
Time to state name	9 ± 4 (4–22)	8 ± 3 (3–18)	7 ± 3* (3–16)	7 ± 3* (2–15)
Time to stand	80 ± 34 (40–200)	86 ± 55 (30–320)	81 ± 38 (35–190)	77 ± 38 (35–200)
Time to walk	110 ± 6 (47–285)	122 ± 85 (37–375)	108 ± 59 (48–220)	108 ± 66 (49–250)
Time to fit for discharge	152 ± 75 (66–375)	157 ± 80 (73–385)	150 ± 66 (68–310)	155 ± 73 (69–325)

*Differences were statistically significant ($p < 0.05$) by Dunnett's procedure comparing all treatments to the propofol-propofol/N_2O (induction and maintenance) group. Results for comparisons greater than one hour after anesthesia show no differences between groups and considerable variability within groups.

EMERGENCE AND RECOVERY TIMES IN OUTPATIENT SURGERY
46 MALES, 42 FEMALES, AGES 19-70
TIMES IN MINUTES: MEAN ± SD (RANGE)

Induction:	Thiopental	Thiopental	Thiopental	Desflurane/O_2
Maintenance:	Isoflurane/N_2O	Desflurane/N_2O	Desflurane/O_2	Desflurane/O_2
Number of Pts:	N = 23	N = 21	N = 23	N = 21
Median age	43 (20–70)	40 (22–67)	43 (19–70)	41 (21–64)
Anesthetic Time	49 ± 23 (11–94)	50 ± 19 (16–80)	50 ± 27 (16–113)	51 ± 23 (19–117)
Time to open eyes	13 ± 7 (5–33)	9 ± 3* (4–16)	12 ± 8 (4–39)	8 ± 2* (4–13)
Time to state name	17 ± 10 (6–44)	11 ± 4* (6–19)	15 ± 10 (6–46)	9 ± 3* (5–14)
Time to walk	195 ± 67 (124–365)	176 ± 60 (101–315)	168 ± 34 (119–258)	181 ± 42 (92–252)
Time to fit for discharge	205 ± 53 (153–365)	202 ± 41 (144–315)	197 ± 35 (155–280)	194 ± 37 (134–288)

*Differences were statistically significant ($p < 0.05$) by Dunnett's procedure comparing all treatments to the thiopental-isoflurane/N_2O (induction and maintenance) group. Results for comparisons greater than one hour after anesthesia show no differences between groups and considerable variability within groups.

RECOVERY TESTS: PERCENT OF PREOPERATIVE BASELINE VALUES
16 MALES, 22 FEMALES, AGES 20-65
PERCENT: MEAN ± SD

	60 minutes After Anesthesia		90 minutes After Anesthesia	
Maintenance:	Desflurane/N_2O	Isoflurane/N_2O	Desflurane/N_2O	Isoflurane/N_2O
Confusion Δ	66±6	47±8	75±7*	56±8
Fatigue Δ	70±9*	33±6	89±12*	47±8
Drowsiness Δ	66±5*	36±8	76±7*	49±9
Clumsiness Δ	65±5	49±8	80±7*	57±9
Comfort Δ	59±7*	30±6	60±8*	31±7
DSST† score	74±4*	50±9	75±4*	55±7
Trieger Tests††	67±5	74±6	90±6	83±7

Δ Visual analog scale (values from 0-100; 100=baseline)
† DSST = Digit Symbol Substitution Test
†† Trieger Test = Dot Connecting Test
* Differences were statistically significant ($p < 0.05$) using a two-sample t-test

Figure 3. $PaCO_2$ During Spontaneous Ventilation in Unstimulated Volunteers

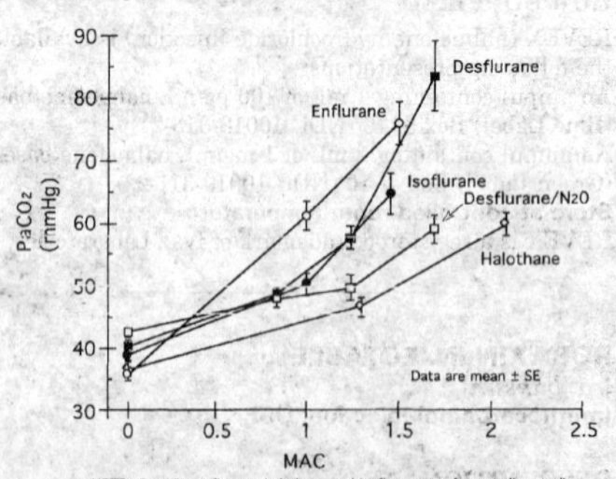

INDUCTION: Anesthetic induction begun with thiopental and continued with desflurane was associated with a 7% incidence of oxyhemoglobin saturation of 90% or less (from pooled data, N = 307) compared with 5% in patients in whom anesthesia was induced with thiopental and isoflurane (from pooled data, N = 152).

MAINTENANCE & RECOVERY: SUPRANE® (desflurane, USP) with or without N_2O or other anesthetics was generally well tolerated. There were no differences between desflurane and the other anesthetics studied in the times that patients were judged fit for discharge.

In one outpatient study, patients received a standardized anesthetic consisting of thiopental 4.2–4.4 mg/kg, fentanyl 3.5–4.0 µg/kg, vecuronium 0.05–0.07 mg/kg, and N_2O 60% in oxygen with either desflurane 3% or isoflurane 0.6%. Emergence times were significantly different; but times to sit up and discharge were not different (see Table).

RECOVERY PROFILES AFTER DESFLURANE 3% IN N_2O 60% vs ISOFLURANE 0.6% IN N_2O 60%
IN OUTPATIENTS
16 MALES, 22 FEMALES, AGES 20-65
MEAN ± SD

	Isoflurane	Desflurane
Number	21	17
Anesthetic time (min)	127 ± 80	98 ± 55
Recovery time to:		
Follow commands (min)	11.1 ± 7.9	6.5 ± 2.3*
Sit up (min)	113 ± 27	95 ± 56

Fit for discharge (min)	231 ± 40	207 ± 54

* Difference was statistically significant from the isoflurane group ($p < 0.05$), unadjusted for multiple comparisons.

Cardiovascular Surgery

Desflurane was compared to isoflurane, sufentanil or fentanyl for the anesthetic management of coronary artery bypass graft (CABG), abdominal aortic aneurysm, peripheral vascular and carotid endarterectomy surgery in 7 studies at 15 centers involving a total of 558 patients. In all patients except the desflurane vs sufentanil study, the volatile anesthetics were supplemented with intravenous opioids, usually fentanyl. Blood pressure and heart rate were controlled by changes in concentration of the volatile anesthetics or opioids and cardiovascular drugs if necessary. Oxygen (100%) was the carrier gas in 253 of 277 desflurane cases (24 of 277 received N_2O/O_2).

[See second table at right]

No differences were found in cardiovascular outcome (death, myocardial infarction, ventricular tachycardia or fibrillation, heart failure) among desflurane and the other anesthetics.

INDUCTION: Desflurane should not be used as the sole agent for anesthetic induction in patients with coronary artery disease or any patients where increases in heart rate or blood pressure are undesirable. In the desflurane vs sufentanil study, anesthetic induction with desflurane without opioids was associated with new transient ischemia in 14 patients vs 0 in the sufentanil group. In the desflurane group, mean heart rate, arterial pressure, and pulmonary blood pressure increased and stroke volume decreased in contrast to no change in the sufentanil group. Cardiovascular drugs were used frequently in both groups: especially esmolol in the desflurane group (56% vs 0%) and phenylephrine in the sufentanil group (43% vs 27%). When 10 µg/kg of fentanyl was used to supplement induction of anesthesia at one other center, continuous 2-lead ECG analysis showed a low incidence of myocardial ischemia and no difference between desflurane and isoflurane. If desflurane is to be used in patients with coronary artery disease, it should be used in combination with other medications for induction of anesthesia, preferably intravenous opioids and hypnotics.

MAINTENANCE & RECOVERY: In studies where desflurane or isoflurane anesthesia was supplemented with fentanyl, there were no differences in hemodynamic variables or the incidence of myocardial ischemia in the patients anesthetized with desflurane compared to those anesthetized with isoflurane.

During the precardiopulmonary bypass period, in the desflurane vs sufentanil study where the desflurane patients received no intravenous opioid, more desflurane patients required cardiovascular adjuvants to control hemodynamics than the sufentanil patients. During this period, the incidence of ischemia detected by ECG or echocardiography was not statistically different between desflurane (18 of 99) and sufentanil (9 of 98) groups. However, the duration and severity of ECG-detected myocardial ischemia was significantly less in the desflurane group. The incidence of myocardial ischemia after cardiopulmonary bypass and in the ICU did not differ between groups.

Geriatric Surgery

SUPRANE® (desflurane, USP) plus N_2O was compared to isoflurane plus N_2O in a multicenter study (6 sites) of 203 ASA physical status II or III elderly patients, aged 57–91 years (median 71).

INDUCTION: Most patients were premedicated with fentanyl (mean 2 µg/kg), preoxygenated, and received thiopental (mean 4.3 mg/kg IV) or thiamylal (mean 4 mg/kg IV) followed by succinylcholine (mean 1.4 mg/kg IV) for intubation.

MAINTENANCE & RECOVERY: Heart rate and arterial blood pressure remained within 20% of preinduction baseline values during administration of SUPRANE® (desflurane, USP) 0.5–7.7% (average 3.6%) with 50–60% N_2O. Induction, maintenance, and recovery cardiovascular measurements did not differ from those during isoflurane/N_2O administration nor did the postoperative incidence of nausea and vomiting differ. The most common cardiovascular adverse event was hypotension occurring in 8% of the SUPRANE® patients and 6% of the isoflurane patients.

Neurosurgery

SUPRANE® (desflurane, USP) was studied in 38 patients aged 26–76 years (median 48 years), ASA physical status II or III undergoing neurosurgical procedures for intracranial lesions.

INDUCTION: Induction consisted of standard neuroanesthetic techniques including hyperventilation and thiopental.

MAINTENANCE: No change in cerebrospinal fluid pressure (CSFP) was observed in 8 patients who had intracranial tumors when the dose of desflurane was 0.5 MAC in N_2O 50%. In another study of 9 patients with intracranial tumors, 0.8 MAC desflurane/air/O_2 did not increase CSFP above postinduction baseline values. In a different study of 10 patients receiving 1.1 MAC desflurane/air/O_2, CSFP increased 7 mm Hg (range 3–13 mm Hg increase, with final values of 11–26 mm Hg) above the predrug values.

HEMODYNAMIC EFFECTS OF DESFLURANE DURING CONTROLLED VENTILATION
12 MALE VOLUNTEERS, AGES 16-26
MEAN ± SD (RANGE)

Total MAC Equivalent	End-Tidal % Des/O_2	End-Tidal %Des/N_2O	Heart Rate (beats/min) O_2	Heart Rate (beats/min) N_2O	Mean Arterial Pressure (mmHg) O_2	Mean Arterial Pressure (mmHg) N_2O	Cardiac Index (L/min/m²) O_2	Cardiac Index (L/min/m²) N_2O
0	0%/21%	0%/0%	69 ± 4 (63–76)	70 ± 6 (62–85)	85 ± 9 (74–102)	85 ± 9 (74–102)	3.7 ± 0.4 (3.0–4.2)	3.7 ± 0.4 (3.0–4.2)
0.8	6%/94%	3%/60%	73 ± 5 (67–80)	77 ± 8 (67–97)	61 ± 5* (55–70)	69 ± 5* (62–80)	3.2 ± 0.5 (2.6–4.0)	3.3 ± 0.5 (2.6–4.1)
1.2	9%/91%	6%/60%	80 ± 5* (72–84)	77 ± 7 (67–90)	59 ± 8* (44–71)	63 ± 8* (47–74)	3.4 ± 0.5 (2.6–4.1)	3.1 ± 0.4* (2.6–3.8)
1.7	12%/88%	9%/60%	94 ± 14* (78–109)	79 ± 9 (61–91)	51 ± 12* (31–66)	59 ± 6* (46–68)	3.5 ± 0.9 (1.7–4.7)	3.0 ± 0.4* (2.4–3.6)

*Differences were statistically significant ($p<0.05$) compared to awake values, Newman-Keul's method of multiple comparison.

CARDIOVASCULAR PATIENTS BY AGENT AND TYPE OF SURGERY
418 MALES, 140 FEMALES, AGES 27-87 (MEDIAN 64)

Type of Surgery	13 Centers: Isoflurane	13 Centers: Desflurane	1 Center: Sufentanil	1 Center: Desflurane	1 Center: Fentanyl	1 Center: Desflurane
CABG	58	57	100	100	25	25
Abd Aorta	29	25	-	-	-	-
Periph Vasc	24	24	-	-	-	-
Carotid Art	45	46	-	-	-	-
Total	156	152	100	100	25	25

All volatile anesthetics may increase intracranial pressure in patients with intracranial space occupying lesions. In such patients, desflurane should be administered at 0.8 MAC or less, and in conjunction with a barbiturate induction and hyperventilation (hypocapnia) in the period before cranial decompression. Appropriate attention must be paid to maintain cerebral perfusion pressure. The use of a lower dose of desflurane and the administration of a barbiturate and mannitol would be predicted to lessen the effect of desflurane on CSFP.

Under hypocapnic conditions ($PaCO_2$ 27 mm Hg) desflurane 1 and 1.5 MAC did not increase cerebral blood flow (CBF) in 9 patients undergoing craniotomies. CBF reactivity to increasing $PaCO_2$ from 27 to 35 mm Hg was also maintained at 1.25 MAC desflurane/air/O_2.

Pediatric Surgery

SUPRANE® (desflurane, USP) or halothane with or without N_2O was used to anesthetize 235 patients aged 2 weeks-12 years (median 2 years), ASA physical status I or II.

INDUCTION: SUPRANE® (desflurane, USP) is not recommended for induction of general anesthesia in infants or pediatric patients because of a high incidence of moderate to severe laryngospasm, coughing, breathholding, and secretions. The occurrence of oxyhemoglobin desaturation was 26%. For incidence, see **ADVERSE REACTIONS**.

MAINTENANCE & RECOVERY: The concentration of SUPRANE® (desflurane, USP) required for maintenance of general anesthesia is age-dependent (see **INDIVIDUALIZATION OF DOSE**). Changes in blood pressure during maintenance of and recovery from anesthesia with desflurane/N_2O/O_2 are similar to those observed with halothane/N_2O/O_2. Heart rate during maintenance of anesthesia is approximately 10 beats per minute faster with desflurane than with halothane. Patients were judged fit for discharge from post-anesthesia care units within one hour with both desflurane and halothane. There were no differences in the incidence of nausea and vomiting between patients receiving desflurane or halothane.

INDIVIDUALIZATION OF DOSE

(Also see **DOSAGE AND ADMINISTRATION**)

Preanesthetic Medication: Issues such as whether or not to premedicate and the choice of premedicant(s) must be individualized. In clinical studies, patients scheduled to be anesthetized with desflurane frequently received IV preanesthetic medication, such as opioid and/or benzodiazepine.

INDUCTION: In adults, some premedicated with opioid, a frequent starting concentration was 3% desflurane, increased in 0.5–1.0% increments every 2 to 3 breaths. End-tidal concentrations of 4–11% SUPRANE® (desflurane, USP) with and without N_2O, produced anesthesia within 2 to 4 minutes. When desflurane was tested as the primary anesthetic induction agent, the incidence of upper airway irritation (apnea, breathholding, laryngospasm, coughing and secretions) was high (see **ADVERSE REACTIONS**). During induction in adults, the overall incidence of oxyhemoglobin desaturation ($SpO_2 < 90\%$) was 6%.

After induction in adults with an intravenous drug such as thiopental or propofol, desflurane can be started at approximately 0.5–1 MAC, whether the carrier gas is O_2 or N_2O/O_2.

MAINTENANCE: Surgical levels of anesthesia in adults may be maintained with concentrations of 2.5–8.5% SUPRANE® (desflurane, USP) with or without the concomitant use of nitrous oxide. In children, surgical levels of anesthesia may be maintained with concentrations of 5.2–10% SUPRANE® with or without the concomitant use of nitrous oxide.

During the maintenance of anesthesia, increasing concentrations of SUPRANE® (desflurane, USP) produce dose-dependent decreases in blood pressure. Excessive decreases in blood pressure may be due to depth of anesthesia and in such instances may be corrected by decreasing the inspired concentration of SUPRANE®.

Concentrations of desflurane exceeding 1 MAC may increase heart rate. Thus with this drug, an increased heart rate may not serve reliably as a sign of inadequate anesthesia. SUPRANE® (desflurane, USP) decreases the doses of neuromuscular blocking agents required (see **PRECAUTIONS, Drug Interactions**).

INDICATIONS AND USAGE

SUPRANE® (desflurane, USP) is indicated as an inhalation agent for induction and/or maintenance of anesthesia for inpatient and outpatient surgery in adults (see **PRECAUTIONS**).

SUPRANE® (desflurane, USP) is not recommended for induction of anesthesia in pediatric patients because of a high incidence of moderate to severe upper airway adverse events (see **WARNINGS**). After induction of anesthesia with agents other than SUPRANE®, and tracheal intubation, SUPRANE® is indicated for maintenance of anesthesia in infants and children.

CONTRAINDICATIONS

SUPRANE® (desflurane, USP) should not be used in patients with a known or suspected genetic susceptibility to malignant hyperthermia.

Known sensitivity to SUPRANE® (desflurane, USP) or to other halogenated agents.

WARNINGS

Pediatric Use: SUPRANE® (desflurane, USP) is not recommended for induction of general anesthesia via mask in infants or children because of the high incidence of moderate to severe laryngospasm in 50% of patients, coughing 72%, breathholding 68%, increase in secretions 21% and oxyhemoglobin desaturation 26%.

SUPRANE® (desflurane, USP) should be administered only by persons trained in the administration of general anesthesia, using a vaporizer specifically designed and designated for use with desflurane. Facilities for maintenance of a patent airway, artificial ventilation, oxygen enrichment, and circulatory resuscitation must be immediately available. Hypotension and respiratory depression increase as anesthesia is deepened.

PRECAUTIONS

During the maintenance of anesthesia, increasing concentrations of SUPRANE® (desflurane, USP) produce dose-dependent decreases in blood pressure. Excessive decreases in blood pressure may be related to depth of anesthesia and in such instances may be corrected by decreasing the inspired concentration of SUPRANE®.

Concentrations of desflurane exceeding 1 MAC may increase heart rate. Thus an increased heart rate may not be a sign of inadequate anesthesia.

In patients with intracranial space occupying lesions, SUPRANE® (desflurane, USP) should be administered at 0.8 MAC or less, in conjunction with a barbiturate induction and hyperventilation (hypocapnia). Appropriate measures should be taken to maintain cerebral perfusion pressure (see **CLINICAL STUDIES, Neurosurgery**).

Continued on next page

Suprane—Cont.

In patients with coronary artery disease, maintenance of normal hemodynamics is important to the avoidance of myocardial ischemia. Desflurane should not be used as the sole agent for anesthetic induction in patients with coronary artery disease or patients where increases in heart rate or blood pressure are undesirable. It should be used with other medications, preferably intravenous opioids and hypnotics (see **CLINICAL STUDIES, Cardiovascular Surgery**).
Inspired concentrations of SUPRANE® (desflurane, USP) greater than 12% have been safely administered to patients, particularly during induction of anesthesia. Such concentrations will proportionately dilute the concentration of oxygen; therefore, maintenance of an adequate concentration of oxygen may require a reduction of nitrous oxide or air if these gases are used concurrently.
The recovery from general anesthesia should be assessed carefully before patients are discharged from the post anesthesia care unit (PACU).
SUPRANE® (desflurane, USP), like some other inhalational anesthetics, can react with desiccated carbon dioxide (CO_2) absorbents to produce carbon monoxide which may result in elevated levels of carboxyhemoglobin in some patients. Case reports suggest that barium hydroxide lime and soda lime become desiccated when fresh gases are passed through the CO_2 absorber cannister at high flow rates over many hours or days. When a clinician suspects that CO_2 absorbent may be desiccated, it should be replaced before the administration of SUPRANE® (desflurane, USP).
As with other halogenated anesthetic agents, SUPRANE® (desflurane, USP) may cause sensitivity hepatitis in patients who have been sensitized by previous exposure to halogenated anesthetics (see **CONTRAINDICATIONS**).

Drug Interactions

No clinically significant adverse interactions with commonly used preanesthetic drugs, or drugs used during anesthesia (muscle relaxants, intravenous agents, and local anesthetic agents) were reported in clinical trials. The effect of desflurane on the disposition of other drugs has not been determined.
Like isoflurane, desflurane does not predispose to premature ventricular arrhythmias in the presence of exogenously infused epinephrine in swine.
BENZODIAZEPINES AND OPIOIDS (MAC REDUCTION): Benzodiazepines (midazolam 25–50 μg/kg) decrease the MAC of desflurane by 16% as do the opioids (fentanyl 3–6 μg/kg) by 50% (see **DOSAGE AND ADMINISTRATION**).
NEUROMUSCULAR BLOCKING AGENTS:
Anesthetic concentrations of desflurane at equilibrium (administered for 15 or more minutes before testing) reduced the ED_{95} of succinylcholine by approximately 30% and that of atracurium and pancuronium by approximately 50% compared to N_2O/opioid anesthesia. The effect of desflurane on duration of nondepolarizing neuromuscular blockade has not been studied.

DOSAGE OF MUSCLE RELAXANT CAUSING 95% DEPRESSION IN NEUROMUSCULAR BLOCKADE

Desflurane	Mean ED_{95} (μg/kg)		
Concentration	Pancuronium	Atracurium	Succinylcholine
0.65 MAC 60% N_2O/O_2	26	123	-
1.25 MAC 60% N_2O/O_2	18	91	-
1.25 MAC O_2	22	120	362

Dosage reduction of neuromuscular blocking agents during induction of anesthesia may result in delayed onset of conditions suitable for endotracheal intubation or inadequate muscle relaxation, because potentiation of neuromuscular blocking agents requires equilibration of muscle with the delivered partial pressure of desflurane.
Among nondepolarizing drugs, only pancuronium and atracurium interactions have been studied. In the absence of specific guidelines:

1. For endotracheal intubation, do not reduce the dose of nondepolarizing muscle relaxants or succinylcholine.
2. During maintenance of anesthesia, the dose of nondepolarizing muscle relaxants is likely to be reduced compared to that during N_2O/opioid anesthesia. Administration of supplemental doses of muscle relaxants should be guided by the response to nerve stimulation.

Malignant Hyperthermia: In susceptible individuals, potent inhalation anesthetic agents may trigger a skeletal muscle hypermetabolic state leading to high oxygen demand and the clinical syndrome known as malignant hyperthermia. In genetically susceptible pigs, desflurane induced malignant hyperthermia. The clinical syndrome is signalled by hypercapnia, and may include muscle rigidity, tachycardia, tachypnea, cyanosis, arrhythmias, and/or unstable blood pressure. Some of these nonspecific signs may also appear during light anesthesia: acute hypoxia, hypercapnia, and hypovolemia.
Treatment of malignant hyperthermia includes discontinuation of triggering agents, administration of intravenous dantrolene sodium, and application of supportive therapy. (Consult prescribing information for dantrolene sodium intravenous for additional information on patient management.) Renal failure may appear later, and urine flow should be monitored and sustained if possible.

Renal or Hepatic Insufficiency

Nine patients receiving SUPRANE® (desflurane, USP) (N=9) were compared to 9 patients receiving isoflurane, all with chronic renal insufficiency (serum creatinine 1.5–6.9 mg/dL). No differences in hematological or biochemical tests, including renal function evaluation, were seen between the two groups. Similarly, no differences were found in a comparison of patients receiving either SUPRANE® (desflurane, USP) (N=28) or isoflurane (N=30) undergoing renal transplant.
Eight patients receiving SUPRANE® (desflurane, USP) were compared to six patients receiving isoflurane, all with chronic hepatic disease (viral hepatitis, alcoholic hepatitis, or cirrhosis). No differences in hematological or biochemical tests, including hepatic enzymes and hepatic function evaluation, were seen.

Carcinogenesis, Mutagenesis, Impairment of Fertility

Animal carcinogenicity studies have not been performed with SUPRANE® (desflurane, USP). *In vitro* and *in vivo* genotoxicity studies did not demonstrate mutagenicity or chromosomal damage by SUPRANE®. Tests for genotoxicity included the Ames mutation assay, the metaphase analysis of human lymphocytes, and the mouse micronucleus assay.
Fertility was not affected after 1 MAC-Hour per day exposure (cumulative 63 and 14 MAC-Hours for males and females, respectively). At higher doses, parental toxicity (mortalities and reduced weight gain) was observed which could affect fertility.

Teratogenic Effects: No teratogenic effect was observed at approximately 10 and 13 cumulative MAC-Hour exposures at 1 MAC-Hour per day during organogenesis in rats or rabbits. At higher doses increased incidences of post-implantation loss and maternal toxicity were observed. However, at 10 MAC-Hours cumulative exposure in rats, about 6% decrease in the weight of male pups was observed at preterm caesarean delivery.

Pregnancy Category B: There are no adequate and well-controlled studies in pregnant women. SUPRANE® (desflurane, USP) should be used during pregnancy only if the potential benefit justifies the potential risk to the fetus.
Rats exposed to desflurane at 1 MAC-hour per day from gestation day 15 to lactation day 21, did not show signs of dystocia. Body weight of pups delivered by these dams at birth and during lactation were comparable to that of control pups. No treatment related behavioral changes were reported in these pups during lactation.

Labor and Delivery: The safety of desflurane during labor or delivery has not been demonstrated.

Nursing Mothers: The concentrations of desflurane in milk are probably of no clinical importance 24 hours after anesthesia. Because of rapid washout, desflurane concentrations in milk are predicted to be below those found with other volatile potent anesthetics.

Geriatric Use: The average MAC for SUPRANE® (desflurane, USP) in a 70 year old patient is two-thirds the MAC for a 20 year old patient (see **DOSAGE AND ADMINISTRATION**).

Pediatric Use: SUPRANE® (desflurane, USP) is not recommended for induction of general anesthesia via mask in pediatric patients because of the high incidence of moderate to severe laryngospasm, coughing, breathholding and increase in secretions and oxyhemoglobin desaturation (see WARNINGS).

Neurosurgical Use: SUPRANE® (desflurane, USP) may produce a dose-dependent increase in cerebrospinal fluid pressure (CSFP) when administered to patients with intracranial space occupying lesions. Desflurane should be administered at 0.8 MAC or less, and in conjunction with a barbiturate induction and hyperventilation (hypocapnia) until cerebral decompression in patients with known or suspected increases in CSFP. Appropriate attention must be paid to maintain cerebral perfusion pressure (see **CLINICAL STUDIES, Neurosurgery**).

ADVERSE REACTIONS

Adverse event information is derived from controlled clinical trials, the majority of which were conducted in the United States. The studies were conducted using a variety of premedications, other anesthetics, and surgical procedures of varying length. Most adverse events reported were mild and transient, and may reflect the surgical procedures, patient characteristics (including disease) and/or medications administered.
Of the 1,843 patients exposed to SUPRANE® (desflurane, USP) in clinical trials, 370 adults and 152 children were induced with desflurane alone and 687 patients were maintained principally with desflurane. The frequencies given reflect the percent of patients with the event. Each patient was counted once for each type of adverse event. They are presented in alphabetical order according to body system.

PROBABLY CAUSALLY RELATED: Incidence greater than 1%.

Induction (use as a mask inhalation agent):

ADULT PATIENTS (N=370):	Coughing 34%, breathholding 30%, apnea 15%, increased secretions*, laryngospasm*, oxyhemoglobin desaturation (SpO_2<90%)* pharyngitis*
PEDIATRIC PATIENTS (N=152):	Coughing 72%, breathholding 68%, laryngospasm 50%, oxyhemoglobin desaturation (SpO_2<90%) 26%, increased secretions 21%, bronchospasm*. (See **WARNINGS**)

Maintenance or Recovery

ADULT AND PEDIATRIC PATIENTS (N=687):

Body as a Whole:	Headache.
Cardiovascular:	Bradycardia, hypertension, nodal arrhythmia, tachycardia.
Digestive:	Nausea 27%, vomiting 16%.
Nervous system:	Increased Salivation.
Respiratory:	Apnea*, breathholding, cough increased*, laryngospasm*, pharyngitis.
Special Senses:	Conjunctivitis (conjunctival hyperemia)

* Incidence of events: 3%–10%

PROBABLY CAUSALLY RELATED: Incidence less than 1% and reported in 3 or more patients, regardless of severity (N=1,843) Adverse reactions reported only from postmarketing experience or in the literature, not seen in clinical trials, are considered rare and are italicized.

Cardiovascular:	Arrhythmia, bigeminy, abnormal electrocardiogram, myocardial ischemia, vasodilation.
Digestive:	*Hepatitis.*
Nervous System:	Agitation, dizziness.
Respiratory:	Asthma, dyspnea, hypoxia.

CAUSAL RELATIONSHIP UNKNOWN: Incidence less than 1% and reported in 3 or more patients, regardless of severity (N=1,843)

Body as a Whole:	Fever.
Cardiovascular:	Hemorrhage, myocardial infarct.
Metabolic and Nutrition:	Increased creatinine phosphokinase.
Musculoskeletal System:	Myalgia.
Skin and Appendages:	Pruritis.

See **PRECAUTIONS** for information regarding pediatric use and malignant hyperthermia.

Laboratory Findings: Transient elevations in glucose and white blood cell count may occur as with use of other anesthetic agents.

DRUG ABUSE AND DEPENDENCE

The potential drug abuse liability, and dependence associated with SUPRANE® (desflurane, USP) have not been studied.

OVERDOSAGE

In the event of overdosage, or suspected overdosage, take the following actions: discontinue administration of SUPRANE® (desflurane, USP), maintain a patent airway, initiate assisted or controlled ventilation with oxygen, and maintain adequate cardiovascular function.

DOSAGE AND ADMINISTRATION

Deliver SUPRANE® (desflurane, USP) from a vaporizer specifically designed and designated for use with desflurane.
The administration of general anesthesia must be individualized based on the patient's response (see **INDIVIDUALIZATION OF DOSE**). The following two tables provide mean relative potency based upon age and drug interaction studies in predominately ASA physical status I or II patients.

EFFECT OF AGE ON MAC OF DESFLURANE MEAN ± SD (percent atmospheres)

Age	N	O_2 100%	N	N_2O 60%
2 weeks	6	9.2 ± 0.0	-	-
10 weeks	5	9.4 ± 0.4	-	-
9 months	4	10.0 ± 0.7	5	7.5 ± 0.8
2 years	3	9.1 ± 0.6	-	-
3 years	-	-	5	6.4 ± 0.4
4 years	4	8.6 ± 0.6	-	-
7 years	5	8.1 ± 0.6	-	-
25 years	4	7.3 ± 0.0	4	4.0 ± 0.3
45 years	4	6.0 ± 0.3	6	2.8 ± 0.6
70 years	6	5.2 ± 0.6	6	1.7 ± 0.4

N = number of crossover pairs (using up-and-down method of quantal response)

Opioids or benzodiazepines decrease the amounts of SUPRANE® (desflurane, USP) required to produce anesthesia. The following table is based on studies of drug interaction (MAC reduction).

SUPRANE® (desflurane, USP) MAC WITH FENTANYL OR MIDAZOLAM
MEAN ± SD (percent reduction)

Dose	18-30 years	31-65 years
No fentanyl	6.4 ± 0.0	6.3 ± 0.4
3 µg/kg fentanyl	3.5 ± 1.9 (46%)	3.1 ± 0.6 (51%)
6 µg/kg fentanyl	3.0 ± 1.2 (53%)	2.3 ± 1.0 (64%)
No midazolam	6.9 ± 0.1	5.9 ± 0.6
25 µg/kg midazolam	-	4.9 ± 0.9 (16%)
50 µg/kg midazolam	-	4.9 ± 0.5 (17%)

SUPRANE® (desflurane, USP) decreases the doses of neuromuscular blocking agents required (see **PRECAUTIONS, Drug Interactions**).
During the maintenance of anesthesia with inflow rates of 2 L/min or more, the alveolar concentration of desflurane will usually be within 10% of the inspired concentration. (F_A/F_I, see **Figure 1** in **Pharmacokinetics** section.)

HOW SUPPLIED

SUPRANE® (desflurane, USP), NDC 10019-641-24, is packaged in amber-colored bottles containing 240 mL desflurane.

SAFETY AND HANDLING

Occupational Caution: There is no specific work exposure limit established for SUPRANE® (desflurane, USP). However, the National Institute for Occupational Safety and Health Administration has recommended an 8-hr, time-weighted average limit of 2 ppm for halogenated anesthetic agents in general (0.5 ppm when coupled with exposure to N_2O).
The predicted effects of acute overexposure by inhalation of SUPRANE® (desflurane, USP) include headache, dizziness or (in extreme cases) unconsciousness.
There are no documented adverse effects of chronic exposure to halogenated anesthetic vapors (Waste Anesthetic Gases or WAGs) in the workplace. Although results of some epidemiological studies suggest a link between exposure to halogenated anesthetics and increased health problems (particularly spontaneous abortion), the relationship is not conclusive. Since exposure to WAGs is one possible factor in the findings for these studies, operating room personnel, and pregnant women in particular, should minimize exposure. Precautions include adequate general ventilation in the operating room, the use of a well-designated and well-maintained scavenging system, work practices to minimize leaks and spills while the anesthetic agent is in use, and routine equipment maintenance to minimize leaks.

STORAGE

Store at room temperature, 15°–30°C (59°–86°F). SUPRANE® (desflurane, USP) has been demonstrated to be stable for the period defined by the expiration dating on the label. The bottle cap should be replaced after each use of SUPRANE®.

BAXTER
Manufactured for
Baxter Healthcare Corporation
Deerfield, IL 60015 USA
by: Baxter Healthcare Corporation of Puerto Rico
Guayama, Puerto Rico 00784 USA
Revised: January 2001
For Product Inquiry 1 800 ANA DRUG
(1-800-262-3784)
400-447-08

Bayer Pharmaceuticals Corporation

400 MORGAN LANE
WEST HAVEN, CT 06516

For Medical Information Contact:
Director, Medical Services
(800) 468-0894
(203) 812-2000

ADALAT® CC ℞

[a'dă-lăt]
(nifedipine)
Extended Release Tablets
For Oral Use

DESCRIPTION

ADALAT® CC is an extended release tablet dosage form of the calcium channel blocker nifedipine. Nifedipine is 3,5-pyridinedicarboxylic acid, 1,4-dihydro-2,6-dimethyl-4-(2-nitrophenyl)-dimethyl ester, $C_{17}H_{18}N_2O_6$, and has the structural formula:
[See chemical structure at top of next column]

CH_3, H, N, CH_3, CH_3OC, O, H, $COCH_3$, O, NO_2

Nifedipine is a yellow crystalline substance, practically insoluble in water but soluble in ethanol. It has a molecular weight of 346.3. ADALAT CC tablets consist of an external coat and an internal core. Both contain nifedipine, the coat as a slow release formulation and the core as a fast release formulation. ADALAT CC tablets contain either 30, 60, or 90 mg of nifedipine for once-a-day oral administration.
Inert ingredients in the formulation are: hydroxypropylcellulose, lactose, corn starch, crospovidone, microcrystalline cellulose, silicon dioxide, and magnesium stearate. The inert ingredients in the film coating are: hypromellose, polyethylene glycol, ferric oxide, and titanium dioxide.

CLINICAL PHARMACOLOGY

Nifedipine is a calcium ion influx inhibitor (slow-channel blocker or calcium ion antagonist) which inhibits the transmembrane influx of calcium ions into vascular smooth muscle and cardiac muscle. The contractile processes of vascular smooth muscle and cardiac muscle are dependent upon the movement of extracellular calcium ions into these cells through specific ion channels. Nifedipine selectively inhibits calcium ion influx across the cell membrane of vascular smooth muscle and cardiac muscle without altering serum calcium concentrations.
Mechanism of Action: The mechanism by which nifedipine reduces arterial blood pressure involves peripheral arterial vasodilatation and consequently, a reduction in peripheral vascular resistance. The increased peripheral vascular resistance that is an underlying cause of hypertension results from an increase in active tension in the vascular smooth muscle. Studies have demonstrated that the increase in active tension reflects an increase in cytosolic free calcium.
Nifedipine is a peripheral arterial vasodilator which acts directly on vascular smooth muscle. The binding of nifedipine to voltage-dependent and possibly receptor-operated channels in vascular smooth muscle results in an inhibition of calcium influx through these channels. Stores of intracellular calcium in vascular smooth muscle are limited and thus dependent upon the influx of extracellular calcium for contraction to occur. The reduction in calcium influx by nifedipine causes arterial vasodilation and decreased peripheral vascular resistance which results in reduced arterial blood pressure.
Pharmacokinetics and Metabolism: Nifedipine is completely absorbed after oral administration. The bioavailability of nifedipine as ADALAT CC relative to immediate release nifedipine is in the range of 84%-89%. After ingestion of ADALAT CC tablets under fasting conditions, plasma concentrations peak at about 2.5-5 hours with a second small peak or shoulder evident at approximately 6-12 hours post dose. The elimination half-life of nifedipine administered as ADALAT CC is approximately 7 hours in contrast to the known 2 hour elimination half-life of nifedipine administered as an immediate release capsule.
When ADALAT CC is administered as multiples of 30 mg tablets over a dose range of 30 mg to 90 mg, the area under the curve (AUC) is dose proportional; however, the peak plasma concentration for the 90 mg dose given as 3 × 30 mg is 29% greater than predicted from the 30 mg and 60 mg doses.
Two 30 mg ADALAT CC tablets may be interchanged with a 60 mg ADALAT CC tablet. Three 30 mg ADALAT CC tablets, however, result in substantially higher C_{max} values than those after a single 90 mg ADALAT CC tablet. Three 30 mg tablets should, therefore, not be considered interchangeable with a 90 mg tablet.
Once daily dosing of ADALAT CC under fasting conditions results in decreased fluctuations in the plasma concentration of nifedipine when compared to t.i.d. dosing with immediate release nifedipine capsules. The mean peak plasma concentration of nifedipine following a 90 mg ADALAT CC tablet, administered under fasting conditions, is approximately 115 ng/mL. When ADALAT CC is given immediately after a high fat meal in healthy volunteers, there is an average increase of 60% in the peak plasma nifedipine concentration, a prolongation in the time to peak concentration, but no significant change in the AUC. Plasma concentrations of nifedipine when ADALAT CC is taken after a fatty meal result in slightly lower peaks compared to the same daily dose of the immediate release formulation administered in three divided doses. This may be, in part, because ADALAT CC is less bioavailable than the immediate release formulation.
Nifedipine is extensively metabolized to highly water soluble, inactive metabolites accounting for 60% to 80% of the dose excreted in the urine. Only traces (less than 0.1% of the dose) of the unchanged form can be detected in the urine. The remainder is excreted in the feces in metabolized form, most likely as a result of biliary excretion.
No studies have been performed with ADALAT CC in patients with renal failure; however, significant alterations in the pharmacokinetics of nifedipine immediate release capsules have not been reported in patients undergoing hemodialysis or chronic ambulatory peritoneal dialysis. Since the absorption of nifedipine from ADALAT CC could be modified by renal disease, caution should be exercised in treating such patients.
Because hepatic biotransformation is the predominant route for the disposition of nifedipine, its pharmacokinetics may be altered in patients with chronic liver disease. ADALAT CC has not been studied in patients with hepatic disease; however, in patients with hepatic impairment (liver cirrhosis) nifedipine has a longer elimination half-life and higher bioavailability than in healthy volunteers.
The degree of protein binding of nifedipine is high (92%–98%). Protein binding may be greatly reduced in patients with renal or hepatic impairment.
After administration of ADALAT CC to healthy elderly men and women (age > 60 years), the mean C_{max} is 36% higher and the average plasma concentration is 70% greater than in younger patients.
In healthy subjects, the elimination half-life of a different sustained release nifedipine formulation was longer in elderly subjects (6.7 h) compared to young subjects (3.8 h) following oral administration. A decreased clearance was also observed in the elderly (348 mL/min) compared to young subjects (519 mL/min) following intravenous administration.
Co-administration of nifedipine with grapefruit juice results in up to a 2-fold increase in AUC and C_{max}, due to inhibition of CYP3A4 related first-pass metabolism.
Clinical Studies: ADALAT CC produced dose-related decreases in systolic and diastolic blood pressure as demonstrated in two double-blind, randomized, placebo-controlled trials in which over 350 patients were treated with ADALAT CC 30, 60 or 90mg once daily for 6 weeks. In the first study, ADALAT CC was given as monotherapy and in the second study, ADALAT CC was added to a beta-blocker in patients not controlled on a beta-blocker alone. The mean trough (24 hours post-dose) blood pressure results from these studies are shown below:

MEAN REDUCTIONS IN TROUGH SUPINE BLOOD PRESSURE (mmHg) SYSTOLIC/DIASTOLIC

STUDY 1		
ADALAT CC DOSE	**N**	**MEAN TROUGH REDUCTION***
30 MG	60	5.3/2.9
60 MG	57	8.0/4.1
90 MG	55	12.5/8.1
STUDY 2		
ADALAT CC DOSE	**N**	**MEAN TROUGH REDUCTION***
30 MG	58	7.6/3.8
60 MG	63	10.1/5.3
90 MG	62	10.2/5.8

*Placebo response subtracted.

The trough/peak ratios estimated from 24 hour blood pressure monitoring ranged from 41%-78% for diastolic and 46%-91% for systolic blood pressure.
Hemodynamics: Like other slow-channel blockers, nifedipine exerts a negative inotropic effect on isolated myocardial tissue. This is rarely, if ever, seen in intact animals or man, probably because of reflex responses to its vasodilating effects. In man, nifedipine decreases peripheral vascular resistance which leads to a fall in systolic and diastolic pressures, usually minimal in normotensive volunteers (less than 5-10 mm Hg systolic), but sometimes larger. With ADALAT CC, these decreases in blood pressure are not accompanied by any significant change in heart rate. Hemodynamic studies of the immediate release nifedipine formulation in patients with normal ventricular function have generally found a small increase in cardiac index without major effects on ejection fraction, left ventricular end-diastolic pressure (LVEDP) or volume (LVEDV). In patients with impaired ventricular function, most acute studies have shown some increase in ejection fraction and reduction in left ventricular filling pressure.
Electrophysiologic Effects: Although, like other members of its class, nifedipine causes a slight depression of sinoatrial node function and atrioventricular conduction in isolated myocardial preparations, such effects have not been seen in studies in intact animals or in man. In formal electrophysiologic studies, predominantly in patients with normal conduction systems, nifedipine administered as the immediate release capsule has had no tendency to prolong atrioventricular conduction or sinus node recovery time, or to slow sinus rate.

INDICATION AND USAGE

ADALAT CC is indicated for the treatment of hypertension. It may be used alone or in combination with other antihypertensive agents.

CONTRAINDICATIONS

Known hypersensitivity to nifedipine.

WARNINGS

Excessive Hypotension: Although in most patients the hypotensive effect of nifedipine is modest and well tolerated, occasional patients have had excessive and poorly tolerated hypotension. These responses have usually occurred during initial titration or at the time of subsequent upward dosage adjustment, and may be more likely in patients using concomitant beta-blockers.

Continued on next page

Adalat CC—Cont.

Severe hypotension and/or increased fluid volume requirements have been reported in patients who received immediate release capsules together with a beta-blocking agent and who underwent coronary artery bypass surgery using high dose fentanyl anesthesia. The interaction with high dose fentanyl appears to be due to the combination of nifedipine and a beta-blocker, but the possibility that it may occur with nifedipine alone, with low doses of fentanyl, in other surgical procedures, or with other narcotic analgesics cannot be ruled out. In nifedipine-treated patients where surgery using high dose fentanyl anesthesia is contemplated, the physician should be aware of these potential problems and, if the patient's condition permits, sufficient time (at least 36 hours) should be allowed for nifedipine to be washed out of the body prior to surgery.

Increased Angina and/or Myocardial Infarction: Rarely, patients, particularly those who have severe obstructive coronary artery disease, have developed well documented increased frequency, duration and/or severity of angina or acute myocardial infarction upon starting nifedipine or at the time of dosage increase. The mechanism of this effect is not established.

Beta-Blocker Withdrawal: When discontinuing a beta-blocker it is important to taper its dose, if possible, rather than stopping abruptly before beginning nifedipine. Patients recently withdrawn from beta blockers may develop a withdrawal syndrome with increased angina, probably related to increased sensitivity to catecholamines. Initiation of nifedipine treatment will not prevent this occurrence and on occasion has been reported to increase it.

Congestive Heart Failure: Rarely, patients (usually while receiving a beta-blocker) have developed heart failure after beginning nifedipine. Patients with tight aortic stenosis may be at greater risk for such an event, as the unloading effect of nifedipine would be expected to be of less benefit to these patients, owing to their fixed impedance to flow across the aortic valve.

PRECAUTIONS

General - Hypotension: Because nifedipine decreases peripheral vascular resistance, careful monitoring of blood pressure during the initial administration and titration of ADALAT CC is suggested. Close observation is especially recommended for patients already taking medications that are known to lower blood pressure (See **WARNINGS**).

Peripheral Edema: Mild to moderate peripheral edema occurs in a dose-dependent manner with ADALAT CC. The placebo subtracted rate is approximately 8% at 30 mg, 12% at 60 mg and 19% at 90 mg daily. This edema is a localized phenomenon, thought to be associated with vasodilation of dependent arterioles and small blood vessels and not due to left ventricular dysfunction or generalized fluid retention. With patients whose hypertension is complicated by congestive heart failure, care should be taken to differentiate this peripheral edema from the effects of increasing left ventricular dysfunction.

Information for Patients: ADALAT CC is an extended release tablet and should be swallowed whole and taken on an empty stomach. It should not be administered with food. Do not chew, divide or crush tablets.

Laboratory Tests: Rare, usually transient, but occasionally significant elevations of enzymes such as alkaline phosphatase, CPK, LDH, SGOT, and SGPT have been noted. The relationship to nifedipine therapy is uncertain in most cases, but probable in some. These laboratory abnormalities have rarely been associated with clinical symptoms; however, cholestasis with or without jaundice has been reported. A small increase (<5%) in mean alkaline phosphatase was noted in patients treated with ADALAT CC. This was an isolated finding and it rarely resulted in values which fell outside the normal range. Rare instances of allergic hepatitis have been reported with nifedipine treatment. In controlled studies, ADALAT CC did not adversely affect serum uric acid, glucose, cholesterol or potassium.

Nifedipine, like other calcium channel blockers, decreases platelet aggregation *in vitro*. Limited clinical studies have demonstrated a moderate but statistically significant decrease in platelet aggregation and increase in bleeding time in some nifedipine patients. This is thought to be a function of inhibition of calcium transport across the platelet membrane. No clinical significance for these findings has been demonstrated.

Positive direct Coombs' test with or without hemolytic anemia has been reported but a causal relationship between nifedipine administration and positivity of this laboratory test, including hemolysis, could not be determined.

Although nifedipine has been used safely in patients with renal dysfunction and has been reported to exert a beneficial effect in certain cases, rare reversible elevations in BUN and serum creatinine have been reported in patients with pre-existing chronic renal insufficiency. The relationship to nifedipine therapy is uncertain in most cases but probable in some.

Drug Interactions: Beta-adrenergic blocking agents: (See **WARNINGS**).

ADALAT® CC was well tolerated when administered in combination with a beta blocker in 187 hypertensive patients in a placebo-controlled clinical trial. However, there have been occasional literature reports suggesting that the combination of nifedipine and beta-adrenergic blocking drugs may increase the likelihood of congestive heart failure, severe hypotension, or exacerbation of angina in patients with cardiovascular disease.

Rifampicin: Rifampicin strongly induces the cytochrome P450 3A4 system. Upon co-administration with rifampicin, the bioavailability of nifedipine is distinctly reduced and its efficacy weakened. The use of rifampicin should be avoided in patients receiving nifedipine.

Digitalis: Since there have been isolated reports of patients with elevated digoxin levels, and there is a possible interaction between digoxin and ADALAT CC, it is recommended that digoxin levels be monitored when initiating, adjusting, and discontinuing ADALAT CC to avoid possible over- or under-digitalization.

Coumarin Anticoagulants: There have been rare reports of increased prothrombin time in patients taking coumarin anticoagulants to whom nifedipine was administered. However, the relationship to nifedipine therapy is uncertain.

Quinidine: There have been rare reports of an interaction between quinidine and nifedipine (with a decreased plasma level of quinidine, or a distinct increase in quinidine plasma concentrations after discontinuation of nifedipine). Monitoring of quinidine plasma concentration and adjustment of quinidine dose are recommended when nifedipine is concomitantly administered or discontinued. In addition, blood pressure should be carefully monitored if quinidine is added to existing nifedipine therapy and, if necessary, the dose of nifedipine should be decreased.

Cimetidine: Both the peak plasma level of nifedipine and the AUC may increase in the presence of cimetidine. Ranitidine produces smaller non-significant increases. This effect of cimetidine may be mediated by its known inhibition of hepatic cytochrome P-450, the enzyme system probably responsible for the first-pass metabolism of nifedipine. If nifedipine therapy is initiated in a patient currently receiving cimetidine, cautious titration is advised.

Cisapride: Concomitant administration of cisapride and nifedipine may lead to increased plasma concentrations of nifedipine. Upon coadministration of both drugs, blood pressure should be monitored and, if necessary, a reduction in nifedipine dose considered.

Diltiazem: Diltiazem decreases the clearance of nifedipine. The combination of both drugs should be administered with caution and a reduction in nifedipine dose may be considered.

Quinupristin/Dalfopristin: Concomitant administration of quinupristin/dalfopristin and nifedipine may lead to increased plasma concentrations of nifedipine. Upon coadministration of both drugs, blood pressure should be monitored and, if necessary, a reduction in nifedipine dose considered.

Phenytoin: Nifedipine is metabolized by CYP3A4. Coadministration of nifedipine 60 mg coat-core tablet with phenytoin, an inducer of CYP3A4, lowered the AUC and C_{max} of nifedipine by approximately 70%. When using nifedipine with phenytoin, the clinical response to nifedipine should be monitored and its dose adjusted if necessary.

Co-administration of nifedipine with other drugs known to inhibit the cytochrome P450 3A4 system, such as erythromycin, fluoxetine, indinavir, ritonavir, saquinavir, amprenavir, nelfinavir, ketoconazole, itraconozole, fluconazole, and nefazodone may cause an increase in nifedipine plasma concentrations. Blood pressure should be monitored and a reduction in nifedipine dose may be considered.

Tacrolimus is also metabolized via the cytochrome P450 3A4 system. If coadministered with nifedipine, the tacrolimus plasma concentrations should be monitored and a reduction of the tacrolimus dose may be considered.

Some drugs, including carbamazepine, and phenobarbitone, have been shown to reduce plasma concentrations of other calcium channel blockers due to enzyme induction. A similar interaction with nifedipine leading to a decrease in nifedipine plasma concentrations and a decrease in efficacy can not be excluded. The opposite effect has been seen with valproic acid and another calcium channel blocker due to enzyme inhibition. Therefore an increase in nifedipine plasma concentrations and an increase in efficacy upon co-administration with valproic acid can not be excluded.

Other Interactions:

Grapefruit Juice: Co-administration of nifedipine with grapefruit juice results in up to a 2-fold increase in AUC and C_{max}, due to inhibition of CYP3A4 related first-pass metabolism. This effect of grapefruit juice may last for at least 3 days. Administration of nifedipine with grapefruit juice is to be avoided.

Carcinogenesis, Mutagenesis, Impairment of Fertility: Nifedipine was administered orally to rats for two years and was not shown to be carcinogenic. When given to rats prior to mating, nifedipine caused reduced fertility at a dose approximately 30 times the maximum recommended human dose. ***There is a literature report of reversible reduction in the ability of human sperm obtained from a limited number of infertile men taking recommended doses of nifedipine to bind to and fertilize an ovum in vitro.*** *In vivo* mutagenicity studies were negative.

Pregnancy: Pregnancy Category C. In rodents, rabbits and monkeys, nifedipine has been shown to have a variety of embryotoxic, placentotoxic and fetotoxic effects, including stunted fetuses (rats, mice and rabbits), digital anomalies (rats and rabbits), rib deformities (mice), cleft palate (mice), small placentas and underdeveloped chorionic villi (monkeys), embryonic and fetal deaths (rats, mice and rabbits), prolonged pregnancy (rats; not evaluated in other species), and decreased neonatal survival (rats; not evaluated in other species). On a mg/kg or mg/m^2 basis, some of the doses associated with these various effects are higher than the maximum recommended human dose and some are lower, but all are within an order of magnitude of it.

The digital anomalies seen in nifedipine-exposed rabbit pups are strikingly similar to those seen in pups exposed to phenytoin, and these are in turn similar to the phalangeal deformities that are the most common malformation seen in human children with *in utero* exposure to phenytoin.

There are no adequate and well-controlled studies in pregnant women. ADALAT CC should generally be avoided during pregnancy and used only if the potential benefit justifies the potential risk to the fetus.

Nursing Mothers: Nifedipine is excreted in human milk. Therefore, a decision should be made to discontinue nursing or to discontinue the drug, taking into account the importance of the drug to the mother.

Geriatric Use: Although small pharmacokinetic studies have identified an increased half-life and increased C_{max} and AUC (See **CLINICAL PHARMACOLOGY: Pharmacokinetics and Metabolism**), clinical studies of nifedipine did not include sufficient numbers of subjects aged 65 and over to determine whether they respond differently from younger subjects. Other reported clinical experience has not identified differences in responses between the elderly and younger patients. In general, dose selection for an elderly patient should be cautious, usually starting at the low end of the dosing range, reflecting the greater frequency of decreased hepatic, renal, or cardiac function, and of concomitant disease or other drug therapy.

ADVERSE EXPERIENCES

The incidence of adverse events during treatment with ADALAT CC in doses up to 90 mg daily were derived from multi-center placebo-controlled clinical trials in 370 hypertensive patients. Atenolol 50 mg once daily was used concomitantly in 187 of the 370 patients on ADALAT CC and in 64 of the 126 patients on placebo. All adverse events reported during ADALAT CC therapy were tabulated independently of their causal relationship to medication.

The most common adverse event reported with ADALAT CC was peripheral edema. This was dose related and the frequency was 18% on ADALAT CC 30 mg daily, 22% on ADALAT CC 60 mg daily and 29% on ADALAT CC 90 mg daily versus 10% on placebo.

Other common adverse events reported in the above placebo-controlled trials include:

Adverse Event	ADALAT CC (%) (n=370)	PLACEBO (%) (n=126)
Headache	19	13
Flushing/heat sensation	4	0
Dizziness	4	2
Fatigue/asthenia	4	4
Nausea	2	1
Constipation	1	0

Where the frequency of adverse events with ADALAT CC and placebo is similar, causal relationship cannot be established.

The following adverse events were reported with an incidence of 3% or less in daily doses up to 90 mg:

Body as a Whole/Systemic: chest pain, leg pain
Central Nervous System: paresthesia, vertigo
Dermatologic: rash
Gastrointestinal: constipation
Musculoskeletal: leg cramps
Respiratory: epistaxis, rhinitis
Urogenital: impotence, urinary frequency

Other adverse events reported with an incidence of less than 1.0% were:

Body as a Whole/Systemic: allergic reaction, asthenia, cellulitis, substernal chest pain, chills, facial edema, lab test abnormal, malaise, neck pain, pelvic pain, pain, photosensitivity reaction

Cardiovascular: atrial fibrillation, bradycardia, cardiac arrest, extrasystole, hypotension, migraine, palpitations, phlebitis, postural hypotension, tachycardia, cutaneous angiectases

Central Nervous System: anxiety, confusion, decreased libido, depression, hypertonia, hypesthesia, insomnia, somnolence

Dermatologic: angioedema, petechial rash, pruritus, sweating

Gastrointestinal: abdominal pain, diarrhea, dry mouth, dysphagia, dyspepsia, eructation, esophagitis, flatulence, gastrointestinal disorder, gastrointestinal hemorrhage, GGT increased, gum disorder, gum hemorrhage, vomiting

Hematologic: eosinophilia, lymphadenopathy

Metabolic: gout, weight loss

Musculoskeletal: arthralgia, arthritis, joint disorder, myalgia, myasthenia

Respiratory: dyspnea, increased cough, rales, pharyngitis, stridor

Special Senses: abnormal vision, amblyopia, conjunctivitis, diplopia, eye disorder, eye hemorrhage, tinnitus

Urogenital/Reproductive: dysuria, kidney calculus, nocturia, breast engorgement, polyuria, urogenital disorder

The following adverse events have been reported rarely in patients given nifedipine in coat core or other formulations: allergenic hepatitis, alopecia, anaphylactic reaction, anemia, arthritis with ANA (+), depression, erythromelalgia, exfoliative dermatitis, fever, gingival hyperplasia, gynecomastia, hyperglycemia, jaundice, leukopenia, mood changes, muscle cramps, nervousness, paranoid syndrome, purpura, shakiness, sleep disturbances, Stevens-Johnson syndrome, syncope, taste perversion, thrombocytopenia, toxic epidermal necrolysis, transient blindness at the peak of plasma level, tremor and urticaria.

OVERDOSAGE

Experience with nifedipine overdosage is limited. Symptoms associated with severe nifedipine overdosage include loss of consciousness, drop in blood pressure, heart rhythm disturbances, metabolic acidosis, hypoxia, cardiogenic shock with pulmonary edema. Generally, overdosage with nifedipine leading to pronounced hypotension calls for active cardiovascular support including monitoring of cardiovascular and respiratory function, elevation of extremities, judicious use of calcium infusion, pressor agents and fluids. Clearance of nifedipine would be expected to be prolonged in patients with impaired liver function. Since nifedipine is highly protein bound, dialysis is not likely to be of any benefit; however, plasmapheresis may be beneficial.

There has been one reported case of massive overdosage with tablets of another extended release formulation of nifedipine. The main effects of ingestion of approximately 4800 mg of nifedipine in a young man attempting suicide as a result of cocaine-induced depression was initial dizziness, palpitations, flushing, and nervousness. Within several hours of ingestion, nausea, vomiting, and generalized edema developed. No significant hypotension was apparent at presentation, 18 hours post ingestion. Blood chemistry abnormalities consisted of a mild, transient elevation of serum creatinine, and modest elevations of LDH and CPK, but normal SGOT. Vital signs remained stable, no electrocardiographic abnormalities were noted and renal function returned to normal within 24 to 48 hours with routine supportive measures alone. No prolonged sequelae were observed.

The effect of a single 900 mg ingestion of nifedipine capsules in a depressed anginal patient on tricyclic antidepressants was loss of consciousness within 30 minutes of ingestion, and profound hypotension, which responded to calcium infusion, pressor agents, and fluid replacement. A variety of ECG abnormalities were seen in this patient with a history of bundle branch block, including sinus bradycardia and varying degrees of AV block. These dictated the prophylactic placement of a temporary ventricular pacemaker, but otherwise resolved spontaneously. Significant hyperglycemia was seen initially in this patient, but plasma glucose levels rapidly normalized without further treatment.

A young hypertensive patient with advanced renal failure ingested 280 mg of nifedipine capsules at one time, with resulting marked hypotension responding to calcium infusion and fluids. No AV conduction abnormalities, arrhythmias, or pronounced changes in heart rate were noted, nor was there any further deterioration in renal function.

DOSAGE AND ADMINISTRATION

Dosage should be adjusted according to each patient's needs. It is recommended that ADALAT CC be administered orally once daily on an empty stomach. ADALAT CC is an extended release dosage form and tablets should be swallowed whole, not bitten or divided. In general, titration should proceed over a 7-14 day period starting with 30 mg once daily. Upward titration should be based on therapeutic efficacy and safety. The usual maintenance dose is 30 mg to 60 mg once daily. Titration to doses above 90 mg daily is not recommended.

If discontinuation of ADALAT CC is necessary, sound clinical practice suggests that the dosage should be decreased gradually with close physician supervision.

Co-administration of nifedipine with grapefruit juice is to be avoided (See **CLINICAL PHARMACOLOGY** and **PRECAUTIONS**).

Care should be taken when dispensing ADALAT CC to assure that the extended release dosage form has been prescribed.

HOW SUPPLIED

ADALAT CC extended release tablets are supplied as 30 mg, 60 mg, and 90 mg round film coated tablets. The different strengths can be identified as follows:

Strength	Color	Markings
30 mg	Pink	30 on one side and ADALAT CC on the other side
60 mg	Salmon	60 on one side and ADALAT CC on the other side
90 mg	Dark Red	90 on one side and ADALAT CC on the other side

ADALAT® CC Tablets are supplied in:

	Strength	NDC Code
Bottles of 100	30 mg	0026-8841-51
	60 mg	0026-8851-51
	90 mg	0026-8861-51
Unit Dose Packages of 100	30 mg	0026-8841-48
	60 mg	0026-8851-48
	90 mg	0026-8861-48

The tablets should be protected from light and moisture and stored below 86°F (30°C). Dispense in tight, light-resistant containers.

Bayer HealthCare
Bayer Pharmaceuticals Corporation
400 Morgan Lane
West Haven, CT 06516
Made in Germany

℞ Only

08753752, R.2 1/04 12220 Printed in USA

Shown in Product Identification Guide, page 307

AVELOX® ℞
[*ă'vĕ-lŏks*]
(moxifloxacin hydrochloride) Tablets
AVELOX® I.V.
(moxifloxacin hydrochloride in sodium chloride injection)

To reduce the development of drug-resistant bacteria and maintain the effectiveness of AVELOX® and other antibacterial drugs, AVELOX should be used only to treat or prevent infections that are proven or strongly suspected to be caused by bacteria.

DESCRIPTION

AVELOX (moxifloxacin hydrochloride) is a synthetic broad spectrum antibacterial agent and is available as AVELOX Tablets for oral administration and as AVELOX I.V. for intravenous administration. Moxifloxacin, a fluoroquinolone, is available as the monohydrochloride salt of 1-cyclopropyl-7-[(S,S)-2,8-diazabicyclo[4.3.0]non-8-yl]-6-fluoro-8-methoxy-1,4-dihydro-4-oxo-3 quinoline carboxylic acid. It is a slightly yellow to yellow crystalline substance with a molecular weight of 437.9. Its empirical formula is $C_{21}H_{24}FN_3O_4$ *HCl and its chemical structure is as follows:

AVELOX Tablets are available as film-coated tablets containing moxifloxacin hydrochloride (equivalent to 400 mg moxifloxacin). The inactive ingredients are microcrystalline cellulose, lactose monohydrate, croscarmellose sodium, magnesium stearate, hypromellose, titanium dioxide, polyethylene glycol and ferric oxide.

AVELOX I.V. is available in ready-to-use 250 mL latex-free flexibags as a sterile, preservative free, 0.8% sodium chloride aqueous solution of moxifloxacin hydrochloride (containing 400 mg moxifloxacin) with pH ranging from 4.1 to 4.6. The appearance of the intravenous solution is yellow. The color does not affect, nor is it indicative of, product stability. The inactive ingredients are sodium chloride, USP, water for Injection, USP, and may include hydrochloric acid and/or sodium hydroxide for pH adjustment.

CLINICAL PHARMACOLOGY

Absorption

Moxifloxacin, given as an oral tablet, is well absorbed from the gastrointestinal tract. The absolute bioavailability of moxifloxacin is approximately 90 percent. Co-administration with a high fat meal (i.e., 500 calories from fat) does not affect the absorption of moxifloxacin.

Consumption of 1 cup of yogurt with moxifloxacin does not significantly affect the extent or rate of systemic absorption (AUC).

The mean (± SD) C_{max} and AUC values following single and multiple doses of 400 mg moxifloxacin given orally are summarized below.

[See first table below]

The mean (± SD) C_{max} and AUC values following single and multiple doses of 400 mg moxifloxacin given by 1 hour I.V. infusion are summarized below.

[See second table below]

Plasma concentrations increase proportionally with dose up to the highest dose tested (1200 mg single oral dose). The mean (± SD) elimination half-life from plasma is 12 ± 1.3 hours; steady-state is achieved after at least three days with a 400 mg once daily regimen.

Mean Steady-State Plasma Concentrations of Moxifloxacin Obtained With Once Daily Dosing of 400 mg Either Orally (n=10) or by I.V. Infusion (n=12)

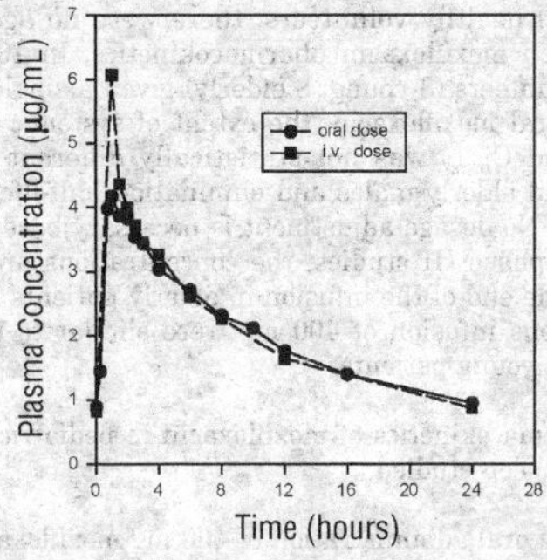

Distribution

Moxifloxacin is approximately 50% bound to serum proteins, independent of drug concentration. The volume of distribution of moxifloxacin ranges from 1.7 to 2.7 L/kg. Moxifloxacin is widely distributed throughout the body, with tissue concentrations often exceeding plasma concentrations. Moxifloxacin has been detected in the saliva, nasal and bronchial secretions, mucosa of the sinuses, skin blister fluid, and subcutaneous tissue, and skeletal muscle following oral or intravenous administration of 400 mg. Concentrations measured at 3 hours post-dose are summarized in the following table. The rates of elimination of moxifloxacin from tissues generally parallel the elimination from plasma.

[See table at top of next page]

Metabolism

Approximately 52% of an oral or intravenous dose of moxifloxacin is metabolized via glucuronide and sulfate conjugation. The cytochrome P450 system is not involved in moxifloxacin metabolism, and is not affected by moxifloxacin. The sulfate conjugate (M1) accounts for approximately 38% of the dose, and is eliminated primarily in the feces. Approximately 14% of an oral or intravenous dose is converted to a glucuronide conjugate (M2), which is excreted exclusively in the urine. Peak plasma concentrations of M2 are approximately 40% those of the parent drug, while plasma concentrations of M1 are generally less than 10% those of moxifloxacin.

In vitro studies with cytochrome (CYP) P450 enzymes indicate that moxifloxacin does not inhibit CYP3A4, CYP2D6, CYP2C9, CYP2C19, or CYP1A2, suggesting that moxifloxacin is unlikely to alter the pharmacokinetics of drugs metabolized by these enzymes.

Excretion

Approximately 45% of an oral or intravenous dose of moxifloxacin is excreted as unchanged drug (~20% in urine and ~25% in feces). A total of 96% ± 4% of an oral dose is ex-

Continued on next page

	C_{max} (mg/L)	AUC (mg•h/L)	Half-life (hr)
Single Dose Oral			
Healthy (n = 372)	3.1 ± 1.0	36.1 ± 9.1	11.5 – 15.6*
Multiple Dose Oral			
Healthy young male/female (n = 15)	4.5 ± 0.5	48.0 ± 2.7	12.7 ± 1.9
Healthy elderly male (n = 8)	3.8 ± 0.3	51.8 ± 6.7	
Healthy elderly female (n = 8)	4.6 ± 0.6	54.6 ± 6.7	
Healthy young male (n = 8)	3.6 ± 0.5	48.2 ± 9.0	
Healthy young female (n = 9)	4.2 ± 0.5	49.3 ± 9.5	

*Range of means from different studies

	C_{max} (mg/L)	AUC (mg•h/L)	Half-life (hr)
Single Dose I.V.			
Healthy young male/female (n = 56)	3.9 ± 0.9	39.3 ± 8.6	8.2 – 15.4*
Patients (n = 118)			
Male (n = 64)	4.4 ± 3.7		
Female (n = 54)	4.5 ± 2.0		
< 65 years (n = 58)	4.6 ± 4.2		
≥ 65 years (n = 60)	4.3 ± 1.3		
Multiple Dose I.V.			
Healthy young male (n = 8)	4.2 ± 0.8	38.0 ± 4.7	14.8 ± 2.2
Healthy elderly (n = 12; 8 male, 4 female)	6.1 ± 1.3	48.2 ± 0.9	10.1 ± 1.6
Patients** (n = 107)			
Male (n = 58)	4.2 ± 2.6		
Female (n = 49)	4.6 ± 1.5		
< 65 years (n = 52)	4.1 ± 1.4		
≥ 65 years (n = 55)	4.7 ± 2.7		

* Range of means from different studies
**Expected C_{max} (concentration obtained around the time of the end of the infusion)

Avelox—Cont.

creted as either unchanged drug or known metabolites. The mean (± SD) apparent total body clearance and renal clearance are 12 ± 2.0 L/hr and 2.6 ± 0.5 L/hr, respectively.

Special Populations

Geriatric

Following oral administration of 400 mg moxifloxacin for 10 days in 16 elderly (8 male; 8 female) and 17 young (8 male; 9 female) healthy volunteers, there were no age-related changes in moxifloxacin pharmacokinetics. In 16 healthy male volunteers (8 young; 8 elderly) given a single 200 mg dose of oral moxifloxacin, the extent of systemic exposure (AUC and C_{max}) was not statistically different between young and elderly males and elimination half-life was unchanged. No dosage adjustment is necessary based on age. In large phase III studies, the concentrations around the time of the end of the infusion in elderly patients following intravenous infusion of 400 mg were similar to those observed in young patients.

Pediatric

The pharmacokinetics of moxifloxacin in pediatric subjects have not been studied.

Gender

Following oral administration of 400 mg moxifloxacin daily for 10 days to 23 healthy males (19–75 years) and 24 healthy females (19–70 years), the mean AUC and C_{max} were 8% and 16% higher, respectively, in females compared to males. There are no significant differences in moxifloxacin pharmacokinetics between male and female subjects when differences in body weight are taken into consideration.

A 400 mg single dose study was conducted in 18 young males and females. The comparison of moxifloxacin pharmacokinetics in this study (9 young females and 9 young males) showed no differences in AUC or C_{max} due to gender. Dosage adjustments based on gender are not necessary.

Race

Steady-state moxifloxacin pharmacokinetics in male Japanese subjects were similar to those determined in Caucasians, with a mean C_{max} of 4.1 μg/mL, an AUC_{24} of 47 μg•h/mL, and an elimination half-life of 14 hours, following 400 mg p.o. daily.

Renal Insufficiency

The pharmacokinetic parameters of moxifloxacin are not significantly altered in mild, moderate, severe, or end-stage renal disease. No dosage adjustment is necessary in patients with renal impairment, including those patients requiring hemodialysis (HD) or continuous ambulatory peritoneal dialysis (CAPD).

In a single oral dose study of 24 patients with varying degrees of renal function from normal to severely impaired, the mean peak concentrations (C_{max}) of moxifloxacin were reduced by 21% and 28% in the patients with moderate ($CL_{CR} \geq 30$ and ≤ 60 mL/min) and severe ($CL_{CR} < 30$ mL/min) renal impairment, respectively. The mean systemic exposure (AUC) in these patients was increased by 13%. In the moderate and severe renally impaired patients, the mean AUC for the sulfate conjugate (M1) increased by 1.7-fold (ranging up to 2.8-fold) and mean AUC and C_{max} for the glucuronide conjugate (M2) increased by 2.8-fold (ranging up to 4.8-fold) and 1.4-fold (ranging up to 2.5-fold), respectively.

The pharmacokinetics of single dose and multiple dose moxifloxacin were studied in patients with $CL_{CR} < 20$ mL/min on either hemodialysis or continuous ambulatory peritoneal dialysis (8 HD, 8 CAPD). Following a single 400 mg oral dose, the AUC of moxifloxacin in these HD and CAPD patients did not vary significantly from the AUC generally found in healthy volunteers. C_{max} values of moxifloxacin were reduced by about 45% and 33% in HD and CAPD patients, respectively, compared to healthy, historical controls. The exposure (AUC) to the sulfate conjugate (M1) increased by 1.4- to 1.5-fold in these patients. The mean AUC of the glucuronide conjugate (M2) increased by a factor of 7.5, whereas the mean C_{max} values of the glucuronide conjugate (M2) increased by a factor of 2.5 to 3, compared to healthy subjects. The sulfate and the glucuronide conjugates of moxifloxacin are not microbiologically active, and the clinical implication of increased exposure to these metabolites in patients with renal disease including those undergoing HD and CAPD has not been studied.

Oral administration of 400 mg QD moxifloxacin for 7 days to patients on HD or CAPD produced mean systemic exposure (AUC_{ss}) to moxifloxacin similar to that generally seen in healthy volunteers. Steady-state C_{max} values were about 22% lower in HD patients but were comparable between CAPD patients and healthy volunteers. Both HD and CAPD removed only small amounts of moxifloxacin from the body (approximately 9% by HD, and 3% by CAPD). HD and CAPD also removed about 4% and 2% of the glucuronide metabolite (M2), respectively.

Hepatic Insufficiency

In 400 mg single oral dose studies in 6 patients with mild (Child Pugh Class A), and 10 patients with moderate (Child Pugh Class B), hepatic insufficiency, moxifloxacin mean systemic exposure (AUC) was 78% and 102%, respectively, of 18 healthy controls and mean peak concentration (C_{max}) was 79% and 84% of controls.

The mean AUC of the sulfate conjugate of moxifloxacin (M1) increased by 3.9-fold (ranging up to 5.9-fold) and 5.7-fold (ranging up to 8.0-fold) in the mild and moderate groups, respectively. The mean C_{max} of M1 increased by approximately 3-fold in both groups (ranging up to 4.7- and 3.9-fold). The mean AUC of the glucuronide conjugate of moxifloxacin (M2) increased by 1.5-fold (ranging up to 2.5-fold) in both groups. The mean C_{max} of M2 increased by 1.6- and 1.3-fold (ranging up to 2.7- and 2.1-fold), respectively. The clinical significance of increased exposure to the sulfate and glucuronide conjugates has not been studied. No dosage adjustment is recommended for mild or moderate hepatic insufficiency (Child Pugh Classes A and B). The pharmacokinetics of moxifloxacin in severe hepatic insufficiency (Child Pugh Class C) have not been studied. (See **DOSAGE AND ADMINISTRATION**.)

Moxifloxacin Concentrations (mean ± SD) After Oral Dosing in Plasma and Tissues Measured 3 Hours After Dosing with 400 mg[§]

Tissue or Fluid	N	Plasma Concentration (μg/mL)	Tissue or Fluid Concentration (μg/mL or μg/g)	Tissue Plasma Ratio:
Respiratory				
Alveolar Macrophages	5	3.3 ± 0.7	61.8 ± 27.3	21.2 ± 10.0
Bronchial Mucosa	8	3.3 ± 0.7	5.5 ± 1.3	1.7 ± 0.3
Epithelial Lining Fluid	5	3.3 ± 0.7	24.4 ± 14.7	8.7 ± 6.1
Sinus				
Maxillary Sinus Mucosa	4	3.7 ± 1.1†	7.6 ± 1.7	2.0 ± 0.3
Anterior Ethmoid Mucosa	3	3.7 ± 1.1†	8.8 ± 4.3	2.2 ± 0.6
Nasal Polyps	4	3.7 ± 1.1†	9.8 ± 4.5	2.6 ± 0.6

§ all moxifloxacin concentrations were measured after a single 400 mg dose, except the sinus concentrations which were measured after 5 days of dosing.
†N = 5

Photosensitivity Potential

A study of the skin response to ultraviolet (UVA and UVB) and visible radiation conducted in 32 healthy volunteers (8 per group) demonstrated that moxifloxacin does not show phototoxicity in comparison to placebo. The minimum erythematous dose (MED) was measured before and after treatment with moxifloxacin (200 mg or 400 mg once daily), lomefloxacin (400 mg once daily), or placebo. In this study, the MED measured for both doses of moxifloxacin were not significantly different from placebo, while lomefloxacin significantly lowered the MED. (See **PRECAUTIONS, Information for Patients.**)

Drug-drug Interactions

The potential for pharmacokinetic drug interactions between moxifloxacin and itraconazole, theophylline, warfarin, digoxin, atenolol, probenecid, morphine, oral contraceptives, ranitidine, glyburide, calcium, iron, and antacids has been evaluated. There was no clinically significant effect of moxifloxacin on itraconazole, theophylline, warfarin, digoxin, atenolol, oral contraceptives, or glyburide kinetics. Itraconazole, theophylline, warfarin, digoxin, probenecid, morphine, ranitidine, and calcium did not significantly affect the pharmacokinetics of moxifloxacin. These results and the data from *in vitro* studies suggest that moxifloxacin is unlikely to significantly alter the metabolic clearance of drugs metabolized by CYP3A4, CYP2D6, CYP2C9, CYP2C19, or CYP1A2 enzymes.

As with all other quinolones, iron and antacids significantly reduced bioavailability of moxifloxacin.

Itraconazole: In a study involving 11 healthy volunteers, there was no significant effect of itraconazole (200 mg once daily for 9 days), a potent inhibitor of cytochrome P4503A4, on the pharmacokinetics of moxifloxacin (a single 400 mg dose given on the 7th day of itraconazole dosing). In addition, moxifloxacin was shown not to affect the pharmacokinetics of itraconazole.

Theophylline: No significant effect of moxifloxacin (200 mg every twelve hours for 3 days) on the pharmacokinetics of theophylline (400 mg every twelve hours for 3 days) was detected in a study involving 12 healthy volunteers. In addition, theophylline was not shown to affect the pharmacokinetics of moxifloxacin. The effect of co-administration of a 400 mg dose of moxifloxacin with theophylline has not been studied, but it is not expected to be clinically significant based on *in vitro* metabolic data showing that moxifloxacin does not inhibit the CYP1A2 isoenzyme.

Warfarin: No significant effect of moxifloxacin (400 mg once daily for eight days) on the pharmacokinetics of R- and S-warfarin (25 mg single dose of warfarin sodium on the fifth day) was detected in a study involving 24 healthy volunteers. No significant change in prothrombin time was observed. (See **PRECAUTIONS, Drug Interactions.**)

Digoxin: No significant effect of moxifloxacin (400 mg once daily for two days) on digoxin (0.6 mg as a single dose) AUC was detected in a study involving 12 healthy volunteers. The mean digoxin C_{max} increased by about 50% during the distribution phase of digoxin. This transient increase in digoxin C_{max} is not viewed to be clinically significant. Moxifloxacin pharmacokinetics were similar in the presence or absence of digoxin. No dosage adjustment for moxifloxacin or digoxin is required when these drugs are administered concomitantly.

Atenolol: In a crossover study involving 24 healthy volunteers (12 male; 12 female), the mean atenolol AUC following a single oral dose of 50 mg atenolol with placebo was similar to that observed when atenolol was given concomitantly with a single 400 mg oral dose of moxifloxacin. The mean C_{max} of single dose atenolol decreased by about 10% following co-administration with a single dose of moxifloxacin.

Morphine: No significant effect of morphine sulfate (a single 10 mg intramuscular dose) on the mean AUC and C_{max} of moxifloxacin (400 mg single dose) was observed in a study of 20 healthy male and female volunteers.

Oral Contraceptives: A placebo-controlled study in 29 healthy female subjects showed that moxifloxacin 400 mg daily for 7 days did not interfere with the hormonal suppression of oral contraception with 0.15 mg levonorgestrel/0.03 mg ethinylestradiol (as measured by serum progesterone, FSH, estradiol, and LH), or with the pharmacokinetics of the administered contraceptive agents.

Probenecid: Probenecid (500 mg twice daily for two days) did not alter the renal clearance and total amount of moxifloxacin (400 mg single dose) excreted renally in a study of 12 healthy volunteers.

Ranitidine: No significant effect of ranitidine (150 mg twice daily for three days as pretreatment) on the pharmacokinetics of moxifloxacin (400 mg single dose) was detected in a study involving 10 healthy volunteers.

Antidiabetic agents: In diabetics, glyburide (2.5 mg once daily for two weeks pretreatment and for five days concurrently) mean AUC and C_{max} were 12% and 21% lower, respectively, when taken with moxifloxacin (400 mg once daily for five days) in comparison to placebo. Nonetheless, blood glucose levels were decreased slightly in patients taking glyburide and moxifloxacin in comparison to those taking glyburide alone, suggesting no interference by moxifloxacin on the activity of glyburide. These interaction results are not viewed as clinically significant.

Calcium: Twelve healthy volunteers were administered concomitant moxifloxacin (single 400 mg dose) and calcium (single dose of 500 mg Ca^{++} dietary supplement) followed by an additional two doses of calcium 12 and 24 hours after moxifloxacin administration. Calcium had no significant effect on the mean AUC of moxifloxacin. The mean C_{max} was slightly reduced and the time to maximum plasma concentration was prolonged when moxifloxacin was given with calcium compared to when moxifloxacin was given alone (2.5 hours versus 0.9 hours). These differences are not considered to be clinically significant.

Antacids: When moxifloxacin (single 400 mg tablet dose) was administered two hours before, concomitantly, or 4 hours after an aluminum/magnesium-containing antacid (900 mg aluminum hydroxide and 600 mg magnesium hydroxide as a single oral dose) to 12 healthy volunteers there was a 26%, 60% and 23% reduction in the mean AUC of moxifloxacin, respectively. Moxifloxacin should be taken at least 4 hours before or 8 hours after antacids containing magnesium or aluminum, as well as sucralfate, metal cations such as iron, and multivitamin preparations with zinc, or VIDEX® (didanosine) chewable/buffered tablets or the pediatric powder for oral solution. (See **PRECAUTIONS, Drug Interactions** and **DOSAGE AND ADMINISTRATION.**)

Iron: When moxifloxacin tablets were administered concomitantly with iron (ferrous sulfate 100 mg once daily for two days), the mean AUC and C_{max} of moxifloxacin was reduced by 39% and 59%, respectively. Moxifloxacin should only be taken more than 4 hours before or 8 hours after iron products. (See **PRECAUTIONS, Drug Interactions** and **DOSAGE AND ADMINISTRATION.**)

Electrocardiogram: Prolongation of the QT interval in the ECG has been observed in some patients receiving moxifloxacin. Following oral dosing with 400 mg of moxifloxacin the mean (± SD) change in QTc from the pre-dose value at the time of maximum drug concentration was 6 msec (± 26) (n = 787). Following a course of daily intravenous dosing (400 mg; 1 hour infusion each day) the mean change in QTc from the Day 1 pre-dose value was 9 msec (± 24) on Day 1 (n = 69) and 3 msec (± 29) on Day 3 (n = 290). (See **WARNINGS.**)

There is limited information available on the potential for a pharmacodynamic interaction in humans between moxifloxacin and other drugs that prolong the QTc interval of the electrocardiogram. Sotalol, a Class III antiarrhythmic, has been shown to further increase the QTc interval when combined with high doses of intravenous (I.V.) moxifloxacin in dogs. Therefore, moxifloxacin should be avoided with Class IA and Class III antiarrhythmics. (See **ANIMAL PHARMACOLOGY, WARNINGS,** and **PRECAUTIONS.**)

MICROBIOLOGY

Moxifloxacin has *in vitro* activity against a wide range of Gram-positive and Gram-negative microorganisms. The bactericidal action of moxifloxacin results from inhibition of the topoisomerase II (DNA gyrase) and topoisomerase IV required for bacterial DNA replication, transcription, repair, and recombination. It appears that the C8-methoxy moiety contributes to enhanced activity and lower selection of resistant mutants of Gram-positive bacteria compared to the C8-H moiety. The presence of the bulky bicycloamine substituent at the C-7 position prevents active efflux, associated with the *NorA* or *pmrA* genes seen in certain Gram-positive bacteria.

The mechanism of action for quinolones, including moxifloxacin, is different from that of macrolides, beta-lactams, aminoglycosides, or tetracyclines; therefore, microorganisms resistant to these classes of drugs may be susceptible to moxifloxacin and other quinolones. There is no known cross-resistance between moxifloxacin and other classes of antimicrobials.

In vitro resistance to moxifloxacin develops slowly via multiple-step mutations. Resistance to moxifloxacin occurs *in vitro* at a general frequency of between 1.8×10^{-9} to $< 1 \times 10^{-11}$ for Gram-positive bacteria.

Cross-resistance has been observed between moxifloxacin and other fluoroquinolones against Gram-negative bacteria. Gram-positive bacteria resistant to other fluoroquinolones may, however, still be susceptible to moxifloxacin.

Moxifloxacin has been shown to be active against most strains of the following microorganisms, both *in vitro* and in clinical infections as described in the **INDICATIONS AND USAGE** section.

Aerobic Gram-positive microorganisms

Staphylococcus aureus (methicillin-susceptible strains only)
Streptococcus pneumoniae (including multi-drug resistant strains [MDRSP]*)
Streptococcus pyogenes

* MDRSP, Multi-drug resistant *Streptococcus pneumoniae* includes isolates previously known as PRSP (Penicillin-resistant *S. pneumoniae*), and are strains resistant to two or more of the following antibiotics: penicillin (MIC ≥ 2 μg/mL 2nd generation cephalosporins (e.g., cefuroxime), macrolides, tetracyclines, and trimethoprim/sulfamethoxazole.

Aerobic Gram-negative microorganisms

Haemophilus influenzae
Haemophilus parainfluenzae
Klebsiella pneumoniae
Moraxella catarrhalis

Other microorganisms

Chlamydia pneumoniae
Mycoplasma pneumoniae

The following *in vitro* data are available, **but their clinical significance is unknown.**

Moxifloxacin exhibits *in vitro* minimum inhibitory concentrations (MICs) of 2 μg/mL or less against most (≥ 90%) strains of the following microorganisms; however, the safety and effectiveness of moxifloxacin in treating clinical infections due to these microorganisms have not been established in adequate and well-controlled clinical trials.

Aerobic Gram-positive microorganisms

Staphylococcus epidermidis (methicillin-susceptible strains only)
Streptococcus agalactiae
Streptococcus viridans group

Aerobic Gram-negative microorganisms

Citrobacter freundii
Enterobacter cloacae
Escherichia coli
Klebsiella oxytoca
Legionella pneumophila
Proteus mirabilis

Anaerobic microorganisms

Fusobacterium species
Peptostreptococcus species
Prevotella species

Susceptibility Tests

Dilution Techniques: Quantitative methods are used to determine antimicrobial minimum inhibitory concentrations (MICs). These MICs provide estimates of the susceptibility of bacteria to antimicrobial compounds. The MICs should be determined using a standardized procedure. Standardized procedures are based on a dilution method[1] (broth or agar) or equivalent with standardized inoculum concentrations and standardized concentrations of moxifloxacin powder. The MIC values should be interpreted according to the following criteria:

For testing Enterobacteriaceae and *Staphylococcus* species:

MIC (μg/mL)	Interpretation	
≤ 2.0	Susceptible	(S)
4.0	Intermediate	(I)
≥ 8.0	Resistant	(R)

For testing *Haemophilus influenzae* and *Haemophilus parainfluenzae*[a]:

MIC (μg/mL)	Interpretation	
≤ 1.0	Susceptible	(S)

[a] This interpretive standard is applicable only to broth microdilution susceptibility tests with *Haemophilus influenzae* and *Haemophilus parainfluenzae* using *Haemophilus* Test Medium[1].

The current absence of data on resistant strains precludes defining any results other than "Susceptible". Strains yielding MIC results suggestive of a "nonsusceptible" category should be submitted to a reference laboratory for further testing.

For testing *Streptococcus* species including *Streptococcus pneumoniae*[b]:

MIC (μg/mL)	Interpretation	
≤ 1.0	Susceptible	(S)
2.0	Intermediate	(I)
≥ 4.0	Resistant	(R)

[b] This interpretive standard is applicable only to broth microdilution susceptibility tests using cation-adjusted Mueller-Hinton broth with 2–5% lysed horse blood.

A report of "Susceptible" indicates that the pathogen is likely to be inhibited if the antimicrobial compound in the blood reaches the concentrations usually achievable. A report of "Intermediate" indicates that the result should be considered equivocal, and, if the microorganism is not fully susceptible to alternative, clinically feasible drugs, the test should be repeated. This category implies possible clinical applicability in body sites where the drug is physiologically concentrated or in situations where a high dosage of drug can be used. This category also provides a buffer zone which prevents small uncontrolled technical factors from causing major discrepancies in interpretation. A report of "Resistant" indicates that the pathogen is not likely to be inhibited if the antimicrobial compound in the blood reaches the concentrations usually achievable; other therapy should be selected.

Standardized susceptibility test procedures require the use of laboratory control microorganisms to control the technical aspects of the laboratory procedures. Standard moxifloxacin powder should provide the following MIC values:

Microorganism		MIC (μg/mL)
Enterococcus faecalis	ATCC 29212	0.06–0.5
Escherichia coli	ATCC 25922	0.008–0.06
Haemophilus influenzae	ATCC 49247[c]	0.008–0.03
Staphylococcus aureus	ATCC 29213	0.015–0.06
Streptococcus pneumoniae	ATCC 49619[d]	0.06–0.25

[c] This quality control range is applicable to only *H. influenzae* ATCC 49247 tested by a broth microdilution procedure using *Haemophilus* Test Medium (HTM)[1].
[d] This quality control range is applicable to only *S. pneumoniae* ATCC 49619 tested by a broth microdilution procedure using cation-adjusted Mueller-Hinton broth with 2–5% lysed horse blood.

Diffusion Techniques: Quantitative methods that require measurement of zone diameters also provide reproducible estimates of the susceptibility of bacteria to antimicrobial compounds. One such standardized procedure[2] requires the use of standardized inoculum concentrations. This procedure uses paper disks impregnated with 5-μg moxifloxacin to test the susceptibility of microorganisms to moxifloxacin. Reports from the laboratory providing results of the standard single-disk susceptibility test with a 5-μg moxifloxacin disk should be interpreted according to the following criteria:

The following zone diameter interpretive criteria should be used for testing Enterobacteriaceae and *Staphylococcus* species:

Zone Diameter (mm)	Interpretation	
≥ 19	Susceptible	(S)
16–18	Intermediate	(I)
≤ 15	Resistant	(R)

For testing *Haemophilus influenzae* and *Haemophilus parainfluenzae*[e]:

Zone Diameter (mm)	Interpretation	
≥ 18	Susceptible	(S)

[e] This zone diameter standard is applicable only to tests with *Haemophilus influenzae* and *Haemophilus parainfluenzae* using *Haemophilus* Test Medium (HTM)[2].

The current absence of data on resistant strains precludes defining any results other than "Susceptible". Strains yielding zone diameter results suggestive of a "nonsusceptible" category should be submitted to a reference laboratory for further testing.

For testing *Streptococcus* species including *Streptococcus pneumoniae*[f]:

Zone Diameter (mm)	Interpretation	
≥ 18	Susceptible	(S)
15–17	Intermediate	(I)
≤ 14	Resistant	(R)

[f] These interpretive standards are applicable only to disk diffusion tests using Mueller-Hinton agar supplemented with 5% sheep blood incubated in 5% CO_2.

Interpretation should be as stated above for results using dilution techniques. Interpretation involves correlation of the diameter obtained in the disk test with the MIC for moxifloxacin.

As with standardized dilution techniques, diffusion methods require the use of laboratory control microorganisms that are used to control the technical aspects of the laboratory procedures. For the diffusion technique, the 5-μg moxifloxacin disk should provide the following zone diameters in these laboratory test quality control strains:

Microorganism		Zone Diameter (mm)
Escherichia coli	ATCC 25922	28–35
Haemophilus influenzae	ATCC 49247[g]	31–39
Staphylococcus aureus	ATCC 25923	28–35
Streptococcus pneumoniae	ATCC 49619[h]	25–31

[g] These quality control limits are applicable to only *H. influenzae* ATCC 49247 testing using *Haemophilus* Test Medium (HTM)[2].
[h] These quality control limits are applicable only to tests conducted with *S. pneumoniae* ATCC 49619 performed by disk diffusion using Mueller-Hinton agar supplemented with 5% defibrinated sheep blood.

INDICATIONS AND USAGE

AVELOX Tablets and I.V. are indicated for the treatment of adults (≥ 18 years of age) with infections caused by susceptible strains of the designated microorganisms in the conditions listed below. (See **DOSAGE AND ADMINISTRATION** for specific recommendations. In addition, for I.V. use see **PRECAUTIONS, Geriatric Use.**)

Acute Bacterial Sinusitis caused by *Streptococcus pneumoniae, Haemophilus influenzae,* or *Moraxella catarrhalis.*

Acute Bacterial Exacerbation of Chronic Bronchitis caused by *Streptococcus pneumoniae, Haemophilus influenzae, Haemophilus parainfluenzae, Klebsiella pneumoniae, Staphylococcus aureus,* or *Moraxella catarrhalis.*

Community Acquired Pneumonia caused by *Streptococcus pneumoniae* (including multi-drug resistant strains*), *Haemophilus influenzae, Moraxella catarrhalis, Staphylococcus aureus, Klebsiella pneumoniae, Mycoplasma pneumoniae,* or *Chlamydia pneumoniae.*

* MDRSP, Multi-drug resistant *Streptococcus pneumoniae* includes isolates previously known as PRSP (Penicillin-resistant *S. pneumoniae*), and are strains resistant to two or more of the following antibiotics: penicillin (MIC ≥ 2 μg/mL), 2nd generation cephalosporins (e.g., cefuroxime), macrolides, tetracyclines, and trimethoprim/sulfamethoxazole.

Uncomplicated Skin and Skin Structure Infections caused by *Staphylococcus aureus* or *Streptococcus pyogenes.*

Appropriate culture and susceptibility tests should be performed before treatment in order to isolate and identify organisms causing infection and to determine their susceptibility to moxifloxacin. Therapy with AVELOX may be initiated before results of these tests are known; once results become available, appropriate therapy should be continued.

To reduce the development of drug-resistant bacteria and maintain the effectiveness of AVELOX and other antibacterial drugs, AVELOX should be used only to treat or prevent infections that are proven or strongly suspected to be caused by susceptible bacteria. When culture and susceptibility information are available, they should be considered in selecting or modifying antibacterial therapy. In the absence of such data, local epidemiology and susceptibility patterns may contribute to the empiric selection of therapy.

CONTRAINDICATIONS

Moxifloxacin is contraindicated in persons with a history of hypersensitivity to moxifloxacin or any member of the quinolone class of antimicrobial agents.

WARNINGS

THE SAFETY AND EFFECTIVENESS OF MOXIFLOXACIN IN PEDIATRIC PATIENTS, ADOLESCENTS (LESS THAN 18 YEARS OF AGE), PREGNANT WOMEN, AND LACTATING WOMEN HAVE NOT BEEN ESTABLISHED. (SEE PRECAUTIONS-PEDIATRIC USE, PREGNANCY AND NURSING MOTHERS SUBSECTIONS.)

Moxifloxacin has been shown to prolong the QT interval of the electrocardiogram in some patients. The drug should be avoided in patients with known prolongation of the QT interval, patients with uncorrected hypokalemia and patients receiving Class IA (e.g., quinidine, procainamide) or Class III (e.g. amiodarone, sotalol) antiarrhythmic agents, due to the lack of clinical experience with the drug in these patient populations.

Continued on next page

Avelox—Cont.

Pharmacokinetic studies between moxifloxacin and other drugs that prolong the QT interval such as cisapride, erythromycin, antipsychotics, and tricyclic antidepressants have not been performed. An additive effect of moxifloxacin and these drugs cannot be excluded, therefore caution should be exercised when moxifloxacin is given concurrently with these drugs. In premarketing clinical trials, the rate of cardiovascular adverse events was similar in 798 moxifloxacin and 702 comparator treated patients who received concomitant therapy with drugs known to prolong the QTc interval. Moxifloxacin should be used with caution in patients with ongoing proarrhythmic conditions, such as clinically significant bradycardia, acute myocardial ischemia. The magnitude of QT prolongation may increase with increasing concentrations of the drug or increasing rates of infusion of the intravenous formulation. Therefore the recommended dose or infusion rate should not be exceeded. QT prolongation may lead to an increased risk for ventricular arrhythmias including torsade de pointes. No cardiovascular morbidity or mortality attributable to QTc prolongation occurred with moxifloxacin treatment in over 7,900 patients in controlled clinical studies, including 223 patients who were hypokalemic at the start of treatment, and there was no increase in mortality in over 18,000 moxifloxacin tablet treated patients in a post-marketing observational study in which ECGs were not performed. (See **CLINICAL PHARMACOLOGY, Electrocardiogram.** For I.V. use see **DOSAGE AND ADMINISTRATION** and **PRECAUTIONS, Geriatric Use.**)

The oral administration of moxifloxacin caused lameness in immature dogs. Histopathological examination of the weight-bearing joints of these dogs revealed permanent lesions of the cartilage. Related quinolone-class drugs also produce erosions of cartilage of weight-bearing joints and other signs of arthropathy in immature animals of various species. (See **ANIMAL PHARMACOLOGY.**)

Convulsions have been reported in patients receiving quinolones. Quinolones may also cause central nervous system (CNS) events including: dizziness, confusion, tremors, hallucinations, depression, and, rarely, suicidal thoughts or acts. These reactions may occur following the first dose. If these reactions occur in patients receiving moxifloxacin, the drug should be discontinued and appropriate measures instituted. As with all quinolones, moxifloxacin should be used with caution in patients with known or suspected CNS disorders (e.g. severe cerebral arteriosclerosis, epilepsy) or in the presence of other risk factors that may predispose to seizures or lower the seizure threshold. (See **PRECAUTIONS: General, Information for Patients,** and **ADVERSE REACTIONS.**)

Serious anaphylactic reactions, some following the first dose, have been reported in patients receiving quinolone therapy, including moxifloxacin. Some reactions were accompanied by cardiovascular collapse, loss of consciousness, tingling, pharyngeal or facial edema, dyspnea, urticaria, and itching. Serious anaphylactic reactions require immediate emergency treatment with epinephrine. Moxifloxacin should be discontinued at the first appearance of a skin rash or any other sign of hypersensitivity. Oxygen, intravenous steroids, and airway management, including intubation, may be administered as indicated.

Severe and sometimes fatal events, some due to hypersensitivity, and some of uncertain etiology, have been reported in patients receiving therapy with all antibiotics. These events may be severe and generally occur following the administration of multiple doses. Clinical manifestations may include one or more of the following: rash, fever, eosinophilia, jaundice, and hepatic necrosis.

Pseudomembranous colitis has been reported with nearly all antibacterial agents and may range in severity from mild to life-threatening. Therefore, it is important to consider this diagnosis in patients who present with diarrhea subsequent to the administration of antibacterial agents.

Treatment with antibacterial agents alters the normal flora of the colon and may permit overgrowth of clostridia. Studies indicate that a toxin produced by *Clostridium difficile* is one primary cause of "antibiotic-associated colitis." After the diagnosis of pseudomembranous colitis has been established, therapeutic measures should be initiated. Mild cases of pseudomembranous colitis usually respond to drug discontinuation alone. In moderate to severe cases, consideration should be given to management with fluids and electrolytes, protein supplementation, and treatment with an antibacterial drug clinically effective against *C. difficile* colitis.

Peripheral neuropathy: Rare cases of sensory or sensorimotor axonal polyneuropathy affecting small and/or large axons resulting in paresthesias, hypoesthesias, dysesthesias and weakness have been reported in patients receiving quinolones.

Tendon Effects: Ruptures of the shoulder, hand, Achilles tendon or other tendons that required surgical repair or resulted in prolonged disability have been reported in patients receiving quinolones, including moxifloxacin. Post-marketing surveillance reports indicate that this risk may be increased in patients receiving concomitant corticosteroids, especially the elderly. Moxifloxacin should be discontinued if the patient experiences pain, inflammation, or rupture of a tendon. Patients should rest and refrain from exercise until the diagnosis of tendonitis or tendon rupture has been excluded. Tendon rupture can occur during or after therapy with quinolones, including moxifloxacin.

PRECAUTIONS

General: Quinolones may cause central nervous system (CNS) events, including: nervousness, agitation, insomnia, anxiety, nightmares or paranoia. (See **WARNINGS** and **Information for Patients.**)

Prescribing AVELOX in the absence of a proven or strongly suspected bacterial infection or a prophylactic indication is unlikely to provide benefit to the patient and increases the risk of the development of drug-resistant bacteria.

Information for Patients:

To assure safe and effective use of moxifloxacin, the following information and instructions should be communicated to the patient when appropriate:

Patients should be advised:

- that antibacterial drugs including AVELOX should only be used to treat bacterial infections. They do not treat viral infections (e.g., the common cold). When AVELOX is prescribed to treat a bacterial infection, patients should be told that although it is common to feel better early in the course of therapy, the medication should be taken exactly as directed. Skipping doses or not completing the full course of therapy may (1) decrease the effectiveness of the immediate treatment and (2) increase the likelihood that bacteria will develop resistance and will not be treatable by AVELOX or other antibacterial drugs in the future.
- that moxifloxacin may produce changes in the electrocardiogram (QTc interval prolongation).
- that moxifloxacin should be avoided in patients receiving Class IA (e.g. quinidine, procainamide) or Class III (e.g. amiodarone, sotalol) antiarrhythmic agents.
- that moxifloxacin may add to the QTc prolonging effects of other drugs such as cisapride, erythromycin, antipsychotics, and tricyclic antidepressants.
- to inform their physician of any personal or family history of QTc prolongation or proarrhythmic conditions such as recent hypokalemia, significant bradycardia, acute myocardial ischemia.
- to inform their physician of any other medications when taken concurrently with moxifloxacin, including over-the-counter medications.
- to contact their physician if they experience palpitations or fainting spells while taking moxifloxacin.
- that moxifloxacin tablets may be taken with or without meals, and to drink fluids liberally.
- that moxifloxacin tablets should be taken at least 4 hours before or 8 hours after multivitamins (containing iron or zinc), antacids (containing magnesium or aluminum), sucralfate, or VIDEX® (didanosine) chewable/buffered tablets or the pediatric powder for oral solution. (See **CLINICAL PHARMACOLOGY, Drug Interactions** and **PRECAUTIONS, Drug Interactions.**)
- that moxifloxacin may be associated with hypersensitivity reactions, including anaphylactic reactions, even following a single dose, and to discontinue the drug at the first sign of a skin rash or other signs of an allergic reaction.
- to discontinue treatment; rest and refrain from exercise; and inform their physician if they experience pain, inflammation, or rupture of a tendon.
- that moxifloxacin may cause dizziness and lightheadedness; therefore, patients should know how they react to this drug before they operate an automobile or machinery or engage in activities requiring mental alertness or coordination.
- that phototoxicity has been reported in patients receiving certain quinolones. There was no phototoxicity seen with moxifloxacin at the recommended dose. In keeping with good medical practice, avoid excessive sunlight or artificial ultraviolet light (e.g. tanning beds). If sunburn-like reaction or skin eruptions occur, contact your physician. (See **CLINICAL PHARMACOLOGY, Photosensitivity Potential.**)
- that convulsions have been reported in patients receiving quinolones, and they should notify their physician before taking this drug if there is a history of this condition.

Drug Interactions:

Antacids, Sucralfate, Metal Cations, Multivitamins: Quinolones form chelates with alkaline earth and transition metal cations. Oral administration of quinolones with antacids containing aluminum or magnesium, with sucralfate, with metal cations such as iron, or with multivitamins containing iron or zinc, or with formulations containing divalent and trivalent cations such as VIDEX® (didanosine) chewable/buffered tablets or the pediatric powder for oral solution, may substantially interfere with the absorption of quinolones, resulting in systemic concentrations considerably lower than desired. Therefore, moxifloxacin should be taken at least 4 hours before or 8 hours after these agents. (See **CLINICAL PHARMACOLOGY, Drug Interactions** and **DOSAGE AND ADMINISTRATION.**)

No clinically significant drug-drug interactions between itraconazole, theophylline, warfarin, digoxin, atenolol, oral contraceptives or glyburide have been observed with moxifloxacin. Itraconazole, theophylline, digoxin, probenecid, morphine, ranitidine, and calcium have been shown not to significantly alter the pharmacokinetics of moxifloxacin. (See **CLINICAL PHARMACOLOGY.**)

Warfarin: No significant effect of moxifloxacin on R- and S-warfarin was detected in a clinical study involving 24 healthy volunteers. No significant changes in prothrombin time were noted in the presence of moxifloxacin. Quinolones, including moxifloxacin, have been reported to enhance the anticoagulant effects of warfarin or its derivatives in the patient population. In addition, infectious disease and its accompanying inflammatory process, age, and general status of the patient are risk factors for increased anticoagulant activity. Therefore the prothrombin time, International Normalized Ratio (INR), or other suitable anticoagulation tests should be closely monitored if a quinolone is administered concomitantly with warfarin or its derivatives.

Drugs metabolized by Cytochrome P450 enzymes: *In vitro* studies with cytochrome P450 isoenzymes (CYP) indicate that moxifloxacin does not inhibit CYP3A4, CYP2D6, CYP2C9, CYP2C19, or CYP1A2, suggesting that moxifloxacin is unlikely to alter the pharmacokinetics of drugs metabolized by these enzymes (e.g. midazolam, cyclosporine, warfarin, theophylline).

Nonsteroidal anti-inflammatory drugs (NSAIDs): Although not observed with moxifloxacin in preclinical and clinical trials, the concomitant administration of a nonsteroidal anti-inflammatory drug with a quinolone may increase the risks of CNS stimulation and convulsions. (See **WARNINGS.**)

Carcinogenesis, Mutagenesis, Impairment of Fertility:

Long term studies in animals to determine the carcinogenic potential of moxifloxacin have not been performed.

Moxifloxacin was not mutagenic in 4 bacterial strains (TA 98, TA 100, TA 1535, TA 1537) used in the Ames *Salmonella* reversion assay. As with other quinolones, the positive response observed with moxifloxacin in strain TA 102 using the same assay may be due to the inhibition of DNA gyrase. Moxifloxacin was not mutagenic in the CHO/HGPRT mammalian cell gene mutation assay. An equivocal result was obtained in the same assay when v79 cells were used. Moxifloxacin was clastogenic in the v79 chromosome aberration assay, but it did not induce unscheduled DNA synthesis in cultured rat hepatocytes. There was no evidence of genotoxicity *in vivo* in a micronucleus test or a dominant lethal test in mice.

Moxifloxacin had no effect on fertility in male and female rats at oral doses as high as 500 mg/kg/day, approximately 12 times the maximum recommended human dose based on body surface area (mg/m^2), or at intravenous doses as high as 45 mg/kg/day, approximately equal to the maximum recommended human dose based on body surface area (mg/m^2). At 500 mg/kg orally there were slight effects on sperm morphology (head-tail separation) in male rats and on the estrous cycle in female rats.

Pregnancy: Teratogenic Effects. Pregnancy Category C:

Moxifloxacin was not teratogenic when administered to pregnant rats during organogenesis at oral doses as high as 500 mg/kg/day or 0.24 times the maximum recommended human dose based on systemic exposure (AUC), but decreased fetal body weights and slightly delayed fetal skeletal development (indicative of fetotoxicity) were observed. Intravenous administration of 80 mg/kg/day (approximately 2 times the maximum recommended human dose based on body surface area (mg/m^2)) to pregnant rats resulted in maternal toxicity and a marginal effect on fetal and placental weights and the appearance of the placenta. There was no evidence of teratogenicity at intravenous doses as high as 80 mg/kg/day. Intravenous administration of 20 mg/kg/day (approximately equal to the maximum recommended human oral dose based upon systemic exposure) to pregnant rabbits during organogenesis resulted in decreased fetal body weights and delayed fetal skeletal ossification. When rib and vertebral malformations were combined, there was an increased fetal and litter incidence of these effects. Signs of maternal toxicity in rabbits at this dose included mortality, abortions, marked reduction of food consumption, decreased water intake, body weight loss and hypoactivity. There was no evidence of teratogenicity when pregnant Cynomolgus monkeys were given oral doses as high as 100 mg/kg/day (2.5 times the maximum recommended human dose based upon systemic exposure). An increased incidence of smaller fetuses was observed at 100 mg/kg/day. In an oral pre- and postnatal development study conducted in rats, effects observed at 500 mg/kg/day included slight increases in duration of pregnancy and prenatal loss, reduced pup birth weight and decreased neonatal survival. Treatment-related maternal mortality occurred during gestation at 500 mg/kg/day in this study.

Since there are no adequate or well-controlled studies in pregnant women, moxifloxacin should be used during pregnancy only if the potential benefit justifies the potential risk to the fetus.

Nursing Mothers:

Moxifloxacin is excreted in the breast milk of rats. Moxifloxacin may also be excreted in human milk. Because of the potential for serious adverse reactions in infants nursing from mothers taking moxifloxacin, a decision should be made whether to discontinue nursing or to discontinue the drug, taking into account the importance of the drug to the mother.

Pediatric Use:

Safety and effectiveness in pediatric patients and adolescents less than 18 years of age have not been established. Moxifloxacin causes arthropathy in juvenile animals. (See **WARNINGS.**)

Geriatric Use:

In controlled multiple-dose clinical trials, 23% of patients receiving oral moxifloxacin were greater than or equal to 65 years of age and 9% were greater than or equal to 75 years of age. The clinical trial data demonstrate that there is no difference in the safety and efficacy of oral moxifloxacin in patients aged 65 or older compared to younger adults.

In intravenous trials in community acquired pneumonia, 45% of moxifloxacin patients were greater than or equal to 65 years of age, and 24% were greater than or equal to 75 years of age. In the pool of 491 elderly (> 65 years) patients, the following ECG abnormalities were reported in moxifloxacin vs. comparator patients: ST-T wave changes (2 events vs. 0 events), QT prolongation (2 vs. 0), ventricular tachycardia (1 vs. 0), atrial flutter (1 vs. 0), tachycardia (2 vs. 1), atrial fibrillation (1 vs. 0), supraventricular tachycardia (1 vs. 0), ventricular extrasystoles (2 vs. 0), and arrhythmia (0 vs. 1). None of the abnormalities was associated with a fatal outcome and a majority of these patients completed a full course of therapy.

ADVERSE REACTIONS

Clinical efficacy trials enrolled over 7,900 moxifloxacin orally and intravenously treated patients, of whom over 6,700 patients received the 400 mg dose. Most adverse events reported in moxifloxacin trials were described as mild to moderate in severity and required no treatment. Moxifloxacin was discontinued due to adverse reactions thought to be drug-related in 3.6% of orally treated patients and 5.7 % of sequentially (intravenous followed by oral) treated patients. The latter studies were conducted in community acquired pneumonia with, in general, a sicker patient population compared to the tablet studies.

Adverse reactions, judged by investigators to be at least possibly drug-related, occurring in greater than or equal to 3% of moxifloxacin treated patients were: nausea (7%), diarrhea (6%), dizziness (3%).

Additional clinically relevant uncommon events, judged by investigators to be at least possibly drug-related, that occurred in greater than or equal to 0.1% and less than 3% of moxifloxacin treated patients were:

BODY AS A WHOLE: headache, abdominal pain, injection site reaction, asthenia, moniliasis, pain, malaise, lab test abnormal (not specified), allergic reaction, leg pain, back pain, chest pain

CARDIOVASCULAR: palpitation, tachycardia, hypertension, peripheral edema, QT interval prolonged

CENTRAL NERVOUS SYSTEM: insomnia, nervousness, anxiety, confusion, somnolence, tremor, vertigo, paresthesia

DIGESTIVE: vomiting, abnormal liver function test, dyspepsia, dry mouth, constipation, oral moniliasis, anorexia, stomatitis, glossitis, flatulence, gastrointestinal disorder, GGTP increased

HEMIC AND LYMPHATIC: prothrombin decrease (prothrombin time prolonged/International Normalized Ratio (INR) increased), thrombocythemia, thrombocytopenia, eosinophilia, leukopenia

METABOLIC AND NUTRITIONAL: amylase increased, lactic dehydrogenase increased

MUSCULOSKELETAL: arthralgia, myalgia

RESPIRATORY: dyspnea

SKIN/APPENDAGES: rash (maculopapular, purpuric, pustular), pruritus, sweating

SPECIAL SENSES: taste perversion

UROGENITAL: vaginal moniliasis, vaginitis

Additional clinically relevant rare events, judged by investigators to be at least possibly drug-related, that occurred in less than 0.1% of moxifloxacin treated patients were:

abnormal dreams, abnormal vision, agitation, amblyopia, amnesia, anemia, aphasia, arthritis, asthma, atrial fibrillation, convulsions, depersonalization, depression, diarrhea (*Clostridium difficile*), dysphagia, ECG abnormal, emotional lability, face edema, gastritis, hallucinations, hyperglycemia, hyperlipidemia, hypertonia, hyperuricemia, hypesthesia, hypotension, incoordination, jaundice (predominantly cholestatic), kidney function abnormal, parosmia, pelvic pain, prothrombin increase (prothrombin time decreased/International Normalized Ratio (INR) decreased), sleep disorders, speech disorders, supraventricular tachycardia, taste loss, tendon disorder, thinking abnormal, thromboplastin decrease, tinnitus, tongue discoloration, urticaria, vasodilatation, ventricular tachycardia

Post-Marketing Adverse Event Reports:

Additional adverse events have been reported from worldwide post-marketing experience with moxifloxacin. Because these events are reported voluntarily from a population of uncertain size, it is not always possible to reliably estimate their frequency or establish a causal relationship to drug exposure. These events, some of them life-threatening, include anaphylactic reaction, anaphylactic shock, angioedema (including laryngeal edema), hepatitis (predominantly cholestatic), pseudomembranous colitis, psychotic reaction, Stevens-Johnson syndrome, syncope, tendon rupture, and ventricular tachyarrhythmias (including in very rare cases cardiac arrest and torsade de pointes, and usually in patients with concurrent severe underlying proarrhythmic conditions).

LABORATORY CHANGES

Changes in laboratory parameters, without regard to drug relationship, which are not listed above and which occurred in ≥ 2% of patients and at an incidence greater than in controls included: increases in MCH, neutrophils, WBCs, PT ratio, ionized calcium, chloride, albumin, globulin, bilirubin; decreases in hemoglobin, RBCs, neutrophils, eosinophils, basophils, PT ratio, glucose, pO_2, bilirubin and amylase. It cannot be determined if any of the above laboratory abnormalities were caused by the drug or the underlying condition being treated.

OVERDOSAGE

Single oral overdoses up to 2.8 g were not associated with any serious adverse events. In the event of acute overdose, the stomach should be emptied and adequate hydration maintained. ECG monitoring is recommended due to the possibility of QT interval prolongation. The patient should be carefully observed and given supportive treatment. The administration of activated charcoal as soon as possible after oral overdose may prevent excessive increase of systemic moxifloxacin exposure. About 3% and 9% of the dose of moxifloxacin, as well as about 2% and 4.5% of its glucuronide metabolite are removed by continuous ambulatory peritoneal dialysis and hemodialysis, respectively.

Single oral moxifloxacin doses of 2000, 500, and 1500 mg/kg were lethal to rats, mice, and Cynomolgus monkeys, respectively. The minimum lethal intravenous dose in mice and rats was 100 mg/kg. Toxic signs after administration of a single high dose of moxifloxacin to these animals included CNS and gastrointestinal effects such as decreased activity, somnolence, tremor, convulsions, vomiting and diarrhea.

DOSAGE AND ADMINISTRATION

The dose of AVELOX is 400 mg (orally or as an intravenous infusion) once every 24 hours. The duration of therapy depends on the type of infection as described below.

Infection*	Daily Dose	Duration
Acute Bacterial Sinusitis	400 mg	10 days
Acute Bacterial Exacerbation of Chronic Bronchitis	400 mg	5 days
Community Acquired Pneumonia	400 mg	7–14 days
Uncomplicated Skin and Skin Structure Infections	400 mg	7 days

*due to the designated pathogens (See **INDICATIONS AND USAGE**.). For I.V. use see **Precautions, Geriatric Use**.

Oral doses of moxifloxacin should be administered at least 4 hours before or 8 hours after antacids containing magnesium or aluminum, as well as sucralfate, metal cations such as iron, and multivitamin preparations with zinc, or VIDEX® (didanosine) chewable/buffered tablets or the pediatric powder for oral solution. (See **CLINICAL PHARMACOLOGY, Drug Interactions** and **PRECAUTIONS, Drug Interactions**.)

Impaired Renal Function

No dosage adjustment is required in renally impaired patients, including those on either hemodialysis or continuous ambulatory peritoneal dialysis.

Impaired Hepatic Function

No dosage adjustment is required in patients with mild or moderate hepatic insufficiency (Child Pugh Classes A and B). The pharmacokinetics of moxifloxacin in patients with severe hepatic insufficiency (Child Pugh Class C) have not been studied. (See **CLINICAL PHARMACOLOGY, Hepatic Insufficiency**.)

When switching from intravenous to oral dosage administration, no dosage adjustment is necessary. Patients whose therapy is started with AVELOX I.V. may be switched to AVELOX Tablets when clinically indicated at the discretion of the physician.

AVELOX I.V. should be administered by INTRAVENOUS infusion only. It is not intended for intra-arterial, intramuscular, intrathecal, intraperitoneal, or subcutaneous administration.

AVELOX I.V. should be administered by intravenous infusion over a period of 60 minutes by direct infusion or through a Y-type intravenous infusion set which may already be in place. CAUTION: RAPID OR BOLUS INTRAVENOUS INFUSION MUST BE AVOIDED.

Since only limited data are available on the compatibility of moxifloxacin intravenous injection with other intravenous substances, additives or other medications should not be added to AVELOX I.V. or infused simultaneously through the same intravenous line. If the same intravenous line or a Y-type line is used for sequential infusion of other drugs, or if the "piggyback" method of administration is used, the line should be flushed before and after infusion of AVELOX I.V. with an infusion solution compatible with AVELOX I.V. as well as with other drug(s) administered via this common line.

AVELOX I.V. is compatible with the following intravenous solutions at ratios from 1:10 to 10:1:

0.9% Sodium Chloride Injection, USP
1M Sodium Chloride Injection
5% Dextrose Injection, USP
Sterile Water for Injection, USP
10% Dextrose for Injection, USP
Lactated Ringer's for Injection

Preparation for administration of AVELOX I.V. injection premix in flexible containers:

1. Close flow control clamp of administration set.
2. Remove cover from port at bottom of container.
3. Insert piercing pin from an appropriate transfer set (e.g. one that does not require excessive force, such as ISO compatible administration set) into port with a gentle twisting motion until pin is firmly seated.

NOTE: Refer to complete directions that have been provided with the administration set.

HOW SUPPLIED

Tablets

AVELOX (moxifloxacin hydrochloride) Tablets are available as oblong, dull red film-coated tablets containing 400 mg moxifloxacin.

The tablet is coded with the word "BAYER" on one side and "M400" on the reverse side.

Package	NDC Code
Bottles of 30:	0026-8581-69
Unit Dose Pack of 50:	0026-8581-88
ABC Pack of 5:	0026-8581-41

Store at 25°C (77°F); excursions permitted to 15–30°C (59–86°F) [see USP Controlled Room Temperature]. Avoid high humidity.

Intravenous Solution – Premix Bags

AVELOX I.V. (moxifloxacin hydrochloride in sodium chloride injection) is available in ready-to-use 250 mL latex-free flexible bags containing 400 mg of moxifloxacin in 0.8% saline. NO FURTHER DILUTION OF THIS PREPARATION IS NECESSARY.

Package	NDC Code
250 mL flexible container	0026-8582-31

Parenteral drug products should be inspected visually for particulate matter prior to administration. Samples containing visible particulates should not be used.

Since the premix flexible containers are for single-use only, any unused portion should be discarded.

Store at 25°C (77°F); excursions permitted to 15–30°C (59–86°F) [see USP Controlled Room Temperature].

DO NOT REFRIGERATE – PRODUCT PRECIPITATES UPON REFRIGERATION.

ANIMAL PHARMACOLOGY

Quinolones have been shown to cause arthropathy in immature animals. In studies in juvenile dogs oral doses of moxifloxacin ≥ 30 mg/kg/day (approximately 1.5 times the maximum recommended human dose based upon systemic exposure) for 28 days resulted in arthropathy. There was no evidence of arthropathy in mature monkeys and rats at oral doses up to 135 and 500 mg/kg, respectively.

Unlike some other members of the quinolone class, crystalluria was not observed in 6 month repeat dose studies in rats and monkeys with moxifloxacin.

No ocular toxicity was observed in a 13 week oral repeat dose study in dogs with a moxifloxacin dose of 60 mg/kg. Ocular toxicity was not observed in 6 month repeat dose studies in rats and monkeys (daily oral doses up to 500 mg/kg and 135 mg/kg, respectively). In beagle dogs, electroretinographic (ERG) changes were observed in a 2 week study at oral doses of 60 and 90 mg/kg. Histopathological changes were observed in the retina from one of four dogs at 90 mg/kg, a dose associated with mortality in this study.

Some quinolones have been reported to have proconvulsant activity that is exacerbated with concomitant use of non-steroidal anti-inflammatory drugs (NSAIDs). Moxifloxacin at an oral dose of 300 mg/kg did not show an increase in acute toxicity or potential for CNS toxicity (e.g. seizures) in mice when used in combination with NSAIDs such as diclofenac, ibuprofen, or fenbufen.

In dog studies, at plasma concentrations about five times the human therapeutic level, a QT-prolonging effect of moxifloxacin was found. Electrophysiological *in vitro* studies suggested an inhibition of the rapid activating component of the delayed rectifier potassium current (I_{Kr}) as an underlying mechanism. In dogs, the combined infusion of sotalol, a Class III antiarrhythmic agent, with moxifloxacin induced a higher degree of QTc prolongation than that induced by the same dose (30 mg/kg) of moxifloxacin alone.

In a local tolerability study performed in dogs, no signs of local intolerability were seen when moxifloxacin was administered intravenously. After intra-arterial injection, inflammatory changes involving the peri-arterial soft tissue were observed suggesting that intra-arterial administration of moxifloxacin should be avoided.

CLINICAL STUDIES

Acute Bacterial Exacerbation of Chronic Bronchitis

AVELOX Tablets (400 mg once daily for five days) were evaluated for the treatment of acute bacterial exacerbation of chronic bronchitis in a large, randomized, double-blind, controlled clinical trial conducted in the US. This study compared AVELOX with clarithromycin (500 mg twice daily for 10 days) and enrolled 629 patients. The primary endpoint for this trial was clinical success at 7–17 days post-therapy. The clinical success for AVELOX was 89% (222/250) compared to 89% (224/251) for clarithromycin.

The following outcomes are the clinical success rates at the follow-up visit for the clinically evaluable patient groups by pathogen:

PATHOGEN	AVELOX	Clarithromycin
Streptococcus pneumoniae	100% (16/16)	87% (20/23)
Haemophilus influenzae	89% (33/37)	88% (36/41)
Haemophilus parainfluenzae	100% (16/16)	100% (14/14)
Moraxella catarrhalis	85% (29/34)	100% (24/24)
Staphylococcus aureus	94% (15/16)	75% (6/8)
Klebsiella pneumoniae	90% (18/20)	91% (10/11)

The microbiological eradication rates (eradication plus presumed eradication) in AVELOX treated patients were *Streptococcus pneumoniae* 100%, *Haemophilus influenzae* 89%,

Continued on next page

Avelox—Cont.

Haemophilus parainfluenzae 100%, *Moraxella catarrhalis* 85%, *Staphylococcus aureus* 94%, and *Klebsiella pneumoniae* 85%.

Community Acquired Pneumonia

A large, randomized, double-blind, controlled clinical trial was conducted in the US to compare the efficacy of AVELOX Tablets (400 mg once daily) to that of high-dose clarithromycin (500 mg twice daily) in the treatment of patients with clinically and radiologically documented community acquired pneumonia. This study enrolled 474 patients (382 of which were valid for the primary efficacy analysis conducted at the 14–35 day follow-up visit). Clinical success for clinically evaluable patients was 95% (184/194) for AVELOX and 95% (178/188) for high dose clarithromycin.

A large, randomized, double-blind, controlled trial was conducted in the US and Canada to compare the efficacy of sequential IV/PO AVELOX 400 mg QD for 7–14 days to an IV/PO fluoroquinolone control (trovafloxacin or levofloxacin) in the treatment of patients with clinically and radiologically documented community acquired pneumonia. This study enrolled 516 patients, 362 of which were valid for the primary efficacy analysis conducted at the 7–30 day post-therapy visit. The clinical success rate was 86% (157/182) for AVELOX therapy and 89% (161/180) for the fluoroquinolone comparators.

An open-label ex-US study that enrolled 628 patients compared AVELOX to sequential IV/PO amoxicillin/clavulanate (1.2 g IV q8h/625 mg PO q8h) with or without high-dose IV/PO clarithromycin (500 mg BID). The intravenous formulations of the comparators are not FDA approved. The clinical success rate at Day 5–7 (the primary efficacy timepoint) for AVELOX therapy was 93% (241/258) and demonstrated superiority to amoxicillin/clavulanate ± clarithromycin (85%, 239/280) [95% C.I. 2.9%, 13.2%]. The clinical success rate at the 21–28 days post-therapy visit for AVELOX was 84% (216/258), which also demonstrated superiority to the comparators (74%, 208/280) [95% C.I. 2.6%, 16.3%].

The clinical success rates by pathogen across four CAP studies are presented below:

Clinical Success Rates By Pathogen (Pooled CAP Studies)

PATHOGEN	AVELOX
Streptococcus pneumoniae	94% (80/85)
Staphylococcus aureus	85% (17/20)
Klebsiella pneumoniae	92% (11/12)
Haemophilus influenzae	92% (56/61)
Chlamydia pneumoniae	93% (119/128)
Mycoplasma pneumoniae	96% (73/76)
Moraxella catarrhalis	92% (11/12)

Community Acquired Pneumonia caused by Multi-Drug Resistant *Streptococcus pneumoniae* (MDRSP)*

Avelox was effective in the treatment of community acquired pneumonia (CAP) caused by multi-drug resistant *Streptococcus pneumoniae* MDRSP* isolates. Of 37 microbiologically evaluable patients with MDRSP isolates, 35 patients (95.0%) achieved clinical and bacteriological success post-therapy. The clinical and bacteriological success rates based on the number of patients treated are shown in the table below.

* MDRSP, Multi-drug resistant *Streptococcus pneumoniae* includes isolates previously known as PRSP (Penicillin-resistant *S. pneumoniae*), and are strains resistant to two or more of the following antibiotics: penicillin (MIC ≥ 2 µg/mL), 2nd generation cephalosporins (e.g., cefuroxime), macrolides, tetracyclines, and trimethoprim/sulfamethoxazole. [See first table below]

Not all isolates were resistant to all antimicrobial classes tested. Success and eradication rates are summarized in the table below:

[See second table below]

Acute Bacterial Sinusitis

In a large, controlled double-blind study conducted in the US, AVELOX Tablets (400 mg once daily for ten days) were compared with cefuroxime axetil (250 mg twice daily for ten days) for the treatment of acute bacterial sinusitis. The trial included 457 patients valid for the primary efficacy determination. Clinical success (cure plus improvement) at the 7 to 21 day post-therapy test of cure visit was 90% for AVELOX and 89% for cefuroxime.

An additional non-comparative study was conducted to gather bacteriological data and to evaluate microbiological eradication in adult patients treated with AVELOX 400 mg once daily for seven days. All patients (n = 336) underwent antral puncture in this study. Clinical success rates and eradication/presumed eradication rates at the 21 to 37 day follow-up visit were 97% (29 out of 30) for *Streptococcus pneumoniae*, 83% (15 out of 18) for *Moraxella catarrhalis*, and 80% (24 out of 30) for *Haemophilus influenzae*.

Uncomplicated Skin and Skin Structure Infections

A randomized, double-blind, controlled clinical trial conducted in the US compared the efficacy of AVELOX 400 mg once daily for seven days with cephalexin HCl 500 mg three times daily for seven days. The percentage of patients treated for uncomplicated abscesses was 30%, furuncles 8%, cellulitis 16%, impetigo 20%, and other skin infections 26%. Adjunctive procedures (incision and drainage or debridement) were performed on 17% of the AVELOX treated patients and 14% of the comparator treated patients. Clinical success rates in evaluable patients were 89% (108/122) for AVELOX and 91% (110/121) for cephalexin HCl.

REFERENCES

1. National Committee for Clinical Laboratory Standards, Methods for Dilution Antimicrobial Susceptibility Tests for Bacteria That Grow Aerobically-Sixth Edition. Approved Standard NCCLS Document M7-A6, Vol. 23, No. 2, NCCLS, Wayne, PA, January, 2003.

2. National Committee for Clinical Laboratory Standards, Performance Standards for Antimicrobial Disk Susceptibility Tests-Eighth Edition. Approved Standard NCCLS Document M2-A8, Vol. 23, No. 1, NCCLS, Wayne, PA, January, 2003.

Patient Information About:
AVELOX®
(moxifloxacin hydrochloride)
400 mg Tablets

This section contains important information about AVELOX (moxifloxacin hydrochloride), and should be read completely before you begin treatment. This section does not take the place of discussions with your doctor or health care professional about your medical condition or your treatment. This section does not list all benefits and risks of AVELOX. The medicine described here can be prescribed only by a licensed health care professional. If you have any questions about AVELOX talk with your health care professional. Only your health care professional can determine if AVELOX is right for you.

What is AVELOX?

AVELOX is an antibiotic used to treat lung, sinus, or skin infections caused by certain germs called bacteria. AVELOX kills many of the types of bacteria that can infect the lungs and sinuses and has been shown in a large number of clinical trials to be safe and effective for the treatment of bacterial infections.

Sometimes viruses rather than bacteria may infect the lungs and sinuses (for example the common cold). AVELOX, like all other antibiotics, does not kill viruses.

You should contact your doctor if you think your condition is not improving while taking AVELOX.

AVELOX Tablets are red and contain 400 mg of active drug.

How and when should I take AVELOX?

AVELOX should be taken once a day for 5–14 days depending on your prescription. It should be swallowed and may be taken with or without food. Try to take the tablet at the same time each day.

You may begin to feel better quickly; however, in order to make sure that all bacteria are killed, you should complete the full course of medication. Do not take more than the prescribed dose of AVELOX even if you missed a dose by mistake. You should not take a double dose.

Who should not take AVELOX?

You should not take AVELOX if you have ever had a severe allergic reaction to any of the group of antibiotics known as "quinolones" such as ciprofloxacin or levofloxacin. If you develop hives, difficulty breathing, or other symptoms of a severe allergic reaction, seek emergency treatment right away. If you develop a skin rash, you should stop taking AVELOX and call your health care professional.

You should avoid AVELOX if you have a rare condition known as congenital prolongation of the QT interval. If you or any of your family members have this condition you should inform your health care professional. You should avoid AVELOX if you are being treated for heart rhythm disturbances with certain medicines such as quinidine, procainamide, amiodarone or sotalol. Inform your health care professional if you are taking a heart rhythm drug.

You should also avoid AVELOX if the amount of potassium in your blood is low. Low potassium can sometimes be caused by medicines called diuretics such as furosemide and hydrochlorothiazide. If you are taking a diuretic medicine you should speak with your health care professional.

If you are pregnant or planning to become pregnant while taking AVELOX, talk to your doctor before taking this medication. AVELOX is not recommended for use during pregnancy or nursing, as the effects on the unborn child or nursing infant are unknown.

AVELOX is not recommended for children.

What are the possible side effects of AVELOX?

AVELOX is generally well tolerated. The most common side effects caused by AVELOX, which are usually mild, include dizziness, nausea, and diarrhea. If diarrhea persists call your health care provider. You should be careful about driving or operating machinery until you are sure AVELOX is not causing dizziness. If you notice any side effects not mentioned in this section or you have any concerns about the side effects you are experiencing, please inform your health care professional.

In some people, AVELOX, as with some other antibiotics, may produce a small effect on the heart that is seen on an electrocardiogram test. Although this has not caused any serious problems in more than 7,900 patients who have already taken the medication in clinical studies, in theory it could result in extremely rare cases of abnormal heartbeat which may be dangerous. Contact your health care professional if you develop heart palpitations (fast beating), or have fainting spells.

Convulsions have been reported in patients receiving quinolone antibiotics. Be sure to let your physician know if you have a history of convulsions. Quinolones, including AVELOX, have been rarely associated with other central nervous system events including confusion, tremors, hallucinations, and depression.

Quinolones, including AVELOX, have been rarely associated with inflammation of tendons. If you experience pain, swelling or rupture of a tendon, you should stop taking AVELOX and call your health care professional.

What about other medicines I am taking?

Tell your doctor about all other prescription and nonprescription medicines or supplements you are taking. You should avoid taking AVELOX with certain medicines used to treat an abnormal heartbeat. These include quinidine, procainamide, amiodarone, and sotalol.

Some medicines also produce an effect on the electrocardiogram test, including cisapride, erythromycin, some antidepressants and some antipsychotic drugs. These may increase the risk of heart beat problems when taken with AVELOX.

Many antacids and multivitamins may interfere with the absorption of AVELOX and may prevent it from working properly. You should take AVELOX either 4 hours before or 8 hours after taking these products.

Remember

Take your dose of AVELOX once a day.

Complete the course of medication even if you are feeling better.

Keep this medication out of the reach of children.

Clinical and Bacteriological Success Rates for Moxifloxacin-Treated MDRSP CAP Patients (Population: Valid for Efficacy):

Screening Susceptibility	Clinical Success		Bacteriological Success	
	n/N[a]	%	n/N[b]	%
Penicillin-resistant	21/21	100%*	21/21	100%*
2nd generation cephalosporin-resistant	25/26	96%*	25/26	96%*
Macrolide-resistant**	22/23	96%	22/23	96%
Trimethoprim/sulfamethoxazole-resistant	28/30	93%	28/30	93%
Tetracycline-resistant	17/18	94%	17/18	94%

[a]n = number of patients successfully treated; N = number of patients with MDRSP (from a total of 37 patients)
[b]n = number of patients successfully treated (presumed eradication or eradication); N = number of patients with MDRSP (from a total of 37 patients)
*One patient had a respiratory isolate that was resistant to penicillin and cefuroxime but a blood isolate that was intermediate to penicillin and cefuroxime. The patient is included in the database based on the respiratory isolate.
**Azithromycin, clarithromycin, and erythromycin were the macrolide antimicrobials tested.

S. pneumoniae with MDRSP	Clinical Success	Bacteriological Eradication Rate
Resistant to 2 antimicrobials	12/13 (92.3 %)	12/13 (92.3 %)
Resistant to 3 antimicrobials	10/11 (90.9 %)*	10/11 (90.9 %)*
Resistant to 4 antimicrobials	6/6 (100%)	6/6 (100%)
Resistant to 5 antimicrobials	7/7 (100%)*	7/7 (100%)*
Bacteremia with MDRSP	9/9 (100%)	9/9 (100%)

*One patient had a respiratory isolate resistant to 5 antimicrobials and a blood isolate resistant to 3 antimicrobials. The patient was included in the category resistant to 5 antimicrobials.

This information does not take the place of discussions with your doctor or health care professional about your medical condition or your treatment.
For more complete information about AVELOX request full prescribing information from your health care professional, pharmacist, or visit our website at www.aveloxusa.com.

Bayer HealthCare
Bayer Pharmaceuticals Corporation
400 Morgan Lane
West Haven, CT 06516
Made in Germany
Rx Only
08753736, R.6 6/04 12344

Printed in U.S.A.
Shown in Product Identification Guide, page 308

CIPRO® ℞
[*sī'prō*]
(ciprofloxacin hydrochloride)
TABLETS

CIPRO® ℞
(ciprofloxacin*)
ORAL SUSPENSION

To reduce the development of drug-resistant bacteria and maintain the effectiveness of CIPRO® Tablets and CIPRO Oral Suspension and other antibacterial drugs, CIPRO Tablets and CIPRO Oral Suspension should be used only to treat or prevent infections that are proven or strongly suspected to be caused by bacteria.

DESCRIPTION

CIPRO (ciprofloxacin hydrochloride) Tablets and CIPRO (ciprofloxacin*) Oral Suspension are synthetic broad spectrum antimicrobial agents for oral administration. Ciprofloxacin hydrochloride, USP, a fluoroquinolone, is the monohydrochloride monohydrate salt of 1-cyclopropyl-6-fluoro-1, 4-dihydro-4-oxo-7-(1-piperazinyl)-3-quinolinecarboxylic acid. It is a faintly yellowish to light yellow crystalline substance with a molecular weight of 385.8. Its empirical formula is $C_{17}H_{18}FN_3O_3 \bullet HCl \bullet H_2O$ and its chemical structure is as follows:

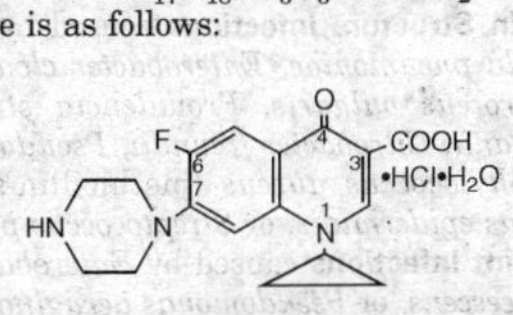

Ciprofloxacin is 1-cyclopropyl-6-fluoro-1,4-dihydro-4-oxo-7-(1-piperazinyl)-3-quinolinecarboxylic acid. Its empirical formula is $C_{17}H_{18}FN_3O_3$ and its molecular weight is 331.4. It is a faintly yellowish to light yellow crystalline substance and its chemical structure is as follows:

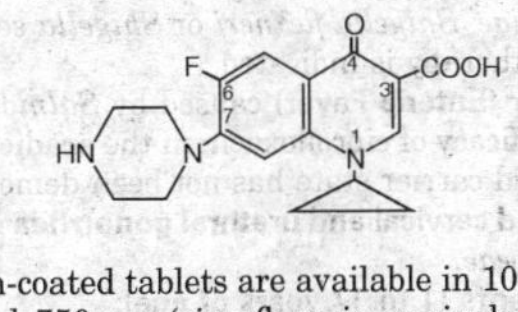

CIPRO film-coated tablets are available in 100 mg, 250 mg, 500 mg and 750 mg (ciprofloxacin equivalent) strengths. Ciprofloxacin tablets are white to slightly yellowish. The inactive ingredients are cornstarch, microcrystalline cellulose, silicon dioxide, crospovidone, magnesium stearate, hypromellose, titanium dioxide, polyethylene glycol and water.
Ciprofloxacin Oral Suspension is available in 5% (5 g ciprofloxacin in 100 mL) and 10% (10 g ciprofloxacin in 100 mL) strengths. Ciprofloxacin Oral Suspension is a white to slightly yellowish suspension with strawberry flavor which may contain yellow-orange droplets. It is composed of ciprofloxacin microcapsules and diluent which are mixed prior to dispensing (See instructions for USE/HANDLING). The components of the suspension have the following compositions:
Microcapsules - ciprofloxacin, povidone, methacrylic acid copolymer, hypromellose, magnesium stearate, and Polysorbate 20.
Diluent - medium-chain triglycerides, sucrose, lecithin, water, and strawberry flavor.
* Does not comply with USP with regards to "loss on drying" and "residue on ignition".

CLINICAL PHARMACOLOGY

Absorption: Ciprofloxacin given as an oral tablet is rapidly and well absorbed from the gastrointestinal tract after oral administration. The absolute bioavailability is approximately 70% with no substantial loss by first pass metabolism. Ciprofloxacin maximum serum concentrations and area under the curve are shown in the chart for the 250 mg to 1000 mg dose range.

Dose (mg)	Maximum Serum Concentration (µg/mL)	Area Under Curve (AUC) (µg•hr/mL)
250	1.2	4.8
500	2.4	11.6
750	4.3	20.2
1000	5.4	30.8

Steady-state Pharmacokinetic Parameters Following Multiple Oral and I.V. Doses

Parameters	500 mg q12h, P.O.	400 mg q12h, I.V.	750 mg q12h, P.O.	400 mg q8h, I.V.
AUC (µg•hr/mL)	13.7[a]	12.7[a]	31.6[b]	32.9[c]
C_{max} (µg/mL)	2.97	4.56	3.59	4.07

[a] AUC_{0-12h}
[b] $AUC\ 24h = AUC_{0-12h} \times 2$
[c] $AUC\ 24h = AUC_{0-8h} \times 3$

Maximum serum concentrations are attained 1 to 2 hours after oral dosing. Mean concentrations 12 hours after dosing with 250, 500, or 750 mg are 0.1, 0.2, and 0.4 µg/mL, respectively. The serum elimination half-life in subjects with normal renal function is approximately 4 hours. Serum concentrations increase proportionately with doses up to 1000 mg.
A 500 mg oral dose given every 12 hours has been shown to produce an area under the serum concentration time curve (AUC) equivalent to that produced by an intravenous infusion of 400 mg ciprofloxacin given over 60 minutes every 12 hours. A 750 mg oral dose given every 12 hours has been shown to produce an AUC at steady-state equivalent to that produced by an intravenous infusion of 400 mg given over 60 minutes every 8 hours. A 750 mg oral dose results in a C_{max} similar to that observed with a 400 mg I.V. dose. A 250 mg oral dose given every 12 hours produces an AUC equivalent to that produced by an infusion of 200 mg ciprofloxacin given every 12 hours.
[See table above]
Distribution: The binding of ciprofloxacin to serum proteins is 20 to 40% which is not likely to be high enough to cause significant protein binding interactions with other drugs.
After oral administration, ciprofloxacin is widely distributed throughout the body. Tissue concentrations often exceed serum concentrations in both men and women, particularly in genital tissue including the prostate. Ciprofloxacin is present in active form in the saliva, nasal and bronchial secretions, mucosa of the sinuses, sputum, skin blister fluid, lymph, peritoneal fluid, bile, and prostatic secretions. Ciprofloxacin has also been detected in lung, skin, fat, muscle, cartilage, and bone. The drug diffuses into the cerebrospinal fluid (CSF); however, CSF concentrations are generally less than 10% of peak serum concentrations. Low levels of the drug have been detected in the aqueous and vitreous humors of the eye.
Metabolism: Four metabolites have been identified in human urine which together account for approximately 15% of an oral dose. The metabolites have antimicrobial activity, but are less active than unchanged ciprofloxacin.
Excretion: The serum elimination half-life in subjects with normal renal function is approximately 4 hours. Approximately 40 to 50% of an orally administered dose is excreted in the urine as unchanged drug. After a 250 mg oral dose, urine concentrations of ciprofloxacin usually exceed 200 µg/mL during the first two hours and are approximately 30 µg/mL at 8 to 12 hours after dosing. The urinary excretion of ciprofloxacin is virtually complete within 24 hours after dosing. The renal clearance of ciprofloxacin, which is approximately 300 mL/minute, exceeds the normal glomerular filtration rate of 120 mL/minute. Thus, active tubular secretion would seem to play a significant role in its elimination. Co-administration of probenecid with ciprofloxacin results in about a 50% reduction in the ciprofloxacin renal clearance and a 50% increase in its concentration in the systemic circulation. Although bile concentrations of ciprofloxacin are several fold higher than serum concentrations after oral dosing, only a small amount of the dose administered is recovered from the bile as unchanged drug. An additional 1 to 2% of the dose is recovered from the bile in the form of metabolites. Approximately 20 to 35% of an oral dose is recovered from the feces within 5 days after dosing. This may arise from either biliary clearance or transintestinal elimination.
With oral administration, a 500 mg dose, given as 10 mL of the 5% CIPRO Suspension (containing 250 mg ciprofloxacin/5mL) is bioequivalent to the 500 mg tablet. A 10 mL volume of the 5% CIPRO Suspension (containing 250 mg ciprofloxacin/5mL) is bioequivalent to a 5 mL volume of the 10% CIPRO Suspension (containing 500 mg ciprofloxacin/5mL).
Drug-drug Interactions: When CIPRO Tablet is given concomitantly with food, there is a delay in the absorption of the drug, resulting in peak concentrations that occur closer to 2 hours after dosing rather than 1 hour whereas there is no delay observed when CIPRO Suspension is given with food. The overall absorption of CIPRO Tablet or CIPRO Suspension, however, is not substantially affected. The pharmacokinetics of ciprofloxacin given as the suspension are also not affected by food. Concurrent administration of antacids containing magnesium hydroxide or aluminum hydroxide may reduce the bioavailability of ciprofloxacin by as much as 90%. (See **PRECAUTIONS**.)
The serum concentrations of ciprofloxacin and metronidazole were not altered when these two drugs were given concomitantly.
Concomitant administration of ciprofloxacin with theophylline decreases the clearance of theophylline resulting in elevated serum theophylline levels and increased risk of a patient developing CNS or other adverse reactions. Ciprofloxacin also decreases caffeine clearance and inhibits the formation of paraxanthine after caffeine administration. (See **PRECAUTIONS**.)
Special Populations: Pharmacokinetic studies of the oral (single dose) and intravenous (single and multiple dose) forms of ciprofloxacin indicate that plasma concentrations of ciprofloxacin are higher in elderly subjects (> 65 years) as compared to young adults. Although the C_{max} is increased 16-40%, the increase in mean AUC is approximately 30%, and can be at least partially attributed to decreased renal clearance in the elderly. Elimination half-life is only slightly (~20%) prolonged in the elderly. These differences are not considered clinically significant. (See **PRECAUTIONS**: **Geriatric Use**.)
In patients with reduced renal function, the half-life of ciprofloxacin is slightly prolonged. Dosage adjustments may be required. (See **DOSAGE AND ADMINISTRATION**.)
In preliminary studies in patients with stable chronic liver cirrhosis, no significant changes in ciprofloxacin pharmacokinetics have been observed. The kinetics of ciprofloxacin in patients with acute hepatic insufficiency, however, have not been fully elucidated.
Following a single oral dose of 10 mg/kg ciprofloxacin suspension to 16 children ranging in age from 4 months to 7 years, the mean C_{max} was 2.4 µg/mL (range: 1.5 – 3.4 µg/mL) and the mean AUC was 9.2 µg*h/mL (range: 5.8 – 14.9 µg*h/mL). There was no apparent age-dependence, and no notable increase in C_{max} or AUC upon multiple dosing (10 mg/kg TID). In children with severe sepsis who were given intravenous ciprofloxacin (10 mg/kg as a 1-hour infusion), the mean C_{max} was 6.1 µg/mL (range: 4.6 – 8.3 µg/mL) in 10 children less than 1 year of age; and 7.2 µg/mL (range: 4.7 – 11.8 µg/mL) in 10 children between 1 and 5 years of age. The AUC values were 17.4 µg*h/mL (range: 11.8 – 32.0 µg*h/mL) and 16.5 µg*h/mL (range: 11.0 – 23.8 µg*h/mL) in the respective age groups. These values are within the range reported for adults at therapeutic doses. Based on population pharmacokinetic analysis of pediatric patients with various infections, the predicted mean half-life in children is approximately 4 - 5 hours, and the bioavailability of the oral suspension is approximately 60%.

MICROBIOLOGY

Ciprofloxacin has *in vitro* activity against a wide range of gram-negative and gram-positive microorganisms. The bactericidal action of ciprofloxacin results from inhibition of the enzymes topoisomerase II (DNA gyrase) and topoisomerase IV, which are required for bacterial DNA replication, transcription, repair, and recombination. The mechanism of action of fluoroquinolones, including ciprofloxacin, is different from that of penicillins, cephalosporins, aminoglycosides, macrolides, and tetracyclines; therefore, microorganisms resistant to these classes of drugs may be susceptible to ciprofloxacin and other quinolones. There is no known cross-resistance between ciprofloxacin and other classes of antimicrobials. *In vitro* resistance to ciprofloxacin develops slowly by multiple step mutations.
Ciprofloxacin is slightly less active when tested at acidic pH. The inoculum size has little effect when tested *in vitro*. The minimal bactericidal concentration (MBC) generally does not exceed the minimal inhibitory concentration (MIC) by more than a factor of 2.
Ciprofloxacin has been shown to be active against most strains of the following microorganisms, both *in vitro* and in clinical infections as described in the **INDICATIONS AND USAGE** section of the package insert for CIPRO (ciprofloxacin hydrochloride) Tablets and CIPRO (ciprofloxacin*) 5% and 10% Oral Suspension.

Aerobic gram-positive microorganisms
Enterococcus faecalis (Many strains are only moderately susceptible.)
Staphylococcus aureus (methicillin-susceptible strains only)
Staphylococcus epidermidis (methicillin-susceptible strains only)
Staphylococcus saprophyticus
Streptococcus pneumoniae (penicillin-susceptible strains only)
Streptococcus pyogenes

Aerobic gram-negative microorganisms
Campylobacter jejuni
Citrobacter diversus
Citrobacter freundii
Enterobacter cloacae
Escherichia coli
Haemophilus influenzae
Haemophilus parainfluenzae
Klebsiella pneumoniae

Continued on next page

Cipro—Cont.

Moraxella catarrhalis
Morganella morganii
Neisseria gonorrhoeae
Proteus mirabilis
Proteus vulgaris
Providencia rettgeri
Providencia stuartii
Pseudomonas aeruginosa
Salmonella typhi
Serratia marcescens
Shigella boydii
Shigella dysenteriae
Shigella flexneri
Shigella sonnei

Ciprofloxacin has been shown to be active against *Bacillus anthracis* both *in vitro* and by use of serum levels as a surrogate marker (see **INDICATIONS AND USAGE** and **INHALATIONAL ANTHRAX – ADDITIONAL INFORMATION**).

The following *in vitro* data are available, **but their clinical significance is unknown.**

Ciprofloxacin exhibits *in vitro* minimum inhibitory concentrations (MICs) of 1 µg/mL or less against most (≥ 90%) strains of the following microorganisms; however, the safety and effectiveness of ciprofloxacin in treating clinical infections due to these microorganisms have not been established in adequate and well-controlled clinical trials.

Aerobic gram-positive microorganisms
Staphylococcus haemolyticus
Staphylococcus hominis
Streptococcus pneumoniae (penicillin-resistant strains only)

Aerobic gram-negative microorganisms
Acinetobacter lwoffi
Aeromonas hydrophila
Edwardsiella tarda
Enterobacter aerogenes
Klebsiella oxytoca
Legionella pneumophila
Pasteurella multocida
Salmonella enteritidis
Vibrio cholerae
Vibrio parahaemolyticus
Vibrio vulnificus
Yersinia enterocolitica

Most strains of *Burkholderia cepacia* and some strains of *Stenotrophomonas maltophilia* are resistant to ciprofloxacin as are most anaerobic bacteria, including *Bacteroides fragilis* and *Clostridium difficile*.

Susceptibility Tests

Dilution Techniques: Quantitative methods are used to determine antimicrobial minimum inhibitory concentrations (MICs). These MICs provide estimates of the susceptibility of bacteria to antimicrobial compounds. The MICs should be determined using a standardized procedure. Standardized procedures are based on a dilution method[1] (broth or agar) or equivalent with standardized inoculum concentrations and standardized concentrations of ciprofloxacin powder. The MIC values should be interpreted according to the following criteria:

For testing aerobic microorganisms other than *Haemophilus influenzae, Haemophilus parainfluenzae,* and *Neisseria gonorrhoeae*[a]:

MIC (µg/mL)	Interpretation
≤1	Susceptible (S)
2	Intermediate (I)
≥4	Resistant (R)

[a] These interpretive standards are applicable only to broth microdilution susceptibility tests with streptococci using cation-adjusted Mueller-Hinton broth with 2-5% lysed horse blood.

For testing *Haemophilus influenzae* and *Haemophilus parainfluenzae*[b]:

MIC (µg/mL)	Interpretation
≤1	Susceptible (S)

[b] This interpretive standard is applicable only to broth microdilution susceptibility tests with *Haemophilus influenzae* and *Haemophilus parainfluenzae* using *Haemophilus* Test Medium[1].

The current absence of data on resistant strains precludes defining any results other than "Susceptible". Strains yielding MIC results suggestive of a "nonsusceptible" category should be submitted to a reference laboratory for further testing.

For testing *Neisseria gonorrhoeae*[c]:

MIC (µg/mL)	Interpretation
≤ 0.06	Susceptible (S)
0.12–0.5	Intermediate (I)
≥1	Resistant (R)

[c] This interpretive standard is applicable only to agar dilution test with GC agar base and 1% defined growth supplement.

A report of "Susceptible" indicates that the pathogen is likely to be inhibited if the antimicrobial compound in the blood reaches the concentrations usually achievable. A report of "Intermediate" indicates that the result should be considered equivocal, and, if the microorganism is not fully susceptible to alternative, clinically feasible drugs, the test should be repeated. This category implies possible clinical applicability in body sites where the drug is physiologically concentrated or in situations where high dosage of drug can be used. This category also provides a buffer zone, which prevents small uncontrolled technical factors from causing major discrepancies in interpretation. A report of "Resistant" indicates that the pathogen is not likely to be inhibited if the antimicrobial compound in the blood reaches the concentrations usually achievable; other therapy should be selected.

Standardized susceptibility test procedures require the use of laboratory control microorganisms to control the technical aspects of the laboratory procedures. Standard ciprofloxacin powder should provide the following MIC values:

Organism		MIC (µg/mL)
E. faecalis	ATCC 29212	0.25 – 2.0
E. coli	ATCC 25922	0.004 – 0.015
H. influenzae[a]	ATCC 49247	0.004 – 0.03
N. gonorrhoeae[b]	ATCC 49226	0.001 – 0.008
P. aeruginosa	ATCC 27853	0.25 – 1.0
S. aureus	ATCC 29213	0.12 – 0.5

[a] This quality control range is applicable to only *H. influenzae* ATCC 49247 tested by a broth microdilution procedure using *Haemophilus* Test Medium (HTM)[1].

[b] This quality control range is applicable to only *N. gonorrhoeae* ATCC 49226 tested by an agar dilution procedure using GC agar base and 1% defined growth supplement.

Diffusion Techniques: Quantitative methods that require measurement of zone diameters also provide reproducible estimates of the susceptibility of bacteria to antimicrobial compounds. One such standardized procedure[2] requires the use of standardized inoculum concentrations. This procedure uses paper disks impregnated with 5-µg ciprofloxacin to test the susceptibility of microorganisms to ciprofloxacin. Reports from the laboratory providing results of the standard single-disk susceptibility test with a 5-µg ciprofloxacin disk should be interpreted according to the following criteria:

For testing aerobic microorganisms other than *Haemophilus influenzae, Haemophilus parainfluenzae,* and *Neisseria gonorrhoeae*[a]:

Zone Diameter (mm)	Interpretation
≥ 21	Susceptible (S)
16 – 20	Intermediate (I)
≤ 15	Resistant (R)

[a] These zone diameter standards are applicable only to tests performed for streptococci using Mueller-Hinton agar supplemented with 5% sheep blood incubated in 5% CO_2.

For testing *Haemophilus influenzae* and *Haemophilus parainfluenzae*[b]:

Zone Diameter (mm)	Interpretation
≥ 21	Susceptible (S)

[b] This zone diameter standard is applicable only to tests with *Haemophilus influenzae* and *Haemophilus parainfluenzae* using *Haemophilus* Test Medium (HTM)[2].

The current absence of data on resistant strains precludes defining any results other than "Susceptible". Strains yielding zone diameter results suggestive of a "nonsusceptible" category should be submitted to a reference laboratory for further testing.

For testing *Neisseria gonorrhoeae*[c]:

Zone Diameter (mm)	Interpretation
≥ 41	Susceptible (S)
28 – 40	Intermediate (I)
≤ 27	Resistant (R)

[c] This zone diameter standard is applicable only to disk diffusion tests with GC agar base and 1% defined growth supplement.

Interpretation should be as stated above for results using dilution techniques. Interpretation involves correlation of the diameter obtained in the disk test with the MIC for ciprofloxacin.

As with standardized dilution techniques, diffusion methods require the use of laboratory control microorganisms that are used to control the technical aspects of the laboratory procedures. For the diffusion technique, the 5-µg ciprofloxacin disk should provide the following zone diameters in these laboratory test quality control strains:

Organism		Zone Diameter (mm)
E. coli	ATCC 25922	30 – 40
H. influenzae[a]	ATCC 49247	34 – 42
N. gonorrhoeae[b]	ATCC 49226	48 – 58
P. aeruginosa	ATCC 27853	25 – 33
S. aureus	ATCC 25923	22 – 30

[a] These quality control limits are applicable to only *H. influenzae* ATCC 49247 testing using *Haemophilus* Test Medium (HTM)[2].

[b] These quality control limits are applicable only to tests conducted with *N. gonorrhoeae* ATCC 49226 performed by disk diffusion using GC agar base and 1% defined growth supplement.

INDICATIONS AND USAGE

CIPRO is indicated for the treatment of infections caused by susceptible strains of the designated microorganisms in the conditions and patient populations listed below. Please see **DOSAGE AND ADMINISTRATION** for specific recommendations.

Adult Patients:

Urinary Tract Infections caused by *Escherichia coli, Klebsiella pneumoniae, Enterobacter cloacae, Serratia marcescens, Proteus mirabilis, Providencia rettgeri, Morganella morganii, Citrobacter diversus, Citrobacter freundii, Pseudomonas aeruginosa, Staphylococcus epidermidis, Staphylococcus saprophyticus,* or *Enterococcus faecalis.*

Acute Uncomplicated Cystitis in females caused by *Escherichia coli* or *Staphylococcus saprophyticus.*

Chronic Bacterial Prostatitis caused by *Escherichia coli* or *Proteus mirabilis.*

Lower Respiratory Tract Infections caused by *Escherichia coli, Klebsiella pneumoniae, Enterobacter cloacae, Proteus mirabilis, Pseudomonas aeruginosa, Haemophilus influenzae, Haemophilus parainfluenzae,* or *Streptococcus pneumoniae.* Also, *Moraxella catarrhalis* for the treatment of acute exacerbations of chronic bronchitis.

NOTE: Although effective in clinical trials, ciprofloxacin is not a drug of first choice in the treatment of presumed or confirmed pneumonia secondary to *Streptococcus pneumoniae.*

Acute Sinusitis caused by *Haemophilus influenzae, Streptococcus pneumoniae,* or *Moraxella catarrhalis.*

Skin and Skin Structure Infections caused by *Escherichia coli, Klebsiella pneumoniae, Enterobacter cloacae, Proteus mirabilis, Proteus vulgaris, Providencia stuartii, Morganella morganii, Citrobacter freundii, Pseudomonas aeruginosa, Staphylococcus aureus* (methicillin-susceptible), *Staphylococcus epidermidis,* or *Streptococcus pyogenes.*

Bone and Joint Infections caused by *Enterobacter cloacae, Serratia marcescens,* or *Pseudomonas aeruginosa.*

Complicated Intra-Abdominal Infections (used in combination with metronidazole) caused by *Escherichia coli, Pseudomonas aeruginosa, Proteus mirabilis, Klebsiella pneumoniae,* or *Bacteroides fragilis.*

Infectious Diarrhea caused by *Escherichia coli* (enterotoxigenic strains), *Campylobacter jejuni, Shigella boydii*[†], *Shigella dysenteriae, Shigella flexneri* or *Shigella sonnei*[†] when antibacterial therapy is indicated.

Typhoid Fever (Enteric Fever) caused by *Salmonella typhi.*

NOTE: The efficacy of ciprofloxacin in the eradication of the chronic typhoid carrier state has not been demonstrated.

Uncomplicated cervical and urethral gonorrhea due to *Neisseria gonorrhoeae.*

Pediatric patients (1 to 17 years of age):

Complicated Urinary Tract Infections and Pyelonephritis due to *Escherichia coli.*

NOTE: Although effective in clinical trials, ciprofloxacin is not a drug of first choice in the pediatric population due to an increased incidence of adverse events compared to controls, including events related to joints and/or surrounding tissues. (See **WARNINGS, PRECAUTIONS, Pediatric Use, ADVERSE REACTIONS** and **CLINICAL STUDIES.**) Ciprofloxacin, like other fluoroquinolones, is associated with arthropathy and histopathological changes in weight-bearing joints of juvenile animals. (See **ANIMAL PHARMACOLOGY.**)

Adult and Pediatric Patients:

Inhalational anthrax (post-exposure): To reduce the incidence or progression of disease following exposure to aerosolized *Bacillus anthracis.*

Ciprofloxacin serum concentrations achieved in humans serve as a surrogate endpoint reasonably likely to predict clinical benefit and provide the basis for this indication.[4] (See also, **INHALATIONAL ANTHRAX – ADDITIONAL INFORMATION**).

[†]Although treatment of infections due to this organism in this organ system demonstrated a clinically significant outcome, efficacy was studied in fewer than 10 patients.

If anaerobic organisms are suspected of contributing to the infection, appropriate therapy should be administered. Appropriate culture and susceptibility tests should be performed before treatment in order to isolate and identify organisms causing infection and to determine their susceptibility to ciprofloxacin. Therapy with CIPRO may be initiated before results of these tests are known; once results become available appropriate therapy should be continued. As with other drugs, some strains of *Pseudomonas aeruginosa* may develop resistance fairly rapidly during treatment with ciprofloxacin. Culture and susceptibility testing performed periodically during therapy will provide information not only on the therapeutic effect of the antimicrobial agent but also on the possible emergence of bacterial resistance.

To reduce the development of drug-resistant bacteria and maintain the effectiveness of CIPRO Tablets and CIPRO Oral Suspension and other antibacterial drugs, CIPRO Tablets and CIPRO Oral Suspension should be used only to treat or prevent infections that are proven or strongly suspected to be caused by susceptible bacteria. When culture and susceptibility information are available, they should be considered in selecting or modifying antibacterial therapy. In the absence of such data, local epidemiology and susceptibility patterns may contribute to the empiric selection of therapy.

CONTRAINDICATIONS

CIPRO (ciprofloxacin hydrochloride) is contraindicated in persons with a history of hypersensitivity to ciprofloxacin or any member of the quinolone class of antimicrobial agents.

WARNINGS

Pregnant Women: THE SAFETY AND EFFECTIVENESS OF CIPROFLOXACIN IN PREGNANT AND LACTATING WOMEN HAVE NOT BEEN ESTABLISHED. (See **PRECAUTIONS: Pregnancy,** and **Nursing Mothers** subsections.)

Pediatrics: Ciprofloxacin should be used in pediatric patients (less than 18 years of age) only for infections listed in the **INDICATIONS AND USAGE** section. An increased incidence of adverse events compared to controls, including events related to joints and/or surrounding tissues, has been observed. (See **ADVERSE REACTIONS.**)

In pre-clinical studies, oral administration of ciprofloxacin caused lameness in immature dogs. Histopathological examination of the weight-bearing joints of these dogs revealed permanent lesions of the cartilage. Related quinolone-class drugs also produce erosions of cartilage of weight-bearing joints and other signs of arthropathy in immature animals of various species. (See **ANIMAL PHARMACOLOGY.**)

Central Nervous System Disorders: Convulsions, increased intracranial pressure, and toxic psychosis have been reported in patients receiving quinolones, including ciprofloxacin. Ciprofloxacin may also cause central nervous system (CNS) events including: dizziness, confusion, tremors, hallucinations, depression, and, rarely, suicidal thoughts or acts. These reactions may occur following the first dose. If these reactions occur in patients receiving ciprofloxacin, the drug should be discontinued and appropriate measures instituted. As with all quinolones, ciprofloxacin should be used with caution in patients with known or suspected CNS disorders that may predispose to seizures or lower the seizure threshold (e.g. severe cerebral arteriosclerosis, epilepsy), or in the presence of other risk factors that may predispose to seizures or lower the seizure threshold (e.g. certain drug therapy, renal dysfunction). (See **PRECAUTIONS: General, Information for Patients, Drug Interactions** and **ADVERSE REACTIONS.**)

Theophylline: SERIOUS AND FATAL REACTIONS HAVE BEEN REPORTED IN PATIENTS RECEIVING CONCURRENT ADMINISTRATION OF CIPROFLOXACIN AND THEOPHYLLINE. These reactions have included cardiac arrest, seizure, status epilepticus, and respiratory failure. Although similar serious adverse effects have been reported in patients receiving theophylline alone, the possibility that these reactions may be potentiated by ciprofloxacin cannot be eliminated. If concomitant use cannot be avoided, serum levels of theophylline should be monitored and dosage adjustments made as appropriate.

Hypersensitivity Reactions: Serious and occasionally fatal hypersensitivity (anaphylactic) reactions, some following the first dose, have been reported in patients receiving quinolone therapy. Some reactions were accompanied by cardiovascular collapse, loss of consciousness, tingling, pharyngeal or facial edema, dyspnea, urticaria, and itching. Only a few patients had a history of hypersensitivity reactions. Serious anaphylactic reactions require immediate emergency treatment with epinephrine. Oxygen, intravenous steroids, and airway management, including intubation, should be administered as indicated.

Severe hypersensitivity reactions characterized by rash, fever, eosinophilia, jaundice, and hepatic necrosis with fatal outcome have also been rarely reported in patients receiving ciprofloxacin along with other drugs. The possibility that these reactions were related to ciprofloxacin cannot be excluded. Ciprofloxacin should be discontinued at the first appearance of a skin rash or any other sign of hypersensitivity.

Pseudomembranous Colitis: Pseudomembranous colitis has been reported with nearly all antibacterial agents, including ciprofloxacin, and may range in severity from mild to life-threatening. Therefore, it is important to consider this diagnosis in patients who present with diarrhea subsequent to the administration of antibacterial agents.

Treatment with antibacterial agents alters the normal flora of the colon and may permit overgrowth of clostridia. Studies indicate that a toxin produced by *Clostridium difficile* is one primary cause of "antibiotic-associated colitis."

After the diagnosis of pseudomembranous colitis has been established, therapeutic measures should be initiated. Mild cases of pseudomembranous colitis usually respond to drug discontinuation alone. In moderate to severe cases, consideration should be given to management with fluids and electrolytes, protein supplementation, and treatment with an antibacterial drug clinically effective against *C. difficile* colitis. Drugs that inhibit peristalsis should be avoided.

Peripheral neuropathy: Rare cases of sensory or sensorimotor axonal polyneuropathy affecting small and/or large axons resulting in paresthesias, hypoesthesias, dysesthesias and weakness have been reported in patients receiving quinolones, including ciprofloxacin. Ciprofloxacin should be discontinued if the patient experiences symptoms of neuropathy including pain, burning, tingling, numbness, and/or weakness, or is found to have deficits in light touch, pain, temperature, position sense, vibratory sensation, and/or motor strength in order to prevent the development of an irreversible condition.

Tendon Effects: Ruptures of the shoulder, hand, Achilles tendon or other tendons that required surgical repair or resulted in prolonged disability have been reported in patients receiving quinolones, including ciprofloxacin. Post-marketing surveillance reports indicate that this risk may be increased in patients receiving concomitant corticosteroids, especially the elderly. Ciprofloxacin should be discontinued if the patient experiences pain, inflammation, or rupture of a tendon. Patients should rest and refrain from exercise until the diagnosis of tendinitis or tendon rupture has been excluded. Tendon rupture can occur during or after therapy with quinolones, including ciprofloxacin.

Syphilis: Ciprofloxacin has not been shown to be effective in the treatment of syphilis. Antimicrobial agents used in high dose for short periods of time to treat gonorrhea may mask or delay the symptoms of incubating syphilis. All patients with gonorrhea should have a serologic test for syphilis at the time of diagnosis. Patients treated with ciprofloxacin should have a follow-up serologic test for syphilis after three months.

PRECAUTIONS

General: Crystals of ciprofloxacin have been observed rarely in the urine of human subjects but more frequently in the urine of laboratory animals, which is usually alkaline. (See **ANIMAL PHARMACOLOGY.**) Crystalluria related to ciprofloxacin has been reported only rarely in humans because human urine is usually acidic. Alkalinity of the urine should be avoided in patients receiving ciprofloxacin. Patients should be well hydrated to prevent the formation of highly concentrated urine.

Central Nervous System: Quinolones, including ciprofloxacin, may also cause central nervous system (CNS) events, including: nervousness, agitation, insomnia, anxiety, nightmares or paranoia. (See **WARNINGS, Information for Patients,** and **Drug Interactions.**)

Renal Impairment: Alteration of the dosage regimen is necessary for patients with impairment of renal function. (See **DOSAGE AND ADMINISTRATION.**)

Phototoxicity: Moderate to severe phototoxicity manifested as an exaggerated sunburn reaction has been observed in patients who are exposed to direct sunlight while receiving some members of the quinolone class of drugs. Excessive sunlight should be avoided. Therapy should be discontinued if phototoxicity occurs.

As with any potent drug, periodic assessment of organ system functions, including renal, hepatic, and hematopoietic function, is advisable during prolonged therapy.

Prescribing CIPRO Tablets and CIPRO Oral Suspension in the absence of a proven or strongly suspected bacterial infection or a prophylactic indication is unlikely to provide benefit to the patient and increases the risk of the development of drug-resistant bacteria.

Information for Patients:

Patients should be advised:

- that antibacterial drugs including CIPRO Tablets and CIPRO Oral Suspension should only be used to treat bacterial infections. They do not treat viral infections (e.g., the common cold). When CIPRO Tablets and CIPRO Oral Suspension is prescribed to treat a bacterial infection, patients should be told that although it is common to feel better early in the course of therapy, the medication should be taken exactly as directed. Skipping doses or not completing the full course of therapy may (1) decrease the effectiveness of the immediate treatment and (2) increase the likelihood that bacteria will develop resistance and will not be treatable by CIPRO Tablets and CIPRO Oral Suspension or other antibacterial drugs in the future.
- that ciprofloxacin may be taken with or without meals and to drink fluids liberally. As with other quinolones, concurrent administration of ciprofloxacin with magnesium/aluminum antacids, or sucralfate, Videx® (didanosine) chewable/buffered tablets or pediatric powder, or with other products containing calcium, iron or zinc should be avoided. Ciprofloxacin may be taken two hours before or six hours after taking these products. Ciprofloxacin should not be taken with dairy products (like milk or yogurt) or calcium-fortified juices alone since absorption of ciprofloxacin may be significantly reduced; however, ciprofloxacin may be taken with a meal that contains these products.
- that ciprofloxacin may be associated with hypersensitivity reactions, even following a single dose, and to discontinue the drug at the first sign of a skin rash or other allergic reaction.
- to avoid excessive sunlight or artificial ultraviolet light while receiving ciprofloxacin and to discontinue therapy if phototoxicity occurs.
- that peripheral neuropathies have been associated with ciprofloxacin use. If symptoms of peripheral neuropathy including pain, burning, tingling, numbness and/or weakness develop, they should discontinue treatment and contact their physicians.
- to discontinue treatment; rest and refrain from exercise; and inform their physician if they experience pain, inflammation, or rupture of a tendon.
- that ciprofloxacin may cause dizziness and lightheadedness; therefore, patients should know how they react to this drug before they operate an automobile or machinery or engage in activities requiring mental alertness or coordination.
- that ciprofloxacin may increase the effects of theophylline and caffeine. There is a possibility of caffeine accumulation when products containing caffeine are consumed while taking quinolones.
- that convulsions have been reported in patients receiving quinolones, including ciprofloxacin, and to notify their physician before taking this drug if there is a history of this condition.
- that ciprofloxacin has been associated with an increased rate of adverse events involving joints and surrounding tissue structures (like tendons) in pediatric patients (less than 18 years of age). Parents should inform their child's physician if the child has a history of joint-related problems before taking this drug. Parents of pediatric patients should also notify their child's physician of any joint-related problems that occur during or following ciprofloxacin therapy. (See **WARNINGS, PRECAUTIONS, Pediatric Use** and **ADVERSE REACTIONS.**)

Drug Interactions: As with some other quinolones, concurrent administration of ciprofloxacin with theophylline may lead to elevated serum concentrations of theophylline and prolongation of its elimination half-life. This may result in increased risk of theophylline-related adverse reactions. (See **WARNINGS.**) If concomitant use cannot be avoided, serum levels of theophylline should be monitored and dosage adjustments made as appropriate.

Some quinolones, including ciprofloxacin, have also been shown to interfere with the metabolism of caffeine. This may lead to reduced clearance of caffeine and a prolongation of its serum half-life.

Concurrent administration of a quinolone, including ciprofloxacin, with multivalent cation-containing products such as magnesium/aluminum antacids, sucralfate, Videx® (didanosine) chewable/buffered tablets or pediatric powder, or products containing calcium, iron, or zinc may substantially decrease its absorption, resulting in serum and urine levels considerably lower than desired. (See **DOSAGE AND ADMINISTRATION** for concurrent administration of these agents with ciprofloxacin.)

Histamine H_2-receptor antagonists appear to have no significant effect on the bioavailability of ciprofloxacin.

Altered serum levels of phenytoin (increased and decreased) have been reported in patients receiving concomitant ciprofloxacin.

The concomitant administration of ciprofloxacin with the sulfonylurea glyburide has, on rare occasions, resulted in severe hypoglycemia.

Some quinolones, including ciprofloxacin, have been associated with transient elevations in serum creatinine in patients receiving cyclosporine concomitantly.

Quinolones, including ciprofloxacin, have been reported to enhance the effects of the oral anticoagulant warfarin or its derivatives. When these products are administered concomitantly, prothrombin time or other suitable coagulation tests should be closely monitored.

Probenecid interferes with renal tubular secretion of ciprofloxacin and produces an increase in the level of ciprofloxacin in the serum. This should be considered if patients are receiving both drugs concomitantly.

Renal tubular transport of methotrexate may be inhibited by concomitant administration of ciprofloxacin potentially leading to increased plasma levels of methotrexate. This might increase the risk of methotrexate associated toxic reactions. Therefore, patients under methotrexate therapy should be carefully monitored when concomitant ciprofloxacin therapy is indicated.

Metoclopramide significantly accelerates the absorption of oral ciprofloxacin resulting in shorter time to reach maximum plasma concentrations. No significant effect was observed on the bioavailability of ciprofloxacin.

Non-steroidal anti-inflammatory drugs (but not acetyl salicylic acid) in combination of very high doses of quinolones have been shown to provoke convulsions in pre-clinical studies.

Carcinogenesis, Mutagenesis, Impairment of Fertility: Eight *in vitro* mutagenicity tests have been conducted with ciprofloxacin, and the test results are listed below:

Salmonella/Microsome Test (Negative)
E. coli DNA Repair Assay (Negative)
Mouse Lymphoma Cell Forward Mutation Assay (Positive)
Chinese Hamster V_{79} Cell HGPRT Test (Negative)
Syrian Hamster Embryo Cell Transformation Assay (Negative)
Saccharomyces cerevisiae Point Mutation Assay (Negative)
Saccharomyces cerevisiae Mitotic Crossover and Gene Conversion Assay (Negative)
Rat Hepatocyte DNA Repair Assay (Positive)

Thus, 2 of the 8 tests were positive, but results of the following 3 *in vivo* test systems gave negative results:

Rat Hepatocyte DNA Repair Assay
Micronucleus Test (Mice)
Dominant Lethal Test (Mice)

Long-term carcinogenicity studies in rats and mice resulted in no carcinogenic or tumorigenic effects due to ciprofloxacin at daily oral dose levels up to 250 and 750 mg/kg to rats and mice, respectively (approximately 1.7- and 2.5- times the highest recommended therapeutic dose based upon mg/m^2).

Results from photo co-carcinogenicity testing indicate that ciprofloxacin does not reduce the time to appearance of UV-induced skin tumors as compared to vehicle control. Hairless (Skh-1) mice were exposed to UVA light for 3.5 hours five times every two weeks for up to 78 weeks while concurrently being administered ciprofloxacin. The time to development of the first skin tumors was 50 weeks in mice

Continued on next page

Cipro—Cont.

treated concomitantly with UVA and ciprofloxacin (mouse dose approximately equal to maximum recommended human dose based upon mg/m^2), as opposed to 34 weeks when animals were treated with both UVA and vehicle. The times to development of skin tumors ranged from 16-32 weeks in mice treated concomitantly with UVA and other quinolones.[3]

In this model, mice treated with ciprofloxacin alone did not develop skin or systemic tumors. There are no data from similar models using pigmented mice and/or fully haired mice. The clinical significance of these findings to humans is unknown.

Fertility studies performed in rats at oral doses of ciprofloxacin up to 100 mg/kg (approximately 0.7-times the highest recommended therapeutic dose based upon mg/m^2) revealed no evidence of impairment.

Pregnancy: Teratogenic Effects. Pregnancy Category C: There are no adequate and well-controlled studies in pregnant women. An expert review of published data on experiences with ciprofloxacin use during pregnancy by TERIS – the Teratogen Information System – concluded that therapeutic doses during pregnancy are unlikely to pose a substantial teratogenic risk (quantity and quality of data=fair), but the data are insufficient to state that there is no risk.[7]

A controlled prospective observational study followed 200 women exposed to fluoroquinolones (52.5% exposed to ciprofloxacin and 68% first trimester exposures) during gestation.[8] In utero exposure to fluoroquinolones during embryogenesis was not associated with increased risk of major malformations. The reported rates of major congenital malformations were 2.2% for the fluoroquinolone group and 2.6% for the control group (background incidence of major malformations is 1-5%). Rates of spontaneous abortions, prematurity and low birth weight did not differ between the groups and there were no clinically significant musculoskeletal dysfunctions up to one year of age in the ciprofloxacin exposed children.

Another prospective follow-up study reported on 549 pregnancies with fluoroquinolone exposure (93% first trimester exposures).[9] There were 70 ciprofloxacin exposures, all within the first trimester. The malformation rates among live-born babies exposed to ciprofloxacin and to fluoroquinolones overall were both within background incidence ranges. No specific patterns of congenital abnormalities were found. The study did not reveal any clear adverse reactions due to in utero exposure to ciprofloxacin.

No differences in the rates of prematurity, spontaneous abortions, or birth weight were seen in women exposed to ciprofloxacin during pregnancy.[7,8] However, these small postmarketing epidemiology studies, of which most experience is from short term, first trimester exposure, are insufficient to evaluate the risk for less common defects or to permit reliable and definitive conclusions regarding the safety of ciprofloxacin in pregnant women and their developing fetuses. Ciprofloxacin should not be used during pregnancy unless the potential benefit justifies the potential risk to both fetus and mother (see **WARNINGS**).

Reproduction studies have been performed in rats and mice using oral doses up to 100 mg/kg (0.6 and 0.3 times the maximum daily human dose based upon body surface area, respectively) and have revealed no evidence of harm to the fetus due to ciprofloxacin. In rabbits, oral ciprofloxacin dose levels of 30 and 100 mg/kg (approximately 0.4- and 1.3-times the highest recommended therapeutic dose based upon mg/m^2) produced gastrointestinal toxicity resulting in maternal weight loss and an increased incidence of abortion, but no teratogenicity was observed at either dose level. After intravenous administration of doses up to 20 mg/kg (approximately 0.3- times the highest recommended therapeutic dose based upon mg/m^2) no maternal toxicity was produced and no embryotoxicity or teratogenicity was observed. (See **WARNINGS.**)

Nursing Mothers: Ciprofloxacin is excreted in human milk. The amount of ciprofloxacin absorbed by the nursing infant is unknown. Because of the potential for serious adverse reactions in infants nursing from mothers taking ciprofloxacin, a decision should be made whether to discontinue nursing or to discontinue the drug, taking into account the importance of the drug to the mother.

Pediatric Use: Ciprofloxacin, like other quinolones, causes arthropathy and histological changes in weight-bearing joints of juvenile animals resulting in lameness. (See **ANIMAL PHARMACOLOGY.**)

Inhalational Anthrax (Post-Exposure)

Ciprofloxacin is indicated in pediatric patients for inhalational anthrax (post-exposure). The risk-benefit assessment indicates that administration of ciprofloxacin to pediatric patients is appropriate. For information regarding pediatric dosing in inhalational anthrax (post-exposure), see **DOSAGE AND ADMINISTRATION** and **INHALATIONAL ANTHRAX – ADDITIONAL INFORMATION.**

Complicated Urinary Tract Infection and Pyelonephritis

Ciprofloxacin is indicated for the treatment of complicated urinary tract infections and pyelonephritis due to *Escherichia coli.* Although effective in clinical trials, ciprofloxacin is not a drug of first choice in the pediatric population due to an increased incidence of adverse events compared to the controls, including events related to joints and/or surrounding tissues. The rates of these events in pediatric patients with complicated urinary tract infection and pyelonephritis within six weeks of follow-up were 9.3% (31/335) versus 6.0% (21/349) for control agents. The rates of these events occurring at any time up to the one year follow-up were 13.7% (46/335) and 9.5% (33/349), respectively. The rate of all adverse events regardless of drug relationship at six weeks was 41% (138/335) in the ciprofloxacin arm compared to 31% (109/349) in the control arm. (See **ADVERSE REACTIONS** and **CLINICAL STUDIES.**)

Cystic Fibrosis

Short-term safety data from a single trial in pediatric cystic fibrosis patients are available. In a randomized, double-blind clinical trial for the treatment of acute pulmonary exacerbations in cystic fibrosis patients (ages 5-17 years), 67 patients received ciprofloxacin I.V. 10 mg/kg/dose q8h for one week followed by ciprofloxacin tablets 20 mg/kg/dose q12h to complete 10-21 days treatment and 62 patients received the combination of ceftazidime I.V. 50 mg/kg/dose q8h and tobramycin I.V. 3 mg/kg/dose q8h for a total of 10-21 days. Patients less than 5 years of age were not studied. Safety monitoring in the study included periodic range of motion examinations and gait assessments by treatment-blinded examiners. Patients were followed for an average of 23 days after completing treatment (range 0-93 days). This study was not designed to determine long term effects and the safety of repeated exposure to ciprofloxacin.

Musculoskeletal adverse events in patients with cystic fibrosis were reported in 22% of the patients in the ciprofloxacin group and 21% in the comparison group. Decreased range of motion was reported in 12% of the subjects in the ciprofloxacin group and 16% in the comparison group. Arthralgia was reported in 10% of the patients in the ciprofloxacin group and 11% in the comparison group. Other adverse events were similar in nature and frequency between treatment arms. One of sixty-seven patients developed arthritis of the knee nine days after a ten day course of treatment with ciprofloxacin. Clinical symptoms resolved, but an MRI showed knee effusion without other abnormalities eight months after treatment. However, the relationship of this event to the patient's course of ciprofloxacin can not be definitively determined, particularly since patients with cystic fibrosis may develop arthralgias/arthritis as part of their underlying disease process.

Geriatric Use: In a retrospective analysis of 23 multiple-dose controlled clinical trials of ciprofloxacin encompassing over 3500 ciprofloxacin treated patients, 25% of patients were greater than or equal to 65 years of age and 10% were greater than or equal to 75 years of age. No overall differences in safety or effectiveness were observed between these subjects and younger subjects, and other reported clinical experience has not identified differences in responses between the elderly and younger patients, but greater sensitivity of some older individuals on any drug therapy cannot be ruled out. Ciprofloxacin is known to be substantially excreted by the kidney, and the risk of adverse reactions may be greater in patients with impaired renal function. No alteration of dosage is necessary for patients greater than 65 years of age with normal renal function. However, since some older individuals experience reduced renal function by virtue of their advanced age, care should be taken in dose selection for elderly patients, and renal function monitoring may be useful in these patients. (See **CLINICAL PHARMACOLOGY** and **DOSAGE AND ADMINISTRATION.**)

ADVERSE REACTIONS

Adverse Reactions in Adult Patients: During clinical investigations with oral and parenteral ciprofloxacin, 49,038 patients received courses of the drug. Most of the adverse events reported were described as only mild or moderate in severity, abated soon after the drug was discontinued, and required no treatment. Ciprofloxacin was discontinued because of an adverse event in 1.0% of orally treated patients. The most frequently reported drug related events, from clinical trials of all formulations, all dosages, all drug-therapy durations, and for all indications of ciprofloxacin therapy were nausea (2.5%), diarrhea (1.6%), liver function tests abnormal (1.3%), vomiting (1.0%), and rash (1.0%).

Additional medically important events that occurred in less than 1% of ciprofloxacin patients are listed below.

BODY AS A WHOLE: headache, abdominal pain/discomfort, foot pain, pain, pain in extremities, injection site reaction (ciprofloxacin intravenous)

CARDIOVASCULAR: palpitation, atrial flutter, ventricular ectopy, syncope, hypertension, angina pectoris, myocardial infarction, cardiopulmonary arrest, cerebral thrombosis, phlebitis, tachycardia, migraine, hypotension

CENTRAL NERVOUS SYSTEM: restlessness, dizziness, lightheadedness, insomnia, nightmares, hallucinations, manic reaction, irritability, tremor, ataxia, convulsive seizures, lethargy, drowsiness, weakness, malaise, anorexia, phobia, depersonalization, depression, paresthesia, abnormal gait, grand mal convulsion

GASTROINTESTINAL: painful oral mucosa, oral candidiasis, dysphagia, intestinal perforation, gastrointestinal bleeding, cholestatic jaundice, hepatitis

HEMIC/LYMPHATIC: lymphadenopathy, petechia

METABOLIC/NUTRITIONAL: amylase increase, lipase increase

MUSCULOSKELETAL: arthralgia or back pain, joint stiffness, achiness, neck or chest pain, flare up of gout

RENAL/UROGENITAL: interstitial nephritis, nephritis, renal failure, polyuria, urinary retention, urethral bleeding, vaginitis, acidosis, breast pain

RESPIRATORY: dyspnea, epistaxis, laryngeal or pulmonary edema, hiccough, hemoptysis, bronchospasm, pulmonary embolism

SKIN/HYPERSENSITIVITY: allergic reaction, pruritus, urticaria, photosensitivity, flushing, fever, chills, angioedema, edema of the face, neck, lips, conjunctivae or hands, cutaneous candidiasis, hyperpigmentation, erythema nodosum, sweating

SPECIAL SENSES: blurred vision, disturbed vision (change in color perception, overbrightness of lights), decreased visual acuity, diplopia, eye pain, tinnitus, hearing loss, bad taste, chromatopsia

In several instances nausea, vomiting, tremor, irritability, or palpitation were judged by investigators to be related to elevated serum levels of theophylline possibly as a result of drug interaction with ciprofloxacin.

In randomized, double-blind controlled clinical trials comparing ciprofloxacin tablets (500 mg BID) to cefuroxime axetil (250 mg - 500 mg BID) and to clarithromycin (500 mg BID) in patients with respiratory tract infections, ciprofloxacin demonstrated a CNS adverse event profile comparable to the control drugs.

Adverse Reactions in Pediatric Patients: Ciprofloxacin, administered I.V. and/or orally, was compared to a cephalosporin for treatment of complicated urinary tract infections (cUTI) or pyelonephritis in pediatric patients 1 to 17 years of age (mean age of 6 ± 4 years). The trial was conducted in the US, Canada, Argentina, Peru, Costa Rica, Mexico, South Africa, and Germany. The duration of therapy was 10 to 21 days (mean duration of treatment was 11 days with a range of 1 to 88 days). The primary objective of the study was to assess musculoskeletal and neurological safety within 6 weeks of therapy and through one year of follow-up in the 335 ciprofloxacin- and 349 comparator-treated patients enrolled.

An Independent Pediatric Safety Committee (IPSC) reviewed all cases of musculoskeletal adverse events as well as all patients with an abnormal gait or abnormal joint exam (baseline or treatment-emergent). These events were evaluated in a comprehensive fashion and included such conditions as arthralgia, abnormal gait, abnormal joint exam, joint sprains, leg pain, back pain, arthrosis, bone pain, pain, myalgia, arm pain, and decreased range of motion in a joint. The affected joints included: knee, elbow, ankle, hip, wrist, and shoulder. Within 6 weeks of treatment initiation, the rates of these events were 9.3% (31/335) in the ciprofloxacin-treated group versus 6.0 % (21/349) in comparator-treated patients. The majority of these events were mild or moderate in intensity. All musculoskeletal events occurring by 6 weeks resolved (clinical resolution of signs and symptoms), usually within 30 days of end of treatment. Radiological evaluations were not routinely used to confirm resolution of the events. The events occurred more frequently in ciprofloxacin-treated patients than control patients, regardless of whether they received I.V. or oral therapy. Ciprofloxacin-treated patients were more likely to report more than one event and on more than one occasion compared to control patients. These events occurred in all age groups and the rates were consistently higher in the ciprofloxacin group compared to the control group. At the end of 1 year, the rate of these events reported at any time during that period was 13.7% (46/335) in the ciprofloxacin-treated group versus 9.5% (33/349) comparator-treated patients.

An adolescent female discontinued ciprofloxacin for wrist pain that developed during treatment. An MRI performed 4 weeks later showed a tear in the right ulnar fibrocartilage. A diagnosis of overuse syndrome secondary to sports activity was made, but a contribution from ciprofloxacin cannot be excluded. The patient recovered by 4 months without surgical intervention.

[See first table at top of next page]

The incidence rates of neurological events within 6 weeks of treatment initiation were 3% (9/335) in the ciprofloxacin group versus 2% (7/349) in the comparator group and included dizziness, nervousness, insomnia, and somnolence.

In this trial, the overall incidence rates of adverse events regardless of relationship to study drug and within 6 weeks of treatment initiation were 41% (138/335) in the ciprofloxacin group versus 31% (109/349) in the comparator group. The most frequent events were gastrointestinal: 15% (50/335) of ciprofloxacin patients compared to 9% (31/349) of comparator patients. Serious adverse events were seen in 7.5% (25/335) of ciprofloxacin-treated patients compared to 5.7% (20/349) of control patients. Discontinuation of drug due to an adverse event was observed in 3% (10/335) of ciprofloxacin-treated patients versus 1.4% (5/349) of comparator patients. Other adverse events that occurred in at least 1% of ciprofloxacin patients were diarrhea 4.8%, vomiting 4.8%, abdominal pain 3.3%, accidental injury 3.0%, rhinitis 3.0%, dyspepsia 2.7%, nausea 2.7%, fever 2.1%, asthma 1.8% and rash 1.8%.

In addition to the events reported in pediatric patients in clinical trials, it should be expected that events reported in adults during clinical trials or post-marketing experience may also occur in pediatric patients.

Post-Marketing Adverse Events: The following adverse events have been reported from worldwide marketing experience with quinolones, including ciprofloxacin. Because these events are reported voluntarily from a population of uncertain size, it is not always possible to reliably estimate their frequency or establish a causal relationship to drug exposure. Decisions to include these events in labeling are typically based on one or more of the following factors: (1) seriousness of the event, (2) frequency of the reporting, or (3) strength of causal connection to the drug.

Agitation, agranulocytosis, albuminuria, anaphylactic reactions, anosmia, candiduria, cholesterol elevation (serum), confusion, constipation, delirium, dyspepsia, dysphagia, erythema multiforme, exfoliative dermatitis, fixed eruption, flatulence, glucose elevation (blood), hemolytic anemia, hepatic failure, hepatic necrosis, hyperesthesia, hypertonia, hypesthesia, hypotension (postural), jaundice, marrow depression (life threatening), methemoglobinemia, moniliasis (oral, gastrointestinal, vaginal), myalgia, myasthenia, myasthenia gravis (possible exacerbation), myoclonus, nystagmus, pancreatitis, pancytopenia (life threatening or fatal outcome), peripheral neuropathy, phenytoin alteration (serum), potassium elevation (serum), prothrombin time prolongation or decrease, pseudomembranous colitis (The onset of pseudomembranous colitis symptoms may occur during or after antimicrobial treatment.), psychosis (toxic), renal calculi, serum sickness like reaction, Stevens-Johnson syndrome, taste loss, tendinitis, tendon rupture, torsade de pointes, toxic epidermal necrolysis, triglyceride elevation (serum), twitching, vaginal candidiasis, and vasculitis. (See **PRECAUTIONS**.)

Adverse Laboratory Changes: Changes in laboratory parameters listed as adverse events without regard to drug relationship are listed below:

Hepatic –Elevations of ALT (SGPT) (1.9%), AST (SGOT) (1.7%), alkaline phosphatase (0.8%), LDH (0.4%), serum bilirubin (0.3%).

Hematologic –Eosinophilia (0.6%), leukopenia (0.4%), decreased blood platelets (0.1%), elevated blood platelets (0.1%), pancytopenia (0.1%).

Renal –Elevations of serum creatinine (1.1%), BUN (0.9%), CRYSTALLURIA, CYLINDRURIA, AND HEMATURIA HAVE BEEN REPORTED.

Other changes occurring in less than 0.1% of courses were: elevation of serum gammaglutamyl transferase, elevation of serum amylase, reduction in blood glucose, elevated uric acid, decrease in hemoglobin, anemia, bleeding diathesis, increase in blood monocytes, leukocytosis.

OVERDOSAGE

In the event of acute overdosage, reversible renal toxicity has been reported in some cases. The stomach should be emptied by inducing vomiting or by gastric lavage. The patient should be carefully observed and given supportive treatment, including monitoring of renal function and administration of magnesium, aluminum, or calcium containing antacids which can reduce the absorption of ciprofloxacin. Adequate hydration must be maintained. Only a small amount of ciprofloxacin (< 10%) is removed from the body after hemodialysis or peritoneal dialysis.

Single doses of ciprofloxacin were relatively non-toxic via the oral route of administration in mice, rats, and dogs. No deaths occurred within a 14-day post treatment observation period at the highest oral doses tested; up to 5000 mg/kg in either rodent species, or up to 2500 mg/kg in the dog. Clinical signs observed included hypoactivity and cyanosis in both rodent species and severe vomiting in dogs. In rabbits, significant mortality was seen at doses of ciprofloxacin > 2500 mg/kg. Mortality was delayed in these animals, occurring 10-14 days after dosing.

In mice, rats, rabbits and dogs, significant toxicity including tonic/clonic convulsions was observed at intravenous doses of ciprofloxacin between 125 and 300 mg/kg.

DOSAGE AND ADMINISTRATION - ADULTS

CIPRO Tablets and Oral Suspension should be administered orally to adults as described in the Dosage Guidelines table.

The determination of dosage for any particular patient must take into consideration the severity and nature of the infection, the susceptibility of the causative organism, the integrity of the patient's host-defense mechanisms, and the status of renal function and hepatic function.

The duration of treatment depends upon the severity of infection. The usual duration is 7 to 14 days; however, for severe and complicated infections more prolonged therapy may be required. Ciprofloxacin should be administered at least 2 hours before or 6 hours after magnesium/aluminum antacids, or sucralfate, Videx® (didanosine) chewable/buffered tablets or pediatric powder for oral solution, or other products containing calcium, iron or zinc.

[See second table at right]

Conversion of I.V. to Oral Dosing in Adults: Patients whose therapy is started with CIPRO I.V. may be switched to CIPRO Tablets or Oral Suspension when clinically indicated at the discretion of the physician (See **CLINICAL PHARMACOLOGY** and table below for the equivalent dosing regimens).

Equivalent AUC Dosing Regimens

Cipro Oral Dosage	Equivalent Cipro I.V. Dosage
250 mg Tablet q 12 h	200 mg I.V. q 12 h
500 mg Tablet q 12 h	400 mg I.V. q 12 h
750 mg Tablet q 12 h	400 mg I.V. q 8 h

Adults with Impaired Renal Function: Ciprofloxacin is eliminated primarily by renal excretion; however, the drug is also metabolized and partially cleared through the biliary system of the liver and through the intestine. These alternative pathways of drug elimination appear to compensate for the reduced renal excretion in patients with renal impairment. Nonetheless, some modification of dosage is recommended, particularly for patients with severe renal dysfunction. The following table provides dosage guidelines for use in patients with renal impairment:

RECOMMENDED STARTING AND MAINTENANCE DOSES FOR PATIENTS WITH IMPAIRED RENAL FUNCTION

Creatinine Clearance (mL/min)	Dose
> 50	See Usual Dosage.
30 – 50	250 – 500 mg q 12 h
5 – 29	250 – 500 mg q 18 h
Patients on hemodialysis or Peritoneal dialysis	250 – 500 mg q 24 h (after dialysis)

When only the serum creatinine concentration is known, the following formula may be used to estimate creatinine clearance.

[See third table above]

The serum creatinine should represent a steady state of renal function.

In patients with severe infections and severe renal impairment, a unit dose of 750 mg may be administered at the intervals noted above. Patients should be carefully monitored.

DOSAGE AND ADMINISTRATION – PEDIATRICS

CIPRO Tablets and Oral Suspension should be administered orally as described in the Dosage Guidelines table. An increased incidence of adverse events compared to controls, including events related to joints and/or surrounding tissues, has been observed. (See **ADVERSE REACTIONS** and **CLINICAL STUDIES**.)

Dosing and initial route of therapy (i.e., I.V. or oral) for complicated urinary tract infection or pyelonephritis should be determined by the severity of the infection. In the clinical trial, pediatric patients with moderate to severe infection were initiated on 6 to 10 mg/kg I.V. every 8 hours and allowed to switch to oral therapy (10 to 20 mg/kg every 12 hours), at the discretion of the physician.

[See first table at top of next page]

Pediatric patients with moderate to severe renal insufficiency were excluded from the clinical trial of complicated urinary tract infection and pyelonephritis. No information is available on dosing adjustments necessary for pediatric patients with moderate to severe renal insufficiency (i.e., creatinine clearance of < 50 mL/min/1.73m²).

HOW SUPPLIED

CIPRO (ciprofloxacin hydrochloride) Tablets are available as round, slightly yellowish film-coated tablets containing 100 mg or 250 mg ciprofloxacin. The 100 mg tablet is coded with the word "CIPRO" on one side and "100" on the reverse side. The 250 mg tablet is coded with the word "CIPRO" on one side and "250" on the reverse side. CIPRO is also available as capsule shaped, slightly yellowish film-coated tablets containing 500 mg or 750 mg ciprofloxacin. The 500 mg tablet is coded with the word "CIPRO" on one side and "500" on the reverse side. The 750 mg tablet is coded with the word "CIPRO" on one side and "750" on the reverse side. CIPRO 250 mg, 500 mg, and 750 mg are available in bottles of 50, 100, and Unit Dose packages of 100. The 100 mg

Continued on next page

Findings Involving Joint or Peri-articular Tissues as Assessed by the IPSC

	Ciprofloxacin	Comparator
All Patients (within 6 weeks)	31/335 (9.3%)	21/349 (6.0%)
95% Confidence Interval*	(-0.8%, +7.2%)	
Age Group		
≥12 months < 24 months	1/36 (2.8%)	0/41
≥ 2 years < 6 years	5/124 (4.0%)	3/118 (2.5%)
≥ 6 years < 12 years	18/143 (12.6%)	12/153 (7.8%)
≥ 12 years to 17 years	7/32 (21.9%)	6/37 (16.2%)
All Patients (within 1 year)	46/335 (13.7%)	33/349 (9.5%)
95% Confidence Interval*	(-0.6%, +9.1%)	

*The study was designed to demonstrate that the arthropathy rate for the ciprofloxacin group did not exceed that of the control group by more than + 6%. At both the 6 week and 1 year evaluations, the 95% confidence interval indicated that it could not be concluded that ciprofloxacin group had findings comparable to the control group.

ADULT DOSAGE GUIDELINES

Infection	Severity	Dose	Frequency	Usual Durations†
Urinary Tract	Acute Uncomplicated	100 mg or 250 mg	q 12 h	3 Days
	Mild/Moderate	250 mg	q 12 h	7 to 14 Days
	Severe/Complicated	500 mg	q 12 h	7 to 14 Days
Chronic Bacterial Prostatitis	Mild/Moderate	500 mg	q 12 h	28 Days
Lower Respiratory Tract	Mild/Moderate	500 mg	q 12 h	7 to 14 Days
	Severe/Complicated	750 mg	q 12 h	7 to 14 Days
Acute Sinusitis	Mild/Moderate	500 mg	q 12 h	10 Days
Skin and Skin Structure	Mild/Moderate	500 mg	q 12 h	7 to 14 Days
	Severe/Complicated	750 mg	q 12 h	7 to 14 Days
Bone and Joint	Mild/Moderate	500 mg	q 12 h	≥ 4 to 6 weeks
	Severe/Complicated	750 mg	q 12 h	≥4 to 6 weeks
Intra-Abdominal*	Complicated	500 mg	q 12 h	7 to 14 Days
Infectious Diarrhea	Mild/Moderate/Severe	500 mg	q 12 h	5 to 7 Days
Typhoid Fever	Mild/Moderate	500 mg	q 12 h	10 Days
Urethral and Cervical Gonococcal Infections	Uncomplicated	250 mg	single dose	single dose
Inhalational anthrax (post-exposure)**		500 mg	q 12 h	60 Days

* used in conjunction with metronidazole

† Generally ciprofloxacin should be continued for at least 2 days after the signs and symptoms of infection have disappeared, except for inhalational anthrax (post-exposure).

** Drug administration should begin as soon as possible after suspected or confirmed exposure. This indication is based on a surrogate endpoint, ciprofloxacin serum concentrations achieved in humans, reasonably likely to predict clinical benefit.[4] For a discussion of ciprofloxacin serum concentrations in various human populations, see **INHALATIONAL ANTHRAX – ADDITIONAL INFORMATION.**

$$\text{Men: Creatinine clearance (mL/min)} = \frac{\text{Weight (kg)} \times (140 - \text{age})}{72 \times \text{serum creatinine (mg/dL)}}$$

Women: 0.85 × the value calculated for men.

Cipro—Cont.

strength is available only as CIPRO Cystitis pack containing 6 tablets for use only in female patients with acute uncomplicated cystitis.

[See second table at right]

Store below 30°C (86°F).

CIPRO Oral Suspension is supplied in 5% and 10% strengths. The drug product is composed of two components (microcapsules containing the active ingredient and diluent) which must be mixed by the pharmacist. See Instructions To The Pharmacist For Use/Handling.

[See third table at right]

Microcapsules and diluent should be stored below 25°C (77°F) and protected from freezing.

Reconstituted product may be stored below 30°C (86°F) for 14 days. Protect from freezing. A teaspoon is provided for the patient.

ANIMAL PHARMACOLOGY

Ciprofloxacin and other quinolones have been shown to cause arthropathy in immature animals of most species tested. (See **WARNINGS**.) Damage of weight bearing joints was observed in juvenile dogs and rats. In young beagles, 100 mg/kg ciprofloxacin, given daily for 4 weeks, caused degenerative articular changes of the knee joint. At 30 mg/kg, the effect on the joint was minimal. In a subsequent study in young beagle dogs, oral ciprofloxacin doses of 30 mg/kg and 90 mg/kg ciprofloxacin (approximately 1.3- and 3.5-times the pediatric dose based upon comparative plasma AUCs) given daily for 2 weeks caused articular changes which were still observed by histopathology after a treatment-free period of 5 months. At 10 mg/kg (approximately 0.6-times the pediatric dose based upon comparative plasma AUCs), no effects on joints were observed. This dose was also not associated with arthrotoxicity after an additional treatment-free period of 5 months. In another study, removal of weight bearing from the joint reduced the lesions but did not totally prevent them.

Crystalluria, sometimes associated with secondary nephropathy, occurs in laboratory animals dosed with ciprofloxacin. This is primarily related to the reduced solubility of ciprofloxacin under alkaline conditions, which predominate in the urine of test animals; in man, crystalluria is rare since human urine is typically acidic. In rhesus monkeys, crystalluria without nephropathy was noted after single oral doses as low as 5 mg/kg. (approximately 0.07-times the highest recommended therapeutic dose based upon mg/m^2). After 6 months of intravenous dosing at 10 mg/kg/day, no nephropathological changes were noted; however, nephropathy was observed after dosing at 20 mg/kg/day for the same duration (approximately 0.2-times the highest recommended therapeutic dose based upon mg/m^2).

In dogs, ciprofloxacin at 3 and 10 mg/kg by rapid I.V. injection (15 sec.) produces pronounced hypotensive effects. These effects are considered to be related to histamine release, since they are partially antagonized by pyrilamine, an antihistamine. In rhesus monkeys, rapid I.V. injection also produces hypotension but the effect in this species is inconsistent and less pronounced.

In mice, concomitant administration of nonsteroidal anti-inflammatory drugs such as phenylbutazone and indomethacin with quinolones has been reported to enhance the CNS stimulatory effect of quinolones.

Ocular toxicity seen with some related drugs has not been observed in ciprofloxacin-treated animals.

CLINICAL STUDIES

Complicated Urinary Tract Infection and Pyelonephritis – Efficacy in Pediatric Patients:

NOTE: Although effective in clinical trials, ciprofloxacin is not a drug of first choice in the pediatric population due to an increased incidence of adverse events compared to controls, including events related to joints and/or surrounding tissues.

Ciprofloxacin, administered I.V. and/or orally, was compared to a cephalosporin for treatment of complicated urinary tract infections (cUTI) and pyelonephritis in pediatric patients 1 to 17 years of age (mean age of 6 ± 4 years). The trial was conducted in the US, Canada, Argentina, Peru, Costa Rica, Mexico, South Africa, and Germany. The duration of therapy was 10 to 21 days (mean duration of treatment was 11 days with a range of 1 to 88 days). The primary objective of the study was to assess musculoskeletal and neurological safety.

Patients were evaluated for clinical success and bacteriological eradication of the baseline organism(s) with no new infection or superinfection at 5 to 9 days post-therapy (Test of Cure or TOC). The Per Protocol population had a causative organism(s) with protocol specified colony count(s) at baseline, no protocol violation, and no premature discontinuation or loss to follow-up (among other criteria).

The clinical success and bacteriologic eradication rates in the Per Protocol population were similar between ciprofloxacin and the comparator group as shown below.

[See fourth table above]

INHALATIONAL ANTHRAX IN ADULTS AND PEDIATRICS – ADDITIONAL INFORMATION

The mean serum concentrations of ciprofloxacin associated with a statistically significant improvement in survival in the rhesus monkey model of inhalational anthrax are reached or exceeded in adult and pediatric patients receiving oral and intravenous regimens. (See **DOSAGE AND ADMINISTRATION**.) Ciprofloxacin pharmacokinetics have been evaluated in various human populations. The mean peak serum concentration achieved at steady-state in human adults receiving 500 mg orally every 12 hours is 2.97 μg/mL, and 4.56 μg/mL following 400 mg intravenously every 12 hours. The mean trough serum concentration at steady-state for both of these regimens is 0.2 μg/mL. In a study of 10 pediatric patients between 6 and 16 years of age, the mean peak plasma concentration achieved is 8.3 μg/mL and trough concentrations range from 0.09 to 0.26 μg/mL, following two 30-minute intravenous infusions of 10 mg/kg administered 12 hours apart. After the second intravenous infusion patients switched to 15 mg/kg orally every 12 hours achieve a mean peak concentration of 3.6 μg/mL after the initial oral dose. Long-term safety data, including effects on cartilage, following the administration of ciprofloxacin to pediatric patients are limited. (For additional information, see **PRECAUTIONS, Pediatric Use.**) Ciprofloxacin serum concentrations achieved in humans serve as a surrogate endpoint reasonably likely to predict clinical benefit and provide the basis for this indication.[4]

A placebo-controlled animal study in rhesus monkeys exposed to an inhaled mean dose of 11 LD_{50} (~5.5 × 10^5 spores (range 5-30 LD_{50}) of *B. anthracis* was conducted. The minimal inhibitory concentration (MIC) of ciprofloxacin for the anthrax strain used in this study was 0.08 μg/mL. In the animals studied, mean serum concentrations of ciprofloxacin achieved at expected T_{max} (1 hour post-dose) following oral dosing to steady-state ranged from 0.98 to 1.69 μg/mL. Mean steady-state trough concentrations at 12 hours post-dose ranged from 0.12 to 0.19 μg/mL[5]. Mortality due to anthrax for animals that received a 30-day regimen of oral ciprofloxacin beginning 24 hours post-exposure was significantly lower (1/9), compared to the placebo group (9/10) [p= 0.001]. The one ciprofloxacin-treated animal that died of anthrax did so following the 30-day drug administration period.[6]

Instructions To The Pharmacist For Use/Handling Of CIPRO Oral Suspension:

CIPRO Oral Suspension is supplied in 5% (5 g ciprofloxacin in 100 mL) and 10% (10 g ciprofloxacin in 100 mL) strengths. The drug product is composed of two components (microcapsules and diluent) which must be combined prior to dispensing.

One teaspoonful (5 mL) of 5% ciprofloxacin oral suspension = 250 mg of ciprofloxacin.

One teaspoonful (5 mL) of 10% ciprofloxacin oral suspension = 500 mg of ciprofloxacin.

Appropriate Dosing Volumes of the Oral Suspensions:

Dose	5%	10%
250 mg	5 mL	2.5 mL
500 mg	10 mL	5 mL
750 mg	15 mL	7.5 mL

PEDIATRIC DOSAGE GUIDELINES

Infection	Route of Administration	Dose (mg/kg)	Frequency	Total Duration
Complicated Urinary Tract or Pyelonephritis (patients from 1 to 17 years of age)	Intravenous	6 to 10 mg/kg (maximum 400 mg per dose; not to be exceeded even in patients weighing >51 kg)	Every 8 hours	10-21 days*
	Oral	10 mg/kg to 20 mg/kg (maximum 750 mg per dose; not to be exceeded even in patients weighing >51 kg)	Every 12 hours	
Inhalational Anthrax (Post-Exposure)**	Intravenous	10 mg/kg (maximum 400 mg per dose)	Every 12 hours	60 days
	Oral	15 mg/kg (maximum 500 mg per dose)	Every 12 hours	

*The total duration of therapy for complicated urinary tract infection and pyelonephritis in the clinical trial was determined by the physician. The mean duration of treatment was 11 days (range 10 to 21 days).

Drug administration should begin as soon as possible after suspected or confirmed exposure to *Bacillus anthracis* spores. This indication is based on a surrogate endpoint, ciprofloxacin serum concentrations achieved in humans, reasonably likely to predict clinical benefit.[4] For a discussion of ciprofloxacin serum concentrations in various human populations, see **INHALATIONAL ANTHRAX – ADDITIONAL INFORMATION.

	Strength	NDC Code	Tablet Identification
Bottles of 50:	750 mg	NDC 0026-8514-50	CIPRO 750
Bottles of 100:	250 mg	NDC 0026-8512-51	CIPRO 250
	500 mg	NDC 0026-8513-51	CIPRO 500
Unit Dose Package of 100:	250 mg	NDC 0026-8512-48	CIPRO 250
	500 mg	NDC 0026-8513-48	CIPRO 500
	750 mg	NDC 0026-8514-48	CIPRO 750
Cystitis Package of 6:	100 mg	NDC 0026-8511-06	CIPRO 100

Strengths	Total volume after reconstitution	Ciprofloxacin Concentration	Ciprofloxacin contents per bottle	NDC Code
5%	100 mL	250 mg/5 mL	5,000 mg	0026-8551-36
10%	100 mL	500 mg/5 mL	10,000 mg	0026-8553-36

Clinical Success and Bacteriologic Eradication at Test of Cure (5 to 9 Days Post-Therapy)

	CIPRO	Comparator
Randomized Patients	337	352
Per Protocol Patients	211	231
Clinical Response at 5 to 9 Days Post-Treatment	95.7% (202/211)	92.6% (214/231)
	95% CI [-1.3%, 7.3%]	
Bacteriologic Eradication by Patient at 5 to 9 Days Post-Treatment*	84.4% (178/211)	78.3% (181/231)
	95% CI [-1.3%, 13.1%]	
Bacteriologic Eradication of the Baseline Pathogen at 5 to 9 Days Post-Treatment		
Escherichia coli	156/178 (88%)	161/179 (90%)

*Patients with baseline pathogen(s) eradicated and no new infections or superinfections/total number of patients. There were 5.5% (6/211) ciprofloxacin and 9.5% (22/231) comparator patients with superinfections or new infections.

Preparation of the suspension:

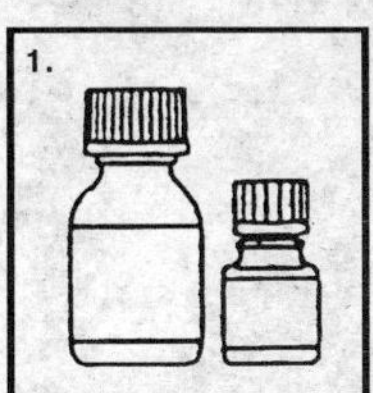

1. The small bottle contains the microcapsules, the large bottle contains the diluent.

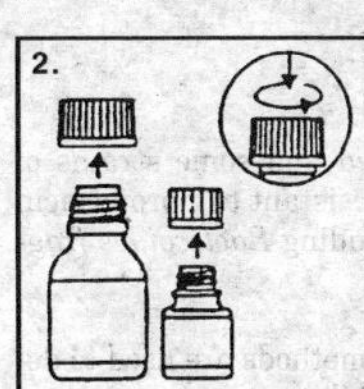

2. Open both bottles. Child-proof cap: Press down according to instructions on the cap while turning to the left.

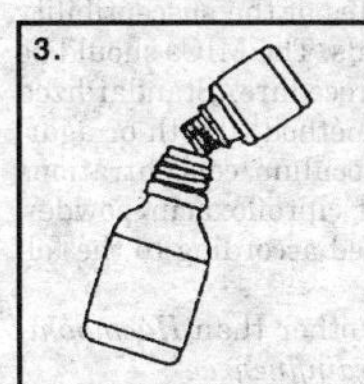

3. Pour the microcapsules completely into the larger bottle of diluent. **Do not add water to the suspension.**

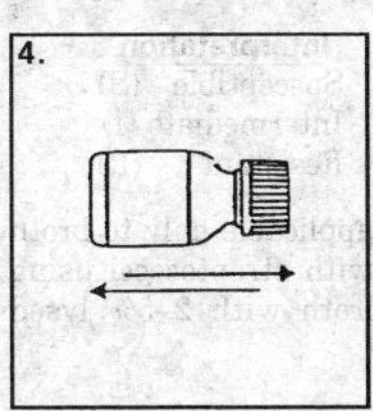

4. Remove the top layer of the diluent bottle label (to reveal the CIPRO Oral Suspension label). Close the large bottle completely according to the directions on the cap and shake vigorously for about 15 seconds. The suspension is ready for use.

CIPRO Oral Suspension should not be administered through feeding tubes due to its physical characteristics. Instruct the patient to shake CIPRO Oral Suspension vigorously each time before use for approximately 15 seconds and not to chew the microcapsules.

References:

1. National Committee for Clinical Laboratory Standards, Methods for Dilution Antimicrobial Susceptibility Tests for Bacteria That Grow Aerobically-Fifth Edition. Approved Standard NCCLS Document M7-A5, Vol. 20, No. 2, NCCLS, Wayne, PA, January, 2000. **2.** National Committee for Clinical Laboratory Standards, Performance Standards for Antimicrobial Disk Susceptibility Tests-Seventh Edition. Approved Standard NCCLS Document M2-A7, Vol. 20, No. 1, NCCLS, Wayne, PA, January, 2000. **3.** Report presented at the FDA's Anti-Infective Drug and Dermatological Drug Product's Advisory Committee meeting, March 31, 1993, Silver Spring, MD. Report available from FDA, CDER, Advisors and Consultants Staff, HFD-21, 1901 Chapman Avenue, Room 200, Rockville, MD 20852, USA. **4.** 21 CFR 314.510 (Subpart H – Accelerated Approval of New Drugs for Life-Threatening Illnesses). **5.** Kelly DJ, et al. Serum concentrations of penicillin, doxycycline, and ciprofloxacin during prolonged therapy in rhesus monkeys. J Infect Dis 1992; 166:1184-7. **6.** Friedlander AM, et al. Postexposure prophylaxis against experimental inhalational anthrax. J Infect Dis 1993; 167:1239-42. **7.** Friedman J, Polifka J. Teratogenic effects of drugs: a resource for clinicians (TERIS). Baltimore, Maryland: Johns Hopkins University Press, 2000:149-195. **8.** Loebstein R, Addis A, Ho E, et al. Pregnancy outcome following gestational exposure to fluoroquinolones: a multicenter prospective controlled study. Antimicrob Agents Chemother. 1998;42(6):1336-1339. **9.** Schaefer C, Amoura-Elefant E, Vial T, et al. Pregnancy outcome after prenatal quinolone exposure. Evaluation of a case registry of the European network of teratology information services (ENTIS). Eur J Obstet Gynecol Reprod Biol. 1996;69:83-89.

Patient Information About:

CIPRO®

(ciprofloxacin hydrochloride) TABLETS

CIPRO®

(ciprofloxacin*) ORAL SUSPENSION

This section contains important patient information about CIPRO (ciprofloxacin hydrochloride) Tablets and CIPRO (ciprofloxacin*) Oral Suspension and should be read completely before you begin treatment. This section does not take the place of discussion with your doctor or health care professional about your medical condition or your treatment. This section does not list all benefits and risks of CIPRO. If you have any concerns about your condition or your medicine, ask your doctor. Only your doctor can determine if CIPRO is right for you.

What is CIPRO?

CIPRO is an antibiotic used to treat bladder, kidney, prostate, cervix, stomach, intestine, lung, sinus, bone, and skin infections caused by certain germs called bacteria. CIPRO kills many types of bacteria that can infect these areas of the body. CIPRO has been shown in a large number of clinical trials to be safe and effective for the treatment of bacterial infections.

Sometimes viruses rather than bacteria may infect the lungs and sinuses (for example the common cold). CIPRO, like all other antibiotics, does not kill viruses. You should contact your doctor if your condition is not improving while taking CIPRO.

CIPRO Tablets are white to slightly yellow in color and are available in 100 mg, 250 mg, 500 mg and 750 mg strengths.

CIPRO Oral Suspension is white to slightly yellow in color and is available in concentrations of 250 mg per teaspoon (5%) and 500 mg per teaspoon (10%).

How and when should I take CIPRO?

CIPRO Tablets:

Unless directed otherwise by your physician, CIPRO should be taken twice a day at approximately the same time, in the morning and in the evening. CIPRO can be taken with food or on an empty stomach. CIPRO should not be taken with dairy products (like milk or yogurt) or calcium-fortified juices alone; however, CIPRO may be taken with a meal that contains these products.

You should take CIPRO for as long as your doctor prescribes it, even after you start to feel better. Stopping an antibiotic too early may result in failure to cure your infection. Do not take a double dose of CIPRO even if you miss a dose by mistake.

CIPRO Oral Suspension:

Take CIPRO Oral Suspension in the same way as above. In addition, remember to **shake the bottle vigorously each time before use for approximately 15 seconds** to make sure the suspension is mixed well. Be sure to swallow the required amount of suspension. Do not chew the microcapsules. Close the bottle completely after use. The product can be used for 14 days when stored in a refrigerator or at room temperature. After treatment has been completed, any remaining suspension should be discarded.

Who should not take CIPRO?

You should not take CIPRO if you have ever had a severe reaction to any of the group of antibiotics known as "quinolones".

CIPRO is not recommended during pregnancy or nursing, as the effects of CIPRO on the unborn child or nursing infant are unknown. If you are pregnant or plan to become pregnant while taking CIPRO talk to your doctor before taking this medication.

Due to possible side effects, CIPRO is not recommended for persons less than 18 years of age except for specific serious infections, such as complicated urinary tract infections.

What are the possible side effects of CIPRO?

CIPRO is generally well tolerated. The most common side effects, which are usually mild, include nausea, diarrhea, vomiting, and abdominal pain/discomfort. If diarrhea persists, call your health care professional.

Rare cases of allergic reactions have been reported in patients receiving quinolones, including CIPRO, even after just one dose. If you develop hives, difficulty breathing, or other symptoms of a severe allergic reaction, seek emergency treatment right away. If you develop a skin rash, you should stop taking CIPRO and call your health care professional.

Some patients taking quinolone antibiotics may become more sensitive to sunlight or ultraviolet light such as that used in tanning salons. You should avoid excessive exposure to sunlight or ultraviolet light while you are taking CIPRO.

You should be careful about driving or operating machinery until you are sure CIPRO is not causing dizziness. Convulsions have been reported in patients receiving quinolone antibiotics including ciprofloxacin. Be sure to let your physician know if you have a history of convulsions. Quinolones, including ciprofloxacin, have been rarely associated with other central nervous system events including confusion, tremors, hallucinations, and depression.

CIPRO has been rarely associated with inflammation of tendons. If you experience pain, swelling or rupture of a tendon, you should stop taking CIPRO and call your health care professional.

CIPRO has been associated with an increased rate of side effects with joints and surrounding structures (like tendons) in pediatric patients (less than 18 years of age). Parents should inform their child's physician if the child has a history of joint-related problems before taking this drug. Parents of pediatric patients should also notify their child's physician of any joint related problems that occur during or following CIPRO therapy.

If you notice any side effects not mentioned in this section, or if you have any concerns about side effects you may be experiencing, please inform your health care professional.

What about other medications I am taking?

CIPRO can affect how other medicines work. Tell your doctor about all other prescription and non-prescription medicines or supplements you are taking. This is especially important if you are taking theophylline. Other medications including warfarin, glyburide, and phenytoin may also interact with CIPRO.

Many antacids, multivitamins, and other dietary supplements containing magnesium, calcium, aluminum, iron or zinc can interfere with the absorption of CIPRO and may prevent it from working. Other medications such as sulcrafate and Videx® (didanosine) chewable/buffered tablets or pediatric powder may also stop CIPRO from working. You should take CIPRO either 2 hours before or 6 hours after taking these products.

What if I have been prescribed CIPRO for possible anthrax exposure?

CIPRO has been approved to reduce the chance of developing anthrax infection following exposure to the anthrax bacteria. In general, CIPRO is not recommended for children; however, it is approved for use in patients younger than 18 years old for anthrax exposure. If you are pregnant, or plan to become pregnant while taking CIPRO, you and your doctor should discuss if the benefits of taking CIPRO for anthrax outweigh the risks.

CIPRO is generally well tolerated. Side effects that may occur during treatment to prevent anthrax might be acceptable due to the seriousness of the disease. You and your doctor should discuss the risks of not taking your medicine against the risks of experiencing side effects.

CIPRO can cause dizziness, confusion, or other similar side effects in some people. Therefore, it is important to know how CIPRO affects you before driving a car or performing other activities that require you to be alert and coordinated such as operating machinery.

Your doctor has prescribed CIPRO only for you. Do not give it to other people. Do not use it for a condition for which it was not prescribed. You should take your CIPRO for as long as your doctor prescribes it; stopping CIPRO too early may result in failure to prevent anthrax.

Remember:

Do not give CIPRO to anyone other than the person for whom it was prescribed.

Take your dose of CIPRO in the morning and in the evening.

Complete the course of CIPRO even if you are feeling better.

Keep CIPRO and all medications out of reach of children.

* Does not comply with USP with regards to "loss on drying" and "residue on ignition".

Bayer HealthCare
Bayer Pharmaceuticals Corporation
400 Morgan Lane
West Haven, CT 06516 USA
℞ Only
08753744, R.4 4/04 Bay o 9867 5202-2-A-U.S.-16
12320

Printed in U.S.A.

CIPRO (ciprofloxacin*) 5% and 10% Oral Suspension Made in Italy.

Cipro (ciprofloxacin HCl) Tablets Made in U.S.A. and Germany

Shown in Product Identification Guide, page 308

CIPRO® I.V. ℞

[*sĭprō*]

(ciprofloxacin)

For Intravenous Infusion

To reduce the development of drug-resistant bacteria and maintain the effectiveness of CIPRO® I.V. and other antibacterial drugs, CIPRO I.V. should be used only to treat or prevent infections that are proven or strongly suspected to be caused by bacteria.

DESCRIPTION

CIPRO I.V. (ciprofloxacin) is a synthetic broad-spectrum antimicrobial agent for intravenous (I.V.) administration. Ciprofloxacin, a fluoroquinolone, is 1-cyclopropyl-6-fluoro-1,4-dihydro-4-oxo-7-(1-piperazinyl)-3-quinolinecarboxylic acid. Its empirical formula is $C_{17}H_{18}FN_3O_3$ and its chemical structure is:

Ciprofloxacin is a faint to light yellow crystalline powder with a molecular weight of 331.4. It is soluble in dilute (0.1N) hydrochloric acid and is practically insoluble in water and ethanol. CIPRO I.V. solutions are available as sterile 1.0% aqueous concentrates, which are intended for dilution prior to administration, and as 0.2% ready-for-use infusion solutions in 5% Dextrose Injection. All formulas contain lactic acid as a solubilizing agent and hydrochloric acid for pH adjustment. The pH range for the 1.0% aqueous concentrates in vials is 3.3 to 3.9. The pH range for the 0.2% ready-for-use infusion solutions is 3.5 to 4.6.

The plastic container is latex-free and is fabricated from a specially formulated polyvinyl chloride. Solutions in contact with the plastic container can leach out certain of its chemical components in very small amounts within the expiration period, e.g., di(2-ethylhexyl) phthalate (DEHP), up to 5 parts per million. The suitability of the plastic has been confirmed in tests in animals according to USP biological tests for plastic containers as well as by tissue culture toxicity studies.

CLINICAL PHARMACOLOGY

Absorption

Following 60-minute intravenous infusions of 200 mg and 400 mg ciprofloxacin to normal volunteers, the mean maximum serum concentrations achieved were 2.1 and 4.6 μg/mL, respectively; the concentrations at 12 hours were 0.1 and 0.2 μg/mL, respectively.

Continued on next page

Cipro I.V.—Cont.

Steady-state Ciprofloxacin Serum Concentrations (μg/mL) After 60-minute I.V. Infusions q 12 h.

	Time after starting the infusion					
Dose	**30 min**	**1 hr**	**3 hr**	**6 hr**	**8 hr**	**12 hr**
200 mg	1.7	2.1	0.6	0.3	0.2	0.1
400 mg	3.7	4.6	1.3	0.7	0.5	0.2

The pharmacokinetics of ciprofloxacin are linear over the dose range of 200 to 400 mg administered intravenously. Comparison of the pharmacokinetic parameters following the 1st and 5th I.V. dose on a q 12 h regimen indicates no evidence of drug accumulation.

The absolute bioavailability of oral ciprofloxacin is within a range of 70–80% with no substantial loss by first pass metabolism. An intravenous infusion of 400-mg ciprofloxacin given over 60 minutes every 12 hours has been shown to produce an area under the serum concentration time curve (AUC) equivalent to that produced by a 500-mg oral dose given every 12 hours. An intravenous infusion of 400 mg ciprofloxacin given over 60 minutes every 8 hours has been shown to produce an AUC at steady-state equivalent to that produced by a 750-mg oral dose given every 12 hours. A 400-mg I.V. dose results in a C_{max} similar to that observed with a 750-mg oral dose. An infusion of 200 mg ciprofloxacin given every 12 hours produces an AUC equivalent to that produced by a 250-mg oral dose given every 12 hours.

[See table below]

Distribution

After intravenous administration, ciprofloxacin is present in saliva, nasal and bronchial secretions, sputum, skin blister fluid, lymph, peritoneal fluid, bile, and prostatic secretions. It has also been detected in the lung, skin, fat, muscle, cartilage, and bone. Although the drug diffuses into cerebrospinal fluid (CSF), CSF concentrations are generally less than 10% of peak serum concentrations. Levels of the drug in the aqueous and vitreous chambers of the eye are lower than in serum.

Metabolism

After I.V. administration, three metabolites of ciprofloxacin have been identified in human urine which together account for approximately 10% of the intravenous dose. The binding of ciprofloxacin to serum proteins is 20 to 40%.

Excretion

The serum elimination half-life is approximately 5–6 hours and the total clearance is around 35 L/hr. After intravenous administration, approximately 50% to 70% of the dose is excreted in the urine as unchanged drug. Following a 200-mg I.V. dose, concentrations in the urine usually exceed 200 μg/mL 0–2 hours after dosing and are generally greater than 15 μg/mL 8–12 hours after dosing. Following a 400-mg I.V. dose, urine concentrations generally exceed 400 μg/mL 0–2 hours after dosing and are usually greater than 30 μg/mL 8–12 hours after dosing. The renal clearance is approximately 22 L/hr. The urinary excretion of ciprofloxacin is virtually complete by 24 hours after dosing. Although bile concentrations of ciprofloxacin are several fold higher than serum concentrations after intravenous dosing, only a small amount of the administered dose (< 1%) is recovered from the bile as unchanged drug. Approximately 15% of an I.V. dose is recovered from the feces within 5 days after dosing.

Special Populations

Pharmacokinetic studies of the oral (single dose) and intravenous (single and multiple dose) forms of ciprofloxacin indicate that plasma concentrations of ciprofloxacin are higher in elderly subjects (> 65 years) as compared to young adults. Although the C_{max} is increased 16–40%, the increase in mean AUC is approximately 30%, and can be at least partially attributed to decreased renal clearance in the elderly. Elimination half-life is only slightly (~20%) prolonged in the elderly. These differences are not considered clinically significant. (See **PRECAUTIONS: Geriatric Use.**)

In patients with reduced renal function, the half-life of ciprofloxacin is slightly prolonged and dosage adjustments may be required. (See **DOSAGE AND ADMINISTRATION.**)

In preliminary studies in patients with stable chronic liver cirrhosis, no significant changes in ciprofloxacin pharmacokinetics have been observed. However, the kinetics of ciprofloxacin in patients with acute hepatic insufficiency have not been fully elucidated.

Following a single oral dose of 10 mg/kg ciprofloxacin suspension to 16 children ranging in age from 4 months to 7 years, the mean C_{max} was 2.4 μg/mL (range: 1.5–3.4 μg/mL) and the mean AUC was 9.2 μg*h/mL (range: 5.8–14.9 μg*h/mL). There was no apparent age-dependence, and no notable increase in C_{max} or AUC upon multiple dosing (10 mg/kg TID). In children with severe sepsis who were given intravenous ciprofloxacin (10 mg/kg as a 1-hour infusion), the mean C_{max} was 6.1 μg/mL (range: 4.6–8.3 μg/mL) in 10 children less than 1 year of age; and 7.2 μg/mL (range: 4.7–11.8 μg/mL) in 10 children between 1 and 5 years of age. The AUC values were 17.4 μg*h/mL (range: 11.8–32.0 μg*h/mL) and 16.5 μg*h/mL (range: 11.0–23.8 μg*h/mL) in the respective age groups. These values are within the range reported for adults at therapeutic doses. Based on population pharmacokinetic analysis of pediatric patients with various infections, the predicted mean half-life in children is approximately 4–5 hours, and the bioavailability of the oral suspension is approximately 60%.

Drug-drug Interactions: The potential for pharmacokinetic drug interactions between ciprofloxacin and theophylline, caffeine, cyclosporins, phenytoin, sulfonylurea glyburide, metronidazole, warfarin, probenecid, and piperacillin sodium has been evaluated. (See **PRECAUTIONS: Drug Interactions.**)

MICROBIOLOGY

Ciprofloxacin has *in vitro* activity against a wide range of gram-negative and gram-positive microorganisms. The bactericidal action of ciprofloxacin results from inhibition of the enzymes topoisomerase II (DNA gyrase) and topoisomerase IV, which are required for bacterial DNA replication, transcription, repair, and recombination. The mechanism of action of fluoroquinolones, including ciprofloxacin, is different from that of penicillins, cephalosporins, aminoglycosides, macrolides, and tetracyclines; therefore, microorganisms resistant to these classes of drugs may be susceptible to ciprofloxacin and other quinolones. There is no known cross-resistance between ciprofloxacin and other classes of antimicrobials. *In vitro* resistance to ciprofloxacin develops slowly by multiple step mutations.

Ciprofloxacin is slightly less active when tested at acidic pH. The inoculum size has little effect when tested *in vitro*. The minimal bactericidal concentration (MBC) generally does not exceed the minimal inhibitory concentration (MIC) by more than a factor of 2.

Ciprofloxacin has been shown to be active against most strains of the following microorganisms, both *in vitro* and in clinical infections as described in the **INDICATIONS AND USAGE** section of the package insert for CIPRO I.V. (ciprofloxacin for intravenous infusion).

Aerobic gram-positive microorganisms

Enterococcus faecalis (Many strains are only moderately susceptible.)
Staphylococcus aureus (methicillin-susceptible strains only)
Staphylococcus epidermidis (methicillin-susceptible strains only)
Staphylococcus saprophyticus
Streptococcus pneumoniae (penicillin-susceptible strains)
Streptococcus pyogenes

Aerobic gram-negative microorganisms

Citrobacter diversus
Citrobacter freundii
Enterobacter cloacae
Escherichia coli
Haemophilus influenzae
Haemophilus parainfluenzae
Klebsiella pneumoniae
Moraxella catarrhalis
Morganella morganii
Proteus mirabilis
Proteus vulgaris
Providencia rettgeri
Providencia stuartii
Pseudomonas aeruginosa
Serratia marcescens

Ciprofloxacin has been shown to be active against *Bacillus anthracis* both *in vitro* and by use of serum levels as a surrogate marker (see **INDICATIONS AND USAGE** and **INHALATIONAL ANTHRAX — ADDITIONAL INFORMATION**).

The following *in vitro* data are available, **but their clinical significance is unknown.**

Ciprofloxacin exhibits *in vitro* minimum inhibitory concentrations (MICs) of 1 μg/mL or less against most (≥ 90%) strains of the following microorganisms; however, the safety and effectiveness of ciprofloxacin intravenous formulations in treating clinical infections due to these microorganisms have not been established in adequate and well-controlled clinical trials.

Aerobic gram-positive microorganisms

Staphylococcus haemolyticus
Staphylococcus hominis
Streptococcus pneumoniae (penicillin-resistant strains)

Aerobic gram-negative microorganisms

Acinetobacter lwoffi
Aeromonas hydrophila
Campylobacter jejuni
Edwardsiella tarda
Enterobacter aerogenes
Klebsiella oxytoca
Legionella pneumophila
Neisseria gonorrhoeae
Pasteurella multocida
Salmonella enteritidis
Salmonella typhi
Shigella boydii
Shigella dysenteriae
Shigella flexneri
Shigella sonnei
Vibrio cholerae
Vibrio parahaemolyticus
Vibrio vulnificus
Yersinia enterocolitica

Most strains of *Burkholderia cepacia* and some strains of *Stenotrophomonas maltophilia* are resistant to ciprofloxacin as are most anaerobic bacteria, including *Bacteroides fragilis* and *Clostridium difficile.*

Susceptibility Tests

Dilution Techniques: Quantitative methods are used to determine antimicrobial minimum inhibitory concentrations (MICs). These MICs provide estimates of the susceptibility of bacteria to antimicrobial compounds. The MICs should be determined using a standardized procedure. Standardized procedures are based on a dilution method[1] (broth or agar) or equivalent with standardized inoculum concentrations and standardized concentrations of ciprofloxacin powder. The MIC values should be interpreted according to the following criteria:

For testing aerobic microorganisms other than *Haemophilus influenzae*, and *Haemophilus parainfluenzae*[a]:

MIC (μg/mL)	Interpretation
≤ 1	Susceptible (S)
2	Intermediate (I)
≥ 4	Resistant (R)

[a]These interpretive standards are applicable only to broth microdilution susceptibility tests with streptococci using cation-adjusted Mueller-Hinton broth with 2–5% lysed horse blood.

For testing *Haemophilus influenzae* and *Haemophilus parainfluenzae*[b]:

MIC (μg/mL)	Interpretation
≤ 1	Susceptible (S)

[b]This interpretive standard is applicable only to broth microdilution susceptibility tests with *Haemophilus influenzae* and *Haemophilus parainfluenzae* using *Haemophilus* Test Medium [1].

The current absence of data on resistant strains precludes defining any results other than "Susceptible". Strains yielding MIC results suggestive of a "nonsusceptible" category should be submitted to a reference laboratory for further testing.

A report of "Susceptible" indicates that the pathogen is likely to be inhibited if the antimicrobial compound in the blood reaches the concentrations usually achievable. A report of "Intermediate" indicates that the result should be considered equivocal, and, if the microorganism is not fully susceptible to alternative, clinically feasible drugs, the test should be repeated. This category implies possible clinical applicability in body sites where the drug is physiologically concentrated or in situations where high dosage of drug can be used. This category also provides a buffer zone, which prevents small uncontrolled technical factors from causing major discrepancies in interpretation. A report of "Resistant" indicates that the pathogen is not likely to be inhibited if the antimicrobial compound in the blood reaches the concentrations usually achievable; other therapy should be selected.

Standardized susceptibility test procedures require the use of laboratory control microorganisms to control the technical aspects of the laboratory procedures. Standard ciprofloxacin powder should provide the following MIC values:

Organism		MIC (μg/mL)
E. faecalis	ATCC 29212	0.25 – 2.0
E. coli	ATCC 25922	0.004 – 0.015
H. influenzae[a]	ATCC 49247	0.004 – 0.03
P. aeruginosa	ATCC 27853	0.25 – 1.0
S. aureus	ATCC 29213	0.12 – 0.5

[a] This quality control range is applicable to only *H. influenzae* ATCC 49247 tested by a broth microdilution procedure using *Haemophilus* Test Medium (HTM)[1].

Diffusion Techniques: Quantitative methods that require measurement of zone diameters also provide reproducible estimates of the susceptibility of bacteria to antimicrobial compounds. One such standardized procedure[2] requires the use of standardized inoculum concentrations. This procedure uses paper disks impregnated with 5-μg ciprofloxacin to test the susceptibility of microorganisms to ciprofloxacin. Reports from the laboratory providing results of the standard single-disk susceptibility test with a 5-μg ciprofloxacin disk should be interpreted according to the following criteria:

For testing aerobic microorganisms other than *Haemophilus influenzae*, and *Haemophilus parainfluenzae*[a]:

Steady-state Pharmacokinetic Parameter Following Multiple Oral and I.V. Doses

Parameters	500 mg q12h, P.O.	400 mg q12h, I.V.	750 mg q12h, P.O.	400 mg q8h, I.V.
AUC (μg•hr/mL)	13.7[a]	12.7[a]	31.6[b]	32.9[c]
C_{max} (μg/mL)	2.97	4.56	3.59	4.07

[a]$AUC_{0\text{-}12h}$
[b]AUC 24h=$AUC_{0\text{-}12h} \times 2$
[c]AUC 24h=$AUC_{0\text{-}8h} \times 3$

Zone Diameter (mm)	Interpretation
≥ 21	Susceptible (S)
16–20	Intermediate (I)
≤ 15	Resistant (R)

[a]These zone diameter standards are applicable only to tests performed for streptococci using Mueller-Hinton agar supplemented with 5% sheep blood incubated in 5% CO_2.

For testing *Haemophilus influenzae* and *Haemophilus parainfluenzae*[b]:

Zone Diameter (mm)	Interpretation
≥ 21	Susceptible (S)

[b]This zone diameter standard is applicable only to tests with *Haemophilus influenzae* and *Haemophilus parainfluenzae*using *Haemophilus* Test Medium (HTM)[2].

The current absence of data on resistant strains precludes defining any results other than "Susceptible". Strains yielding zone diameter results suggestive of a "nonsusceptible" category should be submitted to a reference laboratory for further testing. Interpretation should be as stated above for results using dilution techniques. Interpretation involves correlation of the diameter obtained in the disk test with the MIC for ciprofloxacin.

As with standardized dilution techniques, diffusion methods require the use of laboratory control microorganisms that are used to control the technical aspects of the laboratory procedures. For the diffusion technique, the 5-μg ciprofloxacin disk should provide the following zone diameters in these laboratory test quality control strains:

Organism		Zone Diameter (mm)
E. coli	ATCC 25922	30–40
H. influenzae[a]	ATCC 49247	34–42
P. aeruginosa	ATCC 27853	25–33
S. aureus	ATCC 25923	22–30

[a] These quality control limits are applicable to only *H. influenzae* ATCC 49247 testing using *Haemophilus* Test Medium (HTM)[2].

INDICATIONS AND USAGE

CIPRO I.V. is indicated for the treatment of infections caused by susceptible strains of the designated microorganisms in the conditions and patient populations listed below when the intravenous administration offers a route of administration advantageous to the patient. Please see **DOSAGE AND ADMINISTRATION** for specific recommendations.

Adult Patients:

Urinary Tract Infections caused by *Escherichia coli* (including cases with secondary bacteremia), *Klebsiella pneumoniae* subspecies *pneumoniae, Enterobacter cloacae, Serratia marcescens, Proteus mirabilis, Providencia rettgeri, Morganella morganii, Citrobacter diversus, Citrobacter freundii, Pseudomonas aeruginosa, Staphylococcus epidermidis, Staphylococcus saprophyticus,* or *Enterococcus faecalis.*

Lower Respiratory Infections caused by *Escherichia coli, Klebsiella pneumoniae* subspecies *pneumoniae, Enterobacter cloacae, Proteus mirabilis, Pseudomonas aeruginosa, Haemophilus influenzae, Haemophilus parainfluenzae,* or *Streptococcus pneumoniae.* Also, *Moraxella catarrhalis* for the treatment of acute exacerbations of chronic bronchitis.

NOTE: Although effective in clinical trials, ciprofloxacin is not a drug of first choice in the treatment of presumed or confirmed pneumonia secondary to *Streptococcus pneumoniae.*

Nosocomial Pneumonia caused by *Haemophilus influenzae* or *Klebsiella pneumoniae.*

Skin and Skin Structure Infections caused by *Escherichia coli, Klebsiella pneumoniae* subspecies *pneumoniae, Enterobacter cloacae, Proteus mirabilis, Proteus vulgaris, Providencia stuartii, Morganella morganii, Citrobacter freundii, Pseudomonas aeruginosa, Staphylococcus aureus* (methicillin susceptible), *Staphylococcus epidermidis,* or *Streptococcus pyogenes.*

Bone and Joint Infections caused by *Enterobacter cloacae, Serratia marcescens,* or *Pseudomonas aeruginosa.*

Complicated Intra-Abdominal Infections (used in conjunction with metronidazole) caused by *Escherichia coli, Pseudomonas aeruginosa, Proteus mirabilis, Klebsiella pneumoniae,* or *Bacteroides fragilis.*

Acute Sinusitis caused by *Haemophilus influenzae, Streptococcus pneumoniae,* or *Moraxella catarrhalis.*

Chronic Bacterial Prostatitis caused by *Escherichia coli* or *Proteus mirabilis.*

Empirical Therapy for Febrile Neutropenic Patients in combination with piperacillin sodium. (See **CLINICAL STUDIES.**)

Pediatric patients (1 to 17 years of age):

Complicated Urinary Tract Infections and Pyelonephritis due to *Escherichia coli.*

NOTE: Although effective in clinical trials, ciprofloxacin is not a drug of first choice in the pediatric population due to an increased incidence of adverse events compared to controls, including events related to joints and/or surrounding tissues. (See **WARNINGS, PRECAUTIONS, Pediatric Use, ADVERSE REACTIONS** and **CLINICAL STUDIES.**) Ciprofloxacin, like other fluoroquinolones, is associated with arthropathy and histopathological changes in weight-bearing joints of juvenile animals. (See **ANIMAL PHARMACOLOGY.**)

Adult and Pediatric Patients:

Inhalational anthrax (post-exposure): To reduce the incidence or progression of disease following exposure to aerosolized *Bacillus anthracis.*

Ciprofloxacin serum concentrations achieved in humans serve as a surrogate endpoint reasonably likely to predict clinical benefit and provide the basis for this indication.[4] (See also, **INHALATIONAL ANTHRAX – ADDITIONAL INFORMATION**).

If anaerobic organisms are suspected of contributing to the infection, appropriate therapy should be administered.

Appropriate culture and susceptibility tests should be performed before treatment in order to isolate and identify organisms causing infection and to determine their susceptibility to ciprofloxacin. Therapy with CIPRO I.V. may be initiated before results of these tests are known; once results become available, appropriate therapy should be continued.

As with other drugs, some strains of *Pseudomonas aeruginosa* may develop resistance fairly rapidly during treatment with ciprofloxacin. Culture and susceptibility testing performed periodically during therapy will provide information not only on the therapeutic effect of the antimicrobial agent but also on the possible emergence of bacterial resistance.

To reduce the development of drug-resistant bacteria and maintain the effectiveness of CIPRO I.V. and other antibacterial drugs, CIPRO I.V. should be used only to treat or prevent infections that are proven or strongly suspected to be caused by susceptible bacteria. When culture and susceptibility information are available, they should be considered in selecting or modifying antibacterial therapy. In the absence of such data, local epidemiology and susceptibility patterns may contribute to the empiric selection of therapy.

CONTRAINDICATIONS

CIPRO I.V. (ciprofloxacin) is contraindicated in persons with history of hypersensitivity to ciprofloxacin or any member of the quinolone class of antimicrobial agents.

WARNINGS

Pregnant Women: THE SAFETY AND EFFECTIVENESS OF CIPROFLOXACIN IN PREGNANT AND LACTATING WOMEN HAVE NOT BEEN ESTABLISHED. (See **PRECAUTIONS: Pregnancy**, and **Nursing Mothers** subsections.)

Pediatrics: Ciprofloxacin should be used in pediatric patients (less than 18 years of age) only for infections listed in the **INDICATIONS AND USAGE** section. An increased incidence of adverse events compared to controls, including events related to joints and/or surrounding tissues, has been observed. (See **ADVERSE REACTIONS.**)

In pre-clinical studies, oral administration of ciprofloxacin caused lameness in immature dogs. Histopathological examination of the weight-bearing joints of these dogs revealed permanent lesions of the cartilage. Related quinolone-class drugs also produce erosions of cartilage of weight-bearing joints and other signs of arthropathy in immature animals of various species. (See **ANIMAL PHARMACOLOGY.**)

Central Nervous System Disorders: Convulsions, increased intracranial pressure and toxic psychosis have been reported in patients receiving quinolones, including ciprofloxacin. Ciprofloxacin may also cause central nervous system (CNS) events including: dizziness, confusion, tremors, hallucinations, depression, and, rarely, suicidal thoughts or acts. These reactions may occur following the first dose. If these reactions occur in patients receiving ciprofloxacin, the drug should be discontinued and appropriate measures instituted. As with all quinolones, ciprofloxacin should be used with caution in patients with known or suspected CNS disorders that may predispose to seizures or lower the seizure threshold (e.g. severe cerebral arteriosclerosis, epilepsy), or in the presence of other risk factors that may predispose to seizures or lower the seizure threshold (e.g. certain drug therapy, renal dysfunction). (**See PRECAUTIONS: General, Information for Patients, Drug Interaction** and **ADVERSE REACTIONS.**)

Theophylline: SERIOUS AND FATAL REACTIONS HAVE BEEN REPORTED IN PATIENTS RECEIVING CONCURRENT ADMINISTRATION OF INTRAVENOUS CIPROFLOXACIN AND THEOPHYLLINE. These reactions have included cardiac arrest, seizure, status epilepticus, and respiratory failure. Although similar serious adverse events have been reported in patients receiving theophylline alone, the possibility that these reactions may be potentiated by ciprofloxacin cannot be eliminated. If concomitant use cannot be avoided, serum levels of theophylline should be monitored and dosage adjustments made as appropriate.

Hypersensitivity Reactions: Serious and occasionally fatal hypersensitivity (anaphylactic) reactions, some following the first dose, have been reported in patients receiving quinolone therapy. Some reactions were accompanied by cardiovascular collapse, loss of consciousness, tingling, pharyngeal or facial edema, dyspnea, urticaria, and itching. Only a few patients had a history of hypersensitivity reactions. Serious anaphylactic reactions require immediate emergency treatment with epinephrine and other resuscitation measures, including oxygen, intravenous fluids, intravenous antihistamines, corticosteroids, pressor amines, and airway management, as clinically indicated.

Severe hypersensitivity reactions characterized by rash, fever, eosinophilia, jaundice, and hepatic necrosis with fatal outcome have also been reported extremely rarely in patients receiving ciprofloxacin along with other drugs. The possibility that these reactions were related to ciprofloxacin cannot be excluded. Ciprofloxacin should be discontinued at the first appearance of a skin rash or any other sign of hypersensitivity.

Pseudomembranous Colitis: Pseudomembranous colitis has been reported with nearly all antibacterial agents, including ciprofloxacin, and may range in severity from mild to life-threatening. Therefore, it is important to consider this diagnosis in patients who present with diarrhea subsequent to the administration of antibacterial agents.

Treatment with antibacterial agents alters the normal flora of the colon and may permit overgrowth of clostridia. Studies indicate that a toxin produced by *Clostridium difficile* is one primary cause of "antibiotic-associated colitis."

After the diagnosis of pseudomembranous colitis has been established, therapeutic measures should be initiated. Mild cases of pseudomembranous colitis usually respond to drug discontinuation alone. In moderate to severe cases, consideration should be given to management with fluids and electrolytes, protein supplementation, and treatment with an antibacterial drug clinically effective against *C. difficile* colitis. Drugs that inhibit peristalsis should be avoided.

Peripheral neuropathy: Rare cases of sensory or sensorimotor axonal polyneuropathy affecting small and/or large axons resulting in paresthesias, hypoesthesias, dysesthesias and weakness have been reported in patients receiving quinolones, including ciprofloxacin. Ciprofloxacin should be discontinued if the patient experiences symptoms of neuropathy including pain, burning, tingling, numbness, and/or weakness, or is found to have deficits in light touch, pain, temperature, position sense, vibratory sensation, and/or motor strength in order to prevent the development of an irreversible condition.

Tendon Effects: Ruptures of the shoulder, hand, Achilles tendon or other tendons that required surgical repair or resulted in prolonged disability have been reported in patients receiving quinolones, including ciprofloxacin. Post-marketing surveillance reports indicate that this risk may be increased in patients receiving concomitant corticosteroids, especially the elderly. Ciprofloxacin should be discontinued if the patient experiences pain, inflammation, or rupture of a tendon. Patients should rest and refrain from exercise until the diagnosis of tendonitis or tendon rupture has been excluded. Tendon rupture can occur during or after therapy with quinolones, including ciprofloxacin.

PRECAUTIONS

General: INTRAVENOUS CIPROFLOXACIN SHOULD BE ADMINISTERED BY SLOW INFUSION OVER A PERIOD OF 60 MINUTES. Local I.V. site reactions have been reported with the intravenous administration of ciprofloxacin. These reactions are more frequent if infusion time is 30 minutes or less or if small veins of the hand are used. (See **ADVERSE REACTIONS.**)

Central Nervous System: Quinolones, including ciprofloxacin, may also cause central nervous system (CNS) events, including: nervousness, agitation, insomnia, anxiety, nightmares or paranoia. (See **WARNINGS, Information for Patients,** and **Drug Interactions.**)

Crystals of ciprofloxacin have been observed rarely in the urine of human subjects but more frequently in the urine of laboratory animals, which is usually alkaline. (See **ANIMAL PHARMACOLOGY.**) Crystalluria related to ciprofloxacin has been reported only rarely in humans because human urine is usually acidic. Alkalinity of the urine should be avoided in patients receiving ciprofloxacin. Patients should be well hydrated to prevent the formation of highly concentrated urine.

Renal Impairment: Alteration of the dosage regimen is necessary for patients with impairment of renal function. (See **DOSAGE AND ADMINISTRATION.**)

Phototoxicity: Moderate to severe phototoxicity manifested as an exaggerated sunburn reaction has been observed in some patients who were exposed to direct sunlight while receiving some members of the quinolone class of drugs. Excessive sunlight should be avoided.

As with any potent drug, periodic assessment of organ system functions, including renal, hepatic, and hematopoietic, is advisable during prolonged therapy.

Prescribing CIPRO I.V. in the absence of a proven or strongly suspected bacterial infection or a prophylactic indication is unlikely to provide benefit to the patient and increases the risk of the development of drug-resistant bacteria.

Information For Patients:

Patients should be advised:

- that antibacterial drugs including CIPRO I.V. should only be used to treat bacterial infections. They do not treat viral infections (e.g., the common cold). When CIPRO I.V. is prescribed to treat a bacterial infection, patients should be told that although it is common to feel better early in the course of therapy, the medication should be taken exactly as directed. Skipping doses or not completing the full course of therapy may (1) decrease the effectiveness of the immediate treatment and (2) increase the likelihood that bacteria will develop resistance and will not be treatable by CIPRO I.V. or other antibacterial drugs in the future.
- that ciprofloxacin may be associated with hypersensitivity reactions, even following a single dose, and to discontinue the drug at the first sign of a skin rash or other allergic reaction.

Continued on next page

Cipro I.V.—Cont.

- that ciprofloxacin may cause dizziness and lightheadedness; therefore, patients should know how they react to this drug before they operate an automobile or machinery or engage in activities requiring mental alertness or coordination.
- that ciprofloxacin may increase the effects of theophylline and caffeine. There is a possibility of caffeine accumulation when products containing caffeine are consumed while taking ciprofloxacin.
- that peripheral neuropathies have been associated with ciprofloxacin use. If symptoms of peripheral neuropathy including pain, burning, tingling, numbness and/or weakness develop, they should discontinue treatment and contact their physicians.
- to discontinue treatment; rest and refrain from exercise; and inform their physician if they experience pain, inflammation, or rupture of a tendon.
- that convulsions have been reported in patients taking quinolones, including ciprofloxacin, and to notify their physician before taking this drug if there is a history of this condition.
- that ciprofloxacin has been associated with an increased rate of adverse events involving joints and surrounding tissue structures (like tendons) in pediatric patients (less than 18 years of age). Parents should inform their child's physician if the child has a history of joint-related problems before taking this drug. Parents of pediatric patients should also notify their child's physician of any joint-related problems that occur during or following ciprofloxacin therapy. (See **WARNINGS, PRECAUTIONS, Pediatric Use** and **ADVERSE REACTIONS**.)

Drug Interactions: As with some other quinolones, concurrent administration of ciprofloxacin with theophylline may lead to elevated serum concentrations of theophylline and prolongation of its elimination half-life. This may result in increased risk of theophylline-related adverse reactions. (See **WARNINGS**.) If concomitant use cannot be avoided, serum levels of theophylline should be monitored and dosage adjustments made as appropriate.

Some quinolones, including ciprofloxacin, have also been shown to interfere with the metabolism of caffeine. This may lead to reduced clearance of caffeine and prolongation of its serum half-life.

Some quinolones, including ciprofloxacin, have been associated with transient elevations in serum creatinine in patients receiving cyclosporine concomitantly.

Altered serum levels of phenytoin (increased and decreased) have been reported in patients receiving concomitant ciprofloxacin.

The concomitant administration of ciprofloxacin with the sulfonylurea glyburide has, in some patients, resulted in severe hypoglycemia. Fatalities have been reported.

The serum concentrations of ciprofloxacin and metronidazole were not altered when these two drugs were given concomitantly. Quinolones, including ciprofloxacin, have been reported to enhance the effects of the oral anticoagulant warfarin or its derivatives. When these products are administered concomitantly, prothrombin time or other suitable coagulation tests should be closely monitored.

Probenecid interferes with renal tubular secretion of ciprofloxacin and produces an increase in the level of ciprofloxacin in the serum. This should be considered if patients are receiving both drugs concomitantly.

Renal tubular transport of methotrexate may be inhibited by concomitant administration of ciprofloxacin potentially leading to increased plasma levels of methotrexate. This might increase the risk of methotrexate associated toxic reactions. Therefore, patients under methotrexate therapy should be carefully monitored when concomitant ciprofloxacin therapy is indicated.

Non-steroidal anti-inflammatory drugs (but not acetyl salicylic acid) in combination of very high doses of quinolones have been shown to provoke convulsions in pre-clinical studies.

Following infusion of 400 mg I.V. ciprofloxacin every eight hours in combination with 50 mg/kg I.V. piperacillin sodium every four hours, mean serum ciprofloxacin concentrations were 3.02 µg/mL 1/2 hour and 1.18 µg/mL between 6–8 hours after the end of infusion.

Carcinogenesis, Mutagenesis, Impairment of Fertility: Eight *in vitro* mutagenicity tests have been conducted with ciprofloxacin. Test results are listed below:

- Salmonella/Microsome Test (Negative)
- *E. coli* DNA Repair Assay (Negative)
- Mouse Lymphoma Cell Forward Mutation Assay (Positive)
- Chinese Hamster V_{79} Cell HGPRT Test (Negative)
- Syrian Hamster Embryo Cell Transformation Assay (Negative)
- *Saccharomyces cerevisiae* Point Mutation Assay (Negative)
- *Saccharomyces cerevisiae* Mitotic Crossover and Gene Conversion Assay (Negative)
- Rat Hepatocyte DNA Repair Assay (Positive)

Thus, two of the eight tests were positive, but results of the following three *in vivo* test systems gave negative results:

- Rat Hepatocyte DNA Repair Assay
- Micronucleus Test (Mice)
- Dominant Lethal Test (Mice)

Long-term carcinogenicity studies in rats and mice resulted in no carcinogenic or tumorigenic effects due to ciprofloxacin at daily oral dose levels up to 250 and 750 mg/kg to rats and mice, respectively (approximately 1.7- and 2.5- times the highest recommended therapeutic dose based upon mg/m^2).

Results from photo co-carcinogenicity testing indicate that ciprofloxacin does not reduce the time to appearance of UV-induced skin tumors as compared to vehicle control. Hairless (Skh-1) mice were exposed to UVA light for 3.5 hours five times every two weeks for up to 78 weeks while concurrently being administered ciprofloxacin. The time to development of the first skin tumors was 50 weeks in mice treated concomitantly with UVA and ciprofloxacin (mouse dose approximately equal to maximum recommended human dose based upon mg/m^2), as opposed to 34 weeks when animals were treated with both UVA and vehicle. The times to development of skin tumors ranged from 16–32 weeks in mice treated concomitantly with UVA and other quinolones.[3]

In this model, mice treated with ciprofloxacin alone did not develop skin or systemic tumors. There are no data from similar models using pigmented mice and/or fully haired mice. The clinical significance of these findings to humans is unknown.

Fertility studies performed in rats at oral doses of ciprofloxacin up to 100 mg/kg (approximately 0.7-times the highest recommended therapeutic dose based upon mg/m^2) revealed no evidence of impairment.

Pregnancy: Teratogenic Effects. Pregnancy Category C: There are no adequate and well-controlled studies in pregnant women. An expert review of published data on experiences with ciprofloxacin use during pregnancy by TERIS – the Teratogen Information System - concluded that therapeutic doses during pregnancy are unlikely to pose a substantial teratogenic risk (quantity and quality of data=fair), but the data are insufficient to state that there is no risk.[7]

A controlled prospective observational study followed 200 women exposed to fluoroquinolones (52.5% exposed to ciprofloxacin and 68% first trimester exposures) during gestation.[8] In utero exposure to fluoroquinolones during embryogenesis was not associated with increased risk of major malformations. The reported rates of major congenital malformations were 2.2% for the fluoroquinolone group and 2.6% for the control group (background incidence of major malformations is 1–5%). Rates of spontaneous abortions, prematurity and low birth weight did not differ between the groups and there were no clinically significant musculoskeletal dysfunctions up to one year of age in the ciprofloxacin exposed children.

Another prospective follow-up study reported on 549 pregnancies with fluoroquinolone exposure (93% first trimester exposures).[9] There were 70 ciprofloxacin exposures, all within the first trimester. The malformation rates among live-born babies exposed to ciprofloxacin and to fluoroquinolones overall were both within background incidence ranges. No specific patterns of congenital abnormalities were found. The study did not reveal any clear adverse reactions due to in utero exposure to ciprofloxacin.

No differences in the rates of prematurity, spontaneous abortions, or birth weight were seen in women exposed to ciprofloxacin during pregnancy.[7,8] However, these small postmarketing epidemiology studies, of which most experience is from short term, first trimester exposure, are insufficient to evaluate the risk for less common defects or to permit reliable and definitive conclusions regarding the safety of ciprofloxacin in pregnant women and their developing fetuses. Ciprofloxacin should not be used during pregnancy unless the potential benefit justifies the potential risk to both fetus and mother (see **WARNINGS**).

Reproduction studies have been performed in rats and mice using oral doses up to 100 mg/kg (0.6 and 0.3 times the maximum daily human dose based upon body surface area, respectively) and have revealed no evidence of harm to the fetus due to ciprofloxacin. In rabbits, oral ciprofloxacin dose levels of 30 and 100 mg/kg (approximately 0.4- and 1.3-times the highest recommended therapeutic dose based upon mg/m^2) produced gastrointestinal toxicity resulting in maternal weight loss and an increased incidence of abortion, but no teratogenicity was observed at either dose level. After intravenous administration of doses up to 20 mg/kg (approximately 0.3-times the highest recommended therapeutic dose based upon mg/m^2) no maternal toxicity was produced and no embryotoxicity or teratogenicity was observed. (See **WARNINGS**.)

Nursing Mothers: Ciprofloxacin is excreted in human milk. The amount of ciprofloxacin absorbed by the nursing infant is unknown. Because of the potential for serious adverse reactions in infants nursing from mothers taking ciprofloxacin, a decision should be made whether to discontinue nursing or to discontinue the drug, taking into account the importance of the drug to the mother.

Pediatric Use: Ciprofloxacin, like other quinolones, causes arthropathy and histological changes in weight-bearing joints of juvenile animals resulting in lameness. (See **ANIMAL PHARMACOLOGY**.)

Inhalational Anthrax (Post-Exposure)

Ciprofloxacin is indicated in pediatric patients for inhalational anthrax (post-exposure). The risk-benefit assessment indicates that administration of ciprofloxacin to pediatric patients is appropriate. For information regarding pediatric dosing in inhalational anthrax (post-exposure), see **DOSAGE AND ADMINISTRATION** and **INHALATIONAL ANTHRAX – ADDITIONAL INFORMATION**.

Complicated Urinary Tract Infection and Pyelonephritis

Ciprofloxacin is indicated for the treatment of complicated urinary tract infections and pyelonephritis due to *Escherichia coli*. Although effective in clinical trials, ciprofloxacin is not a drug of first choice in the pediatric population due to an increased incidence of adverse events compared to the controls, including those related to joints and/or surrounding tissues. The rates of these events in pediatric patients with complicated urinary tract infection and pyelonephritis within six weeks of follow-up were 9.3% (31/335) versus 6.0% (21/349) for control agents. The rates of these events occurring at any time up to the one year follow-up were 13.7% (46/335) and 9.5% (33/349), respectively. The rate of all adverse events regardless of drug relationship at six weeks was 41% (138/335) in the ciprofloxacin arm compared to 31% (109/349) in the control arm. (See **ADVERSE REACTIONS** and **CLINICAL STUDIES**.)

Cystic Fibrosis

Short-term safety data from a single trial in pediatric cystic fibrosis patients are available. In a randomized, double-blind clinical trial for the treatment of acute pulmonary exacerbations in cystic fibrosis patients (ages 5–17 years), 67 patients received ciprofloxacin I.V. 10 mg/kg/dose q8h for one week followed by ciprofloxacin tablets 20 mg/kg/dose q12h to complete 10–21 days treatment and 62 patients received the combination of ceftazidime I.V. 50 mg/kg/dose q8h and tobramycin I.V. 3 mg/kg/dose q8h for a total of 10–21 days. Patients less than 5 years of age were not studied. Safety monitoring in the study included periodic range of motion examinations and gait assessments by treatment-blinded examiners. Patients were followed for an average of 23 days after completing treatment (range 0-93 days). This study was not designed to determine long term effects and the safety of repeated exposure to ciprofloxacin.

Musculoskeletal adverse events in patients with cystic fibrosis were reported in 22% of the patients in the ciprofloxacin group and 21% in the comparison group. Decreased range of motion was reported in 12% of the subjects in the ciprofloxacin group and 16% in the comparison group. Arthralgia was reported in 10% of the patients in the ciprofloxacin group and 11% in the comparison group. Other adverse events were similar in nature and frequency between treatment arms. One of sixty-seven patients developed arthritis of the knee nine days after a ten day course of treatment with ciprofloxacin. Clinical symptoms resolved, but an MRI showed knee effusion without other abnormalities eight months after treatment. However, the relationship of this event to the patient's course of ciprofloxacin can not be definitively determined, particularly since patients with cystic fibrosis may develop arthralgias/arthritis as part of their underlying disease process.

Geriatric Use: In a retrospective analysis of 23 multiple-dose controlled clinical trials of ciprofloxacin encompassing over 3500 ciprofloxacin treated patients, 25% of patients were greater than or equal to 65 years of age and 10% were greater than or equal to 75 years of age. No overall differences in safety or effectiveness were observed between these subjects and younger subjects, and other reported clinical experience has not identified differences in responses between the elderly and younger patients, but greater sensitivity of some older individuals on any drug therapy cannot be ruled out. Ciprofloxacin is known to be substantially excreted by the kidney, and the risk of adverse reactions may be greater in patients with impaired renal function. No alteration of dosage is necessary for patients greater than 65 years of age with normal renal function. However, since some older individuals experience reduced renal function by virtue of their advanced age, care should be taken in dose selection for elderly patients, and renal function monitoring may be useful in these patients. (See **CLINICAL PHARMACOLOGY** and **DOSAGE AND ADMINISTRATION**.)

ADVERSE REACTIONS

Adverse Reactions in Adult Patients: During clinical investigations with oral and parenteral ciprofloxacin, 49,038 patients received courses of the drug. Most of the adverse events reported were described as only mild or moderate in severity, abated soon after the drug was discontinued, and required no treatment. Ciprofloxacin was discontinued because of an adverse event in 1.8% of intravenously treated patients.

The most frequently reported drug related events, from clinical trials of all formulations, all dosages, all drug-therapy durations, and for all indications of ciprofloxacin therapy were nausea (2.5%), diarrhea (1.6%), liver function tests abnormal (1.3%), vomiting (1.0%), and rash (1.0%).

In clinical trials the following events were reported, regardless of drug relationship, in greater than 1% of patients treated with intravenous ciprofloxacin: nausea, diarrhea, central nervous system disturbance, local I.V. site reactions, liver function tests abnormal, eosinophilia, headache, restlessness, and rash. Many of these events were described as only mild or moderate in severity, abated soon after the drug was discontinued, and required no treatment. Local I.V. site reactions are more frequent if the infusion time is 30 minutes or less. These may appear as local skin reactions which resolve rapidly upon completion of the infusion. Subsequent intravenous administration is not contraindicated unless the reactions recur or worsen.

Additional medically important events, without regard to drug relationship or route of administration, that occurred in 1% or less of ciprofloxacin patients are listed below:

BODY AS A WHOLE: abdominal pain/discomfort, foot pain, pain, pain in extremities

CARDIOVASCULAR: cardiovascular collapse, cardiopulmonary arrest, myocardial infarction, arrhythmia, tachycardia, palpitation, cerebral thrombosis, syncope, cardiac

murmur, hypertension, hypotension, angina pectoris, atrial flutter, ventricular ectopy, (thrombo)-phlebitis, vasodilation, migraine
CENTRAL NERVOUS SYSTEM: convulsive seizures, paranoia, toxic psychosis, depression, dysphasia, phobia, depersonalization, manic reaction, unresponsiveness, ataxia, confusion, hallucinations, dizziness, lightheadedness, paresthesia, anxiety, tremor, insomnia, nightmares, weakness, drowsiness, irritability, malaise, lethargy, abnormal gait, grand mal convulsion, anorexia
GASTROINTESTINAL: ileus, jaundice, gastrointestinal bleeding, *C. difficile* associated diarrhea, pseudomembranous colitis, pancreatitis, hepatic necrosis, intestinal perforation, dyspepsia, epigastric pain, constipation, oral ulceration, oral candidiasis, mouth dryness, anorexia, dysphagia, flatulence, hepatitis, painful oral mucosa
HEMIC/LYMPHATIC: agranulocytosis, prolongation of prothrombin time, lymphadenopathy, petechia
METABOLIC/NUTRITIONAL: amylase increase, lipase increase
MUSCULOSKELETAL: arthralgia, jaw, arm or back pain, joint stiffness, neck and chest pain, achiness, flare up of gout, myasthenia gravis
RENAL/UROGENITAL: renal failure, interstitial nephritis, nephritis, hemorrhagic cystitis, renal calculi, frequent urination, acidosis, urethral bleeding, polyuria, urinary retention, gynecomastia, candiduria, vaginitis, breast pain. Crystalluria, cylindruria, hematuria and albuminuria have also been reported.
RESPIRATORY: respiratory arrest, pulmonary embolism, dyspnea, laryngeal or pulmonary edema, respiratory distress, pleural effusion, hemoptysis, epistaxis, hiccough, bronchospasm
SKIN/HYPERSENSITIVITY: allergic reactions, anaphylactic reactions, erythema multiforme/Stevens-Johnson syndrome, exfoliative dermatitis, toxic epidermal necrolysis, vasculitis, angioedema, edema of the lips, face, neck, conjunctivae, hands or lower extremities, purpura, fever, chills, flushing, pruritus, urticaria, cutaneous candidiasis, vesicles, increased perspiration, hyperpigmentation, erythema nodosum, thrombophlebitis, burning, paresthesia, erythema, swelling, photosensitivity (See **WARNINGS**.)
SPECIAL SENSES: decreased visual acuity, blurred vision, disturbed vision (flashing lights, change in color perception, overbrightness of lights, diplopia), eye pain, anosmia, hearing loss, tinnitus, nystagmus, chromatopsia, a bad taste.

In several instances, nausea, vomiting, tremor, irritability, or palpitation were judged by investigators to be related to elevated serum levels of theophylline possibly as a result of drug interaction with ciprofloxacin.

In randomized, double-blind controlled clinical trials comparing ciprofloxacin (I.V. and I.V./P.O. sequential) with intravenous beta-lactam control antibiotics, the CNS adverse event profile of ciprofloxacin was comparable to that of the control drugs.

Adverse Reactions in Pediatric Patients: Ciprofloxacin, administered I.V. and/or orally, was compared to a cephalosporin for treatment of complicated urinary tract infections (cUTI) or pyelonephritis in pediatric patients 1 to 17 years of age (mean age of 6 ± 4 years). The trial was conducted in the US, Canada, Argentina, Peru, Costa Rica, Mexico, South Africa, and Germany. The duration of therapy was 10 to 21 days (mean duration of treatment was 11 days with a range of 1 to 88 days). The primary objective of the study was to assess musculoskeletal and neurological safety within 6 weeks of therapy and through one year of follow-up in the 335 ciprofloxacin- and 349 comparator-treated patients enrolled.

An Independent Pediatric Safety Committee (IPSC) reviewed all cases of musculoskeletal adverse events as well as all patients with an abnormal gait or abnormal joint exam (baseline or treatment-emergent). These events were evaluated in a comprehensive fashion and included such conditions as arthralgia, abnormal gait, abnormal joint exam, joint sprains, leg pain, back pain, arthrosis, bone pain, pain, myalgia, arm pain, and decreased range of motion in a joint. The affected joints included: knee, elbow, ankle, hip, wrist, and shoulder. Within 6 weeks of treatment initiation, the rates of these events were 9.3% (31/335) in the ciprofloxacin-treated group versus 6.0 % (21/349) in comparator-treated patients. The majority of these events were mild or moderate in intensity. All musculoskeletal events occurring by 6 weeks resolved (clinical resolution of signs and symptoms), usually within 30 days of end of treatment. Radiological evaluations were not routinely used to confirm resolution of the events. The events occurred more frequently in ciprofloxacin-treated patients than control patients, regardless of whether they received I.V. or oral therapy. Ciprofloxacin-treated patients were more likely to report more than one event and on more than one occasion compared to control patients. These events occurred in all age groups and the rates were consistently higher in the ciprofloxacin group compared to the control group. At the end of 1 year, the rate of these events reported at any time during that period was 13.7% (46/335) in the ciprofloxacin-treated group versus 9.5% (33/349) comparator-treated patients.

An adolescent female discontinued ciprofloxacin for wrist pain that developed during treatment. An MRI performed 4 weeks later showed a tear in the right ulnar fibrocartilage. A diagnosis of overuse syndrome secondary to sports activity was made, but a contribution from ciprofloxacin cannot be excluded. The patient recovered by 4 months without surgical intervention.

ADULT DOSAGE GUIDELINES

Infection†	Severity	Dose	Frequency	Usual Duration
Urinary Tract	Mild/Moderate Severe/Complicated	200 mg 400 mg	q12h q12h	7–14 Days 7–14 Days
Lower Respiratory Tract	Mild/Moderate Severe/Complicated	400 mg 400 mg	q12h q8h	7–14 Days 7–14 Days
Nosocomial Pneumonia	Mild/Moderate/Severe	400 mg	q8h	10–14 Days
Skin and Skin Structure	Mild/Moderate Severe/Complicated	400 mg 400 mg	q12h q8h	7–14 Days 7–14 Days
Bone and Joint	Mild/Moderate Severe/Complicated	400 mg 400 mg	q12h q8h	≥ 4–6 Weeks ≥ 4–6 Weeks
Intra-Abdominal*	Complicated	400 mg	q12h	7–14 Days
Acute Sinusitis	Mild/Moderate	400 mg	q12h	10 Days
Chronic Bacterial Prostatitis	Mild/Moderate	400 mg	q12h	28 Days
Empirical Therapy in Febrile Neutropenic Patients	Severe Ciprofloxacin + Piperacillin	400 mg 50 mg/kg Not to exceed 24 g/day	q8h q4h	7–14 Days
Inhalational anthrax (post-exposure)**		400 mg	q12h	60 Days

* used in conjunction with metronidazole. (See product labeling for prescribing information.)
† DUE TO THE DESIGNATED PATHOGENS (See **INDICATIONS AND USAGE.**)
** Drug administration should begin as soon as possible after suspected or confirmed exposure. This indication is based on a surrogate endpoint, ciprofloxacin serum concentrations achieved in humans, reasonably likely to predict clinical benefit.[4] For a discussion of ciprofloxacin serum concentrations in various human populations, see **INHALATIONAL ANTHRAX — ADDITIONAL INFORMATION**. Total duration of ciprofloxacin administration (I.V. or oral) for inhalational anthrax (post-exposure) is 60 days.

Findings Involving Joint or Peri-articular Tissues as Assessed by the IPSC

	Ciprofloxacin	Comparator
All Patients (within 6 weeks)	31/335 (9.3%)	21/349 (6.0%)
95% Confidence Interval*	(−0.8%, +7.2%)	
Age Group		
≥ 12 months < 24 months	1/36 (2.8%)	0/41
≥ 2 years < 6 years	5/124 (4.0%)	3/118 (2.5%)
≥ 6 years < 12 years	18/143 (12.6%)	12/153 (7.8%)
≥ 12 years to 17 years	7/32 (21.9%)	6/37 (16.2 %)
All Patients (within 1 year)	46/335 (13.7%)	33/349 (9.5%)
95% Confidence Interval*	(−0.6%, +9.1%)	

*The study was designed to demonstrate that the arthropathy rate for the ciprofloxacin group did not exceed that of the control group by more than + 6%. At both the 6 week and 1 year evaluations, the 95% confidence interval indicated that it could not be concluded that the ciprofloxacin group had findings comparable to the control group.

The incidence rates of neurological events within 6 weeks of treatment initiation were 3% (9/335) in the ciprofloxacin group versus 2% (7/349) in the comparator group and included dizziness, nervousness, insomnia, and somnolence.

In this trial, the overall incidence rates of adverse events regardless of relationship to study drug and within 6 weeks of treatment initiation were 41% (138/335) in the ciprofloxacin group versus 31% (109/349) in the comparator group. The most frequent events were gastrointestinal: 15% (50/335) of ciprofloxacin patients compared to 9% (31/349) of comparator patients. Serious adverse events were seen in 7.5% (25/335) of ciprofloxacin-treated patients compared to 5.7% (20/349) of control patients. Discontinuation of drug due to an adverse event was observed in 3% (10/335) of ciprofloxacin-treated patients versus 1.4% (5/349) of comparator patients. Other adverse events that occurred in at least 1% of ciprofloxacin patients were diarrhea 4.8%, vomiting 4.8%, abdominal pain 3.3%, accidental injury 3.0%, rhinitis 3.0%, dyspepsia 2.7%, nausea 2.7%, fever 2.1%, asthma 1.8% and rash 1.8%.

In addition to the events reported in pediatric patients in clinical trials, it should be expected that events reported in adults during clinical trials or post-marketing experience may also occur in pediatric patients.

Post-Marketing Adverse Events: The following adverse events have been reported from worldwide marketing experience with quinolones, including ciprofloxacin. Because these events are reported voluntarily from a population of uncertain size, it is not always possible to reliably estimate their frequency or establish a causal relationship to drug exposure. Decisions to include these events in labeling are typically based on one or more of the following factors: (1) seriousness of the event, (2) frequency of the reporting, or (3) strength of causal connection to the drug.

Agitation, agranulocytosis, albuminuria, anosmia, candiduria, cholesterol elevation (serum), confusion, constipation, delirium, dyspepsia, dysphagia, erythema multiforme, exfoliative dermatitis, fixed eruption, flatulence, glucose elevation (blood), hemolytic anemia, hepatic failure, hepatic necrosis, hyperesthesia, hypertonia, hypesthesia, hypotension (postural), jaundice, marrow depression (life threatening), methemoglobinemia, moniliasis (oral, gastrointestinal, vaginal), myalgia, myasthenia, myasthenia gravis (possible exacerbation), myoclonus, nystagmus, pancreatitis, pancytopenia (life threatening or fatal outcome), peripheral neuropathy, phenytoin alteration (serum), potassium elevation (serum), prothrombin time prolongation or decrease, pseudomembranous colitis (The onset of pseudomembranous colitis symptoms may occur during or after antimicrobial treatment.), psychosis (toxic), renal calculi, serum sickness like reaction, Stevens-Johnson syndrome, taste loss, tendinitis, tendon rupture, torsade de pointes, toxic epidermal necrolysis, triglyceride elevation (serum), twitching, vaginal candidiasis, and vasculitis. (See **PRECAUTIONS.**)

Adverse Laboratory Changes: The most frequently reported changes in laboratory parameters with intravenous ciprofloxacin therapy, without regard to drug relationship are listed below:

Hepatic	—	elevations of AST (SGOT), ALT (SGPT), alkaline phosphatase, LDH, and serum bilirubin
Hematologic	—	elevated eosinophil and platelet counts, decreased platelet counts, hemoglobin and/or hematocrit
Renal	—	elevations of serum creatinine, BUN, and uric acid
Other	—	elevations of serum creatine phosphokinase, serum theophylline (in patients receiving theophylline concomitantly), blood glucose, and triglycerides

Other changes occurring infrequently were: decreased leukocyte count, elevated atypical lymphocyte count, immature WBCs, elevated serum calcium, elevation of serum gamma-glutamyl transpeptidase (γ GT), decreased BUN, decreased uric acid, decreased total serum protein, decreased serum albumin, decreased serum potassium, elevated serum potassium, elevated serum cholesterol. Other changes occurring rarely during administration of ciprofloxacin were: elevation of serum amylase, decrease of blood glucose, pancytopenia, leukocytosis, elevated sedimentation rate, change in serum phenytoin, decreased prothrombin time, hemolytic anemia, and bleeding diathesis.

OVERDOSAGE

In the event of acute overdosage, the patient should be carefully observed and given supportive treatment. Adequate hydration must be maintained. Only a small amount of ciprofloxacin (< 10%) is removed from the body after hemodialysis or peritoneal dialysis.

Continued on next page

Cipro I.V.—Cont.

In mice, rats, rabbits and dogs, significant toxicity including tonic/clonic convulsions was observed at intravenous doses of ciprofloxacin between 125 and 300 mg/kg.

DOSAGE AND ADMINISTRATION - ADULTS

CIPRO I.V. should be administered to adults by intravenous infusion over a period of 60 minutes at dosages described in the Dosage Guidelines table. Slow infusion of a dilute solution into a larger vein will minimize patient discomfort and reduce the risk of venous irritation. (See **Preparation of CIPRO I.V. for Administration** section.)

The determination of dosage for any particular patient must take into consideration the severity and nature of the infection, the susceptibility of the causative microorganism, the integrity of the patient's host-defense mechanisms, and the status of renal and hepatic function.

[See table at top of previous page]

CIPRO I.V. should be administered by intravenous infusion over a period of 60 minutes.

Conversion of I.V. to Oral Dosing in Adults: CIPRO Tablets and CIPRO Oral Suspension for oral administration are available. Parenteral therapy may be switched to oral CIPRO when the condition warrants, at the discretion of the physician. (See **CLINICAL PHARMACOLOGY** and table below for the equivalent dosing regimens.)

Equivalent AUC Dosing Regimens

CIPRO Oral Dosage	Equivalent CIPRO I.V. Dosage
250 mg Tablet q 12 h	200 mg I.V. q 12 h
500 mg Tablet q 12 h	400 mg I.V. q 12 h
750 mg Tablet q 12 h	400 mg I.V. q 8 h

Parenteral drug products should be inspected visually for particulate matter and discoloration prior to administration.

Adults with Impaired Renal Function: Ciprofloxacin is eliminated primarily by renal excretion; however, the drug is also metabolized and partially cleared through the biliary system of the liver and through the intestine. These alternative pathways of drug elimination appear to compensate for the reduced renal excretion in patients with renal impairment. Nonetheless, some modification of dosage is recommended for patients with severe renal dysfunction. The following table provides dosage guidelines for use in patients with renal impairment:

RECOMMENDED STARTING AND MAINTENANCE DOSES FOR PATIENTS WITH IMPAIRED RENAL FUNCTION

Creatinine Clearance (mL/min)	Dosage
> 30	See usual dosage.
5–29	200–400 mg q 18–24 hr

When only the serum creatinine concentration is known, the following formula may be used to estimate creatinine clearance:

[See first table above]

The serum creatinine should represent a steady state of renal function.

For patients with changing renal function or for patients with renal impairment and hepatic insufficiency, careful monitoring is suggested.

DOSAGE AND ADMINISTRATION - PEDIATRICS

CIPRO I.V. should be administered as described in the Dosage Guidelines table. An increased incidence of adverse events compared to controls, including events related to joints and/or surrounding tissues, has been observed. (See **ADVERSE REACTIONS** and **CLINICAL STUDIES**.)

Dosing and initial route of therapy (i.e., I.V. or oral) for complicated urinary tract infection or pyelonephritis should be determined by the severity of the infection. In the clinical trial, pediatric patients with moderate to severe infection were initiated on 6 to 10 mg/kg I.V. every 8 hours and allowed to switch to oral therapy (10 to 20 mg/kg every 12 hours), at the discretion of the physician.

[See second table at right]

Pediatric patients with moderate to severe renal insufficiency were excluded from the clinical trial of complicated urinary tract infection and pyelonephritis. No information is available on dosing adjustments necessary for pediatric patients with moderate to severe renal insufficiency (i.e., creatinine clearance of < 50 mL/min/1.73m^2).

Preparation of CIPRO I.V. for Administration

Vials (Injection Concentrate): THIS PREPARATION MUST BE DILUTED BEFORE USE. The intravenous dose should be prepared by aseptically withdrawing the concentrate from the vial of CIPRO I.V. This should be diluted with a suitable intravenous solution to a final concentration of 1–2mg/mL. (See **COMPATIBILITY AND STABILITY**.) The resulting solution should be infused over a period of 60 minutes by direct infusion or through a Y-type intravenous infusion set which may already be in place.

If the Y-type or "piggyback" method of administration is used, it is advisable to discontinue temporarily the administration of any other solutions during the infusion of CIPRO I.V. If the concomitant use of CIPRO I.V. and another drug is necessary each drug should be given separately in accordance with the recommended dosage and route of administration for each drug.

$$\text{Men: Creatinine clearance (mL/min)} = \frac{\text{Weight (kg)} \times (140 - \text{age})}{72 \times \text{serum creatinine (mg/dL)}}$$

Women: 0.85 × the value calculated for men.

PEDIATRIC DOSAGE GUIDELINES

Infection	Route of Administration	Dose (mg/kg)	Frequency	Total Duration
Complicated Urinary Tract or Pyelonephritis (patients from 1 to 17 years of age)	Intravenous	6 to 10 mg/kg (maximum 400 mg per dose; not to be exceeded even in patients weighing > 51 kg)	Every 8 hours	10–21 days*
	Oral	10 mg/kg to 20 mg/kg (maximum 750 mg per dose; not to be exceeded even in patients weighing > 51 kg)	Every 12 hours	
Inhalational Anthrax (Post-Exposure)**	Intravenous	10 mg/kg (maximum 400 mg per dose)	Every 12 hours	60 days
	Oral	15 mg/kg (maximum 500 mg per dose)	Every 12 hours	

* The total duration of therapy for complicated urinary tract infection and pyelonephritis in the clinical trial was determined by the physician. The mean duration of treatment was 11 days (range 10 to 21 days).

** Drug administration should begin as soon as possible after suspected or confirmed exposure to *Bacillus anthracis* spores. This indication is based on a surrogate endpoint, ciprofloxacin serum concentrations achieved in humans, reasonably likely to predict clinical benefit.[4] For a discussion of ciprofloxacin serum concentrations in various human populations, see **INHALATIONAL ANTHRAX – ADDITIONAL INFORMATION.**

VIAL: manufactured by Bayer Healthcare LLC and Hollister-Stier, Spokane, WA 99220.

SIZE	STRENGTH	NDC NUMBER
20 mL	200 mg, 1%	0026-8562-20
40 mL	400 mg, 1%	0026-8564-64

FLEXIBLE CONTAINER: manufactured for Bayer Pharmaceuticals Corporation by Abbott Laboratories, North Chicago, IL 60064.

SIZE	STRENGTH	NDC NUMBER
100 mL 5% Dextrose	200 mg, 0.2%	0026-8552-36
200 mL 5% Dextrose	400 mg, 0.2%	0026-8554-63

FLEXIBLE CONTAINER: manufactured for Bayer Pharmaceuticals Corporation by Baxter Healthcare Corporation, Deerfield, IL 60015.

SIZE	STRENGTH	NDC NUMBER
100 mL 5% Dextrose	200 mg, 0.2%	0026-8527-36
200 mL 5% Dextrose	400 mg, 0.2%	0026-8527-63

Outcomes	Ciprofloxacin/Piperacillin N = 233 Success (%)	Tobramycin/Piperacillin N = 237 Success (%)
Clinical Resolution of Initial Febrile Episode with No Modifications of Empirical Regimen*	63 (27.0%)	52 (21.9%)
Clinical Resolution of Initial Febrile Episode Including Patients with Modifications of Empirical Regimen	187 (80.3%)	185 (78.1%)
Overall Survival	224 (96.1%)	223 (94.1%)

* To be evaluated as a clinical resolution, patients had to have: (1) resolution of fever; (2) microbiological eradication of infection (if an infection was microbiologically documented); (3) resolution of signs/symptoms of infection; and (4) no modification of empirical antibiotic regimen.

Flexible Containers: CIPRO I.V. is also available as a 0.2% premixed solution in 5% dextrose in flexible containers of 100 mL or 200 mL. The solutions in flexible containers do not need to be diluted and may be infused as described above.

COMPATIBILITY AND STABILITY

Ciprofloxacin injection 1% (10 mg/mL), when diluted with the following intravenous solutions to concentrations of 0.5 to 2.0 mg/mL, is stable for up to 14 days at refrigerated or room temperature storage.

- 0.9% Sodium Chloride Injection, USP
- 5% Dextrose Injection, USP
- Sterile Water for Injection
- 10% Dextrose for Injection
- 5% Dextrose and 0.225% Sodium Chloride for Injection
- 5% Dextrose and 0.45% Sodium Chloride for Injection
- Lactated Ringer's for Injection

HOW SUPPLIED

CIPRO I.V. (ciprofloxacin) is available as a clear, colorless to slightly yellowish solution. CIPRO I.V. is available in 200 mg and 400 mg strengths. The concentrate is supplied in vials while the premixed solution is supplied in latex-free flexible containers as follows:

[See third table above]

STORAGE

Vial: Store between 5–30°C (41–86°F).
Flexible Container: Store between 5–25°C (41–77°F).

Protect from light, avoid excessive heat, protect from freezing.

CIPRO I.V. (ciprofloxacin) is also available in a 120 mL Pharmacy Bulk Package.

Ciprofloxacin is also available as CIPRO (ciprofloxacin HCl) Tablets 100, 250, 500, and 750 mg and CIPRO (ciprofloxacin*) 5% and 10% Oral Suspension.

*Does not comply with USP with regards to "loss on drying" and "residue on ignition".

ANIMAL PHARMACOLOGY

Ciprofloxacin and other quinolones have been shown to cause arthropathy in immature animals of most species tested. (See **WARNINGS**.) Damage of weight bearing joints was observed in juvenile dogs and rats. In young beagles, 100 mg/kg ciprofloxacin, given daily for 4 weeks, caused degenerative articular changes of the knee joint. At 30 mg/kg, the effect on the joint was minimal. In a subsequent study in young beagle dogs, oral ciprofloxacin doses of 30 mg/kg and 90 mg/kg ciprofloxacin (approximately 1.3- and 3.5-times the pediatric dose based upon comparative plasma AUCs) given daily for 2 weeks caused articular changes which were still observed by histopathology after a treatment-free period of 5 months. At 10 mg/kg (approximately 0.6-times the pediatric dose based upon comparative plasma AUCs), no effects on joints were observed. This dose was also not associated with arthrotoxicity after an additional treatment-free period of 5 months. In another study, removal of weight bearing from the joint reduced the lesions but did not totally prevent them.

Crystalluria, sometimes associated with secondary nephropathy, occurs in laboratory animals dosed with ciprofloxacin. This is primarily related to the reduced solubility of ciprofloxacin under alkaline conditions, which predominate in the urine of test animals; in man, crystalluria is rare since human urine is typically acidic. In rhesus monkeys, crystalluria without nephropathy was noted after single oral doses as low as 5 mg/kg (approximately 0.07-times

Clinical Success and Bacteriologic Eradication at Test of Cure (5 to 9 Days Post-Therapy)

	CIPRO	Comparator
Randomized Patients	337	352
Per Protocol Patients	211	231
Clinical Response at 5 to 9 Days Post-Treatment	95.7% (202/211)	92.6% (214/231)
	95% CI [−1.3%, 7.3%]	
Bacteriologic Eradication by Patient at 5 to 9 Days Post-Treatment*	84.4% (178/211)	78.3% (181/231)
	95% CI [−1.3%, 13.1%]	
Bacteriologic Eradication of the Baseline Pathogen at 5 to 9 Days Post-Treatment		
Escherichia coli	156/178 (88%)	161/179 (90%)

* Patients with baseline pathogen(s) eradicated and no new infections or superinfections/total number of patients. There were 5.5% (6/211) ciprofloxacin and 9.5% (22/231) comparator patients with superinfections or new infections.

the highest recommended therapeutic dose based upon mg/m^2). After 6 months of intravenous dosing at 10 mg/kg/day, no nephropathological changes were noted; however, nephropathy was observed after dosing at 20 mg/kg/day for the same duration (approximately 0.2-times the highest recommended therapeutic dose based upon mg/m^2).

In dogs, ciprofloxacin administered at 3 and 10 mg/kg by rapid intravenous injection (15 sec.) produces pronounced hypotensive effects. These effects are considered to be related to histamine release because they are partially antagonized by pyrilamine, an antihistamine. In rhesus monkeys, rapid intravenous injection also produces hypotension, but the effect in this species is inconsistent and less pronounced.

In mice, concomitant administration of nonsteroidal anti-inflammatory drugs, such as phenylbutazone and indomethacin, with quinolones has been reported to enhance the CNS stimulatory effect of quinolones.

Ocular toxicity, seen with some related drugs, has not been observed in ciprofloxacin-treated animals.

INHALATIONAL ANTHRAX – ADDITIONAL INFORMATION

The mean serum concentrations of ciprofloxacin associated with a statistically significant improvement in survival in the rhesus monkey model of inhalational anthrax are reached or exceeded in adult and pediatric patients receiving oral and intravenous regimens. (See **DOSAGE AND ADMINISTRATION**.) Ciprofloxacin pharmacokinetics have been evaluated in various human populations.The mean peak serum concentration achieved at steady-state in human adults receiving 500 mg orally every 12 hours is 2.97 µg/mL, and 4.56 µg/mL following 400 mg intravenously every 12 hours. The mean trough serum concentration at steady-state for both of these regimens is 0.2 µg/mL. In a study of 10 pediatric patients between 6 and 16 years of age, the mean peak plasma concentration achieved is 8.3 µg/mL and trough concentrations range from 0.09 to 0.26 µg/mL, following two 30-minute intravenous infusions of 10 mg/kg administered 12 hours apart. After the second intravenous infusion patients switched to 15 mg/kg orally every 12 hours achieve a mean peak concentration of 3.6 µg/mL after the initial oral dose. Long-term safety data, including effects on cartilage, following the administration of ciprofloxacin to pediatric patients are limited. (For additional information, see **PRECAUTIONS**, **Pediatric Use**.) Ciprofloxacin serum concentrations achieved in humans serve as a surrogate endpoint reasonably likely to predict clinical benefit and provide the basis for this indication.[4]

A placebo-controlled animal study in rhesus monkeys exposed to an inhaled mean dose of 11 LD_{50} (~5.5 × 10^5) spores (range 5–30 LD_{50}) of *B. anthracis* was conducted. The minimal inhibitory concentration (MIC) of ciprofloxacin for the anthrax strain used in this study was 0.08 µg/mL. In the animals studied, mean serum concentrations of ciprofloxacin achieved at expected T_{max} (1 hour post-dose) following oral dosing to steady-state ranged from 0.98 to 1.69 µg/mL. Mean steady-state trough concentrations at 12 hours post-dose ranged from 0.12 to 0.19 µg/mL[5]. Mortality due to anthrax for animals that received a 30-day regimen of oral ciprofloxacin beginning 24 hours post-exposure was significantly lower (1/9), compared to the placebo group (9/10) [p=0.001]. The one ciprofloxacin-treated animal that died of anthrax did so following the 30-day drug administration period.[6]

CLINICAL STUDIES

EMPIRICAL THERAPY IN ADULT FEBRILE NEUTROPENIC PATIENTS

The safety and efficacy of ciprofloxacin, 400 mg I.V. q 8h, in combination with piperacillin sodium, 50 mg/kg I.V. q 4h, for the empirical therapy of febrile neutropenic patients were studied in one large pivotal multicenter, randomized trial and were compared to those of tobramycin, 2 mg/kg I.V. q 8h, in combination with piperacillin sodium, 50 mg/kg I.V. q 4h.

Clinical response rates observed in this study were as follows:

[See fourth table on previous page]

Complicated Urinary Tract Infection and Pyelonephritis – Efficacy in Pediatric Patients:

NOTE: Although effective in clinical trials, ciprofloxacin is not a drug of first choice in the pediatric population due to an increased incidence of adverse events compared to controls, including events related to joints and/or surrounding tissues.

Ciprofloxacin, administered I.V. and/or orally, was compared to a cephalosporin for treatment of complicated urinary tract infections (cUTI) and pyelonephritis in pediatric patients 1 to 17 years of age (mean age of 6 ± 4 years). The trial was conducted in the US, Canada, Argentina, Peru, Costa Rica, Mexico, South Africa, and Germany. The duration of therapy was 10 to 21 days (mean duration of treatment was 11 days with a range of 1 to 88 days). The primary objective of the study was to assess musculoskeletal and neurological safety.

Patients were evaluated for clinical success and bacteriological eradication of the baseline organism(s) with no new infection or superinfection at 5 to 9 days post-therapy (Test of Cure or TOC). The Per Protocol population had a causative organism(s) with protocol specified colony count(s) at baseline, no protocol violation, and no premature discontinuation or loss to follow-up (among other criteria).

The clinical success and bacteriologic eradication rates in the Per Protocol population were similar between ciprofloxacin and the comparator group as shown below.

[See table above]

REFERENCES

1. National Committee for Clinical Laboratory Standards, Methods for Dilution Antimicrobial Susceptibility Tests for Bacteria That Grow Aerobically - Fifth Edition. Approved Standard NCCLS Document M7-A5, Vol. 20, No. 2, NCCLS, Wayne, PA, January, 2000. **2.** National Committee for Clinical Laboratory Standards, Performance Standards for Antimicrobial Disk Susceptibility Tests - Seventh Edition. Approved Standard NCCLS Document M2-A7, Vol. 20, No. 1, NCCLS, Wayne, PA, January, 2000. **3.** Report presented at the FDA's Anti-Infective Drug and Dermatological Drug Products Advisory Committee Meeting, March 31, 1993, Silver Spring, MD. Report available from FDA, CDER, Advisors and Consultants Staff, HFD-21, 1901 Chapman Avenue, Room 200, Rockville, MD 20852, USA. **4.** 21 CFR 314.510 (Subpart H – Accelerated Approval of New Drugs for Life-Threatening Illnesses). **5.** Kelly DJ, et al. Serum concentrations of penicillin, doxycycline, and ciprofloxacin during prolonged therapy in rhesus monkeys. J Infect Dis 1992; 166: 1184–7. **6.** Friedlander AM, et al. Postexposure prophylaxis against experimental inhalational anthrax. J Infect Dis 1993; 167: 1239–42. **7.** Friedman J, Polifka J. Teratogenic effects of drugs: a resource for clinicians (TERIS). Baltimore, Maryland: Johns Hopkins University Press, 2000:149–195. **8.** Loebstein R, Addis A, Ho E, et al. Pregnancy outcome following gestational exposure to fluoroquinolones: a multicenter prospective controlled study. Antimicrob Agents Chemother. 1998;42(6): 1336–1339. **9.** Schaefer C, Amoura-Elefant E, Vial T, et al. Pregnancy outcome after prenatal quinolone exposure. Evaluation of a case registry of the European network of teratology information services (ENTIS). Eur J Obstet Gynecol Reprod Biol. 1996;69:83–89.

Bayer HealthCare
Bayer Pharmaceuticals Corporation
400 Morgan Lane
West Haven, CT 06516 USA

℞ **Only**

08724752, R.6 4/04

EN-0050 BAY q 3939 5202-4-A-U.S.-12
Printed In U.S.A.

Shown in Product Identification Guide, page 308

CIPRO® I.V. ℞

[*sĭ'prō*]

(ciprofloxacin)

For Intravenous Infusion

PHARMACY BULK PACKAGE—NOT FOR DIRECT INFUSION

To reduce the development of drug-resistant bacteria and maintain the effectiveness of CIPRO® I.V. and other antibacterial drugs, CIPRO I.V. should be used only to treat or prevent infections that are proven or strongly suspected to be caused by bacteria.

DESCRIPTION

The pharmacy bulk package is a single-entry container of a sterile preparation for parenteral use that contains many single doses. It contains ciprofloxacin as a 1% aqueous solution concentrate. The contents are intended for use in a pharmacy admixture program and are restricted to the preparation of admixtures for intravenous infusion.

CIPRO I.V. (ciprofloxacin) is a synthetic broad-spectrum antimicrobial agent for intravenous (I.V.) administration. Ciprofloxacin, a fluoroquinolone, is 1-cyclopropyl-6-fluoro-1, 4-dihydro-4-oxo-7-(1-piperazinyl)-3-quinolinecarboxylic acid. Its empirical formula is $C_{17}H_{18}FN_3O_3$ and its chemical structure is:

Ciprofloxacin is a faint to light yellow crystalline powder with a molecular weight of 331.4. It is soluble in dilute (0.1N) hydrochloric acid and is practically insoluble in water and ethanol. CIPRO I.V. solution is available as a sterile 1.0% aqueous concentrate, which is intended for dilution prior to administration. Ciprofloxacin solution contains lactic acid as a solubilizing agent and hydrochloric acid for pH adjustment. The pH range for the 1.0% aqueous concentrate is 3.3 to 3.9.

CLINICAL PHARMACOLOGY

Absorption

Following 60-minute intravenous infusions of 200 mg and 400 mg ciprofloxacin to normal volunteers, the mean maximum serum concentrations achieved were 2.1 and 4.6 µg/mL, respectively; the concentrations at 12 hours were 0.1 and 0.2 µg/mL, respectively.

Steady-state Ciprofloxacin Serum Concentrations (µg/mL) After 60-minute I.V. Infusions q 12 h.

	Time after starting the infusion					
Dose	30 min.	1 hr	3 hr	6 hr	8 hr	12 hr
200 mg	1.7	2.1	0.6	0.3	0.2	0.1
400 mg	3.7	4.6	1.3	0.7	0.5	0.2

The pharmacokinetics of ciprofloxacin are linear over the dose range of 200 to 400 mg administered intravenously. Comparison of the pharmacokinetic parameters following the 1st and 5th I.V. dose on a q 12 h regimen indicates no evidence of drug accumulation.

The absolute bioavailability of oral ciprofloxacin is within a range of 70–80% with no substantial loss by first pass metabolism. An intravenous infusion of 400-mg ciprofloxacin given over 60 minutes every 12 hours has been shown to produce an area under the serum concentration time curve (AUC) equivalent to that produced by a 500-mg oral dose given every 12 hours. An intravenous infusion of 400 mg ciprofloxacin given over 60 minutes every 8 hours has been shown to produce an AUC at steady-state equivalent to that produced by a 750-mg oral dose given every 12 hours. A 400-mg I.V. dose results in a C_{max} similar to that observed with a 750-mg oral dose. An infusion of 200 mg ciprofloxacin given every 12 hours produces an AUC equivalent to that produced by a 250-mg oral dose given every 12 hours.

[See table at top of next page]

Distribution

After intravenous administration, ciprofloxacin is present in saliva, nasal and bronchial secretions, sputum, skin blister fluid, lymph, peritoneal fluid, bile, and prostatic secretions. It has also been detected in the lung, skin, fat, muscle, cartilage, and bone. Although the drug diffuses into cerebrospinal fluid (CSF), CSF concentrations are generally less than 10% of peak serum concentrations. Levels of the drug in the aqueous and vitreous chambers of the eye are lower than in serum.

Metabolism

After I.V. administration, three metabolites of ciprofloxacin have been identified in human urine which together account for approximately 10% of the intravenous dose. The binding of ciprofloxacin to serum proteins is 20 to 40%.

Excretion

The serum elimination half-life is approximately 5–6 hours and the total clearance is around 35 L/hr. After intravenous administration, approximately 50% to 70% of the dose is excreted in the urine as unchanged drug. Following a 200-mg I.V. dose, concentrations in the urine usually exceed 200 µg/mL 0–2 hours after dosing and are generally greater than 15 µg/mL 8–12 hours after dosing. Following a 400-mg I.V. dose, urine concentrations generally exceed 400 µg/mL 0–2 hours after dosing and are usually greater than 30 µg/mL 8–12 hours after dosing. The renal clearance is approximately 22 L/hr. The urinary excretion of ciprofloxacin is virtually complete by 24 hours after dosing. Although bile concentrations of ciprofloxacin are several fold higher than serum concentrations after intravenous dosing, only a small amount of the administered dose (< 1%) is recovered from the bile as unchanged drug. Approximately 15% of an I.V. dose is recovered from the feces within 5 days after dosing.

Continued on next page

Cipro I.V. Bulk—Cont.

Special Populations
Pharmacokinetic studies of the oral (single dose) and intravenous (single and multiple dose) forms of ciprofloxacin indicate that plasma concentrations of ciprofloxacin are higher in elderly subjects (> 65 years) as compared to young adults. Although the C_{max} is increased 16–40%, the increase in mean AUC is approximately 30%, and can be at least partially attributed to decreased renal clearance in the elderly. Elimination half-life is only slightly (~20%) prolonged in the elderly. These differences are not considered clinically significant. (See **PRECAUTIONS: Geriatric Use.**)
In patients with reduced renal function, the half-life of ciprofloxacin is slightly prolonged and dosage adjustments may be required. (See **DOSAGE AND ADMINISTRATION.**)
In preliminary studies in patients with stable chronic liver cirrhosis, no significant changes in ciprofloxacin pharmacokinetics have been observed. However, the kinetics of ciprofloxacin in patients with acute hepatic insufficiency have not been fully elucidated.
Following a single oral dose of 10 mg/kg ciprofloxacin suspension to 16 children ranging in age from 4 months to 7 years, the mean C_{max} was 2.4 µg/mL (range: 1.5 – 3.4 µg/mL) and the mean AUC was 9.2 µg*h/mL (range: 5.8 – 14.9 µg*h/mL). There was no apparent age-dependence, and no notable increase in C_{max} or AUC upon multiple dosing (10 mg/kg TID). In children with severe sepsis who were given intravenous ciprofloxacin (10 mg/kg as a 1-hour infusion), the mean C_{max} was 6.1 µg/mL (range: 4.6 – 8.3 µg/mL) in 10 children less than 1 year of age; and 7.2 µg/mL (range: 4.7 – 11.8 µg/mL) in 10 children between 1 and 5 years of age. The AUC values were 17.4 µg*h/mL (range: 11.8 – 32.0 µg*h/mL) and 16.5 µg*h/mL (range: 11.0 – 23.8 µg*h/mL) in the respective age groups. These values are within the range reported for adults at therapeutic doses. Based on population pharmacokinetic analysis of pediatric patients with various infections, the predicted mean half-life in children is approximately 4 - 5 hours, and the bioavailability of the oral suspension is approximately 60%.
Drug-drug Interactions: The potential for pharmacokinetic drug interactions between ciprofloxacin and theophylline, caffeine, cyclosporins, phenytoin, sulfonylurea glyburide, metronidazole, warfarin, probenecid, and piperacillin sodium has been evaluated. (See **PRECAUTIONS: Drug Interactions.**)

MICROBIOLOGY

Ciprofloxacin has *in vitro* activity against a wide range of gram-negative and gram-positive microorganisms. The bactericidal action of ciprofloxacin results from inhibition of the enzymes topoisomerase II (DNA gyrase) and topoisomerase IV, which are required for bacterial DNA replication, transcription, repair, and recombination. The mechanism of action of fluoroquinolones, including ciprofloxacin, is different from that of penicillins, cephalosporins, aminoglycosides, macrolides, and tetracyclines; therefore, microorganisms resistant to these classes of drugs may be susceptible to ciprofloxacin and other quinolones. There is no known cross-resistance between ciprofloxacin and other classes of antimicrobials. *In vitro* resistance to ciprofloxacin develops slowly by multiple step mutations.
Ciprofloxacin is slightly less active when tested at acidic pH. The inoculum size has little effect when tested *in vitro*. The minimal bactericidal concentration (MBC) generally does not exceed the minimal inhibitory concentration (MIC) by more than a factor of 2.
Ciprofloxacin has been shown to be active against most strains of the following microorganisms, both *in vitro* and in clinical infections as described in the **INDICATIONS AND USAGE** section of the package insert for CIPRO I.V. (ciprofloxacin for intravenous infusion).

Aerobic gram-positive microorganisms
Enterococcus faecalis (Many strains are only moderately susceptible.)
Staphylococcus aureus (methicillin-susceptible strains only)
Staphylococcus epidermidis (methicillin-susceptible strains only)
Staphylococcus saprophyticus
Streptococcus pneumoniae (penicillin-susceptible strains)
Streptococcus pyogenes

Aerobic gram-negative microorganisms
Citrobacter diversus
Citrobacter freundii
Enterobacter cloacae
Escherichia coli
Haemophilus influenzae
Haemophilus parainfluenzae
Klebsiella pneumoniae
Moraxella catarrhalis
Morganella morganii
Proteus mirabilis
Proteus vulgaris
Providencia rettgeri
Providencia stuartii
Pseudomonas aeruginosa
Serratia marcescens

Ciprofloxacin has been shown to be active against *Bacillus anthracis* both *in vitro* and by use of serum levels as a surrogate marker (see **INDICATIONS AND USAGE** and **INHALATIONAL ANTHRAX - ADDITIONAL INFORMATION**).

Steady-state Pharmacokinetic Parameter Following Multiple Oral and I.V. Doses

Parameters	500 mg q12h, P.O.	400 mg q12h, I.V.	750 mg q12h, P.O.	400 mg q8h, I.V.
AUC (µg•hr/mL)	13.7 [a]	12.7 [a]	31.6 [b]	32.9 [c]
C_{max} (µg/mL)	2.97	4.56	3.59	4.07

[a] AUC_{0-12h}
[b] AUC 24h=$AUC_{0-12h} \times 2$
[c] AUC 24h=$AUC_{0-8h} \times 3$

The following *in vitro* data are available, **but their clinical significance is unknown.**
Ciprofloxacin exhibits *in vitro* minimum inhibitory concentrations (MICs) of 1 µg/mL or less against most (≥ 90%) strains of the following microorganisms; however, the safety and effectiveness of ciprofloxacin intravenous formulations in treating clinical infections due to these microorganisms have not been established in adequate and well-controlled clinical trials.

Aerobic gram-positive microorganisms
Staphylococcus haemolyticus
Staphylococcus hominis
Streptococcus pneumoniae (penicillin-resistant strains)

Aerobic gram-negative microorganisms
Acinetobacter Iwoffi
Aeromonas hydrophila
Campylobacter jejuni
Edwardsiella tarda
Enterobacter aerogenes
Klebsiella oxytoca
Legionella pneumophila
Neisseria gonorrhoeae
Pasteurella multocida
Salmonella enteritidis
Salmonella typhi
Shigella boydii
Shigella dysenteriae
Shigella flexneri
Shigella sonnei
Vibrio cholerae
Vibrio parahaemolyticus
Vibrio vulnificus
Yersinia enterocolitica

Most strains of *Burkholderia cepacia* and some strains of *Stenotrophomonas maltophilia* are resistant to ciprofloxacin as are most anaerobic bacteria, including *Bacteroides fragilis* and *Clostridium difficile*.

Susceptibility Tests
Dilution Techniques: Quantitative methods are used to determine antimicrobial minimum inhibitory concentrations (MICs). These MICs provide estimates of the susceptibility of bacteria to antimicrobial compounds. The MICs should be determined using a standardized procedure. Standardized procedures are based on a dilution method[1] (broth or agar) or equivalent with standardized inoculum concentrations and standardized concentrations of ciprofloxacin powder. The MIC values should be interpreted according to the following criteria:
For testing aerobic microorganisms other than *Haemophilus influenzae*, and *Haemophilus parainfluenzae*[a]:

MIC (µg/mL)	Interpretation
≤ 1	Susceptible (S)
2	Intermediate (I)
≥ 4	Resistant (R)

[a] These interpretive standards are applicable only to broth microdilution susceptibility tests with streptococci using cation-adjusted Mueller-Hinton broth with 2–5% lysed horse blood.

For testing *Haemophilus influenzae* and *Haemophilus parainfluenzae*[b]:

MIC (µg/mL)	Interpretation
≤ 1	Susceptible (S)

[b] This interpretive standard is applicable only to broth microdilution susceptibility tests with *Haemophilus influenzae* and *Haemophilus parainfluenzae* using *Haemophilus* Test Medium[1].

The current absence of data on resistant strains precludes defining any results other than "Susceptible". Strains yielding MIC results suggestive of a "nonsusceptible" category should be submitted to a reference laboratory for further testing.
A report of "Susceptible" indicates that the pathogen is likely to be inhibited if the antimicrobial compound in the blood reaches the concentrations usually achievable. A report of "Intermediate" indicates that the result should be considered equivocal, and, if the microorganism is not fully susceptible to alternative, clinically feasible drugs, the test should be repeated. This category implies possible clinical applicability in body sites where the drug is physiologically concentrated or in situations where high dosage of drug can be used. This category also provides a buffer zone, which prevents small uncontrolled technical factors from causing major discrepancies in interpretation. A report of "Resistant" indicates that the pathogen is not likely to be inhibited if the antimicrobial compound in the blood reaches the concentrations usually achievable; other therapy should be selected.
Standardized susceptibility test procedures require the use of laboratory control microorganisms to control the technical aspects of the laboratory procedures. Standard ciprofloxacin powder should provide the following MIC values:

Organism		MIC (µg/mL)
E. faecalis	ATCC 29212	0.25 – 2.0
E. coli	ATCC 25922	0.004 – 0.015
H. influenzae[a]	ATCC 49247	0.004 – 0.03
P. aeruginosa	ATCC 27853	0.25 – 1.0
S. aureus	ATCC 29213	0.12 – 0.5

[a] This quality control range is applicable to only *H. influenzae* ATCC 49247 tested by a broth microdilution procedure using *Haemophilus* Test Medium (HTM)[1].

Diffusion Techniques: Quantitative methods that require measurement of zone diameters also provide reproducible estimates of the susceptibility of bacteria to antimicrobial compounds. One such standardized procedure[2] requires the use of standardized inoculum concentrations. This procedure uses paper disks impregnated with 5-µg ciprofloxacin to test the susceptibility of microorganisms to ciprofloxacin. Reports from the laboratory providing results of the standard single-disk susceptibility test with a 5-µg ciprofloxacin disk should be interpreted according to the following criteria:
For testing aerobic microorganisms other than *Haemophilus influenzae*, and *Haemophilus parainfluenzae*[a]:

Zone Diameter (mm)	Interpretation
≥ 21	Susceptible (S)
16 - 20	Intermediate (I)
≤ 15	Resistant (R)

[a] These zone diameter standards are applicable only to tests performed for streptococci using Mueller-Hinton agar supplemented with 5% sheep blood incubated in 5% CO_2.

For testing *Haemophilus influenzae* and *Haemophilus parainfluenzae*[b]:

Zone Diameter (mm)	Interpretation
≥ 21	Susceptible (S)

[b] This zone diameter standard is applicable only to tests with *Haemophilus influenzae* and *Haemophilus parainfluenzae* using *Haemophilus* Test Medium (HTM)[2].

The current absence of data on resistant strains precludes defining any results other than "Susceptible". Strains yielding zone diameter results suggestive of a "nonsusceptible" category should be submitted to a reference laboratory for further testing.
Interpretation should be as stated above for results using dilution techniques. Interpretation involves correlation of the diameter obtained in the disk test with the MIC for ciprofloxacin.
As with standardized dilution techniques, diffusion methods require the use of laboratory control microorganisms that are used to control the technical aspects of the laboratory procedures. For the diffusion technique, the 5-µg ciprofloxacin disk should provide the following zone diameters in these laboratory test quality control strains:

Organism		Zone Diameter (mm)
E. coli	ATCC 25922	30-40
H. influenzae[a]	ATCC 49247	34-42
P. aeruginosa	ATCC 27853	25-33
S. aureus	ATCC 25923	22-30

[a] These quality control limits are applicable to only *H. influenzae* ATCC 49247 testing using *Haemophilus* Test Medium (HTM)[2].

INDICATIONS AND USAGE

CIPRO I.V. is indicated for the treatment of infections caused by susceptible strains of the designated microorganisms in the conditions and patient populations listed below when the intravenous administration offers a route of administration advantageous to the patient. Please see **DOSAGE AND ADMINISTRATION** for specific recommendations.

Adult Patients:
Urinary Tract Infections caused by *Escherichia coli* (including cases with secondary bacteremia), *Klebsiella pneumoniae* subspecies *pneumoniae, Enterobacter cloacae, Serratia marcescens, Proteus mirabilis, Providencia rettgeri, Morganella morganii, Citrobacter diversus, Citrobacter freundii, Pseudomonas aeruginosa, Staphylococcus epidermidis, Staphylococcus saprophyticus*, or *Enterococcus faecalis*.
Lower Respiratory Infections caused by *Escherichia coli, Klebsiella pneumoniae* subspecies *pneumoniae, Enterobacter cloacae, Proteus mirabilis, Pseudomonas aeruginosa, Haemophilus influenzae, Haemophilus parainfluenzae*, or *Streptococcus pneumoniae*. Also, *Moraxella catarrhalis* for the treatment of acute exacerbations of chronic bronchitis.

NOTE: Although effective in clinical trials, ciprofloxacin is not a drug of first choice in the treatment of presumed or confirmed pneumonia secondary to *Streptococcus pneumoniae*.

Nosocomial Pneumonia caused by *Haemophilus influenzae* or *Klebsiella pneumoniae*.

Skin and Skin Structure Infections caused by *Escherichia coli, Klebsiella pneumoniae* subspecies *pneumoniae, Enterobacter cloacae, Proteus mirabilis, Proteus vulgaris, Providencia stuartii, Morganella morganii, Citrobacter freundii, Pseudomonas aeruginosa, Staphylococcus aureus* (methicillin susceptible), *Staphylococcus epidermidis,* or *Streptococcus pyogenes*.

Bone and Joint Infections caused by *Enterobacter cloacae, Serratia marcescens,* or *Pseudomonas aeruginosa*.

Complicated Intra-Abdominal Infections (used in conjunction with metronidazole) caused by *Escherichia coli, Pseudomonas aeruginosa, Proteus mirabilis, Klebsiella pneumoniae,* or *Bacteroides fragilis*.

Acute Sinusitis caused by *Haemophilus influenzae, Streptococcus pneumoniae,* or *Moraxella catarrhalis*.

Chronic Bacterial Prostatitis caused by *Escherichia coli* or *Proteus mirabilis*.

Empirical Therapy for Febrile Neutropenic Patients in combination with piperacillin sodium. (See **CLINICAL STUDIES.**)

Pediatric patients (1 to 17 years of age):

Complicated Urinary Tract Infections and Pyelonephritis due to *Escherichia coli*.

NOTE: Although effective in clinical trials, ciprofloxacin is not a drug of first choice in the pediatric population due to an increased incidence of adverse events compared to controls, including events related to joints and/or surrounding tissues. (See **WARNINGS, PRECAUTIONS, Pediatric Use, ADVERSE REACTIONS** and **CLINICAL STUDIES**.) Ciprofloxacin, like other fluoroquinolones, is associated with arthropathy and histopathological changes in weight-bearing joints of juvenile animals. (See **ANIMAL PHARMACOLOGY**.)

Adult and Pediatric Patients:

Inhalational anthrax (post-exposure): To reduce the incidence or progression of disease following exposure to aerosolized *Bacillus anthracis*.

Ciprofloxacin serum concentrations achieved in humans serve as a surrogate endpoint reasonably likely to predict clinical benefit and provide the basis for this indication.[4] (See also, **INHALATIONAL ANTHRAX – ADDITIONAL INFORMATION**).

If anaerobic organisms are suspected of contributing to the infection, appropriate therapy should be administered.

Appropriate culture and susceptibility tests should be performed before treatment in order to isolate and identify organisms causing infection and to determine their susceptibility to ciprofloxacin. Therapy with CIPRO I.V. may be initiated before results of these tests are known; once results become available, appropriate therapy should be continued.

As with other drugs, some strains of *Pseudomonas aeruginosa* may develop resistance fairly rapidly during treatment with ciprofloxacin. Culture and susceptibility testing performed periodically during therapy will provide information not only on the therapeutic effect of the antimicrobial agent but also on the possible emergence of bacterial resistance.

To reduce the development of drug-resistant bacteria and maintain the effectiveness of CIPRO I.V. and other antibacterial drugs, CIPRO I.V. should be used only to treat or prevent infections that are proven or strongly suspected to be caused by susceptible bacteria. When culture and susceptibility information are available, they should be considered in selecting or modifying antibacterial therapy. In the absence of such data, local epidemiology and susceptibility patterns may contribute to the empiric selection of therapy.

CONTRAINDICATIONS

CIPRO I.V. (ciprofloxacin) is contraindicated in persons with history of hypersensitivity to ciprofloxacin or any member of the quinolone class of antimicrobial agents.

WARNINGS

Pregnant Women: THE SAFETY AND EFFECTIVENESS OF CIPROFLOXACIN IN PREGNANT AND LACTATING WOMEN HAVE NOT BEEN ESTABLISHED. (See **PRECAUTIONS: Pregnancy,** and **Nursing Mothers** subsections.)

Pediatrics: Ciprofloxacin should be used in pediatric patients (less than 18 years of age) only for infections listed in the **INDICATIONS AND USAGE** section. An increased incidence of adverse events compared to controls, including events related to joints and/or surrounding tissues, has been observed. (See **ADVERSE REACTIONS**.)

In pre-clinical studies, oral administration of ciprofloxacin caused lameness in immature dogs. Histopathological examination of the weight-bearing joints of these dogs revealed permanent lesions of the cartilage. Related quinolone-class drugs also produce erosions of cartilage of weight-bearing joints and other signs of arthropathy in immature animals of various species. (See **ANIMAL PHARMACOLOGY**.)

Central Nervous System Disorders: Convulsions, increased intracranial pressure and toxic psychosis have been reported in patients receiving quinolones, including ciprofloxacin. Ciprofloxacin may also cause central nervous system (CNS) events including: dizziness, confusion, tremors, hallucinations, depression, and, rarely, suicidal thoughts or acts. These reactions may occur following the first dose. If these reactions occur in patients receiving ciprofloxacin, the drug should be discontinued and appropriate measures instituted. As with all quinolones, ciprofloxacin should be used with caution in patients with known or suspected CNS disorders that may predispose to seizures or lower the seizure threshold (e.g. severe cerebral arteriosclerosis, epilepsy), or in the presence of other risk factors that may predispose to seizures or lower the seizure threshold (e.g. certain drug therapy, renal dysfunction). (See **PRECAUTIONS: General, Information for Patients, Drug Interaction** and **ADVERSE REACTIONS**.)

Theophylline: SERIOUS AND FATAL REACTIONS HAVE BEEN REPORTED IN PATIENTS RECEIVING CONCURRENT ADMINISTRATION OF INTRAVENOUS CIPROFLOXACIN AND THEOPHYLLINE. These reactions have included cardiac arrest, seizure, status epilepticus, and respiratory failure. Although similar serious adverse events have been reported in patients receiving theophylline alone, the possibility that these reactions may be potentiated by ciprofloxacin cannot be eliminated. If concomitant use cannot be avoided, serum levels of theophylline should be monitored and dosage adjustments made as appropriate.

Hypersensitivity Reactions: Serious and occasionally fatal hypersensitivity (anaphylactic) reactions, some following the first dose, have been reported in patients receiving quinolone therapy. Some reactions were accompanied by cardiovascular collapse, loss of consciousness, tingling, pharyngeal or facial edema, dyspnea, urticaria, and itching. Only a few patients had a history of hypersensitivity reactions. Serious anaphylactic reactions require immediate emergency treatment with epinephrine and other resuscitation measures, including oxygen, intravenous fluids, intravenous antihistamines, corticosteroids, pressor amines, and airway management, as clinically indicated.

Severe hypersensitivity reactions characterized by rash, fever, eosinophilia, jaundice, and hepatic necrosis with fatal outcome have also been reported extremely rarely in patients receiving ciprofloxacin along with other drugs. The possibility that these reactions were related to ciprofloxacin cannot be excluded. Ciprofloxacin should be discontinued at the first appearance of a skin rash or any other sign of hypersensitivity.

Pseudomembranous Colitis: Pseudomembranous colitis has been reported with nearly all antibacterial agents, including ciprofloxacin, and may range in severity from mild to life-threatening. Therefore, it is important to consider this diagnosis in patients who present with diarrhea subsequent to the administration of antibacterial agents.

Treatment with antibacterial agents alters the normal flora of the colon and may permit overgrowth of clostridia. Studies indicate that a toxin produced by *Clostridium difficile* is one primary cause of "antibiotic-associated colitis."

After the diagnosis of pseudomembranous colitis has been established, therapeutic measures should be initiated. Mild cases of pseudomembranous colitis usually respond to drug discontinuation alone. In moderate to severe cases, consideration should be given to management with fluids and electrolytes, protein supplementation, and treatment with an antibacterial drug clinically effective against *C. difficile* colitis. Drugs that inhibit peristalsis should be avoided.

Peripheral neuropathy: Rare cases of sensory or sensorimotor axonal polyneuropathy affecting small and/or large axons resulting in paresthesias, hypoesthesias, dysesthesias and weakness have been reported in patients receiving quinolones, including ciprofloxacin. Ciprofloxacin should be discontinued if the patient experiences symptoms of neuropathy including pain, burning, tingling, numbness, and/or weakness, or is found to have deficits in light touch, pain, temperature, position sense, vibratory sensation, and/or motor strength in order to prevent the development of an irreversible condition.

Tendon Effects: Ruptures of the shoulder, hand, Achilles tendon or other tendons that required surgical repair or resulted in prolonged disability have been reported in patients receiving quinolones, including ciprofloxacin. Post-marketing surveillance reports indicate that this risk may be increased in patients receiving concomitant corticosteroids, especially the elderly. Ciprofloxacin should be discontinued if the patient experiences pain, inflammation, or rupture of a tendon. Patients should rest and refrain from exercise until the diagnosis of tendonitis or tendon rupture has been excluded. Tendon rupture can occur during or after therapy with quinolones, including ciprofloxacin.

PRECAUTIONS

General: INTRAVENOUS CIPROFLOXACIN SHOULD BE ADMINISTERED BY SLOW INFUSION OVER A PERIOD OF 60 MINUTES. Local I.V. site reactions have been reported with the intravenous administration of ciprofloxacin. These reactions are more frequent if infusion time is 30 minutes or less or if small veins of the hand are used. (See **ADVERSE REACTIONS**.)

Central Nervous System: Quinolones, including ciprofloxacin, may also cause central nervous system (CNS) events, including: nervousness, agitation, insomnia, anxiety, nightmares or paranoia. (See **WARNINGS, Information for Patients,** and **Drug Interactions**.)

Crystals of ciprofloxacin have been observed rarely in the urine of human subjects but more frequently in the urine of laboratory animals, which is usually alkaline. (See **ANIMAL PHARMACOLOGY**.) Crystalluria related to ciprofloxacin has been reported only rarely in humans because human urine is usually acidic. Alkalinity of the urine should be avoided in patients receiving ciprofloxacin. Patients should be well hydrated to prevent the formation of highly concentrated urine.

Renal Impairment: Alteration of the dosage regimen is necessary for patients with impairment of renal function. (See **DOSAGE AND ADMINISTRATION**.)

Phototoxicity: Moderate to severe phototoxicity manifested as an exaggerated sunburn reaction has been observed in some patients who were exposed to direct sunlight while receiving some members of the quinolone class of drugs. Excessive sunlight should be avoided.

As with any potent drug, periodic assessment of organ system functions, including renal, hepatic, and hematopoietic, is advisable during prolonged therapy.

Prescribing CIPRO I.V. in the absence of a proven or strongly suspected bacterial infection or a prophylactic indication is unlikely to provide benefit to the patient and increases the risk of the development of drug-resistant bacteria.

Information For Patients:

Patients should be advised:

- that antibacterial drugs including CIPRO I.V. should only be used to treat bacterial infections. They do not treat viral infections (e.g., the common cold). When CIPRO I.V. is prescribed to treat a bacterial infection, patients should be told that although it is common to feel better early in the course of therapy, the medication should be taken exactly as directed. Skipping doses or not completing the full course of therapy may (1) decrease the effectiveness of the immediate treatment and (2) increase the likelihood that bacteria will develop resistance and will not be treatable by CIPRO I.V. or other antibacterial drugs in the future.
- that ciprofloxacin may be associated with hypersensitivity reactions, even following a single dose, and to discontinue the drug at the first sign of a skin rash or other allergic reaction.
- that ciprofloxacin may cause dizziness and lightheadedness; therefore, patients should know how they react to this drug before they operate an automobile or machinery or engage in activities requiring mental alertness or coordination.
- that ciprofloxacin may increase the effects of theophylline and caffeine. There is a possibility of caffeine accumulation when products containing caffeine are consumed while taking ciprofloxacin.
- that peripheral neuropathies have been associated with ciprofloxacin use. If symptoms of peripheral neuropathy including pain, burning, tingling, numbness and/or weakness develop, they should discontinue treatment and contact their physicians.
- to discontinue treatment; rest and refrain from exercise; and inform their physician if they experience pain, inflammation, or rupture of a tendon.
- that convulsions have been reported in patients taking quinolones, including ciprofloxacin, and to notify their physician before taking this drug if there is a history of this condition.
- that ciprofloxacin has been associated with an increased rate of adverse events involving joints and surrounding tissue structures (like tendons) in pediatric patients (less than 18 years of age). Parents should inform their child's physician if the child has a history of joint-related problems before taking this drug. Parents of pediatric patients should also notify their child's physician of any joint-related problems that occur during or following ciprofloxacin therapy. (See **WARNINGS, PRECAUTIONS, Pediatric Use** and **ADVERSE REACTIONS**.)

Drug Interactions: As with some other quinolones, concurrent administration of ciprofloxacin with theophylline may lead to elevated serum concentrations of theophylline and prolongation of its elimination half-life. This may result in increased risk of theophylline-related adverse reactions. (See **WARNINGS**.) If concomitant use cannot be avoided, serum levels of theophylline should be monitored and dosage adjustments made as appropriate.

Some quinolones, including ciprofloxacin, have also been shown to interfere with the metabolism of caffeine. This may lead to reduced clearance of caffeine and prolongation of its serum half-life.

Some quinolones, including ciprofloxacin, have been associated with transient elevations in serum creatinine in patients receiving cyclosporine concomitantly.

Altered serum levels of phenytoin (increased and decreased) have been reported in patients receiving concomitant ciprofloxacin.

The concomitant administration of ciprofloxacin with the sulfonylurea glyburide has, in some patients, resulted in severe hypoglycemia. Fatalities have been reported.

The serum concentrations of ciprofloxacin and metronidazole were not altered when these two drugs were given concomitantly.

Quinolones, including ciprofloxacin, have been reported to enhance the effects of the oral anticoagulant warfarin or its derivatives. When these products are administered concomitantly, prothrombin time or other suitable coagulation tests should be closely monitored.

Probenecid interferes with renal tubular secretion of ciprofloxacin and produces an increase in the level of ciprofloxacin in the serum. This should be considered if patients are receiving both drugs concomitantly.

Renal tubular transport of methotrexate may be inhibited by concomitant administration of ciprofloxacin potentially leading to increased plasma levels of methotrexate. This

Continued on next page

Cipro I.V. Bulk—Cont.

might increase the risk of methotrexate associated toxic reactions. Therefore, patients under methotrexate therapy should be carefully monitored when concomitant ciprofloxacin therapy is indicated.
Non-steroidal anti-inflammatory drugs (but not acetyl salicylic acid) in combination of very high doses of quinolones have been shown to provoke convulsions in pre-clinical studies.
Following infusion of 400 mg I.V. ciprofloxacin every eight hours in combination with 50 mg/kg I.V. piperacillin sodium every four hours, mean serum ciprofloxacin concentrations were 3.02 μg/mL ½ hour and 1.18 μg/mL between 6–8 hours after the end of infusion.

Carcinogenesis, Mutagenesis, Impairment of Fertility: Eight *in vitro* mutagenicity tests have been conducted with ciprofloxacin. Test results are listed below:

- Salmonella/Microsome Test (Negative)
- *E. coli* DNA Repair Assay (Negative)
- Mouse Lymphoma Cell Forward Mutation Assay (Positive)
- Chinese Hamster V_{79} Cell HGPRT Test (Negative)
- Syrian Hamster Embryo Cell Transformation Assay (Negative)
- *Saccharomyces cerevisiae* Point Mutation Assay (Negative)
- *Saccharomyces cerevisiae* Mitotic Crossover and Gene Conversion Assay (Negative)
- Rat Hepatocyte DNA Repair Assay (Positive)

Thus, two of the eight tests were positive, but results of the following three *in vivo* test systems gave negative results:

- Rat Hepatocyte DNA Repair Assay
- Micronucleus Test (Mice)
- Dominant Lethal Test (Mice)

Long-term carcinogenicity studies in rats and mice resulted in no carcinogenic or tumorigenic effects due to ciprofloxacin at daily oral dose levels up to 250 and 750 mg/kg to rats and mice, respectively (approximately 1.7- and 2.5- times the highest recommended therapeutic dose based upon mg/m^2).
Results from photo co-carcinogenicity testing indicate that ciprofloxacin does not reduce the time to appearance of UV-induced skin tumors as compared to vehicle control. Hairless (Skh-1) mice were exposed to UVA light for 3.5 hours five times every two weeks for up to 78 weeks while concurrently being administered ciprofloxacin. The time to development of the first skin tumors was 50 weeks in mice treated concomitantly with UVA and ciprofloxacin (mouse dose approximately equal to maximum recommended human dose based upon mg/m^2), as opposed to 34 weeks when animals were treated with both UVA and vehicle. The times to development of skin tumors ranged from 16–32 weeks in mice treated concomitantly with UVA and other quinolones.[3]
In this model, mice treated with ciprofloxacin alone did not develop skin or systemic tumors. There are no data from similar models using pigmented mice and/or fully haired mice. The clinical significance of these findings to humans is unknown.
Fertility studies performed in rats at oral doses of ciprofloxacin up to 100 mg/kg (approximately 0.7-times the highest recommended therapeutic dose based upon mg/m^2) revealed no evidence of impairment.

Pregnancy: Teratogenic Effects. Pregnancy Category C: There are no adequate and well-controlled studies in pregnant women. An expert review of published data on experiences with ciprofloxacin use during pregnancy by TERIS – the Teratogen Information System - concluded that therapeutic doses during pregnancy are unlikely to pose a substantial teratogenic risk (quantity and quality of data=fair), but the data are insufficient to state that there is no risk.[7]
A controlled prospective observational study followed 200 women exposed to fluoroquinolones (52.5% exposed to ciprofloxacin and 68% first trimester exposures) during gestation.[8] In utero exposure to fluoroquinolones during embryogenesis was not associated with increased risk of major malformations. The reported rates of major congenital malformations were 2.2% for the fluoroquinolone group and 2.6% for the control group (background incidence of major malformations is 1-5%). Rates of spontaneous abortions, prematurity and low birth weight did not differ between the groups and there were no clinically significant musculoskeletal dysfunctions up to one year of age in the ciprofloxacin exposed children.
Another prospective follow-up study reported on 549 pregnancies with fluoroquinolone exposure (93% first trimester exposures).[9] There were 70 ciprofloxacin exposures, all within the first trimester. The malformation rates among live-born babies exposed to ciprofloxacin and to fluoroquinolones overall were both within background incidence ranges. No specific patterns of congenital abnormalities were found. The study did not reveal any clear adverse reactions due to in utero exposure to ciprofloxacin.
No differences in the rates of prematurity, spontaneous abortions, or birth weight were seen in women exposed to ciprofloxacin during pregnancy.[7,8] However, these small postmarketing epidemiology studies, of which most experience is from short term, first trimester exposure, are insufficient to evaluate the risk for less common defects or to permit reliable and definitive conclusions regarding the safety of ciprofloxacin in pregnant women and their developing fetuses. Ciprofloxacin should not be used during pregnancy unless the potential benefit justifies the potential risk to both fetus and mother (see **WARNINGS**).
Reproduction studies have been performed in rats and mice using oral doses up to 100 mg/kg (0.6 and 0.3 times the maximum daily human dose based upon body surface area, respectively) and have revealed no evidence of harm to the fetus due to ciprofloxacin. In rabbits, oral ciprofloxacin dose levels of 30 and 100 mg/kg (approximately 0.4- and 1.3-times the highest recommended therapeutic dose based upon mg/m^2) produced gastrointestinal toxicity resulting in maternal weight loss and an increased incidence of abortion, but no teratogenicity was observed at either dose level. After intravenous administration of doses up to 20 mg/kg (approximately 0.3-times the highest recommended therapeutic dose based upon mg/m^2) no maternal toxicity was produced and no embryotoxicity or teratogenicity was observed. (See **WARNINGS.**)

Nursing Mothers: Ciprofloxacin is excreted in human milk. The amount of ciprofloxacin absorbed by the nursing infant is unknown. Because of the potential for serious adverse reactions in infants nursing from mothers taking ciprofloxacin, a decision should be made whether to discontinue nursing or to discontinue the drug, taking into account the importance of the drug to the mother.

Pediatric Use: Ciprofloxacin, like other quinolones, causes arthropathy and histological changes in weight-bearing joints of juvenile animals resulting in lameness. (See **ANIMAL PHARMACOLOGY.**)

Inhalational Anthrax (Post-Exposure)
Ciprofloxacin is indicated in pediatric patients for inhalational anthrax (post-exposure). The risk-benefit assessment indicates that administration of ciprofloxacin to pediatric patients is appropriate. For information regarding pediatric dosing in inhalational anthrax (post-exposure), see **DOSAGE AND ADMINISTRATION** and **INHALATIONAL ANTHRAX – ADDITIONAL INFORMATION.**

Complicated Urinary Tract Infection and Pyelonephritis
Ciprofloxacin is indicated for the treatment of complicated urinary tract infections and pyelonephritis due to *Escherichia coli*. Although effective in clinical trials, ciprofloxacin is not a drug of first choice in the pediatric population due to an increased incidence of adverse events compared to the controls, including those related to joints and/or surrounding tissues. The rates of these events in pediatric patients with complicated urinary tract infection and pyelonephritis within six weeks of follow-up were 9.3% (31/335) versus 6.0% (21/349) for control agents. The rates of these events occurring at any time up to the one year follow-up were 13.7% (46/335) and 9.5% (33/349), respectively. The rate of all adverse events regardless of drug relationship at six weeks was 41% (138/335) in the ciprofloxacin arm compared to 31% (109/349) in the control arm. (See **ADVERSE REACTIONS** and **CLINICAL STUDIES.**)

Cystic Fibrosis
Short-term safety data from a single trial in pediatric cystic fibrosis patients are available. In a randomized, double-blind clinical trial for the treatment of acute pulmonary exacerbations in cystic fibrosis patients (ages 5-17 years), 67 patients received ciprofloxacin I.V. 10 mg/kg/dose q8h for one week followed by ciprofloxacin tablets 20 mg/kg/dose q12h to complete 10-21 days treatment and 62 patients received the combination of ceftazidime I.V. 50 mg/kg/dose q8h and tobramycin I.V. 3 mg/kg/dose q8h for a total of 10-21 days. Patients less than 5 years of age were not studied. Safety monitoring in the study included periodic range of motion examinations and gait assessments by treatment-blinded examiners. Patients were followed for an average of 23 days after completing treatment (range 0-93 days). This study was not designed to determine long term effects and the safety of repeated exposure to ciprofloxacin.
Musculoskeletal adverse events in patients with cystic fibrosis were reported in 22% of the patients in the ciprofloxacin group and 21% in the comparison group. Decreased range of motion was reported in 12% of the subjects in the ciprofloxacin group and 16% in the comparison group. Arthralgia was reported in 10% of the patients in the ciprofloxacin group and 11% in the comparison group. Other adverse events were similar in nature and frequency between treatment arms. One of sixty-seven patients developed arthritis of the knee nine days after a ten day course of treatment with ciprofloxacin. Clinical symptoms resolved, but an MRI showed knee effusion without other abnormalities eight months after treatment. However, the relationship of this event to the patient's course of ciprofloxacin can not be definitively determined, particularly since patients with cystic fibrosis may develop arthralgias/arthritis as part of their underlying disease process.

Geriatric Use: In a retrospective analysis of 23 multiple-dose controlled clinical trials of ciprofloxacin encompassing over 3500 ciprofloxacin treated patients, 25% of patients were greater than or equal to 65 years of age and 10% were greater than or equal to 75 years of age. No overall differences in safety or effectiveness were observed between these subjects and younger subjects, and other reported clinical experience has not identified differences in responses between the elderly and younger patients, but greater sensitivity of some older individuals on any drug therapy cannot be ruled out. Ciprofloxacin is known to be substantially excreted by the kidney, and the risk of adverse reactions may be greater in patients with impaired renal function. No alteration of dosage is necessary for patients greater than 65 years of age with normal renal function. However, since some older individuals experience reduced renal function by virtue of their advanced age, care should be taken in dose selection for elderly patients, and renal function monitoring may be useful in these patients. (See **CLINICAL PHARMACOLOGY** and **DOSAGE AND ADMINISTRATION.**)

ADVERSE REACTIONS

Adverse Reactions in Adult Patients: During clinical investigations with oral and parenteral ciprofloxacin, 49,038 patients received courses of the drug. Most of the adverse events reported were described as only mild or moderate in severity, abated soon after the drug was discontinued, and required no treatment. Ciprofloxacin was discontinued because of an adverse event in 1.8% of intravenously treated patients.
The most frequently reported drug related events, from clinical trials of all formulations, all dosages, all drug-therapy durations, and for all indications of ciprofloxacin therapy were nausea (2.5%), diarrhea (1.6%), liver function tests abnormal (1.3%), vomiting (1.0%), and rash (1.0%).
In clinical trials the following events were reported, regardless of drug relationship, in greater than 1% of patients treated with intravenous ciprofloxacin: nausea, diarrhea, central nervous system disturbance, local I.V. site reactions, liver function tests abnormal, eosinophilia, headache, restlessness, and rash. Many of these events were described as only mild or moderate in severity, abated soon after the drug was discontinued, and required no treatment. Local I.V. site reactions are more frequent if the infusion time is 30 minutes or less. These may appear as local skin reactions which resolve rapidly upon completion of the infusion. Subsequent intravenous administration is not contraindicated unless the reactions recur or worsen.
Additional medically important events, without regard to drug relationship or route of administration, that occurred in 1% or less of ciprofloxacin patients are listed below:
BODY AS A WHOLE: abdominal pain/discomfort, foot pain, pain, pain in extremities
CARDIOVASCULAR: cardiovascular collapse, cardiopulmonary arrest, myocardial infarction, arrhythmia, tachycardia, palpitation, cerebral thrombosis, syncope, cardiac murmur, hypertension, hypotension, angina pectoris, atrial flutter, ventricular ectopy, (thrombo)-phlebitis, vasodilation, migraine
CENTRAL NERVOUS SYSTEM: convulsive seizures, paranoia, toxic psychosis, depression, dysphasia, phobia, depersonalization, manic reaction, unresponsiveness, ataxia, confusion, hallucinations, dizziness, lightheadedness, paresthesia, anxiety, tremor, insomnia, nightmares, weakness, drowsiness, irritability, malaise, lethargy, abnormal gait, grand mal convulsion, anorexia
GASTROINTESTINAL: ileus, jaundice, gastrointestinal bleeding, *C. difficile* associated diarrhea, pseudomembranous colitis, pancreatitis, hepatic necrosis, intestinal perforation, dyspepsia, epigastric pain, constipation, oral ulceration, oral candidiasis, mouth dryness, anorexia, dysphagia, flatulence, hepatitis, painful oral mucosa
HEMIC/LYMPHATIC: agranulocytosis, prolongation of prothrombin time, lymphadenopathy, petechia
METABOLIC/NUTRITIONAL: amylase increase, lipase increase
MUSCULOSKELETAL: arthralgia, jaw, arm or back pain, joint stiffness, neck and chest pain, achiness, flare up of gout, myasthenia gravis
RENAL/UROGENITAL: renal failure, interstitial nephritis, nephritis, hemorrhagic cystitis, renal calculi, frequent urination, acidosis, urethral bleeding, polyuria, urinary retention, gynecomastia, candiduria, vaginitis, breast pain. Crystalluria, cylindruria, hematuria and albuminuria have also been reported.
RESPIRATORY: respiratory arrest, pulmonary embolism, dyspnea, laryngeal or pulmonary edema, respiratory distress, pleural effusion, hemoptysis, epistaxis, hiccough, bronchospasm
SKIN/HYPERSENSITIVITY: allergic reactions, anaphylactic reactions, erythema multiforme/Stevens-Johnson syndrome, exfoliative dermatitis, toxic epidermal necrolysis, vasculitis, angioedema, edema of the lips, face, neck, conjunctivae, hands or lower extremities, purpura, fever, chills, flushing, pruritus, urticaria, cutaneous candidiasis, vesicles, increased perspiration, hyperpigmentation, erythema nodosum, thrombophlebitis, burning, paresthesia, erythema, swelling, photosensitivity (See **WARNINGS.**)
SPECIAL SENSES: decreased visual acuity, blurred vision, disturbed vision (flashing lights, change in color perception, overbrightness of lights, diplopia), eye pain, anosmia, hearing loss, tinnitus, nystagmus, chromatopsia, a bad taste
In several instances, nausea, vomiting, tremor, irritability, or palpitation were judged by investigators to be related to elevated serum levels of theophylline possibly as a result of drug interaction with ciprofloxacin.
In randomized, double-blind controlled clinical trials comparing ciprofloxacin (I.V. and I.V./P.O. sequential) with intravenous beta-lactam control antibiotics, the CNS adverse event profile of ciprofloxacin was comparable to that of the control drugs.

Adverse Reactions in Pediatric Patients: Ciprofloxacin, administered I.V. and/or orally, was compared to a cephalosporin for treatment of complicated urinary tract infections (cUTI) or pyelonephritis in pediatric patients 1 to 17 years of age (mean age of 6 ± 4 years). The trial was conducted in the US, Canada, Argentina, Peru, Costa Rica, Mexico, South Africa, and Germany. The duration of therapy was 10 to 21 days (mean duration of treatment was 11 days with a range of 1 to 88 days). The primary objective of the study was to assess musculoskeletal and neurological safety within 6 weeks of therapy and through one year of follow-up in the 335 ciprofloxacin- and 349 comparator-treated patients enrolled.

An Independent Pediatric Safety Committee (IPSC) reviewed all cases of musculoskeletal adverse events as well as all patients with an abnormal gait or abnormal joint exam (baseline or treatment-emergent). These events were evaluated in a comprehensive fashion and included such conditions as arthralgia, abnormal gait, abnormal joint exam, joint sprains, leg pain, back pain, arthrosis, bone pain, pain, myalgia, arm pain, and decreased range of motion in a joint. The affected joints included: knee, elbow, ankle, hip, wrist, and shoulder. Within 6 weeks of treatment initiation, the rates of these events were 9.3% (31/335) in the ciprofloxacin-treated group versus 6.0 % (21/349) in comparator-treated patients. The majority of these events were mild or moderate in intensity. All musculoskeletal events occurring by 6 weeks resolved (clinical resolution of signs and symptoms), usually within 30 days of end of treatment. Radiological evaluations were not routinely used to confirm resolution of the events. The events occurred more frequently in ciprofloxacin-treated patients than control patients, regardless of whether they received I.V. or oral therapy. Ciprofloxacin-treated patients were more likely to report more than one event and on more than one occasion compared to control patients. These events occurred in all age groups and the rates were consistently higher in the ciprofloxacin group compared to the control group. At the end of 1 year, the rate of these events reported at any time during that period was 13.7% (46/335) in the ciprofloxacin-treated group versus 9.5% (33/349) comparator-treated patients.

An adolescent female discontinued ciprofloxacin for wrist pain that developed during treatment. An MRI performed 4 weeks later showed a tear in the right ulnar fibrocartilage. A diagnosis of overuse syndrome secondary to sports activity was made, but a contribution from ciprofloxacin cannot be excluded. The patient recovered by 4 months without surgical intervention.

Findings Involving Joint or Peri-articular Tissues as Assessed by the IPSC

	Ciprofloxacin	Comparator
All Patients (within 6 weeks)	31/335 (9.3%)	21/349 (6.0%)
95% Confidence Interval*	(-0.8%, +7.2%)	
Age Group		
≥ 12 months < 24 months	1/36 (2.8%)	0/41
≥ 2 years < 6 years	5/124 (4.0%)	3/118 (2.5%)
≥ 6 years < 12 years	18/143 (12.6%)	12/153 (7.8%)
≥ 12 years to 17 years	7/32 (21.9%)	6/37 (16.2 %)
All Patients (within 1 year)	46/335 (13.7%)	33/349 (9.5%)
95% Confidence Interval*	(-0.6%, +9.1%)	

*The study was designed to demonstrate that the arthropathy rate for the ciprofloxacin group did not exceed that of the control group by more than + 6%. At both the 6 week and 1 year evaluations, the 95% confidence interval indicated that it could not be concluded that the ciprofloxacin group had findings comparable to the control group.

The incidence rates of neurological events within 6 weeks of treatment initiation were 3% (9/335) in the ciprofloxacin group versus 2% (7/349) in the comparator group and included dizziness, nervousness, insomnia, and somnolence.

In this trial, the overall incidence rates of adverse events regardless of relationship to study drug and within 6 weeks of treatment initiation were 41% (138/335) in the ciprofloxacin group versus 31% (109/349) in the comparator group. The most frequent events were gastrointestinal: 15% (50/335) of ciprofloxacin patients compared to 9% (31/349) of comparator patients. Serious adverse events were seen in 7.5% (25/335) of ciprofloxacin-treated patients compared to 5.7% (20/349) of control patients. Discontinuation of drug due to an adverse event was observed in 3% (10/335) of ciprofloxacin-treated patients versus 1.4% (5/349) of comparator patients. Other adverse events that occurred in at least 1% of ciprofloxacin patients were diarrhea 4.8%, vomiting 4.8%, abdominal pain 3.3%, accidental injury 3.0%, rhinitis 3.0%, dyspepsia 2.7%, nausea 2.7%, fever 2.1%, asthma 1.8% and rash 1.8%.

In addition to the events reported in pediatric patients in clinical trials, it should be expected that events reported in adults during clinical trials or post-marketing experience may also occur in pediatric patients.

Post-Marketing Adverse Events: The following adverse events have been reported from worldwide marketing experience with quinolones, including ciprofloxacin. Because these events are reported voluntarily from a population of uncertain size, it is not always possible to reliably estimate their frequency or establish a causal relationship to drug exposure. Decisions to include these events in labeling are typically based on one or more of the following factors: (1) seriousness of the event, (2) frequency of the reporting, or (3) strength of causal connection to the drug.

Agitation, agranulocytosis, albuminuria, anosmia, candiduria, cholesterol elevation (serum), confusion, constipation, delirium, dyspepsia, dysphagia, erythema multiforme, exfoliative dermatitis, fixed eruption, flatulence, glucose elevation (blood), hemolytic anemia, hepatic failure, hepatic necrosis, hyperesthesia, hypertonia, hypesthesia, hypotension (postural), jaundice, marrow depression (life threatening), methemoglobinemia, moniliasis (oral, gastrointestinal, vaginal), myalgia, myasthenia, myasthenia gravis (possible exacerbation), myoclonus, nystagmus, pancreatitis, pancytopenia (life threatening or fatal outcome), peripheral neuropathy, phenytoin alteration (serum), potassium elevation (serum), prothrombin time prolongation or decrease, pseudomembranous colitis (The onset of pseudomembranous colitis symptoms may occur during or after antimicrobial treatment.), psychosis (toxic), renal calculi, serum sickness like reaction, Stevens-Johnson syndrome, taste loss, tendinitis, tendon rupture, torsade de pointes, toxic epidermal necrolysis, triglyceride elevation (serum), twitching, vaginal candidiasis, and vasculitis. (See **PRECAUTIONS**.)

Adverse Laboratory Changes: The most frequently reported changes in laboratory parameters with intravenous ciprofloxacin therapy, without regard to drug relationship are listed below:

Hepatic	—	elevations of AST (SGOT), ALT (SGPT), alkaline phosphatase, LDH, and serum bilirubin
Hematologic	—	elevated eosinophil and platelet counts, decreased platelet counts, hemoglobin and/or hematocrit
Renal	—	elevations of serum creatinine, BUN, and uric acid
Other	—	elevations of serum creatine phosphokinase, serum theophylline (in patients receiving theophylline concomitantly), blood glucose, and triglycerides

Other changes occurring infrequently were: decreased leukocyte count, elevated atypical lymphocyte count, immature WBCs, elevated serum calcium, elevation of serum gamma-glutamyl transpeptidase (γ GT), decreased BUN, decreased uric acid, decreased total serum protein, decreased serum albumin, decreased serum potassium, elevated serum potassium, elevated serum cholesterol. Other changes occurring rarely during administration of ciprofloxacin were: elevation of serum amylase, decrease of blood glucose, pancytopenia, leukocytosis, elevated sedimentation rate, change in serum phenytoin, decreased prothrombin time, hemolytic anemia, and bleeding diathesis.

OVERDOSAGE

In the event of acute overdosage, the patient should be carefully observed and given supportive treatment. Adequate hydration must be maintained. Only a small amount of ciprofloxacin (< 10%) is removed from the body after hemodialysis or peritoneal dialysis.

In mice, rats, rabbits and dogs, significant toxicity including tonic/clonic convulsions was observed at intravenous doses of ciprofloxacin between 125 and 300 mg/kg.

DOSAGE AND ADMINISTRATION - ADULTS

CIPRO I.V. should be administered to adults by intravenous infusion over a period of 60 minutes at dosages described in the Dosage Guidelines table. Slow infusion of a dilute solution into a larger vein will minimize patient discomfort and reduce the risk of venous irritation. (See **Preparation of CIPRO I.V. for Administration** section.)

The determination of dosage for any particular patient must take into consideration the severity and nature of the infection, the susceptibility of the causative microorganism, the integrity of the patient's host-defense mechanisms, and the status of renal and hepatic function.

[See table above]

CIPRO I.V. should be administered by intravenous infusion over a period of 60 minutes.

ADULT DOSAGE GUIDELINES

Infection†	Severity	Dose	Frequency	Usual Duration
Urinary Tract	Mild/Moderate	200 mg	q12h	7-14 Days
	Severe/Complicated	400 mg	q12h	7-14 Days
Lower Respiratory Tract	Mild/Moderate	400 mg	q12h	7-14 Days
	Severe/Complicated	400 mg	q8h	7-14 Days
Nosocomial Pneumonia	Mild/Moderate/Severe	400 mg	q8h	10-14 Days
Skin and Skin Structure	Mild/Moderate	400 mg	q12h	7-14 Days
	Severe/Complicated	400 mg	q8h	7-14 Days
Bone and Joint	Mild/Moderate	400 mg	q12h	≥ 4-6 Weeks
	Severe/Complicated	400 mg	q8h	≥ 4-6 Weeks
Intra-Abdominal*	Complicated	400 mg	q12h	7-14 Days
Acute Sinusitis	Mild/Moderate	400 mg	q12h	10 Days
Chronic Bacterial Prostatitis	Mild/Moderate	400 mg	q12h	28 Days
Empirical Therapy in Febrile Neutropenic Patients	Severe Ciprofloxacin	400 mg	q8h	
	+ Piperacillin	50 mg/kg Not to exceed 24 g/day	q4h	7-14 Days
Inhalational anthrax (post-exposure)**		400 mg	q12h	60 Days

* used in conjunction with metronidazole. (See product labeling for prescribing information.)

† DUE TO THE DESIGNATED PATHOGENS (See **INDICATIONS AND USAGE**.)

** Drug administration should begin as soon as possible after suspected or confirmed exposure. This indication is based on a surrogate endpoint, ciprofloxacin serum concentrations achieved in humans, reasonably likely to predict clinical benefit.[4] For a discussion of ciprofloxacin serum concentrations in various human populations, see **INHALATIONAL ANTHRAX – ADDITIONAL INFORMATION**. Total duration of ciprofloxacin administration (I.V. or oral) for inhalational anthrax (post-exposure) is 60 days.

Conversion of I.V. to Oral Dosing in Adults: CIPRO Tablets and CIPRO Oral Suspension for oral administration are available. Parenteral therapy may be switched to oral CIPRO when the condition warrants, at the discretion of the physician. (See **CLINICAL PHARMACOLOGY** and table below for the equivalent dosing regimens.)

Equivalent AUC Dosing Regimens

CIPRO Oral Dosage	Equivalent CIPRO I.V. Dosage
250 mg Tablet q 12 h	200 mg I.V. q 12 h
500 mg Tablet q 12 h	400 mg I.V. q 12 h
750 mg Tablet q 12 h	400 mg I.V. q 8 h

Parenteral drug products should be inspected visually for particulate matter and discoloration prior to administration.

Adults with Impaired Renal Function: Ciprofloxacin is eliminated primarily by renal excretion; however, the drug is also metabolized and partially cleared through the biliary system of the liver and through the intestine. These alternative pathways of drug elimination appear to compensate for the reduced renal excretion in patients with renal impairment. Nonetheless, some modification of dosage is recommended for patients with severe renal dysfunction. The following table provides dosage guidelines for use in patients with renal impairment:

RECOMMENDED STARTING AND MAINTENANCE DOSES FOR PATIENTS WITH IMPAIRED RENAL FUNCTION

Creatinine Clearance (mL/min)	Dosage
> 30	See usual dosage.
5 - 29	200-400 mg q 18-24 hr

When only the serum creatinine concentration is known, the following formula may be used to estimate creatinine clearance:

[See first table at top of next page]

Continued on next page

Cipro I.V. Bulk—Cont.

The serum creatinine should represent a steady state of renal function.

For patients with changing renal function or for patients with renal impairment and hepatic insufficiency, careful monitoring is suggested.

DOSAGE AND ADMINISTRATION - PEDIATRICS

CIPRO I.V. should be administered as described in the Dosage Guidelines table. An increased incidence of adverse events compared to controls, including events related to joints and/or surrounding tissues, has been observed. (See **ADVERSE REACTIONS** and **CLINICAL STUDIES**.)

Dosing and initial route of therapy (i.e., I.V. or oral) for complicated urinary tract infection or pyelonephritis should be determined by the severity of the infection. In the clinical trial, pediatric patients with moderate to severe infection were initiated on 6 to 10 mg/kg I.V. every 8 hours and allowed to switch to oral therapy (10 to 20 mg/kg every 12 hours), at the discretion of the physician.

[See second table at right]

Pediatric patients with moderate to severe renal insufficiency were excluded from the clinical trial of complicated urinary tract infection and pyelonephritis. No information is available on dosing adjustments necessary for pediatric patients with moderate to severe renal insufficiency (i.e., creatinine clearance of < 50 mL/min/1.73m^2).

Preparation of CIPRO I.V. for Administration

PHARMACY BULK PACKAGE: The pharmacy bulk package is a single-entry container of a sterile preparation for parenteral use that contains many single doses. It contains ciprofloxacin as a 1% aqueous solution concentrate. The contents are intended for use in a pharmacy admixture program and are restricted to the preparation of admixtures for intravenous infusion. **THE CLOSURE SHALL BE PENETRATED ONLY ONE TIME** with a suitable sterile transfer set or dispensing device which allows measured dispensing of the contents.

The pharmacy bulk package is to be used only in a suitable work area such as laminar flow hood or an equivalent clean air or compounding area. **THIS PREPARATION MUST BE DILUTED BEFORE USE.** The intravenous dose should be prepared by aseptically withdrawing the CIPRO I.V. concentrate from the pharmacy bulk package and diluting the appropriate volume with a suitable intravenous solution to a final concentration of 0.5-2mg/mL. See **COMPATIBILITY AND STABILITY**.) The resulting solution should be infused over a period of 60 minutes by direct infusion or through a Y-type intravenous infusion set which may already be in place.

If the Y-type or "piggyback" method of administration is used, it is advisable to discontinue temporarily the administration of any other solutions during the infusion of CIPRO I.V. If the concomitant use of CIPRO I.V. and another drug is necessary each drug should be given separately in accordance with the recommended dosage and route of administration for each drug.

COMPATIBILITY AND STABILITY

Ciprofloxacin injection 1% (10 mg/mL), when diluted with the following intravenous solutions to concentrations of 0.5 to 2.0 mg/mL, is stable for up to 14 days at refrigerated or room temperature storage.

- 0.9% Sodium Chloride Injection, USP
- 5% Dextrose Injection, USP
- Sterile Water for Injection
- 10% Dextrose for Injection
- 5% Dextrose and 0.225% Sodium Chloride for Injection
- 5% Dextrose and 0.45% Sodium Chloride for Injection
- Lactated Ringer's for Injection

HOW SUPPLIED

CIPRO I.V. (ciprofloxacin) is available as a clear, colorless to slightly yellowish solution supplied in the pharmacy bulk package as follows:

[See third table at right]

CIPRO I.V. (ciprofloxacin) is also available as follows:

[See fourth table at right]

STORAGE

Pharmacy Bulk Package: Store between 5 – 30°C (41 – 86°F).

Protect from light, avoid excessive heat, protect from freezing.

Ciprofloxacin is also available as CIPRO (ciprofloxacin HCl) Tablets 100, 250, 500, and 750 mg and CIPRO (ciprofloxacin*) 5% and 10% Oral Suspension.

* Does not comply with USP with regards to "loss on drying" and "residue on ignition".

ANIMAL PHARMACOLOGY

Ciprofloxacin and other quinolones have been shown to cause arthropathy in immature animals of most species tested. (See **WARNINGS**.) Damage of weight bearing joints was observed in juvenile dogs and rats. In young beagles, 100 mg/kg ciprofloxacin, given daily for 4 weeks, caused degenerative articular changes of the knee joint. At 30 mg/kg, the effect on the joint was minimal. In a subsequent study in young beagle dogs, oral ciprofloxacin doses of 30 mg/kg and 90 mg/kg ciprofloxacin (approximately 1.3- and 3.5-times the pediatric dose based upon comparative plasma AUCs) given daily for 2 weeks caused articular changes which were still observed by histopathology after a treatment-free period of 5 months. At 10 mg/kg (approximately 0.6-times the pediatric dose based upon comparative plasma AUCs), no effects on joints were observed. This dose was also not associated with arthrotoxicity after an additional treatment-free period of 5 months. In another study, removal of weight bearing from the joint reduced the lesions but did not totally prevent them.

Crystalluria, sometimes associated with secondary nephropathy, occurs in laboratory animals dosed with ciprofloxacin. This is primarily related to the reduced solubility of ciprofloxacin under alkaline conditions, which predominate in the urine of test animals; in man, crystalluria is rare since human urine is typically acidic. In rhesus monkeys, crystalluria without nephropathy was noted after single oral doses as low as 5 mg/kg (approximately 0.07-times the highest recommended therapeutic dose based upon mg/m^2). After 6 months of intravenous dosing at 10 mg/kg/day, no nephropathological changes were noted; however, nephropathy was observed after dosing at 20 mg/kg/day for the same duration (approximately 0.2-times the highest recommended therapeutic dose based upon mg/m^2).

In dogs, ciprofloxacin administered at 3 and 10 mg/kg by rapid intravenous injection (15 sec.) produces pronounced hypotensive effects. These effects are considered to be related to histamine release because they are partially antagonized by pyrilamine, an antihistamine. In rhesus monkeys, rapid intravenous injection also produces hypotension, but the effect in this species is inconsistent and less pronounced.

In mice, concomitant administration of nonsteroidal anti-inflammatory drugs, such as phenylbutazone and indomethacin, with quinolones has been reported to enhance the CNS stimulatory effect of quinolones.

Ocular toxicity, seen with some related drugs, has not been observed in ciprofloxacin-treated animals.

INHALATIONAL ANTHRAX – ADDITIONAL INFORMATION

The mean serum concentrations of ciprofloxacin associated with a statistically significant improvement in survival in the rhesus monkey model of inhalational anthrax are reached or exceeded in adult and pediatric patients receiving oral and intravenous regimens. (See **DOSAGE AND ADMINISTRATION**.) Ciprofloxacin pharmacokinetics have been evaluated in various human populations. The mean peak serum concentration achieved at steady-state in human adults receiving 500 mg orally every 12 hours is 2.97 μg/mL, and 4.56 μg/mL following 400 mg intravenously every 12 hours. The mean trough serum concentration at steady-state for both of these regimens is 0.2 μg/mL. In a study of 10 pediatric patients between 6 and 16 years of age, the mean peak plasma concentration achieved is 8.3 μg/mL and trough concentrations range from 0.09 to 0.26 μg/mL, following two 30-minute intravenous infusions of 10 mg/kg administered 12 hours apart. After the second intravenous infusion patients switched to 15 mg/kg orally every 12 hours achieve a mean peak concentration of 3.6 μg/mL after the initial oral dose. Long-term safety data, including effects on cartilage, following the administration of ciprofloxacin to pediatric patients are limited. (For additional information, see **PRECAUTIONS**, **Pediatric Use**.) Ciprofloxacin serum concentrations achieved in humans serve as a surrogate endpoint reasonably likely to predict clinical benefit and provide the basis for this indication.[4]

A placebo-controlled animal study in rhesus monkeys exposed to an inhaled mean dose of 11 LD_{50} (~5.5 × 10^5)

$$\text{Men: Creatinine clearance (mL/min)} = \frac{\text{Weight (kg)} \times (140 - \text{age})}{72 \times \text{serum creatinine (mg/dL)}}$$

Women: 0.85 × the value calculated for men.

PEDIATRIC DOSAGE GUIDELINES

Infection	Route of Administration	Dose (mg/kg)	Frequency	Total Duration
Complicated Urinary Tract or Pyelonephritis (patients from 1 to 17 years of age)	Intravenous	6 to 10 mg/kg (maximum 400 mg per dose; not to be exceeded even in patients weighing > 51 kg)	Every 8 hours	10-21 days*
	Oral	10 mg/kg to 20 mg/kg (maximum 750 mg per dose; not to be exceeded even in patients weighing > 51 kg)	Every 12 hours	
Inhalational Anthrax (Post-Exposure)**	Intravenous	10 mg/kg (maximum 400 mg per dose)	Every 12 hours	60 days
	Oral	15 mg/kg (maximum 500 mg per dose)	Every 12 hours	

* The total duration of therapy for complicated urinary tract infection and pyelonephritis in the clinical trial was determined by the physician. The mean duration of treatment was 11 days (range 10 to 21 days).

** Drug administration should begin as soon as possible after suspected or confirmed exposure to *Bacillus anthracis* spores. This indication is based on a surrogate endpoint, ciprofloxacin serum concentrations achieved in humans, reasonably likely to predict clinical benefit.[4] For a discussion of ciprofloxacin serum concentrations in various human populations, see **INHALATIONAL ANTHRAX – ADDITIONAL INFORMATION**.

CONTAINER	SIZE	STRENGTH	NDC NUMBER
Pharmacy Bulk Package:	120 mL	1200 mg, 1%	0026-8566-65

VIAL: manufactured by Bayer HealthCare LLC and Hollister-Stier, Spokane, WA 99220.

SIZE	STRENGTH	NDC NUMBER
20 mL	200 mg, 1%	0026-8562-20
40 mL	400 mg, 1%	0026-8564-64

FLEXIBLE CONTAINER: manufactured for Bayer Pharmaceuticals Corporation by Abbott Laboratories, North Chicago, IL 60064.

SIZE	STRENGTH	NDC NUMBER
100 mL 5% Dextrose	200 mg, 0.2%	0026-8552-36
200 mL 5% Dextrose	400 mg, 0.2%	0026-8554-63

FLEXIBLE CONTAINER: manufactured for Bayer Pharmaceuticals Corporation by Baxter Healthcare Corporation, Deerfield, IL 60015.

SIZE	STRENGTH	NDC NUMBER
100 mL 5% Dextrose	200 mg, 0.2%	0026-8527-36
200 mL 5% Dextrose	400 mg, 0.2%	0026-8527-63

Outcomes	Ciprofloxacin/Piperacillin N = 233 Success (%)	Tobramycin/Piperacillin N = 237 Success (%)
Clinical Resolution of Initial Febrile Episode with No Modifications of Empirical Regimen*	63 (27.0%)	52 (21.9%)
Clinical Resolution of Initial Febrile Episode Including Patients with Modifications of Empirical Regimen	187 (80.3%)	185 (78.1%)
Overall Survival	224 (96.1%)	223 (94.1%)

* To be evaluated as a clinical resolution, patients had to have: (1) resolution of fever; (2) microbiological eradication of infection (if an infection was microbiologically documented); (3) resolution of signs/symptoms of infection; and (4) no modification of empirical antibiotic regimen.

Clinical Success and Bacteriologic Eradication at Test of Cure (5 to 9 Days Post-Therapy)

	CIPRO	Comparator
Randomized Patients	337	352
Per Protocol Patients	211	231
Clinical Response at 5 to 9 Days Post-Treatment	95.7% (202/211)	92.6% (214/231)
	95% CI [-1.3%, 7.3%]	
Bacteriologic Eradication by Patient at 5 to 9 Days Post-Treatment*	84.4% (178/211)	78.3% (181/231)
	95% CI [-1.3%, 13.1%]	
Bacteriologic Eradication of the Baseline Pathogen at 5 to 9 Days Post-Treatment		
Escherichia coli	156/178 (88%)	161/179 (90%)

* Patients with baseline pathogen(s) eradicated and no new infections or superinfections/total number of patients. There were 5.5% (6/211) ciprofloxacin and 9.5% (22/231) comparator patients with superinfections or new infections.

spores (range 5–30 LD_{50}) of *B. anthracis* was conducted. The minimal inhibitory concentration (MIC) of ciprofloxacin for the anthrax strain used in this study was 0.08 μg/mL. In the animals studied, mean serum concentrations of ciprofloxacin achieved at expected T_{max} (1 hour post-dose) following oral dosing to steady-state ranged from 0.98 to 1.69 μg/mL. Mean steady-state trough concentrations at 12 hours post-dose ranged from 0.12 to 0.19 μg/mL.[5] Mortality due to anthrax for animals that received a 30-day regimen of oral ciprofloxacin beginning 24 hours post-exposure was significantly lower (1/9), compared to the placebo group (9/10) [p=0.001]. The one ciprofloxacin-treated animal that died of anthrax did so following the 30-day drug administration period.[6]

CLINICAL STUDIES

EMPIRICAL THERAPY IN ADULT FEBRILE NEUTROPENIC PATIENTS

The safety and efficacy of ciprofloxacin, 400 mg I.V. q 8h, in combination with piperacillin sodium, 50 mg/kg I.V. q 4h, for the empirical therapy of febrile neutropenic patients were studied in one large pivotal multicenter, randomized trial and were compared to those of tobramycin, 2 mg/kg I.V. q 8h, in combination with piperacillin sodium, 50 mg/kg I.V. q 4h.

Clinical response rates observed in this study were as follows:

[See fifth table on previous page]

Complicated Urinary Tract Infection and Pyelonephritis – Efficacy in Pediatric Patients:

NOTE: Although effective in clinical trials, ciprofloxacin is not a drug of first choice in the pediatric population due to an increased incidence of adverse events compared to controls, including events related to joints and/or surrounding tissues.

Ciprofloxacin, administered I.V. and/or orally, was compared to a cephalosporin for treatment of complicated urinary tract infections (cUTI) and pyelonephritis in pediatric patients 1 to 17 years of age (mean age of 6 ± 4 years). The trial was conducted in the US, Canada, Argentina, Peru, Costa Rica, Mexico, South Africa, and Germany. The duration of therapy was 10 to 21 days (mean duration of treatment was 11 days with a range of 1 to 88 days). The primary objective of the study was to assess musculoskeletal and neurological safety.

Patients were evaluated for clinical success and bacteriological eradication of the baseline organism(s) with no new infection or superinfection at 5 to 9 days post-therapy (Test of Cure or TOC). The Per Protocol population had a causative organism(s) with protocol specified colony count(s) at baseline, no protocol violation, and no premature discontinuation or loss to follow-up (among other criteria).

The clinical success and bacteriologic eradication rates in the Per Protocol population were similar between ciprofloxacin and the comparator group as shown below.

[See table above]

References:

1. National Committee for Clinical Laboratory Standards, Methods for Dilution Antimicrobial Susceptibility Tests for Bacteria That Grow Aerobically - Fifth Edition. Approved Standard NCCLS Document M7-A5, Vol. 20, No. 2, NCCLS, Wayne, PA, January, 2000. 2. National Committee for Clinical Laboratory Standards, Performance Standards for Antimicrobial Disk Susceptibility Tests - Seventh Edition. Approved Standard NCCLS Document M2-A7, Vol. 20, No. 1, NCCLS, Wayne, PA, January, 2000. 3. Report presented at the FDA's Anti-Infective Drug and Dermatological Drug Products Advisory Committee Meeting, March 31, 1993, Silver Spring, MD. Report available from FDA, CDER, Advisors and Consultants Staff, HFD-21, 1901 Chapman Avenue, Room 200, Rockville, MD 20852, USA. 4. 21 CFR 314.510 (Subpart H – Accelerated Approval of New Drugs for Life-Threatening Illnesses). 5. Kelly DJ, et al. Serum concentrations of penicillin, doxycycline, and ciprofloxacin during prolonged therapy in rhesus monkeys. J Infect Dis 1992; 166: 1184-7. 6. Friedlander AM, et al. Postexposure prophylaxis against experimental inhalational anthrax. J Infect Dis 1993; 167: 1239-42. 7. Friedman J, Polifka J. Teratogenic effects of drugs: a resource for clinicians (TERIS). Baltimore, Maryland: Johns Hopkins University Press, 2000:149-195. 8. Loebstein R, Addis A, Ho E, et al. Pregnancy outcome following gestational exposure to fluoroquinolones; a multicenter prospective controlled study. Antimicrob Agents Chemother. 1998;42(6): 1336-1339. 9. Schaefer C, Amoura-Elefant E, Vial T, et al. Pregnancy outcome after prenatal quinolone exposure. Evaluation of a case registry of the European network of teratology information services (ENTIS). Eur J Obstet Gynecol Reprod Biol. 1996;69:83-89.

Bayer HealthCare
Manufactured for:
Bayer Pharmaceuticals Corporation
400 Morgan Lane
West Haven, CT 06516 USA
℞ Only
08709923, R.3 5/04 BAY q 3939

Shown in Product Identification Guide, page 308

CIPRO® XR ℞

[*sĭ′prō*]

(ciprofloxacin* extended-release tablets)

To reduce the development of drug-resistant bacteria and maintain the effectiveness of CIPRO® XR and other antibacterial drugs, CIPRO XR should be used only to treat or prevent infections that are proven or strongly suspected to be caused by bacteria.

DESCRIPTION

CIPRO XR (ciprofloxacin* extended-release tablets) contains ciprofloxacin, a synthetic broad-spectrum antimicrobial agent for oral administration. CIPRO XR tablets are coated, bilayer tablets consisting of an immediate-release layer and an erosion-matrix type controlled-release layer. The tablets contain a combination of two types of ciprofloxacin drug substance, ciprofloxacin hydrochloride and ciprofloxacin betaine (base). Ciprofloxacin hydrochloride is 1-cyclopropyl-6-fluoro-1, 4-dihydro-4-oxo-7-(1-piperazinyl)-3-quinolinecarboxylic acid hydrochloride. It is provided as a mixture of the monohydrate and the sesquihydrate. The empirical formula of the monohydrate is $C_{17}H_{18}FN_3O_3 \bullet HCl \bullet H_2O$ and its molecular weight is 385.8. The empirical formula of the sesquihydrate is $C_{17}H_{18}FN_3O_3 \bullet HCl \bullet 1.5\ H_2O$ and its molecular weight is 394.8. The drug substance is a faintly yellowish to light yellow crystalline substance. The chemical structure of the monohydrate is as follows:

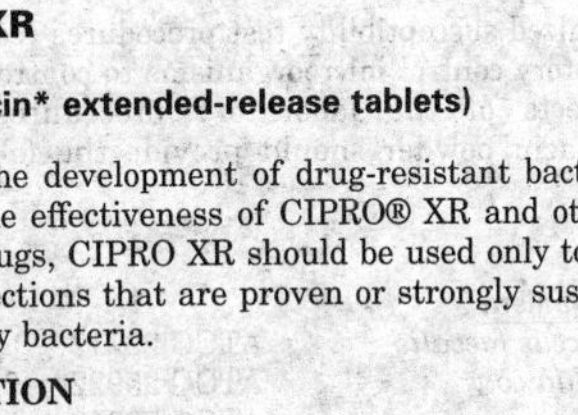

Ciprofloxacin betaine is 1-cyclopropyl-6-fluoro-1, 4-dihydro-4-oxo-7-(1-piperazinyl)-3-quinolinecarboxylic acid. As a hydrate, its empirical formula is $C_{17}H_{18}FN_3O_3 \bullet 3.5\ H_2O$ and its molecular weight is 394.3. It is a pale yellowish to light yellow crystalline substance and its chemical structure is as follows:

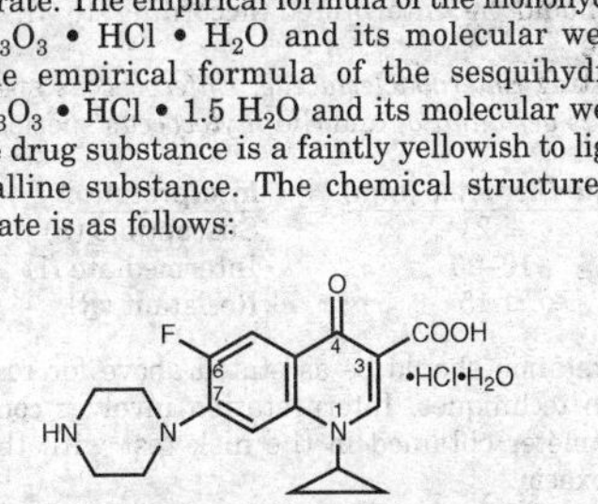

CIPRO XR is available in 500 mg and 1000 mg (ciprofloxacin equivalent) tablet strengths. CIPRO XR tablets are nearly white to slightly yellowish, film-coated, oblong-shaped tablets. Each CIPRO XR 500 mg tablet contains 500 mg of ciprofloxacin as ciprofloxacin HCl (287.5 mg, calculated as ciprofloxacin on the dried basis) and ciprofloxacin[†] (212.6 mg, calculated on the dried basis). Each CIPRO XR 1000 mg tablet contains 1000 mg of ciprofloxacin as ciprofloxacin HCl (574.9 mg, calculated as ciprofloxacin on the dried basis) and ciprofloxacin[†] (425.2 mg, calculated on the dried basis). The inactive ingredients are crospovidone, hypromellose, magnesium stearate, polyethylene glycol, silica colloidal anhydrous, succinic acid, and titanium dioxide.

* as ciprofloxacin [†] and ciprofloxacin hydrochloride
[†] does not comply with the loss on drying test and residue on ignition test of the USP monograph.

CLINICAL PHARMACOLOGY

Absorption

CIPRO XR tablets are formulated to release drug at a slower rate compared to immediate-release tablets. Approximately 35% of the dose is contained within an immediate-release component, while the remaining 65% is contained in a slow-release matrix.

Maximum plasma ciprofloxacin concentrations are attained between 1 and 4 hours after dosing with CIPRO XR. In comparison to the 250 mg and 500 mg ciprofloxacin immediate-release BID treatment, the C_{max} of CIPRO XR 500 mg and 1000 mg once daily are higher than the corresponding BID doses, while the AUCs over 24 hours are equivalent.

The following table compares the pharmacokinetic parameters obtained at steady state for these four treatment regimens (500 mg QD CIPRO XR versus 250 mg BID ciprofloxacin immediate-release tablets and 1000 mg QD CIPRO XR versus 500 mg BID ciprofloxacin immediate-release).

[See table at top of next page]

Results of the pharmacokinetic studies demonstrate that CIPRO XR may be administered with or without food (e.g. high-fat and low-fat meals or under fasted conditions).

Distribution

The volume of distribution calculated for intravenous ciprofloxacin is approximately 2.1–2.7 L/kg. Studies with the oral and intravenous forms of ciprofloxacin have demonstrated penetration of ciprofloxacin into a variety of tissues. The binding of ciprofloxacin to serum proteins is 20% to 40%, which is not likely to be high enough to cause significant protein binding interactions with other drugs. Following administration of a single dose of CIPRO XR, ciprofloxacin concentrations in urine collected up to 4 hours after dosing averaged over 300 mg/L for both the 500 mg and 1000 mg tablets; in urine excreted from 12 to 24 hours after dosing, ciprofloxacin concentration averaged 27 mg/L for the 500 mg tablet, and 58 mg/L for the 1000 mg tablet.

Metabolism

Four metabolites of ciprofloxacin were identified in human urine. The metabolites have antimicrobial activity, but are less active than unchanged ciprofloxacin. The primary metabolites are oxociprofloxacin (M3) and sulfociprofloxacin (M2), each accounting for roughly 3% to 8% of the total dose. Other minor metabolites are desethylene ciprofloxacin (M1), and formylciprofloxacin (M4). The relative proportion of drug and metabolite in serum corresponds to the composition found in urine. Excretion of these metabolites was essentially complete by 24 hours after dosing.

Elimination

The elimination kinetics of ciprofloxacin are similar for the immediate-release and the CIPRO XR tablet. In studies comparing the CIPRO XR and immediate-release ciprofloxacin, approximately 35% of an orally administered dose was excreted in the urine as unchanged drug for both formulations. The urinary excretion of ciprofloxacin is virtually complete within 24 hours after dosing. The renal clearance of ciprofloxacin, which is approximately 300 mL/minute, exceeds the normal glomerular filtration rate of 120 mL/minute. Thus, active tubular secretion would seem to play a significant role in its elimination. Co-administration of probenecid with immediate-release ciprofloxacin results in about a 50% reduction in the ciprofloxacin renal clearance and a 50% increase in its concentration in the systemic circulation. Although bile concentrations of ciprofloxacin are several fold higher than serum concentrations after oral dosing with the immediate-release tablet, only a small amount of the dose administered is recovered from the bile as unchanged drug. An additional 1% to 2% of the dose is recovered from the bile in the form of metabolites. Approximately 20% to 35% of an oral dose of immediate-release ciprofloxacin is recovered from the feces within 5 days after dosing. This may arise from either biliary clearance or transintestinal elimination.

Special Populations

Pharmacokinetic studies of the immediate-release oral tablet (single dose) and intravenous (single and multiple dose) forms of ciprofloxacin indicate that plasma concentrations of ciprofloxacin are higher in elderly subjects (> 65 years) as compared to young adults. C_{max} is increased 16% to 40%, and mean AUC is increased approximately 30%, which can be at least partially attributed to decreased renal clearance in the elderly. Elimination half-life is only slightly (~20%) prolonged in the elderly. These differences are not considered clinically significant. (See **PRECAUTIONS**, **Geriatric Use.**)

In patients with reduced renal function, the half-life of ciprofloxacin is slightly prolonged. No dose adjustment is required for patients with uncomplicated urinary tract infections receiving 500 mg CIPRO XR. For complicated urinary tract infection and acute uncomplicated pyelonephritis, where 1000 mg is the appropriate dose, the dosage of CIPRO XR should be reduced to CIPRO XR 500 mg q24h in patients with creatinine clearance below 30 mL/min. (See **DOSAGE AND ADMINISTRATION.**)

Continued on next page

Cipro XR—Cont.

In studies in patients with stable chronic cirrhosis, no significant changes in ciprofloxacin pharmacokinetics have been observed. The kinetics of ciprofloxacin in patients with acute hepatic insufficiency, however, have not been fully elucidated. (See **DOSAGE AND ADMINISTRATION**.)

Drug-drug Interactions

Previous studies with immediate-release ciprofloxacin have shown that concomitant administration of ciprofloxacin with theophylline decreases the clearance of theophylline resulting in elevated serum theophylline levels and increased risk of a patient developing CNS or other adverse reactions. Ciprofloxacin also decreases caffeine clearance and inhibits the formation of paraxanthine after caffeine administration. Absorption of ciprofloxacin is significantly reduced by concomitant administration of multivalent cation-containing products such as magnesium/aluminum antacids, sucralfate, VIDEX® (didanosine) chewable/buffered tablets or pediatric powder, or products containing calcium, iron, or zinc. (See **PRECAUTIONS, Drug Interactions** and **Information for Patients**, and **DOSAGE AND ADMINISTRATION**.)

Antacids: When CIPRO XR given as a single 1000 mg dose was administered two hours before, or four hours after a magnesium/aluminum-containing antacid (900 mg aluminum hydroxide and 600 mg magnesium hydroxide as a single oral dose) to 18 healthy volunteers, there was a 4% and 19% reduction, respectively, in the mean C_{max} of ciprofloxacin. The reduction in the mean AUC was 24% and 26%, respectively. CIPRO XR should be administered at least 2 hours before or 6 hours after antacids containing magnesium or aluminum, as well as sucralfate, VIDEX® (didanosine) chewable/buffered tablets or pediatric powder, metal cations such as iron, and multivitamin preparations with zinc. Although CIPRO XR may be taken with meals that include milk, concomitant administration with dairy products or with calcium-fortified juices alone should be avoided, since decreased absorption is possible. (See **PRECAUTIONS, Information for Patients** and **Drug Interactions**, and **DOSAGE AND ADMINISTRATION**.)

Omeprazole: When CIPRO XR was administered as a single 1000 mg dose concomitantly with omeprazole (40 mg once daily for three days) to 18 healthy volunteers, the mean AUC and C_{max} of ciprofloxacin were reduced by 20% and 23%, respectively. The clinical significance of this interaction has not been determined. (See **PRECAUTIONS, Drug Interactions**.)

MICROBIOLOGY

Ciprofloxacin has *in vitro* activity against a wide range of gram-negative and gram-positive organisms. The bactericidal action of ciprofloxacin results from inhibition of topoisomerase II (DNA gyrase) and topoisomerase IV (both Type II topoisomerases), which are required for bacterial DNA replication, transcription, repair, and recombination. The mechanism of action of quinolones, including ciprofloxacin, is different from that of other antimicrobial agents such as beta-lactams, macrolides, tetracyclines, or aminoglycosides; therefore, organisms resistant to these drugs may be susceptible to ciprofloxacin. There is no known cross-resistance between ciprofloxacin and other classes of antimicrobials. Resistance to ciprofloxacin *in vitro* develops slowly (multiple-step mutation). Resistance to ciprofloxacin due to spontaneous mutations occurs at a general frequency of between $< 10^{-9}$ to 1×10^{-6}.

Ciprofloxacin is slightly less active when tested at acidic pH. The inoculum size has little effect when tested *in vitro*. The minimal bactericidal concentration (MBC) generally does not exceed the minimal inhibitory concentration (MIC) by more than a factor of 2.

Ciprofloxacin has been shown to be active against most strains of the following microorganisms, both *in vitro* and in clinical infections as described in the **INDICATIONS AND USAGE** section.

Aerobic gram-positive microorganisms

Enterococcus faecalis (Many strains are only moderately susceptible.)
Staphylococcus saprophyticus

Aerobic gram-negative microorganisms

Escherichia coli
Klebsiella pneumoniae
Proteus mirabilis
Pseudomonas aeruginosa

The following *in vitro* data are available, but their clinical significance is unknown.

Ciprofloxacin exhibits *in vitro* minimum inhibitory concentrations (MICs) of 1 µg/mL or less against most (≥ 90%) strains of the following microorganisms; however, the safety and effectiveness of CIPRO XR in treating clinical infections due to these microorganisms have not been established in adequate and well controlled clinical trials.

Aerobic gram-negative microorganisms

Citrobacter koseri
Citrobacter freundii
Edwardsiella tarda
Enterobacter aerogenes
Enterobacter cloacae
Klebsiella oxytoca
Morganella morganii
Proteus vulgaris
Providencia rettgeri
Providencia stuartii
Serratia marcescens

Ciprofloxacin Pharmacokinetics (Mean ± SD) Following CIPRO® and CIPRO XR Administration

	C_{max} (mg/L)	AUC_{0-24h} (mg•h/L)	$T_{1/2}$(hr)	T_{max}(hr)§
CIPRO XR 500 mg QD	1.59 ± 0.43	7.97 ± 1.87	6.6 ± 1.4	1.5 (1.0–2.5)
CIPRO 250 mg BID	1.14 ± 0.23	8.25 ± 2.15	4.8 ± 0.6	1.0 (0.5–2.5)
CIPRO XR 1000 mg QD	3.11 ± 1.08	16.83 ± 5.65	6.31 ± 0.72	2.0 (1–4)
CIPRO 500 mg BID	2.06 ± 0.41	17.04 ± 4.79	5.66 ± 0.89	2.0 (0.5–3.5)

§ median (range)

Susceptibility Tests

Dilution Techniques: Quantitative methods are used to determine antimicrobial minimal inhibitory concentrations (MICs). These MICs provide estimates of the susceptibility of bacteria to antimicrobial compounds. The MICs should be determined using a standardized procedure. Standardized procedures are based on a dilution method[1] (broth or agar) or equivalent with standardized inoculum concentrations and standardized concentrations of ciprofloxacin. The MIC values should be interpreted according to the following criteria:

For testing *Enterobacteriaceae, Enterococcus* species, *Pseudomonas aeruginosa*, and *Staphylococcus* species:

MIC (µg/mL)	Interpretation
≤ 1	Susceptible (S)
2	Intermediate (I)
≥ 4	Resistant (R)

A report of "Susceptible" indicates that the pathogen is likely to be inhibited if the antimicrobial compound in the blood reaches the concentrations usually achievable. A report of "Intermediate" indicates that the result should be considered equivocal, and, if the microorganism is not fully susceptible to alternative, clinically feasible drugs, the test should be repeated. This category implies possible clinical applicability in body sites where the drug is physiologically concentrated or in situations where high dosage of drug can be used. This category also provides a buffer zone which prevents small uncontrolled technical factors from causing major discrepancies in interpretation. A report of "Resistant" indicates that the pathogen is not likely to be inhibited if the antimicrobial compound in the blood reaches the concentrations usually achievable; other therapy should be selected.

Standardized susceptibility test procedures require the use of laboratory control microorganisms to control the technical aspects of the laboratory procedures. Standard ciprofloxacin powder should provide the following MIC values:

Microorganism		MIC Range (µg/mL)
Enterococcus faecalis	ATCC 29212	0.25 – 2.0
Escherichia coli	ATCC 25922	0.004 – 0.015
Staphylococcus aureus	ATCC 29213	0.12 – 0.5
Pseudomonas aeruginosa	ATCC 27853	0.25 – 1

Diffusion Techniques: Quantitative methods that require measurement of zone diameters also provide reproducible estimates of the susceptibility of bacteria to antimicrobial compounds. One such standardized procedure[2] requires the use of standardized inoculum concentrations. This procedure uses paper disks impregnated with 5-µg ciprofloxacin to test the susceptibility of microorganisms to ciprofloxacin. Reports from the laboratory providing results of the standard single-disk susceptibility test with a 5-µg ciprofloxacin disk should be interpreted according to the following criteria:

For testing *Enterobacteriaceae, Enterococcus* species, *Pseudomonas aeruginosa*, and *Staphylococcus* species:

Zone Diameter (mm)	Interpretation
≥ 21	Susceptible (S)
16–20	Intermediate (I)
≤ 15	Resistant (R)

Interpretation should be as stated above for results using dilution techniques. Interpretation involves correlation of the diameter obtained in the disk test with the MIC for ciprofloxacin.

As with standardized dilution techniques, diffusion methods require the use of laboratory control microorganisms that are used to control the technical aspects of the laboratory procedures. For the diffusion technique, the 5-µg ciprofloxacin disk should provide the following zone diameters in these laboratory test quality control strains:

Microorganism		Zone Diameter (mm)
Escherichia coli	ATCC 25922	30 – 40
Staphylococcus aureus	ATCC 25923	22 – 30
Pseudomonas aeruginosa	ATCC 27853	25 – 33

INDICATIONS AND USAGE

CIPRO XR is indicated only for the treatment of urinary tract infections, including acute uncomplicated pyelonephritis, caused by susceptible strains of the designated microorganisms as listed below. CIPRO XR and ciprofloxacin immediate-release tablets are not interchangeable. Please see **DOSAGE AND ADMINISTRATION** for specific recommendations.

Uncomplicated Urinary Tract Infections (Acute Cystitis) caused by *Escherichia coli, Proteus mirabilis, Enterococcus faecalis*, or *Staphylococcus saprophyticus*[a].

Complicated Urinary Tract Infections caused by *Escherichia coli, Klebsiella pneumoniae, Enterococcus faecalis, Proteus mirabilis*, or *Pseudomonas aeruginosa* [a].

Acute Uncomplicated Pyelonephritis caused by *Escherichia coli.*

[a] Treatment of infections due to this organism in the organ system was studied in fewer than 10 patients.

THE SAFETY AND EFFICACY OF CIPRO XR IN TREATING INFECTIONS OTHER THAN URINARY TRACT INFECTIONS HAS NOT BEEN DEMONSTRATED. Appropriate culture and susceptibility tests should be performed before treatment in order to isolate and identify organisms causing infection and to determine their susceptibility to ciprofloxacin. Therapy with CIPRO XR may be initiated before results of these tests are known; once results become available appropriate therapy should be continued. Culture and susceptibility testing performed periodically during therapy will provide information not only on the therapeutic effect of the antimicrobial agent but also on the possible emergence of bacterial resistance.

To reduce the development of drug-resistant bacteria and maintain the effectiveness of CIPRO XR and other antibacterial drugs, CIPRO XR should be used only to treat or prevent infections that are proven or strongly suspected to be caused by susceptible bacteria. When culture and susceptibility information are available, they should be considered in selecting or modifying antibacterial therapy. In the absence of such data, local epidemiology and susceptibility patterns may contribute to the empiric selection of therapy.

CONTRAINDICATIONS

CIPRO XR is contraindicated in persons with a history of hypersensitivity to ciprofloxacin or any member of the quinolone class of antimicrobial agents.

WARNINGS

THE SAFETY AND EFFECTIVENESS OF CIPRO XR IN PEDIATRIC PATIENTS AND ADOLESCENTS (UNDER THE AGE OF 18 YEARS), PREGNANT WOMEN, AND NURSING WOMEN HAVE NOT BEEN ESTABLISHED. (See **PRECAUTIONS: Pediatric Use, Pregnancy,** and **Nursing Mothers** subsections.) The oral administration of ciprofloxacin caused lameness in immature dogs. Histopathological examination of the weight-bearing joints of these dogs revealed permanent lesions of the cartilage. Related quinolone-class drugs also produce erosions of cartilage of weight-bearing joints and other signs of arthropathy in immature animals of various species. (See **ANIMAL PHARMACOLOGY**.)

Convulsions, increased intracranial pressure, and toxic psychosis have been reported in patients receiving quinolones, including ciprofloxacin. Ciprofloxacin may also cause central nervous system (CNS) events including: dizziness, confusion, tremors, hallucinations, depression, and, rarely, suicidal thoughts or acts. These reactions may occur following the first dose. If these reactions occur in patients receiving ciprofloxacin, the drug should be discontinued and appropriate measures instituted. As with all quinolones, ciprofloxacin should be used with caution in patients with known or suspected CNS disorders that may predispose to seizures or lower the seizure threshold (e.g. severe cerebral arteriosclerosis, epilepsy), or in the presence of other risk factors that may predispose to seizures or lower the seizure threshold (e.g. certain drug therapy, renal dysfunction). (See **PRECAUTIONS: General, Information for Patients, Drug Interactions** and **ADVERSE REACTIONS**.)

SERIOUS AND FATAL REACTIONS HAVE BEEN REPORTED IN PATIENTS RECEIVING CONCURRENT ADMINISTRATION OF CIPROFLOXACIN AND THEOPHYLLINE. These reactions have included cardiac arrest, seizure, status epilepticus, and respiratory failure. Although similar serious adverse effects have been reported in patients receiving theophylline alone, the possibility that these reactions may be potentiated by ciprofloxacin cannot be eliminated. If concomitant use cannot be avoided, serum levels of theophylline should be monitored and dosage adjustments made as appropriate.

Serious and occasionally fatal hypersensitivity (anaphylactic) reactions, some following the first dose, have been reported in patients receiving quinolone therapy. Some reactions were accompanied by cardiovascular collapse, loss of consciousness, tingling, pharyngeal or facial edema, dyspnea, urticaria, and itching. Only a few patients had a history of hypersensitivity reactions. Serious anaphylactic reactions require immediate emergency treatment with epinephrine. Oxygen, intravenous steroids, and airway management, including intubation, should be administered as indicated.

Severe hypersensitivity reactions characterized by rash, fever, eosinophilia, jaundice, and hepatic necrosis with fatal outcome have also been rarely reported in patients receiving ciprofloxacin along with other drugs. The possibility that these reactions were related to ciprofloxacin cannot be excluded. Ciprofloxacin should be discontinued at the first appearance of a skin rash or any other sign of hypersensitivity.

Pseudomembranous colitis has been reported with nearly all antibacterial agents, including ciprofloxacin, and may range in severity from mild to life-threatening. Therefore, it is important to consider this diagnosis in patients who present with diarrhea subsequent to the administration of antibacterial agents.

Treatment with antibacterial agents alters the normal flora of the colon and may permit overgrowth of clostridia. Studies indicate that a toxin produced by *Clostridium difficile* is one primary cause of "antibiotic-associated colitis."

If a diagnosis of pseudomembranous colitis is established, therapeutic measures should be initiated. Mild cases of pseudomembranous colitis usually respond to drug discontinuation alone. In moderate to severe cases, consideration should be given to management with fluids and electrolytes, protein supplementation, and treatment with an antibacterial drug clinically effective against *C difficile* colitis. Drugs that inhibit peristalsis should be avoided.

Peripheral neuropathy: Rare cases of sensory or sensorimotor axonal polyneuropathy affecting small and/or large axons resulting in paresthesias, hypoesthesias, dysesthesias and weakness have been reported in patients receiving quinolones, including ciprofloxacin. Ciprofloxacin should be discontinued if the patient experiences symptoms of neuropathy including pain, burning, tingling, numbness, and/or weakness, or is found to have deficits in light touch, pain, temperature, position sense, vibratory sensation, and/or motor strength in order to prevent the development of an irreversible condition.

Tendon Effects: Ruptures of the shoulder, hand, Achilles tendon or other tendons that required surgical repair or resulted in prolonged disability have been reported in patients receiving quinolones, including ciprofloxacin. Post-marketing surveillance reports indicate that this risk may be increased in patients receiving concomitant corticosteroids, especially the elderly. Ciprofloxacin should be discontinued if the patient experiences pain, inflammation, or rupture of a tendon. Patients should rest and refrain from exercise until the diagnosis of tendonitis or tendon rupture has been excluded. Tendon rupture can occur during or after therapy with quinolones, including ciprofloxacin.

PRECAUTIONS

General: Crystals of ciprofloxacin have been observed rarely in the urine of human subjects but more frequently in the urine of laboratory animals, which is usually alkaline. (See **ANIMAL PHARMACOLOGY**.) Crystalluria related to ciprofloxacin has been reported only rarely in humans because human urine is usually acidic. Alkalinity of the urine should be avoided in patients receiving ciprofloxacin. Patients should be well hydrated to prevent the formation of highly concentrated urine.

Quinolones, including ciprofloxacin, may also cause central nervous system (CNS) events, including: nervousness, agitation, insomnia, anxiety, nightmares or paranoia. (See **WARNINGS, Information for Patients**, and **Drug Interactions**.)

Moderate to severe phototoxicity manifested as an exaggerated sunburn reaction has been observed in patients who are exposed to direct sunlight while receiving some members of the quinolone class of drugs. Excessive sunlight should be avoided. Therapy should be discontinued if phototoxicity occurs.

Prescribing CIPRO XR in the absence of a proven or strongly suspected bacterial infection or a prophylactic indication is unlikely to provide benefit to the patient and increases the risk of the development of drug-resistant bacteria.

Information for Patients:

Patients should be advised:

- that antibacterial drugs including CIPRO XR should only be used to treat bacterial infections. They do not treat viral infections (e.g., the common cold). When CIPRO XR is prescribed to treat a bacterial infection, patients should be told that although it is common to feel better early in the course of therapy, the medication should be taken exactly as directed. Skipping doses or not completing the full course of therapy may (1) decrease the effectiveness of the immediate treatment and (2) increase the likelihood that bacteria will develop resistance and will not be treatable by CIPRO XR or other antibacterial drugs in the future.
- that CIPRO XR may be taken with or without meals and to drink fluids liberally. As with other quinolones, concurrent administration with magnesium/aluminum antacids, or sucralfate, VIDEX® (didanosine) chewable/buffered tablets or pediatric powder, or with other products containing calcium, iron, or zinc should be avoided. CIPRO XR may be taken two hours before or six hours after taking these products. (See **CLINICAL PHARMACOLOGY, Drug-drug Interactions, DOSAGE AND ADMINISTRATION**, and **PRECAUTIONS, Drug Interactions**.) CIPRO XR should not be taken with dairy products (like milk or yogurt) or calcium-fortified juices alone since absorption of ciprofloxacin may be significantly reduced; however, CIPRO XR may be taken with a meal that contains these products. (See **CLINICAL PHARMACOLOGY, Drug-drug Interactions, DOSAGE AND ADMINISTRATION**, and **PRECAUTIONS, Drug Interactions**.)
- If the patient should forget to take CIPRO XR at the usual time, he/she may take the dose later in the day. Do not take more than one CIPRO XR tablet per day even if a patient misses a dose. Swallow the CIPRO XR tablet whole. **DO NOT SPLIT, CRUSH, OR CHEW THE TABLET.**
- that ciprofloxacin may be associated with hypersensitivity reactions, even following a single dose, and to discontinue CIPRO XR at the first sign of a skin rash or other allergic reaction.
- to avoid excessive sunlight or artificial ultraviolet light while receiving CIPRO XR and to discontinue therapy if phototoxicity occurs.
- that peripheral neuropathies have been associated with ciprofloxacin use. If symptoms of peripheral neuropathy including pain, burning, tingling, numbness and/or weakness develop, they should discontinue treatment and contact their physicians.
- that if they experience pain, inflammation, or rupture of a tendon to discontinue treatment, to inform their physician, and to rest and refrain from exercise.
- that CIPRO XR may cause dizziness and lightheadedness; therefore, patients should know how they react to this drug before they operate an automobile or machinery or engage in activities requiring mental alertness or coordination.
- that CIPRO XR may increase the effects of theophylline and caffeine. There is a possibility of caffeine accumulation when products containing caffeine are consumed while taking quinolones.
- that convulsions have been reported in patients receiving quinolones, including ciprofloxacin, and to notify their physician before taking CIPRO XR if there is a history of this condition.

Drug Interactions: As with some other quinolones, concurrent administration of ciprofloxacin with theophylline may lead to elevated serum concentrations of theophylline and prolongation of its elimination half-life. This may result in increased risk of theophylline-related adverse reactions. (See **WARNINGS**.) If concomitant use cannot be avoided, serum levels of theophylline should be monitored and dosage adjustments made as appropriate.

Some quinolones, including ciprofloxacin, have also been shown to interfere with the metabolism of caffeine. This may lead to reduced clearance of caffeine and a prolongation of its serum half-life.

Concurrent administration of a quinolone, including ciprofloxacin, with multivalent cation-containing products such as magnesium/aluminum antacids, sucralfate, VIDEX® (didanosine) chewable/buffered tablets or pediatric powder, or products containing calcium, iron, or zinc may substantially interfere with the absorption of the quinolone, resulting in serum and urine levels considerably lower than desired. CIPRO XR should be administered at least 2 hours before or 6 hours after antacids containing magnesium or aluminum, as well as sucralfate, VIDEX® (didanosine) chewable/buffered tablets or pediatric powder, metal cations such as iron, and multivitamin preparations with zinc. (See **CLINICAL PHARMACOLOGY, Drug-drug Interactions, PRECAUTIONS, Information for Patients**, and **DOSAGE AND ADMINISTRATION**.)

Histamine H_2-receptor antagonists appear to have no significant effect on the bioavailability of ciprofloxacin.

Absorption of the CIPRO XR tablet was slightly diminished (20%) when given concomitantly with omeprazole. (See **CLINICAL PHARMACOLOGY, Drug-drug Interactions**.)

Altered serum levels of phenytoin (increased and decreased) have been reported in patients receiving concomitant ciprofloxacin.

The concomitant administration of ciprofloxacin with the sulfonylurea glyburide has, on rare occasions, resulted in severe hypoglycemia.

Some quinolones, including ciprofloxacin, have been associated with transient elevations in serum creatinine in patients receiving cyclosporine concomitantly.

Quinolones, including ciprofloxacin, have been reported to enhance the effects of the oral anticoagulant warfarin or its derivatives. When these products are administered concomitantly, prothrombin time or other suitable coagulation tests should be closely monitored.

Probenecid interferes with renal tubular secretion of ciprofloxacin and produces an increase in the level of ciprofloxacin in the serum. This should be considered if patients are receiving both drugs concomitantly.

Renal tubular transport of methotrexate may be inhibited by concomitant administration of ciprofloxacin potentially leading to increased plasma levels of methotrexate. This might increase the risk of methotrexate associated toxic reactions. Therefore, patients under methotrexate therapy should be carefully monitored when concomitant ciprofloxacin therapy is indicated.

Metoclopramide significantly accelerates the absorption of oral ciprofloxacin resulting in a shorter time to reach maximum plasma concentrations. No significant effect was observed on the bioavailability of ciprofloxacin.

Non-steroidal anti-inflammatory drugs (but not acetyl salicylic acid) in combination of very high doses of quinolones have been shown to provoke convulsions in pre-clinical studies.

Carcinogenesis, Mutagenesis, Impairment of Fertility: Eight *in vitro* mutagenicity tests have been conducted with ciprofloxacin, and the test results are listed below:

Salmonella/Microsome Test (Negative)
E. coli DNA Repair Assay (Negative)
Mouse Lymphoma Cell Forward Mutation Assay (Positive)
Chinese Hamster V_{79} Cell HGPRT Test (Negative)
Syrian Hamster Embryo Cell Transformation Assay (Negative)
Saccharomyces cerevisiae Point Mutation Assay (Negative)
Saccharomyces cerevisiae Mitotic Crossover and Gene Conversion Assay (Negative)
Rat Hepatocyte DNA Repair Assay (Positive)

Thus, 2 of the 8 tests were positive, but results of the following 3 *in vivo* test systems gave negative results:

Rat Hepatocyte DNA Repair Assay
Micronucleus Test (Mice)
Dominant Lethal Test (Mice)

Ciprofloxacin was not carcinogenic or tumorigenic in 2-year carcinogenicity studies with rats and mice at daily oral dose levels of 250 and 750 mg/kg, respectively (approximately 2 and 3 -fold greater than the 1000 mg daily human dose based upon body surface area).

Results from photo co-carcinogenicity testing indicate that ciprofloxacin does not reduce the time to appearance of UV-induced skin tumors as compared to vehicle control. Hairless (Skh-1) mice were exposed to UVA light for 3.5 hours five times every two weeks for up to 78 weeks while concurrently being administered ciprofloxacin. The time to development of the first skin tumors was 50 weeks in mice treated concomitantly with UVA and ciprofloxacin (mouse dose approximately equal to the maximum recommended daily human dose of 1000 mg based upon mg/m^2), as opposed to 34 weeks when animals were treated with both UVA and vehicle. The times to development of skin tumors ranged from 16–32 weeks in mice treated concomitantly with UVA and other quinolones.

In this model, mice treated with ciprofloxacin alone did not develop skin or systemic tumors. There are no data from similar models using pigmented mice and/or fully haired mice. The clinical significance of these findings to humans is unknown.

Fertility studies performed in rats at oral doses of ciprofloxacin up to 100 mg/kg (1.0 times the highest recommended daily human dose of 1000 mg based upon body surface area) revealed no evidence of impairment.

Pregnancy: Teratogenic Effects. Pregnancy Category C: There are no adequate and well-controlled studies in pregnant women. An expert review of published data on experiences with ciprofloxacin use during pregnancy by TERIS - the Teratogen Information System – concluded that therapeutic doses during pregnancy are unlikely to pose a substantial teratogenic risk (quantity and quality of data=fair), but the data are insufficient to state there is no risk.

A controlled prospective observational study followed 200 women exposed to fluoroquinolones (52.5% exposed to ciprofloxacin and 68% first trimester exposures) during gestation. In utero exposure to fluoroquinolones during embryogenesis was not associated with increased risk of major malformations. The reported rates of major congenital malformations were 2.2% for the fluoroquinolone group and 2.6% for the control group (background incidence of major malformations is 1–5%). Rates of spontaneous abortions, prematurity and low birth weight did not differ between the groups and there were no clinically significant musculoskeletal dysfunctions up to one year of age in the ciprofloxacin exposed children.

Another prospective follow-up study reported on 549 pregnancies with fluoroquinolone exposure (93% first trimester exposures). There were 70 ciprofloxacin exposures, all within the first trimester. The malformation rates among live-born babies exposed to ciprofloxacin and to fluoroquinolones overall were both within background incidence ranges. No specific patterns of congenital abnormalities were found. The study did not reveal any clear adverse reactions due to in utero exposure to ciprofloxacin.

No differences in the rates of prematurity, spontaneous abortions, or birth weight were seen in women exposed to ciprofloxacin during pregnancy. However, these small post-marketing epidemiology studies, of which most experience is from short term, first trimester exposure, are insufficient to evaluate the risk for the less common defects or to permit reliable and definitive conclusions regarding the safety of ciprofloxacin in pregnant women and their developing fetuses. Ciprofloxacin should not be used during pregnancy unless potential benefit justifies the potential risk to both fetus and mother (see **WARNINGS**).

Reproduction studies have been performed in rats and mice using oral doses up to 100 mg/kg (0.7 and 0.4 times the maximum daily human dose of 1000 mg based upon body surface area, respectively) and have revealed no evidence of harm to the fetus due to ciprofloxacin. In rabbits, ciprofloxacin (30 and 100 mg/kg orally) produced gastrointestinal disturbances resulting in maternal weight loss and an increased incidence of abortion, but no teratogenicity was observed at either dose. After intravenous administration of doses up to 20 mg/kg, no maternal toxicity was produced in the rabbit, and no embryotoxicity or teratogenicity was observed.

Nursing Mothers: Ciprofloxacin is excreted in human milk. The amount of ciprofloxacin absorbed by the nursing

Continued on next page

Cipro XR—Cont.

infant is unknown. Because of the potential for serious adverse reactions in infants nursing from mothers taking ciprofloxacin, a decision should be made whether to discontinue nursing or to discontinue the drug, taking into account the importance of the drug to the mother.

Pediatric Use: Safety and effectiveness of CIPRO XR in pediatric patients and adolescents less than 18 years of age have not been established. Ciprofloxacin causes arthropathy in juvenile animals. (See **WARNINGS.**)

Geriatric Use: In a large, prospective, randomized CIPRO XR clinical trial in complicated urinary tract infections, 49% (509/1035) of the patients were 65 and over, while 30% (308/1035) were 75 and over. No overall differences in safety or effectiveness were observed between these subjects and younger subjects, and clinical experience with other formulations of ciprofloxacin has not identified differences in responses between the elderly and younger patients, but greater sensitivity of some older individuals cannot be ruled out. Ciprofloxacin is known to be substantially excreted by the kidney, and the risk of adverse reactions may be greater in patients with impaired renal function. No alteration of dosage is necessary for patients greater than 65 years of age with normal renal function. However, since some older individuals experience reduced renal function by virtue of their advanced age, care should be taken in dose selection for elderly patients, and renal function monitoring may be useful in these patients. (See **CLINICAL PHARMACOLOGY** and **DOSAGE AND ADMINISTRATION.**)

ADVERSE REACTIONS

Clinical trials in patients with urinary tract infections enrolled 961 patients treated with 500 mg or 1000 mg CIPRO XR. Most adverse events reported were described as mild to moderate in severity and required no treatment. The overall incidence, type and distribution of adverse events were similar in patients receiving both 500 mg and 1000 mg of CIPRO XR. Because clinical trials are conducted under widely varying conditions, adverse reaction rates observed in clinical trials of a drug cannot be directly compared to rates observed in clinical trials of another drug and may not reflect the rates observed in practice. The adverse reaction information from clinical studies does, however, provide a basis for identifying the adverse events that appear to be related to drug use and for approximating rates.

In the clinical trial of uncomplicated urinary tract infection, CIPRO XR (500 mg once daily) in 444 patients was compared to ciprofloxacin immediate-release tablets (250 mg twice daily) in 447 patients for 3 days. Discontinuations due to adverse reactions thought to be drug-related occurred in 0.2% (1/444) of patients in the CIPRO XR arm and in 0% (0/447) of patients in the control arm.

In the clinical trial of complicated urinary tract infection and acute uncomplicated pyelonephritis, CIPRO XR (1000 mg once daily) in 517 patients was compared to ciprofloxacin immediate-release tablets (500 mg twice daily) in 518 patients for 7 to 14 days. Discontinuations due to adverse reactions thought to be drug-related occurred in 3.1% (16/517) of patients in the CIPRO XR arm and in 2.3% (12/518) of patients in the control arm. The most common reasons for discontinuation in the CIPRO XR arm were nausea/vomiting (4 patients) and dizziness (3 patients). In the control arm the most common reason for discontinuation was nausea/vomiting (3 patients).

In these clinical trials, the following events occurred in ≥2% of all CIPRO XR patients, regardless of drug relationship: nausea (4%), headache (3%), dizziness (2%), diarrhea (2%), vomiting (2%) and vaginal moniliasis (2%).

Adverse events, judged by investigators to be at least possibly drug-related, occurring in greater than or equal to 1% of all CIPRO XR treated patients were: nausea (3%), diarrhea (2%), headache (1%), dyspepsia (1%), dizziness (1%), and vaginal moniliasis (1%). Vomiting (1%) occurred in the 1000 mg group.

Additional uncommon events, judged by investigators to be at least possibly drug-related, that occurred in less than 1% of CIPRO XR treated patients were:

BODY AS A WHOLE: abdominal pain, asthenia, malaise, photosensitivity reaction

CARDIOVASCULAR: bradycardia, migraine, syncope

DIGESTIVE: anorexia, constipation, dry mouth, flatulence, liver function tests abnormal, thirst

HEMIC/LYMPHATIC: prothrombin decrease

CENTRAL NERVOUS SYSTEM: abnormal dreams, depersonalization, depression, hypertonia, incoordination, insomnia, somnolence, tremor, vertigo

METABOLIC: hyperglycemia

SKIN/APPENDAGES: dry skin, maculopapular rash, pruritus, rash, skin disorder, urticaria, vesiculobullous rash

SPECIAL SENSES: diplopia, taste perversion

UROGENITAL: dysmenorrhea, hematuria, kidney function abnormal, vaginitis

The following additional adverse events, some of them life threatening, regardless of incidence or relationship to drug, have been reported during clinical trials and from worldwide post-marketing experience in patients given ciprofloxacin (includes all formulations, all dosages, all drug-therapy durations, and all indications). Because these reactions have been reported voluntarily from a population of uncertain size, it is not always possible to reliably estimate their frequency or a causal relationship to drug exposure. The events in alphabetical order are:

abnormal gait, achiness, acidosis, agitation, agranulocytosis, allergic reactions (ranging from urticaria to anaphylactic reactions), amylase increase, anemia, angina pectoris, angioedema, anosmia, anxiety, arrhythmia, arthralgia, ataxia, atrial flutter, bleeding diathesis, blurred vision, bronchospasm, *C. difficile* associated diarrhea, candidiasis (cutaneous, oral), candiduria, cardiac murmur, cardiopulmonary arrest, cardiovascular collapse, cerebral thrombosis, chills, cholestatic jaundice, chromatopsia, confusion, convulsion, delirium, drowsiness, dysphagia, dysphasia, dyspnea, edema (conjunctivae, face, hands, laryngeal, lips, lower extremities, neck, pulmonary), epistaxis, erythema multiforme, erythema nodosum, exfoliative dermatitis, fever, fixed eruptions, flushing, gastrointestinal bleeding, gout (flare up), grand mal convulsion, gynecomastia, hallucinations, hearing loss, hemolytic anemia, hemoptysis, hemorrhagic cystitis, hepatic failure, hepatic necrosis, hepatitis, hiccup, hyperesthesia, hyperpigmentation, hypertension, hypertonia, hypesthesia, hypotension, ileus, interstitial nephritis, intestinal perforation, jaundice, joint stiffness, lethargy, lightheadedness, lipase increase, lymphadenopathy, manic reaction, marrow depression, migraine, moniliasis (oral, gastrointestinal, vaginal), myalgia, myasthenia, myasthenia gravis (possible exacerbation), myocardial infarction, myoclonus, nephritis, nightmares, nystagmus, oral ulceration, pain (arm, back, breast, chest, epigastric, eye, extremities, foot, jaw, neck, oral mucosa), palpitation, pancreatitis, pancytopenia, paranoia, paresthesia, peripheral neuropathy, perspiration (increased), petechia, phlebitis, phobia, pleural effusion, polyuria, postural hypotension, prothrombin time prolongation, pseudomembranous colitis (the onset of symptoms may occur during or after antimicrobial treatment), pulmonary embolism, purpura, renal calculi, renal failure, respiratory arrest, respiratory distress, restlessness, serum sickness-like reaction, Stevens-Johnson syndrome, sweating, tachycardia, taste loss, tendinitis, tendon rupture, tinnitus, torsade de pointes, toxic epidermal necrolysis, toxic psychosis, twitching, unresponsiveness, urethral bleeding, urinary retention, urination (frequent), vaginal pruritus, vasculitis, ventricular ectopy, vesicles, visual acuity (decreased), visual disturbances (flashing lights, change in color perception, overbrightness of lights).

Laboratory Changes:

The following adverse laboratory changes, in alphabetical order, regardless of incidence or relationship to drug, have been reported in patients given ciprofloxacin (includes all formulations, all dosages, all drug-therapy durations, and all indications):

Decreases in blood glucose, BUN, hematocrit, hemoglobin, leukocyte counts, platelet counts, prothrombin time, serum albumin, serum potassium, total serum protein, uric acid.

Increases in alkaline phosphatase, ALT (SGPT), AST (SGOT), atypical lymphocyte counts, blood glucose, blood monocytes, BUN, cholesterol, eosinophil counts, LDH, platelet counts, prothrombin time, sedimentation rate, serum amylase, serum bilirubin, serum calcium, serum cholesterol, serum creatine phosphokinase, serum creatinine, serum gamma-glutamyl transpeptidase (GGT), serum potassium, serum theophylline (in patients receiving theophylline concomitantly), serum triglycerides, uric acid.

Others: albuminuria, change in serum phenytoin, crystalluria, cylindruria, immature WBCs, leukocytosis, methemoglobinemia, pancytopenia.

OVERDOSAGE

In the event of acute excessive overdosage, reversible renal toxicity has been reported in some cases. The stomach should be emptied by inducing vomiting or by gastric lavage. The patient should be carefully observed and given supportive treatment, including administration of magnesium or calcium containing antacids which can reduce the absorption of ciprofloxacin. Adequate hydration must be maintained. Only a small amount of ciprofloxacin (< 10%) is removed from the body after hemodialysis or peritoneal dialysis.

In mice, rats, rabbits and dogs, significant toxicity including tonic/clonic convulsions was observed at intravenous doses of ciprofloxacin between 125 and 300 mg/kg.

Single doses of ciprofloxacin were relatively non-toxic via the oral route of administration in mice, rats, and dogs. No deaths occurred within a 14-day post treatment observation period at the highest oral doses tested; up to 5000 mg/kg in either rodent species, or up to 2500 mg/kg in the dog. Clinical signs observed included hypoactivity and cyanosis in both rodent species and severe vomiting in dogs. In rabbits, significant mortality was seen at doses of ciprofloxacin > 2500 mg/kg. Mortality was delayed in these animals, occurring 10–14 days after dosing.

DOSAGE AND ADMINISTRATION

CIPRO XR and ciprofloxacin immediate-release tablets are not interchangeable. Cipro XR should be administered orally once daily as described in the following Dosage Guidelines table:

[See table below]

Patients whose therapy is started with CIPRO I.V. for urinary tract infections may be switched to CIPRO XR when clinically indicated at the discretion of the physician.

CIPRO XR should be administered at least 2 hours before or 6 hours after antacids containing magnesium or aluminum, as well as sucralfate, VIDEX® (didanosine) chewable/buffered tablets or pediatric powder, metal cations such as iron, and multivitamin preparations with zinc. Although CIPRO XR may be taken with meals that include milk, concomitant administration with dairy products alone, or with calcium-fortified products should be avoided, since decreased absorption is possible. A 2-hour window between substantial calcium intake (> 800 mg) and dosing with CIPRO XR is recommended. CIPRO XR should be swallowed whole. **DO NOT SPLIT, CRUSH, OR CHEW THE TABLET.** (See **CLINICAL PHARMACOLOGY, Drug-drug Interactions, PRECAUTIONS, Drug Interactions** and **Information for Patients.**)

Impaired Renal Function:

Ciprofloxacin is eliminated primarily by renal excretion; however, the drug is also metabolized and partially cleared through the biliary system of the liver and through the intestine. These alternate pathways of drug elimination appear to compensate for the reduced renal excretion in patients with renal impairment. No dosage adjustment is required for patients with uncomplicated urinary tract infections receiving 500 mg CIPRO XR. In patients with complicated urinary tract infections and acute uncomplicated pyelonephritis, who have a creatinine clearance of ≤ 30 mL/min, the dose of CIPRO XR should be reduced from 1000 mg to 500 mg daily. For patients on hemodialysis or peritoneal dialysis, administer CIPRO XR after the dialysis procedure is completed. (See **CLINICAL PHARMACOLOGY, Special Populations,** and **PRECAUTIONS, Geriatric Use.**)

Impaired Hepatic Function:

No dosage adjustment is required with CIPRO XR in patients with stable chronic cirrhosis. The kinetics of ciprofloxacin in patients with acute hepatic insufficiency, however, have not been fully elucidated. (See **CLINICAL PHARMACOLOGY, Special Populations.**)

HOW SUPPLIED

CIPRO XR is available as nearly white to slightly yellowish, film-coated, oblong-shaped tablets containing 500 mg or 1000 mg ciprofloxacin. The 500 mg tablet is coded with the word "BAYER" on one side and "C500 QD" on the reverse side. The 1000 mg tablet is coded with the word "BAYER" on one side and "C1000 QD" on the reverse side.

	Strength	NDC Code
Bottles of 30	500 mg	0026-8889-69
Bottles of 50	500 mg	0026-8889-50
Bottles of 100	500 mg	0026-8889-51
Bottles of 50	1000 mg	0026-8897-50
Bottles of 100	1000 mg	0026-8897-51
Unit Dose Pack of 30	1000 mg	0026-8897-69

Store at 25°C (77°F); excursions permitted to 15–30°C (59–86°F) [see USP Controlled Room Temperature].

ANIMAL PHARMACOLOGY

Ciprofloxacin and other quinolones have been shown to cause arthropathy in immature animals of most species tested. (See **WARNINGS.**) Damage of weight bearing joints was observed in juvenile dogs and rats. In young beagles, 100 mg/kg ciprofloxacin, given daily for 4 weeks, caused degenerative articular changes of the knee joint. At 30 mg/kg, the effect on the joint was minimal. In a subsequent study in beagles, removal of weight bearing from the joint reduced the lesions but did not totally prevent them.

Crystalluria, sometimes associated with secondary nephropathy, occurs in laboratory animals dosed with ciprofloxacin. This is primarily related to the reduced solubility of ciprofloxacin under alkaline conditions, which predominate in the urine of test animals; in man, crystalluria is rare since human urine is typically acidic. In rhesus monkeys, crystalluria without nephropathy has been noted after single oral doses as low as 5 mg/kg. After 6 months of intravenous dosing at 10 mg/kg/day, no nephropathological changes were noted; however, nephropathy was observed after dosing at 20 mg/kg/day for the same duration.

In mice, concomitant administration of nonsteroidal anti-inflammatory drugs such as phenylbutazone and indomethacin with quinolones has been reported to enhance the CNS stimulatory effect of quinolones.

Ocular toxicity seen with some related drugs has not been observed in ciprofloxacin-treated animals.

CLINICAL STUDIES

Uncomplicated Urinary Tract Infections (acute cystitis)

CIPRO XR was evaluated for the treatment of uncomplicated urinary tract infections (acute cystitis) in a randomized, double-blind, controlled clinical trial conducted in the US. This study compared CIPRO XR (500 mg once daily for

DOSAGE GUIDELINES

Indication	Unit Dose	Frequency	Usual Duration
Uncomplicated Urinary Tract Infection (Acute Cystitis)	500 mg	Q24h	3 Days
Complicated Urinary Tract Infection	1000 mg	Q24h	7–14 Days
Acute Uncomplicated Pyelonephritis	1000 mg	Q24h	7–14 Days

three days) with ciprofloxacin immediate-release tablets (CIPRO® 250 mg BID for three days). Of the 905 patients enrolled, 452 were randomly assigned to the CIPRO XR treatment group and 453 were randomly assigned to the control group. The primary efficacy variable was bacteriologic eradication of the baseline organism(s) with no new infection or superinfection at test-of-cure (Day 4–11 Post-therapy).

The bacteriologic eradication and clinical success rates were similar between CIPRO XR and the control group. The eradication and clinical success rates and their corresponding 95% confidence intervals for the differences between rates (CIPRO XR minus control group) are given in the following table:

[See first table at right]

Complicated Urinary Tract Infections and Acute Uncomplicated Pyelonephritis

CIPRO XR was evaluated for the treatment of complicated urinary tract infections (cUTI) and acute uncomplicated pyelonephritis (AUP) in a randomized, double-blind, controlled clinical trial conducted in the US and Canada. The study enrolled 1,042 patients (521 patients per treatment arm) and compared CIPRO XR (1000 mg once daily for 7 to 14 days) with immediate-release ciprofloxacin (500 mg BID for 7 to 14 days). The primary efficacy endpoint for this trial was bacteriologic eradication of the baseline organism(s) with no new infection or superinfection at 5 to 11 days post-therapy (test-of-cure or TOC) for the Per Protocol and Modified Intent-To-Treat (MITT) populations.

The Per Protocol population was defined as patients with a diagnosis of cUTI or AUP, a causative organism(s) at baseline present at ≥ 10^5 CFU/mL, no inclusion criteria violation, a valid test-of-cure urine culture within the TOC window, an organism susceptible to study drug, no premature discontinuation or loss to follow-up, and compliance with the dosage regimen (among other criteria). More patients in the CIPRO XR arm than in the control arm were excluded from the Per Protocol population and this should be considered in the interpretation of the study results. Reasons for exclusion with the greatest discrepancy between the two arms were no valid test-of-cure urine culture, an organism resistant to the study drug, and premature discontinuation due to adverse events.

An analysis of all patients with a causative organism(s) isolated at baseline and who received study medication, defined as the MITT population, included 342 patients in the CIPRO XR arm and 324 patients in the control arm. Patients with missing responses were counted as failures in this analysis. In the MITT analysis of cUTI patients, bacteriologic eradication was 160/271 (59.0%) versus 156/248 (62.9%) in CIPRO XR and control arm, respectively [97.5% CI* (-13.5%, 5.7%)]. Clinical cure was 184/271 (67.9%) for CIPRO XR and 182/248 (73.4%) for control arm, respectively [97.5% CI* (-14.4%, 3.5%)]. Bacterial eradication in the MITT analysis of patients with AUP at TOC was 47/71 (66.2%) and 58/76 (76.3%) for CIPRO XR and control arm, respectively [97.5% CI* (-26.8%, 6.5%)]. Clinical cure at TOC was 50/71 (70.4%) for CIPRO XR and 58/76 (76.3%) for the control arm [97.5% CI* (-22.0%, 10.4%)].

* confidence interval of the difference in rates (CIPRO XR minus control).

In the Per Protocol population, the differences between CIPRO XR and the control arm in bacteriologic eradication rates at the TOC visit were not consistent between AUP and cUTI patients. The bacteriologic eradication rate for cUTI patients was higher in the CIPRO XR arm than in the control arm. For AUP patients, the bacteriologic eradication rate was lower in the CIPRO XR arm than in the control arm. This inconsistency was not observed between the two treatment groups for clinical cure rates. Clinical cure rates were 96.1% (198/206) and 92.1% (211/229) for CIPRO XR and the control arm, respectively.

The bacterial eradication and clinical cure rates by infection type for CIPRO XR and the control arm at the TOC visit and their corresponding 97.5% confidence intervals for the differences between rates (CIPRO XR minus control arm) are given below for the Per Protocol population analysis:

[See second table at right]

Of the 166 cUTI patients treated with CIPRO XR, 148 (89%) had the causative organism(s) eradicated, 8 (5%) had persistence, 5 (3%) patients developed superinfections and 5 (3%) developed new infections. Of the 177 cUTI patients treated in the control arm, 144 (81%) had the causative organism(s) eradicated, 16 (9%) patients had persistence, 3 (2%) developed superinfections and 14 (8%) developed new infections. Of the 40 patients with AUP treated with CIPRO XR, 35 (87.5%) had the causative organism(s) eradicated, 2 (5%) patients had persistence and 3 (7.5%) developed new infections. Of the 5 CIPRO XR AUP patients without eradication at TOC, 4 were considered clinical cures and did not receive alternative antibiotic therapy. Of the 52 patients with AUP treated in the control arm, 51 (98%) had the causative organism(s) eradicated. One patient (2%) had persistence.

REFERENCES

1. NCCLS, Methods for Dilution Antimicrobial Susceptibility Tests for Bacteria That Grow Aerobically-Sixth Edition. Approved Standard NCCLS Document M7-A6, Vol. 23, No. 2, NCCLS, Wayne, PA, January, 2003.
2. NCCLS, Performance Standards for Antimicrobial Disk Susceptibility Tests-Eighth Edition. Approved Standard NCCLS Document M2-A8, Vol. 23, No. 1, NCCLS, Wayne, PA, January, 2003.

	CIPRO XR 500 mg QD × 3 Days	CIPRO 250 mg BID × 3 Days
Randomized Patients	452	453
Per Protocol Patients†	199	223
Bacteriologic Eradication at TOC (n/N)*	188/199 (94.5%)	209/223 (93.7%)
	CI [−3.5%, 5.1%]	
Bacteriologic Eradication (by organism) at TOC (n/N)**		
E. coli	156/160 (97.5%)	176/181 (97.2%)
E. faecalis	10/11 (90.9%)	17/21 (81.0%)
P. mirabilis	11/12 (91.7%)	7/7 (100%)
S. saprophyticus	6/7 (85.7%)	9/9 (100%)
Clinical Response at TOC (n/N)***	189/199 (95.0%)	204/223 (91.5%)
	CI [−1.1%, 8.1%]	

* n/N = patients with baseline organism(s) eradicated and no new infections or superinfections/total number of patients
** n/N = patients with specified baseline organism eradicated/patients with specified baseline organism
*** n/N = patients with clinical success/total number of patients
† The presence of a pathogen at a level of ≥ 10^5 CFU/mL was required for microbiological evaluability criteria, except for *S. saprophyticus* (≥ 10^4 CFU/mL).

	CIPRO XR 1000 mg QD	CIPRO 500 mg BID
Randomized Patients	521	521
Per Protocol Patient^	206	229
cUTI Patients		
Bacteriologic Eradication at TOC (n/N)*	148/166 (89.2%)	144/177 (81.4%)
	CI [−0.7%, 16.3%]	
Bacteriologic Eradication (by organism) at TOC (n/N)**		
E. coli	91/94 (96.8%)	90/92 (97.8%)
K. pneumoniae	20/21 (95.2%)	19/23 (82.6%)
E. faecalis	17/17 (100%)	14/21 (66.7%)
P. mirabilis	11/12 (91.6%)	10/10 (100%)
P. aeruginosa	3/3 (100%)	3/3 (100%)
Clinical Cure at TOC (n/N)***	159/166 (95.8%)	161/177 (91.0%)
	CI [−1.1%, 10.8%]	
AUP Patients		
Bacteriologic Eradication at TOC (n/N)*	35/40 (87.5%)	51/52 (98.1%)
	CI [−34.8%, 6.2%]	
Bacteriologic Eradication of *E. coli* at TOC (n/N)**	35/36 (97.2%)	41/41 (100%)
Clinical Cure at TOC (n/N)***	39/40 (97.5%)	50/52 (96.2%)
	CI [−15.3%, 21.1%]	

^Patients excluded from the Per Protocol population were primarily those with no causative organism(s) at baseline or no organism present at ≥ 10^5 CFU/mL at baseline, inclusion criteria violation, no valid test-of-cure urine culture within the TOC window, an organism resistant to study drug, premature discontinuation due to an adverse event, lost to follow-up, or non-compliance with dosage regimen (among other criteria).
* n/N = patients with baseline organism(s) eradicated and no new infections or superinfections/total number of patients
**n/N = patients with specified baseline organism eradicated/patients with specified baseline organism
***n/N = patients with clinical success/total number of patients

PATIENT INFORMATION ABOUT CIPRO® XR

(ciprofloxacin extended-release tablets)

This section contains important patient information about CIPRO XR and should be read completely before you begin treatment. This section does not take the place of discussion with your doctor or health care professional about your medical condition or your treatment. This section does not list all benefits and risks of CIPRO XR. CIPRO XR can be prescribed only by a licensed health care professional. Your doctor has prescribed CIPRO XR only for you.

CIPRO XR is intended only to treat urinary tract infections and acute uncomplicated pyelonephritis (also known as a kidney infection). It should not be used to treat other infections. Do not give it to other people even if they have a similar condition. Do not use it for a condition for which it was not prescribed. If you have any concerns about your condition or your medicine, ask your doctor. Only your doctor can determine if CIPRO XR is right for you.

What is CIPRO XR?

CIPRO XR is an antibiotic in the quinolone class that contains the active ingredient ciprofloxacin. CIPRO XR is specifically formulated to be taken just once daily to kill bacteria causing infection in the urinary tract. CIPRO XR has been shown in clinical trials to be effective in the treatment of urinary tract infections. You should contact your doctor if your condition is not improving while taking CIPRO XR.

CIPRO XR tablets are nearly white to slightly yellowish, film-coated, oblong-shaped tablets. CIPRO XR is available in 500 mg and 1000 mg tablet strengths.

How and when should I take CIPRO XR?

CIPRO XR should be taken once a day for three (3) to fourteen (14) days depending on your infection. Take CIPRO XR at approximately the same time each day with food or on an empty stomach. CIPRO XR should not be taken with dairy products (like milk or yogurt) or calcium-fortified juices alone; however, CIPRO XR may be taken with a meal that contains these products. Should you forget to take it at the usual time, you may take your dose later in the day. Do not take more than one CIPRO XR tablet per day even if you missed a dose. Swallow the CIPRO XR tablet whole. **DO NOT SPLIT, CRUSH, OR CHEW THE TABLET.**

Continued on next page

Cipro XR—Cont.

You should take CIPRO XR for as long as your doctor prescribes it, even after you start to feel better. Stopping an antibiotic too early may result in failure to cure your infection.

What should not take CIPRO XR?

You should not take CIPRO XR if you have ever had a severe reaction to any of the group of antibiotics known as "quinolones."

CIPRO XR is not recommended for use during pregnancy or nursing, as the effects on the unborn child or nursing infant are unknown. If you are pregnant or plan to become pregnant while taking CIPRO XR, talk to your doctor before taking this medication.

CIPRO XR is not recommended for persons less than 18 years of age.

What are the possible side effects of CIPRO XR?

CIPRO XR is generally well tolerated. The most common side effects, which are usually mild, include nausea, headache, dyspepsia, dizziness, vaginal yeast infection and diarrhea. If diarrhea persists, call your health care professional. Antibiotics of the quinolone class may also cause vomiting, rash, and abdominal pain/discomfort.

You should be careful about driving or operating machinery until you are sure CIPRO XR is not causing dizziness.

Rare cases of allergic reactions have been reported in patients receiving quinolones, including ciprofloxacin, even after just one dose. If you develop hives, difficulty breathing, or other symptoms of a severe allergic reaction, seek emergency treatment right away. If you develop a skin rash, you should stop taking CIPRO XR and call your health care professional.

Some patients taking quinolone antibiotics may become more sensitive to sunlight or ultraviolet light such as that used in tanning salons. You should avoid excessive exposure to sunlight or ultraviolet light while you are taking CIPRO XR.

Ciprofloxacin has been rarely associated with inflammation of tendons. If you experience pain, swelling or rupture of a tendon, you should stop taking CIPRO XR and call your health care professional.

Convulsions have been reported in patients receiving quinolone antibiotics including ciprofloxacin. If you have experienced convulsions in the past, be sure to let your physician know that you have a history of convulsions. Quinolones, including ciprofloxacin, have been rarely associated with other central nervous system events including confusion, tremors, hallucinations, and depression.

If you notice any side effects not mentioned in this section, or if you have any concerns about side effects you may be experiencing, please inform your health care professional.

What about other medications I am taking?

CIPRO XR can affect how other medicines work. Tell your doctor about all other prescriptions and nonprescription medicines or supplements you are taking. This is especially important if you are taking theophylline or VIDEX® (didanosine) chewable/buffered tablets or pediatric powder. Other medications including warfarin, glyburide, and phenytoin may also interact with CIPRO XR.

Many antacids, multivitamins, and other dietary supplements containing magnesium, calcium, aluminum, iron or zinc can interfere with the absorption of CIPRO XR and may prevent it from working. You should take CIPRO XR either 2 hours before or 6 hours after taking these products.

Remember:

Do not give CIPRO XR to anyone other than the person for whom it was prescribed.

Complete the course of CIPRO XR even if you are feeling better.

Keep CIPRO XR and all medications out of reach of children.

This information does not take the place of discussions with your doctor or health care professional about your medication or treatment.

℞ Only

Bayer HealthCare
Bayer Pharmaceuticals Corporation
400 Morgan Lane
West Haven, CT 06516
Made in Germany
08852106, R.4 Bay o 9867/q 3939 4/04 12313

Printed in U.S.A.

Shown in Product Identification Guide, page 308

DTIC-Dome® ℞
(dacarbazine)
Sterile

> **WARNING**
>
> It is recommended that DTIC-Dome (dacarbazine) be administered under the supervision of a qualified physician experienced in the use of cancer chemotherapeutic agents.
>
> 1. Hemopoietic depression is the most common toxicity with DTIC-Dome (See Warnings).
> 2. Hepatic necrosis has been reported (See Warnings).
> 3. Studies have demonstrated this agent to have a carcinogenic and teratogenic effect when used in animals.
> 4. In treatment of each patient, the physician must weigh carefully the possibility of achieving therapeutic benefit against the risk of toxicity.

DESCRIPTION

DTIC-Dome Sterile (dacarbazine) is a colorless to an ivory colored solid which is light sensitive. Each vial contains 100 mg of dacarbazine, or 200 mg of dacarbazine (the active ingredient), anhydrous citric acid and mannitol. DTIC-Dome is reconstituted and administered intravenously (pH 3–4). DTIC-Dome is an anticancer agent. Chemically, DTIC-Dome is 5-(3,3-dimethyl-l-triazeno)-imidazole-4-carboxamide (DTIC) with the following structural formula:

$(CH_3)_2N{-}N{=}N$ … $H_2N{-}C(=O)$ … $C_6H_{10}N_6O$

CLINICAL PHARMACOLOGY

After intravenous administration of DTIC-Dome, the volume of distribution exceeds total body water content suggesting localization in some body tissue, probably the liver. Its disappearance from the plasma is biphasic with initial half-life of 19 minutes and a terminal half-life of 5 hours.[1] In a patient with renal and hepatic dysfunctions, the half-lives were lengthened to 55 minutes and 7.2 hours.[1] The average cumulative excretion of unchanged DTIC in the urine is 40% of the injected dose in 6 hours.[1] DTIC is subject to renal tubular secretion rather than glomerular filtration. At therapeutic concentrations DTIC is not appreciably bound to human plasma protein.

In man, DTIC is extensively degraded. Besides unchanged DTIC, 5-aminoimidazole -4 carboxamide (AIC) is a major metabolite of DTIC excreted in the urine. AIC is not derived endogenously but from the injected DTIC, because the administration of radioactive DTIC labeled with ^{14}C in the imidazole portion of the molecule (DTIC-2-^{14}C) gives rise to AIC-2-^{14}C.[1]

Although the exact mechanism of action of DTIC-Dome is not known, three hypotheses have been offered:

1. inhibition of DNA synthesis by acting as a purine analog
2. action as an alkylating agent
3. interaction with SH groups

INDICATIONS AND USAGE

DTIC-Dome is indicated in the treatment of metastatic malignant melanoma. In addition, DTIC-Dome is also indicated for Hodgkin's disease as a secondary-line therapy when used in combination with other effective agents.

CONTRAINDICATIONS

DTIC-Dome is contraindicated in patients who have demonstrated a hypersensitivity to it in the past.

WARNINGS

Hemopoietic depression is the most common toxicity with DTIC-Dome and involves primarily the leukocytes and platelets, although, anemia may sometimes occur. Leukopenia and thrombocytopenia may be severe enough to cause death. The possible bone marrow depression requires careful monitoring of white blood cells, red blood cells, and platelet levels. Hemopoietic toxicity may warrant temporary suspension or cessation of therapy with DTIC-Dome.

Hepatic toxicity accompanied by hepatic vein thrombosis and hepatocellular necrosis resulting in death, has been reported. The incidence of such reactions has been low; approximately 0.01% of patients treated. This toxicity has been observed mostly when DTIC-Dome has been administered concomitantly with other anti-neoplastic drugs; however, it has also been reported in some patients treated with DTIC-Dome alone.

Anaphylaxis can occur following the administration of DTIC-Dome.

PRECAUTIONS

Hospitalization is not always necessary but adequate laboratory study capability must be available. Extravasation of the drug subcutaneously during intravenous administration may result in tissue damage and severe pain. Local pain, burning sensation, and irritation at the site of injection may be relieved by locally applied hot packs.

Carcinogenicity of DTIC was studied in rats and mice. Proliferative endocardial lesions, including fibrosarcomas and sarcomas were induced by DTIC in rats. In mice, administration of DTIC resulted in the induction of angiosarcomas of the spleen.

Pregnancy Category C. DTIC-Dome has been shown to be teratogenic in rats when given in doses 20 times the human daily dose on day 12 of gestation. DTIC when administered in 10 times the human daily dose to male rats (twice weekly for 9 weeks) did not affect the male libido, although female rats mated to male rats had higher incidence of resorptions than controls. In rabbits, DTIC daily dose 7 times the human daily dose given on Days 6–15 of gestation resulted in fetal skeletal anomalies. There are no adequate and well controlled studies in pregnant women. DTIC-Dome should be used during pregnancy only if the potential benefit justifies the potential risk to the fetus.

It is not known whether this drug is excreted in human milk. Because many drugs are excreted in human milk and because of the potential for tumorigenicity shown for DTIC-Dome in animal studies, a decision should be made whether to discontinue nursing or to discontinue the drug, taking into account the importance of the drug to the mother.

ADVERSE REACTIONS

Symptoms of anorexia, nausea, and vomiting are the most frequently noted of all toxic reactions. Over 90% of patients are affected with the initial few doses. The vomiting lasts 1–12 hours and is incompletely and unpredictably palliated with phenobarbital and/or prochlorperazine. Rarely, intractable nausea and vomiting have necessitated discontinuance of therapy with DTIC-Dome. Rarely, DTIC-Dome has caused diarrhea. Some helpful suggestions include restricting the patient's oral intake of food for 4–6 hours prior to treatment. The rapid toleration of these symptoms suggests that a central nervous system mechanism may be involved, and usually these symptoms subside after the first 1 or 2 days.

There are a number of minor toxicities that are infrequently noted. Patients have experienced an influenza-like syndrome of fever to 39°C, myalgias and malaise. These symptoms occur usually after large single doses, may last for several days, and they may occur with successive treatments. Alopecia has been noted as has facial flushing and facial paresthesia. There have been few reports of significant liver or renal function test abnormalities in man. However, these abnormalities have been observed more frequently in animal studies.

Erythematous and urticarial rashes have been observed infrequently after administration of DTIC-Dome. Rarely, photosensitivity reactions may occur.

OVERDOSAGE

Give supportive treatment and monitor blood cell counts.

DOSAGE AND ADMINISTRATION

Malignant Melanoma: The recommended dosage is 2 to 4.5mg/kg/day for 10 days. Treatment may be repeated at 4 week intervals.[2]

An alternate recommended dosage is 250mg/square meter body surface/day I.V. for 5 days. Treatment may be repeated every 3 weeks.[3,4]

Hodgkin's Disease: The recommended dosage of DTIC-Dome in the treatment of Hodgkin's disease is 150mg/square meter body surface/day for 5 days, in combination with other effective drugs. Treatment may be repeated every 4 weeks.[5] An alternative recommended dosage is 375mg/square meter body surface on day 1, in combination with other effective drugs, to be repeated every 15 days.[6]

DTIC-Dome (dacarbazine) 100mg/vial and 200mg/vial are reconstituted with 9.9 mL and 19.7 mL, respectively, of Sterile Water for Injection, U.S.P. The resulting solution contains 10mg/mL of dacarbazine having a pH of 3.0 to 4.0. The calculated dose of the resulting solution is drawn into a syringe and administered *only* intravenously.

The reconstituted solution may be further diluted with 5% dextrose injection, U.S.P. or sodium chloride injection, U.S.P. and administered as an intravenous infusion.

After reconstitution and prior to use, the solution in the vial may be stored at 4°C for up to 72 hours or at normal room conditions (temperature and light) for up to 8 hours. If the reconstituted solution is further diluted in 5% dextrose injection, U.S.P. or sodium chloride injection, U.S.P., the resulting solution may be stored at 4°C for up to 24 hours or at normal room conditions for up to 8 hours.

Procedures for proper handling and disposal of anticancer drugs should be considered. Several guidelines on this subject have been published.[7–12] There is no general agreement that all of the procedures recommended in the guidelines are necessary or appropriate.

HOW SUPPLIED

20 mL vials containing 200 mg of DTIC-Dome as sterile dacarbazine in boxes of 12. Store in a refrigerator 2°C to 8°C (36°F to 46°F).

REFERENCES

1. Loo, T.J., *et al.*: Mechanism of action and pharmacology studies with DTIC (NSC-45388). Cancer Treatment Reports 60: 149–152, 1976.
2. Nathanson, L., *et al.*: Characteristics of prognosis and response to an imidazole carboxamide in malignant melanoma. Clinical Pharmacology and Therapeutics 12: 955–962, 1971.
3. Costanza, M.E., *et al.*: Therapy of malignant melanoma with an imidazole carboxamide and bischloroethyl nitrosourea. Cancer 30: 1457–1461, 1972.
4. Luce, J.K., *et al.*: Clinical trials with the antitumor agent 5-(3, 3-dimethyl-l-triazeno) imidazole-4-carboxamide (NSC-45388). Cancer Chemotherapy Reports 54: 119–124, 1970.
5. Bonadonna, G., *et al.*: Combined Chemotherapy (MOPP or ABVD)—radiotherapy approach in advanced Hodgkin's disease. Cancer Treatment Reports 61: 769–777, 1977.
6. Santoro, A., and Bonadonna, G.: Prolonged disease-free survival in MOPP-resistant Hodgkin's disease after treatment with adriamycin, bleomycin, vinblastine and dacarbazine (ABVD). Cancer Chemotherapy Pharmacol. 2: 101–105, 1979.
7. Recommendations for the Safe Handling of Parenteral Antineoplastic Drugs. NIH Publication No. 83-2621. For

sale by the Superintendent of Documents, U.S. Government Printing Office, Washington, D.C. 20402.
8. AMA Council Report. Guidelines for Handling Parenteral Antineoplastics. JAMA, March 15, 1985.
9. National Study Commission on Cytotoxic Exposure—Recommendations for Handling Cytotoxic Agents. Available from Louis P. Jeffrey, Sc. D., Director of Pharmacy Services, Rhode Island Hospital, 593 Eddy Street, Providence, Rhode Island 02902.
10. Clinical Oncological Society of Australia: Guidelines and recommendations for safe handling of antineoplastic agents. Med. J. Australia 1: 426–428, 1983.
11. Jones, R.B., *et al.*: Safe handling of chemotherapeutic agents: A report from the Mount Sinai Medical Center. Ca-A Cancer Journal for Clinicians Sept./Oct. 258–263, 1983.
12. American Society of Hospital Pharmacists technical assistance bulletin on handling cytotoxic drugs in hospitals. Am. J. Hosp. Pharm. 42: 131–137, 1985.

Manufactured by:
Ben Venue Laboratories
Bedford, Ohio 44146
Distributed by:
Bayer Pharmaceuticals Corporation
400 Morgan Lane
West Haven, CT 06516 USA
℞ Only
08844898, R.O 5/03 11778

LEVITRA® ℞

[lĕ-vē-tră]
(vardenafil HCl)
TABLETS

DESCRIPTION

LEVITRA® is an oral therapy for the treatment of erectile dysfunction. This monohydrochloride salt of vardenafil is a selective inhibitor of cyclic guanosine monophosphate (cGMP)-specific phosphodiesterase type 5 (PDE5).

Vardenafil HCl is designated chemically as piperazine, 1-[[3-(1,4-dihydro-5-methyl-4-oxo-7-propylimidazo[5,1-*f*][1,2,4]triazin-2-yl)-4-ethoxyphenyl]sulfonyl]-4-ethyl-, monohydrochloride and has the following structural formula:

x HCl x $3H_2O$

Vardenafil HCl is a nearly colorless, solid substance with a molecular weight of 579.1 g/mol and a solubility of 0.11 mg/mL in water. LEVITRA is formulated as orange, round, film-coated tablets with "BAYER" cross debossed on one side and "2.5", "5", "10", and "20" on the other side corresponding to 2.5 mg, 5 mg, 10 mg, and 20 mg of vardenafil, respectively. In addition to the active ingredient, vardenafil HCl, each tablet contains microcrystalline cellulose, crospovidone, colloidal silicon dioxide, magnesium stearate, hypromellose, polyethylene glycol, titanium dioxide, yellow ferric oxide, and red ferric oxide.

CLINICAL PHARMACOLOGY

Mechanism of Action

Penile erection is a hemodynamic process initiated by the relaxation of smooth muscle in the corpus cavernosum and its associated arterioles. During sexual stimulation, nitric oxide is released from nerve endings and endothelial cells in the corpus cavernosum. Nitric oxide activates the enzyme guanylate cyclase resulting in increased synthesis of cyclic guanosine monophosphate (cGMP) in the smooth muscle cells of the corpus cavernosum. The cGMP in turn triggers smooth muscle relaxation, allowing increased blood flow into the penis, resulting in erection. The tissue concentration of cGMP is regulated by both the rates of synthesis and degradation via phosphodiesterases (PDEs). The most abundant PDE in the human corpus cavernosum is the cGMP-specific phosphodiesterase type 5 (PDE5); therefore, the inhibition of PDE5 enhances erectile function by increasing the amount of cGMP. Because sexual stimulation is required to initiate the local release of nitric oxide, the inhibition of PDE5 has no effect in the absence of sexual stimulation.

In vitro studies have shown that vardenafil is a selective inhibitor of PDE5. The inhibitory effect of vardenafil is more selective on PDE5 than for other known phosphodiesterases (>15-fold relative to PDE6, >130-fold relative to PDE1, >300-fold relative to PDE11, and >1,000-fold relative to PDE2, 3, 4, 7, 8, 9, and 10).

Pharmacokinetics

The pharmacokinetics of vardenafil are approximately dose proportional over the recommended dose range. Vardenafil is eliminated predominantly by hepatic metabolism, mainly by CYP3A4 and to a minor extent, CYP2C isoforms. Concomitant use with strong CYP3A4 inhibitors such as ritonavir, indinavir, ketoconazole, itraconazole as well as moderate CYP3A inhibitors such as erythromycin results in significant increases of plasma levels of vardenafil (see **PRECAUTIONS, WARNINGS** and **DOSAGE AND ADMINISTRATION**). Mean vardenafil plasma concentrations measured after the administration of a single oral dose of 20 mg to healthy male volunteers are depicted in Figure 1.

Figure 1: Plasma Vardenafil Concentration (Mean ± SD) Curve for a Single 20 mg LEVITRA Dose

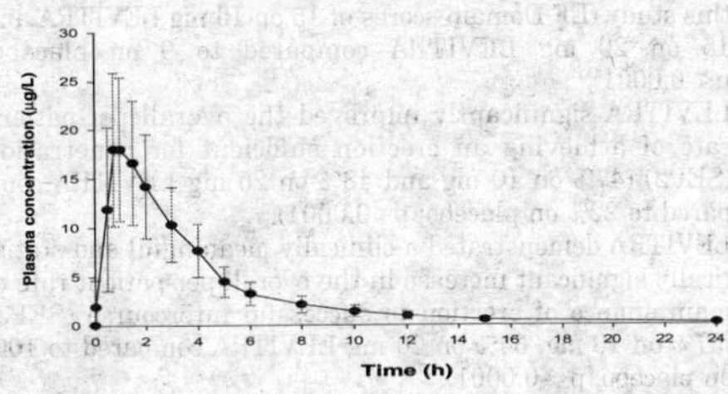

Absorption: Vardenafil is rapidly absorbed with absolute bioavailability of approximately 15%. Maximum observed plasma concentrations after a single 20 mg dose in healthy volunteers are usually reached between 30 minutes and 2 hours (median 60 minutes) after oral dosing in the fasted state. Two food-effect studies were conducted which showed that high-fat meals caused a reduction in C_{max} by 18%-50%.

Distribution: The mean steady-state volume of distribution (Vss) for vardenafil is 208 L, indicating extensive tissue distribution. Vardenafil and its major circulating metabolite, M1, are highly bound to plasma proteins (about 95% for parent drug and M1). This protein binding is reversible and independent of total drug concentrations.

Following a single oral dose of 20 mg vardenafil in healthy volunteers, a mean of 0.00018% of the administered dose was obtained in semen 1.5 hours after dosing.

Metabolism: Vardenafil is metabolized predominantly by the hepatic enzyme CYP3A4, with contribution from the CYP3A5 and CYP2C isoforms. The major circulating metabolite, M1, results from desethylation at the piperazine moiety of vardenafil. M1 is subject to further metabolism. The plasma concentration of M1 is approximately 26% that of the parent compound. This metabolite shows a phosphodiesterase selectivity profile similar to that of vardenafil and an *in vitro* inhibitory potency for PDE5 28% of that of vardenafil. Therefore, M1 accounts for approximately 7% of total pharmacologic activity.

Excretion: The total body clearance of vardenafil is 56 L/h, and the terminal half-life of vardenafil and its primary metabolite (M1) is approximately 4-5 hours. After oral administration, vardenafil is excreted as metabolites predominantly in the feces (approximately 91-95% of administered oral dose) and to a lesser extent in the urine (approximately 2–6% of administered oral dose).

Pharmacokinetics in Special Populations

Pediatrics: Vardenafil trials were not conducted in the pediatric population.

Geriatrics: In a healthy volunteer study of elderly males (≥ 65 years) and younger males (18–45 years), mean C_{max} and AUC were 34% and 52% higher, respectively, in the elderly males (see **PRECAUTIONS, Geriatric Use** and **DOSAGE AND ADMINISTRATION**). Consequently, a lower starting dose of LEVITRA (5 mg) in patients ≥ 65 years of age should be considered.

Renal Insufficiency: In volunteers with mild renal impairment (CL_{cr} = 50–80 ml/min), the pharmacokinetics of vardenafil were similar to those observed in a control group with normal renal function. In the moderate (CL_{cr} = 30–50 ml/min) or severe (CL_{cr} <30 ml/min) renal impairment groups, the AUC of vardenafil was 20–30% higher compared to that observed in a control group with normal renal function (CL_{cr} >80 ml/min). Vardenafil pharmacokinetics have not been evaluated in patients requiring renal dialysis (see **PRECAUTIONS, Renal Insufficiency,** and **DOSAGE AND ADMINISTRATION**).

Hepatic Insufficiency: In volunteers with mild hepatic impairment (Child-Pugh A), the C_{max} and AUC following a 10 mg vardenafil dose were increased by 22% and 17%, respectively, compared to healthy control subjects. In volunteers with moderate hepatic impairment (Child-Pugh B), the C_{max} and AUC following a 10 mg vardenafil dose were increased by 130% and 160%, respectively, compared to healthy control subjects. Consequently, a starting dose of 5 mg is recommended for patients with moderate hepatic impairment, and the maximum dose should not exceed 10 mg (see **PRECAUTIONS** and **DOSAGE AND ADMINISTRATION**). Vardenafil has not been evaluated in patients with severe (Child-Pugh C) hepatic impairment.

Pharmacodynamics

Effects on Blood Pressure: In a clinical pharmacology study of patients with erectile dysfunction, single doses of vardenafil 20 mg caused a mean maximum decrease in supine blood pressure of 7 mm Hg systolic and 8 mm Hg diastolic (compared to placebo), accompanied by a mean maximum increase of heart rate of 4 beats per minute. The maximum decrease in blood pressure occurred between 1 and 4 hours after dosing. Following multiple dosing for 31 days, similar blood pressure responses were observed on Day 31 as on Day 1. Vardenafil may add to the blood pressure lowering effects of antihypertensive agents (see **CONTRAINDICATIONS, PRECAUTIONS, Drug Interactions**).

Effects on Blood Pressure and Heart Rate when LEVITRA is Combined with Nitrates: A study was conducted in which the blood pressure and heart rate response to 0.4 mg nitroglycerin (NTG) sublingually was evaluated in 18 healthy subjects following pretreatment with LEVITRA 20 mg at various times before NTG administration. LEVITRA 20 mg caused an additional time-related reduction in blood pressure and increase in heart rate in association with NTG administration. The blood pressure effects were observed when LEVITRA 20 mg was dosed 1 or 4 hours before NTG and the heart rate effects were observed when 20 mg was dosed 1, 4, or 8 hours before NTG. Additional blood pressure and heart rate changes were not detected when LEVITRA 20 mg was dosed 24 hours before NTG. (See Figure 2.)

Figure 2: Placebo-subtracted point estimates (with 90% CI) of mean maximal blood pressure and heart rate effects of pre-dosing with LEVITRA 20 mg at 24, 8, 4, and 1 hour before 0.4 mg NTG sublingually.

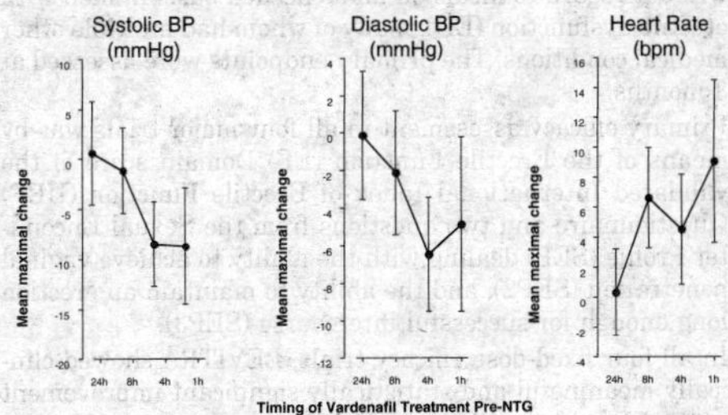

Because the disease state of patients requiring nitrate therapy is anticipated to increase the likelihood of hypotension, the use of vardenafil by patients on nitrate therapy or on nitric oxide donors is contraindicated (see **CONTRAINDICATIONS**).

Electrophysiology: The effect of 10 mg and 80 mg vardenafil on QT interval was evaluated in a single-dose, double-blind, randomized, placebo- and active-controlled (moxifloxacin 400 mg) crossover study in 59 healthy males (81% White, 12% Black, 7% Hispanic) aged 45-60 years. The QT interval was measured at one hour post dose because this time point approximates the average time of peak vardenafil concentration. The 80 mg dose of LEVITRA (four times the highest recommended dose) was chosen because this dose yields plasma concentrations covering those observed upon co-administration of a low-dose of LEVITRA (5 mg) and 600 mg BID of ritonavir. Of the CYP3A4 inhibitors that have been studied, ritonavir causes the most significant drug-drug interaction with vardenafil. Table 1 summarizes the effect on mean uncorrected QT and mean corrected QT interval (QT_c) with different methods of correction (Fridericia and a linear individual correction method) at one hour post-dose. No single correction method is known to be more valid than the other. In this study, the mean increase in heart rate associated with a 10 mg dose of LEVITRA compared to placebo was 5 beats/minute and with an 80 mg dose of LEVITRA the mean increase was 6 beats/minute. [See table 1 above]

Table 1. Mean QT and QT_c changes in msec (90% CI) from baseline relative to placebo at 1 hour post-dose with different methodologies to correct for the effect of heart rate.

Drug/Dose	QT Uncorrected (msec)	Fridericia QT Correction (msec)	Individual QT Correction (msec)
Vardenafil 10 mg	-2 (-4, 0)	8 (6, 9)	4 (3, 6)
Vardenafil 80 mg	-2 (-4, 0)	10 (8, 11)	6 (4, 7)
Moxifloxacin* 400 mg	3 (1, 5)	8 (6, 9)	7 (5, 8)

* Active control (drug known to prolong QT)

Therapeutic and supratherapeutic doses of vardenafil and the active control moxifloxacin produced similar increases

Continued on next page

Levitra—Cont.

in QT_c interval. This study, however, was not designed to make direct statistical comparisons between the drug or the dose levels. The clinical impact of these QT_c changes is unknown (see **PRECAUTIONS**).

Effects on Exercise Treadmill Test in Patients with Coronary Artery Disease (CAD): In two independent trials that assessed 10 mg (n=41) and 20 mg (n=39) vardenafil, respectively, vardenafil did not alter the total treadmill exercise time compared to placebo. The patient population included men aged 40–80 years with stable exercise-induced angina documented by at least one of the following: 1) prior history of MI, CABG, PTCA, or stenting (not within 6 months); 2) positive coronary angiogram showing at least 60% narrowing of the diameter of at least one major coronary artery; or 3) a positive stress echocardiogram or stress nuclear perfusion study.

Results of these studies showed that LEVITRA did not alter the total treadmill exercise time compared to placebo (10 mg LEVITRA vs. placebo: 433±109 and 426±105 seconds, respectively; 20 mg LEVITRA vs. placebo: 414±114 and 411±124 seconds, respectively). The total time to angina was not altered by LEVITRA when compared to placebo (10 mg LEVITRA vs. placebo: 291±123 and 292±110 seconds; 20 mg LEVITRA vs. placebo: 354±137 and 347±143 seconds, respectively). The total time to 1 mm or greater ST-segment depression was similar to placebo in both the 10 mg and the 20 mg LEVITRA groups (10 mg LEVITRA vs. placebo: 380±108 and 334±108 seconds; 20 mg LEVITRA vs. placebo: 364±101 and 366±105 seconds, respectively).

Effects on Vision: Single oral doses of phosphodiesterase inhibitors have demonstrated transient dose-related impairment of color discrimination (blue/green) using the Farnsworth-Munsell 100-hue test and reductions in electroretinogram (ERG) b-wave amplitudes, with peak effects near the time of peak plasma levels. These findings are consistent with the inhibition of PDE6 in rods and cones, which is involved in phototransduction in the retina. The findings were most evident one hour after administration, diminishing but still present 6 hours after administration. In a single dose study in 25 normal males, LEVITRA 40 mg, twice the maximum daily recommended dose, did not alter visual acuity, intraocular pressure, fundoscopic and slit lamp findings.

CLINICAL STUDIES

LEVITRA was evaluated in four major double-blind, randomized, placebo-controlled, fixed-dose, parallel design, multicenter trials in 2431 men aged 20–83 (mean age 57 years; 78% White, 7% Black, 2% Asian, 3% Hispanic and 10% Other/Unknown). The doses of LEVITRA in these studies were 5 mg, 10 mg, and 20 mg. Two of these trials were conducted in the general ED population and two in special ED populations (one in patients with diabetes mellitus and one in post-prostatectomy patients). LEVITRA was dosed without regard to meals on an as needed basis in men with erectile dysfunction (ED), many of whom had multiple other medical conditions. The primary endpoints were assessed at 3 months.

Primary efficacy assessment in all four major trials was by means of the Erectile Function (EF) Domain score of the validated International Index of Erectile Function (IIEF) Questionnaire and two questions from the Sexual Encounter Profile (SEP) dealing with the ability to achieve vaginal penetration (SEP2), and the ability to maintain an erection long enough for successful intercourse (SEP3).

In all four fixed-dose efficacy trials, LEVITRA showed clinically meaningful and statistically significant improvement in the EF Domain, SEP2, and SEP3 scores compared to placebo. The mean baseline EF Domain score in these trials was 11.8 (scores range from 0–30 where lower scores represent more severe disease). LEVITRA (5 mg, 10 mg, and 20 mg) was effective in all age categories (<45, 45 to <65, and ≥65 years) and was also effective regardless of race (White, Black, Other).

Trials in a General Erectile Dysfunction Population: In the major North American fixed-dose trial, 762 patients (mean age 57, range 20–83 years; 79% White, 13% Black, 4% Hispanic, 2% Asian and 2% Other) were evaluated. The mean baseline EF Domain scores were 13, 13, 13, 14 for the LEVITRA 5 mg, 10 mg, 20 mg and placebo groups, respectively. There was significant improvement ($p<0.0001$) at 3 months with LEVITRA (EF Domain scores of 18, 21, 21, for the 5 mg, 10 mg, and 20 mg dose groups, respectively) compared to the placebo group (EF Domain score of 15). The European trial (total N=803) confirmed these results. The improvement in mean score was maintained at all doses at 6 months in the North American trial.

In the North American trial, LEVITRA significantly improved the rates of achieving an erection sufficient for penetration (SEP2) at doses of 5 mg, 10 mg, and 20 mg compared to placebo (65%, 75%, and 80%, respectively, compared to a 52% response in the placebo group at 3 months; $p< 0.0001$). The European trial confirmed these results.

LEVITRA demonstrated a clinically meaningful and statistically significant increase in the overall per-patient rate of maintenance of erection to successful intercourse (SEP3) (51% on 5 mg, 64% on 10 mg, and 65% on 20 mg, respectively, compared to 32% on placebo; $p< 0.0001$) at 3 months in the North American trial. The European trial showed comparable efficacy. This improvement in mean score was maintained at all doses at 6 months in the North American trial.

Trial in Patients with ED and Diabetes Mellitus: LEVITRA demonstrated clinically meaningful and statistically significant improvement in erectile function in a prospective, fixed-dose (10 and 20 mg LEVITRA), double-blind, placebo-controlled trial of patients with diabetes mellitus (n=439; mean age 57 years, range 33–81; 80% White, 9% Black, 8% Hispanic, and 3% Other).

Significant improvements in the EF Domain were shown in this study (EF Domain scores of 17 on 10 mg LEVITRA and 19 on 20 mg LEVITRA compared to 13 on placebo; $p< 0.0001$).

LEVITRA significantly improved the overall per-patient rate of achieving an erection sufficient for penetration (SEP2) (61% on 10 mg and 64% on 20 mg LEVITRA compared to 36% on placebo; $p< 0.0001$).

LEVITRA demonstrated a clinically meaningful and statistically significant increase in the overall per-patient rate of maintenance of erection to successful intercourse (SEP3) (49% on 10 mg, 54% on 20 mg LEVITRA compared to 23% on placebo; $p< 0.0001$).

Trial in Patients with ED after Radical Prostatectomy: LEVITRA demonstrated clinically meaningful and statistically significant improvement in erectile function in a prospective, fixed-dose (10 and 20 mg LEVITRA), double-blind, placebo-controlled trial in post-prostatectomy patients (n=427, mean age 60, range 44-77 years; 93% White, 5% Black, 2% Other).

Significant improvements in the EF Domain were shown in this study (EF Domain scores of 15 on 10 mg LEVITRA and 15 on 20 mg LEVITRA compared to 9 on placebo; $p< 0.0001$).

LEVITRA significantly improved the overall per-patient rate of achieving an erection sufficient for penetration (SEP2) (47% on 10 mg and 48% on 20 mg LEVITRA compared to 22% on placebo; $p<0.0001$).

LEVITRA demonstrated a clinically meaningful and statistically significant increase in the overall per-patient rate of maintenance of erection to successful intercourse (SEP3) (37% on 10 mg, 34% on 20 mg LEVITRA compared to 10% on placebo; $p< 0.0001$).

INDICATIONS AND USAGE

LEVITRA is indicated for the treatment of erectile dysfunction.

CONTRAINDICATIONS

Nitrates: Administration of LEVITRA with nitrates (either regularly and/or intermittently) and nitric oxide donors is contraindicated (see **CLINICAL PHARMACOLOGY, Pharmacodynamics, Effects on Blood Pressure and Heart Rate when LEVITRA is Combined with Nitrates**). Consistent with the effects of PDE5 inhibition on the nitric oxide/cyclic guanosine monophosphate pathway, PDE5 inhibitors may potentiate the hypotensive effects of nitrates. A suitable time interval following LEVITRA dosing for the safe administration of nitrates or nitric oxide donors has not been determined.

Alpha-Blockers: Because the co-administration of alpha-blockers and LEVITRA can produce hypotension, LEVITRA is contraindicated in patients taking alpha-blockers (see **PRECAUTIONS, Drug Interactions**).

Hypersensitivity: LEVITRA is contraindicated for patients with a known hypersensitivity to any component of the tablet.

WARNINGS

Cardiovascular effects

General: Physicians should consider the cardiovascular status of their patients, since there is a degree of cardiac risk associated with sexual activity. In men for whom sexual activity is not recommended because of their underlying cardiovascular status, any treatment for erectile dysfunction, including LEVITRA, generally should not be used.

Left Ventricular Outflow Obstruction: Patients with left ventricular outflow obstruction, e.g., aortic stenosis and idiopathic hypertrophic subaortic stenosis, can be sensitive to the action of vasodilators including Type 5 phosphodiesterase inhibitors.

Blood Pressure Effects: LEVITRA has systemic vasodilatory properties that resulted in transient decreases in supine blood pressure in healthy volunteers (mean maximum decrease of 7 mmHg systolic and 8 mmHg diastolic) (see **CLINICAL PHARMACOLOGY, Pharmacodynamics**). While this normally would be expected to be of little consequence in most patients, prior to prescribing LEVITRA, physicians should carefully consider whether their patients with underlying cardiovascular disease could be affected adversely by such vasodilatory effects.

Effect of Co-administration of Strong CYP3A4 Inhibitors

Long-term safety information is not available on the concomitant administration of vardenafil with HIV protease inhibitors. Concomitant administration with ritonavir or indinavir substantially increases plasma concentrations of vardenafil. To decrease the chance of adverse events in patients concomitantly taking ritonavir or indinavir, which are strong inhibitors of CYP3A4 metabolism, a maximum single dose of 2.5 mg LEVITRA should not be exceeded. Because ritonavir prolongs LEVITRA elimination half-life (5-6-fold), no more than a single 2.5 mg dose of LEVITRA should be taken in a 72-hour period by patients also taking ritonavir. Patients taking indinavir, ketoconazole 400 mg daily, or itraconazole 400 mg daily should not exceed LEVITRA 2.5 mg once daily. For patients taking ketoconazole or itraconazole 200 mg daily, a single dose of 5 mg LEVITRA should not be exceeded in a 24-hour period (see **PRECAUTIONS, Drug Interactions** and **DOSAGE AND ADMINISTRATION**).

Other Effects

There have been rare reports of prolonged erections greater than 4 hours and priapism (painful erections greater than 6 hours in duration) for this class of compounds, including vardenafil. In the event that an erection persists longer than 4 hours, the patient should seek immediate medical assistance. If priapism is not treated immediately, penile tissue damage and permanent loss of potency may result.

Patient Subgroups Not Studied in Clinical Trials

There is no controlled clinical data on the safety or efficacy of LEVITRA in the following patients; and therefore its use is not recommended until further information is available.

- unstable angina; hypotension (resting systolic blood pressure of <90 mm Hg); uncontrolled hypertension (>170/110 mm Hg); recent history of stroke, life-threatening arrhythmia, or myocardial infarction (within the last 6 months); severe cardiac failure
- severe hepatic impairment (Child-Pugh C)
- end stage renal disease requiring dialysis
- known hereditary degenerative retinal disorders, including retinitis pigmentosa

PRECAUTIONS

The evaluation of erectile dysfunction should include a determination of potential underlying causes, a medical assessment, and the identification of appropriate treatment.

Before prescribing LEVITRA, it is important to note the following:

Hepatic Insufficiency: In volunteers with moderate impairment (Child-Pugh B), the C_{max} and AUC following a 10 mg vardenafil dose were increased 130% and 160%, respectively, compared to healthy control subjects. Consequently, a starting dose of 5 mg is recommended for patients with moderate hepatic impairment and the maximum dose should not exceed 10 mg (see **CLINICAL PHARMACOLOGY, Pharmacokinetics in Special Populations,** and **DOSAGE AND ADMINISTRATION**). Vardenafil has not been evaluated in patients with severe hepatic impairment (Child-Pugh C).

Congenital or Acquired QT Prolongation: In a study of the effect of LEVITRA on QT interval in 59 healthy males (see **CLINICAL PHARMACOLOGY, Electrophysiology**), therapeutic (10 mg) and supratherapeutic (80 mg) doses of LEVITRA and the active control moxifloxacin (400 mg) produced similar increases in QT_c interval. This observation should be considered in clinical decisions when prescribing LEVITRA. Patients with congenital QT prolongation and those taking Class IA (e.g., quinidine, procainamide) or Class III (e.g., amiodarone, sotalol) antiarrhythmic medications should avoid using LEVITRA.

Renal Insufficiency: In patients with moderate (CL_{cr} = 30–50 ml/min) to severe (CL_{cr} <30 ml/min) renal impairment, the AUC of vardenafil was 20–30% higher compared to that observed in a control group with normal renal function (CL_{cr} >80 ml/min) (see **CLINICAL PHARMACOLOGY, Pharmacokinetics in Special Populations**). Vardenafil pharmacokinetics have not been evaluated in patients requiring renal dialysis.

General: In humans, vardenafil alone in doses up to 20 mg does not prolong the bleeding time. There is no clinical evidence of any additive prolongation of the bleeding time when vardenafil is administered with aspirin. Vardenafil has not been administered to patients with bleeding disorders or significant active peptic ulceration. Therefore LEVITRA should be administered to these patients after careful benefit-risk assessment.

Treatment for erectile dysfunction should generally be used with caution by patients with anatomical deformation of the penis (such as angulation, cavernosal fibrosis, or Peyronie's disease) or by patients who have conditions that may predispose them to priapism (such as sickle cell anemia, multiple myeloma, or leukemia).

The safety and efficacy of LEVITRA used in combination with other treatments for erectile dysfunction have not been studied. Therefore, the use of such combinations is not recommended.

Information for Patients

Physicians should discuss with patients the contraindication of LEVITRA with regular and/or intermittent use of organic nitrates. Patients should be counseled that concomitant use of LEVITRA with nitrates could cause blood pressure to suddenly drop to an unsafe level, resulting in dizziness, syncope, or even heart attack or stroke.

Physicians should inform their patients that concomitant use of LEVITRA with alpha-blockers is contraindicated because co-administration can produce hypotension.

Physicians should discuss with patients the appropriate use of LEVITRA and its anticipated benefits. It should be explained that sexual stimulation is required for an erection to occur after taking LEVITRA. LEVITRA should be taken approximately 60 minutes before sexual activity. Patients should be counseled regarding the dosing of LEVITRA. Patients should be advised to contact their healthcare provider for dose modification if they are not satisfied with the quality of their sexual performance with LEVITRA or in the case of an unwanted effect. Patients should be advised to contact the prescribing physician if new medications that may interact with LEVITRA are prescribed by another healthcare provider.

Physicians should discuss with patients the potential cardiac risk of sexual activity for patients with preexisting cardiovascular risk factors.

The use of LEVITRA offers no protection against sexually transmitted diseases. Counseling of patients about protective measures necessary to guard against sexually transmitted diseases, including the Human Immunodeficiency Virus (HIV), should be considered.

Physicians should inform patients that there have been rare reports of prolonged erections greater than 4 hours and priapism (painful erections greater than 6 hours in duration) for LEVITRA and this class of compounds. In the event that an erection persists longer than 4 hours, the patient should seek immediate medical assistance. If priapism is not treated immediately, penile tissue damage and permanent loss of potency may result.

Drug Interactions

Effect of other drugs on LEVITRA

In vitro studies: Studies in human liver microsomes showed that vardenafil is metabolized primarily by cytochrome P450 (CYP) isoforms 3A4/5, and to a lesser degree by CYP2C9. Therefore, inhibitors of these enzymes are expected to reduce vardenafil clearance (see **WARNINGS** and **DOSAGE AND ADMINISTRATION**).

In vivo studies: Cytochrome P450 Inhibitors

Cimetidine (400 mg b.i.d.) had no effect on vardenafil bioavailability (AUC) and maximum concentration (C_{max}) of vardenafil when co-administered with 20 mg LEVITRA in healthy volunteers.

Erythromycin (500 mg t.i.d) produced a 4-fold increase in vardenafil AUC and a 3-fold increase in C_{max} when co-administered with LEVITRA 5 mg in healthy volunteers (see **DOSAGE AND ADMINISTRATION**). It is recommended not to exceed a single 5 mg dose of LEVITRA in a 24-hour period when used in combination with erythromycin.

Ketoconazole (200 mg once daily) produced a 10-fold increase in vardenafil AUC and a 4-fold increase in C_{max} when co-administered with LEVITRA (5 mg) in healthy volunteers. A 5-mg LEVITRA dose should not be exceeded when used in combination with 200 mg once daily ketoconazole. Since higher doses of ketoconazole (400 mg daily) may result in higher increases in C_{max} and AUC, a single 2.5 mg dose of LEVITRA should not be exceeded in a 24-hour period when used in combination with ketoconazole 400 mg daily (see **WARNINGS** and **DOSAGE AND ADMINISTRATION**).

HIV Protease Inhibitors:

Indinavir (800 mg t.i.d.) co-administered with LEVITRA 10 mg resulted in a 16-fold increase in vardenafil AUC, a 7-fold increase in vardenafil C_{max} and a 2-fold increase in vardenafil half-life. It is recommended not to exceed a single 2.5 mg LEVITRA dose in a 24-hour period when used in combination with indinavir (see **WARNINGS** and **DOSAGE AND ADMINISTRATION**).

Ritonavir (600 mg b.i.d.) co-administered with LEVITRA 5 mg resulted in a 49-fold increase in vardenafil AUC and a 13-fold increase in vardenafil C_{max}. The interaction is a consequence of blocking hepatic metabolism of vardenafil by ritonavir, a highly potent CYP3A4 inhibitor, which also inhibits CYP2C9. Ritonavir significantly prolonged the half-life of vardenafil to 26 hours. Consequently, it is recommended not to exceed a single 2.5 mg LEVITRA dose in a 72-hour period when used in combination with ritonavir (see **WARNINGS** and **DOSAGE AND ADMINISTRATION**).

Other Drug Interactions: No pharmacokinetic interactions were observed between vardenafil and the following drugs: glyburide, warfarin, digoxin, Maalox, and ranitidine. In the warfarin study, vardenafil had no effect on the prothrombin time or other pharmacodynamic parameters.

Effects of LEVITRA on other drugs

In vitro studies:

Vardenafil and its metabolites had no effect on CYP1A2, 2A6, and 2E1 (Ki > 100μM). Weak inhibitory effects toward other isoforms (CYP2C8, 2C9, 2C19, 2D6, 3A4) were found, but Ki values were in excess of plasma concentrations achieved following dosing. The most potent inhibitory activity was observed for vardenafil metabolite M1, which had a Ki of 1.4 μM toward CYP3A4, which is about 20 times higher than the M1 C_{max} values after an 80 mg LEVITRA dose.

In vivo studies:

Nitrates: The blood pressure lowering effects of sublingual nitrates (0.4 mg) taken 1 and 4 hours after vardenafil and increases in heart rate when taken at 1, 4 and 8 hours were potentiated by a 20 mg dose of LEVITRA in healthy middle-aged subjects. These effects were not observed when LEVITRA 20 mg was taken 24 hours before the NTG. Potentiation of the hypotensive effects of nitrates for patients with ischemic heart disease has not been evaluated, and concomitant use of LEVITRA and nitrates is contraindicated (see **CLINICAL PHARMACOLOGY, Pharmacodynamics, Effects on Blood Pressure and Heart Rate when LEVITRA is Combined with Nitrates; CONTRAINDICATIONS**).

Nifedipine: Vardenafil 20 mg, when co-administered with slow-release nifedipine 30 mg or 60 mg once daily, did not affect the relative bioavailability (AUC) or maximum concentration (C_{max}) of nifedipine, a drug that is metabolized via CYP3A4. Nifedipine did not alter the plasma levels of LEVITRA when taken in combination. In these patients whose hypertension was controlled with nifedipine, LEVITRA 20 mg produced mean additional supine systolic/diastolic blood pressure reductions of 6/5 mm Hg compared to placebo.

Alpha-blockers: When LEVITRA 10 or 20 mg was given to healthy volunteers either simultaneously or 6 hours after a 10 mg dose of terazosin, significant hypotension developed in a substantial number of subjects. With simultaneous dosing of LEVITRA 10 mg and terazosin 10 mg, 6 of 8 subjects experienced a standing systolic blood pressure of less than 85 mm Hg. With simultaneous dosing of LEVITRA 20 mg and terazosin 10 mg, 2 of 9 subjects experienced a standing systolic blood pressure of less than 85 mm Hg. When LEVITRA dosing was separated from terazosin 10 mg by 6 hours, 7 of 28 subjects who received 20 mg of LEVITRA experienced a decrease in standing systolic blood pressure below 85 mm Hg. In a similar study with tamsulosin in healthy volunteers, 1 of 24 subjects dosed with LEVITRA 20 mg and tamsulosin 0.4 mg separated by 6 hours experienced a standing systolic blood pressure below 85 mm Hg. Two of 16 subjects dosed simultaneously with LEVITRA 10 mg and tamsulosin 0.4 mg experienced a standing systolic blood pressure below 85 mm Hg. The administration of lower doses of LEVITRA with alpha-blockers has not been completely evaluated to determine if they can be safely administered together. Based on these data, LEVITRA should not be used in patients on alpha-blocker therapy (see **CONTRAINDICATIONS**).

Ritonavir and indinavir: Upon concomitant administration of 5 mg of LEVITRA with 600 mg BID ritonavir, the C_{max} and AUC of ritonavir were reduced by approximately 20%. Upon administration of 10 mg of LEVITRA with 800 mg TID indinavir, the C_{max} and AUC of indinavir were reduced by 40% and 30%, respectively.

Alcohol: Alcohol (0.5 g/kg body weight: approximately 40 mL of absolute alcohol in a 70 kg person) and vardenafil plasma levels were not altered when dosed simultaneously. LEVITRA (20 mg) did not potentiate the hypotensive effects of alcohol during the 4-hour observation period in healthy volunteers when administered with alcohol (0.5 g/kg body weight).

Aspirin: LEVITRA (10 mg and 20 mg) did not potentiate the increase in bleeding time caused by aspirin (two 81 mg tablets).

Other interactions: LEVITRA had no effect on the pharmacodynamics of glyburide (glucose and insulin concentrations) and warfarin (prothrombin time or other pharmacodynamic parameters).

Carcinogenesis, Mutagenesis, Impairment of Fertility

Vardenafil was not carcinogenic in rats and mice when administered daily for 24 months. In these studies systemic drug exposures (AUCs) for unbound (free) vardenafil and its major metabolite were approximately 400- and 170-fold for male and female rats, respectively, and 21- and 37-fold for male and female mice, respectively, the exposures observed in human males given the Maximum Recommended Human Dose (MRHD) of 20 mg. Vardenafil was not mutagenic as assessed in either the *in vitro* bacterial Ames assay or the forward mutation assay in Chinese hamster V79 cells. Vardenafil was not clastogenic as assessed in either the *in vitro* chromosomal aberration test or the *in vivo* mouse micronucleus test. Vardenafil did not impair fertility in male and female rats administered doses up to 100 mg/kg/day for 28 days prior to mating in male, and for 14 days prior to mating and through day 7 of gestation in females. In a corresponding 1-month rat toxicity study, this dose produced an AUC value for unbound vardenafil 200 fold greater than AUC in humans at the MRHD of 20 mg.

There was no effect on sperm motility or morphology after single 20 mg oral doses of vardenafil in healthy volunteers.

Pregnancy, Nursing Mothers and Pediatric Use

LEVITRA is not indicated for use in women, newborns, or children. Vardenafil was secreted into the milk of lactating rats at concentrations approximately 10-fold greater than found in the plasma. Following a single oral dose of 3 mg/kg, 3.3% of the administered dose was excreted into the milk within 24 hours. It is not known if vardenafil is excreted in human breast milk.

Pregnancy Category B: No evidence of specific potential for teratogenicity, embryotoxicity or fetotoxicity was observed in rats and rabbits that received vardenafil at up to 18 mg/kg/day during organogenesis. This dose is approximately 100 fold (rat) and 29 fold (rabbit) greater than the AUC values for unbound vardenafil and its major metabolite in humans given the MRHD of 20 mg. In the rat pre-and postnatal development study, the NOAEL (no observed adverse effect level) for maternal toxicity was 8 mg/kg/day. Retarded physical development of pups in the absence of maternal effects was observed following maternal exposure to 1 and 8 mg/kg possibly due to vasodilatation and/or secretion of the drug into milk. The number of living pups born to rats exposed pre- and postnatally was reduced at 60 mg/kg/day. Based on the results of the pre- and postnatal study, the developmental NOAEL is less than 1 mg/kg/day. Based on plasma exposures in the rat developmental toxicity study, 1mg/kg/day in the pregnant rat is estimated to produce total AUC values for unbound vardenafil and its major metabolite comparable to the human AUC at the MRHD of 20 mg. There are no adequate and well-controlled trials of vardenafil in pregnant women.

Geriatric Use

Elderly males age 65 years and older have higher vardenafil plasma concentrations than younger males (18 – 45 years), mean C_{max} and AUC were 34% and 52% higher, respectively (see **CLINICAL PHARMACOLOGY, Pharmacokinetics in Special Populations,** and **DOSAGE AND ADMINISTRATION**). Phase 3 clinical trials included more than 834 elderly patients, and no differences in safety or effectiveness of LEVITRA 5, 10, or 20 mg were noted when these elderly patients were compared to younger patients. However, due to increased vardenafil concentrations in the elderly, a starting dose of 5 mg LEVITRA should be considered in patients ≥ 65 years of age.

ADVERSE REACTIONS

LEVITRA was administered to over 4430 men (mean age 56, range 18-89 years; 81% White, 6% Black, 2% Asian, 2% Hispanic and 9% Other) during controlled and uncontrolled clinical trials worldwide. Over 2200 patients were treated for 6 months or longer, and 880 patients were treated for at least 1 year.

In placebo-controlled clinical trials, the discontinuation rate due to adverse events was 3.4% for LEVITRA compared to 1.1% for placebo.

When LEVITRA was taken as recommended in placebo-controlled clinical trials, the following adverse events were reported (see Table 2).

Table 2: Adverse Events Reported By ≥ 2% of Patients Treated with LEVITRA and More Frequent on Drug than Placebo in Fixed and Flexible[γ] Dose Randomized, Controlled Trials of 5 mg, 10 mg, or 20 mg Vardenafil

Adverse Event	Percentage of Patients Reporting Event	
	Placebo N = 1199	LEVITRA N = 2203
Headache	4%	15%
Flushing	1%	11%
Rhinitis	3%	9%
Dyspepsia	1%	4%
Accidental Injury*	2%	3%
Sinusitis	1%	3%
Flu Syndrome	2%	3%
Dizziness	1%	2%
Increased Creatine Kinase	1%	2%
Nausea	1%	2%

* All the events listed in the above table were deemed to be adverse drug reactions with the exception of accidental injury.

γ Flexible dose studies started all patients at LEVITRA 10 mg and allowed decrease in dose to 5 mg or increase in dose to 20 mg based on side effects and efficacy.

Back pain was reported in 2.0% of patients treated with LEVITRA and 1.7% of patients on placebo.

Placebo-controlled trials suggested a dose effect in the incidence of some adverse events (headache, flushing, dyspepsia, nausea, rhinitis) over the 5 mg, 10 mg, and 20 mg doses of LEVITRA. The following section identifies additional, less frequent events (<2%) reported during the clinical development of LEVITRA. Excluded from this list are those events that are infrequent and minor, those events that may be commonly observed in the absence of drug therapy, and those events that are not reasonably associated with the drug.

BODY AS A WHOLE: anaphylactic reaction (including laryngeal edema), asthenia, face edema, pain

AUDITORY: tinnitus

CARDIOVASCULAR: angina pectoris, chest pain, hypertension, hypotension, myocardial ischemia, myocardial infarction, palpitation, postural hypotension, syncope, tachycardia

DIGESTIVE: abdominal pain, abnormal liver function tests, diarrhea, dry mouth, dysphagia, esophagitis, gastritis, gastroesophageal reflux, GGTP increased, vomiting

MUSCULOSKELETAL: arthralgia, back pain, myalgia, neck pain

NERVOUS: hypertonia, hypesthesia, insomnia, paresthesia, somnolence, vertigo

RESPIRATORY: dyspnea, epistaxis, pharyngitis

SKIN AND APPENDAGES: photosensitivity reaction, pruritus, rash, sweating

OPHTHALMOLOGIC: abnormal vision, blurred vision, chromatopsia, changes in color vision, conjunctivitis (increased redness of the eye), dim vision, eye pain, glaucoma, photophobia, watery eyes

UROGENITAL: abnormal ejaculation, priapism (including prolonged or painful erections)

OVERDOSAGE

The maximum dose of LEVITRA for which human data are available is a single 120 mg dose administered to eight healthy male volunteers. The majority of these subjects experienced reversible back pain/myalgia and/or "abnormal vision."

In cases of overdose, standard supportive measures should be taken as required. Renal dialysis is not expected to accelerate clearance because vardenafil is highly bound to plasma proteins and is not significantly eliminated in the urine.

DOSAGE AND ADMINISTRATION

For most patients, the recommended starting dose of LEVITRA is 10 mg, taken orally approximately 60 minutes

Continued on next page

Levitra—Cont.

before sexual activity. The dose may be increased to a maximum recommended dose of 20 mg or decreased to 5 mg based on efficacy and side effects. The maximum recommended dosing frequency is once per day. LEVITRA can be taken with or without food. Sexual stimulation is required for a response to treatment.

Geriatrics: A starting dose of 5 mg LEVITRA should be considered in patients ≥ 65 years of age (see **CLINICAL PHARMACOLOGY, Pharmacokinetics in Special Populations** and **PRECAUTIONS**).

Hepatic Impairment: For patients with mild hepatic impairment (Child-Pugh A), no dose adjustment of LEVITRA is required. Vardenafil clearance is reduced in patients with moderate hepatic impairment (Child-Pugh B), and a starting dose of 5 mg LEVITRA is recommended. The maximum dose in patients with moderate hepatic impairment should not exceed 10 mg. LEVITRA has not been evaluated in patients with severe hepatic impairment (Child-Pugh C) (see **CLINICAL PHARMACOLOGY, Metabolism and Excretion, WARNINGS** and **PRECAUTIONS**).

Renal Impairment: For patients with mild (CL_{cr} = 50-80 ml/min), moderate (CL_{cr} = 30-50 ml/min), or severe (CL_{cr} <30 ml/min) renal impairment, no dose adjustment is required. LEVITRA has not been evaluated in patients on renal dialysis (see **CLINICAL PHARMACOLOGY, Metabolism and Excretion,** and **PRECAUTIONS**).

Concomitant Medications: The dosage of LEVITRA may require adjustment in patients receiving certain CYP3A4 inhibitors (e.g., ketoconazole, itraconazole, ritonavir, indinavir, and erythromycin) (see **WARNINGS, PRECAUTIONS, Drug Interactions**). For ritonavir, a single dose of 2.5 mg LEVITRA should not be exceeded in a 72-hour period. For indinavir, ketoconazole 400 mg daily, and itraconazole 400 mg daily, a single dose of 2.5 mg LEVITRA should not be exceeded in a 24-hour period. For ketoconazole 200 mg daily, itraconazole 200 mg daily, and erythromycin, a single dose of 5 mg LEVITRA should not be exceeded in a 24-hour period.

HOW SUPPLIED

LEVITRA (vardenafil HCl) is formulated as orange, film-coated round tablets with debossed "BAYER" cross on one side and "2.5", "5", "10", and "20" on the other side equivalent to 2.5 mg, 5 mg, 10 mg, and 20 mg of vardenafil, respectively.

Package	Strength	NDC Code
Bottles of 30	2.5 mg	0026-8710-69
	5 mg	0026-8720-69
	10 mg	0026-8730-69
	20 mg	0026-8740-69
Packages of 6	10 mg	0026-8730-05
	20 mg	0026-8740-05

Recommended Storage: Store at 25°C (77°F); excursions permitted to 15-30°C (59-86°F) [see USP Controlled Room Temperature].

Bayer HealthCare
Bayer Pharmaceuticals Corporation
400 Morgan Lane
West Haven, CT 06516
Made in Germany
℞ Only
08669034, R.1 1/04

Patient Information

LEVITRA® (Luh-VEE-Trah)
(vardenafil HCl) Tablets

Read the Patient Information about LEVITRA before you start taking it and again each time you get a refill. There may be new information. You may also find it helpful to share this information with your partner. This leaflet does not take the place of talking with your doctor. You and your doctor should talk about LEVITRA when you start taking it and at regular checkups. If you do not understand the information, or have questions, talk with your doctor or pharmacist.

WHAT IMPORTANT INFORMATION SHOULD YOU KNOW ABOUT LEVITRA?

LEVITRA can cause your blood pressure to drop suddenly to an unsafe level if it is taken with certain other medicines. With a sudden drop in blood pressure, you could get dizzy, faint, or have a heart attack or stroke.

Do not take LEVITRA if you:

- **take any medicines called "nitrates."**
- **use recreational drugs called "poppers" like amyl nitrate and butyl nitrate.**
- **take medicines called alpha-blockers.**

(See "Who Should Not Take LEVITRA?")

Tell all your healthcare providers that you take LEVITRA. If you need emergency medical care for a heart problem, it will be important for your healthcare provider to know when you last took LEVITRA.

WHAT IS LEVITRA?

LEVITRA is a prescription medicine taken by mouth for the treatment of erectile dysfunction (ED) in men.

ED is a condition where the penis does not harden and expand when a man is sexually excited, or when he cannot keep an erection. A man who has trouble getting or keeping an erection should see his doctor for help if the condition bothers him. LEVITRA may help a man with ED get and keep an erection when he is sexually excited.

LEVITRA does not:

- cure ED
- increase a man's sexual desire
- protect a man or his partner from sexually transmitted diseases, including HIV. Speak to your doctor about ways to guard against sexually transmitted diseases.
- serve as a male form of birth control

LEVITRA is only for men with ED. LEVITRA is not for women or children. LEVITRA must be used only under a doctor's care.

HOW DOES LEVITRA WORK?

When a man is sexually stimulated, his body's normal physical response is to increase blood flow to his penis. This results in an erection. LEVITRA helps increase blood flow to the penis and may help men with ED get and keep an erection satisfactory for sexual activity. Once a man has completed sexual activity, blood flow to his penis decreases, and his erection goes away.

WHO CAN TAKE LEVITRA?

Talk to your doctor to decide if LEVITRA is right for you. LEVITRA has been shown to be effective in men over the age of 18 years who have erectile dysfunction, including men with diabetes or who have undergone prostatectomy.

WHO SHOULD NOT TAKE LEVITRA?

Do not take LEVITRA if you:

- **take any medicines called "nitrates"** (See "What important information should you know about LEVITRA?"). Nitrates are commonly used to treat angina. Angina is a symptom of heart disease and can cause pain in your chest, jaw, or down your arm.
  Medicines called nitrates include nitroglycerin that is found in tablets, sprays, ointments, pastes, or patches. Nitrates can also be found in other medicines such as isosorbide dinitrate or isosorbide mononitrate. Some recreational drugs called "poppers" also contain nitrates, such as amyl nitrate and butyl nitrate. Do not use LEVITRA if you are using these drugs. Ask your doctor or pharmacist if you are not sure if any of your medicines are nitrates.
- **take medicines called "alpha-blockers."** Alpha-blockers are sometimes prescribed for prostate problems or high blood pressure. If LEVITRA is taken with alpha-blockers, your blood pressure could suddenly drop to an unsafe level. You could get dizzy and faint.
- **you have been told by your healthcare provider to not have sexual activity because of health problems.** Sexual activity can put an extra strain on your heart, especially if your heart is already weak from a heart attack or heart disease.
- **are allergic to LEVITRA or any of its ingredients.** The active ingredient in LEVITRA is called vardenafil. See the end of this leaflet for a complete list of ingredients.

WHAT SHOULD YOU DISCUSS WITH YOUR DOCTOR BEFORE TAKING LEVITRA?

Before taking LEVITRA, tell your doctor about all your medical problems, including if you:

- **have heart problems** such as angina, heart failure, irregular heartbeats, or have had a heart attack. Ask your doctor if it is safe for you to have sexual activity.
- **have low blood pressure** or have high blood pressure that is not controlled
- **have had a stroke**
- **or any family members have a rare heart condition known as prolongation of the QT interval (long QT syndrome)**
- **have liver problems**
- **have kidney problems and require dialysis**
- **have retinitis pigmentosa,** a rare genetic (runs in families) eye disease
- **have stomach ulcers**
- **have a bleeding problem**
- **have a deformed penis shape** or Peyronie's disease
- **have had an erection that lasted more than 4 hours**
- **have blood cell problems** such as sickle cell anemia, multiple myeloma, or leukemia

CAN OTHER MEDICATIONS AFFECT LEVITRA?

Tell your doctor about all the medicines you take including prescription and non-prescription medicines, vitamins, and herbal supplements. LEVITRA and other medicines may affect each other. Always check with your doctor before starting or stopping any medicines. Especially tell your doctor if you take any of the following:

- medicines called nitrates (See "What important information should you know about LEVITRA?")
- medicines called alpha-blockers. These include Hytrin® (terazosin HCl), Flomax® (tamsulosin HCl), Cardura® (doxazosin mesylate), Minipress® (prazosin HCl) or Uroxatral® (alfuzosin HCl).
- medicines that treat abnormal heartbeat. These include quinidine, procainamide, amiodarone and sotalol.
- ritonavir (Norvir®) or indinavir sulfate (Crixivan®)
- ketoconazole or itraconazole (such as Nizoral® or Sporanox®)
- erythromycin
- other medicines or treatments for ED

HOW SHOULD YOU TAKE LEVITRA?

Take LEVITRA exactly as your doctor prescribes. LEVITRA comes in different doses (2.5 mg, 5 mg, 10 mg, and 20 mg). For most men, the recommended starting dose is 10 mg. **Take LEVITRA no more than once a day.** Doses should be taken at least 24 hours apart. Some men can only take a low dose of LEVITRA because of medical conditions or medicines they take. Your doctor will prescribe the dose that is right for you.

- If you are older than 65 or have liver problems, your doctor may start you on a lower dose of LEVITRA.
- If you are taking certain other medicines your doctor may prescribe a lower starting dose and limit you to one dose of LEVITRA in a 72-hour (3 days) period.

Take 1 LEVITRA tablet about 1 hour (60 minutes) before sexual activity. Some form of sexual stimulation is needed for an erection to happen with LEVITRA. LEVITRA may be taken with or without meals.

Do not change your dose of LEVITRA without talking to your doctor. Your doctor may lower your dose or raise your dose, depending on how your body reacts to LEVITRA.

If you take too much LEVITRA, call your doctor or emergency room right away.

WHAT ARE THE POSSIBLE SIDE EFFECTS OF LEVITRA?

The most common side effects with LEVITRA are headache, flushing, stuffy or runny nose, indigestion, upset stomach, or dizziness. These side effects usually go away after a few hours. Call your doctor if you get a side effect that bothers you or one that will not go away.

LEVITRA may uncommonly cause:

- **an erection that won't go away (priapism).** If you get an erection that lasts more than 4 hours, get medical help right away. Priapism must be treated as soon as possible or lasting damage can happen to your penis including the inability to have erections.
- **vision changes,** such as seeing a blue tinge to objects or having difficulty telling the difference between the colors blue and green.

These are not all the side effects of LEVITRA. For more information, ask your doctor or pharmacist.

HOW SHOULD LEVITRA BE STORED?

- Store LEVITRA at room temperature between 59° and 86° F (15° to 30° C).
- **Keep LEVITRA and all medicines out of the reach of children.**

GENERAL INFORMATION ABOUT LEVITRA.

Medicines are sometimes prescribed for conditions other than those described in patient information leaflets. Do not use LEVITRA for a condition for which it was not prescribed. Do not give LEVITRA to other people, even if they have the same symptoms that you have. It may harm them.

This leaflet summarizes the most important information about LEVITRA. If you would like more information, talk with your healthcare provider. You can ask your doctor or pharmacist for information about LEVITRA that is written for health professionals.

For more information you can also visit www.LEVITRA.com, or call 1-866-LEVITRA.

WHAT ARE THE INGREDIENTS OF LEVITRA?

Active Ingredient: vardenafil hydrochloride

Inactive Ingredients: microcrystalline cellulose, crospovidone, colloidal silicon dioxide, magnesium stearate, hypromellose, polyethylene glycol, titanium dioxide, yellow ferric oxide, and red ferric oxide.

Norvir (ritonavir) is a trademark of Abbott Laboratories
Crixivan (indinavir sulfate) is a trademark of Merck & Co., Inc.
Nizoral (ketoconazole) is a trademark of Johnson & Johnson
Sporanox (itraconazole) is a trademark of Johnson & Johnson
Hytrin (terazosin HCl) is a trademark of Abbott Laboratories
Flomax (tamsulosin HCl) is a trademark of Yamanouchi Pharmaceutical Co., Ltd.
Cardura (doxazosin mesylate) is a trademark of Pfizer Inc.
Minipress (prazosin HCl) is a trademark of Pfizer Inc.
Uroxatral (alfuzosin HCl) is a trademark of Sanofi-Synthelabo

Bayer HealthCare
Bayer Pharmaceuticals Corporation
400 Morgan Lane
West Haven, CT 06516
Made in Germany
℞ Only
08669034IP, R.1 1/04

Shown in Product Identification Guide, page 308

NIMOTOP® ℞

[nī-mō-tŏp]
(nimodipine)
CAPSULES
For Oral Use

DESCRIPTION

Nimotop® (nimodipine) belongs to the class of pharmacological agents known as calcium channel blockers. Nimodipine is isopropyl 2 - methoxyethyl 1, 4 - dihydro - 2, 6 - dimethyl - 4 - (m - nitrophenyl) - 3, 5 - pyridinedicarboxylate It has a molecular weight of 418.5 and a molecular formula of $C_{21}H_{26}N_2O_7$. The structural formula is:

[See chemical structure at top of next column]

Nimodipine is a yellow crystalline substance, practically insoluble in water.

NIMOTOP® capsules are formulated as soft gelatin capsules for oral administration. Each liquid filled capsule contains 30 mg of nimodipine in a vehicle of glycerin, peppermint oil, purified water and polyethylene glycol 400. The soft gelatin capsule shell contains gelatin, glycerin, purified water and titanium dioxide.

CLINICAL PHARMACOLOGY

Mechanism of Action: Nimodipine is a calcium channel blocker. The contractile processes of smooth muscle cells are dependent upon calcium ions, which enter these cells during depolarization as slow ionic transmembrane currents. Nimodipine inhibits calcium ion transfer into these cells and thus inhibits contractions of vascular smooth muscle. In animal experiments, nimodipine had a greater effect on cerebral arteries than on arteries elsewhere in the body perhaps because it is highly lipophilic, allowing it to cross the blood-brain barrier; concentrations of nimodipine as high as 12.5 ng/mL have been detected in the cerebrospinal fluid of nimodipine-treated subarachnoid hemorrhage (SAH) patients.

The precise mechanism of action of nimodipine in humans is unknown. Although the clinical studies described below demonstrate a favorable effect of nimodipine on the severity of neurological deficits caused by cerebral vasospasm following SAH, there is no arteriographic evidence that the drug either prevents or relieves the spasm of these arteries. However, whether or not the arteriographic methodology utilized was adequate to detect a clinically meaningful effect, if any, on vasospasm is unknown.

Pharmacokinetics and Metabolism: In man, nimodipine is rapidly absorbed after oral administration, and peak concentrations are generally attained within one hour. The terminal elimination half-life is approximately 8 to 9 hours but earlier elimination rates are much more rapid, equivalent to a half-life of 1–2 hours; a consequence is the need for frequent (every 4 hours) dosing. There were no signs of accumulation when nimodipine was given three times a day for seven days. Nimodipine is over 95% bound to plasma proteins. The binding was concentration independent over the range of 10 ng/mL to 10 µg/mL. Nimodipine is eliminated almost exclusively in the form of metabolites and less than 1% is recovered in the urine as unchanged drug. Numerous metabolites, all of which are either inactive or considerably less active than the parent compound, have been identified. Because of a high first-pass metabolism, the bioavailability of nimodipine averages 13% after oral administration. The bioavailability is significantly increased in patients with hepatic cirrhosis, with C_{max} approximately double that in normals which necessitates lowering the dose in this group of patients (see Dosage and Administration). In a study of 24 healthy male volunteers, administration of nimodipine capsules following a standard breakfast resulted in a 68% lower peak plasma concentration and 38% lower bioavailability relative to dosing under fasted conditions.

In a single parallel-group study involving 24 elderly subjects (aged 59–79) and 24 younger subjects (aged 22–40), the observed AUC and C_{max} of nimodipine was approximately 2-fold higher in the elderly population compared to the younger study subjects following oral administration (given as a single dose of 30 mg and dosed to steady-state with 30 mg t.i.d. for 6 days). The clinical response to these age-related pharmacokinetic differences, however, was not considered significant. (See **PRECAUTIONS: Geriatric Use**.)

Clinical Trials: Nimodipine has been shown, in 4 randomized, double-blind, placebo-controlled trials, to reduce the severity of neurological deficits resulting from vasospasm in patients who have had a recent subarachnoid hemorrhage (SAH). The trials used doses ranging from 20–30 mg to 90 mg every 4 hours, with drug given for 21 days in 3 studies, and for at least 18 days in the other. Three of the four trials followed patients for 3–6 months. Three of the trials studied relatively well patients, with all or most patients in Hunt and Hess Grades I – III (essentially free of focal deficits after the initial bleed) the fourth studied much sicker patients, Hunt and Hess Grades III – V. Two studies, one U.S., one French, were similar in design, with relatively unimpaired SAH patients randomized to nimodipine or placebo. In each, a judgment was made as to whether any late-developing deficit was due to spasm or other causes, and the deficits were graded. Both studies showed significantly fewer severe deficits due to spasm in the nimodipine group; the second (French) study showed fewer spasm-related deficits of all severities. No effect was seen on deficits not related to spasm.

[See first table above]

A third, large, study was performed in the United Kingdom in SAH patients with all grades of severity (but 89% were in Grades I–III). Nimodipine was dosed 60 mg every 4 hours. Outcomes were not defined as spasm related or not but there was a significant reduction in the overall rate of infarction and severely disabling neurological outcome at 3 months:

	Nimodipine	Placebo
Total patients	278	276
Good Recovery	199*	169
Moderate disability	24	16
Severe disability	12**	31
Death	43***	60

* p = 0.0444 – good and moderate vs severe and dead
** p = 0.001 – severe disability
*** p = 0.056 – death

Study	Dose	Grade*		Patients: Number Analyzed	Any Deficit Due to Spasm	Numbers with Severe Deficit
U.S.	20–30 mg	I–III	Nimodipine	56	13	1
			Placebo	60	16	8**
French	60 mg	I–III	Nimodipine	31	4	2
			Placebo	39	11	10**

* Hunt and Hess Grade
** p=0.03

	Delayed Ischemic Deficits (DID)		Permanent Deficits	
	Nimodipine n (%)	Placebo n (%)	Nimodipine n (%)	Placebo n (%)
DID Spasm Alone	8 (11)*	25 (31)	5 (7) *	22 (27)
DID Spasm Contributing	18 (25)	21 (26)	16 (22)	17 (21)
DID Without Spasm	7 (10)	8 (10)	6 (8)	7 (9)
No DID	39 (54)	28 (34)	45 (63)	36 (44)

*p = 0.001, nimodipine vs placebo

	DOSE q4h Number of Patients (%) Nimodipine					
Sign/Symptom	**0.35 mg/kg (n=82)**	**30 mg (n=71)**	**60 mg (n=494)**	**90 mg (n=172)**	**120 mg (n=4)**	**Placebo (n=479)**
Decreased Blood Pressure	1 (1.2)	0	19 (3.8)	14 (8.1)	2 (50.0)	6 (1.2)
Abnormal Liver Function Test	1 (1.2)	0	2 (0.4)	1 (0.6)	0	7 (1.5)
Edema	0	0	2 (0.4)	2 (1.2)	0	3 (0.6)
Diarrhea	0	3 (4.2)	0	3 (1.7)	0	3 (0.6)
Rash	2 (2.4)	0	3 (0.6)	2 (1.2)	0	3 (0.6)
Headache	0	1 (1.4)	6 (1.2)	0	0	1 (0.2)
Gastrointestinal Symptoms	2 (2.4)	0	0	2 (1.2)	0	0
Nausea	1 (1.2)	1 (1.4)	6 (1.2)	1 (0.6)	0	0
Dyspnea	1 (1.2)	0	0	0	0	0
EKG Abnormalities	0	1 (1.4)	0	1 (0.6)	0	0
Tachycardia	0	1 (1.4)	0	0	0	0
Bradycardia	0	0	5 (1.0)	1 (0.6)	0	0
Muscle Pain/ Cramp	0	1 (1.4)	1 (0.2)	1 (0.6)	0	0
Acne	0	1 (1.4)	0	0	0	0
Depression	0	1 (1.4)	0	0	0	0

A Canadian study entered much sicker patients, (Hunt and Hess Grades III–V), who had a high rate of death and disability, and used a dose of 90 mg every 4 hours, but was otherwise similar to the first two studies. Analysis of delayed ischemic deficits, many of which result from spasm, showed a significant reduction in spasm-related deficits. Among analyzed patients (72 nimodipine, 82 placebo), there were the following outcomes.

[See second table above]

When data were combined for the Canadian and the United Kingdom studies, the treatment difference on success rate (i.e. good recovery) on the Glasgow Outcome Scale was 25.3% (nimodipine) versus 10.9% (placebo) for Hunt and Hess Grades IV or V. The table below demonstrates that nimodipine tends to improve good recovery of SAH patients with poor neurological status post-ictus, while decreasing the numbers with severe disability and vegetative survival.

Glasgow Outcome*	Nimodipine (n=87)	Placebo (n=101)
Good Recovery	22 (25.3%)	11 (10.9%)
Moderate Disability	8 (9.2%)	12 (11.9%)
Severe Disability	6 (6.9%)	15 (14.9%)
Vegetative Survival	4 (4.6%)	9 (8.9%)
Death	47 (54.0%)	54 (53.5%)

* p = 0.045, nimodipine vs placebo

A dose-ranging study comparing 30, 60 and 90 mg doses found a generally low rate of spasm-related neurological deficits but no dose response relationship.

INDICATIONS AND USAGE

Nimotop® (nimodipine) is indicated for the improvement of neurological outcome by reducing the incidence and severity of ischemic deficits in patients with subarachnoid hemorrhage from ruptured intracranial berry aneurysms regardless of their post-ictus neurological condition (i.e., Hunt and Hess Grades I–V).

CONTRAINDICATIONS

None known.

PRECAUTIONS

General: Blood Pressure: Nimodipine has the hemodynamic effects expected of a calcium channel blocker, although they are generally not marked. However, intravenous administration of the contents of Nimotop Capsules has resulted in serious adverse consequences including hypotension, cardiovascular collapse, and cardiac arrest. In patients with subarachnoid hemorrhage given Nimotop® in clinical studies, about 5% were reported to have had lowering of the blood pressure and about 1% left the study because of this (not all could be attributed to nimodipine). Nevertheless, blood pressure should be carefully monitored during treatment with Nimotop® based on its known pharmacology and the known effects of calcium channel blockers.

Hepatic Disease: The metabolism of Nimotop® is decreased in patients with impaired hepatic function. Such patients should have their blood pressure and pulse rate monitored closely and should be given a lower dose (see Dosage and Administration).

Intestinal pseudo-obstruction and ileus have been reported rarely in patients treated with nimodipine. A causal relationship has not been established. The condition has responded to conservative management.

Laboratory Test Interactions: None known.

Drug Interaction: It is possible that the cardiovascular action of other calcium channel blockers could be enhanced by the addition of Nimotop®.

In Europe, Nimotop® was observed to occasionally intensify the effect of antihypertensive compounds taken concomitantly by patients suffering from hypertension; this phenomenon was not observed in North American clinical trials.

Continued on next page

Nimotop—Cont.

A study in eight healthy volunteers has shown a 50% increase in mean peak nimodipine plasma concentrations and a 90% increase in mean area under the curve, after a one-week course of cimetidine at 1,000 mg/day and nimodipine at 90 mg/day. This effect may be mediated by the known inhibition of hepatic cytochrome P-450 by cimetidine, which could decrease first-pass metabolism of nimodipine.

Carcinogenesis, Mutagenesis, Impairment of Fertility: In a two-year study, higher incidences of adenocarcinoma of the uterus and Leydig-cell adenoma of the testes were observed in rats given a diet containing 1800 ppm nimodipine (equivalent to 91 to 121 mg/kg/day nimodipine) than in placebo controls. The differences were not statistically significant, however, and the higher rates were well within historical control range for these tumors in the Wistar strain. Nimodipine was found not to be carcinogenic in a 91-week mouse study but the high dose of 1800 ppm nimodipine-in-feed (546 to 774 mg/kg/day) shortened the life expectancy of the animals. Mutagenicity studies, including the Ames, micronucleus and dominant lethal tests were negative.

Nimodipine did not impair the fertility and general reproductive performance of male and female Wistar rats following oral doses of up to 30 mg/kg/day when administered daily for more than 10 weeks in the males and 3 weeks in the females prior to mating and continued to day 7 of pregnancy. This dose in a rat is about 4 times the equivalent clinical dose of 60 mg q4h in a 50 kg patient.

Pregnancy: Pregnancy Category C. Nimodipine has been shown to have a teratogenic effect in Himalayan rabbits. Incidences of malformations and stunted fetuses were increased at oral doses of 1 and 10 mg/kg/day administered (by gavage) from day 6 through day 18 of pregnancy but not at 3.0 mg/kg/day in one of two identical rabbit studies. In the second study an increased incidence of stunted fetuses was seen at 1.0 mg/kg/day but not at higher doses. Nimodipine was embryotoxic, causing resorption and stunted growth of fetuses, in Long Evans rats at 100 mg/kg/day administered by gavage from day 6 through day 15 of pregnancy. In two other rat studies, doses of 30 mg/kg/day nimodipine administered by gavage from day 16 of gestation and continued until sacrifice (day 20 of pregnancy or day 21 post partum) were associated with higher incidences of skeletal variation, stunted fetuses and stillbirths but no malformations. There are no adequate and well controlled studies in pregnant women to directly assess the effect on human fetuses. Nimodipine should be used during pregnancy only if the potential benefit justifies the potential risk to the fetus.

Nursing Mothers: Nimodipine and/or its metabolites have been shown to appear in rat milk at concentrations much higher than in maternal plasma. It is not known whether the drug is excreted in human milk. Because many drugs are excreted in human milk, nursing mothers are advised not to breast feed their babies when taking the drug.

Pediatric Use: Safety and effectiveness in children have not been established.

Geriatric Use: Clinical studies of nimodipine did not include sufficient numbers of subjects aged 65 and over to determine whether they respond differently from younger subjects. Other reported clinical experience has not identified differences in responses between the elderly and younger patients. In general, dosing in elderly patients should be cautious, reflecting the greater frequency of decreased hepatic, renal or cardiac function, and of concomitant disease or other drug therapy.

ADVERSE REACTIONS

Adverse experiences were reported by 92 of 823 patients with subarachnoid hemorrhage (11.2%) who were given nimodipine. The most frequently reported adverse experience was decreased blood pressure in 4.4% of these patients. Twenty-nine of 479 (6.1%) placebo treated patients also reported adverse experiences. The events reported with a frequency greater than 1% are displayed below by dose.

[See third table on previous page]

There were no other adverse experiences reported by the patients who were given 0.35 mg/kg q4h, 30 mg q4h or 120 mg q4h. Adverse experiences with an incidence rate of less than 1% in the 60 mg q4h dose group were: hepatitis; itching; gastrointestinal hemorrhage; thrombocytopenia; anemia; palpitations; vomiting; flushing; diaphoresis; wheezing; phenytoin toxicity; lightheadedness; dizziness; rebound vasospasm; jaundice; hypertension; hematoma.

Adverse experiences with an incidence rate less than 1% in the 90 mg q4h dose group were: itching; gastrointestinal hemorrhage; thrombocytopenia; neurological deterioration; vomiting; diaphoresis; congestive heart failure; hyponatremia; decreasing platelet count; disseminated intravascular coagulation; deep vein thrombosis.

As can be seen from the table, side effects that appear related to nimodipine use based on increased incidence with higher dose or a higher rate compared to placebo control, included decreased blood pressure, edema and headaches which are known pharmacologic actions of calcium channel blockers. It must be noted, however, that SAH is frequently accompanied by alterations in consciousness which lead to an under reporting of adverse experiences. Patients who received nimodipine in clinical trials for other indications reported flushing (2.1%), headache (4.1%) and fluid retention (0.3%), typical responses to calcium channel blockers. As a calcium channel blocker, nimodipine may have the potential to exacerbate heart failure in susceptible patients or to interfere with A-V conduction, but these events were not observed.

No clinically significant effects on hematologic factors, renal or hepatic function or carbohydrate metabolism have been causally associated with oral nimodipine. Isolated cases of non-fasting elevated serum glucose levels (0.8%), elevated LDH levels (0.4%), decreased platelet counts (0.3%), elevated alkaline phosphatase levels (0.2%) and elevated SGPT levels (0.2%) have been reported rarely.

DRUG ABUSE AND DEPENDENCE

There have been no reported instances of drug abuse or dependence with Nimotop®.

OVERDOSAGE

There have been no reports of overdosage from the oral administration of Nimotop®. Symptoms of overdosage would be expected to be related to cardiovascular effects such as excessive peripheral vasodilation with marked systemic hypotension. Clinically significant hypotension due to Nimotop® overdosage may require active cardiovascular support. Norepinephrine or dopamine may be helpful in restoring blood pressure. Since Nimotop® is highly protein-bound, dialysis is not likely to be of benefit.

DOSAGE AND ADMINISTRATION

Nimotop is given orally in the form of ivory colored, soft gelatin 30 mg capsules for subarachnoid hemorrhage.

The oral dose is 60 mg (two 30 mg capsules) every 4 hours for 21 consecutive days, preferably not less than one hour before or two hours after meals. Oral Nimotop® therapy should commence within 96 hours of the subarachnoid hemorrhage.

If the capsule cannot be swallowed, e.g., at the time of surgery, or if the patient is unconscious, a hole should be made in both ends of the capsule with an 18 gauge needle, and the contents of the capsule extracted into a syringe. The contents should then be emptied into the patient's *in situ* nasogastric tube and washed down the tube with 30 mL of normal saline (0.9%).

The contents of Nimotop Capsules must not be administered by intravenous injection or other parenteral routes.

Patients with hepatic cirrhosis have substantially reduced clearance and approximately doubled C_{max}. Dosage should be reduced to 30 mg every 4 hours, with close monitoring of blood pressure and heart rate.

HOW SUPPLIED

Each ivory colored, soft gelatin NIMOTOP® capsule is imprinted with the word Nimotop and contains 30 mg of nimodipine. The 30 mg capsules are packaged in unit dose foil pouches and supplied in cartons containing 100 capsules. The product is also available in child resistant unit dose safety pak foil pouches containing 30 capsules per carton. The capsules should be stored in the manufacturer's original foil package at 25°C (77°F), excursions permitted to 15–30°C (59–86°F) [See USP controlled Room Temperature.]

Capsules should be protected from light and freezing.

	Strength	NDC Code	Capsule Identification
Unit Dose Package of 100:	30 mg	0026-2855-48	Nimotop
Unit Dose Package of 30:	30 mg	0026-2855-70	Nimotop

Distributed by: Bayer Pharmaceuticals Corporation
400 Morgan Lane
West Haven, CT 06516

Manufactured by: Cardinal Health
St. Petersburg, FL 33716

℞ Only

08897207 4/04 BAY e 9736 5202-7-A-U.S.-10

Printed in USA

Shown in Product Identification Guide, page 308

PRECOSE® ℞

[*prē-cōs*]

(acarbose tablets)

DESCRIPTION

PRECOSE® (acarbose tablets) is an oral alpha-glucosidase inhibitor for use in the management of type 2 diabetes mellitus. Acarbose is an oligosaccharide which is obtained from fermentation processes of a microorganism, *Actinoplanes utahensis*, and is chemically known as *O*-4,6-dideoxy-4-[[(1*S*,4*R*,5*S*,6*S*)-4,5,6-trihydroxy-3-(hydroxymethyl)-2-cyclohexen-1-yl]amino]-α-D-glucopyranosyl-(1 → 4)-*O*-α-D-glucopyranosyl-(1 → 4)-D-glucose. It is a white to off-white powder with a molecular weight of 645.6. Acarbose is soluble in water and has a pK_a of 5.1. Its empirical formula is $C_{25}H_{43}NO_{18}$ and its chemical structure is as follows:

[See chemical structure at top of next column]

PRECOSE® is available as 25 mg, 50 mg and 100 mg tablets for oral use. The inactive ingredients are starch, microcrystalline cellulose, magnesium stearate, and colloidal silicon dioxide.

CLINICAL PHARMACOLOGY

Acarbose is a complex oligosaccharide that delays the digestion of ingested carbohydrates, thereby resulting in a smaller rise in blood glucose concentration following meals. As a consequence of plasma glucose reduction, PRECOSE® reduces levels of glycosylated hemoglobin in patients with type 2 diabetes mellitus. Systemic non-enzymatic protein glycosylation, as reflected by levels of glycosylated hemoglobin, is a function of average blood glucose concentration over time.

Mechanism of Action: In contrast to sulfonylureas, PRECOSE® does not enhance insulin secretion. The antihyperglycemic action of acarbose results from a competitive, reversible inhibition of pancreatic alpha-amylase and membrane-bound intestinal alpha-glucoside hydrolase enzymes. Pancreatic alpha-amylase hydrolyzes complex starches to oligosaccharides in the lumen of the small intestine, while the membrane-bound intestinal alpha-glucosidases hydrolyze oligosaccharides, trisaccharides, and disaccharides to glucose and other monosaccharides in the brush border of the small intestine. In diabetic patients, this enzyme inhibition results in a delayed glucose absorption and a lowering of postprandial hyperglycemia.

Because its mechanism of action is different, the effect of PRECOSE® to enhance glycemic control is additive to that of sulfonylureas, insulin or metformin when used in combination. In addition, PRECOSE® diminishes the insulinotropic and weight-increasing effects of sulfonylureas.

Acarbose has no inhibitory activity against lactase and consequently would not be expected to induce lactose intolerance.

Pharmacokinetics:

Absorption: In a study of 6 healthy men, less than 2% of an oral dose of acarbose was absorbed as active drug, while approximately 35% of total radioactivity from a ^{14}C-labeled oral dose was absorbed. An average of 51% of an oral dose was excreted in the feces as unabsorbed drug-related radioactivity within 96 hours of ingestion. Because acarbose acts locally within the gastrointestinal tract, this low systemic bioavailability of parent compound is therapeutically desired. Following oral dosing of healthy volunteers with ^{14}C-labeled acarbose, peak plasma concentrations of radioactivity were attained 14–24 hours after dosing, while peak plasma concentrations of active drug were attained at approximately 1 hour. The delayed absorption of acarbose-related radioactivity reflects the absorption of metabolites that may be formed by either intestinal bacteria or intestinal enzymatic hydrolysis.

Metabolism: Acarbose is metabolized exclusively within the gastrointestinal tract, principally by intestinal bacteria, but also by digestive enzymes. A fraction of these metabolites (approximately 34% of the dose) was absorbed and subsequently excreted in the urine. At least 13 metabolites have been separated chromatographically from urine specimens. The major metabolites have been identified as 4-methylpyrogallol derivatives (i.e., sulfate, methyl, and glucuronide conjugates). One metabolite (formed by cleavage of a glucose molecule from acarbose) also has alpha-glucosidase inhibitory activity. This metabolite, together with the parent compound, recovered from the urine, accounts for less than 2% of the total administered dose.

Excretion: The fraction of acarbose that is absorbed as intact drug is almost completely excreted by the kidneys. When acarbose was given *intravenously*, 89% of the dose was recovered in the urine as active drug within 48 hours. In contrast, less than 2% of an *oral dose* was recovered in the urine as active (i.e., parent compound and active metabolite) drug. This is consistent with the low bioavailability of the parent drug. The plasma elimination half-life of acarbose activity is approximately 2 hours in healthy volunteers. Consequently, drug accumulation does not occur with three times a day (t.i.d.) oral dosing.

Special Populations: The mean steady-state area under the curve (AUC) and maximum concentrations of acarbose were approximately 1.5 times higher in elderly compared to young volunteers; however, these differences were not statistically significant. Patients with severe renal impairment (Clcr < 25 mL/min/1.73m^2) attained about 5 times higher peak plasma concentrations of acarbose and 6 times larger AUCs than volunteers with normal renal function. No studies of acarbose pharmacokinetic parameters according to race have been performed. In U.S. controlled clinical studies of PRECOSE® in patients with type 2 diabetes mellitus, reductions in glycosylated hemoglobin levels were similar in Caucasians (n=478) and African-Americans (n=167), with a trend toward a better response in Latinos (n=132).

Drug-Drug Interactions: Studies in healthy volunteers have shown that PRECOSE® has no effect on either the pharmacokinetics or pharmacodynamics of nifedipine, propranolol, or ranitidine. PRECOSE® did not interfere with the absorption or disposition of the sulfonylurea glyburide in diabetic patients. PRECOSE® may affect digoxin bioavailability and may require dose adjustment of digoxin by 16% (90% confidence interval: 8–23%), decrease mean C_{max} of digoxin by 26% (90% confidence interval: 16–34%) and decreases mean trough concentrations of digoxin by 9% (90%

confidence limit: 19% decrease to 2% increase). (See **PRECAUTIONS, Drug Interactions**).
The amount of metformin absorbed while taking PRECOSE® was bioequivalent to the amount absorbed when taking placebo, as indicated by the plasma AUC values. However, the peak plasma level of metformin was reduced by approximately 20% when taking PRECOSE® due to a slight delay in the absorption of metformin. There is little if any clinically significant interaction between PRECOSE® and metformin.

CLINICAL TRIALS

Clinical Experience from Dose Finding Studies in Type 2 Diabetes Mellitus Patients on Dietary Treatment Only: Results from six controlled, fixed-dose, monotherapy studies of PRECOSE® in the treatment of type 2 diabetes mellitus, involving 769 PRECOSE®-treated patients, were combined and a weighted average of the difference from placebo in the mean change from baseline in glycosylated hemoglobin (HbA1c) was calculated for each dose level as presented below:
[See table 1 above]
Results from these six fixed-dose, monotherapy studies were also combined to derive a weighted average of the difference from placebo in mean change from baseline for one-hour postprandial plasma glucose levels as shown in the following figure:

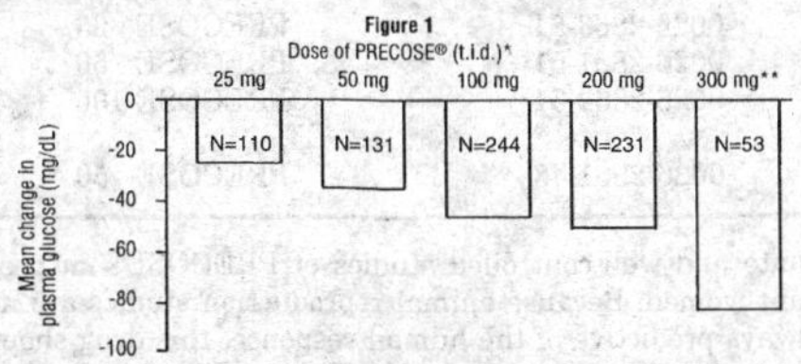

* PRECOSE® was statistically significantly different from placebo at all doses with respect to effect on one-hour postprandial plasma glucose.
**The 300 mg t.i.d. PRECOSE® regimen was superior to lower doses, but there were no statistically significant differences from 50 to 200 mg t.i.d.

Clinical Experience in Type 2 Diabetes Mellitus Patients on Monotherapy, or in Combination with Sulfonylureas, Metformin or Insulin: PRECOSE® was studied as monotherapy and as combination therapy to sulfonylurea, metformin, or insulin treatment. The treatment effects on HbA1c levels and one-hour postprandial glucose levels are summarized for four placebo-controlled, double-blind, randomized studies conducted in the United States in Tables 2 and 3, respectively. The placebo-subtracted treatment differences, which are summarized below, were statistically significant for both variables in all of these studies.
Study 1 (n=109) involved patients on background treatment with diet only. The mean effect of the addition of PRECOSE® to diet therapy was a change in HbA1c of −0.78%, and an improvement of one-hour postprandial glucose of −74.4 mg/dL.
In Study 2 (n=137), the mean effect of the addition of PRECOSE® to maximum sulfonylurea therapy was a change in HbA1c of −0.54%, and an improvement of one-hour postprandial glucose of −33.5 mg/dL.
In Study 3 (n=147), the mean effect of the addition of PRECOSE® to maximum metformin therapy was a change in HbA1c of −0.65%, and an improvement of one-hour postprandial glucose of −34.3 mg/dL.
Study 4 (n=145) demonstrated that PRECOSE® added to patients on background treatment with insulin resulted in a mean change in HbA1c of −0.69%, and an improvement of one-hour postprandial glucose of −36.0 mg/dL.
A one year study of PRECOSE® as monotherapy or in combination with sulfonylurea, metformin or insulin treatment was conducted in Canada in which 316 patients were included in the primary efficacy analysis (Figure 2). In the diet, sulfonylurea and metformin groups, the mean decrease in HbA1c produced by the addition of PRECOSE® was statistically significant at six months, and this effect was persistent at one year. In the PRECOSE®-treated patients on insulin, there was a statistically significant reduction in HbA1c at six months, and a trend for a reduction at one year.
[See table 2 at right]
[See table 3 at right]
[See figure 2 at top of next page]

INDICATIONS AND USAGE

PRECOSE®, as monotherapy, is indicated as an adjunct to diet to lower blood glucose in patients with type 2 diabetes mellitus whose hyperglycemia cannot be managed on diet alone. PRECOSE® may also be used in combination with a sulfonylurea when diet plus either PRECOSE® or a sulfonylurea do not result in adequate glycemic control. Also, PRECOSE® may be used in combination with insulin or metformin. The effect of PRECOSE® to enhance glycemic control is additive to that of sulfonylureas, insulin, or metformin when used in combination, presumably because its mechanism of action is different.
In initiating treatment for type 2 diabetes mellitus, diet should be emphasized as the primary form of treatment. Caloric restriction and weight loss are essential in the obese diabetic patient. Proper dietary management alone may be effective in controlling blood glucose and symptoms of hyperglycemia. The importance of regular physical activity when appropriate should also be stressed. If this treatment program fails to result in adequate glycemic control, the use of PRECOSE® should be considered. The use of PRECOSE® must be viewed by both the physician and patient as a treatment in addition to diet, and not as a substitute for diet or as a convenient mechanism for avoiding dietary restraint.

Table 1

Mean Placebo-Subtracted Change in HbA1c in Fixed-Dose Monotherapy Studies

Dose of PRECOSE*	N	Change in HbA1c %	p-Value
25 mg t.i.d.	110	−0.44	0.0307
50 mg t.i.d.	131	−0.77	0.0001
100 mg t.i.d.	244	−0.74	0.0001
200 mg t.i.d.**	231	−0.86	0.0001
300 mg t.i.d.**	53	−1.00	0.0001

* PRECOSE® was statistically significantly different from placebo at all doses. Although there were no statistically significant differences among the mean results for doses ranging from 50 to 300 mg t.i.d., some patients may derive benefit by increasing the dosage from 50 to 100 mg t.i.d.
**Although studies utilized a maximum dose of 200 or 300 mg t.i.d., the maximum recommended dose for patients < 60 kg is 50 mg t.i.d.; the maximum recommended dose for patients > 60 kg is 100 mg t.i.d.

Table 2: Effect of Precose® on HbA1c

Study	Treatment	HbA1c (%)[a] Mean Baseline	Mean change from baseline[b]	Treatment Difference	p-Value
1	Placebo Plus Diet	8.67	+0.33	—	—
	PRECOSE 100 mg t.i.d. Plus Diet	8.69	−0.45	−0.78	0.0001
2	Placebo Plus SFU[c]	9.56	+0.24	—	—
	PRECOSE 50–300[d] mg t.i.d. Plus SFU[c]	9.64	−0.30	−0.54	0.0096
3	Placebo Plus Metformin[e]	8.17	+0.08[g]	—	—
	PRECOSE 50–100 mg t.i.d. Plus Metformin[e]	8.46	−0.57[g]	−0.65	0.0001
4	Placebo Plus Insulin[f]	8.69	+0.11	—	—
	PRECOSE 50–100 mg t.i.d. Plus Insulin[f]	8.77	−0.58	−0.69	0.0001

[a] HbA1c Normal Range: 4–6%
[b] After four months treatment in Study 1, and six months in Studies 2, 3, and 4
[c] SFU, sulfonylurea, maximum dose
[d] Although studies utilized a maximum dose of up to 300 mg t.i.d., the maximum recommended dose for patients ≤ 60 kg is 50 mg t.i.d.; the maximum recommended dose for patients > 60 kg is 100 mg t.i.d.
[e] Metformin dosed at 2000 mg/day or 2500 mg/day
[f] Mean dose of insulin 61 U/day
[g] Results are adjusted to a common baseline of 8.33%

Table 3: Effect of Precose® on Postprandial Glucose

Study	Treatment	One-Hour Postprandial Glucose (mg/dL) Mean Baseline	Mean change from baseline[a]	Treatment Difference	p-Value
1	Placebo Plus Diet	297.1	+31.8	—	—
	PRECOSE 100 mg t.i.d. Plus Diet	299.1	−42.6	−74.4	0.0001
2	Placebo Plus SFU[b]	308.6	+6.2	—	—
	PRECOSE 50–300[c] mg t.i.d. Plus SFU[b]	311.1	−27.3	−33.5	0.0017
3	Placebo Plus Metformin[d]	263.9	+3.3[f]	—	—
	PRECOSE 50–100 mg t.i.d. Plus Metformin[d]	283.0	−31.0[f]	−34.3	0.0001
4	Placebo Plus Insulin[e]	279.2	+8.0	—	—
	PRECOSE 50–100 mg t.i.d. Plus Insulin[e]	277.8	−28.0	−36.0	0.0178

[a] After four months treatment in Study 1, and six months in Studies 2, 3, and 4
[b] SFU, sulfonylurea, maximum dose
[c] Although studies utilized a maximum dose of up to 300 mg t.i.d., the maximum recommended dose for patients ≤ 60 kg is 50 mg t.i.d.; the maximum recommended dose for patients > 60 kg is 100 mg t.i.d.
[d] Metformin dosed at 2000 mg/day or 2500 mg/day
[e] Mean dose of insulin 61 U/day
[f] Results are adjusted to a common baseline of 273 mg/dL

CONTRAINDICATIONS

PRECOSE® is contraindicated in patients with known hypersensitivity to the drug and in patients with diabetic ketoacidosis or cirrhosis. PRECOSE® is also contraindicated in patients with inflammatory bowel disease, colonic ulceration, partial intestinal obstruction or in patients predisposed to intestinal obstruction. In addition, PRECOSE® is contraindicated in patients who have chronic intestinal diseases associated with marked disorders of digestion or absorption and in patients who have conditions that may deteriorate as a result of increased gas formation in the intestine.

PRECAUTIONS

General

Hypoglycemia: Because of its mechanism of action, PRECOSE® when administered alone should not cause hy-

Continued on next page

Precose—Cont.

poglycemia in the fasted or postprandial state. Sulfonylurea agents or insulin may cause hypoglycemia. Because PRECOSE® given in combination with a sulfonylurea or insulin will cause a further lowering of blood glucose, it may increase the potential for hypoglycemia. Hypoglycemia does not occur in patients receiving metformin alone under usual circumstances of use, and no increased incidence of hypoglycemia was observed in patients when PRECOSE® was added to metformin therapy. Oral glucose (dextrose), whose absorption is not inhibited by PRECOSE®, should be used instead of sucrose (cane sugar) in the treatment of mild to moderate hypoglycemia. Sucrose, whose hydrolysis to glucose and fructose is inhibited by PRECOSE®, is unsuitable for the rapid correction of hypoglycemia. Severe hypoglycemia may require the use of either intravenous glucose infusion or glucagon injection.

Elevated Serum Transaminase Levels: In long-term studies (up to 12 months, and including PRECOSE® doses up to 300 mg t.i.d.) conducted in the United States, treatment-emergent elevations of serum transaminases (AST and/or ALT) above the upper limit of normal (ULN), greater than 1.8 times the ULN, and greater than 3 times the ULN occurred in 14%, 6%, and 3%, respectively, of PRECOSE®-treated patients as compared to 7%, 2%, and 1%, respectively, of placebo-treated patients. Although these differences between treatments were statistically significant, these elevations were asymptomatic, reversible, more common in females, and, in general, were not associated with other evidence of liver dysfunction. In addition, these serum transaminase elevations appeared to be dose related. In US studies including PRECOSE® doses up to the maximum approved dose of 100 mg t.i.d., treatment-emergent elevations of AST and/or ALT at any level of severity were similar between PRECOSE®-treated patients and placebo-treated patients ($p \geq 0.496$).

In approximately 3 million patient-years of international post-marketing experience with PRECOSE®, 62 cases of serum transaminase elevations > 500 IU/L (29 of which were associated with jaundice) have been reported. Forty-one of these 62 patients received treatment with 100 mg t.i.d. or greater and 33 of 45 patients for whom weight was reported weighed < 60 kg. In the 59 cases where follow-up was recorded, hepatic abnormalities improved or resolved upon discontinuation of PRECOSE® in 55 and were unchanged in two. A few cases of fulminant hepatitis with fatal outcome have been reported; the relationship to acarbose is unclear.

Loss of Control of Blood Glucose: When diabetic patients are exposed to stress such as fever, trauma, infection, or surgery, a temporary loss of control of blood glucose may occur. At such times, temporary insulin therapy may be necessary.

Information for Patients: Patients should be told to take PRECOSE® orally three times a day at the start (with the first bite) of each main meal. It is important that patients continue to adhere to dietary instructions, a regular exercise program, and regular testing of urine and/or blood glucose.

PRECOSE® itself does not cause hypoglycemia even when administered to patients in the fasted state. Sulfonylurea drugs and insulin, however, can lower blood sugar levels enough to cause symptoms or sometimes life-threatening hypoglycemia. Because PRECOSE® given in combination with a sulfonylurea or insulin will cause a further lowering of blood sugar, it may increase the hypoglycemic potential of these agents. Hypoglycemia does not occur in patients receiving metformin alone under usual circumstances of use, and no increased incidence of hypoglycemia was observed in patients when PRECOSE® was added to metformin therapy. The risk of hypoglycemia, its symptoms and treatment, and conditions that predispose to its development should be well understood by patients and responsible family members. Because PRECOSE® prevents the breakdown of table sugar, patients should have a readily available source of glucose (dextrose, D-glucose) to treat symptoms of low blood sugar when taking PRECOSE® in combination with a sulfonylurea or insulin.

If side effects occur with PRECOSE®, they usually develop during the first few weeks of therapy. They are most commonly mild-to-moderate gastrointestinal effects, such as flatulence, diarrhea, or abdominal discomfort, and generally diminish in frequency and intensity with time.

Laboratory Tests: Therapeutic response to PRECOSE® should be monitored by periodic blood glucose tests. Measurement of glycosylated hemoglobin levels is recommended for the monitoring of long-term glycemic control.

PRECOSE®, particularly at doses in excess of 50 mg t.i.d., may give rise to elevations of serum transaminases and, in rare instances, hyperbilirubinemia. It is recommended that serum transaminase levels be checked every 3 months during the first year of treatment with PRECOSE® and periodically thereafter. If elevated transaminases are observed, a reduction in dosage or withdrawal of therapy may be indicated, particularly if the elevations persist.

Renal Impairment: Plasma concentrations of PRECOSE® in renally impaired volunteers were proportionally increased relative to the degree of renal dysfunction. Long-term clinical trials in diabetic patients with significant renal dysfunction (serum creatinine > 2.0 mg/dL) have not been conducted. Therefore, treatment of these patients with PRECOSE® is not recommended.

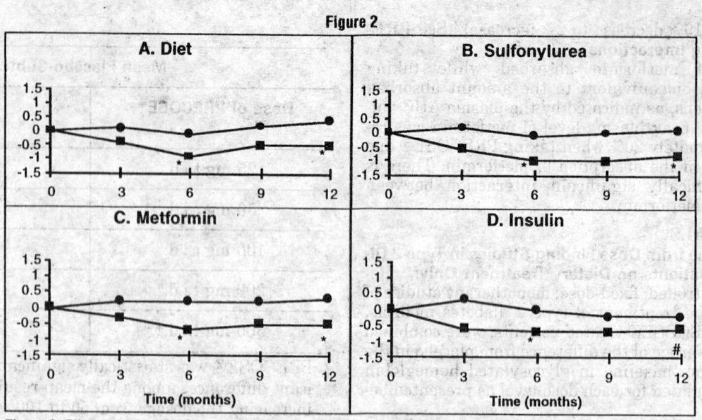

Figure 2: Effects of PRECOSE® (■) and Placebo (●) on mean change in HbA1c levels from baseline throughout a one-year study in patients with type 2 diabetes mellitus when used in combination with: (A) diet alone; (B) sulfonylurea; (C) metformin; or (D) insulin. Treatment differences at 6 and 12 months were tested: * $p < 0.01$; # $p = 0.077$.

	Strength	NDC	Tablet Identification
Bottles of 100:	25 mg	0026-2863-51	PRECOSE 25
	50 mg	0026-2861-51	PRECOSE 50
	100 mg	0026-2862-51	PRECOSE 100
Unit Dose Packages of 100:	50 mg	0026-2861-48	PRECOSE 50

Drug Interactions: Certain drugs tend to produce hyperglycemia and may lead to loss of blood glucose control. These drugs include the thiazides and other diuretics, corticosteroids, phenothiazines, thyroid products, estrogens, oral contraceptives, phenytoin, nicotinic acid, sympathomimetics, calcium channel-blocking drugs, and isoniazid. When such drugs are administered to a patient receiving PRECOSE®, the patient should be closely observed for loss of blood glucose control. When such drugs are withdrawn from patients receiving PRECOSE® in combination with sulfonylureas or insulin, patients should be observed closely for any evidence of hypoglycemia.

Intestinal adsorbents (e.g., charcoal) and digestive enzyme preparations containing carbohydrate-splitting enzymes (e.g., amylase, pancreatin) may reduce the effect of PRECOSE® and should not be taken concomitantly.

PRECOSE ® has been shown to change the bioavailability of digoxin when they are co-administered, which may require digoxin dose adjustment. (See **CLINICAL PHARMACOLOGY, Drug-Drug Interactions**).

Carcinogenesis, Mutagenesis, and Impairment of Fertility: Eight carcinogenicity studies were conducted with acarbose. Six studies were performed in rats (two strains, Sprague-Dawley and Wistar) and two studies were performed in hamsters.

In the first rat study, Sprague-Dawley rats received acarbose in feed at high doses (up to approximately 500 mg/kg body weight) for 104 weeks. Acarbose treatment resulted in a significant increase in the incidence of renal tumors (adenomas and adenocarcinomas) and benign Leydig cell tumors. This study was repeated with a similar outcome. Further studies were performed to separate direct carcinogenic effects of acarbose from indirect effects resulting from the carbohydrate malnutrition induced by the large doses of acarbose employed in the studies. In one study using Sprague-Dawley rats, acarbose was mixed with feed but carbohydrate deprivation was prevented by the addition of glucose to the diet. In a 26-month study of Sprague-Dawley rats, acarbose was administered by daily postprandial gavage so as to avoid the pharmacologic effects of the drug. In both of these studies, the increased incidence of renal tumors found in the original studies did not occur. Acarbose was also given in food and by postprandial gavage in two separate studies in Wistar rats. No increased incidence of renal tumors was found in either of these Wistar rat studies. In two feeding studies of hamsters, with and without glucose supplementation, there was also no evidence of carcinogenicity.

Acarbose did not induce any DNA damage *in vitro* in the CHO chromosomal aberration assay, bacterial mutagenesis (Ames) assay, or a DNA binding assay. *In vivo*, no DNA damage was detected in the dominant lethal test in male mice, or the mouse micronucleus test.

Fertility studies conducted in rats after oral administration produced no untoward effect on fertility or on the overall capability to reproduce.

Pregnancy:

Teratogenic Effects: Pregnancy Category B. The safety of PRECOSE® in pregnant women has not been established. Reproduction studies have been performed in rats at doses up to 480 mg/kg (corresponding to 9 times the exposure in humans, based on drug blood levels) and have revealed no evidence of impaired fertility or harm to the fetus due to acarbose. In rabbits, reduced maternal body weight gain, probably the result of the pharmacodynamic activity of high doses of acarbose in the intestines, may have been responsible for a slight increase in the number of embryonic losses. However, rabbits given 160 mg/kg acarbose (corresponding to 10 times the dose in man, based on body surface area) showed no evidence of embryotoxicity and there was no evidence of teratogenicity at a dose 32 times the dose in man (based on body surface area). There are, however, no adequate and well-controlled studies of PRECOSE® in pregnant women. Because animal reproduction studies are not always predictive of the human response, this drug should be used during pregnancy only if clearly needed. Because current information strongly suggests that abnormal blood glucose levels during pregnancy are associated with a higher incidence of congenital anomalies as well as increased neonatal morbidity and mortality, most experts recommend that insulin be used during pregnancy to maintain blood glucose levels as close to normal as possible.

Nursing Mothers: A small amount of radioactivity has been found in the milk of lactating rats after administration of radiolabeled acarbose. It is not known whether this drug is excreted in human milk. Because many drugs are excreted in human milk, PRECOSE® should not be administered to a nursing woman.

Pediatric Use: Safety and effectiveness of PRECOSE® in pediatric patients have not been established.

Geriatric Use: Of the total number of subjects in clinical studies of PRECOSE® in the United States, 27 percent were 65 and over, while 4 percent were 75 and over. No overall differences in safety and effectiveness were observed between these subjects and younger subjects. The mean steady-state area under the curve (AUC) and maximum concentrations of acarbose were approximately 1.5 times higher in elderly compared to young volunteers; however, these differences were not statistically significant.

ADVERSE REACTIONS

Digestive Tract: Gastrointestinal symptoms are the most common reactions to PRECOSE®. In U.S. placebo-controlled trials, the incidences of abdominal pain, diarrhea, and flatulence were 19%, 31%, and 74% respectively in 1255 patients treated with PRECOSE® 50–300 mg t.i.d., whereas the corresponding incidences were 9%, 12%, and 29% in 999 placebo-treated patients. In a one-year safety study, during which patients kept diaries of gastrointestinal symptoms, abdominal pain and diarrhea tended to return to pretreatment levels over time, and the frequency and intensity of flatulence tended to abate with time. The increased gastrointestinal tract symptoms in patients treated with PRECOSE® are a manifestation of the mechanism of action of PRECOSE® and are related to the presence of undigested carbohydrate in the lower GI tract. Rarely, these gastrointestinal events may be severe and might be confused with paralytic ileus.

Elevated Serum Transaminase Levels: See **PRECAUTIONS**.

Other Abnormal Laboratory Findings: Small reductions in hematocrit occurred more often in PRECOSE®-treated patients than in placebo-treated patients but were not associated with reductions in hemoglobin. Low serum calcium and low plasma vitamin B_6 levels were associated with PRECOSE® therapy but are thought to be either spurious or of no clinical significance.

Hypersensitive Skin Reactions: Rarely, hypersensitive skin reactions such as rash may occur.

Edema: In rare instances edema has been reported.

OVERDOSAGE

Unlike sulfonylureas or insulin, an overdose of PRECOSE® will not result in hypoglycemia. An overdose may result in transient increases in flatulence, diarrhea, and abdominal discomfort which shortly subside.

DOSAGE AND ADMINISTRATION

There is no fixed dosage regimen for the management of diabetes mellitus with PRECOSE® or any other pharmacologic agent. Dosage of PRECOSE® must be individualized on the basis of both effectiveness and tolerance while not exceeding the maximum recommended dose of 100 mg t.i.d. PRECOSE® should be taken three times daily at the start (with the first bite) of each main meal. PRECOSE® should be started at a low dose, with gradual dose escalation as described below, both to reduce gastrointestinal side effects and to permit identification of the minimum dose required for adequate glycemic control of the patient.

During treatment initiation and dose titration (see below), one-hour postprandial plasma glucose may be used to determine the therapeutic response to PRECOSE® and identify the minimum effective dose for the patient. Thereafter, glycosylated hemoglobin should be measured at intervals of approximately three months. The therapeutic goal should be to decrease both postprandial plasma glucose and glycosylated hemoglobin levels to normal or near normal by using the lowest effective dose of PRECOSE®, either as monotherapy or in combination with sulfonylureas, insulin or metformin.

Initial Dosage: The recommended starting dosage of PRECOSE® is 25 mg given orally three times daily at the start (with the first bite) of each main meal. However, some patients may benefit from more gradual dose titration to minimize gastrointestinal side effects. This may be achieved by initiating treatment at 25 mg once per day and subsequently increasing the frequency of administration to achieve 25 mg t.i.d.

Maintenance Dosage: Once a 25 mg t.i.d. dosage regimen is reached, dosage of PRECOSE® should be adjusted at 4–8 week intervals based on one-hour postprandial glucose or glycosylated hemoglobin levels, and on tolerance. The dosage can be increased from 25 mg t.i.d. to 50 mg t.i.d. Some patients may benefit from further increasing the dosage to 100 mg t.i.d. The maintenance dose ranges from 50 mg t.i.d. to 100 mg t.i.d. However, since patients with low body weight may be at increased risk for elevated serum transaminases, only patients with body weight > 60 kg should be considered for dose titration above 50 mg t.i.d. (see **PRECAUTIONS**). If no further reduction in postprandial glucose or glycosylated hemoglobin levels is observed with titration to 100 mg t.i.d., consideration should be given to lowering the dose. Once an effective and tolerated dosage is established, it should be maintained.

Maximum Dosage: The maximum recommended dose for patients ≤ 60 kg is 50 mg t.i.d. The maximum recommended dose for patients > 60 kg is 100 mg t.i.d.

Patients Receiving Sulfonylureas or Insulin: Sulfonylurea agents or insulin may cause hypoglycemia. PRECOSE® given in combination with a sulfonylurea or insulin will cause a further lowering of blood glucose and may increase the potential for hypoglycemia. If hypoglycemia occurs, appropriate adjustments in the dosage of these agents should be made.

HOW SUPPLIED

PRECOSE® is available as 25 mg, 50 mg or 100 mg round, unscored tablets. Each tablet strength is white to yellow-tinged in color. The 25 mg tablet is coded with the word "PRECOSE" on one side and "25" on the other side. The 50 mg tablet is coded with the word "PRECOSE" and "50" on the same side. The 100 mg tablet is coded with the word "PRECOSE" and "100" on the same side. PRECOSE® is available in bottles of 100 and 50 mg strength in unit dose packages of 100.

[See table at top of previous page]

Do not store above 25°C (77°F). Protect from moisture. For bottles, keep container tightly closed.

BAYER HEALTHCARE
BAYER PHARMACEUTICALS CORPORATION
400 Morgan Lane
West Haven, CT 06516 USA
℞ Only
08753825, R.2 8/03 Bay g 5421
PRECOSE®/5202/0/8/USA-12

Shown in Product Identification Guide, page 308

TRASYLOL® ℞
(aprotinin injection)

> Anaphylactic or anaphylactoid reactions are possible when Trasylol® is administered. Hypersensitivity reactions are rare in patients with no prior exposure to aprotinin. The risk of anaphylaxis is increased in patients who are re-exposed to aprotinin-containing products. The benefit of Trasylol® to patients undergoing primary CABG surgery should be weighed against the risk of anaphylaxis should a second exposure to aprotinin be required. (See WARNINGS and PRECAUTIONS).

DESCRIPTION

Trasylol® (aprotinin injection), $C_{284}H_{432}N_{84}O_{79}S_7$, is a natural proteinase inhibitor obtained from bovine lung. Aprotinin (molecular weight of 6512 daltons), consists of 58 amino acid residues that are arranged in a single polypeptide chain, cross-linked by three disulfide bridges. It is supplied as a clear, colorless, sterile isotonic solution for intravenous administration. Each milliliter contains 10,000 KIU (Kallikrein Inhibitor Units) (1.4 mg/mL) and 9 mg sodium chloride in water for injection. Hydrochloric acid and/or sodium hydroxide is used to adjust the pH to 4.5–6.5.

CLINICAL PHARMACOLOGY

Mechanism of Action: Aprotinin is a broad spectrum protease inhibitor which modulates the systemic inflammatory response (SIR) associated with cardiopulmonary bypass (CPB) surgery. SIR results in the interrelated activation of the hemostatic, fibrinolytic, cellular and humoral inflammatory systems. Aprotinin, through its inhibition of multiple mediators [e.g., kallikrein, plasmin] results in the attenuation of inflammatory responses, fibrinolysis, and thrombin generation.

Aprotinin inhibits pro-inflammatory cytokine release and maintains glycoprotein homeostasis. In platelets, aprotinin reduces glycoprotein loss (e.g., GpIb, GpIIb/IIIa), while in granulocytes it prevents the expression of pro-inflammatory adhesive glycoproteins (e.g., CD11b).

The effects of aprotinin use in CPB involves a reduction in inflammatory response which translates into a decreased need for allogeneic blood transfusions, reduced bleeding, and decreased mediastinal re-exploration for bleeding.

Pharmacokinetics: The studies comparing the pharmacokinetics of aprotinin in healthy volunteers, cardiac patients undergoing surgery with cardiopulmonary bypass, and women undergoing hysterectomy suggest linear pharmacokinetics over the dose range of 50,000 KIU to 2 million KIU. After intravenous (IV) injection, rapid distribution of aprotinin occurs into the total extracellular space, leading to a rapid initial decrease in plasma aprotinin concentration. Following this distribution phase, a plasma half-life of about 150 minutes is observed. At later time points, (i.e., beyond 5 hours after dosing) there is a terminal elimination phase with a half-life of about 10 hours.

Average steady state intraoperative plasma concentrations were 137 KIU/mL (n=10) after administration of the following dosage regimen: 1 million KIU IV loading dose, 1 million KIU into the pump prime volume, 250,000 KIU per hour of operation as continuous intravenous infusion (Regimen B). Average steady state intraoperative plasma concentrations were 250 KIU/mL in patients (n=20) treated with aprotinin during cardiac surgery by administration of Regimen A (exactly double Regimen B): 2 million KIU IV loading dose, 2 million KIU into the pump prime volume, 500,000 KIU per hour of operation as continuous intravenous infusion.

Following a single IV dose of radiolabelled aprotinin, approximately 25–40% of the radioactivity is excreted in the urine over 48 hours. After a 30 minute infusion of 1 million KIU, about 2% is excreted as unchanged drug. After a larger dose of 2 million KIU infused over 30 minutes, urinary excretion of unchanged aprotinin accounts for approximately 9% of the dose. Animal studies have shown that aprotinin is accumulated primarily in the kidney. Aprotinin, after being filtered by the glomeruli, is actively reabsorbed by the proximal tubules in which it is stored in phagolysosomes. Aprotinin is slowly degraded by lysosomal enzymes. The physiological renal handling of aprotinin is similar to that of other small proteins, e.g., insulin.

CLINICAL TRIALS

Repeat Coronary Artery Bypass Graft Patients:

Four placebo-controlled, double-blind studies of Trasylol® were conducted in the United States; of 540 randomized patients undergoing repeat coronary artery bypass graft (CABG) surgery, 480 were valid for efficacy analysis. The following treatment regimens were used in the studies: Trasylol® Regimen A (2 million KIU IV loading dose, 2 million KIU into the pump prime volume, and 500,000 KIU per hour of surgery as a continuous intravenous infusion); Trasylol® Regimen B (1 million KIU IV loading dose, 1 million KIU into the pump prime volume, and 250,000 KIU per hour of surgery as a continuous intravenous infusion); a pump prime regimen (2 million KIU into the pump prime volume only); and a placebo regimen (normal saline). All patients valid for efficacy in the above studies were pooled by treatment regimen for analyses of efficacy.

In this pooled analysis, fewer patients receiving Trasylol®, either Regimen A or Regimen B, required any donor blood compared to the pump prime only or placebo regimens. The number of units of donor blood required by patients, the volume (milliliters) of donor blood transfused, the number of units of donor blood products transfused, the thoracic drainage rate, and the total thoracic drainage volumes were also reduced in patients receiving Trasylol® as compared to placebo.

[See table above]

Efficacy Variables: Repeat CABG Patients
Mean (S.D.) or % of Patients

VARIABLE	PLACEBO REGIMEN N=156	Trasylol® PUMP PRIME REGIMEN† N=68	Trasylol® REGIMEN B** N=113	Trasylol® REGIMEN A** N=143
% OF REPEAT CABG PATIENTS WHO REQUIRED DONOR BLOOD	76.3%	72.1%	48.7%	46.9%
UNITS OF DONOR BLOOD TRANSFUSED	3.7 (4.4)	2.5 (2.4)	2.2 (5.0)*	1.6 (2.9)*
mL OF DONOR BLOOD TRANSFUSED	1132 (1443)	756 (807)	723 (1779)*	515 (999)*
PLATELETS TRANSFUSED (Donor Units)	5.0 (10.0)	2.1 (4.6)*	1.3 (4.6)*	0.9 (4.3)*
CRYOPRECIPITATE TRANSFUSED (Donor Units)	0.9 (3.5)	0.0 (0.0)*	0.5 (4.0)	0.1 (0.8)*
FRESH FROZEN PLASMA TRANSFUSED (Donor Units)	1.3 (2.5)	0.5 (1.4)*	0.3 (1.1)*	0.2 (0.9)*
THORACIC DRAINAGE RATE (mL/hr)	89 (77)	73 (69)	66 (244)	40 (36)*
TOTAL THORACIC DRAINAGE VOLUME (mL)[a]	1659 (1226)	1561 (1370)	1103 (2001)*	960 (849)*
REOPERATION FOR DIFFUSE BLEEDING	1.9%	2.9%	0%	0%

† The pump prime regimen was evaluated in only one study in patients undergoing repeat CABG surgery. Note: The pump prime only regimen is not an approved dosage regimen.
* Significantly different from placebo, $p<0.05$ (Transfusion variables analyzed via ANOVA on ranks)
** Differences between Regimen A (high dose) and Regimen B (low dose) in efficacy and safety are not statistically significant.
[a] Excludes patients who required reoperation

Primary Coronary Artery Bypass Graft Patients:

Four placebo-controlled, double-blind studies of Trasylol® were conducted in the United States; of 1745 randomized patients undergoing primary CABG surgery, 1599 were valid for efficacy analysis. The dosage regimens used in these studies were identical to those used in the repeat CABG studies described above (Regimens A, B, pump prime, and placebo). All patients valid for efficacy were pooled by treatment regimen.

In this pooled analysis, fewer patients receiving Trasylol® Regimens A, B, and pump prime required any donor blood in comparison to the placebo regimen. The number of units of donor blood required by patients, the volume of donor blood transfused, the number of units of donor blood products transfused, the thoracic drainage rate, and total thoracic drainage volumes were also reduced in patients receiving Trasylol® as compared to placebo.

[See first table at top of next page]

Additional subgroup analyses showed no diminution in benefit with increasing age. Male and female patients benefited from Trasylol® with a reduction in the average number of units of donor blood transfused. Although male patients did better than female patients in terms of the percentage of patients who required any donor blood transfusions, the number of female patients studied was small.

A double-blind, randomized, Canadian study compared Trasylol® Regimen A (n=28) and placebo (n=23) in primary cardiac surgery patients (mainly CABG) requiring cardiopulmonary bypass who were treated with aspirin within 48 hours of surgery. The mean total blood loss (1209.7 mL vs.

Continued on next page

Trasylol—Cont.

2532.3 mL) and the mean number of units of packed red blood cells transfused (1.6 units vs 4.3 units) were significantly less ($p<0.008$) in the Trasylol® group compared to the placebo group.

In a U.S. randomized study of Trasylol® Regimen A and Regimen B versus the placebo regimen in 212 patients undergoing primary aortic and/or mitral valve replacement or repair, no benefit was found for Trasylol® in terms of the need for transfusion or the number of units of blood required.

INDICATIONS AND USAGE

Trasylol is indicated for prophylactic use to reduce perioperative blood loss and the need for blood transfusion in patients undergoing cardiopulmonary bypass in the course of coronary artery bypass graft surgery.

CONTRAINDICATIONS

Hypersensitivity to aprotinin.

WARNINGS

Anaphylactic or anaphylactoid reactions are possible when Trasylol® is administered. Hypersensitivity reactions are rare in patients with no prior exposure to aprotinin. Hypersensitivity reactions can range from skin eruptions, itching, dyspnea, nausea and tachycardia to fatal anaphylactic shock with circulatory failure. If a hypersensitivity reaction occurs during injection or infusion of Trasylol®, administration should be stopped immediately and emergency treatment should be initiated. It should be noted that severe (fatal) hypersensitivity/anaphylactic reactions can also occur in connection with application of the test dose. Even when a second exposure to aprotinin has been tolerated without symptoms, a subsequent administration may result in severe hypersensitivity/anaphylactic reactions.

Re-exposure to aprotinin: In a retrospective review of 387 European patient records with documented re-exposure to Trasylol®, the incidence of hypersensitivity/anaphylactic reactions was 2.7%. Two patients who experienced hypersensitivity/anaphylactic reactions subsequently died, 24 hours and 5 days after surgery, respectively. The relationship of these 2 deaths to Trasylol® is unclear. This retrospective review also showed that the incidence of a hypersensitivity or anaphylactic reaction following re-exposure is increased when the re-exposure occurs within 6 months of the initial administration (5.0% for re-exposure within 6 months and 0.9% for re-exposure greater than 6 months). Other smaller studies have shown that in case of re-exposure, the incidence of hypersensitivity/anaphylactic reactions may reach the five percent level.

Before initiating treatment with Trasylol® in a patient with a history of prior exposure to aprotinin or products containing aprotinin, the recommendations below should be followed to manage a potential hypersensitivity or anaphylactic reaction: 1) Have standard emergency treatments for hypersensitivity or anaphylactic reactions readily available in the operating room (e.g., epinephrine, corticosteroids). 2) Administration of the test dose and loading dose should be done only when the conditions for rapid cannulation (if necessary) are present. 3) Delay the addition of Trasylol® into the pump prime solution until after the loading dose has been safely administered. Additionally, administration of H1 and H2 blockers 15 minutes before the test dose may be considered.

PRECAUTIONS

General: *Test Dose:* All patients treated with Trasylol® should first receive a test dose to assess the potential for allergic reactions. The test dose of 1 mL Trasylol® should be administered intravenously at least 10 minutes prior to the loading dose. However, even after the uneventful administration of the initial 1 mL test-dose, the therapeutic dose may cause an anaphylactic reaction. If this happens the infusion of aprotinin should immediately be stopped, and standard emergency treatment for anaphylaxis be applied. It should be noted that hypersensitivity/anaphylactic reactions can also occur in connection with application of the test-dose. (see WARNINGS)

Allergic Reactions: Patients with a history of allergic reactions to drugs or other agents may be at greater risk of developing a hypersensitivity or anaphylactic reaction upon exposure to Trasylol®. (see WARNINGS)

Loading Dose: The loading dose of Trasylol® should be given intravenously to patients in the supine position over a 20–30 minute period. Rapid intravenous administration of Trasylol® can cause a transient fall in blood pressure. (see DOSAGE AND ADMINISTRATION).

Use of Trasylol® in patients undergoing deep hypothermic circulatory arrest: Two U.S. case control studies have reported contradictory results in patients receiving Trasylol® while undergoing deep hypothermic circulatory arrest in connection with surgery of the aortic arch.

The first study showed an increase in both renal failure and mortality compared to age-matched historical controls. Similar results were not observed, however, in a second case control study. The strength of this association is uncertain because there are no data from randomized studies to confirm or refute these findings.

Drug Interactions: Trasylol® is known to have antifibrinolytic activity and, therefore, may inhibit the effects of fibrinolytic agents.

Efficacy Variables: Primary CABG Patients Mean (S.D.) or % of Patients

VARIABLE	PLACEBO REGIMEN N=624	Trasylol® PUMP PRIME REGIMEN† N=159	Trasylol® REGIMEN B** N=175	Trasylol® REGIMEN A** N=641
% OF PRIMARY CABG PATIENTS WHO REQUIRED DONOR BLOOD	53.5%	32.7%*	37.1%*	36.8%*
UNITS OF DONOR BLOOD TRANSFUSED	1.7 (2.4)	0.9 (1.6)*	1.0 (1.6)*	0.9 (1.4)*
mL OF DONOR BLOOD TRANSFUSED	584 (840)	286 (518)*	313 (505)*	295 (503)*
PLATELETS TRANSFUSED (Donor Units)	1.3 (3.7)	0.5 (2.4)*	0.3 (1.6)*	0.3 (1.5)*
CRYOPRECIPITATE TRANSFUSED (Donor Units)	0.5 (2.2)	0.0 (0.0)*	0.1 (0.8)*	0.0 (0.0)*
FRESH FROZEN PLASMA TRANSFUSED (Donor Units)	0.6 (1.7)	0.2 (1.7)*	0.2 (0.8)*	0.2 (0.9)*
THORACIC DRAINAGE RATE (mL/hr)	87 (67)	51 (36)*	45 (31)*	39 (32)*
TOTAL THORACIC DRAINAGE VOLUME (mL)	1232 (711)	852 (653)*	792 (465)*	705 (493)*
REOPERATION FOR DIFFUSE BLEEDING	1.4%	0.6%	0%	0%*

† The pump prime regimen was evaluated in only one study in patients undergoing primary CABG surgery. Note: The pump prime only regimen is not an approved dosage regimen.

* Significantly different from placebo, $p<0.05$ (Transfusion variables analyzed via ANOVA on ranks)

** Differences between Regimen A (high dose) and Regimen B (low dose) in efficacy and safety are not statistically significant.

INCIDENCE RATES OF ADVERSE EVENTS (> = 2%) BY BODY SYSTEM AND TREATMENT FOR ALL PATIENTS FROM US PLACEBO-CONTROLLED CLINICAL TRIALS

Adverse Event	Aprotinin (n = 2002) values in %	Placebo (n = 1084) values in %
Any Event	76	77
Body as a Whole		
Fever	15	14
Infection	6	7
Chest Pain	2	2
Asthenia	2	2
Cardiovascular		
Atrial Fibrillation	21	23
Hypotension	8	10
Myocardial Infarct	6	6
Atrial Flutter	6	5
Ventricular Extrasystoles	6	4
Tachycardia	6	7
Ventricular Tachycardia	5	4
Heart Failure	5	4
Pericarditis	5	5
Peripheral Edema	5	5
Hypertension	4	5
Arrhythmia	4	3
Supraventricular Tachycardia	4	3
Atrial Arrhythmia	3	3
Digestive		
Nausea	11	9
Constipation	4	5
Vomiting	3	4
Diarrhea	3	2
Liver Function Tests Abnormal	3	2
Hemic and Lymphatic		
Anemia	2	8
Metabolic & Nutritional		
Creatine Phosphokinase Increased	2	1
Musculoskeletal		
Any Event	2	3
Nervous		
Confusion	4	4
Insomnia	3	4
Respiratory		
Lung Disorder	8	8
Pleural Effusion	7	9
Atelectasis	5	6
Dyspnea	4	4
Pneumothorax	4	4
Asthma	2	3
Hypoxia	2	1
Skin and Appendages		
Rash	2	2
Urogenital		
Kidney Function Abnormal	3	2
Urinary Retention	3	3
Urinary Tract Infection	2	2

In study of nine patients with untreated hypertension, Trasylol® infused intravenously in a dose of 2 million KIU over two hours blocked the acute hypotensive effect of 100mg of captopril.

Trasylol®, in the presence of heparin, has been found to prolong the activated clotting time (ACT) as measured by a celite surface activation method. The kaolin activated clotting time appears to be much less affected. However, Trasylol® should not be viewed as a heparin sparing agent. (see Laboratory Monitoring of Anticoagulation During Cardiopulmonary Bypass).

Carcinogenesis, Mutagenesis, Impairment of Fertility: Long-term animal studies to evaluate the carcinogenic potential of Trasylol® or studies to determine the effect of Trasylol® on fertility have not been performed.

Results of microbial *in vitro* tests using *Salmonella typhimurium* and *Bacillus subtilis* indicate that Trasylol® is not a mutagen.

Pregnancy: Teratogenic Effects: Pregnancy Category B: Reproduction studies have been performed in rats at intravenous doses up to 200,000 KIU/kg/day for 11 days, and in rabbits at intravenous doses up to 100,000 KIU/kg/day for 13 days, 2.4 and 1.2 times the human dose on a mg/kg basis and 0.37 and 0.36 times the human mg/m^2 dose. They have revealed no evidence of impaired fertility or harm to the fetus due to Trasylol®. There are, however, no adequate and well-controlled studies in pregnant women. Because animal reproduction studies are not always predictive of human response, this drug should be used during pregnancy only if clearly needed.

Nursing Mother: Not applicable.

Pediatric Use: Safety and effectiveness in pediatric patient(s) have not been established.

Geriatric Use: Of the total of 3083 subjects in clinical studies of Trasylol®, 1100 (35.7 percent) were 65 and over, while 297 (9.6 percent) were 75 and over. Of patients 65 years and older, 479 (43.5 percent) received Regimen A and 237 (21.5 percent) received Regimen B. No overall differences in safety or effectiveness were observed between these subjects and younger subjects for either dose regimen, and other reported clinical experience has not identified differences in responses between the elderly and younger patients.

Laboratory Monitoring of Anticoagulation during Cardiopulmonary Bypass: Trasylol® prolongs whole blood clotting times by a different mechanism than heparin. In the presence of aprotinin, prolongation is dependent on the type of whole blood clotting test employed. If an activated clotting time (ACT) is used to determine the effectiveness of heparin anticoagulation, the prolongation of the ACT by aprotinin may lead to an overestimation of the degree of anticoagulation, thereby leading to inadequate anticoagulation. During extended extracorporeal circulation, patients may require additional heparin, even in the presence of ACT levels that appear adequate.

In patients undergoing CPB with Trasylol® therapy, one of the following methods may be employed to maintain adequate anticoagulation:

1) ACT - An ACT is not a standardized coagulation test, and different formulations of the assay are affected differently by the presence of aprotinin. The test is further influenced by variable dilution effects and the temperature experienced during cardiopulmonary bypass. It has been observed that Kaolin-based ACTs are not increased to the same degree by aprotinin as are diatomaceous earth-based (celite) ACTs. While protocols vary, a minimal celite ACT of 750 seconds or kaolin-ACT of 480 seconds, independent of the effects of hemodilution and hypothermia, is recommended in the presence of aprotinin. Consult the manufacturer of the ACT test regarding the interpretation of the assay in the presence of Trasylol®.

2) Fixed Heparin Dosing - A standard loading dose of heparin, administered prior to cannulation of the heart, plus the quantity of heparin added to the prime volume of the CPB circuit, should total at least 350 IU/kg. Additional heparin should be administered in a fixed-dose regimen based on patient weight and duration of CPB.

3) Heparin Titration - Protamine titration, a method that is not affected by aprotinin, can be used to measure heparin levels. A heparin dose response, assessed by protamine titration, should be performed prior to administration of aprotinin to determine the heparin loading dose. Additional heparin should be administered on the basis of heparin levels measured by protamine titration. Heparin levels during bypass should not be allowed to drop below 2.7 U/mL (2.0 mg/kg) or below the level indicated by heparin dose response testing performed prior to administration of aprotinin.

Protamine Administration - In patients treated with Trasylol®, the amount of protamine administered to reverse heparin activity should be based on the actual amount of heparin administered, and not on the ACT values.

ADVERSE REACTIONS

Studies of patients undergoing CABG surgery, either primary or repeat, indicate that Trasylol® is generally well tolerated. The adverse events reported are frequent sequelae of cardiac surgery and are not necessarily attributable to Trasylol® therapy. Adverse events reported, up to the time of hospital discharge, from patients in US placebo-controlled trials are listed in the following table. The table lists only those events that were reported in 2% or more of the Trasylol® treated patients without regard to causal relationship.

[See second table on previous page]

In comparison to the placebo group, no increase in mortality in patients treated with Trasylol® was observed. Additional events of particular interest from controlled US trials with an incidence of less than 2%, are listed below:

EVENT	Percentage of patients treated with Trasylol N = 2002	Percentage of patients treated with Placebo N = 1084
Thrombosis	1.0	0.6
Shock	0.7	0.4
Cerebrovascular Accident	0.7	2.1
Thrombophlebitis	0.2	0.5
Deep Thrombophlebitis	0.7	1.0
Lung Edema	1.3	1.5
Pulmonary Embolus	0.3	0.6
Kidney Failure	1.0	0.6
Acute Kidney Failure	0.5	0.6
Kidney Tubular Necrosis	0.8	0.4

Listed below are additional events, from controlled US trials with an incidence between 1 and 2%, and also from uncontrolled, compassionate use trials and spontaneous post-marketing reports. Estimates of frequency cannot be made for spontaneous post-marketing reports *(italicized)*.

Body as a Whole: Sepsis, death, multi-system organ failure, immune system disorder, *hemoperitoneum.*

Cardiovascular: Ventricular fibrillation, heart arrest, bradycardia, congestive heart failure, hemorrhage, bundle branch block, myocardial ischemia, ventricular tachycardia, heart block, pericardial effusion, ventricular arrhythmia, shock, pulmonary hypertension.

Digestive: Dyspepsia, gastrointestinal hemorrhage, jaundice, hepatic failure.

Hematologic and Lymphatic: Although thrombosis was not reported more frequently in aprotinin versus placebo-treated patients in controlled trials, it has been reported in uncontrolled trials, compassionate use trials, and spontaneous post-marketing reporting. These reports of thrombosis encompass the following terms: thrombosis, occlusion, arterial thrombosis, *pulmonary thrombosis*, coronary occlusion, embolus, pulmonary embolus, thrombophlebitis, deep thrombophlebitis, cerebrovascular accident, cerebral embolism. Other hematologic events reported include leukocytosis, thrombocytopenia, coagulation disorder (which includes

Incidence of Graft Closure, Myocardial Infarction and Death by Treatment Group

	Overall Closure Rates*		Incidence of MI**	Incidence of Death***
	All Centers n = 703 %	U.S. Centers n = 381 %	All Centers n = 831 %	All Centers n = 870 %
Trasylol®	15.4	9.4	2.9	1.4
Placebo	10.9	9.5	3.8	1.6
CI for the Difference (%) (Drug - Placebo)	(1.3, 9.6)†	(−3.8, 5.9)†	−3.3 to 1.5‡	−1.9 to 1.4‡

* Population: all patients with assessable saphenous vein grafts
** Population: all patients assessable by blinded consultant
*** All patients
† 90%; per protocol
‡ 95%; not specified in protocol

	TEST DOSE	LOADING DOSE	"PUMP PRIME" DOSE	CONSTANT INFUSION DOSE
TRASYLOL® REGIMEN A	1 mL (1.4 mg, or 10,000 KIU)	200 mL (280 mg, or 2.0 million KIU)	200 mL (280 mg, or 2.0 million KIU)	50 mL/hr (70 mg/hr, or 500,000 KIU/hr)
TRASYLOL® REGIMEN B	1 mL (1.4 mg, or 10,000 KIU)	100 mL (140 mg, or 1.0 million KIU)	100 mL (140 mg, or 1.0 million KIU)	25 mL/hr (35 mg/hr, or 250,000 KIU/hr)

disseminated intravascular coagulation), decreased prothombin.

Metabolic and Nutritional: Hyperglycemia, hypokalemia, hypervolemia, acidosis.

Musculoskeletal: Arthralgia.

Nervous: Agitation, dizziness, anxiety, convulsion.

Respiratory: Pneumonia, apnea, increased cough, lung edema.

Skin: *Skin discoloration.*

Urogenital: Oliguria, kidney failure, acute kidney failure, kidney tubular necrosis.

Myocardial Infarction: In the pooled analysis of all patients undergoing CABG surgery, there was no significant difference in the incidence of investigator-reported myocardial infarction (MI) in Trasylol® treated patients as compared to placebo treated patients. However, because no uniform criteria for the diagnosis of myocardial infarction were utilized by investigators, this issue was addressed prospectively in three later studies (two studies evaluated Regimen A, Regimen B and Pump Prime Regimen; one study evaluated only Regimen A), in which data were analyzed by a blinded consultant employing an algorithm for possible, probable or definite MI. Utilizing this method, the incidence of definite myocardial infarction was 5.9% in the aprotinin-treated patients versus 4.7% in the placebo treated patients. This difference in the incidence rates was not statistically significant. Data from these three studies are summarized below.

Incidence of Myocardial Infarctions by Treatment Group
Population: All CABG Patients Valid for Safety Analysis

Treatment	Definite MI %	Definite or Probable MI %	Definite, Probable or Possible MI %
Pooled Data from Three Studies that Evaluated Regimen A			
Trasylol® Regimen A n = 646	4.6	10.7	14.1
Placebo n = 661	4.7	11.3	13.4
Pooled Data from Two Studies that Evaluated Regimen B and Pump Prime Regimen			
Trasylol® Regimen B n = 241	8.7	15.9	18.7
Trasylol® Pump Prime Regimen n = 239	6.3	15.7	18.1
Placebo n = 240	6.3	15.1	15.8

Graft Patency: In a recently completed multi-center, multi-national study to determine the effects of Trasylol® Regimen A vs. placebo on saphenous vein graft patency in patients undergoing primary CABG surgery, patients were subjected to routine postoperative angiography. Of the 13 study sites, 10 were in the United States and three were non-U.S. centers (Denmark (1), Israel (2)). The results of this study are summarized below.

[See first table above]

Although there was a statistically significantly increased risk of graft closure for Trasylol® treated patients compared to patients who received placebo (p=0.035), further analysis showed a significant treatment by site interaction for one of the non-U.S. sites vs. the U.S. centers. When the analysis of graft closures was repeated for U.S. centers only, there was no statistically significant difference in graft closure rates in patients who received Trasylol® vs. placebo. These results are the same whether analyzed as the proportion of patients who experienced at least one graft closure postoperatively or as the proportion of grafts closed. There were no differences between treatment groups in the incidence of myocardial infarction as evaluated by the blinded consultant (2.9% Trasylol® vs. 3.8% placebo) or of death (1.4% Trasylol® vs. 1.6% placebo) in this study.

Hypersensitivity and Anaphylaxis: See WARNINGS. Hypersensitivity and anaphylactic reactions during surgery were rarely reported in U.S. controlled clinical studies in patients with no prior exposure to Trasylol® (1/1424 patients or <0.1% on Trasylol® vs. 1/861 patients or 0.1% on placebo). In case of re-exposure the incidence of hypersensitivity/anaphylactic reactions has been reported to reach the 5% level. A review of 387 European patient records involving re-exposure to Trasylol® showed that the incidence of hypersensitivity or anaphylactic reactions was 5.0% for re-exposure within 6 months and 0.9% for re-exposure greater than 6 months.

Laboratory Findings

Serum Creatinine: Data pooled from all patients undergoing CABG surgery in U.S. placebo-controlled trials showed no statistically or clinically significant increase in the incidence of postoperative renal dysfunction in patients treated with Trasylol®. The incidence of serum creatinine elevations > 0.5 mg/dL above pre-treatment levels was 9% in the Trasylol® group vs. 8% in the placebo group (p=0.248), while the incidence of elevations >2.0 mg/dL above baseline was only 1% in each group (p=0.883). In the majority of instances, postoperative renal dysfunction was not severe and was reversible. Patients with baseline elevations in serum creatinine were not at increased risk of developing postoperative renal dysfunction following Trasylol® treatment.

Serum Transaminases: Data pooled from all patients undergoing CABG surgery in U.S. placebo-controlled trials showed no evidence of an increase in the incidence of postoperative hepatic dysfunction in patients treated with Trasylol®. The incidence of treatment-emergent increases in ALT (formerly SGPT) > 1.8 times the upper limit of normal was 14% in both the Trasylol® and placebo-treated patients (p=0.687), while the incidence of increases > 3 times the upper limit of normal was 5% in both groups (p=0.847).

Other Laboratory Findings: The incidence of treatment-emergent elevations in plasma glucose, AST (formerly SGOT), LDH, alkaline phosphatase, and CPK-MB was not notably different between Trasylol® and placebo treated patients undergoing CABG surgery. Significant elevations in the partial thromboplastin time (PTT) and celite Activated Clotting Time (celite ACT) are expected in Trasylol® treated patients in the hours after surgery due to circulating concentrations of Trasylol®, which are known to inhibit activation of the intrinsic clotting system by contact with a foreign material (e.g., celite), a method used in these tests. (see Laboratory Monitoring of Anticoagulation During Cardiopulmonary Bypass).

OVERDOSAGE

The maximum amount of Trasylol® that can be safely administered in single or multiple doses has not been determined. Doses up to 17.5 million KIU have been administered within a 24 hour period without any apparent toxicity.

Continued on next page

Trasylol—Cont.

There is one poorly documented case, however, of a patient who received a large, but not well determined, amount of Trasylol® (in excess of 15 million KIU) in 24 hours. The patient, who had pre-existing liver dysfunction, developed hepatic and renal failure postoperatively and died. Autopsy showed hepatic necrosis and extensive renal tubular and glomerular necrosis. The relationship of these findings to Trasylol® therapy is unclear.

DOSAGE AND ADMINISTRATION

Trasylol® given prophylactically in both Regimen A and Regimen B (half Regimen A) to patients undergoing CABG surgery significantly reduced the donor blood transfusion requirement relative to placebo treatment. In low risk patients there is no difference in efficacy between regimen A and B. Therefore, the dosage used (A vs. B) is at the discretion of the practitioner.

Trasylol® is supplied as a solution containing 10,000 KIU/mL, which is equal to 1.4 mg/mL. All intravenous doses of Trasylol® should be administered through a central line. **DO NOT ADMINISTER ANY OTHER DRUG USING THE SAME LINE.** Both regimens include a 1 mL test dose, a loading dose, a dose to be added while **recirculating** the priming fluid of the cardiopulmonary bypass circuit ("pump prime" dose), and a constant infusion dose. To avoid physical incompatibility of Trasylol® and heparin when adding to the pump prime solution, each agent must be added **during recirculation** of the pump prime to assure adequate dilution prior to admixture with the other component. Regimens A and B (both incorporating a 1 mL test dose) are described in the table below:

[See second table at top of previous page]

The 1 mL test dose should be administered intravenously at least 10 minutes before the loading dose. With the patient in a supine position, the loading dose is given slowly over 20–30 minutes, after induction of anesthesia but prior to sternotomy. In patients with known previous exposure to Trasylol®, the loading dose should be given just prior to cannulation. When the loading dose is complete, it is followed by the constant infusion dose, which is continued until surgery is complete and the patient leaves the operating room. The "pump prime" dose is added to the **recirculating** priming fluid of the cardiopulmonary bypass circuit, by replacement of an aliquot of the priming fluid, prior to the institution of cardiopulmonary bypass. Total doses of more than 7 million KIU have not been studied in controlled trials.

Parenteral drug products should be inspected visually for particulate matter and discoloration prior to administration whenever solution and container permit. Discard any unused portion.

Renal and Hepatic Impairment: No formal studies of the pharmacokinetics of aprotinin in patients with pre-existing renal insufficiency have been conducted. However, in the placebo-controlled clinical trials conducted in the United States, patients with mildly elevated pretreatment serum creatinine levels did not have a notably higher incidence of clinically significant post-treatment elevations in serum creatinine following either Trasylol® Regimen A or Regimen B compared to administration of the placebo regimen. Changes in aprotinin pharmacokinetics with age or impaired renal function are not great enough to require any dose adjustment. No pharmacokinetic data from patients with pre-existing hepatic disease treated with Trasylol® are available.

HOW SUPPLIED

Size	Strength	NDC
100 mL vials	1,000,000 KIU	0026-8196-36
200 mL vials	2,000,000 KIU	0026-8197-63

STORAGE

Trasylol® should be stored between 2° and 25°C (36° - 77°F).

Protect from freezing.

Bayer HealthCare
Pharmaceuticals Corporation
400 Morgan Lane
West Haven, CT 06516
Made in Germany

Rx Only

01298181 12/03 ©2003 Bayer Pharmaceuticals Corporation
10350L

Shown in Product Identification Guide, page 309

VIADUR® ℞

[*vī-ă-dūr*]
(leuprolide acetate implant)

DESCRIPTION

Viadur® (leuprolide acetate implant) is a sterile nonbiodegradable, osmotically driven miniaturized implant designed to deliver leuprolide acetate for 12 months at a controlled rate (Figure A). Viadur® incorporates DUROS® technology. The system contains 65 mg of leuprolide (free base). Leuprolide acetate is a synthetic nonapeptide analog of naturally occurring gonadotropin-releasing hormone (GnRH or LH-RH). The analog possesses greater potency than the natural hormone. The implant is inserted subcutaneously in the inner aspect of the upper arm. After 12 months, the implant must be removed. At the time an implant is removed, another implant may be inserted to continue therapy.

Viadur® contains 72 mg of leuprolide acetate (equivalent to 65 mg leuprolide free base) dissolved in 104 mg dimethyl sulfoxide. The 4 mm by 45 mm titanium alloy reservoir houses a polyurethane rate-controlling membrane, an elastomeric piston, and a polyethylene diffusion moderator. The reservoir also contains the osmotic tablets, which are not released with the drug formulation. The osmotic tablets are composed of sodium chloride, sodium carboxymethyl cellulose, povidone, magnesium stearate, and sterile water for injection. Polyethylene glycol fills the space between the osmotic tablets and the reservoir. A minute amount of silicone medical fluid is used during manufacture as a lubricant. The weight of the implant is approximately 1.1g.

Figure A. Viadur® (leuprolide acetate implant) (diagram not to scale)

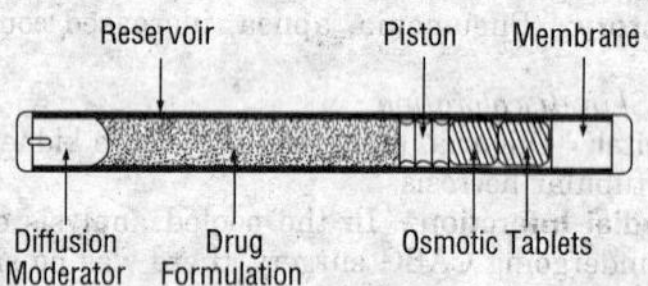

The chemical name is 5-Oxo-L-prolyl-L-histidyl-L-tryptophyl-L-seryl-L-tyrosyl-D-leucyl-L-leucyl-L-arginyl-N-ethyl-L-prolinamide acetate (salt), with the following structural formula:

[See chemical structure above]

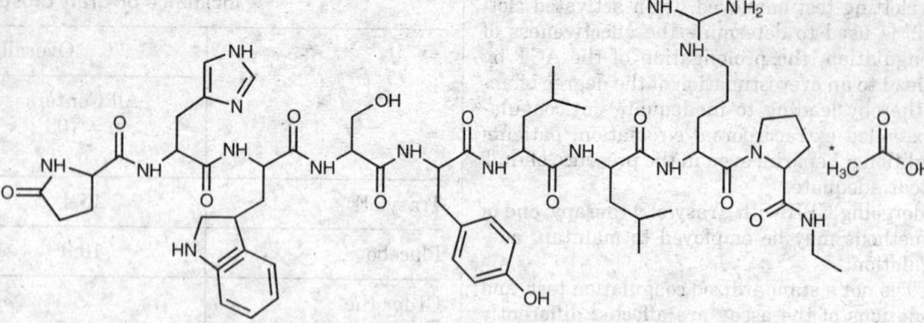

CLINICAL PHARMACOLOGY

Leuprolide acetate, an LH-RH agonist, acts as a potent inhibitor of gonadotropin secretion when given continuously and in therapeutic doses. Animal and human studies indicate that after an initial stimulation, chronic administration of leuprolide acetate results in suppression of ovarian and testicular steroidogenesis.

In humans, administration of leuprolide acetate results in an initial increase in circulating levels of luteinizing hormone (LH) and follicle-stimulating hormone (FSH), leading to a transient increase in concentrations of gonadal steroids (testosterone and dihydrotestosterone in males, and estrone and estradiol in premenopausal females). However, continuous administration of leuprolide acetate results in decreased levels of LH and FSH. In males, testosterone is reduced to castrate levels. These decreases occur within 2 to 4 weeks after initiation of treatment.

One Viadur® Implant nominally delivers 120 micrograms of leuprolide acetate per day over 12 months. Leuprolide acetate is not active when given orally.

PHARMACOKINETICS

Absorption: After insertion of Viadur®, mean serum leuprolide concentrations were 16.9 ng/mL at 4 hours and 2.4 ng/mL at 24 hours. Thereafter, leuprolide was released at a constant rate. Mean serum leuprolide concentrations were maintained at 0.9 ng/mL (0.3 to 3.1 ng/mL; SD = ±0.4) for 12 months. Upon removal and insertion of a new Viadur® at 12 months, steady-state serum leuprolide concentrations were maintained.

Distribution: The mean steady-state volume of distribution of leuprolide following 1 mg intravenous (IV) bolus administration to healthy male volunteers was 27 L. In vitro binding to human plasma proteins ranged from 43% to 49%.[1]

Metabolism: In healthy male volunteers administered a 1 mg IV bolus of leuprolide, the mean systemic clearance was 8.34 L/h, with a terminal elimination half-life of approximately 3 hours, based on a two-compartment model.[1] A pentapeptide (M-1) is the major leuprolide metabolite upon administration with different leuprolide acetate formulations. No drug metabolism study was conducted with Viadur®.

Excretion: No drug excretion study was conducted with Viadur®.

Dose Proportionality: In a study comparing one Viadur® implant to two Viadur® implants, mean serum leuprolide concentrations were proportional to dose.

Special Populations:

Geriatrics: The majority (88%) of the 131 patients studied in clinical trials were age 65 and over.

Pediatrics: The safety and effectiveness of Viadur® in pediatric patients have not been established (see **CONTRAINDICATIONS**).

Race: In the patients studied (80 Caucasian, 23 Black, 3 Hispanic), mean serum leuprolide concentrations were similar.

Renal and Hepatic Insufficiency: The pharmacokinetics of the drug in hepatically and renally impaired patients have not been determined.

Drug-Drug Interactions: No pharmacokinetic drug-drug interaction studies were conducted with Viadur®.

CLINICAL STUDIES

In two open-label, non-comparative, multicenter studies, 131 patients with prostatic cancer were treated with Viadur® and evaluated for up to two years. Two-thirds of the patients had stage C or less advanced disease. The dose-ranging study assessed serum testosterone as the primary efficacy endpoint in 51 patients treated with either one [n=27] or two [n=24] implants for 12 months. The confirmatory study evaluated achievement and maintenance of serum testosterone suppression in 80 patients each treated with one implant for 12 months. Both studies included a removal procedure and insertion of a new implant with evaluation for 12 additional months.

Following the initial insertion in patients receiving one implant, mean serum testosterone concentrations increased from 422 ng/dL at baseline to 690 ng/dL on Day 3, then decreased to below baseline by week two (Figure B). Serum testosterone decreased below the 50 ng/dL castrate threshold by week four in all but one patient [106 of 107 patients, 99%]. Once serum testosterone suppression was achieved [one patient was not continuously suppressed until week 28], testosterone remained suppressed below the castrate threshold for the duration of the treatment phase.

Figure B. Mean (+SD) Serum Total Testosterone Concentrations – All Patients (n=107) Who Received One Implant

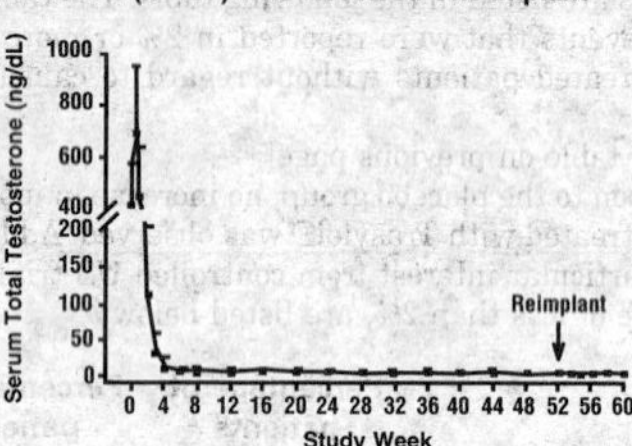

(Diagonal lines [//] indicate change in axis scale)

Most patients [n=118] had a new implant inserted for a second year of therapy following removal of the first implant(s). No patient experienced a clinically significant increase in serum testosterone [acute-on-chronic phenomenon] upon removal of the original implant(s) and insertion of a new implant. Suppression of serum testosterone was maintained in all patients through the two-month follow-up period following removal of the first implant(s) and insertion of a new implant.

Serum Prostate Specific Antigen (PSA) was monitored as a secondary endpoint in the clinical studies with Viadur®. Serum PSA decreased in all patients after they began treatment with Viadur®. At six months, PSA concentrations decreased from baseline by at least 90% in 74.2% of the 97 evaluable patients.

Periodic monitoring of serum testosterone and PSA concentrations is recommended, especially if the anticipated clinical or biochemical response to treatment has not been achieved.

INDICATIONS AND USAGE

Viadur® is indicated in the palliative treatment of advanced prostate cancer.

CONTRAINDICATIONS

1. Viadur® is contraindicated in patients with hypersensitivity to GnRH, GnRH agonist analogs, or any of the components in Viadur®. Anaphylactic reactions to synthetic GnRH or GnRH agonist analogs have been reported in the literature.[2]
2. Viadur® is contraindicated in women and in pediatric patients and was not studied in women or children. Moreover, leuprolide acetate can cause fetal harm when administered to a pregnant woman. Major fetal abnormalities were observed in rabbits but not in rats after administration of leuprolide acetate throughout gestation. There were increased fetal mortality and decreased

fetal weights in rats and rabbits. The effects on fetal mortality are expected consequences of the alterations in hormonal levels brought about by this drug. The possibility exists that spontaneous abortion may occur.

WARNINGS

Viadur®, like other LH-RH agonists, causes a transient increase in serum concentrations of testosterone during the first week of treatment. Patients may experience worsening of symptoms or onset of new symptoms, including bone pain, neuropathy, hematuria, or ureteral or bladder outlet obstruction (see **PRECAUTIONS**).

Cases of ureteral obstruction and spinal cord compression, which may contribute to paralysis with or without fatal complications, have been reported with LH-RH agonists.

If spinal cord compression or renal impairment develops, standard treatment of these complications should be instituted.

PRECAUTIONS

General: Patients with metastatic vertebral lesions and/or with urinary tract obstruction should be closely observed during the first few weeks of therapy (see **WARNINGS**).

X-rays do not affect Viadur® functionality. Viadur® is radio-opaque and is well visualized on X-rays.

The titanium alloy reservoir of Viadur® is nonferromagnetic and is not affected by magnetic resonance imaging (MRI). Slight image distortion around Viadur® may occur during MRI procedures.

Information for Patients: An information leaflet for patients is included with the product.

Laboratory tests: Response to Viadur® should be monitored by measuring serum concentrations of testosterone and prostate-specific antigen periodically.

Results of testosterone determinations are dependent on assay methodology. It is advisable to be aware of the type and precision of the assay methodology to make appropriate clinical and therapeutic decisions.

Drug Interactions: See **PHARMACOKINETICS**.

Drug/Laboratory Test Interactions: Therapy with leuprolide results in suppression of the pituitary-gonadal system. Results of diagnostic tests of pituitary gonadotropic and gonadal functions conducted during and after leuprolide therapy may be affected.

Carcinogenesis, Mutagenesis, Impairment of Fertility: Two-year carcinogenicity studies were conducted in rats and mice. In rats, dose-related increases of benign pituitary hyperplasia and benign pituitary adenomas were noted at 24 months when the drug was administered subcutaneously at high daily doses (4 to 24 mg/m^2, 50 to 300 times the daily human exposure based on body surface area). There were significant but not dose-related increases of pancreatic islet-cell adenomas in females and of testicular interstitial cell adenomas in males (highest incidence in the low dose group). In mice no pituitary abnormalities were observed at up to 180 mg/m^2 (over 2000 times the daily human exposure based on body surface area) for 2 years.

Mutagenicity studies were performed with leuprolide acetate using bacterial and mammalian systems. These studies provided no evidence of a mutagenic potential.

Pregnancy, Teratogenic Effects: Pregnancy Category X (see **CONTRAINDICATIONS**).

Pediatric Use: Viadur® is contraindicated in pediatric patients and was not studied in children (see **CONTRAINDICATIONS**).

ADVERSE REACTIONS

The safety of Viadur® was evaluated in 131 patients with prostate cancer treated for up to 24 months in two clinical trials. Viadur®, like other LHRH analogs, caused a transient increase in serum testosterone concentrations during the first 2 weeks of treatment. Therefore, potential exacerbations of signs and symptoms of the disease during the first few weeks of treatment are of concern in patients with vertebral metastases and/or urinary obstruction or hematuria. If these conditions are aggravated, it may lead to neurological problems such as weakness and/or paresthesia of the lower limbs or worsening of urinary symptoms (see **WARNINGS** and **PRECAUTIONS**).

In the above-described clinical trials, the transient increase in serum testosterone concentrations was associated with an exacerbation of disease symptoms, manifested by pain or bladder outlet obstructive symptoms (urinary retention or frequency) in 6 (4.6%) patients.

The majority of local reactions associated with initial insertion or removal and insertion of a new implant began and resolved within the first two weeks. Reactions persisted in 9.3% of patients. 10.3% of patients developed application-site reactions after the first two weeks following insertion.

Local reactions after initial insertion of a single implant included bruising (34.6%) and burning (5.6%). Other, less frequently reported, reactions included pulling, pressure, itching, erythema, pain, edema, and bleeding.

In these two clinical trials, four patients had local infection/inflammations that resolved after treatment with oral antibiotics.

Local reactions following insertion of a subsequent implant were comparable to those seen after initial insertion.

In the first 12 months after initial insertion of the implant(s), an implant extruded through the incision site in three of 131 patients (see Insertion and Removal Procedures for correct implant placement).

The following possibly or probably related systemic adverse events occurred during clinical trials within 24 months of treatment with Viadur®, and were reported in ≥2% of patients (Table 1).

Table 1: Incidence (%) of Possibly or Probably Related Systemic Adverse Events Reported by ≥ 2% of Patients Treated with Viadur® for up to 24 months

Body System	Adverse Event	Number (%)
Body as a Whole	Asthenia	10 (7.6%)
	Headache	6 (4.6%)
	Extremity pain	4 (3.1%)
Cardiovascular	Vasodilatation (hot flashes)*	89 (67.9%)
Digestive	Diarrhea	3 (2.3%)
Hematology and Lymphatic	Ecchymosis	6 (4.6%)
	Anemia	3 (2.3%)
Metabolic and Nutritional	Peripheral edema	4 (3.1%)
	Weight gain	3 (2.3%)
Nervous	Depression	7 (5.3%)
Respiratory	Dyspnea	3 (2.3%)
Skin	Sweating*	7 (5.3%)
	Alopecia	3 (2.3%)
Urogenital	Gynecomastia/ breast enlargement*	9 (6.9%)
	Nocturia	5 (3.8%)
	Urinary frequency	5 (3.8%)
	Testis atrophy or pain*	5 (3.8%)
	Breast pain*	4 (3.1%)
	Impotence*	3 (2.3%)

*Expected pharmacologic consequences of testosterone suppression.

In addition, the following possibly or probably related systemic adverse events were reported by <2% of patients using Viadur® in clinical studies.

General: General pain, chills, abdominal pain, malaise, dry mucous membranes

Gastrointestinal: Constipation, nausea

Hematologic: Iron deficiency anemia

Metabolic: Edema, weight loss

Musculoskeletal: Bone pain, arthritis

Nervous: Dizziness, insomnia, paresthesia, amnesia, anxiety

Skin: Pruritus, rash, hirsutism

Urogenital: Urinary urgency, prostatic disorder, urinary tract infection, dysuria, urinary incontinence, urinary retention

Changes in Bone Density: Decreased bone density has been reported in the medical literature in men who have had orchiectomy or who have been treated with an LH-RH agonist analog. In a clinical trial, 25 men with prostate cancer, 12 of whom had been treated previously with leuprolide acetate for at least 6 months, underwent bone density studies as a result of pain. The leuprolide-treated group had lower bone density scores than the nontreated control group. It can be anticipated that long periods of medical castration in men will have effects on bone density.

OVERDOSAGE

In clinical trials using daily subcutaneous leuprolide acetate in patients with prostate cancer, doses as high as 20 mg/day for up to 2 years caused no adverse effects differing from those observed with the 1 mg/day dose. The adverse event profiles were similar in patients receiving one or two Viadur® implants.

DOSAGE AND ADMINISTRATION

The recommended dose of Viadur® is one implant for 12 months. Each implant contains 65 mg leuprolide. The implant is inserted subcutaneously in the inner aspect of the upper arm and provides continuous release of leuprolide for 12 months of hormonal therapy.

Viadur® must be removed after 12 months of therapy. At the time an implant is removed, another implant may be inserted to continue therapy. (See Insertion and Removal Procedures.)

INSERTION AND REMOVAL PROCEDURES

Viadur® is supplied in a box containing one sterile Viadur® implant in a sealed vial, one Viadur® sterile implanter, one sealed container of lidocaine HCl USP 2%, 10 mL, and one sterile Viadur® Kit. The Viadur® Kit is designed to provide a sterile field and supplies to facilitate the insertion and/or subsequent removal of the implant.

In addition to the Viadur® Kit, sterile gloves are required for the insertion procedure and subsequent removal of the implant.

INSERTION PROCEDURE

Under aseptic conditions, an implanter is used to place the implant under the skin.

The implant is inserted using the procedure outlined below.

IDENTIFYING THE INSERTION SITE

1. Have the patient lie on his back on the examination table, with his left arm (if the patient is left-handed, the right arm) flexed at the elbow and externally rotated so that his hand is out to his side.

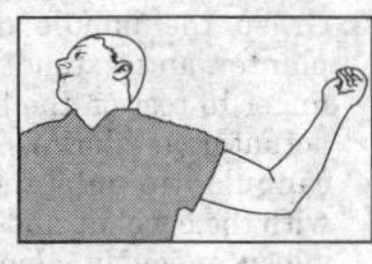

Using a pen and ruler, mark a site on the inner, upper arm approximately 8–10 cm above the elbow crease in the groove between the biceps and triceps muscles. Make sure that the site is unaffected by movement of the muscles.

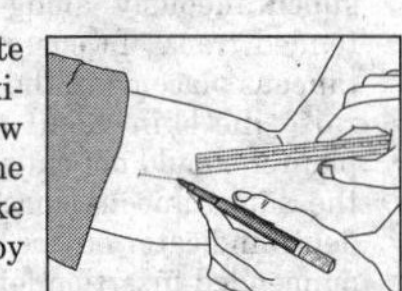

PREPARING THE STERILE FIELD

1. To establish a sterile field, carefully open the sterile Viadur® Kit. The sterile kit contains:
   1 scalpel
   1 forceps
   1 syringe
   1 package povidone-iodine swabs
   1 package wound closure strips
   1-22 Ga × 1.5″ needle
   1-25 Ga × 1.5″ needle
   6 gauze sponges
   2 alcohol prep pads
   1 package skin protectant
   1 bandage
   1 fenestrated drape
   1 marking pen
   1 ruler
   1 mosquito clamp
2. The implant tray contains:
   1 sealed vial, which contains the Viadur® implant
   1 sterile implanter
   1 sealed container of lidocaine HCl USP 2%, 10 mL
   To open the vial, remove the metal band from the bottle and pull up the stopper. Carefully drop the implant from the bottle onto the sterile field. Then, carefully drop the implanter and the container of lidocaine onto the sterile field.

Using sterile technique, remove the protective cap from the implant by pulling the cap straight off. **DO NOT TWIST CAP OFF AS IT MAY UNSCREW THE DIFFUSION MODERATOR, CAUSE ITS REMOVAL, OR OTHERWISE DAMAGE THE IMPLANT. SHOULD DAMAGE OCCUR, DO NOT INSERT THE IMPLANT AS PRODUCT FUNCTION CAN BE IMPAIRED.**

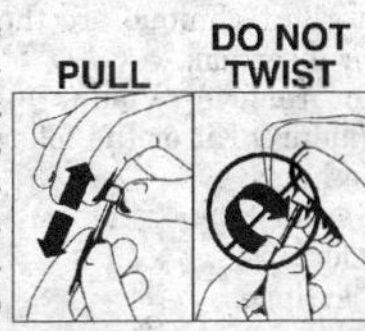

LOADING THE IMPLANTER

1. The implanter is packaged in the correct configuration for implant loading and insertion. Make sure the cannula is fully extended as shown, and the actuator is in its most forward position.

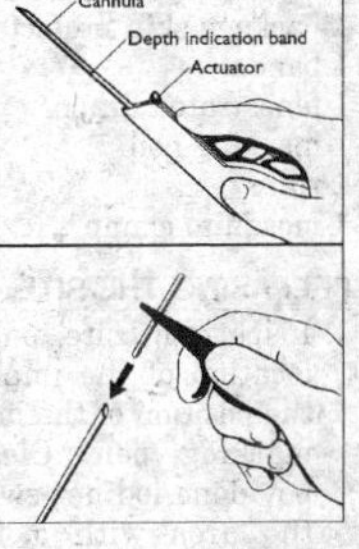

2. Using sterile forceps, slide the implant into the end of the cannula and push until it stops. When properly loaded, the implant should not protrude more than 1 mm past the bottom of the beveled edge.

INSERTING THE IMPLANT

1. Using aseptic technique, cleanse the insertion site, then drape the patient's arm. After determining the absence of known allergies to the anesthetic agent, infiltrate the site with lidocaine. Advance the needle to infiltrate the intended 5 cm track for the implant insertion.

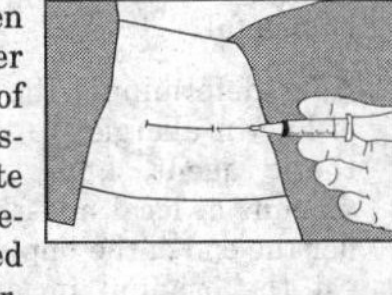

2. Determine that anesthesia is adequate. Make an incision of approximately 5 mm with the scalpel, just through the dermis.

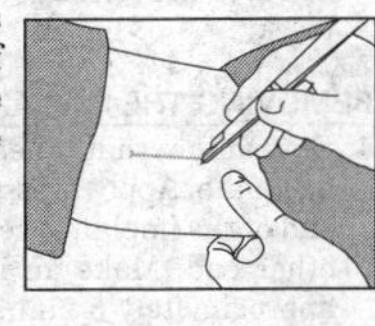

Continued on next page

Viadur—Cont.

3. Grasp the handle of the implanter and extend the index finger to rest on the back of the actuator as shown. Insert the cannula tip into the incision with the bevel up and advance it subcutaneously along the intended track. To ensure subcutaneous placement, the Viadur® implanter should visibly raise the skin at all times during insertion. The implanter should not enter muscle tissue, but be well within the subcutaneous space. Advance the implanter to the depth indicator on the cannula, which indicates the recommended insertion length.

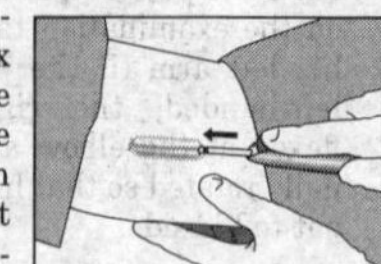

4. Holding the implanter handle in position, use the index finger to slide the actuator slowly back until it stops. (This retracts the actuator cannula into the handle, leaving the implant beneath the skin.). Do not pull back on the implanter handle while sliding the actuator back, as this may lead to incorrect positioning of the implant and subsequent extrusion. Withdraw the implanter from the incision. Release of the implant can be checked by palpation. It is important to keep the implanter steady and not to push the implant into the tissue. After placement, sterile gauze may be used to apply pressure briefly to the insertion site to ensure hemostasis.

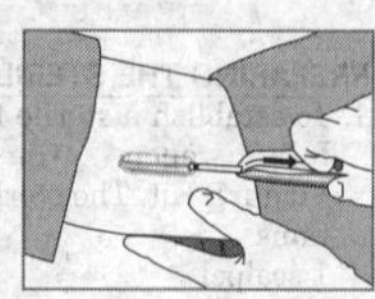

5. Cleanse the insertion area. Press the edges of the incision together, and tightly close the incision with one or two surgical closure strips. Cover with an adhesive bandage. Observe the patient for a few minutes for signs of bleeding from the incision before he is discharged. Instruct the patient to keep the area clean and dry for 24 hours, and to avoid heavy lifting and strenuous physical activity for 48 hours. The surgical closure strip can be removed as soon as the incision has healed, ie, normally in 3 days.

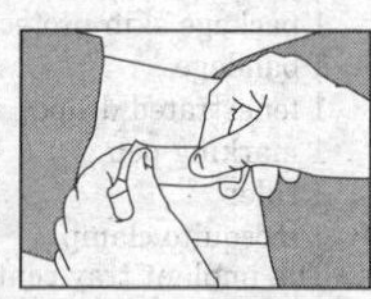

REMOVAL PROCEDURE

Viadur® must be removed following 12 months of therapy.

The position of the patient and the sterile technique are the same as for insertion.

To remove Viadur® use the Viadur® Kit or the following sterile items:

1 scalpel
1 forceps
1 syringe
1 package povidone-iodine swabs
1 package wound closure strips
1-22 Ga × 1.5" needle
1-25 Ga × 1.5" needle
1 sealed container of lidocaine HCl USP 2%, 10 mL
6 gauze sponges
2 alcohol prep pads
1 package skin protectant
1 bandage
1 fenestrated drape
1 marking pen
1 ruler
1 mosquito clamp

PREPARING THE SITE

1. Inspect the site, palpating the location of the implant. Mark the position of the implant with marking pen. Cleanse with povidone-iodine swab. Drape the area with a fenestrated drape.
   Suggestion:
   If unable to locate by palpation, radiological imaging may be helpful.

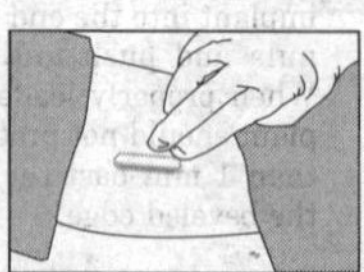

2. After determining the absence of known allergies to the anesthetic agent, apply a small amount of local anesthetic under the end of the implant nearest the original incision site. Then advance the needle to infiltrate the tissue along the track.

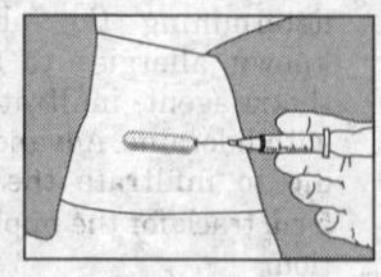

REMOVING THE IMPLANT

1. Determine that anesthesia is adequate. Apply pressure to one end of the implant to elevate the other end. Make an incision of approximately 5 mm at the elevated end of the implant. Do not make a large incision.

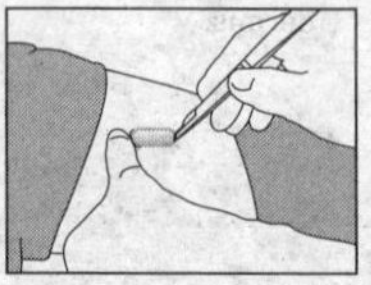

Continue to apply pressure to the end of the implant to encourage expulsion. Push the implant gently towards the incision with the fingers. When the tip is visible or near the incision, grasp it with a clamp and remove.

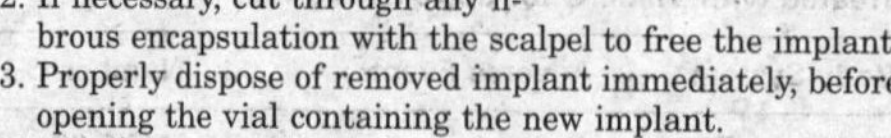

2. If necessary, cut through any fibrous encapsulation with the scalpel to free the implant.
3. Properly dispose of removed implant immediately, before opening the vial containing the new implant.

If inserting a new Viadur®, return to section describing INSERTION PROCEDURE.

The new Viadur® implant may be placed through the same incision site. Alternatively, the contralateral arm may be used.

4. Cleanse insertion site area. Apply pressure to each end of the incision to close the wound. Apply one or two surgical closure strips to close the wound tightly, and cover with an adhesive bandage. Observe the patient for a few minutes for signs of bleeding from the incision before he is discharged. Instruct the patient to keep the area clean and dry for 24 hours, and to avoid strenuous physical activity for 48 hours.

HOW SUPPLIED

Viadur® is supplied in a box containing 2 inner package trays. One tray contains a sterile Viadur® implant in a sealed vial, a sterile Viadur® implanter and a sealed container of lidocaine HCl USP 2%, 10 mL. The other tray constitutes a sterile Viadur® Kit, which includes: 1 scalpel, 1 forceps, 1 syringe, povidone-iodine swabs, 1 package wound closure strips, 1-22 Ga × 1.5" needle, 1-25 Ga × 1.5" needle, 6 gauze sponges, 2 alcohol prep pads, 1 package skin protectant, 1 bandage, 1 fenestrated drape, 1 marking pen, 1 ruler, and 1 mosquito clamp. A physician insert, patient information, and insertion and removal instructions are also provided in the box.

(NDC 0026-9711-01)

℞ Only.

Store at 25°C (77°F); excursions permitted to 15-30°C (59-86°F). [See USP Controlled Room Temperature]

For more information call 1-800-288-8371 or visit www.VIADUR.com.

REFERENCES

1. Sennello LT et al. Single-dose pharmacokinetics of leuprolide in humans following intravenous and subcutaneous administration. *J Pharm Sci* 1986; 75(2):158-160.
2. MacLeod TL et al. Anaphylactic reaction to synthetic luteinizing hormone-releasing hormone. *Fertil Steril* 1987; 48(3):500-502.

An ALZA DUROS®
Technology Product
Manufactured by:
ALZA Corporation
Mountain View, CA 94043 U.S.A.
Bayer HealthCare
Distributed by:
Bayer Pharmaceuticals Corporation
400 Morgan Lane, West Haven, CT 06516 USA

Viadur® and DUROS® are registered trademarks of ALZA Corporation under license to Bayer Pharmaceuticals Corporation. For further information about the product contact Bayer Pharmaceuticals Corporation.

08840302, R.0 7/03

11940 Printed in the U.S.A.

Patient Information About:
Viadur®
(leuprolide acetate implant)

Important Information for Patients Using Viadur® for the treatment of symptoms of advanced prostate cancer.

Please read this information before you start using Viadur®. Each time another Viadur® is inserted, check the patient information leaflet for any new information. Remember, this information does not take the place of your doctor's instructions. Ask your doctor or pharmacist if you have questions or want more information about Viadur®.

What is Viadur®?

Viadur® is a drug-delivery system that contains the drug leuprolide and is placed under the skin. It looks like a small, thin metal tube. After it is placed under the skin, Viadur® delivers leuprolide to your body continuously for 12 months.

How does Viadur® work?

Leuprolide, the active medication in Viadur®, works by reducing the testosterone produced by the testicles. This lowers the amount of testosterone in the body. Testosterone appears to be needed by prostate cancer cells. Usually prostate cancer shrinks or stops growing when the body's supply of testosterone is lowered.

By lowering the amount of testosterone in the body, Viadur® may help relieve the pain, urinary problems, and other symptoms of prostate cancer. However, Viadur® is not a cure for prostate cancer. Once Viadur® is removed by your doctor, your body will start producing testosterone again.

How is Viadur® given?

Viadur® will be placed under the skin of your upper, inner arm. The doctor will numb your arm, make a small incision, and then place Viadur® under the skin. The incision will be closed with special surgical tape and covered with a bandage. You should keep the bandage in place for a few days until the incision heals.

After 12 months, Viadur® must be removed and may be replaced with a new Viadur® by your doctor.

What should I avoid while Viadur® is inserted?

After Viadur® is inserted, keep the site clean and dry for 24 hours. Do not bathe or swim for 24 hours. Avoid heavy lifting and physical activity for 48 hours. Avoid bumping the site for a few days. After the cut has healed, you should be able to go back to your normal activities.

What should I know about using Viadur®?

- If you notice unusual bleeding, redness or pain at the insertion site, contact your doctor.
- In the first few weeks of treatment, if you experience increased pain throughout your body, weakness, or numbness, contact your doctor.
- X-rays and MRI do not affect Viadur®.
- Viadur® is seen on X-rays. Slight image distortion around Viadur® may occur during MRI procedures.
- Viadur® must be removed and may be replaced after 12 months.

Who should NOT use Viadur®?

Do not use Viadur® if you are allergic to the drug leuprolide.

Do not use Viadur® if you are a woman. Viadur® is not approved for use by women of any age. Furthermore, use of Viadur® in a woman who is or may become pregnant may cause harm to the baby. You may lose your baby through a miscarriage if the drug is used while you are pregnant.

Viadur® was not studied in children and should not be used in children.

What are the most common side effects of Viadur®?

The most common side effects related to Viadur® were hot flashes, lack of energy, depression, sweating, headache, bruising, and breast enlargement.

Prostate cancer-related symptoms may become worse during the first few weeks of treatment.

Like other similar treatment options, Viadur® may cause impotence.

There may be some pain and discomfort during and after Viadur® insertion and removal. Bruising may occur. Reactions, such as itching and redness, are usually mild and heal without treatment within two weeks. If they do not heal, contact your doctor.

There is a chance that your bones may become thinner if you use this type of drug for long periods of time. Ask your doctor if this is a risk for you.

This list is not a complete list of all the possible side effects. If you need more information, or are worried about these or other side effects, talk to your doctor or pharmacist.

What tests will my doctor perform during my treatment with Viadur®?

Your doctor may measure blood levels of testosterone and prostate-specific antigen (PSA) during your treatment with Viadur®.

Can I take Viadur® with other medications?

Tell your doctor or pharmacist about any medicines that you are taking, including Viadur®, prescription, non-prescription, and herbal remedies. Do not start taking a new medicine before checking with your doctor or pharmacist.

For more information on Viadur®, talk to your doctor or pharmacist, call 1-800-288-8371 between 8:30 AM and 5 PM Eastern Standard Time, or visit www.VIADUR.com on the Internet.

An ALZA DUROS®
Technology Product
Manufactured by:
ALZA Corporation
Mountain View, CA 94043 U.S.A.
Bayer HealthCare
Distributed by:
Bayer Pharmaceuticals Corporation
400 Morgan Lane, West Haven, CT 06516 USA

Viadur® and DUROS® are registered trademarks of ALZA Corporation under license to Bayer Pharmaceuticals Corporation. For further information about the product contact Bayer Pharmaceuticals Corporation.

08840302IP, R.0 7/03

11940 Printed in the U.S.A.

Shown in Product Identification Guide, page 308

Bayer Corporation
Pharmaceutical Division
Biological Products
ELKHART, IN 46515 USA

For Medical Information Contact:
Director, Clinical Services
(800) 288-8371
(203) 812-6901

BAYGAM® ℞
[*bāy-găm*]
Immune Globulin (Human)
Solvent/Detergent Treated

DESCRIPTION

Immune Globulin (Human) — BayGam® treated with solvent/detergent is a sterile solution of immune globulin for intramuscular administration; it contains no preservative. BayGam is prepared by cold ethanol fractionation from human plasma. The immune globulin is isolated from solubilized Cohn fraction II. The fraction II solution is adjusted to a final concentration of 0.3% tri-n-butyl phosphate (TNBP) and 0.2% sodium cholate. After the addition of solvent (TNBP) and detergent (sodium cholate), the solution is heated to 30°C and maintained at that temperature for not less than 6 hours. After the viral inactivation step, the reactants are removed by precipitation, filtration and finally ultrafiltration and diafiltration. BayGam is formulated as a 15–18% protein solution at a pH of 6.4–7.2 in 0.21–0.32 M glycine. BayGam is then incubated in the final container for 21–28 days at 20–27°C.

The removal and inactivation of spiked model enveloped and non-enveloped viruses during the manufacturing process for BayGam has been validated in laboratory studies. Human Immunodeficiency Virus, Type 1 (HIV-1), was chosen as the relevant virus for blood products; Bovine Viral Diarrhea Virus (BVDV) was chosen to model Hepatitis C virus; Pseudorabies virus (PRV) was chosen to model Hepatitis B virus and the Herpes viruses; and Reo virus type 3 (Reo) was chosen to model non-enveloped viruses and for its resistance to physical and chemical inactivation. Significant removal of model enveloped and non-enveloped viruses is achieved at two steps in the Cohn fractionation process leading to the collection of Cohn Fraction II: the precipitation and removal of Fraction III in the processing of Fraction II + IIIW suspension to Effluent III and the filtration step in the processing of Effluent III to Filtrate III. Significant inactivation of enveloped viruses is achieved at the time of treatment of solubilized Cohn Fraction II with TNBP/sodium cholate.

CLINICAL PHARMACOLOGY

Peak levels of immunoglobulin G are obtained approximately 2 days after intramuscular injection of BayGam.[1] The half-life of IgG in the circulation of individuals with normal IgG levels is 23 days.[2]

Passive immunization with BayGam modifies hepatitis A, prevents or modifies measles, and provides replacement therapy in persons with hypogammaglobulinemia or agammaglobulinemia. BayGam is not standardized with respect to antibody titers against hepatitis B surface antigen (HBsAg) and should not be used for prophylaxis of viral hepatitis type B. Prophylactic treatment to prevent hepatitis B can best be accomplished with use of Hepatitis B Immune Globulin (Human), often in combination with Hepatitis B Vaccine.[3]

BayGam may be of benefit in women who have been exposed to rubella in the first trimester of pregnancy and who will not consider a therapeutic abortion.[4] BayGam may also be considered for use in immunocompromised patients for passive immunization against varicella if Varicella-Zoster Immune Globulin (Human) is not available.[5]

Immune Globulin (Human) is not indicated for routine prophylaxis or treatment of rubella, poliomyelitis, mumps, or varicella. It is not indicated for allergy or asthma in patients who have normal levels of immunoglobulin.[6]

In a clinical study in eight healthy human adults receiving another hyperimmune immune globulin product treated with solvent/detergent, Rabies Immune Globulin (Human), BayRab®, prepared by the same manufacturing process, detectable passive antibody titers were observed in the serum of all subjects by 24 hours post injection and persisted through the 21 day study period. These results suggest that passive immunization with immune globulin products is not affected by the solvent/detergent treatment.

INDICATIONS AND USAGE

Hepatitis A

The prophylactic value of BayGam is greatest when given before or soon after exposure to hepatitis A. BayGam is not indicated in persons with clinical manifestations of hepatitis A or in those exposed more than 2 weeks previously.

Measles (Rubeola)

BayGam should be given to prevent or modify measles in a susceptible person exposed fewer than 6 days previously.[7] A susceptible person is one who has not been vaccinated and has not had measles previously. BayGam may be especially indicated for susceptible household contacts of measles patients, particularly contacts under 1 year of age, for whom the risk of complications is highest.[7] **BayGam and measles vaccine should not be given at the same time.**[7] If a child is older than 12 months and has received BayGam, he should be given measles vaccine about 3 months later when the measles antibody titer will have disappeared.

If a susceptible child exposed to measles is immunocompromised, BayGam should be given immediately.[8] Children who are immunocompromised should not receive measles vaccine or any other live viral vaccine.

Varicella

Passive immunization against varicella in immunosuppressed patients is best accomplished by use of Varicella-Zoster Immune Globulin (Human) [VZIG]. If VZIG is unavailable, BayGam, promptly given, may also modify varicella.[5]

Rubella

The routine use of BayGam for prophylaxis of rubella in early pregnancy is of dubious value and cannot be justified.[6] Some studies suggest that the use of BayGam in exposed, susceptible women can lessen the likelihood of infection and fetal damage; therefore, BayGam may benefit those women who will **not** consider a therapeutic abortion.[4]

Immunoglobulin Deficiency

In patients with immunoglobulin deficiencies, BayGam may prevent serious infection. However, BayGam may not prevent chronic infections of the external secretory tissues such as the respiratory and gastrointestinal tract.

Prophylactic therapy, especially against infections due to encapsulated bacteria, is effective in Bruton-type, sex-linked, congenital agammaglobulinemia, agammaglobulinemia associated with thymoma, and acquired agammaglobulinemia.

CONTRAINDICATIONS

BayGam should not be given to persons with isolated immunoglobulin A (IgA) deficiency. Such persons have the potential for developing antibodies to IgA and could have anaphylactic reactions to subsequent administration of blood products that contain IgA.[9]

BayGam should not be administered to patients who have severe thrombocytopenia or any coagulation disorder that would contraindicate intramuscular injections.

WARNINGS

BayGam is made from human plasma. Products made from human plasma may contain infectious agents, such as viruses, that can cause disease. The risk that such products will transmit an infectious agent has been reduced by screening plasma donors for prior exposure to certain viruses, by testing for the presence of certain current virus infections, and by inactivating and/or removing certain viruses. Despite these measures, such products can still potentially transmit disease. There is also the possibility that unknown infectious agents may be present in such products. Individuals who receive infusions of blood or plasma products may develop signs and/or symptoms of some viral infections, particularly hepatitis C. ALL infections thought by a physician possibly to have been transmitted by this product should be reported by the physician or other healthcare provider to Bayer Corporation [1-800-288-8371].

The physician should discuss the risks and benefits of this product with the patient, before prescribing or administering it to the patient.

BayGam should be given with caution to patients with a history of prior systemic allergic reactions following the administration of human immunoglobulin preparations.[9]

PRECAUTIONS

General

Immune Globulin (Human) should not be administered intravenously because of the potential for serious reactions. Injections should be made intramuscularly, and care should be taken to draw back on the plunger of the syringe before injection in order to be certain that the needle is not in a blood vessel.

Skin tests should not be done. In most human beings the intradermal injection of concentrated gamma globulin solution with its buffers causes a localized area of inflammation which can be misinterpreted as a positive allergic reaction. In actuality, this does not represent an allergy; rather, it is localized tissue irritation of a chemical nature. Misinterpretation of the results of such tests can lead the physician to withhold badly needed human immunoglobulin from a patient who is not actually allergic to this material. True allergic responses to human gamma globulin given in the prescribed intramuscular manner are rare.

Although systemic reactions to intramuscularly administered immunoglobulin preparations are rare, epinephrine should be available for treatment of acute allergic symptoms.

Clinical and Laboratory Tests

None required.

Clinically Significant Product Interactions

Antibodies in the globulin preparation may interfere with the response to live viral vaccines such as measles, mumps, polio and rubella. Therefore, use of such vaccines should be deferred until approximately 3 months after Immune Globulin (Human) — BayGam® administration.

No interactions with other products are known.

Pregnancy Category C

Animal reproduction studies have not been conducted with BayGam. It is also not known whether BayGam can cause fetal harm when administered to a pregnant woman or can affect reproduction capacity. BayGam should be given to a pregnant woman only if clearly needed.

Pediatric Use

Safety and effectiveness in the pediatric population have not been established.

ADVERSE REACTIONS

Local pain and tenderness at the injection site, urticaria, and angioedema may occur. Anaphylactic reactions, although rare, have been reported following the injection of human immune globulin preparations.[6,9] Anaphylaxis is more likely to occur if BayGam is given intravenously; therefore, BayGam must be administered only intramuscularly.

DOSAGE AND ADMINISTRATION

BayGam is administered **intramuscularly** (see PRECAUTIONS), preferably in the anterolateral aspects of the upper thigh and the deltoid muscle of the upper arm. The gluteal region should not be used routinely as an injection site because of the risk of injury to the sciatic nerve. Doses over 10 mL should be divided and injected into several muscle sites to reduce local pain and discomfort. An individual decision as to which muscle is injected must be made for each patient based on the volume of material to be administered. If the gluteal region is used when very large volumes are to be injected or multiple doses are necessary, the central region MUST be avoided; only the upper, outer quadrant should be used.[10]

Parenteral drug products should be inspected visually for particulate matter and discoloration prior to administration, whenever solution and container permit.

A number of factors beyond our control could reduce the efficacy of this product or even result in an ill effect following its use. These include improper storage and handling of the product after it leaves our hands, diagnosis, dosage, method of administration, and biological differences in individual patients. Because of these factors, it is important that this product be stored properly and that the directions be followed carefully during use.

Hepatitis A

BayGam in a dose of 0.01 mL/lb (0.02 mL/kg) is recommended for household and institutional hepatitis A case contacts.

The following doses of BayGam are recommended for persons who plan to travel in areas where hepatitis A is common.[3]

Length of Stay	Dose Volume
Less than 3 months	0.02 mL/kg
3 months or longer	0.06 mL/kg (repeat every 4–6 months)

Measles (Rubeola)

BayGam should be given in a dose of 0.11 mL/lb (0.25 mL/kg) to prevent or modify measles in a susceptible person exposed fewer than 6 days previously.[7]

A susceptible child who is exposed to measles and who is immunocompromised should receive a dose of 0.5 mL/kg (maximum dose, 15 mL) of BayGam immediately.[8]

Varicella

If Varicella-Zoster Immune Globulin (Human) is unavailable, BayGam at a dose of 0.6 to 1.2 mL/kg, promptly given, may also modify varicella.[5]

Rubella

Some studies suggest that the use of BayGam in exposed, susceptible women can lessen the likelihood of infection and fetal damage; therefore, BayGam at a dose of 0.55 mL/kg may benefit those women who will not consider a therapeutic abortion.[4]

Immunoglobulin Deficiency

BayGam may prevent serious infection in patients with immunoglobulin deficiencies if circulating IgG levels of approximately 200 mg/100 mL plasma are maintained. The recommended dosage is 0.66 mL/kg (at least 100 mg/kg) given every 3 to 4 weeks.[6] A double dose is given at onset of therapy; some patients may require more frequent injections.

HOW SUPPLIED

BayGam is supplied in 2 mL and 10 mL single dose vials.

NDC Number	Size
0026-0635-02	2 mL vial (10 pack)
0026-0635-04	2 mL vial
0026-0635-10	10 mL vial (10 pack)
0026-0635-12	10 mL vial

STORAGE

Store at 2–8°C (36–46°F). Do not freeze. Do not use after expiration date.

CAUTION

℞ only

U.S. federal law prohibits dispensing without prescription.

REFERENCES

1. Smith GN, Griffiths B, Mollison D, et al: Uptake of IgG after intramuscular and subcutaneous injection. *Lancet* 1(7762): 1208–12, 1972.
2. Waldmann TA, Strober W, Blaese RM: Variations in the metabolism of immunoglobulins measured by turnover rates. In Merler E (ed.): Immunoglobulins: biologic aspects and clinical uses. Washington DC, Nat Acad Sci, 1970, pp 33–51.

Continued on next page

BayGam—Cont.

3. Recommendation of the Immunization Practices Advisory Committee (ACIP): Postexposure prophylaxis of hepatitis B. *MMWR* 33(21): 285–90, 1984.
4. American Academy of Pediatrics, Committee on Infectious Diseases: Report. ed. 19. Evanston, 1982, p 231.
5. Gershon AA, Piomelli S, Karpatkin M, et al: Antibody to varicella-zoster virus after passive immunization against chickenpox. *J Clin Microbiol* 8(6): 733-5, 1978.
6. American Academy of Pediatrics, Committee on Infectious Diseases: Report. ed. 19. Evanston, 1982, pp 134–5.
7. Recommendation of the Public Health Service Advisory Committee on Immunization Practices: Measles prevention. *MMWR* 27(44): 427–30; 435-7, 1978.
8. American Academy of Pediatrics, Committee on Infectious Diseases: Report. ed. 19. Evanston, 1982, pp 34–6.
9. Fudenberg HH: Sensitization to immunoglobulins and hazards of gamma globulin therapy. In: Merler E (ed.): Immunoglobulins: biologic aspects and clinical uses. Washington DC, Nat Acad Sci, 1970, pp 211–20.
10. Recommendations of the Immunization Practices Advisory Committee (ACIP): General recommendations on immunization. *MMWR* 38(13): 205–14: 219–27, 1989.

Bayer Corporation
Pharmaceutical Division
Elkhart, IN 46515 USA
U.S. License No. 8
08800017 (Rev. January 2003)

BAYHEP B® ℞

[*bā-hĕp*]

Hepatitis B Immune Globulin (Human)
Solvent/Detergent Treated

DESCRIPTION

Hepatitis B Immune Globulin (Human) — BayHep B® treated with solvent/detergent is a sterile solution of hepatitis B hyperimmune immune globulin for intramuscular administration; it contains no preservative. BayHep B is prepared by cold ethanol fractionation from the plasma of donors with high titers of antibody to the hepatitis B surface antigen (anti-HBs). The immune globulin is isolated from solubilized Cohn Fraction II. The Fraction II solution is adjusted to a final concentration of 0.3% tri-n-butyl phosphate (TNBP) and 0.2% sodium cholate. After the addition of solvent (TNBP) and detergent (sodium cholate), the solution is heated to 30°C and maintained at that temperature for not less than 6 hours. After the viral inactivation step, the reactants are removed by precipitation, filtration and finally ultrafiltration and diafiltration. BayHep B is formulated as a 15–18% protein solution at a pH of 6.4–7.2 in 0.21–0.32 M glycine. BayHep B is then incubated in the final container for 21–28 days at 20–27°C. Each vial contains anti-HBs antibody equivalent to or exceeding the potency of anti-HBs in a U.S. reference hepatitis B immune globulin (Center for Biologics Evaluation and Research, FDA). The U.S. reference has been tested against the World Health Organization standard Hepatitis B Immune Globulin and found to be equal to 217 international units (IU) per mL.

The removal and inactivation of spiked model enveloped and non-enveloped viruses during the manufacturing process for BayHep B has been validated in laboratory studies. Human Immunodeficiency Virus, Type 1 (HIV-1), was chosen as the relevant virus for blood products; Bovine Viral Diarrhea Virus (BVDV) was chosen to model Hepatitis C virus; Pseudorabies virus (PRV) was chosen to model Hepatitis B virus and the Herpes viruses; and Reo virus type 3 (Reo) was chosen to model non-enveloped viruses and for its resistance to physical and chemical inactivation. Significant removal of model enveloped and non-enveloped viruses is achieved at two steps in the Cohn fractionation process leading to the collection of Cohn Fraction II: the precipitation and removal of Fraction III in the processing of Fraction II + IIIW suspension to Effluent III and the filtration step in the processing of Effluent III to Filtrate III. Significant inactivation of enveloped viruses is achieved at the time of treatment of solubilized Cohn Fraction II with TNBP/sodium cholate.

CLINICAL PHARMACOLOGY

Hepatitis B Immune Globulin (Human) provides passive immunization for individuals exposed to the hepatitis B virus (HBV) as evidenced by a reduction in the attack rate of hepatitis B following its use.[1–6] The administration of the usual recommended dose of this immune globulin generally results in a detectable level of circulating anti-HBs which persists for approximately 2 months or longer. The highest antibody (IgG) serum levels were seen in the following distribution of subjects studied:[7]

DAY	% OF SUBJECTS
3	38.9%
7	41.7%
14	11.1%
21	8.3%

Mean values for half-life were between 17.5 and 25 days, with the shortest being 5.9 days and the longest 35 days.[7]

Table 1. (adapted from [20])
Recommendations for Hepatitis B Prophylaxis Following Percutaneous or Permucosal Exposure

Source	Exposed Person: Unvaccinated	Exposed Person: Vaccinated
HBsAg-Positive	1. Hepatitis B Immune Globulin (Human)×1 immediately* 2. Initiate HB Vaccine Series†	1. Test exposed person for anti-HBs. 2. If inadequate antibody,‡ Hepatitis B Immune Globulin (Human) (×1) immediately plus HB Vaccine booster dose, or 2 doses of HBIG,* one as soon as possible after exposure and the second 1 month later.
Known Source (High Risk)	1. Initiate HB Vaccine Series 2. Test source for HBsAg. If positive, Hepatitis B Immune Globulin (Human)×1	1. Test Source for HBsAg only if exposed is vaccine nonresponder; if source is HBsAg-positive, give Hepatitis B Immune Globulin (Human)×1 immediately plus HB Vaccine booster dose, or 2 doses of HBIG,* one as soon as possible after exposure and the second 1 month later.
Low Risk HBsAg-Positive	Initiate HB Vaccine series	Nothing required.
Unknown Source	Initiate HB Vaccine series within 7 days of exposure	Nothing required.

* Hepatitis B Immune Globulin (Human), dose 0.06 mL/kg IM.
† HB Vaccine dose 20 µg IM for adults; 10 µg IM for infants or children under 10 years of age. First dose within 1 week; second and third doses, 1 and 6 months later.
‡ Less than 10 sample ratio units (SRU) by radioimmunoassay (RIA), negative by enzyme immunoassay (EIA).

Cases of type B hepatitis are rarely seen following exposure to HBV in persons with preexisting anti-HBs. No confirmed instance of transmission of hepatitis B has been associated with this product.

In a clinical study in eight healthy human adults receiving another hyperimmune immune globulin product treated with solvent/detergent, Rabies Immune Globulin (Human), BayRab®, prepared by the same manufacturing process, detectable passive antibody titers were observed in the serum of all subjects by 24 hours post injection and persisted through the 21 day study period. These results suggest that passive immunization with immune globulin products is not affected by the solvent/detergent treatment.

INDICATIONS AND USAGE

Recommendations on post-exposure prophylaxis are based on available efficacy data and on the likelihood of future HBV exposure for the person requiring treatment. In all exposures, a regimen combining Hepatitis B Immune Globulin (Human) with hepatitis B vaccine will provide both short- and long-term protection, will be less costly than the two-dose Hepatitis B Immune Globulin (Human) treatment alone, and is the treatment of choice.[8]

BayHep B is indicated for post-exposure prophylaxis in the following situations:

Acute Exposure to Blood Containing HBsAg

After either parenteral exposure, e.g., by accidental "needlestick" or direct mucous membrane contact (accidental splash), or oral ingestion (pipetting accident) involving HBsAg-positive materials such as blood, plasma or serum. For inadvertent percutaneous exposure, a regimen of two doses of Hepatitis B Immune Globulin (Human), one given after exposure and one a month later, is about 75% effective in preventing hepatitis B in this setting.

Perinatal Exposure of Infants Born to HBsAg-positive Mothers

Infants born to HBsAg-positive mothers are at risk of being infected with hepatitis B virus and becoming chronic carriers.[5,8–10] This risk is especially great if the mother is HBeAg-positive.[11–13] For an infant with perinatal exposure to an HBsAg-positive and HBeAg-positive mother, a regimen combining one dose of Hepatitis B Immune Globulin (Human) at birth with the hepatitis B vaccine series started soon after birth is 85%–95% effective in preventing development of the HBV carrier state.[8,14] Regimens involving either multiple doses of Hepatitis B Immune Globulin (Human) alone or the vaccine series alone have 70%–90% efficacy, while a single dose of Hepatitis B Immune Globulin (Human) alone has only 50% efficacy.[8,15]

Sexual Exposure to an HBsAg-positive Person

Sex partners of HBsAg-positive persons are at increased risk of acquiring HBV infection. For sexual exposure to a person with acute hepatitis B, a single dose of Hepatitis B Immune Globulin (Human) is 75% effective if administered within 2 weeks of last sexual exposure.[8]

Household Exposure to Persons with Acute HBV Infection

Since infants have close contact with primary care-givers and they have a higher risk of becoming HBV carriers after acute HBV infection, prophylaxis of an infant less than 12 months of age with Hepatitis B Immune Globulin (Human) and hepatitis B vaccine is indicated if the mother or primary care-giver has acute HBV infection.[8]

Administration of Hepatitis B Immune Globulin (Human) either preceding or concomitant with the commencement of active immunization with Hepatitis B Vaccine provides for more rapid achievement of protective levels of hepatitis B antibody, than when the vaccine alone is administered.[16] Rapid achievement of protective levels of antibody to hepatitis B virus may be desirable in certain clinical situations, as in cases of accidental inoculations with contaminated medical instruments.[16] Administration of Hepatitis B Immune Globulin (Human) either 1 month preceding or at the time of commencement of a program of active vaccination with Hepatitis B Vaccine has been shown not to interfere with the active immune response to the vaccine.[16]

CONTRAINDICATIONS

None known.

WARNINGS

BayHep B is made from human plasma. Products made from human plasma may contain infectious agents, such as viruses, that can cause disease. The risk that such products will transmit an infectious agent has been reduced by screening plasma donors for prior exposure to certain viruses, by testing for the presence of certain current virus infections, and by inactivating and/or removing certain viruses. Despite these measures, such products can still potentially transmit disease. There is also the possibility that unknown infectious agents may be present in such products. Individuals who receive infusions of blood or plasma products may develop signs and/or symptoms of some viral infections, particularly hepatitis C. ALL infections thought by a physician possibly to have been transmitted by this product should be reported by the physician or other healthcare provider to Bayer Corporation [1-800-288-8371].

The physician should discuss the risks and benefits of this product with the patient, before prescribing or administering it to the patient.

BayHep B should be given with caution to patients with a history of prior systemic allergic reactions following the administration of human immune globulin preparations. Epinephrine should be available.

In patients who have severe thrombocytopenia or any coagulation disorder that would contraindicate intramuscular injections, Hepatitis B Immune Globulin (Human) should be given only if the expected benefits outweigh the risks.

PRECAUTIONS

General

BayHep B should **not** be administered intravenously because of the potential for serious reactions. Injections should be made intramuscularly, and care should be taken to draw back on the plunger of the syringe before injection in order to be certain that the needle is not in a blood vessel.

Intramuscular injections are preferably administered in the anterolateral aspects of the upper thigh and the deltoid muscle of the upper arm. The gluteal region should not be used routinely as an injection site because of the risk of injury to the sciatic nerve. An individual decision as to which muscle is injected must be made for each patient based on the volume of material to be administered. If the gluteal region is used when very large volumes are to be injected or multiple doses are necessary, the central region MUST be avoided; only the upper, outer quadrant should be used.[17]

Laboratory Tests

None required.

Drug Interactions

Although administration of Hepatitis B Immune Globulin (Human) did not interfere with measles vaccination,[18] it is not known whether Hepatitis B Immune Globulin (Human) may interfere with other live virus vaccines. Therefore, use of such vaccines should be deferred until approximately 3 months after Hepatitis B Immune Globulin (Human) administration. Hepatitis B Vaccine may be administered at the same time, but at a different injection site, without interfering with the immune response.[16] No interactions with other products are known.

Pregnancy Category C

Animal reproduction studies have not been conducted with BayHep B. It is also not known whether BayHep B can cause fetal harm when administered to a pregnant woman or can affect reproduction capacity. BayHep B should be given to a pregnant woman only if clearly needed.

Pediatric Use

Safety and effectiveness in the pediatric population have not been established.

ADVERSE REACTIONS

Local pain and tenderness at the injection site, urticaria and angioedema may occur; anaphylactic reactions, although rare, have been reported following the injection of human immune globulin preparations.[19]

OVERDOSAGE

Although no data are available, clinical experience with other immunoglobulin preparations suggests that the only manifestations would be pain and tenderness at the injection site.

DOSAGE AND ADMINISTRATION

Acute Exposure to Blood Containing HBsAg[15]

Table 1 summarizes prophylaxis for percutaneous (needlestick or bite), ocular, or mucous-membrane exposure to blood according to the source of exposure and vaccination status of the exposed person. For greatest effectiveness, passive prophylaxis with Hepatitis B Immune Globulin (Human) should be given as soon as possible after exposure (its value beyond 7 days of exposure is unclear). If Hepatitis B Immune Globulin (Human) is indicated (see Table 1), an injection of 0.06 mL/kg of body weight should be administered intramuscularly (see PRECAUTIONS) as soon as possible after exposure and within 24 hours, if possible. Consult Hepatitis B Vaccine package insert for dosage information regarding that product.

[See table 1 at top of previous page]

For persons who refuse Hepatitis B Vaccine, a second dose of Hepatitis B Immune Globulin (Human) should be given 1 month after the first dose.

Prophylaxis of Infants Born to HBsAg and HBeAg Positive Mothers

Efficacy of prophylactic Hepatitis B Immune Globulin (Human) in infants at risk depends on administering Hepatitis B Immune Globulin (Human) on the day of birth. It is therefore vital that HBsAg-positive mothers be identified before delivery.

Hepatitis B Immune Globulin (Human) (0.5 mL) should be administered intramuscularly (IM) to the newborn infant after physiologic stabilization of the infant and preferably within 12 hours of birth. Hepatitis B Immune Globulin (Human) efficacy decreases markedly if treatment is delayed beyond 48 hours. Hepatitis B Vaccine should be administered IM in three doses of 0.5 mL of vaccine (10 µg) each. The first dose should be given within 7 days of birth and may be given concurrently with Hepatitis B Immune Globulin (Human) but at a separate site. The second and third doses of vaccine should be given 1 month and 6 months, respectively, after the first. If administration of the first dose of Hepatitis B Vaccine is delayed for as long as 3 months, then a 0.5 mL dose of Hepatitis B Immune Globulin (Human) should be repeated at 3 months. If Hepatitis B Vaccine is refused, the 0.5 mL dose of Hepatitis B Immune Globulin (Human) should be repeated at 3 and 6 months. Hepatitis B Immune Globulin (Human) administered at birth should not interfere with oral polio and diphtheria-tetanus-pertussis vaccines administered at 2 months of age.[15]

Sexual Exposure to an HBsAg-positive Person

All susceptible persons whose sex partners have acute hepatitis B infection should receive a single dose of HBIG (0.06 mL/kg) and should begin the hepatitis B vaccine series if prophylaxis can be started within 14 days of the last sexual contact or if sexual contact with the infected person will continue (see Table 2 below). Administering the vaccine with HBIG may improve the efficacy of postexposure treatment. The vaccine has the added advantage of conferring long-lasting protection.[8]

[See table 2 above]

Table 2. (adapted from [21])
Recommendations for Postexposure Prophylaxis for Sexual Exposure to Hepatitis B

HBIG*		Vaccine	
Dose	Recommended timing	Dose	Recommended timing
0.06 mL/kg IM†	Single dose within 14 days of last sexual contact	1.0 mL IM†	First dose at time of HBIG* treatment¶

* HBIG = Hepatitis B Immune Globulin (Human)
† IM = intramuscularly
¶ The first dose can be administered the same time as the HBIG dose but at a different site; subsequent doses should be administered as recommended for specific vaccine.

Household Exposure to Persons with Acute HBV Infection

Prophylactic treatment with a 0.5 mL dose of Hepatitis B Immune Globulin (Human) and hepatitis B vaccine is indicated for infants <12 months of age who have been exposed to a primary care-giver who has acute hepatitis B. Prophylaxis for other household contacts of persons with acute HBV infection is not indicated unless they have had identifiable blood exposure to the index patient, such as by sharing toothbrushes or razors. Such exposures should be treated like sexual exposures. If the index patient becomes an HBV carrier, all household contacts should receive hepatitis B vaccine.[8]

Hepatitis B Immune Globulin (Human) may be administered at the same time (but at a different site), or up to 1 month preceding Hepatitis B Vaccination without impairing the active immune response from Hepatitis B Vaccination.[16]

Parenteral drug products should be inspected visually for particulate matter and discoloration prior to administration, whenever solution and container permit.

Administer intramuscularly. Do not inject intravenously.

Hepatitis B Immune Globulin (Human) — BayHep B® is supplied with a syringe and an attached UltraSafe® Needle Guard for your protection and convenience. Please follow instructions below for proper use of syringe and UltraSafe® Needle Guard.

Directions for Syringe Usage

1. Remove the prefilled syringe from the package. Lift syringe by barrel, **not** by plunger.
2. Twist the plunger rod clockwise until the threads are seated.
3. With the rubber needle shield secured on the syringe tip, push the plunger rod forward a few millimeters to break any friction seal between the rubber stopper and the glass syringe barrel.
4. Remove the needle shield and expel air bubbles. [Do not remove the rubber needle shield to prepare the product for administration until immediately prior to the anticipated injection time.]
5. Proceed with hypodermic needle puncture.
6. Aspirate prior to injection to confirm that the needle is not in a vein or artery.
7. Inject the medication.
8. Keeping your hands behind the needle, grasp the guard with free hand and slide forward toward needle until it is completely covered and guard clicks into place. If audible click is not heard, guard may not be completely activated. (See Diagrams A and B)
9. Place entire prefilled glass syringe with guard activated into an approved sharps container for proper disposal. (See Diagram C)

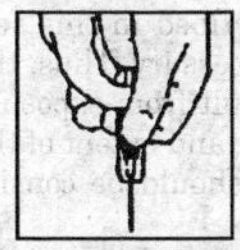
A

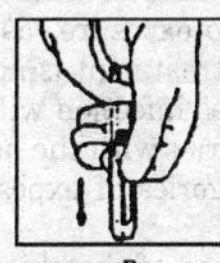
B

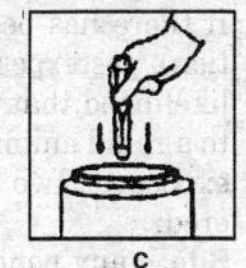
C

A number of factors beyond our control could reduce the efficacy of this product or even result in an ill effect following its use. These include improper storage and handling of the product after it leaves our hands, diagnosis, dosage, method of administration and biological differences in individual patients. Because of these factors, it is important that this product be stored properly and that the directions be followed carefully during use.

HOW SUPPLIED

BayHep B is supplied in a 0.5 mL neonatal single dose syringe with attached needle, a 1 mL single dose syringe with attached needle and a 1 mL and a 5 mL single dose vial.

NDC Number	Size
0026-0636-03	0.5 mL syringe
0026-0636-02	1 mL syringe
0026-0636-01	1 mL vial
0026-0636-05	5 mL vial

STORAGE

Store at 2–8°C (36–46°F). Do not freeze. Do not use after expiration date.

CAUTION

℞ only

U.S. federal law prohibits dispensing without prescription.

REFERENCES

1. Grady GF, Lee VA: Hepatitis B immune globulin — prevention of hepatitis from accidental exposure among medical personnel. *N Engl J Med* 293(21):1067-70, 1975.
2. Seeff LB, Zimmerman HJ, Wright EC, et al: Efficacy of hepatitis B immune serum globulin after accidental exposure. *Lancet* 2(7942):939-41, 1975.
3. Krugman S, Giles JP: Viral hepatitis, type B (MS-2-strain). Further observations on natural history and prevention. *N Engl J Med* 288(15):755-60, 1973.
4. Current trends: Health status of Indochinese refugees: malaria and hepatitis B. *MMWR* 28(39):463-4; 469-70, 1979.
5. Jhaveri R, Rosenfeld W, Salazar JD, et al: High titer multiple dose therapy with HBIG in newborn infants of HBsAg positive mothers. *J Pediatr* 97(2):305-8, 1980.
6. Hoofnagle JH, Seeff LB, Bales ZB, et al: Passive-active immunity from hepatitis B immune globulin. *Ann Intern Med* 91(6):813-8, 1979.
7. Scheiermann N, Kuwert EK: Uptake and elimination of hepatitis B immunoglobulins after intramuscular application in man. *Dev Biol Stand* 54:347-55, 1983.
8. Recommendations of the Immunization Practices Advisory Committee (ACIP): Hepatitis B Virus: A Comprehensive Strategy for Eliminating Transmission in the United States Through Universal Childhood Vaccination. Appendix A: Postexposure Prophylaxis for Hepatitis B. *MMWR* 40(RR-13):21-25, 1991.
9. Stevens CE, Beasley RP, Tsui J, et al: Vertical transmission of hepatitis B antigen in Taiwan. *N Engl J Med* 292(15):771-4, 1975.
10. Shiraki K, Yoshihara N, Kawana T, et al: Hepatitis B surface antigen and chronic hepatitis in infants born to asymptomatic carrier mothers. *Am J Dis Child* 131(6): 644-7, 1977.
11. Recommendation of the Immunization Practices Advisory Committee (ACIP): Immune globulins for protection against viral hepatitis. *MMWR* 30(34):423-8; 433-5, 1981.
12. Okada K, Kamiyama I, Inomata M, et al: e antigen and anti-e in the serum of asymptomatic carrier mothers as indicators of positive and negative transmission of hepatitis B virus to their infants. *N Engl J Med* 294(14): 746-9, 1976.
13. Beasley RP, Trepo C, Stevens CE, et al: The e antigen and vertical transmission of hepatitis B surface antigen. *Am J Epidemiol* 105(2):94-8, 1977.
14. Beasley RP, Hwang LY, Lee GCY, et al: Prevention of perinatally transmitted hepatitis B virus infections with hepatitis B immune globulin and hepatitis B vaccine. *Lancet* 2(8359): 1099-102, 1983.
15. Recommendation of the Immunization Practices Advisory Committee (ACIP): Recommendations for protection against viral hepatitis. *MMWR* 34(22):313-35, 1985.
16. Szmuness W, Stevens CE, Olesko WR, et al: Passive-active immunisation against hepatitis B: immunogenicity studies in adult Americans. *Lancet* 1:575-77, 1981.
17. Recommendations of the Immunization Practices Advisory Committee (ACIP): General recommendations on immunization. *MMWR* 38(13):205-14; 219-27, 1989.
18. Beasley RP, Hwang LY: Measles vaccination not interfered with by hepatitis B immune globulin. *Lancet* 1:161, 1982.
19. Ellis EF, Henney CS: Adverse reactions following administration of human gamma globulin. *J Allerg* 43(1): 45-54, 1969.
20. Recommendations of the Immunization Practices Advisory Committee (ACIP): Update on Adult Immunization. Table 9. Recommendations for postexposure prophylaxis for percutaneous or permucosal exposure to hepatitis B, United States. *MMWR* 40(RR-12):70, 1991.
21. Recommendations of the Immunization Practices Advisory Committee (ACIP): Update on Adult Immunization. Table 10. Recommendations for postexposure prophylaxis for perinatal and sexual exposure to hepatitis B, United States. *MMWR* 40(RR-12):71, 1991.

Bayer
Bayer Corporation
Pharmaceutical Division
Elkhart, IN 46515 USA
U.S. License No. 8
Printed in USA

08895751
(Rev. March 2004)

BAYRAB® ℞

[*bā 'răb*]
Rabies Immune Globulin (Human)
Solvent/Detergent Treated

DESCRIPTION

Rabies Immune Globulin (Human) — BayRab® treated with solvent/detergent is a sterile solution of antirabies immune globulin for intramuscular administration; it contains no preservative. BayRab is prepared by cold ethanol fractionation from the plasma of donors hyperimmunized with rabies vaccine. The immune globulin is isolated from solubilized Cohn Fraction II. The Fraction II solution is adjusted to a final concentration of 0.3% tri-n-butyl phosphate (TNBP) and 0.2% sodium cholate. After the addition of solvent (TNBP) and detergent (sodium cholate), the solution is heated to 30°C and maintained at that temperature for not less than 6 hours. After the viral inactivation step, the reactants are removed by precipitation, filtration and finally ultrafiltration and diafiltration. BayRab is formulated as a 15–18% protein solution at a pH of 6.4–7.2 in 0.21–0.32 M glycine. BayRab is then incubated in the final container for 21–28 days at 20–27°C. The product is standardized against the U.S. Standard Rabies Immune Globulin to contain an average potency value of 150 IU/mL. The U.S. unit of potency is equivalent to the international unit (IU) for rabies antibody.

The removal and inactivation of spiked model enveloped and non-enveloped viruses during the manufacturing pro-

Continued on next page

BayRab—Cont.

cess for BayRab has been validated in laboratory studies. Human Immunodeficiency Virus, Type 1(HIV-1), was chosen as the relevant virus for blood products; Bovine Viral Diarrhea Virus (BVDV) was chosen to model Hepatitis C virus; Pseudorabies virus (PRV) was chosen to model Hepatitis B virus and the Herpes viruses; and Reo virus type 3 (Reo) was chosen to model non-enveloped viruses and for its resistance to physical and chemical inactivation. Significant removal of model enveloped and non-enveloped viruses is achieved at two steps in the Cohn fractionation process leading to the collection of Cohn Fraction II: the precipitation and removal of Fraction III in the processing of Fraction II + IIIW suspension to Effluent III and the filtration step in the processing of Effluent III to Filtrate III. Significant inactivation of enveloped viruses is achieved at the time of treatment of solubilized Cohn Fraction II with TNBP/sodium cholate.

CLINICAL PHARMACOLOGY

The usefulness of prophylactic rabies antibody in preventing rabies in humans when administered immediately after exposure was dramatically demonstrated in a group of persons bitten by a rabid wolf in Iran.[1,2] Similarly, beneficial results were later reported from the U.S.S.R.[3] Studies coordinated by WHO helped determine the optimal conditions under which antirabies serum of equine origin and rabies vaccine can be used in man.[4–7] These studies showed that serum can interfere to a variable extent with the active immunity induced by the vaccine, but could be minimized by booster doses of vaccine after the end of the usual dosage series.

Preparation of rabies immune globulin of human origin with adequate potency was reported by Cabasso et al.[8] In carefully controlled clinical studies, this globulin was used in conjunction with rabies vaccine of duck-embryo origin (DEV).[8,9] These studies determined that a human globulin dose of 20 IU/kg of rabies antibody, given simultaneously with the first DEV dose, resulted in amply detectable levels of passive rabies antibody 24 hours after injection in all recipients. The injections produced minimal, if any, interference with the subject's endogenous antibody response to DEV.

More recently, human diploid cell rabies vaccines (HDCV) prepared from tissue culture fluids containing rabies virus have received substantial clinical evaluation in Europe and the United States.[10–16] In a study in adult volunteers, the administration of Rabies Immune Globulin (Human) did not interfere with antibody formation induced by HDCV when given in a dose of 20 IU per kilogram body weight simultaneously with the first dose of vaccine.[15]

In a clinical study in eight healthy human adults receiving a 20 IU/kg intramuscular dose of Rabies Immune Globulin (Human) treated with solvent/detergent, BayRab®, detectable passive rabies antibody titers were observed in the serum of all subjects by 24 hours post injection and persisted through the 21 day study period. These results are consistent with prior studies[17,18] with non-solvent/detergent treated product.

INDICATIONS AND USAGE

Rabies vaccine and BayRab should be given to all persons suspected of exposure to rabies with one exception: persons who have been previously immunized with rabies vaccine and have a confirmed adequate rabies antibody titer should receive only vaccine. BayRab should be administered as promptly as possible after exposure, but can be administered up to the eighth day after the first dose of vaccine is given.

Recommendations for use of passive and active immunization after exposure to an animal suspected of having rabies have been detailed by the U.S. Public Health Service Advisory Committee on Immunization Practices (ACIP).[19]

Every exposure to possible rabies infection must be individually evaluated. The following factors should be considered before specific antirabies treatment is initiated:

1. Species of Biting Animal

Carnivorous wild animals (especially skunks, foxes, coyotes, raccoons, and bobcats) and bats are the animals most commonly infected with rabies and have caused most of the indigenous cases of human rabies in the United States since 1960.[20] Unless the animal is tested and shown not to be rabid, postexposure prophylaxis should be initiated upon bite or nonbite exposure to these animals (see item 3 below). If treatment has been initiated and subsequent testing in a competent laboratory shows the exposing animal is not rabid, treatment can be discontinued.

In the United States, the likelihood that a domestic dog or cat is infected with rabies varies from region to region; hence, the need for postexposure prophylaxis also varies. However, in most of Asia and all of Africa and Latin America, the dog remains the major source of human exposure; exposures to dogs in such countries represent a special threat. Travelers to those countries should be aware that >50% of the rabies cases among humans in the United States result from exposure to dogs outside the United States.

Rodents (such as squirrels, hamsters, guinea pigs, gerbils, chipmunks, rats, and mice) and lagomorphs (including rabbits and hares) are rarely found to be infected with rabies and have not been known to cause human rabies in the United States. However, from 1971 through 1988, woodchucks accounted for 70% of the 179 cases of rabies among rodents reported to CDC.[21] In these cases, the state or local health department should be consulted before a decision is made to initiate post-exposure antirabies prophylaxis.

2. Circumstances of Biting Incident

An unprovoked attack is more likely to mean that the animal is rabid. (Bites during attempts to feed or handle an apparently healthy animal may generally be regarded as provoked.)

3. Type of Exposure

Rabies is transmitted only when the virus is introduced into open cuts or wounds in skin or mucous membranes. If there has been no exposure (as described in this section), postexposure treatment is not necessary. Thus, the likelihood that rabies infection will result from exposure to a rabid animal varies with the nature and extent of the exposure. Two categories of exposure should be considered:

Bite: any penetration of the skin by teeth. Bites to the face and hands carry the highest risk, but the site of the bite should not influence the decision to begin treatment.[22]

Bat-associated strains of rabies can be transmitted to humans either directly through a bat's bite or indirectly through the bite of an animal previously infected by a bat. Because some bat bites may be less severe, and can go completely undetected, unlike bites inflicted by larger animals, especially mammalian carnivores, rabies postexposure treatment should be considered for any physical contact with bats when bite or mucous membrane contact cannot be excluded.[23]

Nonbite: scratches, abrasions, open wounds or mucous membranes contaminated with saliva or any potentially infectious material, such as brain tissue, from a rabid animal constitute nonbite exposures. If the material containing the virus is dry, the virus can be considered noninfectious. Casual contact, such as petting a rabid animal and contact with the blood, urine, or feces (e.g., guano) of a rabid animal, does not constitute an exposure and is not an indication for prophylaxis. Instances of air-borne rabies have been reported rarely. Adherence to respiratory precautions will minimize the risk of airborne exposure.[24]

The only documented cases of rabies from human-to-human transmission have occurred in patients who received corneas transplanted from persons who died of rabies undiagnosed at the time of death. Stringent guidelines for acceptance of donor corneas have reduced this risk.

Bite and nonbite exposures from humans with rabies theoretically could transmit rabies, although no cases of rabies acquired this way have been documented.

4. Vaccination Status of Biting Animal

A properly immunized animal has only a minimal chance of developing rabies and transmitting the virus.

5. Presence of Rabies in Region

If adequate laboratory and field records indicate that there is no rabies infection in a domestic species within a given region, local health officials are justified in considering this in making recommendations on antirabies treatment following a bite by that particular species. Such officials should be consulted for current interpretations.

Rabies Postexposure Prophylaxis

The following recommendations are only a guide. In applying them, take into account the animal species involved, the circumstances of the bite or other exposure, the vaccination status of the animal, and presence of rabies in the region. Local or state public health officials should be consulted if questions arise about the need for rabies prophylaxis.

Local Treatment of Wounds: Immediate and thorough washing of all bite wounds and scratches with soap and water is perhaps the most effective measure for preventing rabies. In experimental animals, simple local wound cleansing has been shown to reduce markedly the likelihood of rabies.

Tetanus prophylaxis and measures to control bacterial infection should be given as indicated.

Active Immunization: Active immunization should be initiated as soon as possible after exposure (within 24 hours). Many dosage schedules have been evaluated for the currently available rabies vaccines and their respective manufacturers' literature should be consulted.

Passive Immunization: A combination of active and passive immunization (vaccine and immune globulin) is considered the acceptable postexposure prophylaxis except for those persons who have been previously immunized with rabies vaccine and who have documented adequate rabies antibody titer. These individuals should receive vaccine only. For passive immunization, Rabies Immune Globulin (Human) is preferred over antirabies serum, equine.[16,19] It is recommended both for treatment of all bites by animals suspected of having rabies and for nonbite exposure inflicted by animals suspected of being rabid. Rabies Immune Globulin (Human) should be used in conjunction with rabies vaccine and can be administered through the seventh day after the first dose of vaccine is given. Beyond the seventh day, Rabies Immune Globulin (Human) is not indicated since an antibody response to cell culture vaccine is presumed to have occurred.

[See table below]

Rabies Postexposure Prophylaxis Guide[19]

Animal species	Condition of animal at time of exposure/attack	Treatment of exposed person [1]
Dog and cat	Healthy and available for 10 days of observation	None, unless animal develops rabies [2]
	Rabid or suspected rabid	RIGH [3] and HDCV
	Unknown (escaped)	Consult public health officials
Skunk, bat, fox, coyote, raccoon, bobcat, and other carnivores; woodchuck	Regard as rabid unless animal proven negative by laboratory tests [4]	RIGH [3] and HDCV
Livestock, rodents, and lagomorphs (rabbits and hares)	Consider individually. Local and state public health officials should be consulted on questions about the need for rabies prophylaxis. In most geographical areas bites of squirrels, hamsters, guinea pigs, gerbils, chipmunks, rats, mice, other rodents, rabbits, and hares almost never require antirabies postexposure prophylaxis	

[1] ALL POSTEXPOSURE PROPHYLAXIS SHOULD BEGIN WITH IMMEDIATE THOROUGH CLEANSING OF THE WOUND (IF ONE CAN BE DETECTED) WITH SOAP AND WATER. If antirabies treatment is indicated, both Rabies Immune Globulin (Human) [RIGH] and human diploid cell rabies vaccine (HDCV) should be given as soon as possible, REGARDLESS of the interval from exposure.

[2] During the usual holding period of 10 days, begin postexposure prophylaxis at first sign of rabies in a dog or cat that has bitten someone. If the animal exhibits clinical signs of rabies, it should be euthanized immediately and tested.

[3] If RIGH is not available, use antirabies serum, equine (ARS). Do not use more than the recommended dosage.

[4] The animal should be euthanized and tested as soon as possible. Holding for observation is not recommended. Discontinue vaccine if immunofluorescence test results of the animal are negative.

CONTRAINDICATIONS

None known.

WARNINGS

Rabies Immune Globulin (Human) — BayRab® is made from human plasma. Products made from human plasma may contain infectious agents, such as viruses, that can cause disease. The risk that such products will transmit an infectious agent has been reduced by screening plasma donors for prior exposure to certain viruses, by testing for the presence of certain current virus infections, and by inactivating and/or removing certain viruses. Despite these measures, such products can still potentially transmit disease. There is also the possibility that unknown infectious agents may be present in such products. Individuals who receive infusions of blood or plasma products may develop signs and/or symptoms of some viral infections, particularly hepatitis C. ALL infections thought by a physician possibly to have been transmitted by this product should be reported by the physician or other healthcare provider to Bayer Corporation [1-888-765-3203]. The physician should discuss the risks and benefits of this product with the patient, before prescribing or administering it to the patient.

BayRab should be given with caution to patients with a history of prior systemic allergic reactions following the administration of human immunoglobulin preparations.

The attending physician who wishes to administer BayRab to persons with isolated immunoglobulin A (IgA) deficiency must weigh the benefits of immunization against the potential risks of hypersensitivity reactions. Such persons have increased potential for developing antibodies to IgA and could have anaphylactic reactions to subsequent administration of blood products that contain IgA.[25]

As with all preparations administered by the intramuscular route, bleeding complications may be encountered in patients with thrombocytopenia or other bleeding disorders.

PRECAUTIONS

General

BayRab should **not** be administered intravenously because of the potential for serious reactions. Although systemic reactions to immunoglobulin preparations are rare, epinephrine should be available for treatment of acute anaphylactoid symptoms.

Drug Interactions

Repeated doses of BayRab should not be administered once vaccine treatment has been initiated as this could prevent the full expression of active immunity expected from the rabies vaccine.

Rabies postexposure prophylaxis schedule—United States, 1999[19]

Vaccination status	Treatment	Regimen*
Not previously vaccinated	Wound cleansing	All postexposure treatment should begin with immediate thorough cleansing of all wounds with soap and water. If available, a virucidal agent such as povidone-iodine solution should be used to irrigate the wounds.
	RIG	Administer 20 IU/kg body weight. If anatomically feasible, **the full dose** should be infiltrated around the wound(s) and any remaining volume should be administered IM at an anatomical site distant from vaccine administration. Also, RIG should not be administered in the same syringe as vaccine. Because RIG might partially suppress active production of antibody, no more than the recommended dose should be given.
	Vaccine	HDCV, RVA, or PCEC 1.0 mL, IM (deltoid area†), one each on days 0 §, 3, 7, 14, and 28.
Previously vaccinated¶	Wound cleansing	All postexposure treatment should begin with immediate thorough cleansing of all wounds with soap and water. If available, a virucidal agent such as a povidone-iodine solution should be used to irrigate the wounds.
	RIG	RIG should **not** be administered.
	Vaccine	HDCV, RVA, or PCEC 1.0 mL, IM (deltoid area†), one each on days 0§ and 3.

HDCV = human diploid cell vaccine; PCEC = purified chick embryo cell vaccine; RIG = rabies immune globulin; RVA = rabies vaccine adsorbed; IM, intramuscular

*These regimens are applicable for all age groups, including children.

†The deltoid area is the only acceptable site of vaccination for adults and older children. For younger children, the outer aspect of the thigh may be used. Vaccine should never be administered in the gluteal area.

§Day 0 is the day the first dose of vaccine is administered.

¶Any person with a history of preexposure vaccination with HDCV, RVA, or PCEC; prior postexposure prophylaxis with HDCV, RVA, or PCEC; or previous vaccination with any other type of rabies vaccine and a documented history of antibody response to the prior vaccination.

Other antibodies in the BayRab preparation may interfere with the response to live vaccines such as measles, mumps, polio or rubella. Therefore, immunization with live vaccines should not be given within 3 months after BayRab administration.

Pregnancy Category C

Animal reproduction studies have not been conducted with BayRab. It is also not known whether BayRab can cause fetal harm when administered to a pregnant woman or can affect reproduction capacity. BayRab should be given to a pregnant woman only if clearly needed.

Pediatric Use

Safety and effectiveness in the pediatric population have not been established.

ADVERSE REACTIONS

Soreness at the site of injection and mild temperature elevations may be observed at times. Sensitization to repeated injections has occurred occasionally in immunoglobulin-deficient patients. Angioneurotic edema, skin rash, nephrotic syndrome, and anaphylactic shock have rarely been reported after intramuscular injection, so that a causal relationship between immunoglobulin and these reactions is not clear.

DOSAGE AND ADMINISTRATION

The recommended dose for BayRab is 20 IU/kg (0.133 mL/kg) of body weight given preferably at the time of the first vaccine dose.[8,9] It may also be given through the seventh day after the first dose of vaccine is given. If anatomically feasible, up to the full dose of BayRab should be thoroughly infiltrated in the area around the wound and the rest should be administered intramuscularly in the gluteal area or lateral thigh muscle. Because of risk of injury to the sciatic nerve, the central region of the gluteal area MUST be avoided; only the upper, outer quadrant should be used.[26] BayRab should never be administered in the same syringe or needle or in the same anatomical site as vaccine.

Parenteral drug products should be inspected visually for particulate matter and discoloration prior to administration, whenever solution and container permit.

[See table above]

HOW SUPPLIED

BayRab is packaged in 2 mL and 10 mL single dose vials with an average potency value of 150 international units per mL (IU/mL). The 2 mL vial contains a total of 300 IU which is sufficient for a child weighing 15 kg. The 10 mL vial contains a total of 1500 IU which is sufficient for an adult weighing 75 kg.

NDC Number	Size
0026-0618-02	2 mL vial
0026-0618-10	10 mL vial

STORAGE

BayRab should be stored under refrigeration (2–8°C, 36–46°F). Solution that has been frozen should not be used.

CAUTION

℞ only

U.S. federal law prohibits dispensing without prescription.

LIMITED WARRANTY

A number of factors beyond our control could reduce the efficacy of this product or even result in an ill effect following its use. These include improper storage and handling of the product after it leaves our hands, diagnosis, dosage, method of administration, and biological differences in individual patients. Because of these factors, it is important that this product be stored properly and that the directions be followed carefully during use.

No warranty, express or implied, including any warranty of merchantability or fitness is made. Representatives of the Company are not authorized to vary the terms or the contents of the printed labeling, including the package insert for this product, except by printed notice from the Company's headquarters. The prescriber and user of this product must accept the terms hereof.

REFERENCES

1. Baltazard M, Bahmanyar M, Ghodssi M, et al: Essai pratique du sérum antirabique chez les mordus par loups enragés. *Bull WHO* 13:747-72, 1955.
2. Habel K, Koprowski H: Laboratory data supporting the clinical trial of antirabies serum in persons bitten by a rabid wolf. *Bull WHO* 13:773-9, 1955.
3. Selimov M, Boltucij L, Semenova E, et al: [The use of antirabies gamma globulin in subjects severely bitten by rabid wolves or other animals.] *J Hyg Epidemiol Microbiol Immunol (Praha)* 3:168-80, 1959.
4. Atanasiu P, Bahmanyar M, Baltazard M, et al: Rabies neutralizing antibody response to different schedules of serum and vaccine inoculations in non-exposed persons. *Bull WHO* 14:593-611, 1956.
5. Atanasiu P, Bahmanyar M, Baltazard M, et al: Rabies neutralizing antibody response to different schedules of serum and vaccine inoculations in non-exposed persons: Part II. *Bull WHO* 17:911-32, 1957.
6. Atanasiu P, Cannon DA, Dean DJ, et al: Rabies neutralizing antibody response to different schedules of serum and vaccine innoculations in non-exposed persons: Part 3. *Bull WHO* 25:103-14, 1961.
7. Atanasiu P, Dean DJ, Habel K, et al: Rabies neutralizing antibody response to different schedules of serum and vaccine inoculations in non-exposed persons: Part 4. *Bull WHO* 36:361-5, 1967.
8. Cabasso VJ, Loofbourow JC, Roby RE, et al: Rabies immune globulin of human origin: preparation and dosage determination in non-exposed volunteer subjects. *Bull WHO* 45:303-15, 1971.
9. Loofbourow JC, Cabasso VJ, Roby RE, et al: Rabies immune globulin (human): clinical trials and dose determination. *JAMA* 217(13): 1825-31, 1971.
10. Plotkin SA: New rabies vaccine halts disease — without severe reactions. *Mod Med* 45(20):45-8, 1977.
11. Plotkin SA, Wiktor TJ, Koprowski H, et al: Immunization schedules for the new human diploid cell vaccine against rabies. *Am J Epidemiol* 103(1):75-80, 1976.
12. Hafkin B, Hattwick MA, Smith JS, et al: A comparison of a WI-38 vaccine and duck embryo vaccine for preexposure rabies prophylaxis. *Am J Epidemiol* 107(5):439-43, 1978.
13. Kuwert EK, Marcus I, Höher PG: Neutralizing and complement-fixing antibody responses in pre- and postexposure vaccinees to a rabies vaccine produced in human diploid cells. *J Biol Stand* 4(4):249-62, 1976.
14. Grandien M: Evaluation of tests for rabies antibody and analysis of serum responses after administration of three different types of rabies vaccines. *J Clin Microbiol* 5(3):263-7, 1977.
15. Kuwert EK, Marcus I, Werner J, et al: Postexpositionelle Schutzimpfung des Menschen gegen Tollwut mit einer neu-entwickelten Gewebekulturvakzine (HDCS-Impfstoff). *Zentralbl Bakteriol [A]* 239(4):437-58, 1977.
16. Bahmanyar M, Fayaz A, Nour-Salehi S, et al: Successful protection of humans exposed to rabies infection: postexposure treatment with the new human diploid cell rabies vaccine and antirabies serum. *JAMA* 236(24):2751-4, 1976.
17. American Hospital Formulary Service. Drug Information. Section 80:04. Rabies immune globulin. Bethesda, American Society for Health-Systems Pharmacy, 1997, p. 2545-7.
18. Rubin Rh, Sikes RK, Gregg MB: Human rabies immune globulin. Clinical trials and effects on serum anti-globulins. *JAMA* 224:871-4, 1973.
19. Recommendations of the Advisory Committee on Immunization Practices (ACIP): Rabies prevention—United States, 1999. *MMWR* 48(RR-1):1-21, 1999.
20. Reid-Sanden FL, Dobbins JG, Smith JS, et al: Rabies surveillance in the United States during 1989. *J Am Vet Med Assoc* 197(12):1571-83, 1990.
21. Fishbein DB, Belotto AJ, Pacer RE, et al: Rabies in rodents and lagomorphs in the United States, 1971-1984: increased cases in the woodchuck (*Marmota monax*) in mid-Atlantic states. *J Wildl Dis* 22(2):151-5, 1986.
22. Hattwick MAW: Human rabies. *Public Health Rev* 3(3): 229-74, 1974.
23. Epidemiologic Notes and Reports: Human Rabies—California, 1994. *MMWR* 43(25):455-457, 1994.
24. Garner JS, Simmons BP: Guideline for isolation precautions in hospitals. *Infect Control* 4(4 Suppl):245-325, 1983.
25. Fudenberg HH: Sensitization to immunoglobulins and hazards of gamma globulin therapy. In: Merler E (ed.): Immunoglobulins: biologic aspects and clinical uses. Washington, DC, Nat Acad Sci, 1970, pp 211-20.
26. Recommendations of the Immunization Practices Advisory Committee (ACIP): General recommendations on immunization. *MMWR* 38(13):205-14; 219-27, 1989.

Bayer Corporation
Pharmaceutical Division
Elkhart, IN 46515 USA
U.S. License No. 8 14-7618-002
(Rev. April 1999)

BAYRHO-D® MINI-DOSE ℞

[*bāy"rhō-d*]

Rh_o(D) Immune Globulin (Human)
Solvent/Detergent Treated

DESCRIPTION

Rh_o(D) Immune Globulin (Human) — BayRho-D® Mini-Dose treated with solvent/detergent is a sterile solution of immune globulin containing antibodies to Rh_o(D) for intramuscular administration; it contains no preservative. BayRho-D Mini-Dose is prepared by cold ethanol fractionation from human plasma. The immune globulin is isolated from solubilized Cohn Fraction II. The Fraction II solution is adjusted to a final concentration of 0.3% tri-n-butyl phosphate (TNBP) and 0.2% sodium cholate. After the addition of solvent (TNBP) and detergent (sodium cholate), the solution is heated to 30°C and maintained at that temperature for not less than 6 hours. After the viral inactivation step, the reactants are removed by precipitation, filtration and finally ultrafiltration and diafiltration. BayRho-D Mini-Dose is then incubated in the final container for 21–28 days at 20–27°C. BayRho-D Mini-Dose is formulated as a 15–18% protein solution at a pH of 6.4–7.2 in 0.21–0.32 M glycine. One dose of BayRho-D Mini-Dose contains not less than one-sixth the quantity of Rh_o(D) antibody contained in one standard dose of Rh_o(D) Immune Globulin (Human), and it will suppress the immunizing potential of 2.5 mL of Rh_o(D) positive packed red blood cells or the equivalent of whole blood (5 mL). The quantity of Rh_o(D) antibody in BayRho-D Mini-Dose is not less than one-sixth of that contained in 1 mL of the U.S. Food and Drug Administration Reference Rh_o(D) Immune Globulin (Human).

The removal and inactivation of spiked model enveloped and non-enveloped viruses during the manufacturing process for BayRho-D Mini-Dose has been validated in laboratory studies. Human Immunodeficiency Virus, Type 1 (HIV-1), was chosen as the relevant virus for blood products; Bovine Viral Diarrhea Virus (BVDV) was chosen to model Hepatitis C virus; Pseudorabies virus (PRV) was chosen to model Hepatitis B virus and the Herpes viruses; and Reo virus type 3 (Reo) was chosen to model non-enveloped viruses and for its resistance to physical and chemical inactivation. Significant removal of model enveloped and non-enveloped viruses is achieved at two steps in the Cohn fractionation process leading to the collection of Cohn Fraction II: the precipitation and removal of Fraction III in the processing of Fraction II + IIIW suspension to Effluent III and the filtration step in the processing of Effluent III to Filtrate III. Significant inactivation of enveloped viruses is achieved at the time of treatment of solubilized Cohn Fraction II with TNBP/sodium cholate.

CLINICAL PHARMACOLOGY

Rh sensitization may occur in nonsensitized Rh_o(D) negative women following transplacental hemorrhage resulting from spontaneous or induced abortions.[1-2] The risk of sensitization is higher in women undergoing induced abortions than in those aborting spontaneously.[1-3]

BayRho-D Mini-Dose is used to prevent the formation of anti-Rh_o(D) antibody in Rh_o(D) negative women who are exposed to the Rh_o(D) antigen at the time of spontaneous or induced abortion (up to 12 weeks' gestation).[3-5] BayRho-D Mini-Dose suppresses the stimulation of active immunity by

Continued on next page

BayRho-D Mini-Dose—Cont.

$Rh_0(D)$ positive fetal erythrocytes that may enter the maternal circulation at the time of termination of the pregnancy. The amount of anti-$Rh_0(D)$ in BayRho-D Mini-Dose has been shown to effectively prevent maternal isosensitization to the $Rh_0(D)$ antigens following spontaneous or induced abortion occurring up to the 12th week of gestation.[6–8] After the 12th week of gestation, a standard dose of BayRho-D® Full Dose is indicated.

In a clinical study in eight healthy human adults receiving another hyperimmune immune globulin product treated with solvent/detergent, Rabies Immune Globulin (Human), RayRab®, prepared by the same manufacturing process, detectable passive antibody titers were observed in the serum of all subjects by 24 hours post injection and persisted through the 21 day study period. These results suggest that passive immunization with immune globulin products is not affected by the solvent/detergent treatment.

INDICATIONS AND USAGE

BayRho-D Mini-Dose is recommended to prevent the isoimmunization of $Rh_0(D)$ negative women at the time of spontaneous or induced abortion of up to 12 weeks' gestation provided the following criteria are met:

1. The mother must be $Rh_0(D)$ negative and must not already be sensitized to the $Rh_0(D)$ antigen.
2. The father is not known to be $Rh_0(D)$ negative.
3. Gestation is not more than 12 weeks at termination.

Note: $Rh_0(D)$ Immune Globulin (Human) prophylaxis is not indicated if the fetus or father can be determined to be Rh negative. If the Rh status of the fetus is unknown, the fetus must be assumed to be $Rh_0(D)$ positive, and BayRho-D Mini-Dose should be administered to the mother.

FOR ABORTIONS OR MISCARRIAGES OCCURRING AFTER 12 WEEKS' GESTATION, A STANDARD DOSE OF $Rh_0(D)$ IMMUNE GLOBULIN (HUMAN) IS INDICATED.

BayRho-D Mini-Dose should be administered within 3 hours or as soon as possible after spontaneous passage or surgical removal of the products of conception. However, if BayRho-D Mini-Dose is not given within this time period, consideration should still be given to its administration since clinical studies in male volunteers have demonstrated the effectiveness of $Rh_0(D)$ Immune Globulin (Human) in preventing isoimmunization as long as 72 hours after infusion of $Rh_0(D)$ positive red cells.[9]

CONTRAINDICATIONS

None known.

WARNINGS

BayRho-D Mini-Dose is made from human plasma. Products made from human plasma may contain infectious agents, such as viruses, that can cause disease. The risk that such products will transmit an infectious agent has been reduced by screening plasma donors for prior exposure to certain viruses, by testing for the presence of certain current virus infections, and by inactivating and/or removing certain viruses. Despite these measures, such products can still potentially transmit disease. There is also the possibility that unknown infectious agents may be present in such products. Individuals who receive infusions of blood or plasma products may develop signs and/or symptoms of some viral infections, particularly hepatitis C. ALL infections thought by a physician possibly to have been transmitted by this product should be reported by the physician or other healthcare provider to Bayer Corporation [1-888-765-3203].

The physician should discuss the risks and benefits of this product with the patient, before prescribing or administering it to the patient.

NEVER ADMINISTER BAYRHO-D MINI-DOSE INTRAVENOUSLY. INJECT ONLY INTRAMUSCULARLY. ADMINISTER ONLY TO WOMEN POSTABORTION OR POSTMISCARRIAGE OF UP TO 12 WEEKS' GESTATION. NEVER ADMINISTER TO THE NEONATE.

BayRho-D Mini-Dose should be given with caution to patients with a history of prior systemic allergic reactions following the administration of human immune globulin preparations.

The attending physician who wishes to administer BayRho-D Mini-Dose to persons with isolated immunoglobulin A (IgA) deficiency must weigh the benefits of immunization against the potential risks of hypersensitivity reactions. Such persons have increased potential for developing antibodies to IgA and could have anaphylactic reactions to subsequent administration of blood products that contain IgA.

As with all preparations administered by the intramuscular route, bleeding complications may be encountered in patients with thrombocytopenia or other bleeding disorders.

PRECAUTIONS

General

Although systemic reactions to immunoglobulin preparations are rare, epinephrine should be available for treatment of acute anaphylactic symptoms.

Drug Interactions

Other antibodies in the BayRho-D Mini-Dose preparation may interfere with the response to live vaccines such as measles, mumps, polio or rubella. Therefore, immunization with live vaccines should not be given within 3 months after BayRho-D Mini-Dose administration.

Pregnancy Category C

Animal reproduction studies have not been conducted with BayRho-D Mini-Dose. It is also not known whether BayRho-D Mini-Dose can cause fetal harm when administered to a pregnant woman or can affect reproduction capacity.

It should be again noted, however, that BayRho-D Mini-Dose is **not** indicated for use during pregnancy and it should be administered only postabortion or postmiscarriage.

Pediatric Use

Safety and effectiveness in the pediatric population have not been established.

ADVERSE REACTIONS

Reactions to BayRho-D Mini-Dose are infrequent in $Rh_0(D)$ negative individuals and consist primarily of slight soreness at the site of injection and slight temperature elevation. While sensitization to repeated injections of human globulin is extremely rare, it has occurred.

DOSAGE AND ADMINISTRATION

NEVER ADMINISTER BAYRHO-D MINI-DOSE INTRAVENOUSLY. INJECT ONLY INTRAMUSCULARLY. ADMINISTER ONLY TO WOMEN POSTABORTION OR POSTMISCARRIAGE OF UP TO 12 WEEKS' GESTATION. NEVER ADMINISTER TO THE NEONATE.

One syringe of BayRho-D Mini-Dose provides sufficient antibody to prevent Rh sensitization to 2.5 mL $Rh_0(D)$ positive packed red cells or the equivalent (5 mL) of whole blood. This dose is sufficient to provide protection against maternal Rh sensitization for women undergoing spontaneous or induced abortion of up to 12 weeks' gestation.

BayRho-D Mini-Dose should be administered within 3 hours or as soon as possible following spontaneous or induced abortion. If prompt administration is not possible, BayRho-D Mini-Dose should be given within 72 hours following termination of the pregnancy.

BayRho-D Mini-Dose is administered **intramuscularly**, preferably in the anterolateral aspects of the upper thigh and the deltoid muscle of the upper arm. The gluteal region should not be used routinely as an injection site because of the risk of injury to the sciatic nerve. If the gluteal region is used, the central region must be avoided; only the upper, outer quadrant should be used.[10]

Parenteral drug products should be inspected visually for particulate matter and discoloration prior to administration, whenever solution and container permit.

$Rh_0(D)$ Immune Globulin (Human) — BayRho-D® Mini-Dose is supplied with a syringe and an attached UltraSafe® Needle Guard for your protection and convenience. Please follow instructions below for proper use of syringe and UltraSafe® Needle Guard.

Directions for Syringe Usage

1. Remove the prefilled syringe from the package. Lift syringe by barrel, **not** by plunger.
2. Twist the plunger rod clockwise until the threads are seated.
3. With the rubber needle shield secured on the syringe tip, push the plunger rod forward a few millimeters to break any friction seal between the rubber stopper and the glass syringe barrel.
4. Remove the needle shield and expel air bubbles.
5. Proceed with hypodermic needle puncture.
6. Aspirate prior to injection to confirm that the needle is not in a vein or artery.
7. Inject the medication.
8. Keeping your hands behind the needle, grasp the guard with free hand and slide forward toward needle until it is completely covered and guard clicks into place. If audible click is not heard, guard may not be completely activated. (See Diagrams A and B)
9. Place entire prefilled glass syringe with guard activated into an approved sharps container for proper disposal. (See Diagram C)

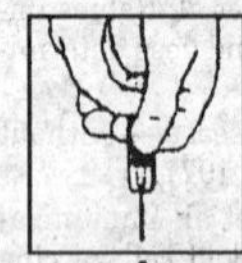
A

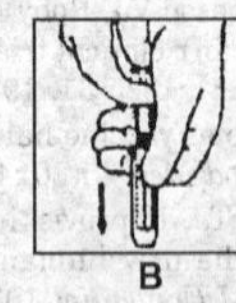
B

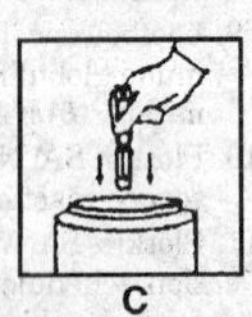
C

A number of factors beyond our control could reduce the efficacy of this product or even result in a ill effect following its use. These include improper storage and handling of the product after it leaves our hands, diagnosis, dosage, method of administration, and biological differences in individual patients. Because of these factors, it is important that this product be stored properly and that the directions be followed carefully during use.

HOW SUPPLIED

BayRho-D Mini-Dose package contains 10 single dose syringes.

NDC Number	Size
0026-0631-06	Syringe (10 pack)

STORAGE

Store at 2–8°C (36–46°F). Do not freeze.

CAUTION

℞ only

U.S. federal law prohibits dispensing without prescription.

REFERENCES

1. Queenan JT, Shah S, Kubarych SF, et al: Role of induced abortion in rhesus immunisation. *Lancet* 1(7704):815–7, 1971.
2. Goldman, JA, Eckerling B: Prevention of Rh immunization after abortion with anti-Rh_0(D)-immunoglobulin. *Obstet Gynecol* 40(3):366–370, 1972.
3. The selective use of $Rh_0(D)$ immune globulin (RhIG). *ACOG Tech Bull* 61, 1981.
4. Prevention of Rh sensitization, *WHO Tech Rep Ser* 468, 1971.
5. Recommendation of the Public Health Service Advisory Committee on Immunization Practices: Rh immune globulin. *MMWR* 21(15):126–7, 1972.
6. Stewart FH, Burnhill MS, Bozorgi N: Reduced dose of Rh immunoglobulin following first trimester pregnancy termination. *Obstet Gynecol* 51(3):318–22, 1978.
7. McMaster conference on prevention of Rh immunization. 28–30 September, 1977. *Vox Sang* 36(1):50–64, 1979.
8. Simonovits I: Efficiency of anti-D IgG prevention after induced abortion. *Vox Sang* 26(4):361–7, 1974.
9. Freda VJ, Gorman JG, Pollack W: Prevention of Rh-hemolytic disease with Rh-immune globulin. *Am J Obstet Gynecol* 128(4):456–60, 1977.
10. Recommendations of the Immunization Practices Advisory Committee (ACIP): General recommendations on immunization. *MMWR* 38(13):205–14; 219–27, 1989.

Bayer Corporation
Pharmaceutical Division
Elkhart, IN 46515 USA
U.S. License No. 8
14-7631-060 (Published October 2000)

The Rh Factor and Your Pregnancy

Information About Pregnancy Protection

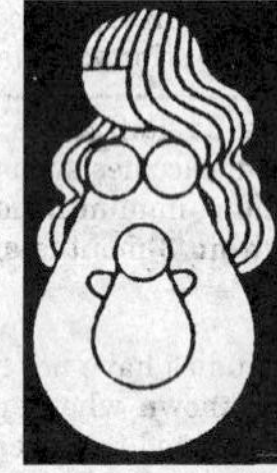

The Rh Factor and When It Is Important

The Rh factor is one of many blood group antigens found on the surface of red blood cells. If you have this antigen you are considered Rh positive. If you don't, then you are considered Rh negative. Everyone is either Rh positive or Rh negative. One type is neither better nor worse than the other, only different.

Your Rh factor is important if you are an Rh negative woman and you become pregnant, or if you receive a blood transfusion.

How the Rh Factor Can Affect Your Future

If you have Rh negative blood, there are two situations that can affect you:

1. If the father of your baby is Rh positive, the baby will probably be Rh positive too. An Rh negative woman carrying an Rh positive baby may have an immune reaction if some of the baby's Rh positive blood cells enter her bloodstream.
   This immune reaction, called isoimmunization, means your body's defense system recognizes Rh positive blood as foreign from your own and produces "antibodies" to destroy the invading Rh positive blood cells.
   The passage of blood from the baby to the mother's bloodstream happens most often at delivery, but can also occur during miscarriage, the termination of pregnancy, amniocentesis (test performed to determine fetal health), or due to an injury or trauma. It is important to note that a small number of women develop antibodies to Rh positive blood cells during pregnancy for no apparent reason.
   Antibodies to Rh positive blood may not be a problem in first pregnancies; however, the antibodies stay in your bloodstream, ready to attack invading Rh positive blood cells, for many years to come. This can lead to problems in future pregnancies by causing miscarriage or a disease known as hemolytic disease of the newborn.
   Babies born to Rh positive mothers, regardless of the father's blood type, will usually be free of the dangers of hemolytic disease.
2. Someday it may become necessary for you to receive a blood transfusion. If Rh positive antibodies already reside in your bloodstream due to isoimmunization and the blood you receive is Rh positive due to error or lifesaving reasons, your Rh positive antibodies will become mobilized and destroy the donor Rh positive cells. As a result, the transfusion could be unsuccessful and possibly harmful to you.

Hemolytic Disease of the Newborn: A Threat to Your Baby

When an Rh negative woman has Rh positive antibodies in her blood and the baby she is carrying is Rh positive, the antibodies could possibly enter the baby's bloodstream, attack the baby's red blood cells and cause hemolytic disease of the newborn. At birth, the infant suffering from hemolytic disease may be jaundiced and anemic or suffer permanent damage of the brain and central nervous system which may result in mental retardation, hearing loss, or cerebral palsy. Extensive medical care can be required, including an exchange transfusion, in which all of the baby's blood is replaced. This usually stops the destruction of the baby's red blood cells and gives the infant a chance to survive.

The risk of hemolytic disease of the newborn is slight with the first baby, but increases with each successive pregnancy.

Preventing Hemolytic Disease

BayRho-D®, Rh_o(D) Immune Globulin (Human) can prevent hemolytic disease of the newborn, provided Rh positive antibodies do not already reside in your bloodstream.

BayRho-D is a specially prepared gamma globulin with a high level of preformed antibodies against Rh positive blood cells. The injection of BayRho-D destroys any Rh positive blood cells that may have entered the mother's bloodstream and prevents the mother's immune system from producing Rh positive antibodies; thus protecting the baby from developing hemolytic disease.

BayRho-D Full Dose — When Prescribed

Pregnancy and Other Obstetric Conditions Pertaining to Rh Negative Women

BayRho-D Full Dose is administered during pregnancy if you fall into a high-risk category. For example, you are at risk of producing Rh positive antibodies if you have an amniocentesis procedure performed, or if you have a miscarriage or other termination of pregnancy at or beyond 13 weeks' gestation.

Laboratory findings have shown that some Rh negative women develop Rh positive antibodies during the last weeks of pregnancy even without an antibody-stimulating event. As a preventive measure, your physician will probably recommend the first injection of BayRho-D Full Dose at the 28th week of pregnancy.

In both of the above situations, if the blood type of the father or baby can be determined to be Rh negative, an injection of BayRho-D is not required.

Another injection of BayRho-D Full Dose is administered within 72 hours of delivery of an Rh positive baby.

Blood Transfusion

BayRho-D Full Dose may be used to prevent isoimmunization in Rh negative individuals who have been transfused with Rh positive red blood cells or blood components containing red blood cells.

BayRho-D Mini-Dose — When Prescribed

A single dose of BayRho-D Mini-Dose may be prescribed for an Rh negative woman instead of BayRho-D Full Dose in the event of miscarriage or other termination of pregnancy occurring **prior** to 13 weeks' gestation. BayRho-D Mini-Dose is not required if the blood type of the father or fetus can be determined to be Rh negative.

Will You Need BayRho-D Again?

BayRho-D provides protection only if you have not already produced Rh positive antibodies. Women who have developed antibodies through previous pregnancy, miscarriage, other termination of pregnancy, or blood transfusion cannot be protected by BayRho-D. This is why with each pregnancy it is important to have BayRho-D injections within the prescribed time period.

Reactions to BayRho-D

You may feel a temporary soreness at the site of the injection. You may also have a slight and temporary change in body temperature. In very rare instances, an allergic type of reaction can occur, for which your physician will take appropriate measures.

Delivering a Sound, Healthy Baby

Your physician can answer any questions you may have about receiving a BayRho-D injection to prevent hemolytic disease of the newborn. If you know that you are Rh negative and you are pregnant, you should discuss your situation with your physician. Today, with BayRho-D, hemolytic disease of the newborn can be reduced to its lowest possible rate of incidence.

14-7631-060 (Published October 2000)

Bayer Corporation
Pharmaceutical Division
Elkhart, IN 46515 USA
U.S. License No. 8

Development of Hemolytic Disease

1
Rh positive (+) father.
Rh negative (−) mother.

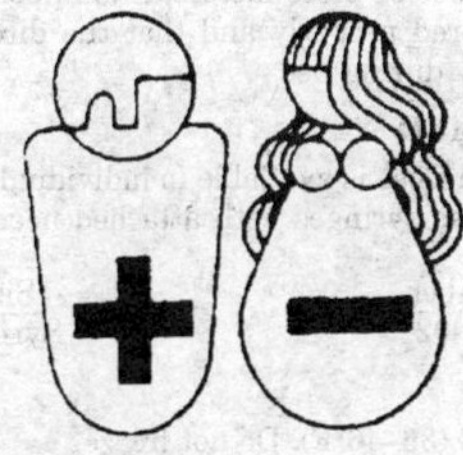

2
Pregnancy: Rh− mother is carrying Rh+ baby.

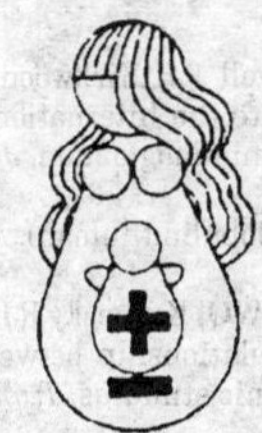

3
The passage of Rh+ blood from the baby to the mother's bloodstream happens most often at delivery, but can also occur during miscarriage, other termination of pregnancy, amniocentesis, or due to injury or trauma.

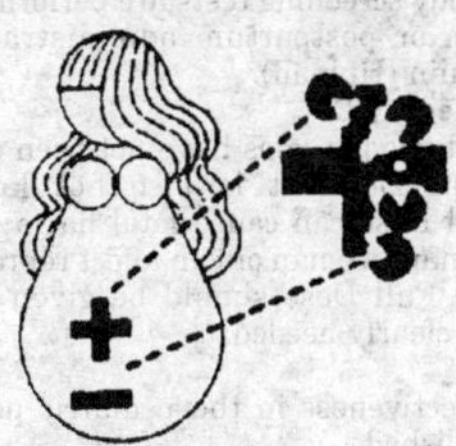

4
Rh+ antibodies stay in your bloodstream, ready to attack invading Rh+ blood cells, for many years to come.

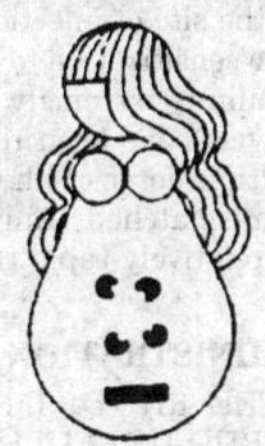

5
Next pregnancy, mother's Rh+ antibodies enter baby's Rh+ bloodstream, attacking baby's blood cells and causing hemolytic disease of the newborn.

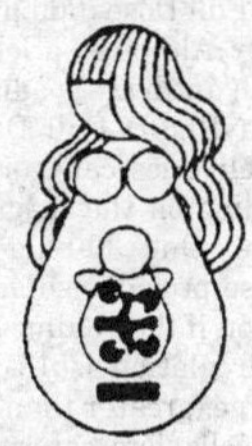

How BayRho-D Immune Globulin Can Prevent Hemolytic Disease

1
You will probably be given two injections of BayRho-D Full Dose, one at the 28th week of your pregnancy and another within 72 hours of delivery, miscarriage or other termination of pregnancy. A single injection of BayRho-D Mini-Dose may be prescribed instead of BayRho-D Full Dose in the event of miscarriage or other termination of pregnancy occurring prior to 13 weeks' gestation.

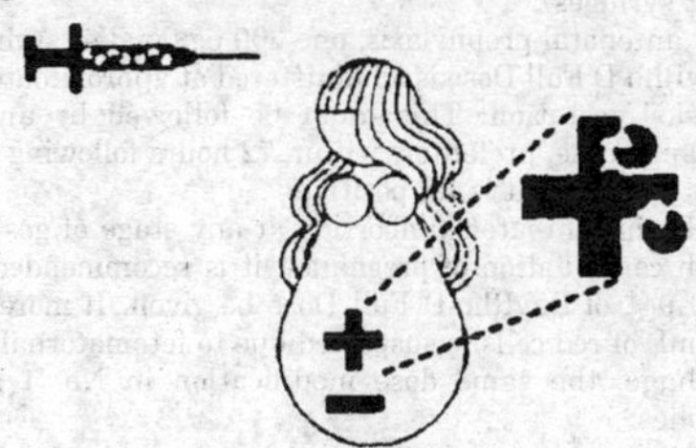

2
BayRho-D immunization prevents formation of mother's own Rh+ antibodies. Mother's bloodstream remains free of Rh+ antibodies.

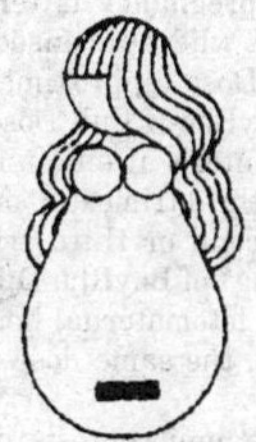

3
Next pregnancy, baby develops normally. BayRho-D should be administered following delivery, miscarriage, or other termination of pregnancy to continue protection if baby is Rh+.

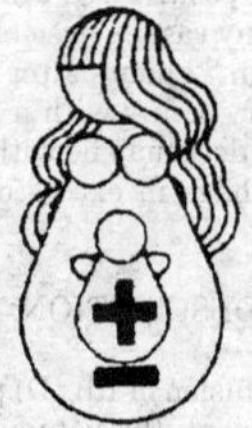

BAYRHO-D® FULL DOSE ℞

[*bāy″rhō-d*]

Rh_o(D) Immune Globulin (Human)
Solvent/Detergent Treated

DESCRIPTION

Rh_o(D) Immune Globulin (Human) — BayRho-D® Full Dose treated with solvent/detergent is a sterile solution of immune globulin containing antibodies to Rh_o(D) for intramuscular administration; it contains no preservative. BayRho-D Full Dose is prepared by cold ethanol fractionation from human plasma. The immune globulin is isolated from solubilized Cohn fraction II. The fraction II solution is adjusted to a final concentration of 0.3% tri-n-butyl phosphate (TNBP) and 0.2% sodium cholate. After the addition of solvent (TNBP) and detergent (sodium cholate), the solution is heated to 30°C and maintained at that temperature for not less than 6 hours. After the viral inactivation step, the reactants are removed by precipitation, filtration and finally ultrafiltration and diafiltration. BayRho-D Full Dose is formulated as a 15–18% protein solution at a pH of 6.4–7.2 in 0.21–0.32 M glycine. BayRho-D Full Dose is then incubated in the final container for 21–28 days at 20–27°C.

The potency is equal to or greater than that of the U.S. Food and Drug Administration Reference Rh_o(D) Immune Globulin. Each single dose vial or syringe contains sufficient anti-Rh_o(D) (approximately 300 μg*) to effectively suppress the immunizing potential of 15 mL of Rh_o(D) positive red blood cells.[2–4]

The removal and inactivation of spiked model enveloped and non-enveloped viruses during the manufacturing process for BayRho-D Full Dose has been validated in laboratory studies. Human Immunodeficiency Virus, Type 1 (HIV-1), was chosen as the relevant virus for blood products; Bovine Viral Diarrhea Virus (BVDV) was chosen to model Hepatitis C virus; Pseudorabies virus (PRV) was chosen to model Hepatitis B virus and the Herpes viruses; and Reo virus type 3 (Reo) was chosen to model non-enveloped viruses and for its resistance to physical and chemical inactivation. Significant removal of model enveloped and non-enveloped viruses is achieved at two steps in the Cohn fractionation process leading to the collection of Cohn Fraction II: the precipitation and removal of Fraction III in the processing of Fraction II + IIIW suspension to Effluent III and the filtration step in the processing of Effluent III to Filtrate III. Significant inactivation of enveloped viruses is achieved at the time of treatment of solubilized Cohn Fraction II with TNBP/sodium cholate.

*A full dose of Rh_o(D) Immune Globulin (Human) has traditionally been referred to as a "300 μg" dose and this usage is employed here for convenience in terminology. It should not be construed as the actual anti-D content. Each full dose of Rh_o(D) Immune Globulin (Human) must contain at least as much anti-D as 1 mL of the U.S. Reference Rh_o(D) Immune Globulin. Studies performed at the FDA have shown that the U.S. Reference contains 820 international units (IU) of anti-D per mL. When the conversion factor determined for the International (WHO) Reference Preparation[1] is used, 820 IU per mL is equivalent to 164 μg per mL of anti-D.

CLINICAL PHARMACOLOGY

BayRho-D Full Dose is used to prevent isoimmunization in the Rh_o(D) negative individual exposed to Rh_o(D) positive blood as a result of a fetomaternal hemorrhage occurring during a delivery of an Rh_o(D) positive infant, abortion (either spontaneous or induced), or following amniocentesis or abdominal trauma. Similarly, immunization resulting in the production of anti-Rh_o(D) following transfusion of Rh positive red cells to an Rh_o(D) negative recipient may be prevented by administering Rh_o(D) Immune Globulin (Human).[5,6]

Rh hemolytic disease of the newborn is the result of the active immunization of an Rh_o(D) negative mother by Rh_o(D) positive red cells entering the maternal circulation during a previous delivery, abortion, amniocentesis, abdominal trauma, or as a result of red cell transfusion.[7,8] BayRho-D Full Dose acts by suppressing the immune response of Rh_o(D) negative individuals to Rh_o(D) positive red blood cells. The mechanism of action of BayRho-D Full Dose is not fully understood.

The administration of Rh_o(D) Immune Globulin (Human) within 72 hours of a full-term delivery of an Rh_o(D) positive infant by an Rh_o(D) negative mother reduces the incidence of Rh isoimmunization from 12%–13% to 1%–2%.[9]

The 1%–2% treatment failures are probably due to isoimmunization occurring during the latter part of pregnancy or following delivery.[10] Bowman and Pollock[11] have reported that the incidence of isoimmunization can be further reduced from approximately 1.6% to less than 0.1% by administering Rh_o(D) Immune Globulin (Human) in two doses, one antenatal at 28 weeks' gestation and another following delivery.

In a clinical study in eight healthy human adults receiving another hyperimmune immune globulin product treated with solvent/detergent, Rabies Immune Globulin (Human), BayRab®, prepared by the same manufacturing process, detectable passive antibody titers were observed in the serum of all subjects by 24 hours post injection and persisted

Continued on next page

BayRho-D Full-Dose—Cont.

through the 21 day study period. These results suggest that passive immunization with immune globulin products is not affected by the solvent/detergent treatment.

INDICATIONS AND USAGE

Pregnancy and Other Obstetric Conditions

BayRho-D Full Dose is recommended for the prevention of Rh hemolytic disease of the newborn by its administration to the Rh_0(D) negative mother within 72 hours after birth of an Rh_0(D) positive infant,[12] providing the following criteria are met:

1. The mother must be Rh_0(D) negative and must not already be sensitized to the Rh_0(D) factor.
2. Her child must be Rh_0(D) positive, and should have a negative direct antiglobulin test (see PRECAUTIONS).

If BayRho-D Full Dose is administered antepartum, it is essential that the mother receive another dose of BayRho-D Full Dose after delivery of an Rh_0(D) positive infant.

If the father can be determined to be Rh_0(D) negative, BayRho-D Full Dose need not be given.

BayRho-D Full Dose should be administered within 72 hours to all nonimmunized Rh_0(D) negative women who have undergone spontaneous or induced abortion, following ruptured tubal pregnancy, amniocentesis or abdominal trauma unless the blood group of the fetus or the father is known to be Rh_0(D) negative.[7,8] If the fetal blood group cannot be determined, one must assume that it is Rh_0(D) positive,[2] and BayRho-D Full Dose should be administered to the mother.

Transfusion

BayRho-D Full Dose may be used to prevent isoimmunization in Rh_0(D) negative individuals who have been transfused with Rh_0(D) positive red blood cells or blood components containing red blood cells.[5,13]

CONTRAINDICATIONS

None known.

WARNINGS

BayRho-D Full Dose is made from human plasma. Products made from human plasma may contain infectious agents, such as viruses, that can cause disease. The risk that such products will transmit an infectious agent has been reduced by screening plasma donors for prior exposure to certain viruses, by testing for the presence of certain current virus infections, and by inactivating and/or removing certain viruses. Despite these measures, such products can still potentially transmit disease. There is also the possibility that unknown infectious agents may be present in such products. Individuals who receive infusions of blood or plasma products may develop signs and/or symptoms of some viral infections, particularly hepatitis C. ALL infections thought by a physician possibly to have been transmitted by this product should be reported by the physician or other healthcare provider to Bayer Corporation [1-888-765-3203].

The physician should discuss the risks and benefits of this product with the patient, before prescribing or administering it to the patient.

NEVER ADMINISTER BAYRHO-D FULL DOSE INTRAVENOUSLY. INJECT ONLY INTRAMUSCULARLY. NEVER ADMINISTER TO THE NEONATE.

Rh_0(D) Immune Globulin (Human) should be given with caution to patients with a history of prior systemic allergic reactions following the administration of human immunoglobulin preparations.

The attending physician who wishes to administer Rh_0(D) Immune Globulin (Human) to persons with isolated immunoglobulin A (IgA) deficiency must weigh the benefits of immunization against the potential risks of hypersensitivity reactions. Such persons have increased potential for developing antibodies to IgA and could have anaphylactic reactions to subsequent administration of blood products that contain IgA.

As with all preparations administered by the intramuscular route, bleeding complications may be encountered in patients with thrombocytopenia or other bleeding disorders.

PRECAUTIONS

General

A large fetomaternal hemorrhage late in pregnancy or following delivery may cause a weak mixed field positive D^u test result. If there is any doubt about the mother's Rh type, she should be given Rh_0(D) Immune Globulin (Human). A screening test to detect fetal red blood cells may be helpful in such cases.

If more than 15 mL of D-positive fetal red blood cells are present in the mother's circulation, more than a single dose of BayRho-D Full Dose is required. Failure to recognize this may result in the administration of an inadequate dose.

Although systemic reactions to human immunoglobulin preparations are rare, epinephrine should be available for treatment of acute anaphylactic reactions.

Drug Interactions

Other antibodies in the Rh_0(D) Immune Globulin (Human) preparation may interfere with the response to live vaccines such as measles, mumps, polio or rubella. Therefore, immunization with live vaccines should not be given within 3 months after Rh_0(D) Immune Globulin (Human) administration.

Drug/Laboratory Interactions

Babies born of women given Rh_0(D) Immune Globulin (Human) antepartum may have a weakly positive direct antiglobulin test at birth.

Passively acquired anti-Rh_0(D) may be detected in maternal serum if antibody screening tests are performed subsequent to antepartum or postpartum administration of Rh_0(D) Immune Globulin (Human).

Pregnancy Category C

Animal reproduction studies have not been conducted with BayRho-D Full Dose. It is also not known whether BayRho-D Full Dose can cause fetal harm when administered to a pregnant woman or can affect reproduction capacity. BayRho-D Full Dose should be given to a pregnant woman only if clearly needed.

Pediatric Use

Safety and effectiveness in the pediatric population have not been established.

ADVERSE REACTIONS

Reactions to Rh_0(D) Immune Globulin (Human) are infrequent in Rh_0(D) negative individuals and consist primarily of slight soreness at the site of injection and slight temperature elevation. While sensitization to repeated injections of human immune globulin is extremely rare, it has occurred. Elevated bilirubin levels have been reported in some individuals receiving multiple doses of Rh_0(D) Immune Globulin (Human) following mismatched transfusions. This is believed to be due to a relatively rapid rate of foreign red cell destruction.

DOSAGE AND ADMINISTRATION

NEVER ADMINISTER RH_O(D) IMMUNE GLOBULIN (HUMAN) — BAYRHO-D® FULL DOSE INTRAVENOUSLY. INJECT ONLY INTRAMUSCULARLY. NEVER ADMINISTER TO THE NEONATE.

Pregnancy and Other Obstetric Conditions

1. For postpartum prophylaxis, administer one vial or syringe of BayRho-D Full Dose (300 µg*), preferably within 72 hours of delivery. Although a lesser degree of protection is afforded if Rh antibody is administered beyond the 72-hour period, BayRho-D Full Dose may still be given.[7,14] Full-term deliveries can vary in their dosage requirements depending on the magnitude of the fetomaternal hemorrhage. One 300 µg* vial or syringe of BayRho-D Full Dose provides sufficient antibody to prevent Rh sensitization if the volume of red blood cells that has entered the circulation is 15 mL or less.[2–4] In instances where a large (greater than 30 mL of whole blood or 15 mL red blood cells) fetomaternal hemorrhage is suspected, a fetal red cell count by an approved laboratory technique (e.g., modified Kleihauer-Betke acid elution stain technique) should be performed to determine the dosage of immune globulin required.[8,15] The red blood cell volume of the calculated fetomaternal hemorrhage is divided by 15 mL to obtain the number of vials or syringes of BayRho-D Full Dose for administration.[3,8,13] If more than 15 mL of red cells is suspected or if the dose calculation results in a fraction, administer the next higher whole number of vials or syringes (e.g., if 1.4, give 2 vials or 2 syringes).
2. For antenatal prophylaxis, one 300 µg* vial or syringe of BayRho-D Full Dose is administered at approximately 28 weeks' gestation. This **must** be followed by another 300 µg* dose, preferably within 72 hours following delivery, if the infant is Rh positive.
3. Following threatened abortion at any stage of gestation with continuation of pregnancy, it is recommended that 300 µg* of BayRho-D Full Dose be given. If more than 15 mL of red cells is suspected due to fetomaternal hemorrhage, the same dose modification in No. 1 above applies.
4. Following miscarriage, abortion, or termination of ectopic pregnancy at or beyond 13 weeks' gestation, it is recommended that 300 µg* of BayRho-D Full Dose be given. If more than 15 mL of red cells is suspected due to fetomaternal hemorrhage, the same dose modification in No. 1 above applies. If pregnancy is terminated prior to 13 weeks' gestation, where licensed, a single dose of BayRho-D® Mini-Dose (approximately 50 µg*) may be used instead of BayRho-D Full Dose.
5. Following amniocentesis at either 15 to 18 weeks' gestation or during the third trimester, or following abdominal trauma in the second or third trimester, it is recommended that 300 µg* of BayRho-D Full Dose be administered. If there is a fetomaternal hemorrhage in excess of 15 mL of red cells, the same dose modification in No. 1 applies.

If abdominal trauma, amniocentesis, or other adverse event requires the administration of BayRho-D Full Dose at 13 to 18 weeks' gestation, another 300 µg* dose should be given at 26 to 28 weeks. To maintain protection throughout pregnancy, the level of passively acquired anti-Rh_0(D) should not be allowed to fall below the level required to prevent an immune response to Rh positive red cells. The half-life of IgG is 23 to 26 days. In any case, a dose of BayRho-D Full Dose should be given within 72 hours after delivery if the baby is Rh positive. If delivery occurs within 3 weeks after the last dose, the postpartum dose may be withheld unless there is a fetomaternal hemorrhage in excess of 15 mL of red blood cells.[16]

*See footnote under DESCRIPTION.

Transfusion

In the case of a transfusion of Rh_0(D) positive red cells to an Rh_0(D) negative recipient, the volume of Rh positive whole blood administered is multiplied by the hematocrit of the donor unit giving the volume of red blood cells transfused. The volume of red blood cells is divided by 15 mL which provides the number of vials or syringes of BayRho-D Full Dose to be administered.

If the dose calculated results in a fraction, the next higher whole number of vials or syringes should be administered (e.g., if 1.4, give 2 vials or 2 syringes). BayRho-D Full Dose should be administered within 72 hours after an incompatible transfusion, but preferably as soon as possible.

Injection Procedure

DO NOT INJECT INTRAVENOUSLY. DO NOT INJECT NEONATE. BayRho-D Full Dose is administered **intramuscularly**, preferably in the anterolateral aspects of the upper thigh and the deltoid muscle of the upper arm. The gluteal region should not be used routinely as an injection site because of the risk of injury to the sciatic nerve. If the gluteal region is used, the central region MUST be avoided; only the upper, outer quadrant should be used.[17]

A. Single Vial or Syringe Dose
   INJECT ENTIRE CONTENTS OF THE VIAL OR SYRINGE INTO THE INDIVIDUAL INTRAMUSCULARLY.

B. Multiple Vial or Syringe Dose
   1. Calculate the number of vials or syringes of BayRho-D Full Dose to be given (see Dosage section).
   2. The total volume of BayRho-D Full Dose can be given in divided doses at different sites at one time or the total dose may be divided and injected at intervals, provided the total dosage is given within 72 hours of the fetomaternal hemorrhage or transfusion. USING STERILE TECHNIQUE, INJECT THE ENTIRE CONTENTS OF THE CALCULATED NUMBER OF VIALS OR SYRINGES INTRAMUSCULARLY INTO THE PATIENT.

Parenteral drug products should be inspected visually for particulate matter and discoloration prior to administration, whenever solution and container permit.

BayRho-D Full Dose is supplied with a syringe and an attached UltraSafe® Needle Guard for your protection and convenience. Please follow instructions below for proper use of syringe and UltraSafe® Needle Guard.

Directions for Syringe Usage

1. Remove the prefilled syringe from the package. Lift syringe by barrel, **not** by plunger.
2. Twist the plunger rod clockwise until the threads are seated.
3. With the rubber needle shield secured on the syringe tip, push the plunger rod forward a few millimeters to break any friction seal between the rubber stopper and the glass syringe barrel.
4. Remove the needle shield and expel air bubbles.
5. Proceed with hypodermic needle puncture.
6. Aspirate prior to injection to confirm that the needle is not in a vein or artery.
7. Inject the medication.
8. Keeping your hands behind the needle, grasp the guard with free hand and slide forward toward needle until it is completely covered and guard clicks into place. If audible click is not heard, guard may not be completely activated. (See Diagrams A and B).
9. Place entire prefilled glass syringe with guard activated into an approved sharps container for proper disposal. (See Diagram C)

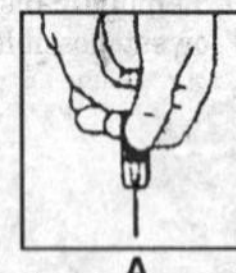
A

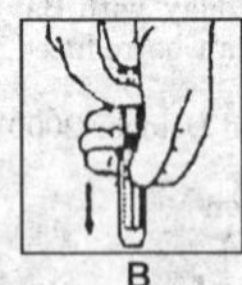
B

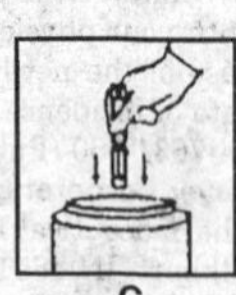
C

A number of factors beyond our control could reduce the efficacy of this product or even result in an ill effect following its use. These include improper storage and handling of the product after it leaves our hands, diagnosis, dosage, method of administration, and biological differences in individual patients. Because of these factors, it is important that this product be stored properly and that the directions be followed carefully during use.

HOW SUPPLIED

BayRho-D Full Dose is available in individual and multiple-pack single dose syringes with attached needles and vials.

NDC Number	Size
0026-0631-02	Syringe

STORAGE

Store at 2–8°C (36–46°F). Do not freeze.

CAUTION

℞ only

U.S. federal law prohibits dispensing without prescription.

REFERENCES

1. Gunson HH, Bowell PJ, Kirkwood TBL: Collaborative study to recalibrate the International Reference Preparation of Anti-D Immunoglobulin. *J Clin Pathol* 33:249–53, 1980.
2. Rh_0(D) immune globulin (human). *Med Lett Drugs Ther* 16(1):3–4, 1974.
3. Pollack W, Ascari WQ, Kochesky RJ, et al: Studies on Rh prophylaxis. I. Relationship between doses of anti-Rh and size of antigenic stimulus. *Transfusion* 11(6):333–9, 1971.

4. Unpublished data in files of Bayer Corporation.
5. Pollack W, Ascari WQ, Crispen JF, et al: Studies on Rh prophylaxis. II. Rh immune prophylaxis after transfusion with Rh-positive blood. *Transfusion* 11 (6):340–4, 1971.
6. Keith LG, Houser GH: Anti-Rh immune globulin after a massive transfusion accident. *Transfusion* 11(3):176, 1971.
7. The selective use of Rh_o(D) immune globulin (RhIG). *ACOG Tech Bull* 61, 1981.
8. Current uses of Rh_o immune globulin and detection of antibodies. *ACOG Tech Bull* 35, 1976.
9. Pollack W: Rh hemolytic disease of the newborn; its cause and prevention. *Prog Clin Biol Res* 70:185–203, 1981.
10. Bowman JM, Chown B, Lewis M, et al: Rh isoimmunization during pregnancy: antenatal prophylaxis. *Can Med Assoc J* 118(6):623–7, 1978.
11. Bowman JM, Pollock JM: Antenatal prophylaxis of Rh isoimmunization: 28-weeks'-gestation service program. *Can Med Assoc J* 118(6):627–30, 1978.
12. Ascari WQ, Allen AE, Baker WJ, et al: Rh_o(D) immune globulin (human): evaluation in women at risk of Rh immunization. *JAMA* 205(1):1–4, 1968.
13. Prevention of Rh sensitization. *WHO Tech Rep Ser* 468: 25, 1971.
14. Samson D, Mollison PL: Effect on primary Rh immunization of delayed administration of anti-Rh. *Immunology* 28:349–57, 1975.
15. Finn R, Harper DT, Stallings, SA, et al: Transplacental hemorrhage. *Transfusion* 3(2):114–24, 1963.
16. Garraty G (ed.): Hemolytic disease of the newborn. Arlington, VA, American Association of Blood Banks, 1984, p 78.
17. Recommendations of the Immunization Practices Advisory Committee (ACIP): General recommendations on immunization. *MMWR* 38(13):205–14; 219–27, 1989.

Bayer Corporation
Pharmaceutical Division
Elkhart, IN 46515 USA
U.S. License No. 8 14-7631-003
(Rev. October 2000)

The Rh Factor and Your Pregnancy

Information About Pregnancy Protection

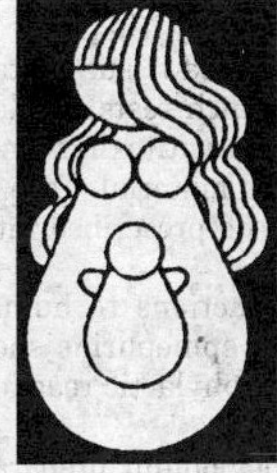

The Rh Factor and When It Is Important

The Rh factor is one of many blood group antigens found on the surface of red blood cells. If you have this antigen you are considered Rh positive. If you don't, then you are considered Rh negative. Everyone is either Rh positive or Rh negative. One type is neither better nor worse than the other, only different.

Your Rh factor is important if you are an Rh negative woman and you become pregnant, or if you receive a blood transfusion.

How the Rh Factor Can Affect Your Future

If you have Rh negative blood, there are two situations that can affect you:

1. If the father of your baby is Rh positive, the baby will probably be Rh positive too. An Rh negative woman carrying an Rh positive baby may have an immune reaction if some of the baby's Rh positive blood cells enter her bloodstream.

   This immune reaction, called isoimmunization, means your body's defense system recognizes Rh positive blood as foreign from your own and produces "antibodies" to destroy the invading Rh positive blood cells.

   The passage of blood from the baby to the mother's bloodstream happens most often at delivery, but can also occur during miscarriage, the termination of pregnancy, amniocentesis (test performed to determine fetal health), or due to an injury or trauma. It is important to note that a small number of women develop antibodies to Rh positive blood cells during pregnancy for no apparent reason.

   Antibodies to Rh positive blood may not be a problem in first pregnancies; however, the antibodies stay in your bloodstream, ready to attack invading Rh positive blood cells, for many years to come. This can lead to problems in future pregnancies by causing miscarriage or a disease known as hemolytic disease of the newborn.

   Babies born to Rh positive mothers, regardless of the father's blood type, will usually be free of the dangers of hemolytic disease.
2. Someday it may become necessary for you to receive a blood transfusion. If Rh positive antibodies already reside in your bloodstream due to isoimmunization and the blood you receive is Rh positive due to error or lifesaving reasons, your Rh positive antibodies will become mobilized and destroy the donor Rh positive cells. As a result, the transfusion could be unsuccessful and possibly harmful to you.

Hemolytic Disease of the Newborn: A Threat to Your Baby

When an Rh negative woman has Rh positive antibodies in her blood and the baby she is carrying is Rh positive, the antibodies could possibly enter the baby's bloodstream, attack the baby's red blood cells and cause hemolytic disease of the newborn. At birth, the infant suffering from hemolytic disease may be jaundiced and anemic or suffer permanent damage of the brain and central nervous system which may result in mental retardation, hearing loss, or cerebral palsy. Extensive medical care can be required, including an exchange transfusion, in which all of the baby's blood is replaced. This usually stops the destruction of the baby's red blood cells and gives the infant a chance to survive.

The risk of hemolytic disease of the newborn is slight with the first baby, but increases with each successive pregnancy.

Preventing Hemolytic Disease

BayRho-D®, Rh_o(D) Immune Globulin (Human) can prevent hemolytic disease of the newborn, provided Rh positive antibodies do not already reside in your bloodstream.

BayRho-D is a specially prepared gamma globulin with a high level of preformed antibodies against Rh positive blood cells. The injection of BayRho-D destroys any Rh positive blood cells that may have entered the mother's bloodstream and prevents the mother's immune system from producing Rh positive antibodies; thus protecting the baby from developing hemolytic disease.

BayRho-D Full Dose — When Prescribed

Pregnancy and Other Obstetric Conditions Pertaining to Rh Negative Women

BayRho-D Full Dose is administered during pregnancy if you fall into a high-risk category. For example, you are at risk of producing Rh positive antibodies if you have an amniocentesis procedure performed, or if you have a miscarriage or other termination of pregnancy at or beyond 13 weeks' gestation.

Laboratory findings have shown that some Rh negative women develop Rh positive antibodies during the last weeks of pregnancy even without an antibody-stimulating event. As a preventive measure, your physician will probably recommend the first injection of BayRho-D Full Dose at the 28th week of pregnancy.

In both of the above situations, if the blood type of the father or baby can be determined to be Rh negative, an injection of BayRho-D is not required.

Another injection of BayRho-D Full Dose is administered within 72 hours of delivery of an Rh positive baby.

Blood Transfusion

BayRho-D Full Dose may be used to prevent isoimmunization in Rh negative individuals who have been transfused with Rh positive red blood cells or blood components containing red blood cells.

BayRho-D Mini-Dose — When Prescribed

A single dose of BayRho-D Mini-Dose may be prescribed for an Rh negative woman instead of BayRho-D Full Dose in the event of miscarriage or other termination of pregnancy occurring **prior** to 13 weeks' gestation. BayRho-D Mini-Dose is not required if the blood type of the father or fetus can be determined to be Rh negative.

Will You Need BayRho-D Again?

BayRho-D provides protection only if you have not already produced Rh positive antibodies. Women who have developed antibodies through previous pregnancy, miscarriage, other termination of pregnancy, or blood transfusion cannot be protected by BayRho-D. This is why with each pregnancy it is important to have BayRho-D injections within the prescribed time period.

Reactions to BayRho-D

You may feel a temporary soreness at the site of the injection. You may also have a slight and temporary change in body temperature. In very rare instances, an allergic type of reaction can occur, for which your physician will take appropriate measures.

Delivering a Sound, Healthy Baby

Your physician can answer any questions you may have about receiving a BayRho-D injection to prevent hemolytic disease of the newborn. If you know that you are Rh negative and you are pregnant, you should discuss your situation with your physician. Today, with BayRho-D, hemolytic disease of the newborn can be reduced to its lowest possible rate of incidence.

14-7631-003 (Rev. October 2000)

Bayer Corporation
Pharmaceutical Division
Elkhart, IN 46515 USA
U.S. License No. 8

Development of Hemolytic Disease

1
Rh positive (+) father.
Rh negative (−) mother.

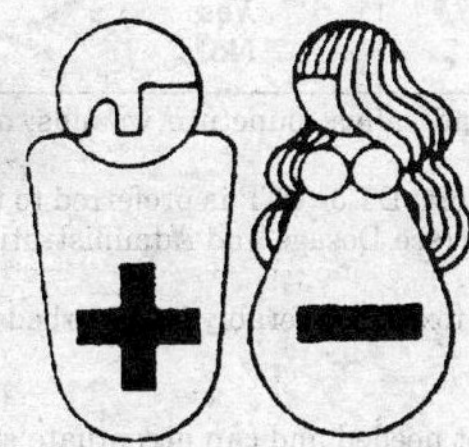

2
Pregnancy: Rh− mother is carrying Rh+ baby.

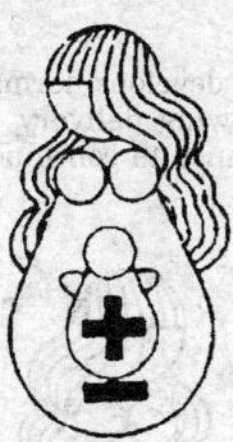

3
The passage of Rh+ blood from the baby to the mother's bloodstream happens most often at delivery, but can also occur during miscarriage, other termination of pregnancy, amniocentesis, or due to injury or trauma.

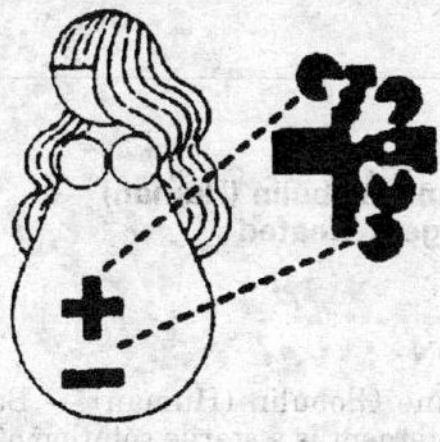

4
Rh+ antibodies stay in your bloodstream, ready to attack invading Rh+ blood cells, for many years to come.

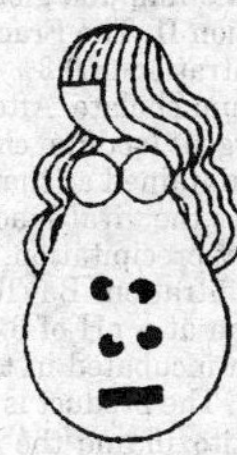

5
Next pregnancy, mother's Rh+ antibodies enter baby's Rh+ bloodstream, attacking baby's blood cells and causing hemolytic disease of the newborn.

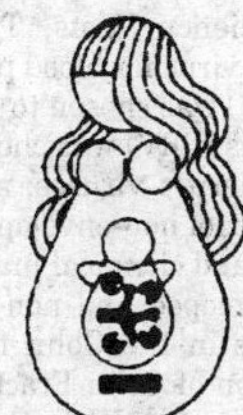

How BayRho-D Immune Globulin Can Prevent Hemolytic Disease

1
You will probably be given two injections of BayRho-D Full Dose, one at the 28th week of your pregnancy and another within 72 hours of delivery, miscarriage or other termination of pregnancy. A single injection of BayRho-D Mini-Dose may be prescribed instead of BayRho-D Full Dose in the event of miscarriage or other termination of pregnancy occurring prior to 13 weeks' gestation.

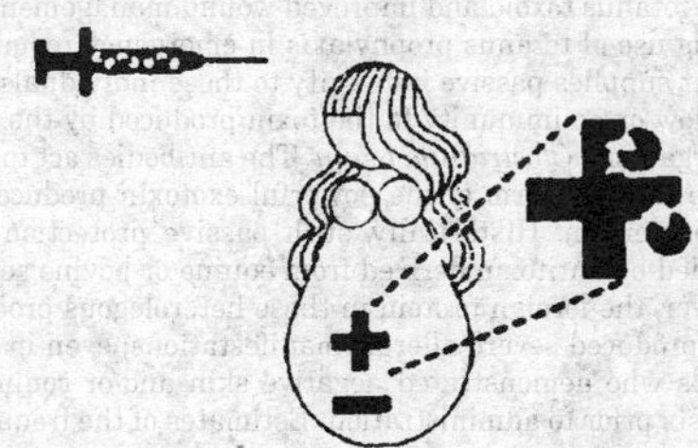

2
BayRho-D immunization prevents formation of mother's own Rh+ antibodies. Mother's bloodstream remains free of Rh+ antibodies.

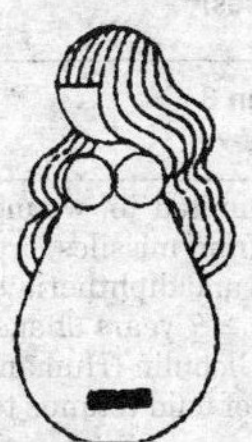

Continued on next page

BayRho-D Full-Dose—Cont.

3
Next pregnancy, baby develops normally. BayRho-D should be administered following delivery, miscarriage, or other termination of pregnancy to continue protection if baby is Rh+.

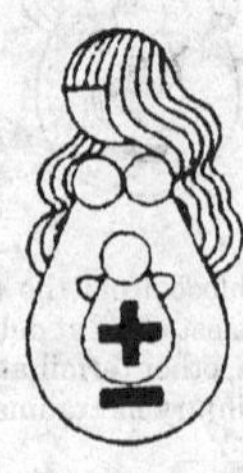

BAYTET® ℞
Tetanus Immune Globulin (Human)
Solvent/Detergent Treated
250 Units

DESCRIPTION
Tetanus Immune Globulin (Human) — BayTet® treated with solvent/detergent is a sterile solution of tetanus hyperimmune immune globulin for intramuscular administration; it contains no preservative. BayTet is prepared by cold ethanol fractionation from the plasma of donors immunized with tetanus toxoid. The immune globulin is isolated from solubilized Cohn Fraction II. The Fraction II solution is adjusted to a final concentration of 0.3% tri-n-butyl phosphate (TNBP) and 0.2% sodium cholate. After the addition of solvent (TNBP) and detergent (sodium cholate), the solution is heated to 30°C and maintained at that temperature for not less than 6 hours. After the viral inactivation step, the reactants are removed by precipitation, filtration and finally ultrafiltration and diafiltration. BayTet is formulated as a 15–18% protein solution at a pH of 6.4–7.2 in 0.21–0.32 M glycine. BayTet is then incubated in the final container for 21–28 days at 20–27°C. The product is standardized against the U.S. Standard Antitoxin and the U.S. Control Tetanus Toxin and contains not less than 250 tetanus antitoxin units per container.
The removal and inactivation of spiked model enveloped and non-enveloped viruses during the manufacturing process for BayTet has been validated in laboratory studies. Human Immunodeficiency Virus, Type 1 (HIV-1), was chosen as the relevant virus for blood products; Bovine Viral Diarrhea Virus (BVDV) was chosen to model Hepatitis C virus; Pseudorabies virus (PRV) was chosen to model Hepatitis B virus and the Herpes viruses; and Reo virus type 3 (Reo) was chosen to model non-enveloped viruses and for its resistance to physical and chemical inactivation. Significant removal of model enveloped and non-enveloped viruses is achieved at two steps in the Cohn fractionation process leading to the collection of Cohn Fraction II: the precipitation and removal of Fraction III in the processing of Fraction II + IIIW suspension to Effluent III and the filtration step in the processing of Effluent III to Filtrate III. Significant inactivation of enveloped viruses is achieved at the time of treatment of solubilized Cohn Fraction II with TNBP/sodium cholate.

CLINICAL PHARMACOLOGY
The occurrence of tetanus in the United States has decreased dramatically from 560 reported cases in 1947, when national reporting began, to a record low of 48 reported cases in 1987[1]. The decline has resulted from widespread use of tetanus toxoid and improved wound management, including use of tetanus prophylaxis in emergency rooms.[2]
BayTet supplies passive immunity to those individuals who have low or no immunity to the toxin produced by the tetanus organism, *Clostridium tetani*. The antibodies act to neutralize the free form of the powerful exotoxin produced by this bacterium. Historically, such passive protection was provided by antitoxin derived from equine or bovine serum; however, the foreign protein in these heterologous products often produced severe allergic manifestations, even in individuals who demonstrated negative skin and/or conjunctival tests prior to administration. Estimates of the frequency of these foreign protein reactions following antitoxin of equine origin varied from 5%–30%.[3–6] If passive immunization is needed, human tetanus immune globulin (TIG) is the product of choice. It provides protection longer than antitoxin of animal origin and causes few adverse reactions.[2]
Several studies suggest the value of human tetanus antitoxin in the treatment of active tetanus.[7,8] In 1961 and 1962, Nation et al,[7] using Hyper-Tet treated 20 patients with tetanus using single doses of 3,000 to 6,000 antitoxin units in combination with other accepted clinical and nursing procedures. Six patients, all over 45 years of age, died of causes other than tetanus. The authors felt that the mortality rate (30%) compared favorably with their previous experience using equine antitoxin in larger doses and that the results were much better than the 60% national death rate for tetanus reported from 1951 to 1954.[9] Blake et al,[10] however, found in a data analysis of 545 cases of tetanus reported to the Centers for Disease Control from 1965 to 1971 that survival was no better with 8,000 units of TIG than with 500 units; however, an optimal dose could not be determined.
Serologic tests indicate that naturally acquired immunity to tetanus toxin does not occur in the United States. Thus, universal primary vaccination, with subsequent maintenance of adequate antitoxin levels by means of appropriately timed boosters, is necessary to protect persons among all age groups. Tetanus toxoid is a highly effective antigen; a completed primary series generally induces protective levels of serum antitoxin that persist for ≥ 10 years.[2]
Passive immunization with BayTet may be undertaken concomitantly with active immunization using tetanus toxoid in those persons who must receive an immediate injection of tetanus antitoxin and in whom it is desirable to begin the process of active immunization. Based on the work of Rubbo,[11] McComb and Dwyer,[12] and Levine et al,[13] the physician may thus supply immediate passive protection against tetanus, and at the same time begin formation of active immunization in the injured individual which upon completion of a **full toxoid series** will preclude future need for antitoxin.
Peak blood levels of IgG are obtained approximately 2 days after intramuscular injection. The half-life of IgG in the circulation of individuals with normal IgG levels is approximately 23 days.[14]
In a clinical study in eight healthy human adults receiving another hyperimmune immune globulin product treated with solvent/detergent, Rabies Immune Globulin (Human), BayRab®, prepared by the same manufacturing process, detectable passive antibody titers were observed in the serum of all subjects by 24 hours post injection and persisted through the 21 day study period. These results suggest that passive immunization with immune globulin products is not affected by the solvent/detergent treatment.

INDICATIONS AND USAGE
BayTet is indicated for prophylaxis against tetanus following injury in patients whose immunization is incomplete or uncertain (see below). It is also indicated, although evidence of effectiveness is limited, in the regimen of treatment of active cases of tetanus.[7,8,15]
A thorough attempt must be made to determine whether a patient has completed primary vaccination. Patients with unknown or uncertain previous vaccination histories should be considered to have had no previous tetanus toxoid doses. Persons who had military service since 1941 can be considered to have received at least one dose, and although most of them may have completed a primary series of tetanus toxoid, this cannot be assumed for each individual. Patients who have not completed a primary series may require tetanus toxoid and passive immunization at the time of wound cleaning and debridement.[2]
The following table is a summary guide to tetanus prophylaxis in wound management:
[See table below]

CONTRAINDICATIONS
None known.

WARNINGS
BayTet is made from human plasma. Products made from human plasma may contain infectious agents, such as viruses, that can cause disease. The risk that such products will transmit an infectious agent has been reduced by screening plasma donors for prior exposure to certain viruses, by testing for the presence of certain current virus infections, and by inactivating and/or removing certain viruses. Despite these measures, such products can still potentially transmit disease. There is also the possibility that unknown infectious agents may be present in such products. Individuals who receive infusions of blood or plasma products may develop signs and/or symptoms of some viral infections, particularly hepatitis C. ALL infections thought by a physician possibly to have been transmitted by this product should be reported by the physician or other healthcare provider to Bayer Corporation [1-800-288-8371].
The physician should discuss the risks and benefits of this product with the patient, before prescribing or administering it to the patient.
BayTet should be given with caution to patients with a history of prior systemic allergic reactions following the administration of human immunoglobulin preparations.
In patients who have severe thrombocytopenia or any coagulation disorder that would contraindicate intramuscular injections, BayTet should be given only if the expected benefits outweigh the risks.

PRECAUTIONS
General
BayTet should not be given intravenously. Intravenous injection of immunoglobulin intended for intramuscular use can, on occasion, cause a precipitous fall in blood pressure, and a picture not unlike anaphylaxis. Injections should only be made **intramuscularly** and care should be taken to draw back on the plunger of the syringe before injection in order to be certain that the needle is not in a blood vessel. Intramuscular injections are preferably administered in the anterolateral aspects of the upper thigh and the deltoid muscle of the upper arm. The gluteal region should not be used routinely as an injection site because of the risk of injury to the sciatic nerve. If the gluteal region is used, the central region MUST be avoided; only the upper, outer quadrant should be used.[16]
Chemoprophylaxis against tetanus is neither practical nor useful in managing wounds. Wound cleaning, debridement when indicated, and proper immunization are important. The need for tetanus toxoid (active immunization), with or without TIG (passive immunization), depends on both the condition of the wound and the patient's vaccination history. Rarely has tetanus occurred among persons with documentation of having received a primary series of toxoid injections.[2] See table under INDICATIONS AND USAGE.
Skin tests should not be done. The intradermal injection of concentrated IgG solutions often causes a localized area of inflammation which can be misinterpreted as a positive allergic reaction. In actuality, this does not represent an allergy; rather, it is localized tissue irritation. Misinterpretation of the results of such tests can lead the physician to withhold needed human antitoxin from a patient who is not actually allergic to this material. True allergic responses to human IgG given in the prescribed intramuscular manner are rare.
Although systemic reactions to human immunoglobulin preparations are rare, epinephrine should be available for treatment of acute anaphylactic reactions.

Drug Interactions
Antibodies in immunoglobulin preparations may interfere with the response to live viral vaccines such as measles, mumps, polio, and rubella. Therefore, use of such vaccines should be deferred until approximately 3 months after Tetanus Immune Globulin (Human) — BayTet® administration.
No interactions with other products are known.

Pregnancy Category C
Animal reproduction studies have not been conducted with BayTet. It is also not known whether BayTet can cause fetal harm when administered to a pregnant woman or can affect reproduction capacity. BayTet should be given to a pregnant woman only if clearly needed.

Pediatric Use
Safety and effectiveness in the pediatric population have not been established.

ADVERSE REACTIONS
Slight soreness at the site of injection and slight temperature elevation may be noted at times. Sensitization to repeated injections of human immunoglobulin is extremely rare.
In the course of routine injections of large numbers of persons with immunoglobulin there have been a few isolated occurrences of angioneurotic edema, nephrotic syndrome, and anaphylactic shock after injection.

OVERDOSAGE
Although no data are available, clinical experience with other immunoglobulin preparations suggests that the only manifestations would be pain and tenderness at the injection site.

DOSAGE AND ADMINISTRATION
Routine prophylactic dosage schedule:
Adults and children 7 years and older: BayTet, 250 units should be given by deep intramuscular injection (see PRECAUTIONS). At the same time, but in a different extremity and with a separate syringe, Tetanus and Diphtheria Toxoids Adsorbed (For Adult Use) (Td) should be administered according to the manufacturer's package insert. Adults with uncertain histories of a complete primary vaccination series should receive a primary series using the combined Td toxoid. To ensure continued protection, booster doses of Td should be given every 10 years.[2]

Guide to Tetanus Prophylaxis in Wound Management[2]

History of Tetanus Immunization (Doses)	Clean, Minor Wounds		All Other Wounds*	
	Td†	TIG‡	Td	TIG
Uncertain or less than 3	Yes	No	Yes	Yes
3 or more §	No ‖	No	No¶	No

* Such as, but not limited to, wounds contaminated with dirt, feces, soil, and saliva; puncture wounds; avulsions; and wounds resulting from missiles, crushing, burns and frostbite.
† Adult type tetanus and diphtheria toxoids. If the patient is less than 7 years old, DT or DTP is preferred to tetanus toxoid alone. For persons ≥ 7 years of age, Td is preferred to tetanus toxoid alone. (see Dosage and Administration)
‡ Tetanus Immune Globulin (Human).
§ If only three doses of fluid tetanus toxoid have been received, a fourth dose of toxoid, preferably an adsorbed toxoid, should be given.
‖ Yes if more than 10 years since the last dose.
¶ Yes if more than 5 years since the last dose. (More frequent boosters are not needed and can accentuate side effects).

Children less than 7 years old: In small children the routine prophylactic dose of BayTet may be calculated by the body weight (4.0 units/kg). However, it may be advisable to administer the entire contents of the vial or syringe of BayTet (250 units) regardless of the child's size, since theoretically the same amount of toxin will be produced in the child's body by the infecting tetanus organism as it will in an adult's body. At the same time but in a different extremity and with a different syringe, Diphtheria and Tetanus Toxoids and Pertussis Vaccine Adsorbed (DTP) or Diphtheria and Tetanus Toxoids Adsorbed (For Pediatric Use) (DT), if pertussis vaccine is contraindicated, should be administered per the manufacturer's package insert.

Note: The single injection of tetanus toxoid only initiates the series for producing active immunity in the recipient. The physician must impress upon the patient the need for further toxoid injections in 1 month and 1 year. Without such, the active immunization series is incomplete. If a contraindication to using tetanus toxoid-containing preparations exists for a person who has not completed a primary series of tetanus toxoid immunization and that person has a wound that is neither clean nor minor, *only* passive immunization should be given using tetanus immune globulin.[2] See table under INDICATIONS AND USAGE.

Available evidence indicates that complete primary vaccination with tetanus toxoid provides long lasting protection ≥ 10 years for most recipients. Consequently, after complete primary tetanus vaccination, boosters–even for wound management–need be given only every 10 years when wounds are minor and uncontaminated. For other wounds, a booster is appropriate if the patient has not received tetanus toxoid within the preceding 5 years. Persons who have received at least two doses of tetanus toxoid rapidly develop antibodies.[2] The prophylactic dosage schedule for these patients and for those with incomplete or uncertain immunity is shown on the table in INDICATIONS AND USAGE.

Since tetanus is actually a local infection, proper initial wound care is of paramount importance. The use of antitoxin is adjunctive to this procedure. However, in approximately 10% of recent tetanus cases, no wound or other breach in skin or mucous membrane could be implicated.[17]

Treatment of active cases of tetanus:

Standard therapy for the treatment of active tetanus including the use of BayTet must be implemented immediately. The dosage should be adjusted according to the severity of the infection.[7,8]

Parenteral drug products should be inspected visually for particulate matter and discoloration prior to administration, whenever solution and container permit. They should not be used if particulate matter and/or discoloration are present.

BayTet is supplied with a syringe and an attached UltraSafe® Needle Guard for your protection and convenience. Please follow instructions below for proper use of syringe and UltraSafe® Needle Guard.

Directions for Syringe Usage

1. Remove the prefilled syringe from the package. Lift syringe by barrel, **not** by plunger.
2. Twist the plunger rod clockwise until the threads are seated.
3. With the rubber needle shield secured on the syringe tip, push the plunger rod forward a few millimeters to break any friction seal between the rubber stopper and the glass syringe barrel.
4. Remove the needle shield and expel air bubbles. [Do not remove the rubber needle shield to prepare the product for administration until immediately prior to the anticipated injection time.]
5. Proceed with hypodermic needle puncture.
6. Aspirate prior to injection to confirm that the needle is not in a vein or artery.
7. Inject the medication.
8. Keeping your hands behind the needle, grasp the guard with free hand and slide forward toward needle until it is completely covered and guard clicks into place. If audible click is not heard, guard may not be completely activated. (See Diagrams A and B)
9. Place entire prefilled glass syringe with guard activated into an approved sharps container for proper disposal. (See Diagram C)

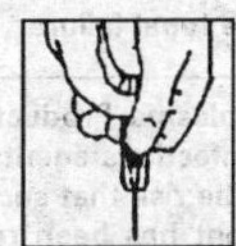
A

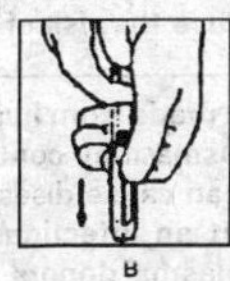
B

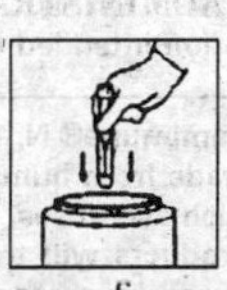
C

A number of factors beyond our control could reduce the efficacy of this product or even result in an ill effect following its use. These include improper storage and handling of the product after it leaves our hands, diagnosis, dosage, method of administration, and biological differences in individual patients. Because of these factors it is important that this product be stored properly and that the directions be followed carefully during use.

HOW SUPPLIED

BayTet is supplied in 250 unit prefilled disposable syringes with attached needles.

NDC Number	Size
0026-0634-02	250 unit syringe

STORAGE

Store at 2–8°C (36–46°F). Solution that has been frozen should not be used.

CAUTION

℞ only

U.S. federal law prohibits dispensing without prescription.

REFERENCES

1. Tetanus — United States, 1987 and 1988, *MMWR* 39(3): 37–41, 1990.
2. Diphtheria, Tetanus, and Pertussis: Recommendations for Vaccine Use and Other Preventive Measures. Recommendations of the Immunization Practices Advisory Committee (ACIP). *MMWR* 40 (RR-10): 1–28, 1991.
3. Moynihan NH: Tetanus prophylaxis and serum sensitivity tests. *Br Med J* 1:260–4, 1956.
4. Scheibel I: The uses and results of active tetanus immunization. *Bull WHO* 13:381–94, 1955.
5. Edsall G: Specific prophylaxis of tetanus. *JAMA* 171(4): 417–27, 1959.
6. Bardenwerper HW: Serum neuritis from tetanus antitoxin. *JAMA* 179(10):763–6, 1962.
7. Nation NS, Pierce NF, Adler SJ, et al: Tetanus: the use of human hyperimmune globulin in treatment. *Calif Med* 98(6):305–6, 1963.
8. Ellis M: Human antitetanus serum in the treatment of tetanus. *Br Med J* 1(5338):1123–6, 1963.
9. Axnick NW, Alexander ER: Tetanus in the United States: A review of the problem. *Am J Public Health* 47(12):1493–1501, 1957.
10. Blake PA, Feldman RA, Buchanan TM, et al: Serologic therapy of tetanus in the United States, 1965–1971. *JAMA* 235(1):42–4, 1976.
11. Rubbo SD: New approaches to tetanus prophylaxis. *Lancet* 2(7461):449–53, 1966.
12. McComb JA, Dwyer RC: Passive-active immunization with tetanus immune globulin (human). *N Engl J Med* 268(16):857–62, 1963.
13. Levine L, McComb JA, Dwyer RC, et al: Active-passive tetanus immunization; choice of toxoid, dose of tetanus immune globulin and timing of injections. *N Engl J Med* 274(4):186–90, 1966.
14. Waldmann TA, Strober W, Blaese RM: Variations in the metabolism of immunoglobulins measured by turnover rates. In Merler E (ed.): Immunoglobulins: biologic aspects and clinical uses. Washington, DC, Nat Acad Sci, 1970, p. 33–51.
15. McCracken GH Jr., Dowell DL, Marshall FN: Double-blind trial of equine antitoxin and human immune globulin in tetanus neonatorum. *Lancet* 1(7710):1146–9, 1971.
16. Recommendations of the Immunization Practices Advisory Committee (ACIP): General recommendations on immunization. *MMWR* 38(13): 205–14; 219–27, 1989.
17. Tetanus-Rates by year, United States, 1955–1984. Annual Summary 1984. *MMWR* 33 (54):61, 1986.

Bayer
Bayer Corporation
Pharmaceutical Division
Elkhart, IN 46515 USA
U.S. License No. 8

08895786
Printed in USA (Rev. March 2004)

GAMIMUNE® N, 10% ℞

Immune Globulin Intravenous (Human), 10%
Solvent/Detergent Treated

DESCRIPTION

Immune Globulin Intravenous (Human), 10% — Gamimune® N, 10% treated with solvent/detergent is a sterile solution of human protein containing no preservative. Gamimune N, 10% consists of 9%–11% protein in 0.16–0.24 M glycine. Not less than 98% of the protein has the electrophoretic mobility of gamma globulin. Not less than 90% of the IgG is monomer. Also present are traces of IgA and of IgM. The distribution of IgG subclasses is similar to that found in normal serum. The measured buffer capacity is 35 mEq/L and the osmolality is 274 mOsmol/kg solvent.

The product is made by cold ethanol fractionation of large pools of human plasma. Part of the fractionation may be performed by another licensed manufacturer. The immunoglobulin is isolated from Cohn Effluent III after limited diafiltration and ultrafiltration. The solution is adjusted to 0.3% tri-n-butyl phosphate (TNBP) and 0.2% sodium cholate. After addition of the solvent (TNBP) and the detergent (sodium cholate), the solution is heated to 30°C and maintained at that temperature for not less than 6 hours. After the viral inactivation step, the reactants are removed by precipitation, filtration, and finally diafiltration and ultrafiltration. The protein is stabilized during the process by adjusting the pH of the solution to 4.0-4.5.[1] Isotonicity is achieved by the addition of glycine. Gamimune N, 10% treated with solvent/detergent is then incubated in the final container (at the low pH of 4.25), for a minimum of 21 days at 20°C. The product is intended for intravenous administration.

The removal and inactivation of spiked model enveloped and non-enveloped viruses during the manufacturing process for Gamimune N, 10% has been validated in laboratory studies. Human Immunodeficiency Virus, Type 1 (HIV-1) was chosen as the relevant virus for blood products; Bovine Viral Diarrhea Virus (BVDV) was chosen to model for Hepatitis C virus; Pseudorabies virus (PRV) was chosen to model for Hepatitis B and the Herpes viruses; and Reo virus type 3 (Reo) was chosen to model non-enveloped viruses and for its resistance to physical and chemical inactivation. Significant removal of model enveloped and non-enveloped viruses is seen between the Fraction II + IIIW and Effluent III steps and between the Effluent III and Filtrate III steps. Significant inactivation of enveloped viruses is achieved at the time of treatment of Filtrate III with TNBP/sodium cholate and also at the time of low pH incubation in the final container.

CLINICAL PHARMACOLOGY

Primary Humoral Immunodeficiency

Gamimune N, 10% supplies a broad spectrum of opsonic and neutralizing IgG antibodies for the prevention or attenuation of a wide variety of infectious diseases. Since Gamimune N, 10% is administered intravenously, essentially 100% of the infused IgG antibodies are immediately available in the recipient's circulation.[2] Studies using a modified intravenous immunoglobulin at pH 6.8 have shown that approximately 30% of the infused IgG disappeared from the circulation in the first 24 hours, due primarily to equilibration of the IgG between the plasma and the extravascular space.[2–5] A further decline to about 40% of the peak level found immediately post-infusion is to be expected during the first week.[2–5] The in vivo half-life of Immune Globulin Intravenous (Human), 5%—Gamimune® N, 5% equals or exceeds the 3-week half-life reported for IgG in the literature, but individual patient variation in half-life has been observed.[2] Thus, this variable as well as the amount of immune globulin administered per dose is important in determining the frequency of administration of the drug for each individual patient. A comparative study of Gamimune N, 10% with Gamimune N, 5% (in 10% maltose) in 18 subjects demonstrated equivalent post-infusion recovery for the two preparations. A comparative study of Gamimune N, 10% treated with solvent/detergent and Gamimune N, 10% in 17 subjects demonstrated bioequivalence.

Idiopathic Thrombocytopenic Purpura

While Gamimune N, 10% has been shown to be effective in some cases of idiopathic thrombocytopenic purpura (ITP) (see INDICATIONS AND USAGE), the mechanism of action has not been fully elucidated.

Bone Marrow Transplantation

Clinical studies with Gamimune N, 5% have shown that it is effective in bone marrow transplant patients ≥ 20 years of age in the first 100 days posttransplant for the following: prevention of systemic and local infections, interstitial pneumonia of infectious and idiopathic etiologies and acute graft-versus-host disease (AGVHD)[6] (see INDICATIONS AND USAGE). Administration of Gamimune N, 5% to bone marrow transplant patients significantly increased IgG and IgG subclass levels while those seen in the control group fell below predicted levels. The mechanism of action of Gamimune N, 5% in reducing the incidence of AGVHD is presently unknown.

Pediatric HIV Infection

Children infected with human immunodeficiency virus (HIV) may display defects in both cellular and humoral immunity.[7–10] As a result, some children with HIV-1 infection experience serious, potentially life-threatening recurrent bacterial infections.[11–13] In one retrospective report, among 71 HIV-infected children observed over 3.5 years, 27 (37%) experienced serious documented bacterial infections.[12] The types of bacterial and viral infections observed in HIV-infected children are similar to those seen in children with primary hypogammaglobulinemia.[14] The replacement of opsonic and neutralizing IgG antibodies has been shown to reduce serious and minor bacterial infection in HIV-infected children.[15,16]

In a randomized, double-blind, placebo-controlled, multicenter study performed between March 7, 1988 and January 15, 1991, the efficacy of Gamimune N, 5% in pediatric HIV disease to decrease the frequency of serious and minor bacterial infections and the frequency of hospitalization, and to increase the time free of serious bacterial infection was documented in children with clinical or immunologic evidence of HIV disease (see INDICATIONS AND USAGE). The primary endpoint of this study was prospectively defined as a significant reduction in the proportion of subjects who develop at least one serious bacterial infection when compared to the control group of HIV-infected children who received placebo. Serious bacterial infections were defined as laboratory-proven and clinically diagnosed (i.e., radiologically proven acute pneumonia and sinusitis) infections. The Data Safety and Monitoring Board (DSMB) recommended early termination of the study based on data presented to them from an interim analysis in December 1990 which showed that treatment with Gamimune N, 5% increased the time free from serious infections in children with CD4 + counts ≥ 200/mm³.

General

Glycine (aminoacetic acid) is a nonessential amino acid normally present in the body.[17] Glycine is a major ingredient in

Continued on next page

Gamimune N, 10%—Cont.

amino acid solutions employed in intravenous alimentation.[18] While toxic effects of glycine administration have been reported,[19] the doses and rates of administration were 3 – 4-fold greater than those for Gamimune N, 10%.

The buffer capacity of Gamimune N, 10% is 35.0 mEq/L (~0.35 mEq/g protein). A dose of 1000 mg/kg body weight therefore represents an acid load of 0.35 mEq/kg body weight. The total buffering capacity of whole blood in a normal individual is 45–50 mEq/L of blood, or 3.6 mEq/kg body weight.[20] Thus, the acid load delivered with a dose of 1000 mg/kg of Gamimune N, 10% would be neutralized by the buffering capacity of whole blood alone, even if the dose was infused instantaneously.

In Phase I human studies comparing Gamimune N, 10% with Gamimune N, 5% (in 10% maltose), venous blood measurements were taken following the intravenous administration of 400 mg/kg body weight in 18 patients. There were no clinically important changes in mean venous pH, bicarbonate, or base excess measurements in these patients receiving either preparation.[2]

In a similar, earlier Phase I study Gamimune N, 5% (in 10% maltose) was compared with a chemically modified 5% intravenous immunoglobulin preparation with a pH of 6.8. No clinically important changes in mean venous pH and bicarbonate measurements were detected following infusions of either preparation at doses of 400 mg/kg body weight in 37 patients.

In patients with limited or compromised acid-base compensatory mechanisms, consideration should be given to the effect of the additional acid load Gamimune N, 10% might present.

INDICATIONS AND USAGE

Primary Humoral Immunodeficiency

Gamimune N, 10% is efficacious in the treatment of primary immunodeficiency states in which severe impairment of antibody forming capacity has been shown, such as: congenital agammaglobulinemias, common variable immunodeficiency, Wiskott-Aldrich syndrome, x-linked immunodeficiency with hyper IgM, and severe combined immunodeficiencies.[5,21–23] Gamimune N, 10% is especially useful when high levels or rapid elevation of circulating antibodies are desired or when intramuscular injections are contraindicated.

Idiopathic Thrombocytopenic Purpura (ITP)

In clinical situations in which a rapid rise in platelet count is needed to control bleeding or to allow a patient with ITP to undergo surgery, administration of Gamimune N, 10% should be considered. Studies with Gamimune N, 5% demonstrate that in patients in whom a response was achieved, the rise of platelets was generally rapid (within 1–5 days), transient (most often lasting from several days to several weeks) and were not considered curative. It is presently not possible to predict which patients with ITP will respond to therapy, although the increase in platelet counts in children seems to be better than that in adults. Childhood ITP may, however, respond spontaneously without treatment.

Gamimune N, 10% has been studied in 31 adult and pediatric subjects with ITP using a dosage of 1,000 mg/kg body weight on either 1 day or 2 consecutive days. Fourteen of 16 children (87.5%) and 9 of 10 adults with platelet follow-up (90%) responded to treatment with clinically significant platelet increments of ≥ 30,000/mm^3. In the 12 children with acute ITP, there was an average increase in platelet count above baseline of 274,000/mm^3 (range 33,000–529,000/mm^3).

Two different dosing regimens of Gamimune N, 5% have been studied in clinical investigations: a regimen consisting of 400 mg/kg body weight daily for 5 consecutive days, and a high dose treatment regimen consisting of 1,000 mg/kg body weight administered on either 1 day or 2 consecutive days (these studies are summarized below).

In clinical studies of Gamimune N, 5%, five of six (83.3%) children and 12 of 16 (75%) adults with acute or chronic ITP treated with 400 mg/kg body weight for 5 consecutive days demonstrated clinically significant platelet increments of ≥ 30,000/mm^3 over baseline. The mean platelet count in children with ITP rose from 27,800/mm^3 at baseline to 297,000/mm^3 (range 50,000–455,000/mm^3) and the mean platelet count in adults with ITP rose from 27,900/mm^3 at baseline to 124,900/mm^3 (range 11,000–341,000/mm^3). Two of three children with acute ITP rapidly went into complete remission.

Thirteen of 14 children (92.9%) and 26 of 29 adults (89.7%) with acute or chronic ITP treated with Gamimune N, 5% 1,000 mg/kg body weight administered on either 1 day or 2 consecutive days responded to treatment with clinically significant platelet increments of ≥ 30,000/mm^3 over baseline. This included three of three patients with ITP that were human immunodeficiency virus (HIV) antibody positive and two of two patients with ITP that were pregnant. The mean platelet count in children with ITP treated with Gamimune N, 5% 1,000 mg/kg body weight on 1 day or 2 consecutive days rose from 44,400/mm^3 at baseline to 285,600/mm^3 (range 89,000–473,000/mm^3) and the mean platelet count in adults with ITP treated with the regimen rose from 23,400/mm^3 at baseline to 173,100/mm^3 (range 28,000–709,000/mm^3). Two patients, one each with acute adult and chronic childhood ITP, entered complete remission with treatment. Six of the 29 adult patients with ITP received Gamimune N, 5% 1,000 mg/kg on 1 day or 2 consecutive days to increase the platelet count prior to splenectomy. Mean platelet counts rose from 14,500/mm^3 at baseline to 129,300/mm^3 (range 51,000–242,000/mm^3) prior to surgery.

The duration of the platelet rise following treatment of ITP with either treatment regimen of Gamimune N, 5% was variable, ranging from several days to 12 months or more. Some ITP patients have demonstrated continuing responsiveness over many months to intermittent infusions of Gamimune N, 5% 400–1,000 mg/kg body weight, administered as a single maintenance dose, at intervals as indicated by the platelet count.

Bone Marrow Transplantation (BMT)

In clinical studies in bone marrow transplant patients ≥ 20 years of age, Gamimune N, 5% decreased the risk of septicemia and other infections, interstitial pneumonia of infectious or idiopathic etiologies and acute graft-versus-host disease (AGVHD) in the first 100 days posttransplant. Gamimune N, 5% is not indicated in bone marrow transplant patients below 20 years of age. In a controlled study of 369 evaluable BMT patients (184 treated and 185 controls) who either did or did not receive Gamimune N, 5% in doses of 500 mg/kg body weight on days –7 and –2 pretransplant, then weekly through day 90 posttransplant, posttransplant complications were evaluated in the entire study group and in patients under age 20 and age 20 or older. For patients ≥ 20 years of age (128 patients in the control group and 119 patients in the treated group), there was a statistically significant reduction in interstitial pneumonia from 21% in the control group to 9% in the treated group (p=0.0032) during the first 100 days posttransplant. Also significantly reduced in this age group were: overall septicemia from 53 infections in the 128 patient control group to 26 infections in the 119 patient treated group (relative risk control:treated [RR] 2.36, p=0.0025); gram-negative septicemia from 24 infections in the 128 patient control group to 9 infections in the 119 patient treated group (RR 2.53, p=0.015); gram-positive septicemia from 16 infections in the 128 patient control group to 8 infections in the 119 patient treated group (RR 2.73, p=0.046); and Grade II to IV AGVHD from an incidence of 58 of 110 in the control group to 38 of 108 in the treated group (p=0.0051).

The given p-values do not take into account multiple endpoints and subset analyses. Therefore, some of the p-values could occur by chance alone. There was no significant improvement in overall mortality in this study.

In patients below age 20, there appeared to be no benefit from treatment with Gamimune N, 5%, either in reducing the incidence of infections or the incidence of AGVHD.

Pediatric HIV Infection

Gamimune N, 5% 400 mg/kg every 28 days significantly decreased the frequency of serious and minor bacterial infections (laboratory-proven and clinically diagnosed) and the frequency of hospitalization, and increased the time free of serious bacterial infection. The effect of Gamimune N, 5% in preventing serious bacterial infections was especially apparent in preventing primary bacteremia (including *Streptococcus pneumoniae* bacteremia) and acute pneumonia.

In a randomized, double-blind, placebo-controlled, multicenter study, 394 HIV-infected, non-hemophilic, children less than 13 years of age were randomized. Of the children randomized, 369 were included in the efficacy analysis and 376 in the safety analysis. The study population had 1) a mean age of 40 months (range 2.4–136.8 months), 2) acquired HIV primarily through vertical transmission (91%), 3) a majority (87%) of CDC Class P-2 (symptomatic), and 4) had a median CD4 + count of 937 cells/mm^3 (range 0–6660 cells/mm^3). At the time of study entry, 14% (52 of 369) were receiving *Pneumocystis carinii* pneumonia (PCP) prophylaxis. During the course of the study, 51% (189 of 369) received PCP prophylaxis and 44% (164 of 369) received zidovudine (ZDV). Children with HIV-1 infection were initially stratified into two groups based upon CD4 + count (< 200 cells/mm^3 versus ≥ 200 cells/mm^3) and CDC classification of pediatric HIV disease (history of opportunistic infections [P-2-D-1] and recurrent serious bacterial infections [P-2-D-2] versus others). Subjects received Gamimune N, 5% (400 mg/kg = 8 mL/kg) (n=185) or an equivalent volume of placebo (0.1% Albumin [Human]) (n=184) every 28 days. The mean follow-up for subjects receiving Gamimune N, 5% was 17.9 months and 17.8 months for patients on placebo.

The number of subjects who had at least one serious bacterial infection was 86 of 184 (47%) in the placebo group and 55 of 185 (30%) in the Gamimune N, 5% group (p=0.0009). All p-values reported are two-sided. Treatment with Gamimune N, 5% compared to placebo was also associated with a significant reduction in both the number of subjects with at least one laboratory-proven infection (36 of 184 vs. 18 of 185, p=0.0081), and the number of subjects with at least one clinically diagnosed infection (71 of 184 vs. 45 of 185, p=0.0036). Efficacy in patients with CD4+ counts < 200/mm^3 was not established, possibly because of the small number of subjects in this category.

The 2-year treatment period defined in the protocol was truncated for some patients by the DSMB based on data from the interim analysis. Rates of serious bacterial infections per 100 patient-years were computed and analyzed to take into account both the unequal duration of treatment and follow-up, as well as recurrent infections in individual subjects. Children treated with Gamimune N, 5% experienced a 50.5% lower frequency of laboratory-proven serious bacterial infection compared to the group treated with placebo (9.1 vs. 18.2 infections per 100 patient-years, p=0.031), a 36.0% lower frequency of clinically diagnosed serious infections (24.0 vs. 37.5 infections per 100 patient-years, p=0.013), a 40.6% reduction in total serious infections (laboratory-proven and clinically diagnosed) (33.1 vs. 55.7 infections per 100 patient-years, p=0.003), a 60% lower frequency of primary bacteremias (5.8 vs. 14.5 infections per 100 patient-years, p=0.009), a 75.6% lower frequency of *Streptococcus pneumoniae* bacteremia (1.1 vs. 4.5 bacteremias per 100 patient-years, p=0.026), a 54.3% lower frequency of clinically diagnosed pneumonia (12.7 vs. 27.8 infections per 100 patient-years, p=0.001), and a 22.5% lower frequency of minor bacterial infections (including otitis media, skin and soft tissue infections, and upper respiratory tract infections) (123.6 vs. 159.5 infections per 100 patient-years, p=0.033).

In addition to a reduced frequency of infection, children treated with Gamimune N, 5% had a 36.8% lower number of hospitalizations per 100 patient-years (72 vs. 114 per 100 patient-years, p=0.002) and a reduced number of hospital days (6.9 vs. 10.5 per patient-year, p=0.030) than patients treated with placebo. Patients treated with Gamimune N, 5% had a higher probability of remaining free of laboratory-proven infections (p=0.0093) and combined laboratory-proven and clinically diagnosed infections (p=0.0015) for 24 months than the group of children treated with placebo. At 24 months, the estimated probabilities of remaining infection-free for the Gamimune N, 5% and placebo arms were 87.8% vs. 76.1%, respectively, for laboratory-proven infections and 63.5% vs. 44.5%, respectively, for combined laboratory-proven and clinically diagnosed infections.

There was no effect of Gamimune N, 5% therapy on mortality, which was low in both treatment groups (17%), or on the frequency of opportunistic or viral infections during the period of study.

Since antibacterial prophylaxis could also account for the observed reduction in the rate of serious bacterial infections, further analysis was performed to evaluate the role of *Pneumocystis carinii* pneumonia (PCP) prophylaxis on the efficacy of Gamimune N, 5%. PCP prophylaxis consisted primarily (96%) of trimethoprim/sulfamethoxazole given 3 successive days each week. This antibiotic combination could be active against the bacteria commonly encountered in this patient population. In the subgroup of patients receiving PCP prophylaxis at study entry, treatment with Gamimune N, 5% was associated with 44.0 infections per 100 patient-years, whereas placebo recipients had 64.7 infections per 100 patient-years (p=0.047). In the subgroup of patients not receiving PCP prophylaxis at study entry, treatment with Gamimune N, 5% was associated with 22.1 infections per 100 patient-years, whereas placebo recipients had 44.9 infections per 100 patient-years on placebo (p=0.024). Thus, Gamimune N, 5% benefitted patients by reducing the rate of serious bacterial infections whether or not they were receiving PCP prophylactic treatment at study entry. However, it should be noted that the use of PCP prophylactic treatment in this study was not randomized and specific guidelines for its administration were not identified.

CONTRAINDICATIONS

Gamimune N, 10% is contraindicated in individuals who are known to have had an anaphylactic or severe systemic response to Immune Globulin (Human). Individuals with selective IgA deficiencies who have known antibody against IgA (anti-IgA antibody) should not receive Gamimune N, 10% since these patients may experience severe reactions to the IgA which may be present.[22]

WARNINGS

Immune Globulin Intravenous (Human) products have been reported to be associated with renal dysfunction, acute renal failure, osmotic nephrosis and death.[24] Patients predisposed to acute renal failure include patients with any degree of pre-existing renal insufficiency, diabetes mellitus, age greater than 65, volume depletion, sepsis, paraproteinemia, or patients receiving known nephrotoxic drugs. Especially in such patients, IGIV products should be administered at the minimum concentration available and the minimum rate of infusion practicable. While these reports of renal dysfunction and acute renal failure have been associated with the use of many of the licensed IGIV products, those containing sucrose as a stabilizer accounted for a disproportionate share of the total number. See PRECAUTIONS and DOSAGE AND ADMINISTRATION sections for important information intended to reduce the risk of acute renal failure.

Gamimune® N, 10% is made from human plasma. Products made from human plasma may contain infectious agents, such as viruses, that can cause disease. The risk that such products will transmit an infectious agent has been reduced by screening plasma donors for prior exposure to certain viruses, by testing for the presence of certain current virus infections, and by inactivating and/or removing certain viruses. Despite these measures, such products can still potentially transmit disease. There is also the possibility that unknown infectious agents may be present in such products. Individuals who receive infusions of blood or plasma products may develop signs and/or symptoms of some viral infections, particularly hepatitis C. ALL infections thought by a physician possibly to have been transmitted by this product should be reported by the physician or other healthcare provider to Bayer Corporation [1-800-288-8371].

The physician should discuss the risks and benefits of this product with the patient, before prescribing or administering it to the patient.

Immune Globulin Intravenous (Human), 10% — Gamimune® N, 10% should be administered only intravenously as the intramuscular and subcutaneous routes have not been evaluated.

Immune Globulin Intravenous (Human), 5% — Gamimune® N, 5% has, on rare occasions, caused a precipitous fall in blood pressure and a clinical picture of anaphylaxis, even when the patient is not known to be sensitive to immune globulin preparations. These reactions may be related to the rate of infusion. Accordingly, the infusion rate given under DOSAGE AND ADMINISTRATION for Gamimune N, 10% should be closely followed, at least until the physician has had sufficient experience with a given patient. The patient's vital signs should be monitored continuously and careful observation made for any symptoms throughout the entire infusion. Epinephrine should be available for the treatment of an acute anaphylactic reaction.

PRECAUTIONS

General

Any vial that has been entered should be used promptly. Partially used vials should be discarded. Do not use if turbid. Solution which has been frozen should not be used.

An aseptic meningitis syndrome (AMS) has been reported to occur infrequently in association with Immune Globulin Intravenous (Human) treatment. The syndrome usually begins within several hours to two days following Immune Globulin Intravenous (Human) treatment. It is characterized by symptoms and signs including severe headache, nuchal rigidity, drowsiness, fever, photophobia, painful eye movements, and nausea and vomiting. Cerebrospinal fluid (CSF) studies are frequently positive with pleocytosis up to several thousand cells per mm^3, predominantly from the granulocytic series, and elevated protein levels up to several hundred mg/dL. Patients exhibiting such symptoms and signs should receive a thorough neurological examination, including CSF studies, to rule out other causes of meningitis. AMS may occur more frequently in association with high dose (2 g/kg) Immune Globulin Intravenous (Human) treatment. Discontinuation of Immune Globulin Intravenous (Human) treatment has resulted in remission of AMS within several days without sequelae.[25-28]

Assure that patients are not volume depleted prior to the initiation of the infusion of IGIV.

Periodic monitoring of renal function tests and urine output is particularly important in patients judged to have a potential increased risk for developing acute renal failure. Renal function, including measurement of blood urea nitrogen (BUN)/serum creatinine, should be assessed prior to the initial infusion of Gamimune N, 10% and again at appropriate intervals thereafter. If renal function deteriorates, discontinuation of the product should be considered. For patients judged to be at risk for developing renal dysfunction, it may be prudent to reduce the amount of product infused per unit time by infusing Gamimune N, 10% at a rate less than 8 mg IG/kg/min (0.08 mL/kg/min).

Information For Patients

Patients should be instructed to immediately report symptoms of decreased urine output, sudden weight gain, fluid retention/edema, and/or shortness of breath (which may suggest kidney damage) to their physicians.

Drug Interactions

Antibodies in Gamimune N, 10% may interfere with the response to live viral vaccines such as measles, mumps and rubella. Therefore, use of such vaccines should be deferred until approximately 6 months after Gamimune N, 10% administration.

Please see DOSAGE AND ADMINISTRATION for other drug interactions.

Pregnancy Category C

Animal reproduction studies have not been conducted with Gamimune N, 10%. It is not known whether Gamimune N, 10% can cause fetal harm when administered to a pregnant woman or can affect reproduction capacity. Gamimune N, 10% should be given to a pregnant woman only if clearly needed.

ADVERSE REACTIONS

General

Increases in creatinine and blood urea nitrogen (BUN) have been observed as soon as one to two days following infusion. Progression to oliguria and anuria requiring dialysis has been observed, although some patients have improved spontaneously following cessation of treatment.[32] Types of severe renal adverse reactions that have been seen following IGIV therapy include: acute renal failure, acute tubular necrosis,[33] proximal tubular nephropathy, and osmotic nephrosis.[24, see also 34–36]

In the studies undertaken to date, other types of reactions have not been reported with Gamimune N, 5% or Gamimune N, 10%. It may be, however, that adverse effects will be similar to those previously reported with intravenous and intramuscular immunoglobulin administration. Potential reactions, therefore, may also include anxiety, flushing, wheezing, abdominal cramps, myalgias, arthralgia, and dizziness; rash has been reported only rarely. Very rarely have there been cases reported of severe injection site reactions. Reactions to intravenous immunoglobulin tend to be related to the rate of infusion.

True anaphylactic reactions to Gamimune N, 10% may occur in recipients with documented prior histories of severe allergic reactions to intramuscular immunoglobulin, but some patients may tolerate cautiously administered intravenous immunoglobulin without adverse effects.[32] Very rarely an anaphylactoid reaction may occur in patients with no prior history of severe allergic reactions to either intramuscular or intravenous immunoglobulin.[2]

Primary Humoral Immunodeficiency

A safety study has been conducted in 20 adult and pediatric subjects with primary immunodeficiency syndrome comparing side effects of Gamimune N, 5% with those of Gamimune N, 10%. The incidence, nature, or severity of reactions with Gamimune N, 10% were not different from those observed with Gamimune N, 5%, and were consistent with those observed in previous studies with Gamimune N, 5%. Symptoms related to the infusion of Gamimune N, 10% were observed in 9 (3.5%) of 255 infusions. These symptoms were all mild to moderate in severity and included chills, fever, headache and emesis.

In a study of 37 patients with immunodeficiency syndromes receiving Gamimune N, 5% in a monthly dose of 400 mg/kg body weight, reactions were seen in 5.2% of the infusions. Symptoms reported included malaise, a feeling of faintness, fever, chills, headache, nausea, vomiting, chest tightness, dyspnea and chest, back or hip pain. Mild erythema following infiltration of Gamimune N, 5% at the infusion site was reported in some cases.

A safety study has been conducted in 17 adult and adolescent subjects with primary immunodeficiency syndrome, comparing side effects and bioequivalency of Gamimune N, 10% with those of Gamimune N, 10% treated with solvent/detergent. The incidence, nature and severity of reactions with Gamimune N, 10% treated with solvent/detergent were not different from those observed with Gamimune N, 10%.

Idiopathic Thrombocytopenic Purpura

An investigation of Gamimune N, 10% in 31 adult and pediatric subjects with ITP encountered side effects in 17 of 119 (14.3%) infusions. The dosage in these studies was 1,000 mg/kg body weight for 1 day or 2 consecutive days. However, in the adult study, an induction dosage of 500 mg/kg body weight for 1 day or 2 consecutive days was associated with 17 of these infusions. Of those 17 infusions, three had adverse events. Overall, side effects included mild chest pain, mild and moderate emesis, moderate fever, mild or moderate headache (severe on one occasion) and a single incidence of hives, pruritus and rash. At least 17 of the 50 infusions in the pediatric study were given at rates of ≥ 0.1 mL/kg body weight per minute as part of a rate escalation investigation. Maximum infusion rates obtained were not limited by or interrupted due to adverse effects.

In studies of Gamimune N, 5% administered at a dose of 400 mg/kg body weight in the treatment of adult and pediatric patients with ITP, systemic reactions were noted in only 4 of 154 (2.6%) infusions, and all but one occurred at rates of infusion greater than 0.04 mL/kg body weight per minute. The symptoms reported included chest tightness, a sense of tachycardia (pulse was 84 beats per minute), and a burning sensation in the head; these symptoms were all mild and transient.

In studies of Gamimune N, 5% administered at a dose of 1,000 mg/kg body weight either as a single dose or as two doses on consecutive days in the treatment of adult and pediatric patients with ITP, adverse reactions were noted in 25 of 251 (10%) infusions. Symptoms reported included headache, nausea, fever, chills, back pain, chest tightness, and shortness of breath. In children, the high dose regimen has been well-tolerated at the highest rates of infusion. In adults, however, the frequency of adverse reactions tended to increase with infusion rates in excess of 0.06 mL/kg body weight per minute. In general, reactions reported with infusion of Gamimune N, 5% in these studies were reported as mild or moderate, and responded to slowing of the infusion rate.

Bone Marrow Transplantation

In studies of Gamimune N, 5% administered to 185 bone marrow transplant recipients at doses of 500 mg/kg (10 mL/kg) body weight on day −7 and day −2 pretransplant, then weekly through day 90 posttransplant, adverse reactions were noted in 12 (6.5%) of the 185 patients that received Gamimune N, 5% and in 14 (0.6%) of 2,176 infusions. All reactions reported were rate-related and classified as mild. Chills were the most common symptom reported, occurring in nine patients. The other symptoms reported included headache, flushing, fever, pruritus and slight back discomfort. All reactions resolved satisfactorily, usually without treatment or decreasing the infusion rate.

Pediatric HIV Infection

Three hundred seventy-six (376) patients, 187 treated with Gamimune N, 5% and 189 treated with placebo (0.1% Albumin [Human]), were included in the safety analysis. Adverse reactions occurred during or within 24 hours of an infusion in 50 of 3,451 (1.4%) infusions of Gamimune N, 5% and 62 of 3,447 (1.8%) infusions of placebo. Fever was the most common adverse reaction and occurred in 30 of 105 (28.6%) patients receiving placebo and 19 of 78 (24.4%) patients treated with Gamimune N, 5%. Irritability was the second most common symptom reported, with 10 of 105 (9.5%) reports for the placebo group and 9 of 78 (11.5%) for the group treated with Gamimune N, 5%. A large number of diverse adverse reactions accounted for the remaining adverse reactions reported in both study groups. In general, the number of adverse events reported was comparable in both the placebo and Gamimune N, 5% treated groups. Three serious adverse reactions were reported. One patient experienced a hypersensitivity reaction and did not receive further Gamimune N, 5% treatment. A second patient developed tachycardia and was admitted to an intensive care unit, but later continued treatment with Gamimune N, 5%. A third patient had skin infiltration during infusion and developed a full thickness skin slough over the dorsum of the hand that required skin grafting.

DOSAGE AND ADMINISTRATION

General

Dosages for specific indications are indicated below, but in general, it is recommended that Gamimune N, 10% be infused by itself at a rate of 0.01 to 0.02 mL/kg body weight per minute for 30 minutes; if well-tolerated, the rate may be **gradually** increased to a maximum of 0.08 mL/kg body weight per minute. Investigations indicate that Gamimune N, 10% is well-tolerated and less likely to produce side effects when infused at the indicated rate. If side effects occur, the rate may be reduced, or the infusion interrupted until symptoms subside. The infusion may then be resumed at the rate which is comfortable for the patient. Parenteral drug products should be inspected visually for particulate matter and discoloration prior to administration, whenever solution and container permit.

It is recommended that infusion of Gamimune N, 10% be given by a separate line, by itself, without mixing with other intravenous fluids or medications the patient might be receiving. Gamimune N, 10% should not be mixed with Immune Globulin Intravenous (Human) from another manufacturer. Gamimune N, 10% is not compatible with saline. If dilution is required, Gamimune N, 10% may be diluted with 5% dextrose in water (D5/W). No other drug interactions or compatibilities have been evaluated.

For patients judged to be at increased risk for developing renal dysfunction, it may be prudent to reduce the amount of product infused per unit time by infusing Gamimune N, 10% at a rate less than 8 mg IG/kg/min (0.08 mL/kg/min). No prospective data are presently available to identify a maximum safe dose, concentration, and rate of infusion in patients determined to be at increased risk of acute renal failure. In the absence of prospective data, recommended doses should not be exceeded and the concentration and infusion rate should be the minimum level practicable. Reduction in dose, concentration, and/or rate of administration in patients at risk of acute renal failure has been proposed in the literature in order to reduce the risk of acute renal failure.[37]

Only 18 gauge needles should be used to penetrate the stopper for dispensing product from 10 mL vial sizes; 16 gauge needles or dispensing pins should only be used with 20 mL vial sizes and larger. Needles or dispensing pins should only be inserted within the stopper area delineated by the raised ring. The stopper should be penetrated perpendicular to the plane of the stopper within the ring.

A number of factors beyond our control could reduce the efficacy of this product or even result in an ill effect following its use. These include improper storage and handling of the product after it leaves our hands, diagnosis, dosage, method of administration, and biological differences in individual patients. Because of these factors, it is important that this product be stored properly and that the directions be followed carefully during use.

Primary Humoral Immunodeficiency

The usual dosage of Gamimune N, 10% for prophylaxis in primary immunodeficiency syndromes is 100–200 mg/kg of body weight administered approximately once a month by intravenous infusion. The dosage may be given more frequently or increased as high as 400 mg/kg body weight, if the clinical response is inadequate, or the level of IgG achieved in the circulation is felt to be insufficient. The minimum level of IgG required for protection has not been determined.

Idiopathic Thrombocytopenic Purpura (ITP)

Induction: An increase in platelet count has been observed in children and some adults with acute or chronic ITP receiving Gamimune N, 5% 400 mg/kg body weight daily for 5 days. Alternatively, studies in adults and children with Gamimune N, 5% and Gamimune N, 10% using a dose of 1,000 mg/kg body weight daily for 1 day or 2 consecutive days have also shown increases in platelet count. In the latter treatment regimen, if an adequate increase in the platelet count is observed at 24 hours, the second dose of 1,000 mg/kg body weight may be withheld. The high dose regimen (1,000 mg/kg × 1–2 days) is not recommended for individuals with expanded fluid volumes or where fluid volume may be a concern. With both treatment regimens, a response usually occurs within several days and is maintained for a variable period of time. In general, a response is seen less often in adults than in children.

Maintenance: In adults and children with ITP, if after induction therapy the platelet count falls to less than 30,000/mm^3 and/or the patient manifests clinically significant bleeding, Gamimune N, 10% 400 mg/kg body weight may be given as a single infusion. If an adequate response does not result, the dose can be increased to 800–1,000 mg/kg of body weight given as a single infusion. Maintenance infusions may be administered intermittently as clinically indicated to maintain a platelet count greater than 30,000/mm^3.

Bone Marrow Transplantation

A reduction in posttransplant complications has been observed in bone marrow transplant patients ≥ 20 years of age receiving Gamimune N, 5%. An equivalent dosage of

Continued on next page

Gamimune N, 10%—Cont.

Gamimune N, 10% is recommended in doses of 500 mg/kg (5 mL/kg) body weight beginning on days −7 and −2 pretransplant (or at the time conditioning therapy for transplantation is begun), then weekly through day 90 posttransplant. Gamimune N, 10% should be administered by itself through a Hickman line while it is in place, and thereafter through a peripheral vein. Please see DOSAGE AND ADMINISTRATION for other drug interactions.

Pediatric HIV Infection

A reduction in bacterial infections has been observed in children infected with HIV-1 receiving Gamimune N, 5%. An equivalent dosage of Gamimune N, 10% is recommended in doses of 400 mg/kg (4 mL/kg) body weight every 28 days.

HOW SUPPLIED

Gamimune N, 10% is supplied in the following sizes:

NDC Number	Size	Grams Protein
0026-0648-12	10 mL	1.0
0026-0648-15	25 mL	2.5
0026-0648-20	50 mL	5.0
0026-0648-71	100 mL	10.0
0026-0648-24	200 mL	20.0

STORAGE

Store at 2–8°C (36–46°F). Do not freeze. Do not use after expiration date.

CAUTION

℞ only

U.S. federal law prohibits dispensing without prescription.

REFERENCES

1. Tenold RA, inventor; Cutter Laboratories, assignee. Intravenously injectable immune serum globulin. U.S. Patent 4,396,608, Aug. 2, 1983.
2. Data on file at Bayer Corporation.
3. Pirofsky B, Campbell SM, Montanaro A: Individual patient variations in the kinetics of intravenous immunoglobulin administration. *J Clin Immunol* 2(2): 7S–14S, 1982.
4. Pirofsky B: Intravenous immune globulin therapy in hypogammaglobulinemia. *Amer J Med* 76(3A):53–60, 1984.
5. Pirofsky B, Anderson CJ, Bardana EJ Jr.: Therapeutic and detrimental effects of intravenous immunoglobulin therapy. In: Alving BM (ed.): *Immunoglobulins: characteristics and uses of intravenous preparations.* Washington, D.C., U.S. Government Printing Office, (1980), pp 15–22.
6. Sullivan KM, Kopecky KJ, Jocom J, et al: Immunomodulatory and antimicrobial efficacy of intravenous immunoglobulin in bone marrow transplantation. *N Engl J Med* 323(11):705–12, 1990.
7. Bernstein LJ, Ochs HD, Wedgwood RJ, et al; Defective humoral immunity in pediatric acquired immune deficiency syndrome. *J Pediatr* 107(3):352–7, 1985.
8. Borkowsky W, Steele CJ, Grubman S, et al: Antibody responses to bacterial toxoids in children infected with human immunodeficiency virus. *J Pediatr* 110(4):563–6, 1987.
9. Blanche S, Le Deist F, Fischer A, et al: Longitudinal study of 18 children with perinatal LAV/HTLV III infection: attempt at prognostic evaluation. *J Pediatr* 109(6): 965–70, 1986.
10. Pahwa S, Fikrig S, Menez R, et al: Pediatric acquired immunodeficiency syndrome demonstration of B-lymphocyte defects in vitro. *Diagn Immunol* 4(1):24–30, 1986.
11. Bernstein LJ, Krieger BZ, Novick B, et al: Bacterial infections in the acquired immunodeficiency syndrome of children. *Pediatr Infect Dis* 4(5):472–5, 1985.
12. Krasinski K, Borkowsky W, Bonk S, et al: Bacterial infections in human immunodeficiency virus-infected children. *Pediatr Infect Dis J* 7(5):323–8, 1988.
13. Scott GB, Buck BE, Leterman JG, et al: Acquired immunodeficiency syndrome in infants. *N Engl J Med* 310(2): 76–81, 1984.
14. Mofenson LM, Willoughby A. Passive immunization. In: Pizzo PA, Wilfert CM, (eds.) *Pediatric AIDS: the challenge of HIV infection in infants, children and adolescents.* Baltimore: Williams & Wilkins (1991) pp 633–50.
15. National Institute of Child Health and Human Development Intravenous Immunoglobulin Study Group. Intravenous immune globulin for the prevention of bacterial infections in children with symptomatic human immunodeficiency virus infection. *N Engl J Med* 325(2):73–80, 1991.
16. Mofenson LM, Moye J Jr, Bethel J, et al: Prophylactic intravenous immunoglobulin in HIV-infected children with CD4 + counts of 0.20 × 10^9/L or more. Effect on viral, opportunistic, and bacterial infections. *JAMA* 268(4):483–88, 1992.
17. Glycine. In: Budavari S, O'Neil MJ, Smith A, et al, eds.: *Merck Index.* 11th ed. Rahway NJ, Merck & Co., 1989. p. 706.
18. Wretlind, A: Complete intravenous nutrition: theoretical and experimental background. *Nutr Metab* 14(Suppl):1–57, 1972.
19. Hahn RG, Stalberg HP, Gustafsson SA: Intravenous infusion of irrigating fluids containing glycine or mannitol with and without ethanol. *J Urol* 142(4):1102–1105, 1989.
20. Guyton AC: *Textbook of Medical Physiology.* 5th ed. Philadelphia, W.B. Saunders, 1976, pp 499–500.
21. Nolte MT, Pirofsky B, Gerritz GA, et al: Intravenous immunoglobulin therapy for antibody deficiency. *Clin Exp Immunol* 36: 237–43, 1979.
22. Buckley RH: Immunoglobulin replacement therapy: indications and contraindications for use and variable IgG levels achieved. In: Alving BM (ed): *Immunoglobulins: characteristics and uses of intravenous preparations.* Washington, D.C., U.S. Government Printing Office, (1980), pp 3–8.
23. Ochs HD: Intravenous immunoglobulin therapy of patients with primary immunodeficiency syndromes: efficacy and safety of a new modified immune globulin preparation. In: Alving BM (ed.): *Immunoglobulins: characteristics and uses of intravenous preparations.* Washington, D.C., U.S. Government Printing Office, (1980), pp 9–14.
24. Cayco AV, Perazella MA, Hayslett JP: Renal insufficiency after intravenous immune globulin therapy: A Report of Two Cases and an Analysis of the Literature. *J Amer Soc Nephrology* 8:1788–1793, 1997.
25. Sekul E, Cupler E, Dalakas M. Aseptic meningitis associated with high-dose intravenous immunoglobulin therapy: Frequency and risk factors. *Ann Int Med* 121: 259–262, 1994.
26. Kato E, Shindo S, Eto Y, et al: Administration of Immune Globulin Associated with Aseptic Meningitis. *JAMA* 259(22):3269–3270, 1988.
27. Casteels-Van Daele M, Wijndaele L, Hunninck K, et al: Intravenous immune globulin and acute aseptic meningitis. *N Engl J Med* 323(9):614–615, 1990.
28. Scribner C, Kapit R, Phillips E, et al: Aseptic meningitis and Intravenous immunoglobulin therapy. *Ann Intern Med* 121(4):305–306, 1994.
29. Schiavotto C, Ruggeri M. Rodeghiero F. Adverse reactions after high-dose intravenous immunoglobulin: incidence in 83 patients treated for idiopathic thrombocytopenic purpura (ITP) and review of the literature. *Haematologica* 78(6:Suppl 2):35–40, 1993.
30. Pasatiempo AM, Kroser JA, Rudnick M, et al: Acute renal failure after intravenous immunoglobulin therapy. *J Rheumatol* 21(2):347–9, 1994.
31. Peerless AG, Stiehm ER: intravenous gammaglobulin for reaction to intramuscular preparation. [letter] *Lancet* 2(8347):461, 1983.
32. Winward DB, Brophy MT: Acute renal failure after administration of intravenous immunoglobulin: review of the literature and case report. *Pharmacotherapy* 15: 765–772, 1995.
33. Phillips AO: Renal failure and intravenous immunoglobulin [letter; comment]. *Clin Nephrol* 36:83–86, 1992.
34. Anderson W, Bethea W: Renal lesions following administration of hypertonic solutions of sucrose. *JAMA* 114: 1983–1987, 1940.
35. Lindberg H, Wald A: Renal changes following the administration of hypertonic solutions. *Arch Intern Med* 63:907–918, 1939.
36. Ridgon RH, Cardwell ES: Renal lesions following the intravenous injection of hypertonic solution of sucrose: A clinical and experimental study. *Arch Intern Med* 69: 670–690, 1942.
37. Tan E, Hajinazarian M, Bay, et al. Acute renal failure resulting from intravenous immunoglobulin therapy. *Arch Neurology* 50:137–139, 1993.

Bayer Corporation
Pharmaceutical Division
Elkhart, IN 46515 USA 08692249
U.S. License No. 8 (Rev. November 2001)

Shown in Product Identification Guide, page 307

GAMUNEX® ℞

[*găm-ew-nĕks*]

Immune Globulin Intravenous (Human), 10% Caprylate/Chromatography Purified

DESCRIPTION

Immune Globulin Intravenous (Human), 10% Caprylate/Chromatography Purified, (GAMUNEX®) is a ready-to-use sterile solution of human immune globulin protein for intravenous administration. GAMUNEX® consists of 9%–11% protein in 0.16–0.24 M glycine. Not less than 98% of the protein has the electrophoretic mobility of gamma globulin. GAMUNEX® contains trace levels of fragments and IgA (average 0.046 mg/mL). IgM levels were at or below the limit of quantitation (0.002 g/L). The distribution of IgG subclasses is similar to that found in normal serum. The measured buffer capacity is 35 mEq/L and the osmolality is 258 mOsmol/kg solvent, which is close to physiological osmolality (285–295 mOsmol/kg). The pH of GAMUNEX® is 4.0–4.5. GAMUNEX® contains no preservative.

GAMUNEX® is made from large pools of human plasma by a combination of cold ethanol fractionation, caprylate precipitation and filtration, and anion-exchange chromatography. Two of the four ethanol fractionation steps of the Cohn-Oncley process have been replaced by tandem anion-exchange chromatography. The IgG proteins are not subjected to heating or chemical or enzymatic modification steps. Fc and Fab functions of the IgG molecule are retained, but do not activate complement or pre-Kallikrein activity in an unspecific manner. The protein is stabilized during the process by adjusting the pH of the solution to 4.0–4.5. Isotonicity is achieved by the addition of glycine. GAMUNEX® is incubated in the final container (at the low pH of 4.0–4.3), for a minimum of 21 days at 23° to 27°C. The product is intended for intravenous administration.

The capacity of the manufacturing process to remove and/or inactivate enveloped and non-enveloped viruses has been validated by laboratory spiking studies on a scaled down process model, using the following enveloped and non-enveloped viruses: human immunodeficiency virus, type I (HIV-1) as the relevant virus for HIV-1 and HIV-2; bovine viral diarrhea virus (BVDV) as a model for hepatitis C virus; pseudorabies virus (PRV) as a model for large DNA viruses (e.g. herpes viruses); Reo virus type 3 (Reo) as a model for non-enveloped viruses and for its resistance to physical and chemical inactivation; hepatitis A virus (HAV) as relevant non-enveloped virus, and porcine parvovirus (PPV) as a model for human parvovirus B19.

The following process steps contribute to virus inactivation and/or removal: caprylate precipitation/cloth filtration, caprylate incubation, column chromatography and final container low pH incubation. Caprylate is the basis of two mechanistically distinct virus clearance steps, the caprylate precipitation/cloth filtration step and the caprylate incubation step. During the caprylate precipitation/cloth filtration step, protein impurities and potential enveloped or non-enveloped viral contaminants are precipitated by caprylate and the precipitate is removed from the product stream by filtration through a cloth filter. In a subsequent step, enveloped viruses are inactivated during incubation with caprylate. The table below presents the contribution of each process step to virus reduction and the overall process reduction. Virus removal steps were evaluated independently and in combination to identify those steps, which were mechanistically distinct. Overall virus reduction was calculated only from steps that were mechanistically independent from each other and truly additive. In addition, each step was verified to provide robust virus reduction across the production range for key operating parameters.

[See first table at top of next page]

CLINICAL PHARMACOLOGY

Primary Humoral Immunodeficiency (PI)

In a double-blind, randomized, parallel group clinical trial with 172 subjects with primary humoral immunodeficiencies (study 100175) GAMUNEX®, Immune Globulin Intravenous (Human), 10% Caprylate/Chromatography Purified, was demonstrated to be at least as efficacious as GAMIMUNE® N, Immune Globulin Intravenous (Human), in the prevention of any infection, i.e. validated plus clinically defined, non-validated infections of any organ system, during a nine month treatment period. Twenty six subjects were excluded from the Per Protocol analysis (2 due to non-compliance and 24 due to protocol violations). The primary efficacy endpoint was the proportion of subjects with at least one of the following validated infections: pneumonia, acute sinusitis and acute exacerbations of chronic sinusitis.

[See second table on next page]

The annual rate of validated infections (Number of Infection/year/subject) was 0.18 in the group treated with GAMUNEX® and 0.43 in the group treated with GAMIMUNE® N, 10% (p=0.023). The annual rates for any infection (validated plus clinically-defined, non-validated infections of any organ system) were 2.88 and 3.38, respectively (p=0.300).[1, 2]

A post hoc analysis of serious infection events during the trial showed five (5) cases of clinically defined pneumonia occurred in 4 GAMUNEX® treated subjects and 11 cases of validated or clinically defined pneumonia occurred in 9 GAMIMUNE® N 10% treated subjects and 1 case of sepsis occurred in a GAMIMUNE® N 10% treated subject. The annual infection rate and 98% confidence interval for serious infections are:

[See third table on next page]

As a secondary endpoint, consequences of infections were recorded and are displayed in the table below:

[See fourth table on next page]

Two randomized pharmacokinetic crossover trials were carried out with GAMUNEX®, Immune Globulin Intravenous (Human), 10% Caprylate/Chromatography Purified, in 38 subjects with Primary Humoral Immunodeficiencies given 3 infusions 3 or 4 weeks apart of test product at a dose of 100–600 mg/kg body weight per infusion. One trial compared the pharmacokinetic characteristics of GAMUNEX® to Gamimune N 10%, Immune Globulin Intravenous (Human), 10% (study 100152) and the other trial compared the pharmacokinetics of GAMUNEX® (10% strength) with a 5% concentration of this product (study 100174). The ratio of the geometric least square means for dose-normalized IgG peak levels of GAMUNEX® and GAMIMUNE® N was 0.996. The corresponding value for the dose-normalized area under the curve (AUC) of IgG levels was 0.990. The results of both PK parameters were within the pre-established limits of 0.080 and 1.25. Similar results were obtained in the comparison of GAMUNEX® 10% to a 5% concentration of GAMUNEX®.[3, 4]

The main pharmacokinetic parameters of GAMUNEX®, measured as total IgG in study 100152 are displayed below:

[See first table at bottom of page 874]

The two pharmacokinetic trials with GAMUNEX® show the IgG concentration/time curve follows a biphasic slope with a distribution phase of about 5 days characterized by a fall in serum IgG levels to about 65–75% of the peak levels achieved immediately post-infusion. This phase is followed by the elimination phase with a half-life of approximately

35 days[3,4]. IgG trough levels were measured over nine months in the therapeutic equivalence trial (100175). Mean trough levels were 7.8 +/− 1.9 mg/mL for the GAMUNEX® treatment group and 8.2 +/− 2.0 mg/mL for the GAMIMUNE® N, 10% control group[1].

Idiopathic Thrombocytopenic Purpura (ITP)

The mechanism of action of high doses of immunoglobulins in the treatment of Idiopathic Thrombocytopenic Purpura (ITP) has not been fully elucidated. Several lines of evidence suggest that Fc-receptor blockade of phagocytes as well as down regulation of auto-reactive B-cells by antiidiotypic antibodies provided by IGIV may constitute the main mechanisms of action[5–10].

A double-blind, randomized, parallel group clinical trial with 97 ITP subjects was carried out to prove the hypothesis that GAMUNEX® was at least as effective as GAMIMUNE® N, 10% in raising platelet counts from less than or equal to 20 $\times 10^9$/L to more than 50 $\times 10^9$/L within 7 days after treatment with 2 g/kg IGIV (study 100176). Twenty-four percent of the subjects were less than or equal to 16 years of age.

GAMUNEX® was demonstrated to be at least as effective as GAMIMUNE® N, 10% in the treatment of adults and children with acute or chronic ITP.[11]

[See second table at bottom of next page]

A trial was conducted to evaluate the clinical response to rapid infusion of GAMUNEX® in patients with ITP. The study involved 28 chronic ITP subjects, wherein the subjects received 1 g/kg GAMUNEX® on three occasions for treatment of relapses. The infusion rate was randomly assigned to 0.08, 0.11, or 0.14 mL/kg/min (8, 11 or 14 mg/kg/min). Pre-medication with corticosteroids to alleviate infusion-related intolerability was not permitted. Pre-treatment with antihistamines, anti-pyretics and analgesics was permitted. The average dose was approximately 1 g/kg body weight at all three prescribed rates of infusion (0.08, 0.11 and 0.14 mL/kg/min). All patients were administered each of the three planned infusions except seven subjects. Based on 21 patients per treatment group, the a posteriori power to detect twice as many drug-related adverse events between groups was 23%. Of the seven subjects that did not complete the study, five did not require additional treatment, one withdrew because he refused to participate without concomitant medication (prednisone) and one experienced an adverse event (hives); however, this was at the lowest dose rate level (0.08 mL/kg/min).

General

GAMUNEX®, Immune Globulin Intravenous (Human), 10% Caprylate/Chromatography Purified, supplies a broad spectrum of opsonic and neutralizing IgG antibodies against bacteria or their toxins, which were demonstrated to be effective in the prevention or attenuation of lethal infections in animal models. GAMUNEX® proved to be effective in preventing severe infections in patients with Primary Humoral Immunodeficiency (PI).

Glycine (aminoacetic acid) is a nonessential amino acid normally present in the body. Glycine is a major ingredient in amino acid solutions employed in intravenous alimentation[12]. While toxic effects of glycine administration have been reported[13], the doses and rates of administration were 3–4 fold greater than those for GAMUNEX®. In another study it was demonstrated that intravenous bolus doses of 0.44 g/kg glycine were not associated with serious adverse effects[14]. GAMUNEX® doses of 1 g/kg correspond to a glycine dose of 0.15 g/kg. 0.2M Glycine stabilizer has been used safely in GAMIMUNE® N since 1992.

Caprylate is a saturated medium-chain (C8) fatty acid of plant origin, which is subjected to rapid beta-oxidation. Medium chain fatty acids are considered to be essentially non-toxic. Human subjects receiving medium chain fatty acids parenterally have tolerated doses of 3.0 to 9.0 g/kg/day for periods of several months without adverse effects[15]. Residual Caprylate concentrations in the final container are no more than 0.216 g/L (1.3 mmol/L).

The buffering capacity of GAMUNEX® is 35.0 mEq/L (0.35 mEq/g protein). A dose of 1000 mg/kg body weight therefore represents an acid load of 0.35 mEq/kg body weight. The total buffering capacity of whole blood in a normal individual is 45–50 mEq/L of blood, or 3.6 mEq/kg body weight[16]. Thus, the acid load delivered with a dose of 1000 mg/kg of GAMUNEX® would be neutralized by the buffering capacity of whole blood alone, even if the dose was infused instantaneously.

INDICATIONS AND USAGE

Primary Humoral Immunodeficiency (PI)

GAMUNEX®, Immune Globulin Intravenous (Human), 10% Caprylate/Chromatography Purified, is indicated as replacement therapy of primary immunodeficiency states in which severe impairment of antibody forming capacity has been shown, such as congenital agammaglobulinemia, common variable immunodeficiency, X-linked immunodeficiency with hyper IgM, Wiskott-Aldrich syndrome, and severe combined immunodeficiencies[17–24].

Idiopathic Thrombocytopenic Purpura (ITP)

GAMUNEX® is indicated in Idiopathic Thrombocytopenic Purpura to rapidly raise platelet counts to prevent bleeding or to allow a patient with ITP to undergo surgery[5–10].

CONTRAINDICATIONS

GAMUNEX®, Immune Globulin Intravenous (Human), 10% Caprylate/Chromatography Purified, is contraindicated in individuals with known anaphylactic or severe systemic response to Immune Globulin (Human). Individuals with severe, selective IgA deficiencies (serum IgA <0.05 g/L) who have known antibody against IgA (anti-IgA antibody) should only receive GAMUNEX® with utmost cautionary measures, due to the risk of severe immediate hypersensitivity reactions including anaphylaxis. No experience is available on tolerability of GAMUNEX® in subjects with selective IgA deficiency since they were excluded from participation in the clinical trials with GAMUNEX®.

Log_{10} Virus Reduction

Process Step	Enveloped Viruses			Non-enveloped Viruses		
	HIV	PRV	BVDV	Reo	HAV	PPV
Caprylate Precipitation/Cloth Filtration	C/I[a]	C/I	2.4 ± 0.3	2.1 ± 0.4	2.6 ± 0.2	2.2 ± 0.1
Caprylate Incubation	≥ 4.5	≥ 4.6	≥ 4.5	NA[b]	NA	NA
Depth Filtration[d]	CAP[c]	CAP	CAP	≥ 4.3	≥ 2.0	3.3 ± 0.3
Column Chromatography	≥ 3.0	≥ 3.3	4.0 ± 0.3	≥ 4.0	≥ 1.4	4.2 ± 0.2
Low pH Incubation (21 days)	≥ 6.5	≥ 4.3	3.5 ± 0.4	NA	NA	NA
Global Reduction	**≥ 14.0**	**≥ 12.2**	**≥ 14.4**	**≥ 6.1**	**≥ 4.0**	**6.4**

[a] C/I — Interference by caprylate precluded determination of virus reduction for this step. Although removal of viruses is likely to occur at the caprylate precipitation/cloth filtration step, BVDV is the only enveloped virus for which reduction is claimed. The presence of caprylate prevents detection of other, less resistant enveloped viruses and therefore their removal cannot be assessed.

[b] Not Applicable — This step has no effect on non-enveloped viruses.

[c] CAP — The presence of caprylate in the process at this step prevents detection of enveloped viruses, and their removal cannot be assessed.

[d] Some mechanistic overlap occurs between depth filtration and other steps. Therefore, Bayer has chosen to exclude this step from the global virus reduction calculations.

Primary Endpoint Per Protocol Analysis (Study 100175)

	GAMUNEX® (n = 73) No. of subjects with at least one infection	GAMIMUNE® N (n = 73) No. of subjects with at least one infection	Mean Difference (90% confidence interval)	p-Value
Validated Infections	9 (12%)	17 (23%)	−0.117 (−0.220, −0.015)	0.06
Acute Sinusitis	4 (5%)	10 (14%)		
Exacerbation of Chronic Sinusitis	5 (7%)	6 (8%)		
Pneumonia	0 (0%)	2 (3%)		
Any Infection (Validated plus Clinically defined non-validated Infections)	56 (77%)	57 (78%)	−0.020 (−0.135, 0.096)	0.78

Post Hoc Analysis of Serious Infections* (Study 100175)

	GAMUNEX® (n = 73) Annual Infection Rate (Infections/year/subject); 98% Confidence Interval	GAMIMUNE® N (n = 73) Annual Infection Rate (Infections/year/subject); 98% Confidence Interval
Serious Infections (Validated and clinically defined Pneumonia, Sepsis)	0.07 (0[1]–0.16)	0.18 (0.06–0.32)

* The definition of Serious Infections was any of the following: validated plus clinically-defined, non-validated pneumonia, bacteremia/sepsis, osteomyelitis/septic arthritis, visceral abscess, bacterial and/or viral meningitis; however, only pneumonia and sepsis were observed.

[1] The actual lower limit was less than 0, but this is not a plausible value.

Secondary Endpoint Clinical Outcomes (Study 100175)

	GAMUNEX® No. of patient days on study: 21479	GAMIMUNE® N No. of patient days on study: 21388
Days on prophylactic antibiotics	3078 (14.4%)	4305 (20.1%)
Days on therapeutic antibiotics	2157 (10.0%)	2494 (11.7%)
Days off school/work	240 (1.1%)	230 (1.1%)
Days with visits of physician's office or emergency room	148 (0.7%)	174 (0.8%)
Hospitalization days	38 (0.2%)	71 (0.3%)

WARNINGS

Immune Globulin Intravenous (Human) products have been reported to be associated with renal dysfunction, acute renal failure, osmotic nephrosis and death.[25] Patients predisposed to acute renal failure include patients with any degree of pre-existing renal insufficiency, diabetes mellitus, age greater than 65, volume depletion, sepsis, paraproteinemia, or patients receiving known nephrotoxic drugs. Especially in such patients, IGIV products should be administered at the minimum concentration available and the minimum rate of infusion practicable. While these reports of renal dysfunction and acute renal failure have been associated with the use of many of the licensed IGIV products, those containing sucrose as a stabilizer accounted for a disproportionate share of the total number. GAMUNEX® does not contain sucrose. Glycine, a natural amino acid, is used as a stabilizer.

See PRECAUTIONS and DOSAGE AND ADMINISTRATION sections for important information intended to reduce the risk of acute renal failure.

Because this product is made from human blood, it may carry a risk of transmitting infectious agents, e.g. viruses that can cause disease. The risk that such products will transmit an infectious agent has been reduced by screening plasma donors for prior exposure to certain viruses, by testing for the presence of certain current virus infections, and by inactivating and/or removing certain viruses. Despite these measures, such products can still potentially transmit disease. There is also the possibility that unknown infectious agents may be present in such products. Individuals who receive infusions of blood or plasma products may develop signs and/or symptoms of some viral infections.

ALL infections thought by a physician possibly to have been transmitted by this product should be reported by the phy-

Continued on next page

Gamunex—Cont.

sician or other healthcare provider to Bayer Corporation [1-800-288-8371]. The physician should discuss the risks and benefits of this product with the patient, before prescribing or administering it to the patient.

GAMUNEX®, Immune Globulin Intravenous (Human), 10% Caprylate/Chromatography Purified, should be administered only intravenously. On rare occasions, treatment with an immune globulin preparation may cause a precipitous fall in blood pressure and a clinical picture of anaphylaxis, even when the patient is not known to be sensitive to immune globulin preparations. Epinephrine and other appropriate supportive care should be available for the treatment of an acute anaphylactic reaction.

PRECAUTIONS

General

Any vial that has been entered should be used promptly. Partially used vials should be discarded. Visually inspect each bottle before use. Do not use if turbid. Solution that has been frozen should not be used.

An aseptic meningitis syndrome (AMS) has been reported to occur infrequently in association with Immune Globulin Intravenous (Human) treatment. The syndrome usually begins within several hours to two days following Immune Globulin Intravenous (Human) treatment. It is characterized by symptoms and signs including severe headache, nuchal rigidity, drowsiness, fever, photophobia, painful eye movements, nausea and vomiting.

AMS may occur more frequently in association with high dose (2 g/kg) and/or rapid infusion of Immune Globulin Intravenous (Human) treatment. Discontinuation of Immune Globulin Intravenous (Human) treatment has resulted in remission of AMS within several days without sequelae[26–28].

Assure that patients are not volume depleted prior to the initiation of the infusion of IGIV. Periodic monitoring of renal function and urine output is particularly important in patients judged to have a potential increased risk for developing acute renal failure. Renal function, including measurement of blood urea nitrogen (BUN)/serum creatinine, should be assessed prior to the initial infusion of GAMUNEX®, Immune Globulin Intravenous (Human), 10% Caprylate/Chromatography Purified, and again at appropriate intervals thereafter. If renal function deteriorates, discontinuation of the product should be considered. For patients judged to be at risk for developing renal dysfunction, it may be prudent to reduce the amount of product infused per unit time by infusing GAMUNEX® at a rate less than 8 mg IG/kg/min (0.08 mL/kg/min).

Information for Patients

Patients should be instructed to immediately report symptoms of decreased urine output, sudden weight gain, fluid retention/edema, and/or shortness of breath (which may suggest kidney damage) to their physicians.

Drug Interactions

Antibodies in GAMUNEX® may interfere with the response to live viral vaccines such as measles, mumps and rubella. Therefore, use of such vaccines should be deferred until approximately 6 months after GAMUNEX® administration. Please see DOSAGE AND ADMINISTRATION for other drug interactions.

Pregnancy Category C

Animal reproduction studies have not been conducted with GAMUNEX®. It is not known whether GAMUNEX® can cause fetal harm when administered to a pregnant woman or can affect reproduction capacity. GAMUNEX® should be given to a pregnant woman only if clearly needed.

ADVERSE REACTIONS

General

Increases in creatinine and blood urea nitrogen (BUN) have been observed as soon as one to two days following infusion with Immune Globulin Intravenous (Human) products, predominantly with products containing sucrose as stabilizer. Progression to oliguria and anuria requiring dialysis has been observed, although some patients have improved spontaneously following cessation of treatment[29]. GAMUNEX®, Immune Globulin Intravenous (Human), 10% Caprylate/Chromatography Purified, does not contain sucrose. Glycine, a natural amino acid, is used as a stabilizer. In the studies undertaken to date with GAMUNEX®, no increase in creatinine and blood urea nitrogen was observed.

Although not necessarily observed for GAMUNEX®, adverse effects similar to those previously reported with administration of intravenous and intramuscular immunoglobulin products may occur. Potential reactions, therefore, may include pyrexia, rigors, dyspnea, cyanosis, hypoxemia, bronchospasm, hepatic dysfunction, leukopenia, pancytopenia, tremor, erythema multiforme, epidermolysis, back pain, abdominal pain, pulmonary edema, seizures, hypotension, thrombosis, transfusion related acute lung injury (TRALI).

True anaphylactic reactions to GAMUNEX® may occur in recipients with documented prior histories of severe allergic reactions to intramuscular immunoglobulin, but some subjects may tolerate cautiously administered intravenous immunoglobulin without adverse effects[30, 31]. Very rarely an anaphylactoid reaction may occur in subjects with no prior history of severe allergic reactions to either intramuscular or intravenous immunoglobulin.[31]

Laboratory Abnormalities

During the course of the clinical program, ALT and AST elevations, similar to those reported for other IGIV products[32, 33], were identified in some subjects. For ALT, in the primary humoral immunodeficiency (PI) study (100175) treatment emergent elevations above the upper limit of normal were transient and observed among 14/80 (18%) of subjects in the GAMUNEX® group versus 5/88 (6%) of subjects in the GAMIMUNE® N group (p = 0.026). In the ITP study which employed a higher dose per infusion, but a maximum of only two infusions, the reverse finding was observed among 3/44 (7%) of subjects in the GAMUNEX® group versus 8/43 (19%) of subjects in the GAMIMUNE® N group (p = 0.118). Elevations of ALT and AST were generally mild (<3 times upper limit of normal), transient, and were not associated with obvious symptoms of liver dysfunction.

GAMUNEX® may contain low levels of anti-Blood Group A and B antibodies primarily of the IgG_4 class. Direct antiglobin tests (DAT or direct Coombs tests), which are carried out in some centers as a safety check prior to red blood cell transfusions, may become positive temporarily. GAMUNEX® does not contain irregular antibodies to Rhesus antigens or other non-ABO RBC antigens. Hemolytic events were not detected in association with positive DAT findings in clinical trials.[1, 3, 4, 11, 34]

PK Parameters of GAMUNEX® and GAMIMUNE® N 10% (Study 100152)

	GAMUNEX®				GAMIMUNE® N 10%			
	N	Mean	SD	Median	N	Mean	SD	Median
Cmax (mg/mL)	17	19.04	3.06	19.71	17	19.31	4.17	19.30
Cmax-norm (kg/mL)	17	0.047	0.007	0.046	17	0.047	0.008	0.047
AUC(0-tn)[a] (mg *hr/mL)	17	6746.48	1348.13	6949.47	17	6854.17	1425.08	7119.86
AUC(0-tn)norm[a] (kg *hr/mL)	17	16.51	1.83	16.95	17	16.69	2.04	16.99
$T_{1/2}$[b] (days)	16	35.74	8.69	33.09	16	34.27	9.28	31.88

[a] Partial AUC: defined as pre-dose concentration to the last concentration common across both treatment periods in the same patient.

[b] only 15 subjects were valid for the analysis of $T_{1/2}$

Platelet Response of Per Protocol Analysis (Study 100176)

	GAMUNEX® (n = 39)	GAMIMUNE® N (n = 42)	Mean Difference (90% confidence interval)
By Day 7	35 (90%)	35 (83%)	0.075 (−0.037, 0.186)
By Day 23	35 (90%)	36 (86%)	0.051 (−0.058, 0.160)
Sustained for 7 days	29 (74%)	25 (60%)	0.164 (0.003, 0.330)

Primary Humoral Immunodeficiencies (PI)

In three randomized clinical trials, 119 subjects with primary humoral immunodeficiencies were exposed to 939 infusions with GAMUNEX®, Immune Globulin Intravenous (Human), 10% Caprylate/Chromatography Purified. The rates of discontinuation from controlled clinical trials of GAMUNEX® due to adverse events were comparable to those of the GAMIMUNE® N, Immune Globulin Intravenous (Human), treatment group. For the Primary Humoral Immunodeficiency studies, 2 subjects (1.4%) treated with GAMUNEX® discontinued due to adverse events (Coombs negative hypochromic anemia, autoimmune pure red cell aplasia). Both events were considered unrelated to study drug as per the investigator.

Two pharmacokinetic trials were carried out in 18–20 subjects each with primary humoral immunodeficiencies, who received 100–600 mg/kg GAMUNEX® or GAMIMUNE® N, 10% for three infusions on a 3 or 4 week infusion interval and then crossed over to three infusions of the alternate product (studies 100152, 100174). In a third trial investigating therapeutic equivalence, 172 subjects were randomized to GAMUNEX® or GAMIMUNE® N for a nine-month double-blinded treatment with either of the two products at a dose between 200 and 600 mg/kg on a 3 or 4 week infusion interval (study 100175). In this trial, only 9 subjects in each treatment group were pretreated with non-steroidal medication prior to infusion. Generally, diphenhydramine and acetaminophen were used. Any adverse events in trial 100175, irrespective of the causality assessment, reported by at least 15% of subjects during the 9-month treatment are given in the table below.

Subjects with At Least One Adverse Event *Irrespective of Causality* (Study 100175)

Adverse Event	GAMUNEX® No. of subjects: 87 No. of subjects with AE (percentage of all subjects)	GAMIMUNE® N No. of subjects: 85 No. of subjects with AE (percentage of all subjects)
Cough increased	47 (54%)	46 (54%)
Rhinitis	44 (51%)	45 (53%)
Pharyngitis	36 (41%)	39 (46%)
Heachache	22 (25%)	28 (33%)
Fever	24 (28%)	27 (32%)
Diarrhea	24 (28%)	27 (32%)
Asthma	25 (29%)	17 (20%)
Nausea	17 (20%)	22 (26%)
Ear Pain	16 (18%)	12 (14%)
Asthenia	9 (10%)	13 (15%)

The severity of the adverse events across the treatment groups is displayed below.

Severity of Adverse Events *Irrespective of Causality* (Study 100175)

	GAMUNEX® No. events with severity statement: 968	GAMIMUNE® N No. events with severity statement: 1083
Mild	558 (58%)	751 (69%)
Moderate	329 (34%)	259 (24%)
Severe	81 (8%)	73 (7%)

The subset of drug related adverse events in trial 100175 reported by at least 3% of subjects during the 9-month treatment are given in the table below.

[See first table at top of next page]

Adverse events, which were reported by at least 5% of subjects, were also analyzed by frequency and in relation to infusions administered. The analysis is displayed below.

[See second table on next page]

The mean number of adverse events per infusion that occurred during or on the same day as an infusion was 0.21 in both the GAMUNEX® and GAMIMUNE® N treatment groups.

In all three trials in primary humoral immunodeficiencies, the maximum infusion rate was 0.08 mL/kg/min (8 mg/kg/min). The actual infusion rate was reduced for 11 of 222 exposed subjects (7 GAMUNEX®, 4 GAMIMUNE® N) at 17 occasions. In most instances, mild to moderate hives/urticaria, itching, pain or reaction at infusion site, anxiety or headache was the main reason. There was one case of severe chills. There were no anaphylactic or anaphylactoid reactions to GAMUNEX® or GAMIMUNE® N.

In trial 100175, serum samples were drawn to monitor the viral safety at baseline and one week after the first infusion (for parvovirus B19), eight weeks after first and fifth infusion, and 16 weeks after the first and fifth infusion of IGIV (for hepatitis C) and at any time of premature discontinuation of the study. Viral markers of hepatitis C, hepatitis B, HIV-1, and parvovirus B19 were monitored by nucleic acid testing (NAT, Polymerase Chain Reaction [PCR]), and serological testing. There were no treatment emergent findings of viral transmission for either GAMUNEX®, or GAMIMUNE® N.[1, 3, 4]

Idiopathic Thrombocytopenic Purpura (ITP)

Two randomized clinical trials in acute or chronic ITP were conducted with GAMUNEX®. Seventy-six subjects with acute or chronic ITP were exposed to 170 infusions with GAMUNEX® (study 100176 and 100213). The rates of discontinuation from controlled clinical trials of GAMUNEX® due to adverse events were comparable to those of the GAMIMUNE® N treatment group. Altogether, 2 subjects (3%) treated with GAMUNEX® discontinued due to adverse events (headache, fever, vomiting, hives).

Study 100176 was a randomized double-blind therapeutic equivalence study, where 97 ITP subjects with acute or chronic ITP were randomized to a single dose of 2 g/kg of GAMUNEX® or GAMIMUNE® N. The total dose was divided into two 1 g/kg doses given on two consecutive days at a maximum infusion rate of 0.08 mL/kg/min. 48 subjects were exposed to 95 infusions with GAMUNEX®. One subject, a 10-year-old boy, died suddenly from myocarditis 50 days after his second infusion of GAMUNEX®. The death was unrelated to GAMUNEX®.

As expected, the adverse event rate of IGIV in this ITP trial was higher than observed in the replacement therapy for Primary Humoral Immunodeficiencies (PI), but was within the range reported earlier for IGIV[35]. It should be noted that the dose per infusion is 2–2.5 fold higher than in Primary Humoral Immunodeficiency and that the total dose was given on two consecutive days. Administration of other IGIV product(s) at 1g/kg/day for 2 consecutive days has been associated with a higher adverse event rate than when the same total dose of product(s) was administered over a 5 day period[5]. Finally, no pre-medication with corticosteroids was permitted by the protocol. Only 12 subjects treated in each treatment group were pretreated with medication prior to infusion. Generally, diphenhydramine and/or acetaminophen were used. More than 90% of the observed drug related adverse events were of mild to moderate severity and of transient nature.

Any adverse events in trial 100176, irrespective of the causality assessment, reported by at least 15% of subjects during the 3-month trial are given in the table below.

[See third table at right]

The severity of the adverse events across the treatment groups is displayed below:

Severity of Adverse Events *Irrespective of Causality* (Study 100176)

	GAMUNEX® No. events with severity statement: 418	GAMIMUNE® N No. events with severity statement: 444
Mild	307 (73%)	326 (73%)
Moderate	97 (23%)	96 (22%)
Severe	14 (3%)	22 (5%)

The subset of drug related adverse events in trial 100176 reported by at least 3% of subjects during the 3-month trial are given in the table below.

[See first table at top of next page]

The actual infusion rate was reduced for only 4 of the 97 exposed subjects (1 GAMUNEX®, 3 GAMIMUNE® N) on 4 occasions. Mild to moderate headache, nausea, and fever were the reported reasons. There were no anaphylactic or anaphylactoid reactions to GAMUNEX® or GAMIMUNE® N.

At baseline, nine days after the first infusion (for parvovirus B19), and 3 months after the first infusion of IGIV and at any time of premature discontinuation of the study, serum samples were drawn to monitor the viral safety of the ITP subjects. Viral markers of hepatitis C, hepatitis B, HIV-1, and parvovirus B19 were monitored by nucleic acid testing (NAT, PCR), and serological testing. There were no treatment related emergent findings of viral transmission for either GAMUNEX®, or GAMIMUNE® N[11].

Although the incidences of abnormal hematocrit, hemoglobin, RBC and glucose were twice as high in the GAMUNEX® group, the actual mean changes from baseline in these parameters were not different between study drugs and the magnitudes of these mean changes were small and clinically insignificant. These changes were attributed to pre-existing differences at baseline for the hematology parameters, which continued through the study with no incremental effect carried forward. For glucose, confounding variables such as non-fasting samples further suggest the finding to be by random chance.

DOSAGE AND ADMINISTRATION

Dosage

General

For patients judged to be at increased risk for developing renal dysfunction, it may be prudent to reduce the amount of product infused per unit time by infusing GAMUNEX®, Immune Globulin Intravenous (Human), 10% Caprylate/Chromatography Purified, at a rate less than 8 mg/kg/min (0.08 mL/kg/min). No prospective data are presently available to identify a maximum safe dose, concentration, and rate of infusion in patients determined to be at increased risk of acute renal failure. In the absence of prospective data, recommended doses should not be exceeded and the concentration and infusion rate should be the minimum level practicable. Reduction in dose, concentration, and/or rate of administration in patients at risk of acute renal failure has been proposed in the literature in order to reduce the risk of acute renal failure[36].

Primary Humoral Immunodeficiency (PI)

GAMUNEX® doses between 300 and 600 mg/kg (3 and 6 mL/kg), which represented the dose range for 92% of the subjects in the therapeutic equivalence trial (100175), may be used for infection prophylaxis. The dose should be individualized taking into account dosing intervals (e.g. 3 or 4 weeks) and GAMUNEX® dose (between 300 and 600 mg/kg). A target serum IgG trough level (i.e. prior to the next infusion) of at least 5 g/L has been proposed in the literature[22, 37], however no randomized controlled trial data are available to validate this recommendation. In a clinical trial with 73 subjects with Primary Immune Deficiencies, treated for nine months with GAMUNEX®, the relationship of validated infections and serum IgG levels at trough are shown in the table below:

[See second table on next page]

Idiopathic Thrombocytopenic Purpura (ITP)

GAMUNEX® may be administered at a total dose of 2 g/kg, divided in two doses of 1 g/kg (10 mL/kg) given on two consecutive days or into five doses of 0.4 g/kg (4 mL/kg) given on five consecutive days. If after administration of the first of two daily 1 g/kg (10 mL/kg) doses, an adequate increase in the platelet count is observed at 24 hours, the second dose of 1g/kg body weight may be withheld.

Forty-eight ITP subjects were treated with 2 g/kg GAMUNEX®, divided in two 1 g/kg doses (10 mL/kg) given on two successive days. With this dose regimen 35/39 subjects (90%) responded with a platelet count from less than or equal to 20 $\times 10^9$/L to more than or equal to 50 $\times 10^9$/L within 7 days after treatment.[11]

The high dose regimen (1 g/kg × 1–2 days) is not recommended for individuals with expanded fluid volumes or where fluid volume may be a concern.

Administration

GAMUNEX® is not compatible with saline. If dilution is required, GAMUNEX® may be diluted with 5% dextrose in water (D5/W). No other drug interactions or compatibilities have been evaluated.

It is recommended that GAMUNEX® should initially be infused at a rate of 0.01 mL/kg per minute (1 mg/kg per min-

Continued on next page

Subjects with At Least One *Drug Related Adverse* Event (Study 100175)

Drug Related Adverse Event	GAMUNEX® No. of subjects: 87 No. of subjects with drug related AE (percentage of all subjects)	GAMIMUNE® N No. of subjects: 85 No. of subjects with drug related AE (percentage of all subjects)
Headache	7 (8%)	8 (9%)
Cough increased	6 (7%)	4 (5%)
Injection site reaction	4 (5%)	7 (8%)
Nausea	4 (5%)	4 (5%)
Pharyngitis	4 (5%)	3 (4%)
Urticaria	4 (5%)	1 (1%)
Asthma	3 (3%)	0 (0%)
Asthenia	3 (3%)	2 (2%)
Fever	1 (1%)	6 (7%)

Adverse Event Frequency (Study 100175)

Adverse Event		GAMUNEX® No. of infusions: 825 No. of AE (percentage of all infusions)	GAMIMUNE® N No. of infusions: 865 No. of AE (percentage of all infusions)
Cough increased	All	154 (18.7%)	148 (17.1%)
	Drug related	*14 (1.7%)*	*11 (1.3%)*
Pharyngitis	All	96 (11.6%)	99 (11.4%)
	Drug related	*7 (0.8%)*	*9 (1.0%)*
Headache	All	57 (6.9%)	69 (8.0%)
	Drug related	*7 (0.8%)*	*11 (1.3%)*
Fever	All	41 (5.0%)	65 (7.5%)
	Drug related	*1 (0.1%)*	*9 (1.0%)*
Nausea	All	31 (3.8%)	43 (5.0%)
	Drug related	*4 (0.5%)*	*4 (0.5%)*
Urticaria	All	5 (0.6%)	8 (0.9%)
	Drug related	*4 (0.5%)*	*5 (0.6%)*

Subjects with At Least One Adverse Event *Irrespective of Causality* (Study 100176)

Adverse Event	GAMUNEX® No. of subjects: 48 No. of subjects with AE (percentage of all subjects)	GAMIMUNE® N No. of subjects: 49 No. of subjects with AE (percentage of all subjects)
Headache	28 (58%)	30 (61%)
Ecchymosis, Purpura	19 (40%)	25 (51%)
Hemorrhage (All systems)	14 (29%)	16 (33%)
Epistaxis	11 (23%)	12 (24%)
Petechiae	10 (21%)	15 (31%)
Fever	10 (21%)	7 (14%)
Vomiting	10 (21%)	10 (20%)
Nausea	10 (21%)	7 (14%)
Thrombocytopenia	7 (15%)	8 (16%)
Accidental injury	6 (13%)	8 (16%)

Gamunex—Cont.

ute) for the first 30 minutes. If well-tolerated, the rate may be gradually increased to a maximum of 0.08 mL/kg per minute (8 mg/kg per minute). If side effects occur, the rate may be reduced, or the infusion interrupted until symptoms subside. The infusion may then be resumed at the rate which is comfortable for the patient.

Parenteral drug products should be inspected visually for particulate matter and discoloration prior to administration, whenever solution and container permit.

Only 18 gauge needles should be used to penetrate the stopper for dispensing product from 10 mL vial sizes; 16 gauge needles or dispensing pins should only be used with 25 mL vial sizes and larger. Needles or dispensing pins should only be inserted within the stopper area delineated by the raised ring. The stopper should be penetrated perpendicular to the plane of the stopper within the ring.

GAMUNEX® vial size	Gauge of needle to penetrate stopper
10 mL	18 gauge
25, 50, 100, 200 mL	16 gauge

Content of vials may be pooled under aseptic conditions into sterile infusion bags and infused within 8 hours after pooling.

It is recommended to infuse GAMUNEX® using a separate line by itself, without mixing with other intravenous fluids or medications the patient might be receiving.

A number of factors could reduce the efficacy of this product or even result in an ill effect following its use. These include improper storage and handling of the product, diagnosis, dosage, method of administration, and biological differences in individual patients. Because of these factors, it is important that this product be stored properly and that the directions be followed carefully during use.

HOW SUPPLIED

GAMUNEX®, Immune Globulin Intravenous (Human), 10% Caprylate/Chromatography Purified, is supplied in the following sizes:

NDC Number	Size	Grams Protein
0026-0645-12	10 mL	1.0
0026-0645-15	25 mL	2.5
0026-0645-20	50 mL	5.0
0026-0645-71	100 mL	10.0
0026-0645-24	200 mL	20.0

STORAGE

GAMUNEX®, Immune Globulin Intravenous (Human), 10% Caprylate/Chromatography Purified, may be stored for 36 months at 2–8°C (36–46°F), AND product may be stored at temperatures not to exceed 25°C (77°F) for up to 5 months during the first 18 months from date of manufacture, after which the product must be immediately used or discarded. Do not freeze. Do not use after expiration date.

Rx only

Subjects with At Least One *Drug Related* Adverse Event (Study 100176)

Drug Related Adverse Event	GAMUNEX® No. of subjects: 48 No. of subjects with drug related AE (percentage of all subjects)	GAMIMUNE® N No. of subjects: 49 No. of subjects with drug related AE (percentage of all subjects)
Headache	24 (50%)	24 (49%)
Vomiting	6 (13%)	8 (16%)
Fever	5 (10%)	5 (10%)
Nausea	5 (10%)	4 (8%)
Back Pain	3 (6%)	2 (4%)
Rash	3 (6%)	0 (0%)
Asthenia	2 (4%)	3 (6%)
Abdominal Pain	2 (4%)	2 (4%)
Pruritus	2 (4%)	0 (0%)
Arthralgia	2 (4%)	0 (0%)
Dizziness	1 (2%)	3 (6%)
Neck Pain	0 (0%)	2 (4%)

Average Serum IgG levels (g/L) Before Next GAMUNEX® Infusion (at Trough)[1]

Average serum IgG levels (g/L)	Number of subjects with validated infections	Number of subjects with any infection (validated plus clinically defined non-validated infections of any organ system)
	GAMUNEX®	GAMUNEX®
≤ 7	3/22 (14%)	19/22 (86%)
> 7 and ≤ 9	5/33 (15%)	24/33 (73%)
> 9	1/18 (6%)	13/18 (72%)
Cochran-Armitage Trend Test	P = 0.46 (NS)	P = 0.27 (NS)

NS = Non-significant

REFERENCES

1. Kelleher J, F.G., Cyrus P, Schwartz L, *A Randomized, Double-Blind, Multicenter, Parallel Group Trial Comparing the Safety and Efficacy of IGIV-Chromatography, 10% (Experimental) with IGIV-Solvent Detergent Treated, 10% (Control) in Patients with Primary Immune Deficiency (PID).* Bayer Report, 2000.
2. *Data on File.*
3. Bayever E, M.F., Sundaresan P, Collins S, *Randomized, Double-Blind, Multicenter, Repeat Dosing, Cross-Over Trial Comparing the Safety, Pharmacokinetics, and Clinical Outcomes of IGIV-Chromatography, 10% (Experimental) with IGIV-Solvent Detergent Treated, 10% (Control) in Patients with Primary Humoral Immune Deficiency (BAY-41-1000-100152).* MMRR-1512/1, 1999.
4. Lathia C, E.B., Sundaresan PR, Schwartz L, *A Randomized, Open-Label, Multicenter, Repeat Dosing, Cross-Over Trial Comparing the Safety, Pharmacokinetics, and Clinical Outcomes of IGIV-Chromatography, 5% with IGIV-Chromatography 10% in Patients with Primary Humoral Immune Deficiency (BAY-41-1000-100174).* 2000.
5. Blanchette, V.S., M.A. Kirby, and Turner, C. *Role of intravenous immunoglobulin G in autoimmune hematologic disorders.* Semin Hematol, 1992. 29(3 Suppl 2): p. 72–82.
6. Lazarus, A.H., Freedman, J. and Semple, J.W. *Intravenous immunoglobulin and anti-D in idiopathic thrombocytopenic purpura (ITP): mechanisms of action.* Transfus Sci, 1998. 19(3): p. 289–94.
7. Semple, J.W., A.H. Lazarus, and J. Freedman, *The cellular immunology associated with autoimmune thrombocytopenic purpura: an update.* Transfus Sci, 1998. 19(3): p. 245–51.
8. Imbach, P.A., *Harmful and beneficial antibodies in immune thrombocytopenic purpura.* Clin Exp Immunol, 1994. 97(Suppl 1): p. 25–30.
9. Bussel, J.B., *Fc receptor blockade and immune thrombocytopenic purpura.* Semin Hematol, 2000. 37(3): p. 261–6.
10. Imbach, P., et al., *Immunthrombocytopenic purpura as a model for pathogenesis and treatment of autoimmunity.* Eur J Pediatr, 1995. 154(9 Suppl 4): p. S60–4.
11. Cyrus P, F.G., Kelleher J, Schwartz L, *A Randomized, Double-Blind, Multicenter, Parallel Group Trial Comparing the Safety, and Efficacy of IGIV-Chromatography, 10% (Experimental) with IGIV-Solvent Detergent Treated, 10% (Control) in Patients with Idiopathic (Immune) Thrombocytopenic Purpura (ITP).* Bayer Report, 2000.
12. Wretlind, A., *Complete intravenous nutrition. Theoretical and experimental background.* Nutr Metab, 1972. 14: p. Suppl:1–57.
13. Hahn, R.G., H.P. Stalberg, and S.A. Gustafsson, *Intravenous infusion of irrigating fluids containing glycine or mannitol with and without ethanol.* J Urol, 1989. 142(4): p. 1102–5.
14. Tai VM, M.E., Lee-Brotherton V, Manley JJ, Nestmann ER, Daniels JM. *Safety Evaluation of Intravenous Glycine in Formulation Development. in J Pharm Pharmaceut Sci* (www.ualberta.ca/-csps). 2000.
15. Traul, K.A., et al., *Review of the toxicologic properties of medium-chain triglycerides.* Food Chem Toxicol, 2000. 38(1): p. 79–98.
16. Guyton, A., *Textbook of Medical Physiology. 5th Edition.* 1976, Philadelphia: W.B. Saunders. 499–500.
17. Ammann, A.J., et al., *Use of intravenous gamma-globulin in antibody immunodeficiency: results of a multicenter controlled trial.* Clin Immunol Immunopathol, 1982. 22(1): p. 60–7.
18. Buckley, R.H. and R.I. Schiff, *The use of intravenous immune globulin in immunodeficiency diseases.* N Engl J Med, 1991. 325(2): p. 110–7.
19. Cunningham-Rundles, C. and C. Bodian, *Common variable immunodeficiency: clinical and immunological features of 248 patients.* Clin Immunol, 1999. 92(1): p. 34–48.
20. Nolte, M.T., et al., *Intravenous immunoglobulin therapy for antibody deficiency.* Clin Exp Immunol, 1979. 36(2): p. 237–43.
21. Pruzanski, W., et al., *Relationship of the dose of intravenous gammaglobulin to the prevention of infections in adults with common variable immunodeficiency.* Inflammation, 1996. 20(4): p. 353–9.
22. Roifman, C.M., H. Levison, and E.W. Gelfand, *High-dose versus low-dose intravenous immunoglobulin in hypogammaglobulinaemia and chronic lung disease.* Lancet, 1987. 1(8541): p. 1075–7.
23. Sorensen, R.U. and S.H. Polmar, *Efficacy and safety of high-dose intravenous immune globulin therapy for antibody deficiency syndromes.* Am J Med, 1984. 76(3A): p. 83–90.
24. Stephan, J.L., et al., *Severe combined immunodeficiency: a retrospective single-center study of clinical presentation and outcome in 117 patients.* J Pediatr, 1993. 123(4): p. 564–72.
25. Cayco, A.V., M.A. Perazella, and J.P. Hayslett, *Renal insufficiency after intravenous immune globulin therapy: a report of two cases and an analysis of the literature.* J Am Soc Nephrol, 1997. 8(11): p. 1788–94.
26. Casteels-Van Daele, M., et al., *Intravenous immune globulin and acute aseptic meningitis [letter].* N Engl J Med, 1990. 323(9): p. 614–5.
27. Kato, E., et al., *Administration of immune globulin associated with aseptic meningitis [letter].* Jama, 1988. 259(22): p. 3269–71.
28. Scribner, C.L., et al., *Aseptic meningitis and intravenous immunoglobulin therapy [editorial; comment].* Ann Intern Med, 1994. 121(4): p. 305–6.
29. Winward, D.B. and M.T. Brophy, *Acute renal failure after administration of intravenous immunoglobulin: review of the literature and case report.* Pharmacotherapy, 1995. 15(6): p. 765–72.
30. Peerless, A.G. and E.R. Stiehm, *Intravenous gammaglobulin for reaction to intramuscular preparation [letter].* Lancet, 1983. 2(8347): p. 461.
31. Corporation, D.o.f.a.B.
32. Stangel, M.M., et al., *Side effects of intravenous immunoglobulins in neurological autoimmune disorders A prospective study.* J Neurol, 2003. 250(7): p. 818–21.
33. Ebeling, F., et al., *Tolerability and kinetics of a solvent-detergent-treated intravenous immunoglobulin preparation in hypogammaglobulinaemia patients.* Vox Sang, 1995. 69(2): p. 91–4.
34. Kelleher J, S.L., *IGIV-C 10% Rapid Infusion Trial in Idiopathic (Immune) Thrombocytopenic Purpura (ITP).* Bayer Report, 2001.
35. George, J.N., et al., *Idiopathic thrombocytopenic purpura: a practice guideline developed by explicit methods for the American Society of Hematology [see comments].* Blood, 1996. 88(1): p. 3–40.
36. Tan, E., et al., *Acute renal failure resulting from intravenous immunoglobulin therapy.* Arch Neurol, 1993. 50(2): p. 137–9.
37. Eijkhout, H.W., et al., *The effect of two different dosages of intravenous immunoglobulin on the incidence of recurrent infections in patients with primary hypogammaglobulinemia. A randomized, double-blind, multicenter crossover trial.* Ann Intern Med, 2001. 135(3): p. 165–74.

08759262 (Issued August 2003)

Bayer

Manufactured by:

Bayer Corporation

Pharmaceutical Division

Elkhart, IN 46515 USA

U.S. License No. 8

KOĀTE®-DVI ℞

[kō āte]

Antihemophilic Factor (Human)
Double Viral Inactivation
Solvent/Detergent Treated and Heated in Final Container at 80°C

DESCRIPTION

Antihemophilic Factor (Human), Koāte®-DVI, is a sterile, stable, purified, dried concentrate of human Antihemophilic Factor (AHF, factor VIII, AHG) which has been treated with tri-n-butyl phosphate (TNBP) and polysorbate 80 and heated in lyophilized form in the final container at 80°C for 72 hours. Koāte-DVI is intended for use in therapy of classical hemophilia (hemophilia A).

Koāte-DVI is purified from the cold insoluble fraction of pooled fresh-frozen plasma by modification and refinements of the methods first described by Hershgold, Pool, and Pappenhagen.[1] Koāte-DVI contains purified and concentrated factor VIII. The factor VIII is 300–1000 times purified over whole plasma. Part of the fractionation may be performed by another licensed manufacturer. When reconstituted as directed, Koāte-DVI contains approximately 50–150 times as much factor VIII as an equal volume of fresh plasma. The specific activity, after addition of Albumin (Human), is in the range of 9–22 IU/mg protein. **Koāte-DVI must be administered by the intravenous route.**

Each bottle of Koāte-DVI contains the labeled amount of antihemophilic factor activity in international units (IU). One IU, as defined by the World Health Organization standard for blood coagulation factor VIII, human, is approximately equal to the level of AHF found in 1.0 mL of fresh pooled human plasma. The final product when reconstituted as directed contains not more than (NMT) 1500 µg/mL polyethylene glycol (PEG), NMT 0.05 M glycine, NMT 25 µg/mL polysorbate 80, NMT 5 µg/g tri-n-butyl phosphate (TNBP), NMT 3 mM calcium, NMT 1 µg/mL aluminum, NMT 0.06 M histidine, and NMT 10 mg/mL Albumin (Human).

CLINICAL PHARMACOLOGY

Hemophilia A is a hereditary bleeding disorder characterized by deficient coagulant activity of the specific plasma protein clotting factor, factor VIII. In afflicted individuals, hemorrhages may occur spontaneously or after only minor trauma. Surgery on such individuals is not feasible without first correcting the clotting abnormality. The administration of Koāte-DVI provides an increase in plasma levels of factor VIII and can temporarily correct the coagulation defect in these patients.

After infusion of Antihemophilic Factor (Human), there is usually an instantaneous rise in the coagulant level followed by an initial rapid decrease in activity, and then a subsequent much slower rate of decrease in activity.[2–4] The early rapid phase may represent the time of equilibration with the extravascular compartment, and the second or slow phase of the survival curve presumably is the result of degradation and reflects the true biologic half-life of the infused Antihemophilic Factor (Human).[3]

The removal and inactivation of spiked relevant and model enveloped and non-enveloped viruses during the manufacturing process for Koāte-DVI have been validated in laboratory studies at Bayer Corporation. Studies performed with the model enveloped viruses indicated that the greatest reduction was achieved by TNBP/polysorbate 80 treatment and 80°C heat. For this reason, VSV (Vesicular Stomatitis Virus, model for RNA enveloped viruses) and HIV-1 (Human Immunodeficiency Virus Type 1) were studied only at these two steps of the manufacturing process. The efficacy of the dry heat treatment was studied using all of the viruses, including BVDV (Bovine Viral Diarrheal Virus, model for hepatitis C virus) and Reo (Reovirus Type 3, model for viruses resistant to physical and chemical agents, such as hepatitis A), and the effect of moisture content on the inactivation of HAV (Hepatitis A Virus), PPV (Porcine Parvovirus, model for parvovirus B19), and PRV (Pseudorabies Virus, model for hepatitis B virus) was investigated.

[See table I above]

Table I. Summary of In Vitro Log_{10}Viral Reduction Studies

	Enveloped Model Viruses				Non-enveloped Model Viruses		
	HIV-I	BVDV	PRV	VSV	Reo	HAV	PPV
Model for	HIV-1/2	HCV	HBV	RNA enveloped viruses	HAV and viruses resistant to chemical and physical agents	HAV	B19
Global Reduction Factor	9.4	10.3	9.5	10.9	9	4.5	3.7

Similar studies have shown that a terminal 80°C heat incubation for 72 hours inactivates non-lipid enveloped viruses such as hepatitis A and canine parvovirus in vitro, as well as lipid enveloped viruses such as hepatitis C.[7]

Koāte-DVI is purified by a gel permeation chromatography step serving the dual purpose of reducing the amount of TNBP and polysorbate 80 as well as increasing the purity of the factor VIII.

A two-stage clinical study using Koāte-DVI was performed in individuals with hemophilia A who had been previously treated with other plasma-derived AHF concentrates. In Stage I of the pharmacokinetic study with 19 individuals, statistical comparisons demonstrated that Koāte-DVI is bioequivalent to the unheated product, Koāte®-HP. The incremental in vivo recovery ten minutes after infusion of Koāte-DVI was 1.90% IU/kg (Koāte-HP 1.82% IU/kg). Mean biologic half-life of Koāte-DVI was 16.12 hours (Koāte-HP 16.13 hours). In Stage II of the study, participants received Koāte-DVI treatments for six months on home therapy with a median of 54 days (range 24–93). No evidence of inhibitor formation was observed, either in the clinical study or in the preclinical investigations.[2]

INDICATIONS AND USAGE

Koāte-DVI is indicated for the treatment of classical hemophilia (hemophilia A) in which there is a demonstrated deficiency of activity of the plasma clotting factor, factor VIII. Koāte-DVI provides a means of temporarily replacing the missing clotting factor in order to control or prevent bleeding episodes, or in order to perform emergency and elective surgery on individuals with hemophilia.

Koāte-DVI contains naturally occurring von Willebrand's factor, which is co-purified as part of the manufacturing process.

Koāte-DVI has not been investigated for efficacy in the treatment of von Willebrand's disease, and hence is not approved for such usage.

CONTRAINDICATIONS

None known.

WARNINGS

Koāte-DVI is made from human plasma. Products made from human plasma may contain infectious agents, such as viruses, that can cause disease. The risk that such products will transmit an infectious agent has been reduced by screening plasma donors for prior exposure to certain viruses, by testing for the presence of certain current virus infections, and by inactivating and/or removing certain viruses. Despite these measures, because this product is made from human blood, it may carry a risk of transmitting infectious agents, e.g., viruses, and theoretically the Creutzfeldt-Jakob disease (CJD) agent. There is also the possibility that unknown infectious agents may be present in such products. ALL infections thought by a physician possibly to have been transmitted by this product should be reported by the physician or other healthcare provider to Bayer Corporation [1-888-765-3203]. The physician should discuss the risks and benefits of this product with the patient, before prescribing or administering it to a patient.

Individuals who receive infusions of blood or plasma products may develop signs and/or symptoms of some viral infections, particularly hepatitis C. It is emphasized that hepatitis B vaccination is essential for patients with hemophilia and it is recommended that this be done at birth or diagnosis.[8,9] Hepatitis A vaccination is also recommended for hemophilic patients who are hepatitis A seronegative.

PRECAUTIONS

General

1. Koāte-DVI is intended for treatment of bleeding disorders arising from a deficiency in factor VIII. This deficiency should be proven prior to administering Koāte-DVI.
2. Administer within 3 hours after reconstitution. Do not refrigerate after reconstitution.
3. **Administer only by the intravenous route.**
4. Filter needle should be used prior to administering.
5. Koāte-DVI contains levels of blood group isoagglutinins which are not clinically significant when controlling relatively minor bleeding episodes. When large or frequently repeated doses are required, patients of blood groups A, B, or AB should be monitored by means of hematocrit for signs of progressive anemia, as well as by direct Coombs' tests.
6. Product administration and handling of the infusion set and needles must be done with caution. Percutaneous puncture with a needle contaminated with blood can transmit infectious viruses including HIV (AIDS) and hepatitis. Obtain immediate medical attention if injury occurs.

   Place needles in sharps container after single use. Discard all equipment including any reconstituted Koāte-DVI product in accordance with biohazard procedures.

Pregnancy Category C

Animal reproduction studies have not been conducted with Koāte-DVI. It is also not known whether Koāte-DVI can cause fetal harm when administered to a pregnant woman or can affect reproduction capacity. Koāte-DVI should be given to a pregnant woman only if clearly needed.

Pediatric Use

Koāte-DVI has not been studied in pediatric patients. Koāte-HP, solvent/detergent treated Antihemophilic Factor (Human), has been used extensively in pediatric patients. Spontaneous adverse event reports with Koāte-HP for pediatric use were within the experience of those reports for adult use.

Information for Patient

Some viruses, such as parvovirus B19 or hepatitis A, are particularly difficult to remove or inactivate at this time. Parvovirus B19 most seriously affects pregnant women, or immune-compromised individuals.

Symptoms of parvovirus B19 infection include fever, drowsiness, chills and runny nose followed about 2 weeks later by a rash and joint pain. Evidence of hepatitis A may include several days to weeks of poor appetite, tiredness, and low-grade fever followed by nausea, vomiting, and pain in the belly. Dark urine and a yellowed complexion are also common symptoms. Patients should be encouraged to consult their physician if such symptoms appear.

ADVERSE REACTIONS

Allergic-type reactions may result from the administration of Antihemophilic Factor (Human) preparations.[10,11]

Ten adverse reactions related to 7 infusions were observed during a total of 1053 infusions performed during the clinical study of Koāte-DVI, for a frequency of 0.7% infusions associated with adverse reactions. All reactions were mild and included tingling in the arm, ear, and face, blurred vision, headache, nausea, stomach ache, and jittery feeling.[2]

DOSAGE AND ADMINISTRATION

Each bottle of Koāte-DVI has the AHF(H) content in international units per bottle stated on the label of the bottle. The reconstituted product must be administered intravenously by either direct syringe injection or drip infusion. The product must be administered within 3 hours after reconstitution.

General Approach to Treatment and Assessment of Treatment Efficacy

The dosages described below are presented as general guidance. It should be emphasized that the dosage of Koāte-DVI required for hemostasis must be individualized according to the needs of the patient, the severity of the deficiency, the severity of the hemorrhage, the presence of inhibitors, and the factor VIII level desired. It is often critical to follow the course of therapy with factor VIII level assays.

The clinical effect of Koāte-DVI is the most important element in evaluating the effectiveness of treatment. It may be necessary to administer more Koāte-DVI than would be estimated in order to attain satisfactory clinical results. If the calculated dose fails to attain the expected factor VIII levels, or if bleeding is not controlled after administration of the calculated dosage, the presence of a circulating inhibitor in the patient should be suspected. Its presence should be substantiated and the inhibitor level quantitated by appropriate laboratory tests.

When an inhibitor is present, the dosage requirement for AHF(H) is extremely variable and the dosage can be determined only by the clinical response. Some patients with low titer inhibitors, (10 Bethesda Units) can be successfully treated with factor VIII without a resultant anamnestic rise in inhibitor titer.[12] Factor VIII levels and clinical response to treatment must be assessed to insure adequate response. Use of alternative treatment products, such as Factor IX Complex concentrates, Antihemophilic Factor (Porcine) or Anti-Inhibitor Coagulant Complex, may be necessary for patients with high titer inhibitors. Immune tolerance therapy using repeated doses of FVIII concentrate administered frequently on a predetermined schedule may result in eradication of the FVIII inhibitor.[13,14] Most successful regimens have employed high doses of FVIII administered at least once daily, but no single dosage regimen has been universally accepted as the most effective. Consultation with a hemophilia expert experienced with the management of immune tolerance regimens is also advisable.

Calculation of Dosage

The in vivo percent elevation in factor VIII level can be estimated by multiplying the dose of AHF(H) per kilogram of body weight (IU/kg) by 2%. This method of calculation is based on clinical findings by Abildgaard et al,[15] and is illustrated in the following examples:

[See table at top of next page]

The dosage necessary to achieve hemostasis depends upon the type and severity of the bleeding episode, according to the following general guidelines:

Mild Hemorrhage

Mild superficial or early hemorrhages may respond to a single dose of 10 IU per kg,[16] leading to an in vivo rise of approximately 20% in the factor VIII level. Therapy need not be repeated unless there is evidence of further bleeding.

Moderate Hemorrhage

For more serious bleeding episodes (e.g., definite hemarthroses, known trauma), the factor VIII level should be raised to 30%–50% by administering approximately 15–25 IU per kg. If further therapy is required, repeated doses of 10–15 IU per kg every 8–12 hours may be given.[17]

Severe Hemorrhage

In patients with life-threatening bleeding or possible hemorrhage involving vital structures (e.g., central nervous system, retropharyngeal and retroperitoneal spaces, iliopsoas sheath), the factor VIII level should be raised to 80%–100% of normal in order to achieve hemostasis. This may be achieved in most patients with an initial AHF [Antihemophilic Factor (Human), Koāte®-DVI] dose of 40–50 IU per kg and a maintenance dose of 20–25 IU per kg every 8–12

Continued on next page

Koāte-DVI—Cont.

hours.[18,19] For major surgical procedures, Factor VIII levels should be checked throughout the perioperative course to ensure adequate replacement therapy.

Surgery

For major surgical procedures, the factor VIII level should be raised to approximately 100% by giving a preoperative dose of 50 IU/kg. The factor VIII level should be checked to assure that the expected level is achieved before the patient goes to surgery. In order to maintain hemostatic levels, repeat infusions may be necessary every 6 to 12 hours initially, and for a total of 10 to 14 days until healing is complete. The intensity of factor VIII replacement therapy required depends on the type of surgery and postoperative regimen employed. For minor surgical procedures, less intensive treatment schedules may provide adequate hemostasis.[18,19]

Prophylaxis

Factor VIII concentrates may also be administered on a regular schedule for prophylaxis of bleeding, as reported by Nilsson et al.[20]

Incorrect diagnosis, inappropriate dosage, method of administration, and biological differences in individual patients, could reduce the efficacy of this product or even result in an ill effect following its use. It is important that this product be stored properly, the directions for use be followed carefully during use, the risk of transmitting viruses be carefully weighed before the product is prescribed, and that plasma factor VIII levels be measured in initial treatment situations or if clinical response appears inadequate.

Reconstitution

Vacuum Transfer

Note: Aseptic technique should be carefully followed. All needles and vial tops that will come into contact with the product to be administered via the intravenous route should not come in contact with any non-sterile surface. Any contaminated needles should be discarded by placing in a puncture proof container, and new equipment should be used.

1. After removing all items from the box, warm the sterile water (diluent) to room temperature (25°C, 77°F).
2. Remove shrink band from product vial.
3. Remove the plastic flip tops from each vial (Fig. A). Cleanse vial tops (grey stoppers) with alcohol swab and allow surface to dry. After cleaning, do not allow anything to touch the latex (rubber) stopper.
4. Carefully remove the plastic sheath from the short end of the transfer needle. Insert the exposed needle into the diluent vial to the hub. (Fig. B)
5. Carefully grip the sheath of the other end of the transfer needle and twist to remove it.
6. Invert the diluent vial and insert the attached needle into the vial of concentrate at a 45° angle (Fig. C). This will direct the stream of diluent against the wall of the concentrate vial and minimize foaming. The vacuum will draw the diluent into the concentrate vial.**
7. Remove the diluent bottle and transfer needle (Fig. D).
8. Immediately after adding the diluent, agitate vigorously for 10–15 seconds, (Fig. E1) then swirl continuously until completely dissolved (Fig. E2). Some foaming will occur, but attempt to avoid excessive foaming. The vial should then be visually inspected for particulate matter and discoloration prior to administration.
9. Clean the top of the vial of reconstituted Koate-DVI again with alcohol swab and let surface dry.
10. Attach the filter needle (from the package) to a sterile syringe. Withdraw the Koate-DVI solution into the syringe through the filter needle (Fig. F).
11. Remove the filter needle from the syringe and replace with an appropriate injection or butterfly needle for administration. Discard filter needle into a puncture proof container.
12. If the same patient is using more than one vial of Koate-DVI, the contents of multiple vials may be drawn into the same syringe through the filter needles provided.

**If vacuum is lost in the concentrate vial, use a sterile syringe and needle to remove the sterile water from the diluent vial and inject it into the concentrate vial, directing the stream of fluid against the wall of the vial.

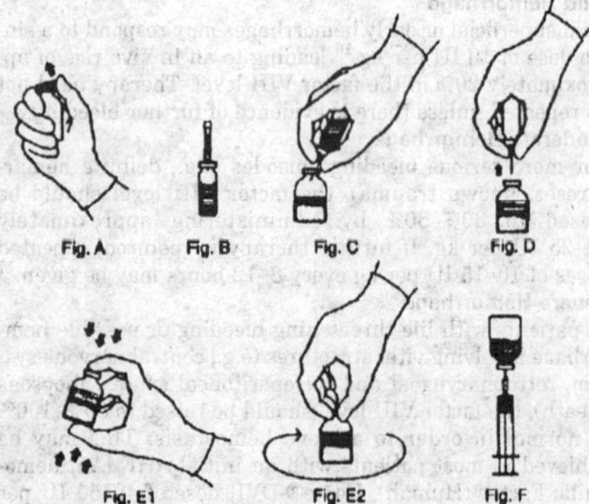

A number of factors beyond our control could reduce the efficacy of this product or even result in an ill effect following

$$\text{Expected \% factor VIII increase} = \frac{\text{\# units administered} \times 2\%/\text{IU/kg}}{\text{body weight (kg)}}$$

$$\text{Example for a 70 kg adult: } \frac{1400 \text{ IU} \times 2\%/\text{IU/kg}}{70 \text{ kg}} = 40\%$$

or

$$\text{Dosage required (IU)} = \frac{\text{body weight (kg)} \times \text{desired \% factor VIII increase}}{2\%/\text{IU/kg}}$$

$$\text{Example for a 15 kg child: } \frac{15 \text{ kg} \times 100\%}{2\%/\text{IU/kg}} = 750 \text{ IU required}$$

its use. These include improper storage and handling of the product after it leaves our hands, diagnosis, dosage, method of administration, and biological differences in individual patients. Because of these factors, it is important that this product be stored properly, that the directions be followed carefully during use, and that the risk of transmitting viruses be carefully weighed before the product is prescribed.

Rate of Administration

The rate of administration should be adapted to the response of the individual patient, but administration of the entire dose in 5 to 10 minutes is generally well-tolerated.

Parenteral drug products should be inspected visually for particulate matter and discoloration prior to administration, whenever solution and container permit.

HOW SUPPLIED

Koāte-DVI is supplied in the following single dose bottles with the total units of factor VIII activity stated on the label of each bottle. A suitable volume of Sterile Water for Injection, USP, a sterile double-ended transfer needle, a sterile filter needle, and a sterile administration set are provided.

NDC Number	Approximate Factor VIII Activity	Diluent
0026-0665-20	250 IU	5 mL
0026-0665-30	500 IU	5 mL
0026-0665-50	1000 IU	10 mL

STORAGE

Koāte-DVI should be stored under refrigeration (2–8°C; 36–46°F). Storage of lyophilized powder at room temperature (up to 25°C or 77°F) for 6 months, such as in home treatment situations, may be done without loss of factor VIII activity. Freezing should be avoided as breakage of the diluent bottle might occur.

CAUTION

℞ only

U.S. federal law prohibits dispensing without prescription.

REFERENCES

1. Hershgold EJ, Pool JG, Pappenhagen AR: The potent antihemophilic globulin concentrate derived from a cold insoluble fraction of human plasma: characterization and further data on preparation and clinical trial. *J Lab Clin Med* 67(1):23–32, 1966.
2. Data on file at Bayer Corporation.
3. Aronson DL: Factor VIII (antihemophilic globulin). *Semin Thromb Hemostas* 6(1):12–27, 1979.
4. Britton M, Harrison J, Abildgaard CF: Early treatment of hemophilic hemarthroses with minimal dose of new factor VIII concentrate. *J Pediatr* 85(2):245–7, 1974.
5. Winkelman L., Feldman PA, Evan DR: Severe heat treatment of lyophilised coagulation factors in Virus Inactivation in Plasma Products. *Curr Stud Hematol Blood Transfus.* Morgenthaler J-J (ed.), Basel, Karger, 1989, No. 56, pp. 55–69.
6. Skidmore SJ, Pasi KJ, Mawson SJ, et al: Serological evidence that dry heating of clotting factor concentrates prevents transmission of non-A, non-B hepatitis. *J. Med Virol.* 30(1):50–2, 1990.
7. Hart HF, Hart WG, Crossley J, et al: Effect of terminal (dry) heat treatment on non-enveloped viruses in coagulation factor concentrates. *Vox Sang* 67(4):345–50, 1994.
8. National Hemophilia Foundation Medical and Scientific Advisory Council. Hemophilia Information Exchange–AIDS Update: Recommendations concerning AIDS and the treatment of hemophilia HIV infection. Section I.G. (Rev. Jan., 1988).
9. Safety of therapeutic products used for hemophilia patients. *MMWR* 37(29):441–4, 449–50, 1988.
10. Eyster ME, Bowman HS, Haverstick JN: Adverse reactions to factor VIII infusions. [letter] *Ann Intern Med* 87(2):248, 1977.
11. Prager D, Djerassi I, Eyster ME, et al: Pennsylvania state-wide hemophilia program: summary of immediate reactions with the use of factor VIII and factor IX concentrate. *Blood* 53(5):1012–3, 1979.
12. Kasper CK: Complications of hemophilia A treatment: factor VIII inhibitors. *Ann NY Acad Sci* 614:97–105, 1991.
13. Mariani G, Hilgartner M, Thompson AR, et al: Immune Tolerance to Factor VIII: International Registry Data. *Adv Exp Med Biol* 386:201–8, 1995.
14. DiMichele D: Hemophilia 1996, New Approach to an Old Disease. *Pediatr Clin North Am* 43(3):709–35, Jun 1995.
15. Abildgaard CF, Simone JV, Corrigan JJ, et al: Treatment of hemophilia with glycine-precipitated factor VIII. *N Engl J Med* 275(9):471–5, 1966.
16. Britton M, Harrison J, Abildgaard CF: Early treatment of hemophilic hemarthroses with minimal dose of new factor VIII concentrate. *J Pediatr* 85(2):245–7, 1974.
17. Abildgaard CF: Current concepts in the management of hemophilia. *Semin Hematol* 12(3):223–32, 1975.
18. Hilgartner MW: Factor replacement therapy. In: Hilgartner MW, Pochedly C, eds.: Hemophilia in the child and adult. New York, Raven Press, 1989, pp 1–26.
19. Kasper CK, Dietrich SL: Comprehensive management of haemophilia. *Clin Haematol* 14(2):489–512, 1985.
20. Nilsson IM, Berntorp E, Löfqvist T, et al: Twenty-five years' experience of prophylactic treatment in severe haemophilia A and B. *J Intern Med* 232(1):25–32, 1992.

Bayer
Bayer Corporation
Pharmaceutical Division
Elkhart, IN 46515 USA
U.S. License No. 8 08848621
Printed in the USA. (Rev. April 2003)

KOGENATE® FS ℞

[kō'jĕn-āt]

Antihemophilic Factor (Recombinant)
Formulated with Sucrose

DESCRIPTION

Kogenate® FS Antihemophilic Factor (Recombinant) is a sterile, stable, purified, nonpyrogenic, dried concentrate that has been manufactured using recombinant DNA technology. Kogenate FS is intended for use in the treatment of classical hemophilia (hemophilia A), and is produced by Baby Hamster Kidney (BHK) cells into which the human factor VIII (FVIII) gene has been introduced.[1] The cell culture medium contains Human Plasma Protein Solution (HPPS) and recombinant insulin, but does not contain any proteins derived from animal sources. Kogenate FS is a highly purified glycoprotein consisting of multiple peptides including an 80 kD and various extensions of the 90 kD subunit. It has the same biological activity as FVIII derived from human plasma. Compared to its predecessor product KOGENATE® Antihemophilic Factor (Recombinant), Kogenate FS incorporates a revised purification and formulation process that eliminates the addition of Albumin (Human).

The purification process includes an effective solvent/detergent virus inactivation step in addition to the use of the classical purification methods of ion exchange chromatography, monoclonal antibody immunoaffinity chromatography, along with other chromatographic steps designed to purify recombinant FVIII and remove contaminating substances. Kogenate FS is formulated with sucrose (0.9–1.3%), glycine (21–25 mg/mL), and histidine (18–23 mM) as stabilizers in the final container in place of Albumin (Human) as used in KOGENATE, and is then lyophilized. The final product also contains calcium chloride (2–3 mM), sodium (27–36 mEq/L), chloride (32–40 mEq/L), polysorbate 80 (not more than [NMT] 96 µg/mL), imidazole (NMT 20 µg/1000 IU), tri-n-butyl phosphate (NMT 5 µg/1000 IU), and copper (NMT 0.6 µg/1000 IU). The product contains no preservatives. The amount of sucrose in each vial is 28 mg. Intravenous administration of sucrose contained in Kogenate FS will not affect blood glucose levels.

Each vial of Kogenate FS contains the labeled amount of recombinant FVIII in international units (IU). One IU, as defined by the World Health Organization standard for blood coagulation FVIII, human, is approximately equal to the level of FVIII activity found in 1 mL of fresh pooled human plasma.

Kogenate FS must be administered by the intravenous route.

CLINICAL PHARMACOLOGY

Pharmacokinetic studies were conducted in 20 patients with severe hemophilia A in North America. In this comparative pharmacokinetic study, Kogenate® FS Antihemophilic Factor (Recombinant) was shown to be similar to its predecessor product KOGENATE® Antihemophilic Factor (Recombinant) (rFVIII). Mean FVIII recovery measured 10 minutes following infusion was 2.1 ± 0.3 %/IU/kg for Kogenate FS and 2.4 ± 0.7 %/IU/kg for KOGENATE. The two recoveries were not statistically different (confidence interval 0.815–1.01). The mean biological half-life of recombinant FVIII formulated with sucrose (rFVIII-FS) is similar to KOGENATE with a mean of approximately 13 hours, which has previously been shown to be similar to plasma-derived Antihemophilic Factor (AHF). The activated partial thromboplastin time shortened appropriately with both rFVIII and rFVIII-FS. The recovery and half-life data for rFVIII-FS were unchanged after 24 weeks of exclusive treatment indicating continued efficacy and no evidence of FVIII inhibition. The mean FVIII recovery measured 10 minutes following a dose of rFVIII-FS in 37 patients (after 24 weeks of treatment with rFVIII-FS) was 2.1%/IU/kg, which was unchanged from FVIII recovery determined at baseline and at weeks 4 and 12.

Seventy-one patients with severe hemophilia A, ages 12–59, who had been previously treated with other recombinant and with plasma-derived AHF products, were enrolled in 6-month studies of home therapy with rFVIII-FS in Europe and North America. A total of 3995 infusions have been administered under this portion of the study, or 7.4 million units of rFVIII-FS. Treatment of 659 bleeding episodes during the study period required 951 infusions of rFVIII-FS. The majority of bleeding episodes (89.5%) were treated successfully with one or two infusions, using a mean dosage of approximately 28 IU/kg per treatment infusion. Regularly scheduled treatment accounted for 76% of infusions administered on study. Nine patients have received rFVIII-FS on 11 occasions for surgical procedures. The procedures included removal of a brain tumor, two total knee replacements, two joint synovectomies (one with Achilles tendon lengthening), two circumcisions, a hernia repair, and three teeth extractions. Hemostasis was satisfactory in all cases.
In clinical studies, Kogenate FS has been used in the treatment of bleeding episodes in previously untreated patients (PUPs) and minimally treated (MTP) pediatric patients. In ongoing studies, 61 PUPs/MTPs have been treated with Kogenate FS. Bleeding episodes were treated effectively with one or two infusions of rFVIII-FS. Ten patients have developed inhibitors. In these trials, approximately half of the patients have achieved 20 or more exposure days, and the incidence of inhibitor formation (16%) is consistent with that observed in other pediatric studies using plasma-derived and recombinant factor VIII products.[2–5]

INDICATIONS AND USAGE

Kogenate FS is indicated for the treatment of classical hemophilia (hemophilia A) in which there is a demonstrated deficiency of activity of the plasma clotting factor FVIII. Kogenate FS provides a means of temporarily replacing the missing clotting factor in order to correct or prevent bleeding episodes, or in order to perform emergency or elective surgery in hemophiliacs.
In clinical studies with the predecessor product KOGENATE, some patients who developed inhibitors on study continued to manifest a clinical response when inhibitor titers were less than 10 Bethesda Units (BU) per mL. When an inhibitor is present, the dosage requirement for FVIII is variable. The dosage can be determined only by clinical response, and by monitoring circulating FVIII levels after treatment (see **DOSAGE AND ADMINISTRATION**).
Because Kogenate FS has similar biological activity to KOGENATE it can be used in the same manner.
Kogenate FS does not contain von Willebrand's factor and therefore is not indicated for the treatment of von Willebrand's disease.

CONTRAINDICATIONS

Known intolerance or allergic reactions to constituents of the preparation.
Known hypersensitivity to mouse or hamster protein may be a contraindication to the use of Kogenate FS.

WARNINGS

None.

PRECAUTIONS

General

Kogenate® FS Antihemophilic Factor (Recombinant) is intended for the treatment of bleeding disorders arising from a deficiency in FVIII. This deficiency should be proven prior to administering Kogenate FS.
The development of circulating neutralizing antibodies to FVIII may occur during the treatment of patients with hemophilia A. Inhibitor formation is especially common in young children with severe hemophilia during their first years of treatment, or in patients of any age who have received little previous treatment with FVIII. Nonetheless, inhibitor formation may occur at any time in the treatment of a patient with hemophilia A. Patients treated with any AHF preparation, including Kogenate FS, should be carefully monitored for the development of antibodies to FVIII by appropriate clinical observation and laboratory tests, according to the recommendation of the patient's hemophilia treatment center.
Among patients treated with antihemophilic factor concentrates, cases of hypotension, urticaria, and chest tightness in association with hypersensitivity reactions have been reported in the literature.[11–13] Very rare cases of allergic and anaphylactic reactions have been reported with the predecessor product KOGENATE® Antihemophilic Factor (Recombinant), particularly in very young patients or patients who have previously reacted to other FVIII concentrates (see ADVERSE REACTIONS—Post-marketing experience). Serious anaphylactic reactions require immediate emergency treatment with resuscitative measures such as the administration of epinephrine and oxygen.

Formation of Antibodies to Mouse and Hamster Protein

Assays to detect seroconversion to mouse and hamster protein were conducted on all patients in clinical studies. No patient has developed specific antibodies to these proteins after commencing study, and no animal protein associated serious allergic reactions have been observed with rFVIII-FS infusions. Although no such reactions were observed, patients should be made aware of the possibility of a hypersensitivity reaction to mouse and/or hamster protein, and alerted to the early signs of such a reaction (e.g., hives, localized or generalized urticaria, wheezing, and hypotension). Patients should be advised to discontinue use of the product and contact their physician if such symptoms occur.

$$\text{Expected \% factor VIII increase} = \frac{\text{\# units administered} \times 2\%/\text{IU/kg}}{\text{body weight (kg)}}$$

$$\text{Example for a 70 kg adult: } \frac{1400\ \text{IU} \times 2\%/\text{IU/kg}}{70\ \text{kg}} = 40\%$$

or

$$\text{Dosage required (IU)} = \frac{\text{body weight (kg)} \times \text{desired \% FVIII increase}}{2\%/\text{IU/kg}}$$

$$\text{Example for a 15 kg child: } \frac{15\ \text{kg} \times 100\%}{2\%/\text{IU/kg}} = 750\ \text{IU required}$$

Carcinogenesis, Mutagenesis, and Impairment of Fertility

In vitro evaluation of the mutagenic potential of rFVIII failed to demonstrate reverse mutation or chromosomal aberrations at doses substantially greater than the maximum expected clinical dose. In vivo evaluation of rFVIII in animals using doses ranging between 10 and 40 times the expected clinical maximum also indicated that rFVIII does not possess a mutagenic potential. Long-term investigations of carcinogenic potential in animals have not been performed.

Pediatric Use

Kogenate FS is appropriate for use in pediatric patients of all ages, including neonates, infants, children, and adolescents. Safety and efficacy studies have been performed in previously untreated and minimally treated pediatric patients (n = 62). Kogenate FS is similar to KOGENATE® Antihemophilic Factor (Recombinant) in its biological activity and may be used in pediatric patients in the same manner as KOGENATE.

Geriatric Use

Clinical studies with Kogenate FS did not include sufficient numbers of patients aged 65 and over to be able to determine whether they respond differently from younger patients. However, clinical experience with KOGENATE and other AHF products has not identified differences between the elderly and younger patients. As with any patient receiving Kogenate FS, dose selection for an elderly patient should be individualized.

Pregnancy Category C

Animal reproduction studies have not been conducted with Kogenate FS. It is also not known whether Kogenate FS can cause fetal harm when administered to a pregnant woman or affect reproduction capacity. Kogenate FS should be used during pregnancy and lactation only if clearly indicated.

ADVERSE REACTIONS

During the clinical studies conducted in previously treated patients (PTPs), 109 adverse events were reported in the course of 4160 infusions (2.6%). Only 13 events were reported by the investigator as at least remotely related to study drug. Another 7 events were nonassessable. Thus 20 events in 11 patients were considered to be either nonassessable or at least remotely related to Kogenate® FS Antihemophilic Factor (Recombinant) administration, for an incidence of 0.5% relative to the number of infusions administered. Events that were at least remotely drug-related included: local injection site reactions (2), dizziness (2), rash (2), unusual taste in the mouth (1), mild increase in blood pressure (1), pruritus (1), depersonalization (1), nausea (1), and rhinitis (1). No FVIII inhibitors have developed in the 72 PTPs with severe hemophilia A who have received Kogenate FS for a mean of 54 exposure days.
In clinical studies with previously untreated patients (PUPs) and minimally treated (MTP) pediatric patients, 18 adverse events were reported by the clinical investigators as at least possibly related to the study drug including the expected complication of inhibitor development in 8 patients (included in the 10 patients discussed under **CLINICAL PHARMACOLOGY**), a forearm bleed following venipuncture, constipation, adenopathy, rash, anemia and pallor in one inhibitor patient with gastroenteritis, and serous otitis media.

Post-marketing experience

The following events are principally derived from post-marketing experience and publications,[14] and accurate rate estimates are generally not possible. Among patients treated with its predecessor product KOGENATE® Antihemophilic Factor (Recombinant), very rare cases of serious allergic reactions and anaphylactic reactions have been reported, particularly in very young patients or patients who had previously reacted to other FVIII concentrates. Individual cases of hypotension have been very rarely reported. Rare cases of urticaria have also been reported. Although such serious reactions have not been reported with the use of Kogenate FS Antihemophilic Factor (Recombinant), Formulated with Sucrose, it is likely that these may also occur. Rare cases of dyspnea have been reported with Kogenate FS.

DOSAGE AND ADMINISTRATION

Each bottle of Kogenate FS has the rFVIII potency in international units stated on the label based on the one-stage assay methodology. The reconstituted product must be administered within 3 hours after reconstitution. It is recommended to use the administration set provided.

GENERAL APPROACH TO TREATMENT AND ASSESSMENT OF TREATMENT EFFICACY

The dosages described below are presented as general guidance. It should be emphasized that the dosage of Kogenate FS required for hemostasis must be individualized according to the needs of the patient, the severity of the deficiency, the severity of the hemorrhage, the presence of inhibitors, and the FVIII level desired. It is often critical to follow the course of therapy with FVIII level assays. The clinical effect of FVIII is the most important element in evaluating the effectiveness of treatment. It may be necessary to administer more FVIII than estimated in order to attain satisfactory clinical results. If the calculated dose fails to attain the expected FVIII levels, or if bleeding is not controlled after administration of the calculated dosage, the presence of a circulating inhibitor in the patient should be suspected. Its presence should be substantiated and the inhibitor level quantitated by appropriate laboratory tests. When an inhibitor is present, the dosage requirement for FVIII could be extremely variable among different patients, and the optimal treatment can be determined only by the clinical response.
Some patients with low-titer inhibitors (< 10 BU) can be successfully treated with FVIII preparations without a resultant anamnestic rise in inhibitor titer.[6] FVIII levels and clinical response to treatment must be assessed to insure adequate response. Use of alternative treatment products, such as Factor IX Complex concentrates, Antihemophilic Factor (Porcine), recombinant Factor VIIa or Anti-Inhibitor Coagulant Complex, may be necessary for patients with anamnestic responses to FVIII treatment and/or high-titer inhibitors.

Calculation of Dosage

The in vivo percent elevation in FVIII level can be estimated by multiplying the dose of Kogenate® FS Antihemophilic Factor (Recombinant) per kilogram of body weight (IU/kg) by 2% per IU per kg. This method of calculation is based on clinical findings with the use of plasma-derived and recombinant AHF products[7–9] and is illustrated in the following examples:
[See table above]
The dosage necessary to achieve hemostasis depends upon the type and severity of the bleeding episode, according to the following general guidelines:

Hemorrhagic event	Therapeutically necessary plasma level of FVIII activity	Dosage necessary to maintain the therapeutic plasma level
Minor hemorrhage (superficial, early hemorrhages, hemorrhages into joints)	20–40%	10–20 IU per kg Repeat dose if evidence of further bleeding.
Moderate to major hemorrhage (hemorrhages into muscles, hemorrhages into the oral cavity, definite hemarthroses, known trauma) **Surgery** (minor surgical procedures)	30–60%	15–30 IU per kg Repeat one dose at 12–24 hours if needed.
Major to life-threatening hemorrhage (intracranial, intraabdominal or intrathoracic hemorrhages, gastrointestinal bleeding, central nervous system bleeding, bleeding in the retropharyngeal or retroperitoneal spaces, or iliopsoas sheath) **Fractures** **Head trauma**	80–100%	Initial dose 40–50 IU per kg Repeat dose 20–25 IU per kg every 8–12 hours.
Surgery Major surgical procedures	~100%	Preoperative dose 50 IU/kg Verify ~100% activity prior to surgery. Repeat as necessary after 6 to 12 hours initially, and for 10 to 14 days until healing is complete.

Prophylaxis

AHF concentrates may also be administered on a regular schedule for prophylaxis of bleeding, as reported by Nilsson et al.[10]

Instructions for Use

Reconstitution, product administration, and handling of the administration set and needles must be done with caution. Percutaneous puncture with a needle contaminated with blood can transmit infectious viruses including HIV (AIDS)

Continued on next page

Kogenate FS—Cont.

and hepatitis. Obtain immediate medical attention if injury occurs. Place needles in a sharps container after single use. Discard all equipment, including any reconstituted Kogenate® FS Antihemophilic Factor (Recombinant) product, in accordance with biohazard procedures.

Reconstitution

Always wash your hands before performing the following procedures:

Vacuum Transfer

1. Warm the unopened diluent and the concentrate to a temperature not to exceed 37°C, 99°F.
2. After removing the plastic flip-top caps (Fig. A), aseptically cleanse the rubber stoppers of both bottles with alcohol, being careful not to handle the rubber stopper.
3. Remove the protective cover from *one end* of the plastic transfer needle cartridge and penetrate the stopper of the diluent bottle (Fig. B).
4. Remove the remaining portion of the *protective cover*, invert the diluent bottle and penetrate the rubber seal on the concentrate bottle (Fig. C) with the needle at an angle.
5. The vacuum will draw the diluent into the concentrate bottle. Hold the diluent bottle at an angle to the concentrate bottle in order to direct the jet of diluent against the wall of the concentrate bottle (Fig. C). Avoid excessive foaming. If the diluent does not get drawn into the bottle, there is insufficient vacuum and the product should not be used.
6. After removing the diluent bottle and transfer needle (Fig. D), swirl until completely dissolved without creating excessive foaming (Fig. E).
7. Re-swab top of reconstituted Kogenate FS bottle with alcohol. Allow the stopper to air dry.
8. After the concentrate powder is completely dissolved, withdraw solution into the syringe through the filter needle that is supplied in the package (Fig. F). Replace the filter needle with the administration set provided and inject intravenously. NOTE: Firmly grasp one or both wings to perform venipuncture; do not use the post-use needle shield for this purpose.
9. After infusion, lock post-use needle shield in place using one of the following methods:
   a) One-hand technique: Hold tubing in hand and advance needle shield with thumb and index finger until locked over needle tip (Fig. G).
   b) Two-hand technique: Hold wing stationary and slide needle shield forward with other hand until locked over needle tip (Fig. H).
10. If the same patient is to receive more than one bottle, the contents of two bottles may be drawn into the same syringe through a separate unused filter needle before attaching the vein needle.
11. Parenteral drug products should be inspected visually for particulate matter and discoloration prior to administration, whenever solution and container permit.

Rate of Administration

The rate of administration should be adapted to the response of the individual patient, but administration of the entire dose in 5 to 10 minutes or less is well tolerated.

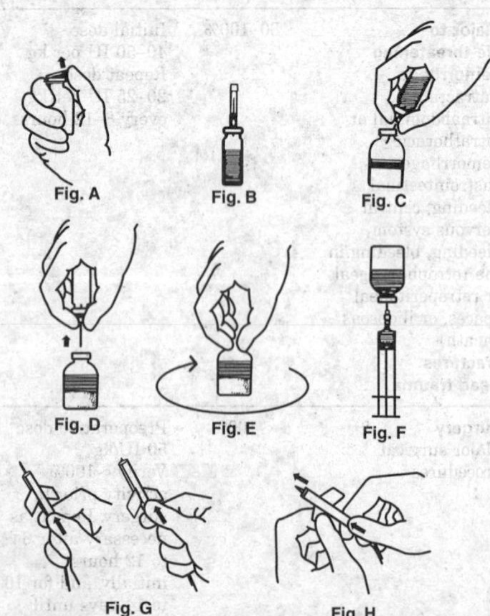

HOW SUPPLIED

Kogenate® FS Antihemophilic Factor (Recombinant) is supplied in the following single use bottles. A suitable volume of Sterile Water for Injection, USP, a sterile double-ended transfer needle, a sterile filter needle, and a sterile administration set are provided.

NDC Number	Approximate FVIII Activity (IU)	Diluent (mL)
0026-0372-20	250	2.5
0026-0372-30	500	2.5
0026-0372-50	1000	2.5

STORAGE

Kogenate FS should be stored under refrigeration (2–8°C; 36–46°F). Freezing must be avoided. Do not use beyond the expiration date indicated on the bottle. Protect from extreme exposure to light and store the lyophilized powder in the carton prior to use.

CAUTION

℞ only

U.S. federal law prohibits dispensing without prescription.

REFERENCES

1. Lawn RM, Vehar GA: The molecular genetics of hemophilia. *Sci Am* 254(3):48–54, 1986.
2. Scharrer I, Bray GL, Neutzling O: Incidence of inhibitors in haemophilia A patients — a review of recent studies of recombinant and plasma-derived factor VIII concentrates. *Haemophilia* 5(3):145–154, 1999.
3. Lusher JM, Arkin S, Abildgaard CF, et al: Recombinant factor VIII for the treatment of previously untreated patients with hemophilia A: safety, efficacy, and development of inhibitors. *N Engl J Med* 328(7):453–459, 1993.
4. Schwarzinger I, Pabinger I, Korninger C, et al: Incidence of inhibitors in patients with severe and moderate hemophilia A treated with factor VIII concentrates. *Am J Hematol* 24(3):241–5, 1987.
5. Ehrenforth S, Kreuz W, Scharrer I, et al: Incidence of development of factor VIII and factor IX inhibitors in hemophiliacs. *Lancet* 339(8793):594–8, 1992.
6. Kasper CK: Complications of hemophilia A treatment: factor VIII inhibitors. *Ann NY Acad Sci* 614:97–105, 1991.
7. Abildgaard CF, Simone JV, Corrigan JJ, et al: Treatment of hemophilia with glycine-precipitated Factor VIII. *N Engl J Med* 275(9):471–5, 1966.
8. Schwartz RS, Abildgaard CF, Aledort LM, et al: Human recombinant DNA-derived antihemophilic factor (factor VIII) in the treatment of hemophilia A. Recombinant Factor VIII Study Group. *N Engl J Med* 323(26):1800–5, 1990.
9. White GC 2nd, Courter S, Bray GL, et al: A multicenter study of recombinant factor VIII (Recombinate) in previously treated patients with hemophilia A. The Recombinate Previously Treated Patient Study Group. *Thromb Haemost* 77(4):660–667, 1997.
10. Nilsson IM, Berntorp E, Löfqvist T, et al: Twenty-five years' experience of prophylactic treatment in severe haemophilia A and B. *J Intern Med* 232(1):25–32, 1992.
11. Brettler DB, Forsberg AD, Levine PH, et al: The use of porcine factor VIII concentrate (Hyate:C) in the treatment of patients with inhibitor antibodies to factor VIII. A multicenter US experience. *Arch Intern Med* 149(6): 1381–5, 1989.
12. Eyster ME, Bowman HS, Haverstick JN: Adverse reactions to factor VIII infusions. *Ann Intern Med* 87(2):248, 1977.
13. Brettler DB, Levine PH: Factor concentrates for treatment of hemophilia: which one to choose? *Blood* 73(8): 2067–73, 1989.
14. Pernod G, Armari C, Barro C, et al: Anaphylaxis following the use of a plasma-derived immunopurified Monoclate-P®, and the recombinant Recombinate® and Kogenate® factor VIII: a therapeutic challenge. *Haemophilia* 5(2):143–4, 1999.

08888054-147378002 (Rev. Jan. 2004)

Bayer

Bayer Corporation
Pharmaceutical Division
Elkhart, IN 46515 USA
U.S. License No. 8

PLASBUMIN®-5 ℞

[*plăs-būmin*]

Albumin (Human) 5%, USP

DESCRIPTION

Albumin (Human) 5%, USP (Plasbumin®-5) is made from pooled human venous plasma using the Cohn cold ethanol fractionation process. Part of the fractionation may be performed by another licensed manufacturer. It is prepared in accordance with the applicable requirements established by the U.S. Food and Drug Administration.

Plasbumin-5 is a 5% sterile solution of albumin in an aqueous diluent. The preparation is stabilized with 0.004 M sodium caprylate and 0.004 M acetyltryptophan. The approximate sodium content of the product is 145 mEq/L. It contains no preservative. Plasbumin-5 must be administered intravenously.

Each vial of Plasbumin-5 is heat-treated at 60°C for 10 hours against the possibility of transmitting the hepatitis viruses.

CLINICAL PHARMACOLOGY

Plasbumin-5 is oncotically equivalent volume for volume to normal human plasma.

When administered intravenously to an adequately hydrated subject, the oncotic (colloid osmotic) effect of Plasbumin-5 is to expand the circulating blood volume by an amount approximately equal to the volume infused. It is primarily used in the treatment of shock associated with hemorrhage, surgery, trauma, burns, bacteremia, renal failure, and cardiovascular collapse.[1]

Albumin is a transport protein and it may be useful in severe jaundice in hemolytic disease of the newborn.[2] This could also be of importance in acute liver failure where albumin might serve the dual role of supporting plasma oncotic pressure, as well as binding excessive plasma bilirubin.[1]

INDICATIONS AND USAGE

Emergency Treatment of Hypovolemic Shock

Plasbumin-5 is iso-oncotic with normal plasma and on intravenous infusion will expand the circulating blood volume by an amount approximately equal to the volume infused. In conditions associated mainly with a volume deficit, albumin is best administered as a 5% solution (Plasbumin-5); but where there is an oncotic deficit, Albumin (Human) 25%, USP (Plasbumin®-25) may be preferred. This is also an important consideration where the treatment of the shock state has been delayed. If Plasbumin-25 is used, appropriate additional crystalloid should be administered.[1]

Crystalloid solutions in volumes several times greater than that of Plasbumin-5 may be effective in treating shock in younger individuals who have no preexisting illness at the time of the incident. Older patients, especially those with preexisting debilitating conditions, or those in whom the shock is caused by a medical disorder, or where the state of shock has existed for some time before active therapy could be instituted, may not tolerate hypoalbuminemia as well.[1]

Removal of ascitic fluid from a patient with cirrhosis may cause changes in cardiovascular function and even result in hypovolemic shock. In such circumstances, the use of albumin infusion may be required to support the blood volume.[1]

Burn Therapy

An optimal therapeutic regimen with respect to the administration of colloids, crystalloids, and water following extensive burns has not been established. During the first 24 hours after sustaining thermal injury, large volumes of crystalloids are infused to restore the depleted extracellular fluid volume. Beyond 24 hours, albumin can be used to maintain plasma colloid osmotic pressure. Plasbumin-25 may be preferred for this purpose.[1]

Cardiopulmonary Bypass[1]

With the relatively small priming volume required with modern pumps, preoperative dilution of the blood using albumin and crystalloid has been shown to be safe and well-tolerated. Although the limit to which the hematocrit and plasma protein concentration can be safely lowered has not been defined, it is common practice to adjust the albumin and crystalloid pump prime to achieve a hematocrit of 20% and a plasma albumin concentration of 2.5 g per 100 mL in the patient.

Acute Liver Failure[1]

In the uncommon situation of rapid loss of liver function, with or without coma, administration of albumin may serve the double purpose of supporting the colloid osmotic pressure of the plasma as well as binding excess plasma bilirubin.

Sequestration of Protein Rich Fluids[2]

This occurs in such conditions as acute peritonitis, pancreatitis, mediastinitis, and extensive cellulitis. The magnitude of loss into the third space may require treatment of reduced volume or oncotic activity with an infusion of albumin.

Situations in Which Albumin Administration is Not Warranted[1]

In chronic nephrosis, infused albumin is promptly excreted by the kidneys with no relief of the chronic edema or effect on the underlying renal lesion. It is of occasional use in the rapid "priming" diuresis of nephrosis. Similarly, in hypoproteinemic states associated with chronic cirrhosis, malabsorption, protein losing enteropathies, pancreatic insufficiency, and undernutrition, the infusion of albumin as a source of protein nutrition is not justified.

CONTRAINDICATIONS

Certain patients, e.g., those with a history of congestive cardiac failure, renal insufficiency or stabilized chronic anemia, are at special risk of developing circulatory overload. A history of allergic reaction to albumin is a specific contraindication for usage.

WARNINGS

Plasbumin-5 is made from human plasma. Products made from human plasma may contain infectious agents, such as viruses, that can cause disease. The risk that such products will transmit an infectious agent has been reduced by screening plasma donors for prior exposure to certain viruses, by testing for the presence of certain current virus infections, and by inactivating and/or removing certain viruses. Despite these measures, such products can still potentially transmit disease. There is also the possibility that unknown infectious agents may be present in such products. Individuals who receive infusions of blood or plasma products may develop signs and/or symptoms of some viral infections, particularly hepatitis C. ALL infections thought by a physician possibly to have been transmitted by this product should be reported by the physician or other healthcare provider to Bayer Corporation [1-800-288-8371].

The physician should discuss the risks and benefits of this product with the patient, before prescribing or administering it to the patient.

Solutions which have been frozen should not be used. Do not use if turbid. Do not begin administration more than 4 hours after the container has been entered. Partially used vials must be discarded. Vials which are cracked or which have been previously entered or damaged should not be used, as this may have allowed the entry of microorganisms. Plasbumin-5 contains no preservative.

PRECAUTIONS

General

Patients should always be monitored carefully in order to guard against the possibility of circulatory overload. Albumin (Human) 5%, USP (Plasbumin®-5) is iso-oncotic with normal plasma and will not tend to aggravate tissue dehydration. Appropriate additional crystalloids should be administered, if required by the patient, to maintain normal fluid balance.

In hemorrhage, the administration of albumin should be supplemented by the transfusion of whole blood to treat the relative anemia associated with hemodilution.[3] When circulating blood volume has been reduced, hemodilution following the administration of albumin persists for many hours. In patients with a normal blood volume, hemodilution lasts for a much shorter period.[4–6] The rapid rise in blood pressure, which may follow the administration of a colloid with positive oncotic activity, necessitates careful observation to detect and treat severed blood vessels which may not have bled at the lower blood pressure.

Drug Interactions

Plasbumin-5 is compatible with whole blood and packed red cells, as well as the standard carbohydrate and electrolyte solutions intended for intravenous use. It should not be mixed with protein hydrolysates, amino acid solutions nor those containing alcohol.

Pregnancy Category C

Animal reproduction studies have not been conducted with Plasbumin-5. It is also not known whether Plasbumin-5 can cause fetal harm when administered to a pregnant woman or can affect reproduction capacity. Plasbumin-5 should be given to a pregnant woman only if clearly needed.

Pediatric Use

Safety and effectiveness in the pediatric population have not been established.

ADVERSE REACTIONS

Adverse reactions to albumin are rare. Such reactions may be allergic in nature or be due to high plasma protein levels from excessive albumin administration. Allergic manifestations include urticaria, chills, fever, and changes in respiration, pulse and blood pressure.

DOSAGE AND ADMINISTRATION

Plasbumin-5 should always be administered by intravenous infusion. The choice between the use of Plasbumin-5 and Albumin (Human) 25%, USP (Plasbumin®-25) depends upon whether the patient requires primarily volume (Plasbumin-5) or primarily colloid osmotic activity (Plasbumin-25). Below a serum oncotic level of 20 mm Hg (equal to a total serum protein concentration of 5.2 g per 100 mL) there is evidence which suggests that the risk of complications increases.[1] When the oncotic pressure drops below this level, the patient should be treated with Plasbumin-25 together with diuretics. This is especially important in high risk patients who have undergone abdominal, cardiovascular, thoracic or urologic surgery or who have acute bacteremia.

The volume administered and the speed of administration should be adapted to the response of the individual patient. A number of factors beyond our control could reduce the efficacy of this product or even result in an ill effect following its use. These include improper storage and handling of the product after it leaves our hands, diagnosis, dosage, method of administration, and biological differences in individual patients. Because of these factors, it is important that this product be stored properly and that the directions be followed carefully during use.

Hypovolemic Shock

The volume infused should be related to the estimated volume deficit and the speed of administration adapted to the response of the patient.

In neonates or infants, Plasbumin-5 may be given in large amounts.[7] The recommended dose is 10 to 20 mL/kg equivalent to 0.5 to 1.0 g albumin/kg body weight.

Burns

After a burn injury (usually beyond 24 hours) there is a close correlation between the amount of albumin infused and the resultant increase in plasma colloid osmotic pressure. The aim should be to maintain the plasma albumin concentration in the region of 2.5 ± 0.5 g per 100 mL with a plasma oncotic pressure of 20 mm Hg (equivalent to a total plasma protein concentration of 5.2 g per 100 mL).[1] This is best achieved by the intravenous administration of Plasbumin, usually as Plasbumin-25. The duration of therapy is decided by the loss of protein from burned areas and in the urine. In addition, oral or parenteral feeding with amino acids should be initiated, as the long-term administration of albumin should not be considered as a source of nutrition.

Other dosage recommendations are given under the specific indications referred to above.

Preparation for Administration

Remove seal to expose stopper. Always swab stopper top immediately with suitable antiseptic prior to entering vial.

Parenteral drug products should be inspected visually for particulate matter and discoloration prior to administration, whenever solution and container permit.

Only 16 gauge needles or dispensing pins should be used with 20 mL vial sizes and larger. Needles or dispensing pins should only be inserted within the stopper area delineated by the raised ring. The stopper should be penetrated perpendicular to the plane of the stopper within the ring.

HOW SUPPLIED

Plasbumin-5 is available in 50 mL, 250 mL and 500 mL rubber-stoppered vials. Each single dose vial contains albumin in the following approximate amounts:

NDC Number	Size	Grams Protein
0026-0685-20	50 mL	2.5
0026-0685-25	250 mL	12.5
0026-0685-27	500 mL	25.0

STORAGE

Store at room temperature not exceeding 30°C (86°F). Do not freeze. Do not use after expiration date.

CAUTION

℞ only

U.S. federal law prohibits dispensing without prescription.

REFERENCES

1. Tullis JL: Albumin. 1. Background and use. 2. Guidelines for clinical use. *JAMA* 237:355–60; 460–3, 1977.
2. Clowes GHA Jr, Vucinic M, Weidner MG: Circulatory and metabolic alterations associated with survivial or death in peritonitis: clinical analysis of 25 cases. *Ann Surg* 163(6):866–85, 1966.
3. Heyl JT, Janeway CA: The use of human albumin in military medicine. I. The theoretical and experimental basis for its use. *US Navy Med Bull* 40:785–91, 1942.
4. Janeway CA, Gibson ST, Woodruff LM, et al: Chemical, clinical, and immunological studies on the products of human plasma fractionation. VII. Concentrated human serum albumin. *J Clin Invest* 23:465–90, 1944.
5. Woodruff LM, Gibson ST: The clinical evaluation of human albumin. *US Navy Med Bull* 40:791–6, 1942.
6. Janeway CA, Berenberg W, Hutchins G: Indications and uses of blood, blood derivatives and blood substitutes. *Med Clin North Am* 29:1069–94, 1945.
7. Bennett EJ: Fluid balance in the newborn. *Anesthesiology* 43:210–24, 1975.

Bayer Corporation
Pharmaceutical Division
Elkhart, IN 46515 USA
U.S. License No. 8
Printed in USA
08705812
(Rev. February 2002)

PLASBUMIN®-25 ℞

[*plăs -būmin*]

Albumin (Human) 25%, USP

DESCRIPTION

Albumin (Human) 25%, USP (Plasbumin®-25) is made from pooled human venous plasma using the Cohn cold ethanol fractionation process. Part of the fractionation may be performed by another licensed manufacturer. It is prepared in accordance with the applicable requirements established by the U.S. Food and Drug Administration.

Plasbumin-25 is a 25% sterile solution of albumin in an aqueous diluent. The preparation is stabilized with 0.02 M sodium caprylate and 0.02 M acetyltryptophan. The approximate sodium content of the product is 145 mEq/L. It contains no preservative. Plasbumin-25 must be administered intravenously.

Each vial of Plasbumin-25 is heat-treated at 60°C for 10 hours against the possibility of transmitting the hepatitis viruses.

CLINICAL PHARMACOLOGY

Each 20 mL vial of Plasbumin-25 supplies the oncotic equivalent of approximately 100 mL citrated plasma; 50 mL supplies the oncotic equivalent of approximately 250 mL citrated plasma.

When administered intravenously to an adequately hydrated subject, the oncotic (colloid osmotic) effect of 20 mL Plasbumin-25 is such that it will draw approximately a further 70 mL of fluid from the extravascular tissues into the circulation within 15 minutes,[1] thus increasing the total blood volume and reducing both hemoconcentration and whole blood viscosity. Accordingly, the main clinical indications are for hypoproteinemic states involving reduced oncotic pressure, with or without accompanying edema.[2] Plasbumin-25 can also be used as a plasma volume expander.

Albumin is a transport protein and it may be useful in severe hemolytic disease in the neonate who is awaiting exchange transfusion. The infused albumin may reduce the level of free bilirubin in the blood.[3]

This could also be of importance in acute liver failure where albumin might serve the dual role of supporting plasma oncotic pressure, as well as binding excessive plasma bilirubin.[2]

INDICATIONS AND USAGE

Emergency Treatment of Hypovolemic Shock

Plasbumin-25 is hyperoncotic and on intravenous infusion will expand the plasma volume by an additional amount, three to four times the volume actually administered, by withdrawing fluid from the interstitial spaces, provided the patient is normally hydrated interstitially or there is interstitial edema.[1] If the patient is dehydrated, additional crystalloids must be given,[4] or alternatively, Albumin (Human) 5%, USP (Plasbumin®-5) should be used. The patient's hemodynamic response should be monitored and the usual precautions against circulatory overload observed. The total dose should not exceed the level of albumin found in the normal individual, i.e., about 2 g per kg body weight in the absence of active bleeding. Although Plasbumin-5 is to be preferred for the usual volume deficits, Plasbumin-25 with appropriate crystalloids may offer therapeutic advantages in oncotic deficits or in long-standing shock where treatment has been delayed.[2]

Removal of ascitic fluid from a patient with cirrhosis may cause changes in cardiovascular function and even result in hypovolemic shock. In such circumstances, the use of an albumin infusion may be required to support the blood volume.[2]

Burn Therapy

An optimal therapeutic regimen with respect to the administration of colloids, crystalloids, and water following extensive burns has not been established. During the first 24 hours after sustaining thermal injury, large volumes of crystalloids are infused to restore the depleted extracellular fluid volume. Beyond 24 hours Plasbumin-25 can be used to maintain plasma colloid osmotic pressure.

Hypoproteinemia With or Without Edema

During major surgery, patients can lose over half of their circulating albumin with the attendant complications of oncotic deficit.[2,4,5] A similar situation can occur in sepsis or intensive care patients. Treatment with Plasbumin-25 may be of value in such cases.[2]

Adult Respiratory Distress Syndrome (ARDS)[2,5]

This is characterized by deficient oxygenation caused by pulmonary interstitial edema complicating shock and postsurgical conditions. When clinical signs are those of hypoproteinemia with a fluid volume overload, Plasbumin-25 together with a diuretic may play a role in therapy.

Cardiopulmonary Bypass[2,6]

With the relatively small priming volume required with modern pumps, preoperative dilution of the blood using albumin and crystalloid has been shown to be safe and well-tolerated. Although the limit to which the hematocrit and plasma protein concentration can be safely lowered has not been defined, it is common practice to adjust the albumin and crystalloid pump prime to achieve a hematocrit of 20% and a plasma albumin concentration of 2.5 g per 100 mL in the patient.

Acute Liver Failure[2]

In the uncommon situation of rapid loss of liver function with or without coma, administration of albumin may serve the double purpose of supporting the colloid osmotic pressure of the plasma as well as binding excess plasma bilirubin.

Neonatal Hemolytic Disease[2,3]

The administration of Plasbumin-25 may be indicated prior to exchange transfusion, in order to bind free bilirubin, thus lessening the risk of kernicterus. A dosage of 1 g/kg body weight is given about 1 hour prior to exchange transfusion. Caution must be observed in hypervolemic infants.

Sequestration of Protein Rich Fluids[7]

This occurs in such conditions as acute peritonitis, pancreatitis, mediastinitis, and extensive cellulitis. The magnitude of loss into the third space may require treatment of reduced volume or oncotic activity with an infusion of albumin.

Erythrocyte Resuspension[2]

Albumin may be required to avoid excessive hypoproteinemia, during certain types of exchange transfusion, or with the use of very large volumes of previously frozen or washed red cells. About 25 g of albumin per liter of erythrocytes is commonly used, although the requirements in preexistent hypoproteinemia or hepatic impairment can be greater. Plasbumin-25 is added to the isotonic suspension of washed red cells immediately prior to transfusion.

Acute Nephrosis[2]

Certain patients may not respond to cyclophosphamide or steroid therapy. The steroids may even aggravate the underlying edema. In this situation a loop diuretic and 100 mL Plasbumin-25 repeated daily for 7 to 10 days may be helpful in controlling the edema and the patient may then respond to steroid treatment.

Renal Dialysis[2]

Although not part of the regular regimen of renal dialysis, Plasbumin-25 may be of value in the treatment of shock or hypotension in these patients. The usual volume administered is about 100 mL, taking particular care to avoid fluid overload as these patients are often fluid overloaded and cannot tolerate substantial volumes of salt solution.

Situations in Which Albumin Administration is Not Warranted[2]

In chronic nephrosis, infused albumin is promptly excreted by the kidneys with no relief of the chronic edema or effect on the underlying renal lesion. It is of occasional use in the rapid "priming" diuresis of nephrosis. Similarly, in hypoproteinemic states associated with chronic cirrhosis, malabsorption, protein losing enteropathies, pancreatic insufficiency, and undernutrition, the infusion of albumin as a source of protein nutrition is not justified.

CONTRAINDICATIONS

Certain patients, e.g., those with a history of congestive cardiac failure, renal insufficiency or stabilized chronic anemia,

Continued on next page

Plasbumin-25—Cont.

are at special risk of developing circulatory overload. A history of an allergic reaction to albumin is a specific contraindication to usage.

WARNINGS

Plasbumin-25 is made from human plasma. Products made from human plasma may contain infectious agents, such as viruses, that can cause disease. The risk that such products will transmit an infectious agent has been reduced by screening plasma donors for prior exposure to certain viruses, by testing for the presence of certain current virus infections, and by inactivating and/or removing certain viruses. Despite these measures, such products can still potentially transmit disease. There is also the possibility that unknown infectious agents may be present in such products. Individuals who receive infusions of blood or plasma products may develop signs and/or symptoms of some viral infections, particularly hepatitis C. ALL infections thought by a physician possibly to have been transmitted by this product should be reported by the physician or other healthcare provider to Bayer Corporation [1-800-288-8371].

The physician should discuss the risks and benefits of this product with the patient, before prescribing or administering it to the patient.

As with any hyperoncotic protein solution likely to be administered in large volumes, severe hemolysis and acute renal failure may result from the inappropriate use of Sterile Water for Injection as a diluent for Albumin (Human), 25%. Acceptable diluents include 0.9% Sodium Chloride or 5% Dextrose in Water. Please refer to the **DOSAGE AND ADMINISTRATION** section for recommended diluents.

Solutions which have been frozen should not be used. Do not use if turbid. Do not begin administration more than 4 hours after the container has been entered. Partially used vials must be discarded. Vials which are cracked or which have been previously entered or damaged should not be used, as this may have allowed the entry of microorganisms. Albumin (Human) 25%, USP (Plasbumin®-25) contains no preservative.

PRECAUTIONS

General

Patients should always be monitored carefully in order to guard against the possibility of circulatory overload. Plasbumin-25 is hyperoncotic, therefore, in the presence of dehydration, albumin must be given with or followed by addition of fluids.[4]

In hemorrhage the administration of albumin should be supplemented by the transfusion of whole blood to treat the relative anemia associated with hemodilution.[8] When circulating blood volume has been reduced, hemodilution following the administration of albumin persists for many hours. In patients with a normal blood volume, hemodilution lasts for a much shorter period.[4,9,10]

The rapid rise in blood pressure which may follow the administration of a colloid with positive oncotic activity necessitates careful observation to detect and treat severed blood vessels which may not have bled at the lower blood pressure.

Drug Interactions

Plasbumin-25 is compatible with whole blood, packed red cells, as well as the standard carbohydrate and electrolyte solutions intended for intravenous use. It should, however, not be mixed with protein hydrolysates, amino acid solutions nor those containing alcohol.

Pregnancy Category C

Animal reproduction studies have not been conducted with Plasbumin-25. It is also not known whether Plasbumin-25 can cause fetal harm when administered to a pregnant woman or can affect reproduction capacity. Plasbumin-25 should be given to a pregnant woman only if clearly needed.

Pediatric Use

Safety and effectiveness in the pediatric population have not been established.

ADVERSE REACTIONS

Adverse reactions to albumin are rare. Such reactions may be allergic in nature or due to high plasma protein levels from excessive albumin administration. Allergic manifestations include urticaria, chills, fever, and changes in respiration, pulse and blood pressure.

DOSAGE AND ADMINISTRATION

Plasbumin-25 should always be administered by intravenous infusion. Plasbumin-25 may be administered either undiluted or diluted in 0.9% Sodium Chloride or 5% Dextrose in Water. If sodium restriction is required, Plasbumin-25 should only be administered either undiluted or diluted in a sodium-free carbohydrate solution such as 5% Dextrose in Water.

A number of factors beyond our control could reduce the efficacy of this product or even result in an ill effect following its use. These include improper storage and handling of the product after it leaves our hands, diagnosis, dosage, method of administration, and biological differences in individual patients. Because of these factors, it is important that this product be stored properly and that the directions be followed carefully during use.

Hypovolemic Shock—For treatment of hypovolemic shock, the volume administered and the speed of infusion should be adapted to the response of the individual patient.

Burns—After a burn injury (usually beyond 24 hours) there is a close correlation between the amount of albumin infused and the resultant increase in plasma colloid osmotic pressure. The aim should be to maintain the plasma albumin concentration in the region of 2.5 ± 0.5 g per 100 mL with a plasma oncotic pressure of 20 mm Hg (equivalent to a total plasma protein concentration of 5.2 g per 100 mL).[2] This is best achieved by the intravenous administration of Plasbumin-25. The duration of therapy is decided by the loss of protein from the burned areas and in the urine. In addition, oral or parenteral feeding with amino acids should be initiated, as the long-term administration of albumin should not be considered as a source of nutrition.

Hypoproteinemia With or Without Edema—Unless the underlying pathology responsible for the hypoproteinemia can be corrected, the intravenous administration of Plasbumin-25 must be considered purely symptomatic or supportive (see section **Situations in Which Albumin Administration is Not Warranted**).[2] The usual daily dose of albumin for adults is 50 to 75 g and for children 25 g. Patients with severe hypoproteinemia who continue to lose albumin may require larger quantities. Since hypoproteinemic patients usually have approximately normal blood volumes, the rate of administration of Plasbumin-25 should not exceed 2 mL per minute, as more rapid injection may precipitate circulatory embarrassment and pulmonary edema.

Other dosage recommendations are given under the specific indications referred to above.

Preparation for Administration

Remove seal to expose stopper. Always swab stopper top immediately with a suitable antiseptic prior to entering vial. Parenteral drug products should be inspected visually for particulate matter and discoloration prior to administration, whenever solution and container permit.

Only 16 gauge needles or dispensing pins should be used with 20 mL vial sizes and larger. Needles or dispensing pins should only be inserted within the stopper area delineated by the raised ring. The stopper should be penetrated perpendicular to the plane of the stopper within the ring.

HOW SUPPLIED

Plasbumin-25 is available in 20 mL, 50 mL, and 100 mL rubber-stoppered vials. Each single dose vial contains albumin in the following approximate amounts:

NDC Number	Size	Grams Protein
0026-0684-16	20 mL	5.0
0026-0684-20	50 mL	12.5
0026-0684-71	100 mL	25.0

STORAGE

Store at room temperature not exceeding 30°C (86°F). Do not freeze. Do not use after expiration date.

CAUTION

℞ only

U.S. federal law prohibits dispensing without prescription.

REFERENCES

1. Heyl JT, Gibson JG II, Janeway CA: Studies on the plasma proteins. V. The effect of concentrated solutions of human and bovine serum albumin on blood volume after acute blood loss in man. *J Clin Invest* 22:763–73, 1943.
2. Tullis JL: Albumin. 1. Background and use. 2. Guidelines for clinical use. *JAMA* 237:355–60; 460–3, 1977.
3. Comley A, Wood B: Albumin administration in exchange transfusion for hyperbilirubinaemia. *Arch Dis Child* 43: 151–4, 1968.
4. Janeway CA, Gibson ST, Woodruff LM, et al: Chemical, clinical, and immunological studies on the products of human plasma fractionation. VII. Concentrated human serum albumin. *J Clin Invest* 23:465–90, 1944.
5. Skillman JJ, Tanenbaum BJ: Unrecognized losses of albumin, plasma, and red cells during abdominal vascular operations. *Curr Top Surg Res* 2:523–33, 1970.
6. Zubiate P, Kay JH, Mendez AM, et al: Coronary artery surgery: a new technique with use of little blood, if any. *J Thorac Cardiovasc Surg* 68(2):263–7, 1974.
7. Clowes GHA Jr, Vucinic M, Weidner MG: Circulatory and metabolic alterations associated with survival or death in peritonitis: clinical analysis of 25 cases. *Ann Surg* 163:866–85, 1966.
8. Heyl JT, Janeway CA: The use of human albumin in military medicine. I. The theoretical and experimental basis for its use. *US Navy Med Bull* 40:785–91, 1942.
9. Woodruff LM, Gibson ST: The clinical evaluation of human albumin. *US Navy Med Bull* 40:791–6, 1942.
10. Janeway CA, Berenberg W, Hutchins G: Indications and uses of blood, blood derivatives and blood substitutes. *Med Clin North Am* 29:1069–94, 1945.

Bayer Corporation
Pharmaceutical Division
Elkhart, IN 46515 USA
U.S. License No. 8

08705898
Printed in USA (Rev. February 2002)

PLASMANATE® ℞

[*plăs'măn-ate*]

Plasma Protein Fraction (Human) 5%, USP

DESCRIPTION

This product has been prepared from large pools of human plasma. Each 100 mL of Plasma Protein Fraction (Human) 5%, USP—Plasmanate® contains 5 g selected plasma proteins buffered with sodium carbonate and stabilized with 0.004 M sodium caprylate and 0.004 M acetyltryptophan. The plasma proteins consist of approximately 88% normal human albumin, 12% alpha and beta globulins and not more than 1% gamma globulin as determined by electrophoresis.[1] The concentration of these proteins is such that this solution is iso-oncotic with normal human plasma and is isotonic. The approximate concentrations of the significant electrolytes in Plasmanate are: sodium 145 mEq/L, potassium 0.25 mEq/L, and chloride 100 mEq/L. Plasmanate must be administered intravenously.

This product is designed to bring to the medical profession a preparation derived from human blood and similar to human plasma. Each vial of Plasmanate is sterile and heat-treated at 60°C for 10 hours against the possibility of transmitting the hepatitis viruses.

The blood group agglutinins and agglutinogens A and B are at such a low level in Plasmanate solution that its use has no effect on routine blood typing procedures. No chemical or microscopic alterations of the urine have been observed with its use.

CLINICAL PHARMACOLOGY

In normal human volunteers, Plasmanate has resulted in an increased blood volume which has lasted up to 48 hours.[2] Clinical experience has indicated that it is an adequate replacement for human plasma in the treatment of shock and is a suitable means of providing human proteins for their osmotic effect.

INDICATIONS AND USAGE

Treatment of Shock—Plasmanate is indicated in the treatment of shock due to burns, crushing injuries, abdominal emergencies, and any other cause where there is a predominant loss of plasma fluids and not red blood cells. It is also effective in the emergency treatment of shock due to hemorrhage.[3,4] Following the emergency phase of therapy, blood transfusions may be indicated depending on the severity of the blood loss.

In infants and small children, Plasmanate has been found to be very useful in the initial therapy of shock due to dehydration and infection.

CONTRAINDICATIONS

Plasmanate is contraindicated for use in patients on cardiopulmonary bypass. Severe hypotension has been reported in such patients when given Plasma Protein Fraction.[4] Plasma Protein Fraction is contraindicated in patients with severe anemia, congestive heart failure, or increased blood volume.

WARNINGS

Plasmanate is made from human plasma. Products made from human plasma may contain infectious agents, such as viruses, that can cause disease. The risk that such products will transmit an infectious agent has been reduced by screening plasma donors for prior exposure to certain viruses, by testing for the presence of certain current virus infections, and by inactivating and/or removing certain viruses. Despite these measures, such products can still potentially transmit disease. There is also the possibility that unknown infectious agents may be present in such products. Individuals who receive infusions of blood or plasma products may develop signs and/or symptoms of some viral infections, particularly hepatitis C. ALL infections thought by a physician possibly to have been transmitted by this product should be reported by the physician or other healthcare provider to Bayer Corporation [1-800-288-8371].

The physician should discuss the risks and benefits of this product with the patient, before prescribing or administering it to the patient.

Solutions which are turbid or which have been frozen should not be used. Do not use if turbid. Do not begin administration more than 4 hours after the container has been entered. Partially used vials must be discarded. Vials which are cracked or which have been previously entered or damaged should not be used, as this may have allowed the entry of microorganisms. Plasmanate contains no preservative.

PRECAUTIONS

General

Rapid infusion of Plasmanate (greater than 10mL/minute) has produced hypotension in patients undergoing surgery or in the preoperative or postoperative period. Blood pressure should be monitored during use and infusion slowed or ceased if sudden hypotension occurs.

Plasmanate does not provide coagulation factors and therefore does not correct coagulation disorders.

Drug Interactions

Plasma Protein Fraction (Human) 5%, USP—Plasmanate® is compatible with whole blood, packed red cells as well as the standard carbohydrate and electrolyte solutions intended for intravenous use. It should, however, not be mixed with protein hydrolysates or solutions containing alcohol.

Pregnancy Category C

Animal reproduction studies have not been conducted with Plasmanate. It is also not known if Plasmanate can cause fetal harm when administered to a pregnant woman or can affect reproduction capacity. Plasmanate should be given to a pregnant woman only if clearly needed.

Pediatric Use

Safety and effectiveness in the pediatric population have not been established.

ADVERSE REACTIONS

Hypotension may occur, particularly following rapid infusion or intraarterial administration to patients on cardiopulmonary bypass. The blood pressure may normalize spontaneously after the slowing or discontinuation of the infusion. Vasopressors will also correct the hypotension.

Flushing, urticaria, back pain, nausea and headache have been occasionally reported by conscious patients.

DOSAGE AND ADMINISTRATION

Dosage is based almost entirely on the nature of the individual case and response to therapy. The usual minimum effective dose in adults is 250–500 mL. As with any plasma expander, the rate should be adjusted or slowed according to the clinical response and rising blood pressure.

Administration should be by vein and preferably through an area of skin at some distance from any site of infection or trauma. Plasmanate is compatible with the usual carbohydrate and electrolyte solutions.

We recommend the following procedure: First swab the stopper with Iodine Tincture, USP followed by a sterile antiseptic swab.

Parenteral drug products should be inspected visually for particulate matter and discoloration prior to administration, whenever solution and container permit.

Only 16 gauge needles or dispensing pins should be used with 20 mL vial sizes and larger. Needles or dispensing pins should only be inserted within the stopper area delineated by the raised ring. The stopper should be penetrated perpendicular to the plane of the stopper within the ring.

A number of factors beyond our control could reduce the efficacy of this product or even result in an ill effect following its use. These include improper storage and handling of the product after it leaves our hands, diagnosis, dosage, method of administration, and biological differences in individual patients. Because of these factors, it is important that this product be stored properly and that the directions be followed carefully during use.

HOW SUPPLIED

Plasmanate is available in 50 mL pediatric size, 250 mL and 500 mL rubber-stoppered vials. Each single dose vial contains plasma protein in the following approximate amounts:

NDC Number	Size	Grams Protein
0026-0613-20	50 mL	2.5
0026-0613-25	250 mL	12.5
0026-0613-27	500 mL	25.0

STORAGE

Store at room temperature not exceeding 30°C (86°F). Solution that has been frozen should not be used. Do not use after expiration date.

CAUTION

℞ only

U.S. federal law prohibits dispensing without prescription.

REFERENCES

1. Hink JH Jr, Hidalgo J, Seeberg VP, et al: Preparation and properties of a heat-treated human plasma protein fraction. *Vox Sang* 2:174–86, 1957.
2. Bertrand JJ, Feichtmeir TV, Kolomeyer N, et al: Clinical investigations with a heat-treated plasma protein fraction—Plasmanate® *Vox Sang* 4:385–402, 1959.
3. Tullis JL: Albumin. 1. Background and use. 2. Guidelines for clinical use. *JAMA* 237:355–60; 460–3, 1977.
4. Bland JHL, Laver MB, Lowenstein E: Vasodilator effect of commercial 5% plasma protein fraction solutions. *JAMA* 224:1721–4, 1973.

Bayer Corporation
Pharmaceutical Division
Elkhart, IN 46515 USA
U.S. License No. 8
Printed in USA
08705065
(Rev. February 2002)

PROLASTIN® ℞

[*prō-lăs-tĭn*]

Alpha$_1$–Proteinase Inhibitor (Human)

FOR INTRAVENOUS USE ONLY

DESCRIPTION

Alpha$_1$-Proteinase Inhibitor (Human), Prolastin® is a sterile, stable, lyophilized preparation of purified human Alpha$_1$-Proteinase Inhibitor (alpha$_1$-PI), also known as alpha$_1$-antitrypsin. Prolastin is intended for use in therapy of congenital alpha$_1$-antitrypsin deficiency.

Prolastin is prepared from pooled human plasma of normal donors by modification and refinements of the cold ethanol method of Cohn.[1] Part of the fractionation may be performed by another licensed manufacturer. In order to reduce the potential risk of transmission of infectious agents, Prolastin has been heat-treated in solution at 60±0.5°C for not less than 10 hours. However, no procedure has been found to be totally effective in removing viral infectivity from plasma fractionation products. *In vitro* studies designed to evaluate the capacity of the Prolastin manufacturing process to remove/inactivate viruses have been conducted to provide additional assurance of the viral safety profile as shown in the table below.

[See table above]

Process Step	Log$_{10}$ Virus Reduction					
	HIV-1*	BVDV**	PRV***	Reo†	HAV††	PPV‡
Fractionation of Effluent I to II + III	3.4	3.5	3.9	2.1	1.4	1.0
PEG Precipitation	4.4	3.2	3.4	3.4	3.1	3.3
Depth Filtration	≥4.7	4.1	≥4.7	≥4.0	≥2.8	≥4.3
Pasteurization	≥6.3	4.8	≥4.8	N/A	N/A	N/A
Accumulated Log$_{10}$ Reduction	≥18.8	15.6	≥16.8	≥9.5	≥7.3	≥8.6

* Human immunodeficiency virus, type 1
** Bovine viral diarrhea virus (BVDV) was chosen to model hepatitis C virus
*** Pseudorabies virus (PRV) was used as a surrogate for hepatitis B virus and the human herpes viruses
† Reovirus type 3 (Reo) was chosen to model non-enveloped viruses
†† Human hepatitis A virus (HAV).
‡ Porcine parvovirus (PPV) was selected as a surrogate for human parvovirus B19

The specific activity of Prolastin is ≥0.35 mg functional alpha$_1$-PI/mg protein and when reconstituted as directed, the concentration of alpha$_1$-PI is ≥20 mg/mL. When reconstituted, Prolastin has a pH of 6.6–7.4, a sodium content of 100–210 mEq/L, a chloride content of 60–180 mEq/L, a sodium phosphate content of 0.015–0.025 M, a polyethylene glycol content of not more than (NMT) 5 ppm, and NMT 0.1% sucrose. Prolastin contains small amounts of other plasma proteins including alpha$_2$-plasmin inhibitor, alpha$_1$-antichymotrypsin, C_1-esterase inhibitor, haptoglobin, antithrombin III, alpha$_1$-lipoprotein, albumin, and IgA.[1]

Each vial of Prolastin contains the labeled amount of functionally active alpha$_1$-PI in milligrams per vial (mg/vial), as determined by capacity to neutralize porcine pancreatic elastase.[1] Prolastin contains no preservative and must be administered by the intravenous route.

CLINICAL PHARMACOLOGY

Alpha$_1$-antitrypsin deficiency is a chronic, hereditary, usually fatal, autosomal recessive disorder in which a low concentration of alpha$_1$-PI (alpha$_1$-antitrypsin) is associated with slowly progressive, severe panacinar emphysema that most often manifests itself in the third to fourth decades of life.[2–9] [Although the terms "Alpha$_1$-Proteinase Inhibitor" and "alpha$_1$-antitrypsin" are used interchangeably in the scientific literature, the hereditary disorder associated with a reduction in the serum level of alpha$_1$-PI is conventionally referred to as "alpha$_1$-antitrypsin deficiency" while the deficient protein is referred to as "Alpha$_1$-Proteinase Inhibitor"[10]]. The emphysema is typically worse in the lower lung zones.[4,8,9] The pathogenesis of development of emphysema in alpha$_1$-antitrypsin deficiency is not well understood at this time. It is believed, however, to be due to a chronic biochemical imbalance between elastase (an enzyme capable of degrading elastin tissues, released by inflammatory cells, primarily neutrophils, in the lower respiratory tract) and alpha$_1$-PI (the principal inhibitor of neutrophil elastase), which is deficient in alpha$_1$-antitrypsin disease.[11–15] As a result, it is believed that alveolar structures are unprotected from chronic exposure to elastase released from a chronic, low-level burden of neutrophils in the lower respiratory tract, resulting in progressive degradation of elastin tissues.[11–15] The eventual outcome is the development of emphysema. Neonatal hepatitis with cholestatic jaundice appears in approximately 10% of newborns with alpha$_1$-antitrypsin deficiency.[15] In some adults, alpha$_1$-antitrypsin deficiency is complicated by cirrhosis.[15]

A large number of phenotypic variants of alpha$_1$-antitrypsin deficiency exists.[15] The most severely affected individuals are those with the PiZZ variant, typically characterized by alpha$_1$-PI serum levels <35% normal.[15] Epidemiologic studies of individuals with various phenotypes of alpha$_1$-antitrypsin deficiency have demonstrated that individuals with endogenous serum levels of alpha$_1$-PI ≤50 mg/dL (based on commercial standards) have a risk of >80% of developing emphysema over a lifetime.[3–6,8,9,16] However, individuals with endogenous alpha$_1$-PI levels >80 mg/dL, in general, do not manifest an increased risk for development of emphysema above the general population background risk.[5,15] From these observations, it is believed that the "threshold" level of alpha$_1$-PI in the serum required to provide adequate anti-elastase activity in the lung of individuals with alpha$_1$-antitrypsin deficiency is about 80 mg/dL (based on commercial standards for immunologic assay of alpha$_1$-PI).[12,15,17]

In clinical studies of Alpha$_1$-Proteinase Inhibitor (Human), Prolastin®, 23 subjects with the PiZZ variant of congenital deficiency of alpha$_1$-antitrypsin deficiency and documented destructive lung disease participated in a study of acute and/or chronic replacement therapy with Prolastin.[18] The mean in vivo recovery of alpha$_1$-PI was 4.2 mg (immunologic)/dL per mg (functional)/kg body weight administered.[18,19] The half-life of alpha$_1$-PI in vivo was approximately 4.5 days.[18,19] Based on these observations, a program of chronic replacement therapy was developed. Nineteen of the subjects in these studies received Prolastin replacement therapy, 60 mg/kg body weight, once weekly for up to 26 weeks (average 24 weeks of therapy). With this schedule of replacement therapy, blood levels of alpha$_1$-PI were maintained above 80 mg/dL (based on the commercial standards for alpha$_1$-PI immunologic assay).[18–20] Within a few weeks of commencing this program, bronchoalveolar lavage studies demonstrated significantly increased levels of alpha$_1$-PI and functional antineutrophil elastase capacity in the epithelial lining fluid of the lower respiratory tract of the lung, as compared to levels prior to commencing the program of chronic replacement therapy with Alpha$_1$-Proteinase Inhibitor (Human), Prolastin®.[18–20]

All 23 individuals who participated in the investigations were immunized with Hepatitis B Vaccine and received a single dose of Hepatitis B Immune Globulin (Human) on entry into the investigation. Although no other steps were taken to prevent hepatitis, neither hepatitis B nor non-A, non-B hepatitis occurred in any of the subjects.[18,19] All subjects remained seronegative for HIV antibody. None of the subjects developed any detectable antibody to alpha$_1$-PI or other serum protein.

Long-term controlled clinical trials to evaluate the effect of chronic replacement therapy with Prolastin on the development of or progression of emphysema in patients with congenital alpha$_1$-antitrypsin deficiency have not been performed. Estimates of the sample size required of this rare disorder and the slow, progressive nature of the clinical course have been considered impediments in the ability to conduct such a trial.[21] Studies to monitor the long-term effects will continue as part of the postapproval process.

INDICATIONS AND USAGE

Congenital Alpha$_1$-Antitrypsin Deficiency

Alpha$_1$-Proteinase Inhibitor (Human), Prolastin® is indicated for chronic replacement therapy of individuals having congenital deficiency of alpha$_1$-PI (alpha$_1$-antitrypsin deficiency) with clinically demonstrable panacinar emphysema. Clinical and biochemical studies have demonstrated that with such therapy, it is possible to increase plasma levels of alpha$_1$-PI, and that levels of functionally active alpha$_1$-PI in the lung epithelial lining fluid are increased proportionately.[18–20] As some individuals with alpha$_1$-antitrypsin deficiency will not go on to develop panacinar emphysema, only those with evidence of such disease should be considered for chronic replacement therapy with Prolastin.[22] Subjects with the PiMZ or PiMS phenotypes of alpha$_1$-antitrypsin deficiency should not be considered for such treatment as they appear to be at small risk for panacinar emphysema.[22] Clinical data are not available as to the long-term effects derived from chronic replacement therapy of individuals with alpha$_1$-antitrypsin deficiency with Prolastin. Only adult subjects have received Prolastin to date.

Prolastin is not indicated for use in patients other than those with PiZZ, PiZ(null) or Pi(null)(null) phenotypes.

CONTRAINDICATIONS

Individuals with selective IgA deficiencies who have known antibody against IgA (anti-IgA antibody) should not receive Alpha$_1$-Proteinase Inhibitor (Human), Prolastin®, since these patients may experience severe reactions, including anaphylaxis, to IgA which may be present.

WARNINGS

Because this product is made from human blood, it may carry a risk of transmitting infectious agents, e.g. viruses, and, theoretically, the Creutzfeldt-Jakob (CJD) agent. The risk that such products will transmit an infectious agent has been reduced by screening plasma donors for prior exposure to certain viruses, by testing for the presence of certain current virus infections, and by inactivating and/or removing certain viruses. Despite these measures, such products can still potentially transmit disease. There is also the possibility that unknown infectious agents may be present in such products. Individuals who receive infusions of blood or plasma products may develop signs and/or symptoms of some viral infections, particularly hepatitis C. ALL infections thought by a physician possibly to have been transmitted by this product should be reported by the physician or other healthcare provider to Bayer Corporation [1-800-288-8371].

The physician should discuss the risks and benefits of this product with the patient, before prescribing or administering it to a patient.

Alpha$_1$-Proteinase Inhibitor (Human), Prolastin® has been heat-treated in solution at 60°C for 10 hours in order to reduce the potential for transmission of infectious agents.[1] No cases of hepatitis, either hepatitis B or hepatitis C, have

Continued on next page

Prolastin—Cont.

been recorded to date in individuals receiving Prolastin.[18] However, as all individuals received prophylaxis against hepatitis B, no conclusion can be drawn at this time regarding potential transmission of hepatitis B virus.

PRECAUTIONS

General

1. Administer within 3 hours after reconstitution. Do not refrigerate after reconstitution.
2. Administer only by the intravenous route.
3. As with any colloid solution, there will be an increase in plasma volume following intravenous administration of Alpha$_1$-Proteinase Inhibitor (Human), Prolastin®.[23] Caution should therefore be used in patients at risk for circulatory overload.
4. Prolastin should be given alone, without mixing with other agents or diluting solutions.
5. Product administration and handling of the needles must be done with caution. Percutaneous puncture with a needle contaminated with blood can transmit infectious virus including HIV (AIDS) and hepatitis. Obtain immediate medical attention if injury occurs.
   Place needles in sharps container after single use. Discard all equipment including any reconstituted Prolastin product in accordance with biohazard procedures.

Carcinogenesis, Mutagenesis, Impairment of Fertility

Long-term studies in animals to evaluate carcinogenesis, mutagenesis, or impairment of fertility have not been conducted.

Pregnancy Category C

Animal reproduction studies have not been conducted with Alpha$_1$-Proteinase Inhibitor (Human), Prolastin®. It is also not known whether Prolastin can cause fetal harm when administered to a pregnant woman or can affect reproduction capacity. Prolastin should be given to a pregnant woman only if clearly needed.

Nursing Mothers

It is not known whether Prolastin is excreted in human milk. Because many drugs are excreted in human milk, caution should be exercised when Prolastin is administered to a nursing woman.

Pediatric Use

Safety and effectiveness in the pediatric population have not been established.

ADVERSE REACTIONS

Therapeutic administration of Alpha$_1$-Proteinase Inhibitor (Human), Prolastin®, 60 mg/kg weekly, has been demonstrated to be well tolerated. In clinical studies, six reactions were observed with 517 infusions of Prolastin, or 1.16%. None of the reactions was severe.[18] The adverse reactions reported included delayed fever (maximum temperature rise was 38.9°C, resolving spontaneously over 24 hours) occurring up to 12 hours following treatment (0.77%), light-headedness (0.19%), and dizziness (0.19%).[18] Mild transient leukocytosis and dilutional anemia several hours after infusion have also been noted.[18] Since market entry, occasional reports of other flu-like symptoms, allergic-like reactions, chills, dyspnea, rash, tachycardia, and, rarely, hypotension have also been received. Rare cases of transient increase in blood pressure or hypertension and chest pain have also been reported.

DOSAGE AND ADMINISTRATION

FOR INTRAVENOUS USE ONLY

Each bottle of Alpha$_1$-Proteinase Inhibitor (Human), Prolastin® has the functional activity, as determined by inhibition of porcine pancreatic elastase,[1] stated on the label of the bottle.

The "threshold" level of alpha$_1$-PI in the serum believed to provide adequate anti-elastase activity in the lung of individuals with alpha$_1$-antitrypsin deficiency is 80 mg/dL (based on commercial standards for alpha$_1$-PI immunologic assay).[12,15,17] However, assays of alpha$_1$-PI based on commercial standards measure antigenic activity of alpha$_1$-PI, whereas the labeled potency value of alpha$_1$-PI is expressed as actual functional activity, i.e., actual capacity to neutralize porcine pancreatic elastase. As functional activity may be less than antigenic activity, serum levels of alpha$_1$-PI determined using commercial immunologic assays may not accurately reflect actual functional alpha$_1$-PI levels. Therefore, although it may be helpful to monitor serum levels of alpha$_1$-PI in individuals receiving Prolastin, using currently available commercial assays of antigenic activity, results of these assays should not be used to determine the required therapeutic dosage.

The recommended dosage of Prolastin is 60 mg/kg body weight administered once weekly. This dose is intended to increase and maintain a level of functional alpha$_1$-PI in the epithelial lining of the lower respiratory tract, providing adequate anti-elastase activity in the lung of individuals with alpha$_1$-antitrypsin deficiency.

Alpha$_1$-Proteinase Inhibitor (Human), Prolastin® may be given at a rate of 0.08 mL/kg/min or greater and must be administered intravenously. The recommended dosage of 60 mg/kg takes approximately 30 minutes to infuse.

Parenteral drug products should be inspected visually for particulate matter and discoloration prior to administration, whenever solution and container permit.

Safety and effectiveness in pediatric patients has not been established.

Reconstitution

Vacuum Transfer

Note: Aseptic technique should be carefully followed. All needles and vial tops that will come into contact with the product to be administered via the intravenous route should not come in contact with any nonsterile surface. Any contaminated needles should be discarded by placing in a puncture-proof container and new equipment should be used.

1. After removing all items from the box, warm the sterile water (diluent) to room temperature (25°C, 77°F)
2. Remove the plastic flip tops from each vial (Fig. A). Cleanse vial tops (grey stoppers) with alcohol swab and allow surface to dry. After cleaning, do not allow anything to touch the latex (rubber) stopper.
3. Carefully remove the plastic sheath from the short end of the transfer needle. Insert the exposed needle into the diluent vial to the hub (Fig. B).
4. Carefully grip the sheath of the other end of the transfer needle and twist to remove it.
5. Invert the diluent vial and insert the attached needle into the vial of concentrate at a 45° angle (Fig. C). This will direct the stream of diluent against the wall of the concentrate vial and minimize foaming. The vacuum will draw the diluent into the concentrate vial.
6. Remove the diluent bottle and transfer needle (Fig. D).
7. Gently swirl the concentrate bottle until the powder is completely dissolved (Fig. E). The vial should then be visually inspected for particulate matter and discoloration prior to administration.
8. Clean the top of the vial of reconstituted Alpha$_1$-Proteinase Inhibitor (Human), Prolastin® again with alcohol swab and let surface dry.
9. Attach the filter needle (from the package) to sterile syringe. Withdraw the Prolastin solution into the syringe through the filter needle (Fig. F).
10. Remove the filter needle from the syringe and replace with an appropriate injection needle for administration. Discard filter needle into a puncture-proof container.
11. The contents of more than one bottle of Prolastin may be drawn into the same syringe before administration. If more than one bottle of Prolastin is used, withdraw contents from bottles using aseptic technique. Place contents into an administration container (plastic minibag or glass bottle) using a syringe. *Avoid pushing an I.V. administration set spike into the product container stopper as this has been known to force the stopper into the vial, with a resulting loss of sterility.

*For a patient of average weight (about 70 kg) the volume needed will exceed the limit of one syringe.

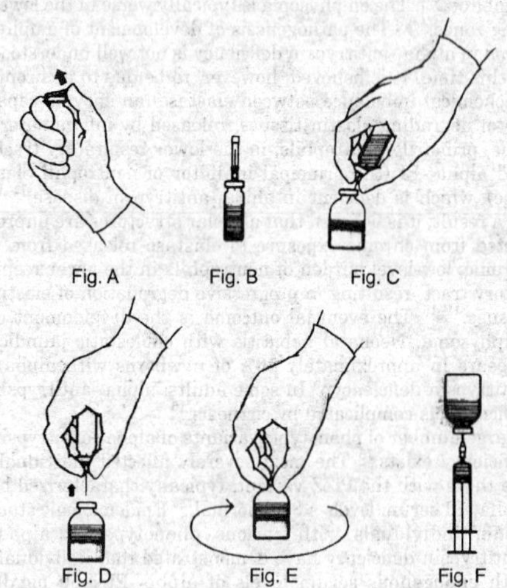

A number of factors beyond our control could reduce the efficacy of this product or even result in an ill effect following its use. These include improper storage and handling of the product after it leaves our hands, diagnosis, dosage, method of administration, and biological differences in individual patients. Because of these factors, it is important that this product be stored properly, that the directions be followed carefully during use, and that the risk of transmitting viruses be carefully weighed before the product is prescribed.

HOW SUPPLIED

Alpha$_1$-Proteinase Inhibitor (Human), Prolastin® is supplied in the following single use vials with the total alpha$_1$-PI functional activity, in milligrams, stated on the label of each vial. A suitable volume of Sterile Water for Injection, USP, is provided.

NDC Number	Approximate Alpha$_1$-PI Functional Activity	Diluent
0026-0601-30	500 mg	20 mL
0026-0601-35	1000 mg	40 mL

STORAGE

Prolastin should be stored at temperatures not to exceed 25°C (77°F). Freezing should be avoided as breakage of the diluent bottle might occur.

℞ only

REFERENCES

1. Coan MH, Brockway WJ, Eguizabal H, et al: Preparation and properties of alpha$_1$-proteinase inhibitor concentrate from human plasma. *Vox Sang* 48(6):333–42, 1985.
2. Laurell CB, Eriksson S: The electrophoretic alpha$_1$-globulin pattern of serum in alpha$_1$-antitrypsin deficiency. *Scand J Clin Lab Invest* 15:132–40, 1963.
3. Eriksson S: Pulmonary emphysema and alpha$_1$-antitrypsin deficiency. *Acta Med Scand* 175(2):197–205, 1964.
4. Eriksson S: Studies in alpha$_1$-antitrypsin deficiency. *Acta Med Scand* Suppl 432:1–85, 1965.
5. Kueppers F, Black LF: Alpha$_1$-antitrypsin and its deficiency. *Am Rev Respir Dis* 110(2):176–94, 1974.
6. Morse JO: Alpha$_1$-antitrypsin deficiency. *N Engl J Med* 299:1045–8; 1099–105, 1978.
7. Black LF, Kueppers F: Alpha$_1$-antitrypsin deficiency in nonsmokers. *Am Rev Respir Dis* 117(3):421–8, 1978.
8. Tobin MJ, Cook PJ, Hutchison DC: Alpha$_1$-antitrypsin deficiency: the clinical and physiological features of pulmonary emphysema in subjects homozygous for Pi type Z. A survey by the British Thoracic Association. *Br J Dis Chest* 77(1):14–27, 1983.
9. Larsson C: Natural history and life expectancy in severe alpha$_1$-antitrypsin deficiency, Pi Z. *Acta Med Scand* 204(5): 345–51, 1978.
10. Pannell R, Johnson D, Travis J: Isolation and properties of human plasma alpha$_1$-proteinase inhibitor. *Biochemistry* 13(26):5439–45, 1974.
11. Lieberman J: Elastase, collagenase, emphysema, and alpha$_1$-antitrypsin deficiency. *Chest* 70(1):62–7, 1976.
12. Gadek JE, Fells GA, Zimmerman RL, et al: Antielastases of the human alveolar structures: implications for the protease-antiprotease theory of emphysema. *J Clin Invest* 68(4):889–98, 1981.
13. Beatty K, Bieth J, Travis J: Kinetics of association of serine proteinases with native and oxidized alpha-1-proteinase inhibitor and alpha-1-antichymotrypsin. *J Biol Chem* 255(9):3931–4, 1980.
14. Janoff A, White R, Carp H, et al: Lung injury induced by leukocytic proteases. *Am J Pathol* 97(1):111–36, 1979.
15. Gadek JE, Crystal RG: Alpha$_1$-antitrypsin deficiency. In: Stanbury JB, Wyngaarden JB, Fredrickson DS, et al, eds.: *The Metabolic Basis of Inherited Disease.* 5th ed. New York, McGraw-Hill, 1983, p. 1450–67.
16. Larsson C, Dirksen H, Sundstrom G, et al: Lung function studies in asymptomatic individuals with moderately (Pi SZ) and severely (Pi Z) reduced levels of alpha$_1$-antitrypsin. *Scand J Respir Dis* 57(6):267–80, 1976.
17. Gadek JE, Klein HG, Holland PV, et al: Replacement therapy of alpha$_1$-antitrypsin deficiency: reversal of protease-antiprotease imbalance within the alveolar structures of PiZ subjects. *J Clin Invest* 68(5):1158–65, 1981.
18. Data on file, Bayer Corporation.
19. Wewers MD, Casolaro MA, Sellers SE, et al: Replacement therapy for alpha$_1$-antitrypsin deficiency associated with emphysema. *N Engl J Med* 316(17):1055–62, 1987.
20. Wewers MD, Casolaro MA, Crystal RG: Comparison of alpha-1-antitrypsin levels and antineutrophil elastase capacity of blood and lung in a patient with the alpha-1-antitrypsin phenotype null-null before and during alpha-1-antitrypsin augmentation therapy. *Am Rev Respir Dis* 135(3):539–43, 1987.
21. Burrows B: A clinical trial of efficacy of antiproteolytic therapy: can it be done? *Am Rev Respir Dis* 127(2:2): S42–3, 1983.
22. Cohen AB: Unraveling the mysteries of alpha$_1$-antitrypsin deficiency. *N Engl J Med* 314(12):778–9, 1986.
23. Finlayson JS: Albumin products. *Semin Thromb Hemost* 6(2):85–120, 1980.

08846114 (Rev. March 2003)

Bayer
Bayer Corporation
Pharmaceutical Division
Elkhart, IN 46515 USA
U.S. License No. 8

ANTITHROMBIN III (HUMAN) ℞
THROMBATE III®

DESCRIPTION

Antithrombin III (Human), THROMBATE III® is a sterile, nonpyrogenic, stable, lyophilized preparation of purified human antithrombin III.

THROMBATE III is prepared from pooled units of human plasma from normal donors by modifications and refinements of the cold ethanol method of Cohn.[1] When reconstituted with Sterile Water for Injection, USP, THROMBATE III has a pH of 6.0–7.5, a sodium content of 110–210 mEq/L, a chloride content of 110–210 mEq/L, an alanine content of 0.075–0.125 M, and a heparin content of not more than 0.004 unit/IU AT-III. THROMBATE III contains no preservative and must be administered by the intravenous route. In addition, THROMBATE III has been heat-treated in solution at 60°C ± 0.5°C for not less than 10 hours.

Each vial of THROMBATE III contains the labeled amount of antithrombin III in international units (IU) per vial. The potency assignment has been determined with a standard calibrated against a World Health Organization (WHO) antithrombin III reference preparation.

CLINICAL PHARMACOLOGY

Antithrombin III (AT-III), an $alpha_2$-glycoprotein of molecular weight 58,000, is normally present in human plasma at a concentration of approximately 12.5 mg/dL[2,3] and is the major plasma inhibitor of thrombin.[4] Inactivation of thrombin by AT-III occurs by formation of a covalent bond resulting in an inactive 1:1 stoichiometric complex between the two, involving an interaction of the active serine of thrombin and an arginine reactive site on AT-III.[4] AT-III is also capable of inactivating other components of the coagulation cascade including factors IXa, Xa, XIa, and XIIa, as well as plasmin.[4]

The neutralization rate of serine proteases by AT-III proceeds slowly in the absence of heparin, but is greatly accelerated in the presence of heparin.[4] As the therapeutic antithrombotic effect in vivo of heparin is mediated by AT-III, heparin is ineffective in the absence or near absence of AT-III.[4-8]

The prevalence of the hereditary deficiency of AT-III is estimated to be one per 2000 to 5000 in the general population.[4-7] The pattern of inheritance is autosomal dominant. In affected individuals, spontaneous episodes of thrombosis and pulmonary embolism may be associated with AT-III levels of 40%–60% of normal.[7] These episodes usually appear after the age of 20, the risk increasing with age and in association with surgery, pregnancy and delivery. The frequency of thromboembolic events in hereditary antithrombin III (AT-III) deficiency during pregnancy has been reported to be 70%, and several studies of the beneficial use of Antithrombin III (Human) concentrates during pregnancy in women with hereditary deficiency have been reported.[9-11] In many cases, however, no precipitating factor can be identified for venous thrombosis or pulmonary embolism.[7] Greater than 85% of individuals with hereditary AT-III deficiency have had at least one thrombotic episode by the age of 50 years.[7] In about 60% of patients thrombosis is recurrent. Clinical signs of pulmonary embolism occur in 40% of affected individuals.[7] In some individuals, treatment with oral anticoagulants leads to an increase of the endogenous levels of AT-III, and treatment with oral anticoagulants may be effective in the prevention of thrombosis in such individuals.[6,7]

In clinical studies of Antithrombin III (Human), THROMBATE III® conducted in 10 asymptomatic subjects with hereditary deficiency of AT-III, the mean in vivo recovery of AT-III was 1.6% per unit per kg administered based on immunologic AT-III assays, and 1.4% per unit per kg administered based on functional AT-III assays.[12] The mean 50% disappearance time (the time to fall to 50% of the peak plasma level following an initial administration) was approximately 22 hours and the biologic half-life was 2.5 days based on immunologic assays and 3.8 days based on functional assays of AT-III.[12] These values are similar to the half-life for radiolabeled Antithrombin III (Human) reported in the literature of 2.8–4.8 days.[13-15]

In clinical studies of THROMBATE III, none of the 13 patients with hereditary AT-III deficiency and histories of thromboembolism treated prophylactically on 16 separate occasions with THROMBATE III for high thrombotic risk situations (11 surgical procedures, 5 deliveries) developed a thrombotic complication. Heparin was also administered in 3 of the 11 surgical procedures and all 5 deliveries. Eight patients with hereditary AT-III deficiency were treated therapeutically with THROMBATE III as well as heparin for major thrombotic or thromboembolic complications, with seven patients recovering. Treatment with THROMBATE III reversed heparin resistance in two patients with hereditary AT-III deficiency being treated for thrombosis or thromboembolism.

During clinical investigation of THROMBATE III, none of 12 subjects monitored for a median of 8 months (range 2–19 months) after receiving THROMBATE III, became antibody positive to human immunodeficiency virus (HIV-1). None of 14 subjects monitored for ≥ 3 months demonstrated any evidence of hepatitis, either non-A, non-B hepatitis or hepatitis B.

INDICATIONS AND USAGE

THROMBATE III is indicated for the treatment of patients with hereditary antithrombin III deficiency in connection with surgical or obstetrical procedures or when they suffer from thromboembolism.

Subjects with AT-III deficiency should be informed about the risk of thrombosis in connection with pregnancy and surgery and about the inheritance of the disease.

The diagnosis of hereditary antithrombin III (AT-III) deficiency should be based on a clear family history of venous thrombosis as well as decreased plasma AT-III levels, and the exclusion of acquired deficiency.

AT-III in plasma may be measured by amidolytic assays using synthetic chromogenic substrates, by clotting assays, or by immunoassays. The latter does not detect all hereditary AT-III deficiencies.[16]

The AT-III level in neonates of parents with hereditary AT-III deficiency should be measured immediately after birth. (Fatal neonatal thromboembolism, such as aortic thrombi in children of women with hereditary antithrombin III deficiency, has been reported.)[17]

Plasma levels of AT-III are lower in neonates than adults, averaging approximately 60% in normal term infants.[18,19] AT-III levels in premature infants may be much lower.[18,19] Low plasma AT-III levels, especially in a premature infant, therefore, do not necessarily indicate hereditary deficiency.

It is recommended that testing and treatment with Antithrombin III (Human), THROMBATE III® of neonates be discussed with an expert on coagulation.[11]

CONTRAINDICATIONS

None known.

WARNINGS

THROMBATE III is made from human plasma. Products made from human plasma may contain infectious agents, such as viruses, that can cause disease. The risk that such products will transmit an infectious agent has been reduced by screening plasma donors for prior exposure to certain viruses, by testing for the presence of certain current virus infections, and by inactivating and/or removing certain viruses. Despite these measures, such products can still potentially transmit disease. There is also the possibility that unknown infectious agents may be present in such products. Individuals who receive infusions of blood or plasma products may develop signs and/or symptoms of some viral infections, particularly hepatitis C. ALL infections thought by a physician possibly to have been transmitted by this product should be reported by the physician or other healthcare provider to Bayer Corporation [1-888-765-3203].

The physician should discuss the risks and benefits of this product with the patient, before prescribing or administering it to a patient.

The anticoagulant effect of heparin is enhanced by concurrent treatment with THROMBATE III in patients with hereditary AT-III deficiency. Thus, in order to avoid bleeding, reduced dosage of heparin is recommended during treatment with THROMBATE III.

PRECAUTIONS

General

1. Administer within 3 hours after reconstitution. Do not refrigerate after reconstitution.
2. Administer only by the intravenous route.
3. THROMBATE III, once reconstituted, should be given alone, without mixing with other agents or diluting solutions.
4. Product administration and handling of the needles must be done with caution. Percutaneous puncture with a needle contaminated with blood can transmit infectious virus including HIV (AIDS) and hepatitis. Obtain immediate medical attention if injury occurs.
   Place needles in sharps container after single use. Discard all equipment including any reconstituted THROMBATE III product in accordance with biohazard procedures.

The diagnosis of hereditary antithrombin III (AT-III) deficiency should be based on a clear family history of venous thrombosis as well as decreased plasma AT-III levels, and the exclusion of acquired deficiency.

Laboratory Tests

It is recommended that AT-III plasma levels be monitored during the treatment period. Functional levels of AT-III in plasma may be measured by amidolytic assays using chromogenic substrates or by clotting assays.

Drug Interactions

The anticoagulant effect of heparin is enhanced by concurrent treatment with Antithrombin III (Human), THROMBATE III® in patients with hereditary AT-III deficiency. Thus, in order to avoid bleeding, reduced dosage of heparin is recommended during treatment with THROMBATE III.

Pregnancy Category B

Reproduction studies have been performed in rats and rabbits at doses up to four times the human dose and have revealed no evidence of impaired fertility or harm to the fetus due to THROMBATE III. It is not known whether THROMBATE III can cause fetal harm when administered to a pregnant woman or can affect reproduction capacity. Because animal reproduction studies are not always predictive of human response, this drug should be used during pregnancy only if clearly needed.

Pediatric Use

Safety and effectiveness in the pediatric population have not been established. The AT-III level in neonates of parents with hereditary AT-III deficiency should be measured immediately after birth. (Fatal neonatal thromboembolism, such as aortic thrombi in children of women with hereditary antithrombin III deficiency, has been reported.)[17]

Plasma levels of AT-III are lower in neonates than adults, averaging approximately 60% in normal term infants.[18,19] AT-III levels in premature infants may be much lower.[18,19] Low plasma AT-III levels, especially in a premature infant, therefore, do not necessarily indicate hereditary deficiency. It is recommended that testing and treatment with THROMBATE III of neonates be discussed with an expert on coagulation.[11]

ADVERSE REACTIONS

In clinical studies involving THROMBATE III, adverse reactions were reported in association with 17 of the 340 infusions during the clinical studies. Included were dizziness (7), chest tightness (3), nausea (3), foul taste in mouth (3), chills (2), cramps (2), shortness of breath (1), chest pain (1), film over eye (1), light-headedness (1), bowel fullness (1), hives (1), fever (1), and oozing and hematoma formation (1). If adverse reactions are experienced, the infusion rate should be decreased, or if indicated, the infusion should be interrupted until symptoms abate.

DOSAGE AND ADMINISTRATION

Each bottle of THROMBATE III has the functional activity, in international units (IU), stated on the label of the bottle. The potency assignment has been determined with a standard calibrated against a World Health Organization antithrombin III reference preparation.

Dosage should be determined on an individual basis based on the pre-therapy plasma antithrombin III (AT-III) level, in order to increase plasma AT-III levels to the level found in normal human plasma (100%). Dosage of THROMBATE III can be calculated from the following formula:

$$\text{units required (IU)} = \frac{[\text{desired - baseline AT-III level*}] \times \text{weight (kg)}}{1.4}$$

*expressed as % normal level based on functional AT-III assay

The above formula is based on an expected incremental in vivo recovery above baseline levels for Antithrombin III (Human), THROMBATE III® of 1.4% per IU per kg administered.[12] Thus, if a 70 kg individual has a baseline AT-III level of 57%, in order to increase plasma AT-III to 120%, the initial THROMBATE III dose would be [(120–57) × 70]/1.4 = 3150 IU total.

However, recovery may vary, and initially levels should be drawn at baseline and 20 minutes postinfusion. Subsequent doses can be calculated based on the recovery of the first dose. These recommendations are intended only as a guide for therapy. The exact loading dose and maintenance intervals should be individualized for each patient.

It is recommended that following an initial dose of THROMBATE III, plasma levels of AT-III be initially monitored at least every 12 hours and before the next infusion of THROMBATE III to maintain plasma AT-III levels greater than 80%. In some situations, e.g., following surgery,[20] hemorrhage or acute thrombosis, and during intravenous heparin administration,[13,21-23] the half-life of Antithrombin III (Human) has been reported to be shortened. In such conditions, plasma AT-III levels should be monitored more frequently, and THROMBATE III administered as necessary. When an infusion of THROMBATE III is indicated for a patient with hereditary deficiency to control an acute thrombotic episode or prevent thrombosis following surgical or obstetrical procedures, it is desirable to raise the AT-III level to normal and maintain this level for 2 to 8 days, depending on the indication for treatment, type and extent of surgery, patient's medical condition, past history and physician's judgment. Concomitant administration of heparin in each of these situations should be based on the medical judgment of the physician.

As a general recommendation, the following therapeutic program may be utilized as a starting program for treatment, modifying the program based on the actual plasma AT-III levels achieved:

a) An initial loading dose of THROMBATE III calculated to elevate the plasma AT-III level to 120%, assuming an expected rise over the baseline plasma AT-III level of 1.4% (functional activity) per IU per kg of THROMBATE III administered. Thus, if an individual has a baseline AT-III level of 57%, the initial THROMBATE III dose would be (120−57)/1.4 = 45 IU/kg.
b) Measure preinfusion and 20 minutes postinfusion (peak) plasma antithrombin III levels following the initial loading dose, plasma antithrombin III level after 12 hours, then preceding the next infusion (trough level). Subsequently measure antithrombin III levels preceding and 20 minutes after each infusion until predictable peak and trough levels have been achieved, generally between 80%–120%. Plasma levels between 80%–120% may be maintained by administration of maintenance doses of 60% of the initial loading dose, administered every 24 hours. Adjustments in the maintenance dose and/or interval between doses should be made based on actual plasma AT-III levels achieved.

The above recommendations for dosing are provided as a general guideline for therapy only. The exact loading and maintenance dosages and dosing intervals should be individualized for each subject, based on the individual clinical conditions, response to therapy, and actual plasma AT-III levels achieved. In some situations, e.g., following surgery,[20] with hemorrhage or acute thrombosis and during intravenous heparin administration,[13,21-23] in vivo survival of infused THROMBATE III has been reported to be shortened, resulting in the need to administer THROMBATE III more frequently.

Antithrombin III (Human), THROMBATE III® should be reconstituted with Sterile Water for Injection, USP and brought to room temperature prior to administration. THROMBATE III should be filtered through a sterile filter needle as supplied in the package prior to use, and should be administered within 3 hours following reconstitution. THROMBATE III may be infused over 10–20 minutes. THROMBATE III must be administered intravenously.

Parenteral drug products should be inspected visually for particulate matter and discoloration prior to administration, whenever solution and container permit.

Reconstitution

Vacuum Transfer

Note: Aseptic technique should be carefully followed. All needles and vial tops that will come into contact with the

Continued on next page

Thrombate III—Cont.

product to be administered via the intravenous route should not come in contact with any nonsterile surface. Any contaminated needles should be discarded by placing in a puncture-proof container and new equipment should be used.

1. After removing all items from the box, warm the sterile water (diluent) to room temperature (25°C, 77°F).
2. Remove the plastic flip tops from each vial (Fig. A). Cleanse vial tops (grey stoppers) with alcohol swab and allow surface to dry. After cleaning, do not allow anything to touch the stopper.
3. Carefully remove the plastic sheath from the short end of the transfer needle. Insert the exposed needle into the diluent vial to the hub (Fig. B).
4. Carefully grip the sheath of the other end of the transfer needle and twist to remove it.
5. Invert the diluent vial and insert the attached needle into the concentrate vial at a 45°angle (Fig. C). This will direct the stream of diluent against the wall of the concentrate vial and minimize foaming. The vacuum will draw the diluent into the concentrate vial.*
6. When diluent transfer is complete, remove the diluent vial and transfer needle (Fig. D).
7. Immediately after adding the diluent, swirl continuously until completely dissolved (Fig. E). Some foaming may occur, but attempt to avoid excessive foaming. The vial should then be visually inspected for particulate matter and discoloration prior to administration.
8. Clean the top of the vial of reconstituted THROMBATE III again with alcohol swab and let surface dry.
9. Attach the filter needle (from the package) to sterile syringe. Withdraw the THROMBATE III solution into the syringe through the filter needle (Fig. F).
10. Remove the filter needle from the syringe and replace with an appropriate injection or butterfly needle for administration. Discard filter needle into a puncture-proof container.
11. If the same patient is using more than one vial of THROMBATE III, the contents of multiple vials may be drawn into the same syringe through the filter needles provided.

*If vacuum is lost in the concentrate vial, use a sterile syringe to remove the sterile water from the diluent vial and inject it into the concentrate vial, directing the stream of fluid against the wall of the vial.

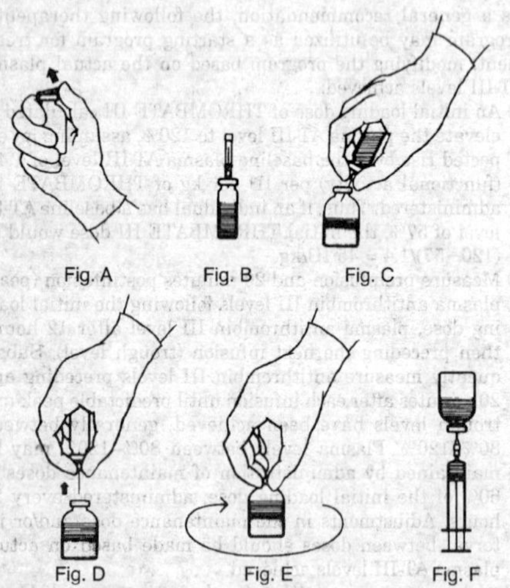

A number of factors beyond our control could reduce the efficacy of this product or even result in an ill effect following its use. These include improper storage and handling of the product after it leaves our hands, diagnosis, dosage, method of administration, and biological differences in individual patients. Because of these factors, it is important that this product is stored properly, that the directions are followed carefully during use, and that the risk of transmitting viruses is carefully weighed before the product is prescribed.

Rate of Administration

The rate of administration should be adapted to the response of the individual patient, but administration of the entire dose in 10 to 20 minutes is generally well tolerated.

HOW SUPPLIED

Antithrombin III (Human), THROMBATE III® is supplied in the following single use vials with the potency in international units stated on the label of each vial. A suitable volume of Sterile Water for Injection, USP, a sterile double-ended transfer needle, and a sterile filter needle are provided.

NDC Number	Approximate Antithrombin III Potency	Diluent
0026-0603-20	500 IU	10 mL
0026-0603-30	1000 IU	20 mL

STORAGE

THROMBATE III should be stored under refrigeration (2–8°C; 36–46°F). Freezing should be avoided as breakage of the diluent bottle might occur.

CAUTION

℞ only

U.S. federal law prohibits dispensing without prescription.

REFERENCES

1. Cohn EJ, Strong LE, Hughes WL Jr, et al: Preparation and properties of serum and plasma proteins. IV. A system for the separation into fractions of the protein and lipoprotein components of biological tissues and fluids. *J Am Chem Soc* 68(3):459–75, 1946.
2. Rosenberg RD, Bauer KA, Marcum JA: Antithrombin III "the heparin-antithrombin system." *Rev Hematol* 2:351–416, 1986.
3. Murano G, Williams L, Miller-Andersson M: Some properties of antithrombin-III and its concentration in human plasma. *Thromb Res* 18(1–2):259–62, 1980.
4. Rosenberg RD: Action and interactions of antithrombin and heparin. *N Engl J Med* 292(3):146–51, 1975.
5. Winter JH, Fenech A, Ridley W, et al: Familial antithrombin III deficiency. *Q J Med* 51(204):373–95, 1982.
6. Marciniak E, Farley CH, DeSimone PA: Familial thrombosis due to antithrombin III deficiency. *Blood* 43(2): 219–31, 1974.
7. Thaler E, Lechner K: Antithrombin III deficiency and thromboembolism. *Clin Haematol* 10(2):369–90, 1981.
8. Blauhut B, Necek S, Kramar H, et al: Activity of antithrombin III and effect of heparin on coagulation in shock. *Thromb Res* 19(6):775–82, 1980.
9. Samson D, Stirling Y, Woolf L, et al: Management of planned pregnancy in a patient with congenital antithrombin III deficiency. *Br J Haematol* 56(2):243–9, 1984.
10. Brandt P: Observations during the treatment of antithrombin-III deficient women with heparin and antithrombin concentrate during pregnancy, parturition, and abortion. *Thromb Res* 22(1–2):15–24, 1981.
11. Hellgren M, Tengborn L, Abildgaard U: Pregnancy in women with congenital antithrombin III deficiency: experience of treatment with heparin and antithrombin. *Gynecol Obstet Invest* 14(2):127–41, 1982.
12. Schwartz RS, Bauer KA, Rosenberg RD, et al: Clinical experience with antithrombin III concentrate in treatment of congenital and acquired deficiency of antithrombin. *Am J Med* 87 (Suppl 3B): 53S–60S, 1989.
13. Collen D, Schetz J, de Cock F, et al: Metabolism of antithrombin III (heparin cofactor) in man: effects of venous thrombosis and of heparin administration. *Eur J Clin Invest* 7(1):27–35, 1977.
14. Knot EAR, de Jong E, ten Cate JW, et al: Purified radiolabeled antithrombin III metabolism in three families with hereditary AT III deficiency: application of a three-compartment model. *Blood* 67(1):93–8, 1986.
15. Tengborn L, Frohm B, Nilsson LE, et al: Antithrombin III concentrate: its catabolism in health and in antithrombin III deficiency. *Scand J Clin Lab Invest* 41(5):469–77, 1981.
16. Sas G, Blasko G, Banhegyi D, et al: Abnormal antithrombin III (antithrombin III "Budapest") as a cause of familial thrombophilia. *Thromb Diath Haemorrh* 32(1):105–15, 1974.
17. Bjarke B, Herin P, Blomback M: Neonatal aortic thrombosis. A possible clinical manifestation of congenital antithrombin III deficiency. *Acta Paediatr Scand* 63: 297–301, 1974.
18. Hathaway WE, Bonnar J: Perinatal coagulation. New York, Grune & Stratton, 1978, p.68.
19. Peters M, Jansen E, ten Cate JW, et al: Neonatal antithrombin III. *Br J Haematol* 58(4):579–87, 1984.
20. Mannucci PM, Boyer C, Wolf M, et al: Treatment of congenital antithrombin III deficiency with concentrates. *Br J Haematol* 50(3):531–5, 1982.
21. Marciniak E, Gockerman JP: Heparin-induced decrease in circulating antithrombin-III. *Lancet* 2(8038):581–4, 1977.
22. O'Brien JR, Etherington MD: Effect of heparin and warfarin on antithrombin III. *Lancet* 2(8050):1232, 1977.
23. Kakkar VV, Bentley PG, Scully MF, et al: Antithrombin III and heparin. *Lancet* 1(8159):103–4, 1980.

14-7603-007 (Rev. Aug. 2001)

Manufactured by:
Bayer Corporation
Pharmaceutical Division
Elkhart, IN 46515 USA

U.S. License No. 8

Distributed in Canada by:
Bayer Inc.
Healthcare Division
Toronto, ON M9W 1G6

Beach Pharmaceuticals

Division of Beach Products, Inc.
5220 SOUTH MANHATTAN AVE.
TAMPA, FL 33611

Direct Inquiries to:
Richard Stephen Jenkins
(813) 839-6565
FAX (813) 837-2511

BEELITH Tablets **OTC**
MAGNESIUM SUPPLEMENT
with PYRIDOXINE HCL
Each tablet supplies 362 mg (30 mEq) of magnesium and 25 mg of pyridoxine hydrochloride.

DESCRIPTION

Each tablet contains magnesium oxide 600 mg and pyridoxine hydrochloride (Vitamin B_6) 25 mg equivalent to Vitamin B_6 20 mg. Each tablet yields 362 mg of magnesium and supplies 90% of the Adult U.S. Recommended Daily Allowance (RDA) for magnesium and 1000% of the Adult RDA for Vitamin B_6.

INDICATIONS

As a dietary supplement for patients with magnesium and/or Vitamin B_6 deficiencies resulting from malnutrition, alcoholism, magnesium depleting drugs, chemotherapy, and inadequate nutritional intake or absorption. Also, increases urinary magnesium levels.

DOSAGE

One tablet daily or as directed by a physician.

DRUG INTERACTION PRECAUTION

Do not take this product if you are presently taking a prescription drug without consulting your physician or other health professional.

WARNINGS

Do not take this product if you are presently taking a prescription drug without consulting your physician or other health professional. Ask a physician before use if you have kidney disease or if you are on a magnesium-restricted diet. Excessive dosage may cause laxation. If pregnant or breastfeeding, ask a health professional before use. Keep out of the reach of children.

HOW SUPPLIED

Golden yellow, film-coated tablet with the letters **BP** and the number **132** imprinted on each tablet. Packaged in bottles of 100 (Item No. 0486-1132-01) tablets.

Shown in Product Identification Guide, page 308

K-PHOS® M.F. ℞
K-PHOS® No.2 ℞
Rx Only

DESCRIPTION

K-PHOS® M.F.: Each tablet contains potassium acid phosphate 155 mg and sodium acid phosphate, anhydrous 350 mg. Each tablet yields approximately 125.6 mg of phosphorus, 44.5 mg of potassium or 1.1 mEq and 67 mg of sodium or 2.9 mEq. **K-PHOS® No.2:** Each tablet contains potassium acid phosphate 305 mg and sodium acid phosphate, anhydrous, 700 mg. Each tablet yields approximately 250 mg of phosphorus, 88 mg of potassium or 2.3 mEq and 134 mg of sodium or 5.8 mEq.

Shown in Product Identification Guide, page 308

K-PHOS® NEUTRAL ℞
Supplies 250 mg of phosphorus per tablet.
Rx Only

DESCRIPTION

Each tablet contains 852 mg dibasic sodium phosphate anhydrous, 155 mg monobasic potassium phosphate, and 130 mg monobasic sodium phosphate monohydrate. Each tablet yields approximately 250 mg of phosphorus, 298 mg of sodium (13.0 mEq) and 45 mg of potassium (1.1 mEq).

CLINICAL PHARMACOLOGY

Phosphorus has a number of important functions in the biochemistry of the body. The bulk of the body's phosphorus is located in the bones, where it plays a key role in osteoblastic and osteoclastic activities. Enzymatically catalyzed phosphate-transfer reactions are numerous and vital in the metabolism of carbohydrate, lipid and protein, and a proper concentration of the anion is of primary importance in assuring an orderly biochemical sequence. In addition, phosphorus plays an important role in modifying steady-state tissue concentrations of calcium. Phosphate ions are important buffers of the intracellular fluid, and also play a primary role in the renal excretion of hydrogen ion.

Oral administration of inorganic phosphates increases serum phosphate levels. Phosphates lower urinary calcium levels in idiopathic hypercalciuria.

In general, in adults, about two thirds of the ingested phosphate is absorbed from the bowel, most of which is rapidly excreted into the urine.

INDICATIONS AND USAGE

K-PHOS® NEUTRAL increases urinary phosphate and pyrophosphate. As a phosphorus supplement, each tablet supplies 25% of the U.S. Recommended Daily Allowance (U.S. RDA) of phosphorus for adults and children over 4 years of age.

CONTRAINDICATIONS

This product is contraindicated in patients with infected phosphate stones, in patients with severely impaired renal function (less than 30% of normal) and in the presence of hyperphosphatemia.

PRECAUTIONS

General: This product contains potassium and sodium and should be used with caution if regulation of these elements is desired. Occasionally, some individuals may experience a mild laxative effect during the first few days of phosphate therapy. If laxation persists to an unpleasant degree, reduce the daily dosage until this effect subsides or, if necessary, discontinue the use of this product.

Caution should be exercised when prescribing this product in the following conditions: Cardiac disease (particularly in digitalized patients); severe adrenal insufficiency (Addison's disease); acute dehydration; severe renal insufficiency; renal function impairment or chronic renal disease; extensive tissue breakdown (such as severe burns); myotonia congenita; cardiac failure; cirrhosis of the liver or severe hepatic disease; peripheral or pulmonary edema; hypernatremia; hypertension; toxemia of pregnancy; hypoparathyroidism; and acute pancreatitis. Rickets may benefit from phosphate therapy, but caution should be exercised. High serum phosphate levels may increase the incidence of extra-skeletal calcification.

Information for Patients: Patients with kidney stones may pass old stones when phosphate therapy is started and should be warned of this possibility. Patients should be advised to avoid the use of antacids containing aluminum, magnesium, or calcium which may prevent the absorption of phosphate.

Laboratory Tests: Careful monitoring of renal function and serum calcium, phosphorus, potassium, and sodium may be required at periodic intervals during phosphate therapy. Other tests may be warranted in some patients, depending on conditions.

Drug Interactions: The use of antacids containing magnesium, aluminum, or calcium in conjunction with phosphate preparations may bind the phosphate and prevent its absorption. Concurrent use of antihypertensives, especially diazoxide, guanethidine, hydralazine, methyldopa, or rauwolfia alkaloid; or corticosteroids, especially mineralocorticoids or corticotropin, with sodium phosphate may result in hypernatremia. Calcium-containing preparations and/or Vitamin D may antagonize the effects of phosphates in the treatment of hypercalcemia. Potassium-containing medications or potassium-sparing diuretics may cause hyperkalemia. Patients should have serum potassium level determinations at periodic intervals.

Carcinogenesis, Mutagenesis, Impairment of Fertility: No long term or reproduction studies in animals or humans have been performed with **K-PHOS® NEUTRAL** to evaluate its carcinogenic, mutagenic, or impairment of fertility potential.

Pregnancy: Teratogenic Effects: Pregnancy Category C. Animal reproduction studies have not been conducted with **K-PHOS® NEUTRAL**. It is also not known whether this product can cause fetal harm when administered to a pregnant woman or can affect reproductive capacity. This product should be given to a pregnant woman only if clearly needed.

Nursing Mothers: It is not known whether this drug is excreted in human milk. Because many drugs are excreted in human milk, caution should be exercised when this product is administered to a nursing woman.

Pediatric Use: See **DOSAGE AND ADMINISTRATION**.

ADVERSE REACTIONS

Gastrointestinal upset (diarrhea, nausea, stomach pain, and vomiting) may occur with phosphate therapy. Also, bone and joint pain (possible phosphate-induced osteomalacia) could occur. The following adverse effects may be observed (primarily from sodium or potassium): headaches; dizziness; mental confusion; seizures; weakness or heaviness of legs; unusual tiredness or weakness; muscle cramps; numbness, tingling, pain, or weakness of hands or feet; numbness or tingling around lips; fast or irregular heartbeat; shortness of breath or troubled breathing; swelling of feet or lower legs; unusual weight gain; low urine output; unusual thirst.

DOSAGE AND ADMINISTRATION

K-PHOS® NEUTRAL tablets should be taken with a full glass of water, with meals and at bedtime. Adults: One or two tablets four times daily; Pediatric Patients over 4 years of age: One tablet four times daily. For Pediatric Patients under 4 years of age, use only as directed by a physician.

HOW SUPPLIED

White, film-coated, capsule-shaped tablet with the name **BEACH** and number **1125** imprinted on each tablet. Bottles of 100 (NDC 0486-1125-01) and 500 (NDC 0486-1125-05) tablets.

Shown in Product Identification Guide, page 308

K–PHOS® ORIGINAL (Sodium Free) ℞

(Potassium Acid Phosphate)
Urinary Acidifier
Supplies 114 mg of phosphorus per tablet.
Rx Only

DESCRIPTION

Each tablet contains potassium acid phosphate 500 mg. Each tablet yields approximately 114 mg of phosphorus and 144 mg of potassium or 3.7 mEq.

ACTIONS

K-PHOS® ORIGINAL (Sodium Free) is a highly effective urinary acidifier.

INDICATIONS AND USAGE

For use in patients with elevated urinary pH. Helps keep calcium soluble and reduces odor and rash caused by ammoniacal urine. Also, by acidifying the urine, it increases the antibacterial activity of methenamine mandelate and methenamine hippurate.

CONTRAINDICATIONS

This product is contraindicated in patients with infected phosphate stones; in patients with severely impaired renal function (less than 30% of normal) and in the presence of hyperphosphatemia and hyperkalemia.

PRECAUTIONS

General: This product contains potassium and should be used with caution if regulation of this element is desired. Occasionally, some individuals may experience a mild laxative effect during the first few days of phosphate therapy. If laxation persists to an unpleasant degree, reduce the daily dosage until this effect subsides or, if necessary, discontinue the use of this product.

Caution should be exercised when prescribing this product in the following conditions: Cardiac disease (particularly in digitalized patients); severe adrenal insufficiency (Addison's disease); acute dehydration; severe renal insufficiency or chronic renal disease; extensive tissue breakdown (such as severe burns); myotonia congenita; hypoparathyroidism; and acute pancreatitis. Rickets may benefit from phosphate therapy, but caution should be exercised. High serum phosphate levels may increase the incidence of extraskeletal calcification.

Information for Patients: Patients with kidney stones may pass old stones when phosphate therapy is started and should be warned of this possibility. Patients should be advised to avoid the use of antacids containing aluminum, calcium, or magnesium which may prevent the absorption of phosphate. To assure against gastrointestinal injury associated with oral ingestion of concentrated potassium salt preparations, patients should be instructed to dissolve tablets completely in an appropriate amount of water before taking.

Laboratory Tests: Careful monitoring of renal function and serum electrolytes (calcium, phosphorus, potassium) may be required at periodic intervals during potassium phosphate therapy. Other tests may be warranted in some patients, depending on conditions.

Drug Interactions: The use of antacids containing magnesium, calcium, or aluminum in conjunction with phosphate preparations may bind the phosphate and prevent its absorption. Potassium-containing medications or potassium-sparing diuretics may cause hyperkalemia when used concurrently with potassium salts. Patients should have serum potassium level determinations at periodic intervals. Concurrent use of salicylates may lead to increased serum salicylate levels since excretion of salicylates is reduced in acidified urine. Serum salicylate levels should be closely monitored to avoid toxicity.

Carcinogenesis, Mutagenesis, Impairment of Fertility: There have been no studies in animals or humans to evaluate the carcinogenesis, mutagenesis, or impairment of fertility for this product.

Pregnancy: Pregnancy Category C. Animal reproduction studies have not been conducted with this product. It is also not known whether this product can cause fetal harm when administered to a pregnant woman or can affect reproductive capacity. This product should be given to a pregnant woman only if clearly needed.

Nursing Mothers: It is not known whether this drug is excreted in human milk. Because many drugs are excreted in human milk, caution should be exercised when this product is administered to a nursing woman.

ADVERSE REACTIONS

Gastrointestinal upset (diarrhea, nausea, stomach pain, and vomiting) may occur with the use of potassium phosphate. Also, bone and joint pain (possible phosphate-induced osteomalacia) could occur. The following adverse effects may be observed with potassium administration: irregular heartbeat; dizziness; mental confusion; weakness or heaviness of legs; unusual tiredness; muscle cramps; numbness, tingling, pain, or weakness in hands or feet; numbness or tingling around lips; shortness of breath or troubled breathing.

DOSAGE AND ADMINISTRATION

Two tablets dissolved in 6–8 oz. of water 4 times daily with meals and at bedtime. For best results, let the tablets soak in water for 2 to 5 minutes, or more if necessary, and stir. If any tablet particles remain undissolved, they may be crushed and stirred vigorously to speed dissolution.

HOW SUPPLIED

White scored tablet with the name **BEACH** and the number **1111** imprinted on each tablet. Bottles of 100 (NDC 0486-1111-01) and bottles of 500 (NDC 0486-1111-05) tablets.

Shown in Product Identification Guide, page 308

UROQID-Acid® No.2 Tablets ℞

Rx Only

DESCRIPTION

Each **UROQID-Acid® No.2** tablet contains methenamine mandelate 500 mg and sodium acid phosphate, monohydrate 500 mg.

CLINICAL PHARMACOLOGY

Methenamine mandelate is rapidly absorbed and excreted in the urine. Formaldehyde is released by acid hydrolysis from methenamine with bactericidal levels rapidly reached at pH 5.0–5.5. Proportionally less formaldehyde is released as urinary pH approaches 6.0 and insufficient quantities are released above this level for therapeutic response. In acid urine, mandelic acid exerts its antibacterial action and also contributes to the acidification of the urine. Mandelic acid is excreted by both glomerular filtration and tubular excretion. In acid urine, there is equally effective antibacterial activity against both gram-positive and gram-negative organisms, since the antibacterial action of mandelic acid and formaldehyde is nonspecific. With Proteus vulgaris and urea splitting strains of Pseudomonas and Aerobacter, results may be discouraging and particular attention is required in monitoring urinary pH and overall management.

INDICATIONS AND USAGE

For the suppression or elimination of bacteriuria associated with chronic and recurrent infections of the urinary tract, including pyelitis, pyelonephritis, cystitis, and infected residual urine accompanying neurogenic bladder. When used as recommended, **UROQID-Acid® No.2** is particularly suitable for long-term therapy because of its relative safety and because resistance to the nonspecific bactericidal action of formaldehyde does not develop. Pathogens resistant to other antibacterial agents may respond because of the nonspecific effect of formaldehyde formed in an acid urine.

Prophylactic Use Rationale: Urine is a good culture medium for many urinary pathogens. Inoculation by a few organisms (relapse or reinfection) may lead to bacteriuria in susceptible individuals. Thus, the rationale of management in recurring urinary tract infection (bacteriuria) is to change the urine from a growth-supporting to a growth-inhibiting medium. There is a growing body of evidence that long-term administration of methenamine can prevent recurrence of bacteriuria in patients with chronic pyelonephritis.

Therapeutic Use Rationale: Helps to sterilize the urine and, in some situations in which underlying pathologic conditions prevent sterilization by any means, can help to suppress bacteriuria. As part of the overall management of the urinary tract infection, a thorough diagnostic evaluation should accompany the use of this product.

CONTRAINDICATIONS

UROQID-Acid® No.2 is contraindicated in patients with renal insufficiency, severe hepatic disease, severe dehydration, hyperphosphatemia, and in patients who have exhibited hypersensitivity to any components of this product.

PRECAUTIONS

General

This product should not be used as the sole therapeutic agent in acute parenchymal infections causing systemic symptoms such as chills and fever.

UROQID-Acid® No.2 contains approximately 83 mg of sodium per tablet and should be used with caution in patients on a sodium-restricted diet.

Sodium phosphates should be used with caution in the following conditions: cardiac failure; peripheral or pulmonary edema; hypernatremia; hypertension; toxemia of pregnancy; hypoparathyroidism; and acute pancreatitis. High serum phosphate levels increase the incidence of extraskeletal calcification.

Large doses of methenamine (8 grams daily for 3 to 4 weeks) have caused bladder irritation, painful and frequent micturition, albuminuria and gross hematuria. Dysuria may occur, although usually at higher than recommended doses, and can be controlled by reducing the dosage. This product contains a urinary acidifier and can cause metabolic acidosis.

Care should be taken to maintain an acidic urinary pH (below 5.5), especially when treating infections due to urea-splitting organisms such as Proteus and strains of Pseudomonas.

Drugs and/or foods which produce an alkaline urine should be restricted. Frequent urine pH tests are essential. If acidification of the urine is contraindicated or unattainable, use of this product should be discontinued.

Information For Patients: To assure an acidic pH, patients should be instructed to restrict or avoid most fruits, milk and milk products, and antacids containing sodium carbonate or bicarbonate.

Laboratory Tests: As with all urinary tract infections, the efficacy of therapy should be monitored by repeated urine

Continued on next page

Uroqid-Acid—Cont.

cultures. During long-term therapy, careful monitoring of renal function, serum phosphorus and sodium may be required at periodic intervals.

Drug Interactions: Formaldehyde and sulfamethizole form an insoluble precipitate in acid urine and increase the risk of crystalluria; therefore, these products should not be used concurrently. Thiazide diuretics, carbonic anhydrase inhibitors, antacids, or urinary alkalinizing agents should not be used concurrently since they may cause the urine to become alkaline and reduce the effectiveness of methenamine by inhibiting its conversion to formaldehyde. Concurrent use of antihypertensives, especially diazoxide, guanethidine, hydralazine, methyldopa, or rauwolfia alkaloids; or corticosteroids, especially mineralocorticoids or corticotropin, with sodium phosphates may lead to hypernatremia. Concurrent use of salicylates may lead to increased serum salicylate levels since excretion of salicylates is reduced in acidified urine. Serum salicylate levels should be closely monitored to avoid toxicity.

Laboratory Test Interactions: Formaldehyde interferes with fluorometric procedures for determination of urinary catecholamines and vanilmandelic acid (VMA) causing erroneously high results. Formaldehyde also causes falsely decreased urine estriol levels by reacting with estriol when acid hydrolysis techniques are used; estriol determinations which use enzymatic hydrolysis are unaffected by formaldehyde. Formaldehyde causes falsely elevated 17-hydroxycorticosteroid levels when the Porter-Silber method is used and falsely decreased 5-hydroxyindoleacetic acid (5HIAA) levels by inhibiting color development when nitrosonaphthol methods are used.

Carcinogenesis, Mutagenesis, Impairment Of Fertility: Long-term animal studies to evaluate the carcinogenic, mutagenic, or impairment of fertility potential of this product have not been performed.

Pregnancy: Teratogenic Effects. Pregnancy Category C. Animal reproduction studies have not been conducted with **UROQID-Acid® No.2.** It is also not known whether this product can cause fetal harm when administered to a pregnant woman or can affect reproductive capacity. Since methenamine is known to cross the placental barrier, this product should be given to a pregnant woman only if clearly needed.

Nursing Mothers: Methenamine is excreted in breast milk. Caution should be exercised when this product is administered to a nursing woman.

ADVERSE REACTIONS

Gastrointestinal disturbances (nausea, stomach upset), generalized skin rash, dysuria, painful or difficult urination may occur occasionally with the use of methenamine preparations. Microscopic and rarely, gross hematuria have also been reported.

Gastrointestinal upset (diarrhea, nausea, stomach pain, and vomiting) may occur with the use of sodium phosphates. Also, bone or joint pain (possible phosphate induced osteomalacia) could occur. The following adverse effects may be observed (primarily from sodium): headaches; dizziness; mental confusion; seizures; weakness or heaviness of legs; unusual tiredness or weakness; muscle cramps; numbness, tingling, pain, or weakness of hands or feet; numbness or tingling around lips; fast or irregular heartbeat; shortness of breath or troubled breathing; swelling of feet or lower legs; unusual weight gain; low urine output, unusual thirst.

DOSAGE AND ADMINISTRATION

UROQID-Acid® No.2: *Adults:* Initially, 2 tablets 4 times daily with a full glass of water. For maintenance, 2 to 4 tablets daily, in divided doses with a full glass of water.

HOW SUPPLIED

UROQID-Acid® No.2 is a yellow, film-coated, capsule-shaped tablet with the name **BEACH** and the number **1114** imprinted on each tablet. Packaged in bottles of 100 tablets (NDC 0486-1114-01).

Shown in Product Identification Guide, page 308

NOTICE
Before prescribing or administering any product described in PHYSICIANS' DESK REFERENCE check the **PDR Supplements** for revised information.

Bedford Laboratories

A Division of Ben Venue Laboratories, Inc.
300 NORTHFIELD ROAD
BEDFORD, OH 44146

Direct Inquiries to:
Customer Service: (800) 562-4797
FAX: (440) 232-6264
Professional Services: (800) 521-5169

ADRIAMYCIN ℞

[ă'dree-a-my-sin]
(DOXOrubicin HCl)
for Injection, USP

ADRIAMYCIN

(DOXOrubicin HCl)
Injection, USP
For Intravenous Use Only
℞ ONLY

WARNINGS

1. Severe local tissue necrosis will occur if there is extravasation during administration (see **DOSAGE AND ADMINISTRATION**). Doxorubicin must not be given by the intramuscular or subcutaneous route.
2. Myocardial toxicity manifested in its most severe form by potentially fatal congestive heart failure may occur either during therapy or months to years after termination of therapy. The probability of developing impaired myocardial function based on a combined index of signs, symptoms and decline in left ventricular ejection fraction (LVEF) is estimated to be 1 to 2% at a total cumulative dose of 300 mg/m^2 of doxorubicin, 3 to 5% at a dose of 400 mg/m^2, 5 to 8% at 450 mg/m^2 and 6 to 20% at 500 mg/m^2.* The risk of developing CHF increases rapidly with increasing total cumulative doses of doxorubicin in excess of 450 mg/m^2. "Risk factors (active or dormant cardiovascular disease, prior or concomitant radiotherapy to the mediastinal/pericardial area, previous therapy with other anthracyclines or anthracenediones, concomitant use of other cardiotoxic drugs) may increase the risk of cardiac toxicity. Cardiac toxicity with doxorubicin may occur at lower cumulative doses whether or not cardiac risk factors are present." Pediatric patients are at increased risk for developing delayed cardiotoxicity.
3. Secondary acute myelogenous leukemia (AML) has been reported in patients treated with anthracyclines, including doxorubicin (see **ADVERSE REACTIONS**). The occurrence of refractory secondary leukemia is more common when such drugs are given in combination with DNA-damaging anti-neoplastic agents, when patients have been heavily pretreated with cytotoxic drugs, or when doses of anthracyclines have been escalated. The rate of developing treatment-related leukemia was estimated in an analysis of 1474 breast cancer patients who received adjuvant treatment with doxorubicin-containing regimens (i.e., FAC) in clinical trials. The estimated risk of developing treatment-related leukemia at 10 years was 2.5% for the 810 patients receiving radiotherapy plus chemotherapy and 0.5% for the 664 patients receiving chemotherapy alone. The overall risk was estimated at 1.5% at 10 years for the entire patient population. Pediatric patients are also at risk of developing secondary AML.
4. Dosage should be reduced in patients with impaired hepatic function.
5. Severe myelosuppression may occur.
6. Doxorubicin should be administered only under the supervision of a physician who is experienced in the use of cancer chemotherapeutic agents.

*Data on file at Pharmacia & Upjohn

DESCRIPTION

Doxorubicin is a cytotoxic anthracycline antibiotic isolated from cultures of *Streptomyces peucetius* var. *caesius*.

Doxorubicin consists of a naphthacenequinone nucleus linked through a glycosidic bond at ring atom 7 to an amino sugar, daunosamine.

Chemically, doxorubicin hydrochloride is (8*S*,10*S*)-10-[(3-Amino-2,3,6-trideoxy-α-L-*lyxo*-hexopyranosyl)-oxy]-8-glycoloyl-7,8,9,10-tetrahydro-6,8,11-trihydroxy-1-methoxy-5,12-naphthacenedione hydrochloride. The structural formula is as follows:

[See chemical structure at top of next column]

Doxorubicin binds to nucleic acids, presumably by specific intercalation of the planar anthracycline nucleus with the DNA double helix. The anthracycline ring is lipophilic, but the saturated end of the ring system contains abundant hydroxyl groups adjacent to the amino sugar, producing a hydrophilic center. The molecule is amphoteric, containing acidic functions in the ring phenolic groups and a basic function in the sugar amino group. It binds to cell membranes, as well as plasma proteins.

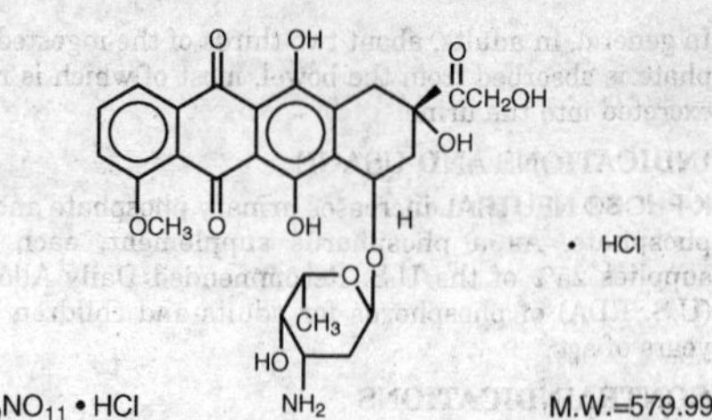

$C_{27}H_{29}NO_{11}$ • HCl M.W.=579.99

It is supplied in the hydrochloride form as a sterile red-orange lyophilized powder containing lactose and as a sterile parenteral, isotonic solution with sodium chloride for intravenous use only.

Adriamycin (DOXOrubicin HCl) for Injection, USP:

Each 10 mg lyophilized vial contains 10 mg of Doxorubicin Hydrochloride, USP and 50 mg of Lactose Monohydrate, NF.

Each 20 mg lyophilized vial contains 20 mg of Doxorubicin Hydrochloride, USP and 100 mg of Lactose Monohydrate, NF.

Each 50 mg lyophilized vial contains 50 mg of Doxorubicin Hydrochloride, USP and 250 mg of Lactose Monohydrate, NF.

Adriamycin (DOXOrubicin HCl) Injection, USP:

Each 2 mg/mL, 5 mL (10 mg) vial contains 10 mg Doxorubicin Hydrochloride, USP; Sodium Chloride 0.9% (to adjust tonicity) and Water for Injection q.s.; pH adjusted to 3 using Hydrochloric Acid.

Each 2 mg/mL, 10 mL (20 mg) vial contains 20 mg Doxorubicin Hydrochloride, USP; Sodium Chloride 0.9% (to adjust tonicity) and Water for Injection q.s.; pH adjusted to 3 using Hydrochloric Acid.

Each 2 mg/mL, 25 mL (50 mg) vial contains 50 mg Doxorubicin Hydrochloride, USP; Sodium Chloride 0.9% (to adjust tonicity) and Water for Injection q.s.; pH adjusted to 3 using Hydrochloric Acid.

Each 2 mg/mL, 100 mL (200 mg) multiple dose vial contains 200 mg Doxorubicin Hydrochloride, USP; Sodium Chloride 0.9% (to adjust tonicity) and Water for Injection q.s.; pH adjusted to 3 using Hydrochloric Acid.

CLINICAL PHARMACOLOGY

The cytotoxic effect of doxorubicin on malignant cells and its toxic effects on various organs are thought to be related to nucleotide base intercalation and cell membrane lipid binding activities of doxorubicin. Intercalation inhibits nucleotide replication and action of DNA and RNA polymerases. The interaction of doxorubicin with topoisomerase II to form DNA-cleavable complexes appears to be an important mechanism of doxorubicin cytocidal activity. Doxorubicin cellular membrane binding may effect a variety of cellular functions. Enzymatic electron reduction of doxorubicin by a variety of oxidases, reductases and dehydrogenases generate highly reactive species including the hydroxyl free radical OH•. Free radical formation has been implicated in doxorubicin cardiotoxicity by means of Cu (II) and Fe (III) reduction at the cellular level. Cells treated with doxorubicin have been shown to manifest the characteristic morphologic changes associated with apoptosis or programmed cell death. Doxorubicin-induced apoptosis may be an integral component of the cellular mechanism of action relating to therapeutic effects, toxicities, or both.

Animal studies have shown activity in a spectrum of experimental tumors, immunosuppression, carcinogenic properties in rodents, induction of a variety of toxic effects, including delayed and progressive cardiac toxicity, myelosuppression in all species and atrophy to testes in rats and dogs.

Pharmacokinetic studies, determined in patients with various types of tumors undergoing either single or multi-agent therapy have shown that doxorubicin follows a multiphasic disposition after intravenous injection. The initial distributive half-life of approximately 5 minutes suggests rapid tissue uptake of doxorubicin, while its slow elimination from tissues is reflected by a terminal half-life of 20 to 48 hours. Steady-state distribution volumes exceed 20 to 30 L/kg and are indicative of extensive drug uptake into tissues. Plasma clearance is in the range of 8 to 20 mL/min/kg and is predominately by metabolism and biliary excretion. Approximately 40% of the dose appears in the bile in 5 days, while only 5 to 12% of the drug and its metabolites appear in the urine during the same time period. Binding of doxorubicin and its major metabolite, doxorubicinol to plasma proteins is about 74 to 76% and is independent of plasma concentration of doxorubicin up to 2 µM. Enzymatic reduction at the 7 position and cleavage of the daunosamine sugar yields aglycones which are accompanied by free radical formation, the local production of which may contribute to the cardiotoxic activity of doxorubicin. Disposition of doxorubicinol (DOX-OL) in patients is formation rate limited. The terminal half-life of DOX-OL is similar to doxorubicin. The relative exposure of DOX-OL, compared to doxorubicin ranges between 0.4 to 0.6. In urine, <3% of the dose was recovered as DOX-OL over 7 days.

A published clinical study involving 6 men and 21 women with no prior anthracycline therapy reported a significantly higher median doxorubicin clearance in the men compared to the women (113 versus 45 L/hr). However, the terminal half-life of doxorubicin was longer in men compared to the women (54 versus 35 hrs).

In four patients, dose-independent pharmacokinetics have been shown for doxorubicin in the dose range of 30 to 70 mg/m^2. Systemic clearance of doxorubicin is significantly reduced in obese women with ideal body weight greater than 130%. There was a significant reduction in clearance without any change in volume of distribution in obese patients when compared with normal patients with less than 115% ideal body weight. The clearance of doxorubicin and doxorubicinol was also reduced in patients with impaired hepatic function. Doxorubicin was excreted in the milk of one lactating patient, with peak milk concentration at 24 hours after treatment being approximately 4.4 -fold greater than the corresponding plasma concentration. Doxorubicin was detectable in the milk up to 72 hours after therapy with 70 mg/m^2 of doxorubicin given as a 15 minute intravenous infusion and 100 mg/m^2 of cisplatin as a 26 hour intravenous infusion. The peak concentration of doxorubicinol in milk at 24 hours was 0.2 μM and AUC up to 24 hours was 16.5 μM.hr while the AUC for doxorubicin was 9.9 μM.hr.
Following administration of 10 to 75-mg/m^2 doses of doxorubicin to 60 children and adolescents ranging from 2 months to 20 years of age, doxorubicin clearance averaged 1443 +/- 114 mL/min/m^2. Further analysis demonstrated that clearance in 52 children greater than 2 years of age (1540 mL/min/m^2) was increased compared with adults. However, clearance in infants younger than 2 years of age (813 mL/min/m^2) was decreased compared with older children and approached the range of clearance values determined in adults.
Doxorubicin does not cross the blood brain barrier.

INDICATIONS AND USAGE

Adriamycin (DOXOrubicin HCl) Injection, USP and Adriamycin (DOXOrubicin HCl) for Injection, USP have been used successfully to produce regression in disseminated neoplastic conditions such as acute lymphoblastic leukemia, acute myeloblastic leukemia, Wilms' tumor, neuroblastoma, soft tissue and bone sarcomas, breast carcinoma, ovarian carcinoma, transitional cell bladder carcinoma, thyroid carcinoma, gastric carcinoma, Hodgkin's disease, malignant lymphoma and bronchogenic carcinoma in which the small cell histologic type is the most responsive compared to other cell types.

CONTRAINDICATIONS

Doxorubicin therapy should not be started in patients who have marked myelosuppression induced by previous treatment with other antitumor agents or by radiotherapy. Doxorubicin treatment is contraindicated in patients who received previous treatment with complete cumulative doses of doxorubicin, daunorubicin, idarubicin, and/or other anthracyclines and anthracenes.

WARNINGS

Special attention must be given to the cardiotoxicity induced by doxorubicin. Irreversible myocardial toxicity, manifested in its most severe form by life-threatening or fatal congestive heart failure, may occur either during therapy or months to years after termination of therapy. The probability of developing impaired myocardial function, based on a combined index of signs, symptoms and decline in left ventricular ejection fraction (LVEF) is estimated to be 1 to 2% at a total cumulative dose of 300 mg/m^2 of doxorubicin, 3 to 5% at a dose of 400 mg/m^2, 5 to 8% at a dose of 450 mg/m^2 and 6 to 20% at a dose of 500 mg/m^2 given in a schedule of a bolus injection once every 3 weeks (data on file at Pharmacia & Upjohn). In a retrospective review by Von Hoff et al, the probability of developing congestive heart failure was reported to be 5/168 (3%) at a cumulative dose of 430 mg/m^2 of doxorubicin, 8/110 (7%) at 575 mg/m^2 and 3/14 (21%) at 728 mg/m^2. The cumulative incidence of CHF was 2.2%. In a prospective study of doxorubicin in combination with cyclophosphamide, fluorouracil and/or vincristine in patients with breast cancer or small cell lung cancer, the cumulative incidence of congestive heart failure was 5 to 6%. The probability of CHF at various cumulative doses of doxorubicin was 1.5% at 300 mg/m^2, 4.9% at 400 mg/m^2, 7.7% at 450 mg/m^2 and 20.5% at 500 mg/m^2.
Cardiotoxicity may occur at lower doses in patients with prior mediastinal irradiation, concurrent cyclophosphamide therapy, exposure at an early age and advanced age. Data also suggest that pre-existing heart disease is a co-factor for increased risk of doxorubicin cardiotoxicity. In such cases, cardiac toxicity may occur at doses lower than the respective recommended cumulative dose of doxorubicin. Studies have suggested that concomitant administration of doxorubicin and calcium channel entry blockers may increase the risk of doxorubicin cardiotoxicity. The total dose of doxorubicin administered to the individual patient should also take into account previous or concomitant therapy with related compounds such as daunorubicin, idarubicin and mitoxantrone. Cardiomyopathy and/or congestive heart failure may be encountered several months or years after discontinuation of doxorubicin therapy.
The risk of congestive heart failure and other acute manifestations of doxorubicin cardiotoxicity in pediatric patients may be as much or lower than in adults. Pediatric patients appear to be at particular risk for developing delayed cardiac toxicity in that doxorubicin induced cardiomyopathy impairs myocardial growth as pediatric patients mature, subsequently leading to possible development of congestive heart failure during early adulthood. As many as 40% of pediatric patients may have subclinical cardiac dysfunction and 5 to 10% of pediatric patients may develop congestive heart failure on long term follow-up. This late cardiac toxicity may be related to the dose of doxorubicin. The longer the length of follow-up the greater the increase in the detection rate.
Treatment of doxorubicin induced congestive heart failure includes the use of digitalis, diuretics, after load reducers such as angiotensin I converting enzyme (ACE) inhibitors, low salt diet, and bed rest. Such intervention may relieve symptoms and improve the functional status of the patient.
Monitoring Cardiac Function: In adult patients severe cardiac toxicity may occur precipitously without antecedent ECG changes. Cardiomyopathy induced by anthracyclines is usually associated with very characteristic histopathologic changes on an endomyocardial biopsy (EM biopsy), and a decrease of left ventricular ejection fraction (LVEF), as measured by multi-gated radionuclide angiography (MUGA scans) and/or echocardiogram (ECHO), from pretreatment baseline values. However, it has not been demonstrated that monitoring of the ejection fraction will predict when individual patients are approaching their maximally tolerated cumulative dose of doxorubicin. Cardiac function should be carefully monitored during treatment to minimize the risk of cardiac toxicity. A baseline cardiac evaluation with an ECG, LVEF, and/or an echocardiogram (ECHO) is recommended especially in patients with risk factors for increased cardiac toxicity (pre-existing heart disease, mediastinal irradiation, or concurrent cyclophosphamide therapy). Subsequent evaluations should be obtained at a cumulative dose of doxorubicin of at least 400 mg/m^2 and periodically thereafter during the course of therapy. Pediatric patients are at increased risk for developing delayed cardiotoxicity following doxorubicin administration and therefore a follow-up cardiac evaluation is recommended periodically to monitor for this delayed cardiotoxicity.
In adults, a 10% decline in LVEF to below the lower limit of normal or an absolute LVEF of 45%, or a 20% decline in LVEF at any level is indicative of deterioration in cardiac function. In pediatric patients, deterioration in cardiac function during or after the completion of therapy with doxorubicin is indicated by a drop in fractional shortening (FS) by an absolute value of ≥10 percentile units or below 29%, and a decline in LVEF of 10 percentile units or an LVEF below 55%. In general, if test results indicate deterioration in cardiac function associated with doxorubicin, the benefit of continued therapy should be carefully evaluated against the risk of producing irreversible cardiac damage.
Acute life-threatening arrhythmias have been reported to occur during or within a few hours after doxorubicin administration.
There is a high incidence of bone marrow depression, primarily of leukocytes, requiring careful hematologic monitoring. With the recommended dosage schedule, leukopenia is usually transient, reaching its nadir at 10 to 14 days after treatment with recovery usually occurring by the 21st day. White blood counts as low as 1000/mm^3 are to be expected during treatment with appropriate doses of doxorubicin. Red blood and platelet levels should also be monitored since they may also be depressed. Hematologic toxicity may require dose reduction or suspension or delay of doxorubicin therapy. Persistent severe myelosuppression may result in superinfection or hemorrhage.
Doxorubicin may potentiate the toxicity of other anticancer therapies. Exacerbation of cyclophosphamide-induced hemorrhagic cystitis and enhancement of the hepatotoxicity of 6-mercaptopurine have been reported. Radiation-induced toxicity to the myocardium, mucosae, skin, and liver have been reported to be increased by the administration of doxorubicin. Pediatric patients receiving concomitant doxorubicin and actinomycin-D have manifested acute 'recall' pneumonitis at variable times after local radiation therapy.
Since metabolism and excretion of doxorubicin occurs predominantly by the hepatobiliary route, toxicity to recommended doses of doxorubicin can be enhanced by hepatic impairment; therefore, prior to the individual dosing, evaluation of hepatic function is recommended using conventional laboratory tests such as SGOT, SGPT, alkaline phosphatase, and bilirubin (see **DOSAGE AND ADMINISTRATION**).
Necrotizing colitis manifested by typhlitis (cecal inflammation), bloody stools and severe and sometimes fatal infections, have been associated with a combination of doxorubicin given by IV push daily for 3 days and cytarabine given by continuous infusion daily for 7 or more days.
On intravenous administration of doxorubicin, extravasation may occur with or without an accompanying stinging or burning sensation, even if blood returns well on aspiration of the infusion needle (see **DOSAGE AND ADMINISTRATION**). If any signs or symptoms of extravasation have occurred the injection or infusion should be immediately terminated and restarted in another vein.
Pregnancy Category D: Safe use of doxorubicin in pregnancy has not been established. Doxorubicin is embryotoxic and teratogenic in rats and embryotoxic and abortifacient in rabbits. There are no adequate and well-controlled studies in pregnant women. If doxorubicin is to be used during pregnancy, or if the patient becomes pregnant during therapy, the patient should be apprised of the potential hazard to the fetus. Women of childbearing age should be advised to avoid becoming pregnant.

PRECAUTIONS

General: Doxorubicin is not an anti-microbial agent.
Information for Patients: Adriamycin (DOXOrubicin HCl) Injection, USP and Adriamycin (DOXOrubicin HCl) for Injection, USP impart a red coloration to the urine for 1 to 2 days after administration, and patients should be advised to expect this during active therapy.
Drug Interactions: Literature contains the following drug interactions with doxorubicin in humans: cyclosporine (Sandimmune) may induce coma and/or seizures, phenobarbital increases the elimination of doxorubicin, phenytoin levels may be decreased by doxorubicin, streptozocin (Zanosar) may inhibit the hepatic metabolism, and administration of live vaccines to immunosuppressed patients, including those undergoing cytotoxic chemotherapy, may be hazardous.
Paclitaxel: Two published studies report that initial administration of paclitaxel infused over 24 hours followed by doxorubicin administered over 48 hours resulted in a significant decrease in doxorubicin clearance with more profound neutropenic and stomatitis episodes than the reverse sequence of administration.
Progesterone: In a published study, progesterone was given intravenously to patients with advanced malignancies (ECOG PS < 2) at high doses (up to 10 g over 24 hours) concomitantly with a fixed doxorubicin dose (60 mg/m^2) via bolus. Enhanced doxorubicin-induced neutropenia and thrombocytopenia were observed.
Verapamil: A study of the effects of verapamil on the acute toxicity of doxorubicin in mice revealed higher intial peak concentrations of doxorubicin in the heart with a higher incidence and severity of degenerative changes in cardiac tissue resulting in a shorter survival.
Cyclosporine: The addition of cyclosporine to doxorubicin may result in increases in AUC for both doxorubicin and doxorubicinol possibly due to a decrease in clearance of parent drug and a decrease in metabolism of doxorubicinol. Literature reports suggest that adding cyclosporine to doxorubicin results in more profound and prolonged hematologic toxicity than doxorubicin alone. Coma and/or seizures have also been described.
Literature reports have also described the following drug interactions: phenobarbital increases the elimination of doxorubicin, phenytoin levels may be decreased by doxorubicin, streptozocin (Zanosar) may inhibit hepatic metabolism of doxorubicin, and administration of live vaccines to immunosuppressed patients including those undergoing cytotoxic chemotherapy may be hazardous.
Laboratory Tests: Initial treatment with doxorubicin requires observation of the patient and periodic monitoring of complete blood counts, hepatic function tests, and radionuclide left ventricular ejection fraction (see **WARNINGS**).
Like other cytotoxic drugs, doxorubicin may induce "tumor lysis syndrome" and hyperuricemia in patients with rapidly growing tumors. Appropriate supportive and pharmacologic measures may prevent or alleviate this complication.
Carcinogenesis, Mutagenesis, Impairment of Fertility: Formal long-term carcinogenicity studies have not been conducted with doxorubicin. Doxorubicin and related compounds have been shown to have mutagenic and carcinogenic properties when tested in experimental models (including bacterial systems, mammalian cells in culture, and female Sprague-Dawley rats).
The possible adverse effect on fertility in males and females in humans or experimental animals have not been adequately evaluated. Testicular atrophy was observed in rats and dogs.
Treatment-related acute myelogenous leukemia has been reported in patients treated with doxorubicin-containing adjuvant chemotherapy regimens (see **ADVERSE REACTIONS, Hematologic**). The exact role of doxorubicin has not been elucidated. Pediatric patients treated with doxorubicin or other topoisomerase II inhibitors are at risk for developing acute myelogenous leukemia and other neoplasms. The extent of increased risk associated with doxorubicin has not been precisely quantified.
Pregnancy Category D: (See **WARNINGS**.)
Nursing Mothers: Because of the potential for serious adverse reactions in nursing infants from doxorubicin, mothers should be advised to discontinue nursing during doxorubicin therapy.
Pediatric Use: Pediatric patients are at increased risk for developing delayed cardiotoxicity. Follow-up cardiac evaluations are recommended periodically to monitor for this delayed cardiotoxicity (see **WARNINGS**).
Doxorubicin, as a component of intensive chemotherapy regimens administered to pediatric patients, may contribute to prepubertal growth failure. It may also contribute to gonadal impairment, which is usually temporary.

ADVERSE REACTIONS

Dose-limiting toxicities of therapy are myelosuppression and cardiotoxicity (see **WARNINGS**). Other reactions reported are:
Cardiotoxicity: (See **WARNINGS**.)
Cutaneous: Reversible complete alopecia occurs in most cases. Hyperpigmentation of nailbeds and dermal creases, primarily in children, and onycholysis have been reported in a few cases. Recall of skin reaction due to prior radiotherapy has occurred with doxorubicin administration.
Gastrointestinal: Acute nausea and vomiting occurs frequently and may be severe. This may be alleviated by antiemetic therapy. Mucositis (stomatitis and esophagitis) may occur 5 to 10 days after administration. The effect may be severe leading to ulceration and represents a site of origin for severe infections. The dosage regimen consisting of administration of doxorubicin on 3 successive days results in

Continued on next page

Adriamycin—Cont.

the greater incidence and severity of mucositis. Ulceration and necrosis of the colon, especially the cecum, may occur leading to bleeding or severe infections which can be fatal. This reaction has been reported in patients with acute nonlymphocytic leukemia treated with a 3-day course of doxorubicin combined with cytarabine. Anorexia and diarrhea have been occasionally reported.

Vascular: Phlebosclerosis has been reported especially when small veins are used or a single vein is used for repeated administration. Facial flushing may occur if the injection is given too rapidly.

Local: Severe cellulitis, vesication and tissue necrosis will occur if extravasation of doxorubicin occurs during administration. Erythematous streaking along the vein proximal to the site of the injection has been reported (see **DOSAGE AND ADMINISTRATION**).

Hematologic: The occurrence of secondary acute myeloid leukemia with or without a preleukemic phase has been reported in patients concurrently treated with doxorubicin in association with DNA-damaging antineoplastic agents. Such cases could have a short (1-3 years) latency period. An analysis of 1474 breast cancer patients who received adjuvant doxorubicin treatment in clinical trials, showed a 10-year estimated risk of developing treatment-related leukemia at 2.5% (95% confidence interval [CI], 1.0% to 5.1%) for the 810 patients receiving radiotherapy plus chemotherapy and 0.5% (95% CI, 0.1% to 2.4%) for the 664 patients receiving chemotherapy alone. The overall risk was 1.5% (95% CI, 0.7%-2.9%) at 10 years for the entire patient population. Pediatric patients are also at risk of developing secondary acute myeloid leukemia.

Hypersensitivity: Fever, chills, and urticaria have been reported occasionally. Anaphylaxis may occur. A case of apparent cross-sensitivity to lincomycin has been reported.

Other: Conjunctivitis and lacrimation occur rarely.

OVERDOSAGE

Acute overdosage with doxorubicin enhances the toxic effects of mucositis, leukopenia, and thrombocytopenia. Treatment of acute overdosage consists of treatment of the severely myelosuppressed patient with hospitalization, antimicrobials, platelet transfusion and symptomatic treatment of mucositis. Use of hemopoietic growth factor (G-CSF, GM-CSF) may be considered.

The 200 mg Adriamycin (DOXOrubicin HCl) Injection, USP is packaged as a multiple dose vial, and caution should be exercised to prevent inadvertent overdosage.

Cumulative dosage with doxorubicin increases the risk of cardiomyopathy and resultant congestive heart failure (see **WARNINGS**). Treatment consists of vigorous management of congestive heart failure with digitalis preparations, diuretics, and afterload reducers such as ACE inhibitors.

DOSAGE AND ADMINISTRATION

Care in the administration of Adriamycin (DOXOrubicin HCl) Injection, USP and Adriamycin (DOXOrubicin HCl) for Injection, USP will reduce the chance of perivenous infiltration (see **WARNINGS**). It may also decrease the chance of local reactions such as urticaria and erythematous streaking. On intravenous administration of doxorubicin, extravasation may occur with or without an accompanying burning or stinging sensation, even if blood returns well on aspiration of the infusion needle. If any signs or symptoms of extravasation have occurred, the injection or infusion should be immediately terminated and restarted in another vein. If extravasation is suspected, intermittent application of ice to the site for 15 min. q.i.d. × 3 days may be useful. The benefit of local administration of drugs has not been clearly established. Because of the progressive nature of extravasation reactions, close observation and plastic surgery consultation is recommended. Blistering, ulceration and/or persistent pain are indications for wide excision surgery, followed by split-thickness skin grafting.[1]

The most commonly used dose schedule when used as a single agent is 60 to 75 mg/m^2 as a single intravenous injection administered at 21-day intervals. The lower dosage should be given to patients with inadequate marrow reserves due to old age, or prior therapy, or neoplastic marrow infiltration. Adriamycin (DOXOrubicin HCl) Injection, USP and Adriamycin (DOXOrubicin HCl) for Injection, USP have been used concurrently with other approved chemotherapeutic agents. Evidence is available that in some types of neoplastic disease, combination chemotherapy is superior to single agents. The benefits and risks of such therapy continue to be elucidated. When used in combination with other chemotherapy drugs, the most commonly used dosage of doxorubicin is 40 to 60 mg/m^2 given as a single intravenous injection every 21 to 28 days. Doxorubicin dosage must be reduced in case of hyperbilirubinemia as follows:

Plasma bilirubin concentration (mg/dL)	Dosage reduction (%)
1.2–3.0	50
3.1–5.0	75

Reconstitution Directions: Adriamycin (DOXOrubicin HCl) for Injection, USP 10 mg, 20 mg, and 50 mg vials should be reconstituted with 5 mL, 10 mL, and 25 mL respectively of 0.9% Sodium Chloride Injection to give a final concentration of 2 mg/mL of doxorubicin hydrochloride. An appropriate volume of air should be withdrawn from the vial during reconstitution to avoid excessive pressure build up. Bacteriostatic diluents are not recommended.

After adding the diluent, the vial should be shaken and the contents allowed to dissolve. The reconstituted solution is stable for 7 days at room temperature and under normal room light (100 foot-candles) and 15 days under refrigeration, 2° to 8°C (36° to 46°F). It should be protected from exposure to sunlight. Discard any unused solution from the 10 mg, 20 mg, and 50 mg single dose vials. Unused solutions of the multiple dose vial remaining beyond the recommended storage times should be discarded.

It is recommended that Adriamycin (DOXOrubicin HCl) Injection, USP and Adriamycin (DOXOrubicin HCl) for Injection, USP be slowly administered into the tubing of a freely running intravenous infusion of Sodium Chloride Injection or 5% Dextrose Injection. The tubing should be attached to a Butterfly® needle inserted preferably into a large vein. If possible, avoid veins over joints or in extremities with compromised venous or lymphatic drainage. The rate of administration is dependent on the size of the vein and the dosage. However, the dose should be administered in not less than 3 to 5 minutes. Local erythematous streaking along the vein as well as facial flushing may be indicative of too rapid an administration. A burning or stinging sensation may be indicative of perivenous infiltration and the infusion should be immediately terminated and restarted in another vein. Perivenous infiltration may occur painlessly.

Doxorubicin should not be mixed with heparin or fluorouracil since it has been reported that these drugs are incompatible to the extent that a precipitate may form. Until specific compatibility data are available, it is not recommended that doxorubicin be mixed with other drugs.

Note: Parenteral drug products should be inspected visually for particulate matter and discoloration prior to administration, whenever solution and container permit.

Handling and Disposal: Skin reactions associated with doxorubicin have been reported. Skin accidently exposed to doxorubicin should be rinsed copiously with soap and warm water, and if the eyes are involved, standard irrigation techniques should be used immediately. The use of goggles, gloves, and protective gowns is recommended during preparation and administration of the drug.

Procedures for proper handling and disposal of anti-cancer drugs should be considered. Several guidelines on this subject have been published.[1-8] There is no general agreement that all of the procedures recommended in the guidelines are necessary or appropriate.

Caregivers of pediatric patients receiving doxorubicin should be counseled to take precautions (such as wearing latex gloves) to prevent contact with the patient's urine and other body fluids for at least 5 days after each treatment.

HOW SUPPLIED

Adriamycin (DOXOrubicin HCl) for Injection, USP is supplied as a sterile red-orange lyophilized powder in single dose flip-top vials in the following package strengths:

NDC 55390-231-10: 10 mg vial; carton of 10.
NDC 55390-232-10: 20 mg vial; carton of 10.
NDC 55390-233-01: 50 mg vial; individually boxed.

Store unreconstituted vial at controlled room temperature, 15° to 30°C (59° to 86°F) [see USP]. **Protect from light.** Retain in carton until time of use. Discard unused portion.

Reconstituted Solution Stability: After adding the diluent, the vial should be shaken and the contents allowed to dissolve. The reconstituted solution is stable for 7 days at room temperature and under normal room light (100 foot-candles) and 15 days under refrigeration (2° to 8°C). It should be protected from exposure to sunlight. Discard any unused solution from the 10 mg, 20 mg and 50 mg single dose vials. Unused solutions of the multiple dose vial remaining beyond the recommended storage times should be discarded.

Adriamycin (DOXOrubicin HCl) Injection, USP is supplied in single-dose, flip-top vials, as a red-orange solution containing Doxorubicin Hydrochloride, USP 2 mg/mL in the following package strengths:

NDC 55390-235-10: 510 mg in 5 mL; carton of 10.
NDC 55390-236-10: 20 mg in 10 mL; carton of 10.
NDC 55390-237-01: 50 mg in 25 mL; individually boxed.

Store refrigerated, 2° to 8°C (36° to 46°F).

Protect from light. Retain in carton until time of use. Discard unused portion.

Adriamycin (DOXOrubicin HCl) Injection, USP is supplied in a sterile, multiple dose, flip-top vial, as a red-orange solution containing Doxorubicin Hydrochloride, USP 2 mg/mL in the following package strength:

NDC 55390-238-01: 200 mg in 100 mL; individually boxed.

Store refrigerated, 2° to 8°C (36° to 46°F).

Protect from light. Retain in carton until contents are used.

REFERENCES

1. Recommendations for the Safe Handling of Parenteral Antineoplastic Drugs. NIH Publication No. 83-2621. For sale by the Superintendent of Documents, U.S. Government Printing Office, Washington, D.C. 20402.
2. AMA Council Report. Guidelines for Handling Parenteral Antineoplastics. *JAMA*, 1985; 253 (11): 1590-1592.
3. National Study Commission on Cytotoxic Exposure — Recommendation for Handling Cytotoxic Agents. Available from Louis P. Jeffrey, ScD, Chairman, National Study Commission on Cytotoxic Exposure, Massachusetts College of Pharmacy and Allied Health Sciences, 179 Longwood Ave., Boston, Massachusetts 02115.
4. Clinical Oncological Society of Australia: Guidelines and Recommendations for Safe Handling of Antineoplastic Agents. *Med J Australia* 1983; *1*:426-428.
5. Jones RB, *et al.* Safe Handling of Chemotherapeutic Agents: A Report From the Mount Sinai Medical Center. *CA-A Cancer Journal for Clinicians* 1983; Sept/Oct, 258-263.
6. American Society of Hospital Pharmacists Technical Assistance Bulletin on Handling Cytotoxic and Hazardous Drugs. *Am J Hosp Pharm* 1990; *47*:1033-1049.
7. Controlling Occupational Exposure to Hazardous Drugs. (OSHA Work-Practice Guidelines), *Am J Healthsyst Pharm*, 1996; *53*: 1669-1685.
8. ONS Clinical Practice Committee. Cancer Chemotherapy Guidelines and Recommendations for Practice Pittsburgh, Pa: Oncology Nursing Society; 1999:32-41.

Manufactured by: Ben Venue Laboratories, Inc. Bedford, OH 44146
Manufactured for: Bedford Laboratories™ Bedford, OH 44146
December 2002 ADR-P00

CERUBIDINE® ℞

[*sy-rew"bĭ 'dēan*]
(Daunorubicin HCl)
FOR INJECTION
Rx ONLY.

WARNING

1. Cerubidine must be given into a rapidly flowing intravenous infusion. It must *never* be given by the intramuscular or subcutaneous route. Severe local tissue necrosis will occur if there is extravasation during administration.
2. Myocardial toxicity manifested in its most severe form by potentially fatal congestive heart failure may occur either during therapy or months to years after termination of therapy. The incidence of myocardial toxicity increases after a total cumulative dose exceeding 400 to 550 mg/m^2 in adults, 300 mg/m^2 in children more than 2 years of age, or 10 mg/kg in children less than 2 years of age.
3. Severe myelosuppression occurs when used in therapeutic doses; this may lead to infection or hemorrhage.
4. It is recommended that Cerubidine be administered only by physicians who are experienced in leukemia chemotherapy and in facilities with laboratory and supportive resources adequate to monitor drug tolerance and protect and maintain a patient compromised by drug toxicity. The physician and institution must be capable of responding rapidly and completely to severe hemorrhagic conditions and/or overwhelming infection.
5. Dosage should be reduced in patients with impaired hepatic or renal function.

DESCRIPTION

Cerubidine (daunorubicin hydrochloride) is the hydrochloride salt of an anthracycline cytotoxic antibiotic produced by a strain of *Streptomyces coeruleorubidus*. It is provided as a sterile reddish lyophilized powder in vials for intravenous administration only. Each vial contains 21.4 mg daunorubicin hydrochloride, (equivalent to 20 mg of daunorubicin), and 100 mg mannitol. It is soluble in water when adequately agitated and produces a reddish solution. It has the following structural formula which may be described with the chemical name of (1*S*,3*S*)-3-Acetyl-1,2,3,4,6,11-hexahydro-3,5,12-trihydroxy-10-methoxy-6,11-dioxo-1-naphthacenyl 3-amino-2,3,6-trideoxy-α-L-*lyxo* -hexopyranoside hydrochloride. Its molecular formula is $C_{27}H_{29}NO_{10}$ •HCl with a molecular weight of 563.99. It is a hygroscopic crystalline powder. The pH of a 5 mg/mL aqueous solution is 4.5 to 6.5. The structural formula is as follows.

CLINICAL PHARMACOLOGY

Mechanism of Action: Cerubidine has antimitotic and cytotoxic activity through a number of proposed mechanisms of action. Cerubidine forms complexes with DNA by intercalation between base pairs. It inhibits topoisomerase II activity by stabilizing the DNA-topoisomerase II complex, preventing the religation portion of the ligation-religation reaction that topoisomerase II catalyzes. Single strand and double strand DNA breaks result.

Cerubidine may also inhibit polymerase activity, affect regulation of gene expression, and produce free radical damage to DNA.

Cerubidine possesses an antitumor effect against a wide spectrum of animal tumors, either grafted or spontaneous.

Pharmacokinetics

General: Following intravenous injection of Cerubidine, plasma levels of daunorubicin decline rapidly, indicating rapid tissue uptake and concentration. Thereafter, plasma levels decline slowly with a half-life of 45 minutes in the initial phase and 18.5 hours in the terminal phase. By 1 hour after drug administration, the predominant plasma species is daunorubicinol, and active metabolite, which disappears with a half-life of 26.7 hours.

Distribution: Cerubidine is rapidly and widely distributed in tissues, with highest levels in the spleen, kidneys, liver, lungs, and heart. The drug binds to many cellular components, particularly nucleic acids. There is no evidence that Cerubidine crosses the blood-brain barrier, but the drug apparently crosses the placenta.

Metabolism and Elimination: Cerubidine is extensively metabolized in the liver and other tissues, mainly by cytoplasmic aldo-keto reductases, producing daunorubicinol, the major metabolite which has antineoplastic activity. Approximately 40% of the drug in the plasma is present as daunorubicinol within 30 minutes and 60% in 4 hours after a dose of daunorubicin. Further metabolism via reduction cleavage of the glycosidic bond, 4-O demethylation, and conjugation with both sulfate and glucuronide have been demonstrated. Simple glycosidic cleavage of daunorubicin or daunorubicinol is not a significant metabolic pathway in man. Twenty-five percent of an administered dose of Cerubidine is eliminated in an active form by urinary excretion and an estimated 40% by biliary excretion.

Special Populations

Pediatric Patients: Although appropriate studies with Cerubidine have not been performed in the pediatric population, cardiotoxicity may be more frequent and occur at lower cumulative doses in children.

Geriatric Patients: Although appropriate studies with Cerubidine have not been performed in the geriatric population, cardiotoxicity may be more frequent in the elderly. Caution should also be used in patients who have inadequate bone marrow reserves due to old age. In addition, elderly patients are more likely to have age-related renal function impairment, which may require reduction of dosage in patients receiving Cerubidine.

Renal and Hepatic Impairment: Doses of Cerubidine should be reduced in patients with hepatic and renal impairment. Patients with serum bilirubin concentrations of 1.2 to 3 mg/dL should receive 75% of the usual daily dose and patients with serum bilirubin concentrations greater than 3 mg/dL should receive 50% of the usual daily dose. Patients with serum creatinine concentrations of greater than 3 mg/dL should receive 50% of the usual daily dose. (See **WARNINGS, Evaluation of Hepatic and Renal Function**).

Clinical Studies: In the treatment of adult acute nonlymphocytic leukemia, Cerubidine, used as a single agent, has produced complete remission rates of 40 to 50%, and in combination with cytarabine, has produced complete remission rates of 53 to 65%.

The addition of Cerubidine to the two-drug induction regimen of vincristine-prednisone in the treatment of childhood acute lymphocytic leukemia does not increase the rate of complete remission. In children receiving identical CNS prophylaxis and maintenance therapy (without consolidation), there is prolongation of complete remission duration (statistically significant, $p<0.02$) in those children induced with the three drug (Cerubidine-vincristine-prednisone) regimen as compared to two drugs. There is no evidence of any impact of Cerubidine on the duration of complete remission when a consolidation (intensification) phase is employed as part of a total treatment program.

In adult acute lymphocytic leukemia, in contrast to childhood acute lymphocytic leukemia, Cerubidine during induction significantly increases the rate of complete remission, but not remission duration, compared to that obtained with vincristine, prednisone, and L-asparaginase alone. The use of Cerubidine in combination with vincristine, prednisone, and L-asparaginase has produced complete remission rates of 83% in contrast to a 47% remission in patients not receiving Cerubidine.

INDICATIONS AND USAGE

Cerubidine in combination with other approved anticancer drugs is indicated for remission induction in acute nonlymphocytic leukemia (myelogenous, monocytic, erythroid) of adults and for remission induction in acute lymphocytic leukemia of children and adults.

CONTRAINDICATIONS

Cerubidine is contraindicated in patients who have shown a hypersensitivity to it.

WARNINGS

Bone Marrow: Cerubidine is a potent bone marrow suppressant. Suppression will occur in all patients given a therapeutic dose of this drug. Therapy with Cerubidine should not be started in patients with pre-existing drug-induced bone marrow suppression unless the benefit from such treatment warrants the risk. Persistent, severe myelosuppression may result in superinfection or hemorrhage.

Cardiac Effects: Special attention must be given to the potential cardiac toxicity of Cerubidine, particularly in infants and children. Pre-existing heart disease and previous therapy with doxorubicin are co-factors of increased risk of Cerubidine-induced cardiac toxicity and the benefit-to-risk ratio of Cerubidine therapy in such patients should be weighed before starting Cerubidine. In adults, at total cumulative doses less than 550 mg/m^2, acute congestive heart failure is seldom encountered. However, rare instances of pericarditis-myocarditis, not dose-related, have been reported.

In adults, at cumulative doses exceeding 550 mg/m^2, there is an increased incidence of drug-induced congestive heart failure. Based on prior clinical experience with doxorubicin, this limit appears lower, namely 400 mg/m^2, in patients who received radiation therapy that encompassed the heart.

In infants and children, there appears to be a greater susceptibility to anthracycline-induced cardiotoxicity compared to that in adults, which is more clearly dose-related. Anthracycline therapy (including daunorubicin) in pediatric patients has been reported to produce impaired left ventricular systolic performance, reduced contractility, congestive heart failure or death. These conditions may occur months to years following cessation of chemotherapy. This appears to be dose-dependent and aggravated by thoracic irradiation. Long-term periodic evaluation of cardiac function in such patients should, thus, be performed. In both children and adults, the total dose of Cerubidine administered should also take into account any previous or concomitant therapy with other potentially cardiotoxic agents or related compounds such as doxorubicin.

There is no absolutely reliable method of predicting the patients in whom acute congestive heart failure will develop as a result of the cardiac toxic effect of Cerubidine. However, certain changes in the electrocardiogram and a decrease in the systolic ejection fraction from pre-treatment baseline may help to recognize those patients at greatest risk to develop congestive heart failure. On the basis of the electrocardiogram, a decrease equal to or greater than 30% in limb lead QRS voltage has been associated with a significant risk of drug-induced cardiomyopathy. Therefore, an electrocardiogram and/or determination of systolic ejection fraction should be performed before each course of Cerubidine. In the event that one or the other of these predictive parameters should occur, the benefit of continued therapy must be weighed against the risk of producing cardiac damage.

Early clinical diagnosis of drug-induced congestive heart failure appears to be essential for successful treatment.

Evaluation of Hepatic and Renal Function: Significant hepatic or renal impairment can enhance the toxicity of the recommended doses of Cerubidine; therefore, prior to administration, evaluation of hepatic function and renal function using conventional clinical laboratory tests is recommended (See **DOSAGE AND ADMINISTRATION** section).

Pregnancy: Cerubidine may cause fetal harm when administered to a pregnant woman. An increased incidence of fetal abnormalities (parieto-occipital cranioschisis, umbilical hernias, or rachischisis) and abortions was reported in rabbits at doses of 0.05 mg/kg/day or approximately 1/100th of the highest recommended human dose on a body surface area basis. Rats showed an increased incidence of esophageal, cardiovascular and urogenital abnormalities as well as rib fusions at doses of 4 mg/kg/day or approximately 1/2 the human dose on a body surface area basis. Decreases in fetal birth weight and post-delivery growth rate were observed in mice. There are no adequate and well-controlled studies in pregnant women. If this drug is used during pregnancy, or if the patient becomes pregnant while taking this drug, the patient should be apprised of the potential hazard to the fetus. Women of childbearing potential should be advised to avoid becoming pregnant.

Secondary leukemias: There have been reports of secondary leukemias in patients exposed to topoisomerase II inhibitors when used in combination with other antineoplastic agents or radiation therapy.

Extravasation at Injection Site: Extravasation of Cerubidine at the site of intravenous administration can cause severe local tissue necrosis. (See **ADVERSE REACTIONS** section.)

PRECAUTIONS

General: Therapy with Cerubidine requires close patient observation and frequent complete blood-count determinations. Cardiac, renal, and hepatic function should be evaluated prior to each course of treatment.

Appropriate measures must be taken to control any systemic infection before beginning therapy with Cerubidine.

Cerubidine may transiently impart a red coloration to the urine after administration, and patients should be advised to expect this.

Laboratory Tests: Cerubidine may induce hyperuricemia secondary to rapid lysis of leukemic cells. As a precaution, allopurinol administration is usually begun prior to initiating antileukemic therapy. Blood uric acid levels should be monitored and appropriate therapy initiated in the event that hyperuricemia develops.

Carcinogenesis, Mutagenesis, Impairment of Fertility: Cerubidine, when injected subcutaneously into mice, causes fibrosarcomas to develop at the injection site. When administered to mice thrice weekly intraperitoneally, no carcinogenic effect was noted after 18 months of observation. In male rats administered Cerubidine thrice weekly for 6 months, at 1/70th the recommended human dose on a body surface area basis, peritoneal sarcomas were found at 18 months. A single IV dose of Cerubidine administered to rats at 1.6 fold the recommended human dose on a body surface area basis caused mammary adenocarcinomas to appear at 1 year. Cerubidine was mutagenic *in vitro* (Ames assay, V79 hamster cell assay), and clastogenic *in vitro* (CCRFCEM human lymphoblasts) and in vivo (SCE assay in mouse bone marrow) tests.

In male dogs at a daily dose of 0.25 mg/kg administered intravenously, testicular atrophy was noted at autopsy. Histologic examination revealed total aplasia of the spermatocyte series in the seminiferous tubules with complete aspermatogenesis.

Pregnancy: Teratogenic Effects — Pregnancy Category D (See **WARNINGS** section.)

Nursing Mothers: It is not known whether this drug is excreted in human milk. Because many drugs are excreted in human milk and because of the potential for serious adverse reactions in nursing infants from Cerubidine, mothers should be advised to discontinue nursing during Cerubidine therapy.

Elderly: See **CLINICAL PHARMACOLOGY, Special Populations, Geriatric Patients** section.

Pediatric Use: See **CLINICAL PHARMACOLOGY, Special Populations, Pediatric Patients** section and **WARNINGS, Cardiac Effects** section.

Drug Interactions: Use of Cerubidine in a patient who has previously received doxorubicin increases the risk of cardiotoxicity. Cerubidine should not be used in patients who have previously received the recommended maximum cumulative doses of doxorubicin or Cerubidine. Cyclophosphamide used concurrently with Cerubidine may also result in increased cardiotoxicity.

Dosage reduction of Cerubidine may be required when used concurrently with other myelosuppressive agents.

Hepatotoxic medications, such as high-dose methotrexate, may impair liver function and increase the risk of toxicity.

ADVERSE REACTIONS

Dose-limiting toxicity includes myelosuppression and cardiotoxicity (See **WARNINGS** section). Other reactions include:

Cutaneous: Reversible alopecia occurs in most patients. Rash, contact dermatitis and urticaria have occurred rarely.

Gastrointestinal: Acute nausea and vomiting occur but are usually mild. Antiemetic therapy may be of some help. Mucositis may occur 3 to 7 days after administration. Diarrhea and abdominal pain have occasionally been reported.

Local: If extravasation occurs during administration, severe local tissue necrosis, severe cellulitis, thrombophlebitis, or painful induration can result.

Acute Reactions: Rarely, anaphylactoid reaction, fever, and chills can occur. Hyperuricemia may occur, especially in patients with leukemia, and serum uric acid levels should be monitored.

DOSAGE AND ADMINISTRATION

Parenteral drug products should be inspected visually for particulate matter prior to administration, whenever solution and container permit.

Principles: In order to eradicate the leukemic cells and induce a complete remission, a profound suppression of the bone marrow is usually required. Evaluation of both the peripheral blood and bone marrow is mandatory in the formulation of appropriate treatment plans.

It is recommended that the dosage of Cerubidine be reduced in instances of hepatic or renal impairment. For example, using serum bilirubin and serum creatinine as indicators of liver and kidney function, the following dose modifications are recommended:

Serum Bilirubin	Serum Creatinine	Dose Reduction
1.2 to 3.0 mg%		25%
>3 mg%		50%
	>3 mg%	50%

Representative Dose Schedules and Combination for the Approved Indication of Remission Induction in Adult Acute Nonlymphocytic Leukemia:

In Combination: For patients under age 60, Cerubidine 45 mg/m^2/day IV on days 1, 2, and 3 of the first course and on days 1, 2 of subsequent courses AND cytosine arabinoside 100 mg/m^2/day IV infusion daily for 7 days for the first course and for 5 days for subsequent courses.

For patients 60 years of age and above, Cerubidine 30 mg/m^2/day IV on days 1, 2, and 3 of the first course and on days 1, 2 of subsequent courses AND cytosine arabinoside 100 mg/m^2/day IV infusion daily for 7 days for the first course and for 5 days for subsequent courses. This Cerubidine dose-reduction is based on a single study and may not be appropriate if optimal supportive care is available.

The attainment of a normal-appearing bone marrow may require up to three courses of induction therapy. Evaluation of the bone marrow following recovery from the previous course of induction therapy determines whether a further course of induction treatment is required.

Representative Dose Schedule and Combination for the Approved Indication of Remission Induction in Pediatric Acute Lymphocytic Leukemia:

In Combination: Cerubidine 25 mg/m^2 IV on day 1 every week, vincristine 1.5 mg/m^2 IV on day 1 every week, prednisone 40 mg/m^2 PO daily. Generally, a complete remission will be obtained within four such courses of therapy; however, if after four courses the patient is in partial remission, an additional one or, if necessary, two courses may be given in an effort to obtain a complete remission.

Continued on next page

Cerubidine—Cont.

In children less than 2 years of age or below 0.5 m^2 body surface area, it has been recommended that the Cerubidine dosage calculation should be based on weight (1 mg/kg) instead of body surface area.

Representative Dose Schedules and Combination for the Approved Indication of Remission Induction in Adult Acute Lymphocytic Leukemia:

In Combination: Cerubidine 45 mg/m^2/day IV on days 1, 2, and 3 AND vincristine 2 mg IV on days 1, 8, and 15; prednisone 40 mg/m^2/day PO on days 1 through 22, then tapered between days 22 to 29; L-asparaginase 500 IU/kg/day x 10 days IV on days 22 through 32.

The contents of a vial should be reconstituted with 4 mL of Sterile Water for Injection and agitated gently until the material has completely dissolved. The sterile vial contents provide 20 mg of daunorubicin, with 5 mg of daunorubicin per mL. The desired dose is withdrawn into a syringe containing 10 mL to 15 mL of 0.9% Sodium Chloride Injection, USP and then injected into the tubing or sidearm in a rapidly flowing IV infusion of 5% Dextrose Injection, USP or 0.9% Sodium Chloride Injection, USP. Cerubidine should not be administered mixed with other drugs or heparin.

Storage and Handling: Store unreconstituted powder at controlled room temperature, 15° to 30° C (59° to 86° F). The reconstituted solution is stable for 24 hours at room temperature and 48 hours under refrigeration. It should be protected from exposure to sunlight. **Protect from light.** Retain in carton until time of use.

If Cerubidine contacts the skin or mucosae, the area should be washed thoroughly with soap and water. Procedures for proper handling and disposal of anticancer drugs should be considered. Several guidelines on this subject have been published.[1-7] There is no general agreement that all of the procedures recommended in the guidelines are necessary or appropriate.

HOW SUPPLIED

Cerubine (daunorubicin HCl) for Injection, is available in butyl-rubber-stoppered vials, each containing 21.4 mg Daunorubicin hydrochloride equivalent to 20 mg of daunorubicin and 100 mg of mannitol, as a sterile reddish lyophilized powder. When reconstituted with 4 mL of Sterile Water for Injection, USP, each mL contains 5 mg daunorubicin activity.

NDC 55390-281-10 20 mg, single dose vials; carton of 10.

REFERENCES

1. Recommendations for the Safe Handling of Parenteral Antineoplastic Drugs. NIH Publication No. 83-2621. For sale by the Superintendent of Documents, U.S. Government Printing Office, Washington, D.C. 20402.
2. AMA Council Report. Guidelines for Handling Parenteral Antineoplastics. *JAMA*, March 15, 1985.
3. National Study Commission on Cytotoxic Exposure Recommendations for Handling Cytotoxic Agents. Available from Louis R Jeffrey, Sc.D., Chairman, National Study Commission on Cytotoxic Exposure, Massachusetts College of Pharmacy and Allied Health Sciences, 179 Longwood Avenue, Boston, Massachusetts 02115.
4. Clinical Oncological Society of Australia: Guidelines and recommendations for safe handling of antineoplastic agents. *Med J Australia* 1:426–428, 1983.
5. Jones RB, et al: Safe handling of chemotherapeutic agents: A report from the Mount Sinai Medical Center, Ca *A Cancer Journal for Clinicians* Sept/Oct, 258–263, 1983.
6. American Society of Hospital Pharmacists technical assistance bulletin on handling cytotoxic and hazardous drugs. *Am J Hosp Pharm* 47:1033–1049, 1990.
7. Controlling Occupational Exposure to Hazardous Drugs. (OSHA Work-Practice Guidelines), *Am J Health-Syst Pharm*, 15:1669–1685, 1996.

Manufactured by:
Ben Venue Laboratories, Inc.
Bedford, OH 44146
Manufactured for:
Bedford Laboratories
Bedford, OH 44146
December 1999 CRD-P03

GLUCAGEN® ℞

[glōō 'ka-gĭn]
[Glucagon (rDNA origin) for injection]

Rx ONLY

DESCRIPTION

GlucaGen® [glucagon (rDNA origin) for injection] manufactured by Novo Nordisk A/S is produced by expression of recombinant DNA in a saccharomyces cerevisiae vector with subsequent purification.

The chemical structure of the glucagon in GlucaGen® is identical to naturally occurring human glucagon and to glucagon extracted from beef and pork pancreas. Glucagon with the empirical formula of $C_{153}H_{225}N_{43}O_{49}S$, and a molecular weight of 3483, is a single-chain polypeptide containing 29 amino acid residues. The structure of glucagon is: [See chemical structure at top of next column]

GlucaGen® 1 mg (1 IU) is supplied as a sterile, lyophilized white powder in a 2 ml vial alone, or accompanied by Sterile Water for Reconstitution (1 ml) also in a 2 ml vial. Glucagon, as supplied at pH 2.5–3.5, is soluble in water.

His-Ser-Gln-Gly-Thr-Phe-Thr-Ser-Asp-Tyr-Ser-
1 2 3 4 5 6 7 8 9 10 11
Lys-Tyr-Leu-Asp-Ser-Arg-Arg-Ala-Gln-Asp-Phe-
12 13 14 15 16 17 18 19 20 21 22
Val-Gln-Trp-Leu-Met-Asn-Thr
23 24 25 26 27 28 29

Active Ingredient in each vial
Glucagon as hydrochloride 1 mg (corresponding to 1 IU).
Other Ingredients
Lactose monohydrate (107 mg)

When the glucagon powder is reconstituted with Sterile Water for Reconstitution, it forms a solution of 1 mg (1 IU)/ml glucagon for subcutaneous (sc), intramuscular (im), or intravenous (iv) injection.

GlucaGen® is an antihypoglycemic agent, and a gastrointestinal motility inhibitor.

CLINICAL PHARMACOLOGY

Intramuscular (IM) injection of GlucaGen® resulted in a mean C_{max} (CV%) of 1686 pg/ml (43%) and a median T_{max} of 12.5 minutes. The mean apparent half-life of 45 minutes after IM injection probably reflects prolonged absorption from the injection site. Glucagon is degraded in the liver, kidney, and plasma.[1]

Antihypoglycemic Action: Glucagon induces liver glycogen breakdown, releasing glucose from the liver. Blood glucose concentration rises within 10 minutes of injection and maximal concentrations are attained at approximately a half hour after injection (see Figure). Hepatic stores of glycogen are necessary for glucagon to produce an antihypoglycemic effect.

Recovery from insulin induced hypoglycemia (mean blood glucose) after i.m. injection of 1 mg GlucaGen® in Type I diabetic men

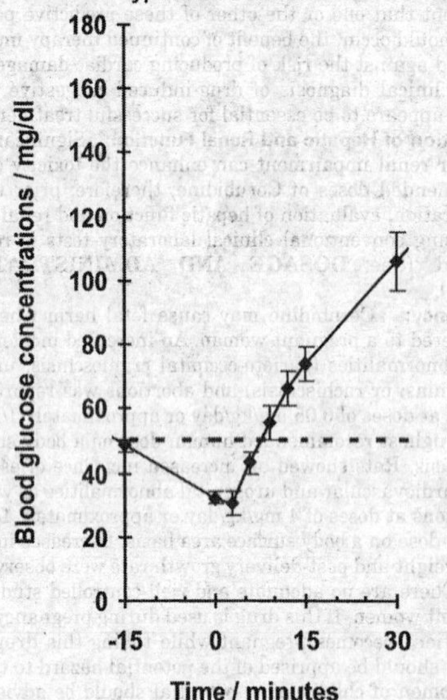

Gastrointestinal Motility Inhibition: Extra hepatic effects of glucagon include relaxation of the smooth muscle of the stomach, duodenum, small bowel, and colon.

INDICATIONS AND USAGE

For the treatment of hypoglycemia: GlucaGen® is used to treat severe hypoglycemic (low blood sugar) reactions which may occur in patients with diabetes treated with insulin.

Because GlucaGen® depletes glycogen stores, the patient should be given supplemental carbohydrates as soon as he/she awakens and is able to swallow, especially children or adolescents.

Medical evaluation is recommended for all patients who experience severe hypoglycemia.

For use as a diagnostic aid: GlucaGen® is indicated for use during radiologic examinations to temporarily inhibit movement of the gastrointestinal tract. Glucagon is as effective for this examination as are the anticholinergic drugs. However, the addition of the anticholinergic agent may result in increased side effects. Because GlucaGen depletes glycogen stores, the patient should be given oral carbohydrates as soon as the procedure is completed.

CONTRAINDICATIONS

Glucagon is contraindicated in patients with known hypersensitivity to glucagon or any constituent in GlucaGen® and in patients with pheochromocytoma or with insulinoma.

WARNINGS

GlucaGen® should be administered cautiously to patients suspected of having pheochromocytoma of insulinoma. Secondary hypoglycemia may occur and should be countered by adequate carbohydrate intake following glucagon treatment.

Glucagon may release catecholamines from pheochromocytomas and is contraindicated in patients with this condition. Allergic reactions may occur and include generalized rash, and in rare cases anaphylactic shock with breathing difficulties, and hypotension. The anaphylactic reactions have generally occurred in association with endoscopic examination during which patients often received other agents including contrast media and local anesthetics. The patients should be given standard treatment for anaphylaxis including an injection of epinephrine if they encounter respiratory difficulties after GlucaGen® injection.

PRECAUTIONS

General—In order for GlucaGen® treatment to reverse hypoglycemia, adequate amounts of glucose must be stored in the liver (as glycogen). Therefore, GlucaGen® should be used with caution in patients with conditions such as prolonged fasting, starvation, adrenal insufficiency or chronic hypoglycemia because these conditions result in low levels of releasable glucose in the liver and an inadequate reversal of hypoglycemia by GlucaGen® treatment. Caution should be observed when glucagon is used in diabetic patients or in elderly patients with known cardiac disease to inhibit gastrointestinal motility.

Information for Patients—Refer patients and family members to the Information for Patients for instructions describing the method of preparing and injecting GlucaGen®. Advise the patient and family members to become familiar with the technique of preparing glucagon before an emergency arises. Instruct patients to use 1 mg for adults or ½ the adult dose (0.5 mg) for children weighing less than 55 lb (25 kg). To prevent severe hypoglycemia, patients and family members should be informed of the symptoms of mild hypoglycemia and how to treat it appropriately. Family members should be informed to arouse the patient as quickly as possible because prolonged hypoglycemia may result in damage to the central nervous system. Patients should be advised to inform their physician when hypoglycemic reactions occur so that the treatment regimen may be adjusted if necessary.

Laboratory Tests—Blood glucose measurements may be considered to monitor the patient's response.

Carcinogenesis, Mutagenesis, Impairment of Fertility—Long term studies in animals to evaluate carcinogenic potential have not been performed. Several studies have been conducted to evaluate the mutagenic potential of glucagon. The mutagenic potential tested in the Ames and human lymphocyte assays, was borderline positive under certain conditions for both glucagon (pancreatic) and glucagon (rDNA) origin. *In vivo*, very high doses (100 and 200 mg/kg) of glucagon (both origins) gave a slightly higher incidence of micronucleus formation in male mice but there was no effect in females. The weight of evidence indicates that GlucaGen® is not different from glucagon pancreatic origin and does not pose a genotoxic risk to humans.

GlucaGen® was not tested in animal fertility studies. Studies in rats have shown that pancreatic glucagon does not cause impaired fertility.[1]

Pregnancy—Pregnancy Category B—Reproduction studies were performed in rats and rabbits at GlucaGen® doses of 0.4, 2.0, and 10 mg/kg. These doses represent exposures of up to 100 and 200 times the human dose based on mg/m^2 for rats and rabbits, respectively, and revealed no evidence of harm to the fetus. There are, however, no adequate and well-controlled studies in pregnant women. Because animal reproduction studies are not always predictive of human response, this drug should be used during pregnancy only if clearly needed.

Nursing Mothers—It is not known whether this drug is excreted in human milk. Because many drugs are excreted in human milk, caution should be exercised when GlucaGen® is administered to a nursing woman.

No clinical studies have been performed in nursing mothers, however, GlucaGen® is a peptide and intact glucagon is not absorbed from the GI tract. Therefore, even if the infant ingested glucagon it would be unlikely to have any effect on the infant. Additionally, GlucaGen® has a short plasma half life thus limiting amounts available to the child.

Pediatric Use—For the treatment of hypoglycemia: The use of glucagon in pediatric patients has been reported to be safe and effective.[2,3,4,5]

For use as a diagnostic aid: Safety and effectiveness in pediatric patients have not been established.

ADVERSE REACTIONS

Severe side effects are very rare, although nausea and vomiting may occur occasionally especially with doses above 1 mg or with rapid injection (less than 1 minute).[1] Glucagon exerts positive inotropic and chronotropic effects (tachycardia). Adverse reactions indicating toxicity of GlucaGen® have not been reported. A transient increase in both blood pressure and pulse rate may occur following the administration of glucagon. Patients taking β-blockers might be expected to have a greater increase in both pulse and blood pressure, an increase of which will be transient because of glucagon's short half-life. The increase in blood pressure and pulse rate may require therapy in patients with pheochromocytoma or coronary artery disease. (see OVERDOSAGE).

Allergic reactions may occur in rare cases (See WARNINGS).

OVERDOSAGE

Signs and Symptoms—No reports of overdosage with GlucaGen® have been reported. It is expected, if overdosage occurred, that the patient may experience nausea, vomiting, inhibition of GI tract motility, increase in blood pressure and pulse rate.[1] In case of suspected overdosing, the serum potassium may decrease and should be monitored and corrected if needed.

The IV and SC LD_{50} for GlucaGen® in rats and mice ranges from 100 to greater than 200 mg/kg body weight.

Treatment—Standard symptomatic treatment may be undertaken if overdosage occurs. If the patient develops a dramatic increase in blood pressure, 5 to 10 mg of phentolamine mesylate has been shown to be effective in lowering blood pressure for the short time that control would be needed. It is unknown whether GlucaGen® is dialyzable, but such a procedure is unlikely to provide any benefit given the short half-life and nature of the symptoms of overdose.

DOSAGE AND ADMINISTRATION

GlucaGen® should be reconstituted with 1 ml of Sterile Water for Reconstitution (if supplied) or with 1 mL Sterile Water for Injection, USP.

Using the syringe, withdraw all of the Sterile Water for Reconstitution (if supplied) or 1 mL Sterile Water for Injection, USP and inject into the GlucaGen® vial. Roll the vial gently until powder is completely dissolved and no particles remain in the fluid. The reconstituted fluid should be clear and of water-like consistency. The reconstituted GlucaGen® gives a concentration of approximately 1 mg/ml Glucagon. The reconstituted GlucaGen® should be used immediately after reconstitution. Discard any unused portion.

For the treatment of hypoglycemia: For adults and for pediatric patients weighing 55 lb (25 kg) or more, administer 1 mg by subcutaneous, intramuscular, or intravenous injection.[1,6] According to the literature, ½ adult dose (0.5 mg) is recommended for pediatric patients weighing less than 55 lb (25 kg) or younger than 6–8 years old.[2,3,4,5,6] Emergency assistance should be sought if the patient fails to respond within 15 minutes after subcutaneous or intramuscular injection of glucagon. The glucagon injection may be repeated while waiting for emergency assistance.[1] Intravenous glucose MUST be administered if the patient fails to respond to glucagon. When the patient has responded to the treatment, give oral carbohydrate to restore the liver glycogen and prevent recurrence of hypoglycemia.

Directions for Use as a Diagnostic Aid: Reconstitute as indicated above. Discard any unused portion. When the diagnostic procedure is over, give oral carbohydrate to restore the liver glycogen and prevent occurrence of secondary hypoglycemia.

Time of maximal glucose concentration

Intravenous: 5 to 20 minutes
Intramuscular: 30 minutes
Subcutaneous: 30 to 45 minutes

Time for GI smooth muscle relaxation[1]

Intravenous: 0.25 to 2 mg (IU)—45 seconds.
Intramuscular:
1 mg (IU)—8 to 10 minutes
2 mg (IU)—4 to 7 minutes

Duration of action—

Hyperglycemic action—60 to 90 minutes
Smooth muscle relaxation—[1]
Intravenous:
0.25 to 0.5 mg (IU)—9 to 17 minutes
2 mg (IU)—22 to 25 minutes
Intramuscular:
1 mg (IU)—12 to 27 minutes
2 mg (IU)—21 to 32 minutes

Stability and storage

Before Reconstitution: The GlucaGen® package may be stored up to 24 months at controlled room temperature 20° to 25°C (68° to 77°F) prior to reconstitution. Avoid freezing and protect from light. GlucaGen® should not be used after the expiry date on the vials.

After Reconstitution: Reconstituted GlucaGen® should be used immediately. Discard any unused portion. If the solution shows any sign of gel formation or particles, it should be discarded.

HOW SUPPLIED

The GlucaGen® Diagnostic Kit includes:
1 vial containing 1 mg (1 IU) GlucaGen® [glucagon (rDNA origin) for injection]
1 vial containing 1 ml Sterile Water for Reconstitution
NDC 55390-004-01
or
The GlucaGen® 10-pack includes:
10×1 vial containing 1 mg (1 IU) GlucaGen® [glucagon (rDNA origin) for injection]
NDC 55390-004-10
Edition March 2001

REFERENCES

1. *Drug Information for the Health Care Professional.* 17th ed. Rockville, Maryland: The United States Pharmacopeial Convention, Inc; 1997; Vol. 1, IA:1516–1518.
2. Gibbs et al: Use of Glucagon to terminate insulin reactions in diabetic children. *Nebr Med J* 1958;43:56–57.
3. Carson MJ, Koch R, Clinical studies with glucagon in children. *J Pediatr* 1955;47:161–170.
4. Shipp JC, et al: Treatment of insulin hypoglycemia in diabetic campers. *Diabetes* 1964; 13:645–648.
5. Aman J, Wranne L: Hypoglycemia in childhood diabetes II: Effect of subcutaneous or intramuscular injection of different doses of glucagon. Acta Pediatr Scand 1988;77: 548–553.
6. Aynsley-Green AS, Eyre JA, and Soltesz G, Hypoglycaemia in diabetic children. In: Frier BM and Fisher BM, eds Hypoglycaemia and Diabetes, Edward Arnold, 1993; 237–238.

Bedford Laboratories™
Bedford, OH 44146

Berlex, Inc.

6 WEST BELT
WAYNE, NJ 07470
www.Berlex.com

Direct Inquiries to:
1-(888) BERLEX-4

BETASERON® ℞

[bay-ta-seer-on]
Interferon beta-1b

DESCRIPTION

Betaseron® (Interferon beta-lb) is a purified, sterile, lyophilized protein product produced by recombinant DNA techniques. Interferon beta-1b is manufactured by bacterial fermentation of a strain of *Escherichia coli* that bears a genetically engineered plasmid containing the gene for human interferon beta$_{ser17}$. The native gene was obtained from human fibroblasts and altered in a way that substitutes serine for the cystine residue found at position 17. Interferon beta-1b has 165 amino acids and an approximate molecular weight of 18,500 daltons. It does not include the carbohydrate side chains found in the natural material.

The specific activity of Betaseron is approximately 32 million international units (IU)/mg Interferon beta-lb. Each vial contains 0.3 mg of Interferon beta-lb. The unit measurement is derived by comparing the antiviral activity of the product to the World Health Organization (WHO) reference standard of recombinant human interferon beta. Mannitol, USP and Albumin (Human), USP (15 mg each/vial) are added as stabilizers.

Lyophilized Betaseron is a sterile, white to off-white powder, for subcutaneous injection after reconstitution with the diluent supplied (Sodium Chloride, 0.54% Solution).

CLINICAL PHARMACOLOGY

General

Interferons (IFNs) are a family of naturally occurring proteins, produced by eukaryotic cells in response to viral infection and other biologic agents. Three major groups of interferons have been distinguished: alpha, beta, and gamma. Interferons alpha and beta comprise the Type I interferons and interferon gamma is a Type II interferon. Type I interferons have considerably overlapping but also distinct biologic activities. The bioactivities of IFNs are mediated by their interactions with specific receptors found on the surfaces of human cells. Differences in bioactivites induced by IFNs likely reflect divergences in the signal transduction process induced by IFN-receptor binding.

Biologic Activities

The mechanism of action of Interferon beta-1b in patients with multiple sclerosis is unknown. Interferon beta-1b receptor binding induces the expression of proteins that are responsible for the pleiotropic bioactivities of Interferon beta-1b. A number of these proteins (including neopterin, β_2-microglobulin, MxA protein, and IL-10) have been measured in blood fractions from Betaseron-treated patients and Betaseron-treated healthy volunteers. Immunomodulatory effects of Interferon beta-1b include the enhancement of suppressor T cell activity, reduction of pro-inflammatory cytokine production, down-regulation of antigen presentation, and inhibition of lymphocyte trafficking into the central nervous system. It is not known if these effects play an important role in the observed clinical activity of Betaseron in multiple sclerosis (MS).

Pharmacokinetics

Because serum concentrations of Interferon beta-1b are low or not detectable following subcutaneous administration of 0.25 mg or less of Betaseron, pharmacokinetic information in patients with MS receiving the recommended dose of Betaseron is not available. Following single and multiple daily subcutaneous administrations of 0.5 mg Betaseron to healthy volunteers (N=12), serum Interferon beta-1b concentrations were generally below 100 IU/mL. Peak serum Interferon beta-1b concentrations occurred between one to eight hours, with a mean peak serum interferon concentration of 40 IU/mL. Bioavailability, based on a total dose of 0.5 mg Betaseron given as two subcutaneous injections at different sites, was approximately 50%.

After intravenous administration of Betaseron (0.006 mg to 2.0 mg), similar pharmacokinetic profiles were obtained from healthy volunteers (N=12) and from patients with diseases other than MS (N=142). In patients receiving single intravenous doses up to 2.0 mg, increases in serum concentrations were dose proportional. Mean serum clearance values ranged from 9.4 mL/min•kg^{-1} to 28.9 mL/min•kg^{-1} and were independent of dose. Mean terminal elimination half-life values ranged from 8.0 minutes to 4.3 hours and mean steady-state volume of distribution values ranged from 0.25 L/kg to 2.88 L/kg. Three-times-a-week intravenous dosing for two weeks resulted in no accumulation of Interferon beta-1b in sera of patients. Pharmacokinetic parameters after single and multiple intravenous doses of Betaseron were comparable.

Following every other day subcutaneous administration of 0.25 mg Betaseron in healthy volunteers, biologic response marker levels (neopterin, β_2-microglobulin, MxA protein, and the immunosuppressive cytokine, IL-10) increased significantly above baseline six-twelve hours after the first Betaseron dose. Biologic response marker levels peaked between 40 and 124 hours and remained elevated above baseline throughout the seven-day (168-hour) study. The relationship between serum Interferon beta-1b levels or induced biologic response marker levels and the clinical effects of Interferon beta-1b in multiple sclerosis is unknown.

CLINICAL STUDIES

The safety and efficacy of Betaseron have been assessed in three multicenter trials. Study 1 evaluated Betaseron in relapsing-remitting MS (RRMS) patients and Studies 2 and 3 assessed Betaseron in secondary progressive MS (SPMS) patients.

The effectiveness of Betaseron in relapsing-remitting MS (Study 1) was evaluated in a double blind, multiclinic, randomized, parallel, placebo controlled clinical investigation of two years duration. The study enrolled MS patients, aged 18 to 50, who were ambulatory (EDSS of ≤ 5.5), exhibited a relapsing-remitting clinical course, met Poser's criteria[1] for clinically definite and/or laboratory supported definite MS and had experienced at least two exacerbations over two years preceding the trial without exacerbation in the preceding month. Patients who had received prior immunosuppressant therapy were excluded.

An exacerbation was defined as the appearance of a new clinical sign/symptom or the clinical worsening of a previous sign/symptom (one that had been stable for at least 30 days) that persisted for a minimum of 24 hours.

Patients selected for study were randomized to treatment with either placebo (N=123), 0.05 mg of Betaseron (N=125), or 0.25 mg of Betaseron (N=124) self-administered subcutaneously every other day. Outcome based on the 372 randomized patients was evaluated after two years.

Patients who required more than three 28-day courses of corticosteroids were removed from the study. Minor analgesics (acetaminophen, codeine), antidepressants, and oral baclofen were allowed ad libitum, but chronic nonsteroidal anti-inflammatory drug (NSAID) use was not allowed.

The primary protocol-defined outcome measures were 1) frequency of exacerbations per patient and 2) proportion of exacerbation free patients. A number of secondary clinical and magnetic resonance imaging (MRI) measures were also employed. All patients underwent annual T2 MRI imaging and a subset of 52 patients at one site had MRIs performed every six weeks for assessment of new or expanding lesions. The study results are shown in **Table 1**.

[See table 1 at top of next page]

Of the 372 RRMS patients randomized, 72 (19%) failed to complete two full years on their assigned treatments.

Over the two-year period, there were 25 MS-related hospitalizations in the 0.25 mg Betaseron-treated group compared to 48 hospitalizations in the placebo group. In comparison, non-MS hospitalizations were evenly distributed among the groups, with 16 in the 0.25 mg Betaseron group and 15 in the placebo group. The average number of days of MS-related steroid use was 41 days in the 0.25 mg Betaseron group and 55 days in the placebo group (p=0.004).

MRI data were also analyzed for patients in this study. A frequency distribution of the observed percent changes in MRI area at the end of two years was obtained by grouping the percentages in successive intervals of equal width. Figure 1 displays a histogram of the proportions of patients, which fell into each of these intervals. The median percent change in MRI area for the 0.25 mg group was -1.1%, which was significantly smaller than the 16.5% observed for the placebo group (p=0.0001).

Distribution of Change in MRI Area

Figure 1

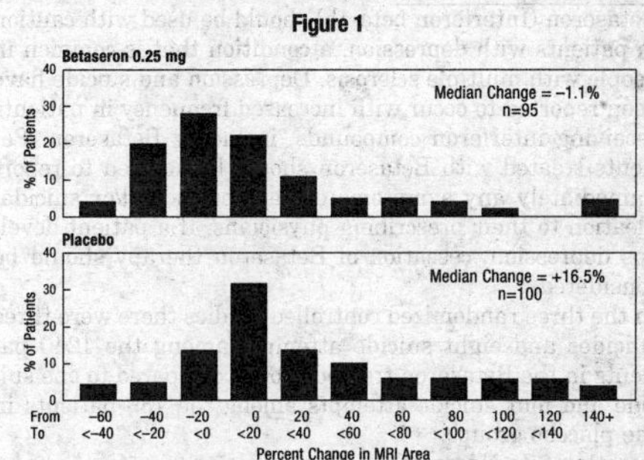

In an evaluation of frequent MRI scans (every six weeks) on 52 patients at one site, the percent of scans with new or expanding lesions was 29% in the placebo group and 6% in the 0.25 mg treatment group (p=0.006).

The exact relationship between MRI findings and clinical status of patients is unknown. Changes in lesion area often do not correlate with changes in disability progression. The prognostic significance of the MRI findings in this study has not been evaluated.

Continued on next page

Information on Berlex products (appearing here) is based on the most current information available at the time of publication closing. Further information for these and other Berlex products can be obtained from Medical & Product Services at Berlex, Inc. by calling 1-888-BERLEX-4.

Betaseron—Cont.

Studies 2 and 3 were multicenter, randomized, double-blind, placebo controlled trials conducted to assess the effect of Betaseron in patients with SPMS. Study 2 was conducted in Europe and Study 3 was conducted in North America. Both studies enrolled patients with clinically definite or laboratory-supported MS in the secondary progressive phase, and who had evidence of disability progression (both Study 2 and 3) or two relapses (Study 2 only) within the previous two years. Baseline Kurtzke expanded disability status scale (EDSS) scores ranged from 3.0 to 6.5.[2] Patients in Study 2 were randomized to receive Betaseron 0.25 mg (n=360) or placebo (n=358). Patients in Study 3 were randomized to Betaseron 0.25 mg (n=317), Betaseron 0.16 mg/m^2 of body surface area (n=314, mean assigned dose 0.30 mg), or placebo (n=308). Test agents were administered subcutaneously, every other day for three years.
The primary outcome measure was progression of disability, defined as a 1.0 point increase in the EDSS score, or a 0.5 point increase for patients with baseline EDSS ≥ 6.0. In Study 2, time to progression in EDSS was longer in the Betaseron treatment group (p=0.005), with estimated annualized rates of progression of 16% and 19% in the Betaseron and placebo groups, respectively. In Study 3, the rates of progression did not differ significantly between treatment groups, with estimated annualized rates of progression of 12%, 14%, and 12% in the Betaseron fixed dose, surface area-adjusted dose, and placebo groups, respectively.
Multiple analyses, including covariate and subset analyses based on sex, age, disease duration, clinical disease activity prior to study enrollment, MRI measures at baseline and early changes in MRI following treatment were evaluated in order to interpret the discordant study results. No demographic or disease-related factors enabled identification of a patient subset where Betaseron treatment was predictably associated with delayed progression of disability.
In Studies 2 and 3, like Study 1, a statistically significant decrease in the incidence of relapses associated with Betaseron treatment was demonstrated. In Study 2, the mean annual relapse rates were 0.42 and 0.63 in the Betaseron and placebo groups, respectively (p<0.001). In Study 3, the mean annual relapse rates were 0.16, 0.20, and 0.28, for the fixed dose, surface area-adjusted dose, and placebo groups, respectively (p<0.02).
MRI endpoints in both Study 2 and Study 3 showed lesser increases in T2 MRI lesion area and decreased number of active MRI lesions in patients in the Betaseron groups. The exact relationship between MRI findings and the clinical status of patients is unknown. Changes in MRI findings often do not correlate with changes in disability progression. The prognostic significance of the MRI findings in these studies is not known.
Safety and efficacy of treatment with Betaseron beyond three years are not known.

INDICATIONS AND USAGE

Betaseron (Interferon beta-1b) is indicated for the treatment of relapsing forms of multiple sclerosis to reduce the frequency of clinical exacerbations.

CONTRAINDICATIONS

Betaseron is contraindicated in patients with a history of hypersensitivity to natural or recombinant interferon beta, Albumin (Human), USP, or any other component of the formulation.

WARNINGS

Depression and Suicide

Betaseron (Interferon beta-1b) should be used with caution in patients with depression, a condition that is common in people with multiple sclerosis. Depression and suicide have been reported to occur with increased frequency in patients receiving interferon compounds, including Betaseron. Patients treated with Betaseron should be advised to report immediately any symptoms of depression and/or suicidal ideation to their prescribing physicians. If a patient develops depression, cessation of Betaseron therapy should be considered.
In the three randomized controlled studies there were three suicides and eight suicide attempts among the 1240 patients in the Betaseron treated groups compared to one suicide and four suicide attempts among the 789 patients in the placebo groups.

Injection Site Necrosis

Injection site necrosis (ISN) has been reported in 5% of patients in controlled clinical trials (see **ADVERSE REACTIONS**). Typically, injection site necrosis occurs within the first four months of therapy, although post-marketing reports have been received of ISN occurring over one year after initiation of therapy. Necrosis may occur at a single or multiple injection sites. The necrotic lesions are typically three cm or less in diameter, but larger areas have been reported. Generally the necrosis has extended only to subcutaneous fat. However, there are also reports of necrosis extending to and including fascia overlying muscle. In some lesions where biopsy results are available, vasculitis has been reported. For some lesions debridement and, infrequently, skin grafting have been required.
As with any open lesion, it is important to avoid infection and, if it occurs, to treat the infection. Time to healing was varied depending on the severity of the necrosis at the time treatment was begun. In most cases healing was associated with scarring.

TABLE 1
Two Year RRMS Study Results
Primary and Secondary Clinical Outcomes

Efficacy Parameters		Treatment Groups			Statistical Comparisons p-value		
Primary End Points		Placebo (N=123)	0.05 mg (N=125)	0.25 mg (N=124)	Placebo vs 0.05 mg	0.05 mg vs 0.25 mg	Placebo vs 0.25 mg
Annual exacerbation rate		1.31	1.14	0.90	0.005	0.113	**0.0001**
Proportion of exacerbation-free patients†		16%	18%	25%	0.609	0.288	**0.094**
Exacerbation frequency per patient	0†	20	22	29	0.151	0.077	**0.001**
	1	32	31	39			
	2	20	28	17			
	3	15	15	14			
	4	15	7	9			
	≥5	21	16	8			
Secondary Endpoints††							
Median number of months to first on-study exacerbation		5	6	9	0.299	0.097	**0.010**
Rate of moderate or severe exacerbations per year		0.47	0.29	0.23	0.020	0.257	**0.001**
Mean number of moderate or severe exacerbation days per patient		44.1	33.2	19.5	0.229	0.064	**0.001**
Mean change in EDSS score‡ at endpoint		0.21	0.21	-0.07	0.995	0.108	**0.144**
Mean change in Scripps score‡‡ at endpoint		-0.53	-0.50	0.66	0.641	0.051	**0.126**
Median duration in days per exacerbation		36	33	35.5	ND	ND	**ND**
% change in mean MRI lesion area at endpoint		21.4%	9.8%	-0.9%	0.015	0.019	**0.0001**

ND Not done
† 14 exacerbation free patients (0 from placebo, six from 0.05 mg, and eight from 0.25 mg) dropped out of the study before completing six months of therapy. These patients are excluded from this analysis.
†† Sequelae and Functional Neurologic Status, both required by protocol, were not analyzed individually but are included as a function of the EDSS.
‡ EDSS scores range from 1-10, with higher scores reflecting greater disability.
‡‡ Scripps neurologic rating scores range from 0-100, with smaller scores reflecting greater disability.

Some patients have experienced healing of necrotic skin lesions while Betaseron therapy continued; others have not. Whether to discontinue therapy following a single site of necrosis is dependent on the extent of necrosis. For patients who continue therapy with Betaseron after injection site necrosis has occurred, Betaseron should not be administered into the affected area until it is fully healed. If multiple lesions occur, therapy should be discontinued until healing occurs.
Patient understanding and use of aseptic self-injection techniques and procedures should be periodically reevaluated, particularly if injection site necrosis has occurred.

Anaphylaxis

Anaphylaxis has been reported as a rare complication of Betaseron use. Other allergic reactions have included dyspnea, bronchospasm, tongue edema, skin rash and urticaria (see **ADVERSE REACTIONS**).

Albumin (Human), USP

This product contains albumin, a derivative of human blood. Based on effective donor screening and product manufacturing processes, it carries an extremely remote risk for transmission of viral diseases. A theoretical risk for transmission of Creutzfeldt-Jakob disease (CJD) also is considered extremely remote. No cases of transmission of viral diseases or CJD have ever been identified for albumin.

PRECAUTIONS

Information for Patients

All patients should be instructed to carefully read the supplied Betaseron Medication Guide. Patients should be cautioned not to change the dose or schedule of administration without medical consultation.
Patients should be made aware that serious adverse reactions during the use of Betaseron have been reported, including depression and suicidal ideation, injection site necrosis, and anaphylaxis (see **WARNINGS**). Patients should be advised of the symptoms of depression or suicidal ideation and be told to report them immediately to their physician. Patients should also be advised of the symptoms of allergic reactions and anaphylaxis.
Patients should be advised to promptly report any break in the skin, which may be associated with blue-black discoloration, swelling, or drainage of fluid from the injection site, prior to continuing their Betaseron therapy.
Patients should be informed that flu-like symptoms are common following initiation of therapy with Betaseron. In the controlled clinical trials, antipyretics and analgesics were permitted for relief of these symptoms. In addition, gradual dose titration during initiation of Betaseron treatment may reduce flu-like symptoms (see **DOSAGE AND ADMINISTRATION**).
Female patients should be cautioned about the abortifacient potential of Betaseron (see **PRECAUTIONS**, **Pregnancy - Teratogenic Effects**).

Instruction on Self-injection Technique and Procedures

Patients should be instructed in the use of aseptic technique when administering Betaseron. Appropriate instruction for reconstitution of Betaseron and self-injection should be provided, including careful review of the Betaseron Medication Guide. The first injection should be performed under the supervision of an appropriately qualified health care professional.
Patients should be cautioned against the re-use of needles or syringes and instructed in safe disposal procedures. A puncture resistant container for disposal of used needles and syringes should be supplied to the patient along with instructions for safe disposal of full containers.
Patients should be advised of the importance of rotating areas of injection with each dose, to minimize the likelihood of severe injection site reactions, including necrosis or localized infection, (see **Picking an Injection Site** section of the **Medication Guide**).

Laboratory Tests

In addition to those laboratory tests normally required for monitoring patients with multiple sclerosis, complete blood and differential white blood cell counts, platelet counts and blood chemistries, including liver function tests, are recommended at regular intervals (one, three, and six months) following introduction of Betaseron therapy, and then periodically thereafter in the absence of clinical symptoms. Thyroid function tests are recommended every six months in patients with a history of thyroid dysfunction or as clinically indicated. Patients with myelosuppression may require more intensive monitoring of complete blood cell counts, with differential and platelet counts.

Drug Interactions

No formal drug interaction studies have been conducted with Betaseron. In the placebo controlled studies in MS, corticosteroids or ACTH were administered for treatment of relapses for periods of up to 28 days in patients (N=664) receiving Betaseron.

Carcinogenesis, Mutagenesis, and Impairment of Fertility

Carcinogenesis: Interferon beta-1b has not been tested for its carcinogenic potential in animals.
Mutagenesis: Betaseron was not mutagenic when assayed for genotoxicity in the Ames bacterial test in the presence or absence of metabolic activation. Interferon beta-1b was not mutagenic to human peripheral blood lymphocytes *in vitro*, in the presence or absence of metabolic inactivation. Betaseron treatment of mouse BALBc-3T3 cells did not re-

sult in increased transformation frequency in an *in vitro* model of tumor transformation.

Impairment of fertility: Studies in normally cycling, female rhesus monkeys at doses up to 0.33 mg/kg/day (32 times the recommended human dose based on body surface area, body surface dose based on 70 kg female) had no apparent adverse effects on either menstrual cycle duration or associated hormonal profiles (progesterone and estradiol) when administered over three consecutive menstrual cycles. The validity of extrapolating doses used in animal studies to human doses is not known. Effects of Betaseron on normally cycling human females are not known.

Pregnancy - Teratogenic Effects

Pregnancy Category C: Betaseron was not teratogenic at doses up to 0.42 mg/kg/day when given to pregnant female rhesus monkeys on gestation days 20 to 70. However, a dose related abortifacient activity was observed in these monkeys when Interferon beta-1b was administered at doses ranging from 0.028 mg/kg/day to 0.42 mg/kg/day (2.8 to 40 times the recommended human dose based on body surface area comparison). The validity of extrapolating doses used in animal studies to human doses is not known. Lower doses were not studied in monkeys. Spontaneous abortions while on treatment were reported in patients (n=4) who participated in the Betaseron RRMS clinical trial. Betaseron given to rhesus monkeys on gestation days 20 to 70 did not cause teratogenic effects; however, it is not known if teratogenic effects exist in humans. There are no adequate and well-controlled studies in pregnant women. If the patient becomes pregnant or plans to become pregnant while taking Betaseron, the patient should be apprised of the potential hazard to the fetus and it should be recommended that the patient discontinue therapy.

Nursing Mothers

It is not known whether Betaseron is excreted in human milk. Because many drugs are excreted in human milk and because of the potential for serious adverse reactions in nursing infants from Betaseron, a decision should be made to either discontinue nursing or discontinue the drug, taking into account the importance of drug to the mother.

Pediatric Use

Safety and efficacy in pediatric patients have not been established.

Geriatric Use

Clinical studies of Betaseron did not include sufficient numbers of patients aged 65 and over to determine whether they respond differently than younger patients.

ADVERSE REACTIONS

In all studies, the most serious adverse reactions with Betaseron were depression, suicidal ideation and injection site necrosis (see **WARNINGS**). The incidence of depression of any severity was approximately 34% in both Betaseron-treated patients and placebo-treated patients. Anaphylaxis and other allergic reactions have been reported in patients using Betaseron (see **WARNINGS**). The most commonly reported adverse reactions were lymphopenia (lymphocytes $<1500/mm^3$), injection site reaction, asthenia, flu-like symptom complex, headache, and pain. The most frequently reported adverse reactions resulting in clinical intervention (e.g., discontinuation of Betaseron, adjustment in dosage, or the need for concomitant medication to treat an adverse reaction symptom) were depression, flu-like symptom complex, injection site reactions, leukopenia, increased liver enzymes, asthenia, hypertonia, and myasthenia.

Because clinical trials are conducted under widely varying conditions and over varying lengths of time, adverse reaction rates observed in the clinical trials of Betaseron cannot be directly compared to rates in clinical trials of other drugs, and may not reflect the rates observed in practice. The adverse reaction information from clinical trials does, however, provide a basis for identifying the adverse events that appear to be related to drug use and for approximating rates.

The data described below reflect exposure to Betaseron in the three placebo controlled trials of 1115 patients with MS treated with 0.25 mg or 0.16 mg/m^2, including 1041 exposed for greater than one year. The population encompassed an age range from 18-65 years. Sixty-five percent (65%) of the patients were female. The percentages of Caucasian, Black, Asian, and Hispanic patients were 94.0%, 4.3%, 0.2%, and 0.8%, respectively.

The safety profiles for Betaseron-treated patients with SPMS and RRMS were similar. Clinical experience with Betaseron in other populations (patients with cancer, HIV positive patients, etc.) provides additional data regarding adverse reactions; however, experience in non-MS populations may not be fully applicable to the MS population.

Injection Site Reactions

In three controlled clinical trials, injection site reactions occurred in 86% of patients receiving Betaseron with injection site necrosis in 5%. Inflammation (53%), pain (18%), hypersensitivity (3%), necrosis (5%), mass (2%), edema (3%) and non-specific reactions were significantly associated with Betaseron treatment (see **WARNINGS** and **PRECAUTIONS**). The incidence of injection site reactions tended to decrease over time, with approximately 76% of patients experiencing the event during the first three months of treatment, compared to approximately 45% at the end of the studies.

Flu-Like Symptom Complex

The rate of flu-like symptom complex was approximately 60% in the three controlled clinical trials. The incidence decreased over time, with only 10% of patients reporting flu-like symptom complex at the end of the studies. For patients who experienced a flu-like symptom complex in Study 1, the median duration was 7.5 days.

Laboratory Abnormalities

In the three clinical trials, leukopenia was reported in 18% and 5% of patients in Betaseron- and placebo-treated groups, respectively. No patients were withdrawn or dose reduced for neutropenia in Study 1. Three percent (3%) of patients in Studies 2 and 3 experienced leukopenia and were dose-reduced. Other laboratory abnormalities included SGPT greater than five times baseline value (10%), and SGOT greater than five times baseline value (3%). In Study 1, two patients were dose reduced for increased liver enzymes; one continued on treatment and one was ultimately withdrawn. In Studies 2 and 3, 1.5% of Betaseron patients were dose-reduced or interrupted treatment for increased liver enzymes. Three (0.3%) patients were withdrawn from treatment with Betaseron for any laboratory abnormality including two (0.2%) patients following dose reduction (see **PRECAUTIONS**, Laboratory Tests).

Menstrual Irregularities

In the three clinical trials, 82 (14%) of the 577 pre-menopausal females treated with Betaseron and 74 (18%) of the 405 pre-menopausal females treated with placebo reported menstrual disorders. One event was reported as severe, all other reports were mild to moderate severity. No patients withdrew from the studies due to menstrual irregularities.

Table 2 enumerates adverse events and laboratory abnormalities that occurred among all patients treated with 0.25 mg or 0.16 mg/m^2 Betaseron every other day for periods of up to three years in the controlled trials at an incidence that was at least 2% more than that observed in the placebo patients.

TABLE 2
Adverse Reactions and Laboratory Abnormalities

Adverse Reaction	Placebo (n=789)	Betaseron (n=1115)
Body as a Whole		
Injection site reaction	29%	85%
Asthenia	54%	61%
Flu-like symptom complex	41%	60%
Headache	48%	57%
Pain	42%	51%
Fever	22%	36%
Chills	11%	25%
Abdominal pain	13%	19%
Chest pain	7%	11%
Malaise	4%	8%
Injection site necrosis	0%	5%
Cardiovascular System		
Peripheral edema	12%	15%
Vasodilation	6%	8%
Hypertension	4%	7%
Peripheral vascular disorder	4%	6%
Palpitation	2%	4%
Tachycardia	2%	4%
Digestive System		
Nausea	25%	27%
Constipation	18%	20%
Diarrhea	16%	19%
Dyspepsia	12%	14%
Hemic and Lymphatic System		
Lymphocytes < $1500/mm^3$	70%	88%
ANC < $1500/mm^3$	5%	14%
WBC < $3000/mm^3$	4%	14%
Lymphadenopathy	4%	8%
Metabolic and Nutritional Disorders		
SGPT > 5 times baseline	4%	10%
SGOT > 5 times baseline	1%	3%
Weight gain	5%	7%
Musculoskeletal System		
Myasthenia	43%	46%
Arthralgia	29%	31%
Myalgia	16%	27%
Leg cramps	2%	4%
Nervous System		
Hypertonia	40%	50%
Dizziness	21%	24%
Insomnia	19%	24%
Incoordination	18%	21%
Anxiety	8%	10%
Nervousness	5%	7%
Respiratory System		
Dyspnea	4%	7%
Skin and Appendages		
Rash	18%	24%
Skin disorder	10%	12%
Sweating	6%	8%
Alopecia	2%	4%
Urogential System		
Urinary urgency	10%	13%
Metrorrhagia*	8%	11%
Menorrhagia*	6%	8%
Impotence**	7%	9%
Urinary frequency	5%	7%
Dysmenorrhea*	5%	7%
Prostatic disorder**	1%	3%

* pre-menopausal women
** male patients

The following adverse events have been observed during postmarketing experience with Betaseron and are classified within body system categories:

Body General: *fatal capillary leak syndrome; Cardiovascular: cardiomyopathy, deep vein thrombosis, pulmonary embolism; Digestive: hepatitis, pancreatitis, vomiting; Endocrine: hypothyroidism, hyperthyroidism, thyroid dysfunction; Hemic and Lymphatic System: anemia, thrombocytopenia; Metabolic and Nutritional: Gamma GT increase, hypocalcemia, hyperuricemia, triglyceride increase; Nervous: ataxia, confusion, convulsion, depersonalization, emotional lability, paresthesia; Respiratory: bronchospasm, pneumonia; Skin and Appendages: pruritus, skin discoloration, urticaria; Urogenital: urinary tract infection, urosepsis.

*The administration of cytokines to patients with a preexisting monoclonal gammopathy has been associated with the development of this syndrome.

Immunogenicity

As with all therapeutic proteins, there is a potential for immunogenicity. Serum samples were monitored for the development of antibodies to Betaseron during the RRMS study. In patients receiving 0.25 mg every other day 56/124 (45%) were found to have serum neutralizing activity at one or more of the time points tested. The relationship between antibody formation and clinical safety or efficacy is not known.

These data reflect the percentage of patients whose test results were considered positive for antibodies to Betaseron using a biological neutralization assay that measures the ability of immune sera to inhibit the production of the interferon-inducible protein, MxA. Neutralization assays are highly dependent on the sensitivity and specificity of the assay. Additionally, the observed incidence of neutralizing activity in an assay may be influenced by several factors including sample handling, timing of sample collection,

Continued on next page

Information on Berlex products (appearing here) is based on the most current information available at the time of publication closing. Further information for these and other Berlex products can be obtained from Medical & Product Services at Berlex, Inc. by calling 1-888-BERLEX-4.

Betaseron—Cont.

concomitant medications, and underlying disease. For these reasons, comparison of the incidence of antibodies to Betaseron with the incidence of antibodies to other products may be misleading.
Anaphylactic reactions have rarely been reported with the use of Betaseron.

DRUG ABUSE AND DEPENDENCE

No evidence or experience suggests that abuse or dependence occurs with Betaseron therapy; however, the risk of dependence has not been systematically evaluated.

OVERDOSAGE

Safety of doses higher than 0.25 mg every other day has not been adequately evaluated. The maximum amount of Betaseron that can be safely administered has not been determined.

DOSAGE AND ADMINISTRATION

The recommended dose of Betaseron is 0.25 mg injected subcutaneously every other day. Generally, patients should be started at 0.0625 mg (0.25 mL) subcutaneously every other day, and increased over a six-week period to 0.25 mg (1.0 mL) every other day (see **Table 3**).

Table 3. Schedule for Dose Titration

	Recommended Titration	Betaseron Dose	Volume
Weeks 1-2	25%	0.0625 mg	0.25 mL
Weeks 3-4	50%	0.125 mg	0.50 mL
Weeks 5-6	75%	0.1875 mg	0.75 mL
Week 7+	100%	0.25 mg	1.0 mL

To reconstitute lyophilized Betaseron for injection, attach the prefilled syringe containing the diluent (Sodium Chloride, 0.54% Solution) to the Betaseron vial using the vial adapter. Slowly inject 1.2 mL of diluent into the Betaseron vial. Gently swirl the vial to dissolve the drug completely; do not shake. Foaming may occur during reconstitution or if the vial is swirled or shaken too vigorously. If foaming occurs, allow the vial to sit undisturbed until the foam settles. Visually inspect the reconstituted product before use; discard the product if it contains particulate matter or is discolored. Keeping the syringe and vial adapter in place, turn the assembly over so that the vial is on top. Withdraw the appropriate dose of Betaseron solution. Remove the vial from the vial adapter before injecting Betaseron. One mL of reconstituted Betaseron solution contains 0.25 mg of Interferon beta-1b/mL.
Betaseron is intended for use under the guidance and supervision of a physician. It is recommended that physicians or qualified medical personnel train patients in the proper technique for self-administering subcutaneous injections. Patients should be advised to rotate sites for subcutaneous injections (see **PRECAUTIONS, Instruction on Self-injection Technique and Procedures**). Concurrent use of analgesics and/or antipyretics may help ameliorate flu-like symptoms on treatment days. Betaseron should be visually inspected for particulate matter and discoloration prior to administration.

Stability and Storage

The reconstituted product contains no preservative. Before reconstitution with diluent, store Betaseron at room temperature 25°C (77°F). Excursions of 15° to 30°C (59° to 86°F) are permitted. After reconstitution, if not used immediately, the product should be refrigerated and used within three hours. Avoid freezing.

HOW SUPPLIED

Betaseron is supplied as a lyophilized powder containing 0.3 mg of Interferon beta-1b, 15 mg Albumin (Human), USP, and 15 mg Mannitol, USP. Drug is packaged in a clear glass, single-use vial (3 mL capacity). A pre-filled single-use syringe containing 1.2 mL of diluent (Sodium Chloride, 0.54% solution), two alcohol prep pads, and one vial adapter with attached 27 gauge needle are included for each vial of drug. Betaseron and the diluent are for single-use only. Unused portions should be discarded. Store at room temperature.
NDC 50419-523-25 15 blister units, 0.3 mg/vial
Rx only

REFERENCES

1. Poser CM, et al. Ann Neurol 1983; 13(3): 227–231. 2. Kurtzke JF. Neurology 1983; 33(11): 1444–1452.
U.S. Patent No. 4,588,585; 4,959,314; 4,737,462; 4,530,787

Medication Guide
Betaseron® (bay-ta-seer-on)
Interferon beta-1b
(in-ter-feer-on beta-one-be)

Please read this leaflet carefully before you start to use Betaseron® and each time your prescription is refilled since there may be new information. The information in this medication guide does not take the place of talking with your doctor or healthcare professional.

What is the most important information I should know about Betaseron?

Betaseron will not cure multiple sclerosis (MS) but it has been shown to decrease the number of flare-ups of the disease. Betaseron can cause serious side effects, so before you start taking Betaseron, you should talk to your doctor about the possible benefits of Betaseron and its possible side effects to decide if Betaseron is right for you. Potential serious side effects include:

- **Depression.** Some patients treated with interferons, including Betaseron, have become seriously depressed (feeling sad). Some patients have thought about or have attempted to kill themselves. Depression (a sinking of spirits or sadness) is not uncommon in people with multiple sclerosis. However, if you are feeling noticeably sadder or helpless, or feel like hurting yourself or others, you should tell a family member or friend right away and call your doctor or health care provider as soon as possible. Your doctor may ask that you stop using Betaseron. Before starting Betaseron, you should also tell your doctor if you have ever had any mental illness, including depression, and if you take any medications for depression.
- **Risk to pregnancy.** If you become pregnant while taking Betaseron you should stop using Betaseron immediately and call your doctor. Betaseron may cause you to lose your baby (miscarriage) or may cause harm to your unborn child. You and your doctor will need to decide whether the potential benefit of taking Betaseron is greater than the potential risks to your unborn child.
- **Allergic reactions.** Some patients taking Betaseron have had severe allergic reactions leading to difficulty breathing and swallowing; these reactions can happen quickly. Allergic reactions can happen after your first dose or may not happen until after you have taken Betaseron many times. Less severe allergic reactions such as rash, itching, skin bumps or swelling of the mouth and tongue can also happen. If you think you are having an allergic reaction, stop using Betaseron immediately and call your doctor.
- **Injection site problems.** Betaseron may cause redness, pain or swelling at the place where an injection was given. A few patients have developed skin infections or areas of severe skin damage (necrosis). If one of your injection sites becomes swollen and painful or the area looks infected and it doesn't heal within a few days, you should call your doctor.

What is Betaseron?

Betaseron is a type of protein called beta interferon that occurs naturally in the body. It is used to treat relapsing forms of multiple sclerosis. It will not cure your MS but may decrease the number of flare-ups of the disease. MS is a life-long disease that affects your nervous system by destroying the protective covering (myelin) that surrounds your nerve fibers. The way Betaseron works in MS is not known.

Who should not take Betaseron?

Do not take Betaseron if you:

- Have had allergic reactions such as difficulty breathing, flushing or hives to another interferon beta or to human albumin.

If you have any of the following conditions or serious medical problems, you should tell your doctor *before* taking Betaseron:

- Depression (a sinking feeling or sadness), anxiety (feeling uneasy, nervous, or fearful for no reason), or trouble sleeping
- Liver diseases
- Problems with your thyroid gland
- Blood problems such as bleeding or bruising easily and anemia (low red blood cells) or low white blood cells
- Epilepsy
- Are pregnant, breast feeding, or planning to become pregnant

You should tell your doctor if you are taking any other prescription or non-prescription medicines. This includes any vitamin or mineral supplements, or herbal products.

How should I take Betaseron?

Betaseron is given by injection under the skin (subcutaneous injection) every other day. Your injections should be approximately 48 hours (two days) apart, so it is best to take them at the same time each day, preferably in the evening just before bedtime.
You may be started on a lower dose when you first start taking Betaseron. Your doctor will tell you what dose of Betaseron to use, and that dose may change based on how your body responds. You should not change your dose without talking with your doctor.
If you miss a dose, you should take your next dose as soon as you remember or are able to take it. Your next injection should be taken about 48 hours (two days) after that dose. **Do not take Betaseron® on two consecutive days.** If you accidentally take more than your prescribed dose, or take it on two consecutive days, call your doctor right away.
You should always follow your doctor's instructions and advice about how to take this medication. If your doctor feels that you, or a family member or friend may give you the injections, then you and/or the other person should be trained by your doctor or healthcare provider in how to give an injection. Do not try to give yourself (or have another person give you) injections at home until you (or both of you) understand and are comfortable with how to prepare your dose and give the injection.
Always use a new, unopened, vial of Betaseron and syringe for each injection. Never reuse vials or syringes.
It is important that you change your injection site each time Betaseron is injected. This will lessen the chance of your having a serious skin reaction at the spot where you inject Betaseron. You should always avoid injecting Betaseron into an area of skin that is sore, reddened, infected or otherwise damaged.
At the end of this leaflet there are detailed instructions on how to prepare and give an injection of Betaseron. You should become familiar with these instructions and follow your doctor's orders before injecting Betaseron.

What should I avoid while taking Betaseron?

- **Pregnancy.** You should avoid becoming pregnant while taking Betaseron until you have talked with your doctor. Betaseron can cause you to lose your baby (miscarry).
- **Breast feeding.** You should talk to your doctor if you are breast feeding an infant. It is not known if the interferon in Betaseron can be passed to an infant in mother's milk, and it is not known whether the drug could harm the infant if it is passed to an infant.

What are the possible side effects of Betaseron?

- **Flu-like symptoms.** Most patients have flu-like symptoms (fever, chills, sweating, muscle aches and tiredness). For many patients, these symptoms will lessen or go away over time. You should talk to your doctor about whether you should take an over the counter medication for pain or fever reduction before or after taking your dose of Betaseron.
- **Skin reactions.** Soreness, redness, pain, bruising or swelling may occur at the place of injection. (***see "What is the most important information I should know about Betaseron?"***).
- **Depression and anxiety.** Some patients taking interferons have become very depressed and/or anxious. There have been patients taking interferons who have had thoughts about killing themselves. If you feel sad or hopeless you should tell a friend or family member right away and call your doctor immediately. (***see "What is the most important information I should know about Betaseron?"***).
- **Liver problems.** Your liver function may be affected. Symptoms of changes in your liver include yellowing of the skin and whites of the eyes and easy bruising.
- **Blood problems.** You may have a drop in the levels of infection-fighting white blood cells, red blood cells, or cells that help you form blood clots. If drops in levels are severe, they can lessen your ability to fight infections, make you feel tired or sluggish or cause you to bruise or bleed easily.
- **Thyroid problems.** Your thyroid function may change. Symptoms of changes in the function of your thyroid include feeling cold or hot much of the time or change in your weight (gain or loss) without a change in your diet or amount of exercise you are getting.
- **Allergic reaction.** Some patients have had hives, rash, skin bumps or itching while they were taking Betaseron. There is also a rare possibility that you can have a life-threatening allergic reaction. (***see "What is the most important information I should know about Betaseron?"***).

Whether you experience any of these side effects or not, you and your doctor should periodically talk about your general health. Your doctor may want to monitor you more closely and ask you to have blood tests done more frequently.

General Information About Prescription Medicines

Medicines are sometimes prescribed for purposes other than those listed in a Medication Guide. This medication has been prescribed for your particular medical condition. Do not use it for another condition or give this drug to anyone else. If you have any questions you should speak with your doctor or health care professional. You may also ask your doctor or pharmacist for a copy of the information provided to them with the product. Keep this and all drugs out of the reach of children.

Instructions for Preparing and Giving Yourself an Injection of Betaseron

1. Find a clean, flat working surface that is well-lit and collect all the supplies you will need to give yourself an injection. You will need:
   - One tray containing Betaseron. Make sure the tray contains: A pre-filled diluent syringe
   - A vial of Betaseron
   - Two (2) alcohol prep pads
   - A vial adapter with a 27 gauge needle attached (in the blister pack)
   - A puncture-resistant sealable container to dispose of used syringes/needles
2. Check the expiration date on the tray label to make sure that it has not expired. **Do not use it if the medication has expired.**
3. Wash your hands thoroughly with soap and water.
4. Open the tray by peeling off the label and take out all the contents. Make sure the blister pack containing the vial adapter is sealed. Check to make sure the rubber cap on the diluent syringe is firmly attached.
5. Turn the tray over, place the Betaseron vial in the well (vial holder) and place the prefilled diluent syringe in the U-shaped trough.

Reconstituting Betaseron

1. Remove the Betaseron vial from the well and take the cap off the vial.
2. Place the vial back into the vial holder. Use an alcohol prep pad to clean the top of the vial. Move the prep pad in one direction. Leave the alcohol prep pad on top of the vial until step 5.
3. Peel the label off the blister pack with the vial adapter in it, but do not remove vial adapter. The vial adapter is sterile; avoid touching the vial adapter.
4. Remove the alcohol prep pad from the top of the Betaseron vial. Keeping the vial adapter in the blister pack, place the adapter on top of the Betaseron vial and push down on the adapter until it pierces the rubber top

of the Betaseron vial and snaps in place (**Figure 1**). Remove the blister packaging from the vial adapter.

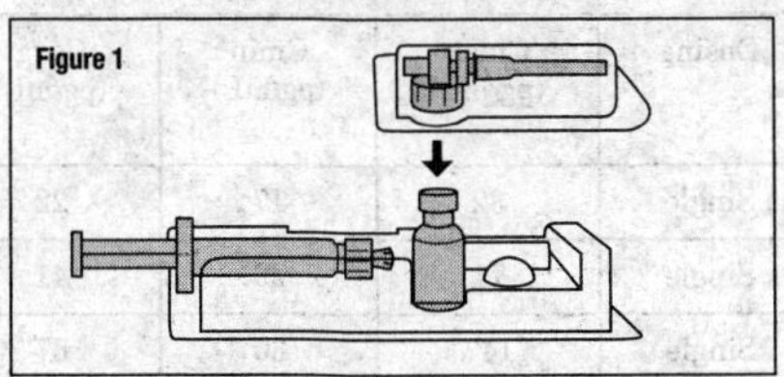

5. Remove the rubber cap from the diluent syringe using a twist and pull motion. Discard the rubber cap.
6. Keeping the syringe assembly attached to the vial, remove the vial from the tray. Be careful not to pull the vial adapter off the top of the vial.
7. Connect the syringe to the vial adapter by turning clockwise and tighten carefully. This will form the *syringe assembly* (**Figure 2**).

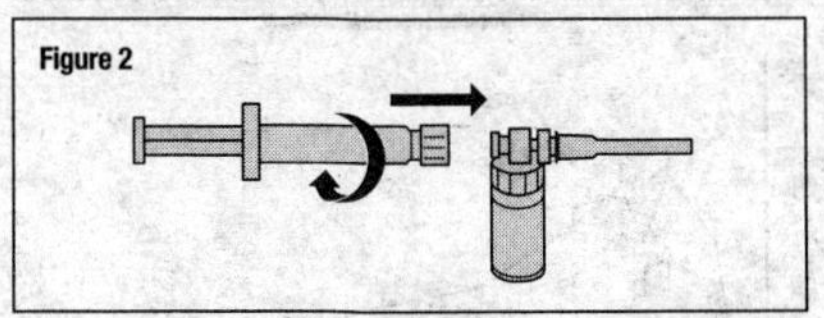

8. Slowly push the plunger of the diluent syringe all the way in. This will transfer all of the diluent in the syringe to the Betaseron vial (**Figure 3**). The plunger may return to its original position after you release it.

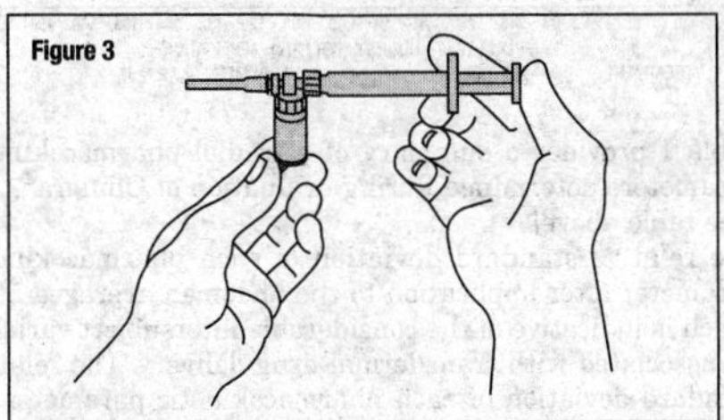

9. Gently swirl the vial to completely dissolve the white cake of Betaseron. Do not shake. Shaking can cause Betaseron to foam; even gently mixing the solution can cause foaming. If there is foam, allow the vial to sit undisturbed until the foam settles.
10. After the cake is dissolved, look closely at the solution to make sure the solution is clear and colorless and does not contain particles. If the mixture contains particles, or is discolored, do not use. Repeat the steps to prepare your dose using a new tray of Betaseron, prefilled syringe, vial adapter and alcohol prep pads. Contact Berlex at 1-800-788-1467 to obtain replacement product.

Preparing the Injection

You have completed the steps to reconstitute your Betaseron and are ready for the injection. The injection should be given immediately after mixing and allowing any foam in the solution to settle. If you must delay giving yourself the injection, you may refrigerate the solution and use within three hours of reconstitution. Do not freeze.

1. Push the plunger in and hold it there; then turn the syringe assembly so that the vial is on top. (The syringe is horizontal.) (**Figure 4**).

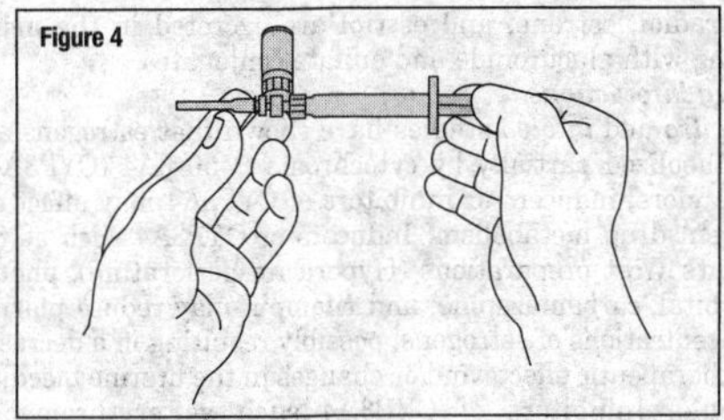

2. Slowly pull the plunger back to withdraw the entire contents of the Betaseron vial into the syringe.
   NOTE: The syringe barrel is marked with numbers from 0.25 to 1.0. If the solution in the vial cannot be drawn up to the 1.0 mark, discard the vial and syringe and start over with a new tray containing a Betaseron vial, prefilled diluent syringe, vial adapter and alcohol prep pads.
3. Turn the syringe assembly so that the needle end is pointing up. Remove any air bubbles by tapping the outer wall of the syringe with your fingers. Slowly push the plunger to the 1 mL mark on the syringe (or to the amount prescribed by your doctor).
   NOTE: If too much solution is pushed into the vial, repeat steps 1, 2, and 3.
4. Remove the vial adapter and the vial from the syringe by twisting the vial adapter as shown in Figure 5. This will remove the vial adapter and the vial from the syringe, but will leave the needle on the syringe (**Figure 5**).

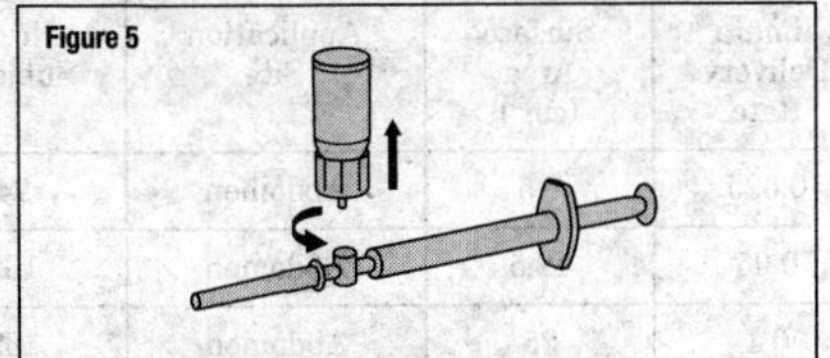

Picking an Injection Site

Betaseron (Interferon beta-1b) is injected under the skin and into the fat layer between the skin and the muscles (subcutaneous tissue). The best areas for injection are where the skin is loose and soft and away from the joints, nerves, and bones. Do not use the area near your navel or waistline. If you are very thin, use only the thigh or outer surface of the arm for injection.

You should pick a different site each time you give yourself an injection. The diagrams show different areas for giving injections. You should not choose the same area for two injections in a row. Keeping a record of your injections will help make sure you rotate your injection sites. You should decide where your injection will be given before you prepare your syringe for injection. If there are any sites that are difficult for you to reach, you can ask someone who has been trained to give injections to help you.

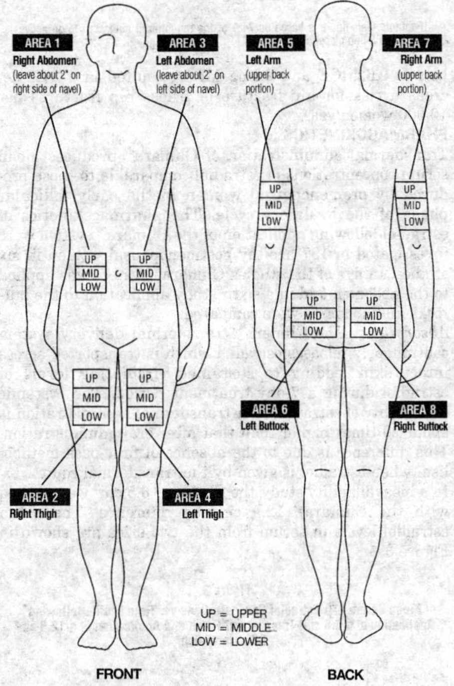

Do not inject in a site where the skin is red, bruised, infected, or scabbed, has broken open, or has lumps, bumps, or pain. Tell your doctor or healthcare provider if you find skin conditions like the ones mentioned here or any other unusual looking areas where you have been given injections.

Using a circular motion, and starting at the injection site and moving outward, clean the injection site with an alcohol wipe. Let the skin area dry before you inject the Betaseron. Remove the cap from the needle.

Hold the syringe like a pencil or dart in one hand.

Gently pinch the skin around the site with the thumb and forefinger of the other hand.

While holding your skin, stick the needle straight into the skin at a 90° angle with a quick, firm motion. Once in your skin, slowly pull back on the plunger. If blood appears in the syringe it means that you have entered a blood vessel. Do not inject Betaseron. Withdraw the needle and repeat the steps to prepare your dose. Choose and clean a new injection site. You should not use the same syringe; discard it in your puncture-proof container.

If no blood appears, slowly push the plunger all the way in until the syringe is empty.

Remove the needle from the skin; then place a dry cotton ball or gauze pad over the injection site.

Gently massage the injection site for a few moments with the dry cotton ball or gauze pad.

Throw away the 1 mL syringe in the disposal container.

Disposing of syringes and needles

Used needles and syringes may be placed in a container made specially for disposing of used syringes and needles (called a "Sharps" container), or a hard plastic container with a screw-on cap or metal container with a plastic lid labeled *"Used Syringes"*. Do not use glass or clear plastic containers. You should always check with your healthcare provider for instructions on how to properly dispose of used vials, needles and syringes. You should follow any special state or local laws regarding the proper disposal of needles and syringes.

DO NOT throw the needle or syringe in the household trash or recycle.

Always keep the disposal container out of the reach of children.

How Should I Store Betaseron?

Betaseron should be stored at room temperature (77°F), but may be stored between 59° and 86°F. Avoid freezing.

This Medication Guide has been approved by the U.S. Food and Drug Administration

Manufactured by:
Chiron Corporation
Emeryville, CA 94608
U.S. License No. 1106
Distributed by:
Berlex Laboratories
Montville, NJ 07045

Printed in U.S.A. on recycled paper
Part Number 10004938 Revision date 10/03
(6052800 BERLEX)

Shown in Product Identification Guide, page 308

CLIMARA® ℞
[*klī-mără*]
(estradiol transdermal system)
Continuous Delivery for Once-Weekly Application

℞ only
PRESCRIBING INFORMATION
Climara® estradiol transdermal system

ESTROGENS INCREASE THE RISK OF ENDOMETRIAL CANCER

Close clinical surveillance of all women taking estrogens is important. Adequate diagnostic measures, including endometrial sampling when indicated, should be undertaken to rule out malignancy in all cases of undiagnosed persistent or recurring abnormal vaginal bleeding. There is no evidence that the use of "natural" estrogens results in a different endometrial risk profile than synthetic estrogens at equivalent estrogen doses.

CARDIOVASCULAR AND OTHER RISKS

Estrogens with and without progestins should not be used for the prevention of cardiovascular disease.

The Women's Health Initiative (WHI) study reported increased risks of myocardial infarction, stroke, invasive breast cancer, pulmonary emboli, and deep vein thrombosis in postmenopausal women during 5 years of treatment with oral conjugated equine estrogens (CE 0.625mg) combined with medroxyprogesterone acetate (MPA 2.5mg) relative to placebo (see **CLINICAL PHARMACOLOGY, Clinical Studies**). Other doses of conjugated estrogens with medroxyprogesterone, and other combinations and dosage forms of estrogens and progestins were not studied in the WHI and, in the absence of comparable data, these risks should be assumed to be similar. Because of these risks, estrogens with or without progestins should be prescribed at the lowest effective doses and for the shortest duration consistent with treatment goals and risks for the individual woman.

DESCRIPTION

Climara®, estradiol transdermal system, is designed to release 17β-estradiol continuously upon application to intact skin. Six (6.5, 9.375, 12.5, 15.0, 18.75 and 25.0 cm^2) systems are available to provide nominal *in vivo* delivery of 0.025, 0.0375, 0.05, 0.060, 0.075 or 0.1 mg respectively of estradiol per day. The period of use is 7 days. Each system has a contact surface area of either 6.5, 9.375, 12.5, 15.0, 18.75 or 25.0 cm^2, and contains 2.0, 2.85, 3.8, 4.55, 5.7 or 7.6 mg of estradiol USP respectively. The composition of the systems per unit area is identical. Estradiol USP (17β-estradiol) is a white, crystalline powder, chemically described as estra-1,3,5(10)-triene-3,17β-diol. It has an empirical formula of $C_{18}H_{24}O_2$ and molecular weight of 272.39. The structural formula is:

[See chemical structure at top of next column]

The Climara® system comprises two layers. Proceeding from the visible surface toward the surface attached to the skin, these layers are (1) a translucent polyethylene film,

Continued on next page

Information on Berlex products (appearing here) is based on the most current information available at the time of publication closing. Further information for these and other Berlex products can be obtained from Medical & Product Services at Berlex, Inc. by calling 1-888-BERLEX-4.

Climara—Cont.

and (2) an acrylate adhesive matrix containing estradiol USP. A protective liner (3) of siliconized or fluoropolymer-coated polyester film is attached to the adhesive surface and must be removed before the system can be used.

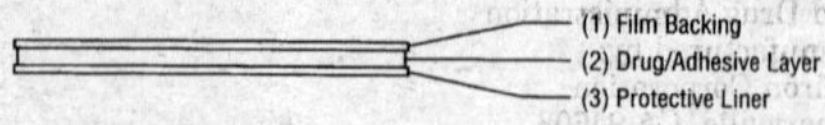

The active component of the system is 17β-estradiol. The remaining components of the system (acrylate copolymer adhesive, fatty acid esters, and polyethylene backing) are pharmacologically inactive.

CLINICAL PHARMACOLOGY

The Climara® system provides systemic estrogen replacement therapy by releasing 17β-estradiol, the major estrogenic hormone secreted by the human ovary.

Endogenous estrogens are largely responsible for the development and maintenance of the female reproductive system and secondary sexual characteristics. Although circulating estrogens exist in a dynamic equilibrium of metabolic interconversions, estradiol is the principal intracellular human estrogen and is substantially more potent than its metabolites, estrone and estriol, at the receptor level.

The primary source of estrogen in normally cycling adult women is the ovarian follicle, which secretes 70 to 500 mcg of estradiol daily, depending on the phase of the menstrual cycle. After menopause, most endogenous estrogen is produced by conversion of androstenedione, secreted by the adrenal cortex, to estrone by peripheral tissues. Thus, estrone and the sulfate conjugated form, estrone sulfate, are the most abundant circulating estrogens in postmenopausal women.

Estrogens act through binding to nuclear receptors in estrogen-responsive tissues. To date, two estrogen receptors have been identified. These vary in proportion from tissue to tissue.

Circulating estrogens modulate the pituitary secretion of the gonadotropins, luteinizing hormone (LH) and follicle-stimulating hormone (FSH), through a negative feedback mechanism. Estrogens act to reduce the elevated levels of these hormones seen in postmenopausal women.

A two-year clinical trial enrolled a total of 175 healthy, hysterectomized, postmenopausal, non-osteoporotic (i.e., lumbar spine bone mineral density > 0.9 gm/cm²) women at 10 study centers in the United States. 129 subjects were allocated to receive active treatment with 4 different doses of 17β-estradiol patches (6.5, 12.5, 15, 25 cm²) and 46 subjects were allocated to receive placebo patches. 77% of the randomized subjects (100 on active drug and 34 on placebo) contributed data to the analysis of percent change of A-P spine bone mineral density (BMD), the primary efficacy variable (see Figure 1). A statistically significant overall treatment effect at each timepoint was noted, implying bone preservation for all active treatment groups at all timepoints, as opposed to bone loss for placebo at all timepoints.

Figure 1
Mean Percent Change from Baseline in Lumbar Spine (A-P View) Bone Mineral Density by Treatment and Time last observation carried forward**

Percent change in BMD of the total hip (see Figure 2) was also statistically significantly different from placebo for all active treatment groups. The results of the measurements of biochemical markers supported the finding of efficacy for all doses of transdermal estradiol. Serum osteocalcin levels decreased, indicative of a decrease in bone formation, at all timepoints for all active treatment doses, statistically significantly different from placebo (which generally rose). Urinary deoxypyridinoline and pyridinoline changes also suggested a decrease in bone turnover for all active treatment groups.

[See figure 2 at top of next column]

Data from the Women's Health Initiative study showed that continuous combined estrogen and progestin (dose equivalent to 0.625 CE and 2.5mg MPA) resulted in a 34% decreased risk for hip fracture or 5 less hip fractures per 10,000 women/year.

Table 1
Pharmacokinetic Summary (Mean Estradiol Values)

Climara® Delivery Rate	Surface Area (cm²)	Application Site	No. of Subjects	Dosing	Cmax (pg/mL)	Cmin (pg/mL)	Cavg (pg/mL)
0.025	6.5	Abdomen	24	Single	32	17	22
0.05	12.5	Abdomen	102	Single	71	29	41
0.1	25	Abdomen	139	Single	147	60	87
0.1	25	Buttock	38	Single	174	71	106

Figure 2
Mean Percent Change from Baseline in Total Hip by Treatment and Time last observation carried forward**

Footnote: This figure is based on 74% of the randomized subjects (95 on active drug and 34 on placebo).

PHARMACOKINETICS

Transdermal administration of Climara® produces mean serum concentrations of estradiol comparable to those produced by premenopausal women in the early follicular phase of the ovulatory cycle. The pharmacokinetics of estradiol following application of the Climara® system were investigated in 197 healthy postmenopausal women in six studies. In five of the studies Climara® system was applied to the abdomen and in a sixth study application to the buttocks and abdomen were compared.

Absorption: The Climara® transdermal delivery system continuously releases estradiol which is transported across intact skin leading to sustained circulating levels of estradiol during a 7-day treatment period. The systemic availability of estradiol after transdermal administration is about 20 times higher than that after oral administration. This difference is due to the absence of first pass metabolism when estradiol is given by the transdermal route.

In a bioavailability study, the Climara® 6.5 cm² was studied with the Climara® 12.5 cm² as reference. The mean estradiol levels in serum from the two sizes are shown in Figure 3.

Figure 3
Mean Serum 17β-Estradiol Concentrations vs. Time Profile following Application of a 6.5 cm² Transdermal Patch and Application of a 12.5 cm² Climara® patch

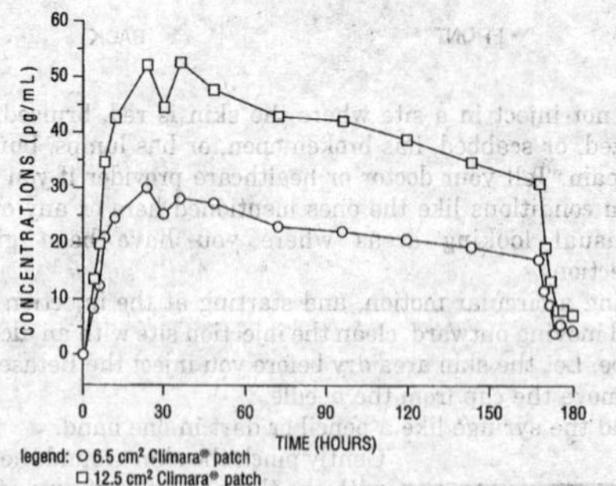

Dose proportionality was demonstrated for the Climara® 6.5 cm² transdermal system as compared to the Climara® 12.5 cm² transdermal system in a 2-week crossover study with a 1-week washout period between the two-transdermal systems in 24 postmenopausal women.

Dose proportionality was also demonstrated for the Climara® system (12.5 cm² and 25 cm²) in a 1-week study conducted in 54 postmenopausal women. The mean steady state levels (Cavg) of the estradiol during the application of Climara® 25 cm² and 12.5 cm² on the abdomen were about 80 and 40 pg/mL, respectively.

In a 3 week multiple application study in 24 postmenopausal women, the 25.0 cm² Climara® system produced average peak estradiol concentrations (Cmax) of approximately 100 pg/mL. Trough values at the end of each wear interval (Cmin) were approximately 35 pg/mL. Nearly identical serum curves were seen each week, indicating little or no accumulation of estradiol in the body. Serum estrone peak and trough levels were 60 and 40 pg/mL, respectively.

In a single dose, randomized, crossover study conducted to compare the effect of site of application, 38 postmenopausal women wore a single Climara® 25 cm² system for 1 week on the abdomen and buttocks. The estradiol serum concentration profiles are shown in Figure 4. Cmax and Cavg values were, respectively, 25% and 17% higher with the buttock application than with the abdomen application.

Figure 4
Observed Mean (± S.E.) Estradiol Serum Concentrations for a One Week Application of the Climara® system (25 cm²) to the abdomen and buttocks of 38 postmenopausal women

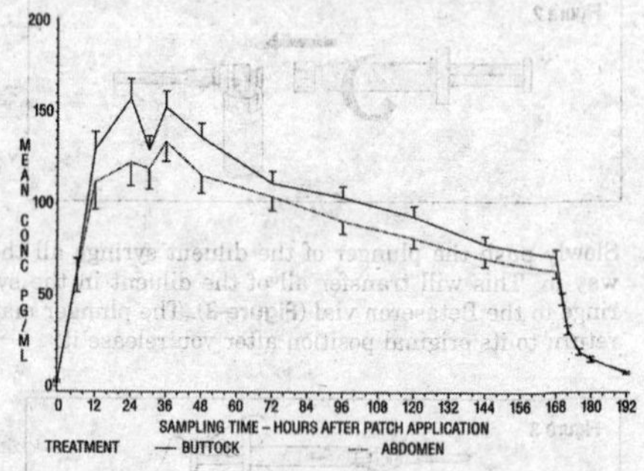

Table 1 provides a summary of estradiol pharmacokinetic parameters determined during evaluation of Climara®.

[See table above]

The relative standard deviation of each pharmacokinetic parameter after application to the abdomen averaged 50%, which is indicative of the considerable intersubject variability associated with transdermal drug delivery. The relative standard deviation of each pharmacokinetic parameter after application to the buttock was lower than that after application to the abdomen (e.g., for Cmax 39% vs 62%, and for Cavg 35% vs 48%).

Distribution

The distribution of exogenous estrogens is similar to that of endogenous estrogens. Estrogens are widely distributed in the body and are generally found in higher concentrations in the sex hormone target organs. Estrogens circulate in the blood largely bound to sex hormone binding globulin (SHBG) and albumin.

Metabolism

Exogenous estrogens are metabolized in the same manner as endogenous estrogens. Circulating estrogens exist in a dynamic equilibrium of metabolic interconversions. These transformations take place mainly in the liver. Estradiol is converted reversibly to estrone, and both can be converted to estriol, which is the major urinary metabolite. Estrogens also undergo enterohepatic recirculation via sulfate and glucuronide conjugation in the liver, biliary secretion of conjugates into the intestine, and hydrolysis in the gut followed by reabsorption. In postmenopausal women, a significant proportion of the circulating estrogens exist as sulfate conjugates, especially estrone sulfate, which serves as a circulating reservoir for the formation of more active estrogens.

Excretion

Estradiol, estrone, and estriol are excreted in the urine along with glucuronide and sulfate conjugates.

Drug Interactions

In vitro and *in vivo* studies have shown that estrogens are metabolized partially by cytochrome P450 3A4 (CYP3A4). Therefore, inducers or inhibitors of CYP3A4 may affect estrogen drug metabolism. Inducers of CYP3A4 such as St. John's Wort preparations (Hypericum perforatum), phenobarbital, carbamazepine, and rifampin may reduce plasma concentrations of estrogens, possibly resulting in a decrease in therapeutic effects and/or changes in the uterine bleeding profile. Inhibitors of CYP3A4 such as erythromycin, clarithromycin, ketoconazole, itraconazole, ritonavir and grapefruit juice may increase plasma concentrations of estrogens and may result in side effects.

Special Populations

Geriatric: There have not been sufficient numbers of geriatric patients involved in clinical studies utilizing Climara® to determine whether those over 65 years of age differ from younger subjects in their response to Climara®.

Pediatric: No pharmacokinetic study for Climara® has been conducted in a pediatric population.

Gender: Climara® is indicated for use in women only.

Race: No studies were done to determine the effect of race on the pharmacokinetics of Climara®.

Patients with Renal Impairment: Total estradiol serum levels are higher in postmenopausal women with end stage renal disease (ESRD) receiving maintenance hemodialysis than in normal subjects at baseline and following oral doses of estradiol. Therefore, conventional transdermal estradiol doses used in individuals with normal renal function may be excessive for postmenopausal women with ESRD receiving maintenance hemodialysis.

Patients with Hepatic Impairment: Estrogens may be poorly metabolized in patients with impaired liver function and should be administered with caution.

Adhesion

An open-label study of adhesion potentials of placebo transdermal systems that correspond to the 6.5 cm^2 and 12.5 cm^2 sizes of Climara® was conducted in 112 healthy women of 45–75 years of age. Each woman applied both transdermal systems weekly, on the upper outer abdomen, for 3 consecutive weeks. It should be noted that lower abdomen and upper quadrant of the buttock are the approved sites of application for Climara®.

The adhesion assessment was done visually on Days 2, 4, 5, 6, 7 of each week of transdermal system wear. A total of 1654 adhesion observations were conducted for 333 transdermal systems of each size.

Of these observations, approximately 90% showed essentially no lift for both the 6.5 cm^2 and 12.5 cm^2 transdermal systems. Of the total number of transdermal systems applied, approximately 5% showed complete detachment for each size. Adhesion potentials of the 18.75 cm^2 and 25.0 cm^2 sizes of transdermal systems (0.075 mg/day and 0.1 mg/day) have not been studied.

Clinical Studies

Climara® is effective in reducing moderate to severe vasomotor symptoms in postmenopausal women.

A total of 214 patients were enrolled in a study to determine the efficacy of Climara® 0.05 mg/day and 0.1 mg/day compared to placebo and an active comparator. Women took drug in a cyclical fashion (three weeks on and one week off).

A study of 214 women 25 to 74 years old met the qualification criteria and were randomly assigned to one of the three treatment groups: 72 to the 0.05 mg estradiol patch, 70 to the 0.1 mg estradiol patch, and 72 to placebo. Potential subjects were postmenopausal women in good general health who experienced vasomotor symptoms. Natural menopause patients had not menstruated for at least 12 months and surgical menopause patients had undergone bilateral oophorectomy at least 4 weeks before evaluation for study entry.

In order to enter the 11-week treatment phase of the study, potential subjects must have experienced a minimum of five moderate to severe hot flushes per week, or a minimum of 15 hot flushes of any severity per week, for 2 consecutive weeks. Women wore the patches in a cyclical fashion (three weeks on and one week off).

During treatment, all subjects used diaries to record the number and severity of hot flushes. Subjects were monitored by clinic visits at the end of weeks 1, 3, 7, and 11 and by telephone at the end of weeks 4, 5, 8, and 9.

Adequate data for the analysis of efficacy was available from 191 subjects. The results are presented as the mean ± SD number of flushes in each of the 3 treatment weeks of each 4-week cycle. In the 0.05 mg estradiol group, the mean weekly hot flush rate across all treatment cycles decreased from 46 ± 6.5 at baseline to 20 ± 3.0 (–67.0%). The 0.1 mg estradiol group had a decline in the mean weekly hot flush rate from 52 ± 4.4 at baseline to 16 ± 2.4 (–72.0%). In the placebo group, the mean weekly hot flush rate declined from 53 ± 4.5 at baseline to 46 ± 6.5 (–18.1%). Compared with placebo, the 0.05 mg and 0.1 mg estradiol groups showed a statistically significantly larger mean decrease in hot flushes across all treatment cycles ($P<0.05$). When the response to treatment was analyzed for each of the three cycles of therapy, similar statistically significant differences were observed between both estradiol treatment groups and the placebo group during all treatment cycles.

In a double-blind, placebo-controlled, randomized study of 187 women receiving Climara® 0.025 mg/day or placebo continuously for up to three 28-day cycles, the Climara® 0.025 mg/day dosage was shown to be statistically better than placebo at weeks 4 and 12 for relief of both the frequency and severity of moderate-to-severe vasomotor symptoms.

Table 2
Mean Change from Baseline in the Number of Moderate-to-Severe Vasomotor Symptoms (ITT)

Treatment Group	Statistics	Week 4	Week 8	Week 12
E_2 TDS	N	82	84	68
	Mean	–6.45	–7.69	–7.56
	SD	4.65	4.76	4.64
Placebo	N	83	71	65
	Mean	–5.11	–5.98	–5.98
	SD	7.43	8.63	9.69
	p-Value	<0.002		<0.003

A second active-control trial of 193 randomized subjects was supportive of the placebo-controlled trial.

Women's Health Initiative Studies

The Women's Health Initiative (WHI) enrolled a total of 27,000 predominantly healthy postmenopausal women to assess the risks and benefits of either the use of 0.625 mg conjugated estrogens (CE) per day alone or the use of 0.625 mg conjugated estrogens plus 2.5 mg medroxyprogesterone acetate (MPA) per day compared to placebo in the prevention of certain chronic diseases. The primary endpoint was the incidence of coronary heart disease (CHD) (nonfatal myocardial infarction and CHD death), with invasive breast cancer as the primary adverse outcome studied. A "global index" included the earliest occurrence of CHD, invasive breast cancer, stroke, pulmonary embolism (PE), endometrial cancer, colorectal cancer, hip fixture, or death due to other cause. The study did not evaluate the effects of CE or CE/MPA on menopausal symptoms.

The CE-only substudy is continuing and results have not been reported. The CE/MPA substudy was stopped early because, according to the predefined stopping rule, the increased risk of breast cancer and cardiovascular events exceeded the specified benefits included in the "global index." Results of the CE/MPA substudy, which included 16,608 women (average age of 63 years, range 50 to 79; 83.9% White, 6.5% Black, 5.5% Hispanic), after an average follow-up of 5.2 years are presented in Table 3 below:

[See table 3 above]

Table 3
Relative and Absolute Risk Seen in the CE/MPA Substudy of WHI[a]

Event[c]	Relative Risk CE/MPA vs placebo at 5.2 Years (95% CI*)	Placebo n = 8102	CE/MPA n = 8506
		Absolute Risk per 10,000 Person-years	
CHD events	1.29 (1.02–1.63)	30	37
Non-fatal MI	*1.32 (1.02–1.72)*	*23*	*30*
CHD death	*1.18 (0.70–1.97)*	*6*	*7*
Invasive breast cancer[b]	1.26 (1.00–1.59)	30	38
Stroke	1.41 (1.07–1.85)	21	29
Pulmonary embolism	2.13 (1.39–3.25)	8	16
Colorectal cancer	0.63 (0.43–0.92)	16	10
Endometrial cancer	0.83 (0.47–1.47)	6	5
Hip fracture	0.66 (0.45–0.98)	15	10
Death due to causes other than the events above	0.92 (0.74–1.14)	40	37
Global Index[c]	1.15 (1.03–1.28)	151	170
Deep vein thrombosis[d]	2.07 (1.49–2.87)	13	26
Vertebral fractures[d]	0.66 (0.44–0.98)	15	9
Other osteoporotic fractures[d]	0.77 (0.69–0.86)	170	131

[a] adapted from JAMA, 2002; 288:321-333
[b] bincludes metastatic and non-metastatic breast cancer with the exception of in situ breast cancer
[c] a subset of the events was combined in a "global index", defined as the earliest occurrence of CHD events, invasive breast cancer, stroke, pulmonary embolism, endometrial cancer, colorectal cancer, hip fracture, or death due to other causes
[d] not included in Global Index
*nominal confidence intervals unadjusted for multiple looks and multiple comparisons

For those outcomes included in the "global index," absolute excess risks per 10,000 person-years in the group treated with CE/MPA were 7 more CHD events, 8 more strokes, 8 more PEs, and 8 more invasive breast cancers, while absolute risk reductions per 10,000 person-years were 6 fewer colorectal cancers and 5 fewer hip fractures. The absolute excess risk of events included in the "global index" was 19 per 10,000 person-years. There was no difference between the groups in terms of all-cause mortality. (See **BOXED WARNINGS, WARNINGS,** and **PRECAUTIONS.**)

INDICATIONS AND USAGE

Climara® is indicated in the:

1. Treatment of moderate to severe vasomotor symptoms associated with the menopause.
2. Treatment of moderate to severe symptoms of vulvar and vaginal atrophy associated with the menopause. When prescribing solely for the treatment of symptoms of vulvar and vaginal atrophy, topical vaginal products should be considered.
3. Treatment of hypoestrogenism due to hypogonadism, castration or primary ovarian failure.
4. Prevention of postmenopausal osteoporosis. When prescribing solely for the prevention of postmenopausal osteoporosis, therapy should only be considered for women at significant risk of osteoporosis and non-estrogen medications should be carefully considered.

The mainstays for decreasing the risk of postmenopausal osteoporosis are weight bearing exercise, adequate calcium and vitamin D intake, and when indicated, pharmacologic therapy. Postmenopausal women require an average of 1500mg/day of elemental calcium. Therefore, when not contraindicated, calcium supplementation may be helpful for women with suboptimal dietary intake. Vitamin D supplementation of 400-800 IU/day may also be required to ensure adequate daily intake in postmenopausal women.

Estrogen therapy reduces bone resorption and retards or halts postmenopausal bone loss. Studies have shown an approximately 60% reduction in hip and wrist fractures in women whose estrogen therapy was begun within a few years of menopause. Studies also suggest that estrogen reduces the rate of vertebral fractures. Even when started as late as 6 years after menopause, estrogen prevents further loss of bone mass for as long as treatment is continued. When estrogen therapy is discontinued, bone mass declines at a rate comparable to the immediate postmenopausal period.

Early menopause is one of the strongest predictors for the development of osteoporosis in all women. Other factors associated with osteoporosis include genetic factors, lifestyle and nutrition.

CONTRAINDICATIONS

Estrogens and estrogen/progestin therapy should not be used in individuals with any of the following conditions:

1. Undiagnosed abnormal genital bleeding.
2. Known, suspected, or history of cancer of the breast.
3. Known or suspected estrogen-dependent neoplasia.
4. Active deep vein thrombosis, pulmonary embolism or a history of these conditions.
5. Active or recent (e.g. within the past year) arterial thromboembolic disease (e.g., stroke, myocardial infarction).
6. Liver dysfunction and disease.
7. Climara® should not be used in patients with known hypersensitivity to its ingredients.
8. Known or suspected pregnancy. There is no indication for Climara® in pregnancy. There appears to be little or no increased risk of birth defects in women who have used estrogens and progestins from oral contraceptives inadvertently during early pregnancy. (See **PRECAUTIONS.**)

WARNINGS

See **BOXED WARNINGS.**

The use of unopposed estrogens in women who have a uterus is associated with an increased risk of endometrial cancer.

1. Cardiovascular disorders.

Estrogen and estrogen/progestin therapy have been associated with an increased risk of cardiovascular events such as myocardial infarction and stroke, as well as venous thrombosis and pulmonary embolism (venous thromboembolism or VTE). Should any of these occur or be suspected, estrogens should be discontinued immediately.

Risk factors for cardiovascular disease (e.g., hypertension, diabetes mellitus, tobacco use, hypercholesterolemia, and obesity) should be managed appropriately.

a. Coronary heart disease and stroke

In the Women's Health Initiative study (WHI), an increase in the number of myocardial infarctions and strokes has been observed in women receiving oral CE compared to placebo. These observations are preliminary, and the study is continuing, (See **CLINICAL PHARMACOLOGY, Clinical Studies.**)

Continued on next page

Information on Berlex products (appearing here) is based on the most current information available at the time of publication closing. Further information for these and other Berlex products can be obtained from Medical & Product Services at Berlex, Inc. by calling 1-888-BERLEX-4.

Climara—Cont.

In the CE/MPA substudy of WHI an increased risk of coronary heart disease (CHD) events (defined as nonfatal myocardial infarction and CHD death) was observed in women receiving CE/MPA compared to women receiving placebo (37 vs 30 per 10,000 person years). The increase in risk was observed in year one and persisted.

In the same substudy of WHI, an increased risk of stroke was observed in women receiving CE/MPA compared to women receiving placebo (29 vs 21 per 10,000 person-years). The increase in risk was observed after the first year and persisted.

In postmenopausal women with documented heart disease (n = 2,763, average age 66.7 years) a controlled clinical trial of secondary prevention of cardiovascular disease (Heart and Estrogen/Progestin Replacement Study; HERS) treatment with CE/MPA-0.625mg/2.5mg per day demonstrated no cardiovascular benefit. During an average follow-up of 4.1 years, treatment with CE/MPA did not reduce the overall rate of CHD events in postmenopausal women with established coronary heart disease. There were more CHD events in the CE/MPA-treated group than in the placebo group in year 1, but not during the subsequent years. Two thousand three hundred and twenty one women from the original HERS trial agreed to participate in an open label extension of HERS, HERS II. Average follow-up in HERS II was an additional 2.7 years, for a total of 6.8 years overall. Rates of CHD events were comparable among women in the CE/MPA group and the placebo group in HERS, HERS II, and overall.

Large doses of estrogen (5 mg conjugated estrogens per day), comparable to those used to treat cancer of the prostate and breast, have been shown in a large prospective clinical trial in men to increase the risks of nonfatal myocardial infarction, pulmonary embolism, and thrombophlebitis.

b. Venous thromboembolism (VTE)

In the Women's Health Initiative study (WHI), an increase in VTE has been observed in women receiving CE compared to placebo. These observations are preliminary, and the study is continuing. (See **CLINICAL PHARMACOLOGY, Clinical Studies.**)

In the CE/MPA substudy of WHI, a 2-fold greater rate of VTE, including deep venous thrombosis and pulmonary embolism, was observed in women receiving CE/MPA compared to women receiving placebo. The rate of VTE was 34 per 10,000 woman-years in the CE/MPA group compared to 16 per 10,000 woman-years in the placebo group. The increase in VTE risk was observed during the first year and persisted.

If feasible, estrogens should be discontinued at least 4 to 6 weeks before surgery of the type associated with an increased risk of thromboembolism, or during periods of prolonged immobilization.

2. Malignant neoplasms

a. Endometrial cancer

The use of unopposed estrogens in women with intact uteri has been associated with an increased risk of endometrial cancer. The reported endometrial cancer risk among unopposed estrogen users is about 2- to 12-fold greater than in non-users, and appears dependent on duration of treatment and on estrogen dose. Most studies show no significant increased risk associated with use of estrogens for less than one year. The greatest risk appears associated with prolonged use, with increased risks of 15- to 24-fold for five to ten years or more and this risk has been shown to persist for at least 8 to 15 years after estrogen therapy is discontinued.

Clinical surveillance of all women taking estrogen/progestin combinations is important. Adequate diagnostic measures, including endometrial sampling when indicated, should be undertaken to rule out malignancy in all cases of undiagnosed persistent or recurring abnormal vaginal bleeding. There is no evidence that the use of natural estrogens results in a different endometrial risk profile than synthetic estrogens of equivalent estrogen dose. Adding a progestin to estrogen therapy has been shown to reduce the risk of endometrial hyperplasia, which may be a precursor to endometrial cancer.

b. Breast cancer

Estrogen and estrogen/progestin therapy in postmenopausal women has been associated with an increased risk of breast cancer. In the CE/MPA substudy of the Women's Health Initiative study (WHI), a 26% increase of invasive breast cancer (38 vs 30 per 10,000 woman-years) after an average of 5.2 years of treatment was observed in women receiving CE/MPA compared to women receiving placebo. The increased risk of breast cancer became apparent after 4 years on CE/MPA. The women reporting prior postmenopausal use of estrogen and/or estrogen with progestin had a higher relative risk for breast cancer associated with CE/MPA than those who had never used these hormones. (See **CLINICAL PHARMACOLOGY, Clinical Studies.**)

In the WHI, no increased risk of breast cancer in CE-treated women compared to placebo was reported after an average of 5.2 years of therapy. These data are preliminary and that substudy of WHI is continuing.

Epidemiologic studies have reported an increased risk of breast cancer in association with increasing duration of postmenopausal treatment with estrogens with or without a progestin. This association was reanalyzed in original data from 51 studies that involved various doses and types of estrogens, with and without progestins. In the reanalysis, an increased risk of having breast cancer diagnosed became apparent after about 5 years of continued treatment, and subsided after treatment had been discontinued for 5 years or longer. Some later studies have suggested that postmenopausal treatment with estrogens and progestin increase the risk of breast cancer more than treatment with estrogen alone.

A postmenopausal woman without a uterus who requires estrogen should receive estrogen-alone therapy, and should not be exposed unnecessarily to progestins. All postmenopausal women should receive yearly breast exams by a health care provider and perform monthly self-examinations. In addition, mammography examinations should be scheduled based on patient age and risk factors.

3. Gallbladder disease

A 2- to 4-fold increase in the risk of gallbladder disease requiring surgery in postmenopausal women receiving estrogens has been reported.

4. Visual abnormalities

Retinal vascular thrombosis has been reported in patients receiving estrogens. Discontinue medication pending examination if there is sudden partial or complete loss of vision, or a sudden onset of proptosis, diplopia, or migraine. If examination reveals papilledema or retinal vascular lesions, estrogens should be discontinued.

PRECAUTIONS

A. GENERAL

1. Addition of a progestin when a woman has not had a hysterectomy.

Studies of the addition of a progestin for 10 or more days of a cycle of estrogen administration, or daily with estrogen in a continuous regimen, have reported a lowered incidence of endometrial hyperplasia than would be induced by estrogen treatment alone. Endometrial hyperplasia may be a precursor to endometrial cancer.

There are, however, possible risks that may be associated with the use of progestins with estrogens compared to estrogen-alone regimens.

These include:

a. A possible increased risk of breast cancer
b. Adverse effects on lipoprotein metabolism (e.g., lowering HDL, raising LDL)
c. Impairment of glucose tolerance

2. Elevated blood pressure

In a small number of case reports, substantial increases in blood pressure have been attributed to idiosyncratic reactions to estrogens. In a large, randomized, placebo-controlled clinical trial, a generalized effect of estrogen therapy on blood pressure was not seen. Blood pressure should be monitored at regular intervals with estrogen use.

3. Familial hyperlipoproteinemia

In patients with familial defects of lipoprotein metabolism, oral estrogen therapy may be associated with elevations of plasma triglycerides leading to pancreatitis and other complications.

4. Impaired liver function

Estrogens may be poorly metabolized in patients with impaired liver function. For patients with a history of cholestatic jaundice associated with past estrogen use or with pregnancy, caution should be exercised and in the case of recurrence, medication should be discontinued.

5. Hypothyroidism

Estrogen administration leads to increased thyroid-binding globulin (TBG) levels. Patients with normal thyroid function can compensate for the increased TBG by making more thyroid hormone, thus maintaining free T_4 and T_3 serum concentrations in the normal range. Patients dependent on thyroid hormone replacement therapy who are also receiving estrogens may require increased doses of their thyroid replacement therapy. These patients should have their thyroid function monitored in order to maintain their free thyroid hormone levels in an acceptable range.

6. Fluid retention

Because estrogens may cause some degree of fluid retention, patients with conditions that might be influenced by this factor, such as a cardiac or renal dysfunction, warrant careful observation when estrogens are prescribed.

7. Hypocalcemia

Estrogens should be used with caution in individuals with severe hypocalcemia.

8. Ovarian cancer

Use of estrogen-only products, in particular for ten or more years, has been associated with an increased risk of ovarian cancer in some epidemiological studies. Other studies did not show a significant association. Data are insufficient to determine whether there is an increased risk with estrogen/progestin combination therapy in post-menopausal women.

9. Exacerbation of endometriosis

Endometriosis may be exacerbated with administration of estrogens.

10. Exacerbation of other conditions

Estrogens may cause an exacerbation of asthma, diabetes mellitus, epilepsy, migraine or porphyria and should be used with caution in women with these conditions.

B. PATIENT INFORMATION

Physicians are advised to discuss the PATIENT INFORMATION leaflet with patients for whom they prescribe Climara®. See text of Patient Information after the **HOW SUPPLIED.**

C. LABORATORY TESTS

Estrogen administration should be initiated at the lowest dose for the approved indication and then guided by clinical response, rather than by serum hormone levels (e.g., estradiol, FSH).

D. DRUG/LABORATORY TEST INTERACTIONS

1. Accelerated prothrombin time, partial thromboplastin time, and platelet aggregation time; increased platelet count; increased factors II, VII antigen, VIII antigen, VIII coagulant activity, IX, X, XII, VII-X complex, II-VII-X complex, and beta-thromboglobulin; decreased levels of antifactor Xa and antithrombin III, decreased antithrombin III activity; increased levels of fibrinogen and fibrinogen activity; increased plasminogen antigen and activity.
2. Increased thyroid-binding globulin (TBG) levels leading to increased circulating total thyroid hormone levels as measured by protein-bound iodine (PBI), T_4 levels (by column or by radioimmunoassay) or T_3 levels by radioimmunoassay. T_3 resin uptake is decreased, reflecting the elevated TBG. Free T_4 and free T_3 concentrations are unaltered. Patients on thyroid replacement therapy may require higher doses of thyroid hormone.
3. Other binding proteins may be elevated in serum (i.e., corticosteroid binding globulin (CBG), sex hormone-binding globulin (SHBG) leading to increased circulating corticosteroids and sex steroids, respectively. Free or biologically active hormone concentrations are unchanged. Other plasma proteins may be increased (angiotensinogen/renin substrate, alpha-l-antitrypsin, ceruloplasmin).
4. Increased plasma HDL and HDL_2 subfraction concentrations, reduced LDL cholesterol concentration, and in oral formulations increased triglyceride levels.
5. Impaired glucose tolerance.
6. Reduced response to metyrapone test.
7. Reduced serum folate concentration.

E. CARCINOGENESES, MUTAGENESIS, AND IMPAIRMENT OF FERTILITY

Long-term continuous administration of natural and synthetic estrogens in certain animal species increases the frequency of carcinomas of the breast, uterus, cervix, vagina, testis, and liver. (See **BOXED WARNINGS, CONTRAINDICATIONS,** and **WARNINGS.**)

F. PREGNANCY

Climara® should not be used during pregnancy. (See **CONTRAINDICATIONS.**)

G. NURSING MOTHERS

Estrogen administration to nursing mothers has been shown to decrease the quantity and quality of the milk. Detectable amounts of estrogens have been identified in the milk of mothers receiving this drug. Caution should be exercised when Climara® is administered to a nursing woman.

H. PEDIATRIC USE

Estrogen replacement therapy has been used for the induction of puberty in adolescents with some forms of pubertal delay. Safety and effectiveness in pediatric patients have not otherwise been established. Large and repeated doses of estrogen over an extended time period have been shown to accelerate epiphyseal closure, which could result in short adult stature if treatment is initiated before the completion of physiologic puberty in normally developing children. If estrogen is administered to patients whose bone growth is not complete, periodic monitoring of bone maturation and effects on epiphyseal centers is recommended during estrogen administration. Estrogen treatment of prepubertal girls also induces premature breast development and vaginal cornification, and may induce vaginal bleeding. In boys, estrogen treatment may modify the normal pubertal process and induce gynecomastia. (See **INDICATIONS** and **DOSAGE AND ADMINISTRATION.**)

I. GERIATRIC USE

There have not been sufficient numbers of geriatric patients involved in clinical studies utilizing Climara® to determine whether those over 65 years of age differ from younger subjects in their response to Climara®.

ADVERSE REACTIONS

See **BOXED WARNINGS, WARNINGS** and **PRECAUTIONS.**

Because clinical trials are conducted under widely varying conditions, adverse reaction rates observed in the clinical trials of a drug cannot be directly compared to rates in the clinical trials of another drug and may not reflect the rates observed in practice. The adverse reaction information from clinical trials does, however, provide a basis for identifying the adverse events that appear to be related to drug use and for approximating rates.

[See table at top of next page]

Summary of Most Frequently Reported Adverse Experiences/Medical Events (≥5%) by Treatment Groups

AE per Body System	Climara® 0.025 mg/day (N=219)	Climara® 0.05 mg/day (N=201)	Climara® 0.1 mg/day (N=194)	Placebo (N=72)
Body as a Whole	21%	39%	37%	29%
Headache	5%	18%	13%	10%
Pain	1%	8%	11%	7%
Back Pain	4%	8%	9%	6%
Edema	0.5%	13%	10%	6%
Gastro-Intestinal	9%	21%	29%	18%
Abdominal Pain	0.0%	11%	16%	8%
Nausea	1%	5%	6%	3%
Flatulence	1%	3%	7%	1%
Musculo-Skeletal	7%	9%	11%	4%
Arthralgia	1%	5%	5%	3%
Psychiatric	13%	10%	11%	1%
Depression	1%	5%	8%	0%
Reproductive	12%	18%	41%	11%
Breast Pain	5%	8%	29%	4%
Leukorrhea	1%	6%	7%	1%
Respiratory	15%	26%	29%	14%
URTI	6%	17%	17%	8%
Pharyngitis	0.5%	3%	7%	3%
Sinusitis	4%	4%	5%	3%
Rhinitis	2%	4%	6%	1%
Skin and Appendages	19%	12%	12%	15%
Pruritus	0.5%	6%	3%	6%

The following additional adverse reactions have been reported with estrogens:

1. Genitourinary system
Changes in vaginal bleeding pattern and abnormal withdrawal bleeding or flow; breakthrough bleeding; spotting; increase in size of uterine leiomyomata; vaginitis, including vaginal candidiasis; change in amount of cervical secretion; changes in cervical ectropion; ovarian cancer; endometrial hyperplasia; endometrial cancer.

2. Breasts
Tenderness, enlargement, pain, nipple discharge, galactorrhea; fibrocystic breast changes; breast cancer.

3. Cardiovascular
Deep and superficial venous thrombosis; pulmonary embolism; thrombophlebitis; myocardial infarction; stroke; increase in blood pressure.

4. Gastrointestinal
Nausea, vomiting; abdominal cramps, bloating; cholestatic jaundice; increased incidence of gall bladder disease; pancreatitis.

5. Skin
Chloasma or melasma, which may persist when drug is discontinued; erythema multiforme; erythema nodosum; hemorrhagic eruption; loss of scalp hair; hirsutism; pruritus, rash.

6. Eyes
Retinal vascular thrombosis; steepening of corneal curvature; intolerance to contact lenses.

7. Central nervous system
Headache; migraine; dizziness; mental depression; chorea; nervousness; mood disturbances; irritability; exacerbation of epilepsy.

8. Miscellaneous
Increase or decrease in weight; reduced carbohydrate tolerance; aggravation of porphyria; edema; arthralgias; leg cramps; changes in libido; anaphylactoid/anaphylactic reactions including urticaria and angioedema; hypocalcemia; exacerbation of asthma; increased triglycerides.

OVERDOSAGE

Overdosage may cause nausea, and withdrawal bleeding may occur in females. Serious ill effects have not been reported following acute ingestion of large doses of estrogen/progestin-containing oral contraceptives by young children.

DOSAGE AND ADMINISTRATION

When estrogen is prescribed for a postmenopausal woman with a uterus, progestin should also be initiated to reduce the risk of endometrial cancer. A woman without a uterus does not need progestin. Use of estrogen, alone or in combination with a progestin, should be limited to the shortest duration consistent with treatment goals and risks for the individual woman. Patients should be reevaluated periodically as clinically appropriate (e.g., 3-month to 6-month intervals) to determine if treatment is still necessary (See **BOXED WARNINGS** and **WARNINGS**.) For women who have a uterus, adequate diagnostic measures, such as endometrial sampling, when indicated, should be undertaken to rule out malignancy in cases of undiagnosed persistent or recurring abnormal vaginal bleeding.

Initiation of Therapy
Patients should be started at the lowest dose. Six (6.5, 9.375, 12.5, 15.0, 18.75 and 25.0 cm2) Climara® systems are available. For the treatment of vasomotor symptoms, treatment should be initiated with the 6.5 cm^2 (0.025 mg/day) Climara® system applied to the skin once weekly. The dose should be adjusted as necessary to control symptoms. Clinical responses (relief of symptoms) at the lowest effective dose should be the guide for establishing administration of the Climara® system, especially in women with an intact uterus. Attempts to taper or discontinue the medication should be made at 3- to 6-month intervals. In women who are not currently taking oral estrogens, treatment with the Climara® system can be initiated at once. In women who are currently taking oral estrogen, treatment with the Climara® system can be initiated 1-week after withdrawal of oral therapy or sooner if symptoms reappear in less than 1-week. For the prevention of postmenopausal osteoporosis, the minimum dose that has been shown to be effective is the 6.5 cm^2 (0.025 mg/day) Climara® system. Response to therapy can be assessed by biochemical markers and measurement of bone mineral density.

Application of the System
The adhesive side of the Climara® system should be placed on a clean, dry area of the lower abdomen or the upper quadrant of the buttock. **The Climara® system should not be applied to or near the breasts.** The sites of application must be rotated, with an interval of at least 1-week allowed between applications to a particular site. The area selected should not be oily, damaged, or irritated. The waistline should be avoided, since tight clothing may rub and remove the system. Application to areas where sitting would dislodge the system should also be avoided. The system should be applied immediately after opening the pouch and removing the protective liner. The system should be pressed firmly in place with the fingers for about 10 seconds, making sure there is good contact, especially around the edges. If the system lifts, apply pressure to maintain adhesion. In the event that a system should fall off, a new system should be applied for the remainder of the 7-day dosing interval. Only one system should be worn at any one time during the 7-day dosing interval. Swimming, bathing, or using a sauna while using the Climara® system has not been studied, and these activities may decrease the adhesion of the system and the delivery of estradiol.

Removal of the System:
Removal of the system should be done carefully and slowly to avoid irritation of the skin. Should any adhesive remain on the skin after removal of the system, allow the area to dry for 15 minutes. Then gently rubbing the area with an oil-based cream or lotion should remove the adhesive residue.

Used patches still contain some active hormones. Each patch should be carefully folded in half so that it sticks to itself before throwing it away.

HOW SUPPLIED

Climara® (estradiol transdermal system), 0.025 mg/day — each 6.5 cm^2 system contains 2.0 mg of estradiol USP
NDC 50419-454-04
Individual Carton of 4 systems
Shelf Pack Carton of 6 Individual Cartons of 4 systems

Climara® (estradiol transdermal system), 0.0375 mg/day — each 9.375 cm^2 system contains 2.85 mg of estradiol USP
NDC 50419-456-04
Individual Carton of 4 systems
Shelf Pack Carton of 6 Individual Cartons of 4 systems

Climara® (estradiol transdermal system), 0.05 mg/day — each 12.5 cm^2 system contains 3.8 mg of estradiol USP
NDC 50419-451-04
Individual Carton of 4 systems
Shelf Pack Carton of 6 Individual Cartons of 4 systems

Climara® (estradiol transdermal system), 0.060 mg/day — each 15.0 cm^2 system contains 4.55 mg of estradiol USP
NDC 50419-459-04
Individual Carton of 4 systems
Shelf Pack Carton of 6 Individual Cartons of 4 systems

Climara® (estradiol transdermal system), 0.075 mg/day — each 18.75 cm^2 system contains 5.7 mg of estradiol USP
NDC 50419-453-04
Individual Carton of 4 systems
Shelf Pack Carton of 6 Individual Cartons of 4 systems

Climara® (estradiol transdermal system), 0.1 mg/day — each 25.0 cm^2 system contains 7.6 mg of estradiol USP
NDC 50419-452-04
Individual Carton of 4 systems
Shelf Pack Carton of 6 Individual Cartons of 4 systems

Do not store above 86°F (30°C). Do not store unpouched. Apply immediately upon removal from the protective pouch.

PATIENT INFORMATION Updated 1/8/04

Climara®
(estradiol transdermal system)

Read this PATIENT INFORMATION before you start taking Climara® and read what you get each time you refill Climara®. There may be new information. This information does not take the place of talking to your health care provider about your medical condition or your treatment.

What is the most important information I should know about Climara® (an estrogen hormone)?

- Estrogens increase the chances of getting cancer of the uterus. Report any unusual vaginal bleeding right away while you are taking estrogens. Vaginal bleeding after menopause may be a warning sign of cancer of the uterus (womb). Your health care provider should check any unusual vaginal bleeding to find out the cause.
- Do not use estrogens with or without progestins to prevent heart disease, heart attacks, or strokes.

Using estrogens with or without progestins may increase your chances of getting heart attack, strokes, breast cancer, and blood clots.You and your healthcare provider should talk regularly about whether you still need treatment with Climara®.

What is Climara®?
Climara® is a medicine that contains estrogen hormones.

What is Climara® used for?
Climara® is used after menopause to:

- **reduce moderate to severe hot flashes.** Estrogens are hormones made by a woman's ovaries. The ovaries normally stop making estrogens when a woman is between 45 to 55 years old. This drop in body estrogen levels causes the "change of life" or menopause (the end of monthly menstrual periods). Sometimes, both ovaries are removed during an operation before natural menopause takes place. The sudden drop in estrogen levels causes "surgical menopause."
  When the estrogen levels begin dropping, some women develop very uncomfortable symptoms, such as feelings of warmth in the face, neck, and chest, or sudden strong feelings of heat and sweating ("hot flashes" or "hot flushes"). In some women, the symptoms are mild, and they will not need estrogens. In other women, symptoms can be more severe. You and your health care provider should talk regularly about whether you still need treatment with Climara®.
- **treat moderate to severe dryness, itching, and burning in or around the vagina.** You and your health care provider should talk regularly about whether you still need treatment with Climara® to control these problems.
- **To treat certain conditions in which a young woman's ovaries do not produce enough estrogen naturally.**
- **help reduce your chances of getting osteoporosis (thin weak bones).** Osteoporosis from menopause is a thinning of the bones that makes them weaker and easier to break. If you use Climara® only to prevent osteoporosis from menopause, talk with your healthcare provider about whether a different treatment or medicine without estrogens might be better for you. You and your healthcare provider should talk regularly about whether you should continue with Climara®.
  Weight-bearing exercise, like walking or running, and taking calcium and vitamin D supplements may also lower your chances of getting postmenopausal osteoporosis. It is important to talk about exercise and supplements with your healthcare provider before starting them.

Who should not take Climara®?
Do not start taking Climara® if you:

- **have unusual vaginal bleeding.**
- **currently have or have had certain cancers.** Estrogens may increase the chances of getting certain types of cancers, including cancer of the breast or uterus. If you have or had cancer, talk with your health care provider about whether you should take Climara®.
- **had a stroke or heart attack in the past year.**
- **currently have or have had blood clots.**

Continued on next page

Information on Berlex products (appearing here) is based on the most current information available at the time of publication closing. Further information for these and other Berlex products can be obtained from Medical & Product Services at Berlex, Inc. by calling 1-888-BERLEX-4.

Climara—Cont.

- **are allergic to Climara® or any of its ingredients.** See the end of this leaflet for a list of ingredients in Climara®
- **think you may be pregnant.**

Tell your health care provider:

- **if you are breastfeeding.** The hormone in Climara® can pass into your milk.
- **about all of your medical problems.** Your health care provider may need to check you more carefully if you have certain conditions, such as asthma (wheezing), epilepsy (seizures), migraine, endometriosis, or problems with your heart, liver, thyroid, kidneys, or have high calcium levels in your blood.
- **about all the medicines you take,** including prescription and nonprescription medicines, vitamins, and herbal supplements. Some medicines may affect how Climara® works. Climara® may also affect how your other medicines work.
- **if you are going to have surgery or will be on bed rest.** You may need to stop taking estrogens.

How the Patch Works

The Climara® patch releases estradiol, which flows through the skin into the bloodstream.

How and Where to Apply the Climara® Patch

Each Climara® patch is individually sealed in a protective pouch. To open the pouch, hold it vertically with the Climara® name facing you. Tear off the top of the pouch using the top tear notch. Tear off the side of the pouch using the side tear notch. Pull the pouch open. The Climara® patch is the see-through plastic film attached to the clear thicker plastic backing. There is a silver foil-sticker attached to the inside of the pouch. Do not remove it from the pouch. The sticker contains a moisture protectant (desiccant). Lift out the Climara® patch. Notice that the patch is attached to a thicker, hard-plastic backing and that the patch itself is oval and see-through.

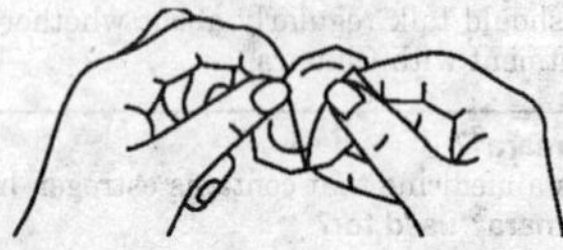

Apply the sticky side of the Climara® patch to a clean, dry area of the lower stomach below your belly button or the top of the buttocks (see diagram below). **Do not apply the Climara® patch to your breasts.** The sites of application on the lower stomach and buttocks must be rotated, allowing at least 1 week between applications to the same site. The site selected should not be oily, damaged, or irritated. Avoid the waistline, since tight clothing may rub and remove the patch. Also, do not put the patch on areas where sitting would rub it off or loosen it. Apply the patch right after opening the pouch and removing the protective liner. Press the patch firmly in place with your fingers for about 10 seconds. Make sure that it sticks all over, especially around the edges.

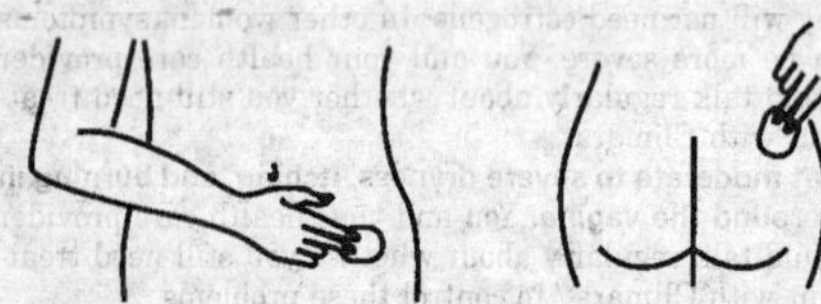

The Climara® patch should be worn continuously for one week. You may wish to try different sites when putting on a new patch, to find ones that are most comfortable for you and where clothing will not rub on the patch or loosen it.

When to Apply the Climara® System?

The Climara® patch should be changed once weekly. Remove the used patch. Carefully fold it in half so that it sticks to itself because used patches still contain active hormones and discard it. Any adhesive that might remain on your skin can be easily rubbed off. Then place the new Climara® patch on a different skin site. (The same skin site should not be used again for at least 1 week after removal of the patch.) Contact with water when you are bathing, swimming, or showering may affect the patch. If the patch falls off, the same patch may be reapplied to another area of the lower abdomen. Make sure that there is good contact, especially around the edges. If the patch will not stick completely to your skin, put a new patch on a different area of the lower abdomen. Do not apply two patches at the same time.

Estrogens should be used only as long as needed. You and your health care provider should talk regularly (for example, every 3 to 6 months) about whether you still need treatment with Climara®.

What are the possible side effects of estrogens?

Less common but serious side effects include:

- Breast cancer
- Cancer of the uterus
- Stroke
- Heart attack
- Blood clots
- Gallbladder disease
- Ovarian cancer

These are some of the warning signs of serious side effects:

- Breast lumps
- Unusual vaginal bleeding
- Dizziness and faintness
- Changes in speech
- Severe headaches
- Chest pain
- Shortness of breath
- Pains in your legs
- Changes in vision
- Vomiting

Call your health care provider right away if you get any of these warning signs, or any other unusual symptom that concerns you.

Common side effects include:

- Headache
- Breast pain
- Irregular vaginal bleeding or spotting
- Stomach/abdominal cramps, bloating
- Nausea and vomiting
- Hair loss

Other side effects include:

- High blood pressure
- Liver problems
- High blood sugar
- Fluid retention
- Enlargement of benign tumors of the uterus ("fibroids")
- Vaginal yeast infection

These are not all the possible side effects of Climara®. For more information, ask your health care provider or pharmacist.

What can I do to lower my chances of a serious side effect with Climara®?

- Talk with your health care provider regularly about whether you should continue using Climara®.
- See your health care provider right away if you get vaginal bleeding while using Climara®.
- Have a breast exam and mammogram (breast X-ray) every year unless your health care provider tells you something else. If members of your family have had breast cancer or if you have ever had breast lumps or an abnormal mammogram, you may need to have breast exams more often.
- If you have high blood pressure, high cholesterol (fat in the blood), diabetes, are overweight, or if you use tobacco, you may have higher chances for getting heart disease.

General information about safe and effective use of Climara®

Medicines are sometimes prescribed for conditions that are not mentioned in patient information leaflets. Do not take Climara® for conditions for which it was not prescribed. Do not give Climara® to other people, even if they have the same symptoms you have. It may harm them.

Keep Climara® out of the reach of children.

This leaflet provides a summary of the most important information about Climara®. If you would like more information, talk with your health care provider or pharmacist. You can ask for information about Climara® that is written for health professionals. You can get more information by calling the toll free number (1-888-237-5394).

What are the ingredients in Climara®?

The active ingredient of Climara® is estradiol. Climara® also contains acrylate copolymer adhesive, fatty acid esters, and polyethylene backing.

Manufactured for:
BERLEX®
Berlex, Montville NJ 07045
Manufactured by 3M Pharmaceuticals, St. Paul, MN 55144
6006500 (3M #629500) March 2004

Shown in Product Identification Guide, page 308

CLIMARA PRO™ ℞

[kli-ma ra]
(Estradiol/Levonorgestrel Transdermal System)
℞ only

> **WARNING**
>
> Estrogens with or without progestins should not be used for the prevention of cardiovascular disease.
>
> The Women's Health Initiative (WHI) study reported increased risks of myocardial infarction, stroke, invasive breast cancer, pulmonary emboli, and deep vein thrombosis in postmenopausal women during 5 years of treatment with oral conjugated estrogens (CE 0.625 mg) combined with medroxyprogesterone acetate (MPA 2.5 mg) relative to placebo (see **CLINICAL PHARMACOLOGY, Clinical Studies**). Other doses of conjugated estrogens with medroxyprogesterone acetate, and other combinations and dosage forms of estrogens and progestins were not studied in the WHI and, in the absence of comparable data, these risks should be assumed to be similar. Because of these risks, estrogens with or without progestins should be prescribed at the lowest effective doses and for the shortest duration consistent with treatment goals and risks for the individual woman.

DESCRIPTION

Climara Pro™ (Estradiol/Levonorgestrel Transdermal System) is an adhesive-based matrix transdermal patch designed to release both estradiol and levonorgestrel, a progestational agent, continuously upon application to intact skin.

The 22 cm² Climara Pro system contains 4.40 mg estradiol and 1.39 mg levonorgestrel and provides a nominal delivery rate (mg per day) of 0.045 estradiol and 0.015 levonorgestrel.

Estradiol USP has a molecular weight of 272.39 and the molecular formula is $C_{18}H_{24}O_2$.

Levonorgestrel USP has a molecular weight of 312.4 and a molecular formula of $C_{21}H_{28}O_2$.

The structural formulas for estradiol and levonorgestrel are:

Estradiol (E_2) Levonorgestrel (LNG)

The Climara Pro system comprises 3 layers. Proceeding from the visible surface towards the surface attached to the skin, these layers are (1) a translucent polyethylene backing film, (2) an acrylate adhesive matrix containing estradiol and levonorgestrel, and (3) a protective liner of either siliconized or fluoropolymer coated polyester film. The protective liner is attached to the adhesive surface and must be removed before the system can be used.

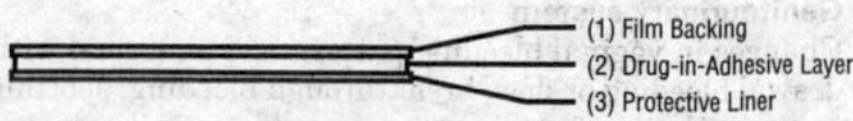

The active components of the system are estradiol and levonorgestrel. The remaining components of the system (acrylate copolymer adhesive and polyvinylpyrrolidone/vinyl acetate copolymer) are pharmacologically inactive.

CLINICAL PHARMACOLOGY

Endogenous estrogens are largely responsible for the development and maintenance of the female reproductive system and secondary sexual characteristics. Although circulating estrogens exist in a dynamic equilibrium of metabolic interconversions, estradiol is the principal intracellular human estrogen and is substantially more potent than its metabolites, estrone and estriol, at the receptor level.

The primary source of estrogen in normally cycling adult women is the ovarian follicle, which secretes 70 to 500 mcg of estradiol daily, depending on the phase of the menstrual cycle. After menopause, most endogenous estrogen is produced by conversion of androstenedione, secreted by the adrenal cortex, to estrone by peripheral tissues. Thus, estrone and the sulfate conjugated form, estrone sulfate, are the most abundant circulating estrogens in postmenopausal women.

Estrogens act through binding to nuclear receptors in estrogen-responsive tissues. To date, two estrogen receptors have been identified. These vary in proportion from tissue to tissue.

Circulating estrogens modulate the pituitary secretion of the gonadotropins, luteinizing hormone (LH) and follicle stimulating hormone (FSH), through a negative feedback mechanism. Estrogens act to reduce the elevated levels of these hormones seen in postmenopausal women.

Levonorgestrel inhibits gonadotropin production resulting in retardation of follicular growth and inhibition of ovulation.

Studies to assess the potency of progestins using estrogen-primed postmenopausal endometrial biochemistry and morphologic features have shown that levonorgestrel counteracts the proliferative effects of estrogens on the endometrium.

Pharmacokinetics

Absorption: Administration of Climara Pro to postmenopausal women produces mean maximum estradiol concentrations in serum in about 2 to 2.5 days. Estradiol concentrations equivalent to the normal ranges observed at the early follicular phase in premenopausal women are achieved within 12-24 hours after the first application.

In one study, steady state estradiol concentrations in serum were measured during week 4 in 44 healthy, postmenopausal women during four consecutive Climara Pro applications of two formulations (0.045 mg estradiol/0.030 mg levonorgestrel and 0.045 mg estradiol/0.015 mg levonorgestrel) to the abdomen (each dose was applied for four 7-day periods). Both formulations were bioequivalent in terms of estradiol and estrone C_{max} and AUC parameters. A summary of Climara Pro single and multiple applications estradiol, estrone and levonorgestrel pharmacokinetic parameters is shown in Table 1.

[See table 1 at top of next page]

All mean parameters are arithmetic means except T_{max} which is expressed as the median.

Table 1: Summary of Mean Pharmacokinetic Parameters

Summary of Mean (± SD) Pharmacokinetic Parameters Following a Single Application of Climara Pro in 24 Healthy Postmenopausal Women

Parameter	Units	Estradiol	Estrone	Levonorgestrel
Single application Week 1 Data				
C_{ave}	Pg/mL	37.7 ± 10.4	41.0 ± 15.0	136 ± 52.7
C_{max}	Pg/mL	54.3 ± 18.9	43.9 ± 14.9	138 ± 51.8
T_{max}	Hours	42	84	90
C_{min}	Pg/mL	27.2 ± 7.66	32.6 ± 14.3	110 ± 41.7
AUC	Pg.h/mL	6340 ± 1740	6890 ± 2520	22900 ± 8860

Summary of Mean (± SD) Pharmacokinetic Parameters (Week 4) Following Four Consecutive Weekly Applications of Climara Pro in 44 Healthy Postmenopausal Women

Multiple application Week 4 Data				
C_{ave}	Pg/mL	35.7 ± 11.4	45.5 ± 62.6	166 ± 97.8
C_{max}	Pg/mL	50.7 ± 28.6	81.6 ± 252	194 ± 111
T_{max}	Hours	36	48	48
C_{min}	Pg/mL	33.8 ± 28.7	72.5 ± 253	153 ± 69.6
AUC	Pg.h/mL	6002 ± 1919	7642 ± 10518	27948 ± 16426

Table 2

Summary of Mean Daily Number of Moderate to Severe Hot Flushes-ITT

		Baseline*	Week 4	Week 8	Week 12
Placebo	n	88	82	73	69
	Mean (SD)	10.80 (5.803)	6.13 (4.311)	5.35 (4.095)	5.59 (4.930)
	Mean Change from baseline (SD)	NA	-4.23 (4.374)	-4.80 (4.448)	-4.55 (5.407)
0.045/.030	n	92	88	80	73
	Mean (SD)	10.13 (3.945)	2.69 (4.455)	1.22 (2.804)	1.06 (3.187)
	Mean Change from baseline (SD)	NA	-7.40 (4.715)	-8.68 (4.146)	-8.82 (4.336)
p-Value[a]		NA	<0.001 [*]	NA	<0.001 [*]

ITT= Intent to Treat population; n= Number of subjects in a treatment group in a cycle; SD= standard deviation
Number of subjects varied from cycle to cycle due to missing data

[a] p-Value for comparison to placebo, adjusted by the method of Bonferroni; [*] p <0.025
*A subject was included at baseline only if the subject had a post-baseline mean score. The post-baseline mean score required 3 days in one week.

Table 3

Summary of Mean Severity of Moderate to Severe Hot Flushes-ITT

		Baseline*	Week 4 (day 7)	Week 8 (day 7)	Week 12 (day 7)
Placebo	n	89	76	68	57
	Mean (SD)	2.42 (0.282)	1.99 (0.875)	1.93 (0.955)	1.80 (1.034)
	Mean Change from baseline (SD)	NA	-0.40 (0.865)	-0.48 (0.922)	-0.57 (1.044)
0.045/.030	n	92	83	72	55
	Mean (SD)	2.48 (0.295)	1.10 (1.191)	0.82 (1.226)	0.44 (0.960)
	Mean Change from baseline (SD)	NA	-1.40 (1.164)	-1.67 (1.245)	-2.06 (1.005)
p-Value[a]		NA	<0.001 [*]	NA	<0.001 [*]

IITT= Intent to Treat population; n= Number of subjects in a treatment group in a cycle; SD= standard deviation
Severity scores are : 1 = Mild, 2 = Moderate, 3 = Severe. Mean severity of hot flushes by day is [(2X number of moderate hot flushes) + (3X number of severe hot flushes)] / total number of moderate to severe hot flushes on that day. If no moderate to severe hot flush was indicated, the mean severity was 0.00.
Number of subjects varied from cycle to cycle due to missing data

[a] p-Value for comparison to placebo, adjusted by the method of Bonferroni; [*] p <0.025
*A subject was included at baseline only if the subject had at least 1 post-baseline value.

At steady state, Climara Pro maintains during the application period an average serum estradiol concentration of 35.7 pg/mL as depicted in Figure 1.
[See figure 1 at top of third column]

Following the application of the Climara Pro transdermal system, levonorgestrel concentrations are maximum in about 2.5 days. At steady state, Climara Pro maintains during the application period an average serum levonorgestrel concentration of 166 pg/mL as depicted in Figure 2. The mean levonorgestrel pharmacokinetic parameters of Climara Pro are summarized in Table 1.

Figure 1: Mean Estradiol Concentration Profile (Week 4) Following Four Consecutive Weekly Applications of Climara Pro

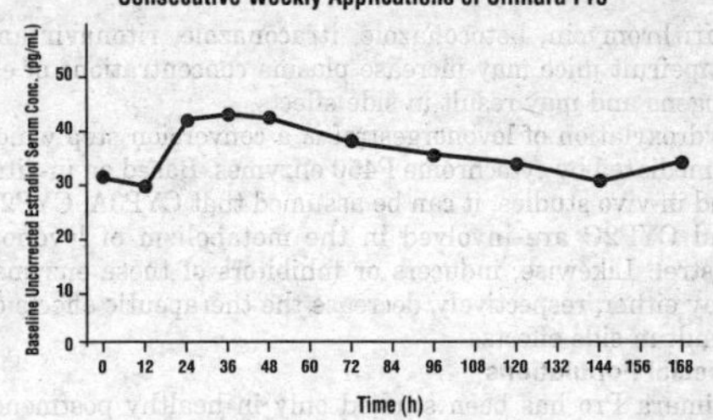

Figure 2: Mean Levonorgestrel Concentration Profile (Week 4) Following Four Consecutive Weekly Applications of Climara Pro

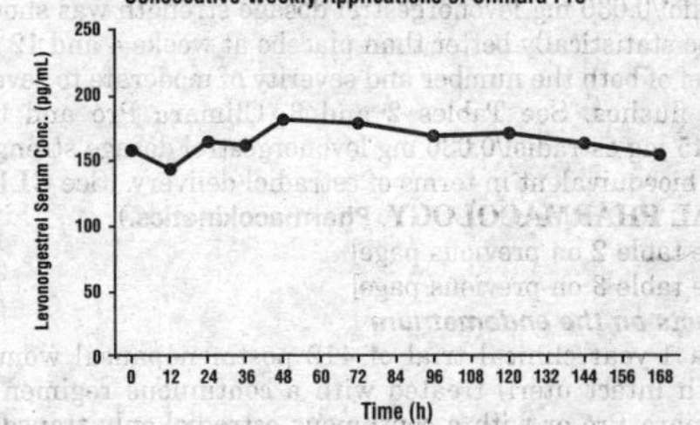

Distribution

The distribution of exogenous estrogens is similar to that of endogenous estrogens. Estrogens are widely distributed in the body and are generally found in higher concentrations in the sex hormone target organs. Estrogens circulate in the blood largely bound to sex hormone binding globulin (SHBG) and albumin.

Levonorgestrel in serum is bound to both SHBG and albumin. Following four consecutive weekly applications of Climara Pro mean (± SD) SHBG concentrations declined from a predose value of 47.5 (25.8) to 41.2 (22.4) nmol/L at week 4.

Metabolism

Exogenous estrogens are metabolized in the same manner as endogenous estrogens. Circulating estrogens exist in a dynamic equilibrium of metabolic interconversions. These transformations take place mainly in the liver. Estradiol is converted reversibly to estrone, and both can be converted to estriol, which is the major urinary metabolite. Estrogens also undergo enterohepatic recirculation via sulfate and glucuronide conjugation in the liver, biliary secretion of conjugates into the intesine, and hydrolysis in the gut followed by reabsorption. In postmenopausal women, a significant proportion of the circulating estrogens exist as sulfate conjugates, especially estrone sulfate, which serves as a circulating reservoir for the formation of more active estrogens. The most important metabolic pathway for levonorgestrel occurs in the reduction of the 4- and the 3-oxo-group as well as hydroxylations at positions 2α, 1β, and 16β, followed by conjugation. Most of the metabolites that circulate in the blood are sulfates of 3, 5β-tetrahydro-levonorgestrel, while excretion occurs predominantly in the form of glucuronides. Some of the parent levonorgestrel also circulates as the 17β-sulfate. In-vitro studies on the biotransformation of levonorgestrel in human skin did not indicate any significant metabolism of levonorgestrel during skin penetration.

Excretion

Estradiol, estrone, and estriol are excreted in the urine along with glucuronide and sulfate conjugates. Following patch removal, serum estradiol concentrations decline rapidly with a mean (± SD) terminal half-life of 3.0 ± 0.67 hours.

Levonorgestrel and its metabolites are primarily excreted in the urine. Mean (± SD) terminal half-life for levonorgestrel was determined to be 28 ± 6.4 hours.

Drug Interactions

In-vitro and in-vivo studies have shown that estrogens are metabolized partially by cytochrome P450 3A4 (CYP3A4). Therefore, inducers or inhibitors of CYP3A4 may affect estrogen drug metabolism. Inducers of CYP3A4 such as St. John's Wort preparations (Hypericum perforatum), phenobarbital, carbamazepine, and rifampin may reduce plasma concentrations of estrogens, possibly resulting in a decrease in therapeutic effects and/or changes in the uterine bleeding profile. Inhibitors of CYP3A4 such as erythromycin,

Continued on next page

Information on Berlex products (appearing here) is based on the most current information available at the time of publication closing. Further information for these and other Berlex products can be obtained from Medical & Product Services at Berlex, Inc. by calling 1-888-BERLEX-4.

Climara Pro—Cont.

clarithromycin, ketoconazole, itraconazole, ritonavir and grapefruit juice may increase plasma concentrations of estrogens and may result in side effects.

Hydroxylation of levonorgestrel is a conversion step which is mediated by cytochrome P450 enzymes. Based on in-vitro and in-vivo studies, it can be assumed that CYP3A, CYP2E and CYP2C are involved in the metabolism of levonorgestrel. Likewise, inducers or inhibitors of these enzymes may either, respectively, decrease the therapeutic effects or result in side effects.

Special Populations

Climara Pro has been studied only in healthy postmenopausal women.

CLINICAL STUDIES

Effects on vasomotor symptoms

The efficacy of 0.045 mg estradiol/0.030 mg levonorgestrel administered weekly versus placebo in the relief of moderate to severe vasomotor symptoms in post-menopausal women was studied in one 12-week clinical trial (n=183, average age 52.1 ± 4.93, 82.0% Caucasian). The 0.045 mg estradiol/0.030 mg levonorgestrel dosage strength was shown to be statistically better than placebo at weeks 4 and 12 for relief of both the number and severity of moderate to severe hot flushes. See Tables 2 and 3. Climara Pro and the 0.045 mg estradiol/0.030 mg levonorgestrel dosage strength are bioequivalent in terms of estradiol delivery. (See **CLINICAL PHARMACOLOGY, Pharmacokinetics.**)

[See table 2 on previous page]
[See table 3 on previous page]

Effects on the endometrium

In a 1-year clinical trial of 412 postmenopausal women (with intact uteri) treated with a continuous regimen of Climara Pro or with a continuous estradiol-only transdermal system, results of evaluable endometrial biopsies show that no hyperplasia was seen with Climara Pro. Table 4 below summarizes these results (Intent-to-Treat populations).

Table 4

Incidence of Endometrial Hyperplasia during Continuous Combined treatment with Climara Pro, Intent-to-Treat Population

	Climara Pro E_2 0.045 mg / LNG 0.015 mg	Estradiol E_2 0.045 mg
	n = 210	n= 202
No. of Patients with Biopsies at ≥6 months[1]	124	139
No. of Patients with Biopsies at 1 year[2]	102	110
No. (%) of Patients with Hyperplasia[3]	0 (0%)[4]	19 (17.3%)
95% Confidence Interval	0-3.55%	9.75-24.79%

n = number of intent-to-treat subjects
[1] Defined as at least 180 days of treatment
[2] Defined as ≥323 days of treatment
[3] Includes hyperplasia occurring at any time after initiation of treatment as a proportion of patients with biopsies at 1 year
[4] $p < 0.0167$ P-value for comparison to unopposed estradiol dose using the Fisher Exact test. P-values were adjusted by the method of Bonferroni.

Effects on uterine bleeding or spotting

The effects of Climara Pro on uterine bleeding or spotting, as recorded using an interactive voice response system, were evaluated in one 12-month clinical trial. Results are shown in Figure 3.

Figure 3: Cumulative proportion of subjects at each cycle with no bleeding/spotting through the end of cycle 13 Last Observation Carried Forward

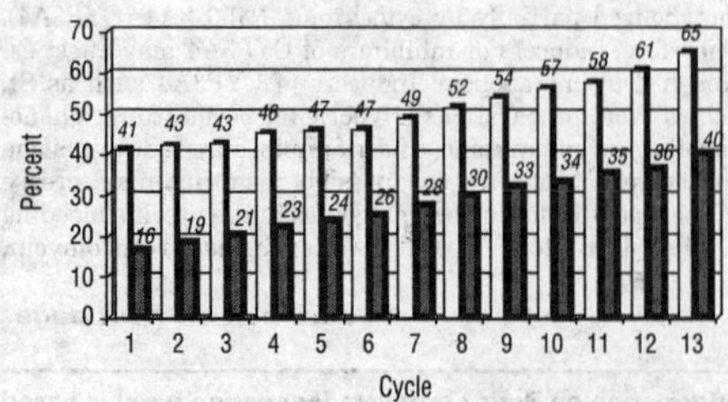

Percent based upon the number of subjects with data
Last non-missing cycle carried forward through cycle 13
Bleeding associated with endometrial biopsies not included

Table 5

RELATIVE AND ABSOLUTE RISK SEEN IN THE CE/MPA SUBSTUDY OF WHI[a]

Event[c]	Relative Risk CE/MPA vs placebo at 5.2 Years (95% CI*)	Placebo n = 8102	CE/MPA n = 8506
		Absolute Risk per 10,000 Person-years	
CHD events	1.29 (1.02-1.63)	30	37
Non-fatal MI	*1.32 (1.02-1.72)*	*23*	*30*
CHD death	*1.18 (0.70-1.97)*	*6*	*7*
Invasive breast cancer[b]	1.26 (1.00-1.59)	30	38
Stroke	1.41 (1.07-1.85)	21	29
Pulmonary embolism	2.13 (1.39-3.25)	8	16
Colorectal cancer	0.63 (0.43-0.92)	16	10
Endometrial cancer	0.83 (0.47-1.47)	6	5
Hip fracture	0.66 (0.45-0.98)	15	10
Death due to causes other than the events above	0.92 (0.74-1.14)	40	37
Global Index[c]	1.15 (1.03-1.28)	151	170
Deep vein thrombosis[d]	2.07 (1.49-2.87)	13	26
Vertebral fractures[d]	0.66 (0.44-0.98)	15	9
Other osteoporotic fractures[d]	0.77 (0.69-0.86)	170	131

[a] adapted from JAMA, 2002; 288:321-33
[b] includes metastatic and non-metastatic breast cancer with the exception of in situ breast cancer
[c] a subset of the events was combined in a "global index", defined as the earliest occurrence of CHD events, invasive breast cancer, stroke, pulmonary embolism, endometrial cancer, colorectal cancer, hip fracture, or death due to other causes
[d] not included in Global Index
*nominal confidence intervals unadjusted for multiple looks and multiple comparisons

Women's Health Initiative Studies

The Women's Health Initiative (WHI) enrolled a total of 27,000 predominantly healthy postmenopausal women to assess the risks and benefits of either the use of 0.625 mg conjugated estrogens (CE) per day alone or the use of 0.625 mg conjugated equine estrogens plus 2.5 mg medroxyprogesterone acetate (MPA) per day compared to placebo in the prevention of certain chronic diseases. The primary endpoint was the incidence of coronary heart disease (CHD) (nonfatal myocardial infarction and CHD death), with invasive breast cancer as the primary adverse outome studied. A "global index" included the earliest occurrence of CHD, invasive breast cancer, stroke, pulmonary embolism (PE), endometrial cancer, colorectal cancer, hip fracture, or death due to other cause. The study did not evaluate the effects of CE or CE/MPA on menopausal symptoms.

The CE-only substudy is continuing and results have not been reported. The CE/MPA substudy was stopped early because, according to the predefined stopping rule, the increased risk of breast cancer and cardiovascular events exceeded the specified benefits included in the "global index." Results of the CE/MPA substudy, which included 16,608 women (average age of 63 years, range 50 to 79; 83.9% White, 6.5% Black, 5.5% Hispanic), after an average follow-up of 5.2 years are presented in Table 5 below:

[See table above]

For those outcomes included in the "global index," absolute excess risks per 10,000 person-years in the group treated with CE/MPA were 7 more CHD events, 8 more strokes, 8 more PEs, and 8 more invasive breast cancers, while absolute risk reductions per 10,000 person-years were 6 fewer colorectal cancers and 5 fewer hip fractures. The absolute excess risk of events included in the "global index" was 19 per 10,000 person-years. There was no difference between the groups in terms of all-cause mortality. (See **BOXED WARNING, WARNINGS,** and **PRECAUTIONS.**)

INDICATIONS AND USAGE

In women with an intact uterus, Climara Pro is indicated for the following:

- Treatment of moderate to severe vasomotor symptoms associated with menopause

CONTRAINDICATIONS

Estrogens/progestins combined should not be used in women with any of the following conditions:

1. Undiagnosed abnormal genital bleeding.
2. Known, suspected, or history of cancer of the breast.
3. Known or suspected estrogen-dependent neoplasia.
4. Active deep vein thrombosis, pulmonary embolism or a history of these conditions.
5. Active or recent (e.g. within the past year) arterial thromboembolic disease (e.g., stroke, myocardial infarction).
6. Liver dysfunction or disease.
7. Climara Pro should not be used in patients with known hypersensitivity to its ingredients.
8. Known or suspected pregnancy. There is no indication for Climara Pro in pregnancy. There appears to be little or no increased risk of birth defects in women who have used estrogens and progestins from oral contraceptives inadvertently during early pregnancy. (See **PRECAUTIONS.**)

WARNINGS

See **BOXED WARNING.**

1. Cardiovascular disorders

Estrogen and estrogen/progestin therapy have been associated with an increased risk of cardiovascular events such as myocardial infarction and stroke, as well as venous thrombosis and pulmonary embolism (venous thromboembolism or VTE). Should any of these occur or be suspected, estrogens should be discontinued immediately.

Risk factors for cardiovascular disease (e.g., hypertension, diabetes mellitus, tobacco use, hypercholesterolemia, and obesity) should be managed appropriately.

a. Coronary heart disease and stroke

In the Women's Health Initiative (WHI) study, an increase in the number of myocardial infarctions and strokes has been observed in women receiving oral CE compared to placebo. These observations are preliminary, and the study is continuing. (See **CLINICAL PHARMACOLOGY, Clinical Studies.**)

In the CE/MPA substudy of WHI an increased risk of coronary heart disease (CHD) events (defined as nonfatal myocardial infarction and CHD death) was observed in women receiving CE/MPA compared to women receiving placebo (37 vs 30 per 10,000 person-years). The increase in risk was observed in year one and persisted.

In the same substudy of WHI, an increased risk of stroke was observed in women receiving CE/MPA compared to women receiving placebo (29 vs 21 per 10,000 person-years). The increase in risk was observed after the first year and persisted.

In postmenopausal women with documented heart disease (n = 2,763, average age 66.7 years) a controlled clinical trial of secondary prevention of cardiovascular disease (Heart and Estrogen/Progestin Replacement Study; HERS) treatment with CE/MPA-0.625 mg/2.5 mg per day demonstrated no cardiovascular benefit. During an average follow-up of 4.1 years, treatment with CE/MPA did not reduce the overall rate of CHD events in postmenopausal women with established coronary heart disease. There were more CHD events in the CE/MPA-treated group than in the placebo group in year 1, but not during the subsequent years. Two thousand three hundred and twenty-one women from the original HERS trial agreed to participate in an open label extension of HERS, HERS II. Average follow-up in HERS II was an additional 2.7 years, for a total of 6.8 years overall. Rates of CHD events were comparable among women in the CE/MPA group and the placebo group in HERS, HERS II, and overall.

Large doses of estrogen (5 mg conjugated estrogens per day), comparable to those used to treat cancer of the prostate and breast, have been shown in a large prospective clinical trial in men to increase the risks of nonfatal myocardial infarction, pulmonary embolism, and thrombophlebitis.

b. Venous thromboembolism

(VTE) In the Women's Health Initiative (WHI) study, an increase in VTE has been observed in women receiving CE compared to placebo. These observations are preliminary, and the study is continuing. (See

CLINICAL PHARMACOLOGY, Clinical Studies.)
In the CE/MPA substudy of WHI, a 2-fold greater rate of VTE, including deep venous thrombosis and pulmonary embolism, was observed in women receiving CE/MPA compared to women receiving placebo. The rate of VTE was 34 per 10,000 woman-years in the CE/MPA group compared to 16 per 10,000 woman-years in the placebo group. The increase in VTE risk was observed during the first year and persisted.
If feasible, estrogens should be discontinued at least 4 to 6 weeks before surgery of the type associated with an increased risk of thromboembolism, or during periods of prolonged immobilization.

2. Malignant neoplasms

a. Endometrial cancer

The use of unopposed estrogens in women with intact uteri has been associated with an increased risk of endometrial cancer. The reported endometrial cancer risk among unopposed estrogen users is about 2- to 12-fold greater than in non-users, and appears dependent on duration of treatment and on estrogen dose. Most studies show no significant increased risk associated with use of estrogens for less than one year. The greatest risk appears associated with prolonged use, with increased risks of 15- to 24-fold for five to ten years or more and this risk has been shown to persist for at least 8 to 15 years after estrogen therapy is discontinued.
Clinical surveillance of all women taking estrogen/progestin combinations is important. Adequate diagnostic measures, including endometrial sampling when indicated, should be undertaken to rule out malignancy in all cases of undiagnosed persistent or recurring abnormal vaginal bleeding. There is no evidence that the use of natural estrogens results in a different endometrial risk profile than synthetic estrogens of equivalent estrogen dose. Adding a progestin to estrogen therapy has been shown to reduce the risk of endometrial hyperplasia, which may be a precursor to endometrial cancer.

b. Breast cancer

Estrogen and estrogen/progestin therapy in postmenopausal women has been associated with an increased risk of breast cancer. In the CE/MPA substudy of the Women's Health Initiative study (WHI), a 26% increase of invasive breast cancer (38 vs 30 per 10,000 woman-years) after an average of 5.2 years of treatment was observed in women receiving CE/MPA compared to women receiving placebo. The increased risk of breast cancer became apparent after 4 years of treatment with CE/MPA. The women reporting prior postmenopausal use of estrogen and/or estrogen with progestin had a higher relative risk for breast cancer associated with CE/MPA than those who had never used these hormones. (See **CLINICAL PHARMACOLOGY, Clinical Studies.**)
In the WHI, no increased risk of breast cancer in CE-treated women compared to placebo was reported after an average of 5.2 years of therapy. These data are preliminary and that substudy of WHI is continuing.
Epidemiologic studies have reported an increased risk of breast cancer in association with increasing duration of postmenopausal treatment with estrogens with or without a progestin. This association was reanalyzed in original data from 51 studies that involved various doses and types of estrogens, with and without progestins. In the reanalysis, an increased risk of having breast cancer diagnosed became apparent after about 5 years of continued treatment, and subsided after treatment had been discontinued for 5 years or longer. Some later studies have suggested that postmenopausal treatment with estrogens and progestin increase the risk of breast cancer more than treatment with estrogen alone.
A postmenopausal woman without a uterus who requires estrogen should receive estrogen-alone therapy, and should not be exposed unnecessarily to progestins.
All postmenopausal women should receive yearly breast exams by a healthcare provider and perform monthly self-examinations. In addition, mammography examinations should be scheduled based on patient age and risk factors.

3. Gallbladder disease

A 2- to 4-fold increase in the risk of gallbladder disease requiring surgery in post-menopausal women receiving estrogens has been reported.

4. Visual abnormalities

Retinal vascular thrombosis has been reported in patients receiving estrogens. Discontinue medication pending examination if there is sudden partial or complete loss of vision, or a sudden onset of proptosis, diplopia, or migraine. If examination reveals papilledema or retinal vascular lesions, estrogens should be discontinued.

PRECAUTIONS

A. GENERAL

1. Addition of a progestin when a woman has not had a hysterectomy

Studies of the addition of a progestin for 10 or more days of a cycle of estrogen administration, or daily with estrogen in a continuous regimen, have reported a lowered incidence of endometrial hyperplasia than would be induced by estrogen treatment alone. Endometrial hyperplasia may be a precursor to endometrial cancer.
There are, however, possible risks that may be associated with the use of progestins with estrogens compared to estrogen-alone regimens. These include a possible increased risk of breast cancer, adverse effects on lipoprotein metabolism (e.g., lowering HDL, raising LDL) and impairment of glucose tolerance.

2. Elevated blood pressure

In a small number of case reports, substantial increases in blood pressure have been attributed to idiosyncratic reactions to estrogens. In a large, randomized, placebo-controlled clinical trial, a generalized effect of estrogen therapy on blood pressure was not seen. Blood pressure should be monitored at regular intervals with estrogen use.

3. Familial hyperlipoproteinemia

In patients with familial defects of lipoprotein metabolism, oral estrogen therapy may be associated with elevations of plasma triglycerides leading to pancreatitis and other complications.

4. Impaired liver function

Estrogens may be poorly metabolized in patients with impaired liver function. For patients with a history of cholestatic jaundice associated with past estrogen use or with pregnancy, caution should be exercised and in the case of recurrence, medication should be discontinued.

5. Hypothyroidism

Estrogen administration leads to increased thyroid-binding globulin (TBG) levels. Patients with normal thyroid function can compensate for the increased TBG by making more thyroid hormone, thus maintaining free T_4 and T_3 serum concentrations in the normal range. Patients dependent on thyroid hormone replacement therapy who are also receiving estrogens may require increased doses of their thyroid replacement therapy. These patients should have their thyroid function monitored in order to maintain their free thyroid hormone levels in an acceptable range.

6. Fluid retention

Because estrogen and estrogen/progestin therapy may cause some degree of fluid retention, patients with conditions that might be influenced by this factor, such as a cardiac or renal dysfunction, warrant careful observation when estrogens are prescribed.

7. Hypocalcemia

Estrogens should be used with caution in individuals with severe hypocalcemia.

8. Ovarian cancer

Use of estrogen-only products, in particular for ten or more years, has been associated with an increased risk of ovarian cancer in some epidemiological studies. Other studies did not show a significant association. Data are insufficient to determine whether there is an increased risk with estrogen/progestin combination therapy in postmenopausal women.

9. Exacerbation of endometriosis

Endometriosis may be exacerbated with administration of estrogens.

10. Exacerbation of other conditions

Estrogens may cause an exacerbation of asthma, diabetes mellitus, epilepsy, migraine or porphyria and should be used with caution in women with these conditions.

B. PATIENT INFORMATION

Physicians are advised to discuss the PATIENT INFORMATION leaflet with patients for whom they prescribe Climara Pro.

C. LABORATORY TESTS

Estrogen administration should be initiated at the lowest dose for the approved indication and then guided by clinical response, rather than by serum hormone levels (e.g., estradiol, FSH).

D. DRUG/LABORATORY TEST INTERACTIONS

1. Accelerated prothrombin time, partial thromboplastin time, and platelet aggregation time; increased platelet count; increased factors II, VII antigen, VIII antigen, VIII coagulant activity, IX, X, XII, VII-X complex, II-VII-X complex, and beta-thromboglobulin; decreased levels of antifactor Xa and antithrombin III, decreased antithrombin III activity; increased levels of fibrinogen and fibrinogen activity; increased plasminogen antigen and activity.
2. Increased thyroid-binding globulin (TBG) levels leading to increased circulating total thyroid hormone levels as measured by protein-bound iodine (PBI), T_4 levels (by column or by radioimmunoassay) or T_3 levels by radioimmunoassay. T_4 resin uptake is decreased, reflecting the elevated TBG. Free T_4 and free T_3 concentrations are unaltered. Patients on thyroid replacement therapy may require higher doses of thyroid hormone.
3. Other binding proteins may be elevated in serum (i.e., corticosteroid binding globulin (CBG), sex hormone-binding globulin (SHBG)) leading to increased circulating corticosteroids and sex steroids, respectively. Free or biologically active hormone concentrations are unchanged. Other plasma proteins may be increased (angiotensinogen/renin substrate, alpha-1-antitrypsin, ceruloplasmin).
4. Increased plasma HDL and HDL_2 subfraction concentrations, reduced LDL cholesterol concentration, and in oral formulations increased triglycerides levels.
5. Impaired glucose tolerance.
6. Reduced response to metyrapone test.
7. Reduced serum folate concentration.

E. CARCINOGENESIS, MUTAGENESIS, IMPAIRMENT OF FERTILITY

Long-term continuous administration of natural and synthetic estrogens in certain animal species increases the frequency of carcinomas of the breast, uterus, cervix, vagina, testis, and liver. (See **BOXED WARNING, CONTRAINDICATIONS**, and **WARNINGS**.)

F. PREGNANCY

Climara Pro should not be used during pregnancy. (See **CONTRAINDICATIONS**.)

G. NURSING MOTHERS

Estrogen administration to nursing mothers has been shown to decrease the quantity and quality of the milk. Detectable amounts of estrogen and progestin have been identified in the milk of mothers receiving these drugs. Caution should be exercised when Climara Pro is administered to a nursing woman.

H. PEDIATRIC USE

Climara Pro is not indicated in children.

I. GERIATRIC USE

There have not been sufficient numbers of geriatric patients involved in studies utilizing Climara Pro to determine whether those over 65 years of age differ from younger subjects in their response to Climara Pro.

ADVERSE REACTIONS

See **BOXED WARNING, WARNINGS** and **PRECAUTIONS**.
Because clinical trials are conducted under widely varying conditions, adverse reaction rates observed in the clinical trials of a drug cannot be directly compared to rates in the clinical trials of another drug and may not reflect the rates observed in practice. The adverse reaction information from clinical trials does, however, provide a basis for identifying the adverse events that appear to be related to drug use and for approximating rates.

Table 6

All Treatment Emergent Events Regardless of Relationship Reported at a Frequency of > 3% with Climara Pro in the 1 year Endometrial Hyperplasia Study

	Climara Pro 0.045 / 0.015 N = 212	E_2 N = 204
Body as a whole		
Abdominal pain	9 (4.2)	11 (5.4)
Accidental Injury	7 (3.3)	6 (2.9)
Back pain	13 (6.1)	12 (5.9)
Flu syndrome	10 (4.7)	13 (6.4)
Infection	7 (3.3)	10 (4.9)
Pain	11 (5.2)	13 (6.4)
Cardiovascular		
Hypertension	7 (3.3)	9 (4.4)
Digestive		
Flatulence	8 (3.8)	11 (5.4)
Metabolic and Nutritional Disorders		
Edema	8 (3.8)	5 (2.5)
Weight gain	6 (2.8)	10 (4.9)
Musculoskeletal		
Arthralgia	9 (4.2)	10 (4.9)
Nervous		
Depression	12 (5.7)	7 (3.4)
Headache	11 (5.2)	14 (6.9)
Respiratory		
Bronchitis	9 (4.2)	7 (3.4)
Sinusitis	8 (3.8)	12 (5.9)
Upper Respiratory Infection	28 (13.2)	26 (12.7)

Continued on next page

Information on Berlex products (appearing here) is based on the most current information available at the time of publication closing. Further information for these and other Berlex products can be obtained from Medical & Product Services at Berlex, Inc. by calling 1-888-BERLEX-4.

Climara Pro—Cont.

Skin and Appendages

Application site reaction	86 (40.6)	69 (33.8)
Breast pain	40 (18.9)	20 (9.8)
Rash	5 (2.4)	10 (4.9)
Urogenital		
Urinary Tract Infection	7 (3.3)	8 (3.9)
Vaginal Bleeding	78 (36.8)	44 (21.6)
Vaginitis	4 (1.9)	6 (2.9)

N = total number of subjects in a treatment group;
n = number of subjects with event

Irritation potential of Climara Pro was assessed in a 3-week irritation study. The study compared the irritation of a Climara Pro placebo patch (22 cm^2) to a Climara® placebo (25 cm^2). Visual assessments of irritation were made on Day 7 of each wear period, approximately 30 minutes after patch removal using a 7-point scale (0 = no evidence of irritation; 1 = minimal erythema, barely perceptible; 2 = definite erythema, readily visible, or minimal edema, or minimal papular response; 3 -7 = erythema and papules, edema, vesicles, strong extensive reaction).

The mean irritation scores were 0.13 (week 1), 0.12 (week 2), and 0.06 (week 3) for the Climara Pro placebo. The mean scores for the Climara placebo were 0.20 (week 1), 0.26 (week 2), 0.12 (week 3). There were no irritation scores greater than 2 at any timepoint in any subject.

In controlled clinical trials, withdrawals due to application site reactions occurred in 6 (2.1%) of subjects in the 12-week symptom study and in 71 (8.5%) of subjects in the 1-year endometrial protection study. The following additional adverse reactions have been reported with estrogen and/or estrogen/progestin therapy:

1. Genitourinary system
Changes in vaginal bleeding pattern and abnormal withdrawal bleeding or flow; breakthrough bleeding; spotting; increase in size of uterine leiomyomata; vaginitis, including vaginal candidiasis; change in amount of cervical secretion; changes in cervical ectropion; ovarian cancer; endometrial hyperplasia; endometrial cancer.

2. Breasts
Tenderness, enlargement, pain, nipple discharge, galactorrhea; fibrocystic breast changes; breast cancer.

3. Cardiovascular
Deep and superficial venous thrombosis; pulmonary embolism; thrombophlebitis; myocardial infarction; stroke; increase in blood pressure.

4. Gastrointestinal
Nausea, vomiting; abdominal cramps, bloating; cholestatic jaundice; increased incidence of gallbladder disease; pancreatitis.

5. Skin
Chloasma or melasma, which may persist when drug is discontinued; erythema multiforme; erythema nodosum; hemorrhagic eruption; loss of scalp hair; hirsutism; pruritus, rash.

6. Eyes
Retinal vascular thrombosis; steepening of corneal curvature; intolerance to contact lenses.

7. Central nervous system
Headache; migraine; dizziness; mental depression; chorea; nervousness; mood disturbances; irritability; exacerbation of epilepsy.

8. Miscellaneous
Increase or decrease in weight; reduced carbohydrate tolerance; aggravation of porphyria; edema; arthalgias; leg cramps; changes in libido; anaphylactoid/anaplylactic reactions including urticaria and angioedema; hypocalcemia; exacerbation of asthma; increased triglycerides.

OVERDOSAGE

Overdosage may cause nausea, and withdrawal bleeding may occur in females. Serious ill effects have not been reported following acute ingestion of large doses of estrogen/progestin-containing oral contraceptives by young children.

DOSAGE AND ADMINISTRATION

When estrogen is prescribed for a postmenopausal woman with a uterus, progestin should also be initiated to reduce the risk of endometrial cancer. A woman without a uterus does not need progestin. Use of estrogen, alone or in combination with a progestin, should be limited to the **lowest effective dose available and for the shortest** duration consistent with treatment goals and risks for the individual woman. Patients should be reevaluated periodically as clinically appropriate (e.g., 3-month to 6-month intervals) to determine if treatment is still necessary. (See **BOXED WARNING** and **WARNINGS.**) For women who have a uterus, adequate diagnostic measures, such as endometrial sampling, when indicated, should be undertaken to rule out malignancy in cases of undiagnosed persistent or recurring abnormal vaginal bleeding.

One Climara Pro transdermal system is available for the treatment of moderate to severe vasomotor symptoms associated with the menopause. Climara Pro delivers 0.045 mg of estradiol per day and 0.015 mg of levonorgestrel per day. The lowest effective estradiol/levonorgestrel dose for the treatment of moderate to severe vasomotor symptoms has not been determined. (See **BOXED WARNING** and **WARNINGS.**)

Initiation of Therapy:
Women not currently using continuous estrogen or combination estrogen/progestin therapy may start therapy with Climara Pro at any time. However, women currently using continuous estrogen or combination estrogen/progestin therapy should complete the current cycle of therapy, before initiating Climara Pro therapy. Women often experience withdrawal bleeding at the completion of the cycle. The first day of this bleeding would be an appropriate time to begin Climara Pro therapy.

Therapeutic Regimen:
A Climara Pro 0.045 mg / 0.015 mg (22 sq cm) matrix transdermal system is worn continuously on the lower abdomen. A new system should be applied weekly during a 28-day cycle.

Application of the System: Site Selection: Climara Pro should be placed on a smooth (fold free), clean, dry area of the skin on the lower abdomen. **Climara Pro should not be applied to or near the breasts.** The area selected should not be oily (which can impair adherence of the system), damaged, or irritated. The waistline should be avoided, since tight clothing may rub the system off or modify drug delivery. The sites of application must be rotated, with an interval of at least one week allowed between applications to the same site.

Application of the system: After opening the pouch, remove one side of the protective liner, taking care not to touch the adhesive part of the transdermal delivery system with the fingers. Immediately apply the transdermal delivery system to a smooth (fold free) area of skin on the lower abdomen. Remove the second side of the protective liner and press the system firmly in place with the hand for at least 10 seconds, making sure there is good contact, especially around the edges.

Care should be taken that the system does not become dislodged during bathing and other activities. If a system should fall off, the same system may be reapplied to another area of the lower abdomen. If necessary, a new transdermal system may be applied, in which case, the original treatment schedule should be continued. Only one system should be worn at any one time during one week dosing interval. Once in place, the transdermal system should not be exposed to the sun for prolonged periods of time.

Removal of the System: Removal of the system should be done carefully and slowly to avoid irritation of the skin. Should any adhesive remain on the skin after removal of the system, allow the area to dry for 15 minutes. Then gently rubbing the area with an oil-based cream or lotion should remove the adhesive residue.

Used patches still contain some active hormones. Each patch should be carefully folded in half so that it sticks to itself before throwing it away.

HOW SUPPLIED

Climara Pro (Estradiol/Levonorgestrel Transdermal System) 0.045 mg/day estradiol and 0.015 mg/day levonorgestrel – each 22 cm^2 system contains 4.40 mg of estradiol and 1.39 mg of levonorgestrel.

NDC 50419-491-04
Individual Carton of 4 systems
Shelf Pack Carton of 6 Individual Cartons of 4 systems

Storage Conditions:
Store at 20-25°C (68-77°F); excursions permitted to 15-30°C (59-86°F) [See USP controlled Room Temperature]. Do not store unpouched.

PATIENT INFORMATION

Updated November 19, 2003
Climara Pro™
(Estradiol/Levonorgestrel Transdermal System)

Read this PATIENT INFORMATION before you start taking Climara Pro and read what you get each time you refill Climara Pro. There may be new information. This information does not take the place of talking to your healthcare provider about your medical condition or your treatment.

What is the most important information I should know about Climara Pro (combination of estrogen and a progestin)?
Do not use estrogens with or without progestins to prevent heart disease, heart attacks, or strokes.
Using estrogens with or without progestins may increase your chances of getting heart attacks, strokes, breast cancer, and blood clots. You and your healthcare provider should talk regularly about whether you still need treatment with Climara Pro.

What is Climara Pro?
Climara Pro is a medicine that contains two kinds of hormones, estrogen and a progestin.

What is Climara Pro used for?
Climara Pro is used after menopause to:
- **reduce moderate to severe hot flashes.** Estrogens are hormones made by a woman's ovaries. The ovaries normally stop making estrogens when a woman is between 45 to 55 years old. This drop in body estrogen levels causes the "change of life" or menopause (the end of monthly menstrual periods). Sometimes, both ovaries are removed during an operation before natural menopause takes place. The sudden drop in estrogen levels causes "surgical menopause."

When the estrogen levels begin dropping, some women develop very uncomfortable symptoms, such as feelings of warmth in the face, neck, and chest, or sudden strong feelings of heat and sweating ("hot flashes" or "hot flushes"). In some women, the symptoms are mild, and they will not need estrogens. In other women, symptoms can be more severe. You and your healthcare provider should talk regularly about whether you still need treatment with Climara Pro.

Who should not use Climara Pro?
Do not use Climara Pro if you have had your uterus removed (hysterectomy).
Climara Pro contains a progestin to decrease the chances of getting cancer of the uterus. If you do not have a uterus, you do not need a progestin and you should not use Climara Pro.

Do not start using Climara Pro if you:
- **have unusual vaginal bleeding.**
- **currently have or have had certain cancers.** Estrogens may increase the chances of getting certain types of cancers, including cancer of the breast or uterus. If you have or had cancer, talk with your healthcare provider about whether you should use Climara Pro.
- **had a stroke or heart attack in the past year.**
- **currently have or have had blood clots.**
- **are allergic to Climara Pro or any of its ingredients.** See the end of this leaflet for a list of ingredients in Climara Pro.
- **think you may be pregnant.**

Tell your healthcare provider:
- **if you are breastfeeding.** The hormones in Climara Pro can pass into your milk.
- **about all of your medical problems.** Your healthcare provider may need to check you more carefully if you have certain conditions, such as asthma (wheezing), epilepsy (seizures), migraine, endometriosis, or problems with your heart, liver, thyroid, kidneys, or have high calcium levels in your blood.
- **about all the medicines you take,** including prescription and nonprescription medicines, vitamins, and herbal supplements. Some medicines may affect how Climara Pro works. Climara Pro may also affect how your other medicines work.
- **if you are going to have surgery or will be on bed rest.** You may need to stop using Climara Pro.

How The Patch Works
The Climara Pro patch releases two hormones, estradiol and levonorgestrel, which flow through the skin into the bloodstream.

How and Where to Apply the Climara Pro Patch
Each Climara Pro patch is individually sealed in a protective pouch. To open the pouch, hold it up with the Climara Pro name facing you. Tear left to right using the top tear notch. Tear from bottom to top using the side tear notch. Pull the pouch open. **Carefully remove the Climara Pro patch.** You will notice that the patch is attached to a thicker, hard-plastic liner and that the patch itself is oval.

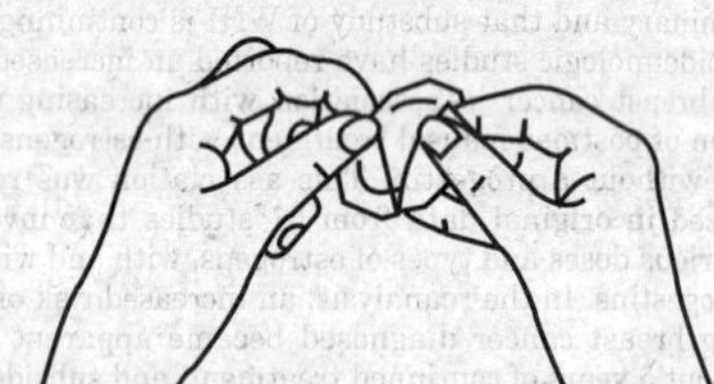

Apply the adhesive side of the Climara Pro patch to a clean, dry area of the lower abdomen. **Do not apply the Climara Pro patch to your breasts.** The sites of application must be rotated, with an interval of at least 1 week allowed between applications to a particular site. The area selected should not be oily, damaged, or irritated. Avoid the waistline, since tight clothing may rub and remove the patch. Application to areas where sitting would dislodge the patch should also be avoided. Apply the patch immediately after opening the pouch and removing the protective liner. Press the patch firmly in place with the fingers for about 10 seconds, making sure there is good contact, especially around the edges.

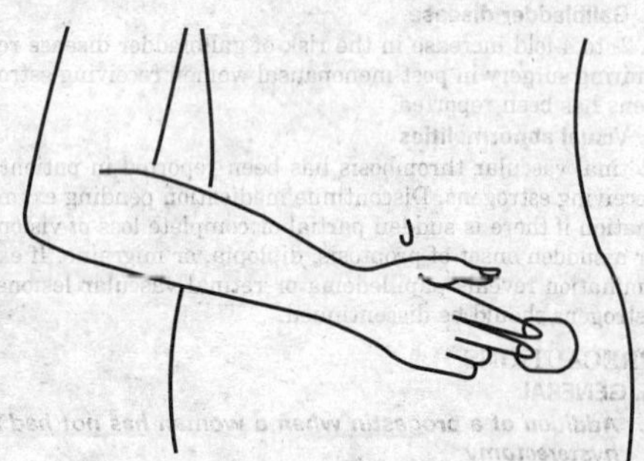

The Climara Pro patch should be worn continuously for one week. You may wish to experiment with different locations when applying a new patch, to find ones that are most comfortable for you and where clothing will not rub on the patch.

When to Apply the Climara Pro Patch
The Climara Pro patch should be changed once weekly. Remove the used patch. Carefully fold it in half so that it sticks to itself because used patches still contain active hormones and discard it. Any adhesive that might remain on your skin can be easily rubbed off. Then place the new Climara Pro patch on a different skin site. (The same skin site should not be used again for at least 1 week after removal of the patch.)
Contact with water when you are bathing, swimming, or showering may affect the patch. If the patch falls off, the same patch may be reapplied to another area of the lower abdomen. Make sure that there is good contact, especially around the edges. If the patch will not stick completely to your skin, put a new patch on a different area of the lower abdomen. Do not apply two patches at the same time.
Once in place, the transdermal system should not be exposed to the sun for prolonged periods of time.
Estrogens should be used only as long as needed. You and your healthcare provider should talk regularly (for example, every 3 to 6 months) about whether you still need treatment with Climara Pro.
What are the possible side effects of estrogens?
Less common but serious side effects include:
- Breast cancer
- Cancer of the uterus
- Stroke
- Heart attack
- Blood clots
- Gallbladder disease
- Ovarian cancer

These are some of the warning signs of serious side effects:
- Breast lumps
- Unusual vaginal bleeding
- Dizziness and faintness
- Changes in speech
- Severe headaches
- Chest pain
- Shortness of breath
- Pains in your legs
- Changes in vision
- Vomiting

Call your healthcare provider right away if you get any of these warning signs, or any other unusual symptom that concerns you.
Common side effects include:
- Headache
- Breast pain
- Irregular vaginal bleeding or spotting
- Stomach/abdominal cramps, bloating
- Nausea and vomiting
- Hair loss

Other side effects include:
- High blood pressure
- Liver problems
- High blood sugar
- Fluid retention
- Enlargement of benign tumors of the uterus ("fibroids")
- Vaginal yeast infection

These are not all the possible side effects of Climara Pro. For more information, ask your healthcare provider or pharmacist.
What can I do to lower my chances of a serious side effect with Climara Pro?
- Talk with your healthcare provider regularly about whether you should continue using Climara Pro.
- See your healthcare provider right away if you get vaginal bleeding while using Climara Pro.
- Have a breast exam and mammogram (breast X-ray) every year unless your healthcare provider tells you something else. If members of your family have had breast cancer or if you have ever had breast lumps or an abnormal mammogram, you may need to have breast exams more often.
- If you have high blood pressure, high cholesterol (fat in the blood), diabetes, are overweight, or if you use tobacco, you may have higher chances for getting heart disease. Ask your healthcare provider for ways to lower your chances for getting heart disease.

General information about safe and effective use of Climara Pro
Medicines are sometimes prescribed for conditions that are not mentioned in patient information leaflets. Do not use Climara Pro for conditions for which it was not prescribed. Do not give Climara Pro to other people, even if they have the same symptoms you have. It may harm them.
Keep Climara Pro out of the reach of children.
This leaflet provides a summary of the most important information about Climara Pro. If you would like more information, talk with your healthcare provider or pharmacist. You can ask for information about Climara Pro that is written for health professionals. You can get more information by calling the toll free number (1-888-237-5394).
What are the ingredients in Climara Pro?
The active ingredients in Climara Pro are estradiol and levonorgestrel. Climara Pro also contains acrylate copolymer adhesive and polyvinylpyrrolidone/vinyl acetate opolymer.
Do not store above 86°F (30°C).
Do not store unpouched.
Made In USA
Manufactured for:
BERLEX
Berlex, Montville, NJ 07045
Manufactured by:
3M Pharmaceuticals
St. Paul, MN 55144
6050700-630000 November 2003
Shown in Product Identification Guide, page 308

FINACEA™ ℞
[*fĭ′nā-shē-ə*]
(azelaic acid) Gel, 15%
For Dermatologic Use Only–Not for Ophthalmic, Oral, or Intravaginal Use
℞ only

DESCRIPTION
FINACEA™ (azelaic acid) Gel, 15%, contains azelaic acid, a naturally occurring saturated dicarboxylic acid. Chemically, azelaic acid is 1,7-heptanedicarboxylic acid, with the molecular formula $C_9H_{16}O_4$, a molecular weight of 188.22, and the structural formula:

[HOOC-$(CH_2)_7$-COOH]

Azelaic acid is a white, odorless crystalline solid that is poorly soluble in water at 20°C (0.24%), but freely soluble in boiling water and in ethanol.
Each gram of FINACEA™ Gel, 15%, contains 0.15 gm azelaic acid (15% w/w) as the active ingredient in an aqueous gel base containing benzoic acid (as a preservative), disodium-EDTA, lecithin, medium-chain triglycerides, polyacrylic acid, polysorbate 80, propylene glycol, purified water, and sodium hydroxide to adjust pH.

CLINICAL PHARMACOLOGY
The mechanism(s) by which azelaic acid interferes with the pathogenic events in rosacea are unknown.
Pharmacokinetics: The percutaneous absorption of azelaic acid after topical application of FINACEA™ Gel, 15%, could not be reliably determined. Mean plasma azelaic acid concentrations in rosacea patients treated with FINACEA™ Gel, 15%, twice daily for at least 8 weeks are in the range of 42 to 63.1 ng/mL. These values are within the maximum concentration range of 24.0 to 90.5 ng/mL observed in rosacea patients treated with vehicle only. This indicates that FINACEA™ Gel, 15%, does not increase plasma azelaic acid concentration beyond the range derived from nutrition and endogenous metabolism.
In vitro and human data suggest negligible cutaneous metabolism of ^{3}H-azelaic acid 20% cream after topical application. Azelaic acid is mainly excreted unchanged in the urine, but undergoes some β-oxidation to shorter chain dicarboxylic acids.

CLINICAL STUDIES
FINACEA™ Gel, 15%, was evaluated for the treatment of mild to moderate papulopustular rosacea in 2 clinical trials comprising a total of 664 (333 active to 331 vehicle). Both trials were multicenter, randomized, double-blind, vehicle-controlled 12-week studies with identical protocols. Overall, 92.5% of patients were Caucasian and 73% of patients were women, and the mean age was 49 (range 21 to 86) years. Enrolled patients had mild to moderate rosacea with a mean lesion count of 18 (range 8 to 60) inflammatory papules and pustules. Subjects without papules and pustules, with nodules, rhinophyma, or ocular involvement, and a history of hypersensitivity to propylene glycol or to any other ingredients of the study drug were excluded. FINACEA™ Gel, 15%, or its vehicle were to be applied twice daily for 12 weeks; no other topical or systemic medication affecting the course of rosacea and/or evaluability was to be used during the studies. Patients were instructed to avoid spicy foods, thermally hot foods and drinks, and alcoholic beverages during the study, and to use only very mild soaps or soapless cleansing lotion for facial cleansing.
The primary efficacy endpoints were both 1) change from baseline in inflammatory lesion counts and 2) success defined as a score of clear or minimal with at least a 2 step reduction from baseline on the Investigator's Global Assessment (IGA):
CLEAR:
No papules and/or pustules; no or residual erythema; no or mild to moderate telangiectasia
MINIMAL:
Rare papules and/or pustules; residual to mild erythema; mild to moderate telangiectasia
MILD:
Few papules and/or pustules; mild erythema; mild to moderate telangiectasia
MILD TO MODERATE:
Distinct number of papules and/or pustules; mild to moderate erythema; mild to moderate telangiectasia
MODERATE:
Pronounced number of papules and/or pustules; moderate erythema; mild to moderate telangiectasia
MODERATE TO SEVERE:
Many papules and/or pustules, occasionally with large inflamed lesions; moderate erythema; moderate degree of telangiectasia
SEVERE:
Numerous papules and/or pustules, occasionally with confluent areas of inflamed lesions; moderate or severe erythema; moderate or severe telangiectasia

Primary efficacy assessment was based on the intent-to-treat (ITT) population with last observation carried forward (LOCF).
Both studies demonstrated a statistically significant difference in favor of FINACEA™ Gel, 15%, over its vehicle in reducing the number of inflammatory papules and pustules associated with rosacea and with success on the IGA in the ITT-LOCF population at the end of treatment.
[See table 1 on next page]
FINACEA™ Gel, 15% was superior to the vehicle with regard to success based on the investigator's global assessment of rosacea on a 7-point static score at the end of treatment, (ITT population; Table 2).
[See table 2 at bottom of next page]

INDICATIONS AND USAGE
FINACEA™ Gel, 15%, is indicated for topical treatment of inflammatory papules and pustules of mild to moderate rosacea. Patients should be instructed to avoid spicy foods, thermally hot foods and drinks, alcoholic beverages and to use only very mild soaps or soapless cleansing lotion for facial cleansing.

CONTRAINDICATIONS
FINACEA™ Gel, 15%, is contraindicated in individuals with a history of hypersensitivity to propylene glycol or any other component of the formulation.

WARNINGS
FINACEA™ Gel, 15%, is for dermatologic use only, and not for ophthalmic, oral or intravaginal use.
There have been isolated reports of hypopigmentation after use of azelaic acid. Since azelaic acid has not been well studied in patients with dark complexion, these patients should be monitored for early signs of hypopigmentation.

PRECAUTIONS
General: Contact with the eyes should be avoided. If sensitivity or severe irritation develops with the use of FINACEA™ Gel, 15%, treatment should be discontinued and appropriate therapy instituted. The safety and efficacy of FINACEA™ Gel, 15%, has not been studied beyond 12 weeks.
Information for Patients: Patients using FINACEA™ Gel, 15%, should receive the following information and instructions:
- FINACEA™ Gel, 15%, is to be used only as directed by the physician.
- FINACEA™ Gel, 15%, is for external use only. It is not to be used orally, intravaginally, or for the eyes.
- Cleanse affected area(s) with a very mild soap or a soapless cleansing lotion and pat dry with a soft towel before applying FINACEA™ Gel, 15%. Avoid alcoholic cleansers, tinctures and astringents, abrasives and peeling agents.
- Avoid contact of FINACEA™ Gel, 15%, with the mouth, eyes and other mucous membranes. If it does come in contact with the eyes, wash the eyes with large amounts of water and consult a physician if eye irritation persists.
- The hands should be washed following application of FINACEA™ Gel, 15%.
- Cosmetics may be applied after FINACEA™ Gel, 15%, has dried.
- Skin irritation (e.g., pruritus, burning, or stinging) may occur during use of FINACEA™ Gel, 15%, usually during the first few weeks of treatment. If irritation is excessive or persists, use of FINACEA™ Gel, 15%, should be discontinued, and patients should consult their physician (See **ADVERSE REACTIONS**).
- Avoid any foods and beverages that might provoke erythema, flushing, and blushing (including spicy food, alcoholic beverages, and thermally hot drinks, including hot coffee and tea).
- Patients should report abnormal changes in skin color to their physician.
- Avoid the use of occlusive dressings or wrappings.

Drug Interactions: There have been no formal studies of the interaction of FINACEA™ Gel, 15%, with other drugs.
Carcinogenesis, Mutagenesis, Impairment of Fertility: Long-term animal studies have not been performed to evaluate the carcinogenic potential of FINACEA™ Gel, 15%. Azelaic acid was not mutagenic or clastogenic in a battery of *in vitro* (Ames assay, HGPRT in V79 cells {Chinese hamster lung cells}, and chromosomal aberration assay in human lymphocytes) and *in vivo* (dominant lethal assay in mice and mouse micronucleus assay) genotoxicity tests.
Oral administration of azelaic acid at dose levels up to 2500 mg/kg/day (162 times the maximum recommended human dose based on body surface area) did not affect fertility or reproductive performance in male or female rats.
Pregnancy: *Teratogenic Effects: Pregnancy Category B*
There are no adequate and well-controlled studies of topically administered azelaic acid in pregnant women. The experience with FINACEA™ Gel, 15%, when used by pregnant women is too limited to permit assessment of the safety of its use during pregnancy.

Continued on next page

Information on Berlex products (appearing here) is based on the most current information available at the time of publication closing. Further information for these and other Berlex products can be obtained from Medical & Product Services at Berlex, Inc. by calling 1-888-BERLEX-4.

Finacea—Cont.

Dermal embryofetal developmental toxicology studies have not been performed with azelaic acid, 15%, gel. Oral embryofetal developmental studies were conducted with azelaic acid in rats, rabbits, and cynomolgus monkeys. Azelaic acid was administered during the period of organogeneisis in all three animal species. Embryotoxicity was observed in rats, rabbits, and monkeys at oral doses of azelaic acid that generated some maternal toxicity. Embryotoxicity was observed in rats given 2500 mg/kg/day (162 times the maximum recommended human dose based on body surface area), rabbits given 150 or 500 mg/kg/day (19 or 65 times the maximum recommended human dose based on body surface area) and cynomolgus monkeys given 500 mg/kg/day (65 times the maximum recommended human dose based on body surface area) azelaic acid. No teratogenic effects were observed in the oral embryofetal developmental studies conducted in rats, rabbits and cynomolgus monkeys.

An oral peri- and post-natal developmental study was conducted in rats. Azelaic acid was administered from gestational day 15 through day 21 postpartum up to a dose level of 2500 mg/kg/day. Embryotoxicity was observed in rats at an oral dose that generated some maternal toxicity (2500 mg/kg/day; 162 times the maximum recommended human dose based on body surface area). In addition, slight disturbances in the postnatal development of fetuses was noted in rats at oral doses that generated some maternal toxicity (500 and 2500 mg/kg/day; 32 and 162 times the maximum recommended human dose based on body surface area). No effects on sexual maturation of the fetuses were noted in this study.

Because animal reproduction studies are not always predictive of human response, this drug should be used only if clearly needed during pregnancy.

Nursing Mothers: Equilibrium dialysis was used to assess human milk partitioning *in vitro*. At an azelaic acid concentration of 25 µg/mL, the milk/plasma distribution coefficient was 0.7 and the milk/buffer distribution was 1.0, indicating that passage of drug into maternal milk may occur. Since less than 4% of a topically applied dose of AZELEX® Cream, 20%, is systemically absorbed, the uptake of azelaic acid into maternal milk is not expected to cause a significant change from baseline azelaic acid levels in the milk. However, caution should be exercised when FINACEA™ Gel, 15%, is administered to a nursing mother.

Pediatric Use: Safety and effectiveness of FINACEA™ Gel, 15%, in pediatric patients have not been established.

Geriatric: Clinical studies of FINACEA™ Gel, 15%, did not include sufficient numbers of subjects aged 65 and over to determine whether they respond differently from younger subjects.

ADVERSE REACTIONS

In the 2 vehicle controlled, identically designed U.S. clinical studies, treatment safety was monitored in 664 patients who used FINACEA™ Gel, 15%, (N=333), or the gel vehicle (N=331), twice daily for 12 weeks.

[See table 3 below]

FINACEA™ Gel, 15%, and its vehicle caused irritant reactions at the application site in human dermal safety studies. FINACEA™ Gel, 15%, caused significantly more irritation than its vehicle in a cumulative irritation study. Some improvement in irritation was demonstrated over the course of the clinical studies, but this improvement might be attributed to subject dropouts. No phototoxicity or photoallergenicity were reported in human dermal safety studies.

In patients using azelaic acid formulations, the following additional adverse experiences have been reported rarely: worsening of asthma, vitiligo depigmentation, small depigmented spots, hypertrichosis, reddening (signs of keratosis pilaris), and exacerbation of recurrent herpes labialis.

OVERDOSAGE

FINACEA™ Gel, 15%, is intended for cutaneous use only. If pronounced local irritation occurs, patients should be directed to discontinue use and appropriate therapy should be instituted (See **PRECAUTIONS**).

DOSAGE AND ADMINISTRATION

A thin layer of FINACEA™ Gel, 15%, should be gently massaged into the affected areas on the face twice daily, in the morning and evening. FINACEA™ Gel, 15%, has only been studied up to 12 weeks in patients with mild to moderate rosacea (See **CLINICAL STUDIES**).

HOW SUPPLIED

FINACEA™ Gel, 15%, is supplied in tubes in the following size:

30 g – NDC 50419-825-01

Storage

Store at 25°C (77°F); excursions permitted between 15°-30°C (59°-86°F) [See USP Controlled Room Temperature].

Distributed under license; *U.S. Patent No 4,713,394*

January 2003

AZELEX® is a registered trademark of Allergan, Inc.

Manufactured by Schering S.p.A., Segrate, Milan, Italy

Distributed by:

BERLEX® Laboratories, Montville, NJ 07045

2189827 6058000

Shown in Product Identification Guide, page 308

Table 1. Inflammatory Papules and Pustules (ITT population)[1]

	Study One FINACEA™ Gel, 15% N = 164	Study One VEHICLE N = 165	Study Two FINACEA™ Gel, 15% N = 169	Study Two VEHICLE N = 166
Mean Lesion Count Baseline	17.5	17.6	17.9	18.5
End of Treatment[1]	6.8	10.5	9.0	12.1
Mean Percent Reduction End of Treatment[1]	57.9%	39.9%	50.0%	38.2%

[1]ITT population with last observation carried forward (LOCF)

Table 2. Investigator's Global Assessment at the End of Treatment[1]

	Study One FINACEA™ Gel, 15%, N = 164	Study One VEHICLE N = 165	Study Two FINACEA™ Gel, 15% N = 169	Study Two VEHICLE N = 166
CLEAR, MINIMAL or MILD at End of Treatment (% of Patients)	61%	40%	62%	48%

[1] ITT population with last observation carried forward (LOCF)

Table 3. Cutaneous Adverse Events Occurring in ≥1% of Subjects in the Rosacea Trials by Treatment Group and Maximum Intensity*

	FINACEA™ Gel, 15% N=333 (100%)			Vehicle N=331 (100%)		
	Mild n=86 (26%)	Moderate n=44 (13%)	Severe n=20 (6%)	Mild N=49 (15%)	Moderate n=27 (8%)	Severe n=5 (2%)
Burning/ stinging/ tingling	66 (20%)	30 (9%)	12 (4%)	8 (2%)	6 (2%)	2 (1%)
Pruritus	24 (7%)	14 (4%)	3 (1%)	9 (3%)	6 (2%)	0 (0%)
Scaling/dry skin/xerosis	21 (6%)	8 (2%)	4 (1%)	33 (10%)	12 (4%)	1 (0%)
Erythema/ irritation	6 (2%)	6 (2%)	1 (0%)	8 (2%)	4 (1%)	2 (1%)
Edema	3 (1%)	2 (1%)	0 (0%)	3 (1%)	0 (0%)	0 (0%)
Contact dermatitis	2 (1%)	2 (1%)	0 (0%)	1 (0%)	0 (0%)	0 (0%)
Acne	2 (1%)	1 (0%)	0 (0%)	1 (0%)	0 (0%)	0 (0%)
Seborrhea	2 (1%)	0 (0%)	0 (0%)	0 (0%)	0 (0%)	0 (0%)
Photo- sensitivity	1 (0%)	0 (0%)	0 (0%)	3 (1%)	1 (0%)	1 (0%)
Skin disease	1 (0%)	0 (0%)	0 (0%)	1 (0%)	2 (1%)	0 (0%)

*Subjects may have >1 cutaneous adverse event; thus, the sum of the frequencies of preferred terms may exceed the number of subjects with at least 1 cutaneous adverse event

LEVLITE® 28 Tablets ℞

[*lĕvlīt*]

(levonorgestrel and ethinyl estradiol tablets, USP)

Rx only

TRI-LEVLEN® 21 ℞

[*trī-lĕvlĕn*]

Tablets

(levonorgestrel and ethinyl estradiol tablets—triphasic regimen)

Rx only

TRI-LEVLEN® 28 ℞

[*trī-lĕvlĕn*]

Tablets

(levonorgestrel and ethinyl estradiol tablets—triphasic regimen)

LEVLEN® 21 ℞

[*lĕvlĕn*]

Tablets

(levonorgestrel and ethinyl estradiol tablets)

LEVLEN® 28 ℞

[*lĕvlĕn*]

Tablets

(levonorgestrel and ethinyl estradiol tablets)

Patients should be counseled that this product does not protect against HIV infection (AIDS) and other sexually transmitted diseases.

DESCRIPTION

LEVLITE® 28 tablets

Each cycle of LEVLITE® 28 (levonorgestrel and ethinyl estradiol tablets, USP) consists of 21 pink active tablets each containing 0.100 mg levonorgestrel and 0.020 mg ethinyl estradiol; and seven white tablets – inert. The inactive ingredients are Calcium Carbonate USP, Corn Starch NF, Ferric Oxide/red/E 172 NF, Ferric Oxide/yellow/E 172 NF, Glycerin 85% Ph. Eur./DAB, Lactose Monohydrate NF, Magnesium Stearate NF, Montanglycol Wax (Wax E) DAB, Polyethylene glycol 6,000 NF, Povidone 25,000 USP, Povidone 700,000 USP, Pregelatinized Starch NF (Modified Starch), Sucrose NF, Talc USP and Titanium Dioxide, E 171 USP.

TRI-LEVLEN® 21 tablets

Each cycle of TRI-LEVLEN® 21 (Levonorgestrel and Ethinyl Estradiol Tablets—Triphasic Regimen) tablets consists of three different drug phases as follows: Phase 1 comprised of 6 brown film-coated tablets, each containing 0.050 mg of levonorgestrel (d)(-)-13 beta-ethyl-17-alpha-ethinyl-17-beta-hydroxygon-4-en-3-one), a totally synthetic progestogen, and 0.030 mg of ethinyl estradiol (19-nor-17α-pregna-1,3,5(10)-trien-20-yne-3, 17-diol); phase 2 comprised of 5 white film-coated tablets, each containing 0.075 mg levonorgestrel and 0.040 mg ethinyl estradiol; and, phase 3 comprised of 10 light-yellow film-coated tablets, each containing 0.125 mg levonorgestrel and 0.030 mg ethinyl estradiol. The inactive ingredients present are cellulose, iron oxides, lactose, magnesium stearate, polacrilin potassium, polyethylene glycol, titanium dioxide, and hydroxypropyl methylcellulose.

TRI-LEVLEN® 28 tablets

Each cycle of TRI-LEVLEN® 28 (Levonorgestrel and Ethinyl Estradiol Tablets—Triphasic Regimen) tablets consists of three different drug phases as follows: Phase 1 comprised of 6 brown film-coated tablets, each containing 0.050 mg of levonorgestrel (d)(-)-13 beta-ethyl-17-alpha-ethinyl-17-beta-hydroxygon-4-en-3-one), a totally synthetic progestogen, and 0.030 mg of ethinyl estradiol (19-nor-17 α-pregna-1,3,5(10)-trien-20-yne-3, 17-diol); phase 2 comprised of 5

TABLE I MEAN (SD) PHARMACOKINETIC PARAMETERS OF LEVLITE® AFTER SINGLE DOSE AND AFTER MULTIPLE DOSING FOR 3 CYCLES

Levonorgestrel

Day (cycle)	Cmax ng/mL	tmax h	AUC ng•h/mL	CL/F mL/min/kg	Vz L	SHBG nmol/L
1	2.36 (0.79)	1.3 (0.4)	29.2 (10.0)	1.0 (0.3)	129 (46)	64.5 (22.0)
			AUC (0–24h) ng•h/mL			
21 (1)	4.04 (2.08)	1.0 (0.3)	43.8 (22.4)	0.73 (0.34)	106 (42)	94.7 (37.4)
21 (3)	4.53 (1.94)	1.0 (0.3)	49.5 (24.5)	0.65 (0.33)	96 (35)	107.4 (45.8)

Ethinyl Estradiol

Day (cycle)	Cmax pg/mL	tmax h	AUC(0–24) pg•h/mL
1	49.5 (13.4)	1.5 (0.4)	298 (215)
21 (1)	66.2 (29.5)	1.4 (0.4)	596 (494)
21 (3)	58.1 (19.3)	1.4 (0.3)	417 (289)

Cmax = maximum concentration
tmax = time to maximum concentration
AUC = area under the drug concentration curve from time 0 to infinity
CL/f = oral clearance
Vz = volume of distribution
SHBG = sex hormone binding globulin
AUC (0–24) = area under the drug concentration time curve from time 0 to 24 hours; this represents the area for one dosing interval at steady state.

white film-coated tablets, each containing 0.075 mg levonorgestrel and 0.040 mg ethinyl estradiol; and phase 3 comprised of 10 light-yellow film-coated tablets, each containing 0.125 mg levonorgestrel and 0.030 mg ethinyl estradiol; then followed by 7 light-green film-coated inert tablets. The inactive ingredients present are cellulose, F D & C Blue 1, iron oxides, lactose, magnesium stearate, polacrilin potassium, polyethylene glycol, titanium dioxide, and hydroxypropyl methylcellulose.

LEVLEN® 21 tablets:
Each LEVLEN® 21 tablet (Levonorgestrel and Ethinyl Estradiol Tablets) contains 0.15 mg of levonorgestrel (d)(-)-13 beta-ethyl-17-alpha-ethinyl-17-beta-hydroxygon-4-en-3-one), a totally synthetic progestogen, and 0.03 mg of ethinyl estradiol (19-nor-17 α-pregna-1,3,5(10)-trien-20-yne-3, 17-diol). The inactive ingredients present are cellulose, FD&C Yellow 6, lactose, magnesium stearate, and polacrillin potassium.

LEVLEN® 28 tablets:
21 light-orange LEVLEN® tablets (Levonorgestrel and Ethinyl Estradiol Tablets), each containing 0.15 mg of levonorgestrel (d)(-)-13 beta-ethyl-17-alpha-ethinyl-17-beta-hydroxygon-4-en-3-one), a totally synthetic progestogen, and 0.03 mg of ethinyl estradiol (19-nor-17 α-pregna-1,3,5(10)-trien-20-yne-3, 17-diol), and 7 pink inert tablets. The inactive ingredients present are cellulose, D&C Red 30, FD&C Yellow 6, lactose, magnesium stearate, and polacrillin potassium.

Levonorgestrel has a molecular weight of 312.4 and a molecular formula of C21H28O2. Ethinyl estradiol has a molecular weight of 296.4 and a molecular formula of C20H24O2. The structural formulas are as follows:

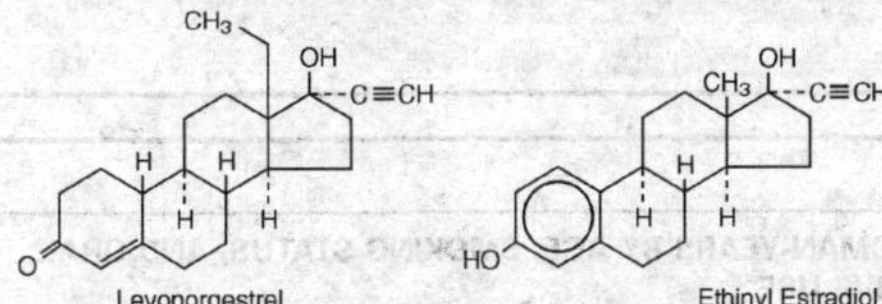

CLINICAL PHARMACOLOGY

Combination oral contraceptives act by suppression of gonadotropins. Although the primary mechanism of this action is inhibition of ovulation, other alterations include changes in the cervical mucus (which increase the difficulty of sperm entry into the uterus) and the endometrium (which reduce the likelihood of implantation).

PHARMACOKINETICS OF LEVLITE®

Absorption

No specific investigation of the absolute bioavailability of levonorgestrel and ethinyl estradiol of LEVLITE® in humans has been conducted. However, literature indicates that levonorgestrel is rapidly and completely absorbed after oral administration and is not subject to first-pass metabolism. Ethinyl estradiol is rapidly and almost completely absorbed from the gastrointestinal tract but, due to first-pass metabolism in gut mucosa and liver, the absolute bioavailability of ethinyl estradiol is about 40%.

After a single dose of three LEVLITE® Tablets to 17 women under fasting conditions, the extent of absorption of levonorgestrel and ethinyl estradiol were 98.6% and 99.0%, respectively, relative to the same dose of the 2 drugs when given as a microcrystalline suspension in water. The effect of food on the bioavailability of LEVLITE® Tablets following oral administration has not been evaluated.

The pharmacokinetics of levonorgestrel and ethinyl estradiol following daily administration of LEVLITE® Tablets for 21 days per cycle for three cycles, were determined in 18 women. Estimates of the pharmacokinetic parameters of levonorgestrel and ethinyl estradiol following single and multiple dose administration of LEVLITE® Tablets are summarized in Table I. Mean levonorgestrel and ethinyl estradiol levels after a single dose and on day 21 at steady state are shown in Figure I.

The pharmacokinetics of total levonorgestrel are non-linear due to an increase in binding to SHBG, which is attributed to increased SHBG levels that are induced by the daily administration of ethinyl estradiol. Increased binding of levonorgestrel to SHBG leads to decreased clearance of levonorgestrel. Observed maximum levonorgestrel concentrations increased from day 1 to day 21 of the 1st and 3rd cycles by 66% and 83%, respectively.

FIGURE I

Mean Levonorgestrel Concentrations in Serum after single dose and on Day 21 of Cycles 1 and 3

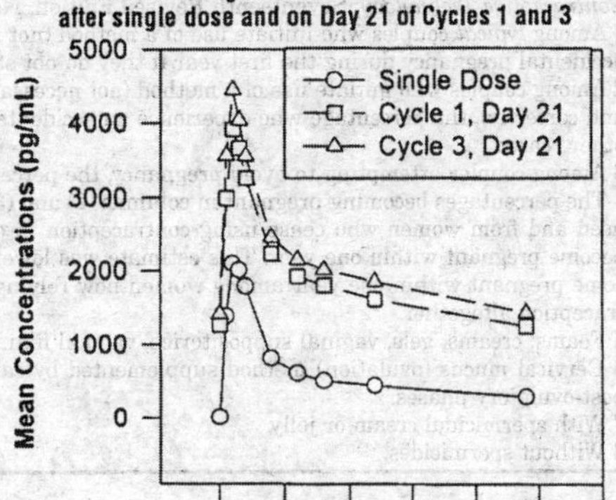

Mean Ethinyl Estradiol Concentrations in Serum after single dose and on Day 21 of Cycles 1 and 3

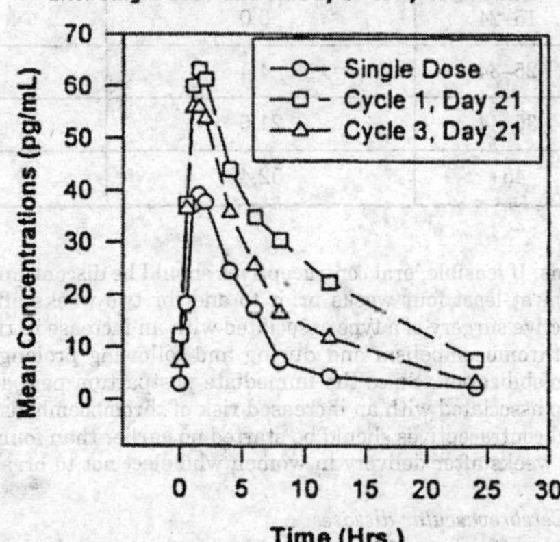

In calculating the mean concentration for ethinyl estradiol, any individual subject value below the quantifiable limit (i.e., 20 pg/mL) was converted to 0; and the 0 values were included for calculation of the mean concentration.

Table I provides a summary of levonorgestrel and ethinyl estradiol pharmacokinetic parameters.
[See table I at left]

Distribution

Levonorgestrel in serum is primarily bound to SHBG. Protein binding values for levonorgestrel are provided in Table II. Ethinyl estradiol is about 97% bound to plasma albumin. Ethinyl estradiol does not bind to SHBG, but induces SHBG synthesis.
[See table II at top of next page]

Metabolism

Levonorgestrel: The most important metabolic pathway occurs in the reduction of the Δ4-3-oxo group and hydroxylation at positions 2α, 1β, and 16β, followed by conjugation. Most of the metabolites that circulate in the blood are sulfates of 3α, 5β-tetrahydro-levonorgestrel, while excretion occurs predominantly in the form of glucuronides. Some of the parent levonorgestrel also circulates as 17β-sulfate. Metabolic clearance rates may differ among individuals by several-fold, and this may account in part for the wide variation in levonorgestrel concentrations among users.

Ethinyl estradiol: Cytochrome P450 enzymes (CYP3A4) in the liver are responsible for the 2-hydroxylation that is the major oxidative reaction. The 2-hydroxy metabolite is further transformed by methylation and glucuronidation prior to urinary and fecal excretion. Levels of Cytochrome P450 (CYP3A) vary widely among individuals and can explain the variation in the rates of ethinyl estradiol 2-hydroxylation. Ethinyl estradiol is excreted in the urine and feces as glucuronide and sulfate conjugates and undergoes enterohepatic circulation.

Excretion

The elimination half-life for levonorgestrel after a single dose of LEVLITE® is 25.4 ± 9.7 hours. Levonorgestrel and its metabolites are primarily excreted in the urine. The elimination half-life of ethinyl estradiol has been reported to be between 15 and 25 hours.

SPECIAL POPULATIONS for LEVLITE®

Hepatic Insufficiency

No formal studies have evaluated the effect of hepatic disease on the disposition of LEVLITE®. However, steroid hormones may be poorly metabolized in patients with impaired liver function.

Renal Insufficiency

No formal studies have evaluated the effect of renal disease on the disposition of LEVLITE®.

Drug-Drug Interactions

Interactions between ethinyl estradiol and other drugs have been reported in the literature.

- *Interactions with Absorption.* Diarrhea may increase gastrointestinal motility and reduce hormone absorption. Similarly, any drug which reduces gut transit time may reduce hormone concentrations in the blood.
- *Interactions with Metabolism*
  Gastrointestinal Wall: Sulfation of ethinyl estradiol has been shown to occur in the gastrointestinal wall. Therefore, drugs which act as competitive inhibitors for sulfation in the gastrointestinal wall may increase ethinyl estradiol bioavailability.
- *Hepatic metabolism:* Interactions can occur with drugs that induce microsomal enzymes which can decrease ethinyl estradiol concentrations (e.g., rifampin, barbiturates, phenylbutazone, phenytoin, griseofulvin).
- *Interference with Enterohepatic Circulation:* Some clinical reports suggest that enteroheptic circulation of estrogens may decrease when certain antibiotic agents are given, which may reduce ethinyl estradiol concentrations (e.g., ampicillin, tetracycline).
- *Interference in the Metabolism of Other Drugs:* Ethinyl estradiol may interfere with the metabolism of other drugs by inhibiting hepatic microsomal enzymes or by inducing hepatic drug conjugation, particularly glucuronidation. Accordingly, plasma and tissue concentrations may either be increased or decreased, respectively (e.g., cyclosporin, theophylline).

INDICATIONS AND USAGE

Oral contraceptives are indicated for the prevention of pregnancy in women who elect to use this product as a method of contraception.

Oral contraceptives are highly effective. Table III lists the typical accidental pregnancy rates for users of combination oral contraceptives and other methods of contraception. The efficacy of these contraceptive methods, except sterilization, depends upon the reliability with which they are used. Correct and consistent use of methods can result in lower failure rates.
[See table III on next page]

CONTRAINDICATIONS

Oral contraceptives should not be used in women with any of the following conditions:

Thrombophlebitis or thromboembolic disorders.

Continued on next page

Information on Berlex products (appearing here) is based on the most current information available at the time of publication closing. Further information for these and other Berlex products can be obtained from Medical & Product Services at Berlex, Inc. by calling 1-888-BERLEX-4.

Levlite/Tri-Levlen/Levlen—Cont.

A past history of deep-vein thrombophlebitis or thromboembolic disorders.
Cerebral-vascular or coronary-artery disease.
Known or suspected carcinoma of the breast.
Carcinoma of the endometrium or other known or suspected estrogen-dependent neoplasia.
Undiagnosed abnormal genital bleeding.
Cholestatic jaundice of pregnancy or jaundice with prior pill use.
Hepatic adenomas or carcinomas.
Known or suspected pregnancy.

WARNINGS

Cigarette smoking increases the risk of serious cardiovascular side effects from oral-contraceptive use. This risk increases with age and with heavy smoking (15 or more cigarettes per day) and is quite marked in women over 35 years of age. Women who use oral contraceptives should be strongly advised not to smoke.

The use of oral contraceptives is associated with increased risks of several serious conditions including myocardial infarction, thromboembolism, stroke, hepatic neoplasia, gallbladder disease, and hypertension, although the risk of serious morbidity or mortality is very small in healthy women without underlying risk factors. The risk of morbidity and mortality increases significantly in the presence of other underlying risk factors such as hypertension, hyperlipidemias, obesity and diabetes.

Practitioners prescribing oral contraceptives should be familiar with the following information relating to these risks.

The information contained in this package insert is based principally on studies carried out in patients who used oral contraceptives with higher formulations of estrogens and progestogens than those in common use today. The effect of long-term use of the oral contraceptives with lower formulations of both estrogens and progestogens remains to be determined.

Throughout this labeling, epidemiologic studies reported are of two types: retrospective or case control studies and prospective or cohort studies. Case control studies provide a measure of the relative risk of a disease, namely, a ratio of the incidence of a disease among oral contraceptive users to that among nonusers. The relative risk does not provide information on the actual clinical occurrence of a disease. Cohort studies provide a measure of attributable risk, which is the difference in the incidence of disease between oral contraceptive users and nonusers. The attributable risk does provide information about the actual occurrence of a disease in the population. For further information, the reader is referred to a text on epidemiologic methods.

1. THROMBOEMBOLIC DISORDERS AND OTHER VASCULAR PROBLEMS

a. *Myocardial infarction*

An increased risk of myocardial infarction has been attributed to oral-contraceptive use. This risk is primarily in smokers or women with other underlying risk factors for coronary-artery disease such as hypertension, hypercholesterolemia, morbid obesity, and diabetes. The relative risk of heart attack for current oral contraceptive users has been estimated to be two to six. The risk is very low under the age of 30.

Smoking in combination with oral contraceptive use has been shown to contribute substantially to the incidence of myocardial infarctions in women in their mid-thirties or older with smoking accounting for the majority of excess cases. Mortality rates associated with circulatory disease have been shown to increase substantially in smokers over the age of 35 and nonsmokers over the age of 40 (Table IV) among women who use oral contraceptives.

[See table IV at right]

Oral contraceptives may compound the effects of well-known risk factors, such as hypertension, diabetes, hyperlipidemias, age and obesity. In particular, some progestogens are known to decrease HDL cholesterol and cause glucose intolerance, while estrogens may create a state of hyperinsulinism. Oral contraceptives have been shown to increase blood pressure among users (see section 9 in "WARNINGS"). Similar effects on risk factors have been associated with an increased risk of heart disease. Oral contraceptives must be used with caution in women with cardiovascular disease risk factors.

b. *Thromboembolism*

An increased risk of thromboembolic and thrombotic disease associated with the use of oral contraceptives is well established. Case control studies have found the relative risk of users compared to nonusers to be 3 for the first episode of superficial venous thrombosis, 4 to 11 for deep vein thrombosis or pulmonary embolism, and 1.5 to 6 for women with predisposing conditions for venous thromboembolic disease. Cohort studies have shown the relative risk to be somewhat lower, about 3 for new cases and about 4.5 for new cases requiring hospitalization. The risk of thromboembolic disease due to oral contraceptives is not related to length of use and disappears after pill use is stopped.

A two- to four-fold increase in the relative risk of postoperative thromboembolic complications has been reported with the use of oral contraceptives. The relative risk of venous thrombosis in women who have predisposing conditions is twice that of women without such medical conditions. If feasible, oral contraceptives should be discontinued from at least four weeks prior to and for two weeks after elective surgery of a type associated with an increase in risk of thromboembolism and during and following prolonged immobilization. Since the immediate postpartum period is also associated with an increased risk of thromboembolism, oral contraceptives should be started no earlier than four to six weeks after delivery in women who elect not to breast-feed.

c. *Cerebrovascular diseases*

Oral contraceptives have been shown to increase both the relative and attributable risks of cerebrovascular events (thrombotic and hemorrhagic strokes), although, in general, the risk is greatest among older (>35 years), hypertensive women who also smoke. Hypertension was found to be a risk factor, for both users and nonusers, for both types of strokes, while smoking interacted to increase the risk for hemorrhagic strokes.

In a large study, the relative risk of thrombotic strokes has been shown to range from 3 for normotensive users to 14 for users with severe hypertension. The relative risk of hemorrhagic stroke is reported to be 1.2 for nonsmokers who used oral contraceptives, 2.6 for smokers who did not use oral contraceptives, 7.6 for smokers who used oral contraceptives, 1.8 for normotensive users and 25.7 for users with severe hypertension. The attributable risk is also greater in older women.

d. *Dose-related risk of vascular disease from oral contraceptives*

A positive association has been observed between the amount of estrogen and progestogen in oral contraceptives

TABLE II. Protein binding (mean ± SD) of levonorgestrel in pools of serum samples collected from 18 women after a single dose of LEVLITE®, and following administration (once daily) over 3x21 days.

Parameter	Single Dose	Cycle 2	Cycle 4
% free	1.11 (0.27)	0.79 (0.22)	0.80 (0.23)
% SHBG-bound	64.5 (8.54)	75.6 (6.59)	74.7 (7.89)
% albumin-bound	34.4 (8.28)	23.6 (6.41)	24.5 (7.67)

TABLE III. Percentage of women experiencing an unintended pregnancy during the first year of typical use and first year of perfect use of contraception and the percentage continuing use at the end of the first year. United States.

	% of Women Experiencing an Accidental Pregnancy within the First Year of Use		% of Women Continuing Use at One Year[3]
Method (1)	Typical Use[1] (2)	Perfect Use[2] (3)	(4)
Chance[4]	85	85	
Spermicides[5]	26	6	40
Periodic abstinence	25		63
Calendar		9	
Ovulation method		3	
Sympto-thermal[6]		2	
Post Ovulation		1	
Withdrawal	19	4	
Cap[7]			
Parous women	40	26	42
Nulliparous women	20	9	56
Sponge			
Parous women	40	20	42
Nulliparous women	20	9	56
Diaphragm[7]	20	6	56
Condom[8]			
Female (Reality)	21	5	56
Male	14	3	61
Pill	5		71
progestin only		0.5	
combined		0.1	
IUD			
Progesterone T	2	1.5	81
Copper T 380A	0.8	0.6	78
Lng 20	0.1	0.1	81
Depo Provera	0.3	0.3	70
Norplant and Norplant-2	0.05	0.05	88
Female sterilization	0.5	0.5	100
Male sterilization	0.15	0.10	100

Source: Trussell J, Contraceptive efficacy. In Hatcher RA, Trussell J, Stewart F, Cates W, Stewart GK, Kowal D, Guest F, *Contraceptive Technology:* Seventeenth Revised Edition. New York NY: Irvington Publishers, 1998, in press.

1 Among *typical* couples who initiate use of a method (not necessarily for the first time), the percentage who experience an accidental pregnancy during the first year if they do not stop use for any other reason.

2 Among couples who initiate use of a method (not necessarily for the first time) and who use it *perfectly* (both consistently and correctly), the percentage who experience an accidental pregnancy during the first year if they do not stop use for any other reason.

3 Among couples attempting to avoid pregnancy, the percentage who continue to use a method for one year.

4 The percentages becoming pregnant in columns (2) and (3) are based on data from populations where contraception is not used and from women who cease using contraception in order to become pregnant. Among such populations, about 89% become pregnant within one year. This estimate was lowered slightly (to 85%) to represent the percentage who would become pregnant within one year among women now relying on reversible methods of contraception if they abandoned contraception altogether.

5 Foams, creams, gels, vaginal suppositories, vaginal film.

6 Cervical mucus (ovulation) method supplemented by calendar in the pre-ovulatory and basal body temperature in the post-ovulatory phases.

7 With spermicidal cream or jelly.

8 Without spermicides.

TABLE IV. (Adapted from P.M. Layde and V. Beral)

CIRCULATORY DISEASE MORTALITY RATES PER 100,000 WOMAN-YEARS BY AGE, SMOKING STATUS, AND ORAL CONTRACEPTIVE USE

AGE	EVER-USERS NON-SMOKERS	EVER-USERS SMOKERS	CONTROLS NON-SMOKERS	CONTROL SMOKERS
15–24	0.0	10.5	0.0	0.0
25–34	4.4	14.2	2.7	4.2
35–44	21.5	63.4	6.4	15.2
45+	52.4	206.7	11.4	27.9

and the risk of vascular disease. A decline in serum high-density lipoproteins (HDL) has been reported with many progestational agents. A decline in serum high-density lipoproteins has been associated with an increased incidence of ischemic heart disease. Because estrogens increase HDL cholesterol, the net effect of an oral contraceptive depends on a balance achieved between doses of estrogen and progestogen and the nature and absolute amount of progestogen used in the contraceptive. The amount of both hormones should be considered in the choice of an oral contraceptive.

Minimizing exposure to estrogen and progestogen is in keeping with good principles of therapeutics. For any particular estrogen/progestogen combination, the dosage regimen prescribed should be one which contains the least amount of estrogen and progestogen that is compatible with a low failure rate and the needs of the individual patient. New acceptors of oral-contraceptive agents should be started on preparations containing the lowest estrogen content which provides satisfactory results in the individual.

e. *Persistence of risk of vascular disease*

There are two studies which have shown persistence of risk of vascular disease for ever-users of oral contraceptives. In a study in the United States, the risk of developing myocardial infarction after discontinuing oral contraceptives persists for at least 9 years for women aged 40–49 years who had used oral contraceptives for five or more years, but this increased risk was not demonstrated in other age groups. In another study in Great Britain, the risk of developing cerebrovascular disease persisted for at least 6 years after discontinuation of oral contraceptives, although excess risk was very small. However, both studies were performed with oral contraceptive formulations containing 50 micrograms or higher of estrogens.

2. ESTIMATES OF MORTALITY FROM CONTRACEPTIVE USE

One study gathered data from a variety of sources which have estimated the mortality rate associated with different methods of contraception at different ages (Table V). These estimates include the combined risk of death associated with contraceptive methods plus the risk attributable to pregnancy in the event of method failure. Each method of contraception has its specific benefits and risks. The study concluded that with the exception of oral contraceptive users 35 and older who smoke and 40 and older who do not smoke, mortality associated with all methods of birth control is less than that associated with childbirth.

The observation of a possible increase in risk of mortality with age for oral-contraceptive users is based on data gathered in the 1970's—but not reported until 1983. However, current clinical practice involves the use of lower estrogen dose formulations combined with careful restriction of oral-contraceptive use to women who do not have the various risk factors listed in this labeling.

Because of these changes in practice and, also, because of some limited new data which suggest that the risk of cardiovascular disease with the use of oral contraceptives may now be less than previously observed, the Fertility and Maternal Health Drugs Advisory Committee was asked to review the topic in 1989. The Committee concluded that although cardiovascular disease risks may be increased with oral-contraceptive use after age 40 in healthy nonsmoking women (even with the newer low-dose formulations), there are greater potential health risks associated with pregnancy in older women and with the alternative surgical and medical procedures which may be necessary if such women do not have access to effective and acceptable means of contraception.

Therefore, the Committee recommended that the benefits of oral-contraceptive use by healthy nonsmoking women over 40 may outweigh the possible risks. Of course, older women, as all women who take oral contraceptives, should take the lowest possible dose formulation that is effective.

[See table V above]

TABLE V—ANNUAL NUMBER OF BIRTH-RELATED OR METHOD-RELATED DEATHS ASSOCIATED WITH CONTROL OF FERTILITY PER 100,000 NONSTERILE WOMEN, BY FERTILITY-CONTROL METHOD ACCORDING TO AGE

Method of control and outcome	15–19	20–24	25–29	30–34	35–39	40–44
No fertility—control methods*	7.0	7.4	9.1	14.8	25.7	28.2
Oral contraceptives nonsmoker**	0.3	0.5	0.9	1.9	13.8	31.6
Oral contraceptives smoker**	2.2	3.4	6.6	13.5	51.1	117.2
IUD**	0.8	0.8	1.0	1.0	1.4	1.4
Condom*	1.1	1.6	0.7	0.2	0.3	0.4
Diaphragm/spermicide*	1.9	1.2	1.2	1.3	2.2	2.8
Periodic abstinence*	2.5	1.6	1.6	1.7	2.9	3.6

* Deaths are birth related
** Deaths are method related

Adapted from H.W. Ory, Family Planning Perspectives *15*:57–63, 1983.

3. CARCINOMA OF THE REPRODUCTIVE ORGANS

Numerous epidemiological studies have been performed on the incidence of breast, endometrial, ovarian and cervical cancer in women using oral contraceptives. The overwhelming evidence in the literature suggests that use of oral contraceptives is not associated with an increase in the risk of developing breast cancer, regardless of the age and parity of first use or with most of the marketed brands and doses. The Cancer and Steroid Hormone (CASH) study also showed no latent effect on the risk of breast cancer for at least a decade following long-term use. A few studies have shown a slightly increased relative risk of developing breast cancer, although the methodology of these studies, which included differences in examination of users and nonusers and differences in age at start of use, has been questioned. Some studies suggest that oral-contraceptive use has been associated with an increase in the risk of cervical intraepithelial neoplasia in some populations of women. However, there continues to be controversy about the extent to which such findings may be due to differences in sexual behavior and other factors.

In spite of many studies of the relationship between oral-contraceptive use and breast and cervical cancers, a cause-and-effect relationship has not been established.

4. HEPATIC NEOPLASIA

Benign hepatic adenomas are associated with oral contraceptive use, although the incidence of benign tumors is rare in the United States. Indirect calculations have estimated the attributable risk to be in the range of 3.3 cases/100,000 for users, a risk that increases after four or more years of use. Rupture of rare, benign, hepatic adenomas may cause death through intra-abdominal hemorrhage.

Studies from Britain have shown an increased risk of developing hepatocellular carcinoma in long-term (>8 years) oral-contraceptive users. However, these cancers are extremely rare in the U.S. and the attributable risk (the excess incidence) of liver cancers in oral contraceptive users approaches less than one per million users.

5. OCULAR LESIONS

There have been clinical case reports of retinal thrombosis associated with the use of oral contraceptives. Oral contraceptives should be discontinued if there is unexplained partial or complete loss of vision; onset of proptosis or diplopia; papilledema; or retinal vascular lesions. Appropriate diagnostic and therapeutic measures should be undertaken immediately.

6. ORAL-CONTRACEPTIVE USE BEFORE OR DURING EARLY PREGNANCY

Extensive epidemiological studies have revealed no increased risk of birth defects in women who have used oral contraceptives prior to pregnancy. Studies also do not suggest a teratogenic effect, particularly insofar as cardiac anomalies and limb-reduction defects are concerned, when taken inadvertently during early pregnancy.

The administration of oral contraceptives to induce withdrawal bleeding should not be used as a test for pregnancy. Oral contraceptives should not be used during pregnancy to treat threatened or habitual abortion.

It is recommended that for any patient who has missed two consecutive periods, pregnancy should be ruled out before continuing oral-contraceptive use. If the patient has not adhered to the prescribed schedule, the possibility of pregnancy should be considered at the time of the first missed period. Oral contraceptive use should be discontinued if pregnancy is confirmed.

7. GALLBLADDER DISEASE

Earlier studies have reported an increased lifetime relative risk of gallbladder surgery in users of oral-contraceptives and estrogens. More recent studies, however, have shown that the relative risk of developing gallbladder disease among oral contraceptive users may be minimal. The recent findings of minimal risk may be related to the use of oral-contraceptive formulations containing lower hormonal doses of estrogens and progestogens.

8. CARBOHYDRATE AND LIPID METABOLIC EFFECTS

Oral contraceptives have been shown to cause glucose intolerance in a significant percentage of users. Oral contraceptives containing greater than 75 micrograms of estrogens cause hyperinsulinism, while lower doses of estrogen cause less glucose intolerance. Progestogens increase insulin secretion and create insulin resistance, this effect varying with different progestational agents. However, in the nondiabetic woman, oral contraceptives appear to have no effect on fasting blood glucose. Because of these demonstrated effects, prediabetic and diabetic women should be carefully observed while taking oral-contraceptives.

A small proportion of women will have persistent hypertriglyceridemia while on the pill. As discussed earlier (see "WARNINGS" 1a. and 1d.), changes in serum triglycerides and lipoprotein levels have been reported in oral-contraceptive users.

9. ELEVATED BLOOD PRESSURE

An increase in blood pressure has been reported in women taking oral-contraceptives and this increase is more likely in older oral-contraceptive users and with continued use. Data from the Royal College of General Practitioners and subsequent randomized trials have shown that the incidence of hypertension increases with increasing quantities of progestogens.

Women with a history of hypertension or hypertension-related diseases, or renal disease should be encouraged to use another method of contraception. If women with hypertension elect to use oral contraceptives, they should be monitored closely, and if significant elevation of blood pressure occurs, oral contraceptives should be discontinued. For most women, elevated blood pressure will return to normal after stopping oral contraceptives, and there is no difference in the occurrence of hypertension among ever- and never-users.

10. HEADACHE

The onset or exacerbation of migraine or development of headache with a new pattern which is recurrent, persistent, or severe requires discontinuation of oral contraceptives and evaluation of the cause.

11. BLEEDING IRREGULARITIES

Breakthrough bleeding and spotting are sometimes encountered in patients on oral contraceptives, especially during the first three months of use. The type and dose of progestogen may be important. Nonhormonal causes should be considered and adequate diagnostic measures taken to rule out malignancy or pregnancy in the event of breakthrough bleeding, as in the case of any abnormal vaginal bleeding. If pathology has been excluded, time or a change to another formulation may solve the problem. In the event of amenorrhea, pregnancy should be ruled out.

Some women may encounter post-pill amenorrhea or oligomenorrhea, especially when such a condition was preexistent.

PRECAUTIONS

1. GENERAL

Patients should be counseled that this product does not protect against HIV infection (AIDS) and other sexually transmitted diseases.

2. PHYSICAL EXAMINATION AND FOLLOW-UP

It is good medical practice for all women to have annual history and physical examinations, including women using oral contraceptives. The physical examination, however, may be deferred until after initiation of oral contraceptives if requested by the woman and judged appropriate by the clinician. The physical examination should include special reference to blood pressure, breasts, abdomen and pelvic organs, including cervical cytology and relevant laboratory tests. In case of undiagnosed, persistent, or recurrent abnormal vaginal bleeding, appropriate diagnostic measures should be conducted to rule out malignancy. Women with a strong family history of breast cancer or who have breast nodules should be monitored with particular care.

3. LIPID DISORDERS

Women who are being treated for hyperlipidemias should be followed closely if they elect to use oral contraceptives. Some progestogens may elevate LDL levels and may render the control of hyperlipidemias more difficult.

4. LIVER FUNCTION

If jaundice develops in any woman receiving such drugs, the medication should be discontinued. Steroid hormones may be poorly metabolized in patients with impaired liver function.

5. FLUID RETENTION

Oral contraceptives may cause some degree of fluid retention. They should be prescribed with caution, and only with careful monitoring, in patients with conditions which might be aggravated by fluid retention.

6. EMOTIONAL DISORDERS

Women with a history of depression should be carefully observed and the drug discontinued if depression recurs to a serious degree.

7. CONTACT LENSES

Contact-lens wearers who develop visual changes or changes in lens tolerance should be assessed by an ophthalmologist.

8. DRUG INTERACTIONS

Reduced efficacy and increased incidence of breakthrough bleeding and menstrual irregularities have been associated with concomitant use of rifampin. A similar association, though less marked, has been suggested with barbiturates, phenylbutazone, phenytoin sodium, and possibly with griseofulvin, ampicillin and tetracyclines.

Continued on next page

Information on Berlex products (appearing here) is based on the most current information available at the time of publication closing. Further information for these and other Berlex products can be obtained from Medical & Product Services at Berlex, Inc. by calling 1-888-BERLEX-4.

Levlite/Tri-Levlen/Levlen—Cont.

9. INTERACTIONS WITH LABORATORY TESTS
Certain endocrine- and liver-function tests and blood components may be affected by oral contraceptives:
a. Increased prothrombin and factors VII, VIII, IX and X; decreased antithrombin 3; increased norepinephrine-induced platelet aggregability.
b. Increased thyroid-binding globulin (TBG) leading to increased circulating total thyroid hormone, as measured by protein-bound iodine (PBI), T4 by column or by radioimmunoassay. Free T3 resin uptake is decreased, reflecting the elevated TBG, free T4 concentration is unaltered.
c. Other binding proteins may be elevated in serum.
d. Sex-binding globulins are increased and result in elevated levels of total circulating sex steroids and corticoids; however, free or biologically active levels remain unchanged.
e. Triglycerides may be increased.
f. Glucose tolerance may be decreased.
g. Serum folate levels may be depressed by oral-contraceptive therapy. This may be of clinical significance if a woman becomes pregnant shortly after discontinuing oral contraceptives.
10. CARCINOGENESIS
See "WARNINGS" section.
11. PREGNANCY
Pregnancy Category X. See "CONTRAINDICATIONS" and "WARNINGS" sections.
12. NURSING MOTHERS
Small amounts of oral-contraceptive steroids have been identified in the milk of nursing mothers, and a few adverse effects on the child have been reported, including jaundice and breast enlargement. In addition, oral contraceptives given in the postpartum period may interfere with lactation by decreasing the quantity and quality of breast milk. If possible, the nursing mother should be advised not to use oral contraceptives but to use other forms of contraception until she has completely weaned her child.
13. PEDIATRIC USE
Safety and efficacy of LEVLITE® have been established in women of reproductive age. Safety and efficacy are expected to be the same for postpubertal adolescents under the age of 16 and for users 16 years and older. Use of this product before menarche is not indicated.

INFORMATION FOR THE PATIENT

See "Patient Labeling" printed below.

ADVERSE REACTIONS

An increased risk of the following serious adverse reactions has been associated with the use of oral contraceptives (see "WARNINGS" section).

- Thrombophlebitis
- Arterial thromboembolism
- Pulmonary embolism
- Myocardial infarction
- Cerebral hemorrhage
- Cerebral thrombosis
- Hypertension
- Gallbladder disease
- Hepatic adenomas or benign liver tumors

There is evidence of an association between the following conditions and the use of oral contraceptives, although additional confirmatory studies are needed:
- Mesenteric thrombosis
- Retinal thrombosis

The following adverse reactions have been reported in patients receiving oral contraceptives and are believed to be drug related:
- Nausea
- Vomiting
- Gastrointestinal symptoms, (such as abdominal cramps and bloating)
- Breakthrough bleeding
- Spotting
- Change in menstrual flow
- Amenorrhea
- Temporary infertility after discontinuation of treatment
- Edema
- Melasma which may persist
- Breast changes: tenderness, enlargement, secretion
- Change in weight (increase or decrease)
- Change in cervical erosion and secretion
- Diminution in lactation when given immediately postpartum
- Cholestatic jaundice
- Migraine
- Rash (allergic)
- Mental depression
- Reduced tolerance to carbohydrates
- Vaginal candidiasis
- Change in corneal curvature (steepening)
- Intolerance to contact lenses

The following adverse reactions have been reported in users of oral contraceptives and the association has been neither confirmed nor refuted:

- Pre-menstrual syndrome
- Cataracts
- Optic neuritis
- Changes in appetite
- Cystitis-like syndrome
- Headache
- Nervousness
- Dizziness
- Hemorrhagic eruption
- Vaginitis
- Porphyria
- Impaired renal function
- Hemolytic uremic syndrome
- Budd-Chiari syndrome
- Acne
- Hirsutism
- Loss of scalp hair
- Erythema multiforme
- Erythema nodosum
- Changes in libido
- Colitis

OVERDOSAGE

Serious ill effects have not been reported following acute ingestion of large doses of oral contraceptives by young children. Overdosage may cause nausea, and withdrawal bleeding may occur in females.

NON-CONTRACEPTIVE HEALTH BENEFITS

The following noncontraceptive health benefits related to the use of oral contraceptives are supported by epidemiological studies which largely utilized oral-contraceptive formulations containing doses exceeding 0.035 mg of ethinyl estradiol or 0.05 mg mestranol.
Effects on menses:
- increased menstrual cycle regularity
- decreased blood loss and decreased incidence of iron-deficiency anemia
- decreased incidence of dysmenorrhea

Effects related to inhibition of ovulation:
- decreased incidence of functional ovarian cysts
- decreased incidence of ectopic pregnancies

Effects from long-term use:
- decreased incidence of fibroadenomas and fibrocystic disease of the breast
- decreased incidence of acute pelvic inflammatory disease
- decreased incidence of endometrial cancer
- decreased incidence of ovarian cancer

DOSAGE AND ADMINISTRATION

LEVLITE® 28 Tablets

To achieve maximum contraceptive effectiveness, LEVLITE® 28 Tablets (levonorgestrel and ethinyl estradiol tablets, USP) must be taken exactly as directed at intervals not exceeding 24-hours.
LEVLITE® 28 Tablets are a monophasic preparation plus 7 inert tablets. The dosage of LEVLITE® 28 Tablets is one tablet daily for 21 consecutive days per menstrual cycle plus 7 white inert tablets according to the prescribed schedule. It is recommended that LEVLITE® 28 Tablets be taken at the same time each day, preferably after the evening meal or at bedtime. During the first cycle of medication, the patient should be instructed to take one pink LEVLITE® 28 Tablet daily and then 7 white inert tablets for twenty-eight (28) consecutive days, beginning on day one (1) of her menstrual cycle. (The first day of menstruation is day one.) Withdrawal bleeding usually occurs within 3 days following the last pink tablet. (If LEVLITE® 28 Tablets are first taken later than the first day of the first menstrual cycle of medication or postpartum, contraceptive reliance should not be placed on LEVLITE® 28 Tablets until after the first 7 consecutive days of administration. The possibility of ovulation and conception prior to initiation of medication should be considered.)
When switching from another oral contraceptive, LEVLITE® 28 Tablets should be started on the first day of bleeding following the last active tablet taken of the previous oral contraceptive.
The patient begins her next and all subsequent 28-day courses of LEVLITE® 28 Tablets on the same day of the week that she began her first course, following the same schedule. She begins taking her pink tablets on the next day after ingestion of the last white tablet, regardless of whether or not a menstrual period has occurred or is still in progress. Anytime a subsequent cycle of LEVLITE® 28 Tablets is started later than the next day, the patient should be protected by another means of contraception until she has taken a tablet daily for seven consecutive days.
If spotting or breakthrough bleeding occurs, the patient is instructed to continue on the same regimen. This type of bleeding is usually transient and without significance, however, if the bleeding is persistent or prolonged, the patient is advised to consult her physician. Although the occurrence of pregnancy is highly unlikely if LEVLITE® 28 Tablets are taken according to directions, if withdrawal bleeding does not occur, the possibility of pregnancy must be considered. If the patient has not adhered to the prescribed schedule (missed one or more active tablets or started taking them on a day later than she should have), the probability of pregnancy should be considered at the time of the first missed period and appropriate diagnostic measures taken before the medication is resumed. If the patient has adhered to the prescribed regimen and misses two consecutive periods, pregnancy should be ruled out before continuing the contraceptive regimen.
The risk of pregnancy increases with each active (pink) tablet missed. For additional patient instructions regarding missed pills, see the "WHAT TO DO IF YOU MISS PILLS" section in the DETAILED PATIENT LABELING below. If breakthrough bleeding occurs following missed tablets, it will usually be transient and of no consequence. If the patient misses one or more white tablets, she is still protected against pregnancy provided she begins taking pink tablets again on the proper day.
In the nonlactating mother, LEVLITE® 28 Tablets may be initiated postpartum, for contraception. When the tablets are administered in the postpartum period, the increased risk of thromboembolic disease associated with the postpartum period must be considered. (See "CONTRAINDICATIONS," "WARNINGS," and "PRECAUTIONS" concerning thromboembolic disease.) It is to be noted that early resumption of ovulation may occur if bromocriptine mesylate has been used for the prevention of lactation.

TRI-LEVLEN® 21 Tablets

To achieve maximum contraceptive effectiveness, TRI-LEVLEN® 21 Tablets (levonorgestrel and ethinyl estradiol tablets—triphasic regimen) should be taken exactly as directed and at intervals not exceeding 24-hours.
TRI-LEVLEN® 21 Tablets are a three-phase preparation. The dosage of TRI-LEVLEN® 21 Tablets is **one tablet** daily for 21 consecutive days per menstrual cycle in the following order: 6 brown tablets (phase 1), followed by 5 white tablets (phase 2), and then followed by the last 10 light-yellow tablets (phase 3), according to the prescribed schedule. Tablets are then discontinued for 7 days (three weeks on, one week off).
It is recommended that TRI-LEVLEN® 21 Tablets be taken at the same time each day. During the first cycle of medication, the patient should be instructed to take one TRI-LEVLEN® 21 Tablet daily in the order of 6 brown, 5 white and, finally, 10 light-yellow tablets for twenty-one (21) consecutive days, beginning on day one (1) of her menstrual cycle. (The first day of menstruation is day one.) The tablets are then discontinued for one week (7 days). Withdrawal bleeding usually occurs within 3 days following discontinuation of TRI-LEVLEN® 21 Tablets. (If an alternate starting regimen is used [Sunday Start or postpartum], contraceptive reliance should not be placed on TRI-LEVLEN® 21 Tablets until after the first 7 consecutive days of administration. The possibility of ovulation and conception prior to initiation of medication should be considered.)
The patient begins her next and all subsequent 21-day courses of TRI-LEVLEN® 21 Tablets on the same day of the week that she began her first course, following the same schedule: 21 days on—7 days off. She begins taking her brown tablets on the 8th day after discontinuance, regardless of whether or not a menstrual period has occurred or is still in progress. Any time the next cycle of TRI-LEVLEN® 21 Tablets is started later than the 8th day, the patient should be protected by another means of contraception until she has taken a tablet daily for seven consecutive days.
If spotting or breakthrough bleeding occurs, the patient is instructed to continue on the same regimen. This type of bleeding is usually transient and without significance; however, if the bleeding is persistent or prolonged, the patient is advised to consult her physician. Although the occurrence of pregnancy is highly unlikely if TRI-LEVLEN® 21 Tablets are taken according to directions, if withdrawal bleeding does not occur, the possibility of pregnancy must be considered. If the patient has not adhered to the prescribed schedule (missed one or more tablets or started taking them on a day later than she should have), the probability of pregnancy should be considered at the time of the first missed period and appropriate diagnostic measures taken before the medication is resumed. If the patient has adhered to the prescribed regimen and misses two consecutive periods, pregnancy should be ruled out before continuing the contraceptive regimen.
The risk of pregnancy increases with each active (brown, white, or light-yellow) tablet missed. For additional patient instructions regarding missed pills, see the "WHAT TO DO IF YOU MISS PILLS" section in the DETAILED PATIENT LABELING below. If breakthrough bleeding occurs following missed active tablets, it will usually be transient and of no consequence. If the patient misses one or more light-green tablets, she is still protected against pregnancy **provided** she begins taking brown tablets again on the proper day.
In the nonlactating mother, TRI-LEVLEN® 21 Tablets may be initiated postpartum, for contraception. When the tablets are administered in the postpartum period, the increased risk of thromboembolic disease associated with the postpartum period must be considered. (See "CONTRAINDICATIONS", "WARNINGS", and "PRECAUTIONS" concerning thromboembolic disease.) It is to be noted that early resumption of ovulation may occur if Parlodel® (bromocriptine mesylate) has been used for the prevention of lactation.

TRI-LEVLEN® 28 Tablets

To achieve maximum contraceptive effectiveness, TRI-LEVLEN® 28 Tablets (levonorgestrel and ethinyl estradiol tablets—triphasic regimen) should be taken exactly as directed and at intervals not exceeding 24-hours.
TRI-LEVLEN® 28 Tablets are a three-phase preparation plus 7 inert tablets. The dosage of TRI-LEVLEN® 28 Tablets is one tablet daily for 28 consecutive days per menstrual cycle in the following order: 6 brown tablets (phase 1), followed by 5 white tablets (phase 2), followed by 10 light-yellow tablets (phase 3), plus 7 light-green inert tablets according to the prescribed schedule.
It is recommended that TRI-LEVLEN® 28 Tablets be taken at the same time each day. During the first cycle of medication, the patient should be instructed to take one TRI-LEVLEN® 28 Tablet daily in the order of 6 brown, 5 white, 10 light-yellow tablets and then 7 light-green inert tablets for twenty-eight (28) consecutive days, beginning on day one (1) of her menstrual cycle. (The first day of menstruation is day one.) Withdrawal bleeding usually occurs within 3 days following the last light-yellow tablets. (If an alternate starting regimen is used [Sunday Start or postpartum], contraceptive reliance should not be placed on TRI-LEVLEN® 28 Tablets until after the first 7 consecutive days of administration. The possibility of ovulation and conception prior to initiation of medication should be considered.)

The patient begins her next and all subsequent 28-day courses of TRI-LEVLEN® 28 Tablets on the same day of the week that she began her first course, following the same schedule: She begins taking her brown tablets on the next day after ingestion of the last light-green tablet, regardless of whether or not a menstrual period has occurred or is still in progress. Any time a subsequent cycle of TRI-LEVLEN® 28 Tablets is started later than the next day, the patient should be protected by another means of contraception until she has taken a tablet daily for seven consecutive days.

If spotting or breakthrough bleeding occurs, the patient is instructed to continue on the same regimen. This type of bleeding is usually transient and without significance; however, if the bleeding is persistent or prolonged, the patient is advised to consult her physician. Although the occurrence of pregnancy is highly unlikely if TRI-LEVLEN® 28 Tablets are taken according to directions, if withdrawal bleeding does not occur, the possibility of pregnancy must be considered. If the patient has not adhered to the prescribed schedule (missed one or more active tablets or started taking them on a day later than she should have), the probability of pregnancy should be considered at the time of the first missed period and appropriate diagnostic measures taken before the medication is resumed. If the patient has adhered to the prescribed regimen and misses two consecutive periods, pregnancy should be ruled out before continuing the contraceptive regimen.

The risk of pregnancy increases with each active (brown, white, or light-yellow) tablet missed. For additional patient instructions regarding missed pills, see the "WHAT TO DO IF YOU MISS PILLS" section in the DETAILED PATIENT LABELING below. If breakthrough bleeding occurs following missed active tablets, it will usually be transient and of no consequence. If the patient misses one or more light-green tablets, she is still protected against pregnancy **provided** she begins taking brown tablets again on the proper day.

In the nonlactating mother, TRI-LEVLEN® 28 Tablets may be initiated postpartum, for contraception. When the tablets are administered in the postpartum period, the increased risk of thromboembolic disease associated with the postpartum period must be considered. (See "CONTRAINDICATIONS", "WARNINGS", and "PRECAUTIONS" concerning thromboembolic disease.) It is to be noted that early resumption of ovulation may occur if Parlodel® (bromocriptine mesylate) has been used for the prevention of lactation.

LEVLEN® 21 Tablets

To achieve maximum contraceptive effectiveness, LEVLEN® 21 Tablets (levonorgestrel and ethinyl estradiol tablets) should be taken exactly as directed and at intervals not exceeding 24-hours.

The dosage of LEVLEN® 21 Tablets is **one tablet** daily for 21 consecutive days per menstrual cycle according to the prescribed schedule. Tablets are then discontinued for 7 days (three weeks on, one week off).

It is recommended that LEVLEN® 21 Tablets be taken at the same time each day. During the first cycle of medication, the patient should be instructed to take one LEVLEN® 21 Tablet daily for twenty-one (21) consecutive days, beginning on day one (1) of her menstrual cycle. (The first day of menstruation is day one.) The tablets are then discontinued for one week (7 days). Withdrawal bleeding usually occurs within 3 days following discontinuation of LEVLEN® 21 Tablets. (If an alternate starting regimen is used [Sunday Start or postpartum], contraceptive reliance should not be placed on LEVLEN® 21 Tablets until after the first 7 consecutive days of administration. The possibility of ovulation and conception prior to initiation of medication should be considered.)

The patient begins her next and all subsequent 21-day courses of LEVLEN® 21 Tablets on the same day of the week that she began her first course, following the same schedule: 21 days on—7 days off. She begins taking her light-orange tablets on the 8th day after discontinuance, regardless of whether or not a menstrual period has occurred or is still in progress. Any time the next cycle of LEVLEN® 21 Tablets is started later than the 8th day, the patient should be protected by another means of contraception until she has taken a tablet daily for seven consecutive days.

If spotting or breakthrough bleeding occurs, the patient is instructed to continue on the same regimen. This type of bleeding is usually transient and without significance; however, if the bleeding is persistent or prolonged, the patient is advised to consult her physician. Although the occurrence of pregnancy is highly unlikely if LEVLEN® 21 Tablets are taken according to directions, if withdrawal bleeding does not occur, the possibility of pregnancy must be considered. If the patient has not adhered to the prescribed schedule (missed one or more tablets or started taking them on a day later than she should have), the probability of pregnancy should be considered at the time of the first missed period and appropriate diagnostic measures taken before the medication is resumed. If the patient has adhered to the prescribed regimen and misses two consecutive periods, pregnancy should be ruled out before continuing the contraceptive regimen.

In the nonlactating mother, LEVLEN® 21 Tablets may be initiated postpartum, for contraception. When the tablets are administered in the postpartum period, the increased risk of thromboembolic disease associated with the postpartum period must be considered. (See "CONTRAINDICATIONS", "WARNINGS", and "PRECAUTIONS" concerning thromboembolic disease.)

LEVLEN® 28 Tablets

To achieve maximum contraceptive effectiveness, LEVLEN® 28 Tablets (levonorgestrel and ethinyl estradiol tablets) should be taken exactly as directed at intervals not exceeding 24-hours.

The dosage of LEVLEN® 28 Tablets is one light-orange tablet daily for 21 consecutive days per menstrual cycle, followed by 7 pink insert tablets according to the prescribed schedule.

It is recommended that LEVLEN® 28 Tablets be taken at the same time each day. During the first cycle of medication, the patient should be instructed to take one TRI-LEVLEN® 28 Tablet daily in the order of 21 light orange and then 7 pink inert tablets for twenty-eight (28) consecutive days, beginning on day one (1) of her menstrual cycle. (The first day of menstruation is day one.) Withdrawal bleeding usually occurs within 3 days following the last light-orange tablet. (If an alternate starting regimen is used [Sunday Start or postpartum], contraceptive reliance should not be placed on LEVLEN® 28 Tablets until after the first 7 consecutive days of administration. The possibility of ovulation and conception prior to initiation of medication should be considered.)

The patient begins her next and all subsequent 28-day courses of LEVLEN® 28 Tablets on the same day of the week that she began her first course, following the same schedule. She begins taking her light-orange tablets on the next day after ingestion of the last pink tablet, regardless of whether or not a menstrual period has occurred or is still in progress. Any time a subsequent cycle of LEVLEN® 28 Tablets is started later than the next day, the patient should be protected by another means of contraception until she has taken a tablet daily for seven consecutive days.

If spotting or breakthrough bleeding occurs, the patient is instructed to continue on the same regimen. This type of bleeding is usually transient and without significance; however, if the bleeding is persistent or prolonged, the patient is advised to consult her physician. Although the occurrence of pregnancy is highly unlikely if LEVLEN® 28 Tablets are taken according to directions, if withdrawal bleeding does not occur, the possibility of pregnancy must be considered. If the patient has not adhered to the prescribed schedule (missed one or more active tablets or started taking them on a day later than she should have), the probability of pregnancy should be considered at the time of the first missed period and appropriate diagnostic measures taken before the medication is resumed. If the patient has adhered to the prescribed regimen and misses two consecutive periods, pregnancy should be ruled out before continuing the contraceptive regimen.

Any time the patient misses two or more tablets, she should also use another method of contraception until she has taken a tablet daily for seven consecutive days. If breakthrough bleeding occurs following missed active tablets, it usually will be transient and of no consequence. If the patient misses one or more pink tablets, she is still protected against pregnancy provided she begins taking the light-orange tablets again on the proper day.

In the nonlactating mother, LEVLEN® 28 Tablets may be initiated postpartum, for contraception. When the tablets are administered in the postpartum period, the increased risk of thromboembolic disease associated with the postpartum period must be considered. (See "CONTRAINDICATIONS", "WARNINGS", and "PRECAUTIONS" concerning thromboembolic disease.)

HOW SUPPLIED

LEVLITE® 28 Tablets (levonorgestrel and ethinyl estradiol tablets, USP), are available in packages of 3 SLIDECASE® dispensers. Each cycle contains 28 round, unscored coated tablets as follows:

In packages of 3 SLIDECASE® dispensers, NDC 50419-408-03

Keep at room temperature, approximately 25° C (77° F).

TRI-LEVLEN® 21 tablets (Levonorgestrel and Ethinyl Estradiol Tablets—Triphasic Regimen), are available in packages of 3 and 6 SLIDECASE® dispensers. Each cycle contains 21 round, film-coated tablets as follows:

NDC 50419-195, six brown tablets marked "B" on one side and "95" on the other side, each containing 0.050 mg levonorgestrel and 0.030 mg ethinyl estradiol;

NDC 50419-196, five white to off-white tablets marked "B" on one side and "96" on the other side, each containing 0.075 mg levonorgestrel and 0.040 mg ethinyl estradiol; and

NDC 50419-197, ten light-yellow tablets marked "B" on one side and "97" on the other side, each containing 0.125 mg levonorgestrel and 0.030 mg ethinyl estradiol.

In packages of:

3 SLIDECASE® dispensers .... NDC 50419-432-03

6 SLIDECASE® dispensers .... NDC 50419-432-06

TRI-LEVLEN® 28 tablets (Levonorgestrel and Ethinyl Estradiol Tablets—Triphasic Regimen), are available in packages of 3 and 6 SLIDECASE® dispensers. Each cycle contains 28 round, film-coated tablets as follows:

NDC 50419-195, six brown tablets marked "B" on one side and "95" on the other side, each containing 0.050 mg levonorgestrel and 0.030 mg ethinyl estradiol;

NDC 50419-196, five white to off-white tablets marked "B" on one side and "96" on the other side, each containing 0.075 mg levonorgestrel and 0.040 mg ethinyl estradiol;

NDC 50419-197, ten light-yellow tablets marked "B" on one side and "97" on the other side, each containing 0.125 mg levonorgestrel and 0.030 mg ethinyl estradiol; and

NDC 50419-111, seven light-green inert tablets marked "B" on one side and "11" on the other side.

In packages of:

3 SLIDECASE® dispensers .... NDC 50419-433-03

6 SLIDECASE® dispensers .... NDC 50419-433-06

LEVLEN® 21 tablets (Levonorgestrel and Ethinyl Estradiol Tablets), are available in packages of 3 SLIDECASE® dispensers. Each cycle contains 21 round, tablets as follows:

NDC 50419-021, 21 active light-orange tablets marked "B" on one side and "21" on the other side, each containing 0.15 mg levonorgestrel and 0.03 mg ethinyl estradiol;

In packages of:

3 SLIDECASE® dispensers .... NDC 50419-410-21

LEVLEN® 28 tablets (Levonorgestrel and Ethinyl Estradiol Tablets), are available in packages of 3 SLIDECASE® dispensers. Each cycle contains 28 round tablets as follows:

NDC 50419-021, 21 active, light-orange tablets marked "B" on one side and "21" on the other side, each containing 0.15 mg levonorgestrel and 0.03 mg ethinyl estradiol;

NDC 50419-028, 7 inert pink tablets marked "B" on one side and "28" on the other side.

In packages of:

3 SLIDECASE® dispensers .... NDC 50419-411-28

REFERENCES

REFERENCES furnished upon request.

BRIEF SUMMARY PATIENT PACKAGE INSERT

This product (like all oral contraceptives) is intended to prevent pregnancy. It does not protect against HIV infection (AIDS) and other sexually transmitted diseases.

Oral contraceptives, also known as "birth-control pills" or "the pill", are taken to prevent pregnancy, and when taken correctly, have a failure rate of less than 1% per year when used without missing any pills. The typical failure rate of large numbers of pill users is less than 3% per year when women who miss pills are included. For most women oral contraceptives are also free of serious or unpleasant side effects. However, forgetting to take pills considerably increases the chances of pregnancy.

For the majority of women, oral contraceptives can be taken safely. But there are some women who are at high risk of developing certain serious diseases that can be life-threatening or may cause temporary or permanent disability or death. The risks associated with taking oral contraceptives increase significantly if you:

- smoke
- have high blood pressure, diabetes, high cholesterol
- have or have had clotting disorders, heart attack, stroke, angina pectoris, cancer of the breast or sex organs, jaundice, or malignant or benign liver tumors.

You should not take the pill if you suspect you are pregnant or have unexplained vaginal bleeding.

Cigarette smoking increases the risk of serious adverse effects on the heart and blood vessels from oral-contraceptive use. This risk increases with age and with heavy smoking (15 or more cigarettes per day) and is quite marked in women over 35 years of age. Women who use oral contraceptives should not smoke.

Most side effects of the pill are not serious. The most common side effects are nausea, vomiting, bleeding between menstrual periods, weight gain, breast tenderness, and difficulty wearing contact lenses. These side effects, especially nausea and vomiting may subside within the first three months of use.

The serious side effects of the pill occur very infrequently, especially if you are in good health and are young. However, you should know that the following medical conditions have been associated with or made worse by the pill:

1. Blood clots in the legs (thrombophlebitis), lungs (pulmonary embolism), stoppage or rupture of a blood vessel in the brain (stroke), blockage of blood vessels in the heart (heart attack and angina pectoris) or other organs of the body. As mentioned above, smoking increases the risk of heart attacks and strokes and subsequent serious medical consequences.
2. Liver tumors, which may rupture and cause severe bleeding. A possible but not definite association has been found with the pill and liver cancer. However, liver cancers are extremely rare. The chance of developing liver cancer from using the pill is thus even rarer.
3. High blood pressure, although blood pressure usually returns to normal when the pill is stopped.

The symptoms associated with these serious side effects are discussed in the detailed leaflet given to you with your supply of pills. Notify your doctor or healthcare provider if you notice any unusual physical disturbances while taking the pill. In addition, drugs such as rifampin, as well as some anticonvulsants and some antibiotics, may decrease oral contraceptive effectiveness.

Studies to date of women taking the pill have not shown an increase in the incidence of cancer of the breast or cervix. There is, however, insufficient evidence to rule out the possibility that pills may cause such cancers.

Continued on next page

Information on Berlex products (appearing here) is based on the most current information available at the time of publication closing. Further information for these and other Berlex products can be obtained from Medical & Product Services at Berlex, Inc. by calling 1-888-BERLEX-4.

Levlite/Tri-Levlen/Levlen—Cont.

Taking the pill provides some important noncontraceptive benefits. These include less painful menstruation, less menstrual blood loss and anemia, fewer pelvic infections, and fewer cancers of the ovary and the lining of the uterus.
Be sure to discuss any medical condition you may have with your healthcare provider. Your healthcare provider will take a medical and family history before prescribing oral contraceptives and will examine you. The physical examination may be delayed to another time if you request it and the healthcare provider believes that it is appropriate to postpone it.
You should be reexamined at least once a year while taking oral contraceptives. The detailed patient information booklet gives you further information which you should read and discuss with your healthcare provider.

DETAILED PATIENT PACKAGE INSERT

This product (like all oral contraceptives) is intended to prevent pregnancy. It does not protect against HIV infection (AIDS) and other sexually transmitted diseases.

INTRODUCTION

Any woman who considers using oral contraceptives (the "birth control pill" or the "pill") should understand the benefits and risks of using this form of birth control. This leaflet will give you much of the information you will need to make this decision and will also help you determine if you are at risk of developing any of the serious side effects of the pill. It will tell you how to use the pill properly so that it will be as effective as possible. However, this leaflet is not a replacement for a careful discussion between you and your healthcare provider. You should discuss the information provided in this leaflet with him or her, both when you first start taking the pill and during your revisits. You should also follow your healthcare provider's advice with regard to regular checks-ups while you are on the pill.

EFFECTIVENESS OF ORAL CONTRACEPTIVES

Oral contraceptives or "birth control pills" or "the pill" are used to prevent pregnancy and are more effective than other nonsurgical methods of birth control. When they are taken correctly, the chance of becoming pregnant is less than 1% when used perfectly, without missing pills. Typical failure rates are less than 3.0% per year. The chance of becoming pregnant increases with each missed pill during the menstrual cycle.
In comparison, typical failure rates for other nonsurgical methods of birth control during the first year of use are as follows:
[See first table below]

WHO SHOULD NOT TAKE ORAL CONTRACEPTIVES

Cigarette smoking increases the risk of serious adverse effects on the heart and blood vessels from oral-contraceptive use. This risk increases with age and with heavy smoking (15 or more cigarettes per day) and is quite marked in women over 35 years of age. Women who use oral contraceptives should not smoke.

Some women should not use the pill. For example, you should not take the pill if you are pregnant or think you may be pregnant. You should also not use the pill if you have had any of the following conditions:

- A history of heart attack or stroke
- Blood clots in the legs (thrombophlebitis), lungs (pulmonary embolism), or eyes
- A history of blood clots in the deep veins of your legs
- Chest pain (angina pectoris)
- Known or suspected breast cancer or cancer of the lining of the uterus, cervix or vagina
- Unexplained vaginal bleeding (until a diagnosis is reached by your doctor)
- Yellowing of the whites of the eyes or of the skin (jaundice) during pregnancy or during previous use of the pill
- Liver tumor (benign or cancerous)
- Known or suspected pregnancy

Tell your health-care provider if you have ever had any of these conditions. Your healthcare provider can recommend another method of birth control.

OTHER CONSIDERATIONS BEFORE TAKING ORAL CONTRACEPTIVES

Tell your healthcare provider if you or any family member has ever had:

- Breast nodules, fibrocystic disease of the breast, an abnormal breast x-ray or mammogram
- Diabetes
- Elevated cholesterol or triglycerides
- High blood pressure
- Migraine or other headaches or epilepsy
- Mental depression
- Gallbladder, heart or kidney disease
- History of scanty or irregular menstrual periods

Women with any of these conditions should be checked often by their healthcare provider if they choose to use oral contraceptives. Also, be sure to inform your doctor or healthcare provider if you smoke or are on any medications.

RISKS OF TAKING ORAL CONTRACEPTIVES

1. RISK OF DEVELOPING BLOOD CLOTS

Blood clots and blockage of blood vessels are the most serious side effects of taking oral contraceptives and can be fatal. In particular, a clot in the legs can cause thrombophlebitis and a clot that travels to the lungs can cause a sudden blocking of the vessel carrying blood to the lungs. Rarely, clots occur in the blood vessels of the eye and may cause blindness, double vision, or impaired vision.
If you take oral contraceptives and need elective surgery, need to stay in bed for a prolonged illness or have recently delivered a baby, you may be at risk of developing blood clots. You should consult your doctor about stopping oral contraceptives three to four weeks before surgery and not taking oral contraceptives for 2 weeks after surgery or during bed rest. You should also not take oral contraceptives soon after delivery of a baby or a midtrimester pregnancy termination. It is advisable to wait for at least 4 weeks after delivery if you are not breast-feeding. If you are breast-feeding, you should wait until you have weaned your child before using the pill. (See also the section on Breast-Feeding in "GENERAL PRECAUTIONS".)

2. HEART ATTACKS AND STROKES

Oral contraceptives may increase the tendency to develop strokes (stoppage or rupture of blood vessels in the brain) and angina pectoris and heart attacks (blockage of blood vessels in the heart). Any of these conditions can cause death or serious disability.
Smoking greatly increases the possibility of suffering heart attacks and strokes. Furthermore, smoking and the use of oral contraceptives greatly increase the chances of developing and dying of heart disease.

3. GALLBLADDER DISEASE

Oral-contraceptive users probably have a greater risk than nonusers of having gallbladder disease, although this risk may be related to pills containing high doses of estrogens.

4. LIVER TUMORS

In rare cases, oral contraceptives can cause benign but dangerous liver tumors. These benign liver tumors can rupture and cause fatal internal bleeding. In addition, a possible but not definite association has been found with the pill and liver cancers in two studies, in which a few women who developed these very rare cancers were found to have used oral contraceptives for long periods. However, liver cancers are extremely rare. The chance of developing liver cancer from using the pill is thus even rarer.

5. CANCER OF THE REPRODUCTIVE ORGANS

There is, at present, no confirmed evidence that oral contraceptives increase the risk of cancer of the reproductive organs in human studies. Several studies have found no overall increase in the risk of developing breast cancer. However, women who use oral contraceptives and have a strong family history of breast cancer or who have breast nodules or abnormal mammograms should be closely followed by their doctors.

Percentage of women experiencing an unintended pregnancy during the first year of typical use and first year of perfect use of contraception and the percentage continuing use at the end of the first year. United States.

	% of Women Experiencing an Accidental Pregnancy within the First Year of Use		% of Women Continuing Use at One Year[3]
Method (1)	Typical Use[1] (2)	Perfect Use[2] (3)	(4)
Chance[4]	85	85	
Spermicides[5]	26	6	40
Periodic abstinence	25		63
Calendar		9	
Ovulation method		3	
Sympto-thermal[6]		2	
Post Ovulation		1	
Withdrawal	19	4	
Cap[7]			
Parous women	40	26	42
Nulliparous women	20	9	56
Sponge			
Parous women	40	20	42
Nulliparous women	20	9	56
Diaphragm[7]	20	6	56
Condom[8]			
Female (Reality)	21	5	56
Male	14	3	61
Pill	5		71
progestin only		0.5	
combined		0.1	
IUD			
Progesterone T	2	1.5	81
Copper T 380A	0.8	0.6	78
Lng 20	0.1	0.1	81
Depo Provera	0.3	0.3	70
Norplant and Norplant-2	0.05	0.05	88
Female sterilization	0.5	0.5	100
Male sterilization	0.15	0.10	100

Source: Trussell J, Contraceptive efficacy. In Hatcher RA, Trussell J, Stewart F, Cates W, Stewart GK, Kowal D, Guest F, *Contraceptive Technology: Seventeenth Revised Edition*. New York NY: Irvington Publishers, 1998, in press.
1 Among *typical* couples who initiate use of a method (not necessarily for the first time), the percentage who experience an accidental pregnancy during the first year if they do not stop use for any other reason.
2 Among couples who initiate use of a method (not necessarily for the first time) and who use it *perfectly* (both consistently and correctly), the percentage who experience an accidental pregnancy during the first year if they do not stop use for any other reason.
3 Among couples attempting to avoid pregnancy, the percentage who continue to use a method for one year.
4 The percentages becoming pregnant in columns (2) and (3) are based on data from populations where contraception is not used and from women who cease using contraception in order to become pregnant. Among such populations, about 89% become pregnant within one year. This estimate was lowered slightly (to 85%) to represent the percentage who would become pregnant within one year among women now relying on reversible methods of contraception if they abandoned contraception altogether.
5 Foams, creams, gels, vaginal suppositories, vaginal film.
6 Cervical mucus (ovulation) method supplemented by calendar in the pre-ovulatory and basal body temperature in the post-ovulatory phases.
7 With spermicidal cream or jelly.
8 Without spermicides.

TABLE V. ANNUAL NUMBER OF BIRTH-RELATED OR METHOD-RELATED DEATHS ASSOCIATED WITH CONTROL OF FERTILITY PER 100,000 NONSTERILE WOMEN, BY FERTILITY-CONTROL METHOD ACCORDING TO AGE

Method of control and outcome	15–19	20–24	25–29	30–34	35–39	40–44
No fertility—control methods*	7.0	7.4	9.1	14.8	25.7	28.2
Oral contraceptives-nonsmoker**	0.3	0.5	0.9	1.9	13.8	31.6
Oral contraceptives-smoker**	2.2	3.4	6.6	13.5	51.1	117.2
IUD**	0.8	0.8	1.0	1.0	1.4	1.4
Condom*	1.1	1.6	0.7	0.2	0.3	0.4
Diaphragm/spermicide*	1.9	1.2	1.2	1.3	2.2	2.8
Periodic abstinence*	2.5	1.6	1.6	1.7	2.9	3.6

* Deaths are birth related
** Deaths are method related

Adapted from H.W. Ory, Family Planning Perspectives *15*:57–63, 1983.

Some studies have found an increase in the incidence of cancer of the cervix in women who use oral contraceptives. However, this finding may be related to factors other than the use of oral contraceptives.

[See table V at bottom of previous page]

In the above table, the risk of death from any birth-control method is less than the risk of childbirth, except for oral contraceptive users over the age of 35 who smoke and pill users over the age of 40 even if they do not smoke. It can be seen in the table that for women aged 15 to 39, the risk of death is highest with pregnancy (7 to 26 deaths per 100,000 women, depending on age). Among pill users who do not smoke, the risk of death was always lower than that associated with pregnancy for any age group, except for those women over the age of 40 when the risk increases to 32 deaths per 100,000 women, compared to 28 associated with pregnancy at that age. However, for pill users who smoke and are over the age of 35, the estimated number of deaths exceeds those for other methods of birth control. If a woman is over the age of 40 and smokes, her estimated risk of death is four times higher (117/100,000 women) than the estimated risk associated with pregnancy (28/100,000 women) in that age group.

The suggestion that women over 40 who don't smoke should not take oral contraceptives is based on information from older high-dose pills and on less-selective use of pills than is practiced today. An Advisory Committee of the FDA discussed this issue in 1989 and recommended that the benefits of oral-contraceptive use by healthy, nonsmoking women over 40 years of age may outweigh the possible risks. However, all women, especially older women, are cautioned to use the lowest-dose pill that is effective.

WARNING SIGNALS

If any of these adverse effects occur while you are taking oral contraceptives, call your doctor immediately:

- Sharp chest pain, coughing of blood, or sudden shortness of breath (indicating a possible clot in the lung).
- Pain in the calf (indicating a possible clot in the leg).
- Crushing chest pain or heaviness in the chest (indicating a possible heart attack).
- Sudden severe headache or vomiting, dizziness or fainting, disturbances of vision or speech, weakness, or numbness in an arm or leg (indicating a possible stroke).
- Sudden partial or complete loss of vision (indicating a possible clot in the eye).
- Breast lumps (indicating possible breast cancer or fibrocystic disease of the breast; ask your doctor or healthcare provider to show you how to examine your breasts).
- Severe pain or tenderness in the stomach area (indicating a possibly ruptured liver tumor).
- Difficulty in sleeping, weakness, lack of energy, fatigue, or change in mood (possibly indicating severe depression).
- Jaundice or a yellowing of the skin or eyeballs, accompanied frequently by fever, fatigue, loss of appetite, dark-colored urine, or light-colored bowel movements (indicating possible liver problems).

SIDE EFFECTS OF ORAL CONTRACEPTIVES

1. VAGINAL BLEEDING

Irregular vaginal bleeding or spotting may occur while you are taking the pills. Irregular bleeding may vary from slight staining between menstrual periods to breakthrough bleeding which is a flow much like a regular period. Irregular bleeding occurs most often during the first few months of oral contraceptive use, but may also occur after you have been taking the pill for some time. Such bleeding may be temporary and usually does not indicate any serious problems. It is important to continue taking your pills on schedule. If the bleeding occurs in more than one cycle or lasts for more than a few days, talk to your doctor or healthcare provider.

2. CONTACT LENSES

If you wear contact lenses and notice a change in vision or an inability to wear your lenses, contact your doctor or healthcare provider.

3. FLUID RETENTION

Oral contraceptives may cause edema (fluid retention) with swelling of the fingers or ankles and may raise your blood pressure. If you experience fluid retention, contact your doctor or healthcare provider.

4. MELASMA

A spotty darkening of the skin is possible, particularly of the face.

5. OTHER SIDE EFFECTS

Other side effects may include change in appetite, headache, nervousness, depression, dizziness, loss of scalp hair, rash, and vaginal infections.

If any of these side effects bother you, call your doctor or healthcare provider.

GENERAL PRECAUTIONS

1. Missed periods and use of oral contraceptives before or during early pregnancy.

There may be times when you may not menstruate regularly after you have completed taking a cycle of pills. If you have taken your pills regularly and miss one menstrual period, continue taking your pills for the next cycle but be sure to inform your healthcare provider before doing so. If you have not taken the pills daily as instructed and missed a menstrual period, or if you missed two consecutive menstrual periods, you may be pregnant. Check with your healthcare provider immediately to determine whether you are pregnant. Do not continue to take oral contraceptives until you are sure you are not pregnant, but continue to use another method of contraception.

There is no conclusive evidence that oral contraceptive use is associated with an increase in birth defects when taken inadvertently during early pregnancy. Previously, a few studies had reported that oral contraceptives might be associated with birth defects, but these studies have not been confirmed. Nevertheless, oral contraceptives or any other drugs should not be used during pregnancy unless clearly necessary and prescribed by your doctor. You should check with your doctor about risks to your unborn child of any medication taken during pregnancy.

2. While breast-feeding

If you are breast-feeding, consult your doctor before starting oral contraceptives. Some of the drug will be passed on to the child in the milk. A few adverse effects on the child have been reported, including yellowing of the skin (jaundice) and breast enlargement. In addition, oral contraceptives may decrease the amount and quality of your milk. If possible, do not use oral contraceptives while breast-feeding. You should use another method of contraception since breast-feeding provides only partial protection from becoming pregnant and this partial protection decreases significantly as you breast-feed for longer periods of time. You should consider starting oral contraceptives only after you have weaned your child completely.

3. Laboratory tests

If you are scheduled for any laboratory tests, tell your doctor you are taking birth-control pills. Certain blood tests may be affected by birth-control pills.

4. Drug interactions

Certain drugs may interact with birth control pills to make them less effective in preventing pregnancy or cause an increase in breakthrough bleeding. Such drugs include rifampin, drugs used for epilepsy such as barbiturates (for example, phenobarbital) and phenytoin (Dilantin is one brand of this drug), phenylbutazone (Butazolidin is one brand) and possibly certain antibiotics. You may need to use an additional method of contraception during any cycle in which you take drugs that can make oral contraceptives less effective.

5. Sexually transmitted diseases

This product (like all oral contraceptives) is intended to prevent pregnancy. It does not protect against transmission of HIV (AIDS) and other sexually transmitted diseases such as chlamydia, genital herpes, genital warts, gonorrhea, hepatitis B, and syphilis.

HOW TO TAKE THE PILL

IMPORTANT POINTS TO REMEMBER

LEVLITE®, TRI-LEVLEN® and LEVLEN® Tablets
BEFORE YOU START TAKING YOUR PILLS:

1. BE SURE TO READ THESE DIRECTIONS:
   Before you start taking your pills.
   Anytime you are not sure what to do.
2. THE RIGHT WAY TO TAKE THE PILL IS TO TAKE ONE PILL EVERY DAY AT THE SAME TIME.
   If you miss pills you could get pregnant. This includes starting the pack late. The more pills you miss, the more likely you are to get pregnant.
3. MANY WOMEN HAVE SPOTTING OR LIGHT BLEEDING, OR MAY FEEL SICK TO THEIR STOMACH DURING THE FIRST 1–3 PACKS OF PILLS.
   If you do feel sick to your stomach, do not stop taking the pill. The problem will usually go away. If it doesn't go away, check with your doctor or clinic.
4. MISSING PILLS CAN ALSO CAUSE SPOTTING OR LIGHT BLEEDING, even when you make up these missed pills.
   On the days you take two pills, to make up for missed pills, you could also feel a little sick to your stomach.
5. IF YOU HAVE VOMITING OR DIARRHEA, for any reason, or IF YOU TAKE SOME MEDICINES, including some antibiotics, your pills may not work as well.
   Use a back-up method (such as condoms, foam, or sponge) until you check with your doctor or clinic.
6. IF YOU HAVE TROUBLE REMEMBERING TO TAKE THE PILL, talk to your doctor or clinic about how to make pill-taking easier or about using another method of birth control.
7. IF YOU HAVE ANY QUESTIONS OR ARE UNSURE ABOUT THE INFORMATION IN THIS LEAFLET, call your doctor or clinic.

BEFORE YOU START TAKING YOUR PILLS

LEVLITE® Tablets

1. DECIDE WHAT TIME OF DAY YOU WANT TO TAKE YOUR PILL.
   It is important to take it at about the same time every day.
2. LOOK AT YOUR PILL PACK.
   The *28-pill* pack has 21 (pink) "active" pills (with hormones) to take for three weeks, followed by 1 week of reminder pills (white) (without hormones).
3. ALSO FIND:
   1) where on the pack to start taking pills,
   2) in what order to take the pills (follow the arrows)
   [See figure at top of next column]
4. BE SURE YOU HAVE READY AT ALL TIMES:
   ANOTHER KIND OF BIRTH CONTROL (such as condoms, foam or sponge) to use as a back-up in case you miss pills.
   AN EXTRA, FULL PILL PACK.

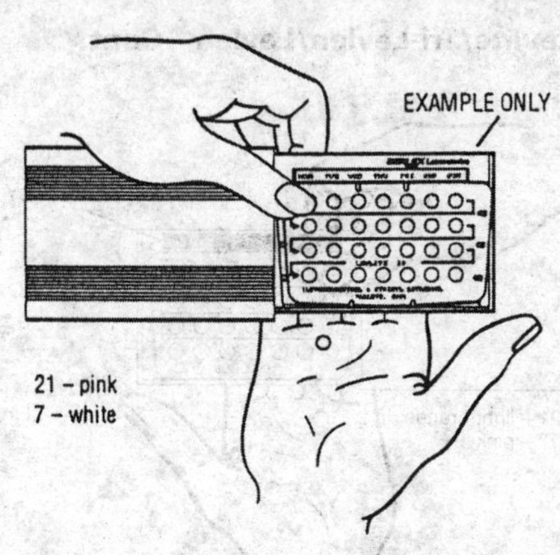

TRI-LEVLEN® Tablets

1. DECIDE WHAT TIME OF DAY YOU WANT TO TAKE YOUR PILL.
   It is important to take it at about the same time every day.
2. LOOK AT YOUR PILL PACK TO SEE IF IT HAS 21 OR 28 PILLS:
   The 21-pill pack has 21 "active" (6 brown, 5 white and 10 light-yellow) pills (with hormones) to take for 3 weeks, followed by 1 week without pills.
   The 28-pill pack has 21 "active" (6 brown, 5 white and 10 light yellow) pills (with hormones) to take for 3 weeks, followed by 1 week of reminder (light-green) pills (without hormones).
3. ALSO FIND:
   1) where on the pack to start taking pills.
   2) in what order to take the pills (follow the arrows)

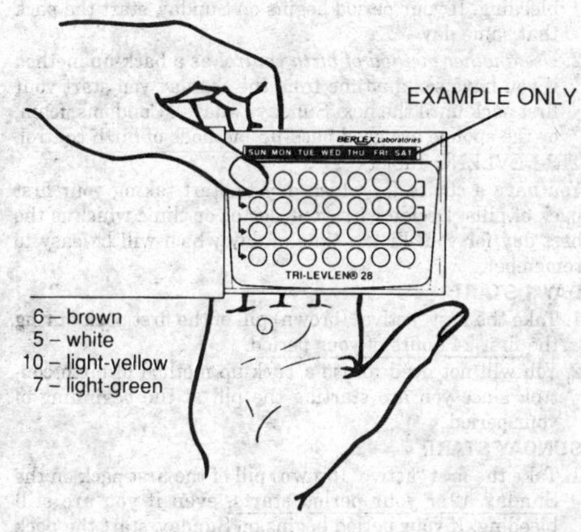

4. BE SURE YOU HAVE READY AT ALL TIMES:
   ANOTHER KIND OF BIRTH CONTROL (such as condoms, foam or sponge) to use as a back-up in case you miss pills.
   AN EXTRA, FULL PILL PACK.

LEVLEN® Tablets

1. DECIDE WHAT TIME OF DAY YOU WANT TO TAKE YOUR PILL.
   It is important to take it at about the same time every day.
2. LOOK AT YOUR PILL PACK TO SEE IF IT HAS 21 OR 28 PILLS:
   The 21-pill pack has 21 "active" (light-orange) pills (with hormones) to take for 3 weeks, followed by 1 week without pills.
   The 28-pill pack has 21 "active" (light-orange) pills (with hormones) to take for 3 weeks, followed by 1 week of reminder (pink) pills (without hormones).
3. ALSO FIND:
   1) where on the pack to start taking pills.
   2) in what order to take the pills (follow the arrows).
   [See figure at top of next column]
4. BE SURE YOU HAVE READY AT ALL TIMES:
   ANOTHER KIND OF BIRTH CONTROL (such as condoms, foam or sponge) to use as a back-up in case you miss pills.
   AN EXTRA, FULL PILL PACK.

Continued on next page

Information on Berlex products (appearing here) is based on the most current information available at the time of publication closing. Further information for these and other Berlex products can be obtained from Medical & Product Services at Berlex, Inc. by calling 1-888-BERLEX-4.

Levlite/Tri-Levlen/Levlen—Cont.

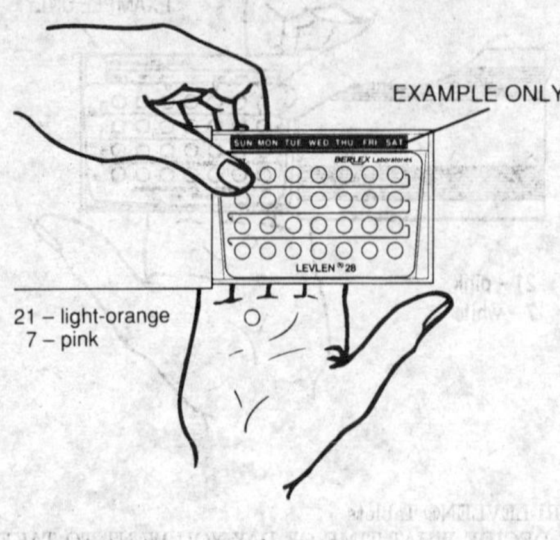

WHEN TO START THE FIRST PACK OF PILLS

LEVLITE® Tablets
You have a choice for which day to start taking your first pack of pills. Decide with your doctor or clinic which is the best day for you. Pick a time of day which will be easy to remember.

DAY 1 START:
1. Take the first (pink) "active" pill of the first pack during the *first 24 hours of your period.*
2. You will not need to use a back-up method of birth control, since you are starting the pill at the beginning of your period.

SUNDAY START:
1. Take the first (pink) "active" pill of the first pack on the *Sunday after your period starts,* even if you are still bleeding. If your period begins on Sunday, start the pack that same day.
2. *Use another method of birth control* as a back-up method if you have sex anytime from the Sunday you start your first pack until the next Sunday (7 days). Condoms, foam, or the sponge are good back-up methods of birth control.

TRI-LEVLEN® Tablets
You have a choice for which day to start taking your first pack of pills. Decide with your doctor or clinic which is the best day for you. Pick a time of day which will be easy to remember.

DAY 1 START:
1. Take the first "active" (brown) pill of the first pack during the first 24 hours of your period.
2. You will not need to use a back-up method of birth control, since you are starting the pill at the beginning of your period.

SUNDAY START:
1. Take the first "active" (brown) pill of the first pack on the Sunday after your period starts, even if you are still bleeding. If your period begins on Sunday, start the pack that same day.
2. Use another method of birth control as a back-up method if you have sex anytime from the Sunday you start your first pack until the next Sunday (7 days). Condoms, foam, or the sponge are good back-up methods of birth control.

LEVLEN® Tablets
You have a choice for which day to start taking your first pack of pills. Decide with your doctor or clinic which is the best day for you. Pick a time of day which will be easy to remember.

DAY 1 START:
1. Take the first "active" (light-orange) pill of the first pack during the first 24 hours of your period.
2. You will not need to use a back-up method of birth control, since you are starting the pill at the beginning of your period.

SUNDAY START:
1. Take the first "active" (light-orange) pill of the first pack on the Sunday after your period starts, even if you are still bleeding. If your period begins on Sunday, start the pack that same day.
2. Use another method of birth control as a back-up method if you have sex anytime from the Sunday you start your first pack until the next Sunday (7 days). Condoms, foam, or the sponge are good back-up methods of birth control.

WHAT TO DO DURING THE MONTH

LEVLITE®, TRI-LEVLEN® and LEVLEN® Tablets
1. **TAKE ONE PILL AT THE SAME TIME EVERY DAY UNTIL THE PACK IS EMPTY**

Do not skip pills even if you are spotting or bleeding between monthly periods or feel sick to your stomach (nausea).
Do not skip pills even if you do not have sex very often.

2. **WHEN YOU FINISH A PACK OR SWITCH YOUR BRAND OF PILLS:**
28 pills: Start the next pack on the day after your last "reminder" pill. Do not wait any days between packs.

WHAT TO DO IF YOU MISS PILLS

LEVLITE® Tablets
If you **MISS 1** (pink) "active" pill:
1. Take it as soon as you remember. Take the next pill at your regular time. This means you may take two pills in one day.
2. You do not need to use a back-up birth control method if you have sex.

If you **MISS 2** (pink) "active" pills in a row in **WEEK 1 OR WEEK 2** of your pack:
1. Take two pills on the day you remember and two pills the next day.
2. Then take one pill a day until you finish the pack.
3. You MAY BECOME PREGNANT if you have sex in the 7 days after you miss pills. You MUST use another birth control method (such as condoms, foam, or sponge) as a back-up for those 7 days.

If you **MISS 2** (pink) "active" pills in a row in **THE 3rd WEEK:**
1. **If you are a Day 1 Starter:**
THROW OUT the rest of the pill pack and start a new pack that same day.
If you are a Sunday Starter:
Keep taking one pill every day until Sunday. On Sunday, THROW OUT the rest of the pack and start a new pack of pills that same day.
2. You may not have your period this month but this is expected. However, if you miss your period two months in a row, call your doctor or clinic because you might be pregnant.
3. You MAY BECOME PREGNANT if you have sex in the 7 days after you miss pills. You MUST use another birth control method (such as condoms, foam, or sponge) as a back-up for those 7 days.

If you **MISS 3 OR MORE** (pink) "active" pills in a row (during the first 3 weeks).
1. **If you are a Day 1 Starter:**
THROW OUT the rest of the pill pack and start a new pack that same day.
If you are a Sunday Starter:
Keep taking 1 pill every day until Sunday. On Sunday, THROW OUT the rest of the pack and start a new pack of pills that same day.
2. You may not have your period this month but this is expected. However, if you miss your period two months in a row, call your doctor or clinic because you might be pregnant.
3. You MAY BECOME PREGNANT if you have sex in the 7 days after you miss pills. You MUST use another birth control method (such as condoms, foam, or sponge) as a back-up for those 7 days.

A REMINDER FOR THOSE ON 28-DAY PACKS:
If you forget any of the 7 (white) "reminder" pills in Week 4:
THROW AWAY the pills you missed.
Keep taking one pill each day until the pack is empty.
You do not need a back-up method.

FINALLY, IF YOU ARE STILL NOT SURE WHAT TO DO ABOUT THE PILLS YOU HAVE MISSED:
Use a BACK-UP METHOD anytime you have sex.
KEEP TAKING ONE ACTIVE PILL EACH DAY until you can reach your doctor or clinic.

TRI-LEVLEN® Tablets
If you **MISS 1** (brown, white or light yellow) "active" pill:
1. Take it as soon as you remember. Take the next pill at your regular time. This means you may take 2 pills in 1 day.
2. You do not need to use a back-up birth control method if you have sex.

If you **MISS 2** (brown or white) "active" pills in a row in **WEEK 1 OR WEEK 2** of your pack:
1. Take 2 pills on the day you remember and 2 pills the next day.
2. Then take 1 pill a day until you finish the pack.
3. YOU MAY BECOME PREGNANT if you have sex in the 7 days after you miss pills. You MUST use another birth control method (such as condoms, foam, or sponge) as a back-up for those 7 days.

If you **MISS 2** (light-yellow) "active" pills in a row in **THE 3rd WEEK:**
1. ***If you are a Day 1 Starter:***
THROW OUT the rest of the pill pack and start a new pack that same day.
If you are a Sunday Starter:
Keep taking 1 pill every day until Sunday. On Sunday, THROW OUT the rest of the pack and start a new pack of pills that same day.
2. You may not have your period this month but this is expected. However, if you miss your period 2 months in a row, call your doctor or clinic because you might be pregnant.
3. You MAY BECOME PREGNANT if you have sex in the 7 days after you miss pills. You MUST use another birth control method (such as condoms, foam, or sponge) as a back-up for those 7 days.

If you **MISS 3 OR MORE** (brown, white or light-yellow) "active" pills in a row (during the first 3 weeks).
1. ***If you are a Day 1 Starter:***
THROW OUT the rest of the pill pack and start a new pack that same day.
If you are a Sunday Starter:
Keep taking 1 pill every day until Sunday. On Sunday, THROW OUT the rest of the pack and start a new pack of pills that same day.
2. You may not have your period this month but this is expected. However, if you miss your period 2 months in a row, call your doctor or clinic because you might be pregnant.
3. You MAY BECOME PREGNANT if you have sex in the 7 days after you miss pills. You MUST use another birth control method (such as condoms, foam, or sponge) as a back-up for those 7 days.

A REMINDER FOR THOSE ON 28-DAY PACKS:
If you forget any of the 7 (light-green) "reminder" pills in Week 4:
THROW AWAY the pills you missed.
Keep taking 1 pill each day until the pack is empty.
You do not need a back-up method if you start your next pack on time.

FINALLY, IF YOU ARE STILL NOT SURE WHAT TO DO ABOUT THE PILLS YOU HAVE MISSED:
Use a BACK-UP METHOD anytime you have sex.
KEEP TAKING ONE "ACTIVE" PILL EACH DAY until you can reach your doctor or clinic.

LEVLEN® Tablets
If you **MISS 1** (light-orange) "active" pill:
1. Take it as soon as you remember. Take the next pill at your regular time. This means you may take 2 pills in 1 day.
2. You do not need to use a back-up birth control method if you have sex.

If you **MISS 2** (light-orange) "active" pills in a row in **WEEK 1 OR WEEK 2** of your pack:
1. Take 2 pills on the day you remember and 2 pills the next day.
2. Then take 1 pill a day until you finish the pack.
3. You MAY BECOME PREGNANT if you have sex in the 7 days after you miss pills. You MUST use another birth control method (such as condoms, foam, or sponge) as a back-up for those 7 days.

If you **MISS 2** (light-orange) "active" pills in a row in **THE 3rd WEEK:**
1. ***If you are a Day 1 Starter:***
THROW OUT the rest of the pill pack and start a new pack that same day.
If you are a Sunday Starter:
Keep taking 1 pill every day until Sunday. On Sunday, THROW OUT the rest of the pack and start a new pack of pills that same day.
2. You may not have your period this month but this is expected. However, if you miss your period 2 months in a row, call your doctor or clinic because you might be pregnant.
3. You MAY BECOME PREGNANT if you have sex in the 7 days after you miss pills. You MUST use another birth control method (such as condoms, foam, or sponge) as a back-up for those 7 days.

If you **MISS 3 OR MORE** (light-orange) "active" pills in a row (during the first 3 weeks).
1. ***If you are a Day 1 Starter:***
THROW OUT the rest of the pill pack and start a new pack that same day.
If you are a Sunday Starter:
Keep taking 1 pill every day until Sunday. On Sunday, THROW OUT the rest of the pack and start a new pack of pills that same day.
2. You may not have your period this month but this is expected. However, if you miss your period 2 months in a row, call your doctor or clinic because you might be pregnant.
3. You MAY BECOME PREGNANT if you have sex in the 7 days after you miss pills. You MUST use another birth control method (such as condoms, foam, or sponge) as a back-up for those 7 days.

A REMINDER FOR THOSE ON 28-DAY PACKS:
If you forget any of the 7 (pink) "reminder" pills in Week 4:
THROW AWAY the pills you missed.
Keep taking 1 pill each day until the pack is empty.
You do not need a back-up method if you start your next pack on time.

FINALLY, IF YOU ARE STILL NOT SURE WHAT TO DO ABOUT THE PILLS YOU HAVE MISSED:
Use a BACK-UP METHOD anytime you have sex.
KEEP TAKING ONE "ACTIVE" PILL EACH DAY until you can reach your doctor or clinic.

PREGNANCY DUE TO PILL FAILURE
The incidence of pill failure resulting in pregnancy is approximately less than 1.0% if taken every day as directed, but more typical failure rates are less than 3.0%. If failure does occur, the risk to the fetus is minimal.
RISKS TO THE FETUS
If you do become pregnant while using oral contraceptives, the risk to the fetus is small, on the order of no more than one per thousand. You should, however, discuss the risks to the developing child with your doctor.
PREGNANCY AFTER STOPPING THE PILL
There may be some delay in becoming pregnant after you stop using oral contraceptives, especially if you had irregular menstrual cycles before you used oral contraceptives. It

may be advisable to postpone conception until you begin menstruating regularly once you have stopped taking the pill and desire pregnancy.
There does not appear to be any increase in birth defects in newborn babies when pregnancy occurs soon after stopping the pill.
OVERDOSAGE
Serious ill effects have not been reported following ingestion of large doses of oral contraceptives by young children. Overdosage may cause nausea and withdrawal bleeding in females. In case of overdosage, contact your healthcare provider or pharmacist.
OTHER INFORMATION
Your healthcare provider will take a medical and family history before prescribing oral contraceptives and will examine you. You should be re-examined at least once a year. Be sure to inform your healthcare provider if there is a family history of any of the conditions listed previously in this leaflet. Be sure to keep all appointments with your healthcare provider, because this is a time to determine if there are early signs of side effects of oral contraceptive use. Do not use the drug for any condition other than the one for which it was prescribed. This drug has been prescribed specifically for you; do not give it to others who may want birth-control pills.

HEALTH BENEFITS FROM ORAL CONTRACEPTIVES

In addition to preventing pregnancy, use of oral contraceptives may provide certain benefits. They are:

- Menstrual cycles may become more regular.
- Blood flow during menstruation may be lighter and less iron may be lost. Therefore, anemia due to iron deficiency is less likely to occur.
- Pain or other symptoms during menstruation may be encountered less frequently.
- Ovarian cysts may occur less frequently.
- Ectopic (tubal) pregnancy may occur less frequently.
- Noncancerous cysts or lumps in the breast may occur less frequently.
- Acute pelvic inflammatory disease may occur less frequently.
- Oral contraceptive use may provide some protection against developing two forms of cancer: cancer of the ovaries and cancer of the lining of the uterus.

If you want more information about birth-control pills, ask your doctor or pharmacist. They have a more technical leaflet called the Prescribing Information which you may wish to read.

Manufactured in Germany
Manufactured for:
BERLEX Laboratories, Wayne, NJ 07470
Revised Jan. 2001 6070002
Revised Feb. 2001 6071903
Revised Sept. 1996 6065802

Shown in Product Identification Guide, page 308

MENOSTAR™ ℞

[*men-ō-star*]
(estradiol transdermal system)
Rx only

PRESCRIBING INFORMATION
Menostar™ (estradiol transdermal system)

ESTROGENS INCREASE THE RISK OF ENDOMETRIAL CANCER

Close clinical surveillance of all women taking estrogens is important. Adequate diagnostic measures, including endometrial sampling when indicated, should be undertaken to rule out malignancy in all cases of undiagnosed persistent or recurring abnormal vaginal bleeding. There is no evidence that the use of "natural" estrogens results in a different endometrial risk profile than synthetic estrogens at equivalent estrogen doses. (See **WARNINGS, Malignant neoplasms, Endometrial cancer.**)

CARDIOVASCULAR AND OTHER RISKS

Estrogens with and without progestins should not be used for the prevention of cardiovascular disease. (See **WARNINGS, Cardiovascular disorders.**)
The Women's Health Initiative (WHI) study reported increased risks of myocardial infarction, stroke, invasive breast cancer, pulmonary emboli, and deep vein thrombosis in postmenopausal women (50 to 79 years of age) during 5 years of treatment with oral conjugated estrogens (CE 0.625mg) combined with medroxyprogesterone acetate (MPA 2.5mg) relative to placebo (see **CLINICAL PHARMACOLOGY, Clinical Studies.**)
The Women's Health Initiative Memory Study (WHIMS), a substudy of WHI, reported increased risk of developing probable dementia in postmenopausal women 65 years of age or older during 4 years of treatment with oral conjugated estrogens plus medroxyprogesterone acetate relative to placebo. It is unknown whether this finding applies to younger postmenopausal women or to women taking estrogen alone therapy. (See **CLINICAL PHARMACOLOGY, Clinical Studies.**)
Other doses of oral conjugated estrogens with medroxyprogesterone acetate, and other combinations and dosage forms of estrogens and progestins were not studied in the WHI clinical trials and, in the absence of comparable data, these risks should be assumed to be similar. Because of these risks, estrogens with or without progestins should be prescribed at the lowest effective doses and for the shortest duration consistent with treatment goals and risks for the individual woman.

Table 1. Summary of Estradiol Pharmacokinetic Parameters (Abdomen Application)

Product	Estradiol Daily Delivery Rate, mcg/day	AUC (0-tlast) pg.h/mL	Cmax pg/mL	Cavg pg/mL	Tmax h	Cmin pg/mL
Menostar™	14	2296	20.6	13.7	42	12.6
Climara® 6.5 cm²	25	4151	37.2	24.7	42	20.4

DESCRIPTION

Menostar™, estradiol transdermal system, is designed to provide nominal *in vivo* delivery of 14 mcg 17β-estradiol per day continuously upon application to intact skin. The period of use is 7 days. The transdermal system has a contact surface area of 3.25 cm², and contains 1.0 mg of estradiol USP. Estradiol USP (17β-estradiol) is a white, crystalline powder, chemically described as estra-1,3,5(10)-triene-3, 17β-diol. It has an empirical formula of $C_{18}H_{24}O_2$ and molecular weight of 272.39. The structural formula is:

The Menostar™ transdermal system comprises three layers. Proceeding from the visible surface toward the surface attached to the skin, these layers are (1) a translucent polyethylene film, and (2) an acrylate adhesive matrix containing estradiol USP. A protective liner (3) of siliconized or fluoropolymer-coated polyester film is attached to the adhesive surface and must be removed before the transdermal system can be used.

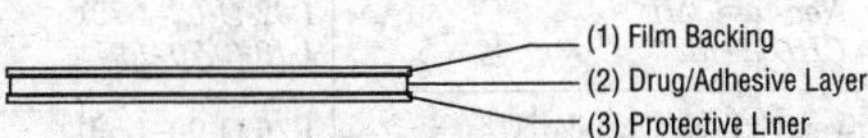

The active component of the transdermal system is 17β-estradiol. The remaining components of the transdermal system (acrylate copolymer adhesive, fatty acid esters, and polyethylene backing) are pharmacologically inactive.

CLINICAL PHARMACOLOGY

The Menostar™ transdermal system provides systemic estrogen therapy by releasing 17β-estradiol, the major estrogenic hormone secreted by the human ovary.
Endogenous estrogens are largely responsible for the development and maintenance of the female reproductive system and secondary sexual characteristics. Although circulating estrogens exist in a dynamic equilibrium of metabolic interconversions, estradiol is the principal intracellular human estrogen and is substantially more potent than its metabolites, estrone and estriol, at the receptor level.
The primary source of estrogen in normally cycling adult women is the ovarian follicle, which secretes 70 to 500 mcg of estradiol daily, depending on the phase of the menstrual cycle. After menopause, most endogenous estrogen is produced by conversion of androstenedione, secreted by the adrenal cortex, to estrone by peripheral tissues. Thus, estrone and the sulfate conjugated form, estrone sulfate, are the most abundant circulating estrogens in postmenopausal women.
Estrogens act through binding to nuclear receptors in estrogen-responsive tissues. To date, two estrogen receptors have been identified. These vary in proportion from tissue to tissue.
Circulating estrogens modulate the pituitary secretion of the gonadotropins, luteinizing hormone (LH) and follicle stimulating hormone (FSH), through a negative feedback mechanism. Estrogens act to reduce the elevated levels of these hormones seen in postmenopausal women.
The decline of ovarian estrogen production that accompanies menopause or oophorectomy results in the acceleration of bone loss and bone resorption. Bone resorption is increased more than bone formation especially in the early years of menopause where bone loss is the greatest. In some women, these changes will eventually lead to decreased bone mass, osteoporosis and increased risk for fractures, particularly that of the spine, hip, and wrist. Vertebral fractures are the most common type of osteoporotic fracture in postmenopausal women.
Postmenopausal women with low serum estradiol concentrations and high serum concentrations of sex hormone-binding globulin (SHBG) have an increased risk of hip and vertebral fractures. Postmenopausal estrogen therapy decreases bone resorption, helping to reestablish balance between resorption and formation. This effect appears to be effective for as long as treatment is continued.

PHARMACOKINETICS

The bioavailability of estradiol following application of a Menostar™ transdermal system, relative to that of a transdermal system delivering 25 mcg/day, was investigated in 18 healthy postmenopausal women mean age 66 years (range 60–80 years). The mean serum estradiol concentrations upon administration of the two patches to the lower abdomen are shown in Figure 1. Transdermal administration of Menostar™ produced geometric mean serum concentration (Cavg) of estradiol of 13.7 pg/mL. No patches failed to adhere during the one week application period of both transdermal systems. Following application of the Menostar™ transdermal system to the abdomen, it is estimated to provide an average nominal *in-vivo* daily delivery of 14 mcg estradiol/day.

Absorption

The Menostar™ transdermal delivery system continuously releases estradiol which is transported across intact skin leading to sustained circulating levels of estradiol during a 7-day treatment period. The systemic availability of estradiol after transdermal administration is about 20 times higher than that after oral administration. This difference is due to the absence of first pass metabolism when estradiol is given by the transdermal route.

Figure 1
Mean Uncorrected Serum 17β-Estradiol Concentrations vs.Time Profile Following Application of Menostar™ and Climara® 6.5 cm² Transdermal System

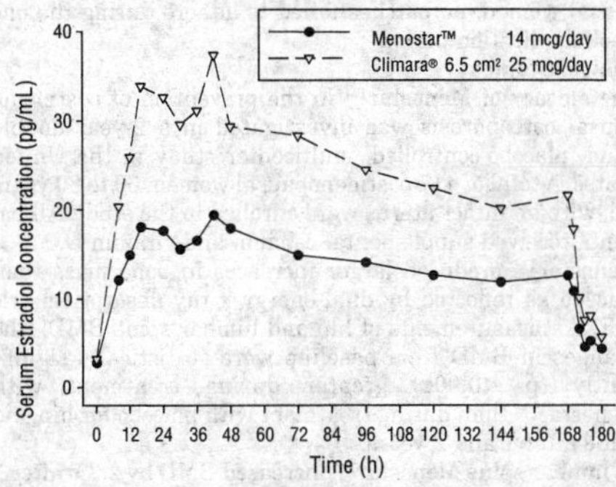

Table 1 provides a summary of estradiol pharmacokinetic parameters determined during evaluation of Menostar™ using baseline uncorrected serum concentrations.
[See table 1 above]
Pharmacokinetic parameters are expressed in geometric means except for the tmax which represents the median estimate and the Cmin which is expressed as the arithmetic mean.
The estimated estradiol daily delivery rate for Climara® 6.5 cm² is quoted from the Climara® labeling.

Distribution

The distribution of exogenous estrogens is similar to that of endogenous estrogens. Estrogens are widely distributed in the body and are generally found in higher concentrations in the sex hormone target organs. Estrogens circulate in the blood largely bound to sex hormone binding globulin (SHBG) and albumin. In the clinical study with 208 patients on Menostar™, SHBG concentration (mean ± SD) remained essentially unchanged over the 2 year period (baseline 45.1 ± 20.1 nmol/L, 24 month visit 46.4 ± 20.9 nmol/L).

Metabolism

Exogenous estrogens are metabolized in the same manner as endogenous estrogens. Circulating estrogens exist in a dynamic equilibrium of metabolic interconversions. These transformations take place mainly in the liver. Estradiol is converted reversibly to estrone, and both can be converted to estriol, which is the major urinary metabolite. Estrogens also undergo enterohepatic recirculation via sulfate and glucuronide conjugation in the liver, biliary secretion of conjugates into the intestine, and hydrolysis in the gut followed by reabsorption. In postmenopausal women, a significant proportion of the circulating estrogens exist as sulfate conjugates, especially estrone sulfate, which serves as a circulating reservoir for the formation of more active estrogens.

Excretion

Estradiol, estrone, and estriol are excreted in the urine along with glucuronide and sulfate conjugates.

Special Populations:

Geriatric: The efficacy and safety of Menostar™ has been studied in women between 60 and 80 years of age, with approximately half over 65 years old.

Continued on next page

Information on Berlex products (appearing here) is based on the most current information available at the time of publication closing. Further information for these and other Berlex products can be obtained from Medical & Product Services at Berlex, Inc. by calling 1-888-BERLEX-4.

Menostar—Cont.

Pediatric: No pharmacokinetic study for Menostar™ has been conducted in a pediatric population.
Gender: Menostar™ is indicated for use in postmenopausal women only.
Race: No studies were done to determine the effect of race on the pharmacokinetics of Menostar™.
Patients with Renal Impairment: Total estradiol serum levels are higher in postmenopausal women with end stage renal disease (ESRD) receiving maintenance hemodialysis than in normal subjects at baseline and following oral doses of estradiol. Therefore, conventional transdermal estradiol doses used in individuals with normal renal function may be excessive for postmenopausal women with ESRD receiving maintenance hemodialysis.
Patients with Hepatic Impairment: Estrogens may be poorly metabolized in patients with impaired liver function and should be administered with caution.

Drug Interactions

In vitro and *in vivo* studies have shown that estrogens are metabolized partially by cytochrome P450 3A4 (CYP3A4). Therefore, inducers or inhibitors of CYP3A4 may affect estrogen drug metabolism. Inducers of CYP3A4 such as St. John's Wort preparations (Hypericum perforatum), phenobarbital, carbamazepine, and rifampin may reduce plasma concentrations of estrogens, possibly resulting in a decrease in therapeutic effects and/or changes in the uterine bleeding profile. Inhibitors of CYP3A4 such as erythromycin, clarithromycin, ketoconazole, itraconazole, ritonavir and grapefruit juice may increase plasma concentrations of estrogens and may result in side effects.

Adhesion

In a Menostar pharmacokinetic study with 18 postmenopausal women, no patches failed to adhere during the one week application period

Clinical Studies

The efficacy of Menostar™ in the prevention of postmenopausal osteoporosis was investigated in a 2-year double blind, placebo-controlled, multicenter study in the United States. A total of 417 postmenopausal women, 60 to 80 years old, with an intact uterus were enrolled in the study. All patients received supplemental calcium and vitamin D.
Menostar™ produced larger increases in bone mass than placebo as reflected by dual-energy x-ray absorptiometric (DEXA) measurements of hip and lumbar spine BMD. The changes in BMD from baseline were statistically significantly ($p < 0.001$) greater during treatment with Menostar™ than during treatment with placebo for hip and spine after 1 and 2 years.
At lumbar spine Menostar™ increased BMD by 2.3% after 1 year and 3.0% after 2 years compared with a 0.5% increase after 1 and 2 years of treatment with placebo. At the hip Menostar™ increased BMD by 0.90% after one year and 0.84% after two years compared with a mean decrease of 0.22% after 1 year and 0.71% after 2 years of placebo treatment (see Table 2 below).
[See table 2 above]

Table 2. Mean Percent BMD Change from Baseline in Lumbar Spine and Total Hip (Full Analysis Set)

Lumbar spine				Total hip			
Time points	Menostar™ N = 208	Placebo N = 209	p-value	Time points	Menostar™ N = 208	Placebo N = 209	p-value
12-month Endpoint	n = 189 +2.29	n = 186 +0.51	< 0.001	12-month Endpoint	n = 189 +0.90	n= 184 -0.22	< 0.001
24-month Endpoint	n = 189 +2.99	n= 186 +0.54	< 0.001	24-month Endpoint	n = 189 +0.84	n = 185 -0.71	< 0.001

N = total number of patients; n = number of patients with data available for each variable

The BMD data of the study were analyzed according to baseline estradiol levels of the patients. Overall, estimated treatment effects on lumbar spine and total hip BMD after 2 years were approximately twice as large in the subgroup with baseline estradiol levels < 5 pg/mL than in the subgroup with baseline estradiol levels ≥ 5.0 pg/mL [Table 3].
[See table 3 above]

Table 3. Mean percent change in lumbar spine and total hip BMD at 24 months by subgroups of baseline estradiol level (< 5 pg/mL, ≥ 5 pg/mL)

	Lumbar spine			Total hip		
Baseline estradiol levels	Menostar™	Placebo	Treatment difference	Menostar™	Placebo	Treatment difference
< 5 pg/mL	n = 101 +3.50	n = 97 +0.29	3.21 (p < 0.001)	n = 101 +1.04	n = 96 -1.09	2.13 (p < 0.001)
≥ 5 pg/mL	n = 88 +2.40	n = 89 +0.81	1.59 (p = 0.002)	n = 88 +0.61	n = 89 -0.31	0.92 (p = 0.045)

n = number of patients with data available for each variable

Menostar™ therapy also resulted in consistent, statistically significant suppression of bone turnover, as reflected by changes in serum and urine markers of bone formation (osteocalcin and bone-specific alkaline phosphatase) and bone resorption (carboxyterminal telopeptide of type 1 collagen (ICTP) and the urinary deoxypyridoline/creatinine ratio).

Women's Health Initiative Studies

The Women's Health Initiative (WHI) enrolled a total of 27,000 predominantly healthy postmenopausal women to assess the risks and benefits of either the use of 0.625 mg conjugated estrogens (CE) per day alone or the use of 0.625 mg conjugated estrogens plus 2.5 mg medroxyprogesterone acetate (MPA) per day compared to placebo in the prevention of certain chronic diseases. The primary endpoint was the incidence of coronary heart disease (CHD) (nonfatal myocardial infarction and CHD death), with invasive breast cancer as the primary adverse outcome studied. A "global index" included the earliest occurrence of CHD, invasive breast cancer, stroke, pulmonary embolism (PE), endometrial cancer, colorectal cancer, hip fracture, or death due to other cause. The study did not evaluate the effects of CE or CE/MPA on menopausal symptoms.
The CE/MPA substudy was stopped early because, according to the predefined stopping rule, the increased risk of breast cancer and cardiovascular events exceeded the specified benefits included in the "global index." Results of the CE/MPA substudy, which included 16,608 women (average age of 63 years, range 50 to 79; 83.9% White, 6.5% Black, 5.5% Hispanic), after an average follow-up of 5.2 years are presented in Table 4 below:
[See table 4 above]

Table 4. RELATIVE AND ABSOLUTE RISK SEEN IN THE CE/MPA SUBSTUDY OF WHI[a]

Event[c]	Relative Risk CE/MPA vs placebo at 5.2 Years (95% CI*)	Placebo n = 8102	CE/MPA n = 8506
		Absolute Risk per 10,000 Person-years	
CHD events	1.29 (1.02–1.63)	30	37
Non-fatal MI	*1.32 (1.02–1.72)*	*23*	*30*
CHD death	*1.18 (0.70–1.97)*	*6*	*7*
Invasive breast cancer[b]	1.26 (1.00–1.59)	30	38
Stroke	1.41 (1.07–1.85)	21	29
Pulmonary embolism	2.13 (1.39–3.25)	8	16
Colorectal cancer	0.63 (0.43–0.92)	16	10
Endometrial cancer	0.83 (0.47–1.47)	6	5
Hip fracture	0.66 (0.45–0.98)	15	10
Death due to causes other than the events above	0.92 (0.74–1.14)	40	37
Global Index[c]	1.15 (1.03–1.28)	151	170
Deep vein thrombosis[d]	2.07 (1.49–2.87)	13	26
Vertebral fractures[d]	0.66 (0.44–0.98)	15	9
Other osteoporotic fractures[d]	0.77 (0.69–0.86)	170	131

[a] adapted from JAMA, 2002; 288:321–333
[b] includes metastatic and non-metastatic breast cancer with the exception of in situ breast cancer
[c] a subset of the events was combined in a "global index", defined as the earliest occurrence of CHD events, invasive breast cancer, stroke, pulmonary embolism, endometrial cancer, colorectal cancer, hip fracture, or death due to other causes
[d] not included in Global Index
*nominal confidence intervals unadjusted for multiple looks and multiple comparisons

For those outcomes included in the "global index," the absolute excess risks per 10,000 women-years in the group treated with CE/MPA were 7 more CHD events, 8 more strokes, 8 more PEs, and 8 more invasive breast cancers, while absolute risk reductions per 10,000 women-years were 6 fewer colorectal cancers and 5 fewer hip fractures. The absolute excess risk of events included in the "global index" was 19 per 10,000 women-years. There was no difference between the groups in terms of all cause mortality. (See **BOXED WARNINGS**, **WARNINGS**, and **PRECAUTIONS**.)

Women's Health Initiative Memory Study

The Women's Health Initiative Memory Study (WHIMS), a substudy of WHI, enrolled 4,532 predominantly postmenopausal women 65 years of age and older (47% were age 65 to 69 years, 35% were 70 to 74 years, and 18% were 75 years of age and older) to evaluate the effects of CE/MPA (0.625 mg conjugated estrogens plus 2.5 mg medroxyprogesterone acetate) on the incidence of probable dementia (primary outcome) compared with placebo.
After an average follow-up of 4 years, 40 women in the estrogen/progestin group (45 per 10,000 women-years) and 21 in the placebo group (22 per 10,000 women-years) were diagnosed with probable dementia. The relative risk of probable dementia in the hormone therapy group was 2.05 (95% CI, 1.21 to 3.48) compared to placebo. Differences between groups became apparent in the first year of treatment. It is unknown whether these findings apply to younger postmenopausal women. (See **BOXED WARNINGS** and **WARNINGS, Dementia.**)

INDICATIONS AND USAGE

Menostar™ is indicated for the prevention of postmenopausal osteoporosis. Therapy should be considered only for women at significant risk of osteoporosis. Non-estrogen medications should be carefully considered.
The mainstays for decreasing the risk of postmenopausal osteoporosis are weight bearing exercise, adequate calcium and vitamin D intake, and when indicated, pharmacologic therapy. Postmenopausal women require an average of 1500mg/day of elemental calcium. Therefore, when not contraindicated, calcium supplementation may be helpful for women with suboptimal dietary intake. Vitamin D supplementation of 400–800 IU/day may also be required to ensure adequate daily intake in postmenopausal women.
Risk factors for osteoporosis include low bone mineral density, low estrogen levels, family history of osteoporosis, previous fracture, small frame (low BMI), light skin color, smoking, and alcohol intake. Response to therapy can be predicted by pre-treatment serum estradiol (see Table 3), and can be assessed during treatment by measuring biochemical markers of bone formation/resorption, and/or bone mineral density.
Estrogen therapy reduces bone resorption and retards or halts postmenopausal bone loss. Studies have shown a risk ratio of about 0.4 for hip and wrist fractures in women whose estrogen therapy was begun within a few years of menopause, compared to women taking calcium and vitamin D alone. Studies also suggest that estrogen reduces the rate of vertebral fractures. Even when started as late as 6 years after menopause, estrogen reduces further loss of bone mass for as long as treatment is continued. When es-

trogen therapy is discontinued, bone mass declines at a rate comparable to the immediate postmenopausal period.

Data from the Women's Health Initiative study showed that use of estrogen (dose equivalent to 0.625 CE) resulted in about 6 less hip fractures per 10,000 women/years, compared to use of placebo (risk ratio about 0.6).

CONTRAINDICATIONS

Menostar™ should not be used in women with any of the following conditions:

1. Undiagnosed abnormal genital bleeding.
2. Known, suspected, or history of cancer of the breast.
3. Known or suspected estrogen-dependent neoplasia.
4. Active deep vein thrombosis, pulmonary embolism or a history of these conditions.
5. Active or recent (e.g. within the past year) arterial thromboembolic disease (e.g., stroke, myocardial infarction).
6. Liver dysfunction or disease.
7. Menostar™ should not be used in patients with known hypersensitivity to its ingredients.
8. Known or suspected pregnancy. There is no indication for Menostar™ in pregnancy. There appears to be little or no increased risk of birth defects in children born to women who have used estrogens and progestins from oral contraceptives inadvertently during early pregnancy (See **PRECAUTIONS**.)

WARNINGS

See BOXED WARNINGS.

1. Cardiovascular disorders.

Estrogen and estrogen/progestin therapy have been associated with an increased risk of cardiovascular events such as myocardial infarction and stroke, as well as venous thrombosis and pulmonary embolism (venous thromboembolism or VTE). Should any of these occur or be suspected, estrogens should be discontinued immediately.

Risk factors for arterial vascular disease (e.g., hypertension, diabetes mellitus, tobacco use, hypercholesterolemia, and obesity) and/or venous thromboembolism (e.g., personal history or family history of VTE, obesity, and systemic lupus erythematosus) should be managed appropriately.

a. *Coronary heart disease and stroke*

In the Women's Health Initiative (WHI) study, an increase in the number of myocardial infarctions and strokes has been observed in women receiving CE compared to placebo. These observations are preliminary (See **CLINICAL PHARMACOLOGY, Clinical Studies.**)

In the CE/MPA substudy of WHI an increased risk of coronary heart disease (CHD) events (defined as nonfatal myocardial infarction and CHD death) was observed in women receiving CE/MPA compared to women receiving placebo (37 vs. 30 per 10,000 women years). The increase in risk was observed in year one and persisted.

In the same substudy of WHI, an increased risk of stroke was observed in women receiving CE/MPA compared to women receiving placebo (29 vs. 21 per 10,000 women-years). The increase in risk was observed after the first year and persisted.

In postmenopausal women with documented heart disease (n = 2,763, average age 66.7 years) a controlled clinical trial of secondary prevention of cardiovascular disease (Heart and Estrogen/Progestin Replacement Study; HERS) treatment with CE/MPA (0.625mg/2.5mg per day) demonstrated no cardiovascular benefit. During an average follow-up of 4.1 years, treatment with CE/MPA did not reduce the overall rate of CHD events in postmenopausal women with established coronary heart disease. There were more CHD events in the CE/MPA-treated group than in the placebo group in year 1, but not during the subsequent years. Two thousand three hundred and twenty one women from the original HERS trial agreed to participate in an open label extension of HERS, HERS II. Average follow-up in HERS II was an additional 2.7 years, for a total of 6.8 years overall. Rates of CHD events were comparable among women in the CE/MPA group and the placebo group in HERS, HERS II, and overall.

Large doses of estrogen (5 mg conjugated estrogens per day), comparable to those used to treat cancer of the prostate and breast, have been shown in a large prospective clinical trial in men to increase the risks of nonfatal myocardial infarction, pulmonary embolism, and thrombophlebitis.

b. *Venous thromboembolism (VTE)*

In the Women's Health Initiative (WHI) study, an increase in VTE has been observed in women receiving CE compared to placebo. These observations are preliminary. (See **CLINICAL PHARMACOLOGY, Clinical Studies.**)

In the CE/MPA substudy of WHI, a 2-fold greater rate of VTE, including deep venous thrombosis and pulmonary embolism, was observed in women receiving CE/MPA compared to women receiving placebo. The rate of VTE was 34 per 10,000 women-years in the CE/MPA group compared to 16 per 10,000 women-years in the placebo group. The increase in VTE risk was observed during the first year and persisted.

If feasible, estrogens should be discontinued at least 4 to 6 weeks before surgery of the type associated with an increased risk of thromboembolism, or during periods of prolonged immobilization.

2. Malignant neoplasms

a. *Endometrial cancer*

The use of unopposed estrogens in women with intact uteri has been associated with an increased risk of endometrial cancer. The reported endometrial cancer risk among unopposed estrogen users is about 2- to 12-fold greater than in non-users, and appears dependent on duration of treatment and on estrogen dose. Most studies show no significant increased risk associated with use of estrogens for less than one year. The greatest risk appears associated with prolonged use, with increased risks of 15- to 24-fold for five to ten years or more and this risk has been shown to persist for at least 8 to 15 years after estrogen therapy is discontinued.

Clinical surveillance of all women taking estrogen/progestin combinations is important. Adequate diagnostic measures, including endometrial sampling when indicated, should be undertaken to rule out malignancy in all cases of undiagnosed persistent or recurring abnormal vaginal bleeding. There is no evidence that the use of natural estrogens results in a different endometrial risk profile than synthetic estrogens of equivalent estrogen dose. Adding a progestin to estrogen therapy has been shown to reduce the risk of endometrial hyperplasia, which may be a precursor to endometrial cancer.

b. *Breast cancer*

The use of estrogens and progestins by postmenopausal women has been reported to increase the risk of breast cancer. The most important randomized clinical trial providing information about this issue is the Women's Health Initiative (WHI) substudy of CE/MPA (see **CLINICAL PHARMACOLOGY, Clinical Studies**). The results from observational studies are generally consistent with those of the WHI clinical trial and report no significant variation in the risk of breast cancer among different estrogens or progestins, doses, or routes of administration.

The CE/MPA substudy of WHI reported an increased risk of breast cancer in women who took CE/MPA for a mean follow-up of 5.6 years. Observational studies have also reported an increased risk for estrogen/progestin combination therapy, and a smaller increased risk for estrogen alone therapy, after several years of use. In the WHI trial and from observational studies, the excess risk increased with duration of use. From observational studies, the risk appeared to return to baseline in about five years after stopping treatment. In addition, observational studies suggest that the risk of breast cancer was greater, and became apparent earlier, with estrogen/progestin combination therapy as compared to estrogen alone therapy.

In the CE/MPA substudy, 26% of the women reported prior use of estrogen alone and/or estrogen/progestin combination hormone therapy. After a mean follow-up of 5.6 years during the clinical trial, the overall relative risk of invasive breast cancer was 1.24 (95% confidence interval 1.01–1.54), and the overall absolute risk was 41 vs. 33 cases per 10,000 women-years, for CE/MPA compared with placebo. Among women who reported prior use of hormone therapy, the relative risk of invasive breast cancer was 1.86, and the absolute risk was 46 vs. 25 cases per 10,000 women-years, for CE/MPA compared with placebo. Among women who reported no prior use of hormone therapy, the relative risk of invasive breast cancer was 1.09, and the absolute risk was 40 vs. 36 cases per 10,000 women-years for CE/MPA compared with placebo. In the same substudy, invasive breast cancers were larger and diagnosed at a more advanced stage in the CE/MPA group compared with the placebo group. Metastatic disease was rare with no apparent difference between the two groups. Other prognostic factors such as histologic subtype, grade and hormone receptor status did not differ between the groups.

The use of estrogen plus progestin has been reported to result in an increase in abnormal mammograms requiring further evaluation. All women should receive yearly breast examinations by a healthcare provider and perform monthly breast self-examinations. In addition, mammography examinations should be scheduled based on patient age, risk factors, and prior mammogram results.

3. Dementia

In the Women's Health Initiative Memory Study (WHIMS), 4,532 generally healthy postmenopausal women 65 years of age and older were studied, of whom 35% were 70 to 74 years of age and 18% were 75 or older. After an average follow-up of 4 years, 40 women being treated with CE/MPA (1.8%, n=2,229) and 21 women in the placebo group (0.9%, n=2,303) received diagnoses of probable dementia. The relative risk for CE/MPA versus placebo was 2.05 (95% confidence interval 1.21 – 3.48), and was similar for women with and without histories of menopausal hormone use before WHIMS. The absolute risk of probable dementia for CE/MPA versus placebo was 45 versus 22 cases per 10,000 women-years, and the absolute excess risk for CE/MPA was 23 cases per 10,000 women-years. It is unknown whether these findings apply to younger postmenopausal women. (See **CLINICAL PHARMACOLOGY, Clinical Studies** and **PRECAUTIONS, Geriatric Use.**)

It is unknown whether these findings apply to estrogen alone therapy.

4. Gallbladder disease

A 2- to 4-fold increase in the risk of gallbladder disease requiring surgery in postmenopausal women receiving estrogens has been reported.

5. Hypercalcemia

Estrogen administration may lead to severe hypercalcemia in patients with breast cancer and bone metastases. If hypercalcemia occurs, use of the drug should be stopped and appropriate measures taken to reduce the serum calcium level.

6. Visual abnormalities

Retinal vascular thrombosis has been reported in patients receiving estrogens. Discontinue medication pending examination if there is sudden partial or complete loss of vision, or a sudden onset of proptosis, diplopia, or migraine. If examination reveals papilledema or retinal vascular lesions, estrogens should be discontinued.

PRECAUTIONS

A. General

1. *Addition of a progestin when a woman has not had a hysterectomy.*

Studies of the addition of a progestin for 10 or more days of a cycle of estrogen administration, or daily with estrogen in a continuous regimen, have reported a lowered incidence of endometrial hyperplasia than would be induced by estrogen treatment alone. Endometrial hyperplasia may be a precursor to endometrial cancer.

There are, however, possible risks that may be associated with the use of progestins with estrogens compared to estrogen-alone regimens. These include a possible increased risk of breast cancer.

2. *Elevated blood pressure*

In a small number of case reports, substantial increases in blood pressure have been attributed to idiosyncratic reactions to estrogens. In a large, randomized, placebo-controlled clinical trial, a generalized effect of estrogen therapy on blood pressure was not seen. Blood pressure should be monitored at regular intervals with estrogen use.

3. *Familial hyperlipoproteinemia*

In patients with familial defects of lipoprotein metabolism, oral estrogen therapy may be associated with elevations of plasma triglycerides leading to pancreatitis and other complications.

4. *Impaired liver function and past history of cholestatis jaundice*

Estrogens may be poorly metabolized in patients with impaired liver function. For patients with a history of cholestatic jaundice associated with past estrogen use or with pregnancy, caution should be exercised and in the case of recurrence, medication should be discontinued.

5. *Hypothyroidism*

Estrogen administration leads to increased thyroid-binding globulin (TBG) levels. Patients with normal thyroid function can compensate for the increased TBG by making more thyroid hormone, thus maintaining free T_4 and T_3 serum concentrations in the normal range. Patients dependent on thyroid hormone replacement therapy who are also receiving estrogens may require increased doses of their thyroid replacement therapy. These patients should have their thyroid function monitored in order to maintain their free thyroid hormone levels in an acceptable range.

6. *Fluid retention*

Because estrogens may cause some degree of fluid retention, patients with conditions that might be influenced by this factor, such as a cardiac or renal dysfunction, warrant careful observation when estrogens are prescribed.

7. *Hypocalcemia*

Estrogens should be used with caution in individuals with severe hypocalcemia.

8. *Ovarian cancer*

The CE/MPA sub-study of WHI reported that estrogen plus progestin increased the risk of ovarian cancer. After an average follow-up of 5.6 years, the relative risk for ovarian cancer for CE/MPA versus placebo was 1.58 (95% confidence interval 0.77–3.24) but was not statistically significant. The absolute risk for CE/MPA versus placebo was 4.2 versus 2.7 cases per 10,000 women-years. In some epidemiological studies, the use of estrogen alone, in particular for ten or more years, has been associated with an increased risk of ovarian cancer. Other epidemiologic studies have not found these associations.

9. *Exacerbation of endometriosis*

Endometriosis may be exacerbated with administration of estrogens. A few cases of malignant transfor-

Continued on next page

Information on Berlex products (appearing here) is based on the most current information available at the time of publication closing. Further information for these and other Berlex products can be obtained from Medical & Product Services at Berlex, Inc. by calling 1-888-BERLEX-4.

Menostar—Cont.

mation of residual endometrial implants have been reported in women treated post-hysterectomy with estrogen alone therapy. For patients known to have residual endometriosis post-hysterectomy, the addition of progestin should be considered.

10. *Exacerbation of other conditions*
Estrogens may cause an exacerbation of asthma, diabetes mellitus, epilepsy, migraine or porphyria, systemic lupus erythematosus, and hepatic hemangiomas and should be used with caution in women with these conditions.

B. PATIENT INFORMATION

Physicians are advised to discuss the PATIENT INFORMATION leaflet with patients for whom they prescribe Menostar™.

C. LABORATORY TESTS

Estrogen administration should be initiated at the lowest dose approved for the indication and then guided by clinical response rather than by serum hormone levels (e.g. estradiol, FSH).

1. Accelerated prothrombin time, partial thromboplastin time, and platelet aggregation time; increased platelet count; increased factors II, VII antigen, VIII antigen, VIII coagulant activity, IX, X, XII, VII-X complex, II-VII-X complex, and beta-thromboglobulin; decreased levels of antifactor Xa and antithrombin III, decreased antithrombin III activity; increased levels of fibrinogen and fibrinogen activity; increased plasminogen antigen and activity.
2. Increased thyroid-binding globulin (TBG) levels leading to increased circulating total thyroid hormone levels as measured by protein-bound iodine (PBI), T_4 levels (by column or by radioimmunoassay) or T_3 levels by radioimmunoassay. T_3 resin uptake is decreased, reflecting the elevated TBG. Free T_4 and free T_3 concentrations are unaltered. Patients on thyroid replacement therapy may require higher doses of thyroid hormone.
3. Other binding proteins may be elevated in serum (i.e., corticosteroid binding globulin (CBG), sex hormone-binding globulin (SHBG) leading to increased circulating corticosteroids and sex steroids, respectively. Free hormone concentrations may be decreased. Other plasma proteins may be increased (angiotensinogen/renin substrate, alpha-1-antitrypsin, ceruloplasmin).
4. Increased plasma HDL and HDL_2 subfraction concentrations, reduced LDL cholesterol concentration, and in oral formulations increased triglyceride levels.
5. Impaired glucose tolerance.
6. Reduced response to metyrapone test.

D. CARCINOGENESES, MUTAGENESIS, AND IMPAIRMENT OF FERTILITY

Long-term continuous administration of estrogen, with and without progestin, in women with and without a uterus, has shown an increased risk of endometrial cancer, breast cancer, and ovarian cancer. (See **BOXED WARNINGS, WARNINGS** and **PRECAUTIONS.**)

Long-term continuous administration of natural and synthetic estrogens in certain animal species increases the frequency of carcinomas of the breast, uterus, cervix, vagina, testis, and liver.

E. PREGNANCY

Menostar™ should not be used during pregnancy. (See **CONTRAINDICATIONS.**)

F. NURSING MOTHERS

Estrogen administration to nursing mothers has been shown to decrease the quantity and quality of the milk. Detectable amounts of estrogens have been identified in the milk of mothers receiving this drug. Caution should be exercised when Menostar™ is administered to a nursing woman.

G. Pediatric Use

The safety and efficacy of Menostar™ in pediatric patients has not been established.

H. Geriatric Use

A total of 417 postmenopausal women 61–79 years old, with an intact uterus, participated in the osteoporosis trial. More than 50% of women receiving study drug, were considered geriatric (65 years or older). Efficacy in older (≥ 65 years) and younger (<65 years) postmenopausal women in the osteoporosis treatment trial was comparable both at 12 and 24 months. Safety in older (≥ 65 years) and younger (<65 years) postmenopausal women in the osteoporosis treatment trial was also comparable throughout the study.

In the Women's Health Initiative Memory Study, including 4,532 women 65 years of age and older, followed for an average of 4 years, 82% (n=3,729) were 65 to 74 while 18% (n=803) were 75 and over. Most women (80%) had no prior hormone therapy use. Women treated with conjugated estrogens plus medroxyprogesterone acetate were reported to have a two-fold increase in the risk of developing probable dementia. Alzheimer's disease was the most common classification of probable dementia in both the conjugated estrogens plus medroxyprogesterone acetate group and the placebo group. Ninety percent of the cases of probable dementia occurred in the 54% of women that were older than 70. (See **WARNINGS, Dementia.**) It is unknown whether these findings apply to estrogen alone therapy.

ADVERSE REACTIONS

See **BOXED WARNINGS, WARNINGS** and **PRECAUTIONS**

Because clinical trials are conducted under widely varying conditions, adverse reaction rates observed in the clinical trials of a drug cannot be directly compared to rates in the clinical trials of another drug and may not reflect the rates observed in practice. The adverse reaction information from clinical trials does, however, provide a basis for identifying the adverse events that appear to be related to drug use and for approximating rates.

[See table below]

The following additional adverse reactions have been reported with estrogens:

1. Genitourinary system

Changes in vaginal bleeding pattern and abnormal withdrawal bleeding or flow; breakthrough bleeding; spotting; dysmenorrhea; increase in size of uterine leiomyomata; vaginitis, including vaginal candidiasis; change in amount of cervical secretion; changes in cervical ectropion; ovarian cancer; endometrial hyperplasia; endometrial cancer.

2. Breasts

Tenderness, enlargement, pain, nipple discharge, galactorrhea; fibrocystic breast changes; breast cancer.

3. Cardiovascular

Deep and superficial venous thrombosis; pulmonary embolism; thrombophlebitis; myocardial infarction; stroke; increase in blood pressure.

4. Gastrointestinal

Nausea, vomiting; abdominal cramps, bloating; cholestatic jaundice; increased incidence of gall bladder disease; pancreatitis; enlargement of hepatic hemangiomas.

5. Skin

Chloasma or melasma, which may persist when drug is discontinued; erythema multiforme; erythema nodosum; hemorrhagic eruption; loss of scalp hair; hirsutism; pruritus, rash.

6. Eyes

Retinal vascular thrombosis; intolerance to contact lenses.

7. Central nervous system

Headache; migraine; dizziness; mental depression; chorea; nervousness; mood disturbances; irritability; exacerbation of epilepsy; dementia.

8. Miscellaneous

Increase or decrease in weight; reduced carbohydrate tolerance; aggravation of porphyria; edema; arthalgias; leg cramps; changes in libido; anaphylactoid/anaphylactic reactions including urticaria and angioedema; hypocalcemia; exacerbation of asthma; increased triglycerides.

Summary of Most Frequently Reported Treatment Emergent Adverse Experiences/Medical Events (≥5%) By Treatment Groups

AE per Body System	Menostar™ 14 mcg/day (N=208)	Placebo (N=209)
Body as a Whole	95 (46%)	100 (48%)
Abdominal Pain	17 (8%)	17 (8%)
Accidental Injury	29 (14%)	23 (11%)
Infection	11 (5%)	10 (5%)
Pain	26 (13%)	26 (12%)
Cardiovascular	20 (10%)	19 (9%)
Digestive System	52 (25%)	44 (21%)
Constipation	11 (5%)	6 (3%)
Dyspepsia	11 (5%)	9 (4%)
Metabolic and Nutritional Disorders	25 (12%)	22 (11%)
Musculoskeletal System	54 (26%)	51 (24%)
Arthralgia	24 (12%)	13 (6%)
Arthritis	11 (5%)	15 (7%)
Myalgia	10 (5%)	6 (3%)
Nervous System	30 (14%)	23 (11%)
Dizziness	11 (5%)	6 (3%)
Respiratory System	62 (30%)	67 (32%)
Bronchitis	12 (6%)	9 (4%)
Upper Respiratory Infection	33 (16%)	35 (17%)
Skin and Appendages	50 (24%)	54 (26%)
Application Site Reaction	18 (9%)	18 (9%)
Breast Pain	10 (5%)	8 (4%)
Urogenital System	66 (32%)	40 (19%)
Cervical polyps	13 (6%)	4 (2%)
Leukorrhea	22 (11%)	3 (1%)

OVERDOSAGE

Overdosage of estrogen may cause nausea, and withdrawal bleeding may occur in females. Serious ill effects have not been reported following acute ingestion of large doses of estrogen-containing drug products by young children.

DOSAGE AND ADMINISTRATION

Menostar™ should only be prescribed to postmenopausal women who are at significant risk of osteoporosis. Non-estrogen medications should be carefully considered. Risk factors for osteoporosis include low bone mineral density, low estrogen levels, family history of osteoporosis, previous fracture, small frame (low BMI), light skin color, smoking, and alcohol intake. Response to therapy can be predicted by pre-treatment serum estradiol (see Table 3), and can be assessed during treatment by measuring biochemical markers of bone formation/resorption, and/or bone mineral density.

When estrogen is prescribed for a postmenopausal woman with a uterus, a progestin should also be used, to reduce the risk of endometrial cancer. A woman without a uterus does not need progestin. For women who have a uterus, adequate diagnostic measures, such as endometrial sampling, when indicated, should be undertaken to rule out malignancy in cases of undiagnosed persistent or recurring abnormal vaginal bleeding.

It is recommended that women who have a uterus and are treated with Menostar™ receive a progestin for 14 days every 6 to 12 months and undergo an endometrial biopsy at yearly intervals or as clinically indicated. (see **BOXED WARNINGS** and **WARNINGS**).

Application of the System

The adhesive side of the Menostar™ transdermal system should be placed on a clean, dry area of the lower abdomen. **Menostar™ should not be applied to or near the breasts.** The sites of application must be rotated, with an interval of at least 1-week allowed between applications to a particular site. The area selected should not be oily, damaged, or irritated. The waistline should be avoided, since tight clothing may rub and remove the transdermal system. Application to areas where sitting would dislodge the transdermal system should also be avoided. The transdermal system should be applied immediately after opening the pouch and removing the protective liner. The transdermal system should be pressed firmly in place with the fingers for about 10 seconds, making sure there is good contact, especially around the edges. If the transdermal system lifts, apply pressure to maintain adhesion. In the event that a transdermal system should fall off, a new transdermal system should be applied for the remainder of the 7-day dosing interval. Only one system should be worn at any one time during the 7-day dosing interval. Swimming, bathing, or using a sauna while using Menostar™ has not been studied, and these activities may decrease the adhesion of the transdermal system and the delivery of estradiol.

Removal of the Transdermal System

Removal of the system should be done carefully and slowly to avoid irritation of the skin. Should any adhesive remain on the skin after removal of the system, allow the area to dry for 15 minutes. Then gently rubbing the area with an oil-based cream or lotion should remove the adhesive residue.

Used patches still contain some active hormones. Each patch should be carefully folded in half so that it sticks to itself before throwing it away.

HOW SUPPLIED

Menostar™ (estradiol transdermal system), 14 mcg/day — each 3.25 cm^2 system contains 1 mg of estradiol USP

NDC 50419-455-04

Individual Carton of 4 systems

Shelf Pack Carton of 6 Individual Cartons of 4 systems

Do not store above 86°F (30°C). Do not store unpouched. Apply immediately upon removal from the protective pouch.

PATIENT INFORMATION
Updated 6/8/04
Menostar™ (Men-ō-star)
(estradiol transdermal system)
Read this before you start taking Menostar™ and read what you get each time you refill Menostar™. There may be new information. This information does not take the place of talking to your health care provider about your medical condition or your treatment.

What is the most important information I should know about Menostar™ (an osteoporosis preventative containing an estrogen hormone)?
- Estrogens increase the chances of getting cancer of the uterus.

Report any unusual vaginal bleeding right away while you are taking estrogens. Vaginal bleeding after menopause may be a warning sign of cancer of the uterus (womb). Your health care provider should check any unusual vaginal bleeding to find out the cause.
- Do not use estrogens with or without progestins to prevent heart disease, heart attacks, or strokes.

Using estrogens with or without progestins may increase your chances of getting heart attacks, strokes, breast cancer, or blood clots. Using estrogens with progestins may increase your risk of dementia. You and your healthcare provider should talk regularly about whether you still need treatment with Menostar.

What is Menostar™?
Menostar™ is a medicine that contains estrogen hormones.
What is Menostar™ used for?
Menostar™ is used after menopause to:
- **help reduce your chances of getting osteoporosis (thin weak bones).**
  Osteoporosis from menopause is a thinning of the bones that makes them weaker and easier to break. Very low doses of estrogen can help keep your bones from becoming weaker. You and your healthcare provider should talk regularly about whether you should continue with Menostar. Weight-bearing exercise, like walking or running, and taking calcium and vitamin D supplements may also lower your chances of getting postmenopausal osteoporosis. It is important to talk about exercise and supplements with your healthcare provider before starting them.

Who should not use Menostar™?
Do not start using Menostar™ if you:
- **have unusual vaginal bleeding**
- **currently have or have had certain cancers.** Estrogens may increase the chances of getting certain types of cancers, including cancer of the breast or uterus. If you have or had cancer, talk with your health care provider about whether you should take Menostar™.
- **had a stroke or heart attack in the past year.**
- **currently have or have had blood clots.**
- **currently have or have had liver problems.**
- **are allergic to Menostar™ or any of its ingredients.** See the end of this leaflet for a list of ingredients in Menostar™. If you are allergic to other estrogen patches, you will likely be allergic to Menostar™.
- **think you may be pregnant**

Tell your health care provider:
- **if you are breastfeeding.** The hormone in Menostar™ can pass into your milk.
- **about all of your medical problems.** Your health care provider may need to check you more carefully if you have certain conditions, such as asthma (wheezing), epilepsy (seizures), migraine, endometriosis, or problems with your heart, liver, thyroid, kidneys, or have high calcium levels in your blood.
- **about all the medicines you take,** including prescription and nonprescription medicines, vitamins, and herbal supplements. Do not use any estrogen pill, patch or injection with Menostar. Some medicines may affect how Menostar™ works. Menostar™ may also affect how your other medicines work.
- **if you are going to have surgery or will be on bed rest.** You may need to stop taking estrogens.

How should I use Menostar™
- Menostar is a patch that you wear on your skin. The estrogen in the Menostar patch passes through your skin. You must change your Menostar patch every 7 days (once a week). See the end of this leaflet for complete instructions for using Menostar.
- Estrogens should be used at the lowest dose possible for your treatment, only as long as needed. You and your healthcare provider should talk regularly about whether you still need treatment with Menostar.

What are the possible side effects of estrogens?
Less common but serious side effects include:
- Breast cancer
- Cancer of the uterus
- Stroke
- Heart attack
- Blood clots
- Gallbladder disease
- Ovarian cancer

These are some of the warning signs of serious side effects:
- Breast lumps
- Unusual vaginal bleeding
- Dizziness and faintness
- Changes in speech
- Severe headaches
- Chest pain
- Shortness of breath
- Pains in your legs
- Changes in vision
- Vomiting

Call your health care provider right away if you get any of these warning signs, or any other unusual symptom that concerns you.
Common side effects include:
- Headache
- Breast pain
- Irregular vaginal bleeding or spotting
- Stomach/abdominal cramps, bloating
- Nausea and vomiting
- Hair loss

Other side effects include:
- High blood pressure
- Liver problems
- High blood sugar
- Fluid retention
- Enlargement of benign tumors of the uterus ("fibroids")
- Vaginal yeast infection

These are not all the possible side effects of Menostar™. For more information, ask your health care provider or pharmacist.
What can I do to lower my chances of a serious side effect with Menostar™?
- Talk with your healthcare provider regularly about whether you should continue taking Menostar. If you have a uterus, talk to your healthcare provider about the recommended use of a progestin.
- See your health care provider right away if you get vaginal bleeding while using Menostar™.
- Have a breast exam and mammogram (breast X-ray) every year unless your health care provider tells you something else. If members of your family have had breast cancer or if you have ever had breast lumps or an abnormal mammogram, you may need to have breast exams more often.
- If you have high blood pressure, high cholesterol (fat in the blood), diabetes, are overweight, or if you use tobacco, you may have higher chances for getting heart disease. Ask your health care provider for ways to lower your chances for getting heart disease.

General information about safe and effective use of Menostar™
Medicines are sometimes prescribed for conditions that are not mentioned in patient information leaflets. Do not take Menostar™ for conditions for which it was not prescribed. Do not give Menostar™ to other people, even if they have the same symptoms you have. It may harm them.
Keep Menostar™ out of the reach of children.
This leaflet provides a summary of the most important information about Menostar™. If you would like more information, talk with your health care provider or pharmacist. You can ask for information about Menostar™ that is written for health professionals. You can get more information by calling the toll free number (1-888-237-5394) or visit www.menostar-us.com.
What are the ingredients in Menostar™?
The active ingredient of Menostar™ is estradiol. Menostar™ also contains acrylate copolymer adhesive, fatty acid esters, and polyethylene backing. Menostar™ does not contain latex.
Instructions for Use
How and where do I apply the Menostar™ patch
- Talk to your healthcare provider or pharmacist if you have questions about applying the Menostar patch.
- 1 Menostar patch is applied and worn for 7 days (1 week). The Menostar patch is changed once a week.
- Each Menostar™ patch is individually sealed in a protective pouch. To open the pouch, hold it upright with the Menostar™ name facing you. Tear off the top of the pouch using the top tear notch. Tear off the side of the pouch using the side tear notch. Pull the pouch open. The Menostar™ patch is the see-through plastic film attached to the clear thicker plastic backing. There is a silver foil-sticker attached to the inside of the pouch. **Do not remove it from the pouch.** The sticker contains a moisture protectant. **Lift out the Menostar™ patch.** Notice that the patch is attached to a thicker, hard-plastic backing and that the patch itself is oval and see-through.

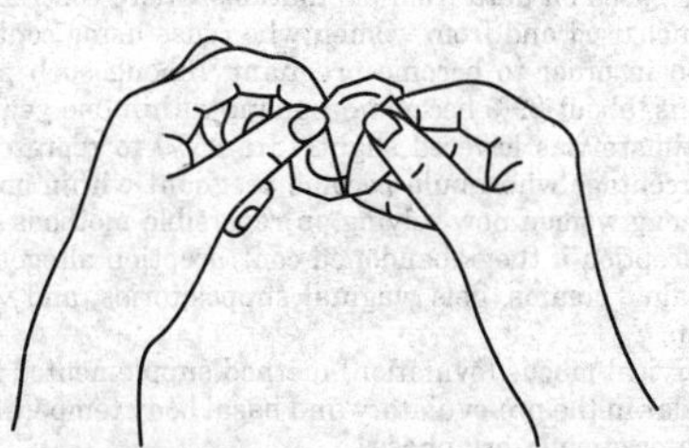

- Apply the sticky side of the Menostar™ patch to a clean, dry area of the lower stomach area below your belly button (see diagram below). **Do not apply the Menostar™ patch to your breasts.** The site selected should not be oily, damaged, or irritated. Avoid the waistline area, since tight clothing may rub and remove the patch. Also, do not put the patch on areas where sitting would rub it off or loosen it. Apply the patch right after opening the pouch and removing the protective liner. Press the patch firmly in place with your fingers for about 10 seconds. Make sure that it sticks all over, especially around the edges.

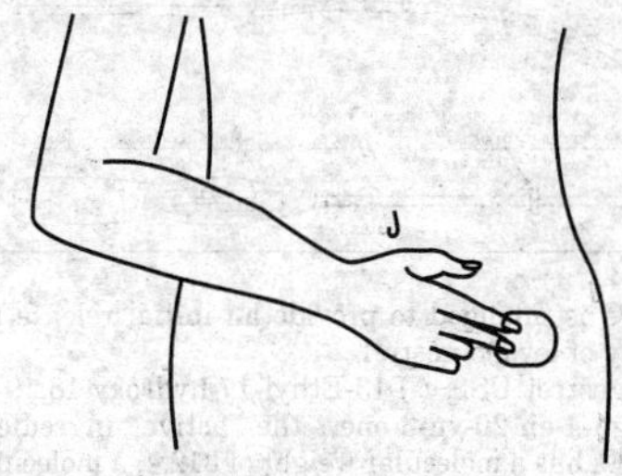

- The Menostar™ patch should be left in place for 7 days (one week). Change the Menostar™ patch every 7 days (once a week). Remove the used patch. Carefully fold it in half so that it sticks to itself and safely throwaway, away from children and pets. Place a new Menostar™ patch on a different clean, dry area of the lower stomach area below your belly button. The same skin site should not be used again for at least 1 week after removal of the patch.
- If the Menostar™ patch falls off, the same patch may be reapplied to another area of your lower stomach. Make sure that Menostar™ patch sticks well to your skin, especially around the edges. If the patch will not stick completely to your skin, remove it and safely throwaway. Apply a new patch on a different area of the lower stomach. Do not wear 2 Menostar™ patches at the same time.
- Bathing, swimming, or showering may affect and loosen the Menostar™ patch.

Manufactured for:
BERLEX®
Berlex, Montville, NJ 07045
Manufactured by 3M Pharmaceuticals, St. Paul, MN 55144
6006000 (3M #630400) June 2004
Shown in Product Identification Guide, page 308

MIRENA® ℞
[*mĭ-rĕ-nä*]
(levonorgestrel-releasing intrauterine system)

PATIENTS SHOULD BE COUNSELED THAT THIS PRODUCT DOES NOT PROTECT AGAINST HIV INFECTION (AIDS) AND OTHER SEXUALLY TRANSMITTED DISEASES
Rx only

DESCRIPTION
MIRENA® (levonorgestrel-releasing intrauterine system) consists of a T-shaped polyethylene frame (T-body) with a steroid reservoir (hormone elastomer core) around the vertical stem. The reservoir consists of a cylinder, made of a mixture of levonorgestrel and silicone (polydimethylsiloxane), containing a total of 52 mg levonorgestrel. The reservoir is covered by a silicone (polydimethylsiloxane) membrane. The T-body is 32 mm in both the horizontal and vertical directions. The polyethylene of the T-body is compounded with barium sulfate, which makes it radiopaque. A monofilament brown polyethylene removal thread is attached to a loop at the end of the vertical stem of the T-body.

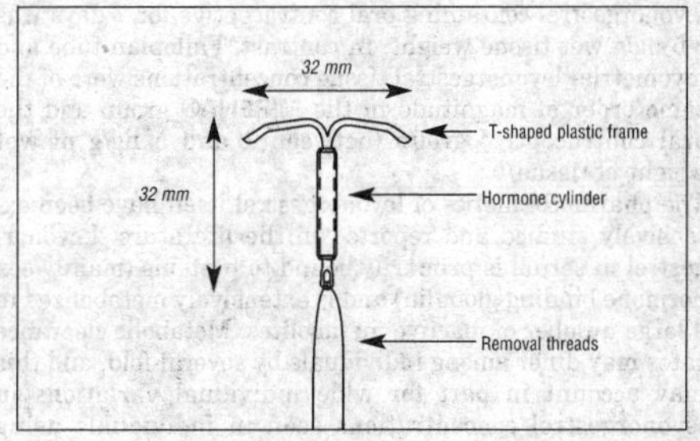

Schematic drawing of **MIRENA®**

INSERTER
MIRENA® is packaged sterile within an inserter. The inserter, which is used for insertion of **MIRENA®** into the uterine cavity, consists of a symmetric two-sided body and slider that are integrated with flange, lock, pre-bent insertion tube

Continued on next page

Information on Berlex products (appearing here) is based on the most current information available at the time of publication closing. Further information for these and other Berlex products can be obtained from Medical & Product Services at Berlex, Inc. by calling 1-888-BERLEX-4.

Mirena—Cont.

and plunger. Once **MIRENA®** is in place, the inserter is discarded.

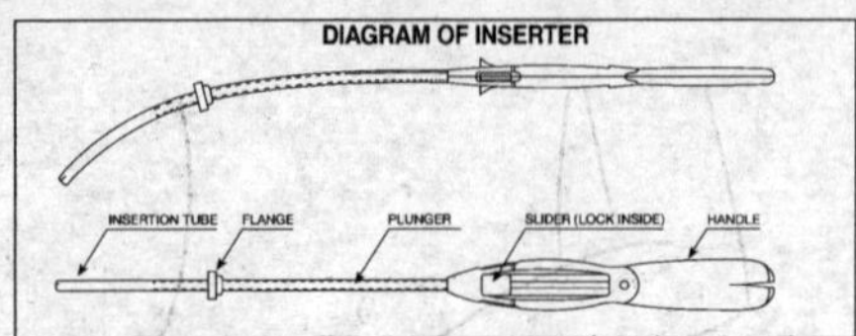

MIRENA® is intended to provide an initial release rate of 20 µg/day of levonorgestrel.
Levonorgestrel USP, (-)-13-Ethyl-17-hydroxy-18,19-dinor-17α-pregn-4-en-20-yn-3-one, the active ingredient in **MIRENA®**, has a molecular weight of 312.4, a molecular formula of $C_{21}H_{28}O_2$, and the following structural formula:

CLINICAL PHARMACOLOGY

Levonorgestrel is a progestogen used in a variety of contraceptive products. Low doses of levonorgestrel can be administered into the uterine cavity with the **MIRENA®** intrauterine delivery system. Initially, levonorgestrel is released at a rate of approximately 20 µg/day. This rate decreases progressively to half that value after 5 years.
MIRENA® has mainly local progestogenic effects in the uterine cavity. Morphological changes of the endometrium are observed, including stromal pseudodecidualization, glandular atrophy, a leucocytic infiltration and a decrease in glandular and stromal mitoses.
Ovulation is inhibited in some women using **MIRENA®**. In a 1-year study approximately 45% of menstrual cycles were ovulatory and in another study after 4 years 75% of cycles were ovulatory.
The local mechanism by which continuously released levonorgestrel enhances contraceptive effectiveness of the IUS has not been conclusively demonstrated. Studies of **MIRENA®** prototypes have suggested several mechanisms that prevent pregnancy: thickening of cervical mucus preventing passage of sperm into the uterus, inhibition of sperm capacitation or survival, and alteration of the endometrium.

Clinical Pharmacokinetics

Following insertion of **MIRENA®**, the initial release of levonorgestrel into the uterine cavity is 20 µg/day. A stable plasma level of levonorgestrel of 150-200 pg/mL occurs after the first few weeks following insertion of **MIRENA®**. Levonorgestrel levels after long term use of 12, 24, and 60 months were 180±66 pg/mL, 192±140 pg/mL, and 159±59 pg/mL, respectively. The plasma concentrations achieved by **MIRENA®** are lower than those seen with levonorgestrel contraceptive implants and with oral contraceptives. Unlike oral contraceptives, plasma levels with **MIRENA®** do not display peaks and troughs.
The mean ± SD levonorgestrel endometrial tissue concentration in four women using levonorgestrel intrauterine systems releasing 30 µg/day of levonorgestrel for 36-49 days was 808 ± 511 ng/g wet tissue weight. The endometrial tissue concentration in 2 women who had been taking a 250 µg levonorgestrel-containing oral contraceptive for 7 days was 3.5 ng/g wet tissue weight. In contrast, Fallopian tube and myometrial levonorgestrel tissue concentrations were of the same order of magnitude in the **MIRENA®** group and the oral contraceptive group (between 1 and 5 ng/g of wet weight of tissue).
The pharmacokinetics of levonorgestrel itself have been extensively studied and reported in the literature. Levonorgestrel in serum is primarily bound to proteins (mainly sex hormone binding globulin) and is extensively metabolized to a large number of inactive metabolites. Metabolic clearance rates may differ among individuals by several-fold, and this may account in part for wide individual variations in levonorgestrel concentrations seen in individuals using levonorgestrel-containing contraceptive products. The elimination half-life of levonorgestrel after daily oral doses is approximately 17 hours; both the parent drug and its metabolites are primarily excreted in the urine.
Pharmacokinetic studies of this product have not been conducted in special populations (pediatric, renal insufficiency, hepatic insufficiency, and different ethnic groups).
Drug-Drug Interactions:
The effect of other drugs on the efficacy of **MIRENA®** has not been studied.

INDICATIONS AND USAGE

MIRENA® is indicated for intrauterine contraception for up to 5 years. Thereafter, if continued contraception is desired, the system should be replaced.

RECOMMENDED PATIENT PROFILE

MIRENA® is recommended for women who have had at least one child, are in a stable, mutually monogamous relationship, have no history of pelvic inflammatory disease, and have no history of ectopic pregnancy or condition that would predispose to ectopic pregnancy.

Clinical Studies

MIRENA® has been studied for safety and efficacy in two large clinical trials in Finland and Sweden. In study sites having verifiable data and informed consent, 1169 women 18 to 35 years of age at enrollment used **MIRENA®** for up to 5 years, for a total of 45,000 women-months of exposure. The study population was predominantly Caucasian, and over 70% of the participants had previously used IUDs. The reported 12-month pregnancy rates were less than or equal to 0.2 per 100 women and the cumulative 5-year pregnancy rate was approximately 0.7 per 100 women. However, due to limitations of the available data a precise estimate of the pregnancy rate is not possible.
The following table provides estimates of the percent of women likely to become pregnant while using a particular contraceptive method for one year. These estimates are based on a variety of studies. In this table, **MIRENA®** is identified as "LNg 20".

TABLE 1: Percentage of women experiencing an unintended pregnancy during the first year of typical use and first year of perfect use of contraception and the percentage continuing use at the end of the first year. United States.

	% of Women Experiencing an Accidental Pregnancy within the First Year of Use		% of Women Continuing Use at One Year[3]
Method (1)	**Typical Use[1] (2)**	**Perfect Use[2] (3)**	**(4)**
Chance[4]	85	85	
Spermicides[5]	26	6	40
Periodic abstinence	25		63
Calendar		9	
Ovulation method		3	
Sympto-thermal[6]		2	
Post-ovulation		1	
Withdrawal	19	4	
Cap[7]			
Parous women	40	26	42
Nulliparous women	20	9	56
Sponge			
Parous women	40	20	42
Nulliparous women	20	9	56
Diaphragm[7]	20	6	56
Condom[8]			
Female (Reality)	21	5	56
Male	14	3	61
Pill	5		71
progestin only		0.5	
combined		0.1	
IUD:			
Progesterone T:	2.0	1.5	81
Copper T 380A	0.8	0.6	78
LNg 20	0.1	0.1	81
Depo Provera	0.3	0.3	70
Norplant and Norplant-2	0.05	0.05	88
Female sterilization	0.5	0.5	100
Male sterilization	0.15	0.10	100

Source: Trussell J. Contraceptive efficacy. In Hatcher RA, Trussell J, Stewart F, Cates W, Steward GK, Kowal D, Guest F, *Contraceptive Technology: Seventeenth Revised Edition*, New York NY: Irvington Publishers, 1998.

1 Among *typical* couples who initiate use of a method (not necessarily for the first time), the percentage who experience an accidental pregnancy during the first year if they do not stop use for any other reason.
2 Among couples who initiate use of a method (not necessarily for the first time) and who use it *perfectly* (both consistently and correctly), the percentage who experience an accidental pregnancy during the first year if they do not stop use for any reason.
3 Among couples attempting to avoid pregnancy, the percentage who continue to use a method for one year.
4 The percents becoming pregnant in columns (2) and (3) are based on data from populations where contraception is not used and from women who cease using contraception in order to become pregnant. Among such populations, about 89% become pregnant within one year. This estimate was lowered slightly (to 85%) to represent the percentage who would become pregnant within one year among women now relying on reversible methods of contraception if they abandoned contraception altogether.
5 Foams, creams, gels, vaginal suppositories, and vaginal film.
6 Cervical mucus (ovulation) method supplemented by calendar in the pre-ovulatory and basal body temperature in the post-ovulatory phases.
7 With spermicidal cream or jelly.
8 Without spermicides.

CONTRAINDICATIONS

MIRENA® insertion is contraindicated when one or more of the following conditions exist:

1. Pregnancy or suspicion of pregnancy.
2. Congenital or acquired uterine anomaly including fibroids if they distort the uterine cavity.
3. Acute pelvic inflammatory disease or a history of pelvic inflammatory disease unless there has been a subsequent intrauterine pregnancy.
4. Postpartum endometritis or infected abortion in the past 3 months.
5. Known or suspected uterine or cervical neoplasia or unresolved, abnormal Pap smear.
6. Genital bleeding of unknown etiology.
7. Untreated acute cervicitis or vaginitis, including bacterial vaginosis or other lower genital tract infections until infection is controlled.
8. Acute liver disease or liver tumor (benign or malignant).
9. Woman or her partner has multiple sexual partners.
10. Conditions associated with increased susceptibility to infections with micro-organisms. Such conditions include, but are not limited to, leukemia, acquired immune deficiency syndrome (AIDS), and I.V. drug abuse.
11. Genital actinomycosis (See WARNINGS)
12. A previously inserted IUD that has not been removed.
13. Hypersensitivity to any component of this product.
14. Known or suspected carcinoma of the breast.
15. History of ectopic pregnancy or condition that would predispose to ectopic pregnancy.

WARNINGS

1. Ectopic Pregnancy

In large clinical trials of **MIRENA®**, half of all pregnancies detected during the studies were ectopic. The per-year incidence of ectopic pregnancy in the clinical trials was approximately 1 ectopic pregnancy per 1000 users per year. The rate of ectopic pregnancies associated with **MIRENA®** use is not significantly different than the rate for sexually active women not using any contraception.
Clinical trials of **MIRENA®** excluded women with a history of ectopic pregnancy. **MIRENA®** is not recommended for use in women with a history of ectopic pregnancy or conditions that increase the risk of ectopic pregnancy. Women who choose **MIRENA®** must be warned about the risks of ectopic pregnancy. They should be taught to recognize and report to their physician promptly any symptoms of ectopic pregnancy. Women should also be informed that ectopic pregnancy has been associated with complications leading to loss of fertility.

2. Intrauterine Pregnancy

In the event of an intrauterine pregnancy with **MIRENA®**, the following should be considered.
a. Septic abortion
In patients becoming pregnant with an IUD in place, septic abortion – with septicemia, septic shock, and death – may occur. If pregnancy should occur with a **MIRENA®** in place, **MIRENA®** should be removed. Removal or manipulation of **MIRENA®** may result in pregnancy loss.
b. Continuation of pregnancy
If a woman becomes pregnant with **MIRENA®** in place and if **MIRENA®** cannot be removed or the woman chooses not to have it removed, she should be warned that failure to remove **MIRENA®** increases the risk of miscarriage, sepsis, premature labor and premature delivery. She should be followed closely and advised to report immediately any flu-like symptoms, fever, chills, cramping, pain, bleeding, vaginal discharge or leakage of fluid.
c. Long-term effects and congenital anomalies
When pregnancy continues with **MIRENA®** in place, long-term effects on the offspring are unknown. Because of the intrauterine administration of levonorgestrel and local exposure to the hormone, the possibility of teratogenicity following exposure to **MIRENA®** cannot be completely excluded. Clinical experience with the outcomes of pregnancies is limited due to the small number of reported pregnancies following exposure to **MIRENA®**.
Congenital anomalies have occurred infrequently when **MIRENA®** has been in place during pregnancy. In these cases the role of **MIRENA®** in the development of the congenital anomalies is unknown. As of September 1999, 32 live births following exposure to **MIRENA®** were reported retrospectively. All but 2 of the infants were healthy at birth. One infant had pulmonary artery hypoplasia and another infant had cystic hypoplastic kidneys. (A sibling of this infant had renal agenesis with no **MIRENA®** exposure.)

3. Sepsis

As of 1999, four cases of Group A streptococcal sepsis (GAS) out of an estimated 1.3 million **MIRENA®** users were reported. All four women experienced the symptom of severe pain within hours of insertion, and this was followed by sepsis within a few days (of insertion). All recovered with treatment. Since death from GAS is more likely if treatment is delayed, it is important to be aware of these rare but serious infections. Aseptic technique during **MIRENA®** insertion is essential. (GAS sepsis can also occur postpartum, after minor surgery, in wounds and in association with other IUDs.)

4. Pelvic Inflammatory Disease (PID)

MIRENA® is contraindicated in the presence of known or suspected PID or in women with a history of PID unless there has been a subsequent intrauterine pregnancy. Use of IUDs has been associated with an increased risk of PID. The highest risk of PID occurs shortly after insertion (usually within the first 20 days thereafter) (see **Insertion Precautions**). A decision to use **MIRENA®** must include consideration of the risks of PID.

a. Women at increased risk for PID
PID is often associated with a sexually transmitted disease, and **MIRENA®** does not protect against sexually transmitted disease. The risk of PID is greater for women who have multiple sexual partners, and also for women whose sexual partner(s) have multiple sexual partners. Women who have ever had PID are at increased risk for a recurrence or re-infection.

b. PID warning to **MIRENA®** users
All women who choose **MIRENA®** must be informed prior to insertion about the possibility of PID and that PID can cause tubal damage leading to ectopic pregnancy or infertility, or in infrequent cases can necessitate hysterectomy, or can cause death. Patients must be taught to recognize and report to their physician promptly any symptoms of pelvic inflammatory disease. These symptoms include development of menstrual disorders (prolonged or heavy bleeding), unusual vaginal discharge, abdominal or pelvic pain or tenderness, dyspareunia, chills, and fever.

c. Asymptomatic PID
PID may be asymptomatic but still result in tubal damage and its sequelae.

d. Treatment of PID
Following a diagnosis of PID, or suspected PID, bacteriologic specimens should be obtained and antibiotic therapy should be initiated promptly. Removal of **MIRENA®** after initiation of antibiotic therapy is usually appropriate. Guidelines for PID treatment are available from the Center for Disease Control (CDC), Atlanta, Georgia. Adequate PID treatment requires the application of current standards of therapy prevailing at the time of occurrence of the infection with reference to prescription labeling.

Actinomycosis has been associated with IUDs. Symptomatic women with IUDs should have the IUD removed and should receive antibiotics. However, the management of the asymptomatic carrier is controversial because actinomycetes can be found normally in the genital tract cultures in healthy women without IUDs. False positive findings of actinomycosis on Pap smears can be a problem. When possible, confirm the Pap smear diagnosis with cultures.

5. Irregular Bleeding and Amenorrhea
MIRENA® can alter the bleeding pattern. During the first three to six months of **MIRENA®** use the number of bleeding and spotting days may be increased and bleeding patterns may be irregular. Thereafter the number of bleeding and spotting days usually decreases but bleeding may remain irregular. If bleeding irregularities develop during prolonged treatment appropriate diagnostic measures should be taken to rule out endometrial pathology.

Amenorrhea develops in approximately 20% of **MIRENA®** users by one year. The possibility of pregnancy should be considered if menstruation does not occur within six weeks of the onset of previous menstruation. Once pregnancy has been excluded, repeated pregnancy tests are not necessary in amenorrheic subjects unless indicated by other signs of pregnancy or by pelvic pain.

6. Embedment
Partial penetration or embedment of **MIRENA®** in the myometrium may decrease contraceptive effectiveness and can result in difficult removal.

7. Perforation
An IUD may perforate the uterus or cervix, most often during insertion although the perforation may not be detected until some time later. If perforation occurs, the IUD must be removed and surgery may be required. Adhesions, peritonitis, intestinal perforations, intestinal obstruction, abscesses and erosion of adjacent viscera have been reported with IUDs.

It is recommended that postpartum **MIRENA®** insertion be delayed until uterine involution is complete to decrease perforation risk. There is an increased risk of perforation in women who are lactating. Inserting **MIRENA®** immediately after first trimester abortion is not known to increase the risk of perforation, but insertion after second trimester abortion should be delayed until uterine involution is complete.

8. Ovarian Cysts
Since the contraceptive effect of **MIRENA®** is mainly due to its local effect, ovulatory cycles with follicular rupture usually occur in women of fertile age using **MIRENA®**. Sometimes atresia of the follicle is delayed and the follicle may continue to grow. Enlarged follicles have been diagnosed in about 12% of the subjects using **MIRENA®**. Most of these follicles are asymptomatic, although some may be accompanied by pelvic pain or dyspareunia. In most cases the enlarged follicles disappear spontaneously during two to three months observation. Surgical intervention is not usually required.

9. Breast Cancer
Women who currently have or have had breast cancer should not use hormonal contraception because breast cancer is a hormone-sensitive tumor.

10. Risks of Mortality
The available data from a variety of sources have been analyzed to estimate the risk of death associated with various methods of contraception. The estimates of risk of death include the combined risk of the contraceptive method plus the risk of pregnancy or abortion in the event of method failure. The findings of the analysis are shown in Table 2.
[See table 2 above]

Table 2: Annual Number of Birth-Related or Method-Related Deaths Associated with Control of Fertility per 100,000 Nonsterile Women, by Fertility Control Method According to Age

	AGE GROUP					
METHODS	15–19	20–24	25–29	30–34	35–39	40–44
No Birth Control Method/Term	4.7	5.4	4.8	6.3	11.7	20.6
No Birth Control Method A/B	2.1	2.0	1.6	1.9	2.8	5.3
IUD	0.2	0.3	0.2	0.1	0.3	0.6
Periodic Abstinence	1.4	1.3	0.7	1.0	1.0	1.9
Withdrawal	0.9	1.7	0.9	1.3	0.8	1.5
Condom	0.6	1.2	0.6	0.9	0.5	1.0
Diaphragm/Cap	0.6	1.1	0.6	0.9	1.6	3.1
Sponge	0.8	1.5	0.8	1.1	2.2	4.1
Spermicides	1.6	1.9	1.4	1.9	1.5	2.7
Oral Contraceptives	0.8	1.3	1.1	1.8	1.0	1.9
Implants/Injectables	0.2	0.6	0.5	0.8	0.5	0.6
Tubal Sterilization	1.3	1.2	1.1	1.1	1.2	1.3
Vasectomy	0.1	0.1	0.1	0.1	0.1	0.2

Harlap S. et al., *Preventing Pregnancy, protecting health: a new look at birth control choices in the US. The Alan Guttmacher Institute 1991: 1–129*

PRECAUTIONS

PATIENTS SHOULD BE COUNSELED THAT THIS PRODUCT DOES NOT PROTECT AGAINST HIV INFECTION (AIDS) AND OTHER SEXUALLY TRANSMITTED DISEASES.

1. PATIENT COUNSELING
Prior to insertion, the physician, nurse, or other trained health professional must provide the patient with the Patient Package Insert. The patient should be given the opportunity to read the information and discuss fully any questions she may have concerning **MIRENA®** as well as other methods of contraception.

Careful and objective counseling of the user prior to insertion regarding the expected bleeding pattern, the possible interindividual variation in changes in bleeding and the etiology of the changes may have an effect on the frequency of removal due to bleeding problems and amenorrhea.

The patient should be told that some bleeding such as irregular or prolonged bleeding and spotting, and/or cramps may occur during the first few weeks after insertion. If her symptoms continue or are severe she should report them to her health care provider. She should also be given instructions on what other symptoms require her to call her health care provider. She should be instructed on how to check after her menstrual period to make certain that the thread still protrudes from the cervix and cautioned not to pull on the thread and displace **MIRENA®**. She should be informed that there is no contraceptive protection if **MIRENA®** is displaced or expelled.

EVALUATION AND CLINICAL CONSIDERATIONS

a. A complete medical and social history, including that of the partner, should be obtained to determine conditions that might influence the selection of an IUD for contraception (see **CONTRAINDICATIONS**). A physical examination should include a pelvic examination, a Pap smear, and appropriate tests for any other forms of genital disease, such as gonorrhea and chlamydia laboratory evaluations, if indicated. **Special attention must be given to ascertaining whether the woman is at increased risk of ectopic pregnancy or PID. MIRENA® is contraindicated in these women.**
b. **The health care provider should determine that the patient is not pregnant.** The possibility of insertion of **MIRENA®** in the presence of an existing undetermined pregnancy is reduced if insertion is performed within 7 days of the onset of a menstrual period. **MIRENA®** can be replaced by a new system at any time in the cycle. **MIRENA®** can be inserted immediately after first trimester abortion.
c. **MIRENA®** should not be inserted until 6 weeks postpartum or until involution of the uterus is complete in order to reduce the incidence of perforation and expulsion.
d. Patients with certain types of valvular or congenital heart disease and surgically constructed systemic-pulmonary shunts are at increased risk of infective endocarditis. Use of **MIRENA®** in these patients may represent a potential source of septic emboli. Patients with known congenital heart disease who may be at increased risk should be treated with appropriate antibiotics at the time of insertion and removal. Patients requiring chronic corticosteroid therapy or insulin for diabetes should be monitored with special care for infection.
e. **MIRENA®** should be used with caution in patients who have a coagulopathy or are receiving anticoagulants.
f. Use of **MIRENA®** in patients with vaginitis or cervicitis should be postponed until proper treatment has eradicated the infection and until it has been shown that the cervicitis is not due to gonorrhea or chlamydia (see **CONTRAINDICATIONS**).

2. Insertion Precautions
Because the presence of organisms capable of establishing PID cannot be determined by appearance, and because IUD insertion may be associated with introduction of vaginal bacteria into the uterus, strict asepsis should be observed at insertion. Administration of antibiotics may be considered, but the utility of this treatment is unknown.

The uterus should be carefully sounded prior to **MIRENA®** insertion to determine the degree of patency of the endocervical canal and the internal os, and the direction and depth of the uterine cavity. In occasional cases, severe cervical stenosis may be encountered. Do not use excessive force to overcome this resistance.

Syncope, bradycardia, or other neurovascular episodes may occur during insertion or removal of **MIRENA®**, especially in patients with a predisposition to these conditions or cervical stenosis. If decreased pulse, perspiration, or pallor are observed, the patient should remain supine until these signs have disappeared.

3. Continuation and Removal
MIRENA® must be replaced every 5 years because contraceptive effectiveness after 5 years has not been established.

a) User complaints of pain, odorous discharge, bleeding, fever, genital lesions or sores should be promptly responded to and prompt examination recommended. (See **WARNINGS** regarding amenorrhea).
b) If examination during visits subsequent to insertion reveals that the length of the threads has changed from the length at time of insertion, and the system is verified as displaced, it should be removed. A new system may be inserted at that time or during the next menses if it is certain that conception has not occurred. If the threads are not visible, location of the **MIRENA®** should be verified, for example with X-ray, ultrasound, or gentle probing of the uterine cavity. If the **MIRENA®** is in place with no evidence of perforation, no intervention is indicated. If expulsion has occurred, it may be replaced within 7 days of a menstrual period after pregnancy has been ruled out.
c) Since **MIRENA®** may be displaced, patients should be reexamined and evaluated shortly after the first postinsertion menses, but definitely within 3 months after insertion. Symptoms of the partial or complete expulsion of any IUD may include bleeding or pain. However, the system can be expelled from the uterine cavity without the woman noticing it. Partial expulsion may decrease the effectiveness of **MIRENA®**. As menstrual flow usually decreases after the first 3 to 6 months of **MIRENA®** use, increase of menstrual flow may be indicative of an expulsion.
d) In the event a pregnancy is confirmed during **MIRENA®** use, the following steps should be taken:
   - Determine whether pregnancy is ectopic and take appropriate measures if it is.
   - Inform patient of the risks of leaving **MIRENA®** in place or removing it during pregnancy and of the lack of data on long-term effects on the offspring of women who have had **MIRENA®** in place during conception or gestation (see **WARNINGS**).

Continued on next page

Mirena—Cont.

- If possible **MIRENA®** should be removed after the patient has been warned of the risks of removal. If removal is difficult, the patient should be counseled and offered pregnancy termination.
- If **MIRENA®** is left in place, the patient's course should be followed closely.

e) Should the patient's relationship cease to be mutually monogamous, or should her partner become HIV positive, or acquire a sexually transmitted disease, she should be instructed to report this change to her clinician immediately. The use of a barrier method as a partial protection against acquiring sexually transmitted diseases should be strongly recommended. Removal of **MIRENA®** should be considered.

f) **MIRENA®** should be removed for the following medical reasons: menorrhagia and/or metrorrhagia producing anemia; acquired immune deficiency syndrome (AIDS); sexually transmitted disease; pelvic infection; endometritis; symptomatic genital actinomycosis; intractable pelvic pain; severe dyspareunia; pregnancy; endometrial or cervical malignancy; uterine or cervical perforation.

g) If the retrieval threads are not visible, they may have retracted into the uterus or have been broken, or **MIRENA®** may have been broken, perforated the uterus, or have been expelled. Location of **MIRENA®** may be determined by sonography, X-ray, or by gentle exploration of the uterine cavity with a probe.

h) Removal of the system should also be considered if any of the following conditions arise for the first time:
- migraine, focal migraine with asymmetrical visual loss or other symptoms indicating transient cerebral ischemia;
- exceptionally severe headache;
- jaundice;
- marked increase of blood pressure;
- severe arterial disease such as stroke or myocardial infarction.

4. Glucose Tolerance

Levonorgestrel may affect glucose tolerance, and the blood glucose concentration should be monitored in diabetic users of **MIRENA®**.

DRUG INTERACTIONS

The effect of hormonal contraceptives may be impaired by drugs which induce liver enzymes. The influence of these drugs on the contraceptive efficacy of **MIRENA®** has not been studied.

CARCINOGENESIS

Long-term studies in animals to assess the carcinogenic potential of levonorgestrel releasing intrauterine system have not been performed. See **"WARNINGS"** section.

PREGNANCY

Pregnancy Category X. See **"WARNINGS"** section.

NURSING MOTHERS

Levonorgestrel has been identified in small quantities in the breast milk of lactating women using **MIRENA®**. In a study of 14 breastfeeding women using a **MIRENA®** prototype during lactation, mean infant serum levels of levonorgestrel were approximately 7% of maternal serum levels. Hormonal contraceptives are not recommended as the contraceptive method of first choice during lactation.

PEDIATRIC USE

Safety and efficacy of **MIRENA®** have been established in women of reproductive age. Use of this product before menarche is not indicated. (See **RECOMMENDED PATIENT PROFILE**)

GERIATRIC USE

MIRENA® has not been studied in women over age 65 and is not currently approved for use in this population.

INFORMATION FOR THE PATIENT See Patient Labeling

Patients should also be advised that the prescribing information is available to them at their request. It is recommended that potential users be fully informed about the risks and benefits associated with the use of **MIRENA®**, with other forms of contraception, and with no contraception at all.

Return to fertility

About 80% of women wishing to become pregnant conceived within 12 months after removal of **MIRENA®**.

ADVERSE REACTIONS

The most serious adverse reactions associated with the use of **MIRENA®** are discussed above in the Warnings section. Others are presented in the Precautions section. Other adverse events reported by 5% or more subjects include:

Abdominal pain	Upper respiratory infection
Leukorrhea	Nausea
Headache	Nervousness
Vaginitis	Dysmenorrhea
Back pain	Weight increase
Breast pain	Skin disorder
Acne	Decreased libido
Depression	Abnormal Pap smear
Hypertension	Sinusitis

Other reported adverse reactions occurring in less than 3% of patients include: failed insertion, migraine, vomiting, anemia, cervicitis, dyspareunia, hair loss, eczema.

HOW SUPPLIED

MIRENA® (levonorgestrel-releasing intrauterine system), containing a total of 52 mg levonorgestrel, is available in a carton of one sterile unit NDC# 50419-421-01. Each **MIRENA®** is packaged in a thermoformed blister package with a peelable lid, together with an insertion tube which is then heat sealed into a secondary pouch.

MIRENA® is supplied sterile. **MIRENA®** is sterilized with ethylene oxide. Do not resterilize. For single use only. Do not use if the inner package is damaged or open. Insert before the end of the month shown on the label.

STORAGE AND HANDLING

Store at 25°C (77°F); with excursions permitted between 15°-30°C (59-86°F) [See USP Controlled Room Temperature]

DIRECTIONS FOR USE

NOTE: Health care providers are advised to become thoroughly familiar with the insertion instructions before attempting insertion of MIRENA®.

Insertion Instructions

MIRENA® is inserted with the provided inserter (figure 1) into the uterine cavity within seven days of the onset of menstruation or immediately after first trimester abortion by carefully following the insertion instructions. It can be replaced by a new system at any time during the menstrual cycle.

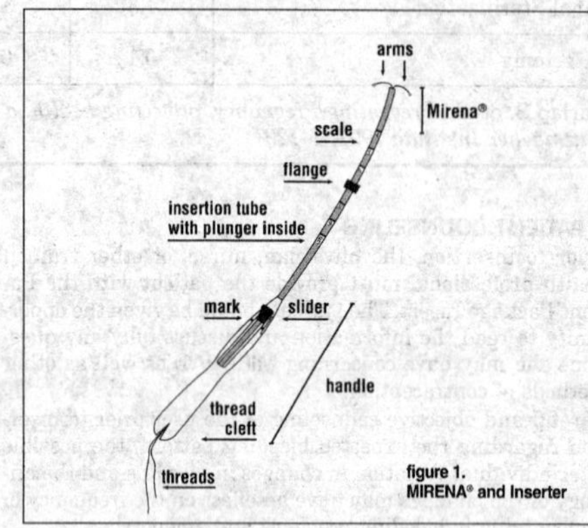

figure 1.
MIRENA® and Inserter

Preparation for insertion

- Confirm that the patient understands the method and alternatives and has signed a consent form.
- Examine the patient to establish the size and position of the uterus, to detect cervicitis or other genital contraindications and to exclude pregnancy.
- Obtain cervical cultures, perform a pregnancy test and give antibiotic prophylaxis if indicated.
- Use aseptic technique during insertion.
- Administer oral analgesics if needed.
- Cleanse the cervix and vagina with an antiseptic solution.
- Administer a paracervical block if needed.
- Grasp the upper lip of the cervix with a tenaculum and apply gentle traction to align the cervical canal with the uterine cavity.
- Carefully sound the uterus to measure its depth and to check the patency of the cervix. If you encounter cervical stenosis, use dilatation, not force, to overcome resistance.
- The uterus should sound to a depth of 6 to 9 cm. Insertion of **MIRENA®** into a uterine cavity less than 6.0 cm by sounding may increase the incidence of expulsion, bleeding, pain, perforation, and possibly, pregnancy.

Insertion Procedure

1.
- Open the sterile package.
- Place sterile gloves on your hands.
- Pick up the inserter containing **MIRENA®**.
- Carefully release the threads from behind the slider, so that they hang freely.
- Make sure that the slider is in the furthest position away from you (positioned at the top of the handle nearest the IUS).
- While looking at the insertion tube, check that the arms of the system are horizontal. If not, align them on a sterile surface (figure 2) or with sterile gloved fingers.

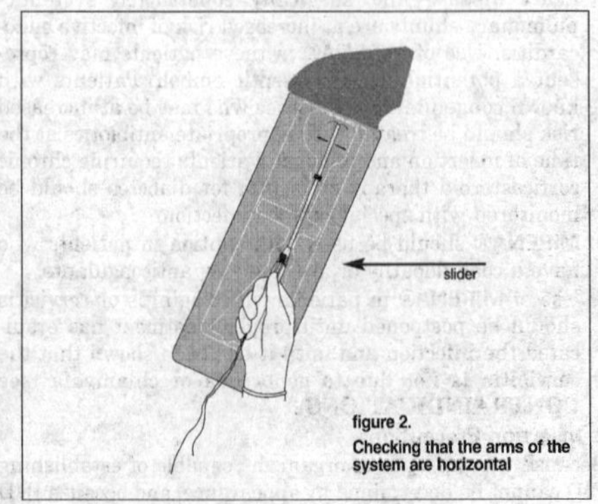

figure 2.
Checking that the arms of the system are horizontal

2.
- Pull on both threads to draw the **MIRENA®** system into the insertion tube (figure 3a).
- Note that the knobs at the ends of the arms now cover the open end of the inserter (figure 3b).

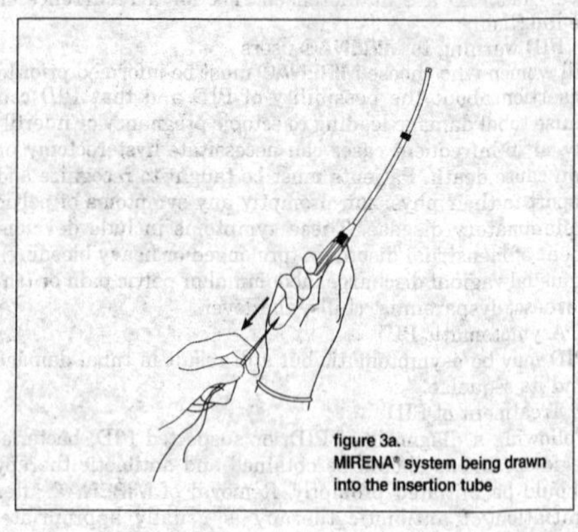
figure 3a.
MIRENA® system being drawn into the insertion tube

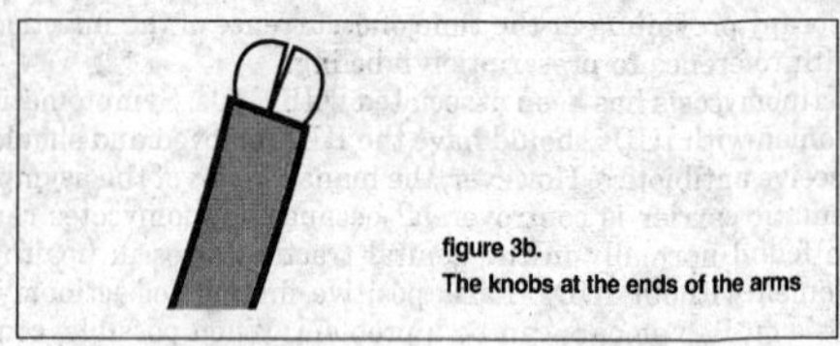
figure 3b.
The knobs at the ends of the arms

3. Fix the threads tightly in the cleft at the end of the handle (figure 4).

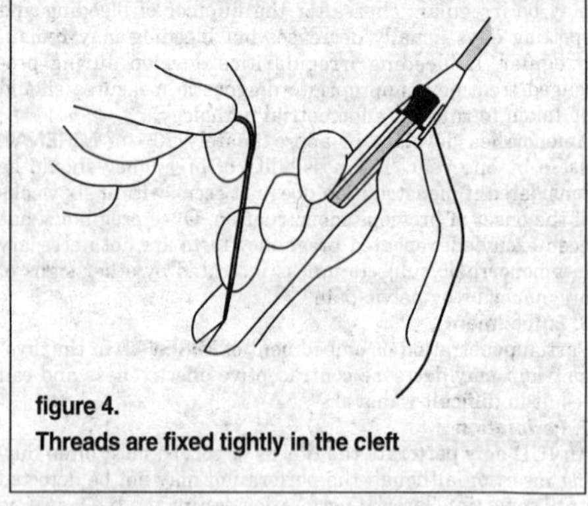
figure 4.
Threads are fixed tightly in the cleft

4. Set the flange to the depth measured by the sound, as indicated in figure 5.

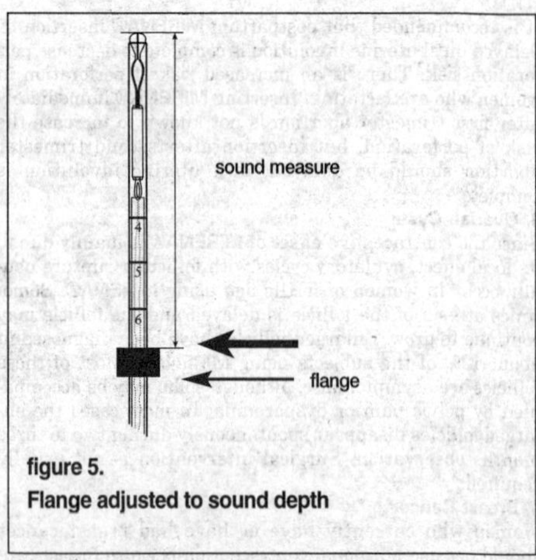

figure 5.
Flange adjusted to sound depth

5. MIRENA® is now ready to be inserted.

Hold the slider firmly in the furthermost position (at the top of the handle). Grasp the cervix with the tenaculum and apply gentle traction to align the cervical canal with the uterine cavity. Gently insert the inserter into the cervical canal and advance the insertion tube into the uterus until the flange is situated at a distance of about 1.5-2 cm from the external cervical os to give sufficient space for the arms to open (figure 6).

NOTE! Do not force the inserter.

[See figure at top of next column]

6. While holding the inserter steady release the arms of **MIRENA®** (figure 7a) by pulling the slider back until the

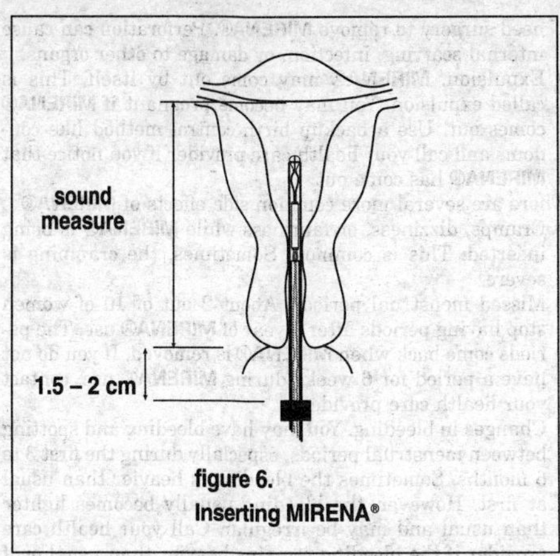

figure 6.
Inserting MIRENA®

top of the slider reaches the mark (raised horizontal line on the handle) (figure 7b).

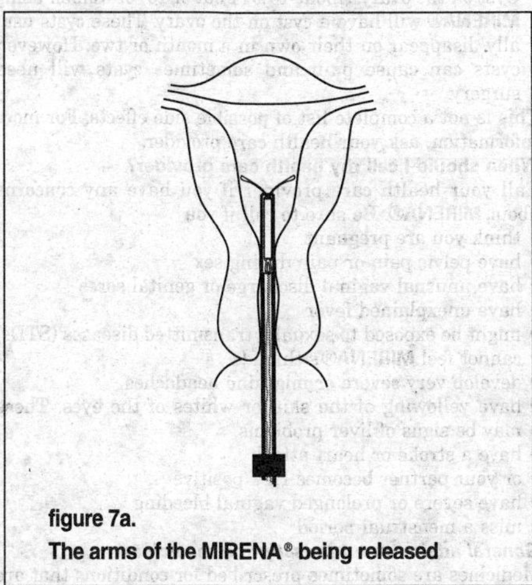
figure 7a.
The arms of the MIRENA® being released

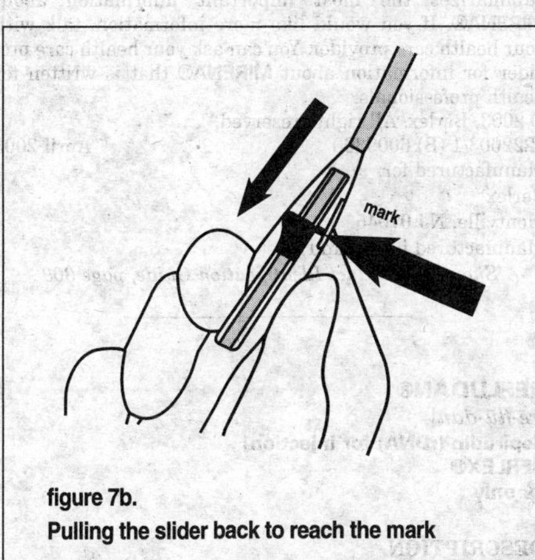

figure 7b.
Pulling the slider back to reach the mark

7. Push the inserter gently into the uterine cavity until the flange touches the cervix. **MIRENA®** should now be in the fundal position (figure 8).

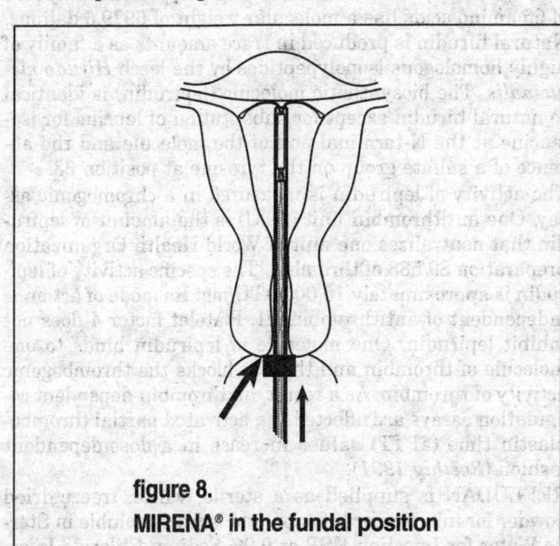
figure 8.
MIRENA® in the fundal position

8. Holding the inserter firmly in position release **MIRENA®** by pulling the slider down all the way. The threads will be released automatically (figure 9).

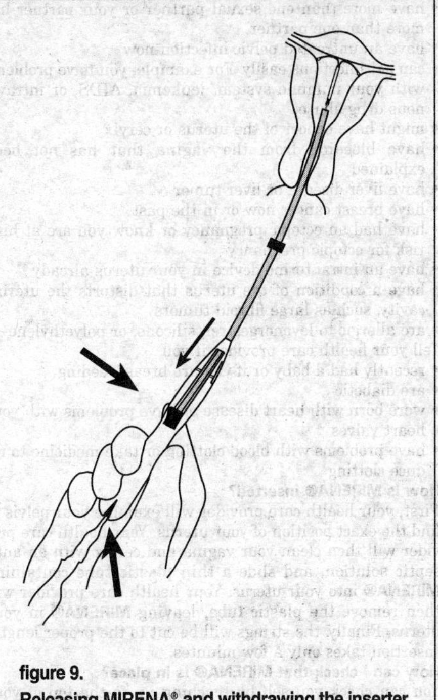
figure 9.
Releasing MIRENA® and withdrawing the inserter

9. Remove the inserter from the uterus. Cut the threads to leave about 2-3 cm visible outside the cervix (figure 10).

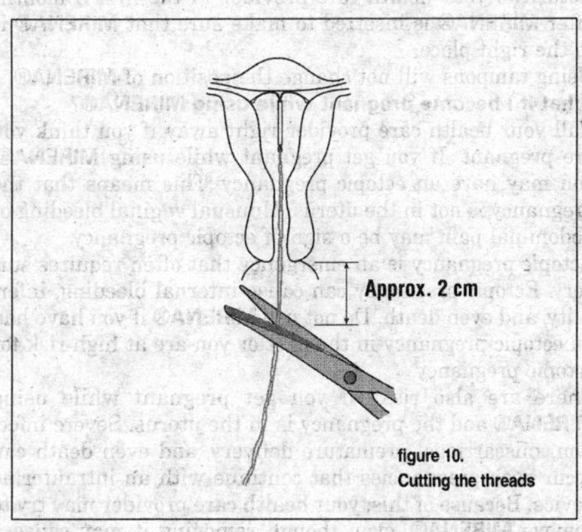

figure 10.
Cutting the threads

IMPORTANT!

If you suspect that the system is not in the correct position, check placement, (with ultrasound, for example). Remove the system if it is not positioned completely within the uterus. Do not reinsert a removed system.

REMOVAL OF MIRENA®

Remove **MIRENA®** by applying gentle traction on the threads with forceps. The arms of the system will fold upward as it is withdrawn from the uterus. The system should not remain in the uterus after 5 years.

SPECIAL NOTES IF A PATIENT WANTS TO CONTINUE CONTRACEPTION AFTER REMOVAL

You may insert a new **MIRENA®** immediately following removal.

If a patient with regular cycles wants to start a different birth control method, remove the system during the first 7 days of the menstrual cycle and start the new method.

If a patient with irregular cycles or amenorrhea wants to start a different birth control method, or if you remove the system after the seventh day of the menstrual cycle, start the new method at least 7 days before removal.

2217966 (B) 6004702 December 2003

PATIENT INFORMATION

MIRENA®

(levonorgestrel-releasing intrauterine system)

MIRENA® (Mur-ĕ-nah) is used to prevent pregnancy. It does not protect against HIV infection (AIDS) and other sexually transmitted diseases (STDs).

Read this information carefully before you decide if **MIRENA®** is right for you. This information does not take the place of talking with your health care provider. If you have any questions about **MIRENA®**, ask your health care provider. You should also learn about other birth control methods to choose the one that is best for you.

WHAT IS MIRENA®?

MIRENA® is a hormone-releasing system placed in your uterus to prevent pregnancy for up to 5 years.

MIRENA® is T-shaped. It contains a hormone called levonorgestrel. Levonorgestrel is a progestin hormone often used in birth control pills. **MIRENA®** releases the hormone into the uterus. Only small amounts of the hormone enter your blood.

Two brown threads are attached to the stem of the T. You can check that **MIRENA®** is in place by feeling for the threads at the top of your vagina with your fingers. Your health care provider can also remove **MIRENA®** at any time by pulling on the threads. The threads are the only part of **MIRENA®** you can feel when **MIRENA®** is in your uterus.

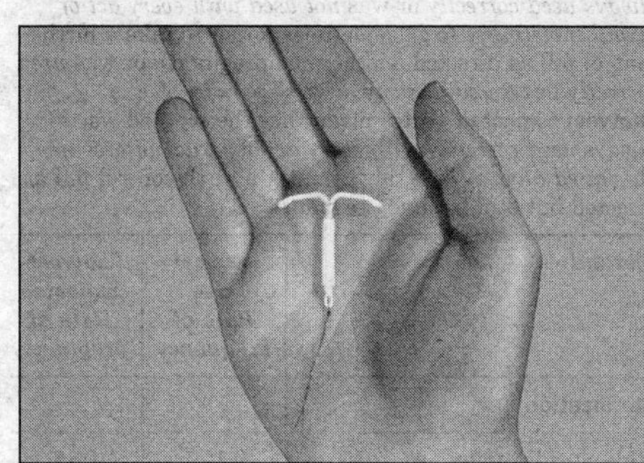
The MIRENA® is small...

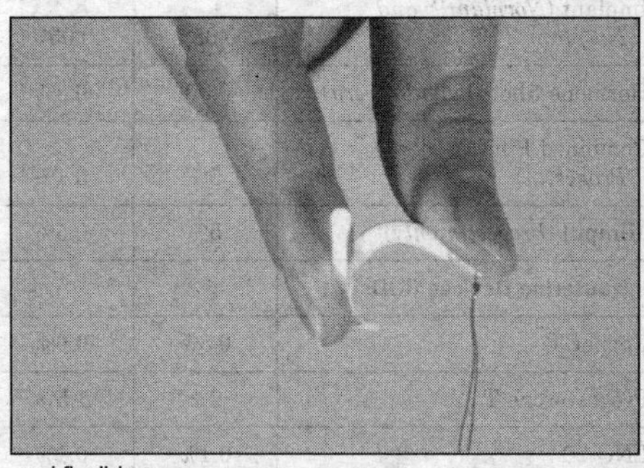
and flexible

What if I need birth control for more than 5 years?

You must have **MIRENA®** removed after 5 years, but your health care provider can insert a new **MIRENA®** then if you choose to continue using **MIRENA®**.

What if I change my mind about birth control and decide to have another baby?

Your health care provider can remove **MIRENA®** at any time by pulling on the threads. You may become pregnant as soon as **MIRENA®** is removed. About 8 out of 10 women who want to become pregnant will become pregnant some time in the first year after **MIRENA®** is removed.

How does MIRENA® work?

There is no single explanation of how **MIRENA®** works. It may stop release of your egg from your ovary, but this is not the way it works in most cases. It may block sperm from reaching or fertilizing your egg. It may make the lining of your uterus thin. We do not know which of these actions is most important for preventing pregnancy and most likely all of them work together.

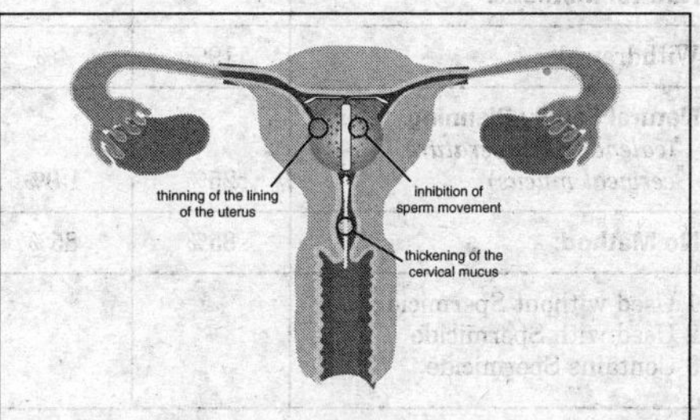

How well does MIRENA® work?

Less than 1 out of 100 women using **MIRENA®** become pregnant during five years of **MIRENA®** use.

The following table shows how **MIRENA®** compares to other birth control methods. In this table **MIRENA®** is identified as "LNG 20".

Continued on next page

Information on Berlex products (appearing here) is based on the most current information available at the time of publication closing. Further information for these and other Berlex products can be obtained from Medical & Product Services at Berlex, Inc. by calling 1-888-BERLEX-4.

Mirena—Cont.

Pregnancy Rates for Birth Control Methods
(For One Year of Use)

The following table provides estimates of the percent of women likely to become pregnant while using a particular contraceptive method for one year. These estimates are based on a variety of studies.

"Typical Use" rates mean that the method either was *not always used correctly* or was *not used with every act of sexual intercourse* (e.g., sometimes forgot to take a birth control pill as directed and became pregnant), or was *used correctly* but *failed anyway*.

"Lowest Expected" rates mean that the method was *always used correctly* with *every act of sexual intercourse* but *failed anyway* (e.g., always took a birth control pill as directed but still became pregnant).

Method	*Typical Use Rate of Pregnancy*	*Lowest Expected Rate of Pregnancy*
Sterilization		
Male Sterilization	0.15%	0.1%
Female Sterilization	0.5%	0.5%
Hormonal Methods:		
Implant (*Norplant™ and Norplant-2™*)	0.05%	0.05%
Hormone Shot (*Depo-Provera*)	0.3%	0.3%
Combined Pill (*Estrogen/ Progestin*)	5%	0.1%
Minipill (*Progestin only*)	5%	0.5%
Intrauterine Devices (IUDs):		
Copper T	0.8%	0.6%
Progesterone T	2%	1.5%
LNG 20	0.1%	0.1%
Barrier Methods:		
Male Latex Condom[1]	14%	3%
Diaphragm[2]	20%	6%
Vaginal Sponge (*no previous births*)[3]	20%	9%
Vaginal Sponge (*previous births*)[3]	40%	20%
Cervical Cap (*no previous births*)[2]	20%	9%
Cervical Cap (*previous births*)[2]	40%	26%
Female Condom	21%	5%
Spermicide: (*gel, foam, suppository, film*)	26%	6%
Natural Methods:		
Withdrawal	19%	4%
Natural Family Planning (*calendar, temperature, cervical mucus*)	25%	1-9%
No Method:	85%	85%
1 Used without Spermicide 2 Used with Spermicide 3 Contains Spermicide		

Data adapted from: Trussell J. Contraceptive efficacy. In Hatcher RA, Trussell J, Stewart F, et al. *Contraceptive Technology: Seventeenth Revised Edition. New York, NY: Ardent Media, 1998.*

Who might use MIRENA®?
You might choose **MIRENA®** if you
- need birth control with a low failure rate
- need birth control that is reversible
- need birth control that is easy to use
- have had at least one baby

Who should not use MIRENA®?
Do not use **MIRENA®** if you
- might be pregnant
- have had a serious pelvic infection called pelvic inflammatory disease (PID)
- have had a serious pelvic infection in the past 3 months after a pregnancy
- have more than one sexual partner or your partner has more than one partner
- have an untreated pelvic infection now
- can get infections easily. For example, you have problems with your immune system, leukemia, AIDS, or intravenous drug abuse.
- might have cancer of the uterus or cervix
- have bleeding from the vagina that has not been explained
- have liver disease or liver tumor
- have breast cancer now or in the past
- have had an ectopic pregnancy or know you are at high risk for ectopic pregnancy
- have an intrauterine device in your uterus already
- have a condition of the uterus that distorts the uterine cavity, such as large fibroid tumors
- are allergic to levonorgestrel, silicone, or polyethylene

Tell your health care provider if you
- recently had a baby or if you are breast feeding
- are diabetic
- were born with heart disease or have problems with your heart valves
- have problems with blood clotting or take medicine to reduce clotting

How is MIRENA® inserted?
First, your health care provider will examine your pelvis to find the exact position of your uterus. Your health care provider will then clean your vagina and cervix with an antiseptic solution, and slide a thin plastic tube containing **MIRENA®** into your uterus. Your health care provider will then remove the plastic tube, leaving **MIRENA®** in your uterus. Finally, the strings will be cut to the proper length. Insertion takes only a few minutes.

How can I check that MIRENA® is in place?
You can check yourself by reaching up to the top of your vagina with clean fingers to feel the threads. Do not pull on the threads. It is a good habit to check **MIRENA®** after each menstrual period. If you feel more of **MIRENA®** than just the threads, **MIRENA®** is not in the right place. Call your health care provider to have it removed. If you cannot feel the threads at all, ask your health care provider to check that **MIRENA®** is still in the right place.
Return to your health care provider in the first 3 months after **MIRENA®** is inserted to make sure that **MIRENA®** is in the right place.
Using tampons will not change the position of **MIRENA®**.

What if I become pregnant while using MIRENA®?
Call your health care provider right away if you think you are pregnant. If you get pregnant while using **MIRENA®**, you may have an ectopic pregnancy. This means that the pregnancy is not in the uterus. Unusual vaginal bleeding or abdominal pain may be a sign of ectopic pregnancy.
Ectopic pregnancy is an emergency that often requires surgery. Ectopic pregnancy can cause internal bleeding, infertility, and even death. Do not use **MIRENA®** if you have had an ectopic pregnancy in the past or you are at high risk for ectopic pregnancy.
There are also risks if you get pregnant while using **MIRENA®** and the pregnancy is in the uterus. Severe infection, miscarriage, premature delivery, and even death can occur with pregnancies that continue with an intrauterine device. Because of this, your health care provider may try to remove **MIRENA®**, even though removing it may cause a miscarriage. If **MIRENA®** cannot be removed, talk with your health care provider about the benefits and risks of continuing the pregnancy.
If you continue your pregnancy, see your health care provider regularly. Call your health care provider right away if you get flu-like symptoms, fever, chills, cramping, pain, bleeding, vaginal discharge, or fluid leaking from your vagina. These may be signs of infection.
We do not know if **MIRENA®** can cause long-term effects on the fetus if it stays in place during a pregnancy.

How will MIRENA® change my periods?
For the first 3 to 6 months, your monthly period may become irregular. You may also have frequent spotting or light bleeding. A few women have heavy bleeding during this time. After your body adjusts, the number of bleeding days is likely to decrease, and you may even find that your periods stop altogether.

What are the possible side effects of using MIRENA®?
The following are serious but uncommon side effects of **MIRENA®**
- Pelvic inflammatory disease (PID). Some IUD users get a serious pelvic infection called pelvic inflammatory disease. PID is usually sexually transmitted. You have a higher chance of getting PID if you or your partner have sex with other partners. PID can cause serious problems such as infertility, ectopic pregnancy or constant pelvic pain.
- PID is usually treated with antibiotics. However, more serious cases of PID may require surgery. A hysterectomy (removal of the uterus) is sometimes needed. In rare cases, infections that start as PID can even cause death. Tell your health care provider right away if you have any of these signs of PID: long-lasting or heavy bleeding, unusual vaginal discharge, low abdominal (stomach area) pain, painful sex, chills, or fever.
- Life-threatening infection. Life-threatening infection occurs rarely within the first few days after **MIRENA®** is inserted. Call your health care provider if you develop severe pain within a few hours after insertion.
- Perforation. **MIRENA®** may go through the uterus. This is called perforation. If your uterus is perforated, you may need surgery to remove **MIRENA®**. Perforation can cause internal scarring, infection, or damage to other organs.
- Expulsion. **MIRENA®** may come out by itself. This is called expulsion. You may become pregnant if **MIRENA®** comes out. Use a backup birth control method like condoms and call your health care provider if you notice that **MIRENA®** has come out.

There are several more common side effects of **MIRENA®**
- Cramps, dizziness, or faintness while **MIRENA®** is being inserted. This is common. Sometimes, the cramping is severe.
- Missed menstrual periods. About 2 out of 10 of women stop having periods after 1 year of **MIRENA®** use. The periods come back when **MIRENA®** is removed. If you do not have a period for 6 weeks during **MIRENA®** use, contact your health care provider.
- Changes in bleeding. You may have bleeding and spotting between menstrual periods, especially during the first 3 to 6 months. Sometimes the bleeding is heavier than usual at first. However, the bleeding usually becomes lighter than usual and may be irregular. Call your health care provider if the bleeding remains heavier than usual or if the bleeding becomes heavy after it has been light for a while.
- Cyst on the ovary. About 10% (1 out of 10) of women using **MIRENA®** will have a cyst on the ovary. These cysts usually disappear on their own in a month or two. However, cysts can cause pain and sometimes cysts will need surgery.

This is not a complete list of possible side effects. For more information, ask your health care provider.

When should I call my health care provider?
Call your health care provider if you have any concerns about **MIRENA®**. Be sure to call if you
- think you are pregnant
- have pelvic pain or pain during sex
- have unusual vaginal discharge or genital sores
- have unexplained fever
- might be exposed to sexually transmitted diseases (STDs)
- cannot feel **MIRENA®**'s threads
- develop very severe or migraine headaches
- have yellowing of the skin or whites of the eyes. These may be signs of liver problems.
- have a stroke or heart attack
- or your partner becomes HIV positive
- have severe or prolonged vaginal bleeding
- miss a menstrual period

General advice about prescription medicines
Medicines are sometimes prescribed for conditions that are not mentioned in patient information leaflets. This leaflet summarizes the most important information about **MIRENA®**. If you would like more information, talk with your health care provider. You can ask your health care provider for information about **MIRENA®** that is written for health professionals.

5222003/1 (B) 6009300 April 2003
Manufactured for:
Berlex
Montville, NJ 07045
Manufactured in Finland

Shown in Product Identification Guide, page 309

REFLUDAN® ℞
[rē-flū-dan]
[lepirudin (rDNA) for injection]
BERLEX®
℞ only

DESCRIPTION
REFLUDAN [lepirudin (rDNA) for injection] is a highly specific direct inhibitor of thrombin. Lepirudin (chemical designation: [Leu[1], Thr[2]]-63-desulfohirudin) is a recombinant hirudin derived from yeast cells. The polypeptide composed of 65 amino acids has a molecular weight of 6979.5 daltons. Natural hirudin is produced in trace amounts as a family of highly homologous isopolypeptides by the leech *Hirudo medicinalis*. The biosynthetic molecule (lepirudin) is identical to natural hirudin except for substitution of leucine for isoleucine at the N-terminal end of the molecule and the absence of a sulfate group on the tyrosine at position 63.
The activity of lepirudin is measured in a chromogenic assay. One antithrombin unit (ATU) is the amount of lepirudin that neutralizes one unit of World Health Organization preparation 89/588 of thrombin. The specific activity of lepirudin is approximately 16,000 ATU/mg. Its mode of action is independent of antithrombin III. Platelet factor 4 does not inhibit lepirudin. One molecule of lepirudin binds to one molecule of thrombin and thereby blocks the thrombogenic activity of thrombin. As a result, all thrombin-dependent coagulation assays are affected, eg, activated partial thromboplastin time (aPTT) values increase in a dose-dependent fashion (*Roethig 1991*).
REFLUDAN is supplied as a sterile, white, freeze-dried powder for injection or infusion and is freely soluble in Sterile Water for Injection USP or 0.9% Sodium Chloride Injection USP.
Each vial of REFLUDAN contains 50 mg lepirudin. Other ingredients are 40 mg mannitol and sodium hydroxide for adjustment of pH to approximately 7.

CLINICAL PHARMACOLOGY

Pharmacokinetic Properties

The pharmacokinetic properties of lepirudin following intravenous administration are well described by a two-compartment model. Distribution is essentially confined to extracellular fluids and is characterized by an initial half-life of approximately 10 minutes. Elimination follows a first-order process and is characterized by a terminal half-life of about 1.3 hours in young healthy volunteers. As the intravenous dose is increased over the range of 0.1 to 0.4 mg/kg, the maximum plasma concentration and the area-under-the-curve increase proportionally.

Lepirudin is thought to be metabolized by release of amino acids via catabolic hydrolysis of the parent drug. However, conclusive data are not available. About 48% of the administration dose is excreted in the urine which consists of unchanged drug (35%) and other fragments of the parent drug. The systemic clearance of lepirudin is proportional to the glomerular filtration rate or creatinine clearance. Dose adjustment based on creatinine clearance is recommended (see **DOSAGE AND ADMINISTRATION**: Monitoring and Adjusting Therapy; Use in Renal Impairment). In patients with marked renal insufficiency (creatinine clearance below 15 mL/min) and on hemodialysis, elimination half-lives are prolonged up to 2 days.

The systemic clearance of lepirudin in women is about 25% lower than in men. In elderly patients, the systemic clearance of lepirudin is 20% lower than in younger patients. This may be explained by the lower creatinine clearance in elderly patients compared to younger patients.

Table 1 summarizes systemic clearance (Cl) and volume of distribution at steady state (Vss) of lepirudin for various study populations.

Table 1: Systemic clearance (Cl) and volume of distribution at steady state (Vss) of lepirudin

	Cl (mL/min) Mean (% CV*)	Vss (L) Mean (% CV*)
Healthy young subjects (n = 18, age 18-60 years)	164 (19.3%)	12.2 (16.4%)
Healthy elderly subjects (n = 10, age 65-80 years)	139 (22.5%)	18.7 (20.6%)
Renally impaired patients (n = 16, creatinine clearance below 80 mL/min)	61 (89.4%)	18.0 (41.1%)
HIT† patients (n = 73)	114 (46.8%)	32.1 (98.9%)

* CV: Coefficient of variation
†HIT: Heparin-induced thrombocytopenia

Pharmacodynamic Properties

The pharmacodynamic effect of REFLUDAN on the proteolytic activity of thrombin was routinely assessed as an increase in aPTT. This was observed with increasing plasma concentrations of lepirudin, with no saturable effect up to the highest tested dose (0.5 mg/kg body weight intravenous bolus). Thrombin time (TT) frequently exceeded 200 seconds even at low plasma concentrations of lepirudin, which renders this test unsuitable for routine monitoring of REFLUDAN therapy.

The pharmacodynamic response defined by the aPTT ratio (aPTT at a time after REFLUDAN administration over an aPTT reference value, usually median of the laboratory normal range for aPTT) depends on plasma drug levels which in turn depend on the individual patient's renal function (see **CLINICAL PHARMACOLOGY**: Pharmacokinetic Properties). For patients undergoing additional thrombolysis, elevated aPTT ratios were already observed at low lepirudin plasma concentrations, and further response to increasing plasma concentrations was relatively flat. In other populations, the response was steeper. At plasma concentrations of 1500 ng/mL, aPTT ratios were nearly 3.0 for healthy volunteers, 2.3 for patients with heparin-induced thrombocytopenia, and 2.1 for patients with deep venous thrombosis.

CLINICAL TRIAL DATA

Heparin-induced thrombocytopenia (HIT) is described as an allergy-like adverse reaction to heparin. It can be found in about 1% to 2% of patients treated with heparin for more than 4 days. The clinical picture of HIT is characterized by thrombocytopenia alone or in combination with thromboembolic complications (TECs). These complications comprise the entire spectrum of venous and arterial thromboembolism including deep venous thrombosis, pulmonary embolism, myocardial infarction, ischemic stroke, and occlusion of limb arteries, which may ultimately result in necroses requiring amputation. Furthermore, there is evidence to suggest that warfarin-induced venous limb gangrene may be associated with HIT. Without further treatment, the mortality in HIT patients with new TECs is about 20% to 30% (*Fondu 1995; Greinacher 1995; Warkentin, Chong, et al., Warkentin, Elavathil, et al. 1997*).

The conclusion that REFLUDAN is an effective treatment for HIT is based upon the data of two prospective, historically controlled clinical trials ("HAT-1" study and "HAT-2" study). The trials were comparable with regard to study design, primary and secondary objectives, and dosing regimens, as well as general study outline and organization. They both used the same historical control group for comparison. This historical control was mainly compiled from a recent retrospective registry of HIT patients.

Overall, 198 (HAT-1: 82, HAT-2: 116) patients were treated with REFLUDAN and 182 historical control patients were treated with other therapies. All except 5 (HAT-1: 1, HAT-2: 4) prospective patients and all historical control patients were diagnosed with HIT using the heparin-induced platelet activation assay (HIPAA) or equivalent assays for testing. In total, 113 (HAT-1: 54, HAT-2: 59) prospective patients ("REFLUDAN") and 91 historical control patients ("historical control") presented with TECs at baseline (day of positive test result) and qualified for direct comparison of clinical endpoints.

The gender distribution was found to be similar in REFLUDAN patients and historical control patients. Overall, REFLUDAN patients tended to be younger than historical control patients. Table 2 summarizes the demographic baseline characteristics of patients presenting with TECs at baseline.

Table 2: Demographic baseline characteristics of patients presenting with TECs

	REFLUDAN		Historical Control
	HAT-1 (n = 54)	HAT-2 (n = 59)	(n = 91)
Males	27.8%	44.1%	35.2%
Females	72.2%	55.9%	64.8%
Age <65 years	63.0%	67.8%	44.0%
Age ≥65 years	37.0%	32.2%	56.0%
Mean age ± SD (years)	57 ± 17	58 ± 12	64 ± 14

The key criteria of efficacy from a laboratory standpoint (n=115 evaluable patients) were platelet recovery (increase in platelet count by at least 30% of nadir to values >100,000) and effective anticoagulation (aPTT ratio >1.5 with a maximum total 40% increase in the initial infusion rate). The proportions of REFLUDAN patients presenting with TECs at baseline who showed platelet recovery, effective anticoagulation, or both (laboratory responders) are shown in Table 3. Comparable rates for the historical control group cannot be given, because (1) platelet counts were not monitored as closely as in the REFLUDAN group, and (2) most historical control patients did not receive therapies affecting aPTT.

Table 3: Proportions of laboratory responders among REFLUDAN patients presenting with TECs

	HAT-1	HAT-2
Number of evaluable patients	55	60
Platelet recovery	90.9%	95.0%
Effective anticoagulation	81.8%	75.0%
Both	72.7%	71.7%

Comparisons of clinical efficacy were made between REFLUDAN patients and historical control patients with regard to the combined and individual incidences of death, limb amputation, or new TEC.

The original main analyses included all events that occurred after laboratory confirmation of HIT. This approach was revealed to be substantially confounded by the relative contribution of the pretreatment period (time between laboratory confirmation of HIT and start of treatment). Although short in duration (mean length 1.5 days in HAT-1 and 2.0 days in HAT-2), the pretreatment period accounted for 45% and 26% of events observed in the main analyses of HAT-1 REFLUDAN patients and HAT-2 REFLUDAN patients, respectively. Therefore, initiation of treatment was set as the starting point for the analyses. For the historical control group, the first treatment selected within 2 days of laboratory confirmation of HIT was used for reference.

Seven days after start of treatment, the cumulative risk of death, limb amputation, or new TEC was 3.7% in the HAT-1 REFLUDAN patients and 16.9% in the HAT-2 REFLUDAN patients, as compared to 24.9% in the historical control group. At 35 days, when approximately 10% of patients were still at risk, the cumulative risk was 13.0% in the HAT-1 REFLUDAN patients and 28.9% in the HAT-2 REFLUDAN patients, as compared to 47.8% in the historical control group.

In an additional meta-analysis, the pooled REFLUDAN patients of the HAT-1 and HAT-2 studies who presented with TECs at baseline were compared to the respective historical control patients. Seven and 35 days after start of treatment, the cumulative risks of death were 4.4% and 8.9% in the REFLUDAN group, as compared to 1.4% and 17.6% in the historical control group. The cumulative risks of limb amputation were 2.7% and 6.5% in the REFLUDAN group, as compared to 2.6% and 10.4% in the historical control group. Most importantly, the cumulative risks of new TEC were 6.3% and 10.1% in the REFLUDAN group, as compared to 22.2% and 27.2% in the historical control group. As shown in Fig 1, the differences in the cumulative risk of death, limb amputation, or new TEC between the groups were statistically significant in favor of REFLUDAN in the analysis of time to event ($P = 0.004$ according to log-rank test).

Fig 1: Cumulative risk of death, limb amputation, or new thromboembolic complication after start of treatment

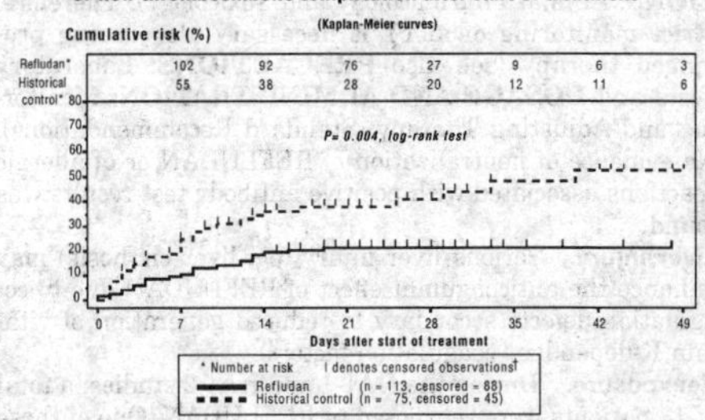

† Censored observations: Patients who did not reach a disease endpoint during their period of follow-up

The immediate impact of treatment on the combined risk of death, limb amputation, or new TEC is demonstrated by comparing pretreatment period and treatment period in regard to average combined event rates per patient day. In the pretreatment period, these rates were found to be 0.075 in the HAT-1 REFLUDAN patients, 0.052 in the HAT-2 REFLUDAN patients, and 0.040 in the historical control group. In the treatment period, the rates showed a marked reduction in the REFLUDAN patients, where they dropped to 0.005 (HAT-1) and to 0.018 (HAT-2), while there was only a moderate decrease to 0.030 in the historical control group. In conclusion, REFLUDAN substantially reduced the risk of serious sequelae of HIT in comparison to a historical control group.

INDICATIONS AND USAGE

REFLUDAN is indicated for anticoagulation in patients with heparin-induced thrombocytopenia (HIT) and associated thromboembolic disease in order to prevent further thromboembolic complications.

CONTRAINDICATIONS

REFLUDAN is contraindicated in patients with known hypersensitivity to hirudins or to any of the components in REFLUDAN [lepirudin (rDNA) for injection].

WARNINGS

Hemorrhagic Events

As with other anticoagulants, hemorrhage can occur at any site in patients receiving REFLUDAN. An unexpected fall in hemoglobin, fall in blood pressure or any unexplained symptom should lead to consideration of a hemorrhagic event. While patients are being anticoagulated with REFLUDAN, the anticoagulation status should be monitored closely using an appropriate measure such as the aPTT (See ADVERSE REACTIONS and DOSAGE AND ADMINISTRATION: Monitoring Section).

Intracranial bleeding following concomitant thrombolytic therapy with rt-PA or streptokinase may be life-threatening. There have been reports of intracranial bleeding with REFLUDAN in the absence of concomitant thrombolytic therapy (see ADVERSE REACTIONS).

For patients with increased risk of bleeding, a careful assessment weighing the risk of REFLUDAN administration vs its anticipated benefit has to be made by the treating physician.

In particular, this includes the following conditions:

- **Recent puncture of large vessels or organ biopsy**
- **Anomaly of vessels or organs**
- **Recent cerebrovascular accident, stroke, intracerebral surgery, or other neuraxial procedures**
- **Severe uncontrolled hypertension**
- **Bacterial endocarditis**
- **Advanced renal impairment (see also WARNINGS: Renal Impairment)**
- **Hemorrhagic diathesis**
- **Recent major surgery**
- **Recent major bleeding (eg, intracranial, gastrointestinal, intraocular, or pulmonary bleeding)**
- **Recent active peptic ulcer**

Renal Impairment

With renal impairment, relative overdose might occur even with standard dosage regimen. Therefore, the bolus dose and the rate of infusion must be reduced in patients with known or suspected renal insufficiency (see **CLINICAL PHARMACOLOGY**: Pharmacokinetic Properties and **DOSAGE AND ADMINISTRATION**: Monitoring and Adjusting Therapy; Use in Renal Impairment).

Continued on next page

Information on Berlex products (appearing here) is based on the most current information available at the time of publication closing. Further information for these and other Berlex products can be obtained from Medical & Product Services at Berlex, Inc. by calling 1-888-BERLEX-4.

Refludan—Cont.

PRECAUTIONS

General

Antibodies. Formation of antihirudin antibodies was observed in about 40% of HIT patients treated with REFLUDAN. This may increase the anticoagulant effect of REFLUDAN possibly due to delayed renal elimination of active lepirudin-antihirudin complexes (see also **PRECAUTIONS**: Animal Pharmacology and Toxicology). Therefore, strict monitoring of aPTT is necessary also during prolonged therapy (see also **PRECAUTIONS**: Laboratory Tests and **DOSAGE AND ADMINISTRATION**: Monitoring and Adjusting Therapy; Standard Recommendations). No evidence of neutralization of REFLUDAN or of allergic reactions associated with positive antibody test results was found.

Liver Injury. Serious liver injury (eg, liver cirrhosis) may enhance the anticoagulant effect of REFLUDAN due to coagulation defects secondary to reduced generation of vitamin K-dependent coagulation factors.

Reexposure. During the HAT-1 and HAT-2 studies, a total of 13 patients were reexposed to REFLUDAN. One of these patients experienced a mild allergic skin reaction during the second treatment cycle. In post marketing experience, anaphylaxis after reexposure has been reported. (see **PRECAUTIONS – Allergic Reactions** below and **ADVERSE REACTIONS – Adverse Events from Post Marketing Reports.**)

Allergic Reactions. There have been reports of allergic and hypersensitivity reactions including anaphylactic reactions. Serious anaphylactic reactions that have resulted in shock or death have been reported. These reactions have been reported during initial administration or upon second or subsequent reexposure(s).

Laboratory Tests

In general, the dosage (infusion rate) should be adjusted according to the aPTT ratio (patient aPTT at a given time over an aPTT reference value, usually median of the laboratory normal range for aPTT); for full information, see **DOSAGE AND ADMINISTRATION**: Monitoring and Adjusting Therapy; Standard Recommendations. Other thrombin-dependent coagulation assays are changed by REFLUDAN (see also **DESCRIPTION**).

Drug Interactions

Concomitant treatment with thrombolytics (eg, rt-PA or streptokinase) may:

- increase the risk of bleeding complications
- considerably enhance the effect of REFLUDAN on aPTT prolongation

(See also **WARNINGS**: Hemorrhagic Events, **ADVERSE REACTIONS**: Adverse Events Reported in Other Populations; Intracranial Bleeding and **DOSAGE AND ADMINISTRATION**: Monitoring and Adjusting Therapy; Concomitant Use With Thrombolytic Therapy). Concomitant treatment with coumarin derivatives (vitamin K antagonists) and drugs that affect platelet function may also increase the risk of bleeding (see also **DOSAGE AND ADMINISTRATION**: Monitoring and Adjusting Therapy; Use in Patients Scheduled for a Switch to Oral Anticoagulation).

Animal Pharmacology and Toxicology

General Toxicity. Lepirudin caused bleeding in animal toxicity studies. Antibodies against hirudin which appeared in several monkeys treated with lepirudin resulted in a prolongation of the terminal half-life and an increase of AUC plasma values of lepirudin.

Carcinogenesis, Mutagenesis, Impairment of Fertility. Long-term animal studies to evaluate the potential for carcinogenesis have not been performed with lepirudin. Lepirudin was not genotoxic in the Ames test, the Chinese hamster cell (V79/HGPRT) forward mutation test, the A549 human cell line unscheduled DNA synthesis (UDS) test, the Chinese hamster V79 cell chromosome aberration test, or the mouse micronucleus test. An effect on fertility and reproductive performance of male and female rats was not seen with lepirudin at intravenous doses up to 30 mg/kg/day (180 mg/m^2/day, 1.2 times the recommended maximum human total daily dose based on body surface area of 1.45m^2 for a 50 kg subject).

Pregnancy

Teratogenic Effects: Category B. Teratology studies with lepirudin performed in pregnant rats at intravenous doses up to 30 mg/kg/day (180 mg/m^2/day, 1.2 times the recommended maximum human total daily dose based on body surface area) and in pregnant rabbits at intravenous doses up to 30 mg/kg/day (360 mg/m^2/day, 2.4 times the recommended maximum human total daily dose based on body surface area) have revealed no evidence of harm to the fetus due to lepirudin. There are, however, no adequate and well-controlled studies in pregnant women. Because animal reproduction studies are not always predictive of human response, this drug should be used during pregnancy only if clearly needed.

Lepirudin (1 mg/kg) by intravenous administration crosses the placental barrier in pregnant rats. It is not known whether the drug crosses the placental barrier in humans. Following intravenous administration of lepirudin at 30 mg/kg/day (180 mg/m^2/day, 1.2 times the recommended maximum human total daily dose based on body surface area) during organogenesis and perinatal-postnatal periods, pregnant rats showed an increased maternal mortality due to undetermined causes.

Table 4: Hemorrhagic Events*

	HAT-1 HAT-2 (All patients) (n = 198)	Patients with TECs REFLUDAN (n = 113)	Patients with TECs Historical control (n = 91)
Bleeding from puncture sites and wounds	14.1%	10.6%	4.4%
Anemia or isolated drop in hemoglobin	13.1%	12.4%	1.1%
Other hematoma and unclassified bleeding	11.1%	10.6%	4.4%
Hematuria	6.6%	4.4%	0
Gastrointestinal and rectal bleeding	5.1%	5.3%	6.6%
Epistaxis	3.0%	4.4%	1.1%
Hemothorax	3.0%	0	1.1%
Vaginal bleeding	1.5%	1.8%	0
Intracranial bleeding	0	0	2.2%

*Patients may have suffered more than one event.

Table 5: Nonhemorrhagic adverse events*

	HAT-1 HAT-2 (All patients) (n = 198)	Patients with TECs REFLUDAN (n = 113)	Patients with TECs Historical control (n = 91)
Fever	6.1%	4.4%	8.8%
Abnormal liver function	6.1%	5.3%	0
Pneumonia	4.0%	4.4%	5.5%
Sepsis	4.0%	3.5%	5.5%
Allergic skin reactions	3.0%	3.5%	1.1%
Heart failure	3.0%	1.8%	2.2%
Abnormal kidney function	2.5%	1.8%	4.4%
Unspecified infections	2.5%	1.8%	1.1%
Multiorgan failure	2.0%	3.5%	0
Pericardial effusion	1.0%	0	1.1%
Ventricular fibrillation	1.0%	0	0

*Patients may have suffered more than one event.

Nursing Mothers

It is not known whether REFLUDAN is excreted in human milk. Because many drugs are excreted in human milk and because of the potential for serious adverse reactions in nursing infants from REFLUDAN, a decision should be made whether to discontinue nursing or to discontinue the drug, taking into account the importance of the drug to the mother.

Pediatric Use

Safety and effectiveness in pediatric patients have not been established. In the HAT-2 study, two children, an 11-year-old girl and a 12-year-old boy, were treated with REFLUDAN. Both children presented with TECs at baseline. REFLUDAN doses given ranged from 0.15 mg/kg/h to 0.22 mg/kg/h for the girl, and from 0.1 mg/kg/h (in conjunction with urokinase) to 0.7 mg/kg/h for the boy. Treatment with REFLUDAN was completed after 8 and 58 days, respectively, without serious adverse events (*Schiffmann 1997*).

ADVERSE REACTIONS

Adverse Events Reported in Clinical Trials in HIT Patients

The following safety information is based on all 198 patients treated with REFLUDAN in the HAT-1 and HAT-2 studies. The safety profile of 113 REFLUDAN patients from these studies who presented with TECs at baseline is compared to 91 such patients in the historical control.

Hemorrhagic Events. Bleeding was the most frequent adverse event observed in patients treated with REFLUDAN. Table 4 gives an overview of all hemorrhagic events which occurred in at least two patients.

[See table 4 above]

Other hemorrhagic events (hemoperitoneum, hemoptysis, liver bleeding, lung bleeding, mouth bleeding, retroperitoneal bleeding) each occurred in one individual among all 198 patients treated with REFLUDAN. Nonhemorrhagic events. Table 5 gives an overview of the most frequently observed nonhemorrhagic events.

[See table 5 above]

Adverse Events Reported in Clinical Trials in Other Populations

The following safety information is based on a total of 2302 individuals who were treated with REFLUDAN in clinical pharmacology studies (n = 323) or for clinical indications other than HIT (n = 1979).

Intracranial Bleeding. Intracranial bleeding was the most serious adverse reaction found in populations other than HIT patients. It occurred in patients with acute myocardial infarction who were started on both REFLUDAN and thrombolytic therapy with rt-PA or streptokinase. The overall frequency of this potentially life-threatening complication among patients receiving both REFLUDAN and thrombolytic therapy was 0.6% (7 out of 1134 patients). Although no intracranial bleeding was observed in 1168 subjects or patients who did not receive concomitant thrombolysis, there have been post marketing reports of intracranial bleeding with REFLUDAN in the absence of concomitant thrombolytic therapy (see **ADVERSE REACTIONS – Adverse Events from Post Marketing Reports** and **WARNINGS**).

Allergic Reactions. (See **PRECAUTIONS**.)

Allergic reactions or suspected allergic reactions in populations other than HIT patients include (in descending order of frequency*):

- Airway reactions (cough, bronchospasm, stridor, dyspnea): common
- Unspecified allergic reactions: uncommon
- Skin reactions (pruritus, urticaria, rash, flushes, chills): uncommon
- General reactions (anaphylactoid or anaphylactic reactions): uncommon
- Edema (facial edema, tongue edema, larynx edema, angioedema): rare

* The CIOMS (Council for International Organization of Medical Sciences) III standard categories are used for classification of frequencies:

very common	10% or more
common (frequent)	1 to <10%
uncommon (infrequent)	0.1 to <1%
rare	0.01 to <0.1%
very rare	0.01% or less

About 53% (n = 46) of all allergic reactions or suspected allergic reactions occurred in patients who concomitantly received thrombolytic therapy (eg, streptokinase) for acute myocardial infarction and/or contrast media for coronary angiography.

Adverse Events from Post Marketing Reports

Serious anaphylactic reactions that have resulted in shock or death have been reported. (See **PRECAUTIONS.**)

Intracranial bleeding has been reported in patients treated with REFLUDAN with or without concomitant thrombolytic therapy. (See **WARNINGS.**) Although no intracranial bleeding was observed in Clinical Trials in those patients who did not receive concomitant thrombolytic therapy (see **Adverse Events Reported in Clinical Trials in HIT Patients** and **Adverse Events Reported in Clinical Trials in Other Populations** below), there have been post marketing reports of intracranial bleeding in patients who received REFLUDAN without concomitant thrombolytic therapy.

OVERDOSAGE

In case of overdose (eg, suggested by excessively high aPTT values) the risk of bleeding is increased.

No specific antidote for REFLUDAN is available. If life-threatening bleeding occurs and excessive plasma levels of lepirudin are suspected, the following steps should be followed:

- Immediately STOP REFLUDAN administration
- Determine aPTT and other coagulation levels as appropriate
- Determine hemoglobin and prepare for blood transfusion
- Follow the current guidelines for treating patients with shock

Individual clinical case reports and in vitro data suggest that either hemofiltration or hemodialysis (using high-flux dialysis membranes with a cutoff point of 50,000 daltons, eg, AN/69) may be useful in this situation.

In studies in pigs, the application of von Willebrand Factor (vWF, 66IU/kg body weight) markedly reduced the bleeding time. The clinical significance of this data is unknown.

DOSAGE AND ADMINISTRATION

Initial Dosage

Anticoagulation in adult patients with HIT and associated thromboembolic disease:

- 0.4 mg/kg body weight (up to 110 kg) slowly intravenously (eg, over 15 to 20 seconds) as a bolus dose,
- followed by 0.15 mg/kg body weight (up to 110 kg)/hour as a continuous intravenous infusion for 2 to 10 days or longer if clinically needed.

Normally the initial dosage depends on the patient's body weight. This is valid up to a body weight of 110kg. In patients with a body weight exceeding 110 kg, the initial dosage should not be increased beyond the 110 kg body weight dose (maximal initial bolus dose of 44 mg, maximal initial infusion dose of 16.5 mg/h; see also **DOSAGE AND ADMINISTRATION**: Administration; Initial Intravenous Bolus, Table 7 and **DOSAGE AND ADMINISTRATION**: Administration; Intravenous Infusion, Table 8).

In general, therapy with REFLUDAN is monitored using the aPTT ratio (patient aPTTat a given time over an aPTT reference value, usually median of the laboratory normal range for aPTT, see **DOSAGE AND ADMINISTRATION**: Monitoring and Adjusting Therapy; Standard Recommendations). A patient baseline aPTT should be determined prior to initiation of therapy with REFLUDAN, since REFLUDAN should not be started in patients presenting with a baseline aPTT ratio of 2.5 or more, in order to avoid initial overdosing.

Monitoring and Adjusting Therapy

Standard Recommendations.

Monitoring.

- **In general, the dosage (infusion rate) should be adjusted according to the aPTT ratio (patient aPTT at a given time over an aPTT reference value, usually median of the laboratory normal range for aPTT).**
- **The target range for the aPTT ratio during treatment (therapeutic window) should be 1.5 to 2.5. Data from clinical trials in HIT patients suggest that with aPTTratios higher than this target range, the risk of bleeding increases, while there is no incremental increase in clinical efficacy.**
- **As stated in DOSAGE AND ADMINISTRATION: Initial Dosage, REFLUDAN should not be started in patients presenting with a baseline aPTT ratio of 2.5 or more, in order to avoid initial overdosing.**
- **The first aPTT determination for monitoring treatment should be done 4 hours after start of the REFLUDAN infusion.**
- **Follow-up aPTT determinations are recommended at least once daily, as long as treatment with REFLUDAN is ongoing.**
- **More frequent aPTT monitoring is highly recommended in patients with renal impairment or serious liver injury (see DOSAGE AND ADMINISTRATION: Monitoring and Adjusting Therapy; Use in Renal Impairment) or with an increased risk of bleeding.**

Dose Modifications.

- **Any aPTT ratio out of the target range is to be confirmed at once before drawing conclusions with respect to dose modifications, unless there is a clinical need to react immediately.**
- **If the confirmed aPTT ratio is above the target range, the infusion should be stopped for two hours. At restart, the infusion rate should be decreased by 50% (no additional intravenous bolus should be administered). The aPTT ratio should be determined again 4 hours later.**
- **If the confirmed aPTT ratio is below the target range, the infusion rate should be increased in steps of 20%. The aPTT ratio should be determined again 4 hours later.**
- **In general, an infusion rate of 0.21 mg/kg/h should not be exceeded without checking for coagulation abnormalities which might be preventive of an appropriate aPTT response.**

Use in Renal Impairment.

As REFLUDAN is almost exclusively excreted in the kidneys (see also **CLINICAL PHARMACOLOGY**: Pharmacokinetic Properties), individual renal function should be considered prior to administration. In case of renal impairment, relative overdose might occur even with the standard dosage regimen. Therefore, the bolus dose and the infusion rate must be reduced in case of known or suspected renal insufficiency (creatinine clearance below 60 mL/min or serum creatinine above 1.5 mg/dL).

There is only limited information on the therapeutic use of REFLUDAN in HIT patients with significant renal impairment. The following dosage recommendations are mainly based on single-dose studies in a small number of patients with renal impairment. Therefore, these recommendations are only tentative and aPTT monitoring should be used along with monitoring of renal status.

Dose adjustments should be based on creatinine clearance values, whenever available, as obtained from a reliable method (24 h urine sampling). If creatinine clearance is not available, the dose adjustments should be based on the serum creatinine.

In all patients with renal insufficiency, the bolus dose is to be reduced to 0.2 mg/kg body weight.

The standard initial infusion rate given in **DOSAGE AND ADMINISTRATION**: Initial Dosage and **DOSAGE AND ADMINISTRATION**: Administration; Intravenous Infusion, Table 8 must be reduced according to the recommendations given in Table 6. Additional aPTT monitoring is highly recommended.

[See table 6 above]

Table 6: Reduction of infusion rate in patients with renal impairment

Creatinine clearance [mL/min]	Serum creatinine [mg/dL]	Adjusted infusion rate [% of standard initial infusion rate]	Adjusted infusion rate [mg/kg/h]
45-60	1.6-2.0	50%	0.075
30-44	2.1-3.0	30%	0.045
15-29	3.1-6.0	15%	0.0225
below 15*	above 6.0*	avoid or STOP infusion!*	

*In hemodialysis patients or in case of acute renal failure (creatinine clearance below 15 mL/min or serum creatinine above 6.0 mg/dL), infusion of REFLUDAN is to be avoided or stopped. Additional intravenous bolus doses of 0.1 mg/kg body weight should be considered every other day only if the aPTT ratio falls below the lower therapeutic limit of 1.5 (see also **DOSAGE AND ADMINISTRATION**: Monitoring and Adjusting Therapy; Standard Recommendations).

Concomitant Use With Thrombolytic Therapy.

Clinical trials in HIT patients have provided only limited information on the combined use of REFLUDAN and thrombolytic agents. The following dosage regimen of REFLUDAN was used in a total of 9 HIT patients in the HAT-1 and HAT-2 studies who presented with TECs at baseline and were started on both REFLUDAN and thrombolytic therapy (rt-PA, urokinase or streptokinase):

- Initial intravenous bolus: 0.2 mg/kg body weight
- Continuous intravenous infusion: 0.1 mg/kg body weight/h

The number of patients receiving combined therapy was too small to identify differences in clinical outcome of patients who were started on both REFLUDAN and thrombolytic therapy as compared to those who were started on REFLUDAN alone. The combined incidences of death, limb amputation, or new TEC were 22.2% and 20.7%, respectively. While there was a 47% relative increase in the overall bleeding rate in patients who were started on both REFLUDAN and thrombolytic therapy (55.6% vs 37.9%), there were no differences in the rates of serious bleeding events (fatal or life-threatening bleeds, bleeds that were permanently or significantly disabling, overt bleeds requiring transfusion of 2 or more units of packed red blood cells, bleeds necessitating surgical intervention, intracranial bleeds) between the groups (11.1% vs 11.2%). Although no intracranial bleeding has been observed in any of these patients, there have been reports of intracranial bleeding in the presence or absence of concomitant thrombolytic therapy. (See **WARNINGS** and **ADVERSE REACTIONS.**)

Special attention should be paid to the fact that thrombolytic agents per se may increase the aPTT ratio. Therefore, aPTT ratios with a given plasma level of lepirudin are usually higher in patients who receive concomitant thrombolysis than in those who do not (see also **CLINICAL PHARMACOLOGY**: Pharmacodynamic Properties).

Use in Patients Scheduled for a Switch to Oral Anticoagulation.

If a patient is scheduled to receive coumarin derivatives (vitamin K antagonists) for oral anticoagulation after REFLUDAN therapy, the dose of REFLUDAN should first be gradually reduced in order to reach an aPTT ratio just above 1.5 before initiating oral anticoagulation. Coumarin derivatives should be initiated only when platelet counts are normalizing. The intended maintenance dose should be started with no loading dose. To avoid prothrombotic effects when initiating coumarin, continue parenteral anticoagulation for 4 to 5 days (see oral anticoagulant package insert for information.) The parenteral agent can be discontinued when the INR stabilizes within the desired target range.

Administration

Directions on Preparation and Dilution.

REFLUDAN should not be mixed with other drugs except for Sterile Water for Injection USP, 0.9% Sodium Chloride Injection USP or 5% Dextrose Injection.

Use REFLUDAN before the expiration date given on the carton and container.

Reconstitution and further dilution are to be carried out under sterile conditions:

- For reconstitution, Sterile Water for Injection USP or 0.9% Sodium Chloride Injection USP are to be used.
- For further dilution, 0.9% Sodium Chloride Injection USP or 5% Dextrose Injection are suitable.
- For rapid, complete reconstitution, inject 1 mL of diluent into the vial and shake it gently. After reconstitution a clear, colorless solution is usually obtained in a few seconds, but definitely in less than 3 minutes.
- Parenteral drug products should be inspected visually for particulate matter and discoloration prior to administration whenever solution and container permit. Do not use solutions that are cloudy or contain particles.
- The reconstituted solution is to be used immediately. It remains stable for up to 24 hours at room temperature (eg, during infusion).
- The preparation should be warmed to room temperature before administration.
- Discard any unused solution appropriately.

Initial Intravenous Bolus.

For intravenous bolus injection, use a solution with a concentration of 5 mg/mL.

Preparation of a REFLUDAN solution with a concentration of 5 mg/mL:

- Reconstitute one vial (50 mg of lepirudin) with 1 mL of Sterile Water for Injection USP or 0.9% Sodium Chloride Injection USP.
- The final concentration of 5mg/mL is obtained by transferring the contents of the vial into a sterile, single-use syringe (of at least 10mL capacity) and diluting the solution to a total volume of 10 mL, using Sterile Water for Injection USP, 0.9% Sodium Chloride Injection USP or 5% Dextrose Injection.
- The final solution is to be administered according to body weight (see Table 7 below and DOSAGE AND ADMINISTRATION: Initial Dosage).

Intravenous injection of the bolus is to be carried out slowly (eg, over 15 to 20 seconds).

Table 7: Standard bolus injection volumes according to body weight for a 5 mg/mL concentration

Body Weight [kg]	Injection volume Dosage 0.4 mg/kg	Injection volume Dosage 0.2 mg/kg*
50	4.0 mL	2.0 mL
60	4.8 mL	2.4 mL
70	5.6 mL	2.8 mL
80	6.4 mL	3.2 mL
90	7.2 mL	3.6 mL
100	8.0 mL	4.0 mL
≥110	8.8 mL	4.4 mL

*Dosage recommended for all patients with renal insufficiency (see **DOSAGE AND ADMINISTRATION**: Monitoring and Adjusting Therapy; Use in Renal Impairment)

Intravenous Infusion

For continuous intravenous infusion, solutions with concentration of 0.2 mg/mL or 0.4 mg/mL may be used.

Continued on next page

Refludan—Cont.

Preparation of a REFLUDAN solution with a concentration of 0.2 or 0.4 mg/mL:

- Reconstitute two vials (each containing 50 mg of lepirudin) with 1 mL each using either Sterile Water for Injection USP or 0.9% Sodium Chloride Injection USP.
- The final concentrations of 0.2 mg/mL or 0.4 mg/mL are obtained by transferring the contents of both vials into an infusion bag containing 500 mL or 250 mL of 0.9% Sodium Chloride Injection USP or 5% Dextrose Injection.

The infusion rate [mL/h] is to be set according to body weight (see Table 8 below and DOSAGE AND ADMINISTRATION: Initial Dosage).

Table 8: Standard infusion rates according to body weight

Body Weight [kg]	Infusion rate at 0.15 mg/kg/h 500-mL infusion bag 0.2 mg/mL	250-mL infusion bag 0.4 mg/mL
50	38 mL/h	19 mL/h
60	45 mL/h	23 mL/h
70	53 mL/h	26 mL/h
80	60 mL/h	30 mL/h
90	68 mL/h	34 mL/h
100	75 mL/h	38 mL/h
≥110	83 mL/h	41 mL/h

HOW SUPPLIED

REFLUDAN [lepirudin (rDNA) for injection] is supplied in boxes of 10 vials, each vial containing 50 mg lepirudin (NDC 50419-150-57). STORE UNOPENED VIALS AT 2 to 25°C (36 to 77°F). USE REFLUDAN BEFORE THE EXPIRATION DATE GIVEN ON THE CARTON AND CONTAINER. ONCE RECONSTITUTED, USE REFLUDAN IMMEDIATELY.

REFERENCES

1. Fondu P. Heparin associated thrombocytopenia: an update. *Acta Clinica Belgica. 1995;50(6):343-357.*
2. Greinacher A. Antigen generation in heparin-associated thrombocytopenia: the nonimmunologic type and the immunologic type are closely linked in their pathogenesis. *Seminars Thromb Hemost. 1995; 21:106-116.*
3. Roethig HJ, Maree JS, Meyer BH. Clinical pharmacology of hirudin (HBW 023). In: Reidenberg, MM ed. *The clinical pharmacology of biotechnology products. Elsevier Publishers; 1991:227-236.*
4. Schiffmann H, Unterhalt M, Harms K, Figula HR, Voelpel H, Greinacher A. Successful treatment of heparin-induced thrombocytopenia (HIT) type II in childhood with recombinant hirudin. *Monatsschr Kinderheilkd. 1997; 145:606-612.*
5. Warkentin TE, Chong BH, Greinacher A. Heparin-induced thrombocytopenia: towards consensus. *Thromb Haemostas. 1998; 79:1-7.*
6. Warkentin TE, Elavathil LJ, Hayward CPM, Johnston MA, Russett JI, Kelton JG. The pathogenesis of venous limb gangrene associated with heparin-induced thrombocytopenia. *Ann Intern Med. 1997; 127:804-812.*

Prescribing Information as of October 2002

revised 10/2002

Manufactured by:
Aventis Behring
Deutschland GmbH
D-35002 Marburg
Germany
Manufactured for:
BERLEX® Laboratories
Wayne, NJ 07470
Made in Germany
www.refludan.com
2222552 (SAG) 6058201 (BERLEX)

Shown in Product Identification Guide, page 309

YASMIN® 28 TABLETS ℞

[*yăz' mĭn*]

(drospirenone and ethinyl estradiol)

Rx only

PATIENTS SHOULD BE COUNSELED THAT THIS PRODUCT DOES NOT PROTECT AGAINST HIV INFECTION (AIDS) AND OTHER SEXUALLY TRANSMITTED DISEASES.

DESCRIPTION

YASMIN provides an oral contraceptive regimen consisting of 21 active film coated tablets each containing 3.0 mg of drospirenone and 0.030 mg of ethinyl estradiol and 7 inert film coated tablets. The inactive ingredients are lactose monohydrate NF, corn starch NF, modified starch NF, povidone 25000 USP, magnesium stearate NF, hydroxylpropylmethyl cellulose USP, macrogol 6000 NF, talc USP, titanium dioxide USP, ferric oxide pigment, yellow NF. The inert film coated tablets contain lactose monohydrate NF, corn starch NF, povidone 25000 USP, magnesium stearate NF, hydroxylpropylmethyl cellulose USP, talc USP, titanium dioxide USP.

Drospirenone (6R,7R,8R,9S,10R,13S,14S,15S,16S,17S)-1,3′,4′,6,6a,7,8,9,10,11,12,13,14,15,15a,16-hexadecahydro-10,13-dimethylspiro-[17H-dicyclopropa-6,7:15,16]cyclo-penta[a]phenanthrene-17,2′(5H)-furan]-3,5′(2H)-dione) is a synthetic progestational compound and has a molecular weight of 366.5 and a molecular formula of $C_{24}H_{30}O_3$. Ethinyl estradiol (19-nor-17•-pregna 1,3,5(10)-triene-20-yne-3,17-diol) is a synthetic estrogenic compound and has a molecular weight of 296.4 and a molecular formula of $C_{20}H_{24}O_2$. The structural formulas are as follows:

Drospirenone

Ethinyl estradiol

TABLE OF MEAN PHARMACOKINETIC PARAMETERS OF YASMIN (Drospirenone 3 mg and Ethinyl Estradiol 0.030 mg)

TABLE I

Drospirenone Mean (%CV) Values

Cycle/Day	No. of Subjects	Cmax (ng/mL)	Tmax (h)	AUC(0-24h) (ng•h/mL)	$t_{1/2}$ (h)
1/1	12	36.9 (13)	1.7 (47)	288 (25)	NA
1/21	12	87.5 (59)	1.7 (20)	827 (23)	30.9 (44)
6/21	12	84.2 (19)	1.8 (19)	930 (19)	32.5 (38)
9/21	12	81.3 (19)	1.6 (38)	957 (23)	31.4 (39)
13/21	12	78.7 (18)	1.6 (26)	968 (24)	31.1 (36)

Ethinyl Estradiol Mean (%CV) Values

Cycle/Day	No. of Subjects	Cmax (pg/mL)	Tmax (h)	AUC(0-24h) (pg•h/mL)	$t_{1/2}$ (h)
1/1	11	53.5 (43)	1.9 (45)	280.3 (87)	NA
1/21	11	92.1 (35)	1.5 (40)	461.3 (94)	NA
6/21	11	99.1 (45)	1.5 (47)	346.4 (74)	NA
9/21	11	87.0 (43)	1.5 (42)	485.3 (92)	NA
13/21	10	90.5 (45)	1.6 (38)	469.5 (83)	NA

NA = Not available

CLINICAL PHARMACOLOGY

PHARMACODYNAMICS

Combination oral contraceptives (COCs) act by suppression of gonadotropins. Although the primary mechanism of this action is inhibition of ovulation, other alterations include changes in the cervical mucus (which increases the difficulty of sperm entry into the uterus) and the endometrium (which reduces the likelihood of implantation).

Drospirenone is a spironolactone analogue with antimineralocorticoid activity. Preclinical studies in animals and *in vitro* have shown that drospirenone has no androgenic, estrogenic, glucocorticoid, and antiglucocorticoid activity. Preclinical studies in animals have also shown that drospirenone has antiandrogenic activity.

PHARMACOKINETICS

Absorption

The absolute bioavailability of drospirenone (DRSP) from a single entity tablet is about 76%. The absolute bioavailability of ethinyl estradiol (EE) is approximately 40% as a result of presystemic conjugation and first-pass metabolism. The absolute bioavailability of **YASMIN** which is a combination tablet of drospirenone and ethinyl estradiol has not been evaluated. Serum concentrations of DRSP and EE reached peak levels within 1-3 hours after administration of **YASMIN**. After single dose administration of **YASMIN**, the relative bioavailability, compared to a suspension, was 107% and 117% for DRSP and EE, respectively.

The pharmacokinetics of DRSP are dose proportional following single doses ranging from 1-10 mg. Following daily dosing of **YASMIN**, steady state DRSP concentrations were observed after 10 days. There was about 2 to 3 fold accumulation in serum Cmax and AUC (0-24h) values of DRSP following multiple dose administration of **YASMIN** (see TABLE I).

For EE, steady-state conditions are reported during the second half of a treatment cycle. Following daily administration of **YASMIN** serum Cmax and AUC(0-24h) values of EE accumulate by a factor of about 1.5 to 2.0.

[See table I above]

Effect of Food

The rate of absorption of DRSP and EE following single administration of two **YASMIN** tablets was slower under fed conditions with the serum Cmax being reduced about 40% for both components. The extent of absorption of DRSP, however, remained unchanged. In contrast the extent of absorption of EE was reduced by about 20% under fed conditions.

Distribution

DRSP and EE serum levels decline in two phases. The apparent volume of distribution of DRSP is approximately 4 L/kg and that of EE is reported to be approximately 4-5 L/kg.

DRSP does not bind to sex hormone binding globulin (SHBG) or corticosteroid binding globulin (CBG) but binds about 97% to other serum proteins. Multiple dosing over 3 cycles resulted in no change in the free fraction (as measured at trough levels). EE is reported to be highly but non-specifically bound to serum albumin (approximately 98.5%) and induces an increase in the serum concentrations of both SHBG and CBG. EE induced effects on SHBG and CBG were not affected by variation of the DRSP dosage in the range of 2 to 3 mg.

Metabolism

The two main metabolites of DRSP found in human plasma were identified to be the acid form of DRSP generated by opening of the lactone ring and the 4,5-dihydrodrospirenone-3-sulfate. These metabolites were shown not to be pharmacologically active. In *in vitro* studies with human liver microsomes, DRSP was metabolized only to a minor extent mainly by cytochrome P450 3A4 (CYP3A4).

EE has been reported to be subject to presystemic conjugation in both small bowel mucosa and the liver. Metabolism occurs primarily by aromatic hydroxylation but a wide variety of hydroxylated and methylated metabolites are formed. These are present as free metabolites and as conjugates with glucuronide and sulfate. CYP3A4 in the liver are responsible for the 2-hydroxylation which is the major oxidative reaction. The 2-hydroxy metabolite is further transformed by methylation and glucuronidation prior to urinary and fecal excretion.

Excretion

DRSP serum levels are characterized by a terminal disposition phase half-life of approximately 30 hours after both single and multiple dose regimens. Excretion of DRSP was nearly complete after ten days and amounts excreted were slightly higher in feces compared to urine. DRSP was extensively metabolized and only trace amounts of unchanged DRSP were excreted in urine and feces. At least 20 different metabolites were observed in urine and feces. About 38-47% of the metabolites in urine were glucuronide and sulfate conjugates. In feces, about 17-20% of the metabolites were excreted as glucuronides and sulfates.

For EE the terminal disposition phase half-life has been reported to be approximately 24 hours. EE is not excreted unchanged. EE is excreted in the urine and feces as glucuronide and sulfate conjugates and undergoes enterohepatic circulation.

Special Populations

Race

The effect of race on the disposition of **YASMIN** has not been evaluated.

Hepatic Dysfunction

YASMIN is contraindicated in patients with hepatic dysfunction **(also see BOLDED WARNING)**. The mean exposure to DRSP in women with moderate liver impairment is approximately three times the exposure in women with normal liver function.

Renal Insufficiency

YASMIN is contraindicated in patients with renal insufficiency **(also see BOLDED WARNING).**

The effect of renal insufficiency on the pharmacokinetics of DRSP (3 mg daily for 14 days) and the effect of DRSP on serum potassium levels were investigated in female subjects (n=28, age 30-65) with normal renal function and mild and moderate renal impairment. All subjects were on a low potassium diet. During the study 7 subjects continued the use of potassium sparing drugs for the treatment of the underlying illness. On the 14th day (steady-state) of DRSP treatment, the serum DRSP levels in the group with mild renal impairment (creatinine clearance CLcr, 50-80 mL/min) were comparable to those in the group with normal renal function (CLcr, >80 mL/min). The serum DRSP levels were on average 37% higher in the group with moderate renal impairment (CLcr, 30-50 mL/min) compared to those in the group with normal renal function. DRSP treatment was well tolerated by all groups. DRSP treatment did not show any clinically significant effect on serum potassium concentration. Although hyperkalemia was not observed in the study, in five of the seven subjects who continued use of potassium sparing drugs during the study, mean serum potassium levels increased by up to 0.33 mEq/L. Therefore, potential exists for hyperkalemia to occur in subjects with renal impairment whose serum potassium is in the upper reference range, and who are concomitantly using potassium sparing drugs.

INDICATIONS AND USAGE

YASMIN is indicated for the prevention of pregnancy in women who elect to use an oral contraceptive.

Oral contraceptives are highly effective. TABLE II lists the typical accidental pregnancy rates for users of combination oral contraceptives and other methods of contraception. The efficacy of these contraceptive methods, except sterilization, depends upon the reliability with which they are used. Correct and consistent use of methods can result in lower failure rates.

[See table II at right]

In clinical efficacy studies of **YASMIN** of up to 2 years duration, 2,629 subjects completed 33,160 cycles of use without any other contraception. The mean age of the subjects was 25.5 ± 4.7 years. The age range was 16 to 37 years. The racial demographic was: 83% Caucasian, 1% Hispanic, 1% Black, <1% Asian, <1% other, <1% missing data, 14% not inquired and <1% unspecified. Pregnancy rates in the clinical trials were less than one per 100 woman-years of use.

CONTRAINDICATIONS

YASMIN should not be used in women who have the following:

- Renal insufficiency
- Hepatic dysfunction
- Adrenal insufficiency
- Thrombophlebitis or thromboembolic disorders
- A past history of deep-vein thrombophlebitis or thromboembolic disorders
- Cerebral-vascular or coronary-artery disease
- Valvular heart disease with thrombogenic complications
- Severe hypertension
- Diabetes with vascular involvement
- Headaches with focal neurological symptoms
- Known or suspected carcinoma of the breast
- Carcinoma of the endometrium or other known or suspected estrogen-dependent neoplasia
- Undiagnosed abnormal genital bleeding
- Cholestatic jaundice of pregnancy or jaundice with prior pill use
- Liver tumor (benign or malignant) or active liver disease
- Known or suspected pregnancy
- Heavy smoking (≥ 15 cigarettes per day) and over age 35

WARNINGS

Cigarette smoking increases the risk of serious cardiovascular side effects from oral contraceptive use. This risk increases with age and with heavy smoking (15 or more cigarettes per day) and is quite marked in women over 35 years of age. Women who use oral contraceptives should be strongly advised not to smoke.

YASMIN contains 3 mg of the progestin drospirenone that has antimineralocorticoid activity, including the potential for hyperkalemia in high-risk patients, comparable to a 25 mg dose of spironolactone. YASMIN should not be used in patients with conditions that predispose to hyperkalemia (i.e. renal insufficiency, hepatic dysfunction and adrenal insufficiency). Women receiving daily, long-term treatment for chronic conditions or diseases with medications that may increase serum potassium, should have their serum potassium level checked during the first treatment cycle. Drugs that may increase serum potassium include ACE inhibitors, angiotensin–II receptor antagonists, potassium-sparing diuretics, heparin, aldosterone antagonists, and NSAIDs.

The use of oral contraceptives is associated with increased risks of several serious conditions including myocardial infarction, thromboembolism, stroke, hepatic neoplasia, gallbladder disease, and hypertension, although the risk of serious morbidity or mortality is very small in healthy women without underlying risk factors. The risk of morbidity and mortality increases significantly in the presence of other underlying risk factors such as hypertension, hyperlipidemias, obesity and diabetes.

TABLE II

Percentage of women experiencing an unintended pregnancy during the first year of typical use and first year of perfect use of contraception and the percentage continuing use at the end of the first year: United States.

Method (1)	% of Women Experiencing an Accidental Pregnancy within the First Year of Use — Typical Use[1] (2)	Perfect Use[2] (3)	% of Women Continuing Use at One Year[3] (4)
Chance[4]	85	85	
Spermicides[5]	26	6	40
Periodic abstinence	25		63
Calendar		9	
Ovulation method		3	
Sympto-thermal[6]		2	
Post-ovulation		1	
Withdrawal	19	4	
Cap[7]			
Parous women	40	26	42
Nulliparous women	20	9	56
Sponge			
Parous women	40	20	42
Nulliparous women	20	9	56
Diaphragm[7]	20	6	56
Condom[8]			
Female (Reality)	21	5	56
Male	14	3	61
Pill	5		71
progestin only		0.5	
combined		0.1	
IUD:			
Progesterone T	2.0	1.5	81
Copper T 380A	0.8	0.6	78
Lng 20	0.1	0.1	81
Depo Provera	0.3	0.3	70
Norplant and Norplant-2	0.05	0.05	88
Female sterilization	0.5	0.5	100
Male sterilization	0.15	0.10	100

Emergency Contraceptive Pills: Treatment initiated within 72 hours after unprotected intercourse reduces the risk of pregnancy by at least 75%.[9]

Lactational Amenorrhea Method: LAM is highly effective, *temporary* method of contraception.[10]

Source: Trussell J, Contraceptive efficacy. In Hatcher RA, Trussell J, Stewart F, Cates W, Stewart GK, Kowal D, Guest F, Contraceptive Technology: Seventeenth Revised Edition. New York NY: Irvington Publishers, 1998.

1 Among *typical* couples who initiate use of a method (not necessarily for the first time), the percentage who experience an accidental pregnancy during the first year if they do not stop use for any other reason.

2 Among couples who initiate use of a method (not necessarily for the first time) and who use it *perfectly* (both consistently and correctly), the percentage who experience an accidental pregnancy during the first year if they do not stop use for any reason.

3 Among couples attempting to avoid pregnancy, the percentage who continue to use a method for one year.

4 The percents becoming pregnant in columns (2) and (3) are based on data from populations where contraception is not used and from women who cease using contraception in order to become pregnant. Among such populations, about 89% become pregnant within one year. This estimate was lowered slightly (to 85%) to represent the percentage who would become pregnant within one year among women now relying on reversible methods of contraception if they abandoned contraception altogether.

5 Foams, creams, gels, vaginal suppositories, and vaginal film.

6 Cervical mucus (ovulation) method supplemented by calendar in the pre-ovulatory and basal body temperature in the post-ovulatory phases.

7 With spermicidal cream or jelly.

8 Without spermicides.

9 The treatment schedule is one dose within 72 hours after unprotected intercourse, and a second dose 12 hours after the first dose. The Food and Drug Administration has declared the following brands of oral contraceptives to be safe and effective for emergency contraception: Ovral (1 dose is 2 white pills), Alesse (1 dose is 5 pink pills), Nordette or Levlen (1 dose is 2 light-orange pills), Lo/Ovral (1 dose is 4 white pills), Triphasil or Tri-Levlen (1 dose is 4 yellow pills).

10 However, to maintain effective protection against pregnancy, another method of contraception must be used as soon as menstruation resumes, the frequency or duration of breastfeeds is reduced, bottle feeds are introduced, or the baby reaches six months of age.

Practitioners prescribing oral contraceptives should be familiar with the following information relating to these risks.

The information contained in this package insert is based principally on studies carried out in patients who used oral contraceptives with higher formulations of estrogens and progestogens than those in common use today. The effect of long-term use of the oral contraceptives with lower formulations of both estrogens and progestogens remains to be determined.

Throughout this labeling, epidemiologic studies reported are of two types: retrospective or case control studies and prospective or cohort studies. Case control studies provide a measure of the relative risk of a disease, namely, a ratio of the incidence of a disease among oral contraceptive users to that among nonusers. The relative risk does not provide information on the actual clinical occurrence of a disease. Cohort studies provide a measure of attributable risk, which is the difference in the incidence of disease between oral contraceptive users and nonusers. The attributable risk does provide information about the actual occurrence of a disease in the population. For further information, the reader is referred to a text on epidemiologic methods.

1. THROMBOEMBOLIC DISORDERS AND OTHER VASCULAR PROBLEMS

a. *Myocardial infarction*

An increased risk of myocardial infarction has been attributed to oral contraceptive use. This risk is primarily in smokers or women with other underlying risk factors for coronary-artery disease such as hypertension, hypercholesterolemia, morbid obesity, and diabetes. The relative risk of heart attack for current oral contraceptive users has been estimated to be two to six. The risk is very low under the age of 30.

Smoking in combination with oral contraceptive use has been shown to contribute substantially to the incidence of myocardial infarctions in women in their mid-thirties or older with smoking accounting for the majority of excess cases. Mortality rates associated with circulatory disease have been shown to increase substantially in smokers over the age of 35 and nonsmokers over the age of 40 (Table III) among women who use oral contraceptives.

[See table III at bottom of next page]

Oral contraceptives may compound the effects of well-known risk factors, such as hypertension, diabetes, hyperlipidemias, age and obesity. In particular, some progestogens are known to decrease HDL cholesterol and cause glucose intolerance, while estrogens may create a state of hyperinsulinism. Oral contraceptives have been shown to increase blood pressure among users (see section 9 in **WARNINGS**). Similar effects on risk factors have been associated with an increased risk of heart disease. Oral contraceptives must be used with caution in women with cardiovascular disease risk factors.

b. *Thromboembolism*

An increased risk of thromboembolic and thrombotic disease associated with the use of oral contraceptives is well

Continued on next page

Information on Berlex products (appearing here) is based on the most current information available at the time of publication closing. Further information for these and other Berlex products can be obtained from Medical & Product Services at Berlex, Inc. by calling 1-888-BERLEX-4.

Yasmin 28—Cont.

established. Case control studies have found the relative risk of users compared to nonusers to be 3 for the first episode of superficial venous thrombosis, 4 to 11 for deep vein thrombosis or pulmonary embolism, and 1.5 to 6 for women with predisposing conditions for venous thromboembolic disease. Cohort studies have shown the relative risk to be somewhat lower, about 3 for new cases and about 4.5 for new cases requiring hospitalization. The risk of thromboembolic disease due to oral contraceptives is not related to length of use and disappears after pill use is stopped.

A two- to four-fold increase in the relative risk of postoperative thromboembolic complications has been reported with the use of oral contraceptives. The relative risk of venous thrombosis in women who have predisposing conditions is twice that of women without such medical conditions. If feasible, oral contraceptives should be discontinued from at least four weeks prior to and for two weeks after elective surgery of a type associated with an increase in risk of thromboembolism and during and following prolonged immobilization. Since the immediate postpartum period is also associated with an increased risk of thromboembolism, oral contraceptives should be started no earlier than four to six weeks after delivery.

c. *Cerebrovascular diseases*

Oral contraceptives have been shown to increase both the relative and attributable risks of cerebrovascular events (thrombotic and hemorrhagic strokes), although, in general, the risk is greatest among older (>35 years), hypertensive women who also smoke. Hypertension was found to be a risk factor, for both users and nonusers, for both types of strokes, while smoking interacted to increase the risk for hemorrhagic strokes.

In a large study, the relative risk of thrombotic strokes has been shown to range from 3 for normotensive users to 14 for users with severe hypertension. The relative risk of hemorrhagic stroke is reported to be 1.2 for nonsmokers who used oral contraceptives, 2.6 for smokers who did not use oral contraceptives, 7.6 for smokers who used oral contraceptives, 1.8 for normotensive users and 25.7 for users with severe hypertension. The attributable risk is also greater in older women.

d. *Dose-related risk of vascular disease from oral contraceptives*

A positive association has been observed between the amount of estrogen and progestogen in oral contraceptives and the risk of vascular disease. A decline in serum high-density lipoproteins (HDL) has been reported with many progestational agents. A decline in serum high-density lipoproteins has been associated with an increased incidence of ischemic heart disease. Because estrogens increase HDL cholesterol, the net effect of an oral contraceptive depends on a balance achieved between doses of estrogen and progestogen and the nature and absolute amount of progestogen used in the contraceptive. The amount of both hormones should be considered in the choice of an oral contraceptive.

Minimizing exposure to estrogen and progestogen is in keeping with good principles of therapeutics. For any particular estrogen/progestogen combination, the dosage regimen prescribed should be one which contains the least amount of estrogen and progestogen that is compatible with a low failure rate and the needs of the individual patient. New acceptors of oral contraceptive agents should be started on preparations containing the lowest estrogen content which provides satisfactory results in the individual.

e. *Persistence of risk of vascular disease*

There are two studies which have shown persistence of risk of vascular disease for ever-users of oral contraceptives. In a study in the United States, the risk of developing myocardial infarction after discontinuing oral contraceptives persists for at least 9 years for women aged 40 to 49 years who had used oral contraceptives for five or more years, but this increased risk was not demonstrated in other age groups. In another study in Great Britain, the risk of developing cerebrovascular disease persisted for at least 6 years after discontinuation of oral contraceptives, although excess risk was very small. However, both studies were performed with oral contraceptive formulations containing 50 micrograms or higher of estrogens.

2. ESTIMATES OF MORTALITY FROM CONTRACEPTIVE USE

One study gathered data from a variety of sources which have estimated the mortality rate associated with different methods of contraception at different ages (Table IV). These estimates include the combined risk of death associated with contraceptive methods plus the risk attributable to pregnancy in the event of method failure. Each method of contraception has its specific benefits and risks. The study concluded that with the exception of oral contraceptive users 35 and older who smoke and 40 and older who do not smoke, mortality associated with all methods of birth control is below that associated with childbirth.

The observation of a possible increase in risk of mortality with age for oral contraceptive users is based on data gathered in the 1970's – but not reported until 1983. However, current clinical practice involves the use of lower estrogen dose formulations combined with careful restriction of oral contraceptive use to women who do not have the various risk factors listed in this labeling.

Because of these changes in practice and, also, because of some limited new data which suggest that the risk of cardiovascular disease with the use of oral contraceptives may now be less than previously observed, the Fertility and Maternal Health Drugs Advisory Committee was asked to review the topic in 1989. The Committee concluded that although cardiovascular disease risks may be increased with oral contraceptive use after age 40 in healthy nonsmoking women (even with the newer low-dose formulations), there are greater potential health risks associated with pregnancy in older women and with the alternative surgical and medical procedures which may be necessary if such women do not have access to effective and acceptable means of contraception.

Therefore, the Committee recommended that the benefits of oral contraceptive use by healthy nonsmoking women over 40 may outweigh the possible risks. Of course, women of all ages who take oral contraceptives, should take the lowest possible dose formulation that is effective.

[See table IV below]

3. CARCINOMA OF THE REPRODUCTIVE ORGANS AND BREASTS

Numerous epidemiological studies have been performed on the incidence of breast, endometrial, ovarian and cervical cancer in women using oral contraceptives.

The risk of having breast cancer diagnosed may be slightly increased among current and recent users of COCs. However, this excess risk appears to decrease over time after COC discontinuation and by 10 years after cessation the increased risk disappears. The risk does not appear to increase with duration of use and no consistent relationships have been found with dose or type of steroid. Most studies show a similar pattern of risk with COC use regardless of a woman's reproductive history or her family breast cancer history. Some studies have found a small increase in risk for women who first use COCs before age 20.

Breast cancers diagnosed in current or previous OC users tend to be less clinically advanced than in nonusers.

Women who currently have or have had breast cancer should not use oral contraceptives because breast cancer is a hormonally-sensitive tumor.

Some studies suggest that oral contraceptive use has been associated with an increase in the risk of cervical intraepithelial neoplasia in some populations of women. However, there continues to be controversy about the extent to which such findings may be due to differences in sexual behavior and other factors.

In spite of many studies of the relationship between oral contraceptive use and breast and cervical cancers, a cause-and-effect relationship has not been established.

4. HEPATIC NEOPLASIA

Benign hepatic adenomas are associated with oral contraceptive use, although the incidence of benign tumors is rare in the United States. Indirect calculations have estimated the attributable risk to be in the range of 3.3 cases/100,000 for users, a risk that increases after four or more years of use. Rupture of rare, benign, hepatic adenomas may cause death through intra-abdominal hemorrhage.

Studies from Britain have shown an increased risk of developing hepatocellular carcinoma in long-term (>8 years) oral contraceptive users. However, these cancers are extremely rare in the U.S. and the attributable risk (the excess incidence) of liver cancers in oral contraceptive users approaches less than one per million users.

5. OCULAR LESIONS

There have been clinical case reports of retinal thrombosis associated with the use of oral contraceptives. Oral contraceptives should be discontinued if there is unexplained partial or complete loss of vision; onset of proptosis or diplopia; papilledema; or retinal vascular lesions. Appropriate diagnostic and therapeutic measures should be undertaken immediately.

6. ORAL CONTRACEPTIVE USE BEFORE OR DURING EARLY PREGNANCY

Extensive epidemiological studies have revealed no increased risk of birth defects in women who have used oral contraceptives prior to pregnancy. Studies also do not suggest a teratogenic effect, particularly in so far as cardiac anomalies and limb-reduction defects are concerned, when taken inadvertently during early pregnancy.

The administration of oral contraceptives to induce withdrawal bleeding should not be used as a test for pregnancy. Oral contraceptives should not be used during pregnancy to treat threatened or habitual abortion.

It is recommended that for any patient who has missed two consecutive periods, pregnancy should be ruled out. If the patient has not adhered to the prescribed dosing schedule, the possibility of pregnancy should be considered at the time of the first missed period. Oral contraceptive use should be discontinued if pregnancy is confirmed.

7. GALLBLADDER DISEASE

Earlier studies have reported an increased lifetime relative risk of gallbladder surgery in users of oral contraceptives and estrogens. More recent studies, however, have shown that the relative risk of developing gallbladder disease among oral contraceptive users may be minimal. The recent findings of minimal risk may be related to the use of oral contraceptive formulations containing lower hormonal doses of estrogens and progestogens.

8. CARBOHYDRATE AND LIPID METABOLIC EFFECTS

Oral contraceptives have been shown to cause glucose intolerance in a significant percentage of users. Oral contraceptives containing greater than 75 micrograms of estrogens cause hyperinsulinism, while lower doses of estrogen cause less glucose intolerance. Progestogens increase insulin secretion and create insulin resistance, this effect varying with different progestational agents. However, in the non-diabetic woman, oral contraceptives appear to have no effect on fasting blood glucose. Because of these demonstrated effects, prediabetic and diabetic women should be carefully observed while taking oral contraceptives.

A small proportion of women will have persistent hypertriglyceridemia while on the pill. As discussed earlier (see **WARNINGS** 1a. and 1d.), changes in serum triglycerides and lipoprotein levels have been reported in oral contraceptive users.

9. ELEVATED BLOOD PRESSURE

An increase in blood pressure has been reported in women taking oral contraceptives and this increase is more likely in older oral contraceptive users and with continued use. Data from the Royal College of General Practitioners and

TABLE III. (Adapted from P.M. Layde and V. Beral)
CIRCULATORY DISEASE MORTALITY RATES PER 100,000 WOMAN-YEARS BY AGE SMOKING STATUS AND ORAL CONTRACEPTIVE USE

AGE	EVER-USERS NON-SMOKERS	EVER-USERS SMOKERS	CONTROL NON-SMOKERS	CONTROL SMOKERS
15-24	0.0	10.5	0.0	0.0
25-34	4.4	14.2	2.7	4.2
35-44	21.5	63.4	6.4	15.2
45+	52.4	206.7	11.4	27.9

TABLE IV
ANNUAL NUMBER OF BIRTH-RELATED OR METHOD-RELATED DEATHS ASSOCIATED WITH CONTROL OF FERTILITY PER 100,000 NONSTERILE WOMEN, BY FERTILITY-CONTROL METHOD ACCORDING TO AGE

Method of Control and Outcome	15-19	20-24	25-29	30-34	35-39	40-44
No fertility control methods[1]	7.0	7.4	9.1	14.8	25.7	28.2
Oral contraceptives non-smoker[2]	0.3	0.5	0.9	1.9	13.8	31.6
Oral contraceptives smoker[2]	2.2	3.4	6.6	13.5	51.1	117.2
IUD[2]	0.8	0.8	1.0	1.0	1.4	1.4
Condom[1]	1.1	1.6	0.7	0.2	0.3	0.4
Diaphragm/spermicide[1]	1.9	1.2	1.2	1.3	2.2	2.8
Periodic abstinence[1]	2.5	1.6	1.6	1.7	2.9	3.6

[1] Deaths are birth related
[2] Deaths are method related

Adapted from H.W. Ory, *Family Planning Perspectives*, 15:57-63, 1983.

subsequent randomized trials have shown that the incidence of hypertension increases with increasing concentrations of progestogens.

Women with a history of hypertension or hypertension-related diseases, or renal disease should be encouraged to use another method of contraception. If women with hypertension elect to use oral contraceptives, they should be monitored closely, and if significant elevation of blood pressure occurs, oral contraceptives should be discontinued. For most women, elevated blood pressure will return to normal after stopping oral contraceptives and there is no difference in the occurrence of hypertension among ever- and never-users.

10. HEADACHE

The onset or exacerbation of migraine or development of headache with a new pattern which is recurrent, persistent or severe requires discontinuation of oral contraceptives and evaluation of the cause.

11. BLEEDING IRREGULARITIES

Breakthrough bleeding and spotting are sometimes encountered in patients on oral contraceptives, especially during the first three months of use. Nonhormonal causes should be considered and adequate diagnostic measures taken to rule out malignancy or pregnancy in the event of breakthrough bleeding, as in the case of any abnormal vaginal bleeding. If pathology has been excluded, time or a change to another formulation may solve the problem. In the event of amenorrhea, pregnancy should be ruled out.

Some women may encounter post-pill amenorrhea or oligomenorrhea, especially when such a condition was preexistent.

PRECAUTIONS

1. GENERAL

Patients should be counseled that this product does not protect against HIV infection (AIDS) and other sexually transmitted diseases.

2. PHYSICAL EXAMINATION AND FOLLOW-UP

It is good medical practice for all women to have annual history and physical examinations, including women using oral contraceptives. The physical examination, however, may be deferred until after initiation of oral contraceptives if requested by the woman and judged appropriate by the clinician. The physical examination should include special reference to blood pressure, breasts, abdomen and pelvic organs, including cervical cytology and relevant laboratory tests. In case of undiagnosed, persistent or recurrent abnormal vaginal bleeding, appropriate measures should be conducted to rule out malignancy. Women with a strong family history of breast cancer or who have breast nodules should be monitored with particular care.

3. LIPID DISORDERS

Women who are being treated for hyperlipidemias should be followed closely if they elect to use oral contraceptives. Some progestogens may elevate LDL levels and may render the control of hyperlipidemias more difficult.

4. LIVER FUNCTION

If jaundice develops in any woman receiving oral contraceptives, the medication should be discontinued. Steroid hormones may be poorly metabolized in patients with impaired liver function.

5. FLUID RETENTION

Oral contraceptives may cause some degree of fluid retention. They should be prescribed with caution, and only with careful monitoring, in patients with conditions which might be aggravated by fluid retention.

6. EMOTIONAL DISORDERS

Women with a history of depression should be carefully observed and the drug discontinued if depression recurs to a serious degree.

7. CONTACT LENSES

Contact-lens wearers who develop visual changes or changes in lens tolerance should be assessed by an ophthalmologist.

8. DRUG INTERACTIONS

Effects of Other Drugs on Combined Hormonal Contraceptives

Rifampin. Metabolism of ethinyl estradiol and some progestins (e.g., norethindrone) is increased by rifampin. A reduction in contraceptive effectiveness and an increase in menstrual irregularities have been associated with concomitant use of rifampin.

Anticonvulsants. Anticonvulsants such as phenobarbital, phenytoin, and carbamazepine have been shown to increase the metabolism of ethinyl estradiol and/or some progestins, which could result in a reduction of contraceptive effectiveness.

Antibiotics. Pregnancy while taking combined hormonal contraceptives has been reported when the combined hormonal contraceptives were administered with antimicrobials such as ampicillin, tetracycline, and griseofulvin. However, clinical pharmacokinetic studies have not demonstrated any consistent effects of antibiotics (other than rifampin) on plasma concentrations of synthetic steroids.

Atorvastatin. Coadministration of atorvastatin and an oral contraceptive increased AUC values for norethindrone and ethinyl estradiol by approximately 30% and 20%, respectively.

St. John's Wort. Herbal products containing St. John's Wort (hypericum perforatum) may induce hepatic enzymes (cytochrome P450) and p-glycoprotein transporter and may reduce the effectiveness of oral contraceptives and emergency contraceptive pills. This may also result in breakthrough bleeding.

Other. Ascorbic acid and acetaminophen may increase plasma concentrations of some synthetic estrogens, possibly by inhibition of conjugation. A reduction in contraceptive effectiveness and an increased incidence of menstrual irregularities has been suggested with phenylbutazone.

Effects of Drospirenone on Other Drugs

- *Metabolic Interactions*

  Metabolism of DRSP and potential effects of DRSP on hepatic cytochrome P450 (CYP) enzymes have been investigated in *in vitro* and *in vivo* studies (see Metabolism). In *in vitro* studies DRSP did not affect turnover of model substrates of CYP1A2 and CYP2D6, but had an inhibitory influence on the turnover of model substrates of CYP1A1, CYP2C9, CYP2C19 and CYP3A4 with CYP2C19 being the most sensitive enzyme. The potential effect of DRSP on CYP2C19 activity was investigated in a clinical pharmacokinetic study using omeprazole as a marker substrate. In the study with 24 postmenopausal women [including 12 women with homozygous (wild type) CYP2C19 genotype and 12 women with heterozygous CYP2C19 genotype] the daily oral administration of 3 mg DRSP for 14 days did not affect the oral clearance of omeprazole (40 mg, single oral dose). Based on the available results of *in vivo* and in *vitro* studies it can be concluded that, at clinical dose level, DRSP shows little propensity to interact to a significant extent with cytochrome P450 enzymes.
- *Interactions With Drugs That Have The Potential To Increase Serum Potassium*

  There is a potential for an increase in serum potassium in women taking **YASMIN** with other drugs **(see BOLDED WARNING)**. Of note, occasional or chronic use of NSAID medication was not restricted in any of the **YASMIN** clinical trials.

  A drug-drug interaction study of DRSP 3 mg/estradiol (E2) 1 mg versus placebo was performed in 24 mildly hypertensive postmenopausal women taking enalapril meleate 10 mg twice daily. Potassium levels were obtained every other day for a total of 2 weeks in all subjects. Mean serum potassium levels in the DRSP/E2 treatment group relative to baseline were 0.22 mEq/L higher than those in the placebo group. Serum potassium concentrations also were measured at multiple timepoints over 24 hours at baseline and on Day 14. On Day 14, the ratios for serum potassium Cmax and AUC in the DRSP/E2 group to those in the placebo group were 0.955 (90% CI: 0.914, 0.999) and 1.010 (90% CI: 0.944, 1.080), respectively. No patient in either treatment group developed hyperkalemia (serum potassium concentrations > 5.5 mEq/L).

Effects of Combined Hormonal Contraceptives on Other Drugs

Combined oral contraceptives containing ethinyl estradiol may inhibit the metabolism of other compounds. Increased plasma concentrations of cyclosporine, prednisolone, and theophylline have been reported with concomitant administration of oral contraceptives. In addition, oral contraceptives may induce the conjugation of other compounds. Decreased plasma concentrations of acetaminophen and increased clearance on temazepam, salicylic acid, morphine, and clofibric acid have been noted when these drugs were administered with oral contraceptives.

9. INTERACTIONS WITH LABORATORY TESTS

Certain endocrine- and liver-function tests and blood components may be affected by oral contraceptives:

a. Increased prothrombin and factors VII, VIII, IX and X; decreased antithrombin 3; increased norepinephrine-induced platelet aggregability.
b. Increased thyroid-binding globulin (TBG) leading to increased circulating total thyroid hormone, as measured by protein-bound iodine (PBI), T4 by column or by radioimmunoassay. Free T3 resin uptake is decreased, reflecting the elevated TBG, free T4 concentration is unaltered.
c. Other binding proteins may be elevated in serum.
d. Sex-hormone-binding globulins are increased and result in elevated levels of total circulating sex steroids and corticoids; however, free or biologically active levels remain unchanged.
e. Triglycerides may be increased.
f. Glucose tolerance may be decreased.
g. Serum folate levels may be depressed by oral contraceptive therapy. This may be of clinical significance if a woman becomes pregnant shortly after discontinuing oral contraceptives.

10. CARCINOGENESIS, MUTAGENESIS, IMPAIRMENT OF FERTILITY

In a 24 month oral carcinogenicity study in mice dosed with 10 mg/kg/day drospirenone alone or 1 + 0.01, 3 + 0.03 and 10 + 0.1 mg/kg/day of drospirenone and ethinyl estradiol, 0.1 to 2 times the exposure (AUC of drospirenone) of women taking a contraceptive dose, there was an increase in carcinomas of the harderian gland in the group that received the high dose of drospirenone alone. In a similar study in rats given 10 mg/kg/day drospirenone alone or 0.3 + 0.003, 3 + 0.03 and 10 + 0.1 mg/kg/day drospirenone and ethinyl estradiol, 0.8 to 10 times the exposure of women taking a contraceptive dose, there was an increased incidence of benign and total (benign and malignant) adrenal gland pheochromocytomas in the group receiving the high dose of drospirenone. Drospirenone was not mutagenic in a number of *in vitro* (Ames, Chinese Hamster Lung gene mutation and chromosomal damage in human lymphocytes) and *in vivo* (mouse micronucleus) genotoxicity tests. Drospirenone increased unscheduled DNA synthesis in rat hepatocytes and formed adducts with rodent liver DNA but not with human liver DNA. See **WARNINGS.**

11. PREGNANCY

Pregnancy category X. See **CONTRAINDICATIONS** and **WARNINGS.**

Estrogens and progestins should not be used during pregnancy. Fourteen pregnancies that occurred with **YASMIN** exposure *in utero* (none with more than a single cycle of exposure) have been identified. One infant was born with esophageal atresia. A causal association with **YASMIN** is unknown.

A teratology study in pregnant rats given drospirenone orally at doses of 5, 15 and 45 mg/kg/day, 6 to 50 times the human exposure based on AUC of drospirenone, resulted in an increased number of fetuses with delayed ossification of bones of the feet in the two higher doses. A similar study in rabbits dosed orally with 1, 30 and 100 mg/kg/day drospirenone, 2 to 27 times the human exposure, resulted in an increase in fetal loss and retardation of fetal development (delayed ossification of small bones, multiple fusions of ribs) at the high dose only. When drospirenone was administered with ethinyl estradiol (100:1) during late pregnancy (the period of genital development) at doses of 5, 15 and 45 mg/kg, there was a dose dependent increase in feminization of male rat fetuses. In a study in 36 cynomolgous monkeys, no teratogenic or feminization effects were observed with orally administered drospirenone and ethinyl estradiol (100:1) at doses up to 10 mg/kg/day drospirenone, 30 times the human exposure.

12. NURSING MOTHERS

Small amounts of oral contraceptive steroids have been identified in the milk of nursing mothers, and a few adverse effects on the child have been reported, including jaundice and breast enlargement. In addition, oral contraceptives given in the postpartum period may interfere with lactation by decreasing the quantity and quality of breast milk. If possible, the nursing mother should be advised not to use oral contraceptives but to use other forms of contraception until she has completely weaned her child.

After oral administration of **YASMIN** about 0.02% of the drospirenone dose was excreted into the breast milk of postpartum women within 24 hours. This results in a maximal daily dose of about 3 mcg drospirenone in an infant.

13. PEDIATRIC USAGE

Safety and efficacy of **YASMIN** have been established in women of reproductive age. Safety and efficacy are expected to be the same for postpubertal adolescents under the age of 16 and for users 16 years and older. Use of this product before menarche is not indicated.

INFORMATION FOR THE PATIENT

See Patient Labeling printed below.

ADVERSE REACTIONS

An increased risk of the following serious adverse reactions has been associated with the use of oral contraceptives (see **WARNINGS**).

- Thrombophlebitis
- Arterial thromboembolism
- Pulmonary embolism
- Myocardial infarction
- Cerebral hemorrhage
- Cerebral thrombosis
- Hypertension
- Gallbladder disease
- Hepatic adenomas or benign liver tumors

There is evidence of an association between the following conditions and the use of oral contraceptives, although additional confirmatory studies are needed:

- Mesenteric thrombosis
- Retinal thrombosis

The following adverse reactions have been reported in patients receiving oral contraceptives and are believed to be drug-related:

- Nausea
- Vomiting
- Gastrointestinal symptoms (such as abdominal cramps and bloating)
- Breakthrough bleeding
- Spotting
- Change in menstrual flow
- Amenorrhea
- Temporary infertility after discontinuation of treatment
- Edema
- Melasma which may persist
- Breast changes: tenderness, enlargement, secretion
- Change in weight (increase or decrease)
- Change in cervical erosion and secretion
- Diminution in lactation when given immediately postpartum
- Cholestatic jaundice
- Migraine
- Rash (allergic)

Continued on next page

Information on Berlex products (appearing here) is based on the most current information available at the time of publication closing. Further information for these and other Berlex products can be obtained from Medical & Product Services at Berlex, Inc. by calling 1-888-BERLEX-4.

Yasmin 28—Cont.

- Mental depression
- Reduced tolerance to carbohydrates
- Vaginal candidiasis
- Change in corneal curvature (steepening)
- Intolerance to contact lenses

The following adverse reactions have been reported in users of oral contraceptives and a causal association has been neither confirmed nor refuted:

- Acne
- Budd-Chiari syndrome
- Cataracts
- Changes in appetite
- Changes in libido
- Colitis
- Cystitis-like syndrome
- Dizziness
- Erythema multiforme
- Erythema nodosum
- Headache
- Hemolytic uremic syndrome
- Hemorrhagic eruption
- Hirsutism
- Impaired renal function
- Loss of scalp hair
- Nervousness
- Porphyria
- Pre-menstrual syndrome
- Vaginitis

The following are the most common adverse events reported with use of **YASMIN** during the clinical trials, occurring in >1% of subjects and which may or may not be drug related: Headache, Menstrual Disorder, Breast Pain, Abdominal Pain, Nausea, Leukorrhea, Flu Syndrome, Acne, Vaginal Moniliasis, Depression, Diarrhea, Asthenia, Dysmenorrhea, Back Pain, Infection, Pharyngitis, Intermenstrual Bleeding, Migraine, Vomiting, Dizziness, Nervousness, Vaginitis, Sinusitis, Cystitis, Bronchitis, Gastroenteritis, Allergic Reaction, Urinary Tract Infection, Pruritus, Emotional Lability, Surgery, Rash, Upper Respiratory Infection.

OVERDOSAGE

Serious ill effects have not been reported following acute ingestion of large doses of other oral contraceptives by young children. Overdosage may cause nausea, and withdrawal bleeding may occur in females. Drospirenone, however, is a spironolactone analogue which has antimineralocorticoid properties. Serum concentration of potassium and sodium, and evidence of metabolic acidosis, should be monitored in cases of overdose.

NON-CONTRACEPTIVE HEALTH BENEFITS

The following non-contraceptive health benefits related to the use of oral contraceptives are supported by epidemiological studies which largely utilized oral contraceptive formulations containing doses exceeding 0.035 mg of ethinyl estradiol or 0.05 mg mestranol.

Effects on menses:

- increased menstrual cycle regularity
- decreased blood loss and decreased incidence of iron-deficiency anemia
- decreased incidence of dysmenorrhea

Effects related to inhibition of ovulation:

- decreased incidence of functional ovarian cysts
- decreased incidence of ectopic pregnancies

Effects from long-term use:

- decreased incidence of fibroadenomas and fibrocystic disease of the breast
- decreased incidence of acute pelvic inflammatory disease
- decreased incidence of endometrial cancer
- decreased incidence of ovarian cancer

DOSAGE AND ADMINISTRATION

YASMIN

To achieve maximum contraceptive effectiveness, **YASMIN** (drospirenone and ethinyl estradiol) must be taken exactly as directed at intervals not exceeding 24 hours.

YASMIN consists of 21 tablets of a monophasic combined hormonal preparation plus 7 inert tablets. The dosage of **YASMIN** is one yellow tablet daily for 21 consecutive days followed by 7 white inert tablets per menstrual cycle. A patient should begin to take **YASMIN** either on the first day of her menstrual period (Day 1 Start) or on the first Sunday after the onset of her menstrual period (Sunday Start).

Day 1 Start. During the first cycle of **YASMIN** use, the patient should be instructed to take one yellow **YASMIN** daily, beginning on day one (1) of her menstrual cycle. (The first day of menstruation is day one.) She should take one yellow **YASMIN** daily for 21 consecutive days, followed by one white inert tablet daily on menstrual cycle days 22 through 28. It is recommended that **YASMIN** be taken at the same time each day, preferably after the evening meal or at bedtime. If **YASMIN** is first taken later than the first day of the menstrual cycle, **YASMIN** should not be considered effective as a contraceptive until after the first 7 consecutive days of product administration. The possibility of ovulation and conception prior to initiation of medication should be considered.

Sunday Start. During the first cycle of **YASMIN** use, the patient should be instructed to take one yellow **YASMIN** daily, beginning on the first Sunday after the onset of her menstrual period. She should take one yellow **YASMIN** daily for 21 consecutive days, followed by one white inert tablet daily on menstrual cycle days 22 through 28. It is recommended that **YASMIN** be taken at the same time each day, preferably after the evening meal or at bedtime. **YASMIN** should not be considered effective as a contraceptive until after the first 7 consecutive days of product administration. The possibility of ovulation and conception prior to initiation of medication should be considered.

The patient should begin her next and all subsequent 28-day regimens of **YASMIN** on the same day of the week that she began her first regimen, following the same schedule. She should begin taking her yellow tablets on the next day after ingestion of the last white tablet, regardless of whether or not a menstrual period has occurred or is still in progress. Anytime a subsequent cycle of **YASMIN** is started later than the day following administration of the last white tablet, the patient should use another method of contraception until she has taken a yellow **YASMIN** daily for seven consecutive days.

When switching from another oral contraceptive, **YASMIN** should be started on the same day that a new pack of the previous oral contraceptive would have been started.

Withdrawal bleeding usually occurs within 3 days following the last yellow tablet. If spotting or breakthrough bleeding occurs while taking **YASMIN**, the patient should be instructed to continue taking her **YASMIN** as instructed and by the regimen described above. She should be instructed that this type of bleeding is usually transient and without significance; however, if the bleeding is persistent or prolonged, the patient should be advised to consult her physician.

Although the occurrence of pregnancy is unlikely if **YASMIN** is taken according to directions, if withdrawal bleeding does not occur, the possibility of pregnancy must be considered. If the patient has not adhered to the prescribed dosing schedule (missed one or more active tablets or started taking them on a day later than she should have), the possibility of pregnancy should be considered at the time of the first missed period and appropriate diagnostic measures taken. If the patient has adhered to the prescribed regimen and misses two consecutive periods, pregnancy should be ruled out. Hormonal contraception should be discontinued if pregnancy is confirmed.

The risk of pregnancy increases with each active yellow tablet missed. For additional patient instructions regarding missed pills, see the "WHAT TO DO IF YOU MISS PILLS" section in the DETAILED PATIENT LABELING which follows. If breakthrough bleeding occurs following missed tablets, it will usually be transient and of no consequence. If the patient misses one or more white tablets, she should still be protected against pregnancy provided she begins taking yellow tablets again on the proper day.

In the nonlactating mother, **YASMIN** may be initiated 4 weeks postpartum, for contraception. When the tablets are administered in the postpartum period, the increased risk of thromboembolic disease associated with the postpartum period must be considered. (See **CONTRAINDICATIONS**, **WARNINGS**, and **PRECAUTIONS** concerning thromboembolic disease.)

HOW SUPPLIED

YASMIN 28 Tablets (drospirenone and ethinyl estradiol) are available in packages of 3 BLISTER packs (NDC 50419-402-03).

Each pack contains 21 active yellow round, unscored, film coated tablets each containing 3 mg drospirenone and 0.03 mg ethinyl estradiol, and 7 inert white round, unscored, film coated tablets.

Store at 25° C (77°F); excursions permitted to 15°-30°C (59°-86°F) [See USP Controlled Room Temperature].

REFERENCES FURNISHED UPON REQUEST

Manufactured for: Berlex Laboratories
Manufactured in: Germany

BRIEF SUMMARY PATIENT PACKAGE INSERT

YASMIN® 28 Tablets
(drospirenone and ethinyl estradiol)

28 tablets containing the following:
21 yellow – "active" tablets
7 white – "inert" tablets

This product (like all oral contraceptives) is intended to prevent pregnancy. It does not protect against HIV infection (AIDS) and other sexually transmitted diseases.

YASMIN is different from other birth-control pills because it contains the progestin drospirenone. Drospirenone may increase potassium. Therefore, you should not take YASMIN if you have kidney, liver or adrenal disease because this could cause serious heart and health problems. Other drugs may also increase potassium. If you are currently on daily, long-term treatment for a chronic condition with any of the medications below, you should consult your healthcare provider about whether YASMIN is right for you, and during the first month that you take YASMIN, you should have a blood test to check your potassium level.

- **NSAIDs (ibuprofen [Motrin®, Advil®], naproxen [Naprosyn®, Aleve® and others] when taken long-term and for treatment of arthritis or other problems)**
- **Potassium-sparing diuretics (spironolactone and others)**
- **Potassium supplementation**
- **ACE inhibitors (Capoten®, Vasotec®, Zestril® and others)**
- **Angiotensin-II receptor antagonists (Cozaar®, Diovan®, Avapro® and others)**
- **Heparin**

Oral contraceptives, also known as "birth-control pills" or "the pill," are taken to prevent pregnancy, and when taken correctly, have a failure rate of less than 1% per year when used without missing any pills. The typical failure rate of large numbers of pill users is less than 5% per year when women who miss pills are included. However, forgetting to take pills considerably increases the chances of pregnancy. For the majority of women, oral contraceptives can be taken safely. But there are some women who are at high risk of developing certain serious diseases that can be life-threatening or may cause temporary or permanent disability or death. The risks associated with taking oral contraceptives increase significantly if you:

- smoke
- have high blood pressure, diabetes, high cholesterol
- have or have had clotting disorders, heart attack, stroke, angina pectoris, cancer of the breast or sex organs, jaundice, or malignant or benign liver tumors.

You should not take the pill if you suspect you are pregnant or have unexplained vaginal bleeding.

Cigarette smoking increases the risk of serious adverse effects on the heart and blood vessels from oral contraceptive use. This risk increases with age and with heavy smoking (15 or more cigarettes per day) and is quite marked in women over 35 years of age. Women who use oral contraceptives should not smoke.

Most side effects of the pill are not serious. The most common such effects are nausea, vomiting, bleeding between menstrual periods, weight gain, breast tenderness, and difficulty wearing contact lenses. These side effects, especially nausea and vomiting may subside within the first three months of use.

The serious side effects of the pill occur very infrequently, especially if you are in good health and are young. However, you should know that the following medical conditions have been associated with or made worse by the pill:

1. Blood clots in the legs (thrombophlebitis), lungs (pulmonary embolism), blockage or rupture of a blood vessel in the brain (stroke), blockage of blood vessels in the heart (heart attack and angina pectoris) or other organs of the body. As mentioned above, smoking increases the risk of heart attacks and strokes and subsequent serious medical consequences.
2. Liver tumors, which may rupture and cause severe bleeding. A possible but not definite association has been found with the pill and liver cancer. However, liver cancers are extremely rare. The chance of developing liver cancer from using the pill is thus even rarer.
3. High blood pressure, although blood pressure usually returns to normal when the pill is stopped.
4. Cancer of the breast. Various studies give conflicting reports on the relationship between breast cancer and oral contraceptive use. Oral contraceptive use may slightly increase your chance of having breast cancer diagnosed, particularly after using hormonal contraceptives at a younger age. After you stop using hormonal contraceptives, the chances of getting breast cancer begin to go back down. You should have regular breast examinations by a healthcare provider and examine your own breasts monthly. Tell your healthcare provider if you have a family history of breast cancer or if you have had breast nodules or an abnormal mammogram. Women who currently have or have had breast cancer should not use oral contraceptives because breast cancer is a hormone-sensitive tumor.

The symptoms associated with these serious side effects are discussed in the detailed leaflet given to you with your supply of pills. Notify your doctor or healthcare provider if you notice any unusual physical disturbances while taking the pill. In addition, drugs such as rifampin, as well as some anticonvulsants, some antibiotics and some herbal products such as St. John's Wort, may decrease oral contraceptive effectiveness.

Taking the pill provides some important non-contraceptive benefits. These include less painful menstruation, less menstrual blood loss and anemia, fewer pelvic infections, and fewer cancers of the ovary and the lining of the uterus.

Be sure to discuss any medical condition you may have with your healthcare provider. Your healthcare provider will take a medical and family history before prescribing oral contraceptives and will examine you. The physical examination may be delayed to another time if you request it and the healthcare provider believes that it is appropriate to postpone it. You should be reexamined at least once a year while taking oral contraceptives. The detailed patient information booklet gives you further information which you should read and discuss with your healthcare provider.

This product (like all oral contraceptives) is intended to prevent pregnancy. It does not protect against transmission of HIV (AIDS) and other sexually transmitted diseases such as chlamydia, genital herpes, genital warts, gonorrhea, hepatitis B, and syphilis.

INSTRUCTIONS TO PATIENTS

HOW TO TAKE THE PILL

IMPORTANT POINTS TO REMEMBER

***BEFORE* YOU START TAKING YOUR PILLS**

1. BE SURE TO READ THESE DIRECTIONS:
   Before you start taking your pills.
   Anytime you are not sure what to do.
2. THE RIGHT WAY TO TAKE THE PILL IS TO TAKE ONE PILL EVERY DAY AT THE SAME TIME.

If you miss pills you could get pregnant. This includes starting the pack late. The more pills you miss, the more likely you are to get pregnant.

3. MANY WOMEN HAVE SPOTTING OR LIGHT BLEEDING, OR MAY FEEL SICK TO THEIR STOMACH DURING THE FIRST 1-3 PACKS OF PILLS.
If you do have spotting or light bleeding or feel sick to your stomach, do not stop taking the pill. The problem will usually go away. If it does not go away, check with your doctor or healthcare provider.
4. MISSING PILLS CAN ALSO CAUSE SPOTTING OR LIGHT BLEEDING, even when you make up these missed pills.
On the days you take two pills, to make up for missed pills, you could also feel a little sick to your stomach.
5. IF YOU HAVE VOMITING OR DIARRHEA, or IF YOU TAKE SOME MEDICINES, including some antibiotics and some herbal products such as St. John's Wort, your pills may not work as well.
Use a back-up method (such as condoms or spermicides) until you check with your doctor or healthcare provider.
6. IF YOU HAVE TROUBLE REMEMBERING TO TAKE THE PILL, talk to your doctor or healthcare provider about how to make pill-taking easier or about using another method of birth control.
7. IF YOU HAVE ANY QUESTIONS OR ARE UNSURE ABOUT THE INFORMATION IN THIS LEAFLET, call your doctor or healthcare provider.

BEFORE YOU START TAKING YOUR PILLS

1. DECIDE WHAT TIME OF DAY YOU WANT TO TAKE YOUR PILL.
It is important to take it at about the same time every day.
2. LOOK AT YOUR PILL PACK — IT HAS 28 PILLS:
The **YASMIN** *pill pack* has 21 yellow "active" pills (with hormones) to be taken for three weeks, followed by 7 white "reminder" pills (without hormones) to be taken for one week.
3. ALSO FIND:
1) where on the pack to start taking pills,
2) in what order to take the pills (follow the arrows)
3) the week numbers as shown in the diagram below

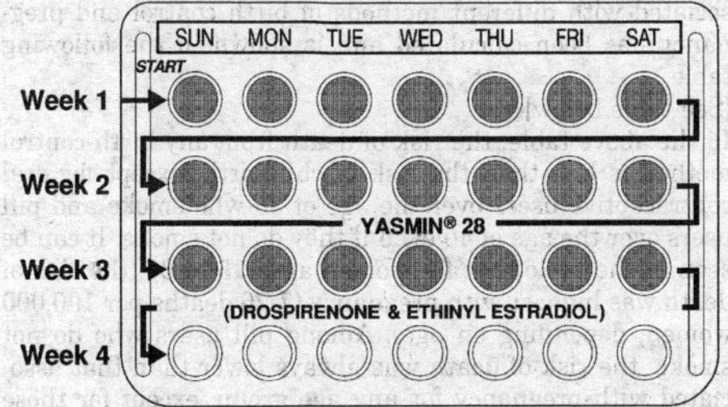

YASMIN 28 TABLETS
(drospirenone and ethinyl estradiol)

4. BE SURE YOU HAVE READY AT ALL TIMES:
ANOTHER KIND OF BIRTH CONTROL (such as condoms or spermicides) to use as a back-up in case you miss pills.
AN EXTRA, FULL PILL PACK.

WHEN TO START THE _FIRST_ PACK OF PILLS

You have a choice for which day to start taking your first pack of pills. Decide with your doctor or healthcare provider which is the best day for you. Pick a time of day which will be easy to remember.

DAY 1 START:

1. Take the first yellow "active" pill of the first pack during the *first 24 hours of your period.*
2. You will not need to use a back-up method of birth control, since you are starting the pill at the beginning of your period.

SUNDAY START:

1. Take the first yellow "active" pill of the first pack on the *Sunday after your period starts*, even if you are still bleeding. If your period begins on Sunday, start the pack that same day.
2. *Use another method of birth control* (such as condoms or spermicides) as a back-up method if you have sex any time from the Sunday you start your first pack until the next Sunday (7 days).

WHAT TO DO DURING THE MONTH

1. **TAKE ONE PILL AT THE SAME TIME EVERY DAY UNTIL THE PACK IS EMPTY**
Do not skip pills even if you are spotting or bleeding between monthly periods or feel sick to your stomach (nausea).
Do not skip pills even if you do not have sex very often.
2. **WHEN YOU FINISH A PACK OR SWITCH YOUR BRAND OF PILLS:**
Start the next pack on the day after your last white "reminder" pill. Do not wait any days between packs.

WHAT TO DO IF YOU MISS PILLS

If you **MISS 1** yellow "active" pill:

1. Take it as soon as you remember. Take the next pill at your regular time. This means you may take two pills in one day.
2. You do not need to use a back-up birth control method if you have sex.

If you **MISS 2** yellow "active" pills in a row in **WEEK 1 OR WEEK 2** of your pack:

Percentage of women experiencing an unintended pregnancy during the first year of typical use and first year of perfect use of contraception and the percentage continuing use at the end of the first year: United States.

	% of Women Experiencing an Accidental Pregnancy within the First Year of Use		% of Women Continuing Use at One Year[3]
Method (1)	Typical Use[1] (2)	Perfect Use[2] (3)	(4)
Chance[4]	85	85	
Spermicides[5]	26	6	40
Periodic abstinence	25		63
Calendar		9	
Ovulation method		3	
Sympto-thermal[6]		2	
Post-ovulation		1	
Withdrawal	19	4	
Cap[7]			
Parous women	40	26	42
Nulliparous women	20	9	56
Sponge			
Parous women	40	20	42
Nulliparous women	20	9	56
Diaphragm[7]	20	6	56
Condom[8]			
Female (Reality)	21	5	56
Male	14	3	61
Pill	5		71
progestin only		0.5	
combined		0.1	
IUD:			
Progesterone T	2.0	1.5	81
Copper T 380A	0.8	0.6	78
Lng 20	0.1	0.1	81
Depo Provera	0.3	0.3	70
Norplant and Norplant-2	0.05	0.05	88
Female sterilization	0.5	0.5	100
Male sterilization	0.15	0.10	100

Emergency Contraceptive Pills: Treatment initiated within 72 hours after unprotected intercourse reduces the risk of pregnancy by at least 75%.[9]
Lactational Amenorrhea Method: LAM is highly effective, *temporary* method of contraception.[10]
Source: Trussell J, Contraceptive efficacy. In Hatcher RA, Trussell J, Stewart F, Cates W, Stewart GK, Kowal D, Guest F, Contraceptive Technology: Seventeenth Revised Edition. New York NY: Irvington Publishers, 1998.

1 Among *typical* couples who initiate use of a method (not necessarily for the first time), the percentage who experience an accidental pregnancy during the first year if they do not stop use for any other reason.
2 Among couples who initiate use of a method (not necessarily for the first time) and who use it *perfectly* (both consistently and correctly), the percentage who experience an accidental pregnancy during the first year if they do not stop use for any reason.
3 Among couples attempting to avoid pregnancy, the percentage who continue to use a method for one year.
4 The percents becoming pregnant in columns (2) and (3) are based on data from populations where contraception is not used and from women who cease using contraception in order to become pregnant. Among such populations, about 89% become pregnant within one year. This estimate was lowered slightly (to 85%) to represent the percentage who would become pregnant within one year among women now relying on reversible methods of contraception if they abandoned contraception altogether.
5 Foams, creams, gels, vaginal suppositories, and vaginal film.
6 Cervical mucus (ovulation) method supplemented by calendar in the pre-ovulatory and basal body temperature in the post-ovulatory phases.
7 With spermicidal cream or jelly.
8 Without spermicides.
9 The treatment schedule is one dose within 72 hours after unprotected intercourse, and a second dose 12 hours after the first dose. The Food and Drug Administration has declared the following brands of oral contraceptives to be safe and effective for emergency contraception: Ovral (1 dose is 2 white pills), Alesse (1 dose is 5 pink pills), Nordette or Levlen (1 dose is 2 light-orange pills), Lo/Ovral (1 dose is 4 white pills), Triphasil or Tri-Levlen (1 dose is 4 yellow pills).
10 However, to maintain effective protection against pregnancy, another method of contraception must be used as soon as menstruation resumes, the frequency or duration of breastfeeds is reduced, bottle feeds are introduced, or the baby reaches six months of age.

1. Take two pills on the day you remember and two pills the next day.
2. Then take one pill a day until you finish the pack.
3. You MAY BECOME PREGNANT if you have sex in the 7 *days* after you miss pills. You MUST use another birth control method (such as condoms or spermicides) as a back-up for those 7 days.

If you **MISS 2** yellow "active" pills in a row in the **3RD WEEK:**

1. ***If you are a Day 1 Starter:***
THROW OUT the rest of the pill pack and start a new pack that same day.
If you are a Sunday Starter:
Keep taking one pill every day until Sunday. On Sunday, THROW OUT the rest of the pack and start a new pack of pills that same day.
2. You may not have your period this month but this is expected. However, if you miss your period two months in a row, call your doctor or healthcare provider because you might be pregnant.
3. You MAY BECOME PREGNANT if you have sex in the 7 *days* after you miss pills. You MUST use another birth control method (such as condoms or spermicides) as a back-up for those 7 days.

If you **MISS 3 OR MORE** yellow "active" pills in a row (during the first 3 weeks).

1. ***If you are a Day 1 Starter:***
THROW OUT the rest of the pill pack and start a new pack that same day.
If you are a Sunday Starter:
Keep taking 1 pill every day until Sunday. On Sunday, THROW OUT the rest of the pack and start a new pack of pills that same day.
2. You may not have your period this month but this is expected. However, if you miss your period two months in a row, call your doctor or healthcare provider because you might be pregnant.
3. You MAY BECOME PREGNANT if you have sex in the 7 *days* after you miss pills. You MUST use another birth control method (such as condoms or spermicides) as a back-up for those 7 days.

If you forget any of the 7 white "reminder" pills in Week 4:
THROW AWAY the pills you missed.
Keep taking one pill each day until the pack is empty.
You do not need a back-up method.

FINALLY, IF YOU ARE STILL NOT SURE WHAT TO DO ABOUT THE PILLS YOU HAVE MISSED:
Use a BACK-UP METHOD (such as condoms or spermicides) anytime you have sex.
KEEP TAKING ONE ACTIVE PILL EACH DAY until you can reach your doctor or healthcare provider.

For additional information see Detailed Patient Labeling

Continued on next page

Information on Berlex products (appearing here) is based on the most current information available at the time of publication closing. Further information for these and other Berlex products can be obtained from Medical & Product Services at Berlex, Inc. by calling 1-888-BERLEX-4.

Yasmin 28—Cont.

DETAILED PATIENT PACKAGE INSERT

This product (like all oral contraceptives) is intended to prevent pregnancy. It does not protect against HIV infection (AIDS) and other sexually transmitted diseases.

YASMIN is different from other birth-control pills because it contains the progestin drospirenone. Drospirenone may increase potassium. Therefore, you should not take YASMIN if you have kidney, liver or adrenal disease because this could cause serious heart and health problems. Other drugs may also increase potassium. If you are currently on daily, long-term treatment for a chronic condition with any of the medications below, you should consult your healthcare provider about whether YASMIN is right for you, and during the first month that you take YASMIN, you should have a blood test to check your potassium level.

- **NSAIDs (ibuprofen [Motrin®, Advil®], naproxen [Naprosyn®, Aleve® and others] when taken long-term and for treatment of arthritis or other problems)**
- **Potassium-sparing diuretics (spironolactone and others)**
- **Potassium supplementation**
- **ACE inhibitors (Capoten®, Vasotec®, Zestril® and others)**
- **Angiotensin-II receptor antagonists (Cozaar®, Diovan®, Avapro® and others)**
- **Heparin**

INTRODUCTION

Any woman who considers using oral contraceptives (the birth-control pill or "the pill") should understand the benefits and risks of using this form of birth control. This leaflet will give you much of the information you will need to make this decision and will also help you determine if you are at risk of developing any of the serious side effects of the pill. It will tell you how to use the pill properly so that it will be as effective as possible. However, this leaflet is not a replacement for a careful discussion between you and your healthcare provider. You should discuss the information provided in this leaflet with him or her, both when you first start taking the pill and during your revisits. You should also follow your healthcare provider's advice with regard to regular check-ups while you are on the pill.

EFFECTIVENESS OF ORAL CONTRACEPTIVES

Oral contraceptives or "birth-control pills" or "the pill" are used to prevent pregnancy and are more effective than other nonsurgical methods of birth control. When they are taken correctly, the chance of becoming pregnant is less than 1.0% (one pregnancy per 100 women per year of use) when used perfectly, without missing any pills. Typical failure rates, including women who don't always follow the instructions exactly, are about 5.0% per year. The chance of becoming pregnant increases with each missed pill during a menstrual cycle.

In comparison, typical failure rates for other nonsurgical methods of birth control during the first year of use are as follows:

[See table at top of previous page]

WHO SHOULD NOT TAKE ORAL CONTRACEPTIVES

Cigarette smoking increases the risk of serious adverse effects on the heart and blood vessels from oral contraceptive use. This risk increases with age and with heavy smoking (15 or more cigarettes per day) and is quite marked in women over 35 years of age. Women who use YASMIN should not smoke.

Some women should not use the pill. For example, you should not take **YASMIN** if you are pregnant or think you may be pregnant. You should also not use **YASMIN** if you have had any of the following conditions:

- A history of heart attack or stroke
- Blood clots in the legs (thrombophlebitis), lungs (pulmonary embolism), brain (stroke) or eyes
- A history of blood clots in the deep veins of your legs
- Chest pain (angina pectoris)
- Known or suspected breast cancer or cancer of the lining of the uterus, cervix or vagina
- Unexplained vaginal bleeding (until a diagnosis is reached by your doctor)
- Yellowing of the whites of the eyes or of the skin (jaundice) during pregnancy or during previous use of the pill
- Liver tumor (benign or cancerous)
- Known or suspected pregnancy

In addition, you should not use **YASMIN** if you have any of the following conditions:

- Kidney Disease
- Liver Disease
- Adrenal Disease

Tell your healthcare provider if you have ever had any of the above conditions (Your healthcare provider can recommend another method of birth control). If you are currently on daily, long-term treatment for a chronic condition with any of the following medications, you should consult your healthcare provider before taking **YASMIN:**

- NSAIDs (ibuprofen, naproxen and others)
- Potassium-sparing diuretics (spironolactone and others)
- Potassium supplementation
- ACE inhibitors (captopril, enalapril, lisinopril and others)
- Angiotensin-II receptor antagonists (Cozaar®, Diovan®, Avapro® and others)
- Heparin

OTHER CONSIDERATIONS BEFORE TAKING ORAL CONTRACEPTIVES

Tell your healthcare provider if you or any family member has ever had:

- Breast nodules, fibrocystic disease of the breast, an abnormal breast X-ray or mammogram
- Diabetes
- Elevated cholesterol or triglycerides
- High blood pressure
- Migraine or other headaches or epilepsy
- Mental depression
- Gallbladder, heart or kidney disease
- History of scanty or irregular menstrual periods

Women with any of these conditions should be checked often by their healthcare provider if they choose to use oral contraceptives.

Also, be sure to inform your doctor or healthcare provider if you smoke or take any medications.

RISKS OF TAKING ORAL CONTRACEPTIVES

1. *RISK OF DEVELOPING BLOOD CLOTS*

Blood clots and blockage of blood vessels are the most serious side effects of taking oral contraceptives and can be fatal. In particular, a clot in the legs can cause thrombophlebitis and a clot that travels to the lungs can cause sudden blocking of the vessel carrying blood to the lungs. Rarely, clots occur in the blood vessels of the eye and may cause blindness, double vision, or impaired vision.

If you take oral contraceptives and need elective surgery, need to stay in bed for a prolonged illness or have recently delivered a baby, you may be at risk of developing blood clots. You should consult your doctor about stopping oral contraceptives three to four weeks before surgery and not taking oral contraceptives for two weeks after surgery or during bed rest. You should also not take oral contraceptives soon after delivery of a baby or a mid-trimester pregnancy loss or termination. It is advisable to wait for at least four weeks after delivery if you are not breast-feeding. If you are breast-feeding, you should wait until you have weaned your child before using the pill. (See also the section on breast-feeding in **GENERAL PRECAUTIONS**.)

2. *HEART ATTACKS AND STROKES*

Oral contraceptives may increase the tendency to develop strokes (stoppage or rupture of blood vessels in the brain) and angina pectoris and heart attacks (blockage of blood vessels in the heart). Any of these conditions can cause death or serious disability.

Smoking greatly increases the possibility of suffering heart attacks and strokes. Furthermore, smoking and the use of oral contraceptives greatly increase the chances of developing and dying of heart disease.

3. *GALLBLADDER DISEASE*

Oral contraceptive users probably have a greater risk than nonusers of having gallbladder disease, although this risk may be related to pills containing high doses of estrogens.

4. *LIVER TUMORS*

In rare cases, oral contraceptives can cause benign but dangerous liver tumors. These benign liver tumors can rupture and cause fatal internal bleeding. In addition, a possible but not definite association has been found with the pill and liver cancers in two studies, in which a few women who developed these very rare cancers were found to have used oral contraceptives for long periods. However, liver cancers are extremely rare. The chance of developing liver cancer from using the pill is thus even rarer.

5. *CANCER OF THE REPRODUCTIVE ORGANS AND BREASTS*

Various studies give conflicting reports on the relationship between breast cancer and oral contraceptive use. Oral contraceptive use may slightly increase your chance of having breast cancer diagnosed, particularly after using hormonal contraceptives at a younger age. After you stop using hormonal contraceptives, the chances of getting breast cancer begin to go back down. You should have regular breast examinations by a healthcare provider and examine your own breasts monthly. Tell your healthcare provider if you have a family history of breast cancer or if you have had breast nodules or an abnormal mammogram. Women who currently have or have had breast cancer should not use oral contraceptives because breast cancer is a hormone-sensitive tumor.

Some studies have found an increase in the incidence of cancer of the cervix in women who use oral contraceptives. However, this finding may be related to factors other than the use of oral contraceptives.

ESTIMATED RISK OF DEATH FROM A BIRTH CONTROL METHOD OR PREGNANCY

All methods of birth control and pregnancy are associated with a risk of developing certain diseases which may lead to disability or death. An estimate of the number of deaths associated with different methods of birth control and pregnancy has been calculated and is shown in the following table.

[See table below]

In the above table, the risk of death from any birth-control method is less than the risk of childbirth, except for oral contraceptive users over the age of 35 who smoke and pill users over the age of 40 even if they do not smoke. It can be seen in the table that for women aged 15 to 39, the risk of death was highest with pregnancy (7-26 deaths per 100,000 women, depending on age). Among pill users who do not smoke, the risk of death was always lower than that associated with pregnancy for any age group, except for those women over the age of 40, when the risk increases to 32 deaths per 100,000 women, compared to 28 associated with pregnancy at that age. However, for pill users who smoke and are over the age of 35, the estimated number of deaths exceeds those for other methods of birth control. If a woman is over the age of 40 and smokes, her estimated risk of death is four times higher (117/100,000 women) than the estimated risk associated with pregnancy (28/100,000 women) in that age group.

The suggestion that women over 40 who do not smoke should not take oral contraceptives is based on information from older high-dose pills and on less-selective use of pills than is practiced today. An Advisory Committee of the FDA discussed this issue in 1989 and recommended that the benefits of oral contraceptive use by healthy, non-smoking women over 40 years of age may outweigh the possible risks. However, all women, especially older women, are cautioned to use the lowest-dose pill that is effective.

WARNING SIGNALS

If any of these adverse effects occur while you are taking oral contraceptives, call your doctor immediately:

- Sharp chest pain, coughing of blood, or sudden shortness of breath (indicating a possible clot in the lung)
- Pain in the calf (indicating a possible clot in the leg)
- Crushing chest pain or heaviness in the chest (indicating a possible heart attack)
- Sudden severe headache or vomiting, dizziness or fainting, disturbances of vision or speech, weakness, or numbness in an arm or leg (indicating a possible stroke)
- Sudden partial or complete loss of vision (indicating a possible clot in the eye)
- Breast lumps (indicating possible breast cancer or fibrocystic disease of the breast; ask your doctor or healthcare provider to show you how to examine your breasts)
- Severe pain or tenderness in the stomach area (indicating a possibly ruptured liver tumor)
- Difficulty in sleeping, weakness, lack of energy, fatigue, or change in mood (possibly indicating severe depression)
- Jaundice or a yellowing of the skin or eyeballs, accompanied frequently by fever, fatigue, loss of appetite, dark-colored urine, or light-colored bowel movements (indicating possible liver problems)

SIDE EFFECTS OF ORAL CONTRACEPTIVES

1. *VAGINAL BLEEDING*

Irregular vaginal bleeding or spotting may occur while you are taking the pills. Irregular bleeding may vary from slight staining between menstrual periods to breakthrough bleeding, which is a flow much like a regular period. Irregular

ANNUAL NUMBER OF BIRTH-RELATED OR METHOD-RELATED DEATHS ASSOCIATED WITH CONTROL OF FERTILITY PER 100,000 NONSTERILE WOMEN, BY FERTILITY-CONTROL METHOD ACCORDING TO AGE

Method of Control and Outcome	15-19	20-24	25-29	30-34	35-39	40-44
No fertility control methods[1]	7.0	7.4	9.1	14.8	25.7	28.2
Oral contraceptives nonsmoker[2]	0.3	0.5	0.9	1.9	13.8	31.6
Oral contraceptives smoker[2]	2.2	3.4	6.6	13.5	51.1	117.2
IUD[2]	0.8	0.8	1.0	1.0	1.4	1.4
Condom[1]	1.1	1.6	0.7	0.2	0.3	0.4
Diaphragm/spermicide[1]	1.9	1.2	1.2	1.3	2.2	2.8
Periodic abstinence[1]	2.5	1.6	1.6	1.7	2.9	3.6

[1] Deaths are birth related
[2] Deaths are method related

Adapted from H.W. Ory, *Family Planning Perspectives* 15:57-63, 1983.

bleeding occurs most often during the first few months of oral contraceptive use, but may also occur after you have been taking the pill for some time. Such bleeding may be temporary and usually does not indicate any serious problems. It is important to continue taking your pills on schedule. If the bleeding occurs in more than one cycle or lasts for more than a few days, talk to your doctor or healthcare provider.

2. *CONTACT LENSES*

If you wear contact lenses and notice a change in vision or an inability to wear your lenses, contact your doctor or healthcare provider.

3. *FLUID RETENTION*

Oral contraceptives may cause edema (fluid retention) with swelling of the fingers or ankles and may raise your blood pressure. If you experience fluid retention, contact your doctor or healthcare provider.

4. *MELASMA*

A spotty darkening of the skin is possible, particularly of the face.

5. *OTHER SIDE EFFECTS*

Other side effects may include nausea, vomiting, change in appetite, headache, nervousness, depression, dizziness, loss of scalp hair, rash, and vaginal infections.

If any of these side effects occur, call your doctor or healthcare provider.

GENERAL PRECAUTIONS

1. *Missed periods and use of oral contraceptives before or during early pregnancy.*

There may be times when you may not menstruate regularly after you have completed taking a cycle of pills. If you have taken your pills regularly and miss one menstrual period, continue taking your pills for the next cycle but be sure to inform your healthcare provider before doing so. If you have not taken the pills daily as instructed and missed a menstrual period, or if you missed two consecutive menstrual periods, you may be pregnant. Check with your healthcare provider immediately to determine whether you are pregnant. Stop taking oral contraceptives if pregnancy is confirmed.

There is no conclusive evidence that oral contraceptive use is associated with an increase in birth defects when taken inadvertently during early pregnancy. Previously, a few studies had reported that oral contraceptives might be associated with birth defects, but these studies have not been confirmed. Nevertheless, oral contraceptives should not be used during pregnancy. You should check with your doctor about risks to your unborn child of any medication taken during pregnancy.

2. *While Breast-Feeding*

If you are breast-feeding, consult your doctor before starting oral contraceptives. Some of the drug will be passed on to the child in the milk. A few adverse effects on the child have been reported, including yellowing of the skin (jaundice) and breast enlargement. In addition, oral contraceptives may decrease the amount and quality of your milk. If possible, do not use oral contraceptives while breast-feeding. You should use another method of contraception since breast-feeding provides only partial protection from becoming pregnant, and this partial protection decreases significantly as you breast-feed for longer periods of time. You should consider starting oral contraceptives only after you have weaned your child completely.

3. *Laboratory Tests*

If you are scheduled for any laboratory tests, tell your doctor you are taking birth-control pills. Certain blood tests may be affected by birth-control pills.

4. *Drug Interactions*

Certain drugs may interact with birth-control pills to make them less effective in preventing pregnancy or cause an increase in breakthrough bleeding. Such drugs include rifampin, drugs used for epilepsy such as barbiturates (for example, phenobarbital) and phenytoin (Dilantin is one brand of this drug), phenylbutazone (Butazolidin is one brand) and possibly certain antibiotics. Herbal products containing St. John's Wort (hypericum perforatum) may reduce the effectiveness of oral contraceptives. This may also result in breakthrough bleeding. You may need to use an additional method of contraception during any cycle in which you take drugs that can make oral contraceptives less effective **(also See BOLDED TEXT AT BEGINNING)**.

5. ***Sexually Transmitted Diseases***

This product (like all oral contraceptives) is intended to prevent pregnancy. It does not protect against transmission of HIV (AIDS) and other sexually transmitted diseases such as chlamydia, genital herpes, genital warts, gonorrhea, hepatitis B, and syphilis.

HOW TO TAKE THE PILL

IMPORTANT POINTS TO REMEMBER

***BEFORE* YOU START TAKING YOUR PILLS**

1. BE SURE TO READ THESE DIRECTIONS:
   Before you start taking your pills.
   Any time you are not sure what to do.
2. THE RIGHT WAY TO TAKE THE PILL IS TO TAKE ONE PILL EVERY DAY AT THE SAME TIME.
   If you miss pills you could get pregnant. This includes starting the pack late. The more pills you miss, the more likely you are to get pregnant.
3. MANY WOMEN HAVE SPOTTING OR LIGHT BLEEDING, OR MAY FEEL SICK TO THEIR STOMACH DURING THE FIRST 1-3 PACKS OF PILLS.
   If you do have spotting or light bleeding or feel sick to your stomach, do not stop taking the pill. The problem will usually go away. If it does not go away, check with your doctor or healthcare provider.
4. MISSING PILLS CAN ALSO CAUSE SPOTTING OR LIGHT BLEEDING, even when you make up these missed pills.
   On the days you take two pills, to make up for missed pills, you could also feel a little sick to your stomach.
5. IF YOU HAVE VOMITING OR DIARRHEA, for any reason, or IF YOU TAKE SOME MEDICINES, including some antibiotics and some herbal products such as St. John's Wort, your pills may not work as well.
   Use a back-up method (such as condoms or spermicides) until you check with your doctor or healthcare provider.
6. IF YOU HAVE TROUBLE REMEMBERING TO TAKE THE PILL, talk to your doctor or healthcare provider about how to make pill-taking easier or about using another method of birth control.
7. IF YOU HAVE ANY QUESTIONS OR ARE UNSURE ABOUT THE INFORMATION IN THIS LEAFLET, call your doctor or healthcare provider.

***BEFORE* YOU START TAKING YOUR PILLS**

1. DECIDE WHAT TIME OF DAY YOU WANT TO TAKE YOUR PILL.
   It is important to take it at about the same time every day.
2. LOOK AT YOUR PILL PACK — IT HAS 28 PILLS:
   The **YASMIN** *pill pack* has 21 yellow "active" pills (with hormones) to be taken for three weeks, followed by 7 white "reminder" pills (without hormones) to be taken for one week.
3. ALSO FIND:
   1) where on the pack to start taking pills,
   2) in what order to take the pills (follow the arrows)
   3) the week numbers as shown in the diagram below

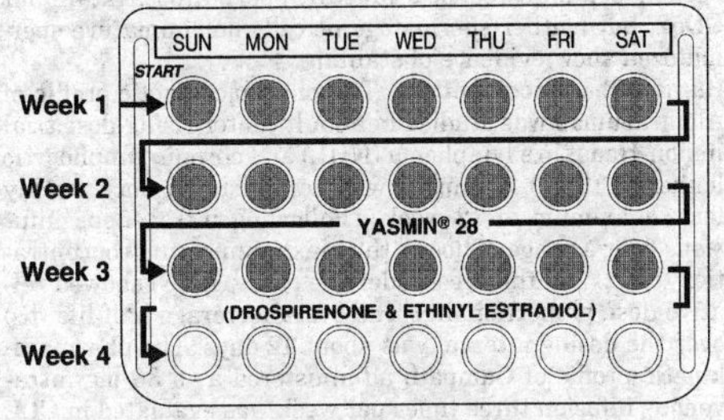

YASMIN 28 TABLETS
(drospirenone and ethinyl estradiol)

4. BE SURE YOU HAVE READY AT ALL TIMES:
   ANOTHER KIND OF BIRTH CONTROL (such as condoms or spermicides) to use as a back-up in case you miss pills.
   AN EXTRA, FULL PILL PACK.

WHEN TO START THE *FIRST* PACK OF PILLS

You have a choice for which day to start taking your first pack of pills. Decide with your doctor or healthcare provider which is the best day for you. Pick a time of day which will be easy to remember.

DAY 1 START:

1. Take the first yellow "active" pill of the first pack during the *first 24 hours of your period*.
2. You will not need to use a back-up method of birth control, since you are starting the pill at the beginning of your period.

SUNDAY START:

1. Take the first yellow "active" pill of the first pack on the *Sunday after your period starts*, even if you are still bleeding. If your period begins on Sunday, start the pack that same day.
2. *Use another method of birth control* (such as condoms or spermicides) as a back-up method if you have sex any time from the Sunday you start your first pack until the next Sunday (7 days).

WHAT TO DO DURING THE MONTH

1. **TAKE ONE PILL AT THE SAME TIME EVERY DAY UNTIL THE PACK IS EMPTY**
   Do not skip pills even if you are spotting or bleeding between monthly periods or feel sick to your stomach (nausea).
   Do not skip pills even if you do not have sex very often.
2. **WHEN YOU FINISH A PACK OR SWITCH YOUR BRAND OF PILLS:**
   Start the next pack on the day after your last white "reminder" pill. Do not wait any days between packs.

WHAT TO DO IF YOU MISS PILLS

If you **MISS 1** yellow "active" pill:

1. Take it as soon as you remember. Take the next pill at your regular time. This means you may take two pills in one day.
2. You do not need to use a back-up birth control method if you have sex.

If you **MISS 2** yellow "active" pills in a row in **WEEK 1 OR WEEK 2** of your pack:

1. Take two pills on the day you remember and two pills the next day.
2. Then take one pill a day until you finish the pack.
3. You MAY BECOME PREGNANT if you have sex in the 7 *days* after you miss pills. You MUST use another birth control method (such as condoms or spermicides) as a back-up for those 7 days.

If you **MISS 2** yellow "active" pills in a row in the **3RD WEEK:**

1. **If you are a Day 1 Starter:**
   THROW OUT the rest of the pill pack and start a new pack that same day.
   If you are a Sunday Starter:
   Keep taking one pill every day until Sunday. On Sunday, THROW OUT the rest of the pack and start a new pack of pills that same day.
2. You may not have your period this month but this is expected. However, if you miss your period two months in a row, call your doctor or healthcare provider because you might be pregnant.
3. You MAY BECOME PREGNANT if you have sex in the 7 *days* after you miss pills. You MUST use another birth control method (such as condoms or spermicides) as a back-up for those 7 days.

If you **MISS 3 OR MORE** yellow "active" pills in a row (during the first 3 weeks).

1. **If you are a Day 1 Starter:**
   THROW OUT the rest of the pill pack and start a new pack that same day.
   If you are a Sunday Starter:
   Keep taking 1 pill every day until Sunday. On Sunday, THROW OUT the rest of the pack and start a new pack of pills that same day.
2. You may not have your period this month but this is expected. However, if you miss your period two months in a row, call your doctor or healthcare provider because you might be pregnant.
3. You MAY BECOME PREGNANT if you have sex in the 7 *days* after you miss pills. You MUST use another birth control method (such as condoms or spermicides) as a back-up for those 7 days.

If you forget any of the 7 white "reminder" pills in Week 4:
THROW AWAY the pills you missed.
Keep taking one pill each day until the pack is empty.
You do not need a back-up method.

FINALLY, IF YOU ARE STILL NOT SURE WHAT TO DO ABOUT THE PILLS YOU HAVE MISSED:
Use a BACK-UP METHOD (such as condoms or spermicides) any time you have sex.
KEEP TAKING ONE ACTIVE PILL EACH DAY until you can reach your doctor or healthcare provider.

PREGNANCY DUE TO PILL FAILURE

The incidence of pill failure resulting in pregnancy is approximately less than 1.0% (one pregnancy per 100 women per year of use) if taken every day as directed, but more typical failure rates are about 5%. If failure does occur with **YASMIN** use, the risk to the fetus is unknown.

PREGNANCY AFTER STOPPING THE PILL

There may be some delay in becoming pregnant after you stop using oral contraceptives, especially if you had irregular menstrual cycles before you used oral contraceptives. It may be advisable to postpone conception until you begin menstruating regularly once you have stopped taking the pill and desire pregnancy.

There does not appear to be any increase in birth defects in newborn babies when pregnancy occurs soon after stopping the pill.

OVERDOSAGE

Serious ill effects have not been reported following ingestion of large doses of other oral contraceptives by young children. Overdosage of **YASMIN** may cause nausea and withdrawal bleeding in females and may increase blood levels of potassium or decrease blood levels of sodium, which could be dangerous. In case of overdosage, contact your healthcare provider.

OTHER INFORMATION

Your healthcare provider will take a medical and family history before prescribing oral contraceptives and will examine you. The physical examination may be delayed to another time if you request it and the healthcare provider believes that it is appropriate to postpone it. You should be re-examined at least once a year. Be sure to inform your healthcare provider if there is a family history of any of the conditions listed previously in this leaflet. Be sure to keep all appointments with your healthcare provider, because this is a time to determine if there are early signs of side effects of oral contraceptive use.

Do not use the drug for any condition other than the one for which it was prescribed. This drug has been prescribed specifically for you; do not give it to others who may want birth-control pills.

HEALTH BENEFITS FROM ORAL CONTRACEPTIVES

In addition to preventing pregnancy, use of oral contraceptives may provide certain benefits. They are:

- Menstrual cycles may become more regular
- Blood flow during menstruation may be lighter and less iron may be lost. Therefore, anemia due to iron deficiency is less likely to occur.

Continued on next page

Information on Berlex products (appearing here) is based on the most current information available at the time of publication closing. Further information for these and other Berlex products can be obtained from Medical & Product Services at Berlex, Inc. by calling 1-888-BERLEX-4.

Yasmin 28—Cont.

- Pain or other symptoms during menstruation may be encountered less frequently
- Ovarian cysts may occur less frequently
- Ectopic (tubal) pregnancy may occur less frequently
- Noncancerous cysts or lumps in the breast may occur less frequently
- Acute pelvic inflammatory disease may occur less frequently
- Oral contraceptive use may provide some protection against developing two forms of cancer: cancer of the ovaries and cancer of the lining of the uterus

If you want more information about birth-control pills, ask your doctor or pharmacist. They have a more technical leaflet called the Prescribing Information which you may wish to read.

Manufactured for
BERLEX® Laboratories, Montville, NJ 07045
Manufactured in Germany

6073303 3159803 June 2003
Shown in Product Identification Guide, page 309

Berlex Laboratories

1191 SECOND AVE, SUITE 1100
SEATTLE, WA 98101-2120

Direct Inquiries to:
888-BERLEX-4

CAMPATH® ℞
(Alemtuzumab)

WARNING
Campath should be administered under the supervision of a physician experienced in the use of antineoplastic therapy.

- **Hematologic Toxicity:** Serious and, in rare instances fatal, pancytopenia/marrow hypoplasia, autoimmune idiopathic thrombocytopenia, and autoimmune hemolytic anemia have occurred in patients receiving Campath therapy. **Single doses of Campath greater than 30 mg or cumulative doses greater than 90 mg per week should not be administered because these doses are associated with a higher incidence of pancytopenia.**
- **Infusion Reactions:** Campath can result in serious infusion reactions. Patients should be carefully monitored during infusions and Campath discontinued if indicated. (See DOSAGE AND ADMINISTRATION.) **Gradual escalation to the recommended maintenance dose is required at the initiation of therapy and after interruption of therapy for 7 or more days.**
- **Infections, Opportunistic Infections:** Serious, sometimes fatal bacterial, viral, fungal, and protozoan infections have been reported in patients receiving Campath therapy. Prophylaxis directed against *Pneumocystis carinii* pneumonia (PCP) and herpes virus infections has been shown to decrease, but not eliminate, the occurrence of these infections.

Campath® (Alemtuzumab) is a recombinant DNA-derived humanized monoclonal antibody (Campath-1H) that is directed against the 21-28 kD cell surface glycoprotein, CD52. CD52 is expressed on the surface of normal and malignant B and T lymphocytes, NK cells, monocytes, macrophages, and tissues of the male reproductive system. The Campath-1H antibody is an IgG1 kappa with human variable framework and constant regions, and complementarity-determining regions from a murine (rat) monoclonal antibody (Campath-1G). The Campath-1H antibody has an approximate molecular weight of 150 kD.

Campath is produced in mammalian cell (Chinese hamster ovary) suspension culture in a medium containing neomycin. Neomycin is not detectable in the final product. Campath is a sterile, clear, colorless, isotonic pH 6.8–7.4 solution for injection. Each single use ampoule of Campath contains 30 mg Alemtuzumab, 24.0 mg sodium chloride, 3.5 mg dibasic sodium phosphate, 0.6 mg potassium chloride, 0.6 mg monobasic potassium phosphate, 0.3 mg polysorbate 80, and 0.056 mg disodium edetate. No preservatives are added.

CLINICAL PHARMACOLOGY

General: Alemtuzumab binds to CD52, a non-modulating antigen that is present on the surface of essentially all B and T lymphocytes, a majority of monocytes, macrophages, and NK cells, and a subpopulation of granulocytes. Analysis of samples collected from multiple volunteers has not identified CD52 expression on erythrocytes or hematopoetic stem cells. The proposed mechanism of action is antibody-dependent lysis of leukemic cells following cell surface binding. Campath-1H Fab binding was observed in lymphoid tissues and the mononuclear phagocyte system. A proportion of bone marrow cells, including some $CD34^+$ cells, express variable levels of CD52. Significant binding was also observed in the skin and male reproductive tract (epididymis, sperm, seminal vesicle). Mature spermatozoa stain for CD52, but neither spermatogenic cells nor immature spermatozoa show evidence of staining.

Human Pharmacokinetics: The pharmacokinetic profile of Alemtuzumab was studied in a multicenter rising-dose trial in non-Hodgkin's lymphoma (NHL) and chronic lymphocytic leukemia (CLL). Campath was administered once weekly for a maximum of 12 weeks. Following intravenous infusions over a range of doses, the maximum serum concentration (C_{max}) and the area under the curve (AUC) showed relative dose proportionality. The overall average half-life ($t_{½}$) over the dosing interval was about 12 days. The pharmacokinetic profile of Campath administered as a 30 mg intravenous infusion three times per week was evaluated in CLL patients. Peak and trough levels of Campath rose during the first few weeks of treatment, and appeared to approach steady state by approximately week 6, although there was marked inter-patient variability. The rise in serum Campath concentration corresponded with the reduction in malignant lymphocytosis.

CLINICAL STUDIES

The safety and efficacy of Campath were evaluated in a multicenter, open-label, noncomparative study (Study 1) of 93 patients with B-cell chronic lymphocytic leukemia (B-CLL) who had been previously treated with alkylating agents and had failed treatment with fludarabine. Fludarabine failure was defined as lack of an objective partial (PR) or complete (CR) response to at least one fludarabine-containing regimen, progressive disease (PD) while on fludarabine treatment, or relapse within 6 months of the last dose of fludarabine. Patients were gradually escalated to a maintenance dose of Campath 30 mg intravenously three times per week for 4 to 12 weeks. Patients received premedication prior to infusion and anti-*Pneumocystis carinii* and anti-herpes prophylaxis while on treatment and for at least 2 months after the last dose of Campath.

Two supportive, multicenter, open-label, noncomparative studies of Campath enrolled a total of 56 patients with B-CLL (Studies 2 and 3). These patients had been previously treated with fludarabine or other chemotherapies. In Studies 2 and 3, the maintenance dose of Campath was 30 mg three times per week with treatment cycles of 8 and 6 weeks respectively. A slightly different dose escalation scheme was used in these trials. Premedication to ameliorate infusional reactions and anti-*Pneumocystis carinii* and anti-herpes prophylaxis were optional.

Objective tumor response rates and duration of response were determined using the NCI Working Group Response Criteria (1996). A comparison of patient characteristics and the results for each of these studies is summarized in Table 1. Time to event parameters, except for duration of response, are calculated from initiation of Campath therapy. Duration of response is calculated from the onset of the response.

[See table 1 below]

INDICATIONS AND USAGE

Campath is indicated for the treatment of B-cell chronic lymphocytic leukemia (B-CLL) in patients who have been treated with alkylating agents and who have failed fludarabine therapy. Determination of the effectiveness of Campath is based on overall response rates. (See CLINICAL STUDIES.) Comparative, randomized trials demonstrating increased survival or clinical benefits such as improvement in disease-related symptoms have not yet been conducted.

CONTRAINDICATIONS

Campath is contraindicated in patients who have active systemic infections, underlying immunodeficiency (e.g., seropositive for HIV), or known Type I hypersensitivity or anaphylactic reactions to Campath or to any one of its components.

WARNINGS (See BOXED WARNING.)

Infusion-Related Events: Campath has been associated with infusion-related events including hypotension, rigors, fever, shortness of breath, bronchospasm, chills, and/or rash. In order to ameliorate or avoid infusion-related events, patients should be premedicated with an oral antihistamine and acetaminophen prior to dosing and monitored closely for infusion-related adverse events. In addition, Campath should be initiated at a low dose with gradual escalation to the effective dose. Careful monitoring of blood pressure and hypotensive symptoms is recommended especially in patients with ischemic heart disease and in patients on antihypertensive medication. If therapy is interrupted for 7 or more days, Campath should be reinstituted with gradual dose escalation. (See ADVERSE EVENTS and DOSAGE AND ADMINISTRATION.)

Immunosuppression/Opportunistic Infections: Campath induces profound lymphopenia. A variety of opportunistic infections have been reported in patients receiving Campath therapy (see ADVERSE EVENTS, Infections). If a serious infection occurs, Campath therapy should be interrupted and may be reinitiated following the resolution of the infection.

Anti-infective prophylaxis is recommended upon initiation of therapy and for a minimum of 2 months following the last dose of Campath or until $CD4^+$ counts are ≥ 200 cells/μL. The median time to recovery of $CD4^+$ counts to ≥ 200/μL was 2 months, however, full recovery (to baseline) of $CD4^+$ and $CD8^+$ counts may take more than 12 months. (See BOXED WARNING and DOSAGE AND ADMINISTRATION.)

Because of the potential for Graft versus Host Disease (GVHD) in severely lymphopenic patients, irradiation of any blood products administered prior to recovery from lymphopenia is recommended.

Hematologic Toxicity: Severe, prolonged, and in rare instances fatal, myelosuppression has occurred in patients with leukemia and lymphoma receiving Campath. Bone marrow aplasia and hypoplasia were observed in the clinical studies at the recommended dose. The incidence of these complications increased with doses above the recommended dose. In addition, severe and fatal autoimmune anemia and thrombocytopenia were observed in patients with CLL. Campath should be discontinued for severe hematologic toxicity (see Table 3 Dose Modification and Reinitiation of Therapy for Hematologic Toxicity) or in any patient with evidence of autoimmune hematologic toxicity. Following resolution of transient, non-immune myelosuppression, Campath may be reinitiated with caution. (See DOSAGE AND ADMINISTRATION.) There is no information on the safety of resumption of Campath in patients with autoimmune cytopenias or marrow aplasia. (See ADVERSE REACTIONS.)

PRECAUTIONS

Laboratory Monitoring: Complete blood counts (CBC) and platelet counts should be obtained at weekly intervals during Campath therapy and more frequently if worsening anemia, neutropenia, or thrombocytopenia is observed on therapy. $CD4^+$ counts should be assessed after treatment until recovery to ≥ 200 cells/μL. (See WARNINGS and ADVERSE REACTIONS.)

Drug/Laboratory Interactions: No formal drug interaction studies have been performed with Campath. An immune response to Campath may interfere with subsequent diagnostic serum tests that utilize antibodies.

Immunization: Patients who have recently received Campath, should not be immunized with live viral vaccines, due to their immunosuppression. The safety of immunization with live viral vaccines following Campath therapy has not been studied. The ability to generate a primary or anamnestic humoral response to any vaccine following Campath therapy has not been studied.

Table 1: Summary of Patient Population and Outcomes

	Study 1 (N = 93)	Study 2 (N = 32)	Study 3 (N = 24)
Median Age in Years (Range)	66 (32–68)	57 (46–75)	62 (44–77)
Median Number of Prior Regimens (Range)	3 (2–7)	3 (1–10)	3 (1–8)
Prior Therapies:			
Alkylating Agents	100%	100%	92%
Fludarabine	100%	34%	100%
Disease Characteristics:			
Rai Stage III/IV Disease	76%	72%	71%
B-Symptoms	42%	31%	21%
Overall Response Rate	33%	21%	29%
(95% Confidence Interval)	(23%, 43%)	(8%, 33%)	(11%, 47%)
Complete Response	2%	0%	0%
Partial Response	31%	21%	29%
Median Duration of Response (months)	7	7	11
(95% Confidence Interval)	(5, 8)	(5, 23)	(6, 19)
Median Time to Response (months)	2	4	4
(95% Confidence Interval)	(1, 2)	(1, 5)	(2, 4)
Progression-Free Survival (months)	4	5	7
(95% Confidence Interval)	(3, 5)	(3, 7)	(3, 9)

Immunogenicity: Four (1.9%) of 211 patients evaluated for development of an immune response were found to have antibodies to Campath. The data reflect the percentage of patients whose test results were considered positive for antibody to Campath in a kinetic enzyme immunoassay, and are highly dependent on the sensitivity and specificity of the assay. The observed incidence of antibody positivity may be influenced by several additional factors including sample handling, concomitant medications and underlying disease. For these reasons, comparison of the incidence of antibodies to Campath with the incidence of antibodies to other products may be misleading. Patients who develop hypersensitivity to Campath may have allergic or hypersensitivity reactions to other monoclonal antibodies.

Carcinogenesis, Mutagenesis, Impairment of Fertility: No long-term studies in animals have been performed to establish the carcinogenic or mutagenic potential of Campath, or to determine its effects on fertility in males or females. Women of childbearing potential and men of reproductive potential should use effective contraceptive methods during treatment and for a minimum of 6 months following Campath therapy.

Pregnancy Category C: Animal reproduction studies have not been conducted with Campath. It is not known whether Campath can affect reproductive capacity or cause fetal harm when administered to a pregnant woman. However, human IgG is known to cross the placental barrier and therefore Campath may cross the placental barrier and cause fetal B and T lymphocyte depletion. Campath should be given to a pregnant woman only if clearly needed.

Nursing Mothers: Excretion of Campath in human breast milk has not been studied. Because many drugs including human IgG are excreted in human milk, breast-feeding should be discontinued during treatment and for at least 3 months following the last dose of Campath.

Pediatric Use: The safety and effectiveness of Campath in children have not been established.

Geriatric Use: Of the 149 patients with B-CLL enrolled in the three clinical studies, 66 (44%) were 65 and over, while 15 (10%) were 75 and over. Substantial differences in safety and efficacy related to age were not observed; however the size of the database is not sufficient to exclude important differences.

ADVERSE REACTIONS

Because clinical trials are conducted under widely varying conditions, adverse reaction rates observed in the clinical trials of a drug cannot be directly compared to rates in the clinical trials of another drug and may not reflect the rates observed in practice. The adverse reaction information from clinical trials does, however, provide a basis for identifying the adverse events that appear to be related to drug use and for approximating rates.

Safety data, except where indicated, are based on 149 patients with B-CLL enrolled in studies of Campath as a single agent administered at a maintenance dose of 30 mg intravenously three times weekly for 4 to 12 weeks. Table 2 lists adverse events including severe or life threatening (NCI-CTC Grade 3 or 4) adverse events reported in > 5% of the patients. More detailed information and follow-up were available for Study 1 (93 patients), therefore the narrative description of certain events, noted below, is based on this study.

Infusion-Related Adverse Events: Infusion-related adverse events resulted in discontinuation of Campath therapy in 6% of the patients enrolled in Study 1. The most commonly reported infusion-related adverse events on this study included rigors in 89% of patients, drug-related fever in 83%, nausea in 47%, vomiting in 33%, and hypotension in 15%. Other frequently reported infusion-related events include, rash in 30% of patients, fatigue in 22%, urticaria in 22%, dyspnea in 17%, pruritis in 14%, headache in 13%, and diarrhea in 13%. Similar types of adverse events were reported on the supporting studies (see Table 2). Acute infusion-related events were most common during the first week of therapy. Antihistamines, acetaminophen, antiemetics, meperidine, and corticosteroids as well as incremental dose escalation were used to prevent or ameliorate infusion-related events. (See WARNINGS and DOSAGE AND ADMINISTRATION.)

Infections: On Study 1, all patients were required to receive anti-herpes and anti-PCP prophylaxis (see DOSAGE AND ADMINISTRATION) and were followed for infections for 6 months. Forty (43%) of 93 patients experienced 59 infections (one or more infections per patient) related to Campath during treatment or within 6 months of the last dose. Of these, 34 (37%) patients experienced 42 infections that were of Grade 3 or 4 severity; 11 (18%) were fatal. Fifty-five percent of the Grade 3 or 4 infections occurred during treatment or within 30 days of last dose. In addition one or more episodes of febrile neutropenia (ANC ≤ 500/μL) were reported in 10% of patients.

The following types of infections were reported in Study 1: Grade 3 or 4 sepsis in 12% of patients with one fatality, Grade 3 or 4 pneumonia in 15% with five fatalities, and opportunistic infections in 17% with four fatalities. Candida infections were reported in 5% of patients; CMV infections in 8% (4% of Grade 3 or 4 severity); Aspergillosis in 2% with fatal Aspergillosis in 1%; fatal Mucormycosis in 2%; fatal Cryptococcal pneumonia in 1%; *Listeria monocytogenes* meningitis in 1%; disseminated *Herpes zoster* in 1%; Grade 3 *Herpes simplex* in 2%; and Torulopsis pneumonia in 1%. PCP pneumonia occurred in one (1%) patient who discontinued PCP prophylaxis.

On Studies 2 and 3 in which anti-herpes and anti-PCP prophylaxis was optional, 37 (66%) patients had 47 infections while or after receiving Campath therapy. In addition to the opportunistic infections reported above, the following types of related events were observed on these studies: interstitial pneumonitis of unknown etiology and progressive multifocal leukoencephalopathy.

Hematologic Adverse Events:

Pancytopenia/Marrow Hypoplasia: Campath therapy was permanently discontinued in six (6%) patients due to pancytopenia/marrow hypoplasia. Two (2%) cases of pancytopenia/marrow hypoplasia were fatal.

Anemia: Forty-four (47%) patients had one or more episodes of new onset NCI-CTC Grade 3 or 4 anemia. Sixty-two (67%) patients required RBC transfusions. In addition, erythropoietin use was reported in nineteen (20%) patients. Autoimmune hemolytic anemia secondary to Campath therapy was reported in 1% of patients. Positive Coombs test without hemolysis was reported in 2% (See BOXED WARNING.)

Neutropenia: Sixty-five (70%) patients had one or more episodes of NCI-CTC Grade 3 or 4 neutropenia. Median duration of Grade 3 or 4 neutropenia was 28 days (range: 2–165 days). (See Infections.)

Thrombocytopenia: Forty-eight (52%) patients had one or more episodes of new onset Grade 3 or 4 thrombocytopenia. Median duration of thrombocytopenia was 21 days (range: 2–165 days). Thirty-five (38%) patients required platelet transfusions for management of thrombocytopenia. Autoimmune thrombocytopenia was reported in 2% of patients with one fatal case of Campath-related autoimmune thrombocytopenia. (See BOXED WARNING.)

Lymphopenia: The median $CD4^+$ count at 4 weeks after initiation of Campath therapy was 2 (two)/μL, at 2 months after discontinuation of Campath therapy, 207/μL, and 6 months after discontinuation, 470/μL. The pattern of change in median $CD8^+$ lymphocyte counts was similar to that of $CD4^+$ cells. In some patients treated with Campath, $CD4^+$ and $CD8^+$ lymphocyte counts had not returned to baseline levels at longer than 1 year post therapy.

Table 2: Adverse Events in >5% of the B-CLL Study Population During Treatment or Within 30 Days (N = 149)

Adverse Event:	B-CLL STUDIES (N = 149) ANY Grade (%)	Grade 3 or 4 (%)
Body As A Whole		
Rigors	86	16
Fever	85	19
Fatigue	34	5
Pain, Skeletal Pain	24	2
Anorexia	20	3
Asthenia	13	4
Edema, Peripheral Edema	13	1
Back Pain	10	3
Chest Pain	10	1
Malaise	9	1
Temperature Change Sensation	5	—
Cardiovascular Disorders, General		
Hypotension	32	5
Hypertension	11	2
Heart Rate & Rhythm Disorders		
Tachycardia, SVT	11	3
Central & Peripheral Nervous System Disorders		
Headache	24	1
Dysthesias	15	—
Dizziness	12	1
Tremor	7	—
Gastrointestinal Disorders		
Nausea	54	2
Vomiting	41	4
Diarrhea	22	1
Stomatitis, Ulcerative Stomatitis, Mucositis	14	1
Abdominal Pain	11	2
Dyspepsia	10	—
Constipation	9	1
Hematologic Disorders		
WBC Disorders: Neutropenia	85	64
RBC Disorders: Anemia	80	38
Pancytopenia	5	3
Platelet, Bleeding & Clotting Disorders		
Thrombocytopenia	72	50
Purpura	8	—
Epistaxis	7	1
Musculoskeletal Disorders		
Myalgias	11	—
Psychiatric Disorders		
Insomnia	10	—
Depression	7	1
Somnolence	5	1
Resistance Mechanism Disorders		
Sepsis	15	10
Herpes Simplex	11	1
Moniliasis	8	1
Infection (other viral or unidentified)	7	1
Respiratory System Disorders		
Dyspnea	26	9
Cough	25	2
Bronchitis, Pneumonitis	21	13
Pneumonia	16	10
Pharyngitis	12	—
Bronchospasm	9	2
Rhinitis	7	—
Skin & Appendage Disorders		
Rash, Maculopapular Rash, Erythematous Rash	40	3
Urticaria	30	5
Pruritus	24	1
Sweating increased	19	1

Serious adverse events:

The following serious adverse events, defined as events which result in death, requiring or prolonging hospitalization, requiring medical intervention to prevent hospitalization, or malignancy, were reported in at least one patient treated on studies where Campath was used as a single agent (and are not reported in Table 2). These studies were conducted in patients with lymphocytic leukemia and lymphoma (N = 745) and in patients with non-malignant diseases (N = 152) such as rheumatoid arthritis, solid organ transplant, or multiple sclerosis.

Body As A Whole: allergic reactions, anaphylactoid reaction, ascites, hypovolemia, influenza-like syndrome, mouth edema, neutropenic fever, syncope

Cardiovascular Disorders: cardiac failure, cyanosis, atrial fibrillation, cardiac arrest, ventricular arrhythmia, ventricular tachycardia, angina pectoris, coronary artery disorder, myocardial infarction, pericarditis

Central and Peripheral Nervous System Disorders: abnormal gait, aphasia, coma, grand mal convulsions, paralysis, meningitis

Endocrine Disorders: hyperthyroidism

Continued on next page

Information on Berlex products (appearing here) is based on the most current information available at the time of publication closing. Further information for these and other Berlex products can be obtained from Medical & Product Services at Berlex, Inc. by calling 1-888-BERLEX-4.

Campath—Cont.

Gastrointestinal System Disorders: duodenal ulcer, esophagitis, gingivitis, gastroenteritis, GI hemorrhage, hematemesis, hemorrhoids, intestinal obstruction, intestinal perforation, melena, paralytic ileus, peptic ulcer, pseudomembranous colitis, colitis, pancreatitis, peritonitis, hyperbilirubinemia, hepatic failure, hepatocellular damage, hypoalbuminemia, biliary pain
Hearing and Vestibular Disorders: decreased hearing
Metabolic and Nutritional Disorders: acidosis, aggravated diabetes mellitus, dehydration, fluid overload, hyperglycemia, hyperkalemia, hypokalemia, hypoglycemia, hyponatremia, increased alkaline phosphatase, respiratory alkalosis
Musculoskeletal System Disorders: arthritis or worsening arthritis, arthropathy, bone fracture, myositis, muscle atrophy, muscle weakness, osteomyelitis, polymyositis
Neoplasms: malignant lymphoma, malignant testicular neoplasm, prostatic cancer, plasma cell dyscrasia, secondary leukemia squamous cell carcinoma, transformation to aggressive lymphoma, transformation to prolymphocytic leukemia
Platelet, Bleeding, and Clotting Disorders: coagulation disorder, disseminated intravascular coagulation, hematoma, pulmonary embolism, thrombocythemia
Psychiatric Disorders: confusion, hallucinations, nervousness, abnormal thinking, apathy
White Cell and RES Disorders: agranulocytosis, aplasia, decreased haptoglobin, lymphadenopathy, marrow depression
Red Blood Cell Disorders: hemolysis, hemolytic anemia, splenic infarction, splenomegaly
Reproductive System Disorders: cervical dysplasia
Resistance Mechanism Disorders: abscess, bacterial infection, *Herpes zoster* infection, *Pneumocystis carinii* infection, otitis media, Tuberculosis infection, viral infection
Respiratory System Disorders: asthma, bronchitis, chronic obstructive pulmonary disease, hemoptysis, hypoxia, pleural effusion pleurisy, pneumothorax, pulmonary edema, pulmonary fibrosis, pulmonary infiltration, respiratory depression, respiratory insufficiency, sinusitis, stridor, throat tightness
Skin and Appendages Disorders: angioedema, bullous eruption, cellulitis, purpuric rash
Special Senses Disorders: taste loss
Urinary System Disorders: abnormal renal function, acute renal failure, anuria, facial edema, hematuria, toxic nephropathy ureteric obstruction, urinary retention, urinary tract infection
Vascular (Extracardiac) Disorders: cerebral hemorrhage, cerebrovascular disorder, deep vein thrombosis, increased capillary fragility, intracranial hemorrhage, phlebitis, subarachnoid hemorrhage, thrombophlebitis
Vision Disorders: endophthalmitis

OVERDOSAGE

Initial doses of Campath of greater than 3 mg are not well-tolerated. One patient who received 80 mg as an initial dose by IV infusion experienced acute bronchospasm, cough, and shortness of breath, followed by anuria and death. A review of the case suggested that tumor lysis syndrome may have played a role.
Single doses of Campath greater than 30 mg or a cumulative weekly dose greater than 90 mg should not be administered as higher doses have been associated with a higher incidence of pancytopenia. (See BOXED WARNING and DOSAGE AND ADMINISTRATION.)
There is no known specific antidote for Campath overdosage. Treatment consists of drug discontinuation and supportive therapy.

DOSAGE AND ADMINISTRATION

Campath should be administered under the supervision of a physician experienced in the use of antineoplastic therapy.
Dosing Schedule and Administration: Campath therapy should be initiated at a dose of 3 mg administered as a 2 hour IV infusion daily. (See ADVERSE EVENTS.) When the Campath 3 mg daily dose is tolerated (e.g., infusion-related toxicities are ≤ Grade 2), the daily dose should be escalated to 10 mg and continued until tolerated. When the 10 mg dose is tolerated, the maintenance dose of Campath 30 mg may be initiated. The maintenance dose of Campath is 30 mg/day administered three times per week on alternate days (i.e., Monday, Wednesday, and Friday) for up to 12 weeks. In most patients, escalation to 30 mg can be accomplished in 3–7 days. **Dose escalation to the recommended maintenance dose of 30 mg administered three times per week is required. Single doses of Campath greater than 30 mg or cumulative weekly doses of greater than 90 mg should not be administered since higher doses are associated with an increased incidence of pancytopenia.** (See BOXED WARNING.) Campath should be administered intravenously only. The infusion should be administered over a 2 hour period. **DO NOT ADMINISTER AS AN INTRAVENOUS PUSH OR BOLUS.**
Recommended Concomitant Medications:
Premedication should be given prior to the first dose, at dose escalations, and as clinically indicated. The premedicaton used in clinical studies was diphenhydramine 50 mg and acetaminophen 650 mg administered 30 minutes prior to Campath infusion. In cases where severe infusion-related events occur, treatment with hydrocortisone 200 mg was used in decreasing the infusion-related events.
Patients should receive anti-infective prophylaxis to minimize the risks of serious opportunistic infections. (See BOXED WARNING.) The anti-infective regimen used on Study 1 consisted of trimethoprim/sulfamethoxazole DS twice daily (BID) three times per week and famciclovir or equivalent 250 mg twice a day (BID) upon initiation of Campath therapy. Prophylaxis should be continued for 2 months after completion of Campath therapy or until the $CD4^+$ count is ≥ 200 cells/µL, whichever occurs later.
Dose Modification and Reinitiation of Therapy: Campath therapy should be discontinued during serious infection, serious hematologic toxicity, or other serious toxicity until the event resolves. (See WARNINGS.) Campath therapy should be permanently discontinued if evidence of autoimmune anemia or thrombocytopenia appears. Table 3 includes recommendations for dose modification for severe neutropenia or thrombocytopenia.
[See table 3 below]
Preparation for Administration:
Parenteral drug products should be inspected for visible particulate matter and discoloration prior to administration. If particulate matter is present or the solution is discolored, the vial should not be used. **DO NOT SHAKE AMPOULE PRIOR TO USE.** As with all parenteral drug products, aseptic technique should be used during the preparation and administration of Campath. Withdraw the necessary amount of Campath from the ampoule into a syringe. Filter with a sterile, low-protein binding, non-fiber releasing 5 µm filter prior to dilution.
Inject into 100 mL sterile 0.9% Sodium Chloride USP or 5% Dextrose in Water USP. **Gently invert the bag to mix the solution.** Discard syringe and any unused drug product.
Campath contains no antimicrobial preservative. Campath should be used within 8 hours after dilution. Campath solutions may be stored at room temperature (15–30°C) or refrigerated. Campath solutions should be protected from light.
Incompatibilities:
No incompatibilities between Campath and polyvinylchloride (PVC) bags, PVC or polyethylene-lined PVC administration sets, or low-protein binding filters have been observed. No data are available concerning the incompatibility of Campath with other drug substances. Other drug substances should not be added or simultaneously infused through the same intravenous line.

HOW SUPPLIED

Campath (Alemtuzumab) is supplied in single-use clear glass ampoules containing 30 mg of Alemtuzumab in 3 mL of solution. Each box contains three Campath ampoules (NDC 50419-355-10).
Campath should be stored at 2–8°C (36–46°F). Do not freeze. DISCARD IF AMPOULE HAS BEEN FROZEN. Protect from direct sunlight.
Rx only.

Table 3: Dose Modification and Reinitiation of Therapy for Hematologic Toxicity

Hematologic Toxicity	Dose Modification and Reinitiation of Therapy
For first occurrence of ANC <250/µL and/or platelet count ≤25,000/µL	Withhold Campath therapy. When ANC ≥500/µL and platelet count ≥50,000/µL, resume Campath therapy at same dose. If delay between dosing is ≥7 days, initiate therapy at Campath 3 mg and escalate to 10 mg and then to 30 mg as tolerated.
For second occurrence of ANC <250/µL and/or platelet count ≤25,000/µL	Withhold Campath therapy. When ANC ≥500/µL and platelet count ≥50,000/µL, resume Campath therapy at **10 mg**. If delay between dosing is ≥7 days, initiate therapy at Campath 3 mg and escalate to **10 mg only**.
For third occurrence of ANC <250/µL and/or platelet count ≤25,000/µL	Discontinue Campath therapy permanently.
For a decrease of ANC and/or platelet count to ≤50% of the baseline value in patients initiating therapy with a baseline ANC ≤500/µL and/or a baseline platelet count ≤25,000/µL	Withhold Campath therapy. When ANC and/or platelet count return to baseline value(s), resume Campath therapy. If the delay between dosing ≥7 days, initiate therapy at Campath 3 mg and escalate to 10 mg and then to 30 mg as tolerated.

U.S. Patents: 5,545,403; 5,545,405; 5,654,403; 5,846,534
Other patents pending
Manufactured by: ILEX Pharmaceuticals, LP., San Antonio, TX 78229
Distributed by:
BERLEX® Laboratories, Richmond, CA 94804
Issued: January 2002
42946/US/1

FLUDARA® ℞

[*flū 'dər-ă*]
(fludarabine phosphate)
FOR INJECTION
FOR INTRAVENOUS USE ONLY
Rx Only

WARNING: FLUDARA FOR INJECTION should be administered under the supervision of a qualified physician experienced in the use of antineoplastic therapy. FLUDARA FOR INJECTION can severely suppress bone marrow function. When used at high doses in dose-ranging studies in patients with acute leukemia, FLUDARA FOR INJECTION was associated with severe neurologic effects, including blindness, coma, and death. This severe central nervous system toxicity occurred in 36% of patients treated with doses approximately four times greater (96 mg/m²/day for 5-7 days) than the recommended dose. Similar severe central nervous system toxicity has been reported rarely (≤0.2%) reported in patients treated at doses in the range of the dose recommended for chronic lymphocytic leukemia.
Instances of life-threatening and sometimes fatal autoimmune hemolytic anemia have been reported to occur after one or more cycles of treatment with FLUDARA FOR INJECTION. Patients undergoing treatment with FLUDARA FOR INJECTION should be evaluated and closely monitored for hemolysis.
In a clinical investigation using FLUDARA FOR INJECTION in combination with pentostatin (deoxycoformycin) for the treatment of refractory chronic lymphocytic leukemia (CLL), there was an unacceptably high incidence of fatal pulmonary toxicity. Therefore, the use of FLUDARA FOR INJECTION in combination with pentostatin is not recommended.

DESCRIPTION

FLUDARA FOR INJECTION contains fludarabine phosphate, a fluorinated nucleotide analog of the antiviral agent vidarabine, 9-β-D-arabinofuranosyladenine (ara-A) that is relatively resistant to deamination by adenosine deaminase. Each vial of sterile lyophilized solid cake contains 50 mg of the active ingredient fludarabine phosphate, 50 mg of mannitol, and sodium hydroxide to adjust pH to 7.7. The pH range for the final product is 7.2-8.2. Reconstitution with 2 mL of Sterile Water for Injection USP results in a solution containing 25 mg/mL of fludarabine phosphate intended for intravenous administration.
The chemical name for fludarabine phosphate is 9H-Purin-6-amine, 2-fluoro-9-(5-O-phosphono-β-D-arabinofuranosyl) (2-fluoro-ara-AMP).
The molecular formula of fludarabine phosphate is $C_{10}H_{13}FN_5O_7P$ (MW 365.2) and the structure is:

NH₂ N N F N N O HO—P—O—CH₂ O OH HO OH

CLINICAL PHARMACOLOGY

Fludarabine phosphate is rapidly dephosphorylated to 2-fluoro-ara-A and then phosphorylated intracellularly by deoxycytidine kinase to the active triphosphate, 2-fluoro-ara-ATP. This metabolite appears to act by inhibiting DNA polymerase alpha, ribonucleotide reductase and DNA primase, thus inhibiting DNA synthesis. The mechanism of action of this antimetabolite is not completely characterized and may be multi-faceted.
Phase I studies in humans have demonstrated that fludarabine phosphate is rapidly converted to the active metabolite, 2-fluoro-ara-A, within minutes after intravenous infusion. Consequently, clinical pharmacology studies have focused on 2-fluoro-ara-A pharmacokinetics. After the five daily doses of 25 mg 2-fluoro-ara-AMP/m² to cancer patients infused over 30 minutes, 2-fluoro-ara-A concentrations show a moderate accumulation. During a 5-day treatment schedule, 2-fluoro-ara-A plasma trough levels increased by a factor of about 2. The terminal half-life of 2-fluoro-ara-A was estimated as approximately 20 hours. *In vitro*, plasma protein binding of fludarabine ranged between 19% and 29%. A correlation was noted between the degree of absolute granulocyte count nadir and increased area under the concentration × time curve (AUC).
Special Populations
Pediatric Patients
Limited pharmacokinetic data for FLUDARA FOR INJECTION are available from a published study of chil-

dren (ages 1-21 years) with refractory acute leukemias or solid tumors (Children's Cancer Group Study 097[1]). When FLUDARA FOR INJECTION was administered as a loading dose over 10 minutes immediately followed by a 5-day continuous infusion, steady-state conditions were reached early.

Patients with Renal Impairment

The total body clearance of the principal metabolite 2-fluoro-ara-A correlated with the creatinine clearance, indicating the importance of the renal excretion pathway for the elimination of the drug. Renal clearance represents approximately 40% of the total body clearance. Patients with moderate renal impairment (17-41 mL/min/m^2) receiving 20% reduced Fludara dose had a similar exposure (AUC; 21 versus 20 nM•h/mL) compared to patients with normal renal function receiving the recommended dose. The mean total body clearance was 172 mL/min for normal and 124 mL/min for patients with moderately impaired renal function.

Clinical Studies

Two single-arm open-label studies of FLUDARA FOR INJECTION have been conducted in adult patients with CLL refractory to at least one prior standard alkylating-agent containing regimen. In a study conducted by M.D. Anderson Cancer Center (MDAH), 48 patients were treated with a dose of 22-40 mg/m^2 daily for 5 days every 28 days. Another study conducted by the Southwest Oncology Group (SWOG) involved 31 patients treated with a dose of 15-25 mg/m^2 daily for 5 days every 28 days. The overall objective response rates were 48% and 32% in the MDAH and SWOG studies, respectively. The complete response rate in both studies was 13%; the partial response rate was 35% in the MDAH study and 19% in the SWOG study. These response rates were obtained using standardized response criteria developed by the National Cancer Institute CLL Working Group[3] and were achieved in heavily pre-treated patients. The ability of FLUDARA FOR INJECTION to induce a significant rate of response in refractory patients suggests minimal cross-resistance with commonly used anti-CLL agents.

The median time to response in the MDAH and SWOG studies was 7 weeks (range of 1 to 68 weeks) and 21 weeks (range of 1 to 53 weeks) respectively. The median duration of disease control was 91 weeks (MDAH) and 65 weeks (SWOG). The median survival of all refractory CLL patients treated with FLUDARA FOR INJECTION was 43 weeks and 52 weeks in the MDAH and SWOG studies, respectively.

Rai stage improved to Stage II or better in 7 of 12 MDAH responders (58%) and in 5 of 7 SWOG responders (71%) who were Stage III or IV at baseline. In the combined studies, mean hemoglobin concentration improved from 9.0 g/dL at baseline to 11.8 g/dL at the time of response in a subgroup of anemic patients. Similarly, average platelet count improved from 63,500/mm^3 to 103,300/mm^3 at the time of response in a subgroup of patients who were thrombocytopenic at baseline.

INDICATIONS AND USAGE

FLUDARA FOR INJECTION is indicated for the treatment of adult patients with B-cell chronic lymphocytic leukemia (CLL) who have not responded to or whose disease has progressed during treatment with at least one standard alkylating-agent containing regimen. The safety and effectiveness of FLUDARA FOR INJECTION in previously untreated or non-refractory patients with CLL have not been established.

CONTRAINDICATIONS

FLUDARA FOR INJECTION is contraindicated in those patients who are hypersensitive to this drug or its components.

WARNINGS

(See boxed warning)

There are clear dose-dependent toxic effects seen with FLUDARA FOR INJECTION. Dose levels approximately 4 times greater (96 mg/m^2/day for 5 to 7 days) than that recommended for CLL (25 mg/m^2/day for 5 days) were associated with a syndrome characterized by delayed blindness, coma and death. Symptoms appeared from 21 to 60 days following the last dose. Thirteen of 36 patients (36%) who received FLUDARA FOR INJECTION at high doses (96 mg/m^2/day for 5 to 7 days) developed this severe neurotoxicity. This syndrome has been reported rarely in patients treated with doses in the range of the recommended CLL dose of 25 mg/m^2/day for 5 days every 28 days. The effect of chronic administration of FLUDARA FOR INJECTION on the central nervous system is unknown; however, patients have received the recommended dose for up to 15 courses of therapy.

Severe bone marrow suppression, notably anemia, thrombocytopenia and neutropenia, has been reported in patients treated with FLUDARA FOR INJECTION. In a Phase I study in adult solid tumor patients, the median time to nadir counts was 13 days (range, 3-25 days) for granulocytes and 16 days (range, 2-32) for platelets. Most patients had hematologic impairment at baseline either as a result of disease or as a result of prior myelosuppressive therapy. Cumulative myelosuppression may be seen. While chemotherapy-induced myelosuppression is often reversible, administration of FLUDARA FOR INJECTION requires careful hematologic monitoring.

Several instances of trilineage bone marrow hypoplasia or aplasia resulting in pancytopenia, sometimes resulting in death, have been reported in adult patients. The duration of clinically significant cytopenia in the reported cases has ranged from approximately 2 months to approximately 1 year. These episodes have occurred both in previously treated or untreated patients.

Instances of life-threatening and sometimes fatal autoimmune hemolytic anemia have been reported to occur after one or more cycles of treatment with FLUDARA FOR INJECTION in patients with or without a previous history of autoimmune hemolytic anemia or a positive Coombs' test and who may or may not be in remission from their disease. Steroids may or may not be effective in controlling these hemolytic episodes. The majority of patients rechallenged with FLUDARA FOR INJECTION developed a recurrence in the hemolytic process. The mechanism(s) which predispose patients to the development of this complication has not been identified. Patients undergoing treatment with FLUDARA FOR INJECTION should be evaluated and closely monitored for hemolysis.

Transfusion-associated graft-versus-host disease has been observed rarely after transfusion of non-irradiated blood in FLUDARA FOR INJECTION treated patients. Consideration should, therefore, be given to the use of irradiated blood products in those patients requiring transfusions while undergoing treatment with FLUDARA FOR INJECTION.

In a clinical investigation using FLUDARA FOR INJECTION in combination with pentostatin (deoxycoformycin) for the treatment of refractory chronic lymphocytic leukemia (CLL) in adults, there was an unacceptably high incidence of fatal pulmonary toxicity. Therefore, the use of FLUDARA FOR INJECTION in combination with pentostatin is not recommended.

Of the 133 adult CLL patients in the two trials, there were 29 fatalities during study. Approximately 50% of the fatalities were due to infection and 25% due to progressive disease.

Pregnancy Category D: FLUDARA FOR INJECTION may cause fetal harm when administered to a pregnant woman. Fludarabine phosphate was teratogenic in rats and in rabbits. Fludarabine phosphate was administered intravenously at doses of 0, 1, 10 or 30 mg/kg/day to pregnant rats on days 6 to 15 of gestation. At 10 and 30 mg/kg/day in rats, there was an increased incidence of various skeletal malformations. Fludarabine phosphate was administered intravenously at doses of 0, 1, 5 or 8 mg/kg/day to pregnant rabbits on days 6 to 15 of gestation. Dose-related teratogenic effects manifested by external deformities and skeletal malformations were observed in the rabbits at 5 and 8 mg/kg/day. Drug-related deaths or toxic effects on maternal and fetal weights were not observed. There are no adequate and well-controlled studies in pregnant women.

If FLUDARA FOR INJECTION is used during pregnancy, or if the patient becomes pregnant while taking this drug, the patient should be apprised of the potential hazard to the fetus. Women of childbearing potential should be advised to avoid becoming pregnant.

PRECAUTIONS

General: FLUDARA FOR INJECTION is a potent antineoplastic agent with potentially significant toxic side effects. Patients undergoing therapy should be closely observed for signs of hematologic and nonhematologic toxicity. Periodic assessment of peripheral blood counts is recommended to detect the development of anemia, neutropenia and thrombocytopenia.

Tumor lysis syndrome associated with FLUDARA FOR INJECTION treatment has been reported in CLL patients with large tumor burdens. Since FLUDARA FOR INJECTION can induce a response as early as the first week of treatment, precautions should be taken in those patients at risk of developing this complication.

There are inadequate data on dosing of patients with renal insufficiency. FLUDARA FOR INJECTION must be administered cautiously in patients with renal insufficiency. The total body clearance of 2-fluoro-ara-A has been shown to be directly correlated with creatinine clearance. Patients with moderate impairment of renal function (creatinine clearance 30-70 mL/min/1.73 m^2) should have their Fludara dose reduced by 20% and be monitored closely. Fludara is not recommended for patients with severely impaired renal function (creatinine clearance less than 30 mL/min/1.73 m^2).

Laboratory Tests: During treatment, the patient's hematologic profile (particularly neutrophils and platelets) should be monitored regularly to determine the degree of hematopoietic suppression.

Drug Interactions: The use of FLUDARA FOR INJECTION in combination with pentostatin is not recommended due to the risk of severe pulmonary toxicity (see WARNINGS section).

Carcinogenesis: No animal carcinogenicity studies with FLUDARA FOR INJECTION have been conducted.

Mutagenesis: Fludarabine phosphate was not mutagenic to bacteria (Ames test) or mammalian cells (HGRPT assay in Chinese hamster ovary cells) either in the presence or absence of metabolic activation. Fludarabine phosphate was clastogenic *in vitro* to Chinese hamster ovary cells (chromosome aberrations in the presence of metabolic activation) and induced sister chromatid exchanges both with and without metabolic activation. In addition, fludarabine phosphate was clastogenic *in vivo* (mouse micronucleus assay) but was not mutagenic to germ cells (dominant lethal test in male mice).

Impairment of Fertility: Studies in mice, rats and dogs have demonstrated dose-related adverse effects on the male reproductive system. Observations consisted of a decrease in mean testicular weights in mice and rats with a trend toward decreased testicular weights in dogs and degeneration and necrosis of spermatogenic epithelium of the testes in mice, rats and dogs. The possible adverse effects on fertility in humans have not been adequately evaluated.

Pregnancy: Pregnancy Category D: (See WARNINGS section).

Nursing Mothers: It is not known whether this drug is excreted in human milk. Because many drugs are excreted in human milk and because of the potential for serious adverse reactions in nursing infants from FLUDARA FOR INJECTION, a decision should be made to discontinue nursing or discontinue the drug, taking into account the importance of the drug for the mother.

Pediatric Use: Data submitted to the FDA was insufficient to establish efficacy in any childhood malignancy. Fludarabine was evaluated in 62 pediatric patients (median age 10, range 1-21) with refractory acute leukemia (45 patients) or solid tumors (17 patients). The fludarabine regimen tested for pediatric acute lymphocytic leukemia (ALL) patients was a loading bolus of 10.5 mg/m^2/day followed by a continuous infusion of 30.5 mg/m^2/day for 5 days. In 12 pediatric patients with solid tumors, dose-limiting myelosuppression was observed with a loading dose of 8 mg/m^2/day followed by a continuous infusion of 23.5 mg/m^2/day for 5 days. The maximum tolerated dose was a loading dose of 7 mg/m^2/day followed by a continuous infusion of 20 mg/m^2/day for 5 days. Treatment toxicity included bone marrow suppression. Platelet counts appeared to be more sensitive to the effects of fludarabine than hemoglobin and white blood cell counts. Other adverse events included fever, chills, asthenia, rash, nausea, vomiting, diarrhea, and infection. There were no reported occurrences of peripheral neuropathy or pulmonary hypersensitivity reaction.

ADVERSE REACTIONS

The most common adverse events include myelosuppression (neutropenia, thrombocytopenia and anemia), fever and chills, infection, and nausea and vomiting. Other commonly reported events include malaise, fatigue, anorexia, and weakness. Serious opportunistic infections have occurred in CLL patients treated with FLUDARA FOR INJECTION. The most frequently reported adverse events and those reactions which are more clearly related to the drug are arranged below according to body system.

Hematopoietic Systems: Hematologic events (neutropenia, thrombocytopenia, and/or anemia) were reported in the majority of CLL patients treated with FLUDARA FOR INJECTION. During FLUDARA FOR INJECTION treatment of 133 patients with CLL, the absolute neutrophil count decreased to less than 500/mm^3 in 59% of patients, hemoglobin decreased from pretreatment values by at least 2 grams percent in 60%, and platelet count decreased from pretreatment values by at least 50% in 55%. Myelosuppression may be severe, cumulative, and may affect multiple cell lines. Bone marrow fibrosis occurred in one CLL patient treated with FLUDARA FOR INJECTION.

Several instances of trilineage bone marrow hypoplasia or aplasia resulting in pancytopenia, sometimes resulting in death, have been reported in postmarketing surveillance. The duration of clinically significant cytopenia in the reported cases has ranged from approximately 2 months to approximately 1 year. These episodes have occurred both in previously treated or untreated patients.

Life-threatening and sometimes fatal autoimmune hemolytic anemia have been reported to occur in patients receiving FLUDARA FOR INJECTION (see WARNINGS section). The majority of patients rechallenged with FLUDARA FOR INJECTION developed a recurrence in the hemolytic process.

Metabolic: Tumor lysis syndrome has been reported in CLL patients treated with FLUDARA FOR INJECTION. This complication may include hyperuricemia, hyperphosphatemia, hypocalcemia, metabolic acidosis, hyperkalemia, hematuria, urate crystalluria, and renal failure. The onset of this syndrome may be heralded by flank pain and hematuria.

Nervous System: (See WARNINGS section) Objective weakness, agitation, confusion, visual disturbances, and coma have occurred in CLL patients treated with FLUDARA FOR INJECTION at the recommended dose. Peripheral neuropathy has been observed in patients treated with FLUDARA FOR INJECTION and one case of wrist-drop was reported.

Pulmonary System: Pneumonia, a frequent manifestation of infection in CLL patients, occurred in 16%, and 22% of those treated with FLUDARA FOR INJECTION in the MDAH and SWOG studies, respectively. Pulmonary hypersensitivity reactions to FLUDARA FOR INJECTION characterized by dyspnea, cough and interstitial pulmonary infiltrate have been observed.

In post-marketing experience, cases of severe pulmonary toxicity have been observed with Fludara use which re-

Continued on next page

Information on Berlex products (appearing here) is based on the most current information available at the time of publication closing. Further information for these and other Berlex products can be obtained from Medical & Product Services at Berlex, Inc. by calling 1-888-BERLEX-4.

Fludara—Cont.

sulted in ARDS, respiratory distress, pulmonary hemorrhage, pulmonary fibrosis, and respiratory failure. After an infectious origin has been excluded, some patients experienced symptom improvement with corticosteroids.

Gastrointestinal System: Gastrointestinal disturbances such as nausea and vomiting, anorexia, diarrhea, stomatitis, and gastrointestinal bleeding have been reported in patients treated with FLUDARA FOR INJECTION.

Cardiovascular: Edema has been frequently reported. One patient developed a pericardial effusion possibly related to treatment with FLUDARA FOR INJECTION. No other severe cardiovascular events were considered to be drug related.

Genitourinary System: Rare cases of hemorrhagic cystitis have been reported in patients treated with FLUDARA FOR INJECTION.

Skin: Skin toxicity, consisting primarily of skin rashes, has been reported in patients treated with FLUDARA FOR INJECTION.

Data in the following table are derived from the 133 patients with CLL who received FLUDARA FOR INJECTION in the MDAH and SWOG studies.

PERCENT OF CLL PATIENTS REPORTING NON-HEMATOLOGIC ADVERSE EVENTS

ADVERSE EVENTS	MDAH (N=101)	SWOG (N=32)
ANY ADVERSE EVENT	88%	91%
BODY AS A WHOLE	72	84
FEVER	60	69
CHILLS	11	19
FATIGUE	10	38
INFECTION	33	44
PAIN	20	22
MALAISE	8	6
DIAPHORESIS	1	13
ALOPECIA	0	3
ANAPHYLAXIS	1	0
HEMORRHAGE	1	0
HYPERGLYCEMIA	1	6
DEHYDRATION	1	0
NEUROLOGICAL	21	69
WEAKNESS	9	65
PARESTHESIA	4	12
HEADACHE	3	0
VISUAL DISTURBANCE	3	15
HEARING LOSS	2	6
SLEEP DISORDER	1	3
DEPRESSION	1	0
CEREBELLAR SYNDROME	1	0
IMPAIRED MENTATION	1	0
PULMONARY	35	69
COUGH	10	44
PNEUMONIA	16	22
DYSPNEA	9	22
SINUSITIS	5	0
PHARYNGITIS	0	9
UPPER RESPIRATORY INFECTION	2	16
ALLERGIC PNEUMONITIS	0	6
EPISTAXIS	1	0
HEMOPTYSIS	1	6
BRONCHITIS	1	0
HYPOXIA	1	0
GASTROINTESTINAL	46	63
NAUSEA/VOMITING	36	31
DIARRHEA	15	13
ANOREXIA	7	34
STOMATITIS	9	0
GI BLEEDING	3	13
ESOPHAGITIS	3	0
MUCOSITIS	2	0
LIVER FAILURE	1	0
ABNORMAL LIVER FUNCTION TEST	1	3
CHOLELITHIASIS	0	3
CONSTIPATION	1	3
DYSPHAGIA	1	0
CUTANEOUS	17	18
RASH	15	15
PRURITUS	1	3
SEBORRHEA	1	0
GENITOURINARY	12	22
DYSURIA	4	3
URINARY INFECTION	2	15
HEMATURIA	2	3
RENAL FAILURE	1	0
ABNORMAL RENAL FUNCTION TEST	1	0
PROTEINURIA	1	0
HESITANCY	0	3
CARDIOVASCULAR	12	38
EDEMA	8	19
ANGINA	0	6
CONGESTIVE HEART FAILURE	0	3
ARRHYTHMIA	0	3
SUPRAVENTRICULAR TACHYCARDIA	0	3
MYOCARDIAL INFARCTION	0	3
DEEP VENOUS THROMBOSIS	1	3
PHLEBITIS	1	3
TRANSIENT ISCHEMIC ATTACK	1	0
ANEURYSM	1	0
CEREBROVASCULAR ACCIDENT	0	3
MUSCULOSKELETAL	7	16
MYALGIA	4	16
OSTEOPOROSIS	2	0
ARTHRALGIA	1	0
TUMOR LYSIS SYNDROME	1	0

More than 3000 adult patients received FLUDARA FOR INJECTION in studies of other leukemias, lymphomas, and other solid tumors. The spectrum of adverse effects reported in these studies was consistent with the data presented above.

OVERDOSAGE

High doses of FLUDARA FOR INJECTION (see WARNINGS section) have been associated with an irreversible central nervous system toxicity characterized by delayed blindness, coma, and death. High doses are also associated with severe thrombocytopenia and neutropenia due to bone marrow suppression. There is no known specific antidote for FLUDARA FOR INJECTION overdosage. Treatment consists of drug discontinuation and supportive therapy.

DOSAGE AND ADMINISTRATION

Usual Dose:

The recommended adult dose of FLUDARA FOR INJECTION is 25 mg/m^2 administered intravenously over a period of approximately 30 minutes daily for five consecutive days. Each 5 day course of treatment should commence every 28 days. Dosage may be decreased or delayed based on evidence of hematologic or nonhematologic toxicity. Physicians should consider delaying or discontinuing the drug if neurotoxicity occurs.

A number of clinical settings may predispose to increased toxicity from FLUDARA FOR INJECTION. These include advanced age, renal insufficiency, and bone marrow impairment. Such patients should be monitored closely for excessive toxicity and the dose modified accordingly.

The optimal duration of treatment has not been clearly established. It is recommended that three additional cycles of FLUDARA FOR INJECTION be administered following the achievement of a maximal response and then the drug should be discontinued.

Renal Insufficiency

Adult with moderate impairment of renal function (creatinine clearance 30-70 mL/min/1.73 m^2) should have a 20% dose reduction of FLUDARA FOR INJECTION. FLUDARA FOR INJECTION should not be administered to patients with severely impaired renal function (creatinine clearance less than 30 mL/min/1.73 m^2).

Preparation of Solutions:

FLUDARA FOR INJECTION should be prepared for parenteral use by aseptically adding Sterile Water for Injection USP. When reconstituted with 2 mL of Sterile Water for Injection, USP, the solid cake should fully dissolve in 15 seconds or less; each mL of the resulting solution will contain 25 mg of fludarabine phosphate, 25 mg of mannitol, and sodium hydroxide to adjust the pH to 7.7. The pH range for the final product is 7.2-8.2. In clinical studies, the product has been diluted in 100 cc or 125 cc of 5% Dextrose Injection USP or 0.9% Sodium Chloride USP.

Reconstituted FLUDARA FOR INJECTION contains no antimicrobial preservative and thus should be used within 8 hours of reconstitution. Care must be taken to assure the sterility of prepared solutions. Parenteral drug products should be inspected visually for particulate matter and discoloration prior to administration.

Handling and Disposal:

Procedures for proper handling and disposal should be considered. Consideration should be given to handling and disposal according to guidelines issued for cytotoxic drugs. Several guidelines on this subject have been published.[1–8] There is no general agreement that all of the procedures recommended in the guidelines are necessary or appropriate.

Caution should be exercised in the handling and preparation of FLUDARA FOR INJECTION solution. The use of latex gloves and safety glasses is recommended to avoid exposure in case of breakage of the vial or other accidental spillage. If the solution contacts the skin or mucous membranes, wash thoroughly with soap and water; rinse eyes thoroughly with plain water. Avoid exposure by inhalation or by direct contact of the skin or mucous membranes.

HOW SUPPLIED

FLUDARA FOR INJECTION is supplied as a white, lyophilized solid cake. Each vial contains 50 mg of fludarabine phosphate, 50 mg of mannitol, and sodium hydroxide to adjust pH to 7.7. The pH range for the final product is 7.2-8.2. Store under refrigeration, between 2°-8°C (36°-46°F).

FLUDARA FOR INJECTION is supplied in a clear glass single dose vial (6 mL capacity) and packaged in a single dose vial carton in a shelf pack of five.

NDC 50419-511-06

Manufactured by: Ben Venue Laboratories, Bedford, OH 44146

Manufactured for: Berlex, Montville, NJ 07045

U.S. Patent Number: 4,357,324

REFERENCES

1. ONS Clinical Practice Committee. Cancer Chemotherapy Guidelines and Recommendations for Practice. Pittsburgh, Pa: Oncology Nursing Society. 1999:32-41.
2. Recommendations for the Safe Handling of Parenteral Antineoplastic Drugs. Washington, DC; Division of Safety, Clinical Center Pharmacy Department and Cancer Nursing Services, National Institute of Health; 1992. US Department of Health and Human Services, Public Health Service Publication NIH 92-2621.
3. AMA Council on Scientific Affairs. Guidelines for Handling Parenteral Antineoplastics. JAMA. 1985;253:1590-1591.
4. National Study Commission on Cytotoxic Exposure—Recommendations for Handling Cytotoxic Agents. 1987. Available from Louis P. Jeffrey, Sc.D., Chairman, National Study Commission on Cytotoxic Exposure, Massachusetts College of Pharmacy and Allied Health Sciences, 179 Longwood Avenue, Boston, MA 02115.
5. Clinical Oncological Society of Australia: Guidelines and Recommendations for Safe Handling of Antineoplastic Agents. Med J Australia. 1983;1:426-428.
6. Jones, R.B, Frank R, Mass T. Safe Handling of Chemotherapeutic Agents: A Report from the Mount Sinai Medical Center. CA Cancer J Clin. 1983; 33:258-263.
7. American Society of Hospital Pharmacists. ASHP Technical Assistance Bulletin on Handling Cytotoxic and Hazardous Drugs. Am J Hosp Pharm. 1990; 47:1033-1049.
8. Controlling Occupational Exposure to Hazardous Drugs (OSHA Work-Practice Guidelines). Am J Health-Syst Pharm. 1996;53:1669-1685.

6063507 Rev. 10/03

Shown in Product Identification Guide, page 308

LEUKINE® ℞

SARGRAMOSTIM

Rx only

DESCRIPTION

LEUKINE® (sargramostim) is a recombinant human granulocyte-macrophage colony stimulating factor (rhu GM-CSF) produced by recombinant DNA technology in a yeast (*S. cerevisiae*) expression system. GM-CSF is a hematopoietic growth factor which stimulates proliferation and differentiation of hematopoietic progenitor cells. LEUKINE is a glycoprotein of 127 amino acids characterized by 3 primary molecular species having molecular masses of 19,500, 16,800 and 15,500 daltons. The amino acid sequence of LEUKINE differs from the natural human GM-CSF by a substitution of leucine at position 23, and the carbohydrate moiety may be different from the native protein. Sargramostim has been selected as the proper name for yeast-derived rhu GM-CSF.

The LEUKINE Liquid presentation is formulated as a sterile, preserved (1.1% benzyl alcohol), injectable solution (500 mcg/mL) in a vial. Lyophilized LEUKINE is a sterile, white, preservative-free powder (250 mcg) that requires reconstitution with 1 mL Sterile Water for Injection, USP or 1 mL Bacteriostatic Water for Injection, USP.

LEUKINE Liquid and reconstituted lyophilized LEUKINE are clear, colorless liquids suitable for subcutaneous injection or intravenous infusion. LEUKINE Liquid contains 500 mcg (2.8 × 10^6 IU/mL) sargramostim and 1.1% benzyl alcohol in a 1 mL solution. The vial of lyophilized LEUKINE contains 250 mcg (1.4 × 10^6 IU/vial) sargramostim. The LEUKINE Liquid vial and reconstituted lyophilized LEUKINE vial also contain 40 mg/mL mannitol, USP; 10 mg/mL sucrose, NF; and 1.2 mg/mL tromethamine, USP, as excipients. Biological potency is expressed in International Units (IU) as tested against the WHO First International Reference Standard. The specific activity of LEUKINE is approximately 5.6 × 10^6 IU/mg.

CLINICAL PHARMACOLOGY

General GM-CSF belongs to a group of growth factors termed colony stimulating factors which support survival, clonal expansion, and differentiation of hematopoietic progenitor cells. GM-CSF induces partially committed progenitor cells to divide and differentiate in the granulocyte-macrophage pathways.

GM-CSF is also capable of activating mature granulocytes and macrophages. GM-CSF is a multilineage factor and, in addition to dose-dependent effects on the myelomonocytic lineage, can promote the proliferation of megakaryocytic and erythroid progenitors.[1] However, other factors are required to induce complete maturation in these two lineages. The various cellular responses (i.e., division, maturation, activation) are induced through GM-CSF binding to specific receptors expressed on the cell surface of target cells.[2]

***In vitro* Studies of LEUKINE in Human Cells** The biological activity of GM-CSF is species-specific. Consequently, *in vitro* studies have been performed on human cells to characterize the pharmacological activity of LEUKINE. *In vitro* exposure of human bone marrow cells to LEUKINE at concentrations ranging from 1–100 ng/mL results in the proliferation of hematopoietic progenitors and in the formation of pure granulocyte, pure macrophage and mixed granulocyte-macrophage colonies.[3] Chemotactic, anti-fungal and anti-parasitic[4] activities of granulocytes and monocytes are increased by exposure to LEUKINE *in vitro*. LEUKINE increases the cytotoxicity of monocytes toward certain neoplastic cell lines[3] and activates polymorphonuclear neutrophils to inhibit the growth of tumor cells.

***In vivo* Primate Studies of LEUKINE** Pharmacology/toxicology studies of LEUKINE were performed in cynomolgus monkeys. An acute toxicity study revealed an absence of treatment-related toxicity following a single IV bolus injection at a dose of 300 mcg/kg. Two subacute studies were performed using IV injection (maximum dose 200 mcg/kg/day × 14 days) and subcutaneous injection (maximum dose 200 mcg/kg/day × 28 days). No major visceral organ toxicity was documented. Notable histopathology findings included increased cellularity in hematologic organs and heart and lung tissues. A dose-dependent increase in leukocyte count, which consisted primarily of segmented neutrophils, occurred during the dosing period; increases in monocytes, basophils, eosinophils and lymphocytes were also noted. Leukocyte counts decreased to pretreatment values over a 1–2 week recovery period.

Pharmacokinetics Pharmacokinetic profiles have been analyzed in controlled studies of 24 normal male volunteers. Liquid and lyophilized LEUKINE, at the recommended dose of 250 mcg/m^2, have been determined to be bioequivalent based on the statistical evaluation of AUC.[5]

When LEUKINE (either liquid or lyophilized) was administered IV over 2 hours to normal volunteers, the mean beta half-life was approximately 60 minutes. Peak concentrations of GM-CSF were observed in blood samples obtained during or immediately after completion of LEUKINE infusion. For LEUKINE Liquid, the mean maximum concentration (Cmax) was 5.0 ng/mL, the mean clearance rate was approximately 420 mL/min/m^2 and the mean AUC (0–inf) was 640 ng/mL•min. Corresponding results for lyophilized LEUKINE in the same subjects were mean Cmax of 5.4 ng/mL, mean clearance rate of 431 mL/min/m^2, and mean AUC (0-inf) of 677 ng/mL•min. GM-CSF was last detected in blood samples obtained at 3 or 6 hours.

When LEUKINE (either liquid or lyophilized) was administered SC to normal volunteers, GM-CSF was detected in the serum at 15 minutes, the first sample point. The mean beta half-life was approximately 162 minutes. Peak levels occurred at 1 to 3 hours post injection, and LEUKINE remained detectable for up to 6 hours after injection. The mean Cmax was 1.5 ng/mL. For LEUKINE Liquid, the mean clearance was 549 mL/min/m^2 and the mean AUC (0–inf) was 549 ng/mL•min. For lyophilized LEUKINE, the mean clearance was 529 mL/min/m^2 and the mean AUC (0-inf) was 501 ng/mL•min.

Antibody Formation Serum samples collected before and after LEUKINE treatment from 214 patients with a variety of underlying diseases have been examined for the presence of antibodies. Neutralizing antibodies were detected in 5 of 214 patients (2.3%) after receiving LEUKINE by continuous IV infusion (3 patients) or subcutaneous injection (2 patients) for 28 to 84 days in multiple courses. All 5 patients had impaired hematopoiesis before the administration of LEUKINE and consequently the effect of the development of anti-GM-CSF antibodies on normal hematopoiesis could not be assessed. Drug-induced neutropenia, neutralization of endogenous GM-CSF activity and diminution of the therapeutic effect of LEUKINE secondary to formation of neutralizing antibody remain a theoretical possibility.

INDICATIONS AND USAGE

Use Following Induction Chemotherapy in Acute Myelogenous Leukemia LEUKINE is indicated for use following induction chemotherapy in older adult patients with acute myelogenous leukemia (AML) to shorten time to neutrophil recovery and to reduce the incidence of severe and life-threatening infections and infections resulting in death. The safety and efficacy of LEUKINE have not been assessed in patients with AML under 55 years of age.

The term acute myelogenous leukemia, also referred to as acute non-lymphocytic leukemia (ANLL), encompasses a heterogeneous group of leukemias arising from various non-lymphoid cell lines which have been defined morphologically by the French-American-British (FAB) system of classification.

Use in Mobilization and Following Transplantation of Autologous Peripheral Blood Progenitor Cells LEUKINE is indicated for the mobilization of hematopoietic progenitor cells into peripheral blood for collection by leukapheresis. Mobilization allows for the collection of increased numbers of progenitor cells capable of engraftment as compared with collection without mobilization. After myeloablative chemotherapy, the transplantation of an increased number of progenitor cells can lead to more rapid engraftment, which may result in a decreased need for supportive care. Myeloid reconstitution is further accelerated by administration of LEUKINE following peripheral blood progenitor cell transplantation.

Use in Myeloid Reconstitution After Autologous Bone Marrow Transplantation LEUKINE is indicated for acceleration of myeloid recovery in patients with non-Hodgkin's lymphoma (NHL), acute lymphoblastic leukemia (ALL) and Hodgkin's disease undergoing autologous bone marrow transplantation (BMT). After autologous BMT in patients with NHL, ALL, or Hodgkin's disease, LEUKINE has been found to be safe and effective in accelerating myeloid engraftment, decreasing median duration of antibiotic administration, reducing the median duration of infectious episodes and shortening the median duration of hospitalization. Hematologic response to LEUKINE can be detected by complete blood count (CBC) with differential performed twice per week.

Hematological Recovery (in Days): Induction

Dataset	sargramostim n=52* Median (25%, 75%)	Placebo n=47 Median (25%, 75%)	p-value**
ANC>500/mm^3 [a]	13 (11, 16)	17 (13, 25)	0.009
ANC>1000/mm^3 [b]	14 (12, 18)	21 (13, 34)	0.003
PLT>20,000/mm^3 [c]	11 (7, 14)	12 (9, >42)	0.10
RBC [d]	12 (9, 24)	14 (9, 42)	0.53

* *Patients with missing data censored.*
[a] *2 Patients on sargramostim and 4 patients on placebo had missing values.*
[b] *2 Patients on sargramostim and 3 patients on placebo had missing values.*
[c] *4 Patients on placebo had missing values.*
[d] *3 Patients on sargramostim and 4 patients on placebo had missing values.*
** *p=Generalized Wilcoxon*

Use in Myeloid Reconstitution After Allogeneic Bone Marrow Transplantation LEUKINE is indicated for acceleration of myeloid recovery in patients undergoing allogeneic BMT from HLA-matched related donors. LEUKINE has been found to be safe and effective in accelerating myeloid engraftment, reducing the incidence of bacteremia and other culture positive infections, and shortening the median duration of hospitalization.

Use in Bone Marrow Transplantation Failure or Engraftment Delay LEUKINE is indicated in patients who have undergone allogeneic or autologous bone marrow transplantation (BMT) in whom engraftment is delayed or has failed. LEUKINE has been found to be safe and effective in prolonging survival of patients who are experiencing graft failure or engraftment delay, in the presence or absence of infection, following autologous or allogeneic BMT. Survival benefit may be relatively greater in those patients who demonstrate one or more of the following characteristics: autologous BMT failure or engraftment delay, no previous total body irradiation, malignancy other than leukemia or a multiple organ failure (MOF) score ≤ 2 (See CLINICAL EXPERIENCE). Hematologic response to LEUKINE can be detected by complete blood count (CBC) with differential performed twice per week.

CLINICAL EXPERIENCE

Acute Myelogenous Leukemia The safety and efficacy of sargramostim in patients with AML who are younger than 55 years of age have not been determined. Based on Phase II data suggesting the best therapeutic effects could be achieved in patients at highest risk for severe infections and mortality while neutropenic, the Phase III clinical trial was conducted in older patients. The safety and efficacy of LEUKINE in the treatment of AML were evaluated in a multi-center, randomized, double-blind placebo-controlled trial of 99 newly diagnosed adult patients, 55–70 years of age, receiving induction with or without consolidation.[6] A combination of standard doses of daunorubicin (days 1–3) and ara-C (days 1–7) was administered during induction and high dose ara-C was administered days 1–6 as a single course of consolidation, if given. Bone marrow evaluation was performed on day 10 following induction chemotherapy. If hypoplasia with <5% blasts was not achieved, patients immediately received a second cycle of induction chemotherapy. If the bone marrow was hypoplastic with <5% blasts on day 10 or 4 days following the second cycle of induction chemotherapy, LEUKINE (250 mcg/m^2/day) or placebo was given IV over 4 hours each day, starting 4 days after the completion of chemotherapy. Study drug was continued until an ANC ≥1500/mm^3 for three consecutive days was attained or a maximum of 42 days. LEUKINE or placebo was also administered after the single course of consolidation chemotherapy if delivered (ara-C 3–6 weeks after induction following neutrophil recovery). Study drug was discontinued immediately if leukemic regrowth occurred.

[See table above]

LEUKINE (sargramostim) significantly shortened the median duration of ANC <500/mm^3 by 4 days and <1000/mm^3 by 7 days following induction (see table at right). 75% of patients receiving LEUKINE achieved ANC >500/mm^3 by day 16, compared to day 25 for patients receiving placebo. The proportion of patients receiving 1 cycle (70%) or 2 cycles (30%) of induction was similar in both treatment groups; LEUKINE significantly shortened the median times to neutrophil recovery whether one cycle (12 versus 15 days) or two cycles (14 versus 23 days) of induction chemotherapy was administered. Median times to platelet (>20,000/mm^3) and RBC transfusion independence were not significantly different between treatment groups.

During the consolidation phase of treatment, LEUKINE did not shorten the median time to recovery of ANC to 500/mm^3 (13 days) or 1000/mm^3 (14.5 days) compared to placebo. There were no significant differences in time to platelet and RBC transfusion independence.

The incidence of severe infections and deaths associated with infections was significantly reduced in patients who received LEUKINE. During induction or consolidation, 27 of 52 patients receiving LEUKINE and 35 of 47 patients receiving placebo had at least one grade 3, 4 or 5 infection (p=0.02). Twenty-five patients receiving LEUKINE and 30 patients receiving placebo experienced severe and fatal infections during induction only. There were significantly fewer deaths from infectious causes in the sargramostim arm (3 versus 11, p=0.02). The majority of deaths in the placebo group were associated with fungal infections with pneumonia as the primary infection.

Disease outcomes were not adversely affected by the use of LEUKINE. The proportion of patients achieving complete remission (CR) was higher in the LEUKINE group (69% as compared to 55% for the placebo group), but the difference was not significant (p=0.21). There was no significant difference in relapse rates; 12 of 36 patients who received LEUKINE and 5 of 26 patients who received placebo relapsed within 180 days of documented CR (p=0.26). The overall median survival was 378 days for patients receiving LEUKINE and 268 days for those on placebo (p=0.17). The study was not sized to assess the impact of LEUKINE treatment on response or survival.

Mobilization and Engraftment of PBPC A retrospective review was conducted of data from patients with cancer undergoing collection of peripheral blood progenitor cells (PBPC) at a single transplant center. Mobilization of PBPC and myeloid reconstitution post-transplant were compared between four groups of patients (n=196) receiving LEUKINE for mobilization and a historical control group who did not receive any mobilization treatment [progenitor cells collected by leukapheresis without mobilization (n=100)]. Sequential cohorts received LEUKINE. The cohorts differed by dose (125 or 250 mcg/m^2/day), route (IV over 24 hours or SC) and use of LEUKINE post-transplant. Leukaphereses were initiated for all mobilization groups after the WBC reached 10,000/mm^3. Leukaphereses continued until both a minimum number of mononucleated cells (MNC) were collected (6.5 or 8.0 × 10^8/kg body weight) and a minimum number of phereses (5–8) were performed. Both minimum requirements varied by treatment cohort and planned conditioning regimen. If subjects failed to reach a WBC of 10,000 cells/mm^3 by day 5, another cytokine was substituted for LEUKINE; these subjects were all successfully leukapheresed and transplanted. The most marked mobilization and post-transplant effects were seen in patients administered the higher dose of LEUKINE (250 mcg/m^2) either IV (n=63) or SC (n=41).

PBPCs from patients treated at the 250 mcg/m^2/day dose had significantly higher number of granulocyte-macrophage colony-forming units (CFU-GM) than those collected without mobilization. The mean value after thawing was 11.41 × 10^4 CFU-GM/kg for all LEUKINE-mobilized patients, compared to 0.96 × 10^4/kg for the non-mobilized group. A similar difference was observed in the mean number of erythrocyte burst-forming units (BFU-E) collected (23.96 × 10^4/kg for patients mobilized with 250 mcg/m^2 doses of LEUKINE administered SC vs. 1.63 × 10^4/kg for non-mobilized patients).

[See first table at top of next page]

After transplantation, mobilized subjects had shorter times to myeloid engraftment and fewer days between transplantation and the last platelet transfusion compared to non-mobilized subjects. Neutrophil recovery (ANC >500/mm^3) was more rapid in patients administered LEUKINE following PBPC transplantation with LEUKINE-mobilized cells (see table at right). Mobilized patients also had fewer days to the last platelet transfusion and last RBC transfusion, and a shorter duration of hospitalization than did non-mobilized subjects.

A second retrospective review of data from patients undergoing PBPC at another single transplant center was also conducted. LEUKINE was given SC at 250 mcg/m^2/day once a day (n=10) or twice a day (n=21) until completion of the phereses. Phereses were begun on day 5 of LEUKINE administration and continued until the targeted MNC count of 9 × 10^8/kg or CD34+ cell count of 1 × 10^6/kg was reached. There was no difference in CD34+ cell count in patients receiving LEUKINE once or twice a day. The median time to ANC>500/mm^3 was 12 days and to platelet recovery (>25,000/mm^3) was 23 days.

Survival studies comparing mobilized study patients to the non-mobilized patients and to an autologous historical bone marrow transplant group showed no differences in median survival time.

Continued on next page

Information on Berlex products (appearing here) is based on the most current information available at the time of publication closing. Further information for these and other Berlex products can be obtained from Medical & Product Services at Berlex, Inc. by calling 1-888-BERLEX-4.

Leukine—Cont.

Autologous Bone Marrow Transplantation[7] Following a dose-ranging Phase I/II trial in patients undergoing autologous BMT for lymphoid malignancies,[8, 9] three single center, randomized, placebo-controlled and double-blinded studies were conducted to evaluate the safety and efficacy of LEUKINE for promoting hematopoietic reconstitution following autologous BMT. A total of 128 patients (65 LEUKINE, 63 placebo) were enrolled in these 3 studies. The majority of the patients had lymphoid malignancy (87 NHL, 17 ALL), 23 patients had Hodgkin's disease, and 1 patient had acute myeloblastic leukemia (AML). In 72 patients with NHL or ALL, the bone marrow harvest was purged prior to storage with one of several monoclonal antibodies. No chemical agent was used for *in vitro* treatment of the bone marrow. Preparative regimens in the 3 studies included cyclophosphamide (total dose 120–150 mg/kg) and total body irradiation (total dose 1,200–1,575 rads). Other regimens used in patients with Hodgkin's disease and NHL without radiotherapy consisted of 3 or more of the following in combination (expressed as total dose): cytosine arabinoside (400 mg/m^2) and carmustine (300 mg/m^2), cyclophosphamide (140–150 mg/kg), hydroxyurea (4.5 grams/m^2) and etoposide (375-450 mg/m^2).

Compared to placebo, administration of LEUKINE in 2 studies (n=44 and 47) significantly improved the following hematologic and clinical endpoints: time to neutrophil engraftment, duration of hospitalization and infection experience or antibacterial usage. In the third study (n=37) there was a positive trend toward earlier myeloid engraftment in favor of LEUKINE. This latter study differed from the other 2 in having enrolled a large number of patients with Hodgkin's disease who had also received extensive radiation and chemotherapy prior to harvest of autologous bone marrow. A subgroup analysis of the data from all 3 studies revealed that the median time to engraftment for patients with Hodgkin's disease, regardless of treatment, was 6 days longer when compared to patients with NHL and ALL, but that the overall beneficial LEUKINE treatment effect was the same. In the following combined analysis of the 3 studies, these 2 subgroups (NHL and ALL vs. Hodgkin's disease) are presented separately.

Patients with Lymphoid Malignancy (Non-Hodgkin's Lymphoma and Acute Lymphoblastic Leukemia): Myeloid engraftment (absolute neutrophil count [ANC] ≥ 500 cells/mm^3) in 54 patients receiving LEUKINE was observed 6 days earlier than in 50 patients treated with placebo (see table at right). Accelerated myeloid engraftment was associated with significant clinical benefits. The median duration of hospitalization was 6 days shorter for the LEUKINE group than for the placebo group. Median duration of infectious episodes (defined as fever and neutropenia; or 2 positive cultures of the same organism; or fever >38°C and 1 positive blood culture; or clinical evidence of infection) was 3 days less in the group treated with LEUKINE. The median duration of antibacterial administration in the post-transplantation period was 4 days shorter for the patients treated with LEUKINE than for placebo-treated patients. The study was unable to detect a significant difference between the treatment groups in rate of disease relapse 24 months post-transplantation. As a group, leukemic subjects receiving LEUKINE derived less benefit than NHL subjects. However, both the leukemic and NHL groups receiving LEUKINE engrafted earlier than controls.

[See second table above]

Patients with Hodgkin's Disease: If patients with Hodgkin's disease are analyzed separately, a trend toward earlier myeloid engraftment is noted. LEUKINE-treated patients engrafted earlier (by 5 days) than the placebo-treated patients (p=0.189, Wilcoxon) but the number of patients was small (n=22). Studies are in progress to confirm statistically the trend toward earlier engraftment with LEUKINE in patients with Hodgkin's disease.

Allogeneic Bone Marrow Transplantation A multi-center, randomized, placebo-controlled, and double-blinded study was conducted to evaluate the safety and efficacy of LEUKINE for promoting hematopoietic reconstitution following allogeneic BMT. A total of 109 patients (53 LEUKINE, 56 placebo) were enrolled in the study. Twenty-three patients (11 LEUKINE, 12 placebo) were 18 years old or younger. Sixty-seven patients had myeloid malignancies (33 AML, 34 CML), 17 had lymphoid malignancies (12 ALL, 5 NHL), 3 patients had Hodgkin's disease, 6 had multiple myeloma, 9 had myelodysplastic disease, and 7 patients had aplastic anemia. In 22 patients at one of the seven study sites, bone marrow harvests were depleted of T cells. Preparative regimens included cyclophosphamide, busulfan, cytosine arabinoside, etoposide, methotrexate, corticosteroids, and asparaginase. Some patients also received total body, splenic, or testicular irradiation. Primary graft-versus-host disease (GVHD) prophylaxis was cyclosporine A and a corticosteroid.

Accelerated myeloid engraftment was associated with significant laboratory and clinical benefits. Compared to placebo, administration of LEUKINE significantly improved the following: time to neutrophil engraftment, duration of hospitalization, number of patients with bacteremia and overall incidence of infection (see table at right).

[See third table above]

Median time to myeloid engraftment (ANC ≥ 500 cells/mm^3) in 53 patients receiving LEUKINE (sargramostim) was 4 days less than in 56 patients treated with placebo (see table at right). The number of patients with bacteremia and infection was significantly lower in the LEUKINE group compared to the placebo group (9/53 versus 19/56 and 30/53 versus 42/56, respectively). There were a number of secondary laboratory and clinical endpoints. Of these, only the incidence of severe (grade 3/4) mucositis was significantly improved in the LEUKINE group (4/53) compared to the placebo group (16/56) at p<0.05. LEUKINE-treated patients also had a shorter median duration of post-transplant IV antibiotic infusions, and shorter median number of days to last platelet and RBC transfusions compared to placebo patients, but none of these differences reached statistical significance.

Bone Marrow Transplantation Failure or Engraftment Delay A historically controlled study was conducted in patients experiencing graft failure following allogeneic or autologous BMT to determine whether LEUKINE improved survival after BMT failure.

Three categories of patients were eligible for this study:

1) patients displaying a delay in engraftment (ANC ≤ 100 cells/mm^3 by day 28 post-transplantation);
2) patients displaying a delay in engraftment (ANC ≤ 100 cells/mm^3 by day 21 post-transplantation) and who had evidence of an active infection; and
3) patients who lost their marrow graft after a transient engraftment (manifested by an average of ANC ≥ 500 cells/mm^3 for at least one week followed by loss of engraftment with ANC < 500 cells/mm^3 for at least one week beyond day 21 post-transplantation).

A total of 140 eligible patients from 35 institutions were treated with LEUKINE and evaluated in comparison to 103 historical control patients from a single institution. One hundred sixty-three patients had lymphoid or myeloid leukemia, 24 patients had non-Hodgkin's lymphoma, 19 patients had Hodgkin's disease and 37 patients had other diseases, such as aplastic anemia, myelodysplasia or non-hematologic malignancy. The majority of patients (223 out of 243) had received prior chemotherapy with or without radiotherapy and/or immunotherapy prior to preparation for transplantation.

One hundred day survival was improved in favor of the patients treated with LEUKINE after graft failure following either autologous or allogeneic BMT. In addition, the median survival was improved by greater than 2-fold. The median survival of patients treated with LEUKINE after autologous failure was 474 days versus 161 days for the historical patients. Similarly, after allogeneic failure, the median survival was 97 days with LEUKINE treatment and 35 days for the historical controls. Improvement in survival was better in patients with fewer impaired organs.

The MOF score is a simple clinical and laboratory assessment of 7 major organ systems: cardiovascular, respiratory, gastrointestinal, hematologic, renal, hepatic and neurologic.[10] Assessment of the MOF score is recommended as an additional method of determining the need to initiate treatment with LEUKINE in patients with graft failure or delay in engraftment following autologous or allogeneic BMT.

[See fourth table above]

Factors that Contribute to Survival: The probability of survival was relatively greater for patients with any one of the following characteristics: autologous BMT failure or delay in engraftment, exclusion of total body irradiation from the preparative regimen, a non-leukemic malignancy or MOF score ≤ 2 (0, 1 or 2 dysfunctional organ systems). Leukemic subjects derived less benefit than other subjects.

CONTRAINDICATIONS

LEUKINE is contraindicated:

1) in patients with excessive leukemic myeloid blasts in the bone marrow or peripheral blood (≥ 10%);
2) in patients with known hypersensitivity to GM-CSF, yeast-derived products or any component of the product;
3) for concomitant use with chemotherapy and radiotherapy.

Due to the potential sensitivity of rapidly dividing hematopoietic progenitor cells, LEUKINE should not be administered simultaneously with cytotoxic chemotherapy or radiotherapy or within 24 hours preceding or following chemotherapy or radiotherapy. In one controlled study, patients with small cell lung cancer received LEUKINE and concurrent thoracic radiotherapy and chemotherapy or the identical radiotherapy and chemotherapy without LEUKINE. The patients randomized to LEUKINE had significantly higher incidence of adverse events, including higher mortality and a higher incidence of grade 3 and 4 infections and grade 3 and 4 thrombocytopenia.[11]

WARNINGS

Pediatric Use Benzyl alcohol is a constituent of LEUKINE Liquid and Bacteriostatic Water for Injection diluent. Benzyl alcohol has been reported to be associated with a fatal

ANC and Platelet Recovery after PBPC Transplant

	Route for Mobilization	Post-transplant LEUKINE	ENGRAFTMENT (median value in days) ANC>500/mm^3	Last platelet transfusion
No Mobilization	—	no	29	28
LEUKINE 250 mcg/m^2	IV	no	21	24
	IV	yes	12	19
	SC	yes	12	17

Autologous BMT: Combined Analysis from Placebo-Controlled Clinical Trials of Responses in Patients with NHL and ALL
Median Values (days)

	ANC ≥500/mm^3	ANC ≥1000/mm^3	Duration of Hospitalization	Duration of Infection	Duration of Antibacterial Therapy
LEUKINE (n=54)	18*#	24*#	25*	1*	21*
Placebo (n=50)	24	32	31	4	25

* *p <0.05 Wilcoxon or CMH ridit chi-squared*
 # p <0.05 Log rank
Note: The single AML patient was not included.

Allogeneic BMT: Analysis of Data from Placebo-Controlled Clinical Trial
Median Values (days or number of patients)

	ANC ≥ 500/mm^3	ANC ≥ 1000/mm^3	Number of Patients with Infections	Number of Patients with Bacteremia	Days of Hospitalization
LEUKINE (n=53)	13*	14*	30*	9**	25*
Placebo (n=56)	17	19	42	19	26

* *p <0.05 generalized Wilcoxon test*
*** p <0.05 simple chi-square test*

Median Survival by Multiple Organ Failure (MOF) Category
Median Survival (days)

	MOF ≤ 2 Organs	MOF > 2 Organs	MOF (Composite of Both Groups)
Autologous BMT			
LEUKINE	474 (n=58)	78.5 (n=10)	474 (n=68)
Historical	165 (n=14)	39 (n=3)	161 (n=17)
Allogeneic BMT			
LEUKINE	174 (n=50)	27 (n=22)	97 (n=72)
Historical	52.5 (n=60)	15.5 (n=26)	35 (n=86)

"Gasping Syndrome" in premature infants. **Liquid solutions containing benzyl alcohol (including LEUKINE Liquid) or lyophilized LEUKINE reconstituted with Bacteriostatic Water for Injection, USP (0.9% benzyl alcohol) should not be administered to neonates** (see PRECAUTIONS and DOSAGE AND ADMINISTRATION).

Fluid Retention Edema, capillary leak syndrome, pleural and/or pericardial effusion have been reported in patients after LEUKINE administration. In 156 patients enrolled in placebo-controlled studies using LEUKINE at a dose of 250 mcg/m^2/day by 2-hour IV infusion, the reported incidences of fluid retention (LEUKINE vs. placebo) were as follows: peripheral edema, 11% vs. 7%; pleural effusion, 1% vs. 0%; and pericardial effusion, 4% vs. 1%. Capillary leak syndrome was not observed in this limited number of studies; based on other uncontrolled studies and reports from users of marketed LEUKINE, the incidence is estimated to be less than 1%. In patients with preexisting pleural and pericardial effusions, administration of LEUKINE may aggravate fluid retention; however, fluid retention associated with or worsened by LEUKINE has been reversible after interruption or dose reduction of LEUKINE with or without diuretic therapy. LEUKINE should be used with caution in patients with preexisting fluid retention, pulmonary infiltrates or congestive heart failure.

Respiratory Symptoms Sequestration of granulocytes in the pulmonary circulation has been documented following LEUKINE infusion,[12] and dyspnea has been reported occasionally in patients treated with LEUKINE. Special attention should be given to respiratory symptoms during or immediately following LEUKINE infusion, especially in patients with preexisting lung disease. In patients displaying dyspnea during LEUKINE administration, the rate of infusion should be reduced by half. If respiratory symptoms worsen despite infusion rate reduction, the infusion should be discontinued. Subsequent IV infusions may be administered following the standard dose schedule with careful monitoring. LEUKINE should be administered with caution in patients with hypoxia.

Cardiovascular Symptoms Occasional transient supraventricular arrhythmia has been reported in uncontrolled studies during LEUKINE administration, particularly in patients with a previous history of cardiac arrhythmia. However, these arrhythmias have been reversible after discontinuation of LEUKINE. LEUKINE should be used with caution in patients with preexisting cardiac disease.

Renal and Hepatic Dysfunction In some patients with preexisting renal or hepatic dysfunction enrolled in uncontrolled clinical trials, administration of LEUKINE has induced elevation of serum creatinine or bilirubin and hepatic enzymes. Dose reduction or interruption of LEUKINE administration has resulted in a decrease to pretreatment values. However, in controlled clinical trials the incidences of renal and hepatic dysfunction were comparable between LEUKINE (250 mcg/m^2/day by 2-hour IV infusion) and placebo-treated patients. Monitoring of renal and hepatic function in patients displaying renal or hepatic dysfunction prior to initiation of treatment is recommended at least every other week during LEUKINE administration.

PRECAUTIONS

General Parenteral administration of recombinant proteins should be attended by appropriate precautions in case an allergic or untoward reaction occurs. Serious allergic or anaphylactic reactions have been reported. If any serious allergic or anaphylactic reaction occurs, LEUKINE therapy should immediately be discontinued and appropriate therapy initiated.

A syndrome characterized by respiratory distress, hypoxia, flushing, hypotension, syncope, and/or tachycardia has been reported following the first administration of LEUKINE (sargramostim) in a particular cycle. These signs have resolved with symptomatic treatment and usually do not recur with subsequent doses in the same cycle of treatment.

Stimulation of marrow precursors with LEUKINE may result in a rapid rise in white blood cell (WBC) count. If the ANC exceeds 20,000 cells/mm^3 or if the platelet count exceeds 500,000/mm^3, LEUKINE administration should be interrupted or the dose reduced by half. The decision to reduce the dose or interrupt treatment should be based on the clinical condition of the patient. Excessive blood counts have returned to normal or baseline levels within 3 to 7 days following cessation of LEUKINE therapy. Twice weekly monitoring of CBC with differential (including examination for the presence of blast cells) should be performed to preclude development of excessive counts.

Growth Factor Potential LEUKINE is a growth factor that primarily stimulates normal myeloid precursors. However, the possibility that LEUKINE can act as a growth factor for any tumor type, particularly myeloid malignancies, cannot be excluded. Because of the possibility of tumor growth potentiation, precaution should be exercised when using this drug in any malignancy with myeloid characteristics.

Should disease progression be detected during LEUKINE treatment, LEUKINE therapy should be discontinued.

LEUKINE has been administered to patients with myelodysplastic syndromes (MDS) in uncontrolled studies without evidence of increased relapse rates.[13, 14, 15] Controlled studies have not been performed in patients with MDS.

Use in Patients Receiving Purged Bone Marrow LEUKINE is effective in accelerating myeloid recovery in patients receiving bone marrow purged by anti-B lymphocyte monoclonal antibodies. Data obtained from uncontrolled studies suggest that if *in vitro* marrow purging with chemical agents causes a significant decrease in the number of responsive hematopoietic progenitors, the patient may not respond to LEUKINE. When the bone marrow purging process preserves a sufficient number of progenitors (>1,2 × 10^4/kg), a beneficial effect of LEUKINE on myeloid engraftment has been reported.[16]

Percent of AuBMT Patients Reporting Events

Events by Body System	LEUKINE (n=79)	Placebo (n=77)	Events by Body System	LEUKINE (n=79)	Placebo (n=77)
Body, General			**Metabolic, Nutritional Disorder**		
Fever	95	96	Edema	34	35
Mucous membrane disorder	75	78	Peripheral edema	11	7
Asthenia	66	51	**Respiratory System**		
Malaise	57	51	Dyspnea	28	31
Sepsis	11	14	Lung disorder	20	23
Digestive System			**Hemic and Lymphatic System**		
Nausea	90	96	Blood dyscrasia	25	27
Diarrhea	89	82	**Cardiovascular System**		
Vomiting	85	90	Hemorrhage	23	30
Anorexia	54	58	**Urogenital System**		
GI disorder	37	47	Urinary tract disorder	14	13
GI hemorrhage	27	33	Kidney function abnormal	8	10
Stomatitis	24	29	**Nervous System**		
Liver damage	13	14	CNS disorder	11	16
Skin and Appendages					
Alopecia	73	74			
Rash	44	38			

Percent of Allogeneic BMT Patients Reporting Events

Events by Body System	LEUKINE (n=53)	Placebo (n=56)	Events by Body System	LEUKINE (n=53)	Placebo (n=56)
Body, General			**Metabolic/Nutritional Disorders**		
Fever	77	80	Bilirubinemia	30	27
Abdominal pain	38	23	Hyperglycemia	25	23
Headache	36	36	Peripheral edema	15	21
Chills	25	20	Increased creatinine	15	14
Pain	17	36	Hypomagnesemia	15	9
Asthenia	17	20	Increased SGPT	13	16
Chest pain	15	9	Edema	13	11
Back pain	9	18	Increased alk. phosphatase	8	14
Digestive System			**Respiratory System**		
Diarrhea	81	66	Pharyngitis	23	13
Nausea	70	66	Epistaxis	17	16
Vomiting	70	57	Dyspnea	15	14
Stomatitis	62	63	Rhinitis	11	14
Anorexia	51	57	**Hemic and Lymphatic System**		
Dyspepsia	17	20	Thrombocytopenia	19	34
Hematemesis	13	7	Leukopenia	17	29
Dysphagia	11	7	Petechia	6	11
GI hemorrhage	11	5	Agranulocytosis	6	11
Constipation	8	11	**Urogenital System**		
Skin and Appendages			Hematuria	9	21
Rash	70	73	**Nervous System**		
Alopecia	45	45	Paresthesia	11	13
Pruritis	23	13	Insomnia	11	9
Musculo-skeletal System			Anxiety	11	2
Bone pain	21	5	**Laboratory Abnormalities***		
Arthralgia	11	4	High glucose	41	49
Special Senses			Low albumin	27	36
Eye hemorrhage	11	0	High BUN	23	17
Cardiovascular System			Low calcium	2	7
Hypertension	34	32	High cholesterol	17	8
Tachycardia	11	9			

**Grade 3 and 4 laboratory abnormalities only. Denominators may vary due to missing laboratory measurements.*

Use in Patients Previously Exposed to Intensive Chemotherapy/Radiotherapy In patients who before autologous BMT, have received extensive radiotherapy to hematopoietic sites for the treatment of primary disease in the abdomen or chest, or have been exposed to multiple myelotoxic agents (alkylating agents, anthracycline antibiotics and antimetabolites), the effect of LEUKINE on myeloid reconstitution may be limited.

Use in Patients with Malignancy Undergoing LEUKINE-Mobilized PBPC Collection When using LEUKINE to mobilize PBPC, the limited *in vitro* data suggest that tumor cells may be released and reinfused into the patient in the leukapheresis product. The effect of reinfusion of tumor cells has not been well studied and the data are inconclusive.

Patient Monitoring LEUKINE can induce variable increases in WBC and/or platelet counts. In order to avoid potential complications of excessive leukocytosis (WBC >50,000 cells/mm^3; ANC >20,000 cells/mm^3), a CBC is recommended twice per week during LEUKINE therapy. Monitoring of renal and hepatic function in patients displaying renal or hepatic dysfunction prior to initiation of treatment is recommended at least biweekly during LEUKINE administration. Body weight and hydration status should be carefully monitored during LEUKINE administration.

Drug Interaction Interactions between LEUKINE and other drugs have not been fully evaluated. Drugs which may potentiate the myeloproliferative effects of LEUKINE, such as lithium and corticosteroids, should be used with caution.

Carcinogenesis, Mutagenesis, Impairment of Fertility Animal studies have not been conducted with LEUKINE to evaluate the carcinogenic potential or the effect on fertility.

Pregnancy (Category C) Animal reproduction studies have not been conducted with LEUKINE. It is not known whether LEUKINE can cause fetal harm when administered to a pregnant woman or can affect reproductive capability. LEUKINE should be given to a pregnant woman only if clearly needed.

Nursing Mothers It is not known whether LEUKINE is excreted in human milk. Because many drugs are excreted in human milk, LEUKINE should be administered to a nursing woman only if clearly needed.

Pediatric Use Safety and effectiveness in pediatric patients have not been established; however, available safety data indicate that LEUKINE does not exhibit any greater toxicity in pediatric patients than in adults. A total of 124 pediatric subjects between the ages of 4 months and 18 years have been treated with LEUKINE in clinical trials at doses ranging from 60–1,000 mcg/m^2/day intravenously and 4–1,500 mcg/m^2/day subcutaneously. In 53 pediatric patients enrolled in controlled studies at a dose of 250 mcg/m^2/day by 2-hour IV infusion, the type and frequency of adverse events were comparable to those reported for the adult population. **Liquid solutions containing benzyl alcohol (including LEUKINE Liquid) or lyophilized LEUKINE reconstituted with Bacteriostatic Water for Injection, USP (0.9% benzyl alcohol) should not be administered to neonates** (see WARNINGS).

Geriatric Use In the clinical trials, experience in older patients (age ≥65 years), was limited to the acute myelogenous leukemia (AML) study. Of the 52 patients treated with

Continued on next page

Leukine—Cont.

LEUKINE in this randomized study, 22 patients were age 65–70 years and 30 patients were age 55–64 years. The number of placebo patients in each age group were 13 and 33 patients respectively. This was not an adequate database from which determination of differences in efficacy endpoints or safety assessments could be reliably made and this clinical study was not designed to evaluate difference between these two age groups. Analyses of general trends in safety and efficacy were undertaken and demonstrate similar patterns for older (65–70 yrs) vs younger patients (55–64 yrs). Greater sensitivity of some older individuals cannot be ruled out.

ADVERSE REACTIONS

Autologous and Allogeneic Bone Marrow Transplantation LEUKINE is generally well tolerated. In 3 placebo-controlled studies enrolling a total of 156 patients after autologous BMT or peripheral blood progenitor cell transplantation, events reported in at least 10% of patients who received IV LEUKINE or placebo were as reported at right:
[See first table at top of previous page]
No significant differences were observed between LEUKINE and placebo-treated patients in the type or frequency of laboratory abnormalities, including renal and hepatic parameters. In some patients with preexisting renal or hepatic dysfunction enrolled in uncontrolled clinical trials, administration of LEUKINE has induced elevation of serum creatinine or bilirubin and hepatic enzymes (see WARNINGS). In addition, there was no significant difference in relapse rate and 24 month survival between the LEUKINE and placebo-treated patients.
In the placebo-controlled trial of 109 patients after allogeneic BMT, events reported in at least 10% of patients who received IV LEUKINE or placebo were as reported at right:
[See second table at top of previous page]
There were no significant differences in the incidence or severity of GVHD, relapse rates and survival between the LEUKINE and placebo-treated patients.
Adverse events observed for the patients treated with LEUKINE (sargramostim) in the historically controlled BMT failure study were similar to those reported in the placebo-controlled studies. In addition, headache (26%), pericardial effusion (25%), arthralgia (21%) and myalgia (18%) were also reported in patients treated with LEUKINE in the graft failure study.
In uncontrolled Phase I/II studies with LEUKINE in 215 patients, the most frequent adverse events were fever, asthenia, headache, bone pain, chills and myalgia. These systemic events were generally mild or moderate and were usually prevented or reversed by the administration of analgesics and antipyretics such as acetaminophen. In these uncontrolled trials, other infrequent events reported were dyspnea, peripheral edema, and rash.
Reports of events occurring with marketed LEUKINE include arrhythmia, fainting, eosinophilia, dizziness, hypotension, injection site reactions, pain (including abdominal, back, chest, and joint pain), tachycardia, thrombosis, and transient liver function abnormalities.
In patients with preexisting edema, capillary leak syndrome, pleural and/or pericardial effusion, administration of LEUKINE may aggravate fluid retention (see WARNINGS). Body weight and hydration status should be carefully monitored during LEUKINE administration.
Adverse events observed in pediatric patients in controlled studies were comparable to those observed in adult patients.

Acute Myelogenous Leukemia Adverse events reported in at least 10% of patients who received LEUKINE or placebo were as reported at right:
[See table below]
Nearly all patients reported leukopenia, thrombocytopenia and anemia. The frequency and type of adverse events observed following induction were similar between LEUKINE and placebo groups. The only significant difference in the rates of these adverse events was an increase in skin associated events in the LEUKINE group (p=0.002). No significant differences were observed in laboratory results, renal or hepatic toxicity. No significant differences were observed between the LEUKINE- and placebo-treated patients for adverse events following consolidation. There was no significant difference in response rate or relapse rate.
In a historically controlled study of 86 patients with acute myelogenous leukemia (AML), the LEUKINE treated group exhibited an increased incidence of weight gain (p=0.007), low serum proteins and prolonged prothrombin time (p=0.02) when compared to the control group. Two LEUKINE treated patients had progressive increase in circulating monocytes and promonocytes and blasts in the marrow which reversed when LEUKINE was discontinued. The historical control group exhibited an increased incidence of cardiac events (p=0.018), liver function abnormalities (p=0.008), and neurocortical hemorrhagic events (p=0.025).[15]

OVERDOSAGE

The maximum amount of LEUKINE that can be safely administered in single or multiple doses has not been determined. Doses up to 100 mcg/kg/day (4,000 mcg/m²/day or 16 times the recommended dose) were administered to 4 patients in a Phase I uncontrolled clinical study by continuous IV infusion for 7 to 18 days. Increases in WBC up to 200,000 cells/mm³ were observed. Adverse events reported were dyspnea, malaise, nausea, fever, rash, sinus tachycardia, headache and chills. All these events were reversible after discontinuation of LEUKINE.
In case of overdosage, LEUKINE therapy should be discontinued and the patient carefully monitored for WBC increase and respiratory symptoms.

DOSAGE AND ADMINISTRATION

Neutrophil Recovery Following Chemotherapy in Acute Myelogenous Leukemia The recommended dose is 250 mcg/m²/day administered intravenously over a 4 hour period starting approximately on day 11 or 4 days following the completion of induction chemotherapy, if the day 10 bone marrow is hypoplastic with <5% blasts. If a second cycle of induction chemotherapy is necessary, LEUKINE should be administered approximately 4 days after the completion of chemotherapy if the bone marrow is hypoplastic with <5% blasts. LEUKINE should be continued until an ANC >1500 cells/mm³ for 3 consecutive days or a maximum of 42 days. LEUKINE should be discontinued immediately if leukemic regrowth occurs. If a severe adverse reaction occurs, the dose can be reduced by 50% or temporarily discontinued until the reaction abates.
In order to avoid potential complications of excessive leukocytosis (WBC > 50,000 cells/mm³ or ANC > 20,000 cells/mm³) a CBC with differential is recommended twice per week during LEUKINE therapy. LEUKINE treatment should be interrupted or the dose reduced by half if the ANC exceeds 20,000 cells/mm³.

Mobilization of Peripheral Blood Progenitor Cells The recommended dose is 250 mcg/m²/day administered IV over 24 hours or SC once daily. Dosing should continue at the same dose through the period of PBPC collection. The optimal schedule for PBPC collection has not been established. In clinical studies, collection of PBPC was usually begun by day 5 and performed daily until protocol specified targets were achieved (see CLINICAL EXPERIENCE, Mobilization and Engraftment of PBPC). If WBC > 50,000 cells/mm³, the LEUKINE dose should be reduced by 50%. If adequate numbers of progenitor cells are not collected, other mobilization therapy should be considered.

Post Peripheral Blood Progenitor Cell Transplantation The recommended dose is 250 mcg/m²/day administered IV over 24 hours or SC once daily beginning immediately following infusion of progenitor cells and continuing until an ANC>1500 cells/mm³ for 3 consecutive days is attained.

Myeloid Reconstitution After Autologous or Allogeneic Bone Marrow Transplantation The recommended dose is 250 mcg/m²/day administered IV over a 2-hour period beginning 2 to 4 hours after bone marrow infusion, and not less than 24 hours after the last dose of chemotherapy or radiotherapy. Patients should not receive LEUKINE until the post marrow infusion ANC is less than 500 cells/mm³. LEUKINE should be continued until an ANC >1500 cells/mm³ for 3 consecutive days is attained. If a severe adverse reaction occurs, the dose can be reduced by 50% or temporarily discontinued until the reaction abates. LEUKINE should be discontinued immediately if blast cells appear or disease progression occurs.
In order to avoid potential complications of excessive leukocytosis (WBC > 50,000 cells/mm³, ANC > 20,000 cells/mm³) a CBC with differential is recommended twice per week during LEUKINE therapy. LEUKINE treatment should be interrupted or the dose reduced by 50% if the ANC exceeds 20,000 cells/mm³.

Bone Marrow Transplantation Failure or Engraftment Delay The recommended dose is 250 mcg/m²/day for 14 days as a 2-hour IV infusion. The dose can be repeated after 7 days off therapy if engraftment has not occurred. If engraftment still has not occurred, a third course of 500 mcg/m²/day for 14 days may be tried after another 7 days off therapy. If there is still no improvement, it is unlikely that further dose escalation will be beneficial. If a severe adverse reaction occurs, the dose can be reduced by 50% or temporarily discontinued until the reaction abates. LEUKINE should be discontinued immediately if blast cells appear or disease progression occurs.
In order to avoid potential complications of excessive leukocytosis (WBC > 50,000 cells/mm³, ANC > 20,000 cells/mm³) a CBC with differential is recommended twice per week during LEUKINE therapy. LEUKINE treatment should be interrupted or the dose reduced by half if the ANC exceeds 20,000 cells/mm³.

Preparation of LEUKINE

1. LEUKINE Liquid is formulated as a sterile, preserved (1.1% benzyl alcohol), injectable solution (500 mcg/mL) in a vial. Lyophilized LEUKINE is a sterile, white, preservative-free powder (250 mcg) that requires reconstitution with 1 mL Sterile Water for Injection, USP, or 1 mL Bacteriostatic Water for Injection, USP.
2. LEUKINE Liquid may be stored for up to 20 days at 2–8°C once the vial has been entered. Discard any remaining solution after 20 days.
3. Lyophilized LEUKINE (250 mcg) should be reconstituted aseptically with 1.0 mL of diluent (see below). The contents of vials reconstituted with different diluents should not be mixed together.
   Sterile Water for Injection, USP (without preservative): Lyophilized LEUKINE vials contain no antibacterial preservative, and therefore solutions prepared with Sterile Water for Injection, USP should be administered as soon as possible, and within 6 hours following reconstitution and/or dilution for IV infusion. The vial should not be reentered or reused. Do not save any unused portion for administration more than 6 hours following reconstitution.
   Bacteriostatic Water for Injection, USP (0.9% benzyl alcohol): Reconstituted solutions prepared with Bacteriostatic Water for Injection, USP (0.9% benzyl alcohol) may be stored for up to 20 days at 2–8°C prior to use. Discard reconstituted solution after 20 days. Previously reconstituted solutions mixed with freshly reconstituted solutions must be administered within 6 hours following mixing. **Preparations containing benzyl alcohol (including LEUKINE Liquid and lyophilized LEUKINE reconstituted with Bacteriostatic Water for Injection) should not be used in neonates** (see WARNINGS).
4. During reconstitution of lyophilized LEUKINE the diluent should be directed at the side of the vial and the contents gently swirled to avoid foaming during dissolution. Avoid excessive or vigorous agitation; do not shake.
5. LEUKINE should be used for SC injection without further dilution. Dilution for IV infusion should be performed in 0.9% Sodium Chloride Injection, USP. If the final concentration of LEUKINE is below 10 mcg/mL, Albumin (Human) at a final concentration of 0.1% should be added to the saline prior to addition of LEUKINE to prevent adsorption to the components of the drug delivery system. To obtain a final concentration of 0.1% Albumin (Human), add 1 mg Albumin (Human) per 1 mL 0.9% Sodium Chloride Injection, USP (e.g., use 1 mL 5% Albumin [Human] in 50 mL 0.9% Sodium Chloride Injection, USP).
6. An in-line membrane filter should NOT be used for intravenous infusion of LEUKINE.
7. Store LEUKINE Liquid and reconstituted lyophilized LEUKINE solutions under refrigeration at 2–8°C (36–46°F); DO NOT FREEZE.
8. In the absence of compatibility and stability information, no other medication should be added to infusion solutions containing LEUKINE. Use only 0.9% Sodium Chloride Injection, USP to prepare IV infusion solutions.
9. Aseptic technique should be employed in the preparation of all LEUKINE solutions. To assure correct concentration following reconstitution, care should be exercised to eliminate any air bubbles from the needle hub of the syringe used to prepare the diluent. Parenteral drug products should be inspected visually for particulate matter and discoloration prior to administration whenever solution and container permit.

Percent of AML Patients Reporting Events

Events by Body System	LEUKINE (n=52)	Placebo (n=47)
Body, General		
Fever (no infection)	81	74
Infection	65	68
Weight loss	37	28
Weight gain	8	21
Chills	19	26
Allergy	12	15
Sweats	6	13
Digestive System		
Nausea	58	55
Liver	77	83
Diarrhea	52	53
Vomiting	46	34
Stomatitis	42	43
Anorexia	13	11
Abdominal distention	4	13
Skin and Appendages		
Skin	77	45
Alopecia	37	51
Metabolic/Nutritional Disorder		
Metabolic	58	49
Edema	25	23
Respiratory System		
Pulmonary	48	64
Hemic and Lymphatic System		
Coagulation	19	21
Cardiovascular System		
Hemorrhage	29	43
Hypertension	25	32
Cardiac	23	32
Hypotension	13	26
Urogenital System		
GU	50	57
Nervous System		
Neuro-clinical	42	53
Neuro-motor	25	26
Neuro-psych	15	26
Neuro-sensory	6	11

HOW SUPPLIED

LEUKINE Liquid is available in vials containing 500 mcg/mL (2.8×10^6 IU/mL) sargramostim. Lyophilized LEUKINE is available in vials containing 250 mcg (1.4×10^6 IU/vial) sargramostim. Each dosage form is supplied as follows:

Carton of 5 vials of lyophilized LEUKINE 250 mcg (NDC 50419-002-33).

Carton of 5 multiple-dose vials; each vial contains 1 mL of preserved 500 mcg/mL LEUKINE Liquid (NDC 50419-050-30).

STORAGE

LEUKINE should be refrigerated at 2–8°C (36–46°F). Do not freeze or shake. Do not use beyond the expiration date printed on the vial.

REFERENCES

1. Metcalf D. The molecular biology and functions of the granulocyte-macrophage colony-stimulating factors. Blood 1986; 67(2):257–267.
2. Park LS, Friend D, Gillis S, Urdal DL. Characterization of the cell surface receptor for human granulocyte/macrophage colony stimulating factor. J Exp Med 1986; 164: 251–262.
3. Grabstein KH, Urdal DL, Tushinski RJ, *et al.* Induction of macrophage tumoricidal activity by granulocyte-macrophage colony-stimulating factors. Science 1986; 232: 506–508.
4. Reed SG, Nathan CF, Pihl DL, *et al.* Recombinant granulocyte/macrophage colony-stimulating factor activates macrophages to inhibit *Trypanosoma cruzi* and release hydrogen peroxide. J Exp Med 1987; 166:1734–1746.
5. Data on file Berlex Laboratories, Inc. Richmond, CA
6. Rowe JM, Andersen JW, Mazza JJ, *et al.* A randomized placebo-controlled phase III study of granulocyte-macrophage colony-stimulating factor in adult patients (>55 to 70 years of age) with acute myelogenous leukemia: a study of the Eastern Cooperative Oncology Group (E1490). Blood 1995; 86(2):457–462.
7. Nemunaitis J, Rabinowe SN, Singer JW, *et al.* Recombinant human granulocyte-macrophage colony-stimulating factor after autologous bone marrow transplantation for lymphoid malignancy: Pooled results of a randomized, double-blind, placebo controlled trial. NEJM 1991; 324(25):1773–1778.
8. Nemunaitis J, Singer JW, Buckner CD, *et al.* Use of recombinant human granulocyte-macrophage colony stimulating factor in autologous bone marrow transplantation for lymphoid malignancies. Blood 1988; 72(2): 834–836.
9. Nemunaitis J, Singer JW, Buckner CD, *et al.* Long-term follow-up of patients who received recombinant human granulocyte-macrophage colony stimulating factor after autologous bone marrow transplantation for lymphoid malignancy. BMT 1991; 7:49–52.
10. Goris RJA, Boekhorst TPA, Nuytinck JKS, *et al.* Multiple organ failure: Generalized auto-destructive inflammation? Arch Surg 1985; 120:1109–1115.
11. Bunn P, Crowley J, Kelly K, *et al.* Chemoradiotherapy with or without granulocyte-macrophage colony-stimulating factor in the treatment of limited-stage small-cell lung cancer: a prospective phase III randomized study of the southwest oncology group. JCO 1995; 13(7): 1632–1641.
12. Herrmann F, Schulz G, Lindemann A, *et al.* Yeast-expressed granulocyte-macrophage colony-stimulating factor in cancer patients: A phase Ib clinical study. In Behring Institute Research Communications, Colony Stimulating Factors-CSF. International Symposium, Garmisch-Partenkirchen, West Germany. 1988; 83: 107–118.
13. Estey EH, Dixon D, Kantarjian H, *et al.* Treatment of poor-prognosis, newly diagnosed acute myeloid leukemia with Ara-C and recombinant human granulocyte-macrophage colony-stimulating factor. Blood 1990; 75(9):1766–1769.
14. Vadhan-Raj S, Keating M, LeMaistre A, *et al.* Effects of recombinant human granulocyte-macrophage colony-stimulating factor in patients with myelodysplastic syndromes. NEJM 1987; 317:1545–1552.
15. Buchner T, Hiddemann W, Koenigsmann M, *et al.* Recombinant human granulocyte-macrophage colony stimulating factor after chemotherapy in patients with acute myeloid leukemia at higher age or after relapse. Blood 1991; 78(5):1190–1197.
16. Blazar BR, Kersey JH, McGlave PB, *et al.* *In vivo* administration of recombinant human granulocyte/macrophage colony-stimulating factor in acute lymphoblastic leukemia patients receiving purged autografts. Blood 1989; 73(3):849–857.

Berlex Laboratories, Inc. U.S. Patent Nos. 5,391,485; 5,393,870; and 5,229,496. Licensed under Research Corporation Technologies U.S. Patent No. 5,602,007, and under Novartis Corporation U.S. Patent Nos. 5,942,221; 5,908,763; 5,895,646; 5,891,429; and 5,720,952.

Manufactured by:
BERLEX™
Berlex Laboratories, Inc., Richmond, CA 94804
U.S. License No. 1650
6052400 Revised June 2002

Berna Products, Corp. an Acambis Company

4216 PONCE DE LEON BLVD.
CORAL GABLES, FL 33146

Direct Inquiries to:
Gregory Koppel
(305) 443-2900
(800) 533-5899

For Medical Information Contact: Andres Murai, Jr
In Emergencies: Andres Murai, Jr.
(305) 443-2900
(800) 533-5899

VIVOTIF® ℞

[*vī-vō-tĭf*]
Typhoid Vaccine Live Oral Ty21a

DESCRIPTION

Vivotif® (Typhoid Vaccine Live Oral Ty21a) is a live attenuated vaccine for oral administration only. The vaccine contains the attenuated strain *Salmonella typhi* Ty21a (1,2).

Vivotif® is manufactured by the Berna Biotech Ltd. The vaccine strain is grown in fermentors under controlled conditions in medium containing a digest of yeast extract, an acid digest of casein, dextrose and galactose. The bacteria are collected by centrifugation, mixed with a stabilizer containing sucrose, ascorbic acid and amino acids, and lyophilized. The lyophilized bacteria are mixed with lactose and magnesium stearate and filled into gelatin capsules which are coated with an organic solution to render them resistant to dissolution in stomach acid. The enteric-coated, salmon/white capsules are then packaged in 4-capsule blisters for distribution. The contents of each enteric-coated capsule are shown in Table 1.

Table 1: Contents of one enteric-coated capsule of Vivotif® (typhoid Vaccine Live Oral Ty21a)

Viable *S. typhi* Ty21a	$2\text{-}6 \times 10^9$ colony-forming units*
Non-viable *S. typhi* Ty21a	$5\text{-}50 \times 10^9$ bacterial cells
Sucrose	26-130 mg
Ascorbic acid	1-5 mg
Amino acid mixture	1.4-7 mg
Lactose	100-180 mg
Magnesium stearate	3.6-4.4 mg

*Vaccine potency (viable cell counts per capsule) is determined by inoculation of agar plates with appropriate dilutions of the vaccine suspended in physiological saline.

CLINICAL PHARMACOLOGY

Salmonella typhi is the etiological agent of typhoid fever, an acute, febrile enteric disease. Typhoid fever continues to be an important disease in many parts of the world. Travelers entering infected areas are at risk of contracting typhoid fever following the ingestion of contaminated food or water. Typhoid fever is considered to be endemic in most areas of Central and South America, the African continent, the Near East and the Middle East, Southeast Asia and the Indian subcontinent (3). There are approximately 500 cases of typhoid fever per year diagnosed in the United States (4). In 62% of these patients (data from 1975–1984) the disease was acquired outside of the United States while in 38% of the patients the disease was acquired within the United States (5). Of 340 cases acquired in the United States between 1977 and 1979, 23% of the cases were associated with typhoid carriers, 24% were due to food outbreaks, 23% were associated with the ingestion of contaminated food or water, 6% due to household contact with an infected person and 4% following exposure to *S. typhi* in a laboratory setting (6).

The majority of typhoid cases respond favorably to antibiotic therapy. However, the emergence of multi-drug resistant strains has greatly complicated therapy and cases of typhoid fever that are treated with ineffective drugs can be fatal (7). Approximately 2-4% of acute typhoid cases result in the development of a chronic carrier state (8). These non-symptomatic carriers are the natural reservoir for *S. typhi* and can serve to maintain the disease in its endemic state or to directly infect individuals (3).

Virulent strains of *S. typhi* upon ingestion are able to pass through the stomach acid barrier, colonize the intestinal tract, penetrate the lumen and enter the lymphatic system and blood stream, thereby causing disease. One possible mechanism by which disease may be prevented is by evoking a local immune response in the intestinal tract. Such local immunity may be induced by oral ingestion of a live attenuated strain of *S. typhi* undergoing an aborted infection. The ability of *S. typhi* to cause disease and to induce a protective immune response is dependent upon the bacteria possessing a complete lipopolysaccharide (1). The *S. typhi* Ty21a vaccine strain, by virtue of a reduction in enzymes essential for lipopolysaccharide biosynthesis, is restricted in its ability to produce complete lipopolysaccharide (1,2). However, a sufficient quantity of complete lipopolysaccharide is synthesized to evoke a protective immune response. Despite low levels of lipopolysaccharide synthesis, the cells lyse before regaining a virulent phenotype due to the intracellular build-up of intermediates during lipopolysaccharide synthesis (1,2).

Results from clinical studies indicate that adults and children greater than 6 years of age may be protected against typhoid fever following the oral ingestion of 4 doses of Vivotif ® (Typhoid Vaccine Live Oral Ty21a). The efficacy of the *S. typhi* Ty21a strain has been evaluated in a series of randomized, double-blind, controlled field trials. Suspected typhoid cases, detected by passive surveillance, were confirmed bacteriologically either by blood or bone marrow culture. The first trial was performed in Alexandria, Egypt with a study population of 32,388 children aged 6 to 7 years. Three doses of vaccine, in the form of a freshly reconstituted suspension administered after ingestion of 1 g of bicarbonate, were given on alternate days. Immunization resulted in a 95% decrease [95% confidence interval (CI) = 77%-99%] in the incidence of typhoid fever over a 3-year period of surveillance (9). A series of field trials were subsequently performed in Santiago, Chile to evaluate efficacy when the vaccine strain was administered in the form of an acid-resistant enteric-coated capsule. The initial trial involved 82,543 school-aged children, and compared 1 or 2 doses of vaccine given one week apart. After 24 months of surveillance vaccine efficacy was 29% (95% CI = 4%-47%) for the single dose schedule and 59% (95% CI = 41%-71%) for the 2-dose schedule (10). A further field trial was performed in Santiago, Chile involving 109,594 school-aged children (11). Three doses of enteric-coated capsules were administered either on alternate days (short immunization schedule) or 21 days apart (long immunization schedule). Following 36 months of surveillance vaccination resulted in a 67% (95% CI = 47%-79%) decrease in the incidence of typhoid fever in the short immunization schedule group and a 49% reduction (95% CI = 24%-66%) in the long immunization schedule group. After 48 months of surveillance the short immunization schedule resulted in a 69% (95% CI = 55%-80%) decrease in typhoid fever (12). An undiminished level of protection was observed during the fifth year of surveillance. A field trial was next conducted in Santiago, Chile to determine the relative efficacy of 2, 3 and 4 doses of enteric-coated vaccine administered on alternate days to school-aged children. Relative vaccine efficacy as determined by comparison of disease incidence within the three vaccinated groups was highest for the four dose regimen (13). The incidence of typhoid fever per 105 study subjects was 160.5 (95% CI = 130-191) for the three dose regimen versus 95.8 (95% CI = 71-121) for the four dose regimen ($p<0.004$). An additional field trial to determine vaccine efficacy was conducted in Plaju, Indonesia involving 20,543 individuals approximately 3 to 44 years of age (14). Due to logistical considerations three doses of enteric-coated capsules were administered at weekly intervals, a schedule known to provide suboptimal protection (11). After 30 months of surveillance vaccine efficacy for all age groups was 42% (95% CI = 23%-57%).

Vaccine organisms can be shed transiently in the stool of vaccine recipients (16). However, secondary transmission of vaccine organisms has not been documented. Ty21a has not been isolated from blood cultures following immunization. At present, the precise mechanism(s) by which Vivotif® confers protection against typhoid fever is unknown. However, it is known that immunization of adult subjects can elicit a humoral anti-*S. typhi* LPS antibody response. Taking advantage of this fact, the seroconversion rate (defined as a ³0.15 increase in optical density units over baseline determined in an ELISA) was compared in an open study between adults living in an endemic area (Chile) and non-endemic areas (United States and Switzerland) after the ingestion of 3 doses of vaccine. Comparable seroconversion rates were seen between these groups (15). *S. typhi* Ty21a cultured in medium not containing BHI induced an anti-*S. typhi* LPS antibody response comparable to that obtained with vaccine organisms cultured in medium containing BHI (15). Challenge studies in North American volunteers have shown that the Ty21a strain is capable of providing significant protection to an experimental challenge of *S. typhi* (16). Because of the very low incidence of typhoid fever in United States citizens, efficacy studies are not currently feasible in this population. However, the above observations support the expectation that Vivotif® will provide protection to recipients from non-typhoid endemic areas such as the United States.

INDICATIONS AND USAGE

Vivotif® (Typhoid Vaccine Live Oral Ty21a) is indicated for immunization of adults and children greater than 6 years of age against disease caused by *Salmonella typhi*. Routine typhoid vaccination is not recommended in the United States of America. Selective immunization against typhoid fever is recommended for the following groups: 1) travelers to areas in which there is a recognized risk of exposure to *S. typhi*, 2) persons with intimate exposure (e.g. household contact) to a *S. typhi* carrier, and 3) microbiology laboratorians who work frequently with *S. typhi* (7). There is no evidence to support the use of typhoid vaccine to control common source outbreaks, disease following natural disasters or in persons attending rural summer camps.

Not all recipients of Vivotif® will be fully protected against typhoid fever. Vaccinated individuals should continue to take personal precautions against exposure to typhoid organisms. The vaccine will not afford protection against spe-

Continued on next page

Vivotif—Cont.

cies of *Salmonella* other than *Salmonella typhi* or other bacteria that cause enteric disease. The vaccine is not suitable for treatment of acute infections with *S. typhi*.

CONTRAINDICATIONS

Hypersensitivity to any component of the vaccine or the enteric-coated capsule. The vaccine should not be administered to persons during an acute febrile illness. Safety of the vaccine has not been demonstrated in persons deficient in their ability to mount a humoral or cell-mediated immune response, due to either a congenital or acquired immunodeficient state including treatment with immunosuppressive or antimitotic drugs. The vaccine should not be administered to these persons regardless of benefits.

WARNINGS

Vivotif® (Typhoid Vaccine Live Oral Ty21a) is not to be taken during an acute gastrointestinal illness. The vaccine should not be administered to individuals receiving sulfonamides and antibiotics since these agents may be active against the vaccine strain and prevent a sufficient degree of multiplication to occur in order to induce a protective immune response. Postpone taking the vaccine if persistent diarrhea or vomiting is occurring. Unless a complete immunization schedule is followed, an optimum immune response may not be achieved. Not all recipients of Vivotif® will be fully protected against typhoid fever. Vaccinated individuals should continue to take personal precautions against exposure to typhoid organisms, i.e. travelers should take all necessary precautions to avoid contact or ingestion of potentially contaminated food or water.

Drug-Interactions

Several anti-malaria drugs, such as mefloquine, chloroquine and proguanil (not approved for use in US) possess antibacterial activity which may interfere with the immunogenicity of Vivotif® (17,18). To determine the effect of these anti-malaria drugs on the humoral IgG or IgA anti-*S. typhi* immune response, healthy adult subjects were given mefloquine (250 mg at weekly intervals; N = 30) chloroquine (500 mg at weekly intervals; N = 30) or proguanil (200 mg daily; N = 30) together with the *S. typhi* Ty21a vaccine strain (19). Concomitant treatment with mefloquine or chloroquine did not result in a significant reduction in the serum anti-*S. typhi* immune response compared to subjects receiving vaccine strain only (N = 45). The simultaneous administration of proguanil did effect a significant decrease in the immune response rate. These findings indicate that mefloquine and chloroquine can be administered together with Vivotif®. Proguanil should be administered only if 10 days or more have elapsed since the final dose of Vivotif® was ingested. The concomitant administration of oral polio vaccine or yellow fever vaccine does not suppress the immune response elicited by the Ty21a vaccine strain (19). There are no data regarding simultaneous administration of other parenteral vaccines or immunoglobulins with Vivotif®.

PRECAUTIONS

General

The health care provider should take all necessary precautions to ensure the safe and effective use of the vaccine. Patients should be questioned about previous reactions to this or similar products. The previous immunization history of the patient and current antibiotic usage should be obtained by the health care provider.

Information for Patients

It is essential that all 4 doses of vaccine be taken at the prescribed alternate day interval to obtain a maximal protective immune response. Vaccine potency is dependent upon storage under refrigeration [between 2°C and 8°C (35.6°F-46.4°F)]. The vaccine should be stored under refrigeration at all times. It is essential to replace unused vaccine in the refrigerator between doses. The vaccine capsule should be swallowed approximately 1 hour before a meal with a cold or luke-warm [temperature not to exceed body temperature, e.g., 37 °C (98.6 °F)] drink. Care should be taken not to chew the vaccine capsule. The vaccine capsule should be swallowed as soon after placing in the mouth as possible.

Not all recipients of Vivotif® (Typhoid Vaccine Live Oral Ty21a) will be fully protected against typhoid fever. Travelers should take all necessary precautions to avoid contact or ingestion of potentially contaminated food or water. Several anti-malaria drugs, such as mefloquine, chloroquine and proguanil (not approved for use in US) possess antibacterial activity which may interfere with the immunogenicity of Vivotif®. Clinical results (see Warnings – Drug-Interactions) indicate that mefloquine and chloroquine can be administered together with Vivotif®. Proguanil should be administered only if 10 days or more have elapsed since the final dose of Vivotif® was ingested. Any serious adverse reactions related to the administration of the vaccine should be reported to your health care provider. You may also report an adverse reaction directly to the Vaccine Adverse Event Reporting System (1–800–822–7967) (20). Your health care provider should inform you of the benefits and risks of the vaccine, the importance of taking all 4 capsules in the correct schedule, and the importance of proper storage temperature of the capsules.

Carcinogenesis, Mutagenesis, Impairment of Fertility

Long-term studies in animals with Vivotif® have not been performed to evaluate carcinogenic potential, mutagenic potential or impairment of fertility.

Pregnancy
Category C

Animal reproduction studies have not been conducted with Vivotif®. It is not known whether Vivotif® can cause fetal harm when administered to pregnant women or can affect reproduction capacity. Vivotif® should be given to a pregnant woman only if clearly needed.

Nursing Mothers

There is no data to warrant the use of this product in nursing mothers. It is not known if Vivotif® is excreted in human milk.

Pediatric Use

The safety and efficacy of Vivotif® has not been established in children under 6 years of age. This product is not indicated for use in children under 6 years of age.

ADVERSE REACTIONS

More than 1.4 million doses of Ty21a have been administered in controlled clinical trials and more than 150 million doses of Vivotif® (Typhoid Vaccine Live Oral Ty21a) have been marketed world-wide. Active surveillance for adverse reactions of enteric-coated capsules was performed in a pilot study (21) and in a subgroup of a large field trial (14) involving a total of 483 individuals receiving three vaccine doses. The overall symptom rates from both studies when vaccinated with capsules were combined and shown to be: abdominal pain (6.4%), nausea (5.8%), headache (4.8%), fever (3.3%), diarrhea (2.9%), vomiting (1.5%) and skin rash (1.0%). Only the incidence of nausea occured at a statistically higher frequency in the vaccinated group as compared to the placebo group (14). Administration of vaccine doses more than 5-fold higher than the currently recommended dose caused only mild reactions in an open study involving 155 healthy adult males (16).

Post-marketing surveillance has revealed that adverse reactions are infrequent and mild (17). Adverse reactions reported to the manufacturer during 1991–1995, during which time over 60 million doses (capsules) were administered, included: diarrhea (N = 45), abdominal pain (N = 42), nausea (N = 35), fever (N = 34), headache (N = 26), skin rash (N = 26), vomiting (N = 18), or urticaria in the trunk and/or extremities (N = 13). One isolated, non-fatal anaphylactic shock considered to be an allergic reaction to the vaccine was reported.

DOSAGE AND ADMINISTRATION

One capsule is to be swallowed approximately 1 hour before a meal with a cold or luke-warm [temperature not to exceed body temperature, e.g., 37 °C (98.6 °F)] drink on alternate days, e.g., days 1, 3, 5 and 7. Immunization (ingestion of all 4 doses of Vivotif® (Typhoid Vaccine Live Oral Ty21a) should be completed at least 1 week prior to potential exposure to *S. typhi*.

The blister containing the vaccine capsules should be inspected to ensure that the foil seal and capsules are intact. The vaccine capsule should not be chewed and should be swallowed as soon after placing in the mouth as possible. A complete immunization schedule is the ingestion of 4 vaccine capsules as described above.

Re-immunization

The optimum booster schedule for Vivotif® has not been determined. Efficacy has been shown to persist for at least 5 years. Further, there is no experience with Vivotif® as a booster in persons previously immunized with parenteral typhoid vaccine. It is recommended that a re-immunization dose consisting of four vaccine capsules taken on alternate days be given every 5 years under conditions of repeated or continued exposure to typhoid fever (7).

HOW SUPPLIED

A single foil blister contains 4 doses of vaccine in a single package.

STORAGE

Vivotif® (Typhoid Vaccine Live Oral Ty21a) is not stable when exposed to ambient temperatures. Vivotif® should therefore be shipped and stored between 2 °C and 8 °C (35.6 °F-46.4 °F). Each package of vaccine shows an expiration date. This expiration date is valid only if the product has been maintained at 2 °C-8 °C (35.6 °F-46.4 °F).

Manufactured by
Berna Biotech Ltd, Berne, Switzerland
US-Licence No. 1632
Distributed by
Berna Products Corp., Coral Gables, FL 33146
℞ only

REFERENCES

1. Germanier R., E. Fürer. Isolation and characterisation of Gal E mutant Ty21a of *Salmonella typhi*: a candidate strain for a live, oral typhoid vaccine. J. Infect. Dis. 131: 553-558, 1975.
2. Germanier R., E. Fürer. Characteristics of the attenuated oral vaccine strain *S. typhi* Ty21a. Develop. Biol. Standard 53: 3-7, 1983.
3. Miller S.I., E.L. Hohmann, D.A. Pegues. *Salmonella* (including *Salmonella typhi*). In: Principles and practice of infectious diseases. G.L. Mandell, J.E. Bennett, R. Dolin (ed.) fourth edition, Churchill Livingstone Inc. 2013-2033, 1995.
4. Centers for Disease Control. Summary of notifiable diseases, United States 1995. MMWR 44 (Supplement), 1996.
5. Ryan C.A., N.T. Hargrett-Bean, P.A. Blake. *Salmonella typhi* infections in the United States, 1975-1984: Increasing role of foreign travel. Rev. Infect. Dis. 11: 1-8, 1989.
6. Taylor D.N., R.A. Pollard, P.A. Blake. Typhoid in the United States and the Risk to the International Traveler. J. Infect. Dis. 148: 599-602, 1983.
7. Recommendations of the Advisory Committee on Immunization Practices (ACIP): Typhoid Immunization. MMWR 43 (RR-14), 1994.
8. Ames W.R., M. Robbins. Age and sex as factors in the development of the typhoid carrier state, and a model for estimating carrier prevalence. Am. J. Public Health 33: 221-230, 1943.
9. Wahdan M.H., C. Sérié, Y. Cerisier, S. Sallam, R. Germanier. A controlled field trial of live Salmonella typhi strain Ty21a oral vaccine against typhoid: three-year results. J. Infect. Dis. 145: 292-296, 1982.
10. Black R.E., M.M. Levine, C. Ferreccio, M.L. Clements, C. Lanata, J. Rooney, R. Germanier, Chilean Typhoid Committee. Efficacy of one or two doses of Ty21a *Salmonella typhi* vaccine in enteric-coated capsules in a controlled field trial. Vaccine 8: 81-84, 1990.
11. Levine M.M., C. Ferreccio, R.E. Black, R. Germanier, Chilean Typhoid Committee. Large-Scale Field Trial of Ty21a Typhoid Vaccine Live Oral Ty21a in Enteric-Coated Capsule Formulation. Lancet 1: 1049-1052, 1987.
12. Levine M.M., C. Ferreccio, R.E. Black, C.O. Tacket, R. Germanier, Chilean Typhoid Committee. Progress in vaccines against typhoid fever. Rev. Infect. Dis. 11 (Supplement 3): S552-S567, 1989.
13. Ferreccio C., M.M. Levine, H. Rodriguez, R. Contreras, Chilean Typhoid Committee. Comparative efficacy of two, three, or four doses of Ty21a live oral typhoid vaccine in enteric-coated capsules: a field trial in endemic area. J. Infect. Dis. 159: 766-769, 1989.
14. Simanjuntak C.H., F.P. Paleologo, N.H. Punjabi, R. Darmowigoto, Soeprawoto, H. Totosudirjo, P. Haryanto, E. Suprijanto, N.D. Witham, S.L. Hoffman. Oral immunisation against typhoid fever in Indonesia with Ty21a vaccine. Lancet 338: 1055-1059, 1991.
15. Data on File, Swiss Serum and Vaccine Institute Berne, Switzerland.
16. Gilman R.H., R.B. Hornick, W.E. Woodward, H.L. DuPont, M.J. Snyder, M.M. Levine, J.P. Libonati. Evaluation of a UDP-glucose-4-epimeraseless mutant of *Salmonella typhi* as a live oral vaccine. J. Infect. Dis. 136: 717-723, 1977.
17. Cryz S.J. Jr., Post-marketing experience with live oral Ty21a Vaccine. Lancet; 341: 49-50, 1993. Data on File, Swiss Serum and Vaccine Institute Berne, Switzerland.
18. Horowitz H., CA. Carbonaro, Inhibition of the *Salmonella typhi* oral vaccine strain Ty21a, by mefloquine and chloroquine. J. Infect. Dis. 166: 1462-1464, 1992.
19. Kollaritsch H., J.U. Que, C. Kunz, G. Wiedermann, C. Herzog, S.J. Cryz Jr. Safety and immunogenicity of live oral cholera and typhoid vaccines administered alone or in combination with anti-malarial drugs, oral polio vaccine or yellow fever vaccine. J. Infect. Dis. 175: 871-875, 1997.
20. Vaccine Adverse Event Reporting System – United States. MMWR 39: 730-733, 1990.
21. Levine M.M., R.E. Black, C. Ferreccio, M.L. Clements, C. Lanata, J. Rooney, R. Gemanier. The efficacy of attenuated *Salmonella typhi* oral vaccine strain Ty21a evaluated in controlled field trials. In: Development of Vaccines and Drugs against Diarrhea. 11th Noble Conference, Stockholm, 1985, p. 90-101. J. Holmgren, A. Lindberg and R. Möllby (eds.), Studentlitteratur, Lund, Sweden, 1986.

Version:
March 2003

Shown in Product Identification Guide, page 309

Bertek Pharmaceuticals, Inc.

for further product information see Mylan Bertek Pharmaceuticals Inc.

Beutlich LP Pharmaceuticals

1541 SHIELDS DRIVE
WAUKEGAN, IL 60085-8304

Direct Inquiries to:
847-473-1100
800-238-8542
FAX 847-473-1122
E-mail beutlich@beutlich.com
World Wide Web http://www.beutlich.com

HURRICAINE® TOPICAL ANESTHETIC — OTC

COMPOSITION

HURRICAINE contains 20% benzocaine in a flavored, water soluble polyethylene glycol base.

PACKAGING AVAILABLE

Gel
1 oz. Jar Wild Cherry NDC #0283-0871-31
1 oz. Jar Fresh Mint NDC #0283-0998-31
1 oz. Jar Pina Colada NDC #0283-0886-31
1 oz. Jar Watermelon NDC #0283-0293-31
1/6 oz. Tube Wild Cherry NDC #0283-0871-75
Liquid
1 fl. oz. Jar Wild Cherry NDC #0283-0569-31
1 fl. oz. Jar Pina Colada NDC #0283-1886-31
.25 ml Swab Applicator Wild Cherry NDC #0283-0569-01

5 mL Snap N Go tubes NDC #0283-0569-70
Spray
2 oz. Aerosol Wild Cherry NDC #0283-0679-02
Spray Kit
2 oz. Aerosol Wild Cherry NDC #0283-0679-60 with 200 Disposable Extension Tubes

(See PDR For Nonprescription Drugs and Dietary Supplements)

PERIDIN-C® **OTC**

COMPOSITION Each orange colored sugar free tablet contains 2 popular antioxidants; Vitamin C and Bioflavonoids.
Ascorbic Acid 200 mg.
Hesperidin Complex 150 mg.
Hesperidin Methyl Chalcone 50 mg. F.D. & C. #6.

DOSAGE 1 tablet daily or as directed.

HOW SUPPLIED In bottles of:
100 tablets #0283-0597-01
500 tablets #0283-0597-05

Biogen Idec

14 CAMBRIDGE CENTER
CAMBRIDGE, MA 02142

Direct Inquiries to:
AMEVIVE Customer Service:
Tel: 866-263-8483
Fax: 866-420-8888
AVONEX Customer Service:
Tel: 800-456-2255
Fax: 617-679-8100
RITUXAN Customer Service:
Tel: 800-821-8590
ZEVALIN Customer Service:
Tel: 877-433-4332

AMEVIVE® ℞
[ă' mē-vēv]
(alefacept)

DESCRIPTION
AMEVIVE® (alefacept) is an immunosuppressive dimeric fusion protein that consists of the extracellular CD2-binding portion of the human leukocyte function antigen-3 (LFA-3) linked to the Fc (hinge, C_H2 and C_H3 domains) portion of human IgG1. Alefacept is produced by recombinant DNA technology in a Chinese Hamster Ovary (CHO) mammalian cell expression system. The molecular weight of alefacept is 91.4 kilodaltons.
AMEVIVE® is supplied as a sterile, white-to-off-white, preservative-free, lyophilized powder for parenteral administration. After reconstitution with 0.6 mL of the supplied Sterile Water for Injection, USP, the solution of AMEVIVE® is clear, with a pH of approximately 6.9.
AMEVIVE® is available in two formulations. AMEVIVE® for intramuscular injection contains 15 mg alefacept per 0.5 mL of reconstituted solution. AMEVIVE® for intravenous injection contains 7.5 mg alefacept per 0.5 mL of reconstituted solution. Both formulations also contain 12.5 mg sucrose, 5.0 mg glycine, 3.6 mg sodium citrate dihydrate, and 0.06 mg citric acid monohydrate per 0.5 mL.

CLINICAL PHARMACOLOGY
AMEVIVE® interferes with lymphocyte activation by specifically binding to the lymphocyte antigen, CD2, and inhibiting LFA-3/CD2 interaction. Activation of T lymphocytes involving the interaction between LFA-3 on antigen-presenting cells and CD2 on T lymphocytes plays a role in the pathophysiology of chronic plaque psoriasis. The majority of T lymphocytes in psoriatic lesions are of the memory effector phenotype characterized by the presence of the CD45RO marker[1], express activation markers (e.g., CD25, CD69) and release inflammatory cytokines, such as interferon γ.
AMEVIVE® also causes a reduction in subsets of CD2+ T lymphocytes (primarily CD45RO+), presumably by bridging between CD2 on target lymphocytes and immunoglobulin Fc receptors on cytotoxic cells, such as natural killer cells. Treatment with AMEVIVE® results in a reduction in circulating total CD4+ and CD8+ T lymphocyte counts. CD2 is also expressed at low levels on the surface of natural killer cells and certain bone marrow B lymphocytes. Therefore, the potential exists for AMEVIVE® to affect the activation and numbers of cells other than T lymphocytes. In clinical studies of AMEVIVE®, minor changes in the numbers of circulating cells other than T lymphocytes have been observed.

Pharmacokinetics
In patients with moderate to severe plaque psoriasis, following a 7.5 mg intravenous (IV) administration, the mean volume of distribution of alefacept was 94 mL/kg, the mean clearance was 0.25 mL/h/kg, and the mean elimination half-life was approximately 270 hours. Following an intramuscular (IM) injection, bioavailability was 63%.

Table 2. Percentage of Patients Responding to the First Course of Treatment in Study 1 (the Intravenous Study) and Study 2 (the Intramuscular Study) Two Weeks Post Dosing

Treatment response: (reduction in disease activity from baseline)	Study 1 Placebo (N=186)	Study 1 AMEVIVE® 7.5 mg IV (N=367)[1]	Study 1 Difference (95% CI)	Study 2 Placebo (N=168)	Study 2 AMEVIVE® 15 mg IM (N=166)	Study 2 Difference (95% CI)
≥75% reduction PASI	4%	14%	10* (6, 15)	5%	21%	16* (9, 23)
≥50% reduction PASI	10%	38%	28* (22, 35)	18%	42%	24* (14, 33)
PGA "almost clear" or "clear"	4%	11%	7⁺(3, 12)	5%	14%	9$(3, 15)

[1]Cohorts 1 and 2 are combined.
*p values <0.001
⁺p value 0.004
$p value 0.006

The pharmacokinetics of alefacept in pediatric patients have not been studied. The effects of renal or hepatic impairment on the pharmacokinetics of alefacept have not been studied.

Pharmacodynamics
At doses tested in clinical trials, AMEVIVE® therapy resulted in a dose-dependent decrease in circulating total lymphocytes[2]. This reduction predominantly affected the memory effector subset of the CD4+ and CD8+ T lymphocyte compartments (CD4+CD45RO+ and CD8+CD45RO+), the predominant phenotype in psoriatic lesions. Circulating naïve T lymphocyte and natural killer cell counts appeared to be only minimally susceptible to AMEVIVE® treatment, while circulating B lymphocyte counts appeared not to be affected by AMEVIVE® (see **ADVERSE REACTIONS, Effect on Lymphocyte Counts**).

CLINICAL STUDIES
AMEVIVE® was evaluated in two randomized, double-blind, placebo-controlled studies in adults with chronic (≥1 year) plaque psoriasis and a minimum body surface area involvement of 10% who were candidates for or had previously received systemic therapy or phototherapy. Each course consisted of once-weekly administration for 12 weeks (IV for Study 1, IM for Study 2) of placebo or AMEVIVE®. Patients could receive concomitant low potency topical steroids. Concomitant phototherapy or systemic therapy was not allowed.
In Study 1, patients were randomized to receive one or two courses of AMEVIVE® 7.5 mg administered by IV bolus. The first and second courses in the two-course cohort were separated by at least a 12-week post-dosing interval. A total of 553 patients were randomized into three cohorts (Table 1).

Table 1. Treatment Group and Number of Patients Dosed in Study 1

	Course 1 (No. of patients)	Course 2 (No. of patients)
Cohort 1	AMEVIVE® (183)	AMEVIVE® (154)
Cohort 2	AMEVIVE® (184)	Placebo (142)
Cohort 3	Placebo (186)	AMEVIVE®(153)

Study 2 provided a basis for comparison of patients treated with either 10 mg or 15 mg AMEVIVE® IM. One hundred seventy-three patients were randomized to receive 10 mg of AMEVIVE® IM, 166 to receive 15 mg of AMEVIVE® IM, and 168 to receive placebo.
In Studies 1 and 2, 77% of patients had previously received systemic therapy and/or phototherapy for psoriasis. Of these, 23% and 19%, respectively, had failed to respond to at least one of these previous therapies.
Table 2 shows the treatment response in the first course of Study 1 and Study 2. Response to treatment in both studies was defined as the proportion of patients with a reduction in score on the Psoriasis Area and Severity Index (PASI)[3] of at least 75% from baseline at two weeks following the 12-week treatment period.
Other treatment responses included the proportion of patients who achieved a scoring of "almost clear" or "clear" by Physician Global Assessment (PGA) and the proportion of patients with a reduction in PASI of at least 50% from baseline two weeks after the 12-week treatment period.
[See table 2 above]
In Study 2, the proportion of responders to the 10 mg IM dose was higher than placebo, but the difference was not statistically significant.
In both studies, onset of response to AMEVIVE® treatment (at least a 50% reduction of baseline PASI) began 60 days after the start of therapy.
With one course of therapy in Study 1 (IV route), the median duration of response (defined as maintenance of a 75% or greater reduction in PASI) was 3.5 months for AMEVIVE®-treated patients and 1 month for placebo-treated patients. In Study 2 (IM route), the median duration of response was approximately 2 months for both AMEVIVE®-treated patients and placebo-treated patients.
Most patients who had responded to either AMEVIVE® or placebo maintained a 50% or greater reduction in PASI through the 3-month observation period.
The responders (n=52) in a subset of patients in Study 1 who crossed over to placebo for course 2 (Cohort 2) maintained a 50% or greater reduction in PASI for a median of 7 months.
Some patients achieved their maximal response beyond 2 weeks post-dosing. In Studies 1 and 2, an additional 11% (42/367) and 7% (12/166) of patients treated with AMEVIVE®, respectively, achieved a 75% reduction from baseline PASI score at one or more visits after the first 2 weeks of the follow-up period.

Retreatment
Patients in Study 1 who had completed the first IV treatment course were eligible to receive a second treatment course if their psoriasis was less than "clear" by PGA and their CD4+ T lymphocyte count was above the lower limit of normal. The level of response (decrease in median PASI score) over the two courses of IV treatment is shown in Figure 1. The median reduction in PASI score was greater in patients who received a second course of AMEVIVE® treatment (see Cohort 1) compared to patients who received placebo (see Cohort 2).
[See figure 1 at top of next page]
Data on the safety and efficacy of AMEVIVE® treatment beyond two courses are limited.

INDICATIONS AND USAGE
AMEVIVE® is indicated for the treatment of adult patients with moderate to severe chronic plaque psoriasis who are candidates for systemic therapy or phototherapy.

CONTRAINDICATIONS
AMEVIVE® should not be administered to patients with known hypersensitivity to AMEVIVE® or any of its components.

WARNINGS
LYMPHOPENIA
AMEVIVE® INDUCES DOSE-DEPENDENT REDUCTIONS IN CIRCULATING CD4+ AND CD8+ T LYMPHOCYTE COUNTS.

A COURSE OF AMEVIVE® THERAPY SHOULD NOT BE INITIATED IN PATIENTS WITH A CD4+ T LYMPHOCYTE COUNT BELOW NORMAL. THE CD4+ T LYMPHOCYTE COUNTS OF PATIENTS RECEIVING AMEVIVE® SHOULD BE MONITORED WEEKLY THROUGHOUT THE COURSE OF THE 12-WEEK DOSING REGIMEN. DOSING SHOULD BE WITHHELD IF CD4+ T LYMPHOCYTE COUNTS ARE BELOW 250 CELLS/μL. THE DRUG SHOULD BE DISCONTINUED IF THE COUNTS REMAIN BELOW 250 CELLS/μL FOR ONE MONTH (SEE DOSAGE AND ADMINISTRATION).

Malignancies
AMEVIVE® may increase the risk of malignancies. Some patients who received AMEVIVE® in clinical studies developed malignancies (**see ADVERSE REACTIONS, Malignancies**). In preclinical studies, animals developed B cell hyperplasia, and one animal developed a lymphoma (**see PRECAUTIONS, Carcinogenesis, Mutagenesis, and Fertility**). AMEVIVE® should not be administered to patients with a history of systemic malignancy. Caution should be exercised when considering the use of AMEVIVE® in patients at high risk for malignancy. If a patient develops a malignancy, AMEVIVE® should be discontinued.

Serious Infections
AMEVIVE® is an immunosuppressive agent and, therefore, has the potential to increase the risk of infection and reactivate latent, chronic infections. AMEVIVE® should not be administered to patients with a clinically important infection. Caution should be exercised when considering the use of AMEVIVE® in patients with chronic infections or a history of recurrent infection. Patients should be monitored for signs and symptoms of infection during or after a course of AMEVIVE®. New infections should be closely monitored. If a patient develops a serious infection, AMEVIVE® should be discontinued (see **ADVERSE REACTIONS, Infections**).

Continued on next page

Amevive—Cont.

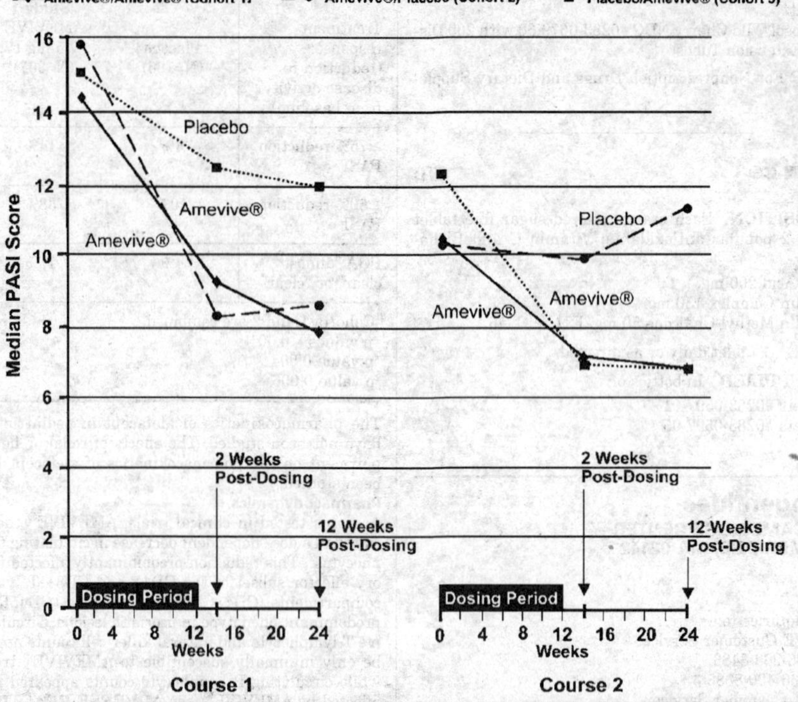

PRECAUTIONS

Effects on the Immune System

Patients receiving other immunosuppressive agents or phototherapy should not receive concurrent therapy with AMEVIVE® because of the possibility of excessive immunosuppression. The duration of the period following treatment with AMEVIVE® before one should consider starting other immunosuppressive therapy has not been evaluated.

The safety and efficacy of vaccines, specifically live or live-attenuated vaccines, administered to patients being treated with AMEVIVE® have not been studied. In a study of 46 patients with chronic plaque psoriasis, the ability to mount immunity to tetanus toxoid (recall antigen) and an experimental neo-antigen was preserved in those patients undergoing AMEVIVE® therapy.

Allergic Reactions

Hypersensitivity reactions (urticaria, angioedema) were associated with the administration of AMEVIVE®. If an anaphylactic reaction or other serious allergic reaction occurs, administration of AMEVIVE® should be discontinued immediately and appropriate therapy initiated.

Information for Patients

Patients should be informed of the need for regular monitoring of white blood cell (lymphocyte) counts during therapy and that AMEVIVE® must be administered under the supervision of a physician. Patients should also be informed that AMEVIVE® reduces lymphocyte counts, which could increase their chances of developing an infection or a malignancy. Patients should be advised to inform their physician promptly if they develop any signs of an infection or malignancy while undergoing a course of treatment with AMEVIVE®.

Female patients should also be advised to notify their physicians if they become pregnant while taking AMEVIVE® (or within 8 weeks of discontinuing AMEVIVE®) and be advised of the existence of and encouraged to enroll in the Pregnancy Registry. Call 1-866-AMEVIVE (1-866-263-8483) to enroll into the Registry (see **PRECAUTIONS, Pregnancy**).

Laboratory Tests

CD4+ T lymphocyte counts should be monitored weekly during the 12-week dosing period and used to guide dosing. Patients should have normal CD4+ T lymphocyte counts prior to an initial or a subsequent course of treatment with AMEVIVE®. Dosing should be withheld if CD4+ T lymphocyte counts are below 250 cells/µL. AMEVIVE® should be discontinued if CD4+ T lymphocyte counts remain below 250 cells/µL for one month.

Drug Interactions

No formal interaction studies have been performed. The duration of the period following treatment with AMEVIVE® before one should consider starting other immunosuppressive therapy has not been evaluated.

Carcinogenesis, Mutagenesis, and Fertility

In a chronic toxicity study, cynomolgus monkeys were dosed weekly for 52 weeks with intravenous alefacept at 1 mg/kg/dose or 20 mg/kg/dose. One animal in the high dose group developed a B-cell lymphoma that was detected after 28 weeks of dosing. Additional animals in both dose groups developed B-cell hyperplasia of the spleen and lymph nodes.

All animals in the study were positive for an endemic primate gammaherpes virus also known as lymphocryptovirus (LCV). Latent LCV infection is generally asymptomatic, but can lead to B-cell lymphomas when animals are immune suppressed.

In a separate study, baboons given 3 doses of alefacept at 1 mg/kg every 8 weeks were found to have centroblast proliferation in B-cell dependent areas in the germinal centers of the spleen following a 116-day washout period.

The role of AMEVIVE® in the development of the lymphoid malignancy and the hyperplasia observed in non-human primates and the relevance to humans is unknown. Immunodeficiency-associated lymphocyte disorders (plasmacytic hyperplasia, polymorphic proliferation, and B-cell lymphomas) occur in patients who have congenital or acquired immunodeficiencies including those resulting from immunosuppressive therapy.

No carcinogenicity or fertility studies were conducted.

Mutagenicity studies were conducted *in vitro* and *in vivo*; no evidence of mutagenicity was observed.

Pregnancy (Category B)

Women of childbearing potential make up a considerable segment of the patient population affected by psoriasis. Since the effect of AMEVIVE® on pregnancy and fetal development, including immune system development, is not known, health care providers are encouraged to enroll patients currently taking AMEVIVE® who become pregnant into the Biogen Pregnancy Registry by calling 1-866-AMEVIVE (1-866-263-8483).

Reproductive toxicology studies have been performed in cynomolgus monkeys at doses up to 5 mg/kg/week (about 62 times the human dose based on body weight) and have revealed no evidence of impaired fertility or harm to the fetus due to AMEVIVE®. No abortifacient or teratogenic effects were observed in cynomolgus monkeys following intravenous bolus injections of AMEVIVE® administered weekly during the period of organogenesis to gestation. AMEVIVE® underwent trans-placental passage and produced *in utero* exposure in the developing monkeys. *In utero*, serum levels of exposure in these monkeys were 23% of maternal serum levels. No evidence of fetal toxicity including adverse effects on immune system development was observed in any of these animals.

Animal reproduction studies, however, are not always predictive of human response and there are no adequate and well-controlled studies in pregnant women. Because the risk to the development of the fetal immune system and postnatal immune function in humans is unknown, AMEVIVE® should be used during pregnancy only if clearly needed. If pregnancy occurs while taking AMEVIVE®, continued use of the drug should be assessed.

Nursing Mothers

It is not known whether AMEVIVE® is excreted in human milk. Because many drugs are excreted in human milk, and because there exists the potential for serious adverse reactions in nursing infants from AMEVIVE®, a decision should be made whether to discontinue nursing while taking the drug or to discontinue the use of the drug, taking into account the importance of the drug to the mother.

Geriatric Use

Of the 1357 patients who received AMEVIVE® in clinical trials, a total of 100 patients were ≥ 65 years of age and 13 patients were ≥ 75 years of age. No differences in safety or efficacy were observed between older and younger patients, but there were not sufficient data to exclude important differences. Because the incidence of infections and certain malignancies is higher in the elderly population, in general, caution should be used in treating the elderly.

Pediatric Use

The safety and efficacy of AMEVIVE® in pediatric patients have not been studied. AMEVIVE® is not indicated for pediatric patients.

ADVERSE REACTIONS

The most serious adverse reactions were:

- Lymphopenia (see **WARNINGS**)
- Malignancies (see **WARNINGS**)
- Serious Infections requiring hospitalization (see **WARNINGS**)
- Hypersensitivity Reactions (see **PRECAUTIONS, Allergic Reactions**)

Commonly observed adverse events seen in the first course of placebo-controlled clinical trials with at least a 2% higher incidence in the AMEVIVE®-treated patients compared to placebo-treated patients were: pharyngitis, dizziness, increased cough, nausea, pruritus, myalgia, chills, injection site pain, injection site inflammation, and accidental injury. The only adverse event that occurred at a 5% or higher incidence among AMEVIVE®-treated patients compared to placebo-treated patients was chills (1% placebo *vs.* 6% AMEVIVE®), which occurred predominantly with intravenous administration.

The adverse reactions which most commonly resulted in clinical intervention were cardiovascular events including coronary artery disorder in <1% of patients and myocardial infarct in <1% of patients. These events were not observed in any of the 413 placebo-treated patients. The total number of patients hospitalized for cardiovascular events in the AMEVIVE®-treated group was 1.2% (11/876).

The most common events resulting in discontinuation of treatment with AMEVIVE® were CD4+ T lymphocyte levels below 250 cells/µL (see **WARNINGS**, and **ADVERSE REACTIONS, Effect on Lymphocyte Counts**), headache (0.2%), and nausea (0.2%).

Because clinical trials are conducted under widely varying conditions, adverse event rates observed in the clinical trials of a drug cannot be directly compared to rates in the clinical trials of another drug and may not reflect the rates observed in practice. The adverse reaction information does, however, provide a basis for identifying the adverse events that appear to be related to drug use and a basis for approximating rates.

The data described below reflect exposure to AMEVIVE® in a total of 1357 psoriasis patients, 85% of whom received 1 to 2 courses of therapy and the rest received 3 to 6 courses and were followed for up to three years. Of the 1357 total patients, 876 received their first course in placebo-controlled studies. The population studied ranged in age from 16 to 84 years, and included 69% men and 31% women. The patients were mostly Caucasian (89%), reflecting the general psoriatic population. Disease severity at baseline was moderate to severe psoriasis.

Effect on Lymphocyte Counts

In the intramuscular study (Study 2), 4% of patients temporarily discontinued treatment and no patients permanently discontinued treatment due to CD4+ T lymphocyte counts below the specified threshold of 250 cells/µL. In Study 2, 10%, 28%, and 42% of patients had total lymphocyte, CD4+, and CD8+ T lymphocyte counts below normal, respectively. Twelve weeks after a course of therapy (12 weekly doses), 2%, 8%, and 21% of patients had total lymphocyte, CD4+, and CD8+ T cell counts below normal.

In the first course of the intravenous study (Study 1), 10% of patients temporarily discontinued treatment and 2% permanently discontinued treatment due to CD4+ T lymphocyte counts below the specified threshold of 250 cells/µL. During the first course of Study 1, 22% of patients had total lymphocyte counts below normal, 48% had CD4+ T lymphocyte counts below normal and 59% had CD8+ T lymphocyte counts below normal. The maximal effect on lymphocytes was observed within 6 to 8 weeks of initiation of treatment. Twelve weeks after a course of therapy (12 weekly doses), 4% of patients had total lymphocyte counts below normal, 19% had CD4+ T lymphocyte counts below normal, and 36% had CD8+ T lymphocyte counts below normal.

For patients receiving a second course of AMEVIVE® in Study 1, 17% of patients had total lymphocyte counts below normal, 44% had CD4+ T lymphocyte counts below normal, and 56% had CD8+ T lymphocyte counts below normal. Twelve weeks after completing dosing, 3% of patients had total lymphocyte counts below normal, 17% had CD4+ T lymphocyte counts below normal, and 35% had CD8+ T lymphocyte counts below normal (see **WARNINGS**, and **PRECAUTIONS, Laboratory Tests**).

Malignancies

In the 24-week period constituting the first course of placebo-controlled studies, 13 malignancies were diagnosed in 11 AMEVIVE®-treated patients. The incidence of malignancies was 1.3% (11/876) for AMEVIVE®-treated patients compared to 0.5% (2/413) in the placebo group.

Among 1357 patients who received AMEVIVE®, 25 patients were diagnosed with 35 treatment-emergent malignancies. The majority of these malignancies (23 cases) were basal (6) or squamous cell cancers (17) of the skin. Three cases of lymphoma were observed; one was classified as non-Hodgkin's follicle-center cell lymphoma and two were classified as Hodgkin's disease.

Infections

In the 24-week period constituting the first course of placebo-controlled studies, serious infections (infections requiring hospitalization) were seen at a rate of 0.9% (8/876) in AMEVIVE®-treated patients and 0.2% (1/413) in the placebo group. In patients receiving repeated courses of AMEVIVE® therapy, the rates of serious infections were 0.7% (5/756) and 1.5% (3/199) in the second and third course of therapy, respectively. Serious infections among 1357 AMEVIVE®-treated patients included necrotizing cellulitis, peritonsillar abscess, post-operative and burn wound infection, toxic shock, pneumonia, appendicitis, preseptal cellulitis, cholecystitis, gastroenteritis and herpes simplex infection.

Hypersensitivity Reactions

In clinical studies two patients were reported to experience angioedema, one of whom was hospitalized. In the 24-week period constituting the first course of placebo-controlled studies, urticaria was reported in 6 (<1%) AMEVIVE®-treated patients *vs.* 1 patient in the control group. Urticaria resulted in discontinuation of therapy in one of the AMEVIVE®-treated patients.

Hepatic Events

In post-marketing surveillance hepatic events, including a case of hepatitis associated with transient coagulopathy and hyperbilirubinemia, have been reported.

Injection Site Reactions

In the intramuscular study (Study 2), 16% of AMEVIVE®-treated patients and 8% of placebo-treated patients reported injection site reactions. Reactions at the site of injection were generally mild, typically occurred on single occasions, and included either pain (7%), inflammation (4%), bleeding (4%), edema (2%), non-specific reaction (2%), mass (1%), or skin hypersensitivity (<1%). In the clinical trials, a single case of injection site reaction led to the discontinuation of AMEVIVE®.

Immunogenicity

Approximately 3% (35/1306) of patients receiving AMEVIVE® developed low-titer antibodies to alefacept. No apparent correlation of antibody development and clinical response or adverse events was observed. The long-term immunogenicity of AMEVIVE® is unknown.

The data reflect the percentage of patients whose test results were considered positive for antibodies to alefacept in an ELISA assay, and are highly dependent on the sensitivity and specificity of the assay. Additionally, the observed incidence of antibody positivity in an assay may be influenced by several factors including sample handling, timing of sample collection, concomitant medications, and underlying disease. For these reasons, comparison of the incidence of antibodies to alefacept with the incidence of antibodies to other products may be misleading.

Other Observed Adverse Reactions from Clinical Trials

Less common events that were observed at a higher rate in AMEVIVE®-treated patients include rare cases (9) of transaminase elevations to 5 to 10 times the upper limit of normal.

OVERDOSAGE

The highest dose tested in humans (0.75 mg/kg IV) was associated with chills, headache, arthralgia, and sinusitis within one day of dosing. Patients who have been inadvertently administered an excess of the recommended dose should be closely monitored for effects on total lymphocyte count and CD4+ T lymphocyte count.

DOSAGE AND ADMINISTRATION

AMEVIVE® should only be used under the guidance and supervision of a physician.

The recommended dose of AMEVIVE® is 7.5 mg given once weekly as an IV bolus or 15 mg given once weekly as an IM injection. The recommended regimen is a course of 12 weekly injections. Retreatment with an additional 12-week course may be initiated provided that CD4+ T lymphocyte counts are within the normal range, and a minimum of a 12-week interval has passed since the previous course of treatment. Data on retreatment beyond two cycles are limited.

The CD4+ T lymphocyte counts of patients receiving AMEVIVE® should be monitored weekly before initiating dosing and throughout the course of the 12-week dosing regimen. Dosing should be withheld if CD4+ T lymphocyte counts are below 250 cells/μL. The drug should be discontinued if the counts remain below 250 cells/μL for one month (see **PRECAUTIONS, Laboratory Tests**).

Preparation Instructions

AMEVIVE® should be reconstituted by a health care professional using aseptic technique. Each vial is intended for single patient use only.

Do not use an AMEVIVE® dose tray beyond the date stamped on the carton, dose tray lid, AMEVIVE® vial label, or diluent container label.

AMEVIVE® 15 mg lyophilized powder for IM administration should be reconstituted with 0.6 mL of the supplied diluent (Sterile Water for Injection, USP). 0.5 mL of the reconstituted solution contains 15 mg of alefacept.

AMEVIVE® 7.5 mg lyophilized powder for IV administration should be reconstituted with 0.6 mL of the supplied diluent. 0.5 mL of the reconstituted solution contains 7.5 mg of alefacept.

Do not add other medications to solutions containing AMEVIVE®. Do not reconstitute AMEVIVE® with other diluents. Do not filter reconstituted solution during preparation or administration.

All procedures require the use of aseptic technique. Using the supplied syringe and one of the supplied needles, withdraw **only 0.6 mL** of the supplied diluent, (Sterile Water for Injection, USP). Keeping the needle pointed at the sidewall of the vial, slowly inject the diluent into the vial of AMEVIVE®. Some foaming will occur, which is normal. To avoid excessive foaming, do not shake or vigorously agitate. The contents should be swirled gently during dissolution. Generally, dissolution of AMEVIVE® takes less than two minutes. The solution should be used as soon as possible after reconstitution.

The reconstituted solution should be clear and colorless to slightly yellow. Visually inspect the solution for particulate matter and discoloration prior to administration. The solution should not be used if discolored or cloudy, or if undissolved material remains.

Following reconstitution, the product should be used immediately or within 4 hours if stored in the vial at 2–8°C (36–46°F). AMEVIVE® NOT USED WITHIN 4 HOURS OF RECONSTITUTION SHOULD BE DISCARDED.

Remove the needle used for reconstitution and attach the other supplied needle. Withdraw 0.5 mL of the AMEVIVE® solution into the syringe. Some foam or bubbles may remain in the vial.

Administration Instructions

For intramuscular use, inject the full 0.5 mL of solution. Rotate injection sites so that a different site is used for each new injection. New injections should be given at least 1 inch from an old site and never into areas where the skin is tender, bruised, red, or hard.

For intravenous use,

- Prepare 2 syringes with 3.0 mL Normal Saline, USP for pre- and post-administration flush.
- Prime the winged infusion set with 3.0 mL saline and insert the set into the vein.
- Attach the AMEVIVE®-filled syringe to the infusion set and administer the solution over no more than 5 seconds.
- Flush the infusion set with 3.0 mL saline, USP.

HOW SUPPLIED

AMEVIVE® for IV administration is supplied in either a carton containing four administration dose packs, or in a carton containing one administration dose pack. Each dose pack contains one 7.5-mg single-use vial of AMEVIVE®, one 10 mL single-use diluent vial (Sterile Water for Injection, USP), one syringe, one 23 gauge, ¾ inch winged infusion set, and two 23 gauge, 1 ¼ inch needles. The NDC number for the four administration dose pack carton is 59627-020-01 The NDC number for the one administration dose pack carton is 59627-020-02.

AMEVIVE® for IM administration is supplied in either a carton containing four administration dose packs, or in a carton containing one administration dose pack. Each dose pack contains one 15-mg single-use vial of AMEVIVE®, one 10 mL single-use diluent vial (Sterile Water for Injection, USP), one syringe, and two 23 gauge, 1 ¼ inch needles. The NDC number for the four administration dose pack carton is 59627-021-03. The NDC number for the one administration dose pack carton is 59627-021-04

AMEVIVE® is reconstituted with 0.6 mL of the 10 mL single-use diluent.

Storage

The dose tray containing AMEVIVE® (lyophilized powder) should be stored at controlled room temperature (15–30°C; 59–86°F). PROTECT FROM LIGHT. Retain in carton until time of use.

Rx only

REFERENCES

1. Bos JD, Hagenaars C, Das PK, et al. Predominance of "memory" T cells (CD4+, CDw29+) over "naïve" T cells (CD4+, CD45R+) in both normal and diseased human skin. Arch Dermatol Res 1989; 281:24–30.
2. Ellis C, Krueger GG. Treatment of chronic plaque psoriasis by selective targeting of memory effector T lymphocytes. N Engl J Med 2001; 345:248–255.
3. Fredriksson T, Pettersson U. Severe psoriasis–oral therapy with a new retinoid. Dermatologica 1978; 157:238–244.

Issued: May/2004
AMEVIVE® (alefacept)
Manufactured by:
BIOGEN, INC.
14 Cambridge Center
Cambridge, MA 02142 USA

1-866-263-8483
U.S. Patents:
4,956,281
5,547,853
5,728,677
5,914,111
5,928,643
6,162,432
Additional U.S. Patents Pending
I63007-2

AVONEX® ℞

[*a-vuh-necks*]

(Interferon beta-1a)

IM Injection

DESCRIPTION

AVONEX® (Interferon beta-1a) is a 166 amino acid glycoprotein with a predicted molecular weight of approximately 22,500 daltons. It is produced by recombinant DNA technology using genetically engineered Chinese Hamster Ovary cells into which the human interferon beta gene has been introduced. The amino acid sequence of AVONEX® is identical to that of natural human interferon beta.

Using the World Health Organization (WHO) natural interferon beta standard, Second International Standard for Interferon, Human Fibroblast (Gb-23-902-531), AVONEX® has a specific activity of approximately 200 million international units (IU) of antiviral activity per mg of Interferon beta-1a determined specifically by an *in vitro* cytopathic effect bioassay using lung carcinoma cells (A549) and Encephalomyocarditis virus (ECM). AVONEX® 30 mcg contains approximately 6 million IU of antiviral activity using this method. The activity against other standards is not known. Comparison of the activity of AVONEX® with other Interferon betas is not appropriate, because of differences in the reference standards and assays used to measure activity.

30 mcg Lyophilized Powder Vial

A vial of AVONEX® is formulated as a sterile, white to off-white lyophilized powder for intramuscular injection after reconstitution with supplied diluent (Sterile Water for Injection, USP). Each vial of reconstituted AVONEX® contains 30 mcg of Interferon beta-1a; 15 mg Albumin (Human), USP; 5.8 mg Sodium Chloride, USP; 5.7 mg Dibasic Sodium Phosphate, USP; and 1.2 mg Monobasic Sodium Phosphate, USP, in 1.0 mL at a pH of approximately 7.3.

30 mcg Prefilled Syringe

A prefilled syringe of AVONEX® is formulated as a sterile liquid for intramuscular injection. Each 0.5 mL (30 mcg dose) of AVONEX® in a prefilled glass syringe contains 30 mcg of Interferon beta-1a, 0.79 mg Sodium Acetate Trihydrate, USP; 0.25 mg Glacial Acetic Acid, USP; 15.8 mg Arginine Hydrochloride, USP; and 0.025 mg Polysorbate 20 in Water for Injection, USP at a pH of approximately 4.8.

CLINICAL PHARMACOLOGY

General

Interferons are a family of naturally occurring proteins and glycoproteins that are produced by eukaryotic cells in response to viral infection and other biological inducers. Interferon beta, one member of this family, is produced by various cell types including fibroblasts and macrophages. Natural interferon beta and Interferon beta-1a are glycosylated, with each containing a single N-linked complex carbohydrate moiety. Glycosylation of other proteins is known to affect their stability, activity, aggregation, biodistribution, and half-life in blood. However, the effects of glycosylation of interferon beta on these properties have not been fully defined.

Biologic Activities

Interferons are cytokines that mediate antiviral, antiproliferative and immunomodulatory activities in response to viral infection and other biological inducers. Three major interferons have been distinguished: alpha, beta, and gamma. Interferons alpha and beta form the Type I class of interferons, and interferon gamma is a Type II interferon. These interferons have overlapping but clearly distinct biological activities.

Interferon beta exerts its biological effects by binding to specific receptors on the surface of human cells. This binding initiates a complex cascade of intracellular events that leads to the expression of numerous interferon-induced gene products and markers. These include 2′, 5′-oligoadenylate synthetase, β_2-microglobulin, and neopterin. These products have been measured in the serum and cellular fractions of blood collected from patients treated with AVONEX®.

The specific interferon-induced proteins and mechanisms by which AVONEX® exerts its effects in multiple sclerosis have not been fully defined. Clinical studies conducted in multiple sclerosis patients showed that interleukin 10 (IL-10) levels in cerebrospinal fluid were increased in patients treated with AVONEX® compared to placebo. Serum IL-10 levels were increased 48 hours after intramuscular (IM) injection of AVONEX® and remained elevated for 1 week. However, no relationship has been established between absolute levels of IL-10 and clinical outcome in multiple sclerosis.

Pharmacokinetics

Pharmacokinetics of AVONEX® in multiple sclerosis patients have not been evaluated. The pharmacokinetic and pharmacodynamic profiles of AVONEX® in healthy subjects following doses of 30 mcg through 75 mcg have been investigated. Serum levels of AVONEX® as measured by antiviral activity are slightly above detectable limits following a 30 mcg IM dose, and increase with higher doses.

After an IM dose, serum levels of AVONEX® typically peak between 3 and 15 hours and then decline at a rate consistent with a 10 hour elimination half-life. Serum levels of AVONEX® may be sustained after IM administration due to prolonged absorption from the IM site. Systemic exposure, as determined by AUC and C_{max} values, is greater following IM than subcutaneous (SC) administration.

Subcutaneous administration of AVONEX® should not be substituted for intramuscular administration. Subcutaneous and intramuscular administration have been observed to have non-equivalent pharmacokinetic and pharmacodynamic parameters following administration to healthy volunteers.

Biological response markers (e.g., neopterin and β_2-microglobulin) are induced by AVONEX® following parenteral doses of 15 mcg through 75 mcg in healthy subjects and

Continued on next page

Avonex—Cont.

treated patients. Biological response marker levels increase within 12 hours of dosing and remain elevated for at least 4 days. Peak biological response marker levels are typically observed 48 hours after dosing. The relationship of serum AVONEX® levels or levels of these induced biological response markers to the mechanisms by which AVONEX® exerts its effects in multiple sclerosis is unknown.

Clinical Studies

The clinical effects of AVONEX® in multiple sclerosis were studied in two randomized, multicenter, double-blind, placebo-controlled studies in patients with multiple sclerosis.[1,2] Safety and efficacy of treatment with AVONEX® beyond 3 years is not known.

In Study 1, 301 patients received either 30 mcg of AVONEX® (n=158) or placebo (n=143) by IM injection once weekly. Patients were entered into the trial over a 2½ year period, received injections for up to 2 years, and continued to be followed until study completion. Two hundred eighty-two patients completed 1 year on study, and 172 patients completed 2 years on study. There were 144 patients treated with AVONEX® for more than 1 year, 115 patients for more than 18 months and 82 patients for 2 years.

All patients had a definite diagnosis of multiple sclerosis of at least 1 year duration and had at least 2 exacerbations in the 3 years prior to study entry (or 1 per year if the duration of disease was less than 3 years). At entry, study participants were without exacerbation during the prior 2 months and had Kurtzke Expanded Disability Status Scale (EDSS[3]) scores ranging from 1.0 to 3.5. Patients with chronic progressive multiple sclerosis were excluded from this study.

The primary outcome assessment was time to progression in disability, measured as an increase in the EDSS score of at least 1.0 point that was sustained for at least 6 months. An increase in EDSS score reflects accumulation of disability. This endpoint was used to ensure that progression reflected permanent increase in disability rather than a transient effect due to an exacerbation.

Secondary outcomes included exacerbation frequency and results of magnetic resonance imaging (MRI) scans including gadolinium (Gd)-enhanced lesion number and volume and T2-weighted (proton density) lesion volume. Additional secondary endpoints included 2 upper limb (tested in both arms) and 3 lower limb function tests.

Twenty-three of the 301 patients (8%) discontinued treatment prematurely. Of these, 1 patient treated with placebo (1%) and 6 patients treated with AVONEX® (4%) discontinued treatment due to adverse events. Thirteen of these 23 patients remained on study and were evaluated for clinical endpoints.

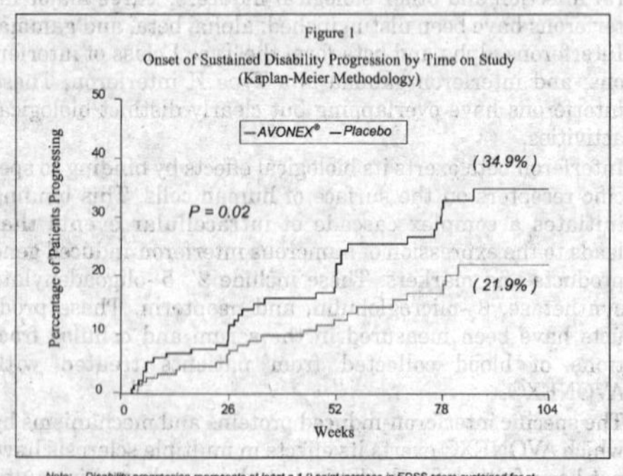

Time to onset of sustained progression in disability was significantly longer in patients treated with AVONEX® than in patients receiving placebo (p = 0.02). The Kaplan-Meier plots of these data are presented in Figure 1. The Kaplan-Meier estimate of the percentage of patients progressing by the end of 2 years was 34.9% for placebo-treated patients and 21.9% for AVONEX®-treated patients, indicating a slowing of the disease process. This represents a 37% relative reduction in the risk of accumulating disability in the AVONEX®-treated group compared to the placebo-treated group.

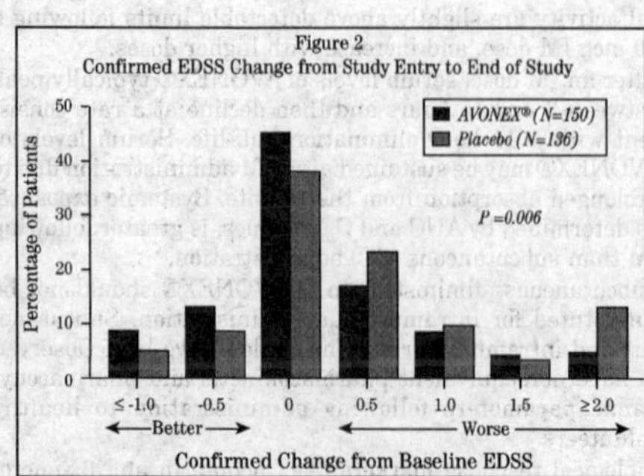

The distribution of confirmed EDSS change from study entry (baseline) to the end of the study is shown in Figure 2. There was a statistically significant difference between

Table 1
Clinical and MRI Endpoints in Study 1

Endpoint	Placebo	AVONEX®	P-Value
PRIMARY ENDPOINT:			
Time to sustained progression in disability (N: 143, 158)[1]	–See Figure 1–		0.02[2]
Percentage of patients progressing in disability at 2 years (Kaplan-Meier estimate)[1]	34.9%	21.9%	
SECONDARY ENDPOINTS:			
DISABILITY			
Mean confirmed change in EDSS from study entry to end of study (N: 136, 150)[1]	0.50	0.20	0.006[3]
EXACERBATIONS			
Number of exacerbations in subset completing 2 years (N: 87, 85)			0.03[3]
0	26%	38%	
1	30%	31%	
2	11%	18%	
3	14%	7%	
≥4	18%	7%	
Percentage of patients exacerbation-free in subset completing 2 years (N: 87, 85)	26%	38%	0.10[4]
Annual exacerbation rate (N: 143, 158)[1]	0.82	0.67	0.04[5]
MRI			
Number of Gd-enhanced lesions:			
At study entry (N: 132, 141)			
Mean (Median)	2.3 (1.0)	3.2 (1.0)	
Range	0-23	0-56	
Year 1 (N: 123, 134)			
Mean (Median)	1.6 (0)	1.0 (0)	0.02[3]
Range	0-22	0-28	
Year 2 (N: 82, 83)			
Mean (Median)	1.6 (0)	0.8 (0)	0.05[3]
Range	0-34	0-13	
T2 lesion volume:			
Percentage change from study entry to Year 1 (N: 116, 123)			
Median	-3.3%	-13.1%	0.02[3]
Percentage change from study entry to Year 2 (N: 83, 81)			
Median	-6.5%	-13.2%	0.36[3]

Note: (N: ,) denotes the number of evaluable placebo and AVONEX® patients, respectively.
[1] *Patient data included in this analysis represent variable periods of time on study.*
[2] *Analyzed by Mantel-Cox (logrank) test.*
[3] *Analyzed by Mann-Whitney rank-sum test.*
[4] *Analyzed by Cochran-Mantel-Haenszel test.*
[5] *Analyzed by likelihood ratio test.*

treatment groups in confirmed change for patients with at least 2 scheduled visits (136 placebo-treated and 150 AVONEX®-treated patients; p = 0.006; see Table 1).

The rate and frequency of exacerbations were determined as secondary outcomes. For all patients included in the study, irrespective of time on study, the annual exacerbation rate was 0.67 per year in the AVONEX®-treated group and 0.82 per year in the placebo-treated group (p = 0.04).

AVONEX® treatment significantly decreased the frequency of exacerbations in the subset of patients who were enrolled in the study for at least 2 years (87 placebo-treated patients and 85 AVONEX®-treated patients; p = 0.03; see Table 1).

Gd-enhanced and T2-weighted (proton density) MRI scans of the brain were obtained in most patients at baseline and at the end of 1 and 2 years of treatment. Gd-enhancing lesions seen on brain MRI scans represent areas of breakdown of the blood brain barrier thought to be secondary to inflammation. Patients treated with AVONEX® demonstrated significantly lower Gd-enhanced lesion number after 1 and 2 years of treatment ($p \leq 0.05$; see Table 1). The volume of Gd-enhanced lesions was also analyzed, and showed similar treatment effects ($p \leq 0.03$). Percentage change in T2-weighted lesion volume from study entry to Year 1 was significantly lower in AVONEX®-treated than placebo-treated patients (p = 0.02). A significant difference in T2-weighted lesion volume change was not seen between study entry and Year 2.

The exact relationship between MRI findings and the clinical status of patients is unknown. The prognostic significance of MRI findings in these studies has not been evaluated.

Of the limb function tests, only 1 demonstrated a statistically significant difference between treatment groups (favoring AVONEX®). A summary of the effects of AVONEX® on the clinical and MRI endpoints of this study is presented in Table 1.

[See table 1 above]

In Study 2, 383 patients who had recently experienced an isolated demyelinating event involving the optic nerve, spinal cord, or brainstem/cerebellum, and who had lesions typical of multiple sclerosis on brain MRI, received either 30 mcg AVONEX® (n = 193) or placebo (n = 190) by IM injection once weekly. All patients received intravenous steroid treatment for the initiating clinical exacerbation. Patients were enrolled into the study over a two-year period and followed for up to three years or until they developed a second clinical exacerbation in an anatomically distinct region of the central nervous system. Sixteen percent of subjects on AVONEX® and 14% of subjects on placebo withdrew from the study for a reason other than the development of a second exacerbation[2].

The primary outcome measure was time to development of a second exacerbation in an anatomically distinct region of the central nervous system. Secondary outcomes were brain MRI measures, including the cumulative increase in the number of new or enlarging T2 lesions, T2 lesion volume compared to baseline at 18 months, and the number of Gd-enhancing lesions at 6 months.

Time to development of a second exacerbation was significantly delayed in patients treated with AVONEX® compared to placebo (p = 0.002). The Kaplan-Meier estimates of the percentage of patients developing an exacerbation within 24 months were 38.6% in the placebo group and 21.1% in the AVONEX® group (Figure 3). The relative rate of developing a second exacerbation in the AVONEX® group was 0.56 of the rate in the placebo group (95% confidence interval 0.38 to 0.81). The brain MRI findings are described in Table 2.

[See figure 3 at top of next page]
[See table 2 on next page]

INDICATIONS AND USAGE

AVONEX® (Interferon beta-1a) is indicated for the treatment of patients with relapsing forms of multiple sclerosis to slow the accumulation of physical disability and decrease the frequency of clinical exacerbations. Patients with multiple sclerosis in whom efficacy has been demonstrated include patients who have experienced a first clinical episode and have MRI features consistent with multiple sclerosis. Safety and efficacy in patients with chronic progressive multiple sclerosis have not been established.

CONTRAINDICATIONS

AVONEX® is contraindicated in patients with a history of hypersensitivity to natural or recombinant interferon beta, or any other component of the formulation.

The lyophilized vial formulation of AVONEX® is contraindicated in patients with a history of hypersensitivity to albumin (human).

WARNINGS

Depression and Suicide

AVONEX® should be used with caution in patients with depression or other mood disorders, conditions that are common with multiple sclerosis. Depression and suicide have been reported to occur with increased frequency in patients receiving interferon compounds, including AVONEX®. Patients treated with AVONEX® should be advised to report immediately any symptoms of depression and/or suicidal ideation to their prescribing physicians. If a patient develops depression or other severe psychiatric symptoms, cessation of AVONEX® therapy should be considered. In Study 2, AVONEX®-treated patients were more likely to experience depression than placebo-treated patients. An equal incidence of depression was seen in the placebo-treated and AVONEX®-treated patients in Study 1. Additionally, there have been post-marketing reports of depression, suicidal ideation and/or development of new or worsening of pre-existing other psychiatric disorders, including psychosis. Some of these patients improved upon cessation of AVONEX® dosing.

Anaphylaxis

Anaphylaxis has been reported as a rare complication of AVONEX® use. Other allergic reactions have included dyspnea, orolingual edema, skin rash and urticaria (see ADVERSE REACTIONS).

Decreased Peripheral Blood Counts

Decreased peripheral blood counts in all cell lines, including rare pancytopenia and thrombocytopenia, have been reported from post-marketing experience (see ADVERSE REACTIONS). Some cases of thrombocytopenia have had nadirs below 10,000/µL. Some cases reoccur with rechallenge (see ADVERSE REACTIONS). Patients should be monitored for signs of these disorders (see Precautions: Laboratory Tests).

Albumin (Human)

The lyophilized vial of AVONEX® contains albumin, a derivative of human blood. Based on effective donor screening and product manufacturing processes, it carries an extremely remote risk for transmission of viral diseases. A theoretical risk for transmission of Creutzfeldt-Jakob disease (CJD) also is considered extremely remote. No cases of transmission of viral diseases or CJD have been identified for albumin. The prefilled syringe of AVONEX® does not contain albumin.

PRECAUTIONS

Seizures

Caution should be exercised when administering AVONEX® to patients with pre-existing seizure disorders. In the two placebo-controlled studies in multiple sclerosis, 4 patients receiving AVONEX® experienced seizures, while no seizures occurred in the placebo group. Three of these 4 patients had no prior history of seizure (see ADVERSE REACTIONS). It is not known whether these events were related to the effects of multiple sclerosis alone, to AVONEX®, or to a combination of both. The effect of AVONEX® administration on the medical management of patients with seizure disorder is unknown.

Cardiomyopathy and Congestive Heart Failure

Patients with cardiac disease, such as angina, congestive heart failure, or arrhythmia, should be closely monitored for worsening of their clinical condition during initiation and continued treatment with AVONEX®. While AVONEX® does not have any known direct-acting cardiac toxicity, during the post-marketing period infrequent cases of congestive heart failure, cardiomyopathy, and cardiomyopathy with congestive heart failure have been reported in patients without known predisposition to these events, and without other known etiologies being established. In rare cases, these events have been temporally related to the administration of AVONEX®. In some of these instances recurrence upon rechallenge was observed.

Autoimmune Disorders

Autoimmune disorders of multiple target organs have been reported post-marketing including idiopathic thrombocytopenia, hyper- and hypothyroidism, and rare cases of autoimmune hepatitis have also been reported. Patients should be monitored for signs of these disorders (see Precautions: Laboratory Tests) and appropriate treatment implemented when observed.

Hepatic Injury

Hepatic injury including elevated serum hepatic enzyme levels and hepatitis, some of which have been severe, has been reported post-marketing. In some patients a recurrence of elevated serum levels of hepatic enzymes has occurred upon AVONEX® rechallenge. In some cases, these events have occurred in the presence of other drugs that have been associated with hepatic injury. The potential of additive effects from multiple drugs or other hepatotoxic agents (e.g., alcohol) has not been determined. Patients should be monitored for signs of hepatic injury (see Precautions: Laboratory Tests) and caution exercised when AVONEX® is used concomitantly with other drugs associated with hepatic injury.

Information to Patients

All patients should be instructed to read the AVONEX® Medication Guide supplied to them. Patients should be cautioned not to change the dosage or the schedule of administration without medical consultation.

Patients should be informed of the most serious (see WARNINGS) and the most common adverse events associated with AVONEX® administration, including symptoms associated with flu syndrome (see ADVERSE REACTIONS). Symptoms of flu syndrome are most prominent at the initiation of therapy and decrease in frequency with continued treatment. Concurrent use of analgesics and/or antipyretics may help ameliorate flu-like symptoms on treatment days. Patients should be cautioned to report depression or suicidal ideation (see WARNINGS).

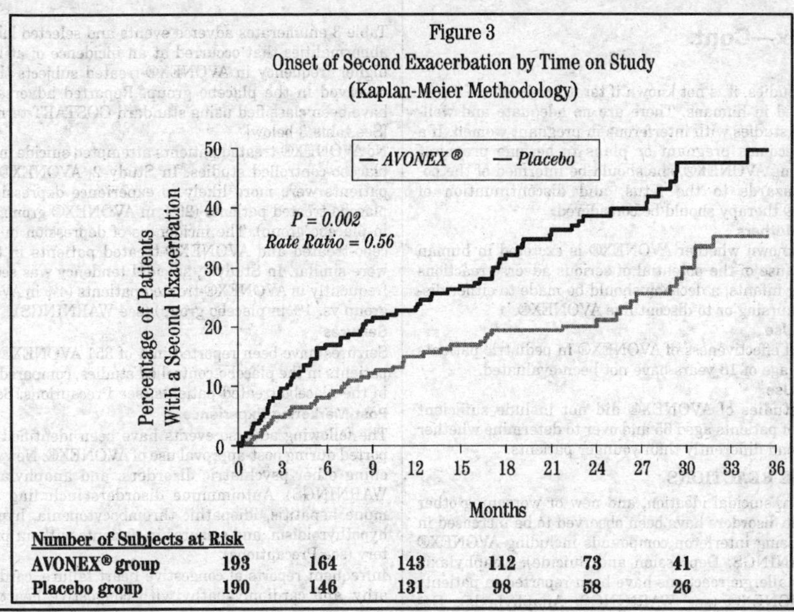

Number of Subjects at Risk						
AVONEX® group	193	164	143	112	73	41
Placebo group	190	146	131	98	58	26

Table 2
Brain MRI Data According to Treatment Group

	AVONEX®	Placebo
CHANGE IN T2 VOLUME @18 MONTHS:	N = 119	N = 109
Actual Change (mm^3)[1]*		
Median ($25^{th}\%$, $75^{th}\%$)	28 (-576, 397)	313 (5, 1140)
Percentage Change[1]*		
Median ($25^{th}\%$, $75^{th}\%$)	1 (-24, 29)	16 (0, 53)
NUMBER OF NEW OR ENLARGING	N = 132	N = 119
T2 LESIONS @ 18 MONTHS[1]*:	N (%)	N (%)
0	62 (47)	22 (18)
1–3	41 (31)	47 (40)
≥4	29 (22)	50 (42)
Mean (SD)	2.13 (3.19)	4.97 (7.71)
NUMBER OF GD-ENHANCING	N = 165	N = 152
LESIONS @ 6 MONTHS[2]*:	N (%)	N (%)
0	115 (70)	93 (61)
1	27 (16)	16 (11)
>1	23 (14)	43 (28)
Mean (SD)	0.87 (2.28)	1.49 (3.14)

[1]P value <0.001
[2]P value <0.03
*P value from a Mann-Whitney rank-sum test

Patients should be advised about the abortifacient potential of AVONEX® (see Precautions: Pregnancy—Teratogenic Effects).

The prefilled syringe cap contains dry natural rubber.

When a physician determines that AVONEX® can be used outside of the physician's office, persons who will be administering AVONEX® should receive instruction in reconstitution and injection, including the review of the injection procedures. If a patient is to self-administer, the physical ability of that patient to self-inject intramuscularly should be assessed. The first injection should be performed under the supervision of a qualified health care professional. A puncture-resistant container for disposal of needles and syringes should be used. Patients should be instructed in the technique and importance of proper syringe and needle disposal and be cautioned against reuse of these items.

Laboratory Tests

In addition to those laboratory tests normally required for monitoring patients with multiple sclerosis, complete blood and differential white blood cell counts, platelet counts, and blood chemistries, including liver function tests, are recommended during AVONEX® therapy (see WARNINGS: Decreased Peripheral Blood Counts and PRECAUTIONS: Cardiomyopathy and Congestive Heart Failure, and Autoimmune Disorders). During the placebo-controlled studies in multiple sclerosis, these tests were performed at least every 6 months. There were no significant differences between the placebo and AVONEX® groups in the incidence of liver enzyme elevation, leukopenia, or thrombocytopenia. However, these are known to be dose-related laboratory abnormalities associated with the use of interferons. Patients with myelosuppression may require more intensive monitoring of complete blood cell counts, with differential and platelet counts. Thyroid function should be monitored periodically. If patients have or develop symptoms of thyroid dysfunction (hypo- or hyperthyroidism), thyroid function tests should be performed according to standard medical practice.

Drug Interactions

No formal drug interaction studies have been conducted with AVONEX®. In the placebo-controlled studies in multiple sclerosis, corticosteroids or ACTH were administered for treatment of exacerbations in some patients concurrently receiving AVONEX®. In addition, some patients receiving AVONEX® were also treated with anti-depressant therapy and/or oral contraceptive therapy. No unexpected adverse events were associated with these concomitant therapies.

Carcinogenesis, Mutagenesis, and Impairment of Fertility

Carcinogenesis: No carcinogenicity data for AVONEX® are available in animals or humans.

Mutagenesis: AVONEX® was not mutagenic when tested in the Ames bacterial test and in an *in vitro* cytogenetic assay in human lymphocytes in the presence and absence of metabolic activation. These assays are designed to detect agents that interact directly with and cause damage to cellular DNA. AVONEX® is a glycosylated protein that does not directly bind to DNA.

Impairment of Fertility: No studies were conducted to evaluate the effects of AVONEX® on fertility in normal women or women with multiple sclerosis. It is not known whether AVONEX® can affect human reproductive capacity. Menstrual irregularities were observed in monkeys administered AVONEX® at a dose 100 times the recommended weekly human dose (based upon a body surface area comparison). Anovulation and decreased serum progesterone levels were also noted transiently in some animals. These effects were reversible after discontinuation of drug.

Treatment of monkeys with AVONEX® at 2 times the recommended weekly human dose (based upon a body surface area comparison) had no effects on cycle duration or ovulation.

The accuracy of extrapolating animal doses to human doses is not known. In the placebo-controlled studies in multiple sclerosis, 5% of patients receiving placebo and 6% of patients receiving AVONEX® experienced menstrual disorder. If menstrual irregularities occur in humans, it is not known how long they will persist following treatment.

Pregnancy—Teratogenic Effects

Pregnancy Category C: The reproductive toxicity of AVONEX® has not been studied in animals or humans. In pregnant monkeys given AVONEX® at 100 times the recommended weekly human dose (based upon a body surface area comparison), no teratogenic or other adverse effects on fetal development were observed. Abortifacient activity was evident following 3 to 5 doses at this level. No abortifacient effects were observed in monkeys treated at 2 times the recommended weekly human dose (based upon a body surface area comparison). Although no teratogenic effects were seen

Continued on next page

Avonex—Cont.

in these studies, it is not known if teratogenic effects would be observed in humans. There are no adequate and well-controlled studies with interferons in pregnant women. If a woman becomes pregnant or plans to become pregnant while taking AVONEX®, she should be informed of the potential hazards to the fetus, and discontinuation of AVONEX® therapy should be considered.

Nursing Mothers

It is not known whether AVONEX® is excreted in human milk. Because of the potential of serious adverse reactions in nursing infants, a decision should be made to either discontinue nursing or to discontinue AVONEX®.

Pediatric Use

Safety and effectiveness of AVONEX® in pediatric patients below the age of 18 years have not been evaluated.

Geriatric Use

Clinical studies of AVONEX® did not include sufficient numbers of patients aged 65 and over to determine whether they respond differently than younger patients.

ADVERSE REACTIONS

Depression, suicidal ideation, and new or worsening other psychiatric disorders have been observed to be increased in patients using interferon compounds including AVONEX® (see WARNINGS: Depression and Suicide). Anaphylaxis and other allergic reactions have been reported in patients using AVONEX® (see WARNINGS: Anaphylaxis). Decreased peripheral blood counts have been reported in patients using AVONEX® (see WARNINGS: Decreased Peripheral Blood Counts). Seizures, cardiovascular adverse events, and autoimmune disorders also have been reported in association with the use of AVONEX® (see Precautions).

The adverse reactions most commonly reported in patients associated with the use of AVONEX® were flu-like and other symptoms occurring within hours to days following an injection. Symptoms can include myalgia, fever, fatigue, headaches, chills, nausea, and vomiting. Some patients have experienced paresthesias, hypertonia and myasthenia.

The most frequently reported adverse reactions resulting in clinical intervention (e.g., discontinuation of AVONEX®, or the need for concomitant medication to treat an adverse reaction symptom) were flu-like symptoms and depression.

Because clinical trials are conducted under widely varying conditions, adverse reaction rates observed in the clinical trials of AVONEX® cannot be directly compared to rates in clinical trials of other drugs and may not reflect the rates observed in practice.

The data described below reflect exposure to AVONEX® in 351 patients, including 319 patients exposed for 6 months, and 288 patients exposed for greater than one year in placebo-controlled trials. The mean age of patients receiving AVONEX® was 35 years, 74% were women and 89% were Caucasian. Patients received either 30 mcg AVONEX® or placebo.

Table 3 enumerates adverse events and selected laboratory abnormalities that occurred at an incidence of at least 2% higher frequency in AVONEX®-treated subjects than was observed in the placebo group. Reported adverse events have been classified using standard COSTART terms.

[See table 3 below]

No AVONEX®-treated patients attempted suicide in the two placebo-controlled studies. In Study 2, AVONEX®-treated patients were more likely to experience depression than placebo-treated patients (20% in AVONEX® group vs. 13% in placebo group). The incidences of depression in the placebo-treated and AVONEX®-treated patients in Study 1 were similar. In Study 1, suicidal tendency was seen more frequently in AVONEX®-treated patients (4% in AVONEX® group vs. 1% in placebo group) (see WARNINGS).

Seizures

Seizures have been reported in 4 of 351 AVONEX®-treated patients in the placebo-controlled studies, compared to none in the placebo-treated patients (see Precautions: Seizures).

Post-Marketing Experience

The following adverse events have been identified and reported during post-approval use of AVONEX®: New or worsening other psychiatric disorders, and anaphylaxis (see WARNINGS). Autoimmune disorders including autoimmune hepatitis, idiopathic thrombocytopenia, hyper- and hypothyroidism, and seizures in patients without prior history (see Precautions).

Infrequent reports of congestive heart failure, cardiomyopathy, and cardiomyopathy with congestive heart failure with rare cases being temporally related to the administration of AVONEX® (see Precautions: Cardiomyopathy and Congestive Heart Failure).

Decreased peripheral blood counts in all cell lines, including rare pancytopenia and thrombocytopenia (see WARNINGS: Decreased Peripheral Blood Counts). Some cases of thrombocytopenia have had nadirs below 10,000/µL. Some of these cases reoccur upon rechallenge.

Hepatic injury including elevated serum hepatic enzyme levels and hepatitis, some of which have been severe, has been reported post-marketing (see Precautions: Hepatic Injury).

Meno- and metrorrhagia, rash (including vesicular rash), rare cases of injection site abscess or cellulitis that may require surgical intervention have also been reported in post-marketing experience.

Because reports of these reactions are voluntary and the population is of an uncertain size, it is not always possible to reliably estimate the frequency of the event or establish a causal relationship to drug exposure.

Adverse Reactions Associated with Subcutaneous Use

AVONEX® has also been evaluated in 290 patients with diseases other than multiple sclerosis, primarily chronic viral hepatitis B and C, in which the doses studied ranged from 15 mcg to 75 mcg, given SC, 3 times a week, for up to 6 months. Inflammation at the site of the subcutaneous injection was observed in 52% of treated patients in these studies. Subcutaneous injections were also associated with the following local reactions: injection site necrosis, injection site atrophy, injection site edema and injection site hemorrhage. None of the above was observed in the multiple sclerosis patients participating in Study 1. Injection site edema and injection site hemorrhage were observed in multiple sclerosis patients participating in Study 2.

Immunogenicity

As with all therapeutic proteins, there is a potential for immunogenicity. In recent studies assessing immunogenicity in multiple sclerosis patients administered AVONEX® for at least 1 year, 5% (21 of 390 patients) showed the presence of neutralizing antibodies at one or more times. The clinical significance of neutralizing antibodies to AVONEX® is unknown.

These data reflect the percentage of patients whose test results were considered positive for antibodies to AVONEX® using a two-tiered assay (ELISA binding assay followed by an antiviral cytopathic effect assay), and are highly dependent on the sensitivity and specificity of the assay. Additionally, the observed incidence of neutralizing activity in an assay may be influenced by several factors including sample handling, timing of sample collection, concomitant medications, and underlying disease. For these reasons, comparison of the incidence of antibodies to AVONEX® with the incidence of antibodies to other products may be misleading.

Anaphylaxis has been reported as a rare complication of AVONEX® use. Other allergic reactions have included dyspnea, orolingual edema, skin rash and urticaria (see WARNINGS: Anaphylaxis).

DRUG ABUSE AND DEPENDENCE

There is no evidence that abuse or dependence occurs with AVONEX® therapy. However, the risk of dependence has not been systematically evaluated.

OVERDOSAGE

Safety of doses higher than 60 mcg once a week have not been adequately evaluated. The maximum amount of AVONEX® that can be safely administered has not been determined.

DOSAGE AND ADMINISTRATION

The recommended dosage of AVONEX® (Interferon beta-1a) is 30 mcg injected intramuscularly once a week.

AVONEX® is intended for use under the guidance and supervision of a physician. Patients may self-inject only if their physician determines that it is appropriate and with medical follow-up, as necessary, after proper training in intramuscular injection technique. Sites for injection include the thigh or upper arm (see Medication Guide).

Reconstitution of AVONEX® Vials

Use appropriate aseptic technique during the preparation of AVONEX®. To reconstitute lyophilized AVONEX®, use a sterile syringe and MICRO PIN® to inject 1.1 mL of the supplied diluent, Sterile Water for Injection, USP, into the AVONEX® vial. Gently swirl the vial of AVONEX® to dissolve the drug completely. **DO NOT SHAKE.** The reconstituted solution should be clear to slightly yellow without particles. Inspect the reconstituted product visually prior to use. Discard the product if it contains particulate matter or is discolored. Each vial of reconstituted solution contains 30 mcg/1.0 mL Interferon beta-1a.

Withdraw 1.0 mL of reconstituted solution from the vial into a sterile syringe. Replace the cover on the MICRO PIN® and attach the sterile 23 gauge, 1¼ inch needle and inject the solution intramuscularly. The AVONEX® and diluent vials are for single-use only; unused portions should be discarded.

Using Avonex® Prefilled Syringes

The AVONEX® prefilled syringe should be held upright (rubber cap faces up). Remove the protective cover by turning and gently pulling the rubber cap in a clockwise motion. Attach the 23 gauge, 1¼ inch needle and inject the solution intramuscularly. The AVONEX® prefilled syringe is for single-use only.

HOW SUPPLIED

30 mcg Lyophilized Powder Vial

A vial of AVONEX® is supplied as a lyophilized powder in a single-use vial containing 33 mcg (6.6 million IU) of Interferon beta-1a; 16.5 mg Albumin (Human), USP; 6.4 mg Sodium Chloride, USP; 6.3 mg Dibasic Sodium Phosphate, USP; and 1.3 mg Monobasic Sodium Phosphate, USP, and is preservative-free. Diluent is supplied in a single-use vial (Sterile Water for Injection, USP).

AVONEX® lyophilized vials are available in the following package configuration (NDC 59627-001-03): A package containing four Administration Dose Packs (each containing one vial of AVONEX®, one 10 mL diluent vial, two alcohol wipes, one gauze pad, one 3 mL syringe, one MICRO PIN®* vial access pin, one 23 gauge, 1¼ inch needle, and one adhesive bandage).

30 mcg Prefilled Syringe

A prefilled syringe of AVONEX® is supplied as a sterile liquid albumin-free formulation containing 30 mcg of Interferon beta-1a, 0.79 mg Sodium Acetate Trihydrate, USP; 0.25 mg Glacial Acetic Acid, USP; 15.8 mg Arginine Hydrochloride, USP; and 0.025 mg Polysorbate 20 in Water for Injection, USP. Each prefilled glass syringe contains 0.5 mL for IM injection.

AVONEX® prefilled syringes are available in the following package configuration (NDC 59627-002-05): A package containing four Administration Dose Packs (each containing

Table 3
Adverse Events and Selected Laboratory Abnormalities in the Placebo-Controlled Studies

Adverse Event	Placebo (N = 333)	AVONEX® (N = 351)
Body as a Whole		
Headache	55%	58%
Flu-like symptoms (otherwise unspecified)	29%	49%
Pain	21%	23%
Asthenia	18%	24%
Fever	9%	20%
Chills	5%	19%
Abdominal pain	6%	8%
Injection site pain	6%	8%
Infection	4%	7%
Injection site inflammation	2%	6%
Chest pain	2%	5%
Injection site reaction	1%	3%
Toothache	1%	3%
Nervous System		
Depression	14%	18%
Dizziness	12%	14%
Respiratory System		
Upper respiratory tract infection	12%	14%
Sinusitis	12%	14%
Bronchitis	5%	8%
Digestive System		
Nausea	19%	23%
Musculoskeletal System		
Myalgia	22%	29%
Arthralgia	6%	9%
Urogenital		
Urinary tract infection	15%	17%
Urine constituents abnormal	0%	3%
Skin and Appendages		
Alopecia	2%	4%
Special Senses		
Eye disorder	2%	4%
Hemic and Lymphatic System		
Injection site ecchymosis	4%	6%
Anemia	1%	4%
Cardiovascular System		
Migraine	3%	5%
Vasodilation	0%	2%

one single-use syringe of AVONEX® and one 23 gauge, 1¼ inch needle), and a recloseable accessory pouch containing 4 alcohol wipes, 4 gauze pads, and 4 adhesive bandages.

Stability and Storage

30 mcg Lyophilized Powder Vial

Vials of AVONEX® must be stored in a 2–8°C (36–46°F) refrigerator. Should refrigeration be unavailable, vials of AVONEX® can be stored at 25°C (77°F) for a period of up to 30 days. DO NOT EXPOSE TO HIGH TEMPERATURES. DO NOT FREEZE. Protect from light. Do not use beyond the expiration date stamped on the vial. Following reconstitution, it is recommended the product be used as soon as possible within 6 hours stored at 2–8°C (36–46°F). DO NOT FREEZE RECONSTITUTED AVONEX®.

30 mcg Prefilled Syringe

AVONEX® in prefilled syringes must be stored in a 2–8°C (36–46°F) refrigerator. Once removed from the refrigerator, AVONEX® in a prefilled syringe should be allowed to warm to room temperature (about 30 minutes) and used within 12 hours. Do not use external heat sources such as hot water to warm AVONEX® in a prefilled syringe. DO NOT EXPOSE TO HIGH TEMPERATURES. DO NOT FREEZE. Protect from light. Do not use beyond the expiration date stamped on the syringe.

REFERENCES

1. Jacobs LD, et al. Intramuscular interferon beta-1a for disease progression in relapsing multiple sclerosis. Ann Neurol 1996;39(3):285–294.
2. Jacobs LD, et al. Intramuscular interferon beta-1a initiated during a first demyelinating event in multiple sclerosis. NEJM 2000;343:898–904.
3. Kurtzke JF. Rating neurologic impairment in multiple sclerosis: an expanded disability status scale (EDSS). Neurology 1983;33:1444–1452.

AVONEX® (Interferon beta-1a)

Manufactured by:

BIOGEN, INC.

14 Cambridge Center

Cambridge, MA 02142 USA

1-800-456-2255

U.S. Patent Pending

I61018-4 (Issue date 03/2004)

Rx only

**Micro Pin® is the trademark of B. Braun Medical Inc.*

MEDICATION GUIDE

AVONEX®

Interferon beta-1a

(Including appendix with instructions for using AVONEX® Prefilled Syringe or the AVONEX® vials)

Please read this guide carefully before you start to use AVONEX® (a-vuh-necks) and each time your prescription is refilled since there may be new information. The information in this guide does not take the place of talking with your doctor or healthcare professional.

What is the most important information I should know about AVONEX®?

AVONEX® will not cure multiple sclerosis (MS) but it has been shown to decrease the number of flare-ups and slow the occurrence of some of the physical disability that is common in people with MS. AVONEX® can cause serious side effects, so before you start taking AVONEX®, you should talk with your doctor about the possible benefits of AVONEX® and its possible side effects to decide if AVONEX® is right for you. Potential serious side effects include:

- **Depression**—Some people treated with interferons, including AVONEX®, have become depressed (feeling sad, feeling low or feeling bad about oneself). Some people have thought about killing themselves and a few have committed suicide. Depression is common in people with MS. If you are noticeably sadder or feeling more hopeless, you should tell a family member or friend right away and call your doctor as soon as possible. You should tell the doctor if you have ever had any mental illness, including depression, and if you take any medicines for depression.
- **Risk to pregnancy**—If you become pregnant while taking AVONEX®, you should stop using AVONEX® immediately and call your doctor. AVONEX® may cause you to lose your baby (miscarry) or may cause harm to your unborn child. You and your doctor will need to decide whether the potential benefit of taking AVONEX® is greater than the risks are to your unborn child.
- **Allergic reactions**—Some patients taking AVONEX® have had severe allergic reactions leading to difficulty breathing. Allergic reactions can happen after your first dose or may not happen until after you have taken AVONEX® many times. Less severe allergic reactions such as rash, itching, skin bumps or swelling of the mouth and tongue can also happen. If you think you are having an allergic reaction, stop using AVONEX® immediately and call your doctor.
- **Blood problems**—You may have a drop in the levels of infection-fighting blood cells, red blood cells or cells that help to form blood clots. If the drop in levels are severe, they can lessen your ability to fight infections, make you feel tired or sluggish or cause you to bruise or bleed easily.
- **Seizures**—Some patients have had seizures while taking AVONEX®, including some patients who have never had seizures before. It is not known whether the seizures were related to the effects of their MS, to AVONEX®, or to a combination of both. If you have a seizure while taking AVONEX®, you should stop taking AVONEX® and call your doctor right away.
- **Heart problems**—While AVONEX® is not known to have direct effects on the heart, a few patients who did not have a history of heart problems developed heart muscle problems or congestive heart failure after taking AVONEX®. Some of the symptoms of heart problems are swollen ankles, shortness of breath, decreased ability to exercise, fast heartbeat, tightness in chest, increased need to urinate at night, and not being able to lay flat in bed. If you develop these symptoms or any heart problems while taking AVONEX®, you should call your doctor right away.

For more information on possible side effects with AVONEX®, please read the section on **"What are the possible side effects of AVONEX®?"** in this Medication Guide.

What is AVONEX®?

AVONEX® is a form of a protein called beta interferon that occurs naturally in the body. It is used to treat relapsing forms of multiple sclerosis. It will not cure your MS but may decrease the number of flare-ups of the disease and slow the occurrence of some of the physical disability that is common in people with MS. MS is a life-long disease that affects your nervous system by destroying the protective covering (myelin) that surrounds your nerve fibers. The way AVONEX® works in MS is not known.

Who should not take AVONEX®?

Do not take AVONEX® if you have had an allergic reaction (difficulty breathing, itching, flushing or skin bumps spread widely over the body) to interferon beta.

Do not take the vial formulation of AVONEX® if you have a history of hypersensitivity to albumin (human).

If you have ever had any of the following conditions or serious medical problems, you should tell your doctor before taking AVONEX®:

- Depression (sinking feeling or sadness), anxiety (feeling uneasy or fearful for no reason), or trouble sleeping
- Problems with your thyroid gland
- Blood problems such as bleeding or bruising easily and anemia (low red blood cells) or low white blood cells
- Seizures (for example, epilepsy)
- Heart problems
- Liver disease
- Are planning to become pregnant

You should tell your doctor if you are taking any other prescription or nonprescription medicines. This includes any vitamin or mineral supplements, or herbal products.

You should tell your doctor if you have had a natural rubber sensitivity since the AVONEX® prefilled syringe cap contains dry natural rubber, which may cause allergic reactions.

How should I take AVONEX®?

To get the most benefit from this medicine, it is important that you take AVONEX® exactly as your doctor tells you.

AVONEX® is given by injection into the muscle (intramuscular injection) once a week, on the same day (for example, every Monday right before bedtime). If you miss a dose, you should take your next dose as soon as you remember. You should continue your regular schedule the following week. **Do not take AVONEX® on two consecutive days.** Take only the dose your doctor has prescribed for you. Do not change your dose unless you are told to by your doctor. If you take more than your prescribed dose, call your healthcare provider right away. Your doctor may want to monitor you more closely.

You should always follow your doctor's instructions and advice about how to take this medication. If your doctor feels that you, or a family member or friend, may give you the injections, then you and/or the other person should be instructed by your doctor or other healthcare provider in how to prepare and inject your dose of AVONEX®. Do not try to give yourself injections at home until you are sure that you (or the person who will be giving you the injections) fully understands and is comfortable with how to prepare and inject the product. At the end of this guide there are detailed instructions on how to prepare and give yourself an injection of AVONEX® that will help remind you of the instructions from your doctor or healthcare provider.

Always use a new, unopened AVONEX® vial or prefilled syringe for each injection. Never reuse the vials or syringes. It is important to keep your work area, your hands, and your injection site clean to minimize risk of infection. You should wash your hands prior to handling the syringe.

It is important that you change your injection site each week.

Do not inject into an area of the body where the skin is irritated, reddened, bruised, infected or scarred in any way. Use the alcohol wipe to **thoroughly** clean the skin at the injection site you haven chosen. Using a circular motion, and starting at the injection site and moving outward, clean the injection site with an alcohol wipe. Let the skin area dry before you inject the AVONEX.

AVONEX® comes in two different forms (a powder in a single-use vial and a liquid in a prefilled syringe). **See the attached appendix for detailed instructions for preparing and giving a dose of AVONEX®. These instructions are specific to the form of AVONEX® chosen for you by your healthcare provider.**

What should I avoid while taking AVONEX®?

- **Pregnancy**—You should avoid becoming pregnant while taking AVONEX® until you have talked with your doctor. AVONEX® can cause you to lose your baby (miscarry).
- **Breast-feeding**—You should talk to your doctor if you are breast-feeding an infant. It is not known if the interferon in AVONEX® gets into the breast milk, or if it could harm your nursing baby.

What are the possible side effects of AVONEX®?

- **Flu-like symptoms**—Most people who take AVONEX® have flu-like symptoms (fever, chills, sweating, muscle aches, and tiredness) early during the course of therapy. Usually, these symptoms last for a day after the injection. You may be able to manage these flu-like symptoms by injecting your AVONEX® dose at bedtime and taking over-the-counter pain and fever reducers. For many people, these symptoms lessen or go away over time. Talk to your doctor if these symptoms continue longer than the first few months of therapy, or if they are difficult to manage.
- **Depression**—Some patients taking interferons have become severely depressed and/or anxious. If you feel sad or hopeless you should tell a friend or family member right away and call your doctor immediately. Your doctor or healthcare provider may ask that you stop taking AVONEX®, and/or may recommend that you take a medication to treat your depression. **(See "What is the most important information I should know about AVONEX®?")**
- **Blood problems**—A drop in the levels of white (infection-fighting) blood cells, red blood cells, or a part of your blood that helps to form blood clots (platelets) can happen. If this drop in blood levels is severe, it can lessen your ability to fight infections, make you feel very tired or sluggish, or cause you to bruise or bleed easily. Your doctor may ask you to have periodic blood tests. **(See "What is the most important information I should know about AVONEX®?")**
- **Liver problems**—Your liver function may be affected. Symptoms of changes in your liver include yellowing of the skin and whites of the eyes and easy bruising.
- **Thyroid problems**—Some people taking AVONEX® develop changes in the function of their thyroid. Symptoms of these changes include feeling cold or hot all the time, a change in your weight (gain or loss) without a change in your diet or amount of exercise you get, or feeling emotional.
- **Seizures**—Some patients have had seizures while taking AVONEX®, including patients who have never had seizures before. It is not known whether the seizures were related to the effects of their MS, to AVONEX®, or to a combination of both. If you have a seizure while taking AVONEX®, you should call your doctor right away. **(See "What is the most important information I should know about AVONEX®?")**
- **Heart problems**—While AVONEX® is not known to have any direct effects on the heart, a few patients who did not have a history of heart problems developed heart muscle problems or congestive heart failure after taking AVONEX®. Some of the symptoms of heart problems are swollen ankles, shortness of breath, decreased ability to exercise, fast heartbeat, tightness in chest, increased need to urinate at night, and not being able to lay flat in bed. If you develop these symptoms or any heart problems while taking AVONEX®, you should call your doctor right away. **(See "What is the most important information I should know about AVONEX®?")**

If you get any of the symptoms listed in this section or any listed in the section **"What is the most important information I should know about AVONEX®?"**, you should call your doctor right away. Whether you experience any side effects or not, you and your doctor should periodically discuss your general health. Your doctor may want to monitor you more closely or may ask you to have blood tests more frequently.

General advice about prescription medicines

Medicines are sometimes prescribed for purposes other than those listed in a Medication Guide. This medication has been prescribed for your particular condition. Do not use it for another condition or give this drug to anyone else. If you have questions you should speak with your doctor or healthcare professional. You may also ask your doctor or pharmacist for a copy of the information provided to them with the product.

Keep this and all drugs out of the reach of children.

This Medication Guide has been approved by the U.S. Food and Drug Administration.

Manufactured by:

Biogen, Inc.

14 Cambridge Center

Cambridge, MA 02142 USA

1-800-456-2255

I61018- 3(Issue date03/2004)

Medication Guide Appendix: Instructions for Preparing and Giving a Dose with an AVONEX® Prefilled Syringe

Storing AVONEX® Prefilled Syringes

AVONEX® in prefilled syringes should be refrigerated (36–46°F or 2–8°C). Once removed from the refrigerator, AVONEX® in a prefilled syringe should be allowed to warm to room temperature (about 30 minutes) and used within 12

Continued on next page

Avonex—Cont.

hours. Do not use external heat sources such as hot water to warm AVONEX® in a prefilled syringe. Do not expose to high temperatures. Do not freeze. Protect from light.

How do I prepare and inject a dose of AVONEX®?

Find a well lit, clean, flat work surface like a table and collect all the supplies you will need to give yourself or receive an injection. Take one AVONEX® Administration Dose Pack out of the refrigerator about 30 minutes before you plan on injecting your dose to allow it to reach room temperature. A room temperature solution is more comfortable to inject.

You will need the following supplies:

- single-use prefilled syringe
- sterile needle
- alcohol wipe
- gauze pad
- adhesive bandage
- a puncture resistant container for disposal of used syringes and needles
- 1 syringe diagram card

Preparing the AVONEX® prefilled syringe

It is important to keep your work area, your hands, and your injection site clean to minimize risk of infection. You should wash your hands prior to handling the syringe.

1. Check the expiration date. The expiration date is printed on the AVONEX® prefilled syringe, syringe package and the carton. Do not use if the medication is expired.
2. Check the contents of the syringe. The solution in the syringe should be clear and colorless. If the solution is colored or cloudy, do not use the syringe. Get a new syringe.
3. Hold the syringe so the rubber cap is facing down. Take the card with the drawing of the syringe and hold it next to the real syringe so the drawing and the real syringe are side-by-side. Check to make sure the amount of liquid in the syringe is the same or very close to the 0.5 mL arrow shown on the card with the drawing of the prefilled syringe. The top of the liquid may be curved as shown in the drawing. The 0.5 mL arrow should point near the middle of the curved liquid. If the real syringe does not have the correct amount of liquid, DO NOT USE THAT SYRINGE. Call your pharmacist.
4. Hold the AVONEX® prefilled syringe upright (rubber cap facing up).

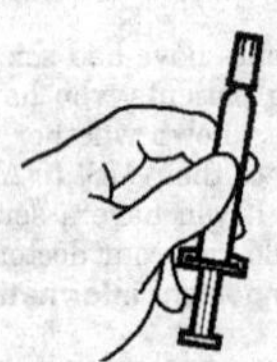

5. Remove the protective rubber cap by turning and gently pulling the cap in a clockwise motion.

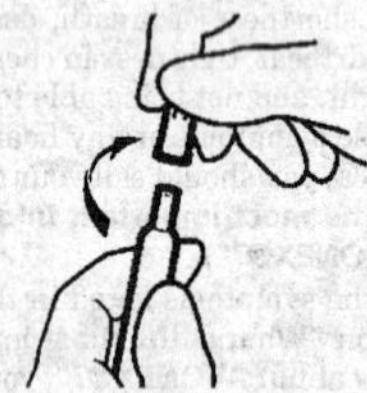

6. Open the package with the 23 gauge 1¼ inch needle. Attach the needle by firmly pressing it onto the syringe and turning it a half turn clockwise.

NOTE: If you do not firmly attach the needle to the syringe, it may leak so you may not get your full dose of AVONEX®.

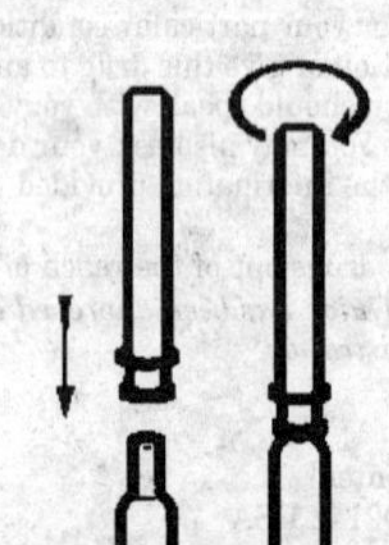

Selecting an injection site

You should use a different site each time you inject. This can be as simple as switching between thighs (if you are always injecting yourself), or if another person is helping you, you can rotate between your upper arms and your thighs. Keeping a record of the date and location of each injection will help you.

Do not inject into an area of the body where the skin is irritated, reddened, bruised, infected or scarred in any way. The best sites for intramuscular injection are the thigh and upper arm:

- thigh

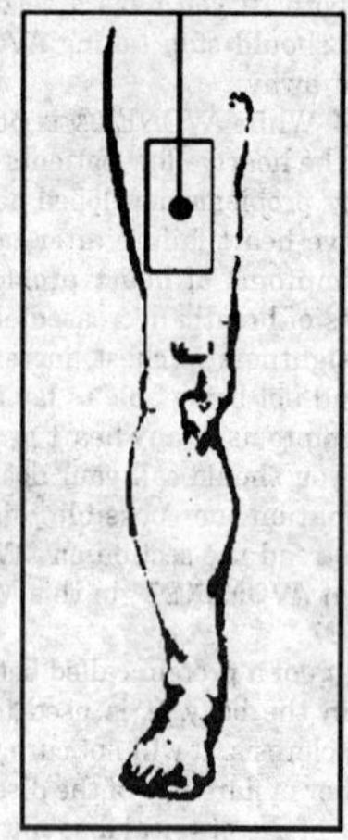

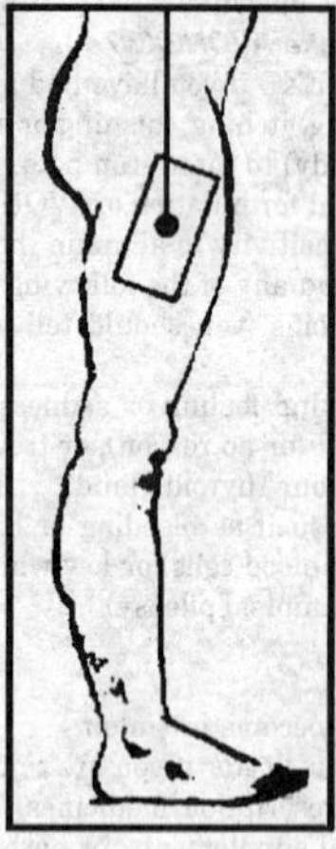

- upper arm

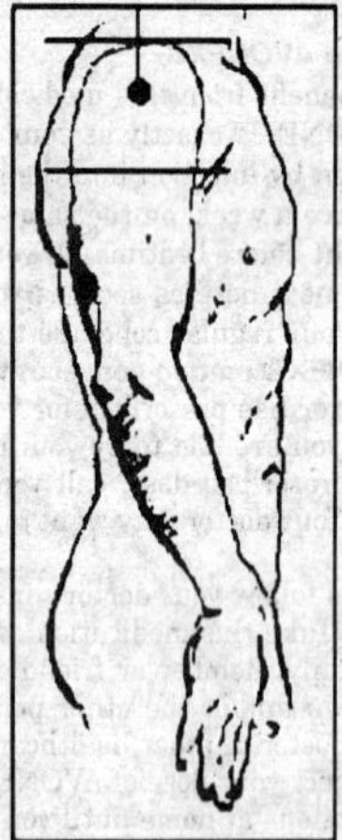

Injecting the AVONEX® dose

1. Use the alcohol wipe to clean the skin at the injection site you choose. Then, pull the protective cover **straight** off the needle; do not twist the cover off.
2. With one hand, stretch the skin out around the injection site. Hold the syringe like a pencil with the other hand, and using a quick motion insert the needle at a 90° angle, through the skin and into the muscle.
3. Once the needle is in, let go of the skin and slowly push the plunger down until the syringe is empty.

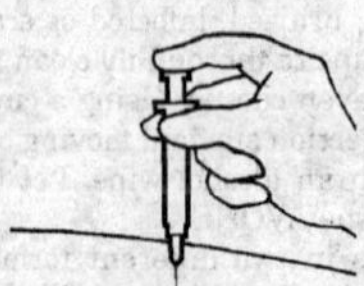

4. Take the gauze pad and hold it near the needle at the injection site and pull the needle straight out. Use the gauze pad to apply pressure to the site for a few seconds or rub gently in a circular motion.

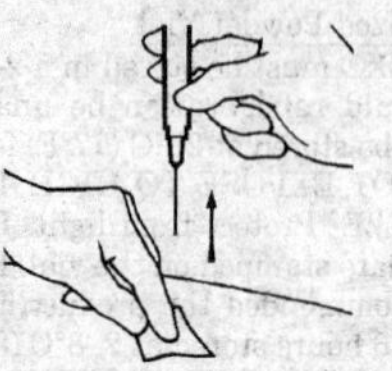

5. If there is bleeding at the site, wipe it off and, if necessary, apply an adhesive bandage.
6. After 2 hours, check the injection site for redness, swelling or tenderness. If you have a skin reaction and it does not clear up in a few days, contact your doctor or nurse.
7. Dispose of the used syringe and needle in your puncture resistant container. This is a single-use syringe. DO NOT USE a syringe or needle more than once.

Disposal of syringes and needles

There may be special state and/or local laws for disposing of used needles and syringes. Your doctor, nurse or pharmacist should provide you with instructions on how to dispose of your used needles and syringes.

- **Always keep your disposal container out of the reach of children.**
- DO NOT throw used needles and syringes into the household trash and DO NOT RECYCLE.

Appendix Revision Date: 05/2003

Medication Guide Appendix: Instructions for Preparing and Giving a Dose with an AVONEX® <u>Vial</u>

Storing AVONEX® Vials

Prior to use, AVONEX® should be refrigerated (36–46°F or 2–8°C) but can be kept for up to 30 days at room temperature (77°F or 25°C). You should avoid exposing AVONEX® to high temperatures and freezing. After mixing, AVONEX® solution should be used immediately, within 6 hours when stored refrigerated at 36–46°F or 2–8°C. Do not freeze the AVONEX® solution.

How do I prepare and inject a dose of AVONEX®?

Find a well-lit, clean, flat work surface like a table and collect all the supplies you will need to give yourself or receive an injection. You may want to take one AVONEX® Administration Dose Pack out of the refrigerator about 30 minutes before you plan on injecting your dose to allow it to reach room temperature. A room temperature solution is more comfortable to inject.

You will need the following supplies:

- vial of AVONEX® (white to off-white powder or cake)
- vial of diluent, single-use (Sterile Water for Injection, USP)
- 3 mL syringe
- blue MICRO PIN® (vial access pin)
- sterile needle
- alcohol wipes
- gauze pad
- adhesive bandage
- a puncture resistant container for disposal of used syringes, needles, and MICRO PINS.

Preparing the AVONEX® solution

It is important to keep your work area, your hands, and your injection site clean to minimize risk of infection. You should wash your hands prior to preparing the medication.

1. Check the expiration date on the AVONEX® vial and the vial of diluent; do not use if the medication or diluent is expired.
2. Remove the caps from the vial of AVONEX® and the vial of diluent, and clean the rubber stopper on the top of each vial with an alcohol wipe.

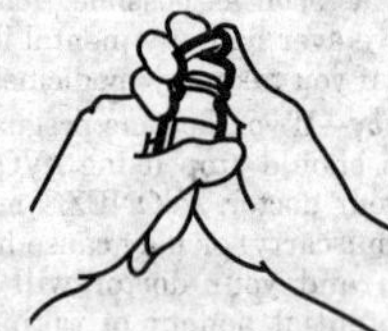

3. Remove the small light blue protective cover from the end of the syringe barrel with a counterclockwise turn.

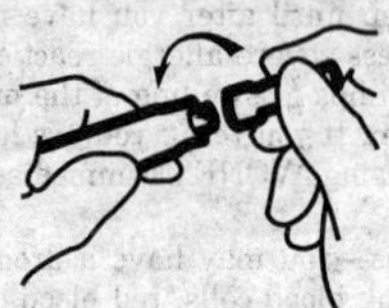

4. Attach the blue MICRO PIN® to the syringe by turning clockwise until secure. *NOTE: Over-tightening can make the MICRO PIN® difficult to remove.*

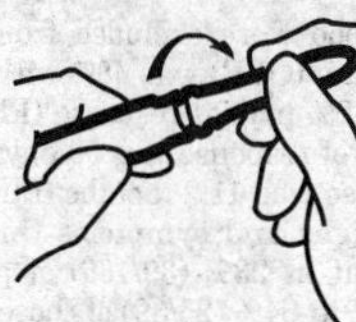

5. Pull the MICRO PIN® cover straight off; do not twist. Save the cover for later use.

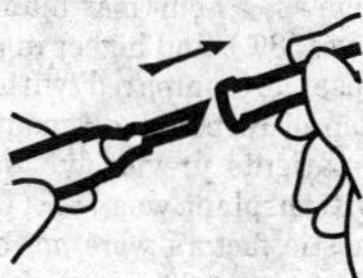

6. Pull back the syringe plunger to the 1.1 mL mark.

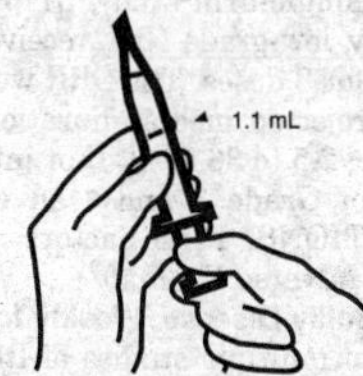

7. Firmly push the MICRO PIN® down through the **center** of the rubber stopper of the diluent vial.

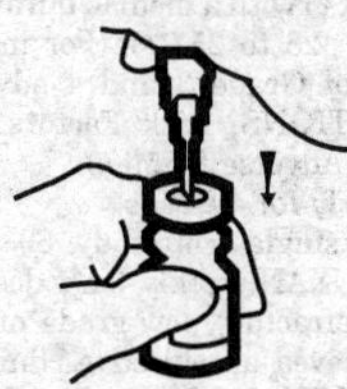

8. Inject the air in the syringe into the diluent vial by pushing down on the plunger until it cannot be pushed any further.
9. Keeping the MICRO PIN® in the vial, turn the diluent vial and syringe upside down.
10. While keeping the MICRO PIN® in the fluid, slowly pull back on the plunger to withdraw 1.1 mL of diluent into the syringe.

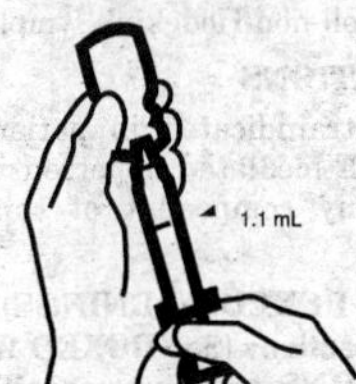

11. Gently tap the syringe with your finger to make any air bubbles rise to the top. If bubbles are present, slowly press the plunger in (to push just the bubbles out through the needle). Make sure there is still 1.1 mL of diluent in the syringe.

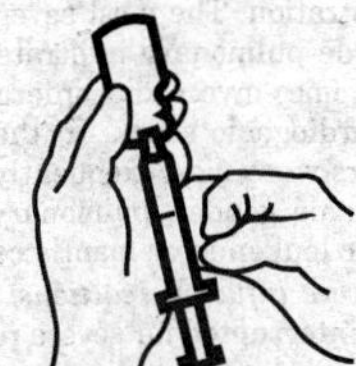

12. Slowly pull the MICRO PIN® out of the diluent vial.
13. Carefully insert the MICRO PIN® through the **center** of the rubber stopper of the vial of AVONEX®. *NOTE: Off-center punctures can push the stopper into the vial. If the stopper falls into the vial, do not use.*
14. **Slowly** inject the diluent into the vial of AVONEX®. DO NOT aim the stream of diluent directly on the AVONEX® powder. Too direct or forceful a stream of diluent onto the powder may cause foaming, and make it difficult to withdraw AVONEX®.

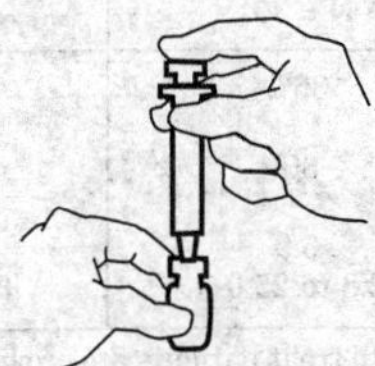

15. Without removing the syringe, **gently** swirl the vial until the AVONEX® is dissolved. ***DO NOT SHAKE.***

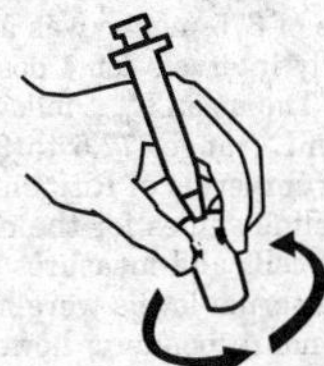

16. Check to see that all of the AVONEX® is dissolved. Check the solution in the vial of AVONEX®. It should be clear to slightly yellow in color and should not have any particles. Do not use the vial if the solution is cloudy, has particles in it or is a color other than clear to slightly yellow.
17. Turn the vial and syringe upside down. Slowly pull back on the plunger to withdraw 1.0 mL of AVONEX®. If bubbles appear, push solution slowly back into the vial and withdraw the solution again.

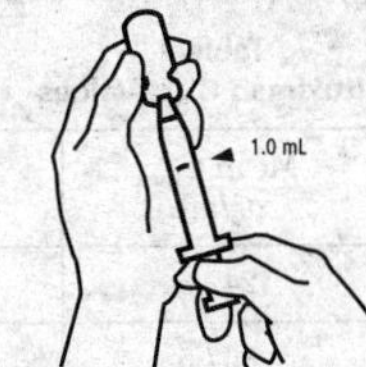

18. With the vial still upside down, tap the syringe **gently** to make any air bubbles rise to the top. Then press the plunger in until the AVONEX® is at the top of the syringe. Check the volume (should be 1.0 mL) and withdraw more medication if necessary. Withdraw the MICRO PIN® and syringe from the vial.
19. Replace the cover on the MICRO PIN® and remove from the syringe with a counterclockwise turn.
20. Attach the sterile needle for injection to the syringe turning clockwise until the needle is secure. A secure attachment will prevent leakage during the injection.

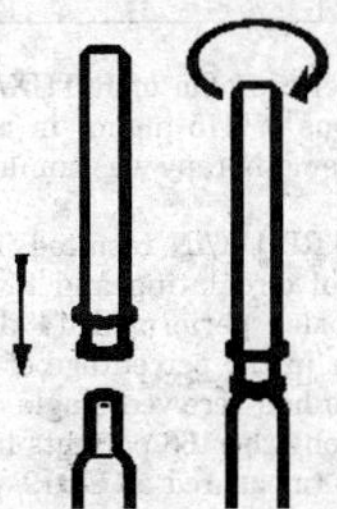

Selecting an injection site

You should use a different site each time you inject. This can be as simple as switching between thighs (if you are always injecting yourself), or if another person is helping you, you can rotate between your upper arms and your thighs. Keeping a record of the date and location of each injection will help you.

Do not inject into an area of the body where the skin is irritated, reddened, bruised, infected or scarred in any way. The best sites for intramuscular injection are the thigh and upper arm:

• thigh

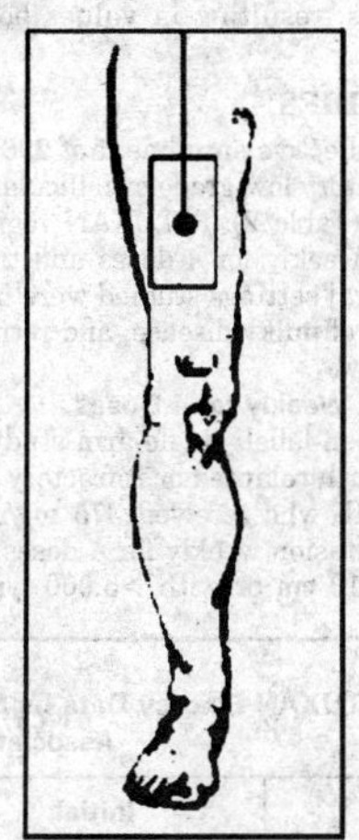

[See first figure at top of next column]

• upper arm

[See second figure at top of next column]

You should rotate injection sites each week. This can be as simple as switching between thighs (if you are always injecting yourself). If another person is helping you, you can rotate among your thighs and upper arms. Make sure that the site you choose is free from any skin irritations.

Injecting the AVONEX® dose

1. Use a new alcohol wipe to clean the skin at one of the recommended intramuscular injection sites. Then, pull the protective cover **straight** off the needle; do not twist the cover off.

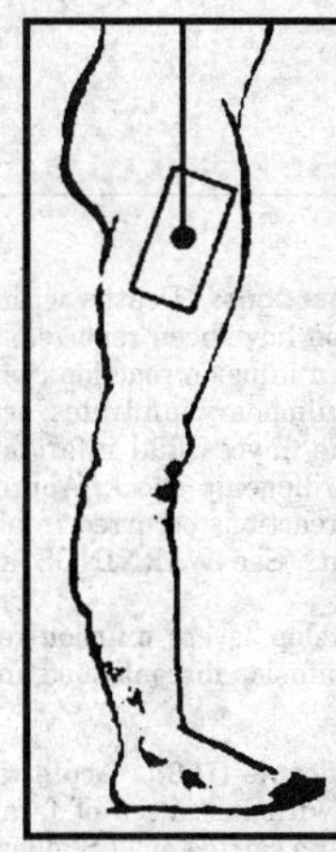

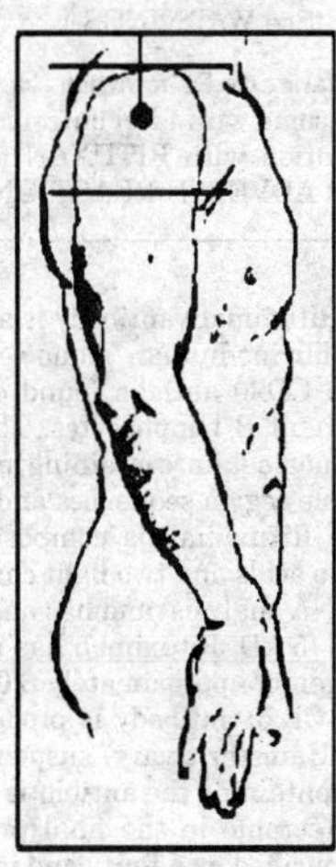

2. With one hand, stretch the skin out around the injection site. Hold the syringe like a pencil with the other hand, and using a quick motion insert the needle at a 90° angle, through the skin and into the muscle.
3. Once the needle is in, let go of the skin and slowly push the plunger down until the syringe is empty.

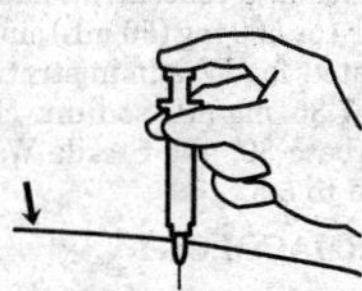

4. Hold a gauze pad near the needle at the injection site and pull the needle straight out. Use the pad to apply pressure to the site for a few seconds or rub gently in a circular motion.

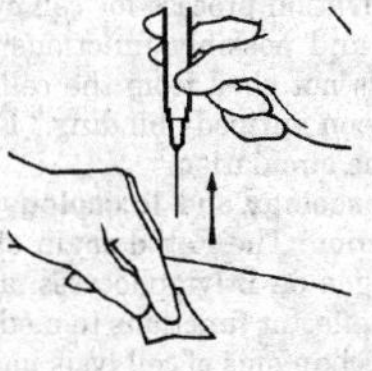

5. If there is bleeding at the site, wipe it off and, if necessary, apply an adhesive bandage.
6. Dispose of the used syringe, needle and blue MICRO PIN® in your puncture resistant container. DO NOT USE a syringe, MICRO PIN®, or needle more than once. The AVONEX® and diluent vials should be put in the trash.

Disposal of syringes and needles

There may be special state and/or local laws for disposing of used needles and syringes. Your doctor, nurse or pharmacist should provide you with instructions on how to dispose of your used needles and syringes.

- **Always keep your disposal container out of the reach of children.**
- DO NOT throw used needles and syringes into the household trash and DO NOT RECYCLE.

Appendix Revision Date: 03/2004

Continued on next page

RITUXAN® ℞
[rĭ-tŭk-sĭn]
Rituximab

WARNINGS

Fatal Infusion Reactions: Deaths within 24 hours of RITUXAN infusion have been reported. These fatal reactions followed an infusion reaction complex which included hypoxia, pulmonary infiltrates, acute respiratory distress syndrome, myocardial infarction, ventricular fibrillation or cardiogenic shock. Approximately 80% of fatal infusion reactions occurred in association with the first infusion. (See WARNINGS and ADVERSE REACTIONS.)
Patients who develop severe infusion reactions should have RITUXAN infusion discontinued and receive medical treatment.

Tumor Lysis Syndrome (TLS): Acute renal failure requiring dialysis with instances of fatal outcome has been reported in the setting of TLS following treatment with RITUXAN. (See WARNINGS.)

Severe Mucocutaneous Reactions: Severe mucocutaneous reactions, some with fatal outcome, have been reported in association with RITUXAN treatment. (See WARNINGS and ADVERSE REACTIONS.)

DESCRIPTION

The RITUXAN® (Rituximab) antibody is a genetically engineered chimeric murine/human monoclonal antibody directed against the CD20 antigen found on the surface of normal and malignant B lymphocytes. The antibody is an IgG_1 kappa immunoglobulin containing murine light- and heavy-chain variable region sequences and human constant region sequences. Rituximab is composed of two heavy chains of 451 amino acids and two light chains of 213 amino acids (based on cDNA analysis) and has an approximate molecular weight of 145 kD. Rituximab has a binding affinity for the CD20 antigen of approximately 8.0 nM.
The chimeric anti-CD20 antibody is produced by mammalian cell (Chinese Hamster Ovary) suspension culture in a nutrient medium containing the antibiotic gentamicin. Gentamicin is not detectable in the final product. The anti-CD20 antibody is purified by affinity and ion exchange chromatography. The purification process includes specific viral inactivation and removal procedures. Rituximab drug product is manufactured from either bulk drug substance manufactured by Genentech, Inc. (US License No. 1048) or utilizing formulated bulk Rituximab supplied by IDEC Pharmaceuticals Corporation (US License No. 1235) under a shared manufacturing arrangement.
RITUXAN is a sterile, clear, colorless, preservative-free liquid concentrate for intravenous (IV) administration. RITUXAN is supplied at a concentration of 10 mg/mL in either 100 mg (10 mL) or 500 mg (50 mL) single-use vials. The product is formulated for IV administration in 9.0 mg/mL sodium chloride, 7.35 mg/mL sodium citrate dihydrate, 0.7 mg/mL polysorbate 80, and Sterile Water for Injection. The pH is adjusted to 6.5.

CLINICAL PHARMACOLOGY

General
Rituximab binds specifically to the antigen CD20 (human B-lymphocyte-restricted differentiation antigen, Bp35), a hydrophobic transmembrane protein with a molecular weight of approximately 35 kD located on pre-B and mature B lymphocytes.[1,2] The antigen is also expressed on > 90% of B-cell non-Hodgkin's lymphomas (NHL),[3] but is not found on hematopoietic stem cells, pro-B cells, normal plasma cells or other normal tissues.[4] CD20 regulates an early step(s) in the activation process for cell cycle initiation and differentiation,[4] and possibly functions as a calcium ion channel.[5] CD20 is not shed from the cell surface and does not internalize upon antibody binding.[6] Free CD20 antigen is not found in the circulation.[2]

Preclinical Pharmacology and Toxicology
Mechanism of Action: The Fab domain of Rituximab binds to the CD20 antigen on B lymphocytes, and the Fc domain recruits immune effector functions to mediate B-cell lysis *in vitro*. Possible mechanisms of cell lysis include complement-dependent cytotoxicity (CDC)[7] and antibody-dependent cell mediated cytotoxicity (ADCC). The antibody has been shown to induce apoptosis in the DHL-4 human B-cell lymphoma line.[8]
Normal Tissue Cross-reactivity: Rituximab binding was observed on lymphoid cells in the thymus, the white pulp of the spleen, and a majority of B lymphocytes in peripheral blood and lymph nodes. Little or no binding was observed in the non-lymphoid tissues examined.

Human Pharmacokinetics/Pharmacodynamics
In patients given single doses at 10, 50, 100, 250 or 500 mg/m² as an IV infusion, serum levels and the half-life of Rituximab were proportional to dose.[9] In 14 patients given 375 mg/m² as an IV infusion for 4 weekly doses, the mean serum half-life was 76.3 hours (range, 31.5 to 152.6 hours) after the first infusion and 205.8 hours (range, 83.9 to 407.0 hours); after the fourth infusion.[10,11,12] The wide range of half-lives may reflect the variable tumor burden among patients and the changes in CD20-positive (normal and malignant) B-cell populations upon repeated administrations.
RITUXAN at a dose of 375 mg/m² was administered as an IV infusion at weekly intervals for 4 doses to 203 patients naive to RITUXAN. The mean C_{max} following the fourth infusion was 486 µg/mL (range, 77.5 to 996.6 µg/mL). The peak and trough serum levels of Rituximab were inversely correlated with baseline values for the number of circulating CD20-positive B cells and measures of disease burden. Median steady-state serum levels were higher for responders compared with nonresponders; however, no difference was found in the rate of elimination as measured by serum half-life. Serum levels were higher in patients with International Working Formulation (IWF) subtypes B, C, and D as compared with those with subtype A. Rituximab was detectable in the serum of patients 3 to 6 months after completion of treatment.
RITUXAN at a dose of 375 mg/m² was administered as an IV infusion at weekly intervals for 8 doses to 37 patients. The mean C_{max} after 8 infusions was 550 µg/mL (range, 171 to 1177 µg/mL). The mean C_{max} increased with each successive infusion through the eighth infusion (Table 1).

Table 1
Rituximab C_{max} Values

Infusion Number	Mean C_{max} µg/mL	Range µg/mL
1	242.6	16.1–581.9
2	357.5	106.8–948.6
3	381.3	110.5–731.2
4	460.0	138.0–835.8
5	475.3	156.0–929.1
6	515.4	152.7–865.2
7	544.6	187.0–936.8
8	550.0	170.6–1177.0

The pharmacokinetic profile of RITUXAN when administered as 6 infusions of 375 mg/m² in combination with 6 cycles of CHOP chemotherapy was similar to that seen with RITUXAN alone.
Administration of RITUXAN resulted in a rapid and sustained depletion of circulating and tissue-based B cells. Lymph node biopsies performed 14 days after therapy showed a decrease in the percentage of B cells in seven of eight patients who had received single doses of Rituximab ≥100 mg/m².[9] Among the 166 patients in the pivotal study, circulating B cells (measured as CD19–positive cells) were depleted within the first three doses with sustained depletion for up to 6 to 9 months post-treatment in 83% of patients. Of the responding patients assessed (n = 80), 1% failed to show significant depletion of CD19– positive cells after the third infusion of Rituximab as compared to 19% of the nonresponding patients. B-cell recovery began at approximately 6 months following completion of treatment. Median B-cell levels returned to normal by 12 months following completion of treatment.
There were sustained and statistically significant reductions in both IgM and IgG serum levels observed from 5 through 11 months following Rituximab administration. However, only 14% of patients had reductions in IgM and/or IgG serum levels, resulting in values below the normal range.

CLINICAL STUDIES

Studies with a collective enrollment of 296 patients having relapsed or refractory low-grade or follicular B-cell NHL are described below (Table 2). RITUXAN regimens tested include treatment weekly for 4 doses and treatment weekly for 8 doses. Clinical settings studied were initial treatment, initial treatment of bulky disease, and retreatment.
[See table 2 below]

Initial Treatment, Weekly for 4 Doses
A multicenter, open-label, single-arm study was conducted in 166 patients with relapsed or refractory low-grade or follicular B-cell NHL who received 375 mg/m² of RITUXAN given as an IV infusion weekly for 4 doses.[13] Patients with tumor masses >10 cm or with >5,000 lymphocytes/µL in the peripheral blood were excluded from the study. The overall response rate (ORR) was 48% with 6% complete response (CR) and 42% partial response (PR) rates. The median time to onset of response was 50 days and the median duration of response was 11.2 months (range, 1.9 to 42.1+). Disease-related signs and symptoms (including B-symptoms) were present in 23% (39/166) of patients at study entry and resolved in 64% (25/39) of those patients.
In a multivariate analysis, the ORR was higher in patients with IWF B, C, and D histologic subtypes as compared to IWF subtype A (58% vs. 12%), higher in patients whose largest lesion was <5 cm vs. >7 cm (maximum, 21 cm) in greatest diameter (53% vs. 38%), and higher in patients with chemosensitive relapse as compared with chemoresistant (defined as duration of response <3 months) relapse (53% vs. 36%). ORR in patients previously treated with autologous bone marrow transplant was 78% (18/23). The following adverse prognostic factors were *not* associated with a lower response rate: age ≥60 years, extranodal disease, prior anthracycline therapy, and bone marrow involvement.

Initial Treatment, Weekly for 8 Doses
In a multicenter, single-arm study, 37 patients with relapsed or refractory, low-grade NHL received 375 mg/m² of RITUXAN weekly for 8 doses. The ORR was 57% (CR 14%, PR 43%) with a projected median duration of response of 13.4 months (range, 2.5 to 36.5+).[14] (For information on the higher incidence of Grade 3 and 4 adverse events, see ADVERSE REACTIONS, Risk Factors Associated with Increased Rates of Adverse Events.)

Initial Treatment, Bulky Disease, Weekly for 4 Doses
In pooled data from multiple studies of RITUXAN, 39 patients with relapsed or refractory, bulky disease (single lesion >10 cm in diameter), low-grade NHL received 375 mg/m² of RITUXAN weekly for 4 doses. The ORR was 36% (CR 3%, PR 33%) with a median duration of response of 6.9 months (range 2.8 to 25.0+). (For information on the higher incidence of Grade 3 and 4 adverse events, see ADVERSE REACTIONS, Risk Factors Associated with Increased Rates of Adverse Events.)

Retreatment, Weekly for 4 Doses
In a multi-center, single-arm study, 60 patients received 375 mg/m² of RITUXAN weekly for 4 doses.[15] All patients had relapsed or refractory, low-grade or follicular B-cell NHL and had achieved an objective clinical response to a prior course of RITUXAN. Of these 60 patients, 55 received their second course of RITUXAN, 3 patients received their third course and 2 patients received their second and third courses of RITUXAN in this study. The ORR was 38% (10% CR and 28% PR) with a projected median duration of response of 15 months (range, 3.0 to 25.1+ months).

INDICATIONS AND USAGE

RITUXAN® (Rituximab) is indicated for the treatment of patients with relapsed or refractory, low-grade or follicular, CD20-positive, B-cell non-Hodgkin's lymphoma.

CONTRAINDICATIONS

RITUXAN is contraindicated in patients with known anaphylaxis or IgE-mediated hypersensitivity to murine proteins or to any component of this product. (See WARNINGS.)

WARNINGS (See BOXED WARNINGS)

Severe Infusion Reactions (See BOXED WARNINGS, ADVERSE REACTIONS and Hypersensitivity Reactions): RITUXAN has caused severe infusion reactions. In some cases, these reactions were fatal. These severe reactions typically occurred during the first infusion with time to onset of 30 to 120 minutes. Signs and symptoms of severe infusion reactions may include hypotension, angioedema, hypoxia or bronchospasm, and may require interruption of RITUXAN administration. The most severe manifestations and sequelae include pulmonary infiltrates, acute respiratory distress syndrome, myocardial infarction, ventricular fibrillation, and cardiogenic shock. In the reported cases, the following factors were more frequently associated with fatal outcomes: female gender, pulmonary infiltrates, and chronic lymphocytic leukemia or mantle cell lymphoma.
Management of severe infusion reactions: The RITUXAN infusion should be interrupted for severe reactions and supportive care measures instituted as medically indicated (e.g., intravenous fluids, vasopressors, oxygen, bronchodilators, diphenhydramine, and acetaminophen). In most cases, the infusion can be resumed at a 50% reduction in rate (e.g., from 100 mg/hr to 50 mg/hr) when symptoms have com-

Table 2
Summary of RITUXAN Efficacy Data by Schedule and Clinical Setting (See ADVERSE REACTIONS for Risk Factors Associated with Increased Rates of Adverse Events.)

	Initial, Weekly × 4 N = 166	Initial, Weekly × 8 N = 37	Initial, Bulky, Weekly × 4 N = 39[1]	Retreatment, Weekly × 4 N = 60
Overall Response Rate	48%	57%	36%	38%
Complete Response Rate	6%	14%	3%	10%
Median Duration Of Response[2,3,4] (Months)	11.2	13.4	6.9	15.0
[Range]	[1.9 to 42.1+]	[2.5 to 36.5+]	[2.8 to 25.0+]	[3.0 to 25.1+]

[1]Six of these patients are included in the first column. Thus, data from 296 intent to treat patients are provided in this table.
[2]Kaplan-Meier projected with observed range.
[3]"+" indicates an ongoing response.
[4]Duration of response: interval from the onset of response to disease progression.

pletely resolved. Patients requiring close monitoring during first and all subsequent infusions include those with preexisting cardiac and pulmonary conditions, those with prior clinically significant cardiopulmonary adverse events and those with high numbers of circulating malignant cells ($\geq$ 25,000/mm^3) with or without evidence of high tumor burden.

Tumor Lysis Syndrome [TLS] (See BOXED WARNINGS and ADVERSE REACTIONS): Rapid reduction in tumor volume followed by acute renal failure, hyperkalemia, hypocalcemia, hyperuricemia, or hyperphosphatasemia, have been reported within 12 to 24 hours after the first RITUXAN infusion. Rare instances of fatal outcome have been reported in the setting of TLS following treatment with RITUXAN. The risks of TLS appear to be greater in patients with high numbers of circulating malignant cells ($\geq$ 25,000/mm^3) or high tumor burden. Prophylaxis for TLS should be considered for patients at high risk. Correction of electrolyte abnormalities, monitoring of renal function and fluid balance, and administration of supportive care, including dialysis, should be initiated as indicated. Following complete resolution of the complications of TLS, RITUXAN has been tolerated when re-administered in conjunction with prophylactic therapy for TLS in a limited number of cases.

Hepatitis B Reactivation with Related Fulminant Hepatitis: Hepatitis B virus (HBV) reactivation with fulminant hepatitis, hepatic failure, and death has been reported in some patients with hematologic malignancies treated with RITUXAN. The majority of patients received RITUXAN in combination with chemotherapy. The median time to the diagnosis of hepatitis was approximately 4 months after the initiation of RITUXAN and approximately one month after the last dose.

Persons at high risk of HBV infection should be screened before initiation of RITUXAN. Carriers of hepatitis B should be closely monitored for clinical and laboratory signs of active HBV infection and for signs of hepatitis during and for up to several months following RITUXAN therapy.

In patients who develop viral hepatitis, RITUXAN and any concomitant chemotherapy should be discontinued and appropriate treatment including antiviral therapy initiated. There are insufficient data regarding the safety of resuming RITUXAN therapy in patients who develop hepatitis subsequent to HBV reactivation.

Hypersensitivity Reactions:

RITUXAN has been associated with hypersensitivity reactions (non-IgE-mediated reactions) which may respond to adjustments in the infusion rate and in medical management. Hypotension, bronchospasm, and angioedema have occurred in association with RITUXAN infusion (see Severe Infusion Reactions). RITUXAN infusion should be interrupted for severe hypersensitivity reactions and can be resumed at a 50% reduction in rate (e.g., from 100 mg/hr to 50 mg/hr) when symptoms have completely resolved. Treatment of these symptoms with diphenhydramine and acetaminophen is recommended; additional treatment with bronchodilators or IV saline may be indicated. In most cases, patients who have experienced non-life-threatening hypersensitivity reactions have been able to complete the full course of therapy. (See DOSAGE and ADMINISTRATION.) Medications for the treatment of hypersensitivity reactions, e.g., epinephrine, antihistamines and corticosteroids, should be available for immediate use in the event of a reaction during administration.

Cardiovascular: Infusions should be discontinued in the event of serious or life-threatening cardiac arrhythmias. Patients who develop clinically significant arrhythmias should undergo cardiac monitoring during and after subsequent infusions of RITUXAN. Patients with pre-existing cardiac conditions including arrhythmias and angina have had recurrences of these events during RITUXAN therapy and should be monitored throughout the infusion and immediate post-infusion period.

Renal: RITUXAN administration has been associated with severe renal toxicity including acute renal failure requiring dialysis and in some cases, has led to a fatal outcome. Renal toxicity has occurred in patients with high numbers of circulating malignant cells (>25,000/mm^3) or high tumor burden who experience tumor lysis syndrome (see Tumor Lysis Syndrome) and in patients administered concomitant cisplatin therapy during clinical trials. The combination of cisplatin and RITUXAN is not an approved treatment regimen. If this combination is used in clinical trials *extreme caution* should be exercised; patients should be monitored closely for signs of renal failure. Discontinuation of RITUXAN should be considered for those with rising serum creatinine or oliguria.

Severe Mucocutaneous Reactions (See BOXED WARNINGS and ADVERSE REACTIONS): Mucocutaneous reactions, some with fatal outcome, have been reported in patients treated with RITUXAN. These reports include paraneoplastic pemphigus (an uncommon disorder which is a manifestation of the patient's underlying malignancy),[16] Stevens-Johnson syndrome, lichenoid dermatitis, vesiculobullous dermatitis, and toxic epidermal necrolysis. The onset of the reaction in the reported cases has varied from 1 to 13 weeks following RITUXAN exposure. Patients experiencing a severe mucocutaneous reaction should not receive any further infusions and seek prompt medical evaluation. Skin biopsy may help to distinguish among different mucocutaneous reactions and guide subsequent treatment. The safety of readministration of RITUXAN to patients with any of these mucocutaneous reactions has not been determined.

PRECAUTIONS

Laboratory Monitoring: Because RITUXAN targets all CD20-positive B lymphocytes, malignant and nonmalignant, complete blood counts (CBC) and platelet counts should be obtained at regular intervals during RITUXAN therapy and more frequently in patients who develop cytopenias (see ADVERSE REACTIONS). The duration of cytopenias caused by RITUXAN can extend well beyond the treatment period.

Drug/Laboratory Interactions: There have been no formal drug interaction studies performed with RITUXAN. However, renal toxicity was seen with this drug in combination with cisplatin in clinical trials. (See WARNINGS, Renal.)

HACA Formation: Human antichimeric antibody (HACA) was detected in 4 of 356 patients and 3 had an objective clinical response. The data reflect the percentage of patients whose test results were considered positive for antibodies to RITUXAN using an enzyme-linked immunosorbant assay (limit of detection = 7 ng/mL). The observed incidence of antibody positivity in an assay is highly dependent on the sensitivity and specificity of the assay and may be influenced by several factors including sample handling, concomitant medications, and underlying disease. For these reasons, comparison of the incidence of antibodies to RITUXAN with the incidence of antibodies to other products may be misleading.

Immunization: The safety of immunization with live viral vaccines following RITUXAN therapy has not been studied. The ability to generate a primary or anamnestic humoral response to vaccination is currently being studied.

Carcinogenesis, Mutagenesis, Impairment of Fertility: No long-term animal studies have been performed to establish the carcinogenic or mutagenic potential of RITUXAN, or to determine its effects on fertility in males or females. Individuals of childbearing potential should use effective contraceptive methods during treatment and for up to 12 months following RITUXAN therapy.

Pregnancy Category C: Animal reproduction studies have not been conducted with RITUXAN. It is not known whether RITUXAN can cause fetal harm when administered to a pregnant woman or whether it can affect reproductive capacity. Human IgG is known to pass the placental barrier, and thus may potentially cause fetal B-cell depletion; therefore, RITUXAN should be given to a pregnant woman only if clearly needed.

Nursing Mothers: It is not known whether RITUXAN is excreted in human milk. Because human IgG is excreted in human milk and the potential for absorption and immunosuppression in the infant is unknown, women should be advised to discontinue nursing until circulating drug levels are no longer detectable. (See CLINICAL PHARMACOLOGY.)

Pediatric Use: The safety and effectiveness of RITUXAN in pediatric patients have not been established.

Geriatric Use: Among the 331 patients enrolled in clinical studies of single agent RITUXAN, 24% were 65 to 75 years old and 5% were 75 years old and older. The overall response rates were higher in older (age $\geq$ 65 years) vs. younger (age < 65 years) patients (52% vs. 44%, respectively). However, the median duration of response, based on Kaplan-Meier estimates, was shorter in older vs. younger patients: 10.1 months (range, 1.9 to 36.5+) vs. 11.4 months (range, 2.1 to 42.1+), respectively. This shorter duration of response was not statistically significant. Adverse reactions, including incidence, severity and type of adverse reaction were similar between older and younger patients.

ADVERSE REACTIONS

The most serious adverse reactions caused by RITUXAN include infusion reactions, tumor lysis syndrome, mucocutaneous reactions, hypersensitivity reactions, cardiac arrhythmias and angina, and renal failure. Please refer to the BOXED WARNINGS and WARNINGS sections for detailed descriptions of these reactions. Infusion reactions and lymphopenia are the most commonly occurring adverse reactions.

Because clinical trials are conducted under widely varying conditions, adverse reaction rates observed in the clinical trials of a drug cannot be directly compared to rates in the clinical trials of another drug and may not reflect the rates observed in practice. The adverse reaction information from clinical trials does, however, provide a basis for identifying the adverse events that appear to be related to drug use and for approximating rates.

Additional adverse reactions have been identified during postmarketing use of RITUXAN. Because these reactions are reported voluntarily from a population of uncertain size, it is not always possible to reliably estimate their frequency or establish a causal relationship to RITUXAN exposure. Decisions to include these reactions in labeling are typically based on one or more of the following factors: (1) seriousness of the reaction, (2) frequency of reporting, or (3) strength of causal connection to RITUXAN.

Where specific percentages are noted, these data are based on 356 patients treated in nonrandomized, single-arm studies of RITUXAN administered as a single agent. Most patients received RITUXAN 375 mg/m^2 weekly for 4 doses. These include 39 patients with bulky disease (lesions $\geq$ 10 cm) and 60 patients who received more than 1 course of RITUXAN. Thirty-seven patients received 375 mg/m^2 for 8 doses and 25 patients received doses other than 375 mg/m^2 for 4 doses and up to 500 mg/m^2 single dose in the Phase 1 setting. Adverse events of greater severity are referred to as "Grade 3 and 4 events" defined by the commonly used National Cancer Institute Common Toxicity Criteria.[17]

Table 3

Incidence of Adverse Events $\geq$ 5% of Patients in Clinical Trials (N = 356) (Adverse Events were followed for a period of 12 months following RITUXAN therapy)

	All Grades (%)	Grade 3 and 4 (%)
Any Adverse Events	**99**	**57**
Body as a Whole	**86**	**10**
Fever	53	1
Chills	33	3
Infection	31	4
Asthenia	26	1
Headache	19	1
Abdominal Pain	14	1
Pain	12	1
Back Pain	10	1
Throat Irritation	9	0
Flushing	5	0
Cardiovascular System	**25**	**3**
Hypotension	10	1
Hypertension	6	1
Digestive System	**37**	**2**
Nausea	23	1
Diarrhea	10	1
Vomiting	10	1
Hemic and Lymphatic System	**67**	**48**
Lymphopenia	48	40
Leukopenia	14	4
Neutropenia	14	6
Thrombocytopenia	12	2
Anemia	8	3
Metabolic and Nutritional Disorders	**38**	**3**
Angioedema	11	1
Hyperglycemia	9	1
Peripheral Edema	8	0
LDH Increase	7	0
Musculoskeletal System	**26**	**3**
Myalgia	10	1
Arthralgia	10	1
Nervous System	**32**	**1**
Dizziness	10	1
Anxiety	5	1
Respiratory System	**38**	**4**
Increased Cough	13	1
Rhinitis	12	1
Bronchospasm	8	1
Dyspnea	7	1
Sinusitis	6	0
Skin and Appendages	**44**	**2**
Night Sweats	15	1
Rash	15	1
Pruritus	14	1
Urticaria	8	1

Risk Factors Associated with Increased Rates of Adverse Events: Administration of RITUXAN weekly for 8 doses resulted in higher rates of Grade 3 and 4 adverse events[17] overall (70%) compared with administration weekly for 4 doses (57%). The incidence of Grade 3 or 4 adverse events was similar in patients retreated with RITUXAN compared with initial treatment (58% and 57%, respectively). The incidence of the following clinically significant adverse events was higher in patients with bulky disease (lesions $\geq$10 cm) (N = 39) versus patients with lesions < 10 cm (N = 195): abdominal pain, anemia, dyspnea, hypotension, and neutropenia.

Infusion Reactions (See BOXED WARNINGS and WARNINGS): Mild to moderate infusion reactions consisting of fever and chills/rigors occurred in the majority of patients during the first RITUXAN infusion. Other frequent infusion reaction symptoms included nausea, pruritus, angioedema, asthenia, hypotension, headache, bronchospasm, throat irritation, rhinitis, urticaria, rash, vomiting, myalgia, dizziness, and hypertension. These reactions generally occurred within 30 to 120 minutes of beginning the first infusion, and resolved with slowing or interruption of the RITUXAN infusion and with supportive care (diphenhydramine, acetaminophen, IV saline, and vasopressors). In an analysis of data from 356 patients with relapsed or refractory, low-grade NHL who received 4 (N = 319) or 8 (N = 37) weekly infusions of RITUXAN, the incidence of infusion reactions was highest during the first infusion (77%) and decreased with each subsequent infusion (30% with fourth infusion and 14% with eighth infusion).

Infectious Events: RITUXAN induced B-cell depletion in 70% to 80% of patients and was associated with decreased serum immunoglobulins in a minority of patients; the lymphopenia lasted a median of 14 days (range, 1 to 588 days). Infectious events occurred in 31% of patients: 19% of patients had bacterial infections, 10% had viral infections, 1% had fungal infections, and 6% were unknown infections. Incidence is not additive because a single patient may have had more than one type of infection. Serious infectious

Continued on next page

Rituxan—Cont.

events (Grade 3 or 4),[17] including sepsis, occurred in 2% of patients.

Hematologic Events: In clinical trials, Grade 3 and 4 cytopenias[17] were reported in 48% of patients treated with RITUXAN; these include: lymphopenia (40%), neutropenia (6%), leukopenia (4%), anemia (3%), and thrombocytopenia (2%). The median duration of lymphopenia was 14 days (range, 1 to 588 days) and of neutropenia was 13 days (range, 2 to 116 days). A single occurrence of transient aplastic anemia (pure red cell aplasia) and two occurrences of hemolytic anemia following RITUXAN therapy were reported.

In addition, there have been a limited number of postmarketing reports of prolonged pancytopenia, marrow hypoplasia, and late onset neutropenia (defined as occurring 40 days after the last dose of RITUXAN) in patients with hematologic malignancies. In reported cases of late onset neutropenia (NCI-CTC Grade 3 and 4), the median duration of neutropenia was 10 days (range 3 to 148 days). Documented resolution of the neutropenia was described in approximately one-half of the reported cases; of those with documented recovery, approximately half received growth factor support. In the remaining cases, information on resolution was not provided. More than half of the reported cases of delayed onset neutropenia occurred in patients who had undergone a prior autologous bone marrow transplantation. In an adequately designed, controlled, clinical trial, the reported incidence of NCI-CTC Grade 3 and 4 neutropenia was higher in patients receiving RITUXAN in combination with fludarabine as compared to those receiving fludarabine alone (76% [39/51] vs.39% [21/53]).[18]

Cardiac Events (See BOXED WARNINGS): Grade 3 or 4 cardiac-related events include hypotension. Rare, fatal cardiac failure with symptomatic onset weeks after RITUXAN has also been reported. Patients who develop clinically significant cardiopulmonary events should have RITUXAN infusion discontinued.

Pulmonary Events (See BOXED WARNINGS): 135 patients (38%) experienced pulmonary events in clinical trials. The most common respiratory system adverse events experienced were increased cough, rhinitis, bronchospasm, dyspnea, and sinusitis. In both clinical studies and postmarketing surveillance, there have been a limited number of reports of bronchiolitis obliterans presenting up to 6 months post-RITUXAN infusion and a limited number of reports of pneumonitis (including interstitial pneumonitis) presenting up to 3 months post-RITUXAN infusion, some of which resulted in fatal outcomes. The safety of resumption or continued administration of RITUXAN in patients with pneumonitis or bronchiolitis obliterans is unknown.

Immune/Autoimmune Events: Immune/autoimmune events have been reported, including uveitis, optic neuritis in a patient with systemic vasculitis, pleuritis in a patient with a lupus-like syndrome, serum sickness with polyarticular arthritis, and vasculitis with rash.

Less Commonly Observed Events: In clinical trials, < 5% and > 1% of the patients experienced the following events regardless of causality assessment: agitation, anorexia, arthritis, conjunctivitis, depression, dyspepsia, edema, hyperkinesia, hypertonia, hypesthesia, hypoglycemia, injection site pain, insomnia, lacrimation disorder, malaise, nervousness, neuritis, neuropathy, paresthesia, somnolence, vertigo, weight decrease.

OVERDOSAGE

There has been no experience with overdosage in human clinical trials. Single doses of up to 500 mg/m^2 have been given in controlled clinical trials.[10]

DOSAGE AND ADMINISTRATION

Initial Therapy:

RITUXAN is given at 375 mg/m^2 IV infusion once weekly for 4 or 8 doses.

Retreatment Therapy: Patients who subsequently develop progressive disease may be safely retreated with RITUXAN 375 mg/m^2 IV infusion once weekly for 4 doses. Currently there are limited data concerning more than 2 courses.

RITUXAN as a Component of Zevalin™ (Ibritumomab Tiuxetan) Therapeutic Regimen: As a required component of the Zevalin therapeutic regimen, RITUXAN 250 mg/m^2 should be infused within 4 hours prior to the administration of Indium-111- (In-111-) Zevalin and within 4 hours prior to the administration of Yttrium-90- (Y-90-) Zevalin. Administration of RITUXAN and In-111-Zevalin should precede RITUXAN and Y-90-Zevalin by 7–9 days. Refer to the Zevalin package insert for full prescribing information regarding the Zevalin therapeutic regimen.

RITUXAN may be administered in an outpatient setting. **DO NOT ADMINISTER AS AN INTRAVENOUS PUSH OR BOLUS. (See Administration.)**

Instructions for Administration

Preparation for Administration: Use appropriate aseptic technique. Withdraw the necessary amount of RITUXAN and dilute to a final concentration of 1 to 4 mg/mL into an infusion bag containing either 0.9% Sodium Chloride, USP, or 5% Dextrose in Water, USP. Gently invert the bag to mix the solution. Discard any unused portion left in the vial. Parenteral drug products should be inspected visually for particulate matter and discoloration prior to administration.

RITUXAN solutions for infusion may be stored at 2–8°C (36–46°F) for 24 hours. RITUXAN solutions for infusion have been shown to be stable for an additional 24 hours at room temperature. However, since RITUXAN solutions do not contain a preservative, diluted solutions should be stored refrigerated (2–8°C). No incompatibilities between RITUXAN and polyvinylchloride or polyethylene bags have been observed.

Administration: DO NOT ADMINISTER AS AN INTRAVENOUS PUSH OR BOLUS.

Infusion and hypersensitivity reactions may occur (see BOXED WARNINGS, WARNINGS, and ADVERSE REACTIONS). Premedication consisting of acetaminophen and diphenhydramine should be considered before each infusion of RITUXAN. Premedication may attenuate infusion reactions. Since transient hypotension may occur during RITUXAN infusion, consideration should be given to withholding antihypertensive medications 12 hours prior to RITUXAN infusion.

First Infusion: The RITUXAN solution for infusion should be administered intravenously at an initial rate of 50 mg/hr. RITUXAN should not be mixed or diluted with other drugs. If hypersensitivity or infusion reactions do not occur, escalate the infusion rate in 50 mg/hr increments every 30 minutes, to a maximum of 400 mg/hr. If a hypersensitivity (non-IgE-mediated) or an infusion reaction develops, the infusion should be temporarily slowed or interrupted (see BOXED WARNINGS and WARNINGS). The infusion can continue at one-half the previous rate upon improvement of patient symptoms.

Subsequent Infusions: If the patient tolerated the first infusion well, subsequent RITUXAN infusions can be administered at an initial rate of 100 mg/hr, and increased by 100 mg/hr increments at 30-minute intervals, to a maximum of 400 mg/hr as tolerated. If the patient did not tolerate the first infusion well, follow the guidelines under First Infusion.

Stability and Storage: RITUXAN vials are stable at 2–8°C (36–46°F). Do not use beyond expiration date stamped on carton. RITUXAN vials should be protected from direct sunlight. Refer to the "Preparation and Administration" section for information on the stability and storage of solutions of RITUXAN diluted for infusion.

HOW SUPPLIED

RITUXAN® (Rituximab) is supplied as 100 mg and 500 mg of sterile, preservative-free, single-use vials.

Single unit 100 mg carton: Contains one 10 mL vial of RITUXAN (10 mg/mL).
NDC 50242-051-21

Single unit 500 mg carton: Contains one 50 mL vial of RITUXAN (10 mg/mL).
NDC 50242-053-06

REFERENCES

1. Valentine MA, Meier KE, Rossie S, et al. Phosphorylation of the CD20 phosphoprotein in resting B lymphocytes. *J Biol Chem* 1989 264(19):11282–11287.
2. Einfeld DA, Brown JP, Valentine MA, et al. Molecular cloning of the human B cell CD20 receptor predicts a hydrophobic protein with multiple transmembrane domains. *EMBO J* 1988 7(3):711–717.
3. Anderson KC, Bates MP, Slaughenhoupt BL, et al. Expression of human B cell-associated antigens on leukemias and lymphomas: A model of human B cell differentiation. *Blood* 1984 63(6):1424–1433.
4. Tedder TF, Boyd AW, Freedman AS, et al. The B cell surface molecule B1 is functionally linked with B cell activation and differentiation. *J Immunol* 1985 135(2):973–979.
5. Tedder TF, Zhou LJ, Bell PD, et al. The CD20 surface molecule of B lymphocytes functions as a calcium channel. *J Cell Biochem* 1990 14D:195.
6. Press OW, Applebaum F, Ledbetter JA, Martin PJ, Zarling J, Kidd P, et al. Monoclonal antibody 1F5 (anti-CD20) serotherapy of human B-cell lymphomas. *Blood* 1987 69(2):584–591.
7. Reff ME, Carner C, Chambers KS, Chinn PC, Leonard JE, Raab R, et al. Depletion of B cells in vivo by a chimeric mouse human monoclonal antibody to CD20. *Blood* 1994 83(2):435–445.
8. Demidem A, Lam T, Alas S, Hariharan K, Hanna N, and Bonavida B. Chimeric anti-CD20 (IDEC-C2B8) monoclonal antibody sensitizes a B cell lymphoma cell line to cell killing by cytotoxic drugs. *Cancer Biotherapy & Radiopharmaceuticals* 1997 12(3):177–186.
9. Maloney DG, Liles TM, Czerwinski C, Waldichuk J, Rosenberg J, Grillo-López A, et al. Phase I clinical trial using escalating single-dose infusion of chimeric anti-CD20 monoclonal antibody (IDEC-C2B8) in patients with recurrent B-cell lymphoma. *Blood* 1994 84(8):2457–2466.
10. Berinstein NL, Grillo-López AJ, White CA, Bence-Bruckler I, Maloney D, Czuczman M, et al. Association of serum Rituximab (IDEC-C2B8) concentration and anti-tumor response in the treatment of recurrent low-grade or follicular non-Hodgkin's lymphoma. *Annals of Oncology* 1998, 9:995–1001.
11. Maloney DG, Grillo-López AJ, Bodkin D, White CA, Liles T-M, Royston I, et al. IDEC-C2B8: Results of a phase I multiple-dose trial in patients with relapsed non-Hodgkin's lymphoma. *J Clin Oncol* 1997 15(10):3266–3274.
12. Maloney DG, Grillo-López AJ, White CA, Bodkin D, Schilder RJ, Neidhart JA, et al. IDEC-C2B8 (Rituximab) anti-CD20 monoclonal antibody therapy in patients with relapsed low-grade non-Hodgkin's lymphoma. *Blood* 1997 90(6):2188–2195.
13. McLaughlin P, Grillo-López AJ, Link BK, Levy R, Czuczman MS, Williams ME, et al. Rituximab chimeric anti-CD20 monoclonal antibody therapy for relapsed indolent lymphoma: half of patients respond to a four-dose treatment program. *J Clin Oncol* 1998 16(8):2825–2833.
14. Piro LD, White CA, Grillo-López AJ, Janakiraman N, Saven A, Beck TM, et al. Extended Rituximab (anti-CD20 monoclonal antibody) therapy for relapsed or refractory low-grade or follicular non-Hodgkin's lymphoma. *Annals of Oncology* 1999 10:655–661.
15. Davis TA, Grillo-López AJ, White CA, McLaughlin P, Czuczman MS, Link BK, Maloney DG, Weaver RL, Rosenberg J, Levy R. Rituximab anti-CD20 monoclonal antibody therapy in non-hodgkin's lymphoma: safety and efficacy of re-treatment. *J Clin Oncol* 2000 18(17):3135–3143.
16. Anhalt GJ, Kim SC, Stanley JR, Korman NJ, Jabs DA, Kory M, Izumi H, Ratrie H, Mutasim D, Ariss-Abdo L, Labib RS. Paraneoplastic Pemphigus, an autoimmune mucocutaneous disease associated with neoplasia. *NEJM* 1990 323(25):1729–1735.
17. National Institutes of Health (US), National Cancer Institute. Common Toxicity Criteria. [Bethesda, MD.]: National Institutes of Health, National Cancer Institute; c1998. 73p.
18. Byrd JC, Peterson BL, Morrison VA, Park K, Jacobson R, Hoke E, Vardiman JW, Rai K, Schiffer CA, Larson RA. Randomized phase 2 study of fludarabine with concurrent versus sequential treatment with rituximab in symptomatic, untreated patients with B-cell chronic lymphocytic leukemia: results from Cancer and Leukemia Group B 9712 (CALGB 9712). *Blood* 2003 101(1):6–14.

Jointly Marketed by:
IDEC Pharmaceuticals Corporation
11011 Torreyana Road
San Diego, CA 92121
Genentech, Inc.
1 DNA Way
South San Francisco, CA 94080-4990
4809705
Revised June 2004

ZEVALIN® ℞

[*zĕ-vă-lĭn*]

Ibritumomab Tiuxetan

Kits for the Preparation of Indium-111 (In-111) Ibritumomab Tiuxetan (In-111 ZEVALIN) and Yttrium-90 (Y-90) Ibritumomab Tiuxetan (Y-90 ZEVALIN)

In-111 Ibritumomab Tiuxetan and Y-90 Ibritumomab Tiuxetan are components of the ZEVALIN therapeutic regimen (See Description).

WARNINGS

Fatal Infusion Reactions: Deaths have occurred within 24 hours of Rituximab infusion, an essential component of the ZEVALIN therapeutic regimen. These fatalities were associated with an infusion reaction symptom complex that included hypoxia, pulmonary infiltrates, acute respiratory distress syndrome, myocardial infarction, ventricular fibrillation, or cardiogenic shock. Approximately 80% of fatal infusion reactions occurred in association with the first Rituximab infusion (See WARNINGS and ADVERSE REACTIONS). Patients who develop severe infusion reactions should have Rituximab, In-111 ZEVALIN, and Y-90 ZEVALIN infusions discontinued and receive medical treatment.

Prolonged and Severe Cytopenias: Y-90 ZEVALIN administration results in severe and prolonged cytopenias in most patients. The ZEVALIN therapeutic regimen should not be administered to patients with ≥ 25% lymphoma marrow involvement and/or impaired bone marrow reserve (See WARNINGS and ADVERSE REACTIONS).

Dosing

- The prescribed, measured, and administered dose of Y-90 ZEVALIN should not exceed the absolute maximum allowable dose of 32.0 mCi (1184 MBq).
- Y-90 ZEVALIN should not be administered to patients with altered biodistribution as determined by imaging with In-111 ZEVALIN.

In-111 ZEVALIN and Y-90 ZEVALIN are radiopharmaceuticals and should be used only by physicians and other professionals qualified by training and experienced in the safe use and handling of radionuclides.

DESCRIPTION

ZEVALIN®

ZEVALIN (Ibritumomab Tiuxetan) is the immunoconjugate resulting from a stable thiourea covalent bond between the monoclonal antibody Ibritumomab and the linker-chelator tiuxetan [N-[2-bis(carboxymethyl)amino]-3-(p-isothiocyanatophenyl)-propyl]-[N-[2-bis(carboxymethyl)amino]-2-(methyl)-ethyl]glycine. This linker-chelator provides a high affinity, conformationally restricted chelation site for Indium-111 or Yttrium-90. The approximate molecular weight of Ibritumomab Tiuxetan is 148 kD.

The antibody moiety of ZEVALIN is Ibritumomab, a murine IgG_1 kappa monoclonal antibody directed against the CD20 antigen, which is found on the surface of normal and malignant B lymphocytes. Ibritumomab is produced in Chinese hamster ovary cells and is composed of two murine gamma 1 heavy chains of 445 amino acids each and two kappa light chains of 213 amino acids each.

ZEVALIN Therapeutic Regimen

The ZEVALIN therapeutic regimen is administered in two steps: Step 1 includes one infusion of Rituximab preceding In-111 ZEVALIN. Step 2 follows Step 1 by seven to nine days and consists of a second infusion of Rituximab followed by Y-90 ZEVALIN.

ZEVALIN is supplied as two separate and distinctly labeled kits that contain all of the non-radioactive ingredients necessary to produce a single dose of In-111 ZEVALIN and a single dose of Y-90 ZEVALIN, both essential components of the ZEVALIN therapeutic regimen. Indium-111 chloride and Rituximab must be ordered separately from the ZEVALIN kit. Yttrium-90 Chloride Sterile Solution is supplied by MDS Nordion when the Y-90 ZEVALIN kit is ordered.

ZEVALIN Kits

Each of the two ZEVALIN kits contains four vials that are used to produce a single dose of either In-111 ZEVALIN or Y-90 ZEVALIN, as indicated on the outer container label:

(1) One (1) ZEVALIN vial containing 3.2 mg of Ibritumomab Tiuxetan in 2 mL of 0.9% sodium chloride solution; a sterile, pyrogen-free, clear, colorless solution that may contain translucent particles; no preservative present.

(2) One (1) 50 mM Sodium Acetate Vial containing 13.6 mg of sodium acetate trihydrate in 2 mL of Water for Injection; a sterile, pyrogen-free, clear, colorless solution; no preservative present.

(3) One (1) Formulation Buffer Vial containing 750 mg of Albumin (Human), 76 mg of sodium chloride, 21 mg of sodium phosphate dibasic heptahydrate, 4 mg of pentetic acid, 2 mg of potassium phosphate monobasic and 2 mg of potassium chloride in 10 mL of Water for Injection adjusted to pH 7.1 with either sodium hydroxide or hydrochloric acid; a sterile, pyrogen-free, clear yellow to amber colored solution; no preservative present.

(4) One (1) empty Reaction Vial, sterile, pyrogen-free.

Physical/Radiochemical Characteristics of In-111

Indium-111 decays by electron capture, with a physical half-life of 67.3 hours (2.81 days)[1]. The product of radioactive decay is nonradioactive cadmium-111. Radiation emission data for In-111 are summarized in Table 1.

Table 1.
Principal In-111 Radiation Emission Data

Radiation	Mean % per Disintegration	Mean Energy (keV)
Gamma-2	90.2	171.3
Gamma-3	94.0	245.4

External Radiation

The exposure rate constant for 37 MBq (1 mCi) of In-111 is 8.3×10^{-4} C/kg/hr (3.2 R/hr) at 1 cm. Adequate shielding should be used with this gamma-emitter, in accordance with institutional good radiation safety practices.

To allow correction for physical decay of In-111, the fractions that remain at selected intervals before and after the time of calibration are shown in Table 2.

Table 2.
Physical Decay Chart: In-111
Half-life 2.81 Days (67.3 Hours)

Calibration Time (Hrs.)	Fraction Remaining
-48	1.64
-42	1.54
-36	1.45
-24	1.28
-12	1.13
-6	1.06
0	1.00
6	0.94
12	0.88
24	0.78
36	0.69
42	0.65
48	0.61

Physical/Radiochemical Characteristics of Y-90

Yttrium-90 decays by emission of beta particles, with a physical half-life of 64.1 hours (2.67 days)[1]. The product of radioactive decay is non-radioactive zirconium-90. The range of beta particles in soft tissue (χ_{90}) is 5 mm. Radiation emission data for Y-90 are summarized in Table 3.

Table 3.
Principal Y-90 Radiation Emission Data

Radiation	Mean % per Disintegration	Mean Energy (keV)
Beta minus	100	750-935

External Radiation

The exposure rate for 37 MBq (1 mCi) of Y-90 is 8.3×10^{-3} C/kg/hr (32 R/hr) at the mouth of an open Y-90 vial. Adequate shielding should be used with this beta-emitter, in accordance with institutional good radiation safety practices.

To allow correction for physical decay of Y-90, the fractions that remain at selected intervals before and after the time of calibration are shown in Table 4.

Table 4.
Physical Decay Chart: Y-90
Half-life 2.67 Days (64.1 Hours)

Calibration Time (Hrs.)	Fraction Remaining	Calibration Time (Hrs.)	Fraction Remaining
-36	1.48	0	1.00
-24	1.30	1	0.99
-12	1.14	2	0.98
-8	1.09	3	0.97
-7	1.08	4	0.96
-6	1.07	5	0.95
-5	1.06	6	0.94
-4	1.04	7	0.93
-3	1.03	8	0.92
-2	1.02	12	0.88
-1	1.01	24	0.77
0	1.00	36	0.68

CLINICAL PHARMACOLOGY

General Pharmacology

Ibritumomab Tiuxetan binds specifically to the CD20 antigen (human B-lymphocyte-restricted differentiation antigen, Bp35)[2,3]. The apparent affinity (K_D) of Ibritumomab Tiuxetan for the CD20 antigen ranges between approximately 14 to 18 nM. The CD20 antigen is expressed on pre-B and mature B lymphocytes and on > 90% of B-cell non-Hodgkin's lymphomas (NHL)[4,5]. The CD20 antigen is not shed from the cell surface and does not internalize upon antibody binding[6].

Mechanism of Action: The complementarity-determining regions of Ibritumomab bind to the CD20 antigen on B lymphocytes. Ibritumomab, like Rituximab, induces apoptosis in CD20+ B-cell lines *in vitro*[6]. The chelate tiuxetan, which tightly binds In-111 or Y-90, is covalently linked to the amino groups of exposed lysines and arginines contained within the antibody. The beta emission from Y-90 induces cellular damage by the formation of free radicals in the target and neighboring cells[7].

Normal Human Tissue Cross-Reactivity: Ibritumomab Tiuxetan binding was observed *in vitro* on lymphoid cells of the bone marrow, lymph node, thymus, red and white pulp of the spleen, and lymphoid follicles of the tonsil, as well as lymphoid nodules of other organs such as the large and small intestines. Binding was not observed on the nonlymphoid tissues or gonadal tissues (see **CLINICAL PHARMACOLOGY, Radiation Dosimetry**)

Pharmacokinetics / Pharmacodynamics

Pharmacokinetic and biodistribution studies were performed using In-111 ZEVALIN (5 mCi [185 MBq] In-111, 1.6 mg Ibritumomab Tiuxetan). In an early study designed to assess the need for pre-administration of unlabeled antibody, only 18% of known sites of disease were imaged when In-111 ZEVALIN was administered without unlabeled Ibritumomab. When preceded by unlabeled Ibritumomab (1.0 mg/kg or 2.5 mg/kg), In-111 ZEVALIN detected 56% and 92% of known disease sites, respectively. These studies were conducted with a ZEVALIN therapeutic regimen that included unlabeled Ibritumomab.

In pharmacokinetic studies of patients receiving the ZEVALIN therapeutic regimen, the mean effective half-life for Y-90 activity in blood was 30 hours, and the mean area under the fraction of injected activity (FIA) vs. time curve in blood was 39 hours. Over 7 days, a median of 7.2% of the injected activity was excreted in urine.

In clinical studies, administration of the ZEVALIN therapeutic regimen resulted in sustained depletion of circulating B cells. At four weeks, the median number of circulating B cells was zero (range, 0-1084 cell/mm^3). B-cell recovery began at approximately 12 weeks following treatment, and the median level of B cells was within the normal range (32 to 341 cells/mm^3) by 9 months after treatment. Median serum levels of IgG and IgA remained within the normal range throughout the period of B-cell depletion. Median IgM serum levels dropped below normal (median 49 mg/dL, range 13-3990 mg/dL) after treatment and recovered to normal values by 6-month post therapy.

Radiation Dosimetry

Estimations of radiation-absorbed doses for In-111 ZEVALIN and Y-90 ZEVALIN were performed using sequential whole body images and the MIRDOSE 3 software program[8,9]. The estimated radiation absorbed doses to organs and marrow from a course of the ZEVALIN therapeutic regimen are summarized in Table 5. Absorbed dose estimates for the lower large intestine, upper large intestine, and small intestine have been modified from the standard MIRDOSE 3 output to account for the assumption that activity is within the intestine wall rather than the intestine contents.

[See table 5 at top of next page]

CLINICAL STUDIES

The safety and efficacy of the ZEVALIN therapeutic regimen were evaluated in two multi-center trials enrolling a total of 197 subjects. The ZEVALIN therapeutic regimen was administered in two steps (see DOSAGE AND ADMINISTRATION). The activity and toxicity of a variation of the ZEVALIN therapeutic regimen employing a reduced dose of Y-90 ZEVALIN was further defined in a third study enrolling a total of 30 patients who had mild thrombocytopenia (platelet count 100,000 to 149,000 cells/mm^3).

Study 1 was a single arm study of 54 patients with relapsed follicular lymphoma refractory to Rituximab treatment. Patients were considered refractory if their last prior treatment with Rituximab did not result in a complete or partial response, or if time to disease progression (TTP) was < 6 months[11]. The primary efficacy endpoint of the study was the overall response rate (ORR) using the International Workshop Response Criteria (IWRC)[12]. Secondary efficacy endpoints included time to disease progression (TTP) and duration of response (DR). In a secondary analysis comparing objective response to the ZEVALIN therapeutic regimen with that observed with the most recent treatment with Rituximab, the median duration of response following the ZEVALIN therapeutic regimen was 6 vs. 4 months. Table 6 summarizes efficacy data from this study.

Study 2 was a randomized, controlled, multicenter study comparing the ZEVALIN therapeutic regimen to treatment with Rituximab. The trial was conducted in 143 patients with relapsed or refractory low-grade or follicular non-Hodgkin's lymphoma (NHL), or transformed B-cell NHL. A total of 73 patients received the ZEVALIN therapeutic regimen, and 70 patients received Rituximab given as an IV infusion at 375 mg/m^2 weekly times 4 doses. The primary efficacy endpoint of the study was to determine the ORR using the IWRC[12] (see Table 6). The ORR was significantly higher (80% vs. 56%, p = 0.002)[13] for patients treated with the ZEVALIN therapeutic regimen. The secondary endpoints, duration of response and time to progression, were not significantly different between the two treatment arms.

[See table 6 on next page]

Study 3 was a single arm study of 30 patients with relapsed or refractory low-grade, follicular, or transformed B-cell NHL who had mild thrombocytopenia (platelet count 100,000 to 149,000 cells/mm^3). Excluded from the study were patients with ≥ 25% lymphoma marrow involvement and/or impaired bone marrow reserve. Patients were considered to have impaired bone marrow reserve if they had any of the following: prior myeloablative therapy with stem cell support; prior external beam radiation to > 25% of active marrow; a platelet count <100,000 cells/mm^3; or neutrophil count <1,500 cells/mm^3. In this study, a modification of the ZEVALIN therapeutic regimen with a lower Y-90 ZEVALIN dose [Y-90 ZEVALIN at 0.3 mCi/kg (11.1 MBq/kg)] was used. Objective, durable clinical responses were observed [67% ORR (95% CI: 48-85%)[14], 11.8 months median DR (range: 4-17 months)] and resulted in a greater incidence of hematologic toxicity (see ADVERSE REACTIONS) than in Studies 1 and 2.

INDICATIONS AND USAGE

ZEVALIN, as part of the ZEVALIN therapeutic regimen (see DOSAGE AND ADMINISTRATION), is indicated for the treatment of patients with relapsed or refractory low-grade, follicular, or transformed B-cell non-Hodgkin's lymphoma, including patients with Rituximab refractory follicular non-Hodgkin's lymphoma. Determination of the effectiveness of the ZEVALIN therapeutic regimen in a relapsed or refractory patient population is based on overall response rates (see CLINICAL STUDIES). The effects of the ZEVALIN therapeutic regimen on survival are not known.

CONTRAINDICATIONS

The ZEVALIN therapeutic regimen is contraindicated in patients with known Type I hypersensitivity or anaphylactic reactions to murine proteins or to any component of this product, including Rituximab, yttrium chloride, and indium chloride.

WARNINGS (SEE BOXED WARNING)

Altered Biodistribution: Y-90 ZEVALIN should not be administered to patients with altered biodistribution of In-111 ZEVALIN. The expected biodistribution of In-111 ZEVALIN includes easily detectable uptake in the blood pool areas on the first day image, with less activity in the blood pool areas on the second or third day image; moderately high to high uptake in normal liver and spleen during the first day and the second or third day image; and moderately low or very low uptake in normal kidneys, urinary bladder, and normal bowel on the first day image and the second or third day image. Altered biodistribution of In-111 ZEVALIN can be characterized by diffuse uptake in normal lung more intense than the cardiac blood pool on the first day image or more intense than the liver on the second or third day image; kidneys with greater intensity than the liver on the posterior view of the second or third day image; or intense

Continued on next page

Zevalin—Cont.

areas of uptake throughout the normal bowel comparable to uptake by the liver on the second or third day images.

Severe Infusion Reactions (See PRECAUTIONS, Hypersensitivity): The ZEVALIN therapeutic regimen may cause severe, and potentially fatal, infusion reactions. These severe reactions typically occur during the first Rituximab infusion with time to onset of 30 to 120 minutes. Signs and symptoms of severe infusion reaction may include hypotension, angioedema, hypoxia, or bronchospasm, and may require interruption of Rituximab, In-111 ZEVALIN, or Y-90 ZEVALIN administration. The most severe manifestations and sequelae may include pulmonary infiltrates, acute respiratory distress syndrome, myocardial infarction, ventricular fibrillation, and cardiogenic shock. **Because the ZEVALIN therapeutic regimen includes the use of Rituximab, see also prescribing information for RITUXAN (Rituximab).**

Cytopenias (See ADVERSE REACTIONS, Hematologic Events):

The most common severe adverse events reported with the ZEVALIN therapeutic regimen were thrombocytopenia (61% of patients with platelet counts <50,000 cells/mm^3) and neutropenia (57% of patients with absolute neutrophil count (ANC) <1,000 cells/mm^3) in patients with ≥150,000 platelets/mm^3 prior to treatment. Both incidences of severe thrombocytopenia and neutropenia increased to 78% and 74% for patients with mild thrombocytopenia at baseline (platelet count of 100,000 to 149,000 cells/mm^3). For all patients, the median time to nadir was 7-9 weeks and the median duration of cytopenias was 22-35 days. In <5% of cases, patients experienced severe cytopenia that extended beyond the prospectively defined protocol treatment period of 12 weeks following administration of the ZEVALIN therapeutic regimen. Some of these patients eventually recovered from cytopenia, while others experienced progressive disease, received further anti-cancer therapy, or died of their lymphoma without having recovered from cytopenia. The cytopenias may have influenced subsequent treatment decisions.

Hemorrhage, including fatal cerebral hemorrhage, and severe infections have occurred in a minority of patients in clinical studies. Careful monitoring for and management of cytopenias and their complications (e.g., febrile neutropenia, hemorrhage) for up to 3 months after use of the ZEVALIN therapeutic regimen are necessary. Caution should be exercised in treating patients with drugs that interfere with platelet function or coagulation following the ZEVALIN therapeutic regimen and patients receiving such agents should be closely monitored.

The ZEVALIN therapeutic regimen should not be administered to patients with ≥ 25% lymphoma marrow involvement and/or impaired bone marrow reserve, e.g., prior myeloablative therapies; platelet count <100,000 cells/mm^3; neutrophil count <1,500 cells/mm^3; hypocellular bone marrow (≤ 15% cellularity or marked reduction in bone marrow precursors); or to patients with a history of failed stem cell collection.

Secondary Malignancies: Out of 349 patients treated with the ZEVALIN therapeutic regimen, three cases of acute myelogenous leukemia and two cases of myelodysplastic syndrome have been reported following the ZEVALIN therapeutic regimen (see ADVERSE REACTIONS).

Pregnancy Category D: Y-90 ZEVALIN can cause fetal harm when administered to a pregnant woman. There are no adequate and well-controlled studies in pregnant women. If this drug is used during pregnancy, or if the patient becomes pregnant while receiving this drug, the patient should be apprised of the potential hazard to the fetus. Women of childbearing potential should be advised to avoid becoming pregnant.

Creutzfeldt-Jakob disease (CJD): This product contains albumin, a derivative of human blood. Based on effective donor screening and product manufacturing processes, it carries an extremely remote risk for transmission of viral diseases. A theoretical risk for transmission of Creutzfeldt-Jakob disease (CJD) also is considered extremely remote. No cases of transmission of viral diseases or CJD have ever been identified for albumin.

PRECAUTIONS

The ZEVALIN therapeutic regimen is intended as a single course treatment. The safety and toxicity profile from multiple courses of the ZEVALIN therapeutic regimen or of other forms of therapeutic irradiation preceding, following, or in combination with the ZEVALIN therapeutic regimen have not been established.

Radionuclide Precautions: The contents of the ZEVALIN kit are not radioactive. However, during and after radiolabeling ZEVALIN with In-111 or Y-90, care should be taken to minimize radiation exposure to patients and to medical personnel, consistent with institutional good radiation safety practices and patient management procedures.

Hypersensitivity: Anaphylactic and other hypersensitivity reactions have been reported following the intravenous administration of proteins to patients. Medications for the treatment of hypersensitivity reactions, e.g., epinephrine, antihistamines and corticosteroids, should be available for immediate use in the event of an allergic reaction during administration of ZEVALIN. Patients who have received murine proteins should be screened for human anti-mouse antibodies (HAMA). Patients with evidence of HAMA have not been studied and may be at increased risk of allergic or serious hypersensitivity reactions during ZEVALIN therapeutic regimen administrations.

Immunization: The safety of immunization with live viral vaccines following the ZEVALIN therapeutic regimen has not been studied. Also, the ability of patients who received the ZEVALIN therapeutic regimen to generate a primary or anamnestic humoral response to any vaccine has not been studied.

Laboratory Monitoring: Complete blood counts (CBC) and platelet counts should be obtained weekly following the ZEVALIN therapeutic regimen and should continue until levels recover. CBC and platelet counts should be monitored more frequently in patients who develop severe cytopenia, or as clinically indicated.

Drug Interactions: No formal drug interaction studies have been performed with ZEVALIN. Due to the frequent occurrence of severe and prolonged thrombocytopenia, the potential benefits of medications which interfere with platelet function and/or anticoagulation should be weighed against the potential increased risks of bleeding and hemorrhage. Patients receiving medications that interfere with platelet function or coagulation should have more frequent laboratory monitoring for thrombocytopenia. In addition, the transfusion practices for such patients may need to be modified given the increased risk of bleeding.

Table 5.
Estimated Radiation Absorbed Doses From Y-90 ZEVALIN and In-111 ZEVALIN

	Y-90 ZEVALIN mGy/MBq		In-111 ZEVALIN mGy/MBq	
Organ	**Median**	**Range**	**Median**	**Range**
Spleen[1]	9.4	1.8-14.4	0.9	0.2-1.2
Testes[1]	9.1	5.4-11.4	0.6	0.4-0.8
Liver[1]	4.8	2.3-8.1	0.7	0.3-1.1
Lower Large Intestinal Wall[1]	4.8	3.1-8.2	0.4	0.2-0.6
Upper Large Intestinal Wall[1]	3.6	2.0-6.7	0.3	0.2-0.6
Heart Wall[1]	2.8	1.5-3.2	0.4	0.2-0.5
Lungs[1]	2.0	1.2-3.4	0.2	0.1-0.4
Small Intestine[1]	1.4	0.8-2.1	0.2	0.1-0.3
Red Marrow[2]	1.3	0.7-1.8	0.2	0.1-0.2
Urinary Bladder Wall[3]	0.9	0.7-2.1	0.2	0.1-0.2
Bone Surfaces[2]	0.9	0.5-1.2	0.2	0.1-0.2
Ovaries[3]	0.4	0.3-0.5	0.2	0.2-0.2
Uterus[3]	0.4	0.3-0.5	0.2	0.1-0.2
Adrenals[3]	0.3	0.0-0.5	0.2	0.1-0.3
Brain[3]	0.3	0.0-0.5	0.1	0.0-0.1
Breasts[3]	0.3	0.0-0.5	0.1	0.0-0.1
Gallbladder Wall[3]	0.3	0.0-0.5	0.3	0.1-0.4
Muscle[3]	0.3	0.0-0.5	0.1	0.0-0.1
Pancreas[3]	0.3	0.0-0.5	0.2	0.1-0.3
Skin[3]	0.3	0.0-0.5	0.1	0.0-0.1
Stomach[3]	0.3	0.0-0.5	0.1	0.1-0.2
Thymus[3]	0.3	0.0-0.5	0.1	0.1-0.2
Thyroid[3]	0.3	0.0-0.5	0.1	0.0-0.1
Kidneys[1]	0.1	0.0-0.2	0.2	0.1-0.2
Total Body[3]	0.5	0.2-0.7	0.1	0.1-0.2

[1] Organ region of interest
[2] Sacrum region of interest[10]
[3] Whole body region of interest

Table 6.
Summary of Efficacy Data[1]

	Study 1	Study 2	
	ZEVALIN therapeutic regimen N = 54	**ZEVALIN therapeutic regimen N = 73**	**Rituximab N = 70**
Overall Response Rate (%)	74	80	56
Complete Response Rate (%)	15	30	16
CRu Rate[2] (%)	0	4	4
Median DR[3,4] (Months) [Range[5]]	6.4 [0.5-24.9+]	13.9 [1.0-30.1+]	11.8 [1.2-24.5]
Median TTP[3,6] (Months) [Range[5]]	6.8 [1.1-25.9+]	11.2 [0.8-31.5+]	10.1 [0.7-26.1]

[1]IWRC: International Workshop response criteria
[2]CRu: Unconfirmed complete response
[3]Estimated with observed range.
[4]Duration of response: interval from the onset of response to disease progression.
[5]"+" indicates an ongoing response.
[6]Time to Disease Progression: interval from the first infusion to disease progression.

Carcinogenesis, Mutagenesis, Impairment of Fertility: No long-term animal studies have been performed to establish the carcinogenic or mutagenic potential of the ZEVALIN therapeutic regimen, or to determine its effects on fertility in males or females. However, radiation is a potential carcinogen and mutagen. The ZEVALIN therapeutic regimen results in a significant radiation dose to the testes. The radiation dose to the ovaries has not been established. There have been no studies to evaluate whether the ZEVALIN therapeutic regimen causes hypogonadism, premature menopause, azoospermia and/or mutagenic alterations to germ cells. There is a potential risk that the ZEVALIN therapeutic regimen could cause toxic effects on the male and female gonads. Effective contraceptive methods should be used during treatment and for up to 12 months following the ZEVALIN therapeutic regimen.

Pregnancy Category D: SEE WARNINGS.

Nursing Mothers: It is not known whether ZEVALIN is excreted in human milk. Because human IgG is excreted in human milk and the potential for ZEVALIN exposure in the infant is unknown, women should be advised to discontinue nursing and formula feeding should be substituted for breast feedings (see CLINICAL PHARMACOLOGY).

Geriatric Use: Of 349 patients treated with the ZEVALIN therapeutic regimen in clinical studies, 38% (132 patients) were age 65 years and over, while 12% (41 patients) were age 75 years and over. No overall differences in safety or effectiveness were observed between these subjects and younger subjects, but greater sensitivity of some older individuals cannot be ruled out.

Pediatric Use: The safety and effectiveness of the ZEVALIN therapeutic regimen in children have not been established.

ADVERSE REACTIONS

Safety data, except where indicated, are based upon 349 patients treated in 5 clinical studies with the ZEVALIN therapeutic regimen (see DOSAGE AND ADMINISTRATION). Because the ZEVALIN therapeutic regimen includes the use of Rituximab, also see prescribing information for RITUXAN (Rituximab).

The most serious adverse reactions caused by the ZEVALIN therapeutic regimen include infections (predominantly bacterial in origin), allergic reactions (bronchospasm and angioedema), and hemorrhage while thrombocytopenic (resulting in deaths). In addition, patients who have received the ZEVALIN therapeutic regimen have developed myeloid malignancies and dysplasias. Fatal infusion reactions have occurred following the infusion of Rituximab. Please refer to the BOXED WARNINGS and WARNINGS sections for detailed descriptions of these reactions.

The most common toxicities reported were neutropenia, thrombocytopenia, anemia, gastrointestinal symptoms (nausea, vomiting, abdominal pain, and diarrhea), increased cough, dyspnea, dizziness, arthralgia, anorexia, anxiety, and ecchymosis. Hematologic toxicity was often severe and prolonged, whereas most non-hematologic toxicity was mild in severity. Table 7 lists adverse events that occurred in ≥ 5% of patients. A more detailed description of the incidence and duration of hematologic toxicities, according to baseline platelet count (as an indicator of bone marrow reserve) is provided in Table 8, Hematologic Toxicity.

Table 7.
Incidence of Adverse Events in ≥ 5% of Patients Receiving the ZEVALIN therapeutic regimen†
(N = 349)

	All Grades %	Grade 3/4 %
Any Adverse Event	**99**	**89**
Body as a Whole	**80**	**12**
Asthenia	43	3
Infection	29	5
Chills	24	<1
Fever	17	1
Abdominal Pain	16	3
Pain	13	1
Headache	12	1
Throat Irritation	10	0
Back Pain	8	1
Flushing	6	0
Cardiovascular System	**17**	**3**
Hypotension	6	1
Digestive System	**48**	**3**
Nausea	31	1
Vomiting	12	0
Diarrhea	9	<1
Anorexia	8	0
Abdominal enlargement	5	0
Constipation	5	0
Hemic and Lymphatic System	**98**	**86**
Thrombocytopenia	95	63
Neutropenia	77	60
Anemia	61	17
Ecchymosis	7	<1
Metabolic and Nutritional Disorders	**23**	**3**
Peripheral Edema	8	1
Angioedema	5	<1
Musculoskeletal System	**18**	**1**
Arthralgia	7	1
Myalgia	7	<1
Nervous System	**27**	**2**
Dizziness	10	<1
Insomnia	5	0
Respiratory System	**36**	**3**
Dyspnea	14	2
Increased Cough	10	0
Rhinitis	6	0
Bronchospasm	5	0
Skin and Appendages	**28**	**1**
Pruritus	9	<1
Rash	8	<1
Special Senses	**7**	**<1**
Urogenital System	**6**	**<1**

† Adverse events were followed for a period of 12 weeks following the first Rituximab infusion of the ZEVALIN therapeutic regimen

Note: All adverse events are included, regardless of relationship.

Table 8.
Severe Hematologic Toxicity

	ZEVALIN therapeutic regimen using 0.4 mCi/kg Y-90 Dose (14.8 MBq/kg)	Modified ZEVALIN therapeutic regimen using 0.3 mCi/kg Y-90 dose (11.1 MBq/kg)
ANC		
Median nadir (cells/mm^3)	800	600
Per Patient Incidence ANC <1000 cells/mm^3	57%	74%
Per Patient Incidence ANC <500 cells/mm^3	30%	35%
Median Duration (Days)* ANC <1000 cells/mm^3	22	29
Platelets		
Median nadir (cells/mm^3)	41,000	24,000
Per Patient Incidence Platelets <50,000 cells/mm^3	61%	78%
Per Patient Incidence Platelets <10,000 cells/mm^3	10%	14%
Median Duration (Days)# Platelets <50,000 cells/mm^3	24	35

*Median duration of neutropenia for patients with ANC <1000 cells/mm^3 (Date from last laboratory value showing ANC ≥1000 cells/mm^3 to date of first laboratory value following nadir showing ANC ≥1000 cells/mm^3, censored at initiation of next treatment or death)

Median duration of thrombocytopenia for patients with platelets <50,000 cells/mm^3 (Date from last laboratory value showing platelet count ≥50,000 cells/mm^3 to date of first laboratory value following nadir showing platelet count ≥50,000 cells/mm^3, censored at initiation of next treatment or death)

The following adverse events (except for those noted in Table 7) occurred in between 1 and 4% of patients during the treatment period: urticaria (4%), anxiety (4%), dyspepsia (4%), sweats (4%), petechia (3%), epistaxis (3%), allergic reaction (2%), and melena (2%).

Severe or life-threatening adverse events occurring in 1-5% of patients (except for those noted in Table 7) consisted of pancytopenia (2%), allergic reaction (1%), gastrointestinal hemorrhage (1%), melena (1%), tumor pain (1%), and apnea (1%). The following severe or life threatening events occurred in <1% of patients: angioedema, tachycardia, urticaria, arthritis, lung edema, pulmonary embolus, encephalopathy, hematemesis, subdural hematoma, and vaginal hemorrhage.

Hematologic Events: Hematologic toxicity was the most frequently observed adverse event in clinical trials. Table 8 presents the incidence and duration of severe hematologic toxicity for patients with normal baseline platelet count (≥ 150,000 cells/mm^3) treated with the ZEVALIN therapeutic regimen and patients with mild thrombocytopenia (platelet count 100,000 to 149,000 cells/mm^3) at baseline who were treated with a modified ZEVALIN therapeutic regimen that included a lower Y-90 ZEVALIN dose at 0.3 mCi/kg (11.1 MBq/kg).

[See table 8 above]

Median time to ANC nadir was 62 days, to platelet nadir was 53 days, and to hemoglobin nadir was 68 days. Information on growth factor use and platelet transfusions is based on 211 patients for whom data were collected. Filgrastim was given to 13% of patients and erythropoietin to 8%. Platelet transfusions were given to 22% of patients and red blood cell transfusions to 20%.

Infectious Events: During the first 3 months after initiating the ZEVALIN therapeutic regimen, 29% of patients developed infections. Three percent of patients developed serious infections comprising urinary tract infection, febrile neutropenia, sepsis, pneumonia, cellulitis, colitis, diarrhea, osteomyelitis, and upper respiratory tract infection. Life threatening infections were reported for 2% of patients that included sepsis, empyema, pneumonia, febrile neutropenia, fever, and biliary stent-associated cholangitis. During follow-up from 3 months to 4 years after the start of treatment with ZEVALIN, 6% of patients developed infections. Two percent of patients had serious infections comprising urinary tract infection, bacterial or viral pneumonia, febrile neutropenia, perihilar infiltrate, pericarditis, and intravenous drug-associated viral hepatitis. One percent of patients had life threatening infections that included bacterial pneumonia, respiratory disease, and sepsis.

Secondary Malignancies: A total of 2% of patients developed secondary malignancies following the ZEVALIN therapeutic regimen. One patient developed a Grade 1 meningioma, three developed acute myelogenous leukemia, and two developed a myelodysplastic syndrome. The onset of a second cancer was 8-34 months following the ZEVALIN therapeutic regimen and 4 to 14 years following the patients' diagnosis of NHL.

Immunogenicity: Of 211 patients who received the ZEVALIN therapeutic regimen in clinical trials and who were followed for 90 days, there were eight (3.8%) patients with evidence of human anti-mouse antibody (HAMA) (n=5) or human anti-chimeric antibody (HACA) (n=4) at any time during the course of the study. Two patients had low titers of HAMA prior to initiation of the ZEVALIN therapeutic regimen; one remained positive without an increase in titer while the other had a negative titer post-treatment. Three patients had evidence of HACA responses prior to initiation of the ZEVALIN therapeutic regimen; one had a marked increase in HACA titer while the other two had negative titers post-treatment. Of the three patients who had negative HAMA or HACA titers prior to the ZEVALIN therapeutic regimen, two developed HAMA in absence of HACA titers, and one had both HAMA and HACA positive titers post-treatment. Evidence of immunogenicity may be masked in patients who are lymphopenic. There has not been adequate evaluation of HAMA and HACA at delayed timepoints, concurrent with the recovery from lymphopenia at 6-12 months, to establish whether masking of the immunogenicity at early timepoints occurs. The data reflect the percentage of patients whose test results were considered positive for antibodies to Ibritumomab or Rituximab using kinetic enzyme immunoassays to Ibritumomab and Rituximab. The observed incidence of antibody positivity in an assay is highly dependent on the sensitivity and specificity of the assay and may be influenced by several factors including sample handling and concomitant medications. Comparisons of the incidence of HAMA/HACA to the ZEVALIN therapeutic regimen with the incidence of antibodies to other products may be misleading.

OVERDOSAGE

Doses as high as 0.52 mCi/kg (19.2 MBq/kg) of Y-90 ZEVALIN were administered in ZEVALIN therapeutic regimen clinical trials and severe hematological toxicities were observed. No fatalities or second organ injury resulting from overdosage administrations were documented. However, single doses up to 50 mCi (1850 MBq) of Y-90 ZEVALIN, and multiple doses of 20 mCi (740 MBq) followed by 40 mCi (1480 MBq) of Y-90 ZEVALIN were studied in a limited number of subjects. In these trials, some patients required autologous stem cell support to manage hematological toxicity.

DOSAGE AND ADMINISTRATION

The ZEVALIN therapeutic regimen is administered in two steps: Step 1 includes a single infusion of 250 mg/m^2 Ritux-

Continued on next page

Zevalin—Cont.

imab (not included in the ZEVALIN kits) preceding a fixed dose of 5.0 mCi (1.6 mg total antibody dose) of In-111 ZEVALIN administered as a 10 minute IV push. Step 2 follows step 1 by seven to nine days and consists of a second infusion of 250 mg/m^2 of Rituximab prior to 0.4 mCi/kg of Y-90 ZEVALIN administered as a 10 minute IV push.

Rituximab Administration: NOTE THAT THE DOSE OF RITUXIMAB IS LOWER WHEN USED AS PART OF THE ZEVALIN THERAPEUTIC REGIMEN, AS COMPARED TO THE DOSE OF RITUXIMAB WHEN USED AS A SINGLE AGENT. DO NOT ADMINISTER RITUXIMAB AS AN INTRAVENOUS PUSH OR BOLUS. Hypersensitivity reactions may occur (see WARNINGS). Premedication, consisting of acetaminophen and diphenhydramine, should be considered before each infusion of Rituximab.

ZEVALIN Therapeutic Regimen Dose Modification in Patients with Mild Thrombocytopenia: The Y-90 ZEVALIN dose should be reduced to 0.3 mCi/kg (11.1 MBq/kg) for patients with a baseline platelet count between 100,000 and 149,000 cells/mm^3.

Two separate and distinctly-labeled kits are ordered for the preparation of a single dose each of In-111 ZEVALIN and Y-90 ZEVALIN. In-111 ZEVALIN and Y-90 ZEVALIN are radiopharmaceuticals and should be used only by physicians and other professionals qualified by training and experienced in the safe use and handling of radionuclides. **Changing the ratio of any of the reactants in the radiolabeling process may adversely impact therapeutic results. In-111 ZEVALIN and Y-90 ZEVALIN should not be used in the absence of the Rituximab pre-dose.**

Overview of Dosing Schedule:

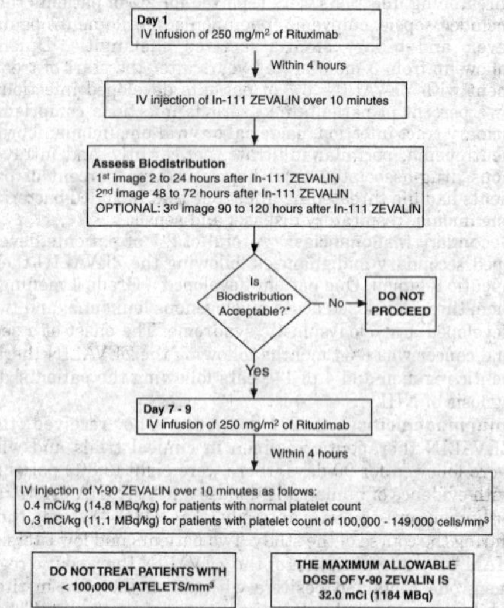

ZEVALIN Therapeutic Regimen Administration

Step 1:

First Rituximab Infusion: Rituximab at a dose of 250 mg/m^2 should be administered intravenously at an initial rate of 50 mg/hr. Rituximab should not be mixed or diluted with other drugs. If hypersensitivity or infusion-related events do not occur, escalate the infusion rate in 50 mg/hr increments every 30 minutes, to a maximum of 400 mg/hr. If hypersensitivity or an infusion-related event develops, the infusion should be temporarily slowed or interrupted (see WARNINGS). The infusion can continue at one-half the previous rate upon improvement of patient symptoms.

In-111 ZEVALIN Injection: Within 4 hours following completion of the Rituximab dose, 5.0 mCi (1.6 mg total antibody dose) of In-111 ZEVALIN is injected intravenously (I.V.) over a period of 10 minutes. A 0.22 micrometer low-protein-binding filter should be in-line between the syringe and the infusion port prior to injection of In-111 ZEVALIN. After injection, the line should be flushed with at least 10 mL of normal saline.

Step 2:

Step 2 of the ZEVALIN therapeutic regimen is initiated seven to nine days following Step 1 administrations.

Second Rituximab Infusion: Rituximab at a dose of 250 mg/m^2 is administered I.V. at an initial rate of 100 mg/hr (50 mg/hr if infusion related events were documented during the first Rituximab administration) and increased by 100 mg/hr increments at 30 minute intervals, to a maximum of 400 mg/hr, as tolerated.

Y-90 ZEVALIN Injection:

Within 4 hours following completion of the Rituximab dose, Y-90 ZEVALIN at a dose of 0.4 mCi/kg (14.8 MBq/kg) actual body weight for patients with a platelet count $\geq$150,000 cells/mm^3, and 0.3 mCi/kg (11.1 MBq/kg) actual body weight for patients with a platelet count of 100,000-149,000 cells/mm^3 is injected intravenously (I.V.) over a period of 10 minutes. A 0.22 micrometer low-protein-binding filter should be in-line between the syringe and the infusion port prior to injection of Y-90 ZEVALIN. After injection, the line should be flushed with at least 10 mL of normal saline.

Precautions should be taken to avoid extravasation. A free flowing I.V. line should be established prior to Y-90 ZEVALIN injection. Close monitoring for evidence of extravasation during the injection of Y-90 ZEVALIN is required. If any signs or symptoms of extravasation have occurred, the infusion should be immediately terminated and restarted in another vein. **The prescribed, measured, and administered dose of Y-90 ZEVALIN must not exceed the absolute maximum allowable dose of 32.0 mCi (1184 MBq), regardless of the patient's body weight. Do not give Y-90 ZEVALIN to patients with a platelet count <100,000/mm^3 (see WARNINGS).**

DIRECTIONS FOR PREPARATION OF RADIOLABELED ZEVALIN

A. PREPARATION OF THE IN-111 ZEVALIN DOSE

GENERAL:

Read all directions thoroughly and assemble all materials before starting the radiolabeling procedure. Important, significant differences exist in the preparation of the In-111 ZEVALIN dose and the Y-90 ZEVALIN dose.

The patient dose should be measured by a suitable radioactivity calibration system immediately prior to administration. The dose calibrator must be operated in accordance with the manufacturer's specifications and quality control for the measurement of In-111.

Proper aseptic technique and precautions for handling radioactive materials should be employed. Waterproof gloves should be utilized in the preparation and during the determination of radiochemical purity of In-111 ZEVALIN. Appropriate shielding should be used during radiolabeling, and use of a syringe shield is recommended during administration to the patient. The radiolabeling of ZEVALIN shall be done according to the following directions.

Required materials not supplied in the kit:

A. Indium-111 Chloride Sterile Solution (In-111 Chloride) from Amersham Health, Inc. or Mallinckrodt, Inc.
B. Three sterile 1 mL syringes
C. One sterile 3 mL syringe
D. Two sterile 10 mL syringes with 18-20 G needles
E. Instant thin-layer chromatographic silica gel strips
F. 0.9% sodium chloride aqueous solution for the chromatography solvent
G. Developing chamber for chromatography
H. Suitable radioactivity counting apparatus
I. Filter, 0.22 micrometer, low-protein-binding (see DOSAGE AND ADMINISTRATION, Zevalin Therapeutic Regimen Administration)
J. Vial and syringe shield

Method:

1. Sterile, pyrogen-free In-111 chloride must be used for the preparation of In-111 ZEVALIN. The use of high purity In-111 chloride manufactured by Amersham Health, Inc. or Mallinckrodt, Inc. is required.
2. Before radiolabeling, allow contents of the refrigerated carton to reach room temperature. Note: The ZEVALIN vial contains a protein solution that may develop translucent particulates. These particulates will be removed by filtration prior to administration.
3. Clean the rubber stoppers of all of the vials in the kit and the In-111 chloride vial with a suitable alcohol swab and allow to air dry.
4. Place the empty Reaction Vial in a suitable dispensing shield (pre-warmed to room temperature). To avoid the buildup of excessive pressure during the procedure, use a 10 mL syringe to withdraw 10 mL of air from the Reaction Vial.
5. Prior to initiating the radiolabeling reaction, determine the amount of each component needed according to the directions below:
   a. Calculate the volume of In-111 chloride that is equivalent to 5.5 mCi based on the activity concentration of the In-111 chloride stock.
   b. The volume of 50 mM sodium acetate solution needed is 1.2 times the volume of In-111 chloride solution determined in step 5.a., above. (The 50 mM sodium acetate is used to adjust the pH for the radiolabeling reaction.)
   c. Calculate the volume of Formulation Buffer needed to bring the Reaction Vial contents to a final volume of 10 mL. This is the volume of Formulation Buffer needed to protect the labeled product from radiolysis and to terminate the labeling reaction. For example, if volumes of 0.5 mL of In-111 chloride, 0.6 mL of sodium acetate and 1.0 mL of ZEVALIN were used, then the amount of formulation buffer would be 10-(0.5 + 0.6 + 1.0) = 7.9 mL.
6. With a sterile 1 mL syringe, transfer the calculated volume of 50 mM of sodium acetate to the empty Reaction Vial. Coat the entire inner surface of the Reaction Vial by gentle inversion or rolling.
7. Transfer 5.5 mCi of In-111 chloride to the Reaction Vial with a sterile 1 mL syringe. Mix the two solutions and coat the entire inner surface of the Reaction Vial by gentle inversion or rolling.
8. With a sterile 3 mL syringe, transfer 1.0 mL of ZEVALIN (Ibritumomab Tiuxetan) to the Reaction Vial. Coat the entire surface of the Reaction Vial by gentle inversion or rolling. **Do not shake or agitate the vial contents, since this will cause foaming and denaturation of the protein.**
9. Allow the labeling reaction to proceed at room temperature for 30 minutes. Allowing the labeling reaction to proceed for a longer or shorter time may result in inadequate labeling.
10. **Immediately** after the 30-minute incubation period, using a sterile 10 mL syringe with a large bore needle (18 G-20 G), transfer the calculated volume of Formulation Buffer from step 5.c. to the Reaction Vial. Gently add the Formulation Buffer down the side of the Reaction Vial. If necessary, to normalize air pressure, withdraw an equal volume of air. Coat the entire inner surface of the Reaction Vial by gentle inversion or rolling. Do not shake or agitate the vial contents. Avoid foaming.
11. Using the supplied labels, record the patient identification, the date and time of preparation, the total activity and volume, and the date and time of expiration, and affix these labels to the reaction vial and shielded reaction vial container.
12. Calculate the volume required for an In-111 ZEVALIN dose of 5 mCi. Withdraw the required volume from the Reaction Vial contents into a sterile 10 mL syringe with a large bore needle (18 G-20 G). Assay the syringe and contents in a dose calibrator. The syringe should contain the dose of In-111 ZEVALIN to be administered to the patient. Using the supplied labels, record the patient identification, the date and time of preparation, the total activity and volume added, and the date and time of expiration, and affix these labels to the syringe and shielded unit dose container.
13. Determine Radiochemical purity. See Section C: Procedure for Determining Radiochemical Purity Section that follows DIRECTIONS FOR PREPARATION OF THE Y-90 ZEVALIN DOSE.
14. Indium-111 ZEVALIN should be stored at 2-8°C (36-46°F) until use and administered within 12 hours of radiolabeling.
15. See DOSAGE AND ADMINISTRATION: ZEVALIN Therapeutic Regimen Administration: Step 1
16. Discard vials, needles and syringes in accordance with local, state, and federal regulations governing radioactive and biohazardous waste.

B. PREPARATION OF THE Y-90 ZEVALIN DOSE

GENERAL:

Read all directions thoroughly and assemble all materials before starting the radiolabeling procedure. Important, significant differences exist in the preparation of the In-111 ZEVALIN dose and the Y-90 ZEVALIN dose.

The patient dose should be measured by a suitable radioactivity calibration system immediately prior to administration. The dose calibrator must be operated in accordance with the manufacturer's specifications and quality control for the measurement of Y-90.

Proper aseptic technique and precautions for handling radioactive materials should be employed. Waterproof gloves should be utilized in the preparation and during the determination of radiochemical purity of Y-90 ZEVALIN. Appropriate shielding should be used during radiolabeling, and use of a syringe shield is recommended during administration to the patient. The radiolabeling of ZEVALIN shall be done according to the following directions.

Required materials not supplied in the kit:

A. Yttrium-90 Chloride Sterile Solution from MDS Nordion (shipped directly from MDS Nordion upon placement of an order for the Y-90 ZEVALIN kit)
B. Three sterile 1 mL syringes
C. One sterile 3 mL syringe
D. Two sterile 10 mL syringes with 18-20 G needles
E. Instant thin-layer chromatographic silica gel strips (ITLC-SG)
F. 0.9% sodium chloride aqueous solution for the chromatography solvent
G. Suitable radioactivity counting apparatus
H. Developing chamber for chromatography
I. Filter, 0.22 micrometer, low-protein-binding (see DOSAGE AND ADMINISTRATION, Zevalin Therapeutic Regimen Administration)
J. Vial and syringe shield

Method:

1. Sterile, pyrogen-free Y-90 chloride must be used for the preparation of Y-90 ZEVALIN. The use of high purity Y-90 chloride manufactured by MDS Nordion is required.
2. Before radiolabeling, allow the contents of the refrigerated carton to reach room temperature. Note: The ZEVALIN vial contains a protein solution that may develop translucent particulates. These particulates will be removed by filtration prior to administration.
3. Clean the rubber stoppers of all of the vials in the kit and the Y-90 chloride vial with a suitable alcohol swab and allow to air dry.
4. Place the empty Reaction Vial in a suitable dispensing shield (pre-warmed to room temperature). To avoid the buildup of excessive pressure during the procedure, use a 10 mL syringe to withdraw 10 mL of air from the Reaction Vial.
5. Prior to initiating the radiolabeling reaction, determine the amount of each component needed according to the directions below:
   a. Calculate the volume of Y-90 chloride that is equivalent to 40 mCi based on the activity concentration of the Y-90 chloride stock.
   b. The volume of 50 mM sodium acetate solution needed is 1.2 times the volume of Y-90 chloride so-

lution determined in step 5.a., above. (The 50 mM sodium acetate is used to adjust the pH for the radiolabeling reaction.)

c. Calculate the volume of Formulation Buffer needed to bring the Reaction Vial contents to a final volume of 10 mL. This is the volume of Formulation Buffer needed to protect the labeled product from radiolysis and to terminate the labeling reaction. For example if the volumes were 0.5 mL of Y-90 chloride, 0.6 mL of sodium acetate and 1.3 mL of ZEVALIN, then the amount of formulation buffer would be 10-(0.5 + 0.6 + 1.3) = 7.6 mL.

6. With a sterile 1 mL syringe, transfer the calculated volume of 50 mM sodium acetate to the empty Reaction Vial. Coat the entire inner surface of the Reaction Vial by gentle inversion or rolling.
7. Transfer 40 mCi of Y-90 chloride to the Reaction Vial with a sterile 1 mL syringe. Mix the two solutions and coat the entire inner surface of the Reaction Vial by gentle inversion or rolling.
8. With a sterile 3 mL syringe, transfer 1.3 mL of ZEVALIN (Ibritumomab Tiuxetan) to the Reaction Vial. Coat the entire surface of the Reaction Vial by gentle inversion or rolling. **Do not shake or agitate the vial contents, since this will cause foaming and denaturation of the protein.**
9. Allow the labeling reaction to proceed at room temperature for 5 minutes. Allowing the labeling reaction to proceed for a longer or shorter time may result in inadequate labeling.
10. **Immediately** after the 5-minute incubation period, using a sterile 10 mL syringe with a large bore needle (18 G-20 G), transfer the calculated volume of Formulation Buffer from step 5.c. to the Reaction Vial, terminating incubation. Gently add the Formulation Buffer down the side of the Reaction Vial. If necessary to normalize air pressure, withdraw an equal volume of air. Coat the entire inner surface of the Reaction Vial by gentle inversion or rolling. Do not shake or agitate the vial contents. Avoid foaming.
11. Using the supplied labels, record the patient identification, the date and time of preparation, the total activity and volume, and the date and time of expiration and affix these labels to the reaction vial and shielded reaction vial container.
12. Calculate the volume required for a Y-90 ZEVALIN dose of 0.4 mCi/kg (14.8 MBq/kg) actual body weight for patients with normal platelet count, and 0.3 mCi/kg (11.1 MBq/kg) actual body weight for patients with platelet count of 100,000-149,000 cells/mm^3. **The prescribed, measured, and administered dose of Y-90 ZEVALIN must not exceed the absolute maximum allowable dose of 32.0 mCi (1184 MBq), regardless of the patient's body weight.** Withdraw the required volume from the Reaction Vial contents into a sterile 10 mL syringe with a large bore needle (18 G-20 G). Assay the syringe and contents in a dose calibrator. The dose calibrator must be operated in accordance with the manufacturer's specifications and quality control for the measurement of Y-90. The syringe should contain the dose of Y-90 ZEVALIN to be administered to the patient, and should be within 10% of the actual prescribed dose of Y-90 ZEVALIN, not to exceed a maximum dose of 32.0 mCi. Do not exceed ± 10% of the prescribed dose. Using the supplied labels, record the patient identification, the date and time of preparation, the total activity and volume added, and the date and time of expiration and affix these labels to the syringe and shielded unit dose container.
13. Determine Radiochemical Purity. See Section C: Procedure for Determining Radiochemical Purity Section that follows these DIRECTIONS FOR PREPARATION OF THE Y-90 ZEVALIN DOSE.
14. Yttrium-90 ZEVALIN should be stored at 2-8°C (36-46°F) until use and administered within 8 hours of radiolabeling.
15. See DOSAGE AND ADMINISTRATION: ZEVALIN Therapeutic Regimen Administration: Step 2.
16. Discard vials, needles and syringes in accordance with local, state, and federal regulations governing radioactive and biohazardous waste.

Yttrium-90 ZEVALIN is suitable for administration on an outpatient basis. Beyond the use of vial and syringe shields for preparation and injection, no special shielding is necessary.

C. PROCEDURE FOR DETERMINING RADIOCHEMICAL PURITY (RCP)

The following procedure should be used for both In-111 ZEVALIN and Y-90 ZEVALIN:

A. At room temperature, place a small drop of either In-111 ZEVALIN or Y-90 ZEVALIN at the origin of an ITLC-SG strip.
B. Place the ITLC-SG strip into a chromatography chamber with the origin at the bottom and the solvent front at the top. Allow the solvent (0.9% NaCl) to migrate at least 5 cm from the bottom of the strip. Remove the strip from the chamber and cut the strip in half. Count each half of the ITLC-SG strip for one minute (CPM) with a suitable counting apparatus.
C. Calculate the percent RCP as follows:

$$\% \text{ RCP} = \frac{\text{CPM bottom half}}{\text{CPM bottom half} + \text{CPM top half}} \times 100$$

D. If the radiochemical purity is <95%, the ITLC procedure should be repeated. If repeat testing confirms that radiochemical purity is <95%, the preparation should not be administered.

IMAGE ACQUISITION AND INTERPRETATION

The biodistribution of In-111 ZEVALIN should be assessed by a visual evaluation of whole body planar view anterior and posterior gamma images at 2-24 hours and 48-72 hours after injection. To resolve ambiguities, a third image at 90-120 hours may be necessary. Images should be acquired using a large field of view gamma camera equipped with a medium energy collimator. Whole body anterior/posterior planar images should be acquired using a large field-of-view gamma camera and medium energy collimators. Suggested gamma camera settings: 256 × 1024 matrix; dual energy photopeaks set at 172 and 247 keV; 15% symmetric window; scan speed of 10 cm/min for the 2-24 hour scan, 7-10 cm/min for the 48-72 hour scan and 5 cm/min for the optional 90-120 hour scan.

The radiopharmaceutical is expected to be easily detectable in the blood pool areas at the first time point, with less activity in the blood pool on later images. Moderately high to high uptake is seen in the normal liver and spleen, with low uptake in the lungs, kidneys, and urinary bladder. Localization to lymphoid aggregates in the bowel wall has been reported. Tumor uptake may be visualized in soft tissue as areas of increased intensity, and tumor-bearing areas in normal organs may be seen as areas of increased or decreased intensity.

If a visual inspection of the gamma images reveals an altered biodistribution, the patient should not proceed to the Y-90 ZEVALIN dose. The patient may be considered to have an altered biodistribution if the blood pool is not visualized on the first image indicating rapid clearance of the radiopharmaceutical by the reticuloendothelial system to the liver, spleen, and/or marrow. Other potential examples of altered biodistribution may include diffuse uptake in the normal lungs or kidneys more intense than the liver on the second or third image.

During ZEVALIN clinical development, individual tumor radiation absorbed dose estimates as high as 778 cGy/mCi have been reported. Although solid organ toxicity has not been directly attributed to radiation from adjacent tumors, careful consideration should be applied before proceeding with treatment in patients with very high tumor uptake next to critical organs or structures.

HOW SUPPLIED

The In-111 ZEVALIN kit provides for the radiolabeling of Ibritumomab Tiuxetan with In-111. The Y-90 ZEVALIN kit provides for the radiolabeling of Ibritumomab Tiuxetan with Y-90.

The kit for the preparation of a single dose of In-111 ZEVALIN includes four vials: one ZEVALIN vial containing 3.2 mg of Ibritumomab Tiuxetan in 2 mL of 0.9% sodium chloride solution; one 50 mM Sodium Acetate vial; one Formulation Buffer vial; one empty Reaction vial and four identification labels.

The kit for the preparation of a single dose of Y-90 ZEVALIN includes four vials: one ZEVALIN vial containing 3.2 mg of Ibritumomab Tiuxetan in 2 mL of 0.9% sodium chloride solution; one 50 mM Sodium Acetate vial; one Formulation Buffer vial; one empty Reaction vial and four identification labels.

The contents of all vials are sterile, pyrogen-free and contain no preservatives.

The Indium-111 Chloride Sterile Solution (In-111 Chloride) must be ordered separately from either Amersham Health, Inc. or Mallinckrodt, Inc. at the time the In-111 ZEVALIN kit is ordered. The Yttrium-90 Chloride Sterile Solution will be shipped directly from MDS Nordion upon placement of an order for the Y-90 ZEVALIN kit.

Storage

Store at 2-8°C (36-46°F). Do not freeze.

REFERENCES

1. Kocher DC. Radioactive Decay Data Tables - A Handbook of Decay Data for Application to Radiation Dosimetry and Radiological Assessments: U.S. Department of Energy 1981; DOE/TIC-11026.
2. Valentine MA, Meier KE, Rossie S, Clark EA. Phosphorylation of the CD20 phosphoprotein in resting B lymphocytes. Regulation by protein kinase C. J Biol Chem 1989;264(19):11282-7.
3. Einfeld D, Brown J, Valentine M, Clark E, Ledbetter J. Molecular cloning of the human B cell CD20 receptor predicts a hydrophobic protein with multiple transmembrane domains. EMBO J 1988;7(3):711-7.
4. Anderson KC, Bates MP, Slaughenhoupt BL, Pinkus GS, Schlossman SF, Nadler LM. Expression of human B cell-associated antigens on leukemias and lymphomas: a model of human B cell differentiation. Blood 1984;63(6):1424-33.
5. Tedder T, Boyd A, Freedman A, Nadler L, Schlossman S. The B cell surface molecule B1 is functionally linked with B cell activation and differentiation. J Immunol 1985;135(2):973-9.
6. Press O, Appelbaum F, Ledbetter J, Martin P, Zarling J, Kidd P, et al. Monoclonal antibody 1F5 (anti-CD20) serotherapy of human B-cell lymphomas. Blood 1987;69(2):584-91.
7. Chakrabarti MC, Le N, Paik CH, De Graff WG, Carrasquillo JA. Prevention of radiolysis of monoclonal antibody during labeling. J Nucl Med 1996;37(8):1384-8.
8. Wiseman GA, White CA, Stabin M, Dunn WL, Erwin W, Dahlbom M, et al. Phase I/II 90Y ZevalinTM (90yttrium ibritumomab tiuxetan, IDEC-Y2B8) radioimmunotherapy dosimetry results in relapsed or refractory non-Hodgkin's lymphoma. Eur J Nucl Med 2000;27(7):766-77.
9. Wiseman GA, White CA, Sparks RB, Erwin WD, Podoloff DA, Lamonica DA, et al. Biodistribution and dosimetry results from a phase III prospectively randomized controlled trial of Zevalin radioimmunotherapy for low-grade, follicular, or transformed B-cell non-Hodgkin's lymphoma. Crit Rev Oncol Hematol 2001;39(1-2):181-94.
10. Siegel J, Lee R, Pawlyk D, Horowitz J, Sharkey R, Goldenberg D. Sacral scintigraphy for bone marrow dosimetry in radioimmunotherapy. Int J Appl Radiat Instr 1989;16(Part B):553-9.
11. Witzig TE, Flinn IW, Gordon LI, Emmanouilides C, Czuczman MS, Saleh MN, et al. Treatment with ibritumomab tiuxetan radioimmunotherapy in patients with rituximab-refractory follicular non-Hodgkin's Lymphoma. J. Clin Oncol 2002 in press.
12. Cheson BD, Horning SJ, Coiffier B, Shipp MA, Fisher RI, Connors JM, et al. Report of an international workshop to standardize response criteria for non-Hodgkin's lymphoma. J Clin Oncol 1999;17(4):1244-53.
13. Witzig TE, Gordon LI, Cabanillas F, Czuczman MS, Emmanouilides C, Joyce R, et al. Randomized controlled trial of yttrium-90-labeled ibritumomab tiuxetan radioimmunotherapy versus rituximab immunotherapy for patients with relapsed or refractory low-grade, follicular, or transformed B-cell non-hodgkins lymphoma. J Clin Oncol. 2002;20(10):2453-63.
14. Wiseman GA, Gordon LI, Multani PS, Witzig TE, Spies S, Bartlett NL, et al. Ibritumomab tiuxetan radioimmunotherapy for relapsed or refractory non-hodgkins lymphoma patients with mild thrombocytopenia: a phase II multicenter trial. Blood 2002; 99(12):4336-4342.

Rx Only

In-111 ZEVALIN kit, NDC 64406-104-04
Y-90 ZEVALIN kit, NDC 64406-103-03

3030 Callan Road
San Diego, CA 92121
U.S. License Number 1235
Protected by one or more U.S. Patents.
Issue date: January 2003

Biogen Inc. Dermatology

Please see Biogen Idec

Biogen Inc - Neurology

Please see Biogen Idec

Bioglan Pharmaceuticals Company

7 GREAT VALLEY PARKWAY
SUITE 301
MALVERN PA 19355

Direct Inquiries to:
Phone (888) 246-4526
Fax (610) 232-2020

ADOXA® ℞
DOXYCYCLINE TABLETS

DESCRIPTION

Doxycycline is a broad-spectrum antibiotic synthetically derived from oxytetracycline. Doxycycline 100 mg, 75 mg and 50 mg tablets contain doxycycline monohydrate equivalent to 100 mg, 75 mg or 50 mg of doxycycline for oral administration. Inactive ingredients include colloidal silicon dioxide, FD&C yellow #6, magnesium stearate, microcrystalline cellulose, sodium starch glycolate, and titanium dioxide. In addition, Doxycycline 100 mg and 50 mg tablets contain hypromellose 3cP, hypromellose 6cP, D&C yellow #10 lake, polyethylene glycol 400, polysorbate 80; Doxycycline 75 mg tablets contain hydroxypropyl methylcellulose, lactose monohydrate, synthetic yellow iron oxide and triethyl citrate. Its molecular weight is 462.46. The chemical designation of the light-yellow crystalline powder is alpha-6-deoxy-5-oxytetracycline.

Continued on next page

Adoxa—Cont.

Structural formula:

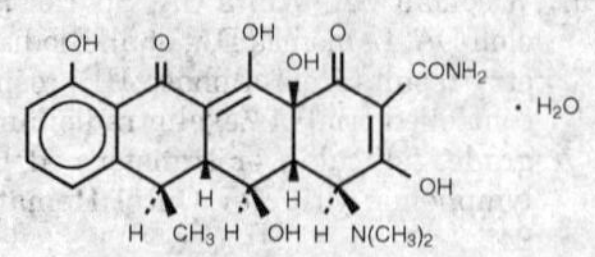

$C_{22}H_{24}N_2O_8H_2O$

Doxycycline has a high degree of lipid solubility and a low affinity for calcium binding. It is highly stable in normal human serum. Doxycycline will not degrade into an epianhydro form.

HOW SUPPLIED

Doxycycline Tablets 50 mg are a yellow, film coated, round, biconvex tablet, debossed "B" on one side and "728" on the other side. Each tablet contains doxycycline monohydrate equivalent to 50 mg of doxycycline. They are supplied as follows:

Bottles of 100	NDC 62436-728-01

Doxycycline Tablets 75 mg are a light orange, film coated, round, biconvex tablet, debossed "B" on one side and "730" on the other side. Each tablet contains doxycycline monohydrate equivalent to 75 mg of doxycycline. They are supplied as follows:

Bottles of 100	NDC 62436-730-01
Bottles of 500	NDC 62436-730-05

Doxycycline Tablets 100 mg are a yellow, film coated, round, biconvex tablet, debossed "B" on one side and "729" on the other side. Each tablet contains doxycycline monohydrate equivalent to 100 mg of doxycycline. They are supplied as follows:

Bottles of 50	NDC 62436-729-03
Bottles of 250	NDC 62436-729-04

Store at controlled room temperature 15°–30°C (59°–86°F). (See USP).
PROTECT FROM LIGHT.

SOLARAZE™ GEL ℞

Diclofenac Sodium-3%
FOR DERMATOLOGIC USE ONLY.
NOT FOR OPHTHALMIC USE.
Rx Only

DESCRIPTION

Solaraze™ (diclofenac sodium) Gel, 3%, contains the active ingredient, diclofenac sodium, in a clear, transparent, colorless to slightly yellow gel base. Diclofenac sodium is a white to slightly yellow crystalline powder. It is freely soluble in methanol, soluble in ethanol, sparingly soluble in water, slightly soluble in acetone, and partially insoluble in ether.
The chemical name for diclofenac sodium is:
Sodium [o-(2,6-dichloranilino) phenyl] acetate
Diclofenac sodium has a molecular weight of 318.13.
The CAS number is CAS-15307-79-6. The structural formula is represented below:

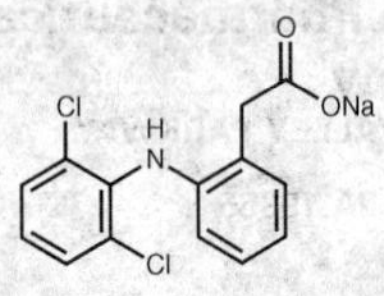

Solaraze™ Gel also contains benzyl alcohol, hyaluronate sodium, polyethylene glycol monomethyl ether, and purified water.
1 g of Solaraze™ (diclofenac sodium) Gel contains 30 mg of the active substance, diclofenac sodium.

HOW SUPPLIED

Available in tubes of 50 g (NDC 62436-003-50) and 100 g (NDC 62436-003-01). Each gram of gel contains 30 mg of diclofenac sodium.
Storage: Store at controlled room temperature 20°–25°C (68°–77°F), excursions permitted between 15–30°C (59–86°F). Protect from heat. Avoid freezing.

ZONALON® CREAM, 5% ℞

(doxepin hydrochloride)
FOR TOPICAL DERMATOLOGIC USE ONLY—
NOT FOR OPHTHALMIC, ORAL, OR INTRAVAGINAL USE.

DESCRIPTION

Zonalon (doxepin hydrochloride) Cream, 5% is a topical cream. Each gram contains: 50 mg of doxepin hydrochloride (equivalent to 44.3 mg of doxepin).
Doxepin hydrochloride is one of a class of agents known as dibenzoxepin tricyclic antidepressant compounds. It is an isomeric mixture of N,N-dimethyldibenz[*b,e*]oxepin-$\Delta^{11(6H),\gamma}$-propylamine hydrochloride. Doxepin hydrochloride has an empirical formula of $C_{19}H_{21}NO \cdot HCl$ and a molecular weight of 316.

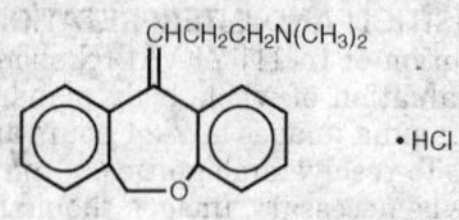

Zonalon Cream also contains sorbitol, cetyl alcohol, isopropyl myristate, glyceryl stearate, PEG-100 stearate, petrolatum, benzyl alcohol, titanium dioxide and purified water.

HOW SUPPLIED

Zonalon Cream is available in 30 g (NDC 62436-523-30) and 45 g (NDC 62436-523-45) tubes. Store at or below 27° C (80° F).

Biomarin™ Pharmaceutical Inc.

371 BEL MARIN KEYS BLVD
SUITE 210
NOVATO, CA 94949

PH# 415-506-6700
FAX# 415-382-7889
www.BMRN.com

ORAPRED® ℞

[*ōr əprĕd*]
(prednisolone sodium phosphate oral solution)
Rx only

DESCRIPTION

Orapred Solution is a dye free, pale to light yellow solution. Each 5 mL (teaspoonful) of Orapred contains 20.2 mg prednisolone sodium phosphate (15 mg prednisolone base) in a palatable, aqueous vehicle.
Inactive Ingredients: Orapred Solution equivalent to 15 mg prednisolone per 5 mL contains the following inactive ingredients: alcohol 2%, fructose, glycerin, monoammonium glycyrrhizinate, povidone, sodium benzoate, sorbitol, and flavor. Orapred may contain citric acid and/or sodium hydroxide for pH adjustment.
Prednisolone sodium phosphate occurs as white or slightly yellow, friable granules or powder. It is freely soluble in water; soluble in methanol; slightly soluble in alcohol and in chloroform; and very slightly soluble in acetone and in dioxane. The chemical name of prednisolone sodium phosphate is pregna-1,4-diene-3,20-dione,11,17-dihydroxy-21-(phosphonooxy)-, disodium salt, (11β)-. The empirical formula is $C_{21}H_{27}Na_2O_8P$; the molecular weight is 484.39. Its chemical structure is:

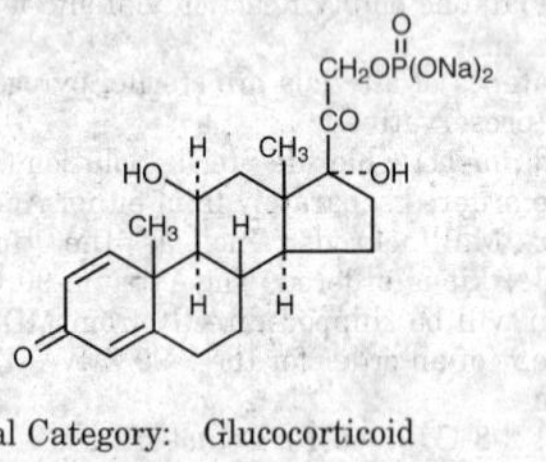

Pharmacological Category: Glucocorticoid

CLINICAL PHARMACOLOGY

Naturally occurring glucocorticoids (hydrocortisone), which also have salt-retaining properties, are used as replacement therapy in adrenocortical deficiency states. Their synthetic analogs are primarily used for their potent anti-inflammatory effects in disorders of many organ systems.
Prednisolone is a synthetic adrenocortical steroid drug with predominantly glucocorticoid properties. Some of these properties reproduce the physiological actions of endogenous glucocorticosteroids, but others do not necessarily reflect any of the adrenal hormones' normal functions; they are seen only after administration of large therapeutic doses of the drug. The pharmacological effects of prednisolone which are due to its glucocorticoid properties include: promotion of gluconeogenesis; increased deposition of glycogen in the liver; inhibition of the utilization of glucose; anti-insulin activity; increased catabolism of protein; increased lipolysis; stimulation of fat synthesis and storage; increased glomerular filtration rate and resulting increase in urinary excretion of urate (creatinine excretion remains unchanged); and increased calcium excretion.
Depressed production of eosinophils and lymphocytes occurs, but erythropoiesis and production of polymorphonuclear leukocytes are stimulated. Inflammatory processes (edema, fibrin deposition, capillary dilatation, migration of leukocytes and phagocytosis) and the later stages of wound healing (capillary proliferation, deposition of collagen, cicatrization) are inhibited.
Prednisolone can stimulate secretion of various components of gastric juice. Suppression of the production of corticotropin may lead to suppression of endogenous corticosteroids. Prednisolone has slight mineralocorticoid activity, whereby entry of sodium into cells and loss of intracellular potassium is stimulated. This is particularly evident in the kidney, where rapid ion exchange leads to sodium retention and hypertension.
Prednisolone is rapidly and well absorbed from the gastrointestinal tract following oral administration. Orapred Solution produces a 14% higher peak plasma level of prednisolone which occurs 20% faster than the peak seen with tablets. Prednisolone is 70–90% protein-bound in the plasma and it is eliminated from the plasma with a half-life of 2 to 4 hours. It is metabolized mainly in the liver and excreted in the urine as sulfate and glucuronide conjugates.

INDICATIONS AND USAGE

Orapred Solution is indicated in the following conditions:

1. Endocrine Disorders
Primary or secondary adrenocortical insufficiency (hydrocortisone or cortisone is the first choice; synthetic analogs may be used in conjunction with mineralocorticoids where applicable; in infancy mineralocorticoid supplementation is of particular importance); congenital adrenal hyperplasia; hypercalcemia associated with cancer; nonsuppurative thyroiditis.

2. Rheumatic Disorders
As adjunctive therapy for short term administration (to tide the patient over an acute episode or exacerbation) in: psoriatic arthritis; rheumatoid arthritis, including juvenile rheumatoid arthritis (selected cases may require low dose maintenance therapy); ankylosing spondylitis; acute and subacute bursitis; acute nonspecific tenosynovitis; acute gouty arthritis; epicondylitis. For the treatment of systemic lupus erythematosus, dermatomyositis (polymyositis), polymyalgia rheumatica, Sjogren's syndrome, relapsing polychondritis, and certain cases of vasculitis.

3. Dermatologic Diseases
Pemphigus; bullous dermatitis herpetiformis; severe erythema multiforme (Stevens-Johnson syndrome); exfoliative erythroderma; mycosis fungoides.

4. Allergic States
Control of severe or incapacitating allergic conditions intractable to adequate trials of conventional treatment in adult and pediatric populations with: seasonal or perennial allergic rhinitis; asthma; contact dermatitis; atopic dermatitis; serum sickness; drug hypersensitivity reactions.

5. Ophthalmic Diseases
Uveitis and ocular inflammatory conditions unresponsive to topical corticosteroids; temporal arteritis; sympathetic ophthalmia.

6. Respiratory Diseases
Symptomatic sarcoidosis; idiopathic eosinophilic pneumonias; fulminating or disseminated pulmonary tuberculosis when used concurrently with appropriate antituberculous chemotherapy; asthma (as distinct from allergic asthma listed above under "Allergic States"), hypersensitivity pneumonitis, idiopathic pulmonary fibrosis, acute exacerbations of chronic obstructive pulmonary disease (COPD), and Pneumocystis carinii pneumonia (PCP) associated with hypoxemia occurring in an HIV (+) individual who is also under treatment with appropriate anti-PCP antibiotics. Studies support the efficacy of systemic corticosteroids for the treatment of these conditions: allergic bronchopulmonary aspergillosis, idiopathic bronchiolitis obliterans with organizing pneumonia.

7. Hematologic Disorders
Idiopathic thrombocytopenic purpura in adults; selected cases of secondary thrombocytopenia; acquired (autoimmune) hemolytic anemia; pure red cell aplasia; Diamond-Blackfan anemia.

8. Neoplastic Diseases
For the treatment of acute leukemia and aggressive lymphomas in adults and children.

9. Edematous States
To induce diuresis or remission of proteinuria in nephrotic syndrome in adults with lupus erythematosus and in adults and pediatric populations, with idiopathic nephrotic syndrome, without uremia.

10. Gastrointestinal Diseases
To tide the patient over a critical period of the disease in: ulcerative colitis; regional enteritis.

11. Nervous System
Acute exacerbations of multiple sclerosis.

12. Miscellaneous
Tuberculous meningitis with subarachnoid block or impending block, tuberculosis with enlarged mediastinal lymph nodes causing respiratory difficulty, and tuberculosis with pleural or pericardial effusion (appropriate antituberculous chemotherapy must be used concurrently when treating any tuberculosis complications); trichinosis with neurologic or myocardial involvement; acute or chronic solid organ rejection (with or without other agents).

CONTRAINDICATIONS

Systemic fungal infections.
Hypersensitivity to the drug or any of its components.

WARNINGS

General:
In patients on corticosteroid therapy subjected to unusual stress, increased dosage of rapidly acting corticosteroids before, during and after the stressful situation is indicated.
Endocrine:
Corticosteroids can produce reversible hypothalamic-pituitary adrenal (HPA) axis suppression with the potential for glucocorticosteroid insufficiency after withdrawal of treatment.

Metabolic clearance of corticosteroids is decreased in hypothyroid patients and increased in hyperthyroid patients. Changes in thyroid status of the patient may necessitate adjustment in dosage.

Infections (general):
Persons who are on drugs which suppress the immune system are more susceptible to infections than healthy individuals. There may be decreased resistance and inability to localize infection when corticosteroids are used. Infection with any pathogen including viral, bacterial, fungal, protozoan or helminthic infection, in any location of the body, may be associated with the use of corticosteroids alone or in combination with other immunosuppressive agents that affect humoral or cellular immunity, or neutrophil function. These infections may be mild to severe, and, with increasing doses of corticosteroids, the rate of occurrence of infectious complications increases. Corticosteroids may also mask some signs of infection after it has already started.

Viral infections:
Chicken pox and measles for example, can have a more serious or even fatal course in non-immune children or adults on corticosteroids. In such children or adults who have not had the diseases, particular care should be taken to avoid exposure. How the dose, route and duration of corticosteroid administration affect the risk of developing a disseminated infection is not known. The contribution of the underlying disease and/or prior corticosteroid treatment to the risk is also not known. If exposed to chicken pox, prophylaxis with varicella zoster immune globulin (VZIG) may be indicated. If exposed to measles, prophylaxis with immunoglobulin (IG) may be indicated. (See the respective package inserts for complete VZIG and IG prescribing information). If chicken pox develops, treatment with antiviral agents should be considered.

Special pathogens:
Latent disease may be activated or there may be an exacerbation of intercurrent infections due to pathogens, including those caused by Candida, Mycobacterium, Ameba, Toxoplasma, Pneumocystis, Cryptococcus, Nocardia, etc.
Corticosteroids may activate latent amebiasis. Therefore, it is recommended that latent or active amebiasis be ruled out before initiating corticosteroid therapy in any patient who has spent time in the tropics or in any patient with unexplained diarrhea.
Similarly, corticosteroids should be used with great care in patients with known or suspected Strongyloides (threadworm) infestation. In such patients, corticosteroid-induced immunosuppression may lead to Strongyloides hyperinfection and dissemination with widespread larval migration, often accompanied by severe enterocolitis and potentially fatal gram-negative septicemia.
Corticosteroids should not be used in cerebral malaria.

Tuberculosis:
The use of prednisolone in active tuberculosis should be restricted to those cases of fulminating or disseminated tuberculosis in which the corticosteroid is used for the management of the disease in conjunction with an appropriate antituberculous regimen.
If corticosteroids are indicated in patients with latent tuberculosis or tuberculin reactivity, close observation is necessary as reactivation of the disease may occur. During prolonged corticosteroid therapy these patients should receive chemoprophylaxis.

Vaccination:
Administration of live or live, attenuated vaccines is contraindicated in patients receiving immunosuppressive doses of corticosteroids. Killed or inactivated vaccines may be administered, however, the response to such vaccines can not be predicted. Immunization procedures may be undertaken in patients who are receiving corticosteroids as replacement therapy, e.g., for Addison's disease.

Ophthalmic:
Use of corticosteroids may produce posterior subcapsular cataracts, glaucoma with possible damage to the optic nerves, and may enhance the establishment of secondary ocular infections due to bacteria, fungi or viruses. The use of oral corticosteroids is not recommended in the treatment of optic neuritis and may lead to an increase in the risk of new episodes. Corticosteroids should not be used in active ocular herpes simplex.

Cardio-renal:
Average and large doses of hydrocortisone or cortisone can cause elevation of blood pressure, salt and water retention, and increased excretion of potassium. These effects are less likely to occur with the synthetic derivatives except when used in large doses. Dietary salt restriction and potassium supplementation may be necessary. All corticosteroids increase calcium excretion.

PRECAUTIONS

General:
The lowest possible dose of corticosteroid should be used to control the condition under treatment, and when reduction in dosage is possible, the reduction should be gradual.
Since complications of treatment with glucocorticoids are dependent on the size of the dose and the duration of treatment, a risk/benefit decision must be made in each individual case as to dose and duration of treatment and as to whether daily or intermittent therapy should be used.
There is an enhanced effect of corticosteroids in patients with hypothyroidism and in those with cirrhosis.
Kaposi's sarcoma has been reported to occur in patients receiving corticosteroid therapy, most often for chronic conditions. Discontinuation of corticosteroids may result in clinical improvement.

Endocrine:
Drug-induced secondary adrenocortical insufficiency may be minimized by gradual reduction of dosage. This type of relative insufficiency may persist for months after discontinuation of therapy; therefore, in any situation of stress occurring during that period, hormone therapy should be reinstituted. Since mineralocorticoid secretion may be impaired, salt and/or a mineralocorticoid should be administered concurrently.

Ophthalmic:
Intraocular pressure may become elevated in some individuals. If steroid therapy is continued for more than 6 weeks, intraocular pressure should be monitored.

Neuro-psychiatric:
Although controlled clinical trials have shown corticosteroids to be effective in speeding the resolution of acute exacerbations of multiple sclerosis, they do not show that they affect the ultimate outcome or natural history of the disease. The studies do show that relatively high doses of corticosteroids are necessary to demonstrate a significant effect. (See DOSAGE AND ADMINISTRATION.)
An acute myopathy has been observed with the use of high doses of corticosteroids, most often occurring in patients with disorders of neuromuscular transmission (e.g., myasthenia gravis), or in patients receiving concomitant therapy with neuromuscular blocking drugs (e.g., pancuronium). This acute myopathy is generalized, may involve ocular and respiratory muscles, and may result in quadriparesis. Elevation of creatinine kinase may occur. Clinical improvement or recovery after stopping corticosteroids may require weeks to years.
Psychic derangements may appear when corticosteroids are used, ranging from euphoria, insomnia, mood swings, personality changes, and severe depression, to frank psychotic manifestations. Also, existing emotional instability or psychotic tendencies may be aggravated by corticosteroids.

Gastrointestinal:
Steroids should be used with caution in nonspecific ulcerative colitis, if there is a probability of impending perforation, abscess or other pyogenic infection: diverticulitis; fresh intestinal anastomoses; active or latent peptic ulcer.
Signs of peritoneal irritation following gastrointestinal perforation in patients receiving corticosteroids may be minimal or absent.

Cardio-renal:
As sodium retention with resultant edema and potassium loss may occur in patients receiving corticosteroids, these agents should be used with caution in patients with hypertension, congestive heart failure, or renal insufficiency.

Musculoskeletal:
Corticosteroids decrease bone formation and increase bone resorption both through their effect on calcium regulation (i.e., decreasing absorption and increasing excretion) and inhibition of osteoblast function. This, together with a decrease in the protein matrix of the bone secondary to an increase in protein catabolism, and reduced sex hormone production, may lead to inhibition of bone growth in children and adolescents and the development of osteoporosis at any age. Special consideration should be given to patients at increased risk of osteoporosis (i.e., post-menopausal women) before initiating corticosteroid therapy.

Information for Patients:
Patients should be warned not to discontinue the use of Orapred abruptly or without medical supervision, to advise any medical attendants that they are taking Orapred and to seek medical advice at once should they develop fever or other signs of infection.
Persons who are on immunosuppressant doses of corticosteroids should be warned to avoid exposure to chickenpox or measles. Patients should also be advised that if they are exposed, medical advice should be sought without delay.

Drug Interactions:
Drugs such as barbiturates, phenytoin, ephedrine, and rifampin, which induce hepatic microsomal drug metabolizing enzyme activity may enhance metabolism of prednisolone and require that the dosage of Orapred be increased.
Increased activity of both cyclosporin and corticosteroids may occur when the two are used concurrently. Convulsions have been reported with this concurrent use.
Estrogens may decrease the hepatic metabolism of certain corticosteroids thereby increasing their effect.
Ketoconazole has been reported to decrease the metabolism of certain corticosteroids by up to 60% leading to an increased risk of corticosteroid side effects.
Coadministration of corticosteroids and warfarin usually results in inhibition of response to warfarin, although there have been some conflicting reports. Therefore, coagulation indices should be monitored frequently to maintain the desired anticoagulant effect.
Concomitant use of aspirin (or other non-steroidal anti-inflammatory agents) and corticosteroids increases the risk of gastrointestinal side effects. Aspirin should be used cautiously in conjunction with corticosteroids in hypoprothrombinemia. The clearance of salicylates may be increased with concurrent use of corticosteroids.
When corticosteroids are administered concomitantly with potassium-depleting agents (i.e., diuretics, amphotericin-B), patients should be observed closely for development of hypokalemia. Patients on digitalis glycosides may be at increased risk of arrhythmias due to hypokalemia.
Concomitant use of anticholinesterase agents and corticosteroids may produce severe weakness in patients with myasthenia gravis. If possible, anticholinesterase agents should be withdrawn at least 24 hours before initiating corticosteroid therapy.
Due to inhibition of antibody response, patients on prolonged corticosteroid therapy may exhibit a diminished response to toxoids and live or inactivated vaccines. Corticosteroids may also potentiate the replication of some organisms contained in live attenuated vaccines. If possible, routine administration of vaccines or toxoids should be deferred until corticosteroid therapy is discontinued.
Because corticosteroids may increase blood glucose concentrations, dosage adjustment of antidiabetic agents may be required.
Corticosteroids may suppress reactions to skin tests.

Pregnancy: Teratogenic effects: Pregnancy Category C.
Prednisolone has been shown to be teratogenic in many species when given in doses equivalent to the human dose. Animal studies in which prednisolone has been given to pregnant mice, rats, and rabbits have yielded an increased incidence of cleft palate in the offspring. There are no adequate and well-controlled studies in pregnant women. Orapred should be used during pregnancy only if the potential benefit justifies the potential risk to the fetus. Infants born to mothers who have received corticosteroids during pregnancy should be carefully observed for signs of hypoadrenalism.

Nursing Mothers:
Systemically administered corticosteroids appear in human milk and could suppress growth, interfere with endogenous corticosteroid production, or cause other untoward effects. Caution should be exercised when Orapred is administered to a nursing woman.

Pediatric Use:
The efficacy and safety of prednisolone in the pediatric population are based on the well-established course of effect of corticosteroids which is similar in pediatric and adult populations. Published studies provide evidence of efficacy and safety in pediatric patients for the treatment of nephrotic syndrome (>2 years of age), and aggressive lymphomas and leukemias (>1 month of age). However, some of these conclusions and other indications for pediatric use of corticosteroid, e.g., severe asthma and wheezing, are based on adequate and well-controlled trials conducted in adults, on the premises that the course of the diseases and their pathophysiology are considered to be substantially similar in both populations.
The adverse effects of prednisolone in pediatric patients are similar to those in adults (see ADVERSE REACTIONS). Like adults, pediatric patients should be carefully observed with frequent measurements of blood pressure, weight, height, intraocular pressure, and clinical evaluation for the presence of infection, psychosocial disturbances, thromboembolism, peptic ulcers, cataracts, and osteoporosis. Children who are treated with corticosteroids by any route, including systemically administered corticosteroids, may experience a decrease in their growth velocity. This negative impact of corticosteroids on growth has been observed at low systemic doses and in the absence of laboratory evidence of HPA axis suppression (i.e., cosyntropin stimulation and basal cortisol plasma levels). Growth velocity may therefore be a more sensitive indicator of systemic corticosteroid exposure in children than some commonly used tests of HPA axis function. The linear growth of children treated with corticosteroids by any route should be monitored, and the potential growth effects of prolonged treatment should be weighed against clinical benefits obtained and the availability of other treatment alternatives. In order to minimize the potential growth effects of corticosteroids, children should be *titrated* to the lowest effective dose.

ADVERSE REACTIONS

(listed alphabetically under each subsection)

Fluid and Electrolyte Disturbances: Congestive heart failure in susceptible patients; fluid retention; hypertension; hypokalemic alkalosis; potassium loss; sodium retention.

Cardiovascular: Hypertrophic cardiomyopathy in premature infants.

Musculoskeletal: Aseptic necrosis of femoral and humeral heads; loss of muscle mass; muscle weakness; osteoporosis; pathologic fracture of long bones; steroid myopathy; tendon rupture; vertebral compression fractures.

Gastrointestinal: Abdominal distention; elevation in serum liver enzyme levels (usually reversible upon discontinuation); pancreatitis; peptic ulcer with possible perforation and hemorrhage; ulcerative esophagitis.

Dermatologic: Facial erythema; increased sweating; impaired wound healing; may suppress reactions to skin tests; petechiae and ecchymoses; thin fragile skin; urticaria; edema.

Metabolic: Negative nitrogen balance due to protein catabolism.

Neurological: Convulsions; headache; increased intracranial pressure with papilledema (pseudotumor cerebri), usually following discontinuation of treatment; psychic disorders; vertigo.

Endocrine: Decreased carbohydrate tolerance; development of cushingoid state; hirsutism; increased requirements for insulin or oral hypoglycemic agents in diabetes; manifestations of latent diabetes mellitus; menstrual irregularities; secondary adrenocortical and pituitary unresponsiveness, particularly in times of stress, as in trauma, surgery or illness; suppression of growth in children.

Continued on next page

Orapred—Cont.

Ophthalmic: Exophthalmos; glaucoma; increased intraocular pressure; posterior subcapsular cataracts.
Other: Increased appetite; malaise; nausea; weight gain.

OVERDOSAGE

The effects of accidental ingestion of large quantities of prednisolone over a very short period of time have not been reported, but prolonged use of the drug can produce mental symptoms, moon face, abnormal fat deposits, fluid retention, excessive appetite, weight gain, hypertrichosis, acne, striae, ecchymosis, increased sweating, pigmentation, dry scaly skin, thinning scalp hair, increased blood pressure, tachycardia, thrombophlebitis, decreased resistance to infection, negative nitrogen balance with delayed bone and wound healing, headache, weakness, menstrual disorders, accentuated menopausal symptoms, neuropathy, fractures, osteoporosis, peptic ulcer, decreased glucose tolerance, hypokalemia, and adrenal insufficiency. Hepatomegaly and abdominal distention have been observed in children.
Treatment of acute overdosage is by immediate gastric lavage or emesis followed by supportive and symptomatic therapy. For chronic overdosage in the face of severe disease requiring continuous steroid therapy the dosage of prednisolone may be reduced only temporarily, or alternate day treatment may be introduced.

DOSAGE AND ADMINISTRATION

The initial dose of Orapred may vary from 1.67 mL to 20 mL (5 to 60 mg prednisolone base) per day depending on the specific disease entity being treated. In situations of less severity, lower doses will generally suffice while in selected patients higher initial doses may be required. The initial dosage should be maintained or adjusted until a satisfactory response is noted. If after a reasonable period of time, there is a lack of satisfactory clinical response, Orapred should be discontinued and the patient placed on other appropriate therapy. **IT SHOULD BE EMPHASIZED THAT DOSAGE REQUIREMENTS ARE VARIABLE AND MUST BE INDIVIDUALIZED ON THE BASIS OF THE DISEASE UNDER TREATMENT AND THE RESPONSE OF THE PATIENT.** After a favorable response is noted, the proper maintenance dosage should be determined by decreasing the initial drug dosage in small decrements at appropriate time intervals until the lowest dosage which will maintain an adequate clinical response is reached. It should be kept in mind that constant monitoring is needed in regard to drug dosage. Included in the situations which may make dosage adjustments necessary are changes in clinical status secondary to remissions or exacerbations in the disease process, the patient's individual drug responsiveness, and the effect of patient exposure to stressful situations not directly related to the disease entity under treatment; in this latter situation it may be necessary to increase the dosage of Orapred for a period of time consistent with the patient's condition. If after long term therapy the drug is to be stopped, it is recommended that it be withdrawn gradually rather than abruptly.
In the treatment of acute exacerbations of multiple sclerosis daily doses of 200 mg of prednisolone for a week followed by 80 mg every other day or 4 to 8 mg dexamethasone every other day for one month have been shown to be effective.
In pediatric patients, the initial dose of Orapred may vary depending on the specific disease entity being treated. The range of initial doses is 0.14 to 2 mg/kg/day in three or four divided doses (4 to 60 mg/m^{2}bsa/day).
The standard regimen used to treat nephrotic syndrome in pediatric patients is 60 mg/m^2/day given in three divided doses for 4 weeks, followed by 4 weeks of single dose alternate-day therapy at 40 mg/m^2/day.
The National Heart, Lung, and Blood Institute (NHLBI) recommended dosing for systemic *prednisone, prednisolone* or *methylprednisolone* in children whose asthma is uncontrolled by inhaled corticosteroids and long-acting bronchodilators is 1–2 mg/kg/day in single or divided doses. It is further recommended that short course, or "burst" therapy, be continued until a child achieves a peak expiratory flow rate of 80% of his or her personal best or symptoms resolve. This usually requires 3 to 10 days of treatment, although it can take longer. There is no evidence that tapering the dose after improvement will prevent a relapse.
For the purpose of comparison, 5 mL of Orapred (20.2 mg prednisolone sodium phosphate) is equivalent to the following milligram dosage of the various glucocorticoids:

Cortisone, 75	*Triamcinolone, 12*
Hydrocortisone, 60	*Paramethasone, 6*
Prednisolone, 15	*Betamethasone, 2.25*
Prednisone, 15	*Dexamethasone, 2.25*
Methylprednisolone, 12	

These dose relationships apply only to oral or intravenous administration of these compounds. When these substances or their derivatives are injected intramuscularly or into joint spaces, their relative properties may be greatly altered.

HOW SUPPLIED

Each 5 mL (teaspoonful) of grape flavored solution contains 20.2 mg prednisolone sodium phosphate (15 mg prednisolone base).
Available as:
8 fl oz (237 mL) NDC 68135-455-02
Dispense in tight, light-resistant glass or PET plastic containers as defined in USP.
Store refrigerated, 2–8°C (36–46°F)
Keep tightly closed and out of the reach of children.
Revised June 2004.
Manufactured for Ascent Pediatrics
Novato, CA 94949
by Lyne Laboratories, Inc., Brockton, MA 02301
ASCENT® PEDIATRICS
BIOMARIN™ Pharmaceutical Inc.

Biovail Pharmaceuticals, Inc.

700 ROUTE 202-206 NORTH
BRIDGEWATER, NJ USA 08807-0980

For direct inquiries contact:
Phone: 1-866-BIOVAIL
1-866-246-8245

CARDIZEM® LA ℞

[kăr-dĭ-zĕm]
(Diltiazem Hydrochloride)
Extended Release Tablets
℞ only
Once-a-Day Dosage

DESCRIPTION

Diltiazem hydrochloride is a calcium ion cellular influx inhibitor (slow channel blocker or calcium antagonist). Chemically, diltiazem hydrochloride is 1,5-benzothiazepin-4(5H)one,3-(acetyloxy)-5-[2-(dimethylamino)ethyl]-2, 3-dihydro-2-(4-methoxyphenyl)-, monohydrochloride, (+)-cis-. The structural formula is:

OCH_3 • HCl H S H N $OCOCH_3$ O $CH_2CH_2N(CH_3)_2$

Diltiazem hydrochloride is a white to off-white crystalline powder with a bitter taste. It is soluble in water, methanol and chloroform. It has a molecular weight of 450.99. CARDIZEM® LA Tablets, for oral administration, are formulated as a once-a-day extended release tablet containing either 120 mg, 180 mg, 240 mg, 300 mg, 360 mg or 420 mg of diltiazem hydrochloride.
Also contains: Carnauba Wax NF, Colloidal Silicon Dioxide NF, Croscarmellose Sodium NF, Hydrogenated Vegetable Oil NF, Hypromellose USP, Magnesium Stearate NF, Microcrystalline Cellulose NF, Microcrystalline Wax NF, Pregelatinized Starch NF, Polyacrylate Dispersion 30%, Polyethylene Glycol NF, Polydextrose, Polysorbate NF, Povidone USP, Simethicone USP, Sodium Starch Glycolate NF, Sucrose Stearate, Talc USP, Titanium Dioxide USP.

CLINICAL PHARMACOLOGY

The therapeutic effects of diltiazem are believed to be related to its ability to inhibit the influx of calcium ions during membrane depolarization of cardiac and vascular smooth muscle.

Mechanisms of Action

Hypertension. Diltiazem produces its antihypertensive effect primarily by relaxation of vascular smooth muscle and the resultant decrease in peripheral vascular resistance. The magnitude of blood pressure reduction is related to the degree of hypertension; thus hypertensive individuals experience an antihypertensive effect, whereas there is only a modest fall in blood pressure in normotensives.
Angina. Diltiazem has been shown to produce increases in exercise tolerance, probably due to its ability to reduce myocardial oxygen demand. This is accomplished via reductions in heart rate and systemic blood pressure at submaximal and maximal work loads. Diltiazem has been shown to be a potent dilator of coronary arteries, both epicardial and subendocardial. Spontaneous and ergonovine-induced coronary artery spasms are inhibited by diltiazem.
In animal models, diltiazem interferes with the slow inward (depolarizing) current in excitable tissues. It causes excitation-contraction uncoupling in various myocardial tissues without changes in the configuration of the action potential. Diltiazem causes relaxation of coronary smooth muscle and dilation of both large and small coronary arteries at drug levels which cause little or no negative inotropic effect. The resultant increases in coronary blood flow (epicardial and subendocardial) occur in ischemic and non-ischemic models and are accompanied by dose-dependent decreases in systemic blood pressure and decreases in peripheral resistance.

Pharmacokinetics and Metabolism

Diltiazem is well absorbed from the gastrointestinal tract and is subject to an extensive first-pass effect, giving an absolute bioavailability (compared to intravenous administration) of about 40%. Diltiazem undergoes extensive metabolism in which only 2% to 4% of the unchanged drug appears in the urine. Drugs which induce or inhibit hepatic microsomal enzymes may alter diltiazem disposition.
Total radioactivity measurement following short IV administration in healthy volunteers suggests the presence of other unidentified metabolites, which attain higher concentrations than those of diltiazem and are more slowly eliminated; half-life of total radioactivity is about 20 hours compared to 2 to 5 hours for diltiazem.
In vitro binding studies show diltiazem is 70% to 80% bound to plasma proteins. Competitive *in vitro* ligand binding studies have also shown diltiazem hydrochloride binding is not altered by therapeutic concentrations of digoxin, hydrochlorothiazide, phenylbutazone, propranolol, salicylic acid, or warfarin. The plasma elimination half-life following single or multiple drug administration is approximately 3.0 to 4.5 hours. Desacetyl diltiazem is also present in the plasma at levels of 10% to 20% of the parent drug and is 25% to 50% as potent as a coronary vasodilator as diltiazem. Minimum therapeutic plasma diltiazem concentrations appear to be in the range of 50 to 200 ng/mL. There is a departure from linearity when dose strengths are increased; the half-life is slightly increased with dose. A study that compared patients with normal hepatic function to patients with cirrhosis found an increase in half-life and a 69% increase in bioavailability in the hepatically impaired patients. A single study in patients with severely impaired renal function showed no difference in the pharmacokinetic profile of diltiazem compared to patients with normal renal function.
CARDIZEM LA Tablets. A single 360 mg dose of CARDIZEM LA results in detectable plasma levels within 3 to 4 hours and peak plasma levels between 11 and 18 hours; absorption occurs throughout the dosing interval. The apparent elimination half-life for CARDIZEM LA Tablets after single or multiple dosing is 6 to 9 hours. When CARDIZEM LA Tablets were coadministered with a high fat content breakfast, diltiazem peak and systemic exposures were not affected indicating that the tablet can be administered without regard to food. As the dose of CARDIZEM LA Tablets is increased from 120 to 240 mg, area-under-the-curve increases 2.5-fold.

Pharmacodynamics and Clinical Studies

Like other calcium channel antagonists, diltiazem decreases sinoatrial and atrioventricular conduction in isolated tissues and has a negative inotropic effect in isolated preparations. In the intact animal, prolongation of the AH interval can be seen at higher doses.
In man, diltiazem prevents spontaneous and ergonovine-provoked coronary artery spasm. It causes a decrease in peripheral vascular resistance and a modest fall in blood pressure in normotensive individuals and, in exercise tolerance studies in patients with ischemic heart disease, reduces the heart rate-blood pressure product for any given work load. Studies to date, primarily in patients with good ventricular function, have not revealed evidence of a negative inotropic effect; cardiac output, ejection fraction, and left ventricular end diastolic pressure have not been affected. Such data has no predictive value with respect to effects in patients with poor ventricular function, and increased heart failure has been reported in patients with preexisting impairment of ventricular function. There are as yet few data on the interaction of diltiazem and beta-blockers in patients with poor ventricular function. Resting heart rate is usually slightly reduced by diltiazem. Diltiazem decreases vascular resistance, increases cardiac output (by increasing stroke volume), and produces a slight decrease or no change in heart rate.
During dynamic exercise, increases in diastolic pressure are inhibited, while maximum achievable systolic pressure is usually reduced. Chronic therapy with diltiazem produces no change or an increase in plasma catecholamines. No increased activity of the renin-angiotensin-aldosterone axis has been observed. Diltiazem reduces the renal and peripheral effects of angiotensin II. Hypertensive animal models respond to diltiazem with reductions in blood pressure and increased urinary output and natriuresis without a change in urinary sodium/potassium ratio.
Intravenous diltiazem hydrochloride in doses of 20 mg prolongs AH conduction time and AV node functional and effective refractory periods by approximately 20%. In a study involving single oral doses of 300 mg of diltiazem hydrochloride in six normal volunteers, the average maximum PR prolongation was 14% with no instances of greater than first-degree AV block. Diltiazem associated prolongation of the AH interval is not more pronounced in patients with first-degree heart block. In patients with sick sinus syndrome, diltiazem significantly prolongs sinus cycle length (up to 50% in some cases).
Chronic oral administration of diltiazem hydrochloride to patients in doses of up to 540 mg/day has resulted in small increases in PR interval, and on occasion produces abnormal prolongation (see WARNINGS).
Hypertension. In a randomized, double-blind, parallel-group, dose-response study involving 478 patients with essential hypertension, evening doses of CARDIZEM LA 120, 240, 360, and 540 mg were compared to placebo and to 360 mg administered in the morning. The mean reductions in diastolic blood pressure by ABPM at roughly 24 hours after the morning (4 AM - 8AM) or evening (6 PM -10 PM) administration (i.e., the time corresponding to expected trough serum concentrations) are shown in the table below:

Mean Change in Trough Diastolic Pressure by ABPM

Evening Dosing				Morning Dosing
120 mg	240 mg	360 mg	540 mg	360 mg
−2.0	−4.4	−4.4	−8.1	−6.4

A second randomized, double-blind, parallel-group, dose-response study (N=258) evaluated CARDIZEM LA following morning doses of placebo or 120, 180, 300, or 540 mg. Diastolic blood pressure measured by supine office cuff sphygmomanometer at trough (7 AM to 9 AM) decreased in an apparently linear manner over the dosage range studied. Group mean changes for placebo, 120 mg, 180 mg, 300 mg and 540 mg were −2.6, −1.9, −5.4, −6.1 and −8.6 mm Hg respectively.

Whether the time of administration impacts the clinical benefits of antihypertensive treatment is not known.

Postural hypotension is infrequently noted upon suddenly assuming an upright position. No reflex tachycardia is associated with the chronic antihypertensive effects.

Angina. The effects of Cardizem LA on angina were evaluated in a randomized, double-blind, parallel-group, dose-response trial of 311 patients with chronic stable angina. Evening doses of 180, 360 and 420 mg were compared to placebo and to 360 mg administered in the morning. All doses of Cardizem LA administered at night increased exercise tolerance when compared with placebo after 21 hours. The mean effect, placebo-subtracted, was 20 to 28 seconds for all three doses, and no dose-response was demonstrated. Cardizem LA, 360 mg, given in the morning, also improved exercise tolerance when measured 25 hours later. As expected, the effect was smaller than the effects measured only 21 hours following nighttime administration. Cardizem LA had a larger effect to increase exercise tolerance at peak serum concentrations than at trough.

INDICATIONS AND USAGE

CARDIZEM LA is indicated for the treatment of hypertension. It may be used alone or in combination with other antihypertensive medications.

CARDIZEM LA is indicated for the management of chronic stable angina.

CONTRAINDICATIONS

Diltiazem is contraindicated in (1) patients with sick sinus syndrome except in the presence of a functioning ventricular pacemaker, (2) patients with second- or third-degree AV block except in the presence of a functioning ventricular pacemaker, (3) patients with hypotension (less than 90 mm Hg systolic), (4) patients who have demonstrated hypersensitivity to the drug, and (5) patients with acute myocardial infarction and pulmonary congestion documented by x-ray on admission.

WARNINGS

1. **Cardiac Conduction.** Diltiazem prolongs AV node refractory periods without significantly prolonging sinus node recovery time, except in patients with sick sinus syndrome. This effect may rarely result in abnormally slow heart rates (particularly in patients with sick sinus syndrome) or second- or third-degree AV block (13 of 3290 patients or 0.40%). Concomitant use of diltiazem with beta-blockers or digitalis may result in additive effects on cardiac conduction. A patient with Prinzmetal's angina developed periods of asystole (2 to 5 seconds) after a single dose of 60 mg of diltiazem (see ADVERSE REACTIONS section).
2. **Congestive Heart Failure.** Although diltiazem has a negative inotropic effect in isolated animal tissue preparations, hemodynamic studies in humans with normal ventricular function have not shown a reduction in cardiac index nor consistent negative effects on contractility (dp/dt). An acute study of oral diltiazem in patients with impaired ventricular function (ejection fraction 24% ± 6%) showed improvement in indices of ventricular function without significant decrease in contractile function (dp/dt). Worsening of congestive heart failure has been reported in patients with preexisting impairment of ventricular function. Experience with the use of diltiazem in combination with beta-blockers in patients with impaired ventricular function is limited. Caution should be exercised when using this combination.
3. **Hypotension.** Decreases in blood pressure associated with diltiazem therapy may occasionally result in symptomatic hypotension.
4. **Acute Hepatic Injury.** Mild elevations of transaminases with and without concomitant elevation in alkaline phosphatase and bilirubin have been observed in clinical studies. Such elevations were usually transient and frequently resolved even with continued diltiazem treatment. In rare instances, significant elevations in enzymes such as alkaline phosphatase, LDH, SGOT, SGPT, and other phenomena consistent with acute hepatic injury have been noted. These reactions tended to occur early after therapy initiation (1 to 8 weeks) and have been reversible upon discontinuation of drug therapy. The relationship to diltiazem is uncertain in some cases, but probable in some (see PRECAUTIONS).

PRECAUTIONS

General

Diltiazem hydrochloride is extensively metabolized by the liver and excreted by the kidneys and in bile. As with any drug given over prolonged periods, laboratory parameters of renal and hepatic function should be monitored at regular intervals. The drug should be used with caution in patients with impaired renal or hepatic function.

In subacute and chronic dog and rat studies designed to produce toxicity, high doses of diltiazem were associated with hepatic damage. In special subacute hepatic studies, oral doses of 125 mg/kg and higher in rats were associated with histological changes in the liver, which were reversible when the drug was discontinued. In dogs, doses of 20 mg/kg were also associated with hepatic changes; however, these changes were reversible with continued dosing.

Dermatological events (see ADVERSE REACTIONS section) may be transient and may disappear despite continued use of diltiazem. However, skin eruptions progressing to erythema multiforme and/or exfoliative dermatitis have also been infrequently reported. Should a dermatologic reaction persist, the drug should be discontinued.

Drug Interactions. Due to the potential for additive effects, caution and careful titration are warranted in patients receiving diltiazem concomitantly with other agents known to affect cardiac contractility and/or conduction (see WARNINGS). Pharmacologic studies indicate that there may be additive effects in prolonging AV conduction when using beta-blockers or digitalis concomitantly with diltiazem (see WARNINGS).

As with all drugs, care should be exercised when treating patients with multiple medications. Diltiazem is both a substrate and an inhibitor of the cytochrome P-450 3A4 enzyme system. Other drugs that are specific substrates, inhibitors, or inducers of this enzyme system may have a significant impact on the efficacy and side effect profile of diltiazem. Patients taking other drugs that are substrates of CYP450, especially patients with renal and/or hepatic impairment, may require dosage adjustment when starting or stopping concomitantly administered diltiazem in order to maintain optimum therapeutic blood levels.

Beta-Blockers. Controlled and uncontrolled domestic studies suggest that concomitant use of diltiazem and beta-blockers is usually well tolerated, but available data are not sufficient to predict the effects of concomitant treatment in patients with left ventricular dysfunction or cardiac conduction abnormalities.

Administration of diltiazem concomitantly with propranolol in five normal volunteers resulted in increased propranolol levels in all subjects and bioavailability of propranolol was increased approximately 50%. *In vitro*, propranolol appears to be displaced from its binding sites by diltiazem. If combination therapy is initiated or withdrawn in conjunction with propranolol, an adjustment in the propranolol dose may be warranted (see WARNINGS).

Cimetidine. A study in six healthy volunteers has shown a significant increase in peak diltiazem plasma levels (58%) and area-under-the-curve (53%) after a 1-week course of cimetidine at 1200 mg per day and a single dose of diltiazem 60 mg. Ranitidine produced smaller, nonsignificant increases. The effect may be mediated by cimetidine's known inhibition of hepatic cytochrome P-450, the enzyme system responsible for the first-pass metabolism of diltiazem. Patients currently receiving diltiazem therapy should be carefully monitored for a change in pharmacological effect when initiating and discontinuing therapy with cimetidine. An adjustment in the diltiazem dose may be warranted.

Digitalis. Administration of diltiazem with digoxin in 24 healthy male subjects increased plasma digoxin concentrations approximately 20%. Another investigator found no increase in digoxin levels in 12 patients with coronary artery disease. Since there have been conflicting results regarding the effect of digoxin levels, it is recommended that digoxin levels be monitored when initiating, adjusting, and discontinuing diltiazem therapy to avoid possible over- or under-digitalization (see WARNINGS).

Anesthetics. The depression of cardiac contractility, conductivity, and automaticity as well as the vascular dilation associated with anesthetics may be potentiated by calcium channel blockers. When used concomitantly, anesthetics and calcium blockers should be titrated carefully.

Benzodiazepines Studies showed that diltiazem increased the AUC of midazolam and triazolam by 3- to 4-fold and the C_{max} by 2-fold, compared to placebo. The elimination half-life of midazolam and triazolam also increase (1.5- to 2.5 fold) during coadministration with diltiazem. These pharmacokinetic effects seen during diltiazem coadministration can result in increased clinical effects (e.g., prolonged sedation) of both midazolam and triazolam.

Cyclosporine. A pharmacokinetic interaction between diltiazem and cyclosporine has been observed during studies involving renal and cardiac transplant patients. In renal and cardiac transplant recipients, a reduction of cyclosporine dose ranging from 15% to 48% was necessary to maintain cyclosporine trough concentrations similar to those seen prior to the addition of diltiazem. If these agents are to be administered concurrently, cyclosporine concentrations should be monitored, especially when diltiazem therapy is initiated, adjusted, or discontinued.

The effect of cyclosporine on diltiazem plasma concentrations has not been evaluated.

Carbamazepine. Concomitant administration of diltiazem with carbamazepine has been reported to result in elevated serum levels of carbamazepine (40% to 72% increase), resulting in toxicity in some cases. Patients receiving these drugs concurrently should be monitored for a potential drug interaction.

Lovastatin. In a ten-subject study, coadministration of diltiazem (120 mg bid diltiazem SR) with lovastatin resulted in a 3–4 times increase in mean lovastatin AUC and C_{max} versus lovastatin alone; no change in pravastatin AUC and C_{max} was observed during diltiazem coadministration.

Diltiazem plasma levels were not significantly affected by lovastatin or pravastatin.

Rifampin. Coadministration of rifampin with diltiazem lowered the diltiazem plasma concentrations to undetectable levels. Coadministration of diltiazem with rifampin or any known CYP 3A4 inducer should be avoided when possible, and alternative therapy considered.

Carcinogenesis, Mutagenesis, Impairment of Fertility. A 24-month study in rats at oral dosage levels of up to 100 mg/kg/day, and a 21-month study in mice at oral dosage levels of up to 30 mg/kg/day showed no evidence of carcinogenicity. There was also no mutagenic response *in vitro* or *in vivo* in mammalian cell assays or in vitro in bacteria. No evidence of impaired fertility was observed in a study performed in male and female rats at oral dosages of up to 100 mg/kg/day.

Pregnancy. Category C. Reproduction studies have been conducted in mice, rats, and rabbits. Administration of doses ranging from 4 to 6 times (depending on species) the upper limit of the optimum dosage range in clinical trials (480 mg q.d. or 8 mg/kg q.d. for a 60 kg patient) resulted in embryo and fetal lethality. These studies revealed, in one species or another, a propensity to cause fetal abnormalities of the skeleton, heart, retina, and tongue. Also observed were reductions in early individual pup weights, pup survival, as well as prolonged delivery times and an increased incidence of stillbirths.

There are no well-controlled studies in pregnant women; therefore, use diltiazem in pregnant women only if the potential benefit justifies the potential risk to the fetus.

Nursing Mothers. Diltiazem is excreted in human milk. One report suggests that concentrations in breast milk may approximate serum levels. If use of diltiazem is deemed essential, an alternative method of infant feeding should be instituted.

Pediatric Use Safety and effectiveness in pediatric patients have not been established.

Geriatric Use Clinical studies of diltiazem did not include sufficient numbers of subjects aged 65 and over to determine whether they respond differently from younger subjects. Other reported clinical experience has not identified differences in responses between the elderly and younger patients. In general, dose selection for an elderly patient should be cautious, usually starting at the low end of the dosing range, reflecting the greater frequency of decreased hepatic, renal, or cardiac function, and of concomitant disease or other drug therapy.

ADVERSE REACTIONS

Serious adverse reactions have been rare in studies carried out to date, but it should be recognized that patients with impaired ventricular function and cardiac conduction abnormalities have usually been excluded from these studies.

In the hypertension study, the following table presents adverse reactions more common on diltiazem than on placebo (but excluding events with no plausible relationship to treatment), as reported in placebo-controlled hypertension trials in patients receiving a diltiazem hydrochloride extended-release formulation (once-a-day dosing) up to 540 mg.

	Placebo	Diltiazem hydrochloride extended-release	
Adverse Reactions (MedDRA Term)	**n = 120 # pts (%)**	**120–360 mg n = 501 # pts (%)**	**540 mg n = 123 # pts (%)**
Oedema lower limb	4 (3)	24 (5)	10 (8)
Sinus congestion	0 (0)	2 (1)	2 (2)
Rash NOS	0 (0)	3 (1)	2 (2)

In the angina study, the adverse event profile of CARDIZEM LA was consistent with what has been previously described for CARDIZEM LA and other formulations of diltiazem HCl. The most frequent adverse effects experienced by CARDIZEM LA-treated patients were edema lower-limb (6.8%), dizziness (6.4%), fatigue (4.8%), bradycardia (3.6%), first-degree atrioventricular block (3.2%), and cough (2%).

In clinical trials of other diltiazem formulations involving over 3200 patients, the most common events (i.e. greater than 1%) were edema (4.6%), headache (4.6%), dizziness (3.5%), asthenia (2.6%), first-degree AV block (2.4%), bradycardia (1.7%), flushing (1.4%), nausea (1.4%) and rash (1.2%).

In addition, the following events have been reported infrequently (less than 2%) in hypertension trials with other diltiazem products:

Cardiovascular: Angina, arrhythmia, AV block (second- or third-degree), bundle branch block, congestive heart failure, ECG abnormalities, hypotension, palpitations, syncope, tachycardia, ventricular extrasystoles.

Nervous System: Abnormal dreams, amnesia, depression, gait abnormality, hallucinations, insomnia, nervousness,

Continued on next page

Cardizem LA—Cont.

paresthesia, personality change, somnolence, tinnitus, tremor.

Gastrointestinal: Anorexia, constipation, diarrhea, dry mouth, dysgeusia, mild elevations of SGOT, SGPT, LDH, and alkaline phosphatase (see hepatic warnings), nausea, thirst, vomiting, weight increase.

Dermatological: Petechiae, photosensitivity, pruritus.

Other: Albuminuria, allergic reaction, amblyopia, asthenia, CPK increase, crystalluria, dyspnea, ecchymosis, edema, epistaxis, eye irritation, headache, hyperglycemia, hyperuricemia, impotence, muscle cramps, nasal congestion, neck rigidity, nocturia, osteoarticular pain, pain, polyuria, rhinitis, sexual difficulties, gynecomastia.

The following postmarketing events have been reported infrequently in patients receiving diltiazem: allergic reactions, alopecia, angioedema (including facial or periorbital edema), asystole, erythema multiforme (including Stevens-Johnson syndrome, toxic epidermal necrolysis), exfoliative dermatitis, extrapyramidal symptoms, gingival hyperplasia, hemolytic anemia, increased bleeding time, leukopenia, purpura, retinopathy, and thrombocytopenia. In addition, events such as myocardial infarction have been observed which are not readily distinguishable from the natural history of the disease in these patients. A number of well-documented cases of generalized rash, some characterized as leukocytoclastic vasculitis, have been reported. However, a definitive cause and effect relationship between these events and diltiazem therapy is yet to be established.

OVERDOSAGE

The oral LD_{50}'s in mice and rats range from 415 to 740 mg/kg and from 560 to 810 mg/kg, respectively. The intravenous LD_{50}'s in these species were 60 and 38 mg/kg, respectively. The oral LD_{50} in dogs is considered to be in excess of 50 mg/kg, while lethality was seen in monkeys at 360 mg/kg.

The toxic dose in man is not known. Due to extensive metabolism, blood levels after a standard dose of diltiazem can vary over tenfold, limiting the usefulness of blood levels in overdose cases.

There have been 29 reports of diltiazem overdose in doses ranging from less than 1 g to 10.8 g. Sixteen of these reports involved multiple drug ingestions.

Twenty-two reports indicated patients had recovered from diltiazem overdose ranging from less than 1 g to 10.8 g. There were seven reports with a fatal outcome; although the amount of diltiazem ingested was unknown, multiple drug ingestions were confirmed in six of the seven reports.

Events observed following diltiazem overdose included bradycardia, hypotension, heart block, and cardiac failure. Most reports of overdose described some supportive medical measure and/or drug treatment. Bradycardia frequently responded favorably to atropine as did heart block, although cardiac pacing was also frequently utilized to treat heart block. Fluids and vasopressors were used to maintain blood pressure, and in cases of cardiac failure, inotropic agents were administered. In addition, some patients received treatment with ventilatory support, gastric lavage, activated charcoal, and/or intravenous calcium. Evidence of the effectiveness of intravenous calcium administration to reverse the pharmacological effects of diltiazem overdose was conflicting.

In the event of overdose or exaggerated response, appropriate supportive measures should be employed in addition to gastrointestinal decontamination. Diltiazem does not appear to be removed by peritoneal or hemodialysis. Limited data suggest that plasmapheresis or charcoal hemoperfusion may hasten diltiazem eliminiation following overdose. Based on the known pharmacological effects of diltiazem and/or reported clinical experiences, the following measures may be considered:

Bradycardia: Administer atropine (0.60 to 1 mg). If there is no response to vagal blockage, administer isoproterenol cautiously.

High-Degree AV Block: Treat as for bradycardia above. Fixed high-degree AV block should be treated with cardiac pacing.

Cardiac Failure: Administer inotropic agents (isoproterenol, dopamine, or dobutamine) and diuretics.

Hypotension Vasopressors (e.g., dopamine or norepinephrine).

Actual treatment and dosage should depend on the severity of the clinical situation and the judgment and experience of the treating physician.

DOSAGE AND ADMINISTRATION

CARDIZEM LA Tablets are an extended release formulation intended for once-a-day administration.

Patients controlled on diltiazem alone or in combination with other medications may be switched to CARDIZEM LA Tablets once-a-day at the nearest equivalent total daily dose. Higher doses of CARDIZEM LA Tablets once-a-day dosage may be needed in some patients. Patients should be closely monitored. Subsequent titration to higher or lower doses may be necessary and should be initiated as clinically warranted. There is limited general clinical experience with doses above 360 mg, but the safety and efficacy of doses as high as 540 mg have been studied in clinical trials. The incidence of side effects increases as the dose increases with first-degree AV block, dizziness, and sinus bradycardia bearing the strongest relationship to dose.

The tablet should be swallowed whole and not chewed or crushed.

Hypertension

Dosage needs to be adjusted by titration to individual patient needs. When used as monotherapy, reasonable starting doses are 180 to 240 mg once daily, although some patients may respond to lower doses. Maximum antihypertensive effect is usually observed by 14 days of chronic therapy; therefore, dosage adjustments should be scheduled accordingly. The dosage range studied in clinical trials was 120 to 540 mg once daily. The dosage may be titrated to a maximum of 540 mg daily.

CARDIZEM LA Tablets should be taken about the same time once each day either in the morning or at bedtime. The time of dosing should be considered when making dose adjustments based on trough effects.

Angina

Dosage for the treatment of angina should be individualized based on response. The initial dose of 180 mg once daily may be increased at intervals of 7 - 14 days if adequate response is not obtained. CARDIZEM LA doses above 360 mg appear to confer no additional benefit.

CARDIZEM LA can be given once daily, either in the evening or in the morning.

Concomitant Use with Other Cardiovascular Agents

1. **Sublingual NTG.** May be taken as required to abort acute anginal attacks during Diltiazem Hydrochloride Extended release therapy.
2. **Prophylactic Nitrate Therapy.** Diltiazem Hydrochloride Extended Release Tablets may be safely coadministered with short-and and long-acting nitrates.
3. **Beta-blockers.** (See WARNINGS and PRECAUTIONS.)
4. **Antihypertensives.** CARDIZEM LA has an additive antihypertensive effect when used with other antihypertensive agents. Therefore, the dosage of Diltiazem Hydrochloride Extended Release Tablets or the concomitant antihypertensives may need to be adjusted when adding one to the other.

HOW SUPPLIED

CARDIZEM LA is supplied as white, capsule-shaped tablets debossed with "B" on one side and the diltiazem content (mg) on the other.

NDC # 64455-xxx-yy

Strength	Qty 7	Qty 30	Qty 90	Qty 1000
120 mg	100-07	100-30	100-90	100-10
180 mg	101-07	101-30	101-90	101-10
240 mg	102-07	102-30	102-90	102-10
300 mg	103-07	103-30	103-90	103-10
360 mg	104-07	104-30	104-90	104-10
420 mg	105-07	105-30	105-90	105-10

Storage conditions: Store at 25°C (77°F); excursions permitted to 15-30°C (59-86°F) [see USP Controlled Room Temperature].
Avoid excessive humidity and temperatures above 30°C (86°F).

Dispense in tight, light resistant container as defined in USP.

Rx Only.

® Cardizem is a registered trademark of
Biovail Laboratories Incorporated.
Manufactured by:
Biovail Corporation
Mississauga, ON, L5N 8M5
Canada
BIOVAIL
Pharmaceuticals, Inc.
Distributed by:
Biovail Pharmaceuticals, Inc.
Bridgewater, New Jersey, 08807, USA
Made in Canada
PR0024-04
Rev. 04/04

TEVETEN® ℞

[tĕ vĕ tĕn]

(eprosartan mesylate)
400 mg
600 mg

PRESCRIBING INFORMATION

USE IN PREGNANCY

When used in pregnancy during the second and third trimesters, drugs that act directly on the renin-angiotensin system can cause injury and even death to the developing fetus. When pregnancy is detected, TEVETEN® should be discontinued as soon as possible. See WARNINGS: Fetal/Neonatal Morbidity and Mortality.

DESCRIPTION

TEVETEN® (eprosartan mesylate) is a non-biphenyl nontetrazole angiotensin II receptor (AT_1) antagonist. A selective non-peptide molecule, TEVETEN® is chemically described as the monomethanesulfonate of (*E*)-2-butyl-1-(*p*-carboxybenzyl)-α-2-thienylmethylimidazole-5-acrylic acid. Its empirical formula is $C_{23}H_{24}N_2O_4S \bullet CH_4O_3S$ and molecular weight is 520.625. Its structural formula is:

·$HOSO_2CH_3$

Eprosartan mesylate is a white to off-white free-flowing crystalline powder that is insoluble in water, freely soluble in ethanol, and melts between 248°C and 250°C.

TEVETEN® is available as aqueous film-coated tablets containing eprosartan mesylate equivalent to 400 mg or 600 mg eprosartan zwitterion (pink, oval, non-scored tablets or white, non-scored, capsule-shaped tablets, respectively).

Inactive Ingredients

The 400 mg tablet contains the following: croscarmellose sodium, hypromellose, iron oxide red, iron oxide yellow, lactose monohydrate, magnesium stearate, microcrystalline cellulose, polyethylene glycol, polysorbate 80, pregelatinized starch, and titanium dioxide. The 600 mg tablet contains crospovidone, hypromellose, lactose monohydrate, magnesium stearate, microcrystalline cellulose, polyethylene glycol, polysorbate 80, pregelatinized starch, and titanium dioxide.

CLINICAL PHARMACOLOGY

Mechanism of Action

Angiotensin II (formed from angiotensin I in a reaction catalyzed by angiotensin-converting enzyme [kininase II]), a potent vasoconstrictor, is the principal pressor agent of the renin-angiotensin system. Angiotensin II also stimulates aldosterone synthesis and secretion by the adrenal cortex, cardiac contraction, renal resorption of sodium, activity of the sympathetic nervous system, and smooth muscle cell growth. Eprosartan blocks the vasoconstrictor and aldosterone-secreting effects of angiotensin II by selectively blocking the binding of angiotensin II to the AT_1 receptor found in many tissues (e.g., vascular smooth muscle, adrenal gland). There is also an AT_2 receptor found in many tissues but it is not known to be associated with cardiovascular homeostasis. Eprosartan does not exhibit any partial agonist activity at the AT_1 receptor. Its affinity for the AT_1 receptor is 1,000 times greater than for the AT_2 receptor. *In vitro* binding studies indicate that eprosartan is a reversible, competitive inhibitor of the AT_1 receptor.

Blockade of the AT_1 receptor removes the negative feedback of angiotensin II on renin secretion, but the resulting increased plasma renin activity and circulating angiotensin II do not overcome the effect of eprosartan on blood pressure.

TEVETEN® does not inhibit kininase II, the enzyme that converts angiotensin I to angiotensin II and degrades bradykinin; whether this has clinical relevance is not known. It does not bind to or block other hormone receptors or ion channels known to be important in cardiovascular regulation.

Pharmacokinetics

General

Absolute bioavailability following a single 300 mg oral dose of eprosartan is approximately 13%. Eprosartan plasma concentrations peak at 1 to 2 hours after an oral dose in the fasted state. Administering eprosartan with food delays absorption, and causes variable changes (<25%) in C_{max} and AUC values which do not appear clinically important.

Plasma concentrations of eprosartan increase in a slightly less than dose-proportional manner over the 100 mg to 800 mg dose range. The mean terminal elimination half-life of eprosartan following multiple oral doses of 600 mg was approximately 20 hours. Eprosartan does not significantly accumulate with chronic use.

Metabolism and Excretion

Eprosartan is eliminated by biliary and renal excretion, primarily as unchanged compound. Less than 2% of an oral dose is excreted in the urine as a glucuronide. There are no active metabolites following oral and intravenous dosing with [^{14}C] eprosartan in human subjects. Eprosartan was the only drug-related compound found in the plasma and feces. Following intravenous [^{14}C] eprosartan, about 61% of the material is recovered in the feces and about 37% in the urine. Following an oral dose of [^{14}C] eprosartan, about 90% is recovered in the feces and about 7% in the urine. Approximately 20% of the radioactivity excreted in the urine was an acyl glucuronide of eprosartan with the remaining 80% being unchanged eprosartan.

Distribution

Plasma protein binding of eprosartan is high (approximately 98%) and constant over the concentration range achieved with therapeutic doses.

The pooled population pharmacokinetic analysis from two Phase 3 trials of 299 men and 172 women with mild to moderate hypertension (aged 20 to 93 years) showed that eprosartan exhibited a population mean oral clearance (CL/F) for an average 60-year-old patient of 48.5 L/hr. The population mean steady-state volume of distribution (Vss/F) was 308 L. Eprosartan pharmacokinetics were not influenced by weight, race, gender or severity of hypertension at baseline. Oral clearance was shown to be a linear function of age with CL/F decreasing 0.62 L/hr for every year increase.

Special Populations

Pediatric

Eprosartan pharmacokinetics have not been investigated in patients younger than 18 years of age.

Geriatric

Following single oral dose administration of eprosartan to healthy elderly men (aged 68 to 78 years), AUC, C_{max}, and T_{max} eprosartan values increased, on average by approximately twofold, compared to healthy young men (aged 20 to 39 years) who received the same dose. The extent of plasma protein binding was not influenced by age.

Gender

There was no difference in the pharmacokinetics and plasma protein binding between men and women following single oral dose administration of eprosartan.

Race

A pooled population pharmacokinetic analysis of 442 Caucasian and 29 non-Caucasian hypertensive patients showed that oral clearance and steady-state volume of distribution were not influenced by race.

Renal Insufficiency

Following administration of 600 mg once daily, there was a 70–90% increase in AUC, and a 30–50% increase in C_{max} in moderate or severe renal impairment. The unbound eprosartan fractions increased by 35% and 59% in patients with moderate and severe renal impairment, respectively. No initial dosing adjustment is generally necessary in patients with moderate or severe renal impairment, with maximum dose not exceeding 600 mg daily. Eprosartan was poorly removed by hemodialysis (CL_{HD}<1 L/hr) (see DOSAGE AND ADMINISTRATION).

Hepatic Insufficiency

Eprosartan AUC (but not C_{max}) values increased, on average, by approximately 40% in men with decreased hepatic function compared to healthy men after a single 100 mg oral dose of eprosartan. Hepatic disease was defined as a documented clinical history of chronic hepatic abnormality diagnosed by liver biopsy, liver/spleen scan or clinical laboratory tests. The extent of eprosartan plasma protein binding was not influenced by hepatic dysfunction. No dosage adjustment is necessary for patients with hepatic impairment (see DOSAGE AND ADMINISTRATION).

Drug Interactions

Concomitant administration of eprosartan and digoxin had no effect on single oral-dose digoxin pharmacokinetics. Concomitant administration of eprosartan and warfarin had no effect on steady-state prothrombin time ratios (INR) in healthy volunteers. Concomitant administration of eprosartan and glyburide in diabetic patients did not affect 24-hour plasma glucose profiles. Eprosartan pharmacokinetics were not affected by concomitant administration of ranitidine. Eprosartan did not inhibit human cytochrome P450 enzymes CYP1A, 2A6, 2C9/8, 2C19, 2D6, 2E and 3A *in vitro*. Eprosartan is not metabolized by the cytochrome P450 system; eprosartan steady-state concentrations were not affected by concomitant administration of ketoconazole or fluconazole, potent inhibitors of CYP3A and 2C9, respectively.

Pharmacodynamics and Clinical Effects

Eprosartan inhibits the pharmacologic effects of angiotensin II infusions in healthy adult men. Single oral doses of eprosartan from 10 mg to 400 mg have been shown to inhibit the vasopressor, renal vasoconstrictive and aldosterone-secretory effects of infused angiotensin II with complete inhibition evident at doses of 350 mg and above. Eprosartan inhibits the pressor effects of angiotensin II infusions. A single oral dose of 350 mg of eprosartan inhibits pressor effects by approximately 100% at peak, with approximately 30% inhibition persisting for 24 hours. The absence of angiotensin II AT_1 agonist activity has been demonstrated in healthy adult men. In hypertensive patients treated chronically with eprosartan, there was a twofold rise in angiotensin II plasma concentration and a twofold rise in plasma renin activity, while plasma aldosterone levels remained unchanged. Serum potassium levels also remained unchanged in these patients.

Achievement of maximal blood pressure response to a given dose in most patients may take 2 to 3 weeks of treatment. Onset of blood pressure reduction is seen within 1 to 2 hours of dosing with few instances of orthostatic hypotension. Blood pressure control is maintained with once- or twice-daily dosing over a 24-hour period. Discontinuing treatment with eprosartan does not lead to a rapid rebound increase in blood pressure.

There was no change in mean heart rate in patients treated with eprosartan in controlled clinical trials.

Eprosartan increases mean effective renal plasma flow (ERPF) in salt-replete and salt-restricted normal subjects. A dose-related increase in ERPF of 25% to 30% occurred in salt-restricted normal subjects, with the effect plateauing between the 200 mg and 400 mg doses. There was no change in ERPF in hypertensive patients and patients with renal insufficiency on normal salt diets. Eprosartan did not reduce glomerular filtration rate in patients with renal insufficiency or in patients with hypertension, after 7 days and 28 days of dosing, respectively. In hypertensive patients and patients with chronic renal insufficiency, eprosartan did not change fractional excretion of sodium and potassium.

Eprosartan (1200 mg once daily for 7 days or 300 mg twice daily for 28 days) had no effect on the excretion of uric acid in healthy men, patients with essential hypertension or those with varying degrees of renal insufficiency.

There were no effects on mean levels of fasting triglycerides, total cholesterol, HDL cholesterol, LDL cholesterol or fasting glucose.

Clinical Trials

The safety and efficacy of TEVETEN® have been evaluated in controlled clinical trials worldwide that enrolled predominantly hypertensive patients with sitting DBP ranging from 95 mmHg to ≤115 mmHg.

There is also some experience with use of eprosartan together with other anti-hypertensive drugs in more severe hypertension.

The antihypertensive effects of TEVETEN® were demonstrated principally in five placebo-controlled trials (4 to 13 weeks' duration) including dosages of 400 mg to 1200 mg given once daily (two studies), 25 mg to 400 mg twice daily (two studies), and one study comparing total daily doses of 400 mg to 800 mg given once daily or twice daily. The five studies included 1,111 patients randomized to eprosartan and 395 patients randomized to placebo. The studies showed dose-related antihypertensive responses.

At study endpoint, patients treated with TEVETEN® at doses of 600 mg to 1200 mg given once daily experienced significant decreases in sitting systolic and diastolic blood pressure at trough, with differences from placebo of approximately 5-10/3-6 mmHg. Limited experience is available with the dose of 1200 mg administered once daily. In a direct comparison of 200 mg to 400 mg b.i.d. with 400 mg to 800 mg q.d. of TEVETEN®, effects at trough were similar. Patients treated with TEVETEN® at doses of 200 mg to 400 mg given twice daily experienced significant decreases in sitting systolic and diastolic blood pressure at trough, with differences from placebo of approximately 7–10/4–6 mmHg.

Peak (1 to 3 hours) effects were uniformly, but moderately, larger than trough effects with b.i.d. dosing, with the trough-to-peak ratio for diastolic blood pressure 65% to 80%. In the once-daily dose-response study, trough-to-peak responses of ≤50% were observed at some doses (including 1200 mg), suggesting attenuation of effect at the end of the dosing interval.

The antihypertensive effect of TEVETEN® was similar in men and women, but was somewhat smaller in patients over 65. There were too few black subjects to determine whether their response was similar to Caucasians. In general, blacks (usually a low renin population) have had smaller responses to ACE inhibitors and angiotensin II inhibitors than Caucasian populations.

Angiotensin-converting enzyme (ACE) inhibitor-induced cough (a dry, persistent cough) can lead to discontinuation of ACE inhibitor therapy. In one study, patients who had previously coughed while taking an ACE inhibitor were treated with eprosartan, an ACE inhibitor (enalapril) or placebo for six weeks. The incidence of dry, persistent cough was 2.2% on eprosartan, 4.4% on placebo, and 20.5% on the ACE inhibitor; P=0.008 for the comparison of eprosartan with enalapril. In a second study comparing the incidence of cough in 259 patients treated with eprosartan to 261 patients treated with the ACE inhibitor enalapril, the incidence of dry, persistent cough in eprosartan-treated patients (1.5%) was significantly lower (P=0.018) than that observed in patients treated with the ACE inhibitor (5.4%). In addition, analysis of overall data from six double-blind clinical trials involving 1,554 patients showed an incidence of spontaneously reported cough in patients treated with eprosartan of 3.5%, similar to placebo (2.6%).

INDICATIONS AND USAGE

TEVETEN® is indicated for the treatment of hypertension. It may be used alone or in combination with other antihypertensives such as diuretics and calcium channel blockers.

CONTRAINDICATIONS

TEVETEN® is contraindicated in patients who are hypersensitive to this product or any of its components.

WARNINGS

Fetal/Neonatal Morbidity and Mortality

Drugs that act directly on the renin-angiotensin system can cause fetal and neonatal morbidity and death when administered to pregnant women. Several dozen cases have been reported in the world literature in patients who were taking angiotensin-converting enzyme inhibitors. When pregnancy is detected, TEVETEN® should be discontinued as soon as possible.

The use of drugs that act directly on the renin-angiotensin system during the second and third trimesters of pregnancy has been associated with fetal and neonatal injury, including hypotension, neonatal skull hypoplasia, anuria, reversible or irreversible renal failure, and death. Oligohydramnios has also been reported, presumably resulting from decreased fetal renal function; oligohydramnios in this setting has been associated with fetal limb contractures, craniofacial deformation, and hypoplastic lung development. Prematurity, intrauterine growth retardation, and patent ductus arteriosus have also been reported, although it is not clear whether these occurrences were due to exposure to the drug.

These adverse effects do not appear to have resulted from intrauterine drug exposure that has been limited to the first trimester. Mothers whose embryos and fetuses are exposed to an angiotensin II receptor antagonist only during the first trimester should be so informed. Nonetheless, when patients become pregnant, physicians should advise the patient to discontinue the use of eprosartan as soon as possible.

Rarely (probably less often than once in every thousand pregnancies), no alternative to a drug acting on the renin-angiotensin system will be found. In these rare cases, the mothers should be apprised of the potential hazards to their fetuses, and serial ultrasound examinations should be performed to assess the intra-amniotic environment.

If oligohydramnios is observed, TEVETEN® should be discontinued unless it is considered life-saving for the mother. Contraction stress testing (CST), a nonstress test (NST) or biophysical profiling (BPP) may be appropriate, depending upon the week of pregnancy. Patients and physicians should be aware, however, that oligohydramnios may not appear until after the fetus has sustained irreversible injury.

Infants with histories of *in utero* exposure to an angiotensin II receptor antagonist should be closely observed for hypotension, oliguria, and hyperkalemia. If oliguria occurs, attention should be directed toward support of blood pressure and renal perfusion. Exchange transfusion or dialysis may be required as means of reversing hypotension and/or substituting for disordered renal function.

Eprosartan mesylate has been shown to produce maternal and fetal toxicities (maternal and fetal mortality, low maternal body weight and food consumption, resorptions, abortions and litter loss) in pregnant rabbits given oral doses as low as 10 mg eprosartan/kg/day. No maternal or fetal adverse effects were observed at 3 mg/kg/day; this oral dose yielded a systemic exposure (AUC) to unbound eprosartan 0.8 times that achieved in humans given 400 mg b.i.d. No adverse effects on *in utero* or postnatal development and maturation of offspring were observed when eprosartan mesylate was administered to pregnant rats at oral doses up to 1000 mg eprosartan/kg/day (the 1000 mg eprosartan/kg/day dose in non-pregnant rats yielded systemic exposure to unbound eprosartan approximately 0.6 times the exposure achieved in humans given 400 mg b.i.d.).

Hypotension in Volume- and/or Salt-Depleted Patients

In patients with an activated renin-angiotensin system, such as volume- and/or salt-depleted patients (e.g., those being treated with diuretics), symptomatic hypotension may occur. These conditions should be corrected prior to administration of TEVETEN®, or the treatment should start under close medical supervision. If hypotension occurs, the patient should be placed in the supine position and, if necessary, given an intravenous infusion of normal saline. A transient hypotensive response is not a contraindication to further treatment, which usually can be continued without difficulty once the blood pressure has stabilized.

PRECAUTIONS

Risk of Renal Impairment

As a consequence of inhibiting the renin-angiotensin-aldosterone system, changes in renal function have been reported in susceptible individuals treated with angiotensin II antagonists; in some patients, these changes in renal function were reversible upon discontinuation of therapy. In patients whose renal function may depend on the activity of the renin-angiotensin-aldosterone system (e.g., patients with severe congestive heart failure), treatment with angiotensin-converting enzyme inhibitors and angiotensin II receptor antagonists has been associated with oliguria and/or progressive azotemia and (rarely) with acute renal failure and/or death. TEVETEN® would be expected to behave similarly.

In studies of ACE inhibitors in patients with unilateral or bilateral renal artery stenosis, increases in serum creatinine or BUN have been reported. Similar effects have been reported with angiotensin II antagonists; in some patients, these effects were reversible upon discontinuation of therapy.

Information for Patients

Pregnancy

Female patients of childbearing age should be told about the consequences of second- and third-trimester exposure to drugs that act on the renin-angiotensin system, and they should also be told that these consequences do not appear to have resulted from intrauterine drug exposure that has been limited to the first trimester. These patients should be asked to report pregnancies to their physicians as soon as possible so that treatment may be discontinued under medical supervision.

Drug Interactions

Eprosartan has been shown to have no effect on the pharmacokinetics of digoxin and the pharmacodynamics of warfarin and glyburide. Thus, no dosing adjustments are necessary during concomitant use with these agents. Because eprosartan is not metabolized by the cytochrome P450 system, inhibitors of CYP450 enzyme would not be expected to affect its metabolism, and ketoconazole and fluconazole, potent inhibitors of CYP3A and 2C9, respectively, have been shown to have no effect on eprosartan pharmacokinetics. Ranitidine also has no effect on eprosartan pharmacokinetics.

Eprosartan (up to 400 mg b.i.d. or 800 mg q.d.) doses have been safely used concomitantly with a thiazide diuretic (hydrochlorothiazide). Eprosartan doses of up to 300 mg b.i.d. have been safely used concomitantly with sustained-release calcium channel blockers (sustained-release nifedipine) with no clinically significant adverse interactions.

Carcinogenesis, Mutagenesis, Impairment of Fertility

Eprosartan mesylate was not carcinogenic in dietary restricted rats or *ad libitum* fed mice dosed at 600 mg and 2000 mg eprosartan/kg/day, respectively, for up to 2 years.

Continued on next page

Teveten—Cont.

In male and female rats, the systemic exposure (AUC) to unbound eprosartan at the dose evaluated was only approximately 20% of the exposure achieved in humans given 400 mg b.i.d. In mice, the systemic exposure (AUC) to unbound eprosartan was approximately 25 times the exposure achieved in humans given 400 mg b.i.d.

Eprosartan mesylate was not mutagenic *in vitro* in bacteria or mammalian cells (mouse lymphoma assay). Eprosartan mesylate also did not cause structural chromosomal damage *in vivo* (mouse micronucleus assay). In human peripheral lymphocytes *in vitro*, eprosartan mesylate was equivocal for clastogenicity with metabolic activation, and was negative without metabolic activation. In the same assay, eprosartan mesylate was positive for polyploidy with metabolic activation and equivocal for polyploidy without metabolic activation.

Eprosartan mesylate had no adverse effects on the reproductive performance of male or female rats at oral doses up to 1000 mg eprosartan/kg/day. This dose provided systemic exposure (AUC) to unbound eprosartan approximately 0.6 times the exposure achieved in humans given 400 mg b.i.d.

Pregnancy

Pregnancy Category C (first trimester) and D (second and third trimesters): See WARNINGS: Fetal/Neonatal Morbidity and Mortality.

Nursing Mothers

Eprosartan is excreted in animal milk; it is not known whether eprosartan is excreted in human milk. Because many drugs are excreted in human milk and because of the potential for serious adverse reactions in nursing infants from eprosartan, a decision should be made whether to discontinue nursing or to discontinue the drug, taking into account the importance of the drug to the mother.

Pediatric Use

Safety and effectiveness in pediatric patients have not been established.

Geriatric Use

Of the total number of patients receiving TEVETEN® in clinical studies, 29% (681 of 2,334) were 65 years and over, while 5% (124 of 2,334) were 75 years and over. Based on the pooled data from randomized trials, the decrease in diastolic blood pressure and systolic blood pressure with TEVETEN® was slightly less in patients (≥65 years of age compared to younger patients. In a study of only patients over the age of 65, TEVETEN® at 200 mg twice daily (and increased optionally up to 300 mg twice daily) decreased diastolic blood pressure on average by 3 mmHg (placebo corrected). Adverse experiences were similar in younger and older patients.

ADVERSE REACTIONS

TEVETEN® has been evaluated for safety in more than 3,300 healthy volunteers and patients worldwide, including more than 1,460 patients treated for more than 6 months, and more than 980 patients treated for 1 year or longer. TEVETEN® was well tolerated at doses up to 1200 mg daily. Most adverse events were of mild or moderate severity and did not require discontinuation of therapy. The overall incidence of adverse experiences and the incidences of specific adverse events reported with eprosartan were similar to placebo.

Adverse experiences were similar in patients regardless of age, gender, or race. Adverse experiences were not dose-related.

In placebo-controlled clinical trials, about 4% of 1,202 patients treated with TEVETEN® discontinued therapy due to clinical adverse experiences, compared to 6.5% of 352 patients given placebo.

Adverse Events Occurring at an Incidence of 1% or More Among Eprosartan-treated Patients

The following table lists adverse events that occurred at an incidence of 1% or more among eprosartan-treated patients who participated in placebo-controlled trials of 8 to 13 weeks' duration, using doses of 25 mg to 400 mg twice daily, and 400 mg to 1200 mg once daily. The overall incidence of adverse events reported with TEVETEN® (54.4%) was similar to placebo (52.8%).

Table 1. Adverse Events Reported by ≥1% of Patients Receiving TEVETEN® (eprosartan mesylate) and Were More Frequent on Eprosartan than Placebo

Event	Eprosartan (n=1,202) %	Placebo (n=352) %
Body as a Whole		
Infection viral	2	1
Injury	2	1
Fatigue	2	1
Gastrointestinal		
Abdominal pain	2	1
Metabolic and Nutritional		
Hypertriglyceridemia	1	0
Musculoskeletal		
Arthralgia	2	1
Nervous System		
Depression	1	0
Respiratory		
Upper respiratory tract infection	8	5
Rhinitis	4	3
Pharyngitis	4	3
Coughing	4	3
Urogenital		
Urinary tract infection	1	0

The following adverse events were also reported at a rate of 1% or greater in patients treated with eprosartan, but were as, or more, frequent in the placebo group: headache, myalgia, dizziness, sinusitis, diarrhea, bronchitis, dependent edema, dyspepsia, and chest pain.

Facial edema was reported in 5 patients receiving eprosartan. Angioedema has been reported with other angiotensin II antagonists.

Rare cases of rhabdomyolysis have been reported in patients receiving angiotensin II receptor blockers.

In addition to the adverse events above, potentially important events that occurred in at least two patients/subjects exposed to eprosartan or other adverse events that occurred in <1% of patients in clinical studies are listed below. It cannot be determined whether events were causally related to eprosartan:

Body as a Whole: alcohol intolerance, asthenia, substernal chest pain, peripheral edema, fatigue, fever, hot flushes, influenza-like symptoms, malaise, rigors, pain;

Cardiovascular: angina pectoris, bradycardia, abnormal ECG, specific abnormal ECG, extrasystoles, atrial fibrillation, hypotension (including orthostatic hypotension), tachycardia, palpitations;

Gastrointestinal: anorexia, constipation, dry mouth, esophagitis, flatulence, gastritis, gastroenteritis, gingivitis, nausea, periodontitis, toothache, vomiting;

Hematologic: anemia, purpura;

Liver and Biliary: increased SGOT, increased SGPT;

Metabolic and Nutritional: increased creatine phosphokinase, diabetes mellitus, glycosuria, gout, hypercholesterolemia, hyperglycemia, hyperkalemia, hypokalemia, hyponatremia;

Musculoskeletal: arthritis, aggravated arthritis, arthrosis, skeletal pain, tendinitis, back pain;

Nervous System/Psychiatric: anxiety, ataxia, insomnia, migraine, neuritis, nervousness, paresthesia, somnolence, tremor, vertigo;

Resistance Mechanism: herpes simplex, otitis externa, otitis media, upper respiratory tract infection;

Respiratory: asthma, epistaxis;

Skin and Appendages: eczema, furunculosis, pruritus, rash, maculopapular rash, increased sweating;

Special Senses: conjunctivitis, abnormal vision, xerophthalmia, tinnitus;

Urinary: albuminuria, cystitis, hematuria, micturition frequency, polyuria, renal calculus, urinary incontinence;

Vascular: leg cramps, peripheral ischemia.

Laboratory Test Findings

In placebo-controlled studies, clinically important changes in standard laboratory parameters were rarely associated with administration of TEVETEN®. Patients were rarely withdrawn from TEVETEN® because of laboratory test results.

Creatinine, Blood Urea Nitrogen

Minor elevations in creatinine and in BUN occurred in 0.6% and 1.3%, respectively, of patients taking TEVETEN® and 0.9% and 0.3%, respectively, of patients given placebo in controlled clinical trials. Two patients were withdrawn from clinical trials for elevations in serum creatinine and BUN, and three additional patients were withdrawn for increases in serum creatinine.

Liver Function Tests

Minor elevations of ALAT, ASAT, and alkaline phosphatase occurred for comparable percentages of patients taking TEVETEN® or placebo in controlled clinical trials. An elevated ALAT of >3.5 × ULN occurred in 0.1% of patients taking TEVETEN® (one patient) and in no patient given placebo in controlled clinical trials. Four patients were withdrawn from clinical trials for an elevation in liver function tests.

Hemoglobin

A greater than 20% decrease in hemoglobin was observed in 0.1% of patients taking TEVETEN® (one patient) and in no patient given placebo in controlled clinical trials. Two patients were withdrawn from clinical trials for anemia.

Leukopenia

A WBC count of $\leq 3.0 \times 10^3/mm^3$ occurred in 0.3% of patients taking TEVETEN® and in 0.3% of patients given placebo in controlled clinical trials. One patient was withdrawn from clinical trials for leukopenia.

Neutropenia

A neutrophil count of $\leq 1.5 \times 10^3/mm^3$ occurred in 1.3% of patients taking TEVETEN® and in 1.4% of patients given placebo in controlled clinical trials. No patient was withdrawn from any clinical trial for neutropenia.

Thrombocytopenia

A platelet count of $\leq 100 \times 10^9/L$ occurred in 0.3% of patients taking TEVETEN® (one patient) and in no patient given placebo in controlled clinical trials. Four patients receiving TEVETEN® in clinical trials were withdrawn for thrombocytopenia. In one case, thrombocytopenia was present prior to dosing with TEVETEN®.

Serum Potassium

A potassium value of ≥5.6 mmol/L occurred in 0.9% of patients taking TEVETEN® and 0.3% of patients given placebo in controlled clinical trials. One patient was withdrawn from clinical trials for hyperkalemia and three for hypokalemia.

OVERDOSAGE

Limited data are available regarding overdosage. Appropriate symptomatic and supportive therapy should be given if overdosage should occur. There was no mortality in rats and mice receiving oral doses of up to 3000 mg eprosartan/kg and in dogs receiving oral doses of up to 1000 mg eprosartan/kg.

DOSAGE AND ADMINISTRATION

The usual recommended starting dose of TEVETEN® is 600 mg once daily when used as monotherapy in patients who are not volume-depleted (see WARNINGS, Hypotension in Volume- and/or Salt-Depleted Patients). TEVETEN® can be administered once or twice daily with total daily doses ranging from 400 mg to 800 mg. There is limited experience with doses beyond 800 mg/day.

If the antihypertensive effect measured at trough using once-daily dosing is inadequate, a twice-a-day regimen at the same total daily dose or an increase in dose may give a more satisfactory response. Achievement of maximum blood pressure reduction in most patients may take 2 to 3 weeks.

TEVETEN® may be used in combination with other antihypertensive agents such as thiazide diuretics or calcium channel blockers if additional blood-pressure-lowering effect is required. Discontinuation of treatment with eprosartan does not lead to a rapid rebound increase in blood pressure.

Elderly, Hepatically Impaired or Renally Impaired Patients

No initial dosing adjustment is generally necessary for elderly or hepatically impaired patients or those with renal impairment. No initial dosing adjustment is generally necessary in patients with moderate and severe renal impairment, with maximum dose not exceeding 600 mg daily.

TEVETEN® may be taken with or without food.

HOW SUPPLIED

TEVETEN® is available as aqueous film-coated tablets as follows:

400 mg pink, non-scored, oval tablets, debossed with "SOLVAY" on one side and "5044" on the other.
NDC 64455-130-01 (bottles of 100)

600 mg white, non-scored, capsule-shaped tablets, debossed with "SOLVAY" on one side and "5046" on the other.
NDC 64455-131-01 (bottles of 100)

STORAGE

Store at controlled room temperature 20° to 25°C (68° to 77°F) [see USP Controlled Room Temperature].

Rx only

Manufactured by:
Solvay Pharmaceuticals, BV
Olst, The Netherlands
Tablets made in The Netherlands.
Marketed by:
Biovail Pharmaceuticals, Inc.
Bridgewater, NJ, 08807, USA
©2003 Biovail Pharmaceuticals, Inc.
LB0029-00 January 2004

TEVETEN® HCT ℞

[tĕ vĕ tĕn]

(eprosartan mesylate/hydrochlorothiazide)
600/12.5mg
600/25mg

PRESCRIBING INFORMATION

USE IN PREGNANCY

When used in pregnancy during the second and third trimesters, drugs that act directly on the renin-angiotensin system can cause injury and even death to the developing fetus. When pregnancy is detected, TEVETEN® HCT Tablets should be discontinued as soon as possible. See WARNINGS: Fetal/Neonatal Morbidity and Mortality.

DESCRIPTION

TEVETEN® HCT 600/12.5 and TEVETEN® HCT 600/25 (eprosartan mesylate-hydrochlorothiazide) combine an angiotensin II receptor (AT_1 subtype) antagonist and a diuretic, hydrochlorothiazide. TEVETEN® (eprosartan mesylate) is a non-biphenyl non-tetrazole angiotensin II receptor (AT_1) antagonist. A selective non-peptide molecule, TEVETEN® is chemically described as the monomethanesulfonate of (*E*)-2-butyl-1-(*p*-carboxybenzyl)-α-2-thienylmethylimidazole-5-acrylic acid. Its empirical formula is $C_{23}H_{24}N_2O_4S{\bullet}CH_4O_3S$ and molecular weight is 520.625. Its structural formula is:

[See chemical structure at top of next column]

Eprosartan mesylate is a white to off-white free-flowing crystalline powder that is insoluble in water, freely soluble in ethanol, and melts between 248°C and 250°C. Hydrochlorothiazide is 6-chloro-3,4-dihydro-2 *H* 1,2,4-benzothiadiazine-7-sulfonamide 1,1-dioxide. Its empirical formula is $C_7H_8ClN_3O_4S_2$ and its structural formula is:

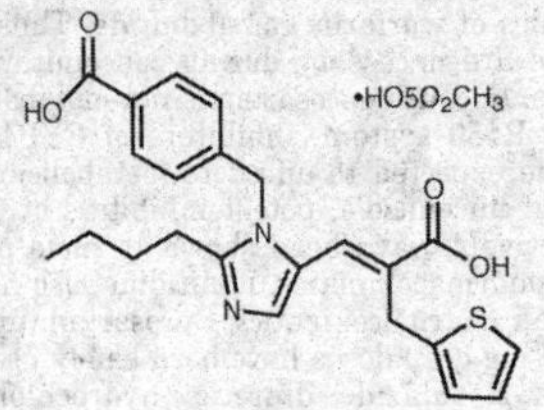

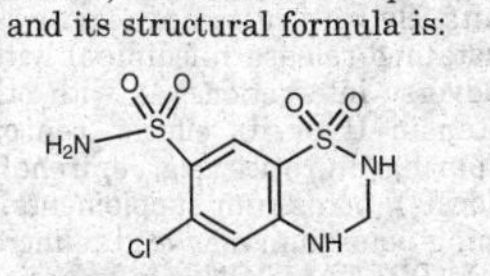

Hydrochlorothiazide is a white, or practically white, crystalline powder with a molecular weight of 297.74, which is slightly soluble in water, but freely soluble in sodium hydroxide solution. TEVETEN® HCT is available for oral administration in film-coated, non-scored, capsule-shaped tablet combinations of eprosartan mesylate and hydrochlorothiazide. TEVETEN® HCT 600/12.5 contains 735.8 mg of eprosartan mesylate (equivalent to 600 mg eprosartan) and 12.5 mg hydrochlorothiazide in a butterscotch-colored tablet. TEVETEN® HCT 600/25 contains 735.8 mg of eprosartan mesylate (equivalent to 600 mg eprosartan) and 25 mg hydrochlorothiazide in a brick-red tablet. Inactive ingredients of both tablets: microcrystalline cellulose, lactose monohydrate, pregelatinized starch, crospovidone, magnesium stearate, and purified water. Ingredients of the OPADRY® OY-R-3736 butterscotch film coating: hypromellose, polyethylene glycol 400, titanium dioxide, iron oxide black, and iron oxide yellow. Ingredients of the OPADRY® II 33G24616 pink film coating: hypromellose, lactose monohydrate, macrogol/PEG 3000, triacetin, titanium dioxide, iron oxide red, and iron oxide yellow.

CLINICAL PHARMACOLOGY

Mechanism of Action

Eprosartan: Angiotensin II (formed from angiotensin I in a reaction catalyzed by angiotensin-converting enzyme [kininase II]), a potent vasoconstrictor, is the principal pressor agent of the renin-angiotensin system. Angiotensin II also stimulates aldosterone synthesis and secretion by the adrenal cortex, cardiac contraction, renal resorption of sodium, activity of the sympathetic nervous system, and smooth muscle cell growth. Eprosartan blocks the vasoconstrictor and aldosterone-secreting effects of angiotensin II by selectively blocking the binding of angiotensin II to the AT_1 receptor found in many tissues (e.g., vascular smooth muscle, adrenal gland). There is also an AT_2 receptor found in many tissues but it is not known to be associated with cardiovascular homeostasis. Eprosartan does not exhibit any partial agonist activity at the AT_1 receptor. Its affinity for the AT_1 receptor is 1,000 times greater than for the AT_2 receptor. *In vitro* binding studies indicate that eprosartan is a reversible, competitive inhibitor of the AT_1 receptor. Blockade of the AT_1 receptor removes the negative feedback of angiotensin II on renin secretion, but the resulting increased plasma renin activity and circulating angiotensin II do not overcome the effect of eprosartan on blood pressure. TEVETEN® HCT does not inhibit kininase II, the enzyme that converts angiotensin I to angiotensin II and degrades bradykinin; whether this has clinical relevance is not known. It does not bind to or block other hormone receptors or ion channels known to be important in cardiovascular regulation.

Hydrochlorothiazide: Hydrochlorothiazide is a thiazide diuretic. Thiazides affect the renal tubular mechanisms of electrolyte reabsorption, directly increasing excretion of sodium and chloride in approximately equivalent amounts. Indirectly, the diuretic action of hydrochlorothiazide reduces plasma volume, with consequent increases in plasma renin activity, increases in aldosterone secretion, increases in urinary potassium loss, and decreases in serum potassium. The renin-aldosterone link is mediated by angiotensin II, so coadministration of an angiotensin II receptor antagonist tends to reverse the potassium loss associated with these diuretics. The mechanism of the antihypertensive effect of thiazides is unknown.

Pharmacokinetics

General

Eprosartan: Absolute bioavailability following a single 300-mg oral dose of eprosartan is approximately 13%. Eprosartan plasma concentrations peak at 1 to 2 hours after an oral dose in the fasted state. Administering eprosartan with food delays absorption, and causes variable changes (<25%) in C_{max} and AUC values which do not appear clinically important. Plasma concentrations of eprosartan increase in a slightly less than dose-proportional manner over the 100 mg to 800 mg dose range. The mean terminal elimination half-life of eprosartan following multiple oral doses of 600 mg was approximately 20 hours. Eprosartan does not significantly accumulate with chronic use.

Hydrochlorothiazide: When hydrochlorothiazide plasma levels have been followed for at least 24 hours, the plasma half-life has been observed to vary between 5.6 and 14.8 hours.

Metabolism and Excretion

Eprosartan: Eprosartan is eliminated by biliary and renal excretion, primarily as unchanged compound. Less than 2% of an oral dose is excreted in the urine as a glucuronide. There are no active metabolites following oral and intravenous dosing with [^{14}C] eprosartan in human subjects. Eprosartan was the only drug-related compound found in the plasma and feces. Following intravenous [^{14}C] eprosartan, about 61% of the material is recovered in the feces and about 37% in the urine. Following an oral dose of [^{14}C] eprosartan, about 90% is recovered in the feces and about 7% in the urine. Approximately 20% of the radioactivity excreted in the urine was an acyl glucuronide of eprosartan with the remaining 80% being unchanged eprosartan. Eprosartan is not metabolized by cytochrome P450 enzymes.

Hydrochlorothiazide: Hydrochlorothiazide is not metabolized but is eliminated rapidly by the kidney. At least 61% of the oral dose is eliminated unchanged within 24 hours.

Distribution

Eprosartan: Plasma protein binding of eprosartan is high (approximately 98%) and constant over the concentration range achieved with therapeutic doses. The pooled population pharmacokinetic analysis from two Phase 3 trials of 299 men and 172 women with mild to moderate hypertension (aged 20 to 93 years) showed that eprosartan exhibited a population mean oral clearance (CL/F) for an average 60-year-old patient of 48.5 L/hr. The population mean steady-state volume of distribution (Vss/F) was 308 L. Eprosartan pharmacokinetics were not influenced by weight, race, gender or severity of hypertension at baseline. Oral clearance was shown to be a linear function of age with CL/F decreasing 0.62 L/hr for every year increase.

Hydrochlorothiazide: Hydrochlorothiazide crosses the placental but not the blood-brain barrier and it is excreted in breast milk.

Special Populations

Pediatric: Eprosartan pharmacokinetics have not been investigated in patients younger than 18 years of age.

Geriatric: Following single oral dose administration of eprosartan to healthy elderly men, (aged 68 to 78 years), AUC, C_{max}, and T_{max} eprosartan values increased, on average, by approximately twofold, compared to healthy young men (aged 20 to 38 years) who received the same dose. The extent of plasma protein binding is not influenced by age.

Gender: There was no difference in the pharmacokinetics and plasma protein binding between men and women following single oral dose administration of eprosartan.

Race: A pooled population pharmacokinetic analysis of 442 Caucasian and 29 non-Caucasian hypertensive patients showed that oral clearance and steady-state volume of distribution were not influenced by race.

Renal Insufficiency: Following administration of 600 mg once daily, there was a 70-90% increase in AUC, and a 30-50% increase in C_{max} in moderate or severe renal impairment. The unbound eprosartan fractions increased by 35% and 59% in patients with moderate and severe renal impairment, respectively. No initial dosing adjustment is generally necessary in patients with moderate or severe renal impairment, with maximum dose not exceeding 600 mg daily. Eprosartan was poorly removed by hemodialysis (CL_{HD}<1L/hr) (see DOSAGE AND ADMINISTRATION).

Hepatic Insufficiency: Eprosartan AUC (but not C_{max}) values increased, on average, by approximately 40% in men with decreased hepatic function compared to healthy men after a single 100 mg oral dose of eprosartan. The extent of eprosartan plasma protein binding was not influenced by hepatic dysfunction. No dosage adjustment is necessary for patients with hepatic impairment.

Drug Interactions

Eprosartan: Concomitant administration of eprosartan with digoxin had no effect on a single oral-dose digoxin pharmacokinetics. Concomitant administration of eprosartan and warfarin had no effect on steady-state prothrombin time ratios (INR) in healthy volunteers. Concomitant administration of eprosartan and glyburide in diabetic patients did not affect 24-hour plasma glucose profiles. Eprosartan pharmacokinetics were not affected by concomitant administration of ranitidine. Eprosartan did not inhibit human cytochrome P450 enzymes CYP1A, 2A6, 2C9/8, 2C19, 2D6, 2E, and 3A *in vitro*. Eprosartan steady-state plasma concentrations were not affected by concomitant administration of ketoconazole or fluconazole, potent inhibitors of CYP3A and 2C9, respectively.

Eprosartan-Hydrochlorothiazide: There is no pharmacokinetic interaction between 600 mg eprosartan and 12.5 mg hydrochlorothiazide.

Pharmacodynamics and Clinical Effects

Eprosartan: Eprosartan inhibits the pharmacologic effects of angiotensin II infusions in healthy adult men. Single oral doses of eprosartan from 10 mg to 400 mg have been shown to inhibit the vasopressor, renal vasoconstrictive and aldosterone secretory effects of infused angiotensin II with complete inhibition evident at doses of 350 mg and above. Eprosartan inhibits the pressor effects of angiotensin II infusions. A single oral dose of 350 mg of eprosartan inhibits pressor effects by approximately 100% at peak, with approximately 30% inhibition persisting for 24 hours. The absence of angiotensin II AT_1 agonist activity has been demonstrated in healthy adult men. In hypertensive patients treated chronically with eprosartan, there was a twofold rise in angiotensin II plasma concentration and a twofold rise in plasma renin activity, while plasma aldosterone levels remained unchanged. Serum potassium levels also remained unchanged in these patients. Achievement of maximal blood pressure response to a given dose in most patients may take 2 to 3 weeks of treatment. Onset of blood pressure reduction is seen within 1 to 2 hours of dosing with few instances of orthostatic hypotension. Blood pressure control is maintained with once- or twice-daily dosing over a 24-hour period. Discontinuing treatment with eprosartan does not lead to a rapid rebound increase in blood pressure. There was no change in mean heart rate in patients treated with eprosartan in controlled clinical trials. Eprosartan increases mean effective renal plasma flow (ERPF) in salt-replete and salt-restricted normal subjects. A dose-related increase in ERPF of 25% to 30% occurred in salt-restricted normal subjects, with the effect plateauing between 200 mg and 400 mg doses. There was no change in ERPF in hypertensive patients and patients with renal insufficiency on normal salt diets. Eprosartan did not reduce glomerular filtration rate in patients with renal insufficiency or in patients with hypertension, after 7 days and 28 days of dosing, respectively. In hypertensive patients and patients with chronic renal insufficiency, eprosartan did not change fractional excretion of sodium and potassium. Eprosartan (1200 mg once daily for 7 days or 300 mg twice daily for 28 days) had no effect on the excretion of uric acid in healthy men, patients with essential hypertension or those with varying degrees of renal insufficiency. There were no effects on mean levels of fasting triglycerides, total cholesterol, HDL cholesterol, LDL cholesterol or fasting glucose.

Clinical Trials

Eprosartan Mesylate: The safety and efficacy of TEVETEN® has been evaluated in controlled clinical trials worldwide that enrolled predominantly hypertensive patients with sitting DBP ranging from 95 mmHg to ≤115 mmHg. There is also some experience with use of eprosartan together with other antihypertensive drugs in more severe hypertension. The antihypertensive effects of TEVETEN® were demonstrated principally in five placebo-controlled trials (4 to 13 weeks' duration) including dosages of 400 mg to 1200 mg given once daily (two studies), 25 mg to 400 mg twice daily (two studies), and one study comparing total daily doses of 400 mg to 800 mg given once daily or twice daily. The five studies included 1,111 patients randomized to eprosartan and 395 patients randomized to placebo. The studies showed dose-related antihypertensive responses. At study endpoint, patients treated with TEVETEN® at doses of 600 mg to 1200 mg given once daily experienced significant decreases in sitting systolic and diastolic blood pressure at trough, with differences from placebo of approximately 5-10/3-6 mmHg. Limited experience is available with the dose of 1200 mg administered once daily. In a direct comparison of 200 mg to 400 mg b.i.d. with 400 mg to 800 mg q.d. of TEVETEN®, effects at trough were similar. Patients treated with TEVETEN® at doses of 200 mg to 400 mg given twice daily experienced significant decreases in sitting systolic and diastolic blood pressure at trough, with differences from placebo of approximately 7-10/4-6 mmHg. Peak (1 to 3 hours) effects were uniformly, but moderately, larger than trough effects with b.i.d. dosing, with the trough-to-peak ratio for diastolic blood pressure 65% to 80%. In the once-daily dose-response study, trough-to-peak responses of ≤50% were observed at some doses (including 1200 mg), suggesting attenuation of effect at the end of the dosing interval. The antihypertensive effect of TEVETEN® was similar in men and women, but was somewhat smaller in patients over 65. There were too few black subjects to determine whether their response was similar to Caucasians. In general, blacks (usually a low renin population) have had smaller responses to ACE inhibitors and angiotensin II inhibitors than Caucasian populations. Angiotensin-converting enzyme (ACE) inhibitor-induced cough (a dry, persistent cough) can lead to discontinuation of ACE inhibitor therapy. In one study, patients who had previously coughed while taking an ACE inhibitor were treated with eprosartan, an ACE inhibitor (enalapril) or placebo for six weeks. The incidence of dry, persistent cough was 2.2% on eprosartan, 4.4% on placebo, and 20.5% on the ACE inhibitor; *P*=0.008 for the comparison of eprosartan with enalapril. In a second study comparing the incidence of cough in 259 patients treated with eprosartan to 261 patients treated with the ACE inhibitor enalapril, the incidence of dry, persistent cough in eprosartan-treated patients (1.5%) was significantly lower (*P*=0.018) than that observed in patients treated with the ACE inhibitor (5.4%). In addition, analysis of overall data from six double-blind clinical trials involving 1,554 patients showed an incidence of spontaneously reported cough in patients treated with eprosartan of 3.5%, similar to placebo (2.6%).

Hydrochlorothiazide: After oral administration of hydrochlorothiazide, diuresis begins within 2 hours, peaks in about 4 hours, and lasts about 6 to 12 hours.

Eprosartan Mesylate – Hydrochlorothiazide: Four adequate and well-controlled studies were conducted to assess the antihypertensive effectiveness of TEVETEN®/ hydrochlorothiazide in 1457 patients with mild-to-moderate essential hypertension. In a 2×2 factorial study with 112-119 hypertensive patients per arm, the mean baseline- and placebo-subtracted reductions in blood pressure at 8 weeks were 3.6/2.1 mmHg on eprosartan 600 mg, 5.6/1.9 mmHg on hydrochlorothiazide 12.5 mg, and 10.0/5.0 mmHg on the combination.

INDICATIONS AND USAGE

TEVETEN® HCT is indicated for the treatment of hypertension. It may be used alone or in combination with other antihypertensives such as calcium channel blockers. This fixed dose combination is not indicated for initial therapy (see DOSAGE AND ADMINISTRATION).

Continued on next page

Teveten HCT—Cont.

CONTRAINDICATIONS

TEVETEN® HCT is contraindicated in patients who are hypersensitive to this product or any of its components. Because of the hydrochlorothiazide component, this product is contraindicated in patients with anuria or hypersensitivity to other sulfonamide-derived drugs.

WARNINGS

Fetal/Neonatal Morbidity and Mortality

Drugs that act directly on the renin-angiotensin system can cause fetal and neonatal morbidity and death when administered to pregnant women. Several dozen cases have been reported in the world literature in patients who were taking angiotensin-converting enzyme inhibitors. When pregnancy is detected, TEVETEN® HCT should be discontinued as soon as possible. The use of drugs that act directly on the renin-angiotensin system during the second and third trimesters of pregnancy has been associated with fetal and neonatal injury, including hypotension, neonatal skull hypoplasia, anuria, reversible or irreversible renal failure, and death. Oligohydramnios has also been reported, presumably resulting from decreased fetal renal function; oligohydramnios in this setting has been associated with fetal limb contractures, craniofacial deformation, and hypoplastic lung development. Prematurity, intrauterine growth retardation, and patent ductus arteriosus have also been reported, although it is not clear whether these occurrences were due to exposure to the drug. These adverse effects do not appear to have resulted from intrauterine drug exposure that has been limited to the first trimester. Mothers whose embryos and fetuses are exposed to an angiotensin II receptor antagonist only during the first trimester should be so informed. Nonetheless, when patients become pregnant, physicians should advise the patient to discontinue the use of eprosartan as soon as possible. Rarely (probably less often than once in every thousand pregnancies), no alternative to a drug acting on the renin-angiotensin system will be found. In these rare cases, the mothers should be apprised of the potential hazards to their fetuses, and serial ultrasound examinations should be performed to assess the intra-amniotic environment. If oligohydramnios is observed, TEVETEN® HCT should be discontinued unless it is considered life-saving for the mother. Contraction stress testing (CST), a nonstress test (NST) or biophysical profiling (BPP) may be appropriate, depending upon the week of pregnancy. Patients and physicians should be aware, however, that oligohydramnios may not appear until after the fetus has sustained irreversible injury. Infants with histories of *in utero* exposure to an angiotensin II receptor antagonist should be closely observed for hypotension, oliguria, and hyperkalemia. If oliguria occurs, attention should be directed toward support of blood pressure and renal perfusion. Exchange transfusion or dialysis may be required as means of reversing hypotension and/or substituting for disordered renal function. Eprosartan mesylate, alone or in combination with hydrochlorothiazide, has been shown to produce maternal and fetal toxicities (maternal and fetal mortality, low maternal body weight and food consumption, resorptions, abortions and litter loss) in pregnant rabbits given oral doses as low as 10 mg eprosartan/kg/day and 3 mg hydrochlorothiazide/kg/day. No maternal or fetal adverse effects were observed in rabbits at 3 mg eprosartan/kg/day alone or in combination with 1 mg/kg/day of hydrochlorothiazide; this oral dose yielded a systemic exposure (AUC) to unbound eprosartan approximately equal to the human systemic exposure achieved with the dose of eprosartan mesylate contained in the maximum recommended human dose of TEVETEN® HCT (600 mg eprosartan/day). No adverse effects on *in utero* or postnatal development and maturation of offspring were observed when eprosartan mesylate was administered to pregnant rats at oral doses up to 1000 mg eprosartan/kg/day (the 1000 mg eprosartan/kg/day dose in non-pregnant rats yielded systemic exposure to unbound eprosartan approximately 0.8 times the exposure achieved in humans given 600 mg/day). Thiazides cross the placental barrier and appear in cord blood. There is a risk of fetal or neonatal jaundice, thrombocytopenia, and possibly other adverse reactions that have occurred in adults.

Hypotension in Volume- and/or Salt-Depleted Patients

In patients with an activated renin-angiotensin system, such as volume- and/or salt-depleted patients (e.g., those being treated with diuretics), symptomatic hypotension may occur. These conditions should be corrected prior to administration of TEVETEN® HCT, or the treatment should start under close medical supervision. If hypotension occurs, the patient should be placed in the supine position and, if necessary, given an intravenous infusion of normal saline. A transient hypotensive response is not a contraindication to further treatment, which usually can be continued without difficulty once the blood pressure has stabilized.

Hydrochlorothiazide

Impaired Hepatic Function: Thiazides should be used with caution in patients with impaired hepatic function or progressive liver disease, since minor alterations of fluid and electrolyte balance may precipitate hepatic coma.

Hypersensitivity Reactions: Hypersensitivity reactions to hydrochlorothiazide may occur in patients with or without a history of allergy or bronchial asthma, but are more likely in patients with such a history.

Systemic Lupus Erythematosus: Thiazide diuretics have been reported to cause exacerbation or activation of systemic lupus erythematosus. Lithium Interaction: Lithium generally should not be given with thiazides (see PRECAUTIONS, Drug Interactions, *Hydrochlorothiazide*, *Lithium*).

PRECAUTIONS

General

Hyperuricemia may occur or frank gout may be precipitated in certain patients receiving thiazide therapy. Thiazides have been shown to increase the urinary excretion of magnesium; this may result in hypomagnesemia. Thiazides may decrease urinary calcium excretion. Thiazides may cause intermittent and slight elevation of serum calcium in the absence of known disorders of calcium metabolism. Marked hypercalcemia may be evidence of hidden hyperparathyroidism. Thiazides should be discontinued before carrying out tests for parathyroid function. In diabetic patients, dosage adjustment of insulin or oral hypoglycemic agents may be required. Hyperglycemia may occur with thiazide diuretics. Thus, latent diabetes mellitus may become manifest during thiazide therapy. The antihypertensive effects of hydrochlorothiazide may be enhanced in postsympathectomy patients.

Electrolyte Imbalance

Periodic determination of serum electrolytes to detect possible electrolyte imbalance should be performed at appropriate intervals. All patients receiving thiazide therapy should be observed for clinical signs of fluid or electrolyte imbalance: hyponatremia, hypochloremic alkalosis, and hypokalemia. Serum and urine electrolyte determinations are particularly important when the patient is vomiting excessively or receiving parenteral fluids. Warning signs or symptoms of fluid and electrolyte imbalance, irrespective of cause, include: dryness of mouth, thirst, weakness, lethargy, drowsiness, restlessness, confusion, seizures, muscle pains or cramps, muscular fatigue, hypotension, oliguria, tachycardia, and gastrointestinal disturbances such as nausea and vomiting. Hypokalemia may develop, especially with brisk diuresis, when severe cirrhosis is present, or after prolonged therapy. Interference with adequate oral electrolyte intake will also contribute to hypokalemia. Hypokalemia may cause cardiac arrhythmia and may also sensitize or exaggerate the response of the heart to the toxic effects of digitalis (e.g., increased ventricular irritability). Although any chloride deficit is generally mild and usually does not require specific treatment except under extraordinary circumstances (as in liver disease or renal disease), chloride replacement may be required in the treatment of metabolic alkalosis. Dilutional hyponatremia may occur in edematous patients in hot weather; appropriate therapy is water restriction, rather than administration of salt except in rare instances when the hyponatremia is life-threatening. In actual salt depletion, appropriate replacement is the therapy of choice.

Risk of Renal Impairment

As a consequence of inhibiting the renin-angiotensin-aldosterone system, changes in renal function have been reported in susceptible individuals treated with angiotensin II antagonists; in some patients, these changes in renal function were reversible upon discontinuation of therapy. In patients whose renal function may depend on the activity of the renin-angiotensin-aldosterone system (e.g., patients with severe congestive heart failure), treatment with angiotensin-converting enzyme inhibitors and angiotensin II receptor antagonists has been associated with oliguria and/or progressive azotemia and (rarely) with acute renal failure and/or death. TEVETEN® HCT would be expected to behave similarly. In studies of ACE inhibitors in patients with unilateral or bilateral renal artery stenosis, increases in serum creatinine or BUN have been reported. Similar effects have been reported with angiotensin II antagonists; in some patients, these effects were reversible upon discontinuation of therapy. Thiazides should be used with caution in severe renal disease. In patients with renal disease, thiazides may precipitate azotemia. Cumulative effects of the drug may develop in patients with impaired renal function. If progressive renal impairment becomes evident, consider withholding or discontinuing diuretic therapy.

Information for Patients

Pregnancy: Female patients of childbearing age should be told about the consequences of second- and third-trimester exposure to drugs that act on the renin-angiotensin system, and they should also be told that these consequences do not appear to have resulted from intrauterine drug exposure that has been limited to the first trimester. These patients should be asked to report pregnancies to their physicians as soon as possible so that treatment may be discontinued under medical supervision.

Symptomatic Hypotension: A patient receiving TEVETEN® HCT should be cautioned that lightheadedness can occur, especially during the first days of therapy, and that it should be reported to the prescribing physician. The patient should be told that if syncope occurs, TEVETEN® HCT should be discontinued until the physician has been consulted. All patients should be cautioned that inadequate fluid intake, excessive perspiration, diarrhea, or vomiting can lead to an excessive fall in blood pressure, with the same consequences of light-headedness and possible syncope.

Potassium Supplements: A patient receiving TEVETEN® HCT should be told not to use potassium supplements or salt substitutes containing potassium without consulting the prescribing physician (see PRECAUTIONS, Drug Interactions, *Eprosartan Mesylate*).

Drug Interactions

Eprosartan Mesylate: Eprosartan has been shown to have no effect on the pharmacokinetics of digoxin and the pharmacodynamics of warfarin and glyburide. Thus, no dosing adjustments are necessary during concomitant use with these agents. Because eprosartan is not metabolized by the cytochrome P450 system, inhibitors of CYP450 enzyme would not be expected to affect its metabolism, and ketoconazole and fluconazole, potent inhibitors of CYP3A and 2C9, respectively, have been shown to have no effect on eprosartan pharmacokinetics. Ranitidine also has no effect on eprosartan pharmacokinetics. Eprosartan (up to 400 mg b.i.d. or 800 mg q.d.) doses have been safely used concomitantly with a thiazide diuretic (hydrochlorothiazide). Eprosartan doses of up to 300 mg b.i.d. have been safely used concomitantly with sustained-release calcium channel blockers (sustained-release nifedipine) with no clinically significant adverse interactions. As with other drugs that block angiotensin II or its effects, concomitant use of potassium-sparing diuretics (e.g., spironolactone, triamterene, amiloride), potassium supplements or salt substitutes containing potassium may lead to increases in serum potassium (see PRECAUTIONS, Information for Patients, *Potassium Supplements*).

Hydrochlorothiazide: When administered concurrently the following drugs may interact with thiazide diuretics: *Alcohol, barbiturates, or narcotics* – potentiation of orthostatic hypotension may occur. *Antidiabetic drug (oral agents and insulin)* – dosage adjustment of the antidiabetic drug may be required. *Other antihypertensive drugs* – additive effect or potentiation. *Cholestyramine and colestipol resins* – Absorption of hydrochlorothiazide is impaired in the presence of anionic exchange resins. Single doses of either cholestyramine or colestipol resins bind the hydrochlorothiazide and reduce its absorption from the gastrointestinal tract by up to 85% and 43%, respectively. *Corticosteroids, ACTH* – intensified electrolyte depletion, particularly hypokalemia. *Pressor amines (e.g., norepinephrine)* – possible decreased response to pressor amines but not sufficient to preclude their use. *Skeletal muscle relaxants, nondepolarizing (e.g., tubocurarine)* – possible increased responsiveness to the muscle relaxant. *Lithium* – should not generally be given with diuretics. Diuretic agents reduce the renal clearance of lithium and add a high risk of lithium toxicity. Refer to the package insert for lithium preparations before use of such preparations with TEVETEN® HCT. *Nonsteroidal Anti-Inflammatory Drugs* – in some patients, the administration of a nonsteroidal anti-inflammatory agent can reduce the diuretic, natriuretic, and antihypertensive effects of loop, potassium-sparing and thiazide diuretics. Therefore, when TEVETEN® HCT and nonsteroidal anti-inflammatory agents are used concomitantly, the patient should be observed closely to determine if the desired effect of the diuretic is obtained.

Carcinogenesis, Mutagenesis, Impairment of Fertility

No carcinogenicity studies have been conducted with eprosartan mesylate in combination with hydrochlorothiazide. Eprosartan mesylate was not carcinogenic in dietary restricted rats or *ad libitum* fed mice dosed at 600 mg and 2000 mg eprosartan/kg/day, respectively, for up to 2 years. In male and female rats, the systemic exposure (AUC) to unbound eprosartan at the dose evaluated was only approximately 25% of the exposure achieved in humans given TEVETEN® HCT. In mice, the systemic exposure (AUC) to unbound eprosartan was approximately 35 times the exposure achieved in humans given TEVETEN® HCT. Two-year feeding studies in mice and rats conducted under the auspices of the National Toxicology Program (NTP) uncovered no evidence of a carcinogenic potential of hydrochlorothiazide in female mice (at doses of up to approximately 600 mg/kg/day) or in male and female rats (at doses of up to approximately 100 mg/kg/day). The NTP, however, found equivocal evidence for hepatocarcinogenicity in male mice. Eprosartan mesylate was not mutagenic *in vitro* in mammalian cells (mouse lymphoma assay). Eprosartan mesylate alone or in combination with hydrochlorothiazide was not mutagenic *in vitro* in bacteria (Ames test) and did not cause structural chromosomal damage *in vivo* (mouse micronucleus assay). In human peripheral lymphocytes *in vitro*, eprosartan mesylate in combination with hydrochlorothiazide was positive for clastogenicity with and without metabolic activation. In the same assay, eprosartan mesylate alone was associated with polyploidy but there was only equivocal evidence of structural chromosomal damage. Hydrochlorothiazide was not genotoxic *in vitro* in the Ames test and in the Chinese Hamster Ovary (CHO) test for chromosomal aberrations, or *in vivo* in assays using mouse germinal cell chromosomes, Chinese hamster bone marrow chromosomes, and the *Drosophila* sex-linked recessive lethal trait gene. Positive test results were obtained in the *in vitro* CHO Sister Chromatid Exchange (clastogenicity) and Mouse Lymphoma Cell (mutagenicity) assays and in the *Aspergillus nidulans* non-disjunction assay. No fertility studies have been conducted with eprosartan mesylate in combination with hydrochlorothiazide. Eprosartan mesylate had no adverse effects on the reproductive performance of male or female rats at oral doses up to 1000 mg eprosartan/kg/day. Hydrochlorothiazide had no adverse effects on the fertility of mice and rats of either sex in studies wherein these species were exposed, via their diet, to doses of up to 100 and 4 mg/kg/day, respectively, prior to conception and throughout gestation.

Pregnancy

Pregnancy Category C (first trimester) and D (second and third trimesters): See WARNINGS: Fetal/Neonatal Morbidity and Mortality.

Nursing Mothers

Eprosartan is excreted in animal milk; it is not known whether eprosartan is excreted in human milk. Because many drugs are excreted in human milk and because of the potential for serious adverse reactions in nursing infants from eprosartan, a decision should be made whether to discontinue nursing or to discontinue the drug, taking into account the importance of the drug to the mother. Thiazides appear in human milk. Because of the potential for adverse effects on the nursing infant, a decision should be made whether to discontinue nursing or discontinue the drug, taking into account the importance of the drug to the mother.

Pediatric Use

Safety and effectiveness in pediatric patients have not been established.

Geriatric Use

In the controlled clinical trials where patients received eprosartan/hydrochlorothiazide combination therapy, 15% to 33% of the patients were 65 years of age or greater. There was no difference in the effect of TEVETEN® HCT 600/12.5 treatment according to age. However, following single oral dose administration of eprosartan to healthy elderly men, (aged 68 to 78 years), AUC, C_{max}, and T_{max} eprosartan values increased, on average, by approximately twofold, compared to healthy young men (aged 20 to 38 years) who received the same dose. (See Pharmacokinetics, Special Populations).

ADVERSE REACTIONS

TEVETEN® HCT 600/12.5 has been evaluated for safety in 268 patients in double-blind, controlled clinical trials. Most of these patients were treated with TEVETEN® HCT 600/12.5 for 29 to 60 days. Eprosartan/hydrochlorothiazide combination therapy has been evaluated for safety in 890 patients in open-label, long-term clinical trials. Approximately 50% of these patients were treated with eprosartan/hydrochlorothiazide for over 2 years. Eprosartan/hydrochlorothiazide combination therapy was well tolerated. Most adverse events were of mild or moderate severity and did not require discontinuation of therapy. Adverse experiences were similar in patients regardless of age, gender, or race. In the controlled clinical trials, about 3% of the 268 patients treated with TEVETEN® HCT 600/12.5 discontinued therapy due to clinical adverse experiences.

Adverse Events Occurring at an Incidence of Greater Than 3% Among TEVETEN® HCT Treated Patients

The following table lists adverse events that occurred at an incidence of >3% among TEVETEN® HCT 600/12.5- or monotherapy-treated patients who participated in the controlled clinical trials. Of the 268 patients who received TEVETEN® HCT 600/12.5 during the double-blind treatment period in the controlled trials, 110 patients were reported to have adverse events.

[See table 1 above]

Table 1
Incidence of Adverse Events >3% During the Double-Blind Treatment Period by Preferred Term and Treatment Grouping: Controlled Studies

Preferred Term	Placebo (N=246)		Eprosartan 600 mg (N=275)		HCTZ 12.5 mg (N=117)		HCTZ 25 mg (N=52)		Eprosartan 600 mg/HCTZ 12.5 mg (N=268)	
	n	(%)	n	(%)	n	(%)	n	(%)	n	(%)
Dizziness	4	(1.6)	5	(1.8)	2	(1.7)	2	(3.8)	11	(4.1)
Headache	22	(8.9)	10	(3.6)	4	(3.4)	3	(5.8)	9	(3.4)
Back pain	6	(2.4)	7	(2.5)	2	(1.7)	2	(3.8)	7	(2.6)
Fatigue	6	(2.4)	5	(1.8)	1	(0.9)	2	(3.8)	5	(1.9)
Myalgia	8	(3.3)	2	(0.7)	3	(2.6)	0	(0.0)	1	(0.4)
Upper Respiratory Tract Infection	8	(3.3)	2	(0.7)	0	(0.0)	2	(3.8)	1	(0.4)
Sinusitis	4	(1.6)	1	(0.4)	0	(0.0)	2	(3.8)	0	(0.0)
Viral Infection	4	(1.6)	0	(0.0)	2	(1.7)	2	(3.8)	0	(0.0)

Eprosartan (mg)	HCTZ (mg)	Color	NDC 64455
600	12.5	Butterscotch	132-01
600	25	Brick red	133-01

The adverse events reported in over 600 patients that received TEVETEN®/hydrochlorothiazide combination therapy for at least 1 year in the open-label, long-term clinical trials were comparable to those reported in the controlled trials.

Eprosartan Mesylate: In addition to the adverse events above, potentially important adverse events that are included in the current labeling for TEVETEN® monotherapy are listed below. Most of these adverse events occurred in <1% of patients, or were as frequent or more frequent in the placebo group. It is not known if these events were related to eprosartan usage: ***Body as a Whole:*** alcohol intolerance, asthenia, substernal chest pain, dependent edema, peripheral edema, facial edema, fatigue, fever, hot flushes, influenza-like symptoms, injury, malaise, pain, rigors, viral infection; ***Cardiovascular:*** angina pectoris, bradycardia, abnormal ECG, specific abnormal ECG, extrasystoles, atrial fibrillation, hypotension (including orthostatic hypotension), tachycardia, palpitations; ***Gastrointestinal:*** abdominal pain, anorexia, constipation, diarrhea, dry mouth, dyspepsia, esophagitis, flatulence, gastritis, gastroenteritis, gingivitis, nausea, periodontitis, toothache, vomiting; ***Hematologic:*** anemia, purpura; ***Liver and Biliary:*** increased SGOT, increased SGPT; ***Metabolic and Nutritional:*** increased creatine phosphokinase, diabetes mellitus, glycosuria, gout, hypercholesterolemia, hyperglycemia, hyperkalemia, hypokalemia, hyponatremia, hypertriglyceridemia; ***Musculoskeletal:*** arthralgia, arthritis, aggravated arthritis, arthrosis, skeletal pain, tendinitis; ***Nervous System/Psychiatric:*** anxiety, ataxia, depression, dizziness, insomnia, migraine, neuritis, nervousness, paresthesia, somnolence, tremor, vertigo; ***Resistance Mechanism:*** herpes simplex, otitis externa, otitis media, upper respiratory tract infection; ***Respiratory:*** asthma, bronchitis, coughing, epistaxis, pharyngitis, rhinitis; ***Skin and Appendages:*** eczema, furunculosis, pruritus, rash, maculopapular rash, increased sweating; ***Special Senses:*** conjunctivitis, abnormal vision, xerophthalmia, tinnitus; ***Urinary:*** albuminuria, cystitis, hematuria, micturition frequency, polyuria, renal calculus, urinary incontinence, urinary tract infection; ***Vascular:*** leg cramps, peripheral ischemia.

Hydrochlorothiazide: Other adverse events that have been reported for hydrochlorothiazide, without regard to causality, are listed below: ***Body as a Whole:*** weakness; ***Cardiovascular:*** hypotension (including orthostatic hypotension); ***Digestive:*** pancreatitis, jaundice (intrahepatic cholestatic jaundice), diarrhea, vomiting, sialadenitis, cramping, constipation, gastric irritation, nausea, anorexia; ***Hematologic:*** aplastic anemia, agranulocytosis, leukopenia, hemolytic anemia, thrombocytopenia; ***Hypersensitivity:*** anaphylactic reactions, necrotizing angiitis (vasculitis and cutaneous vasculitis), respiratory distress including pneumonitis, and pulmonary edema, photosensitivity, fever, urticaria, rash, purpura; ***Metabolic:*** electrolyte imbalance including hyponatremia, hypokalemia, and hypochloremic alkalosis, hyperglycemia, glycosuria, hyperuricemia; ***Musculoskeletal:*** muscle spasm; ***Nervous System/Psychiatric:*** vertigo, paresthesias, restlessness; ***Renal:*** renal failure, renal dysfunction, interstitial nephritis, azotemia; ***Skin:*** erythema multiform, including Stevens-Johnson syndrome, exfoliative dermatitis, including toxic epidermal necrolysis, alopecia; ***Special Senses:*** transient blurred vision, xanthopsia; ***Urogenital:*** impotence.

Laboratory Test Findings

In placebo-controlled studies, clinically important changes in standard laboratory parameters were rarely associated with administration of TEVETEN®. Patients were rarely withdrawn from TEVETEN® because of laboratory test results. Laboratory test findings that have been reported for TEVETEN® are listed below: ***Creatinine, Blood Urea Nitrogen:*** Minor elevations in creatinine and in BUN occurred in 0.6% and 1.3%, respectively, of patients taking TEVETEN® and 0.9% and 0.3%, respectively, of patients given placebo in controlled clinical trials. Two patients were withdrawn from clinical trials for elevations in serum creatinine and BUN, and three additional patients were withdrawn for increases in serum creatinine. ***Liver Function Tests:*** Minor elevations of ALAT, ASAT, and alkaline phosphatase occurred for comparable percentages of patients taking TEVETEN® or placebo in controlled clinical trials. An elevated ALAT of >3.5 × ULN occurred in 0.1% of patients taking TEVETEN® (one patient) and in no patient given placebo in controlled clinical trials. Four patients were withdrawn from clinical trials for an elevation in liver function tests. ***Hemoglobin:*** A greater than 20% decrease in hemoglobin was observed in 0.1% of patients taking TEVETEN® (one patient) and in no patient given placebo in controlled clinical trials. Two patients were withdrawn from clinical trials for anemia. ***Leukopenia:*** A WBC count of $\leq 3.0 \times 10^3/mm^3$ occurred in 0.3% of patients taking TEVETEN® and in 0.3% of patients given placebo in controlled clinical trials. One patient was withdrawn from clinical trials for leukopenia. ***Neutropenia:*** A neutrophil count of $\leq 1.5 \times 10^3/mm^3$ occurred in 1.3% of patients taking TEVETEN® and in 1.4% of patients given placebo in controlled clinical trials. No patient was withdrawn from any clinical trials for neutropenia. ***Thrombocytopenia:*** A platelet count of $\leq 100 \times 10^9/L$ occurred in 0.3% of patients taking TEVETEN® (one patient) and in no patient given placebo in controlled clinical trials. Four patients receiving TEVETEN® in clinical trials were withdrawn for thrombocytopenia. In one case, thrombocytopenia was present prior to dosing with TEVETEN®. ***Serum Potassium:*** A potassium value of ≥ 5.6 mmol/L occurred in 0.9% of patients taking TEVETEN® and 0.3% of patients given placebo in controlled clinical trials. One patient was withdrawn from clinical trials for hyperkalemia and three for hypokalemia.

Additional Information

Among the adverse events reported for patients receiving either TEVETEN® monotherapy or TEVETEN®/hydrochlorothiazide combination therapy in the TEVETEN® HCT clinical trials, some adverse events are not included in the current labeling for either TEVETEN® or hydrochlorothiazide monotherapy. The adverse events which are not currently included in the labeling for TEVETEN® or hydrochlorothiazide monotherapy include the following: angioedema, bilirubinemia, blood urea nitrogen increased, edema periorbital, eosinophilia, and NPN increased. The majority of these adverse events were reported in the open-label, long-term trials and were reported in small numbers of patients receiving TEVETEN® alone or TEVETEN® in combination with hydrochlorothiazide. All of these adverse events were either not reported in patients receiving TEVETEN® monotherapy or combination therapy with hydrochlorothiazide during the double-blind period of the controlled trials, or were reported at an incidence of ≤1% or in only one patient per treatment group in the controlled trials. The overall safety profile of the TEVETEN®/hydrochlorothiazide combination treatment is as expected based on the safety profile of each of the components and what is generally known about the patient population.

OVERDOSAGE

Eprosartan Mesylate: Limited data are available regarding overdosage. Appropriate symptomatic and supportive therapy should be given if overdosage should occur. There was no mortality in rats and mice receiving oral doses of up to 3000 mg eprosartan/kg and in dogs receiving oral doses of up to 1000 mg eprosartan/kg.

Hydrochlorothiazide: The most common signs and symptoms observed are those caused by electrolyte depletion (hypokalemia, hypochloremia, and hyponatremia) and dehydration resulting from excessive diuresis. If digitalis has also been administered, hypokalemia may accentuate cardiac arrhythmias. The degree to which hydrochlorothiazide is removed by hemodialysis has not been established. The oral LD_{50} of hydrochlorothiazide is greater than 10 g/kg in both mice and rats.

DOSAGE AND ADMINISTRATION

The usual recommended starting dose of eprosartan is 600 mg once daily when used as monotherapy in patients who are not volume-depleted (see WARNINGS, Hypotension in Volume- and/or Salt-Depleted Patients). Eprosartan can be administered once or twice daily and total daily doses ranging from 400 mg to 800 mg. There is limited experience with doses beyond 800 mg/day. If the antihypertensive effect measured at trough using once-daily monotherapy dosing is inadequate, a twice-a-day regimen at the same total daily dose or an increase in dose may give a more satisfactory response. Achievement of maximum blood pressure reduction in most patients may take 2 to 3 weeks. Hydrochlorothiazide is effective in doses of 12.5 mg to 50 mg once daily. To minimize dose-independent side effects, it is usually appropriate to begin combination therapy only after a patient has failed to achieve the desired effect with monotherapy. The side effects (see WARNINGS) of eprosartan are generally rare and apparently independent of dose; those of hydrochlorothiazide are a mixture of dose-dependent (primarily hypokalemia) and dose-independent (e.g., pancreatitis) phenomena, the former much more common than the latter. Therapy with any combination of eprosartan and hydrochlorothiazide will be associated with both sets of dose-independent side effects.

Replacement Therapy

TEVETEN® HCTmay be substituted for the individual components. The usual recommended dose of TEVETEN® HCT is 600 mg/12.5 mg once daily when used as combination therapy in patients who are not volume-depleted (see WARNINGS, Hypotension in Volume-and/or Salt-Depleted Patients). If the antihypertensive effect measured at trough using TEVETEN® HCT 600/12.5 is inadequate, patients may be titrated to TEVETEN® HCT 600/25 once daily. Higher doses have not been studied in combination. Achievement of maximum blood pressure reduction in most patients may take 2 to 3 weeks. If the patient under treatment with TEVETEN® HCT requires additional blood pressure control at trough, or to maintain a twice a day dosing schedule of monotherapy, 300 mg TEVETEN® may be added as evening dose. TEVETEN® HCT may be used in combination with other antihypertensive agents such

Continued on next page

Teveten HCT—Cont.

as calcium channel blockers if additional blood-pressure-lowering effect is required. Discontinuation of treatment with eprosartan does not lead to a rapid rebound increase in blood pressure.

Elderly, Hepatically Impaired or Renally Impaired Patients: No initial dosing adjustment is generally necessary for elderly or hepatically impaired patients or those with renal impairment. No initial dosing adjustment is generally necessary in patients with moderate and severe renal impairment with maximum dose not exceeding 600 mg daily. TEVETEN® HCT may be taken with or without food.

HOW SUPPLIED

TEVETEN® HCT is available as film-coated, capsule-shaped tablets, debossed with "SOLVAY" on one side and "5147" or "5150" on the other, supplied as bottles of 100 tablets as follows:

[See second table at top of previous page]

STORAGE

Store at controlled room temperature 20° to 25°C (68° to 77°F) [see USP Controlled Room Temperature].

Rx only

Manufactured by:

Solvay Pharmaceuticals, BV
Olst, The Netherlands
Tablets made in The Netherlands.

Marketed by:

BIOVAIL Pharmaceuticals, Inc.
Biovail Pharmaceuticals, Inc.
Bridgewater, NJ, 08807, USA

LB0031-00
January 2004

ZOVIRAX® ℞

[zō'vī-răks]
(acyclovir)
Cream 5%
USE ONLY FOR COLD SORES
PRESCRIBING INFORMATION

DESCRIPTION

ZOVIRAX is the brand name for acyclovir, a synthetic nucleoside analogue active against herpesviruses. ZOVIRAX Cream 5% is a formulation for topical administration. Each gram of ZOVIRAX Cream 5% contains 50 mg of acyclovir and the following inactive ingredients: cetostearyl alcohol, mineral oil, poloxamer 407, propylene glycol, sodium lauryl sulfate, water, and white petrolatum.

Acyclovir is a white, crystalline powder with the molecular formula $C_8H_{11}N_5O_3$ and a molecular weight of 225. The maximum solubility in water at 37°C is 2.5 mg/mL. The pKa's of acyclovir are 2.27 and 9.25.

The chemical name of acyclovir is 2-amino-1,9-dihydro-9-[(2-hydroxyethoxy)methyl]-6*H*-purin-6-one; it has the following structural formula:

VIROLOGY

Mechanism of Antiviral Action: Acyclovir is a synthetic purine nucleoside analogue with in vitro and in vivo inhibitory activity against herpes simplex virus types 1 (HSV-1), 2 (HSV-2), and varicella-zoster virus (VZV).

The inhibitory activity of acyclovir is highly selective due to its affinity for the enzyme thymidine kinase (TK) encoded by HSV and VZV. This viral enzyme converts acyclovir into acyclovir monophosphate, a nucleotide analogue. The monophosphate is further converted into diphosphate by cellular guanylate kinase and into triphosphate by a number of cellular enzymes. In vitro, acyclovir triphosphate stops replication of herpes viral DNA. This is accomplished in 3 ways: 1) competitive inhibition of viral DNA polymerase, 2) incorporation into and termination of the growing viral DNA chain, and 3) inactivation of the viral DNA polymerase. The greater antiviral activity of acyclovir against HSV compared with VZV is due to its more efficient phosphorylation by the viral TK.

Antiviral Activities: The quantitative relationship between the in vitro susceptibility of herpes viruses to antivirals and the clinical response to therapy has not been established in humans, and virus sensitivity testing has not been standardized. Sensitivity testing results, expressed as the concentration of drug required to inhibit by 50% the growth of virus in cell culture (IC_{50}), vary greatly depending upon a number of factors. Using plaque-reduction assays, the IC_{50} against herpes simplex virus isolates ranges from 0.02 to 13.5 mcg/mL for HSV-1 and from 0.01 to 9.9 mcg/mL for HSV-2. The IC_{50} for acyclovir against most laboratory strains and clinical isolates of VZV ranges from 0.12 to 10.8 mcg/mL. Acyclovir also demonstrates activity against the Oka vaccine strain of VZV with a mean IC_{50} of 1.35 mcg/mL.

Drug Resistance: Resistance of HSV and VZV to acyclovir can result from qualitative and quantitative changes in the viral TK and/or DNA polymerase. Clinical isolates of HSV and VZV with reduced susceptibility to acyclovir have been recovered from immunocompromised patients, especially with advanced HIV infection. While most of the acyclovir-resistant mutants isolated thus far from immunocompromised patients have been found to be TK-deficient mutants, other mutants involving the viral TK gene (TK partial and TK altered) and DNA polymerase have been isolated. TK-negative mutants may cause severe disease in infants and immunocompromised adults. The possibility of viral resistance to acyclovir should be considered in patients who show poor clinical response during therapy.

CLINICAL PHARMACOLOGY

Pharmacokinetics: *Adults:* A clinical pharmacology study was performed with ZOVIRAX Cream in adult volunteers to evaluate the percutaneous absorption of acyclovir. In this study, which included 6 male volunteers, the cream was applied to an area of 710 cm^2 on the backs of the volunteers 5 times daily at intervals of 2 hours for a total of 4 days. The weight of cream applied and urinary excretion of acyclovir were measured daily. Plasma concentration of acyclovir was assayed 1 hour after the final application. The average daily urinary excretion of acyclovir was approximately 0.04% of the daily applied dose. Plasma acyclovir concentrations were below the limit of detection (0.01 μM) in 5 subjects and barely detectable (0.014 μM) in 1 subject. Systemic absorption of acyclovir from ZOVIRAX Cream is minimal in adults.

Pediatric Patients: The systemic absorption of acyclovir following topical application of cream has not been evaluated in patients <18 years of age.

CLINICAL TRIALS

Adults: ZOVIRAX Cream was evaluated in 2 double-blind, randomized, placebo (vehicle)-controlled trials for the treatment of recurrent herpes labialis. The average patient had 5 episodes of herpes labialis in the previous 12 months. In the first study, median age was 37 years (range 18 to 81 years), 74% were female, and 94% were Caucasian. In the second study, median age was 38 years (range 18 to 87 years), 73% were female, and 94% were Caucasian. Subjects were instructed to initiate treatment within 1 hour of noticing signs or symptoms and continue treatment for 4 days, with application of study medication 5 times per day. In both studies, the mean duration of the recurrent herpes labialis episode was approximately one-half day shorter in the subjects treated with ZOVIRAX Cream (n = 682) compared with subjects treated with placebo (n = 703) (approximately 4.5 days versus 5 days, respectively). No significant difference was observed between subjects receiving ZOVIRAX Cream or vehicle in the prevention of progression of cold sore lesions.

Pediatric Patients: An open-label, uncontrolled trial with ZOVIRAX Cream 5% was conducted in 113 patients aged 12 to 17 years with herpes labialis. In this study, therapy was applied using the same dosing regimen as in adults and subjects were followed for adverse events. The safety profile was similar to that observed in adults.

INDICATIONS AND USAGE

ZOVIRAX Cream is indicated for the treatment of recurrent herpes labialis (cold sores) in adults and adolescents (12 years of age and older).

CONTRAINDICATIONS

ZOVIRAX Cream is contraindicated in patients with known hypersensitivity to acyclovir, valacyclovir, or any component of the formulation.

PRECAUTIONS

General: ZOVIRAX Cream is intended for cutaneous use only and should not be used in the eye or inside the mouth or nose. ZOVIRAX Cream should only be used on herpes labialis on the affected external aspects of the lips and face. Because no data are available, application to human mucous membranes is not recommended. ZOVIRAX Cream has a potential for irritation and contact sensitization (see ADVERSE REACTIONS). The effect of ZOVIRAX Cream has not been established in immunocompromised patients.

Information for Patients: Please see **Patient Information About ZOVIRAX Cream.**

Drug Interactions: Clinical experience has identified no interactions resulting from topical or systemic administration of other drugs concomitantly with ZOVIRAX Cream.

Carcinogenesis, Mutagenesis, Impairment of Fertility: Systemic exposure following topical administration of acyclovir is minimal. Dermal carcinogenicity studies were not conducted. Results from the studies of carcinogenesis, mutagenesis and fertility are not included in the full prescribing information for ZOVIRAX Cream due to the minimal exposures of acyclovir that result from dermal application. Information on these studies is available in the full prescribing information for ZOVIRAX Capsules, Tablets, and Suspension and ZOVIRAX for Injection.

Pregnancy: *Teratogenic Effects:* Pregnancy Category B. Acyclovir was not teratogenic in the mouse, rabbit, or rat at exposures greatly in excess of human exposure. There are no adequate and well-controlled studies of systemic acyclovir in pregnant women. A prospective epidemiologic registry of acyclovir use during pregnancy was established in 1984 and completed in April 1999. There were 749 pregnancies followed in women exposed to systemic acyclovir during the first trimester of pregnancy resulting in 756 outcomes. The occurrence rate of birth defects approximates that found in the general population. However, the small size of the registry is insufficient to evaluate the risk for less common defects or to permit reliable or definitive conclusions regarding the safety of acyclovir in pregnant women and their developing fetuses. Systemic acyclovir should be used during pregnancy only if the potential benefit justifies the potential risk to the fetus.

Nursing Mothers: It is not known whether topically applied acyclovir is excreted in breast milk. Systemic exposure following topical administration is minimal.

After oral administration of ZOVIRAX, acyclovir concentrations have been documented in breast milk in 2 women and ranged from 0.6 to 4.1 times the corresponding plasma levels. These concentrations would potentially expose the nursing infant to a dose of acyclovir up to 0.3 mg/kg/day. Nursing mothers who have active herpetic lesions near or on the breast should avoid nursing.

Geriatric Use: Clinical studies of acyclovir cream did not include sufficient numbers of subjects aged 65 and over to determine whether they respond differently from younger subjects. Other reported clinical experience has not identified differences in responses between the elderly and younger patients. Systemic absorption of acyclovir after topical administration is minimal (see CLINICAL PHARMACOLOGY).

Pediatric Use: Safety and effectiveness in pediatric patients less than 12 years of age have not been established.

ADVERSE REACTIONS

In 5 double-blind, placebo-controlled trials, 1,124 patients were treated with ZOVIRAX Cream and 1,161 with placebo (vehicle) cream. ZOVIRAX Cream was well tolerated; 5% of patients on ZOVIRAX Cream and 4% of patients on placebo reported local application site reactions.

The most common adverse reactions at the site of topical application were dry lips, desquamation, dryness of skin, cracked lips, burning skin, pruritus, flakiness of skin, and stinging on skin; each event occurred in less than 1% of patients receiving ZOVIRAX Cream and vehicle. Three patients on ZOVIRAX Cream and 1 patient on placebo discontinued treatment due to an adverse event.

An additional study, enrolling 22 healthy adults, was conducted to evaluate the dermal tolerance of ZOVIRAX Cream compared with vehicle using single occluded and semi-occluded patch testing methodology. Both ZOVIRAX Cream and vehicle showed a high and cumulative irritation potential. Another study, enrolling 251 healthy adults, was conducted to evaluate the contact sensitization potential of ZOVIRAX Cream using repeat insult patch testing methodology. Of 202 evaluable subjects, possible cutaneous sensitization reactions were observed in the same 4 (2%) subjects with both ZOVIRAX Cream and vehicle, and these reactions to both ZOVIRAX Cream and vehicle were confirmed in 3 subjects upon rechallenge. The sensitizing ingredient(s) has not been identified.

The safety profile in patients 12 to 17 years of age was similar to that observed in adults.

Observed During Clinical Practice: In addition to adverse events reported from clinical trials, the following events have been identified during post-approval use of acyclovir cream. Because they are reported voluntarily from a population of unknown size, estimates of frequency cannot be made. These events have been chosen for inclusion due to a combination of their seriousness, frequency of reporting, or potential causal connection to acyclovir cream

General: Angioedema, anaphylaxis.

Skin: Contact dermatitis, eczema, application site reactions including signs and symptoms of inflammation.

OVERDOSAGE

Overdosage by topical application of ZOVIRAX Cream is unlikely because of minimal systemic exposure (see CLINICAL PHARMACOLOGY).

DOSAGE AND ADMINISTRATION

ZOVIRAX Cream should be applied 5 times per day for 4 days. Therapy should be initiated as early as possible following onset of signs and symptoms (i.e., during the prodrome or when lesions appear). For adolescents 12 years of age and older, the dosage is the same as in adults.

HOW SUPPLIED

Each gram of ZOVIRAX Cream 5% contains 50 mg acyclovir in an aqueous cream base. ZOVIRAX Cream is supplied as follows:

2-g tubes (NDC 64455-994-42).
5-g tubes (NDC 64455-994-45).

Store at or below 25°C (77°F); excursions permitted to 15° to 30°C (59° to 86°F) (see USP Controlled Room Temperature).

Manufactured by
GlaxoSmithKline
Research Triangle Park, NC 27709
for
Biovail Pharmaceuticals, Inc.
Bridgewater, NJ 08807

January 2004
RL-2061
A005174

PATIENT INFORMATION ABOUT ZOVIRAX® (ACYCLOVIR) CREAM 5%

USE ONLY FOR COLD SORES. FOR EXTERNAL USE ONLY.

Read this information before you start using ZOVIRAX (acyclovir) Cream and each time you refill your prescription. There may be new information. This summary is not meant to take the place of your doctor's advice.

What is ZOVIRAX Cream?

ZOVIRAX Cream is a prescription medicine that is applied to the skin to treat cold sores (herpes labialis) that occur on the face or lips. However, ZOVIRAX Cream is not a cure for cold sores.

Who should not use ZOVIRAX Cream?

Do not use ZOVIRAX Cream if you are allergic to ZOVIRAX (also known as acyclovir), VALTREX® (also known as valacyclovir), or any of the ingredients of ZOVIRAX Cream. Ask your doctor or pharmacist about the inactive ingredients.

Before you start using ZOVIRAX Cream, tell your doctor if you are pregnant, planning to become pregnant, or are breast feeding.

The safety and efficacy of ZOVIRAX Cream have not been studied in patients younger than 12 years of age or in patients whose immune system is not normal.

How do I use ZOVIRAX Cream?

ZOVIRAX Cream is most effective when used early, at the start of a cold sore. For best results, apply the cream at the first sign of a cold sore (such as tingle, redness, bump, or itch).

- Wash your hands before using ZOVIRAX Cream.
- Apply ZOVIRAX Cream to clean, dry skin.
- Apply a layer of ZOVIRAX Cream to cover only the cold sore or cover only the area of tingling (or other symptoms) before the cold sore appears. Rub the cream in until it disappears.
- Apply the cream 5 times a day for 4 days.
- Wash your hands with soap and water after applying ZOVIRAX Cream. This should remove any cream left on the hands.

What Should I Avoid While Using ZOVIRAX Cream?

- Use ZOVIRAX Cream only on your affected skin. Do not swallow ZOVIRAX Cream. Do not apply ZOVIRAX Cream to the eyes, inside the mouth or nose, or on unaffected skin. Do not use ZOVIRAX Cream for genital herpes.
- Do not cover the cold sore area with a bandage or dressing unless otherwise instructed by your doctor.
- Do not apply another type of skin product (for example, cosmetics, sun screens, or lip balms) or other skin medication to the cold sore area while using ZOVIRAX Cream unless otherwise instructed by your doctor.
- Avoid irritation of the cold sore area while using ZOVIRAX Cream.
- Do not bathe, shower, or swim right after applying ZOVIRAX Cream. This could wash off the medicine.

What Are the Possible Side Effects of ZOVIRAX Cream?

ZOVIRAX Cream was well tolerated in studies in patients with cold sores. The most common skin-related side effects of ZOVIRAX Cream are dry or cracked lips, flakiness or dryness of skin, a burning or stinging feeling, or itching of the skin. Each event occurred in fewer than 1 in 100 patients in clinical studies. Ask a doctor or pharmacist about any concerns about ZOVIRAX Cream.

How Should I Store ZOVIRAX Cream?

Store ZOVIRAX Cream at room temperature (59° to 86°F). Never leave ZOVIRAX Cream in your car in cold or hot weather. Make sure the cap on the tube is tightly closed. Keep ZOVIRAX Cream out of the reach of children.

General Advice about Prescription Medicines

Do not use ZOVIRAX Cream for a condition for which it was not prescribed. Do not give ZOVIRAX Cream to other people, even if they have the same symptoms you have. If you have any concerns about ZOVIRAX Cream, ask your doctor. Your doctor or pharmacist can give you additional information about ZOVIRAX Cream that was written for healthcare professionals.

Manufactured by
GlaxoSmithKline
Research Triangle Park, NC 27709
for
Biovail
Pharmaceuticals, Inc.
Bridgewater, NJ 08807

January 2004
RL-2061
A005174

ZOVIRAX® ℞
[*zō-vī 'răx*]
(acyclovir)
Ointment 5%
PRESCRIBING INFORMATION

DESCRIPTION

ZOVIRAX is the brand name for acyclovir, a synthetic nucleoside analogue active against herpes viruses. ZOVIRAX Ointment 5% is a formulation for topical administration. Each gram of ZOVIRAX Ointment 5% contains 50 mg of acyclovir in a polyethylene glycol (PEG) base.

Acyclovir is a white, crystalline powder with the molecular formula $C_8H_{11}N_5O_3$ and a molecular weight of 225. The maximum solubility in water at 37°C is 2.5 mg/mL. The pka's of acyclovir are 2.27 and 9.25.

The chemical name of acyclovir is 2-amino-1,9-dihydro-9-[(2-hydroxyethoxy)methyl]-6*H*-purin-6-one; it has the following structural formula:

VIROLOGY

Mechanism of Antiviral Action: Acyclovir is a synthetic purine nucleoside analogue with in vitro and in vivo inhibitory activity against herpes simplex virus types 1 (HSV-1), 2 (HSV-2), and varicella-zoster virus (VZV).

The inhibitory activity of acyclovir is highly selective due to its affinity for the enzyme thymidine kinase (TK) encoded by HSV and VZV. This viral enzyme converts acyclovir into acyclovir monophosphate, a nucleotide analogue. The monophosphate is further converted into diphosphate by cellular guanylate kinase and into triphosphate by a number of cellular enzymes. In vitro, acyclovir triphosphate stops replication of herpes viral DNA. This is accomplished in 3 ways: 1) competitive inhibition of viral DNA polymerase, 2) incorporation into and termination of the growing viral DNA chain, and 3) inactivation of the viral DNA polymerase. The greater antiviral activity of acyclovir against HSV compared to VZV is due to its more efficient phosphorylation by the viral TK.

Antiviral Activities: The quantitative relationship between the in vitro susceptibility of herpes viruses to antivirals and the clinical response to therapy has not been established in humans, and virus sensitivity testing has not been standardized. Sensitivity testing results, expressed as the concentration of drug required to inhibit by 50% the growth of virus in cell culture (IC_{50}), vary greatly depending upon a number of factors. Using plaque-reduction assays, the IC_{50} against herpes simplex virus isolates ranges from 0.02 to 13.5 mcg/mL for HSV-1 and from 0.01 to 9.9 mcg/mL for HSV-2. The IC_{50} for acyclovir against most laboratory strains and clinical isolates of VZV ranges from 0.12 to 10.8 mcg/mL. Acyclovir also demonstrates activity against the Oka vaccine strain of VZV with a mean IC_{50} of 1.35 mcg/mL.

Drug Resistance: Resistance of HSV and VZV to acyclovir can result from qualitative and quantitative changes in the viral TK and/or DNA polymerase. Clinical isolates of HSV and VZV with reduced susceptibility to acyclovir have been recovered from immunocompromised patients, especially with advanced HIV infection. While most of the acyclovir-resistant mutants isolated thus far from immunocompromised patients have been found to be TK-deficient mutants, other mutants involving the viral TK gene (TK partial and TK altered) and DNA polymerase have been isolated. TK-negative mutants may cause severe disease in infants and immunocompromised adults. The possibility of viral resistance to acyclovir should be considered in patients who show poor clinical response during therapy.

CLINICAL PHARMACOLOGY

Two clinical pharmacology studies were performed with ZOVIRAX Ointment 5% in immunocompromised adults at risk of developing mucocutaneous Herpes simplex virus infections or with localized varicella-zoster infections. These studies were designed to evaluate the dermal tolerance, systemic toxicity, and percutaneous absorption of acyclovir.

In 1 of these studies, which included 16 inpatients, the complete ointment or its vehicle were randomly administered in a dose of 1-cm strips (25 mg acyclovir) 4 times a day for 7 days to an intact skin surface area of 4.5 square inches. No local intolerance, systemic toxicity, or contact dermatitis were observed. In addition, no drug was detected in blood and urine by radioimmunoassay (sensitivity, 0.01 mcg/mL).

The other study included 11 patients with localized varicella-zoster infections. In this uncontrolled study, acyclovir was detected in the blood of 9 patients and in the urine of all patients tested. Acyclovir levels in plasma ranged from <0.01 to 0.28 mcg/mL in 8 patients with normal renal function, and from <0.01 to 0.78 mcg/mL in 1 patient with impaired renal function. Acyclovir excreted in the urine ranged from <0.02% to 9.4% of the daily dose. Therefore, systemic absorption of acyclovir after topical application is minimal.

CLINICAL TRIALS

In clinical trials of initial genital herpes infections, ZOVIRAX Ointment 5% has shown a decrease in healing time and, in some cases, a decrease in duration of viral shedding and duration of pain. In studies in immunocompromised patients mainly with herpes labialis, there was a decrease in duration of viral shedding and a slight decrease in duration of pain.

In studies of recurrent genital herpes and of herpes labialis in nonimmunocompromised patients, there was no evidence of clinical benefit; there was some decrease in duration of viral shedding.

INDICATIONS AND USAGE

ZOVIRAX (acyclovir) Ointment 5% is indicated in the management of initial genital herpes and in limited non-life-threatening mucocutaneous Herpes simplex virus infections in immunocompromised patients.

CONTRAINDICATIONS

ZOVIRAX Ointment 5% is contraindicated in patients who develop hypersensitivity to the components of the formulation.

WARNINGS

ZOVIRAX Ointment 5% is intended for cutaneous use only and should not be used in the eye.

PRECAUTIONS

General: The recommended dosage, frequency of applications, and length of treatment should not be exceeded (see DOSAGE AND ADMINISTRATION). There are no data to support the use of ZOVIRAX Ointment 5% to prevent transmission of infection to other persons or prevent recurrent infections when applied in the absence of signs and symptoms. ZOVIRAX Ointment 5% should not be used for the prevention of recurrent HSV infections. Although clinically significant viral resistance associated with the use of ZOVIRAX Ointment 5% has not been observed, this possibility exists.

Drug Interactions: Clinical experience has identified no interactions resulting from topical or systemic administration of other drugs concomitantly with ZOVIRAX Ointment 5%.

Carcinogenesis, Mutagenesis, Impairment of Fertility: Systemic exposure following topical administration of acyclovir is minimal. Dermal carcinogenicity studies were not conducted. Results from the studies of carcinogenesis, mutagenesis, and fertility are not included in the full prescribing information for ZOVIRAX Ointment 5% due to the minimal exposures of acyclovir that result from dermal application. Information on these studies is available in the full prescribing information for ZOVIRAX Capsules, Tablets, and Suspension and ZOVIRAX for Injection.

Pregnancy: ***Teratogenic Effects:*** Pregnancy Category B. Acyclovir was not teratogenic in the mouse, rabbit, or rat at exposures greatly in excess of human exposure. There are no adequate and well-controlled studies of systemic acyclovir in pregnant women. A prospective epidemiologic registry of acyclovir use during pregnancy was established in 1984 and completed in April 1999. There were 749 pregnancies followed in women exposed to systemic acyclovir during the first trimester of pregnancy resulting in 756 outcomes. The occurrence rate of birth defects approximates that found in the general population. However, the small size of the registry is insufficient to evaluate the risk for less common defects or to permit reliable or definitive conclusions regarding the safety of acyclovir in pregnant women and their developing fetuses. Systemic acyclovir should be used during pregnancy only if the potential benefit justifies the potential risk to the fetus.

Nursing Mothers: It is not known whether topically applied acyclovir is excreted in breast milk. Systemic exposure following topical administration is minimal. After oral administration of ZOVIRAX, acyclovir concentrations have been documented in breast milk in 2 women and ranged from 0.6 to 4.1 times the corresponding plasma levels. These concentrations would potentially expose the nursing infant to a dose of acyclovir up to 0.3 mg/kg per day. Nursing mothers who have active herpetic lesions near or on the breast should avoid nursing.

Geriatric Use: Clinical studies of ZOVIRAX Ointment did not include sufficient numbers of subjects aged 65 and over to determine whether they respond differently from younger subjects. Other reported clinical experience has not identified differences in responses between the elderly and younger patients. Systemic absorption of acyclovir after topical administration is minimal (see CLINICAL PHARMACOLOGY).

Pediatric Use: Safety and effectiveness in pediatric patients have not been established.

ADVERSE REACTIONS

In the controlled clinical trials, mild pain (including transient burning and stinging) was reported by about 30% of patients in both the active and placebo arms; treatment was discontinued in 2 of these patients. Local pruritus occurred in 4% of these patients. In all studies, there was no significant difference between the drug and placebo group in the rate or type of reported adverse reactions nor were there any differences in abnormal clinical laboratory findings.

Observed During Clinical Practice: Based on clinical practice experience in patients treated with ZOVIRAX Ointment in the US, spontaneously reported adverse events are uncommon. Data are insufficient to support an estimate of their incidence or to establish causation. These events may also occur as part of the underlying disease process. Voluntary reports of adverse events that have been received since market introduction include:

General: Edema and/or pain at the application site.

Skin: Pruritus, rash.

OVERDOSAGE

Overdosage by topical application of ZOVIRAX Ointment 5% is unlikely because of limited transcutaneous absorption (see CLINICAL PHARMACOLOGY).

DOSAGE AND ADMINISTRATION

Apply sufficient quantity to adequately cover all lesions every 3 hours, 6 times per day for 7 days. The dose size per application will vary depending upon the total lesion area

Continued on next page

Zovirax Ointment—Cont.

but should approximate a one-half inch ribbon of ointment per 4 square inches of surface area. A finger cot or rubber glove should be used when applying ZOVIRAX to prevent autoinoculation of other body sites and transmission of infection to other persons. **Therapy should be initiated as early as possible following onset of signs and symptoms.**

HOW SUPPLIED

Each gram of ZOVIRAX Ointment 5% contains 50 mg acyclovir in a polyethylene glycol base. It is supplied as follows:
15-g tubes (NDC 64455-993-94)
3-g tubes (NDC 64455-993-41).
Store at 15° to 25°C (59° to 77°F) in a dry place.
Manufactured by
GlaxoSmithKline,
Research Triangle Park, NC 27709
for
BIOVAIL
Pharmaceuticals, Inc.
Bridgewater, NJ 08807

January 2004
RL-2062
A005180

Blaine Pharmaceuticals

1515 PRODUCTION DRIVE
BURLINGTON, KY 41005

Inquiries or Medical Information Contact:
(859) 372-8080
(800) 633-9353
FAX: (859) 283-9460
Website: www.MagOx.com

MAG-OX 400® — OTC

DESCRIPTION

EACH TABLET CONTAINS: Magnesium Oxide, 400 mg [241.3 mg elemental magnesium (19.86 mEq)].
Mag-Ox 400 tablets meet USP 24 disintegration test <701> and dissolution test <711>.

INDICATIONS

As a dietary supplement to increase daily intake of magnesium; for relief of acid indigestion and upset stomach.

DIRECTIONS

As an Adult Dietary Supplement - Take 2 tablets per day with food or as directed by your physician.
As an Adult Antacid - Take 2 tablets per day with food or as directed by your physician.
DRUG INTERACTION PRECAUTION: Consult a physician before use if you are taking a prescription drug. If you are pregnant, nursing a baby, or have kidney disease, consult a physician. May have a laxative effect. Antacids may interact with certain prescription drugs.

WARNINGS

As an Adult Dietary Supplement - Do not take more than 2 tablets in a 24-hr period, except under the advice and supervision of a physician. If you have a kidney disease, are pregnant, or are nursing a baby, consult a physician before using this product. May have a laxative effect. **As an Adult Antacid** - Do not take more than 2 tablets in a 24-hour period, except under the advice and supervision of a physician. May have a laxative effect. As with any drug, if you are pregnant or nursing a baby, seek the advice of a health professional before using this product. Keep this and all drugs out of the reach of children. Store in a dry place at 20°–25°C (68°–77°F).

HOW SUPPLIED

Bottles of 60, 120, 1000 and Hospital Unit Dose (UD).

URO-MAG® — OTC

DESCRIPTION

EACH CAPSULE CONTAINS: Magnesium Oxide 140 mg 84.5 mg [elemental Magnesium (6.93 mEq)].

INDICATIONS

As an adult dietary supplement to increase daily intake of magnesium.

DIRECTIONS

Take 4 or 5 capsules daily or as directed by a physician.

WARNINGS

Not recommended for use in amounts over the Recommended Daily Intake (RDI) of 400 mg per day (4 or 5 capsules). If you have a kidney disease, are pregnant, or are nursing a baby, consult a physician before using this product. May have a laxative effect. Keep this and all drugs out of the reach of children. Store at controlled room temperature 15°–30°C (59°–86°F).

HOW SUPPLIED

Bottles of 100 and 1000 and Hospital Unit Dose (UD).

EDUCATIONAL MATERIAL

Professional samples available to physicians upon request.
(800) 633-9353
Website: www.MagOx.com

Blansett Pharmacal

P.O. BOX 638
N. LITTLE ROCK, AR 72115

Direct Inquiries to:
Customer Service
(501) 758-8635
FAX: (501) 758-5369
Direct ProctoFoam HC Inquiries to:
Schwarz Pharma
Professional Services
(800) 558-5114
FAX: (262) 238-0311

CORTANE-B® *Aqueous* Ear Drops — ℞
(chloroxylenol, pramoxine HCl, hydrocortisone)

Each 1 mL contains:

Chloroxylenol	1 mg
Pramoxine HCl	10 mg
Hydrocortisone	10 mg

In a bland *Aqueous* Vehicle

HOW SUPPLIED

Plastic dropper bottles of 10 mL.

CORTANE-B® OTIC — ℞
(chloroxylenol, hydrocortisone, pramoxine HCl)

Each 1 mL contains:

Chloroxylenol	1 mg
Pramoxine HCl	10 mg
Hydrocortisone	10 mg

HOW SUPPLIED

Plastic dropper bottles of 10 mL.

NALEX®-A 12 SUSPENSION — ℞
[*nā-lĕx-ā*]

DESCRIPTION

Each 5 mL raspberry flavored suspension contains:

Phenylephrine Tannate	5 mg
Chlorpheniramine Tannate	2 mg
Pyrilamine Tannate	12.5 mg

HOW SUPPLIED

Bottles of 4 oz.

PROCTOFOAM®-HC — ℞
(hydrocortisone acetate, pramoxine hydrochloride)

Each aerosol container contains:

Hydrocortisone Acetate	1%
Pramoxine Hydrochloride	1%

HOW SUPPLIED

10 g topical aerosol with anal applicator
See Schwarz Pharma for full prescribing information.

RELAGARD® Therapeutic Vaginal Gel — ℞
[*rĕl-ă-gărd*]

DESCRIPTION

Each application contains:

Glacial Acetic Acid	0.9%
Oxyquinoline Sulfate	0.025%

HOW SUPPLIED

50g tube with applicator

Boehringer Ingelheim Pharmaceuticals, Inc.

A subsidiary of Boehringer Ingelheim Corporation
900 RIDGEBURY ROAD
POST OFFICE BOX 368
RIDGEFIELD, CT 06877-0368

For Medical Information Contact:
1-800-542-6257
or email:
druginfo@rdg.boehringer-ingelheim.com

AGGRENOX® — ℞
(aspirin/extended-release dipyridamole)
25 mg/200 mg capsules
Prescribing Information

DESCRIPTION

AGGRENOX® (aspirin/extended-release dipyridamole) is a combination antiplatelet agent intended for oral administration. Each hard gelatin capsule contains 200 mg dipyridamole in an extended-release form and 25 mg aspirin, as an immediate-release sugar-coated tablet. In addition, each capsule contains the following inactive ingredients: acacia, aluminum stearate, colloidal silicon dioxide, corn starch, dimethicone, hydroxypropyl methylcellulose, hydroxypropyl methylcellulose phthalate, lactose monohydrate, methacrylic acid copolymer, microcrystalline cellulose, povidone, stearic acid, sucrose, talc, tartaric acid, titanium dioxide and triacetin.
Each capsule shell contains gelatin, red iron oxide and yellow iron oxide, titanium dioxide and water.

Dipyridamole

Dipyridamole is an antiplatelet agent chemically described as 2,2′,2″,2‴-[(4,8-Dipiperidinopyrimido[5,4-*d*]pyrimidine-2,6-diyl)dinitrilo]-tetraethanol. It has the following structural formula:

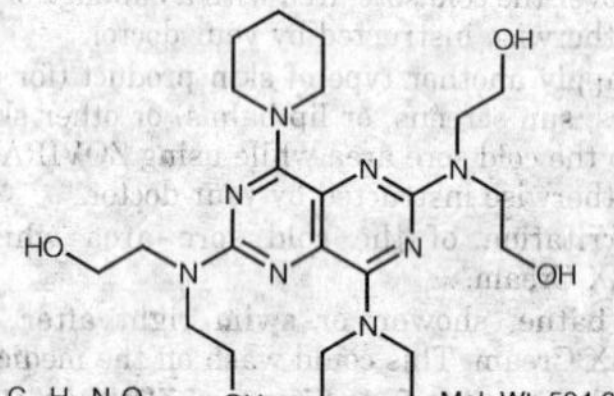

$C_{24}H_{40}N_8O_4$ Mol. Wt. 504.63

Dipyridamole is an odorless yellow crystalline substance, having a bitter taste. It is soluble in dilute acids, methanol and chloroform, and is practically insoluble in water.

Aspirin

The antiplatelet agent aspirin (acetylsalicylic acid) is chemically known as benzoic acid, 2-(acetyloxy)-, and has the following structural formula:

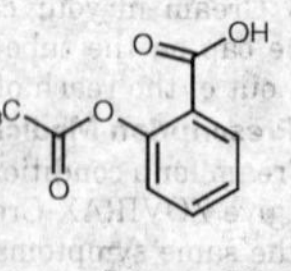

$C_9H_8O_4$ Mol. Wt. 180.16

Aspirin is an odorless white needle-like crystalline or powdery substance. When exposed to moisture, aspirin hydrolyzes into salicylic and acetic acids, and gives off a vinegary odor. It is highly lipid soluble and slightly soluble in water.

CLINICAL PHARMACOLOGY

Mechanism of Action

The antithrombotic action of AGGRENOX (aspirin/extended-release dipyridamole) is the result of the additive antiplatelet effects of dipyridamole and aspirin.

Dipyridamole

Dipyridamole inhibits the uptake of adenosine into platelets, endothelial cells and erythrocytes *in vitro* and *in vivo*; the inhibition occurs in a dose-dependent manner at therapeutic concentrations (0.5–1.9 μg/mL). This inhibition results in an increase in local concentrations of adenosine which acts on the platelet A_2-receptor thereby stimulating platelet adenylate cyclase and increasing platelet cyclic-3′,5′-adenosine monophosphate (cAMP) levels. Via this mechanism, platelet aggregation is inhibited in response to various stimuli such as platelet activating factor (PAF), collagen and adenosine diphosphate (ADP).
Dipyridamole inhibits phosphodiesterase (PDE) in various tissues. While the inhibition of cAMP-PDE is weak, therapeutic levels of dipyridamole inhibit cyclic-3′,5′-guanosine monophosphate-PDE (cGMP-PDE), thereby augmenting the increase in cGMP produced by EDRF (endothelium-derived relaxing factor, now identified as nitric oxide).

Aspirin

Aspirin inhibits platelet aggregation by irreversible inhibition of platelet cyclooxygenase and thus inhibits the generation of thromboxane A_2, a powerful inducer of platelet aggregation and vasoconstriction.

Table 1: Summary of First Stroke (Fatal or Nonfatal): ESPS2: Intent-to-Treat Population

	Total Number of Patients n	Number of Patients With Stroke Within 2 Years n (%)	Kaplan-Meier Estimate of Survival at 2 Years (95% C.I.)	Gehan-Wilcoxon Test P-value	Risk Reduction at 2 Years	Odds Ratio (95% C.I.)
Individual Treatment Group						
AGGRENOX	1650	157 (9.5%)	89.9% (88.4%, 91.4%)	-	-	-
ER-DP	1654	211 (12.8%)	86.7% (85.0%, 88.4%)	-	-	-
ASA	1649	206 (12.5%)	87.1% (85.4%, 88.7%)	-	-	-
Placebo	1649	250 (15.2%)	84.1% (82.2%, 85.9%)	-	-	-
Pairwise Treatment Group Comparisons						
AGGRENOX vs. ER-DP	-	-	-	0.002**	24.4%	0.72 (0.58, 0.90)
AGGRENOX vs. ASA	-	-	-	0.008**	22.1%	0.74 (0.59, 0.92)
AGGRENOX vs. Placebo	-	-	-	<0.001**	36.8%	0.59 (0.48, 0.73)
ER-DP vs. Placebo	-	-	-	0.036*	16.5%	0.82 (0.67, 1.00)
ASA vs. Placebo	-	-	-	0.009**	18.9%	0.80 (0.66, 0.97)

*0.010 < p-value ≤0.050; **p-value ≤0.010.
Note: ER-DP = extended-release dipyridamole 200 mg; ASA = aspirin 25 mg. The dosage regimen for all treatment groups is b.i.d.

Pharmacokinetics
There are no significant interactions between aspirin and dipyridamole. The kinetics of the components are unchanged by their co-administration as AGGRENOX.

Dipyridamole
Absorption: Peak plasma levels of dipyridamole are achieved 2 hours (range 1–6 hours) after administration of a daily dose of 400 mg AGGRENOX (given as 200 mg b.i.d.). The peak plasma concentration at steady-state is 1.98 µg/mL (1.01–3.99 µg/mL) and the steady-state trough concentration is 0.53 µg/mL (0.18–1.01 µg/mL).
Effect of Food: When AGGRENOX capsules were taken with a high fat meal, dipyridamole peak plasma levels (C_{max}) and total absorption (AUC) were decreased at steady-state by 20–30% compared to fasting. Due to the similar degree of inhibition of adenosine uptake at these plasma concentrations, this food effect is not considered clinically relevant.
Distribution: Dipyridamole is highly lipophilic (log P=3.71, pH=7); however, it has been shown that the drug does not cross the blood-brain barrier to any significant extent in animals. The steady-state volume of distribution of dipyridamole is about 92 L. Approximately 99% of dipyridamole is bound to plasma proteins, predominantly to alpha 1-acid glycoprotein and albumin.
Metabolism and Elimination: Dipyridamole is metabolized in the liver, primarily by conjugation with glucuronic acid, of which monoglucuronide which has low pharmacodynamic activity is the primary metabolite. In plasma, about 80% of the total amount is present as parent compound and 20% as monoglucuronide. Most of the glucuronide metabolite (about 95%) is excreted via bile into the feces, with some evidence of enterohepatic circulation. Renal excretion of parent compound is negligible and urinary excretion of the glucuronide metabolite is low (about 5%). With intravenous (i.v.) treatment of dipyridamole, a triphasic profile is obtained: a rapid alpha phase, with a half-life of about 3.4 minutes, a beta phase, with a half-life of about 39 minutes, (which, together with the alpha phase accounts for about 70% of the total area under the curve, AUC) and a prolonged elimination phase λ_z with a half-life of about 15.5 hours. Due to the extended absorption phase of the dipyridamole component, only the terminal phase is apparent from oral treatment with AGGRENOX which, in trial 9.123 was 13.6 hours.
Special Populations:
Geriatric Patients: In ESPS2 (See **CLINICAL PHARMACOLOGY, Clinical Trials**), plasma concentrations (determined as AUC) of dipyridamole in healthy elderly subjects (>65 years) were about 40% higher than in subjects younger than 55 years receiving treatment with AGGRENOX.
Hepatic Dysfunction: No study has been conducted with the AGGRENOX formulation in patients with hepatic dysfunction.
In a study conducted with an intravenous formulation of dipyridamole, patients with mild to severe hepatic insufficiency showed no change in plasma concentrations of dipyridamole but showed an increase in the pharmacologically inactive monoglucuronide metabolite. Dipyridamole can be dosed without restriction as long as there is no evidence of hepatic failure.
Renal Dysfunction: No study has been conducted with the AGGRENOX formulation in patients with renal dysfunction.
In ESPS2 patients (See **CLINICAL PHARMACOLOGY, Clinical Trials**), with creatinine clearances ranging from about 15 mL/min to >100 mL/min, no changes were observed in the pharmacokinetics of dipyridamole or its glucuronide metabolite if data were corrected for differences in age.

Aspirin
Absorption: Peak plasma levels of aspirin are achieved 0.63 hours (0.5–1 hour) after administration of a 50 mg aspirin daily dose from AGGRENOX (given as 25 mg b.i.d.). The peak plasma concentration at steady-state is 319 ng/mL (175–463 ng/mL). Aspirin undergoes moderate hydrolysis to salicylic acid in the liver and the gastrointestinal wall, with 50%–75% of an administered dose reaching the systemic circulation as intact aspirin.
Effect of Food: When AGGRENOX capsules were taken with a high fat meal, there was no difference for aspirin in AUC at steady-state, and the approximately 50% decrease in C_{max} was not considered clinically relevant based on a similar degree of cyclooxygenase inhibition comparing the fed and fasted state.
Distribution: Aspirin is poorly bound to plasma proteins and its apparent volume of distribution is low (10 L). Its metabolite, salicylic acid, is highly bound to plasma proteins, but its binding is concentration-dependent (nonlinear). At low concentrations (<100 µg/mL), approximately 90% of salicylic acid is bound to albumin. Salicylic acid is widely distributed to all tissues and fluids in the body, including the central nervous system, breast milk, and fetal tissues. Early signs of salicylate overdose (salicylism), including tinnitus (ringing in the ears), occur at plasma concentrations approximating 200 µg/mL (See **ADVERSE REACTIONS; OVERDOSAGE**).
Metabolism and Elimination: Aspirin is rapidly hydrolyzed in plasma to salicylic acid, with a half-life of 20 minutes. Plasma levels of aspirin are essentially undetectable 2–2.5 hours after dosing and peak salicylic acid concentrations occur 1 hour (range: 0.5–2 hours) after administration of aspirin. Salicylic acid is primarily conjugated in the liver to form salicyluric acid, a phenolic glucuronide, an acyl glucuronide, and a number of minor metabolites. Salicylate metabolism is saturable and total body clearance decreases at higher serum concentrations due to the limited ability of the liver to form both salicyluric acid and phenolic glucuronide. Following toxic doses (10–20 g), the plasma half-life may be increased to over 20 hours.
The elimination of acetylsalicylic acid follows first-order kinetics with AGGRENOX and has a half-life of 0.33 hours. The half-life of salicylic acid is 1.71 hours. Both values correspond well with data from the literature at lower doses which state a resultant half-life of approximately 2–3 hours. At higher doses, the elimination of salicylic acid follows zero-order kinetics (i.e., the rate of elimination is constant in relation to plasma concentration), with an apparent half-life of 6 hours or higher. Renal excretion of unchanged drug depends upon urinary pH. As urinary pH rises above 6.5, the renal clearance of free salicylate increases from <5% to >80%. Alkalinization of the urine is a key concept in the management of salicylate overdose (See **OVERDOSAGE**). Following therapeutic doses, about 10% is excreted as salicylic acid and 75% as salicyluric acid, as the phenolic and acyl glucuronides, in urine.
Special Populations:
Hepatic Dysfunction: Aspirin is to be avoided in patients with severe hepatic insufficiency.
Renal Dysfunction: Aspirin is to be avoided in patients with severe renal failure (glomerular filtration rate less than 10 mL/min).

Clinical Trials
AGGRENOX® was studied in a double-blind, placebo-controlled, 24-month study (European Stroke Prevention Study 2, ESPS2) in which 6602 patients had an ischemic stroke (76%) or transient ischemic attack (TIA, 24%) within three months prior to entry. Patients were randomized to one of four treatment groups: AGGRENOX (aspirin/extended-release dipyridamole) 25 mg/200 mg; extended-release dipyridamole (ER-DP) 200 mg alone; aspirin (ASA) 25 mg alone; or placebo. Patients received one capsule twice daily (morning and evening). Efficacy assessments included analyses of stroke (fatal or nonfatal) and death (from all causes) as confirmed by a blinded morbidity and mortality assessment group.
Stroke Endpoint:
AGGRENOX reduced the risk of stroke by 22.1% compared to aspirin 50 mg/day alone (p =0.008) and reduced the risk of stroke by 24.4% compared to extended-release dipyridamole 400 mg/day alone (p = 0.002) (Table 1). AGGRENOX reduced the risk of stroke by 36.8% compared to placebo (p <0.001).
[See table 1 above]

ESPS2: Cumulative Stroke Rate (Fatal or Nonfatal) Over 24 Months Of Follow-Up

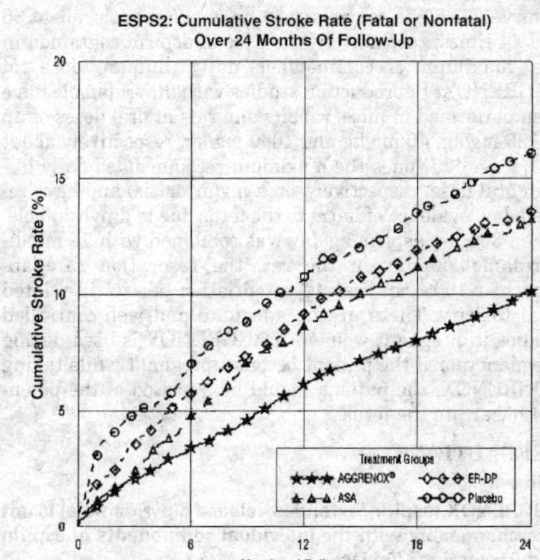

Note: ER-DP - extended-release dipyridamole 200 mg; ASA - aspirin 25 mg.
Note: The dosage regimen for all treatment groups is b.i.d.

Combined Stroke or Death Endpoint
In ESPS2, AGGRENOX reduced the risk of stroke or death by 12.1% compared to aspirin alone and by 10.3% compared to extended-release dipyridamole alone. These results were not statistically significant. AGGRENOX reduced the risk of stroke or death by 24.2% compared to placebo.
Death Endpoint
The incidence rate of all cause mortality was 11.3% for AGGRENOX, 11.0% for aspirin alone, 11.4% for extended-release dipyridamole alone and 12.3% for placebo alone. The differences between the AGGRENOX, aspirin alone and extended-release dipyridamole alone treatment groups were not statistically significant. These incidence rates for AGGRENOX and aspirin alone are consistent with previous aspirin studies in stroke and TIA patients.

INDICATIONS AND USAGE
AGGRENOX (aspirin/extended-release dipyridamole) is indicated to reduce the risk of stroke in patients who have had transient ischemia of the brain or completed ischemic stroke due to thrombosis.

CONTRAINDICATIONS
AGGRENOX (aspirin/extended-release dipyridamole) is contraindicated in patients with hypersensitivity to dipyridamole, aspirin or any of the other product components.
Allergy: Aspirin is contraindicated in patients with known allergy to nonsteroidal anti-inflammatory drug products and in patients with the syndrome of asthma, rhinitis, and nasal polyps. Aspirin may cause severe urticaria, angioedema or bronchospasm (asthma).
Reye's Syndrome: Aspirin should not be used in children or teenagers for viral infections, with or without fever, because of the risk of Reye's syndrome with concomitant use of aspirin in certain viral illnesses.

Continued on next page

Aggrenox—Cont.

WARNINGS

Alcohol Warning: Patients who consume three or more alcoholic drinks every day should be counseled about the bleeding risks involved with chronic, heavy alcohol use while taking aspirin.

Coagulation Abnormalities: Even low doses of aspirin can inhibit platelet function leading to an increase in bleeding time. This can adversely affect patients with inherited or acquired (liver disease or vitamin K deficiency) bleeding disorders.

Gastrointestinal (GI) Side Effects: GI side effects include stomach pain, heartburn, nausea, vomiting, and gross GI bleeding. Although minor upper GI symptoms, such as dyspepsia, are common and can occur anytime during therapy, physicians should remain alert for signs of ulceration and bleeding, even in the absence of previous GI symptoms. Physicians should inform patients about the signs and symptoms of GI side effects and what steps to take if they occur.

Peptic Ulcer Disease: Patients with a history of active peptic ulcer disease should avoid using aspirin, which can cause gastric mucosal irritation, and bleeding.

Pregnancy: AGGRENOX can cause fetal harm when administered to a pregnant woman. Maternal aspirin use during later stages of pregnancy may cause low birth weight, increased incidence for intracranial hemorrhage in premature infants, stillbirths and neonatal death. Because of the above and because of the known effects of nonsteroidal anti-inflammatory drugs (NSAIDs) on the fetal cardiovascular system (closure of the ductus arteriosus), AGGRENOX should be avoided in the third trimester of pregnancy.

Aspirin has been shown to be teratogenic in rats (spina bifida, exencephaly, microphthalmia and coelosomia) and rabbits (congested fetuses, agenesis of skull and upper jaw, generalized edema with malformation of the head, and diaphanous skin) at oral doses of 330 mg/kg/day and 110 mg/kg/day, respectively. These doses, which also resulted in a high resorption rate in rats (63% of implantations versus 5% in controls), are, on a mg/m^2 basis, about 66 and 44 times, respectively, the dose of aspirin contained in the maximum recommended daily human dose of AGGRENOX. Reproduction studies with dipyridamole have been performed in mice, rabbits and rats at oral doses of up to 125 mg/kg, 40 mg/kg and 1000 mg/kg, respectively about 1 ½, 2 and 25 times the maximum recommended daily human oral dose, respectively, on a mg/m^2 basis) and have revealed no evidence of harm to the fetus due to dipyridamole. When 330 mg aspirin/kg/day was combined with 75 mg dipyridamole/kg/day in the rat, the resorption rate approached 100%, indicating potentiation of aspirin-related fetal toxicity. There are no adequate and well-controlled studies in pregnant women. If AGGRENOX is used during pregnancy, or if the patient becomes pregnant while taking AGGRENOX, the patient should be apprised of the potential hazard to the fetus.

PRECAUTIONS

General

AGGRENOX (aspirin/extended-release dipyridamole) is not interchangeable with the individual components of aspirin and Persantine® Tablets.

Coronary Artery Disease: Dipyridamole has a vasodilatory effect and should be used with caution in patients with severe coronary artery disease (e.g., unstable angina or recently sustained myocardial infarction). Chest pain may be aggravated in patients with underlying coronary artery disease who are receiving dipyridamole.

For stroke or TIA patients for whom aspirin is indicated to prevent recurrent myocardial infarction (MI) or angina pectoris, the aspirin in this product may not provide adequate treatment for the cardiac indications.

Hepatic Insufficiency: Elevations of hepatic enzymes and hepatic failure have been reported in association with dipyridamole administration.

Hypotension: Dipyridamole should be used with caution in patients with hypotension since it can produce peripheral vasodilation.

Renal Failure: Avoid aspirin in patients with severe renal failure (glomerular filtration rate less than 10 mL/minute).

Risk of Bleeding: In ESPS2 the incidence of gastrointestinal bleeding was 68 patients (4.1%) in the AGGRENOX group, 36 patients (2.2%) in the extended-release dipyridamole group, 52 patients (3.2%) in the aspirin group, and 34 patients (2.1%) in the placebo groups.

The incidence of intracranial hemorrhage was 9 patients (0.6%) in the AGGRENOX group, 6 patients (0.5%) in the extended-release dipyridamole group, 6 patients (0.4%) in the aspirin group and 7 patients (0.4%) in the placebo groups.

Laboratory Tests

Aspirin has been associated with elevated hepatic enzymes, blood urea nitrogen and serum creatinine, hyperkalemia, proteinuria and prolonged bleeding time.

Dipyridamole has been associated with elevated hepatic enzymes.

Drug Interactions

No pharmacokinetic drug-drug interaction studies were conducted with the AGGRENOX formulation. The following information was obtained from the literature.

Table 2: Incidence of Adverse Events in ESPS2*

Body System/Preferred Term	Indivdual Treatment Group			
	AGGRENOX	**ER-DP Alone**	**ASA Alone**	**Placebo**
Total Number of Patients	1650	1654	1649	1649
Total Number (%) of Patients With at Least One On-Treatment Adverse Event	1319 (79.9%)	1305 (78.9%)	1323 (80.2%)	1304 (79.1%)
Central & Peripheral Nervous System Disorders				
Headache	647 (39.2%)	634 (38.3%)	558 (33.8%)	543 (32.9%)
Convulsions	28 (1.7%)	15 (0.9%)	28 (1.7%)	26 (1.6%)
Gastro-Intestinal System Disorders				
Dyspepsia	303 (18.4%)	288 (17.4%)	299 (18.1%)	275 (16.7%)
Abdominal Pain	289 (17.5%)	255 (15.4%)	262 (15.9%)	239 (14.5%)
Nausea	264 (16.0%)	254 (15.4%)	210 (12.7%)	232 (14.1%)
Diarrhea	210 (12.7%)	257 (15.5%)	112 (6.8%)	161 (9.8%)
Vomiting	138 (8.4%)	129 (7.8%)	101 (6.1%)	118 (7.2%)
Hemorrhage Rectum	26 (1.6%)	22 (1.3%)	16 (1.0%)	13 (0.8%)
Melena	31 (1.9%)	10 (0.6%)	20 (1.2%)	13 (0.8%)
Hemorrhoids	16 (1.0%)	13 (0.8%)	10 (0.6%)	10 (0.6%)
GI Hemorrhage	20 (1.2%)	5 (0.3%)	15 (0.9%)	7 (0.4%)
Body as a Whole - General Disorders				
Pain	105 (6.4%)	88 (5.3%)	103 (6.2%)	99 (6.0%)
Fatigue	95 (5.8%)	93 (5.6%)	97 (5.9%)	90 (5.5%)
Back Pain	76 (4.6%)	77 (4.7%)	74 (4.5%)	65 (3.9%)
Accidental Injury	42 (2.5%)	24 (1.5%)	51 (3.1%)	37 (2.2%)
Malaise	27 (1.6%)	23 (1.4%)	26 (1.6%)	22 (1.3%)
Asthenia	29 (1.8%)	19 (1.1%)	17 (1.0%)	18 (1.1%)
Syncope	17 (1.0%)	13 (0.8%)	16 (1.0%)	8 (0.5%)
Psychiatric Disorders				
Amnesia	39 (2.4%)	40 (2.4%)	57 (3.5%)	34 (2.1%)
Confusion	18 (1.1%)	9 (0.5%)	22 (1.3%)	15 (0.9%)
Anorexia	19 (1.2%)	17 (1.0%)	10 (0.6%)	15 (0.9%)
Somnolence	20 (1.2%)	13 (0.8%)	18 (1.1%)	9 (0.5%)
Musculoskeletal System Disorders				
Arthralgia	91 (5.5%)	75 (4.5%)	91 (5.5%)	76 (4.6%)
Arthritis	34 (2.1%)	25 (1.5%)	17 (1.0%)	19 (1.2%)
Arthrosis	18 (1.1%)	22 (1.3%)	13 (0.8%)	14 (0.8%)
Myalgia	20 (1.2%)	16 (1.0%)	11 (0.7%)	11 (0.7%)
Respiratory System Disorders				
Coughing	25 (1.5%)	18 (1.1%)	32 (1.9%)	21 (1.3%)
Upper Respiratory Tract Infection	16 (1.0%)	9 (0.5%)	16 (1.0%)	14 (0.8%)
Cardiovascular Disorders, General				
Cardiac Failure	26 (1.6%)	17 (1.0%)	30 (1.8%)	25 (1.5%)
Platelet, Bleeding & Clotting Disorders				
Hemorrhage NOS	52 (3.2%)	24 (1.5%)	46 (2.8%)	24 (1.5%)
Epistaxis	39 (2.4%)	16 (1.0%)	45 (2.7%)	25 (1.5%)
Purpura	23 (1.4%)	8 (0.5%)	9 (0.5%)	7 (0.4%)
Neoplasm				
Neoplasm NOS	28 (1.7%)	16 (1.0%)	23 (1.4%)	20 (1.2%)
Red Blood Cell Disorders				
Anemia	27 (1.6%)	16 (1.0%)	19 (1.2%)	9 (0.5%)

*Reported by ≥1% of patients during AGGRENOX treatment where the incidence was greater than in those treated with placebo.

Note: ER-DP = extended-release dipyridamole 200 mg; ASA = aspirin 25 mg. The dosage regimen for all treatment groups is b.i.d. NOS = not otherwise specified.

Adenosine: Dipyridamole has been reported to increase the plasma levels and cardiovascular effects of adenosine. Adjustment of adenosine dosage may be necessary.

Angiotensin Converting Enzyme (ACE) Inhibitors: Due to the indirect effect of aspirin on the renin-angiotensin conversion pathway, the hyponatremic and hypotensive effects of ACE inhibitors may be diminished by concomitant administration of aspirin.

Acetazolamide: Concurrent use of aspirin and acetazolamide can lead to high serum concentrations of acetazolamide (and toxicity) due to competition at the renal tubule for secretion.

Anticoagulant Therapy (heparin and warfarin): Patients on anticoagulation therapy are at increased risk for bleeding because of drug-drug interactions and effects on platelets. Aspirin can displace warfarin from protein binding sites, leading to prolongation of both the prothrombin time and the bleeding time. Aspirin can increase the anticoagulant activity of heparin, increasing bleeding risk.

Anticonvulsants: Salicylic acid can displace protein-bound phenytoin and valproic acid, leading to a decrease in the total concentration of phenytoin and an increase in serum valproic acid levels.

Beta Blockers: The hypotensive effects of beta blockers may be diminished by the concomitant administration of aspirin due to inhibition of renal prostaglandins, leading to decreased renal blood flow and salt and fluid retention.

Cholinesterase Inhibitors: Dipyridamole may counteract

the anticholinesterase effect of cholinesterase inhibitors, thereby potentially aggravating myasthenia gravis.
Diuretics: The effectiveness of diuretics in patients with underlying renal or cardiovascular disease may be diminished by the concomitant administration of aspirin due to inhibition of renal prostaglandins, leading to decreased renal blood flow and salt and fluid retention.
Methotrexate: Salicylate can inhibit renal clearance of methotrexate, leading to bone marrow toxicity, especially in the elderly or renal impaired.
Nonsteroidal Anti-Inflammatory Drugs (NSAIDs): The concurrent use of aspirin with other NSAIDs may increase bleeding or lead to decreased renal function.
Oral Hypoglycemics: Moderate doses of aspirin may increase the effectiveness of oral hypoglycemic drugs, leading to hypoglycemia.
Uricosuric Agents (probenecid and sulfinpyrazone): Salicylates antagonize the uricosuric action of uricosuric agents.

Carcinogenesis, Mutagenesis, Impairment of Fertility
In studies in which dipyridamole was administered in the feed to mice (up to 111 weeks in males and females) and rats (up to 128 weeks in males and up to 142 weeks in females), there was no evidence of drug-related carcinogenesis. The highest dose administered in these studies (75 mg/kg/day) was, on a mg/m^2 basis, about equivalent to the maximum recommended daily human oral dose (MRHD) in mice and about twice the MRHD in rats.
Combinations of dipyridamole and aspirin (1:5 ratio) tested negative in the Ames test, *in vivo* chromosome aberration tests (in mice and hamsters), oral micronucleus tests (in mice and hamsters) and oral dominant lethal test (in mice). Aspirin, alone, induced chromosome aberrations in cultured human fibroblasts. Mutagenicity tests of dipyridamole alone with bacterial and mammalian cell systems were negative.
Combinations of dipyridamole and aspirin have not been evaluated for effects on fertility and reproductive performance. There was no evidence of impaired fertility when dipyridamole was administered to male and female rats at oral doses up to 500 mg/kg/day (about 12 times the MRHD on a mg/m^2 basis). A significant reduction in number of corpora lutea with consequent reduction in implantations and live fetuses was, however, observed at 1250 mg/kg (more than 30 times the MRHD on a mg/m^2 basis). Aspirin inhibits ovulation in rats.

Pregnancy
Teratogenic Effects: PREGNANCY CATEGORY D. See **WARNINGS**

Labor and Delivery
Aspirin can result in excessive blood loss at delivery as well as prolonged gestation and prolonged labor. Because of these effects on the mother and because of adverse fetal effects seen with aspirin during the later stages of pregnancy (see **WARNINGS/Pregnancy** subsection), AGGRENOX should be avoided in the third trimester of pregnancy and during labor and delivery.

Nursing Mothers
Both dipyridamole and aspirin are excreted in human milk. Caution should be exercised when AGGRENOX is administered to a nursing woman.

Pediatric Use
Safety and effectiveness of AGGRENOX in pediatric patients have not been studied. Due to the aspirin component, use of this product in the pediatric population is not recommended (See **CONTRAINDICATIONS**).

ADVERSE REACTIONS

A 24-month, multicenter, double-blind, randomized study (ESPS2) was conducted to compare the efficacy and safety of AGGRENOX (aspirin/extended-release dipyridamole) with placebo, extended-release dipyridamole alone and aspirin alone. The study was conducted in a total of 6602 male and female patients who had experienced a previous ischemic stroke or transient ischemia of the brain within three months prior to randomization.
Table 2 presents the incidence of adverse events that occurred in 1% or more of patients treated with AGGRENOX where the incidence was also greater than in those patients treated with placebo. There is no clear benefit of the dipyridamole/aspirin combination over aspirin with respect to safety.
[See table 2 at top of previous page]
Discontinuation due to adverse events in ESPS2 was 25% for AGGRENOX, 25% for extended-release dipyridamole, 19% for aspirin, and 21% for placebo (refer to Table 3).
[See table 3 above]

Table 3: Incidence of Adverse Events that Led to the Discontinuation of Treatment: Adverse Events with an Incidence of ≥1% in the AGGRENOX group

	Treatment Groups			
	AGGRENOX®	ER-DP	ASA	Placebo
Total Number of Patients	1650	1654	1649	1649
Patients with at least one Adverse Event that led to treatment discontinuation	417 (25%)	419 (25%)	318 (19%)	352 (21%)
Headache	165 (10%)	166 (10%)	57 (3%)	69 (4%)
Dizziness	85 (5%)	97 (6%)	69 (4%)	68 (4%)
Nausea	91 (6%)	95 (6%)	51 (3%)	53 (3%)
Abdominal Pain	74 (4%)	64 (4%)	56 (3%)	52 (3%)
Dyspepsia	59 (4%)	61 (4%)	49 (3%)	46 (3%)
Vomiting	53 (3%)	52 (3%)	28 (2%)	24 (1%)
Diarrhea	35 (2%)	41 (2%)	9 (<1%)	16 (<1%)
Stroke	39 (2%)	48 (3%)	57 (3%)	73 (4%)
Transient Ischemic Attack	35 (2%)	40 (2%)	26 (2%)	48 (3%)
Angina Pectoris	23 (1%)	20 (1%)	16 (<1%)	26 (2%)

Note: ER-DP = extended-release dipyridamole 200 mg; ASA = aspirin 25 mg. The dosage regimen for all treatment groups is b.i.d.

Other adverse events:
Adverse reactions that occurred in less than 1% of patients treated with AGGRENOX in the ESPS2 study and that were medically judged to be possibly related to either dipyridamole or aspirin are listed below (See **WARNINGS**). *Body as a Whole:* Allergic reaction, fever. *Cardiovascular:* Hypotension. *Central Nervous System:* Coma, dizziness, paresthesia, cerebral hemorrhage, intracranial hemorrhage, subarachnoid hemorrhage. *Gastrointestinal:* Gastritis, ulceration and perforation. *Hearing & Vestibular Disorders:* Tinnitus, and deafness. Patients with high frequency hearing loss may have difficulty perceiving tinnitus. In these patients, tinnitus cannot be used as a clinical indicator of salicylism. *Heart Rate and Rhythm Disorders:* Tachycardia, palpitation, arrhythmia, supraventricular tachycardia. *Liver and Biliary System Disorders:* Cholelithiasis, jaundice, hepatic function abnormal. *Metabolic & Nutritional Disorders:* Hyperglycemia, thirst. *Platelet, Bleeding and Clotting Disorders:* Hematoma, gingival bleeding. *Psychiatric Disorders:* Agitation. *Reproductive:* Uterine hemorrhage. *Respiratory:* Hyperpnea, asthma, bronchospasm, hemoptysis, pulmonary edema. *Special Senses Other Disorders:* Taste loss. *Skin and Appendages Disorders:* Pruritus, urticaria. *Urogenital:* Renal insufficiency and failure, hematuria. *Vascular (Extracardiac) Disorders:* Flushing.
The following is a list of additional adverse reactions that have been reported either in the literature or are from postmarketing spontaneous reports for either dipyridamole or aspirin. *Body as a Whole:* Hypothermia, chest pain. *Cardiovascular:* Angina pectoris. *Central Nervous System:* Cerebral edema. *Fluid and Electrolyte:* Hyperkalemia, metabolic acidosis, respiratory alkalosis, hypokalemia. *Gastrointestinal:* Pancreatitis, Reye's syndrome, hematemesis. *Hearing and Vestibular Disorders:* Hearing loss. *Hypersensitivity:* Acute anaphylaxis, laryngeal edema. *Liver and Biliary System Disorders:* Hepatitis, hepatic failure. *Musculoskeletal:* Rhabdomyolysis. *Metabolic & Nutritional Disorders:* Hypoglycemia, dehydration. *Platelet, Bleeding and Clotting Disorders:* Prolongation of the prothrombin time, disseminated intravascular coagulation, coagulopathy, thrombocytopenia. *Reproductive:* Prolonged pregnancy and labor, stillbirths, lower birth weight infants, antepartum and postpartum bleeding. *Respiratory:* Tachypnea, dyspnea. *Skin and Appendages Disorders:* Rash, alopecia, angioedema, Stevens-Johnson syndrome. *Urogenital:* Interstitial nephritis, papillary necrosis, proteinuria. *Vascular (Extracardiac Disorders):* Allergic vasculitis.
The following is a list of additional adverse events that have been reported either in the literature or are from postmarketing spontaneous reports for either dipyridamole or aspirin. The causal relationship of these adverse events has not been established: anorexia, aplastic anemia, pancytopenia, thrombocytosis.

Laboratory Changes
Over the course of the 24-month study (ESPS2), patients treated with AGGRENOX showed a decline (mean change from baseline) in hemoglobin of 0.25 g/dL, hematocrit of 0.75%, and erythrocyte count of 0.13×10^6/mm^3.

OVERDOSAGE

Because of the dose ratio of dipyridamole to aspirin, overdosage of AGGRENOX (aspirin/extended-release dipyridamole) is likely to be dominated by signs and symptoms of dipyridamole overdose. In case of real or suspected overdose, seek medical attention or contact a Poison Control Center immediately. Careful medical management is essential.

Dipyridamole
Based upon the known hemodynamic effects of dipyridamole, symptoms such as warm feeling, flushes, sweating, restlessness, feeling of weakness and dizziness may occur. A drop in blood pressure and tachycardia might also be observed.
Symptomatic treatment is recommended, possibly including a vasopressor drug. Gastric lavage should be considered. Administration of xanthine derivatives (e.g. aminophylline) may reverse the hemodynamic effects of dipyridamole overdose. Since dipyridamole is highly protein bound, dialysis is not likely to be of benefit.

Aspirin
Salicylate toxicity may result from acute ingestion (overdose) or chronic intoxication. The early signs of salicylic overdose (salicylism), including tinnitus (ringing in the ears), occur at plasma concentrations approaching 200 μg/mL. Plasma concentrations of aspirin above 300 μg/mL are clearly toxic. Severe toxic effects are associated with levels above 400 μg/mL. A single lethal dose of aspirin in adults is not known with certainty but death may be expected at 30 g.
Treatment consists primarily of supporting vital functions, increasing salicylate elimination, and correcting the acid-base disturbance. Gastric emptying and/or lavage are recommended as soon as possible after ingestion, even if the patient has vomited spontaneously. After lavage and/or emesis, administration of activated charcoal, as a slurry, is beneficial, if less than 3 hours have passed since ingestion. Charcoal absorption should not be employed prior to emesis and lavage.
Severity of aspirin intoxication is determined by measuring the blood salicylate level. Acid-base status should be closely followed with serial blood gas and serum pH measurements. Fluid and electrolyte balance should also be maintained.
In severe cases, hyperthermia and hypovolemia are the major immediate threats to life. Children should be sponged with tepid water. Replacement fluid should be administered intravenously and augmented with correction of acidosis. Plasma electrolytes and pH should be monitored to promote alkaline diuresis of salicylate if renal function is normal. Infusion of glucose may be required to control hypoglycemia. Hemodialysis and peritoneal dialysis can be performed to reduce the body drug content. In patients with renal insufficiency or in cases of life-threatening intoxication, dialysis is usually required. Exchange transfusion may be indicated in infants and young children.

DOSAGE AND ADMINISTRATION

The recommended dose of AGGRENOX (aspirin/extended-release dipyridamole) is one capsule given orally twice daily, one in the morning and one in the evening. The capsules should be swallowed whole without chewing. AGGRENOX capsules may be administered with or without food.
AGGRENOX is not interchangeable with the individual components of aspirin and Persantine® Tablets.

HOW SUPPLIED

AGGRENOX (aspirin/extended-release dipyridamole) is available as a hard gelatin capsule, with a red cap and an ivory-colored body, 24.0 mm in length, containing yellow extended-release pellets incorporating dipyridamole and a round white tablet incorporating immediate-release aspirin. The capsule body is imprinted in red with the Boehringer Ingelheim logo and with "01A".
AGGRENOX is supplied in unit-of-use bottles of 60 capsules (NDC 0597-0001-60).
Store at 25°C (77°F); excursions permitted to 15-30°C (59-86°F) [see USP Controlled Room Temperature]. Protect from excessive moisture.
℞ only
Marketed by: Boehringer Ingelheim Pharmaceuticals Inc., Ridgefield, CT 06877 USA
Manufactured by: Boehringer Ingelheim Pharma GmbH & Co KG, Biberach, Germany
Licensed from: Boehringer Ingelheim International GmbH

Patent No. 6,015,577
Revised:05/08/03
42633/US/4
Shown in Product Identification Guide, page 309

Continued on next page

ALUPENT® ℞

[al' u-pent]

(metaproterenol sulfate USP)
Inhalation Aerosol
Bronchodilator
100 and 200 Inhalations

Prescribing Information

DESCRIPTION

Alupent® (metaproterenol sulfate USP) Inhalation Aerosol is a bronchodilator administered by oral inhalation. The Alupent Inhalation Aerosol containing 75 mg of metaproterenol sulfate as micronized powder is sufficient medication for 100 inhalations. The Alupent Inhalation Aerosol containing 150 mg of metaproterenol sulfate as micronized powder is sufficient medication for 200 inhalations. Each metered dose delivers through the mouthpiece 0.65 mg of metaproterenol sulfate (each ml contains 15 mg). The inert ingredients are dichlorodifluoromethane, dichlorotetrafluoroethane and trichloromonofluoromethane as propellants, and sorbitan trioleate.

Alupent, 1-(3,5-dihydroxyphenyl)-2-isopropylaminoethanol sulfate, is a white, crystalline, racemic mixture of two optically active isomers. It has the following chemical structure:

metaproterenol sulfate (Alupent)
$(C_{11}H_{17}NO_3)_2 \cdot H_2SO_4$
Mol. Wt. 520.59

CLINICAL PHARMACOLOGY

In vitro studies and *in vivo* pharmacologic studies have demonstrated that Alupent® (metaproterenol sulfate USP) has a preferential effect on beta-2 adrenergic receptors compared with isoproterenol. While it is recognized that beta-2 adrenergic receptors are the predominant receptors in bronchial smooth muscle, recent data indicate that there is a population of beta-2 receptors in the human heart existing in a concentration between 10–50%. The precise function of these, however, is not yet established (see WARNINGS section).

The pharmacologic effects of beta adrenergic agonist drugs, including Alupent, are at least in part attributable to stimulation through beta adrenergic receptors of intracellular adenyl cyclase, the enzyme which catalyzes the conversion of adenosine triphosphate (ATP) to cyclic-3',5'-adenosine monophosphate (c-AMP). Increased c-AMP levels are associated with relaxation of bronchial smooth muscle and inhibition of release of mediators of immediate hypersensitivity from cells, especially from mast cells.

Pharmacokinetics Absorption, biotransformation and excretion studies in humans following administration by inhalation have shown that approximately 3 percent of the actuated dose is absorbed intact through the lungs. The major metabolite, metaproterenol-3-0-sulfate, is produced in the gastrointestinal tract. Alupent is not metabolized by catechol-0-methyltransferase nor have glucuronide conjugates been isolated to date.

Pulmonary function tests performed concomitantly usually show improvement following aerosol Alupent administration, e.g. an increase in the one-second forced expiratory volume (FEV_1), maximum expiratory flow rate, forced vital capacity, and/or a decrease in airway resistance. The resultant decrease in airway obstruction may relieve the dyspnea associated with bronchospasm.

Controlled single- and multiple-dose studies have been performed with pulmonary function monitoring. The duration of effect of a single dose of two to three inhalations of Alupent (that is, the period of time during which there is a 20 percent or greater increase in FEV_1) has varied from 1 to 5 hours.

In repetitive-dosing studies (up to q.i.d.) the duration of effect for a similar dose of Alupent has ranged from about 1 to 2.5 hours. Present studies are inadequate to explain the divergence in duration of the FEV_1 effect between single- and repetitive-dosing studies, respectively.

Recent studies in laboratory animals (minipigs, rodents and dogs) recorded the occurrence of cardiac arrhythmias and sudden death (with histologic evidence of myocardial necrosis) when beta agonists and methylxanthines were administered concurrently. The significance of these findings when applied to humans is currently unknown.

INDICATIONS AND USAGE

Alupent® (metaproterenol sulfate USP) is indicated as a bronchodilator for bronchial asthma and for reversible bronchospasm which may occur in association with bronchitis and emphysema.

CONTRAINDICATIONS

Use in patients with cardiac arrhythmias associated with tachycardia is contraindicated.

Although rare, immediate hypersensitivity reactions can occur. Therefore, Alupent® (metaproterenol sulfate USP) Inhalation Aerosol is contraindicated in patients with a history of hypersensitivity to any of its components.

WARNINGS

Fatalities have been reported following excessive use of Alupent® (metaproterenol sulfate USP) as with other sympathomimetic inhalation preparations, and the exact cause is unknown. Cardiac arrest was noted in several cases.

Alupent, like other beta adrenergic agonists, can produce a significant cardiovascular effect in some patients, as measured by pulse rate, blood pressure, symptoms, and/or ECG changes. As with other beta adrenergic aerosols, Alupent can produce paradoxical bronchospasm (which can be life threatening). If it occurs, the preparation should be discontinued immediately and alternative therapy instituted.

Alupent should not be used more often than prescribed. Patients should be advised to contact their physician in the event that they do not respond to their usual dose of a sympathomimetic amine aerosol.

PRECAUTIONS

General Extreme care must be exercised with respect to the administration of additional sympathomimetic agents. Since metaproterenol is a sympathomimetic amine, it should be used with caution in patients with cardiovascular disorders, including ischemic heart disease, hypertension or cardiac arrhythmias, in patients with hyperthyroidism or diabetes mellitus, and in patients who are unusually responsive to sympathomimetic amines or who have convulsive disorders. Significant changes in systolic and diastolic blood pressure could be expected to occur in some patients after use of any beta adrenergic bronchodilator.

Information for Patients Appropriate care should be exercised when considering the administration of additional sympathomimetic agents. A sufficient interval of time should elapse prior to administration of another sympathomimetic agent.

Drug Interactions Other beta adrenergic aerosol bronchodilators should not be used concomitantly with Alupent® (metaproterenol sulfate USP) because they may have additive effects. Beta adrenergic agonists should be administered with caution to patients being treated with monoamine oxidase inhibitors or tricyclic antidepressants, since the action of beta adrenergic agonists on the vascular system may be potentiated.

Carcinogenesis/Mutagenesis/Impairment of Fertility In an 18-month study in mice, Alupent produced an increase in benign ovarian tumors in females at doses corresponding to 320 and 640 times the maximum recommended dose (based on a 50 kg individual). In a two-year study in rats, a nonsignificant incidence of benign leiomyomata of the mesovarium was noted at 640 times the maximum recommended dose. The relevance of these findings to man is not known. Mutagenic studies with Alupent have not been conducted. Reproduction studies in rats revealed no evidence of impaired fertility.

Pregnancy/Teratogenic Effects *PREGNANCY CATEGORY C:* Alupent has been shown to be teratogenic and embryotoxic in rabbits when given in doses corresponding to 640 times the maximum recommended dose. These effects included skeletal abnormalities, hydrocephalus and skull bone separation. Results of other studies in rabbits, rats or mice have not revealed any teratogenic, embryocidal or fetotoxic effects. There are no adequate and well-controlled studies in pregnant women. Alupent should be used during pregnancy only if the potential benefit justifies the potential risk to the fetus.

Nursing Mothers It is not known whether Alupent is excreted in human milk; therefore, Alupent should be used during nursing only if the potential benefit justifies the possible risk to the newborn.

Pediatric Use Safety and effectiveness in the pediatric population below the age of 12 have not been established. Studies are currently under way in this age group.

ADVERSE REACTIONS

Adverse reactions are similar to those noted with other sympathomimetic agents. The most frequent adverse reaction to Alupent® (metaproterenol sulfate USP) administered by metered-dose inhaler among 251 patients in 90-day controlled clinical trials was nervousness. This was reported in 6.8% of patients. Less frequent adverse experiences, occurring in 1-4% of patients were headache, dizziness, palpitations, gastrointestinal distress, tremor, throat irritation, nausea, vomiting, cough and asthma exacerbation. Tachycardia occurred in less than 1% of patients.

OVERDOSAGE

The expected symptoms with overdosage are those of excessive beta-stimulation and/or any of the symptoms listed under adverse reactions, e.g. angina, hypertension or hypotension, arrhythmias, nervousness, headache, tremor, dry mouth, palpitation, nausea, dizziness, fatigue, malaise and insomnia.

Treatment consists of discontinuation of metaproterenol together with appropriate symptomatic therapy.

DOSAGE AND ADMINISTRATION

The usual single dose is two to three inhalations. With repetitive dosing, inhalation should usually not be repeated more often than about every three to four hours. Total dosage per day should not exceed 12 inhalations.

Alupent® (metaproterenol sulfate USP) Inhalation Aerosol is not recommended for children under 12 years of age.

It is recommended that the physician titrate dosage according to each individual patient's response to therapy.

HOW SUPPLIED

Each 100 inhalations of Alupent® (metaproterenol sulfate USP) Inhalation Aerosol contains 75 mg of metaproterenol sulfate as a micronized powder in inert propellants. Each metered dose delivers through the mouthpiece 0.65 mg metaproterenol sulfate (each ml contains 15 mg). Alupent Inhalation Aerosol with Mouthpiece (NDC 0597-0070-08), net contents 7g (5 ml). The mouthpiece is white with a clear, colorless sleeve and a blue protective cap.

Each 200 inhalations of Alupent Inhalation Aerosol contains 150 mg of metaproterenol sulfate as a micronized powder in inert propellants. Each metered dose delivers through the mouthpiece 0.65 mg metaproterenol sulfate (each ml contains 15 mg). Alupent Inhalation Aerosol with Mouthpiece (NDC 0597-0070-17), net contents 14g (10 ml). The mouthpiece is white with a clear, colorless sleeve and a blue protective cap. Alupent Inhalation Aerosol Refill (NDC 0597-0070-18), net contents 14g (10 ml).

Note: The indented statement below is required by the Federal government's Clean Air Act for all products containing or manufactured with chlorofluorocarbons (CFCs):

> WARNING: Contains trichloromonofluoromethane (CFC-11), dichlorodifluoromethane (CFC-12) and dichlorotetrafluoroethane (CFC-114), substances which harm public health and the environment by destroying ozone in the upper atmosphere.

A notice similar to the above WARNING has been placed in the information for the patient of this product under the Environmental Protection Agency's (EPA's) regulations. The patient's warning states that the patient should consult his or her physician if there are questions about alternatives.

Store between 59°F (15°C) and 77°F (25°C). Avoid excessive humidity.

Rx only.

Boehringer
Ingelheim

Distributed by Boehringer Ingelheim Pharmaceuticals, Inc., Ridgefield, CT 06877

Licensed from Boehringer Ingelheim International GmbH

Manufactured by 3M Pharmaceuticals, St. Paul, MN 55144-1000

Printed in U.S.A. Revised 2/99 029
4041090

Shown in Product Identification Guide, page 309

ATROVENT® ℞

[ă' trō" vĕnt]

(ipratropium bromide)
Inhalation Aerosol
Bronchodilator Aerosol
For Oral Inhalation Only

Prescribing Information

DESCRIPTION

The active ingredient in ATROVENT® (ipratropium bromide) Inhalation Aerosol is ipratropium bromide. It is an anticholinergic bronchodilator chemically described as 8-azoniabicyclo[3.2.1]-octane, 3-(3-hydroxy-1-oxo-2-phenylpropoxy)-8-methyl-8-(1- methylethyl)-, bromide, monohydrate (*endo,syn*)-,(±): a synthetic quaternary ammonium compound chemically related to atropine. The structural formula is:

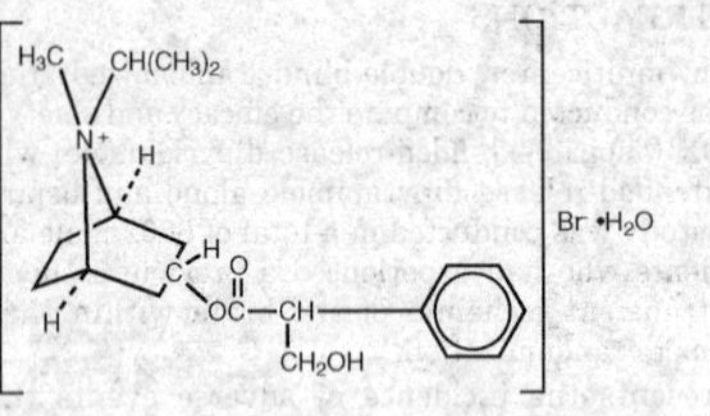

$C_{20}H_{30}BrNO_3 \cdot H_2O$ ipratropium bromide Mol. Wt. 430.4

Ipratropium bromide is a white to off-white crystalline substance, freely soluble in water and lower alcohols but insoluble in lipophilic solvents such as ether, chloroform, and fluorocarbons.

ATROVENT Inhalation Aerosol contains a microcrystalline suspension of ipratropium bromide in a pressurized metered-dose aerosol unit for oral inhalation administration. The net weight is at least 14.7 grams; it yields 200 inhalations. Each actuation meters 21 mcg of ipratropium bromide from the valve and delivers 18 mcg of ipratropium bromide from the mouthpiece. The excipients are dichlorodifluoromethane, dichlorotetrafluoroethane, and trichloromonofluoromethane as propellants and soya lecithin.

CLINICAL PHARMACOLOGY

Mechanism of Action

Ipratropium bromide is an anticholinergic (parasympatholytic) agent which, based on animal studies, appears to inhibit vagally mediated reflexes by antagonizing the action of acetylcholine, the transmitter agent released from the vagus nerve. Anticholinergics prevent the increases in intracellular concentration of cyclic guanosine monophosphate (cyclic GMP) which are caused by interaction of acetylcholine with the muscarinic receptor on bronchial smooth muscle.

Pharmacokinetics

The bronchodilation following inhalation of ipratropium bromide is primarily a local, site-specific effect, not a systemic one. Much of an administered dose is swallowed as shown by fecal excretion studies. Ipratropium bromide is a quaternary amine. It is not readily absorbed into the systemic circulation either from the surface of the lung or from the gastrointestinal tract as confirmed by blood level and renal excretion studies.

The half-life of elimination is about 2 hours after inhalation or intravenous administration. Ipratropium bromide is minimally bound (0 to 9% *in vitro*) to plasma albumin and α_1-acid glycoprotein. It is partially metabolized to inactive ester hydrolysis products. Following intravenous administration, approximately one-half of the dose is excreted unchanged in the urine. Autoradiographic studies in rats have shown that ipratropium bromide does not penetrate the blood-brain barrier.

In controlled 90 day studies in patients with bronchospasm associated with chronic obstructive pulmonary disease (chronic bronchitis and emphysema) significant improvements in pulmonary function (FEV_1 and $FEF_{25-75\%}$ increases of 15% or more) occurred within 15 minutes, reached a peak in 1–2 hours, and persisted for periods of 3 to 4 hours in the majority of patients and up to 6 hours in some patients. In addition, significant increases in Forced Vital Capacity (FVC) have been demonstrated.

Controlled clinical studies have demonstrated that ATROVENT (ipratropium bromide) Inhalation Aerosol does not alter either mucociliary clearance or the volume or viscosity of respiratory secretions. In studies without a positive control ATROVENT Inhalation Aerosol did not alter pupil size, accommodation or visual acuity (See ADVERSE REACTIONS). Ventilation/perfusion studies have shown no clinically significant effects on pulmonary gas exchange or arterial oxygen tension. At recommended doses, ATROVENT Inhalation Aerosol does not produce clinically significant changes in pulse rate or blood pressure.

INDICATIONS AND USAGE

ATROVENT (ipratropium bromide) Inhalation Aerosol is indicated as a bronchodilator for maintenance treatment of bronchospasm associated with chronic obstructive pulmonary disease, including chronic bronchitis and emphysema.

CONTRAINDICATIONS

ATROVENT (ipratropium bromide) Inhalation Aerosol is contraindicated in patients with a history of hypersensitivity to soya lecithin or related food products such as soybean and peanut. ATROVENT Inhalation Aerosol should also not be taken by patients hypersensitive to any other components of the drug product or to atropine or its derivatives.

WARNINGS

ATROVENT (ipratropium bromide) Inhalation Aerosol is not indicated for the initial treatment of acute episodes of bronchospasm where rapid response is required.

1. Immediate Hypersensitivity Reactions: Immediate hypersensitivity reactions may occur after administration of ipratropium bromide, as demonstrated by rare cases of urticaria, angioedema, rash, bronchospasm, anaphylaxis and oropharyngeal edema.
2. Storage Conditions: The contents of ATROVENT Inhalation Aerosol are under pressure. Do not puncture. Do not use or store near heat or open flame. Exposure to temperatures above 120° F may cause bursting. Never throw the container into a fire or incinerator. Keep out of reach of children.

PRECAUTIONS

General

1. Effects Seen with Anticholinergic Drugs: ATROVENT (ipratropium bromide) Inhalation Aerosol should be used with caution in patients with narrow-angle glaucoma, prostatic hyperplasia or bladder-neck obstruction.

Information for Patients

Patients should be cautioned to avoid spraying the aerosol into their eyes and be advised that this may result in precipitation or worsening of narrow-angle glaucoma, mydriasis, eye pain or discomfort, temporary blurring of vision, visual halos or colored images in association with red eyes from conjunctival and corneal congestion. Patients should also be advised that should any combination of these symptoms develop, they should consult their physician immediately.

ATROVENT Inhalation Aerosol should not be used more frequently than recommended. The dose or frequency of ATROVENT Inhalation Aerosol should not be increased without patients consulting their physician. If treatment with ATROVENT Inhalation Aerosol becomes less effective for symptomatic relief, their symptoms become worse, and/or patients need to use the product more frequently than usual, medical attention should be sought immediately. The patient, if pregnant or nursing, should be advised to contact their physician about the use of ATROVENT Inhalation Aerosol. Appropriate use of ATROVENT Inhalation Aerosol includes an understanding of the way it should be administered (See Patient's Instructions for Use).

Drug Interactions

ATROVENT Inhalation Aerosol has been used concomitantly with other drugs, including sympathomimetic bronchodilators, methylxanthines, and steroids, commonly used in the treatment of chronic obstructive pulmonary disease. With the exception of albuterol, there are no formal studies fully evaluating the interaction effects of ATROVENT Inhalation Aerosol and these drugs with respect to effectiveness.

Anticholinergic agents: Although ipratropium bromide is minimally absorbed into the systemic circulation, there is some potential for an additive interaction with concomitantly used anticholinergic medications. Caution is therefore advised in the co-administration of ATROVENT Inhalation Aerosol with other anticholinergic-containing drugs.

Carcinogenesis, Mutagenesis, Impairment of Fertility

Two-year oral carcinogenicity studies in rats and mice have revealed no carcinogenic potential at doses up to 6 mg/kg/day. This dose corresponds to approximately 360 and 180 times the maximum recommended human daily inhalation dose of ipratropium bromide in rats and mice respectively, on a mg/m^2 basis. Results of various mutagenicity studies (Ames test, mouse dominant lethal test, mouse micronucleus test and chromosome aberration of bone marrow in Chinese hamsters) were negative.

Fertility of male or female rats at oral doses up to 50 mg/kg/day (approximately 3000 times the maximum recommended human daily inhalation dose on a mg/m^2 basis) was unaffected by ipratropium bromide administration. At doses above 90 mg/kg/day (approximately 5400 times the maximum recommended human daily inhalation dose on a mg/m^2 basis), increased resorption and decreased conception rates were observed.

Pregnancy

TERATOGENIC EFFECTS Pregnancy Category B

Oral reproduction studies were performed at doses of 10 mg/kg in mice, 100 mg/kg in rats and 125 mg/kg in rabbits. These doses correspond, in each species, respectively, to approximately 300, 6000 and 15,000 times the maximum recommended human daily inhalation dose of ipratropium bromide on a mg/m^2 basis. Inhalation reproduction studies were conducted in rats and rabbits at doses of 1.5 and 1.8 mg/kg/day (approximately 90 and 210 times the maximum recommended human daily inhalation dose on a mg/m^2 basis). These studies have demonstrated no evidence of teratogenic effects as a result of ipratropium bromide. However, no adequate or well controlled studies have been conducted in pregnant women. Because animal reproduction studies are not always predictive of human response, ATROVENT Inhalation Aerosol should be used during pregnancy only if clearly needed.

Nursing Mothers

It is not known whether ATROVENT Inhalation Aerosol is excreted in human milk. Although lipid-insoluble quaternary bases pass into breast milk, it is unlikely that the active component, ipratropium bromide, would reach the infant to an important extent, especially when taken by aerosol. However, because many drugs are excreted in human milk, caution should be exercised when ATROVENT Inhalation Aerosol is administered to a nursing mother.

Pediatric Use

Safety and effectiveness in the pediatric population below the age of 12 years have not been established.

ADVERSE REACTIONS

Adverse reaction information concerning ATROVENT (ipratropium bromide) Inhalation Aerosol is derived from 90 day controlled clinical trials (N=254), other controlled clinical trials using recommended doses of ATROVENT Inhalation Aerosol (N=377) and an uncontrolled study (N=1924). Additional information is derived from the post-marketing experience and the published literature.

Adverse reactions occurring in greater than one percent of patients in the 90 day controlled clinical trials appear in Table 1.

Table 1 Adverse Reactions Occurring in >1% of COPD Patients

	Percent of Patients	
	Ipratropium Bromide	Metaproterenol Sulfate
	N = 254	N = 249
Reaction		
Cardiovascular		
Palpitations	1.8	1.6
Central Nervous System		
Nervousness	3.1	6.8
Dizziness	2.4	2.8
Headache	2.4	2.0
Dermatological		
Rash	1.2	0.4
Gastrointestinal		
Nausea	2.8	1.2
Gastrointestinal distress	2.4	2.8
Vomiting	0	1.2
Musculoskeletal		
Tremor	0	2.4
Ophthalmological		
Blurred vision	1.2	0.8
Oro-Otolaryngeal		
Dry mouth	2.4	0.8
Irritation from aerosol	1.6	1.6
Respiratory		
Cough	5.9	1.2
Exacerbation of symptoms	2.4	3.6

Additional adverse reactions reported in less than one percent of the patients considered possibly due to ATROVENT Inhalation Aerosol include urinary difficulty, fatigue, insomnia and hoarseness.

The large uncontrolled, open-label study included seriously ill patients. About 7% of patients treated discontinued the program because of adverse events.

Of the 2301 patients treated in the large uncontrolled study and in clinical trials other than the 90 day studies, the most common adverse reactions reported were: dryness of the oropharynx, about 5 in 100; cough, exacerbation of symptoms and irritation from aerosol, each about 3 in 100; headache, about 2 in 100; nausea, dizziness, blurred vision/difficulty in accommodation, and drying of secretions, each about 1 in 100. Less frequently reported adverse reactions that were possibly due to ATROVENT (ipratropium bromide) Inhalation Aerosol include tachycardia, paresthesia, drowsiness, coordination difficulty, itching, hives, flushing, alopecia, constipation, tremor, and mucosal ulcers.

Cases of precipitation or worsening of narrow-angle glaucoma, acute eye pain, and hypotension, have been reported.

In a 5-year placebo-controlled trial, hospitalizations for supraventricular tachycardia and atrial fibrillation occurred with an incidence rate of 0.5% in patients receiving ATROVENT Inhalation Aerosol.

Post-Marketing Experience

Allergic-type reactions such as skin rash, angioedema of tongue, lips and face, urticaria (including giant urticaria), laryngospasm and anaphylactic reaction have been reported, with positive rechallenge in some cases. Many of the patients had a history of allergies to other drugs and/or foods, including soybean. (See CONTRAINDICATIONS).

Additionally, urinary retention, mydriasis, and bronchospasm, including paradoxical bronchospasm, have been reported during the post-marketing period.

OVERDOSAGE

Acute overdosage by inhalation is unlikely since ipratropium bromide is not well absorbed systemically after aerosol or oral administration. The oral median lethal dose of ipratropium bromide ranged between 1001 and 2010 mg/kg in mice (approximately 30,000 and 60,000 times the maximum recommended human daily inhalation dose on a mg/m^2 basis, respectively); between 1667 and 4000 mg/kg in rats (approximately 100,000 and 240,000 times the maximum recommended human daily inhalation dose, respectively, on a mg/m^2 basis); and between 400 and 1300 mg/kg in dogs (approximately 80,000 and 260,000 times the maximum recommended human daily inhalation dose, respectively, on a mg/m^2 basis).

DOSAGE AND ADMINISTRATION

The usual starting dose of ATROVENT (ipratropium bromide) Inhalation Aerosol is two inhalations (36 mcg) four times a day. Patients may take additional inhalations as required; however, the total number of inhalations should not exceed 12 in 24 hours. It is recommended to "test-spray" three times before using for the first time and in cases where the aerosol has not been used for more than 24 hours. ***Avoid spraying into eyes.***

HOW SUPPLIED

ATROVENT (ipratropium bromide) Inhalation Aerosol is supplied as a metered dose inhaler with a white mouthpiece which has a clear, colorless sleeve and a green protective cap. The ATROVENT Inhalation Aerosol canister is to be used with the ATROVENT Inhalation Aerosol mouthpiece only. This mouthpiece should not be used with other aerosol medications. Similarly, the canister should not be used with other mouthpieces. Each actuation meters 21 mcg of ipratropium bromide from the valve and delivers 18 mcg of ipratropium bromide from the mouthpiece. Each 14.7 gram canister provides sufficient medication for 200 inhalations (NDC 0597-0082-14).

Note: The indented statement below is required by the Federal government's Clean Air Act for all products containing or manufactured with chlorofluorocarbons (CFCs):

Warning: Contains trichloromonofluoromethane (CFC-11), dichlorodifluoromethane (CFC-12) and dichlorotet-

Continued on next page

Atrovent Inh. Aero.—Cont.

rafluoroethane (CFC-114), substances which harm public health and the environment by destroying ozone in the upper atmosphere.

A notice similar to the above **Warning** has been placed in the information for the patient of this product under the Environmental Protection Agency's (EPA's) regulations. The patient's warning states that the patient should consult with his or her physician if there are questions about alternatives.

Store between 59°F (15°C) and 86°F (30°C). Avoid excessive humidity.

Keep out of children's reach. **Shake the canister well before using.** Patients should be reminded to read and follow the accompanying "Patient's Instructions for Use", which should be dispensed with the product. For optimal results, the canister should be at room temperature before use.

Warning: Discard the canister after you have used the labeled number of inhalations. The correct amount of medication in each inhalation cannot be assured after this point.

℞ Only

Distributed by:
Boehringer Ingelheim Pharmaceuticals, Inc.
Ridgefield, CT 06877 USA

Manufactured by:
3M Pharmaceuticals
St. Paul, MN 55144 USA

Licensed from:
Boehringer Ingelheim International GmbH

Revised 3/27/02
10001403/US/1
10001403/01

Shown in Product Identification Guide, page 309

ATROVENT® ℞

[*ă 'trō "vĕnt*]
(ipratropium bromide)
Inhalation Solution .... BI-Code 80

Prescribing Information

DESCRIPTION

The active ingredient in Atrovent® (ipratropium bromide) Inhalation Solution is ipratropium bromide monohydrate. It is an anticholinergic bronchodilator chemically described as 8-azoniabicyclo[3.2.1]-octane, 3-(3-hydroxy-1-oxo-2-phenylpropoxy)-8-methyl-8-(1-methylethyl)-, bromide, monohydrate *(endo, syn)*-, (±)-; a synthetic quaternary ammonium compound, chemically related to atropine.

ipratropium bromide monohydrate (Atrovent) $C_{20}H_{30}BrNO_3 \cdot H_2O$ Mol. Wt. 430.4

Ipratropium bromide is a white crystalline substance, freely soluble in water and lower alcohols. It is a quaternary ammonium compound and thus exists in an ionized state in aqueous solutions. It is relatively insoluble in non-polar media.

Atrovent Inhalation Solution is administered by oral inhalation with the aid of a nebulizer. It contains ipratropium bromide 0.02% (anhydrous basis) in a sterile, isotonic saline solution, pH-adjusted to 3.4 (3 to 4) with hydrochloric acid.

CLINICAL PHARMACOLOGY

Atrovent® (ipratropium bromide) is an anticholinergic (parasympatholytic) agent that, based on animal studies, appears to inhibit vagally-mediated reflexes by antagonizing the action of acetylcholine, the transmitter agent released from the vagus nerve.

Anticholinergics prevent the increases in intracellular concentration of cyclic guanosine monophosphate (cyclic GMP) that are caused by interaction of acetylcholine with the muscarinic receptor on bronchial smooth muscle.

The bronchodilation following inhalation of Atrovent is primarily a local, site-specific effect, not a systemic one. Much of an administered dose is swallowed but not absorbed, as shown by fecal excretion studies. Following nebulization of a 2 mg dose, a mean 7% of the dose was absorbed into the systemic circulation either from the surface of the lung or from the gastrointestinal tract. The half-life of elimination is about 1.6 hours after intravenous administration. Ipratropium bromide is minimally (0 to 9% in vitro) bound to plasma albumin and α_1-acid glycoproteins. It is partially metabolized. Autoradiographic studies in rats have shown that Atrovent does not penetrate the blood-brain barrier. Atrovent has not been studied in patients with hepatic or renal insufficiency. It should be used with caution in those patient populations.

All Adverse Events, from a Double-blind, Parallel, 12-week Study of Patients with COPD*

	PERCENT OF PATIENTS				
	Atrovent® (500 mcg t.i.d) n=219	Alupent® 15 mg t.i.d) n=212	Atrovent®/Alupent® (500 mcg t.i.d/ 15 mg t.i.d) n=108	Albuterol (2.5 mg t.i.d) n=205	Atrovent®/ Albuterol (500 mcg t.i.d/ 2.5 mg t.i.d) n=100
Body as a Whole-General Disorders					
Headache	6.4	5.2	6.5	6.3	9.0
Pain	4.1	3.3	0.9	2.9	5.0
Influenza-like symptoms	3.7	4.7	6.5	0.5	1.0
Back pain	3.2	1.9	1.9	2.4	0.0
Chest pain	3.2	4.2	5.6	2.0	1.0
Cardiovascular Disorders					
Hypertension/Hypertension Aggravated	0.9	1.9	0.9	1.5	4.0
Central & Peripheral Nervous System					
Dizziness	2.3	3.3	1.9	3.9	4.0
Insomnia	0.9	0.5	4.6	1.0	1.0
Tremor	0.9	7.1	8.3	1.0	0.0
Nervousness	0.5	4.7	6.5	1.0	1.0
Gastrointestinal System Disorders					
Mouth Dryness	3.2	0.0	1.9	2.0	3.0
Nausea	4.1	3.8	1.9	2.9	2.0
Constipation	0.9	0.0	3.7	1.0	1.0
Musculo-skeletal System Disorders					
Arthritis	0.9	1.4	0.9	0.5	3.0
Respiratory System Disorders (Lower)					
Coughing	4.6	8.0	6.5	5.4	6.0
Dyspnea	9.6	13.2	16.7	12.7	9.0
Bronchitis	14.6	24.5	15.7	16.6	20.0
Bronchospasm	2.3	2.8	4.6	5.4	5.0
Sputum Increased	1.4	1.4	4.6	3.4	0.0
Respiratory Disorder	0.0	6.1	6.5	2.0	4.0
Respiratory System Disorders (Upper)					
Upper Respiratory Tract Infection	13.2	11.3	9.3	12.2	16.0
Pharyngitis	3.7	4.2	5.6	2.9	4.0
Rhinitis	2.3	4.2	1.9	2.4	0.0
Sinusitis	2.3	2.8	0.9	5.4	4.0

* All adverse events, regardless of drug relationship, reported by three percent or more patients in the 12-week controlled clinical trials.

In controlled 12-week studies in patients with bronchospasm associated with chronic obstructive pulmonary disease (chronic bronchitis and emphysema) significant improvements in pulmonary function (FEV_1 increases of 15% or more) occurred within 15 to 30 minutes, reached a peak in 1–2 hours, and persisted for periods of 4–5 hours in the majority of patients, with about 25–38% of the patients demonstrating increases of 15% or more for at least 7–8 hours. Continued effectiveness of Atrovent Inhalation Solution was demonstrated throughout the 12-week period. In addition, significant increases in forced vital capacity (FVC) have been demonstrated. However, Atrovent did not consistently produce significant improvement in subjective symptom scores nor in quality of life scores over the 12-week duration of study.

Additional controlled 12-week studies were conducted to evaluate the safety and effectiveness of Atrovent Inhalation Solution administered concomitantly with the beta adrenergic bronchodilator solutions metaproterenol and albuterol compared with the administration of each of the beta agonists alone. Combined therapy produced significant additional improvement in FEV_1 and FVC. On combined therapy, the median duration of 15% improvement in FEV_1 was 5–7 hours, compared with 3–4 hours in patients receiving a beta agonist alone.

INDICATIONS AND USAGE

Atrovent® (ipratropium bromide) Inhalation Solution administered either alone or with other bronchodilators, especially beta adrenergics, is indicated as a bronchodilator for maintenance treatment of bronchospasm associated with chronic obstructive pulmonary disease, including chronic bronchitis and emphysema.

CONTRAINDICATIONS

Atrovent® (ipratropium bromide) is contraindicated in known or suspected cases of hypersensitivity to ipratropium bromide, or to atropine and its derivatives.

WARNINGS

The use of Atrovent® (ipratropium bromide) Inhalation Solution as a single agent for the relief of bronchospasm in acute COPD exacerbation has not been adequately studied. Drugs with faster onset of action may be preferable as initial therapy in this situation. Combination of Atrovent and beta agonists has not been shown to be more effective than either drug alone in reversing the bronchospasm associated with acute COPD exacerbation.

Immediate hypersensitivity reactions may occur after administration of ipratropium bromide, as demonstrated by rare cases of urticaria, angioedema, rash, bronchospasm and oropharyngeal edema.

PRECAUTIONS

General Atrovent® (ipratropium bromide) should be used with caution in patients with narrow-angle glaucoma, prostatic hypertrophy or bladder-neck obstruction.

Information for Patients Patients should be advised that temporary blurring of vision, precipitation or worsening of narrow-angle glaucoma or eye pain may result if the solution comes into direct contact with the eyes. Use of a nebulizer with mouthpiece rather than face mask may be preferable, to reduce the likelihood of the nebulizer solution reaching the eyes. Patients should be advised that Atrovent Inhalation Solution can be mixed in the nebulizer with albuterol or metaproterenol if used within one hour. Drug stability and safety of Atrovent Inhalation Solution when mixed with other drugs in a nebulizer have not been established. Patients should be reminded that Atrovent Inhalation Solution should be used consistently as prescribed throughout the course of therapy.

Drug Interactions Atrovent has been shown to be a safe and effective bronchodilator when used in conjuction with beta-adrenergic bronchodilators. Atrovent has also been used with other pulmonary medications, including methylxanthines and corticosteroids, without adverse drug interactions.

Carcinogenesis, Mutagenesis, Impairment of Fertility Two-year oral carcinogenicity studies in rats and mice have revealed no carcinogenic potential at dietary doses up to 6 mg/kg/day of Atrovent.

Results of various mutagenicity studies (Ames test, mouse dominant lethal test, mouse micronucleus test and chromosome aberration of bone marrow in Chinese hamsters) were negative.

Fertility of male or female rats at oral doses up to 50 mg/kg/day was unaffected by Atrovent administration. At doses above 90 mg/kg, increased resorption and decreased conception rates were observed.

Pregnancy *TERATOGENIC EFFECTS*

Pregnancy Category B. Oral reproduction studies were performed in mice, rats and rabbits at doses of 10, 100, and 125 mg/kg respectively, and inhalation reproduction studies in rats and rabbits at doses of 1.5 and 1.8 mg/kg (or approximately 38 and 45 times the recommended human daily dose) respectively, have demonstrated no evidence of teratogenic effects as a result of Atrovent. However, no adequate or well-controlled studies have been conducted in pregnant women. Because animal reproduction studies are not always predictive of human response, Atrovent should be used during pregnancy only if clearly needed.

Nursing Mothers It is not known whether Atrovent is excreted in human milk. Although lipid-insoluble quaternary bases pass into breast milk, it is unlikely that Atrovent®

(ipratropium bromide) would reach the infant to a significant extent, especially when taken by inhalation since Atrovent is not well absorbed systemically after inhalation or oral administration. However, because many drugs are excreted in human milk, caution should be exercised when Atrovent is administered to a nursing woman.

Pediatric Use Safety and effectiveness in the pediatric population below the age of 12 have not been established.

ADVERSE REACTIONS

Adverse reaction information concerning Atrovent® (ipratropium bromide) Inhalation Solution is derived from 12-week active-controlled clinical trials. Additional information is derived from foreign post-marketing experience and the published literature.

All adverse events, regardless of drug relationship, reported by three percent or more patients in the 12-week controlled clinical trials appear in the table below:

[See table at top of previous page]

Additional adverse reactions reported in less than three percent of the patients treated with Atrovent include tachycardia, palpitations, eye pain, urinary retention, urinary tract infection and urticaria. Cases of precipitation or worsening of narrow-angle glaucoma and acute eye pain have been reported.

Lower respiratory adverse reactions (bronchitis, dyspnea and bronchospasm) were the most common events leading to discontinuation of Atrovent therapy in the 12-week trials. Headache, mouth dryness and aggravation of COPD symptoms are more common when the total daily dose of Atrovent equals or exceeds 2,000 mcg.

Allergic-type reactions such a skin rash, angioedema of tongue, lips and face, urticaria, laryngospasm and anaphylactic reaction have been reported. Many of the patients had a history of allergies to other drugs and/or foods.

OVERDOSAGE

Acute systemic overdosage by inhalation is unlikely since Atrovent® (ipratropium bromide) is not well absorbed after inhalation at up to four-fold the recommended dose, or after oral administration at up to forty-fold the recommended dose. The oral LD_{50} of Atrovent ranged between 1001 and 2010 mg/kg in mice; between 1667 and more than 4000 mg/kg in rats; and between 400 and 1300 mg/kg in dogs.

DOSAGE AND ADMINISTRATION

The usual dosage of Atrovent® (ipratropium bromide) Inhalation Solution is 500 mcg (1 Unit-Dose Vial) administered three to four times a day by oral nebulization, with doses 6 to 8 hours apart. Atrovent Inhalation Solution Unit-Dose Vials contain 500 mcg ipratropium bromide anhydrous in 2.5 ml normal saline. Atrovent Inhalation Solution can be mixed in the nebulizer with albuterol or metaproterenol if used within one hour. Drug stability and safety of Atrovent Inhalation Solution when mixed with other drugs in a nebulizer have not been established.

HOW SUPPLIED

Atrovent® (ipratropium bromide) Inhalation Solution Unit Dose Vial is supplied as a 0.02% clear, colorless solution containing 2.5 ml with 5 Unit Dose Vials per pouch, 5 pouches per carton (NDC 0597-0080-62).

Each vial is made from a low density polyethylene (LDPE) resin.

Store between 59°F (15°C) and 86°F (30°C). Protect from light.

Store unused vials in the foil pouch.

ATTENTION PHARMACIST: Detach "Patient's Instructions for Use" from Package Insert and dispense with solution.

Rx only

830885-R Revised 10/98

Shown in Product Identification Guide, page 309

ATROVENT® ℞

(ipratropium bromide)
Nasal Spray
0.03%

21mcg/spray

Prescribing Information

DESCRIPTION

The active ingredient in ATROVENT® Nasal Spray is ipratropium bromide monohydrate. It is an anticholinergic agent chemically described as 8-azoniabicyclo (3.2.1) octane,3-(3-hydroxy-1-oxo-2-phenylpropoxy)-8-methyl-8-(1-methylethyl)-, bromide, monohydrate (endo,syn)-, (±)-: a synthetic quaternary ammonium compound, chemically related to atropine. Its structural formula is:

[See chemical structure at top of next column]

Ipratropium bromide is a white to off-white, crystalline substance. It is freely soluble in lower alcohols and water, existing in an ionized state in aqueous solutions, and relatively insoluble in non-polar media.

ATROVENT (ipratropium bromide) Nasal Spray 0.03% is a metered-dose, manual pump spray unit which delivers 21 mcg (70µL) ipratropium bromide per spray on an anhydrous basis in an isotonic, aqueous solution with pH adjusted to 4.7. It also contains benzalkonium chloride, ede-

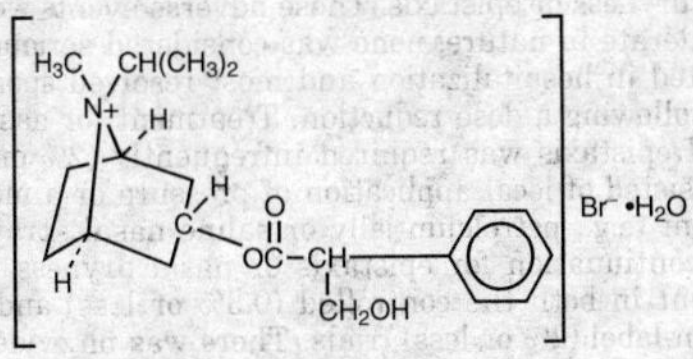

ipratropium bromide monohydrate $C_{20}H_{30}BrNO_3 \bullet H_2O$ Mol. Wt. 430.4

tate disodium, sodium chloride, sodium hydroxide, hydrochloric acid, and purified water. Each bottle contains 345 sprays.

CLINICAL PHARMACOLOGY

Mechanism of Action

Ipratropium bromide is an anticholinergic agent that inhibits vagally-mediated reflexes by antagonizing the action of acetylcholine at the cholinergic receptor. In humans, ipratropium bromide has antisecretory properties and, when applied locally, inhibits secretions from the serous and seromucous glands lining the nasal mucosa. Ipratropium bromide is a quaternary amine that minimally crosses the nasal and gastrointestinal membrane and the blood-brain barrier, resulting in a reduction of the systemic anticholinergic effects (e.g., neurologic, ophthalmic, cardiovascular, and gastrointestinal effects) that are seen with tertiary anticholinergic amines.

Pharmacokinetics

Absorption: Ipratropium bromide is poorly absorbed into the systemic circulation following oral administration (2–3%). Less than 20% of an 84 mcg per nostril dose was absorbed from the nasal mucosa of normal volunteers, induced-cold patients, or perennial rhinitis patients.

Distribution: Ipratropium bromide is minimally bound (0 to 9% *in vitro*) to plasma albumin and α_1-acid glycoprotein. Its blood/plasma concentration ratio was estimated to be about 0.89. Studies in rats have shown that ipratropium bromide does not penetrate the blood-brain barrier.

Metabolism: Ipratropium bromide is partially metabolized to ester hydrolysis products, tropic acid and tropane. These metabolites appear to be inactive on *in vitro* receptor affinity studies using rat brain tissue homogenates.

Elimination: After intravenous administration of 2 mg ipratropium bromide to 10 healthy volunteers, the terminal half-life of ipratropium was approximately 1.6 hours. The total body clearance and renal clearance were estimated to be 2,505 and 1,019 ml/min, respectively. The amount of the total dose excreted unchanged in the urine (Ae) within 24 hours was approximately one-half of the administered dose.

Pediatrics: Following administration of 42 mcg of ipratropium bromide per nostril two or three times a day in perennial rhinitis patients 6-18 years old, the mean amounts of the total dose excreted unchanged in the urine (8.6 to 11.1%) were higher than those reported in adult volunteers or adult perennial rhinitis patients (3.7 to 5.6%). Plasma ipratropium concentrations were relatively low (ranging from undetectable up to 0.49 ng/ml). No correlation of the amount of the total dose excreted unchanged in the urine (Ae) with age or gender was observed in the pediatric population.

Special Populations: Gender does not appear to influence the absorption or excretion of nasally administered ipratropium bromide. The pharmacokinetics of ipratropium bromide have not been studied in patients with hepatic or renal insufficiency or in the elderly.

Drug-Drug Interaction: No specific pharmacokinetic studies were conducted to evaluate potential drug-drug interactions.

Pharmacodynamics: In two single-dose trials (n=17), doses up to 336 mcg of ipratropium bromide did not significantly affect pupillary diameter, heart rate, or systolic/diastolic blood pressure. Similarly, in patients with induced-colds, ATROVENT (ipratropium bromide) Nasal Spray 0.06% (84 mcg/nostril four times a day), had no significant effects on pupillary diameter, heart rate or systolic/diastolic blood pressure.

Two nasal provocation trials in perennial rhinitis patients (n=44) using ipratropium bromide nasal spray showed a dose dependent increase in inhibition of methacholine induced nasal secretion with an onset of action within 15 minutes (time of first observation).

Controlled clinical trials demonstrated that intranasal fluorocarbon-propelled ipratropium bromide does not alter physiologic nasal functions (e.g., sense of smell, ciliary beat frequency, mucociliary clearance, or the air conditioning capacity of the nose).

Clinical Trials

The clinical trials for ATROVENT (ipratropium bromide) Nasal Spray 0.03% were conducted in patients with nonallergic perennial rhinitis (NAPR) and in patients with allergic perennial rhinitis (APR). APR patients were those who experienced symptoms of nasal hypersecretion and nasal congestion or sneezing when exposed to specific perennial allergens (e.g., dust mites, molds) and were skin test positive to these allergens. NAPR patients were those who experienced symptoms of nasal hypersecretion and nasal congestion or sneezing throughout the year, but were skin test negative to common perennial allergens.

In four controlled, four- and eight-week comparisons of ATROVENT (ipratropium bromide) Nasal Spray 0.03% (42 mcg per nostril, two or three times daily) with its vehicle, in patients with allergic or nonallergic perennial rhinitis, there was a statistically significant decrease in the severity and duration of rhinorrhea in the ATROVENT group throughout the entire study period. An effect was seen as early as the first day of therapy.

There was no effect of ATROVENT (ipratropium bromide) Nasal Spray 0.03% on degree of nasal congestion, sneezing, or postnasal drip. The response to ATROVENT (ipratropium bromide) Nasal Spray 0.03% did not appear to be affected by the type of perennial rhinitis (NAPR or APR), age, or gender. No controlled clinical trials directly compared the efficacy of BID versus TID treatment.

INDICATIONS AND USAGE

ATROVENT® (ipratropium bromide) Nasal Spray 0.03% is indicated for the symptomatic relief of rhinorrhea associated with allergic and nonallergic perennial rhinitis in adults and children age 6 years and older. ATROVENT (ipratropium bromide) Nasal Spray 0.03% does not relieve nasal congestion, sneezing, or postnasal drip associated with allergic or nonallergic perennial rhinitis.

CONTRAINDICATIONS

ATROVENT® (ipratropium bromide) Nasal Spray 0.03% is contraindicated in patients with a history of hypersensitivity to atropine or its derivatives, or to any of the other ingredients.

WARNINGS

Immediate hypersensitivity reactions may occur after administration of ipratropium bromide, as demonstrated by rare cases of urticaria, angioedema, rash, bronchospasm, and oropharyngeal edema.

PRECAUTIONS

General

ATROVENT® (ipratropium bromide) Nasal Spray 0.03% should be used with caution in patients with narrow-angle glaucoma, prostatic hypertrophy, or bladder neck obstruction, particularly if they are receiving an anticholinergic by another route. Cases of precipitation or worsening of narrow-angle glaucoma and acute eye pain have been reported with direct eye contact of ipratropium bromide administered by oral inhalation.

Information for Patients

Patients should be advised that temporary blurring of vision, precipitation or worsening or narrow-angle glaucoma, or eye pain may result if ATROVENT (ipratropium bromide) Nasal Spray 0.03% comes into direct contact with the eyes. Patients should be instructed to avoid spraying ATROVENT (ipratropium bromide) Nasal Spray 0.03% in or around their eyes. Patients who experience eye pain, blurred vision, excessive nasal dryness, or episodes of nasal bleeding should be instructed to contact their doctor. Patients should be reminded to carefully read and follow the accompanying Patient's Instructions for Use.

Drug Interactions

No controlled clinical trials were conducted to investigate drug-drug interactions. ATROVENT (ipratropium bromide) Nasal Spray 0.03% is minimally absorbed into the systemic circulation; nonetheless, there is some potential for an additive interaction with other concomitantly administered anticholinergic medications, including ATROVENT for oral inhalation.

Carcinogenesis, Mutagenesis, Impairment of Fertility

In two-year carcinogenicity studies in rats and mice, ipratropium bromide at oral doses up to 6 mg/kg (approximately 190 and 95 times the maximum recommended daily intranasal dose in adults, respectively, and approximately 110 and 60 times the maximum recommended daily intranasal dose in children, respectively on a mg/m^2 basis) showed no carcinogenic activity. Results of various mutagenicity studies (Ames test, mouse dominant lethal test, mouse micronucleus test, and chromosome aberration of bone marrow in Chinese hamsters) were negative.

Fertility of male or female rats was unaffected by ipratropium bromide at oral doses up to 50 mg/kg (approximately 1,600 times the maximum recommended daily intranasal dose in adults on a mg/m^2 basis). At an oral dose of 500 mg/kg (approximately 16,000 times the maximum recommended daily intranasal dose in adults on a mg/m^2 basis), ipratropium bromide produced a decrease in the conception rate.

Pregnancy

TERATOGENIC EFFECTS Pregnancy Category B.

Oral reproduction studies were performed at doses of 10 mg/kg in mice, 1000 mg/kg in rats and 125 mg/kg in rabbits. These doses correspond, in each species respectively, to approximately 160, 32,000, and 8,000 times the maximum recommended daily intranasal dose in adults on a mg/m^2 basis. Inhalation reproduction studies were conducted in rats and rabbits at doses of 1.5 and 1.8 mg/kg respectively, (approximately 50 and 120 times, respectively, the maximum recommended daily intranasal dose in adults on a mg/m^2 basis). These studies demonstrated no evidence of teratogenic effects as a result of ipratropium bromide. At oral doses above 90 mg/kg in rats (approximately 2,900 times the maximum recommended daily intranasal dose in adults on a mg/m^2 basis) embryotoxicity was observed as increased resorption. This effect is not considered relevant to human use due to the large doses at which it was observed and the difference in route of administration. However, no adequate or well controlled studies have been conducted in

Continued on next page

Atrovent Nasal Spray 0.03%—Cont.

pregnant women. Because animal reproduction studies are not always predictive of human response, ATROVENT (ipratropium bromide) Nasal Spray 0.03% should be used during pregnancy only if clearly needed.

Nursing Mothers

It is known that some ipratropium bromide is systemically absorbed following nasal administration; however the portion which may be excreted in human milk is unknown. Although lipid-insoluble quaternary bases pass into breast milk, the minimal systemic absorption makes it unlikely that ipratropium bromide would reach the infant in an amount sufficient to cause a clinical effect. However, because many drugs are excreted in human milk, caution should be exercised when ATROVENT (ipratropium bromide) Nasal Spray 0.03% is administered to a nursing woman.

Pediatric Use

The safety of ATROVENT (ipratropium bromide) Nasal Spray 0.03% at a dose of two sprays (42 mcg) per nostril two or three times daily (total dose 168 to 252 mcg/day) has been demonstrated in 77 pediatric patients 6-12 years of age in placebo-controlled, 4-week trials and 55 pediatric patients in active-controlled, 6 month trials. The effectiveness of ATROVENT (ipratropium bromide) Nasal Spray 0.03% for the treatment of rhinorrhea associated with allergic and nonallergic perennial rhinitis in this pediatric age group is based on an extrapolation of the demonstrated efficacy of ATROVENT (ipratropium bromide) Nasal Spray 0.03% in adults with these conditions and the likelihood that the disease course, pathophysiology, and the drug's effects are substantially similar to that of the adults. The recommended dose for the pediatric population is based on within and cross-study comparisons of the efficacy of ATROVENT (ipratropium bromide) Nasal Spray 0.03% in adults and pediatric patients on its safety profile in both adults and pediatric patients. The safety and effectiveness of ATROVENT (ipratropium bromide) Nasal Spray 0.03% in patients under 6 years of age have not been established.

ADVERSE REACTIONS

Adverse reaction information on ATROVENT (ipratropium bromide) Nasal Spray 0.03% in patients with perennial rhinitis was derived from four multicenter, vehicle-controlled clinical trials involving 703 patients (356 patients on ATROVENT and 347 patients on vehicle), and a one-year, open-label, follow-up trial. In three of the trials, patients received ATROVENT (ipratropium bromide) Nasal Spray 0.03% three times daily, for eight weeks. In the other trial, ATROVENT (ipratropium bromide) Nasal Spray 0.03% was given to patients two times daily for four weeks. Of the 285 patients who entered the open-label, follow-up trial, 232 were treated for 3 months, 200 for 6 months, and 159 up to one year. The majority (>86%) of patients treated for one year were maintained on 42 mcg per nostril, two or three times daily, of ATROVENT (ipratropium bromide) Nasal Spray 0.03%.

The following table shows adverse events, and the frequency that these adverse events led to the discontinuation of treatment, reported for patients who received ATROVENT (ipratropium bromide) Nasal Spray 0.03% at the recommended dose of 42 mcg per nostril, or vehicle two or three times daily for four or eight weeks. Only adverse events reported with an incidence of at least 2.0% in the ATROVENT group and higher in the ATROVENT group than in the vehicle group are shown.

[See table below]

ATROVENT (ipratropium bromide) Nasal Spray 0.03% was well tolerated by most patients. The most frequently reported nasal adverse events were transient episodes of nasal dryness or epistaxis. These adverse events were mild or moderate in nature, none was considered serious, none resulted in hospitalization and most resolved spontaneously or following a dose reduction. Treatment for nasal dryness and epistaxis was required infrequently (2% or less) and consisted of local application of pressure or a moisturizing agent (e.g., petroleum jelly or saline nasal spray). Patient discontinuation for epistaxis or nasal dryness was infrequent in both the controlled (0.3% or less) and one-year, open-label (2% or less) trials. There was no evidence of nasal rebound (i.e., a clinically significant increase in rhinorrhea, posterior nasal drip, sneezing or nasal congestion severity compared to baseline) upon discontinuation of double-blind therapy in these trials.

Adverse events reported by less than 2% of the patients receiving ATROVENT (ipratropium bromide) Nasal Spray 0.03% during the controlled clinical trials or during the open-label follow-up trial, which are potentially related to ATROVENT's local effects or systemic anticholinergic effects include: dry mouth/throat, dizziness, ocular irritation, blurred vision, conjunctivitis, hoarseness, cough, and taste perversion.

Additional anticholinergic effects noted with other ATROVENT dosage forms (ATROVENT Inhalation Solution, ATROVENT Inhalation Aerosol, and ATROVENT Nasal Spray 0.06%) include: precipitation or worsening of narrow angle glaucoma, urinary retention, prostatic disorders, tachycardia, constipation, and bowel obstruction.

There were infrequent reports of skin rash in both the controlled and uncontrolled clinical studies. Allergic-type reactions such as skin rash, angioedema of the throat, lips and face, generalized urticaria, laryngospasm, and anaphylactic reactions have been reported with ATROVENT Nasal Spray 0.03% and other ipratropium bromide products.

OVERDOSAGE

Acute overdosage by intranasal administration is unlikely since ipratropium bromide is not well absorbed systemically after intranasal or oral administration. Following administration of a 20 mg oral dose (equivalent to ingesting more than four bottles of ATROVENT® Nasal Spray 0.03%) to 10 male volunteers, no change in heart rate or blood pressure was noted. Following a 2 mg intravenous infusion over 15 minutes to the same 10 male volunteers, plasma ipratropium concentrations of 22-45 ng/mL were observed (>100 times the concentrations observed following intranasal administration). Following intravenous infusion these 10 volunteers had a mean increase of heart rate of 50 bpm and less than 20 mmHg change in systolic or diastolic blood pressure at the time of peak ipratropium levels.

Oral median lethal doses of ipratropium bromide were greater than 1,000 mg/kg in mice (approximately 16,000 and 9,500 times the maximum recommended daily intranasal dose in adults and children, respectively, on a mg/m^2 basis), 1,700 mg/kg in rats (approximately 55,000 and 32,000 times the maximum recommended daily intranasal dose in adults and children, respectively, on a mg/m^2 basis), and 400 mg/kg in dogs (approximately 43,000 and 25,000 times the maximum recommended daily intranasal dose in adults and children, respectively, on a mg/m^2 basis).

DOSAGE AND ADMINISTRATION

The recommended dose of ATROVENT® (ipratropium bromide) Nasal Spray 0.03% is two sprays (42 mcg) per nostril two or three times daily (total dose 168 to 252 mcg/day) for the symptomatic relief of rhinorrhea associated with allergic and nonallergic perennial rhinitis in adults and children age 6 years and older. Optimum dosage varies with the response of the individual patient. Initial pump priming requires seven sprays of the pump. If used regularly as recommended, no further priming is required. If not used for more than 24 hours, the pump will require two sprays, or if not used for more than seven days, the pump will require seven sprays to reprime.

% of Patients Reporting Events+

	ATROVENT Nasal Spray 0.03% (n=356)		Vehicle Control (n=347)	
	Incidence %	Discontinued %	Incidence %	Discontinued %
Headache	9.8	0.6	9.2	0
Upper respiratory tract infection	9.8	1.4	7.2	1.4
Epistaxis[1]	9.0	0.3	4.6	0.3
Rhinitis*				
Nasal dryness	5.1	0	0.9	0.3
Nasal irritation[2]	2.0	0	1.7	0.6
Other nasal symptoms[3]	3.1	1.1	1.7	0.3
Pharyngitis	8.1	0.3	4.6	0
Nausea	2.2	0.3	0.9	0

+ This table includes adverse events which occurred at an incidence rate of at least 2.0% in the ATROVENT group and more frequently in the ATROVENT group than in the vehicle group.

1 Epistaxis reported by 7.0% of ATROVENT patients and 2.3% of vehicle patients, blood-tinged mucus by 2.0% of ATROVENT patients and 2.3% of vehicle patients.

2 Nasal irritation includes reports of nasal itching, nasal burning, nasal irritation, and ulcerative rhinitis.

3 Other nasal symptoms include reports of nasal congestion, increased rhinorrhea, increased rhinitis, posterior nasal drip, sneezing, nasal polyps, and nasal edema.

* All events are listed by their WHO term; rhinitis has been presented by descriptive terms for clarification.

HOW SUPPLIED

ATROVENT® (ipratropium bromide) Nasal Spray 0.03% is supplied in a white high density polyethylene (HDPE) bottle fitted with a white and clear metered nasal spray pump, a green safety clip to prevent accidental discharge of the spray, and a clear plastic dust cap. It contains 31.1g of product formulation, 345 sprays, each delivering 21 mcg (70µL) of ipratropium per spray, or 28 days of therapy at the maximum recommended dose (two sprays per nostril three times a day).

Store tightly closed between 59°F (15°C) and 86°F (30°C). Avoid freezing. Keep out of reach of children. Do not spray in the eyes.

Patients should be reminded to read and follow the accompanying Patient's Instructions for Use, which should be dispensed with the product.

Rx only

Boehringer Ingelheim Pharmaceuticals, Inc.
Ridgefield, CT 06877
Licensed from: Boehringer Ingelheim International GmbH
U.S. Patent No. 4,385,048
Rev. May 29, 2003
10001900/US/2 10001900/02

Shown in Product Identification Guide, page 309

ATROVENT®
(ipratropium bromide)
Nasal Spray 0.06%

42 mcg/spray

Prescribing Information

DESCRIPTION

The active ingredient in ATROVENT® Nasal Spray is ipratropium bromide monohydrate. It is an anticholinergic agent chemically described as 8-azoniabicyclo (3.2.1) octane, 3-(3-hydroxy-1-oxo-2-phenylpropoxy)-8-methyl-8- (1-methylethyl)-, bromide, monohydrate *(endo,syn)*-, (±)-: a synthetic quaternary ammonium compound, chemically related to atropine. Its structural formula is:

ipratropium bromide monohydrate

$C_{20}H_{30}BrNO_3 \cdot H_2O$
Mol. Wt. 430.4

Ipratropium bromide is a white to off-white, crystalline substance. It is freely soluble in lower alcohols and water, existing in an ionized state in aqueous solutions, and relatively insoluble in non-polar media.

ATROVENT (ipratropium bromide) Nasal Spray 0.06% is a metered-dose, manual pump spray unit which delivers 42 mcg ipratropium bromide (on an anhydrous basis) per spray (70µL) in an isotonic, aqueous solution with pH-adjusted to 4.7. It also contains benzalkonium chloride, edetate disodium, sodium chloride, sodium hydroxide, hydrochloric acid, and purified water. Each bottle contains 165 sprays.

CLINICAL PHARMACOLOGY

Mechanism of Action

Ipratropium bromide is an anticholinergic agent that inhibits vagally-mediated reflexes by antagonizing the action of acetylcholine at the cholinergic receptor. In humans, ipratropium bromide has anti-secretory properties and, when applied locally, inhibits secretions from the serous and seromucous glands lining the nasal mucosa. Ipratropium bromide is a quaternary amine that minimally crosses the nasal and gastrointestinal membranes and the blood-brain barrier, resulting in a reduction of the systemic anticholinergic effects (e.g., neurologic, ophthalmic, cardiovascular, and gastrointestinal effects) that are seen with tertiary anticholinergic amines.

Pharmacokinetics

Absorption: Ipratropium bromide is poorly absorbed into the systemic circulation following oral administration (2-3%). Less than 20% of an 84 mcg per nostril dose was absorbed from the nasal mucosa of normal volunteers, induced-cold adult volunteers, naturally acquired common cold pediatric patients, or perennial rhinitis adult patients.

Distribution: Ipratropium bromide is minimally bound (0 to 9% *in vitro*) to plasma albumin and α_1-acid glycoprotein. Its blood/plasma concentration ratio was estimated to be about 0.89. Studies in rats have shown that ipratropium bromide does not penetrate the blood-brain barrier.

Metabolism: Ipratropium bromide is partially metabolized to ester hydrolysis products, tropic acid, and tropane. These metabolites appear to be inactive based on *in vitro* receptor affinity studies using rat brain tissue homogenates.

Elimination: After intravenous administration of 2 mg ipratropium bromide to 10 healthy volunteers, the terminal half-life of ipratropium bromide was approximately 1.6 hours. The total body clearance and renal clearance were estimated to be 2,505 and 1,019 mL/min, respectively. The amount of the total dose excreted unchanged in the urine

(Ae) within 24 hours was approximately one-half of the administered dose.

Pediatrics: Following administration of 84 mcg of ipratropium bromide per nostril three times a day in patients 5-18 years old (n=42) with a naturally acquired common cold, the mean amount of the total dose excreted unchanged in the urine of 7.8% was comparable to 84 mcg per nostril four times a day in an adult induced common cold population (n=22) of 7.3 to 8.1%. Plasma ipratropium concentrations were relatively low (ranging from undetectable up to 0.62 ng/mL). No correlation of the amount of the total dose excreted unchanged in the urine (Ae) with age or gender was observed in the pediatric population.

Special Populations: Gender does not appear to influence the absorption or excretion of nasally administered ipratropium bromide. The pharmacokinetics of ipratropium bromide have not been studied in patients with hepatic or renal insufficiency or in the elderly.

Drug-Drug Interactions: No specific pharmacokinetic studies were conducted to evaluate potential drug-drug interactions.

Pharmacodynamics: In two single dose trials (n=17), doses up to 336 mcg of ipratropium bromide did not significantly affect pupillary diameter, heart rate, or systolic/diastolic blood pressure. Similarly, ATROVENT Nasal Spray 0.06% in adult patients (n=22) with induced-colds (84 mcg/nostril four times a day) and in pediatric patients (n=45) with naturally acquired common cold (84 mcg/nostril three times a day) had no significant effects on pupillary diameter, heart rate, or systolic/diastolic blood pressure.

Controlled clinical trials demonstrated that intranasal fluorocarbon-propelled ipratropium bromide does not alter physiologic nasal functions (e.g., sense of smell, ciliary beat frequency, mucociliary clearance, or the air conditioning capacity of the nose).

Clinical Trials

Clinical trials for ATROVENT (ipratropium bromide) Nasal Spray 0.06% were conducted in patients with rhinorrhea associated with naturally occurring common colds. In two controlled four day comparisons of ATROVENT (ipratropium bromide) Nasal Spray 0.06% (84 mcg per nostril, administered three or four times daily; n=352) with its vehicle (n=351), there was a statistically significant reduction of rhinorrhea, as measured by both nasal discharge weight and the patients' subjective assessment of severity of rhinorrhea using a visual analog scale. These significant differences were evident within one hour following dosing. There was no effect of ATROVENT (ipratropium bromide) Nasal Spray 0.06% on degree of nasal congestion or sneezing. The response to ATROVENT (ipratropium bromide) Nasal Spray 0.06% did not appear to be affected by age or gender. No controlled clinical trials directly compared the efficacy of three times daily versus four times daily treatment.

One clinical trial was conducted with ATROVENT Nasal Spray 0.06%, administered four times daily for three weeks, in 218 patients with rhinorrhea associated with Seasonal Allergic Rhinitis (SAR), compared to its vehicle in 211 patients. Patients in this trial were adults and adolescents 12 years of age and above. ATROVENT (ipratropium bromide) Nasal Spray 0.06% was significantly more effective in reducing the severity and duration of rhinorrhea over the three weeks of the study, as measured by daily patient symptom scores. There was no difference between treatment groups in the effect on nasal congestion, sneezing or itching eyes.

INDICATIONS AND USAGE

ATROVENT® (ipratropium bromide) Nasal Spray 0.06% is indicated for the symptomatic relief of rhinorrhea associated with the common cold or seasonal allergic rhinitis for adults and children age 5 years and older. ATROVENT (ipratropium bromide) Nasal Spray 0.06% does not relieve nasal congestion or sneezing associated with the common cold or seasonal allergic rhinitis.

The safety and effectiveness of the use of ATROVENT (ipratropium bromide) Nasal Spray 0.06% beyond four days in patients with the common cold or beyond three weeks in patients with seasonal allergic rhinitis has not been established.

CONTRAINDICATIONS

ATROVENT® (ipratropium bromide) Nasal Spray 0.06% is contraindicated in patients with a history of hypersensitivity to atropine or its derivatives, or to any of the other ingredients.

WARNINGS

Immediate hypersensitivity reactions may occur after administration of ipratropium bromide, as demonstrated by rare cases of urticaria, angioedema, rash, bronchospasm and oropharyngeal edema.

PRECAUTIONS

General

ATROVENT® (ipratropium bromide) Nasal Spray 0.06% should be used with caution in patients with narrow-angle glaucoma, prostatic hypertrophy or bladder neck obstruction, particularly if they are receiving an anticholinergic by another route. Cases of precipitation or worsening of narrow-angle glaucoma and acute eye pain have been reported with direct eye contact of ipratropium bromide administered by oral inhalation.

Information for Patients

Patients should be advised that temporary blurring of vision, precipitation or worsening of narrow-angle glaucoma or eye pain may result if ATROVENT® (ipratropium bromide) Nasal Spray 0.06% comes into direct contact with the eyes. Patients should be instructed to avoid spraying ATROVENT (ipratropium bromide) Nasal Spray 0.06% in or around the eyes. Patients who experience eye pain, blurred vision, excessive nasal dryness or episodes of nasal bleeding should be instructed to contact their doctor. Patients should be reminded to carefully read and follow the accompanying Patient's Instructions for Use.

Drug Interactions

No controlled clinical trials were conducted to investigate potential drug-drug interactions. ATROVENT (ipratropium bromide) Nasal Spray 0.06% is minimally absorbed into the systemic circulation; nonetheless, there is some potential for an additive interaction with other concomitantly administered medications with anticholinergic properties, including ATROVENT for oral inhalation.

Carcinogenesis, Mutagenesis, Impairment of Fertility

In two-year carcinogenicity studies in rats and mice, ipratropium bromide at oral doses up to 6 mg/kg (approximately 70 and 35 times the maximum recommended daily intranasal dose in adults, respectively, and approximately 45 and 25 times the maximum recommended daily intranasal dose in children, respectively, on a mg/m^2 basis) showed no carcinogenic activity. Results of various mutagenicity studies (Ames test, mouse dominant lethal test, mouse micronucleus test, and chromosome aberration of bone marrow in Chinese hamsters) were negative.

Fertility of male or female rats was unaffected by ipratropium bromide at oral doses up to 50 mg/kg (approximately 600 times the maximum recommended daily intranasal dose in adults on a mg/m^2 basis). At an oral dose of 500 mg/kg (approximately 16,000 times the maximum recommended daily intranasal dose in adults on a mg/m^2 basis), ipratropium bromide produced a decrease in the conception rate.

Pregnancy

TERATOGENIC EFFECTS Pregnancy Category B.

Oral reproduction studies were performed at doses of 10 mg/kg in mice, 1,000 mg/kg in rats and 125 mg/kg in rabbits. These doses correspond, in each species respectively, to approximately 60, 12,000, and 3,000 times the maximum recommended daily intranasal dose in adults on a mg/m^2 basis. Inhalation reproduction studies were conducted in rats and rabbits at doses of 1.5 and 1.8 mg/kg, respectively, (approximately 20 and 45 times, respectively, the maximum recommended daily intranasal dose in adults on a mg/m^2 basis). These studies demonstrated no evidence of teratogenic effects as a result of ipratropium bromide. At oral doses above 90 mg/kg in rats (approximately 1,100 times the maximum recommended daily intranasal dose in adults on a mg/m^2 basis) embryotoxicity was observed as increased resorption. This effect is not considered relevant to human use due to the large doses at which it was observed and the difference in route of administration. However, no adequate or well controlled studies have been conducted in pregnant women. Because animal reproduction studies are not always predictive of human response, ipratropium bromide should be used during pregnancy only if clearly needed.

Nursing Mothers

It is known that some ipratropium bromide is systemically absorbed following nasal administration; however the portion which may be excreted in human milk is unknown. Although lipid-insoluble quaternary bases pass into breast milk, the minimal systemic absorption makes it unlikely that ipratropium bromide would reach the infant in an amount sufficient to cause a clinical effect. However, because many drugs are excreted in human milk, caution should be exercised when ATROVENT® (ipratropium bromide) Nasal Spray 0.06% is administered to a nursing woman.

Pediatric Use

The safety of ATROVENT (ipratropium bromide) Nasal Spray 0.06% at a dose of two sprays (84 mcg) per nostril three times a day (total dose 504 mcg/day) for two to four days has been demonstrated in two clinical trials involving 362 pediatric patients 5-11 years of age with naturally acquired common colds. In this pediatric population ATROVENT (ipratropium bromide) Nasal Spray 0.06% had an adverse event profile similar to that observed in adolescent and adult patients. When ATROVENT was concomitantly administered with an oral decongestant (pseudoephedrine HCl) in 122 children ages 5-12 years, and concomitantly administered with an oral decongestant/antihistamine combination (pseudoephedrine HCl/chlorpheniramine maleate) in 123 children ages 5-12 years, adverse event profiles were similar to ATROVENT alone. The safety of ATROVENT (ipratropium bromide) Nasal Spray 0.06% at a dose of two sprays (84 mcg) per nostril four times a day (total dose 672 mcg/day) for three weeks in pediatric seasonal allergic rhinitis patients down to 5 years is based upon the safety demonstrated in the pediatric common cold trials and the trial in adult and adolescent patients 12 to 75 years of age with seasonal allergic rhinitis. The effectiveness of ATROVENT (ipratropium bromide) Nasal Spray 0.06% for the treatment of rhinorrhea associated with the common cold and seasonal allegic rhinitis in this pediatric age group is based on extrapolation of the demonstrated efficacy of ATROVENT (ipratropium bromide) Nasal Spray 0.06% in adolescents and adults with the conditions and the likelihood that the disease course, pathophysiology, and the drug's effects are substantially similar to that of adults. The recommended dose for common cold for the pediatric population is based on cross-study comparisons of the efficacy of ATROVENT (ipratropium bromide) Nasal Spray 0.06% in adult and pediatric patients and on its safety profile in both adults and pediatric common cold patients. The recommended dose for seasonal allergic rhinitis for the pediatric population down to 5 years is based upon the efficacy and safety of ATROVENT (ipratropium bromide) Nasal Spray in adults and adolescents 12 years of age and above with seasonal allergic rhinitis and the safety profile of this dose in both adult and pediatric common cold patients. The safety and effectiveness of ATROVENT (ipratropium bromide) Nasal Spray 0.06% in pediatric patients under 5 years of age have not been established.

ADVERSE REACTIONS

Adverse reaction information on ATROVENT® (ipratropium bromide) Nasal Spray 0.06% in patients with the common cold was derived from two multicenter, vehicle-controlled clinical trials involving 1,276 patients (195 patients on ATROVENT® (ipratropium bromide) Nasal Spray 0.03%, 352 patients on ATROVENT (ipratropium bromide) Nasal Spray 0.06%, 189 patients on ATROVENT (ipratropium bromide) Nasal Spray 0.12%, 351 patients on vehicle and 189 patients receiving no treatment).

Table 1 shows adverse events reported for patients who received ATROVENT (ipratropium bromide) Nasal Spray 0.06% at the recommended dose of 84 mcg per nostril, or vehicle, administered three or four times daily, where the incidence is 1% or greater in the ATROVENT group and higher in the ATROVENT® group than in the vehicle group.

Table 1 % of Patients with Common Cold Reporting Events[1]

	ATROVENT Nasal Spray 0.06%	Vehicle Control
No. of Patients	352	351
Epistaxis[2]	8.2%	2.3%
Nasal Dryness	4.8%	2.8%
Dry Mouth/Throat	1.4%	0.3%
Nasal Congestion	1.1%	0.0%

[1] This table includes adverse events for which the incidence was 1% or greater in the ATROVENT group and higher in the ATROVENT group than in the vehicle group.

[2] Epistaxis reported by 5.4% of ATROVENT patients and 1.4% of vehicle patients, blood tinged nasal mucus by 2.8% of ATROVENT patients and 0.9% of vehicle patients.

ATROVENT (ipratropium bromide) Nasal Spray 0.06% was well tolerated by most patients. The most frequently reported adverse events were transient episodes of nasal dryness or epistaxis. The majority of these adverse events (96%) were mild or moderate in nature, none was considered serious, and none resulted in hospitalization. No patient required treatment for nasal dryness, and only three patients (<1%) required treatment for epistaxis, which consisted of local application of pressure or a moisturizing agent (e.g., petroleum jelly). No patient receiving ATROVENT (ipratropium bromide) Nasal Spray 0.06% was discontinued from the trial due to either nasal dryness or bleeding.

Adverse events reported by less than 1% of the patients receiving ATROVENT (ipratropium bromide) Nasal Spray 0.06% during the controlled clinical trials that are potentially related to ATROVENT's local effects or systemic anticholinergic effects include: taste perversion, nasal burning, conjunctivitis, coughing, dizziness, hoarseness, palpitation, pharyngitis, tachycardia, thirst, tinnitus, and blurred vision. No controlled trial was conducted to address the relative incidence of adverse events for three times daily versus four times daily therapy.

Nasal adverse events seen in the clinical trial with seasonal allergic rhinitis (SAR) patients (see Table 2) were similar to those seen in the common cold trials. Additional events were reported at a higher rate in the SAR trial due in part to the longer duration of the trial and the inclusion of upper respiratory tract infection (URI) as an adverse event. In common cold trials, URI was the disease under study and not an adverse event.

Table 2 % of Patients with SAR Reporting Events[1]

	ATROVENT® Nasal Spray 0.06%	Vehicle Control
No. of Patients	218	211
Epistaxis[2]	6.0%	3.3%
Pharyngitis	5.0%	3.8%
URI	5.0%	3.3%
Nasal Dryness	4.6%	0.9%

Continued on next page

Atrovent Nasal Spray 0.06%—Cont.

Headache	4.1%	0.5%
Dry Mouth/Throat	4.1%	0.0%
Taste Perversion	3.7%	1.4%
Sinusitis	2.8%	2.8%
Pain	1.8%	0.9%
Diarrhea	1.8%	0.5%

[1] This table includes adverse events for which the incidence was 1% or greater in the ATROVENT group and higher in the ATROVENT group than in the vehicle group.

[2] Epistaxis reported by 3.7% of ATROVENT patients and 2.4% of vehicle patients, blood tinged nasal mucus by 2.3% of ATROVENT patients and 1.9% of vehicle patients.

Additional anticholinergic effects noted with other ATROVENT dosage forms (ATROVENT Inhalation Solution, ATROVENT Inhalation Aerosol and ATROVENT Nasal Spray 0.03%) include: precipitation or worsening of narrow-angle glaucoma, urinary retention, prostate disorders, constipation, and bowel obstruction.

There were no reports of allergic-type reactions in the controlled clinical trials. Allergic-type reactions such as skin rash, angioedema of the throat, tongue, lips and face, generalized urticaria, laryngospasm and anaphylactic reactions have been reported with ATROVENT Nasal Spray 0.06% and other ipratropium bromide products.

OVERDOSAGE

Acute overdosage by intranasal administration is unlikely since ipratropium bromide is not well absorbed systemically after intranasal or oral administration. Following administration of a 20 mg oral dose (equivalent to ingesting more than two bottles of ATROVENT® Nasal Spray 0.06%) to 10 male volunteers, no change in heart rate or blood pressure was noted. Following a 2 mg intravenous infusion over 15 minutes to the same 10 male volunteers, plasma ipratropium concentrations of 22-45 ng/mL were observed (>100 times the concentrations observed following intranasal administration). Following intravenous infusion these 10 volunteers had a mean increase of heart rate of 50 bpm and less than 20 mm Hg change in systolic or diastolic blood pressure at the time of peak ipratropium levels.

Oral median lethal doses of ipratropium bromide were greater than 1,000 mg/kg in mice (approximately 6,000 and 3,800 times the maximum recommended daily intranasal dose in adults and children, respectively, on a mg/m^2 basis), 1,700 mg/kg in rats (approximately 21,000 and 13,000 times the maximum recommended daily intranasal dose in adults and children, respectively, on a mg/m^2 basis) and 400 mg/kg in dogs (approximately 16,000 and 10,000 times the maximum recommended daily intranasal dose in adults and children, respectively, on a mg/m^2 basis).

DOSAGE AND ADMINISTRATION

For Symptomatic Relief of Rhinorrhea Associated with the Common Cold

The recommended dose of ATROVENT® (ipratropium bromide) Nasal Spray 0.06% is two sprays (84 mcg) per nostril three or four times daily (total dose 504 to 672 mcg/day) in adults and children age 12 years and older. Optimum dosage varies with response of the individual patient. The recommended dose of ATROVENT (ipratropium bromide) Nasal Spray 0.06% for children age 5-11 years is two sprays (84 mcg) per nostril three times daily (total dose of 504 mcg/day).

The safety and effectiveness of the use of ATROVENT (ipratropium bromide) Nasal Spray 0.06% beyond four days in patients with the common cold have not been established.

For Symptomatic Relief of Rhinorrhea Associated with Seasonal Allergic Rhinitis

The recommended dose of ATROVENT (ipratropium bromide) Nasal Spray 0.06% is two sprays (84 mcg) per nostril four times daily (total dose 672 mcg/day) in adults and children age 5 years and older.

The safety and effectiveness of the use of ATROVENT (ipratropium bromide) Nasal Spray 0.06% beyond three weeks in patients with seasonal allergic rhinitis have not been established.

Initial pump priming requires seven sprays of the pump. If used regularly as recommended, no further priming is required. If not used for more than 24 hours, the pump will require two sprays, or if not used for more than seven days, the pump will require seven sprays to reprime.

HOW SUPPLIED

ATROVENT® (ipratropium bromide) Nasal Spray 0.06% is supplied in a white high density polyethylene (HDPE) bottle fitted with a metered nasal spray pump, a green safety clip to prevent accidental discharge of the spray, and a clear plastic dust cap. It contains 16.6 g of product formulation, 165 sprays, each delivering 42 mcg of ipratropium bromide per spray (70 µL), or 10 days of therapy at the maximum recommended dose (two sprays per nostril four times a day).

Store tightly closed between 59°F (15°C) and 86°F (30°C). Avoid freezing. Keep out of reach of children. Do not spray in the eyes.

Patients should be reminded to read and follow the accompanying Patient's Instructions for Use, which should be dispensed with the product.

Rx only

Boehringer Ingelheim Pharmaceuticals, Inc.
Ridgefield, CT 06877
Licensed from: Boehringer Ingelheim International GmbH
U.S. Patent No. 4,385,048
Rev. May 29, 2003
4042182/US/4 4042182//04

Shown in Product Identification Guide, page 309

CATAPRES® ℞

[kah 'tah-pres]
(clonidine hydrochloride USP)
Oral Antihypertensive
Tablets of 0.1, 0.2 and 0.3 mg

Prescribing Information

DESCRIPTION

CATAPRES® (clonidine hydrochloride USP) is a centrally acting alpha-agonist hypotensive agent available as tablets for oral administration in three dosage strengths: 0.1 mg, 0.2 mg and 0.3 mg. The 0.1 mg tablet is equivalent to 0.087 mg of the free base.

The inactive ingredients are colloidal silicon dioxide, cornstarch, dibasic calcium phosphate, FD&C Yellow No. 6, gelatin, glycerin, lactose, magnesium stearate, methylparaben, propylparaben. The CATAPRES 0.1 mg tablet also contains FD&C Blue No. 1 and FD&C Red No. 3.

Clonidine hydrochloride is an imidazoline derivative and exists as a mesomeric compound. The chemical name is 2-(2,6-dichlorophenylamino)-2-imidazoline hydrochloride. The following is the structural formula:

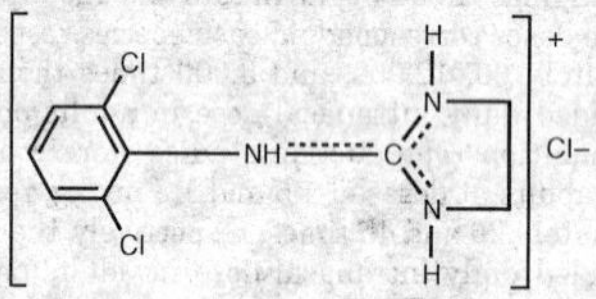

$C_9H_9Cl_2N_3 \cdot HCl$ Mol. Wt. 266.56

Clonidine hydrochloride is an odorless, bitter, white, crystalline substance soluble in water and alcohol.

CLINICAL PHARMACOLOGY

Clonidine stimulates alpha-adrenoreceptors in the brain stem. This action results in reduced sympathetic outflow from the central nervous system and in decreases in peripheral resistance, renal vascular resistance, heart rate, and blood pressure. CATAPRES (clonidine hydrochloride USP) acts relatively rapidly. The patient's blood pressure declines within 30 to 60 minutes after an oral dose, the maximum decrease occurring within 2 to 4 hours. Renal blood flow and glomerular filtration rate remain essentially unchanged. Normal postural reflexes are intact; therefore, orthostatic symptoms are mild and infrequent.

Acute studies with clonidine hydrochloride in humans have demonstrated a moderate reduction (15% to 20%) of cardiac output in the supine position with no change in the peripheral resistance: at a 45° tilt there is a smaller reduction in cardiac output and a decrease of peripheral resistance. During long-term therapy, cardiac output tends to return to control values, while peripheral resistance remains decreased. Slowing of the pulse rate has been observed in most patients given clonidine, but the drug does not alter normal hemodynamic response to exercise.

Tolerance to the antihypertensive effect may develop in some patients, necessitating a reevaluation of therapy.

Other studies in patients have provided evidence of a reduction in plasma renin activity and in the excretion of aldosterone and catecholamines. The exact relationship of these pharmacologic actions to the antihypertensive effect of clonidine has not been fully elucidated.

Clonidine acutely stimulates growth hormone release in both children and adults, but does not produce a chronic elevation of growth hormone with long-term use.

Pharmacokinetics: The plasma level of clonidine peaks in approximately 3 to 5 hours and the plasma half-life ranges from 12 to 16 hours. The half-life increases up to 41 hours in patients with severe impairment of renal function. Following oral administration about 40–60% of the absorbed dose is recovered in the urine as unchanged drug in 24 hours. About 50% of the absorbed dose is metabolized in the liver.

INDICATIONS AND USAGE

CATAPRES® (clonidine hydrochloride USP) is indicated in the treatment of hypertension. CATAPRES may be employed alone or concomitantly with other antihypertensive agents.

CONTRAINDICATIONS

CATAPRES® (clonidine hydrochloride USP) Tablets should not be used in patients with known hypersensitivity to clonidine (see PRECAUTIONS).

WARNINGS

Withdrawal Patients should be instructed not to discontinue therapy without consulting their physician. Sudden cessation of clonidine treatment has, in some cases, resulted in symptoms such as nervousness, agitation, headache, and tremor accompanied or followed by a rapid rise in blood pressure and elevated catecholamine concentrations in the plasma. The likelihood of such reactions to discontinuation of clonidine therapy appears to be greater after administration of higher doses or continuation of concomitant beta-blocker treatment and special caution is therefore advised in these situations. Rare instances of hypertensive encephalopathy, cerebrovascular accidents and death have been reported after clonidine withdrawal. When discontinuing therapy with CATAPRES®, the physician should reduce the dose gradually over 2 to 4 days to avoid withdrawal symptomatology.

An excessive rise in blood pressure following discontinuation of CATAPRES therapy can be reversed by administration of oral clonidine hydrochloride or by intravenous phentolamine. If therapy is to be discontinued in patients receiving a beta-blocker and clonidine concurrently, the beta-blocker should be withdrawn several days before the gradual discontinuation of CATAPRES.

Because children commonly have gastrointestinal illnesses that lead to vomiting, they may be particularly susceptible to hypertensive episodes resulting from abrupt inability to take medication.

PRECAUTIONS

General: In patients who have developed localized contact sensitization to CATAPRES-TTS® (clonidine), continuation of CATAPRES-TTS or substitution of oral clonidine hydrochloride therapy may be associated with the development of a generalized skin rash.

In patients who develop an allergic reaction to CATAPRES-TTS, substitution of oral clonidine hydrochloride may also elicit an allergic reaction (including generalized rash, urticaria, or angioedema).

CATAPRES® (clonidine hydrochloride) should be used with caution in patients with severe coronary insufficiency, conduction disturbances, recent myocardial infarction, cerebrovascular disease or chronic renal failure.

Perioperative Use: Administration of CATAPRES should be continued to within four hours of surgery and resumed as soon as possible thereafter. Blood pressure should be carefully monitored during surgery and additional measures to control blood pressure should be available if required.

Information for Patients: Patients should be cautioned against interruption of CATAPRES therapy without their physician's advice.

Patients who engage in potentially hazardous activities, such as operating machinery or driving, should be advised of a possible sedative effect of clonidine. They should also be informed that this sedative effect may be increased by concomitant use of alcohol, barbiturates, or other sedating drugs.

Drug Interactions: Clonidine may potentiate the CNS-depressive effects of alcohol, barbiturates or other sedating drugs. If a patient receiving clonidine hydrochloride is also taking tricyclic antidepressants, the hypotensive effect of clonidine may be reduced, necessitating an increase in the clonidine dose.

Due to a potential for additive effects such as bradycardia and AV block, caution is warranted in patients receiving clonidine concomitantly with agents known to affect sinus node function or AV nodal conduction, e.g. digitalis, calcium channel blockers and beta-blockers.

Amitriptyline in combination with clonidine enhances the manifestation of corneal lesions in rats (See TOXICOLOGY).

Toxicology: In several studies with oral clonidine hydrochloride, a dose-dependent increase in the incidence and severity of spontaneous retinal degeneration was seen in albino rats treated for six months or longer. Tissue distribution studies in dogs and monkeys showed a concentration of clonidine in the choroid.

In view of the retinal degeneration seen in rats, eye examinations were performed during clinical trials in 908 patients before, and periodically after, the start of clonidine therapy. In 353 of these 908 patients, the eye examinations were carried out over periods of 24 months or longer. Except for some dryness of the eyes, no drug-related abnormal ophthalmological findings were recorded and, according to specialized tests such as electroretinography and macular dazzle, retinal function was unchanged.

In combination with amitriptyline, clonidine hydrochloride administration led to the development of corneal lesions in rats within 5 days.

Carcinogenesis, Mutagenesis, Impairment of Fertility: Chronic dietary administration of clonidine was not carcinogenic to rats (132 weeks) or mice (78 weeks) dosed, respectively, at up to 46 or 70 times the maximum recommended daily human dose as mg/kg (9 or 6 times the MRDHD on a mg/m^2 basis). There was no evidence of genotoxicity in the Ames test for mutagenicity or mouse micronucleus test for clastogenicity.

Fertility of male or female rats was unaffected by clonidine doses as high as 150 mcg/kg (approximately 3 times MRDHD). In a separate experiment, fertility of female rats appeared to be affected at dose levels of 500 to 2000 mcg/kg (10 to 40 times the oral MRDHD on a mg/kg basis; 2 to 8 times the MRDHD on a mg/m^2 basis).

Usage in Pregnancy: *TERATOGENIC EFFECTS Pregnancy Category C* Reproduction studies performed in rabbits at doses up to approximately 3 times the oral maximum recommended daily human dose (MRDHD) of

Dose (mg)	Color	Marking	Bottle of 100	Bottle of 1000	Unit Dose of 100
0.1	Tan	BI 6	NDC0597-0006-01	NDC0597-0006-10	NDC0597-0006-61
0.2	Orange	BI 7	NDC0597-0007-01	NDC0597-0007-10	NDC0597-0007-61
0.3	Peach	BI 11	NDC0597-0011-01		

CATAPRES (clonidine hydrochloride) produced no evidence of a teratogenic or embryotoxic potential in rabbits. In rats, however, doses as low as $^1/_3$ the oral MRDHD ($^1/_{15}$ the MRDHD on a mg/m^2 basis) of clonidine were associated with increased resorptions in a study in which dams were treated continuously from 2 months prior to mating. Increased resorptions were not associated with treatment at the same time or at higher dose levels (up to 3 times the oral MRDHD) when the dams were treated on gestation days 6–15. Increases in resorption were observed at much higher dose levels (40 times the oral MRDHD on a mg/kg basis; 4 to 8 times the MRDHD on a mg/m^2 basis) in mice and rats treated on gestation days 1–14 (lowest dose employed in the study was 500 mcg/kg).

No adequate, well-controlled studies have been conducted in pregnant women. Because animal reproduction studies are not always predictive of human response, this drug should be used during pregnancy only if clearly needed.

Nursing Mothers: As clonidine hydrochloride is excreted in human milk, caution should be exercised when CATAPRES® (clonidine hydrochloride USP) is administered to a nursing woman.

Pediatric Use: Safety and effectiveness in pediatric patients below the age of twelve have not been established (See Warnings on Withdrawal).

ADVERSE REACTIONS

Most adverse effects are mild and tend to diminish with continued therapy. The most frequent (which appear to be dose-related) are dry mouth, occurring in about 40 of 100 patients; drowsiness, about 33 in 100; dizziness, about 16 in 100; constipation and sedation, each about 10 in 100.

The following less frequent adverse experiences have also been reported in patients receiving CATAPRES® (clonidine hydrochloride USP), but in many cases patients were receiving concomitant medication and a causal relationship has not been established.

Body as a Whole: Weakness, about 10 in 100 patients; fatigue, about 4 in 100; headache and withdrawal syndrome each about 1 in 100. Also reported were pallor; a weakly positive Coombs' test; increased sensitivity to alcohol; and fever.

Cardiovascular: Orthostatic symptoms, about 3 in 100 patients; palpitations and tachycardia, and bradycardia, each about 5 in 1000. Syncope, Raynaud's phenomenon, congestive heart failure, and electrocardiographic abnormalities (i.e., sinus node arrest, junctional bradycardia, high degree AV block and arrhythmias) have been reported rarely. Rare cases of sinus bradycardia and atrioventricular block have been reported, both with and without the use of concomitant digitalis.

Central Nervous System: Nervousness and agitation, about 3 in 100 patients; mental depression, about 1 in 100 and insomnia, about 5 in 1000. Other behavioral changes, vivid dreams or nightmares, restlessness, anxiety, visual and auditory hallucinations and delirium have rarely been reported.

Dermatological: Rash, about 1 in 100 patients; pruritus, about 7 in 1000; hives, angioneurotic edema and urticaria, about 5 in 1000; alopecia, about 2 in 1000.

Gastrointestinal: Nausea and vomiting, about 5 in 100 patients; anorexia and malaise, each about 1 in 100; mild transient abnormalities in liver function tests, about 1 in 100; hepatitis, parotitis, constipation, pseudo-obstruction, and abdominal pain, rarely.

Genitourinary: Decreased sexual activity, impotence and loss of libido, about 3 in 100 patients; nocturia, about 1 in 100; difficulty in micturition, about 2 in 1000; urinary retention, about 1 in 1000.

Hematologic: Thrombocytopenia, rarely.

Metabolic: Weight gain, about 1 in 100 patients; gynecomastia, about 1 in 1000; transient elevation of blood glucose or serum creatine phosphokinase, rarely.

Musculoskeletal: Muscle or joint pain, about 6 in 1000 and leg cramps, about 3 in 1000.

Oro-otolaryngeal: Dryness of the nasal mucosa was rarely reported.

Ophthalmological: Dryness of the eyes, burning of the eyes and blurred vision were reported.

OVERDOSAGE

Hypertension may develop early and may be followed by hypotension, bradycardia, respiratory depression, hypothermia, drowsiness, decreased or absent reflexes, weakness, irritability and miosis. The frequency of CNS depression may be higher in children than adults. Large overdoses may result in reversible cardiac conduction defects or dysrhythmias, apnea, coma and seizures. Signs and symptoms of overdose generally occur within 30 minutes to two hours after exposure. As little as 0.1 mg of clonidine has produced signs of toxicity in children.

There is no specific antidote for clonidine overdose. Clonidine overdosage may result in the rapid development of CNS depression; therefore, induction of vomiting with ipecac syrup is not recommended. Gastric lavage may be indicated following recent and/or large ingestions. Administration of activated charcoal and/or a cathartic may be beneficial. Supportive care may include atropine sulfate for bradycardia, intravenous fluids and/or vasopressor agents for hypotension and vasodilators for hypertension. Naloxone may be a useful adjunct for the management of clonidine-induced respiratory depression, hypotension and/or coma; blood pressure should be monitored since the administration of naloxone has occasionally resulted in paradoxical hypertension. Tolazoline administration has yielded inconsistent results and is not recommended as first-line therapy. Dialysis is not likely to significantly enhance the elimination of clonidine.

The largest overdose reported to date involved a 28-year old male who ingested 100 mg of clonidine hydrochloride powder. This patient developed hypertension followed by hypotension, bradycardia, apnea, hallucinations, semicoma, and premature ventricular contractions. The patient fully recovered after intensive treatment. Plasma clonidine levels were 60 ng/ml after 1 hour, 190 ng/ml after 1.5 hours, 370 ng/ml after 2 hours, and 120 ng/ml after 5.5 and 6.5 hours. In mice and rats, the oral LD_{50} of clonidine is 206 and 465 mg/kg, respectively.

DOSAGE AND ADMINISTRATION

Adults: The dose of CATAPRES® (clonidine hydrochloride USP) must be adjusted according to the patient's individual blood pressure response. The following is a general guide to its administration.

Initial Dose: 0.1 mg tablet twice daily (morning and bedtime). Elderly patients may benefit from a lower initial dose.

Maintenance Dose: Further increments of 0.1 mg per day may be made at weekly intervals if necessary until the desired response is achieved. Taking the larger portion of the oral daily dose at bedtime may minimize transient adjustment effects of dry mouth and drowsiness. The therapeutic doses most commonly employed have ranged from 0.2 mg to 0.6 mg per day given in divided doses. Studies have indicated that 2.4 mg is the maximum effective daily dose, but doses as high as this have rarely been employed.

Renal Impairment: Dosage must be adjusted according to the degree of impairment, and patients should be carefully monitored. Since only a minimal amount of clonidine is removed during routine hemodialysis, there is no need to give supplemental clonidine following dialysis.

HOW SUPPLIED

CATAPRES® (clonidine hydrochloride USP) is supplied in scored oval tablets containing 0.1 mg, 0.2 mg or 0.3 mg of clonidine hydrochloride.

[See table above]

Store at 25°C (77°F).

Excursions permitted to 15–30°C (59–86°F).

(See USP controlled room temperature).

Dispense in tight, light-resistant container.

Rx only

Revised 4/98 340066/US/2

Shown in Product Identification Guide, page 309

CATAPRES-TTS® ℞

[*căt-a'prĕs*]

(clonidine)

Catapres-TTS® -1

Catapres-TTS® -2

Catapres-TTS® -3

Transdermal Therapeutic System

Programmed delivery *in vivo* of 0.1, 0.2, or 0.3 mg clonidine per day, for one week.

Prescribing Information

DESCRIPTION

CATAPRES-TTS® (clonidine) is a transdermal system providing continuous systemic delivery of clonidine for 7 days at an approximately constant rate. Clonidine is a centrally acting alpha-agonist hypotensive agent. It is an imidazoline derivative with the chemical name 2, 6-dichloro-N-2-imidazolidinylidenebenzenamine and has the following chemical structure:

(clonidine)

System Structure and Components

CATAPRES-TTS is a multi-layered film, 0.2 mm thick, containing clonidine as the active agent.

The system areas are 3.5 cm^2 (CATAPRES-TTS-1), 7.0 cm^2 (CATAPRES-TTS-2) and 10.5 cm^2 (CATAPRES-TTS-3) and the amount of drug released is directly proportional to the area (See Release Rate Concept). The composition per unit area is the same for all three doses.

Proceeding from the visible surface towards the surface attached to the skin, there are four consecutive layers: 1) a backing layer of pigmented polyester film; 2) a drug reservoir of clonidine, mineral oil, polyisobutylene, and colloidal silicon dioxide; 3) a microporous polypropylene membrane that controls the rate of delivery of clonidine from the system to the skin surface; 4) an adhesive formulation of clonidine, mineral oil, polyisobutylene, and colloidal silicon dioxide. Prior to use, a protective slit release liner of polyester that covers the adhesive layer is removed.

Cross Section of the System:

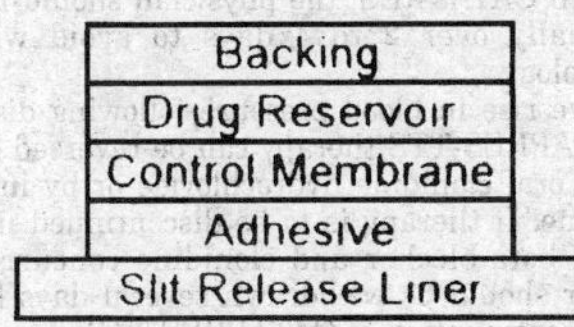

Release Rate Concept

CATAPRES-TTS is programmed to release clonidine at an approximately constant rate for 7 days. The energy for drug release is derived from the concentration gradient existing between a saturated solution of drug in the system and the much lower concentration prevailing in the skin. Clonidine flows in the direction of the lower concentration at a constant rate, limited by the rate-controlling membrane, so long as a saturated solution is maintained in the drug reservoir.

Following system application to intact skin, clonidine in the adhesive layer saturates the skin site below the system. Clonidine from the drug reservoir then begins to flow through the rate-controlling membrane and the adhesive layer of the system into the systemic circulation via the capillaries beneath the skin. Therapeutic plasma clonidine levels are achieved 2 to 3 days after initial application of CATAPRES-TTS.

The 3.5, 7.0, and 10.5 cm^2 systems deliver 0.1, 0.2, and 0.3 mg of clonidine per day, respectively. To ensure constant release of drug for 7 days, the total drug content of the system is higher than the total amount of drug delivered. Application of a new system to a fresh skin site at weekly intervals continuously maintains therapeutic plasma concentrations of clonidine. If the CATAPRES-TTS is removed and not replaced with a new system, therapeutic plasma clonidine levels will persist for about 8 hours and then decline slowly over several days. Over this time period, blood pressure returns gradually to pretreatment levels.

CLINICAL PHARMACOLOGY

Clonidine stimulates alpha-adrenoreceptors in the brain stem. This action results in reduced sympathetic outflow from the central nervous system and in decreases in peripheral resistance, renal vascular resistance, heart rate, and blood pressure. Renal blood flow and glomerular filtration rate remain essentially unchanged. Normal postural reflexes are intact; therefore, orthostatic symptoms are mild and infrequent.

Acute studies with clonidine hydrochloride in humans have demonstrated a moderate reduction (15%-20%) of cardiac output in the supine position with no change in the peripheral resistance; at a 45° tilt there is a smaller reduction in cardiac output and a decrease of peripheral resistance.

During long-term therapy, cardiac output tends to return to control values, while peripheral resistance remains decreased. Slowing of the pulse rate has been observed in most patients given clonidine, but the drug does not alter normal hemodynamic responses to exercise.

Tolerance to the antihypertensive effect may develop in some patients, necessitating a reevaluation of therapy.

Other studies in patients have provided evidence of a reduction in plasma renin activity and in the excretion of aldosterone and catecholamines. The exact relationship of these pharmacologic actions to the antihypertensive effect of clonidine has not been fully elucidated.

Clonidine acutely stimulates the release of growth hormone in children as well as adults but does not produce a chronic elevation of growth hormone with long-term use.

Pharmacokinetics The plasma half-life of clonidine is 12.7 ± 7 hours. Following oral administration, about 40-60% of the absorbed dose is recovered in the urine as unchanged drug within 24 hours. The remainder of the absorbed dose is metabolized in the liver.

INDICATIONS AND USAGE

CATAPRES-TTS (clonidine) is indicated in the treatment of hypertension. It may be employed alone or concomitantly with other antihypertensive agents.

CONTRAINDICATIONS

CATAPRES-TTS (clonidine) should not be used in patients with known hypersensitivity to clonidine or to any other component of the therapeutic system.

WARNINGS

Withdrawal

Patients should be instructed not to discontinue therapy without consulting their physician. Sudden cessation of clonidine treatment has, in come cases, resulted in symptoms such as nervousness, agitation, headache, and confusion accompanied or followed by a rapid rise in blood pressure and elevated catecholamine concentrations in the plasma. The likelihood of such reactions to discontinuation of clonidine therapy appears to be greater after administration of higher doses or continuation of concomitant beta-blocker treatment and special caution is therefore advised

Continued on next page

Catapres-TTS—Cont.

in these situations. Rare instances of hypertensive encephalopathy, cerebrovascular accidents and death have been reported after clonidine withdrawal. When discontinuing therapy with CATAPRES, the physician should reduce the dose gradually over 2 to 4 days to avoid withdrawal symptomatology.

An excessive rise in blood pressure following discontinuation of CATAPRES-TTS therapy can be reversed by administration of oral clonidine hydrochloride or by intravenous phentolamine. If therapy is to be discontinued in patients receiving a beta-blocker and clonidine concurrently, the beta-blocker should be withdrawn several days before the gradual discontinuation of CATAPRES-TTS.

PRECAUTIONS

General

In patients who have developed localized contact sensitization to (CATAPRES-TTS clonidine) continuation of CATAPRES-TTS or substitution of oral clonidine hydrochloride therapy may be associated with development of a generalized skin rash.

In patients who develop an allergic reaction to CATAPRES-TTS, substitution of oral clonidine hydrochloride may also elicit an allergic reaction (including generalized rash, urticaria, or angioedema).

CATAPRES-TTS should be used with caution in patients with severe coronary insufficiency, conduction disturbances, recent myocardial infarction, cerebrovascular disease, or chronic renal failure.

In rare instances, loss of blood pressure control has been reported in patients using CATAPRES-TTS according to the instructions for use.

Perioperative Use

CATAPRES-TTS therapy should not be interrupted during the surgical period. Blood pressure should be carefully monitored during surgery and additional measures to control blood pressure should be available if required. Physicians considering starting CATAPRES-TTS therapy during the perioperative period must be aware that therapeutic plasma clonidine levels are not achieved until 2 to 3 days after initial application of CATAPRES-TTS (see DOSAGE AND ADMINISTRATION).

Defibrillation or Cardioversion

The transdermal clonidine systems should be removed before attempting defibrillation or cardioversion because of the potential for altered electrical conductivity which may increase the risk of arcing, a phenomenon associated with the use of defibrillators.

Information for Patients

Patients should be cautioned against interruption of CATAPRES-TTS therapy without their physician's advice.

Patients who engage in potentially hazardous activities, such as operating machinery or driving, should be advised of a possible sedative effect of clonidine. They should also be informed that this sedative effect may be increased by concomitant use of alcohol, barbiturates, or other sedating drugs.

Patients should be instructed to consult their physicians promptly about the possible need to remove the patch if they observe moderate to severe localized erythema and/or vesicle formation at the site of application or generalized skin rash.

If a patient experiences isolated, mild localized skin irritation before completing 7 days of use, the system may be removed and replaced with a new system applied to a fresh skin site.

If the system should begin to loosen from the skin after application, the patient should be instructed to place the adhesive overlay directly over the system to ensure adhesion during its 7-day use.

Used CATAPRES-TTS patches contain a substantial amount of their initial drug content which may be harmful to infants and children if accidentally applied or ingested. THEREFORE, PATIENTS SHOULD BE CAUTIONED TO KEEP BOTH USED AND UNUSED CATAPRES-TTS PATCHES OUT OF THE REACH OF CHILDREN. After use, CATAPRES-TTS should be folded in half with the adhesive sides together and discarded away from children's reach.

Instructions for use, storage and disposal of the system are provided at the end of this monograph. These instructions are also included in each box of CATAPRES-TTS.

Drug Interactions

Clonidine may potentiate the CNS-depressive effects of alcohol, barbiturates or other sedating drugs. If a patient receiving clonidine is also taking tricyclic antidepressants, the hypotensive effect of clonidine may be reduced, necessitating an increase in the clonidine dose.

Due to a potential for additive effects such as bradycardia and AV block, caution is warranted in patients receiving clonidine concomitantly with agents known to affect sinus node function or AV nodal conduction e.g., digitalis, calcium channel blockers and beta-blockers.

Amitriptyline in combination with clonidine enhances the manifestation of corneal lesions in rats. (See TOXICOLOGY.)

Toxicology

In several studies with oral clonidine hydrochloride, a dose-dependent increase in the incidence and severity of spontaneous retinal degeneration was seen in albino rats treated for six months or longer. Tissue distribution studies in dogs and monkeys showed a concentration of clonidine in the choroid.

		Programmed Delivery Clonidine *in vivo* Per Day Over 1 Week	Clonidine Content	Size	Code
Catapres-TTS®-1	(clonidine)	0.1 mg	2.5 mg	3.5 cm^2	BI-31
Catapres-TTS®-2	(clonidine)	0.2 mg	5.0 mg	7.0 cm^2	BI-32
Catapres-TTS®-3	(clonidine)	0.3 mg	7.5 mg	10.5 cm^2	BI-33

In view of the retinal degeneration seen in rats, eye examinations were performed during clinical trials in 908 patients before, and periodically after, the start of clonidine therapy. In 353 of these 908 patients, the eye examinations were carried out over periods of 24 months or longer. Except for some dryness of the eyes, no drug-related abnormal ophthalmological findings were recorded and, according to specialized tests such as electroretinography and macular dazzle, retinal function was unchanged.

In combination with amitriptyline, clonidine hydrochloride administration led to the development of corneal lesions in rats within 5 days.

Carcinogenesis, Mutagenesis, Impairment of Fertility

Chronic dietary administration of clonidine was not carcinogenic to rats (132 weeks) or mice (78 weeks) dosed, respectively, at up to 46 to 70 times the maximum recommended daily human dose as mg/kg (9 or 6 times the MRDHD on a mg/m^2 basis). There was no evidence of genotoxicity in the Ames test for mutagenicity or mouse micronucleus test for clastogenicity.

Fertility of male and female rats was unaffected by clonidine doses as high as 150 mcg/kg (approximately 3 times the MRDHD). In a separate experiment, fertility of female rats appeared to be affected at dose levels of 500 to 2000 mcg/kg (10 to 40 times the oral MRDHD on a mg/kg basis; 2 to 8 times the MRDHD on a mg/m^2 basis).

Pregnancy

TERATOGENIC EFFECTS Pregnancy Category C

Reproduction studies performed in rabbits at doses up to approximately 3 times the oral maximum recommended daily human dose (MRDHD) of CATAPRES (clonidine hydrochloride) produced no evidence of a teratogenic or embryotoxic potential in rabbits. In rats, however, doses as low as 1/3 the oral MRDHD (1/15 the MRDHD on a mg/m^2 basis) of clonidine were associated with increased resorptions in a study in which dams were treated continuously from 2 months prior to mating. Increased resorptions were not associated with treatment at the same or at higher dose levels (up to 3 times the oral MRDHD) when the dams were treated on gestation days 6-15. Increases in resorption were observed at much higher dose levels (40 times the oral MRDHD on mg/kg basis; 4 to 8 times the MRDHD on a mg/m^2 basis) in mice and rats treated on gestation days 1-14 (lowest dose employed in the study was 500 mcg/kg).

No adequate well-controlled studies have been conducted in pregnant women. Because animal reproduction studies are not always predictive of human response, this drug should be used during pregnancy only if clearly needed.

Nursing Mothers

As clonidine is excreted in human milk, caution should be exercised when CATAPRES-TTS is administered to a nursing woman.

Pediatric Use

Safety and effectiveness in pediatric patients below the age of twelve have not been established (See Warnings on Withdrawal).

ADVERSE REACTIONS

Clinical trial experience with CATAPRES-TTS

Most systemic adverse effects during CATAPRES-TTS therapy have been mild and have tended to diminish with continued therapy. In a 3-month multiclinic trial of CATAPRES-TTS in 101 hypertensive patients, the systemic adverse reactions were, dry mouth (25 patients) and drowsiness (12), fatigue (6), headache (5), lethargy and sedation (3 each), insomnia, dizziness, impotence/sexual dysfunction, dry throat (2 each) and constipation, nausea, change in taste and nervousness (1 each).

In the above mentioned 3-month controlled clinical trial, as well as other uncontrolled clinical trials, the most frequent adverse reactions were dermatological and are described below.

In the 3-month trial, 51 of the 101 patients had localized skin reactions such as erythema (26 patients) and/or pruritus, particularly after using an adhesive overlay throughout the 7-day dosage interval. Allergic contact sensitization to CATAPRES-TTS was observed in 5 patients. Other skin reactions were localized vesiculation (7 patients), hyperpigmentation (5), edema (3), excoriation (3), burning (3), papules (1), throbbing (1), blanching (1), and a generalized macular rash (1).

In additional clinical experience, contact dermatitis resulting in treatment discontinuation was observed in 128 of 673 patients (about 19 in 100) after a mean duration of treatment of 37 weeks. The incidence of contact dermatitis was about 34 in 100 among white women, about 18 in 100 in white men, about 14 in 100 in black women, and approximately 8 in 100 in black men. Analysis of skin reaction data showed that the risk of having to discontinue CATAPRES-TTS treatment because of contact dermatitis was greatest between treatment weeks 6 and 26, although sensitivity may develop either earlier or later in treatment.

In a large-scale clinical applicability and safety study by 451 physicians in a total of 3539 patients, other allergic reactions were recorded for which a causal relationship to CATAPRES-TTS was not established: maculopapular rash (10 cases); urticaria (2 cases); and angioedema of the face (2 cases), which also affected the tongue in one of the patients.

Marketing Experience with CATAPRES-TTS

Other adverse effects reported since the drug has been marketed are listed below by body system. In this setting, an incidence or causal relationship cannot always be accurately determined. However, none of the events listed below occurred in a frequency greater than 0.5%.

Body as a Whole Fever; malaise; weakness; pallor; and withdrawal syndrome.

Cardiovascular Congestive heart failure; cerebrovascular accident; electrocardiographic abnormalities (i.e., bradycardia, sick sinus syndrome disturbances and arrhythmias); chest pain; orthostatic symptoms; syncope, increases in blood pressure; sinus bradycardia and atrioventricular block with and without the use of concomitant digitalis; Raynaud's phenomenon; tachycardia; bradycardia; and palpitations.

Central and Peripheral Nervous System/Psychiatric Delirium; mental depression; visual and auditory hallucinations; localized numbness; vivid dreams or nightmares; restlessness; anxiety; agitation; irritability; other behavioral changes; and drowsiness.

Dermatological Angioneurotic edema; localized or generalized rash; hives; urticaria; contact dermatitis; pruritus; alopecia; and localized hypo or hyper pigmentation.

Gastrointestinal Anorexia and vomiting.

Genitourinary Difficult micturition; loss of libido; and decreased sexual activity.

Metabolic Gynecomastia or breast enlargement and weight gain.

Musculoskeletal Muscle or joint pain; and leg cramps.

Ophthalmological Blurred vision; burning of the eyes and dryness of the eyes.

Adverse Events Associated with Oral CATAPRES Therapy:

Most adverse events are mild and tend to diminish with continued therapy. The most frequent (which appear to be dose-related) are dry mouth, occurring in about 40 of 100 patients; drowsiness, about 33 in 100; dizziness, about 16 in 100; constipation and sedation, each about 10 in 100. The following less frequent adverse experiences have also been reported in patients receiving CATAPRES (clonidine hydrochloride USP), but in many cases patients were receiving concomitant medication and a causal relationship has not been established.

Body as a Whole Weakness, about 10 in 100 patients; fatigue, about 4 in 100; headache and withdrawal syndrome each about 1 in 100. Also reported were pallor; a weakly positive Coombs' test; increased sensitivity to alcohol; and fever.

Cardiovascular Orthostatic symptoms, about 3 in 100 patients; palpitations and tachycardia, and bradycardia, each about 5 in 1000. Syncope, Raynaud's phenomenon, congestive heart failure, and electrocardiographic abnormalities (i.e., sinus node arrest, functional bradycardia, high degree AV block and arrhythmias) have been reported rarely. Rare cases of sinus bradycardia and AV block have been reported, both with and without the use of concomitant digitalis.

Central Nervous System Nervousness and agitation, about 3 in 100 patients, mental depression, about 1 in 100 and insomnia, about 5 in 1000. Other behavioral changes, vivid dreams or nightmares, restlessness, anxiety, visual and auditory hallucinations and delirium have rarely been reported.

Dermatological Rash, about 1 in 100 patients; pruritus, about 7 in 1000; hives, angioneurotic edema and urticaria, about 5 in 1000; alopecia, about 2 in 1000.

Gastrointestinal Nausea and vomiting, about 5 in 100 patients; anorexia and malaise, each about 1 in 100; mild transient abnormalities in liver function tests, about 1 in 100; hepatitis, parotitis, constipation, pseudo-obstruction, and abdominal pain, rarely.

Genitourinary Decreased sexual activity, impotence and loss of libido, about 3 in 100 patients; nocturia, about 1 in 100; difficulty in micturition, about 2 in 1000; urinary retention, about 1 in 1000.

Hematologic Thrombocytopenia, rarely.

Metabolic Weight gain, about 1 in 100 patients; gynecomastia, about 1 in 1000; transient elevation of blood glucose or serum creatine phosphokinase, rarely.

Musculoskeletal Muscle or joint pain, about 6 in 1000 and leg cramps, about 3 in 1000.

Oro-otolaryngeal Dryness of the nasal mucosa was rarely reported.

Ophthalmological Dryness of the eyes, burning of the eyes and blurred vision were reported.

OVERDOSAGE

Hypertension may develop early and may be followed by hypotension, bradycardia, respiratory depression, hypothermia, drowsiness, decreased or absent reflexes, weakness, irritability and miosis. The frequency of CNS depression may be higher in children than adults. Large overdoses may result in reversible cardiac conduction defects or dysrhythmias, apnea, coma and seizures. Signs and symptoms of overdose generally occur within 30 minutes to two hours after exposure. As little as 0.1 mg of clonidine has produced signs of toxicity in children.

If symptoms of poisoning occur following dermal exposure, remove all CATAPRES-TTS systems. After their removal, the plasma clonidine levels will persist for about 8 hours,

then decline slowly over a period of several days. Rare cases of CATAPRES-TTS poisoning due to accidental or deliberate mouthing or ingestion of the patch have been reported, many of them involving children.
There is no specific antidote for clonidine overdosage. Ipecac syrup-induced vomiting and gastric lavage would not be expected to remove significant amounts of clonidine following dermal exposure. If the patch is ingested, whole bowel irrigation may be considered and the administration of activated charcoal and/or cathartic may be beneficial. Supportive care may include atropine sulfate for bradycardia, intravenous fluids and/or vasopressor agents for hypotension and vasodilators for hypertension. Naloxone may be a useful adjunct for the management of clonidine-induced respiratory depression, hypotension and/or coma; blood pressure should be monitored since the administration of naloxone has occasionally resulted in paradoxical hypertension. Tolazoline administration has yielded inconsistent results and is not recommended as first-line therapy. Dialysis is not likely to significantly enhance the elimination of clonidine.
The largest overdose reported to date, involved a 28-year old male who ingested 100 mg of clonidine hydrochloride powder. This patient developed hypertension followed by hypotension, bradycardia, apnea, hallucinations, semicoma, and premature ventricular contractions. The patient fully recovered after intensive treatment. Plasma clonidine levels were 60 ng/mL after 1 hour, 190 ng/mL after 1.5 hours, 370 ng/mL after 2 hours, and 120 ng/mL after 5.5 and 6.5 hours. In mice and rats, the oral LD_{50} of clonidine is 206 and 465 mg/kg, respectively.

DOSAGE AND ADMINISTRATION

Apply CATAPRES-TTS (clonidine) once every 7 days to a hairless area of intact skin on the upper outer arm or chest. Each new application of CATAPRES-TTS should be on a different skin site from the previous location. If the system loosens during 7-day wearing, the adhesive overlay should be applied directly over the system to ensure good adhesion. There have been rare reports of the need for patch changes prior to 7 days to maintain blood pressure control.
To initiate therapy, CATAPRES-TTS dosage should be titrated according to individual therapeutic requirements, starting with CATAPRES-TTS-1. If after one or two weeks the desired reduction in blood pressure is not achieved, increase the dosage by adding another CATAPRES-TTS-1 or changing to a larger system. An increase in dosage above two CATAPRES-TTS-3 is usually not associated with additional efficacy.
When substituting CATAPRES-TTS for oral clonidine or for other antihypertensive drugs, physicians should be aware that the antihypertensive effect of CATAPRES-TTS may not commence until 2-3 days after initial application. Therefore, gradual reduction of prior drug dosage is advised. Some or all previous antihypertensive treatment may have to be continued, particularly in patients with more severe forms of hypertension.

Renal Impairment

Dosage must be adjusted according to the degree of impairment, and patients should be carefully monitored. Since only a minimal amount of clonidine is removed during routine hemodialysis, there is no need to give supplemental clonidine following dialysis.

HOW SUPPLIED

CATAPRES-TTS-1 (clonidine) and CATAPRES-TTS-2 are supplied as 4 pouched systems and 4 adhesive overlays per carton, 3 cartons per shipper (NDC 0597-0031-12 and 0597-0032-12, respectively). CATAPRES-TTS-3 is supplied as 4 pouched systems and 4 adhesive overlays per carton (NDC 0597-0033-34). See chart below.
[See table at top of previous page]

STORAGE AND HANDLING

Store below 86° F (30° C).

Rx only

Manufactured by:
ALZA Corporation, Mountain View, California 94043 USA
Distributed by:
Boehringer Ingelheim Pharmaceuticals, Inc., Ridgefield, CT 06877 USA
Licensed from:
Boehringer Ingelheim International GmbH

Revised October 2003
4044415/US/3 4144415//03
Shown in Product Identification Guide, page 309

COMBIVENT® ℞

(ipratropium bromide and albuterol sulfate)
Inhalation Aerosol
Bronchodilator Aerosol
For Oral Inhalation Only

Prescribing Information

DESCRIPTION

Combivent® Inhalation Aerosol is a combination of ipratropium bromide and albuterol sulfate. Ipratropium bromide is an anticholinergic bronchodilator chemically described as 8-azoniabicyclo[3.2.1]octane, 3-(3-hydroxy-1-oxo-2-phenylpropoxy)-8-methyl-8-(1-methylethyl)-, bromide, monohydrate *(endo,syn)*-,(±): a synthetic quaternary ammonium compound chemically related to atropine. Ipratropium bromide is a white to off-white crystalline substance, freely soluble in water and lower alcohols but insoluble in lipophilic solvents such as ether, chloroform and fluorocarbons. The structural formula is:

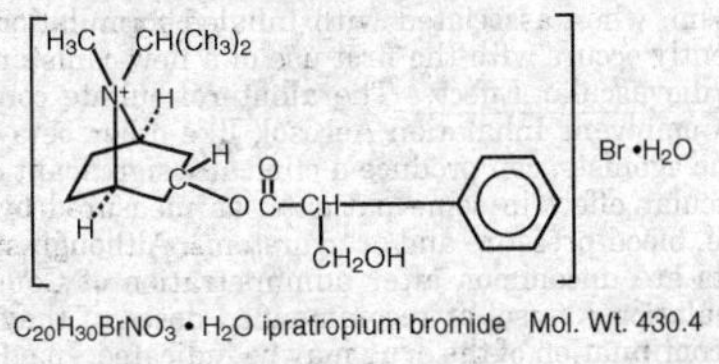

$C_{20}H_{30}BrNO_3 \cdot H_2O$ ipratropium bromide Mol. Wt. 430.4

Albuterol sulfate, chemically known as (1,3-benzenedimethanol, α′-[[(1,1-dimethylethyl) amino] methyl]-4-hydroxy, sulfate (2:1)(salt), (±)- is a relatively selective $beta_2$-adrenergic bronchodilator.
Albuterol is the official generic name in the United States. The World Health Organization recommended name for the drug is salbutamol. Albuterol sulfate is a white to off-white crystalline powder, soluble in water and slightly soluble in ethanol. The structural formula is:

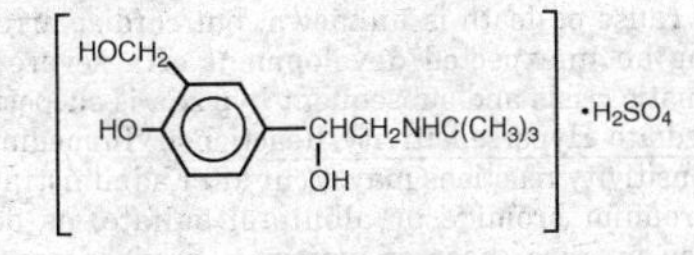

$(C_{13}H_{21}NO_3)_2 \cdot H_2SO_4$ albuterol sulfate Mol. Wt. 576.7

Combivent Inhalation Aerosol contains a microcrystalline suspension of ipratropium bromide and albuterol sulfate in a pressurized metered-dose aerosol unit for oral inhalation administration. The 200 inhalation unit has a net weight of 14.7 grams. Each actuation meters 21 mcg of ipratropium bromide and 120 mcg of albuterol sulfate from the valve and delivers 18 mcg of ipratropium bromide and 103 mcg of albuterol sulfate (equivalent to 90 mcg albuterol base) from the mouthpiece. The excipients are dichlorodifluoromethane, dichlorotetrafluoroethane, and trichloromonofluoromethane as propellants and soya lecithin.

CLINICAL PHARMACOLOGY

Combivent Inhalation Aerosol is a combination of the anticholinergic bronchodilator, ipratropium bromide, and the $beta_2$-adrenergic bronchodilator, albuterol sulfate.

Ipratropium Bromide:

Mechanism of Action

Ipratropium bromide is an anticholinergic (parasympatholytic) agent which, based on animal studies, appears to inhibit vagally mediated reflexes by antagonizing the action of acetylcholine, the transmitter agent released from the vagus nerve. Anticholinergics prevent the increases in intracellular concentration of cyclic guanosine monophosphate (cyclic GMP) which are caused by interaction of acetylcholine with the muscarinic receptor on bronchial smooth muscle.

Pharmacokinetics

The bronchodilation following inhalation of ipratropium bromide is primarily a local, site-specific effect, not a systemic one. Much of an administered dose is swallowed as shown by fecal excretion studies. Ipratropium bromide is a quaternary amine. It is not readily absorbed into the systemic circulation either from the surface of the lung or from the gastrointestinal tract as confirmed by blood level and renal excretion studies. Plasma levels of ipratropium bromide were below the assay sensitivity limit of 100 pg/mL.
The half-life of elimination is about 2 hours after inhalation or intravenous administration. Ipratropium bromide is minimally bound (0 to 9% *in vitro*) to plasma albumin and α_1-acid glycoprotein. It is partially metabolized to inactive ester hydrolysis products. Following intravenous administration, approximately one-half of the dose is excreted unchanged in the urine. Studies in rats have shown that ipratropium bromide does not penetrate the blood-brain barrier. The pharmacokinetics of Combivent Inhalation Aerosol or ipratropium bromide have not been studied in patients with hepatic or renal insufficiency or in the elderly (See PRECAUTIONS).
Controlled clinical studies have demonstrated that ipratropium bromide does not alter either mucociliary clearance or the volume or viscosity of respiratory secretions. In studies without a positive control, ipratropium bromide did not alter pupil size, accommodation or visual acuity (See ADVERSE REACTIONS). Ventilation/perfusion studies have shown no clinically significant effects on pulmonary gas exchange or arterial oxygen tension. At recommended doses, ipratropium bromide does not produce clinically significant changes in pulse rate or blood pressure.

Albuterol Sulfate:

Mechanism of Action

In vitro studies and *in vivo* pharmacologic studies have demonstrated that albuterol has a preferential effect on $beta_2$-adrenergic receptors compared with isoproterenol. While it is recognized that $beta_2$-adrenergic receptors are the predominant receptors on bronchial smooth muscle, recent data indicate that there is a population of $beta_2$-receptors in the human heart which comprise between 10% and 50% of cardiac beta-adrenergic receptors. The precise function of these receptors, however, is not yet established (See WARNINGS).
Activation of $beta_2$-adrenergic receptors on airway smooth muscle leads to the activation of adenylyl cyclase and to an increase in the intracellular concentration of cyclic-3′,5′-adenosine monophosphate (cyclic AMP). This increase of cyclic AMP leads to the activation of protein kinase A, which inhibits the phosphorylation of myosin and lowers intracellular ionic calcium concentrations, resulting in relaxation. Albuterol relaxes the smooth muscles of all airways, from the trachea to the terminal bronchioles. Albuterol acts as a functional antagonist to relax the airway irrespective of the spasmogen involved, thus protecting against all bronchoconstrictor challenges. Increased cyclic AMP concentrations are also associated with the inhibition of release of mediators from mast cells in the airway.
Albuterol has been shown in most clinical trials to have more bronchial smooth muscle relaxation effect than isoproterenol at comparable doses while producing fewer cardiovascular effects. However, all beta-adrenergic drugs, including albuterol sulfate, can produce a significant cardiovascular effect in some patients (See PRECAUTIONS).

Pharmacokinetics Albuterol is longer acting than isoproterenol in most patients because it is not a substrate for the cellular uptake processes for catecholamines nor for metabolism by catechol-O-methyl transferase. Instead, the drug is conjugatively metabolized to albuterol 4′-O-sulfate.
In a pharmacokinetic study in 12 healthy male volunteers of two inhalations of albuterol sulfate, 103 mcg dose/inhalation through the mouthpiece, peak plasma albuterol concentrations ranging from 419 to 802 pg/mL (mean 599 ± 122 pg/mL) were obtained within three hours post-administration. Following this single-dose administration, 30.8 ± 10.2% of the estimated mouthpiece dose was excreted unchanged in the 24 hour urine. Since albuterol sulfate is rapidly and completely absorbed, this study could not distinguish between pulmonary and gastrointestinal absorption.
Intravenous pharmacokinetics of albuterol were studied in a comparable group of 16 healthy male volunteers; the mean terminal half-life following a 30-minute infusion of 1.5 mg was 3.9 hours with a mean clearance of 439 mL/min/1.73 m^2.
Intravenous albuterol studies in rats demonstrated that albuterol crossed the blood-brain barrier and reached brain concentrations amounting to about 5% of the plasma concentrations. In structures outside the blood-brain barrier (pineal and pituitary glands), the drug achieved concentrations more than 100 times those in whole brain.
Studies in pregnant rats with tritiated albuterol demonstrated that approximately 10% of the circulating maternal drug was transferred to the fetus. Disposition in fetal lungs was comparable to maternal lungs, but fetal liver disposition was 1% of maternal liver levels.
Studies in laboratory animals (minipigs, rodents, and dogs) have demonstrated the occurrence of cardiac arrhythmias and sudden death (with histologic evidence of myocardial necrosis) when beta-agonists and methylxanthines were administered concurrently. The significance of these findings when applied to humans is unknown.

Combivent Inhalation Aerosol:

Mechanism of Action Combivent Inhalation Aerosol is expected to maximize the response to treatment in patients with chronic obstructive pulmonary disease (COPD) by reducing bronchospasm through two distinctly different mechanisms, anticholinergic (parasympatholytic) and sympathomimetic. Simultaneous administration of both an anticholinergic (ipratropium bromide) and a $beta_2$-sympathomimetic (albuterol sulfate) is designed to benefit the patient by producing a greater bronchodilator effect than when either drug is utilized alone at its recommended dosage.

Pharmacokinetics In a crossover pharmacokinetic study in 12 healthy male volunteers comparing the pattern of absorption and excretion of two inhalations of Combivent Inhalation Aerosol to the two active components individually, the co-administration of ipratropium bromide and albuterol sulfate from a single canister did not significantly alter the systemic absorption of either component.
Ipratropium bromide levels remained below detectable limits (<100 pg/mL). Peak albuterol level obtained within 3 hours post-administration was 492 ± 132 pg/mL. Following this single administration, 27.1 ± 5.7% of the estimated mouthpiece dose was excreted unchanged in the 24 hour urine. From a pharmacokinetic perspective, the synergistic efficacy of Combivent Inhalation Aerosol is likely to be due to a local effect on the muscarinic and $beta_2$-adrenergic receptors in the lung.

Clinical Trials In two 12-week randomized, double-blind, active-controlled clinical trials, 1067 patients with chronic obstructive pulmonary disease (COPD) were evaluated for the bronchodilator efficacy of Combivent Inhalation Aerosol (358 patients) in comparison to its components, ipratropium bromide (362 patients) and albuterol sulfate (347 patients). Serial FEV_1 measurements (shown below as a percent change from test-day baseline) demonstrated that Combivent Inhalation Aerosol produced significantly greater improvement in pulmonary function than either ipratropium bromide or albuterol sulfate when given separately. The median time to onset of a 15% increase in FEV_1 was 15 minutes and the median time to peak FEV_1 was one hour for Combivent Inhalation Aerosol and its components. The median duration of effect as measured by FEV_1 was 4–5 hours for Combivent Inhalation Aerosol compared to 4

Continued on next page

Combivent—Cont.

hours for ipratropium bromide and 3 hours for albuterol sulfate.

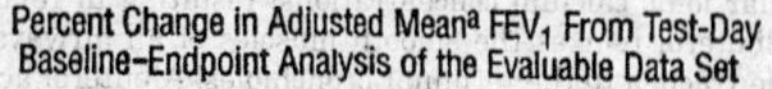

Percent Change in Adjusted Mean[a] FEV1 From Test-Day
Baseline–Endpoint Analysis of the Evaluable Data Set

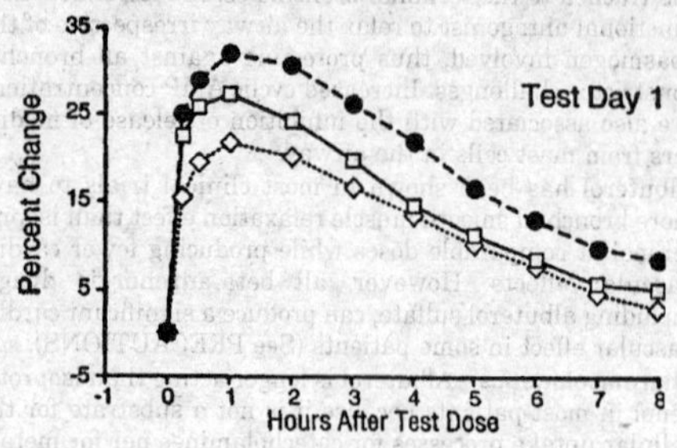

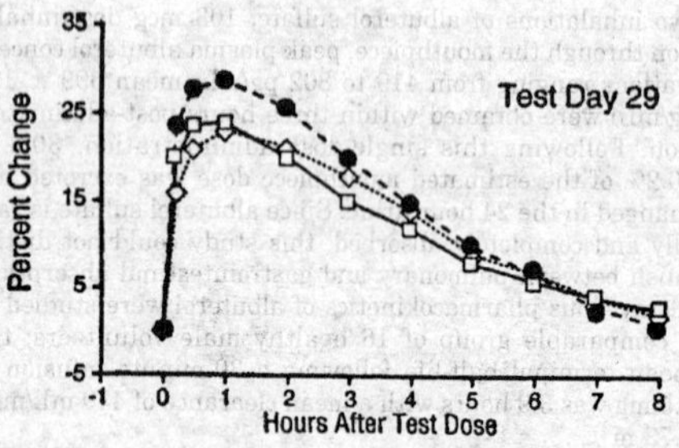

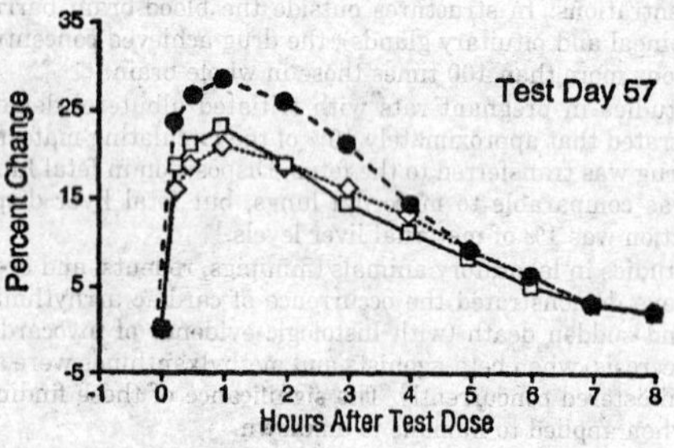

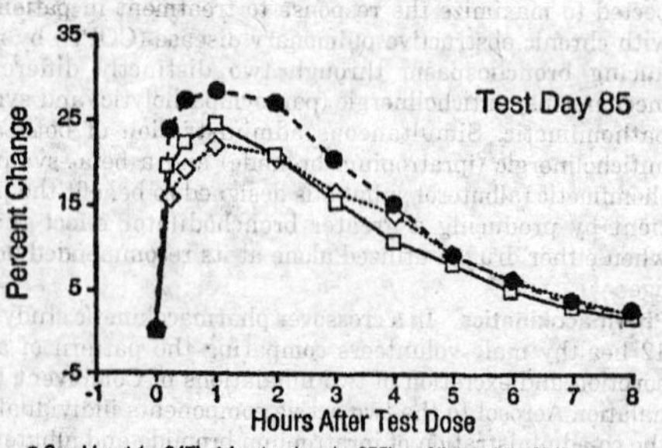

● Combivent (n=347) ◇ Ipratropium (n=355) □ Albuterol (n=331)
[a] Adjusted for test-day baseline FEV_1, center and treatment-by-center interaction

These studies demonstrated that each component of Combivent Inhalation Aerosol contributed to the improvement in pulmonary function produced by the combination, especially during the first 4–5 hours after dosing, and that Combivent Inhalation Aerosol was significantly more effective than ipratropium bromide or albuterol sulfate administered alone.

In the two controlled twelve-week studies, Combivent Inhalation Aerosol did not produce any change in the secondary efficacy parameters including symptom scores, physician global assessments and morning PEFR, all of which were monitored throughout the study period.

INDICATIONS AND USAGE

Combivent Inhalation Aerosol is indicated for use in patients with chronic obstructive pulmonary disease (COPD) on a regular aerosol bronchodilator who continue to have evidence of bronchospasm and who require a second bronchodilator.

CONTRAINDICATIONS

Combivent Inhalation Aerosol is contraindicated in patients with a history of hypersensitivity to soya lecithin or related food products such as soybean and peanut. Combivent Inhalation Aerosol is also contraindicated in patients hypersensitive to any other components of the drug product or to atropine or its derivatives.

WARNINGS

1. Paradoxical Bronchospasm: Combivent Inhalation Aerosol can produce paradoxical bronchospasm that can be life threatening. If it occurs, the preparation should be discontinued immediately and alternative therapy instituted. It should be recognized that paradoxical bronchospasm, when associated with inhaled formulations, frequently occurs with the first use of a new canister.
2. Cardiovascular Effect: The albuterol sulfate contained in Combivent Inhalation Aerosol, like other beta-adrenergic agonists, can produce a clinically significant cardiovascular effect in some patients, as measured by pulse rate, blood pressure and/or symptoms. Although such effects are uncommon after administration of Combivent Inhalation Aerosol at recommended doses, if they occur, discontinuation of the drug may be indicated. In addition, beta-adrenergic agents have been reported to produce ECG changes, such as flattening of the T wave, prolongation of the QTc interval, and ST segment depression. Therefore, Combivent Inhalation Aerosol should be used with caution in patients with cardiovascular disorders, especially coronary insufficiency, cardiac arrhythmias and hypertension.
3. Do Not Exceed Recommended Dose: Fatalities have been reported in association with excessive use of inhaled sympathomimetic drugs, in patients with asthma. The exact cause of death is unknown, but cardiac arrest following an unexpected development of a severe acute asthmatic crisis and subsequent hypoxia is suspected.
4. Immediate Hypersensitivity Reactions: Immediate hypersensitivity reactions may occur after administration of ipratropium bromide or albuterol sulfate, as demonstrated by rare cases of urticaria, angioedema, rash, bronchospasm, anaphylaxis and oropharyngeal edema.
5. Storage Conditions: The contents of Combivent Inhalation Aerosol are under pressure. Do not puncture. Do not use or store near heat or open flame. Exposure to temperatures above 120°F may cause bursting. Never throw the container into a fire or incinerator. Keep out of reach of children.

PRECAUTIONS

General

1. Effects Seen with Anticholinergic Drugs: Combivent Inhalation Aerosol contains ipratropium bromide and, therefore, should be used with caution in patients with narrow-angle glaucoma, prostatic hypertrophy or bladder-neck obstruction.
2. Effects Seen with Sympathomimetic Drugs: Preparations containing sympathomimetic amines such as albuterol sulfate should be used with caution in patients with convulsive disorders, hyperthyroidism, or diabetes mellitus and in patients who are unusually responsive to sympathomimetic amines. Beta-adrenergic agents may also produce significant hypokalemia in some patients (possibly through intracellular shunting) which has the potential to produce adverse cardiovascular effects. The decrease in serum potassium is usually transient, not requiring supplementation.
3. Use in Hepatic or Renal Disease: Combivent Inhalation Aerosol has not been studied in patients with hepatic or renal insufficiency. It should be used with caution in those patient populations.

Information for Patients

Patients should be cautioned to avoid spraying the aerosol into their eyes and be advised that this may result in precipitation or worsening of narrow-angle glaucoma, eye pain or discomfort, temporary blurring of vision, visual halos or colored images in association with red eyes from conjunctival and corneal congestion. Should any combination of these symptoms develop, consult your physician immediately.

The action of Combivent Inhalation Aerosol should last 4–5 hours or longer. Combivent Inhalation Aerosol should not be used more frequently than recommended. Do not increase the dose or frequency of Combivent Inhalation Aerosol without consulting your physician. If you find that treatment with Combivent Inhalation Aerosol becomes less effective for symptomatic relief, your symptoms become worse, and/or you need to use the product more frequently than usual, medical attention should be sought immediately. While you are taking Combivent Inhalation Aerosol, other inhaled drugs should be taken only as directed by your physician. If you are pregnant or nursing, contact your physician about use of Combivent Inhalation Aerosol. Appropriate use of Combivent Inhalation Aerosol includes an understanding of the way it should be administered (See Patient's Instructions for Use).

Drug Interactions

Combivent Inhalation Aerosol has been used concomitantly with other drugs, including sympathomimetic bronchodilators, methylxanthines and steroids, commonly used in the treatment of COPD, without adverse drug reactions. No formal drug interaction studies have been performed with Combivent Inhalation Aerosol and these or other medications commonly used in the treatment of COPD.

Anticholinergic agents: Although ipratropium bromide is minimally absorbed into the systemic circulation, there is some potential for an additive interaction with concomitantly used anticholinergic medications. Caution is therefore advised in the co-administration of Combivent Inhalation Aerosol with other anticholinergic-containing drugs.

Beta-adrenergic agents: Caution is advised in the co-administration of Combivent Inhalation Aerosol and other sympathomimetic agents due to the increased risk of adverse cardiovascular effects.

Beta-receptor blocking agents and albuterol inhibit the effect of each other. Beta-receptor blocking agents should be used with caution in patients with hyperreactive airways.

Diuretics: The ECG changes and/or hypokalemia which may result from the administration of non-potassium sparing diuretics (such as loop or thiazide diuretics) can be acutely worsened by beta-agonists, especially when the recommended dose of the beta agonist is exceeded. Although the clinical significance of these effects is not known, caution is advised in the co-administration of beta agonist-containing drugs, such as Combivent Inhalation Aerosol, with non-potassium sparing diuretics.

Monoamine oxidase inhibitors or tricyclic antidepressants: Combivent Inhalation Aerosol should be administered with extreme caution to patients being treated with monoamine oxidase inhibitors or tricyclic antidepressants or within two weeks of discontinuation of such agents because the action of albuterol on the cardiovascular system may be potentiated.

Carcinogenesis, Mutagenesis, Impairment of Fertility

Ipratropium bromide: Two-year oral carcinogenicity studies in rats and mice have revealed no carcinogenic potential at doses up to 6 mg/kg/day. This dose corresponds to approximately 360 and 180 times the maximum recommended human daily inhalation dose in rats and mice respectively, on a mg/m^2 basis. Results of various mutagenicity studies (Ames test, mouse dominant lethal test, mouse micronucleus test and chromosome aberration of bone marrow in Chinese hamsters) were negative. Fertility of male or female rats at oral doses up to 50 mg/kg/day (approximately 3000 times the maximum recommended human daily inhalation dose on a mg/m^2 basis) was unaffected by ipratropium bromide administration. At doses above 90 mg/kg/day (approximately 5400 times the maximum recommended human daily inhalation dose on a mg/m^2 basis), increased resorption and decreased conception rates were observed.

Albuterol: Like other agents in its class, albuterol caused a significant dose-related increase in the incidence of benign leiomyomas of the mesovarium in a two-year study in the rat at dietary doses of 2, 10 and 50 mg/kg/day (approximately 20, 100 and 500 times the maximum recommended human daily inhalation dose on a mg/m^2 basis). In another study this effect was blocked by the co-administration of propranolol. The relevance of these findings to humans is not known. An 18-month study in mice at dietary doses up to 500 mg/kg/day (approximately 2500 times the maximum recommended human daily inhalation dose on a mg/m^2 basis) and a 99-week study in hamsters at oral doses up to 50 mg/kg/day (approximately 375 times the maximum recommended human daily inhalation dose on a mg/m^2 basis) revealed no evidence of tumorigenicity. Studies with albuterol revealed no evidence of mutagenesis. Reproduction studies in rats with albuterol sulfate revealed no evidence of impaired fertility.

Pregnancy

TERATOGENIC EFFECTS Pregnancy Category C.

Ipratropium bromide: *Pregnancy Category B.* Oral reproduction studies were performed at doses of 10 mg/kg in mice, 100 mg/kg in rats and 125 mg/kg in rabbits. These doses correspond, in each species, respectively, to approximately 300, 600 and 15,000 times the maximum recommended human daily inhalation dose on a mg/m^2 basis. Inhalation reproduction studies were conducted in rats and rabbits at doses of 1.5 and 1.8 mg/kg/day (approximately 90 and 210 times the maximum recommended human daily inhalation dose on a mg/m^2 basis). These studies have demonstrated no evidence of teratogenic effects as a result of ipratropium bromide.

Albuterol: *Pregnancy Category C.* Albuterol has been shown to be teratogenic in mice. A reproduction study in CD-1 mice given albuterol subcutaneously (0.025, 0.25 and 2.5 mg/kg) showed cleft palate formation in 5 of 111 (4.5%) fetuses at 0.25 mg/kg (equivalent to the maximum recommended human daily inhalation dose on a mg/m^2 basis) and in 10 of 108 (9.3%) fetuses at 2.5 mg/kg (approximately 10 times the maximum recommended human daily inhalation dose on a mg/m^2 basis). None was observed at 0.025 mg/kg (approximately one-tenth the maximum recommended human daily inhalation dose). Cleft palate also occurred in 22 of 72 (30.5%) fetuses treated with 2.5 mg/kg isoproterenol (positive control). A reproduction study with oral albuterol in Stride Dutch rabbits revealed cranioschisis in 7 of 19 (37%) fetuses at 50 mg/kg (approximately 1000 times the maximum recommended human daily inhalation dose on a mg/m^2 basis).

There are, however, no adequate and well-controlled studies of Combivent Inhalation Aerosol, ipratropium bromide or albuterol sulfate, in pregnant women. Because animal reproduction studies are not always predictive of human response, Combivent Inhalation Aerosol should be used during pregnancy only if the potential benefit justifies the potential risk to the fetus.

Labor and Delivery

Because of the potential for beta-agonist interference with uterine contractility, use of Combivent Inhalation Aerosol for the treatment of COPD during labor should be restricted to those patients in whom the benefits clearly outweigh the risk.

Nursing Mothers

It is not known whether the components of Combivent Inhalation Aerosol are excreted in human milk.

Ipratropium bromide: Although lipid-insoluble quaternary bases pass into breast milk, it is unlikely that the active component, ipratropium bromide, would reach the infant to an important extent, especially when taken by aerosol. However, because many drugs are excreted in human milk, caution should be exercised when Combivent Inhalation Aerosol is administered to a nursing mother.

Albuterol: Because of the potential for tumorigenicity shown for albuterol in animal studies, a decision should be made whether to discontinue nursing or to discontinue the drug, taking into account the importance of the drug to the mother.

Pediatric Use

Safety and effectiveness of Combivent Inhalation Aerosol in pediatric patients have not been established.

ADVERSE REACTIONS

Adverse reaction information concerning Combivent Inhalation Aerosol is derived from two 12-week controlled clinical trials (N=358 for Combivent Inhalation Aerosol). [See table above]

Additional adverse reactions, reported in less than two percent of the patients in the Combivent Inhalation Aerosol treatment group include edema, fatigue, hypertension, dizziness, nervousness, paresthesia, tremor, dysphonia, insomnia, diarrhea, dry mouth, dyspepsia, vomiting, arrhythmia, palpitation, tachycardia, arthralgia, angina, increased sputum, taste perversion, and urinary tract infection/dysuria. Allergic-type reactions such as skin rash, angioedema of tongue, lips and face, urticaria (including giant urticaria), laryngospasm and anaphylactic reaction have been reported, with positive rechallenge in some cases. Many of these patients had a history of allergies to other drugs and/or foods including soybean (See CONTRAINDICATIONS).

Additional information derived from the published literature and post-marketing surveillance on the use of ipratropium or albuterol inhalation aerosol singly or in combination that is not included in the lists above includes: cases of precipitation or worsening of narrow-angle glaucoma, acute eye pain, blurred vision, nasal congestion, drying of secretions, mucosal ulcers, irritation from aerosol, paradoxical bronchospasm, wheezing, exacerbation of COPD symptoms, heartburn, drowsiness, CNS stimulation, coordination difficulty, weakness, itching, flushing, alopecia, hypotension, gastrointestinal distress, constipation, and urinary difficulties.

OVERDOSAGE

The effects of overdosage are expected to be related primarily to albuterol sulfate. Acute overdosage with ipratropium bromide is unlikely since ipratropium bromide is not well absorbed systemically after aerosol or oral administration. The oral median lethal dose of ipratropium bromide ranged between 1001 and 2010 mg/kg in mice (approximately 30,000 and 60,000 times the maximum recommended human daily inhalation dose on a mg/m^2 basis, respectively); between 1667 and 4000 mg/kg in rats approximately 100,000 and 240,000 times the maximum recommended human daily inhalation dose, respectively, on a mg/m^2 basis); and between 400 and 1300 mg/kg (approximately 80,000 and 260,000 times the maximum recommended human daily inhalation dose, respectively, on a mg/m^2 basis) in dogs. Whereas the oral median lethal dose of albuterol sulfate in mice and rats was greater than 2,000 mg/kg (approximately 10,000 and 20,000 times the maximum recommended human daily inhalation dose, respectively, on a mg/m^2 basis), the inhalational median lethal dose could not be determined. Manifestations of overdosage with albuterol may include anginal pain, hypertension, hypokalemia, tachycardia with rates up to 200 beats per minute and exaggeration of the pharmacologic effects listed in ADVERSE REACTIONS. As with all sympathomimetic aerosol medications, cardiac arrest and even death may be associated with abuse. Dialysis is not appropriate treatment for overdosage of albuterol as an inhalation aerosol; the judicious use of a cardiovascular beta-receptor blocker, such as metoprolol tartrate may be indicated.

DOSAGE AND ADMINISTRATION

The dose of Combivent Inhalation Aerosol is two inhalations four times a day. Patients may take additional inhalations as required; however, the total number of inhalations should not exceed 12 in 24 hours. Safety and efficacy of additional doses of Combivent Inhalation Aerosol beyond 12 puffs/24 hours have not been studied. Also, safety and efficacy of extra doses of ipratropium or albuterol in addition to the recommended doses of Combivent Inhalation Aerosol have not been studied. It is recommended to "test-spray" three times before using for the first time and in cases where the aerosol has not been used for more than 24 hours.

HOW SUPPLIED

Combivent® Inhalation Aerosol is supplied as a metered-dose inhaler with a white mouthpiece which has a clear, colorless sleeve and an orange protective cap. The Combivent Inhalation Aerosol canister should be used with the Combivent Inhalation Aerosol actuator only. The actuator should not be used with other aerosol medications. Each actuation meters 21 mcg of ipratropium bromide and 120 mcg of albuterol sulfate from the valve and delivers 18 mcg of ipratropium bromide and 103 mcg of albuterol sulfate (equivalent to 90 mcg albuterol base) from the mouthpiece. Each 14.7 gram canister provides sufficient medication for 200 inhalations (NDC 0597-0013-14).

The canister should be discarded after the labeled number of actuations have been used. The amount of medication in each actuation cannot be assured after this point.

All Adverse Events (in percentages), from Two Large Double-Blind, Parallel, 12-Week Studies of Patients with COPD*

	Combivent Ipratropium Bromide 36 mcg/Albuterol Sulfate 206 mcg q.i.d. N=358	Ipratropium Bromide 36 mcg q.i.d. N=362	Albuterol Sulfate 206 mcg q.i.d. N=347
Body as A Whole—General Disorders			
Headache	5.6	3.9	6.6
Pain	2.5	1.9	1.2
Influenza	1.4	2.2	2.9
Chest Pain	0.3	1.4	2.9
Gastrointestinal System Disorders			
Nausea	2.0	2.5	2.6
Respiratory System Disorders (Lower)			
Bronchitis	12.3	12.4	17.9
Dyspnea	4.5	3.9	4.0
Coughing	4.2	2.8	2.6
Respiratory Disorders	2.5	1.7	2.3
Pneumonia	1.4	2.5	0.6
Bronchospasm	0.3	3.9	1.7
Respiratory System Disorders (Upper)			
Upper Resp. Tract Infection	10.9	12.7	13.0
Pharyngitis	2.2	3.3	2.3
Sinusitis	2.3	1.9	0.9
Rhinitis	1.1	2.5	2.3

*All adverse events, regardless of drug relationship, reported by two percent or more patients in one or more treatment group in the 12-week controlled clinical trials.

Store between 59°F (15° C) and 86° F (30° C). Avoid excessive humidity. For optimal results, the canister should be at room temperature before use. **Shake well before using.**

Note: The indented statement below is required by the Federal government's Clean Air Act for all products containing or manufactured with chlorofluorocarbons (CFCs):

> **Warning:** Contains trichloromonofluoromethane (CFC-11), dichlorodifluoromethane (CFC-12) and dichlorotetrafluoroethane (CFC-114), substances which harm public health and the environment by destroying ozone in the upper atmosphere.

A notice similar to the above **Warning** has been placed in the information for the patient of this product under the Environmental Protection Agency's (EPA's) regulations. The patient's warning states that the patient should consult his or her physician if there are any questions about alternatives.

℞ only

Manufactured by: Boehringer Ingelheim Pharmaceuticals, Inc. Ridgefield, CT 06877, USA

Ipratropium bromide licensed from: Boehringer Ingelheim International GmbH

Revised 9/01

10000291/03 10000291/US/03

Patient's Instructions for Use

Combivent®
(ipratropium bromide and albuterol sulfate)
Inhalation Aerosol

Read complete instructions carefully before using

1. Insert metal canister into clear end of mouthpiece. Make sure the canister is fully and firmly inserted into the actuator. The Combivent® canister is to be used only with the Combivent Inhalation Aerosol mouthpiece. This mouthpiece should not be used with other aerosol medications. Similarly, the canister should not be used with other mouthpieces.
2. Remove orange protective cap, hold canister as illustrated in Figure 1 and ***shake well*** before each use. If the cap is not present on the mouthpiece, the mouthpiece should be inspected for the presence of foreign objects before use. For optimal results, the canister should be at room temperature before use.

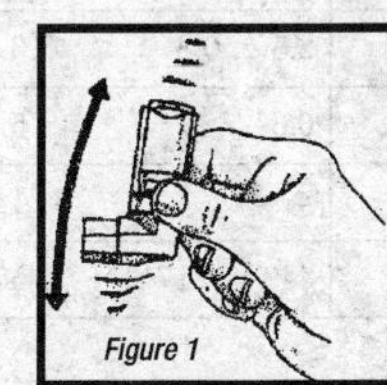

Figure 1

3. It is recommended to "test-spray" three times before using for the first time and in cases where the aerosol has not been used for more than 24 hours. ***Avoid spraying in eyes.***
4. ***Exhale deeply*** through the mouth. Holding the canister as illustrated in Figure 2, enclose mouthpiece with the lips. Keep the eyes closed because temporary blurring of vision, precipitation or worsening of narrow-angle glaucoma or eye pain may result if the aerosol is sprayed into the eyes.

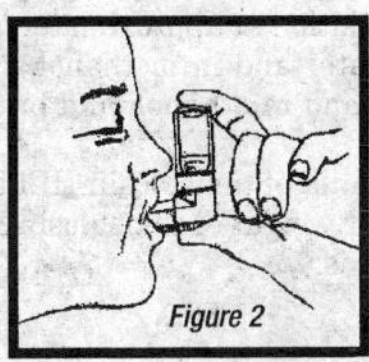

Figure 2

5. ***Inhale slowly*** through the mouth ***and at the same time*** firmly ***press once*** on the upended canister base as in Figure 3; continue to inhale deeply.

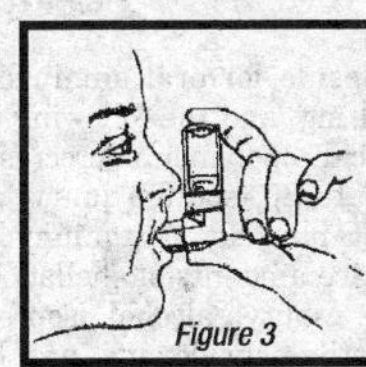

Figure 3

6. ***Hold your breath*** for ten seconds and then remove the mouthpiece from the mouth and exhale slowly, as in Figure 4. ***Wait approximately two minutes, shake the inhaler again and repeat previous steps 4–6.***

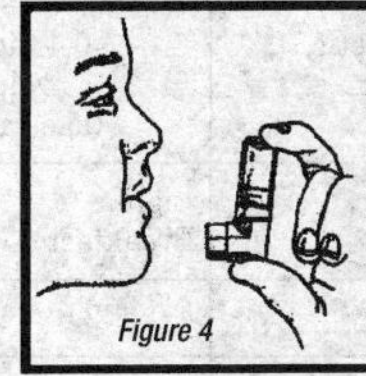

Figure 4

7. Replace protective cap after use.
8. ***Keep the mouthpiece clean.*** Wash with hot water. If soap is used, rinse thoroughly with plain water. Dry thoroughly before use. When dry, replace cap on the mouthpiece when not using the drug product.
9. ***Track the number of sprays used and discard after 200 sprays.*** The amount of medication in each inhalation cannot be assured after 200 sprays.
10. While taking Combivent® Inhalation Aerosol, other inhaled drugs should be taken only as directed by your physician.
11. If the recommended dosage does not provide relief or symptoms become worse, patients should seek immedi-

Continued on next page

Combivent—Cont.

ate medical attention. Do not increase the dose or frequency of Combivent Inhalation Aerosol without consulting your physician.

12. Note: The indented statement below is required by the Federal government's Clean Air Act for all products containing or manufactured with chlorofluorocarbons (CFCs):

    This product contains trichloromonofluoromethane (CFC-11), dichlorodifluoromethane (CFC12) and dichlorotetrafluoroethane (CFC-114), substances which harm the environment by destroying ozone in the upper atmosphere.

    Your physician has determined that this product is likely to help your personal health. **USE THIS PRODUCT AS DIRECTED, UNLESS INSTRUCTED TO DO OTHERWISE BY YOUR PHYSICIAN.** If you have any questions about alternatives, consult with your physician.

13. The contents of Combivent Inhalation Aerosol are under pressure. Do not puncture. Do not use or store near heat or open flame. Exposure to temperatures above 120°F may cause bursting. Never throw the container into a fire or incinerator. Keep out of reach of children. Avoid spraying in eyes.

Store between 59°F (15°C) and 86°F (30°C). Avoid excessive humidity.

Manufactured by: Boehringer Ingelheim Pharmaceuticals, Inc., Ridgefield, CT 06877, USA

Ipratropium bromide licensed from:
Boehringer Ingelheim International GmbH

Revised 9/01
10000291/03 10000291/US/03

Shown in Product Identification Guide, page 309

FLOMAX® ℞

[flō-măx]
(tamsulosin hydrochloride)
Capsules
Prescribing Information

DESCRIPTION

Tamsulosin hydrochloride is an antagonist of alpha$_{1A}$ adrenoceptors in the prostate.

Tamsulosin HCl is (-)-(*R*)-5-[2-[[2-(0-ethoxyphenoxy) ethyl]amino]propyl]-2-methoxybenzenesulfonamide, monohydrochloride. Tamsulosin HCl occurs as white crystals that melt with decomposition at approximately 230°C. It is sparingly soluble in water and in methanol, slightly soluble in glacial acetic acid and in ethanol, and practically insoluble in ether.

The empirical formula of tamsulosin HCl is $C_{20}H_{28}N_2O_5S \cdot HCl$. The molecular weight of tamsulosin HCl is 444.98. Its structural formula is:

Each FLOMAX capsule for oral administration contains tamsulosin HCl 0.4 mg, and the following inactive ingredients: methacrylic acid copolymer, microcrystalline cellulose, triacetin, polysorbate 80, sodium lauryl sulfate, calcium stearate, talc, FD&C blue No. 2, titanium dioxide, ferric oxide, gelatin, and trace amounts of shellac, industrial methylated spirit 74 OP, *n*-butyl, alcohol, isopropyl alcohol, propylene glycol, dimethylpolysiloxane, and black iron oxide E172.

CLINICAL PHARMACOLOGY

The symptoms associated with benign prostatic hyperplasia (BPH) are related to bladder outlet obstruction, which is comprised of two underlying components: static and dynamic. The static component is related to an increase in prostate size caused, in part, by a proliferation of smooth muscle cells in the prostatic stroma. However, the severity of BPH symptoms and the degree of urethral obstruction do not correlate well with the size of the prostate. The dynamic component is a function of an increase in smooth muscle tone in the prostate and bladder neck leading to constriction of the bladder outlet. Smooth muscle tone is mediated by the sympathetic nervous stimulation of alpha$_1$ adrenoceptors, which are abundant in the prostate, prostatic capsule, prostatic urethra, and bladder neck. Blockade of these adrenoceptors can cause smooth muscles in the bladder neck and prostate to relax, resulting in an improvement in urine flow rate and a reduction in symptoms of BPH.

Tamsulosin, an alpha$_1$ adrenoceptor blocking agent, exhibits its selectivity for alpha$_1$ receptors in the human prostate. At least three discrete alpha$_1$-adrenoceptor subtypes have been identified: alpha$_{1A}$, alpha$_{1B}$ and alpha$_{1D}$; their distribution differs between human organs and tissue. Approximately 70% of the alpha$_1$-receptors in human prostate are of the alpha$_{1A}$ subtype.

FLOMAX capsules are not intended for use as an antihypertensive drug.

Pharmacokinetics

The pharmacokinetics of tamsulosin HCl have been evaluated in adult healthy volunteers and patients with BPH after single and/or multiple administration with doses ranging from 0.1 mg to 1 mg.

Absorption: Absorption of tamsulosin HCl from FLOMAX capsules 0.4 mg is essentially complete (>90%) following oral administration under fasting conditions. Tamsulosin HCl exhibits linear kinetics following single and multiple dosing, with achievement of steady-state concentrations by the fifth day of once-a-day dosing.

Effect of Food: The time to maximum concentration (T_{max}) is reached by four to five hours under fasting conditions and by six to seven hours when FLOMAX capsules are administered with food. Taking FLOMAX capsules under fasted conditions results in a 30% increase in bioavailability (AUC) and 40% to 70% increase in peak concentrations (C_{max}) compared to fed conditions (Figure 1).

Figure 1: Mean Plasma Tamsulosin HCl Concentrations Following Single-Dose Administration of FLOMAX capsules 0.4 mg Under Fasted and Fed Conditions (n=8).

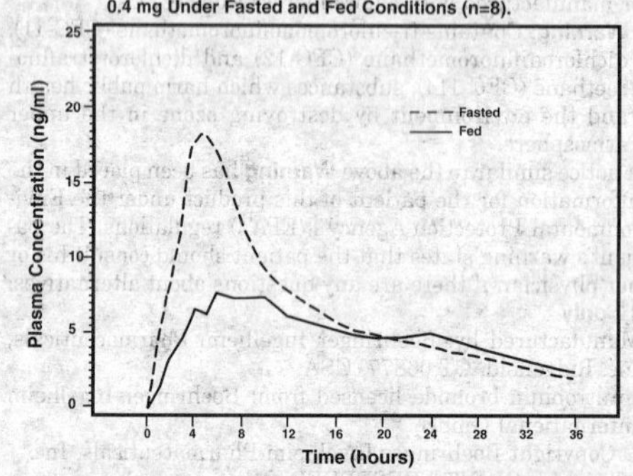

The effects of food on the pharmacokinetics of tamsulosin HCl are consistent regardless of whether a FLOMAX capsule is taken with a light breakfast or a high-fat breakfast (Table 1).

[See table 1 below]

Distribution: The mean steady-state apparent volume of distribution of tamsulosin HCl after intravenous administration to ten healthy male adults was 16L, which is suggestive of distribution into extracellular fluids in the body. Additionally, whole body autoradiographic studies in mice and rats and tissue distribution in rats and dogs indicate that tamsulosin HCl is widely distributed to most tissues including kidney, prostate, liver, gall bladder, heart, aorta, and brown fat, and minimally distributed to the brain, spinal cord, and testes.

Tamsulosin HCl is extensively bound to human plasma proteins (94% to 99%), primarily alpha-1 acid glycoprotein (AAG), with linear binding over a wide concentration range (20 to 600 ng/mL). The results of two-way *in vitro* studies indicate that the binding of tamsulosin HCl to human plasma proteins is not affected by amitriptyline, diclofenac, glyburide, simvastatin plus simvastatin-hydroxy acid metabolite, warfarin, diazepam, propranolol, trichlormethiazide, or chlormadinone. Likewise, tamsulosin HCl had no effect on the extent of binding of these drugs.

Metabolism: There is no enantiometric bioconversion from tamsulosin HCl [R(-) isomer] to the S(+) isomer in humans. Tamsulosin HCl is extensively metabolized by cytochrome P450 enzymes in the liver and less than 10% of the dose is excreted in urine unchanged. However, the pharmacokinetic profile of the metabolites in humans has not been established. Additionally, the cytochrome P450 enzymes that primarily catalyze the Phase I metabolism of tamsulosin HCl have not been conclusively identified. Therefore, possible interactions with other cytochrome P450 metabolized compounds cannot be discerned with current information. The metabolites of tamsulosin HCl undergo extensive conjugation to glucuronide or sulfate prior to renal excretion.

Incubations with human liver microsomes showed no evidence of clinically significant metabolic interactions between tamsulosin HCl and amitriptyline, albuterol (beta agonist), glyburide (glibenclamide) and finasteride (5alpha-reductase inhibitor for treatment of BPH). However, results of the *in vitro* testing of the tamsulosin HCl interaction with diclofenac and warfarin were equivocal.

Excretion: On administration of the radiolabeled dose of tamsulosin HCl to four healthy volunteers, 97% of the administered radioactivity was recovered, with urine (76%) representing the primary route of excretion compared to feces (21%) over 168 hours.

Following intravenous or oral administration of an immediate-release formulation, the elimination half-life of tamsulosin HCl in plasma range from five to seven hours. Because of absorption rate-controlled pharmacokinetics with FLOMAX capsules, the apparent half-life of tamsulosin HCl is approximately 9 to 13 hours in healthy volunteers and 14 to 15 hours in the target population.

Tamsulosin HCl undergoes restrictive clearance in humans, with a relatively low systemic clearance (2.88 L/h).

Special Populations: Geriatrics (Age): Cross-study comparison of FLOMAX capsules overall exposure (AUC) and half-life indicate that the pharmacokinetic disposition of tamsulosin HCl may be slightly prolonged in geriatric males compared to young, healthy male volunteers. Intrinsic clearance is independent of tamsulosin HCl binding to AAG, but diminishes with age, resulting in a 40% overall higher exposure (AUC) in subjects of age 55 to 75 years compared to subjects of age 20 to 32 years.

Renal Dysfunction: The pharmacokinetics of tamsulosin HCl have been compared in 6 subjects with mild-moderate ($30 \leq CL_{cr} < 70$ mL/min/1.73m^2) or moderate-severe ($10 \leq CL_{cr} < 30$ mL/min/1.73m^2) renal impairment and 6 normal subjects ($CL_{cr} < 90$ mL/min/1.73m^2). While a change in the overall plasma concentration of tamsulosin HCl was observed as the result of altered binding to AAG, the unbound (active) concentration of tamsulosin HCl, as well as the intrinsic clearance, remained relatively constant. Therefore, patients with renal impairment do not require an adjustment in FLOMAX capsules dosing. However, patients with endstage renal disease ($CL_{cr} < 10$ mL/min/1.73m^2) have not been studied.

Hepatic Dysfunction: The pharmacokinetics of tamsulosin HCl have been compared in 8 subjects with moderate hepatic dysfunction (Child-Pugh's classification: Grades A and B) and 8 normal subjects. While a change in the overall plasma concentration of tamsulosin HCl was observed as the result of altered binding to AAG, the unbound (active) concentration of tamsulosin HCl does not change significantly with only a modest (32%) change in intrinsic clearance of unbound tamsulosin HCl. Therefore, patients with moderate hepatic dysfunction do not require an adjustment in FLOMAX capsules dosage.

Drug-Drug Interactions: Nifedipine, Atenolol, Enalapril: In three studies in hypertensive subjects (age range 47–79 years) whose blood pressure was controlled with stable doses of Procardia XL®, atenolol, or enalapril for at least three months, FLOMAX capsules 0.4 mg for seven days followed by FLOMAX capsules 0.8 mg for another seven days (n=8 per study) resulted in no clinically significant effects on blood pressure and pulse rate compared to placebo (n=4 per study). Therefore, dosage adjustments are not necessary when FLOMAX capsules are administered concomitantly with Procardia XL®, atenolol, or enalapril.

Warfarin: A definitive drug-drug interaction study between tamsulosin HCl and warfarin was not conducted. Results from limited *in vitro* and *in vivo* studies are inconclusive. Therefore, caution should be exercised with concomitant administration of warfarin and FLOMAX capsules.

Digoxin and Theophylline: In two studies in healthy volunteers (n=10 per study; age range 19-39 years) receiving

TABLE 1 Mean (± S.D.) Pharmacokinetic Parameters Following FLOMAX capsules 0.4 mg Once Daily or 0.8 mg Once Daily with a Light Breakfast, High-Fat Breakfast or Fasted

Pharmacokinetic Parameter	0.4 mg q.d. to healthy volunteers; n=33 (age range 18-32 years)		0.8 mg q.d. to healthy volunteers; n=22 (age range 55-75 years)		
	Light Breakfast	Fasted	Light Breakfast	High-Fat Breakfast	Fasted
Cmin (ng/mL)	4.0 ± 2.6	3.8 ± 2.5	12.3 ± 6.7	13.5 ± 7.6	13.3 ± 13.3
Cmax (ng/mL)	10.1 ± 4.8	17.1 ± 17.1	29.8 ± 10.3	29.1 ± 11.0	41.6 ± 15.6
Cmax/Cmin Ratio	3.1 ± 1.0	5.3 ± 2.2	2.7 ± 0.7	2.5 ± 0.8	3.6 ± 1.1
Tmax (hours)	6.0	4.0	7.0	6.6	5.0
T1/2 (hours)	–	–	–	–	14.9 ± 3.9
AUCτ (ng•hr/mL)	151 ± 81.5	199 ± 94.1	440 ± 195	449 ± 217	557 ± 257

Cmin = observed minimum concentration
Cmax = observed maximum tamsulosin HCl plasma concentration
Tmax = median time-to-maximum concentration
T1/2 = observed half-life
AUCτ = Area under the tamsulosin HCl plasma time curve over the dosing interval

FLOMAX capsules 0.4 mg/day for two days, followed by FLOMAX capsules 0.8 mg/day for five to eight days, single intravenous doses of digoxin 0.5 mg or theophylline 5 mg/kg resulted in no change in the pharmacokinetics of digoxin or theophylline. Therefore, dosage adjustments are not necessary when a FLOMAX capsule is administered concomitantly with digoxin or theophylline.

Furosemide: The pharmacokinetic and pharmacodynamic interaction between FLOMAX capsules 0.8 mg/day (steady-state) and furosemide 20 mg intravenously (single dose) was evaluated in ten healthy volunteers (age range 21-40 years). FLOMAX capsules had no effect on the pharmacodynamics (excretion of electrolytes) of furosemide. While furosemide produced an 11% to 12% reduction in tamsulosin HCl Cmax and AUC, these changes are expected to be clinically insignificant and do not require adjustment of the FLOMAX capsules dosage.

Cimetidine: The effects of cimetidine at the highest recommended dose (400 mg every six hours for six days) on the pharmacokinetics of a single FLOMAX capsule 0.4 mg dose was investigated in ten healthy volunteers (age range 21-38 years). Treatment with cimetidine resulted in a significant decrease (26%) in the clearance of tamsulosin HCl which resulted in a moderate increase in tamsulosin HCl AUC (44%). Therefore, FLOMAX capsules should be used with caution in combination with cimetidine, particularly at doses higher than 0.4 mg.

Clinical Studies

Four placebo-controlled clinical studies and one active-controlled clinical study enrolled a total of 2296 patients (1003 received FLOMAX capsules 0.4 mg once daily, 491 received FLOMAX capsules 0.8 mg once daily, and 802 were control patients) in the U.S. and Europe.

In the two U.S. placebo-controlled, double-blind, 13-week, multicenter studies [Study 1 (US92-03A) and Study 2 (US93-01)], 1486 men with the signs and symptoms of BPH were enrolled. In both studies, patients were randomized to either placebo, FLOMAX capsules 0.4 mg once daily, or FLOMAX capsules 0.8 mg once daily. Patients in FLOMAX capsules 0.8 mg once daily treatment groups received a dose of 0.4 mg once daily for one week before increasing to the 0.8 mg once daily dose. The primary efficacy assessments included: 1) total American Urological Association (AUA) Symptom Score questionnaire, which evaluated irritative (frequency, urgency, and nocturia), and obstructive (hesitancy, incomplete emptying, intermittency, and weak stream) symptoms, where a decrease in score is consistent with improvement in symptoms; and 2) peak urine flow rate, where an increased peak urine flow rate value over baseline is consistent with decreased urinary obstruction.

Mean changes from baseline to week 13 in total AUA Symptom Score were significantly greater for groups treated with FLOMAX capsules 0.4 mg and 0.8 mg once daily compared to placebo in both U.S. studies (Table 2, Figures 2A and 2B). The changes from baseline to week 13 in peak urine flow rate were also significantly greater for the FLOMAX capsules 0.4 mg and 0.8 mg once daily groups compared to placebo in Study 1, and for the FLOMAX capsules 0.8 mg once daily group in Study 2 (Table 2, Figures 3A and 3B). Overall there were no significant differences in improvement observed in total AUA Symptom Scores or peak urine flow rates between the 0.4 mg and the 0.8 mg dose groups with the exception that the 0.8 mg dose in Study 1 had a significantly greater improvement in total AUA Symptom Score compared to the 0.4 mg dose.

[See table 2 above]

Mean total AUA Symptom Scores for both FLOMAX capsules 0.4 mg and 0.8 mg once daily groups showed a rapid decrease starting at one week after dosing and remained decreased through 13 weeks in both studies (Figures 2A and 2B).

In Study 1, 400 patients (53% of the originally randomized group) elected to continue in their originally assigned treatment groups in a double-blind, placebo controlled, 40 week extension trial (138 patients on 0.4 mg, 135 patients on 0.8 mg and 127 patients on placebo). Three hundred and twenty-three patients (43% of the originally randomized group) completed one year. Of these, 81% (97 patients) on 0.4 mg, 74% (75 patients) on 0.8 mg and 56% (57 patients) on placebo had a response ≥25% above baseline in total AUA Symptom Score at one year.

[See figure 2A above]
[See figure 2B at right]
[See figure 3A at top of next page]
[See figure 3B on next page]

TABLE 2 MEAN (±S.D.) CHANGES FROM BASELINE TO WEEK 13 IN TOTAL AUA SYMPTOM SCORE ** AND PEAK URINE FLOW RATE (ML/SEC)

	Total AUA Symptom Score		Peak Urine Flow Rate	
	Mean Baseline Value	Mean Change	Mean Baseline Value	Mean Change
Study 1 †				
FLOMAX capsules 0.8 mg once daily	19.9±4.9 n=247	−9.6*±6.7 n=237	9.57±2.51 n=247	1.78*±3.35 n=247
FLOMAX capsules 0.4 mg once daily	19.8±5.0 n=254	−8.3*±6.5 n=246	9.46±2.49 n=254	1.75*±3.57 n=254
Placebo	19.6±4.9 n=254	−5.5±6.6 n=246	9.75±2.54 n=254	0.52±3.39 n=253
Study 2 ‡				
FLOMAX capsules 0.8 mg once daily	18.2±5.6 n=244	−5.8*±6.4 n=238	9.96±3.16 n=244	1.79*±3.36 n=237
FLOMAX capsules 0.4 mg once daily	17.9±5.8 n=248	−5.1*±6.4 n=244	9.94±3.14 n=248	1.52±3.64 n=244
Placebo	19.2±6.0 n=239	−3.6±5.7 n=235	9.95±3.12 n=239	0.93±3.28 n=235

* Statistically significant difference from placebo (p-value ≤0.050; Bonferroni-Holm multiple test procedure);
**Total AUA Symptom Scores ranged from 0 to 35
† Peak urine flow rate measured 4 to 8 hours post dose at week 13
‡ Peak urine flow rate measured 24 to 27 hours post dose at week 13
Week 13: For patients not completing the 13 week study the last observation was carried forward.

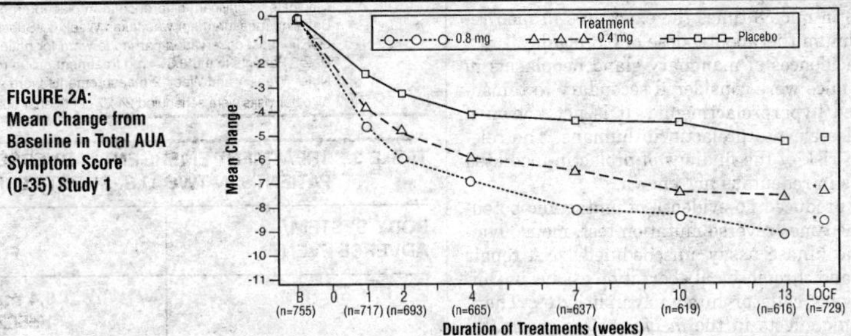

FIGURE 2A: Mean Change from Baseline in Total AUA Symptom Score (0-35) Study 1

* indicates significant difference from placebo (p-value ≤ 0.050).
B = Baseline determined approximately one week prior to the initial dose of double-blind medication at Week 0. Subsequent values are observed cases.
LOCF = Last observation carried forward for patients not completing the 13-week study.
Note: Patients in the 0.8 – mg treatment group received 0.4 mg for the first week.
Note: Total AUA Symptom Scores range from 0 to 35.

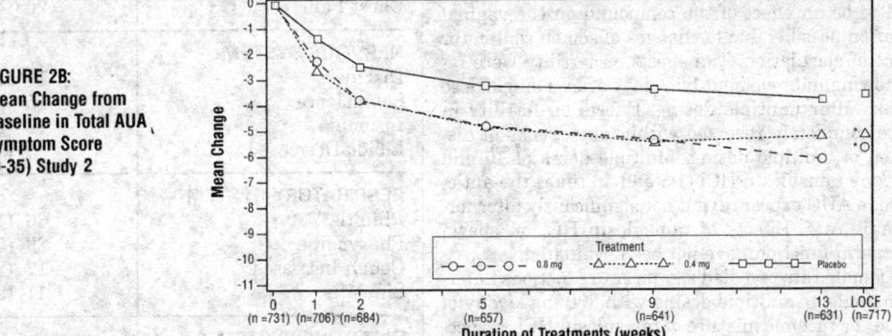

FIGURE 2B: Mean Change from Baseline in Total AUA Symptom Score (0-35) Study 2

* indicates significant difference from placebo (p-value ≤ 0.050).
Baseline measurement was taken Week 0. Subsequent values are observed cases.
LOCF = Last observation carried forward for patients not completing the 13-week study.
Note: Patients in the 0.8 – mg treatment group received 0.4 mg for the first week.
Note: Total AUA Symptom Scores range from 0 to 35.

INDICATIONS AND USAGE

FLOMAX® (tamsulosin HCl) capsules are indicated for the treatment of the signs and symptoms of benign prostatic hyperplasia (BPH). FLOMAX capsules are not indicated for the treatment of hypertension.

CONTRAINDICATIONS

FLOMAX capsules are contraindicated in patients known to be hypersensitive to tamsulosin HCl or any component of FLOMAX capsules.

WARNINGS

The signs and symptoms of orthostasis (postural hypotension, dizziness and vertigo) were detected more frequently in FLOMAX capsule treated patients than in placebo recipients. As with other alpha-adrenergic blocking agents there is a potential risk of syncope (see ADVERSE REACTIONS).

Patients beginning treatment with FLOMAX capsules should be cautioned to avoid situations where injury could result should syncope occur.

Rarely (probably less than one in fifty thousand patients), tamsulosin, like other alpha$_1$ antagonists, has been associated with priapism (persistent painful penile erection unrelated to sexual activity). Because this condition can lead to permanent impotence if not properly treated, patients must be advised about the seriousness of the condition (see Precautions: Information for Patients).

PRECAUTIONS

General

1) Carcinoma of the prostate: Carcinoma of the prostate and BPH cause many of the same symptoms. These two diseases frequently co-exist. Patients should be evaluated prior to the start of FLOMAX capsules therapy to rule out the presence of carcinoma of the prostate.

2) Drug-Drug Interactions: The pharmacokinetic and pharmacodynamic interactions between FLOMAX capsules and other alpha-adrenergic blocking agents have not been determined. However, interactions may be expected and FLOMAX capsules should NOT be used in combination with other alpha-adrenergic blocking agents.

The pharmacokinetic interaction between cimetidine and FLOMAX capsules was investigated. The results indicate significant changes in tamsulosin HCl clearance (26% decrease) and AUC (44% increase). Therefore, FLOMAX capsules should be used with caution in combination with cimetidine, particularly at doses higher than 0.4 mg.

Results from limited *in vitro* and *in vivo* drug-drug interaction studies between tamsulosin HCl and warfarin are inconclusive. Therefore, caution should be exercised with concomitant administration of warfarin and FLOMAX capsules.

(See also drug-drug interaction studies in CLINICAL PHARMACOLOGY, Pharmacokinetics subsection.)

Information for Patients (see Patient Package Insert)

Patients should be told about the possible occurrence of symptoms related to postural hypotension such as dizziness when taking FLOMAX capsules, and they should be cautioned about driving, operating machinery or performing hazardous tasks.

Patients should be advised not to crush, chew or open the FLOMAX capsules.

Patients should be advised about the possibility of priapism as a result of treatment with FLOMAX Capsules and other similar medications. Patients should be informed that this reaction is extremely rare, but if not brought to immediate medical attention, can lead to permanent erectile dysfunction (impotence).

Laboratory Tests

No laboratory test interactions with FLOMAX capsules are known. Treatment with FLOMAX capsules for up to 12 months had no significant effect on prostate-specific antigen (PSA).

Continued on next page

Flomax—Cont.

Pregnancy

Teratogenic Effects, Pregnancy Category B.

Administration of tamsulosin HCl to pregnant female rats at dose levels up to 300 mg/kg/day (approximately 50 times the human therapeutic AUC exposure) revealed no evidence of harm to the fetus. Administration of tamsulosin HCl to pregnant rabbits at dose levels up to 50 mg/kg/day produced no evidence of fetal harm. FLOMAX capsules are not indicated for use in women.

Nursing Mothers

FLOMAX capsules are not indicated for use in women.

Pediatric Use

FLOMAX capsules are not indicated for use in pediatric populations.

Carcinogenesis, Mutagenesis, and Impairment of Fertility

Rats administered doses up to 43 mg/kg/day in males and 52 mg/kg/day in females had no increases in tumor incidence with the exception of a modest increase in the frequency of mammary gland fibroadenomas in female rats receiving doses ≥ 5.4 mg/kg ($P < 0.015$). The highest doses of tamsulosin HCl evaluated in the rat carcinogenicity study produced systemic exposures (AUC) in rats 3 times the exposures in men receiving the maximum therapeutic dose of 0.8 mg/day.

Mice were administered doses up to 127 mg/kg/day in males and 158 mg/kg/day in females. There were no significant tumor findings in male mice. Female mice treated for 2 years with the two highest doses of 45 and 158 mg/kg/day had statistically significant increases in the incidence of mammary gland fibroadenomas ($P < 0.0001$) and adenocarcinomas ($P < 0.0075$). The highest dose levels of tamsulosin HCl evaluated in the mice carcinogenicity study produced systemic exposures (AUC) in mice 8 times the exposures in men receiving the maximum therapeutic dose of 0.8 mg/day.

The increased incidences of mammary gland neoplasms in female rats and mice were considered secondary to tamsulosin HCl-induced hyperprolactinemia. It is not known if FLOMAX capsules elevate prolactin in humans. The relevance for human risk of the findings of prolactin-mediated endocrine tumors in rodents is not known.

Tamsulosin HCl produced no evidence of mutagenic potential *in vitro* in the Ames reverse mutation test, mouse lymphoma thymidine kinase assay, unscheduled DNA repair synthesis assay, and chromosomal aberration assays in Chinese hamster ovary cells or human lymphocytes. There were no mutagenic effects in the *in vivo* sister chromatid exchange and mouse micronucleus assay.

Studies in rats revealed significantly reduced fertility in males dosed with single or multiple daily doses of 300 mg/kg/day of tamsulosin HCl (AUC exposure in rats about 50 times the human exposure with the maximum therapeutic dose). The mechanism of decreased fertility in male rats is considered to be an effect of the compound on the vaginal plug formation possibly due to changes of semen content or impairment of ejaculation. The effects on fertility were reversible showing improvement by 3 days after a single dose and 4 weeks after multiple dosing. Effects on fertility in males were completely reversed within nine weeks of discontinuation of multiple dosing. Multiple doses of 10 and 100 mg/kg/day tamsulosin HCl (1/5 and 16 times the anticipated human AUC exposure) did not significantly alter fertility in male rats. Effects of tamsulosin HCl on sperm counts or sperm function have not been evaluated.

Studies in female rats revealed significant reductions in fertility after single or multiple dosing with 300 mg/kg/day of the R-isomer or racemic mixture of tamsulosin HCl, respectively. In female rats, the reductions in fertility after single doses were considered to be associated with impairments in fertilization. Multiple dosing with 10 or 100 mg/kg/day of the racemic mixture did not significantly alter fertility in female rats.

ADVERSE REACTIONS

The incidence of treatment-emergent adverse events has been ascertained from six short-term U.S. and European placebo-controlled clinical trials in which daily doses of 0.1 to 0.8 mg FLOMAX capsules were used. These studies evaluated safety in 1783 patients treated with FLOMAX capsules and 798 patients administered placebo. Table 3 summarizes the treatment-emergent adverse events that occurred in ≥ 2% of patients receiving either FLOMAX capsules 0.4 mg, or 0.8 mg and at an incidence numerically higher than that in the placebo group during two 13-week U.S. trials (US92-03A and US93-01) conducted in 1487 men.

[See table 3 at right]

Signs and Symptoms of Orthostasis In the two U.S. studies, symptomatic postural hypotension was reported by 0.2% of patients (1 of 502) in the 0.4 mg group, 0.4% of patients (2 of 492) in the 0.8 mg group, and by no patients in the placebo group. Syncope was reported by 0.2% of patients (1 of 502) in the 0.4 mg group, 0.4% of patients (2 of 492) in the 0.8 mg group and 0.6% of patients (3 of 493) in the placebo group. Dizziness was reported by 15% of patients (75 of 502) in the 0.4 mg group, 17% of patients (84 of 492) in the 0.8 mg group, and 10% of patients (50 of 493) in the placebo group. Vertigo was reported by 0.6% of patients (3 of 502) in the 0.4 mg group, 1% of patients (5 of 492) in the 0.8 mg group and by 0.6% of patients (3 of 493) in the placebo group.

Multiple testing for orthostatic hypotension was conducted in a number of studies. Such a test was considered positive if it met one or more of the following criteria: (1) a decrease in systolic blood pressure of ≥20 mmHg upon standing from the supine position during the orthostatic tests; (2) a decrease in diastolic blood pressure ≥10 mmHg upon standing, with the standing diastolic blood pressure <65 mmHg during the orthostatic test; (3) an increase in pulse rate of ≥20 bpm upon standing with a standing pulse rate ≥100 bpm during the orthostatic test; and (4) the presence of clinical symptoms (faintness, lightheadedness/lightheaded, dizziness, spinning sensation, vertigo, or postural hypotension) upon standing during the orthostatic test.

Following the first dose of double-blind medication in Study 1, a positive orthostatic test result at 4 hours post-dose was observed in 7% of patients (37 of 498) who received FLOMAX capsules 0.4 mg once daily and in 3% of the patients (8 of 253) who received placebo. At 8 hours post-dose, a positive orthostatic test result was observed for 6% of the patients (31 of 498) who received FLOMAX capsules 0.4 mg once daily and 4% (9 of 250) who received placebo (Note: patients in the 0.8 mg group received 0.4 mg once daily for the first week of Study 1).

In Studies 1 and 2, at least one positive orthostatic test result was observed during the course of these studies for 81 of the 502 patients (16%) in the FLOMAX capsules 0.4 mg once daily group, 92 of the 491 patients (19%) in the FLOMAX capsules 0.8 mg once daily group and 54 of the 493 patients (11%) in the placebo group.

Because orthostasis was detected more frequently in FLOMAX capsule-treated patients than in placebo recipients, there is a potential risk of syncope (see WARNINGS).

Abnormal Ejaculation: Abnormal ejaculation includes ejaculation failure, ejaculation disorder, retrograde ejaculation and ejaculation decrease. As shown in Table 3, abnormal ejaculation was associated with FLOMAX capsules ad-

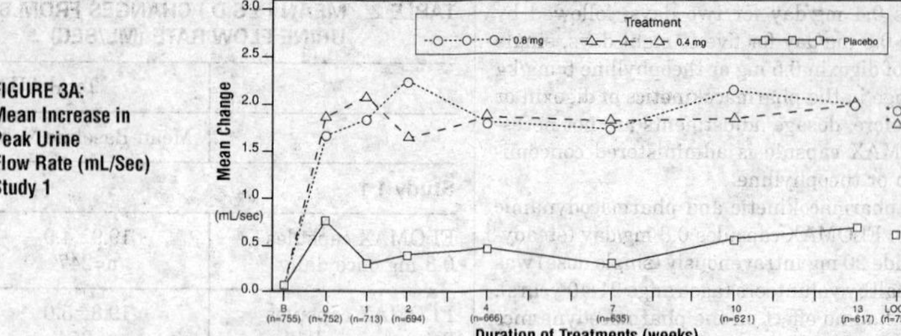

* indicates significant difference from placebo (p-value ≤0.050).
B = Baseline determined approximately one week prior to the initial dose of double-blind medication at Week 0. Subsequent values are observed cases.
LOCF = last observation carried forward for patients not completing the 13-week study.
Note: The uroflowmetry assessments at week 0 were recorded 4-8 hours after patients received the first dose of double-blind medication.
Measurements at each visit were scheduled 4-8 hours after dosing (approximately peak plasma tamsulosin concentration).
Note: Patients in the 0.8 mg treatment groups received 0.4 mg for the first week.

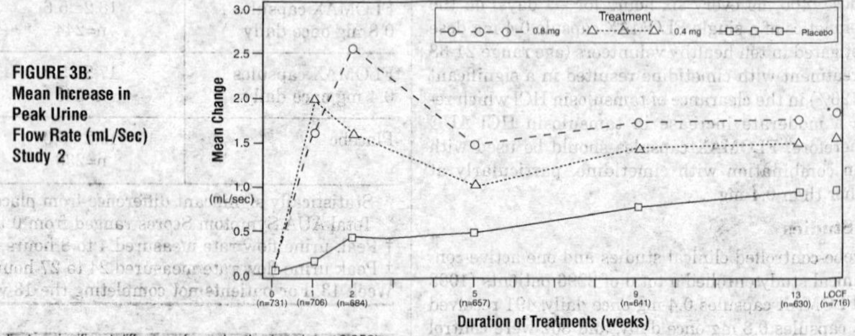

* indicates significant difference from placebo (p-value ≤0.050).
Baseline measurement was taken Week 0. Subsequent values are observed cases.
LOCF = Last observation carried forward for patients not completing the 13-week study.
Note: Patients in the 0.8 mg treatment group received 0.4 mg for the first week.
Note: Week 1 and Week 2 measurements were scheduled 4-8 hours after dosing (approximate peak plasma tamsulosin concentration).
All other visits were scheduled 24-27 hours after dosing (approximate trough tamsulosin concentration).

TABLE 3. TREATMENT EMERGENT[1] ADVERSE EVENTS OCCURRING IN ≥2% OF FLOMAX CAPSULES OR PLACEBO PATIENTS IN TWO U.S. SHORT-TERM PLACEBO-CONTROLLED CLINICAL STUDIES

BODY SYSTEM/ ADVERSE EVENT	FLOMAX CAPSULES GROUPS		PLACEBO
	0.4 mg n=502	0.8 mg n=492	n=493
BODY AS WHOLE			
Headache	97 (19.3%)	104 (21.1%)	99 (20.1%)
Infection	45 (9.0%)	53 (10.8%)	37 (7.5%)
Asthenia	39 (7.8%)	42 (8.5%)	27 (5.5%)
Back Pain	35 (7.0%)	41 (8.3%)	27 (5.5%)
Chest Pain	20 (4.0%)	20 (4.1%)	18 (3.7%)
NERVOUS SYSTEM			
Dizziness	75 (14.9%)	84 (17.1%)	50 (10.1%)
Somnolence	15 (3.0%)	21 (4.3%)	8 (1.6%)
Insomnia	12 (2.4%)	7 (1.4%)	3 (0.6%)
Libido Decreased	5 (1.0%)	10 (2.0%)	6 (1.2%)
RESPIRATORY SYSTEM			
Rhinitis	66 (13.1%)	88 (17.9%)	41 (8.3%)
Pharyngitis	29 (5.8%)	25 (5.1%)	23 (4.7%)
Cough Increased	17 (3.4%)	22 (4.5%)	12 (2.4%)
Sinusitis	11 (2.2%)	18 (3.7%)	8 (1.6%)
DIGESTIVE SYSTEM			
Diarrhea	31 (6.2%)	21 (4.3%)	22 (4.5%)
Nausea	13 (2.6%)	19 (3.9%)	16 (3.2%)
Tooth Disorder	6 (1.2%)	10 (2.0%)	7 (1.4%)
UROGENITAL SYSTEM			
Abnormal Ejaculation	42 (8.4%)	89 (18.1%)	1 (0.2%)
SPECIAL SENSES			
Amblyopia	1 (0.2%)	10 (2.0%)	2 (0.4%)

[1]A treatment-emergent adverse event was defined as any event satisfying one of the following criteria:
- The adverse event occurred for the first time after initial dosing with double-blind study medication.
- The adverse event was present prior to or at the time of initial dosing with double-blind study medication and subsequently increased in severity during double-blind treatment;

or
- The adverse event was present prior to or at the time of initial dosing with double-blind study medication, disappeared completely, and then reappeared during double-blind treatment.

ministration and was dose-related in the U.S. studies. Withdrawal from these clinical studies of FLOMAX capsules because of abnormal ejaculation was also dose-dependent with 8 of 492 patients (1.6%) in the 0.8 mg group, and no patients in the 0.4 mg or placebo groups discontinuing treatment due to abnormal ejaculation.

Post-Marketing Experience: Allergic-type reactions such as skin rash, pruritus, angioedema of tongue, lips and face and urticaria have been reported with positive rechallenge in some cases. Priapism has been reported rarely. Infrequent reports of palpitations, constipation and vomiting have been received during the post-marketing period.

OVERDOSAGE

Should overdosage of FLOMAX capsules lead to hypotension (See WARNINGS and ADVERSE REACTIONS), support of the cardiovascular system is of first importance. Restoration of blood pressure and normalization of heart rate may be accomplished by keeping the patient in the supine position. If this measure is inadequate, then administration of intravenous fluids should be considered. If necessary, vasopressors should then be used and renal function should be monitored and supported as needed. Laboratory data indicate that tamsulosin HCl is 94% to 99% protein bound; therefore, dialysis is unlikely to be of benefit.

One patient reported an overdose of thirty 0.4 mg FLOMAX capsules. Following the ingestion of the capsules, the patient reported a severe headache.

DOSAGE AND ADMINISTRATION

FLOMAX capsules 0.4 mg once daily is recommended as the dose for the treatment of the signs and symptoms of BPH. It should be administered approximately one-half hour following the same meal each day.

For those patients who fail to respond to the 0.4 mg dose after two to four weeks of dosing, the dose of FLOMAX capsules can be increased to 0.8 mg once daily. If FLOMAX capsules administration is discontinued or interrupted for several days at either the 0.4 mg or 0.8 mg dose, therapy should be started again with the 0.4 mg once daily dose.

HOW SUPPLIED

FLOMAX capsules 0.4 mg are supplied in high-density polyethylene bottles containing 100 or 1000 hard gelatin capsules with olive green opaque cap and orange opaque body. The capsules are imprinted on one side with "Flomax 0.4 mg" and on the other side with "BI 58."

FLOMAX Capsules 0.4 mg, 100 capsules (NDC 0597-0058-01)

FLOMAX Capsules 0.4 mg, 1000 capsules (NDC 0597-0058-10)

Store at 25°C (77°F); excursions permitted to 15–30°C (59–86°).

Keep FLOMAX capsules and all medicines out of reach of children.

℞ only.

Marketed by:
Boehringer Ingelheim Pharmaceuticals, Inc.
Ridgefield, CT 06877
and
Abbott Laboratories Inc.
North Chicago, IL 60064
Licensed from and Manufactured by:
Yamanouchi Pharmaceutical Co., Ltd.
3–11 Nihonbashi-Honcho 2-Chome
Chuo-ku, Tokyo 103-8411, Japan
SRT16/US/1 08/02

Shown in Product Identification Guide, page 309

MICARDIS® ℞

(telmisartan)
Tablets, 20 mg, 40 mg and 80 mg
Prescribing Information

> **USE IN PREGNANCY**
> **When used in pregnancy during the second and third trimesters, drugs that act directly on the renin-angiotensin system can cause injury and even death to the developing fetus.** When pregnancy is detected, MICARDIS® tablets should be discontinued as soon as possible.
> **See WARNINGS: Fetal/Neonatal Morbidity and Mortality**

DESCRIPTION

MICARDIS® (telmisartan) is a nonpeptide angiotensin II receptor (type AT_1) antagonist.

Telmisartan is chemically described as 4′-[(1,4′-dimethyl-2′-propyl[2,6′-bi-1H-benzimidazol]-1′-yl)methyl]-[1,1′-biphenyl]-2-carboxylic acid. Its empirical formula is $C_{33}H_{30}N_4O_2$, its molecular weight is 514.63, and its structural formula is:

[See chemical structure at top of next column]

Telmisartan is a white to slightly yellowish solid. It is practically insoluble in water and in the pH range of 3 to 9, sparingly soluble in strong acid (except insoluble in hydrochloric acid), and soluble in strong base.

MICARDIS is available as tablets for oral administration, containing 20 mg, 40 mg or 80 mg of telmisartan. The tablets contain the following inactive ingredients: sodium hy-

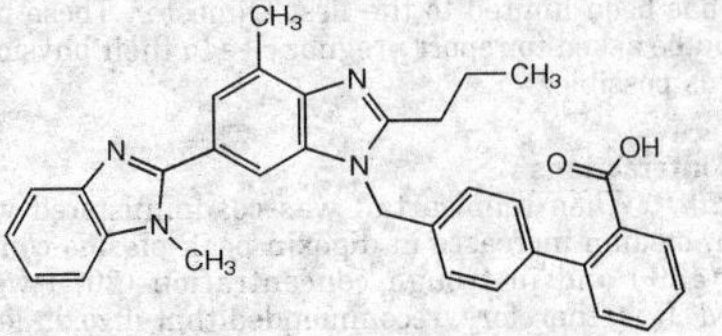

droxide, meglumine, povidone, sorbitol, and magnesium stearate. MICARDIS tablets are hygroscopic and require protection from moisture.

CLINICAL PHARMACOLOGY

Mechanism of Action

Angiotensin II is formed from angiotensin I in a reaction catalyzed by angiotensin-converting enzyme (ACE, kininase II). Angiotensin II is the principal pressor agent of the renin-angiotensin system, with effects that include vasoconstriction, stimulation of synthesis and release of aldosterone, cardiac stimulation, and renal reabsorption of sodium. Telmisartan blocks the vasoconstrictor and aldosterone-secreting effects of angiotensin II by selectively blocking the binding of angiotensin II to the AT_1 receptor in many tissues, such as vascular smooth muscle and the adrenal gland. Its action is therefore independent of the pathways for angiotensin II synthesis.

There is also an AT_2 receptor found in many tissues, but AT_2 is not known to be associated with cardiovascular homeostasis. Telmisartan has much greater affinity (>3,000 fold) for the AT_1 receptor than for the AT_2 receptor.

Blockade of the renin-angiotensin system with ACE inhibitors, which inhibit the biosynthesis of angiotensin II from angiotensin I, is widely used in the treatment of hypertension. ACE inhibitors also inhibit the degradation of bradykinin, a reaction also catalyzed by ACE. Because telmisartan does not inhibit ACE (kininase II), it does not affect the response to bradykinin. Whether this difference has clinical relevance is not yet known. Telmisartan does not bind to or block other hormone receptors or ion channels known to be important in cardiovascular regulation.

Blockade of the angiotensin II receptor inhibits the negative regulatory feedback of angiotensin II on renin secretion, but the resulting increased plasma renin activity and angiotensin II circulating levels do not overcome the effect of telmisartan on blood pressure.

Pharmacokinetics

General

Following oral administration, peak concentrations (C_{max}) of telmisartan are reached in 0.5-1 hour after dosing. Food slightly reduces the bioavailability of telmisartan, with a reduction in the area under the plasma concentration-time curve (AUC) of about 6% with the 40 mg tablet and about 20% after a 160 mg dose. The absolute bioavailability of telmisartan is dose dependent. At 40 and 160 mg the bioavailability was 42% and 58%, respectively. The pharmacokinetics of orally administered telmisartan are nonlinear over the dose range 20-160 mg, with greater than proportional increases of plasma concentrations (C_{max} and AUC) with increasing doses. Telmisartan shows bi-exponential decay kinetics with a terminal elimination half life of approximately 24 hours. Trough plasma concentrations of telmisartan with once daily dosing are about 10-25% of peak plasma concentrations. Telmisartan has an accumulation index in plasma of 1.5 to 2.0 upon repeated once daily dosing.

Metabolism and Elimination

Following either intravenous or oral administration of ^{14}C-labeled telmisartan, most of the administered dose (>97%) was eliminated unchanged in feces via biliary excretion; only minute amounts were found in the urine (0.91% and 0.49% of total radioactivity, respectively).

Telmisartan is metabolized by conjugation to form a pharmacologically inactive acylglucuronide; the glucuronide of the parent compound is the only metabolite that has been identified in human plasma and urine. After a single dose, the glucuronide represents approximately 11% of the measured radioactivity in plasma. The cytochrome P450 isoenzymes are not involved in the metabolism of telmisartan.

Total plasma clearance of telmisartan is >800 mL/min. Terminal half-life and total clearance appear to be independent of dose.

Distribution

Telmisartan is highly bound to plasma proteins (>99.5%), mainly albumin and α_1-acid glycoprotein. Plasma protein binding is constant over the concentration range achieved with recommended doses. The volume of distribution for telmisartan is approximately 500 liters indicating additional tissue binding.

Special Populations

Pediatric: Telmisartan pharmacokinetics have not been investigated in patients <18 years of age.

Geriatric: The pharmacokinetics of telmisartan do not differ between the elderly and those younger than 65 years (see DOSAGE AND ADMINISTRATION).

Gender: Plasma concentrations of telmisartan are generally 2-3 times higher in females than in males. In clinical trials, however, no significant increases in blood pressure response or in the incidence of orthostatic hypotension were found in women. No dosage adjustment is necessary.

Renal Insufficiency: Renal excretion does not contribute to the clearance of telmisartan. Based on modest experience in patients with mild-to-moderate renal impairment (creatinine clearance of 30-80 mL/min, mean clearance approximately 50 mL/min), no dosage adjustment is necessary in patients with decreased renal function. Telmisartan is not removed from blood by hemofiltration (see PRECAUTIONS, and DOSAGE AND ADMINISTRATION).

Hepatic Insufficiency: In patients with hepatic insufficiency, plasma concentrations of telmisartan are increased, and absolute bioavailability approaches 100% (see PRECAUTIONS, and DOSAGE AND ADMINISTRATION).

Drug Interactions: See PRECAUTIONS, Drug Interactions.

Pharmacodynamics

In normal volunteers, a dose of telmisartan 80 mg inhibited the pressor response to an intravenous infusion of angiotensin II by about 90% at peak plasma concentrations with approximately 40% inhibition persisting for 24 hours.

Plasma concentration of angiotensin II and plasma renin activity (PRA) increased in a dose-dependent manner after single administration of telmisartan to healthy subjects and repeated administration to hypertensive patients. The once-daily administration of up to 80 mg telmisartan to healthy subjects did not influence plasma aldosterone concentrations. In multiple dose studies with hypertensive patients, there were no clinically significant changes in electrolytes (serum potassium or sodium), or in metabolic function (including serum levels of cholesterol, triglycerides, HDL, LDL, glucose, or uric acid).

In 30 hypertensive patients with normal renal function treated for 8 weeks with telmisartan 80 mg or telmisartan 80 mg in combination with hydrochlorothiazide 12.5 mg, there were no clinically significant changes from baseline in renal blood flow, glomerular filtration rate, filtration fraction, renovascular resistance, or creatinine clearance.

Clinical Trials

The antihypertensive effects of MICARDIS (telmisartan) have been demonstrated in six principal placebo-controlled clinical trials, studying a range of 20-160 mg; one of these examined the antihypertensive effects of telmisartan and hydrochlorothiazide in combination. The studies involved a total of 1773 patients with mild to moderate hypertension (diastolic blood pressure of 95-114 mmHg), 1031 of whom were treated with telmisartan. Following once daily administration of telmisartan, the magnitude of blood pressure reduction from baseline after placebo subtraction was approximately (SBP/DBP) 6-8/6 mmHg for 20 mg, 9-13/6-8 mmHg for 40 mg, and 12-13/7-8 mmHg for 80 mg. Larger doses (up to 160 mg) did not appear to cause a further decrease in blood pressure.

Upon initiation of antihypertensive treatment with telmisartan, blood pressure was reduced after the first dose, with a maximal reduction by about 4 weeks. With cessation of treatment with MICARDIS tablets, blood pressure gradually returned to baseline values over a period of several days to one week. During long term studies (without placebo control) the effect of telmisartan appeared to be maintained for up to at least one year. The antihypertensive effect of telmisartan is not influenced by patient age, gender, weight or body mass index. Blood pressure response in black patients (usually a low-renin population) is noticeably less than that in Caucasian patients. This has been true for most, but not all, angiotensin II antagonists and ACE inhibitors.

In a controlled study, the addition of telmisartan to hydrochlorothiazide produced an additional dose-related reduction in blood pressure that was similar in magnitude to the reduction achieved with telmisartan monotherapy. Hydrochlorothiazide also had an added blood pressure effect when added to telmisartan.

The onset of antihypertensive activity occurs within 3 hours after administration of a single oral dose. At doses of 20, 40, and 80 mg, the antihypertensive effect of once daily administration of telmisartan is maintained for the full 24-hour dose interval. With automated ambulatory blood pressure monitoring and conventional blood pressure measurements, the 24-hour trough-to-peak ratio for 40-80 mg doses telmisartan was 70-100% for both systolic and diastolic blood pressure. The incidence of symptomatic orthostasis after the first dose in all controlled trials was low (0.04%).

There were no changes in the heart rate of patients treated with telmisartan in controlled trials.

INDICATIONS AND USAGE

MICARDIS (telmisartan) is indicated for the treatment of hypertension. It may be used alone or in combination with other antihypertensive agents.

CONTRAINDICATIONS

MICARDIS (telmisartan) is contraindicated in patients who are hypersensitive to any component of this product.

WARNINGS

Fetal/Neonatal Morbidity and Mortality

Drugs that act directly on the renin-angiotensin system can cause fetal and neonatal morbidity and death when administered to pregnant women. Several dozen cases have been reported in the world literature in patients who were taking angiotensin converting enzyme inhibitors. When pregnancy is detected, MICARDIS (telmisartan) tablets should be discontinued as soon as possible.

The use of drugs that act directly on the renin-angiotensin system during the second and third trimesters of pregnancy has been associated with fetal and neonatal injury, including hypotension, neonatal skull hypoplasia, anuria, reversible or irreversible renal failure, and death. Oligohydramnios has also been reported, presumably resulting from decreased fetal renal function; oligohydramnios in this setting has been associated with fetal limb contractures, cra-

Continued on next page

Micardis—Cont.

niofacial deformation, and hypoplastic lung development. Prematurity, intrauterine growth retardation, and patent ductus arteriosus have also been reported, although it is not clear whether these occurrences were due to exposure to the drug.

These adverse effects do not appear to have resulted from intrauterine drug exposure that has been limited to the first trimester. Mothers whose embryos and fetuses are exposed to an angiotensin II receptor antagonist only during the first trimester should be so informed. Nonetheless, when patients become pregnant, physicians should have the patient discontinue the use of MICARDIS tablets as soon as possible.

Rarely (probably less often than once in every thousand pregnancies), no alternative to an angiotensin II receptor antagonist will be found. In these rare cases, the mothers should be apprised of the potential hazards to their fetuses, and serial ultrasound examinations should be performed to assess the intra-amniotic environment.

If oligohydramnios is observed, MICARDIS tablets should be discontinued unless they are considered life-saving for the mother. Contraction stress testing (CST), a non-stress test (NST), or biophysical profiling (BPP) may be appropriate, depending upon the week of pregnancy. Patients and physicians should be aware, however, that oligohydramnios may not appear until after the fetus has sustained irreversible injury.

Infants with histories of *in utero* exposure to an angiotensin II receptor antagonist should be closely observed for hypotension, oliguria, and hyperkalemia. If oliguria occurs, attention should be directed toward support of blood pressure and renal perfusion. Exchange transfusion or dialysis may be required as a means of reversing hypotension and/or substituting for disordered renal function.

There is no clinical experience with the use of MICARDIS tablets in pregnant women. No teratogenic effects were observed when telmisartan was administered to pregnant rats at oral doses of up to 50 mg/kg/day and to pregnant rabbits at oral doses up to 45 mg/kg/day. In rabbits, embryolethality associated with maternal toxicity (reduced body weight gain and food consumption) was observed at 45 mg/kg/day [about 12 times the maximum recommended human dose (MRHD) of 80 mg on a mg/m^2 basis]. In rats, maternally toxic (reduction in body weight gain and food consumption) telmisartan doses of 15 mg/kg/day (about 1.9 times the MRHD on a mg/m^2 basis), administered during late gestation and lactation, were observed to produce adverse effects in neonates, including reduced viability, low birth weight, delayed maturation, and decreased weight gain. Telmisartan has been shown to be present in rat fetuses during late gestation and in rat milk. The no observed effect doses for developmental toxicity in rats and rabbits, 5 and 15 mg/kg/day, respectively, are about 0.64 and 3.7 times, on a mg/m^2 basis, the maximum recommended human dose of telmisartan (80 mg/day).

Hypotension in Volume-Depleted Patients

In patients with an activated renin-angiotensin system, such as volume- and/or salt-depleted patients (e.g., those being treated with high doses of diuretics), symptomatic hypotension may occur after initiation of therapy with MICARDIS tablets. This condition should be corrected prior to administration of MICARDIS tablets, or treatment should start under close medical supervision with a reduced dose.

If hypotension does occur, the patient should be placed in the supine position, and if necessary, given an intravenous infusion of normal saline. A transient hypotensive response is not a contraindication to further treatment, which usually can be continued without difficulty once the blood pressure has stabilized.

PRECAUTIONS

General

Impaired Hepatic Function: As the majority of telmisartan is eliminated by biliary excretion, patients with biliary obstructive disorders or hepatic insufficiency can be expected to have reduced clearance. MICARDIS (telmisartan) tablets should be used with caution in these patients.

Impaired Renal Function: As a consequence of inhibiting the renin-angiotensin-aldosterone system, changes in renal function may be anticipated in susceptible individuals. In patients whose renal function may depend on the activity of the renin-angiotensin-aldosterone system (e.g., patients with severe congestive heart failure), treatment with angiotensin-converting enzyme inhibitors and angiotensin receptor antagonists has been associated with oliguria and/or progressive azotemia and (rarely) with acute renal failure and/or death. Similar results may be anticipated in patients treated with MICARDIS® tablets.

In studies of ACE inhibitors in patients with unilateral or bilateral renal artery stenosis, increases in serum creatinine or blood urea nitrogen were observed. There has been no long term use of MICARDIS tablets in patients with unilateral or bilateral renal artery stenosis but an effect similar to that seen with ACE inhibitors should be anticipated.

Information for Patients

Pregnancy: Female patients of childbearing age should be told about the consequences of second- and third-trimester exposure to drugs that act on the renin-angiotensin system, and they should also be told that these consequences do not appear to have resulted from intrauterine drug exposure that has been limited to the first trimester. These patients should be asked to report pregnancies to their physicians as soon as possible.

Drug Interactions

Digoxin: When telmisartan was coadministered with digoxin, median increases in digoxin peak plasma concentration (49%) and in trough concentration (20%) were observed. It is, therefore, recommended that digoxin levels be monitored when initiating, adjusting, and discontinuing telmisartan to avoid possible over- or under-digitalization.

Warfarin: Telmisartan administered for 10 days slightly decreased the mean warfarin trough plasma concentration; this decrease did not result in a change in International Normalized Ratio (INR).

Other Drugs: Coadministration of telmisartan did not result in a clinically significant interaction with acetaminophen, amlodipine, glibenclamide, simvastatin, hydrochlorothiazide or ibuprofen. Telmisartan is not metabolized by the cytochrome P450 system and had no effects *in vitro* on cytochrome P450 enzymes, except for some inhibition of CYP2C19. Telmisartan is not expected to interact with drugs that inhibit cytochrome P450 enzymes; it is also not expected to interact with drugs metabolized by cytochrome P450 enzymes, except for possible inhibition of the metabolism of drugs metabolized by CYP2C19.

Carcinogenesis, Mutagenesis, Impairment of Fertility

There was no evidence of carcinogenicity when telmisartan was administered in the diet to mice and rats for up to 2 years. The highest doses administered to mice (1000 mg/kg/day) and rats (100 mg/kg/day) are, on a mg/m^2 basis, about 59 and 13 times respectively, the maximum recommended human dose (MRHD) of telmisartan. These same doses have been shown to provide average systemic exposures to telmisartan >100 times and >25 times, respectively, the systemic exposure in humans receiving the MRHD (80 mg/day).

Genotoxicity assays did not reveal any telmisartan-related effects at either the gene or chromosome level. These assays included bacterial mutagenicity tests with Salmonella and *E coli* (Ames), a gene mutation test with Chinese hamster V79 cells, a cytogenetic test with human lymphocytes, and a mouse micronucleus test.

No drug-related effects on the reproductive performance of male and female rats were noted at 100 mg/kg/day (the highest dose administered), about 13 times, on a mg/m^2 basis, the MRHD of telmisartan. This dose in the rat resulted in an average systemic exposure (telmisartan AUC is determined on day 6 of pregnancy) at least 50 times the average systemic exposure in humans at the MRHD (80 mg/day).

Pregnancy

Pregnancy Categories C (first trimester) and D (second and third trimesters). See WARNINGS: Fetal/Neonatal Morbidity and Mortality.

Nursing Mothers

It is not known whether telmisartan is excreted in human milk, but telmisartan was shown to be present in the milk of lactating rats. Because of the potential for adverse effects on the nursing infant, a decision should be made whether to discontinue nursing or discontinue the drug, taking into account the importance of the drug to the mother.

Pediatric Use

Safety and effectiveness in pediatric patients have not been established.

Geriatric Use

Of the total number of patients receiving MICARDIS in clinical studies, 551 (18.6%) were 65 to 74 years of age and 130 (4.4%) were 75 years or older. No overall differences in effectiveness and safety were observed in these patients compared to younger patients and other reported clinical experience has not identified differences in responses between the elderly and younger patients, but greater sensitivity of some older individuals cannot be ruled out.

ADVERSE REACTIONS

MICARDIS (telmisartan) has been evaluated for safety in more than 3700 patients, including 1900 treated for over six months and more than 1300 for over one year. Adverse experiences have generally been mild and transient in nature and have only infrequently required discontinuation of therapy.

In placebo-controlled trials involving 1041 patients treated with various doses of telmisartan (20-160mg) monotherapy for up to 12 weeks, an overall incidence of adverse events similar to that of placebo was observed.

Adverse events occurring at an incidence of 1% or more in patients treated with telmisartan and at a greater rate than in patients treated with placebo, irrespective of their causal association, are presented in the following table.

	Telmisartan n = 1455 %	Placebo n = 380 %
Upper respiratory tract infection	7	6
Back pain	3	1
Sinusitis	3	2
Diarrhea	3	2
Pharyngitis	1	0

In addition to the adverse events in the table, the following events occurred at a rate of 1% but were at least as frequent in the placebo group: influenza-like symptoms, dyspepsia, myalgia, urinary tract infection, abdominal pain, headache, dizziness, pain, fatigue, coughing, hypertension, chest pain, nausea and peripheral edema. Discontinuation of therapy due to adverse events was required in 2.8% of 1455 patients treated with MICARDIS tablets and 6.1% of 380 placebo patients in placebo-controlled clinical trials.

The incidence of adverse events was not dose-related and did not correlate with gender, age, or race of patients.

The incidence of cough occurring with telmisartan in six placebo-controlled trials was identical to that noted for placebo-treated patients (1.6%).

In addition to those listed above, adverse events that occurred in more than 0.3% of 3500 patients treated with MICARDIS monotherapy in controlled or open trials are listed below. It cannot be determined whether these events were causally related to MICARDIS tablets:

Autonomic Nervous System: impotence, increased sweating, flushing; *Body as a Whole:* allergy, fever, leg pain, malaise; *Cardiovascular:* palpitation, dependent edema, angina pectoris, tachycardia, leg edema, abnormal ECG; *CNS:* insomnia, somnolence, migraine, vertigo, paresthesia, involuntary muscle contractions, hypoaesthesia; *Gastrointestinal:* flatulence, constipation, gastritis, vomiting, dry mouth, hemorrhoids, gastroenteritis, enteritis, gastroesophageal reflux, toothache, non-specific gastrointestinal disorders; *Metabolic:* gout, hypercholesterolemia, diabetes mellitus; *Musculoskeletal:* arthritis, arthralgia, leg cramps; *Psychiatric:* anxiety, depression, nervousness; *Resistance Mechanism:* infection, fungal infection, abscess, otitis media; *Respiratory:* asthma, bronchitis, rhinitis, dyspnea, epistaxis; *Skin:* dermatitis, rash, eczema, pruritus; *Urinary:* micturition frequency, cystitis; *Vascular:* cerebrovascular disorder; and *Special Senses:* abnormal vision, conjunctivitis, tinnitus, earache.

During initial clinical studies, a single case of angioedema was reported (among a total of 3781 patients treated).

Clinical Laboratory Findings

In placebo-controlled clinical trials, clinically relevant changes in standard laboratory test parameters were rarely associated with administration of MICARDIS tablets.

Hemoglobin: A greater than 2 g/dL decrease in hemoglobin was observed in 0.8% telmisartan patients compared with 0.3% placebo patients. No patients discontinued therapy due to anemia.

Creatinine: A 0.5 mg/dL rise or greater in creatinine was observed in 0.4% telmisartan patients compared with 0.3% placebo patients. One telmisartan-treated patient discontinued therapy due to increases in creatinine and blood urea nitrogen.

Liver Enzymes: Occasional elevations of liver chemistries occurred in patients treated with telmisartan; all marked elevations occurred at a higher frequency with placebo. No telmisartan-treated patients discontinued therapy due to abnormal hepatic function.

Post-Marketing Experience

The following adverse reactions have been identified during post-approval use of MICARDIS tablets. Because these reactions are reported voluntarily from a population of uncertain size, it is not always possible to reliably estimate their frequency or establish a causal relationship to drug exposure. Decisions to include these reactions in labeling are typically based on one or more of the following factors: (1) seriousness of the reaction, (2) frequency of reporting, or (3) strength of causal connection to MICARDIS tablets. The most frequently spontaneously reported events include: headache, dizziness, asthenia, coughing, nausea, fatigue, weakness, edema, face edema, lower limb edema, angioneurotic edema, urticaria, hypersensitivity, sweating increased, erythema, chest pain, atrial fibrillation, congestive heart failure, myocardial infarction, blood pressure increased, hypertension aggravated, hypotension (including postural hypotension), hyperkalemia, syncope, dyspepsia, diarrhea, pain, urinary tract infection, erectile dysfunction, back pain, abdominal pain, muscle cramps (including leg cramps), and myalgia.

Rare cases of rhabdomyolysis have been reported in patients receiving angiotensin II receptor blockers, including MICARDIS.

OVERDOSAGE

Limited data are available with regard to overdosage in humans. The most likely manifestation of overdosage with MICARDIS (telmisartan) tablets would be hypotension, dizziness and tachycardia; bradycardia could occur from parasympathetic (vagal) stimulation. If symptomatic hypotension should occur, supportive treatment should be instituted. Telmisartan is not removed by hemodialysis.

DOSAGE AND ADMINISTRATION

Dosage must be individualized. The usual starting dose of MICARDIS (telmisartan) tablets is 40 mg once a day. Blood pressure response is dose related over the range of 20-80 mg (see CLINICAL PHARMACOLOGY, Clinical Trials).

Special Populations: Patients with depletion of intravascular volume should have the condition corrected or MICARDIS tablets should be initiated under close medical supervision (see WARNINGS, Hypotension in Volume-Depleted Patients). Patients with biliary obstructive disorders or hepatic insufficiency should have treatment started under close medical supervision (see PRECAUTIONS, General, *Impaired Hepatic Function*, and *Impaired Renal Function*).

Most of the antihypertensive effect is apparent within two weeks and maximal reduction is generally attained after four weeks. When additional blood pressure reduction beyond that achieved with 80 mg MICARDIS is required, a diuretic may be added.
No initial dosing adjustment is necessary for elderly patients or patients with mild-to-moderate renal impairment. Patients on dialysis may develop orthostatic hypotension; their blood pressure should be closely monitored.
MICARDIS tablets may be administered with other antihypertensive agents.
MICARDIS tablets may be administered with or without food.

HOW SUPPLIED

MICARDIS (telmisartan) is available as white or off-white, uncoated tablets containing telmisartan 20 mg, 40 mg or 80 mg. Tablets are marked with the BOEHRINGER INGELHEIM logo on one side, and on the other side, with either 50H, 51H or 52H for the 20 mg, 40 mg, and 80 mg strengths respectively. Tablets are provided as follows:
MICARDIS (telmisartan) tablets 20 mg are round and individually blister-sealed in cartons of 28 tablets as 4 × 7 cards (NDC 0597-0039-28).
MICARDIS (telmisartan) tablets 40 mg are oblong shaped and individually blister-sealed in cartons of 28 tablets as 4 × 7 cards (NDC 0597-0040-28).
MICARDIS (telmisartan) tablets 80 mg are oblong shaped and individually blister-sealed in cartons of 28 tablets as 4 × 7 cards (NDC 0597-0041-28).

Storage

Store at 25°C (77°F); excursions permitted to 15-30°C (59-86°F) [see USP Controlled Room Temperature]. Tablets should not be removed from blisters until immediately before administration.

Rx only

Manufactured by: Boehringer Ingelheim Pharma GmbH & Co. KG Ingelheim, Germany

Licensed from: Boehringer Ingelheim International GmbH, Ingelheim, Germany

Marketed by:

Boehringer Ingelheim Pharmaceuticals, Inc., Ridgefield, CT 06877 USA

and

Abbott Laboratories, North Chicago, IL 60064 USA

Revised 11/5/03 or Revised 11/5/03
340138/US/2 553206/US/8

Shown in Product Identification Guide, page 309

MICARDIS® HCT ℞

(telmisartan and hydrochlorothiazide)
Tablets, 40 mg/12.5 mg
80 mg/12.5 mg and 80 mg/25 mg

Prescribing Information

USE IN PREGNANCY
When used in pregnancy during the second and third trimesters, drugs that act directly on the renin-angiotensin system can cause injury and even death to the developing fetus. When pregnancy is detected, MICARDIS® HCT (telmisartan/hydrochlorothiazide) tablets should be discontinued as soon as possible (see WARNINGS, Fetal/Neonatal Morbidity and Mortality).

DESCRIPTION

MICARDIS® HCT (telmisartan/hydrochlorothiazide) is a combination of telmisartan, an orally active angiotensin II antagonist acting on the AT_1 receptor subtype, and hydrochlorothiazide, a diuretic.
Telmisartan, a nonpeptide molecule, is chemically described as 4′-[(1,4′-dimethyl-2′-propyl[2,6′-bi-1H-benzimidazol]-1′-yl)methyl]-[1,1′-biphenyl]-2-carboxylic acid. Its empirical formula is $C_{33}H_{30}N_4O_2$, its molecular weight is 514.63, and its structural formula is:

Telmisartan is a white to slightly yellowish solid. It is practically insoluble in water and in the pH range of 3 to 9, sparingly soluble in strong acid (except insoluble in hydrochloric acid), and soluble in strong base.
Hydrochlorothiazide is a white, or practically white, practically odorless, crystalline powder with a molecular weight of 297.74. It is slightly soluble in water, and freely soluble in sodium hydroxide solution. Hydrochlorothiazide is chemically described as 6-chloro-3,4-dihydro-2*H*-1,2,4-benzothiadiazine-7-sulfonamide 1,1-dioxide. Its empirical formula is $C_7H_8ClN_3O_4S_2$, and its structural formula is:

MICARDIS HCT tablets are formulated for oral administration in three combinations of 40 mg/12.5 mg, 80 mg/12.5 mg, and 80 mg/25 mg telmisartan and hydrochlorothiazide, respectively. The tablets contain the following inactive ingredients: sodium hydroxide, meglumine, povidone, sorbitol, magnesium stearate, lactose monohydrate, microcrystalline cellulose, maize starch, sodium starch glycolate. As coloring agents, the 40 mg/12.5 mg and 80 mg/12.5 mg tablets contain iron oxide red, and the 80 mg/25 mg tablets contain iron oxide yellow. MICARDIS HCT tablets are hygroscopic and require protection from moisture.

CLINICAL PHARMACOLOGY

Mechanism of Action

Angiotensin II is formed from angiotensin I in a reaction catalyzed by angiotensin-converting enzyme (ACE, kininase II). Angiotensin II is the principal pressor agent of the renin-angiotensin system, with effects that include vasoconstriction, stimulation of synthesis and release of aldosterone, cardiac stimulation, and renal reabsorption of sodium. Telmisartan blocks the vasoconstrictor and aldosterone-secreting effects of angiotensin II by selectively blocking the binding of angiotensin II to the AT_1 receptor in many tissues, such as vascular smooth muscle and the adrenal gland. Its action is therefore independent of the pathways for angiotensin II synthesis.
There is also an AT_2 receptor found in many tissues, but AT_2 is not known to be associated with cardiovascular homeostasis. Telmisartan has much greater affinity (>3,000 fold) for the AT_1 receptor than for the AT_2 receptor.
Blockade of the renin-angiotensin system with ACE inhibitors, which inhibit the biosynthesis of angiotensin II from angiotensin I, is widely used in the treatment of hypertension. ACE inhibitors also inhibit the degradation of bradykinin, a reaction also catalyzed by ACE. Because telmisartan does not inhibit ACE (kininase II), it does not affect the response to bradykinin. Whether this difference has clinical relevance is not yet known. Telmisartan does not bind to or block other hormone receptors or ion channels known to be important in cardiovascular regulation.
Blockade of the angiotensin II receptor inhibits the negative regulatory feedback of angiotensin II on renin secretion, but the resulting increased plasma renin activity and angiotensin II circulating levels do not overcome the effect of telmisartan on blood pressure.
Hydrochlorothiazide is a thiazide diuretic. Thiazides affect the renal tubular mechanisms of electrolyte reabsorption, directly increasing excretion of sodium salt and chloride in approximately equivalent amounts. Indirectly, the diuretic action of hydrochlorothiazide reduces plasma volume, with consequent increases in plasma renin activity, increases in aldosterone secretion, increases in urinary potassium loss, and decreases in serum potassium. The renin-aldosterone link is mediated by angiotensin II, so coadministration of an angiotensin II receptor antagonist tends to reverse the potassium loss associated with these diuretics.
The mechanism of the antihypertensive effect of thiazides is not fully understood.

Pharmacokinetics

General

Telmisartan:
Following oral administration, peak concentrations (C_{max}) of telmisartan are reached in 0.5-1 hour after dosing. Food slightly reduces the bioavailability of telmisartan, with a reduction in the area under the plasma concentration-time curve (AUC) of about 6% with the 40 mg tablet and about 20% after a 160 mg dose. The absolute bioavailability of telmisartan is dose dependent. At 40 and 160 mg the bioavailability was 42% and 58%, respectively. The pharmacokinetics of orally administered telmisartan are nonlinear over the dose range 20-160 mg, with greater than proportional increases of plasma concentrations (C_{max} and AUC) with increasing doses. Telmisartan shows bi-exponential decay kinetics with a terminal elimination half-life of approximately 24 hours. Trough plasma concentrations of telmisartan with once daily dosing are about 10-25% of peak plasma concentrations. Telmisartan has an accumulation index in plasma of 1.5 to 2.0 upon repeated once daily dosing.
Hydrochlorothiazide:
When plasma levels have been followed for at least 24 hours, the plasma half-life has been observed to vary between 5.6 and 14.8 hours.

Metabolism and Elimination

Telmisartan:
Following either intravenous or oral administration of ^{14}C-labeled telmisartan, most of the administered dose (>97%) was eliminated unchanged in feces via biliary excretion; only minute amounts were found in the urine (0.91% and 0.49% of total radioactivity, respectively).
Telmisartan is metabolized by conjugation to form a pharmacologically inactive acylglucuronide; the glucuronide of the parent compound is the only metabolite that has been identified in human plasma and urine. After a single dose, the glucuronide represents approximately 11% of the measured radioactivity in plasma. The cytochrome P450 isoenzymes are not involved in the metabolism of telmisartan.
Total plasma clearance of telmisartan is >800 mL/min. Terminal half-life and total clearance appear to be independent of dose.
Hydrochlorothiazide:
Hydrochlorothiazide is not metabolized but is eliminated rapidly by the kidney. At least 61% of the oral dose is eliminated as unchanged drug within 24 hours.

Distribution

Telmisartan:
Telmisartan is highly bound to plasma proteins (>99.5%), mainly albumin and α_1-acid glycoprotein. Plasma protein binding is constant over the concentration range achieved with recommended doses. The volume of distribution for telmisartan is approximately 500 liters, indicating additional tissue binding.
Hydrochlorothiazide:
Hydrochlorothiazide crosses the placental but not the blood-brain barrier and is excreted in breast milk.

Special Populations

Pediatric: Telmisartan pharmacokinetics have not been investigated in patients <18 years of age.
Geriatric: The pharmacokinetics of telmisartan do not differ between the elderly and those younger than 65 years (see DOSAGE AND ADMINISTRATION).
Gender: Plasma concentrations of telmisartan are generally 2-3 times higher in females than in males. In clinical trials, however, no significant increases in blood pressure response or in the incidence of orthostatic hypotension were found in women. No dosage adjustment is necessary.
Renal Insufficiency: Renal excretion does not contribute to the clearance of telmisartan. Based on modest experience in patients with mild-to-moderate renal impairment (creatinine clearance of 30-80 mL/min, mean clearance approximately 50 mL/min), no dosage adjustment is necessary in patients with decreased renal function. Telmisartan is not removed from blood by hemofiltration (see PRECAUTIONS, and DOSAGE AND ADMINISTRATION).
Hepatic Insufficiency: In patients with hepatic insufficiency, plasma concentrations of telmisartan are increased, and absolute bioavailability approaches 100% (see PRECAUTIONS, and DOSAGE AND ADMINISTRATION).

Drug Interactions: See PRECAUTIONS, Drug Interactions.

Pharmacodynamics

Telmisartan:
In normal volunteers, a dose of telmisartan 80 mg inhibited the pressor response to an intravenous infusion of angiotensin II by about 90% at peak plasma concentrations with approximately 40% inhibition persisting for 24 hours.
Plasma concentration of angiotensin II and plasma renin activity (PRA) increased in a dose-dependent manner after single administration of telmisartan to healthy subjects and repeated administration to hypertensive patients. The once-daily administration of up to 80 mg telmisartan to healthy subjects did not influence plasma aldosterone concentrations. In multiple dose studies with hypertensive patients, there were no clinically significant changes in electrolytes (serum potassium or sodium), or in metabolic function (including serum levels of cholesterol, triglycerides, HDL, LDL, glucose, or uric acid).
In 30 hypertensive patients with normal renal function treated for 8 weeks with telmisartan 80 mg or telmisartan 80 mg in combination with hydrochlorothiazide 12.5 mg, there were no clinically significant changes from baseline in renal blood flow, glomerular filtration rate, filtration fraction, renovascular resistance, or creatinine clearance.
Hydrochlorothiazide:
After oral administration of hydrochlorothiazide, diuresis begins within 2 hours, peaks in about 4 hours and lasts about 6 to 12 hours.

Clinical Trials

Telmisartan:
The antihypertensive effects of telmisartan have been demonstrated in six principal placebo-controlled clinical trials, studying a range of 20-160 mg; one of these examined the antihypertensive effects of telmisartan and hydrochlorothiazide in combination. The studies involved a total of 1773 patients with mild to moderate hypertension (diastolic blood pressure of 95-114 mmHg), 1031 of whom were treated with telmisartan. Following once daily administration of telmisartan, the magnitude of blood pressure reduction from baseline after placebo subtraction was approximately (SBP/DBP) 6-8/6 mmHg for 20 mg, 9-13/6-8 mmHg for 40 mg, and 12-13/7-8 mmHg for 80 mg. Larger doses (up to 160 mg) did not appear to cause a further decrease in blood pressure.
Upon initiation of antihypertensive treatment with telmisartan, blood pressure was reduced after the first dose, with a maximal reduction by about 4 weeks. With cessation of treatment with telmisartan tablets, blood pressure gradually returned to baseline values over a period of several days to one week. During long-term studies (without placebo control) the effect of telmisartan appeared to be maintained for up to at least one year. The antihypertensive effect of telmisartan is not influenced by patient age, gender, weight or body mass index. Blood pressure response in black patients (usually a low-renin population) is noticeably less than that in Caucasian patients. This has been true for most, but not all, angiotensin II antagonists and ACE inhibitors.

Continued on next page

Micardis HCT—Cont.

The onset of antihypertensive activity occurs within 3 hours after administration of a single oral dose. At doses of 20, 40, and 80 mg, the antihypertensive effect of once daily administration of telmisartan is maintained for the full 24-hour dose interval. With automated ambulatory blood pressure monitoring and conventional blood pressure measurements, the 24-hour trough-to-peak ratio for 40-80 mg doses of telmisartan was 70-100% for both systolic and diastolic blood pressure. The incidence of symptomatic orthostasis after the first dose in all controlled trials was low (0.04%).
There were no changes in the heart rate of patients treated with telmisartan in controlled trials.
Telmisartan & Hydrochlorothiazide:
In controlled clinical trials with over 2500 patients, 1017 patients were exposed to telmisartan (20 to 160 mg) and concomitant hydrochlorothiazide (6.25 to 25 mg). These trials included one factorial trial with combinations of telmisartan (20, 40, 80, 160 mg, or placebo) and hydrochlorothiazide (6.25, 12.5, 25 mg and placebo). Four other studies of at least six months duration allowed add-on of hydrochlorothiazide for patients who either were not adequately controlled on the randomized monotherapy dose or had not achieved adequate response after completing the up-titration of telmisartan.
The combination of telmisartan and hydrochlorothiazide resulted in additive placebo-adjusted decreases in systolic and diastolic blood pressure at trough of 16-21/9-11 mmHg for doses between 40/12.5 mg and 80/25 mg, compared to 9-13/7-8 mmHg for telmisartan 40 mg to 80 mg and 4/4 mmHg for hydrochlorothiazide 12.5 mg alone.
In active controlled studies, the addition of 12.5 mg hydrochlorothiazide to titrated doses of telmisartan in patients who did not achieve or maintain adequate response with telmisartan monotherapy further reduced systolic and diastolic blood pressure.
The antihypertensive effect was independent of age or gender.
There was essentially no change in heart rate in patients treated with the combination of telmisartan and hydrochlorothiazide in the placebo controlled trial.

INDICATIONS AND USAGE

MICARDIS® HCT (telmisartan/hydrochlorothiazide) is indicated for the treatment of hypertension. This fixed dose combination is not indicated for initial therapy (see DOSAGE AND ADMINISTRATION).

CONTRAINDICATIONS

MICARDIS HCT (telmisartan/hydrochlorothiazide) is contraindicated in patients who are hypersensitive to any component of this product.
Because of the hydrochlorothiazide component, this product is contraindicated in patients with anuria or hypersensitivity to other sulfonamide-derived drugs.

WARNINGS

Fetal/Neonatal Morbidity and Mortality

Drugs that act directly on the renin-angiotensin system can cause fetal and neonatal morbidity and death when administered to pregnant women. Several dozen cases have been reported in the world literature in patients who were taking anigotensin converting enzyme inhibitors. When pregnancy is detected, MICARDIS HCT (telmisartan/hydrochlorothiazide) tablets should be discontinued as soon as possible.
The use of drugs that act directly on the renin-angiotensin system during the second and third trimesters of pregnancy has been associated with fetal and neonatal injury, including hypotension, neonatal skull hypoplasia, anuria, reversible or irreversible renal failure, and death. Oligohydramnios has also been reported, presumably resulting from decreased fetal renal function; oligohydramnios in this setting has been associated with fetal limb contractures, craniofacial deformation, and hypoplastic lung development. Prematurity, intrauterine growth retardation, and patent ductus arteriosus have also been reported, although it is not clear whether these occurrences were due to exposure to the drug.
These adverse effects do not appear to have resulted from intrauterine drug exposure that has been limited to the first trimester. Mothers whose embryos and fetuses are exposed to an angiotensin II receptor antagonist only during the first trimester should be so informed. Nonetheless, when patients become pregnant, physicians should have the patient discontinue the use of MICARDIS HCT tablets as soon as possible.
Rarely (probably less often than once in every thousand pregnancies), no alternative to an angiotensin II receptor antagonist will be found. In these rare cases, the mothers should be apprised of the potential hazards to their fetuses, and serial ultrasound examinations should be performed to assess the intra-amniotic environment.
If oligohydramnios is observed, MICARDIS HCT tablets should be discontinued unless they are considered lifesaving for the mother. Contraction stress testing (CST), a non-stress test (NST), or biophysical profiling (BPP) may be appropriate, depending upon the week of pregnancy. Patients and physicians should be aware, however, that oligohydramnios may not appear until after the fetus has sustained irreversible injury.
Infants with histories of *in utero* exposure to an angiotensin II receptor antagonist should be closely observed for hypotension, oliguria, and hyperkalemia. If oliguria occurs, attention should be directed toward support of blood pressure and renal perfusion. Exchange transfusion or dialysis may be required as a means of reversing hypotension and/or substituting for disordered renal function.
A developmental toxicity study was performed in rats with telmisartan/hydrochlorothiazide doses of 3.2/1.0, 15/4.7, 50/15.6, and 0/15.6 mg/kg/day. Although the two higher dose combinations appeared to be more toxic (significant decrease in body weight gain) to the dams than either drug alone, there did not appear to be an increase in toxicity to the developing embryos.
No teratogenic effects were observed when telmisartan was administered to pregnant rats at oral doses of up to 50 mg/kg/day and to pregnant rabbits at oral doses up to 45 mg/kg/day. In rabbits, embryolethality associated with maternal toxicity (reduced body weight gain and food consumption) was observed at 45 mg/kg/day [about 12 times the maximum recommended human dose (MRHD) of 80 mg on a mg/m^2 basis]. In rats, maternally toxic (reduction in body weight gain and food consumption) telmisartan doses of 15 mg/kg/day (about 1.9 times the MRHD on a mg/m^2 basis), administered during late gestation and lactation, were observed to produce adverse effects in neonates, including reduced viability, low birth weight, delayed maturation, and decreased weight gain. Telmisartan has been shown to be present in rat fetuses during late gestation and in rat milk. The no observed effect doses for developmental toxicity in rats and rabbits, 5 and 15 mg/kg/day, respectively, are about 0.64 and 3.7 times, on a mg/m^2 basis, the maximum recommended human dose of telmisartan (80 mg/day).
Studies in which hydrochlorothiazide was administered to pregnant mice and rats during their respective periods of major organogenesis at doses up to 3000 and 1000 mg/kg/day, respectively, provided no evidence of harm to the fetus. Thiazides cross the placental barrier and appear in cord blood. There is a risk of fetal or neonatal jaundice, thrombocytopenia, and possibly other adverse reactions that have occurred in adults.

Hypotension in Volume-Depleted Patients

Initiation of antihypertensive therapy in patients whose renin-angiotensin system are activated such as patients who are intravascular volume- or sodium-depleted, e.g., in patients treated vigorously with diuretics, should only be approached cautiously. These conditions should be corrected prior to administration of MICARDIS HCT. Treatment should be started under close medical supervision (see DOSAGE AND ADMINISTRATION). If hypotension occurs, the patients should be placed in the supine position and, if necessary, given an intravenous infusion of normal saline. A transient hypotensive response is not a contraindication to further treatment which usually can be continued without difficulty once the blood pressure has stabilized.

Hydrochlorothiazide

Hepatic Impairment: Thiazide diuretics should be used with caution in patients with impaired hepatic function or progressive liver disease, since minor alterations of fluid and electrolyte balance may precipitate hepatic coma.
Hypersensitivity Reaction: Hypersensitivity reactions to hydrochlorothiazide may occur in patients with or without a history of allergy or bronchial asthma, but are more likely in patients with such a history.
Systemic Lupus Erythematosus: Thiazide diuretics have been reported to cause exacerbation or activation of systemic lupus erythematosis.
Lithium Interaction: Lithium generally should not be given with thiazides (see PRECAUTIONS, Drug Interactions, Hydrochlorothiazide, *Lithium*).

PRECAUTIONS

Serum Electrolytes

Telmisartan & Hydrochlorothiazide:
In controlled trials using the telmisartan/hydrochlorothiazide combination treatment, no patient administered 40/12.5 mg, 80/12.5 mg or 80/25 mg had a decrease in potassium ≥1.4 mEq/L, and no patient experienced hyperkalemia. No discontinuations due to hypokalemia occurred during treatment with the telmisartan/hydrochlorothiazide combination. The absence of significant changes in serum potassium levels may be due to the opposing mechanisms of action of telmisartan and hydrochlorothiazide on potassium excretion on the kidney.
Hydrochlorothiazide:
Periodic determinations of serum electrolytes to detect possible electrolyte imbalance should be performed at appropriate intervals. All patients receiving thiazide therapy should be observed for clinical signs of fluid or electrolyte imbalance: hyponatremia, hypochloremic alkalosis, and hypokalemia. Serum and urine electrolyte determinations are particularly important when the patient experiences excessive vomiting or receives parenteral fluids. Warning signs or symptoms of fluid and electrolyte imbalance, irrespective of cause, include dryness of mouth, thirst, weakness, lethargy, drowsiness, restlessness, confusion, seizures, muscle pains or cramps, muscular fatigue, hypotension, oliguria, tachycardia, and gastrointestinal disturbances such as nausea and vomiting.
Hypokalemia may develop, especially with brisk diuresis, when severe cirrhosis is present, or after prolonged therapy. Interference with adequate oral electrolyte intake will also contribute to hypokalemia. Hypokalemia may cause cardiac arrhythmia and may also sensitize or exaggerate the response of the heart to the toxic effects of digitalis (e.g., increased ventricular irritability).
Although any chloride deficit is generally mild and usually does not require specific treatment except under extraordinary circumstances (as in liver disease or renal disease), chloride replacement may be required in the treatment of metabolic alkalosis.
Dilutional hyponatremia may occur in edematous patients in hot weather; appropriate therapy is water restriction, rather than administration of salt except in rare instances when the hyponatremia is life-threatening. In actual salt depletion, appropriate replacement is the therapy of choice.
Hyperuricemia may occur or frank gout may be precipitated in certain patients receiving thiazide therapy.
In diabetic patients dosage adjustment of insulin or oral hypoglycemic agents may be required. Hyperglycemia may occur with thiazide diuretics. Thus latent diabetes mellitus may become manifest during thiazide therapy.
The antihypertensive effects of the drug may be enhanced in the post sympathectomy patient.
If progressive renal impairment becomes evident consider withholding or discontinuing diuretic therapy.
Thiazides have been shown to increase the urinary excretion of magnesium; this may result in hypomagnesemia.
Thiazides may decrease urinary calcium excretion. Thiazides may cause intermittent and slight elevation of serum calcium in the absence of known disorders of calcium metabolism. Marked hypercalcemia may be evidence of hidden hyperparathyroidism. Thiazides should be discontinued before carrying out tests for parathyroid function.
Increases in cholesterol and triglyceride levels may be associated with thiazide diuretic therapy.

Impaired Hepatic Function

Telmisartan:
As the majority of telmisartan is eliminated by biliary excretion, patients with biliary obstructive disorders or hepatic insufficiency can be expected to have reduced clearance. MICARDIS® HCT tablets should therefore be used with caution in these patients.

Impaired Renal Function

Telmisartan:
As a consequence of inhibiting the renin-angiotensin-aldosterone system, changes in renal function may be anticipated in susceptible individuals. In patients whose renal function may depend on the activity of the renin-angiotensin-aldosterone system (e.g., patients with severe congestive heart failure), treatment with angiotensin-converting enzyme inhibitors and angiotensin receptor antagonists has been associated with oliguria and/or progressive azotemia and (rarely) with acute renal failure and/or death. Similar results may be anticipated in patients treated with telmisartan.
In studies of ACE inhibitors in patients with unilateral or bilateral renal artery stenosis, increases in serum creatinine or blood urea nitrogen were observed. There has been no long-term use of telmisartan in patients with unilateral or bilateral renal artery stenosis but an effect similar to that seen with ACE inhibitors should be anticipated.
Hydrochlorothiazide:
Thiazides should be used with caution in severe renal disease. In patients with renal disease, thiazides may precipitate azotemia. Cumulative effects of the drug may develop in patients with impaired renal function.

Information for Patients

Pregnancy: Female patients of childbearing age should be told about the consequences of second- and third-trimester exposure to drugs that act on the renin-angiotensin system, and they should also be told that these consequences do not appear to have resulted from intrauterine drug exposure that has been limited to the first trimester. These patients should be asked to report pregnancies to their physicians as soon as possible.
Symptomatic Hypotension: A patient receiving MICARDIS HCT should be cautioned that lightheadedness can occur, especially during the first days of therapy, and that it should be reported to the prescribing physician. The patients should be told that if syncope occurs, MICARDIS HCT should be discontinued until the physician has been consulted.
All patients should be cautioned that inadequate fluid intake, excessive perspiration, diarrhea, or vomiting can lead to an excessive fall in blood pressure, with the same consequences of lightheadedness and possible syncope.
Potassium Supplements: A patient receiving MICARDIS HCT should be told not to use potassium supplements or salt substitutes that contain potassium without consulting the prescribing physician.

Drug Interactions

Telmisartan:
Digoxin: When telmisartan was coadministered with digoxin, median increases in digoxin peak plasma concentration (49%) and in trough concentration (20%) were observed. It is, therefore, recommended that digoxin levels be monitored when initiating, adjusting, and discontinuing telmisartan to avoid possible over- or under-digitalization.
Warfarin: Telmisartan administered for 10 days slightly decreased the mean warfarin trough plasma concentration; this decrease did not result in a change in International Normalized Ratio (INR).
Other Drugs: Coadministration of telmisartan did not result in a clinically significant interaction with acetaminophen, amlodipine, glibenclamide, simvastatin, hydrochlorothiazide or ibuprofen. Telmisartan is not metabolized by the cytochrome P450 system and had no effects *in vitro* on cytochrome P450 enzymes, except for some inhibition of CYP2C19. Telmisartan is not expected to interact with

drugs that inhibit cytochrome P450 enzymes; it is also not expected to interact with drugs metabolized by cytochrome P450 enzymes, except for possible inhibition of the metabolism of drugs metabolized by CYP2C19.
Hydrochlorothiazide:
When administered concurrently, the following drugs may interact with thiazide diuretics:
Alcohol, barbiturates, or narcotics: Potentiation of orthostatic hypotension may occur.
Antidiabetic drugs (oral agents and insulin): Dosage adjustment of the antidiabetic drug may be required.
Other antihypertensive drugs: Additive effect or potentiation.
Cholestyramine and colestipol resins: Absorption of hydrochlorothiazide is impaired in the presence of anionic exchange resins. Single doses of either cholestyramine or colestipol resins bind the hydrochlorothiazide and reduce its absorption from the gastrointestinal tract by up to 85% and 43%, respectively.
Corticosteroids, ACTH: Intensified electrolyte depletion, particularly hypokalemia.
Pressor amines (e.g., norepinephrine): Possible decreased response to pressure amines but not sufficient to preclude their use.
Skeletal muscle relaxants, nondepolarizing (e.g., tubocurarine): Possible increased responsiveness to the muscle relaxant.
Lithium: Should not generally be given with diuretics. Diuretic agents reduce the renal clearance of lithium and add a high risk of lithium toxicity. Refer to the package insert for lithium preparations before use of such preparations with MICARDIS HCT.
Non-steroidal anti-inflammatory drugs: In some patients, the administration of a non-steroidal anti-inflammatory agent can reduce the diuretic, natriuretic, and antihypertensive effects of loop, potassium-sparing and thiazide diuretics. Therefore, when MICARDIS HCT and non-steroidal anti-inflammatory agents are used concomitantly, the patient should be observed closely to determine if the desired effect of the diuretic is obtained.

Carcinogenesis, Mutagenesis, Impairment of Fertility

Telmisartan & Hydrochlorothiazide:
No carcinogenicity, mutagenicity, or fertility studies have been conducted with the combination of telmisartan and hydrochlorothiazide.
Telmisartan:
There was no evidence of carcinogenicity when telmisartan was administered in the diet to mice and rats for up to 2 years. The highest doses administered to mice (1000 mg/kg/day) and rats (100 mg/kg/day) are, on a mg/m^2 basis, about 59 and 13 times, respectively, the maximum recommended human dose (MRHD) of telmisartan. These same doses have been shown to provide average systemic exposures to telmisartan >100 times and >25 times, respectively, the systemic exposure in humans receiving the MRHD (80 mg/day).
Genotoxicity assays did not reveal any telmisartan-related effects at either the gene or chromosome level. These assays included bacterial mutagenicity tests with Salmonella and *E coli* (Ames), a gene mutation test with Chinese hamster V79 cells, a cytogenetic test with human lymphocytes, and a mouse micronucleus test.
No drug-related effects on the reproductive performance of male and female rats were noted at 100 mg/kg/day (the highest dose administered), about 13 times, on a mg/m^2 basis, the MRHD of telmisartan. This dose in the rat resulted in an average systemic exposure (telmisartan AUC as determined on day 6 of pregnancy) at least 50 times the average systemic exposure in humans at the MRHD (80 mg/day).
Hydrochlorothiazide:
Two-year feeding studies in mice and rats conducted under the auspices of the National Toxicology Program (NTP) uncovered no evidence of a carcinogenic potential of hydrochlorothiazide in female mice (at doses of up to approximately 600 mg/kg/day) or in male and female rats (at doses of up to approximately 100 mg/kg/day). The NTP, however, found equivocal evidence for hepatocarcinogenicity in male mice.
Hydrochlorothiazide was not genotoxic *in vitro* in the Ames mutagenicity assay of *Salmonella typhimurium* strains TA 98, TA 100, TA 1535, TA 1537, and TA 1538 and in the Chinese Hamster Ovary (CHO) test for chromosomal aberrations, or *in vivo* in assays using mouse germinal cell chromosomes, Chinese hamster bone marrow chromosomes, and the *Drosophila* sex-linked recessive lethal trait gene. Positive test results were obtained in the *in vitro* CHO Sister Chromatid Exchange (clastogenicity) assay, in the Mouse Lymphoma Cell (mutagenicity) assay, and in the *Aspergillus nidulans* non-disjunction assay.
Hydrochlorothiazide had no adverse effects on the fertility of mice and rats of either sex in studies wherein these species were exposed, via their diet, to doses of up to 100 and 4 mg/kg, respectively, prior to mating and throughout gestation.

Pregnancy

Pregnancy Categories C (first trimester) and D (second and third trimesters) (See WARNINGS, Fetal/Neonatal Morbidity and Mortality).

Nursing Mothers

It is not known whether telmisartan is excreted in human milk, but telmisartan was shown to be present in the milk of lactating rats. Thiazides appear in human milk. Because of the potential for adverse effects on the nursing infant, a decision should be made whether to discontinue nursing or discontinue the drug, taking into account the importance of the drug to the mother.

Pediatric Use

Safety and effectiveness in pediatric patients have not been established.

Geriatric Use

In the controlled clinical trials (n=1017), approximately 20% of patients treated with telmisartan/hydrochlorothiazide were 65 years of age or older, and 5% were 75 years of age or older. No overall differences in effectiveness and safety of telmisartan/hydrochlorothiazide were observed in these patients compared to younger patients. Other reported clinical experience has not identified differences in responses between the elderly and younger patients, but greater sensitivity of some older individuals cannot be ruled out.

ADVERSE REACTIONS

MICARDIS HCT (telmisartan/hydrochlorothiazide) has been evaluated for safety in over 1700 patients, including 716 treated for over six months and 420 for over one year. In clinical trials with MICARDIS HCT, no unexpected adverse events have been observed. Adverse experiences have been limited to those that have been previously reported with telmisartan and/or hydrochlorothiazide. The overall incidence of adverse experiences reported with the combination was comparable to placebo. Most adverse experiences were mild in intensity and transient in nature and did not require discontinuation of therapy.
Adverse events occurring at an incidence of 2% or more in patients treated with telmisartan/hydrochlorothiazide and at a greater rate than in patients treated with placebo, irrespective of their causal association, are presented in Table 1.

TABLE 1 Adverse Events Occurring in ≥ 2% of Telmisartan/Hydrochlorothiazide (HCTZ) Patients*

	Telm/HCTZ (N=414) (%)	Placebo (N=74) (%)	Telm (N=209) (%)	HCTZ (N=121) (%)
Body as a whole				
Fatigue	3	1	3	3
Influenza-like symptoms	2	1	2	3
Central/peripheral nervous system				
Dizziness	5	1	4	6
Gastrointestinal system				
Diarrhea	3	0	5	2
Nausea	2	0	1	2
Respiratory system disorder				
Sinusitis	4	3	3	6
Upper respiratory tract infection	8	7	7	10

**includes all doses of telmisartan (20-160 mg), hydrochlorothiazide (6.25-25 mg), and combinations thereof*

The following adverse events were reported at a rate less than 2% in patients treated with telmisartan/hydrochlorothiazide and at a greater rate than in patients treated with placebo: back pain, dyspepsia, vomiting, tachycardia, hypokalemia, bronchitis, pharyngitis, rash, hypotension postural, abdominal pain.
Finally, the following adverse events were reported at a rate of 2% or greater in patients treated with telmisartan/hydrochlorothiazide, but were as, or more common in the placebo group: pain, headache, cough, urinary tract infection.
Adverse events occurred at approximately the same rates in men and women, older and younger patients, and black and non-black patients.
In controlled trials (n=1017), 0.3% of patients treated with MICARDIS® HCT 40/12.5 mg, 80/12.5 mg or 80/25 mg discontinued due to orthostatic hypotension, and the incidence of dizziness was 4%, 7%, and 1% respectively.

Telmisartan:

Other adverse experiences that have been reported with telmisartan, without regard to causality, are listed below:
Autonomic Nervous System: impotence, increased sweating, flushing;
Body as a Whole: allergy, fever, leg pain, malaise, chest pain;
Cardiovascular: palpitation, dependent edema, angina pectoris, leg edema, abnormal ECG, hypertension, peripheral edema;
CNS: insomnia, somnolence, migraine, vertigo, paresthesia, involuntary muscle contractions, hypoaesthesia;
Gastrointestinal: flatulence, constipation, gastritis, dry mouth, hemorrhoids, gastroenteritis, enteritis, gastroesophageal reflux, toothache, non-specific gastrointestinal disorders;
Metabolic: gout, hypercholesterolemia, diabetes mellitus;
Musculoskeletal: arthritis, arthralgia, leg cramps, myalgia;
Psychiatric: anxiety, depression, nervousness;
Resistance Mechanism: infection, fungal infection, abscess, otitis media;
Respiratory: asthma, rhinitis, dyspnea, epistaxis;
Skin: dermatitis, eczema, pruritus;
Urinary: micturition frequency, cystitis;
Vascular: cerebrovascular disorder;
Special Senses: abnormal vision, conjunctivitis, tinnitus, earache.
A single case of angioedema was reported (among a total of 3781 patients treated with telmisartan). In post-marketing experience, additional cases of angioedema and urticaria have been noted.

Hydrochlorothiazide:

Other adverse experiences that have been reported with hydrochlorothiazide, without regard to causality, are listed below:
Body as a whole: weakness;
Digestive: pancreatitis, jaundice (intrahepatic cholestatic jaundice), sialadenitis, cramping, gastric irritation;
Hematologic: aplastic anemia, agranulocytosis, leukopenia, hemolytic anemia, thrombocytopenia;
Hypersensitivity: purpura, photosensitivity, urticaria, necrotizing angiitis (vasculitis and cutaneous vasculitis), fever, respiratory distress including pneumonitis and pulmonary edema, anaphylactic reactions;
Metabolic: hyperglycemia, glycosuria, hyperuricemia;
Musculoskeletal: muscle spasm;
Nervous System/Psychiatric: restlessness;
Renal: renal failure, renal dysfunction, interstitial nephritis;
Skin: erythema multiforme including Stevens-Johnson syndrome, exfoliative dermatitis including toxic epidermal necrolysis;
Special Senses: transient blurred vision, xanthopsia.

Clinical Laboratory Findings

In controlled trials, clinically relevant changes in standard laboratory test parameters were rarely associated with administration of MICARDIS HCT tablets.
Hemoglobin and Hematocrit: Decreases in hemoglobin (≥ 2 g/dL) and hematocrit (≥ 9%) were observed in 1.2% and 0.6% of telmisartan/hydrochlorothiazide patients, respectively, in controlled trials. Changes in hemoglobin and hematocrit were not considered clinically significant and there were no discontinuations due to anemia.
Creatinine, Blood Urea Nitrogen (BUN): Increases in BUN (≥ 11.2 mg/dL) and serum creatinine (≥ 0.5 mg/dL) were observed in 2.8% and 1.4%, respectively, of patients with essential hypertension treated with MICARDIS HCT in controlled trials. No patient discontinued treatment with MICARDIS HCT due to an increase in BUN or creatinine.
Liver Function Tests: Occasional elevations of liver enzymes and/or serum bilirubin have occurred. No telmisartan/hydrochlorothiazide treated patients discontinued therapy due to abnormal hepatic function.
Serum Electrolytes: See PRECAUTIONS.

OVERDOSAGE

Telmisartan:
Limited data are available with regard to overdosage in humans. The most likely manifestations of overdosage with telmisartan would be hypotension, dizziness and tachycardia; bradycardia could occur from parasympathetic (vagal) stimulation. If symptomatic hypotension should occur, supportive treatment should be instituted. Telmisartan is not removed by hemodialysis.
Hydrochlorothiazide:
The most common signs and symptoms observed in patients are those caused by electrolyte depletion (hypokalemia, hypochloremia, hyponatremia) and dehydration resulting from excessive diuresis. If digitalis has also been administered, hypokalemia may accentuate cardiac arrhythmias. The degree to which hydrochlorothiazide is removed by hemodialysis has not been established. The oral LD_{50} of hydrochlorothiazide is greater than 10 g/kg in both mice and rats.

DOSAGE AND ADMINISTRATION

The usual starting dose of telmisartan is 40 mg once a day; blood pressure response is dose related over the range of 20-80 mg. Patients with depletion of intravascular volume should have the condition corrected or telmisartan tablets should be initiated under close medical supervision (see WARNINGS, Hypotension in Volume Depleted Patients). Patients with biliary obstructive disorders or hepatic insufficiency should have treatment started under close medical supervision (see PRECAUTIONS).
Hydrochlorothiazide is effective in doses of 12.5 mg to 50 mg once daily.
To minimize dose-independent side effects, it is usually appropriate to begin combination therapy only after a patient has failed to achieve the desired effect with monotherapy. The side effects (see WARNINGS) of telmisartan are generally rare and apparently independent of dose; those of hydrochlorothiazide are a mixture of dose-dependent phenomena (primarily hypokalemia) and dose-independent phenomena (e.g., pancreatitis), the former much more common than the latter. Therapy with any combination of telmisartan and hydrochlorothiazide will be associated with both sets of dose-independent side effects.
MICARDIS HCT tablets may be administered with other antihypertensive agents.
MICARDIS HCT tablets may be administered with or without food.

Continued on next page

Micardis HCT—Cont.

Replacement Therapy
The combination may be substituted for the titrated components.
Dose Titration by Clinical Effect
MICARDIS HCT is available as tablets containing either telmisartan 40 mg and hydrochlorothiazide 12.5 mg, or telmisartan 80 mg and hydrochlorothiazide 12.5 mg or 25 mg. A patient whose blood pressure is not adequately controlled with telmisartan monotherapy 80 mg (see above) may be switched to MICARDIS HCT, telmisartan 80 mg/hydrochlorothiazide 12.5 mg once daily, and finally titrated up to 160/25 mg, if necessary.
A patient whose blood pressure is inadequately controlled by 25 mg once daily of hydrochlorothiazide may be switched to MICARDIS HCT (telmisartan 80 mg/hydrochlorothiazide 12.5 mg or telmisartan 80 mg/hydrochlorothiazide 25 mg) once daily. The clinical response to MICARDIS HCT should be subsequently evaluated and if blood pressure remains uncontrolled after 2-4 weeks of therapy, the dose may be titrated up to 160/25 mg, if necessary. Those patients controlled by 25 mg hydrochlorothiazide but who experience hypokalemia with this regimen, may be switched to MICARDIS HCT (telmisartan 80 mg/hydrochlorothiazide 12.5 mg) once daily, reducing the dose of hydrochlorothiazide without reducing the overall expected antihypertensive response.
Patients with Renal Impairment
The usual regimens of therapy with MICARDIS HCT may be followed as long as the patient's creatinine clearance is >30 mL/min. In patients with more severe renal impairment, loop diuretics are preferred to thiazides, so MICARDIS HCT is not recommended.
Patients with Hepatic Impairment
MICARDIS HCT is not recommended for patients with severe hepatic impairment. Patients with biliary obstructive disorders or hepatic insufficiency should have treatment started under close medical supervision using the 40/12.5 mg combination (see PRECAUTIONS).

HOW SUPPLIED

MICARDIS HCT (telmisartan/hydrochlorothiazide) is available in three strengths as biconvex two-layered, oblong-shaped, uncoated tablets in three combinations of 40 mg/12.5 mg, 80 mg/12.5 mg and 80 mg/25 mg telmisartan and hydrochlorothiazide, respectively. The hydrochlorothiazide layer is red in the 40 mg/12.5 mg and 80 mg/12.5 mg tablets, and yellow in the 80 mg/25 mg tablets, and all are unmarked. The telmisartan layer for all three strengths is white, but may contain red specks in the 40 mg/12.5 mg and 80 mg/12.5 mg tablets and yellow specks in the 80 mg/25 mg tablets. The telmisartan layer is marked with the BOEHRINGER INGELHEIM logo and H4 for the 40 mg/12.5 mg dose strength, H8 for the 80 mg/12.5 mg dose strength and H9 for the 80 mg/25 mg dose strength.
Tablets are provided as follows:
MICARDIS HCT tablets 40 mg/12.5 mg are individually blister-sealed in cartons of 28 tablets as 4 × 7 cards (NDC 0597-0043-28).
MICARDIS HCT tablets 80 mg/12.5 mg are individually blister-sealed in cartons of 28 tablets as 4 × 7 cards (NDC 0597-0044-28).
MICARDIS HCT tablets 80 mg/25 mg are individually blister-sealed in cartons of 28 tablets as 4 × 7 cards (NDC 0597-0042-28).
Storage
Store at 25°C (77°F); excursions permitted to 15–30°C (59–86°F) [see USP Controlled Room Temperature]. Tablets should not be removed from blisters until immediately before administration.
Rx only
553449/US/3
Manufactured by: Boehringer Ingelheim Pharma GmbH & Co. KG, Ingelheim, Germany
Marketed by: Boehringer Ingelheim Pharmaceuticals, Inc., Ridgefield, CT, 06877 USA
and Abbott Laboratories, North Chicago, IL 60064 USA
Licensed from: Boehringer Ingelheim International GmbH, Ingelheim, Germany

Rev April 19, 2004 553449/US/6 or 553446/US/6
Shown in Product Identification Guide, page 309

MIRAPEX® ℞
[mĭ-ră-pĕks]
(pramipexole dihydrochloride)
0.125 mg, 0.25 mg, 0.5 mg, 1 mg, and 1.5 mg Tablets

DESCRIPTION

MIRAPEX® (pramipexole dihydrochloride) Tablets contain pramipexole, a dopamine agonist indicated for the treatment of the signs and symptoms of idiopathic Parkinson's disease. The chemical name of pramipexole dihydrochloride is (S)-2-amino-4,5,6,7-tetrahydro-6-(propylamino)benzothiazole dihydrochloride monohydrate. Its empirical formula is $C_{10}H_{17}N_3S \cdot 2\,HCl \cdot H_2O$, and its molecular weight is 302.27. The structural formula is:

H_2N … $\cdot$ 2 HCl $\cdot$ H_2O

Pramipexole dihydrochloride is a white to off-white powder substance. Melting occurs in the range of 296°C to 301°C, with decomposition. Pramipexole dihydrochloride is more than 20% soluble in water, about 8% in methanol, about 0.5% in ethanol, and practically insoluble in dichloromethane.
MIRAPEX (pramipexole dihydrochloride) Tablets, for oral administration, contain 0.125 mg, 0.25 mg, 0.5 mg, 1.0 mg, or 1.5 mg of pramipexole dihydrochloride monohydrate. Inactive ingredients consist of mannitol, corn starch, colloidal silicon dioxide, povidone, and magnesium stearate.

CLINICAL PHARMACOLOGY

Pramipexole is a nonergot dopamine agonist with high relative in vitro specificity and full intrinsic activity at the D_2 subfamily of dopamine receptors, binding with higher affinity to D_3 than to D_2 or D_4 receptor subtypes. The relevance of D_3 receptor binding in Parkinson's disease is unknown.
The precise mechanism of action of pramipexole as a treatment for Parkinson's disease is unknown, although it is believed to be related to its ability to stimulate dopamine receptors in the striatum. This conclusion is supported by electrophysiologic studies in animals that have demonstrated that pramipexole influences striatal neuronal firing rates via activation of dopamine receptors in the striatum and the substantia nigra, the site of neurons that send projections to the striatum.
Pharmacokinetics
Pramipexole is rapidly absorbed, reaching peak concentrations in approximately 2 hours. The absolute bioavailability of pramipexole is greater than 90%, indicating that it is well absorbed and undergoes little presystemic metabolism. Food does not affect the extent of pramipexole absorption, although the time of maximum plasma concentration (T_{max}) is increased by about 1 hour when the drug is taken with a meal.
Pramipexole is extensively distributed, having a volume of distribution of about 500 L (coefficient of variation [CV]=20%). It is about 15% bound to plasma proteins. Pramipexole distributes into red blood cells as indicated by an erythrocyte-to-plasma ratio of approximately 2.
Pramipexole displays linear pharmacokinetics over the clinical dosage range. Its terminal half-life is about 8 hours in young healthy volunteers and about 12 hours in elderly volunteers (see CLINICAL PHARMACOLOGY, Pharmacokinetics in Special Populations). Steady-state concentrations are achieved within 2 days of dosing.
Metabolism and elimination: Urinary excretion is the major route of pramipexole elimination, with 90% of a pramipexole dose recovered in urine, almost all as unchanged drug. Nonrenal routes may contribute to a small extent to pramipexole elimination, although no metabolites have been identified in plasma or urine. The renal clearance of pramipexole is approximately 400 mL/min (CV=25%), approximately three times higher than the glomerular filtration rate. Thus, pramipexole is secreted by the renal tubules, probably by the organic cation transport system.
Pharmacokinetics in Special Populations
Because therapy with pramipexole is initiated at a subtherapeutic dosage and gradually titrated upward according to clinical tolerability to obtain the optimum therapeutic effect, adjustment of the initial dose based on gender, weight, or age is not necessary. However, renal insufficiency, which can cause a large decrease in the ability to eliminate pramipexole, may necessitate dosage adjustment (see CLINICAL PHARMACOLOGY, Renal Insufficiency).
Gender: Pramipexole clearance is about 30% lower in women than in men, but most of this difference can be accounted for by differences in body weight. There is no difference in half-life between males and females.
Age: Pramipexole clearance decreases with age as the half-life and clearance are about 40% longer and 30% lower, respectively, in elderly (aged 65 years or older) compared with young healthy volunteers (aged less than 40 years). This difference is most likely due to the well-known reduction in renal function with age, since pramipexole clearance is correlated with renal function, as measured by creatinine clearance (see CLINICAL PHARMACOLOGY, Renal Insufficiency).
Parkinson's disease patients: A cross-study comparison of data suggests that the clearance of pramipexole may be reduced by about 30% in Parkinson's disease patients compared with healthy elderly volunteers. The reason for this difference appears to be reduced renal function in Parkinson's disease patients, which may be related to their poorer general health. The pharmacokinetics of pramipexole were comparable between early and advanced Parkinson's disease patients.
Pediatric: The pharmacokinetics of pramipexole in the pediatric population have not been evaluated.
Hepatic insufficiency: The influence of hepatic insufficiency on pramipexole pharmacokinetics has not been evaluated. Because approximately 90% of the recovered dose is excreted in the urine as unchanged drug, hepatic impairment would not be expected to have a significant effect on pramipexole elimination.
Renal insufficiency: The clearance of pramipexole was about 75% lower in patients with severe renal impairment (creatinine clearance approximately 20 mL/min) and about 60% lower in patients with moderate impairment (creatinine clearance approximately 40 mL/min) compared with healthy volunteers. A lower starting and maintenance dose is recommended in these patients (see PRECAUTIONS and DOSAGE AND ADMINISTRATION). In patients with varying degrees of renal impairment, pramipexole clearance correlates well with creatinine clearance. Therefore, creatinine clearance can be used as a predictor of the extent of decrease in pramipexole clearance. Pramipexole clearance is extremely low in dialysis patients, as a negligible amount of pramipexole is removed by dialysis. Caution should be exercised when administering pramipexole to patients with renal disease.

CLINICAL STUDIES

The effectiveness of MIRAPEX (pramipexole dihydrochloride) Tablets in the treatment of Parkinson's disease was evaluated in a multinational drug development program consisting of seven randomized, controlled trials. Three were conducted in patients with early Parkinson's disease who were not receiving concomitant levodopa, and four were conducted in patients with advanced Parkinson's disease who were receiving concomitant levodopa. Among these seven studies, three studies provide the most persuasive evidence of pramipexole's effectiveness in the management of patients with Parkinson's disease who were and were not receiving concomitant levodopa. Two of these three trials enrolled patients with early Parkinson's disease (not receiving levodopa), and one enrolled patients with advanced Parkinson's disease who were receiving maximally tolerated doses of levodopa. In all studies, the Unified Parkinson's Disease Rating Scale (UPDRS), or one or more of its subparts, served as the primary outcome assessment measure. The UPDRS is a four-part multi-item rating scale intended to evaluate mentation (part I), activities of daily living (part II), motor performance (part III), and complications of therapy (part IV).
Part II of the UPDRS contains 13 questions relating to activities of daily living (ADL), which are scored from 0 (normal) to 4 (maximal severity) for a maximum (worst) score of 52. Part III of the UPDRS contains 27 questions (for 14 items) and is scored as described for part II. It is designed to assess the severity of the cardinal motor findings in patients with Parkinson's disease (eg, tremor, rigidity, bradykinesia, postural instability, etc), scored for different body regions, and has a maximum (worst) score of 108.
Studies In Patients With Early Parkinson's Disease
Patients (N=599) in the two studies of early Parkinson's disease had a mean disease duration of 2 years, limited or no prior exposure to levodopa (generally none in the preceding 6 months), and were not experiencing the "on-off" phenomenon and dyskinesia characteristic of later stages of the disease.
One of the two early Parkinson's disease studies (N=335) was a double-blind, placebo-controlled, parallel trial consisting of a 7-week dose-escalation period and a 6-month maintenance period. Patients could be on selegiline, anticholinergics, or both, but could not be on levodopa products or amantadine. Patients were randomized to MIRAPEX (pramipexole dihydrochloride) or placebo. Patients treated with MIRAPEX (pramipexole dihydrochloride) had a starting daily dose of 0.375 mg and were titrated to a maximally tolerated dose, but no higher than 4.5 mg/day in three divided doses. At the end of the 6-month maintenance period, the mean improvement from baseline on the UPDRS part II (ADL) total score was 1.9 in the group receiving MIRAPEX (pramipexole dihydrochloride) and –0.4 in the placebo group, a difference that was statistically significant. The mean improvement from baseline on the UPDRS part III total score was 5.0 in the group receiving MIRAPEX (pramipexole dihydrochloride) and –0.8 in the placebo group, a difference that was also statistically significant. A statistically significant difference between groups in favor of MIRAPEX (pramipexole dihydrochloride) was seen beginning at week 2 of the UPDRS part II (maximum dose 0.75 mg/day) and at week 3 of the UPDRS part III (maximum dose 1.5 mg/day).
The second early Parkinson's disease study (N=264) was a double-blind, placebo-controlled, parallel trial consisting of a 6-week dose-escalation period and a 4-week maintenance period. Patients could be on selegiline, anticholinergics, amantadine, or any combination of these, but could not be on levodopa products. Patients were randomized to 1 of 4 fixed doses of MIRAPEX (pramipexole dihydrochloride) (1.5 mg, 3.0 mg, 4.5 mg, or 6.0 mg per day) or placebo. At the end of the 4-week maintenance period, the mean improvement from baseline on the UPDRS part II total score was 1.8 in the patients treated with MIRAPEX (pramipexole dihydrochloride), regardless of assigned dose group, and 0.3 in placebo-treated patients. The mean improvement from baseline on the UPDRS part III total score was 4.2 in patients treated with MIRAPEX (pramipexole dihydrochloride) and 0.6 in placebo-treated patients. No dose-response relationship was demonstrated. The between-treatment differences on both parts of the UPDRS were statistically significant in favor of MIRAPEX (pramipexole dihydrochloride) for all doses.
No differences in effectiveness based on age or gender were detected. There were too few non-Caucasian patients to

evaluate the effect of race. Patients receiving selegiline or anticholinergics had responses similar to patients not receiving these drugs.

Studies In Patients With Advanced Parkinson's Disease

In the advanced Parkinson's disease study, the primary assessments were the UPDRS and daily diaries that quantified amounts of "on" and "off" time.

Patients in the advanced Parkinson's disease study (N=360) had a mean disease duration of 9 years, had been exposed to levodopa for long periods of time (mean 8 years), used concomitant levodopa during the trial, and had "on-off" periods. The advanced Parkinson's disease study was a double-blind, placebo-controlled, parallel trial consisting of a 7-week dose-escalation period and a 6-month maintenance period. Patients were all treated with concomitant levodopa products and could additionally be on concomitant selegiline, anticholinergics, amantadine, or any combination. Patients treated with MIRAPEX (pramipexole dihydrochloride) had a starting dose of 0.375 mg/day and were titrated to a maximally tolerated dose, but no higher than 4.5 mg/day in three divided doses. At selected times during the 6-month maintenance period, patients were asked to record the amount of "off," "on," or "on with dyskinesia" time per day for several sequential days. At the end of the 6-month maintenance period, the mean improvement from baseline on the UPDRS part II total score was 2.7 in the group treated with MIRAPEX (pramipexole dihydrochloride) and 0.5 in the placebo group, a difference that was statistically significant. The mean improvement from baseline on the UPDRS part III total score was 5.6 in the group treated with MIRAPEX (pramipexole dihydrochloride) and 2.8 in the placebo group, a difference that was statistically significant. A statistically significant difference between groups in favor of MIRAPEX (pramipexole dihydrochloride) was seen at week 3 of the UPDRS part II (maximum dose 1.5 mg/day) and at week 2 of the UPDRS part III (maximum dose 0.75 mg/day). Dosage reduction of levodopa was allowed during this study if dyskinesia (or hallucinations) developed; levodopa dosage reduction occurred in 76% of patients treated with MIRAPEX (pramipexole dihydrochloride) versus 54% of placebo patients. On average, the levodopa dose was reduced 27%.

The mean number of "off" hours per day during baseline was 6 hours for both treatment groups. Throughout the trial, patients treated with MIRAPEX (pramipexole dihydrochloride) had a mean of 4 "off" hours per day, while placebo-treated patients continued to experience 6 "off" hours per day.

No differences in effectiveness based on age or gender were detected. There were too few non-Caucasian patients to evaluate the effect of race.

INDICATIONS AND USAGE

MIRAPEX (pramipexole dihydrochloride) Tablets are indicated for the treatment of the signs and symptoms of idiopathic Parkinson's disease.

The effectiveness of MIRAPEX (pramipexole dihydrochloride) was demonstrated in randomized, controlled trials in patients with early Parkinson's disease who were not receiving concomitant levodopa therapy as well as in patients with advanced disease on concomitant levodopa (see CLINICAL STUDIES).

CONTRAINDICATIONS

MIRAPEX (pramipexole dihydrochloride) Tablets are contraindicated in patients who have demonstrated hypersensitivity to the drug or its ingredients.

WARNINGS

Falling Asleep During Activities of Daily Living:

Patients treated with MIRAPEX (pramipexole dihydrochloride) have reported falling asleep while engaged in activities of daily living, including the operation of motor vehicles which sometimes resulted in accidents. Although many of these patients reported somnolence while on MIRAPEX (pramipexole dihydrochloride), some perceived that they had no warning signs such as excessive drowsiness, and believed that they were alert immediately prior to the event. Some of these events have been reported as late as one year after the initiation of treatment.

Somnolence is a common occurrence in patients receiving MIRAPEX (pramipexole dihydrochloride) at doses above 1.5 mg/day. Many clinical experts believe that falling asleep while engaged in activities of daily living always occurs in a setting of pre-existing somnolence, although patients may not give such a history. For this reason, prescribers should continually reassess patients for drowsiness or sleepiness, especially since some of the events occur well after the start of treatment. Prescribers should also be aware that patients may not acknowledge drowsiness or sleepiness until directly questioned about drowsiness or sleepiness during specific activities.

Before initiating treatment with MIRAPEX (pramipexole dihydrochloride), patients should be advised of the potential to develop drowsiness and specifically asked about factors that may increase the risk with MIRAPEX (pramipexole dihydrochloride) such as concomitant sedating medications, the presence of sleep disorders, and concomitant medications that increase pramipexole plasma levels (e.g., cimetidine — see PRECAUTIONS, Drug Interactions). If a patient develops significant daytime sleepiness or episodes of falling asleep during activities that require active participation (e.g., conversations, eating, etc.), MIRAPEX (pramipexole dihydrochloride) should ordinarily be discontinued. If a decision is made to continue MIRAPEX (pramipexole dihydrochloride), patients should be advised to not drive and to avoid other potentially dangerous activities. While dose reduction clearly reduces the degree of somnolence, there is insufficient information to establish that dose reduction will eliminate episodes of falling asleep while engaged in activities of daily living.

Symptomatic Hypotension: Dopamine agonists, in clinical studies and clinical experience, appear to impair the systemic regulation of blood pressure, with resulting orthostatic hypotension, especially during dose escalation. Parkinson's disease patients, in addition, appear to have an impaired capacity to respond to an orthostatic challenge. For these reasons, Parkinson's disease patients being treated with dopaminergic agonists ordinarily require careful monitoring for signs and symptoms of orthostatic hypotension, especially during dose escalation, and should be informed of this risk (see PRECAUTIONS, Information for Patients).

In clinical trials of pramipexole, however, and despite clear orthostatic effects in normal volunteers, the reported incidence of clinically significant orthostatic hypotension was not greater among those assigned to MIRAPEX (pramipexole dihydrochloride) Tablets than among those assigned to placebo. This result is clearly unexpected in light of the previous experience with the risks of dopamine agonist therapy.

While this finding could reflect a unique property of pramipexole, it might also be explained by the conditions of the study and the nature of the population enrolled in the clinical trials. Patients were very carefully titrated, and patients with active cardiovascular disease or significant orthostatic hypotension at baseline were excluded.

Hallucinations: In the three double-blind, placebo-controlled trials in early Parkinson's disease, hallucinations were observed in 9% (35 of 388) of patients receiving MIRAPEX (pramipexole dihydrochloride), compared with 2.6% (6 of 235) of patients receiving placebo. In the four double-blind, placebo-controlled trials in advanced Parkinson's disease, where patients received MIRAPEX (pramipexole dihydrochloride) and concomitant levodopa, hallucinations were observed in 16.5% (43 of 260) of patients receiving MIRAPEX (pramipexole dihydrochloride) compared with 3.8% (10 of 264) of patients receiving placebo. Hallucinations were of sufficient severity to cause discontinuation of treatment in 3.1% of the early Parkinson's disease patients and 2.7% of the advanced Parkinson's disease patients compared with about 0.4% of placebo patients in both populations.

Age appears to increase the risk of hallucinations attributable to pramipexole. In the early Parkinson's disease patients, the risk of hallucinations was 1.9 times greater than placebo in patients younger than 65 years and 6.8 times greater than placebo in patients older than 65 years. In the advanced Parkinson's disease patients, the risk of hallucinations was 3.5 times greater than placebo in patients younger than 65 years and 5.2 times greater than placebo in patients older than 65 years.

PRECAUTIONS

Rhabdomyolysis: A single case of rhabdomyolysis occurred in a 49-year-old male with advanced Parkinson's disease treated with MIRAPEX (pramipexole dihydrochloride) Tablets. The patient was hospitalized with an elevated CPK (10,631 IU/L). The symptoms resolved with discontinuation of the medication.

Renal: Since pramipexole is eliminated through the kidneys, caution should be exercised when prescribing MIRAPEX (pramipexole dihydrochloride) to patients with renal insufficiency (see DOSAGE AND ADMINISTRATION).

Dyskinesia: MIRAPEX (pramipexole dihydrochloride) may potentiate the dopaminergic side effects of levodopa and may cause or exacerbate preexisting dyskinesia. Decreasing the dose of levodopa may ameliorate this side effect.

Retinal pathology in albino rats: Pathologic changes (degeneration and loss of photoreceptor cells) were observed in the retina of albino rats in the 2-year carcinogenicity study. While retinal degeneration was not diagnosed in pigmented rats treated for 2 years, a thinning in the outer nuclear layer of the retina was slightly greater in rats given drug compared with controls. Evaluation of the retinas of albino mice, monkeys, and minipigs did not reveal similar changes. The potential significance of this effect in humans has not been established, but cannot be disregarded because disruption of a mechanism that is universally present in vertebrates (ie, disk shedding) may be involved (see ANIMAL TOXICOLOGY).

Events Reported With Dopaminergic Therapy

Although the events enumerated below have not been reported in association with the use of pramipexole in its development program, they are associated with the use of other dopaminergic drugs. The expected incidence of these events, however, is so low that even if pramipexole caused these events at rates similar to those attributable to other dopaminergic therapies, it would be unlikely that even a single case would have occurred in a cohort of the size exposed to pramipexole in studies to date.

Withdrawal-emergent hyperpyrexia and confusion: Although not reported with pramipexole in the clinical development program, a symptom complex resembling the neuroleptic malignant syndrome (characterized by elevated temperature, muscular rigidity, altered consciousness, and autonomic instability), with no other obvious etiology, has been reported in association with rapid dose reduction, withdrawal of, or changes in antiparkinsonian therapy.

Fibrotic complications: Although not reported with pramipexole in the clinical development program, cases of retroperitoneal fibrosis, pulmonary infiltrates, pleural effusion, and pleural thickening have been reported in some patients treated with ergot-derived dopaminergic agents. While these complications may resolve when the drug is discontinued, complete resolution does not always occur.

Although these adverse events are believed to be related to the ergoline structure of these compounds, whether other, nonergot derived dopamine agonists can cause them is unknown.

Information for Patients: Patients should be instructed to take MIRAPEX (pramipexole dihydrochloride) only as prescribed.

Patients should be alerted to the potential sedating effects associated with MIRAPEX (pramipexole dihydrochloride), including somnolence and the possibility of falling asleep while engaged in activities of daily living. Since somnolence is a frequent adverse event with potentially serious consequences, patients should neither drive a car nor engage in other potentially dangerous activities until they have gained sufficient experience with MIRAPEX (pramipexole dihydrochloride) to gauge whether or not it affects their mental and/or motor performance adversely. Patients should be advised that if increased somnolence or new episodes of falling asleep during activities of daily living (e.g., watching television, passenger in a car, etc.) are experienced at any time during treatment, they should not drive or participate in potentially dangerous activities until they have contacted their physician. Because of possible additive effects, caution should be advised when patients are taking other sedating medications or alcohol in combination with MIRAPEX (pramipexole dihydrochloride) and when taking concomitant medications that increase plasma levels of pramipexole (e.g., cimetidine).

Patients should be informed that hallucinations can occur and that the elderly are at a higher risk than younger patients with Parkinson's disease.

Patients may develop postural (orthostatic) hypotension, with or without symptoms such as dizziness, nausea, fainting or blackouts, and sometimes, sweating. Hypotension may occur more frequently during initial therapy. Accordingly, patients should be cautioned against rising rapidly after sitting or lying down, especially if they have been doing so for prolonged periods and especially at the initiation of treatment with MIRAPEX (pramipexole dihydrochloride).

Because the teratogenic potential of pramipexole has not been completely established in laboratory animals, and because experience in humans is limited, patients should be advised to notify their physicians if they become pregnant or intend to become pregnant during therapy (see PRECAUTIONS, Pregnancy).

Because of the possibility that pramipexole may be excreted in breast milk, patients should be advised to notify their physicians if they intend to breast-feed or are breast-feeding an infant.

If patients develop nausea, they should be advised that taking MIRAPEX (pramipexole dihydrochloride) with food may reduce the occurrence of nausea.

Laboratory Tests: During the development of MIRAPEX (pramipexole dihydrochloride), no systematic abnormalities on routine laboratory testing were noted. Therefore, no specific guidance is offered regarding routine monitoring; the practitioner retains responsibility for determining how best to monitor the patient in his or her care.

Drug Interactions

Carbidopa/levodopa: Carbidopa/levodopa did not influence the pharmacokinetics of pramipexole in healthy volunteers (N=10). Pramipexole did not alter the extent of absorption (AUC) or the elimination of carbidopa/levodopa, although it caused an increase in levodopa C_{max} by about 40% and a decrease in T_{max} from 2.5 to 0.5 hours.

Selegiline: In healthy volunteers (N=11), selegiline did not influence the pharmacokinetics of pramipexole.

Amantadine: Population pharmacokinetic analysis suggests that amantadine is unlikely to alter the oral clearance of pramipexole (N=54).

Cimetidine: Cimetidine, a known inhibitor of renal tubular secretion of organic bases via the cationic transport system, caused a 50% increase in pramipexole AUC and a 40% increase in half-life (N=12).

Probenecid: Probenecid, a known inhibitor of renal tubular secretion of organic acids via the anionic transporter, did not noticeably influence pramipexole pharmacokinetics (N=12).

Other drugs eliminated via renal secretion: Population pharmacokinetic analysis suggests that coadministration of drugs that are secreted by the cationic transport system (eg, cimetidine, ranitidine, diltiazem, triamterene, verapamil, quinidine, and quinine) decreases the oral clearance of pramipexole by about 20%, while those secreted by the anionic transport system (eg, cephalosporins, penicillins, indomethacin, hydrochlorothiazide, and chlorpropamide) are likely to have little effect on the oral clearance of pramipexole.

CYP interactions: Inhibitors of cytochrome P450 enzymes would not be expected to affect pramipexole elimination because pramipexole is not appreciably metabolized by these enzymes in vivo or in vitro. Pramipexole does not inhibit

Continued on next page

Mirapex—Cont.

CYP enzymes CYP1A2, CYP2C9, CYP2C19, CYP2E1, and CYP3A4. Inhibition of CYP2D6 was observed with an apparent Ki of 30 μM, indicating that pramipexole will not inhibit CYP enzymes at plasma concentrations observed following the highest recommended clinical dose (1.5 mg tid).

Dopamine antagonists: Since pramipexole is a dopamine agonist, it is possible that dopamine antagonists, such as the neuroleptics (phenothiazines, butyrophenones, thioxanthenes) or metoclo- pramide, may diminish the effectiveness of MIRAPEX (pramipexole dihydrochloride).

Drug/Laboratory Test Interactions: There are no known interactions between MIRAPEX (pramipexole dihydrochloride) and laboratory tests.

Carcinogenesis, Mutagenesis, Impairment of Fertility: Two-year carcinogenicity studies with pramipexole have been conducted in mice and rats. Pramipexole was administered in the diet to Chbb:NMRI mice at doses of 0.3, 2, and 10 mg/kg/day (0.3, 2.2, and 11 times the highest recommended clinical dose [1.5 mg tid] on a mg/m^2 basis). Pramipexole was administered in the diet to Wistar rats at 0.3, 2, and 8 mg/kg/day (plasma AUCs equal to 0.3, 2.5, and 12.5 times the AUC in humans receiving 1.5 mg tid). No significant increases in tumors occurred in either species.

Pramipexole was not mutagenic or clastogenic in a battery of assays, including the in vitro Ames assay, V79 gene mutation assay for HGPRT mutants, chromosomal aberration assay in Chinese hamster ovary cells, and in vivo mouse micronucleus assay.

In rat fertility studies, pramipexole at a dose of 2.5 mg/kg/day (5.4 times the highest clinical dose on a mg/m^2 basis), prolonged estrus cycles and inhibited implantation. These effects were associated with reductions in serum levels of prolactin, a hormone necessary for implantation and maintenance of early pregnancy in rats.

Pregnancy: Pregnancy Category C. When pramipexole was given to female rats throughout pregnancy, implantation was inhibited at a dose of 2.5 mg/kg/day (5.4 times the highest clinical dose on a mg/m^2 basis). Administration of 1.5 mg/kg/day of pramipexole to pregnant rats during the period of organogenesis (gestation days 7 through 16) resulted in a high incidence of total resorption of embryos. The plasma AUC in rats dosed at this level was 4.3 times the AUC in humans receiving 1.5 mg tid. These findings are thought to be due to the prolactin-lowering effect of pramipexole, since prolactin is necessary for implantation and maintenance of early pregnancy in rats (but not rabbits or humans). Because of pregnancy disruption and early embryonic loss in these studies, the teratogenic potential of pramipexole could not be adequately evaluated. There was no evidence of adverse effects on embryo-fetal development following administration of up to 10 mg/kg/day to pregnant rabbits during organogenesis (plasma AUC was 71 times that in humans receiving 1.5 mg tid). Postnatal growth was inhibited in the offspring of rats treated with 0.5 mg/kg/day (approximately equivalent to the highest clinical dose on a mg/m^2 basis) or greater during the latter part of pregnancy and throughout lactation.

There are no studies of pramipexole in human pregnancy. Because animal reproduction studies are not always predictive of human response, pramipexole should be used during pregnancy only if the potential benefit outweighs the potential risk to the fetus.

Nursing Mothers: A single-dose, radio-labeled study showed that drug-related materials were excreted into the breast milk of lactating rats. Concentrations of radioactivity in milk were three to six times higher than concentrations in plasma at equivalent time points.

Other studies have shown that pramipexole treatment resulted in an inhibition of prolactin secretion in humans and rats.

It is not known whether this drug is excreted in human milk. Because many drugs are excreted in human milk and because of the potential for serious adverse reactions in nursing infants from pramipexole, a decision should be made as to whether to discontinue nursing or to discontinue the drug, taking into account the importance of the drug to the mother.

Pediatric Use: The safety and efficacy of MIRAPEX® (pramipexole dihydrochloride) in pediatric patients has not been established.

Geriatric Use: Pramipexole total oral clearance was approximately 30% lower in subjects older than 65 years compared with younger subjects, because of a decline in pramipexole renal clearance due to an age-related reduction in renal function. This resulted in an increase in elimination half-life from approximately 8.5 hours to 12 hours. In clinical studies, 38.7% of patients were older than 65 years. There were no apparent differences in efficacy or safety between older and younger patients, except that the relative risk of hallucination associated with the use of MIRAPEX (pramipexole dihydrochloride) was increased in the elderly.

ADVERSE EVENTS

During the premarketing development of pramipexole, patients with either early or advanced Parkinson's disease were enrolled in clinical trials. Apart from the severity and duration of their disease, the two populations differed in their use of concomitant levodopa therapy. Patients with early disease did not receive concomitant levodopa therapy during treatment with pramipexole; those with advanced Parkinson's disease all received concomitant levodopa treatment. Because these two populations may have differential risks for various adverse events, this section will, in general, present adverse-event data for these two populations separately.

Because the controlled trials performed during premarketing development all used a titration design, with a resultant confounding of time and dose, it was impossible to adequately evaluate the effects of dose on the incidence of adverse events.

Early Parkinson's Disease

In the three double-blind, placebo-controlled trials of patients with early Parkinson's disease, the most commonly observed adverse events (>5%) that were numerically more frequent in the group treated with MIRAPEX (pramipexole dihydrochloride) Tablets were nausea, dizziness, somnolence, insomnia, constipation, asthenia, and hallucinations.

Approximately 12% of 388 patients with early Parkinson's disease and treated with MIRAPEX (pramipexole dihydrochloride) who participated in the double-blind, placebo-controlled trials discontinued treatment due to adverse events compared with 11% of 235 patients who received placebo. The adverse events most commonly causing discontinuation of treatment were related to the nervous system (hallucinations [3.1% on MIRAPEX (pramipexole dihydrochloride) vs 0.4% on placebo]; dizziness [2.1% on MIRAPEX (pramipexole dihydrochloride) vs 1% on placebo]; somnolence [1.6% on MIRAPEX (pramipexole dihydrochloride) vs 0% on placebo]; extrapyramidal syndrome [1.6% on MIRAPEX (pramipexole dihydrochloride) vs 6.4% on placebo]; headache and confusion [1.3% and 1.0%, respectively, on MIRAPEX (pramipexole dihydrochloride) vs 0% on placebo]); and gastrointestinal system (nausea [2.1% on MIRAPEX (pramipexole dihydrochloride) vs 0.4% on placebo]).

Adverse-event incidence in controlled clinical studies in early Parkinson's disease: Table 1 lists treatment-emergent adverse events that occurred in the double-blind, placebo-controlled studies in early Parkinson's disease that were reported by ≥1% of patients treated with MIRAPEX (pramipexole dihydrochloride) and were numerically more frequent than in the placebo group. In these studies, patients did not receive concomitant levodopa. Adverse events were usually mild or moderate in intensity.

The prescriber should be aware that these figures cannot be used to predict the incidence of adverse events in the course of usual medical practice where patient characteristics and other factors differ from those that prevailed in the clinical studies. Similarly, the cited frequencies cannot be compared with figures obtained from other clinical investigations involving different treatments, uses, and investigators. However, the cited figures do provide the prescribing physician with some basis for estimating the relative contribution of drug and nondrug factors to the adverse-event incidence rate in the population studied.

Table 1: Treatment-Emergent Adverse-Event* Incidence in Double-Blind, Placebo-Controlled Trials in Early Parkinson's Disease (Events ≥ 1% of Patients Treated With MIRAPEX (pramipexole dihydrochloride) and Numerically More Frequent Than in the Placebo Group)

Body System/ Adverse Event	MIRAPEX (pramipexole (dihydrochloride) N=388	Placebo N=235
Body as a Whole		
Asthenia	14	12
General edema	5	3
Malaise	2	1
Reaction unevaluable	2	1
Fever	1	0
Digestive System		
Nausea	28	18
Constipation	14	6
Anorexia	4	2
Dysphagia	2	0
Metabolic & Nutritional System		
Peripheral edema	5	4
Decreased weight	2	0
Nervous System		
Dizziness	25	24
Somnolence	22	9
Insomnia	17	12
Hallucinations	9	3
Confusion	4	1
Amnesia	4	2
Hypesthesia	3	1
Dystonia	2	1
Akathisia	2	0
Thinking abnormalities	2	0
Decreased libido	1	0
Myoclonus	1	0
Special Senses		
Vision abnormalities	3	0
Urogenital System		
Impotence	2	1

* Patients may have reported multiple adverse experiences during the study or at discontinuation; thus, patients may be included in more than one category.

Other events reported by 1% or more of patients with early Parkinson's disease and treated with MIRAPEX (pramipexole dihydrochloride) but reported equally or more frequently in the placebo group were infection, accidental injury, headache, pain, tremor, back pain, syncope, postural hypotension, hypertonia, depression, abdominal pain, anxiety, dyspepsia, flatulence, diarrhea, rash, ataxia, dry mouth, extrapyramidal syndrome, leg cramps, twitching, pharyngitis, sinusitis, sweating, rhinitis, urinary tract infection, vasodilation, flu syndrome, increased saliva, tooth disease, dyspnea, increased cough, gait abnormalities, urinary frequency, vomiting, allergic reaction, hypertension, pruritis, hypokinesia, increased creatine PK, nervousness, dream abnormalities, chest pain, neck pain, paresthesia, tachycardia, vertigo, voice alteration, conjunctivitis, paralysis, accommodation abnormalities, tinnitus, diplopia, and taste perversions.

In a fixed-dose study in early Parkinson's disease, occurrence of the following events increased in frequency as the dose increased over the range from 1.5 mg/day to 6 mg/day: postural hypotension, nausea, constipation, somnolence, and amnesia. The frequency of these events was generally 2-fold greater than placebo for pramipexole doses greater than 3 mg/day. The incidence of somnolence with pramipexole at a dose of 1.5 mg/day was comparable to that reported for placebo.

Advanced Parkinson's Disease

In the four double-blind, placebo-controlled trials of patients with advanced Parkinson's disease, the most commonly observed adverse events (>5%) that were numerically more frequent in the group treated with MIRAPEX (pramipexole dihydrochloride) and concomitant levodopa were postural (orthostatic) hypotension, dyskinesia, extrapyramidal syndrome, insomnia, dizziness, hallucinations, accidental injury, dream abnormalities, confusion, constipation, asthenia, somnolence, dystonia, gait abnormality, hypertonia, dry mouth, amnesia, and urinary frequency.

Approximately 12% of 260 patients with advanced Parkinson's disease who received MIRAPEX (pramipexole dihydrochloride) and concomitant levodopa in the double-blind, placebo-controlled trials discontinued treatment due to adverse events compared with 16% of 264 patients who received placebo and concomitant levodopa. The events most commonly causing discontinuation of treatment were related to the nervous system (hallucinations [2.7% on MIRAPEX (pramipexole dihydrochloride) vs 0.4% on placebo]; dyskinesia [1.9% on MIRAPEX (pramipexole dihydrochloride) vs 0.8% on placebo]; extrapyramidal syndrome [1.5% on MIRAPEX (pramipexole dihydrochloride) vs 4.9% on placebo]; dizziness [1.2% on MIRAPEX (pramipexole dihydrochloride) vs 1.5% on placebo]; confusion [1.2% on MIRAPEX (pramipexole dihydrochloride) vs 2.3% on placebo]); and cardiovascular system (postural [orthostatic] hypotension [2.3% on MIRAPEX (pramipexole dihydrochloride) vs 1.1% on placebo]).

Adverse-event incidence in controlled clinical studies in advanced Parkinson's disease: Table 2 lists treatment-emergent adverse events that occurred in the double-blind, placebo-controlled studies in advanced Parkinson's disease that were reported by ≥1% of patients treated with MIRAPEX (pramipexole dihydrochloride) and were numerically more frequent than in the placebo group. In these studies, MIRAPEX (pramipexole dihydrochloride) or placebo was administered to patients who were also receiving concomitant levodopa. Adverse events were usually mild or moderate in intensity.

The prescriber should be aware that these figures cannot be used to predict the incidence of adverse events in the course of usual medical practice where patient characteristics and other factors differ from those that prevailed in the clinical studies. Similarly, the cited frequencies cannot be compared with figures obtained from other clinical investigations involving different treatments, uses, and investigators. However, the cited figures do provide the prescribing physician with some basis for estimating the relative contribution of drug and nondrug factors to the adverse-events incidence rate in the population studied.

Table 2: Treatment-Emergent Adverse-Event* Incidence in Double-Blind, Placebo-Controlled Trials in Advanced Parkinson's Disease (Events ≥ 1% of Patients Treated With MIRAPEX (pramipexole dihydrochloride) and Numerically More Frequent Than in the Placebo Group)

Body System/ Adverse Event	MIRAPEX† (pramipexole (dihydrochloride) N=260	Placebo† N=264
Body as a Whole		
Accidental injury	17	15
Asthenia	10	8
General edema	4	3
Chest pain	3	2
Malaise	3	2
Cardiovascular System		
Postural hypotension	53	48
Digestive System		
Constipation	10	9
Dry mouth	7	3
Metabolic & Nutritional System		
Peripheral edema	2	1
Increased creatine PK	1	0
Musculoskeletal System		
Arthritis	3	1
Twitching	2	0
Bursitis	2	0
Myasthenia	1	0
Nervous System		
Dyskinesia	47	31
Extrapyramidal syndrome	28	26
Insomnia	27	22
Dizziness	26	25
Hallucinations	17	4
Nervous System		
Dream abnormalities	11	10
Confusion	10	7
Somnolence	9	6
Dystonia	8	7
Gait abnormalities	7	5
Hypertonia	7	6
Amnesia	6	4
Akathisia	3	2
Thinking abnormalities	3	2
Paranoid reaction	2	0
Delusions	1	0
Sleep disorders	1	0
Respiratory System		
Dyspnea	4	3
Rhinitis	3	1
Pneumonia	2	0
Skin & Appendages		
Skin disorders	2	1
Special Senses		
Accommodation abnormalities	4	2
Vision abnormalities	3	1
Diplopia	1	0
Urogenital System		
Urinary frequency	6	3
Urinary tract infection	4	3
Urinary incontinence	2	1

* Patients may have reported multiple adverse experiences during the study or at discontinuation; thus, patients may be included in more than one category.
† Patients received concomitant levodopa.

Other events reported by 1% or more of patients with advanced Parkinson's disease and treated with MIRAPEX (pramipexole dihydrochloride) but reported equally or more frequently in the placebo group were nausea, pain, infection, headache, depression, tremor, hypokinesia, anorexia, back pain, dyspepsia, flatulence, ataxia, flu syndrome, sinusitis, diarrhea, myalgia, abdominal pain, anxiety, rash, paresthesia, hypertension, increased saliva, tooth disorder, apathy, hypotension, sweating, vasodilation, vomiting, increased cough, nervousness, pruritus, hypesthesia, neck pain, syncope, arthralgia, dysphagia, palpitations, pharyngitis, vertigo, leg cramps, conjunctivitis, and lacrimation disorders.

Adverse Events; Relationship to Age, Gender, and Race: Among the treatment-emergent adverse events in patients treated with MIRAPEX (pramipexole dihydrochloride), hallucination appeared to exhibit a positive relationship to age. No gender-related differences were observed. Only a small percentage (4%) of patients enrolled were non-Caucasian, therefore, an evaluation of adverse events related to race is not possible.

Other Adverse Events Observed During All Phase 2 and 3 Clinical Trials: MIRAPEX (pramipexole dihydrochloride) has been administered to 1,408 individuals during all clinical trials (Parkinson's disease and other patient populations), 648 of whom were in seven double-blind, placebo-controlled Parkinson's disease trials. During these trials, all adverse events were recorded by the clinical investigators using terminology of their own choosing. To provide a meaningful estimate of the proportion of individuals having adverse events, similar types of events were grouped into a smaller number of standardized categories using modified COSTART dictionary terminology. These categories are used in the listing below. The events listed below occurred in less than 1% of the 1,408 individuals exposed to MIRAPEX (pramipexole dihydrochloride) and occurred on at least two occasions (on one occasion if the event was serious). All reported events, except those already listed above, are included, without regard to determination of a causal relationship to MIRAPEX (pramipexole dihydrochloride).

Events are listed within body-system categories in order of decreasing frequency.

Body as a whole: enlarged abdomen, death, fever, suicide attempt.

Cardiovascular system: peripheral vascular disease, myocardial infarction, angina pectoris, atrial fibrillation, heart failure, arrhythmia, atrial arrhythmia, pulmonary embolism.

Digestive system: thirst.

Musculoskeletal system: joint disorder, myasthenia.

Nervous system: agitation, CNS stimulation, hyperkinesia, psychosis, convulsions.

Respiratory system: pneumonia.

Special senses: cataract, eye disorder, glaucoma.

Urogenital system: dysuria, abnormal ejaculation, prostate cancer, hematuria, prostate disorder.

Falling Asleep During Activities of Daily Living: Patients treated with MIRAPEX (pramipexole dihydrochloride) have reported falling asleep while engaged in activities of daily living, including operation of a motor vehicle which sometimes resulted in accidents (see bolded WARNING).

DRUG ABUSE AND DEPENDENCE

Pramipexole is not a controlled substance. Pramipexole has not been systematically studied in animals or humans for its potential for abuse, tolerance, or physical dependence. However, in a rat model on cocaine self-administration, pramipexole had little or no effect.

OVERDOSAGE

There is no clinical experience with massive overdosage. One patient, with a 10-year history of schizophrenia, took 11 mg/day of pramipexole for 2 days; this is two to three times the protocol recommended daily dose. No adverse events were reported related to the increased dose. Blood pressure remained stable although pulse rate increased to between 100 and 120 beats/minute. The patient withdrew from the study at the end of week 2 due to lack of efficacy. There is no known antidote for overdosage of a dopamine agonist. If signs of central nervous system stimulation are present, a phenothiazine or other butyrophenone neuroleptic agent may be indicated; the efficacy of such drugs in reversing the effects of overdosage has not been assessed. Management of overdose may require general supportive measures along with gastric lavage, intravenous fluids, and electrocardiogram monitoring.

DOSAGE AND ADMINISTRATION

In all clinical studies, dosage was initiated at a subtherapeutic level to avoid intolerable adverse effects and orthostatic hypotension. MIRAPEX (pramipexole dihydrochloride) should be titrated gradually in all patients. The dosage should be increased to achieve a maximum therapeutic effect, balanced against the principal side effects of dyskinesia, hallucinations, somnolence, and dry mouth.

Dosing in Patients With Normal Renal Function

Initial Treatment: Dosages should be increased gradually from a starting dose of 0.375 mg/day given in three divided doses and should not be increased more frequently than every 5 to 7 days. A suggested ascending dosage schedule that was used in clinical studies is shown in the following table:

Table 3: Ascending Dosage Schedule of MIRAPEX (pramipexole dihydrochloride)

Week	Dosage (mg)	Total Daily Dose (mg)
1	0.125 tid	0.375
2	0.25 tid	0.75
3	0.5 tid	1.50
4	0.75 tid	2.25
5	1.0 tid	3.0
6	1.25 tid	3.75
7	1.5 tid	4.50

Maintenance Treatment: MIRAPEX (pramipexole dihydrochloride) Tablets were effective and well tolerated over a dosage range of 1.5 to 4.5 mg/day administered in equally divided doses three times per day with or without concomitant levodopa (approximately 800 mg/day).

In a fixed-dose study in early Parkinson's disease patients, doses of 3 mg, 4.5 mg, and 6 mg per day of MIRAPEX (pramipexole dihydrochloride) were not shown to provide any significant benefit beyond that achieved at a daily dose of 1.5 mg/day. However, in the same fixed-dose study, the following adverse events were dose related: postural hypotension, nausea, constipation, somnolence, and amnesia. The frequency of these events was generally 2-fold greater than placebo for pramipexole doses greater than 3 mg/day. The incidence of somnolence reported with pramipexole at a dose of 1.5 mg/day was comparable to placebo.

When MIRAPEX (pramipexole dihydrochloride) is used in combination with levodopa, a reduction of the levodopa dosage should be considered. In a controlled study in advanced Parkinson's disease, the dosage of levodopa was reduced by an average of 27% from baseline.

Table 4: Patients with Renal Impairment

Pramipexole Dosage in the Renally Impaired		
Renal Status	Starting Dose (mg)	Maximum Dose (mg)
Normal to mild impairment (creatinine Cl > 60 mL/min)	0.125 tid	1.5 tid
Moderate impairment (creatinine Cl = 35 to 59 mL/min)	0.125 bid	1.5 bid
Severe impairment (creatinine Cl = 15 to 34 mL/min)	0.125 qd	1.5 qd
Very severe impairment (creatinine Cl < 15 mL/min and hemodialysis patients)	The use of MIRAPEX (pramipexole dihydrochloride) has not been adequately studied in this group of patients.	

Discontinuation of Treatment: It is recommended that MIRAPEX (pramipexole dihydrochloride) be discontinued over a period of 1 week; in some studies, however, abrupt discontinuation was uneventful.

HOW SUPPLIED

MIRAPEX (pramipexole dihydrochloride) Tablets are available as follows:

0.125 mg: white, round tablet with "U" on one side and "2" on the reverse side.

Bottles of 63 NDC 0597-0083-53

Continued on next page

Mirapex—Cont.

0.25 mg: white, oval, scored tablet with "U" twice on one side and "4" twice on the reverse side.

Bottles of 90 NDC 0597-0084-90
Unit dose packages of 100 NDC 0597-0084-61

0.5 mg: white, oval, scored tablet with "U" twice on one side and "8" twice on the reverse side.

Bottles of 90 NDC 0597-0085-90
Unit dose packages of 100 NDC 0597-0085-61

1 mg: white, round, scored tablet with "U" twice on one side and "6" twice on the reverse side.

Bottles of 90 NDC 0597-0090-90
Unit dose packages of 100 NDC 0597-0090-61

1.5 mg: white, round, scored tablet with "U" twice on one side and "37" twice on the reverse side.

Bottles of 90 NDC 0597-0091-90
Unit dose packages of 100 NDC 0597-0091-61

Store at 25°C (77°F); excursions permitted to 15°–30°C (59°–86°F) [see USP Controlled Room Temperature]. Protect from light.

℞ only

ANIMAL TOXICOLOGY

Retinal Pathology in Albino Rats

Pathologic changes (degeneration and loss of photoreceptor cells) were observed in the retina of albino rats in the 2-year carcinogenicity study with pramipexole. These findings were first observed during week 76 and were dose dependent in animals receiving 2 or 8 mg/kg/day (plasma AUCs equal to 2.5 and 12.5 times the AUC in humans that received 1.5 mg tid). In a similar study of pigmented rats with 2 years exposure to pramipexole at 2 or 8 mg/kg/day, retinal degeneration was not diagnosed. Animals given drug had thinning in the outer nuclear layer of the retina that was only slightly greater than that seen in control rats utilizing morphometry.

Investigative studies demonstrated that pramipexole reduced the rate of disk shedding from the photoreceptor rod cells of the retina in albino rats, which was associated with enhanced sensitivity to the damaging effects of light. In a comparative study, degeneration and loss of photoreceptor cells occurred in albino rats after 13 weeks of treatment with 25 mg/kg/day of pramipexole (54 times the highest clinical dose on a mg/m^2 basis) and constant light (100 lux) but not in pigmented rats exposed to the same dose and higher light intensities (500 lux). Thus, the retina of albino rats is considered to be uniquely sensitive to the damaging effects of pramipexole and light. Similar changes in the retina did not occur in a 2-year carcinogenicity study in albino mice treated with 0.3, 2, or 10 mg/kg/day (0.3, 2.2 and 11 times the highest clinical dose on a mg/m^2 basis). Evaluation of the retinas of monkeys given 0.1, 0.5, or 2.0 mg/kg/day of pramipexole (0.4, 2.2, and 8.6 times the highest clinical dose on a mg/m^2 basis) for 12 months and minipigs given 0.3, 1, or 5 mg/kg/day of pramipexole for 13 weeks also detected no changes.

The potential significance of this effect in humans has not been established, but cannot be disregarded because disruption of a mechanism that is universally present in vertebrates (ie, disk shedding) may be involved.

Fibro-osseous Proliferative Lesions in Mice

An increased incidence of fibro-osseous proliferative lesions occurred in the femurs of female mice treated for 2 years with 0.3, 2.0, or 10 mg/kg/day (0.3, 2.2, and 11 times the highest clinical dose on a mg/m^2 basis). Lesions occurred at a lower rate in control animals. Similar lesions were not observed in male mice or rats and monkeys of either sex that were treated chronically with pramipexole. The significance of this lesion to humans is not known.

Distributed by: Boehringer Ingelheim Pharmaceuticals, Inc. Ridgefield, CT 06877 USA

Co-marketed by: Boehringer Ingelheim Pharmaceuticals, Inc. and Pfizer Inc, New York, NY 10017

Licensed from: Boehringer Ingelheim International GmbH

Trademark under license from:
Boehringer Ingelheim International GmbH
U.S. Patent Nos. 4,886,812 and 4,843,086

Revised October 2003 819898001/US/1

MOBIC® ℞

[*mō-bĭc*]

(meloxicam)

Tablets 7.5 mg and 15 mg

Prescribing Information

DESCRIPTION

MOBIC® (meloxicam), an oxicam derivative, is a member of the enolic acid group of nonsteroidal anti-inflammatory drugs (NSAIDs). Each pastel yellow tablet contains meloxicam 7.5 mg or 15 mg for oral administration. It is chemically designated as 4-hydroxy-2-methyl-*N*-(5-methyl-2-thiazolyl)-2*H*-1,2-benzothiazine-3-carboxamide 1,1-dioxide. The molecular weight is 351.4. Its empirical formula is $C_{14}H_{13}N_3O_4S_2$ and it has the following structural formula.

Table 1 Single Dose and Steady State Pharmacokinetic Parameters for Oral 7.5 mg and 15 mg Meloxicam (Mean and % CV)[1]

Pharmcokinetic Parameters (% CV)		Steady State			Single Dose	
		Healthy male adults (Fed)[2]	Elderly males (Fed)[2]	Elderly females (Fed)[2]	Renal failure (Fasted)	Hepatic insufficiency (Fasted)
		7.5 mg[3] tablets	15 mg capsules	15 mg capsules	15 mg capsules	15 mg capsules
N		18	5	8	12	12
C_{max}	[μg/mL]	1.05 (20)	2.3 (59)	3.2 (24)	0.59 (36)	0.84 (29)
t_{max}	[h]	4.9 (8)	5 (12)	6 (27)	4 (65)	10 (87)
$t_{½}$	[h]	20.1 (29)	21 (34)	24 (34)	18 (46)	16 (29)
CL/f	[mL/min]	8.8 (29)	9.9 (76)	5.1 (22)	19 (43)	11 (44)
V_z/f[4]	[L]	14.7 (32)	15 (42)	10 (30)	26 (44)	14 (29)

[1]The parameter values in the Table are from various studies;
[2]not under high fat conditions;
[3]MOBIC tablets;
[4]V_z/f =Dose/(AUC•K_{el})

Meloxicam is a pastel yellow solid, practically insoluble in water, with higher solubility observed in strong acids and bases. It is very slightly soluble in methanol. Meloxicam has an apparent partition coefficient (log P)$_{app}$ = 0.1 in *n*-octanol/buffer pH 7.4. Meloxicam has pKa values of 1.1 and 4.2.

MOBIC is available as a tablet for oral administration containing 7.5 mg or 15 mg meloxicam.

The inactive ingredients in MOBIC include colloidal silicon dioxide, crospovidone, lactose monohydrate, magnesium stearate, microcrystalline cellulose, povidone and sodium citrate dihydrate.

CLINICAL PHARMACOLOGY

Mechanism of Action

Meloxicam is a nonsteroidal anti-inflammatory drug (NSAID) that exhibits anti-inflammatory, analgesic, and antipyretic activities in animal models. The mechanism of action of meloxicam, like that of other NSAIDs, may be related to prostaglandin synthetase (cyclooxygenase) inhibition.

Pharmacokinetics

Absorption

The absolute bioavailability of meloxicam capsules was 89% following a single oral dose of 30 mg compared with 30 mg IV bolus injection. Meloxicam capsules have been shown to be bioequivalent to MOBIC tablets. Following single intravenous doses, dose-proportional pharmacokinetics were shown in the range of 5 mg to 60 mg. After multiple oral doses the pharmacokinetics of meloxicam capsules were dose-proportional over the range of 7.5 mg to 15 mg. Mean C_{max} was achieved within four to five hours after a 7.5 mg meloxicam tablet was taken under fasted conditions, indicating a prolonged drug absorption. The rate or extent of absorption was not affected by multiple dose administration, suggesting linear pharmacokinetics. With multiple dosing, steady state conditions were reached by day 5. A second meloxicam concentration peak occurs around 12 to 14 hours post-dose suggesting gastrointestinal recirculation.

[See table 1 above]

Food and Antacid Effects

Drug intake after a high fat breakfast (75 g of fat) did not affect extent of absorption of meloxicam capsules, but led to 22% higher C_{max} values. Mean C_{max} values were achieved between five and six hours. No pharmacokinetic interaction was detected with concomitant administration of antacids. MOBIC tablets can be administered without regard to timing of meals and antacids.

Distribution

The mean volume of distribution (Vss) of meloxicam is approximately 10 L. Meloxicam is ~ 99.4% bound to human plasma proteins (primarily albumin) within the therapeutic dose range. The fraction of protein binding is independent of drug concentration, over the clinically relevant concentration range, but decreases to ~ 99% in patients with renal disease. Meloxicam penetration into human red blood cells, after oral dosing, is less than 10%. Following a radiolabeled dose, over 90% of the radioactivity detected in the plasma was present as unchanged meloxicam.

Meloxicam concentrations in synovial fluid, after a single oral dose, range from 40% to 50% of those in plasma. The free fraction in synovial fluid is 2.5 times higher than in plasma, due to the lower albumin content in synovial fluid as compared to plasma. The significance of this penetration is unknown.

Metabolism

Meloxicam is almost completely metabolized to four pharmacologically inactive metabolites. The major metabolite, 5'-carboxy meloxicam (60% of dose), from P-450 mediated metabolism was formed by oxidation of an intermediate metabolite 5'-hydroxymethyl meloxicam which is also excreted to a lesser extent (9% of dose). *In vitro* studies indicate that cytochrome P-450 2C9 plays an important role in this metabolic pathway with a minor contribution of the CYP 3A4 isozyme. Patients' peroxidase activity is probably responsible for the other two metabolites which account for 16% and 4% of the administered dose, respectively.

Excretion

Meloxicam excretion is predominantly in the form of metabolites, and occurs to equal extents in the urine and feces. Only traces of the unchanged parent compound are excreted in the urine (0.2%) and feces (1.6%). The extent of the urinary excretion was confirmed for unlabeled multiple 7.5 mg doses: 0.5%, 6% and 13% of the dose were found in urine in the form of meloxicam, and the 5'-hydroxymethyl and 5'-carboxy metabolites, respectively. There is significant biliary and/or enteral secretion of the drug. This was demonstrated when oral administration of cholestyramine following a single IV dose of meloxicam decreased the AUC of meloxicam by 50%.

The mean elimination half-life ($t_{½}$) ranges from 15 hours to 20 hours. The elimination half-life is constant across dose levels indicating linear metabolism within the therapeutic dose range. Plasma clearance ranges from 7 to 9 mL/min.

Special Populations

Pediatric

The pharmacokinetics of MOBIC in pediatric patients under 18 years of age have not been investigated.

Geriatric

Elderly males (≥ 65 years of age) exhibited meloxicam plasma concentrations and steady state pharmacokinetics similar to young males. Elderly females (≥ 65 years of age) had a 47% higher AUC_{ss} and 32% higher $C_{max\ ss}$ as compared to younger females (≤ 55 years of age) after body weight normalization. Despite the increased total concentrations in the elderly females, the adverse event profile was comparable for both elderly patient populations. A smaller free fraction was found in elderly female patients in comparison to elderly male patients.

Gender

Young females exhibited slightly lower plasma concentrations relative to young males. After single doses of 7.5 mg MOBIC, the mean elimination half-life was 19.5 hours for the female group as compared to 23.4 hours for the male group. At steady state, the data were similar (17.9 hours vs. 21.4 hours). This pharmacokinetic difference due to gender is likely to be of little clinical importance. There was linearity of pharmacokinetics and no appreciable difference in the C_{max} or T_{max} across genders.

Hepatic Insufficiency

Following a single 15 mg dose of meloxicam there was no marked difference in plasma concentrations in subjects with mild (Child-Pugh Class I) and moderate (Child-Pugh Class II) hepatic impairment compared to healthy volunteers. Protein binding of meloxicam was not affected by hepatic insufficiency. No dose adjustment is necessary in mild to moderate hepatic insufficiency. Patients with severe hepatic impairment (Child-Pugh Class III) have not been adequately studied.

Renal Insufficiency

Meloxicam pharmacokinetics have been investigated in subjects with different degrees of renal insufficiency. Total drug plasma concentrations decreased with the degree of renal impairment while free AUC values were similar. Total clearance of meloxicam increased in these patients probably due to the increase in free fraction leading to an increased metabolic clearance. There is no need for dose adjustment in patients with mild to moderate renal failure (CrCL >15 mL/min). Patients with severe renal insufficiency have not been adequately studied. The use of MOBIC in subjects with severe renal impairment is not recommended (see WARNINGS, Advanced Renal Disease).

Hemodialysis

Following a single dose of meloxicam, the free C_{max} plasma concentrations were higher in patients with renal failure on chronic hemodialysis (1% free fraction) in comparison to healthy volunteers (0.3% free fraction). Hemodialysis did not lower the total drug concentration in plasma; therefore, additional doses are not necessary after hemodialysis. Meloxicam is not dialyzable.

CLINICAL TRIALS

The use of MOBIC for the treatment of the signs and symptoms of osteoarthritis of the knee and hip was evaluated in a double-blind controlled trial in the U.S. involving 464 patients treated with MOBIC for 12 weeks. MOBIC (3.75 mg, 7.5 mg and 15 mg daily) was compared to placebo. The four primary endpoints were investigator's global assessment, patient global assessment, patient pain assessment, and total WOMAC score (a self-administered questionnaire addressing pain, function and stiffness). Patients on MOBIC 7.5 mg daily and MOBIC 15 mg daily showed significant improvement in each of these endpoints compared with placebo.

The use of MOBIC for the management of signs and symptoms of osteoarthritis was evaluated in six double-blind, active-controlled trials outside the U.S. in which a total of 9589 patients were treated for 4 weeks to 6 months. In these trials, the efficacy of MOBIC, in doses of 7.5 mg/day and 15 mg/day, was comparable to piroxicam 20 mg/day and diclofenac SR 100 mg/day and consistent with the efficacy seen in the U.S. trial.

INDICATIONS AND USAGE

MOBIC is indicated for relief of the signs and symptoms of osteoarthritis.

CONTRAINDICATIONS

MOBIC is contraindicated in patients with known hypersensitivity to meloxicam or any excipient of the product. It should not be given to patients who have experienced asthma, urticaria, or allergic-type reactions after taking aspirin or other NSAIDs. Severe, rarely fatal, anaphylactic-like reactions to NSAIDs have been reported in such patients (see WARNINGS, Anaphylactoid Reactions, and PRECAUTIONS, Pre-existing Asthma).

WARNINGS

Gastrointestinal (GI) Effects - Risk of GI Ulceration, Bleeding, and Perforation:

Serious gastrointestinal toxicity, such as inflammation, bleeding, ulceration, and perforation of the stomach, small intestine or large intestine, can occur at any time, with or without warning symptoms, in patients treated with nonsteroidal anti-inflammatory drugs (NSAIDs). Minor upper gastrointestinal problems, such as dyspepsia, are common and may also occur at any time during NSAID therapy. Therefore, physicians and patients should remain alert for ulceration and bleeding, even in the absence of previous GI symptoms. Patients should be informed about the signs and/or symptoms of serious GI toxicity and the steps to take if they occur. The utility of periodic laboratory monitoring has not been demonstrated, nor has it been adequately assessed. Only one in five patients who develop a serious upper GI adverse event on NSAID therapy is symptomatic. It has been demonstrated that upper GI ulcers, gross bleeding or perforation, caused by NSAIDs, appear to occur in approximately 1% of the patients treated for 3-6 months, and in about 2-4% of patients treated for one year. These trends continue thus, increasing the likelihood of developing a serious GI event at some time during the course of therapy. However, even short-term therapy is not without risk.

NSAIDs should be prescribed with extreme caution in those with a prior history of ulcer disease or gastrointestinal bleeding. Most spontaneous reports of fatal GI events are in elderly or debilitated patients and therefore special care should be taken in treating this population. **To minimize the potential risk for an adverse GI event, the lowest effective dose should be used for the shortest possible duration.** For high-risk patients, alternate therapies that do not involve NSAIDs should be considered.

Studies have shown that patients with a *prior history of peptic ulcer disease and/or gastrointestinal bleeding* and who use NSAIDs, have a greater than 10-fold risk for developing a GI bleed than patients with neither of these risk factors. In addition to a past history of ulcer disease, pharmacoepidemiological studies have identified several other co-therapies or co-morbid conditions that may increase the risk for GI bleeding such as: treatment with oral corticosteroids, treatment with anticoagulants, longer duration of NSAID therapy, smoking, alcoholism, older age, and poor general health status.

Anaphylactoid Reactions

As with other NSAIDs, anaphylactoid reactions have occurred in patients without known prior exposure to MOBIC. MOBIC should not be given to patients with the aspirin triad. This symptom complex typically occurs in asthmatic patients who experience rhinitis with or without nasal polyps, or who exhibit severe, potentially fatal bronchospasm after taking aspirin or other NSAIDs (see CONTRAINDICATIONS and PRECAUTIONS, Pre-existing Asthma). Emergency help should be sought in cases where an anaphylactoid reaction occurs.

Advanced Renal Disease

In cases with advanced kidney disease, treatment with MOBIC is not recommended. If NSAID therapy must be initiated, close monitoring of the patient's kidney function is advisable (see PRECAUTIONS, Renal Effects).

Pregnancy

In late pregnancy, as with other NSAIDs, MOBIC should be avoided because it may cause premature closure of the ductus arteriosus.

PRECAUTIONS

General

MOBIC cannot be expected to substitute for corticosteroids or to treat corticosteroid insufficiency. Abrupt discontinuation of corticosteroids may lead to disease exacerbation. Patients on prolonged corticosteroid therapy should have their therapy tapered slowly if a decision is made to discontinue corticosteroids.

The pharmacological activity of MOBIC in reducing inflammation and possibly fever may diminish the utility of these diagnostic signs in detecting complications of presumed noninfectious, painful conditions.

Table 2 Adverse Events (%) Occurring in ≥ 2% of MOBIC Patients in a 12-Week Osteoarthritis Placebo and Active-Controlled Trial

	Placebo	MOBIC 7.5 mg daily	MOBIC 15 mg daily	Diclofenac 100 mg daily
No. of Patients	**157**	**154**	**156**	**153**
Gastrointestinal	17.2	20.1	17.3	28.1
Abdominal Pain	2.5	1.9	2.6	1.3
Diarrhea	3.8	7.8	3.2	9.2
Dyspepsia	4.5	4.5	4.5	6.5
Flatulence	4.5	3.2	3.2	3.9
Nausea	3.2	3.9	3.8	7.2
Body as a Whole				
Accident Household	1.9	4.5	3.2	2.6
Edema[1]	2.5	1.9	4.5	3.3
Fall	0.6	2.6	0.0	1.3
Influenza-Like Symptoms	5.1	4.5	5.8	2.6
Central and Peripheral Nervous System				
Dizziness	3.2	2.6	3.8	2.0
Headache	10.2	7.8	8.3	5.9
Respiratory				
Pharyngitis	1.3	0.6	3.2	1.3
Upper Respiratory Tract Infection	1.9	3.2	1.9	3.3
Skin				
Rash[2]	2.5	2.6	0.6	2.0

[1]WHO preferred terms edema, edema dependent, edema peripheral and edema legs combined
[2]WHO preferred terms rash, rash erythematous and rash maculo-papular combined

Hepatic Effects

Borderline elevations of one or more liver tests may occur in up to 15% of patients taking NSAIDs, including MOBIC. These laboratory abnormalities may progress, may remain unchanged, or may be transient with continuing therapy. Notable elevations of ALT or AST (approximately three or more times the upper limit of normal) have been reported in approximately 1% of patients in clinical trials with NSAIDs. In addition, rare cases of severe hepatic reactions, including jaundice and fatal fulminant hepatitis, liver necrosis and hepatic failure, some of them with fatal outcomes, have been reported with NSAIDs.

Patients with signs and/or symptoms suggesting liver dysfunction, or in whom an abnormal liver test has occurred, should be evaluated for evidence of the development of a more severe hepatic reaction while on therapy with MOBIC. If clinical signs and symptoms consistent with liver disease develop, or if systemic manifestations occur (e.g., eosinophilia, rash, etc.), MOBIC should be discontinued.

Renal Effects

Caution should be used when initiating treatment with MOBIC in patients with considerable dehydration. It is advisable to rehydrate patients first and then start therapy with MOBIC. Caution is also recommended in patients with pre-existing kidney disease (see WARNINGS, Advanced Renal Disease).

Long-term administration of NSAIDs has resulted in renal papillary necrosis and other renal medullary changes. Renal toxicity has also been seen in patients in whom renal prostaglandins have a compensatory role in the maintenance of renal perfusion. In these patients, administration of NSAIDs may cause dose-dependent reduction in prostaglandin formation and, secondarily, in renal blood flow, which may precipitate overt renal decompensation. Patients at greatest risk of this reaction are those with impaired renal function, heart failure, liver dysfunction, those taking diuretics and ACE inhibitors, and the elderly. Discontinuation of NSAID therapy is usually followed by recovery to the pretreatment state.

The extent to which metabolites may accumulate in patients with renal failure has not been studied with MOBIC. Because some MOBIC metabolites are excreted by the kidney, patients with significantly impaired renal function should be more closely monitored.

Hematological Effects

Anemia is sometimes seen in patients receiving NSAIDs, including MOBIC. This may be due to fluid retention, GI blood loss, or an incompletely described effect upon erythropoiesis. Patients on long-term treatment with NSAIDs, including MOBIC, should have their hemoglobin or hematocrit checked if they exhibit any signs or symptoms of anemia.

Drugs which inhibit the biosynthesis of prostaglandins may interfere to some extent with platelet function and vascular responses to bleeding.

NSAIDs inhibit platelet aggregation and have been shown to prolong bleeding time in some patients. Unlike aspirin their effect on platelet function is quantitatively less, or of shorter duration, and reversible. MOBIC does not generally affect platelet counts, prothrombin time (PT), or partial thromboplastin time (PTT). Patients receiving MOBIC who may be adversely affected by alterations in platelet function, such as those with coagulation disorders or patients receiving anticoagulants, should be carefully monitored.

Fluid Retention and Edema

Fluid retention and edema have been observed in some patients taking NSAIDs, including MOBIC. Therefore, as with other NSAIDs, MOBIC should be used with caution in patients with fluid retention, hypertension, or heart failure.

Pre-existing Asthma

Patients with asthma may have aspirin-sensitive asthma. The use of aspirin in patients with aspirin-sensitive asthma has been associated with severe bronchospasm which can be fatal. Since cross reactivity, including bronchospasm, between aspirin and other nonsteroidal anti-inflammatory drugs has been reported in such aspirin-sensitive patients, MOBIC should not be administered to patients with this form of aspirin sensitivity and should be used with caution in patients with pre-existing asthma.

Information for Patients

MOBIC, like other drugs of its class, can cause discomfort and, rarely, more serious side effects, such as gastrointestinal bleeding, which may result in hospitalization and even fatal outcomes. Although serious GI tract ulcerations and bleeding can occur without warning symptoms, patients should be alert for the signs and symptoms of ulcerations and bleeding, and should ask for medical advice when observing any indicative signs or symptoms. Patients should be made aware of the importance of this follow-up (see WARNINGS, Gastrointestinal (GI) Effects - Risk of GI Ulceration, Bleeding and Perforation).

Patients should report to their physicians signs or symptoms of gastrointestinal ulceration or bleeding, skin rash, weight gain, or edema.

Patients should be informed of the warning signs and symptoms of hepatotoxicity (e.g., nausea, fatigue, lethargy, pruritus, jaundice, right upper quadrant tenderness, and "flu-like" symptoms). If these occur, patients should be instructed to stop therapy and seek immediate medical therapy.

Patients should also be instructed to seek immediate emergency help in the case of an anaphylactoid reaction (see WARNINGS, Anaphylactoid Reactions).

In late pregnancy, as with other NSAIDs, MOBIC should be avoided because it may cause premature closure of the ductus arteriosus.

Laboratory Tests

Patients on long-term treatment with NSAIDs should have their CBC and a chemistry profile checked periodically. If clinical signs and symptoms consistent with liver or renal disease develop, systemic manifestations occur (e.g., eosinophilia, rash, etc.) or if abnormal liver tests persist or worsen, MOBIC should be discontinued.

Drug Interactions

ACE inhibitors

Reports suggest that NSAIDs may diminish the antihypertensive effect of angiotensin-converting enzyme (ACE) inhibitors. This interaction should be given consideration in patients taking NSAIDs concomitantly with ACE inhibitors.

Aspirin

Concomitant administration of aspirin (1000 mg TID) to healthy volunteers tended to increase the AUC (10%) and C_{max} (24%) of meloxicam. The clinical significance of this interaction is not known; however, as with other NSAIDs, concomitant administration of meloxicam and aspirin is not generally recommended because of the potential for increased adverse effects. Concomitant administration of low-dose aspirin with MOBIC may result in an increased rate of GI ulceration or other complications, compared to use of MOBIC alone. MOBIC is not a substitute for aspirin for cardiovascular prophylaxis.

Cholestyramine

Pretreatment for four days with cholestyramine significantly increased the clearance of meloxicam by 50%. This

Continued on next page

Mobic—Cont.

resulted in a decrease in $t_{1/2}$, from 19.2 hours to 12.5 hours, and a 35% reduction in AUC. This suggests the existence of a recirculation pathway for meloxicam in the gastrointestinal tract. The clinical relevance of this interaction has not been established.

Cimetidine

Concomitant administration of 200 mg cimetidine QID did not alter the single-dose pharmacokinetics of 30 mg meloxicam.

Digoxin

Meloxicam 15 mg once daily for 7 days did not alter the plasma concentration profile of digoxin after β-acetyldigoxin administration for 7 days at clinical doses. *In vitro* testing found no protein binding drug interaction between digoxin and meloxicam.

Furosemide

Clinical studies, as well as post-marketing observations, have shown that NSAIDs can reduce the natriuretic effect of furosemide and thiazide diuretics in some patients. This effect has been attributed to inhibition of renal prostaglandin synthesis. Studies with furosemide agents and meloxicam have not demonstrated a reduction in natriuretic effect. Furosemide single and multiple dose pharmacodynamics and pharmacokinetics are not affected by multiple doses of meloxicam. Nevertheless, during concomitant therapy with furosemide and MOBIC, patients should be observed closely for signs of declining renal function (see PRECAUTIONS, Renal Effects), as well as to assure diuretic efficacy.

Lithium

In clinical trials, NSAIDs have produced an elevation of plasma lithium levels and a reduction in renal lithium clearance. In a study conducted in healthy subjects, mean pre-dose lithium concentration and AUC were increased by 21% in subjects receiving lithium doses ranging from 804 to 1072 mg BID with meloxicam 15 mg QD as compared to subjects receiving lithium alone. These effects have been attributed to inhibition of renal prostaglandin synthesis by MOBIC. Patients on lithium treatment should be closely monitored when MOBIC is introduced, adjusted, or withdrawn.

Methotrexate

A study in 13 rheumatoid arthritis (RA) patients evaluated the effects of multiple doses of meloxicam on the pharmacokinetics of methotrexate taken once weekly. Meloxicam did not have a significant effect on the pharmacokinetics of single doses of methotrexate. *In vitro*, methotrexate did not displace meloxicam from its human serum binding sites.

Warfarin

Anticoagulant activity should be monitored, particularly in the first few days after initiating or changing MOBIC therapy in patients receiving warfarin or similar agents, since these patients are at an increased risk of bleeding. The effect of meloxicam on the anticoagulant effect of warfarin was studied in a group of healthy subjects receiving daily doses of warfarin that produced an INR (International Normalized Ratio) between 1.2 and 1.8. In these subjects, meloxicam did not alter warfarin pharmacokinetics and the average anticoagulant effect of warfarin as determined by prothrombin time. However, one subject showed an increase in INR from 1.5 to 2.1. Caution should be used when administering MOBIC with warfarin since patients on warfarin may experience changes in INR and an increased risk of bleeding complications when a new medication is introduced.

Carcinogenesis, Mutagenesis, Impairment of Fertility

No carcinogenic effect of meloxicam was observed in rats given oral doses up to 0.8 mg/kg/day (approximately 0.4-fold the human dose at 15 mg/day for a 50 kg adult based on body surface area conversion) for 104 weeks or in mice given oral doses up to 8.0 mg/kg/day (approximately 2.2-fold the human dose, as noted above) for 99 weeks.

Meloxicam was not mutagenic in an Ames assay, or clastogenic in a chromosome aberration assay with human lymphocytes and an *in vivo* micronucleus test in mouse bone marrow.

Meloxicam did not impair male and female fertility in rats at oral doses up to 9 and 5 mg/kg/day, respectively (4.9-fold and 2.5-fold the human dose, as noted above). However, an increased incidence of embryolethality at oral doses ≥ 1 mg/kg/day (0.5-fold the human dose, as noted above) was observed in rats when dams were given meloxicam 2 weeks prior to mating and during early embryonic development.

Pregnancy

Teratogenic Effects: Pregnancy Category C.

Meloxicam caused an increased incidence of septal defect of the heart, a rare event, at an oral dose of 60 mg/kg/day (64.5-fold the human dose at 15 mg/day for a 50 kg adult based on body surface area conversion) and embryolethality at oral doses ≥ 5 mg/kg/day (5.4-fold the human dose, as noted above) when rabbits were treated throughout organogenesis. Meloxicam was not teratogenic in rats up to an oral dose of 4 mg/kg/day (approximately 2.2-fold the human dose, as noted above) throughout organogenesis. An increased incidence of stillbirths was observed when rats were given oral doses ≥ 1 mg/kg/day throughout organogenesis. Meloxicam crosses the placental barrier. There are no adequate and well-controlled studies in pregnant women. MOBIC should be used during pregnancy only if the potential benefit justifies the potential risk to the fetus.

Table 3 Adverse Events (%) Occurring in ≥ 2% of MOBIC Patients in 4 to 6 Weeks and 6 Month Active-Controlled Osteoarthritis Trials

	4–6 Weeks Controlled Trials		6 Month Controlled Trials	
	MOBIC 7.5 mg daily	MOBIC 15 mg daily	MOBIC 7.5 mg daily	MOBIC 15 mg daily
No. of Patients	8955	256	169	306
Gastrointestinal	11.8	18.0	26.6	24.2
Abdominal Pain	2.7	2.3	4.7	2.9
Constipation	0.8	1.2	1.8	2.6
Diarrhea	1.9	2.7	5.9	2.6
Dyspepsia	3.8	7.4	8.9	9.5
Flatulence	0.5	0.4	3.0	2.6
Nausea	2.4	4.7	4.7	7.2
Vomiting	0.6	0.8	1.8	2.6
Body as a Whole				
Edema[1]	0.6	2.0	2.4	1.6
Pain	0.9	2.0	3.6	5.2
Central and Peripheral Nervous System				
Dizziness	1.1	1.6	2.4	2.6
Headache	2.4	2.7	3.6	2.6
Hematologic				
Anemia	0.1	0.0	4.1	2.9
Musculo-Skeletal				
Arthralgia	0.5	0.0	5.3	1.3
Back Pain	0.5	0.4	3.0	0.7
Psychiatric				
Insomnia	0.4	0.0	3.6	1.6
Respiratory				
Coughing	0.2	0.8	2.4	1.0
Upper Respiratory Tract Infection	0.2	0.0	8.3	7.5
Skin				
Pruritus	0.4	1.2	2.4	0.0
Rash[2]	0.3	1.2	3.0	1.3
Urinary				
Micturition Frequency	0.1	0.4	2.4	1.3
Urinary Tract Infection	0.3	0.4	4.7	6.9

[1]WHO preferred terms edema, edema dependent, edema peripheral and edema legs combined
[2]WHO preferred terms rash, rash erythematous and rash maculo-papular combined

Body as a Whole:	allergic reaction, *anaphylactoid reactions including shock,* face edema, fatigue, fever, hot flushes, malaise, syncope, weight decrease, weight increase
Cardiovascular:	angina pectoris, cardiac failure, hypertension, hypotension, myocardial infarction, vasculitis
Central and Peripheral Nervous System:	convulsions, paresthesia, tremor, vertigo
Gastrointestinal:	colitis, dry mouth, duodenal ulcer, eructation, esophagitis, gastric ulcer, gastritis, gastroesophageal reflux, gastrointestinal hemorrhage, hematemesis, hemorrhagic duodenal ulcer, hemorrhagic gastric ulcer, intestinal perforation, melena, pancreatitis, perforated duodenal ulcer, perforated gastric ulcer, stomatitis ulcerative
Heart Rate and Rhythm:	arrhythmia, palpitation, tachycardia
Hematologic:	*agranulocytosis,* leukopenia, purpura, thrombocytopenia
Liver and Biliary System:	ALT increased, AST increased, bilirubinemia, GGT increased, hepatitis, *jaundice, liver failure*
Metabolic and Nutritional:	dehydration
Psychiatric Disorders:	abnormal dreaming, anxiety, appetite increased, confusion, depression, nervousness, somnolence
Respiratory:	asthma, bronchospasm, dyspnea
Skin and Appendages:	alopecia, angioedema, bullous eruption, *erythema multiforme,* photosensitivity reaction, pruritus, *Stevens-Johnson syndrome,* sweating increased, *toxic epidermal necrolysis,* urticaria
Special Senses:	abnormal vision, conjunctivitis, taste perversion, tinnitus
Urinary System:	albuminuria, BUN increased, creatinine increased, hematuria, *interstitial nephritis,* renal failure

Nonteratogenic Effects:

Meloxicam caused a reduction in birth index, live births, and neonatal survival at oral doses ≥ 0.125 mg/kg/day (approximately 0.07-fold the human dose at 15 mg/day for a 50 kg adult based on body surface area conversion) when rats were treated during the late gestation and lactation period. No studies have been conducted to evaluate the effect of meloxicam on the closure of the ductus arteriosus in humans; use of meloxicam during the third trimester of pregnancy should be avoided.

Labor and Delivery

Studies in rats with meloxicam, as with other drugs known to inhibit prostaglandin synthesis, showed an increased incidence of stillbirths, increased length of delivery time, and delayed parturition at oral dosages ≥ 1 mg/kg/day (approximately 0.5-fold the human dose at 15 mg/day for a 50 kg adult based on body surface area conversion), and decreased pup survival at an oral dose of 4 mg/kg/day (approximately 2.1-fold the human dose, as noted above) throughout organogenesis. Similar findings were observed in rats receiving oral dosages ≥ 0.125 mg/kg/day (approximately 0.07-fold the human dose, as noted above) during late gestation and the lactation period.

Nursing Mothers

Studies of meloxicam excretion in human milk have not been conducted; however, meloxicam was excreted in the milk of lactating rats at concentrations higher than those in plasma. Because of the potential for serious adverse reactions in nursing infants from MOBIC, a decision should be made whether to discontinue nursing or to discontinue the drug, taking into account the importance of the drug to the mother.

Pediatric Use

Safety and effectiveness in pediatric patients under 18 years of age have not been established.

Geriatric Use

As with any NSAID, caution should be exercised in treating the elderly (65 years and older).

ADVERSE REACTIONS

The MOBIC phase 2/3 clinical trial database includes 10,122 patients treated with MOBIC 7.5 mg/day and 3,505 patients treated with MOBIC 15 mg/day. MOBIC at these doses was administered to 661 patients for at least 6 months and to 312 patients for at least one year. Approximately 10,500 of these patients were treated in ten placebo and/or active-controlled osteoarthritis trials. Gastrointestinal (GI) adverse events were the most frequently reported adverse events in all treatment groups across MOBIC trials.

A 12-week multicenter, double-blind, randomized trial was conducted in patients with osteoarthritis of the knee or hip to compare the efficacy and safety of MOBIC with placebo and with an active control. Table 2 depicts adverse events that occurred in ≥ 2% of the MOBIC treatment groups.

[See table 2 at top of page 1007]

The adverse events that occurred with MOBIC in ≥ 2% of patients treated short-term (4-6 weeks) and long-term (6 months) in active-controlled osteoarthritis trials are presented in Table 3.

[See table 3 at top of previous page]

As with other NSAIDs, higher doses of MOBIC (e.g., chronic daily 30 mg dose) were associated with an increased risk of serious GI events, therefore the daily dose of MOBIC should not exceed 15 mg.

The following is a list of adverse drug reactions occurring in < 2% of patients receiving MOBIC in clinical trials involving approximately 15,400 patients. Adverse reactions reported only in worldwide post-marketing experience or the literature are shown in italics and are considered rare (< 0.1%).

[See second table on previous page]

OVERDOSAGE

There is limited experience with meloxicam overdose. Four cases have taken 6 to 11 times the highest recommended dose; all recovered. Cholestyramine is known to accelerate the clearance of meloxicam.

Symptoms following acute NSAID overdose are usually limited to lethargy, drowsiness, nausea, vomiting, and epigastric pain, which are generally reversible with supportive care. Gastrointestinal bleeding can occur. Severe poisoning may result in hypertension, acute renal failure, hepatic dysfunction, respiratory depression, coma, convulsions, cardiovascular collapse, and cardiac arrest. Anaphylactoid reactions have been reported with therapeutic ingestion of NSAIDs, and may occur following an overdose.

Patients should be managed with symptomatic and supportive care following an NSAID overdose. In cases of acute overdose, gastric lavage followed by activated charcoal is recommended. Gastric lavage performed more than one hour after overdose has little benefit in the treatment of overdose. Administration of activated charcoal is recommended for patients who present 1-2 hours after overdose. For substantial overdose or severely symptomatic patients, activated charcoal may be administered repeatedly.

Accelerated removal of meloxicam by 4 g oral doses of cholestyramine given three times a day was demonstrated in a clinical trial. Administration of cholestyramine may be useful following an overdose. Forced diuresis, alkalinization of urine, hemodialysis, or hemoperfusion may not be useful due to high protein binding.

DOSAGE AND ADMINISTRATION

The lowest dose of MOBIC should be sought for each patient. For the treatment of osteoarthritis the recommended starting and maintenance oral dose of MOBIC is 7.5 mg once daily. Some patients may receive additional benefit by increasing the dose to 15 mg once daily. The maximum recommended daily oral dose of MOBIC is 15 mg.

MOBIC may be taken without regard to timing of meals.

HOW SUPPLIED

MOBIC is available as a pastel yellow, round, biconvex, uncoated tablet containing meloxicam 7.5 mg or as a pastel yellow, oblong, biconvex, uncoated tablet containing meloxicam 15 mg. The 7.5 mg tablet is impressed with the Boehringer Ingelheim logo on one side, and on the other side, the letter "M". The 15 mg tablet is impressed with the tablet code "15" on one side and the letter "M" on the other.

MOBIC Tablets 7.5 mg are available as follows:

NDC 0597-0029-30; Bottles of 30
NDC 0597-0029-01; Bottles of 100

MOBIC Tablets 15 mg are available as follows:

NDC 0597-0030-01; Bottles of 100

Store at 25°C (77°F); excursions permitted to 15°C-30°C (59°F-86°F). Keep in a dry place.

Dispense in a tight container.

℞ only

Mobic Tablets 7.5 mg and 15 mg

Manufactured by:
Boehringer Ingelheim Pharma GmbH & Co. KG
Ingelheim, Germany
and
Boehringer Ingelheim Promeco
S.A. de C.V., Mexico City, Mexico

Marketed by:
Boehringer Ingelheim Pharmaceuticals, Inc.
Ridgefield, CT 06877 USA
and
Abbott Laboratories
North Chicago, IL 60064 USA
Licensed from:
Boehringer Ingelheim International GmbH

4057500/10 4057500/10
Rev. January 15, 2003
Shown in Product Identification Guide, page 309

PERSANTINE® ℞

[*pər'săn-tīn*]

(dipyridamole USP)

25 mg, 50 mg, and 75 mg tablets

Prescribing Information

DESCRIPTION

PERSANTINE® (dipyridamole USP) is a platelet inhibitor chemically described as 2,2′,2″,2‴-[(4,8-Dipiperidinopyrimido[5,4-*d*]pyrimidine-2,6-diyl)dinitrilo]-tetraethanol. It has the following structural formula:

$C_{24}H_{40}N_8O_4$ Mol. Wt. 504.63

Dipyridamole is an odorless-yellow crystalline powder, having a bitter taste. It is soluble in dilute acids, methanol and chloroform, and practically insoluble in water.

PERSANTINE tablets for oral administration contain:

Active Ingredient *TABLETS 25 mg, 50 mg, and 75 mg*: dipyridamole USP 25 mg, 50 mg and 75 mg, respectively.

Inactive Ingredients *TABLETS 25 mg, 50 mg, and 75 mg*: acacia, carnauba wax, corn starch, edible white ink, lactose monohydrate, magnesium stearate, Opalux® AS-2578 orange, polyethylene glycol, povidone, sucrose, talc, titanium dioxide, and white wax.

CLINICAL PHARMACOLOGY

It is believed that platelet reactivity and interaction with prosthetic cardiac valve surfaces, resulting in abnormally shortened platelet survival time, is a significant factor in thromboembolic complications occurring in connection with prosthetic heart valve replacement.

PERSANTINE (dipyridamole USP) tablets have been found to lengthen abnormally shortened platelet survival time in a dose-dependent manner.

In three randomized controlled clinical trials involving 854 patients who had undergone surgical placement of a prosthetic heart valve, PERSANTINE tablets, in combination with warfarin, decreased the incidence of postoperative thromboembolic events by 62 to 91% compared to warfarin treatment alone. The incidence of thromboembolic events in patients receiving the combination of PERSANTINE tablets and warfarin ranged from 1.2 to 1.8%. In three additional studies involving 392 patients taking PERSANTINE tablets and coumarin-like anticoagulants, the incidence of thromboembolic events ranged from 2.3 to 6.9%.

In these trials, the coumarin anticoagulant was begun between 24 hours and 4 days postoperatively, and the PERSANTINE tablets were begun between 24 hours and 10 days postoperatively. The length of follow-up in these trials varied from 1 to 2 years.

PERSANTINE tablets do not influence prothrombin time or activity measurements when administered with warfarin.

Mechanism of Action

Dipyridamole inhibits the uptake of adenosine into platelets, endothelial cells and erythrocytes *in vitro* and *in vivo*; the inhibition occurs in a dose-dependent manner at therapeutic concentrations (0.5–1.9 µg/mL). This inhibition results in an increase in local concentrations of adenosine which acts on the platelet A_2-receptor thereby stimulating platelet adenylate cyclase and increasing platelet cyclic-3′,5′-adenosine monophosphate (cAMP) levels. Via this mechanism, platelet aggregation is inhibited in response to various stimuli such as platelet activating factor (PAF), collagen and adenosine diphosphate (ADP).

Dipyridamole inhibits phosphodiesterase (PDE) in various tissues. While the inhibition of cAMP-PDE is weak, therapeutic levels of dipyridamole inhibit cyclic-3′,5′-guanosine monophosphate-PDE (cGMP-PDE), thereby augmenting the increase in cGMP produced by EDRF (endothelium-derived relaxing factor, now identified as nitric oxide).

Hemodynamics

In dogs intraduodenal doses of dipyridamole of 0.5 to 4.0 mg/kg produced dose-related decreases in systemic and coronary vascular resistance leading to decreases in systemic blood pressure and increases in coronary blood flow. Onset of action was in about 24 minutes and effects persisted for about 3 hours.

Similar effects were observed following IV PERSANTINE® in doses ranging from 0.025 to 2.0 mg/kg.

In man the same qualitative hemodynamic effects have been observed. However, acute intravenous administration of PERSANTINE may worsen regional myocardial perfusion distal to partial occlusion of coronary arteries.

Pharmacokinetics and Metabolism

Following an oral dose of PERSANTINE tablets, the average time to peak concentration is about 75 minutes. The decline in plasma concentration following a dose of PERSANTINE tablets fits a two-compartment model. The alpha half-life (the initial decline following peak concentration) is approximately 40 minutes. The beta half-life (the terminal decline in plasma concentration) is approximately 10 hours. Dipyridamole is highly bound to plasma proteins. It is metabolized in the liver where it is conjugated as a glucuronide and excreted with the bile.

INDICATIONS AND USAGE

PERSANTINE (dipyridamole USP) tablets are indicated as an adjunct to coumarin anticoagulants in the prevention of postoperative thromboembolic complications of cardiac valve replacement.

CONTRAINDICATIONS

Hypersensitivity to dipyridamole and any of the other components.

PRECAUTIONS

General

Coronary Artery Disease: Dipyridamole has a vasodilatory effect and should be used with caution in patients with severe coronary artery disease (e.g., unstable angina or recently sustained myocardial infarction). Chest pain may be aggravated in patients with underlying coronary artery disease who are receiving dipyridamole.

Hepatic Insufficiency: Elevations of hepatic enzymes and hepatic failure have been reported in association with dipyridamole administration.

Hypotension: Dipyridamole should be used with caution in patients with hypotension since it can produce peripheral vasodilation.

Laboratory Tests

Dipyridamole has been associated with elevated hepatic enzymes.

Drug Interactions

No pharmacokinetic drug-drug interaction studies were conducted with PERSANTINE® (dipyridamole USP) Tablets. The following information was obtained from the literature.

Adenosine: Dipyridamole has been reported to increase the plasma levels and cardiovascular effects of adenosine. Adjustment of adenosine dosage may be necessary.

Cholinesterase Inhibitors: Dipyridamole may counteract the anticholinesterase effect of cholinesterase inhibitors, thereby potentially aggravating myasthenia gravis.

Carcinogenesis, Mutagenesis, Impairment of Fertility

In studies in which dipyridamole was administered in the feed to mice (up to 111 weeks in males and females) and rats (up to 128 weeks in males and up to 142 weeks in females), there was no evidence of drug-related carcinogenesis. The highest dose administered in these studies (75 mg/kg/day) was, on a mg/m^2 basis, about equivalent to the maximum recommended daily human oral dose (MRHD) in mice and about twice the MRHD in rats. Mutagenicity tests of dipyridamole with bacterial and mammalian cell systems were negative. There was no evidence of impaired fertility when dipyridamole was administered to male and female rats at oral doses up to 500 mg/kg/day (about 12 times the MRHD on a mg/m^2 basis). A significant reduction in number of corpora lutea with consequent reduction in implantations and live fetuses was, however, observed at 1250 mg/kg (more than 30 times the MRHD on a mg/m^2 basis).

Pregnancy

Teratogenic Effects: PREGNANCY CATEGORY B.

Reproduction studies have been performed in mice, rabbits and rats at oral dipyridamole doses up of up to 125 mg/kg, 40 mg/kg and 1000 mg/kg, respectively (about 1 ½, 2 and 25 times the maximum recommended daily human oral dose, respectively, on a mg/m^2 basis) and have revealed no evidence of harm to the fetus due to dipyridamole. There are, however, no adequate and well-controlled studies in pregnant women. Because animal reproduction studies are not always predictive of human response, PERSANTINE should be used during pregnancy only if clearly needed.

Nursing Mothers

As dipyridamole is excreted in human milk, caution should be exercised when PERSANTINE tablets are administered to a nursing woman.

Continued on next page

Persantine—Cont.

Pediatric Use
Safety and effectiveness in the pediatric population below the age of 12 years have not been established.

ADVERSE REACTIONS

Adverse reactions at therapeutic doses are usually minimal and transient. On long-term use of PERSANTINE (dipyridamole USP) tablets initial side effects usually disappear. The following reactions in Table 1 were reported in two heart valve replacement trials comparing PERSANTINE tablets and warfarin therapy to either warfarin alone or warfarin and placebo:

Table 1 **Adverse Reactions Reported in 2 Heart Valve Replacement Trials**

Adverse Reaction	PERSANTINE Tablets/ Warfarin	Placebo/ Warfarin
Number of patients	147	170
Dizziness	13.6%	8.2%
Abdominal distress	6.1%	3.5%
Headache	2.3%	0.0%
Rash	2.3%	1.1%

Other reactions from uncontrolled studies include diarrhea, vomiting, flushing and pruritus. In addition, angina pectoris has been reported rarely and there have been rare reports of liver dysfunction. On those uncommon occasions when adverse reactions have been persistent or intolerable, they have ceased on withdrawal of the medication.

When PERSANTINE tablets were administered concomitantly with warfarin, bleeding was no greater in frequency or severity than that observed when warfarin was administered alone.

In post-marketing reporting experience, there have been rare reports of hypersensitivity reactions (such as rash, urticaria, severe bronchospasm, and angioedema), larynx edema, fatigue, malaise, myalgia, arthritis, nausea, dyspepsia, paresthesia, hepatitis, thrombocytopenia, alopecia, cholelithiasis, hypotension, palpitation, and tachycardia.

OVERDOSAGE

In case of real or suspected overdose, seek medical attention or contact a Poison Control Center immediately. Careful medical management is essential. Based upon the known hemodynamic effects of dipyridamole, symptoms such as warm feeling, flushes, sweating, restlessness, feeling of weakness and dizziness may occur. A drop in blood pressure and tachycardia might also be observed.

Symptomatic treatment is recommended, possibly including a vasopressor drug. Gastric lavage should be considered. Administration of xanthine derivatives (e.g., aminophylline) may reverse the haemodynamic effects of dipyridamole overdose. Since dipyridamole is highly protein bound, dialysis is not likely to be of benefit.

DOSAGE AND ADMINISTRATION

Adjunctive Use in Prophylaxis of Thromboembolism after Cardiac Valve Replacement. The recommended dose is 75-100 mg four times daily as an adjunct to the usual warfarin therapy. Please note that aspirin is not to be administered concomitantly with coumarin anticoagulants.

HOW SUPPLIED

PERSANTINE (dipyridamole USP) tablets are available as round, orange, sugar-coated tablets of 25 mg, 50 mg and 75 mg coded BI/17, BI/18 and BI/19, respectively.

They are available in bottles of 100 tablets as indicated below:

25 mg Tablets	(NDC 0597-0017-01)
50 mg Tablets	(NDC 0597-0018-01)
75 mg Tablets	(NDC 0597-0019-01)

Store at 25°C (77°F); excursions permitted to 15-30°C (59°-86°F) [see USP Controlled Room Temperature]. Keep out of reach of children.
Rx only

Distributed by:
Boehringer Ingelheim Pharmaceuticals, Inc.
Ridgefield, CT 06877 USA

Licensed from:
Boehringer Ingelheim
International GmbH

Manufactured by:
Boehringer Ingelheim Promeco, S.A. de C.V.
Mexico City, Mexico

340067/US/5 Revised 05/14/03
Shown in Product Identification Guide, page 309

SPIRIVA® HANDIHALER® ℞

[spĭ-rī-vă]
(tiotropium bromide inhalation powder)
For Oral Inhalation Only

Prescribing Information

DESCRIPTION

SPIRIVA® HandiHaler® (tiotropium bromide inhalation powder) consists of a capsule dosage form containing a dry powder formulation of SPIRIVA (tiotropium bromide) intended for oral inhalation only with the HandiHaler inhalation device.
Each light green, hard gelatin capsule contains 18 mcg tiotropium (equivalent to 22.5 mcg tiotropium bromide monohydrate) blended with lactose monohydrate as the carrier.
The dry powder formulation within the capsule is intended for oral inhalation only.
The active component of SPIRIVA is tiotropium. The drug substance, tiotropium bromide monohydrate, is an anticholinergic with specificity for muscarinic receptors. It is chemically described as (1α, 2β, 4β, 5α, 7β)-7-[(Hydroxydi-2-thienylacetyl)oxy]-9,9-dimethyl-3-oxa-9-azoniatricyclo [3.3.1.0^{2,4}]nonane bromide monohydrate. It is a synthetic, non-chiral, quaternary ammonium compound. Tiotropium bromide is a white or yellowish white powder. It is sparingly soluble in water and soluble in methanol.
The structural formula is:

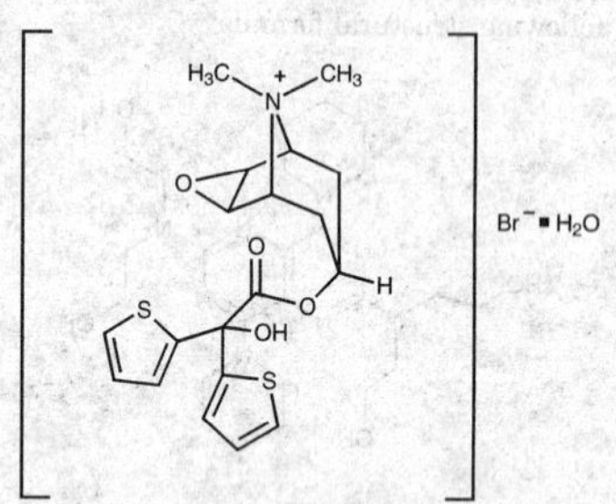

Tiotropium bromide (monohydrate) has a molecular mass of 490.4 and a molecular formula of $C_{19}H_{22}NO_4S_2Br \bullet H_2O$.
The HandiHaler is an inhalation device used to inhale the dry powder contained in the SPIRIVA capsule. The dry powder is delivered from the HandiHaler device at flow rates as low as 20 L/min. Under standardized *in vitro* testing, the HandiHaler device delivers a mean of 10.4 mcg tiotropium when tested at a flow rate of 39 L/min for 3.1 seconds (2L total). In a study of 26 adult patients with chronic obstructive pulmonary disease (COPD) and severely compromised lung function [mean FEV_1 1.02 L (range 0.45 to 2.24 L); 37.6% of predicted (range 16%–65%)], the median peak inspiratory flow (PIF) through the HandiHaler device was 30.0 L/min (range 20.4 to 45.6 L/min). The amount of drug delivered to the lungs will vary depending on patient factors such as inspiratory flow and peak inspiratory flow through the HandiHaler device, which may vary from patient to patient, and may vary with the exposure time of the capsule outside the blister pack.
For administration of SPIRIVA, a capsule is placed into the center chamber of the HandiHaler device. The capsule is pierced by pressing and releasing the button on the side of the inhalation device. The tiotropium formulation is dispersed into the air stream when the patient inhales through the mouthpiece. (see **Patient's Instructions For Use**)

CLINICAL PHARMACOLOGY

Mechanism of Action
Tiotropium is a long-acting, antimuscarinic agent, which is often referred to as an anticholinergic. It has similar affinity to the subtypes of muscarinic receptors, M_1 to M_5. In the airways, it exhibits pharmacological effects through inhibition of M_3-receptors at the smooth muscle leading to bronchodilation. The competitive and reversible nature of antagonism was shown with human and animal origin receptors and isolated organ preparations. In preclinical *in vitro* as well as *in vivo* studies prevention of methacholine-induced bronchoconstriction effects were dose-dependent and lasted longer than 24 hours. The bronchodilation following inhalation of tiotropium is predominantly a site-specific effect.

Pharmacokinetics
Tiotropium is administered by dry powder inhalation. In common with other inhaled drugs, the majority of the delivered dose is deposited in the gastrointestinal tract and, to a lesser extent, in the lung, the intended organ. Many of the pharmacokinetic data described below were obtained with higher doses than recommended for therapy.

Absorption:
Following dry powder inhalation by young healthy volunteers, the absolute bioavailability of 19.5% suggests that the fraction reaching the lung is highly bioavailable. It is expected from the chemical structure of the compound (quaternary ammonium compound) that tiotropium is poorly absorbed from the gastrointestinal tract. Food is not expected to influence the absorption of tiotropium for the same reason. Oral solutions of tiotropium have an absolute bioavailability of 2–3%. Maximum tiotropium plasma concentrations were observed five minutes after inhalation.

Distribution:
Tiotropium shows a volume of distribution of 32 L/kg indicating that the drug binds extensively to tissues. The drug is bound by 72% to plasma proteins. At steady state, peak tiotropium plasma levels in COPD patients were 17–19 pg/mL when measured 5 minutes after dry powder inhalation of an 18 mcg dose and decreased rapidly in a multi-compartmental manner. Steady state trough plasma concentrations were 3–4 pg/mL. Local concentrations in the lung are not known, but the mode of administration suggests substantially higher concentrations in the lung. Studies in rats have shown that tiotropium does not readily penetrate the blood-brain barrier.

Biotransformation:
The extent of biotransformation appears to be small. This is evident from a urinary excretion of 74% of unchanged substance after an intravenous dose to young healthy volunteers. Tiotropium, an ester, is nonenzymatically cleaved to the alcohol *N*-methylscopine and dithienylglycolic acid, neither of which bind to muscarinic receptors.
In vitro experiments with human liver microsomes and human hepatocytes suggest that a fraction of the administered dose (74% of an intravenous dose is excreted unchanged in the urine, leaving 25% for metabolism) is metabolized by cytochrome P450-dependent oxidation and subsequent glutathione conjugation to a variety of Phase II metabolites. This enzymatic pathway can be inhibited by CYP450 2D6 and 3A4 inhibitors, such as quinidine, ketoconazole, and gestodene. Thus, CYP450 2D6 and 3A4 are involved in the metabolic pathway that is responsible for the elimination of a small part of the administered dose. *In vitro* studies using human liver microsomes showed that tiotropium in supra-therapeutic concentrations does not inhibit CYP450 1A1, 1A2, 2B6, 2C9, 2C19, 2D6, 2E1, or 3A4.

Elimination:
The terminal elimination half-life of tiotropium is between 5 and 6 days following inhalation. Total clearance was 880 mL/min after an intravenous dose in young healthy volunteers with an inter-individual variability of 22%. Intravenously administered tiotropium is mainly excreted unchanged in urine (74%). After dry powder inhalation, urinary excretion is 14% of the dose, the remainder being mainly non-absorbed drug in the gut which is eliminated via the feces. The renal clearance of tiotropium exceeds the creatinine clearance, indicating active secretion into the urine. After chronic once-daily inhalation by COPD patients, pharmacokinetic steady state was reached after 2–3 weeks with no accumulation thereafter.

Drug Interactions:
An interaction study with tiotropium (14.4 mcg intravenous infusion over 15 minutes) and cimetidine 400 mg three times daily or ranitidine 300 mg once daily was conducted. Concomitant administration of cimetidine with tiotropium resulted in a 20% increase in the AUC_{0-4h}, a 28% decrease in the renal clearance of tiotropium and no significant change in the C_{max} and amount excreted in urine over 96 hours. Co-administration of tiotropium with ranitidine did not affect the pharmacokinetics of tiotropium. Therefore, no clinically significant interaction occurred between tiotropium and cimetidine or ranitidine.

Electrophysiology:
In a multicenter, randomized, double-blind trial that enrolled 198 patients with COPD, the number of subjects with changes from baseline-corrected QT interval of 30–60 msec was higher in the SPIRIVA group as compared with placebo. This difference was apparent using both the Bazett (QTcB) [20 (20%) patient vs. 12 (12%) patients] and Fredericia (QTcF) [16 (16%) patients vs. 1 (1%) patient] corrections of QT for heart rate. No patients in either group had either QTcB or QTcF of >500 msec. Other clinical studies with SPIRIVA did not detect an effect of the drug on QTc intervals.

Special Populations:
Elderly Patients:
As expected for drugs predominantly excreted renally, advanced age was associated with a decrease of tiotropium renal clearance (326 mL/min in COPD patients <58 years to 163 mL/min in COPD patients >70 years), which may be explained by decreased renal function. Tiotropium excretion in urine after inhalation decreased from 14% (young healthy volunteers) to about 7% (COPD patients). Plasma concentrations were numerically increased with advancing age within COPD patients (43% increase in AUC_{0-4} after dry powder inhalation), which was not significant when considered in relation to inter- and intra-individual variability. (See **DOSAGE AND ADMINISTRATION SECTION**)
Hepatically-impaired Patients:
The effects of hepatic impairment on the pharmacokinetics of tiotropium were not studied. However, hepatic insufficiency is not expected to have relevant influence on tiotropium pharmacokinetics. Tiotropium is predominantly cleared by renal elimination (74% in young healthy volunteers) and by simple non-enzymatic ester cleavage to products that do not bind to muscarinic receptors. (See **DOSAGE AND ADMINISTRATION SECTION**)
Renally-impaired Patients:
Since tiotropium is predominantly renally excreted, renal impairment was associated with increased plasma drug concentrations and reduced drug clearance after both intravenous infusion and dry powder inhalation. Mild renal impairment (CrCl 50–80 mL/min), which is often seen in elderly patients, increased tiotropium plasma concentrations (39% increase in AUC_{0-4} after intravenous infusion). In COPD patients with moderate to severe renal impairment

(CrCl <50 mL/min), the intravenous administration of tiotropium resulted in doubling of the plasma concentrations (82% increase in AUC_{0-4}), which was confirmed by plasma concentrations after dry powder inhalation. (See **DOSAGE AND ADMINISTRATION** and **PRECAUTIONS Sections**)

CLINICAL STUDIES

The SPIRIVA HandiHaler clinical development program consisted of six phase 3 studies in 2,663 patients with COPD (1,308 receiving SPIRIVA): two 1-year, placebo-controlled studies, two 6-month, placebo-controlled studies and two 1-year, ipratropium-controlled studies. These studies enrolled patients who had a clinical diagnosis of COPD, were 40 years of age or older, had a history of smoking greater than 10 pack-years, had an FEV_1 less than or equal to 60 or 65% of predicted, and a ratio of FEV_1/FVC of less than or equal to 0.7.

In these studies, SPIRIVA, administered once-daily in the morning, provided improvement in lung function (forced expiratory volume in one second, FEV_1), with peak effect occurring within 3 hours following the first dose.

In the 1-year, placebo controlled trials, the mean improvement in FEV_1 at 30 minutes was 0.13 liters (13%) with a peak improvement of 0.24 liters (24%) relative to baseline after the first dose (day 1). Further improvements in FEV_1 and FVC were observed with pharmacodynamic steady state reached by day 8 with once-daily treatment. The mean peak improvement in FEV_1, relative to baseline, was 0.28 to 0.31 liters (28% to 31%), after 1 week (day 8) of once-daily treatment. Improvement of lung function was maintained for 24 hours after a single dose and consistently maintained over the 1-year treatment period with no evidence of tolerance.

In the two 6-month, placebo-controlled trials, serial spirometric evaluations were performed throughout daytime hours in Trial A (12 hours) and limited to 3 hours in Trial B. The serial FEV_1 values over 12 hours (Trial A) are displayed in Figure 1. These trials further support the improvement in pulmonary function (FEV_1) with SPIRIVA, which persisted over the spirometric observational period. Effectiveness was maintained for 24 hours after administration over the 6-month treatment period.

[See figure 1 at right]

Results of each of the one-year ipratropium-controlled trials were similar to the results of the one-year placebo-controlled trials. The results of one of these trials are shown in Figure 2.

[See figure 2 at right]

Figure 1: Mean FEV_1 Over Time (prior to and after administration of study drug) on Days 1 and 169 for Trial A (a Six-Month Placebo-Controlled Study)*

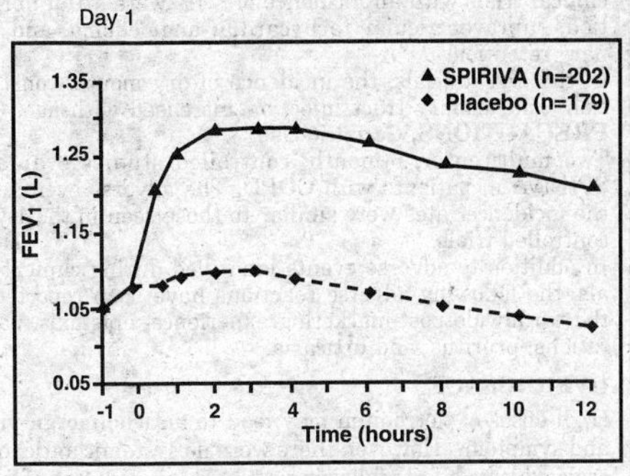

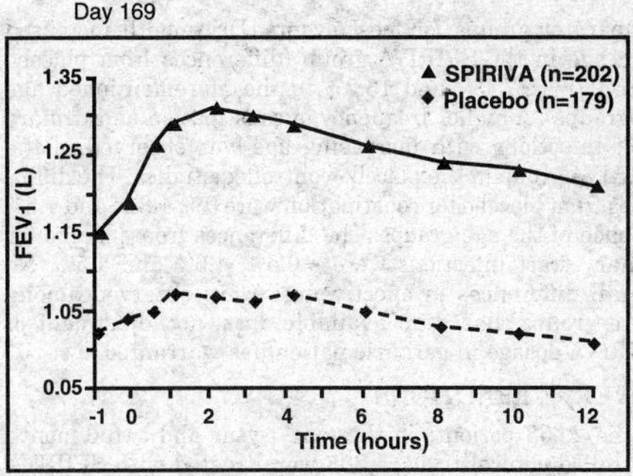

*Means adjusted for center, treatment, and baseline effect. On Day 169, a total of 183 and 149 patients in the SPIRIVA and placebo groups, respectively, completed the trial. The data for the remaining patients were imputed using last observation or least favorable observation carried forward.

Figure 2: Mean FEV_1 Over Time (0 to 6 hours postdose) on Days 1 and 92, respectively for one of the two Ipratropium-Controlled Studies*

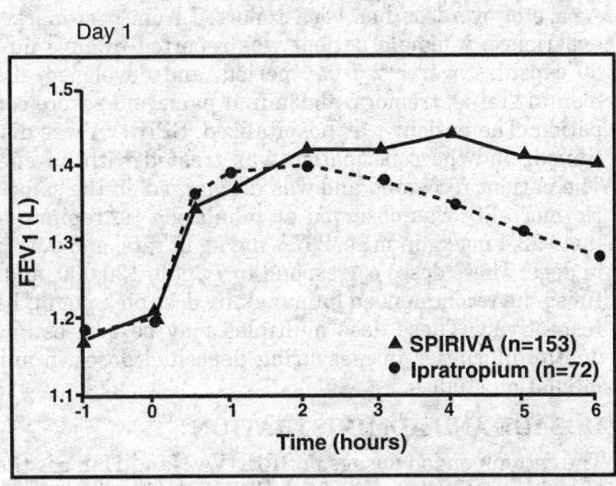

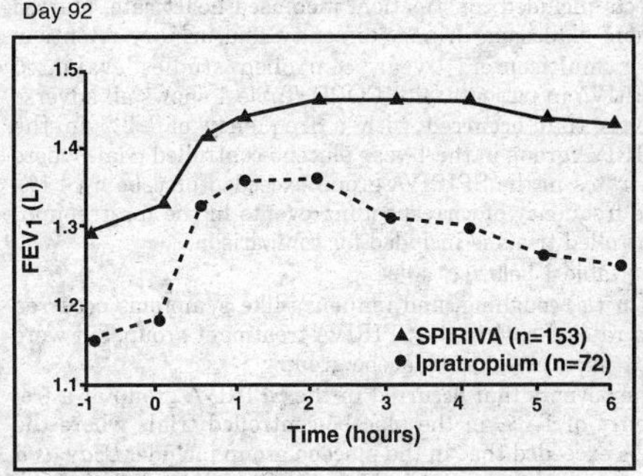

*Means adjusted for center, treatment, and baseline effect. On Day 92 (primary endpoint), a total of 151 and 69 patients in the SPIRIVA and ipratropium groups, respectively, completed through three months of observation.The data for the remaining patients were imputed using last observation or least favorable observation carried forward.

A randomized, placebo-controlled clinical study in 105 patients with COPD demonstrated that bronchodilation was maintained throughout the 24-hour dosing interval in comparison to placebo, regardless of whether SPIRIVA was administered in the morning or in the evening.

Throughout each week of the one-year treatment period in the two placebo-controlled trials, patients taking SPIRIVA had a reduced requirement for the use of rescue short-acting $beta_2$-agonists. Reduction in the use of rescue short-acting $beta_2$-agonists, as compared to placebo, was demonstrated in one of the two 6-month studies.

INDICATIONS AND USAGE

SPIRIVA HandiHaler is indicated for the long-term, once-daily, maintenance treatment of bronchospasm associated with chronic obstructive pulmonary disease (COPD), including chronic bronchitis and emphysema.

CONTRAINDICATIONS

SPIRIVA HandiHaler is contraindicated in patients with a history of hypersensitivity to atropine or its derivatives, including ipratropium, or to any component of this product.

WARNINGS

SPIRIVA HandiHaler is intended as a once-daily maintenance treatment for COPD and is not indicated for the initial treatment of acute episodes of bronchospasm, i.e., rescue therapy.

Immediate hypersensitivity reactions, including angioedema, may occur after administration of SPIRIVA. If such a reaction occurs, therapy with SPIRIVA should be stopped at once and alternative treatments should be considered.

Inhaled medicines, including SPIRIVA, may cause paradoxical bronchospasm. If this occurs, treatment with SPIRIVA should be stopped and other treatments considered.

PRECAUTIONS

General

As an anticholinergic drug, SPIRIVA may potentially worsen symptoms and signs associated with narrow-angle glaucoma, prostatic hyperplasia or bladder-neck obstruction and should be used with caution in patients with any of these conditions.

As a predominantly renally excreted drug, patients with moderate to severe renal impairment (creatinine clearance of ≤50 mL/min) treated with SPIRIVA should be monitored closely. (See **CLINICAL PHARMACOLOGY, Pharmacokinetics,** Special Populations: *Renally-impaired Patients*)

Information for Patients

It is important for patients to understand how to correctly administer SPIRIVA capsules using the HandiHaler inhalation device. (See **Patient's Instructions for Use**) SPIRIVA capsules should only be administered via the HandiHaler device and the HandiHaler device should not be used for administering other medications.

Capsules should always be stored in sealed blisters and only removed immediately before use. The blister strip should be carefully opened to expose only one capsule at a time. Open the blister foil as far as the *STOP* line to remove only one capsule at a time. The drug should be used immediately after the packaging over an individual capsule is opened, or else its effectiveness may be reduced. Capsules that are inadvertently exposed to air (i.e., not intended for immediate use) should be discarded.

Eye pain or discomfort, blurred vision, visual halos or colored images in association with red eyes from conjunctival congestion and corneal edema may be signs of acute narrow-angle glaucoma. Should any of these signs and symptoms develop, consult a physician immediately. Miotic eye drops alone are not considered to be effective treatment.

Care must be taken not to allow the powder to enter into the eyes as this may cause blurring of vision and pupil dilation.

SPIRIVA HandiHaler is a once-daily maintenance bronchodilator and should not be used for immediate relief of breathing problems, i.e., as a rescue medication.

Drug Interactions

SPIRIVA has been used concomitantly with other drugs commonly used in COPD without increases in adverse drug reactions. These include sympathomimetic bronchodilators, methylxanthines, and oral and inhaled steroids. However, the co-administration of SPIRIVA with other anticholinergic-containing drugs (e.g., ipratropium) has not been studied and is therefore not recommended.

Drug/Laboratory Test Interactions

None known.

Carcinogenesis, Mutagenesis, Impairment of Fertility

No evidence of tumorigenicity was observed in a 104-week inhalation study in rats at tiotropium doses up to 0.059 mg/kg/day, in an 83-week inhalation study in female mice at doses up to 0.145 mg/kg/day, and in a 101-week inhalation study in male mice at doses up to 0.002 mg/kg/day. These doses correspond to 25, 35, and 0.5 times the Recommended Human Daily Dose (RHDD) on a mg/m^2 basis, respectively. These dose multiples may be over-estimated due to difficulties in measuring deposited doses in animal inhalation studies.

Tiotropium bromide demonstrated no evidence of mutagenicity or clastogenicity in the following assays: the bacterial gene mutation assay, the V79 Chinese hamster cell mutagenesis assay, the chromosomal aberration assays in human lymphocytes *in vitro* and mouse micronucleus formation *in vivo*, and the unscheduled DNA synthesis in primary rat hepatocytes *in vitro* assay.

In rats, decreases in the number of corpora lutea and the percentage of implants were noted at inhalation tiotropium doses of 0.078 mg/kg/day or greater (approximately 35 times the RHDD on a mg/m^2 basis). No such effects were observed at 0.009 mg/kg/day (approximately 4 times than the RHDD on a mg/m^2 basis). The fertility index, however, was not affected at inhalation doses up to 1.689 mg/kg/day (approximately 760 times the RHDD on a mg/m^2 basis). These dose multiples may be over-estimated due to difficulties in measuring deposited doses in animal inhalation studies.

Pregnancy

Pregnancy Category C

No evidence of structural alterations was observed in rats and rabbits at inhalation tiotropium doses of up to 1.471 and 0.007 mg/kg/day, respectively. These doses correspond to approximately 660 and 6 times the recommended human daily dose (RHDD) on a mg/m^2 basis. However, in rats, fetal resorption, litter loss, decreases in the number of live pups at birth and the mean pup weights, and a delay in pup sexual maturation were observed at inhalation tiotropium doses of ≥ 0.078 mg/kg (approximately 35 times the RHDD on a mg/m^2 basis). In rabbits, an increase in post-implantation loss was observed at an inhalation dose of 0.4 mg/kg/day (approximately 360 times the RHDD on a mg/m^2 basis). Such effects were not observed at inhalation doses of 0.009 and up to 0.088 mg/kg/day in rats and rabbits, respectively. These doses correspond to approximately 4 and 80 times the RHDD on a mg/m^2 basis, respectively. These dose multiples may be over-estimated due to difficulties in measuring deposited doses in animal inhalation studies.

There are no adequate and well-controlled studies in pregnant women. SPIRIVA should be used during pregnancy only if the potential benefit justifies the potential risk to the fetus.

Use in Labor and Delivery

The safety and effectiveness of SPIRIVA has not been studied during labor and delivery.

Nursing Mothers

Clinical data from nursing women exposed to tiotropium are not available. Based on lactating rodent studies, tiotropium is excreted into breast milk. It is not known whether tiotropium is excreted in human milk, but because many drugs are excreted in human milk and given these findings in rats, caution should be exercised if SPIRIVA is administered to a nursing woman.

Pediatric Use

SPIRIVA HandiHaler is approved for use in the maintenance treatment of bronchospasm associated with chronic obstructive pulmonary disease, including chronic bronchitis and emphysema. This disease does not normally occur in children. The safety and effectiveness of SPIRIVA in pediatric patients have not been established.

Geriatric Use

Of the total number of patients who received SPIRIVA in the 1-year clinical trials, 426 were <65 years, 375 were 65–74 years and 105 were ≥75 years of age. Within each age subgroup, there were no differences between the proportion of patients with adverse events in the SPIRIVA and the

Continued on next page

Spiriva—Cont.

comparator groups for most events. Dry mouth increased with age in the SPIRIVA group (differences from placebo were 9.0%, 17.1%, and 16.2% in the aforementioned age subgroups). A higher frequency of constipation and urinary tract infections with increasing age was observed in the SPIRIVA group in the placebo-controlled studies. The differences from placebo for constipation were 0%, 1.8%, and 7.8% for each of the age groups. The differences from placebo for urinary tract infections were −0.6%, 4.6% and 4.5%. No overall differences in effectiveness were observed among these groups. Based on available data, no adjustment of SPIRIVA dosage in geriatric patients is warranted.

ADVERSE REACTIONS

Of the 2,663 patients in the four 1-year and two 6-month controlled clinical trials, 1,308 were treated with SPIRIVA at the recommended dose of 18 mcg once a day. Patients with narrow angle glaucoma, or symptomatic prostatic hypertrophy or bladder outlet obstruction were excluded from these trials.

The most commonly reported adverse drug reaction was dry mouth. Dry mouth was usually mild and often resolved during continued treatment. Other reactions reported in individual patients and consistent with possible anticholinergic effects included constipation, increased heart rate, blurred vision, glaucoma, urinary difficulty, and urinary retention.

Four multicenter, 1-year, controlled studies evaluated SPIRIVA in patients with COPD. Table 1 shows all adverse events that occurred with a frequency of ≥3% in the SPIRIVA group in the 1-year placebo-controlled trials where the rates in the SPIRIVA group exceeded placebo by ≥1%. The frequency of corresponding events in the ipratropium-controlled trials is included for comparison.

[See table 1 below]

Arthritis, coughing, and influenza-like symptoms occurred at a rate of ≥3% in the SPIRIVA treatment group, but were <1% in excess of the placebo group.

Other events that occurred in the SPIRIVA group at a frequency of 1–3% in the placebo-controlled trials where the rates exceeded that in the placebo group include: *Body as a Whole:* allergic reaction, leg pain; *Central and Peripheral Nervous System:* dysphonia, paresthesia; *Gastrointestinal System Disorders:* gastrointestinal disorder not otherwise specified (NOS), gastroesophageal reflux, stomatitis (including ulcerative stomatitis); *Metabolic and Nutritional Disorders:* hypercholesterolemia, hyperglycemia; *Musculoskeletal System Disorders:* skeletal pain: *Cardiac Events:* angina pectoris (including aggravated angina pectoris); *Psychiatric Disorder:* depression; *Infections:* herpes zoster; *Respiratory System Disorder (Upper):* laryngitis; *Vision Disorder:* cataract. In addition, among the adverse events observed in the clinical trials with an incidence of <1% were atrial fibrillation, supraventricular tachycardia, angioedema, and urinary retention.

In the 1-year trials, the incidence of dry mouth, constipation, and urinary tract infection increased with age. (See **PRECAUTIONS, Geriatric Use**)

Two multicenter, 6-month, controlled studies evaluated SPIRIVA in patients with COPD. The adverse events and the incidence rates were similar to those seen in the 1-year controlled trials.

In addition to adverse events identified during clinical trials, the following adverse reactions have been reported in the worldwide post-marketing experience: epistaxis, palpitations, pruritus, and urticaria.

OVERDOSAGE

High doses of tiotropium may lead to anticholinergic signs and symptoms. However, there were no systemic anticholinergic adverse effects following a single inhaled dose of up to 282 mcg tiotropium in 6 healthy volunteers. In a study of 12 healthy volunteers, bilateral conjunctivitis and dry mouth were seen following repeated once-daily inhalation of 141 mcg of tiotropium.

Acute intoxication by inadvertent oral ingestion of SPIRIVA capsules is unlikely since it is not well-absorbed systemically.

A case of overdose has been reported from post-marketing experience. A female patient was reported to have inhaled 30 capsules over a 2.5 day period, and developed altered mental status, tremors, abdominal pain, and severe constipation. The patient was hospitalized, SPIRIVA was discontinued, and the constipation was treated with an enema. The patient recovered and was discharged on the same day.

No mortality was observed at inhalation tiotropium doses up to 32.4 mg/kg in mice, 267.7 mg/kg in rats, and 0.6 mg/kg in dogs. These doses correspond to 7,3000, 120,000, and 850 times the recommended human daily dose on a mg/m^2 basis, respectively. These dose multiples may be over-estimated due to difficulties in measuring deposited doses in animal inhalation studies.

DOSAGE AND ADMINISTRATION

The recommended dosage of SPIRIVA HandiHaler is the inhalation of the contents of one SPIRIVA capsule, once-daily, with the HandiHaler inhalation device. (See **Patient's Instructions for Use**)

No dosage adjustment is required for geriatric, hepatically-impaired, or renally-impaired patients. However, patients with moderate to severe renal impairment given SPIRIVA should be monitored closely. (See **CLINICAL PHARMACOLOGY, Pharmacokinetics,** Special Populations and **PRECAUTIONS**)

Table 1: Adverse Experience Incidence (% Patients) in One-Year-COPD Clinical Trials

Body System (Event)	Placebo-Controlled Trials SPIRIVA [n=550]	Placebo [n=371]	Ipratropium-Controlled Trials SPIRIVA [n=356]	Ipratropium [n=179]
Body as a Whole				
Accidents	13	11	5	8
Chest Pain (non-specific)	7	5	5	2
Edema, Dependent	5	4	3	5
Gastrointestinal System Disorders				
Abdominal Pain	5	3	6	6
Constipation	4	2	1	1
Dry Mouth	16	3	12	6
Dyspepsia	6	5	1	1
Vomiting	4	2	1	2
Musculoskeletal System				
Myalgia	4	3	4	3
Resistance Mechanism Disorders				
Infection	4	3	1	3
Moniliasis	4	2	3	2
Respiratory System (upper)				
Epistaxis	4	2	1	1
Pharyngitis	9	7	7	3
Rhinitis	6	5	3	2
Sinusitis	11	9	3	2
Upper Respiratory Tract Infection	41	37	43	35
Skin and Appendage Disorders				
Rash	4	2	2	2
Urinary System				
Urinary Tract Infection	7	5	4	2

SPIRIVA capsules are for inhalation only and must not be swallowed.

HOW SUPPLIED

SPIRIVA capsules, containing 18 mcg tiotropium, are light green, with TI01 printed on one side of the capsule and the Boehringer Ingelheim company logo on the other side.

The HandiHaler inhalation device is gray colored with a green button. It is imprinted with SPIRIVA HandiHaler (tiotropium bromide inhalation powder), the Boehringer Ingelheim company logo, and the Pfizer company logo. It is also imprinted to indicate that SPIRIVA capsules should not be stored in the HandiHaler device and that the HandiHaler device is only to be used with SPIRIVA capsules.

Six SPIRIVA capsules are packaged in an Aluminum/PVC/Aluminum blister card. One blister card consists of two blister strips, each containing 3 capsules and joined along a perforated-cut line. After using the first capsule, the 2 remaining capsules should be used over the next 2 consecutive days. Capsules should always be stored in the blister and only removed immediately before use. The foil lidding should only be peeled back as far as the *STOP* line printed on the blister foil to prevent exposure of more than one capsule. The drug should be used immediately after the packaging over an individual capsule is opened.

The following packages are available:

carton containing 6 SPIRIVA capsules (1 blister card) and 1 HandiHaler inhalation device (NDC 0597-0075-06)

carton containing 30 SPIRIVA capsules (5 blister cards) and 1 HandiHaler inhalation device (NDC 0597-0075-37)

Storage

Store at 25°C (77°F); excursions permitted to 15–30°C (59–86°F) [see USP Controlled Room Temperature].

The capsules should not be exposed to extreme temperature or moisture. Do not store capsules in the HandiHaler device.

℞ only

Manufactured by:
Boehringer Ingelheim Pharma GmbH & Co. KG
Ingelheim, Germany

Marketed by:
Boehringer Ingelheim Pharmaceuticals, Inc.
Ridgefield, CT 06877 USA
and
Pfizer Inc.
New York, NY 10017 USA

Address Medical Inquiries to:
www.Spiriva.com or (800) 542-6257

Licensed from Boehringer Ingelheim International GmbH.

SPIRIVA® and HandiHaler® are registered trademarks and are used under license from Boehringer Ingelheim International GmbH

Tiotropium bromide is covered by U.S. Patent No. 5,610,163 with other Patents Pending. The HandiHaler inhalation device is covered by U.S. Design Patent No. 355,029.

59873/US/1 January 2004

PATIENT'S INSTRUCTIONS FOR USE

Spiriva®
HandiHaler®
(tiotropium bromide inhalation powder)

FOR ORAL INHALATION ONLY

Read all instructions before use.

This leaflet provides summary information about SPIRIVA capsules and the HandiHaler inhalation device. Before you start to take SPIRIVA or use the HandiHaler, read this leaflet carefully and keep it for future use. You should read the leaflet that comes with your prescription every time you refill it because there may be new information.

For more information, ask your health-care provider or pharmacist.

What should you know about SPIRIVA and HandiHaler?

Each SPIRIVA capsule contains a dry powder blend of active drug (18 mcg tiotropium) and lactose monohydrate as the carrier. The dry powder in the capsule is inhaled from the HandiHaler inhalation device. SPIRIVA capsules contain only a small amount of powder and as a result the capsule is only partially filled. When disposing of the capsule, you may notice that a tiny amount of this powder is left in the capsule. This is normal.

SPIRIVA is a once daily maintenance bronchodilator medicine that opens narrowed airways and helps keep them open for 24 hours. SPIRIVA HandiHaler should not be used for immediate relief of breathing problems, i.e., as a rescue medication.

SPIRIVA CAPSULES ARE INTENDED FOR ORAL INHALATION ONLY AND ARE TO BE USED ONLY WITH THE HANDIHALER INHALATION DEVICE.

SPIRIVA CAPSULES SHOULD NOT BE SWALLOWED.

The HandiHaler is an inhalation device that has been specially designed for use with SPIRIVA capsules. It must not be used to take any other medication.

Care must be taken not to allow the powder to enter into the eyes. If symptoms of eye pain, eye discomfort, blurred vision, visual halos, or colored images in association with red eyes occur, consult a physician immediately.

How do you take your dose of SPIRIVA using the HandiHaler?

Taking your dose of SPIRIVA, requires four main steps: Open the blister and the HandiHaler device, insert the

SPIRIVA capsule, press the HandiHaler button, and inhale your medication. (See below for details.)

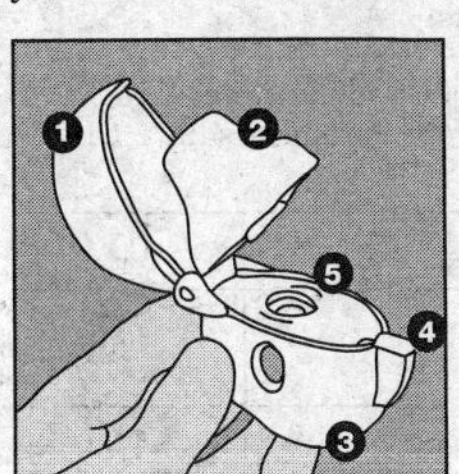

Become familiar with the components of the HandiHaler inhalation device:

1. dust cap
2. mouthpiece
3. base
4. piercing button
5. center chamber

Removing the SPIRIVA capsule from the blister.

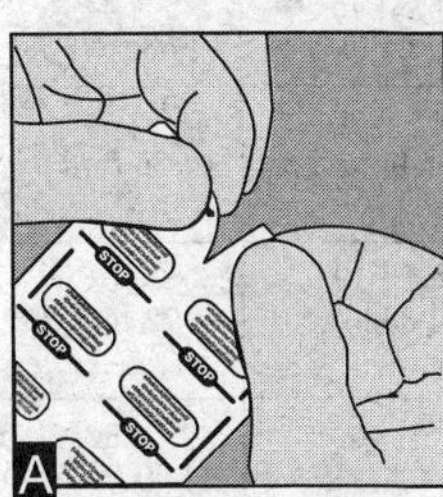

A) SPIRIVA capsules are packaged in a blister card. Each blister card consists of two blister strips, each containing 3 capsules and joined along a perforated-cut line. Prior to removing the first capsule from the blister card, separate the blister strips by tearing along the perforation. (Figure A)

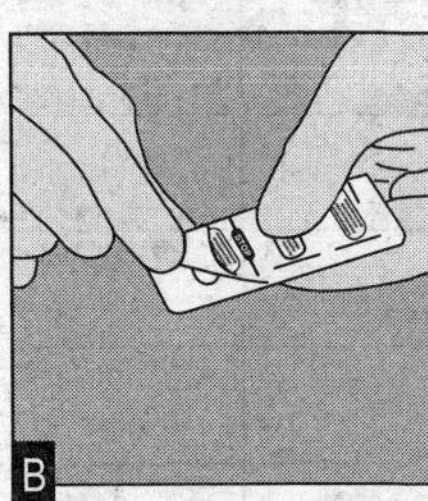

B) The blister should be carefully opened to expose only one capsule at a time. Immediately before you are ready to use your dose of SPIRIVA, peel back the aluminum foil using the tab until one capsule is fully visible. The foil lidding should only be peeled back as far as the ***STOP*** line printed on the blister foil to prevent exposure of more than one capsule. (Figure B)

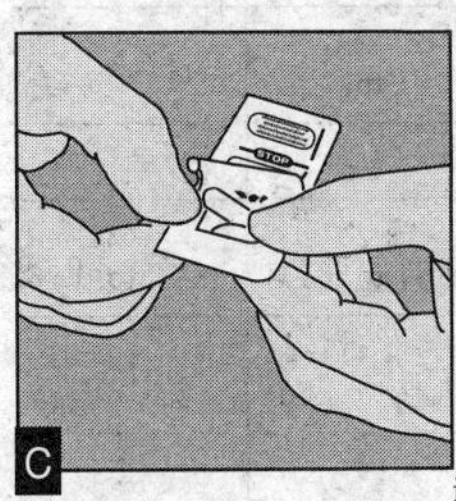

C) **Capsules should always be stored in the sealed blisters and only removed immediately before use. The drug should be used immediately after the packaging over an individual capsule is opened, or else its effectiveness may be reduced.** The blister strip should be carefully opened to expose one capsule at a time. After using the first capsule, the 2 remaining capsules should be used over the next 2 consecutive days. SPIRIVA capsules should always be stored in the blister. The blister should only be opened and the capsule removed immediately before use. If additional capsules are inadvertently exposed to air, they should not be used and should be discarded. (Figure C)

Do not store capsules in the HandiHaler device.

Opening the HandiHaler device and inserting the SPIRIVA capsule.

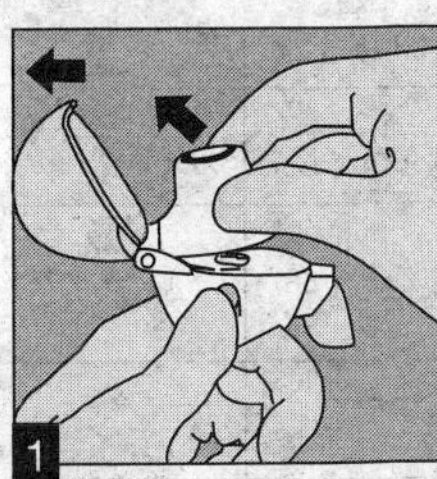

1) **OPEN:** Open the dust cap by pulling it upwards. Then open the mouthpiece. (Figure 1)

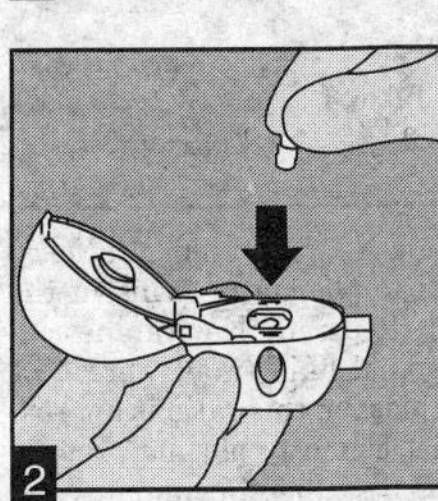

2) **INSERT:** Place the capsule in the center chamber. It does not matter which end of the capsule is placed in the chamber. (Figure 2)

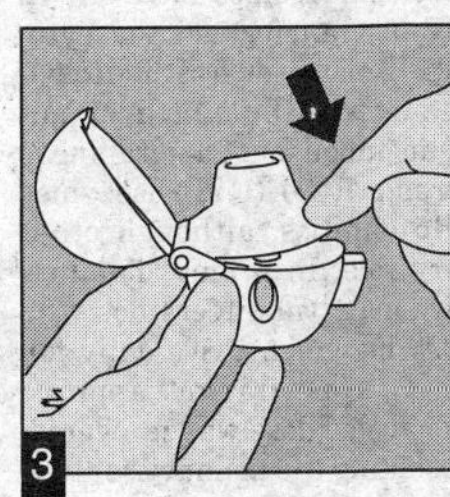

3) Close the mouthpiece **firmly until you hear a click,** leaving the dust cap open. (Figure 3)

Taking your dose of SPIRIVA.

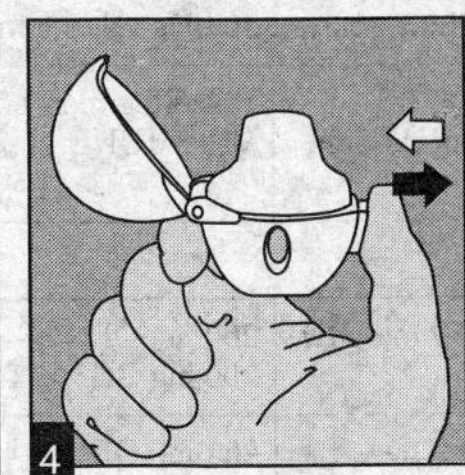

4) **PRESS: Hold the HandiHaler device with the mouthpiece upwards and press the piercing button completely in once, and release.** This makes holes in the capsule and allows the medication to be released when you breathe in. (Figure 4)

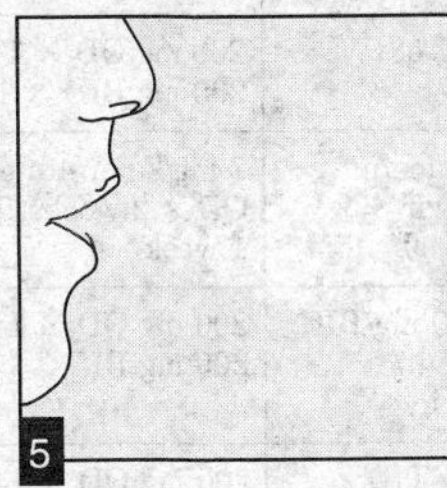

5) **Breathe out completely.** (Figure 5)

Important: Do not breathe into the mouthpiece at any time.

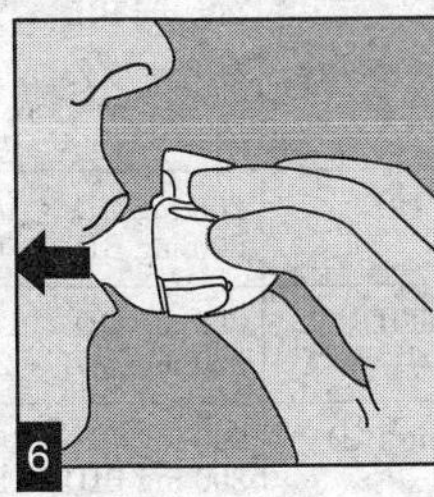

6) **INHALE:** Raise the HandiHaler device to your mouth and close your lips tightly around the mouthpiece. Keep your head in an upright position and breathe in slowly and deeply but at a rate **sufficient to hear the capsule vibrate.** Breathe in until your lungs are full; then hold your breath as long as is comfortable and at the same time take the HandiHaler device out of your mouth. Resume normal breathing. (Figure 6)

To ensure you get the full dose of SPIRIVA, you must repeat steps 5 and 6 once again.

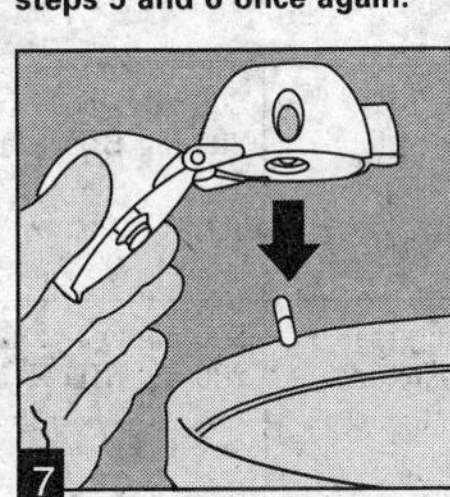

7) After you have finished taking your daily dose of SPIRIVA, open the mouthpiece again. Tip out the used capsule and dispose. (Figure 7)

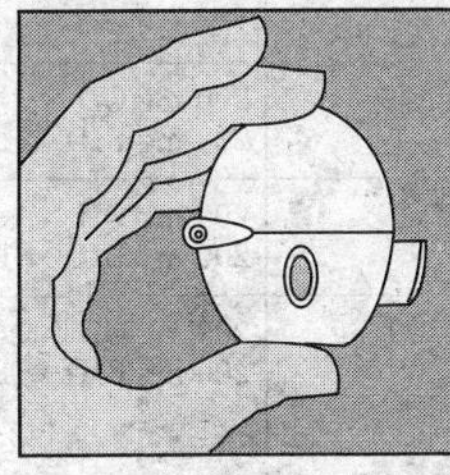

Close the mouthpiece and dust cap for storage of your HandiHaler device.

When and how should you clean your HandiHaler Device?

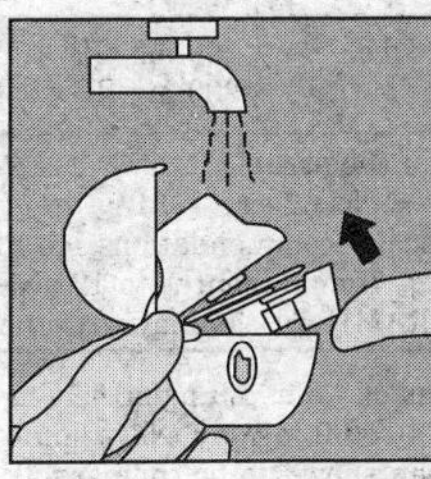

Normally, during a one-month period of use, the HandiHaler device does not need to be cleaned. However, if cleaning is needed the HandiHaler device can be cleaned as described below:

Open the dust cap and mouthpiece. Open the base by lifting the piercing button. Rinse the complete inhaler with warm water to remove any powder. Do not use cleaning agents or detergents.

Dry the HandiHaler device thoroughly by tipping the excess water out on a paper towel and air-dry afterwards, leaving the dust cap, mouthpiece and base open. **It takes 24 hours to air dry, so clean it right after you use it and it will be ready for your next dose.** Do not use the HandiHaler device when it is wet.

If needed, the outside of the mouthpiece may be cleaned with a moist, but not wet tissue.

The HandiHaler device should not be placed in the dishwasher for cleaning.

Where should you store SPIRIVA capsules and the HandiHaler Device?

Store at 25°C (77°F); excursions permitted to 15–30°C (59–86°F) [see USP Controlled Room Temperature].

The capsules should not be exposed to extreme temperature or moisture. Do not store capsules in the HandiHaler.

As with all prescription medications, keep this out of the reach of children.

Tell your doctor before you use SPIRIVA HandiHaler:

if you may be pregnant or wish to become pregnant;
if you are a breastfeeding mother;
if you are taking any medications including eye drops, this includes those you can buy without a prescription;
if you have any other medical problems such as difficulty urinating or an enlarged prostate;
if you are allergic to any medications.

USE THIS PRODUCT AS DIRECTED, UNLESS INSTRUCTED TO DO OTHERWISE BY YOUR PHYSICIAN.

Manufactured by:
Boehringer Ingelheim Pharma GmbH & Co. KG
Ingelheim, Germany
Marketed by:
Boehringer Ingelheim Pharmaceuticals, Inc.
Ridgefield, CT 06877 USA
and
Pfizer Inc.
New York, NY 10017 USA
Licensed from Boehringer Ingelheim International GmbH.
SPIRIVA® and HandiHaler® are registered trademarks and are used under license from Boehringer Ingelheim International GmbH

Tiotropium bromide is covered by U.S. Patent No. 5,610,163 with other Patents Pending. The HandiHaler inhalation device is covered by U.S. Design Patient No. 355,029.
59873/US/1
January 2004

Shown in Product Identification Guide, page 309

VIRAMUNE® ℞
(nevirapine) Tablets
VIRAMUNE®
(nevirapine) Oral Suspension
℞ only

> **WARNING**
> **Severe, life-threatening, and in some cases fatal hepatotoxicity, including fulminant and cholestatic hepatitis, hepatic necrosis and hepatic failure, has been reported in patients treated with VIRAMUNE®. In some cases, patients presented with non-specific prodromal signs or symptoms of hepatitis and progressed to hepatic failure. These events are often associated with rash. Women, and patients with higher CD4 counts, are at increased risk of these hepatic events. Women with CD4 counts >250 cells/mm^3, including pregnant women receiving chronic treatment for HIV infection, are at considerably higher risk of these events. Patients with signs or symptoms of hepatitis must discontinue VIRAMUNE and seek medical evaluation immediately. (See WARNINGS)**
> **Severe, life-threatening skin reactions, including fatal cases, have occurred in patients treated with VIRAMUNE. These have included cases of Stevens-Johnson syndrome, toxic epidermal necrolysis, and hypersensitivity reactions characterized by rash, constitutional findings, and organ dysfunction. Patients developing signs or symptoms of severe skin reactions or hypersensitivity reactions must discontinue VIRAMUNE and seek medical evaluation immediately. (See WARNINGS)**
> **It is essential that patients be monitored intensively during the first 18 weeks of therapy with VIRAMUNE to detect potentially life-threatening hepatotoxicity or skin reactions. The greatest risk of severe rash or hepatic events (often associated with rash) occurs in the first 6 weeks of therapy. However, the risk of any hepatic event, with or without rash, continues past this period and monitoring should continue at frequent intervals. In some cases, hepatic injury has progressed despite discontinuation of treatment. VIRAMUNE should not be restarted following severe hepatic, skin or hypersensitivity reactions. In addition, the 14-day lead-in period with VIRAMUNE 200 mg daily dosing must be strictly followed. (See WARNINGS)**

DESCRIPTION

VIRAMUNE is the brand name for nevirapine (NVP), a non-nucleoside reverse transcriptase inhibitor with activity against Human Immunodeficiency Virus Type 1 (HIV-1). Nevirapine is structurally a member of the dipyridodiazepinone chemical class of compounds.

VIRAMUNE Tablets are for oral administration. Each tablet contains 200 mg of nevirapine and the inactive ingredients microcrystalline cellulose, lactose monohydrate, povidone, sodium starch glycolate, colloidal silicon dioxide and magnesium stearate.

Continued on next page

Viramune—Cont.

VIRAMUNE Oral Suspension is for oral administration. Each 5 mL of VIRAMUNE suspension contains 50 mg of nevirapine (as nevirapine hemihydrate). The suspension also contains the following excipients: carbomer 934P, methylparaben, propylparaben, sorbitol, sucrose, polysorbate 80, sodium hydroxide and purified water.

The chemical name of nevirapine is 11-cyclopropyl-5,11-dihydro-4-methyl-6H-dipyrido [3,2-b:2',3'-e][1,4] diazepin-6-one. Nevirapine is a white to off-white crystalline powder with the molecular weight of 266.30 and the molecular formula $C_{15}H_{14}N_4O$. Nevirapine has the following structural formula:

MICROBIOLOGY

Mechanism of Action:

Nevirapine is a non-nucleoside reverse transcriptase inhibitor (NNRTI) of HIV-1. Nevirapine binds directly to reverse transcriptase (RT) and blocks the RNA-dependent and DNA-dependent DNA polymerase activities by causing a disruption of the enzyme's catalytic site. The activity of nevirapine does not compete with template or nucleoside triphosphates. HIV-2 RT and eukaryotic DNA polymerases (such as human DNA polymerases α, β, γ, or δ) are not inhibited by nevirapine.

In Vitro HIV Susceptibility:

The *in vitro* antiviral activity of nevirapine was measured in peripheral blood mononuclear cells, monocyte derived macrophages, and lymphoblastoid cell lines. IC_{50} values (50% inhibitory concentration) ranged from 10-100 nM against laboratory and clinical isolates of HIV-1. In cell culture, nevirapine demonstrated additive to synergistic activity against HIV-1 in drug combination regimens with zidovudine (ZDV), didanosine (ddI), stavudine (d4T), lamivudine (3TC), saquinavir, and indinavir. The relationship between *in vitro* susceptibility of HIV-1 to nevirapine and the inhibition of HIV-1 replication in humans has not been established.

Resistance:

HIV-1 isolates with reduced susceptibility (100-250-fold) to nevirapine emerge *in vitro*. Genotypic analysis showed mutations in the HIV-1 RT gene Y181C and/or V106A depending upon the virus strain and cell line employed. Time to emergence of nevirapine resistance *in vitro* was not altered when selection included nevirapine in combination with several other NNRTIs.

Phenotypic and genotypic changes in HIV-1 isolates from patients treated with either nevirapine (n=24) or nevirapine and ZDV (n=14) were monitored in Phase I/II trials over 1 to ≥12 weeks. After 1 week of nevirapine monotherapy, isolates from 3/3 patients had decreased susceptibility to nevirapine *in vitro*; one or more of the RT mutations K103N, V106A, V108I, Y181C, Y188C and G190A were detected in HIV-1 isolates from some patients as early as 2 weeks after therapy initiation. By week eight of nevirapine monotherapy, 100% of the patients tested (n=24) had HIV-1 isolates with a >100-fold decrease in susceptibility to nevirapine *in vitro* compared to baseline, and had one or more of the nevirapine-associated RT resistance mutations; 19 of 24 patients (80%) had isolates with Y181C mutations regardless of dose. Nevirapine+ZDV combination therapy did not alter the emergence rate of nevirapine-resistant virus or the magnitude of nevirapine resistance *in vitro*. The clinical relevance of phenotypic and genotypic changes associated with nevirapine therapy has not been established.

Cross-resistance:

Rapid emergence of HIV-1 strains which are cross-resistant to NNRTIs has been observed *in vitro*. Nevirapine-resistant HIV-1 isolates were cross-resistant to the NNRTIs efavirenz and delavirdine. However, nevirapine-resistant isolates were susceptible to the nucleoside analogues ZDV and ddI. Similarly, ZDV-resistant isolates were susceptible to nevirapine *in vitro*.

ANIMAL PHARMACOLOGY

Animal studies have shown that nevirapine is widely distributed to nearly all tissues and readily crosses the blood-brain barrier.

CLINICAL PHARMACOLOGY

Pharmacokinetics in Adults:

Absorption and Bioavailability: Nevirapine is readily absorbed (>90%) after oral administration in healthy volunteers and in adults with HIV-1 infection. Absolute bioavailability in 12 healthy adults following single-dose administration was 93 ± 9% (mean ± SD) for a 50 mg tablet and 91 ± 8% for an oral solution. Peak plasma nevirapine concentrations of 2 ± 0.4 μg/mL (7.5 μM) were attained by 4 hours following a single 200 mg dose. Following multiple doses, nevirapine peak concentrations appear to increase linearly in the dose range of 200 to 400 mg/day. Steady state trough nevirapine concentrations of 4.5 ± 1.9 μg/mL (17 ± 7 μM), (n = 242) were attained at 400 mg/day. Nevirapine tablets and suspension have been shown to be comparably bioavailable and interchangeable at doses up to 200 mg. When VIRAMUNE (200 mg) was administered to 24 healthy adults (12 female, 12 male), with either a high fat breakfast (857 kcal, 50 g fat, 53% of calories from fat) or antacid (Maalox® 30 mL), the extent of nevirapine absorption (AUC) was comparable to that observed under fasting conditions. In a separate study in HIV-1 infected patients (n=6), nevirapine steady-state systemic exposure (AUCτ) was not significantly altered by didanosine, which is formulated with an alkaline buffering agent. VIRAMUNE may be administered with or without food, antacid or didanosine.

Distribution: Nevirapine is highly lipophilic and is essentially nonionized at physiologic pH. Following intravenous administration to healthy adults, the apparent volume of distribution (Vdss) of nevirapine was 1.21 ± 0.09 L/kg, suggesting that nevirapine is widely distributed in humans. Nevirapine readily crosses the placenta and is also found in breast milk. (See PRECAUTIONS, *Nursing Mothers*) Nevirapine is about 60% bound to plasma proteins in the plasma concentration range of 1–10 μg/mL. Nevirapine concentrations in human cerebrospinal fluid (n=6) were 45% (± 5%) of the concentrations in plasma; this ratio is approximately equal to the fraction not bound to plasma protein.

Metabolism/Elimination: *In vivo* studies in humans and *in vitro* studies with human liver microsomes have shown that nevirapine is extensively biotransformed via cytochrome P450 (oxidative) metabolism to several hydroxylated metabolites. *In vitro* studies with human liver microsomes suggest that oxidative metabolism of nevirapine is mediated primarily by cytochrome P450 (CYP) isozymes from the CYP3A4 and CYP2B6 families, although other isozymes may have a secondary role. In a mass balance/excretion study in eight healthy male volunteers dosed to steady state with nevirapine 200 mg given twice daily followed by a single 50 mg dose of ^{14}C-nevirapine, approximately 91.4 ± 10.5% of the radiolabeled dose was recovered, with urine (81.3 ± 11.1%) representing the primary route of

Table 1: Drug Interactions:
Changes in Pharmacokinetic Parameters for Co-administered Drug in the Presence of VIRAMUNE
(All interaction studies were conducted in HIV-1 positive patients)

Co-administered Drug	Dose of Co-administered Drug	Dose Regimen of VIRAMUNE	n	% Change of Co-administered Drug Pharmacokinetic Parameters (90% CI)		
Antiretrovirals				AUC	C_{max}	C_{min}
Didanosine	100–150 mg BID	200 mg QD × 14 days; 200 mg BID × 14 days	18	↔	↔	§
Efavirenz[a]	600 mg QD	200 mg QD × 14 days; 400 mg QD × 14 days	17	↓28 (↓34 to ↓14)	↓12 (↓23 to ↑1)	↓32 (↓35 to ↓19)
Indinavir[a]	800 mg q8H	200 mg QD × 14 days; 200 mg BID × 14 days	19	↓31 (↓39 to ↓22)	↓15 (↓24 to ↓4)	↓44 (↓53 to ↓33)
Lopinavir[a,b]	300/75 mg/m² (lopinavir/ ritonavir)[b]	7 mg/kg or 4 mg/kg QD × 2 weeks; BID × 1 week	12, 15[c]	↓14 (↓36 to ↑16)	↓22 (↓44 to ↑9)	↓55 (↓75 to ↓9)
Lopinavir[a]	400/100 mg BID (lopinavir/ ritonavir)	200 mg QD × 14 days; 200 mg BID > 1 year	22, 19[c]	↓27 (↓47 to ↓2)	↓19 (↓38 to ↑5)	↓51 (↓72 to ↓26)
Nelfinavir[a]	750 mg TID	200 mg QD × 14 days; 200 mg BID × 14 days	23	↔	↔	↓32 (↓50 to ↑5)
Nelfinavir-M8 metabolite				↓62 (↓70 to ↓53)	↓59 (↓68 to ↓48)	↓66 (↓74 to ↓55)
Ritonavir	600 mg BID	200 mg QD × 14 days; 200 mg BID × 14 days	18	↔	↔	↔
Saquinavir[a]	600 mg TID	200 mg QD × 14 days; 200 mg BID × 21 days	23	↓38 (↓47 to ↓11)	↓32 (↓44 to ↓6)	§
Stavudine	30–40 mg BID	200 mg QD × 14 days; 200 mg BID × 14 days	22	↔	↔	§
Zalcitabine	0.125–0.25 mg TID	200 mg QD × 14 days; 200 mg BID × 14 days	6	↔	↔	§
Zidovudine	100–200 mg TID	200 mg QD × 14 days; 200 mg BID × 14 days	11	↓28 (↓40 to ↓4)	↓30 (↓51 to ↑14)	§
Other Medications				AUC	C_{max}	C_{min}
Clarithromycin[a]	500 mg BID	200 mg QD × 14 days; 200 mg BID × 14 days	15	↓31 (↓38 to ↓24)	↓23 (↓31 to ↓14)	↓57 (↓70 to ↓36)
Metabolite 14-OH-clarithromycin				↑42 (↑16 to ↑73)	↑47 (↑21 to ↑80)	↔
Ethinyl estradiol[a]	0.035 mg (as Ortho-Novum® 1/35)	200 mg QD × 14 days; 200 mg BID × 14 days	10	↓20 (↓33 to ↓3)	↔	§
and						
Norethindrone[a]	1 mg (as Ortho-Novum® 1/35)			↓19 (↓30 to ↓7)	↓16 (↓27 to ↓3)	§
Fluconazole	200 mg QD	200 mg QD × 14 days; 200 mg BID × 14 days	19	↔	↔	↔
Ketoconazole[a]	400 mg QD	200 mg QD × 14 days; 200 mg BID × 14 days	21	↓72 (↓80 to ↓60)	↓44 (↓58 to ↓27)	§
Rifabutin[a]	150 or 300 mg QD	200 mg QD × 14 days; 200 mg BID × 14 days	19	↑17 (↓2 to ↑40)	↑28 (↑9 to ↑51)	↔
Metabolite 25-O-desacetyl-rifabutin				↑24 (↓16 to ↑84)	↑29 (↓2 to ↑68)	↑22 (↓14 to ↑74)
Rifampin[a]	600 mg QD	200 mg QD × 14 days; 200 mg BID × 14 days	14	↑11 (↓4 to ↑28)	↔	§

§ = C_{min} below detectable level of the assay
↑ = Increase, ↓ = Decrease, ↔ = No Effect
[a]For information regarding clinical recommendations see PRECAUTIONS, *Drug Interactions*, Table 3
[b]Pediatric subjects ranging in age from 6 months to 12 years
[c]Parallel group design; n for VIRAMUNE +lopinavir/ritonavir, n for lopinavir/ritonavir alone

excretion compared to feces (10.1 ± 1.5%). Greater than 80% of the radioactivity in urine was made up of glucuronide conjugates of hydroxylated metabolites. Thus cytochrome P450 metabolism, glucuronide conjugation, and urinary excretion of glucuronidated metabolites represent the primary route of nevirapine biotransformation and elimination in humans. Only a small fraction (<5%) of the radioactivity in urine (representing <3% of the total dose) was made up of parent compound; therefore, renal excretion plays a minor role in elimination of the parent compound.
Nevirapine is an inducer of hepatic cytochrome P450 (CYP) metabolic enzymes 3A4 and 2B6. Nevirapine induces CYP3A4 and CYP2B6 by approximately 20–25%, as indicated by erythromycin breath test results and urine metabolites. Autoinduction of CYP3A4 and CYP2B6 mediated metabolism leads to an approximately 1.5 to 2 fold increase in the apparent oral clearance of nevirapine as treatment continues from a single dose to two-to-four weeks of dosing with 200–400 mg/day. Autoinduction also results in a corresponding decrease in the terminal phase half-life of nevirapine in plasma, from approximately 45 hours (single dose) to approximately 25–30 hours following multiple dosing with 200–400 mg/day.

Pharmacokinetics in Special Populations:

Renal Impairment: HIV seronegative adults with mild (CrCL 50-79 mL/min; n=7), moderate (CrCL 30-49 mL/min; n=6), or severe (CrCL <30 mL/min; n=4) renal impairment received a single 200 mg dose of nevirapine in a pharmacokinetic study. These subjects did not require dialysis. The study included six additional subjects with renal failure requiring dialysis.
In subjects with renal impairment (mild, moderate or severe), there were no significant changes in the pharmacokinetics of nevirapine. However, subjects requiring dialysis exhibited a 44% reduction in nevirapine AUC over a one-week exposure period. There was also evidence of accumulation of nevirapine hydroxy-metabolites in plasma in subjects requiring dialysis. An additional 200 mg dose following each dialysis treatment is indicated. (See DOSAGE and ADMINISTRATION; PRECAUTIONS)

Hepatic Impairment: HIV seronegative adults with mild (Child-Pugh Class A; n=6) or moderate (Child-Pugh Class B; n=4) hepatic impairment received a single 200 mg dose of nevirapine in a pharmacokinetic study.
In the majority of patients with mild or moderate hepatic impairment, no significant changes were seen in the pharmacokinetics of nevirapine. However, a significant increase in the AUC of nevirapine observed in one patient with Child-Pugh Class B and ascites suggests that patients with worsening hepatic function and ascites may be at risk of accumulating nevirapine in the systemic circulation. Because nevirapine induces its own metabolism with multiple dosing, a single dose study may not reflect the impact of hepatic impairment on multiple dose pharmacokinetics. (See PRECAUTIONS) Nevirapine should not be administered to patients with severe hepatic impairment. (See WARNINGS)

Gender: In one Phase I study in healthy volunteers (15 females, 15 males), the weight-adjusted apparent volume of distribution (Vdss/F) of nevirapine was higher in the female subjects (1.54 L/kg) compared to the males (1.38 L/kg), suggesting that nevirapine was distributed more extensively in the female subjects. However, this difference was offset by a slightly shorter terminal-phase half-life in the females resulting in no significant gender difference in nevirapine oral clearance (24.6±7.7 mL/kg/hr in females vs. 19.9±3.9 mL/kg/hr in males after single dose) or plasma concentrations following either single- or multiple-dose administration(s).

Race: An evaluation of nevirapine plasma concentrations (pooled data from several clinical trials) from HIV-1-infected patients (27 Black, 24 Hispanic, 189 Caucasian) revealed no marked difference in nevirapine steady-state trough concentrations (median C_{minss} = 4.7 µg/mL Black, 3.8 µg/mL Hispanic, 4.3 µg/mL Caucasian) with long-term nevirapine treatment at 400 mg/day. However, the pharmacokinetics of nevirapine have not been evaluated specifically for the effects of ethnicity.

Geriatric Patients: Nevirapine pharmacokinetics in HIV-1 infected adults do not appear to change with age (range 18–68 years); however, nevirapine has not been extensively evaluated in patients beyond the age of 55 years.

Pediatric Patients: The pharmacokinetics of nevirapine have been studied in two open-label studies in children with HIV-1 infection. In one study (BI 853; ACTG 165), nine HIV-1-infected children ranging in age from 9 months to 14 years were administered a single dose (7.5 mg, 30 mg, or 120 mg per m^2; n=3 per dose) of nevirapine suspension after an overnight fast. The mean nevirapine apparent clearance adjusted for body weight was greater in children compared to adults.
In a multiple dose study (BI 882; ACTG 180), nevirapine suspension or tablets (240 or 400 mg/m^2/day) were administered as monotherapy or in combination with ZDV or ZDV+ddI to 37 HIV-1-infected pediatric patients with the following demographics: male (54%), racial minority groups (73%), median age of 11 months (range: 2 months–15 years). The majority of these patients received 120 mg/m^2/day of nevirapine for approximately 4 weeks followed by 120 mg/m^2/b.i.d. (patients > 9 years of age) or 200 mg/m^2/b.i.d. (patients ≤ 9 years of age). Nevirapine apparent clearance adjusted for body weight reached maximum values by age 1 to 2 years and then decreased with increasing age. Nevirapine apparent clearance adjusted for body weight was at least two-fold greater in children younger than 8 years compared to adults. The relationship between nevirapine clearance with long term drug administration and age is shown in Figure 1. The pediatric dosing regimens were selected in order to achieve steady-state plasma concentrations in pediatric patients that approximate those in adults. (See DOSAGE AND ADMINISTRATION, *Pediatric Patients*)

Figure 1: Nevirapine Apparent Clearance (mL/kg/hr) in Pediatric Patients

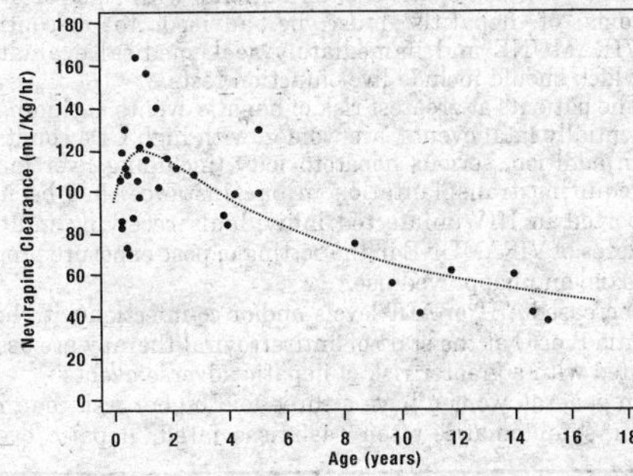

Drug Interactions: (See PRECAUTIONS, *Drug Interactions*) Nevirapine induces hepatic cytochrome P450 metabolic isoenzymes 3A4 and 2B6. Co-administration of VIRAMUNE and drugs primarily metabolized by CYP3A4 or CYP2B6 may result in decreased plasma concentrations of these drugs and attenuate their therapeutic effects.
While primarily an inducer of cytochrome P450 3A4 and 2B6 enzymes, nevirapine may also inhibit this system. Among human hepatic cytochrome P450s, nevirapine was capable in vitro of inhibiting the 10-hydroxylation of (R)-warfarin (CYP3A4). The estimated K_i for the inhibition of CYP3A4 was 270 µM, a concentration that is unlikely to be achieved in patients as the therapeutic range is <25 µM. Therefore, nevirapine may have minimal inhibitory effect on other substrates of CYP3A4.
Nevirapine does not appear to affect the plasma concentrations of drugs that are substrates of other CYP450 enzyme systems, such as 1A2, 2D6, 2A6, 2E1, 2C9 or 2C19.
Table 1 (see below) contains the results of drug interaction studies performed with VIRAMUNE and other drugs likely to be co-administered. The effects of VIRAMUNE on the AUC, C_{max}, and C_{min} of co-administered drugs are summarized. To measure the full potential pharmacokinetic interaction effect following induction, patients on the concomitant drug at steady state were administered 28 days of VIRAMUNE (200 mg QD for 14 days followed by 200 mg BID for 14 days) followed by a steady state reassessment of the concomitant drug.
[See table 1 at top of previous page]
Because of the design of the drug interaction trials (addition of 28 days of VIRAMUNE therapy to existing HIV therapy) the effect of the concomitant drug on plasma nevirapine steady state concentrations was estimated by comparison to historical controls.
Administration of rifampin had a clinically significant effect on nevirapine pharmacokinetics, decreasing AUC and C_{max} by greater than 50%. Administration of fluconazole resulted in an approximate 100% increase in nevirapine exposure, based on a comparison to historic data. (See PRECAUTIONS, *Drug Interactions*, Table 3). The effect of other drugs listed in Table 1 on nevirapine pharmacokinetics was not significant.

INDICATIONS AND USAGE

VIRAMUNE (nevirapine) is indicated for use in combination with other antiretroviral agents for the treatment of HIV-1 infection. This indication is based on one principal clinical trial that demonstrated prolonged suppression of HIV-RNA and two smaller supportive studies, one of which is described below.

Description of Clinical Studies:

Trial BI 1090, was a placebo-controlled, double-blind, randomized trial in 2249 HIV-1 infected patients with <200 CD4+ cells at screening. Initiated in 1995, BI 1090 compared treatment with VIRAMUNE + lamivudine + background therapy versus lamivudine + background therapy in NNRTI naïve patients. Treatment doses were VIRAMUNE, 200 mg daily for two weeks followed by 200 mg twice daily or placebo, and lamivudine 150 mg twice daily. Other antiretroviral agents were given at approved doses. Initial background therapy (in addition to lamivudine) was one NRTI in 1309 patients (58%), two or more NRTIs in 771 (34%), and PIs and NRTIs in 169 (8%). The patients (median age 36.5 years, 70% Caucasian, 79% male) had advanced HIV infection, with a median baseline CD4+ cell count of 96 cells/mm^3 and a baseline HIV RNA of 4.58 log_{10} copies/mL (38,291 copies/mL). Prior to entering the trial, 45% had previously experienced an AIDS-defining clinical event. Eighty-nine percent had antiretroviral treatment prior to entering the trial. BI 1090 was originally designed as a clinical endpoint study. Prior to unblinding the trial, the primary endpoint was changed to proportion of patients with HIV RNA <50 copies/mL and not previously failed at 48 weeks. Treatment response and outcomes are shown in Figure 2 and Table 2.
[See figure at top of next column]
Total number of patients with HIV-RNA data at specified time point, plus number of patients who previously reached a failure endpoint:

Figure 2: BI 1090: Percent Responders by Visit (LOQ=50 copies/mL)

Percent Responders (%)
VIRAMUNE + lamivudine + background therapy
Placebo + lamivudine + background therapy
Weeks in study

	8 Weeks	48 Weeks	96 Weeks
VIRAMUNE:	1120	1097	941
Placebo:	1128	1120	1105

Table 2: BI 1090 Outcomes through 48 weeks

Outcome	VIRAMUNE (N=1121) %	Placebo (N=1128) %
Responders at 48 weeks: HIV RNA <50 copies/mL	18.0	1.6
Treatment Failure	82.0	98.4
Never suppressed viral load	44.6	66.4
Virologic failure after response	7.2	4.3
CDC category C event or death	9.6	11.2
Added antiretroviral therapy[1] while <50 copies/mL	5.0	0.9
Discontinued trial therapy due to AE	7.0	5.9
Discontinued trial <48 weeks[2]	8.5	9.8

[1] including change to open-label NVP
[2] includes withdrawal of consent, lost to follow-up, non-compliance with protocol, other administrative reasons

The change from baseline in CD4+ cell count through one year of therapy was significantly greater for the VIRAMUNE group compared to the placebo group for the overall study population (64 cells/mm^3 vs 22 cells/mm^3, respectively), as well as for patients who entered the trial as treatment naïve or having received only ZDV (85 cells/mm^3 vs 25 cells/mm^3, respectively).
At two years into the study, 16% of subjects on VIRAMUNE had experienced class C CDC events as compared to 21% of subjects on the control arm.

Trial BI 1046 (INCAS) was a double-blind, placebo-controlled, randomized, three arm trial with 151 HIV-1 infected patients with CD4+ cell counts of 200–600 at baseline. BI 1046 compared treatment with VIRAMUNE+zidovudine+didanosine to VIRAMUNE+zidovudine and zidovudine+didanosine. Treatment doses were VIRAMUNE at 200 mg daily for two weeks followed by 200 mg twice daily or placebo, zidovudine at 200 mg three times daily, and didanosine at 125 or 200 mg twice daily (depending on body weight). The patients had mean baseline HIV RNA of 4.41 log_{10} copies/mL (25,704 copies/mL) and mean baseline CD4+ cell count of 376 cells/mm^3. The primary endpoint was the proportion of patients with HIV-RNA < 400 copies/mL and not previously failed at 48 weeks. The virologic responder rates at 48 weeks were 45% for patients treated with VIRAMUNE+zidovudine+didanosine, 19% for patients treated with zidovudine+didanosine, and 0% for patients treated with VIRAMUNE+zidovudine.
CD4+ cell counts in the VIRAMUNE+ZDV+ddI group increased above baseline by a mean of 139 cells/mm^3 at one year, significantly greater than the increase of 87 cells/mm^3 in the ZDV+ddI patients. The VIRAMUNE+ZDV group mean decreased by 6 cells/mm^3 below baseline.

CONTRAINDICATIONS

VIRAMUNE (nevirapine) is contraindicated in patients with clinically significant hypersensitivity to any of the components contained in the tablet or the oral suspension.

WARNINGS

General:

The first 18 weeks of therapy with VIRAMUNE are a critical period during which intensive monitoring of patients is required to detect potentially life-threatening hepatic events and skin reactions. The optimal frequency of monitoring during this time period has not been established. Some experts recommend clinical and laboratory monitoring more often than once per month, and in particular, would include monitoring of liver function tests at baseline, prior to dose

Continued on next page

Viramune—Cont.

escalation and at two weeks post-dose escalation. After the initial 18 week period, frequent clinical and laboratory monitoring should continue throughout VIRAMUNE treatment. In addition, the 14-day lead-in period with VIRAMUNE 200 mg daily dosing has been demonstrated to reduce the frequency of rash.

Resistant virus emerges rapidly and uniformly when VIRAMUNE is administered as monotherapy. Therefore, VIRAMUNE should always be administered in combination with other antiretroviral agents for the treatment of HIV-1 infection.

Hepatic Events:

Severe, life-threatening, and in some cases fatal hepatotoxicity, including fulminant and cholestatic hepatitis, hepatic necrosis and hepatic failure, have been reported in patients treated with VIRAMUNE. In clinical trials, the risk of hepatic events regardless of severity was greatest in the first 6 weeks of therapy. The risk continued to be greater in the VIRAMUNE groups compared to controls through 18 weeks of treatment. However, hepatic events may occur at any time during treatment. In some cases, patients presented with non-specific, prodromal signs or symptoms of fatigue, malaise, anorexia, nausea, jaundice, liver tenderness or hepatomegaly, with or without initially abnormal serum transaminase levels. Some of these events have progressed to hepatic failure with transaminase elevation, with or without hyperbilirubinemia, prolonged partial thromboplastin time, or eosinophilia. Rash and fever accompanied some of these hepatic events. Patients with signs or symptoms of hepatitis must be advised to discontinue VIRAMUNE and immediately seek medical evaluation, which should include liver function tests.

The patients at greatest risk of hepatic events, including potentially fatal events, are women with high CD4 counts.

In addition, serious hepatotoxicity (including liver failure requiring transplantation in one instance) has been reported in HIV-uninfected individuals receiving multiple doses of VIRAMUNE in the setting of post-exposure prophylaxis, an unapproved use.

Increased AST or ALT levels and/or co-infection with hepatitis B or C at the start of antiretroviral therapy are associated with a greater risk of hepatic adverse events.

In general, women have a three fold higher risk than men for symptomatic, often rash-associated, hepatic events (5.8% versus 2.2%), and patients with higher CD4 counts at initiation of VIRAMUNE therapy are at higher risk for symptomatic hepatic events with VIRAMUNE. In a retrospective review, women with CD4 counts >250 cells/mm^3 had a 12 fold higher risk of symptomatic hepatic adverse events compared to women with CD4 counts <250 cells/mm^3 (11.0% versus 0.9%). An increased risk was observed in men with CD4 counts >400 cells/mm^3 (6.3% versus 2.3% for men with CD4 counts <400 cells/mm^3).

Because increased nevirapine levels and nevirapine accumulation may be observed in patients with serious liver disease, VIRAMUNE should not be administered to patients with severe hepatic impairment. (See CLINICAL PHARMACOLOGY, *Pharmacokinetics in Special Populations*: *Hepatic Impairment*; PRECAUTIONS, *General*).

Intensive clinical and laboratory monitoring, including liver function tests, is essential at baseline and during the first 18 weeks of treatment. (See WARNINGS, *General*) Monitoring should continue at frequent intervals thereafter. Liver function tests should be performed immediately if a patient experiences signs or symptoms suggestive of hepatitis and/or hypersensitivity reaction. Liver function tests should also be obtained for all patients who develop a rash in the first 18 weeks of treatment. Physicians and patients should be vigilant for the appearance of signs or symptoms of hepatitis, such as fatigue, malaise, anorexia, nausea, jaundice, bilirubinuria, acholic stools, liver tenderness or hepatomegaly. The diagnosis of hepatotoxicity should be considered in this setting, even if liver function tests are initially normal or alternative diagnoses are possible. (See PRECAUTIONS, *Information for Patients*; ADVERSE REACTIONS; DOSAGE AND ADMINISTRATION).

If clinical hepatitis occurs, VIRAMUNE should be permanently discontinued and not restarted after recovery. In some cases, hepatic injury progresses despite discontinuation of treatment.

Skin Reactions:

Severe, life-threatening skin reactions, including fatal cases, have been reported with VIRAMUNE treatment, occurring most frequently during the first 6 weeks of therapy. These have included cases of Stevens-Johnson syndrome, toxic epidermal necrolysis, and hypersensitivity reactions characterized by rash, constitutional findings, and organ dysfunction. Patients developing signs or symptoms of severe skin reactions or hypersensitivity reactions (including, but not limited to, severe rash or rash accompanied by fever, general malaise, fatigue, muscle or joint aches, blisters, oral lesions, conjunctivitis, facial edema, and/or hepatitis, eosinophilia, granulocytopenia, lymphadenopathy, and renal dysfunction) must permanently discontinue VIRAMUNE and seek medical evaluation immediately. (See PRECAUTIONS, *Information for Patients*; ADVERSE REACTIONS) VIRAMUNE should not be restarted following severe skin rash or hypersensitivity reaction. Some of the risk factors for developing serious cutaneous reactions include failure to follow the initial dosing of 200 mg daily during the 14-day lead-in period and delay in stopping the VIRAMUNE treatment after the onset of the initial symptoms.

If patients present with a suspected VIRAMUNE-associated rash, liver function tests should be performed. Patients with rash-associated AST or ALT elevations should be permanently discontinued from VIRAMUNE.

Therapy with VIRAMUNE must be initiated with a 14-day lead-in period of 200 mg/day (4 mg/kg/day in pediatric patients), which has been shown to reduce the frequency of rash. If rash is observed during this lead-in period, dose escalation should not occur until the rash has resolved. (See DOSAGE AND ADMINISTRATION) Patients should be monitored closely if isolated rash of any severity occurs.

Women appear to be at higher risk than men of developing rash with VIRAMUNE.

In a clinical trial, concomitant prednisone use (40 mg/day for the first 14 days of VIRAMUNE administration) was associated with an increase in incidence and severity of rash during the first 6 weeks of VIRAMUNE therapy. Therefore, use of prednisone to prevent VIRAMUNE-associated rash is not recommended.

St. John's wort:

Concomitant use of St. John's wort (hypericum perforatum) or St. John's wort containing products and VIRAMUNE is not recommended. Co-administration of Non-Nucleoside Reverse Transcriptase Inhibitors (NNRTIs), including VIRAMUNE, with St. John's wort is expected to substantially decrease NNRTI concentrations and may result in sub-optimal levels of VIRAMUNE and lead to loss of virologic response and possible resistance to VIRAMUNE or to the class of NNRTIs.

PRECAUTIONS

General:

Nevirapine is extensively metabolized by the liver and nevirapine metabolites are extensively eliminated by the kidney. No adjustment in nevirapine dosing is required in patients with CrCL ≥20 mL/min. In patients undergoing chronic hemodialysis, an additional 200 mg dose following each dialysis treatment is indicated. Nevirapine metabolites may accumulate in patients receiving dialysis; however, the clinical significance of this accumulation is not known. (See CLINICAL PHARMACOLOGY, *Pharmacokinetics in Special Populations*: *Renal Impairment*; DOSAGE AND ADMINISTRATION, *Dosage Adjustment*)

It is not clear whether a dosing adjustment is needed for patients with mild to moderate hepatic impairment, because multiple dose pharmacokinetic data are not available

Table 3

***Established* Drug Interactions: Alteration in Dose or Regimen May Be Recommended Based on Drug Interaction Studies (See CLINICAL PHARMACOLOGY, Table 1 for Magnitude of Interaction)**

Drug Name	Effect on Concentration of Nevirapine or Concomitant Drug	Clinical Comment
Clarithromycin	↓ Clarithromycin ↑ 14-OH clarithromycin	Clarithromycin exposure was significantly decreased by nevirapine; however, 14-OH metabolite concentrations were increased. Because clarithromycin active metabolite has reduced activity against *Mycobacterium avium-intracellulare complex*, overall activity against this pathogen may be altered. Alternatives to clarithromycin, such as azithromycin, should be considered.
Efavirenz	↓ Efavirenz	Appropriate doses for this combination are not established.
Ethinyl estradiol and Norethindrone	↓ Ethinyl estradiol ↓ Norethindrone	Oral contraceptives and other hormonal methods of birth control should not be used as the sole method of contraception in women taking nevirapine, since nevirapine may lower the plasma levels of these medications. An alternative or additional method of contraception is recommended.
Fluconazole	↑ Nevirapine	Because of the risk of increased exposure to nevirapine, caution should be used in concomitant administration, and patients should be monitored closely for nevirapine-associated adverse events.
Indinavir	↓ Indinavir	Appropriate doses for this combination are not established, but an increase in the dosage of indinavir may be required.
Ketoconazole	↓ Ketoconazole	Nevirapine and ketoconazole should not be administered concomitantly because decreases in ketoconazole plasma concentrations may reduce the efficacy of the drug.
Lopinavir/Ritonavir	↓ Lopinavir	A dose increase of lopinavir/ritonavir to 533/133 mg twice daily with food is recommended in combination with nevirapine.
Methadone	↓ Methadone[a]	Methadone levels may be decreased; increased dosages may be required to prevent symptoms of opiate withdrawal. Methadone maintained patients beginning nevirapine therapy should be monitored for evidence of withdrawal and methadone dose should be adjusted accordingly.
Nelfinavir	↓ Nelfinavir M8 Metabolite ↓ Nelfinavir C_{min}	The appropriate dose for nelfinavir in combination with nevirapine, with respect to safety and efficacy, has not been established.
Rifabutin	↑ Rifabutin	Rifabutin and its metabolite concentrations were moderately increased. Due to high intersubject variability, however, some patients may experience large increases in rifabutin exposure and may be at higher risk for rifabutin toxicity. Therefore, caution should be used in concomitant administration.
Rifampin	↓ Nevirapine	Nevirapine and rifampin should not be administered concomitantly because decreases in nevirapine plasma concentrations may reduce the efficacy of the drug. Physicians needing to treat patients co-infected with tuberculosis and using a nevirapine containing regimen may use rifabutin instead.
Saquinavir	↓ Saquinavir	Appropriate doses for this combination are not established, but an increase in the dosage of saquinavir may be required.

[a]Based on reports of narcotic withdrawal syndrome in patients treated with nevirapine and methadone concurrently, and evidence of decreased plasma concentrations of methadone.

for this population. However, patients with moderate hepatic impairment and ascites may be at risk of accumulating nevirapine in the systemic circulation. Caution should be exercised when nevirapine is administered to patients with moderate hepatic impairment. Nevirapine should not be administered to patients with severe hepatic impairment. (See WARNINGS; CLINICAL PHARMACOLOGY, *Pharmacokinetics in Special Populations*: *Hepatic Impairment*)

The duration of clinical benefit from antiretroviral therapy may be limited. Patients receiving VIRAMUNE or any other antiretroviral therapy may continue to develop opportunistic infections and other complications of HIV infection, and therefore should remain under close clinical observation by physicians experienced in the treatment of patients with associated HIV diseases.

When administering VIRAMUNE as part of an antiretroviral regimen, the complete product information for each therapeutic component should be consulted before initiation of treatment.

Drug Interactions:

Nevirapine is principally metabolized by the liver via the cytochrome P450 isoenzymes, 3A4 and 2B6. Nevirapine is known to be an inducer of these enzymes. As a result, drugs that are metabolized by these enzyme systems may have lower than expected plasma levels when co-administered with nevirapine.

The specific pharmacokinetic changes that occur with co-administration of nevirapine and other drugs are listed in CLINICAL PHARMACOLOGY, Table 1. Clinical comments about possible dosage modifications based on these pharmacokinetic changes are listed in Table 3. The data in Tables 1 and 3 are based on the results of drug interaction studies conducted in HIV-1 seropositive subjects unless otherwise indicated.

In addition to established drug interactions, there may be potential pharmacokinetic interactions between nevirapine and other drug classes that are metabolized by the cytochrome P450 system. These potential drug interactions are listed in Table 4. Although specific drug interaction studies in HIV-1 seropositive subjects have not been conducted for the classes of drugs listed in Table 4, additional clinical monitoring may be warranted when co-administering these drugs.

The *in vitro* interaction between nevirapine and the antithrombotic agent warfarin is complex. As a result, when giving these drugs concomitantly, plasma warfarin levels may change with the potential for increases in coagulation time. When warfarin is co-administered with nevirapine, anticoagulation levels should be monitored frequently.

[See table 3 on previous page]

Table 4
***Potential* Drug Interactions: Use With Caution, Dose Adjustment of Co-administered Drug May Be Needed due to Possible Decrease in Clinical Effect**

Examples of Drugs in Which Plasma Concentrations May Be Decreased By Co-administration With Nevirapine

Drug Class	Examples of Drugs
Antiarrhythmics	Amiodarone, disopyramide, lidocaine
Anticonvulsants	Carbamazepine, clonazepam, ethosuximide
Antifungals	Itraconazole
Calcium channel blockers	Diltiazem, nifedipine, verapamil
Cancer chemotherapy	Cyclophosphamide
Ergot alkaloids	Ergotamine
Immunosuppressants	Cyclosporin, tacrolimus, sirolimus
Motility agents	Cisapride
Opiate agonists	Fentanyl
Examples of Drugs in Which Plasma Concentrations May Be Increased By Co-administration With Nevirapine	
Antithrombotics	Warfarin Potential effect on anticoagulation. Monitoring of anticoagulation levels is recommended.

Fat redistribution: Redistribution/accumulation of body fat including central obesity, dorsocervical fat enlargement (buffalo hump), peripheral wasting, facial wasting, breast enlargement, and "cushingoid appearance" have been observed in patients receiving antiretroviral therapy. The mechanism and long-term consequences of these events are currently unknown. A causal relationship has not been established.

Table 5: Risk of Rash (%) in Adult Placebo Controlled Trials[1] – Regardless of Causality

		VIRAMUNE	Placebo
		n=1374 %	n=1331 %
Through 6 weeks of treatment[2]			
Rash events of all grades[3]		14.8	5.9
Grade 1	Erythema, pruritus	8.5	4.2
Grade 2	Diffuse maculopapular rash, dry desquamation	4.8	1.6
Grade 3 or 4	Grade 3: vesiculation, moist desquamation, ulceration; Grade 4: erythema multiforme, Stevens Johnson syndrome, toxic epidermal necrolysis, necrosis requiring surgery, exfoliative dermatitis	1.5	0.1
Through 52 weeks of treatment[2]			
Rash events of all grades[3]		24.0	14.9
Grade 1	See above	15.5	10.8
Grade 2	See above	7.1	3.9
Grade 3 or 4	See above	1.7	0.2
Proportion of Patients who Discontinued Treatment Due to Rash			
		4.3	1.2

[1] Trials 1037, 1038, 1046 and 1090
[2] % based on Kaplan-Meier probability estimates
[3] NCI grading system

Information for Patients:

Patients should be informed of the possibility of severe liver disease or skin reactions associated with VIRAMUNE that may result in death. Patients developing signs or symptoms of liver disease or severe skin reactions should be instructed to discontinue VIRAMUNE and seek medical attention immediately, including performance of laboratory monitoring. Symptoms of liver disease include fatigue, malaise, anorexia, nausea, jaundice, acholic stools, liver tenderness or hepatomegaly. Symptoms of severe skin or hypersensitivity reactions include rash accompanied by fever, general malaise, fatigue, muscle or joint aches, blisters, oral lesions, conjunctivitis, facial edema and/or hepatitis.

Intensive clinical and laboratory monitoring, including liver function tests, is essential during the first 18 weeks of therapy with VIRAMUNE to detect potentially life-threatening hepatotoxicity. However, liver disease can occur after this period, therefore monitoring should continue at frequent intervals throughout VIRAMUNE treatment. Extra vigilance is warranted during the first 6 weeks of therapy, which is the period of greatest risk of hepatic events and skin reactions. Patients with signs and symptoms of hepatitis should discontinue VIRAMUNE and seek medical evaluation immediately. If VIRAMUNE is discontinued due to hepatitis, it should not be restarted. Patients should be advised that co-infection with hepatitis B or C and/or increased liver function tests at the start of antiretroviral therapy are associated with a greater risk of hepatic events with VIRAMUNE. Patients, particularly women, with increased CD4+ cell count at initiation of VIRAMUNE therapy (>250 cells/mm^3 in women and >400 cells/mm^3 in men) may be at substantially higher risk for development of hepatic events, often associated with rash. (See WARNINGS, *Hepatic Events*)

The majority of rashes associated with VIRAMUNE occur within the first 6 weeks of initiation of therapy. Patients should be instructed that if any rash occurs during the two-week lead-in period, the VIRAMUNE dose should not be escalated until the rash resolves. Any patient experiencing severe rash or hypersensitivity reactions should discontinue VIRAMUNE and consult a physician. VIRAMUNE should not be restarted following severe skin rash or hypersensitivity reaction. Women tend to be at higher risk for development of VIRAMUNE associated rash.

Oral contraceptives and other hormonal methods of birth control should not be used as the sole method of contraception in women taking VIRAMUNE, since nevirapine may lower the plasma levels of these medications. Additionally, when oral contraceptives are used for hormonal regulation during VIRAMUNE therapy, the therapeutic effect of the hormonal therapy should be monitored. (See PRECAUTIONS, *Drug Interactions*)

Patients should be informed that VIRAMUNE therapy has not been shown to reduce the risk of transmission of HIV-1 to others through sexual contact or blood contamination. The long-term effects of VIRAMUNE are unknown at this time.

VIRAMUNE is not a cure for HIV-1 infection; patients may continue to experience illnesses associated with advanced HIV-1 infection, including opportunistic infections. Patients should be advised to remain under the care of a physician when using VIRAMUNE.

Patients should be informed to take VIRAMUNE every day as prescribed. Patients should not alter the dose without consulting their doctor. If a dose is missed, patients should take the next dose as soon as possible. However, if a dose is skipped, the patient should not double the next dose. Patients should be advised to report to their doctor the use of any other medications. Based on the known metabolism of methadone, nevirapine may decrease plasma concentrations of methadone by increasing its hepatic metabolism. Narcotic withdrawal syndrome has been reported in patients treated with VIRAMUNE and methadone concomitantly. Methadone-maintained patients beginning nevirapine therapy should be monitored for evidence of withdrawal and methadone dose should be adjusted accordingly.

VIRAMUNE may interact with some drugs, therefore, patients should be advised to report to their doctor the use of any other prescription, non-prescription medication or herbal products, particularly St. John's wort.

Patients should be informed that redistribution or accumulation of body fat may occur in patients receiving antiretroviral therapy and that the cause and long term health effects of these conditions are not known at this time.

The Patient Package Insert provides written information for the patient, and should be dispensed with each new prescription and refill.

Carcinogenesis, Mutagenesis, Impairment of Fertility:

Long-term carcinogenicity studies in mice and rats were carried out with nevirapine. Mice were dosed with 0, 50, 375 or 750 mg/kg/day for two years. Hepatocellular adenomas and carcinomas were increased at all doses in males and at the two high doses in females. In studies in which rats were administered nevirapine at doses of 0, 3.5, 17.5 or 35 mg/kg/day for two years, an increase in hepatocellular adenomas was seen in males at all doses and in females at the high dose. The systemic exposure (based on AUCs) at all doses in the two animal studies were lower than that measured in humans at the 200 mg bid dose. The mechanism of the carcinogenic potential is unknown. However, in genetic toxicology assays, nevirapine showed no evidence of mutagenic or clastogenic activity in a battery of *in vitro* and *in vivo* studies. These included microbial assays for gene mutation (Ames: Salmonella strains and *E. coli*), mammalian cell gene mutation assay (CHO/HGPRT), cytogenetic assays using a Chinese hamster ovary cell line and a mouse bone marrow micronucleus assay following oral administration. Given the lack of genotoxic activity of nevirapine, the relevance to humans of hepatocellular neoplasms in nevirapine treated mice and rats is not known. In reproductive toxicology studies, evidence of impaired fertility was seen in female rats at doses providing systemic exposure, based on AUC, approximately equivalent to that provided with the recommended clinical dose of VIRAMUNE.

Pregnancy: Pregnancy Category C

No observable teratogenicity was detected in reproductive studies performed in pregnant rats and rabbits. In rats, a significant decrease in fetal body weight occurred at doses providing systemic exposure approximately 50% higher, based on AUC, than that seen at the recommended human clinical dose.

The maternal and developmental no-observable-effect level dosages in rats and rabbits produced systemic exposures approximately equivalent to or approximately 50% higher,

Continued on next page

Viramune—Cont.

respectively, than those seen at the recommended daily human dose, based on AUC. There are no adequate and well-controlled studies in pregnant women. VIRAMUNE should be used during pregnancy only if the potential benefit justifies the potential risk to the fetus. Severe hepatic events, including fatalities, have been reported in pregnant women receiving chronic VIRAMUNE therapy as part of combination treatment of HIV infection. It is unclear if pregnancy augments the already increased risk observed in non-pregnant women. (see Boxed WARNING)

Antiretroviral Pregnancy Registry:

To monitor maternal-fetal outcomes of pregnant women exposed to VIRAMUNE, an Antiretroviral Pregnancy Registry has been established. Physicians are encouraged to register patients by calling (800) 258-4263.

Nursing Mothers:

The Centers for Disease Control and Prevention recommend that HIV-infected mothers not breast-feed their infants to avoid risking postnatal transmission of HIV. Nevirapine is excreted in breast milk. Because of both the potential for HIV transmission and the potential for serious adverse reactions in nursing infants, mothers should be instructed not to breast-feed if they are receiving VIRAMUNE.

Pediatric Use:

The pharmacokinetics of nevirapine have been studied in two open-label studies in children with HIV-1 infection. (See CLINICAL PHARMACOLOGY, *Pharmacokinetics in Special Populations*) For dose recommendations for pediatric patients see DOSAGE AND ADMINISTRATION. The most frequently reported adverse events related to VIRAMUNE in pediatric patients were similar to those observed in adults, with the exception of granulocytopenia, which was more commonly observed in children. (See ADVERSE REACTIONS, *Pediatric Patients*) The evaluation of the antiviral activity of VIRAMUNE in pediatric patients is ongoing.

Geriatric Use:

Clinical studies of VIRAMUNE did not include sufficient numbers of subjects aged 65 and older to determine whether elderly subjects respond differently from younger subjects. In general, dose selection for an elderly patient should be cautious, reflecting the greater frequency of decreased hepatic, renal or cardiac function, and of concomitant disease or other drug therapy.

ADVERSE REACTIONS

Adults:

Clinical practice has shown that the most serious adverse reactions associated with VIRAMUNE are clinical hepatitis/hepatic failure, Stevens-Johnson syndrome, toxic epidermal necrolysis, and hypersensitivity reactions. Clinical hepatitis/hepatic failure may be isolated or associated with signs of hypersensitivity which may include severe rash or rash accompanied by fever, general malaise, fatigue, muscle or joint aches, blisters, oral lesions, conjunctivitis, facial edema, and/or hepatitis, eosinophilia, granulocytopenia, lymphadenopathy, and renal dysfunction.

Severe and life-threatening hepatotoxicity, and fatal fulminant hepatitis have been reported in patients treated with VIRAMUNE. Hepatic adverse events have been reported to occur more frequently during the first 18 weeks of treatment, but such events may occur at any time during treatment.

In controlled clinical trials, clinical hepatic events regardless of severity occurred in 4.0% (range 2.5% to 11.0%) of patients who received VIRAMUNE and 1.2% of patients in control groups. Transaminase elevations (ALT or AST > 5× ULN) were observed in 8.8% of patients receiving VIRAMUNE and 6.2% of patients in control groups in clinical trials. In a retrospective analysis of controlled and uncontrolled clinical trials, patients with higher CD4 counts at initiation of VIRAMUNE therapy, particularly women, were at greater risk for acute symptomatic hepatic events, including death, especially in the first six weeks of therapy. Patients with chronic hepatitis B or C infection were at higher risk for later hepatic events. (See WARNINGS)

The most common clinical toxicity of VIRAMUNE is rash. Severe or life-threatening rash occurred in approximately 2% of VIRAMUNE-treated patients, most frequently within the first 6 weeks of therapy. (See Table 5) Rashes are usually mild to moderate, maculopapular erythematous cutaneous eruptions, with or without pruritus, located on the trunk, face and extremities. Women tend to be at higher risk for development of VIRAMUNE associated rash.

[See table 5 at top of previous page]

Treatment related, adverse experiences of moderate or severe intensity observed in >2% of patients receiving VIRAMUNE in placebo-controlled trials are shown in Table 6.

[See table 6 above]

Table 6: Percentage of Patients with Moderate or Severe Drug Related Events in Adult Placebo Controlled Trials

	Trial 1090[1]		Trials 1037, 1038, 1046[2]	
	VIRAMUNE (n=1121)	**Placebo (n=1128)**	**VIRAMUNE (n=253)**	**Placebo (n=203)**
Median exposure (weeks)	58	52	28	28
Any adverse event	14.5%	11.1%	31.6%	13.3%
Rash	5.1	1.8	6.7	1.5
Abnormal LFTs	1.2	0.9	6.7	1.5
Nausea	0.5	1.1	8.7	3.9
Granulocytopenia	1.8	2.8	0.4	0
Headache	0.7	0.4	3.6	0.5
Fatigue	0.2	0.3	4.7	3.9
Diarrhea	0.2	0.8	2.0	0.5
Abdominal pain	0.1	0.4	2.0	0
Myalgia	0.2	0	1.2	2.0

[1] Background therapy included 3TC for all patients and combinations of NRTIs and PIs. Patients had CD4+ cell counts <200 cells/mm^3.

[2] Background therapy included ZDV and ZDV+ddI; VIRAMUNE monotherapy was administered in some patients. Patients had CD4+ cell count ≥200 cells/mm^3.

Laboratory Abnormalities: Liver function test abnormalities (AST, ALT) were observed more frequently in patients receiving VIRAMUNE than in controls. (Table 7) Asymptomatic elevations in GGT occur frequently but are not a contraindication to continue VIRAMUNE therapy in the absence of elevations in other liver function tests. Other laboratory abnormalities (bilirubin, anemia, neutropenia, thrombocytopenia) were observed with similar frequencies in clinical trials comparing VIRAMUNE and control regimens. (See Table 7)

[See table 7 above]

Table 7: Percentage of Adult Patients with Laboratory Abnormalities

	Trial 1090[1]		Trials 1037, 1038, 1046[2]	
	VIRAMUNE	**Placebo**	**VIRAMUNE**	**Placebo**
Laboratory Abnormality	**n=1121**	**n=1128**	**n=253**	**n=203**
Blood Chemistry				
SGPT (ALT) >250 U/L	5.3%	4.4%	14.0%	4.0%
SGOT (AST) >250 U/L	3.7	2.5	7.6	1.5
Bilirubin >2.5 mg/dL	1.7	2.2	1.7	1.5
Hematology				
Hemoglobin <8.0 g/dL	3.2	4.1	0	0
Platelets <50,000/mm^3	1.3	1.0	0.4	1.5
Neutrophils <750/mm^3	13.3	13.5	3.6	1.0

[1] Background therapy included 3TC for all patients and combinations of NRTIs and PIs. Patients had CD4+ cell counts <200 cells/mm^3.

[2] Background therapy included ZDV and ZDV+ddI; VIRAMUNE monotherapy was administered in some patients. Patients had CD4+ cell count ≥200 cells/mm^3.

Because clinical hepatitis has been reported in VIRAMUNE-treated patients, intensive clinical and laboratory monitoring, including liver function tests, is essential at baseline and during the first 18 weeks of treatment. Monitoring should continue at frequent intervals thereafter, depending on the patient's clinical status. (See WARNINGS)

Post Marketing Surveillance: In addition to the adverse events identified during clinical trials, the following events have been reported with the use of VIRAMUNE in clinical practice:

Body as a Whole: fever, somnolence, drug withdrawal (See PRECAUTIONS: *Drug Interactions*), redistribution/accumulation of body fat (see PRECAUTIONS, Fat redistribution).

Gastrointestinal: vomiting

Liver and Biliary: jaundice, fulminant and cholestatic hepatitis, hepatic necrosis, hepatic failure

Hematology: anemia, eosinophilia, neutropenia

Musculoskeletal: arthralgia

Neurologic: paraesthesia

Skin and Appendages: allergic reactions including anaphylaxis, angioedema, bullous eruptions, ulcerative stomatitis and urticaria have all been reported. In addition, hypersensitivity syndrome and hypersensitivity reactions with rash associated with constitutional findings such as fever, blistering, oral lesions, conjunctivitis, facial edema, muscle or joint aches, general malaise, fatigue or significant hepatic abnormalities (See WARNINGS) plus one or more of the following: hepatitis, eosinophilia, granulocytopenia, lymphadenopathy and/or renal dysfunction have been reported with the use of VIRAMUNE.

Pediatric Patients:

Safety was assessed in trial BI 882 in which patients were followed for a mean duration of 33.9 months (range: 6.8 months to 5.3 years, including long-term follow-up in 29 of these patients in trial BI 892). The most frequently reported adverse events related to VIRAMUNE in pediatric patients were similar to those observed in adults, with the exception of granulocytopenia, which was more commonly observed in children. Serious adverse events were assessed in ACTG 245, a double-blind, placebo-controlled trial of VIRAMUNE (n = 305) in which pediatric patients received combination treatment with VIRAMUNE. In this trial two patients were reported to experience Stevens-Johnson syndrome or Stevens-Johnson/toxic epidermal necrolysis transition syndrome. Cases of allergic reaction, including one case of anaphylaxis, were also reported.

Table 8 summarizes the marked laboratory abnormalities occurring in pediatric patients in Trial BI 882 and in follow-up Trial BI 892.

Table 8: Number of Pediatric Patients (%) with Laboratory Abnormalities In Trials BI 882 and BI 892 Combined

	No. (%) of Patients n=37
Blood Chemistry	
Increased ALT (>250 U/L)	4 (11)
Increased AST (>250 U/L)	5 (14)
Increased GGT (>450 U/L)	4 (11)
Increased total bilirubin (>2.5 mg/dL)	1 (3)
Increased alkaline phosphatase (>2× ULN)	19 (51)
Increased amylase (>2× ULN)	6 (16)
Hematology	
Decreased Hg (<8.0 g/dL)	7 (19)
Decreased platelets (<50,000/mm^3)	4 (11)
Decreased neutrophils (<750/mm^3)	14 (38)
Increased MCV (>100 F/L)	13 (35)

OVERDOSAGE

There is no known antidote for VIRAMUNE overdosage. Cases of VIRAMUNE overdose at doses ranging from 800 to 1800 mg per day for up to 15 days have been reported. Patients have experienced events including edema, erythema nodosum, fatigue, fever, headache, insomnia, nausea, pulmonary infiltrates, rash, vertigo, vomiting and weight decrease. All events subsided following discontinuation of VIRAMUNE.

DOSAGE AND ADMINISTRATION

Adults:

The recommended dose for VIRAMUNE is one 200 mg tablet daily for the first 14 days **(this lead-in period should be used because it has been found to lessen the frequency of rash),** followed by one 200 mg tablet twice daily, in combination with other antiretroviral agents. For concomitantly administered antiretroviral therapy, the manufacturer's recommended dosage and monitoring should be followed.

Pediatric Patients:

The recommended oral dose of VIRAMUNE for pediatric patients 2 months up to 8 years of age is 4 mg/kg once daily for the first 14 days followed by 7 mg/kg twice daily thereafter. For patients 8 years and older the recommended dose is 4 mg/kg once daily for two weeks followed by 4 mg/kg twice daily thereafter. The total daily dose should not exceed 400 mg for any patient.

VIRAMUNE suspension should be shaken gently prior to administration. It is important to administer the entire measured dose of suspension by using an oral dosing syringe or dosing cup. An oral dosing syringe is recommended, particularly for volumes of 5 mL or less. If a dosing cup is used, it should be thoroughly rinsed with water and the rinse should also be administered to the patient.

Monitoring of Patients:

Intensive clinical and laboratory monitoring, including liver function tests, is essential at baseline and during the first 18 weeks of treatment with VIRAMUNE. The optimal frequency of monitoring during this period has not been established. Some experts recommend clinical and laboratory monitoring more often than once per month, and in particular, would include monitoring of liver function tests at baseline, prior to dose escalation, and at two weeks post dose escalation. After the initial 18 week period, frequent clinical and laboratory monitoring should continue throughout VIRAMUNE treatment. (See WARNINGS) In some cases, hepatic injury has progressed despite discontinuation of treatment.

Dosage Adjustment:

VIRAMUNE should be discontinued if patients experience severe rash or a rash accompanied by constitutional findings. (See WARNINGS) Patients experiencing rash during the 14-day lead-in period of 200 mg/day (4 mg/kg/day in pediatric patients) should not have their VIRAMUNE dose increased until the rash has resolved. (See PRECAUTIONS, *Information for Patients*)

If clinical hepatitis occurs, VIRAMUNE should be permanently discontinued and not restarted after recovery.

Patients who interrupt VIRAMUNE dosing for more than 7 days should restart the recommended dosing, using one 200 mg tablet daily (4 mg/kg/day in pediatric patients) for the first 14 days (lead-in) followed by one 200 mg tablet twice daily (4 or 7 mg/kg twice daily, according to age, for pediatric patients).

An additional 200 mg dose of VIRAMUNE following each dialysis treatment is indicated in patients requiring dialysis. Nevirapine metabolites may accumulate in patients receiving dialysis; however, the clinical significance of this accumulation is not known. (See CLINICAL PHARMACOLOGY, *Pharmacokinetics in Special Populations*: Renal Impairment) Patients with CrCL ≥20 mL/min do not require an adjustment in VIRAMUNE dosing.

HOW SUPPLIED

VIRAMUNE (nevirapine) Tablets, 200 mg, are white, oval, biconvex tablets, 9.3 mm × 19.1 mm. One side is embossed with "54 193", with a single bisect separating the "54" and "193". The opposite side has a single bisect.

VIRAMUNE Tablets are supplied in bottles of 60 (NDC 0597-0046-60),

VIRAMUNE (nevirapine) Oral Suspension is a white to off-white preserved suspension containing 50 mg nevirapine (as nevirapine hemihydrate) in each 5 mL. VIRAMUNE suspension is supplied in plastic bottles with child-resistant closures containing 240 mL of suspension (NDC 0597-0047-24).

VIRAMUNE Tablets and VIRAMUNE Oral Suspension should be stored at 25°C (77°F); excursions permitted to 15°–30°C (59°F–86°F). [see USP Controlled Room Temperature] Store in a safe place out of the reach of children.

Boehringer Ingelheim Pharmaceuticals, Inc.
Ridgefield, CT 06877 USA
Boehringer Ingelheim

(01/04)
Revised 01/23/04
4077435/US/11

Shown in Product Identification Guide, page 309

Bone Care International, Inc.

BONE CARE CENTER
1600 ASPEN COMMONS
MIDDLETON, WI 53562

Direct Inquiries to:
Professional Services Department
TELEPHONE: (888)-389-4242
FAX: 608-662-7870

HECTOROL® CAPSULES ℞

[*heck-tŏrŏl*]
(doxercalciferol)

DESCRIPTION

Doxercalciferol, the active ingredient in Hectorol®, is a synthetic vitamin D_2 analog that undergoes metabolic activation *in vivo* to form 1α,25-dihydroxyvitamin D_2 (1α,25-$(OH)_2D_2$), a naturally occurring, biologically active form of vitamin D_2. Hectorol® is available as soft gelatin capsules containing 0.5 mcg or 2.5 mcg doxercalciferol. Each capsule also contains fractionated triglyceride of coconut oil, ethanol, and butylated hydroxyanisole (BHA). The capsule shells contain gelatin, glycerin, titanium dioxide, and D&C Yellow No. 10 with or without FD&C Red No. 40.

Doxercalciferol is a colorless crystalline compound with a calculated molecular weight of 412.66 and a molecular formula of $C_{28}H_{44}O_2$. It is soluble in oils and organic solvents, but is relatively insoluble in water. Chemically, doxercalciferol is (1α,3β,5Z,7E,22E)-9,10-secoergosta-5,7,10(19),22-tetraene-1,3-diol and has the following structural formula:

Other names frequently used for doxercalciferol are 1α-hydroxyvitamin D_2, 1α-OH-D_2, and 1α-hydroxyergocalciferol.

CLINICAL PHARMACOLOGY

Vitamin D levels in humans depend on two sources: (1) exposure to the ultraviolet rays of the sun for conversion of 7-dehydrocholesterol in the skin to vitamin D_3 (cholecalciferol) and (2) dietary intake of either vitamin D_2 (ergocalciferol) or vitamin D_3. Vitamin D_2 and vitamin D_3 must be metabolically activated in the liver and the kidney before becoming fully active on target tissues. The initial step in the activation process is the introduction of a hydroxyl group in the side chain at C-25 by the hepatic enzyme, CYP 27 (a vitamin D-25-hydroxylase). The products of this reaction are 25-$(OH)D_2$ and 25-$(OH)D_3$, respectively. Further hydroxylation of these metabolites occurs in the mitochondria of kidney tissue, catalyzed by renal 25-hydroxyvitamin D-1-α-hydroxylase to produce 1α,25-$(OH)_2D_2$, the primary biologically active form of vitamin D_2, and 1α,25-$(OH)_2D_3$ (calcitriol), the biologically active form of vitamin D_3.

Mechanism of Action

Calcitriol (1α,25-$(OH)_2D_3$) and 1α,25-$(OH)_2D_2$ regulate blood calcium at levels required for essential body functions. Specifically, the biologically active vitamin D metabolites control the intestinal absorption of dietary calcium, the tubular reabsorption of calcium by the kidney and, in conjunction with parathyroid hormone (PTH), the mobilization of calcium from the skeleton. They act directly on bone cells (osteoblasts) to stimulate skeletal growth, and on the parathyroid glands to suppress PTH synthesis and secretion. These functions are mediated by the interaction of these biologically active metabolites with specific receptor proteins in the various target tissues. In patients with chronic kidney disease (CKD), deficient production of biologically active vitamin D metabolites (due to lack of or insufficient 25-hydroxyvitamin D-1-alpha-hydroxylase activity) leads to secondary hyperparathyroidism, which contributes to the development of metabolic bone disease.

Pharmacokinetics and Metabolism

Doxercalciferol is absorbed from the gastrointestinal tract and activated by CYP 27 in the liver to form 1α,25-$(OH)_2D_2$ (major metabolite) and 1α,24-dihydroxyvitamin D_2 (minor metabolite). Activation of doxercalciferol does not require the involvement of the kidneys.

In healthy volunteers, peak blood levels of 1α,25-$(OH)_2D_2$, the major metabolite of doxercalciferol, are attained at 11–12 hours after repeated oral doses of 5 to 15 mcg of Hectorol® and the mean elimination half-life of 1α,25-$(OH)_2D_2$ is approximately 32 to 37 hours with a range of up to 96 hours. The mean elimination half-life in patients with end-stage renal disease (ESRD) on dialysis appears to be similar. Hemodialysis causes a temporary increase in 1α,25-$(OH)_2D_2$ mean concentrations, presumably due to volume contraction. 1α,25-$(OH)_2D_2$ is not removed from blood during hemodialysis.

Clinical Studies

Dialysis: The safety and effectiveness of Hectorol® were evaluated in two double-blind, placebo-controlled, multicentered clinical studies (Study A and Study B) in a total of 138 patients with chronic kidney disease on hemodialysis (Stage 5 CKD). Patients in Study A were an average age of 52 years (range: 22–75), were 55% male, and were 58% African-American, 31% Caucasian, and 11% Hispanic, and had been on hemodialysis for an average of 53 months. Patients in Study B were an average of 52 years (range: 27–75), were 45% male, and 99% African-American, and 1% Caucasian, and had been on hemodialysis for an average of 56 months. After randomization to two groups, eligible patients underwent an 8-week washout period during which no vitamin D derivatives were administered to either group. Subsequently, all patients received Hectorol® in an open-label fashion for 16 weeks followed by a double-blind period of 8 weeks during which patients received either Hectorol® or placebo. The initial dose of Hectorol® during the open-label phase was 10 micrograms after each dialysis session (3 times weekly) for a total of 30 mcg per week. The dosage of Hectorol® was adjusted as necessary by the investigator in an attempt to achieve intact parathyroid hormone (iPTH) levels within a targeted range of 150 to 300 pg/mL. The maximum dosage was limited to 20 mcg after each dialysis session (60 mcg/week). If at any time during the trial iPTH fell below 150 pg/mL, Hectorol® was immediately suspended and restarted at a lower dosage the following week.

Results: One hundred and six of the 138 patients who were treated with Hectorol® during the 16-week open-label phase achieved iPTH levels ≤ 300 pg/mL. Ninety-four of these patients exhibited plasma iPTH levels ≤ 300 pg/mL on at least 3 occasions. Eighty-seven patients had plasma iPTH levels < 150 pg/mL on at least one occasion during the open-label phase of study participation.

Mean weekly doses during the 16-week open-label period in Study A ranged from 14.8 mcg to 28.7 mcg. In Study B, the mean weekly doses during the 16-week open-label period ranged from 19.2 mcg to 28.0 mcg.

Continued on next page

		iPTH (pg/mL) means ± s.d. (n*) p Value *v.* Baseline p Value *v.* Placebo	
		Hectorol®	Placebo
Study A	Baseline	797.2 ± 443.8 (30) n.a. 0.97	847.1 ± 765.5 (32)
	Week 16 (open-label)	384.3 ± 397.8 (24) <.001 0.72	526.5 ± 872.2 (29) <.001
	Week 24 (double-blind)	404.4 ± 262.9 (21) <.001 0.008	672.6 ± 356.9 (24) 0.70
Study B	Baseline	973.9 ± 567.0 (41) n.a. 0.81	990.4 ± 488.3 (35)
	Week 16 (open-label)	476.1 ± 444.5 (37) <.001 0.91	485.9 ± 443.4 (32) <.001
	Week 24 (double-blind)	459.8 ± 443.0 (35) <.001 <.001	871.9 ± 623.6 (30) <.065

* all subjects; last value carried to discontinuation

Hectorol Capsules—Cont.

Decreases in plasma iPTH from baseline values were calculated, using, as baseline, the average of the last 3 values obtained during the 8-week washout phase and are displayed in the table below.
[See table at bottom of previous page]
In both studies, iPTH levels increased progressively and significantly in 65.9% of the patients during the 8-week washout (control) period during which no vitamin D derivatives were administered. In contrast, Hectorol® treatment resulted in a statistically significant reduction from baseline in mean iPTH levels during the 16-week open-label treatment period in more than 93.5% of the 138 treated patients. During the double-blind period (weeks 17 to 24), the reduction in mean iPTH levels was maintained in the Hectorol® treatment group compared to a return to near baseline in the placebo group.
In the clinical trials, the values for iPTH varied widely from patient to patient and from week to week for individual patients. The following table shows the numbers of patients within each group who achieved and maintained iPTH levels below 300 pg/mL during the open-label and double-blind phases. Seventy-four of 138 patients (53.6%) had plasma iPTH levels within the target range (150–300 pg/mL) during Weeks 14–16.
[See first table below]
During the 8-week double-blind phase, more patients achieved and maintained the target range of values for iPTH with Hectorol® than with placebo.
Pre-dialysis: The safety and effectiveness of Hectorol® were evaluated in two clinical studies in 55 patients with Stage 3 or Stage 4 chronic kidney disease. Eighty-two percent of the patients were male, the average age was 64.6 years, 51% were Caucasian, 40% African-American, and the average serum iPTH level at baseline was 194.6 pg/ml. While levels of 25-(OH) vitamin D were not evaluated at baseline, retrospective assessments of stored serum revealed that the mean ± SD serum 25-(OH) vitamin D was 18.5 ± 8.1 ng/mL (range: <5 to 54 ng/mL) in the study population.
After randomization to two groups, eligible patients underwent an 8-week washout period during which no vitamin D derivatives were administered to either group. Subsequently, one group received Hectorol® and the other placebo during a double-blind period of 24 weeks. The initial dose of Hectorol® was 1.0 mcg per day. The dosage of Hectorol® was adjusted as necessary by the investigator in order to reduce intact parathyroid hormone (iPTH) levels to a target of ≥30% below post-washout baseline. The maximum dosage was limited to 3.5 mcg per day. If at any time during the trial iPTH fell below 15 pg/mL, Hectorol® was immediately suspended and restarted at a lower dosage the following week.
Results: Decreases in the mean plasma iPTH from baseline values were calculated using as baseline the average of the last 2 values obtained during the 8-week washout phase. In analyses of pooled data from the two studies, iPTH levels decreased from baseline by an average of 101.4 pg/mL in the Hectorol® group and by 4.4 pg/mL in the placebo group (p<0.001). Greater reductions of iPTH with Hectorol® compared to placebo were observed in each study. Twenty (74%) of 27 subjects in the Hectorol® group achieved mean plasma iPTH suppression of ≥30% from baseline for the last four weeks of treatment; whereas two (7%) of the 28 subjects treated with placebo achieved this level of iPTH suppression. In the Hectorol®-treated patients, the reductions in plasma iPTH were associated with a reduction in serum bone-specific alkaline phosphatase.

INDICATIONS AND USAGE

Dialysis Patients: Hectorol® is indicated for the treatment of secondary hyperparathyroidism in patients with chronic kidney disease on dialysis.
Pre-Dialysis Patients: Hectorol® is indicated for the treatment of secondary hyperparathyroidism in patients with Stage 3 or Stage 4 chronic kidney disease.

CONTRAINDICATIONS

Hectorol® should not be given to patients with a tendency towards hypercalcemia or evidence of vitamin D toxicity.

WARNINGS

Overdosage of any form of vitamin D, including Hectorol®, is dangerous (see **OVERDOSAGE**). Progressive hypercalcemia due to overdosage of vitamin D and its metabolites may be so severe as to require emergency attention. Acute hypercalcemia may exacerbate tendencies for cardiac arrhythmias and seizures and may potentiate the action of digitalis drugs. Chronic hypercalcemia can lead to generalized vascular calcification and other soft-tissue calcification. The serum calcium times serum phosphorus (Ca X P) product should be maintained at <55 mg^2/dL^2 in patients with chronic kidney disease. Radiographic evaluation of suspect anatomical regions may be useful in the early detection of this condition.
Since doxercalciferol is a precursor for 1α,25-$(OH)_2D_2$, a potent metabolite of vitamin D_2, pharmacologic doses of vitamin D and its derivatives should be withheld during Hectorol® treatment to avoid possible additive effects and hypercalcemia.
Oral calcium-based or other non-aluminum-containing phosphate binders and a low phosphate diet should be used to control serum phosphorus levels in patients with chronic kidney disease. Uncontrolled serum phosphorus exacerbates secondary hyperparathyroidism and can lessen the effectiveness of Hectorol® in reducing blood PTH levels. If hypercalcemia occurs after initiating Hectorol® therapy, the dose of Hectorol® and/or calcium containing-phosphate binders should be decreased. If hyperphosphatemia occurs after initiating Hectorol®, the dose of Hectorol® should be decreased and/or the dose of phosphate binders increased. (See dosing recommendations for Hectorol® under **DOSAGE AND ADMINISTRATION** section.)
Magnesium-containing antacids and Hectorol® should not be used concomitantly in patients on chronic renal dialysis because such use may lead to the development of hypermagnesemia.

PRECAUTIONS

General

Active vitamin D sterols should not be used as initial treatment of nutritional vitamin D deficiency (as defined by low 25-hydroxy vitamin D). Patients should be checked and treated for nutritional vitamin D deficiency prior to initiating treatment with Hectorol®.
The principal adverse effects of treatment with Hectorol® are hypercalcemia, hyperphosphatemia, hypercalciuria, and oversuppression of iPTH. Prolonged hypercalcemia can lead to calcification of soft tissues, including the heart and arteries, and hyperphosphatemia can exacerbate hyperparathyroidism. Hypercalciuria can accelerate the onset of renal failure through nephrocalcinosis. Oversuppression of iPTH may lead to adynamic bone syndrome. All of these potential adverse effects should be managed by regular patient monitoring and appropriate dosage adjustments. During treatment with Hectorol®, patients usually require dose titration, as well as adjustment in co-therapy (i.e., dietary phosphate binders) in order to effect and sustain PTH suppression while maintaining serum calcium and phosphorus within prescribed ranges.
Dialysis: In four adequate and well-controlled studies, the incidence of hypercalcemia and hyperphosphatemia increased during therapy with Hectorol®. The observed increases during Hectorol® treatment, although occurring at a low rate, underscore the importance of regular safety monitoring of serum calcium and phosphorus levels throughout treatment. Patients with higher pre-treatment serum levels of calcium (>10.5 mg/dL) or phosphorus (>6.9 mg/dL) were more likely to experience hypercalcemia or hyperphosphatemia. Therefore, Hectorol® should not be given to patients with a recent history of hypercalcemia or hyperphosphatemia, or evidence of vitamin D toxicity.
Pre-dialysis: In two clinical studies, the incidences of hypercalcemia and hyperphosphatemia during therapy with Hectorol® were similar to placebo therapy, and no episodes of hypercalciuria were observed. The baseline median 25-(OH) vitamin D levels of patients enrolled in these studies was 17.2 ng/mL. Ninety-three percent of patients had 25-(OH) vitamin D levels less than 30 ng/mL; 26% had 25-(OH) vitamin D levels ≥20 to <30 ng/mL; 58% had levels >10 to <20 ng/mL; and 7% had levels >5 to <10 ng/mL and 2% had levels <5 ng/mL. The incidences of hypercalcemia, hyperphosphatemia, and hypercalciuria in patients treated with Hectorol® for hyperparathyroidism related to pre-dialysis renal insufficiency has not been fully studied when 25-OH vitamin D levels are greater than or equal to 30 ng/mL.

Information for the Patient

The patient, spouse, or guardian should be informed about compliance with dosage instructions, adherence to instructions about diet, calcium supplementation, and avoidance of the use of nonprescription drugs without prior approval from their physician. Patients should also be carefully informed about the symptoms of hypercalcemia (see **ADVERSE REACTIONS** section).
Patients should have a combined (dietary and calcium based phosphate binder) daily intake of 1.5 to 2 gm.

Laboratory Tests

Serum or plasma iPTH and serum calcium, phosphorus, and alkaline phosphatase should be determined periodically. In the early phase of treatment for dialysis patients, iPTH, serum calcium, and serum phosphorus should be determined prior to initiation of Hectorol® treatment and weekly thereafter. For pre-dialysis patients, serum levels of calcium and phosphorus and plasma levels of iPTH should be monitored at least every two weeks for 3 months after initiation of Hectorol® therapy or following dose-adjustments in Hectorol® therapy, then monthly for 3 months, and every 3 months thereafter.

Drug Interactions

Specific drug interaction studies have not been conducted. Cholestyramine has been reported to reduce intestinal absorption of fat-soluble vitamins; therefore, it may impair intestinal absorption of doxercalciferol. Magnesium-containing antacids and Hectorol® should not be used concomitantly, because such use may lead to the develop-

		Number of times iPTH ≤ 300 pg/mL					
		1		2		≥ 3	
		Hectorol®	Placebo	Hectorol®	Placebo	Hectorol®	Placebo
Study A	Weeks 1–16 (open-label)	2/30	2/32	0/30	0/32	22/30	23/32
	Weeks 17–24 (double-blind)	0/24	9/29	3/24	1/29	17/24	5/29
Study B	Weeks 1–16 (open-label)	2/41	4/35	1/41	0/35	29/41	21/35
	Weeks 17–24 (double-blind)	2/37	6/32	1/37	4/32	26/37	4/32

Adverse Events Reported by ≥2% of Hectorol® Treated Patients and More Frequently Than Placebo During the Double-blind Phase of Two Clinical Studies

Adverse Event	Hectorol® (n=61) %	Placebo (n=61) %
Body as a Whole		
Abscess	3.3	0.0
Headache	27.9	18.0
Malaise	27.9	19.7
Cardiovascular System		
Bradycardia	6.6	4.9
Digestive System		
Anorexia	4.9	3.3
Constipation	3.3	3.3
Dyspepsia	4.9	1.6
Nausea/Vomiting	21.3	19.7
Musculo-Skeletal System		
Arthralgia	4.9	0.0
Metabolic and Nutritional		
Edema	34.4	21.3
Weight increase	4.9	0.0
Nervous System		
Dizziness	11.5	9.8
Sleep disorder	3.3	0.0
Respiratory System		
Dyspnea	11.5	6.6
Skin		
Pruritus	8.2	6.6

A patient who reported the same medical term more than once was counted only once for that medical term.

ment of hypermagnesemia (see **WARNINGS**). The use of mineral oil or other substances that may affect absorption of fat may influence the absorption and availability of Hectorol®. Although not examined specifically, both enzyme inducers (such as glutethimide and phenobarbital) may affect the 25-hydroxylation of Hectorol® and may necessitate dosage adjustments.

Carcinogenesis, Mutagenesis, Impairment of Fertility

Long-term studies in animals to evaluate the carcinogenic potential of doxercalciferol have not been conducted. No evidence of genetic toxicity was observed in an *in vitro* bacterial mutagenicity assay (Ames test) or a mouse lymphoma gene mutation assay. Doxercalciferol caused structural chromatid and chromosome aberrations in an *in vitro* human lymphocyte clastogenicity assay with metabolic activation. However, doxercalciferol was negative in an *in vivo* mouse micronucleus clastogenicity assay. Doxercalciferol had no effect on male or female fertility in rats at oral doses up to 2.5 mcg/kg/day (approximately 3 times the maximum recommended human dose of 60 mcg/week based on mcg/m^2 body surface area).

Use in Pregnancy

Pregnancy Category B

Reproduction studies in rats and rabbits, at doses up to 20 mcg/kg/day and 0.1 mcg/kg/day (approximately 25 times and less than the maximum recommended human dose of 60 mcg/week based on mcg/m^2 body surface area, respectively) have revealed no teratogenic or fetotoxic effects due to doxercalciferol. There are, however, no adequate and well-controlled studies in pregnant women. Because animal reproduction studies are not always predictive of human response, this drug should be used during pregnancy only if clearly needed.

Nursing Mothers

It is not known whether doxercalciferol is excreted in human milk. Because other vitamin D derivatives are excreted in human milk and because of the potential for serious adverse reactions in nursing infants from doxercalciferol, a decision should be made whether to discontinue nursing or to discontinue the drug, taking into account the importance of the drug to the mother.

Pediatric Use

Safety and efficacy of Hectorol® in pediatric patients have not been established.

Geriatric Use

Of the 138 patients treated with Hectorol® Capsules in two Phase 3 clinical studies, 30 patients were 65 years or over. In these studies, no overall differences in efficacy or safety were observed between patients 65 years or older and younger patients.

Hepatic Insufficiency

Since patients with hepatic insufficiency may not metabolize Hectorol® appropriately, the drug should be used with caution in patients with impaired hepatic function. More frequent monitoring of iPTH, calcium, and phosphorus levels should be done in such individuals.

ADVERSE REACTIONS

Dialysis: Hectorol® has been evaluated for safety in clinical studies in 165 patients with chronic kidney disease on hemodialysis. In two placebo-controlled, double-blind, multicenter studies, discontinuation of therapy due to any adverse event occurred in 2.9% of 138 patients treated with Hectorol® for four to six months (dosage titrated to achieve target iPTH levels, see **CLINICAL PHARMACOLOGY/ Clinical Studies**) and in 3.3% of 61 patients treated with placebo for two months. Adverse events occurring in the Hectorol® group at a frequency of 2% or greater and more frequently than in the placebo group are presented in the following table:

[See second table at bottom of previous page]

Predialysis: Hectorol® has been evaluated for safety in clinical studies in 55 patients (27 active and 28 placebo) with chronic kidney disease, Stages 3 or 4. In two placebo-controlled, double-blind, multicenter studies, discontinuation of therapy due to any adverse event occurred in one (3.7%) of 27 patients treated with Hectorol® for 24 weeks (dosage titrated to achieve target iPTH levels, see **CLINICAL PHARMACOLOGY/Clinical Studies**) and in three (10.7%) of 28 patients treated with placebo for 24 weeks. Adverse events occurring in the Hectorol® group at a frequency of 5% or greater and more frequently than in the placebo group are as follows: **Body as a Whole** – Infection, Pain chest; **Digestive System** – Constipation, Dyspepsia; **Hematologic and Lymphatic** – Anemia; **Metabolic and Nutritional** – Dehydration; **Nervous System** – Depression, Hypertonia, Insomnia, Paresthesia; **Respiratory System** – Cough increased, Dyspnea, Rhinitis.

Potential adverse effects of Hectorol are, in general, similar to those encountered with excessive vitamin D intake. The early and late signs and symptoms of vitamin D intoxication associated with hypercalcemia include:

Early

Weakness, headache, somnolence, nausea, vomiting, dry mouth, constipation, muscle pain, bone pain, metallic taste, and anorexia.

Late

Polyuria, polydipsia, anorexia, weight loss, nocturia, conjunctivitis (calcific), pancreatitis, photophobia, rhinorrhea, pruritus, hyperthermia, decreased libido, elevated blood urea nitrogen (BUN), albuminuria, hypercholesterolemia, elevated serum aspartate transaminase (AST) and alanine transaminase (ALT), ectopic calcification, hypertension, cardiac arrhythmias, sensory disturbances, dehydration, apathy, arrested growth, urinary tract infections, and, rarely, overt psychosis.

OVERDOSAGE

Administration of Hectorol® to patients in excess doses can cause hypercalcemia, hypercalciuria, hyperphosphatemia, and oversuppression of PTH secretion leading in certain cases to adynamic bone disease. High intake of calcium and phosphate concomitant with Hectorol® may lead to similar abnormalities. High levels of calcium in the dialysate bath may contribute to hypercalcemia.

Treatment of Hypercalcemia and Overdosage

General treatment of hypercalcemia (greater than 1 mg/dL above the upper limit of the normal range in dialysis patients; >10.7 mg/dL in pre-dialysis patients) consists of immediate suspension of Hectorol® therapy, institution of a low calcium diet, and withdrawal of calcium supplements. Serum calcium levels should be determined at least weekly until normocalcemia ensues. Hypercalcemia usually resolves in 2 to 7 days. When serum calcium levels have returned to within normal limits, Hectorol® therapy may be reinstituted at a dose that is lower (at least 2.5 mcg in dialysis patients and 0.5 mcg in pre-dialysis patients) than prior therapy. In dialysis patients, serum calcium levels should be obtained weekly after all dosage changes and during subsequent dosage titration. Persistent or markedly elevated serum calcium levels may be corrected by dialysis against a reduced calcium or calcium-free dialysate.

Treatment of Accidental Overdosage of Doxercalciferol

The treatment of acute accidental overdosage of Hectorol® should consist of general supportive measures. If drug ingestion is discovered within a relatively short time (10 minutes), induction of emesis or gastric lavage may be of benefit in preventing further absorption. If drug ingestion is discovered later than 10 minutes post-ingestion, the administration of mineral oil may promote its fecal elimination. Serial serum electrolyte determinations (especially calcium), rate of urinary calcium excretion, and assessment of electrocardiographic abnormalities due to hypercalcemia should be obtained. Such monitoring is critical in patients receiving digitalis. Discontinuation of supplemental calcium and institution of a low calcium diet are also indicated in accidental overdosage. If persistent and markedly elevated serum calcium levels occur, there are a variety of therapeutic alternatives that may be considered. These include the use of drugs such as phosphates and corticosteroids as well as measures to induce diuresis. Also, one may consider dialysis against a calcium-free dialysate.

DOSAGE AND ADMINISTRATION

Adult Administration:

The optimal dose of Hectorol® must be carefully determined for each patient. The following table provides the current recommended therapeutic target levels for iPTH in patients with chronic kidney disease:

Target Range of Intact Plasma PTH by Stage of CKD

CKD Stage	GFR (mL/min/1.73 m^2)	Target "intact" PTH (pg/mL)
3	30–59	35–70
4	15–29	70–110
5	<15 (or dialysis)	150–300

From Table 15 of National Kidney Foundation. *K/DOQI Clinical Practice Guidelines for Bone Metabolism and Disease in Chronic Kidney Disease.* Am J Kidney Dis 42:S1-S202, 2003 (suppl 3)

Dialysis: The recommended initial dose of Hectorol® is 10.0 mcg administered three times weekly at dialysis (approximately every other day). The initial dose should be adjusted, as needed, in order to lower blood iPTH into the range of 150 to 300 pg/mL. The dose may be increased at 8-week intervals by 2.5 mcg if iPTH is not lowered by 50% and fails to reach the target range. The maximum recommended dose of Hectorol® is 20 mcg administered three times a week at dialysis for a total of 60 mcg per week. Drug administration should be suspended if iPTH falls below 100 pg/mL and restarted one week later at a dose that is at least 2.5 mcg lower than the last administered dose. During titration, iPTH, serum calcium, and serum phosphorus levels should be obtained weekly. If hypercalcemia, hyperphosphatemia, or a serum calcium times serum phosphorus product greater than 55 mg^2/dL^2 is noted, the dose of Hectorol® should be decreased or suspended and/or the dose of phosphate binders should be appropriately adjusted. If suspended, the drug should be restarted at a dose that is at least 2.5 mcg lower.

Dosing must be individualized and based on iPTH levels with monitoring of serum calcium and serum phosphorus levels. The following is a suggested approach in dose titration:

[See first table above]

Initial Dosing

iPTH Level	Hectorol® Dose
> 400 pg/mL	10.0 mcg three times per week at dialysis

Dose Titration

iPTH Level	Hectorol® Dose
Above 300 pg/mL	Increase by 2.5 mcg at eight-week intervals as necessary
150–300 pg/mL	Maintain
< 100 pg/mL	Suspend for one week, then resume at a dose that is at least 2.5 mcg lower

Pre-dialysis: The recommended initial dose of Hectorol® is 1.0 mcg administered once daily. The initial dose should be adjusted, as needed, in order to lower blood iPTH to within target ranges (see table below). The dose may be increased at 2-week intervals by 0.5 mcg to achieve the target range of iPTH. The maximum recommended dose of Hectorol® is 3.5 mcg administered once per day.

Serum levels of calcium and phosphorus and plasma levels of iPTH should be monitored at least every two weeks for 3 months after initiation of Hectorol® therapy or following dose-adjustments in Hectorol® therapy, then monthly for 3 months, and every 3 months thereafter. If hypercalcemia, hyperphosphatemia, or a serum calcium times phosphorus product greater than 55 mg^2/dL^2 is noted, the dose of Hectorol® should be decreased or suspended and/or the dose of phosphate binders should be appropriately adjusted. If suspended, the drug should be restarted at a dose that is at least 0.5 mcg lower.

Dosing must be individualized and based on iPTH levels with monitoring of serum calcium and serum phosphorus levels. The following is a suggested approach in dose titration:

[See second table above]

Initial Dosing

iPTH Level	Hectorol® Dose
> 70 pg/mL (Stage 3) > 110 pg/mL (Stage 4)	1.0 mcg once per day

Dose Titration

iPTH Level	Hectorol® Dose
Above 70 pg/mL (Stage 3) 110 pg/mL (Stage 4)	Increase by 0.5 mcg at two-week intervals as necessary
35–70 pg/mL (Stage 3) 70–110 pg/mL (Stage 4)	Maintain
< 35 pg/mL (Stage 3) <70 pg/mL (Stage 4)	Suspend for one week, then resume at a dose that is at least 0.5 mcg lower

HOW SUPPLIED

NDC 64894-825-50

NDC 64894-805-50

2.5 mcg doxercalciferol in soft gelatin, sunshine yellow, oval capsules, imprinted **BCI**; bottles of 50.

0.5 mcg doxercalciferol in soft gelatin, citrus orange, oval capsules, imprinted **BCI**; bottles of 50.

Store at controlled room temperature 20° to 25°C (68° to 77°F) [see USP].

Manufactured by Cardinal Health 409, Inc. for
Bone Care International, Inc., Middleton, WI 53562
888-389-4242

PI-001-02 04/04

Shown in Product Identification Guide, page 309

HECTOROL® INJECTION ℞

[*heck-tŏrŏl*]
(doxercalciferol)

DESCRIPTION

Doxercalciferol, the active ingredient in Hectorol, is a synthetic vitamin D analog that undergoes metabolic activation *in vivo* to form 1α,25-dihydroxyvitamin D_2 (1α,25-$(OH)_2D_2$),

Continued on next page

Hectorol Injection—Cont.

a naturally occurring, biologically active form of vitamin D_2. Hectorol is available as a sterile, clear, essentially colorless to faint yellow, aqueous solution for intravenous injection. Each milliliter (mL) of solution contains doxercalciferol, 2 mcg; TWEEN® Polysorbate 20, 4 mg; sodium chloride, 1.5 mg; sodium ascorbate, 10 mg; sodium phosphate, dibasic, 7.6 mg; sodium phosphate, monobasic, 1.8 mg; and disodium edetate, 1.1 mg.

Doxercalciferol is a colorless crystalline compound with a calculated molecular weight of 412.66 and a molecular formula of $C_{28}H_{44}O_2$. It is soluble in oils and organic solvents, but is relatively insoluble in water. Chemically, doxercalciferol is (1α,3β,5Z,7E,22E)-9,10-secoergosta-5,7,10(19),22-tetraene-1,3-diol and has the following structural formula:

Other names frequently used for doxercalciferol are 1α-hydroxyvitamin D_2, 1α-OH-D_2, and 1α-hydroxyergocalciferol.

CLINICAL PHARMACOLOGY

Vitamin D levels in humans depend on two sources: (1) exposure to the ultraviolet rays of the sun for conversion of 7-dehydrocholesterol in the skin to vitamin D_3 (cholecalciferol) and (2) dietary intake of either vitamin D_2 (ergocalciferol) or vitamin D_3. Vitamin D_2 and vitamin D_3 must be metabolically activated in the liver and kidney before becoming fully active on target tissues. The initial step in the activation process is the introduction of an hydroxyl group in the side chain at C-25 by an hepatic enzyme, CYP 27 (a vitamin D-25-hydroxylase). The products of this reaction are 25-$(OH)D_2$ and 25-$(OH)D_3$, respectively. Further hydroxylation of these metabolites occurs in the mitochondria of kidney tissue, catalyzed by renal 25-hydroxyvitamin D-1-α-hydroxylase to produce 1α,25-$(OH)_2D_2$, the primary biologically active form of vitamin D_2, and 1α,25-$(OH)_2D_3$ (calcitriol), the biologically active form of vitamin D_3.

Mechanism of Action

Calcitriol (1α,25-$(OH)_2D_3$) and 1α,25-$(OH)_2D_2$ regulate blood calcium at levels required for essential body functions. Specifically, the biologically active vitamin D metabolites control the intestinal absorption of dietary calcium, the tubular reabsorption of calcium by the kidney and, in conjunction with parathyroid hormone (PTH), the mobilization of calcium from the skeleton. They act directly on bone cells (osteoblasts) to stimulate skeletal growth, and on the parathyroid glands to suppress PTH synthesis and secretion. These functions are mediated by the interaction of these biologically active metabolites with specific receptor proteins in the various target tissues. In uremic patients, deficient production of biologically active vitamin D metabolites (due to lack of or insufficient 25-hydroxyvitamin D-1-alpha-hydroxylase activity) leads to secondary hyperparathyroidism, which contributes to the development of metabolic bone disease in patients with renal failure.

Pharmacokinetics and Metabolism

After intravenous administration, doxercalciferol is activated by CYP 27 in the liver to form 1α,25-$(OH)_2D_2$ (major metabolite) and 1α,24-dihydroxyvitamin D_2 (minor metabolite). Activation of doxercalciferol does not require the involvement of the kidneys.

Peak blood levels of 1α,25-$(OH)_2D_2$ are reached at 8+/−5.9 hours (mean +/−SD) after a single intravenous dose of 5 µg of doxercalciferol. The mean elimination half-life of 1α,25-$(OH)_2D_2$ after an oral dose is approximately 32 to 37 hours with a range of up to 96 hours. The mean elimination half-life in patients with end stage renal disease (ESRD) and in healthy volunteers appears to be similar following an oral dose. Hemodialysis causes a temporary increase in 1α,25-$(OH)_2D_2$ mean concentrations presumably due to volume contraction. 1α,25-$(OH)_2D_2$ is not removed from blood during hemodialysis.

Clinical Studies

The safety and effectiveness of Hectorol Injection were evaluated in two open-label, single-arm, multi-centered clinical studies (Study C and Study D) in a total of 70 patients with chronic renal disease on hemodialysis. Patients in Study C were an average age of 54 years (range: 23–73), were 50% male, and were 61% Black, 25% Caucasian, and 14% Hispanic, and had been on hemodialysis for an average of 65 months. Patients in Study D were an average age of 51 years (range: 28–76), were 48% male, and 100% Black and had been on hemodialysis for an average of 61 months. This group of 70 of the 138 patients who had been treated with Hectorol Capsules in prior clinical studies (Study A and Study B) received Hectorol Injection in an open-label fashion for 12 weeks following an 8-week washout (control) period. Dosing of Hectorol Injection was initiated at the rate of 4.0 mcg administered at the end of each dialysis session (3 times weekly) for a total of 12.0 mcg per week. The dosage of Hectorol was adjusted in an attempt to achieve iPTH levels within a targeted range of 150 to 300 pg/mL. The dosage was increased by 2.0 mcg per dialysis session after 8 weeks of treatment if the iPTH levels remained above 300 pg/mL and were greater than 50% of baseline levels. The maximum dosage was limited to 18.0 mcg per week. If at any time during the trial iPTH fell below 150 pg/mL, Hectorol Injection was immediately suspended and restarted at a lower dosage the following week.

Results:

Fifty-two of the 70 patients who were treated with Hectorol Injection achieved iPTH levels ≤ 300 pg/mL. Forty-one of these patients exhibited plasma iPTH levels ≤ 300 pg/mL on at least 3 occasions. Thirty-six patients had plasma iPTH levels < 150 pg/mL on at least one occasion during study participation.

Mean weekly doses in Study C ranged from 8.9 mcg to 12.5 mcg. In Study D, the mean weekly doses ranged from 9.1 mcg to 11.6 mcg.

Decreases in plasma iPTH from baseline values were calculated, using, as baseline, the average of the last 3 values obtained during the 8-week washout period and are displayed in the table below. Plasma iPTH levels were measured weekly during the 12-week study.

[See first table above]

iPTH summary data for patients receiving Hectorol Injection

iPTH Level	Study C (n=28)	Study D (n=42)	Combined protocols (n=70)
Baseline (Mean of Weeks −2, −1 and 0)			
Mean (SE)	698 (60)	762 (65)	736 (46)
Median	562	648	634
On-treatment (Week 12[1])			
Mean (SE)	406 (63)	426 (60)	418 (43)
Median	311	292	292
Change from Baseline[2]			
Mean (SE)	−292 (55)	−336 (41)	−318 (33)
Median	−274	−315	−304
P-value[3]	.004	.001	<.001

[1] Values were carried forward for the two patients on study for 10 weeks
[2] Treatment iPTH minus baseline iPTH
[3] Wilcoxon one-sample test

In both studies, iPTH levels increased progressively and significantly in 62.9% of patients during the 8-week washout (control) period during which no vitamin D derivatives were administered. In contrast, Hectorol Injection treatment resulted in a clinically significant reduction (at least 30%) from baseline in mean iPTH levels during the 12-week open-label treatment period in more than 92% of the 70 treated patients.

The following table shows the numbers of patients who achieved iPTH levels below 300 pg/mL on one, two, or three or more non-consecutive occasions during the 12-week treatment period. Thirty-seven of 70 patients (53%) had plasma iPTH levels within the targeted range (150–300 pg/mL) during Weeks 10–12.

	Number of times iPTH ≤ 300 pg/mL		
	1	2	≥ 3
Study C	3/28	0/28	16/28
Study D	4/42	4/42	25/42

INDICATIONS AND USAGE

Hectorol is indicated for the reduction of elevated iPTH levels in the management of secondary hyperparathyroidism in patients undergoing chronic renal dialysis.

CONTRAINDICATIONS

Hectorol should not be given to patients with a tendency towards hypercalcemia or current evidence of vitamin D toxicity.

WARNINGS

Overdosage of any form of vitamin D, including Hectorol, is dangerous (see **OVERDOSAGE**). Progressive hypercalcemia due to overdosage of vitamin D and its metabolites may be so severe as to require emergency attention. Acute hypercalcemia may exacerbate tendencies for cardiac arrhythmias and seizures and may potentiate the action of digitalis drugs. Chronic hypercalcemia can lead to generalized vascular calcification and other soft-tissue calcification. The serum calcium times serum phosphorus (Ca X P) product should not be allowed to exceed 70. Radiographic evaluation of suspect anatomical regions may be useful in the early detection of this condition.

Since doxercalciferol is a precursor for 1α,25-$(OH)_2D_2$, a potent metabolite of vitamin D, pharmacologic doses of vitamin D and its derivatives should be withheld during doxercalciferol treatment to avoid possible additive effects and hypercalcemia.

Oral calcium-based or other nonaluminum-containing phosphate binders and a low phosphate diet should be used to control serum phosphorus levels in patients undergoing dialysis. Uncontrolled serum phosphorus exacerbates secondary hyperparathyroidism and can lessen the effectiveness of doxercalciferol in reducing blood PTH levels. After initiating doxercalciferol therapy, the dose of phosphate binders should be decreased to correct persistent mild hypercalcemia (10.6 to 11.2 mg/dL for 3 consecutive determinations), or increased to correct persistent mild hyperphosphatemia (7.0 to 8.0 mg/dL for 3 consecutive determinations).

Magnesium-containing antacids and Hectorol should not be used concomitantly in patients on chronic renal dialysis because such use may lead to the development of hypermagnesemia.

PRECAUTIONS

General

The principal adverse effects of treatment with Hectorol Injection are hypercalcemia, hyperphosphatemia, and oversuppression of iPTH (less than 150 pg/mL). Prolonged hypercalcemia can lead to calcification of soft tissues, including the heart and arteries, and hyperphosphatemia can exacerbate hyperparathyroidism. Oversuppression of iPTH may lead to adynamic bone syndrome. All of these potential adverse effects should be managed by regular patient monitoring and appropriate dosage adjustments. During treatment with Hectorol, patients usually require dose titration, as well as adjustment in co-therapy (i.e., dietary phosphate binders) in order to maximize iPTH suppression while maintaining serum calcium and phosphorus levels within prescribed ranges.

In two open-label, single-arm, multi-centered studies, the incidence of hypercalcemia and hyperphosphatemia increased during therapy with Hectorol Injection (see **ADVERSE REACTIONS** section). The observed increases during Hectorol treatment underscore the importance of regular safety monitoring of serum calcium and phosphorus levels throughout treatment. Patients with higher pretreatment serum levels of calcium (> 10.5 mg/dL) or phosphorus (> 6.9 mg/dL) were more likely to experience hypercalcemia or hyperphosphatemia. Therefore, Hectorol should not be given to patients with a recent history of hypercalcemia or hyperphosphatemia, or evidence of vitamin D toxicity.

[See second table above]

Incidence Rates of Hypercalcemia and Hyperphosphatemia in Two Phase 3 Studies with Hectorol Injection

Study	Hypercalcemia (per 100 patient weeks)		Hyperphosphatemia (per 100 patient weeks)	
	Washout (Off Treatment)	Open-Label (Treatment)	Washout (Off Treatment)	Open-Label (Treatment)
Study C	0.9	0.9	0.9	2.4
Study D	0.3	1.0	1.2	3.7

Information for the Patient

The patient, spouse, or guardian should be informed about adherence to instructions about diet, calcium supplementation, and avoidance of the use of nonprescription drugs without prior approval from their physician. Patients should also be carefully informed about the symptoms of hypercalcemia (see **ADVERSE REACTIONS** section).

Laboratory Tests

Serum levels of iPTH, calcium, and phosphorus should be determined prior to initiation of Hectorol treatment. During the early phase of treatment (i.e., first 12 weeks), serum iPTH, calcium, and phosphorus levels should be determined weekly. For dialysis patients in general, serum or plasma iPTH and serum calcium, phosphorus, and alkaline phosphatase should be determined periodically.

Drug Interactions

Specific drug interaction studies have not been conducted. Magnesium-containing antacids and Hectorol should not be used concomitantly, because such use may lead to the development of hypermagnesemia (see **WARNINGS**). Although not examined specifically, enzyme inducers (such as glutethimide and phenobarbital) may affect the 25-hydroxylation of Hectorol and may necessitate dosage adjustments.

Carcinogenesis, Mutagenesis, Impairment of Fertility

Long-term studies in animals to evaluate the carcinogenic potential of doxercalciferol have not been conducted. No evidence of genetic toxicity was observed in an *in vitro* bacterial mutagenicity assay (Ames test) or a mouse lymphoma gene mutation assay. Doxercalciferol caused structural chromatid and chromosome aberrations in an *in vitro* human lymphocyte clastogenicity assay with metabolic activation. However, doxercalciferol was negative in an *in vivo* mouse micronucleus clastogenicity assay. Doxercalciferol had no effect on male or female fertility in rats at oral doses up to 2.5 mcg/kg/day (approximately 3 times the maximum recommended human oral dose of 60 mcg/wk based on mcg/m^2 body surface area).

Use in Pregnancy

Pregnancy Category B

Reproduction studies in rats and rabbits, at doses up to 20 mcg/kg/day and 0.1 mcg/kg/day (approximately 25 times and less than the maximum recommended human oral dose of 60 mcg/week based on mcg/m^2 body surface area, respectively) have revealed no teratogenic or fetotoxic effects due to doxercalciferol. There are, however, no adequate and well-controlled studies in pregnant women. Because animal reproduction studies are not always predictive of human response, this drug should be used during pregnancy only if clearly needed.

Nursing Mothers

It is not known whether doxercalciferol is excreted in human milk. Because other vitamin D derivatives are excreted in human milk and because of the potential for serious adverse reactions in nursing infants from doxercalciferol, a decision should be made whether to discontinue nursing or to discontinue the drug, taking into account the importance of the drug to the mother.

Pediatric Use

Safety and efficacy of Hectorol in pediatric patients have not been established.

Geriatric Use

Of the 70 patients treated with Hectorol Injection in the two Phase 3 clinical studies, 12 patients were 65 years or over. In these studies, no overall differences in efficacy or safety were observed between patients 65 years or older and younger patients.

Hepatic Insufficiency

Studies examining the influence of hepatic insufficiency on the metabolism of Hectorol were inconclusive. Since patients with hepatic insufficiency may not metabolize doxercalciferol appropriately, the drug should be used with caution in patients with impaired hepatic function. More frequent monitoring of iPTH, calcium, and phosphorus levels should be done in such individuals.

ADVERSE REACTIONS

Hectorol Injection has been evaluated for safety in 70 patients with chronic renal disease on hemodialysis (who had been previously treated with oral Hectorol) from two 12-week, open-label, single-arm, multi-centered studies. (Dosage titrated to achieve target plasma iPTH levels, see **CLINICAL PHARMACOLOGY/Clinical Studies.**)

Because there was no placebo group included in the studies of Hectorol Injection, the table below provides the adverse event incidence rates from placebo-controlled studies of oral Hectorol.

Adverse Events Reported by ≥2% of Hectorol Treated Patients and More Frequently Than Placebo During the Double-blind Phase of Two Clinical Studies

Adverse Event	Hectorol (n=61) %	Placebo (n=61) %
Body as a Whole		
Abscess	3.3	0.0
Headache	27.9	18.0
Malaise	27.9	19.7
Cardiovascular System		
Bradycardia	6.6	4.9
Digestive System		
Anorexia	4.9	3.3
Constipation	3.3	3.3
Dyspepsia	4.9	1.6
Nausea/Vomiting	21.3	19.7
Musculo-Skeletal System		
Arthralgia	4.9	0.0
Metabolic and Nutritional		
Edema	34.4	21.3
Weight increase	4.9	0.0
Nervous System		
Dizziness	11.5	9.8
Sleep disorder	3.3	0.0
Respiratory System		
Dyspnea	11.5	6.6
Skin		
Pruritus	8.2	6.6

A patient who reported the same medical term more than once was counted only once for that medical term.

Potential adverse effects of Hectorol are, in general, similar to those encountered with excessive vitamin D intake. The early and late signs and symptoms of vitamin D intoxication associated with hypercalcemia include:

Early

Weakness, headache, somnolence, nausea, vomiting, dry mouth, constipation, muscle pain, bone pain, and metallic taste.

Late

Polyuria, polydipsia, anorexia, weight loss, nocturia, conjunctivitis (calcific), pancreatitis, photophobia, rhinorrhea, pruritus, hyperthermia, decreased libido, elevated blood urea nitrogen (BUN), albuminuria, hypercholesterolemia, elevated serum aspartate transaminase (AST) and alanine transaminase (ALT), ectopic calcification, hypertension, cardiac arrhythmias and, rarely, overt psychosis.

OVERDOSAGE

Administration of Hectorol to patients in excess doses can cause hypercalcemia, hypercalciuria, hyperphosphatemia, and over-suppression of PTH secretion leading in certain cases to adynamic bone disease. High intake of calcium and phosphate concomitant with Hectorol may lead to similar abnormalities. High levels of calcium in the dialysate bath may contribute to hypercalcemia.

Treatment of Hypercalcemia and Overdosage

General treatment of hypercalcemia (greater than 1 mg/dL above the upper limit of the normal range) consists of immediate suspension of Hectorol therapy, institution of a low calcium diet, and withdrawal of calcium supplements. Serum calcium levels should be determined at least weekly until normocalcemia ensues. Hypercalcemia usually resolves in 2 to 7 days. When serum calcium levels have returned to within normal limits, Hectorol therapy may be reinstituted at a dose that is at least 1.0 mcg lower than prior therapy. Serum calcium levels should be obtained weekly after all dosage changes and during subsequent dosage titration. Persistent or markedly elevated serum calcium levels may be corrected by dialysis against a reduced calcium or calcium-free dialysate.

Treatment of Accidental Overdosage of Hectorol

The treatment of acute accidental overdosage of Hectorol should consist of general supportive measures. Serial serum electrolyte determinations (especially calcium), rate of urinary calcium excretion, and assessment of electrocardiographic abnormalities due to hypercalcemia should be obtained. Such monitoring is critical in patients receiving digitalis. Discontinuation of supplemental calcium and institution of a low calcium diet are also indicated in accidental overdosage. If persistent and markedly elevated serum calcium levels occur, there are a variety of therapeutic alternatives which may be considered. These include the use of drugs such as phosphates and corticosteroids as well as measures to induce diuresis. Also, one may consider dialysis against a calcium-free dialysate.

DOSAGE AND ADMINISTRATION

Adult Administration:

The optimal dose of Hectorol must be carefully determined for each patient.

The recommended initial dose of Hectorol is 4.0 mcg administered as a bolus dose three times weekly at the end of dialysis (approximately every other day). The initial dose should be adjusted, as needed, in order to lower blood iPTH into the range of 150 to 300 pg/mL. The dose may be increased at 8-week intervals by 1.0 – 2.0 mcg if iPTH is not lowered by 50% and fails to reach the target range. Dosages higher than 18 mcg weekly have not been studied. Drug administration should be suspended if iPTH falls below 100 pg/mL and restarted one week later at a dose which is at least 1.0 mcg lower than the last administered dose. During titration, iPTH, serum calcium, and serum phosphorus levels should be obtained weekly. If hypercalcemia, hyperphosphatemia, or a serum calcium times phosphorus product greater than 70 is noted, the drug should be immediately suspended until these parameters are appropriately lowered. Then, the drug should be restarted at a dose which is 1.0 mcg lower.

Dosing must be individualized and based on iPTH levels with monitoring of serum calcium and serum phosphorus levels. The following is a suggested approach in dose titration:

Initial Dosing

iPTH Level	Hectorol Dose
> 400 pg/mL	4.0 mcg three times per week at the end of dialysis, or approximately every other day

Dose Titration

iPTH Level	Hectorol Dose
Decreased by < 50% and above 300 pg/mL	Increase by 1.0 to 2.0 mcg at eight-week intervals as necessary
150–300 pg/mL	Maintain
< 100 pg/mL	Suspend for one week, then resume at a dose that is at least 1.0 mcg lower

Discard unused portion.

HOW SUPPLIED

Hectorol (doxercalciferol) Injection is supplied in pre-scored amber glass ampules

NDC number	Volume	mcg/ampule
64894-840-50	2 mL	4.0

Store at 15° to 25° C (59° to 77° F). Protect from light.

Manufactured by Draxis Pharma, Inc. for
Bone Care International, Inc., Middleton, WI 53562
888-389-4242

PI-002A-02 12/03

Shown in Product Identification Guide, page 309

Braintree Laboratories, Inc.

P.O. BOX 850929
BRAINTREE, MA 02185-0929

Direct Inquiries to:
Harry P. Keegan, President
(781) 843-2202

For Medical Information Contact:
In Emergencies:
Jack DiPalma, M.D.
(800) 874-6756

GoLYTELY® ℞
[*go-līt 'lē*]
(PEG-3350 and Electrolytes For Oral Solution)

NuLYTELY® ℞
[*new-līt 'lē*]
(PEG-3350, Sodium Chloride, Sodium Bicarbonate and Potassium Chloride for Oral Solution)

DESCRIPTION

GoLYTELY®

A white powder in a 4 liter jug for reconstitution, containing 236 g polyethylene glycol 3350, 22.74 g sodium sulfate (anhydrous), 6.74 g sodium bicarbonate, 5.86 g sodium chloride, 2.97 g potassium chloride. When dissolved in water to a volume of 4 liters, GoLYTELY (PEG-3350 and electrolytes for oral solution) is an isosmotic solution having a mildly salty taste. GoLYTELY is administered orally or via nasogastric tube as a gastrointestinal lavage.

NuLYTELY®

A white powder for reconstitution containing 420 g polyethylene glycol 3350, 5.72 g sodium bicarbonate, 11.2 g sodium chloride, 1.48 g potassium chloride. When dissolved in water to a volume of 4 liters, NuLYTELY (PEG-3350, sodium chloride, sodium bicarbonate and potassium chloride for oral solution) is an isosmotic solution having a pleasant mineral water taste. NuLYTELY is administered orally or via nasogastric tube as a gastrointestinal lavage.

CLINICAL PHARMACOLOGY

GoLYTELY and NuLYTELY induce a diarrhea which rapidly cleanses the bowel, usually within four hours. The osmotic activity of polyethylene glycol 3350 and the electrolyte concentration result in virtually no net absorption or excretion of ions or water. Accordingly, large volumes may be administered without significant changes in fluid or electrolyte balance.

INDICATIONS AND USAGE

GoLYTELY®

GoLYTELY is indicated for bowel cleansing prior to colonoscopy and barium enema X-ray examination.

NuLYTELY®

NuLYTELY is indicated for bowel cleansing prior to colonoscopy.

CONTRAINDICATIONS

GoLYTELY and NuLYTELY are contraindicated in patients known to be hypersensitive to any of the components. GoLYTELY and NuLYTELY are contraindicated in patients with gastrointestinal obstruction, gastric retention, bowel perforation, toxic colitis, toxic megacolon or ileus.

Continued on next page

GoLytely/NuLytely—Cont.

WARNINGS

GoLYTELY®
No additional ingredients, e.g. flavorings, should be added to the solution. GoLYTELY should be used with caution in patients with severe ulcerative colitis.

NuLYTELY®
No additional ingredients, e.g. flavorings, should be added to the solution. NuLYTELY should be used with caution in patients with severe ulcerative colitis. Use of NuLYTELY in children younger than 2 years of age should be carefully monitored for occurrence of possible hypoglycemia, as this solution has no caloric substrate. Dehydration has been reported in 1 child and hypokalemia has been reported in 3 children.

PRECAUTIONS

General: Patients with impaired gag reflex, unconscious, or semiconscious patients, and patients prone to regurgitation or aspiration should be observed during the administration of GoLYTELY or NuLYTELY, especially if it is administered via nasogastric tube. If a patient experiences severe bloating, distention or abdominal pain, administration should be slowed or temporarily discontinued until the symptoms abate. If gastrointestinal obstruction or perforation is suspected, appropriate studies should be performed to rule out these conditions before administration of GoLYTELY or NuLYTELY.

Information for Patients: GoLYTELY and NuLYTELY produce a watery stool which cleanses the bowel before examination. Prepare the solution according to the instructions on the bottle. It is more palatable if chilled. For best results, no solid food should be consumed during the 3 to 4 hour period before drinking the solution, but in no case should solid foods be eaten within 2 hours of taking GoLYTELY or NuLYTELY.

GoLYTELY®: Drink 240 mL (8 oz.) every 10 minutes. Rapid drinking of each portion is better than drinking small amounts continuously.

NuLYTELY®: Adults drink 240 mL (8 oz.) every 10 minutes. Continue drinking until the watery stool is clear and free of solid matter. This usually requires at least 3 liters and it is best to drink all of the solution. Any unused portion should be discarded. Pediatric patients (aged 6 months or greater) drink 25 mL/kg/hour. Continue drinking until the watery stool is clear and free of solid matter. Any unused portion should be discarded. Use of NuLYTELY in children younger than 2 years of age should be carefully monitored for occurrence of possible hypoglycemia, as this solution has no caloric substrate. Dehydration has been reported in 1 child and hypokalemia has been reported in 3 children.

The first bowel movement should occur approximately one hour after the start of GoLYTELY or NuLYTELY administration. You may experience some abdominal bloating and distention before the bowels start to move. If severe discomfort or distention occur, stop drinking temporarily or drink each portion at longer intervals until these symptoms disappear.

Drug Interactions: Oral medication administered within one hour of the start of administration of GoLYTELY or NuLYTELY may be flushed from the gastrointestinal tract and not absorbed.

Carcinogenesis, Mutagenesis, Impairment of Fertility:
Carcinogenic and reproductive studies with animals have not been performed.

Pregnancy: Category C. Animal reproduction studies have not been conducted with GoLYTELY and NuLYTELY. It is also not known whether GoLYTELY and NuLYTELY can cause fetal harm when administered to a pregnant woman or can affect reproductive capacity. GoLYTELY and NuLYTELY should be given to a pregnant woman only if clearly needed.

Pediatric Use:

GoLYTELY®
Safety and effectiveness in children have not been established.

NuLYTELY®
Safety and effectiveness of NuLYTELY in pediatric patients aged 6 months and older is supported by evidence from adequate and well-controlled clinical trials of NuLYTELY in adults with additional safety and efficacy data from published studies of similar formulations.

ADVERSE REACTIONS

Nausea, abdominal fullness and bloating are the most common adverse reactions (occurring in up to 50% of patients) to administration of GoLYTELY or NuLYTELY. Abdominal cramps, vomiting and anal irritation occur less frequently. These adverse reactions are transient and subside rapidly. Isolated cases of urticaria, rhinorrhea, dermatitis and (rarely) anaphylactic reaction have been reported which may represent allergic reactions.

Published literature contains isolated reports of serious adverse reactions following the administration of PEG-ELS products in patients over 60 years of age. These adverse events include upper GI bleeding from Mallory-Weiss Tear, esophageal perforation, asystole, sudden dyspnea with pulmonary edema, and "butterfly-like" infiltrate on chest X-ray after vomiting and aspirating PEG.

DOSAGE AND ADMINISTRATION

GoLYTELY®
The recommended dose for adults is 4 liters of GoLYTELY solution prior to gastrointestinal examination, as ingestion of this dose produces a satisfactory preparation in over 95% of patients. Ideally, the patient should fast for approximately three or four hours prior to GoLYTELY administration, but in no case should solid food be given for at least two hours before the solution is given.

GoLYTELY is usually administered orally, but may be given via nasogastric tube to patients who are unwilling or unable to drink the solution. **Oral administration** is at a rate of 240 mL (8 oz.) every 10 minutes, until 4 liters are consumed or the rectal effluent is clear. Rapid drinking of each portion is preferred to drinking small amounts continuously. **Nasogastric tube administration** is at the rate of 20–30 mL per minute (1.2–1.8 liters per hour). The first bowel movement should occur approximately one hour after the start of GoLYTELY administration.

Various regimens have been used. One method is to schedule patients for examination in midmorning or later, allowing the patients three hours for drinking and an additional one hour period for complete bowel evacuation. Another method is to administer GoLYTELY on the evening before the examination, particularly if the patient is to have a barium enema.

NuLYTELY®
NuLYTELY is usually administered orally, but may be given via nasogastric tube to patients who are unwilling or unable to drink the solution. Ideally, the patient should fast for approximately three or four hours prior to NuLYTELY administration, but in no case should solid food be given for at least two hours before the solution is given.

Oral administration:

Adults: At a rate of 240 mL (8 oz.) every 10 minutes, until the rectal effluent is clear or 4 liters are consumed.

Pediatric Patients (aged 6 months or greater): At a rate of 25 mL/kg/hour, until the rectal effluent is clear.

Rapid drinking of each portion is preferred to drinking small amounts continuously.

Nasogastric tube administration:

Adults: At a rate of 20–30 mL per minute (1.2–1.8 liters per hour).

Pediatric Patients (aged 6 months or greater): At a rate of 25 mL/kg/hour, until the rectal effluent is clear.

The first bowel movement should occur approximately one hour after the start of NuLYTELY administration. Ingestion of 4 liters of NuLYTELY solution prior to gastrointestinal examination produces satisfactory preparation in over 95% of patients.

Various regimens have been used. One method is to schedule patients for examination in midmorning or later, allowing the patients three hours for drinking and an additional one hour period for complete bowel evacuation. Another method is to administer NuLYTELY on the evening before the examination.

Preparation of the solution:

GoLYTELY® solution is prepared by filling the container to the 4 liter mark with water and shaking vigorously several times to insure that the ingredients are dissolved. Dissolution is facilitated by using lukewarm water. The solution is more palatable if chilled before administration. The reconstituted solution should be refrigerated and used within 48 hours. Discard any unused portion.

NuLYTELY® solution is prepared by filling the container to the 4 liter mark with water and shaking vigorously several times to insure that the ingredients are dissolved. Dissolution is facilitated by using lukewarm water. The solution is more palatable if chilled before administration. However, chilled solution is not recommended for infants. The reconstituted solution should be refrigerated and used within 48 hours. Discard any unused portion.

HOW SUPPLIED

GoLYTELY®
In powdered form, for oral administration as a solution following reconstitution.

GoLYTELY® is available in a disposable jug and a packet in powdered form containing: **Disposable Jug:** polyethylene glycol 3350 236 g, sodium sulfate (anhydrous) 22.74 g, sodium bicarbonate 6.74 g, sodium chloride 5.86 g, potassium chloride 2.97 g. When made up to 4 liters volume with water, the solution contains PEG-3350 17.6 mmol/L, sodium 125 mmol/L, sulfate 40 mmol/L, chloride 35 mmol/L, bicarbonate 20 mmol/L and potassium 10 mmol/L. **Packet:** polyethylene glycol 3350 227.1 g, anhydrous sodium sulfate 21.5 g, sodium bicarbonate 6.36 g, sodium chloride 5.53 g, potassium chloride 2.82 g. When made up to 1 gallon volume with water, the solution contains PEG-3350 60g/L, sodium sulfate 5.68 g/L, sodium bicarbonate 1.68 g/L, sodium chloride 1.46 g/L and potassium chloride 0.745 g/L.

Pineapple Flavor GoLYTELY is available in a disposable jug in powdered form containing: polyethylene glycol 3350 236 g, sodium sulfate (anhydrous) 22.74 g, sodium bicarbonate 6.74 g, sodium chloride 5.86 g, potassium chloride 2.97 g, flavoring ingredients 3.0 g. When made up to 4 liters volume with water, the solution contains PEG-3350 17.6 mmol/L, sodium 125 mmol/L, sulfate 40 mmol/L, chloride 35 mmol/L, bicarbonate 20 mmol/L and potassium 10 mmol/L.

NuLYTELY®
NuLYTELY, Cherry NuLYTELY, Lemon-Lime NuLYTELY and Orange NuLYTELY are available in a disposable jug, in powdered form, for oral administration as a solution following reconstitution.

Each jug contains:

NuLYTELY: polyethylene glycol 3350 420 g, sodium bicarbonate 5.72 g, sodium chloride 11.2 g, potassium chloride 1.48 g. When made up to 4 liters volume with water, the solution contains PEG-3350 31.3 mmol/L, sodium 65 mmol/L, chloride 53 mmol/L, bicarbonate 17 mmol/L and potassium 5 mmol/L.

Cherry NuLYTELY: polyethylene glycol 3350 420 g, sodium bicarbonate 5.72 g, sodium chloride 11.2 g, potassium chloride 1.48 g and flavoring ingredients 2.0 g. When made up to 4 liters volume with water, the solution contains PEG-3350 31.3 mmol/L, sodium 65 mmol/L, chloride 53 mmol/L, bicarbonate 17 mmol/L and potassium 5 mmol/L.

Lemon-Lime NuLYTELY: polyethylene glycol 3350 420 g, sodium bicarbonate 5.72 g, sodium chloride 11.2 g, potassium chloride 1.48 g and flavoring ingredients 2.0 g. When made up to 4 liters volume with water, the solution contains PEG-3350 31.3 mmol/L, sodium 65 mmol/L, chloride 53 mmol/L, bicarbonate 17 mmol/L and potassium 5 mmol/L.

Orange NuLYTELY: polyethylene glycol 3350 420 g, sodium bicarbonate 5.72 g, sodium chloride 11.2 g, potassium chloride 1.48 g and flavoring ingredients 2.0 g. When made up to 4 liters volume with water, the solution contains PEG-3350 31.3 mmol/L, sodium 65 mmol/L, chloride 53 mmol/L, bicarbonate 17 mmol/L and potassium 5 mmol/L.

STORAGE: Store in sealed container at 25°C. When reconstituted, keep solution refrigerated. Use within 48 hours. Discard unused portion.

GoLYTELY	NDC 52268-100-01
GoLYTELY 1 Gallon Packet	NDC 52268-700-01
Pineapple Flavor GoLYTELY	NDC 52268-101-01
NuLYTELY	NDC 52268-300-01
Cherry Flavor NuLYTELY	NDC 52268-301-01
Lemon-Lime Flavor NuLYTELY	NDC 52268-302-01
Orange Flavor NuLYTELY	NDC 52268-303-01

Rx only

Distributed by Braintree Laboratories, Inc., Braintree, MA 02185

Shown in Product Identification Guide, page 309

HALFLYTELY® AND BISACODYL TABLETS ℞

[hăf-līt-le]

Bowel Prep Kit

Rx Only

PEG-3350, sodium chloride, sodium bicarbonate and potassium chloride for oral solution and bisacodyl delayed release tablets

DESCRIPTION

Each **HalfLytely® and Bisacodyl Tablets Bowel Prep Kit** (Polyethylene glycol 3350, sodium chloride, sodium bicarbonate and potassium chloride for oral solution and bisacodyl delayed release tablets) consists of:

One pack of 4 bisacodyl delayed release tablets: Each pink, round, enteric coated delayed release tablet (stamped "BRA") contains 5 mg bisacodyl, USP ($C_{22}H_{19}NO_4$); MW=361.40. **Inactive ingredients:** lactose (anhydrous) NF, microcrystalline cellulose NF, croscarmellose sodium NF, magnesium stearate NF, eudragit L 30-55, polyethylene glycol 400, talc USP, gelatin, calcium sulfate (anhydrous) NF, confections sugar, kaolin USP, sucrose NF, opalux pink, beeswax, carnuba wax.

The bisacodyl delayed release tablets are administered orally prior to drinking the solution.

One 2 liter bottle of HalfLytely® (PEG-3350, sodium chloride, sodium bicarbonate and potassium chloride for oral solution): A white powder for reconstitution containing 210 g polyethylene glycol 3350, 2.86 g sodium bicarbonate, 5.6 g sodium chloride, 0.74 g potassium chloride and 1.0 g flavoring ingredient (if applicable). When dissolved in water to a volume of 2 liters, the solution is isosmotic. The solution is administered orally as a gastrointestinal lavage in combination with four bisacodyl delayed release tablets. All solutions are clear and colorless.

CLINICAL PHARMACOLOGY

HalfLytely and Bisacodyl Tablets Bowel Prep Kit induces a diarrhea which cleanses the bowel. Bisacodyl is a contact stimulant laxative. After being hydrolyzed by intestinal brush border enzymes and colonic bacteria, its active metabolite, bis-(p-hydroxyphenyl)-pyridyl-2 methane (BHPM) acts directly on the colonic mucosa to produce peristalsis throughout the large intestine.

The osmotic activity of polyethylene glycol 3350 and electrolytes result in virtually no net absorption or excretion of ions or water.

INDICATIONS AND USAGE

HalfLytely and Bisacodyl Tablets Bowel Prep Kit is indicated for bowel cleansing prior to colonoscopy.

CONTRAINDICATIONS

HalfLytely and Bisacodyl Tablets Bowel Prep Kit is contraindicated in patients known to be hypersensitive to any of the components. HalfLytely and Bisacodyl Tablets Bowel Prep Kit is contraindicated in patients with ileus, gastrointestinal obstruction, gastric retention, bowel perforation, toxic colitis or toxic megacolon.

WARNINGS
No additional ingredients, e.g. flavorings, should be added to the solution. HalfLytely and Bisacodyl Tablets Bowel Prep Kit should be used with caution in patients with severe ulcerative colitis. Do NOT chew or crush the bisacodyl delayed release tablets.

PRECAUTIONS
General: Patients with impaired gag reflex and patients prone to regurgitation or aspiration should be observed during the administration of the solution. If a patient experiences severe bloating, distention or abdominal pain, administration of the solution should be slowed or temporarily discontinued until the symptoms abate. If gastrointestinal obstruction or perforation is suspected, appropriate studies should be performed to rule out these conditions before administration of HalfLytely and Bisacodyl Tablets Bowel Prep Kit.
Patients should avoid consumption of large quantities of water during or after preparation or colonoscopy. Patients with impaired water handling (renal insufficiency or patients taking diuretics) that experience severe vomiting or nausea should be closely monitored including measurement of electrolytes.
Information for patients: HalfLytely and Bisacodyl Tablets Bowel Prep Kit produces a watery stool which cleanses the bowel before examination. Prepare the solution according to the instructions on the kit. For best results, no solid food or milk (clear liquids only) should be consumed on the day of the preparation. No antacids should be taken within one hour of taking the bisacodyl delayed release tablets.
Adults swallow all four bisacodyl delayed release tablets with water (do **NOT** chew or crush). The first bowel movement should occur in approximately 1–6 hours after taking the bisacodyl delayed release tablets. Wait for a bowel movement (or maximum of 6 hours) then drink the solution, 1 (8 oz) glass every 10 minutes (approximately 8 glasses). **Drink ALL of the solution.** Rapid drinking of each portion is better than drinking small amounts continuously. A watery bowel movement should occur in approximately 1 hour after drinking the solution. You may experience some abdominal bloating and distention before the bowels start to move. If severe discomfort or distention occurs, stop drinking the solution temporarily or drink each portion at longer intervals until these symptoms disappear.
Drug Interactions: Oral medication administered within one hour of the start of administration of the solution may be flushed from the gastrointestinal tract and not absorbed. Do not take the bisacodyl delayed release tablets within one hour of taking an antacid.
Carcinogenesis, Mutagenesis, Impairment of Fertility: Long-term studies in animals have not been performed to evaluate the carcinogenic potential of HalfLytely and Bisacodyl Tablets Bowel Prep Kit. Studies to evaluate its potential for impairment of fertility or its mutagenic potential have not been performed.
Pregnancy: Category C. Animal reproduction studies have not been conducted with HalfLytely and Bisacodyl Tablets Bowel Prep Kit. It is also not known whether HalfLytely and Bisacodyl Tablets Bowel Prep Kit can cause fetal harm when administered to a pregnant woman or can affect reproductive capacity. HalfLytely and Bisacodyl Tablets Bowel Prep Kit should be given to a pregnant or nursing woman only if clearly needed.
Nursing Mothers: It is not known whether HalfLytely and Bisacody Tablets Bowel Prep Kit is excreted in human milk, caution should be exercised when HalfLytely and Bisacodyl Tablets Bowel Prep Kit is administered to a nursing woman.
Pediatric Use: Safety and effectiveness in pediatric patients has not been established.
Geriatric Use: There is no evidence for special consideration when administered to elderly patients. Of the total number of subjects in clinical studies (n=186), 28 percent were aged 65 or older, while 9.1 percent were over 75. No overall differences in safety or effectiveness were observed.

ADVERSE REACTIONS
Nausea, cramping and abdominal fullness are the most common adverse reactions (occurring in up to 50% of patients) to administration of HalfLytely and Bisacodyl Tablets Bowel Prep Kit. Vomiting occurs less frequently (approximately 2.7% of patients versus 6.7% of patients taking large volume PEG solutions). In clinical studies, most of these complaints were significantly reduced when compared to the 4 liter preparation. Table 1 shows patient rating of symptoms associated with the preparation from 2 clinical studies (n= 400). These adverse reactions are transient and subside rapidly. Isolated cases of urticaria, rhinorrhea, dermatitis and (rarely) anaphylactic reaction have been reported with PEG based products which may represent allergic reactions

Table 1: Patient Symptom Rating
Bothersome-Severe Complaints

	HalfLytely and Bisacodyl Tablets Bowel Prep Kit	4 liters of PEG electrolyte solution
Nausea	17.1%	31.8%
Cramping	9.1%	17.4%
Fullness	22.3%	44.1%
Vomiting	5.9%	13.7%
Overall Discomfort	19.1%	37.3%

Published literature contains isolated reports of serious adverse reactions following the administration of (4L) PEG-ELS products in patients over 60 years of age. These adverse events include upper GI bleeding from Mallory-Weiss syndrome esophageal perforation, asystole, sudden dyspnea with pulmonary edema, and "butterfly-like" infiltrate on chest X-ray after vomiting and aspirating PEG.
In addition, during administration of 4L PEG-3350 bowel cleansing preparations the following serious adverse events were seen: two deaths in end-stage renal failure patients who developed diarrhea, vomiting, dysnatremia; tonic-clonic seizures in patients with and without prior history of seizures. These adverse events have not been reported in HalfLytely and Bisacodyl Tablets Bowel Prep Kit clinical trials.

DOSAGE AND ADMINISTRATION
HalfLytely and Bisacodyl Tablets Bowel Prep Kit is administered orally. Ideally, the patient should only consume clear liquids (no solid food, no milk) prior to HalfLytely and Bisacodyl Tablets Bowel Prep Kit administration. No antacids should be given for at least one hour before beginning the regimen.
Oral administration: Swallow all four bisacodyl delayed release tablets with water (do **NOT** chew or crush). The first bowel movement should occur in approximately 1–6 hours after taking the bisacodyl delayed release tablets. Wait for a bowel movement (or maximum of 6 hours) then drink the solution at a rate of 1 (8 oz) glass every 10 minutes (approximately 8 glasses). **Drink ALL of the solution.** Rapid drinking of each portion is preferred to drinking small amounts continuously. A watery bowel movement should occur in approximately 1 hour after drinking the solution.
The recommended regimen is to consume clear liquids only (no solid food, no milk) the day of the preparation, take all four bisacodyl delayed release tablets at noon, following the first bowel movement or a maximum of 6 hours, begin drinking the solution.
Preparation of the solution: The solution is prepared by filling the container to the 2 liter mark with water, cap the bottle and shake to dissolve ingredients. Dissolution is facilitated by using lukewarm water. The reconstituted solution may be refrigerated and should be used within 48 hours. All reconstituted solutions are clear and colorless.

HOW SUPPLIED
HalfLytely and Bisacodyl Tablets Bowel Prep Kit is available in Lemon-Lime flavor. Each foil lined blister pack contains 4 (5 mg each) bisacodyl delayed release tablets for ingestion prior to drinking of the solution. Each disposable bottle contains powder for oral administration as a solution following reconstitution.
Each HalfLytely and Bisacodyl Tablets Bowel Prep Kit contains:
One pack bisacodyl delayed release tablets: Four (5 mg each) bisacodyl delayed release tablets.
One 2 liter bottle of HalfLytely® (PEG-3350, sodium chloride, sodium bicarbonate and potassium chloride for oral solution): polyethylene glycol 3350 210 g, sodium bicarbonate 2.86 g, sodium chloride 5.60 g, potassium chloride 0.74 g, and 1.0 g flavoring ingredient (if applicable). When made up to 2 liters volume with water, the solution contains PEG-3350 31.3 mmol/L, sodium 65 mmol/L, chloride 53 mmol/L, bicarbonate 17 mmol/L and potassium 5 mmol/L.
All reconstituted solutions are clear and colorless.
STORAGE: Store at 20–25°C (68–77°F). Excursions permitted between 15–30°C (59–86°F). When reconstituted, you may keep solution refrigerated. Use within 48 hours.
Lemon-Lime HalfLytely and Bisacodyl Tablets
Bowel Prep Kit **NDC 52268-502-01**
Distributed by Braintree Laboratories, Inc.
Braintree, MA 02185 **H 5/04**
Shown in Product Identification Guide, page 309

MIRALAX™ ℞
[mĭrä 'lăx]
Polyethylene Glycol 3350, NF Powder for Solution
Full Prescribing Information

DESCRIPTION
A white powder for reconstitution. MiraLax (polyethylene glycol 3350, NF powder for solution) is a synthetic polyglycol having an average molecular weight of 3350. The actual molecular weight is not less than 90.0 percent and not greater than 110.0 percent of the nominal value. The chemical formula is $HO(C_2H_4O)_nH$ in which n represents the average number of oxyethylene groups. Below 55°C it is a free flowing white powder freely soluble in water. MiraLax is an osmotic agent for the treatment of constipation.

CLINICAL PHARMACOLOGY
Pharmacology: MiraLax is an osmotic agent which causes water to be retained with the stool. Essentially, complete recovery of MiraLax was shown in normal subjects without constipation. Attempts at recovery of MiraLax in constipated patients resulted in incomplete and highly variable recovery. In vitro study showed indirectly that MiraLax was not fermented into hydrogen or methane by the colonic microflora in human feces. MiraLax appears to have no effect on the active absorption or secretion of glucose or electrolytes. There is no evidence of tachyphylaxis.

CLINICAL TRIALS
In one study, patients with less than 3 bowel movements per week were randomized to MiraLax, 17 grams, or placebo for 14 days. An increase in bowel movement frequency was observed for both treatment groups during the first week of treatment. MiraLax was statistically superior to placebo during the second week of treatment.
In another study, patients with 3 bowel movements or less per week and/or less than 300 grams of stool per week were randomized to 2 dose levels of MiraLax or placebo for 10 days each. Success was defined by an increase in both bowel movement frequency and daily stool weight. For both parameters, superiority of the 17 gram dose of MiraLax over placebo was demonstrated.

INDICATIONS AND USAGE
For the treatment of occasional constipation. This product should be used for 2 weeks or less or as directed by a physician.

CONTRAINDICATIONS
MiraLax is contraindicated in patients with known or suspected bowel obstruction and patients known to be allergic to polyethylene glycol.

WARNINGS
Patients with symptoms suggestive of bowel obstruction (nausea, vomiting, abdominal pain or distention) should be evaluated to rule out this condition before initiating MiraLax therapy.

PRECAUTIONS
General: Patients presenting with complaints of constipation should have a thorough medical history and physical examination to detect associated metabolic, endocrine and neurogenic conditions, and medications. A diagnostic evaluation should include a structural examination of the colon. Patients should be educated about good defecatory and eating habits (such as high fiber diets) and lifestyle changes (adequate dietary fiber and fluid intake, regular exercise) which may produce more regular bowel habits.
MiraLax should be administered after being dissolved in approximately 8 ounces of water, juice, soda, coffee, or tea.
Information for Patients: MiraLax softens the stool and increases the frequency of bowel movements by retaining water in the stool. It should always be taken by mouth after being dissolved in 8 ounces of water, juice, soda, coffee, or tea. Should unusual cramps, bloating, or diarrhea occur, consult your physician.
Two to 4 days may be required to produce a bowel movement. This product should be used for 2 weeks or less or as directed by a physician. Prolonged, frequent or excessive use of MiraLax may result in electrolyte imbalance and dependence on laxatives.
Laboratory Tests: No clinically significant effects on laboratory tests have been demonstrated.
Drug Interactions: No specific drug interactions have been demonstrated.
Carcinogenesis, Mutagenesis, Impairment of Fertility: Long term carcinogenicity studies, genetic toxicity studies and reproductive toxicity studies in animals have not been performed with MiraLax.
Pregnancy: Category C. Animal reproductive studies have not been performed with MiraLax. It is also not known whether MiraLax can cause fetal harm when administered to a pregnant woman, or can effect reproductive capacity. MiraLax should only be administered to a pregnant woman if clearly needed.
Pediatric Use: Safety and effectiveness in pediatric patients has not been established.
Geriatric Use: There is no evidence for special considerations when MiraLax is administered to elderly patients.
In geriatric nursing home patients a higher incidence of diarrhea occurred at the recommended 17 gram dose. If diarrhea occurs MiraLax should be discontinued.

ADVERSE REACTIONS
Nausea, abdominal bloating, cramping and flatulence may occur. High doses may produce diarrhea and excessive stool frequency, particularly in elderly nursing home patients.
Patients taking other medications containing polyethylene glycol have occasionally developed urticaria suggestive of an allergic reaction.

OVERDOSAGE
There have been no reports of accidental overdosage. In the event of overdosage diarrhea would be the expected major event. If an overdose of drug occurred without concomitant ingestion of fluid, dehydration due to diarrhea may result. Medication should be terminated and free water administered. The oral LD_{50} is >50 gm/Kg in mice, rats and rabbits.

DOSAGE AND ADMINISTRATION
The usual dose is 17 grams (about 1 heaping tablespoon) of powder per day (or as directed by physician) in 8 ounces of

Continued on next page

Miralax—Cont.

water, juice, soda, coffee, or tea. Each bottle of MiraLax is supplied with a measuring cap marked to contain 17 grams of laxative powder when filled to the indicated line.
Two to 4 days (48 to 96 hours) may be required to produce a bowel movement.

HOW SUPPLIED

In powdered form, for oral administration after dissolution in water, juice, soda, coffee, or tea. MiraLax is available in three package sizes; a 14 oz. container of 255 grams of laxative powder, a 26 oz. container of 527 grams of laxative powder, and a carton of 12 individual packets containing a single 17 g dose.
The cap on each bottle is marked with a measuring line and may be used to measure a single MiraLax dose of 17 grams (about 1 heaping tablespoon).
Each individual packet contains a single MiraLax dose of 17 grams (about 1 heaping tablespoon).

Rx only

STORAGE

Store at 25 degrees C (77 degrees F); excursions permitted to 15–30 degrees C (59–86 degrees F). See USP "Controlled Room Temperature."

Distributed by Braintree Laboratories, Inc., Braintree, MA 02185

D 6/01

Shown in Product Identification Guide, page 309

Bristol-Myers Squibb Company

P.O. BOX 4500
PRINCETON, NJ 08543-4500

For Medical Information Contact:
Generally:
Bristol-Myers Squibb Drug Information Department
P.O. Box 4500
Princeton, NJ 08543-4500
(800) 321–1335

Adverse Drug Experiences
and Product Defects Reporting call
between 8:30 AM–4:30 PM EST:
(609) 818-3737

Sales and Ordering:
Orders may be placed by:
1. Calling your purchase orders toll-free between 8:30 AM–5:00 PM EST:
(800) 631-5244
2. Mailing your purchase orders to:
Bristol-Myers Squibb U.S. Pharmaceuticals
Attn: Customer Service
P.O. Box 5250
Princeton, NJ 08543-5250
3. Faxing your purchase orders to:
(800) 523-2965
4. Transmitting computer-to-computer on the NWDA and UCS formats through Ordernet Services use: DEA#PE0048579

ABILIFY® ℞

[ā-bĭl-ĭ-fī]
(aripiprazole) Tablets
℞ only

DESCRIPTION

ABILIFY® (aripiprazole) is a psychotropic drug that is available as tablets for oral administration. Aripiprazole is 7-[4-[4-(2,3-dichlorophenyl)-1-piperazinyl]butoxy]-3,4-dihydrocarbostyril. The empirical formula is $C_{23}H_{27}Cl_2N_3O_2$ and its molecular weight is 448.38. The chemical structure is:

ABILIFY tablets are available in 5-mg, 10-mg, 15-mg, 20-mg, and 30-mg strengths. Inactive ingredients include lactose monohydrate, cornstarch, microcrystalline cellulose, hydroxypropyl cellulose, and magnesium stearate. Colorants include ferric oxide (yellow or red) and FD&C Blue No. 2 Aluminum Lake.

CLINICAL PHARMACOLOGY

Pharmacodynamics

Aripiprazole exhibits high affinity for dopamine D_2 and D_3, serotonin $5\text{-}HT_{1A}$ and $5\text{-}HT_{2A}$ receptors (K_i values of 0.34, 0.8, 1.7, and 3.4 nM, respectively), moderate affinity for dopamine D_4, serotonin $5\text{-}HT_{2C}$ and $5\text{-}HT_7$, $alpha_1$-adrenergic and histamine H_1 receptors (K_i values of 44, 15, 39, 57, and 61 nM, respectively), and moderate affinity for the serotonin reuptake site (K_i=98 nM). Aripiprazole has no appreciable affinity for cholinergic muscarinic receptors (IC_{50} >1000 nM). Aripiprazole functions as a partial agonist at the dopamine D_2 and the serotonin $5\text{-}HT_{1A}$ receptors, and as an antagonist at serotonin $5\text{-}HT_{2A}$ receptor.
The mechanism of action of aripiprazole, as with other drugs having efficacy in schizophrenia, is unknown. However, it has been proposed that the efficacy of aripiprazole is mediated through a combination of partial agonist activity at D_2 and $5\text{-}HT_{1A}$ receptors and antagonist activity at $5\text{-}HT_{2A}$ receptors. Actions at receptors other than D_2, $5\text{-}HT_{1A}$, and $5\text{-}HT_{2A}$ may explain some of the other clinical effects of aripiprazole, e.g., the orthostatic hypotension observed with aripiprazole may be explained by its antagonist activity at adrenergic $alpha_1$ receptors.

Pharmacokinetics

ABILIFY activity is presumably primarily due to the parent drug, aripiprazole, and to a lesser extent, to its major metabolite, dehydro-aripiprazole, which has been shown to have affinities for D_2 receptors similar to the parent drug and represents 40% of the parent drug exposure in plasma. The mean elimination half-lives are about 75 hours and 94 hours for aripiprazole and dehydro-aripiprazole, respectively. Steady-state concentrations are attained within 14 days of dosing for both active moieties. Aripiprazole accumulation is predictable from single-dose pharmacokinetics. At steady state, the pharmacokinetics of aripiprazole are dose-proportional. Elimination of aripiprazole is mainly through hepatic metabolism involving two P450 isozymes, CYP2D6 and CYP3A4.

Absorption

Aripiprazole is well absorbed, with peak plasma concentrations occurring within 3 to 5 hours; the absolute oral bioavailability of the tablet formulation is 87%. ABILIFY (aripiprazole) can be administered with or without food. Administration of a 15-mg ABILIFY tablet with a standard high-fat meal did not significantly affect the C_{max} or AUC of aripiprazole or its active metabolite, dehydro-aripiprazole, but delayed T_{max} by 3 hours for aripiprazole and 12 hours for dehydro-aripiprazole.

Distribution

The steady-state volume of distribution of aripiprazole following intravenous administration is high (404 L or 4.9 L/kg), indicating extensive extravascular distribution. At therapeutic concentrations, aripiprazole and its major metabolite are greater than 99% bound to serum proteins, primarily to albumin. In healthy human volunteers administered 0.5 to 30 mg/day aripiprazole for 14 days, there was dose-dependent D_2-receptor occupancy indicating brain penetration of aripiprazole in humans.

Metabolism and Elimination

Aripiprazole is metabolized primarily by three biotransformation pathways: dehydrogenation, hydroxylation, and N-dealkylation. Based on *in vitro* studies, CYP3A4 and CYP2D6 enzymes are responsible for dehydrogenation and hydroxylation of aripiprazole, and N-dealkylation is catalyzed by CYP3A4. Aripiprazole is the predominant drug moiety in the systemic circulation. At steady state, dehydro-aripiprazole, the active metabolite, represents about 40% of aripiprazole AUC in plasma.
Approximately 8% of Caucasians lack the capacity to metabolize CYP2D6 substrates and are classified as poor metabolizers (PM), whereas the rest are extensive metabolizers (EM). PMs have about an 80% increase in aripiprazole exposure and about a 30% decrease in exposure to the active metabolite compared to EMs, resulting in about a 60% higher exposure to the total active moieties from a given dose of aripiprazole compared to EMs. Coadministration of ABILIFY with known inhibitors of CYP2D6, like quinidine in EMs, results in a 112% increase in aripiprazole plasma exposure, and dosing adjustment is needed (see **PRECAUTIONS: Drug-Drug Interactions**). The mean elimination half-lives are about 75 hours and 146 hours for aripiprazole in EMs and PMs, respectively. Aripiprazole does not inhibit or induce the CYP2D6 pathway.
Following a single oral dose of [^{14}C]-labeled aripiprazole, approximately 25% and 55% of the administered radioactivity was recovered in the urine and feces, respectively. Less than 1% of unchanged aripiprazole was excreted in the urine and approximately 18% of the oral dose was recovered unchanged in the feces.

Special Populations

In general, no dosage adjustment for ABILIFY (aripiprazole) is required on the basis of a patient's age, gender, race, smoking status, hepatic function, or renal function (see **DOSAGE AND ADMINISTRATION: Dosage in Special Populations**). The pharmacokinetics of aripiprazole in special populations are described below.

Hepatic Impairment

In a single-dose study (15 mg of aripiprazole) in subjects with varying degrees of liver cirrhosis (Child-Pugh Classes A, B, and C) the AUC of aripiprazole, compared to healthy subjects, increased 31% in mild HI, increased 8% in moderate HI, and decreased 20% in severe HI. None of these differences would require dose adjustment.

Renal Impairment

In patients with severe renal impairment (creatinine clearance <30 mL/min), C_{max} of aripiprazole (given in a single dose of 15 mg) and dehydro-aripiprazole increased by 36% and 53%, respectively, but AUC was 15% lower for aripiprazole and 7% higher for dehydro-aripiprazole. Renal excretion of both unchanged aripiprazole and dehydro-aripiprazole is less than 1% of the dose. No dosage adjustment is required in subjects with renal impairment.

Elderly

In formal single-dose pharmacokinetic studies (with aripiprazole given in a single dose of 15 mg), aripiprazole clearance was 20% lower in elderly (≥65 years) subjects compared to younger adult subjects (18 to 64 years). There was no detectable age effect, however, in the population pharmacokinetic analysis in schizophrenia patients. Also, the pharmacokinetics of aripiprazole after multiple doses in elderly patients appeared similar to that observed in young, healthy subjects. No dosage adjustment is recommended for elderly patients (see **PRECAUTIONS: Geriatric Use**).

Gender

C_{max} and AUC of aripiprazole and its active metabolite, dehydro-aripiprazole, are 30 to 40% higher in women than in men, and correspondingly, the apparent oral clearance of aripiprazole is lower in women. These differences, however, are largely explained by differences in body weight (25%) between men and women. No dosage adjustment is recommended based on gender.

Race

Although no specific pharmacokinetic study was conducted to investigate the effects of race on the disposition of aripiprazole, population pharmacokinetic evaluation revealed no evidence of clinically significant race-related differences in the pharmacokinetics of aripiprazole. No dosage adjustment is recommended based on race.

Smoking

Based on studies utilizing human liver enzymes *in vitro*, aripiprazole is not a substrate for CYP1A2 and also does not undergo direct glucuronidation. Smoking should, therefore, not have an effect on the pharmacokinetics of aripiprazole. Consistent with these *in vitro* results, population pharmacokinetic evaluation did not reveal any significant pharmacokinetic differences between smokers and nonsmokers. No dosage adjustment is recommended based on smoking status.

Drug-Drug Interactions

Potential for Other Drugs to Affect ABILIFY (aripiprazole)

Aripiprazole is not a substrate of CYP1A1, CYP1A2, CYP2A6, CYP2B6, CYP2C8, CYP2C9, CYP2C19, or CYP2E1 enzymes. Aripiprazole also does not undergo direct glucuronidation. This suggests that an interaction of aripiprazole with inhibitors or inducers of these enzymes, or other factors, like smoking, is unlikely.
Both CYP3A4 and CYP2D6 are responsible for aripiprazole metabolism. Agents that induce CYP3A4 (e.g., carbamazepine) could cause an increase in aripiprazole clearance and lower blood levels. Inhibitors of CYP3A4 (e.g., ketoconazole) or CYP2D6 (e.g., quinidine, fluoxetine, or paroxetine) can inhibit aripiprazole elimination and cause increased blood levels.

Potential for ABILIFY (aripiprazole) to Affect Other Drugs

Aripiprazole is unlikely to cause clinically important pharmacokinetic interactions with drugs metabolized by cytochrome P450 enzymes. In *in vivo* studies, 10- to 30-mg/day doses of aripiprazole had no significant effect on metabolism by CYP2D6 (dextromethorphan), CYP2C9 (warfarin), CYP2C19 (omeprazole, warfarin), and CYP3A4 (dextromethorphan) substrates. Additionally, aripiprazole and dehydro-aripiprazole did not show potential for altering CYP1A2-mediated metabolism *in vitro* (see **PRECAUTIONS: Drug-Drug Interactions**).

Aripiprazole had no clinically important interactions with the following drugs:

Famotidine: Coadministration of aripiprazole (given in a single dose of 15 mg) with a 40-mg single dose of the H_2 antagonist famotidine, a potent gastric acid blocker, decreased the solubility of aripiprazole and, hence, its rate of absorption, reducing by 37% and 21% the C_{max} of aripiprazole and dehydro-aripiprazole, respectively, and by 13% and 15%, respectively, the extent of absorption (AUC). No dosage adjustment of aripiprazole is required when administered concomitantly with famotidine.

Valproate: When valproate (500–1500 mg/day) and aripiprazole (30 mg/day) were coadministered at steady state, the C_{max} and AUC of aripiprazole were decreased by 25%. No dosage adjustment of aripiprazole is required when administered concomitantly with valproate.

Lithium: A pharmacokinetic interaction of aripiprazole with lithium is unlikely because lithium is not bound to plasma proteins, is not metabolized, and is almost entirely excreted unchanged in urine. Coadministration of therapeutic doses of lithium (1200–1800 mg/day) for 21 days with aripiprazole (30 mg/day) did not result in clinically significant changes in the pharmacokinetics of aripiprazole or its active metabolite, dehydro-aripiprazole (C_{max} and AUC increased by less than 20%). No dosage adjustment of aripiprazole is required when administered concomitantly with lithium.

Dextromethorphan: Aripiprazole at doses of 10 to 30 mg per day for 14 days had no effect on dextromethorphan's O-dealkylation to its major metabolite, dextrorphan, a pathway known to be dependent on CYP2D6 activity. Aripiprazole also had no effect on dextromethorphan's N-demethylation to its metabolite 3-methyoxymorphan, a pathway known to be dependent on CYP3A4 activity. No dosage adjustment of dextromethorphan is required when administered concomitantly with aripiprazole.

Warfarin: Aripiprazole 10 mg per day for 14 days had no effect on the pharmacokinetics of R- and S-warfarin or on the pharmacodynamic end point of International Normalized Ratio, indicating the lack of a clinically relevant effect of aripiprazole on CYP2C9 and CYP2C19 metabolism or the binding of highly protein-bound warfarin. No dosage adjustment of warfarin is required when administered concomitantly with aripiprazole.

Omeprazole: Aripiprazole 10 mg per day for 15 days had no effect on the pharmacokinetics of a single 20-mg dose of omeprazole, a CYP2C19 substrate, in healthy subjects. No dosage adjustment of omeprazole is required when administered concomitantly with aripiprazole.

Clinical Studies

The efficacy of ABILIFY (aripiprazole) in the treatment of schizophrenia was evaluated in four short-term (4- and 6-week), placebo-controlled trials of acutely relapsed inpatients who predominantly met DSM-III/IV criteria for schizophrenia. Three of the four trials were able to distinguish aripiprazole from placebo, but one study, the smallest, did not. Three of these studies also included an active control group consisting of either risperidone (one trial) or haloperidol (two trials), but they were not designed to allow for a comparison of ABILIFY and the active comparators.

In the three positive trials for ABILIFY, four primary measures were used for assessing psychiatric signs and symptoms. The Positive and Negative Syndrome Scale (PANSS) is a multi-item inventory of general psychopathology used to evaluate the effects of drug treatment in schizophrenia. The PANSS positive subscale is a subset of items in the PANSS that rates seven positive symptoms of schizophrenia (delusions, conceptual disorganization, hallucinatory behavior, excitement, grandiosity, suspiciousness/persecution, and hostility). The PANSS negative subscale is a subset of items in the PANSS that rates seven negative symptoms of schizophrenia (blunted affect, emotional withdrawal, poor rapport, passive apathetic withdrawal, difficulty in abstract thinking, lack of spontaneity/flow of conversation, stereotyped thinking). The Clinical Global Impression (CGI) assessment reflects the impression of a skilled observer, fully familiar with the manifestations of schizophrenia, about the overall clinical state of the patient.

In a 4-week trial (n=414) comparing two fixed doses of ABILIFY (15 or 30 mg/day) and haloperidol (10 mg/day) to placebo, both doses of ABILIFY were superior to placebo in the PANSS total score, PANSS positive subscale, and CGI-severity score. In addition, the 15-mg dose was superior to placebo in the PANSS negative subscale.

In a 4-week trial (n=404) comparing two fixed doses of ABILIFY (20 or 30 mg/day) and risperidone (6 mg/day) to placebo, both doses of ABILIFY were superior to placebo in the PANSS total score, PANSS positive subscale, PANSS negative subscale, and CGI-severity score.

In a 6-week trial (n=420) comparing three fixed doses of ABILIFY (10, 15, or 20 mg/day) to placebo, all three doses of ABILIFY were superior to placebo in the PANSS total score, PANSS positive subscale, and the PANSS negative subscale.

In a fourth study, a 4-week trial (n=103) comparing ABILIFY in a range of 5 to 30 mg/day or haloperidol 5 to 20 mg/day to placebo, haloperidol was superior to placebo, in the Brief Psychiatric Rating Scale (BPRS), a multi-item inventory of general psychopathology traditionally used to evaluate the effects of drug treatment in psychosis, and in a responder analysis based on the CGI-severity score, the primary outcomes for that trial. ABILIFY was only significantly different compared to placebo in a responder analysis based on the CGI-severity score.

Thus, the efficacy of 15-mg, 20-mg, and 30-mg daily doses was established in two studies for each dose, whereas the efficacy of the 10-mg dose was established in one study. There was no evidence in any study that the higher dose groups offered any advantage over the lowest dose group.

An examination of population subgroups did not reveal any clear evidence of differential responsiveness on the basis of age, gender, or race.

A longer-term trial enrolled 310 inpatients or outpatients meeting DSM-IV criteria for schizophrenia who were, by history, symptomatically stable on other antipsychotic medications for periods of 3 months or longer. These patients were discontinued from their antipsychotic medications and randomized to ABILIFY 15 mg or placebo for up to 26 weeks of observation for relapse. Relapse during the double-blind phase was defined as CGI-Improvement score of ≥5 (minimally worse), scores ≥5 (moderately severe) on the hostility or uncooperativeness items of the PANSS, or ≥20% increase in the PANSS total score. Patients receiving ABILIFY 15 mg experienced a significantly longer time to relapse over the subsequent 26 weeks compared to those receiving placebo.

INDICATIONS AND USAGE

ABILIFY (aripiprazole) is indicated for the treatment of schizophrenia. The efficacy of ABILIFY in the treatment of schizophrenia was established in short-term (4- and 6-week) controlled trials of schizophrenic inpatients (see **CLINICAL PHARMACOLOGY: Clinical Studies**).

The efficacy of ABILIFY in maintaining stability in patients with schizophrenia who had been symptomatically stable on antipsychotic medications for periods of 3 months or longer, were discontinued from those other medications, and were then administered ABILIFY 15 mg/day and observed for relapse during a period of up 26 weeks was demonstrated in a placebo-controlled trial (see **CLINICAL PHARMACOLOGY: Clinical Studies**). The physician who elects to use ABILIFY for extended periods should periodically re-evaluate the long-term usefulness of the drug for the individual patient (see **DOSAGE AND ADMINISTRATION**).

CONTRAINDICATIONS

ABILIFY is contraindicated in patients with a known hypersensitivity to the product.

WARNINGS

Neuroleptic Malignant Syndrome (NMS)

A potentially fatal symptom complex sometimes referred to as Neuroleptic Malignant Syndrome (NMS) has been reported in association with administration of antipsychotic drugs, including aripiprazole. Two possible cases of NMS occurred during aripiprazole treatment in the premarketing worldwide clinical database. Clinical manifestations of NMS are hyperpyrexia, muscle rigidity, altered mental status, and evidence of autonomic instability (irregular pulse or blood pressure, tachycardia, diaphoresis, and cardiac dysrhythmia). Additional signs may include elevated creatine phosphokinase, myoglobinuria (rhabdomyolysis), and acute renal failure.

The diagnostic evaluation of patients with this syndrome is complicated. In arriving at a diagnosis, it is important to exclude cases where the clinical presentation includes both serious medical illness (e.g., pneumonia, systemic infection, etc) and untreated or inadequately treated extrapyramidal signs and symptoms (EPS). Other important considerations in the differential diagnosis include central anticholinergic toxicity, heat stroke, drug fever, and primary central nervous system pathology.

The management of NMS should include: 1) immediate discontinuation of antipsychotic drugs and other drugs not essential to concurrent therapy; 2) intensive symptomatic treatment and medical monitoring; and 3) treatment of any concomitant serious medical problems for which specific treatments are available. There is no general agreement about specific pharmacological treatment regimens for uncomplicated NMS.

If a patient requires antipsychotic drug treatment after recovery from NMS, the potential reintroduction of drug therapy should be carefully considered. The patient should be carefully monitored, since recurrences of NMS have been reported.

Tardive Dyskinesia

A syndrome of potentially irreversible, involuntary, dyskinetic movements may develop in patients treated with antipsychotic drugs. Although the prevalence of the syndrome appears to be highest among the elderly, especially elderly women, it is impossible to rely upon prevalence estimates to predict, at the inception of antipsychotic treatment, which patients are likely to develop the syndrome. Whether antipsychotic drug products differ in their potential to cause tardive dyskinesia is unknown.

The risk of developing tardive dyskinesia and the likelihood that it will become irreversible are believed to increase as the duration of treatment and the total cumulative dose of antipsychotic drugs administered to the patient increase. However, the syndrome can develop, although much less commonly, after relatively brief treatment periods at low doses.

There is no known treatment for established cases of tardive dyskinesia, although the syndrome may remit, partially or completely, if antipsychotic treatment is withdrawn. Antipsychotic treatment, itself, however, may suppress (or partially suppress) the signs and symptoms of the syndrome and, thereby, may possibly mask the underlying process. The effect that symptomatic suppression has upon the long-term course of the syndrome is unknown.

Given these considerations, ABILIFY (aripiprazole) should be prescribed in a manner that is most likely to minimize the occurrence of tardive dyskinesia. Chronic antipsychotic treatment should generally be reserved for patients who suffer from a chronic illness that (1) is known to respond to antipsychotic drugs, and (2) for whom alternative, equally effective, but potentially less harmful treatments are not available or appropriate. In patients who do require chronic treatment, the smallest dose and the shortest duration of treatment producing a satisfactory clinical response should be sought. The need for continued treatment should be reassessed periodically.

If signs and symptoms of tardive dyskinesia appear in a patient on ABILIFY, drug discontinuation should be considered. However, some patients may require treatment with ABILIFY despite the presence of the syndrome.

Hyperglycemia and Diabetes Mellitus

Hyperglycemia, in some cases extreme and associated with ketoacidosis or hyperosmolar coma or death, has been reported in patients treated with atypical antipsychotics. There have been few reports of hyperglycemia in patients treated with ABILIFY (aripiprazole). Although fewer patients have been treated with ABILIFY, it is not known if this more limited experience is the sole reason for the paucity of such reports. Assessment of the relationship between atypical antipsychotic use and glucose abnormalities is complicated by the possibility of an increased background risk of diabetes mellitus in patients with schizophrenia and the increasing incidence of diabetes mellitus in the general population. Given these confounders, the relationship between atypical antipsychotic use and hyperglycemia-related adverse events is not completely understood. However, epidemiological studies which did not include ABILIFY suggest an increased risk of treatment-emergent hyperglycemia-related adverse events in patients treated with the atypical antipsychotics included in these studies. Because ABILIFY was not marketed at the time these studies were performed, it is not known if ABILIFY is associated with this increased risk. Precise risk estimates for hyperglycemia-related adverse events in patients treated with atypical antipsychotics are not available.

Patients with an established diagnosis of diabetes mellitus who are started on atypical antipsychotics should be monitored regularly for worsening of glucose control. Patients with risk factors for diabetes mellitus (e.g., obesity, family history of diabetes) who are starting treatment with atypical antipsychotics should undergo fasting blood glucose testing at the beginning of treatment and periodically during treatment. Any patient treated with atypical antipsychotics should be monitored for symptoms of hyperglycemia including polydipsia, polyuria, polyphagia, and weakness. Patients who develop symptoms of hyperglycemia during treatment with atypical antipsychotics should undergo fasting blood glucose testing. In some cases, hyperglycemia has resolved when the atypical antipsychotic was discontinued; however, some patients required continuation of anti-diabetic treatment despite discontinuation of the suspect drug.

PRECAUTIONS

General

Orthostatic Hypotension

Aripiprazole may be associated with orthostatic hypotension, perhaps due to its α_1-adrenergic receptor antagonism. The incidence of orthostatic hypotension associated events from five short-term, placebo-controlled trials in schizophrenia (n=926) on ABILIFY included: orthostatic hypotension (placebo 1%, aripiprazole 1.9%); orthostatic lightheadedness (placebo 1%, aripiprazole 0.9%), and syncope (placebo 1%, aripiprazole 0.6%). The incidence of a significant orthostatic change in blood pressure (defined as a decrease of at least 30 mmHg in systolic blood pressure when changing from a supine to standing position) for aripiprazole was not statistically different from placebo (14% among aripiprazole-treated patients and 12% among placebo-treated patients).

Aripiprazole should be used with caution in patients with known cardiovascular disease (history of myocardial infarction or ischemic heart disease, heart failure or conduction abnormalities), cerebrovascular disease, or conditions which would predispose patients to hypotension (dehydration, hypovolemia, and treatment with antihypertensive medications).

Seizure

Seizures occurred in 0.1% (1/926) of aripiprazole-treated patients in short-term, placebo-controlled trials. As with other antipsychotic drugs, aripiprazole should be used cautiously in patients with a history of seizures or with conditions that lower the seizure threshold, e.g., Alzheimer's dementia. Conditions that lower the seizure threshold may be more prevalent in a population of 65 years or older.

Potential for Cognitive and Motor Impairment

In short-term, placebo-controlled trials, somnolence was reported in 11% of patients on ABILIFY (aripiprazole) compared to 8% of patients on placebo; somnolence led to discontinuation in 0.1% (1/926) of patients on ABILIFY (aripiprazole) in short-term, placebo-controlled trials. Despite the relatively modest increased incidence of somnolence compared to placebo, ABILIFY, like other antipsychotics, may have the potential to impair judgment, thinking, or motor skills. Patients should be cautioned about operating hazardous machinery, including automobiles, until they are reasonably certain that therapy with ABILIFY does not affect them adversely.

Body Temperature Regulation

Disruption of the body's ability to reduce core body temperature has been attributed to antipsychotic agents. Appropriate care is advised when prescribing aripiprazole for patients who will be experiencing conditions which may contribute to an elevation in core body temperature, e.g., exercising strenuously, exposure to extreme heat, receiving concomitant medication with anticholinergic activity, or being subject to dehydration.

Dysphagia

Esophageal dysmotility and aspiration have been associated with antipsychotic drug use. Aspiration pneumonia is a common cause of morbidity and mortality in elderly patients, in particular those with advanced Alzheimer's dementia. Aripiprazole and other antipsychotic drugs should be used cautiously in patients at risk for aspiration pneumonia (see **PRECAUTIONS:** *Use in Patients with Concomitant Illness*).

Suicide

The possibility of a suicide attempt is inherent in psychotic illnesses, and close supervision of high-risk patients should accompany drug therapy. Prescriptions for ABILIFY should be written for the smallest quantity of tablets consistent with good patient management in order to reduce the risk of overdose.

Use in Patients with Concomitant Illness

Safety Experience in Elderly Patients with Psychosis Associated with Alzheimer's Disease:

In a flexible dose (2 to 15 mg/day), 10-week, placebo-controlled study of aripiprazole in elderly patients (mean age: 81.5 years; range: 56 to 95 years) with psychosis associated with Alzheimer's dementia, 4 of 105 patients (3.8%) who received ABILIFY (aripiprazole) died compared to no deaths among 102 patients who received placebo during or within 30 days after termination of the double blind portion of the study. Three of the patients (age 92, 91, and 87 years) died following the discontinuation of ABILIFY in the double-blind phase of the study (causes of death were pneumonia, heart failure, and shock). The fourth patient (age 78 years) died following hip surgery while in the double-blind portion of the study. The treatment-emergent adverse events that were reported at an incidence of ≥5% and having a greater incidence than placebo in this study were accidental injury, somnolence, and bronchitis. Eight percent of the ABILIFY-treated patients reported somnolence com-

Continued on next page

Abilify—Cont.

pared to one percent of placebo patients. In a small pilot, open-label, ascending-dose cohort study (n=30) in elderly patients with dementia, ABILIFY was associated in a dose-related fashion with somnolence.

The safety and efficacy of ABILIFY in the treatment of patients with psychosis associated with dementia have not been established. If the prescriber elects to treat such patients with ABILIFY, vigilance should be exercised, particularly for the emergence of difficulty swallowing or excessive somnolence, which could predispose to accidental injury or aspiration.

Clinical experience with ABILIFY in patients with certain concomitant systemic illnesses (see **CLINICAL PHARMACOLOGY: Special Populations:** *Renal Impairment* and *Hepatic Impairment*) is limited.

ABILIFY has not been evaluated or used to any appreciable extent in patients with a recent history of myocardial infarction or unstable heart disease. Patients with these diagnoses were excluded from premarketing clinical studies.

Information for Patients

Physicians are advised to discuss the following issues with patients for whom they prescribe ABILIFY:

Interference with Cognitive and Motor Performance

Because aripiprazole may have the potential to impair judgment, thinking, or motor skills, patients should be cautioned about operating hazardous machinery, including automobiles, until they are reasonably certain that aripiprazole therapy does not affect them adversely.

Pregnancy

Patients should be advised to notify their physician if they become pregnant or intend to become pregnant during therapy with ABILIFY.

Nursing

Patients should be advised not to breast-feed an infant if they are taking ABILIFY.

Concomitant Medication

Patients should be advised to inform their physicians if they are taking, or plan to take, any prescription or over-the-counter drugs, since there is a potential for interactions.

Alcohol

Patients should be advised to avoid alcohol while taking ABILIFY.

Heat Exposure and Dehydration

Patients should be advised regarding appropriate care in avoiding overheating and dehydration.

Drug-Drug Interactions

Given the primary CNS effects of aripiprazole, caution should be used when ABILIFY is taken in combination with other centrally acting drugs and alcohol. Due to its α_1-adrenergic receptor antagonism, aripiprazole has the potential to enhance the effect of certain antihypertensive agents.

Potential for Other Drugs to Affect ABILIFY (aripiprazole)

Aripiprazole is not a substrate of CYP1A1, CYP1A2, CYP2A6, CYP2B6, CYP2C8, CYP2C9, CYP2C19, or CYP2E1 enzymes. Aripiprazole also does not undergo direct glucuronidation. This suggests that an interaction of aripiprazole with inhibitors or inducers of these enzymes, or other factors, like smoking, is unlikely.

Both CYP3A4 and CYP2D6 are responsible for aripiprazole metabolism. Agents that induce CYP3A4 (e.g., carbamazepine) could cause an increase in aripiprazole clearance and lower blood levels. Inhibitors of CYP3A4 (e.g., ketoconazole) or CYP2D6 (e.g., quinidine, fluoxetine, or paroxetine) can inhibit aripiprazole elimination and cause increased blood levels.

Ketoconazole: Coadministration of ketoconazole (200 mg/day for 14 days) with a 15-mg single dose of aripiprazole increased the AUC of aripiprazole and its active metabolite by 63% and 77%, respectively. The effect of a higher ketoconazole dose (400 mg/day) has not been studied. When concomitant administration of ketoconazole with aripiprazole occurs, aripiprazole dose should be reduced to one-half of its normal dose. Other strong inhibitors of CYP3A4 (itraconazole) would be expected to have similar effects and need similar dose reductions; weaker inhibitors (erythromycin, grapefruit juice) have not been studied. When the CYP3A4 inhibitor is withdrawn from the combination therapy, aripiprazole dose should then be increased.

Quinidine: Coadministration of a 10-mg single dose of aripiprazole with quinidine (166 mg/day for 13 days), a potent inhibitor of CYP2D6, increased the AUC of aripiprazole by 112% but decreased the AUC of its active metabolite, dehydro-aripiprazole, by 35%. Aripiprazole dose should be reduced to one-half of its normal dose when concomitant administration of quinidine with aripiprazole occurs. Other significant inhibitors of CYP2D6, such as fluoxetine or paroxetine, would be expected to have similar effects and, therefore, should be accompanied by similar dose reductions. When the CYP2D6 inhibitor is withdrawn from the combination therapy, aripiprazole dose should then be increased.

Carbamazepine: Coadministration of carbamazepine (200 mg BID), a potent CYP3A4 inducer, with aripiprazole (30 mg QD) resulted in an approximate 70% decrease in C_{max} and AUC values of both aripiprazole and its active metabolite, dehydro-aripiprazole. When carbamazepine is added to aripiprazole therapy, aripiprazole dose should be doubled. Additional dose increases should be based on clinical evaluation. When carbamazepine is withdrawn from the combination therapy, aripiprazole dose should then be reduced.

No clinically significant effect of famotidine, valproate, or lithium was seen on the pharmacokinetics of aripiprazole (see **CLINICAL PHARMACOLOGY: Drug-Drug Interactions**).

Potential for ABILIFY (aripiprazole) to Affect Other Drugs

Aripiprazole is unlikely to cause clinically important pharmacokinetic interactions with drugs metabolized by cytochrome P450 enzymes. In *in vivo* studies, 10- to 30-mg/day doses of aripiprazole had no significant effect on metabolism by CYP2D6 (dextromethorphan), CYP2C9 (warfarin), CYP2C19 (omeprazole, warfarin), and CYP3A4 (dextromethorphan) substrates. Additionally, aripiprazole and dehydro-aripiprazole did not show potential for altering CYP1A2-mediated metabolism *in vitro* (see **CLINICAL PHARMACOLOGY: Drug-Drug Interactions**).

Alcohol: There was no significant difference between aripiprazole coadministered with ethanol and placebo coadministered with ethanol on performance of gross motor skills or stimulus response in healthy subjects. As with most psychoactive medications, patients should be advised to avoid alcohol while taking ABILIFY.

Carcinogenesis, Mutagenesis, Impairment of Fertility

Carcinogenesis

Lifetime carcinogenicity studies were conducted in ICR mice and in Sprague-Dawley (SD) and F344 rats. Aripiprazole was administered for 2 years in the diet at doses of 1, 3, 10, and 30 mg/kg/day to ICR mice and 1, 3, and 10 mg/kg/day to F344 rats (0.2 to 5 and 0.3 to 3 times the maximum recommended human dose [MRHD] based on mg/m^2, respectively). In addition, SD rats were dosed orally for 2 years at 10, 20, 40, and 60 mg/kg/day (3 to 19 times the MRHD based on mg/m^2). Aripiprazole did not induce tumors in male mice or rats. In female mice, the incidences of pituitary gland adenomas and mammary gland adenocarcinomas and adenoacanthomas were increased at dietary doses of 3 to 30 mg/kg/day (0.1 to 0.9 times human exposure at MRHD based on AUC and 0.5 to 5 times the MRHD based on mg/m^2). In female rats, the incidence of mammary gland fibroadenomas was increased at a dietary dose of 10 mg/kg/day (0.1 times human exposure at MRHD based on AUC and 3 times the MRHD based on mg/m^2); and the incidences of adrenocortical carcinomas and combined adrenocortical adenomas/carcinomas were increased at an oral dose of 60 mg/kg/day (14 times human exposure at MRHD based on AUC and 19 times the MRHD based on mg/m^2).

Proliferative changes in the pituitary and mammary gland of rodents have been observed following chronic administration of other antipsychotic agents and are considered prolactin-mediated. Serum prolactin was not measured in the aripiprazole carcinogenicity studies. However, increases in serum prolactin levels were observed in female mice in a 13-week dietary study at the doses associated with mammary gland and pituitary tumors. Serum prolactin was not increased in female rats in 4- and 13-week dietary studies at the dose associated with mammary gland tumors. The relevance for human risk of the findings of prolactin-mediated endocrine tumors in rodents is unknown.

Mutagenesis

The mutagenic potential of aripiprazole was tested in the *in vitro* bacterial reverse-mutation assay, the *in vitro* bacterial DNA repair assay, the *in vitro* forward gene mutation assay in mouse lymphoma cells, the *in vitro* chromosomal aberration assay in Chinese hamster lung (CHL) cells, the *in vivo* micronucleus assay in mice, and the unscheduled DNA synthesis assay in rats. Aripiprazole and a metabolite (2,3-DCPP) were clastogenic in the *in vitro* chromosomal aberration assay in CHL cells with and without metabolic activation. The metabolite, 2,3-DCPP, produced increases in numerical aberrations in the *in vitro* assay in CHL cells in the absence of metabolic activation. A positive response was obtained in the *in vivo* micronucleus assay in mice, however, the response was shown to be due to a mechanism not considered relevant to humans.

Impairment of Fertility

Female rats were treated with oral doses of 2, 6, and 20 mg/kg/day (0.6, 2, and 6 times the maximum recommended human dose [MRHD] on a mg/m^2 basis) of aripiprazole from 2 weeks prior to mating through day 7 of gestation. Estrus cycle irregularities and increased corpora lutea were seen at all doses, but no impairment of fertility was seen. Increased pre-implantation loss was seen at 6 and 20 mg/kg, and decreased fetal weight was seen at 20 mg/kg.

Male rats were treated with oral doses of 20, 40, and 60 mg/kg/day (6, 13, and 19 times the MRHD on a mg/m^2 basis) of aripiprazole from 9 weeks prior to mating through mating. Disturbances in spermatogenesis were seen at 60 mg/kg, and prostate atrophy was seen at 40 and 60 mg/kg, but no impairment of fertility was seen.

Pregnancy

Pregnancy Category C

In animal studies, aripiprazole demonstrated developmental toxicity, including possible teratogenic effects in rats and rabbits.

Pregnant rats were treated with oral doses of 3, 10, and 30 mg/kg/day (1, 3, and 10 times the maximum recommended human dose [MRHD] on a mg/m^2 basis) of aripiprazole during the period of organogenesis. Gestation was slightly prolonged at 30 mg/kg. Treatment caused a slight delay in fetal development, as evidenced by decreased fetal weight (30 mg/kg), undescended testes (30 mg/kg), and delayed skeletal ossification (10 and 30 mg/kg). There were no adverse effects on embryofetal or pup survival. Delivered offspring had decreased bodyweights (10 and 30 mg/kg), and increased incidences of hepatodiaphragmatic nodules and diaphragmatic hernia at 30 mg/kg (the other dose groups were not examined for these findings). (A low incidence of diaphragmatic hernia was also seen in the fetuses exposed to 30 mg/kg.) Postnatally, delayed vaginal opening was seen at 10 and 30 mg/kg and impaired reproductive performance (decreased fertility rate, corpora lutea, implants, and live fetuses, and increased post-implantation loss, likely mediated through effects on female offspring) was seen at 30 mg/kg. Some maternal toxicity was seen at 30 mg/kg, however, there was no evidence to suggest that these developmental effects were secondary to maternal toxicity.

Pregnant rabbits were treated with oral doses of 10, 30, and 100 mg/kg/day (2, 3, and 11 times human exposure at MRHD based on AUC and 6, 19, and 65 times the MRHD based on mg/m^2) of aripiprazole during the period of organogenesis. Decreased maternal food consumption and increased abortions were seen at 100 mg/kg. Treatment caused increased fetal mortality (100 mg/kg), decreased fetal weight (30 and 100 mg/kg), increased incidence of skeletal abnormality (fused sternebrae at 30 and 100 mg/kg) and minor skeletal variations (100 mg/kg).

In a study in which rats were treated with oral doses of 3, 10, and 30 mg/kg/day (1, 3, and 10 times the MRHD on a mg/m^2 basis) of aripiprazole perinatally and postnatally (from day 17 of gestation through day 21 postpartum), slight maternal toxicity and slightly prolonged gestation were seen at 30 mg/kg. An increase in stillbirths, and decreases in pup weight (persisting into adulthood) and survival, were seen at this dose.

There are no adequate and well-controlled studies in pregnant women. It is not known whether aripiprazole can cause fetal harm when administered to a pregnant woman or can affect reproductive capacity. Aripiprazole should be used during pregnancy only if the potential benefit outweighs the potential risk to the fetus.

Labor and Delivery

The effect of aripiprazole on labor and delivery in humans is unknown.

Nursing Mothers

Aripiprazole was excreted in milk of rats during lactation. It is not known whether aripiprazole or its metabolites are excreted in human milk. It is recommended that women receiving aripiprazole should not breast-feed.

Pediatric Use

Safety and effectiveness in pediatric and adolescent patients have not been established.

Geriatric Use

Of the 5592 patients treated with aripiprazole in premarketing clinical trials, 659 (12%) were ≥65 years old and 525 (9%) were ≥75 years old. The majority (91%) of the 659 patients were diagnosed with dementia of the Alzheimer's type.

Placebo-controlled studies of aripiprazole in schizophrenia did not include sufficient numbers of subjects aged 65 and over to determine whether they respond differently from younger subjects. There was no effect of age on the pharmacokinetics of a single 15-mg dose of aripiprazole. Aripiprazole clearance was decreased by 20% in elderly subjects (≥65 years) compared to younger adult subjects (18 to 64 years), but there was no detectable effect of age in the population pharmacokinetic analysis in schizophrenia patients.

Studies of elderly patients with psychosis associated with Alzheimer's disease, have suggested that there may be a different tolerability profile in this population compared to younger patients with schizophrenia (see **PRECAUTIONS:** *Use in Patients with Concomitant Illness*). The safety and efficacy of ABILIFY (aripiprazole) in the treatment of patients with psychosis associated with Alzheimer's disease has not been established. If the prescriber elects to treat such patients with ABILIFY, vigilance should be exercised.

ADVERSE REACTIONS

Aripiprazole has been evaluated for safety in 5592 patients who participated in multiple-dose, premarketing trials in schizophrenia, bipolar mania, and dementia of the Alzheimer's type, and who had approximately 3639 patient-years of exposure. A total of 1887 aripiprazole-treated patients were treated for at least 180 days and 1251 aripiprazole-treated patients had at least 1 year of exposure.

The conditions and duration of treatment with aripiprazole included (in overlapping categories) double-blind, comparative and noncomparative open-label studies, inpatient and outpatient studies, fixed- and flexible-dose studies, and short- and longer-term exposure.

Adverse events during exposure were obtained by collecting volunteered adverse events, as well as results of physical examinations, vital signs, weights, laboratory analyses, and ECG. Adverse experiences were recorded by clinical investigators using terminology of their own choosing. In the tables and tabulations that follow, modified COSTART dictionary terminology has been used initially to classify reported adverse events into a smaller number of standardized event categories, in order to provide a meaningful estimate of the proportion of individuals experiencing adverse events.

The stated frequencies of adverse events represent the proportion of individuals who experienced at least once, a treatment-emergent adverse event of the type listed. An event was considered treatment emergent if it occurred for the first time or worsened while receiving therapy following baseline evaluation. There was no attempt to use investigator causality assessments; ie, all reported events are included.

The prescriber should be aware that the figures in the tables and tabulations cannot be used to predict the incidence of side effects in the course of usual medical practice where patient characteristics and other factors differ from those that prevailed in the clinical trials. Similarly, the cited frequencies cannot be compared with figures obtained from other clinical investigations involving different treatment, uses, and investigators. The cited figures, however, do provide the prescribing physician with some basis for estimating the relative contribution of drug and nondrug factors to the adverse event incidence in the population studied.

Adverse Findings Observed in Short-Term, Placebo-Controlled Trials of Patients with Schizophrenia

The following findings are based on a pool of five placebo-controlled trials (four 4-week and one 6-week) in which aripiprazole was administered in doses ranging from 2 to 30 mg/day.

Adverse Events Associated with Discontinuation of Treatment in Short-Term, Placebo-Controlled Trials

Overall, there was no difference in the incidence of discontinuation due to adverse events between aripiprazole-treated (7%) and placebo-treated (9%) patients. The types of adverse events that led to discontinuation were similar between the aripiprazole and placebo-treated patients.

Adverse Events Occurring at an Incidence of 2% or More Among Aripiprazole-Treated Patients and Greater than Placebo in Short-Term Placebo-Controlled Trials

Table 1 enumerates the incidence, rounded to the nearest percent, of treatment-emergent adverse events that occurred during acute therapy (up to 6 weeks), including only those events that occurred in 2% or more of patients treated with aripiprazole (doses ≥2 mg/day) and for which the incidence in patients treated with aripiprazole was greater than the incidence in patients treated with placebo.

Table 1: Treatment-Emergent Adverse Events in Short-Term, Placebo-Controlled Trials

Body System / Adverse Event	Percentage of Patients Reporting Event[a] Aripiprazole (n=926)	Placebo (n=413)
Body as a Whole		
Headache	32	25
Asthenia	7	5
Fever	2	1
Digestive System		
Nausea	14	10
Vomiting	12	7
Constipation	10	8
Nervous System		
Anxiety	25	24
Insomnia	24	19
Lightheadedness	11	7
Somnolence	11	8
Akathisia	10	7
Tremor	3	2
Respiratory System		
Rhinitis	4	3
Coughing	3	2
Skin and Appendages		
Rash	6	5
Special Senses		
Blurred vision	3	1

[a] Events reported by at least 2% of patients treated with aripiprazole, except the following events, which had an incidence equal to or less than placebo: abdominal pain, accidental injury, back pain, dental pain, dyspepsia, diarrhea, dry mouth, myalgia, agitation, psychosis, extrapyramidal syndrome, hypertonia, pharyngitis, upper respiratory tract infection, dysmenorrhea, vaginitis.

An examination of population subgroups did not reveal any clear evidence of differential adverse event incidence on the basis of age, gender, or race.

Dose-Related Adverse Events

Dose response relationships for the incidence of treatment-emergent adverse events were evaluated from four trials comparing various fixed doses (2, 10, 15, 20, and 30 mg/day) of aripiprazole to placebo. This analysis, stratified by study, indicated that the only adverse event to have a possible dose response relationship, and then most prominent only with 30 mg, was somnolence (placebo, 7.7%; 15 mg, 8.7%; 20 mg, 7.5%; 30 mg, 15.3%).

Extrapyramidal Symptoms

In the short-term, placebo-controlled trials, the incidence of reported EPS for aripiprazole-treated patients was 6% vs. 6% for placebo. Objectively collected data from those trials on the Simpson Angus Rating Scale (for EPS), the Barnes Akathisia Scale (for akathisia), and the Assessments of Involuntary Movement Scales (for dyskinesias) also did not show a difference between aripiprazole and placebo, with the exception of the Barnes Akathisia Scale (aripiprazole, 0.08; placebo, −0.05).

Similarly, in a long-term (26-week), placebo-controlled trial, objectively collected data on the Simpson Angus Rating Scale (for EPS), the Barnes Akathisia Scale (for akathisia), and the Assessments of Involuntary Movement Scales (for dyskinesias) did not show a difference between aripiprazole and placebo.

Laboratory Test Abnormalities

A between group comparison for 4- to 6-week placebo-controlled trials revealed no medically important differences between the aripiprazole and placebo groups in the proportions of patients experiencing potentially clinically significant changes in routine serum chemistry, hematology, or urinalysis parameters. Similarly, there were no aripiprazole/placebo differences in the incidence of discontinuations for changes in serum chemistry, hematology, or urinalysis.

In a long-term (26-week), placebo-controlled trial there were no medically important differences between the aripiprazole and placebo patients in the mean change from baseline in prolactin, fasting glucose, triglyceride, HDL, LDL, and total cholesterol measurements.

Weight Gain

In short-term trials, there was a slight difference in mean weight gain between aripiprazole and placebo patients (+0.7 kg vs. −0.05 kg, respectively), and also a difference in the proportion of patients meeting a weight gain criterion of ≥7% of body weight [aripiprazole (8%) compared to placebo (3%)].

Table 2 provides the weight change results from a long-term (26-week), placebo-controlled study of aripiprazole, both mean change from baseline and proportions of patients meeting a weight gain criterion of ≥7% of body weight relative to baseline, categorized by BMI at baseline:

[See table 2 above]

Table 2: Weight Change Results Categorized by BMI at Baseline: Placebo-Controlled Study in Schizophrenia, Safety Sample

	BMI <23		BMI 23–27		BMI >27	
	Placebo	Aripiprazole	Placebo	Aripiprazole	Placebo	Aripiprazole
Mean change from baseline (kg)	-0.5	-0.5	-0.6	-1.3	-1.5	-2.1
% with ≥7% increase BW	3.7%	6.8%	4.2%	5.1%	4.1%	5.7%

Table 3 provides the weight change results from a long-term (52-week), study of aripiprazole, both mean change from baseline and proportions of patients meeting a weight gain criterion of ≥7% of body weight relative to baseline, categorized by BMI at baseline:

Table 3: Weight Change Results Categorized by BMI at Baseline

	BMI <23	BMI 23-27	BMI >27
Mean change from baseline (kg)	2.6	1.4	-1.2
% with ≥7% increase BW	30%	19%	8%

ECG Changes

Between group comparisons for pooled, placebo-controlled trials revealed no significant differences between aripiprazole and placebo in the proportion of patients experiencing potentially important changes in ECG parameters; in fact, within the dose range of 10 to 30 mg/day, aripiprazole tended to slightly shorten the QT_c interval. Aripiprazole was associated with a median increase in heart rate of 4 beats per minute compared to a 1 beat per minute increase among placebo patients.

Additional Findings Observed in Clinical Trials

Adverse Events in a Long-Term, Double-Blind, Placebo-Controlled Trial

The adverse events reported in a 26-week, double-blind trial comparing ABILIFY (aripiprazole) and placebo were generally consistent with those reported in the short-term, placebo-controlled trials, except for a higher incidence of tremor [9% (13/153) for ABILIFY vs. 1% (2/153) for placebo]. In this study, the majority of the cases of tremor were of mild intensity (9/13 mild and 4/13 moderate), occurred early in therapy (9/13 ≤49 days), and were of limited duration (9/13 ≤10 days). Tremor infrequently led to discontinuation (<1%) of ABILIFY. In addition, in a long-term (52-week), active-controlled study, the incidence of tremor for ABILIFY was 4% (34/859).

Other Adverse Events Observed During the Premarketing Evaluation of Aripiprazole

Following is a list of modified COSTART terms that reflect treatment-emergent adverse events as defined in the introduction to the **ADVERSE REACTIONS** section reported by patients treated with aripiprazole at multiple doses ≥2 mg/day during any phase of a trial within the database of 5592 patients. All reported events are included except those already listed in Table 1, or other parts of the **ADVERSE REACTIONS** section, those considered in the **WARNINGS** or **PRECAUTIONS**, those event terms which were so general as to be uninformative, events reported with an incidence of <0.05% and which did not have a substantial probability of being acutely life-threatening, events that are otherwise common as background events, and events considered unlikely to be drug related. It is important to emphasize that, although the events reported occurred during treatment with aripiprazole, they were not necessarily caused by it.

Events are further categorized by body system and listed in order of decreasing frequency according to the following definitions: frequent adverse events are those occurring in at least 1/100 patients (only those not already listed in the tabulated results from placebo-controlled trials appear in this listing); infrequent adverse events are those occurring in 1/100 to 1/1000 patients; rare events are those occurring in fewer than 1/1000 patients.

Body as a Whole: Frequent – flu syndrome, peripheral edema, chest pain, neck pain, neck rigidity; *Infrequent* – pelvic pain, suicide attempt, face edema, malaise, photosensitivity, arm rigidity, jaw pain, chills, bloating, jaw tightness, enlarged abdomen, chest tightness; *Rare* – throat pain, back tightness, head heaviness, moniliasis, throat tightness, leg rigidity, neck tightness, Mendelson's syndrome, heat stroke.

Cardiovascular System: Frequent – hypertension, tachycardia, hypotension, bradycardia; *Infrequent* – palpitation, hemorrhage, myocardial infarction, prolonged QT interval, cardiac arrest, atrial fibrillation, heart failure, AV block, myocardial ischemia, phlebitis, deep vein thrombosis, angina pectoris, extrasystoles; *Rare* – vasovagal reaction, cardiomegaly, atrial flutter, thrombophlebitis.

Digestive System: Frequent – anorexia, nausea and vomiting; *Infrequent* – increased appetite, gastroenteritis, dysphagia, flatulence, gastritis, tooth caries, gingivitis, hemorrhoids, gastroesophageal reflux, gastrointestinal hemorrhage, periodontal abscess, tongue edema, fecal incontinence, colitis, rectal hemorrhage, stomatitis, mouth ulcer, cholecystitis, fecal impaction, oral moniliasis, cholelithiasis, eructation, intestinal obstruction, peptic ulcer; *Rare* – esophagitis, gum hemorrhage, glossitis, hematemesis, melena, duodenal ulcer, cheilitis, hepatitis, hepatomegaly, pancreatitis, intestinal perforation.

Endocrine System: Infrequent – hypothyroidism; *Rare* – goiter, hyperthyroidism.

Hemic/Lymphatic System: Frequent – ecchymosis, anemia; *Infrequent* – hypochromic anemia, leukopenia, leukocytosis, lymphadenopathy, thrombocytopenia; *Rare* – eosinophilia, thrombocythemia, macrocytic anemia.

Metabolic and Nutritional Disorders: Frequent – weight loss, creatine phosphokinase increased; *Infrequent* – dehydration, edema, hypercholesteremia, hyperglycemia, hypokalemia, diabetes mellitus, SGPT increased, hyperlipemia, hypoglycemia, thirst, BUN increased, hyponatremia, SGOT increased, alkaline phosphatase increased, iron deficiency anemia, creatinine increased, bilirubinemia, lactic dehydrogenase increased, obesity; *Rare* – hyperkalemia, gout, hypernatremia, cyanosis, hyperuricemia, hypoglycemic reaction.

Musculoskeletal System: Frequent – muscle cramp; *Infrequent* – arthralgia, bone pain, myasthenia, arthritis, arthrosis, muscle weakness, spasm, bursitis; *Rare* – rhabdomyolysis, tendonitis, tenosynovitis, rheumatoid arthritis, myopathy.

Nervous System: Frequent – depression, nervousness, increased salivation, hostility, suicidal thought, manic reaction, abnormal gait, confusion, cogwheel rigidity; *Infrequent* – dystonia, twitch, impaired concentration, paresthesia, vasodilation, hypesthesia, extremity tremor, impotence, bradykinesia, decreased libido, panic attack, apathy, dyskinesia, hypersomnia, vertigo, dysarthria, tardive dyskinesia, ataxia, impaired memory, stupor, increased libido, amnesia, cerebrovascular accident, hyperactivity, depersonalization, hypokinesia, restless leg, myoclonus, dysphoria, neuropathy, increased reflexes, slowed thinking, hyperkinesia, hyperesthesia, hypotonia, oculogyric crisis; *Rare* – delirium, euphoria, buccoglossal syndrome, akinesia, blunted affect, decreased consciousness, incoordination, cerebral ischemia, decreased reflexes, obsessive thought, intracranial hemorrhage.

Respiratory System: Frequent – dyspnea, pneumonia; *Infrequent* – asthma, epistaxis, hiccup, laryngitis; *Rare* – hemoptysis, aspiration pneumonia, increased sputum, dry nasal passages, pulmonary edema, pulmonary embolism, hypoxia, respiratory failure, apnea.

Skin and Appendages: Frequent – dry skin, pruritis, sweating, skin ulcer; *Infrequent* – acne, vesiculobullous rash, eczema, alopecia, psoriasis, seborrhea; *Rare* – maculopapular rash, exfoliative dermatitis, urticaria.

Special Senses: Frequent – conjunctivitus, ear pain; *Infrequent* – dry eye, eye pain, tinnitus, otitis media, cataract, altered taste, blepharitis; *Rare* – increased lacrimation, frequent blinking, otitis externa, amblyopia, deafness, diplopia, eye hemorrhage, photophobia.

Urogenital System: Frequent – urinary incontinence; *Infrequent* – cystitis, urinary frequency, leukorrhea, urinary retention, hematuria, dysuria, amenorrhea, abnormal ejaculation, vaginal hemorrhage, vaginal moniliasis, kidney failure, uterus hemorrhage, menorrhagia, albuminuria, kidney calculus, nocturia, polyuria, urinary urgency; *Rare* – breast pain, cervicitis, female lactation, anorgasmy, urinary burning, glycosuria, gynecomastia, urolithiasis, priapism.

Other Events Observed During the Postmarketing Evaluation of Aripiprazole

Voluntary reports of adverse events in patients taking aripiprazole that have been received since market introduction

Continued on next page

Abilify—Cont.

and not listed above that may have no causal relationship with the drug include rare occurrences of allergic reaction (e.g., anaphylactic reaction, angioedema, laryngospasm, pruritis, or urticaria).

DRUG ABUSE AND DEPENDENCE

Controlled Substance

ABILIFY (aripiprazole) is not a controlled substance.

Abuse and Dependence

Aripiprazole has not been systematically studied in humans for its potential for abuse, tolerance, or physical dependence. In physical dependence studies in monkeys, withdrawal symptoms were observed upon abrupt cessation of dosing. While the clinical trials did not reveal any tendency for any drug-seeking behavior, these observations were not systematic and it is not possible to predict on the basis of this limited experience the extent to which a CNS-active drug will be misused, diverted, and/or abused once marketed. Consequently, patients should be evaluated carefully for a history of drug abuse, and such patients should be observed closely for signs of ABILIFY (aripiprazole) misuse or abuse (e.g., development of tolerance, increases in dose, drug-seeking behavior).

OVERDOSAGE

Human Experience

In clinical studies, accidental or intentional acute overdosage of aripiprazole was identified in patients with estimated doses up to1080 mg with no fatalities. The reported signs and symptoms observed with aripiprazole overdose include nausea, vomiting, asthenia, diarrhea, and somnolence. In the patients who were evaluated in hospital settings, there were no reported observations indicating clinically significant adverse changes in vital signs, laboratory assessments, or ECG.

During postmarketing experience, the reported signs and symptoms observed in adult patients who overdosed with aripiprazole alone at doses up to 450 mg included tachycardia. In addition, reports of accidental overdose with aripiprazole (up to 195 mg) in children have been received. The potentially medically serious signs and symptoms reported include extrapyramidal symptoms and transient loss of consciousness with recovery.

Management of Overdosage

No specific information is available on the treatment of overdose with aripiprazole. An electrocardiogram should be obtained in case of overdosage and, if QT_c interval prolongation is present, cardiac monitoring should be instituted. Otherwise, management of overdose should concentrate on supportive therapy, maintaining an adequate airway, oxygenation and ventilation, and management of symptoms. Close medical supervision and monitoring should continue until the patient recovers.

Charcoal: In the event of an overdose of ABILIFY (aripiprazole), an early charcoal administration may be useful in partially preventing the absorption of aripiprazole. Administration of 50 g of activated charcoal, one hour after a single 15-mg oral dose of aripiprazole, decreased the mean AUC and C_{max} of aripiprazole by 50%.

Hemodialysis: Although there is no information on the effect of hemodialysis in treating an overdose with aripiprazole, hemodialysis is unlikely to be useful in overdose management since aripiprazole is highly bound to plasma proteins.

DOSAGE AND ADMINISTRATION

Usual Dose

The recommended starting and target dose for ABILIFY is 10 or 15 mg/day administered on a once-a-day schedule without regard to meals. ABILIFY has been systematically evaluated and shown to be effective in a dose range of 10 to 30 mg/day; however, doses higher than 10 or 15 mg/day, the lowest doses in these trials, were not more effective than 10 or 15 mg/day. Dosage increases should not be made before 2 weeks, the time needed to achieve steady state.

Dosage in Special Populations

Dosage adjustments are not routinely indicated on the basis of age, gender, race, or renal or hepatic impairment status (see **CLINICAL PHARMACOLOGY: Special Populations**).

Dosage adjustment for patients taking aripiprazole concomitantly with potential CYP3A4 inhibitors: When concomitant administration of ketoconazole with aripiprazole occurs, aripiprazole dose should be reduced to one-half of the usual dose. When the CYP3A4 inhibitor is withdrawn from the combination therapy, aripiprazole dose should then be increased.

Dosage adjustment for patients taking aripiprazole concomitantly with potential CYP2D6 inhibitors: When concomitant administration of potential CYP2D6 inhibitors such as quinidine, fluoxetine, or paroxetine with aripiprazole occurs, aripiprazole dose should be reduced at least to one-half of its normal dose. When the CYP2D6 inhibitor is withdrawn from the combination therapy, aripiprazole dose should then be increased.

Dosage adjustment for patients taking potential CYP3A4 inducers: When a potential CYP3A4 inducer such as carbamazepine is added to aripiprazole therapy, the aripiprazole dose should be doubled (to 20 to 30 mg). Additional dose increases should be based on clinical evaluation. When carbamazepine is withdrawn from the combination therapy, the aripiprazole dose should be reduced to 10 to 15 mg.

Maintenance Therapy

While there is no body of evidence available to answer the question of how long a patient treated with aripiprazole should remain on it, systematic evaluation of patients with schizophrenia who had been symptomatically stable on other antipsychotic medications for periods of 3 months or longer, were discontinued from those medications, and were then administered ABILIFY 15 mg/day and observed for relapse during a period of up to 26 weeks, demonstrated a benefit of such maintenance treatment (see **CLINICAL PHARMACOLOGY: Clinical Studies**). Patients should be periodically reassessed to determine the need for maintenance treatment.

Switching from Other Antipsychotics

There are no systematically collected data to specifically address switching patients with schizophrenia from other antipsychotics to ABILIFY or concerning concomitant administration with other antipsychotics. While immediate discontinuation of the previous antipsychotic treatment may be acceptable for some patients with schizophrenia, more gradual discontinuation may be most appropriate for others. In all cases, the period of overlapping antipsychotic administration should be minimized.

ANIMAL TOXICOLOGY

Aripiprazole produced retinal degeneration in albino rats in a 26-week chronic toxicity study at a dose of 60 mg/kg and in a 2-year carcinogenicity study at doses of 40 and 60 mg/kg. The 40- and 60-mg/kg doses represent 13 and 19 times the maximum recommended human dose (MRHD) based on mg/m^2 and 7 to 14 times human exposure at MRHD based on AUC. Evaluation of the retinas of albino mice and monkeys did not reveal evidence of retinal degeneration. Additional studies to further evaluate the mechanism have not been performed. The relevance of this finding to human risk is unknown.

HOW SUPPLIED

ABILIFY® (aripiprazole) Tablets are available in the following strengths and packages.

The 5-mg ABILIFY tablets are blue, modified rectangular tablets, debossed on one side with "A-007" and "5".

Bottles of 30	NDC 59148-007-13
Blister of 100	NDC 59148-007-35

The 10-mg ABILIFY tablets are pink, modified rectangular tablets, debossed on one side with "A-008" and "10".

Bottles of 30	NDC 59148-008-13
Blister of 100	NDC 59148-008-35

The 15-mg ABILIFY tablets are yellow, round tablets, debossed on one side with "A-009" and "15".

Bottles of 30	NDC 59148-009-13
Blister of 100	NDC 59148-009-35

The 20-mg ABILIFY tablets are white, round tablets, debossed on one side with "A-010" and "20".

Bottles of 30	NDC 59148-010-13
Blister of 100	NDC 59148-010-35

The 30-mg ABILIFY tablets are pink, round tablets, debossed on one side with "A-011" and "30".

Bottles of 30	NDC 59148-011-13
Blister of 100	NDC 59148-011-35

Storage

Store at 25° C (77° F); excursions permitted to 15-30° C (59-86° F) [see USP Controlled Room Temperature].

Marketed by Otsuka America Pharmaceutical, Inc, Rockville, MD 20850 USA

and Bristol-Myers Squibb Co, Princeton, NJ 08543 USA

Manufactured and Distributed by Bristol-Myers Squibb Co, Princeton, NJ 08543 USA

U.S. Patent Nos. 4,734,416 and 5,006,528

Bristol-Myers Squibb Company
Princeton, NJ 08543 U.S.A.
Otsuka America
Pharmaceutical, Inc.

D6-B0001-05-04 Revised: May 2004
1152082A3 AP4114/06-04

Shown in Product Identification Guide, page 310

AVALIDE® ℞

[avă-līde]
(irbesartan-hydrochlorothiazide)
Tablets
Rx only

> **USE IN PREGNANCY**
> **When used in pregnancy during the second and third trimesters, drugs that act directly on the renin-angiotensin system can cause injury and even death to the developing fetus.** When pregnancy is detected, AVALIDE should be discontinued as soon as possible. (See **WARNINGS: Fetal/Neonatal Morbidity and Mortality.**)

DESCRIPTION

AVALIDE®* (irbesartan-hydrochlorothiazide) Tablets is a combination of an angiotensin II receptor antagonist (AT_1 subtype), irbesartan, and a thiazide diuretic, hydrochlorothiazide (HCTZ).

Irbesartan is a non-peptide compound, chemically described as a 2-butyl-3-[*p*-(*o*-1*H*-tetrazol-5-ylphenyl)benzyl]-1,3-diazaspiro [4.4]non-1-en-4-one. Its empirical formula is $C_{25}H_{28}N_6O$, and its structural formula is:

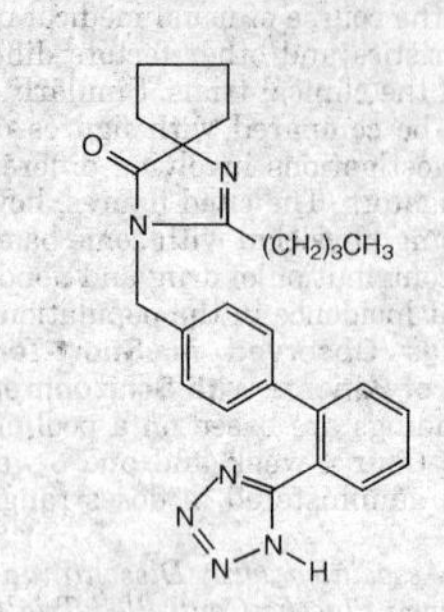

Irbesartan is a white to off-white crystalline powder with a molecular weight of 428.5. It is a nonpolar compound with a partition coefficient (octanol/water) of 10.1 at pH of 7.4. Irbesartan is slightly soluble in alcohol and methylene chloride and practically insoluble in water.

Hydrochlorothiazide is 6-chloro-3,4-dihydro-2*H*-1,2,4-benzothiadiazine-7-sulfonamide 1,1-dioxide. Its empirical formula is $C_7H_8ClN_3O_4S_2$ and its structural formula is:

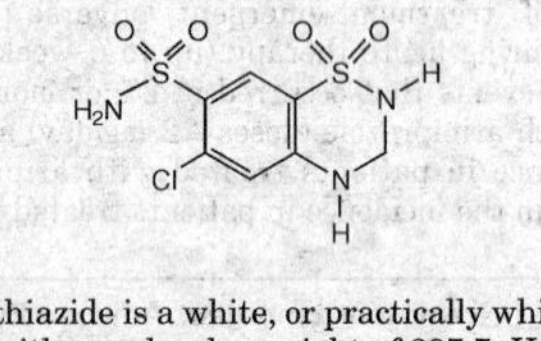

Hydrochlorothiazide is a white, or practically white, crystalline powder with a molecular weight of 297.7. Hydrochlorothiazide is slightly soluble in water and freely soluble in sodium hydroxide solution.

AVALIDE is available for oral administration in tablets containing 150 mg or 300 mg of irbesartan combined with 12.5 mg of hydrochlorothiazide. Inactive ingredients include: lactose monohydrate, microcrystalline cellulose, pregelatinized starch, croscarmellose sodium, ferric oxide red, ferric oxide yellow, silicon dioxide, and magnesium stearate.

CLINICAL PHARMACOLOGY

Mechanism Of Action

Irbesartan

Angiotensin II is a potent vasoconstrictor formed from angiotensin I in a reaction catalyzed by angiotensin-converting enzyme (ACE, kininase II). Angiotensin II is the principal pressor agent of the renin-angiotensin system (RAS) and also stimulates aldosterone synthesis and secretion by adrenal cortex, cardiac contraction, renal resorption of sodium, activity of the sympathetic nervous system, and smooth muscle cell growth. Irbesartan blocks the vasoconstrictor and aldosterone-secreting effects of angiotensin II by selectively binding to the AT_1 angiotensin II receptor. There is also an AT_2 receptor in many tissues, but it is not involved in cardiovascular homeostasis.

Irbesartan is a specific competitive antagonist of AT_1 receptors with a much greater affinity (more than 8500-fold) for the AT_1 receptor than for the AT_2 receptor, and no agonist activity.

Blockade of the AT_1 receptor removes the negative feedback of angiotensin II on renin secretion, but the resulting increased plasma renin activity and circulating angiotensin II do not overcome the effects of irbesartan on blood pressure.

Irbesartan does not inhibit ACE or renin or affect other hormone receptors or ion channels known to be involved in the cardiovascular regulation of blood pressure and sodium homeostasis. Because irbesartan does not inhibit ACE, it does not affect the response to bradykinin; whether this has clinical relevance is not known.

Hydrochlorothiazide

Hydrochlorothiazide is a thiazide diuretic. Thiazides affect the renal tubular mechanisms of electrolyte reabsorption, directly increasing excretion of sodium and chloride in approximately equivalent amounts. Indirectly, the diuretic action of hydrochlorothiazide reduces plasma volume, with consequent increases in plasma renin activity, increases in aldosterone secretion, increases in urinary potassium loss, and decreases in serum potassium. The renin-aldosterone link is mediated by angiotensin II, so coadministration of an angiotensin II receptor antagonist tends to reverse the potassium loss associated with these diuretics.

The mechanism of the antihypertensive effect of thiazides is not fully understood.

Pharmacokinetics

Irbesartan

Irbesartan is an orally active agent that does not require biotransformation into an active form. The oral absorption of irbesartan is rapid and complete with an average absolute bioavailability of 60–80%. Following oral administration of irbesartan, peak plasma concentrations of irbesartan are attained at 1.5–2 hours after dosing. Food does not affect the bioavailability of irbesartan.

Irbesartan exhibits linear pharmacokinetics over the therapeutic dose range.

The terminal elimination half-life of irbesartan averaged 11–15 hours. Steady-state concentrations are achieved within 3 days. Limited accumulation of irbesartan (<20%) is observed in plasma upon repeated once-daily dosing.

Hydrochlorothiazide
When plasma levels have been followed for at least 24 hours, the plasma half-life has been observed to vary between 5.6 and 14.8 hours.

Metabolism and Elimination
Irbesartan
Irbesartan is metabolized via glucuronide conjugation and oxidation. Following oral or intravenous administration of ^{14}C-labeled irbesartan, more than 80% of the circulating plasma radioactivity is attributable to unchanged irbesartan. The primary circulating metabolite is the inactive irbesartan glucuronide conjugate (approximately 6%). The remaining oxidative metabolites do not add appreciably to irbesartan's pharmacologic activity.
Irbesartan and its metabolites are excreted by both biliary and renal routes. Following either oral or intravenous administration of ^{14}C-labeled irbesartan, about 20% of radioactivity is recovered in the urine and the remainder in the feces, as irbesartan or irbesartan glucuronide.
In vitro studies of irbesartan oxidation by cytochrome P450 isoenzymes indicated irbesartan was oxidized primarily by 2C9; metabolism by 3A4 was negligible. Irbesartan was neither metabolized by, nor did it substantially induce or inhibit, isoenzymes commonly associated with drug metabolism (1A1, 1A2, 2A6, 2B6, 2D6, 2E1). There was no induction or inhibition of 3A4.
Hydrochlorothiazide
Hydrochlorothiazide is not metabolized but is eliminated rapidly by the kidney. At least 61 percent of the oral dose is eliminated unchanged within 24 hours.

Distribution
Irbesartan
Irbesartan is 90% bound to serum proteins (primarily albumin and α_1-acid glycoprotein) with negligible binding to cellular components of blood. The average volume of distribution is 53–93 liters. Total plasma and renal clearances are in the range of 157–176 and 3.0–3.5 mL/min, respectively. With repetitive dosing, irbesartan accumulates to no clinically relevant extent.
Studies in animals indicate that radiolabeled irbesartan weakly crosses the blood brain barrier and placenta. Irbesartan is excreted in the milk of lactating rats.
Hydrochlorothiazide
Hydrochlorothiazide crosses the placental but not the blood-brain barrier and is excreted in breast milk.

Special Populations
Pediatric: Irbesartan pharmacokinetics have not been investigated in patients <18 years of age.
Gender: No gender related differences in pharmacokinetics were observed in healthy elderly (age 65–80 years) or in healthy young (age 18–40 years) subjects. In studies of hypertensive patients, there was no gender difference in half-life or accumulation, but somewhat higher plasma concentrations of irbesartan were observed in females (11–44%). No gender-related dosage adjustment is necessary.
Geriatric: In elderly subjects (age 65–80 years), irbesartan elimination half-life was not significantly altered, but AUC and C_{max} values were about 20–50% greater than those of young subjects (age 18–40 years). No dosage adjustment is necessary in the elderly.
Race: In healthy black subjects, irbesartan AUC values were approximately 25% greater than whites; there were no differences in C_{max} values.
Renal Insufficiency: The pharmacokinetics of irbesartan were not altered in patients with renal impairment or in patients on hemodialysis. Irbesartan is not removed by hemodialysis. No dosage adjustment is necessary in patients with mild to severe renal impairment unless a patient with renal impairment is also volume depleted. (See **WARNINGS: Hypotension in Volume- or Salt-depleted Patients** and **DOSAGE AND ADMINISTRATION**.)
Hepatic Insufficiency: The pharmacokinetics of irbesartan following repeated oral administration were not significantly affected in patients with mild to moderate cirrhosis of the liver. No dosage adjustment is necessary in patients with hepatic insufficiency.
Drug Interactions: (See **PRECAUTIONS: Drug Interactions.**)

Pharmacodynamics
Irbesartan
In healthy subjects, single oral irbesartan doses of up to 300 mg produced dose-dependent inhibition of the pressor effect of angiotensin II infusions. Inhibition was complete (100%) 4 hours following oral doses of 150 mg or 300 mg and partial inhibition was sustained for 24 hours (60% and 40% at 300 mg and 150 mg, respectively).
In hypertensive patients, angiotensin II receptor inhibition following chronic administration of irbesartan causes a 1.5–2 fold rise in angiotensin II plasma concentration and a 2–3 fold increase in plasma renin levels. Aldosterone plasma concentrations generally decline following irbesartan administration, but serum potassium levels are not significantly affected at recommended doses.
In hypertensive patients, chronic oral doses of irbesartan (up to 300 mg) had no effect on glomerular filtration rate, renal plasma flow or filtration fraction. In multiple dose studies in hypertensive patients, there were no clinically important effects on fasting triglycerides, total cholesterol, HDL-cholesterol, or fasting glucose concentrations. There was no effect on serum uric acid during chronic oral administration and no uricosuric effect.

Hydrochlorothiazide
After oral administration of hydrochlorothiazide, diuresis begins within 2 hours, peaks in about 4 hours and lasts about 6 to 12 hours.

Clinical Studies
Irbesartan
The antihypertensive effects of irbesartan were examined in seven (7) major placebo-controlled 8–12 week trials in patients with baseline diastolic blood pressures of 95–110 mmHg. Doses of 1–900 mg were included in these trials in order to fully explore the dose-range of irbesartan. These studies allowed a comparison of once- or twice-daily regimens at 150 mg/day, comparisons of peak and trough effects, and comparisons of response by gender, age, and race. Two of the seven placebo-controlled trials identified above and two additional placebo-controlled studies examined the antihypertensive effects of irbesartan and hydrochlorothiazide in combination.
The seven (7) studies of irbesartan monotherapy included a total of 1915 patients randomized to irbesartan (1–900 mg) and 611 patients randomized to placebo. Once-daily doses of 150 to 300 mg provided statistically and clinically significant decreases in systolic and diastolic blood pressure with trough (24 hour post-dose) effects after 6–12 weeks of treatment compared to placebo, of about 8–10/5–6 and 8–12/5–8 mmHg, respectively. No further increase in effect was seen at dosages greater than 300 mg. The dose-response relationships for effects on systolic and diastolic pressure are shown in Figures 1 and 2.

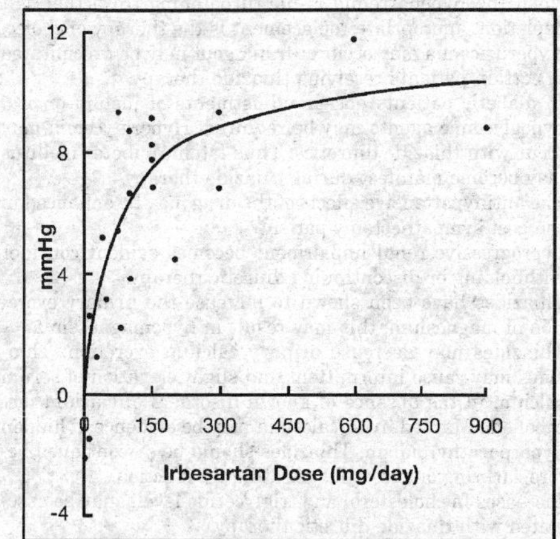

Figure 1. Placebo-subtracted reduction in trough SeSBP; integrated analysis

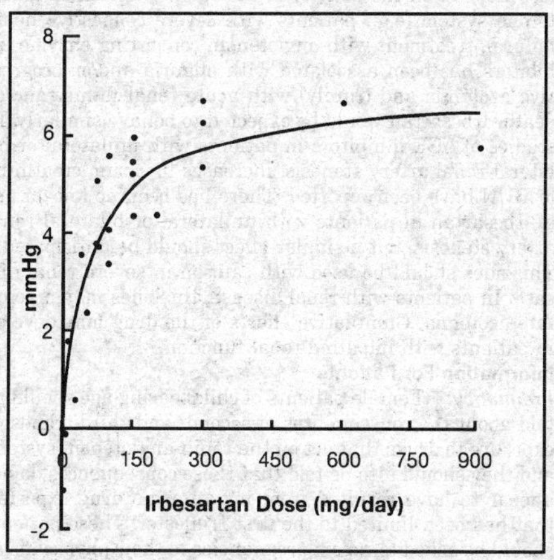

Figure 2. Placebo-subtracted reduction in trough SeDBP; integrated analysis

Once-daily administration of therapeutic doses of irbesartan gave peak effects at around 3–6 hours and, in one continuous ambulatory blood pressure monitoring study, and again around 14 hours. This was seen with both once-daily and twice-daily dosing. Trough-to-peak ratios for systolic and diastolic response were generally between 60–70%. In a continuous ambulatory blood pressure monitoring study, once-daily dosing with 150 mg gave trough and mean 24-hour responses similar to those observed in patients receiving twice-daily dosing at the same total daily dose.
Analysis of age, gender, and race subgroups of patients showed that men and women, and patients over and under 65 years of age, had generally similar responses. Irbesartan was effective in reducing blood pressure regardless of race, although the effect was somewhat less in blacks (usually a low-renin population). Black patients typically show an improved response with the addition of a low dose diuretic (e.g., 12.5 mg hydrochlorothiazide).
The effect of irbesartan is apparent after the first dose and is close to the full observed effect at 2 weeks. At the end of the 8-week exposure, about 2/3 of the antihypertensive effect was still present 1 week after the last dose. Rebound hypertension was not observed. There was essentially no change in average heart rate in irbesartan-treated patients in controlled trials.

Irbesartan-Hydrochlorothiazide
The antihypertensive effects of AVALIDE (irbesartan-hydrochlorothiazide) Tablets were examined in 4 placebo-controlled studies of 8–12 weeks in patients with mild-moderate hypertension. These trials included 1914 patients randomized to fixed doses of irbesartan (37.5 to 300 mg) and concomitant hydrochlorothiazide (6.25 to 25 mg). One factorial study compared all combinations of irbesartan (37.5, 100 and 300 mg or placebo) and hydrochlorothiazide (6.25, 12.5, and 25 mg or placebo). The irbesartan-hydrochlorothiazide combinations of 75/12.5 mg and 150/12.5 mg were compared to their individual components and placebo in a separate study. A third study investigated the ambulatory blood pressure responses to irbesartan-hydrochlorothiazide (75/12.5 mg and 150/12.5 mg) and placebo after 8 weeks of dosing. Another trial investigated the effects of the addition of irbesartan (75 mg) in patients not controlled on hydrochlorothiazide (25 mg) alone.
In controlled trials, the addition of irbesartan 150–300 mg to hydrochlorothiazide doses of 6.25, 12.5 or 25 mg produced further dose-related reductions in blood pressure of 8–10/3–6 mmHg, comparable to those achieved with the same monotherapy dose of irbesartan. The addition of hydrochlorothiazide to irbesartan produced further dose-related reductions in blood pressure at trough (24 hours post-dose) of 5–6/2–3 mmHg (12.5 mg) and 7–11/4–5 mmHg (25 mg), also comparable to effects achieved with hydrochlorothiazide alone. Once-daily dosing with 150 mg irbesartan and 12.5 mg hydrochlorothiazide, 300 mg irbesartan and 12.5 mg hydrochlorothiazide, or 300 mg irbesartan and 25 mg hydrochlorothiazide produced mean placebo-adjusted blood pressure reductions at trough (24 hours post-dosing) of about 13–15/7–9, 14/9–12, and 19–21/11–12 mmHg, respectively. Peak effects occurred at 3–6 hours, with the trough-to-peak ratios >65%.
In another study, irbesartan (75–150 mg) or placebo was added on a background of 25 mg hydrochlorothiazide in patients not adequately controlled (SeDBP 93–120 mmHg) on hydrochlorothiazide (25 mg) alone. The addition of irbesartan (75–150 mg) gave an additive effect (systolic/diastolic) at trough (24 hours post-dosing) of 11/7 mmHg.
There was no difference in response for men and women or in patients over or under 65 years of age. Black patients had a larger response to hydrochlorothiazide than non-black patients and a smaller response to irbesartan. The overall response to the combination was similar for black and non-black patients.

*Registered trademark of Sanofi-Synthelabo, Inc.

INDICATIONS AND USAGE

AVALIDE (irbesartan-hydrochlorothiazide) Tablets is indicated for the treatment of hypertension. This fixed dose combination is not indicated for initial therapy (see **DOSAGE AND ADMINISTRATION**).

CONTRAINDICATIONS

AVALIDE is contraindicated in patients who are hypersensitive to any component of this product.
Because of the hydrochlorothiazide component, this product is contraindicated in patients with anuria or hypersensitivity to other sulfonamide-derived drugs.

WARNINGS

Fetal/Neonatal Morbidity and Mortality
Drugs that act directly on the renin-angiotensin system can cause fetal and neonatal morbidity and death when administered to pregnant women. Several dozen cases have been reported in the world literature in patients who were taking angiotensin converting enzyme inhibitors. When pregnancy is detected, AVALIDE (irbesartan-hydrochlorothiazide) Tablets should be discontinued as soon as possible.
The use of drugs that act directly on the renin-angiotensin system during the second and third trimesters of pregnancy has been associated with fetal and neonatal injury, including hypotension, neonatal skull hypoplasia, anuria, reversible or irreversible renal failure, and death. Oligohydramnios has also been reported, presumably resulting from decreased fetal renal function; oligohydramnios in this setting has been associated with fetal limb contractures, craniofacial deformation, and hypoplastic lung development. Prematurity, intrauterine growth retardation, and patent ductus arteriosus have also been reported, although it is not clear whether these occurrences were due to exposure to the drug.
These adverse effects do not appear to have resulted from intrauterine drug exposure that has been limited to the first trimester.
Mothers whose embryos and fetuses are exposed to an angiotensin II receptor antagonist only during the first trimester should be so informed. Nonetheless, when patients become pregnant, physicians should have the patient discontinue the use of AVALIDE as soon as possible.
Rarely (probably less often than once in every thousand pregnancies), no alternative to a drug acting on the renin-angiotensin system will be found. In these rare cases, the mothers should be apprised of the potential hazards to their fetuses, and serial ultrasound examinations should be performed to assess the intraamniotic environment.

Continued on next page

Avalide—Cont.

If oligohydramnios is observed, AVALIDE (irbesartan-hydrochlorothiazide) Tablets should be discontinued unless it is considered life-saving for the mother. Contraction stress testing (CST), a non-stress test (NST), or biophysical profiling (BPP) may be appropriate depending upon the week of pregnancy. Patients and physicians should be aware, however, that oligohydramnios may not appear until after the fetus has sustained irreversible injury.

Infants with histories of *in utero* exposure to an angiotensin II receptor antagonist should be closely observed for hypotension, oliguria, and hyperkalemia. If oliguria occurs, attention should be directed toward support of blood pressure and renal perfusion. Exchange transfusion or dialysis may be required as a means of reversing hypotension and/or substituting for disordered renal function.

When pregnant rats were treated with irbesartan from day 0 to day 20 of gestation (oral doses of 50, 180, and 650 mg/kg/day), increased incidences of renal pelvic cavitation, hydroureter and/or absence of renal papilla were observed in fetuses at doses ≥50 mg/kg/day [approximately equivalent to the maximum recommended human dose (MRHD), 300 mg/day, on a body surface area basis]. Subcutaneous edema was observed in fetuses at doses ≥180 mg/kg/day (about 4 times the MRHD on a body surface area basis). As these anomalies were not observed in rats in which irbesartan exposure (oral doses of 50, 150 and 450 mg/kg/day) was limited to gestation days 6–15, they appear to reflect late gestational effects of the drug. In pregnant rabbits, oral doses of 30 mg irbesartan/kg/day were associated with maternal mortality and abortion. Surviving females receiving this dose (about 1.5 times the MRHD on a body surface area basis) had a slight increase in early resorptions and a corresponding decrease in live fetuses. Irbesartan was found to cross the placental barrier in rats and rabbits.

Radioactivity was present in the rat and rabbit fetus during late gestation and in rat milk following oral doses of radiolabeled irbesartan.

Studies in which hydrochlorothiazide was administered to pregnant mice and rats during their respective periods of major organogenesis at doses up to 3000 and 1000 mg/kg/day, respectively, provided no evidence of harm to the fetus.

A development toxicity study was performed in rats with doses of 50/50 and 150/150 mg/kg/day irbesartan-hydrochlorothiazide. Although the high dose combination appeared to be more toxic to the dams than either drug alone, there did not appear to be an increase in toxicity to the developing embryos.

Thiazides cross the placental barrier and appear in cord blood. There is a risk of fetal or neonatal jaundice, thrombocytopenia, and possibly other adverse reactions that have occurred in adults.

Hypotension in Volume- or Salt-depleted Patients

Excessive reduction of blood pressure was rarely seen in patients with uncomplicated hypertension treated with irbesartan alone (<0.1%) or with irbesartan-hydrochlorothiazide (approximately 1%). Initiation of antihypertensive therapy may cause symptomatic hypotension in patients with intravascular volume- or sodium-depletion, e.g., in patients treated vigorously with diuretics or in patients on dialysis. Such volume depletion should be corrected prior to administration of antihypertensive therapy.

If hypotension occurs, the patient should be placed in the supine position and, if necessary, given an intravenous infusion of normal saline. A transient hypotensive response is not a contraindication to further treatment, which usually can be continued without difficulty once the blood pressure has stabilized.

Hydrochlorothiazide

Hepatic Impairment

Thiazides should be used with caution in patients with impaired hepatic function or progressive liver disease, since minor alterations of fluid and electrolyte balance may precipitate hepatic coma.

Hypersensitivity Reaction

Hypersensitivity reactions to hydrochlorothiazide may occur in patients with or without a history of allergy or bronchial asthma, but are more likely in patients with such a history.

Systemic Lupus Erythematosus

Thiazide diuretics have been reported to cause exacerbation or activation of systemic lupus erythematosus.

Lithium Interaction

Lithium generally should not be given with thiazides (see **PRECAUTIONS: Drug Interactions; Hydrochlorothiazide**, *Lithium*).

PRECAUTIONS

General

Irbesartan-Hydrochlorothiazide

In double-blind clinical trials of various doses of irbesartan and hydrochlorothiazide, the incidence of hypertensive patients who developed hypokalemia (serum potassium <3.5 mEq/L) was 7.5% versus 6.0% for placebo; the incidence of hyperkalemia (serum potassium >5.7 mEq/L) was <1.0% versus 1.7% for placebo. No patient discontinued due to increases or decreases in serum potassium. Overall, the combination of irbesartan and hydrochlorothiazide had no effect on serum potassium. Higher doses of irbesartan ameliorated the hypokalemic response to hydrochlorothiazide.

Hydrochlorothiazide

Periodic determination of serum electrolytes to detect possible electrolyte imbalance should be performed at appropriate intervals. All patients receiving thiazide therapy should be observed for clinical signs of fluid or electrolyte imbalance: hyponatremia, hypochloremic alkalosis, and hypokalemia. Serum and urine electrolyte determinations are particularly important when the patient is vomiting excessively or receiving parenteral fluids. Warning signs or symptoms of fluid and electrolyte imbalance, irrespective of cause, include dryness of mouth, thirst, weakness, lethargy, drowsiness, restlessness, confusion, seizures, muscle pains or cramps, muscular fatigue, hypotension, oliguria, tachycardia, and gastrointestinal disturbances such as nausea and vomiting.

Hypokalemia may develop, especially with brisk diuresis, when severe cirrhosis is present, or after prolonged therapy. Interference with adequate oral electrolyte intake will also contribute to hypokalemia. Hypokalemia may cause cardiac arrhythmia and may also sensitize or exaggerate the response of the heart to the toxic effects of digitalis (e.g., increased ventricular irritability).

Although any chloride deficit is generally mild and usually does not require specific treatment except under extraordinary circumstances (as in liver disease or renal disease), chloride replacement may be required in the treatment of metabolic alkalosis.

Dilutional hyponatremia may occur in edematous patients in hot weather; appropriate therapy is water restriction, rather than administration of salt except in rare instances when the hyponatremia is life-threatening. In actual salt depletion, appropriate replacement is the therapy of choice.

Hyperuricemia may occur or frank gout may be precipitated in certain patients receiving thiazide therapy.

In diabetic patients dosage adjustments of insulin or oral hypoglycemic agents may be required. Hyperglycemia may occur with thiazide diuretics. Thus latent diabetes mellitus may become manifest during thiazide therapy.

The antihypertensive effects of the drug may be enhanced in the post sympathectomy patient.

If progressive renal impairment becomes evident consider withholding or discontinuing diuretic therapy.

Thiazides have been shown to increase the urinary excretion of magnesium; this may result in hypomagnesemia.

Thiazides may decrease urinary calcium excretion. Thiazides may cause intermittent and slight elevation of serum calcium in the absence of known disorders of calcium metabolism. Marked hypercalcemia may be evidence of hidden hyperparathyroidism. Thiazides should be discontinued before carrying out tests for parathyroid function.

Increases in cholesterol and triglyceride levels may be associated with thiazide diuretic therapy.

Impaired Renal Function

As a consequence of inhibiting the renin-angiotensin-aldosterone system, changes in renal function may be anticipated in susceptible individuals. In patients whose renal function may depend on the activity of the renin-angiotensin-aldosterone system (e.g., patients with severe congestive heart failure), treatment with angiotensin converting enzyme inhibitors has been associated with oliguria and/or progressive azotemia and (rarely) with acute renal failure and/or death. Irbesartan would be expected to behave similarly. In studies of ACE inhibitors in patients with unilateral or bilateral renal artery stenosis, increases in serum creatinine or BUN have been reported. There has been no known use of irbesartan in patients with unilateral or bilateral renal artery stenosis, but a similar effect should be anticipated.

Thiazides should be used with caution in severe renal disease. In patients with renal disease, thiazides may precipitate azotemia. Cumulative effects of the drug may develop in patients with impaired renal function.

Information For Patients

Pregnancy: Female patients of childbearing age should be told about the consequences of second- and third-trimester exposure to drugs that act on the renin-angiotensin system, and they should also be told that these consequences do not appear to have resulted from intrauterine drug exposure that has been limited to the first trimester. These patients should be asked to report pregnancies to their physicians as soon as possible.

Symptomatic Hypotension: A patient receiving AVALIDE (irbesartan-hydrochlorothiazide) Tablets should be cautioned that lightheadedness can occur, especially during the first days of therapy, and that it should be reported to the prescribing physician. The patients should be told that if syncope occurs, AVALIDE should be discontinued until the physician has been consulted.

All patients should be cautioned that inadequate fluid intake, excessive perspiration, diarrhea, or vomiting can lead to an excessive fall in blood pressure, with the same consequences of lightheadedness and possible syncope.

Drug Interactions

Irbesartan

No significant drug-drug pharmacokinetic (or pharmacodynamic) interactions have been found in interaction studies with hydrochlorothiazide, digoxin, warfarin, and nifedipine. *In vitro* studies show significant inhibition of the formation of oxidized irbesartan metabolites with the known cytochrome CYP 2C9 substrates/inhibitors sulphenazole, tolbutamide and nifedipine. However, in clinical studies the consequences of concomitant irbesartan on the pharmacodynamics of warfarin were negligible. Concomitant nifedipine or hydrochlorothiazide had no effect on irbesartan pharmacokinetics. Based on *in vitro* data, no interaction would be expected with drugs whose metabolism is dependent upon cytochrome P450 isozymes 1A1, 1A2, 2A6, 2B6, 2D6, 2E1, or 3A4.

In separate studies of patients receiving maintenance doses of warfarin, hydrochlorothiazide, or digoxin, irbesartan administration for 7 days had no effect on the pharmacodynamics of warfarin (prothrombin time) or the pharmacokinetics of digoxin. The pharmacokinetics of irbesartan were not affected by coadministration of nifedipine or hydrochlorothiazide.

Hydrochlorothiazide

When administered concurrently the following drugs may interact with thiazide diuretics:

Alcohol, Barbiturates, Or Narcotics—potentiation of orthostatic hypotension may occur.

Antidiabetic Drugs (oral agents and insulin)—dosage adjustment of the antidiabetic drug may be required.

Other Antihypertensive Drugs—additive effect or potentiation.

Cholestyramine And Colestipol Resins —absorption of hydrochlorothiazide is impaired in the presence of anionic exchange resins. Single doses of either cholestyramine or colestipol resins bind the hydrochlorothiazide and reduce its absorption from the gastrointestinal tract by up to 85 and 43 percent, respectively.

Corticosteroids, ACTH—intensified electrolyte depletion, particularly hypokalemia.

Pressor Amines (e.g., Norepinephrine)—possible decreased response to pressor amines but not sufficient to preclude their use.

Skeletal Muscle Relaxants, Nondepolarizing (e.g., Tubocurarine)—possible increased responsiveness to the muscle relaxant.

Lithium—should not generally be given with diuretics. Diuretic agents reduce the renal clearance of lithium and add a high risk of lithium toxicity. Refer to the package insert for lithium preparations before use of such preparations with AVALIDE.

Non-steroidal Anti-inflammatory Drugs—in some patients, the administration of a non-steroidal anti-inflammatory agent can reduce the diuretic, natriuretic, and antihypertensive effects of loop, potassium-sparing and thiazide diuretics. Therefore, when AVALIDE (irbesartan-hydrochlorothiazide) Tablets and non-steroidal anti-inflammatory agents are used concomitantly, the patient should be observed closely to determine if the desired effect of the diuretic is obtained.

Carcinogenesis, Mutagenesis, Impairment Of Fertility

Irbesartan-Hydrochlorothiazide

No carcinogenicity studies have been conducted with the irbesartan-hydrochlorothiazide combination.

Irbesartan-hydrochlorothiazide was not mutagenic in standard *in vitro* tests (Ames microbial test and Chinese hamster mammalian-cell forward gene-mutation assay). Irbesartan-hydrochlorothiazide was negative in tests for induction of chromosomal aberrations (*in vitro*—human lymphocyte assay; *in vivo*—mouse micronucleus study).

The combination of irbesartan and hydrochlorothiazide has not been evaluated in definitive studies of fertility.

Irbesartan

No evidence of carcinogenicity was observed when irbesartan was administered at doses of up to 500/1000 mg/kg/day (males/females, respectively) in rats and 1000 mg/kg/day in mice for up to two years. For male and female rats, 500 mg/kg/day provided an average systemic exposure to irbesartan ($AUC_{0-24hours}$, bound plus unbound) about 3 and 11 times, respectively, the average systemic exposure in humans receiving the maximum recommended dose (MRD) of 300 mg irbesartan/day, whereas 1000 mg/kg/day (administered to females only) provided an average systemic exposure about 21 times that reported for humans at the MRD. For male and female mice, 1000 mg/kg/day provided an exposure to irbesartan about 3 and 5 times, respectively, the human exposure at 300 mg/day.

Irbesartan was not mutagenic in a battery of *in vitro* tests (Ames microbial test, rat hepatocyte DNA repair test, V79 mammalian-cell forward gene-mutation assay). Irbesartan was negative in several tests for induction of chromosomal aberrations (*in vitro*-human lymphocyte assay; *in vivo*-mouse micronucleus study).

Irbesartan had no adverse effects on fertility or mating of male or female rats at oral doses ≤650 mg/kg/day, the highest dose providing a systemic exposure to irbesartan ($AUC_{0-24hours}$, bound plus unbound) about 5 times that found in humans receiving the maximum recommended dose of 300 mg/day.

Hydrochlorothiazide

Two-year feeding studies in mice and rats conducted under the auspices of the National Toxicology Program (NTP) uncovered no evidence of a carcinogenic potential of hydrochlorothiazide in female mice (at doses of up to approximately 600 mg/kg/day) or in male and female rats (at doses of up to approximately 100 mg/kg/day). The NTP, however, found equivocal evidence for hepatocarcinogenicity in male mice. Hydrochlorothiazide was not genotoxic *in vitro* in the Ames mutagenicity assay of *Salmonella typhimurium* strains TA 98, TA 100, TA 1535, TA 1537, and TA 1538 and in the Chinese Hamster Ovary (CHO) test for chromosomal aberrations, or *in vivo* in assays using mouse germinal cell chromosomes, Chinese hamster bone marrow chromosomes, and the *Drosophila* sex-linked recessive lethal trait gene. Positive test results were obtained only in the *in vitro* CHO Sister Chromatid Exchange (clastogenicity) and in the Mouse Lymphoma Cell (mutagenicity) assays, using concentrations of hydrochlorothiazide from 43 to 1300 μg/mL, and in the *Aspergillus nidulans* non-disjunction assay at an unspecified concentration.

Hydrochlorothiazide had no adverse effects on the fertility of mice and rats of either sex in studies wherein these species were exposed, via their diet, to doses of up to 100 and 4 mg/kg, respectively, prior to mating and throughout gestation.

Pregnancy

Pregnancy Categories C (first trimester) and D (second and third trimesters)

(See **WARNINGS: Fetal/Neonatal Morbidity and Mortality**.)

Nursing Mothers

It is not known whether irbesartan is excreted in human milk, but irbesartan or some metabolite of irbesartan is secreted at low concentration in the milk of lactating rats. Because of the potential for adverse effects on the nursing infant, a decision should be made whether to discontinue nursing or discontinue the drug, taking into account the importance of the drug to the mother.

Thiazides appear in human milk. Because of the potential for adverse effects on the nursing infant, a decision should be made whether to discontinue nursing or discontinue the drug, taking into account the importance of the drug to the mother.

Pediatric Use

Safety and effectiveness in pediatric patients have not been established.

Geriatric Use

Clinical studies of AVALIDE did not include sufficient numbers of subjects aged 65 and over to determine whether they respond differently from younger subjects. Other reported clinical experience has not identified differences in responses between the elderly and younger patients. In general, dose selection for an elderly patient should be cautious, usually starting at the low end of the dosing range, reflecting the greater frequency of deceased hepatic, renal or cardiac function, and of concomitant disease or other drug therapy.

ADVERSE REACTIONS

Irbesartan-hydrochlorothiazide

AVALIDE (irbesartan-hydrochlorothiazide) Tablets has been evaluated for safety in 898 patients treated for essential hypertension. In clinical trials with AVALIDE, no adverse experiences peculiar to this combination drug product have been observed. Adverse experiences have been limited to those that were reported previously with irbesartan and/or hydrochlorothiazide (HCTZ). The overall incidence of adverse experiences reported with the combination was comparable to placebo. In general, treatment with AVALIDE was well tolerated. For the most part, adverse experiences have been mild and transient in nature and have not required discontinuation of therapy. In controlled clinical trials, discontinuation of AVALIDE therapy due to clinical adverse experiences was required in only 3.6%. This incidence was significantly less (p=0.023) than the 6.8% of patients treated with placebo who discontinued therapy.

In these double-blind controlled clinical trials, the following adverse experiences reported with AVALIDE occurred in ≥1% of patients, and more often on the irbesartan-hydrochlorothiazide combination then on placebo, regardless of drug relationship:

[See table above]

	Irbesartan/HCTZ (n=898) (%)	Placebo (n=236) (%)	Irbesartan (n=400) (%)	HCTZ (n=380) (%)
Body as a Whole				
Chest Pain	2	1	2	2
Fatigue	7	3	4	3
Influenza	3	1	2	2
Cardiovascular				
Edema	3	3	2	2
Tachycardia	1	0	1	1
Gastrointestinal				
Abdominal Pain	2	1	2	2
Dyspepsia/heartburn	2	1	0	2
Nausea/vomiting	3	0	2	0
Immunology				
Allergy	1	0	1	1
Musculoskeletal				
Musculoskeletal Pain	7	5	6	10
Nervous System				
Dizziness	8	4	6	5
Dizziness Orthostatic	1	0	1	1
Renal / Genitourinary				
Abnormality Urination	2	1	1	2

The following adverse events were also reported at a rate of 1% or greater, but were as, or more, common in the placebo group: headache, sinus abnormality, cough, URI, pharyngitis, diarrhea, rhinitis, urinary tract infection, rash, anxiety/nervousness, and muscle cramp.

Adverse events occurred at about the same rates in men and women, older and younger patients, and black and non-black patients.

Irbesartan

Other adverse experiences that have been reported with irbesartan, without regard to causality are listed below:

Body as a Whole: fever, chills, orthostatic effects, facial edema, upper extremity edema

Cardiovascular: flushing, hypertension, cardiac murmur, myocardial infarction, angina pectoris, hypotension, syncope, arrhythmic/conduction disorder, cardio-respiratory arrest, heart failure, hypertensive crisis

Dermatologic: pruritus, dermatitis, ecchymosis, erythema face, urticaria

Endocrine / Metabolic / Electrolyte Imbalances: sexual dysfunction, libido change, gout

Gastrointestinal: diarrhea, constipation, gastroenteritis, flatulence, abdominal distention

Musculoskeletal / Connective Tissue: musculoskeletal trauma, extremity swelling, muscle cramp, arthritis, muscle ache, musculoskeletal chest pain, joint stiffness, bursitis, muscle weakness

Nervous System: anxiety/nervousness, sleep disturbance, numbness, somnolence, vertigo, emotional disturbance, depression, paresthesia, tremor, transient ischemic attack, cerebrovascular accident

Renal / Genitourinary: prostate disorder

Respiratory: cough, upper respiratory infection, epistaxis, tracheobronchitis, congestion, pulmonary congestion, dyspnea, wheezing

Special Senses: vision disturbance, hearing abnormality, ear infection, ear pain, conjunctivitis.

Hydrochlorothiazide

Other adverse experiences that have been reported with hydrochlorothiazide, without regard to causality, are listed below:

Body As A Whole: weakness

Digestive: pancreatitis, jaundice (intrahepatic cholestatic jaundice), sialadenitis, cramping, gastric irritation

Hematologic: aplastic anemia, agranulocytosis, leukopenia, hemolytic anemia, thrombocytopenia

Hypersensitivity: purpura, photosensitivity, urticaria, necrotizing angiitis (vasculitis and cutaneous vasculitis), fever, respiratory distress including pneumonitis and pulmonary edema, anaphylactic reactions

Metabolic: hyperglycemia, glycosuria, hyperuricemia

Musculoskeletal: muscle spasm

Nervous System / Psychiatric: restlessness

Renal: renal failure, renal dysfunction, interstitial nephritis

Skin: erythema multiforme including Stevens-Johnson syndrome, exfoliative dermatitis including toxic epidermal necrolysis

Special Senses: transient blurred vision, xanthopsia

Post-Marketing Experience

The following have been very rarely reported in post-marketing experience: urticaria; angioedema (involving swelling of the face, lips, pharynx, and/or tongue). Hyperkalemia has been rarely reported.

Very rare cases of jaundice have been reported with irbesartan.

Laboratory Test Findings

In controlled clinical trials, clinically important changes in standard laboratory parameters were rarely associated with administration of AVALIDE (irbesartan-hydrochlorothiazide) Tablets.

Creatinine, Blood Urea Nitrogen: Minor increases in blood urea nitrogen (BUN) or serum creatinine were observed in 2.3 and 1.1 percent, respectively, of patients with essential hypertension treated with AVALIDE alone. No patient discontinued taking AVALIDE due to increased BUN. One patient discontinued taking AVALIDE due to a minor increase in serum creatinine.

Hemoglobin: Mean decreases of approximately 0.2 g/dL occurred in patients treated with AVALIDE alone, but were rarely of clinical importance. This compared to a mean of 0.4 g/dL in patients receiving placebo. No patients were discontinued due to anemia.

Liver Function Tests: Occasional elevations of liver enzymes and/or serum bilirubin have occurred. In patients with essential hypertension treated with AVALIDE alone, one patient was discontinued due to elevated liver enzymes.

Serum Electrolytes: (See **PRECAUTIONS**.)

OVERDOSAGE

Irbesartan

No data are available in regard to overdosage in humans. However, daily doses of 900 mg for 8 weeks were well-tolerated. The most likely manifestations of overdosage are expected to be hypotension and tachycardia; bradycardia might also occur from overdose. Irbesartan is not removed by hemodialysis.

To obtain up-to-date information about the treatment of overdosage, a good resource is a certified Regional Poison-Control Center. Telephone numbers of certified poison-control centers are listed in the *Physicians' Desk Reference* (PDR). In managing overdose, consider the possibilities of multiple-drug interactions, drug-drug interactions, and unusual drug kinetics in the patient.

Laboratory determinations of serum levels of irbesartan are not widely available, and such determinations have, in any event, no established role in the management of irbesartan overdose.

Acute oral toxicity studies with irbesartan in mice and rats indicated acute lethal doses were in excess of 2000 mg/kg, about 25- and 50-fold the maximum recommended human dose (300 mg) on a mg/m^2 basis, respectively.

Hydrochlorothiazide

The most common signs and symptoms of overdose observed in humans are those caused by electrolyte depletion (hypokalemia, hypochloremia, hyponatremia) and dehydration resulting from excessive diuresis. If digitalis has also been administered, hypokalemia may accentuate cardiac arrhythmias. The degree to which hydrochlorothiazide is removed by hemodialysis has not been established. The oral LD_{50} of hydrochlorothiazide is greater than 10 g/kg in both mice and rats.

DOSAGE AND ADMINISTRATION

The recommended initial dose of irbesartan is 150 mg once daily. Patients requiring further reduction in blood pressure should be titrated to 300 mg once daily.

A lower initial dose of irbesartan (75 mg) is recommended in patients with depletion of intravascular volume (e.g., patients treated vigorously with diuretics or on hemodialysis) (see **WARNING: Hypotension in Volume- or Salt-depleted Patients**). Patients not adequately treated by the maximum dose of 300 mg once daily are unlikely to derive additional benefit from a higher dose or twice-daily dosing.

Hydrochlorothiazide is effective in doses of 12.5 to 50 mg once daily.

To minimize dose-independent side effects, it is usually appropriate to begin combination therapy only after a patient has failed to achieve the desired effect with monotherapy.

The side effects (see **WARNINGS**) of irbesartan are generally rare and apparently independent of dose; those of hydrochlorothiazide are a mixture of dose-dependent (primarily hypokalemia) and dose-independent phenomena (e.g., pancreatitis), the former much more common than the latter. Therapy with any combination of irbesartan and hydrochlorothiazide will be associated with both sets of dose-independent side effects.

AVALIDE (irbesartan and hydrochlorothiazide) may be administered with other antihypertensive agents.

AVALIDE may be administered with or without food.

Replacement Therapy

The combination may be substituted for the titrated components.

Dose Titration by Clinical Effect

A patient whose blood pressure is inadequately controlled by irbesartan or hydrochlorothiazide alone may be switched to once daily AVALIDE. Recommended doses of AVALIDE, in order of increasing mean effect, are (irbesartan-hydrochlorothiazide) 150/12.5 mg, 300/12.5 mg, and 300/25 mg (two 150/12.5 mg tablets). The largest incremental effect will likely be in the transition from monotherapy to 150/12.5 mg. (See **CLINICAL PHARMACOLOGY: Clinical Studies**). It takes 2–4 weeks for the blood pressure to stabilize after a change in the dose of AVALIDE.

The usual dose of AVALIDE is one tablet once daily. More than two tablets once daily is not recommended. The maximal antihypertensive effect is attained about 2–4 weeks after initiation of therapy.

Use in Patients with Renal Impairment

The usual regimens of therapy with AVALIDE may be followed as long as the patient's creatinine clearance is >30 mL/min. In patients with more severe renal impairment, loop diuretics are preferred to thiazides, so AVALIDE is not recommended.

Patients with Hepatic Impairment

No dosage adjustment is necessary in patients with hepatic impairment.

HOW SUPPLIED

AVALIDE® (irbesartan-hydrochlorothiazide) Tablets are peach, biconvex, and oval with a heart debossed on one side and 2775 or 2776 on the reverse, supplied as follows:

Irbesartan (mg)	HCTZ (mg)	NDC 0087-xxxx-xx for unit of use	
		Bottle of	
		30	90
150	12.5	2775-31	2775-32
300	12.5	2776-31	2776-32

Continued on next page

Avalide—Cont.

Storage

Store at 25°C (77°F); excursions permitted to 15°C–30°C (59°F–86°F) [see USP Controlled Room Temperature].

Distributed by:
Bristol-Myers Squibb Sanofi-Synthelabo Partnership
New York, NY 10016
1030329A5 Revised May 2004
B4-B0001-05-04

Bristol-Myers Squibb Company
Sanofi-Synthelabo

Shown in Product Identification Guide, page 310

AVAPRO® ℞

[*ă-vă-prō*]
(irbesartan) Tablets
Rx only

> **USE IN PREGNANCY**
> **When used in pregnancy during the second and third trimesters, drugs that act directly on the renin-angiotensin system can cause injury and even death to the developing fetus.** When pregnancy is detected, AVAPRO should be discontinued as soon as possible. See **WARNINGS: Fetal/Neonatal Morbidity and Mortality.**

DESCRIPTION

AVAPRO* (irbesartan) is an angiotensin II receptor (AT_1 subtype) antagonist.

Irbesartan is a non-peptide compound, chemically described as a 2-butyl-3-[*p*-(*o*-1*H*-tetrazol-5-ylphenyl)benzyl]-1,3-diazaspiro[4,4]non-1-en-4-one.

Its empirical formula is $C_{25}H_{28}N_6O$, and the structural formula:

Irbesartan is a white to off-white crystalline powder with a molecular weight of 428.5. It is a nonpolar compound with a partition coefficient (octanol/water) of 10.1 at pH of 7.4. Irbesartan is slightly soluble in alcohol and methylene chloride and practically insoluble in water.

AVAPRO is available for oral administration in unscored tablets containing 75 mg, 150 mg, or 300 mg of irbesartan. Inactive ingredients include: lactose, microcrystalline cellulose, pregelatinized starch, croscarmellose sodium, poloxamer 188, silicon dioxide and magnesium stearate.

*Registered trademark of Sanofi-Synthelabo, Inc.

CLINICAL PHARMACOLOGY

Mechanism of Action

Angiotensin II is a potent vasoconstrictor formed from angiotensin I in a reaction catalyzed by angiotensin-converting enzyme (ACE, kininase II). Angiotensin II is the principal pressor agent of the renin-angiotensin system (RAS) and also stimulates aldosterone synthesis and secretion by adrenal cortex, cardiac contraction, renal resorption of sodium, activity of the sympathetic nervous system, and smooth muscle cell growth. Irbesartan blocks the vasoconstrictor and aldosterone-secreting effects of angiotensin II by selectively binding to the AT_1 angiotensin II receptor. There is also an AT_2 receptor in many tissues, but it is not involved in cardiovascular homeostasis.

Irbesartan is a specific competitive antagonist of AT_1 receptors with a much greater affinity (more than 8500-fold) for the AT_1 receptor than for the AT_2 receptor and no agonist activity.

Blockade of the AT_1 receptor removes the negative feedback of angiotensin II on renin secretion, but the resulting increased plasma renin activity and circulating angiotensin II do not overcome the effects of irbesartan on blood pressure.

Irbesartan does not inhibit ACE or renin or affect other hormone receptors or ion channels known to be involved in the cardiovascular regulation of blood pressure and sodium homeostasis. Because irbesartan does not inhibit ACE, it does not affect the response to bradykinin; whether this has clinical relevance is not known.

Pharmacokinetics

Irbesartan is an orally active agent that does not require biotransformation into an active form. The oral absorption of irbesartan is rapid and complete with an average absolute bioavailability of 60–80%. Following oral administration of AVAPRO, peak plasma concentrations of irbesartan are attained at 1.5–2 hours after dosing. Food does not affect the bioavailability of AVAPRO.

Irbesartan exhibits linear pharmacokinetics over the therapeutic dose range.

The terminal elimination half-life of irbesartan averaged 11–15 hours. Steady-state concentrations are achieved within 3 days. Limited accumulation of irbesartan (<20%) is observed in plasma upon repeated once-daily dosing.

Metabolism and Elimination

Irbesartan is metabolized via glucuronide conjugation and oxidation. Following oral or intravenous administration of ^{14}C-labeled irbesartan, more than 80% of the circulating plasma radioactivity is attributable to unchanged irbesartan. The primary circulating metabolite is the inactive irbesartan glucuronide conjugate (approximately 6%). The remaining oxidative metabolites do not add appreciably to irbesartan's pharmacologic activity.

Irbesartan and its metabolites are excreted by both biliary and renal routes. Following either oral or intravenous administration of ^{14}C-labeled irbesartan, about 20% of radioactivity is recovered in the urine and the remainder in the feces, as irbesartan or irbesartan glucuronide.

In vitro studies of irbesartan oxidation by cytochrome P450 isoenzymes indicated irbesartan was oxidized primarily by 2C9; metabolism by 3A4 was negligible. Irbesartan was neither metabolized by, nor did it substantially induce or inhibit, isoenzymes commonly associated with drug metabolism (1A1, 1A2, 2A6, 2B6, 2D6, 2E1). There was no induction or inhibition of 3A4.

Distribution

Irbesartan is 90% bound to serum proteins (primarily albumin and α_1-acid glycoprotein) with negligible binding to cellular components of blood. The average volume of distribution is 53–93 liters. Total plasma and renal clearances are in the range of 157–176 and 3.0–3.5 mL/min, respectively. With repetitive dosing, irbesartan accumulates to no clinically relevant extent.

Studies in animals indicate that radiolabeled irbesartan weakly crosses the blood brain barrier and placenta. Irbesartan is excreted in the milk of lactating rats.

Special Populations

Pediatric: The pharmacokinetics of irbesartan were studied in hypertensive children (age 6-12, n=9) and adolescents (age 13-16, n=12) following single and multiple daily doses of 2 mg/kg (maximum dose of 150 mg per day) for 4 weeks. Accumulation with repeated doses was limited (18%) in both age groups. Clearance rates, AUC values, and C_{max} values were comparable to adults receiving 150 mg daily. Irbesartan pharmacokinetics have not been investigated in patients <6 years of age.

Gender: No gender related differences in pharmacokinetics were observed in healthy elderly (age 65–80 years) or in healthy young (age 18–40 years) subjects. In studies of hypertensive patients, there was no gender difference in half-life or accumulation, but somewhat higher plasma concentrations of irbesartan were observed in females (11–44%). No gender-related dosage adjustment is necessary.

Geriatric: In elderly subjects (age 65–80 years), irbesartan elimination half-life was not significantly altered, but AUC and C_{max} values were about 20–50% greater than those of young subjects (age 18–40 years). No dosage adjustment is necessary in the elderly.

Race: In healthy black subjects, irbesartan AUC values were approximately 25% greater than whites; there were no differences in C_{max} values.

Renal Insufficiency: The pharmacokinetics of irbesartan were not altered in patients with renal impairment or in patients on hemodialysis. Irbesartan is not removed by hemodialysis. No dosage adjustment is necessary in patients with mild to severe renal impairment unless a patient with renal impairment is also volume depleted. (See **WARNINGS: Hypotension in Volume- or Salt-depleted Patients** and **DOSAGE AND ADMINISTRATION**.)

Hepatic Insufficiency: The pharmacokinetics of irbesartan following repeated oral administration were not significantly affected in patients with mild to moderate cirrhosis of the liver. No dosage adjustment is necessary in patients with hepatic insufficiency.

Drug Interactions: (See **PRECAUTIONS: Drug Interactions.**)

Pharmacodynamics

In healthy subjects, single oral irbesartan doses of up to 300 mg produced dose-dependent inhibition of the pressor effect of angiotensin II infusions. Inhibition was complete (100%) 4 hours following oral doses of 150 mg or 300 mg and partial inhibition was sustained for 24 hours (60% and 40% at 300 mg and 150 mg, respectively).

In hypertensive patients, angiotensin II receptor inhibition following chronic administration of irbesartan causes a 1.5–2 fold rise in angiotensin II plasma concentration and a 2–3 fold increase in plasma renin levels. Aldosterone plasma concentrations generally decline following irbesartan administration, but serum potassium levels are not significantly affected at recommended doses.

In hypertensive patients, chronic oral doses of irbesartan (up to 300 mg) had no effect on glomerular filtration rate, renal plasma flow or filtration fraction. In multiple dose studies in hypertensive patients, there were no clinically important effects on fasting triglycerides, total cholesterol, HDL-cholesterol, or fasting glucose concentrations. There was no effect on serum uric acid during chronic oral administration, and no uricosuric effect.

Clinical Studies

Hypertension

The antihypertensive effects of AVAPRO (irbesartan) were examined in seven (7) major placebo-controlled 8–12 week trials in patients with baseline diastolic blood pressures of 95–110 mmHg. Doses of 1–900 mg were included in these trials in order to fully explore the dose-range of irbesartan. These studies allowed comparison of once- or twice-daily regimens at 150 mg/day, comparisons of peak and trough effects, and comparisons of response by gender, age, and race. Two of the seven placebo-controlled trials identified above examined the antihypertensive effects of irbesartan and hydrochlorothiazide in combination.

The seven (7) studies of irbesartan monotherapy included a total of 1915 patients randomized to irbesartan (1–900 mg) and 611 patients randomized to placebo. Once-daily doses of 150 and 300 mg provided statistically and clinically significant decreases in systolic and diastolic blood pressure with trough (24 hours post-dose) effects after 6–12 weeks of treatment compared to placebo, of about 8–10/5–6 and 8–12/5–8 mmHg, respectively. No further increase in effect was seen at dosages greater than 300 mg. The dose-response relationships for effects on systolic and diastolic pressure are shown in Figures 1 and 2.

Figure 1. Placebo-subtracted reduction in trough SeSBP; integrated analysis

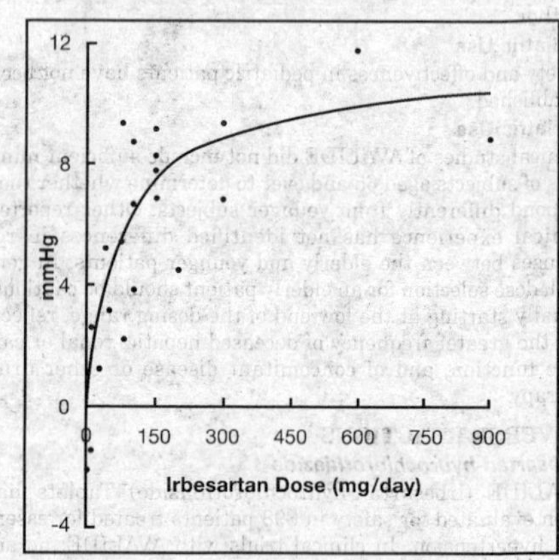

Figure 2. Placebo-subtracted reduction in trough SeDBP; integrated analysis

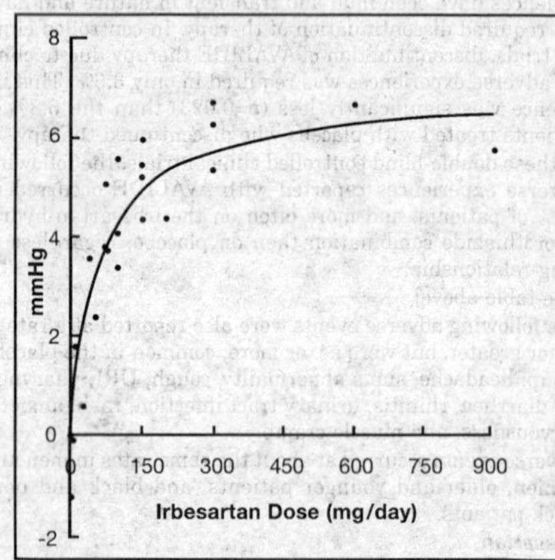

Once-daily administration of therapeutic doses of irbesartan gave peak effects at around 3–6 hours and, in one ambulatory blood pressure monitoring study, again around 14 hours. This was seen with both once-daily and twice-daily dosing. Trough-to-peak ratios for systolic and diastolic response were generally between 60–70%. In a continuous ambulatory blood pressure monitoring study, once-daily dosing with 150 mg gave trough and mean 24-hour responses similar to those observed in patients receiving twice-daily dosing at the same total daily dose.

In controlled trials, the addition of irbesartan to hydrochlorothiazide doses of 6.25, 12.5, or 25 mg produced further dose-related reductions in blood pressure similar to those achieved with the same monotherapy dose of irbesartan. HCTZ also had an approximately additive effect.

Analysis of age, gender, and race subgroups of patients showed that men and women, and patients over and under 65 years of age, had generally similar responses. Irbesartan was effective in reducing blood pressure regardless of race, although the effect was somewhat less in blacks (usually a low-renin population).

The effect of irbesartan is apparent after the first dose and it is close to its full observed effect at 2 weeks. At the end of an 8-week exposure, about 2/3 of the antihypertensive effect was still present one week after the last dose. Rebound hypertension was not observed. There was essentially no change in average heart rate in irbesartan-treated patients in controlled trials.

Nephropathy in Type 2 Diabetic Patients:
The Irbesartan Diabetic Nephropathy Trial (IDNT) was a randomized, placebo- and active-controlled, double-blind multicenter study, conducted worldwide in 1715 patients with type 2 diabetes, hypertension (SeSBP >135 mmHg or SeDBP >85 mmHg), and nephropathy (serum creatinine 1.0 to 3.0 mg/dL in females or 1.2 to 3.0 mg/dL in males and proteinuria ≥900 mg/day). Patients were randomized to receive AVAPRO (irbesartan) 75 mg, amlodipine 2.5 mg, or matching placebo once-daily. Patients were titrated to a maintenance dose of AVAPRO 300 mg, or amlodipine 10 mg, as tolerated. Additional antihypertensive agents (excluding ACE inhibitors, angiotensin II receptor antagonists and calcium channel blockers) were added as needed to achieve blood pressure goal (≤135/85 or 10 mmHg reduction in systolic blood pressure if higher than 160 mmHg) for patients in all groups.
The study population was 66.5% male, 72.9% below 65 years of age and 72% White, (Asian/Pacific Islander 5.0%, Black 13.3%, Hispanic 4.8%). The mean baseline seated systolic and diastolic blood pressure were 159 mmHg and 87 mmHg, respectively. The patients entered the trial with a mean serum creatinine of 1.7 mg/dL and mean proteinuria of 4144 mg/day.
The mean blood pressure achieved was 142/77 mmHg for AVAPRO (irbesartan), 142/76 mmHg for amlodipine, and 145/79 mmHg for placebo. Overall, 83.0% of patients received the target dose of irbesartan more than 50% of the time. Patients were followed for a mean duration of 2.6 years.
The primary composite endpoint was the time to occurrence of any one of the following events: doubling of baseline serum creatinine, end-stage renal disease (ESRD; defined by serum creatinine ≥6 mg/dL, dialysis, or renal transplantation) or death. Treatment with AVAPRO resulted in a 20% risk reduction versus placebo (p=0.0234) (see Figure 3 and Table 1). Treatment with AVAPRO also reduced the occurrence of sustained doubling of serum creatinine as a separate endpoint (33%), but had no significant effect on ESRD alone and no effect on overall mortality (See Table 1).

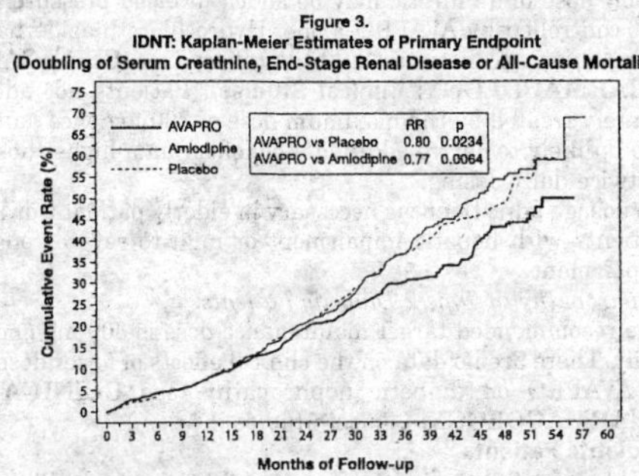

Figure 3.
IDNT: Kaplan-Meier Estimates of Primary Endpoint (Doubling of Serum Creatinine, End-Stage Renal Disease or All-Cause Mortality)

The percentages of patients experiencing an event during the course of the study can be seen in **Table 1** below.
[See table 1 above]
The secondary endpoint of the study was a composite of cardiovascular mortality and morbidity (myocardial infarction, hospitalization for heart failure, stroke with permanent neurological deficit, amputation). There were no statistically significant differences among treatment groups in these endpoints. Compared with placebo, AVAPRO (irbesartan) significantly reduced proteinuria by about 27%, an effect that was evident within 3 months of starting therapy. AVAPRO significantly reduced the rate of loss of renal function (glomerular filtration rate), as measured by the reciprocal of the serum creatinine concentration, by 18.2%.
Table 2 presents results for demographic subgroups. Subgroup analyses are difficult to interpret and it is not known whether these observations represent true differences or chance effects. For the primary endpoint, AVAPRO's favorable effects were seen in patients also taking other antihypertensive medications (angiotensin II receptor antagonists, angiotensin converting enzyme inhibitors and calcium channel blockers were not allowed), oral hypoglycemic agents, and lipid-lowering agents.
[See table 2 above]

Table 1.
IDNT: Components of Primary Composite Endpoint

	AVAPRO	Comparison with placebo			Comparison with amlodipine		
	N=579 (%)	Placebo N=569 (%)	Hazard Ratio	95% CI	Amlodipine N=567 (%)	Hazard Ratio	95% CI
Primary Composite Endpoint	32.6	39.0	0.80	0.66-0.97 (p=0.0234)	41.1	0.77	0.63-0.93
Breakdown of first occurring event contributing to primary endpoint							
2× creatinine	14.2	19.5	—	—	22.8	—	—
ESRD	7.4	8.3	—	—	8.8	—	—
Death	11.1	11.2	—	—	9.5	—	—
Incidence of total events over entire period of follow-up							
2× creatinine	16.9	23.7	0.67	0.52–0.87	25.4	0.63	0.49–0.81
ESRD	14.2	17.8	0.77	0.57–1.03	18.3	0.77	0.57–1.03
Death	15.0	16.3	0.92	0.69–1.23	14.6	1.04	0.77–1.40

Table 2.
IDNT: Primary Efficacy Outcome Within Subgroups

Baseline Factors	AVAPRO N=579 (%)	Comparison with placebo		
		Placebo N=569 (%)	Hazard Ratio	95% CI
Gender				
Male	27.5	36.7	0.68	0.53–0.88
Female	42.3	44.6	0.98	0.72–1.34
Race				
White	29.5	37.3	0.75	0.60–0.95
Non-White	42.6	43.5	0.95	0.67–1.34
Age (years)				
<65	31.8	39.9	0.77	0.62–0.97
≥65	35.1	36.8	0.88	0.61–1.29

INDICATIONS AND USAGE

Hypertension
AVAPRO (irbesartan) is indicated for the treatment of hypertension. It may be used alone or in combination with other antihypertensive agents.

Nephropathy in Type 2 Diabetic Patients
AVAPRO is indicated for the treatment of diabetic nephropathy with an elevated serum creatinine and proteinuria (>300 mg/day) in patients with type 2 diabetes and hypertension. In this population, AVAPRO reduces the rate of progression of nephropathy as measured by the occurrence of doubling of serum creatinine or end-stage renal disease (need for dialysis or renal transplantation) (see **CLINICAL PHARMACOLOGY: Clinical Studies**).

CONTRAINDICATIONS

AVAPRO is contraindicated in patients who are hypersensitive to any component of this product.

WARNINGS

Fetal/Neonatal Morbidity and Mortality
Drugs that act directly on the renin-angiotensin system can cause fetal and neonatal morbidity and death when administered to pregnant women. Several dozen cases have been reported in the world literature in patients who were taking angiotensin-converting-enzyme inhibitors. When pregnancy is detected, AVAPRO should be discontinued as soon as possible.
The use of drugs that act directly on the renin-angiotensin system during the second and third trimesters of pregnancy has been associated with fetal and neonatal injury, including hypotension, neonatal skull hypoplasia, anuria, reversible or irreversible renal failure, and death. Oligohydramnios has also been reported, presumably resulting from decreased fetal renal function; oligohydramnios in this setting has been associated with fetal limb contractures, craniofacial deformation, and hypoplastic lung development. Prematurity, intrauterine growth retardation, and patent ductus arteriosus have also been reported, although it is not clear whether these occurrences were due to exposure to the drug.
These adverse effects do not appear to have resulted from intrauterine drug exposure that has been limited to the first trimester.
Mothers whose embryos and fetuses are exposed to an angiotensin II receptor antagonist only during the first trimester should be so informed. Nonetheless, when patients become pregnant, physicians should have the patient discontinue the use of AVAPRO as soon as possible.
Rarely (probably less often than once in every thousand pregnancies), no alternative to a drug acting on the renin-angiotensin system will be found. In these rare cases, the mothers should be apprised of the potential hazards to their fetuses, and serial ultrasound examinations should be performed to assess the intraamniotic environment.
If oligohydramnios is observed, AVAPRO (irbesartan) should be discontinued unless it is considered life-saving for the mother. Contraction stress testing (CST), a non-stress test (NST), or biophysical profiling (BPP) may be appropriate depending upon the week of pregnancy. Patients and physicians should be aware, however, that oligohydramnios may not appear until after the fetus has sustained irreversible injury.
Infants with histories of *in utero* exposure to an angiotensin II receptor antagonist should be closely observed for hypotension, oliguria, and hyperkalemia. If oliguria occurs, attention should be directed toward support of blood pressure and renal perfusion. Exchange transfusion or dialysis may be required as means of reversing hypotension and/or substituting for disordered renal function.
When pregnant rats were treated with irbesartan from day 0 to day 20 of gestation (oral doses of 50, 180, and 650 mg/kg/day), increased incidences of renal pelvic cavitation, hydroureter and/or absence of renal papilla were observed in fetuses at doses ≥50 mg/kg/day [approximately equivalent to the maximum recommended human dose (MRHD), 300 mg/day, on a body surface area basis]. Subcutaneous edema was observed in fetuses at doses ≥180 mg/kg/day (about 4 times the MRHD on a body surface area basis). As these anomalies were not observed in rats in which irbesartan exposure (oral doses of 50, 150 and 450 mg/kg/day) was limited to gestation days 6–15, they appear to reflect late gestational effects of the drug. In pregnant rabbits, oral doses of 30 mg irbesartan/kg/day were associated with maternal mortality and abortion. Surviving females receiving this dose (about 1.5 times the MRHD on a body surface area basis) had a slight increase in early resorptions and a corresponding decrease in live fetuses. Irbesartan was found to cross the placental barrier in rats and rabbits.
Radioactivity was present in the rat and rabbit fetus during late gestation and in rat milk following oral doses of radiolabeled irbesartan.

Hypotension in Volume- or Salt-depleted Patients
Excessive reduction of blood pressure was rarely seen (<0.1%) in patients with uncomplicated hypertension. Initiation of antihypertensive therapy may cause symptomatic hypotension in patients with intravascular volume- or sodium-depletion, e.g., in patients treated vigorously with diuretics or in patients on dialysis. Such volume depletion should be corrected prior to administration of AVAPRO (irbesartan), or a low starting dose should be used (see **DOSAGE AND ADMINISTRATION**).
If hypotension occurs, the patient should be placed in the supine position and, if necessary, given an intravenous infusion of normal saline. A transient hypotensive response is not a contraindication to further treatment, which usually can be continued without difficulty once the blood pressure has stabilized.

PRECAUTIONS

Impaired Renal Function
As a consequence of inhibiting the renin-angiotensin-aldosterone system, changes in renal function may be anticipated in susceptible individuals. In patients whose renal function may depend on the activity of the renin-angiotensin-aldosterone system (e.g., patients with severe congestive heart failure), treatment with angiotensin-converting-enzyme inhibitors has been associated with oli-

Continued on next page

Avapro—Cont.

guria and/or progressive azotemia and (rarely) with acute renal failure and/or death. AVAPRO would be expected to behave similarly.
In studies of ACE inhibitors in patients with unilateral or bilateral renal artery stenosis, increases in serum creatinine or BUN have been reported. There has been no known use of AVAPRO in patients with unilateral or bilateral renal artery stenosis, but a similar effect should be anticipated.

Information for Patients

Pregnancy: Female patients of childbearing age should be told about the consequences of second- and third-trimester exposure to drugs that act on the renin-angiotensin system, and they should also be told that these consequences do not appear to have resulted from intrauterine drug exposure that has been limited to the first trimester. These patients should be asked to report pregnancies to their physicians as soon as possible.

Drug Interactions

No significant drug-drug pharmacokinetic (or pharmacodynamic) interactions have been found in interaction studies with hydrochlorothiazide, digoxin, warfarin, and nifedipine.
In vitro studies show significant inhibition of the formation of oxidized irbesartan metabolites with the known cytochrome CYP 2C9 substrates/inhibitors sulphenazole, tolbutamide and nifedipine. However, in clinical studies the consequences of concomitant irbesartan on the pharmacodynamics of warfarin were negligible. Based on *in vitro* data, no interaction would be expected with drugs whose metabolism is dependent upon cytochrome P450 isozymes 1A1, 1A2, 2A6, 2B6, 2D6, 2E1, or 3A4.
In separate studies of patients receiving maintenance doses of warfarin, hydrochlorothiazide, or digoxin, irbesartan administration for 7 days had no effect on the pharmacodynamics of warfarin (prothrombin time) or pharmacokinetics of digoxin. The pharmacokinetics of irbesartan were not affected by coadministration of nifedipine or hydrochlorothiazide.

Carcinogenesis, Mutagenesis, Impairment of Fertility

No evidence of carcinogenicity was observed when irbesartan was administered at doses of up to 500/1000 mg/kg/day (males/females, respectively) in rats and 1000 mg/kg/day in mice for up to two years. For male and female rats, 500 mg/kg/day provided an average systemic exposure to irbesartan (AUC_{0-24h}, bound plus unbound) about 3 and 11 times, respectively, the average systemic exposure in humans receiving the maximum recommended dose (MRD) of 300 mg irbesartan/day, whereas 1000 mg/kg/day (administered to females only) provided an average systemic exposure about 21 times that reported for humans at the MRD. For male and female mice, 1000 mg/kg/day provided an exposure to irbesartan about 3 and 5 times, respectively, the human exposure at 300 mg/day.
Irbesartan was not mutagenic in a battery of *in vitro* tests (Ames microbial test, rat hepatocyte DNA repair test, V79 mammalian-cell forward gene-mutation assay). Irbesartan was negative in several tests for induction of chromosomal aberrations (*in vitro*-human lymphocyte assay; *in vivo*-mouse micronucleus study).
Irbesartan had no adverse effects on fertility or mating of male or female rats at oral doses ≤650 mg/kg/day, the highest dose providing a systemic exposure to irbesartan (AUC_{0-24h}, bound plus unbound) about 5 times that found in humans receiving the maximum recommended dose of 300 mg/day.

Pregnancy

Pregnancy Categories C (first trimester) and D (second and third trimester).
See **WARNINGS: Fetal/Neonatal Morbidity and Mortality.**

Nursing Mothers

It is not known whether irbesartan is excreted in human milk, but irbesartan or some metabolite of irbesartan is secreted at low concentration in the milk of lactating rats. Because of the potential for adverse effects on the nursing infant, a decision should be made whether to discontinue nursing or discontinue the drug, taking into account the importance of the drug to the mother.

Pediatric Use

Safety and effectiveness in pediatric patients have not been established.
Pharmacokinetic parameters in pediatric subjects (age 6-16, n=21) were comparable to adults. At doses up to 150 mg daily for 4 weeks, AVAPRO was well tolerated in hypertensive children and adolescents (see **CLINICAL PHARMACOLOGY: Special Populations**). Blood pressure reductions were comparable to adults receiving 150 mg daily; however, greater sensitivity in some patients cannot be ruled out (see **DOSAGE AND ADMINISTRATION: Pediatric Patients**). AVAPRO has not been studied in pediatric patients less than 6 years old.

Geriatric Use

Of 4925 subjects receiving AVAPRO (irbesartan) in controlled clinical studies of hypertension, 911 (18.5%) were 65 years and over, while 150 (3.0%) were 75 years and over. No overall differences in effectiveness or safety were observed between these subjects and younger subjects, but greater sensitivity of some older individuals cannot be ruled out. (See **Pharmacokinetics, Special Populations,** and **Clinical Studies.**)

ADVERSE REACTIONS

Hypertension

AVAPRO (irbesartan) has been evaluated for safety in more than 4300 patients with hypertension and about 5000 subjects overall. This experience includes 1303 patients treated for over 6 months and 407 patients for 1 year or more. Treatment with AVAPRO was well-tolerated, with an incidence of adverse events similar to placebo. These events generally were mild and transient with no relationship to the dose of AVAPRO.
In placebo-controlled clinical trials, discontinuation of therapy due to a clinical adverse event was required in 3.3% of patients treated with AVAPRO, versus 4.5% of patients given placebo.
In placebo-controlled clinical trials, the following adverse event experiences reported in at least 1% of patients treated with AVAPRO (n=1965) and at a higher incidence versus placebo (n=641), excluding those too general to be informative and those not reasonably associated with the use of drug because they were associated with the condition being treated or are very common in the treated population include: diarrhea (3% vs. 2%), dyspepsia/heartburn (2% vs. 1%), and fatigue (4% vs. 3%).
The following adverse events occurred at an incidence of 1% or greater in patients treated with irbesartan, but were at least as frequent or more frequent in patients receiving placebo: abdominal pain, anxiety/nervousness, chest pain, dizziness, edema, headache, influenza, musculoskeletal pain, pharyngitis, nausea/vomiting, rash, rhinitis, sinus abnormality, tachycardia and urinary tract infection.
Irbesartan use was not associated with an increased incidence of dry cough, as is typically associated with ACE inhibitor use. In placebo controlled studies, the incidence of cough in irbesartan treated patients was 2.8% versus 2.7% in patients receiving placebo.
The incidence of hypotension or orthostatic hypotension was low in irbesartan treated patients (0.4%), unrelated to dosage, and similar to the incidence among placebo treated patients (0.2%). Dizziness, syncope, and vertigo were reported with equal or less frequency in patients receiving irbesartan compared with placebo.
In addition, the following potentially important events occurred in less than 1% of the 1965 patients and at least 5 patients (0.3%) receiving irbesartan in clinical studies, and those less frequent, clinically significant events (listed by body system). It cannot be determined whether these events were causally related to irbesartan:
Body as a Whole: fever, chills, facial edema, upper extremity edema;
Cardiovascular: flushing, hypertension, cardiac murmur, myocardial infarction, angina pectoris, arrhythmic/conduction disorder, cardio-respiratory arrest, heart failure, hypertensive crisis;
Dermatologic: pruritus, dermatitis, ecchymosis, erythema face, urticaria;
Endocrine/Metabolic/Electrolyte Imbalances: sexual dysfunction, libido change, gout;
Gastrointestinal: constipation, oral lesion, gastroenteritis, flatulence, abdominal distention;
Musculoskeletal/Connective Tissue: extremity swelling, muscle cramp, arthritis, muscle ache, musculoskeletal chest pain, joint stiffness, bursitis, muscle weakness;
Nervous System: sleep disturbance, numbness, somnolence, emotional disturbance, depression, paresthesia, tremor, transient ischemic attack, cerebrovascular accident;
Renal/Genitourinary: abnormal urination, prostate disorder;
Respiratory: epistaxis, tracheobronchitis, congestion, pulmonary congestion, dyspnea, wheezing;
Special Senses: vision disturbance, hearing abnormality, ear infection, ear pain, conjunctivitis, other eye disturbance, eyelid abnormality, ear abnormality.

Nephropathy in Type 2 Diabetic Patients

In clinical studies in patients with hypertension and type 2 diabetic renal disease, the adverse drug experiences were similar to those seen in patients with hypertension with the exception of an increased incidence of orthostatic symptoms (dizziness, orthostatic dizziness, and orthostatic hypotension) observed in IDNT (proteinuria ≥900 mg/day, and serum creatinine ranging from 1.0-3.0 mg/dL). In this trial, orthostatic symptoms occurred more frequently in the AVAPRO group (dizziness 10.2%, orthostatic dizziness 5.4%, orthostatic hypotension 5.4%) than in the placebo group (dizziness 6.0%, orthostatic dizziness 2.7%, orthostatic hypotension 3.2%).

Post-Marketing Experience

The following have been very rarely reported in post-marketing experience: urticaria; angioedema (involving swelling of the face, lips, pharynx, and/or tongue); increased liver function tests; jaundice. Hyperkalemia has been rarely reported.

Laboratory Test Findings

Hypertension

In controlled clinical trials, clinically important differences in laboratory tests were rarely associated with administration of AVAPRO (irbesartan).
Creatinine, Blood Urea Nitrogen: Minor increases in blood urea nitrogen (BUN) or serum creatinine were observed in less than 0.7% of patients with essential hypertension treated with AVAPRO alone versus 0.9% on placebo. (See **PRECAUTIONS: Impaired Renal Function.**)
Hematologic: Mean decreases in hemoglobin of 0.2 g/dL were observed in 0.2% of patients receiving AVAPRO compared to 0.3% of placebo treated patients. Neutropenia (<1000 cells/mm^3) occurred at similar frequencies among patients receiving AVAPRO (0.3%) and placebo treated patients (0.5%).

Nephropathy in Type 2 Diabetic Patients

Hyperkalemia: In IDNT (proteinuria ≥900 mg/day, and serum creatinine ranging from 1.0–3.0 mg/dL), the percent of patients with hyperkalemia (>6 mEq/L) was 18.6% in the AVAPRO group vs. 6.0% in the placebo group. Discontinuations due to hyperkalemia in the AVAPRO group were 2.1% vs. 0.4% in the placebo group.

OVERDOSAGE

No data are available in regard to overdosage in humans. However, daily doses of 900 mg for 8 weeks were well-tolerated. The most likely manifestations of overdosage are expected to be hypotension and tachycardia; bradycardia might also occur from overdose. Irbesartan is not removed by hemodialysis.
To obtain up-to-date information about the treatment of overdosage, a good resource is a certified Regional Poison-Control Center. Telephone numbers of certified poison-control centers are listed in the *Physicians' Desk Reference* (PDR). In managing overdose, consider the possibilities of multiple-drug interactions, drug-drug interactions, and unusual drug kinetics in the patient.
Laboratory determinations of serum levels of irbesartan are not widely available, and such determinations have, in any event, no known established role in the management of irbesartan overdose.
Acute oral toxicity studies with irbesartan in mice and rats indicated acute lethal doses were in excess of 2000 mg/kg, about 25- and 50-fold the maximum recommended human dose (300 mg) on a mg/m^2 basis, respectively.

DOSAGE AND ADMINISTRATION

AVAPRO (irbesartan) may be administered with other antihypertensive agents and with or without food.
Hypertension
The recommended initial dose of AVAPRO is 150 mg once daily. Patients requiring further reduction in blood pressure should be titrated to 300 mg once daily.
A low dose of a diuretic may be added, if blood pressure is not controlled by AVAPRO alone. Hydrochlorothiazide has been shown to have an additive effect (see **CLINICAL PHARMACOLOGY: Clinical Studies**). Patients not adequately treated by the maximum dose of 300 mg once daily are unlikely to derive additional benefit from a higher dose or twice-daily dosing.
No dosage adjustment is necessary in elderly patients, or in patients with hepatic impairment or mild to severe renal impairment.
Nephropathy in Type 2 Diabetic Patients
The recommended target maintenance dose is 300 mg once daily. There are no data on the clinical effects of lower doses of AVAPRO on diabetic nephropathy (see **CLINICAL PHARMACOLOGY: Clinical Studies**).

Pediatric Patients

Children (<6 years): Safety and effectiveness have not been established.
Children (6-12 years): An initial dose of 75 mg once daily is reasonable. Patients requiring further reduction in blood pressure should be titrated to 150 mg once daily (see **PRECAUTIONS: Pediatric Use**).
Adolescent patients (13-16 years): An initial dose of 150 mg once daily is reasonable. Patients requiring further reduction in blood pressure should be titrated to 300 mg once daily. Higher doses are not recommended (see **PRECAUTIONS: Pediatric Use**).

Volume- and Salt-depleted Patients

A lower initial dose of AVAPRO (75 mg) is recommended in patients with depletion of intravascular volume or salt (e.g., patients treated vigorously with diuretics or on hemodialysis) (see **WARNINGS: Hypotension in Volume- or Salt-depleted Patients**).

HOW SUPPLIED

AVAPRO® (irbesartan) is available as white to off-white biconvex oval tablets, debossed with a heart shape on one side and a portion of the NDC code on the other. Unit-of-use bottles contain 30, 90, or 500 tablets and blister packs contain 100 tablets, as follows:

	75 mg	150 mg	300 mg
Debossing	2771	2772	2773
Bottle of 30	0087-2771-31	0087-2772-31	0087-2773-31
Bottle of 90	0087-2771-32	0087-2772-32	0087-2773-32
Bottle of 500	—	0087-2772-15	0087-2773-15
Blister of 100	—	0087-2772-35	—

Storage

Store at 25° C (77° F); excursions permitted to 15° C-30° C (59° F–86° F) [see USP Controlled Room Temperature].
Distributed by:
Bristol-Myers Squibb Sanofi-Synthelabo Partnership
New York, NY 10016
Bristol-Myers Squibb Company sanofi~synthelabo
Revised May 2004 1017108A9
B2-B0001-05-04
Shown in Product Identification Guide, page 310

CEFZIL® ℞
[sef-zil]
(cefprozil) Tablets
250 mg and 500 mg

CEFZIL® ℞
(cefprozil)
for Oral Suspension
125 mg/5 mL and 250 mg/5 mL
Rx only

To reduce the development of drug-resistant bacteria and maintain the effectiveness of CEFZIL® (cefprozil) and other antibacterial drugs, CEFZIL should be used only to treat or prevent infections that are proven or strongly suspected to be caused by bacteria.

DESCRIPTION

CEFZIL is a semi-synthetic broad-spectrum cephalosporin antibiotic.

Cefprozil is a cis and trans isomeric mixture (≥90% cis). The chemical name for the monohydrate is (6R, 7R)-7-[(R)-2-amino-2-(p-hydroxyphenyl)acetamido]-8-oxo-3-propenyl-5-thia-1-azabicyclo[4.2.0]oct-2-ene-2-carboxylic acid monohydrate, and the structural formula is:

NH_2 H N S N O O HO $\bullet H_2O$ CO_2H

Cefprozil is a white to yellowish powder with a molecular formula for the monohydrate of $C_{18}H_{19}N_3O_5S \bullet H_2O$ and a molecular weight of 407.45.

CEFZIL tablets and CEFZIL for oral suspension are intended for oral administration.

CEFZIL tablets contain cefprozil equivalent to 250 mg or 500 mg of anhydrous cefprozil. In addition, each tablet contains the following inactive ingredients: cellulose, hypromellose, magnesium stearate, methylcellulose, simethicone, sodium starch glycolate, polyethylene glycol, polysorbate 80, sorbic acid, and titanium dioxide. The 250 mg tablets also contain FD&C Yellow No. 6.

CEFZIL for oral suspension contains cefprozil equivalent to 125 mg or 250 mg anhydrous cefprozil per 5 mL constituted suspension. In addition, the oral suspension contains the following inactive ingredients: aspartame, cellulose, citric acid, colloidal silicone dioxide, FD&C Red No. 3, flavors (natural and artificial), glycine, polysorbate 80, simethicone, sodium benzoate, sodium carboxymethylcellulose, sodium chloride, and sucrose.

CLINICAL PHARMACOLOGY

The pharmacokinetic data were derived from the capsule formulation; however, bioequivalence has been demonstrated for the oral solution, capsule, tablet, and suspension formulations under fasting conditions.

Following oral administration of cefprozil to fasting subjects, approximately 95% of the dose was absorbed. The average plasma half-life in normal subjects was 1.3 hours, while the steady-state volume of distribution was estimated to be 0.23 L/kg. The total body clearance and renal clearance rates were approximately 3 mL/min/kg and 2.3 mL/min/kg, respectively.

Average peak plasma concentrations after administration of 250 mg, 500 mg, or 1 g doses of cefprozil to fasting subjects were approximately 6.1, 10.5, and 18.3 μg/mL, respectively, and were obtained within 1.5 hours after dosing. Urinary recovery accounted for approximately 60% of the administered dose. (See Table.)

[See first table above]

Dosage (mg)	Mean Plasma Cefprozil Concentrations (μg/mL)* Peak appx. 1.5 h	4 h	8 h	8-hour Urinary Excretion (%)
250 mg	6.1	1.7	0.2	60%
500 mg	10.5	3.2	0.4	62%
1000 mg	18.3	8.4	1.0	54%

* Data represent mean values of 12 healthy volunteers.

During the first 4-hour period after drug administration, the average urine concentrations following 250 mg, 500 mg, and 1 g doses were approximately 700 μg/mL, 1000 μg/mL, and 2900 μg/mL, respectively.

Administration of CEFZIL tablet or suspension formulation with food did not affect the extent of absorption (AUC) or the peak plasma concentration (C_{max}) of cefprozil. However, there was an increase of 0.25 to 0.75 hours in the time to maximum plasma concentration of cefprozil (T_{max}).

The bioavailability of the capsule formulation of cefprozil was not affected when administered 5 minutes following an antacid.

Plasma protein binding is approximately 36% and is independent of concentration in the range of 2 μg/mL to 20 μg/mL.

There was no evidence of accumulation of cefprozil in the plasma in individuals with normal renal function following multiple oral doses of up to 1000 mg every 8 hours for 10 days.

In patients with reduced renal function, the plasma half-life may be prolonged up to 5.2 hours depending on the degree of the renal dysfunction. In patients with complete absence of renal function, the plasma half-life of cefprozil has been shown to be as long as 5.9 hours. The half-life is shortened during hemodialysis. Excretion pathways in patients with markedly impaired renal function have not been determined. (See **PRECAUTIONS** and **DOSAGE AND ADMINISTRATION**.)

In patients with impaired hepatic function, the half-life increases to approximately 2 hours. The magnitude of the changes does not warrant a dosage adjustment for patients with impaired hepatic function.

Healthy geriatric volunteers (≥65 years old) who received a single 1-g dose of cefprozil had 35-60% higher AUC and 40% lower renal clearance values compared with healthy adult volunteers 20-40 years of age. The average AUC in young and elderly female subjects was approximately 15-20% higher than in young and elderly male subjects. The magnitude of these age- and gender-related changes in the pharmacokinetics of cefprozil is not sufficient to necessitate dosage adjustments.

Adequate data on CSF levels of cefprozil are not available. Comparable pharmacokinetic parameters of cefprozil are observed between pediatric patients (6 months–12 years) and adults following oral administration of selected matched doses. The maximum concentrations are achieved at 1–2 hours after dosing. The plasma elimination half-life is approximately 1.5 hours. In general, the observed plasma concentrations of cefprozil in pediatric patients at the 7.5, 15, and 30 mg/kg doses are similar to those observed within the same time frame in normal adult subjects at the 250, 500 and 1000 mg doses, respectively. The comparative plasma concentrations of cefprozil in pediatric patients and adult subjects at the equivalent dose level are presented in the table below.

[See second table above]

Population	Dose	Mean (SD) Plasma Cefprozil Concentrations (μg/mL) 1 h	2 h	4 h	6 h	$T_{1/2}$ (h)
children (n = 18)	7.5 mg/kg	4.70 (1.57)	3.99 (1.24)	0.91 (0.30)	0.23[a] (0.13)	0.94 (0.32)
adults (n =12)	250 mg	4.82 (2.13)	4.92 (1.13)	1.70[b] (0.53)	0.53 (0.17)	1.28 (0.34)
children (n = 19)	15 mg/kg	10.86 (2.55)	8.47 (2.03)	2.75 (1.07)	0.61[c] (0.27)	1.24 (0.43)
adults (n = 12)	500 mg	8.39 (1.95)	9.42 (0.98)	3.18[d] (0.76)	1.00[d] (0.24)	1.29 (0.14)
children (n = 10)	30 mg/kg	6.69 (4.26)	17.61 (6.39)	8.66 (2.70)	–	2.06 (0.21)
adults (n = 12)	1000 mg	11.99 (4.67)	16.95 (4.07)	8.36 (4.13)	2.79 (1.77)	1.27 (0.12)

[a]n = 11; [b]n = 5; [c]n = 9; [d]n = 11.

Microbiology

Cefprozil has *in vitro* activity against a broad range of gram-positive and gram-negative bacteria. The bactericidal action of cefprozil results from inhibition of cell-wall synthesis. Cefprozil has been shown to be active against most strains of the following microorganisms both *in vitro* and in clinical infections as described in the **INDICATIONS AND USAGE** section.

Aerobic gram-positive microorganisms:

Staphylococcus aureus (including β-lactamase-producing strains)

NOTE: Cefprozil is inactive against methicillin-resistant staphylococci.

Streptococcus pneumoniae
Streptococcus pyogenes

Aerobic gram-negative microorganisms:

Haemophilus influenzae (including β-lactamase-producing strains)
Moraxella (Branhamella) catarrhalis (including β-lactamase-producing strains)

The following *in vitro* data are available; however, their clinical significance is unknown. Cefprozil exhibits *in vitro* minimum inhibitory concentrations (MICs) of 8 μg/mL or less against most (≥90%) strains of the following microorganisms; however, the safety and effectiveness of cefprozil in treating clinical infections due to these microorganisms have not been established in adequate and well-controlled clinical trials.

Aerobic gram-positive microorganisms:

Enterococcus durans
Enterococcus faecalis
Listeria monocytogenes
Staphylococcus epidermidis
Staphylococcus saprophyticus
Staphylococcus warneri
Streptococcus agalactiae
Streptococci (Groups C, D, F, and G)
viridans group Streptococci

NOTE: Cefprozil is inactive against *Enterococcus faecium.*

Aerobic gram-negative microorganisms:

Citrobacter diversus
Escherichia coli
Klebsiella pneumoniae
Neisseria gonorrhoeae (including β-lactamase-producing strains)
Proteus mirabilis
Salmonella spp.
Shigella spp.
Vibrio spp.

NOTE: Cefprozil is inactive against most strains of *Acinetobacter, Enterobacter, Morganella morganii, Proteus vulgaris, Providencia, Pseudomonas,* and *Serratia.*

Anaerobic microorganisms:

Prevotella (Bacteroides) melaninogenicus
Clostridium difficile
Clostridium perfringens
Fusobacterium spp.
Peptostreptococcus spp.
Propionibacterium acnes

NOTE: Most strains of the *Bacteroides fragilis* group are resistant to cefprozil.

Susceptibility Tests

Dilution Techniques: Quantitative methods are used to determine antimicrobial minimal inhibitory concentrations (MICs). These MICs provide estimates of the susceptibility of bacteria to antimicrobial compounds. The MICs should be determined using a standardized procedure. Standardized procedures are based on a dilution method[1,2] (broth or agar) or equivalent with standardized inoculum concentrations and standardized concentrations of cefprozil powder. The MIC values should be interpreted according to the following criteria:

MIC (μg/mL)	Interpretation
≤ 8	Susceptible (S)
16	Intermediate (I)
≥ 32	Resistant (R)

A report of "Susceptible" indicates that the pathogen is likely to be inhibited if the antimicrobial compound in the blood reaches the concentrations usually achievable. A report of "Intermediate" indicates that the result should be considered equivocal, and, if the microorganism is not fully susceptible to alternative, clinically feasible drugs, the test should be repeated. This category implies possible clinical applicability in body sites where the drug is physiologically concentrated or in situations where high dosage of drug can be used. This category also provides a buffer zone which prevents small uncontrolled technical factors from causing major discrepancies in interpretation. A report of "Resistant" indicates that the pathogen is not likely to be inhibited if the antimicrobial compound in the blood reaches the concentrations usually achievable; other therapy should be selected.

Standardized susceptibility test procedures require the use of laboratory control microorganisms to control the technical aspects of the laboratory procedures. Standard cefprozil powder should provide the following MIC values:

Microorganism	MIC (μg/mL)
Enterococcus faecalis ATCC 29212	4–16
Escherichia coli ATCC 25922	1–4
Haemophilus influenzae ATCC 49766	1–4
Staphylococcus aureus ATCC 29213	0.25–1
Streptococcus pneumoniae ATCC 49619	0.25–1

Diffusion Techniques: Quantitative methods that require measurement of zone diameters also provide reproducible estimates of the susceptibility of bacteria to antimicrobial compounds. One such standardized procedure[3] requires the use of standardized inoculum concentrations. This procedure uses paper disks impregnated with 30 μg cefprozil to test the susceptibility of microorganisms to cefprozil.

Reports from the laboratory providing results of the standard single-disk susceptibility test with a 30 μg cefprozil disk should be interpreted according to the following criteria:

Continued on next page

Cefzil—Cont.

Zone diameter (mm)	Interpretation
≥ 18	Susceptible (S)
15–17	Intermediate (I)
≤ 14	Resistant (R)

Interpretation should be as stated above for results using dilution techniques. Interpretation involves correlation of the diameter obtained in the disk test with the MIC for cefprozil.

As with standardized dilution techniques, diffusion methods require the use of laboratory control microorganisms that are used to control the technical aspects of the laboratory procedures. For the diffusion technique, the 30 µg cefprozil disk should provide the following zone diameters in these laboratory test quality control strains.

Microorganism	Zone diameter (mm)
Escherichia coli ATCC 25922	21–27
Haemophilus influenzae ATCC 49766	20–27
Staphylococcus aureus ATCC 25923	27–33
Streptococcus pneumoniae ATCC 49619	25–32

INDICATIONS AND USAGE

CEFZIL (cefprozil) is indicated for the treatment of patients with mild to moderate infections caused by susceptible strains of the designated microorganisms in the conditions listed below:

UPPER RESPIRATORY TRACT

Pharyngitis/tonsillitis caused by *Streptococcus pyogenes*.

NOTE: The usual drug of choice in the treatment and prevention of streptococcal infections, including the prophylaxis of rheumatic fever, is penicillin given by the intramuscular route. Cefprozil is generally effective in the eradication of *Streptococcus pyogenes* from the nasopharynx; however, substantial data establishing the efficacy of cefprozil in the subsequent prevention of rheumatic fever are not available at present.

Otitis Media caused by *Streptococcus pneumoniae, Haemophilus influenzae* (including β-lactamase-producing strains), and *Moraxella (Branhamella) catarrhalis* (including β-lactamase-producing strains). (See **CLINICAL STUDIES**.)

NOTE: In the treatment of otitis media due to β-lactamase producing organisms, cefprozil had bacteriologic eradication rates somewhat lower than those observed with a product containing a specific β-lactamase inhibitor. In considering the use of cefprozil, lower overall eradication rates should be balanced against the susceptibility patterns of the common microbes in a given geographic area and the increased potential for toxicity with products containing β-lactamase inhibitors.

Acute Sinusitis caused by *Streptococcus pneumoniae, Haemophilus influenzae* (including β-lactamase-producing strains), and *Moraxella (Branhamella) catarrhalis* (including β-lactamase-producing strains).

LOWER RESPIRATORY TRACT

Secondary Bacterial Infection of Acute Bronchitis and Acute Bacterial Exacerbation of Chronic Bronchitis caused by *Streptococcus pneumoniae, Haemophilus influenzae* (including β-lactamase-producing strains), and *Moraxella (Branhamella) catarrhalis* (including β-lactamase-producing strains).

SKIN AND SKIN STRUCTURE

Uncomplicated Skin and Skin-Structure Infections caused by *Staphylococcus aureus* (including penicillinase-producing strains) and *Streptococcus pyogenes*. Abscesses usually require surgical drainage.

To reduce the development of drug-resistant bacteria and maintain the effectiveness of CEFZIL and other antibacterial drugs, CEFZIL should be used only to treat or prevent infections that are proven or strongly suspected to be caused by susceptible bacteria. When culture susceptibility information are available, they should be considered in selecting or modifying antibacterial therapy. In the absence of such data, local epidemiology and susceptibility patterns may contribute to the empiric selection of therapy.

CONTRAINDICATIONS

CEFZIL (cefprozil) is contraindicated in patients with known allergy to the cephalosporin class of antibiotics.

WARNINGS

BEFORE THERAPY WITH CEFZIL IS INSTITUTED, CAREFUL INQUIRY SHOULD BE MADE TO DETERMINE WHETHER THE PATIENT HAS HAD PREVIOUS HYPERSENSITIVITY REACTIONS TO CEFZIL, CEPHALOSPORINS, PENICILLINS, OR OTHER DRUGS. IF THIS PRODUCT IS TO BE GIVEN TO PENICILLIN-SENSITIVE PATIENTS, CAUTION SHOULD BE EXERCISED BECAUSE CROSS-SENSITIVITY AMONG β-LACTAM ANTIBIOTICS HAS BEEN CLEARLY DOCUMENTED AND MAY OCCUR IN UP TO 10% OF PATIENTS WITH A HISTORY OF PENICILLIN ALLERGY. IF AN ALLERGIC REACTION TO CEFZIL OCCURS, DISCONTINUE THE DRUG. SERIOUS ACUTE HYPERSENSITIVITY REACTIONS MAY REQUIRE TREATMENT WITH EPINEPHRINE AND OTHER EMERGENCY MEASURES, INCLUDING OXYGEN, INTRAVENOUS FLUIDS, INTRAVENOUS ANTIHISTAMINES, CORTICOSTEROIDS, PRESSOR AMINES, AND AIRWAY MANAGEMENT, AS CLINICALLY INDICATED.

Pseudomembranous colitis has been reported with nearly all antibacterial agents, including cefprozil, and may range in severity from mild to life threatening. Therefore, it is important to consider this diagnosis in patients who present with diarrhea subsequent to the administration of antibacterial agents.

Treatment with antibacterial agents alters the normal flora of the colon and may permit overgrowth of clostridia. Studies indicate that a toxin produced by *Clostridium difficile* is one primary cause of "antibiotic-associated" colitis.

After the diagnosis of pseudomembranous colitis has been established, appropriate therapeutic measures should be initiated. Mild cases of pseudomembranous colitis usually respond to drug discontinuation alone. In moderate to severe cases, consideration should be given to management with fluids and electrolytes, protein supplementation, and treatment with an antibacterial drug clinically effective against *Clostridium difficile* colitis.

PRECAUTIONS

General

Prescribing CEFZIL (cefprozil) in the absence of proven or strongly suspected bacterial infection or a prophylactic indication is unlikely to provide benefit to the patient and increases the risk of the development of drug-resistant bacteria.

In patients with known or suspected renal impairment (see **DOSAGE AND ADMINISTRATION**), careful clinical observation and appropriate laboratory studies should be done prior to and during therapy. The total daily dose of CEFZIL should be reduced in these patients because high and/or prolonged plasma antibiotic concentrations can occur in such individuals from usual doses. Cephalosporins, including CEFZIL, should be given with caution to patients receiving concurrent treatment with potent diuretics since these agents are suspected of adversely affecting renal function.

Prolonged use of CEFZIL may result in the overgrowth of nonsusceptible organisms. Careful observation of the patient is essential. If superinfection occurs during therapy, appropriate measures should be taken.

Cefprozil should be prescribed with caution in individuals with a history of gastrointestinal disease particularly colitis.

Positive direct Coombs' tests have been reported during treatment with cephalosporin antibiotics.

Information for Patients

Phenylketonurics: CEFZIL (cefprozil) for oral suspension contains phenylalanine 28 mg per 5 mL (1 teaspoonful) constituted suspension for both the 125 mg/5 mL and 250 mg/5 mL dosage forms.

Patients should be counseled that antibacterial drugs including CEFZIL should only be used to treat bacterial infections. They do not treat viral infections (e.g., the common cold). When CEFZIL is prescribed to treat a bacterial infection, patients should be told that although it is common to feel better early in the course of therapy, the medication should be taken exactly as directed. Skipping doses or not completing the full course of therapy may (1) decrease the effectiveness of the immediate treatment and (2) increase the likelihood that bacteria will develop resistance and will not be treatable by CEFZIL or other antibacterial drugs in the future.

Drug Interactions

Nephrotoxicity has been reported following concomitant administration of aminoglycoside antibiotics and cephalosporin antibiotics. Concomitant administration of probenecid doubled the AUC for cefprozil.

The bioavailability of the capsule formulation of cefprozil was not affected when administered 5 minutes following an antacid.

Drug/Laboratory Interactions

Cephalosporin antibiotics may produce a false positive reaction for glucose in the urine with copper reduction tests (Benedict's or Fehling's solution or with Clinitest® tablets), but not with enzyme-based tests for glycosuria (e.g., Clinistix®). A false negative reaction may occur in the ferricyanide test for blood glucose. The presence of cefprozil in the blood does not interfere with the assay of plasma or urine creatinine by the alkaline picrate method.

Carcinogenesis, Mutagenesis, and Impairment of Fertility

Long term *in vivo* studies have not been performed to evaluate the carcinogenic potential of cefprozil.

Cefprozil was not found to be mutagenic in either the Ames *Salmonella* or *E. coli* WP2 urvA reversion assays or the Chinese hamster ovary cell HGPRT forward gene mutation assay and it did not induce chromosomal abnormalities in Chinese hamster ovary cells or unscheduled DNA synthesis in rat hepatocytes *in vitro*. Chromosomal aberrations were not observed in bone marrow cells from rats dosed orally with over 30 times the highest recommended human dose based upon mg/m^2.

Impairment of fertility was not observed in male or female rats given oral doses of cefprozil up to 18.5 times the highest recommended human dose based upon mg/m^2.

Pregnancy: Teratogenic Effects. Pregnancy Category B

Reproduction studies have been performed in rabbits, mice, and rats using oral doses of cefprozil of 0.8, 8.5, and 18.5 times the maximum daily human dose (1000 mg) based upon mg/m^2, and have revealed no harm to the fetus. There are, however, no adequate and well-controlled studies in pregnant women. Because animal reproduction studies are not always predictive of human response, this drug should be used during pregnancy only if clearly needed.

Labor and Delivery

Cefprozil has not been studied for use during labor and delivery. Treatment should only be given if clearly needed.

Nursing Mothers

Small amounts of cefprozil (<0.3% of dose) have been detected in human milk following administration of a single 1 gram dose to lactating women. The average levels over 24 hours ranged from 0.25 to 3.3 µg/mL. Caution should be exercised when CEFZIL is administered to a nursing woman, since the effect of cefprozil on nursing infants is unknown.

Pediatric Use: (See **INDICATIONS AND USAGE** and **DOSAGE AND ADMINISTRATION**.)

The safety and effectiveness of cefprozil in the treatment of otitis media have been established in the age groups 6 months to 12 years. Use of CEFZIL (cefprozil) for the treatment of otitis media is supported by evidence from adequate and well-controlled studies of cefprozil in pediatric patients. (See **CLINICAL STUDIES**.)

The safety and effectiveness of cefprozil in the treatment of pharyngitis/tonsillitis or uncomplicated skin and skin structure infections have been established in the age groups 2 to 12 years. Use of CEFZIL for the treatment of these infections is supported by evidence from adequate and well-controlled studies of cefprozil in pediatric patients.

The safety and effectiveness of cefprozil in the treatment of acute sinusitis have been established in the age groups 6 months to 12 years. Use of CEFZIL in these age groups is supported by evidence from adequate and well-controlled studies of cefprozil in adults.

Safety and effectiveness in pediatric patients below the age of 6 months have not been established for the treatment of otitis media or acute sinusitis or below the age of 2 years for the treatment of pharyngitis/tonsillitis or uncomplicated skin and skin structure infections. However, accumulation of other cephalosporin antibiotics in newborn infants (resulting from prolonged drug half-life in this age group) has been reported.

Geriatric Use

Of the more than 4500 adults treated with CEFZIL in clinical studies, 14% were 65 years and older, while 5% were 75 years and older. When geriatric patients received the usual recommended adult doses, their clinical efficacy and safety were comparable to clinical efficacy and safety in nongeriatric adult patients. Other reported clinical experience has not identified differences in responses between elderly and younger patients, but greater sensitivity of some older individuals to the effects of CEFZIL cannot be excluded (see **CLINICAL PHARMACOLOGY**).

CEFZIL is known to be substantially excreted by the kidney, and the risk of toxic reactions to this drug may be greater in patients with impaired renal function. Because elderly patients are more likely to have decreased renal function, care should be taken in dose selection and it may be useful to monitor renal function. See **DOSAGE AND ADMINISTRATION** for dosing recommendations for patients with impaired renal function.

ADVERSE REACTIONS

The adverse reactions to cefprozil are similar to those observed with other orally administered cephalosporins. Cefprozil was usually well tolerated in controlled clinical trials. Approximately 2% of patients discontinued cefprozil therapy due to adverse events.

The most common adverse effects observed in patients treated with cefprozil are:

Gastrointestinal: Diarrhea (2.9%), nausea (3.5%), vomiting (1%), and abdominal pain (1%).

Hepatobiliary: Elevations of AST (SGOT) (2%), ALT (SGPT) (2%), alkaline phosphatase (0.2%), and bilirubin values (<0.1%). As with some penicillins and some other cephalosporin antibiotics, cholestatic jaundice has been reported rarely.

Hypersensitivity: Rash (0.9%), urticaria (0.1%). Such reactions have been reported more frequently in children than in adults. Signs and symptoms usually occur a few days after initiation of therapy and subside within a few days after cessation of therapy.

CNS: Dizziness (1%). Hyperactivity, headache, nervousness, insomnia, confusion, and somnolence have been reported rarely (<1%). All were reversible.

Hematopoietic: Decreased leukocyte count (0.2%), eosinophilia (2.3%).

Renal: Elevated BUN (0.1%), serum creatinine (0.1%).

Other: Diaper rash and superinfection (1.5%), genital pruritus and vaginitis (1.6%).

The following adverse events, regardless of established causal relationship to CEFZIL (cefprozil), have been rarely reported during postmarketing surveillance: anaphylaxis, angioedema, colitis (including pseudomembranous colitis), erythema multiforme, fever, serum-sickness like reactions, Stevens-Johnson syndrome, and thrombocytopenia.

Cephalosporin class paragraph

In addition to the adverse reactions listed above which have been observed in patients treated with cefprozil, the following adverse reactions and altered laboratory tests have been reported for cephalosporin-class antibiotics:

Aplastic anemia, hemolytic anemia, hemorrhage, renal dysfunction, toxic epidermal necrolysis, toxic nephropathy, prolonged prothrombin time, positive Coombs' test, elevated LDH, pancytopenia, neutropenia, agranulocytosis.

Clinitest® and Clinistix® are registered trademarks of Bayer HealthCare LLC.

Several cephalosporins have been implicated in triggering seizures, particularly in patients with renal impairment, when the dosage was not reduced. (See **DOSAGE AND ADMINISTRATION** and **OVERDOSAGE**.) If seizures associated with drug therapy occur, the drug should be discontinued. Anticonvulsant therapy can be given if clinically indicated.

OVERDOSAGE

Single 5000 mg/kg oral doses of cefprozil caused no mortality or signs of toxicity in adult, weanling, or neonatal rats, or adult mice. A single oral dose of 3000 mg/kg caused diarrhea and loss of appetite in cynomolgus monkeys, but no mortality.
Cefprozil is eliminated primarily by the kidneys. In case of severe overdosage, especially in patients with compromised renal function, hemodialysis will aid in the removal of cefprozil from the body.

DOSAGE AND ADMINISTRATION

CEFZIL (cefprozil) is administered orally.
[See first table at right]

Renal Impairment

Cefprozil may be administered to patients with impaired renal function. The following dosage schedule should be used.

Creatinine Clearance (mL/min)	Dosage (mg)	Dosing Interval
30–120	standard	standard
0–29*	50% of standard	standard

* Cefprozil is in part removed by hemodialysis; therefore, cefprozil should be administered after the completion of hemodialysis.

Hepatic Impairment

No dosage adjustment is necessary for patients with impaired hepatic function.

HOW SUPPLIED

CEFZIL® (cefprozil) Tablets
Each light orange film-coated tablet, imprinted with "7720" on one side and "250" on the other, contains the equivalent of 250 mg anhydrous cefprozil.
Bottles of 100 Tablets **NDC** 0087-7720-60
Each white film-coated tablet, imprinted with "7721" on one side and "500" on the other, contains the equivalent of 500 mg anhydrous cefprozil.
Bottles of 50 Tablets **NDC** 0087-7721-50
Bottles of 100 Tablets **NDC** 0087-7721-60
Store at controlled room temperature, 59° to 86° F (15° to 30° C).
CEFZIL® (cefprozil) For Oral Suspension
Each 5 mL of constituted suspension contains the equivalent of 125 mg anhydrous cefprozil.
50 mL Bottle **NDC** 0087-7718-40
75 mL Bottle **NDC** 0087-7718-62
100 mL Bottle **NDC** 0087-7718-64
Each 5 mL of constituted suspension contains the equivalent of 250 mg anhydrous cefprozil.
50 mL Bottle **NDC** 0087-7719-40
75 mL Bottle **NDC** 0087-7719-62
100 mL Bottle **NDC** 0087-7719-64
All powder formulations for oral suspension contain cefprozil in a bubble-gum flavored mixture.
Reconstitution Directions for Oral Suspension
Prepare the suspension at the time of dispensing; for ease in preparation, add water in two portions and shake well after each aliquot.
[See second table at right]
After mixing, store in a refrigerator and discard unused portion after 14 days.
Store at 59° to 77° F (15° to 25° C) prior to constitution.
U.S. Patent No. 4,520,022

CLINICAL STUDIES

Study One:

In a controlled clinical study of **acute otitis media** performed in the United States where significant rates of β-lactamase-producing organisms were found, cefprozil was compared to an oral antimicrobial agent that contained a specific β-lactamase inhibitor. In this study, using very strict evaluability criteria and microbiologic and clinical response criteria at the 10-16 days post-therapy follow-up, the following presumptive bacterial eradication/clinical cure outcomes (i.e. clinical success) and safety results were obtained:
[See third table at right]
SAFETY:
The incidences of adverse events, primarily diarrhea and rash*, were clinically and statistically significantly higher in the control arm versus the cefprozil arm.

Age Group	Cefprozil	Control
6 months-2 years	21%	41%
3-12 years	10%	19%

*The majority of these involved the diaper area in young children.

Study Two:

In a controlled clinical study of **acute otitis media** performed in Europe, cefprozil was compared to an oral antimicrobial agent that contained a specific β-lactamase inhibitor. As expected in a European population, this study population had a lower incidence of β-lactamase-producing organisms than usually seen in U.S. trials. In this study, using very strict evaluability criteria and microbiologic and clinical response criteria at the 10-16 days post-therapy follow-up, the following presumptive bacterial eradication/clinical cure outcomes (i.e. clinical success) were obtained:
[See fourth table above]
SAFETY:
The incidence of adverse events in the cefprozil arm was comparable to the incidence of adverse events in the control arm (agent that contained a specific β-lactamase inhibitor).

Population/Infection	Dosage (mg)	Duration (days)
ADULTS (13 years and older)		
UPPER RESPIRATORY TRACT		
Pharyngitis/Tonsillitis	500 q24h	10[a]
Acute Sinusitis (For moderate to severe infections, the higher dose should be used)	250 q12h or 500 q12h	10
LOWER RESPIRATORY TRACT		
Secondary Bacterial Infection of Acute Bronchitis and Acute Bacterial Exacerbation of Chronic Bronchitis	500 q12h	10
SKIN AND SKIN STRUCTURE		
Uncomplicated Skin and Skin Structure Infections	250 q12h or 500 q24h or 500 q12h	10
CHILDREN (2 years - 12 years)		
UPPER RESPIRATORY TRACT[b]		
Pharyngitis/Tonsillitis	7.5 mg/kg q12h	10[a]
SKIN AND SKIN STRUCTURE[b]		
Uncomplicated Skin and Skin Structure Infections	20 mg/kg q24h	10
INFANTS & CHILDREN (6 months - 12 years)		
UPPER RESPIRATORY TRACT[b]		
Otitis Media (See **INDICATIONS AND USAGE** and **CLINICAL STUDIES**)	15 mg/kg q12h	10
Acute Sinusitis (For moderate to severe infections, the higher dose should be used)	7.5 mg/kg q12h or 15 mg/kg	10

[a] In the treatment of infections due to *Streptococcus pyogenes*, CEFZIL should be administered for at least 10 days.
[b] Not to exceed recommended adult doses.

Bottle Size	Total Amount of Water Required for Reconstitution: Final Concentration 125 mg/5 mL	Final Concentration 250 mg/5 mL
50 mL	36 mL	36 mL
75 mL	54 mL	54 mL
100 mL	72 mL	72 mL

U.S. Acute Otitis Media Study
Cefprozil vs β-lactamase inhibitor-containing control drug

EFFICACY:

Pathogen	% of Cases with Pathogen (n = 155)	Outcome
S. pneumoniae	48.4%	cefprozil success rate 5% better than control
H. influenzae	35.5%	cefprozil success rate 17% less than control
M. catarrhalis	13.5%	cefprozil success rate 12% less than control
S. pyogenes	2.6%	cefprozil equivalent to control
Overall	100.0%	cefprozil success rate 5% less than control

European Acute Otitis Media Study
Cefprozil vs β-lactamase inhibitor-containing control drug

EFFICACY:

Pathogen	% of Cases with Pathogen (n = 47)	Outcome
S. pneumoniae	51.0%	cefprozil equivalent to control
H. influenzae	29.8%	cefprozil equivalent to control
M. catarrhalis	6.4%	cefprozil equivalent to control
S. pyogenes	12.8%	cefprozil equivalent to control
Overall	100.0%	cefprozil equivalent to control

REFERENCES

1. National Committee for Clinical Laboratory Standards. *Methods for Dilution Antimicrobial Susceptibility Tests for Bacteria that Grow Aerobically*—Third Edition. Approved Standard NCCLS Document M7-A3, Vol. 13, No. 25, NCCLS, Villanova, PA, December 1993.
2. National Committee for Clinical Laboratory Standards. *Methods for Antimicrobial Susceptibility Testing of Anaerobic Bacteria*—Third Edition. Approved Standard NCCLS Document M11-A3, Vol. 13, No. 26, NCCLS, Villanova, PA, December 1993.
3. National Committee for Clinical Laboratory Standards. *Performance Standards for Antimicrobial Disk Susceptibility Tests*—Fifth Edition. Approved Standard NCCLS Document M2-A5, Vol. 13, No. 24, NCCLS, Villanova, PA, December 1993.

E2-B0001-12-03 7718DIM-14
Revised December 2003
Bristol-Myers Squibb Company
Princeton, NJ 08543 U.S.A.
Shown in Product Identification Guide, page 310

COUMADIN® TABLETS ℞
[*coo-ma-din*]
(Warfarin Sodium Tablets, USP) Crystalline
COUMADIN® FOR INJECTION
(Warfarin Sodium for Injection, USP)
ANTICOAGULANT
Rx only

DESCRIPTION

COUMADIN (crystalline warfarin sodium) is an anticoagulant which acts by inhibiting vitamin K-dependent coagulation factors. Chemically, it is 3-(α-acetonylbenzyl)-4-

Continued on next page

Coumadin—Cont.

hydroxycoumarin and is a racemic mixture of the R- and S-enantiomers. Crystalline warfarin sodium is an isopropanol clathrate. The crystallization of warfarin sodium virtually eliminates trace impurities present in amorphous warfarin. Its empirical formula is C_{19} H_{15} NaO_4, and its structural formula may be represented by the following:

Crystalline warfarin sodium occurs as a white, odorless, crystalline powder, is discolored by light and is very soluble in water; freely soluble in alcohol; very slightly soluble in chloroform and in ether.

COUMADIN Tablets for oral use also contain:

All strengths:	Lactose, starch and magnesium stearate
1 mg:	D&C Red No. 6 Barium Lake
2 mg:	FD&C Blue No. 2 Aluminum Lake and FD&C Red No. 40 Aluminum Lake
2-1/2 mg:	D&C Yellow No. 10 Aluminum Lake and FD&C Blue No. 1 Aluminum Lake
3 mg:	FD&C Yellow No. 6 Aluminum Lake, FD&C Blue No. 2 Aluminum Lake and FD&C Red No. 40 Aluminum Lake
4 mg:	FD&C Blue No. 1 Aluminum Lake
5 mg:	FD&C Yellow No. 6 Aluminum Lake
6 mg:	FD&C Yellow No. 6 Aluminum Lake and FD&C Blue No. 1 Aluminum Lake
7-1/2 mg:	D&C Yellow No. 10 Aluminum Lake and FD&C Yellow No. 6 Aluminum Lake
10 mg:	Dye Free

COUMADIN for Injection is supplied as a sterile, lyophilized powder, which, after reconstitution with 2.7 mL sterile Water for Injection, contains:

Warfarin Sodium	2 mg/mL
Sodium Phosphate, Dibasic, Heptahydrate	4.98 mg/mL
Sodium Phosphate, Monobasic, Monohydrate	0.194 mg/mL
Sodium Chloride	0.1 mg/mL
Mannitol	38.0 mg/mL
Sodium Hydroxide, as needed for pH adjustment to	8.1 to 8.3

CLINICAL PHARMACOLOGY

COUMADIN and other coumarin anticoagulants act by inhibiting the synthesis of vitamin K dependent clotting factors, which include Factors II, VII, IX and X, and the anticoagulant proteins C and S. Half-lives of these clotting factors are as follows: Factor II - 60 hours, VII - 4-6 hours, IX - 24 hours, and X - 48-72 hours. The half-lives of proteins C and S are approximately 8 hours and 30 hours, respectively. The resultant *in vivo* effect is a sequential depression of Factors VII, IX, X and II activities. Vitamin K is an essential cofactor for the post ribosomal synthesis of the vitamin K dependent clotting factors. The vitamin promotes the biosynthesis of ∝-carboxyglutamic acid residues in the proteins which are essential for biological activity. Warfarin is thought to interfere with clotting factor synthesis by inhibition of the regeneration of vitamin K_1 epoxide. The degree of depression is dependent upon the dosage administered. Therapeutic doses of warfarin decrease the total amount of the active form of each vitamin K dependent clotting factor made by the liver by approximately 30% to 50%.

An anticoagulation effect generally occurs within 24 hours after drug administration. However, peak anticoagulant effect may be delayed 72 to 96 hours. The duration of action of a single dose of racemic warfarin is 2 to 5 days. The effects of COUMADIN may become more pronounced as effects of daily maintenance doses overlap. Anticoagulants have no direct effect on an established thrombus, nor do they reverse ischemic tissue damage. However, once a thrombus has occurred, the goal of anticoagulant treatment is to prevent further extension of the formed clot and prevent secondary thromboembolic complications which may result in serious and possibly fatal sequelae.

Pharmacokinetics: COUMADIN is a racemic mixture of the R- and S-enantiomers. The S-enantiomer exhibits 2-5 times more anticoagulant activity than the R-enantiomer in humans, but generally has a more rapid clearance.

Absorption: COUMADIN is essentially completely absorbed after oral administration with peak concentration generally attained within the first 4 hours.

Distribution: There are no differences in the apparent volumes of distribution after intravenous and oral administration of single doses of warfarin solution. Warfarin distributes into a relatively small apparent volume of distribution of about 0.14 liter/kg. A distribution phase lasting 6 to 12 hours is distinguishable after rapid intravenous or oral administration of an aqueous solution. Using a one compartment model, and assuming complete bioavailability, estimates of the volumes of distribution of R- and S-warfarin are similar to each other and to that of the racemate. Concentrations in fetal plasma approach the maternal values, but warfarin has not been found in human milk (see **WARNINGS: Lactation**). Approximately 99% of the drug is bound to plasma proteins.

Metabolism: The elimination of warfarin is almost entirely by metabolism. COUMADIN is stereoselectively metabolized by hepatic microsomal enzymes (cytochrome P-450) to inactive hydroxylated metabolites (predominant route) and by reductases to reduced metabolites (warfarin alcohols). The warfarin alcohols have minimal anticoagulant activity. The metabolites are principally excreted into the urine; and to a lesser extent into the bile. The metabolites of warfarin that have been identified include dehydrowarfarin, two diastereoisomer alcohols. 4-, 6-, 7-, 8- and 10-hydroxywarfarin. The cytochrome P-450 isozymes involved in the metabolism of warfarin include 2C9, 2C19, 2C8, 2C18, 1A2, and 3A4. 2C9 is likely to be the principal form of human liver P-450 which modulates the *in vivo* anticoagulant activity of warfarin.

Excretion: The terminal half-life of warfarin after a single dose is approximately one week; however, the effective half-life ranges from 20 to 60 hours, with a mean of about 40 hours. The clearance of R-warfarin is generally half that of S-warfarin, thus as the volumes of distribution are similar, the half-life of R-warfarin is longer than that of S-warfarin. The half-life of R-warfarin ranges from 37 to 89 hours, while that of S-warfarin ranges from 21 to 43 hours. Studies with radiolabeled drug have demonstrated that up to 92% of the orally administered dose is recovered in urine. Very little warfarin is excreted unchanged in urine. Urinary excretion is in the form of metabolites.

Elderly: Patients 60 years or older appear to exhibit greater than expected prothrombin time (PT)/International Normalized Ratio (INR) response to the anticoagulant effects of warfarin. The cause of the increased sensitivity to the anticoagulant effects of warfarin in this age group is unknown. This increased anticoagulant effect from warfarin may be due to a combination of pharmacokinetic and pharmacodynamic factors. Racemic warfarin clearance may be unchanged or reduced with increasing age. Limited information suggests there is no difference in the clearance of S-warfarin in the elderly versus young subjects. However, there may be a slight decrease in the clearance of R-warfarin in the elderly as compared to the young. Therefore, as patient age increases, a lower dose of warfarin is usually required to produce a therapeutic level of anticoagulation.

Asians: Asian patients may require lower initiation and maintenance doses of warfarin. One non-controlled study conducted in 151 Chinese outpatients reported a mean daily warfarin requirement of 3.3 ± 1.4 mg to achieve an INR of 2 to 2.5. These patients were stabilized on warfarin for various indications. Patient age was the most important determinant of warfarin requirement in Chinese patients with a progressively lower warfarin requirement with increasing age.

Renal Dysfunction: Renal clearance is considered to be a minor determinant of anticoagulant response to warfarin. No dosage adjustment is necessary for patients with renal failure.

Hepatic Dysfunction: Hepatic dysfunction can potentiate the response to warfarin through impaired synthesis of clotting factors and decreased metabolism of warfarin.

The administration of COUMADIN (Warfarin Sodium) via the intravenous (IV) route should provide the patient with the same concentration of an equal oral dose, but maximum plasma concentration will be reached earlier. However, the full anticoagulant effect of a dose of warfarin may not be achieved until 72-96 hours after dosing, indicating that the administration of IV COUMADIN (Warfarin Sodium) should not provide any increased biological effect or earlier onset of action.

Clinical Trials

Atrial Fibrillation (AF): In five prospective randomized controlled clinical trials involving 3711 patients with non-rheumatic AF, warfarin significantly reduced the risk of systemic thromboembolism including stroke (See Table 1). The risk reduction ranged from 60% to 86% in all except one trial (CAFA: 45%) which stopped early due to published positive results from two of these trials. The incidence of major bleeding in these trials ranged from 0.6 to 2.7% (See Table 1). Meta-analysis findings of these studies revealed that the effects of warfarin in reducing thromboembolic events including stroke were similar at either moderately high INR (2.0-4.5) or low INR (1.4-3.0). There was a significant reduction in minor bleeds at the low INR. Similar data from clinical studies in valvular atrial fibrillation patients are not available.

[See table 1 at left]

Myocardial Infarction: WARIS (The Warfarin Re-Infarction Study) was a double-blind, randomized study of 1214 patients 2 to 4 weeks post-infarction treated with warfarin to a target INR of 2.8 to 4.8. [But note that a lower INR was achieved and increased bleeding was associated with INR's above 4.0; (see **DOSAGE AND ADMINISTRATION**)]. The primary endpoint was a combination of total mortality and recurrent infarction. A secondary endpoint of cerebrovascular events was assessed. Mean follow-up of the patients was 37 months. The results for each endpoint separately, including an analysis of vascular death, are provided in the following table:

[See table 2 at left]

Mechanical and Bioprosthetic Heart Valves: In a prospective, randomized, open label, positive-controlled study (Mok et al, 1985) in 254 patients, the thromboembolic-free interval was found to be significantly greater in patients with mechanical prosthetic heart valves treated with warfarin alone compared with dipyridamole-aspirin ($p<0.005$) and pentoxifylline-aspirin ($p<0.05$) treated patients. Rates of thromboembolic events in these groups were 2.2, 8.6, and 7.9/100 patient years, respectively. Major bleeding rates were 2.5, 0.0, and 0.9/100 patient years, respectively.

In a prospective, open label, clinical trial (Saour et al, 1990) comparing moderate (INR 2.65) vs. high intensity (INR 9.0) warfarin therapies in 258 patients with mechanical prosthetic heart valves, thromboembolism occurred with similar frequency in the two groups (4.0 and 3.7 events/100 patient years, respectively). Major bleeding was more common in the high intensity group (2.1 events/100 patient years) vs. 0.95 events/100 patient years in the moderate intensity group.

In a randomized trial (Turpie et al, 1988) in 210 patients comparing two intensities of warfarin therapy (INR 2.0-2.25 vs. INR 2.5-4.0) for a three-month period following tissue heart valve replacement, thromboembolism occurred with similar frequency in the two groups (major embolic events 2.0% vs. 1.9%, respectively and minor embolic events 10.8% vs. 10.2%, respectively). Major bleeding complications were more frequent with the higher intensity (major hemorrhages 4.6%) vs. none in the lower intensity.

INDICATIONS AND USAGE

COUMADIN (Warfarin Sodium) is indicated for the prophylaxis and/or treatment of venous thrombosis and its extension, and pulmonary embolism.

COUMADIN is indicated for the prophylaxis and/or treatment of the thromboembolic complications associated with atrial fibrillation and/or cardiac valve replacement.

TABLE 1. CLINICAL STUDIES OF WARFARIN IN NON-RHEUMATIC AF PATIENTS*

Study	n				Thromboembolism		% Major Bleeding	
	Warfarin-Treated Patients	Control Patients	PT Ratio	INR	% Risk Reduction	*p*-value	Warfarin-Treated Patients	Control Patients
AFASAK	335	336	1.5-2.0	2.8-4.2	60	0.027	0.6	0.0
SPAF	210	211	1.3-1.8	2.0-4.5	67	0.01	1.9	1.9
BAATAF	212	208	1.2-1.5	1.5-2.7	86	<0.05	0.9	0.5
CAFA	187	191	1.3-1.6	2.0-3.0	45	0.25	2.7	0.5
SPINAF	260	265	1.2-1.5	1.4-2.8	79	0.001	2.3	1.5

* All study results of warfarin vs. control are based on intention-to-treat analysis and include ischemic stroke and systemic thromboembolism, excluding hemorrhage and transient ischemic attacks.

TABLE 2

Event	Warfarin (N=607)	Placebo (N=607)	RR (95% CI)	% Risk Reduction (*p*-value)
Total Patient Years of Follow-up	2018	1944		
Total Mortality	94 (4.7/100 py)	123 (6.3/100 py)	0.76 (0.60, 0.97)	24 (p=0.030)
Vascular Death	82 (4.1/100 py)	105 (5.4/100 py)	0.78 (0.60, 1.02)	22 (p=0.068)
Recurrent MI	82 (4.1/100 py)	124 (6.4/100 py)	0.66 (0.51, 0.85)	34 (p=0.001)
Cerebrovascular Event	20 (1.0/100 py)	44 (2.3/100 py)	0.46 (0.28, 0.75)	54 (p=0.002)

RR=Relative risk; Risk reduction=(I - RR); CI=Confidence interval; MI=Myocardial infarction; py=patient years

COUMADIN is indicated to reduce the risk of death, recurrent myocardial infarction, and thromboembolic events such as stroke or systemic embolization after myocardial infarction.

CONTRAINDICATIONS

Anticoagulation is contraindicated in any localized or general physical condition or personal circumstance in which the hazard of hemorrhage might be greater than the potential clinical benefits of anticoagulation, such as:

Pregnancy: COUMADIN (Warfarin Sodium) is contraindicated in women who are or may become pregnant because the drug passes through the placental barrier and may cause fatal hemorrhage to the fetus *in utero*. Furthermore, there have been reports of birth malformations in children born to mothers who have been treated with warfarin during pregnancy.

Embryopathy characterized by nasal hypoplasia with or without stippled epiphyses (chondrodysplasia punctata) has been reported in pregnant women exposed to warfarin during the first trimester. Central nervous system abnormalities also have been reported, including dorsal midline dysplasia characterized by agenesis of the corpus callosum, Dandy-Walker malformation, and midline cerebellar atrophy. Ventral midline dysplasia, characterized by optic atrophy, and eye abnormalities have been observed. Mental retardation, blindness, and other central nervous system abnormalities have been reported in association with second and third trimester exposure. Although rare, teratogenic reports following *in utero* exposure to warfarin include urinary tract anomalies such as single kidney, asplenia, anencephaly, spina bifida, cranial nerve palsy, hydrocephalus, cardiac defects and congenital heart disease, polydactyly, deformities of toes, diaphragmatic hernia, corneal leukoma, cleft palate, cleft lip, schizencephaly, and microcephaly.

Spontaneous abortion and stillbirth are known to occur and a higher risk of fetal mortality is associated with the use of warfarin. Low birth weight and growth retardation have also been reported.

Women of childbearing potential who are candidates for anticoagulant therapy should be carefully evaluated and the indications critically reviewed with the patient. If the patient becomes pregnant while taking this drug, she should be apprised of the potential risks to the fetus, and the possibility of termination of the pregnancy should be discussed in light of those risks.

Hemorrhagic tendencies or blood dyscrasias.

Recent or contemplated surgery of: (1) central nervous system; (2) eye; (3) traumatic surgery resulting in large open surfaces.

Bleeding tendencies associated with active ulceration or overt bleeding of: (1) gastrointestinal, genitourinary or respiratory tracts; (2) cerebrovascular hemorrhage; (3) aneurysms-cerebral, dissecting aorta; (4) pericarditis and pericardial effusions; (5) bacterial endocarditis.

Threatened abortion, eclampsia and preeclampsia.

Inadequate laboratory facilities.

Unsupervised patients with senility, alcoholism, or psychosis or other lack of patient cooperation.

Spinal puncture and other diagnostic or therapeutic procedures with potential for uncontrollable bleeding.

Miscellaneous: major regional, lumbar block anesthesia, malignant hypertension and known hypersensitivity to warfarin or to any other components of this product.

WARNINGS

The most serious risks associated with anticoagulant therapy with warfarin sodium are hemorrhage in any tissue or organ and, less frequently (<0.1%), necrosis and/or gangrene of skin and other tissues. The risk of hemorrhage is related to the level of intensity and the duration of anticoagulant therapy. Hemorrhage and necrosis have in some cases been reported to result in death or permanent disability. Necrosis appears to be associated with local thrombosis and usually appears within a few days of the start of anticoagulant therapy. In severe cases of necrosis, treatment through debridement or amputation of the affected tissue, limb, breast or penis has been reported. Careful diagnosis is required to determine whether necrosis is caused by an underlying disease. Warfarin therapy should be discontinued when warfarin is suspected to be the cause of developing necrosis and heparin therapy may be considered for anticoagulation. Although various treatments have been attempted, no treatment for necrosis has been considered uniformly effective. See below for information on predisposing conditions. These and other risks associated with anticoagulant therapy must be weighed against the risk of thrombosis or embolization in untreated cases.

It cannot be emphasized too strongly that treatment of each patient is a highly individualized matter. COUMADIN (Warfarin Sodium), a narrow therapeutic range (index) drug, may be affected by factors such as other drugs and dietary Vitamin K. Dosage should be controlled by periodic determinations of PT/INR or other suitable coagulation tests. Determinations of whole blood clotting and bleeding times are not effective measures for control of therapy. Heparin prolongs the one-stage PT. When heparin and COUMADIN are administered concomitantly, refer below to CONVERSION FROM HEPARIN THERAPY for recommendations.

Caution should be observed when COUMADIN is administered in any situation or in the presence of any predisposing condition where added risk of hemorrhage, necrosis, and/or gangrene is present.

Anticoagulation therapy with COUMADIN may enhance the release of atheromatous plaque emboli, thereby increasing the risk of complications from systemic cholesterol microembolization, including the "purple toes syndrome." Discontinuation of COUMADIN therapy is recommended when such phenomena are observed.

ENDOGENOUS FACTORS:

blood dyscrasias— see CONTRAINDICATIONS	diarrhea	hyperthyroidism
cancer	elevated temperature	poor nutritional state
collagen vascular disease	hepatic disorders	steatorrhea
congestive heart failure	infectious hepatitis	vitamin K deficiency
	jaundice	

EXOGENOUS FACTORS:

Potential drug interactions with COUMADIN are listed below by drug class and by specific drugs.

Classes of Drugs

5-lipoxygenase Inhibitor	Antineoplastics†	Fibric Acid Derivatives
Adrenergic Stimulants, Central	Antiparasitic/Antimicrobials	HMG-CoA Reductase Inhibitors†
Alcohol Abuse Reduction Preparations	Antiplatelet Drugs/Effects	Leukotriene Receptor Antagonist
Analgesics	Antithyroid Drugs†	Monoamine Oxidase Inhibitors
Anesthetics, Inhalation	Beta-Adrenergic Blockers	Narcotics, prolonged
Antiandrogen	Cholelitholytic Agents	Nonsteroidal Anti-Inflammatory Agents
Antiarrhythmics†	Diabetes Agents, Oral	Psychostimulants
Antibiotics†	Diuretics†	Pyrazolones
Aminoglycosides (oral)	Fungal Medications, Intravaginal, Systemic†	Salicylates
Cephalosporins, parenteral	Gastric Acidity and Peptic Ulcer Agents†	Selective Serotonin Reuptake Inhibitors
Macrolides	Gastrointestinal	Steroids, Adrenocortical†
Miscellaneous	Prokinetic Agents	Steroids, Anabolic (17-Alkyl Testosterone Derivatives)
Penicillins, intravenous, high dose	Ulcerative Colitis Agents	Thrombolytics
Quinolones (fluoroquinolones)	Gout Treatment Agents	Thyroid Drugs
Sulfonamides, long acting	Hemorrheologic Agents	Tuberculosis Agents†
Tetracyclines	Hepatotoxic Drugs	Uricosuric Agents
Anticoagulants	Hyperglycemic Agents	Vaccines
Anticonvulsants†	Hypertensive Emergency Agents	Vitamins†
Antidepressants†	Hypnotics†	
Antimalarial Agents	Hypolipidemics†	
	Bile Acid-Binding Resins†	

Specific Drugs Reported

acetaminophen	fluconazole	penicillin G, intravenous
alcohol†	fluorouracil	pentoxifylline
allopurinol	fluoxetine	phenylbutazone
aminosalicylic acid	flutamide	phenytoin†
amiodarone HCl	fluvastatin	piperacillin
aspirin	fluvoxamine	piroxicam
atorvastatin†	gemfibrozil	pravastatin†
azithromycin	glucagon	prednisone†
capecitabine	halothane	propafenone
cefamandole	heparin	propoxyphene
cefazolin	ibuprofen	propranolol
cefoperazone	ifosfamide	propylthiouracil†
cefotetan	indomethacin	quinidine
cefoxitin	influenza virus vaccine	quinine
ceftriaxone	itraconazole	ranitidine†
celecoxib	ketoprofen	rofecoxib
cerivastatin	ketorolac	sertraline
chenodiol	levamisole	simvastatin
chloramphenicol	levofloxacin	stanozolol
chloral hydrate†	levothyroxine	streptokinase
chlorpropamide	liothyronine	sulfamethizole
cholestyramine†	lovastatin	sulfamethoxazole
cimetidine	mefenamic acid	sulfinpyrazone
ciprofloxacin	methimazole†	sulfisoxazole
cisapride	methyldopa	sulindac
clarithromycin	methylphenidate	tamoxifen
clofibrate	methylsalicylate ointment (topical)	tetracycline
COUMADIN overdose	metronidazole	thyroid
cyclophosphamide†	miconazole (intravaginal, systemic)	ticarcillin
danazol	moricizine hydrochloride†	ticlopidine
dextran	nalidixic acid	tissue plasminogen activator (t-PA)
dextrothyroxine	naproxen	tolbutamide
diazoxide	neomycin	tramadol
diclofenac	norfloxacin	trimethoprim/sulfamethoxazole
dicumarol	ofloxacin	urokinase
diflunisal	olsalazine	valproate
disulfiram	omeprazole	vitamin E
doxycycline	oxaprozin	zafirlukast
erythromycin	oxymetholone	zileuton
ethacrynic acid	paroxetine	
fenofibrate		
fenoprofen		

also: other medications affecting blood elements which may modify hemostasis
dietary deficiencies
prolonged hot weather
unreliable PT/INR determinations

†Increased and decreased PT/INR responses have been reported.

Systemic atheroemboli and cholesterol microemboli can present with a variety of signs and symptoms including purple toes syndrome, livedo reticularis, rash, gangrene, abrupt and intense pain in the leg, foot, or toes, foot ulcers, myalgia, penile gangrene, abdominal pain, flank or back pain, hematuria, renal insufficiency, hypertension, cerebral ischemia, spinal cord infarction, pancreatitis, symptoms simulating polyarteritis, or any other sequelae of vascular compromise due to embolic occlusion. The most commonly involved visceral organs are the kidneys followed by the pancreas, spleen, and liver. Some cases have progressed to necrosis or death.

Purple toes syndrome is a complication of oral anticoagulation characterized by a dark, purplish or mottled color of the toes, usually occurring between 3-10 weeks, or later, after the initiation of therapy with warfarin or related compounds. Major features of this syndrome include purple color of plantar surfaces and sides of the toes that blanches on moderate pressure and fades with elevation of the legs; pain and tenderness of the toes; waxing and waning of the color over time. While the purple toes syndrome is reported to be reversible, some cases progress to gangrene or necrosis which may require debridement of the affected area, or may lead to amputation.

Continued on next page

Coumadin—Cont.

Heparin-induced thrombocytopenia: COUMADIN (Warfarin Sodium) should be used with caution in patients with heparin-induced thrombocytopenia and deep venous thrombosis. Cases of venous limb ischemia, necrosis, and gangrene have occurred in patients with heparin-induced thrombocytopenia and deep venous thrombosis when heparin treatment was discontinued and warfarin therapy was started or continued. In some patients sequelae have included amputation of the involved area and/or death (Warkentin et al, 1997).

A severe elevation (>50 seconds) in activated partial thromboplastin time (aPTT) with a PT/INR in the desired range has been identified as an indication of increased risk of postoperative hemorrhage.

The decision to administer anticoagulants in the following conditions must be based upon clinical judgment in which the risks of anticoagulant therapy are weighed against the benefits:

Lactation: Based on very limited published data, warfarin has not been detected in the breast milk of mothers treated with warfarin. The same limited published data reports that some breast-fed infants, whose mothers were treated with warfarin, had prolonged prothrombin times, although not as prolonged as those of the mothers. The decision to breast-feed should be undertaken only after careful consideration of the available alternatives. Women who are breast-feeding and anticoagulated with warfarin should be very carefully monitored so that recommended PT/INR values are not exceeded. It is prudent to perform coagulation tests and to evaluate vitamin K status in infants at risk for bleeding tendencies before advising women taking warfarin to breast-feed. Effects in premature infants have not been evaluated.

Severe to moderate hepatic or renal insufficiency.

Infectious diseases or disturbances of intestinal flora: sprue, antibiotic therapy.

Trauma which may result in internal bleeding.

Surgery or trauma resulting in large exposed raw surfaces.

Indwelling catheters.

Severe to moderate hypertension.

Known or suspected deficiency in protein C mediated anticoagulant response: Hereditary or acquired deficiencies of protein C or its cofactor, protein S, have been associated with tissue necrosis following warfarin administration. Not all patients with these conditions develop necrosis, and tissue necrosis occurs in patients without these deficiencies. Inherited resistance to activated protein C has been described in many patients with venous thromboembolic disorders but has not yet been evaluated as a risk factor for tissue necrosis. The risk associated with these conditions, both for recurrent thrombosis and for adverse reactions, is difficult to evaluate since it does not appear to be the same for everyone. Decisions about testing and therapy must be made on an individual basis. It has been reported that concomitant anticoagulation therapy with heparin for 5 to 7 days during initiation of therapy with COUMADIN may minimize the incidence of tissue necrosis. Warfarin therapy should be discontinued when warfarin is suspected to be the cause of developing necrosis and heparin therapy may be considered for anticoagulation.

Miscellaneous: polycythemia vera, vasculitis, and severe diabetes.

Minor and severe allergic/hypersensitivity reactions and anaphylactic reactions have been reported.

In patients with acquired or inherited warfarin resistance, decreased therapeutic responses to COUMADIN have been reported. Exaggerated therapeutic responses have been reported in other patients.

Patients with congestive heart failure may exhibit greater than expected PT/INR response to COUMADIN, thereby requiring more frequent laboratory monitoring, and reduced doses of COUMADIN (Warfarin Sodium).

Concomitant use of anticoagulants with streptokinase or urokinase is not recommended and may be hazardous. (Please note recommendations accompanying these preparations.)

PRECAUTIONS

Periodic determination of PT/INR or other suitable coagulation test is essential.

Numerous factors, alone or in combination, including travel, changes in diet, environment, physical state and medications, including botanicals, may influence response of the patient to anticoagulants. It is generally good practice to monitor the patient's response with additional PT/INR determinations in the period immediately after discharge from the hospital, and whenever other medications, including botanicals, are initiated, discontinued or taken irregularly. The following factors are listed for reference; however, other factors may also affect the anticoagulant response.

Drugs may interact with COUMADIN through pharmacodynamic or pharmacokinetic mechanisms. Pharmacodynamic mechanisms for drug interactions with COUMADIN are synergism (impaired hemostasis, reduced clotting factor synthesis), competitive antagonism (vitamin K), and altered physiologic control loop for vitamin K metabolism (hereditary resistance). Pharmacokinetic mechanisms for drug interactions with COUMADIN are mainly enzyme induction, enzyme inhibition, and reduced plasma protein binding. It is important to note that some drugs may interact by more than one mechanism.

The following factors, alone or in combination, may be responsible for INCREASED PT/INR response:

[See table at top of previous page]

The following factors, alone or in combination, may be responsible for DECREASED PT/INR response:

ENDOGENOUS FACTORS:

edema	hypothyroidism
hereditary coumarin resistance	nephrotic syndrome
hyperlipemia	

EXOGENOUS FACTORS:

Potential drug interactions with COUMADIN (Warfarin Sodium) are listed below by drug class and by specific drugs.

[See table below]

Because a patient may be exposed to a combination of the above factors, the net effect of COUMADIN (Warfarin Sodium) on PT/INR response may be unpredictable. More frequent PT/INR monitoring is therefore advisable. Medications of unknown interaction with coumarins are best regarded with caution. When these medications are started or stopped, more frequent PT/INR monitoring is advisable.

It has been reported that concomitant administration of warfarin and ticlopidine may be associated with cholestatic hepatitis.

Botanical (Herbal) Medicines: Caution should be exercised when botanical medicines (botanicals) are taken concomitantly with COUMADIN (Warfarin Sodium). Few adequate, well-controlled studies exist evaluating the potential for metabolic and/or pharmacologic interactions between botanicals and COUMADIN. Due to a lack of manufacturing standardization with botanical medicinal preparations, the amount of active ingredients may vary. This could further confound the ability to assess potential interactions and effects on anticoagulation. It is good practice to monitor the patient's response with additional PT/INR determinations when initiating or discontinuing botanicals.

Specific botanicals reported to affect COUMADIN therapy include the following:

- Bromelains, danshen, dong quai *(Angelica sinensis)*, garlic, Ginkgo biloba, and ginseng are associated most often with an INCREASE in the effects of COUMADIN.
- Coenzyme Q_{10} (ubidecarenone) and St. John's wort are associated most often with a DECREASE in the effects of COUMADIN.

Some botanicals may cause bleeding events when taken alone (e.g., garlic and Ginkgo biloba) and may have anticoagulant, antiplatelet, and/or fibrinolytic properties. These effects would be expected to be additive to the anticoagulant effects of COUMADIN. Conversely, other botanicals may have coagulant properties when taken alone or may decrease the effects of COUMADIN.

Some botanicals that may affect coagulation are listed below for reference; however, this list should not be considered all-inclusive. Many botanicals have several common names and scientific names. The most widely recognized common botanical names are listed.

[See first table at top of next page]

Effect on Other Drugs: Coumarins may also affect the action of other drugs. Hypoglycemic agents (chlorpropamide and tolbutamide) and anticonvulsants (phenytoin and phenobarbital) may accumulate in the body as a result of interference with either their metabolism or excretion.

Special Risk Patients: COUMADIN (Warfarin Sodium) is a narrow therapeutic range (index) drug, and caution should be observed when warfarin sodium is administered to certain patients such as the elderly or debilitated or when administered in any situation or physical condition where added risk of hemorrhage is present.

Intramuscular (I.M.) injections of concomitant medications should be confined to the upper extremities which permits easy access for manual compression, inspections for bleeding and use of pressure bandages.

Caution should be observed when COUMADIN (or warfarin) is administered concomitantly with nonsteroidal anti-inflammatory drugs (NSAIDs), including aspirin, to be certain that no change in anticoagulation dosage is required. In addition to specific drug interactions that might affect PT/INR, NSAIDs, including aspirin, can inhibit platelet aggregation, and can cause gastrointestinal bleeding, peptic ulceration and/or perforation.

Acquired or inherited warfarin resistance should be suspected if large daily doses of COUMADIN (Warfarin Sodium) are required to maintain a patient's PT/INR within a normal therapeutic range.

Information for Patients: The objective of anticoagulant therapy is to decrease the clotting ability of the blood so that thrombosis is prevented, while avoiding spontaneous bleeding. Effective therapeutic levels with minimal complications are in part dependent upon cooperative and well-instructed patients who communicate effectively with their physician. Patients should be advised: Strict adherence to prescribed dosage schedule is necessary. Do not take or discontinue any other medication, including salicylates (e.g., aspirin and topical analgesics), other over-the-counter medications, and botanical (herbal) products (e.g., bromelains, coenzyme Q_{10}, danshen, dong quai, garlic, Ginkgo biloba, ginseng, and St. John's wort) except on advice of the physician. Avoid alcohol consumption. Do not take COUMADIN during pregnancy and do not become pregnant while taking it (see **CONTRAINDICATIONS**). Avoid any activity or sport that may result in traumatic injury. Prothrombin time tests and regular visits to physician or clinic are needed to monitor therapy. Carry identification stating that COUMADIN is being taken. If the prescribed dose of COUMADIN is forgotten, notify the physician immediately. Take the dose as soon as possible on the same day but do not take a double dose of COUMADIN the next day to make up for missed doses. The amount of vitamin K in food may affect therapy with COUMADIN. Eat a normal, balanced diet maintaining a consistent amount of vitamin K. Avoid drastic changes in dietary habits, such as eating large amounts of green leafy vegetables. Contact physician to report any illness, such as diarrhea, infection or fever. Notify physician immediately if any unusual bleeding or symptoms occur. Signs and symptoms of bleeding include: pain, swelling or discomfort, prolonged bleeding from cuts, increased menstrual flow or vaginal bleeding, nosebleeds, bleeding of gums from brushing, unusual bleeding or bruising, red or dark brown urine, red or tar black stools, headache, dizziness, or weakness. If therapy with COUMADIN is discontinued, patients should be cautioned that the anticoagulant effects of COUMADIN may persist for about 2 to 5 days. **Patients should be informed that all warfarin sodium, USP, products represent the same medication, and should not be taken concomitantly, as overdosage may result.**

Carcinogenesis, Mutagenesis, Impairment of Fertility: Carcinogenicity and mutagenicity studies have not been performed with COUMADIN. The reproductive effects of COUMADIN have not been evaluated.

Classes of Drugs

Adrenal Corticol Steroid Inhibitors	Antithyroid Drugs†	HMG-CoA Reductase Inhibitors†
Antacids	Barbiturates	Immunosuppressives
Antianxiety Agents	Diuretics†	Oral Contraceptives, Estrogen Containing
Antiarrhythmics†	Enteral Nutritional Supplements	Selective Estrogen Receptor Modulators
Antibiotics†	Fungal Medications, Systemic†	Steroids, Adrenocortical†
Anticonvulsants†	Gastric Acidity and Peptic Ulcer Agents†	Tuberculosis Agents†
Antidepressants†	Hypnotics†	Vitamins†
Antihistamines	Hypolipidemics†	
Antineoplastics†	Bile Acid-Binding Resins†	
Antipsychotic Medications		

Specific Drugs Reported

alcohol†	COUMADIN underdosage	phenytoin†
aminoglutethimide	cyclophosphamide†	pravastatin†
amobarbital	dicloxacillin	prednisone†
atorvastatin†	ethchlorvynol	primidone
azathioprine	glutethimide	propylthiouracil†
butabarbital	griseofulvin	raloxifene
butalbital	haloperidol	ranitidine†
carbamazepine	meprobamate	rifampin
chloral hydrate†	6-mercaptopurine	secobarbital
chlordiazepoxide	methimazole†	spironolactone
chlorthalidone	moricizine hydrochloride†	sucralfate
cholestyramine†	nafcillin	trazodone
clozapine	paraldehyde	vitamin C (high dose)
corticotropin	pentobarbital	vitamin K
cortisone	phenobarbital	

also: diet high in vitamin K
unreliable PT/INR determinations

†Increased and decreased PT/INR responses have been reported.

Use in Pregnancy: Pregnancy Category X—See **CONTRAINDICATIONS.**

Pediatric Use: Safety and effectiveness in pediatric patients below the age of 18 have not been established, in randomized, controlled clinical trials. However, the use of COUMADIN in pediatric patients is well-documented for the prevention and treatment of thromboembolic events. Difficulty achieving and maintaining therapeutic PT/INR ranges in the pediatric patient has been reported. More frequent PT/INR determinations are recommended because of possible changing warfarin requirements.

Geriatric Use: Patients 60 years or older appear to exhibit greater than expected PT/INR response to the anticoagulant effects of warfarin (see **CLINICAL PHARMACOLOGY**). COUMADIN is contraindicated in any unsupervised patient with senility. Caution should be observed with administration of warfarin sodium to elderly patients in any situation or physical condition where added risk of hemorrhage is present. Lower initiation and maintenance doses of COUMADIN are recommended for elderly patients (see **DOSAGE AND ADMINISTRATION**).

ADVERSE REACTIONS

Potential adverse reactions to COUMADIN (Warfarin Sodium) may include:

- Fatal or nonfatal hemorrhage from any tissue or organ. This is a consequence of the anticoagulant effect. The signs, symptoms, and severity will vary according to the location and degree or extent of the bleeding. Hemorrhagic complications may present as paralysis; paresthesia; headache, chest, abdomen, joint, muscle or other pain; dizziness; shortness of breath, difficult breathing or swallowing; unexplained swelling; weakness; hypotension; or unexplained shock. Therefore, the possibility of hemorrhage should be considered in evaluating the condition of any anticoagulated patient with complaints which do not indicate an obvious diagnosis. Bleeding during anticoagulant therapy does not always correlate with PT/INR. (See **OVERDOSAGE: Treatment.**)
- Bleeding which occurs when the PT/INR is within the therapeutic range warrants diagnostic investigation since it may unmask a previously unsuspected lesion, e.g., tumor, ulcer, etc.
- Necrosis of skin and other tissues. (See **WARNINGS.**)
- Adverse reactions reported infrequently include: hypersensitivity/allergic reactions, systemic cholesterol microembolization, purple toes syndrome, hepatitis, cholestatic hepatic injury, jaundice, elevated liver enzymes, vasculitis, edema, fever, rash, dermatitis, including bullous eruptions, urticaria, abdominal pain including cramping, flatulence/bloating, fatigue, lethargy, malaise, asthenia, nausea, vomiting, diarrhea, pain, headache, dizziness, taste perversion, pruritus, alopecia, cold intolerance, and paresthesia including feeling cold and chills.

Rare events of tracheal or tracheobronchial calcification have been reported in association with long-term warfarin therapy. The clinical significance of this event is unknown. Priapism has been associated with anticoagulant administration, however, a causal relationship has not been established.

OVERDOSAGE

Signs and Symptoms: Suspected or overt abnormal bleeding (e.g., appearance of blood in stools or urine, hematuria, excessive menstrual bleeding, melena, petechiae, excessive bruising or persistent oozing from superficial injuries) are early manifestations of anticoagulation beyond a safe and satisfactory level.

Treatment: Excessive anticoagulation, with or without bleeding, may be controlled by discontinuing COUMADIN therapy and if necessary, by administration of oral or parenteral vitamin K_1. (Please see recommendations accompanying vitamin K_1 preparations prior to use.)

Such use of vitamin K_1 reduces response to subsequent COUMADIN therapy. Patients may return to a pretreatment thrombotic status following the rapid reversal of a prolonged PT/INR. Resumption of COUMADIN (Warfarin Sodium) administration reverses the effect of vitamin K, and a therapeutic PT/INR can again be obtained by careful dosage adjustment. If rapid anticoagulation is indicated, heparin may be preferable for initial therapy.

If minor bleeding progresses to major bleeding, give 5 to 25 mg (rarely up to 50 mg) parenteral vitamin K_1. In emergency situations of severe hemorrhage, clotting factors can be returned to normal by administering 200 to 500 mL of fresh whole blood or fresh frozen plasma, or by giving commercial Factor IX complex.

A risk of hepatitis and other viral diseases is associated with the use of these blood products; Factor IX complex is also associated with an increased risk of thrombosis. Therefore, these preparations should be used only in exceptional or life-threatening bleeding episodes secondary to COUMADIN (Warfarin Sodium) overdosage.

Purified Factor IX preparations should not be used because they cannot increase the levels of prothrombin, Factor VII and Factor X which are also depressed along with the levels of Factor IX as a result of COUMADIN treatment. Packed red blood cells may also be given if significant blood loss has occurred. Infusions of blood or plasma should be monitored carefully to avoid precipitating pulmonary edema in elderly patients or patients with heart disease.

DOSAGE AND ADMINISTRATION

The dosage and administration of COUMADIN must be individualized for each patient according to the particular pa-

Botanicals that contain coumarins with potential anticoagulant effects:

Alfalfa	Celery	Parsley
Angelica (Dong Quai)	Chamomile (German and Roman)	Passion Flower
Aniseed	Dandelion[3]	Prickly Ash (Northern)
Arnica	Fenugreek	Quassia
Asa Foetida	Horse Chestnut	Red Clover
Bogbean[1]	Horseradish	Sweet Clover
Boldo	Licorice[3]	Sweet Woodruff
Buchu	Meadowsweet[1]	Tonka Beans
Capsicum[2]	Nettle	Wild Carrot
Cassia[3]		Wild Lettuce

Miscellaneous botanicals with anticoagulant properties:

Bladder Wrack (*Fucus*)	Pau d'arco	

Botanicals that contain salicylate and/or have antiplatelet properties:

Agrimony[4]	Dandelion[3]	Meadowsweet[1]
Aloe Gel	Feverfew	Onion[5]
Aspen	Garlic[5]	Policosanol
Black Cohosh	German Sarsaparilla	Poplar
Black Haw	Ginger	Senega
Bogbean[1]	Ginkgo Biloba	Tamarind
Cassia[3]	Ginseng (*Panax*)[5]	Willow
Clove	Licorice[3]	Wintergreen

Botanicals with fibrinolytic properties:

Bromelains	Garlic[5]	Inositol Nicotinate
Capsicum[2]	Ginseng (*Panax*)[5]	Onion[5]

Botanicals with coagulant properties:

Agrimony[4]	Mistletoe	Yarrow
Goldenseal		

[1]Contains coumarins and salicylate.
[2]Contains coumarins and has fibrinolytic properties.
[3]Contains coumarins and has antiplatelet properties.
[4]Contains salicylate and has coagulant properties.
[5]Has antiplatelet and fibrinolytic properties.

TABLE 3
Relationship Between INR and PT Ratios For Thromboplastins With Different ISI Values (Sensitivities)

	PT RATIOS				
	ISI 1.0	ISI 1.4	ISI 1.8	ISI 2.3	ISI 2.8
INR = 2.0-3.0	2.0-3.0	1.6-2.2	1.5-1.8	1.4-1.6	1.3-1.5
INR = 2.5-3.5	2.5-3.5	1.9-2.4	1.7-2.0	1.5-1.7	1.4-1.6

tient's PT/INR response to the drug. The dosage should be adjusted based upon the patient's PT/INR. (See **LABORATORY CONTROL** below for full discussion on INR.)

Venous Thromboembolism (including pulmonary embolism): Available clinical evidence indicates that an INR of 2.0-3.0 is sufficient for prophylaxis and treatment of venous thromboembolism and minimizes the risk of hemorrhage associated with higher INRs. In patients with risk factors for recurrent venous thromboembolism including venous insufficiency, inherited thrombophilia, idiopathic venous thromboembolism, and a history of thrombotic events, consideration should be given to longer term therapy (Schulman et al, 1995 and Schulman et al, 1997).

Atrial Fibrillation: Five recent clinical trials evaluated the effects of warfarin in patients with non-valvular atrial fibrillation (AF). Meta-analysis findings of these studies revealed that the effects of warfarin in reducing thromboembolic events including stroke were similar at either moderately high INR (2.0-4.5) or low INR (1.4-3.0). There was a significant reduction in minor bleeds at the low INR. Similar data from clinical studies in valvular atrial fibrillation patients are not available. The trials in non-valvular atrial fibrillation support the American College of Chest Physicians' (ACCP) recommendation that an INR of 2.0-3.0 be used for long term warfarin therapy in appropriate AF patients.

Post-Myocardial Infarction: In post-myocardial infarction patients, COUMADIN (Warfarin Sodium) therapy should be initiated early (2-4 weeks post-infarction) and dosage should be adjusted to maintain an INR of 2.5-3.5 long-term. The recommendation is based on the results of the WARIS study in which treatment was initiated 2 to 4 weeks after the infarction. In patients thought to be at an increased risk of bleeding complications or on aspirin therapy, maintenance of COUMADIN therapy at the lower end of this INR range is recommended.

Mechanical and Bioprosthetic Heart Valves: In patients with mechanical heart valve(s), long term prophylaxis with warfarin to an INR of 2.5-3.5 is recommended. In patients with bioprosthetic heart valve(s), based on limited data, the American College of Chest Physicians recommends warfarin therapy to an INR of 2.0-3.0 for 12 weeks after valve insertion. In patients with additional risk factors such as atrial fibrillation or prior thromboembolism, consideration should be given for longer term therapy.

Recurrent Systemic Embolism: In cases where the risk of thromboembolism is great, such as in patients with recurrent systemic embolism, a higher INR may be required.

An INR of greater than 4.0 appears to provide no additional therapeutic benefit in most patients and is associated with a higher risk of bleeding.

Initial Dosage: The dosing of COUMADIN must be individualized according to patient's sensitivity to the drug as indicated by the PT/INR. Use of a large loading dose may increase the incidence of hemorrhagic and other complications, does not offer more rapid protection against thrombi formation, and is not recommended. Lower initiation and maintenance doses are recommended for elderly and/or debilitated patients and patients with potential to exhibit greater than expected PT/INR response to COUMADIN (see **PRECAUTIONS**). Based on limited data, Asian patients may also require lower initiation and maintenance doses of COUMADIN (see **CLINICAL PHARMACOLOGY**). It is recommended that COUMADIN therapy be initiated with a dose of 2 to 5 mg per day with dosage adjustments based on the results of PT/INR determinations.

Maintenance: Most patients are satisfactorily maintained at a dose of 2 to 10 mg daily. Flexibility of dosage is provided by breaking scored tablets in half. The individual dose and interval should be gauged by the patient's prothrombin response.

Duration of Therapy: The duration of therapy in each patient should be individualized. In general, anticoagulant therapy should be continued until the danger of thrombosis and embolism has passed.

Missed Dose: The anticoagulant effect of COUMADIN persists beyond 24 hours. If the patient forgets to take the prescribed dose of COUMADIN at the scheduled time, the dose should be taken as soon as possible on the same day. The patient should not take the missed dose by doubling the daily dose to make up for missed doses, but should refer back to his or her physician.

Intravenous Route of Administration: COUMADIN for Injection provides an alternate administration route for patients who cannot receive oral drugs. The IV dosages would be the same as those that would be used orally if the patient could take the drug by the oral route. COUMADIN (Warfarin Sodium) for Injection should be administered as a slow

Continued on next page

	100's	1000's	Hospital Unit-Dose Blister Package of 100
1 mg pink	NDC 0056-0169-70	NDC 0056-0169-90	NDC 0056-0169-75
2 mg lavender	NDC 0056-0170-70	NDC 0056-0170-90	NDC 0056-0170-75
2-1/2 mg green	NDC 0056-0176-70	NDC 0056-0176-90	NDC 0056-0176-75
3 mg tan	NDC 0056-0188-70	NDC 0056-0188-90	NDC 0056-0188-75
4 mg blue	NDC 0056-0168-70	NDC 0056-0168-90	NDC 0056-0168-75
5 mg peach	NDC 0056-0172-70	NDC 0056-0172-90	NDC 0056-0172-75
6 mg teal	NDC 0056-0189-70	NDC 0056-0189-90	NDC 0056-0189-75
7-1/2 mg yellow	NDC 0056-0173-70		NDC 0056-0173-75
10 mg white (Dye Free)	NDC 0056-0174-70		NDC 0056-0174-75

Coumadin—Cont.

bolus injection over 1 to 2 minutes into a peripheral vein. It is not recommended for intramuscular administration. The vial should be reconstituted with 2.7 mL of sterile Water for Injection and inspected for particulate matter and discoloration immediately prior to use. Do not use if either particulate matter and/or discoloration is noted. After reconstitution, COUMADIN for Injection is chemically and physically stable for 4 hours at room temperature. It does not contain any antimicrobial preservative and, thus, care must be taken to assure the sterility of the prepared solution. The vial is not recommended for multiple use and unused solution should be discarded.

LABORATORY CONTROL: The PT reflects the depression of vitamin K dependent Factors VII, X and II. There are several modifications of the one-stage PT and the physician should become familiar with the specific method used in his laboratory. The degree of anticoagulation indicated by any range of PTs may be altered by the type of thromboplastin used; the appropriate therapeutic range must be based on the experience of each laboratory. The PT should be determined daily after the administration of the initial dose until PT/INR results stabilize in the therapeutic range. Intervals between subsequent PT/INR determinations should be based upon the physician's judgment of the patient's reliability and response to COUMADIN in order to maintain the individual within the therapeutic range. Acceptable intervals for PT/INR determinations are normally within the range of one to four weeks after a stable dosage has been determined. To ensure adequate control, it is recommended that additional PT tests are done when other warfarin products are interchanged with warfarin sodium tablets, USP, as well as whenever other medications are initiated, discontinued, or taken irregularly (see **PRECAUTIONS**).

Different thromboplastin reagents vary substantially in their sensitivity to sodium warfarin-induced effects on PT. To define the appropriate therapeutic regimen it is important to be familiar with the sensitivity of the thromboplastin reagent used in the laboratory and its relationship to the International Reference Preparation (IRP), a sensitive thromboplastin reagent prepared from human brain.

A system of standardizing the PT in oral anticoagulant control was introduced by the World Health Organization in 1983. It is based upon the determination of an International Normalized Ratio (INR) which provides a common basis for communication of PT results and interpretations of therapeutic ranges. The INR system of reporting is based on a logarithmic relationship between the PT ratios of the test and reference preparation. The INR is the PT ratio that would be obtained if the International Reference Preparation (IRP), which has an ISI of 1.0, was used to perform the test. Early clinical studies of oral anticoagulants, which formed the basis for recommended therapeutic ranges of 1.5 to 2.5 times control mean normal PT, used sensitive human brain thromboplastin. When using the less sensitive rabbit brain thromboplastins commonly employed in PT assays today, adjustments must be made to the targeted PT range that reflect this decrease in sensitivity.

The INR can be calculated as: $INR = (\text{observed PT ratio})^{ISI}$ where the ISI (International Sensitivity Index) is the correction factor in the equation that relates the PT ratio of the local reagent to the reference preparation and is a measure of the sensitivity of a given thromboplastin to reduction of vitamin K-dependent coagulation factors; the lower the ISI, the more "sensitive" the reagent and the closer the derived INR will be to the observed PT ratio.[1]

The proceedings and recommendations of the 1992 National Conference on Antithrombotic Therapy[2-4] review and evaluate issues related to oral anticoagulant therapy and the sensitivity of thromboplastin reagents and provide additional guidelines for defining the appropriate therapeutic regimen. The conversion of the INR to PT ratios for the less-intense (INR 2.0–3.0) and more intense (INR 2.5-3.5) therapeutic range recommended by the ACCP for thromboplastins over a range of ISI values is shown in Table 3.[5]

[See table 3 on previous page]

TREATMENT DURING DENTISTRY AND SURGERY The management of patients who undergo dental and surgical procedures requires close liaison between attending physicians, surgeons and dentists. PT/INR determination is recommended just prior to any dental or surgical procedure. In patients undergoing minimal invasive procedures who must be anticoagulated prior to, during, or immediately following these procedures, adjusting the dosage of COUMADIN (Warfarin Sodium) to maintain the PT/INR at the low end of the therapeutic range may safely allow for continued anticoagulation. The operative site should be sufficiently limited and accessible to permit the effective use of local procedures for hemostasis. Under these conditions, dental and minor surgical procedures may be performed without undue risk of hemorrhage. Some dental or surgical procedures may necessitate the interruption of COUMADIN therapy. When discontinuing COUMADIN even for a short period of time, the benefits and risks should be strongly considered.

CONVERSION FROM HEPARIN THERAPY Since the anticoagulant effect of COUMADIN is delayed, heparin is preferred initially for rapid anticoagulation. Conversion to COUMADIN may begin concomitantly with heparin therapy or may be delayed 3 to 6 days. To ensure continuous anticoagulation, it is advisable to continue full dose heparin therapy and that COUMADIN therapy be overlapped with heparin for 4 to 5 days, until COUMADIN (Warfarin Sodium) has produced the desired therapeutic response as determined by PT/INR. When COUMADIN has produced the desired PT/INR or prothrombin activity, heparin may be discontinued.

COUMADIN may increase the aPTT test, even in the absence of heparin. During initial therapy with COUMADIN, the interference with heparin anticoagulation is of minimal clinical significance.

As heparin may affect the PT/INR, patients receiving both heparin and COUMADIN should have blood for PT/INR determination drawn at least:

- 5 hours after the last IV bolus dose of heparin, or
- 4 hours after cessation of a continuous IV infusion of heparin, or
- 24 hours after the last subcutaneous heparin injection.

HOW SUPPLIED

Tablets: For oral use, single scored with one face imprinted numerically with 1, 2, 2-1/2, 3, 4, 5, 6, 7-1/2 or 10 superimposed and inscribed with "COUMADIN" and with the opposite face plain. COUMADIN is available in bottles and Hospital Unit-Dose Blister Packages with potencies and colors as follows:

[See table above]

Protect from light. Store at controlled room temperature (59°-86°F, 15°-30°C). Dispense in a tight, light-resistant container as defined in the USP.

Hospital Unit-Dose Blister Packages are to be stored in carton until contents have been used.

Injection: Available for intravenous use only. Not recommended for intramuscular administration. Reconstitute with 2.7 mL of sterile Water for Injection to yield 2 mg/mL. Net contents 5.4 mg lyophilized powder. Maximum yield 2.5 mL.

5 mg vial (box of 6) NDC 0590-0324-35

Protect from light. Keep vial in box until used. Store at controlled room temperature (59°-86°F, 15°-30°C).

After reconstitution, store at controlled room temperature (59°-86°F, 15°-30°C) and use within 4 hours. Do not refrigerate. Discard any unused solution.

REFERENCES

1. Poller, L.: Laboratory Control of Anticoagulant Therapy. Seminars in Thrombosis and Hemostasis, Vol. 12, No. 1, pp. 13–19, 1986. **2.** Hirsh, J.: Is the Dose of Warfarin Prescribed by American Physicians Unnecessarily High? *Arch Int Med*, Vol. 147, pp. 769–771, 1987. **3.** Cook, D.J., Guyatt, H.G., Laupacis, A., Sackett, D.L.: Rules of Evidence and Clinical Recommendations on the Use of Antithrombotic Agents. Chest ACCP Consensus Conference on Antithrombotic Therapy. *Chest*, Vol. 102(Suppl), pp. 305S-311S, 1992. **4.** Hirsh, J., Dalen, J., Deykin, D., Poller, L.: Oral Anticoagulants Mechanism of Action, Clinical Effectiveness, and Optimal Therapeutic Range. Chest ACCP Consensus Conference on Antithrombotic Therapy. *Chest*, Vol. 102(Suppl), pp. 312S-326S, 1992. **5.** Hirsh, J., M.D., F.C.C.P.: Hamilton Civic Hospitals Research Center, Hamilton, Ontario, Personal Communication.

Distributed by:
Bristol-Myers Squibb Company
Princeton, NJ 08543 U.S.A.

T1-B001-07-02 6572-01/Rev. June, 2002
Printed in U.S.A.

Shown in Product Identification Guide, page 310

ERBITUX™ ℞

[*ər-bĭ-tŭks*]
(Cetuximab)
℞ ONLY
For intravenous use only.

> **WARNING**
>
> **Infusion Reactions:** Severe infusion reactions occurred with the administration of ERBITUX in approximately 3% of patients, rarely with fatal outcome (<1 in 1000). Approximately 90% of severe infusion reactions were associated with the first infusion of ERBITUX. Severe infusion reactions are characterized by rapid onset of airway obstruction (bronchospasm, stridor, hoarseness), urticaria, and hypotension (see **WARNINGS** and **ADVERSE REACTIONS**). Severe infusion reactions require immediate interruption of the ERBITUX infusion and permanent discontinuation from further treatment. (See **WARNINGS: Infusion Reactions** and **DOSAGE AND ADMINISTRATION: Dose Modifications.**)

DESCRIPTION

ERBITUX™ (Cetuximab) is a recombinant, human/mouse chimeric monoclonal antibody that binds specifically to the extracellular domain of the human epidermal growth factor receptor (EGFR). ERBITUX is composed of the Fv regions of a murine anti-EGFR antibody with human IgG1 heavy and kappa light chain constant regions and has an approximate molecular weight of 152 kDa. ERBITUX is produced in mammalian (murine myeloma) cell culture.

ERBITUX is a sterile, clear, colorless liquid of pH 7.0 to 7.4, which may contain a small amount of easily visible, white, amorphous, Cetuximab particulates. Each single-use, 50-mL vial contains 100 mg of Cetuximab at a concentration of 2 mg/mL and is formulated in a preservative-free solution containing 8.48 mg/mL sodium chloride, 1.88 mg/mL sodium phosphate dibasic heptahydrate, 0.42 mg/mL sodium phosphate monobasic monohydrate, and Water for Injection, USP.

CLINICAL PHARMACOLOGY

General

ERBITUX binds specifically to the epidermal growth factor receptor (EGFR, HER1, c-ErbB-1) on both normal and tumor cells, and competitively inhibits the binding of epidermal growth factor (EGF) and other ligands, such as transforming growth factor–alpha. Binding of ERBITUX to the EGFR blocks phosphorylation and activation of receptor-associated kinases, resulting in inhibition of cell growth, induction of apoptosis, and decreased matrix metalloproteinase and vascular endothelial growth factor production. The EGFR is a transmembrane glycoprotein that is a member of a subfamily of type I receptor tyrosine kinases including EGFR (HER1), HER2, HER3, and HER4. The EGFR is constitutively expressed in many normal epithelial tissues, including the skin and hair follicle. Over-expression of EGFR is also detected in many human cancers including those of the colon and rectum.

In vitro assays and *in vivo* animal studies have shown that ERBITUX inhibits the growth and survival of tumor cells that over-express the EGFR. No anti-tumor effects of ERBITUX were observed in human tumor xenografts lacking EGFR expression. The addition of ERBITUX to irinotecan or irinotecan plus 5-fluorouracil in animal studies resulted in an increase in anti-tumor effects compared to chemotherapy alone.

Human Pharmacokinetics

ERBITUX administered as monotherapy or in combination with concomitant chemotherapy or radiotherapy exhibits nonlinear pharmacokinetics. The area under the concentration time curve (AUC) increased in a greater than dose proportional manner as the dose increased from 20 to 400 mg/m^2. ERBITUX clearance (CL) decreased from 0.08 to 0.02 L/h/m^2 as the dose increased from 20 to 200 mg/m^2, and at doses >200 mg/m^2, it appeared to plateau. The volume of the distribution (Vd) for ERBITUX appeared to be independent of dose and approximated the vascular space of 2-3 L/m^2.

Following a 2-hour infusion of 400 mg/m^2 of ERBITUX, the maximum mean serum concentration (C_{max}) was 184 µg/mL (range: 92-327 µg/mL) and the mean elimination half-life was 97 hours (range 41-213 hours). A 1-hour infusion of 250 mg/m^2 produced a mean C_{max} of 140 µg/mL (range 120-170 µg/mL). Following the recommended dose regimen (400 mg/m^2 initial dose/250 mg/m^2 weekly dose), ERBITUX concentrations reached steady-state levels by the third weekly infusion with mean peak and trough concentrations across studies ranging from 168 to 235 and 41 to 85 µg/mL, respectively. The mean half-life was 114 hours (range 75-188 hours).

Special Populations

A population pharmacokinetic analysis was performed to explore the potential effects of selected covariates including race, gender, age, and hepatic and renal function on ERBITUX pharmacokinetics.

Female patients had a 25% lower intrinsic ERBITUX clearance than male patients. The toxicity profile was similar in males and females. Definitive conclusions regarding the comparability in efficacy cannot be made given the small number of patients with objective tumor response.

ERBITUX has not been studied in pediatric populations.

CLINICAL STUDIES

The efficacy and safety of ERBITUX alone or in combination with irinotecan were studied in a randomized, controlled trial (329 patients) and in combination with irinotecan in an open-label, single-arm trial (138 patients). ERBITUX was further evaluated as a single agent in a third clinical trial (57 patients). Safety data from 111 patients treated with single-agent ERBITUX was also evaluated. All trials studied patients with EGFR-expressing metastatic colorectal cancer, whose disease had progressed after receiving an irinotecan-containing regimen.

Randomized, Controlled Trial

A multicenter, randomized, controlled clinical trial was conducted in 329 patients randomized to receive either ERBITUX plus irinotecan (218 patients) or ERBITUX monotherapy (111 patients). In both arms of the study, ERBITUX was administered as a 400 mg/m^2 initial dose, followed by 250 mg/m^2 weekly until disease progression or unacceptable toxicity. All patients received a 20-mg test dose on Day 1. In the ERBITUX plus irinotecan arm, irinotecan was added to ERBITUX using the same dose and schedule for irinotecan as the patient had previously failed. Acceptable irinotecan schedules were 350 mg/m^2 every 3 weeks, 180 mg/m^2 every 2 weeks, or 125 mg/m^2 weekly times four doses every 6 weeks. An Independent Radiographic Review Committee (IRC), blinded to the treatment arms, assessed both the progression on prior irinotecan and the response to protocol treatment for all patients.

Of the 329 randomized patients, 206 (63%) were male. The median age was 59 years (range 26-84), and the majority was Caucasian (323, 98%). Eighty-eight percent of patients had baseline Karnofsky Performance Status ≥80. Fifty-eight percent of patients had colon cancer and 40% rectal cancer. Approximately two-thirds (63%) of patients had previously failed oxaliplatin treatment.

The efficacy of ERBITUX plus irinotecan or ERBITUX monotherapy was evaluated in all randomized patients.

Analyses were also conducted in two pre-specified subpopulations: irinotecan refractory and irinotecan and oxaliplatin failures. The irinotecan refractory population was defined as randomized patients who had received at least two cycles of irinotecan-based chemotherapy prior to treatment with ERBITUX, and had independent confirmation of disease progression within 30 days of completion of the last cycle of irinotecan-based chemotherapy.

The irinotecan and oxaliplatin failure population was defined as irinotecan refractory patients who had previously been treated with and failed an oxaliplatin-containing regimen.

The objective response rates (ORR) in these populations are presented in Table 1.

[See table 1 above]

Table 1: Objective Response Rates per Independent Review

	ERBITUX + Irinotecan		ERBITUX Monotherapy		Difference (95% CI[a])	
Populations	n	ORR (%)	n	ORR (%)	%	p-value CMH[b]
All Patients	218	22.9	111	10.8	12.1 (4.1 - 20.2)	0.007
• Irinotecan-Oxaliplatin Failure	80	23.8	44	11.4	12.4 (-0.8 - 25.6)	0.09
• Irinotecan Refractory	132	25.8	69	14.5	11.3 (0.1 - 22.4)	0.07

[a] 95% confidence interval for the difference in objective response rates.
[b] Cochran-Mantel-Haenszel test.

The median duration of response in the overall population was 5.7 months in the combination arm and 4.2 months in the monotherapy arm. Compared with patients randomized to ERBITUX alone, patients randomized to ERBITUX and irinotecan experienced a significantly longer median time to disease progression (see Table 2).

[See table 2 above]

Table 2: Time to Progression per Independent Review

Populations	ERBITUX + Irinotecan (median)	ERBITUX Monotherapy (median)	Hazard Ratio (95% CI[a])	Log-rank p-value
All Patients	4.1 mo	1.5 mo	0.54 (0.42 - 0.71)	<0.001
• Irinotecan-Oxaliplatin Failure	2.9 mo	1.5 mo	0.48 (0.31 - 0.72)	<0.001
• Irinotecan Refractory	4.0 mo	1.5 mo	0.52 (0.37 - 0.73)	<0.001

[a] Hazard ratio of ERBITUX + irinotecan: ERBITUX monotherapy with 95% confidence interval.

Single-Arm Trials

ERBITUX, in combination with irinotecan, was studied in a single-arm, multicenter, open-label clinical trial in 138 patients with EGFR-expressing metastatic colorectal cancer who had progressed following an irinotecan-containing regimen. Patients received a 20-mg test dose of ERBITUX on day 1, followed by a 400-mg/m^2 initial dose, and 250 mg/m^2 weekly until disease progression or unacceptable toxicity. Patients received the same dose and schedule for irinotecan as the patient had previously failed. Acceptable irinotecan schedules were 350 mg/m^2 every 3 weeks or 125 mg/m^2 weekly times four doses every 6 weeks. Of 138 patients enrolled, 74 patients had documented progression to irinotecan as determined by an IRC. The overall response rate was 15% for the overall population and 12% for the irinotecan-failure population. The median durations of response were 6.5 and 6.7 months, respectively.

ERBITUX was studied as a single agent in a multicenter, open-label, single-arm clinical trial in patients with EGFR-expressing metastatic colorectal cancer who progressed following an irinotecan-containing regimen. Of 57 patients enrolled, 28 patients had documented progression to irinotecan. The overall response rate was 9% for the all-treated group and 14% for the irinotecan-failure group. The median times to progression were 1.4 and 1.3 months, respectively. The median duration of response was 4.2 months for both groups.

EGFR Expression and Response

Patients enrolled in the clinical studies were required to have immunohistochemical evidence of positive EGFR expression. Primary tumor or tumor from a metastatic site was tested with the DakoCytomation EGFR pharmDx™ test kit. Specimens were scored based on the percentage of cells expressing EGFR and intensity (barely/faint, weak to moderate, and strong). Response rate did not correlate with either the percentage of positive cells or the intensity of EGFR expression.

INDICATIONS AND USAGE

ERBITUX, used in combination with irinotecan, is indicated for the treatment of EGFR-expressing, metastatic colorectal carcinoma in patients who are refractory to irinotecan-based chemotherapy.

ERBITUX (Cetuximab) administered as a single agent is indicated for the treatment of EGFR-expressing, metastatic colorectal carcinoma in patients who are intolerant to irinotecan-based chemotherapy.

The effectiveness of ERBITUX is based on objective response rates (see **CLINICAL STUDIES**). Currently, no data are available that demonstrate an improvement in disease-related symptoms or increased survival with ERBITUX.

CONTRAINDICATIONS

None.

WARNINGS

Infusion Reactions (See BOXED WARNING: Infusion Reactions, ADVERSE REACTIONS: Infusion Reactions, and DOSAGE AND ADMINISTRATION: Dose Modifications.)

Severe infusion reactions occurred with the administration of ERBITUX in approximately 3% (20/774) of patients, rarely with fatal outcome (<1 in 1000). Approximately 90% of severe infusion reactions were associated with the first infusion of ERBITUX despite the use of prophylactic antihistamines. These reactions were characterized by the rapid onset of airway obstruction (bronchospasm, stridor, hoarseness), urticaria, and/or hypotension. Caution must be exercised with every ERBITUX infusion, as there were patients who experienced their first severe infusion reaction during later infusions.

Severe infusion reactions require the immediate interruption of ERBITUX therapy and permanent discontinuation from further treatment. Appropriate medical therapy including epinephrine, corticosteroids, intravenous antihistamines, bronchodilators, and oxygen should be available for use in the treatment of such reactions. Patients should be carefully observed until the complete resolution of all signs and symptoms.

In clinical trials, mild to moderate infusion reactions were managed by slowing the infusion rate of ERBITUX and by continued use of antihistamine medications (eg, diphenhydramine) in subsequent doses (see **DOSAGE AND ADMINISTRATION: Dose Modifications**).

Pulmonary Toxicity

Interstitial lung disease (ILD) was reported in 3 of 774 (<0.5%) patients with advanced colorectal cancer receiving ERBITUX. Interstitial pneumonitis with non-cardiogenic pulmonary edema resulting in death was reported in one case. Two patients had pre-existing fibrotic lung disease and experienced an acute exacerbation of their disease while receiving ERBITUX in combination with irinotecan. In the clinical investigational program, an additional case of interstitial pneumonitis was reported in a patient with head and neck cancer treated with ERBITUX and cisplatin. The onset of symptoms occurred between the fourth and eleventh doses of treatment in all reported cases.

In the event of acute onset or worsening pulmonary symptoms, ERBITUX therapy should be interrupted and a prompt investigation of these symptoms should occur. If ILD is confirmed, ERBITUX should be discontinued and the patient should be treated appropriately.

Dermatologic Toxicity (See ADVERSE REACTIONS: Dermatologic Toxicity and DOSAGE AND ADMINISTRATION: Dose Modifications.)

In cynomolgus monkeys, ERBITUX, when administered at doses of approximately 0.4 to 4 times the weekly human exposure (based on total body surface area), resulted in dermatologic findings, including inflammation at the injection site and desquamation of the external integument. At the highest dose level, the epithelial mucosa of the nasal passage, esophagus, and tongue were similarly affected, and degenerative changes in the renal tubular epithelium occurred. Deaths due to sepsis were observed in 50% (5/10) of the animals at the highest dose level beginning after approximately 13 weeks of treatment.

In clinical studies of ERBITUX, dermatologic toxicities, including acneform rash, skin drying and fissuring, and inflammatory and infectious sequelae (eg, blepharitis, cheilitis, cellulitis, cyst) were reported. In patients with advanced colorectal cancer, acneform rash was reported in 89% (686/774) of all treated patients, and was severe (Grade 3 or 4) in 11% (84/774) of these patients. Subsequent to the development of severe dermatologic toxicities, complications including *S. aureus* sepsis and abscesses requiring incision and drainage were reported.

Patients developing dermatologic toxicities while receiving ERBITUX should be monitored for the development of inflammatory or infectious sequelae, and appropriate treatment of these symptoms initiated. Dose modifications of any future ERBITUX infusions should be instituted in case of severe acneform rash (see **DOSAGE AND ADMINISTRATION**, Table 4). Treatment with topical and/or oral antibiotics should be considered; topical corticosteroids are not recommended.

PRECAUTIONS

General

ERBITUX therapy should be used with caution in patients with known hypersensitivity to Cetuximab, murine proteins, or any component of this product.

It is recommended that patients wear sunscreen and hats and limit sun exposure while receiving ERBITUX as sunlight can exacerbate any skin reactions that may occur.

EGF Receptor Testing

Patients enrolled in the clinical studies were required to have immunohistochemical evidence of positive EGFR expression using the DakoCytomation EGFR pharmDx™ test kit. Assessment for EGFR expression should be performed by laboratories with demonstrated proficiency in the specific technology being utilized. Improper assay performance, including use of suboptimally fixed tissue, failure to utilize specified reagents, deviation from specific assay instructions, and failure to include appropriate controls for assay validation, can lead to unreliable results. Refer to the DakoCytomation test kit package insert for full instructions on assay performance. (See **CLINICAL STUDIES: EGFR Expression and Response.**)

Drug Interactions

A drug interaction study was performed in which ERBITUX was administered in combination with irinotecan. There was no evidence of any pharmacokinetic interactions between ERBITUX and irinotecan.

Immunogenicity

As with all therapeutic proteins, there is potential for immunogenicity. Potential immunogenic responses to ERBITUX were assessed using either a double antigen radiometric assay or an enzyme-linked immunosorbant assay. Due to limitations in assay performance and sampling timing, the incidence of antibody development in patients receiving ERBITUX has not been adequately determined. The incidence of antibodies to ERBITUX was measured by collecting and analyzing serum pre-study, prior to selected infusions and during treatment follow-up. Patients were considered evaluable if they had a negative pre-treatment sample and a post-treatment sample. Non-neutralizing anti-ERBITUX antibodies were detected in 5% (28 of 530) of evaluable patients. In patients positive for anti-ERBITUX antibody, the median time to onset was 44 days (range 8-281 days). Although the number of sero-positive patients is limited, there does not appear to be any relationship between the appearance of antibodies to ERBITUX and the safety or antitumor activity of the molecule.

The observed incidence of anti-ERBITUX antibody responses may be influenced by the low sensitivity of available assays, inadequate to reliably detect lower antibody titers. Other factors which might influence the incidence of anti-ERBITUX antibody response include sample handling, timing of sample collection, concomitant medications, and underlying disease. For these reasons, comparison of the incidence of antibodies to ERBITUX with the incidence of antibodies to other products may be misleading.

Carcinogenesis, Mutagenesis, Impairment of Fertility

Long-term animal studies have not been performed to test ERBITUX for carcinogenic potential. No mutagenic or clastogenic potential of ERBITUX was observed in the *Salmonella-Escherichia coli* (Ames) assay or in the *in vivo* rat micronucleus test. A 39-week toxicity study in cynomol-

Continued on next page

Erbitux—Cont.

gus monkeys receiving 0.4 to 4 times the human dose of ERBITUX (based on total body surface area) revealed a tendency for impairment of menstrual cycling in treated female monkeys, including increased incidences of irregularity or absence of cycles, when compared to control animals, and beginning from week 25 of treatment and continuing through the 6-week recovery period. Serum testosterone levels and analysis of sperm counts, viability, and motility were not remarkably different between ERBITUX-treated and control male monkeys. It is not known if ERBITUX can impair fertility in humans.

Pregnancy Category C

Animal reproduction studies have not been conducted with ERBITUX. However, the EGFR has been implicated in the control of prenatal development and may be essential for normal organogenesis, proliferation, and differentiation in the developing embryo. In addition, human IgG1 is known to cross the placental barrier; therefore, ERBITUX has the potential to be transmitted from the mother to the developing fetus. It is not known whether ERBITUX can cause fetal harm when administered to a pregnant woman or whether ERBITUX can affect reproductive capacity. There are no adequate and well-controlled studies of ERBITUX in pregnant women. ERBITUX should only be given to a pregnant woman, or any woman not employing adequate contraception if the potential benefit justifies the potential risk to the fetus. All patients should be counseled regarding the potential risk of ERBITUX treatment to the developing fetus prior to initiation of therapy. If the patient becomes pregnant while receiving this drug, she should be apprised of the potential hazard to the fetus and/or the potential risk for loss of the pregnancy.

Nursing Mothers

It is not known whether ERBITUX (Cetuximab) is secreted in human milk. Because human IgG1 is secreted in human milk, the potential for absorption and harm to the infant after ingestion is unknown. Based on the mean half-life of ERBITUX after multiple dosing of 114 hours [range 75-188 hours] (see **CLINICAL PHARMACOLOGY: Human Pharmacokinetics**), women should be advised to discontinue nursing during treatment with ERBITUX and for 60 days following the last dose of ERBITUX.

Pediatric Use

The safety and effectiveness of ERBITUX in pediatric patients have not been established.

Geriatric Use

Of the 774 patients who received ERBITUX with irinotecan or ERBITUX monotherapy in four advanced colorectal cancer studies, 253 patients (33%) were 65 years of age or older. No overall differences in safety or efficacy were observed between these patients and younger patients.

ADVERSE REACTIONS

Except where indicated, the data described below reflect exposure to ERBITUX in 774 patients with advanced metastatic colorectal cancer. ERBITUX was studied in combination with irinotecan (n=354) or as monotherapy (n=420). Patients receiving ERBITUX plus irinotecan received a median of 12 doses (with 88/354 [25%] treated for over 6 months), and patients receiving ERBITUX monotherapy received a median of 7 doses (with 36/420 [9%] treated for over 6 months). The population had a median age of 59 and was 59% male and 91% Caucasian. The range of dosing for patients receiving ERBITUX plus irinotecan was 1-84 infusions, and the range of dosing for patients receiving ERBITUX monotherapy was 1-63 infusions.

The most **serious adverse reactions** associated with ERBITUX were:

- Infusion reaction (3%) (see **BOXED WARNING, WARNINGS,** and **DOSAGE AND ADMINISTRATION: Dose Modifications**);
- Dermatologic toxicity (1%) (see **WARNINGS** and **DOSAGE AND ADMINISTRATION: Dose Modifications**);
- Interstitial lung disease (0.4%) (see **WARNINGS**);
- Fever (5%);
- Sepsis (3%);
- Kidney failure (2%);
- Pulmonary embolus (1%);
- Dehydration (5%) in patients receiving ERBITUX plus irinotecan, 0.2% in patients receiving ERBITUX monotherapy;
- Diarrhea (6%) in patients receiving ERBITUX plus irinotecan, 0.2% in patients receiving ERBITUX monotherapy.

Thirty-seven (10%) patients receiving ERBITUX plus irinotecan and 17 (4%) patients receiving ERBITUX monotherapy discontinued treatment primarily because of adverse events.

Table 3: Incidence of Adverse Events (≥10%) in Patients with Advanced Colorectal Carcinoma

	ERBITUX plus Irinotecan (n=354)		ERBITUX Monotherapy (n=420)	
Body System	Grades 1 - 4	Grades 3 and 4	Grades 1 - 4	Grades 3 and 4
Preferred Term[1]	% of Patients			
Body as a Whole				
Asthenia/Malaise[2]	73	16	48	10
Abdominal Pain	45	8	26	9
Fever[3]	34	4	26	<1
Pain	23	6	17	5
Infusion Reaction[4]	19	3	21	2
Infection	16	1	14	1
Back Pain	16	3	10	2
Headache	14	2	16	2
Digestive				
Diarrhea	72	22	25	2
Nausea	55	6	29	2
Vomiting	41	7	25	3
Anorexia	36	4	23	2
Constipation	30	2	26	2
Stomatitis	26	2	10	<1
Dyspepsia	14	0	6	0
Hematic/Lymphatic				
Leukopenia	25	17	<1	0
Anemia	16	5	9	3
Metabolic/Nutritional				
Weight Loss	21	0	7	1
Peripheral Edema	16	1	10	1
Dehydration	15	6	10	3
Nervous				
Insomnia	12	0	10	<1
Depression	10	0	7	0
Respiratory				
Dyspnea[3]	23	2	17	7
Cough Increased	20	0	11	1
Skin/Appendages				
Acneform Rash[5]	88	14	90	8
Alopecia	21	0	4	0
Skin Disorder	15	1	4	0
Nail Disorder	12	<1	16	<1
Pruritus	10	1	11	<1
Conjunctivitis	14	1	7	<1

[1] Adverse events that occurred (toxicity Grades 1 through 4) in ≥10% of patients with refractory colorectal carcinoma treated with ERBITUX plus irinotecan or in ≥10% of patients with refractory colorectal carcinoma treated with ERBITUX monotherapy.

[2] Asthenia/malaise is defined as any event described as "asthenia", "malaise", or "somnolence".

[3] Includes cases reported as infusion reaction.

[4] Infusion reaction is defined as any event described at any time during the clinical study as "allergic reaction" or "anaphylactoid reaction", or any event occurring on the first day of dosing described as "allergic reaction", "anaphylactoid reaction", "fever", "chills", "chills and fever", or "dyspnea".

[5] Acneform rash is defined as any event described as "acne", "rash", "maculopapular rash", "pustular rash", "dry skin", or "exfoliative dermatitis".

The most common adverse events seen in 354 patients receiving ERBITUX plus irinotecan were acneform rash (88%), asthenia/malaise (73%), diarrhea (72%), nausea (55%), abdominal pain (45%), and vomiting (41%).

The most common adverse events seen in 420 patients receiving ERBITUX monotherapy were acneform rash (90%), asthenia/malaise (48%), nausea (29%), fever (27%), constipation (26%), abdominal pain (26%), headache (26%), and diarrhea (25%).

Because clinical trials are conducted under widely varying conditions, adverse reaction rates observed in the clinical trials of a drug cannot be directly compared to rates in the clinical trials of another drug and may not reflect the rates observed in practice. The adverse reaction information from clinical trials does, however, provide a basis for identifying the adverse events that appear to be related to drug use and for approximating rates.

Data in patients with advanced colorectal carcinoma in Table 3 are based on the experience of 354 patients treated with ERBITUX plus irinotecan and 420 patients treated with ERBITUX monotherapy.

[See table 3 below]

Infusion Reactions (see BOXED WARNING: Infusion Reactions.)

In clinical trials, severe, potentially fatal infusion reactions were reported. These events include the rapid onset of airway obstruction (bronchospasm, stridor, hoarseness), urticaria, and/or hypotension. In studies in advanced colorectal cancer, severe infusion reactions were observed in 3% of patients receiving ERBITUX plus irinotecan and 2% of patients receiving ERBITUX monotherapy. Grade 1 and 2 infusion reactions, including chills, fever, and dyspnea usually occurring on the first day of initial dosing, were observed in 16% of patients receiving ERBITUX plus irinotecan and 19% of patients receiving ERBITUX monotherapy. (See **WARNINGS: Infusion Reactions** and **DOSAGE AND ADMINISTRATION: Dose Modifications.**)

In the clinical studies described above, a 20-mg test dose was administered intravenously over 10 minutes prior to the loading dose to all patients. The test dose did not reliably identify patients at risk for severe allergic reactions.

Dermatologic Toxicity and Related Disorders

Non-suppurative acneform rash described as "acne", "rash", "maculopapular rash", "pustular rash", "dry skin", or "exfoliative dermatitis" was observed in patients receiving ERBITUX (Cetuximab) plus irinotecan or ERBITUX monotherapy. One or more of the dermatological adverse events were reported in 88% (14% Grade 3) of patients receiving ERBITUX plus irinotecan and in 90% (8% Grade 3) of patients receiving ERBITUX monotherapy. Acneform rash most commonly occurred on the face, upper chest, and back, but could extend to the extremities and was characterized by multiple follicular- or pustular-appearing lesions. Skin drying and fissuring were common in some instances, and were associated with inflammatory and infectious sequelae (eg, blepharitis, cellulitis, cyst). Two cases of *S. aureus* sepsis were reported. The onset of acneform rash was generally within the first two weeks of therapy. Although in a majority of the patients the event resolved following cessation of treatment, in nearly half of the cases, the event continued beyond 28 days. (See **WARNINGS: Dermatologic Toxicity** and **DOSAGE AND ADMINISTRATION: Dose Modifications.**)

A related nail disorder, occurring in 14% of patients (0.4% Grade 3), was characterized as a paronychial inflammation with associated swelling of the lateral nail folds of the toes and fingers, with the great toes and thumbs as the most commonly affected digits.

Use with Radiation Therapy

In a study of 21 patients with locally advanced squamous cell cancer of the head and neck, patients treated with ERBITUX, cisplatin, and radiation had a 95% incidence of rash (19% Grade 3). The incidence and severity of cutaneous reactions with combined modality therapy appears to be additive, particularly within the radiation port. The addition of radiation to ERBITUX therapy in patients with colorectal cancer should be done with appropriate caution.

OVERDOSAGE

Single doses of ERBITUX higher than 500 mg/m^2 have not been tested. There is no experience with overdosage in human clinical trials.

DOSAGE AND ADMINISTRATION

The recommended dose of ERBITUX, in combination with irinotecan or as monotherapy, is 400 mg/m^2 as an initial loading dose (first infusion) administered as a 120-minute IV infusion (maximum infusion rate 5 mL/min). The recommended weekly maintenance dose (all other infusions) is 250 mg/m^2 infused over 60 minutes (maximum infusion rate 5 mL/min). Premedication with an H_1 antagonist (eg, 50 mg of diphenhydramine IV) is recommended. Appropriate medical resources for the treatment of severe infusion reactions should be available during ERBITUX infusions. (See **WARNINGS: Infusion Reactions.**)

Dose Modifications

Infusion Reactions

If the patient experiences a mild or moderate (Grade 1 or 2) infusion reaction, the infusion rate should be permanently reduced by 50%.

ERBITUX should be immediately and permanently discontinued in patients who experience severe (Grade 3 or 4) infusion reactions. (See **WARNINGS** and **ADVERSE REACTIONS.**)

Table 4: ERBITUX Dose Modification Guidelines

Severe Acneform Rash	ERBITUX	Outcome	ERBITUX Dose Modification
1st occurrence	Delay infusion 1 to 2 weeks	Improvement No Improvement	Continue at 250 mg/m^2 Discontinue ERBITUX
2nd occurrence	Delay infusion 1 to 2 weeks	Improvement No Improvement	Reduce dose to 200 mg/m^2 Discontinue ERBITUX
3rd occurrence	Delay infusion 1 to 2 weeks	Improvement No Improvement	Reduce dose to 150 mg/m^2 Discontinue ERBITUX
4th occurrence	Discontinue ERBITUX		

Dermatologic Toxicity and Related Disorders
If a patient experiences severe acneform rash, ERBITUX treatment adjustments should be made according to Table 4. In patients with mild and moderate skin toxicity, treatment should continue without dose modification. (See **WARNINGS** and **ADVERSE REACTIONS**.)
[See table 4 above]

Preparation for Administration
DO NOT ADMINISTER ERBITUX AS AN IV PUSH OR BOLUS.
ERBITUX must be administered with the use of a low protein binding 0.22-micrometer in-line filter.
ERBITUX is supplied as a 50-mL, single-use vial containing 100 mg of Cetuximab at a concentration of 2 mg/mL in phosphate buffered saline. The solution should be clear and colorless and may contain a small amount of easily visible, white, amorphous, Cetuximab particulates. **DO NOT SHAKE OR DILUTE.**
ERBITUX CAN BE ADMINISTERED VIA INFUSION PUMP OR SYRINGE PUMP.
Infusion Pump:
- Draw up the volume of a vial using a sterile syringe attached to an appropriate needle (a vented spike or other appropriate transfer device may be used).
- Fill ERBITUX into a sterile evacuated container or bag such as glass containers, polyolefin bags (eg, Baxter Intravia), ethylene vinyl acetate bags (eg, Baxter Clintec), DEHP plasticized PVC bags (eg, Abbott Lifecare), or PVC bags.
- Repeat procedure until the calculated volume has been put into the container. Use a new needle for each vial.
- Administer through a low protein binding 0.22-micrometer in-line filter (placed as proximal to the patient as practical).
- Affix the infusion line and prime it with ERBITUX before starting the infusion.
- Maximum infusion rate should not exceed 5 mL/min.
- Use 0.9% saline solution to flush line at the end of infusion.

Syringe Pump:
- Draw up the volume of a vial using a sterile syringe attached to an appropriate needle (a vented spike may be used).
- Place the syringe into the syringe driver of a syringe pump and set the rate.
- Administer through a low protein binding 0.22-micrometer in-line filter rated for syringe pump use (placed as proximal to the patient as practical).
- Connect up the infusion line and start the infusion after priming the line with ERBITUX.
- Repeat procedure until the calculated volume has been infused.
- Use a new needle and filter for each vial.
- Maximum infusion rate should not exceed 5 mL/min.
- Use 0.9% saline solution to flush line at the end of infusion.

ERBITUX should be piggybacked to the patient's infusion line.
Following the ERBITUX infusion, a 1-hour observation period is recommended.

HOW SUPPLIED
ERBITUX™ (Cetuximab) is supplied as a single-use, 50-mL vial containing 100 mg of Cetuximab as a sterile, preservative-free, injectable liquid. Each carton contains one ERBITUX vial (NDC 66733-948-23).
Stability and Storage
Store vials under refrigeration at 2° C to 8° C (36° F to 46° F). **DO NOT FREEZE.** Increased particulate formation may occur at temperatures at or below 0° C. This product contains no preservatives. Preparations of ERBITUX in infusion containers are chemically and physically stable for up to 12 hours at 2° C to 8° C (36° F to 46° F) and up to 8 hours at controlled room temperature (20° C to 25° C; 68° F to 77° F). Discard any remaining solution in the infusion container after 8 hours at controlled room temperature or after 12 hours at 2° to 8° C. Discard any unused portion of the vial.
US Patent No. 6,217,866
ERBITUX™ is a trademark of ImClone Systems Incorporated.
Manufactured by ImClone Systems Incorporated, Branchburg, NJ 08876
Distributed and Marketed by Bristol-Myers Squibb Company, Princeton, NJ 08543
ImClone Systems Incorporated
Bristol-Myers Squibb Company

ER-B0001-06-04 Issued June 2004
Based on 51-022606-00, 1169848
Shown in Product Identification Guide, page 310

METAGLIP™ ℞
[*mĕ-tă-glīp*]
(glipizide and metformin HCl) Tablets
℞ only
2.5 mg/250 mg
2.5 mg/500 mg
5 mg/500 mg

DESCRIPTION
METAGLIP™ (glipizide and metformin HCl) Tablets contains two oral antihyperglycemic drugs used in the management of type 2 diabetes, glipizide and metformin hydrochloride.
Glipizide is an oral antihyperglycemic drug of the sulfonylurea class. The chemical name for glipizide is 1-cyclohexyl-3-[[*p*-[2-(5-methylpyrazinecarboxamido)ethyl]phenyl]sulfonyl]urea. Glipizide is a whitish, odorless powder with a molecular formula of $C_{21}H_{27}N_5O_4S$, a molecular weight of 445.55 and a pK_a of 5.9. It is insoluble in water and alcohols, but soluble in 0.1 *N* NaOH; it is freely soluble in dimethylformamide. The structural formula is represented below.

Glipizide

Metformin hydrochloride is an oral antihyperglycemic drug used in the management of type 2 diabetes. Metformin hydrochloride (*N,N*-dimethylimidodicarbonimidic diamide mono-hydrochloride) is not chemically or pharmacologically related to sulfonylureas, thiazolidinediones, or α-glucosidase inhibitors. It is a white to off-white crystalline compound with a molecular formula of $C_4H_{12}ClN_5$ (monohydrochloride) and a molecular weight of 165.63. Metformin hydrochloride is freely soluble in water and is practically insoluble in acetone, ether, and chloroform. The pK_a of metformin is 12.4. The pH of a 1% aqueous solution of metformin hydrochloride is 6.68. The structural formula is as shown:

Metformin Hydrochloride

METAGLIP is available for oral administration in tablets containing 2.5 mg glipizide with 250 mg metformin hydrochloride, 2.5 mg glipizide with 500 mg metformin hydrochloride, and 5 mg glipizide with 500 mg metformin hydrochloride. In addition, each tablet contains the following inactive ingredients: microcrystalline cellulose, povidone, croscarmellose sodium, and magnesium stearate. The tablets are film coated, which provides color differentiation.

CLINICAL PHARMACOLOGY
Mechanism of Action
METAGLIP (glipizide and metformin HCl) combines glipizide and metformin hydrochloride, two antihyperglycemic agents with complementary mechanisms of action, to improve glycemic control in patients with type 2 diabetes.
Glipizide appears to lower blood glucose acutely by stimulating the release of insulin from the pancreas, an effect dependent upon functioning beta cells in the pancreatic islets. Extrapancreatic effects may play a part in the mechanism of action of oral sulfonylurea hypoglycemic drugs. The mechanism by which glipizide lowers blood glucose during long-term administration has not been clearly established. In man, stimulation of insulin secretion by glipizide in response to a meal is undoubtedly of major importance. Fasting insulin levels are not elevated even on long-term glipizide administration, but the postprandial insulin response continues to be enhanced after at least 6 months of treatment.
Metformin hydrochloride is an antihyperglycemic agent that improves glucose tolerance in patients with type 2 diabetes, lowering both basal and postprandial plasma glucose. Metformin hydrochloride decreases hepatic glucose production, decreases intestinal absorption of glucose, and improves insulin sensitivity by increasing peripheral glucose uptake and utilization.
Pharmacokinetics
Absorption and Bioavailability
METAGLIP
In a single dose study in healthy subjects, the glipizide and metformin components of METAGLIP 5 mg/500 mg were bioequivalent to coadministered GLUCOTROL® and GLUCOPHAGE® (metformin hydrochloride). Following administration of a single METAGLIP 5 mg/500 mg tablet in healthy subjects with either a 20% glucose solution or a 20% glucose solution with food, there was a small effect of food on peak plasma concentration (C_{max}) and no effect of food on area under the curve (AUC) of the glipizide component. Time to peak plasma concentration (T_{max}) for the glipizide component was delayed 1 hour with food relative to the same tablet strength administered fasting with a 20% glucose solution. C_{max} for the metformin component was reduced approximately 14% by food whereas AUC was not affected. T_{max} for the metformin component was delayed 1 hour after food.
Glipizide
Gastrointestinal absorption of glipizide is uniform, rapid, and essentially complete. Peak plasma concentrations occur 1-3 hours after a single oral dose. Glipizide does not accumulate in plasma on repeated oral administration. Total absorption and disposition of an oral dose was unaffected by food in normal volunteers, but absorption was delayed by about 40 minutes.
Metformin hydrochloride
The absolute bioavailability of a 500 mg metformin hydrochloride tablet given under fasting conditions is approximately 50-60%. Studies using single oral doses of metformin tablets of 500 mg and 1500 mg, and 850 mg to 2550 mg, indicate that there is a lack of dose proportionality with increasing doses, which is due to decreased absorption rather than an alteration in elimination. Food decreases the extent of and slightly delays the absorption of metformin, as shown by approximately a 40% lower peak concentration and a 25% lower AUC in plasma and a 35-minute prolongation of time to peak plasma concentration following administration of a single 850 mg tablet of metformin with food, compared to the same tablet strength administered fasting. The clinical relevance of these decreases is unknown.
Distribution
Glipizide
Protein binding was studied in serum from volunteers who received either oral or intravenous glipizide and found to be 98-99% one hour after either route of administration. The apparent volume of distribution of glipizide after intravenous administration was 11 liters, indicative of localization within the extracellular fluid compartment. In mice, no glipizide or metabolites were detectable autoradiographically in the brain or spinal cord of males or females, nor in the fetuses of pregnant females. In another study, however, very small amounts of radioactivity were detected in the fetuses of rats given labeled drug.
Metformin hydrochloride
The apparent volume of distribution (V/F) of metformin following single oral doses of 850 mg averaged 654 ± 358 L. Metformin is negligibly bound to plasma proteins. Metformin partitions into erythrocytes, most likely as a function of time. At usual clinical doses and dosing schedules of metformin, steady state plasma concentrations of metformin are reached within 24-48 hours and are generally <1 μg/mL. During controlled clinical trials, maximum metformin plasma levels did not exceed 5 μg/mL, even at maximum doses.
Metabolism and Elimination
Glipizide
The metabolism of glipizide is extensive and occurs mainly in the liver. The primary metabolites are inactive hydroxylation products and polar conjugates and are excreted mainly in the urine. Less than 10% unchanged glipizide is found in the urine. The half-life of elimination ranges from 2-4 hours in normal subjects, whether given intravenously or orally. The metabolic and excretory patterns are similar with the two routes of administration, indicating that first-pass metabolism is not significant.
Metformin hydrochloride
Intravenous single-dose studies in normal subjects demonstrate that metformin is excreted unchanged in the urine and does not undergo hepatic metabolism (no metabolites have been identified in humans) nor biliary excretion. Renal clearance (see **Table 1**) is approximately 3.5 times greater than creatinine clearance, which indicates that tubular secretion is the major route of metformin elimination. Following oral administration, approximately 90% of the absorbed drug is eliminated via the renal route within the first 24 hours, with a plasma elimination half-life of approximately 6.2 hours. In blood, the elimination half-life is approximately 17.6 hours, suggesting that the erythrocyte mass may be a compartment of distribution.
Special Populations
Patients With Type 2 Diabetes
In the presence of normal renal function, there are no differences between single- or multiple-dose pharmacokinetics of metformin between patients with type 2 diabetes and normal subjects (see **Table 1**), nor is there any accumulation of metformin in either group at usual clinical doses.

Continued on next page

Metaglip—Cont.

Hepatic Insufficiency

The metabolism and excretion of glipizide may be slowed in patients with impaired hepatic function (see **PRECAUTIONS**). No pharmacokinetic studies have been conducted in patients with hepatic insufficiency for metformin.

Renal Insufficiency

The metabolism and excretion of glipizide may be slowed in patients with impaired renal function (see **PRECAUTIONS**).

In patients with decreased renal function (based on creatinine clearance), the plasma and blood half-life of metformin is prolonged and the renal clearance is decreased in proportion to the decrease in creatinine clearance (see **Table 1**; also, see **WARNINGS**).

Geriatrics

There is no information on the pharmacokinetics of glipizide in elderly patients.

Limited data from controlled pharmacokinetic studies of metformin in healthy elderly subjects suggest that total plasma clearance is decreased, the half-life is prolonged, and C_{max} is increased, compared to healthy young subjects. From these data, it appears that the change in metformin pharmacokinetics with aging is primarily accounted for by a change in renal function (see **Table 1**). Metformin treatment should not be initiated in patients ≥80 years of age unless measurement of creatinine clearance demonstrates that renal function is not reduced.

[See table 1 at right]

Pediatrics

No data from pharmacokinetic studies in pediatric subjects are available for either glipizide or metformin.

Gender

There is no information on the effect of gender on the pharmacokinetics of glipizide.

Metformin pharmacokinetic parameters did not differ significantly in subjects with or without type 2 diabetes when analyzed according to gender (males = 19, females = 16). Similarly, in controlled clinical studies in patients with type 2 diabetes, the antihyperglycemic effect of metformin was comparable in males and females.

Race

No information is available on race differences in the pharmacokinetics of glipizide.

No studies of metformin pharmacokinetic parameters according to race have been performed. In controlled clinical studies of metformin in patients with type 2 diabetes, the antihyperglycemic effect was comparable in whites (n=249), blacks (n=51), and Hispanics (n=24).

CLINICAL STUDIES

Initial Therapy

In a 24-week, double-blind, active-controlled, multicenter international clinical trial, patients with type 2 diabetes, whose hyperglycemia was not adequately controlled with diet and exercise alone (hemoglobin A_{1c} [HbA_{1c}] >7.5% and ≤12% and fasting plasma glucose [FPG] <300 mg/dL) were randomized to receive initial therapy with glipizide 5 mg, metformin 500 mg, METAGLIP 2.5 mg/250 mg, or METAGLIP 2.5 mg/500 mg. After two weeks, the dose was progressively increased (up to the 12-week visit) to a maximum of four tablets daily in divided doses as needed to reach a target mean daily glucose (MDG) of ≤130 mg/dL. Trial data at 24 weeks are summarized in **Table 2**.

[See table 2 at right]

After 24 weeks, treatment with METAGLIP (glipizide and metformin HCl) Tablets 2.5 mg/250 mg and 2.5 mg/500 mg resulted in significantly greater reduction in HbA_{1c} compared to glipizide and to metformin therapy. Also, METAGLIP 2.5 mg/250 mg therapy resulted in significant reductions in FPG versus metformin therapy.

Increases above fasting glucose and insulin levels were determined at baseline and final study visits by measurement of plasma glucose and insulin for three hours following a standard mixed liquid meal. Treatment with METAGLIP lowered the three-hour postprandial glucose AUC, compared to baseline, to a significantly greater extent than did the glipizide and the metformin therapies. Compared to baseline, METAGLIP enhanced the postprandial insulin response, but did not significantly affect fasting insulin levels.

There were no clinically meaningful differences in changes from baseline for all lipid parameters between METAGLIP (glipizide and metformin HCl) therapy and either metformin therapy or glipizide therapy. The adjusted mean changes from baseline in body weight were: METAGLIP 2.5 mg/250 mg, -0.4 kg; METAGLIP 2.5 mg/500 mg, -0.5 kg; glipizide, -0.2 kg; and metformin, -1.9 kg. Weight loss was greater with metformin than with METAGLIP.

Second-Line Therapy

In an 18-week, double-blind, active-controlled U.S. clinical trial, a total of 247 patients with type 2 diabetes not adequately controlled (HbA_{1c} ≥7.5% and ≤12% and FPG <300 mg/dL) while being treated with at least one-half the maximum labeled dose of a sulfonylurea (e.g., glyburide 10 mg, glipizide 20 mg) were randomized to receive glipizide (fixed dose, 30 mg), metformin (500 mg), or METAGLIP 5 mg/500 mg. The doses of metformin and METAGLIP were titrated (up to the eight-week visit) to a maximum of four tablets daily as needed to achieve MDG ≤130 mg/dL. Trial data at 18 weeks are summarized in **Table 3**.

Table 1: Select Mean (±S.D.) Metformin Pharmacokinetic Parameters Following Single or Multiple Oral Doses of Metformin

Subject Groups: Metformin Dose[a] (Number of Subjects)	C_{max}[b] (μg/mL)	T_{max}[c] (hrs)	Renal Clearance (mL/min)
Healthy, Nondiabetic Adults:			
500 mg SD[d] (24)	1.03 (±0.33)	2.75 (±0.81)	600 (±132)
850 mg SD (74)[e]	1.60 (±0.38)	2.64 (±0.82)	552 (±139)
850 mg t.i.d. for 19 doses[f] (9)	2.01 (±0.42)	1.79 (±0.94)	642 (±173)
Adults with Type 2 Diabetes:			
850 mg SD (23)	1.48 (±0.5)	3.32 (±1.08)	491 (±138)
850 mg t.i.d. for 19 doses[f] (9)	1.90 (±0.62)	2.01 (±1.22)	550 (±160)
Elderly[g], Healthy Nondiabetic Adults:			
850 mg SD (12)	2.45 (±0.70)	2.71 (±1.05)	412 (±98)
Renal-impaired Adults: 850 mg SD			
Mild (CL_{cr}[h] 61-90 mL/min) (5)	1.86 (±0.52)	3.20 (±0.45)	384 (±122)
Moderate (CL_{cr} 31-60 mL/min) (4)	4.12 (±1.83)	3.75 (±0.50)	108 (±57)
Severe (CL_{cr} 10-30 mL/min) (6)	3.93 (±0.92)	4.01 (±1.10)	130 (± 90)

[a] All doses given fasting except the first 18 doses of the multiple-dose studies
[b] Peak plasma concentration
[c] Time to peak plasma concentration
[d] SD = single dose
[e] Combined results (average means) of five studies: mean age 32 years (range 23-59 years)
[f] Kinetic study done following dose 19, given fasting
[g] Elderly subjects, mean age 71 years (range 65-81 years)
[h] CL_{cr} = creatinine clearance normalized to body surface area of 1.73 m^2

Table 2: Active-Controlled Trial of METAGLIP as Initial Therapy: Summary of Trial Data at 24 Weeks

	Glipizide 5 mg tablets	Metformin 500 mg tablets	METAGLIP 2.5 mg/250 mg tablets	METAGLIP 2.5 mg/500 mg tablets
Mean Final Dose	16.7 mg	1749 mg	7.9 mg/ 791 mg	7.4 mg/ 1477 mg
Hemoglobin A_{1c} (%)	N=168	N=171	N=166	N=163
Baseline Mean	9.17	9.15	9.06	9.10
Final Mean	7.36	7.67	6.93	6.95
Adjusted Mean Change from Baseline	-1.77	-1.46	-2.15	-2.14
Difference from Glipizide			-0.38[a]	-0.37[a]
Difference from Metformin			-0.70[a]	-0.69[a]
% Patients with Final HbA_{1c} <7%	43.5%	35.1%	59.6%	57.1%
Fasting Plasma Glucose (mg/dL)	N=169	N=176	N=170	N=169
Baseline Mean	210.7	207.4	206.8	203.1
Final Mean	162.1	163.8	152.1	148.7
Adjusted Mean Change from Baseline	-46.2	-42.9	-54.2	-56.5
Difference from Glipizide			-8.0	-10.4
Difference from Metformin			-11.3	-13.6

[a] $p < 0.001$

Table 3: METAGLIP as Second-Line Therapy: Summary of Trial Data at 18 Weeks

	Glipizide 5 mg tablets	Metformin 500 mg tablets	METAGLIP 5 mg/500 mg tablets
Mean Final Dose	30.0 mg	1927 mg	17.5 mg/1747 mg
Hemoglobin A_{1c} (%)	N=79	N=71	N=80
Baseline Mean	8.87	8.61	8.66
Final Adjusted Mean	8.45	8.36	7.39
Difference from Glipizide			-1.06[a]
Difference from Metformin			-0.98[a]
% Patients with Final HbA_{1c}<7%	8.9%	9.9%	36.3%
Fasting Plasma Glucose (mg/dL)	N=82	N=75	N=81
Baseline Mean	203.6	191.3	194.3
Adjusted Mean Change from Baseline	7.0	6.7	-30.4
Difference from Glipizide			-37.4
Difference from Metformin			-37.2

[a] $p < 0.001$

[See table 3 above]

After 18 weeks, treatment with METAGLIP at doses up to 20 mg/2000 mg per day resulted in significantly lower mean final HbA_{1c} and significantly greater mean reductions in FPG compared to glipizide and to metformin therapy. Treatment with METAGLIP lowered the three-hour postprandial glucose AUC, compared to baseline, to a significantly greater extent than did the glipizide and the metformin therapies. METAGLIP did not significantly affect fasting insulin levels.

There were no clinically meaningful differences in changes from baseline for all lipid parameters between METAGLIP (glipizide and metformin HCl) therapy and either metformin therapy or glipizide therapy. The adjusted mean changes from baseline in body weight were: METAGLIP 5 mg/500 mg, -0.3 kg; glipizide, -0.4 kg; and metformin, -2.7 kg. Weight loss was greater with metformin than with METAGLIP.

INDICATIONS AND USAGE

METAGLIP (glipizide and metformin HCl) Tablets is indicated as initial therapy, as an adjunct to diet and exercise, to improve glycemic control in patients with type 2 diabetes whose hyperglycemia cannot be satisfactorily managed with diet and exercise alone.

METAGLIP is indicated as second-line therapy when diet, exercise, and initial treatment with a sulfonylurea or metformin do not result in adequate glycemic control in patients with type 2 diabetes.

CONTRAINDICATIONS

METAGLIP is contraindicated in patients with:

1. Renal disease or renal dysfunction (e.g., as suggested by serum creatinine levels ≥1.5 mg/dL [males], ≥1.4 mg/dL [females], or abnormal creatinine clearance) which may also result from conditions such as cardiovascular collapse (shock), acute myocardial infarction, and septicemia (see **WARNINGS** and **PRECAUTIONS**).
2. Congestive heart failure requiring pharmacologic treatment.
3. Known hypersensitivity to glipizde or metformin hydrochloride.
4. Acute or chronic metabolic acidosis, including diabetic ketoacidosis, with or without coma. Diabetic ketoacidosis should be treated with insulin.

METAGLIP should be temporarily discontinued in patients undergoing radiologic studies involving intravascular administration of iodinated contrast materials, because use of such products may result in acute alteration of renal function. (See also **PRECAUTIONS**.)

WARNINGS

Metformin Hydrochloride

Lactic acidosis:

Lactic acidosis is a rare, but serious, metabolic complication that can occur due to metformin accumulation during treatment with METAGLIP; when it occurs, it is fatal in approximately 50% of cases. Lactic acidosis may also occur in association with a number of pathophysiologic conditions, including diabetes mellitus, and whenever there is significant tissue hypoperfusion and hypoxemia. Lactic acidosis is characterized by elevated blood lactate levels (>5 mmol/L), decreased blood pH, electrolyte disturbances with an increased anion gap, and an increased lactate/pyruvate ratio. When metformin is implicated as the cause of lactic acidosis, metformin plasma levels >5 µg/mL are generally found.

The reported incidence of lactic acidosis in patients receiving metformin hydrochloride is very low (approximately 0.03 cases/1000 patient-years, with approximately 0.015 fatal cases/1000 patient-years). Reported cases have occurred primarily in diabetic patients with significant renal insufficiency, including both intrinsic renal disease and renal hypoperfusion, often in the setting of multiple concomitant medical/surgical problems and multiple concomitant medications. Patients with congestive heart failure requiring pharmacologic management, in particular those with unstable or acute congestive heart failure who are at risk of hypoperfusion and hypoxemia, are at increased risk of lactic acidosis. The risk of lactic acidosis increases with the degree of renal dysfunction and the patient's age. The risk of lactic acidosis may, therefore, be significantly decreased by regular monitoring of renal function in patients taking metformin and by use of the minimum effective dose of metformin. In particular, treatment of the elderly should be accompanied by careful monitoring of renal function. METAGLIP (glipizide and metformin HCl) treatment should not be initiated in patients ≥80 years of age unless measurement of creatinine clearance demonstrates that renal function is not reduced, as these patients are more susceptible to developing lactic acidosis. In addition, METAGLIP should be promptly withheld in the presence of any condition associated with hypoxemia, dehydration, or sepsis. Because impaired hepatic function may significantly limit the ability to clear lactate, METAGLIP should generally be avoided in patients with clinical or laboratory evidence of hepatic disease. Patients should be cautioned against excessive alcohol intake, either acute or chronic, when taking METAGLIP, since alcohol potentiates the effects of metformin hydrochloride on lactate metabolism. In addition, METAGLIP should be temporarily discontinued prior to any intravascular radiocontrast study and for any surgical procedure (see also PRECAUTIONS).

The onset of lactic acidosis often is subtle, and accompanied only by nonspecific symptoms such as malaise, myalgias, respiratory distress, increasing somnolence, and nonspecific abdominal distress. There may be associated hypothermia, hypotension, and resistant bradyarrhythmias with more marked acidosis. The patient and the patient's physician must be aware of the possible importance of such symptoms and the patient should be instructed to notify the physician immediately if they occur (see also PRECAUTIONS). METAGLIP should be withdrawn until the situation is clarified. Serum electrolytes, ketones, blood glucose, and if indicated, blood pH, lactate levels, and even blood metformin levels may be useful. Once a patient is stabilized on any dose level of METAGLIP, gastrointestinal symptoms, which are common during initiation of therapy with metformin, are unlikely to be drug related. Later occurrence of gastrointestinal symptoms could be due to lactic acidosis or other serious disease. Levels of fasting venous plasma lactate above the upper limit of normal but less than 5 mmol/L in patients taking METAGLIP do not necessarily indicate impending lactic acidosis and may be explainable by other mechanisms, such as poorly controlled diabetes or obesity, vigorous physical activity, or technical problems in sample handling. (See also PRECAUTIONS).

Lactic acidosis should be suspected in any diabetic patient with metabolic acidosis lacking evidence of ketoacidosis (ketonuria and ketonemia).

Lactic acidosis is a medical emergency that must be treated in a hospital setting. In a patient with lactic acidosis who is taking METAGLIP, the drug should be discontinued immediately and general supportive measures promptly instituted. Because metformin hydrochloride is dialyzable (with a clearance of up to 170 mL/min under good hemodynamic conditions), prompt hemodialysis is recommended to correct the acidosis and remove the accumulated metformin. Such management often results in prompt reversal of symptoms and recovery. (See also CONTRAINDICATIONS and PRECAUTIONS.)

SPECIAL WARNING ON INCREASED RISK OF CARDIOVASCULAR MORTALITY

The administration of oral hypoglycemic drugs has been reported to be associated with increased cardiovascular mortality as compared to treatment with diet alone or diet plus insulin. This warning is based on the study conducted by the University Group Diabetes Program (UGDP), a long-term prospective clinical trial designed to evaluate the effectiveness of glucose-lowering drugs in preventing or delaying vascular complications in patients with non-insulin-dependent diabetes. The study involved 823 patients who were randomly assigned to one of four treatment groups (*Diabetes* 19 (Suppl. 2):747-830, 1970).

UGDP reported that patients treated for 5 to 8 years with diet plus a fixed dose of tolbutamide (1.5 grams per day) had a rate of cardiovascular mortality approximately 2½ times that of patients treated with diet alone. A significant increase in total mortality was not observed, but the use of tolbutamide was discontinued based on the increase in cardiovascular mortality, thus limiting the opportunity for the study to show an increase in overall mortality. Despite controversy regarding the interpretation of these results, the findings of the UGDP study provide an adequate basis for this warning. The patient should be informed of the potential risks and benefits of glipizide and of alternative modes of therapy.

Although only one drug in the sulfonylurea class (tolbutamide) was included in this study, it is prudent from a safety standpoint to consider that this warning may also apply to other hypoglycemic drugs in this class, in view of their close similarities in mode of action and chemical structure.

PRECAUTIONS

General

METAGLIP

Hypoglycemia

METAGLIP (glipizide and metformin HCl) Tablets is capable of producing hypoglycemia, therefore, proper patient selection, dosing, and instructions are important to avoid potential hypoglycemic episodes. The risk of hypoglycemia is increased when caloric intake is deficient, when strenuous exercise is not compensated by caloric supplementation, or during concomitant use with other glucose-lowering agents or ethanol. Renal insufficiency may cause elevated drug levels of both glipizide and metformin hydrochloride. Hepatic insufficiency may increase drug levels of glipizide and may also diminish gluconeogenic capacity, both of which increase the risk of hypoglycemic reactions. Elderly, debilitated, or malnourished patients and those with adrenal or pituitary insufficiency or alcohol intoxication are particularly susceptible to hypoglycemic effects. Hypoglycemia may be difficult to recognize in the elderly, and in people who are taking beta-adrenergic blocking drugs.

Glipizide

Renal and hepatic disease

The metabolism and excretion of glipizide may be slowed in patients with impaired renal and/or hepatic function. If hypoglycemia should occur in such patients, it may be prolonged and appropriate management should be instituted.

Metformin Hydrochloride

Monitoring of renal function

Metformin is known to be substantially excreted by the kidney, and the risk of metformin accumulation and lactic acidosis increases with the degree of impairment of renal function. Thus, patients with serum creatinine levels above the upper limit of normal for their age should not receive METAGLIP (glipizide and metformin HCl). In patients with advanced age, METAGLIP should be carefully titrated to establish the minimum dose for adequate glycemic effect, because aging is associated with reduced renal function. In elderly patients, particularly those ≥80 years of age, renal function should be monitored regularly and, generally, METAGLIP should not be titrated to the maximum dose (see **WARNINGS** and **DOSAGE AND ADMINISTRATION**). Before initiation of METAGLIP therapy and at least annually thereafter, renal function should be assessed and verified as normal. In patients in whom development of renal dysfunction is anticipated, renal function should be assessed more frequently and METAGLIP discontinued if evidence of renal impairment is present.

Use of concomitant medications that may affect renal function or metformin disposition

Concomitant medication(s) that may affect renal function or result in significant hemodynamic change or may interfere with the disposition of metformin, such as cationic drugs that are eliminated by renal tubular secretion (see **PRECAUTIONS: Drug Interactions**), should be used with caution.

Radiologic studies involving the use of intravascular iodinated contrast materials (for example, intravenous urogram, intravenous cholangiography, angiography, and computed tomography (CT) scans with intravascular contrast materials)

Intravascular contrast studies with iodinated materials can lead to acute alteration of renal function and have been associated with lactic acidosis in patients receiving metformin (see **CONTRAINDICATIONS**). Therefore, in patients in whom any such study is planned, METAGLIP should be temporarily discontinued at the time of or prior to the procedure, and withheld for 48 hours subsequent to the procedure and reinstituted only after renal function has been re-evaluated and found to be normal.

Hypoxic states

Cardiovascular collapse (shock) from whatever cause, acute congestive heart failure, acute myocardial infarction, and other conditions characterized by hypoxemia have been associated with lactic acidosis and may also cause prerenal azotemia. When such events occur in patients on METAGLIP therapy, the drug should be promptly discontinued.

Surgical procedures

METAGLIP therapy should be temporarily suspended for any surgical procedure (except minor procedures not associated with restricted intake of food and fluids) and should not be restarted until the patient's oral intake has resumed and renal function has been evaluated as normal.

Alcohol intake

Alcohol is known to potentiate the effect of metformin on lactate metabolism. Patients, therefore, should be warned against excessive alcohol intake, acute or chronic, while receiving METAGLIP. Due to its effect on the gluconeogenic capacity of the liver, alcohol may also increase the risk of hypoglycemia.

Impaired hepatic function

Since impaired hepatic function has been associated with some cases of lactic acidosis, METAGLIP should generally be avoided in patients with clinical or laboratory evidence of hepatic disease.

Vitamin B_{12} levels

In controlled clinical trials with metformin of 29 weeks duration, a decrease to subnormal levels of previously normal serum Vitamin B_{12}, without clinical manifestations, was observed in approximately 7% of patients. Such decrease, possibly due to interference with B_{12} absorption from the B_{12}-intrinsic factor complex, is, however, very rarely associated with anemia and appears to be rapidly reversible with discontinuation of metformin or Vitamin B_{12} supplementation. Measurement of hematologic parameters on an annual basis is advised in patients on metformin and any apparent abnormalities should be appropriately investigated and managed (see **PRECAUTIONS: Laboratory Tests**).

Certain individuals (those with inadequate Vitamin B_{12} or calcium intake or absorption) appear to be predisposed to developing subnormal Vitamin B_{12} levels. In these patients, routine serum Vitamin B_{12} measurements at two- to three-year intervals may be useful.

Change in clinical status of patients with previously controlled type 2 diabetes

A patient with type 2 diabetes previously well-controlled on metformin who develops laboratory abnormalities or clinical illness (especially vague and poorly defined illness) should be evaluated promptly for evidence of ketoacidosis or lactic acidosis. Evaluation should include serum electrolytes and ketones, blood glucose and, if indicated, blood pH, lactate, pyruvate, and metformin levels. If acidosis of either form occurs, METAGLIP (glipizide and metformin HCl) Tablets must be stopped immediately and other appropriate corrective measures initiated (see also **WARNINGS**).

Information for Patients

METAGLIP

Patients should be informed of the potential risks and benefits of METAGLIP and of alternative modes of therapy. They should also be informed about the importance of adherence to dietary instructions, of a regular exercise program, and of regular testing of blood glucose, glycosylated hemoglobin, renal function, and hematologic parameters.

The risks of lactic acidosis associated with metformin therapy, its symptoms, and conditions that predispose to its development, as noted in the **WARNINGS** and **PRECAUTIONS** sections, should be explained to patients. Patients

Continued on next page

Metaglip—Cont.

should be advised to discontinue METAGLIP (glipizide and metformin HCl) immediately and to promptly notify their health practitioner if unexplained hyperventilation, myalgia, malaise, unusual somnolence, or other nonspecific symptoms occur. Once a patient is stabilized on any dose level of METAGLIP, gastrointestinal symptoms, which are common during initiation of metformin therapy, are unlikely to be drug related. Later occurrence of gastrointestinal symptoms could be due to lactic acidosis or other serious disease.

The risks of hypoglycemia, its symptoms and treatment, and conditions that predispose to its development should be explained to patients and responsible family members.

Patients should be counseled against excessive alcohol intake, either acute or chronic, while receiving METAGLIP. (See **Patient Information** printed below.)

Laboratory Tests

Periodic fasting blood glucose and glycosylated hemoglobin (HbA_{1c}) measurements should be performed to monitor therapeutic response.

Initial and periodic monitoring of hematologic parameters (e.g., hemoglobin/hematocrit and red blood cell indices) and renal function (serum creatinine) should be performed, at least on an annual basis. While megaloblastic anemia has rarely been seen with metformin therapy, if this is suspected, Vitamin B_{12} deficiency should be excluded.

Drug Interactions

METAGLIP

Certain drugs tend to produce hyperglycemia and may lead to loss of blood glucose control. These drugs include the thiazides and other diuretics, corticosteroids, phenothiazines, thyroid products, estrogens, oral contraceptives, phenytoin, nicotinic acid, sympathomimetics, calcium channel blocking drugs, and isoniazid. When such drugs are administered to a patient receiving METAGLIP, the patient should be closely observed for loss of blood glucose control. When such drugs are withdrawn from a patient receiving METAGLIP, the patient should be observed closely for hypoglycemia. Metformin is negligibly bound to plasma proteins and is, therefore, less likely to interact with highly protein-bound drugs such as salicylates, sulfonamides, chloramphenicol, and probenecid as compared to sulfonylureas, which are extensively bound to serum proteins.

Glipizide

The hypoglycemic action of sulfonylureas may be potentiated by certain drugs including nonsteroidal anti-inflammatory agents, some azoles, and other drugs that are highly protein bound, salicylates, sulfonamides, chloramphenicol, probenecid, coumarins, monoamine oxidase inhibitors, and beta adrenergic blocking agents. When such drugs are administered to a patient receiving METAGLIP, the patient should be observed closely for hypoglycemia. When such drugs are withdrawn from a patient receiving METAGLIP, the patient should be observed closely for loss of blood glucose control. *In vitro* binding studies with human serum proteins indicate that glipizide binds differently than tolbutamide and does not interact with salicylate or dicumarol. However, caution must be exercised in extrapolating these findings to the clinical situation and in the use of METAGLIP (glipizide and metformin HCl) Tablets with these drugs.

A potential interaction between oral miconazole and oral hypoglycemic agents leading to severe hypoglycemia has been reported. Whether this interaction also occurs with the intravenous, topical, or vaginal preparations of miconazole is not known. The effect of concomitant administration of fluconazole and glipizide has been demonstrated in a placebo-controlled crossover study in normal volunteers. All subjects received glipizide alone and following treatment with 100 mg of fluconazole as a single oral daily dose for 7 days, the mean percent increase in the glipizide AUC after fluconazole administration was 56.9% (range: 35 to 81%).

Metformin Hydrochloride

Furosemide

A single-dose, metformin-furosemide drug interaction study in healthy subjects demonstrated that pharmacokinetic parameters of both compounds were affected by co-administration. Furosemide increased the metformin plasma and blood C_{max} by 22% and blood AUC by 15%, without any significant change in metformin renal clearance. When administered with metformin, the C_{max} and AUC of furosemide were 31% and 12% smaller, respectively, than when administered alone, and the terminal half-life was decreased by 32%, without any significant change in furosemide renal clearance. No information is available about the interaction of metformin and furosemide when co-administered chronically.

Nifedipine

A single-dose, metformin-nifedipine drug interaction study in normal healthy volunteers demonstrated that co-administration of nifedipine increased plasma metformin C_{max} and AUC by 20% and 9%, respectively, and increased the amount excreted in the urine. T_{max} and half-life were unaffected. Nifedipine appears to enhance the absorption of metformin. Metformin had minimal effects on nifedipine.

Cationic drugs

Cationic drugs (e.g., amiloride, digoxin, morphine, procainamide, quinidine, quinine, ranitidine, triamterene, trimethoprim, or vancomycin) that are eliminated by renal tubular secretion theoretically have the potential for interaction with metformin by competing for common renal tubular transport systems. Such interaction between metformin and oral cimetidine has been observed in normal healthy volunteers in both single- and multiple-dose, metformin-cimetidine drug interaction studies, with a 60% increase in peak metformin plasma and whole blood concentrations and a 40% increase in plasma and whole blood metformin AUC. There was no change in elimination half-life in the single-dose study. Metformin had no effect on cimetidine pharmacokinetics. Although such interactions remain theoretical (except for cimetidine), careful patient monitoring and dose adjustment of METAGLIP (glipizide and metformin HCl) Tablets and/or the interfering drug is recommended in patients who are taking cationic medications that are excreted via the proximal renal tubular secretory system.

Other

In healthy volunteers, the pharmacokinetics of metformin and propranolol and metformin and ibuprofen were not affected when co-administered in single-dose interaction studies.

Carcinogenesis, Mutagenesis, Impairment of Fertility

No animal studies have been conducted with the combined products in METAGLIP (glipizide and metformin HCl). The following data are based on findings in studies performed with the individual products.

Glipizide

A 20-month study in rats and an 18-month study in mice at doses up to 75 times the maximum human dose revealed no evidence of drug-related carcinogenicity. Bacterial and *in vivo* mutagenicity tests were uniformly negative. Studies in rats of both sexes at doses up to 75 times the human dose showed no effects on fertility.

Metformin Hydrochloride

Long-term carcinogenicity studies were performed with metformin alone in rats (dosing duration of 104 weeks) and mice (dosing duration of 91 weeks) at doses up to and including 900 mg/kg/day and 1500 mg/kg/day, respectively. These doses are both approximately four times the maximum recommended human daily dose of 2000 mg of the metformin component of METAGLIP based on body surface area comparisons. No evidence of carcinogenicity with metformin alone was found in either male or female mice. Similarly, there was no tumorigenic potential observed with metformin alone in male rats. There was, however, an increased incidence of benign stromal uterine polyps in female rats treated with 900 mg/kg/day of metformin alone.

There was no evidence of a mutagenic potential of metformin alone in the following *in vitro* tests: Ames test (*S. typhimurium*), gene mutation test (mouse lymphoma cells), or chromosomal aberrations test (human lymphocytes). Results in the *in vivo* mouse micronucleus test were also negative.

Fertility of male or female rats was unaffected by metformin alone when administered at doses as high as 600 mg/kg/day, which is approximately three times the maximum recommended human daily dose of the metformin component of METAGLIP based on body surface area comparisons.

Pregnancy

Teratogenic Effects: Pregnancy Category C

Recent information strongly suggests that abnormal blood glucose levels during pregnancy are associated with a higher incidence of congenital abnormalities. Most experts recommend that insulin be used during pregnancy to maintain blood glucose as close to normal as possible. Because animal reproduction studies are not always predictive of human response, METAGLIP should not be used during pregnancy unless clearly needed. (See below.)

There are no adequate and well-controlled studies in pregnant women with METAGLIP or its individual components. No animal studies have been conducted with the combined products in METAGLIP. The following data are based on findings in studies performed with the individual products.

Glipizide

Glipizide was found to be mildly fetotoxic in rat reproductive studies at all dose levels (5-50 mg/kg). This fetotoxicity has been similarly noted with other sulfonylureas, such as tolbutamide and tolazamide. The effect is perinatal and believed to be directly related to the pharmacologic (hypoglycemic) action of glipizide. In studies in rats and rabbits, no teratogenic effects were found.

Metformin hydrochloride

Metformin alone was not teratogenic in rats or rabbits at doses up to 600 mg/kg/day. This represents an exposure of about two and six times the maximum recommended human daily dose of 2000 mg of the metformin component of METAGLIP (glipizide and metformin HCl) Tablets based on body surface area comparisons for rats and rabbits, respectively. Determination of fetal concentrations demonstrated a partial placental barrier to metformin.

Nonteratogenic Effects

Prolonged severe hypoglycemia (4 to 10 days) has been reported in neonates born to mothers who were receiving a sulfonylurea drug at the time of delivery. This has been reported more frequently with the use of agents with prolonged half-lives. It is not recommended that METAGLIP be used during pregnancy. However, if it is used, METAGLIP should be discontinued at least one month before the expected delivery date. (See **Pregnancy; Teratogenic Effects: Pregnancy Category C.**)

Nursing Mothers

Although it is not known whether glipizide is excreted in human milk, some sulfonylurea drugs are known to be excreted in human milk. Studies in lactating rats show that metformin is excreted into milk and reaches levels comparable to those in plasma. Similar studies have not been conducted in nursing mothers. Because the potential for hypoglycemia in nursing infants may exist, a decision should be made whether to discontinue nursing or to discontinue METAGLIP, taking into account the importance of the drug to the mother. If METAGLIP is discontinued, and if diet alone is inadequate for controlling blood glucose, insulin therapy should be considered.

Pediatric Use

Safety and effectiveness of METAGLIP in pediatric patients have not been established.

Geriatric Use

Of the 345 patients who received METAGLIP 2.5 mg/250 mg and 2.5 mg/500 mg in the initial therapy trial, 67 (19.4%) were aged 65 and older while 5 (1.4%) were aged 75 and older. Of the 87 patients who received METAGLIP in the second-line therapy trial, 17 (19.5%) were aged 65 and older while one (1.1%) was at least aged 75. No overall differences in effectiveness or safety were observed between these patients and younger patients in either the initial therapy trial or the second-line therapy trial, and other reported clinical experience has not identified differences in response between the elderly and younger patients, but greater sensitivity of some older individuals cannot be ruled out.

Metformin hydrochloride is known to be substantially excreted by the kidney and because the risk of serious adverse reactions to the drug is greater in patients with impaired renal function, METAGLIP should only be used in patients with normal renal function (see **CONTRAINDICATIONS, WARNINGS**, and **CLINICAL PHARMACOLOGY: Pharmacokinetics**). Because aging is associated with reduced renal function, METAGLIP should be used with caution as age increases. Care should be taken in dose selection and should be based on careful and regular monitoring of renal function. Generally, elderly patients should not be titrated to the maximum dose of METAGLIP (see also **WARNINGS** and **DOSAGE AND ADMINISTRATION**).

ADVERSE REACTIONS

METAGLIP

In a double-blind 24-week clinical trial involving METAGLIP (glipizide and metformin HCl) Tablets as initial therapy, a total of 172 patients received METAGLIP 2.5 mg/250 mg, 173 received METAGLIP 2.5 mg/500 mg, 170 received glipizide, and 177 received metformin. The most common clinical adverse events in these treatment groups are listed in **Table 4**.

[See table 4 at left]

In a double-blind 18-week clinical trial involving METAGLIP as second-line therapy, a total of 87 patients received METAGLIP, 84 received glipizide, and 75 received metformin. The most common clinical adverse events in this clinical trial are listed in **Table 5**.

[See table 5 at top of next page]

Hypoglycemia

In a controlled initial therapy trial of METAGLIP (glipizide and metformin HCl) Tablets 2.5 mg/250 mg and 2.5 mg/500 mg the numbers of patients with hypoglycemia documented by symptoms (such as dizziness, shakiness, sweating, and hunger) and a fingerstick blood glucose measurement ≤50 mg/dL were 5 (2.9%) for glipizide, 0 (0%)

Table 4: Clinical Adverse Events >5% in any Treatment Group, by Primary Term, in Initial Therapy Study

	Number (%) of Patients			
Adverse Event	Glipizide 5 mg tablets N=170	Metformin 500 mg tablets N=177	METAGLIP 2.5 mg/250 mg tablets N=172	METAGLIP 2.5 mg/500 mg tablets N=173
Upper respiratory infection	12 (7.1)	15 (8.5)	17 (9.9)	14 (8.1)
Diarrhea	8 (4.7)	15 (8.5)	4 (2.3)	9 (5.2)
Dizziness	9 (5.3)	2 (1.1)	3 (1.7)	9 (5.2)
Hypertension	17 (10.0)	10 (5.6)	5 (2.9)	6 (3.5)
Nausea/vomiting	6 (3.5)	9 (5.1)	1 (0.6)	3 (1.7)

for metformin, 13 (7.6%) for METAGLIP 2.5 mg/250 mg, and 16 (9.3%) for METAGLIP 2.5 mg/500 mg. Among patients taking either METAGLIP 2.5 mg/250 mg or METAGLIP 2.5 mg/500 mg, nine (2.6%) patients discontinued METAGLIP due to hypoglycemic symptoms and one required medical intervention due to hypoglycemia. In a controlled second-line therapy trial of METAGLIP 5 mg/500 mg, the numbers of patients with hypoglycemia documented by symptoms and a fingerstick blood glucose measurement $\leq$50 mg/dL were 0 (0%) for glipizide, 1 (1.3%) for metformin, and 11 (12.6%) for METAGLIP. One (1.1%) patient discontinued METAGLIP therapy due to hypoglycemic symptoms and none required medical intervention due to hypoglycemia. (See **PRECAUTIONS** section.)

Gastrointestinal Reactions

Among the most common clinical adverse events in the initial therapy trial were diarrhea and nausea/vomiting; the incidences of these events were lower with both METAGLIP dosage strengths than with metformin therapy. There were 4 (1.2%) patients in the initial therapy trial who discontinued METAGLIP therapy due to GI adverse events. Gastrointestinal symptoms of diarrhea, nausea/vomiting, and abdominal pain were comparable among METAGLIP, glipizide and metformin in the second-line therapy trial. There were 4 (4.6%) patients in the second-line therapy trial who discontinued METAGLIP therapy due to GI adverse events.

OVERDOSAGE

Glipizide

Overdosage of sulfonylureas, including glipizide, can produce hypoglycemia. Mild hypoglycemic symptoms, without loss of consciousness or neurological findings, should be treated aggressively with oral glucose and adjustments in drug dosage and/or meal patterns. Close monitoring should continue until the physician is assured that the patient is out of danger. Severe hypoglycemic reactions with coma, seizure, or other neurological impairment occur infrequently, but constitute medical emergencies requiring immediate hospitalization. If hypoglycemic coma is diagnosed or suspected, the patient should be given a rapid intravenous injection of concentrated (50%) glucose solution. This should be followed by a continuous infusion of a more dilute (10%) glucose solution at a rate that will maintain the blood glucose at a level above 100 mg/dL. Patients should be closely monitored for a minimum of 24 to 48 hours, since hypoglycemia may recur after apparent clinical recovery. Clearance of glipizide from plasma would be prolonged in persons with liver disease. Because of the extensive protein binding of glipizide, dialysis is unlikely to be of benefit.

Metformin Hydrochloride

Among cases of overdosage of metformin hydrochloride, including ingestion of amounts greater than 100 grams, hypoglycemia was reported in approximately 10%, but no causal association with metformin hydrochloride has been established, although lactic acidosis has occurred in such circumstances (see **WARNINGS**). Metformin is dialyzable with a clearance of up to 170 mL/min under good hemodynamic conditions. Therefore, hemodialysis may be useful for removal of accumulated drug from patients in whom metformin overdosage is suspected.

DOSAGE AND ADMINISTRATION

General Considerations

Dosage of METAGLIP (glipizide and metformin HCl) Tablets must be individualized on the basis of both effectiveness and tolerance while not exceeding the maximum recommended daily dose of 20 mg glipizide/2000 mg metformin. METAGLIP should be given with meals and should be initiated at a low dose, with gradual dose escalation as described below, in order to avoid hypoglycemia (largely due to glipizide), to reduce GI side effects (largely due to metformin), and to permit determination of the minimum effective dose for adequate control of blood glucose for the individual patient.

With initial treatment and during dose titration, appropriate blood glucose monitoring should be used to determine the therapeutic response to METAGLIP and to identify the minimum effective dose for the patient. Thereafter, HbA_{1c} should be measured at intervals of approximately 3 months to assess the effectiveness of therapy. The therapeutic goal in all patients with type 2 diabetes is to decrease FPG, PPG, and HbA_{1c} to normal or as near normal as possible. Ideally, the response to therapy should be evaluated using HbA_{1c} (glycosylated hemoglobin), which is a better indicator of long-term glycemic control than FPG alone.

No studies have been performed specifically examining the safety and efficacy of switching to METAGLIP therapy in patients taking concomitant glipizide (or other sulfonylurea) plus metformin. Changes in glycemic control may occur in such patients, with either hyperglycemia or hypoglycemia possible. Any change in therapy of type 2 diabetes should be undertaken with care and appropriate monitoring.

METAGLIP as Initial Therapy

For patients with type 2 diabetes whose hyperglycemia cannot be satisfactorily managed with diet and exercise alone, the recommended starting dose of METAGLIP (glipizide and metformin HCl) Tablets is 2.5 mg/250 mg once a day with a meal. For patients whose FPG is 280 to 320 mg/dL a starting dose of METAGLIP 2.5 mg/500 mg twice daily should be considered. The efficacy of METAGLIP in patients whose FPG exceeds 320 mg/dL has not been established. Dosage increases to achieve adequate glycemic control should be made in increments of one tablet per day every two weeks up to maximum of 10 mg/1000 mg or 10 mg/2000 mg METAGLIP per day given in divided doses. In clinical trials of METAGLIP as initial therapy, there was no experience with total daily doses greater than 10 mg/2000 mg per day.

Table 5: Clinical Adverse Events >5% in any Treatment Group, by Primary Term, in Second-line Therapy Study

Adverse Event	Number (%) of Patients		
	Glipizide 5 mg tablets[a] N=84	Metformin 500 mg tablets[a] N=75	METAGLIP 5 mg/500 mg tablets[a] N=87
Diarrhea	11 (13.1)	13 (17.3)	16 (18.4)
Headache	5 (6.0)	4 (5.3)	11 (12.6)
Upper respiratory infection	11 (13.1)	8 (10.7)	9 (10.3)
Musculoskeletal pain	6 (7.1)	5 (6.7)	7 (8.0)
Nausea/vomiting	5 (6.0)	6 (8.0)	7 (8.0)
Abdominal pain	7 (8.3)	5 (6.7)	5 (5.7)
UTI	4 (4.8)	6 (8.0)	1 (1.1)

[a] The dose of glipizide was fixed at 30 mg daily; doses of metformin and METAGLIP were titrated.

METAGLIP as Second-Line Therapy

For patients not adequately controlled on either glipizide (or another sulfonylurea) or metformin alone, the recommended starting dose of METAGLIP is 2.5 mg/500 mg or 5 mg/500 mg twice daily with the morning and evening meals. In order to avoid hypoglycemia, the starting dose of METAGLIP should not exceed the daily doses of glipizide or metformin already being taken. The daily dose should be titrated in increments of no more than 5 mg/500 mg up to the minimum effective dose to achieve adequate control of blood glucose or to a maximum dose of 20 mg/2000 mg per day.

Patients previously treated with combination therapy of glipizide (or another sulfonylurea) plus metformin may be switched to METAGLIP 2.5 mg/500 mg or 5 mg/500 mg; the starting dose should not exceed the daily dose of glipizide (or equivalent dose of another sulfonylurea) and metformin already being taken. The decision to switch to the nearest equivalent dose or to titrate should be based on clinical judgment. Patients should be monitored closely for signs and symptoms of hypoglycemia following such a switch and the dose of METAGLIP should be titrated as described above to achieve adequate control of blood glucose.

Specific Patient Populations

METAGLIP is not recommended for use during pregnancy or for use in pediatric patients. The initial and maintenance dosing of METAGLIP should be conservative in patients with advanced age, due to the potential for decreased renal function in this population. Any dosage adjustment requires a careful assessment of renal function. Generally, elderly, debilitated, and malnourished patients should not be titrated to the maximum dose of METAGLIP to avoid the risk of hypoglycemia. Monitoring of renal function is necessary to aid in prevention of metformin-associated lactic acidosis, particularly in the elderly. (See **WARNINGS**.)

HOW SUPPLIED

METAGLIP™ (glipizide and metformin HCl) Tablets

METAGLIP **2.5 mg/250 mg** tablet is a pink oval-shaped, biconvex film-coated tablet with "**BMS**" debossed on one side and "**6081**" debossed on the opposite side.

METAGLIP **2.5 mg/500 mg** tablet is a white oval-shaped, biconvex film-coated tablet with "**BMS**" debossed on one side and "**6077**" debossed on the opposite side.

METAGLIP **5 mg/500 mg** tablet is a pink oval-shaped, biconvex film-coated tablet with "**BMS**" debossed on one side and "**6078**" debossed on the opposite side.

METAGLIP		NDC 0087-xxxx-xx for unit of use
Glipizide (mg)	Metformin HCl (mg)	Bottle of 100
2.5	250	6081-31
2.5	500	6077-31
5.0	500	6078-31

STORAGE

Store at 20° C–25° C (68° F–77° F); excursions permitted to 15° C–30° C (59° F–86° F). [See USP Controlled Room Temperature.]

METAGLIP™ is a trademark of Merck Santé S.A.S., an associate of Merck KGaA of Darmstadt, Germany. Licensed to Bristol-Myers Squibb Company.

GLUCOPHAGE® is a registered trademark of Merck Santé S.A.S., an associate of Merck KGaA of Darmstadt, Germany. Licensed to Bristol-Myers Squibb Company.

GLUCOTROL® is a registered trademark of Pfizer Inc.

PATIENT INFORMATION ABOUT

METAGLIP™

(glipizide and metformin HCl) Tablets

WARNING: A small number of people who have taken metformin hydrochloride have developed a serious condition called lactic acidosis. Properly functioning kidneys are needed to help prevent lactic acidosis. Most people with kidney problems should not take METAGLIP. (See Question Nos. 9–13.)

Q1. WHY DO I NEED TO TAKE METAGLIP?

Your doctor has prescribed METAGLIP (glipizide and metformin HCl) to treat your type 2 diabetes. This is also known as non-insulin-dependent diabetes mellitus.

Q2. WHAT IS TYPE 2 DIABETES?

People with diabetes are not able to make enough insulin and/or respond normally to the insulin their body does make. When this happens, sugar (glucose) builds up in the blood. This can lead to serious medical problems including kidney damage, amputations, and blindness. Diabetes is also closely linked to heart disease. The main goal of treating diabetes is to lower your blood sugar to a normal level.

Q3. WHY IS IT IMPORTANT TO CONTROL TYPE 2 DIABETES?

The main goal of treating diabetes is to lower your blood sugar to a normal level. Studies have shown that good control of blood sugar may prevent or delay complications such as heart disease, kidney disease, or blindness.

Q4. HOW IS TYPE 2 DIABETES USUALLY CONTROLLED?

High blood sugar can be lowered by diet and exercise, by a number of oral medications, and by insulin injections. Before taking METAGLIP (glipizide and metformin HCl) Tablets you should first try to control your diabetes by exercise and weight loss. Even if you are taking METAGLIP, you should still exercise and follow the diet recommended for your diabetes.

Q5. DOES METAGLIP WORK DIFFERENTLY FROM OTHER GLUCOSE-CONTROL MEDICATIONS?

Yes it does. METAGLIP combines two glucose lowering drugs, glipizide and metformin. These two drugs work together to improve the different metabolic defects found in type 2 diabetes. Glipizide lowers blood sugar primarily by causing more of the body's own insulin to be released, and metformin lowers blood sugar, in part, by helping your body use your own insulin more effectively. Together, they are efficient in helping you achieve better glucose control.

Q6. WHAT HAPPENS IF MY BLOOD SUGAR IS STILL TOO HIGH?

When blood sugar cannot be lowered enough by METAGLIP your doctor may prescribe injectable insulin or take other measures to control your diabetes.

Q7. CAN METAGLIP CAUSE SIDE EFFECTS?

METAGLIP, like all blood sugar-lowering medications, can cause side effects in some patients. Most of these side effects are minor. However, there are also serious, but rare, side effects related to METAGLIP (see **Question Nos. 9-13**).

Q8. WHAT ARE THE MOST COMMON SIDE EFFECTS OF METAGLIP?

The most common side effects of METAGLIP are normally minor ones such as diarrhea, nausea, and upset stomach. If these side effects occur, they usually occur during the first few weeks of therapy. Taking your METAGLIP with meals can help reduce these side effects.

Symptoms of hypoglycemia (low blood sugar), such as lightheadedness, dizziness, shakiness, or hunger may occur. The risk of hypoglycemic symptoms increases when meals are skipped, too much alcohol is consumed, or heavy exercise occurs without enough food. Following the advice of your doctor can help you to avoid these symptoms.

Q9. ARE THERE ANY SERIOUS SIDE EFFECTS THAT METAGLIP CAN CAUSE?

METAGLIP rarely causes serious side effects. The most serious side effect that METAGLIP can cause is called lactic acidosis.

Continued on next page

Metaglip—Cont.

Q10. WHAT IS LACTIC ACIDOSIS AND CAN IT HAPPEN TO ME?

Lactic acidosis is caused by a buildup of lactic acid in the blood. Lactic acidosis associated with metformin is rare and has occurred mostly in people whose kidneys were not working normally. Lactic acidosis has been reported in about one in 33,000 patients taking metformin over the course of a year. Although rare, if lactic acidosis does occur, it can be fatal in up to half the cases.

It's also important for your liver to be working normally when you take METAGLIP. Your liver helps remove lactic acid from your bloodstream.

Your doctor will monitor your diabetes and may perform blood tests on you from time to time to make sure your kidneys and your liver are functioning normally.

There is no evidence that METAGLIP causes harm to the kidneys or liver.

Q11. ARE THERE OTHER RISK FACTORS FOR LACTIC ACIDOSIS?

Your risk of developing lactic acidosis from taking METAGLIP (glipizide and metformin HCl) Tablets is very low as long as your kidneys and liver are healthy. However, some factors can increase your risk because they can affect kidney and liver function. You should discuss your risk with your physician.

You should not take METAGLIP if:

- You have chronic kidney or liver problems
- You have congestive heart failure which is treated with medications, e.g., digoxin (Lanoxin®) or furosemide (Lasix®)
- You drink alcohol excessively (all the time or short-term "binge" drinking)
- You are seriously dehydrated (have lost a large amount of body fluids)
- You are going to have certain X-ray procedures with injectable contrast agents
- You are going to have surgery
- You develop a serious condition such as a heart attack, severe infection, or a stroke
- You are ≥80 years of age and have NOT had your kidney function tested

Q12. WHAT ARE THE SYMPTOMS OF LACTIC ACIDOSIS?

Some of the symptoms include: feeling very weak, tired or uncomfortable; unusual muscle pain, trouble breathing, unusual or unexpected stomach discomfort, feeling cold, feeling dizzy or lightheaded, or suddenly developing a slow or irregular heartbeat.

If you notice these symptoms, or if your medical condition has suddenly changed, stop taking METAGLIP tablets and call your doctor right away. Lactic acidosis is a medical emergency that must be treated in a hospital.

Q13. WHAT DOES MY DOCTOR NEED TO KNOW TO DECREASE MY RISK OF LACTIC ACIDOSIS?

Tell your doctor if you have an illness that results in severe vomiting, diarrhea, and/or fever, or if your intake of fluids is significantly reduced. These situations can lead to severe dehydration, and it may be necessary to stop taking METAGLIP temporarily.

You should let your doctor know if you are going to have any surgery or specialized x-ray procedures that require injection of contrast agents. METAGLIP therapy will need to be stopped temporarily in such instances.

Q14. CAN I TAKE METAGLIP WITH OTHER MEDICATIONS?

Remind your doctor that you are taking METAGLIP when any new drug is prescribed or a change is made in how you take a drug already prescribed.

METAGLIP may interfere with the way some drugs work and some drugs may interfere with the action of METAGLIP.

Q15. WHAT IF I BECOME PREGNANT WHILE TAKING METAGLIP?

Tell your doctor if you plan to become pregnant or have become pregnant. As with other oral glucose-control medications, you should not take METAGLIP (glipizide and metformin HCl) Tablets during pregnancy.

Usually your doctor will prescribe insulin while you are pregnant. As with all medications, you and your doctor should discuss the use of METAGLIP if you are nursing a child.

Q16. HOW DO I TAKE METAGLIP?

Your doctor will tell you how many METAGLIP tablets to take and how often.

This should also be printed on the label of your prescription. You will probably be started on a low dose of METAGLIP and your dosage will be increased gradually until your blood sugar is controlled.

Q17. WHERE CAN I GET MORE INFORMATION ABOUT METAGLIP?

This leaflet is a summary of the most important information about METAGLIP.

If you have any questions or problems, you should talk to your doctor or other healthcare provider about type 2 diabetes as well as METAGLIP and its side effects. There is also a leaflet (package insert) written for health professionals that your pharmacist can let you read.

METAGLIP™ is a trademark of Merck Santé S.A.S., an associate of Merck KGaA of Darmstadt, Germany. Licensed to Bristol-Myers Squibb Company.

Bristol-Myers Squibb Company

Distributed by
Bristol-Myers Squibb Company
Princeton, NJ 08543 USA
M1-B0001-10-02 Issued: October 2002

Shown in Product Identification Guide, page 310

PLAVIX® ℞

[plă-vĭcks]

(clopidogrel bisulfate tablets)

DESCRIPTION

PLAVIX (clopidogrel bisulfate) is an inhibitor of ADP-induced platelet aggregation acting by direct inhibition of adenosine diphosphate (ADP) binding to its receptor and of the subsequent ADP-mediated activation of the glycoprotein GPIIb/IIIa complex. Chemically it is methyl (+)-(*S*)-α-(2-chlorophenyl)-6,7-dihydrothieno[3,2-c]pyridine-5(4*H*)-acetate sulfate (1:1). The empirical formula of clopidogrel bisulfate is $C_{16}H_{16}Cl\ NO_2S{\bullet}H_2SO_4$ and its molecular weight is 419.9.

The structural formula is as follows:

Clopidogrel bisulfate is a white to off-white powder. It is practically insoluble in water at neutral pH but freely soluble at pH 1. It also dissolves freely in methanol, dissolves sparingly in methylene chloride, and is practically insoluble in ethyl ether. It has a specific optical rotation of about +56°.

PLAVIX for oral administration is provided as pink, round, biconvex, debossed film-coated tablets containing 97.875 mg of clopidogrel bisulfate which is the molar equivalent of 75 mg of clopidogrel base.

Each tablet contains hydrogenated castor oil, hydroxypropylcellulose, mannitol, microcrystalline cellulose and polyethylene glycol 6000 as inactive ingredients. The pink film coating contains ferric oxide, hydroxypropylmethylcellulose 2910, lactose monohydrate, titanium dioxide and triacetin. The tablets are polished with Carnauba wax.

CLINICAL PHARMACOLOGY

Mechanism of Action

Clopidogrel is an inhibitor of platelet aggregation. A variety of drugs that inhibit platelet function have been shown to decrease morbid events in people with established cardiovascular atherosclerotic disease as evidenced by stroke or transient ischemic attacks, myocardial infarction, unstable angina or the need for vascular bypass or angioplasty. This indicates that platelets participate in the initiation and/or evolution of these events and that inhibiting them can reduce the event rate.

Pharmacodynamic Properties

Clopidogrel selectively inhibits the binding of adenosine diphosphate (ADP) to its platelet receptor and the subsequent ADP-mediated activation of the glycoprotein GPIIb/IIIa complex, thereby inhibiting platelet aggregation. Biotransformation of clopidogrel is necessary to produce inhibition of platelet aggregation, but an active metabolite responsible for the activity of the drug has not been isolated. Clopidogrel also inhibits platelet aggregation induced by agonists other than ADP by blocking the amplification of platelet activation by released ADP. Clopidogrel does not inhibit phosphodiesterase activity.

Clopidogrel acts by irreversibly modifying the platelet ADP receptor. Consequently, platelets exposed to clopidogrel are affected for the remainder of their lifespan.

Dose dependent inhibition of platelet aggregation can be seen 2 hours after single oral doses of PLAVIX. Repeated doses of 75 mg PLAVIX (clopidogrel bisulfate) per day inhibit ADP-induced platelet aggregation on the first day, and inhibition reaches steady state between Day 3 and Day 7. At steady state, the average inhibition level observed with a dose of 75 mg PLAVIX per day was between 40% and 60%. Platelet aggregation and bleeding time gradually return to baseline values after treatment is discontinued, generally in about 5 days.

Pharmacokinetics and Metabolism

After repeated 75-mg oral doses of clopidogrel (base), plasma concentrations of the parent compound, which has no platelet inhibiting effect, are very low and are generally below the quantification limit (0.00025 mg/L) beyond 2 hours after dosing. Clopidogrel is extensively metabolized by the liver. The main circulating metabolite is the carboxylic acid derivative, and it too has no effect on platelet aggregation. It represents about 85% of the circulating drug-related compounds in plasma.

Following an oral dose of ^{14}C-labeled clopidogrel in humans, approximately 50% was excreted in the urine and approximately 46% in the feces in the 5 days after dosing. The elimination half-life of the main circulating metabolite was 8 hours after single and repeated administration. Covalent binding to platelets accounted for 2% of radiolabel with a half-life of 11 days.

Effect of Food: Administration of PLAVIX with meals did not significantly modify the bioavailability of clopidogrel as assessed by the pharmacokinetics of the main circulating metabolite.

Absorption and Distribution: Clopidogrel is rapidly absorbed after oral administration of repeated doses of 75 mg clopidogrel (base), with peak plasma levels (≅3 mg/L) of the main circulating metabolite occurring approximately 1 hour after dosing. The pharmacokinetics of the main circulating metabolite are linear (plasma concentrations increased in proportion to dose) in the dose range of 50 to 150 mg of clopidogrel. Absorption is at least 50% based on urinary excretion of clopidogrel-related metabolites.

Clopidogrel and the main circulating metabolite bind reversibly *in vitro* to human plasma proteins (98% and 94%, respectively). The binding is nonsaturable *in vitro* up to a concentration of 100 µg/mL.

Metabolism and Elimination: *In vitro* and *in vivo*, clopidogrel undergoes rapid hydrolysis into its carboxylic acid derivative. In plasma and urine, the glucuronide of the carboxylic acid derivative is also observed.

Special Populations

Geriatric Patients: Plasma concentrations of the main circulating metabolite are significantly higher in elderly (≥75 years) compared to young healthy volunteers but these higher plasma levels were not associated with differences in platelet aggregation and bleeding time. No dosage adjustment is needed for the elderly.

Renally Impaired Patients: After repeated doses of 75 mg PLAVIX (clopidogrel bisulfate) per day, plasma levels of the main circulating metabolite were lower in patients with severe renal impairment (creatinine clearance from 5 to 15 mL/min) compared to subjects with moderate renal impairment (creatinine clearance 30 to 60 mL/min) or healthy subjects. Although inhibition of ADP-induced platelet aggregation was lower (25%) than that observed in healthy volunteers, the prolongation of bleeding time was similar to healthy volunteers receiving 75 mg of PLAVIX per day.

Gender: No significant difference was observed in the plasma levels of the main circulating metabolite between males and females. In a small study comparing men and women, less inhibition of ADP-induced platelet aggregation was observed in women, but there was no difference in prolongation of bleeding time. In the large, controlled clinical study (Clopidogrel vs. Aspirin in Patients at Risk of Ischemic Events; CAPRIE), the incidence of clinical outcome events, other adverse clinical events, and abnormal clinical laboratory parameters was similar in men and women.

Race: Pharmacokinetic differences due to race have not been studied.

CLINICAL STUDIES

The clinical evidence for the efficacy of PLAVIX is derived from two double-blind trials: the CAPRIE study (Clopidogrel vs. Aspirin in Patients at Risk of Ischemic Events), a comparison of PLAVIX to aspirin, and the CURE study (Clopidogrel in Unstable Angina to Prevent Recurrent Ischemic Events), a comparison of PLAVIX to placebo, both given in combination with aspirin and other standard therapy.

The CAPRIE trial was a 19,185-patient, 304-center, international, randomized, double-blind, parallel-group study comparing PLAVIX (75 mg daily) to aspirin (325 mg daily). The patients randomized had: 1) recent histories of myocardial infarction (within 35 days); 2) recent histories of ischemic stroke (within 6 months) with at least a week of residual neurological signs; or 3) objectively established peripheral arterial disease. Patients received randomized treatment for an average of 1.6 years (maximum of 3 years).

The trial's primary outcome was the time to first occurrence of new ischemic stroke (fatal or not), new myocardial infarction (fatal or not), or other vascular death. Deaths not easily attributable to nonvascular causes were all classified as vascular.

Table 1: Outcome Events in the CAPRIE Primary Analysis

Patients	PLAVIX 9599	aspirin 9586
IS (fatal or not)	438 (4.6%)	461 (4.8%)
MI (fatal or not)	275 (2.9%)	333 (3.5%)
Other vascular death	226 (2.4%)	226 (2.4%)
Total	939 (9.8%)	1020 (10.6%)

As shown in the table, PLAVIX was associated with a lower incidence of outcome events of every kind. The overall risk reduction (9.8% vs. 10.64%) was 8.7%, P=0.045. Similar results were obtained when all-cause mortality and all-cause strokes were counted instead of vascular mortality and ischemic strokes (risk reduction 6.9%). In patients who survived an on-study stroke or myocardial infarction, the incidence of subsequent events was again lower in the PLAVIX group.

The curves showing the overall event rate are shown in Figure 1. The event curves separated early and continued to diverge over the 3-year follow-up period.

[See figure 1 at top of next column]

Although the statistical significance favoring PLAVIX (clopidogrel bisulfate) over aspirin was marginal (P=0.045), and represents the result of a single trial that has not been replicated, the comparator drug, aspirin, is itself effective (vs. placebo) in reducing cardiovascular events in patients with recent myocardial infarction or stroke. Thus, the difference between PLAVIX and placebo, although not measured directly, is substantial.

The CAPRIE trial included a population that was randomized on the basis of 3 entry criteria. The efficacy of PLAVIX relative to aspirin was heterogeneous across these randomized subgroups (P=0.043). It is not clear whether this differ-

Figure 1: Fatal or Non-Fatal Vascular Events in the CAPRIE Study

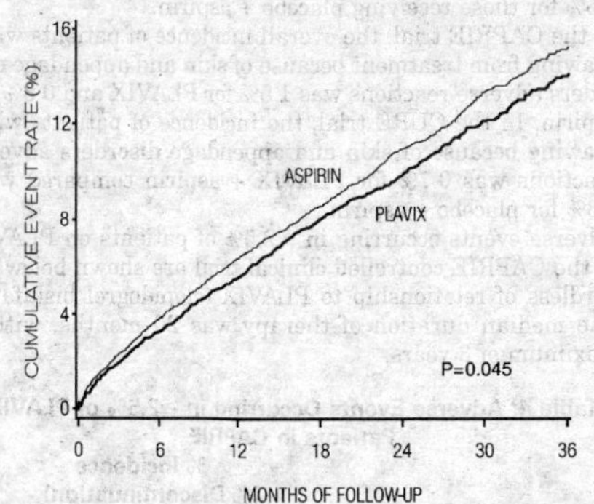

ence is real or a chance occurrence. Although the CAPRIE trial was not designed to evaluate the relative benefit of PLAVIX over aspirin in the individual patient subgroups, the benefit appeared to be strongest in patients who were enrolled because of peripheral vascular disease (especially those who also had a history of myocardial infarction) and weaker in stroke patients. In patients who were enrolled in the trial on the sole basis of a recent myocardial infarction, PLAVIX was not numerically superior to aspirin.

In the meta-analyses of studies of aspirin vs. placebo in patients similar to those in CAPRIE, aspirin was associated with a reduced incidence of thrombotic events. There was a suggestion of heterogeneity in these studies too, with the effect strongest in patients with a history of myocardial infarction, weaker in patients with a history of stroke, and not discernible in patients with a history of peripheral vascular disease. With respect to the inferred comparison of PLAVIX to placebo, there is no indication of heterogeneity.

The CURE study included 12,562 patients with acute coronary syndrome without ST segment elevation (unstable angina or non-Q-wave myocardial infarction) and presenting within 24 hours of onset of the most recent episode of chest pain or symptoms consistent with ischemia. Patients were required to have either ECG changes compatible with new ischemia (without ST segment elevation) or elevated cardiac enzymes or troponin I or T to at least twice the upper limit of normal. The patient population was largely Caucasian (82%) and included 38% women, and 52% patients ≥65 years of age.

Patients were randomized to receive PLAVIX (clopidogrel bisulfate) (300 mg loading dose followed by 75 mg/day) or placebo, and were treated for up to one year. Patients also received aspirin (75-325 mg once daily) and other standard therapies such as heparin. The use of GPIIb/IIIa inhibitors was not permitted for three days prior to randomization.

The number of patients experiencing the primary outcome (CV death, MI, or stroke) was 582 (9.30%) in the PLAVIX-treated group and 719 (11.41%) in the placebo-treated group, a 20% relative risk reduction (95% CI of 10%-28%; p=0.00009) for the PLAVIX-treated group (see Table 2).

At the end of 12 months, the number of patients experiencing the co-primary outcome (CV death, MI, stroke or refractory ischemia) was 1035 (16.54%) in the PLAVIX-treated group and 1187 (18.83%) in the placebo-treated group, a 14% relative risk reduction (95% CI of 6%-21%; p=0.0005) for the PLAVIX-treated group (see Table 2).

In the PLAVIX-treated group, each component of the two primary endpoints (CV death, MI, stroke, refractory ischemia) occurred less frequently than in the placebo-treated group.

[See table 2 above]

The benefits of PLAVIX were maintained throughout the course of the trial (up to 12 months).

Figure 2: Cardiovascular Death, Myocardial Infarction, and Stroke in the CURE Study

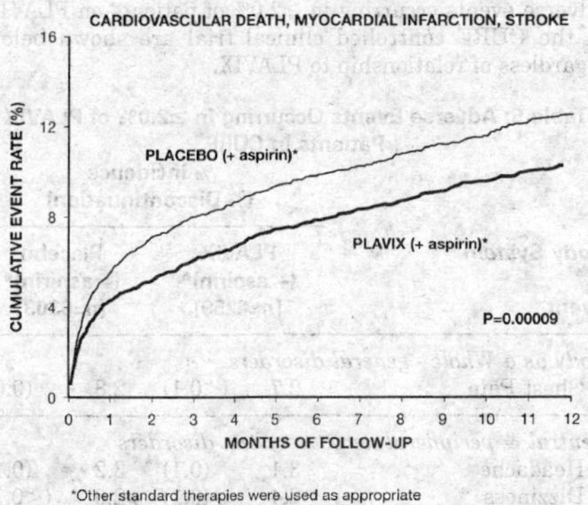

*Other standard therapies were used as appropriate

In CURE, the use of PLAVIX (clopidogrel bisulfate) was associated with a lower incidence of CV death, MI or stroke in patient populations with different characteristics, as shown in Figure 3. The benefits associated with PLAVIX were independent of the use of other acute and long-term cardiovascular therapies, including heparin/LMWH (low molecu-

Table 2: Outcome Events in the CURE Primary Analysis

Outcome	PLAVIX (+ aspirin)* (n=6259)		Placebo (+ aspirin)* (n=6303)		Relative Risk Reduction (%) (95% CI)
Primary outcome (Cardiovascular death, MI, Stroke)	582	(9.3%)	719	(11.4%)	20% (10.3, 27.9) P=0.00009
Co-primary outcome (Cardiovascular death, MI, Stroke, Refractory Ischemia)	1035	(16.5%)	1187	(18.8%)	14% (6.2, 20.6) P=0.00052
All Individual Outcome Events:†					
CV death	318	(5.1%)	345	(5.5%)	7% (-7.7, 20.6)
MI	324	(5.2%)	419	(6.6%)	23% (11.0, 33.4)
Stroke	75	(1.2%)	87	(1.4%)	14% (-17.7, 36.6)
Refractory ischemia	544	(8.7%)	587	(9.3%)	7% (-4.0, 18.0)

* Other standard therapies were used as appropriate.
† The individual components do not represent a breakdown of the primary and co-primary outcomes, but rather the total number of subjects experiencing an event during the course of the study.

lar weight heparin), IV glycoprotein IIb/IIIa (GPIIb/IIIa) inhibitors, lipid-lowering drugs, beta-blockers, and ACE-inhibitors. The efficacy of PLAVIX was observed independently of the dose of aspirin (75-325 mg once daily). The use of oral anticoagulants, non-study anti-platelet drugs and chronic NSAIDs was not allowed in CURE.

Figure 3: Hazard Ratio for Patient Baseline Characteristics and On-Study Concomitant Medications/Interventions for the CURE Study

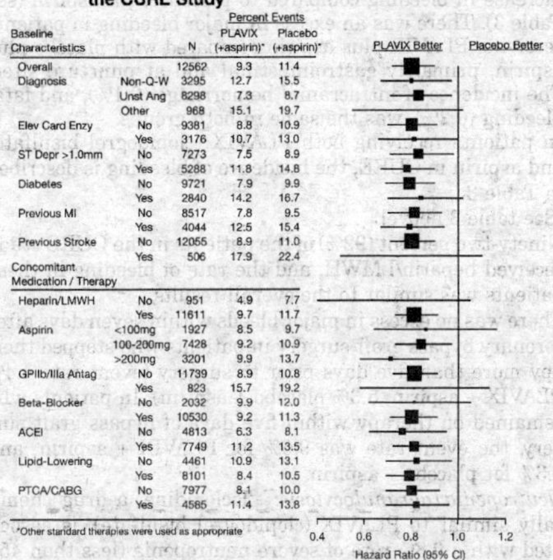

The use of PLAVIX in CURE was associated with a decrease in the use of thrombolytic therapy (71 patients [1.1%] in the PLAVIX group, 126 patients [2.0%] in the placebo group; relative risk reduction of 43%, P=0.0001), and GPIIb/IIIa inhibitors (369 patients [5.9%] in the PLAVIX group, 454 patients [7.2%] in the placebo group; relative risk reduction of 18%, P=0.003). The use of PLAVIX in CURE did not impact the number of patients treated with CABG or PCI (with or without stenting), (2253 patients [36.0%] in the PLAVIX group, 2324 patients [36.9%] in the placebo group; relative risk reduction of 4.0%, P=0.1658).

INDICATIONS AND USAGE

PLAVIX (clopidogrel bisulfate) is indicated for the reduction of thrombotic events as follows:

- **Recent MI, Recent Stroke or Established Peripheral Arterial Disease**
  For patients with a history of recent myocardial infarction (MI), recent stroke, or established peripheral arterial disease, PLAVIX has been shown to reduce the rate of a combined endpoint of new ischemic stroke (fatal or not), new MI (fatal or not), and other vascular death.
- **Acute Coronary Syndrome**
  For patients with acute coronary syndrome (unstable angina/non-Q-wave MI) including patients who are to be managed medically and those who are to be managed with percutaneous coronary intervention (with or without stent) or CABG, PLAVIX has been shown to decrease the rate of a combined endpoint of cardiovascular death, MI, or stroke as well as the rate of a combined endpoint of cardiovascular death, MI, stroke, or refractory ischemia.

CONTRAINDICATIONS

The use of PLAVIX is contraindicated in the following conditions:

- Hypersensitivity to the drug substance or any component of the product.
- Active pathological bleeding such as peptic ulcer or intracranial hemorrhage.

WARNINGS

Thrombotic thrombocytopenic purpura (TTP): TTP has been reported rarely following use of PLAVIX, sometimes after a short exposure (<2weeks). TTP is a serious condition requiring prompt treatment. It is characterized by thrombocytopenia, microangiopathic hemolytic anemia (schistocytes [fragmented RBCs] seen on peripheral smear), neurological findings, renal dysfunction, and fever. TTP was not seen during clopidogrel's clinical trials, which included over 17,500 clopidogrel-treated patients. In world-wide postmarketing experience, however, TTP has been reported at a rate of about four cases per million patients exposed, or about 11 cases per million patient-years. The background rate is thought to be about four cases per million person-years.

PRECAUTIONS

General

PLAVIX prolongs the bleeding time and therefore should be used with caution in patients who may be at risk of increased bleeding from trauma, surgery, or other pathological conditions (particularly gastrointestinal and intraocular). If a patient is to undergo elective surgery and an antiplatelet effect is not desired, PLAVIX should be discontinued 5 days prior to surgery.

Due to the risk of bleeding and undesirable hematological effects, blood cell count determination and/or other appropriate testing should be promptly considered, whenever such suspected clinical symptoms arise during the course of treatment (see **ADVERSE REACTIONS**).

GI Bleeding: In CAPRIE, PLAVIX was associated with a rate of gastrointestinal bleeding of 2.0%, vs. 2.7% on aspirin. In CURE, the incidence of major gastrointestinal bleeding was 1.3% vs. 0.7% (PLAVIX + aspirin vs. placebo + aspirin, respectively.) PLAVIX should be used with caution in patients who have lesions with a propensity to bleed (such as ulcers). Drugs that might induce such lesions should be used with caution in patients taking PLAVIX.

Use in Hepatically-Impaired Patients: Experience is limited in patients with severe hepatic disease, who may have bleeding diatheses. PLAVIX should be used with caution in this population.

Use in Renally-Impaired Patients: Experience is limited in patients with severe renal impairment. PLAVIX should be used with caution in this population.

Information for Patients

Patients should be told that it may take them longer than usual to stop bleeding when they take PLAVIX, and that they should report any unusual bleeding to their physician. Patients should inform physicians and dentists that they are taking PLAVIX before any surgery is scheduled and before any new drug is taken.

Drug Interactions

Study of specific drug interactions yielded the following results:

Aspirin: Aspirin did not modify the clopidogrel-mediated inhibition of ADP-induced platelet aggregation. Concomitant administration of 500 mg of aspirin twice a day for 1 day did not significantly increase the prolongation of bleeding time induced by PLAVIX. PLAVIX (clopidogrel bisulfate) potentiated the effect of aspirin on collagen-induced platelet aggregation. PLAVIX and aspirin have been administered together for up to one year.

Heparin: In a study in healthy volunteers, PLAVIX did not necessitate modification of the heparin dose or alter the effect of heparin on coagulation. Coadministration of heparin had no effect on inhibition of platelet aggregation induced by PLAVIX.

Nonsteroidal Anti-Inflammatory Drugs (NSAIDs): In healthy volunteers receiving naproxen, concomitant administration of PLAVIX was associated with increased occult gastrointestinal blood loss. NSAIDs and PLAVIX should be coadministered with caution.

Warfarin: Because of the increased risk of bleeding, the concomitant administration of warfarin with PLAVIX should be undertaken with caution. (See **Precautions-General**).

Continued on next page

Table 3: CURE Incidence of Bleeding Complications (% Patients)

Event	PLAVIX (+ aspirin)* (n=6259)	Placebo (+ aspirin)* (n=6303)	P-value
Major bleeding†	3.7‡	2.7§	0.001
Life threatening bleeding	2.2	1.8	0.13
Fatal	0.2	0.2	
5 g/dL hemoglobin drop	0.9	0.9	
Requiring surgical intervention	0.7	0.7	
Hemorrhagic strokes	0.1	0.1	
Requiring inotropes	0.5	0.5	
Requiring transfusion (≥ 4 units)	1.2	1.0	
Other major bleeding	1.6	1.0	0.005
Significantly disabling	0.4	0.3	
Intraocular bleeding with significant loss of vision	0.05	0.03	
Requiring 2-3 units of blood	1.3	0.9	
Minor bleeding¶	5.1	2.4	<0.001

* Other standard therapies were used as appropriate.
† Life threatening and other major bleeding.
‡ Major bleeding event rate for PLAVIX + aspirin was dose-dependent on aspirin: < 100 mg=2.6%; 100-200 mg=3.5%; >200 mg=4.9%
§ Major bleeding event rate for placebo + aspirin was dose-dependent on aspirin: < 100 mg=2.0%; 100-200 mg=2.3%; >200 mg=4.0%
¶ Led to interruption of study medication.

Plavix—Cont.

Other Concomitant Therapy: No clinically significant pharmacodynamic interactions were observed when PLAVIX was coadministered with **atenolol, nifedipine,** or both atenolol and nifedipine. The pharmacodynamic activity of PLAVIX was also not significantly influenced by the coadministration of **phenobarbital, cimetidine** or **estrogen.**
The pharmacokinetics of **digoxin** or **theophylline** were not modified by the coadministration of PLAVIX.
At high concentrations *in vitro,* clopidogrel inhibits P_{450} (2C9). Accordingly, PLAVIX (clopidogrel bisulfate) may interfere with the metabolism of **phenytoin, tamoxifen, tolbutamide, warfarin, torsemide, fluvastatin,** and many **non-steroidal anti-inflammatory agents,** but there are no data with which to predict the magnitude of these interactions. Caution should be used when any of these drugs is coadministered with PLAVIX.
In addition to the above specific interaction studies, patients entered into clinical trials with PLAVIX received a variety of concomitant medications including **diuretics, beta-blocking agents, angiotensin converting enzyme inhibitors, calcium antagonists, cholesterol lowering agents, coronary vasodilators, antidiabetic agents,** (including **insulin), antiepileptic agents, hormone replacement therapy, heparins** (unfractionated and LMWH) and **GPIIb/IIIa antagonists** without evidence of clinically significant adverse interactions. The use of oral anticoagulants, non-study anti-platelet drug and chronic NSAIDs was not allowed in CURE and there are no data on their concomitant use with clopidogrel.

Drug/Laboratory Test Interactions
None known.

Carcinogenesis, Mutagenesis, Impairment of Fertility
There was no evidence of tumorigenicity when clopidogrel was administered for 78 weeks to mice and 104 weeks to rats at dosages up to 77 mg/kg per day, which afforded plasma exposures >25 times that in humans at the recommended daily dose of 75 mg.
Clopidogrel was not genotoxic in four *in vitro* tests (Ames test, DNA-repair test in rat hepatocytes, gene mutation assay in Chinese hamster fibroblasts, and metaphase chromosome analysis of human lymphocytes) and in one *in vivo* test (micronucleus test by oral route in mice).
Clopidogrel was found to have no effect on fertility of male and female rats at oral doses up to 400 mg/kg per day (52 times the recommended human dose on a mg/m^2 basis).

Pregnancy
Pregnancy Category B. Reproduction studies performed in rats and rabbits at doses up to 500 and 300 mg/kg/day (respectively, 65 and 78 times the recommended daily human dose on a mg/m^2 basis), revealed no evidence of impaired fertility or fetotoxicity due to clopidogrel. There are, however, no adequate and well-controlled studies in pregnant women. Because animal reproduction studies are not always predictive of a human response, PLAVIX should be used during pregnancy only if clearly needed.

Nursing Mothers
Studies in rats have shown that clopidogrel and/or its metabolites are excreted in the milk. It is not known whether this drug is excreted in human milk. Because many drugs are excreted in human milk and because of the potential for serious adverse reactions in nursing infants, a decision should be made whether to discontinue nursing or to discontinue the drug, taking into account the importance of the drug to the nursing woman.

Pediatric Use
Safety and effectiveness in the pediatric population have not been established.

ADVERSE REACTIONS

PLAVIX has been evaluated for safety in more than 17,500 patients, including over 9,000 patients treated for 1 year or more. The overall tolerability of PLAVIX in CAPRIE was similar to that of aspirin regardless of age, gender and race, with an approximately equal incidence (13%) of patients withdrawing from treatment because of adverse reactions. The clinically important adverse events observed in CAPRIE and CURE are discussed below.
Hemorrhagic: In CAPRIE patients receiving PLAVIX, gastrointestinal hemorrhage occurred at a rate of 2.0%, and required hospitalization in 0.7%. In patients receiving aspirin, the corresponding rates were 2.7% and 1.1%, respectively. The incidence of intracranial hemorrhage was 0.4% for PLAVIX compared to 0.5% for aspirin.
In CURE, PLAVIX use with aspirin was associated with an increase in bleeding compared to placebo with aspirin (see Table 3). There was an excess in major bleeding in patients receiving PLAVIX plus aspirin compared with placebo plus aspirin, primarily gastrointestinal and at puncture sites. The incidence of intracranial hemorrhage (0.1%), and fatal bleeding (0.2%), was the same in both groups.
In patients receiving both PLAVIX (clopidogrel bisulfate) and aspirin in CURE, the incidence of bleeding is described in Table 3.
[See table 3 above]
Ninety-two percent (92%) of the patients in the CURE study received heparin/LMWH, and the rate of bleeding in these patients was similar to the overall results.
There was no excess in major bleeds within seven days after coronary bypass graft surgery in patients who stopped therapy more than five days prior to surgery (event rate 4.4% PLAVIX + aspirin; 5.3% placebo + aspirin). In patients who remained on therapy within five days of bypass graft surgery, the event rate was 9.6% for PLAVIX + aspirin, and 6.3% for placebo + aspirin.
Neutropenia/agranulocytosis: Ticlopidine, a drug chemically similar to PLAVIX (clopidogrel bisulfate), is associated with a 0.8% rate of severe neutropenia (less than 450 neutrophils/μL). In CAPRIE, severe neutropenia was observed in six patients, four on PLAVIX and two on aspirin. Two of the 9599 patients who received PLAVIX and none of the 9586 patients who received aspirin had neutrophil counts of zero. One of the four PLAVIX patients in CAPRIE was receiving cytotoxic chemotherapy, and another recovered and returned to the trial after only temporarily interrupting treatment with PLAVIX. In CURE, the numbers of patients with thrombocytopenia (19 PLAVIX + aspirin vs 24 placebo + aspirin) or neutropenia (3 vs 3) were similar.
Although the risk of myelotoxicity with PLAVIX thus appears to be quite low, this possibility should be considered when a patient receiving PLAVIX demonstrates fever or other sign of infection.
Gastrointestinal: Overall, the incidence of gastrointestinal events (e.g. abdominal pain, dyspepsia, gastritis and constipation) in patients receiving PLAVIX was 27.1%, compared to 29.8% in those receiving aspirin in the CAPRIE trial. In the CURE trial, the incidence of these gastrointestinal events for patients receiving PLAVIX + aspirin was 11.7% compared to 12.5% for those receiving placebo + aspirin.
In the CAPRIE trial, the incidence of peptic, gastric or duodenal ulcers was 0.7% for PLAVIX and 1.2% for aspirin. In the CURE trial, the incidence of peptic, gastric or duodenal ulcers was 0.4% for PLAVIX + aspirin and 0.3% for placebo + aspirin.
Cases of diarrhea were reported in the CAPRIE trial in 4.5% of patients in the PLAVIX group compared to 3.4% in the aspirin group. However, these were rarely severe (PLAVIX=0.2% and aspirin=0.1%). In the CURE trial, the incidence of diarrhea for patients receiving PLAVIX + aspirin was 2.1% compared to 2.2% for those receiving placebo + aspirin.
In the CAPRIE trial, the incidence of patients withdrawing from treatment because of gastrointestinal adverse reactions was 3.2% for PLAVIX and 4.0% for aspirin. In the CURE trial, the incidence of patients withdrawing from treatment because of gastrointestinal adverse reactions was 0.9% for PLAVIX + aspirin compared with 0.8% for placebo + aspirin.
Rash and Other Skin Disorders: In the CAPRIE trial, the incidence of skin and appendage disorders in patients receiving PLAVIX was 15.8% (0.7% serious); the corresponding rate in aspirin patients was 13.1% (0.5% serious). In the CURE trial, the incidence of rash or other skin disorders in patients receiving PLAVIX + aspirin was 4.0% compared to 3.5% for those receiving placebo + aspirin.
In the CAPRIE trial, the overall incidence of patients withdrawing from treatment because of skin and appendage disorders adverse reactions was 1.5% for PLAVIX and 0.8% for aspirin. In the CURE trial, the incidence of patients withdrawing because of skin and appendage disorders adverse reactions was 0.7% for PLAVIX + aspirin compared with 0.3% for placebo + aspirin.
Adverse events occurring in ≥2.5% of patients on PLAVIX in the CAPRIE controlled clinical trial are shown below regardless of relationship to PLAVIX (clopidogrel bisulfate). The median duration of therapy was 20 months, with a maximum of 3 years.

Table 4: Adverse Events Occurring in ≥2.5% of PLAVIX Patients in CAPRIE

Body System Event	PLAVIX [n=9599] % Incidence	(% Discontinuation)	Aspirin [n=9586] % Incidence	(% Discontinuation)
Body as a Whole - general disorders				
Chest Pain	8.3	(0.2)	8.3	(0.3)
Accidental/Inflicted Injury	7.9	(0.1)	7.3	(0.1)
Influenza-like symptoms	7.5	(<0.1)	7.0	(<0.1)
Pain	6.4	(0.1)	6.3	(0.1)
Fatigue	3.3	(0.1)	3.4	(0.1)
Cardiovascular disorders, general				
Edema	4.1	(<0.1)	4.5	(<0.1)
Hypertension	4.3	(<0.1)	5.1	(<0.1)
Central & peripheral nervous system disorders				
Headache	7.6	(0.3)	7.2	(0.2)
Dizziness	6.2	(0.2)	6.7	(0.3)
Gastrointestinal system disorders				
Abdominal pain	5.6	(0.7)	7.1	(1.0)
Dyspepsia	5.2	(0.6)	6.1	(0.7)
Diarrhea	4.5	(0.4)	3.4	(0.3)
Nausea	3.4	(0.5)	3.8	(0.4)
Metabolic & nutritional disorders				
Hypercholesterolemia	4.0	(0)	4.4	(<0.1)
Musculo-skeletal system disorders				
Arthralgia	6.3	(0.1)	6.2	(0.1)
Back Pain	5.8	(0.1)	5.3	(<0.1)
Platelet, bleeding, & clotting disorders				
Purpura/Bruise	5.3	(0.3)	3.7	(0.1)
Epistaxis	2.9	(0.2)	2.5	(0.1)
Psychiatric disorders				
Depression	3.6	(0.1)	3.9	(0.2)
Respiratory system disorders				
Upper resp tract infection	8.7	(<0.1)	8.3	(<0.1)
Dyspnea	4.5	(0.1)	4.7	(0.1)
Rhinitis	4.2	(0.1)	4.2	(<0.1)
Bronchitis	3.7	(0.1)	3.7	(0)
Coughing	3.1	(<0.1)	2.7	(<0.1)
Skin & appendage disorders				
Rash	4.2	(0.5)	3.5	(0.2)
Pruritus	3.3	(0.3)	1.6	(0.1)
Urinary system disorders				
Urinary tract infection	3.1	(0)	3.5	(0.1)

Incidence of discontinuation, regardless of relationship to therapy, is shown in parentheses.
Adverse events occurring in ≥2.0% of patients on PLAVIX in the CURE controlled clinical trial are shown below regardless of relationship to PLAVIX.

Table 5: Adverse Events Occurring in ≥2.0% of PLAVIX Patients in CURE

Body System Event	PLAVIX (+ aspirin)* [n=6259] % Incidence	(% Discontinuation)	Placebo (+ aspirin)* [n=6303] % Incidence	(% Discontinuation)
Body as a Whole - general disorders				
Chest Pain	2.7	(<0.1)	2.8	(0.0)
Central & peripheral nervous system disorders				
Headache	3.1	(0.1)	3.2	(0.1)
Dizziness	2.4	(0.1)	2.0	(<0.1)
Gastrointestinal system disorders				
Abdominal pain	2.3	(0.3)	2.8	(0.3)
Dyspepsia	2.0	(0.1)	1.9	(<0.1)
Diarrhea	2.1	(0.1)	2.2	(0.1)

* Other standard therapies were used as appropriate.

Other adverse experiences of potential importance occurring in 1% to 2.5% of patients receiving PLAVIX (clopidogrel bisulfate) in the CAPRIE or CURE controlled clinical trials are listed below regardless of relationship to PLAVIX. In general, the incidence of these events was similar to that in patients receiving aspirin (in CAPRIE) or placebo + aspirin (in CURE).

Autonomic Nervous System Disorders: Syncope, Palpitation. *Body as a Whole - general disorders:* Asthenia, Fever, Hernia. *Cardiovascular disorders:* Cardiac failure. *Central and peripheral nervous system disorders:* Cramps legs, Hypoaesthesia, Neuralgia, Paresthesia, Vertigo. *Gastrointestinal system disorders:* Constipation, Vomiting. *Heart rate and rhythm disorders:* Fibrillation atrial. *Liver and biliary system disorders:* Hepatic enzymes increased. *Metabolic and nutritional disorders:* Gout, hyperuricemia, non-protein nitrogen (NPN) increased. *Musculo-skeletal system disorders:* Arthritis, Arthrosis. *Platelet, bleeding & clotting disorders:* GI hemorrhage, hematoma, platelets decreased. *Psychiatric disorders:* Anxiety, Insomnia. *Red blood cell disorders:* Anemia. *Respiratory system disorders:* Pneumonia, Sinusitis. *Skin and appendage disorders:* Eczema, Skin ulceration. *Urinary system disorders:* Cystitis. *Vision disorders:* Cataract, Conjunctivitis.

Other potentially serious adverse events which may be of clinical interest but were rarely reported (<1%) in patients who received PLAVIX in the CAPRIE or CURE controlled clinical trials are listed below regardless of relationship to PLAVIX (clopidogrel bisulfate). In general, the incidence of these events was similar to that in patients receiving aspirin (in CAPRIE) or placebo + aspirin (in CURE).

Body as a whole: Allergic reaction, necrosis ischemic. *Cardiovascular disorders:* Edema generalized. *Gastrointestinal system disorders:* Gastric ulcer perforated, gastritis hemorrhagic, upper GI ulcer hemorrhagic. *Liver and Biliary system disorders:* Bilirubinemia, hepatitis infectious, liver fatty. *Platelet, bleeding and clotting disorders:* hemarthrosis, hematuria, hemoptysis, hemorrhage intracranial, hemorrhage retroperitoneal, hemorrhage of operative wound, ocular hemorrhage, pulmonary hemorrhage, purpura allergic, Thrombocytopenia. *Red blood cell disorders:* Anemia aplastic, anemia hypochromic. *Reproductive disorders, female:* Menorrhagia. *Respiratory system disorders:* Hemothorax. *Skin and appendage disorders:* Bullous eruption, rash erythematous, rash maculopapular, urticaria. *Urinary system disorders:* Abnormal renal function, acute renal failure. *White cell and reticuloendothelial system disorders:* Agranulocytosis, granulocytopenia, leukemia, leukopenia, neutrophils decreased.

Postmarketing Experience

The following events have been reported spontaneously from worldwide postmarketing experience:

- *Body as a whole:*
  — hypersensitivity reactions, anaphylactoid reactions
- *Central and Peripheral Nervous System disorders:*
  — confusion, hallucinations, taste disorders
- *Liver and Biliary system disorders:*
  — abnormal liver function test, hepatitis (non-infectious)
- *Platelet, Bleeding and Clotting disorders:*
  — cases of bleeding with fatal outcome (especially intracranial, gastrointestinal and retroperitoneal hemorrhage)
  — agranulocytosis, aplastic anemia/pancytopenia, thrombotic thrombocytopenic purpura (TTP) — see WARNINGS.
  — conjunctival, ocular and retinal bleeding
- *Respiratory system disorders:*
  — bronchospasm
- *Skin and Appendage disorders:*
  — angioedema, erythema multiforme
- *Urinary system disorders:*
  — glomerulopathy, abnormal creatinine levels
- *Collagen disorders:*
  — vasculitis
- *Gastrointestinal disorders*
  — colitis (including ulcerative or lymphatic colitis)

OVERDOSAGE

One case of deliberate overdosage with PLAVIX was reported in the large, CAPRIE controlled clinical study. A 34-year-old woman took a single 1,050-mg dose of PLAVIX (equivalent to 14 standard 75-mg tablets). There were no associated adverse events. No special therapy was instituted, and she recovered without sequelae.

No adverse events were reported after single oral administration of 600 mg (equivalent to 8 standard 75-mg tablets) of PLAVIX in healthy volunteers. The bleeding time was prolonged by a factor of 1.7, which is similar to that typically observed with the therapeutic dose of 75 mg of PLAVIX per day.

A single oral dose of clopidogrel at 1500 or 2000 mg/kg was lethal to mice and to rats and at 3000 mg/kg to baboons. Symptoms of acute toxicity were vomiting (in baboons), prostration, difficult breathing, and gastrointestinal hemorrhage in all species.

Recommendations About Specific Treatment:

Based on biological plausibility, platelet transfusion may be appropriate to reverse the pharmacological effects of PLAVIX if quick reversal is required.

DOSAGE AND ADMINISTRATION

Recent MI, Recent Stroke, or Established Peripheral Arterial Disease

The recommended daily dose of PLAVIX is 75 mg once daily.

Acute Coronary Syndrome

For patients with acute coronary syndrome (unstable angina/non-Q-wave MI), PLAVIX should be initiated with a single 300 mg loading dose and then continued at 75 mg once daily. Aspirin (75 mg-325 mg once daily) should be initiated and continued in combination with PLAVIX. In CURE, most patients with Acute Coronary Syndrome also received heparin acutely (see **CLINICAL STUDIES**).

PLAVIX can be administered with or without food.

No dosage adjustment is necessary for elderly patients or patients with renal disease. (See **Clinical Pharmacology: Special Populations.**)

HOW SUPPLIED

PLAVIX (clopidogrel bisulfate) is available as a pink, round, biconvex, film-coated tablet debossed with "75" on one side and "1171" on the other. Tablets are provided as follows:

NDC 63653-1171-6 bottles of 30
NDC 63653-1171-1 bottles of 90
NDC 63653-1171-5 bottles of 500
NDC 63653-1171-3 blisters of 100

Storage

Store at 25° C (77° F); excursions permitted to 15°–30° C (59°–86° F) [See USP Controlled Room Temperature]

Distributed by:
Bristol-Myers Squibb/Sanofi Pharmaceuticals Partnership
New York, NY 10016
sanofi~synthelabo
Bristol-Myers Squibb Company
PLAVIX® is a registered trademark of Sanofi-Synthelabo
Revised: May 2003 J4-643P
B1-B0001-10-03 51-021345-04

Shown in Product Identification Guide, page 310

PRAVACHOL® ℞

[*prā-vā-kōl*]
(pravastatin sodium) Tablets
Rx only

DESCRIPTION

PRAVACHOL® (pravastatin sodium) is one of a new class of lipid-lowering compounds, the HMG-CoA reductase inhibitors, which reduce cholesterol biosynthesis. These agents are competitive inhibitors of 3-hydroxy-3-methylglutaryl-coenzyme A (HMG-CoA) reductase, the enzyme catalyzing the early rate-limiting step in cholesterol biosynthesis, conversion of HMG-CoA to mevalonate.

Pravastatin sodium is designated chemically as 1-Naphthalene-heptanoic acid, 1,2,6,7,8,8a-hexahydro-β,δ,6-trihydroxy-2-methyl-8-(2-methyl-1-oxobutoxy)-, monosodium salt, [1S-[1α(βS*,δS*),2α,6α,8β(R*),8aα]]-. Structural formula:

NaOOC OH HO O O CH₃ H CH₃ HO

$C_{23}H_{35}NaO_7$ MW 446.52

Pravastatin sodium is an odorless, white to off-white, fine or crystalline powder. It is a relatively polar hydrophilic compound with a partition coefficient (octanol/water) of 0.59 at a pH of 7.0. It is soluble in methanol and water (>300 mg/mL), slightly soluble in isopropanol, and practically insoluble in acetone, acetonitrile, chloroform, and ether.

PRAVACHOL is available for oral administration as 10 mg, 20 mg, 40 mg, and 80 mg tablets. Inactive ingredients include: croscarmellose sodium, lactose, magnesium oxide, magnesium stearate, microcrystalline cellulose, and povidone. The 10 mg tablet also contains Red Ferric Oxide, the 20 mg and 80 mg tablets also contain Yellow Ferric Oxide, and the 40 mg tablet also contains Green Lake Blend (mixture of D&C Yellow No. 10-Aluminum Lake and FD&C Blue No. 1-Aluminum Lake).

CLINICAL PHARMACOLOGY

Cholesterol and triglycerides in the bloodstream circulate as part of lipoprotein complexes. These complexes can be separated by density ultracentrifugation into high (HDL), intermediate (IDL), low (LDL), and very low (VLDL) density lipoprotein fractions. Triglycerides (TG) and cholesterol synthesized in the liver are incorporated into very low density lipoproteins (VLDLs) and released into the plasma for delivery to peripheral tissues. In a series of subsequent steps, VLDLs are transformed into intermediate density lipoproteins (IDLs), and cholesterol-rich low density lipoproteins (LDLs). High density lipoproteins (HDLs), containing apolipoprotein A, are hypothesized to participate in the reverse transport of cholesterol from tissues back to the liver.

PRAVACHOL (pravastatin sodium) produces its lipid -lowering effect in two ways. First, as a consequence of its reversible inhibition of HMG-CoA reductase activity, it effects modest reductions in intracellular pools of cholesterol. This results in an increase in the number of LDL-receptors on cell surfaces and enhanced receptor-mediated catabolism and clearance of circulating LDL. Second, pravastatin inhibits LDL production by inhibiting hepatic synthesis of VLDL, the LDL precursor.

Clinical and pathologic studies have shown that elevated levels of total cholesterol (Total-C), low density lipoprotein cholesterol (LDL-C), and apolipoprotein B (Apo B - a membrane transport complex for LDL) promote human atherosclerosis. Similarly, decreased levels of HDL-cholesterol (HDL-C) and its transport complex, apolipoprotein A, are associated with the development of atherosclerosis. Epidemiologic investigations have established that cardiovascular morbidity and mortality vary directly with the level of Total-C and LDL-C and inversely with the level of HDL-C. Like LDL, cholesterol-enriched triglyceride-rich lipoproteins, including VLDL, IDL, and remnants, can also promote atherosclerosis. Elevated plasma TG are frequently found in a triad with low HDL-C levels and small LDL particles, as well as in association with non-lipid metabolic risk factors for coronary heart disease. As such, total plasma TG has not consistently been shown to be an independent risk factor for CHD. Furthermore, the independent effect of raising HDL or lowering TG on the risk of coronary and cardiovascular morbidity and mortality has not been determined.

In both normal volunteers and patients with hypercholesterolemia, treatment with PRAVACHOL reduced Total-C, LDL-C, and apolipoprotein B. PRAVACHOL also reduced VLDL-C and TG and produced increases in HDL-C and apolipoprotein A. The effects of pravastatin on Lp (a), fibrinogen, and certain other independent biochemical risk markers for coronary heart disease are unknown. Although pravastatin is relatively more hydrophilic than other HMG-CoA reductase inhibitors, the effect of relative hydrophilicity, if any, on either efficacy or safety has not been established.

In one primary (West of Scotland Coronary Prevention Study – WOS)[1] and two secondary (Long-term Intervention with Pravastatin in Ischemic Disease – LIPID[2] and the Cholesterol and Recurrent Events – CARE[3]) prevention studies, PRAVACHOL has been shown to reduce cardiovascular morbidity and mortality across a wide range of cholesterol levels (see **Clinical Studies**).

Pharmacokinetics/Metabolism

PRAVACHOL is administered orally in the active form. In clinical pharmacology studies in man, pravastatin is rapidly absorbed, with peak plasma levels of parent compound attained 1 to 1.5 hours following ingestion. Based on urinary recovery of radiolabeled drug, the average oral absorption of pravastatin is 34% and absolute bioavailability is 17%. While the presence of food in the gastrointestinal tract reduces systemic bioavailability, the lipid-lowering effects of the drug are similar whether taken with, or 1 hour prior, to meals.

Pravastatin undergoes extensive first-pass extraction in the liver (extraction ratio 0.66), which is its primary site of action, and the primary site of cholesterol synthesis and of LDL-C clearance. *In vitro* studies demonstrated that pravastatin is transported into hepatocytes with substantially less uptake into other cells. In view of pravastatin's apparently extensive first-pass hepatic metabolism, plasma levels may not necessarily correlate perfectly with lipid-lowering efficacy. Pravastatin plasma concentrations [including: area under the concentration-time curve (AUC), peak (C_{max}), and steady-state minimum (C_{min})] are directly proportional to administered dose. Systemic bioavailability of pravastatin administered following a bedtime dose was decreased 60% compared to that following an AM dose. Despite this decrease in systemic bioavailability, the efficacy of pravastatin administered once daily in the evening, although not statistically significant, was marginally more effective than that after a morning dose. This finding of lower systemic bioavailability suggests greater hepatic extraction of the drug following the evening dose. Steady-state AUCs, C_{max} and C_{min} plasma concentrations showed no evidence of pravastatin accumulation following once or twice daily administration of PRAVACHOL (pravastatin sodium) tablets. Approximately 50% of the circulating drug is bound to plasma proteins. Following single dose administration of ^{14}C- pravastatin, the elimination half-life (t½) for total radioactivity (pravastatin plus metabolites) in humans is 77 hours.

Pravastatin, like other HMG-CoA reductase inhibitors, has variable bioavailability. The coefficient of variation (CV), based on between-subject variability, was 50% to 60% for AUC. Pravastatin 20 mg was administered under fasting conditions in adults. The geometric means of C_{max} and AUC ranged from 23.3 to 26.3 ng/mL and from 54.7 to 62.2 ng*hr/mL, respectively.

Approximately 20% of a radiolabeled oral dose is excreted in urine and 70% in the feces. After intravenous administration of radiolabeled pravastatin to normal volunteers, approximately 47% of total body clearance was via renal excretion and 53% by non-renal routes (i.e., biliary excretion and biotransformation). Since there are dual routes of elimination, the potential exists both for compensatory excretion by the alternate route as well as for accumulation of drug and/or metabolites in patients with renal or hepatic insufficiency.

In a study comparing the kinetics of pravastatin in patients with biopsy confirmed cirrhosis (N=7) and normal subjects (N=7), the mean AUC varied 18-fold in cirrhotic patients and 5-fold in healthy subjects. Similarly, the peak pravastatin values varied 47-fold for cirrhotic patients compared to 6-fold for healthy subjects.

Biotransformation pathways elucidated for pravastatin include: (a) isomerization to 6-epi pravastatin and the 3α-

Continued on next page

Pravachol—Cont.

hydroxyisomer of pravastatin (SQ 31,906), (b) enzymatic ring hydroxylation to SQ 31,945, (c) ω-1 oxidation of the ester side chain, (d) β-oxidation of the carboxy side chain, (e) ring oxidation followed by aromatization, (f) oxidation of a hydroxyl group to a keto group, and (g) conjugation. The major degradation product is the 3α-hydroxy isomeric metabolite, which has one-tenth to one-fortieth the HMG-CoA reductase inhibitory activity of the parent compound.

In a single oral dose study using pravastatin 20 mg, the mean AUC for pravastatin was approximately 27% greater and the mean cumulative urinary excretion (CUE) approximately 19% lower in elderly men (65 to 75 years old) compared with younger men (19 to 31 years old). In a similar study conducted in women, the mean AUC for pravastatin was approximately 46% higher and the mean CUE approximately 18% lower in elderly women (65 to 78 years old) compared with younger women (18 to 38 years old). In both studies, C_{max}, T_{max} and t½ values were similar in older and younger subjects.

After two weeks of once-daily 20 mg oral pravastatin administration, the geometric means of AUC were 80.7 (CV 44%) and 44.8 (CV 89%) ng*hr/mL for children (8-11 years, n=14) and adolescents (12-16 years, n=10), respectively. The corresponding values for C_{max} were 42.4 (CV 54%) and 18.6 ng/mL (CV 100%) for children and adolescents, respectively. No conclusion can be made based on these findings due to the small number of samples and large variability.

Clinical Studies

Prevention of Coronary Heart Disease

In the Pravastatin Primary Prevention Study (West of Scotland Coronary Prevention Study – WOS),[1] the effect of PRAVACHOL (pravastatin sodium) on fatal and nonfatal coronary heart disease (CHD) was assessed in 6595 men 45-64 years of age, without a previous myocardial infarction (MI), and with LDL-C levels between 156-254 mg/dL (4-6.7 mmol/L). In this randomized, double-blind, placebo-controlled study, patients were treated with standard care, including dietary advice, and either PRAVACHOL 40 mg daily (N=3302) or placebo (N=3293) and followed for a median duration of 4.8 years. Median (25th, 75th percentile) percent changes from baseline after 6 months of pravastatin treatment in Total C, LDL-C, TG, and HDL were -20.3 (-26.9, -11.7), -27.7 (-36.0, -16.9), -9.1 (-27.6, 12.5), and 6.7 (-2.1, 15.6), respectively.

PRAVACHOL significantly reduced the rate of first coronary events (either coronary heart disease [CHD] death or nonfatal MI) by 31% [248 events in the placebo group (CHD death=44, nonfatal MI=204) vs 174 events in the PRAVACHOL group (CHD death=31, nonfatal MI=143), p=0.0001 (see figure below)]. The risk reduction with PRAVACHOL was similar and significant throughout the entire range of baseline LDL cholesterol levels. This reduction was also similar and significant across the age range studied with a 40% risk reduction for patients younger than 55 years and a 27% risk reduction for patients 55 years and older. The Pravastatin Primary Prevention Study included only men and therefore it is not clear to what extent these data can be extrapolated to a similar population of female patients.

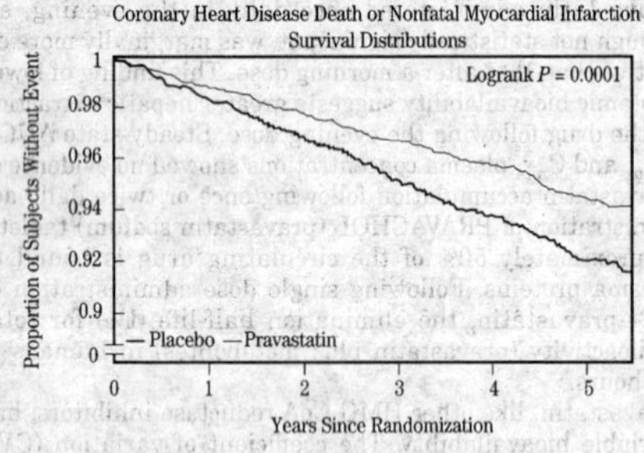

PRAVACHOL also significantly decreased the risk for undergoing myocardial revascularization procedures (coronary artery bypass graft [CABG] surgery or percutaneous transluminal coronary angioplasty [PTCA]) by 37% (80 vs 51 patients, p=0.009) and coronary angiography by 31% (128 vs 90, p=0.007). Cardiovascular deaths were decreased by 32% (73 vs 50, p=0.03) and there was no increase in death from non-cardiovascular causes.

Secondary Prevention of Cardiovascular Events

In the Long-term Intervention with Pravastatin in Ischemic Disease (LIPID)[2] study, the effect of PRAVACHOL (pravastatin sodium), 40 mg daily, was assessed in 9014 patients (7498 men; 1516 women; 3514 elderly patients [age ≥65 years]; 782 diabetic patients) who had experienced either an MI (5754 patients) or had been hospitalized for unstable angina pectoris (3260 patients) in the preceding 3–36 months. Patients in this multicenter, double-blind, placebo-controlled study participated for an average of 5.6 years (median of 5.9 years) and at randomization had total cholesterol between 114 and 563 mg/dL (mean 219 mg/dL), LDL-C between 46 and 274 mg/dL (mean 150 mg/dL), triglycerides between 35 and 2710 mg/dL (mean 160 mg/dL), and HDL-C between 1 and 103 mg/dL (mean 37 mg/dL). At baseline, 82% of patients were receiving aspirin and 76%

Table 1: LIPID – Primary and Secondary Endpoints

Event	Pravastatin 40 mg (N=4512)	Placebo (N=4502)	Risk Reduction	*P*-value
	Number (%) of Subjects			
Primary Endpoint				
CHD mortality	287 (6.4)	373 (8.3)	24%	0.0004
Secondary Endpoints				
Total mortality	498 (11.0)	633 (14.1)	23%	<0.0001
CHD mortality or non-fatal MI	557 (12.3)	715 (15.9)	24%	<0.0001
Myocardial revascularization procedures (CABG or PTCA)	584 (12.9)	706 (15.7)	20%	<0.0001
Stroke				
All-cause	169 (3.7)	204 (4.5)	19%	0.0477
Non-hemorrhagic	154 (3.4)	196 (4.4)	23%	0.0154
Cardiovascular mortality	331 (7.3)	433 (9.6)	25%	<0.0001

Table 2: CARE – Primary and Secondary Endpoints

Event	Pravastatin 40 mg (N=2081)	Placebo (N=2078)	Risk Reduction	*P*-value
	Number (%) of Subjects			
Primary Endpoint				
CHD mortality or non-fatal MI*	212 (10.2)	274 (13.2)	24%	0.003
Secondary Endpoints				
Myocardial revascularization procedures (CABG or PTCA)	294 (14.1)	391 (18.8)	27%	<0.001
Stroke or TIA	93 (4.5)	124 (6.0)	26%	0.029

* The risk reduction due to treatment with PRAVACHOL was consistent in both sexes.

were receiving antihypertensive medication. Treatment with PRAVACHOL significantly reduced the risk for total mortality by reducing coronary death (see **Table 1**). The risk reduction due to treatment with PRAVACHOL on CHD mortality was consistent regardless of age. PRAVACHOL significantly reduced the risk for total mortality (by reducing CHD death) and CHD events (CHD mortality or nonfatal MI) in patients who qualified with a history of either MI or hospitalization for unstable angina pectoris.

[See table 1 above]

In the Cholesterol and Recurrent Events (CARE)[3] study the effect of PRAVACHOL (pravastatin sodium), 40 mg daily, on coronary heart disease death and nonfatal MI was assessed in 4159 patients (3583 men and 576 women) who had experienced a myocardial infarction in the preceding 3-20 months and who had normal (below the 75th percentile of the general population) plasma total cholesterol levels. Patients in this double-blind, placebo controlled study participated for an average of 4.9 years and had a mean baseline total cholesterol of 209 mg/dL. LDL cholesterol levels in this patient population ranged from 101 mg/dL-180 mg/dL (mean=139 mg/dL). At baseline, 84% of patients were receiving aspirin and 82% were taking antihypertensive medications. Median (25th, 75th percentile) percent changes from baseline after 6 months of pravastatin treatment in Total C, LDL-C, TG, and HDL were -22.0 (-28.4, -14.9), -32.4 (-39.9, -23.7), -11.0 (-26.5, 8.6), and 5.1 (-2.9, 12.7), respectively. Treatment with PRAVACHOL significantly reduced the rate of first recurrent coronary events (either CHD death or nonfatal MI), the risk of undergoing revascularization procedures (PTCA, CABG), and the risk for stroke or transient ischemic attack (TIA) (**see Table 2**).

[See table 2 above]

In the Pravastatin Limitation of Atherosclerosis in the Coronary Arteries (PLAC I)[4] study, the effect of pravastatin therapy on coronary atherosclerosis was assessed by coronary angiography in patients with coronary disease and moderate hypercholesterolemia (baseline LDL-C range= 130-190 mg/dL). In this double-blind, multicenter, controlled clinical trial angiograms were evaluated at baseline and at three years in 264 patients. Although the difference between pravastatin and placebo for the primary endpoint (per-patient change in mean coronary artery diameter) and one of two secondary endpoints (change in percent lumen diameter stenosis) did not reach statistical significance, for the secondary endpoint of change in minimum lumen diameter, statistically significant slowing of disease was seen in the pravastatin treatment group (p=0.02).

In the Regression Growth Evaluation Statin Study (REGRESS)[5], the effect of pravastatin on coronary atherosclerosis was assessed by coronary angiography in 885 patients with angina pectoris, angiographically documented coronary artery disease and hypercholesterolemia (baseline total cholesterol range=160-310 mg/dL). In this double-blind, multicenter, controlled clinical trial, angiograms were evaluated at baseline and at two years in 653 patients (323 treated with pravastatin). Progression of coronary atherosclerosis was significantly slowed in the pravastatin group as assessed by changes in mean segment diameter (p=0.037) and minimum obstruction diameter (p=0.001).

Analysis of pooled events from PLAC I, the Pravastatin, Lipids and Atherosclerosis in the Carotids Study (PLAC II)[6], REGRESS, and the Kuopio Atherosclerosis Prevention Study (KAPS)[7] (combined N=1891) showed that treatment with pravastatin was associated with a statistically significant reduction in the composite event rate of fatal and nonfatal myocardial infarction (46 events or 6.4% for placebo versus 21 events or 2.4% for pravastatin, p=0.001). The predominant effect of pravastatin was to reduce the rate of nonfatal myocardial infarction.

Primary Hypercholesterolemia (Fredrickson Type IIa and IIb)

PRAVACHOL (pravastatin sodium) is highly effective in reducing Total-C, LDL-C and Triglycerides (TG) in patients with heterozygous familial, presumed familial combined and non-familial (non-FH) forms of primary hypercholesterolemia, and mixed dyslipidemia. A therapeutic response is seen within 1 week, and the maximum response usually is achieved within 4 weeks. This response is maintained during extended periods of therapy. In addition, PRAVACHOL is effective in reducing the risk of acute coronary events in hypercholesterolemic patients with and without previous myocardial infarction.

A single daily dose is as effective as the same total daily dose given twice a day. In multicenter, double-blind, placebo-controlled studies of patients with primary hypercholesterolemia, treatment with pravastatin in daily doses ranging from 10 mg to 40 mg consistently and significantly decreased Total-C, LDL-C, TG, and Total-C/HDL-C and LDL-C/HDL-C ratios (see **Table 3**).

In a pooled analysis of two multicenter, double-blind, placebo-controlled studies of patients with primary hypercholesterolemia, treatment with pravastatin at a daily dose of 80 mg (N=277) significantly decreased Total-C, LDL-C, and TG. The 25th and 75th percentile changes from baseline in LDL-C for pravastatin 80 mg were -43% and -30%. The efficacy results of the individual studies were consistent with the pooled data (see **Table 3**).

Treatment with PRAVACHOL modestly decreased VLDL-C and PRAVACHOL across all doses produced variable increases in HDL-C (see **Table 3**).

Table 3: Primary Hypercholesterolemia Studies: Dose Response of PRAVACHOL Once Daily Administration

Dose	Total-C	LDL-C	HDL-C	TG
Mean Percent Changes From Baseline After 8 Weeks*				
Placebo (N=36)	-3%	-4%	+1%	-4%
10 mg (N=18)	-16%	-22%	+7%	-15%
20 mg (N=19)	-24%	-32%	+2%	-11%
40 mg (N=18)	-25%	-34%	+12%	-24%
Mean Percent Changes From Baseline After 6 Weeks**				
Placebo (N=162)	0%	-1%	-1%	+1%
80 mg (N=277)	-27%	-37%	+3%	-19%

*a multicenter, double-blind, placebo-controlled study

**pooled analysis of 2 multicenter, double-blind, placebo-controlled studies

In another clinical trial, patients treated with pravastatin in combination with cholestyramine (70% of patients were taking cholestyramine 20 or 24 g per day) had reductions equal to or greater than 50% in LDL-C. Furthermore, pravastatin attenuated cholestyramine-induced increases in TG levels (which are themselves of uncertain clinical significance).

Hypertriglyceridemia (Fredrickson Type IV)

The response to pravastatin in patients with Type IV hyperlipidemia (baseline TG >200 mg/dL and LDL-C <160 mg/dL) was evaluated in a subset of 429 patients from the Cholesterol and Recurrent Events (CARE) study. For pravastatin-treated subjects, the median (min, max) baseline triglyceride level was 246.0 (200.5, 349.5) mg/dL (see **Table 4**).

Table 4: Patients With Fredrickson Type IV Hyperlipidemia Median (25th, 75th percentile) Percent Change From Baseline

	Pravastatin 40 mg (N=429)	Placebo (N=430)
Triglycerides	-21.1 (-34.8, 1.3)	-6.3 (-23.1, 18.3)
Total-C	-22.1 (-27.1, -14.8)	0.2 (-6.9, 6.8)
LDL-C	-31.7 (-39.6, -21.5)	0.7 (-9.0, 10.0)
HDL-C	7.4 (-1.2, 17.7)	2.8 (-5.7, 11.7)
Non-HDL-C	-27.2 (-34.0, -18.5)	-0.8 (-8.2, 7.0)

Dysbetalipoproteinemia (Fredrickson Type III)

The response to pravastatin in two double-blind crossover studies of 46 patients with genotype E2/E2 and Fredrickson Type III dysbetalipoproteinemia is shown in **Table 5.**

[See table 5 at right]

Pediatric Clinical Study

A double-blind placebo-controlled study in 214 patients (100 boys and 114 girls) with heterozygous familial hypercholesterolemia (HeFH), aged 8-18 years was conducted for two (2) years. The children (aged 8-13 years) were randomized to placebo (n=63) or 20 mg of pravastatin daily (n=65) and the adolescents (aged 14-18 years) were randomized to placebo (n=45) or 40 mg of pravastatin daily (n=41). Inclusion in the study required LDL-C level >95th percentile for age and sex and one parent with either a clinical or molecular diagnosis of familial hypercholesterolemia. The mean baseline LDL-C value was 239 mg/dL and 237 mg/dL in the pravastatin (range: 151-405 mg/dL) and placebo (range: 154-375 mg/dL) groups, respectively.

Pravastatin significantly decreased plasma levels of LDL-C, Total-C, and apolipoprotein B in both children and adolescents (see **Table 6**). The effect of pravastatin treatment in the two age groups was similar.

[See table 6 at right]

The mean achieved LDL-C was 186 mg/dL (range: 67-363 mg/dL) in the pravastatin group compared to 236 mg/dL (range: 105-438 mg/dL) in the placebo group.

The safety and efficacy of pravastatin doses above 40 mg daily have not been studied in children. The long-term efficacy of pravastatin therapy in childhood to reduce morbidity and mortality in adulthood has not been established.

INDICATIONS AND USAGE

Therapy with PRAVACHOL (pravastatin sodium) should be considered in those individuals at increased risk for atherosclerosis-related clinical events as a function of cholesterol level, the presence or absence of coronary heart disease, and other risk factors.

Primary Prevention of Coronary Events

In hypercholesterolemic patients without clinically evident coronary heart disease, PRAVACHOL is indicated to:

– Reduce the risk of myocardial infarction
– Reduce the risk of undergoing myocardial revascularization procedures
– Reduce the risk of cardiovascular mortality with no increase in death from non-cardiovascular causes.

Secondary Prevention of Cardiovascular Events

In patients with clinically evident coronary heart disease, PRAVACHOL is indicated to:

– Reduce the risk of total mortality by reducing coronary death
– Reduce the risk of myocardial infarction
– Reduce the risk of undergoing myocardial revascularization procedures
– Reduce the risk of stroke and stroke/transient ischemic attack (TIA)
– Slow the progression of coronary atherosclerosis.

Hyperlipidemia

PRAVACHOL is indicated as an adjunct to diet to reduce elevated Total-C, LDL-C, Apo B, and TG levels and to increase HDL-C in patients with primary hypercholesterolemia and mixed dyslipidemia (Fredrickson Type IIa and IIb).[8]

PRAVACHOL is indicated as adjunctive therapy to diet for the treatment of patients with elevated serum triglyceride levels (Fredrickson Type IV).

PRAVACHOL is indicated for the treatment of patients with primary dysbetalipoproteinemia (Fredrickson Type III) who do not respond adequately to diet.

PRAVACHOL is indicated as an adjunct to diet and lifestyle modification for treatment of HeFH in children and adolescent patients ages 8 years and older if after an adequate trial of diet the following findings are present.

1. LDL-C remains ≥190 mg/dL or
2. LDL C remains ≥160 mg/dL and;
   – there is a positive family history of premature cardiovascular disease or
   – two or more other CVD risk factors are present in the patient.

Lipid-altering agents should be used in addition to a diet restricted in saturated fat and cholesterol when the response to diet and other nonpharmacological measures alone has been inadequate (see NCEP Guidelines below).

Prior to initiating therapy with pravastatin, secondary causes for hypercholesterolemia (e.g., poorly controlled diabetes mellitus, hypothyroidism, nephrotic syndrome, dysproteinemias, obstructive liver disease, other drug therapy, alcoholism) should be excluded, and a lipid profile performed to measure Total-C, HDL-C, and TG. For patients with triglycerides (TG) <400 mg/dL (<4.5 mmol/L), LDL-C can be estimated using the following equation:

$$LDL\text{-}C = Total\text{-}C - HDL\text{-}C - \frac{1}{5}\,TG$$

For TG levels >400 mg/dL (>4.5 mmol/L), this equation is less accurate and LDL-C concentrations should be determined by ultracentrifugation. In many hypertriglyceridemic patients, LDL-C may be low or normal despite elevated Total-C. In such cases, HMG-CoA reductase inhibitors are not indicated.

Lipid determinations should be performed at intervals of no less than four weeks and dosage adjusted according to the patient's response to therapy.

The National Cholesterol Education Program's Treatment Guidelines are summarized below:

[See third table above]

After the LDL-C goal has been achieved, if the TG is still ≥200 mg/dL, non-HDL-C (Total-C minus HDL-C) becomes a secondary target of therapy. Non-HDL-C goals are set 30 mg/dL higher than LDL-C goals for each risk category.

At the time of hospitalization for an acute coronary event, consideration can be given to initiating drug therapy at discharge if the LDL-C is ≥130 mg/dL (see NCEP Treatment Guidelines, above).

Since the goal of treatment is to lower LDL-C, the NCEP recommends that LDL C levels be used to initiate and assess treatment response. Only if LDL-C levels are not available, should the Total-C be used to monitor therapy.

As with other lipid-lowering therapy, PRAVACHOL (pravastatin sodium) is not indicated when hypercholesterolemia is due to hyperalphalipoproteinemia (elevated HDL-C).

The NCEP classification of cholesterol levels in pediatric patients with a familial history of hypercholesterolemia or premature cardiovascular disease is summarized below:

Continued on next page

Table 5: Patients With Fredrickson Type III Dysbetalipoproteinemia Median (min, max) Percent Change From Baseline

	Median (min, max) at Baseline (mg/dL)	Median % Change (min, max) Pravastatin 40 mg (N=20)
Study 1		
Total-C	386.5 (245.0, 672.0)	-32.7 (-58.5, 4.6)
Triglycerides	443.0 (275.0, 1299.0)	-23.7 (-68.5, 44.7)
VLDL-C*	206.5 (110.0, 379.0)	-43.8 (-73.1, -14.3)
LDL-C*	117.5 (80.0, 170.0)	-40.8 (-63.7, 4.6)
HDL-C	30.0 (18.0, 88.0)	6.4 (-45.0, 105.6)
Non-HDL-C	344.5 (215.0, 646.0)	-36.7 (-66.3, 5.8)
*N=14		
	Median (min, max) at Baseline (mg/dL)	**Median % Change (min, max) Pravastatin 40 mg (N=26)**
Study 2		
Total-C	340.3 (230.1, 448.6)	-31.4 (-54.5, -13.0)
Triglycerides	343.2 (212.6, 845.9)	-11.9 (-56.5, 44.8)
VLDL-C	145.0 (71.5, 309.4)	-35.7 (-74.7, 19.1)
LDL-C	128.6 (63.8, 177.9)	-30.3 (-52.2, 13.5)
HDL-C	38.7 (27.1, 58.0)	5.0 (-17.7, 66.7)
Non-HDL-C	295.8 (195.3, 421.5)	-35.5 (-81.0, -13.5)

Table 6: Lipid-Lowering Effects of Pravastatin in Pediatric Patients with Heterozygous Familial Hypercholesterolemia: Least-Squares Mean Percent Change from Baseline at Month 24 (Last Observation Carried Forward: Intent-to-Treat)*

	Pravastatin 20 mg (Aged 8-13 years) N=65	Pravastatin 40 mg (Aged 14-18 years) N=41	Combined Pravastatin (Aged 8-18 years) N=106	Combined Placebo (Aged 8-18 years) N=108	95% CI of the Difference Between Combined Pravastatin and Placebo
LDL-C	-26.04**	-21.07**	-24.07**	-1.52	(-26.74, -18.86)
TC	-20.75**	-13.08**	-17.72**	-0.65	(-20.40, -13.83)
HDL-C	1.04	13.71	5.97	3.13	(-1.71, 7.43)
TG	-9.58	-0.30	-5.88	-3.27	(-13.95, 10.01)
ApoB (N)	-23.16** (61)	-18.08** (39)	-21.11** (100)	-0.97 (106)	(-24.29, -16.18)

*The above least-squares mean values were calculated based on log-transformed lipid values.
**Significant at p≤0.0001 when compared with placebo.

NCEP Treatment Guidelines: LDL-C Goals and Cutpoints for Therapeutic Lifestyle Changes and Drug Therapy in Different Risk Categories

Risk Category	LDL Goal (mg/dL)	LDL Levels at Which to Initiate Therapeutic Lifestyle Changes (mg/dL)	LDL Level at Which to Consider Drug Therapy (mg/dL)
CHD[a] or CHD Risk equivalents (10-year risk >20%)	<100	≥100	≥130 (100-129: drug optional)[b]
2+ Risk factors (10-year risk ≤20%)	<130	≥130	10-year risk 10%-20%: ≥130 10-year risk <10%: ≥160
0-1 Risk factor[c]	<160	≥160	≥190 (160-189: LDL-lowering drug optional)

[a] CHD, coronary heart disease.
[b] Some authorities recommend the use of LDL-lowering drugs in this category if an LDL-C level of <100 mg/dL cannot be achieved by therapeutic lifestyle changes. Others prefer use of drugs that primarily modify triglycerides and HDL-C, e.g., nicotinic acid or fibrate. Clinical judgement also may call for deferring drug therapy in this subcategory.
[c] Almost all people with 0-1 risk factor have 10-year risk <10%; thus, 10-year risk assessment in people with 0-1 risk factor is not necessary.

Pravachol—Cont.

Category	Total-C (mg/dL)	LDL-C (mg/dL)
Acceptable	<170	<110
Borderline	170-199	110-129
High	≥200	≥130

CONTRAINDICATIONS

Hypersensitivity to any component of this medication.

Active liver disease or unexplained, persistent elevations in liver function tests (see **WARNINGS**).

Pregnancy and Lactation. Atherosclerosis is a chronic process and discontinuation of lipid-lowering drugs during pregnancy should have little impact on the outcome of long-term therapy of primary hypercholesterolemia. Cholesterol and other products of cholesterol biosynthesis are essential components for fetal development (including synthesis of steroids and cell membranes). Since HMG-CoA reductase inhibitors decrease cholesterol synthesis and possibly the synthesis of other biologically active substances derived from cholesterol, they are contraindicated during pregnancy and in nursing mothers. **Pravastatin should be administered to women of childbearing age only when such patients are highly unlikely to conceive and have been informed of the potential hazards.** If the patient becomes pregnant while taking this class of drug, therapy should be discontinued immediately and the patient apprised of the potential hazard to the fetus (see **PRECAUTIONS: Pregnancy**).

WARNINGS

Liver Enzymes

HMG-CoA reductase inhibitors, like some other lipid-lowering therapies, have been associated with biochemical abnormalities of liver function. In three long-term (4.8-5.9 years), placebo-controlled clinical trials (WOS, LIPID, CARE; see **CLINICAL PHARMACOLOGY: Clinical Studies**), 19,592 subjects (19,768 randomized), were exposed to pravastatin or placebo. In an analysis of serum transaminase values (ALT, AST), incidences of marked abnormalities were compared between the pravastatin and placebo treatment groups; a marked abnormality was defined as a post-treatment test value greater than three times the upper limit of normal for subjects with pretreatment values less than or equal to the upper limit of normal, or four times the pretreatment value for subjects with pretreatment values greater than the upper limit of normal but less than 1.5 times the upper limit of normal. Marked abnormalities of ALT or AST occurred with similar low frequency (≤1.2%) in both treatment groups. Overall, clinical trial experience showed that liver function test abnormalities observed during pravastatin therapy were usually asymptomatic, not associated with cholestasis, and did not appear to be related to treatment duration.

It is recommended that liver function tests be performed prior to the initiation of therapy, prior to the elevation of the dose, and when otherwise clinically indicated.

Active liver disease or unexplained persistent transaminase elevations are contraindications to the use of pravastatin (see **CONTRAINDICATIONS**). Caution should be exercised when pravastatin is administered to patients who have a recent history of liver disease, have signs that may suggest liver disease (e.g., unexplained aminotransferase elevations, jaundice), or are heavy users of alcohol (see **CLINICAL PHARMACOLOGY: Pharmacokinetics/Metabolism**). Such patients should be closely monitored, started at the lower end of the recommended dosing range, and titrated to the desired therapeutic effect.

Patients who develop increased transaminase levels or signs and symptoms of liver disease should be monitored with a second liver function evaluation to confirm the finding and be followed thereafter with frequent liver function tests until the abnormality(ies) return to normal. Should an increase in AST or ALT of three times the upper limit of normal or greater persist, withdrawal of pravastatin therapy is recommended.

Skeletal Muscle

Rare cases of rhabdomyolysis with acute renal failure secondary to myoglobinuria have been reported with pravastatin and other drugs in this class. Uncomplicated myalgia has also been reported in pravastatin-treated patients (see **ADVERSE REACTIONS**). Myopathy, defined as muscle aching or muscle weakness in conjunction with increases in creatine phosphokinase (CPK) values to greater than 10 times the upper normal limit, was rare (<0.1%) in pravastatin clinical trials. Myopathy should be considered in any patient with diffuse myalgias, muscle tenderness or weakness, and/or marked elevation of CPK. Patients should be advised to report promptly unexplained muscle pain, tenderness or weakness, particularly if accompanied by malaise or fever. **Pravastatin therapy should be discontinued if markedly elevated CPK levels occur or myopathy is diagnosed or suspected. Pravastatin therapy should also be temporarily withheld in any patient experiencing an acute or serious condition predisposing to the development of renal failure secondary to rhabdomyolysis, e.g., sepsis; hypotension; major surgery; trauma; severe metabolic, endocrine, or electrolyte disorders; or uncontrolled epilepsy.**

The risk of myopathy during treatment with another HMG-CoA reductase inhibitor is increased with concurrent therapy with either erythromycin, cyclosporine, niacin, or fibrates. However, neither myopathy nor significant increases in CPK levels have been observed in three reports involving a total of 100 post-transplant patients (24 renal and 76 cardiac) treated for up to two years concurrently with pravastatin 10-40 mg and cyclosporine. Some of these patients also received other concomitant immunosuppressive therapies. Further, in clinical trials involving small numbers of patients who were treated concurrently with pravastatin and niacin, there were no reports of myopathy. Also, myopathy was not reported in a trial of combination pravastatin (40 mg/day) and gemfibrozil (1200 mg/day), although 4 of 75 patients on the combination showed marked CPK elevations versus one of 73 patients receiving placebo. There was a trend toward more frequent CPK elevations and patient withdrawals due to musculoskeletal symptoms in the group receiving combined treatment as compared with the groups receiving placebo, gemfibrozil, or pravastatin monotherapy (see **PRECAUTIONS: Drug Interactions**). **The use of fibrates alone may occasionally be associated with myopathy. The combined use of pravastatin and fibrates should be avoided unless the benefit of further alterations in lipid levels is likely to outweigh the increased risk of this drug combination.**

PRECAUTIONS

General

PRAVACHOL (pravastatin sodium) may elevate creatine phosphokinase and transaminase levels (see **ADVERSE REACTIONS**). This should be considered in the differential diagnosis of chest pain in a patient on therapy with pravastatin.

Homozygous Familial Hypercholesterolemia

Pravastatin has not been evaluated in patients with rare homozygous familial hypercholesterolemia. In this group of patients, it has been reported that HMG-CoA reductase inhibitors are less effective because the patients lack functional LDL receptors.

Renal Insufficiency

A single 20 mg oral dose of pravastatin was administered to 24 patients with varying degrees of renal impairment (as determined by creatinine clearance). No effect was observed on the pharmacokinetics of pravastatin or its 3α-hydroxy isomeric metabolite (SQ 31,906). A small increase was seen in mean AUC values and half-life (t½) for the inactive enzymatic ring hydroxylation metabolite (SQ 31,945). Given this small sample size, the dosage administered, and the degree of individual variability, patients with renal impairment who are receiving pravastatin should be closely monitored.

Information for Patients

Patients should be advised to report promptly unexplained muscle pain, tenderness or weakness, particularly if accompanied by malaise or fever (see **WARNINGS: Skeletal Muscle**).

Drug Interactions

Immunosuppressive Drugs, Gemfibrozil, Niacin (Nicotinic Acid), Erythromycin: See **WARNINGS: Skeletal Muscle.**

Cytochrome P450 3A4 Inhibitors: In vitro and *in vivo* data indicate that pravastatin is not metabolized by cytochrome P450 3A4 to a clinically significant extent. This has been shown in studies with known cytochrome P450 3A4 inhibitors (see diltiazem and itraconazole below). Other examples of cytochrome P450 3A4 inhibitors include ketoconazole, mibefradil, and erythromycin.

Diltiazem: Steady-state levels of diltiazem (a known, weak inhibitor of P450 3A4) had no effect on the pharmacokinetics of pravastatin. In this study, the AUC and C_{max} of another HMG-CoA reductase inhibitor which is known to be metabolized by cytochrome P450 3A4 increased by factors of 3.6 and 4.3, respectively.

Itraconazole: The mean AUC and C_{max} for pravastatin were increased by factors of 1.7 and 2.5, respectively, when given with itraconazole (a potent P450 3A4 inhibitor which also inhibits p-glycoprotein transport) as compared to placebo. The mean t½ was not affected by itraconazole, suggesting that the relatively small increases in C_{max} and AUC were due solely to increased bioavailability rather than a decrease in clearance, consistent with inhibition of p-glycoprotein transport by itraconazole. This drug transport system is thought to affect bioavailability and excretion of HMG-CoA reductase inhibitors, including pravastatin. The AUC and C_{max} of another HMG-CoA reductase inhibitor which is known to be metabolized by cytochrome P450 3A4 increased by factors of 19 and 17, respectively, when given with itraconazole.

Antipyrine: Since concomitant administration of pravastatin had no effect on the clearance of antipyrine, interactions with other drugs metabolized via the same hepatic cytochrome isozymes are not expected.

Cholestyramine/Colestipol: Concomitant administration resulted in an approximately 40 to 50% decrease in the mean AUC of pravastatin. However, when pravastatin was administered 1 hour before or 4 hours after cholestyramine or 1 hour before colestipol and a standard meal, there was no clinically significant decrease in bioavailability or therapeutic effect. (See **DOSAGE AND ADMINISTRATION: Concomitant Therapy**.)

Warfarin: Concomitant administration of 40 mg pravastatin had no clinically significant effect on prothrombin time when administered in a study to normal elderly subjects who were stabilized on warfarin.

Cimetidine: The AUC_{0-12hr} for pravastatin when given with cimetidine was not significantly different from the AUC for pravastatin when given alone. A significant difference was observed between the AUC's for pravastatin when given with cimetidine compared to when administered with antacid.

Digoxin: In a crossover trial involving 18 healthy male subjects given 20 mg pravastatin and 0.2 mg digoxin concurrently for 9 days, the bioavailability parameters of digoxin were not affected. The AUC of pravastatin tended to increase, but the overall bioavailability of pravastatin plus its metabolites SQ 31,906 and SQ 31,945 was not altered.

Cyclosporine: Some investigators have measured cyclosporine levels in patients on pravastatin (up to 20 mg), and to date, these results indicate no clinically meaningful elevations in cyclosporine levels. In one single-dose study, pravastatin levels were found to be increased in cardiac transplant patients receiving cyclosporine.

Gemfibrozil: In a crossover study in 20 healthy male volunteers given concomitant single doses of pravastatin and gemfibrozil, there was a significant decrease in urinary excretion and protein binding of pravastatin. In addition, there was a significant increase in AUC, C_{max}, and T_{max} for the pravastatin metabolite SQ 31,906. Combination therapy with pravastatin and gemfibrozil is generally not recommended. (See **WARNINGS: Skeletal Muscle**.)

In interaction studies with *aspirin, antacids* (1 hour prior to PRAVACHOL), *cimetidine, nicotinic acid,* or *probucol,* no statistically significant differences in bioavailability were seen when PRAVACHOL (pravastatin sodium) was administered.

Endocrine Function

HMG-CoA reductase inhibitors interfere with cholesterol synthesis and lower circulating cholesterol levels and, as such, might theoretically blunt adrenal or gonadal steroid hormone production. Results of clinical trials with pravastatin in males and post-menopausal females were inconsistent with regard to possible effects of the drug on basal steroid hormone levels. In a study of 21 males, the mean testosterone response to human chorionic gonadotropin was significantly reduced ($p<0.004$) after 16 weeks of treatment with 40 mg of pravastatin. However, the percentage of patients showing a ≥50% rise in plasma testosterone after human chorionic gonadotropin stimulation did not change significantly after therapy in these patients. The effects of HMG-CoA reductase inhibitors on spermatogenesis and fertility have not been studied in adequate numbers of patients. The effects, if any, of pravastatin on the pituitary-gonadal axis in pre-menopausal females are unknown. Patients treated with pravastatin who display clinical evidence of endocrine dysfunction should be evaluated appropriately. Caution should also be exercised if an HMG-CoA reductase inhibitor or other agent used to lower cholesterol levels is administered to patients also receiving other drugs (e.g., ketoconazole, spironolactone, cimetidine) that may diminish the levels or activity of steroid hormones.

In a placebo-controlled study of 214 pediatric patients with HeFH, of which 106 were treated with pravastatin (20 mg in the children aged 8-13 years and 40 mg in the adolescents aged 14-18 years) for two years, there were no detectable differences seen in any of the endocrine parameters [ACTH, cortisol, DHEAS, FSH, LH, TSH, estradiol (girls) or testosterone (boys)] relative to placebo. There were no detectable differences seen in height and weight changes, testicular volume changes, or Tanner score relative to placebo.

CNS Toxicity

CNS vascular lesions, characterized by perivascular hemorrhage and edema and mononuclear cell infiltration of perivascular spaces, were seen in dogs treated with pravastatin at a dose of 25 mg/kg/day. These effects in dogs were observed at approximately 59 times the human dose of 80 mg/day, based on AUC. Similar CNS vascular lesions have been observed with several other drugs in this class. A chemically similar drug in this class produced optic nerve degeneration (Wallerian degeneration of retinogeniculate fibers) in clinically normal dogs in a dose-dependent fashion starting at 60 mg/kg/day, a dose that produced mean plasma drug levels about 30 times higher than the mean drug level in humans taking the highest recommended dose (as measured by total enzyme inhibitory activity). This same drug also produced vestibulocochlear Wallerian-like degeneration and retinal ganglion cell chromatolysis in dogs treated for 14 weeks at 180 mg/kg/day, a dose which resulted in a mean plasma drug level similar to that seen with the 60 mg/kg/day dose.

Carcinogenesis, Mutagenesis, Impairment of Fertility

In a 2-year study in rats fed pravastatin at doses of 10, 30, or 100 mg/kg body weight, there was an increased incidence of hepatocellular carcinomas in males at the highest dose ($p<0.01$). These effects in rats were observed at approximately 12 times the human dose (HD) of 80 mg, based on body surface area mg/m^2 and at approximately 4 times the human dose, based on AUC.

In a 2-year study in mice fed pravastatin at doses of 250 and 500 mg/kg/day, there was an increased incidence of hepatocellular carcinomas in males and females at both 250 and 500 mg/kg/day ($p<0.0001$). At these doses, lung adenomas in females were increased ($p=0.013$). These effects in mice were observed at approximately 15 times (250 mg/kg/day) and 23 times (500 mg/kg/day) the human dose of 80 mg, based on AUC. In another 2-year study in mice with doses up to 100 mg/kg/day (producing drug exposures approximately 2 times the human dose of 80 mg, based on AUC), there were no drug-induced tumors.

No evidence of mutagenicity was observed *in vitro*, with or without rat-liver metabolic activation, in the following studies: microbial mutagen tests, using mutant strains of *Salmonella typhimurium* or *Escherichia coli*; a forward mutation assay in L5178Y TK +/- mouse lymphoma cells; a chromosomal aberration test in hamster cells; and a gene conversion assay using *Saccharomyces cerevisiae*. In addition, there was no evidence of mutagenicity in either a dominant lethal test in mice or a micronucleus test in mice.

In a study in rats, with daily doses up to 500 mg/kg, pravastatin did not produce any adverse effects on fertility or general reproductive performance. However, in a study with another HMG-CoA reductase inhibitor, there was decreased fertility in male rats treated for 34 weeks at 25 mg/kg body weight, although this effect was not observed in a subsequent fertility study when this same dose was administered for 11 weeks (the entire cycle of spermatogenesis, including epididymal maturation). In rats treated with this same reductase inhibitor at 180 mg/kg/day, seminiferous tubule degeneration (necrosis and loss of spermatogenic epithelium) was observed. Although not seen with pravastatin, two similar drugs in this class caused drug-related testicular atrophy, decreased spermatogenesis, spermatocytic degeneration, and giant cell formation in dogs. The clinical significance of these findings is unclear.

Pregnancy

Pregnancy Category X.

See **CONTRAINDICATIONS.**

Safety in pregnant women has not been established. Pravastatin was not teratogenic in rats at doses up to 1000 mg/kg daily or in rabbits at doses of up to 50 mg/kg daily. These doses resulted in 10X (rabbit) or 120X (rat) the human exposure based on surface area (mg/meter^2). Rare reports of congenital anomalies have been received following intrauterine exposure to other HMG-CoA reductase inhibitors. In a review[9] of approximately 100 prospectively followed pregnancies in women exposed to simvastatin or lovastatin, the incidences of congenital anomalies, spontaneous abortions and fetal deaths/stillbirths did not exceed what would be expected in the general population. The number of cases is adequate only to exclude a three-to-fourfold increase in congenital anomalies over the background incidence. In 89% of the prospectively followed pregnancies, drug treatment was initiated prior to pregnancy and was discontinued at some point in the first trimester when pregnancy was identified. As safety in pregnant women has not been established and there is no apparent benefit to therapy with PRAVACHOL (pravastatin sodium) during pregnancy (see **CONTRAINDICATIONS**), treatment should be immediately discontinued as soon as pregnancy is recognized. PRAVACHOL should be administered to women of childbearing potential only when such patients are highly unlikely to conceive and have been informed of the potential hazards.

Nursing Mothers

A small amount of pravastatin is excreted in human breast milk. Because of the potential for serious adverse reactions in nursing infants, women taking PRAVACHOL should not nurse (see **CONTRAINDICATIONS**).

Pediatric Use

The safety and effectiveness of PRAVACHOL in children and adolescents from 8-18 years of age have been evaluated in a placebo-controlled study of two years duration. Patients treated with pravastatin had an adverse experience profile generally similar to that of patients treated with placebo with influenza and headache commonly reported in both treatment groups. (See **ADVERSE REACTIONS: Pediatric Patients.**) **Doses greater than 40 mg have not been studied in this population.** Children and adolescent females of childbearing potential should be counseled on appropriate contraceptive methods while on pravastatin therapy (see **CONTRAINDICATIONS** and **PRECAUTIONS: Pregnancy**). For dosing information see **DOSAGE AND ADMINISTRATION: Adult Patients and Pediatric Patients.**

Double-blind, placebo-controlled pravastatin studies in children less than 8 years of age have not been conducted.

Geriatric Use

Two secondary prevention trials with pravastatin (CARE and LIPID) included a total of 6,593 subjects treated with pravastatin 40 mg for periods ranging up to 6 years. Across these two studies, 36.1% of pravastatin subjects were aged 65 and older and 0.8% were aged 75 and older. The beneficial effect of pravastatin in elderly subjects in reducing cardiovascular events and in modifying lipid profiles was similar to that seen in younger subjects. The adverse event profile in the elderly was similar to that in the overall population. Other reported clinical experience has not identified differences in responses to pravastatin between elderly and younger patients.

Mean pravastatin AUCs are slightly (25-50%) higher in elderly subjects than in healthy young subjects, but mean C_{max}, T_{max} and t½ values are similar in both age groups and substantial accumulation of pravastatin would not be expected in the elderly (see **CLINICAL PHARMACOLOGY: Pharmacokinetics/Metabolism**).

ADVERSE REACTIONS

Pravastatin is generally well tolerated; adverse reactions have usually been mild and transient. In 4-month long placebo-controlled trials, 1.7% of pravastatin-treated patients and 1.2% of placebo-treated patients were discontinued from treatment because of adverse experiences attributed to study drug therapy; this difference was not statistically significant. (See also **PRECAUTIONS: Geriatric Use** section).

Adverse Clinical Events

Short-Term Controlled Trials

All adverse clinical events (regardless of attribution) reported in more than 2% of pravastatin-treated patients in placebo-controlled trials of up to four months duration are identified in **Table 7**; also shown are the percentages of patients in whom these medical events were believed to be related or possibly related to the drug:

[See table 7 above]

Table 7: Adverse Events in >2 Percent of Patients Treated with Pravastatin 10-40 mg in Short-Term Placebo-Controlled Trials

	All Events		Events Attributed to Study Drug	
Body System/Event	**Pravastatin (N=900) % of patients**	**Placebo (N=411) % of patients**	**Pravastatin (N=900) % of patients**	**Placebo (N=411) % of patients**
Cardiovascular				
Cardiac Chest Pain	4.0	3.4	0.1	0.0
Dermatologic				
Rash	4.0*	1.1	1.3	0.9
Gastrointestinal				
Nausea/Vomiting	7.3	7.1	2.9	3.4
Diarrhea	6.2	5.6	2.0	1.9
Abdominal Pain	5.4	6.9	2.0	3.9
Constipation	4.0	7.1	2.4	5.1
Flatulence	3.3	3.6	2.7	3.4
Heartburn	2.9	1.9	2.0	0.7
General				
Fatigue	3.8	3.4	1.9	1.0
Chest Pain	3.7	1.9	0.3	0.2
Influenza	2.4*	0.7	0.0	0.0
Musculoskeletal				
Localized Pain	10.0	9.0	1.4	1.5
Myalgia	2.7	1.0	0.6	0.0
Nervous System				
Headache	6.2	3.9	1.7*	0.2
Dizziness	3.3	3.2	1.0	0.5
Renal / Genitourinary				
Urinary Abnormality	2.4	2.9	0.7	1.2
Respiratory				
Common Cold	7.0	6.3	0.0	0.0
Rhinitis	4.0	4.1	0.1	0.0
Cough	2.6	1.7	0.1	0.0

*Statistically significantly different from placebo.

The safety and tolerability of PRAVACHOL (pravastatin sodium) at a dose of 80 mg in two controlled trials with a mean exposure of 8.6 months was similar to that of PRAVACHOL at lower doses except that 4 out of 464 patients taking 80 mg of pravastatin had a single elevation of CK >10X ULN compared to 0 out of 115 patients taking 40 mg of pravastatin.

Long-Term Controlled Morbidity and Mortality Trials

Adverse event data were pooled from seven double-blind, placebo-controlled trials (West of Scotland Coronary Prevention study [WOS]; Cholesterol and Recurrent Events study [CARE]; Long-term Intervention with Pravastatin in Ischemic Disease study [LIPID]; Pravastatin Limitation of Atherosclerosis in the Coronary Arteries study [PLAC I]; Pravastatin, Lipids and Atherosclerosis in the Carotids study [PLAC II]; Regression Growth Evaluation Statin Study [REGRESS]; and Kuopio Atherosclerosis Prevention Study [KAPS]) involving a total of 10,764 patients treated with pravastatin 40 mg and 10,719 patients treated with placebo. The safety and tolerability profile in the pravastatin group was comparable to that of the placebo group. Patients were exposed to pravastatin for a mean of 4.0 to 5.1 years in WOS, CARE, and LIPID and 1.9 to 2.9 years in PLAC I, PLAC II, KAPS, and REGRESS. In these long-term trials, the most common reasons for discontinuation were mild, non-specific gastrointestinal complaints. Collectively, these seven trials represent 47,613 patient-years of exposure to pravastatin. Events believed to be of probable, possible, or uncertain relationship to study drug, occurring in at least 1% of patients treated with pravastatin in these studies are identified in **Table 8.**

Table 8: Adverse Events in ≥1 Percent of Patients Treated with Pravastatin 40 mg in Long-Term Placebo-Controlled Trials

Body System/Event	**Pravastatin (N=10,764) % of patients**	**Placebo (N=10,719) % of patients**
Cardiovascular		
Angina Pectoris	3.1	3.4
Dermatologic		
Rash	2.1	2.2
Gastrointestinal		
Dyspepsia/Heartburn	3.5	3.7
Abdominal Pain	2.4	2.5
Nausea/Vomiting	1.6	1.6
Flatulence	1.2	1.1
Constipation	1.2	1.3
General		
Fatigue	3.4	3.3
Chest Pain	2.6	2.6
Musculoskeletal		
Musculoskeletal Pain (includes arthralgia)	6.0	5.8
Muscle Cramp	2.0	1.8
Myalgia	1.4	1.4
Nervous System		
Dizziness	2.2	2.1
Headache	1.9	1.8
Sleep Disturbance	1.0	0.9
Depression	1.0	1.0
Anxiety/Nervousness	1.0	1.2
Renal / Genitourinary		
Urinary Abnormality (includes dysuria, frequency, nocturia)	1.0	0.8
Respiratory		
Dyspnea	1.6	1.6
Upper Respiratory Infection	1.3	1.3
Cough	1.0	1.0
Special Senses		
Vision Disturbance (includes blurred vision, diplopia)	1.6	1.3

Events of probable, possible, or uncertain relationship to study drug that occurred in <1.0% of pravastatin-treated patients in the long-term trials included the following; frequencies were similar in placebo-treated patients:

Dermatologic: pruritus, dermatitis, dryness of skin, scalp hair abnormality (including alopecia), urticaria.

Endocrine / Metabolic: sexual dysfunction, libido change.

Gastrointestinal: decreased appetite.

General: fever, flushing.

Immunologic: allergy, edema head/neck.

Musculoskeletal: muscle weakness.

Nervous System: paresthesia, vertigo, insomnia, memory impairment, tremor, neuropathy (including peripheral neuropathy).

Special Senses: lens opacity, taste disturbance.

Postmarketing Experience

In addition to the events reported above, as with other drugs in this class, the following events have been reported rarely during postmarketing experience with PRAVACHOL (pravastatin sodium), regardless of causality assessment:

Musculoskeletal: myopathy, rhabdomyolysis.

Nervous System: dysfunction of certain cranial nerves (including alteration of taste, impairment of extra-ocular movement, facial paresis), peripheral nerve palsy.

Hypersensitivity: anaphylaxis, lupus erythematosus-like syndrome, polymyalgia rheumatica, dermatomyositis, vasculitis, purpura, hemolytic anemia, positive ANA, ESR increase, arthritis, arthralgia, asthenia, photosensitivity, chills, malaise, toxic epidermal necrolysis, erythema multiforme, including Stevens-Johnson syndrome.

Gastrointestinal: pancreatitis, hepatitis, including chronic active hepatitis, cholestatic jaundice, fatty change in liver, cirrhosis, fulminant hepatic necrosis, hepatoma.

Dermatologic: A variety of skin changes (e.g., nodules, discoloration, dryness of mucous membranes, changes to hair/nails).

Reproductive: gynecomastia.

Laboratory Abnormalities: elevated alkaline phosphatase and bilirubin; thyroid function abnormalities.

Laboratory Test Abnormalities

Increases in serum transaminase (ALT, AST) values and CPK have been observed (see **WARNINGS**).

Continued on next page

Pravachol—Cont.

Transient, asymptomatic eosinophilia has been reported. Eosinophil counts usually returned to normal despite continued therapy. Anemia, thrombocytopenia, and leukopenia have been reported with HMG-CoA reductase inhibitors.

Concomitant Therapy

Pravastatin has been administered concurrently with cholestyramine, colestipol, nicotinic acid, probucol and gemfibrozil. Preliminary data suggest that the addition of either probucol or gemfibrozil to therapy with lovastatin or pravastatin is **not** associated with greater reduction in LDL-cholesterol than that achieved with lovastatin or pravastatin alone. No adverse reactions unique to the combination or in addition to those previously reported for each drug alone have been reported. Myopathy and rhabdomyolysis (with or without acute renal failure) have been reported when another HMG-CoA reductase inhibitor was used in combination with immunosuppressive drugs, gemfibrozil, erythromycin, or lipid-lowering doses of nicotinic acid. Concomitant therapy with HMG-CoA reductase inhibitors and these agents is generally not recommended. (See **WARNINGS: Skeletal Muscle** and **PRECAUTIONS: Drug Interactions.**)

Pediatric Patients

In a two year double-blind placebo-controlled study involving 100 boys and 114 girls with HeFH, the safety and tolerability profile of pravastatin was generally similar to that of placebo. (See **CLINICAL PHARMACOLOGY, Pediatric Clinical Study** and **PRECAUTIONS, Pediatric Use.**)

OVERDOSAGE

To date, there has been limited experience with overdosage of pravastatin. If an overdose occurs, it should be treated symptomatically with laboratory monitoring and supportive measures should be instituted as required. (See **WARNINGS.**)

DOSAGE AND ADMINISTRATION

The patient should be placed on a standard cholesterol-lowering diet before receiving PRAVACHOL (pravastatin sodium) and should continue on this diet during treatment with PRAVACHOL (see NCEP Treatment Guidelines for details on dietary therapy).

PRAVACHOL can be administered orally as a single dose at any time of the day, with or without food. Since the maximal effect of a given dose is seen within 4 weeks, periodic lipid determinations should be performed at this time and dosage adjusted according to the patient's response to therapy and established treatment guidelines.

Adult Patients

The recommended starting dose is 40 mg once daily. If a daily dose of 40 mg does not achieve desired cholesterol levels, 80 mg once daily is recommended. In patients with a history of significant renal or hepatic dysfunction, a starting dose of 10 mg daily is recommended.

Pediatric Patients

Children (Ages 8 to 13 Years, Inclusive)

The recommended dose is 20 mg once daily in children 8 to 13 years of age. Doses greater than 20 mg have not been studied in this patient population.

Adolescents (Ages 14 to 18 Years)

The recommended starting dose is 40 mg once daily in adolescents 14 to 18 years of age. Doses greater than 40 mg have not been studied in this patient population.

Children and adolescents treated with pravastatin should be reevaluated in adulthood and appropriate changes made to their cholesterol-lowering regimen to achieve adult goals for LDL-C (see **INDICATIONS AND USAGE, Hyperlipidemia, NCEP Treatment Guidelines**).

In patients taking immunosuppressive drugs such as cyclosporine (see **WARNINGS: Skeletal Muscle**) concomitantly with pravastatin, therapy should begin with 10 mg of pravastatin once-a-day at bedtime and titration to higher doses should be done with caution. Most patients treated with this combination received a maximum pravastatin dose of 20 mg/day.

Concomitant Therapy

The lipid-lowering effects of PRAVACHOL on total and LDL cholesterol are enhanced when combined with a bile-acid-binding resin. When administering a bile-acid-binding resin (e.g., cholestyramine, colestipol) and pravastatin, PRAVACHOL should be given either 1 hour or more before or at least 4 hours following the resin. (See also **ADVERSE REACTIONS: Concomitant Therapy.**)

HOW SUPPLIED

PRAVACHOL® (pravastatin sodium) Tablets are supplied as:

10 mg tablets: Pink to peach, rounded, rectangular-shaped, biconvex with a P embossed on one side and PRAVACHOL 10 engraved on the opposite side. They are supplied in bottles of 90 (NDC 0003-5154-05). Bottles contain a desiccant canister.

20 mg tablets: Yellow, rounded, rectangular-shaped, biconvex with a P embossed on one side and PRAVACHOL 20 engraved on the opposite side. They are supplied in bottles of 90 (NDC 0003-5178-05), bottles of 1000 (NDC 0003-5178-75), and hospital unit-dose packages of 100 tablets (NDC 0003-5178-06). Bottles contain a desiccant canister.

40 mg tablets: Green, rounded, rectangular-shaped, biconvex with a P embossed on one side and PRAVACHOL 40 engraved on the opposite side. They are supplied in bottles of 90 (NDC 0003-5194-10) and hospital unit-dose packages of 100 tablets (NDC 0003-5194-33). Bottles contain a desiccant canister.

80 mg tablets: Yellow, oval-shaped, biconvex with BMS embossed on one side and 80 engraved on the opposite side. They are supplied in bottles of 90 (NDC 0003-5195-10), bottles of 500 (NDC 0003-5195-12), and hospital unit-dose packages of 100 tablets (NDC 0003-5195-33). Bottles contain a desiccant canister.

STORAGE

Store at 25°C (77°F); excursions permitted to 15°-30°C (59°-86°F) [see USP Controlled Room Temperature]. Keep tightly closed (protect from moisture). Protect from light.

REFERENCES

1. Shepherd J, et al. Prevention of coronary heart disease with pravastatin in men with hypercholesterolemia (WOS). *N Engl J Med* 1995;333:1301-7.
2. The Long-term Intervention with Pravastatin in Ischemic Disease Group. Prevention of cardiovascular events and death with pravastatin in patients with coronary heart disease and a broad range of initial cholesterol levels (LIPID). *N Engl J Med* 1998;339:1349-1357.
3. Sacks FM, et al. The effect of pravastatin on coronary events after myocardial infarction in patients with average cholesterol levels (CARE). *N Engl J Med*. 1996;335:1001-9.
4. Pitt B, et al. Pravastatin Limitation of Atherosclerosis in the Coronary Arteries (PLAC I): Reduction in Atherosclerosis Progression and Clinical Events. *J Am Coll Cardiol* 1995;26:1133-9.
5. Jukema JW, et al. Effects of Lipid Lowering by Pravastatin on Progression and Regression of Coronary Artery Disease in Symptomatic Man With Normal to Moderately Elevated Serum Cholesterol Levels. The Regression Growth Evaluation Statin Study (REGRESS). *Circulation* 1995;91:2528-2540.
6. Crouse JR, et al. Pravastatin, lipids, and atherosclerosis in the carotid arteries: design features of a clinical trial with carotid atherosclerosis outcome (PLAC II). *Controlled Clinical Trials* 1992;13:495.
7. Salonen R, et al. Kuopio Atherosclerosis Prevention Study (KAPS). A population-based primary preventive trial of the effect of LDL lowering on atherosclerotic progression in carotid and femoral arteries. Research Institute of Public Health, University of Kuopio, Finland. *Circulation* 1995;92:1758.
8. Fredrickson DS, et al. Fat transport in lipoproteins–an integrated approach to mechanisms and disorders. *N Engl J Med* 1967; 276:34-42, 94-102, 148-156, 215-224, 273-281.
9. Manson JM, Freyssinges C, Ducrocq MB, Stephenson WP. Postmarketing Surveillance of Lovastatin and Simvastatin Exposure During Pregnancy. *Reproductive Toxicology* 1996;10(6):439-446.

US Patent Nos.: 4,346,227; 5,030,447; 5,180,589; 5,622,985

Bristol-Myers Squibb Company
Princeton, NJ 08543 U.S.A.

D3-B0001-01-04
Revised November 2003 5154DIM-23

Shown in Product Identification Guide, page 310

REYATAZ® ℞

[rā'ă-tăz]

(atazanavir sulfate) Capsules

℞ ONLY

(Patient Information Leaflet Included)

DESCRIPTION

REYATAZ® (atazanavir sulfate) is an azapeptide inhibitor of HIV-1 protease.

The chemical name for atazanavir sulfate is (3*S*,8*S*,9*S*,12*S*)-3,12-Bis(1,1-dimethylethyl)-8-hydroxy-4,11-dioxo-9-(phenylmethyl)-6-[[4-(2-pyridinyl)phenyl]methyl]-2,5,6,10,13-pentaazatetradecanedioic acid dimethyl ester, sulfate (1:1). Its molecular formula is $C_{38}H_{52}N_6O_7 \bullet H_2SO_4$, which corresponds to a molecular weight of 802.9 (sulfuric acid salt). The free base molecular weight is 704.9. Atazanavir sulfate has the following structural formula:

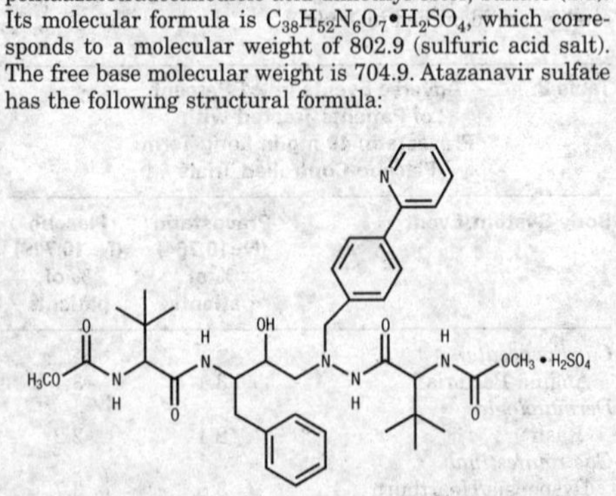

Atazanavir sulfate is a white to pale yellow crystalline powder. It is slightly soluble in water (4-5 mg/mL, free base equivalent) with the pH of a saturated solution in water being about 1.9 at 24 ± 3° C.

REYATAZ Capsules are available for oral administration in strengths containing the equivalent of 100 mg, 150 mg, or 200 mg of atazanavir as atazanavir sulfate and the following inactive ingredients: crospovidone, lactose monohydrate, and magnesium stearate. The capsule shells contain the following inactive ingredients: gelatin, FD&C Blue #2, and titanium dioxide. The capsules are printed with ink containing shellac, titanium dioxide, FD&C Blue #2, isopropyl alcohol, ammonium hydroxide, propylene glycol, n-butyl alcohol, simethicone, and dehydrated alcohol.

CLINICAL PHARMACOLOGY

Microbiology

Mechanism of Action

Atazanavir (ATV) is an azapeptide HIV-1 protease inhibitor (PI). The compound selectively inhibits the virus-specific processing of viral Gag and Gag-Pol polyproteins in HIV-1 infected cells, thus preventing formation of mature virions.

Antiviral Activity In Vitro

Atazanavir exhibits anti-HIV-1 activity with a mean 50% inhibitory concentration (IC_{50}) in the absence of human serum of 2 to 5 nM against a variety of laboratory and clinical HIV-1 isolates grown in peripheral blood mononuclear cells, macrophages, CEM-SS cells, and MT-2 cells. Two-drug combination studies with ATV showed additive to antagonistic antiviral activity *in vitro* with abacavir and the NNRTIs (delavirdine, efavirenz, and nevirapine) and additive antiviral activity *in vitro* with the PIs (amprenavir, indinavir, lopinavir, nelfinavir, ritonavir, and saquinavir), NRTIs (didanosine, emtricitabine, lamivudine, stavudine, tenofovir, zalcitabine, and zidovudine), the HIV-1 fusion inhibitor enfuvirtide, and two compounds used in the treatment of viral hepatitis, adefovir and ribavirin, without enhanced cytotoxicity.

Resistance

In vitro: HIV-1 isolates with a decreased susceptibility to ATV have been selected *in vitro* and obtained from patients treated with ATV or atazanavir/ritonavir (ATV/RTV). HIV-1 isolates that were 93- to 183-fold resistant to ATV from three different viral strains were selected *in vitro* by 5 months. The mutations in these HIV-1 viruses that contributed to ATV resistance included I50L, N88S, I84V, A71V, and M46I. Changes were also observed at the protease cleavage sites following drug selection. Recombinant viruses containing the I50L mutation were growth impaired and displayed increased *in vitro* susceptibility to other PIs (amprenavir, indinavir, lopinavir, nelfinavir, ritonavir, and saquinavir). The I50L and I50V substitutions yielded selective resistance to ATV and amprenavir, respectively, and did not appear to be cross-resistant.

Clinical Studies of Treatment-Naive Patients: ATV-resistant clinical isolates from treatment-naive patients who experienced virologic failure developed an I50L mutation (after an average of 50 weeks of ATV therapy), often in combination with an A71V mutation. In treatment-naive patients, viral isolates that developed the I50L mutation showed phenotypic resistance to ATV but retained *in vitro* susceptibility to other PIs (amprenavir, indinavir, lopinavir, nelfinavir, ritonavir, and saquinavir); however, there are no clinical data available to demonstrate the effect of the I50L mutation on the efficacy of subsequently administered PIs.

Clinical Studies of Treatment-Experienced Patients: In contrast, from studies of treatment-experienced patients treated with ATV or ATV/RTV, most ATV-resistant isolates from patients who experienced virologic failure developed mutations that were associated with resistance to multiple PIs and displayed decreased susceptibility to multiple PIs. The most common protease mutations to develop in the viral isolates of patients who failed treatment with ATV 300 mg once daily and RTV 100 mg once daily (together with tenofovir and an NRTI) included V32I, L33F/V/I, E35D/G, M46I/L, I50L, F53L/V, I54V, A71V/T/I, G73S/T/C, V82A/T/L, I85V, and L89V/Q/M/T. Other mutations that developed on ATV/RTV treatment including E34K/A/Q, G48V, I84V, N88S/D/T, and L90M occurred in less than 10% of patient isolates. Generally, if multiple PI resistance mutations were present in the HIV-1 of the patient at baseline, ATV resistance developed through mutations associated with resistance to other PIs and could include the development of the I50L mutation.

Cross-Resistance

Cross-resistance among PIs has been observed. Baseline phenotypic and genotypic analyses of clinical isolates from ATV clinical trials of PI-experienced subjects showed that isolates cross-resistant to multiple PIs were cross-resistant to ATV. Greater than 90% of the isolates with mutations that included I84V or G48V were resistant to ATV. Greater than 60% of isolates containing L90M, G73S/T/C, A71V/T, I54V, M46I/L, or a change at V82 were resistant to ATV, and 38% of isolates containing a D30N mutation in addition to other changes were resistant to ATV. Isolates resistant to ATV were also cross-resistant to other PIs with >90% of the isolates resistant to indinavir, lopinavir, nelfinavir, ritonavir, and saquinavir, and 80% resistant to amprenavir. In treatment-experienced patients, PI-resistant viral isolates that developed the I50L mutation in addition to other PI resistance-associated mutations were also cross-resistant to other PIs.

Genotypic and/or phenotypic analysis of baseline virus may aid in determining ATV susceptibility before initiation of ATV/RTV therapy. An association between virologic response at 48 weeks and the number and type of primary PI-resistance-associated mutations detected in baseline HIV-1 isolates from antiretroviral-experienced patients receiving ATV/RTV once daily or lopinavir (LPV)/RTV twice daily in Study AI424-045 is shown in Table 1.

Overall, both the number and type of baseline PI mutations affected response rates in treatment-experienced patients. In the ATV/RTV group, patients had lower response rates when 3 or more baseline PI mutations including a mutation at position 36, 71, 77, 82 or 90 were present compared to patients with 1-2 PI mutations including one of these mutations.

Table 1: HIV RNA Response by Number and Type of Baseline PI Mutation, Antiretroviral-Experienced Patients in Study AI424-045, As-Treated Analysis

Number and Type of Baseline PI Mutations[a]	Virologic Response = HIV RNA <400 copies/mL[b] ATV/RTV (n=110)	LPV/RTV (n=113)
3 or more primary PI mutations including[c]:		
D30N	75% (6/8)	50% (3/6)
M36I/V	19% (3/16)	33% (6/18)
M46I/L/T	24% (4/17)	23% (5/22)
I54V/L/T/M/A	31% (5/16)	31% (5/16)
A71V/T/I/G	34% (10/29)	39% (12/31)
G73S/A/C/T	14% (1/7)	38% (3/8)
V77I	47% (7/15)	44% (7/16)
V82A/F/T/S/I	29% (6/21)	27% (7/26)
I84V/A	11% (1/9)	33% (2/6)
N88D	63% (5/8)	67% (4/6)
L90M	10% (2/21)	44% (11/25)
Number of baseline primary PI mutations[a]		
All patients, as-treated	58% (64/110)	59% (67/113)
0–2 PI mutations	75% (50/67)	75% (50/67)
3–4 PI mutations	41% (14/34)	43% (12/28)
5 or more PI mutations	0% (0/9)	28% (5/18)

[a] Primary mutations include any change at D30, V32, M36, M46, I47, G48, I50, I54, A71, G73, V77, V82, I84, N88, and L90.
[b] Results should be interpreted with caution because the subgroups were small.
[c] There were insufficient data (n<3) for PI mutations V32I, I47V, G48V, I50V, and F53L.

The response rates of antiretroviral-experienced patients in Study AI424-045 were analyzed by baseline phenotype (shift in *in vitro* susceptibility relative to reference, Table 2). The analyses are based on a select patient population with 62% of patients receiving an NNRTI-based regimen before study entry compared to 35% receiving a PI-based regimen. Additional data are needed to determine clinically relevant break points for REYATAZ (atazanavir sulfate).

Table 2: Baseline Phenotype by Outcome, Antiretroviral-Experienced Patients in Study AI424-045, As-Treated Analysis

Baseline Phenotype[a]	Virologic Response = HIV RNA <400 copies/mL[b] ATV/RTV (n=111)	LPV/RTV (n=111)
0–2	71% (55/78)	70% (56/80)
>2–5	53% (8/15)	44% (4/9)
>5–10	13% (1/8)	33% (3/9)
>10	10% (1/10)	23% (3/13)

[a] Fold change in *in vitro* susceptibility relative to the wild-type reference.
[b] Results should be interpreted with caution because the subgroups were small.

Pharmacokinetics

The pharmacokinetics of atazanavir were evaluated in healthy adult volunteers and in HIV-infected patients after administration of REYATAZ 400 mg once daily and after administration of REYATAZ 300 mg with ritonavir 100 mg once daily (see Table 3).

[See table 3 above]

Figure 1 displays the mean plasma concentrations of atazanavir at steady state after REYATAZ (atazanavir sulfate) 400 mg once daily (as two 200-mg capsules) with a light meal and after REYATAZ 300 mg (as two 150-mg capsules) with ritonavir 100 mg once daily with a light meal in HIV-infected adults patients.

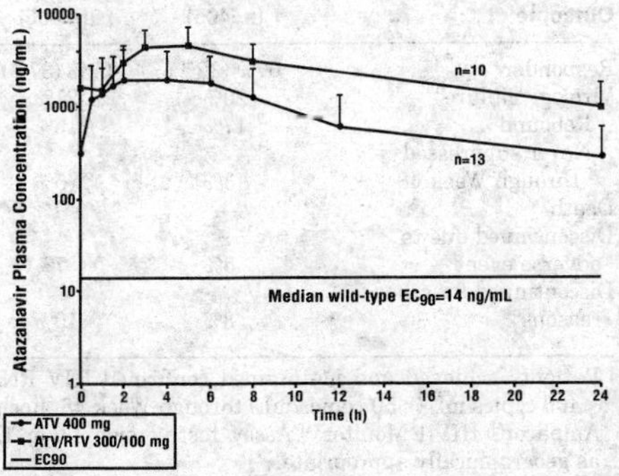

Figure 1: Mean (SD) Steady-State Plasma Concentrations of Atazanavir 400 mg (n=13) and 300 mg with Ritonavir (n=10) for HIV-Infected Adult Patients

Table 3: Steady-State Pharmacokinetics of Atazanavir in Healthy Subjects or HIV-Infected Patients in the Fed State

Parameter	400 mg once daily: Healthy Subjects (n=14)	400 mg once daily: HIV-Infected Patients (n=13)	300 mg with ritonavir 100 mg once daily: Healthy Subjects (n=28)	300 mg with ritonavir 100 mg once daily: HIV-Infected Patients (n=10)
C_{max} (ng/mL)				
Geometric mean (CV%)	5199 (26)	2298 (71)	6129 (31)	4422 (58)
Mean (SD)	5358 (1371)	3152 (2231)	6450 (2031)	5233 (3033)
T_{max} (h)				
Median	2.5	2.0	2.7	3.0
AUC (ng•h/mL)				
Geometric mean (CV%)	28132 (28)	14874 (91)	57039 (37)	46073 (66)
Mean (SD)	29303 (8263)	22262 (20159)	61435 (22911)	53761 (35294)
T-half (h)				
Mean (SD)	7.9 (2.9)	6.5 (2.6)	18.1 (6.2)[a]	8.6 (2.3)
C_{min} (ng/mL)				
Geometric mean (CV%)	159 (88)	120 (109)	1227 (53)	636 (97)
Mean (SD)	218 (191)	273 (298)[b]	1441 (757)	862 (838)

[a] n=26.
[b] n=12.

Table 4: Drug Interactions: Pharmacokinetic Parameters for Atazanavir in the Presence of Coadministered Drugs[a]

Coadministered Drug	Coadministered Drug Dose/Schedule	REYATAZ Dose/Schedule	n	Ratio (90% Confidence Interval) of Atazanavir Pharmacokinetic Parameters with/without Coadministered Drug; No Effect = 1.00: C_{max}	AUC	C_{min}
atenolol	50 mg QD, d 7-11 and d 19-23	400 mg QD, d 1-11	19	1.00 (0.89, 1.12)	0.93 (0.85, 1.01)	0.74 (0.65, 0.86)
clarithromycin	500 mg BID, d 7-10 and d 18-21	400 mg QD, d 1-10	29	1.06 (0.93, 1.20)	1.28 (1.16, 1.43)	1.91 (1.66, 2.21)
didanosine (ddl) (buffered tablets) plus stavudine (d4T)[b]	ddl: 200 mg × 1 dose, d4T: 40 mg × 1 dose	400 mg × 1 dose simultaneously with ddl and d4T	32[c]	0.11 (0.06, 0.18)	0.13 (0.08, 0.21)	0.16 (0.10, 0.27)
	ddl: 200 mg × 1 dose, d4T: 40 mg × 1 dose	400 mg × 1 dose 1 h after ddl + d4T	32[c]	1.12 (0.67, 1.18)	1.03 (0.64, 1.67)	1.03 (0.61, 1.73)
diltiazem	180 mg QD, d 7-11 and d 19-23	400 mg QD, d 1-11	30	1.04 (0.96, 1.11)	1.00 (0.95, 1.05)	0.98 (0.90, 1.07)
efavirenz	600 mg QD, d 7-20	400 mg QD, d 1-20	27	0.41 (0.33, 0.51)	0.26 (0.22, 0.32)	0.07 (0.05, 0.10)
	600 mg QD d 7-20	400 mg QD, d 1-6 then 300 mg/ritonavir 100 mg QD, 2h before efavirenz, d 7-20	13	1.14 (0.83, 1.58)	1.39 (1.02, 1.88)	1.48 (1.24, 1.76)
ketoconazole	200 mg QD, d 7-13	400 mg QD, d 1-13	14	0.99 (0.77, 1.28)	1.10 (0.89, 1.37)	1.03 (0.53, 2.01)
rifabutin	150 mg QD, d 15-28	400 mg QD, d 1-28	7	1.34 (1.14, 1.59)	1.15 (0.98, 1.34)	1.13 (0.68, 1.87)
ritonavir[d]	100 mg QD, d 11-20	300 mg QD, d 1-20	28	1.86 (1.69, 2.05)	3.38 (3.13, 3.63)	11.89 (10.23, 13.82)
tenofovir[e]	300 mg QD, d 9-16	400 mg QD, d 2-16	34	0.79 (0.73, 0.86)	0.75 (0.70, 0.81)	0.60 (0.52, 0.68)
	300 mg QD, d 15-42	300 mg/ ritonavir 100 mg QD, d1-42	10	0.72[f] (0.50, 1.05)	0.75[f] (0.58, 0.97)	0.77[f] (0.54, 1.10)

[a] Data provided are under fed conditions unless otherwise noted.
[b] All drugs were given under fasted conditions.
[c] One subject did not receive REYATAZ (atazanavir sulfate).
[d] Compared with atazanavir 400 mg QD historical data, administration of atazanavir/ritonavir 300/100 mg QD increased the atazanavir geometric mean values of C_{max}, AUC, and C_{min} by 18%, 103%, and 671%, respectively.
[e] tenofovir disoproxil fumarate.
[f] Ratio of atazanavir plus ritonavir plus tenofovir to atazanavir plus ritonavir. Atazanavir 300 mg plus ritonavir 100 mg results in higher atazanavir exposure than atazanavir 400 mg (see footnote[d]). The geometric mean values of atazanavir pharmacokinetic parameters when coadministered with ritonavir and tenofovir were: C_{max} = 3190 ng/mL AUC = 34459 ng•h/mL, and C_{min} = 491 ng/mL.

Absorption

Atazanavir is rapidly absorbed with a T_{max} of approximately 2.5 hours. Atazanavir demonstrates nonlinear pharmacokinetics with greater than dose-proportional increases in AUC and C_{max} values over the dose range of 200–800 mg once daily. Steady-state is achieved between Days 4 and 8, with an accumulation of approximately 2.3-fold.

Food Effect

Administration of REYATAZ with food enhances bioavailability and reduces pharmacokinetic variability. Administration of a single 400-mg dose of REYATAZ with a light meal (357 kcal, 8.2 g fat, 10.6 g protein) resulted in a 70% increase in AUC and 57% increase in C_{max} relative to the fasting state. Administration of a single 400-mg dose of REYATAZ with a high-fat meal (721 kcal, 37.3 g fat, 29.4 g protein) resulted in a mean increase in AUC of 35% with no change in C_{max} relative to the fasting state. Administration of REYATAZ with either a light meal or high-fat meal decreased the coefficient of variation of AUC and C_{max} by approximately one half compared to the fasting state.

Distribution

Atazanavir is 86% bound to human serum proteins and protein binding is independent of concentration. Atazanavir binds to both alpha-1-acid glycoprotein (AAG) and albumin to a similar extent (89% and 86%, respectively). In a multiple-dose study in HIV-infected patients dosed with REYATAZ 400 mg once daily with a light meal for 12 weeks, atazanavir was detected in the cerebrospinal fluid and semen. The cerebrospinal fluid/plasma ratio for atazanavir (n=4) ranged between 0.0021 and 0.0226 and seminal fluid/plasma ratio (n=5) ranged between 0.11 and 4.42.

Metabolism

Atazanavir is extensively metabolized in humans. The major biotransformation pathways of atazanavir in humans consisted of monooxygenation and (atazanavir sulfate) dioxygenation. Other minor biotransformation pathways for atazanavir or its metabolites consisted of glucuronidation, N-dealkylation, hydrolysis, and oxygenation with dehydro-

Continued on next page

Reyataz—Cont.

genation. Two minor metabolites of atazanavir in plasma have been characterized. Neither metabolite demonstrated *in vitro* antiviral activity. *In vitro* studies using human liver microsomes suggested that atazanavir is metabolized by CYP3A.

Elimination

Following a single 400-mg dose of ^{14}C-atazanavir, 79% and 13% of the total radioactivity was recovered in the feces and urine, respectively. Unchanged drug accounted for approximately 20% and 7% of the administered dose in the feces and urine, respectively. The mean elimination half-life of atazanavir in healthy volunteers (n=214) and HIV-infected adult patients (n=13) was approximately 7 hours at steady state following a dose of 400 mg daily with a light meal.

Effects on Electrocardiogram

Concentration- and dose-dependent prolongation of the PR interval in the electrocardiogram has been observed in healthy volunteers receiving atazanavir. In a placebo-controlled study (AI424-076), the mean (±SD) maximum change in PR interval from the predose value was 24 (±15) msec following oral dosing with 400 mg of atazanavir (n=65) compared to 13 (±11) msec following dosing with placebo (n=67). The PR interval prolongations in this study were asymptomatic. There is limited information on the potential for a pharmacodynamic interaction in humans between atazanavir and other drugs that prolong the PR interval of the electrocardiogram. (See **WARNINGS**.)

Electrocardiographic effects of atazanavir were determined in a clinical pharmacology study of 72 healthy subjects. Oral doses of 400 mg and 800 mg were compared with placebo; there was no concentration-dependent effect of atazanavir on the QTc interval (using Fridericia's correction). In 1793 HIV-infected patients receiving antiretroviral regimens, QTc prolongation was comparable in the atazanavir and comparator regimens. No atazanavir-treated healthy subject or HIV-infected patient had a QTc interval >500 msec.

Special Populations

Age/Gender

A study of the pharmacokinetics of atazanavir was performed in young (n=29; 18–40 years) and elderly (n=30; ≥65 years) healthy subjects. There were no clinically important pharmacokinetic differences observed due to age or gender.

Race

There are insufficient data to determine whether there are any effects of race on the pharmacokinetics of atazanavir.

Pediatrics

The pharmacokinetics of atazanavir in pediatric patients are under investigation. There are insufficient data at this time to recommend a dose.

Impaired Renal Function

In healthy subjects, the renal elimination of unchanged atazanavir was approximately 7% of the administered dose. There are no pharmacokinetic data available on patients with impaired renal function.

Impaired Hepatic Function

Atazanavir is metabolized and eliminated primarily by the liver. REYATAZ has been studied in adult subjects with moderate to severe hepatic impairment (14 Child-Pugh B and 2 Child-Pugh C subjects) after a single 400-mg dose. The mean AUC (0–∞) was 42% greater in subjects with impaired hepatic function than in healthy volunteers. The mean half-life of atazanavir in hepatically impaired subjects was 12.1 hours compared to 6.4 hours in healthy volunteers. Increased concentrations of atazanavir are expected in patients with moderately or severely impaired hepatic function (see **PRECAUTIONS** and **DOSAGE AND ADMINISTRATION**). The pharmacokinetics of REYATAZ in combination with ritonavir have not been studied in subjects with hepatic impairment.

Drug-Drug Interactions (see also **CONTRAINDICATIONS, WARNINGS,** and **PRECAUTIONS: Drug Interactions**)

Atazanavir is metabolized in the liver by CYP3A. Atazanavir inhibits CYP3A and UGT1A1 at clinically relevant concentrations with K_i of 2.35 µM (CYP3A4 isoform) and 1.9 µM, respectively. REYATAZ (atazanavir sulfate) should not be administered concurrently with medications with narrow therapeutic windows that are substrates of CYP3A or UGT1A1 (see **CONTRAINDICATIONS**).

Atazanavir competitively inhibits CYP1A2 and CYP2C9 with K_i values of 12 µM and a C_{max}/K_i ratio of ~0.25. There is a potential drug-drug interaction between atazanavir and CYP1A2 or CYP2C9 substrates. Atazanavir does not inhibit CYP2C19 or CYP2E1 at clinically relevant concentrations.

Atazanavir has been shown *in vivo* not to induce its own metabolism, nor to increase the biotransformation of some drugs metabolized by CYP3A. In a multiple-dose study, REYATAZ decreased the urinary ratio of endogenous 6β-OH cortisol to cortisol versus baseline, indicating that CYP3A production was not induced.

Drugs that induce CYP3A activity may increase the clearance of atazanavir, resulting in lowered plasma concentrations. Coadministration of REYATAZ (atazanavir sulfate) and other drugs that inhibit CYP3A may increase atazanavir plasma concentrations.

Drug interaction studies were performed with REYATAZ (atazanavir sulfate) and other drugs likely to be coadministered and some drugs commonly used as probes for pharmacokinetic interactions. The effects of coadministration of REYATAZ (atazanavir sulfate) on the AUC, C_{max}, and C_{min} are summarized in Tables 4 and 5. For information regarding clinical recommendations, see **PRECAUTIONS: Drug Interactions**, Tables 10 and 11.

[See table 4 on previous page]

[See table 5 at left]

Table 5: Drug Interactions: Pharmacokinetic Parameters for Coadministered Drugs in the Presence of REYATAZ[a]

Coadministered Drug	Coadministered Drug Dose/ Schedule	REYATAZ Dose/Schedule	n	Ratio (90% Confidence Interval) of Coadministered Drug Pharmacokinetic Parameters with/without REYATAZ; No Effect = 1.00 C_{max}	AUC	C_{min}
atenolol	50 mg QD, d 7-11 and d 19-23	400 mg QD, d 1-11	19	1.34 (1.26, 1.42)	1.25 (1.16, 1.34)	1.02 (0.88, 1.19)
clarithromycin	500 mg BID, d 7-10 and d 18-21	400 mg QD, d 1-10	21	1.50 (1.32, 1.71) OH-clarithromycin: 0.28 (0.24, 0.33)	1.94 (1.75, 2.16) OH-clarithromycin: 0.30 (0.26, 0.34)	0.38 (0.35, 0.43) OH-clarithromycin: 2.64 (2.36, 2.94)
didanosine (ddl) (buffered tablets) plus stavudine (d4T)[b]	ddl: 200 mg × 1 dose, d4T: 40 mg × 1 dose	400 mg × 1 dose simultaneous with ddl and d4T	32[c]	ddl: 0.92 (0.84, 1.02) d4T: 1.08 (0.96, 1.22)	ddl: 0.98 (0.92, 1.05) d4T: 1.00 (0.97, 1.03)	NA d4T: 1.04 (0.94, 1.16)
diltiazem	180 mg QD, d 7-11 and d 19-23	400 mg QD, d 1-11	28	1.98 (1.78, 2.19) desacetyl-diltiazem: 2.72 (2.44, 3.03)	2.25 (2.09, 2.16) desacetyl-diltiazem: 2.65 (2.45, 2.87)	0.41 (0.37, 0.47) desacetyl-diltiazem: 0.45 (0.41, 0.49)
ethinyl estradiol & norethindrone	Ortho-Novum® 7/7/7 QD, d 1-29	400 mg QD, d 16-29	19	ethinyl estradiol: 1.15 (0.99, 1.32) norethindrone: 1.67 (1.42, 1.96)	ethinyl estradiol: 1.48 (1.31, 1.68) norethindrone: 2.10 (1.68, 2.62)	ethinyl estradiol: 1.91 (1.57, 2.33) norethindrone: 3.62 (2.57, 5.09)
rifabutin	300 mg QD, d 1-10 then 150 mg QD, d 11-20	600 mg QD[d], d 11-20	3	1.18 (0.94, 1.48) 25-O-desacetyl-rifabutin: 8.20 (5.90, 11.40)	2.10 (1.57, 2.79) 25-O-desacetyl-rifabutin: 22.01 (15.97, 30.34)	3.43 (1.98, 5.96) 25-O-desacetyl-rifabutin: 75.6 (30.1, 190.0)
saquinavir (soft gelatin capsules)[e]	1200 mg QD, d 1-13	400 mg QD, d 7-13	7	4.39 (3.24, 5.95)	5.49 (4.04, 7.47)	6.86 (5.29, 8.91)
tenofovir[f]	300 mg QD, d 9-16 and d 24-30	400 mg QD, d 2-16	33	1.14 (1.08, 1.20)	1.24 (1.21, 1.28)	1.22 (1.15, 1.30)
lamivudine + zidovudine	150 mg lamivudine + 300 mg zidovudine BID, d 1-12	400 mg QD, d 7-12	19	lamivudine: 1.04 (0.92, 1.16) zidovudine: 1.05 (0.88, 1.24) zidovudine glucuronide: 0.95 (0.88, 1.02)	lamivudine: 1.03 (0.98, 1.08) zidovudine: 1.05 (0.96, 1.14) zidovudine glucuronide: 1.00 (0.97, 1.03)	lamivudine: 1.12 (1.04, 1.21) zidovudine: 0.69 (0.57, 0.84) zidovudine glucuronide: 0.82 (0.62, 1.08)

[a] Data provided are under fed conditions unless otherwise noted.
[b] All drugs were given under fasted conditions.
[c] One subject did not receive REYATAZ (atazanavir sulfate).
[d] Not the recommended therapeutic dose of atazanavir.
[e] The combination of atazanavir and saquinavir 1200 mg QD produced daily saquinavir exposures similar to the values produced by the standard therapeutic dosing of saquinavir at 1200 mg TID. However, the C_{max} is about 79% higher than that for the standard dosing of saquinavir (soft gelatin capsules) alone at 1200 mg TID.
[f] tenofovir disoproxil fumarate.
NA=not available.

INDICATIONS AND USAGE

REYATAZ (atazanavir sulfate) is indicated in combination with other antiretroviral agents for the treatment of HIV-1 infection.

This indication is based on analyses of plasma HIV-1 RNA levels and CD4+ cell counts from controlled studies of 48 weeks duration in antiretroviral-naive and antiretroviral-treatment-experienced patients.

The following points should be considered when initiating therapy with REYATAZ:

- In antiretroviral-experienced patients with prior virologic failure, coadministration of REYATAZ/ritonavir is recommended.
- In Study AI424-045 REYATAZ/ritonavir and lopinavir/ritonavir were similar for the primary efficacy outcome measure of time-averaged difference in change from baseline in HIV RNA level. This study was not large enough to reach a definitive conclusion that REYATAZ/ritonavir and lopinavir/ritonavir are equivalent on the secondary efficacy outcome measure of proportions below the HIV RNA lower limit of detection (see **Description of Clinical Studies**).
- The number of baseline primary protease inhibitor mutations affects the virologic response to REYATAZ/ritonavir (see **CLINICAL PHARMACOLOGY: Microbiology**).
- There are no data regarding the use of REYATAZ/ritonavir in therapy-naive patients.

Description of Clinical Studies

Patients Without Prior Antiretroviral Therapy

Study AI424-034: REYATAZ once daily compared to efavirenz once daily, each in combination with fixed-dose lamivudine + zidovudine twice daily. Study AI424-034 was a randomized, double-blind, multicenter trial comparing REYATAZ (atazanavir sulfate) (400 mg once daily) to efavirenz (600 mg once daily), each in combination with a fixed-dose combination of lamivudine (3TC) (150 mg) and zidovudine (ZDV) (300 mg) given twice daily, in 810 antiretroviral treatment-naive patients. Patients had a mean age of 34 years (range: 18 to 73), 36% were Hispanic, 33% were Caucasian, and 65% were male. The mean baseline CD4+ cell count was 321 cells/mm^3 (range: 64 to 1424 cells/mm^3) and the mean baseline plasma HIV-1 RNA level was 4.8 $\log_{10}$ copies/mL (range: 2.2 to 5.9 $\log_{10}$ copies/mL). Treatment response and outcomes through Week 48 are presented in Table 6.

Table 6: Outcomes of Randomized Treatment Through Week 48 (Study AI424-034)

Outcome	REYATAZ 400 mg once daily + lamivudine + zidovudine[d] (n=405)	efavirenz 600 mg once daily + lamivudine + zidovudine[d] (n=405)
Responder[a]	67% (32%)	62% (37%)
Virologic failure[b]	20%	21%
Rebound	17%	16%
Never suppressed through Week 48	3%	5%
Death	—	<1%
Discontinued due to adverse event	5%	7%
Discontinued for other reasons[c]	8%	10%

[a] Patients achieved and maintained confirmed HIV RNA <400 copies/mL (<50 copies/mL) through Week 48. Roche Amplicor® HIV-1 Monitor™ Assay, test version 1.0 or 1.5 as geographically appropriate.

[b] Includes confirmed viral rebound and failure to achieve confirmed HIV RNA <400 copies/mL through Week 48.
[c] Includes lost to follow-up, patient's withdrawal, noncompliance, protocol violation, and other reasons.
[d] As a fixed dose combination: 150 mg lamivudine, 300 mg zidovudine twice daily.

Through 48 weeks of therapy, the proportion of responders among patients with high viral loads (ie, baseline HIV RNA ≥100,000 copies/mL) was comparable for the REYATAZ and efavirenz arms. The mean increase from baseline in CD4+ cell count was 176 cells/mm^3 for the REYATAZ arm and 160 cells/mm^3 for the efavirenz arm.

Study AI424-008: REYATAZ 400 mg once daily compared to REYATAZ 600 mg once daily, and compared to nelfinavir 1250 mg twice daily, each in combination with stavudine and lamivudine twice daily. Study AI424-008 was a 48-week, randomized, multi-center trial, blinded to dose of REYATAZ (atazanavir sulfate), comparing REYATAZ at two dose levels (400 mg and 600 mg once daily) to nelfinavir (1250 mg twice daily), each in combination with stavudine (40 mg) and lamivudine (150 mg) given twice daily, in 467 antiretroviral treatment-naive patients. Patients had a mean age of 35 years (range: 18 to 69), 55% were Caucasian, and 63% were male. The mean baseline CD4+ cell count was 295 cells/mm^3 (range: 4 to 1003 cells/mm^3) and the mean baseline plasma HIV-1 RNA level was 4.7 $\log_{10}$ copies/mL (range: 1.8 to 5.9 $\log_{10}$ copies/mL). Treatment response and outcomes through Week 48 are presented in Table 7.

Table 7: Outcomes of Randomized Treatment Through Week 48 (Study AI424-008)

Outcome	REYATAZ 400 mg once daily + lamivudine + stavudine (n=181)	nelfinavir 1250 mg twice daily + lamivudine + stavudine (n=91)
Responder[a]	67% (33%)	59% (38%)
Virologic failure[b]	24%	27%
Rebound	14%	14%
Never suppressed through Week 48	10%	13%
Death	<1%	–
Discontinued due to adverse event	1%	3%
Discontinued for other reasons[c]	7%	10%

[a] Patients achieved and maintained confirmed HIV RNA <400 copies/mL (<50 copies/mL) through Week 48. Roche Amplicor® HIV-1 Monitor™ Assay, test version 1.0 or 1.5 as geographically appropriate.
[b] Includes confirmed viral rebound and failure to achieve confirmed HIV RNA <400 copies/mL through Week 48.
[c] Includes lost to follow-up, patient's withdrawal, noncompliance, protocol violation, and other reasons.

Through 48 weeks of therapy, the mean increase from baseline in CD4+ cell count was 234 cells/mm^3 for the REYATAZ 400-mg arm and 211 cells/mm^3 for the nelfinavir arm.

Patients With Prior Antiretroviral Therapy

Study AI424-045: REYATAZ (atazanavir sulfate) once daily + ritonavir once daily compared to REYATAZ once daily + saquinavir (soft gelatin capsules) once daily, and compared to lopinavir + ritonavir twice daily, each in combination with tenofovir + one NRTI. Study AI424-045 is an ongoing, randomized, multicenter trial comparing REYATAZ (300 mg once daily) with ritonavir (100 mg once daily) to REYATAZ (400 mg once daily) with saquinavir soft gelatin capsules (1200 mg once daily), and to lopinavir + ritonavir (400/100 mg twice daily), each in combination with tenofovir and one NRTI, in 347 (of 358 randomized) patients who experienced virologic failure on HAART (atazanavir sulfate) regimens containing PIs, NRTIs, and NNRTIs. The mean time of prior exposure to antiretrovirals was 139 weeks for PIs, 283 weeks for NRTIs, and 85 weeks for NNRTIs. The mean age was 41 years (range: 24 to 74); 60% were Caucasian, and 78% were male. The mean baseline CD4+ cell count was 338 cells/mm^3 (range: 14 to 1543 cells/mm^3) and the mean baseline plasma HIV-1 RNA level was 4.4 $\log_{10}$ copies/mL (range: 2.6 to 5.88 $\log_{10}$ copies/mL).

Treatment outcomes through Week 48 for the REYATAZ/ritonavir and lopinavir/ritonavir treatment arms are presented in Table 8. **REYATAZ/ritonavir and lopinavir/ritonavir were similar for the primary efficacy outcome measure of time-averaged difference in change from baseline in HIV RNA level. Study AI424-045 was not large enough to reach a definitive conclusion that REYATAZ/ritonavir and lopinavir/ritonavir are equivalent on the secondary efficacy outcome measure of proportions below the HIV RNA lower limit of detection.** See also Tables 1 and 2 in **CLINICAL PHARMACOLOGY: Microbiology.**

[See table 8 above]

Table 8: Outcomes of Treatment Through Week 48 in Study AI424-045 (Patients with Prior Antiretroviral Experience)

Outcome	REYATAZ 300 mg + ritonavir 100 mg once daily + tenofovir + 1 NRTI (n=119)	lopinavir/ritonavir (400/100 mg) twice daily+ tenofovir + 1 NRTI (n=118)	Difference[a] (REYATAZ-lopinavir/ritonavir) (CI)
HIV RNA Change from Baseline ($\log_{10}$ copies/mL)[b]	−1.58	−1.70	+0.12[c] (−0.17, 0.41)
CD4+ Change from Baseline (cells/mm^3)[d]	116	123	−7 (−67, 52)
Percent of Patients Responding[e]			
HIV RNA <400 copies/mL[b]	55%	57%	−2.2% (−14.8%, 10.5%)
HIV RNA <50 copies/mL[b]	38%	45%	−7.1% (−19.6%, 5.4%)

[a] Time-averaged difference through Week 48 for HIV RNA; Week 48 difference in HIV RNA percentages and CD4+ mean changes, REYATAZ (atazanavir sulfate)/ritonavir vs lopinavir/ritonavir; CI = 97.5% confidence interval for change in HIV RNA; 95% confidence interval otherwise.
[b] Roche Amplicor® HIV-1 MonitorTM Assay, test version 1.5.
[c] Protocol-defined primary efficacy outcome measure.
[d] Based on patients with baseline and Week 48 CD4+ cell count measurements (REYATAZ/ritonavir, n=85; lopinavir/ritonavir, n=93).
[e] Patients achieved and maintained confirmed HIV-1 RNA <400 copies/mL (<50 copies/mL) through Week 48.

No patients in the REYATAZ/ritonavir treatment arm and three patients in the lopinavir/ritonavir treatment arm experienced a new-onset CDC Category C event during the study.

In Study AI424-045, the mean change from baseline in plasma HIV-1 RNA for REYATAZ (atazanavir sulfate) 400 mg with saquinavir (n=115) was −1.55 $\log_{10}$ copies/mL, and the time-averaged difference in change in HIV-1 RNA levels versus lopinavir/ritonavir was 0.33. The corresponding mean increase in CD4+ cell count was 72 cells/mm^3. Through 48 weeks of treatment, the proportion of patients in this treatment arm with plasma HIV-1 RNA <400 (<50) copies/mL was 38% (26%). In this study, coadministration of REYATAZ and saquinavir did not provide adequate efficacy (see **PRECAUTIONS: Drug Interactions**, Table 11).

Study AI424-045 also compared changes from baseline in lipid values (see **ADVERSE REACTIONS**, Table 17).

Study AI424-043: Study AI424-043 was a randomized, open-label, multicenter trial comparing REYATAZ (400 mg once daily) to lopinavir/ritonavir (400/100 mg twice daily), each in combination with two NRTIs, in 300 patients who experienced virologic failure to only one prior PI-containing regimen. Through 48 weeks, the proportion of patients with plasma HIV-1 RNA <400 (<50) copies/mL was 49% (35%) for patients randomized to REYATAZ (n=144) and 69% (53%) for patients randomized to lopinavir/ritonavir (n=146). The mean change from baseline was -1.59 $\log_{10}$ copies/mL in the REYATAZ treatment arm and −2.02 $\log_{10}$ copies/mL in the lopinavir/ritonavir arm. Based on the results of this study, REYATAZ without ritonavir is inferior to lopinavir/ritonavir in PI-experienced patients with prior virologic failure and is not recommended for such patients.

CONTRAINDICATIONS

REYATAZ (atazanavir sulfate) is contraindicated in patients with known hypersensitivity to any of its ingredients, including atazanavir.

Coadministration of REYATAZ is contraindicated with drugs that are highly dependent on CYP3A for clearance and for which elevated plasma concentrations are associated with serious and/or life-threatening events. These drugs are listed in Table 9.

Table 9: Drugs That Are Contraindicated with REYATAZ Due to Potential CYP450-Mediated Interactions*

Drug class	Drugs within class that are contraindicated with REYATAZ
Benzodiazepines	midazolam, triazolam
Ergot Derivatives	dihydroergotamine, ergotamine, ergonovine, methylergonovine
GI Motility Agent	cisapride
Neuroleptic	pimozide

*Please see Table 10 for additional drugs that should not be coadministered with REYATAZ.

WARNINGS

ALERT: Find out about medicines that should NOT be taken with REYATAZ. This statement is included on the product's bottle label. (See **CONTRAINDICATIONS, WARNINGS: Drug Interactions,** and **PRECAUTIONS: Drug Interactions.**)

Drug Interactions

Atazanavir is an inhibitor of CYP3A and UGT1A1. Coadministration of REYATAZ (atazanavir sulfate) and drugs primarily metabolized by CYP3A [eg, calcium channel blockers, HMG-CoA reductase inhibitors, immunosuppressants, and phosphodiesterase (PDE5) inhibitors] or UGT1A1 (eg, irinotecan) may result in increased plasma concentrations of the other drug that could increase or prolong its therapeutic and adverse effects. (Also see **PRECAUTIONS: Drug Interactions,** Tables 10 and 11.)

Particular caution should be used when prescribing PDE5 inhibitors for erectile dysfunction (eg, sildenafil, tadalafil, or vardenafil) for patients receiving protease inhibitors, including REYATAZ. Coadministration of a protease inhibitor with a PDE5 inhibitor is expected to substantially increase the PDE5 inhibitor concentration and may result in an increase in PDE5 inhibitor-associated adverse events, including hypotension, visual changes, and priapism. (See **PRECAUTIONS: Drug Interactions** and **Information for Patients,** and the complete prescribing information for the PDE5 inhibitor.)

Concomitant use of REYATAZ with lovastatin or simvastatin is not recommended. Caution should be exercised if HIV protease inhibitors, including REYATAZ, are used concurrently with other HMG-CoA reductase inhibitors that are also metabolized by the CYP3A pathway (eg, atorvastatin). The risk of myopathy, including rhabdomyolysis, may be increased when HIV protease inhibitors, including REYATAZ, are used in combination with these drugs.

Concomitant use of REYATAZ (atazanavir sulfate) and St. John's wort (*Hypericum perforatum*), or products containing St. John's wort, is not recommended. Coadministration of protease inhibitors, including REYATAZ (atazanavir sulfate), with St. John's wort is expected to substantially decrease concentrations of the protease inhibitor and may result in suboptimal levels of atazanavir and lead to loss of virologic response and possible resistance to atazanavir or to the class of protease inhibitors.

PR Interval Prolongation

Atazanavir has been shown to prolong the PR interval of the electrocardiogram in some patients. In healthy volunteers and in patients, abnormalities in atrioventricular (AV) conduction were asymptomatic and generally limited to first-degree AV block. There have been rare reports of second-degree AV block and other conduction abnormalities and no reports of third-degree AV block (see **OVERDOSAGE**). In clinical trials, asymptomatic first-degree AV block was observed in 5.9% of atazanavir-treated patients (n=920), 5.2% of lopinavir/ritonavir-treated patients (n=252), 10.4% of nelfinavir-treated patients (n=48), and 3.0% of efavirenz-treated patients (n=329). In Study AI424-045, asymptomatic first-degree AV block was observed in 5% (6/118) of atazanavir/ritonavir-treated patients and 5% (6/116) of lopinavir/ritonavir-treated patients who had on-study electrocardiogram measurements. Because of limited clinical experience, atazanavir should be used with caution in patients with preexisting conduction system disease (eg, marked first-degree AV block or second- or third-degree AV block). (See **CLINICAL PHARMACOLOGY: Effects on Electrocardiogram.**)

In a pharmacokinetic study between atazanavir 400 mg once daily and diltiazem 180 mg once daily, a CYP3A substrate, there was a 2–fold increase in the diltiazem plasma concentration and an additive effect on the PR interval. When used in combination with atazanavir, a dose reduction of diltiazem by one half should be considered and ECG monitoring is recommended. In a pharmacokinetic study between atazanavir 400 mg once daily and atenolol 50 mg once daily, there was no substantial additive effect of atazanavir and atenolol on the PR interval. When used in combination with atazanavir, there is no need to adjust the dose of atenolol. (See **PRECAUTIONS: Drug Interactions.**)

Pharmacokinetic studies between atazanavir and other drugs that prolong the PR interval including beta blockers (other than atenolol), verapamil, and digoxin have not been performed. An additive effect of atazanavir and these drugs cannot be excluded; therefore, caution should be exercised when atazanavir is given concurrently with these drugs, especially those that are metabolized by CYP3A (eg, verapamil). (See **PRECAUTIONS: Drug Interactions.**)

Diabetes Mellitus/Hyperglycemia

New-onset diabetes mellitus, exacerbation of preexisting diabetes mellitus, and hyperglycemia have been reported during postmarketing surveillance in HIV-infected patients receiving protease inhibitor therapy. Some patients required either initiation or dose adjustments of insulin or oral hypoglycemic agents for treatment of these events. In some cases, diabetic ketoacidosis has occurred. In those patients who discontinued protease inhibitor therapy, hyperglycemia persisted in some cases. Because these events have been reported voluntarily during clinical practice, estimates of frequency cannot be made and a causal relationship between protease inhibitor therapy and these events has not been established.

PRECAUTIONS

General

Hyperbilirubinemia

Most patients taking REYATAZ (atazanavir sulfate) experience asymptomatic elevations in indirect (unconjugated)

Continued on next page

Reyataz—Cont.

bilirubin related to inhibition of UDP-glucuronosyl transferase (UGT). This hyperbilirubinemia is reversible upon discontinuation of REYATAZ. Hepatic transaminase elevations that occur with hyperbilirubinemia should be evaluated for alternative etiologies. No long-term safety data are available for patients experiencing persistent elevations in total bilirubin >5 times ULN. Alternative antiretroviral therapy to REYATAZ may be considered if jaundice or scleral icterus associated with bilirubin elevations presents cosmetic concerns for patients. Dose reduction of atazanavir is not recommended since long-term efficacy of reduced doses has not been established. (See **ADVERSE REACTIONS: Laboratory Abnormalities**, Tables 14 and 16.)

Rash

In controlled clinical trials (n=1597), rash (all grades, regardless of causality) occurred in 21% of patients treated with REYATAZ. The median time to onset of rash was 8 weeks after initiation of REYATAZ and the median duration of rash was 1.3 weeks. Rashes were generally mild-to-moderate maculopapular skin eruptions. Dosing with REYATAZ was often continued without interruption in patients who developed rash. The discontinuation rate for rash in clinical trials was 0.4%. REYATAZ should be discontinued if severe rash develops. Cases of Stevens-Johnson syndrome and erythema multiforme have been reported in patients receiving REYATAZ.

Hepatic Impairment and Toxicity

Atazanavir is principally metabolized by the liver; caution should be exercised when administering this drug to patients with hepatic impairment because atazanavir concentrations may be increased (see **DOSAGE AND ADMINISTRATION**). Patients with underlying hepatitis B or C viral infections or marked elevations in transaminases prior to treatment may be at increased risk for developing further transaminase elevations or hepatic decompensation. There are no clinical trial data on the use of REYATAZ/ritonavir in patients with any degree of hepatic impairment.

Resistance / Cross-Resistance

Various degrees of cross-resistance among protease inhibitors have been observed. Resistance to atazanavir may not preclude the subsequent use of other protease inhibitors. (See **CLINICAL PHARMACOLOGY: Microbiology**.)

Hemophilia

There have been reports of increased bleeding, including spontaneous skin hematomas and hemarthrosis, in patients with hemophilia type A and B treated with protease inhibitors. In some patients, additional factor VIII was given. In more than half of the reported cases, treatment with protease inhibitors was continued or reintroduced. A causal relationship between protease inhibitor therapy and these events has not been established.

Fat Redistribution

Redistribution/accumulation of body fat, including central obesity, dorsocervical fat enlargement (buffalo hump), peripheral wasting, facial wasting, breast enlargement, and "cushingoid appearance" have been observed in patients receiving anti-retroviral therapy. The mechanism and long-term consequences of these events are currently unknown. A causal relationship has not been established.

Immune Reconstitution Syndrome

Immune reconstitution syndrome has been reported in patients treated with combination antiretroviral therapy, including REYATAZ (atazanavir sulfate). During the initial phase of combination antiretroviral treatment, patients whose immune system responds may develop an inflammatory response to indolent or residual opportunistic infections (such as *Mycobacterium avium* infection, cytomegalovirus, *Pneumocystis carinii* pneumonia, or tuberculosis), which may necessitate further evaluation and treatment.

Information for Patients

A statement to patients and healthcare providers is included on the product's bottle label: **ALERT: Find out about medicines that should NOT be taken with REYATAZ.** A Patient Package Insert (PPI) for REYATAZ is available for patient information.

Patients should be told that sustained decreases in plasma HIV RNA have been associated with a reduced risk of progression to AIDS and death. Patients should remain under the care of a physician while using REYATAZ. Patients should be advised to take REYATAZ with food every day and take other concomitant antiretroviral therapy as prescribed. REYATAZ must always be used in combination with other antiretroviral drugs. Patients should not alter the dose or discontinue therapy without consulting with their doctor. If a dose of REYATAZ is missed, patients should take the dose as soon as possible and then return to their normal schedule. However, if a dose is skipped, the patient should not double the next dose.

Patients should be informed that REYATAZ is not a cure for HIV infection and that they may continue to develop opportunistic infections and other complications associated with HIV disease. Patients should be told that there are currently no data demonstrating that therapy with REYATAZ can reduce the risk of transmitting HIV to others through sexual contact.

REYATAZ may interact with some drugs; therefore, patients should be advised to report to their doctor the use of any other prescription, nonprescription medication, or herbal products, particularly St. John's wort.

Table 10: Drugs That Should Not Be Administered with REYATAZ (atazanavir sulfate)

Drug class: Specific Drugs	Clinical Comment
Antimycobacterials: rifampin	Decreases plasma concentrations and AUC of most protease inhibitors by about 90%. This may result in loss of therapeutic effect and development of resistance.
Antineoplastics: irinotecan	Atazanavir inhibits UGT and may interfere with the metabolism of irinotecan, resulting in increased irinotecan toxicities.
Benzodiazepines: (atazanavir sulfate) midazolam, triazolam	CONTRAINDICATED due to potential for serious and/or life-threatening events such as prolonged or increased sedation or respiratory depression.
Ergot Derivatives: dihydroergotamine, ergotamine, ergonovine, methylergonovine	CONTRAINDICATED due to potential for serious and/or life-threatening events such as acute ergot toxicity characterized by peripheral vasospasm and ischemia of the extremities and other tissues.
GI Motility Agent: cisapride	CONTRAINDICATED due to potential for serious and/or life-threatening reactions such as cardiac arrhythmias.
HMG-CoA Reductase Inhibitors: lovastatin, simvastatin	Potential for serious reactions such as myopathy including rhabdomyolysis.
Neuroleptic: pimozide	CONTRAINDICATED due to potential for serious and/or life-threatening reactions such as cardiac arrhythmias.
Protease Inhibitors: indinavir	Both REYATAZ and indinavir are associated with indirect (unconjugated) hyperbilirubinemia. Combinations of these drugs have not been studied and coadministration of REYATAZ and indinavir is not recommended.
Proton-Pump Inhibitors	Concomitant use of REYATAZ and proton-pump inhibitors is not recommended. Coadministration of REYATAZ with proton-pump inhibitors is expected to substantially decrease REYATAZ plasma concentrations and reduce its therapeutic effect.
Herbal Products: St. John's wort (*Hypericum perforatum*)	Patients taking REYATAZ should not use products containing St. John's wort (*Hypericum perforatum*) because coadministration may be expected to reduce plasma concentrations of atazanavir. This may result in loss of therapeutic effect and development of resistance.

Table 11: Established and Other Potentially Significant Drug Interactions: Alteration in Dose or Regimen May Be Recommended Based on Drug Interaction Studies[a] or Predicted Interactions (Information in the table applies to REYATAZ with or without ritonavir, unless otherwise indicated)

Concomitant Drug Class: Specific Drugs	Effect on Concentration of Atazanavir or Concomitant Drug	Clinical Comment
HIV Antiviral Agents		
Nucleoside Reverse Transcriptase Inhibitors (NRTIs): didanosine buffered formulations	↓ atazanavir	Coadministration of REYATAZ (atazanavir sulfate) with didanosine buffered tablets did not alter exposure to didanosine; however, exposure to atazanavir was markedly decreased (presumably due to the increase in gastric pH caused by buffers in the didanosine tablets). In addition, it is recommended that didanosine be administered on an empty stomach; therefore, REYATAZ should be given (with food) 2 h before or 1 h after didanosine buffered formulations (see **CLINICAL PHARMACOLOGY: Drug-Drug Interactions**). Because didanosine EC capsules are to be given on an empty stomach and REYATAZ is to be given with food, they should be administered at different times.
Nucleotide Reverse Transcriptase Inhibitors: tenofovir disoproxil fumarate	↓ atazanavir ↑ tenofovir	Tenofovir may decrease the AUC and C_{min} of atazanavir. When coadministered with tenofovir, it is recommended that REYATAZ 300 mg be given with ritonavir 100 mg and tenofovir 300 mg (all as a single daily dose with food). **REYATAZ without ritonavir should not be coadministered with tenofovir.** REYATAZ increases tenofovir concentrations. The mechanism of this interaction is unknown. Higher tenofovir concentrations could potentiate tenofovir-associated adverse events, including renal disorders. Patients receiving REYATAZ and tenofovir should be monitored for tenofovir-associated adverse events.
Non-nucleoside Reverse Transcriptase Inhibitors (NNRTIs): efavirenz	↓ atazanavir	In treatment-naive patients who receive efavirenz and REYATAZ, the recommended dose is REYATAZ 300 mg with ritonavir 100 mg and efavirenz 600 mg (all once daily), as this combination results in atazanavir exposure that approximates the mean exposure to atazanavir produced by 400 mg of REYATAZ alone. Dosing recommendations for efavirenz and REYATAZ in treatment-experienced patients have not been established.
Non-nucleoside Reverse Transcriptase Inhibitors: nevirapine	↓ atazanavir	***REYATAZ/ritonavir:*** The effects of coadministration have not been studied. Nevirapine, an inducer of CYP3A, is expected to decrease atazanavir exposure. In the absence of data, coadministration is not recommended.
Protease Inhibitors: saquinavir (soft gelatin capsules)	↑ saquinavir	Appropriate dosing recommendations for this combination, with or without ritonavir, with respect to efficacy and safety, have not been established. In a clinical study, saquinavir 1200 mg coadministered with REYATAZ 400 mg and tenofovir 300 mg (all given once daily) plus nucleoside analogue reverse transcriptase inhibitors did not provide adequate efficacy (see **Description of Clinical Studies**).

(Table continued on next page)

Patients receiving a PDE5 inhibitor and atazanavir should be advised that they may be at an increased risk of PDE5 inhibitor-associated adverse events including hypotension, visual changes, and prolonged penile erection, and should promptly report any symptoms to their doctor.
Patients should be informed that atazanavir may produce changes in the electrocardiogram (PR prolongation). Patients should consult their physician if they are experiencing symptoms such as dizziness or lightheadedness.
REYATAZ (atazanavir sulfate) should be taken with food to enhance absorption.
Patients should be informed that asymptomatic elevations in indirect bilirubin have occurred in patients receiving REYATAZ. This may be accompanied by yellowing of the skin or whites of the eyes and alternative antiretroviral therapy may be considered if the patient has cosmetic concerns.
Patients should be informed that redistribution or accumulation of body fat may occur in patients receiving antiretroviral therapy including protease inhibitors and that the cause and long-term health effects of these conditions are not known at this time. It is unknown whether long-term use of REYATAZ (atazanavir sulfate) will result in a lower incidence of lipodystrophy than with other protease inhibitors.

Drug Interactions

Atazanavir is an inhibitor of CYP3A and UGT1A1. Coadministration of REYATAZ and drugs primarily metabolized by CYP3A (eg, calcium channel blockers, HMG-CoA reductase inhibitors, immunosuppressants, and PDE5 inhibitors) or UGT1A1 (eg, irinotecan) may result in increased plasma concentrations of the other drug that could increase or prolong both its therapeutic and adverse effects, (see Tables 10 and 11). Atazanavir is metabolized in the liver by the cytochrome P450 enzyme system. Coadministration of REYATAZ and drugs that induce CYP3A, such as rifampin, may decrease atazanavir plasma concentrations and reduce its therapeutic effect. Coadministration of REYATAZ and drugs that inhibit CYP3A may increase atazanavir plasma concentrations.
The potential for drug interactions with REYATAZ changes when REYATAZ is coadministered with the potent CYP3A inhibitor ritonavir. The magnitude of CYP3A-mediated drug interactions (effect on atazanavir or effect on coadministered drug) may change when REYATAZ is coadministered with ritonavir. See the complete prescribing information for Norvir® (ritonavir) for information on drug interactions with ritonavir.
Atazanavir solubility decreases as pH increases. Reduced plasma concentrations of atazanavir are expected if antacids, buffered medications, H_2-receptor antagonists, and proton-pump inhibitors are administered with atazanavir.
Atazanavir has the potential to prolong the PR interval of the electrocardiogram in some patients. Caution should be used when coadministering REYATAZ with medicinal products known to induce PR interval prolongation (eg, atenolol, diltiazem [see Table 11]).
Drugs that are contraindicated or not recommended for coadministration with REYATAZ are included in Table 10. These recommendations are based on either drug interaction studies or predicted interactions due to the expected magnitude of interaction and potential for serious events or loss of efficacy.

[See table 10 at top of previous page]
[See table 11 on pages 1064 through 1066]

Based on known metabolic profiles, clinically significant drug interactions are not expected between REYATAZ (atazanavir sulfate) and fluvastatin, pravastatin, dapsone, trimethoprim/sulfamethoxazole, azithromycin, erythromycin, or fluconazole. REYATAZ does not interact with substrates of CYP2D6 (eg, nortriptyline, desipramine, metoprolol).

Carcinogenesis, Mutagenesis, and Impairment of Fertility

Long-term carcinogenicity studies of atazanavir in animals have not been completed. Atazanavir tested positive in an *in vitro* clastogenicity test using primary human lymphocytes, in the absence and presence of metabolic activation. Atazanavir tested negative in the *in vitro* Ames reverse-mutation assay, *in vivo* micronucleus and DNA repair tests in rats, and *in vivo* DNA damage test in rat duodenum (comet assay).
At the systemic drug exposure levels (AUC) equal to (in male rats) or two times (in female rats) those at the human clinical dose (400 mg once daily), atazanavir did not produce significant effects on mating, fertility, or early embryonic development.

Pregnancy

Pregnancy Category B

At maternal doses producing the systemic drug exposure levels equal to (in rabbits) or two times (in rats) those at the human clinical dose (400 mg once daily), atazanavir did not produce teratogenic effects. In the pre- and post-natal development assessment in rats, atazanavir, at maternally toxic drug exposure levels two times those at the human clinical dose, caused body weight loss or weight gain suppression in the offspring. Offspring were unaffected at a lower dose that produced maternal exposure equivalent to that observed in humans given 400 mg once daily.
Hyperbilirubinemia occurred frequently during treatment with REYATAZ. It is not known whether REYATAZ administered to the mother during pregnancy will exacerbate physiological hyperbilirubinemia and lead to kernicterus in neonates and young infants. In the prepartum period, additional monitoring and alternative therapy to REYATAZ should be considered.

Table 11 *(cont.)*: Established and Other Potentially Significant Drug Interactions: Alteration in Dose or Regimen May Be Recommended Based on Drug Interaction Studies[a] or Predicted Interactions (Information in the table applies to REYATAZ with or without ritonavir, unless otherwise indicated)

Concomitant Drug Class: **Specific Drugs**	**Effect on Concentration of Atazanavir or Concomitant Drug**	**Clinical Comment**
Protease Inhibitors: ritonavir	↑ atazanavir	If REYATAZ (atazanavir sulfate) is coadministered with ritonavir, it is recommended that REYATAZ 300 mg once daily be given with ritonavir 100 mg once daily with food. See the complete prescribing information for Norvir® (ritonavir) for information on drug interactions with ritonavir.
Protease Inhibitors: others	↑ other protease inhibitor	***REYATAZ/ritonavir:*** Although not studied, the coadministration of REYATAZ/ritonavir and other protease inhibitors would be expected to increase exposure to the other protease inhibitor. Such coadministration is not recommended.
Other Agents		
Antacids and buffered medications	↓ atazanavir	Reduced plasma concentrations of atazanavir are expected if antacids, including buffered medications, are administered with REYATAZ. REYATAZ should be administered 2 h before or 1 h after these medications.
Antiarrhythmics: amiodarone, bepridil, lidocaine (systemic), quinidine	↑ amiodarone, bepridil, lidocaine (systemic), quinidine	Coadministration with REYATAZ has the potential to produce serious and/or life-threatening adverse events and has not been studied. Caution is warranted and therapeutic concentration monitoring of these drugs is recommended if they are used concomitantly with REYATAZ.
Anticoagulants: warfarin	↑ warfarin	Coadministration with REYATAZ has the potential to produce serious and/or life-threatening bleeding and has not been studied. It is recommended that INR (International Normalized Ratio) be monitored.
Antidepressants: tricyclic antidepressants	↑ tricyclic antidepressants	Coadministration with REYATAZ has the potential to produce serious and/or life-threatening adverse events and has not been studied. Concentration monitoring of these drugs is recommended if they are used concomitantly with REYATAZ.
Antifungals: ketoconazole, itraconazole	**REYATAZ/ritonavir:** ketoconazole ↑ ↑ itraconazole	Coadministration of ketoconazole has only been studied with REYATAZ without ritonavir (negligible increase in atazanavir AUC and C_{max}). Due to the effect of ritonavir on ketoconazole, high doses of ketoconazole and itraconazole (>200 mg/day) should be used cautiously with REYATAZ/ritonavir.
Antifungals: voriconazole	Effect is unknown	Coadministration of voriconazole with REYATAZ, with or without ritonavir, has not been studied. However, administration of voriconazole with ritonavir 400 mg every 12 hours decreased voriconazole steady-state AUC by an average of 82%. The effect of lower ritonavir doses on voriconazole is not known at this time. Until data are available, voriconazole should not be administered to patients receiving REYATAZ/ritonavir. Codaministration of voriconazole with REYATAZ (without ritonavir) may increase atazanavir concentrations; however, no data are available.
Antimycobacterials: rifabutin	↑ rifabutin	A rifabutin dose reduction of up to 75% (eg, 150 mg every other day or 3 times per week) is recommended.
Calcium channel blockers: diltiazem	↑ diltiazem and desacetyl-diltiazem	Caution is warranted. A dose reduction of diltiazem by 50% should be considered. ECG monitoring is recommended. Coadministration of REYATAZ/ritonavir with diltiazem has not been studied.
eg, felodipine, nifedipine, nicardipine, and verapamil	↑ calcium channel blocker	Caution is warranted. Dose titration of the calcium channel blocker should be considered. ECG monitoring is recommended.
HMG-CoA reductase inhibitors: atorvastatin	↑ atorvastatin	The risk of myopathy including rhabdomyolysis may be increased when protease inhibitors, including REYATAZ, are used in combination with atorvastatin. Caution should be exercised.
H_2-Receptor antagonists	↓ atazanavir	Reduced plasma concentrations of atazanavir are expected if H_2-receptor antagonists are administered with REYATAZ. This may result in loss of therapeutic effect and development of resistance. To lessen the effect of H_2-receptor antagonists on atazanavir exposure, it is recommended that an H_2-receptor antagonist and REYATAZ be administered as far apart as possible, preferably 12 hours apart.

(Table continued on next page)

There are no adequate and well-controlled studies in pregnant women. Cases of lactic acidosis syndrome, sometimes fatal, and symptomatic hyperlactatemia have been reported in patients (including pregnant women) receiving REYATAZ in combination with nucleoside analogues, which are known to be associated with increased risk of lactic acidosis syndrome. REYATAZ should be used during pregnancy only if the potential benefit justifies the potential risk to the fetus. (See **PRECAUTIONS: Lactic Acidosis Syndrome.**)
Antiretroviral Pregnancy Registry: To monitor maternal-fetal outcomes of pregnant women exposed to REYATAZ, an Antiretroviral Pregnancy Registry has been established. Physicians are encouraged to register patients by calling 1-800-258-4263.

Nursing Mothers

The Centers for Disease Control and Prevention recommend that HIV-infected mothers not breast-feed their infants to avoid risking postnatal transmission of HIV. It is not known whether atazanavir is secreted in human milk. A study in lactating rats has demonstrated that atazanavir is

Continued on next page

Reyataz—Cont.

secreted in milk. Because of both the potential for HIV transmission and the potential for serious adverse reactions in nursing infants, **mothers should be instructed not to breast-feed if they are receiving REYATAZ.**

Pediatric Use

The optimal dosing regimen for use of REYATAZ (atazanavir sulfate) in pediatric patients has not been established. REYATAZ should not be administered to pediatric patients below the age of 3 months due to the risk of kernicterus.

Geriatric Use

Clinical studies of REYATAZ did not include sufficient numbers of patients aged 65 and over to determine whether they respond differently from younger patients. Based on a comparison of mean single dose pharmacokinetic values for C_{max} and AUC, a dose adjustment based upon age is not recommended. In general, appropriate caution should be exercised in the administration and monitoring of REYATAZ in elderly patients reflecting the greater frequency of decreased hepatic, renal, or cardiac function, and of concomitant disease or other drug therapy.

ADVERSE REACTIONS

Adult Patients

Treatment-Emergent Adverse Events in Treatment-Naive Patients

Selected drug-related clinical adverse events of moderate or severe intensity reported in ≥2% of treatment-naive patients receiving combination therapy including REYATAZ are presented in Table 12. For other information regarding observed or potentially serious adverse events, see **WARNINGS** and **PRECAUTIONS.**

[See table 12 at right]

Treatment-Emergent Adverse Events in Treatment-Experienced Patients

Selected drug-related clinical adverse events of moderate-severe intensity in ≥2% of treatment-experienced patients receiving REYATAZ/ritonavir are presented in Table 13. For other information regarding observed or potentially serious adverse events, see **WARNINGS** and **PRECAUTIONS.**

Table 13: Selected Treatment-Emergent Adverse Events[a] of Moderate or Severe Intensity Reported in ≥2% of Adult Treatment-Experienced Patients[b], Study AI424-045

	48 weeks[c] REYATAZ/ritonavir 300/100 mg once daily + tenofovir + NRTI (n=119)	48 weeks[c] lopinavir/ritonavir 400/100 mg twice daily[d] + tenofovir + NRTI (n=118)
Body as a Whole		
Fever	2%	*
Digestive System		
Jaundice/scleral icterus	9%	*
Diarrhea	3%	11%
Nausea	3%	2%
Nervous System		
Depression	2%	<1%
Musculoskeletal System		
Myalgia	4%	*

*None reported in this treatment arm.
[a] Includes events of possible, probable, certain, or unknown relationship to treatment regimen.
[b] Based on the regimen containing REYATAZ (atazanavir sulfate).
[c] Median time on therapy.
[d] As a fixed-dose combination.

Laboratory Abnormalities

Treatment-Naive Patients

The percentages of adult treatment-naive patients treated with combination therapy including REYATAZ with Grade 3-4 laboratory abnormalities are presented in Table 14.

[See table 14 at top of next page]

Lipids, Change from Baseline

For Study AI424-034, changes from baseline in fasting LDL-cholesterol, HDL-cholesterol, total cholesterol, and fasting triglycerides are shown in Table 15.

[See table 15 on next page]

Treatment-Experienced Patients

The percentages of adult treatment-experienced patients treated with combination therapy including REYATAZ/ritonavir with Grade 3-4 laboratory abnormalities are presented in Table 16.

[See table 16 on next page]

Lipids, Change from Baseline

For Study AI424-045, changes from baseline in fasting LDL-cholesterol, HDL-cholesterol, total cholesterol, and fasting triglycerides are shown in Table 17. The observed magnitude of dyslipidemia was less with REYATAZ/ritonavir than with lopinavir/ritonavir. However, the clinical impact of such findings has not been demonstrated.

[See table 17 at bottom of next page]

Table 11 (*cont.*): Established and Other Potentially Significant Drug Interactions: Alteration in Dose or Regimen May Be Recommended Based on Drug Interaction Studies[a] or Predicted Interactions (Information in the table applies to REYATAZ with or without ritonavir, unless otherwise indicated)

Concomitant Drug Class: Specific Drugs	Effect on Concentration of Atazanavir or Concomitant Drug	Clinical Comment
Immunosuppressants: cyclosporine, sirolimus, tacrolimus	↑ immunosuppressants	Therapeutic concentration monitoring is recommended for immunosuppressant agents when coadministered with REYATAZ (atazanavir sulfate).
Macrolide antibiotics: clarithromycin	↑ clarithromycin ↓ 14-OH clarithromycin ↑ atazanavir	Increased concentrations of clarithromycin may cause QTc prolongations; therefore, a dose reduction of clarithromycin by 50% should be considered when it is coadministered with REYATAZ. In addition, concentrations of the active metabolite 14-OH clarithromycin are significantly reduced; consider alternative therapy for indications other than infections due to *Mycobacterium avium* complex. Coadministration of REYATAZ/ritonvair with clarithromycin has not been studied.
Hormonal contraceptives: ethinyl estradiol and norethindrone	↑ ethinyl estradiol ↑ norethindrone	Coadministration of REYATAZ/ritonavir with hormonal contraceptives has not been studied. However, higher doses of ritonavir, without REYATAZ, decrease contraceptive steroid concentrations. Because contraceptive steroid concentrations may be altered when REYATAZ or REYATAZ/ritonavir is coadministered with oral contraceptives or with the contraceptive patch, alternate methods of nonhormonal contraception are recommended.
PDE5 inhibitors: sildenafil tadalafil vardenafil	↑ sildenafil ↑ tadalafil ↑ vardenafil	Coadministration with REYATAZ has not been studied but may result in an increase in PDE5 inhibitor-associated adverse events, including hypotension, visual changes, and priapism. Use sildenafil with caution at reduced doses of 25 mg every 48 hours with increased monitoring for adverse events. Use tadalafil with caution at reduced doses of 10 mg every 72 hours with increased monitoring for adverse events. Use vardenafil with caution at reduced doses of no more than 2.5 mg every 72 hours with increased monitoring for adverse events.

[a] For magnitude of interactions, see **CLINICAL PHARMACOLOGY**: Tables 4 and 5.

Table 12: Selected Treatment-Emergent Adverse Events[a] of Moderate or Severe Intensity Reported in ≥2% of Adult Treatment-Naive Patients[b]

	Phase III Study AI424-034		Phase II Studies AI424-007, -008	
	64 weeks[c] REYATAZ 400 mg once daily + lamivudine + zidovudine[e] (n=404)	64 weeks[c] efavirenz 600 mg once daily + lamivudine + zidovudine[e] (n=401)	120 weeks[c,d] REYATAZ 400 mg once daily + stavudine + lamivudine or didanosine (n=279)	73 weeks[c,d] nelfinavir 750 mg TID or 1250 mg BID + stavudine + lamivudine or didanosine (n=191)
Body as a Whole				
Headache	6%	6%	1%	2%
Digestive System				
Nausea	14%	12%	6%	4%
Jaundice/scleral icterus	7%	*	7%	*
Vomiting	4%	7%	3%	3%
Diarrhea	1%	2%	3%	16%
Abdominal pain	4%	4%	4%	2%
Nervous System				
Dizziness	2%	7%	<1%	*
Insomnia	3%	3%	<1%	*
Peripheral neurologic symptoms	<1%	1%	4%	3%
Skin and Appendages				
Rash	7%	10%	5%	1%

*None reported in this treatment arm.
[a] Includes events of possible, probable, certain, or unknown relationship to treatment regimen.
[b] Based on regimens containing REYATAZ (atazanavir sulfate).
[c] Median time on therapy.
[d] Includes long-term follow-up.
[e] As a fixed dose combination: 150 mg lamivudine, 300 mg zidovudine twice daily.

Patients Co-infected With Hepatitis B and/or Hepatitis C Virus

Liver function tests should be monitored in patients with a history of hepatitis B or C. In studies AI424-008 and AI424-034, 74 patients treated with 400 mg of REYATAZ once daily, 58 who received efavirenz, and 12 who received nelfinavir were seropositive for hepatitis B and/or C at study entry. ALT levels >5 times the upper limit of normal (ULN) developed in 15% of the REYATAZ-treated patients, 14% of the efavirenz-treated patients, and 17% of the nelfinavir-treated patients. AST levels >5 times ULN developed in 9% of the REYATAZ-treated patients, 5% of the efavirenz-treated patients, and 17% of the nelfinavir-treated patients. Within atazanavir and control regimens, no difference in frequency of bilirubin elevations was noted between seropositive and seronegative patients.

In study AI424-045, 20 patients treated with REYATAZ/ritonavir 300 mg/100 mg once daily and 18 patients treated with lopinavir/ritonavir 400 mg/100 mg twice daily were seropositive for hepatitis B and/or C at study entry. ALT levels >5 times ULN developed in 25% (5/20) of the REYATAZ/ritonavir-treated patients and 6% (1/18) of the lopinavir/ritonavir-treated patients. AST levels >5 times ULN developed in 10% (2/20) of the REYATAZ/ritonavir-treated patients and 6% (1/18) of the lopinavir/ritonavir-treated patients (see **PRECAUTIONS: General**).

OVERDOSAGE

Human experience of acute overdose with REYATAZ is limited. Single doses up to 1200 mg have been taken by healthy volunteers without symptomatic untoward effects. A single self-administered overdose of 29.2 g of REYATAZ in an HIV-infected patient (73 times the 400-mg recommended dose) was associated with asymptomatic bifascicular block and PR interval prolongation. These events resolved spontaneously. At high doses that lead to high drug exposures, jaundice due to indirect (unconjugated) hyperbilirubinemia (without associated liver function test changes) or PR interval prolongation may be observed. (See **WARNINGS, PRECAUTIONS,** and **CLINICAL PHARMACOLOGY: Effects on Electrocardiogram.**)

Treatment of overdosage with REYATAZ (atazanavir sulfate) should consist of general supportive measures, including monitoring of vital signs and ECG, and observations of the patient's clinical status. If indicated, elimination of unabsorbed atazanavir should be achieved by emesis or gas-

Table 14: Grade 3-4 Laboratory Abnormalities Reported in ≥2% of Adult Treatment-Naive Patients[a]

Variable	Limit[d]	Phase III Study AI424-034: 64 weeks[b] REYATAZ 400 mg once daily + lamivudine + zidovudine[e] (n=404)	64 weeks[b] efavirenz 600 mg once daily + lamivudine + zidovudine[e] (n=401)	Phase II Studies AI424-007, -008: 120 weeks[b,c] REYATAZ 400 mg once daily + stavudine + lamivudine or + stavudine + didanosine (n=279)	73 weeks[b,c] nelfinavir 750 mg TID or 1250 mg BID + stavudine + lamivudine or + stavudine + didanosine (n=191)
Chemistry	High				
SGOT/AST	≥5.1 × ULN	2%	2%	7%	5%
SGPT/ALT	≥5.1 × ULN	4%	3%	9%	7%
Total Bilirubin	≥2.6 × ULN	35%	<1%	47%	3%
Amylase	≥2.1 × ULN	*	*	14%	10%
Lipase	≥2.1 × ULN	<1%	1%	4%	5%
Creatinine Kinase	≥5.1 × ULN	6%	6%	11%	9%
Total Cholesterol	≥240 mg/dL	6%	24%	19%	48%
Triglycerides	≥751 mg/dL	<1%	3%	4%	2%
Hematology	Low				
Hemoglobin	<8.0 g/dL	5%	3%	<1%	4%
Neutrophils	<750 cells/mm^3	7%	9%	3%	7%

*None reported in this treatment arm.
[a] Based on regimen(s) containing REYATAZ.
[b] Median time on therapy.
[c] Includes long-term follow-up.
[d] ULN=upper limit of normal.
[e] As a fixed-dose combination: 150 mg lamivudine, 300 mg zidovudine twice daily.

Table 15: Lipid Values, Mean Change from Baseline, Study AI424-034

	REYATAZ[a,b] Baseline mg/dL (n=383[e])	Week 48 mg/dL (n=283[e])	Change[d] (n=272[e])	efavirenz[b,c] Baseline mg/dL (n=378[e])	Week 48 mg/dL (n=264[e])	Change[d] (n=253[e])
LDL-Cholesterol[f]	98	98	+1%	98	114	+18%
HDL-Cholesterol	39	43	+13%	38	46	+24%
Total Cholesterol	164	168	+2%	162	195	+21%
Triglycerides[f]	138	124	−9%	129	168	+23%

[a] REYATAZ 400 mg once daily with the fixed-dose combination: 150 mg lamivudine, 300 mg zidovudine twice daily.
[b] Values obtained after initiation of serum lipid-reducing agents were not included in these analyses. Use of serum lipid-reducing agents was more common in the efavirenz treatment arm (3%) than in the REYATAZ arm (1%).
[c] Efavirenz 600 mg once daily with the fixed-dose combination: 150 mg lamivudine, 300 mg zidovudine twice daily.
[d] The change from baseline is the mean of within-patient changes from baseline for patients with both baseline and Week 48 values and is not a simple difference of the baseline and Week 48 mean values.
[e] Number of patients with LDL-cholesterol measured.
[f] Fasting.

Table 16: Grade 3-4 Laboratory Abnormalities Reported in ≥2% of Adult Treatment-Experienced Patients, Study AI424-045[a]

Variable	Limit[c]	48 weeks[b] REYATAZ/ritonavir 300/100 mg once daily + tenofovir + NRTI (n=119)	48 weeks[b] lopinavir/ritonavir 400/100 mg twice daily[d] + tenofovir + NRTI (n=118)
Chemistry	High		
SGOT/AST	≥5.1 × ULN	3%	3%
SGPT/ALT	≥5.1 × ULN	4%	3%
Total Bilirubin	≥2.6 × ULN	49%	<1%
Lipase	≥2.1 × ULN	5%	6%
Creatine Kinase	≥5.1 × ULN	8%	8%
Total Cholesterol	≥240 mg/dL	25%	26%
Triglycerides	≥751 mg/dL	8%	12%
Glucose	≥251 mg/dL	5%	<1%
Hematology	Low		
Platelets	<50,000 cells/mm^3	2%	3%
Neutrophils	<750 cells/mm^3	7%	8%

[a] Based on regimen(s) containing REYATAZ (atazanavir sulfate).
[b] Median time on therapy.
[c] ULN = upper limit of normal.
[d] As a fixed-dose combination.

Table 17: Lipid Values, Mean Change from Baseline, Study A1424-045

	REYATAZ/ritonavir[a,b] Baseline mg/dL (n=111[e])	Week 48 mg/dL (n=75[e])	Change[d] (n=74[e])	lopinavir/ritonavir[b,c] Baseline mg/dL (n=108[e])	Week 48 mg/dL (n=76[e])	Change[d] (n=73[e])
LDL-Cholesterol[f]	108	98	−10%	104	103	+1%
HDL-Cholesterol	40	39	−7%	39	41	+2%
Total Cholesterol	188	177	−8%	181	187	+6%
Triglycerides[f]	215	161	−4%	196	224	+30%

[a] REYATAZ (atazanavir sulfate) 300 mg once daily + ritonavir + tenofovir + 1 NRTI.
[b] Values obtained after initiation of serum lipid-reducing agents were not included in these analyses. Use of serum lipid-reducing agents was more common in the lopinavir/ritonavir treatment arm (19%) than in the REYATAZ/ritonavir arm (8%).
[c] Lopinavir/ritonavir (400/100 mg) BID + tenofovir + 1 NRTI.
[d] The change from baseline is the mean of within-patient changes from baseline for patients with both baseline and Week 48 values and is not a simple difference of the baseline and Week 48 mean values.
[e] Number of patients with LDL-cholesterol measured.
[f] Fasting.

tric lavage. Administration of activated charcoal may also be used to aid removal of unabsorbed drug. There is no specific antidote for overdose with REYATAZ. Since atazanavir is extensively metabolized by the liver and is highly protein bound, dialysis is unlikely to be beneficial in significant removal of this medicine.

DOSAGE AND ADMINISTRATION

Adults

REYATAZ Capsules must be taken with food.

The recommended oral dose of REYATAZ is as follows:

Therapy-Naive Patients

- REYATAZ 400 mg (two 200-mg capsules) once daily taken with food.
  There are no data regarding the use of REYATAZ/ritonavir in therapy-naive patients.

Therapy-Experienced Patients

- REYATAZ 300 mg (two 150-mg capsules) once daily plus ritonavir 100 mg once daily taken with food.
  REYATAZ without ritonavir is not recommended for treatment-experienced patients with prior virologic failure (see **Description of Clinical Studies**).

Efficacy and safety of REYATAZ with ritonavir in doses greater than 100 mg once daily have not been established. The use of higher ritonavir doses might alter the safety profile of atazanavir (cardiac effects, hyperbilirubinemia) and, therefore, is not recommended. Prescribers should consult the complete prescribing information for NORVIR® (ritonavir) when using this agent.

Important dosing information:

Efavirenz. In treatment-naive patients who receive efavirenz and REYATAZ, the recommended dose is REYATAZ 300 mg with ritonavir 100 mg and efavirenz 600 mg (all once daily). Dosing recommendations for efavirenz and REYATAZ in treatment-experienced patients have not been established.

Didanosine. When coadministered with didanosine buffered formulations, REYATAZ should be given (with food) 2 hours before or 1 hour after didanosine.

Tenofovir disoproxil fumarate. When coadministered with tenofovir, it is recommended that REYATAZ 300 mg be given with ritonavir 100 mg and tenofovir 300 mg (all as a single daily dose with food). **REYATAZ without ritonavir should not be coadministered with tenofovir.**

For these drugs and other antiretroviral agents for which dosing modification may be appropriate, see **CLINICAL PHARMACOLOGY: Drug-Drug Interactions** and **PRECAUTIONS**, Table 11.

Patients with Renal Impairment

There are insufficient data to recommend a dosage adjustment for patients with renal impairment (see **CLINICAL PHARMACOLOGY: Special Populations,** *Impaired Renal Function*).

Patients with Hepatic Impairment

REYATAZ should be used with caution in patients with mild to moderate hepatic impairment. For patients with moderate hepatic impairment (Child-Pugh Class B) who have not experienced prior virologic failure, a dose reduction to 300 mg once daily should be considered. REYATAZ should not be used in patients with severe hepatic impairment (Child-Pugh Class C). REYATAZ/ritonavir has not been studied in subjects with hepatic impairment and is not recommended. (See **PRECAUTIONS** and **CLINICAL PHARMACOLOGY: Special Populations,** *Impaired Hepatic Function.*)

HOW SUPPLIED

REYATAZ® (atazanavir sulfate) Capsules are available in the following strengths and configurations of plastic bottles with child-resistant closures.

[See table at top of next page]

REYATAZ (atazanavir sulfate) Capsules should be stored at 25°C (77°F); excursions permitted to 15–30°C (59–86°F) [see USP Controlled Room Temperature].

US Patent Nos: 5,849,911 and 6,087,383.

Bristol-Myers Squibb Company
Princeton, NJ 08543 USA

F1-B0001-07-04 Revised July 2004
based on 1168954A2

PATIENT INFORMATION ℞ ONLY

REYATAZ® (RAY-ah-taz)
(generic name = **atazanavir sulfate**) **Capsules**

ALERT: Find out about medicines that should NOT be taken with REYATAZ. Read the section "What important information should I know about taking REYATAZ with other medicines?"

Read the Patient Information that comes with REYATAZ before you start using it and each time you get a refill. There may be new information. This leaflet provides a summary about REYATAZ and does not include everything there is to know about your medicine. This information does not take the place of talking with your healthcare provider about your medical condition or treatment.

What is REYATAZ?

REYATAZ (atazanavir sulfate) is a prescription medicine used with other anti-HIV medicines to treat people who are infected with the human immunodeficiency virus (HIV). HIV is the virus that causes acquired immune deficiency syndrome (AIDS). REYATAZ is a type of anti-HIV medicine called a protease inhibitor. HIV infection destroys CD4+ (T) cells, which are important to the immune system. The immune system helps fight infection. After a large number of T

Continued on next page

Reyataz—Cont.

cells are destroyed, AIDS develops. REYATAZ helps to block HIV protease, an enzyme that is needed for the HIV virus to multiply. REYATAZ may lower the amount of HIV in your blood, help your body keep its supply of CD4+ (T) cells, and reduce the risk of death and illness associated with HIV.

Does REYATAZ cure HIV or AIDS?

REYATAZ does not cure HIV infection or AIDS. At present there is no cure for HIV infection. People taking REYATAZ may still get opportunistic infections or other conditions that happen with HIV infection. Opportunistic infections are infections that develop because the immune system is weak. Some of these conditions are pneumonia, herpes virus infections, and Mycobacterium avium complex (MAC) infections. **It is very important that you see your healthcare provider regularly while taking REYATAZ.**

REYATAZ does not lower your chance of passing HIV to other people through sexual contact, sharing needles, or being exposed to your blood. For your health and the health of others, it is important to always practice safer sex by using a latex or polyurethane condom or other barrier to lower the chance of sexual contact with semen, vaginal secretions, or blood. Never use or share dirty needles.

Who should not take REYATAZ?

Do not take REYATAZ if you:

- **are taking certain medicines.** (See "What important information should I know about taking REYATAZ with other medicines?") Serious life-threatening side effects or death may happen. Before you take REYATAZ, tell your healthcare provider about all medicines you are taking or planning to take. These include other prescription and nonprescription medicines, vitamins, and herbal supplements.
- **are allergic to REYATAZ or to any of its ingredients.** The active ingredient is atazanavir sulfate. See the end of this leaflet for a complete list of ingredients in REYATAZ. Tell your healthcare provider if you think you have had an allergic reaction to any of these ingredients.

What should I tell my healthcare provider before I take REYATAZ?

Tell your healthcare provider:

- **If you are pregnant or planning to become pregnant.** It is not known if REYATAZ can harm your unborn baby. Pregnant women have experienced serious side effects when taking REYATAZ with other HIV medicines called nucleoside analogues. You and your healthcare provider will need to decide if REYATAZ is right for you. If you use REYATAZ while you are pregnant, talk to your healthcare provider about the Antiretroviral Pregnancy Registry.
- **If you are breast-feeding.** You should not breast-feed if you are HIV-positive because of the chance of passing HIV to your baby. Also, it is not known if REYATAZ can pass into your breast milk and if it can harm your baby. If you are a woman who has or will have a baby, talk with your healthcare provider about the best way to feed your baby.
- **If you have liver problems or are infected with the hepatitis B or C virus.** See "What are the possible side effects of REYATAZ?"
- **If you have diabetes.** See "What are the possible side effects of REYATAZ?"
- **If you have hemophilia.** See "What are the possible side effects of REYATAZ?"
- **About all the medicines you take,** including prescription and nonprescription medicines, vitamins, and herbal supplements. Keep a list of your medicines with you to show your healthcare provider. For more information, see "What important information should I know about taking REYATAZ with other medicines?" and "Who should not take REYATAZ?" Some medicines can cause serious side effects if taken with REYATAZ (atazanavir sulfate).

How should I take REYATAZ?

- **Take REYATAZ once every day exactly as instructed by your healthcare provider.** Your healthcare provider will prescribe the amount of REYATAZ that is right for you.
  - For adults who have never taken anti-HIV medicines before, the usual does is 400 mg (two 200-mg capsules) once daily taken with food.
  - For adults who have taken anti-HIV medicines in the past, the usual dose is 300 mg (two 150-mg capsules) plus 100 mg of NORVIR® (ritonavir) once daily taken with food.

  Your dose will depend on your liver function and on the other anti-HIV medicines that you are taking. REYATAZ is always used with other anti-HIV medicines. If you are taking REYATAZ with SUSTIVA® (efavirenz) or with VIREAD® (tenofovir disoproxil fumarate), you should also be taking NORVIR® (ritonavir).
- **Always take REYATAZ with food** (a meal or snack) to help it work better. Swallow the capsules whole. **Do not open the capsules.** Take REYATAZ at the same time each day.
- **If you are taking antacids or VIDEX® (didanosine) Chewable/Dispersible Buffered Tablets,** take REYATAZ 2 hours before or 1 hour after these medicines.
- **Do not change your dose or stop taking REYATAZ without first talking with your healthcare provider.** It is important to stay under a healthcare provider's care while taking REYATAZ.
- **When your supply of REYATAZ starts to run low,** get more from your healthcare provider or pharmacy. It is important not to run out of REYATAZ. The amount of HIV in your blood may increase if the medicine is stopped for even a short time.

Product Strength*	Capsule Shell Color (cap/body)	Markings on Capsule (ink color)		Capsules per Bottle	NDC Number
		cap	body		
100 mg	blue/white	BMS 100 mg (white)	3623 (blue)	60	0003-3623-12
150 mg	blue/powder blue	BMS 150 mg (white)	3624 (blue)	60	0003-3624-12
200 mg	blue/blue	BMS 200 mg (white)	3631 (white)	60	0003-3631-12

*atazanavir equivalent as atazanavir sulfate.

- **If you miss a dose of REYATAZ,** take it as soon as possible and then take your next scheduled dose at its regular time. If, however, it is within 6 hours of your next dose, do not take the missed dose. Wait and take the next dose at the regular time. Do not double the next dose. **It is important that you do not miss any doses of REYATAZ or your other anti-HIV medicines.**
- **If you take more than the prescribed dose of REYATAZ,** call your healthcare provider or poison control center right away.

Can children take REYATAZ?

REYATAZ has not been fully studied in children under 16 years of age. REYATAZ should not be used in babies under the age of 3 months.

What are the possible side effects of REYATAZ?

The following list of side effects is **not** complete. Report any new or continuing symptoms to your healthcare provider. If you have questions about side effects, ask your healthcare provider. Your healthcare provider may be able to help you manage these side effects.

The following side effects have been reported with REYATAZ (atazanavir sulfate):

- **rash** (redness and itching) sometimes occurs in patients taking REYATAZ, most often in the first few weeks after the medicine is started. Rashes usually go away within 2 weeks with no change in treatment. Tell your healthcare provider if rash occurs.
- **yellowing of the skin or eyes.** These effects may be due to increases in bilirubin levels in the blood (bilirubin is made by the liver). Call your healthcare provider if your skin or the white part of your eyes turn yellow. Although these effects may not be damaging to your liver, skin, or eyes, it is important to tell your healthcare provider promptly if they occur.
- **a change in the way your heart beats (heart rhythm change).** Call your healthcare provider right away if you get dizzy or lightheaded. These could be symptoms of a heart problem.
- **diabetes and high blood sugar (hyperglycemia)** sometimes happen in patients taking protease inhibitor medicines like REYATAZ. Some patients had diabetes before taking protease inhibitors while others did not. Some patients may need changes in their diabetes medicine.
- **if you have liver disease** including hepatitis B or C, your liver disease may get worse when you take anti-HIV medicines like REYATAZ.
- **some patients with hemophilia** have increased bleeding problems with protease inhibitors like REYATAZ.
- **changes in body fat.** These changes may include an increased amount of fat in the upper back and neck ("buffalo hump"), breast, and around the trunk. Loss of fat from the legs, arms, and face may also happen. The cause and long-term health effects of these conditions are not known at this time.

Other common side effects of REYATAZ taken with other anti-HIV medicines include nausea; headache; stomach pain; vomiting; diarrhea; depression; fever; dizziness; trouble sleeping; numbness, tingling, or burning of hands or feet; and muscle pain.

What important information should I know about taking REYATAZ with other medicines*?

Do not take REYATAZ if you take the following medicines (not all brands may be listed; tell your healthcare provider about all the medicines you take). REYATAZ may cause serious, life-threatening side effects or death when used with these medicines.

- Ergot medicines: dihydroergotamine, ergonovine, ergotamine, and methylergonovine such as CAFERGOT®, MIGRANAL®, D.H.E. 45®, ergotrate maleate, METHERGINE®, and others (used for migraine headaches).
- HALCION® (triazolam, used for insomnia).
- VERSED® (midazolam, used for sedation).
- ORAP® (pimozide, used for Tourette's disorder).
- PROPULSID® (cisapride, used for certain stomach problems).

Do not take the following medicines with REYATAZ (atazanavir sulfate) because of possible serious side effects:

- CAMPTOSAR® (irinotecan, used for cancer).
- CRIXIVAN® (indinavir, used for HIV infection). Both REYATAZ and CRIXIVAN sometimes cause increased levels of bilirubin in the blood.
- Cholesterol-lowering medicines MEVACOR® (lovastatin) or ZOCOR® (simvastatin).

Do not take the following medicines with REYATAZ because they may lower the amount of REYATAZ in your blood. This may lead to an increased HIV viral load. Resistance to REYATAZ or cross-resistance to other HIV medicines may develop:

- Rifampin (also known as RIMACTANE®, RIFADIN®, RIFATER®, or RIFAMATE®, used for tuberculosis).
- St. John's wort (Hypericum perforatum), an herbal product sold as a dietary supplement, or products containing St. John's wort.
- "Proton-pump inhibitors" used for indigestion, heartburn, or ulcers such as AcipHex® (rabeprazole), NEXIUM® (esomeprazole), PREVACID® (lansoprazole), PRILOSEC® (omeprazole), or PROTONIX® (pantoprazole).

Do not take the following medicines if you are taking REYATAZ and NORVIR® together:

- VFEND® (voriconazole).

The following medicines may require your healthcare provider to monitor your therapy more closely:

- CIALIS® (tadalafil), LEVITRA® (vardenafil), or VIAGRA® (sildenafil). REYATAZ may increase the chances of serious side effects that can happen with CIALIS, LEVITRA, or VIAGRA. Do not use CIALIS, LEVITRA, or VIAGRA while you are taking REYATAZ unless your healthcare provider tells you it is okay.
- LIPITOR® (atorvastatin). There is an increased chance of serious side effects if you take REYATAZ with this cholesterol-lowering medicine.
- Medicines for abnormal heart rhythm: CORDARONE® (amiodarone), lidocaine, quinidine (also known as CARDIOQUIN®, QUINIDEX®, and others).
- VASCOR® (bedridil, used for chest pain).
- COUMADIN® (warfarin).
- Tricyclic antidepressants such as ELAVIL® (amitriptyline), NORPRAMIN® (desipramine), SINEQUAN® (doxepin), SURMONTIL® (trimipramine), TOFRANIL® (imipramine), or VIVACTIL® (protriptyline).
- Medicines to prevent organ transplant rejection: SANDIMMUNE® or NEORAL® (cyclosporine), RAPAMUNE® (sirolimus), or PROGRAF® (tacrolimus).

The following medicines may require a change in the dose or dose schedule of either REYATAZ or the other medicine:

- FORTOVASE®, INVIRASE® (saquinavir).
- NORVIR® (ritonavir).
- SUSTIVA® (efavirenz).
- VIDEX® (didanosine) or antacids.
- VIREAD® (tenofovir disoproxil fumarate).
- MYCOBUTIN® (rifabutin).
- Calcium channel blockers such as CARDIZEM® or TIAZAC® (diltiazem), COVERA-HS® or ISOPTIN SR® (verapamil) and others.
- BIAXIN® (clarithromycin).
- Medicines for indigestion, heartburn, or ulcers such as AXID® (nizatidine), PEPCID AC® (famotidine), TAGAMET® (cimetidine), or ZANTAC® (ranitidine).

Women who use birth control pills or "the patch" should choose a different kind of contraception. REYATAZ may affect the safety and effectiveness of birth control pills or the patch. Talk to your healthcare provider about choosing an effective contraceptive.

Remember:

1. **Know all the medicines you take.**
2. **Tell your healthcare provider about all the medicines you take.**
3. **Do not start a new medicine without talking to your healthcare provider.**

How should I store REYATAZ?

- Store REYATAZ (atazanavir sulfate) Capsules at room temperature, 59° to 86° F (15° to 30° C). Do **not** store this medicine in a damp place such as a bathroom medicine cabinet or near the kitchen sink.
- Keep your medicine in a tightly closed container.
- Throw away REYATAZ when it is outdated or no longer needed by flushing it down the toilet or pouring it down the sink.

General information about REYATAZ

This medicine was prescribed for your particular condition. Do not use REYATAZ for another condition. Do not give REYATAZ to other people, even if they have the same symptoms you have. It may harm them. **Keep REYATAZ and all medicines out of the reach of children and pets.**

This summary does not include everything there is to know about REYATAZ. Medicines are sometimes prescribed for conditions that are not mentioned in patient information leaflets. Remember, no written summary can replace careful discussion with your healthcare provider. If you would like more information, talk with your healthcare provider or you can call 1-800-426-7644.

What are the ingredients in REYATAZ?

Active Ingredient: atazanavir sulfate

Inactive Ingredients: Crospovidone, lactose monohydrate (milk sugar), magnesium stearate, gelatin, FD&C Blue #2, and titanium dioxide.

*VIDEX® is a registered trademark of Bristol-Myers Squibb Company. COUMADIN® and SUSTIVA® are registered trademarks of Bristol-Myers Squibb Pharma Company. Other brands listed are the trademarks of their respective owners and are not trademarks of Bristol-Myers Squibb Company.

Bristol-Myers Squibb Company
Princeton, NJ 08543 USA

This Patient Information Leaflet has been approved by the U.S. Food and Drug Administration.

F1-B0001-07-04

Based on package insert dated July 2004, 1168954A2

Revised July 2004

Shown in Product Identification Guide, page 310

SUSTIVA® ℞

[*sus-TEE-vah*]

(efavirenz) capsules and tablets

℞ Only

DESCRIPTION

SUSTIVA® (efavirenz) is a human immunodeficiency virus type 1 (HIV-1) specific, non-nucleoside, reverse transcriptase inhibitor (NNRTI).

Capsules: SUSTIVA is available as capsules for oral administration containing either 50 mg, 100 mg, or 200 mg of efavirenz and the following inactive ingredients: lactose monohydrate, magnesium stearate, sodium lauryl sulfate, and sodium starch glycolate. The capsule shell contains the following inactive ingredients and dyes: gelatin, sodium lauryl sulfate, titanium dioxide, and/or yellow iron oxide. The capsule shells may also contain silicon dioxide. The capsules are printed with ink containing carmine 40 blue, FD&C Blue No. 2, and titanium dioxide.

Tablets: SUSTIVA is available as film-coated tablets for oral administration containing 600 mg of efavirenz and the following inactive ingredients: croscarmellose sodium, hydroxypropyl cellulose, lactose monohydrate, magnesium stearate, microcrystalline cellulose, and sodium lauryl sulfate. The film coating contains Opadry® Yellow and Opadry® Clear. The tablets are polished with carnauba wax and printed with purple ink, Opacode® WB.

Efavirenz is chemically described as (S)-6-chloro-(cyclopropylethynyl)-1,4-dihydro-4-(trifluoromethyl)-2H-3,1-benzoxazin-2-one.

Its empirical formula is $C_{14}H_9ClF_3NO_2$ and its structural formula is:

Efavirenz is a white to slightly pink crystalline powder with a molecular mass of 315.68. It is practically insoluble in water (<10 μg/mL).

Opadry® and Opacode® are registered trademarks of BPSI.

MICROBIOLOGY

Mechanism of Action: Efavirenz is a non-nucleoside reverse transcriptase (RT) inhibitor of human immunodeficiency virus type 1 (HIV-1). Efavirenz activity is mediated predominantly by noncompetitive inhibition of HIV-1 RT. HIV-2 RT and human cellular DNA polymerases alpha, beta, gamma, and delta are not inhibited by efavirenz.

***In vitro* HIV Susceptibility:** The clinical significance of *in vitro* susceptibility of HIV-1 to efavirenz has not been established. The *in vitro* antiviral activity of efavirenz was assessed in lymphoblastoid cell lines, peripheral blood mononuclear cells (PBMCs), and macrophage/monocyte cultures. The 90–95% inhibitory concentration (IC_{90-95}) of efavirenz for wild-type laboratory adapted strains and clinical isolates ranged from 1.7 to 25 nM. Efavirenz demonstrated synergistic activity against HIV-1 in cell culture when combined with zidovudine (ZDV), didanosine, or indinavir (IDV).

Resistance: HIV-1 isolates with reduced susceptibility to efavirenz (>380-fold increase in IC_{90}) compared to baseline can emerge *in vitro*. Phenotypic (n=26) changes in evaluable HIV-1 isolates and genotypic (n=104) changes in plasma virus from selected patients treated with efavirenz in combination with IDV, or with ZDV plus lamivudine were monitored. One or more RT mutations at amino acid positions 98, 100, 101, 103, 106, 108, 188, 190, and 225, were observed in 102 of 104 patients with a frequency of at least 9% compared to baseline. The mutation at RT amino acid position 103 (lysine to asparagine) was the most frequently observed (≥90%). A mean loss in susceptibility (IC_{90}) to efavirenz of 47-fold was observed in 26 clinical isolates. Five clinical isolates were evaluated for both genotypic and phenotypic changes from baseline. Decreases in efavirenz susceptibility (range from 9 to >312-fold increase in IC_{90}) were observed for these isolates *in vitro* compared to baseline. All five isolates possessed at least one of the efavirenz-associated RT mutations. The clinical relevance of phenotypic and genotypic changes associated with efavirenz therapy is under evaluation.

Cross-Resistance: Rapid emergence of HIV-1 strains that are cross-resistant to non-nucleoside RT inhibitors has been observed *in vitro*. Thirteen clinical isolates previously characterized as efavirenz-resistant were also phenotypically resistant to nevirapine and delavirdine *in vitro* compared to baseline. Clinically derived ZDV-resistant HIV-1 isolates tested *in vitro* retained susceptibility to efavirenz. Cross-resistance between efavirenz and HIV protease inhibitors is unlikely because of the different enzyme targets involved.

Table 1: Effect of Efavirenz on Coadministered Drug Plasma C_{max} and AUC

Coadministered Drug	Dose	Efavirenz Dose	Number of Subjects	Coadministered Drug (% change) C_{max} (mean [90% CI])	Coadministered Drug (% change) AUC (mean [90% CI])
Indinavir	1000 mg q8h× 10 days	600 mg × 10 days	20		
After morning dose				↔[a]	↓ (33%)[a] [26–39%]
After afternoon dose				↔[a]	↓ (37%)[a] [(26–46%]
After evening dose				↓ (29%)[a] [11–43%]	↓ (46%)[a] [37–54%]
Lopinavir/ ritonavir	400/100 mg q12h × 9 days	600 mg × 9 days	11,7[b]	↔[c]	↓ (19%)[c] [↓ 36– ↑ 3%]
Nelfinavir	750 mg q8h× 7 days	600 mg × 7 days	10	↑ (21%) [10–33%]	↑ (20%) [8–34%]
Metabolite AG -1402				↓ (40%) [30–48%]	↓ (37%) [25–48%]
Ritonavir	500 mg q12h× 8 days	600 mg × 10 days	11		
	After AM dose			↑ (24%) [12–38%]	↑ (18%) [6–33%]
	After PM dose			↔	↔
Saquinavir SGC[d]	1200 mg q8h × 10 days	600 mg × 10 days	12	↓ (50%) [28–66%]	↓ (62%) [45–74%]
Lamivudine	150 mg q12h× 14 days	600 mg × 14 days	9	↔	↔
Zidovudine	300 mg q12h× 14 days	600 mg × 14 days	9	↔	↔
Azithromycin	600 mg single dose	400 mg × 7 days	14	↑ (22%) [4–42%]	↔
Clarithromycin	500 mg q12h× 7 days	400 mg × 7 days	11	↓ (26%) [15–35%]	↓ (39%) [30–46%]
14-OH metabolite				↑ (49%) [32–69%]	↑ (34%) [18–53%]
Fluconazole	200 mg × 7 days	400 mg × 7 days	10	↔	↔
Rifabutin	300 mg qd× 14 days	600 mg × 14 days	9	↓ (32%) [15–46%]	↓ (38%) [28–47%]
Cetirizine	10 mg single dose	600 mg × 10 days	11	↓ (24%) [18–30%]	↔
Ethinyl estradiol	50 μg single dose	400 mg × 10 days	13	↔	↑ (37%) [25–51%]
Lorazepam	2 mg single dose	600 mg × 10 days	12	↑ (16%) [2–32%]	↑ (7%) [1–14%]
Methadone	Stable maintenance 35–100 mg daily	600 mg × 14–21 days	11	↓ (45%) [25–59%]	↓ (52%) [33–66%]
Paroxetine	200 mg qd × 14 days	600 mg × 14 days	16	↔	↔
Sertraline	50 mg qd × 14 days	600 mg × 14 days	13	↓ (29%) [25–40%]	↓ (39%) [27–50%]

↑ Indicates increase
↓ Indicates decrease
↔ Indicates no change

[a] Comparator dose of indinavir was 800 mg q8h × 10 days. Mean decreases in the C_{min} of indinavir ranged from 39 to 57%.
[b] Parallel-group design; n for efavirenz + lopinavir/ritonavir, n for lopoinavir/ritonavir alone.
[c] C_{min} of lopinavir was significantly decreased by 39%. The pharmacokinetics of ritonavir 100 mg q12h are unaffected by concurrent efavirenz.
[d] Soft Gelatin Capsule.

CLINICAL PHARMACOLOGY

Pharmacokinetics

Absorption—Peak efavirenz plasma concentrations of 1.6–9.1 μM were attained by 5 hours following single oral doses of 100 mg to 1600 mg administered to uninfected volunteers. Dose-related increases in C_{max} and AUC were seen for doses up to 1600 mg; the increases were less than proportional suggesting diminished absorption at higher doses.

In HIV-infected patients at steady state mean C_{max}, mean C_{min}, and mean AUC were dose proportional following 200-mg, 400-mg, and 600-mg daily doses. Time-to-peak plasma concentrations were approximately 3–5 hours and steady state plasma concentrations were reached in 6–10 days. In 35 patients receiving SUSTIVA 600 mg once daily, steady-state C_{max} was 12.9 ± 3.7 μM (mean ± SD), steady state C_{min} was 5.6 ± 3.2 μM, and AUC was 184 ± 73 μM•h.

Effect of Food on Oral Absorption-

Capsules—Administration of a single 600-mg dose of efavirenz capsules with a high-fat/high-caloric meal (894 kcal, 54 g fat, 54% calories from fat) or a reduced-fat/normal-caloric meal (440 kcal, 2 g fat, 4% calories from fat) was associated with a mean increase of 22% and 17% in efavirenz AUC_∞ and a mean increase of 39% and 51% in efavirenz C_{max}, respectively, relative to the exposures achieved when given under fasted conditions. (See **DOSAGE AND ADMINISTRATION** and **PRECAUTIONS: Information for Patients.**)

Tablets—Administration of a single 600-mg efavirenz tablet with a high-fat/high-caloric meal (approximately 1000 kcal, 500–600 kcal from fat) was associated with a 28% increase in mean AUC_∞ of efavirenz and a 79% increase in mean

Continued on next page

Sustiva—Cont.

C_{max} of efavirenz relative to the exposures achieved under fasted conditions. (See **DOSAGE AND ADMINISTRATION** and **PRECAUTIONS: Information for Patients.**)

Distribution—Efavirenz is highly bound (approximately 99.5–99.75%) to human plasma proteins, predominantly albumin. In HIV-1 infected patients (n=9) who received SUSTIVA (efavirenz) 200 to 600 mg once daily for at least one month, cerebrospinal fluid concentrations ranged from 0.26 to 1.19% (mean 0.69%) of the corresponding plasma concentration. This proportion is approximately 3-fold higher than the non-protein-bound (free) fraction of efavirenz in plasma.

Metabolism—Studies in humans and *in vitro* studies using human liver microsomes have demonstrated that efavirenz is principally metabolized by the cytochrome P450 system to hydroxylated metabolites with subsequent glucuronidation of these hydroxylated metabolites. These metabolites are essentially inactive against HIV-1. The *in vitro* studies suggest that CYP3A4 and CYP2B6 are the major isozymes responsible for efavirenz metabolism.

Efavirenz has been shown to induce P450 enzymes, resulting in the induction of its own metabolism. Multiple doses of 200–400 mg per day for 10 days resulted in a lower than predicted extent of accumulation (22–42% lower) and a shorter terminal half-life of 40–55 hours (single dose half-life 52–76 hours).

Elimination—Efavirenz has a terminal half-life of 52–76 hours after single doses and 40–55 hours after multiple doses. A one-month mass balance/excretion study was conducted using 400 mg per day with a ^{14}C-labeled dose administered on Day 8. Approximately 14–34% of the radiolabel was recovered in the urine and 16–61% was recovered in the feces. Nearly all of the urinary excretion of the radiolabeled drug was in the form of metabolites. Efavirenz accounted for the majority of the total radioactivity measured in feces.

Special Populations:

Hepatic Impairment—The pharmacokinetics of efavirenz have not been adequately studied in patients with hepatic impairment (see **PRECAUTIONS: General**).

Renal Impairment—The pharmacokinetics of efavirenz have not been studied in patients with renal insufficiency; however, less than 1% of efavirenz is excreted unchanged in the urine, so the impact of renal impairment on efavirenz elimination should be minimal.

Gender and Race—The pharmacokinetics of efavirenz in patients appear to be similar between men and women and among the racial groups studied.

Geriatric—See **PRECAUTIONS: Geriatric Use.**

Pediatrics—See **PRECAUTIONS: Pediatric Use.**

Drug Interactions (see also **CONTRAINDICATIONS** and **PRECAUTIONS: Drug Interactions)** Efavirenz has been shown *in vivo* to cause hepatic enzyme induction, thus increasing the biotransformation of some drugs metabolized by CYP3A4. *In vitro* studies have shown that efavirenz inhibited P450 isozymes 2C9, 2C19, and 3A4 with K_i values (8.5–17 µM) in the range of observed efavirenz plasma concentrations. In *in vitro* studies, efavirenz did not inhibit CYP2E1 and inhibited CYP2D6 and CYP1A2 (K_i values 82–160 µM) only at concentrations well above those achieved clinically. The effects on CYP3A4 activity are expected to be similar between 200-mg, 400-mg, and 600-mg doses of efavirenz. Coadministration of efavirenz with drugs primarily metabolized by 2C9, 2C19, and 3A4 isozymes may result in altered plasma concentrations of the coadministered drug. Drugs which induce CYP3A4 activity would be expected to increase the clearance of efavirenz resulting in lowered plasma concentrations.

Drug interaction studies were performed with efavirenz and other drugs likely to be coadministered or drugs commonly used as probes for pharmacokinetic interaction. The effects of coadministration of efavirenz on the AUC and C_{max} are summarized in Table 1 (effect of efavirenz on other drugs) and Table 2 (effect of other drugs on efavirenz). For information regarding clinical recommendations see **PRECAUTIONS: Drug Interactions.**

[See table 1 at top of previous page]

[See table 2 below]

Table 2: Effect of Coadministered Drug on Efavirenz Plasma C_{max} and AUC

Coadministered Drug	Dose	Efavirenz Dose	Number of Subjects	Efavirenz (% change) C_{max} (mean [90% CI])	Efavirenz (% change) AUC (mean [90% CI])
Indinavir	800 mg q8h× 14 days	200 mg × 14 days	11	↔	↔
Lopinavir/ ritonavir	400/100 mg q12h × 9 days	600 mg × 9 days	11,12[a]	↔	↓(16%) [↓38–↑15%]
Nelfinavir	750 mg q8h× 7 days	600 mg × 7 days	10	↔	↔
Ritonavir	500 mg q12h× 8 days	600 mg × 10 days	9	↑ (14%) [4–26%]	↑ (21%) [10–34%]
Saquinavir SGC[b]	1200 mg q8h × 10 days	600 mg × 10 days	13	↓ (13%) [5–20%]	↓ (12%) [4–19%]
Azithromycin	600 mg single dose	400 mg × 7 days	14	↔	↔
Clarithromycin	500 mg q12h× 7 days	400 mg × 7 days	12	↑ (11%) [3–19%]	↔
Fluconazole	200 mg × 7 days	400 mg × 7 days	10	↔	↑ (16%) [6–26%]
Rifabutin	300 mg qd× 14 days	600 mg × 14 days	11	↔	↔
Rifampin	600 mg × 7 days	600 mg × 7 days	12	↓ (20%) [11–28%]	↓ (26%) [15–36%]
Aluminum hydroxide 400 mg, magnesium hydroxide 400 mg, plus simethicone 40 mg	30 mL single dose	400 mg single dose	17	↔	↔
Cetirizine	10 mg single dose	600 mg × 10 days	11	↔	↓(8%) [4–11%]
Ethinyl estradiol	50 µg single dose	400 mg × 10 days	13	↔	↔
Famotidine	40 mg single dose	400 mg single dose	17	↔	↔
Paroxetine	20 mg qd× 14 days	600 mg × 14 days	17	↔	↔
Sertraline	50 mg qd× 14 days	600 mg × 14 days	13	↑(11%) [6–16%]	↔

↑ Indicates increase
↓ Indicates decrease
↔ Indicates no change
[a]Parallel-group design; n for efavirenz + lopinavir/ritonavir, n for efavirenz alone.
[b]Soft Gelatin Capsule.

INDICATIONS AND USAGE

SUSTIVA (efavirenz) in combination with other antiretroviral agents is indicated for the treatment of HIV-1 infection. This indication is based on two clinical trials of at least one year duration that demonstrated prolonged suppression of HIV RNA.

Description of Studies: In the two principal studies described as follows (Study 006 and ACTG 364), the response was measured as the time to treatment failure (TTF). Plasma HIV-RNA levels were quantified using the AMPLICOR HIV-1 MONITOR® (assay limit 400 copies/mL in Study 006 and 500 copies/mL in ACTG 364).

Study 006, an ongoing, randomized, open-label trial, compares SUSTIVA (600 mg once daily) + indinavir (IDV, 1000 mg q8h) or SUSTIVA (600 mg once daily) + zidovudine (ZDV, 300 mg q12h) + lamivudine (LAM, 150 mg q12h) with indinavir (800 mg q8h) + zidovudine (300 mg q12h) + lamivudine (150 mg q12h). Twelve hundred sixty-six patients (mean age 36.5 years [range 18–81], 60% Caucasian, 83% male) were enrolled. All patients were efavirenz-, lamivudine-, NNRTI-, and PI-naive at study entry. The mean baseline CD4 cell count was 341 cells/mm^3 and the mean baseline HIV-RNA level was 60,250 copies/mL. There was no significant difference in mean CD4 cell count among the treatment groups; the overall mean increase was approximately 200 cells at 48 weeks among patients who continued on study regimens. Treatment response and outcomes through 48 weeks are shown in Figure 1 and Table 3, respectively.

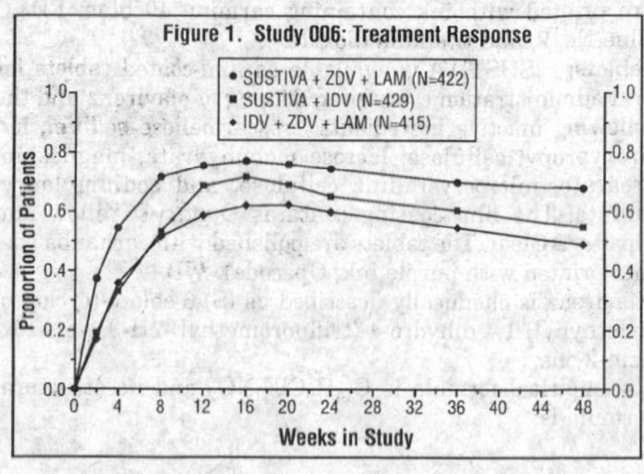

Figure 1. Study 006: Treatment Response

• Proportion of patients at each time point who have HIV RNA <400 copies, who are on their original study medication, and who have not experienced an AIDS-defining event.

[See table 3 at top of next page]

In addition to the complete 48-week follow-up data reported above, longer-term data are shown in Figure 2. This analysis allows for the inclusion of data beyond 48 weeks as Kaplan-Meier estimates by accounting for patients who have not reached 112 weeks of follow-up.

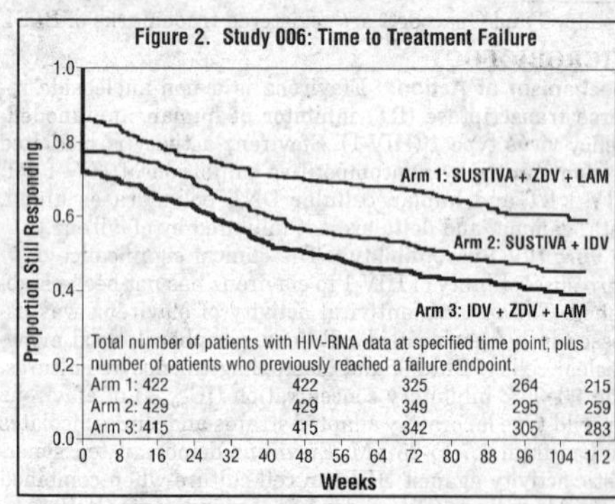

Figure 2. Study 006: Time to Treatment Failure

• Subjects were considered to have reached the study endpoint at the first time they either experienced virologic rebound (two HIV RNA values ≥400 copies), had an AIDS-defining clinical event, or discontinued study medication.
• Subjects who did not respond to initial treatment (no HIV RNA values <400 copies) were considered to have reached this endpoint at time zero.

ACTG 364 is a randomized, double-blind, placebo-controlled 48-week study in NRTI-experienced patients who had completed two prior ACTG studies. One hundred ninety-six patients (mean age 41 years [range 18–76], 74% Caucasian, 88% male) received NRTIs in combination with SUSTIVA (efavirenz) (600 mg once daily), or nelfinavir (NFV, 750 mg TID), or SUSTIVA (600 mg once daily) + nelfinavir in a randomized, double-blinded manner. The mean baseline CD4 cell count was 389 cells/mm^3 and mean baseline HIV RNA level was 8130 copies/mL. Upon entry into the study, all patients were assigned a new open-label NRTI regimen, which was dependent on their previous NRTI treatment experience. There was no significant difference in the mean CD4 cell count among treatment groups; the overall mean increase was approximately 100 cells at 48 weeks among patients who continued on study regimens. Treatment response and outcomes are shown in Figure 3 and Table 4, respectively.

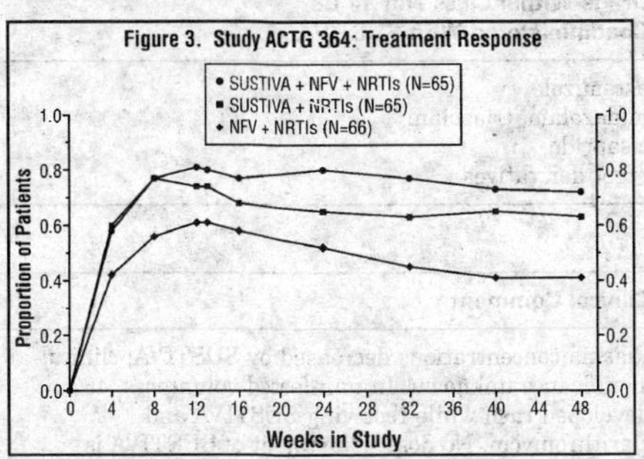

- Proportion of patients at each time point who have HIV RNA <500 copies confirmed by two consecutive observations and are on their original study medication and who have not experienced an AIDS-defining event.

[See table 4 above]

In addition to the complete 48-week data reported above, longer-term data are shown in Figure 4. This analysis allows for the inclusion of data beyond 48 weeks as Kaplan-Meier estimates by accounting for patients who have not reached 72 weeks of follow-up.

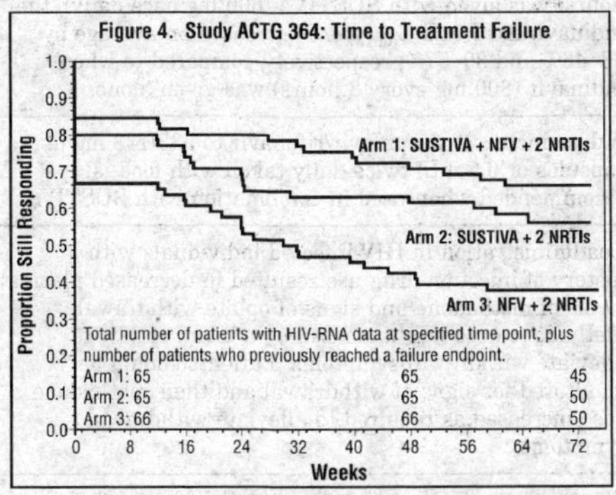

- Subjects were considered to have reached the study endpoint at the first time they either experienced virologic rebound (two HIV RNA values ≥500 copies), had an AIDS-defining clinical event, or discontinued study medication.
- Subjects who did not respond to initial treatment (no HIV RNA values ≤500 copies) were considered to have reached this endpoint at time zero.
- The initial plateaus through Week 12 are due to the virologic testing schedule and the lack of dropouts during this interval.

AMPLICOR HIV-1 MONITOR® is a registered trademark of a member of the Roche Group

Table 3: Study 006 - Outcomes of Randomized Treatment Through 48 Weeks

Outcome	SUSTIVA+ ZDV+LAM n=422	SUSTIVA+ IDV n=429	IDV+ ZDV+LAM n=415
HIV RNA <400 copies/mL (<50[a] copies/mL)	68% (62%)	55% (49%)	49% (43%)
HIV RNA ≥400 copies/mL[b]	6%	14%	11%
CDC Category C event[b]	3%	2%	2%
Discontinuations for adverse events[b,c]	8%	8%	17%
Discontinuations for other reasons[b,d]	15%	22%	21%

[a] Ultrasensitive HIV-1 MONITOR assay.
[b] These rates reflect events that were counted as the initial reason for treatment failure in the analysis.
[c] See **ADVERSE REACTIONS** for a description of the safety profile of these regimens.
[d] Consent withdrawn, lost to follow-up, missing data or protocol violation.

Table 4: Study ACTG 364 - Outcomes of Randomized Treatment Through 48 Weeks*

Outcome	SUSTIVA+ NFV+NRTIs n=65	SUSTIVA+ NRTIs n=65	NFV+ NRTIs n=66
HIV RNA <500 copies/mL[a]	71%	63%	41%
HIV RNA ≥500 copies/mL[b]	17%	34%	54%
CDC Category C Event	2%	0%	0%
Discontinuations for adverse events[c]	3%	3%	5%
Discontinuations for other reasons[d]	8%	0%	0%

* For some patients, Week 56 data were used to confirm the status at Week 48.
[a] Subjects achieved virologic response (two consecutive viral loads <500 copies/mL) and maintained it through Week 48.
[b] Includes viral rebound and failure to achieve confirmed <500 copies/mL by Week 48.
[c] See **ADVERSE REACTIONS** for a safety profile of these regimens.
[d] Includes loss to follow-up, consent withdrawn, non-compliance.

CONTRAINDICATIONS

SUSTIVA (efavirenz) is contraindicated in patients with clinically significant hypersensitivity to any of its components.

SUSTIVA should not be administered concurrently with astemizole, cisapride, midazolam, triazolam, or ergot derivatives because competition for CYP3A4 by efavirenz could result in inhibition of metabolism of these drugs and create the potential for serious and/or life-threatening adverse events (eg, cardiac arrhythmias, prolonged sedation, or respiratory depression).

WARNINGS

ALERT: Find out about medicines that should NOT be taken with SUSTIVA. This statement is also included on the product's bottle labels. (See **CONTRAINDICATIONS** and **PRECAUTIONS: Drug Interactions.**)

SUSTIVA must not be used as a single agent to treat HIV or added on as a sole agent to a failing regimen. As with all other non-nucleoside reverse transcriptase inhibitors, resistant virus emerges rapidly when efavirenz is administered as monotherapy. The choice of new antiretroviral agents to be used in combination with efavirenz should take into consideration the potential for viral cross-resistance.

Psychiatric Symptoms: Serious psychiatric adverse experiences have been reported in patients treated with SUSTIVA. In controlled trials of 1008 patients treated with regimens containing SUSTIVA for an average of 1.6 years and 635 patients treated with control regimens for an average of 1.3 years, the frequency of specific serious psychiatric events among patients who received SUSTIVA or control regimens, respectively, were: severe depression (1.6%, 0.6%), suicidal ideation (0.6%, 0.3%), nonfatal suicide attempts (0.4%, 0%), aggressive behavior (0.4%, 0.3%), paranoid reactions (0.4%, 0.3%), and manic reactions (0.1%, 0%). Patients with a history of psychiatric disorders appear to be at greater risk of these serious psychiatric adverse experiences, with the frequency of each of the above events ranging from 0.3% for manic reactions to 2.0% for both severe depression and suicidal ideation. There have also been occasional post-marketing reports of death by suicide, delusions, and psychosis-like behavior, although a causal relationship to the use of SUSTIVA cannot be determined from these reports. Patients with serious psychiatric adverse experiences should seek immediate medical evaluation to assess the possibility that the symptoms may be related to the use of SUSTIVA, and if so, to determine whether the risks of continued therapy outweigh the benefits (see **ADVERSE REACTIONS**).

Nervous System Symptoms: Fifty-three percent of patients receiving SUSTIVA in controlled trials reported central nervous system symptoms compared to 25% of patients receiving control regimens. These symptoms included, but were not limited to, dizziness (28.1%), insomnia (16.3%), impaired concentration (8.3%), somnolence (7.0%), abnormal dreams (6.2%), and hallucinations (1.2%). These symptoms were severe in 2.0% of patients, and 2.1% of patients discontinued therapy as a result. These symptoms usually begin during the first or second day of therapy and generally resolve after the first 2–4 weeks of therapy. After 4 weeks of therapy, the prevalence of nervous system symptoms of at least moderate severity ranged from 5% to 9% in patients treated with regimens containing SUSTIVA and from 3% to 5% in patients treated with a control regimen. Patients should be informed that these common symptoms were likely to improve with continued therapy and were not predictive of subsequent onset of the less frequent psychiatric symptoms (see **WARNINGS: Psychiatric Symptoms**). Dosing at bedtime may improve the tolerability of these nervous system symptoms (see **ADVERSE REACTIONS** and **DOSAGE AND ADMINISTRATION**).

Patients receiving SUSTIVA should be alerted to the potential for additive central nervous system effects when SUSTIVA is used concomitantly with alcohol or psychoactive drugs.

Patients who experience central nervous system symptoms such as dizziness, impaired concentration, and/or drowsiness should avoid potentially hazardous tasks such as driving or operating machinery.

Drug Interactions: Concomitant use of SUSTIVA and St. John's wort (*Hypericum perforatum*) or St. John's wort-containing products is not recommended. Coadministration of non-nucleoside reverse transcriptase inhibitors (NNRTIs), including SUSTIVA, with St. John's wort is expected to substantially decrease NNRTI concentrations and may result in suboptimal levels of efavirenz and lead to loss of virologic response and possible resistance to efavirenz or to the class of NNRTIs.

Reproductive Risk Potential: Malformations have been observed in fetuses from efavirenz-treated monkeys that received doses which resulted in plasma drug concentrations similar to those in humans given 600 mg/day (see **PRECAUTIONS: Pregnancy**); therefore, pregnancy should be avoided in women receiving SUSTIVA. Barrier contraception should always be used in combination with other methods of contraception (eg, oral or other hormonal contraceptives). Women of childbearing potential should undergo pregnancy testing prior to initiation of SUSTIVA.

PRECAUTIONS

General:

Skin Rash—In controlled clinical trials, 26% (266/1008) of patients treated with 600 mg SUSTIVA experienced new-onset skin rash compared with 17% (111/635) of patients treated in control groups. Rash associated with blistering, moist desquamation, or ulceration occurred in 0.9% (9/1008) of patients treated with SUSTIVA. The incidence of Grade 4 rash (eg, erythema multiforme, Stevens-Johnson syndrome) in patients treated with SUSTIVA in all studies and expanded access was 0.1%. The median time to onset of rash in adults was 11 days and the median duration, 16 days. The discontinuation rate for rash in clinical trials was 1.7% (17/1008). SUSTIVA should be discontinued in patients developing severe rash associated with blistering, desquamation, mucosal involvement, or fever. Appropriate antihistamines and/or corticosteroids may improve the tolerability and hasten the resolution of rash.

Rash was reported in 26 of 57 pediatric patients (46%) treated with SUSTIVA capsules. One pediatric patient experienced Grade 3 rash (confluent rash with fever), and two patients had Grade 4 rash (erythema multiforme). The median time to onset of rash in pediatric patients was 8 days. Prophylaxis with appropriate antihistamines prior to initiating therapy with SUSTIVA in pediatric patients should be considered (see **ADVERSE REACTIONS**).

Liver Enzymes—In patients with known or suspected history of hepatitis B or C infection and in patients treated with other medications associated with liver toxicity, monitoring of liver enzymes is recommended. In patients with persistent elevations of serum transaminases to greater than five times the upper limit of the normal range, the benefit of continued therapy with SUSTIVA needs to be weighed against the unknown risks of significant liver toxicity (see **ADVERSE REACTIONS: Laboratory Abnormalities**).

Because of the extensive cytochrome P450-mediated metabolism of efavirenz and limited clinical experience in patients with hepatic impairment, caution should be exercised in administering SUSTIVA to these patients.

Convulsions—Convulsions have been observed infrequently in patients receiving efavirenz, generally in the presence of known medical history of seizures. Patients who are receiving concomitant anticonvulsant medications primarily metabolized by the liver, such as phenytoin, carbamazepine, and phenobarbital, may require periodic monitoring of plasma levels. Caution must be taken in any patient with a history of seizures.

Animal Toxicology—Nonsustained convulsions were observed in 6 of 20 monkeys receiving efavirenz at doses yielding plasma AUC values 4- to 13- fold greater than those in humans given the recommended dose.

Cholesterol—Monitoring of cholesterol and triglycerides should be considered in patients treated with SUSTIVA (see **ADVERSE REACTIONS**).

Fat Redistribution—Redistribution/accumulation of body fat including central obesity, dorsocervical fat enlargement (buffalo hump), peripheral wasting, facial wasting, breast enlargement, and "cushingoid appearance" have been observed in patients receiving antiretroviral therapy. The mechanism and long-term consequences of these events are currently unknown. A causal relationship has not been established.

Information for Patients: A statement to patients and healthcare providers is included on the product's bottle la-

Continued on next page

Sustiva—Cont.

bels: **ALERT: Find out about medicines that should NOT be taken with SUSTIVA (efavirenz).** A Patient Package Insert (PPI) for SUSTIVA is available for patient information.

Patients should be informed that SUSTIVA is not a cure for HIV infection and that they may continue to develop opportunistic infections and other complications associated with HIV disease. Patients should be told that there are currently no data demonstrating that SUSTIVA therapy can reduce the risk of transmitting HIV to others through sexual contact or blood contamination.

Patients should be advised to take SUSTIVA every day as prescribed. SUSTIVA must always be used in combination with other antiretroviral drugs. Patients should be advised to take SUSTIVA on an empty stomach, preferably at bedtime. Taking SUSTIVA with food increases efavirenz concentrations and may increase the frequency of adverse events. Dosing at bedtime may improve the tolerability of nervous system symptoms (see **ADVERSE REACTIONS** and **DOSAGE AND ADMINISTRATION**). Patients should remain under the care of a physician while taking SUSTIVA.

Patients should be informed that central nervous system symptoms including dizziness, insomnia, impaired concentration, drowsiness, and abnormal dreams are commonly reported during the first weeks of therapy with SUSTIVA. Dosing at bedtime may improve the tolerability of these symptoms, and these symptoms are likely to improve with continued therapy. Patients should be alerted to the potential for additive central nervous system effects when SUSTIVA is used concomitantly with alcohol or psychoactive drugs. Patients should be instructed that if they experience these symptoms they should avoid potentially hazardous tasks such as driving or operating machinery (see **WARNINGS: Nervous System Symptoms**). In clinical trials, patients who develop central nervous system symptoms were not more likely to subsequently develop psychiatric symptoms (see **WARNINGS: Psychiatric Symptoms**).

Patients should also be informed that serious psychiatric symptoms including severe depression, suicide attempts, aggressive behavior, delusions, paranoia, and psychosis-like symptoms have also been infrequently reported in patients receiving SUSTIVA. Patients should be informed that if they experience severe psychiatric adverse experiences they should seek immediate medical evaluation to assess the possibility that the symptoms may be related to the use of SUSTIVA, and if so, to determine whether discontinuation of SUSTIVA may be required. Patients should also inform their physician of any history of mental illness or substance abuse (see **WARNINGS: Psychiatric Symptoms**).

Patients should be informed that another common side effect is rash. These rashes usually go away without any change in treatment. In a small number of patients, rash may be serious. Patients should be advised that they should contact their physician promptly if they develop a rash.

Because malformations have been observed in fetuses from efavirenz-treated animals, instructions should be given to avoid pregnancy in women receiving SUSTIVA (efavirenz). Women should be advised to notify their physician if they become pregnant while taking SUSTIVA. A reliable form of barrier contraception should always be used in combination with other methods of contraception, including oral or other hormonal contraception, because the effects of efavirenz on hormonal contraceptives are not fully characterized.

SUSTIVA may interact with some drugs; therefore, patients should be advised to report to their doctor the use of any other prescription, nonprescription medication, or herbal products, particularly St. John's wort.

Patients should be informed that redistribution or accumulation of body fat may occur in patients receiving antiretroviral therapy and that the cause and long-term health effects of these conditions are not known at this time.

Drug Interactions (see also **CONTRAINDICATIONS** and **CLINICAL PHARMACOLOGY: Drug Interactions**)

Efavirenz has been shown *in vivo* to induce CYP3A4. Other compounds that are substrates of CYP3A4 may have decreased plasma concentrations when coadministered with SUSTIVA. *In vitro* studies have demonstrated that efavirenz inhibits 2C9, 2C19, and 3A4 isozymes in the range of observed efavirenz plasma concentrations. Coadministration of efavirenz with drugs primarily metabolized by these isozymes may result in altered plasma concentrations of the coadministered drug. Therefore, appropriate dose adjustments may be necessary for these drugs.

Drugs which induce CYP3A4 activity (eg, phenobarbital, rifampin, rifabutin) would be expected to increase the clearance of efavirenz resulting in lowered plasma concentrations. Drug interactions with SUSTIVA are summarized in Table 5.

[See table 5 at right]

Other Drugs—Based on the results of drug interaction studies (see Tables 1 and 2), no dosage adjustment is recommended when SUSTIVA (efavirenz) is given with the following: aluminum/magnesium hydroxide antacids, azithromycin, cetirizine, famotidine, fluconazole, lamivudine, lorazepam, nelfinavir, paroxetine, and zidovudine.

Specific drug interaction studies have not been performed with SUSTIVA and NRTIs other than lamivudine and zidovudine. Clinically significant interactions would not be expected since the NRTIs are metabolized via a different route than efavirenz and would be unlikely to compete for the same metabolic enzymes and elimination pathways.

Table 5[a]: Drugs That Should Not Be Coadministered With SUSTIVA

Drug Class	Drugs Within Class Not To Be Coadministered With SUSTIVA
Antihistamines	astemizole
Benzodiazepines	midazolam, triazolam
GI Motility Agents	cisapride
Anti-Migraine	ergot derivatives

Established Drug Interactions

Drug Name	Effect	Clinical Comment
Clarithromycin	↓ clarithromycin concentration ↑ 14-OH metabolite concentration	Plasma concentrations decreased by SUSTIVA; clinical significance unknown. In uninfected volunteers, 46% developed rash while receiving SUSTIVA and clarithromycin. No dose adjustment of SUSTIVA is recommended when given with clarithromycin. Alternatives to clarithromycin, such as azithromycin, should be considered (see **Other Drugs**, following table). Other macrolide antibiotics, such as erythromycin, have not been studied in combination with SUSTIVA.
Indinavir	↓ indinavir concentration	The optimal dose of indinavir, when given in combination with SUSTIVA, is not known. Increasing the indinavir dose to 1000 mg every 8 hours does not compensate for the increased indinavir metabolism due to SUSTIVA. When indinavir at an increased dose (1000 mg every 8 hours) was given with SUSTIVA (600 mg once daily), the indinavir AUC and C_{min} were decreased on average by 33–46% and 39–57%, respectively, compared to when indinavir (800 mg every 8 hours) was given alone.
Lopinavir/ritonavir	↓ lopinavir concentration	A dose increase of lopinavir/ritonavir to 533/133 mg (4 capsules or 6.5 mL) twice daily taken with food is recommended when used in combination with SUSTIVA.
Methadone	↓ methadone concentration	Coadministration in HIV-infected individuals with a history of injection drug use resulted in decreased plasma levels of methadone and signs of opiate withdrawal. Methadone dose was increased by a mean of 22% to alleviate withdrawal symptoms. Patients should be monitored for signs of withdrawal and their methadone dose increased as required to alleviate withdrawal symptoms.
Ethinyl estradiol	↑ ethinyl estradiol concentration	Plasma concentrations increased by SUSTIVA (efavirenz); clinical significance unknown. Because the potential interaction of efavirenz with oral contraceptives has not been fully characterized, a reliable method of barrier contraception should be used in addition to oral contraceptives.
Rifabutin	↓ rifabutin concentration	Increase daily dose of rifabutin by 50%. Consider doubling the rifabutin dose in regimens where rifabutin is given 2 or 3 times a week.
Rifampin	↓ efavirenz concentration	Clinical significance of reduced efavirenz concentrations unknown.
Ritonavir	↑ ritonavir concentration ↑ efavirenz concentration	Combination was associated with a higher frequency of adverse clinical experiences (eg, dizziness, nausea, paresthesia) and laboratory abnormalities (elevated liver enzymes). Monitoring of liver enzymes is recommended when SUSTIVA is used in combination with ritonavir.
Saquinavir	↓ saquinavir concentration	Should not be used as sole protease inhibitor in combination with SUSTIVA (efavirenz).
Sertraline	↓ sertraline concentration	Increases in sertraline dose should be guided by clinical response.

Other Potentially Clinically Significant Drug or Herbal Product Interactions With SUSTIVA[b]

Drug	Clinical Comment
Anticoagulants: Warfarin	Plasma concentrations and effects potentially increased or decreased by SUSTIVA.
Anticonvulsants: Phenytoin Phenobarbital Carbamazepine	Potential for reduction in anticonvulsant and/or efavirenz plasma levels; periodic monitoring of anticonvulsant plasma levels should be conducted.
Antifungals: Itraconazole Ketoconazole	Drug interaction studies with SUSTIVA and these imidazole and triazole antifungals have not been conducted. SUSTIVA has the potential to decrease plasma concentrations of itraconazole and ketoconazole.
Anti-HIV protease inhibitors: Saquinavir/ritonavir combination	No pharmacokinetic data are available.
Amprenavir	SUSTIVA has the potential to decrease serum concentrations of amprenavir.
Non-nucleoside reverse transcriptase inhibitors	No studies have been performed with other NNRTIs.
St. John's wort *(hypericum perforatum)*	Expected to substantially decrease plasma levels of efavirenz; has not been studied in combination with SUSTIVA.

[a] See Tables 1 and 2.
[b] This table is not all-inclusive.

Carcinogenesis, Mutagenesis, and Impairment of Fertility

Long-term carcinogenicity studies in mice and rats were carried out with efavirenz. Mice were dosed with 0, 25, 75, 150, or 300 mg/kg/day for 2 years. Incidences of hepatocellular adenomas and carcinomas and pulmonary alveolar/bronchiolar adenomas were increased above background in females. No increases in tumor incidence above background were seen in males. In studies in which rats were administered efavirenz at doses of 0, 25, 50, or 100 mg/kg/day for 2 years, no increases in tumor incidence above background were observed. The systemic exposure (based on AUCs) in mice was approximately 1.7-fold that in humans receiving the 600-mg/day dose. The exposure in rats was lower than that in humans. The mechanism of the carcinogenic potential is unknown. However, in genetic toxicology assays, efavirenz showed no evidence of mutagenic or clastogenic activity in a battery of *in vitro* and *in vivo* studies. These included bacterial mutation assays in *S. typhimurium* and *E. coli*, mammalian mutation assays in Chinese hamster ovary cells, chromosome aberration assays in human peripheral blood lymphocytes or Chinese hamster ovary cells, and an *in vivo* mouse bone marrow micronucleus assay. Given the lack of genotoxic activity of efavirenz, the relevance to humans of neoplasms in efavirenz-treated mice is not known.

Efavirenz did not impair mating or fertility of male or female rats, and did not affect sperm of treated male rats. The reproductive performance of offspring born to female rats given efavirenz was not affected. As a result of the rapid clearance of efavirenz in rats, systemic drug exposures achieved in these studies were equivalent to or below those achieved in humans given therapetuic doses of efavirenz.

Pregnancy:

Pregnancy "Category C"—Pregnancy should be avoided in women receiving SUSTIVA. Barrier contraception should always be used in combination with other methods of contraception (eg, oral or other hormonal contraceptives). Women of childbearing potential should undergo pregnancy testing prior to initiation of SUSTIVA (see **WARNINGS: Reproductive Risk Potential**).

Antiretroviral Pregnancy Registry: To monitor fetal outcomes of pregnant women exposed to SUSTIVA, an Antiretroviral Pregnancy Registry has been established. Physicians are encouraged to register patients by calling (800) 258-4263.

There are no adequate and well-controlled studies in pregnant women. SUSTIVA should be used during pregnancy only if the potential benefit justifies the potential risk to the fetus, such as in pregnant women without other therapeutic options. As of July 2003, the Antiretroviral Pregnancy Registry has received reports of 165 pregnancies exposed to efavirenz-containing regimens, the majority of which were first-trimester exposures (160 pregnancies). Birth defects occurred in 4 of 142 live births (first-trimester exposure) and 0 of 11 live births (second-/third-trimester exposure). In addition, there has been one report of multiple defects including abnormalities consistent with Dandy-Walker syndrome in a fetus from a spontaneous abortion, one report of neural tube defect in a fetus from a pregnancy electively terminated in the second trimester, and one report of meningomyelocele in an infant. All three mothers were exposed to efavirenz-containing regimens in the first trimester. A causal relationship of these events to the use of SUSTIVA (efavirenz) cannot be established.

Malformations have been observed in 3 of 20 fetuses/infants from efavirenz-treated cynomolgus monkeys (versus 0 of 20 concomitant controls) in a developmental toxicity study. The pregnant monkeys were dosed throughout pregnancy (postcoital days 20–150) with efavirenz 60 mg/kg daily, a dose which resulted in plasma drug concentrations similar to those in humans given 600 mg/day of SUSTIVA. Anencephaly and unilateral anophthalmia were observed in one fetus, microophthalmia was observed in another fetus, and cleft palate was observed in a third fetus. Efavirenz crosses the placenta in cynomolgus monkeys and produces fetal blood concentrations similar to maternal blood concentrations. Efavirenz has been shown to cross the placenta in rats and rabbits and produces fetal blood concentrations of efavirenz similar to maternal concentrations. An increase in fetal resorptions was observed in rats at efavirenz doses that produced peak plasma concentrations and AUC values in female rats equivalent to or lower than those achieved in humans given 600 mg once daily of SUSTIVA. Efavirenz produced no reproductive toxicities when given to pregnant rabbits at doses that produced peak plasma concentrations similar to and AUC values approximately half of those achieved in humans given 600 mg once daily of SUSTIVA.

Nursing Mothers: The Centers for Disease Control and Prevention recommend that HIV-infected mothers not breast-feed their infants to avoid risking postnatal transmission of HIV. Although it is not known if efavirenz is secreted in human milk, efavirenz is secreted into the milk of lactating rats. Because of the potential for HIV transmission and the potential for serious adverse effects in nursing infants, **mothers should be instructed not to breast-feed if they are receiving SUSTIVA.**

Pediatric Use: ACTG 382 is an ongoing, open-label study in 57 NRTI-experienced pediatric patients to characterize the safety, pharmacokinetics, and antiviral activity of SUSTIVA in combination with nelfinavir (20–30 mg/kg TID) and NRTIs. Mean age was 8 years (range 3–16). SUSTIVA has not been studied in pediatric patients below 3 years of age or who weigh less than 13 kg. At 48 weeks, the type and frequency of adverse experiences was generally similar to that of adult patients with the exception of a higher incidence of rash, which was reported in 46% (26/57) of pediatric patients compared to 26% of adults, and a higher frequency of Grade 3 or 4 rash reported in 5% (3/57) of

Table 6: Percent of Patients with One or More Selected Nervous System Symptoms[a,b]

Percent of Patients with:	SUSTIVA 600 mg Once Daily (n=1008) %	Control Groups (n=635) %
Symptoms of any severity	52.7	24.6
Mild symptoms[c]	33.3	15.6
Moderate symptoms[d]	17.4	7.7
Severe symptoms[e]	2.0	1.3
Treatment discontinuation as a result of symptoms	2.1	1.1

[a] Includes events reported regardless of causality.
[b] Data from Study 006 and three Phase 2/3 studies.
[c] "Mild" = Symptoms which do not interfere with patient's daily activities.
[d] "Moderate" = Symptoms which may interfere with daily activities.
[e] "Severe" = Events which interrupt patient's usual daily activities.

Table 7: Percent of Patients with Treatment-Emergent Rash[a,b]

Percent of Patients with:	Description of Rash Grade[c]	SUSTIVA 600 mg Once Daily Adults (n=1008) %	SUSTIVA Pediatric Patients (n=57) %	Control Groups Adults (n=635) %
Rash of any grade	—	26.3	45.6	17.5
Grade 1 Rash	Erythema, pruritus	10.7	8.8	9.8
Grade 2 Rash	Diffuse maculopapular rash, dry desquamation	14.7	31.6	7.4
Grade 3 Rash	Vesiculation, moist desquamation, ulceration	0.8	1.8	0.3
Grade 4 Rash	Erythema multiforme, Stevens-Johnson Syndrome, toxic epidermal necrolysis, necrosis requiring surgery, exfoliative dermatitis	0.1	3.5	0.0
Treatment discontinuation as a result of rash	—	1.7	8.8	0.3

[a] Includes events reported regardless of causality.
[b] Data from Study 006 and three Phase 2/3 studies.
[c] NCI Grading System.

pediatric patients compared to 0.9% of adults (see **ADVERSE REACTIONS**, Table 7).

The starting dose of SUSTIVA (efavirenz) was 600 mg once daily adjusted to body size, based on weight, targeting AUC levels in the range of 190–380 μM•h. The pharmacokinetics of efavirenz in pediatric patients were similar to the pharmacokinetics in adults who received 600-mg daily doses of SUSTIVA. In 48 pediatric patients receiving the equivalent of a 600-mg dose of SUSTIVA, steady state C_{max} was 14.2 ± 5.8 μM (mean ± SD), steady state C_{min} was 5.6 ± 4.1 μM, and AUC was 218 ± 104 μM•h.

Geriatric Use: Clinical studies of SUSTIVA (efavirenz) did not include sufficient numbers of subjects aged 65 years and over to determine whether they respond differently from younger subjects. In general, dose selection for an elderly patient should be cautious, reflecting the greater frequency of decreased hepatic, renal, or cardiac function and of concomitant disease or other therapy.

ADVERSE REACTIONS

The most significant adverse events observed in patients treated with SUSTIVA are nervous system symptoms, psychiatric symptoms, and rash.

Nervous System Symptoms: Fifty-three percent of patients receiving SUSTIVA reported central nervous system symptoms (see **WARNINGS: Nervous System Symptoms**). Table 6 lists the frequency of the symptoms of different degrees of severity and gives the discontinuation rates in clinical trials for one or more of the following nervous system symptoms: dizziness, insomnia, impaired concentration, somnolence, abnormal dreaming, euphoria, confusion, agitation, amnesia, hallucinations, stupor, abnormal thinking, and depersonalization. The frequencies of specific central and peripheral nervous system symptoms are provided in Table 8.

[See table 6 above]

Psychiatric Symptoms: Serious psychiatric adverse experiences have been reported in patients treated with SUSTIVA. In controlled trials, the frequency of specific serious psychiatric symptoms among patients who received SUSTIVA or control regimens, respectively, were: severe depression (1.6%, 0.6%), suicidal ideation (0.6%, 0.3%), nonfatal suicide attempts (0.4%, 0%), aggressive behavior (0.4%, 0.3%), paranoid reactions (0.4%, 0.3%), and manic reactions (0.1%, 0%) (see **WARNINGS: Psychiatric Symptoms**). Additional psychiatric symptoms observed at a frequency of >2% among patients treated with SUSTIVA or control regimens, respectively, in controlled clinical trials were depression (15.8%, 13.1%), anxiety (11.1%, 7.6%), and nervousness (6.3%, 2.0%).

Skin Rash: Rashes are usually mild-to-moderate maculopapular skin eruptions that occur within the first 2 weeks of initiating therapy with SUSTIVA. In most patients, rash resolves with continuing SUSTIVA (efavirenz) therapy within one month. SUSTIVA can be reinitiated in patients interrupting therapy because of rash. Use of appropriate antihistamines and/or corticosteroids may be considered when SUSTIVA is restarted. SUSTIVA should be discontinued in patients developing severe rash associated with blistering, desquamation, mucosal involvement, or fever. The frequency of rash by NCI grade and the discontinuation rates as a result of rash are provided in Table 7.

[See table 7 above]

As seen in Table 7, rash is more common in pediatric patients and more often of higher grade (ie, more severe) (see **PRECAUTIONS: General**).

Experience with SUSTIVA in patients who discontinued other antiretroviral agents of the NNRTI class is limited. Nineteen patients who discontinued nevirapine because of rash have been treated with SUSTIVA. Nine of these patients developed mild-to-moderate rash while receiving therapy with SUSTIVA, and two of these patients discontinued because of rash.

A few cases of pancreatitis have been described, although a causal relationship with efavirenz has not been established. Asymptomatic increases in serum amylase levels were observed in a significantly higher number of patients treated with efavirenz 600 mg than in control patients (see **ADVERSE REACTIONS: Laboratory Abnormalities**).

Drug-related clinical adverse experiences of moderate or severe intensity observed in ≥2% of patients in two controlled clinical trials are presented in Table 8.

[See table 8 at top of next page]

In Study 006, lipodystrophy was reported in 2.3% of patients treated with SUSTIVA+indinavir, 0.7% of patients

Continued on next page

Sustiva—Cont.

treated with SUSTIVA+zidovudine+lamivudine, and 1.0% of patients treated with indinavir+zidovudine+lamivudine. Clinical adverse experiences observed in ≥10% of 57 pediatric patients aged 3 to 16 years who received SUSTIVA (efavirenz) capsules, nelfinavir, and one or more NRTIs were: rash (46%), diarrhea/loose stools (39%), fever (21%), cough (16%), dizziness/lightheaded/fainting (16%), ache/pain/discomfort (14%), nausea/vomiting (12%), and headache (11%). The incidence of nervous system symptoms was 18% (10/57). One patient experienced Grade 3 rash, two patients had Grade 4 rash, and five patients (9%) discontinued because of rash (see also **PRECAUTIONS: Skin Rash** and **Pediatric Use**).

Postmarketing Experience:

Body as a Whole—allergic reactions, asthenia, redistribution/accumulation of body fat (see **PRECAUTIONS: Fat Redistribution**).

Central and Peripheral Nervous System—abnormal coordination, ataxia, convulsions, hypoesthesia, paresthesia, neuropathy, tremor

Endocrine—gynecomastia

Gastrointestinal—constipation, malabsorption

Cardiovascular—flushing, palpitations

Liver and Biliary System—hepatic enzyme increase, hepatic failure, hepatitis

Metabolic and Nutritional—hypercholesterolemia, hypertriglyceridemia

Musculoskeletal—arthralgia, myalgia, myopathy

Psychiatric—aggressive reactions, agitation, delusions, emotional lability, mania, neurosis, paranoia, psychosis, suicide

Respiratory—dyspnea

Skin and Appendages—erythema multiforme, nail disorders, skin discoloration, Stevens-Johnson syndrome

Special Senses—abnormal vision, tinnitus

Laboratory Abnormalities

Liver Enzymes—Among 1008 patients treated with 600 mg efavirenz in controlled clinical trials, 3% developed AST levels and 3% developed ALT levels greater than five times the upper limit of normal. Similar elevations of AST and ALT were seen in patients treated with control regimens.

Liver function tests should be monitored in patients with a prior history of hepatitis B and/or C. In 156 patients treated with 600 mg of SUSTIVA (efavirenz) who were seropositive for hepatitis B and/or C, 7% developed AST levels and 8% developed ALT levels greater than five times the upper limit of normal. In 91 patients seropositive for hepatitis B and/or C treated with control regimens, 5% developed AST elevations and 4% developed ALT elevations to these levels. Elevations of GGT to greater than five times the upper limit of the normal range were observed in 4% of all patients treated with 600 mg of SUSTIVA and in 10% of patients seropositive for hepatitis B or C. In patients treated with control regimens, the incidence of GGT elevations to this level was 1.5–2%, irrespective of hepatitis B or C serology. Isolated elevations of GGT in patients receiving SUSTIVA may reflect enzyme induction not associated with liver toxicity (see **PRECAUTIONS: General**).

Lipids—Increases in total cholesterol of 10–20% have been observed in some uninfected volunteers receiving SUSTIVA. In patients treated with SUSTIVA+ zidovudine+ lamivudine, increases in nonfasting total cholesterol and HDL of approximately 20% and 25%, respectively, were observed. In patients treated with SUSTIVA+indinavir, increases in nonfasting cholesterol and HDL of approximately 40% and 35%, respectively, were observed. The effects of SUSTIVA on triglycerides and LDL were not well characterized since samples were taken from nonfasting patients. The clinical significance of these findings is unknown (see **PRECAUTIONS: General**).

Serum Amylase—Asymptomatic elevations in serum amylase greater than 1.5 times the upper limit of normal were seen in 10% of patients treated with SUSTIVA and in 6% of patients treated with control regimens. The clinical significance of asymptomatic increases in serum amylase is unknown (see **ADVERSE REACTIONS**).

Cannabinoid Test Interaction—Efavirenz does not bind to cannabinoid receptors. False-positive urine cannabinoid test results have been observed in non-HIV-infected volunteers receiving SUSTIVA when the Microgenics CEDIA® DAU Multi-Level THC assay was used for screening. Negative results were obtained when more specific confirmatory testing was performed with gas chromatography/mass spectrometry.

Of the three assays analyzed (Microgenics CEDIA DAU Multi-Level THC assay, Cannabinoid Enzyme Immunoassay [Diagnostic Reagents, Inc.], and AxSYM® Cannabinoid Assay), only the Microgenics CEDIA DAU Multi-Level THC assay showed false-positive results. The other two assays provided true-negative results. The effects of SUSTIVA on cannabinoid screening tests other than these three are unknown. The manufacturers of cannabinoid assays should be contacted for additional information regarding the use of their assays with patients receiving efavirenz.

CEDIA® is a registered trademark of Roche Diagnostics.
AxSYM® is a registered trademark of Abbott Laboratories.

Table 8: Percent of Patients with Treatment-Emergent[a] Adverse Events of Moderate or Severe Intensity Reported in ≥2% of Patients in Studies 006 and ACTG 364

Adverse Events	Study 006 LAM, NNRTI, and Protease Inhibitor-Naive Patients			Study ACTG 364 NRTI-experienced NNRTI-, and Protease Inhibitor-Naive Patients		
	SUSTIVA[b] + ZDV/LAM (n=412) %	SUSTIVA[b] + Indinavir (n=415) %	Indinavir + ZDV/LAM (n=401) %	SUSTIVA[b] + Nelfinavir + NRTIs (n=64) %	SUSTIVA[b] + NRTIs (n=65) %	Nelfinavir + NRTIs (n=66) %
Body as a Whole						
Fatigue	7	5	8	0	2	3
Pain	1	1	5	13	6	17
Central and Peripheral Nervous System						
Dizziness	8	8	3	2	6	6
Headache	7	4	4	5	2	3
Concentration Impaired	5	2	0	0	0	0
Insomnia	6	7	3	0	0	2
Abnormal Dreams	3	1	0	—	—	—
Somnolence	3	2	2	0	0	0
Anorexia	1	0	1	0	2	2
Gastrointestinal						
Nausea	12	7	25	3	2	2
Vomiting	7	6	14	—	—	—
Diarrhea	6	8	6	14	3	9
Dyspepsia	3	3	5	0	0	2
Abdominal Pain	1	2	4	3	3	3
Psychiatric						
Anxiety	1	3	0	—	—	—
Depression	2	1	0	3	0	5
Nervousness	2	2	0	2	0	2
Skin & Appendages						
Rash	13	20	7	9	5	9
Pruritus	0	1	1	9	5	9
Increased Sweating	2	1	0	0	0	0

[a] Includes adverse events at least possibly related to study drug or of unknown relationship for Study 006. Includes all adverse events regardless of relationship to study drug for Study ACTG 364.
[b] SUSTIVA provided as 600 mg once daily.
—= Not Specified.
ZDV = zidovudine, LAM = lamivudine

OVERDOSAGE

Some patients accidentally taking 600 mg twice daily have reported increased nervous system symptoms. One patient experienced involuntary muscle contractions.

Treatment of overdose with SUSTIVA (enfavirenz) should consist of general supportive measures, including monitoring of vital signs and observation of the patient's clinical status. Administration of activated charcoal may be used to aid removal of unabsorbed drug. There is no specific antidote for overdose with SUSTIVA. Since efavirenz is highly protein bound, dialysis is unlikely to significantly remove the drug from blood.

DOSAGE AND ADMINISTRATION

Adults

The recommended dosage of SUSTIVA is 600 mg orally, once daily, in combination with a protease inhibitor and/or nucleoside analogue reverse transcriptase inhibitors (NRTIs). It is recommended that SUSTIVA be taken on an empty stomach, preferably at bedtime. The increased efavirenz concentrations observed following administration of SUSTIVA with food may lead to an increase in frequency of adverse events (see **CLINICAL PHARMACOLOGY: Effect of Food on Oral Absorption**). Dosing at bedtime may improve the tolerability of nervous system symptoms (see **WARNINGS: Nervous System Symptoms, PRECAUTIONS: Information for Patients,** and **ADVERSE REACTIONS**).

Concomitant Antiretroviral Therapy: SUSTIVA must be given in combination with other antiretroviral medications (see **CLINICAL PHARMACOLOGY: Drug Interactions** and **PRECAUTIONS: Drug Interactions** and **INDICATIONS AND USAGE**).

Pediatric Patients

It is recommended that SUSTIVA be taken on an empty stomach, preferably at bedtime. Table 9 describes the recommended dose of SUSTIVA for pediatric patients 3 years of age or older and weighing between 10 and 40 kg. The recommended dosage of SUSTIVA for pediatric patients weighing greater than 40 kg is 600 mg, once daily.

Table 9: Pediatric Dose To Be Administered Once Daily

Body Weight kg	Body Weight lbs	SUSTIVA Dose (mg)
10 to <15	22 to <33	200
15 to <20	33 to <44	250
20 to <25	44 to <55	300
25 to <32.5	55 to <71.5	350
32.5 to <40	71.5 to <88	400
≥40	≥88	600

HOW SUPPLIED

Capsules: SUSTIVA® (efavirenz) capsules are available as follows:

Capsules 200 mg are gold color, reverse printed with "SUSTIVA" on the body and imprinted "200 mg" on the cap.

Bottles of 90 **NDC** 0056-0474-92

Capsules 100 mg are white, reverse printed with "SUSTIVA" on the body and imprinted "100 mg" on the cap.

Bottles of 30 **NDC** 0056-0473-30

Capsules 50 mg are gold color and white, printed with "SUSTIVA" on the gold color cap and reverse printed "50 mg" on the white body.

Bottles of 30 **NDC** 0056-0470-30

Tablets: SUSTIVA® (efavirenz) tablets are available as follows:

Tablets 600 mg are yellow, capsular-shaped, film-coated tablets, with "SUSTIVA" printed on both sides.

Bottles of 30 **NDC** 0056-0510-30

SUSTIVA capsules and SUSTIVA tablets should be stored at 25°C (77°F); excursions permitted to 15°–30°C (59°–86°F) [see USP Controlled Room Temperature].

Distributed by Bristol-Myers Squibb Company Princeton, NJ 08543 USA

SUSTIVA® is a registered trademark of Bristol-Myers Squibb Pharma Company.

T4-B0001-03-04 Revised March 2004

PATIENT INFORMATION

SUSTIVA® (sus-TEE-vah)

[efavirenz (eh-FAH-vih-rehnz)]

℞ only

capsules and tablets

ALERT: Find out about medicines that should NOT be taken with SUSTIVA.

Please also read the section **"MEDICINES YOU SHOULD NOT TAKE WITH SUSTIVA."**

Read this information before you start taking SUSTIVA (efavirenz). Read it again each time you refill your prescription, in case there is any new information. This leaflet provides a summary about SUSTIVA and does not include everything there is to know about your medicine. This information is not meant to take the place of talking with your doctor.

What is SUSTIVA?

SUSTIVA is a medicine used in combination with other medicines to help treat infection with Human Immunodeficiency Virus (HIV), the virus that causes AIDS (acquired immune deficiency syndrome). SUSTIVA is a type of anti-HIV drug called a "non-nucleoside reverse transcriptase inhibitor" (NNRTI).

SUSTIVA works by lowering the amount of HIV in the blood (viral load). SUSTIVA must be taken with other anti-HIV medicines. When taken with other anti-HIV medicines, SUSTIVA has been shown to reduce viral load and increase the number of CD4 cells, a type of immune cell in blood. SUSTIVA may not have these effects in every patient.

SUSTIVA does not cure HIV or AIDS. People taking SUSTIVA may still develop other infections and complications. Therefore, it is very important that you stay under the care of your doctor.

SUSTIVA has not been shown to reduce the risk of passing HIV to others. Therefore, continue to practice safe sex, and do not use or share dirty needles.

What are the possible side effects of SUSTIVA?

Serious psychiatric problems. A small number of patients experience severe depression, strange thoughts, or angry behavior while taking SUSTIVA. Some patients have thoughts of suicide and a few have actually committed suicide. These problems tend to occur more often in patients who have had mental illness. Contact your doctor right away if you think you are having these psychiatric symptoms, so your doctor can decide if you should continue to take SUSTIVA.

Common side effects. Many patients have dizziness, trouble sleeping, drowsiness, trouble concentrating, and/or unusual dreams during treatment with SUSTIVA. These side effects may be reduced if you take SUSTIVA at bedtime on an empty stomach. They also tend to go away after you have taken the medicine for a few weeks. If you have these common side effects, such as dizziness, it does not mean that you will also have serious psychiatric problems, such as severe depression, strange thoughts, or angry behavior. Tell your doctor right away if any of these side effects continue or if they bother you. It is possible that these symptoms may be more severe if SUSTIVA is used with alcohol or mood altering (street) drugs.

If you are dizzy, have trouble concentrating, or are drowsy, avoid activities that may be dangerous, such as driving or operating machinery.

Rash is common. Rashes usually go away without any change in treatment. In a small number of patients, rash may be serious. If you develop a rash, call your doctor right away. **Rash may be a serious problem in some children.** Tell your child's doctor right away if you notice rash or any other side effects while your child is taking SUSTIVA.

Other common side effects include tiredness, upset stomach, vomiting, and diarrhea.

Changes in body fat. Changes in body fat develop in some patients taking anti-HIV medicine. These changes may include an increased amount of fat in the upper back and neck ("buffalo hump"), in the breasts, and around the trunk. Loss of fat from the legs, arms, and face may also happen. The cause and long-term health effects of these fat changes are not known.

Tell your doctor or healthcare provider if you notice any side effects while taking SUSTIVA.

Contact your doctor before stopping SUSTIVA because of side effects or for any other reason.

This is not a complete list of side effects possible with SUSTIVA. Ask your doctor or pharmacist for a more complete list of side effects of SUSTIVA and all the medicines you will take.

How should I take SUSTIVA (efavirenz)?

General Information

- You should take SUSTIVA on an empty stomach, preferably at bedtime.
- Swallow SUSTIVA with water.
- Taking SUSTIVA with food increases the amount of medicine in your body, which may increase the frequency of side effects.
- Taking SUSTIVA at bedtime may make some side effects less bothersome.
- SUSTIVA must be taken in combination with other anti-HIV medicines. If you take only SUSTIVA, the medicine may stop working.
- Do not miss a dose of SUSTIVA. If you forget to take SUSTIVA, take the missed dose right away, unless it is almost time for your next dose. Do not double the next dose. Carry on with your regular dosing schedule. If you need help in planning the best times to take your medicine, ask your doctor or pharmacist.
- Take the exact amount of SUSTIVA your doctor prescribes. Never change the dose on your own. Do not stop this medicine unless your doctor tells you to stop.
- If you believe you took more than the prescribed amount of SUSTIVA, contact your local Poison Control Center or emergency room right away.
- Tell your doctor if you start any new medicine or change how you take old ones. Your doses may need adjustment.
- When your SUSTIVA supply starts to run low, get more from your doctor or pharmacy. This is very important because the amount of virus in your blood may increase if the medicine is stopped for even a short time. The virus may develop resistance to SUSTIVA and become harder to treat.
- Your doctor may want to do blood tests to check for certain side effects while you take SUSTIVA.

Capsules

- The dose of SUSTIVA capsules for adults is 600 mg (three 200-mg capsules, taken together) once a day by mouth. The dose of SUSTIVA for children may be lower (see **Can children take SUSTIVA?**).

Tablets

- The dose of SUSTIVA tablets for adults is 600 mg (one tablet) once a day by mouth.

Can children take SUSTIVA?

Yes, children who are able to swallow capsules can take SUSTIVA. Rash may be a serious problem in some children. Tell your child's doctor right away if you notice rash or any other side effects while your child is taking SUSTIVA. The dose of SUSTIVA for children may be lower than the dose for adults. Capsules containing lower doses of SUSTIVA are available. Your child's doctor will determine the right dose based on your child's weight.

Who should not take SUSTIVA?

Do not take SUSTIVA if you are allergic to the active ingredient, efavirenz, or to any of the inactive ingredients. Your doctor and pharmacist have a list of the inactive ingredients.

What should I avoid while taking SUSTIVA (efavirenz)?

- **Women taking SUSTIVA should not become pregnant.** Serious birth defects have been seen in animals treated with SUSTIVA. It is not known whether this could happen in humans. **Tell your doctor right away if you are pregnant.** Also talk with your doctor if you want to become pregnant.
- Women should not rely only on hormone-based birth control, such as pills, injections, or implants, because SUSTIVA may make these contraceptives ineffective. Women must use a reliable form of barrier contraception, such as a condom or diaphragm, even if they also use other methods of birth control.
- **Do not breast-feed if you are taking SUSTIVA.** The Centers for Disease Control and Prevention recommend that mothers with HIV not breast-feed because they can pass the HIV through their milk to the baby. Also, SUSTIVA may pass through breast milk and cause serious harm to the baby. Talk with your doctor if you are breast-feeding. You may need to stop breast-feeding or use a different medicine.
- Taking SUSTIVA with alcohol or other medicines causing similar side effects as SUSTIVA, such as drowsiness, may increase those side effects.
- Do not take any other medicines without checking with your doctor. These medicines include prescription and nonprescription medicines and herbal products, especially St. John's wort.

Before using SUSTIVA, tell your doctor if you

- **have problems with your liver or have hepatitis.** Your doctor may want to do tests to check your liver while you take SUSTIVA.
- **have ever had mental illness or are using drugs or alcohol.**
- **have ever had seizures or are taking medicine for seizures** [for example, Dilantin® (phenytoin), Tegretol® (carbamazepine), or phenobarbital]. Your doctor may want to check drug levels in your blood from time to time.

What important information should I know about taking other medicines with SUSTIVA?

SUSTIVA (efavirenz) may change the effect of other medicines, including ones for HIV, and cause serious side effects. Your doctor may change your other medicines or change their doses. Other medicines, including herbal products, may affect SUSTIVA. For this reason, **it is very important to:**

- let all your doctors and pharmacists know that you take SUSTIVA.
- tell your doctors and pharmacists about all medicines you take. This includes those you buy over-the-counter and herbal or natural remedies.

Bring all your prescription and nonprescription medicines as well as any herbal remedies that you are taking when you see a doctor, or make a list of their names, how much you take, and how often you take them. This will give your doctor a complete picture of the medicines you use. Then he or she can decide the best approach for your situation.

Taking SUSTIVA with St. John's wort *(Hypericum perforatum)*, an herbal product sold as a dietary supplement, or products containing St. John's wort is not recommended. Talk with your doctor if you are taking or are planning to take St. John's wort. Taking St. John's wort may decrease SUSTIVA levels and lead to increased viral load and possible resistance to SUSTIVA or cross-resistance to other anti-HIV drugs.

MEDICINES YOU SHOULD NOT TAKE WITH SUSTIVA

The following medicines may cause serious and life-threatening side effects when taken with SUSTIVA. You should not take any of these medicines while taking SUSTIVA:

- Hismanal® (astemizole)
- Propulsid® (cisapride)
- Versed® (midazolam)
- Halcion® (triazolam)
- Ergot medications (for example, Wigraine® and Cafergot®)

The following medicines may need to be replaced with another medicine when taken with SUSTIVA (efavirenz):

- Fortovase®, Invirase® (saquinavir)
- Biaxin® (clarithromycin)

The following medicines may need to have their dose changed when taken with SUSTIVA:

- Crixivan® (indinavir)
- Kaletra® (lopinavir/ritonavir)
- Methadone
- Mycobutin® (rifabutin)
- Zoloft® (sertraline)

These are not all the medicines that may cause problems if you take SUSTIVA. Be sure to tell your doctor about all medicines that you take.

General advice about SUSTIVA:

Medicines are sometimes prescribed for conditions that are not mentioned in patient information leaflets. Do not use SUSTIVA for a condition for which it was not prescribed. Do not give SUSTIVA to other people, even if they have the same symptoms you have. It may harm them.

Keep SUSTIVA at room temperature (77°F) in the bottle given to you by your pharmacist. The temperature can range from 59° to 86°F.

Keep SUSTIVA out of the reach of children.

This leaflet summarizes the most important information about SUSTIVA. If you would like more information, talk with your doctor. You can ask your pharmacist or doctor for the full prescribing information about SUSTIVA (efavirenz), or you can visit the SUSTIVA website at http://www.sustiva.com or call 1-800-426-7644.

Dilantin® is a registered trademark of Parke-Davis, division of Warner-Lambert Co.

Tegretol® is a registered trademark of Novartis Pharmaceuticals Corporation.

Hismanal® and Propulsid® are registered trademarks of Janssen Pharmaceutica Products, LP.

Versed®, Fortovase®,and Invirase® are registered trademarks of Roche Pharmaceuticals.

Halcion® and Mycobutin® are registered trademarks of Pharmacia & Upjohn.

Wigraine® is a registered trademark of Organon.

Cafergot® is a registered trademark of Novartis Pharmaceuticals Corporation.

Biaxin® and Kaletra® are registered trademarks of Abbott Laboratories.

Crixivan® is a registered trademark of Merck & Co., Inc.

Zoloft® is a registered trademark of Pfizer, Inc.

*SUSTIVA® is a registered trademark of Bristol-Myers Squibb Pharma Company.

Distributed by:
Bristol-Myers Squibb Company
Princeton, NJ 08543
U.S.A.

T4-B0001-03-04
Based on: 51-022486-02
Based on package insert dated March 2004
Revised June 2003

Shown in Product Identification Guide, page 310

TEQUIN® ℞

[tĕ kwĭn]
(gatifloxacin)
Tablets

TEQUIN®

(gatifloxacin)
Injection

TEQUIN®

(gatifloxacin in 5% dextrose)
Injection
(Patient Information Included)
℞ only

TEQUIN® is available as TEQUIN (gatifloxacin) Tablets for oral administration and TEQUIN (gatifloxacin) Injection and TEQUIN (gatifloxacin in 5% dextrose) Injection for intravenous administration.

To reduce the development of drug-resistant bacteria and maintain the effectiveness of TEQUIN and other antibacterial drugs, TEQUIN should be used only to treat or prevent infections that are proven or strongly suspected to be caused by bacteria.

DESCRIPTION

TEQUIN contains gatifloxacin, a synthetic broad-spectrum 8-methoxyfluoroquinolone antibacterial agent for oral or intravenous administration. Chemically, gatifloxacin is (±) -1-cyclopropyl-6-fluoro-1, 4-dihydro-8-methoxy-7-(3-methyl-1-piperazinyl)-4-oxo-3-quinolinecarboxylic acid sesquihydrate.

The chemical structure is:

Its empirical formula is $C_{19}H_{22}FN_3O_4 \cdot 1.5\ H_2O$ and its molecular weight is 402.42. Gatifloxacin is a sesquihydrate crystalline powder and is white to pale yellow in color. It exists as a racemate, with no net optical rotation. The solubility of the compound is pH dependent. The maximum aqueous solubility (40-60 mg/mL) occurs at a pH range of 2 to 5.

TEQUIN Tablets

TEQUIN Tablets are available as 200 mg and 400 mg white, film-coated tablets and contain the following inactive ingredients: hypromellose, magnesium stearate, methylcellulose, microcrystalline cellulose, polyethylene glycol, polysorbate 80, simethicone, sodium starch glycolate, sorbic acid, and titanium dioxide.

TEQUIN Injection for Intravenous Administration

TEQUIN Injection is available in 40 mL (400 mg) single-use vials as a sterile, preservative-free aqueous solution of gatifloxacin with pH ranging from 3.5 to 5.5. TEQUIN (gatifloxacin in 5% dextrose) Injection is also available in ready-to-use 100 mL (200 mg) and 200 mL (400 mg) flexible

Continued on next page

Tequin—Cont.

bags as a sterile, preservative-free aqueous solution of gatifloxacin with pH ranging from 3.5 to 5.5. The appearance of the intravenous solution may range from light yellow to greenish-yellow in color. The color does not affect nor is it indicative of product stability.
The intravenous formulation contains dextrose, anhydrous, USP or dextrose, monohydrate, USP and Water for Injection, USP, and may contain hydrochloric acid and/or sodium hydroxide for pH adjustment.

CLINICAL PHARMACOLOGY

Gatifloxacin is administered as a racemate, with the disposition and antibacterial activity of the R- and S-enantiomers virtually identical.

Absorption

Gatifloxacin is well absorbed from the gastrointestinal tract after oral administration and can be given without regard to food. The absolute bioavailability of gatifloxacin is 96%. Peak plasma concentrations of gatifloxacin usually occur 1-2 hours after oral dosing.
The oral and intravenous routes of administration for TEQUIN (gatifloxacin) can be considered interchangeable, since the pharmacokinetics of gatifloxacin after 1-hour intravenous administration are similar to those observed for orally administered gatifloxacin when equal doses are administered (Figure 1) (see **DOSAGE AND ADMINISTRATION**).

Figure 1.
Mean Plasma Concentration-Time Profiles of Gatifloxacin Following Intravenous (IV) and Oral (PO) Administration of a Single 400 mg Dose to Healthy Subjects.

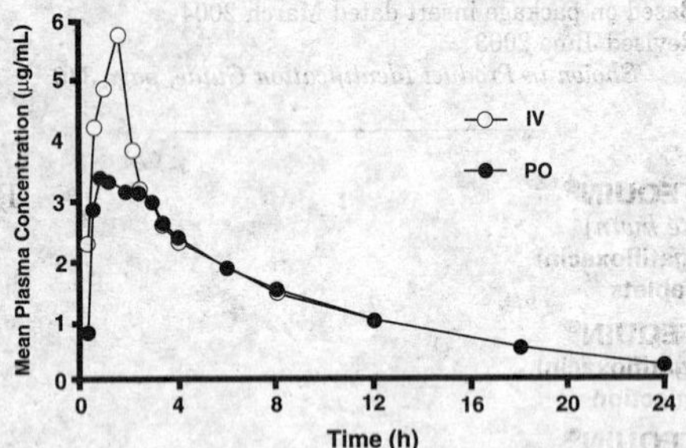

Pharmacokinetics

The mean (SD) pharmacokinetic parameters of gatifloxacin following oral administration to healthy subjects with bacterial infections and subjects with renal insufficiency are listed in Table 1. The mean (SD) pharmacokinetic parameters of gatifloxacin following intravenous administration to healthy subjects are listed in Table 2.
[See table 1 below]
[See table 2 below]

Gatifloxacin pharmacokinetics are linear and time-independent at doses ranging from 200 to 800 mg administered over a period of up to 14 days. Steady-state concentrations are achieved by the third daily oral or intravenous dose of gatifloxacin. The mean steady-state peak and trough plasma concentrations attained following a dosing regimen of 400 mg once daily are approximately 4.2 µg/mL and 0.4 µg/mL, respectively, for oral administration and 4.6 µg/mL and 0.4 µg/mL, respectively, for intravenous administration.

Distribution

Serum protein binding of gatifloxacin is approximately 20% in volunteers and is concentration independent. Consistent with the low protein binding, concentrations of gatifloxacin in saliva were approximately equal to those in plasma (mean [range] saliva:plasma ratio was 0.88 [0.46-1.57]). The mean volume of distribution of gatifloxacin at steady-state (Vd_{ss}) ranged from 1.5 to 2.0 L/kg. Gatifloxacin is widely distributed throughout the body into many body tissues and fluids. Rapid distribution of gatifloxacin into tissues results in higher gatifloxacin concentrations in most target tissues than in serum (Table 3).

Table 3: Gatifloxacin Tissue — Fluid/Serum Ratio (Range)[a]

Fluid or Tissue	Tissue-Fluid/ Serum Ratio (Range)[a]
Respiratory	
Alveolar macrophages	26.5 (10.9-61.1)
Bronchial mucosa	1.65 (1.12-2.22)
Lung epithelial lining fluid	1.67 (0.81-4.46)
Lung parenchyma	4.09 (0.50-9.22)
Sinus mucosa	1.78 (1.17-2.49)
Sputum (Multiple dose)	1.28 (0.49-2.38)
Skin	
Skin blister fluid	1.00 (0.50-1.47)
Reproductive	
Ejaculate	1.07 (0.86-1.32)
Seminal fluid	1.01 (0.81-1.21)
Vagina	1.22 (0.57-1.63)
Cervix	1.45 (0.56-2.64)

[a] Mean of individual ratios collected over 24 hours following single (100, 150, 200, 300, or 400 mg) or multiple (150 or 200 mg BID) doses of gatifloxacin except for skin blister fluid, where mean AUC ratio is presented.

Metabolism

Gatifloxacin undergoes limited biotransformation in humans with less than 1% of the dose excreted in the urine as ethylenediamine and methylethylenediamine metabolites.
In vitro studies with cytochrome P450 isoenzymes (CYP) indicate that gatifloxacin does not inhibit CYP3A4, CYP2D6, CYP2C9, CYP2C19, or CYP1A2, suggesting that gatifloxacin is unlikely to alter the pharmacokinetics of drugs metabolized by these enzymes (e.g., midazolam, cyclosporine, warfarin, theophylline).
In vivo studies in animals and humans indicate that gatifloxacin is not an enzyme inducer; therefore, gatifloxacin is unlikely to alter the metabolic elimination of itself or other coadministered drugs.

Excretion

Gatifloxacin is excreted as unchanged drug primarily by the kidney. More than 70% of an administered TEQUIN (gatifloxacin) dose was recovered as unchanged drug in the urine within 48 hours following oral and intravenous administration, and 5% was recovered in the feces. Less than 1% of the dose is recovered in the urine as two metabolites. Crystals of gatifloxacin have not been observed in the urine of normal, healthy human subjects following administration of intravenous or oral doses up to 800 mg.
The mean elimination half-life of gatifloxacin ranges from 7 to 14 hours and is independent of dose and route of administration. Renal clearance is independent of dose with mean value ranging from 124 to 161 mL/min. The magnitude of this value, coupled with the significant decrease in the elimination of gatifloxacin seen with concomitant probenecid administration, indicates that gatifloxacin undergoes both glomerular filtration and tubular secretion. Gatifloxacin may also undergo minimal biliary and/or intestinal elimination, since 5% of dose was recovered in the feces as unchanged drug. This finding is supported by the 5-fold higher concentration of gatifloxacin in the bile compared to the plasma (mean bile:plasma ratio [range] 5.34 [0.33-14.0]).

Special Populations

Patients with Bacterial Infections

The pharmacokinetics of gatifloxacin were similar between healthy volunteers and patients with infection, when underlying renal function was taken into account (see Table 1).

Geriatric

Following a single oral 400 mg dose of gatifloxacin in young (18-40 years) and elderly (≥65 years) male and female subjects, there were only modest differences in the pharmacokinetics of gatifloxacin noted in female subjects; elderly females had a 21% increase in C_{max} and a 32% increase in $AUC_{(0-\infty)}$ compared to young females. These differences were mainly due to decreasing renal function with increasing age and are not thought to be clinically important. No dosage adjustment based on age alone is necessary for elderly subjects when administering TEQUIN (gatifloxacin).

Pediatric

The pharmacokinetics of gatifloxacin in pediatric populations (<18 years of age) have not been established.

Gender

Following a single oral 400 mg dose of gatifloxacin in male and female subjects, there were only modest differences in the pharmacokinetics of gatifloxacin, mainly confined to elderly subjects. Elderly females had a 21% increase in C_{max} and a 33% increase in $AUC_{(0-\infty)}$ compared to elderly males. Both results were accounted for by gender-related differences in body weight and are not thought to be clinically important. Dosage adjustment of TEQUIN is not necessary based on gender.

Chronic Hepatic Disease

Following a single oral 400 mg dose of gatifloxacin in healthy subjects and in subjects with moderate hepatic impairment (Child-Pugh B classification of cirrhosis), C_{max} and $AUC_{(0-\infty)}$ values for gatifloxacin were modestly higher (32% and 23% respectively). Due to the concentration-dependent antimicrobial activity associated with quino-

Table 1: Gatifloxacin Pharmacokinetic Parameters — Oral Administration

	C_{max} (µg/mL)	T_{max}[a] (h)	AUC[b] (µg·h/mL)	$T_{1/2}$ (h)	Cl/F (mL/min)	Cl_R (mL/min)	UR (%)
200 mg — Healthy Volunteers							
Single dose (n=12)	2.0 ± 0.4	1.00 (0.50, 2.50)	14.2 ± 0.4	—	241 ± 40	—	73.8 ± 10.9
400 mg — Healthy Volunteers							
Single dose (n=202)[c]	3.8 ± 1.0	1.00 (0.50, 6.00)	33.0 ± 6.2	7.8 ± 1.3	210 ± 44	151 ± 46	72.4 ± 18.1
Multiple dose (n=18)	4.2 ± 1.3	1.50 (0.50, 4.00)	34.4 ± 5.7	7.1 ± 0.6	199 ± 31	159 ± 34	80.2 ± 12.1
400 mg — Patients with Infection							
Multiple dose (n=140)[d]	4.2 ± 1.9	—	51.3 ± 20.4	—	147 ± 48	—	—
400 mg — Single Dose Subjects with Renal Insufficiency							
Cl_{cr} 50-89 mL/min (n=8)	4.4 ± 1.1	1.13 (0.75, 2.00)	48.0 ± 12.7	11.2 ± 2.8	148 ± 41	124 ± 38	83.7 ± 7.8
Cl_{cr} 30-49 mL/min (n=8)	5.1 ± 1.8	0.75 (0.50, 6.00)	74.9 ± 12.6	17.2 ± 8.5	92 ± 17	67 ± 24	71.1 ± 17.4
Cl_{cr} <30 mL/min (n=8)	4.5 ± 1.2	1.50 (0.50, 6.00)	149.3 ± 35.6	30.7 ± 8.4	48 ± 16	23 ± 13	44.7 ± 13.0
Hemodialysis (n=8)	4.7 ± 1.0	1.50 (1.00, 3.00)	180.3 ± 34.4	35.7 ± 7.0	38 ± 8	—	—
CAPD (n=8)	4.7 ± 1.3	1.75 (0.50, 3.00)	227.0 ± 60.0	40.3 ± 8.3	31 ± 8	—	—

[a] Median (Minimum, Maximum)
[b] Single dose: $AUC_{(0-\infty)}$, Multiple dose: $AUC_{(0-24)}$
[c] n=184 for Cl/F, n=134 for Cl_R, and n=132 for UR
[d] Based on the patient population pharmacokinetic modeling, n=103 for C_{max}
C_{max}: Maximum serum concentration; T_{max}: Time to C_{max}; AUC: Area under concentration versus time curve; $T_{1/2}$: Serum half-life; Cl/F: Apparent total clearance; Cl_R: Renal clearance; UR: Urinary recovery

Table 2: Gatifloxacin Pharmacokinetic Parameters — Intravenous Administration

	C_{max} (µg/mL)	T_{max}[a] (h)	AUC[b] (µg·h/mL)	$T_{1/2}$ (h)	Vd_{ss} (L/kg)	Cl (mL/min)	Cl_R (mL/min)	UR (%)
200 mg — Healthy Volunteers								
Single dose (n=12)	2.2 ± 0.3	1.00 (0.67, 1.50)	15.9 ± 2.6	11.1 ± 4.1	1.9 ± 0.1	214 ± 36	155 ± 32	71.7 ± 6.8
Multiple dose (n=8)[c]	2.4 ± 0.4	1.00 (0.67, 1.00)	16.8 ± 3.6	12.3 ± 4.6	2.0 ± 0.3	207 ± 44	155 ± 55	72.4 ± 16.4
400 mg — Healthy Volunteers								
Single dose (n=30)	5.5 ± 1.0	1.00 (0.50, 1.00)	35.1 ± 6.7	7.4 ± 1.6	1.5 ± 0.2	196 ± 33	124 ± 41	62.3 ± 16.7
Multiple dose (n=5)	4.6 ± 0.6	1.00 (1.00, 1.00)	35.4 ± 4.6	13.9 ± 3.9	1.6 ± 0.5	190 ± 24	161 ± 43	83.5 ± 13.8

[a] Median (Minimum, Maximum)
[b] Single dose: $AUC_{(0-\infty)}$, Multiple dose: $AUC_{(0-24)}$
[c] n=7 for Cl_R and UR
C_{max}: Maximum serum concentration; T_{max}: Time to C_{max}; AUC: Area under concentration versus time curve; $T_{1/2}$: Serum half-life; Vd_{ss}: Volume of distribution; Cl: Total clearance; Cl_R: Renal clearance; UR: Urinary recovery

lones, the modestly higher C_{max} values in the subjects with moderate hepatic impairment are not expected to negatively impact the outcome of TEQUIN therapy in this population. Dosage adjustment of TEQUIN is not necessary in patients with moderate hepatic impairment. The effect of severe hepatic impairment on the pharmacokinetics of TEQUIN is unknown.

Renal Insufficiency

Following administration of a single oral 400 mg dose of gatifloxacin to subjects with varying degrees of renal impairment, apparent total clearance of gatifloxacin (Cl/F) was reduced and systemic exposure (AUC) was increased commensurate with the decrease in renal function (see Table 1). Total gatifloxacin clearance was reduced 57% in moderate renal insufficiency (Cl_{cr} 30-49 mL/min) and 77% in severe renal insufficiency (Cl_{cr} <30 mL/min). Systemic exposure to gatifloxacin was approximately 2 times higher in moderate renal insufficiency and approximately 4 times higher in severe renal insufficiency, compared to subjects with normal renal function. Mean C_{max} values were modestly increased. A reduced dosage of TEQUIN (gatifloxacin) is recommended in patients with creatinine clearance <40 mL/min, including patients requiring hemodialysis or continuous ambulatory peritoneal dialysis (CAPD) (see **PRECAUTIONS: General** and **DOSAGE AND ADMINISTRATION: Impaired Renal Function**).

Diabetes Mellitus

The pharmacokinetics of gatifloxacin in patients with type 2 diabetes (non–insulin-dependent diabetes mellitus), following TEQUIN (gatifloxacin) 400 mg orally for 10 days, were comparable to those in healthy subjects.

Glucose Homeostasis

Disturbances of blood glucose, including symptomatic hyper- and hypoglycemia, have been reported with TEQUIN, usually in diabetic patients. Therefore, careful monitoring of blood glucose is recommended when TEQUIN is administered to patients with diabetes (see **WARNINGS**, **PRECAUTIONS: Information for Patients**, and **Drug Interactions**, and **ANIMAL PHARMACOLOGY**).

In a postmarketing study conducted in non-infected patients (n=70) with type 2 diabetes mellitus controlled primarily with either the combination of glyburide and metformin or metformin alone, daily administration of gatifloxacin 400 mg orally for 14 days was associated with initial hypoglycemia followed by hyperglycemia. Upon initiation of gatifloxacin dosing (i.e., first two days of treatment), there were increases in serum insulin concentrations and resulting decreases in serum glucose, as compared to baseline glucose values, despite ingestion of dietary restricted meals. In some patients, the reductions in glucose produced signs and symptoms of hypoglycemia (asthenia, sweating, dizziness) and necessitated administration of additional food. With continued gatifloxacin dosing (i.e., from the third day of treatment and throughout the dosing period) fasting serum glucose concentrations were increased compared to baseline. The serum glucose concentrations returned to baseline in most of these uninfected patients by 28 days after the cessation of gatifloxacin treatment. Single doses of insulin were administered to 3 patients in this study to correct the hyperglycemia during continued gatifloxacin administration.

In two premarketing studies, no clinically significant changes in glucose tolerance (via measurement of oral glucose challenge) and glucose homeostasis (via measurement of fasting serum glucose, serum insulin and c-peptide) were observed following single or multiple intravenous infusion doses of 200 to 800 mg TEQUIN in healthy volunteers (n=30), or 400 mg oral doses of TEQUIN for 10 days in patients (n=16) with type 2 (non–insulin-dependent) diabetes mellitus controlled on diet and exercise. Compared to placebo, transient modest increases in serum insulin of approximately 20-40% and decreases in glucose concentrations of approximately 30% were noted with the first dose of intravenous or oral gatifloxacin.

In another premarketing study, following administration of single oral 400 mg doses of TEQUIN (gatifloxacin) for 10 days in patients (n=16) with type 2 diabetes mellitus controlled with glyburide, decreases in serum insulin concentrations of approximately 30-40%, as compared to placebo, were noted following oral glucose challenge; however, these decreases were not accompanied by statistically significant changes in serum glucose levels. In this study, modest increases in fasting glucose (average increases of 40 mg/dL) were also noted by day 4 of continued gatifloxacin administration, although these changes did not reach statistical significance.

Photosensitivity Potential

In a study of the skin response to ultraviolet and visible radiation conducted in 48 healthy, male Caucasian volunteers (12 per group), the minimum erythematous dose was measured for ciprofloxacin (500 mg BID), lomefloxacin (400 mg QD), gatifloxacin (400 mg QD), and placebo before and after drug administration for 7 days. In this study, gatifloxacin was comparable to placebo at all wavelengths tested and had a lower potential for producing delayed photosensitivity skin reactions than ciprofloxacin or lomefloxacin.

Electrocardiogram

In premarketing studies of volunteer subjects with pre- and post-dose ECGs obtained in 55 male volunteers receiving oral or IV TEQUIN doses of 200 to 800 mg, the mean change in the post-dose QTc interval was <10 msec and there were no subjects with prolonged post-dose QTc intervals of >450 msec. In a postmarketing study of 34 healthy male and female volunteers receiving single oral doses of TEQUIN 400, 800, and 1200 mg and placebo, an association between increases in post-dose QTc interval changes from baseline and increases in gatifloxacin plasma concentrations were observed. At the therapeutic dose of 400 mg, the mean change in the post-dose QTc interval from baseline was <10 msec. There were no subjects with prolonged post-dose QTc intervals of >450 msec for males and >470 msec for females.

In a postmarketing clinical trial of 262 patients with respiratory tract infections receiving repeated 400 mg oral doses of TEQUIN who were studied with pre- and post-dose ECGs, the mean change in the post-dose QTc interval was <10 msec following the first 400 mg dose. In another postmarketing study of patients, with an acute coronary syndrome occurring within 4 weeks prior to TEQUIN administration, pre- and post-dose ECGs were obtained in patients who were administered TEQUIN 400 mg orally after single (n=372) and repeated (steady state; n=36) dosing. The mean changes in the post-dose QTc interval in these patients were <10 msec after both single and repeated dosing.

There is limited information available on the potential for a pharmacodynamic interaction in humans between gatifloxacin and drugs that prolong the QTc interval of an electrocardiogram. Therefore, gatifloxacin should not be used with Class IA and Class III antiarrhythmics (see **WARNINGS** and **PRECAUTIONS: Information for Patients**).

Spirometry

No clinically significant changes in spirometry were observed following single or multiple 200 mg, 400 mg, 600 mg, and 800 mg intravenous infusion doses of TEQUIN (gatifloxacin) in healthy volunteers.

Drug-Drug Interactions

Systemic exposure to TEQUIN (gatifloxacin) is increased following concomitant administration of TEQUIN and probenecid, and is reduced by concomitant administration of TEQUIN and ferrous sulfate or antacids containing aluminum or magnesium salts. TEQUIN (gatifloxacin) can be administered 4 hours before the administration of dietary supplements containing zinc, magnesium, or iron (such as multivitamins).

Probenecid: Concomitant administration of TEQUIN (single oral 200 mg dose) with probenecid (500 mg BID x 1 day) resulted in a 42% increase in AUC and a 44% longer half-life of gatifloxacin.

Iron: When TEQUIN (single oral 400 mg dose) was administered concomitantly with ferrous sulfate (single oral 325 mg dose), bioavailability of gatifloxacin was reduced (54% reduction in mean C_{max} and 35% reduction in mean AUC). Administration of TEQUIN (single oral 400 mg dose) 2 hours after or 2 hours before ferrous sulfate (single oral 325 mg dose) did not significantly alter the oral bioavailability of gatifloxacin (see **DOSAGE AND ADMINISTRATION**).

Antacids: When TEQUIN (single oral 400 mg dose) was administered 2 hours before, concomitantly, or 2 hours after an aluminum/magnesium-containing antacid (1800 mg of aluminum oxide and 1200 mg of magnesium hydroxide single oral dose), there was a 15%, 69%, and 47% reduction in C_{max} and a 17%, 64%, and 40% reduction in AUC of gatifloxacin, respectively. An aluminum/magnesium-containing antacid did not have a clinically significant effect on the pharmacokinetics of gatifloxacin when administered 4 hours after gatifloxacin administration (single oral 400 mg dose) (see **DOSAGE AND ADMINISTRATION**).

Milk, Calcium, and Calcium-containing Antacids: No significant pharmacokinetic interactions occur when milk or calcium carbonate is administered concomitantly with TEQUIN. Concomitant administration of 200 mL of milk or 1000 mg of calcium carbonate with TEQUIN (200 mg gatifloxacin dose for the milk study and 400 mg gatifloxacin dose for the calcium carbonate study) had no significant effect on the pharmacokinetics of gatifloxacin. TEQUIN can be administered 4 hours before the administration of dietary supplements containing zinc, magnesium, or iron (such as multivitamins).

Minor pharmacokinetic interactions occur following concomitant administration of gatifloxacin and digoxin; a priori dosage adjustments of either drug are not warranted.

Digoxin: Overall, only modest increases in C_{max} and AUC of digoxin were noted (12% and 19% respectively) in 8 of 11 healthy volunteers who received concomitant administration of TEQUIN (400 mg oral tablet, once daily for 7 days) and digoxin (0.25 mg orally, once daily for 7 days). In 3 of 11 subjects, however, a significant increase in digoxin concentrations was observed. In these 3 subjects, digoxin C_{max} increased by 18%, 29%, and 58% while digoxin AUC increased by 66%, 104%, and 79%, and digoxin clearance decreased by 40%, 51%, and 45%. Although dose adjustments for digoxin are not warranted with initiation of gatifloxacin treatment, patients taking digoxin should be monitored for signs and/or symptoms of toxicity. In patients who display signs and/or symptoms of digoxin intoxication, serum digoxin concentrations should be determined, and digoxin dosage should be adjusted as appropriate. The pharmacokinetics of gatifloxacin was not altered by digoxin.

No significant pharmacokinetic interactions occur when cimetidine, midazolam, theophylline, warfarin, or glyburide is administered concomitantly with TEQUIN (gatifloxacin). These results and the data from *in vitro* studies suggest that gatifloxacin is unlikely to significantly alter the metabolic clearance of drugs metabolized by CYP3A, CYP1A2, CYP2C9, CYP2C19, and CYP2D6 isoenzymes.

Cimetidine: Administration of TEQUIN (single oral dose of 200 mg) 1 hour after cimetidine (single oral dose of 200 mg) had no significant effect on the pharmacokinetics of gatifloxacin. These results suggest that absorption of gatifloxacin is expected to be unaffected by H_2-receptor antagonists like cimetidine.

Midazolam: TEQUIN administration had no significant effect on the systemic clearance of intravenous midazolam. A single intravenous dose of midazolam (0.0145 mg/kg) had no effect on the steady-state pharmacokinetics of gatifloxacin (once daily oral doses of 400 mg for 5 days). These results are consistent with the lack of effect of TEQUIN in *in vitro* studies with the human CYP3A4 isoenzyme.

Theophylline: Concomitant administration of TEQUIN (once daily oral doses of 400 mg for 5 days) and theophylline (300 mg BID oral dose for 10 days) had no significant effect on the pharmacokinetics of either drug. These results are consistent with the lack of effect of TEQUIN in *in vitro* studies with the human CYP1A2 isoenzyme.

Warfarin: Concomitant administration of TEQUIN (once daily oral doses of 400 mg for 11 days) and warfarin (single oral dose of 25 mg) had no significant effect on the pharmacokinetics of either drug nor was the prothrombin time significantly altered. These results are consistent with the lack of effect of TEQUIN in *in vitro* studies with the human CYP2C9, CYP1A2, CYP3A4 and CYP2C19 isoenzymes (see **PRECAUTIONS: Drug Interactions**).

Glyburide: Pharmacodynamic changes in glucose homeostasis were seen with concomitant administration of TEQUIN (once daily oral doses of 400 mg for 10 days) and glyburide (steady-state once daily regimen) in patients with type 2 diabetes mellitus. This was not associated with significant effects on the pharmacokinetic disposition of either drug. These latter results are consistent with the lack of effect of TEQUIN in *in vitro* studies with the human CYP3A4 isoenzyme (see **CLINICAL PHARMACOLOGY: Glucose Homeostasis** and **WARNINGS**).

Microbiology

Gatifloxacin is an 8-methoxyfluoroquinolone with *in vitro* activity against a wide range of gram-negative and gram-positive microorganisms. The antibacterial action of gatifloxacin results from inhibition of DNA gyrase and topoisomerase IV. DNA gyrase is an essential enzyme that is involved in the replication, transcription and repair of bacterial DNA. Topoisomerase IV is an enzyme known to play a key role in the partitioning of the chromosomal DNA during bacterial cell division. It appears that the C-8-methoxy moiety contributes to enhanced activity and lower selection of resistant mutants of gram-positive bacteria compared to the non-methoxy C-8 moiety.

The mechanism of action of fluoroquinolones including gatifloxacin is different from that of penicillins, cephalosporins, aminoglycosides, macrolides, and tetracyclines. Therefore, fluoroquinolones may be active against pathogens that are resistant to these antibiotics. There is no cross-resistance between gatifloxacin and the mentioned classes of antibiotics.

From *in vitro* synergy tests, gatifloxacin, as with other fluoroquinolones, is antagonistic with rifampin against enterococci.

Resistance to gatifloxacin *in vitro* develops slowly via multiple-step mutations. Resistance to gatifloxacin *in vitro* occurs at a general frequency of between 1×10^{-7} to 10^{-10}. Although cross-resistance has been observed between gatifloxacin and some other fluoroquinolones, some microorganisms resistant to other fluoroquinolones may be susceptible to gatifloxacin.

Gatifloxacin has been shown to be active against most strains of the following microorganisms, both *in vitro* and in clinical infections as described in the **INDICATIONS AND USAGE** section:

Aerobic gram-positive microorganisms
- *Staphylococcus aureus* (methicillin-susceptible strains only)
- *Streptococcus pneumoniae* (penicillin-susceptible strains)
- *Streptococcus pyogenes*

Aerobic gram-negative microorganisms
- *Escherichia coli*
- *Haemophilus influenzae*
- *Haemophilus parainfluenzae*
- *Klebsiella pneumoniae*
- *Moraxella catarrhalis*
- *Neisseria gonorrhoeae*
- *Proteus mirabilis*

Other microorganisms
- *Chlamydia pneumoniae*
- *Legionella pneumophila*
- *Mycoplasma pneumoniae*

The following *in vitro* data are available, **but their clinical significance is unknown.**

Gatifloxacin exhibits *in vitro* minimum inhibitory concentrations (MICs) of ≤2 µg/mL (≤1 µg/mL for *Streptococcus pneumoniae*) against most (≥90%) strains of the following microorganisms; however, the safety and effectiveness of gatifloxacin in treating clinical infections due to these microorganisms have not been established in adequate and well-controlled clinical trials.

Aerobic gram-positive microorganisms
- *Staphylococcus epidermidis* (methicillin-susceptible strains only)

Continued on next page

Tequin—Cont.

Staphylococcus saprophyticus
Streptococcus (Group C/G/F)
Streptococcus agalactiae
Streptococcus pneumoniae (penicillin-resistant strains)
Streptococcus (viridans group)

Aerobic gram-negative microorganisms
Acinetobacter lwoffii
Citrobacter freundii
Citrobacter koseri
Enterobacter aerogenes
Enterobacter cloacae
Klebsiella oxytoca
Morganella morganii
Proteus vulgaris

Anaerobic microorganisms
Peptostreptococcus species

NOTE: The activity of gatifloxacin against *Treponema pallidum* has not been evaluated; however, other quinolones are not active against *Treponema pallidum* (see **WARNINGS**).

NOTE: Extended-spectrum β-lactamase producing gram-negative microorganisms may have reduced susceptibility to quinolones.

Susceptibility Tests

Dilution techniques: Quantitative methods are used to determine antimicrobial minimum inhibitory concentrations (MICs). These MICs provide estimates of the susceptibility of bacteria to antimicrobial compounds. The MICs should be determined using a standardized procedure. Standardized procedures are based on a dilution method[1] (broth or agar) or equivalent with standardized inoculum concentrations and standardized concentrations of gatifloxacin powder. The MIC values should be interpreted according to the following criteria:

For testing *Enterobacteriaceae* and *Staphylococcus* species:

MIC (μg/mL)	Interpretation
≤2.0	Susceptible (S)
4.0	Intermediate (I)
≥8.0	Resistant (R)

For testing *Haemophilus influenzae* and *Haemophilus parainfluenzae*[a]:

MIC (μg/mL)	Interpretation
≤1.0	Susceptible (S)

[a] This interpretive standard is applicable only to broth microdilution susceptibility tests with *Haemophilus influenzae* and *Haemophilus parainfluenzae* using *Haemophilus* Test Medium (HTM).[1]

The current absence of data on resistant strains precludes defining any results other than "Susceptible". Strains yielding MIC results suggestive of a "nonsusceptible" category should be submitted to a reference laboratory for further testing.

For testing *Streptococcus pneumoniae*[b]:

MIC (μg/mL)	Interpretation
≤1.0	Susceptible (S)
2.0	Intermediate (I)
≥4.0	Resistant (R)

For testing *Streptococcus* species other than *Streptococcus pneumoniae*[b]:

MIC (μg/mL)	Interpretation
≤2.0	Susceptible (S)
4.0	Intermediate (I)
≥8.0	Resistant (R)

[b] These interpretive standards are applicable only to broth microdilution susceptibility tests using cation-adjusted Mueller-Hinton broth with 2-5% lysed horse blood.

For testing *Neisseria gonorrhoeae*[c]:

MIC (μg/mL)	Interpretation
≤0.125	Susceptible (S)
0.25	Intermediate (I)
≥0.5	Resistant (R)

[c] These interpretive standards are applicable to agar dilution tests with GC agar base and 1% defined growth supplement.

A report of "Susceptible" indicates that the pathogen is likely to be inhibited if the antimicrobial compound in the blood reaches the concentration usually achievable. A report of "Intermediate" indicates that the result should be considered equivocal, and if the microorganism is not fully susceptible to alternative, clinically feasible drugs, the test should be repeated. This category implies possible clinical applicability in body sites where the drug is physiologically concentrated or in situations where high dosage of drug can be used. This category also provides a buffer zone, which prevents small uncontrolled technical factors from causing major discrepancies in interpretation. A report of "Resistant" indicates that the pathogen is not likely to be inhibited if the antimicrobial compound in the blood reaches the concentration usually achievable; other therapy should be selected.

Standardized susceptibility test procedures require the use of laboratory control microorganisms to control the technical aspects of the laboratory procedures. Standard gatifloxacin powder should provide the following MIC values:

Microorganism	MIC Range (μg/mL)
Enterococcus faecalis ATCC 29212	0.12-1.0
Escherichia coli ATCC 25922	0.008-0.03
Haemophilus influenzae ATCC 49247[d]	0.004-0.03
Neisseria gonorrhoeae ATCC 49226[e]	0.002-0.016
Pseudomonas aeruginosa ATCC 27853	0.5-2.0
Staphylococcus aureus ATCC 29213	0.03-0.12
Streptococcus pneumoniae ATCC 49619[f]	0.12-0.5

[d] This quality control range is applicable to only *H. influenzae* ATCC 49247 tested by a broth microdilution procedure using HTM.[1]

[e] This quality control range is applicable to only *N. gonorrhoeae* ATCC 49226 tested by an agar dilution procedure using GC agar base with 1% defined growth supplement.[1]

[f] This quality control range is applicable to only *S. pneumoniae* ATCC 49619 tested by a microdilution procedure using cation-adjusted Mueller-Hinton broth with 2-5% lysed horse blood.[1]

Diffusion techniques: Quantitative methods that require measurement of zone diameters also provide reproducible estimates of the susceptibility of bacteria to antimicrobial compounds. One such standardized procedure[2] requires the use of standardized inoculum concentrations. This procedure uses paper disks impregnated with 5 μg gatifloxacin to test the susceptibility of microorganisms to gatifloxacin.

Reports from the laboratory providing results of the standard single-disk susceptibility test with a 5 μg gatifloxacin disk should be interpreted according to the following criteria:

The following zone diameter interpretive criteria should be used for testing *Enterobacteriaceae* and *Staphylococcus* species:

Zone Diameter (mm)	Interpretation
≥18	Susceptible (S)
15-17	Intermediate (I)
≤14	Resistant (R)

For testing *Haemophilus influenzae* and *Haemophilus parainflenzae*[g]:

Zone Diameter (mm)	Interpretation
≥18	Susceptible (S)

[g] This zone diameter standard is applicable only to tests with *Haemophilus influenzae* and *Haemophilus parainfluenzae* using *Haemophilus* Test Medium (HTM).[2]

The current absence of data on resistant strains precludes defining any results other than "Susceptible". Strains yielding MIC results suggestive of a "nonsusceptible" category should be submitted to a reference laboratory for further testing.

For testing *Streptococcus pneumoniae*[h]:

Zone Diameter (mm)	Interpretation
≥21	Susceptible (S)
18-20	Intermediate (I)
≤17	Resistant (R)

For testing *Streptococcus* species other than *Streptococcus pneumoniae*[h]:

Zone Diameter (mm)	Interpretation
≥18	Susceptible (S)
15-17	Intermediate (I)
≤14	Resistant (R)

[h] These zone diameter standards only apply to tests performed using Mueller-Hinton agar supplemented with 5% sheep blood incubated in 5% CO_2.[2]

For testing *Neisseria gonorrhoeae*[i]:

Zone Diameter (mm)	Interpretation
≥38	Susceptible (S)
34-37	Intermediate (I)
≤33	Resistant (R)

[i] These interpretive standards are applicable to disk diffusion tests with GC agar base and 1% defined growth supplement incubated in 5% CO_2.

Interpretation should be as stated above for results using dilution techniques. Interpretation involves correlation of the diameter obtained in the disk test with the MIC for gatifloxacin.[2]

As with standardized dilution techniques, methods require the use of laboratory control microorganisms that are used to control the technical aspects of the laboratory procedures. For the diffusion technique, the 5 μg gatifloxacin disk should provide the following zone diameters in these laboratory quality control strains:

Microorganism	Zone Diameter Range (mm)
Escherichia coli ATCC 25922	30-37
Haemophilus influenzae ATCC 49247[j]	33-41
Neisseria gonorrhoeae ATCC 49226[k]	45-56
Pseudomonas aeruginosa ATCC 27853	20-28
Staphylococcus aureus ATCC 25923	27-33
Streptococcus pneumoniae ATCC 49619[l]	24-31

[j] This quality control range applies to tests conducted with *Haemophilus influenzae* ATCC 49247 using *Haemophilus* Test Medium (HTM).[2]

[k] This quality control range is only applicable to tests conducted with *N. gonorrhoeae* ATCC 49226 performed by disk diffusion using GC agar base and 1% defined growth supplement.[2]

[l] This quality control range is applicable only to tests conducted with *S. pneumoniae* ATCC 49619 performed by disk diffusion using Mueller-Hinton agar supplemented with 5% defibrinated sheep blood.

INDICATIONS AND USAGE

TEQUIN (gatifloxacin) is indicated for the treatment of infections due to susceptible strains of the designated microorganisms in the conditions listed below (see **DOSAGE AND ADMINISTRATION**).

Acute bacterial exacerbation of chronic bronchitis due to *Streptococcus pneumoniae, Haemophilus influenzae, Haemophilus parainfluenzae, Moraxella catarrhalis*, or *Staphylococcus aureus*.

Acute sinusitis due to *Streptococcus pneumoniae* or *Haemophilus influenzae*.

Community-acquired pneumonia due to *Streptococcus pneumoniae, Haemophilus influenzae, Haemophilus parainfluenzae, Moraxella catarrhalis, Staphylococcus aureus, Mycoplasma pneumoniae, Chlamydia pneumoniae*, or *Legionella pneumophila*.

Uncomplicated skin and skin structure infections (i.e., simple abscesses, furuncles, folliculitis, wound infections, and cellulitis) due to *Staphylococcus aureus* (methicillin-susceptible strains only) or *Streptococcus pyogenes*.

NOTE: An insufficient number of patients with the diagnosis of impetiginous lesions were available for evaluation.

Uncomplicated urinary tract infections (cystitis) due to *Escherichia coli, Klebsiella pneumoniae*, or *Proteus mirabilis*.

Complicated urinary tract infections due to *Escherichia coli, Klebsiella pneumoniae*, or *Proteus mirabilis*.

Pyelonephritis due to *Escherichia coli*.

Uncomplicated urethral and cervical gonorrhea due to *Neisseria gonorrhoeae*. **Acute, uncomplicated rectal infections in women** due to *Neisseria gonorrhoeae* (see **WARNINGS**).

To reduce the development of drug-resistant bacteria and maintain the effectiveness of TEQUIN and other antibacterial drugs, TEQUIN should be used only to treat or prevent infections that are proven or strongly suspected to be caused by susceptible bacteria. When culture and susceptibility information are available, they should be considered in selecting or modifying antibacterial therapy. In the absence of such data, local epidemiology and susceptibility patterns may contribute to the empiric selection of therapy.

CONTRAINDICATIONS

TEQUIN (gatifloxacin) is contraindicated in persons with a history of hypersensitivity to gatifloxacin or any member of the quinolone class of antimicrobial agents.

WARNINGS

THE SAFETY AND EFFECTIVENESS OF GATIFLOXACIN IN PEDIATRIC PATIENTS, ADOLESCENTS (LESS THAN 18 YEARS OF AGE), PREGNANT WOMEN, AND LACTATING WOMEN HAVE NOT BEEN ESTABLISHED (see PRECAUTIONS: Pediatric Use, Pregnancy, and Nursing Mothers).

Prolongation of the QTc Interval

GATIFLOXACIN HAS THE POTENTIAL TO PROLONG THE QTc INTERVAL OF THE ELECTROCARDIOGRAM IN SOME PATIENTS. DUE TO THE LACK OF CLINICAL EXPERIENCE IN PATIENTS WITH KNOWN PROLONGATION OF THE QTc INTERVAL, PATIENTS WITH UNCORRECTED HYPOKALEMIA, AND PATIENTS RECEIVING CLASS IA (E.G., QUINIDINE, PROCAINAMIDE) OR CLASS III (E.G., AMIODARONE, SOTALOL) ANTIARRHYTHMIC AGENTS, GATIFLOXACIN SHOULD BE AVOIDED IN THESE PATIENT POPULATIONS.

Pharmacokinetic and pharmacodynamic studies between gatifloxacin and drugs that prolong the QTc interval such as cisapride, erythromycin, antipsychotics, and tricyclic antidepressants have not been performed. Gatifloxacin should be used with caution when given concurrently with these drugs, as well as in patients with ongoing proarrhythmic conditions, such as clinically significant bradycardia or acute myocardial ischemia.

The magnitude of QTc prolongation increases with increasing concentrations of the drug; therefore, the recommended dose and the recommended intravenous infusion rate should not be exceeded (see **DOSAGE AND ADMINISTRATION** for dosing recommendations for patients with or without renal impairment). QTc prolongation may lead to

an increased risk for ventricular arrhythmias including torsades de pointes (see **CLINICAL PHARMACOLOGY: Electrocardiogram**).
No cardiovascular morbidity or mortality attributable to QTc prolongation has occurred in over 44,000 patients treated with gatifloxacin in clinical trials; these include 118 patients concurrently receiving drugs known to prolong the QTc interval and 139 patients known to have uncorrected hypokalemia (ECG monitoring was not performed). During postmarketing surveillance, rare cases of torsades de pointes have been reported in patients taking gatifloxacin. These cases have occurred primarily in elderly patients with underlying medical problems for which they were receiving concomitant medications known to prolong the QTc interval; the contribution, if any, of gatifloxacin to the development of torsades de pointes in these patients is unknown.

Disturbances in Blood Glucose
Disturbances of blood glucose, including symptomatic hyper- and hypoglycemia, have been reported with TEQUIN, usually in diabetic patients. Therefore, careful monitoring of blood glucose is recommended when TEQUIN is administered to patients with diabetes (see **CLINICAL PHARMACOLOGY, PRECAUTIONS: Information for Patients** and **Drug Interactions**, and **ANIMAL PHARMACOLOGY**).
Studies conducted in non-infected patients with type 2 diabetes mellitus controlled on oral hypoglycemic agents have demonstrated that TEQUIN (gatifloxacin) is associated with disturbances in glucose homeostasis including an increase in serum insulin and decrease in serum glucose usually following administration of initial doses (i.e., first 2 days of treatment) and sometimes associated with symptomatic hypoglycemia. Increases in fasting serum glucose were also observed, usually after the third day of TEQUIN administration continuing throughout the duration of treatment, and returning to baseline by 28 days after the cessation of gatifloxacin treatment in most patients.
During the postmarketing period, there have been reports of serious disturbances of glucose homeostasis in patients being treated with TEQUIN. Hypoglycemic episodes, in some cases severe, have been reported in patients with diabetes mellitus treated with either sulfonylurea or non-sulfonylurea oral hypoglycemic medications. These events frequently occurred on the first day of therapy and usually within 3 days following the initiation of TEQUIN. Hyperglycemic episodes, in some cases severe and associated with hyperosmolar non-ketotic hyperglycemic coma, were reported in diabetic patients, mostly between 4 and 10 days following the initiation of TEQUIN therapy. Some of the hyperglycemic and hypoglycemic events were life-threatening and many required hospitalization, although these events were reversible when appropriately managed. Many of these patients had other underlying medical problems and were receiving concomitant medications that may have contributed to the glucose abnormality. Episodes of hyperglycemia, including hyperosmolar non-ketotic hyperglycemic coma, also occurred in patients not previously diagnosed with diabetes mellitus. Elderly patients who may have unrecognized diabetes, age-related decrease in renal function, underlying medical problems, and/or are taking concomitant medications associated with hyperglycemia may be at particular risk for serious hyperglycemia.
The dose of TEQUIN should be adjusted based on underlying renal function (see **DOSAGE AND ADMINISTRATION**). When TEQUIN is used in diabetic patients, blood glucose should be closely monitored. Signs and symptoms of hypoglycemia should be monitored, especially during the first 3 days of therapy, and signs and symptoms of hyperglycemia should be monitored in diabetics and patients who may be at risk for hyperglycemia, especially with continued treatment with TEQUIN beyond 3 days. If signs and symptoms of either hypoglycemia or hyperglycemia occur in any patient being treated with TEQUIN, appropriate therapy must be initiated immediately and TEQUIN should be discontinued.

Other
As with other members of the quinolone class, gatifloxacin has caused arthropathy and/or chondrodysplasia in immature dogs. The relevance of these findings to the clinical use of gatifloxacin is unknown (see **ANIMAL PHARMACOLOGY**).
Convulsions, increased intracranial pressure, and psychosis have been reported in patients receiving quinolones. Quinolones may also cause central nervous system (CNS) stimulation, which may lead to tremors, restlessness, lightheadedness, confusion, hallucinations, paranoia, depression, nightmares and insomnia. These reactions may occur following the first dose. If these reactions occur in patients receiving gatifloxacin, the drug should be discontinued and appropriate measures instituted (see **ADVERSE REACTIONS**).
As with other quinolones, TEQUIN (gatifloxacin) should be used with caution in patients with known or suspected CNS disorders, such as severe cerebral atherosclerosis, epilepsy, and other factors that predispose to seizures.
Serious and occasionally fatal hypersensitivity and/or anaphylactic reactions have been reported in patients receiving therapy with quinolones. These reactions may occur following the first dose. Some reactions have been accompanied by cardiovascular collapse, hypotension/shock, seizure, loss of consciousness, tingling, angioedema (including tongue, laryngeal, throat or facial edema/swelling), airway obstruction (including bronchospasm, shortness of breath, and acute respiratory distress), dyspnea, urticaria, itching and other serious skin reactions.
TEQUIN should be discontinued at the first appearance of a skin rash or any other sign of hypersensitivity. Serious acute hypersensitivity reactions may require treatment with epinephrine and other resuscitative measures, including oxygen, intravenous fluids, antihistamines, corticosteroids, pressor amines, and airway management, as clinically indicated (see **PRECAUTIONS**).
Serious and sometimes fatal events, some due to hypersensitivity and some due to uncertain etiology, have been reported in patients receiving antibacterial therapy. These events may be severe and generally occur following the administration of multiple doses. Clinical manifestations may include one or more of the following: fever, rash or severe dermatologic reactions (e.g., toxic epidermal necrolysis, Stevens-Johnson syndrome); vasculitis, arthralgia, myalgia, serum sickness; allergic pneumonitis, interstitial nephritis; acute renal insufficiency or failure; hepatitis, jaundice, acute hepatic necrosis or failure; anemia, including hemolytic and aplastic; thrombocytopenia, including thrombotic thrombocytopenic purpura; leukopenia; agranulocytosis; pancytopenia; and/or other hematologic abnormalities.
Pseudomembranous colitis has been reported with nearly all antibacterial agents, including TEQUIN, and may range in severity from mild to life-threatening. It is important, therefore, to consider this diagnosis in patients who present with diarrhea subsequent to the administration of any antibacterial agent.
Treatment with antibacterial agents alters the flora of the colon and may permit overgrowth of clostridia. Studies indicate that a toxin produced by *Clostridium difficile* is the primary cause of "antibiotic-associated colitis."
After the diagnosis of pseudomembranous colitis has been established, therapeutic measures should be initiated. Mild cases of pseudomembranous colitis usually respond to drug discontinuation alone. In moderate to severe cases, consideration should be given to management with fluids and electrolytes, protein supplementation, and treatment with an antibacterial drug clinically effective against *C. difficile* colitis.
Ruptures of the shoulder, hand, and Achilles tendons that required surgical repair or resulted in prolonged disability have been reported in patients receiving quinolones. TEQUIN (gatifloxacin) should be discontinued if the patient experiences pain, inflammation or rupture of a tendon. Patients should rest and refrain from exercise until the diagnosis of tendonitis or tendon rupture has been confidently excluded. Tendon rupture can occur during or after therapy with quinolones.
Gatifloxacin has not been shown to be effective in the treatment of syphilis. Antimicrobial agents used in high doses for short periods of time to treat gonorrhea may mask or delay the symptoms of incubating syphilis. All patients with gonorrhea should have a serologic test for syphilis at the time of diagnosis.

PRECAUTIONS

General
Prescribing TEQUIN in the absence of proven or strongly suspected bacterial infection or a prophylactic indication is unlikely to provide benefit to the patient and increases the risk of the development of drug-resistant bacteria.
Quinolones may cause central nervous system (CNS) events including nervousness, agitation, insomnia, anxiety, nightmares, or paranoia (see **WARNINGS** and **PRECAUTIONS: Information for Patients**).
Administer gatifloxacin with caution in the presence of renal insufficiency. Careful clinical observation and appropriate laboratory studies should be performed prior to and during therapy since elimination of gatifloxacin may be reduced. In patients with impaired renal function (creatinine clearance <40 mL/min), adjustment of the dosage regimen is necessary to avoid the accumulation of gatifloxacin due to decreased clearance (see **CLINICAL PHARMACOLOGY** and **DOSAGE AND ADMINISTRATION**).
Because a hypotonic solution results, Water for Injection should not be used as a diluent when preparing a 2 mg/mL solution from the concentrated solution of gatifloxacin (10 mg/mL) (see **DOSAGE AND ADMINISTRATION**).
Disturbances of blood glucose homeostasis have been reported during the postmarketing period (see **CLINICAL PHARMACOLOGY, WARNINGS,** and **ANIMAL PHARMACOLOGY**).

Information for Patients (See **Patient Information** Section.)
To assure safe and effective use of TEQUIN, the following information and instructions should be communicated to the patient when appropriate.
Patients should be advised:

- that antibacterial drugs including TEQUIN should only be used to treat bacterial infections. They do not treat viral infections (e.g., the common cold). When TEQUIN is prescribed to treat a bacterial infection, patients should be told that although it is common to feel better early in the course of therapy, the medication should be taken exactly as directed. Skipping doses or not completing the full course of therapy may (1) decrease the effectiveness of the immediate treatment and (2) increase the likelihood that bacteria will develop resistance and will not be treatable by TEQUIN or other antibacterial drugs in the future;
- that TEQUIN may produce changes in the electrocardiogram (QTc interval prolongation);
- that TEQUIN should be avoided in patients receiving Class IA (e.g., quinidine, procainamide) or Class III (e.g., amiodarone, sotalol) antiarrhythmic agents;
- that TEQUIN should be used with caution in patients receiving drugs that may effect the QTc interval such as cisapride, erythromycin, antipsychotics, and tricyclic antidepressants;
- to inform their physician of any personal or family history of QTc prolongation or proarrhythmic conditions such as recent hypokalemia, significant bradycardia, or recent myocardial ischemia;
- that disturbances of blood glucose, including symptomatic hyper- and hypoglycemia, have been reported with TEQUIN (gatifloxacin), usually in diabetic patients or in patients at risk for hyperglycemia. If a hypoglycemic reaction or symptoms of hyperglycemia occur, patients should initiate appropriate therapy immediately, discontinue TEQUIN, and contact their physician (see **CLINICAL PHARMACOLOGY** and **WARNINGS**);
- to inform their physician of any other medications when taken concurrently with TEQUIN, including over-the-counter medications;
- to contact their physician if they experience palpitations or fainting spells while taking TEQUIN;
- that TEQUIN Tablets may be taken with or without meals;
- that TEQUIN Tablets should be taken 4 hours before any aluminum- or magnesium-based antacids (see **PRECAUTIONS: Drug Interactions**);
- that TEQUIN Tablets should be taken at least 4 hours before the administration of ferrous sulfate or dietary supplements containing zinc, magnesium, or iron (such as multivitamins) (see **PRECAUTIONS: Drug Interactions**);
- that TEQUIN should be taken 4 hours before VIDEX® (didanosine) buffered tablets or pediatric powder for oral solution;
- that TEQUIN may be associated with hypersensitivity reactions, even following the first dose, and to discontinue the drug at the first sign of a skin rash, hives or other skin reactions, difficulty in swallowing or breathing, any swelling suggesting angioedema (e.g., swelling of the lips, tongue, face, tightness of the throat, hoarseness), or other symptoms of an allergic reaction (see **WARNINGS** and **ADVERSE REACTIONS**);
- to discontinue treatment; rest and refrain from exercise; and inform their physician if they experience pain, inflammation, or rupture of a tendon;
- that TEQUIN may cause dizziness and lightheadedness; therefore, patients should know how they react to this drug before they operate an automobile or machinery or engage in activities requiring mental alertness or coordination;
- that phototoxicity has been reported in patients receiving certain quinolones. There was no phototoxicity seen with gatifloxacin at the recommended dose. In keeping with good medical practice, avoid excessive sunlight or artificial ultraviolet light (e.g., tanning beds). If sunburn-like reaction or skin eruptions occur, contact their physician (see **CLINICAL PHARMACOLOGY: Photosensitivity Potential**);
- that convulsions have been reported in patients receiving quinolones, and they should notify their physician before taking this drug if there is a history of this condition.

Drug Interactions
TEQUIN (gatifloxacin) can be taken 4 hours before ferrous sulfate, dietary supplements containing zinc, magnesium, or iron (such as multivitamins), or aluminum/magnesium-containing antacids without any significant pharmacokinetic interactions (see **CLINICAL PHARMACOLOGY**).
Milk, calcium carbonate, cimetidine, theophylline, warfarin, or midazolam: No significant interactions have been observed when administered concomitantly with TEQUIN. No dosage adjustments are necessary when these drugs are administered concomitantly with TEQUIN (see **CLINICAL PHARMACOLOGY**).
Antidiabetic agents: Pharmacodynamic changes in glucose homeostasis have been seen with concomitant glyburide use. However, no significant pharmacokinetic interactions have been observed when glyburide was administered concomitantly with TEQUIN (see **CLINICAL PHARMACOLOGY: Glucose Homeostasis** and **WARNINGS**).
Digoxin: Concomitant administration of TEQUIN and digoxin did not produce significant alteration of the pharmacokinetics of gatifloxacin; however, an increase in digoxin concentrations was observed for 3 of 11 subjects. Patients taking digoxin should therefore be monitored for signs and/or symptoms of toxicity. In patients who display signs and/or symptoms of digoxin intoxication, serum digoxin concentrations should be determined, and digoxin dosage should be adjusted as appropriate (see **CLINICAL PHARMACOLOGY**).
Probenecid: The systemic exposure of TEQUIN is significantly increased following the concomitant administration of TEQUIN and probenecid (see **CLINICAL PHARMACOLOGY**).
Warfarin: In subjects receiving warfarin, no significant change in clotting time was observed when gatifloxacin was coadministered. However, because some quinolones have been reported to enhance the effects of warfarin or its derivatives, prothrombin time or other suitable anticoagulation test should be monitored closely if a quinolone antimicrobial is administered with warfarin or its derivatives.
Nonsteroidal anti-inflammatory drugs (NSAIDs): Although not observed with gatifloxacin in preclinical and clinical tri-

Continued on next page

Tequin—Cont.

als, the concomitant administration of nonsteroidal anti-inflammatory drugs with a quinolone may increase the risks of CNS stimulation and convulsions (see **WARNINGS**).

Laboratory Test Interactions

There are no reported laboratory test interactions.

Carcinogenesis, Mutagenesis, Impairment of Fertility

B6C3F1 mice given gatifloxacin in the diet for 18 months at doses with an average intake up to 81 mg/kg/day in males and 90 mg/kg/day in females showed no increases in neoplasms. These doses are approximately 0.13 and 0.18 times the maximum recommended human dose based upon daily systemic exposure (AUC).

In a 2-year dietary carcinogenicity study in Fischer 344 rats, no increases in neoplasms were seen in males given doses up to 47 mg/kg/day and females given up to 139 mg/kg/day. These doses are approximately 0.36 (males) and 0.81 (females) times the maximum recommended human dose based upon daily systemic exposure. A statistically significant increase in the incidence of large granular lymphocyte (LGL) leukemia was seen in males treated with a high dose of 100 mg/kg/day (approximately 0.74 times the maximum recommended human dose based upon daily systemic exposure) versus controls. Although Fischer 344 rats have a high spontaneous background rate of LGL leukemia, the incidence in high-dose males slightly exceeded the historical control range established for this strain. The findings in high-dose males are not considered a concern with regard to the safe use of gatifloxacin in humans.

In genetic toxicity tests, gatifloxacin was not mutagenic in several strains of bacteria used in the Ames test; however, it was mutagenic to *Salmonella* strain TA102. Gatifloxacin was negative in four *in vivo* assays that included oral and intravenous micronucleus tests in mice, an oral cytogenetics test in rats, and an oral DNA repair test in rats. Gatifloxacin was positive in *in vitro* gene-mutation assays in Chinese hamster V-79 cells and *in vitro* cytogenetics assays in Chinese hamster CHL/IU cells. These findings were not unexpected; similar findings have been seen with other quinolones and may be due to the inhibitory effects of high concentrations on eukaryotic type II DNA topoisomerase.

There were no adverse effects on fertility or reproduction in rats given gatifloxacin orally at doses up to 200 mg/kg/day (approximately equivalent to the maximum human dose based on systemic exposure [AUC]).

Pregnancy: Category C

There were no teratogenic effects observed in rats or rabbits at oral gatifloxacin doses up to 150 or 50 mg/kg, respectively (approximately 0.7 and 1.9 times the maximum human dose based on systemic exposure). However, skeletal malformations were observed in fetuses from rats given 200 mg/kg/day orally or 60 mg/kg/day intravenously during organogenesis. Developmental delays in skeletal ossification, including wavy ribs, were observed in fetuses from rats given oral doses of ≥150 mg/kg or intravenous doses of ≥30 mg/kg daily during organogenesis, suggesting that gatifloxacin is slightly fetotoxic at these doses. Similar findings have been seen with other quinolones. These changes were not seen in rats or rabbits given oral doses of gatifloxacin up to 50 mg/kg (approximately 0.2 and 1.9 times the maximum human dose, respectively, based on systemic exposure).

When rats were given oral doses of 200 mg/kg of gatifloxacin beginning in late pregnancy and continuing throughout lactation, late postimplantation loss increased, as did neonatal and perinatal mortalities. These observations also suggest fetotoxicity. Similar findings have been seen with other quinolones.

Because there are no adequate and well-controlled studies in pregnant women, TEQUIN (gatifloxacin) should be used during pregnancy only if the potential benefit outweighs the potential risk to the fetus.

Nursing Mothers

Gatifloxacin is excreted in the breast milk of rats. It is not known whether this drug is excreted in human milk. Because many drugs are excreted in human milk, caution should be exercised when gatifloxacin is administered to a nursing woman.

Pediatric Use

The safety and effectiveness of gatifloxacin in pediatric populations (<18 years of age) have not been established. Quinolones, including gatifloxacin, cause arthropathy and osteochondrotoxicity in juvenile animals (rats and dogs).

Geriatric Use

During the postmarketing period, serious disturbances of glucose homeostasis have been reported in elderly patients being treated with TEQUIN (gatifloxacin) (see **WARNINGS, PRECAUTIONS: Drug Interactions** and **ANIMAL PHARMACOLOGY**).

In multiple-dose clinical trials of gatifloxacin (n = 2891), 22% of patients were ≥65 years of age and 10% were ≥75 years of age. No overall differences in safety or efficacy were observed in clinical trials between these subjects and younger subjects, and other reported clinical experience has not identified differences in responses between the elderly and younger patients, but greater sensitivity of some older individuals cannot be ruled out.

This drug is known to be substantially excreted by the kidney, and the risk of toxic reactions to this drug may be greater in patients with impaired renal function. Because elderly patients are more likely to have decreased renal function, care should be taken in dose selection, and it may be useful to monitor renal function (see **DOSAGE AND ADMINISTRATION**).

ADVERSE REACTIONS

Over 5000 patients have been treated with gatifloxacin in single- and multiple-dose clinical efficacy trials worldwide.

In gatifloxacin studies, the majority of adverse reactions were described as mild in nature. Gatifloxacin was discontinued for adverse events thought related to drug in 2.7% of patients.

Drug-related adverse events classified as possibly, probably, or definitely related with a frequency of ≥3% in patients receiving gatifloxacin in single- and multiple-dose clinical trials are as follows: nausea 8%, vaginitis 6%, diarrhea 4%, headache 3%, dizziness 3%.

In patients who were treated with either intravenous gatifloxacin or with intravenous followed by oral therapy, the incidence of adverse events was similar to those who received oral therapy alone. Local injection site reactions (redness at injection site) were noted in 5% of patients.

Additional drug-related adverse events (possibly, probably, or definitely related) considered clinically relevant that occurred in ≥0.1% to <3% of patients receiving gatifloxacin in single- and multiple-dose clinical trials are as follows:

Body as a Whole: allergic reaction, asthenia, back pain, chest pain, chills, face edema, fever

Cardiovascular System: hypertension, palpitation

Digestive System: abdominal pain, anorexia, constipation, dyspepsia, flatulence, gastritis, glossitis, mouth ulcer, oral moniliasis, stomatitis, vomiting

Metabolic/Nutritional System: hyperglycemia, peripheral edema, thirst

Musculoskeletal System: arthralgia, leg cramp

Nervous System: abnormal dream, agitation, anxiety, confusion, insomnia, nervousness, paresthesia, somnolence, tremor, vasodilatation, vertigo

Respiratory System: dyspnea, pharyngitis

Skin/Appendages: dry skin, pruritus, rash, sweating

Special Senses: abnormal vision, taste perversion, tinnitus

Urogenital System: dysuria

Additional drug-related adverse events considered clinically relevant that occurred in <0.1% (rare adverse events) of patients receiving gatifloxacin in single- and multiple-dose clinical trials are as follows: abnormal thinking, alcohol intolerance, arthritis, asthma (bronchospasm), ataxia, bone pain, bradycardia, breast pain, cheilitis, colitis, convulsion, cyanosis, depersonalization, depression, diabetes mellitus, dysphagia, ear pain, ecchymosis, edema, epistaxis, euphoria, eye pain, eye photosensitivity, gastrointestinal hemorrhage, generalized edema, gingivitis, halitosis, hallucination, hematemesis, hematuria, hostility, hyperesthesia, hypertonia, hyperventilation, hypoglycemia, lymphadenopathy, maculopapular rash, metrorrhagia, migraine, mouth edema, myalgia, myasthenia, neck pain, panic attack, paranoia, parosmia, photophobia, pseudomembranous colitis, psychosis, ptosis, rectal hemorrhage, stress, substernal chest pain, tachycardia, taste loss, tongue edema, vesiculobullous rash.

Laboratory Changes

Clinically relevant changes in laboratory parameters, without regard to drug relationship, occurred in fewer than 1% of TEQUIN-treated patients. These included the following: neutropenia, increased ALT or AST levels, alkaline phosphatase, bilirubin, serum amylase, and electrolytes abnormalities. It is not known whether these abnormalities were caused by the drug or the underlying condition being treated.

Postmarketing Adverse Event Reports

The following events have been reported during postapproval use of TEQUIN (gatifloxacin). Because these events are reported voluntarily from a population of uncertain size, it is not always possible to reliably estimate their frequency or establish a causal relationship to drug exposure.

Abnormal renal function (including acute renal failure), acute allergic reaction including anaphylactic reaction and angioneurotic edema, hepatitis, hypotension, increased International Normalized Ratio (INR)/prothrombin time, pancreatitis, severe hyperglycemia (including hyperosmolar nonketotic hyperglycemia), severe hypoglycemia (including hypoglycemic coma), Stevens-Johnson syndrome, syncope, tendon rupture, thrombocytopenia, and torsades de pointes.

OVERDOSAGE

Gatifloxacin exhibits a low potential for acute toxicity in animal studies. The minimum lethal oral doses in rats and dogs were greater than 2000 mg/kg and 1000 mg/kg, respectively. The minimum lethal intravenous dose was 144 mg/kg in rats and greater than 45 mg/kg in dogs. Clinical signs observed included decreased activity and respiratory rate, vomiting, tremors, and convulsions.

In the event of acute oral overdose, the stomach should be emptied by inducing vomiting or by gastric lavage. The patient should be carefully observed (including ECG monitoring) and given symptomatic and supportive treatment. Adequate hydration should be maintained. Gatifloxacin is not efficiently removed from the body by hemodialysis (approximately 14% recovered over 4 hours) or by chronic ambulatory peritoneal dialysis (CAPD) (approximately 11% recovered over 8 days).

DOSAGE AND ADMINISTRATION

The recommended dosage for TEQUIN (gatifloxacin) Tablets or TEQUIN Injection is described in Table 4. Doses of TEQUIN are administered once every 24 hours. These recommendations apply to all patients with a creatinine clearance ≥40 mL/min. For patients with a creatinine clearance <40 mL/min, see the **Impaired Renal Function** subsection.

TEQUIN can be administered without regard to food, including milk and dietary supplements containing calcium.

Oral doses of TEQUIN should be administered at least 4 hours before the administration of ferrous sulfate, dietary supplements containing zinc, magnesium, or iron (such as multivitamins), aluminum/magnesium-containing antacids, or VIDEX® (didanosine) buffered tablets or pediatric powder for oral solution.

TEQUIN can be administered without regard to gender or age (≥18 years). Consideration should be given to the possibility that the elderly may have impaired renal function (see **PRECAUTIONS: Geriatric Use**).

When switching from intravenous to oral dosage administration, no dosage adjustment is necessary. Patients whose therapy is started with TEQUIN Injection may be switched to TEQUIN Tablets when clinically indicated at the discretion of the physician.

TEQUIN (gatifloxacin) Injection should be administered by INTRAVENOUS infusion only. It is not intended for intramuscular, intrathecal, intraperitoneal, or subcutaneous administration.

Single-use vials require dilution prior to administration. (See *Preparation of Gatifloxacin for Intravenous Administration.*)

TEQUIN Injection should be administered by intravenous infusion over a period of 60 minutes. CAUTION: RAPID OR BOLUS INTRAVENOUS INFUSION SHOULD BE AVOIDED.

Table 4: Gatifloxacin — Dosage Guidelines

INFECTION[a]	DAILY DOSE[b]	DURATION
Acute Bacterial Exacerbation of Chronic Bronchitis	400 mg	5 days
Acute Sinusitis	400 mg	10 days
Community-acquired Pneumonia	400 mg	7-14 days
Uncomplicated Skin and Skin Structure Infections	400 mg	7-10 days
Uncomplicated Urinary Tract Infections (cystitis)	400 mg or 200 mg	Single dose 3 days
Complicated Urinary Tract Infections	400 mg	7-10 days
Acute Pyelonephritis	400 mg	7-10 days
Uncomplicated Urethral Gonorrhea in Men; Endocervical and Rectal Gonorrhea in Women	400 mg	Single dose

[a] Due to the designated pathogens (see **INDICATIONS AND USAGE**).

[b] For either the oral or intravenous routes of administration for TEQUIN (see **CLINICAL PHARMACOLOGY**).

Impaired Renal Function

Since gatifloxacin is eliminated primarily by renal excretion, a dosage modification of TEQUIN is recommended for patients with creatinine clearance <40 mL/min, including patients on hemodialysis and on CAPD. The recommended dosage of TEQUIN is:

Table 5: Recommended Dosage of TEQUIN in Adult Patients with Renal Impairment

Creatinine Clearance	Initial Dose	Subsequent Dose[a]
≥40 mL/min	400 mg	400 mg every day
<40 mL/min	400 mg	200 mg every day
Hemodialysis	400 mg	200 mg every day
Continuous peritoneal dialysis	400 mg	200 mg every day

[a] Start subsequent dose on Day 2 of dosing.

Administer TEQUIN (gatifloxacin) after a dialysis session for patients on hemodialysis.

Single 400 mg dose TEQUIN regimen (for the treatment of uncomplicated urinary tract infections and gonorrhea) and 200 mg once daily for 3 days TEQUIN regimen (for the treatment of uncomplicated urinary tract infections) require no dosage adjustment in patients with impaired renal function.

The following formula may be used to estimate creatinine clearance:

[See table at top of next page]

Chronic Hepatic Disease

No adjustment in the dosage of TEQUIN is necessary in patients with moderate hepatic impairment (Child-Pugh Class B). There are no data in patients with severe hepatic impairment (Child-Pugh Class C) (see **CLINICAL PHARMACOLOGY**).

Intravenous Administration

Preparation of Gatifloxacin for Intravenous Administration

TEQUIN solution in single-use vials: TEQUIN Injection is supplied in single-use 40 mL vials (10 mg/mL) containing a concentrated solution of gatifloxacin in 5% dextrose (400 mg of gatifloxacin) (see **HOW SUPPLIED**). THESE TEQUIN INJECTION SINGLE-USE VIALS MUST BE FURTHER DILUTED WITH AN APPROPRIATE SOLUTION PRIOR TO INTRAVENOUS ADMINISTRATION. The concentration of the resulting diluted solution should be 2 mg/mL prior to administration.

Compatible intravenous solutions: Because a hypotonic solution results, Water for Injection should not be used as a diluent when preparing a 2 mg/mL solution from the concentrated solution of gatifloxacin (10 mg/mL) (see **PRECAUTIONS**). Any of the following intravenous solutions may be used to prepare a 2 mg/mL gatifloxacin solution:

5% Dextrose Injection, USP
0.9% Sodium Chloride Injection, USP
5% Dextrose and 0.9% Sodium Chloride Injection, USP
Lactated Ringer's and 5% Dextrose Injection, USP
5% Sodium Bicarbonate Injection, USP
Plasma-Lyte® 56 and 5% Dextrose Injection (Multiple Electrolytes and Dextrose Injection, Type 1, USP)
M/6 Sodium Lactate Injection, USP

Plasma-Lyte® is a registered trademark of Baxter International, Inc.

Gatifloxacin solutions at 2 mg/mL also have been shown to be compatible with 20 mEq/L Potassium Chloride in 5% Dextrose and 0.45% Sodium Chloride Injection, USP.

This intravenous drug product should be inspected visually for particulate matter prior to dilution and administration. Samples containing visible particles should be discarded. Since no preservative or bacteriostatic agent is present in this product, aseptic technique must be used in preparation of the final intravenous solution. Since the vials are for single-use only, any unused portion remaining in the vial should be discarded.

Since only limited data are available on the compatibility of gatifloxacin intravenous injection with other intravenous substances, additives or other medications should not be added to TEQUIN (gatifloxacin) Injection in single-use vials or infused simultaneously through the same intravenous line.

If the same intravenous line is used for sequential infusion of different drugs, the line should be flushed before and after infusion of TEQUIN Injection with an infusion solution compatible with TEQUIN Injection and with any other drug(s) administered via this common line.

If TEQUIN Injection is to be given concomitantly with another drug, each drug should be given separately in accordance with the recommended dosage and route of administration for each drug.

TEQUIN Injection premix in single-use flexible containers: TEQUIN Injection is also available in ready-to-use 100 and 200 mL flexible bags containing a dilute solution of 200 or 400 mg gatifloxacin in 5% dextrose. NO FURTHER DILUTION OF THIS PREPARATION IS NECESSARY.

This intravenous drug product should be inspected visually for particulate matter prior to administration. Samples containing visible particles should be discarded.

Since the premix flexible bags are for single use only, any unused portion should be discarded.

Since only limited data are available on the compatibility of gatifloxacin intravenous injection with other intravenous substances, additives or other medications should not be added to TEQUIN Injection in flexible containers or infused simultaneously through the same intravenous line. If the same intravenous line is used for sequential infusion of different drugs, the line should be flushed before and after infusion of TEQUIN (gatifloxacin) Injection with an infusion solution compatible with TEQUIN Injection and with any other drug(s) administered via this common line.

Instructions for the use of TEQUIN (gatifloxacin in 5% dextrose) Injection premix in flexible containers:

To open:

1. Tear outer wrap at the notch and remove solution container.
2. Check the container for minute leaks by squeezing the inner bag firmly. If leaks are found, or if the seal is not intact, discard the solution, as the sterility may be compromised.
3. Use only if solution is clear and light yellow to greenish-yellow in color.
4. Use sterile equipment.
5. **WARNING: Do not use flexible containers in series connections.** Such use could result in air embolism due to residual air being drawn from the primary container before administration of the fluid from the secondary container is complete.

Preparation for administration:

1. Close flow control clamp of administration set.
2. Remove cover from port at bottom of container.

$$\text{Men: Creatinine Clearance (mL/min)} = \frac{\text{Weight (kg)} \times (140 - \text{age})}{72 \times \text{serum creatinine (mg/dL)}}$$

Women: 0.85 × the value calculated for men.

3. Insert piercing pin of administration set into port with a twisting motion until the pin is firmly seated. **NOTE: See full directions on administration set carton.**
4. Suspend container from hanger.
5. Squeeze and release drip chamber to establish proper fluid level in chamber during infusion of TEQUIN Injection premix in flexible containers.
6. Open flow control clamp to expel air from set. Close clamp.
7. Regulate rate of administration with flow control clamp.

Stability of TEQUIN Injection as Supplied

When stored under recommended conditions, TEQUIN Injection, as supplied in 20 mL and 40 mL vials and in 100 mL and 200 mL flexible containers, is stable through the expiration date printed on the label.

Stability of TEQUIN Injection Following Dilution

TEQUIN Injection, when diluted in a compatible intravenous fluid to a concentration of 2 mg/mL, is stable for 14 days when stored between 20°C to 25°C or when stored under refrigeration between 2°C to 8°C.

TEQUIN Injection, when diluted to a concentration of 2 mg/mL in a compatible intravenous fluid EXCEPT FOR 5% SODIUM BICARBONATE INJECTION, USP, may be stored for up to 6 months at -25°C to -10°C (-13°F to 14°F). Frozen solutions may be thawed at controlled room temperature. Solutions that have been thawed are stable for 14 days after removal from the freezer when stored between 20°C to 25°C or when stored under refrigeration between 2°C to 8°C. Solutions should not be refrozen.

HOW SUPPLIED

Tablets

TEQUIN® (gatifloxacin) Tablets are available as 200 mg and 400 mg white, film-coated tablets. The tablets are almond shaped and biconvex and contain gatifloxacin sesquihydrate equivalent to either 200 mg or 400 mg gatifloxacin.

TEQUIN Tablets are packaged in bottles, unit dose blister strips, and multidose blister packs of 5 tablets (TEQUIN Teq-Paqs™) in the following configurations:

200 mg tablets — color: white; shape: biconvex; debossing: "BMS" on one side and "TEQUIN" and "200" on the other.
Bottles of 30 (NDC 0015-1117-50)
Blister pack of 100 (NDC 0015-1117-80)
400 mg tablets — color: white; shape: biconvex; debossing: "BMS" on one side and "TEQUIN" and "400" on the other.
Bottles of 50 (NDC 0015-1177-60)
Blister pack of 100 (NDC 0015-1177-80)
Carton of 3 TEQUIN Teq-Paqs™ (5 tablets each) (NDC 0015-1177-21)

Storage

Store at 25°C (77°F); excursions permitted to 15° to 30°C (59° to 86°F) [see USP Controlled Room Temperature].

Intravenous Solution — Single-Use Vials

TEQUIN® (gatifloxacin) Injection is available for intravenous administration in the following configuration:

Single-use vials containing a clear, light yellow to greenish-yellow solution at a concentration of 10 mg/mL gatifloxacin.
10 mg/mL (400 mg), 40 mL vials (NDC 0015-1179-80)

Storage

Store at 25°C (77°F); excursions permitted to 15° to 30°C (59° to 86°F) [see USP Controlled Room Temperature].

Intravenous Solution — Premix Bags

TEQUIN® (gatifloxacin in 5% dextrose) Injection is available in ready-to-use flexible bags containing a dilute solution of 200 mg or 400 mg of gatifloxacin in 5% dextrose. Premix bags are manufactured by Abbott Laboratories in North Chicago, IL.

2 mg/mL (200 mg), 100 mL flexible container (NDC 0015-1180-80)
Carton of 24 (NDC 0015-1180-79)
2 mg/mL (400 mg), 200 mL flexible container (NDC 0015-1181-80)
Carton of 24 (NDC 0015-1181-79)

Storage

Store at 25°C (77°F); excursions permitted to 15° to 30°C (59° to 86°F) [see USP Controlled Room Temperature].
Do not freeze.

ANIMAL PHARMACOLOGY

In three animal species (rats, beagle dogs, and cynomolgus monkeys) given oral gatifloxacin doses approximately 1.0- to 19-times the approved human dose (based on body surface area) from one to six months, electron microscopy showed vesiculation of rough endoplasmic reticulum and decreased secretory granules in pancreatic β-cells of all three species. These ultrastructural changes correlated with vacuolation of pancreatic β-cells seen by light microscopy in dogs given a dose level for one or six months that was approximately equivalent to the human dose (based upon body surface area and plasma AUC). Following a 4-week recovery period without gatifloxacin, partial recovery from these pancreatic changes was seen in the rat, and complete recovery was evident in beagle dogs and cynomologus monkeys (see **WARNINGS** and **CLINICAL PHARMACOLOGY**).

In contrast to some other quinolone antibacterials, there was no evidence of phototoxicity when gatifloxacin was evaluated in the hairless mouse or guinea pig models using simulated sunlight or UVA radiation, respectively.

Unlike some other members of the quinolone class, crystalluria, ocular toxicity, and testicular degeneration were not observed in 6-month repeat dose studies with rats or dogs given gatifloxacin.

While some quinolone antibacterials have proconvulsant activity that is exacerbated with concomitant use of nonsteroidal anti-inflammatory drugs (NSAIDs), gatifloxacin did not produce an increase in seizure activity when administered intravenously to mice at doses up to 100 mg/kg in combination with the NSAID fenbufen.

Quinolone antibacterials have been shown to cause arthropathy in immature animals. There is no evidence of arthropathy in fully mature rats and dogs given gatifloxacin for 6 months at doses of 240 or 24 mg/kg, respectively (approximately 1.5 times the maximum human dose in both species based on systemic exposure). Arthropathy and chondrodysplasia were observed in immature dogs given 10 mg/kg gatifloxacin orally for 7 days (approximately equal to the maximum human dose based upon systemic exposure) [see **WARNINGS**]. The relevance of these findings to the clinical use of gatifloxacin is unknown.

Some other members of the quinolone class have been shown to cause prolongation of the QT interval in dogs. Intravenous 10 mg/kg bolus doses of gatifloxacin had no effect on QT interval in anesthetized dogs.

REFERENCES

1. National Committee for Clinical Laboratory Standards. *Methods for Dilution Antimicrobial Susceptibility Tests for Bacteria That Grows Aerobically* - Fifth Edition; Approved Standard, NCCLS Document M7-A5, Vol. 20, No. 2, NCCLS, Wayne, PA, January 2000.
2. National Committee for Clinical Laboratory Standards. *Performance Standards for Antimicrobial Disk Susceptibility Tests* - Seventh Edition; Approved Standard, NCCLS Document M2-A7, Vol. 20, No. 1, NCCLS, Wayne, PA, January 2000.

Patient Information About:

TEQUIN® (gatifloxacin)

200 mg and 400 mg Tablets

This section contains important information about TEQUIN (gatifloxacin) that you should read before you begin treatment. This section does not list all the benefits and risks of TEQUIN and does not take the place of discussions with your doctor or healthcare professional about your medical condition or your treatment. If you have questions, talk with your healthcare professional. The medicine described here can only be prescribed by a licensed healthcare professional. Only your healthcare professional can determine if TEQUIN is right for you.

What is TEQUIN?

TEQUIN (*pronounced TEK win*) is an antibiotic used to treat lung, sinus, skin, or urinary tract infections, and also to treat certain sexually transmitted diseases caused by germs called bacteria. TEQUIN kills many of the kinds of bacteria that can infect the lungs, sinus, skin, and urinary tract and that cause certain sexually transmitted diseases. TEQUIN has been shown in a large number of clinical trials to be safe and effective for the treatment of bacterial infections.

Sometimes viruses, rather than bacteria, may infect the lungs and sinuses (for example, the common cold). TEQUIN, like all other antibiotics, does not kill viruses.

The sexually transmitted disease called gonorrhea is treated by TEQUIN. Other diseases called syphilis or non-gonococcal disease are not treated by TEQUIN.

You should contact your doctor if you think your condition is not improving while taking TEQUIN. TEQUIN Tablets are white and contain either 200 mg or 400 mg of active drug.

How and when should I take TEQUIN?

TEQUIN should be taken once a day for 1 to 14 days depending on your prescription. It should be swallowed whole and may be taken with or without food. Try to take the tablet at the same time each day.

You may begin to feel better quickly; however, in order to make sure that all bacteria are killed, you should complete the full course of medication. Do not take more than the prescribed dose of TEQUIN. Try not to miss a dose, but if you do, take it as soon as possible. If it is almost time for the next dose, skip the missed dose and continue your regular dose.

Who should not take TEQUIN?

You should avoid TEQUIN (gatifloxacin) if you have ever had a severe allergic reaction to any medicine in the group of antibiotics known as "quinolones" such as CIPRO® (ciprofloxacin) or LEVAQUIN® (levofloxacin).

Continued on next page

Tequin—Cont.

You should avoid TEQUIN if you have a rare condition known as congenital prolongation of the QTc interval. If any of your family members have this condition, you should inform your healthcare professional.
You should avoid TEQUIN if you are being treated for heart rhythm disturbances with certain medicines such as quinidine, procainamide, amiodarone, or sotalol. Inform your healthcare professional if you are taking a heart rhythm drug.
You should avoid TEQUIN if you have a condition known as hypokalemia (low blood potassium). Hypokalemia may be caused by medicines called diuretics such as furosemide and hydrochlorothiazide. If you are taking a diuretic you should speak with your healthcare professional.
If you are pregnant or planning to become pregnant while taking TEQUIN, talk to your doctor before taking this medication. TEQUIN is not recommended for use during pregnancy or nursing, as the effects on the unborn child or nursing infant are unknown.
TEQUIN is not recommended for children.

What about other medications I am taking?

It is important to let your healthcare provider know all of the medicines that you are using.

- It is important to let your healthcare provider know if you are taking certain medicines that can have an effect on an electrocardiogram test, such as cisapride, erythromycin, some antidepressants, and some antipsychotic drugs.
- You should tell your healthcare professional if you are taking medicines called diuretics (also sometimes called water pills) such as furosemide and hydrochlorothiazide, because diuretics can sometimes cause low potassium.
- If you have diabetes, it is important to let your healthcare provider know that you have this condition and what medications you are taking for it.
- Many antacids and multivitamins may interfere with the absorption of TEQUIN and may prevent it from working properly. You should take TEQUIN 4 hours before taking these products.

What are the possible side effects of TEQUIN?

TEQUIN (gatifloxacin) is generally well tolerated. The most common side effects that can occur while taking TEQUIN are usually mild and include nausea, vomiting, stomach pain, diarrhea, dizziness, and headache. You should be careful about driving or operating machinery until you are sure TEQUIN does not cause dizziness. If you notice any side effects not mentioned in this section or if you have any questions or concerns about the side effects you are experiencing, please discuss them with your healthcare professional.
In a few people, TEQUIN, like some other antibiotics, may produce a small effect on the heart that is seen on an electrocardiogram test. Although this has not caused any problems in more than 4000 patients who have taken TEQUIN in premarketing clinical trials, in theory, it could result in extremely rare cases of abnormal heartbeat, which may be dangerous. Contact your healthcare professional if you develop heart palpitations (fast beating) or have fainting spells.
Disturbances of blood sugar, including high blood sugar (hyperglycemia) and low blood sugar (hypoglycemia), have been reported with TEQUIN in diabetic patients. Elderly patients with additional medical problems or taking additional medications may also be at risk for high blood sugar. If you develop low blood sugar while on TEQUIN, you should take immediate measures to increase your blood sugar, stop taking TEQUIN, and contact your healthcare professional at once. If you develop high blood sugar while on TEQUIN, you should contact your healthcare professional at once before taking additional TEQUIN. If you have diabetes or suspect that you may have diabetes, discuss how to detect changes in your blood sugar with your healthcare professional at once before taking additional TEQUIN.

Where can I get more information about TEQUIN?

This section is a summary of the most important information about TEQUIN. It does not include everything there is to know about TEQUIN. If you have any questions or problems, you should talk to your doctor or healthcare provider. There is also a leaflet (Package Insert) written for healthcare professionals that your pharmacist can let you read. You may want to read this information and discuss it with your doctor or healthcare professional. Remember, no written information can replace careful discussion with your doctor.

Remember

- Take your dose of TEQUIN once a day.
- Complete the course of medication (take all of the pills) even if you are feeling better.
- Do not use TEQUIN for another condition or give it to others.
- Store TEQUIN tablets at room temperature in a tightly sealed container.
- Throw away TEQUIN when it is outdated or no longer needed by flushing it down the toilet.
- Keep this and all medications out of reach of children.

CIPRO® (ciprofloxacin) is a registered trademark of the Bayer Corporation.
LEVAQUIN® (levofloxacin) is a registered trademark of Ortho-McNeil Pharmaceutical, Inc.

Bristol-Myers Squibb Company
Princeton, NJ 08543 U.S.A.
E5-B001-10-03 Revised October 2003
J4-677M 117880DIM-16
Licensed from Kyorin Pharmaceutical Company, Limited. Tokyo, Japan.
Shown in Product Identification Guide, page 310

VIDEX® EC ℞

[*vī-dĕks*]
(didanosine)
℞ ONLY
VIDEX® EC (didanosine) Delayed-Release Capsules Enteric-Coated Beadlets
(Patient Information Leaflet Included)

WARNING
FATAL AND NONFATAL PANCREATITIS HAVE OCCURRED DURING THERAPY WITH DIDANOSINE USED ALONE OR IN COMBINATION REGIMENS IN BOTH TREATMENT-NAIVE AND TREATMENT-EXPERIENCED PATIENTS, REGARDLESS OF DEGREE OF IMMUNOSUPPRESSION. VIDEX EC SHOULD BE SUSPENDED IN PATIENTS WITH SUSPECTED PANCREATITIS AND DISCONTINUED IN PATIENTS WITH CONFIRMED PANCREATITIS (SEE WARNINGS).
LACTIC ACIDOSIS AND SEVERE HEPATOMEGALY WITH STEATOSIS, INCLUDING FATAL CASES, HAVE BEEN REPORTED WITH THE USE OF NUCLEOSIDE ANALOGUES ALONE OR IN COMBINATION, INCLUDING DIDANOSINE AND OTHER ANTIRETROVIRALS. FATAL LACTIC ACIDOSIS HAS BEEN REPORTED IN PREGNANT WOMEN WHO RECEIVED THE COMBINATION OF DIDANOSINE AND STAVUDINE WITH OTHER ANTIRETROVIRAL AGENTS. THE COMBINATION OF DIDANOSINE AND STAVUDINE SHOULD BE USED WITH CAUTION DURING PREGNANCY AND IS RECOMMENDED ONLY IF THE POTENTIAL BENEFIT CLEARLY OUTWEIGHS THE POTENTIAL RISK (SEE WARNINGS AND PRECAUTIONS: PREGNANCY).

DESCRIPTION

VIDEX® EC (didanosine) is the brand name for an enteric-coated formulation of didanosine (ddI), a synthetic purine nucleoside analogue active against the Human Immunodeficiency Virus (HIV). VIDEX EC (didanosine) Delayed-Release Capsules, containing enteric-coated beadlets, are available for oral administration in strengths of 125, 200, 250, and 400 mg of didanosine. The inactive ingredients in the beadlets include carboxymethylcellulose sodium 12, diethyl phthalate, methacrylic acid copolymer, sodium hydroxide, sodium starch glycolate, and talc. The capsule shells contain colloidal silicon dioxide, gelatin, sodium lauryl sulfate, and titanium dioxide. The capsules are imprinted with edible inks.
Didanosine is also available as buffered formulations. Please consult the prescribing information for VIDEX (didanosine) Chewable/Dispersible Buffered Tablets and Pediatric Powder for Oral Solution for additional information.
The chemical name for didanosine is 2′,3′-dideoxyinosine. The structural formula is:

Didanosine is a white crystalline powder with the molecular formula $C_{10}H_{12}N_4O_3$ and a molecular weight of 236.2. The aqueous solubility of didanosine at 25°C and pH of approximately 6 is 27.3 mg/mL. Didanosine is unstable in acidic solutions. For example, at pH <3 and 37°C, 10% of didanosine decomposes to hypoxanthine in less than 2 minutes. In VIDEX EC (didanosine), an enteric coating is used to protect didanosine from degradation by stomach acid.

MICROBIOLOGY

Mechanism of Action: Didanosine is a synthetic nucleoside analogue of the naturally occurring nucleoside deoxyadenosine in which the 3′-hydroxyl group is replaced by hydrogen. Intracellularly, didanosine is converted by cellular enzymes to the active metabolite, dideoxyadenosine 5′-triphosphate. Dideoxyadenosine 5′-triphosphate inhibits the activity of HIV-1 reverse transcriptase both by competing with the natural substrate, deoxyadenosine 5′-triphosphate, and by its incorporation into viral DNA causing termination of viral DNA chain elongation.

***In Vitro* HIV Susceptibility:** The *in vitro* anti-HIV-1 activity of didanosine was evaluated in a variety of HIV-1 infected lymphoblastic cell lines and monocyte/macrophage cell cultures. The concentration of drug necessary to inhibit viral replication by 50% (IC_{50}) ranged from 2.5 to 10 μM (1 μM = 0.24 μg/mL) in lymphoblastic cell lines and 0.01 to 0.1 μM in monocyte/macrophage cell cultures. The relationship between *in vitro* susceptibility of HIV to didanosine and the inhibition of HIV replication in humans has not been established.

Drug Resistance: HIV-1 isolates with reduced sensitivity to didanosine have been selected *in vitro* and were also obtained from patients treated with didanosine. Genetic analysis of isolates from didanosine-treated patients showed mutations in the reverse transcriptase gene that resulted in the amino acid substitutions K65R, L74V, and M184V. The L74V mutation was most frequently observed in clinical isolates. Phenotypic analysis of HIV-1 isolates from 60 patients (some with prior zidovudine treatment) receiving 6 to 24 months of didanosine monotherapy showed that isolates from 10 of 60 patients exhibited an average of a 10-fold decrease in susceptibility to didanosine *in vitro* compared to baseline isolates. Clinical isolates that exhibited a decrease in didanosine susceptibility harbored one or more didanosine-associated mutations. The clinical relevance of genotypic and phenotypic changes associated with didanosine therapy has not been established.

Cross-resistance: HIV-1 isolates from 2 of 39 patients receiving combination therapy for up to 2 years with zidovudine and didanosine exhibited decreased susceptibility to zidovudine, didanosine, zalcitabine, stavudine, and lamivudine *in vitro* These isolates harbored five mutations (A62V, V75I, F77L, F116Y, and Q151M) in the reverse transcriptase gene. The clinical relevance of these observations has not been established.

CLINICAL PHARMACOLOGY

Animal Toxicology: Evidence of a dose-limiting skeletal muscle toxicity has been observed in mice and rats (but not in dogs) following long-term (greater than 90 days) dosing with didanosine at doses that were approximately 1.2 to 12 times the estimated human exposure. The relationship of this finding to the potential of didanosine to cause myopathy in humans is unclear. However, human myopathy has been associated with administration of didanosine and other nucleoside analogues.

Pharmacokinetics: The pharmacokinetic parameters of didanosine are summarized in Table 1. Didanosine is rapidly absorbed, with peak plasma concentrations generally observed from 0.25 to 1.50 hours following oral dosing with a buffered formulation. Increases in plasma didanosine concentrations were dose proportional over the range of 50 to 400 mg. Steady-state pharmacokinetic parameters did not differ significantly from values obtained after a single dose. Binding of didanosine to plasma proteins *in vitro* was low (<5%). Based on data from *in vitro* and animal studies, it is presumed that the metabolism of didanosine in man occurs by the same pathways responsible for the elimination of endogenous purines.

Table 1
Pharmacokinetic Parameters for Didanosine in Adults

Parameter	Mean ± SD	n
Oral bioavailability[a]	42±12%	6
Apparent volume of distribution[b]	1.08±0.22 L/kg	6

Table 2
Mean ± SD Pharmacokinetic Parameters for Didanosine Following a Single Oral Dose of a Buffered Formulation

Parameter	Creatinine Clearance (mL/min) ≥ 90 (n=12)	60–90 (n=6)	30–59 (n=6)	10–29 (n=3)	Dialysis Patients (n=11)
CL_{cr}(mL/min)	112±22	68±8	46±8	13±5	ND
CL/F (mL/min)	2164±638	1566±833	1023±378	628±104	543±174
CL_R(mL/min)	458±164	247±153	100±44	20±8	<10
$T_{1/2}$ (h)	1.42±0.33	1.59±0.13	1.75±0.43	2.0±0.3	4.1±1.2

ND = not determined due to anuria.
CL_{cr} = creatinine clearance.
CL/F = apparent oral clearance.
CL_R = renal clearance.

Table 3
Results of Drug Interaction Studies with VIDEX EC: Effects of Coadministered Drug on Didanosine Plasma AUC and C_{MAX} Values[a]

Drug	Didanosine Dosage	n	AUC of Didanosine (90% CI)	C_{MAX} of Didanosine (90% CI)
tenofovir,[b] 300 mg once daily with a light meal[c]	400 mg single dose fasting 2 h before tenofovir	26	↑48% (31, 67%)	↑48% (25, 76%)
tenofovir,[b] 300 mg once daily with a light meal[c]	400 mg single dose with tenofovir and a light meal	25	↑60% (44, 79%)	↑64% (41, 89%)
tenofovir,[b] 300 mg once daily with a light meal[c]	200 mg single dose with tenofovir and a light meal	33	↑16% (6, 27%)[d]	↓12% (-25, 3%)
	250 mg single dose with tenofovir and a light meal	33	↔ (-13, 5%)[e]	↓20% (-32, -7%)[e]
	325 mg single dose with tenofovir and a light meal	33	↑13% (3, 24%)[e]	↓11% (-24, 4%)[e]

↑ indicates increase.
↓ indicates decrease.
↔ indicates no change, or mean increase or decrease of <10%.
[a] All studies conducted in healthy volunteers ≥60 kg with creatinine clearance ≥60 mL/min.
[b] tenofovir disoproxil fumarate.
[c] 373 kcalories, 8.2 grams fat.
[d] Compared with VIDEX EC 250 mg administered alone under fasting conditions.
[e] Compared with VIDEX EC 400 mg administered alone under fasting conditions.

Table 4
Results of Drug Interaction Studies with VIDEX EC (didanosine): Effects of Didanosine on Coadministered Drug Plasma AUC and C_{MAX} Values[a]

Drug	Didanosine Dosage	n	AUC of Coadministered Drug	C_{MAX} of Coadministered Drug
ciprofloxacin, 750 mg single dose	400 mg single dose	16	↔	↔
indinavir, 800 mg single dose	400 mg single dose	23	↔	↔
ketoconazole, 200 mg single dose	400 mg single dose	21	↔	↔
tenofovir,[b] 300 mg once daily with a light meal[c]	400 mg single dose fasting 2 h before tenofovir	25	↔	↔
tenofovir,[b] 300 mg once daily with a light meal[c]	400 mg single dose with tenofovir and a light meal	25	↔	

↔ indicates no change, or mean increase or decrease of <10%.
[a] All studies conducted in healthy volunteers ≥60 kg with creatinine clearance ≥60 mL/min.
[b] tenofovir disoproxil fumarate.
[c] 373 kcalories, 8.2 grams fat.

Table 5
Results of Drug Interaction Studies with Buffered Formulations of Didanosine: Effects of Coadministered Drug on Didanosine Plasma AUC and C_{MAX} Values

Drugs With Clinical Recommendations Regarding Coadministration *(see* **PRECAUTIONS: Drug Interactions***)*

Drug	Didanosine Dosage	n	AUC of Didanosine (95% CI)	C_{MAX} of Didanosine (95% CI)
allopurinol, renally impaired, 300 mg/day	200 mg single dose	2	↑312%	↑232%
healthy volunteer, 300 mg/day for 7 days	400 mg single dose	14	↑113%	↑69%
ganciclovir, 1000 mg q8h, 2 h after didanosine	200 mg q12h	12	↑111%	NA
methadone, chronic maintenance dose	200 mg single dose	16, 10[a]	↓57%	↓66%
tenofovir,[b] 300 mg once daily 1 h after didanosine	250[c] or 400 mg once daily for 7 days	14	↑44% (31, 59%)[d]	↑28% (11, 48%)[d]

(Table continued on next page)

CSF-plasma ratio[b]	21±0.03%[c]	5
Systemic clearance[b]	13.0±1.6 mL/min/kg	6
Renal clearance[a]	5.5±2.1 mL/min/kg	6
Elimination half-life[a]	1.5±0.4 h	6
Urinary recovery of didanosine[a]	18±8%	6

CSF = cerebrospinal fluid.
[a] following oral administration of a buffered formulation.
[b] following I.V. administration.
[c] mean ± SE.

Comparison of Didanosine Formulations—In VIDEX EC (didanosine) the active ingredient, didanosine, is protected against degradation by stomach acid by the use of an enteric coating on the beadlets in the capsule. The enteric coating dissolves when the beadlets empty into the small intestine, the site of drug absorption. With buffered formulations of didanosine, administration with antacid provides protection from degradation by stomach acid.

In healthy volunteers, as well as subjects infected with HIV, the area under the plasma concentration time curve (AUC) is equivalent for didanosine administered as the VIDEX EC (didanosine) formulation relative to a buffered tablet formulation. The peak plasma concentration (C_{MAX} of didanosine, administered as VIDEX EC, is reduced approximately 40% relative to didanosine buffered tablets. The time to the peak concentration (T_{MAX}) increases from approximately 0.67 hours for didanosine buffered tablets to 2.0 hours for VIDEX EC (didanosine).

Effect of Food on Absorption of Didanosine—In the presence of food, the C_{MAX} and AUC for VIDEX EC were reduced by approximately 46% and 19%, respectively, compared to the fasting state. VIDEX EC should be taken on an empty stomach.

Special Populations:

Renal Insufficiency—It is recommended that the VIDEX EC dose be modified in patients with reduced creatinine clearance and in patients receiving maintenance hemodialysis (see **DOSAGE AND ADMINISTRATION**). Data from two studies using a buffered formulation of didanosine indicated that the apparent oral clearance of didanosine decreased and the terminal elimination half-life increased as creatinine clearance decreased (see Table 2). Following oral administration, didanosine was not detectable in peritoneal dialysate fluid (n=6); recovery in hemodialysate (n=5) ranged from 0.6% to 7.4% of the dose over a 3–4 hour dialysis period. The absolute bioavailability of didanosine was not affected in patients requiring dialysis.

[See table 2 at bottom of previous page]

Pediatric Patients—The pharmacokinetics of didanosine administered as VIDEX EC have not been studied in pediatric patients.

Geriatric Patients—Didanosine pharmacokinetics have not been studied in patients over 65 years of age (see **PRECAUTIONS: Geriatric Use**).

Gender—The effects of gender on didanosine pharmacokinetics have not been studied.

Drug Interactions: (See also **PRECAUTIONS: Drug Interactions.**)

Ribavirin has been shown *in vitro* to increase intracellular triphosphate levels of didanosine, which could cause or worsen clinical toxicities (see **PRECAUTIONS: Drug Interactions**).

VIDEX EC (didanosine)—Tables 3 and 4 summarize the effects on AUC and C_{MAX}, with a 90% confidence interval (CI) when available, following coadministration of VIDEX EC with a variety of drugs. Clinical recommendations based on drug interaction studies for drugs in bold font are included in **PRECAUTIONS: Drug Interactions** and **DOSAGE AND ADMINISTRATION.**

[See table 3 at left]
[See table 4 at left]

Didanosine Buffered Formulations—Tables 5 and 6 summarize the effects on AUC and C_{MAX}, with a 90% or 95% CI when available, following coadministration of buffered formulations of didanosine with a variety of drugs. Except as noted in table footnotes, the results of these studies may be expected to apply to VIDEX EC. For most of the listed drugs, no clinically significant pharmacokinetic interactions were noted. Clinical recommendations based on drug interaction studies for drugs in bold font are included in **PRECAUTIONS: Drug Interactions** and **DOSAGE AND ADMINISTRATION** (for tenofovir).

[See table 5 at left and on next page]
[See table 6 at top of page 1085]

INDICATIONS AND USAGE

VIDEX EC (didanosine) in combination with other antiretroviral agents is indicated for the treatment of HIV-1 infection in adults. (See Clinical Studies.)

Clinical Studies: Study AI454-152 was a 48-week, randomized, open-label study comparing VIDEX EC (didanosine) (400 mg once daily) plus stavudine (40 mg twice daily) plus nelfinavir (750 mg three times daily) to zidovudine (300 mg) plus lamivudine (150 mg) combination tablets twice daily plus nelfinavir (750 mg three times daily) in 511 treatment-naive patients, with a mean CD4 cell count of 411 cells/mm³ (range 39 to 1105 cells/mm³) and a mean plasma HIV-1 RNA of 4.71 $\log_{10}$ copies/mL (range 2.8 to 5.9 $\log_{10}$ copies/mL) at baseline. Patients were primarily males (72%) and Caucasian (53%) with a mean age of 35 years (range 18 to 73 years). The percentages of patients with HIV RNA <400 and <50 copies/mL and outcomes of patients through 48 weeks are summarized in Figure 1 and Table 7, respectively.

Figure 1. Treatment Response Through Week 48*, AI454-152

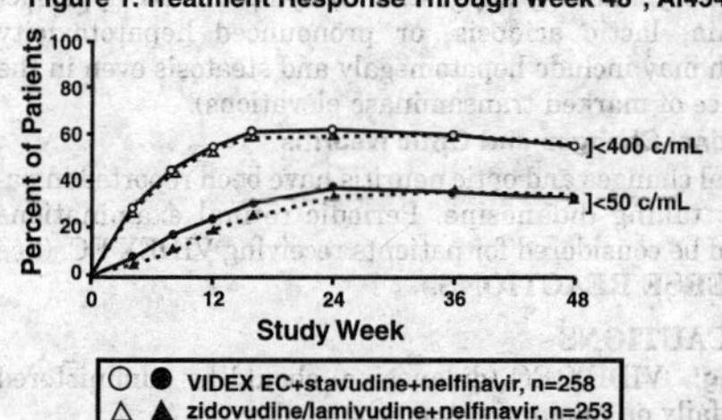

***Percent of patients at each time point who have HIV RNA <400 or <50 copies/mL and do not meet any criteria for treatment failure (e.g., virologic failure or discontinuation for any reason).**

Continued on next page

Videx EC—Cont.

Table 7
Outcomes of Randomized Treatment Through Week 48, AI454-152

Outcome	Percent of Patients with HIV RNA <400 copies/mL (<50 copies/mL) VIDEX EC +stavudine+ nelfinavir n=258	zidovudine/ lamivudine[a]+ nelfinavir n=253
Responder[b,c]	55% (33%)	56% (33%)
Virologic failure[d]	22% (45%)	21% (43%)
Death or discontinued due to disease progression	1% (1%)	2% (2%)
Discontinued due to adverse event	6% (6%)	7% (7%)
Discontinued due to other reasons[e]	16% (16%)	15% (16%)

[a] Zidovudine/lamivudine combination tablet.
[b] Corresponds to rates at Week 48 in Figure 1.
[c] Subjects achieved and maintained confirmed HIV RNA <400 copies/mL (<50 copies/mL) through Week 48.
[d] Includes viral rebound at or before Week 48 and failure to achieve confirmed HIV RNA <400 copies/mL (<50 copies/mL) through Week 48.
[e] Includes lost to follow-up, subject's withdrawal, discontinuation due to physician's decision, never treated, and other reasons.

Table 5 *(cont.)*
Results of Drug Interaction Studies with Buffered Formulations of Didanosine: Effects of Coadministered Drug on Didanosine Plasma AUC and C_{MAX} Values

No Clinically Significant Interaction Observed

Drug	Didanosine Dosage	n	AUC of Didanosine (95% CI)	C_{MAX} of Didanosine (95% CI)
ciprofloxacin, 750 mg q12h for 3 days, 2 h before didanosine	200 mg q12h for 3 days	8[e]	↓16%	↓28%
indinavir, 800 mg single dose simultaneous	200 mg single dose	16	↔	↔
1 h before didanosine	200 mg single dose	16	↓17% (−27, −7%)[d]	↓13% (−28, 5%)[d]
ketoconazole, 200 mg/day for 4 days, 2 h before didanosine	375 mg q12h for 4 days	12[e]	↔	↓12%
loperamide, 4 mg q6h for 1 day	300 mg single dose	12[e]	↔	↓23%
metoclopramide, 10 mg single dose	300 mg single dose	12[e]	↔	↑13%
ranitidine, 150 mg single dose, 2 h before didanosine	375 mg single dose	12[e]	↑14%	↑13%
rifabutin, 300 or 600 mg/day for 12 days	167 or 250 mg q12h for 12 days	11	↑13% (−1, 27%)	↑17% (−4, 38%)
ritonavir, 600 mg q12h for 4 days	200 mg q12h for 4 days	12	↓13% (0, 23%)	↓16% (5, 26%)
stavudine, 40 mg q12h for 4 days	100 mg q12h for 4 days	10	↔	
sulfamethoxazole, 1000 mg single dose	200 mg single dose	8[e]	↔	↔
trimethoprim, 200 mg single dose	200 mg single dose	8[e]	↔	↑17% (−23, 77%)
zidovudine, 200 mg q8h for 3 days	200 mg q12h for 3 days	6[e]	↔	↔

↑ indicates increase.
↓ indicates decrease.
↔indicates no change, or mean increase or decrease of <10%.
[a] Parallel-group design; entries are subjects receiving combination and control regimens, respectively.
[b] tenofovir disoproxil fumarate.
[c] patients <60 kg with creatinine clearance ≥60 mL/min.
[d] 90% CI.
[e] HIV-infected patients.
NA Not available.

CONTRAINDICATION

VIDEX EC (didanosine) is contraindicated in patients with previously demonstrated clinically significant hypersensitivity to any component of the formulation.

WARNINGS

1. Pancreatitis

FATAL AND NONFATAL PANCREATITIS HAVE OCCURRED DURING THERAPY WITH DIDANOSINE USED ALONE OR IN COMBINATION REGIMENS IN BOTH TREATMENT-NAIVE AND TREATMENT-EXPERIENCED PATIENTS, REGARDLESS OF DEGREE OF IMMUNOSUPPRESSION. VIDEX EC SHOULD BE SUSPENDED IN PATIENTS WITH SIGNS OR SYMPTOMS OF PANCREATITIS AND DISCONTINUED IN PATIENTS WITH CONFIRMED PANCREATITIS. PATIENTS TREATED WITH VIDEX EC IN COMBINATION WITH STAVUDINE, WITH OR WITHOUT HYDROXYUREA, MAY BE AT INCREASED RISK FOR PANCREATITIS.

When treatment with life-sustaining drugs known to cause pancreatic toxicity is required, suspension of VIDEX EC therapy is recommended. In patients with risk factors for pancreatitis, VIDEX EC should be used with extreme caution and only if clearly indicated. Patients with advanced HIV infection, especially the elderly, are at increased risk of pancreatitis and should be followed closely. Patients with renal impairment may be at greater risk for pancreatitis if treated without dose adjustment.

The frequency of pancreatitis is dose related. In phase 3 studies with buffered formulations of didanosine, incidence ranged from 1% to 10% with doses higher than are currently recommended and 1% to 7% with recommended dose.

2. Lactic Acidosis/Severe Hepatomegaly with Steatosis

Lactic acidosis and severe hepatomegaly with steatosis, including fatal cases, have been reported with the use of nucleoside analogues alone or in combination, including didanosine and other antiretrovirals. A majority of these cases have been in women. Obesity and prolonged nucleoside exposure may be risk factors. Fatal lactic acidosis has been reported in pregnant women who received the combination of didanosine and stavudine with other antiretroviral agents. The combination of didanosine and stavudine should be used with caution during pregnancy and is recommended only if the potential benefit clearly outweighs the potential risk (see **PRECAUTIONS: Pregnancy**). Particular caution should be exercised when administering VIDEX EC to any patient with known risk factors for liver disease; however, cases have also been reported in patients with no known risk factors. Treatment with VIDEX EC should be suspended in any patient who develops clinical or laboratory findings suggestive of symptomatic hyperlactatemia, lactic acidosis, or pronounced hepatotoxicity (which may include hepatomegaly and steatosis even in the absence of marked transaminase elevations).

3. Retinal Changes and Optic Neuritis

Retinal changes and optic neuritis have been reported in patients taking didanosine. Periodic retinal examinations should be considered for patients receiving VIDEX EC. (See **ADVERSE REACTIONS**.)

PRECAUTIONS

Dosing: VIDEX EC (didanosine) should be administered once daily on an empty stomach.

Peripheral Neuropathy: Peripheral neuropathy, manifested by numbness, tingling, or pain in the hands or feet, has been reported in patients receiving didanosine therapy. Peripheral neuropathy has occurred more frequently in patients with advanced HIV disease, in patients with a history of neuropathy, or in patients being treated with neurotoxic drug therapy, including stavudine (see **ADVERSE REACTIONS**).

Fat Redistribution: Redistribution/accumulation of body fat including central obesity, dorsocervical fat enlargement (buffalo hump), peripheral wasting, facial wasting, breast enlargement, and "cushingoid appearance" have been observed in patients receiving antiretroviral therapy. The mechanism and long-term consequences of these events are currently unknown. A causal relationship has not been established.

General:

Patients with Renal Impairment—Patients with renal impairment (creatinine clearance <60 mL/min) may be at greater risk of toxicity from didanosine due to decreased drug clearance (see **CLINICAL PHARMACOLOGY**). A dose reduction is recommended in these patients (see **DOSAGE AND ADMINISTRATION**).

Patients with Hepatic Impairment—It is unknown if hepatic impairment significantly affects didanosine pharmacokinetics. Therefore, these patients should be monitored closely for evidence of didanosine toxicity.

Hyperuricemia—Didanosine has been associated with asymptomatic hyperuricemia; treatment suspension may be necessary if clinical measures aimed at reducing uric acid levels fail.

Information for Patients (See Patient Information Leaflet.): Patients should be informed that a serious toxicity of didanosine, used alone and in combination regimens, is pancreatitis, which may be fatal.

Patients should also be aware that peripheral neuropathy, manifested by numbness, tingling, or pain in hands or feet, may develop during therapy with VIDEX EC (didanosine). Patients should be counseled that peripheral neuropathy occurs with greatest frequency in patients with advanced HIV disease or a history of peripheral neuropathy, and that dose modification and/or discontinuation of VIDEX EC may be required if toxicity develops.

Patients should be informed that when didanosine is used in combination with other agents with similar toxicities, the incidence of adverse events may be higher than when didanosine is used alone. These patients should be followed closely.

Patients should be cautioned about the use of medications or other substances, including alcohol, that may exacerbate VIDEX EC toxicities.

VIDEX EC (didanosine) is not a cure for HIV infection, and patients may continue to develop HIV-associated illnesses, including opportunistic infection. Therefore, patients should remain under the care of a physician when using VIDEX EC. Patients should be advised that VIDEX EC therapy has not been shown to reduce the risk of transmission of HIV to others through sexual contact or blood contamination. Patients should be informed that the long-term effects of VIDEX EC (didanosine) are unknown at this time. Patients should be informed that redistribution or accumulation of body fat may occur in patients receiving antiretroviral therapy and that the cause and long-term health effects of these conditions are not known at this time.

Drug Interactions (see also CLINICAL PHARMACOLOGY: Drug Interactions): Drug interactions that have been established based on drug interaction studies are listed with the pharmacokinetic results in **CLINICAL PHARMACOLOGY: Drug Interactions** (Tables 3–6). The clinical recommendations based on the results of these studies are listed in Table 8.

[See table 8 on next page]

Coadministration of VIDEX EC with drugs that are known to cause pancreatitis may increase the risk of this toxicity (see WARNINGS: Pancreatitis). Predicted drug interactions with VIDEX EC are listed in Table 9.

[See table 9 at top of page 1086]

Nucleoside/nucleotide analogues

Tenofovir disoproxil fumarate. Exposure to didanosine is increased when coadministered with tenofovir (see Tables 3, 5, and 8). **Increased exposure may cause or worsen didanosine-related clinical toxicities, including pancreatitis, symptomatic hyperlactatemia/lactic acidosis, and peripheral neuropathy. Coadministration of tenofovir with VIDEX EC should be undertaken with caution, and patients should be monitored closely for didanosine-related toxicities. VIDEX EC should be suspended if signs or symptoms of pancreatitis, symptomatic hyperlactatemia, or lactic acidosis develop (see WARNINGS).** Administration of reduced doses of VIDEX EC with tenofovir and a light meal resulted in didanosine exposures (AUC) similar to the recommended doses of VIDEX EC given alone in the fasted state (see Table 3). Therefore, when administered with tenofovir, a dose reduction of VIDEX EC to 250 mg (adults weighing ≥60 kg with creatinine clearance ≥60 mL/min) or 200 mg (adults weighing <60 kg with creatinine clearance ≥60 mL/min) once daily is recommended and both drugs may be taken together with a light meal (≤400 kcalories, ≤20% fat) or in the fasted state (see **DOSAGE AND ADMINISTRATION**). Coadministration of didanosine with food decreases didanosine concentrations. Thus, although not studied, it is possible that coadministration with heavier meals could reduce didanosine concentrations further.

Table 6
Results of Drug Interaction Studies with Buffered Formulations of Didanosine: Effects of Didanosine on Coadministered Drug Plasma AUC and C_{MAX} Values

No Clinically Significant Interaction Observed

Drug	Didanosine Dosage	n	AUC of Coadministered Drug (95% CI)	C_{MAX} of Coadministered Drug (95% CI)
dapsone, 100 mg single dose	200 mg q12h for 14 days	6[a]	↔	↔
delavirdine, 400 mg single dose				
simultaneous	125 or 200 mg q12h	12[a]	↓32%[b]	↓53%[b]
1 hr before didanosine	125 or 200 mg q12h	12[a]	↑20%	↑18%
ganciclovir, 1000 mg q8h, 2 h after didanosine	200 mg q12h	12[a]	↓21%	NA
nelfinavir, 750 mg single dose, 1 h after didanosine	200 mg single dose	10[a]	↑12%	↔
ranitidine, 150 mg single dose, 2 h before didanosine	375 mg single dose	12[a]	↓16%	↔
ritonavir, 600 mg q12h for 4 days	200 mg q12h for 4 days	12	↔	↔
stavudine, 40 mg q12h for 4 days	100 mg q12h for 4 days	10[a]	↔	↑17%
sulfamethoxazole, 1000 mg single dose	200 mg single dose	8[a]	↓11% (−17, −4%)	↓12% (−28, 8%)
tenofovir,[c] 300 mg once daily 1 h after didanosine	250[d] or 400 mg once daily for 7 days	14	↔	↔
trimethoprim, 200 mg single dose	200 mg single dose	8[a]	↑10% (−9, 34%)	↓22% (−59, 49%)
zidovudine, 200 mg q8h for 3 days	200 mg q12h for 3 days	6[a]	↓10% (−27, 11%)	↓16.5% (−53, 47%)

↑ indicates increase.
↓ indicates decrease.
↔indicates no change, or mean increase or decrease of <10%.
[a] HIV-infected patients.
[b] This result is probably related to the buffer and is not expected to occur with VIDEX EC.
[c] tenofovir disoproxil fumarate.
[d] patients <60 kg with creatinine clearance ≥60 mL min.
NA Not available.

Table 8
Established Drug Interactions Based on Studies with VIDEX EC or Studies with Buffered Formulations of Didanosine and Expected to Occur with VIDEX EC

***Coadministration Not Recommended Based on Drug Interaction Studies** (see **CLINICAL PHARMACOLOGY: Drug Interactions** for Magnitude of Interaction)*

Drug	Effect	Clinical Comment
allopurinol	↑didanosine concentration	Coadministration not recommended.

***Alteration in Dose or Regimen Recommended Based on Drug Interaction Studies** (see **CLINICAL PHARMACOLOGY: Drug Interactions** for Magnitude of Interaction)*

Drug	Effect	Clinical Comment
ganciclovir	↑didanosine concentration	Appropriate doses for this combination, with respect to efficacy and safety, have not been established.
methadone	↓didanosine concentration	Appropriate doses for this combination, with respect to efficacy and safety, have not been established.
tenofovir disoproxil fumarate	↑didanosine concentration	A dose reduction of VIDEX EC to 250 mg (adults weighing ≥60 kg with creatinine clearance ≥60 mL/min) or 200 mg (adults weighing <60 kg with creatinine clearance ≥60 mL/min) once daily taken together with tenofovir and a light meal (≤400 kcalories and ≤20% fat) or in the fasted state is recommended. Patients should be monitored for didanosine-associated toxicities (see below).

↑ indicates increase.
↓ indicates decrease.

Ribavirin: Exposure to the active metabolite of didanosine (dideoxyadenosine 5′-triphosphate) is increased when didanosine is coadministered with ribavirin (see Table 9). Fatal hepatic failure, as well as peripheral neuropathy, pancreatitis, and symptomatic hyperlactatemia/lactic acidosis have been reported in patients receiving both didanosine and ribavirin. Coadministration of didanosine and ribavirin is not recommended.

Carcinogenesis and Mutagenesis: Lifetime carcinogenicity studies were conducted in mice and rats for 22 and 24 months, respectively. In the mouse study, initial doses of 120, 800, and 1200 mg/kg/day for each sex were lowered after 8 months to 120, 210, and 210 mg/kg/day for females and 120, 300, and 600 mg/kg/day for males. The two higher doses exceeded the maximally tolerated dose in females and the high dose exceeded the maximally tolerated dose in males. The low dose in females represented 0.68-fold maximum human exposure and the intermediate dose in males represented 1.7-fold maximum human exposure based on relative AUC comparisons. In the rat study, initial doses were 100, 250, and 1000 mg/kg/day, and the high dose was lowered to 500 mg/kg/day after 18 months. The upper dose in male and female rats represented 3-fold maximum human exposure.

Didanosine induced no significant increase in neoplastic lesions in mice or rats at maximally tolerated doses.

Didanosine was positive in the following genetic toxicology assays: 1) the *Escherichia coli* tester strain WP2 uvrA bacterial mutagenicity assay; 2) the L5178Y/TK+/-mouse lymphoma mammalian cell gene mutation assay; 3) the *in vitro* chromosomal aberrations assay in cultured human peripheral lymphocytes; 4) the *in vitro* chromosomal aberrations assay in Chinese Hamster Lung cells; and 5) the BALB/c 3T3 *in vitro* transformation assay. No evidence of mutagenicity was observed in an Ames *Salmonella* bacterial mutagenicity assay or in rat and mouse *in vivo* micronucleus assays.

Pregnancy, Reproduction, and Fertility: Pregnancy Category B. Reproduction studies have been performed in rats and rabbits at doses up to 12 and 14.2 times the estimated human exposure (based upon plasma levels), respectively, and have revealed no evidence of impaired fertility or harm to the fetus due to didanosine. At approximately 12 times the estimated human exposure, didanosine was slightly toxic to female rats and their pups during mid and late lactation. These rats showed reduced food intake and body weight gains but the physical and functional development of the offspring was not impaired and there were no major changes in the F2 generation. A study in rats showed that didanosine and/or its metabolites are transferred to the fetus through the placenta. Animal reproduction studies are not always predictive of human response.

There are no adequate and well-controlled studies of didanosine in pregnant women. Didanosine should be used during pregnancy only if the potential benefit justifies the potential risk.

Fatal lactic acidosis has been reported in pregnant women who received the combination of didanosine and stavudine with other antiretroviral agents. It is unclear if pregnancy augments the risk of lactic acidosis/hepatic steatosis syndrome reported in nonpregnant individuals receiving nucleoside analogues (see **WARNINGS: Lactic Acidosis/Severe Hepatomegaly with Steatosis). The combination of didanosine and stavudine should be used with caution during pregnancy and is recommended only if the potential benefit clearly outweighs the potential risk.** Health care providers caring for HIV-infected pregnant women receiving didanosine should be alert for early diagnosis of lactic acidosis/hepatic steatosis syndrome.

Antiretroviral Pregnancy Registry: To monitor maternal-fetal outcomes of pregnant women exposed to didanosine and other antiretroviral agents, an Antiretroviral Pregnancy Registry has been established. Physicians are encouraged to register patients by calling 1-800-258-4263.

Nursing Mothers: The Centers for Disease Control and Prevention recommend that HIV-infected mothers not breast-feed their infants to avoid risking postnatal transmission of HIV. A study in rats showed that following oral administration, didanosine and/or its metabolites were excreted into the milk of lactating rats. It is not known if didanosine is excreted in human milk. Because of both the potential for HIV transmission and the potential for serious adverse reactions in nursing infants, **mothers should be instructed not to breast-feed if they are receiving VIDEX EC (didanosine).**

Pediatric Use: The safety and efficacy of VIDEX EC in pediatric patients have not been established. Please consult the complete prescribing information for VIDEX (didanosine) Chewable/Dispersible Buffered Tablets and Pediatric Powder for Oral Solution for dosage and administration of didanosine to pediatric patients.

Geriatric Use: In an Expanded Access Program using a buffered formulation of didanosine for the treatment of advanced HIV infection, patients aged 65 years and older had a higher frequency of pancreatitis (10%) than younger patients (5%) (see **WARNINGS**). Clinical studies of didanosine, including those for VIDEX EC, did not include sufficient numbers of subjects aged 65 years and over to determine whether they respond differently than younger subjects. Didanosine is known to be substantially excreted by the kidney, and the risk of toxic reactions to this drug may be greater in patients with impaired renal function. Because elderly patients are more likely to have decreased renal function, care should be taken in dose selection. In addition, renal function should be monitored and dosage adjustments should be made accordingly (see **DOSAGE AND ADMINISTRATION: Dose Adjustment**).

ADVERSE REACTIONS

A SERIOUS TOXICITY OF DIDANOSINE IS PANCREATITIS, WHICH MAY BE FATAL (see **WARNINGS**). OTHER IMPORTANT TOXICITIES INCLUDE LACTIC ACIDOSIS/ SEVERE HEPATOMEGALY WITH STEATOSIS; RETINAL CHANGES AND OPTIC NEURITIS; AND PERIPHERAL NEUROPATHY (see **WARNINGS** and **PRECAUTIONS**).

When didanosine is used in combination with other agents with similar toxicities, the incidence of these toxicities may be higher than when didanosine is used alone. Thus, patients treated with VIDEX EC in combination with stavudine, with or without hydroxyurea, may be at increased risk for pancreatitis, which may be fatal, and hepatotoxicity (see WARNINGS). Patients treated with VIDEX EC in combination with stavudine may also be at increased risk for peripheral neuropathy (see PRECAUTIONS).

Selected clinical adverse events that occurred in a study of VIDEX EC in combination with other antiretroviral agents are provided in Table 10.

Table 10
Selected Clinical Adverse Events, Study AI454-152[a]

	Percent of Patients[b]	
Adverse Events	**VIDEX EC+ stavudine+ nelfinavir n=258**	**zidovudine/ lamivudine[c]+ nelfinavir n=253**
Diarrhea	57	58

Continued on next page

Videx EC—Cont.

Peripheral Neurologic Symptoms/Neuropathy	25	11
Nausea	24	36
Headache	22	17
Rash	14	12
Vomiting	14	19
Pancreatitis (see below)	<1	*

[a] Median duration of treatment was 62 weeks in the VIDEX EC (didanosine) + stavudine + nelfinavir group and 61 weeks in the zidovudine/lamivudine + nelfinavir group.
[b] Percentages based on treated patients.
[c] Zidovudine/lamivudine combination tablet.
*This event was not observed in this study arm.

In clinical trials using a buffered formulation of didanosine, pancreatitis resulting in death was observed in one patient who received didanosine plus stavudine plus nelfinavir, one patient who received didanosine plus stavudine plus indinavir, and 2 of 68 patients who received didanosine plus stavudine plus indinavir plus hydroxyurea. In an early access program, pancreatitis resulting in death was observed in one patient who received VIDEX EC (didanosine) plus stavudine plus hydroxyurea plus ritonavir plus indinavir plus efavirenz (see WARNINGS).

The frequency of pancreatitis is dose related. In phase 3 studies with buffered formulations of didanosine, incidence ranged from 1% to 10% with doses higher than are currently recommended and 1% to 7% with recommended dose.

Selected laboratory abnormalities that occurred in a study of VIDEX EC in combination with other antiretroviral agents are shown in Table 11.

Table 11
Selected Laboratory Abnormalities, Study AI454-152[a]

	Percent of Patients[b]			
	VIDEX EC+ stavudine+ nelfinavir n=258		zidovudine/ lamivudine[c]+ nelfinavir n=253	
Parameter	Grades 3–4[d]	All Grades	Grades 3–4[d]	All Grades
SGOT (AST)	5	46	5	19
SGPT (ALT)	6	44	5	22
Lipase	5	23	2	13
Bilirubin	<1	9	<1	3

[a] Median duration of treatment was 62 weeks in the VIDEX EC (didanosine) + stavudine + nelfinavir group and 61 weeks in the zidovudine/lamivudine + nelfinavir group.
[b] Percentages based on treated patients.
[c] Zidovudine/lamivudine combination tablet.
[d] >5 × ULN for SGOT and SGPT, ≥2.1 × ULN for lipase, and ≥2.6 × ULN for bilirubin (ULN = upper limit of normal).

Observed During Clinical Practice: The following events have been identified during postapproval use of didanosine buffered formulations. Because they are reported voluntarily from a population of unknown size, estimates of frequency cannot be made. These events have been chosen for inclusion due to their seriousness, frequency of reporting, causal connection to didanosine, or a combination of these factors.

Body as a Whole—abdominal pain, alopecia, anaphylactoid reaction, asthenia, chills/fever, pain, and redistribution/accumulation of body fat (see **PRECAUTIONS: Fat Redistribution**).

Digestive Disorders—anorexia, dyspepsia, and flatulence.

Exocrine Gland Disorders—pancreatitis (including fatal cases) (see **WARNINGS**), sialoadenitis, parotid gland enlargement, dry mouth, and dry eyes.

Hematologic Disorders—anemia, leukopenia, and thrombocytopenia.

Liver—symptomatic hyperlactatemia/lactic acidosis and hepatic steatosis (see **WARNINGS**); hepatitis and liver failure.

Metabolic Disorders—diabetes mellitus, elevated serum alkaline phosphatase level, elevated serum amylase level, elevated serum gamma-glutamyltransferase level, elevated serum uric acid level, hypoglycemia, and hyperglycemia.

Musculoskeletal Disorders—myalgia (with or without increases in creatine kinase), rhabdomyolysis including acute renal failure and hemodialysis, arthralgia, and myopathy.

Ophthalmologic Disorders—retinal depigmentation and optic neuritis (see **WARNINGS**).

OVERDOSAGE

There is no known antidote for didanosine overdosage. In phase 1 studies, in which buffered formulations of didanosine were initially administered at doses ten times the currently recommended dose, toxicities included: pancreatitis, peripheral neuropathy, diarrhea, hyperuricemia, and hepatic dysfunction. Didanosine is not dialyzable by peritoneal dialysis, although there is some clearance by hemodialysis (see **CLINICAL PHARMACOLOGY: Pharmacokinetics**).

Table 9
Predicted Drug Interactions with VIDEX EC (didanosine)

Drug or Drug Class	Effect	Clinical Comment
Drugs that may cause pancreatic toxicity	↑ risk of pancreatitis	Use only with extreme caution.[a]
Neurotoxic drugs	↑ risk of neuropathy	Use with caution.[b]
Ribavirin	↑ risk of toxicity	Ribavirin has been shown *in vitro* to increase intracellular triphosphate levels of didanosine. Coadministration is not recommended (see below).

↑ indicates increase.
[a] Only if other drugs are not available and if clearly indicated. If treatment with life-sustaining drugs that cause pancreatic toxicity is required, suspension of VIDEX EC is recommended (see **WARNINGS: Pancreatitis**).
[b] See **PRECAUTIONS: Peripheral Neuropathy.**

DOSAGE AND ADMINISTRATION

Dosage:

***Adults*—VIDEX EC (didanosine) should be administered on an empty stomach.**

VIDEX EC Delayed-Release Capsules should be swallowed intact.

The recommended daily dose is dependent on body weight and is administered as one capsule given on a once-daily schedule as outlined in Table 12.

Table 12
Dosing of VIDEX EC (didanosine) Delayed-Release Capsules

Patient Weight	Dosage
≥60 kg	400 mg once daily
<60 kg	250 mg once daily

Pediatric Patients—VIDEX EC has not been studied in pediatric patients. Please consult the complete prescribing information for VIDEX (didanosine) Chewable/Dispersible Buffered Tablets and Pediatric Powder for Oral Solution for dosage and administration of didanosine to pediatric patients.

Dose Adjustment: Clinical and laboratory signs suggestive of pancreatitis should prompt dose suspension and careful evaluation of the possibility of pancreatitis. VIDEX EC use should be discontinued in patients with confirmed pancreatitis (see WARNINGS and PRECAUTIONS: Drug Interactions).

Based on data with buffered didanosine formulations, patients with symptoms of peripheral neuropathy may tolerate a reduced dose of VIDEX EC after resolution of the symptoms of peripheral neuropathy upon drug interruption. If neuropathy recurs after resumption of VIDEX EC, permanent discontinuation of VIDEX EC should be considered.

Concomitant Therapy—Tenofovir disoproxil fumarate. A dose reduction of VIDEX EC to 250 mg (adults weighing ≥60 kg with creatinine clearance ≥60 mL/min) or 200 mg (adults weighing <60 kg with creatinine clearance ≥60 mL/min) once daily taken together with tenofovir and a light meal (≤400 kcalories, ≤20% fat) or in the fasted state is recommended. **The appropriate dose of VIDEX EC coadministered with tenofovir in patients with creatinine clearance <60 mL/min has not been established.** (See **CLINICAL PHARMACOLOGY: Drug Interactions** and **PRECAUTIONS: Drug Interactions.**)

Renal Impairment—Dosing recommendations for VIDEX EC and VIDEX buffered formulations are different for patients with renal impairment. Please consult the complete prescribing information on administration of VIDEX buffered formulations to patients with renal impairment.

In adult patients with impaired renal function, the dose of VIDEX EC should be adjusted to compensate for the slower rate of elimination. The recommended doses and dosing intervals of VIDEX EC in adult patients with renal insufficiency are presented in Table 13.

Table 13
Recommended Dosage of VIDEX EC in Renal Impairment by Body Weight[a]

Creatinine Clearance (mL/min)	Dosage (mg)	
	≥60 kg	<60 kg
≥60	400 once daily	250 once daily
30–59	200 once daily	125 once daily
10–29	125 once daily	125 once daily
<10	125 once daily	[b]

[a] Based on studies using a buffered formulation of didanosine.
[b] Not suitable for use in patients <60 kg with CL_{CR} <10 mL/min. An alternate formulation of didanosine should be used.

Patients Requiring Continuous Ambulatory Peritoneal Dialysis (CAPD) or Hemodialysis—For patients requiring CAPD or hemodialysis, follow dosing recommendations for patients with creatinine clearance less than 10 mL/min, shown in Table 13. It is not necessary to administer a supplemental dose of didanosine following hemodialysis.

Hepatic Impairment—(See **WARNINGS** and **PRECAUTIONS**).

HOW SUPPLIED

VIDEX® EC (didanosine) Delayed-Release Capsules are white, opaque capsules that are packaged in bottles with child-resistant closures as described in Table 14.

Table 14
VIDEX EC Delayed-Release Capsules

125 mg capsule imprinted with BMS 125 mg 6671 in Tan	
NDC No. 0087-6671-17	30 capsules/bottle
200 mg capsule imprinted with BMS 200 mg 6672 in Green	
NDC No. 0087-6672-17	30 capsules/bottle
250 mg capsule imprinted with BMS 250 mg 6673 in Blue	
NDC No. 0087-6673-17	30 capsules/bottle
400 mg capsule imprinted with BMS 400 mg 6674 in Red	
NDC No. 0087-6674-17	30 capsules/bottle

The capsules should be stored in tightly closed containers at 25°C (77°F). Excursions between 15° and 30°C (59° and 86°F) are permitted [see USP Controlled Room Temperature].

HANDLING AND DISPOSAL

Disposal options include incineration, landfill, or sewer as dictated by specific circumstances and relevant national, state, and local regulations.

US Patent Nos: 4,861,759 and 5,254,539, and 5,880,106 (didanosine). Patent also Pending (didanosine capsules).

PATIENT INFORMATION ℞ ONLY

VIDEX® EC

(generic name = **didanosine** also known as **ddl**)

VIDEX® EC (didanosine) Delayed-Release Capsules Enteric-Coated Beadlets

What is VIDEX EC?

VIDEX EC (pronounced *VY dex ee see*) is a prescription medicine used in combination with other drugs to treat adults who are infected with HIV (the human immunodeficiency virus, the virus that causes AIDS). VIDEX EC belongs to a class of drugs called nucleoside analogues. By reducing the growth of HIV, VIDEX EC helps your body maintain its supply of CD4 cells, which are important for fighting HIV and other infections.

VIDEX EC will not cure your HIV infection. At present there is no cure for HIV infection. Even while taking VIDEX EC (didanosine), you may continue to have HIV-related illnesses, including infections with other disease-producing organisms. Continue to see your doctor regularly and report any medical problems that occur.

VIDEX EC does not prevent a patient infected with HIV from passing the virus to other people. To protect others, you must continue to practice safe sex and take precautions to prevent others from coming in contact with your blood and other body fluids.

There is limited information on the antiviral response of long-term use of VIDEX EC.

In VIDEX EC, an enteric coating is used to protect the medicine while it is in your stomach since stomach acids can break it down. The enteric coating dissolves when the medicine reaches your small intestine.

Who should not take VIDEX EC?

Do not take VIDEX EC if you are allergic to any of its ingredients, including its active ingredient, didanosine, and the inactive ingredients. (See **Inactive Ingredients** at the end of this leaflet.) Tell your doctor if you think you have had an allergic reaction to any of these ingredients.

Because it has only been studied in adults, VIDEX EC is not recommended for children.

How should I take VIDEX EC?
How should I store it?

VIDEX EC (didanosine) should only be taken once daily. Your doctor will determine your dose based on your body weight, kidney and liver function, other medicines you are taking, and any side effects that you may have had with VIDEX EC or other medicines. Take VIDEX EC **on an empty stomach. Do not take VIDEX EC with food.** Swallow the capsule whole; do not open it. Try not to miss a dose, but if you do, take it as soon as possible. If it is almost time for the next dose, skip the missed dose and continue your regular dosing schedule.

Store capsules in a tightly closed container at room temperature away from heat and out of the reach of children and pets.

If you have kidney disease: If your kidneys are not working properly, your doctor will need to do regular tests to check how they are working while you take VIDEX EC. Your doctor may also lower your dosage of VIDEX EC.

What should I do if someone takes an overdose of VIDEX EC?

If someone may have taken an overdose of VIDEX EC, get medical help right away. Contact their doctor or a poison control center.

What should I avoid while taking VIDEX EC?

Alcohol. Do not drink alcohol while taking VIDEX EC since alcohol may increase your risk of pancreatitis (pain and inflammation of the pancreas) or liver damage.

Other medicines. Other medicines, including those you can buy without a prescription, may interfere with the actions of VIDEX EC or may increase the possibility or severity of side effects. **Do not take any medicine, vitamin supplement, or other health preparation without first checking with your doctor.**

Pregnancy. It is not known if VIDEX EC can harm a human fetus. Also, pregnant women have experienced serious side effects when taking didanosine (the active ingredient in VIDEX EC (didanosine) in combination with ZERIT (stavudine), also known as d4T, and other HIV medicines. VIDEX EC should be used during pregnancy only after discussion with your doctor. **Tell your doctor if you become pregnant or plan to become pregnant while taking VIDEX EC.**

Nursing. Studies have shown didanosine (the active ingredient in VIDEX EC) is in the breast milk of animals getting the drug. It may also be in human breast milk. The Centers for Disease Control and Prevention (CDC) recommends that HIV-infected mothers **not** breast-feed. This should reduce the risk of passing HIV infection to their babies and the potential for serious adverse reactions in nursing infants. Therefore, do not nurse a baby while taking VIDEX EC.

What are the possible side effects of VIDEX EC?

Pancreatitis. Pancreatitis is a dangerous inflammation of the pancreas that may cause death. ***Tell your doctor right away if you develop stomach pain, nausea, or vomiting. These can be signs of pancreatitis.*** Before starting VIDEX EC therapy, let your doctor know if you have ever had pancreatitis. This condition is more likely to happen in people who have had it before. It is also more likely in people with advanced HIV disease. However, it can occur at any stage of HIV disease. It may be more common in patients with kidney problems, those who drink alcohol, and those who are also treated with stavudine or hydroxyurea. If you get pancreatitis, your doctor will tell you to stop taking VIDEX EC.

Lactic acidosis, severe liver enlargement, and **liver failure** including deaths, have been reported among patients taking VIDEX EC (including pregnant women). Symptoms that may indicate a liver problem are:

- feeling very weak, tired, or uncomfortable,
- unusual or unexpected stomach discomfort,
- feeling cold,
- feeling dizzy or lightheaded,
- suddenly developing a slow or irregular heartbeat.

Lactic acidosis is a medical emergency that must be treated in a hospital.

If you notice any of these symptoms or if your medical condition changes, stop taking VIDEX EC and **call your doctor right away** Women, overweight patients, and those who have been treated for a long time with other medicines used to treat HIV infection are more likely to develop lactic acidosis. Your doctor should check your liver function periodically while you are taking VIDEX EC. You should be especially careful if you have a history of heavy alcohol use or a liver problem.

Vision changes. VIDEX EC may affect the nerves in your eyes. Because of this, you should have regular eye examinations. You should also report any changes in vision to your doctor right away. This includes, for example, seeing colors abnormally or blurred vision.

Peripheral neuropathy. This is a problem with the nerves in your hands or feet. The nerve problem may be serious. ***Tell your doctor right away if you have continuing numbness, tingling, or pain in the feet or hands.***

Before starting VIDEX EC therapy, let your doctor know if you have ever had peripheral neuropathy. This condition is more likely to happen in people who have had it before. It is also more likely in patients taking medicines that affect the nerves and in people with advanced HIV disease. However, it can occur at any stage of HIV disease. If you get peripheral neuropathy, your doctor will tell you to stop taking VIDEX EC (didanosine). After stopping VIDEX EC, the symptoms may get worse for a short time and then get better. Once symptoms of peripheral neuropathy go away completely, you and your doctor should decide if starting VIDEX EC is right for you. If so, you might be started at a lower dose.

Special note about other medicines. If you take VIDEX EC along with other medicines with similar side effects, you may increase the chance of having these side effects. For example, using VIDEX EC in combination with other medicines that may cause pancreatitis, peripheral neuropathy, or liver problems (including stavudine and hydroxyurea) may increase your chance of having these side effects.

Other side effects: The most common side effects in adults taking VIDEX EC in combination with other HIV drugs included diarrhea, nausea, headache, vomiting, and rash. Changes in body fat have been seen in some patients taking antiretroviral therapy. These changes may include increased amount of fat in the upper back and neck ("buffalo hump"), breast, and around the trunk. Loss of fat from the legs, arms, and face may also happen. The cause and long-term health effects of these conditions are not known at this time.

Inactive Ingredients: Carboxymethylcellulose sodium 12, diethyl phthalate, methacrylic acid copolymer, sodium hydroxide, sodium starch glycolate, talc, colloidal silicon dioxide, gelatin, sodium lauryl sulfate, and titanium dioxide.

This medicine was prescribed for your particular condition. Do not use VIDEX EC for another condition or give it to others. Keep VIDEX EC and all medicines out of the reach of children. Throw away VIDEX EC when it is outdated or no longer needed by flushing it down the toilet or pouring it down the sink.

This summary does not include everything there is to know about VIDEX EC. Medicines are sometimes prescribed for purposes other than those listed in a Patient Information Leaflet. If you have questions or concerns, or want more information about VIDEX EC, your physician and pharmacist have the complete prescribing information upon which this leaflet is based. You may want to read it and discuss it with your doctor or other healthcare professional. Remember, no written summary can replace careful discussion with your doctor.

BMS Virology™
Bristol-Myers Squibb Company
Princeton, NJ 08543
U.S.A.

This Patient Information Leaflet has been approved by the U.S. Food and Drug Administration.

N3522-09 1116303A9
F3-B0001-01-04 Revised January 2004
Based on Package Insert dated January 2004

Shown in Product Identification Guide, page 310

ZERIT® (stavudine) ℞
ZERIT® (stavudine) Capsules
ZERIT® (stavudine) for Oral Solution
(Patient Information Leaflet Included)

> **WARNING**
> **LACTIC ACIDOSIS AND SEVERE HEPATOMEGALY WITH STEATOSIS, INCLUDING FATAL CASES, HAVE BEEN REPORTED WITH THE USE OF NUCLEOSIDE ANALOGUES ALONE OR IN COMBINATION, INCLUDING STAVUDINE AND OTHER ANTIRETROVIRALS. FATAL LACTIC ACIDOSIS HAS BEEN REPORTED IN PREGNANT WOMEN WHO RECEIVED THE COMBINATION OF STAVUDINE AND DIDANOSINE WITH OTHER ANTIRETROVIRAL AGENTS. THE COMBINATION OF STAVUDINE AND DIDANOSINE SHOULD BE USED WITH CAUTION DURING PREGNANCY AND IS RECOMMENDED ONLY IF THE POTENTIAL BENEFIT CLEARLY OUTWEIGHS THE POTENTIAL RISK (SEE WARNINGS AND PRECAUTIONS: PREGNANCY).**
> **FATAL AND NONFATAL PANCREATITIS HAVE OCCURRED DURING THERAPY WHEN ZERIT (stavudine) WAS PART OF A COMBINATION REGIMEN THAT INCLUDED DIDANOSINE, WITH OR WITHOUT HYDROXYUREA,**
> **IN BOTH TREATMENT-NAIVE AND TREATMENT-EXPERIENCED PATIENTS, REGARDLESS OF DEGREE OF IMMUNOSUPPRESSION (SEE WARNINGS).**

DESCRIPTION

ZERIT® is the brand name for stavudine (d4T), a synthetic thymidine nucleoside analogue, active against the Human Immunodeficiency Virus (HIV).

ZERIT (stavudine) Capsules are supplied for oral administration in strengths of 15, 20, 30, and 40 mg of stavudine. Each capsule also contains inactive ingredients microcrystalline cellulose, sodium starch glycolate, lactose, and magnesium stearate. The hard gelatin shell consists of gelatin, silicon dioxide, sodium lauryl sulfate, titanium dioxide, and iron oxides.

ZERIT (stavudine) for Oral Solution is supplied as a dye-free, fruit-flavored powder in bottles with child-resistant closures providing 200 mL of a 1 mg/mL stavudine solution upon constitution with water per label instructions. The powder for oral solution contains the following inactive ingredients: methylparaben, propylparaben, sodium carboxymethylcellulose, sucrose, and antifoaming and flavoring agents.

The chemical name for stavudine is 2′,3′-didehydro-3′-deoxythymidine. Stavudine has the following structural formula:

[See chemical structure at top of next column]

Stavudine is a white to off-white crystalline solid with the molecular formula $C_{10}H_{12}N_2O_4$ and a molecular weight of 224.2. The solubility of stavudine at 23°C is approximately 83 mg/mL in water and 30 mg/mL in propylene glycol. The n-octanol/water partition coefficient of stavudine at 23°C is 0.144.

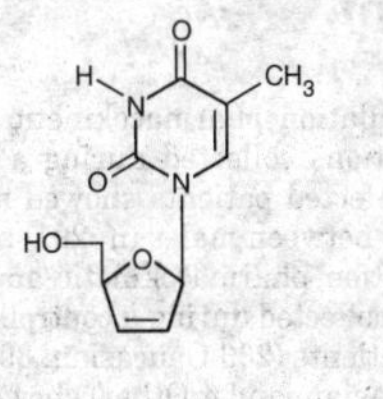

MICROBIOLOGY

Mechanism of Action: Stavudine, a nucleoside analogue of thymidine, inhibits the replication of HIV in human cells *in vitro*. Stavudine is phosphorylated by cellular kinases to the active metabolite stavudine triphosphate. Stavudine triphosphate inhibits the activity of HIV reverse transcriptase both by competing with the natural substrate deoxythymidine triphosphate (K_i=0.0083 to 0.032 µM), and by its incorporation into viral DNA causing a termination of DNA chain elongation because stavudine lacks the essential 3′-OH group. Stavudine triphosphate inhibits cellular DNA polymerase beta and gamma, and markedly reduces the synthesis of mitochondrial DNA.

***In vitro* HIV Susceptibility:** The *in vitro* antiviral activity of stavudine was measured in peripheral blood mononuclear cells, monocytic cells, and lymphoblastoid cell lines. The concentration of drug necessary to inhibit viral replication by 50% (ED_{50}) ranged from 0.009 to 4 µM against laboratory and clinical isolates of HIV-1. Stavudine had additive and synergistic activity in combination with didanosine and zalcitabine, respectively, *in vitro*. Stavudine combined with zidovudine had additive or antagonistic activity *in vitro* depending upon the molar ratios of the agents tested. The relationship between *in vitro* susceptibility of HIV to stavudine and the inhibition of HIV replication in humans has not been established.

Drug Resistance: HIV isolates with reduced susceptibility to stavudine have been selected *in vitro* and were also obtained from patients treated with stavudine. Phenotypic analysis of HIV isolates from stavudine-treated patients revealed, in 3 of 20 paired isolates, a 4- to 12-fold decrease in susceptibility to stavudine *in vitro*. The genetic basis for these susceptibility changes has not been identified. The clinical relevance of changes in stavudine susceptibility has not been established.

Cross-resistance: Five of 11 stavudine post-treatment isolates developed moderate resistance to zidovudine (9- to 176-fold) and 3 of those 11 isolates developed moderate resistance to didanosine (7- to 29-fold). The clinical relevance of these findings is unknown.

CLINICAL PHARMACOLOGY

Pharmacokinetics: The pharmacokinetics of stavudine have been evaluated in HIV-infected adult and pediatric patients (Tables 1 and 2). Peak plasma concentrations (C_{max}) and area under the plasma concentration-time curve (AUC) increased in proportion to dose after both single and multiple doses ranging from 0.03 to 4 mg/kg. There was no significant accumulation of stavudine with repeated administration every 6, 8, or 12 hours.

***Absorption*-** Following oral administration, stavudine is rapidly absorbed, with peak plasma concentrations occurring within 1 hour after dosing. The systemic exposure to stavudine is the same following administration as capsules or solution.

***Distribution*-** Binding of stavudine to serum proteins was negligible over the concentration range of 0.01 to 11.4 µg/mL. Stavudine distributes equally between red blood cells and plasma.

***Metabolism*-** The metabolic fate of stavudine has not been elucidated in humans.

***Excretion*-** Renal elimination accounted for about 40% of the overall clearance regardless of the route of administration. The mean renal clearance was about twice the average endogenous creatinine clearance, indicating active tubular secretion in addition to glomerular filtration.

[See table 1 at top of next page]

Special Populations:

***Pediatric*-** For pharmacokinetic properties of stavudine in pediatric patients, see Table 2.

[See table 2 on next page]

***Renal Insufficiency*-** Data from two studies in adults indicated that the apparent oral clearance of stavudine decreased and the terminal elimination half-life increased as creatinine clearance decreased (see Table 3). C_{max} and T_{max} were not significantly altered by renal insufficiency. The mean ± SD hemodialysis clearance value of stavudine was 120 ± 18 mL/min (n=12); the mean ± SD percentage of the stavudine dose recovered in the dialysate, timed to occur between 2-6 hours post-dose, was 31 ± 5%. Based on these observations, it is recommended that ZERIT (stavudine) dosage be modified in patients with reduced creatinine clearance and in patients receiving maintenance hemodialysis (see **DOSAGE AND ADMINISTRATION**).

[See table 3 on next page]

***Hepatic Insufficiency*-** Stavudine pharmacokinetics were not altered in 5 non-HIV-infected patients with hepatic impairment secondary to cirrhosis (Child-Pugh classification B or C) following the administration of a single 40-mg dose.

***Geriatric*-** Stavudine pharmacokinetics have not been studied in patients >65 years of age. (See **PRECAUTIONS: Geriatric Use.**)

Continued on next page

Zerit—Cont.

Gender- A population pharmacokinetic analysis of stavudine concentrations collected during a controlled clinical study in HIV-infected patients showed no clinically important differences between males (n=291) and females (n=27).
Race- A population pharmacokinetic analysis of stavudine concentrations collected during a controlled clinical study in HIV-infected patients (233 Caucasian, 39 African American, 41 Hispanic, 1 Asian, and 4 Other) showed no clinically important differences associated with race.
Drug Interactions- Drug interaction studies have demonstrated that there are no clinically significant interactions between stavudine and the following: didanosine, lamivudine, or nelfinavir.
Zidovudine may competitively inhibit the intracellular phosphorylation of stavudine. Therefore, use of zidovudine in combination with ZERIT (stavudine) is not recommended.

Table 1
Pharmacokinetic Parameters of Stavudine in Adult HIV-Infected Patients

Parameter	Mean ± SD	n
Oral bioavailability	86.4 ± 18.2%	25
Volume of distribution[a]	58 ± 21 L	44
Apparent oral volume of distribution[b]	66 ± 22 L	71
Total body clearance[a]	8.3 ± 2.3 mL/min/kg	44
Apparent oral clearance[b]	8.0 ± 2.6 mL/min/kg	113
Elimination half-life, I.V. dose[a]	1.15 ± 0.35 h	44
Elimination half-life, oral dose[b]	1.44 ± 0.30 h	115
Urinary recovery of stavudine (% of dose)[b]	39 ± 23%	88

[a] following 1 hour I.V. infusion.
[b] following single oral dose.

Table 2
Pharmacokinetic Parameters (Mean ± SD) of Stavudine in HIV Exposed or -Infected Pediatric Patients

Parameter	Ages 5 weeks to 15 years	n	Ages 14 to 28 days	n	Day of Birth	n
Oral bioavailability (%)	76.9 ± 31.7	20	ND		ND	
Volume of distribution[a] (L/kg)	0.73 ± 0.32	21	ND		ND	
Ratio of CSF:plasma concentrations (as %)[b]	59 ± 35	8	ND		ND	
Total body clearance[a] (mL/min/kg)	9.75 ± 3.76	21	ND		ND	
Apparent oral clearance[c] (mL/min/kg)	13.75 ± 4.29	20	11.52 ± 5.93	30	5.08 ± 2.80	17
Elimination half-life, I.V. dose[a] (h)	1.11 ± 0.28	21	ND		ND	
Elimination half-life, oral dose[c] (h)	0.96 ± 0.26	20	1.59 ± 0.29	30	5.27 ± 2.01	17
Urinary recovery of stavudine (% of dose)[c]	34 ± 16	19	ND		ND	

[a] following 1 hour I.V. infusion.
[b] following multiple oral doses.
[c] following single oral dose.
ND=not determined.

Table 3
Mean ± SD Pharmacokinetic Parameter Values Single 40-mg Oral Dose of ZERIT (stavudine)

	Creatinine Clearance			
	>50 mL/min (n=10)	26-50 mL/min (n=5)	9-25 mL/min (n=5)	Hemodialysis Patients* (n=11)
CL_{cr}(mL/min)	104 ± 28	41 ± 5	17 ± 3	NA
CL/F (mL/min)	335 ± 57	191 ± 39	116 ± 25	105 ± 17
CL_R(mL/min)	167 ± 65	73 ± 18	17 ± 3	NA
$T_{1/2}$ (h)	1.7 ± 0.4	3.5 ± 2.5	4.6 ± 0.9	5.4 ± 1.4

CL_{cr} = creatinine clearance.
CL/F = apparent oral clearance.
CL_R = renal clearance.
$T_{1/2}$ = terminal elimination half-life.
NA = not applicable.
*Determined while patients were off dialysis.

INDICATIONS AND USAGE

ZERIT (stavudine), in combination with other antiretroviral agents, is indicated for the treatment of HIV-1 infection (see Clinical Studies).

Clinical Studies:
Combination Therapy- The combination use of ZERIT (stavudine) is based on the results of clinical studies in HIV-infected patients in double- and triple-combination regimens with other antiretroviral agents.
One of these studies (START 1) was a multicenter, randomized, open-label study comparing ZERIT (stavudine) (40 mg twice daily) plus lamivudine plus indinavir to zidovudine plus lamivudine plus indinavir in 202 treatment-naive patients. Both regimens resulted in a similar magnitude of inhibition of HIV RNA levels and increases in CD4 cell counts through 48 weeks.
Monotherapy- The efficacy of ZERIT (stavudine) was demonstrated in a randomized, double-blind study (AI455-019, conducted 1992-1994) comparing ZERIT (stavudine) with zidovudine in 822 patients with a spectrum of HIV-related symptoms. The outcome in terms of progression of HIV disease and death was similar for both drugs.

CONTRAINDICATIONS

ZERIT (stavudine) is contraindicated in patients with clinically significant hypersensitivity to stavudine or to any of the components contained in the formulation.

WARNINGS

1. Lactic Acidosis/Severe Hepatomegaly with Steatosis/Hepatic Failure: Lactic acidosis and severe hepatomegaly with steatosis, including fatal cases, have been reported with the use of nucleoside analogues alone or in combination, including stavudine and other antiretrovirals. Although relative rates of lactic acidosis have not been assessed in prospective well-controlled trials, longitudinal cohort and retrospective studies suggest that this infrequent event may be more often associated with antiretroviral combinations containing stavudine. Female gender, obesity, and prolonged nucleoside exposure may be risk factors. Fatal lactic acidosis has been reported in pregnant women who received the combination of stavudine and didanosine with other antiretroviral agents. The combination of stavudine and didanosine should be used with caution during pregnancy and is recommended only if the potential benefit clearly outweighs the potential risk (see **PRECAUTIONS: Pregnancy**).
Particular caution should be exercised when administering ZERIT (stavudine) to any patient with known risk factors for liver disease; however, cases of lactic acidosis have also been reported in patients with no known risk factors. Generalized fatigue, digestive symptoms (nausea, vomiting, abdominal pain, and sudden unexplained weight loss); respiratory symptoms (tachypnea and dyspnea); or neurologic symptoms (including motor weakness, see **2. Neurologic Symptoms**) might be indicative of lactic acidosis development.
Treatment with ZERIT (stavudine) should be suspended in any patient who develops clinical or laboratory findings suggestive of lactic acidosis or pronounced hepatotoxicity (which may include hepatomegaly and steatosis even in the absence of marked transaminase elevations).
An increased risk of hepatotoxicity may occur in patients treated with ZERIT (stavudine) in combination with didanosine and hydroxyurea compared to when ZERIT (stavudine) is used alone. Deaths attributed to hepatotoxicity have occurred in patients receiving this combination. Patients treated with this combination should be closely monitored for signs of liver toxicity.
2. Neurologic Symptoms: Motor weakness has been reported rarely in patients receiving combination antiretroviral therapy including ZERIT (stavudine). Most of these cases occurred in the setting of lactic acidosis. The evolution of motor weakness may mimic the clinical presentation of Guillain-Barré syndrome (including respiratory failure). Symptoms may continue or worsen following discontinuation of therapy.
Peripheral neuropathy, manifested by numbness, tingling, or pain in the hands or feet, has been reported in patients receiving ZERIT (stavudine) therapy. Peripheral neuropathy has occurred more frequently in patients with advanced HIV disease, a history of neuropathy, or concurrent neurotoxic drug therapy, including didanosine (see **ADVERSE REACTIONS**).
3. Pancreatitis: Fatal and nonfatal pancreatitis have occurred during therapy when ZERIT (stavudine) was part of a combination regimen that included didanosine, with or without hydroxyurea, in both treatment-naive and treatment-experienced patients, regardless of degree of immunosuppression. The combination of ZERIT (stavudine) and didanosine (with or without hydroxyurea) and any other agents that are toxic to the pancreas should be suspended in patients with suspected pancreatitis. Reinstitution of ZERIT (stavudine) after a confirmed diagnosis of pancreatitis should be undertaken with particular caution and close patient monitoring. The new regimen should contain neither didanosine nor hydroxyurea.

PRECAUTIONS

Fat Redistribution: Redistribution/accumulation of body fat including central obesity, dorsocervical fat enlargement (buffalo hump), peripheral wasting, facial wasting, breast enlargement, and "cushingoid appearance" have been observed in patients receiving antiretroviral therapy. The mechanism and long-term consequences of these events are currently unknown. A causal relationship has not been established.

Information for Patients (See **Patient Information Leaflet.**): Patients should be informed of the importance of early recognition of symptoms of lactic acidosis, which include abdominal discomfort, nausea, vomiting, fatigue, dyspnea, and motor weakness. Patients in whom these symptoms develop should seek medical attention immediately. Discontinuation of ZERIT (stavudine) therapy may be required.
Patients should be informed that an important toxicity of ZERIT (stavudine) is peripheral neuropathy. Patients should be aware that peripheral neuropathy is manifested by numbness, tingling, or pain in hands or feet, and that these symptoms should be reported to their physicians. Patients should be counseled that peripheral neuropathy occurs with greatest frequency in patients who have advanced HIV disease or a history of peripheral neuropathy, and that dose modification and/or discontinuation of ZERIT (stavudine) may be required if toxicity develops.
Caregivers of young children receiving ZERIT (stavudine) therapy should be instructed regarding detection and reporting of peripheral neuropathy.
Patients should be informed that when ZERIT (stavudine) is used in combination with other agents with similar toxicities, the incidence of adverse events may be higher than

when ZERIT (stavudine) is used alone. An increased risk of pancreatitis, which may be fatal, may occur in patients treated with the combination of ZERIT (stavudine) and didanosine, with or without hydroxyurea. Patients treated with this combination should be closely monitored for symptoms of pancreatitis. An increased risk of hepatotoxicity, which may be fatal, may occur in patients treated with ZERIT (stavudine) in combination with didanosine and hydroxyurea. Patients treated with this combination should be closely monitored for signs of liver toxicity.

Patients should be informed that ZERIT (stavudine) is not a cure for HIV infection, and that they may continue to acquire illnesses associated with HIV infection, including opportunistic infections. Patients should be advised to remain under the care of a physician when using ZERIT (stavudine). They should be advised that ZERIT (stavudine) therapy has not been shown to reduce the risk of transmission of HIV to others through sexual contact or blood contamination. Patients should be informed that the long-term effects of ZERIT (stavudine) are unknown at this time.

Patients should be informed that the Centers for Disease Control and Prevention (CDC) recommend that HIV-infected mothers not nurse newborn infants to reduce the risk of postnatal transmission of HIV infection.

Patients should be informed that redistribution or accumulation of body fat may occur in patients receiving antiretroviral therapy and that the cause and long-term health effects of these conditions are not known at this time.

Drug Interactions: Zidovudine may competitively inhibit the intracellular phosphorylation of stavudine. Therefore, use of zidovudine in combination with ZERIT (stavudine) is not recommended (see **CLINICAL PHARMACOLOGY**.)

Carcinogenesis, Mutagenesis, Impairment of Fertility: In 2-year carcinogenicity studies in mice and rats, stavudine was noncarcinogenic at doses which produced exposures (AUC) 39 and 168 times, respectively, human exposure at the recommended clinical dose. Benign and malignant liver tumors in mice and rats and malignant urinary bladder tumors in male rats occurred at levels of exposure 250 (mice) and 732 (rats) times human exposure at the recommended clinical dose.

Stavudine was not mutagenic in the Ames, *E. coli* reverse mutation, or the CHO/HGPRT mammalian cell forward gene mutation assays, with and without metabolic activation. Stavudine produced positive results in the *in vitro* human lymphocyte clastogenesis and mouse fibroblast assays, and in the *in vivo* mouse micronucleus test. In the *in vitro* assays, stavudine elevated the frequency of chromosome aberrations in human lymphocytes (concentrations of 25 to 250 µg/mL, without metabolic activation) and increased the frequency of transformed foci in mouse fibroblast cells (concentrations of 25 to 2500 µg/mL, with and without metabolic activation). In the *in vivo* micronucleus assay, stavudine was clastogenic in bone marrow cells following oral stavudine administration to mice at dosages of 600 to 2000 mg/kg/day for 3 days.

No evidence of impaired fertility was seen in rats with exposures (based on C_{max}) up to 216 times that observed following a clinical dosage of 1 mg/kg/day.

Pregnancy: Pregnancy "Category C". Reproduction studies have been performed in rats and rabbits with exposures (based on C_{max}) up to 399 and 183 times, respectively, of that seen at a clinical dosage of 1 mg/kg/day and have revealed no evidence of teratogenicity. The incidence in fetuses of a common skeletal variation, unossified or incomplete ossification of sternebra, was increased in rats at 399 times human exposure, while no effect was observed at 216 times human exposure. A slight post-implantation loss was noted at 216 times the human exposure with no effect noted at approximately 135 times the human exposure. An increase in early rat neonatal mortality (birth to 4 days of age) occurred at 399 times the human exposure, while survival of neonates was unaffected at approximately 135 times the human exposure. A study in rats showed that stavudine is transferred to the fetus through the placenta. The concentration in fetal tissue was approximately one-half the concentration in maternal plasma. Animal reproduction studies are not always predictive of human response.

There are no adequate and well-controlled studies of stavudine in pregnant women. Stavudine should be used during pregnancy only if the potential benefit justifies the potential risk.

Fatal lactic acidosis has been reported in pregnant women who received the combination of stavudine and didanosine with other antiretroviral agents. It is unclear if pregnancy augments the risk of lactic acidosis/hepatic steatosis syndrome reported in nonpregnant individuals receiving nucleoside analogues (see **WARNINGS: Lactic Acidosis/Severe Hepatomegaly with Steatosis/Hepatic Failure). The combination of stavudine and didanosine should be used with caution during pregnancy and is recommended only if the potential benefit clearly outweighs the potential risk.** Healthcare providers caring for HIV-infected pregnant women receiving stavudine should be alert for early diagnosis of lactic acidosis/hepatic steatosis syndrome.

Antiretroviral Pregnancy Registry: To monitor maternal-fetal outcomes of pregnant women exposed to stavudine and other antiretroviral agents, an Antiretroviral Pregnancy Registry has been established. Physicians are encouraged to register patients by calling 1-800-258-4263.

Nursing Mothers: The Centers for Disease Control and Prevention recommend that HIV-infected mothers not breast-feed their infants to avoid risking postnatal transmission of HIV. Studies in lactating rats demonstrated that stavudine is excreted in milk. Although it is not known whether stavudine is excreted in human milk, there exists the potential for adverse effects from stavudine in nursing infants. Because of both the potential for HIV transmission and the potential for serious adverse reactions in nursing infants, **mothers should be instructed not to breast-feed if they are receiving ZERIT (stavudine)**.

Pediatric Use: Use of stavudine in pediatric patients from birth through adolescence is supported by evidence from adequate and well-controlled studies of stavudine in adults with additional pharmacokinetic and safety data in pediatric patients.

Adverse events and laboratory abnormalities reported to occur in pediatric patients in clinical studies were generally consistent with the safety profile of stavudine in adults. These studies include ACTG 240, where 105 pediatric patients ages 3 months to 6 years received ZERIT (stavudine) 2 mg/kg/day for a median of 6.4 months; a controlled clinical trial where 185 newborns received ZERIT (stavudine) 2 mg/kg/day either alone or in combination with didanosine from birth through 6 weeks of age; and a clinical trial where 8 newborns received ZERIT (stavudine) 2 mg/kg/day in combination with didanosine and nelfinavir from birth through 4 weeks of age.

Stavudine pharmacokinetics have been evaluated in 25 HIV-infected pediatric patients ranging in age from 5 weeks to 15 years and in weight from 2 to 43 kg after I.V. or oral administration of single doses and twice-daily regimens and in 30 HIV-exposed or -infected newborns ranging in age from birth to 4 weeks after oral administration of twice-daily regimens (see **CLINICAL PHARMACOLOGY**, Table 2).

Geriatric Use: Clinical studies of ZERIT (stavudine) did not include sufficient numbers of patients aged 65 years and over to determine whether they respond differently than younger patients. Greater sensitivity of some older individuals to the effects of ZERIT (stavudine) cannot be ruled out.

In a monotherapy Expanded Access Program for patients with advanced HIV infection, peripheral neuropathy or peripheral neuropathic symptoms were observed in 15 of 40 (38%) elderly patients receiving 40 mg twice daily and 8 of 51 (16%) elderly patients receiving 20 mg twice daily. Of the approximately 12,000 patients enrolled in the Expanded Access Program, peripheral neuropathy or peripheral neuropathic symptoms developed in 30% of patients receiving 40 mg twice daily and 25% of patients receiving 20 mg twice daily. Elderly patients should be closely monitored for signs and symptoms of peripheral neuropathy.

ZERIT (stavudine) is known to be substantially excreted by the kidney, and the risk of toxic reactions to this drug may be greater in patients with impaired renal function. Because elderly patients are more likely to have decreased renal function, it may be useful to monitor renal function. Dose adjustment is recommended for patients with renal impairment (see **DOSAGE AND ADMINISTRATION: Dosage Adjustment**).

ADVERSE REACTIONS

Adults: Fatal lactic acidosis has occurred in patients treated with ZERIT (stavudine) in combination with other antiretroviral agents. Patients with suspected lactic acidosis should immediately suspend therapy with ZERIT (stavudine). Permanent discontinuation of ZERIT (stavudine) should be considered for patients with confirmed lactic acidosis.

ZERIT (stavudine) therapy has rarely been associated with motor weakness, occurring predominantly in the setting of lactic acidosis. If motor weakness develops, ZERIT (stavudine) should be discontinued.

ZERIT (stavudine) therapy has also been associated with peripheral sensory neuropathy, which can be severe, is dose related, and occurs more frequently in patients being treated with neurotoxic drug therapy, including didanosine, in patients with advanced HIV infection, or in patients who have previously experienced peripheral neuropathy.

Patients should be monitored for the development of neuropathy, which is usually manifested by numbness, tingling, or pain in the feet or hands. Stavudine-related peripheral neuropathy may resolve if therapy is withdrawn promptly. In some cases, symptoms may worsen temporarily following discontinuation of therapy. If symptoms resolve completely, patients may tolerate resumption of treatment at one-half the dose (see **DOSAGE AND ADMINISTRATION**). If neuropathy recurs after resumption, permanent discontinuation of ZERIT (stavudine) should be considered.

When ZERIT (stavudine) is used in combination with other agents with similar toxicities, the incidence of adverse events may be higher than when ZERIT (stavudine) is used alone. Pancreatitis, peripheral neuropathy, and liver function abnormalities occur more frequently in patients treated with the combination of ZERIT (stavudine) and didanosine, with or without hydroxyurea. Fatal pancreatitis and hepatotoxicity may occur more frequently in patients treated with ZERIT (stavudine) in combination with didanosine and hydroxyurea (see **WARNINGS** and **PRECAUTIONS**).

Selected clinical adverse events that occurred in adult patients receiving ZERIT (stavudine) in a controlled monotherapy study (Study AI455-019) are provided in Table 4.

Table 4
Selected Clinical Adverse Events in Study AI455-019[a] (Monotherapy)

	Percent (%)	
Adverse Events	**ZERIT (stavudine) (40 mg twice daily) (n=412)**	**zidovudine (200 mg 3 times daily) (n=402)**
Headache	54	49
Diarrhea	50	44
Peripheral Neurologic Symptoms/Neuropathy	52	39
Rash	40	35
Nausea and Vomiting	39	44

[a] Median duration of stavudine therapy = 79 weeks; median duration of zidovudine therapy = 53 weeks.

Pancreatitis was observed in 3 of the 412 adult patients who received ZERIT (stavudine) in a controlled monotherapy study.

Selected clinical adverse events that occurred in antiretroviral naive adult patients receiving ZERIT (stavudine) from two controlled combination studies are provided in Table 5. [See table 5 above]

Table 5
Selected Clinical Adverse Events in START 1 and START 2[a] Studies (Combination Therapy)

	Percent (%)			
	START 1		START 2	
Adverse Events	**ZERIT (stavudine) + lamivudine+ indinavir (n=100[b])**	**zidovudine+ lamivudine+ indinavir (n=102)**	**ZERIT (stavudine) + didanosine+ indinavir (n=102[b])**	**zidovudine+ lamivudine+ indinavir (n=103)**
Nausea	43	63	53	67
Diarrhea	34	16	45	39
Headache	25	26	46	37
Rash	18	13	30	18
Vomiting	18	33	30	35
Peripheral Neurologic Symptoms/Neuropathy	8	7	21	10

[a] START 2 compared two triple-combination regimens in 205 treatment-naive patients. Patients received either ZERIT (stavudine) (40 mg twice daily) plus didanosine plus indinavir or zidovudine plus lamivudine plus indinavir.
[b] Duration of stavudine therapy = 48 weeks.

Pancreatitis resulting in death was observed in patients treated with ZERIT (stavudine) plus didanosine, with or without hydroxyurea, in controlled clinical studies and in postmarketing reports.

Selected laboratory abnormalities reported in a controlled monotherapy study (Study AI455-019) are provided in Table 6.

Table 6
Selected Adult Laboratory Abnormalities in Study AI455-019[a,b]

	Percent (%)	
Parameter	**ZERIT (stavudine) (40 mg twice daily) (n=412)**	**zidovudine (200 mg 3 times daily) (n=402)**
AST (SGOT) (>5.0 × ULN)	11	10
ALT (SGPT) (>5.0 × ULN)	13	11
Amylase (≥1.4 × ULN)	14	13

[a] Data presented for patients for whom laboratory evaluations were performed.

Continued on next page

Zerit—Cont.

[b] Median duration of stavudine therapy = 79 weeks; median duration of zidovudine therapy = 53 weeks.
ULN = upper limit of normal.

Selected laboratory abnormalities reported in two controlled combination studies are provided in Tables 7 and 8.
[See table 7 at right]
[See table 8 at right]

Observed During Clinical Practice: The following events have been identified during post-approval use of ZERIT (stavudine). Because they are reported voluntarily from a population of unknown size, estimates of frequency cannot be made. These events have been chosen for inclusion due to their seriousness, frequency of reporting, causal connection to ZERIT (stavudine), or a combination of these factors.

Body as a Whole- abdominal pain, allergic reaction, chills/fever, and redistribution/accumulation of body fat (see **PRECAUTIONS: Fat Redistribution**).
Digestive Disorders- anorexia.
Exocrine Gland Disorders- pancreatitis [including fatal cases (see **WARNINGS**)].
Hematologic Disorders- anemia, leukopenia, and thrombocytopenia.
Liver- lactic acidosis and hepatic steatosis (see **WARNINGS**), hepatitis and liver failure.
Musculoskeletal- myalgia.
Nervous System- insomnia, severe motor weakness (most often reported in the setting of lactic acidosis, see **WARNINGS**).

Pediatric Patients: Adverse reactions and serious laboratory abnormalities in pediatric patients from birth through adolescence were similar in type and frequency to those seen in adult patients (see **PRECAUTIONS: Pediatric Use**).

OVERDOSAGE

Experience with adults treated with 12 to 24 times the recommended daily dosage revealed no acute toxicity. Complications of chronic overdosage include peripheral neuropathy and hepatic toxicity. Stavudine can be removed by hemodialysis; the mean ± SD hemodialysis clearance of stavudine is 120 ± 18 mL/min. Whether stavudine is eliminated by peritoneal dialysis has not been studied.

DOSAGE AND ADMINISTRATION

The interval between doses of ZERIT (stavudine) should be 12 hours. ZERIT (stavudine) may be taken without regard to meals.

Adults: The recommended dose based on body weight is as follows:

40 mg twice daily for patients ≥60 kg.
30 mg twice daily for patients <60 kg.

Pediatrics: The recommended dose for newborns from birth to 13 days old is 0.5 mg/kg/dose given every 12 hours (see **CLINICAL PHARMACOLOGY**). The recommended dose for pediatric patients at least 14 days old and weighing less than 30 kg is 1 mg/kg/dose, given every 12 hours. Pediatric patients weighing 30 kg or greater should receive the recommended adult dosage.

Dosage Adjustment: Patients should be monitored for the development of peripheral neuropathy, which is usually manifested by numbness, tingling, or pain in the feet or hands. These symptoms may be difficult to detect in young children (see **WARNINGS**). If these symptoms develop during treatment, stavudine therapy should be interrupted. Symptoms may resolve if therapy is withdrawn promptly. In some cases, symptoms may worsen temporarily following discontinuation of therapy. If symptoms resolve completely, patients may tolerate resumption of treatment at one-half the recommended dose:

20 mg twice daily for patients ≥60 kg.
15 mg twice daily for patients <60 kg.

If peripheral neuropathy recurs after resumption of ZERIT (stavudine), permanent discontinuation should be considered.

Renal Impairment- ZERIT (stavudine) may be administered to adult patients with impaired renal function with adjustment in dose as shown in Table 9.

Table 9
Recommended Dosage Adjustment for Renal Impairment

Creatinine Clearance (mL/min)	Recommended ZERIT (stavudine) Dose by Patient Weight	
	≥60 kg	**<60 kg**
>50	40 mg every 12 hours	30 mg every 12 hours
26-50	20 mg every 12 hours	15 mg every 12 hours
10-25	20 mg every 24 hours	15 mg every 24 hours

Since urinary excretion is also a major route of elimination of stavudine in pediatric patients, the clearance of stavudine may be altered in children with renal impairment. Although there are insufficient data to recommend a specific dose adjustment of ZERIT (stavudine) in this patient population, a reduction in the dose and/or an increase in the interval between doses should be considered.

Hemodialysis Patients- The recommended dose is 20 mg every 24 hours (≥60 kg) or 15 mg every 24 hours (<60 kg), administered after the completion of hemodialysis and at the same time of day on non-dialysis days.

Method of Preparation:
ZERIT (stavudine) for Oral Solution
Prior to dispensing, the pharmacist must constitute the dry powder with purified water to a concentration of 1 mg stavudine per mL of solution, as follows:
1. Add 202 mL of purified water to the container.
2. Shake container vigorously until the powder dissolves completely. Constitution in this way produces 200 mL (deliverable volume) of 1 mg/mL stavudine solution. The solution may appear slightly hazy.
3. Dispense solution in original container with measuring cup provided. Instruct patient to shake the container vigorously prior to measuring each dose and to store the tightly closed container in a refrigerator, 36° to 46°F (2° to 8°C). Discard any unused portion after 30 days.

Table 7
Selected Laboratory Abnormalities in START 1 and START 2 Studies (Grades 3-4)

Parameter	START 1: ZERIT (stavudine) + lamivudine+ indinavir (n=100)	START 1: zidovudine+ lamivudine+ indinavir (n=102)	START 2: ZERIT (stavudine) + didanosine+ indinavir (n=102)	START 2: zidovudine+ lamivudine+ indinavir (n=103)
	Percent (%)			
Bilirubin (>2.6 × ULN)	7	6	16	8
SGOT (AST) (>5 × ULN)	5	2	7	7
SGPT (ALT) (>5 × ULN)	6	2	8	5
GGT (>5 × ULN)	2	2	5	2
Lipase (>2 × ULN)	6	3	5	5
Amylase (>2 × ULN)	4	<1	8	2

ULN = upper limit of normal.

Table 8
Selected Laboratory Abnormalities in START 1 and START 2 Studies (All Grades)

Parameter	START 1: ZERIT (stavudine) + lamivudine+ indinavir (n=100)	START 1: zidovudine+ lamivudine+ indinavir (n=102)	START 2: ZERIT (stavudine) + didanosine+ indinavir (n=102)	START 2: zidovudine+ lamivudine+ indinavir (n=103)
	Percent (%)			
Total Bilirubin	65	60	68	55
SGOT (AST)	42	20	53	20
SGPT (ALT)	40	20	50	18
GGT	15	8	28	12
Lipase	27	12	26	19
Amylase	21	19	31	17

Table 10
Capsule Strength/Configuration

Product Strength	Capsule Shell Color	Markings on Capsule (in Black Ink)	Capsules per Bottle	NDC No.
15 mg	Light yellow & dark red	BMS 1964 15	60	0003-1964-01
20 mg	Light brown	BMS 1965 20	60	0003-1965-01
30 mg	Light orange & dark orange	BMS 1966 30	60	0003-1966-01
40 mg	Dark orange	BMS 1967 40	60	0003-1967-01

HOW SUPPLIED

ZERIT® Capsules are available in the following strengths and configurations of plastic bottles with child-resistant closures:
[See table 10 above]

ZERIT® (stavudine) for Oral Solution is a dye-free, fruit-flavored powder that provides 1 mg of stavudine per mL of solution upon constitution with water. Directions for solution preparation are included on the product label and in the **DOSAGE AND ADMINISTRATION** section of this insert. ZERIT (stavudine) for Oral Solution (**NDC** No. 0003-1968-01) is available in child-resistant containers that provide 200 mL of solution after constitution with water.
US Patent No.: 4,978,655

Storage: ZERIT (stavudine) Capsules should be stored in tightly closed containers at controlled room temperature, 59° to 86°F (15° to 30°C).

ZERIT (stavudine) for Oral Solution should be protected from excessive moisture and stored in tightly closed containers at controlled room temperature, 59° to 86°F (15° to 30°C). After constitution, store tightly closed containers of ZERIT (stavudine) for Oral Solution in a refrigerator, 36° to 46°F (2° to 8°C). Discard any unused portion after 30 days.

BMS Virology™
Bristol-Myers Squibb Company
Princeton, NJ 08543
U.S.A.

F9-B001-62-02 1099813A5
J4673E 1967DIM-7
Revised April 2002

PATIENT INFORMATION

ZERIT® ℞ **ONLY**
(generic name = **stavudine**, also known as **d4T**)
ZERIT® (stavudine) Capsules
ZERIT® (stavudine) for Oral Solution

What is ZERIT (stavudine)?

ZERIT (pronounced ZER it) (stavudine) is a prescription medicine used in combination with other drugs to treat adults and children who are infected with HIV (the human immunodeficiency virus), the virus that causes AIDS. ZERIT (stavudine) belongs to a class of drugs called nucleoside analogues. By reducing the growth of HIV, ZERIT (stavudine) helps your body maintain its supply of CD4 cells, which are important for fighting HIV and other infections.

ZERIT (stavudine) will not cure your HIV infection. At present there is no cure for HIV infection. Even while taking ZERIT (stavudine), you may continue to have HIV-related illnesses, including infections caused by other disease-producing organisms. Continue to see your doctor regularly and report any medical problems that occur.

ZERIT (stavudine) does not prevent a patient infected with HIV from passing the virus to other people. To protect others, you must continue to practice safe sex and take precautions to prevent others from coming in contact with your blood and other body fluids.

There is limited information on the long-term use of ZERIT (stavudine).

Who should not take ZERIT (stavudine)?

Do not take ZERIT (stavudine) if you are allergic to any of its ingredients, including its active ingredient, stavudine, and the inactive ingredients. (See **Inactive Ingredients** at the end of this leaflet.) Tell your doctor if you think you have had an allergic reaction to any of these ingredients.

How should I take ZERIT (stavudine)? How should I store it?

Your doctor will determine your dose (the amount in each capsule or spoonful) based on your body weight, kidney and liver function, and any side effects that you may have had with other medicines. Take ZERIT (stavudine) exactly as instructed. Try not to miss a dose, but if you do, take it as soon as possible. If it is almost time for the next dose, skip the missed dose and continue your regular dosing schedule. ZERIT (stavudine) may be taken with food or on an empty stomach.

- ***Capsules:*** ZERIT (stavudine) capsules are usually taken twice a day (every 12 hours). Store ZERIT (stavudine) capsules in a tightly closed container at room temperature away from heat and out of the reach of children and pets. Do NOT store this medicine in a damp place such as a bathroom medicine cabinet or near the kitchen sink.
- ***Oral solution (for children):*** ZERIT (stavudine) for Oral Solution is taken twice a day (every 12 hours). If your child will be taking ZERIT (stavudine), the doctor should give you written instructions on how to give this medicine. Before measuring each dose, shake the bottle well. Store ZERIT (stavudine) for Oral Solution in a tightly closed container in a refrigerator and throw away any unused portion after 30 days.

If you have a kidney problem: If your kidneys are not working properly, your doctor may monitor your kidney function while you take ZERIT (stavudine). Also, your dosage of ZERIT (stavudine) may be adjusted.

What should I do if someone takes an overdosage of ZERIT (stavudine)?

If you suspect that someone has taken an overdose of ZERIT (stavudine), get medical help right away. Contact their doctor or a poison control center.

What should I avoid while taking ZERIT (stavudine)?

Other medicines. Other medicines, including those you can buy without a prescription, may interfere with the actions of ZERIT (stavudine). You should not use ZERIT (stavudine) in combination with zidovudine (AZT). **Do not take any medicine, vitamin, supplement, or other health preparation without first checking with your doctor.** (Taking ZERIT (stavudine) with other drugs that also may cause peripheral neuropathy may increase your risk of getting this serious side effect.)

Pregnancy: It is not known if ZERIT (stavudine) can harm a human fetus. Also, pregnant women have experienced serious side effects when taking ZERIT (stavudine) in combination with didanosine and other HIV medicines. ZERIT (stavudine) should be used during pregnancy only after discussion with your doctor. **Tell your doctor if you become pregnant or plan to become pregnant while taking ZERIT (stavudine).**

Nursing: Because studies have shown ZERIT (stavudine) is in the breast milk of animals receiving the drug, it may be present in human breast milk. The Centers for Disease Control and Prevention (CDC) recommends that HIV-infected mothers **not** breast-feed to reduce the risk of passing HIV infection to their babies and the potential for serious adverse reactions in nursing infants. Therefore, do not nurse a baby while taking ZERIT (stavudine).

What are the possible side effects of ZERIT (stavudine)?

Serious side effects of ZERIT (stavudine) may include:

- **Lactic acidosis**, severe increase of lactic acid in the blood, **severe liver enlargement**, including inflammation (pain and swelling) of the liver, and **liver failure**, which can cause death.
- **Peripheral neuropathy**, a nerve disorder of the hands and feet.

People who take ZERIT (stavudine) along with other medicines that may cause similar side effects may have a higher chance of developing these side effects than if they took ZERIT (stavudine) alone. For example, if you use ZERIT (stavudine) in combination with other drugs (including didanosine, with or without hydroxyurea) that may be associated with liver enlargement, peripheral neuropathy, or pancreatitis, you may be at increased risk for these side effects. Children experience side effects that are similar to those experienced by adults.

Lactic acidosis and severe liver enlargement: Lactic acidosis and severe liver enlargement, including deaths, have been reported among patients taking ZERIT (stavudine) (including pregnant women). ***Symptoms of lactic acidosis may include:***

- ***nausea, vomiting, or unusual or unexpected stomach discomfort;***
- ***feeling very weak and tired;***
- ***shortness of breath;***
- ***weakness in arms and legs.***

If you notice these symptoms or if your medical condition has suddenly changed, stop taking ZERIT (stavudine) and call your doctor right away. Lactic acidosis is a medical emergency that must be treated in a hospital. Women, overweight patients, and those who have had lengthy treatment with nucleoside medicines are more likely to develop lactic acidosis. Your doctor should check your liver function periodically while you are taking ZERIT (stavudine), especially if you have a history of heavy alcohol use or a liver problem. The combination of ZERIT (stavudine), didanosine, and hydroxyurea may increase your risk for liver damage, which may be fatal. Your doctor should closely monitor your liver function if you are taking this combination.

Peripheral neuropathy: This nerve disorder is rare, but may be serious. ***Tell your doctor right away*** *if you or a child taking ZERIT (stavudine) has continuing numbness, tingling, burning, or pain in the feet and/or hands.* A child may not recognize these symptoms or know to tell you that his or her feet or hands are numb, burning, tingling, or painful. Ask your child's doctor for instructions on how to find out if your child develops peripheral neuropathy.

Let your doctor know if you or a child taking ZERIT (stavudine) has ever had peripheral neuropathy, because this condition occurs more often in patients who have had it previously. Peripheral neuropathy is also more likely to occur in patients taking drugs that affect the nerves and in patients with advanced HIV disease, but it can occur at any disease stage. If you develop peripheral neuropathy, your doctor may tell you to stop taking ZERIT (stavudine). In some cases the symptoms worsen for a short time before getting better. Once symptoms of peripheral neuropathy go away completely, ZERIT (stavudine) may be started again at a lower dose.

Pancreatitis: Pancreatitis is a dangerous inflammation of the pancreas. It may cause death. ***Tell your doctor right away if you develop stomach pain, nausea, or vomiting. These can be signs of pancreatitis.*** Let your doctor know if you have ever had pancreatitis, regularly drink alcoholic beverages, or have gallstones. Pancreatitis occurs more often in patients with these conditions. It is also more likely in people with advanced HIV disease, but can occur at any disease stage. The combination of ZERIT (stavudine) and didanosine, with or without hydroxyurea, may increase your risk for pancreatitis.

Other side effects: In addition to peripheral neuropathy, the most frequent side effects observed in studies of adults taking the recommended dose of ZERIT (stavudine) were headache, diarrhea, rash, and nausea and vomiting. Other side effects may include abdominal pain, muscle pain, insomnia, loss of appetite, chills or fever, allergic reactions, and blood disorders.

Changes in body fat have been seen in some patients taking antiretroviral therapy. These changes may include increased amount of fat in the upper back and neck ("buffalo hump"), breast, and around the trunk. Loss of fat from the legs, arms, and face may also happen. The cause and long-term health effects of these conditions are not known at this time.

What else should I know about ZERIT (stavudine)?

If you have diabetes mellitus: ZERIT (stavudine) for Oral Solution

contains 50 mg of sucrose (sugar) per mL.

Inactive Ingredients:

ZERIT (stavudine) Capsules: microcrystalline cellulose, sodium starch glycolate, lactose (milk sugar), and magnesium stearate in a hard gelatin shell.

ZERIT (stavudine) for Oral Solution: methylparaben, propylparaben, sodium carboxymethylcellulose, sucrose (table sugar), and flavoring agents.

This medicine was prescribed for your particular condition. Do not use ZERIT (stavudine) for another condition or give it to others. Keep ZERIT (stavudine) and all other medicines out of the reach of children. Throw away ZERIT (stavudine) when it is outdated or no longer needed by flushing it down the toilet or pouring it down the sink.

This summary does not include everything there is to know about ZERIT (stavudine). Medicines are sometimes prescribed for purposes other than those listed in a Patient Information Leaflet. If you have questions or concerns, or want more information about ZERIT (stavudine), your physician and pharmacist have the complete prescribing information upon which this leaflet was based. You may want to read it and discuss it with your doctor or other healthcare professional. Remember, no written summary can replace careful discussion with your doctor.

BMS Virology™
Bristol-Myers Squibb Company
Princeton, NJ 08543
U.S.A.

This Patient Information Leaflet has been approved by the U.S. Food and Drug Administration.

F9-B001B-6-02 Based on 1099813A5
Revised April 2002

Shown in Product Identification Guide, page 310

J.R. Carlson Laboratories, Inc.

15 COLLEGE DR.
ARLINGTON HEIGHTS, IL 60004-1985

Direct Inquiries to:
Customer Service
(847) 255-1600
FAX: (847) 255-1605
www.carlsonlabs.com

For Medical Information Contact:
In Emergencies:
Customer Service
(847) 255-1600
FAX: (847) 255-1605

ACES® OTC

DESCRIPTION

ACES provides four natural antioxidant nutrients.

Two Soft Gels Contain:		% U.S. RDA
Beta-Carotene (Pro-Vitamin A)	10,000 IU	200%
Vitamin C (Calcium Ascorbate)	1000 mg	1667%
Vitamin E (d-Alpha Tocopherol)	400 IU	1333%
Selenium (L-selenomethionine)	100 mcg	*

RDA: Recommended Daily Allowance—Adults
*U.S. RDA not determined

The nutrients in ACES are: Beta Carotene—(Pro-vitamin A) derived from tiny sea plants or algae (*D. salina*) grown in the fresh ocean waters off southern Australia; Vitamin C provided as the gentle, buffered calcium ascorbate; Vitamin E 100% natural-source from soy, the most biologically active form; And Selenium—organically bound with the essential nutrient methionine to promote assimilation.

Suggested Use: For dietary supplementation, take two soft gels daily, preferably at mealtime.

Corn-free. Wheat-free. Milk-free. Sugar-free. Yeast-free. Preservative-free. Soft Gel Contents: Nutrients listed above, soybean oil, vegetable stearin, lecithin, beeswax. Soft Gel Shell: Beef gelatin, glycerin, water, carob.

HOW SUPPLIED

In bottles of 50, 90, 200, and 360.
Also available as *ACES ® plus ZINC.*

E-GEMS® OTC

DESCRIPTION

100% natural-source vitamin E (d-alpha tocopheryl acetate) soft gels. Available in 8 strengths: 30 IU, 100 IU, 200 IU, 400 IU, 600 IU, 800 IU, 1000 IU, 1200 IU.

HOW SUPPLIED

Supplied in a variety of bottle sizes.

CARLSON NORWEGIAN COD LIVER OIL OTC

Each Teaspoonful of Carlson Norwegian Cod Liver Oil provides:

Total Omega 3 Fatty Acids	1100 mg
DHA (Docosahexaenoic Acid)	500 mg
EPA (Eicosapentaenoic Acid)	460 mg
ALA (Alpha-linolenic Acid)	45 mg
Vitamin A	1100 IU
Vitamin D	400 IU
Vitamin E	10 IU

DESCRIPTION

Carlson Norwegian Cod Liver oil comes from the livers of fresh cod fish found in the North Atlantic waters near Norway. Medical scientists are encouraging people to eat more fish, as fish oil is the only major source of the long chain polyunsaturated omega-3's, EPA and DHA. Cod liver oil is a naturally rich source of these important Omega-3's

Suggested Use: Take one teaspoonful one or two times daily at mealtime.

This product is regularly tested using AOAC international protocols for potency and purity by an independent FDA registered laboratory and found to be free of detectable levels of mercury, cadmium, lead, PCB's and 28 other contaminants.

HOW SUPPLIED

Supplied in bottles of 250ml and 500ml. Lemon or regular flavor.

SUPER OMEGA-3 OTC

DESCRIPTION

Carlson Super Omega-3 soft gels contain a special concentrate of fish body oils from deep cold-water fish, which are rich in EPA & DHA. Tested to AOAC International protocols for potency and purity.

Continued on next page

Super Omega-3—Cont.

Each soft gelatin capsule provides 1000 mg of omega-3 fish oils consisting of:

EPA (eicosanpentaenoic acid)	300 mg
DHA (docosahexaenoic acid)	200 mg
Vitamin E (d-alpha tocopherol)	10 IU

HOW SUPPLIED

In bottles of 50, 100, 250.

Celgene Corporation

7 POWDER HORN DRIVE
WARREN, NJ 07059

Direct Inquiries to:
(732) 271-1001
(800) 890-4619
Customer Service
888-4-CELGENE
888-423-5436
Medical Services
732-805-3905
(732) 805-3671 fax
Drug Safety
732-805-3667
732-271-4115 fax

ALKERAN® ℞

[*ăl'-kur-ăn*]
(melphalan hydrochloride)
for Injection

> **WARNING**
> Melphalan should be administered under the supervision of a qualified physician experienced in the use of cancer chemotherapeutic agents. Severe bone marrow suppression with resulting infection or bleeding may occur. Controlled trials comparing intravenous (IV) to oral melphalan have shown more myelosuppression with the IV formulation. Hypersensitivity reactions, including anaphylaxis, have occurred in approximately 2% of patients who received the IV formulation. Melphalan is leukemogenic in humans. Melphalan produces chromosomal aberrations in vitro and in vivo and, therefore, should be considered potentially mutagenic in humans.

DESCRIPTION

Melphalan, also known as L-phenylalanine mustard, phenylalanine mustard, L-PAM, or L-sarcolysin, is a phenylalanine derivative of nitrogen mustard. Melphalan is a bifunctional alkylating agent that is active against selected human neoplastic diseases. It is known chemically as 4-[bis(2-chloroethyl)amino]-*L*-phenylalanine. The molecular formula is $C_{13}H_{18}Cl_2N_2O_2$ and the molecular weight is 305.20. The structural formula is:

$$(ClCH_2CH_2)_2N-C_6H_4-CH_2-CH(NH_2)-COOH$$

Melphalan is the active L-isomer of the compound and was first synthesized in 1953 by Bergel and Stock; the D-isomer, known as medphalan, is less active against certain animal tumors, and the dose needed to produce effects on chromosomes is larger than that required with the L-isomer. The racemic (DL-) form is known as merphalan or sarcolysin.

Melphalan is practically insoluble in water and has a pKa_1 of ~2.5.

ALKERAN for Injection is supplied as a sterile, nonpyrogenic, freeze-dried powder. Each single-use vial contains melphalan hydrochloride equivalent to 50 mg melphalan and 20 mg povidone. ALKERAN for Injection is reconstituted using the sterile diluent provided. Each vial of sterile diluent contains sodium citrate 0.2 g, propylene glycol 6.0 mL, ethanol (96%) 0.52 mL, and Water for Injection to a total of 10 mL. ALKERAN for Injection is administered intravenously.

CLINICAL PHARMACOLOGY

Melphalan is an alkylating agent of the bischloroethylamine type. As a result, its cytotoxicity appears to be related to the extent of its interstrand cross-linking with DNA, probably by binding at the N^7 position of guanine. Like other bifunctional alkylating agents, it is active against both resting and rapidly dividing tumor cells.

Pharmacokinetics: The pharmacokinetics of melphalan after IV administration has been extensively studied in adult patients. Following injection, drug plasma concentrations declined rapidly in a biexponential manner with distribution phase and terminal elimination phase half-lives of approximately 10 and 75 minutes, respectively. Estimates of average total body clearance varied among studies, but typical values of approximately 7 to 9 mL/min/kg (250 to 325 mL/min/m²) were observed. One study has reported that on repeat dosing of 0.5 mg/kg every 6 weeks, the clearance of melphalan decreased from 8.1 mL/min/kg after the first course, to 5.5 mL/min/kg after the third course, but did not decrease appreciably after the third course. Mean (±SD) peak melphalan plasma concentrations in myeloma patients given IV melphalan at doses of 10 or 20 mg/m² were 1.2 ± 0.4 and 2.8 ± 1.9 mcg/mL, respectively.

The steady-state volume of distribution of melphalan is 0.5 L/kg. Penetration into cerebrospinal fluid (CSF) is low. The extent of melphalan binding to plasma proteins ranges from 60% to 90%. Serum albumin is the major binding protein, while α_1-acid glycoprotein appears to account for about 20% of the plasma protein binding. Approximately 30% of the drug is (covalently) irreversibly bound to plasma proteins. Interactions with immunoglobulins have been found to be negligible.

Melphalan is eliminated from plasma primarily by chemical hydrolysis to monohydroxymelphalan and dihydroxymelphalan. Aside from these hydrolysis products, no other melphalan metabolites have been observed in humans. Although the contribution of renal elimination to melphalan clearance appears to be low, one study noted an increase in the occurrence of severe leukopenia in patients with elevated BUN after 10 weeks of therapy.

Clinical Trial: A randomized trial compared prednisone plus IV melphalan to prednisone plus oral melphalan in the treatment of myeloma. As discussed below, overall response rates at week 22 were comparable; however, because of changes in trial design, conclusions as to the relative activity of the 2 formulations after week 22 are impossible to make.

Both arms received oral prednisone starting at 0.8 mg/kg/day with doses tapered over 6 weeks. Melphalan doses in each arm were:

Arm 1 Oral melphalan 0.15 mg/kg/day × 7 followed by 0.05 mg/kg/day when WBC began to rise.
Arm 2 IV melphalan 16 mg/m² q 2 weeks × 4 (over 6 weeks) followed by the same dose every 4 weeks.

Doses of melphalan were adjusted according to the following criteria:

Table 1: Criteria for Dosage Adjustment in a Randomized Clinical Trial

WBC/mm³	Platelets	Percent of Full Dose
≥4,000	≥100,000	100
≥3,000	≥75,000	75
≥2,000	≥50,000	50
<2,000	<50,000	0

One hundred seven patients were randomized to the oral melphalan arm and 203 patients to the IV melphalan arm. More patients had a poor-risk classification (58% versus 44%) and high tumor load (51% versus 34%) on the oral compared to the IV arm (P<0.04). Response rates at week 22 are shown in the following table:

Table 2: Response Rates at Week 22

Initial Arm	Evaluable Patients	Responders n (%)	*P*
Oral melphalan	100	44 (44%)	*P*>0.2
IV melphalan	195	74 (38%)	

Because of changes in protocol design after week 22, other efficacy parameters such as response duration and survival cannot be compared.

Severe myelotoxicity (WBC ≤1,000 and/or platelets ≤25,000) was more common in the IV melphalan arm (28%) than in the oral melphalan arm (11%).

An association was noted between poor renal function and myelosuppression; consequently, an amendment to the protocol required a 50% reduction in IV melphalan dose if the BUN was ≥30 mg/dL. The rate of severe leukopenia in the IV arm in the patients with BUN over 30 mg/dL decreased from 50% (8/16) before protocol amendment to 11% (3/28) (P = 0.01) after the amendment.

Before the dosing amendment, there was a 10% (8/77) incidence of drug-related death in the IV arm. After the dosing amendment, this incidence was 3% (3/108). This compares to an overall 1% (1/100) incidence of drug-related death in the oral arm.

INDICATIONS AND USAGE

ALKERAN for Injection is indicated for the palliative treatment of patients with multiple myeloma for whom oral therapy is not appropriate.

CONTRAINDICATIONS

Melphalan should not be used in patients whose disease has demonstrated prior resistance to this agent. Patients who have demonstrated hypersensitivity to melphalan should not be given the drug.

WARNINGS

Melphalan should be administered in carefully adjusted dosage by or under the supervision of experienced physicians who are familiar with the drug's actions and the possible complications of its use.

As with other nitrogen mustard drugs, excessive dosage will produce marked bone marrow suppression. Bone marrow suppression is the most significant toxicity associated with ALKERAN for Injection in most patients. Therefore, the following tests should be performed at the start of therapy and prior to each subsequent dose of ALKERAN: platelet count, hemoglobin, white blood cell count, and differential. Thrombocytopenia and/or leukopenia are indications to withhold further therapy until the blood counts have sufficiently recovered. Frequent blood counts are essential to determine optimal dosage and to avoid toxicity. Dose adjustment on the basis of blood counts at the nadir and day of treatment should be considered.

Hypersensitivity reactions including anaphylaxis have occurred in approximately 2% of patients who received the IV formulation (see ADVERSE REACTIONS). These reactions usually occur after multiple courses of treatment. Treatment is symptomatic. The infusion should be terminated immediately, followed by the administration of volume expanders, pressor agents, corticosteroids, or antihistamines at the discretion of the physician. If a hypersensitivity reaction occurs, IV or oral melphalan should not be readministered since hypersensitivity reactions have also been reported with oral melphalan.

Carcinogenesis: Secondary malignancies, including acute nonlymphocytic leukemia, myeloproliferative syndrome, and carcinoma, have been reported in patients with cancer treated with alkylating agents (including melphalan). Some patients also received other chemotherapeutic agents or radiation therapy. Precise quantitation of the risk of acute leukemia, myeloproliferative syndrome, or carcinoma is not possible. Published reports of leukemia in patients who have received melphalan (and other alkylating agents) suggest that the risk of leukemogenesis increases with chronicity of treatment and with cumulative dose. In one study, the 10-year cumulative risk of developing acute leukemia or myeloproliferative syndrome after oral melphalan therapy was 19.5% for cumulative doses ranging from 730 to 9,652 mg. In this same study, as well as in an additional study, the 10-year cumulative risk of developing acute leukemia or myeloproliferative syndrome after oral melphalan therapy was less than 2% for cumulative doses under 600 mg. This does not mean that there is a cumulative dose below which there is no risk of the induction of secondary malignancy. The potential benefits from melphalan therapy must be weighed on an individual basis against the possible risk of the induction of a second malignancy.

Adequate and well-controlled carcinogenicity studies have not been conducted in animals. However, intraperitoneal (IP) administration of melphalan in rats (5.4 to 10.8 mg/m²) and in mice (2.25 to 4.5 mg/m²) 3 times per week for 6 months followed by 12 months post-dose observation produced peritoneal sarcoma and lung tumors, respectively.

Mutagenesis: Melphalan has been shown to cause chromatid or chromosome damage in humans. Intramuscular administration of melphalan at 6 and 60 mg/m² produced structural aberrations of the chromatid and chromosomes in bone marrow cells of Wistar rats.

Impairment of Fertility: Melphalan causes suppression of ovarian function in premenopausal women, resulting in amenorrhea in a significant number of patients. Reversible and irreversible testicular suppression have also been reported.

Pregnancy: Pregnancy Category D. Melphalan may cause fetal harm when administered to a pregnant woman. While adequate animal studies have not been conducted with IV melphalan, oral (6 to 18 mg/m²/day for 10 days) and IP (18 mg/m²) administration in rats was embryolethal and teratogenic. Malformations resulting from melphalan included alterations of the brain (underdevelopment, deformation, meningocele, and encephalocele) and eye (anophthalmia and microphthalmos), reduction of the mandible and tail, as well as hepatocele (exomphaly). There are no adequate and well-controlled studies in pregnant women. If this drug is used during pregnancy, or if the patient becomes pregnant while taking this drug, the patient should be apprised of the potential hazard to the fetus. Women of childbearing potential should be advised to avoid becoming pregnant.

PRECAUTIONS

General: In all instances where the use of ALKERAN for Injection is considered for chemotherapy, the physician must evaluate the need and usefulness of the drug against the risk of adverse events. Melphalan should be used with extreme caution in patients whose bone marrow reserve may have been compromised by prior irradiation or chemotherapy or whose bone marrow function is recovering from previous cytotoxic therapy.

Dose reduction should be considered in patients with renal insufficiency receiving IV melphalan. In one trial, increased bone marrow suppression was observed in patients with BUN levels ≥30 mg/dL. A 50% reduction in the IV melphalan dose decreased the incidence of severe bone marrow suppression in the latter portion of this study.

Information for Patients: Patients should be informed that the major acute toxicities of melphalan are related to bone marrow suppression, hypersensitivity reactions, gastrointestinal toxicity, and pulmonary toxicity. The major long-term toxicities are related to infertility and secondary malignancies. Patients should never be allowed to take the drug without close medical supervision and should be advised to consult their physicians if they experience skin rash, signs or symptoms of vasculitis, bleeding, fever, persistent cough, nausea, vomiting, amenorrhea, weight loss, or unusual lumps/masses. Women of childbearing potential should be advised to avoid becoming pregnant.

Laboratory Tests: Periodic complete blood counts with differentials should be performed during the course of treatment with melphalan. At least 1 determination should be obtained prior to each dose. Patients should be observed closely for consequences of bone marrow suppression, which include severe infections, bleeding, and symptomatic anemia (see WARNINGS).

Drug Interactions: The development of severe renal failure has been reported in patients treated with a single dose of IV melphalan followed by standard oral doses of cyclosporine. Cisplatin may affect melphalan kinetics by inducing renal dysfunction and subsequently altering melphalan clearance. IV melphalan may also reduce the threshold for BCNU lung toxicity. When nalidixic acid and IV melphalan are given simultaneously, the incidence of severe hemorrhagic necrotic enterocolitis has been reported to increase in pediatric patients.

Carcinogenesis, Mutagenesis, Impairment of Fertility: See WARNINGS section.

Pregnancy: ***Teratogenic Effects:*** Pregnancy Category D: See WARNINGS section.

Nursing Mothers: It is not known whether this drug is excreted in human milk. IV melphalan should not be given to nursing mothers.

Pediatric Use: The safety and effectiveness in pediatric patients have not been established.

Geriatric Use: Clinical studies of ALKERAN for Injection did not include sufficient numbers of subjects aged 65 and over to determine whether they respond differently from younger subjects. Other reported clinical experience has not identified differences in responses between the elderly and younger patients. In general, dose selection for an elderly patient should be cautious, usually starting at the low end of the dosing range, reflecting the greater frequency of decreased hepatic, renal, or cardiac function, and of concomitant disease or other drug therapy.

ADVERSE REACTIONS (see OVERDOSAGE)

The following information on adverse reactions is based on data from both oral and IV administration of melphalan as a single agent, using several different dose schedules for treatment of a wide variety of malignancies.

Hematologic: The most common side effect is bone marrow suppression. White blood cell count and platelet count nadirs usually occur 2 to 3 weeks after treatment, with recovery in 4 to 5 weeks after treatment. Irreversible bone marrow failure has been reported.

Gastrointestinal: Gastrointestinal disturbances such as nausea and vomiting, diarrhea, and oral ulceration occur infrequently. Hepatic disorders ranging from abnormal liver function tests to clinical manifestations such as hepatitis and jaundice have been reported. Hepatic veno-occlusive disease has been reported.

Hypersensitivity: Acute hypersensitivity reactions including anaphylaxis were reported in 2.4% of 425 patients receiving ALKERAN for Injection for myeloma (see WARNINGS). These reactions were characterized by urticaria, pruritus, edema, and in some patients, tachycardia, bronchospasm, dyspnea, and hypotension. These patients appeared to respond to antihistamine and corticosteroid therapy. If a hypersensitivity reaction occurs, IV or oral melphalan should not be readministered since hypersensitivity reactions have also been reported with oral melphalan.

Miscellaneous: Other reported adverse reactions include skin hypersensitivity, skin ulceration at injection site, skin necrosis rarely requiring skin grafting, vasculitis, alopecia, hemolytic anemia, allergic reaction, pulmonary fibrosis, and interstitial pneumonitis.

OVERDOSAGE

Overdoses resulting in death have been reported. Overdoses, including doses up to 290 mg/m^2, have produced the following symptoms: severe nausea and vomiting, decreased consciousness, convulsions, muscular paralysis, and cholinomimetic effects. Severe mucositis, stomatitis, colitis, diarrhea, and hemorrhage of the gastrointestinal tract occur at high doses (>100 mg/m^2). Elevations in liver enzymes and veno-occlusive disease occur infrequently. Significant hyponatremia caused by an associated inappropriate secretion of ADH syndrome has been observed. Nephrotoxicity and adult respiratory distress syndrome have been reported rarely. The principal toxic effect is bone marrow suppression. Hematologic parameters should be closely followed for 3 to 6 weeks. An uncontrolled study suggests that administration of autologous bone marrow or hematopoietic growth factors (i.e., sargramostim, filgrastim) may shorten the period of pancytopenia. General supportive measures together with appropriate blood transfusions and antibiotics should be instituted as deemed necessary by the physician. This drug is not removed from plasma to any significant degree by hemodialysis or hemoperfusion. A pediatric patient survived a 254-mg/m^2 overdose treated with standard supportive care.

DOSAGE AND ADMINISTRATION

The usual IV dose is 16 mg/m^2. Dosage reduction of up to 50% should be considered in patients with renal insufficiency (BUN ≥30 mg/dL) (see PRECAUTIONS: General). The drug is administered as a single infusion over 15 to 20 minutes. Melphalan is administered at 2-week intervals for 4 doses, then, after adequate recovery from toxicity, at 4-week intervals. Available evidence suggests about one third to one half of the patients with multiple myeloma show a favorable response to the drug. Experience with oral melphalan suggests that repeated courses should be given since improvement may continue slowly over many months, and the maximum benefit may be missed if treatment is abandoned prematurely. Dose adjustment on the basis of blood cell counts at the nadir and day of treatment should be considered.

Administration Precautions: As with other toxic compounds, caution should be exercised in handling and preparing the solution of ALKERAN. Skin reactions associated with accidental exposure may occur. The use of gloves is recommended. If the solution of ALKERAN contacts the skin or mucosa, immediately wash the skin or mucosa thoroughly with soap and water.

Procedures for proper handling and disposal of anticancer drugs should be considered. Several guidelines on this subject have been published.[1–8] There is no general agreement that all of the procedures recommended in the guidelines are necessary or appropriate.

Parenteral drug products should be visually inspected for particulate matter and discoloration prior to administration whenever solution and container permit. If either occurs, do not use this product.

Preparation for Administration/Stability

1. ALKERAN for Injection must be reconstituted by rapidly injecting 10 mL of the supplied diluent directly into the vial of lyophilized powder using a sterile needle (20-gauge or larger needle diameter) and syringe. Immediately shake vial vigorously until a clear solution is obtained. This provides a 5-mg/mL solution of melphalan. Rapid addition of the diluent followed by immediate vigorous shaking is important for proper dissolution.
2. **Immediately** dilute the dose to be administered in 0.9% Sodium Chloride Injection, USP, to a concentration not greater than 0.45 mg/mL.
3. Administer the diluted product over a minimum of 15 minutes.
4. Complete administration within 60 minutes of reconstitution.

The time between reconstitution/dilution and administration of ALKERAN should be kept to a minimum because reconstituted and diluted solutions of ALKERAN are unstable. Over as short a time as 30 minutes, a citrate derivative of melphalan has been detected in reconstituted material from the reaction of ALKERAN with Sterile Diluent for ALKERAN. Upon further dilution with saline, nearly 1% label strength of melphalan hydrolyzes every 10 minutes.

A precipitate forms if the reconstituted solution is stored at 5°C. DO NOT REFRIGERATE THE RECONSTITUTED PRODUCT.

HOW SUPPLIED

ALKERAN for Injection is supplied in a carton containing one single-use clear glass vial of freeze-dried melphalan hydrochloride equivalent to 50 mg melphalan and one 10-mL clear glass vial of sterile diluent (NDC 59572-301-01).

Store at controlled room temperature 15° to 30°C (59° to 86°F) and protect from light.

REFERENCES

1. ONS Clinical Practice Committee. Cancer Chemotherapy Guidelines and Recommendations for Practice. Pittsburgh, PA: Oncology Nursing Society; 1999:32-41.
2. Recommendations for the safe handling of parenteral antineoplastic drugs. Washington, DC: Division of Safety, Clinical Center Pharmacy Department and Cancer Nursing Services, National Institutes of Health; 1982. US Dept of Health and Human Services, Public Health Service publication NIH 92-2621.
3. AMA Council on Scientific Affairs. Guidelines for handling parenteral antineoplastics. *JAMA.* 1985;253:1590-1591.
4. National Study Commission on Cytotoxic Exposure. Recommendations for handling cytotoxic agents. 1987. Available from Louis P. Jeffrey, Chairman, National Study Commission on Cytotoxic Exposure. Massachusetts College of Pharmacy and Allied Health Sciences, 179 Longwood Avenue, Boston, MA 02115.
5. Clinical Oncological Society of Australia. Guidelines and recommendations for safe handling of antineoplastic agents. *Med J Australia.* 1983;1:426-428.
6. Jones RB, Frank R, Mass T. Safe handling of chemotherapeutic agents: a report from the Mount Sinai Medical Center. *CA-A Cancer J for Clin.* 1983;33:258-263.
7. American Society of Hospital Pharmacists. ASHP technical assistance bulletin on handling cytotoxic and hazardous drugs. *Am J Hosp Pharm.* 1990;47:1033-1049.
8. Controlling Occupational Exposure to Hazardous Drugs. (OSHA Work-Practice Guidelines.) *Am J Health-Syst Pharm.* 1996;53:1669-1685.

Manufactured by
Cardinal Health
Albuquerque, NM 87107
Celgene®
Distributed by
Celgene Corporation
Warren, NJ 07059
7-CGSAUSA-01
June 2003 RL-2012 4155564

Shown in Product Identification Guide, page 310

ALKERAN® ℞

[*ăl'kər'ăn*]
(melphalan)
Tablets

WARNING

ALKERAN (melphalan) should be administered under the supervision of a qualified physician experienced in the use of cancer chemotherapeutic agents. Severe bone marrow suppression with resulting infection or bleeding may occur. Melphalan is leukemogenic in humans. Melphalan produces chromosomal aberrations in vitro and in vivo and, therefore, should be considered potentially mutagenic in humans.

DESCRIPTION

ALKERAN (melphalan), also known as L-phenylalanine mustard, phenylalanine mustard, L-PAM, or L-sarcolysin, is a phenylalanine derivative of nitrogen mustard. Melphalan is a bifunctional alkylating agent which is active against selective human neoplastic diseases. It is known chemically as 4-[bis(2-chloroethyl)amino]-*L*-phenylalanine. The molecular formula is $C_{13}H_{18}Cl_2N_2O_2$ and the molecular weight is 305.20. The structural formula is:

$(ClCH_2CH_2)_2N$–[benzene ring]–CH_2–C(H)(NH_2)–COOH

Melphalan is the active L-isomer of the compound and was first synthesized in 1953 by Bergel and Stock; the D-isomer, known as medphalan, is less active against certain animal tumors, and the dose needed to produce effects on chromosomes is larger than that required with the L-isomer. The racemic (DL–) form is known as merphalan or sarcolysin. Melphalan is practically insoluble in water and has a pK_{a1} of ~2.5.

ALKERAN (melphalan) is available in tablet form for oral administration. Each film-coated tablet contains 2 mg melphalan and the inactive ingredients colloidal silicon dioxide, crospovidone, hypromellose, macrogol/PEG 400, magnesium stearate, microcrystalline cellulose, and titanium dioxide.

CLINICAL PHARMACOLOGY

Melphalan is an alkylating agent of the bischloroethylamine type. As a result, its cytotoxicity appears to be related to the extent of its interstrand cross-linking with DNA, probably by binding at the N^7 position of guanine. Like other bifunctional alkylating agents, it is active against both resting and rapidly dividing tumor cells.

Pharmacokinetics: The pharmacokinetics of ALKERAN after oral administration has been extensively studied in adult patients. Plasma melphalan levels are highly variable after oral dosing, both with respect to the time of the first appearance of melphalan in plasma (range approximately 0 to 6 hours) and to the peak plasma concentration (C_{max}) (range 70 to 4,000 ng/mL, depending upon the dose) achieved. These results may be due to incomplete intestinal absorption, a variable "first pass" hepatic metabolism, or to rapid hydrolysis. Five patients were studied after both oral and intravenous (IV) dosing with 0.6 mg/kg as a single bolus dose by each route. The areas under the plasma concentration-time curves (AUC) after oral administration averaged 61% ± 26% (± standard deviation [SD]; range 25% to 89%) of those following IV administration. In 18 patients given a single oral dose of 0.6 mg/kg of ALKERAN, the terminal elimination plasma half-life ($t_{1/2}$) of parent drug was 1.5 ± 0.83 hours. The 24-hour urinary excretion of parent drug in these patients was 10% ± 4.5%, suggesting that renal clearance is not a major route of elimination of parent drug. In a separate study in 18 patients given single oral doses of 0.2 to 0.25 mg/kg of ALKERAN, C_{max} and AUC, when dose adjusted to a dose of 14 mg, were (mean ± SD) 212 ± 74 ng/mL and 498 ± 137 ng•h/mL, respectively. Elimination phase $t_{1/2}$ in these patients was approximately 1 hour and the median t_{max} was 1 hour.

One study using universally labeled ^{14}C-melphalan, found substantially less radioactivity in the urine of patients given the drug by mouth (30% of administered dose in 9 days) than in the urine of those given it intravenously (35% to 65% in 7 days). Following either oral or IV administration, the pattern of label recovery was similar, with the majority being recovered in the first 24 hours. Following oral administration, peak radioactivity occurred in plasma at 2 hours and then disappeared with a half-life of approximately 160 hours. In 1 patient where parent drug (rather than just radiolabel) was determined, the melphalan half-disappearance time was 67 minutes.

The steady-state volume of distribution of melphalan is 0.5 L/kg. Penetration into cerebrospinal fluid (CSF) is low. The extent of melphalan binding to plasma proteins ranges from 60% to 90%. Serum albumin is the major binding protein, while α_1-acid glycoprotein appears to account for about 20% of the plasma protein binding. Approximately 30% of melphalan is (covalently) irreversibly bound to plasma proteins. Interactions with immunoglobulins have been found to be negligible.

Melphalan is eliminated from plasma primarily by chemical hydrolysis to monohydroxymelphalan and dihydroxymel-

Continued on next page

Alkeran Tablets—Cont.

phalan. Aside from these hydrolysis products, no other melphalan metabolites have been observed in humans. Although the contribution of renal elimination to melphalan clearance appears to be low, one pharmacokinetic study showed a significant positive correlation between the elimination rate constant for melphalan and renal function and a significant negative correlation between renal function and the area under the plasma melphalan concentration/time curve.

INDICATIONS AND USAGE

ALKERAN Tablets are indicated for the palliative treatment of multiple myeloma and for the palliation of non-resectable epithelial carcinoma of the ovary.

CONTRAINDICATIONS

ALKERAN should not be used in patients whose disease has demonstrated a prior resistance to this agent. Patients who have demonstrated hypersensitivity to melphalan should not be given the drug.

WARNINGS

ALKERAN should be administered in carefully adjusted dosage by or under the supervision of experienced physicians who are familiar with the drug's actions and the possible complications of its use.

As with other nitrogen mustard drugs, excessive dosage will produce marked bone marrow suppression. Bone marrow suppression is the most significant toxicity associated with ALKERAN in most patients. Therefore, the following tests should be performed at the start of therapy and prior to each subsequent course of ALKERAN: platelet count, hemoglobin, white blood cell count, and differential. Thrombocytopenia and/or leukopenia are indications to withhold further therapy until the blood counts have sufficiently recovered. Frequent blood counts are essential to determine optimal dosage and to avoid toxicity (see PRECAUTIONS: Laboratory Tests). Dose adjustment on the basis of blood counts at the nadir and day of treatment should be considered.

Hypersensitivity reactions, including anaphylaxis, have occurred rarely (see ADVERSE REACTIONS). These reactions have occurred after multiple courses of treatment and have recurred in patients who experienced a hypersensitivity reaction to IV ALKERAN. If a hypersensitivity reaction occurs, oral or IV ALKERAN should not be readministered.

Carcinogenesis: Secondary malignancies, including acute nonlymphocytic leukemia, myeloproliferative syndrome, and carcinoma have been reported in patients with cancer treated with alkylating agents (including melphalan). Some patients also received other chemotherapeutic agents or radiation therapy. Precise quantitation of the risk of acute leukemia, myeloproliferative syndrome, or carcinoma is not possible. Published reports of leukemia in patients who have received melphalan (and other alkylating agents) suggest that the risk of leukemogenesis increases with chronicity of treatment and with cumulative dose. In one study, the 10-year cumulative risk of developing acute leukemia or myeloproliferative syndrome after melphalan therapy was 19.5% for cumulative doses ranging from 730 mg to 9,652 mg. In this same study, as well as in an additional study, the 10-year cumulative risk of developing acute leukemia or myeloproliferative syndrome after melphalan therapy was less than 2% for cumulative doses under 600 mg. This does not mean that there is a cumulative dose below which there is no risk of the induction of secondary malignancy. The potential benefits from melphalan therapy must be weighed on an individual basis against the possible risk of the induction of a second malignancy.

Adequate and well-controlled carcinogenicity studies have not been conducted in animals. However, i.p. administration of melphalan in rats (5.4 to 10.8 mg/m^2) and in mice (2.25 to 4.5 mg/m^2) 3 times per week for 6 months followed by 12 months post-dose observation produced peritoneal sarcoma and lung tumors, respectively.

Mutagenesis: ALKERAN has been shown to cause chromatid or chromosome damage in humans. Intramuscular administration of ALKERAN at 6 and 60 mg/m^2 produced structural aberrations of the chromatid and chromosomes in bone marrow cells of Wistar rats.

Impairment of Fertility: ALKERAN causes suppression of ovarian function in premenopausal women, resulting in amenorrhea in a significant number of patients. Reversible and irreversible testicular suppression have also been reported.

Pregnancy: Pregnancy Category D. ALKERAN may cause fetal harm when administered to a pregnant woman. Melphalan was embryolethal and teratogenic in rats following oral (6 to 18 mg/m^2/day for 10 days) and intraperitoneal (18 mg/m^2) administration. Malformations resulting from melphalan included alterations of the brain (underdevelopment, deformation, meningocele, and encephalocele) and eye (anophthalmia and microphthalmos), reduction of the mandible and tail, as well as hepatocele (exomphaly).

There are no adequate and well-controlled studies in pregnant women. If this drug is used during pregnancy, or if the patient becomes pregnant while taking this drug, the patient should be apprised of the potential hazard to the fetus. Women of childbearing potential should be advised to avoid becoming pregnant.

PRECAUTIONS

General: In all instances where the use of ALKERAN is considered for chemotherapy, the physician must evaluate the need and usefulness of the drug against the risk of adverse events. ALKERAN should be used with extreme caution in patients whose bone marrow reserve may have been compromised by prior irradiation or chemotherapy, or whose marrow function is recovering from previous cytotoxic therapy. If the leukocyte count falls below 3,000 cells/mcL, or the platelet count below 100,000 cells/mcL, ALKERAN should be discontinued until the peripheral blood cell counts have recovered.

A recommendation as to whether or not dosage reduction should be made routinely in patients with renal insufficiency cannot be made because:

a) There is considerable inherent patient-to-patient variability in the systemic availability of melphalan in patients with normal renal function.

b) Only a small amount of the administered dose appears as parent drug in the urine of patients with normal renal function.

Patients with azotemia should be closely observed, however, in order to make dosage reductions, if required, at the earliest possible time.

Information for Patients: Patients should be informed that the major toxicities of ALKERAN are related to bone marrow suppression, hypersensitivity reactions, gastrointestinal toxicity, and pulmonary toxicity. The major long-term toxicities are related to infertility and secondary malignancies. Patients should never be allowed to take the drug without close medical supervision and should be advised to consult their physician if they experience skin rash, vasculitis, bleeding, fever, persistent cough, nausea, vomiting, amenorrhea, weight loss, or unusual lumps/masses. Women of childbearing potential should be advised to avoid becoming pregnant.

Laboratory Tests: Periodic complete blood counts with differentials should be performed during the course of treatment with ALKERAN. At least one determination should be obtained prior to each treatment course. Patients should be observed closely for consequences of bone marrow suppression, which include severe infections, bleeding, and symptomatic anemia (see WARNINGS).

Drug Interactions: There are no known drug/drug interactions with oral ALKERAN.

Carcinogenesis, Mutagenesis, Impairment of Fertility: See WARNINGS section.

Pregnancy: ***Teratogenic Effects:*** Pregnancy Category D: See WARNINGS section.

Nursing Mothers: It is not known whether this drug is excreted in human milk. ALKERAN should not be given to nursing mothers.

Pediatric Use: The safety and effectiveness of ALKERAN in pediatric patients have not been established.

Geriatric Use: Clinical studies of ALKERAN Tablets did not include sufficient numbers of subjects aged 65 and over to determine whether they respond differently from younger subjects. Other reported clinical experience has not identified differences in responses between the elderly and younger patients. In general, dose selection for an elderly patient should be cautious, usually starting at the low end of the dosing range, reflecting the greater frequency of decreased hepatic, renal, or cardiac function, and of concomitant disease or other drug therapy.

ADVERSE REACTIONS

Hematologic: The most common side effect is bone marrow suppression. Although bone marrow suppression frequently occurs, it is usually reversible if melphalan is withdrawn early enough. However, irreversible bone marrow failure has been reported.

Gastrointestinal: Gastrointestinal disturbances such as nausea and vomiting, diarrhea, and oral ulceration occur infrequently. Hepatic disorders ranging from abnormal liver function tests to clinical manifestations such as hepatitis and jaundice have been reported.

Miscellaneous: Other reported adverse reactions include: pulmonary fibrosis and interstitial pneumonitis, skin hypersensitivity, vasculitis, alopecia, and hemolytic anemia. Allergic reactions, including rare anaphylaxis, have occurred after multiple courses of treatment.

OVERDOSAGE

Overdoses, including doses up to 50 mg/day for 16 days, have been reported. Immediate effects are likely to be vomiting, ulceration of the mouth, diarrhea, and hemorrhage of the gastrointestinal tract. The principal toxic effect is bone marrow suppression. Hematologic parameters should be closely followed for 3 to 6 weeks. An uncontrolled study suggests that administration of autologous bone marrow or hematopoietic growth factors (i.e., sargramostim, filgrastim) may shorten the period of pancytopenia. General supportive measures, together with appropriate blood transfusions and antibiotics, should be instituted as deemed necessary by the physician. This drug is not removed from plasma to any significant degree by hemodialysis.

DOSAGE AND ADMINISTRATION

Multiple Myeloma: The usual oral dose is 6 mg (3 tablets) daily. The entire daily dose may be given at one time. The dose is adjusted, as required, on the basis of blood counts done at approximately weekly intervals. After 2 to 3 weeks of treatment, the drug should be discontinued for up to 4 weeks, during which time the blood count should be followed carefully. When the white blood cell and platelet counts are rising, a maintenance dose of 2 mg daily may be instituted. Because of the patient-to-patient variation in melphalan plasma levels following oral administration of the drug, several investigators have recommended that the dosage of ALKERAN be cautiously escalated until some myelosuppression is observed in order to assure that potentially therapeutic levels of the drug have been reached.

Other dosage regimens have been used by various investigators. Osserman and Takatsuki have used an initial course of 10 mg/day for 7 to 10 days. They report that maximal suppression of the leukocyte and platelet counts occurs within 3 to 5 weeks and recovery within 4 to 8 weeks. Continuous maintenance therapy with 2 mg/day is instituted when the white blood cell count is greater than 4,000 cells/mcL and the platelet count is greater than 100,000 cells/mcL. Dosage is adjusted to between 1 and 3 mg/day depending upon the hematological response. It is desirable to try to maintain a significant degree of bone marrow depression so as to keep the leukocyte count in the range of 3,000 to 3,500 cells/mcL.

Hoogstraten et al have started treatment with 0.15 mg/kg/day for 7 days. This is followed by a rest period of at least 14 days, but it may be as long as 5 to 6 weeks. Maintenance therapy is started when the white blood cell and platelet counts are rising. The maintenance dose is 0.05 mg/kg/day or less and is adjusted according to the blood count.

Available evidence suggests that about one third to one half of the patients with multiple myeloma show a favorable response to oral administration of the drug.

One study by Alexanian et al has shown that the use of ALKERAN in combination with prednisone significantly improves the percentage of patients with multiple myeloma who achieve palliation. One regimen has been to administer courses of ALKERAN at 0.25 mg/kg/day for 4 consecutive days (or, 0.20 mg/kg/day for 5 consecutive days) for a total dose of 1 mg/kg/course. These 4- to 5-day courses are then repeated every 4 to 6 weeks if the granulocyte count and the platelet count have returned to normal levels.

It is to be emphasized that response may be very gradual over many months; it is important that repeated courses or continuous therapy be given since improvement may continue slowly over many months, and the maximum benefit may be missed if treatment is abandoned too soon.

In patients with moderate to severe renal impairment, currently available pharmacokinetic data do not justify an absolute recommendation on dosage reduction to those patients, but it may be prudent to use a reduced dose initially.

Epithelial Ovarian Cancer: One commonly employed regimen for the treatment of ovarian carcinoma has been to administer ALKERAN at a dose of 0.2 mg/kg daily for 5 days as a single course. Courses are repeated every 4 to 5 weeks depending upon hematologic tolerance.

Administration Precautions: Procedures for proper handling and disposal of anticancer drugs should be considered. Several guidelines on this subject have been published.[1–8] There is no general agreement that all of the procedures recommended in the guidelines are necessary or appropriate.

HOW SUPPLIED

ALKERAN is supplied as white, film-coated, round, biconvex tablets containing 2 mg melphalan in amber glass bottles with child-resistant closures. One side is engraved with "GX EH3" and the other side is engraved with an "A." Bottle of 50 (NDC 59572-302-50).

Store in a refrigerator, 2° to 8°C (36° to 46°F). Protect from light.

REFERENCES

1. ONS Clinical Practice Committee. Cancer Chemotherapy Guidelines and Recommendations for Practice. Pittsburgh, PA: Oncology Nursing Society;1999:32–41.
2. Recommendations for the safe handling of parenteral antineoplastic drugs. Washington, DC: Division of Safety, Clinical Center Pharmacy Department and Cancer Nursing Services, National Institutes of Health; 1992. US Dept of Health and Human Services. Public Health Service publication NIH 92-2621.
3. AMA Council on Scientific Affairs. Guidelines for handling parenteral antineoplastics. *JAMA.* 1985;253:1590–1591.
4. National Study Commission on Cytotoxic Exposure. Recommendations for handling cytotoxic agents. 1987. Available from Louis P. Jeffrey, Chairman, National Study Commission on Cytotoxic Exposure. Massachusetts College of Pharmacy and Allied Health Sciences, 179 Longwood Avenue, Boston, MA 02115.
5. Clinical Oncological Society of Australia. Guidelines and recommendations for safe handling of antineoplastic agents. *Med J Australia.* 1983;1:426–428.
6. Jones RB, Frank R, Mass T. Safe handling of chemotherapeutic agents: a report from the Mount Sinai Medical Center. *CA-A Cancer J for Clin.* 1983;33:258–263.
7. American Society of Hospital Pharmacists. ASHP technical assistance bulletin on handling cytotoxic and hazardous drugs. *Am J Hosp Pharm.* 1990;47:1033–1049.
8. Controlling Occupational Exposure to Hazardous Drugs. (OSHA Work-Practice Guidelines.) *Am J Health-Syst Pharm.* 1996;53:1669–1685.

GlaxoSmithKline
Research Triangle Park, NC 27709
Distributed by
Celgene Corporation
Warren, NJ 07059

May 2003 RL-2014
Shown in Product Identification Guide, page 310

THALOMID® ℞
[*thă-lō-mĭd*]
(thalidomide) Capsules
50 mg, 100 mg, & 200 mg

WARNING: SEVERE, LIFE-THREATENING HUMAN BIRTH DEFECTS.
IF THALIDOMIDE IS TAKEN DURING PREGNANCY, IT CAN CAUSE SEVERE BIRTH DEFECTS OR DEATH TO AN UNBORN BABY. THALIDOMIDE SHOULD NEVER BE USED BY WOMEN WHO ARE PREGNANT OR WHO COULD BECOME PREGNANT WHILE TAKING THE DRUG. EVEN A SINGLE DOSE [1 CAPSULE (50 mg, 100 mg or 200 mg)] TAKEN BY A PREGNANT WOMAN DURING HER PREGNANCY CAN CAUSE SEVERE BIRTH DEFECTS.
BECAUSE OF THIS TOXICITY AND IN AN EFFORT TO MAKE THE CHANCE OF FETAL EXPOSURE TO THALOMID® (thalidomide) AS NEGLIGIBLE AS POSSIBLE, THALOMID® (thalidomide) IS APPROVED FOR MARKETING ONLY UNDER A SPECIAL RESTRICTED DISTRIBUTION PROGRAM APPROVED BY THE FOOD AND DRUG ADMINISTRATION. THIS PROGRAM IS CALLED THE "SYSTEM FOR THALIDOMIDE EDUCATION AND PRESCRIBING SAFETY *(S.T.E.P.S.®)*."
UNDER THIS RESTRICTED DISTRIBUTION PROGRAM, ONLY PRESCRIBERS AND PHARMACISTS REGISTERED WITH THE PROGRAM ARE ALLOWED TO PRESCRIBE AND DISPENSE THE PRODUCT. IN ADDITION, PATIENTS MUST BE ADVISED OF, AGREE TO, AND COMPLY WITH THE REQUIREMENTS OF THE *S.T.E.P.S.®* PROGRAM IN ORDER TO RECEIVE PRODUCT.
PLEASE SEE THE FOLLOWING BOXED WARNINGS CONTAINING SPECIAL INFORMATION FOR PRESCRIBERS, FEMALE PATIENTS, AND MALE PATIENTS ABOUT THIS RESTRICTED DISTRIBUTION PROGRAM.

PRESCRIBERS

THALOMID® (thalidomide) may be prescribed only by licensed prescribers who are registered in the *S.T.E.P.S.®* program and understand the risk of teratogenicity if thalidomide is used during pregnancy.
Major human fetal abnormalities related to thalidomide administration during pregnancy have been documented: amelia (absence of limbs), phocomelia (short limbs), hypoplasticity of the bones, absence of bones, external ear abnormalities (including anotia, micro pinna, small or absent external auditory canals), facial palsy, eye abnormalities (anophthalmos, microphthalmos), and congenital heart defects. Alimentary tract, urinary tract, and genital malformations have also been documented.[1] Mortality at or shortly after birth has been reported at about 40%.[2]
Effective contraception (see **CONTRAINDICATIONS**) must be used for at least 4 weeks before beginning thalidomide therapy, during thalidomide therapy, and for 4 weeks following discontinuation of thalidomide therapy. Reliable contraception is indicated even where there has been a history of infertility, unless due to hysterectomy or because the patient has been postmenopausal for at least 24 months. Two reliable forms of contraception must be used simultaneously unless continuous abstinence from heterosexual sexual contact is the chosen method. Women of childbearing potential should be referred to a qualified provider of contraceptive methods, if needed. Sexually mature women who have not undergone a hysterectomy or who have not been postmenopausal for at least 24 consecutive months (i.e., who have had menses at some time in the preceding 24 consecutive months) are considered to be women of childbearing potential.
Before starting treatment, women of childbearing potential should have a pregnancy test (sensitivity of at least 50 mIU/mL). The test should be performed within the 24 hours prior to beginning thalidomide therapy. A prescription for thalidomide for a woman of childbearing potential must not be issued by the prescriber until a written report of a negative pregnancy test has been obtained by the prescriber.
Male Patients: Because thalidomide is present in the semen of patients receiving the drug, males receiving thalidomide must always use a latex condom during any sexual contact with women of childbearing potential even if they have undergone a successful vasectomy.
Once treatment has started, pregnancy testing should occur weekly during the first 4 weeks of use, then pregnancy testing should be repeated at 4 weeks in women with regular menstrual cycles. If menstrual cycles are irregular, the pregnancy testing should occur every 2 weeks. Pregnancy testing and counseling should be performed if a patient misses her period or if there is any abnormality in menstrual bleeding.
If pregnancy does occur during thalidomide treatment, thalidomide must be discontinued immediately.
Any suspected fetal exposure to THALOMID® (thalidomide) must be reported immediately to the FDA *via* the MedWatch number at 1-800-FDA-1088 and also to Celgene Corporation. The patient should be referred to an obstetrician/gynecologist experienced in reproductive toxicity for further evaluation and counseling.

Table 1
Pharmacokinetic Parameter Values for THALOMID® (thalidomide)
Mean (%CV)

Population/ Single Dose	$AUC_{0-\infty}$ µg•hr/mL	C_{max} µg/mL	T_{max} (hrs)	Half-life (hrs)
Healthy Subjects (n=14)				
50 mg	4.9 (16%)	0.62 (52%)	2.9 (66%)	5.52 (37%)
200 mg	18.9 (17%)	1.76 (30%)	3.5 (57%)	5.53 (25%)
400 mg	36.4 (26%)	2.82 (28%)	4.3 (37%)	7.29 (36%)
Patients with Hansen's Disease (n=6)				
400 mg	46.4 (44.1%)	3.44 (52.6%)	5.7 (27%)	6.86 (17%)

FEMALE PATIENTS

Thalidomide is contraindicated in WOMEN of childbearing potential unless alternative therapies are considered inappropriate AND the patient MEETS ALL OF THE FOLLOWING CONDITIONS (i.e., she is essentially unable to become pregnant while on thalidomide therapy):

- she understands and can reliably carry out instructions.
- she is capable of complying with the mandatory contraceptive measures, pregnancy testing, patient registration, and patient survey as described in the System for Thalidomide Education and Prescribing Safety (*S.T.E.P.S.®*) program.
- she has received both oral and written warnings of the hazards of taking thalidomide during pregnancy and of exposing a fetus to the drug.
- she has received both oral and written warnings of the risk of possible contraception failure and of the need to use two reliable forms of contraception simultaneously (see **CONTRAINDICATIONS**), unless continuous abstinence from heterosexual sexual contact is the chosen method. Sexually mature women who have not undergone a hysterectomy or who have not been postmenopausal for at least 24 consecutive months (i.e., who have had menses at some time in the preceding 24 consecutive months) are considered to be women of childbearing potential.
- she acknowledges, in writing, her understanding of these warnings and of the need for using two reliable methods of contraception for 4 weeks prior to beginning thalidomide therapy, during thalidomide therapy, and for 4 weeks after discontinuation of thalidomide therapy.
- she has had a negative pregnancy test with a sensitivity of at least 50 mIU/mL, within the 24 hours prior to beginning therapy. (See **PRECAUTIONS, CONTRAINDICATIONS.**)
- if the patient is between 12 and 18 years of age, her parent or legal guardian must have read this material and agreed to ensure compliance with the above.

MALE PATIENTS

Thalidomide is contraindicated in sexually mature MALES unless the PATIENT MEETS ALL OF THE FOLLOWING CONDITIONS:

- he understands and can reliably carry out instructions.
- he is capable of complying with the mandatory contraceptive measures that are appropriate for men, patient registration, and patient survey as described in the *S.T.E.P.S.®* program.
- he has received both oral and written warnings of the hazards of taking thalidomide and exposing a fetus to the drug.
- he has received both oral and written warnings of the risk of possible contraception failure and of the presence of thalidomide in semen. He has been instructed that he must always use a latex condom during any sexual contact with women of childbearing potential, even if he has undergone a successful vasectomy.
- he acknowledges, in writing, his understanding of these warnings and of the need to use a latex condom during any sexual contact with women of childbearing potential, even if he has undergone a successful vasectomy. Sexually mature women who have not undergone a hysterectomy or who have not been postmenopausal for at least 24 consecutive months (i.e., who have had menses at any time in the preceding 24 consecutive months) are considered to be women of childbearing potential.
- if the patient is between 12 and 18 years of age, his parent or legal guardian must have read this material and agreed to ensure compliance with the above.

DESCRIPTION

THALOMID® (thalidomide), α-(N-phthalimido)glutarimide, is an immunomodulatory agent. The empirical formula for thalidomide is $C_{13}H_{10}N_2O_4$ and the gram molecular weight is 258.2. The CAS number of thalidomide is 50-35-1.

Chemical Structure of thalidomide

Note: • = asymmetric carbon atom

Thalidomide is an off-white to white, odorless, crystalline powder that is soluble at 25°C in dimethyl sulfoxide and sparingly soluble in water and ethanol. The glutarimide moiety contains a single asymmetric center and, therefore, may exist in either of two optically active forms designated S-(-) or R-(+). THALOMID® (thalidomide) is an equal mixture of the S-(-) and R-(+) forms and, therefore, has a net optical rotation of zero.
THALOMID® (thalidomide) is available in 50 mg, 100 mg and 200 mg capsules for oral administration. Active ingredient: thalidomide. Inactive ingredients: pregelatinized starch and magnesium stearate. The 50 mg capsule shell contains gelatin, titanium dioxide, and black ink. The 100 mg capsule shell contains black iron oxide, yellow iron oxide, titanium dioxide, gelatin, and black ink. The 200 mg capsule shell contains FD&C blue #2, titanium dioxide, gelatin, and white ink.

CLINICAL PHARMACOLOGY

Mechanism of Action

Thalidomide is an immunomodulatory agent with a spectrum of activity that is not fully characterized. In patients with erythema nodosum leprosum (ENL) the mechanism of action is not fully understood.
Available data from *in vitro* studies and preliminary clinical trials suggest that the immunologic effects of this compound can vary substantially under different conditions, but may be related to suppression of excessive tumor necrosis factor-alpha (TNF-α) production and down-modulation of selected cell surface adhesion molecules involved in leukocyte migration.[3–6] For example, administration of thalidomide has been reported to decrease circulating levels of TNF-α in patients with ENL,[3] however, it has also been shown to increase plasma TNF-α levels in HIV-seropositive patients.[7]

Pharmacokinetics and Drug Metabolism

Absorption

The absolute bioavailability of thalidomide from THALOMID® (thalidomide) capsules has not yet been characterized in human subjects due to its poor aqueous solubility. In studies of both healthy volunteers and subjects with Hansen's disease, the mean time to peak plasma concentrations (T_{max}) of THALOMID® (thalidomide) ranged from 2.9 to 5.7 hours indicating that THALOMID® (thalidomide) is slowly absorbed from the gastrointestinal tract. While the extent of absorption (as measured by area under the curve [AUC]) is proportional to dose in healthy subjects, the observed peak concentration (C_{max}) increased in a less than proportional manner (see Table 1 below). This lack of C_{max} dose proportionality, coupled with the observed increase in T_{max} values, suggests that the poor solubility of thalidomide in aqueous media may be hindering the rate of absorption. [See table 1 above]
Coadministration of THALOMID® (thalidomide) with a high fat meal causes minor (<10%) changes in the observed AUC and C_{max} values; however, it causes an increase in T_{max} to approximately 6 hours.

Distribution

In human blood plasma, the geometric mean plasma protein binding was 55% and 66%, respectively, for (+)-(R)- and (-)-(S)-thalidomide.[8] In a pharmacokinetic study of thalidomide in HIV-seropositive adult male subjects receiving thalidomide 100 mg/day, thalidomide was detectable in the semen.

Metabolism

At the present time, the exact metabolic route and fate of thalidomide is not known in humans. Thalidomide itself does not appear to be hepatically metabolized to any large extent, but appears to undergo non-enzymatic hydrolysis in plasma to multiple metabolites. In a repeat dose study in which THALOMID® (thalidomide) 200 mg was administered to 10 healthy females for 18 days, thalidomide displayed similar pharmacokinetic profiles on the first and last day of dosing. This suggests that thalidomide does not induce or inhibit its own metabolism.

Continued on next page

Thalomid—Cont.

Elimination
As indicated in Table 1 (above) the mean half-life of elimination ranges from approximately 5 to 7 hours following a single dose and is not altered upon multiple dosing. As noted in the metabolism subsection, the precise metabolic fate and route of elimination of thalidomide in humans is not known at this time. Thalidomide itself has a renal clearance of 1.15 mL/minute with less than 0.7% of the dose excreted in the urine as unchanged drug. Following a single dose, urinary levels of thalidomide were undetectable 48 hrs after dosing. Although thalidomide is thought to be hydrolyzed to a number of metabolites,[9] only a very small amount (0.02% of the administered dose) of 4-OH-thalidomide was identified in the urine of subjects 12 to 24 hours after dosing.

Pharmacokinetic Data in Special Populations
HIV-seropositive Subjects: There is no apparent significant difference in measured pharmacokinetic parameter values between healthy human subjects and HIV-seropositive subjects following single dose administration of THALOMID® (thalidomide) capsules.
Patients with Hansen's Disease: Analysis of data from a small study in Hansen's patients suggests that these patients, relative to healthy subjects, may have an increased bioavailability of THALOMID® (thalidomide). The increase is reflected both in an increased area under the curve and in increased peak plasma levels. The clinical significance of this increase is unknown.
Patients with Renal Insufficiency: The pharmacokinetics of thalidomide in patients with renal dysfunction have not been determined.
Patients with Hepatic Disease: The pharmacokinetics of thalidomide in patients with hepatic impairment have not been determined.
Age: Analysis of the data from pharmacokinetic studies in healthy volunteers and patients with Hansen's disease ranging in age from 20 to 69 years does not reveal any age-related changes.
Pediatric: No pharmacokinetic data are available in subjects below the age of 18 years.
Gender: While a comparative trial of the effects of gender on thalidomide pharmacokinetics has not been conducted, examination of the data for thalidomide does not reveal any significant gender differences in pharmacokinetic parameter values.
Race: Pharmacokinetic differences due to race have not been studied.

Clinical Studies
The primary data demonstrating the efficacy of thalidomide in the treatment of the cutaneous manifestations of moderate to severe ENL are derived from the published medical literature and from a retrospective study of 102 patients treated by the U.S. Public Health Service.
Two double-blind, randomized, controlled trials reported the dermatologic response to a 7-day course of 100 mg thalidomide (four times daily) or control. Dosage was lower for patients under 50 kg in weight.
[See table 2 above]

Table 2
Double-Blind, Controlled Clinical Trials of Thalidomide in Patients with ENL: Cutaneous Response

Reference	No. of Patients	No. Treatment Courses*	Percent Responding**	
Iyer *et al.*[10]			Thalidomide	Aspirin
Bull World Health Organization 1971;45:719	92	204	75%	25%
Sheskin *et al.*[11]			Thalidomide	Placebo
Int J Lep 1969;37:135	52	173	66%	10%

*In patients with cutaneous lesions
**Iyer: Complete response or lesions absent
**Sheskin: Complete improvement + "striking" improvement (i.e., >50% improvement)

Waters[12] reported the results of two studies, both double-blind, randomized, placebo-controlled, crossover trials in a total of 10 hospitalized, steroid-dependent patients with chronic ENL treated with 100 mg thalidomide or placebo (three times daily). All patients also received dapsone. The primary endpoint was reduction in weekly steroid dosage.
[See table 3 above]

Table 3
Double-Blind, Controlled Trial of Thalidomide in Patients with ENL: Reduction in Steroid Dosage

Reference	Duration of Treatment	No. of Patients	Number Responding	
			Thalidomide	Placebo
Waters[12]	4 weeks	9	4/5	0/4
Lep Rev 1971;42:26	6 weeks (crossover)	8	8/8	1/8

Data on the efficacy of thalidomide in prevention of ENL relapse were derived from a retrospective evaluation of 102 patients treated under the auspices of the U.S. Public Health Service. A subset of patients with ENL controlled on thalidomide demonstrated repeated relapse upon drug withdrawal and remission with reinstitution of therapy.
Twenty U.S. patients between the ages of 11 and 17 years were treated with thalidomide, generally at 100 mg daily. Response rates and safety profiles were similar to that observed in the adult population.
Thirty-two other published studies containing over 1600 patients consistently report generally successful treatment of the cutaneous manifestations of moderate to severe ENL with thalidomide.

INDICATIONS AND USAGE
THALOMID® (thalidomide) is indicated for the acute treatment of the cutaneous manifestations of moderate to severe erythema nodosum leprosum (ENL). THALOMID® (thalidomide) is not indicated as monotherapy for such ENL treatment in the presence of moderate to severe neuritis.
THALOMID® (thalidomide) is also indicated as maintenance therapy for prevention and suppression of the cutaneous manifestations of ENL recurrence.

CONTRAINDICATIONS (See BOXED WARNINGS.)
Pregnancy: Category X
Due to its known human teratogenicity, even following a single dose, thalidomide is contraindicated in pregnant women and women capable of becoming pregnant. (See **BOXED WARNINGS.**) When there is no alternative treatment, women of childbearing potential may be treated with thalidomide provided adequate precautions are taken to avoid pregnancy. Women must commit either to abstain continuously from heterosexual sexual contact or to use two methods of reliable birth control, including at least one highly effective method (e.g., IUD, hormonal contraception, tubal ligation, or partner's vasectomy) and one additional effective method (e.g., latex condom, diaphragm, or cervical cap), beginning 4 weeks prior to initiating treatment with thalidomide, during therapy with thalidomide, and continuing for 4 weeks following discontinuation of thalidomide therapy. If hormonal or IUD contraception is medically contraindicated (see also **PRECAUTIONS: Drug Interactions),** two other effective or highly effective methods may be used. Women of childbearing potential being treated with thalidomide should have a pregnancy test (sensitivity of at least 50 mIU/mL). The test should be performed within the 24 hours prior to beginning thalidomide therapy and then weekly during the first 4 weeks of thalidomide therapy, then at 4 week intervals in women with regular menstrual cycles or every 2 weeks in women with irregular menstrual cycles. Pregnancy testing and counseling should be performed if a patient misses her period or if there is any abnormality in menstrual bleeding. If pregnancy occurs during thalidomide treatment, thalidomide must be discontinued immediately. Under these conditions, the patient should be referred to an obstetrician/gynecologist experienced in reproductive toxicity for further evaluation and counseling.
Because thalidomide is present in the semen of patients receiving the drug, males receiving thalidomide must always use a latex condom during any sexual contact with women of childbearing potential. The risk to the fetus from the semen of male patients taking thalidomide is unknown.
THALOMID® (thalidomide) is contraindicated in patients who have demonstrated hypersensitivity to the drug and its components.

WARNINGS (See BOXED WARNINGS.)
Birth defects:
Thalidomide can cause severe birth defects in humans. (See **BOXED WARNINGS** and **CONTRAINDICATIONS.**) Patients should be instructed to take thalidomide only as prescribed and not to share their thalidomide with anyone else. Because thalidomide is present in the semen of patients receiving the drug, males receiving thalidomide must always use a latex condom during any sexual contact with women of childbearing potential. The risk to the fetus from the semen of male patients taking thalidomide is unknown.
Drowsiness and Somnolence:
Thalidomide frequently causes drowsiness and somnolence. Patients should be instructed to avoid situations where drowsiness may be a problem and not to take other medications that may cause drowsiness without adequate medical advice. Patients should be advised as to the possible impairment of mental and/or physical abilities required for the performance of hazardous tasks, such as driving a car or operating other complex or dangerous machinery.
Peripheral Neuropathy:
Thalidomide is known to cause nerve damage that may be permanent. Peripheral neuropathy is a common, potentially severe, side effect of treatment with thalidomide that may be irreversible. Peripheral neuropathy generally occurs following chronic use over a period of months; however, reports following relatively short-term use also exist. The correlation with cumulative dose is unclear. Symptoms may occur some time after thalidomide treatment has been stopped and may resolve slowly or not at all. Few reports of neuropathy have arisen in the treatment of ENL despite long-term thalidomide treatment. However, the inability clinically to differentiate thalidomide neuropathy from the neuropathy often seen in Hansen's disease makes it difficult to determine accurately the incidence of thalidomide-related neuropathy in ENL patients treated with thalidomide.
Patients should be examined at monthly intervals for the first 3 months of thalidomide therapy to enable the clinician to detect early signs of neuropathy, which include numbness, tingling or pain in the hands and feet. Patients should be evaluated periodically thereafter during treatment. Patients should be regularly counseled, questioned, and evaluated for signs or symptoms of peripheral neuropathy. Consideration should be given to electrophysiological testing, consisting of measurement of sensory nerve action potential (SNAP) amplitudes at baseline and thereafter every 6 months in an effort to detect asymptomatic neuropathy. If symptoms of drug-induced neuropathy develop, thalidomide should be discontinued immediately to limit further damage, if clinically appropriate. Usually, treatment with thalidomide should only be reinitiated if the neuropathy returns to baseline status. Medications known to be associated with neuropathy should be used with caution in patients receiving thalidomide.
Thrombotic Events:
Thrombotic events have been reported in patients treated with THALOMID® (thalidomide). Patients with neoplastic and various inflammatory conditions being treated with THALOMID® (thalidomide) may have an increased incidence of pulmonary embolism, deep vein thrombophlebitis, thrombophlebitis, or thrombosis. It is not known if concomitant therapy with other medications, including anticancer agents, are a contributing factor.
Dizziness and Orthostatic Hypotension:
Patients should also be advised that thalidomide may cause dizziness and orthostatic hypotension and that, therefore, they should sit upright for a few minutes prior to standing up from a recumbent position.
Neutropenia:
Decreased white blood cell counts, including neutropenia, have been reported in association with the clinical use of thalidomide. Treatment should not be initiated with an absolute neutrophil count (ANC) of <750/mm^3. White blood cell count and differential should be monitored on an ongoing basis, especially in patients who may be more prone to neutropenia, such as patients who are HIV-seropositive. If ANC decreases to below 750/mm^3 while on treatment, the patient's medication regimen should be re-evaluated and, if the neutropenia persists, consideration should be given to withholding thalidomide if clinically appropriate.
Increased HIV Viral Load:
In a randomized, placebo-controlled trial of thalidomide in an HIV-seropositive patient population, plasma HIV RNA levels were found to increase (median change = 0.42 $\log_{10}$ copies HIV RNA/mL, p = 0.04 compared to placebo).[7] A similar trend was observed in a second, unpublished study conducted in patients who were HIV-seropositive.[13] The clinical significance of this increase is unknown. Both studies were conducted prior to availability of highly active antiretroviral therapy. Until the clinical significance of this finding is further understood, in HIV-seropositive patients, viral load should be measured after the first and third months of treatment and every 3 months thereafter.

PRECAUTIONS
General:
The only type of thalidomide exposure known to result in drug-associated birth defects is as a result of direct oral ingestion of thalidomide. Currently no specific data are available regarding the cutaneous absorption or inhalation of thalidomide in women of childbearing potential and whether these exposures may result in any birth defects. Patients should be instructed to not extensively handle or open THALOMID® (thalidomide) Capsules and to maintain storage of capsules in blister packs until ingestion. If there is contact with non-intact thalidomide capsules or the powder contents, the exposed area should be washed with soap and water.
Thalidomide has been shown to be present in the serum and semen of patients receiving thalidomide. If healthcare providers or other caregivers are exposed to body fluids from patients receiving THALOMID® (thalidomide), appropriate precautions should be utilized, such as wearing gloves to prevent the potential cutaneous exposure to THALOMID® (thalidomide) or washing the exposed area with soap and water.
Hypersensitivity:
Hypersensitivity to THALOMID® (thalidomide) has been reported. Signs and symptoms have included the occurrence of erythematous macular rash, possibly associated with fever, tachycardia, and hypotension, and if severe, may necessitate interruption of therapy. If the reaction recurs when dosing is resumed, THALOMID® (thalidomide) should be discontinued.
Bradycardia:
Bradycardia in association with thalidomide use has been reported. Cases of bradycardia have been reported, some required medical interventions. The clinical significance and underlying etiology of the bradycardia noted in some thalidomide-treated patients are presently unknown.

Stevens-Johnson Syndrome and Toxic Epidermal Necrolysis:
Serious dermatologic reactions including Stevens-Johnson syndrome and toxic epidermal necrolysis, which may be fatal, have been reported. THALOMID® (thalidomide) should be discontinued if a skin rash occurs and only resumed following appropriate clinical evaluation. If the rash is exfoliative, purpuric, or bullous or if Stevens-Johnson syndrome or toxic epidermal necrolysis is suspected, use of THALOMID® (thalidomide) should not be resumed.

Seizures:
Although not reported from pre-marketing controlled clinical trials, seizures, including grand mal convulsions, have been reported during post-approval use of THALOMID® (thalidomide) in clinical practice. Because these events are reported voluntarily from a population of unknown size, estimates of frequency cannot be made. Most patients had disorders that may have predisposed them to seizure activity, and it is not currently known whether thalidomide has any epileptogenic influence. During therapy with thalidomide, patients with a history of seizures or with other risk factors for the development of seizures should be monitored closely for clinical changes that could precipitate acute seizure activity.

Information for Patients (See BOXED WARNINGS.)
Patients should be instructed about the potential teratogenicity of thalidomide and the precautions that must be taken to preclude fetal exposure as per the *S.T.E.P.S.*® program and boxed warnings in this package insert. Patients should be instructed to take thalidomide only as prescribed in compliance with all of the provisions of the *S.T.E.P.S.*® Restricted Distribution Program.
Patients should be instructed to not extensively handle or open THALOMID® (thalidomide) Capsules and to maintain storage of capsules in blister packs until ingestion.
Patients should be instructed not to share medication with anyone else.
Patients should be instructed that thalidomide frequently causes drowsiness and somnolence. Patients should be instructed to avoid situations where drowsiness may be a problem and not to take other medications that may cause drowsiness without adequate medical advice. Patients should be advised as to the possible impairment of mental and/or physical abilities required for the performance of hazardous tasks, such as driving a car or operating other complex machinery. Patients should be instructed that thalidomide may potentiate the somnolence caused by alcohol.
Patients should be instructed that thalidomide can cause peripheral neuropathies that may be initially signaled by numbness, tingling, or pain or a burning sensation in the feet or hands. Patients should be instructed to report such occurrences to their prescriber immediately.
Patients should also be instructed that thalidomide may cause dizziness and orthostatic hypotension and that, therefore, they should sit upright for a few minutes prior to standing up from a recumbent position.
Patients should be instructed that they are not permitted to donate blood while taking thalidomide. In addition, male patients should be instructed that they are not permitted to donate sperm while taking thalidomide.

Laboratory Tests
Pregnancy Testing: **(See BOXED WARNINGS.)** Women of childbearing potential should have a pregnancy test performed (sensitivity of at least 50 mIU/mL). The test should be performed within the 24 hours prior to beginning thalidomide therapy and then weekly during the first 4 weeks of use, then at 4 week intervals in women with regular menstrual cycles or every 2 weeks in women with irregular menstrual cycles. Pregnancy testing and counseling should be performed if a patient misses her period or if there is any abnormality in menstrual bleeding.
Neutropenia: **(See WARNINGS.)**
Increased HIV Viral Load: **(See WARNINGS.)**

Drug Interactions
Thalidomide has been reported to enhance the sedative activity of barbiturates, alcohol, chlorpromazine, and reserpine.
Peripheral Neuropathy: Medications known to be associated with peripheral neuropathy should be used with caution in patients receiving thalidomide.
Oral Contraceptives: In 10 healthy women, the pharmacokinetic profiles of norethindrone and ethinyl estradiol following administration of a single dose containing 1.0 mg of norethindrone acetate and 75 µg of ethinyl estradiol were studied. The results were similar with and without coadministration of thalidomide 200 mg/day to steady-state levels.

Important Non-Thalidomide Drug Interactions
Drugs That Interfere with Hormonal Contraceptives: Concomitant use of HIV-protease inhibitors, griseofulvin, modafinil, penicillins, rifampin, rifabutin, phenytoin, carbamazepine, or certain herbal supplements such as St. John's Wort with hormonal contraceptive agents may reduce the effectiveness of the contraception and up to one month after discontinuation of these concomitant therapies. Therefore, women requiring treatment with one or more of these drugs must use two OTHER effective or highly effective methods of contraception or abstain from heterosexual sexual contact while taking thalidomide.

Carcinogenesis, Mutagenesis, Impairment of Fertility
Long-term carcinogenicity tests have not been conducted using thalidomide. Thalidomide gave no evidence of mutagenic effects when assayed in *in vitro* bacterial (*Salmonella typhimurium* and *Escherichia coli;* Ames mutagenicity test), *in vitro* mammalian (AS52 Chinese hamster ovary cells; AS52/XPRT mammalian cell forward gene mutation assay) and *in vivo* mammalian (CD-1 mice; *in vivo* micronucleus test) test systems.
Animal studies to characterize the effects of thalidomide on fertility have not been conducted.

Pregnancy
Pregnancy Category X **(See BOXED WARNING and CONTRAINDICATIONS.)**
Because of the known human teratogenicity of thalidomide, thalidomide is contraindicated in women who are or may become pregnant and who are not using the two required types of birth control or who are not continually abstaining from heterosexual sexual contact. If thalidomide is taken during pregnancy, it can cause severe birth defects or death to an unborn baby. Thalidomide should never be used by women who are pregnant or who could become pregnant while taking the drug. Even a single dose [1 capsule (50 mg, 100 mg, or a 200 mg)] taken by a pregnant woman can cause birth defects. If pregnancy does occur during treatment, the drug should be immediately discontinued. Under these conditions, the patient should be referred to an obstetrician/gynecologist experienced in reproductive toxicity for further evaluation and counseling. Any suspected fetal exposure to THALOMID® (thalidomide) must be reported to the FDA *via* the MedWatch program at 1-800-FDA-1088 and also to Celgene Corporation.
Because thalidomide is present in the semen of patients receiving the drug, males receiving thalidomide must always use a latex condom during any sexual contact with women of childbearing potential. The risk to the fetus from the semen of male patients taking thalidomide is unknown.
Animal studies to characterize the effects of thalidomide on late-stage pregnancy have not been conducted.

Use in Nursing Mothers
It is not known whether thalidomide is excreted in human milk. Because many drugs are excreted in human milk and because of the potential for serious adverse reactions in nursing infants from thalidomide, a decision should be made whether to discontinue nursing or to discontinue the drug, taking into account the importance of the drug to the mother.

Pediatric Use
Safety and effectiveness in pediatric patients below the age of 12 years have not been established.

Geriatric Use
No systematic studies in geriatric patients have been conducted. Thalidomide has been used in clinical trials in patients up to 90 years of age. Adverse events in patients over the age of 65 years did not appear to differ in kind from those reported for younger individuals.

ADVERSE REACTIONS

The most serious toxicity associated with thalidomide is its documented human teratogenicity. (See **BOXED WARNINGS** and **CONTRAINDICATIONS.**) The risk of severe birth defects, primarily phocomelia or death to the fetus, is extremely high during the critical period of pregnancy. The critical period is estimated, depending on the source of information, to range from 35 to 50 days after the last menstrual period. The risk of other potentially severe birth defects outside this critical period is unknown, but may be significant. Based on present knowledge, thalidomide must not be used at any time during pregnancy.
Because thalidomide is present in the semen of patients receiving the drug, males receiving thalidomide must always use a latex condom during any sexual contact with women of childbearing potential.
Thalidomide is associated with drowsiness/somnolence, peripheral neuropathy, dizziness/orthostatic hypotension, neutropenia, and HIV viral load increase. (See **WARNINGS.**)
Hypersensitivity to THALOMID® (thalidomide) and bradycardia in patients treated with thalidomide have been reported. (See **PRECAUTIONS.)**
Somnolence, dizziness, and rash are the most commonly observed adverse events associated with the use of thalidomide. Thalidomide has been studied in controlled and uncontrolled clinical trials in patients with ENL and in people who are HIV-seropositive. In addition, thalidomide has been administered investigationally for more than 20 years in numerous indications. Adverse event profiles from these uses are summarized in the sections that follow.

Other Adverse Events
Due to the nature of the longitudinal data that form the basis of this product's safety evaluation, no determination has been made of the causal relationship between the reported adverse events listed below and thalidomide. These lists are of various adverse events noted by investigators in patients to whom they had administered thalidomide under various conditions. The use of thalidomide may not limit disease progression and/or death.

Incidence in Controlled Clinical Trials
Table 4 lists treatment-emergent signs and symptoms that occurred in THALOMID® (thalidomide)-treated patients in controlled clinical trials in ENL. Doses ranged from 50 to 300 mg/day. All adverse events were mild to moderate in severity, and none resulted in discontinuation. Table 4 also lists treatment-emergent adverse events that occurred in at least three of the THALOMID® (thalidomide)-treated HIV-seropositive patients who participated in an 8-week, placebo-controlled clinical trial. Events that were more frequent in the placebo-treated group are not included. **(See WARNINGS, PRECAUTIONS and Drug interactions.)**
[See table 4 at top of next page]

Other Adverse Events Observed in ENL Patients
Thalidomide in doses up to 400 mg/day has been administered investigationally in the United States over a 19-year period in 1465 patients with ENL. The published literature describes the treatment of an additional 1678 patients. To provide a meaningful estimate of the proportion of the individuals having adverse events, similar types of events were grouped into a smaller number of standardized categories using a modified COSTART dictionary/terminology. These categories are used in the listing below. All reported events are included except those already listed in the previous table. Due to the fact that these data were collected from uncontrolled studies, the incidence rate cannot be determined. As mentioned previously, **no causal relationship between thalidomide and these events can be conclusively determined at this time.** These are reports of all adverse events noted by investigators in patients to whom they had administered thalidomide.
Body as a Whole: Abdomen enlarged, fever, photosensitivity, upper extremity pain.
Cardiovascular System: Bradycardia, hypertension, hypotension, peripheral vascular disorder, tachycardia, vasodilation.
Digestive System: Anorexia, appetite increase/weight gain, dry mouth, dyspepsia, enlarged liver, eructation, flatulence, increased liver function tests, intestinal obstruction, vomiting.
Hemic and Lymphatic: ESR decrease, eosinophilia, granulocytopenia, hypochromic anemia, leukemia, leukocytosis, leukopenia, MCV elevated, RBC abnormal, spleen palpable, thrombocytopenia.
Metabolic and Endocrine: ADH inappropriate, amyloidosis, bilirubinemia, BUN increased, creatinine increased, cyanosis, diabetes, edema, electrolyte abnormalities, hyperglycemia, hyperkalemia, hyperuricemia, hypocalcemia, hypoproteinemia, LDH increased, phosphorus decreased, SGPT increased.
Muscular Skeletal: Arthritis, bone tenderness, hypertonia, joint disorder, leg cramps, myalgia, myasthenia, periosteal disorder.
Nervous System: Abnormal thinking, agitation, amnesia, anxiety, causalgia, circumoral paresthesia, confusion, depression, euphoria, hyperesthesia, insomnia, nervousness, neuralgia, neuritis, neuropathy, paresthesia, peripheral neuritis, psychosis.
Respiratory System: Cough, emphysema, epistaxis, pulmonary embolus, rales, upper respiratory infection, voice alteration.
Skin and Appendages: Acne, alopecia, dry skin, eczematous rash, exfoliative dermatitis, ichthyosis, perifollicular thickening, skin necrosis, seborrhea, sweating, urticaria, vesiculobullous rash.
Special Senses: Amblyopia, deafness, dry eye, eye pain, tinnitus.
Urogenital: Decreased creatinine clearance, hematuria, orchitis, proteinuria, pyuria, urinary frequency.

Other Adverse Events Observed in HIV-seropositive Patients
In addition to controlled clinical trials, THALOMID® (thalidomide) has been used in uncontrolled studies in 145 patients. Less frequent adverse events that have been reported in these HIV-seropositive patients treated with THALOMID® (thalidomide) were grouped into a smaller number of standardized categories using modified COSTART dictionary/terminology and these categories are used in the listing below. Adverse events that have already been included in the tables and narrative above, or that are too general to be informative, are not listed.
Body as a Whole: Ascites, AIDS, allergic reaction, cellulitis, chest pain, chills and fever, cyst, decreased CD4 count, facial edema, flu syndrome, hernia, thyroid hormone level altered, moniliasis, photosensitivity reaction, sarcoma, sepsis, viral infection.
Cardiovascular System: Angina pectoris, arrhythmia, atrial fibrillation, bradycardia, cerebral ischemia, cerebrovascular accident, congestive heart failure, deep thrombophlebitis, heart arrest, heart failure, hypertension, hypotension, murmur, myocardial infarct, palpitation, pericarditis, peripheral vascular disorder, postural hypotension, syncope, tachycardia, thrombophlebitis, thrombosis.
Digestive System: Cholangitis, cholestatic jaundice, colitis, dyspepsia, dysphagia, esophagitis, gastroenteritis, gastrointestinal disorder, gastrointestinal hemorrhage, gum disorder, hepatitis, pancreatitis, parotid gland enlargement, periodontitis, stomatitis, tongue discoloration, tooth disorder.
Hemic and Lymphatic: Aplastic anemia, macrocytic anemia, megaloblastic anemia, microcytic anemia.
Metabolic and Endocrine: Avitaminosis, bilirubinemia, dehydration, hypercholesteremia, hypoglycemia, increased alkaline phosphatase, increased lipase, increased serum creatinine, peripheral edema.
Muscular Skeletal: Myalgia, myasthenia.
Nervous System: Abnormal gait, ataxia, decreased libido, decreased reflexes, dementia, dysesthesia, dyskinesia, emo-

Continued on next page

Thalomid—Cont.

tional lability, hostility, hypalgesia, hyperkinesia, incoordination, meningitis, neurologic disorder, tremor, vertigo.

Respiratory System: Apnea, bronchitis, lung disorder, lung edema, pneumonia (including *Pneumocystis carinii* pneumonia), rhinitis.

Skin and Appendages: Angioedema, benign skin neoplasm, eczema, herpes simplex, incomplete Stevens-Johnson syndrome, nail disorder, pruritus, psoriasis, skin discoloration, skin disorder.

Special Senses: Conjunctivitis, eye disorder, lacrimation disorder, retinitis, taste perversion.

Other Adverse Events Observed in Post-Marketing Use

Cardiovascular System: Cardiac arrhythmias including atrial fibrillation, bradycardia, tachycardia, sick sinus syndrome and EKG abnormalities.

Digestive System: Intestinal perforation.

Metabolic and Endocrine: Electrolyte imbalance, including hypercalcemia or hypocalcemia, hyperkalemia and hypokalemia, hyponatremia, hypothyroidism, and increased alkaline phosphatase, tumor lysis syndrome.

Nervous System: Changes in mental status or mood including depression and suicide attempts, disturbances in consciousness including lethargy, syncope, loss of consciousness or stupor, seizures including grand mal convulsions and status epilepicus.

Skin and Appendages: Erythema multiforme.

Hemic and Lymphatic: Decreased white blood cell counts including neutropenia and febrile neutropenia, changes in prothrombin time.

Respiratory System: Pleural effusion.

Other Adverse Events in the Published Literature or Reported from Other Sources

The following additional events have been identified either in the published literature or from spontaneous reports from other sources: acute renal failure, amenorrhea, aphthous stomatitis, bile duct obstruction, carpal tunnel, chronic myelogenous leukemia, diplopia, dysesthesia, dyspnea, enuresis, erythema nodosum, erythroleukemia, foot drop, galactorrhea, gynecomastia, hangover effect, hypomagnesemia, hypothyroidism, lymphedema, lymphopenia, metrorrhagia, migraine, myxedema, nodular sclerosing Hodgkin's disease, nystagmus, oliguria, pancytopenia, petechiae, purpura, Raynaud's syndrome, stomach ulcer, and suicide attempt.

DRUG ABUSE AND DEPENDENCE

Physical and psychological dependence has not been reported in patients taking thalidomide. However, as with other tranquilizers/hypnotics, thalidomide too has been reported to create in patients habituation to its soporific effects.

OVERDOSAGE

There have been three cases of overdose reported, all attempted suicides. There have been no reported fatalities in doses of up to 14.4 grams, and all patients recovered without reported sequelae.

DOSAGE AND ADMINISTRATION

THALOMID® (thalidomide) MUST ONLY BE ADMINISTERED IN COMPLIANCE WITH ALL OF THE TERMS OUTLINED IN THE *S.T.E.P.S.®* PROGRAM. THALOMID® (thalidomide) MAY ONLY BE PRESCRIBED BY PRESCRIBERS REGISTERED WITH THE *S.T.E.P.S.®* PROGRAM AND MAY ONLY BE DISPENSED BY PHARMACISTS REGISTERED WITH THE *S.T.E.P.S.®* PROGRAM.

Drug prescribing to women of childbearing potential should be contingent upon initial and continued confirmed negative results of pregnancy testing.

For an episode of cutaneous ENL, THALOMID® (thalidomide) dosing should be initiated at 100 to 300 mg/day, administered once daily with water, preferably at bedtime and at least 1 hour after the evening meal. Patients weighing less than 50 kilograms should be started at the low end of the dose range.

In patients with a severe cutaneous ENL reaction, or in those who have previously required higher doses to control the reaction, THALOMID® (thalidomide) dosing may be initiated at higher doses up to 400 mg/day once daily at bedtime or in divided doses with water, at least 1 hour after meals.

In patients with moderate to severe neuritis associated with a severe ENL reaction, corticosteroids may be started concomitantly with THALOMID® (thalidomide). Steroid usage can be tapered and discontinued when the neuritis has ameliorated.

Dosing with THALOMID® (thalidomide) should usually continue until signs and symptoms of active reaction have subsided, usually a period of at least 2 weeks. Patients may then be tapered off medication in 50 mg decrements every 2 to 4 weeks.

Patients who have a documented history of requiring prolonged maintenance treatment to prevent the recurrence of cutaneous ENL or who flare during tapering, should be maintained on the minimum dose necessary to control the reaction. Tapering off medication should be attempted every 3 to 6 months, in decrements of 50 mg every 2 to 4 weeks.

HOW SUPPLIED

(THIS PRODUCT IS ONLY SUPPLIED TO PHARMACISTS REGISTERED WITH THE *S.T.E.P.S.®* PROGRAM - See BOXED WARNINGS.)

Table 4
Summary of Adverse Events (AEs)
Reported in Celgene-sponsored Controlled Clinical Trials

Body System/Adverse Event	All AEs Reported in ENL Patients	AEs Reported in ≥3 HIV-seropositive Patients Thalidomide		Placebo
	50 to 300 mg/day (N=24)	100 mg/day (N=36)	200 mg/day (N=32)	(N=35)
Body as a Whole	**16 (66.7%)**	**18 (50.0%)**	**19 (59.4%)**	**13 (37.1%)**
Abdominal pain	1 (4.2%)	1 (2.8%)	1 (3.1%)	4 (11.4%)
Accidental injury	1 (4.2%)	2 (5.6%)	0	1 (2.9%)
Asthenia	2 (8.3%)	2 (5.6%)	7 (21.9%)	1 (2.9%)
Back pain	1 (4.2%)	2 (5.6%)	0	0
Chills	1 (4.2%)	0	3 (9.4%)	4 (11.4%)
Facial edema	1 (4.2%)	0	0	0
Fever	0	7 (19.4%)	7 (21.9%)	6 (17.1%)
Headache	3 (12.5%)	6 (16.7%)	6 (18.7%)	4 (11.4%)
Infection	0	3 (8.3%)	2 (6.3%)	1 (2.9%)
Malaise	2 (8.3%)	0	0	0
Neck pain	1 (4.2%)	0	0	0
Neck rigidity	1 (4.2%)	0	0	0
Pain	2 (8.3%)	0	1 (3.1%)	2 (5.7%)
Digestive System	**5 (20.8%)**	**16 (44.4%)**	**16 (50.0%)**	**15 (42.9%)**
Anorexia	0	1 (2.8%)	3 (9.4%)	2 (5.7%)
Constipation	1 (4.2%)	1 (2.8%)	3 (9.4%)	0
Diarrhea	1 (4.2%)	4 (11.1%)	6 (18.7%)	6 (17.1%)
Dry mouth	0	3 (8.3%)	3 (9.4%)	2 (5.7%)
Flatulence	0	3 (8.3%)	0	2 (5.7%)
Liver function tests multiple abnormalities	0	0	3 (9.4%)	0
Nausea	1 (4.2%)	0	4 (12.5%)	1 (2.9%)
Oral moniliasis	1 (4.2%)	4 (11.1%)	2 (6.3%)	0
Tooth pain	1 (4.2%)	0	0	0
Hemic and Lymphatic	**0**	**8 (22.2%)**	**13 (40.6%)**	**10 (28.6%)**
Anemia	0	2 (5.6%)	4 (12.5%)	3 (8.6%)
Leukopenia	0	6 (16.7%)	8 (25.0%)	3 (8.6%)
Lymphadenopathy	0	2 (5.6%)	4 (12.5%)	3 (8.6%)
Metabolic and Endocrine Disorders	**1 (4.2%)**	**8 (22.2%)**	**12 (37.5%)**	**8 (22.9%)**
Edema peripheral	1 (4.2%)	3 (8.3%)	1 (3.1%)	0
Hyperlipemia	0	2 (5.6%)	3 (9.4%)	1 (2.9%)
SGOT increased	0	1 (2.8%)	4 (12.5%)	2 (5.7%)
Nervous System	**13 (54.2%)**	**19 (52.8%)**	**18 (56.3%)**	**12 (34.3%)**
Agitation	0	0	3 (9.4%)	0
Dizziness	1 (4.2%)	7 (19.4%)	6 (18.7%)	0
Insomnia	0	0	3 (9.4%)	2 (5.7%)
Nervousness	0	1 (2.8%)	3 (9.4%)	0
Neuropathy	0	3 (8.3%)	0	0
Paresthesia	0	2 (5.6%)	5 (15.6%)	4 (11.4%)
Somnolence	9 (37.5%)	13 (36.1%)	12 (37.5%)	4 (11.4%)
Tremor	1 (4.2%)	0	0	0
Vertigo	2 (8.3%)	0	0	0
Respiratory System	**3 (12.5%)**	**9 (25.0%)**	**6 (18.7%)**	**9 (25.7%)**
Pharyngitis	1 (4.2%)	3 (8.3%)	2 (6.3%)	2 (5.7%)
Rhinitis	1 (4.2%)	0	0	4 (11.4%)
Sinusitis	1 (4.2%)	3 (8.3%)	1 (3.1%)	2 (5.7%)
Skin and Appendages	**10 (41.7%)**	**17 (47.2%)**	**18 (56.3%)**	**19 (54.3%)**
Acne	0	4 (11.1%)	1 (3.1%)	0
Dermatitis fungal	1 (4.2%)	2 (5.6%)	3 (9.4%)	0
Nail disorder	1 (4.2%)	0	1 (3.1%)	0
Pruritus	2 (8.3%)	1 (2.8%)	2 (6.3%)	2 (5.7%)
Rash	5 (20.8%)	9 (25.0%)	8 (25.0%)	11 (31.4%)
Rash maculo-papular	1 (4.2%)	6 (16.7%)	6 (18.7%)	2 (5.7%)
Sweating	0	0	4 (12.5%)	4 (11.4%)
Urogenital System	**2 (8.3%)**	**6 (16.7%)**	**2 (6.3%)**	**4 (11.4%)**
Albuminuria	0	3 (8.3%)	1 (3.1%)	2 (5.7%)
Hematuria	0	4 (11.1%)	0	1 (2.9%)
Impotence	2 (8.3%)	1 (2.8%)	0	0

THALOMID® (thalidomide) Capsules are supplied in the following dosages:

50 mg capsules [white opaque], imprinted "Celgene / 50 mg" with a "Do Not Get Pregnant" logo.

Individual blister packs of 28 capsules (NDC 59572-205-14).

Boxes of 280 containing 10 prescription packs of 28 capsules each (NDC 59572-205-94).

100 mg capsules [tan], imprinted "Celgene / 100 mg" with a "Do Not Get Pregnant" logo.

Individual blister packs of 28 capsules (NDC 59572-210-15).

Boxes of 140 containing 5 prescription packs of 28 capsules each (NDC 59572-210-95).

200 mg capsules [blue], imprinted "Celgene / 200 mg" with a "Do Not Get Pregnant" logo.

Individual blister packs of 28 capsules (NDC 59572-220-16).

Boxes of 84 containing 3 prescription packs of 28 capsules each (NDC 59572-220-96).

STORAGE AND DISPENSING

PHARMACISTS NOTE:

BEFORE DISPENSING THALOMID® (thalidomide), YOU MUST ACTIVATE THE AUTHORIZATION NUMBER ON EVERY PRESCRIPTION BY CALLING THE CELGENE CUSTOMER CARE CENTER AT 1-888-4-CELGENE (1-888-423-5436) AND OBTAINING A CONFIRMATION NUMBER. YOU MUST ALSO WRITE THE CONFIRMATION NUMBER ON THE PRESCRIPTION. YOU SHOULD ACCEPT A PRESCRIPTION ONLY IF IT HAS BEEN ISSUED WITHIN THE PREVIOUS 7 DAYS (TELEPHONE PRESCRIPTIONS ARE NOT PERMITTED); DISPENSE NO MORE THAN A 4-WEEK (28-DAY) SUPPLY. A NEW PRESCRIPTION IS REQUIRED FOR FURTHER DISPENSING. DISPENSE BLISTER PACKS INTACT (CAPSULES CANNOT BE REPACKAGED); DISPENSE SUBSEQUENT PRESCRIPTIONS ONLY IF FEWER THAN 7 DAYS OF THERAPY REMAIN ON THE PREVIOUS PRESCRIPTION; AND EDUCATE ALL STAFF PHARMACISTS ABOUT THE DISPENSING PROCEDURE FOR THALOMID® (thalidomide).

This drug must not be repackaged.

Store at 25°C (77°F); excursions permitted to 15-30°C (59-86°F). [See USP Controlled Room Temperature].

Protect from light.

Rx only and only able to be prescribed and dispensed under the terms of the *S.T.E.P.S.®* Restricted Distribution Program

Manufactured for Celgene Corporation
7 Powder Horn Drive
Warren, New Jersey 07059
1-(888) 423-5436

Important Information and Warnings for All Patients Taking THALOMID® (thalidomide)

WARNING: SEVERE, LIFE-THREATENING HUMAN BIRTH DEFECTS.
IF THALIDOMIDE IS TAKEN DURING PREGNANCY, IT CAN CAUSE SEVERE BIRTH DEFECTS OR DEATH TO AN UNBORN BABY. THALIDOMIDE SHOULD NEVER BE USED BY WOMEN WHO ARE PREGNANT OR WHO COULD BECOME PREGNANT WHILE TAKING THE DRUG. EVEN A SINGLE DOSE [1 CAPSULE (50 mg, 100 mg or 200 mg)] TAKEN BY A PREGNANT WOMAN CAN CAUSE SEVERE BIRTH DEFECTS.

All Patients

- The patient understands that severe birth defects can occur with the use of THALOMID® (thalidomide).
- The patient has been warned by his/her doctor that an unborn baby will almost certainly have severe birth defects and can even die, if a woman is pregnant or becomes pregnant while taking THALOMID® (thalidomide).
- THALOMID® (thalidomide) will be prescribed ONLY for the patient and must NOT be shared with ANYONE, even someone who has similar symptoms.

- THALOMID® (thalidomide) must be kept out of the reach of children and should NEVER be given to women who are able to have children.
- The patient cannot donate blood while taking THALOMID® (thalidomide).
- The patient has read the THALOMID® (thalidomide) patient brochure and/or viewed the videotape, "Important Information for Men and Women Taking THALOMID® (thalidomide)" and understands the contents, including other possible health problems from THALOMID® (thalidomide), "side effects."
- The patient's doctor has answered any questions the patient has asked.
- The patient must participate in a telephone survey and patient registry, while taking THALOMID® (thalidomide).

Female Patients of Childbearing Potential

- The patient must not take THALOMID® (thalidomide) if she is pregnant, breast-feeding a baby, or able to get pregnant and not using the required two methods of birth control.
- The patient confirms that she is not now pregnant, nor will she try to become pregnant during THALOMID® (thalidomide) therapy and for at least 4 weeks after she has completely finished taking THALOMID® (thalidomide).
- If the patient is able to become pregnant, she must use at least one highly effective method and one additional effective method of birth control (contraception) AT THE SAME TIME:

At least one highly effective method	AND	One additional effective method
IUD		Latex condom
Hormonal (birth control pills, injections, or implants)		Diaphragm
Tubal ligation		Cervical cap
Partner's vasectomy		

- These birth control methods must be used for at least 4 weeks before beginning THALOMID® (thalidomide) therapy, during THALOMID® (thalidomide) therapy, and for 4 weeks following discontinuation THALOMID® (thalidomide) therapy.
- The patient must use these birth control methods unless she completely abstains from heterosexual sexual contact.
- If a hormonal method (birth control pills, injections, or implants) or IUD is not medically possible for the patient, she may use another highly effective method or two barrier methods AT THE SAME TIME.
- The patient must have a pregnancy test done by her doctor within the 24 hours prior to starting THALOMID® (thalidomide) therapy, then every week during the first 4 weeks of THALOMID® (thalidomide) therapy.
- Thereafter, the patient must have a pregnancy test every 4 weeks if she has regular menstrual cycles, or every 2 weeks if her cycles are irregular while she is taking THALOMID® (thalidomide).
- The patient must immediately stop taking THALOMID® (thalidomide) and inform her doctor:
  If she becomes pregnant while taking the drug
  If she misses her menstrual period, or experiences unusual menstrual bleeding
  If she stops using birth control
  If she thinks FOR ANY REASON that she may be pregnant

The patient understands that if her doctor is not available, she can call 1-888-668-2528 for information on emergency contraception

Female Patients Not of Childbearing Potential

- The patient certifies that she is not now pregnant, nor of childbearing potential as she has been postmenopausal for at least 24 months (been through the change of life); or she has had a hysterectomy.
- The patient or guardian certifies that a prepubertal female child is not now pregnant, or is of childbearing potential as menstruation has not yet begun, and/or the child will not be engaging in heterosexual sexual contact for at least 4 weeks before THALOMID® (thalidomide) therapy, during THALOMID® (thalidomide) therapy, and for at least 4 weeks after stopping therapy.

Male Patients

- The patient has been told by his doctor that he must NEVER have unprotected sexual contact with a woman who can become pregnant.
- Because THALOMID® (thalidomide) is present in semen, his doctor has explained that he must either completely abstain from sexual contact with women who are pregnant or able to become pregnant, or he must use a latex condom EVERY TIME he engages in any sexual contact with women who are pregnant or may become pregnant while he is taking THALOMID® (thalidomide) and for 4 weeks after he stops taking the drug, even if he has had a successful vasectomy.
- The patient must inform his doctor:
  If he has had unprotected sexual contact with a woman who can become pregnant
  If he thinks FOR ANY REASON, that his sexual partner may be pregnant

The patient understands that if his doctor is not available, he can call 1-888-668-2528 for information on emergency contraception.

- The patient cannot donate semen or sperm while taking THALOMID® (thalidomide).

Authorization:

This information has been read aloud to me in the language of my choice. I understand that if I do not follow all of my doctor's instructions, I will not be able to receive THALOMID® (thalidomide).

I now authorize my doctor to begin my treatment with THALOMID® (thalidomide).

Patient Signature ______________________

Date ______________________

I have fully explained to the patient the nature, purpose, and risks of the treatment described above, especially the risks to women of childbearing potential. I have asked the patient if he/she has any questions regarding his/her treatment with THALOMID® (thalidomide) and have answered those questions to the best of my ability. I will comply with all of my obligations and responsibilities as a prescriber registered under the *S.T.E.P.S.*® restricted distribution program.

Prescriber Name (please type): ______________________

DEA Number: ______________________

Social Security Number if PA or NP: ______________________

Street Address: ______________________

City: __________ State: __________ Zip: __________

Prescriber Signature ______________________

REFERENCES

1. Manson JM. 1986. Teratogenicity. Cassarett and Doull's Toxicology: The Basic Science of Poisons. Third Edition. Pages 195-220. New York: MacMillan Publishing Co.
2. Smithels RW and Newman CG. 1992. J. Med. Genet. 29(10):716-723.
3. Sampaio EP, Kaplan G, Miranda A, *et al.* 1993. J. Infect. Dis. 168(2):408-414.
4. Sarno EN, Grau GE, Vieira LM, *et al.* 1991. Clin. Exp. Immunol. 84:103-108.
5. Sampaio EP, Moreira AL, Sarno EN, *et al.* 1992. J. Exp. Med. 175:1729-1737.
6. Nogueira AC, Neubert R, Helge H, *et al.* 1994. Life Sciences. 55(2):77-92.
7. Jacobson JM, Greenspan JS, Spritzler J, *et al.* 1997. New Eng. J. Med. 336(21):1487-1493
8. Eriksson T, Björkman S, Roth B, *et al.* 1998. Chirality. 10(3): 223-228.
9. Schumaker H, Smith RL, and Williams RT. 1965. Br. J. Pharmacol. 25:324-337.
10. Iyer CGS, Languillon J, Ramanujam K, *et al.* 1971. Bull. WHO. 45:719-732.
11. Sheskin J and Convit J. 1969. Intl. J. Leprosy. 37:135-146.
12. Waters MFR. 1971. Lepr. Rev. 42:26-42.
13. Unpublished data, on file at Celgene.

S.T.E.P.S.® is a registered trademark of Celgene Corporation.

U.S. Pat. Nos. 6,045,501 & 6,315,720.

THALPI.008 02/04 CG

Shown in Product Identification Guide, page 310

Cell Therapeutics, Inc.

501 ELLIOTT AVE W. #400
SEATTLE, WA 98119

Direct Inquiries to:
Medical Information
(800) 715-0944
(510) 985-9750
Customer Service
(888) 305-2289

TRISENOX® ℞

[trī-sĕ-nŏks]
(arsenic trioxide) injection
For Intravenous Use Only
10 mg/10 mL (1 mg/mL) ampule
Rx only

WARNING

Experienced Physician and Institution: TRISENOX® (arsenic trioxide) injection should be administered under the supervision of a physician who is experienced in the management of patients with acute leukemia.

APL Differentiation Syndrome: Some patients with APL treated with TRISENOX® have experienced symptoms similar to a syndrome called the retinoic-acid-Acute Promyelocytic Leukemia (RA-APL) or APL differentiation syndrome, characterized by fever, dyspnea, weight gain, pulmonary infiltrates and pleural or pericardial effusions, with or without leukocytosis. This syndrome can be fatal. The management of the syndrome has not been fully studied, but high-dose steroids have been used at the first suspicion of the APL differentiation syndrome and appear to mitigate signs and symptoms. At the first signs that could suggest the syndrome (unexplained fever, dyspnea and/or weight gain, abnormal chest auscultatory findings or radiographic abnormalities), high-dose steroids (dexamethasone 10 mg intravenously BID) should be immediately initiated, irrespective of the leukocyte count, and continued for at least 3 days or longer until signs and symptoms have abated. The majority of patients do not require termination of TRISENOX® therapy during treatment of the APL differentiation syndrome.

ECG Abnormalities: Arsenic trioxide can cause QT interval prolongation and complete atrioventricular block. QT prolongation can lead to a torsade de pointes-type ventricular arrhythmia, which can be fatal. The risk of torsade de pointes is related to the extent of QT prolongation, concomitant administration of QT prolonging drugs, a history of torsade de pointes, preexisting QT interval prolongation, congestive heart failure, administration of potassium-wasting diuretics, or other conditions that result in hypokalemia or hypomagnesemia. One patient (also receiving amphotericin B) had torsade de pointes during induction therapy for relapsed APL with arsenic trioxide.

ECG and Electrolyte Monitoring Recommendations: Prior to initiating therapy with TRISENOX®, a 12-lead ECG should be performed and serum electrolytes (potassium, calcium, and magnesium) and creatinine should be assessed; preexisting electrolyte abnormalities should be corrected and, if possible, drugs that are known to prolong the QT interval should be discontinued. For QTc greater than 500 msec, corrective measures should be completed and the QTc reassessed with serial ECGs prior to considering using TRISENOX®. During therapy with TRISENOX®, potassium concentrations should be kept above 4 mEq/L and magnesium concentrations should be kept above 1.8 mg/dL. Patients who reach an absolute QT interval value > 500 msec should be reassessed and immediate action should be taken to correct concomitant risk factors, if any, while the risk/benefit of continuing versus suspending TRISENOX® therapy should be considered. If syncope, rapid or irregular heartbeat develops, the patient should be hospitalized for monitoring, serum electrolytes should be assessed, TRISENOX® therapy should be temporarily discontinued until the QTc interval regresses to below 460 msec, electrolyte abnormalities are corrected, and the syncope and irregular heartbeat cease. There are no data on the effect of TRISENOX® on the QTc interval during the infusion.

DESCRIPTION

TRISENOX® is a sterile injectable solution of arsenic trioxide. The molecular formula of the drug substance in the solid state is As_2O_3, with a molecular weight of 197.8 g. TRISENOX® is available in 10 mL, single-use ampules containing 10 mg of arsenic trioxide. TRISENOX® is formulated as a sterile, nonpyrogenic, clear solution of arsenic trioxide in water for injection using sodium hydroxide and dilute hydrochloric acid to adjust to pH 8. TRISENOX® is preservative-free. Arsenic trioxide, the active ingredient, is present at a concentration of 1.0 mg/mL. Inactive ingredients and their respective approximate concentrations are sodium hydroxide (1.2 mg/mL) and hydrochloric acid, which is used to adjust the pH to 7.5-8.5.

CLINICAL PHARMACOLOGY

Mechanism of Action

The mechanism of action of TRISENOX® is not completely understood. Arsenic trioxide causes morphological changes and DNA fragmentation characteristic of apoptosis in NB4 human promyelocytic leukemia cells *in vitro*. Arsenic trioxide also causes damage or degradation of the fusion protein PML/RAR-alpha.

Pharmacokinetics

The pharmacokinetics of trivalent arsenic, the active species of TRISENOX®, have not been characterized.

Metabolism

The metabolism of arsenic trioxide involves reduction of pentavalent arsenic to trivalent arsenic by arsenate reductase and methylation of trivalent arsenic to monomethylarsonic acid and monomethylarsonic acid to dimethylarsinic acid by methyltransferases. The main site of methylation reactions appears to be the liver. Arsenic is stored mainly in liver, kidney, heart, lung, hair and nails.

In vitro enzymatic studies with human liver microsomes revealed that arsenic trioxide has no inhibitory activity on substrates of the major cytochrome P450 enzymes such as 1A2, 2A6, 2B6, 2C8, 2C9, 2C19, 2D6, 2E1, 3A4/5, 4A9/11.

Continued on next page

Trisenox—Cont.

Excretion
Disposition of arsenic following intravenous administration has not been studied. Trivalent arsenic is mostly methylated in humans and excreted in urine.

Special Populations
The effects of renal or hepatic impairment or gender, age and race on the pharmacokinetics of TRISENOX® have not been studied (see PRECAUTIONS).

Drug Interactions
No formal assessments of pharmacokinetic drug-drug interactions between TRISENOX® and other drugs have been conducted. The methyltransferases responsible for metabolizing arsenic trioxide are not members of the cytochrome P450 family of isoenzymes (see PRECAUTIONS).

Clinical Studies

TRISENOX® has been investigated in 40 relapsed or refractory APL patients, previously treated with an anthracycline and a retinoid regimen, in an open-label, single-arm, non-comparative study. Patients received 0.15 mg/kg/day intravenously over 1 to 2 hours until the bone marrow was cleared of leukemic cells or up to a maximum of 60 days. The CR (absence of visible leukemic cells in bone marrow and peripheral recovery of platelets and white blood cells with a confirmatory bone marrow ≥ 30 days later) rate in this population of previously treated patients was 28 of 40 (70%). Among the 22 patients who had relapsed less than one year after treatment with ATRA, there were 18 complete responders (82%). Of the 18 patients receiving TRISENOX® ≥ one year from ATRA treatment, there were 10 complete responders (55%). The median time to bone marrow remission was 44 days and to onset of CR was 53 days. Three of 5 children, 5 years or older, achieved CR. No children less than 5 years old were treated.

Three to six weeks following bone marrow remission, 31 patients received consolidation therapy with TRISENOX®, at the same dose, for 25 additional days over a period up to 5 weeks. In follow-up treatment, 18 patients received further arsenic trioxide as a maintenance course. Fifteen patients had bone marrow transplants. At last follow-up, 27 of 40 patients were alive with a median follow-up time of 484 days (range 280 to 755) and 23 of 40 patients remained in complete response with a median follow-up time of 483 days (range 280 to 755).

Cytogenetic conversion to no detection of the APL chromosome rearrangement was observed in 24 of 28 (86%) patients who met the response criteria defined above, in 5 of 5 (100%) patients who met some but not all of the response criteria, and 3 of 7 (43%) of patients who did not respond.

Reverse Transcriptase – Polymerase Chain Reaction conversions to no detection of the APL gene rearrangement were demonstrated in 22 of 28 (79%) of patients who met the response criteria, in 3 of 5 (60%) of patients who met some but not all of the response criteria, and in 2 of 7 (29%) of patients who did not respond.

Responses were seen across all age groups tested, ranging from 6 to 72 years. The ability to achieve a CR was similar for both genders. There were insufficient patients of Black, Hispanic or Asian derivation to estimate relative response rates in these groups, but responses were seen in members of each group.

Another single center study in 12 patients with relapsed or refractory APL, where patients received TRISENOX® doses generally similar to the recommended dose, had similar results with 9 of 12 (75%) patients attaining a CR.

INDICATIONS

TRISENOX® is indicated for induction of remission and consolidation in patients with acute promyelocytic leukemia (APL) who are refractory to, or have relapsed from, retinoid and anthracycline chemotherapy, and whose APL is characterized by the presence of the t(15;17) translocation or PML/RAR-alpha gene expression.

The response rate of other acute myelogenous leukemia subtypes to TRISENOX® has not been examined.

CONTRAINDICATIONS

TRISENOX® is contraindicated in patients who are hypersensitive to arsenic.

WARNINGS (see boxed WARNING)

TRISENOX® should be administered under the supervision of a physician who is experienced in the management of patients with acute leukemia.

APL Differentiation Syndrome (see boxed WARNING): Nine of 40 patients with APL treated with TRISENOX®, at a dose of 0.15 mg/kg, experienced the APL differentiation syndrome (see boxed WARNING and ADVERSE REACTIONS).

Hyperleukocytosis: Treatment with TRISENOX® has been associated with the development of hyperleukocytosis (≥ 10 × 10^3/μL) in 20 of 40 patients. A relationship did not exist between baseline WBC counts and development of hyperleukocytosis nor baseline WBC counts and peak WBC counts. Hyperleukocytosis was not treated with additional chemotherapy. WBC counts during consolidation were not as high as during induction treatment.

QT Prolongation (see boxed WARNING): QT/QTc prolongation should be expected during treatment with arsenic trioxide and torsade de pointes as well as complete heart block has been reported. Over 460 ECG tracings from 40 patients with refractory or relapsed APL treated with TRISENOX® were evaluated for QTc prolongation. Sixteen of 40 patients (40%) had at least one ECG tracing with a QTc interval greater than 500 msec. Prolongation of the QTc was observed between 1 and 5 weeks after TRISENOX® infusion, and then returned towards baseline by the end of 8 weeks after TRISENOX® infusion. In these ECG evaluations, women did not experience more pronounced QT prolongation than men, and there was no correlation with age.

Adverse Events (any grade) Occurring in ≥ 5% of 40 Patients with APL who Received TRISENOX® at a dose of 0.15 mg/kg/day

System organ class/Adverse Event	All Adverse Events, Any Grade		Grade 3 & 4 Events	
	n	%	n	%
General disorders and administration site conditions				
Fatigue	25	63	2	5
Pyrexia (Fever)	25	63	2	5
Edema—non-specific	16	40		
Rigors	15	38		
Chest pain	10	25	2	5
Injection site pain	8	20		
Pain—non specific	6	15	1	3
Injection site erythema	5	13		
Injection site edema	4	10		
Weakness	4	10	2	5
Hemorrhage	3	8		
Weight gain	5	13		
Weight loss	3	8		
Drug hypersensitivity	2	5	1	3
Gastrointestinal disorders				
Nausea	30	75		
Anorexia	9	23		
Appetite decreased	6	15		
Diarrhea	21	53		
Vomiting	23	58		
Abdominal pain (lower & upper)	23	58	4	10
Sore throat	14	35		
Constipation	11	28	1	3
Loose stools	4	10		
Dyspepsia	4	10		
Oral blistering	3	8		
Fecal incontinence	3	8		
Gastrointestinal hemorrhage	3	8		
Dry mouth	3	8		
Abdominal tenderness	3	8		
Diarrhea hemorrhagic	3	8		
Abdominal distension	3	8		
Metabolism and nutrition disorders				
Hypokalemia	20	50	5	13
Hypomagnesemia	18	45	5	13
Hyperglycemia	18	45	5	13
ALT increased	8	20	2	5
Hyperkalemia	7	18	2	5
AST increased	5	13	1	3
Hypocalcemia	4	10		
Hypoglycemia	3	8		
Acidosis	2	5		
Nervous system disorders				
Headache	24	60	1	3
Insomnia	17	43	1	3

(Table continued on next page)

Adverse Events (any grade) Occurring in ≥ 5% of 40 Patients with APL who Received TRISENOX® at a dose of 0.15 mg/kg/day *(cont.)*

System organ class/Adverse Event	All Adverse Events, Any Grade		Grade 3 & 4 Events	
	n	%	n	%
Paresthesia	13	33	2	5
Dizziness (excluding vertigo)	9	23		
Tremor	5	13		
Convulsion	3	8	2	5
Somnolence	3	8		
Coma	2	5	2	5
Respiratory				
Cough	26	65		
Dyspnea	21	53	4	10
Epistaxis	10	25		
Hypoxia	9	23	4	10
Pleural effusion	8	20	1	3
Post nasal drip	5	13		
Wheezing	5	13		
Decreased breath sounds	4	10		
Crepitations	4	10		
Rales	4	10		
Hemoptysis	3	8		
Tachypnea	3	8		
Rhonchi	3	8		
Skin & subcutaneous tissue disorders				
Dermatitis	17	43		
Pruritus	13	33	1	3
Ecchymosis	8	20		
Dry Skin	6	15		
Erythema—non-specific	5	13		
Increased sweating	5	13		
Facial edema	3	8		
Night sweats	3	8		
Petechiae	3	8		
Hyperpigmentation	3	8		
Non-specific skin lesions	3	8		
Urticaria	3	8		
Local exfoliation	2	5		
Eyelid edema	2	5		
Cardiac disorders				
Tachycardia	22	55		
ECG QT corrected interval prolonged > 500 msec	16	40		
Palpitations	4	10		
ECG abnormal other than QT interval prolongation	3	8		
Infections and infestations				
Sinusitis	8	20		
Herpes simplex	5	13		
Upper respiratory tract infection	5	13	1	3
Bacterial infection—non-specific	3	8	1	3
Herpes zoster	3	8		

(Table continued on next page)

Complete AV block: Complete AV block has been reported with arsenic trioxide in the published literature including a case of a patient with APL.

Carcinogenesis: Carcinogenicity studies have not been conducted with TRISENOX® by intravenous administration. The active ingredient of TRISENOX®, arsenic trioxide is a human carcinogen.

Pregnancy: TRISENOX® may cause fetal harm when administered to a pregnant woman. Studies in pregnant mice, rats, hamsters, and primates have shown that inorganic arsenicals cross the placental barrier when given orally or by injection. The reproductive toxicity of arsenic trioxide has been studied in a limited manner. An increase in resorptions, neural-tube defects, anophthalmia and microphthalmia were observed in rats administered 10 mg/kg of arsenic trioxide on gestation day 9 (approximately 10 times the recommended human daily dose on a mg/m^2 basis). Similar findings occurred in mice administered a 10 mg/kg dose of a related trivalent arsenic, sodium arsenite, (approximately 5 times the projected human dose on a mg/m^2 basis) on gestation days 6, 7, 8 or 9. Intravenous injection of 2 mg/kg sodium arsenite (approximately equivalent to the projected human daily dose on a mg/m^2 basis) on gestation day 7 (the lowest dose tested) resulted in neural-tube defects in hamsters.

There are no studies in pregnant women using TRISENOX®. If this drug is used during pregnancy or if the patient becomes pregnant while taking this drug, the patient should be apprised of the potential harm to the fetus. One patient who became pregnant while receiving arsenic trioxide had a miscarriage. Women of childbearing potential should be advised to avoid becoming pregnant.

PRECAUTIONS

Laboratory Tests: The patient's electrolyte, hematologic and coagulation profiles should be monitored at least twice weekly, and more frequently for clinically unstable patients during the induction phase and at least weekly during the consolidation phase. ECGs should be obtained weekly, and more frequently for clinically unstable patients, during induction and consolidation.

Drug Interactions: No formal assessments of pharmacokinetic drug-drug interactions between TRISENOX® and other agents have been conducted. Caution is advised when TRISENOX® is coadministered with other medications that can prolong the QT interval (e.g. certain antiarrhythmics or thioridazine) or lead to electrolyte abnormalities (such as diuretics or amphotericin B).

Carcinogenesis, Mutagenesis, Impairment of Fertility: See WARNINGS section for information on carcinogenesis. Arsenic trioxide and trivalent arsenite salts have not been demonstrated to be mutagenic to bacteria, yeast or mammalian cells. Arsenite salts are clastogenic *in vitro* (human fibroblast, human lymphocytes, Chinese hamster ovary cells, Chinese hamster V79 lung cells). Trivalent arsenic produced an increase in the incidence of chromosome aberrations and micronuclei in bone marrow cells of mice. The effect of arsenic on fertility has not been adequately studied.

Pregnancy: Pregnancy Category D. See WARNINGS section.

Nursing Mothers: Arsenic is excreted in human milk. Because of the potential for serious adverse reactions in nursing infants from TRISENOX®, a decision should be made whether to discontinue nursing or to discontinue the drug, taking into account the importance of the drug to the mother.

Pediatric Use: There are limited clinical data on the pediatric use of TRISENOX®. Of 5 patients below the age of 18 years (age range: 5 to 16 years) treated with TRISENOX®, at the recommended dose of 0.15 mg/kg/day, 3 achieved a complete response.

Safety and effectiveness in pediatric patients below the age of 5 years have not been studied.

Patients with Renal or Hepatic Impairment: Safety and effectiveness of TRISENOX® in patients with renal and hepatic impairment have not been studied. Particular caution is needed in patients with renal failure receiving TRISENOX®, as renal excretion is the main route of elimination of arsenic.

ADVERSE REACTIONS

Safety information was available for 52 patients with relapsed or refractory APL who participated in clinical trials of TRISENOX®. Forty patients in the Phase 2 study received the recommended dose of 0.15 mg/kg of which 28 completed both induction and consolidation treatment cycles. An additional 12 patients with relapsed or refractory APL received doses generally similar to the recommended dose. Most patients experienced some drug-related toxicity, most commonly leukocytosis, gastrointestinal (nausea, vomiting, diarrhea, and abdominal pain), fatigue, edema, hyperglycemia, dyspnea, cough, rash or itching, headaches, and dizziness. These adverse effects have not been observed to be permanent or irreversible nor do they usually require interruption of therapy.

Serious adverse events (SAEs), grade 3 or 4 according to version 2 of the NCI Common Toxicity Criteria, were common. Those SAEs attributed to TRISENOX® in the Phase 2 study of 40 patients with refractory or relapsed APL included APL differentiation syndrome (n=3), hyperleukocytosis (n=3), QTc interval ≥ 500 msec (n=16, 1 with torsade de pointes), atrial dysrhythmias (n=2), and hyperglycemia (n=2).

The following table describes the adverse events that were observed in patients treated for APL with TRISENOX® at the recommended dose at a rate of 5% or more. Similar adverse event profiles were seen in the other patient populations who received TRISENOX®.

[See table on pages 1100 through 1102]

OVERDOSAGE

If symptoms suggestive of serious acute arsenic toxicity (e.g., convulsions, muscle weakness and confusion) appear,

Continued on next page

Adverse Events (any grade) Occurring in ≥ 5% of 40 Patients with APL who Received TRISENOX® at a dose of 0.15 mg/kg/day *(cont.)*

System organ class/Adverse Event	All Adverse Events, Any Grade		Grade 3 & 4 Events	
	n	%	n	%
Nasopharyngitis	2	5		
Oral candidiasis	2	5		
Sepsis	2	5	2	5
Musculoskeletal, connective tissue and bone disorders				
Arthralgia	13	33	3	8
Myalgia	10	25	2	5
Bone pain	9	23	4	10
Back pain	7	18	1	3
Neck Pain	5	13		
Pain in limb	5	13	2	5
Hematologic disorders				
Leukocytosis	20	50	1	3
Anemia	8	20	2	5
Thrombocytopenia	7	18	5	13
Febrile neutropenia	5	13	3	8
Neutropenia	4	10	4	10
Disseminated intravascular coagulation	3	8	3	8
Lymphadenopathy	3	8		
Vascular disorders				
Hypotension	10	25	2	5
Flushing	4	10		
Hypertension	4	10		
Pallor	4	10		
Psychiatric disorders				
Anxiety	12	30		
Depression	8	20		
Agitation	2	5		
Confusion	2	5		
Ocular disorders				
Eye irritation	4	10		
Blurred vision	4	10		
Dry eye	3	8		
Painful red eye	2	5		
Renal and urinary disorders				
Renal failure	3	8	1	3
Renal impairment	3	8		
Oliguria	2	5		
Incontinence	2	5		
Reproductive system disorders				
Vaginal hemorrhage	5	13		
Intermenstrual bleeding	3	8		
Ear Disorders				
Earache	3	8		
Tinnitus	2	5		

Trisenox—Cont.

TRISENOX® should be immediately discontinued and chelation therapy should be considered. A conventional protocol for acute arsenic intoxication includes dimercaprol administered at a dose of 3 mg/kg intramuscularly every 4 hours until immediate life-threatening toxicity has subsided. Thereafter, penicillamine at a dose of 250 mg orally, up to a maximum frequency of four times per day (≤ 1 g per day), may be given.

DOSAGE AND ADMINISTRATION

TRISENOX® should be diluted with 100 to 250 mL 5% Dextrose Injection, USP or 0.9% Sodium Chloride Injection, USP, using proper aseptic technique, immediately after withdrawal from the ampule. The TRISENOX® ampule is single-use and does not contain any preservatives. Unused portions of each ampule should be discarded properly. Do not save any unused portions for later administration. Do not mix TRISENOX® with other medications.

TRISENOX® should be administered intravenously over 1-2 hours. The infusion duration may be extended up to 4 hours if acute vasomotor reactions are observed. A central venous catheter is not required.

Stability

After dilution, TRISENOX® is chemically and physically stable when stored for 24 hours at room temperature and 48 hours when refrigerated.

Dosing Regimen

TRISENOX® is recommended to be given according to the following schedule:

Induction Treatment Schedule: TRISENOX® should be administered intravenously at a dose of 0.15 mg/kg daily until bone marrow remission. Total induction dose should not exceed 60 doses.

Consolidation Treatment Schedule: Consolidation treatment should begin 3 to 6 weeks after completion of induction therapy. TRISENOX® should be administered intravenously at a dose of 0.15 mg/kg daily for 25 doses over a period up to 5 weeks.

HANDLING AND DISPOSAL

Procedures for proper handling and disposal of anticancer drugs should be considered. Several guidelines on this subject have been published.[1-7] There is no general agreement that all of the procedures recommended in the guidelines are necessary or appropriate.

HOW SUPPLIED

TRISENOX® (arsenic trioxide) injection is supplied as a sterile, clear, colorless solution in 10 mL glass, single-use ampules.

NDC 60553-111-10 10 mg/10 mL (1 mg/mL) ampule in packages of ten ampules.

Store at 25°C (77°F); excursions permitted to 15-30°C (59-86°F). Do not freeze.

Do not use beyond expiration date printed on the label.

REFERENCES

1. *Recommendations for the Safe Handling of Parenteral Antineoplastic Drugs.* Publication NIH 83-2621. For sale by the Superintendent of Documents, U.S. Government Printing Office, Washington, DC 20402.
2. Council on Scientific Affairs. Guidelines for handling parenteral antineoplastics. *JAMA.* 1985;253:1590-1592.
3. National Study Commission on Cytotoxic Exposure. *Recommendations for handling cytotoxic agents.* Available from Louis P. Jeffrey, ScD, Chairman, National Study Commission on Cytotoxic Exposure, Massachusetts College of Pharmacy and Allied Health Sciences, 179 Longwood Avenue, Boston, Massachusetts 02115.
4. Clinical Oncological Society of Australia. Guidelines and recommendations for safe handling of antineoplastic agents. *Med J Australia.* 1983;1:426-428.
5. Jones RB, et al. Safe handling of chemotherapeutic agents: a report from the Mount Sinai Medical Center. *CA J Clin.* 1983;33:258-263.
6. American Society of Hospital Pharmacists Technical Assistance Bulletin on Handling Cytotoxic and Hazardous Drugs. *Am J Hosp Pharm.* 1990;47:1033-1049.
7. Controlling Occupational Exposure to Hazardous Drugs (OSHA Work-Practice Guidelines). *Am J Health-Syst Pharm.* 1996;53:1669-1685.

Rx only

For additional information, contact Cell Therapeutics, Inc.
Professional Services at 1-800-715-0944
Customer Service at 1-888-305-2289.

Manufactured for:
Cell Therapeutics, Inc.
Seattle, WA 98119

June 2003

Shown in Product Identification Guide, page 310

Celltech Pharmaceuticals, Inc.

755 JEFFERSON ROAD
ROCHESTER, NY 14623

Direct Inquiries to:
Customer Service Department
P.O. Box 31766
Rochester, NY 14603
(585) 274-5300
(888) 963-3382

In Emergencies:
(800) 932-1950 (24 hours)

AMERICAINE®
ANESTHETIC LUBRICANT ℞
[*uh-mer 'ĭ-kān "*]
(benzocaine)
R531
Rev. 7/01
℞ only

DESCRIPTION

AMERICAINE Anesthetic Lubricant contains benzocaine 20% with benzethonium chloride 0.1% as a preservative in a water soluble base of polyethylene glycol 300 and 3350.

Benzocaine, a local anesthetic, is chemically ethyl *p*-aminobenzoate, $C_9H_{11}NO_2$, with a molecular weight of 165.19 and has the following structural formula:

CLINICAL PHARMACOLOGY

Benzocaine reversibly stabilizes the neuronal membrane which decreases its permeability to sodium ions. Depolarization of the neuronal membrane is inhibited thereby blocking the initiation and conduction of nerve impulses.

INDICATIONS AND USAGE

AMERICAINE Anesthetic Lubricant is indicated for general use as a lubricant and topical anesthetic on intratracheal catheters and pharyngeal and nasal airways to obtund the pharyngeal and tracheal reflexes; on nasogastric and endoscopic tubes; urinary catheters; laryngoscopes; proctoscopes; sigmoidoscopes and vaginal specula.

CONTRAINDICATIONS

Known allergy or hypersensitivity to benzocaine.

PRECAUTIONS

General: Medication should be discontinued if sensitivity or irritation occurs.

Carcinogenesis, Mutagenesis, Impairment of Fertility: Long-term studies in animals or humans to evaluate the carcinogenic and mutagenic potential or the effect on fertility have not been conducted.

Pregnancy: Pregnancy Category C. Animal reproduction studies have not been conducted with AMERICAINE Anesthetic Lubricant. It is also not known whether AMERICAINE Anesthetic Lubricant can cause fetal harm when administered to a pregnant woman or can affect reproduction capacity. AMERICAINE Anesthetic Lubricant should be given to a pregnant woman only if clearly needed.

Nursing Mothers: It is not known whether this drug is excreted in human milk. Because many drugs are excreted in human milk, caution should be exercised when AMERICAINE Anesthetic Lubricant is administered to a nursing woman.

Pediatric Use: Do not use in infants under 1 year of age.

ADVERSE REACTIONS

Contact dermatitis and/or hypersensitivity to benzocaine can cause burning, stinging, pruritus, tenderness, erythema, rash, urticaria and edema. Rarely, benzocaine may induce methemoglobinemia causing respiratory distress and cyanosis. Intravenous methylene blue is the specific therapy for this condition.

DOSAGE AND ADMINISTRATION

Apply evenly to exterior of tube or instrument prior to use.

HOW SUPPLIED

AMERICAINE Anesthetic Lubricant (benzocaine) is available in:

NDC 53014-376-16	28 g tube
NDC 53014-376-62	2.5 g unit dose foil packs, 144 per carton

Store at 15°–25°C (59°–77°F).

Celltech Pharmaceuticals, Inc.
Rochester, NY 14623 USA
®Ciba-Geigy Corporation

Rev. 7/01
R531

DIPENTUM®

(olsalazine sodium capsules)
250 mg
℞ only

℞

DESCRIPTION

The active ingredient in DIPENTUM Capsules (olsalazine sodium) is the sodium salt of a salicylate, disodium 3,3′-azobis (6-hydroxybenzoate) a compound that is effectively bioconverted to 5-aminosalicylic acid (5-ASA), which has anti-inflammatory activity in ulcerative colitis. Its empirical formula is $C_{14}H_8N_2Na_2O_6$ with a molecular weight of 346.21.

The structural formula is:

Olsalazine sodium is a yellow crystalline powder which melts with decomposition at 240°C. It is the sodium salt of a weak acid, soluble in water and DMSO, and practically insoluble in ethanol, chloroform and ether. Olsalazine sodium has acceptable stability under acidic or basic conditions.

DIPENTUM is supplied in hard gelatin capsules for oral administration. The inert ingredient in each 250 mg capsule of olsalazine sodium is magnesium stearate. The capsule shell has the following inactive ingredients: black iron oxide, caramel, gelatin, and titanium dioxide.

CLINICAL PHARMACOLOGY

After oral administration, olsalazine has limited systemic bioavailability. Based on oral and intravenous dosing studies, approximately 2.4% of a single 1.0 g oral dose is absorbed. Less than 1% of olsalazine is recovered in the urine. The remaining 98 to 99% of an oral dose will reach the colon where each molecule is rapidly converted into two molecules of 5-aminosalicylic acid (5-ASA) by colonic bacteria and the low prevailing redox potential found in this environment. The liberated 5-ASA is absorbed slowly resulting in very high local concentrations in the colon.

The conversion of olsalazine to mesalamine (5-ASA) in the colon is similar to that of sulfasalazine, which is converted into sulfapyridine and mesalamine. It is thought that the mesalamine component is therapeutically active in ulcerative colitis (A.K. Azad-Kahn et al, *LANCET,* 2:892-895, 1977). The usual dose of sulfasalazine for maintenance of remission in patients with ulcerative colitis is 2 grams daily, which would provide approximately 0.8 gram of mesalamine to the colon. More than 0.9 gram of mesalamine would usually be made available in the colon from 1 gram of olsalazine.

The mechanism of action of mesalamine (and sulfasalazine) is unknown, but appears to be topical rather than systemic. Mucosal production of arachidonic acid (AA) metabolites, both through the cyclooxygenase pathways, i.e., prostanoids, and through the lipoxygenase pathways, i.e., leukotrienes (LTs) and hydroxyeicosatetraenoic acids (HETEs) is increased in patients with chronic inflammatory bowel disease, and it is possible that mesalamine diminishes inflammation by blocking cyclooxygenase and inhibiting prostaglandin (PG) production in the colon.

Pharmacokinetics

The pharmacokinetics of olsalazine are similar in both healthy volunteers and in patients with ulcerative colitis. Maximum serum concentrations of olsalazine appear after approximately 1 hour, and, even after a 1.0 g single dose, are low, e.g., 1.6 to 6.2 μmol/L. Olsalazine has a very short serum half-life, approximately 0.9 hours. Olsalazine is more than 99% bound to plasma proteins. It does not interfere with protein binding of warfarin. The urinary recovery of olsalazine is below 1%. Total recovery of oral ^{14}C-labeled olsalazine in animals and humans ranges from 90 to 97%.

Approximately 0.1% of an oral dose of olsalazine is metabolized in the liver to olsalazine-O-sulfate (olsalazine-S). Olsalazine-S, in contrast to olsalazine has a half-life of 7 days. Olsalazine-S accumulates to steady state within 2 to 3 weeks.

Patients on daily doses of 1.0 g olsalazine for 2 to 4 years show a stable plasma concentration of olsalazine-S (3.3 to 12.4 μmol/L). Olsalazine-S is more than 99% bound to plasma proteins. Its long half-life is mainly due to slow dissociation from the protein binding site. Less than 1% of both olsalazine and olsalazine-S appears undissociated in plasma.

5-aminosalicylic acid (5-ASA): Serum concentrations of 5-ASA are detected after 4 to 8 hours. The peak levels of 5-ASA after an oral dose of 1.0 g olsalazine are low, i.e., 0 to 4.3 μmol/L. Of the total 5-ASA found in the urine, more than 90% is in the form of N-acetyl-5-ASA (Ac-5-ASA). Only small amounts of 5-ASA are detected.

N-acetyl-5-ASA (Ac-5-ASA), the major metabolite of 5-ASA found in plasma and urine, is acetylated (deactivated) in at least two sites, the colonic epithelium and the liver. Ac-5-ASA is found in the serum, with peak values of 1.7 to 8.7 μmol/L after a single 1.0 g dose. Approximately 20% of the total 5-ASA is recovered in the urine, where it is found almost exclusively as Ac-5-ASA. The remaining 5-ASA is partially acetylated and is excreted in the feces. From fecal dialysis, the concentration of 5-ASA in the colon following olsalazine has been calculated to be 18 to 49 mmol/L. No accumulation of 5-ASA or Ac-5-ASA in plasma has been detected. 5-ASA and Ac-5-ASA are 74 and 81%, respectively, bound to plasma proteins.

ANIMAL TOXICOLOGY

Preclinical subacute and chronic toxicity studies in rats have shown the kidney to be the major target organ of olsalazine toxicity. At an oral daily dose of 400 mg/kg or higher, olsalazine treatment produced nephritis and tubular necrosis in a 4-week study; interstitial nephritis and tubular calcinosis in a 6-month study, and renal fibrosis, mineralization and transitional cell hyperplasia in a 1-year study.

CLINICAL STUDIES

Two controlled studies have demonstrated the efficacy of olsalazine as maintenance therapy in patients with ulcerative colitis. In the first, ulcerative colitis patients in remission were randomized to olsalazine 500 mg B.I.D. or placebo, and relapse rates for a six month period of time were compared. For the 52 patients randomized to olsalazine, 12 relapses occurred, while for the 49 placebo patients, 22 relapses occurred. This difference in relapse rates was significant ($p<.02$).

In the second study, 164 ulcerative colitis patients in remission were randomized to olsalazine 500 mg B.I.D. or sulfasalazine 1 gram B.I.D., and relapse rates were compared after six months. The relapse rate for olsalazine was 19.5% while that for sulfasalazine was 12.2%, a non-significant difference.

INDICATIONS AND USAGE

Olsalazine is indicated for the maintenance of remission of ulcerative colitis in patients who are intolerant of sulfasalazine.

CONTRAINDICATIONS

Hypersensitivity to salicylates.

PRECAUTIONS

General

Overall, approximately 17% of subjects receiving olsalazine in clinical studies reported diarrhea sometime during therapy. This diarrhea resulted in withdrawal of treatment in 6% of patients. This diarrhea appears to be dose related, although it may be difficult to distinguish from the underlying symptoms of the disease.

Exacerbation of the symptoms of colitis thought to have been caused by mesalamine or sulfasalazine has been noted. Although renal abnormalities were not reported in clinical trials with olsalazine, there have been rare reports from post-marketing experience (see under ADVERSE REACTIONS). Therefore, the possibility of renal tubular damage due to absorbed mesalamine or its n-acetylated metabolite, as noted in the ANIMAL TOXICOLOGY section must be kept in mind, particularly for patients with pre-existing renal disease. In these patients, monitoring with urinalysis, BUN and creatinine determinations is advised.

Information for Patients

Patients should be instructed to take olsalazine with food. The drug should be taken in evenly divided doses. Patients should be informed that about 17% of subjects receiving olsalazine during clinical studies reported diarrhea sometime during therapy. If diarrhea occurs, patients should contact their physician.

Drug Interactions: Increased prothrombin time in patients taking concomitant warfarin has been reported.

Drug/Laboratory Test Interactions: None known.

Carcinogenesis, Mutagenesis, Impairment of Fertility

In a two year oral rat carcinogenicity study, olsalazine was tested in male and female Wistar rats at daily doses of 200, 400 and 800 mg/kg/day (approximately 10 to 40 times the human maintenance dose, based on a patient weight of 50 kg and a human dose of 1 g). Urinary bladder transitional cell carcinomas were found in three male rats (6%, p=0.022, exact trend test) receiving 40 times the human dose and were not found in untreated male controls. In the same study, urinary bladder transitional cell carcinoma and papilloma occurred in 2 untreated control female rats (2%). No such tumors were found in any of the female rats treated at doses up to 40 times the human dose.

In an eighteen month oral mouse carcinogenicity study, olsalazine was tested in male and female CD-1 mice at daily doses of 500, 1000 and 2000 mg/kg/day (approximately 25 to 100 times the human maintenance dose). Liver hemangiosarcomata were found in two male mice (4%) receiving olsalazine at 100 times the human dose, while no such tumor occurred in the other treated male mice groups or any of the treated female mice. The observed incidence of this tumor is within the 4% incidence in historical controls.

Olsalazine was not mutagenic in *in vitro* Ames tests, mouse lymphoma cell mutation assays, human lymphocyte chromosomal aberration tests and the *in vivo* rat bone marrow cell chromosomal aberration test.

Olsalazine in a dose range of 100 to 400 mg/kg/day (approximately 5 to 20 times the human maintenance dose) did not influence the fertility of male or female rats. The oligospermia and infertility in men associated with sulfasalazine have not been reported with olsalazine.

Pregnancy. Teratogenic Effects. Pregnancy Category C.

Olsalazine has been shown to produce fetal developmental toxicity as indicated by reduced fetal weights, retarded ossifications and immaturity of the fetal visceral organs when given during organogenesis to pregnant rats in doses 5 to 20 times the human dose (100 to 400 mg/kg). There are no adequate and well-controlled studies in pregnant women. Olsalazine should be used during pregnancy only if the potential benefit justifies the potential risk to the fetus.

Nursing Mothers

Oral administration of olsalazine to lactating rats in doses 5 to 20 times the human dose produced growth retardation in their pups. It is not known whether this drug is excreted in human milk. Because many drugs are excreted in human milk, caution should be exercised when olsalazine is administered to a nursing woman.

Pediatric Use

Safety and effectiveness in a pediatric population have not been established.

Geriatric Use

Clinical studies of DIPENTUM did not include sufficient numbers of subjects aged 65 and over to determine whether they respond differently from younger subjects. Other reported clinical experience has not identified differences in responses between the elderly and younger patients. In general, elderly patients should be treated with caution due to the greater frequency of decreased hepatic, renal, or cardiac function, co-existence of other disease, as well as concomitant drug therapy.

ADVERSE REACTIONS

Olsalazine has been evaluated in ulcerative colitis patients in remission as well as those with acute disease. Both sulfasalazine-tolerant and intolerant patients have been studied in controlled clinical trials. Overall, 10.4% of pa-

Continued on next page

Information on the Celltech Pharmaceuticals, Inc. products listed on these pages contains the full prescribing information from product circulars in use as of July 2004. For further information, please consult the package insert currently accompanying the product.

Dipentum—Cont.

tients discontinued olsalazine because of an adverse experience compared with 6.7% of placebo patients. The most commonly reported adverse reactions leading to treatment withdrawal were diarrhea or loose stools (olsalazine 5.9%; placebo 4.8%), abdominal pain and rash or itching (slightly more than 1% of patients receiving olsalazine). Other adverse reactions to olsalazine leading to withdrawal occurred in fewer than 1% of patients (TABLE 1).

TABLE 1
Adverse Reactions Resulting in Withdrawal From Controlled Studies

	Total Olsalazine (N = 441)	Placebo (N = 208)
Diarrhea/Loose Stools	26 (5.9%)	10 (4.8%)
Nausea	3	2
Abdominal Pain	5 (1.1%)	0
Rash/Itching	5 (1.1%)	0
Headache	3	0
Heartburn	2	0
Rectal Bleeding	1	0
Insomnia	1	0
Dizziness	1	0
Anorexia	1	0
Light Headedness	1	0
Depression	1	0
Miscellaneous	4 (0.9%)	3 (1.4%)
Total Number of Patients Withdrawn	46 (10.4%)	14 (6.7%)

For those controlled studies, the comparative incidences of adverse reactions reported in 1% or more patients treated with olsalazine or placebo are provided in TABLE 2.

TABLE 2: COMPARATIVE INCIDENCE (%) OF ADVERSE EFFECTS REPORTED BY ONE PERCENT OR MORE OF ULCERATIVE COLITIS PATIENTS TREATED WITH OLSALAZINE OR PLACEBO IN DOUBLE BLIND CONTROLLED STUDIES

ADVERSE EVENT	Olsalazine (N = 441) %	Placebo (N = 208) %
Digestive System		
Diarrhea	11.1	6.7
Abdominal Pain/Cramps	10.1	7.2
Nausea	5.0	3.9
Dyspepsia	4.0	4.3
Bloating	1.5	1.4
Anorexia	1.3	1.9
Vomiting	1.0	–
Stomatitis	1.0	–
Increased Blood in Stool	–	3.4
CNS/Psychiatric		
Headache	5.0	4.8
Fatigue/Drowsiness/Lethargy	1.8	2.9
Depression	1.5	–
Vertigo/Dizziness	1.0	–
Insomnia	–	2.4
Skin		
Rash	2.3	1.4
Itching	1.3	–
Musculoskeletal		
Arthralgia/Joint Pain	4.0	2.9
Miscellaneous		
Upper Respiratory Infection	1.5	–

Over 2,500 patients have been treated with olsalazine in various controlled and uncontrolled clinical studies. In these as well as in the post-marketing experience, olsalazine was administered mainly to patients intolerant to sulfasalazine. There have been rare reports of the following adverse effects in patients receiving olsalazine. These were often difficult to distinguish from possible symptoms of the underlying disease or from the effects of prior and/or concomitant therapy.

A causal relationship to the drug has not been demonstrated for some of these reactions.

Digestive: Pancreatitis, diarrhea with dehydration, increased blood in stool, rectal bleeding, flare in symptoms, rectal discomfort, epigastric discomfort, flatulence.

In a double-blind, placebo-controlled study, increased frequency and severity of diarrhea were reported in patients randomized to olsalazine 500 mg B.I.D. with concomitant pelvic radiation.

Rare cases of granulomatous hepatitis and nonspecific, reactive hepatitis have been reported in patients receiving olsalazine. Additionally, a patient developed mild cholestatic hepatitis during treatment with sulfasalazine and experienced the same symptoms two weeks later after the treatment was changed to olsalazine. Withdrawal of olsalazine led to complete recovery in these cases.

Neurologic: Paresthesia, tremors, insomnia, mood swings, irritability, fever chills, rigors.

Dermatologic: Erythema nodosum, photosensitivity, erythema, hot flashes, alopecia.

Musculoskeletal: Muscle cramps.

Cardiovascular/Pulmonary: Pericarditis, second degree heart block, interstitial pulmonary disease, hypertension, orthostatic hypotension, peripheral edema, chest pains, tachycardia, palpitations, bronchospasm, shortness of breath.

A patient who developed thyroid disease 9 days after starting DIPENTUM was given propranolol and radioactive iodine and subsequently developed shortness of breath and nausea. The patient died 5 days later with signs and symptoms of acute diffuse myocarditis.

Genitourinary: Frequency, dysuria, hematuria, proteinuria, nephrotic syndrome, interstitial nephritis, impotence, menorrhagia.

Hematologic: Leucopenia, neutropenia, lymphopenia, eosinophilia, thrombocytopenia, anemia, hemolytic anemia, reticulocytosis.

Laboratory: ALT (SGPT) or AST (SGOT) elevated beyond the normal range.

Special Senses: Tinnitus, dry mouth, dry eyes, watery eyes, blurred vision.

Postmarketing Reports

The following events have been identified during post-approval use of products which contain (or are metabolized to) mesalamine in clinical practice. Because they are reported voluntarily from a population of unknown size, estimates of frequency cannot be made. These events have been chosen for inclusion due to a combination of seriousness, frequency of reporting, or potential causal connection to mesalamine:

Gastrointestinal: Reports of hepatotoxicity, including elevated liver function tests (SGOT/AST, SGPT/ALT, GGT, LDH, alkaline phosphatase, bilirubin), jaundice, cholestatic jaundice, cirrhosis, and possible hepatocellular damage including liver necrosis and liver failure. Some of these cases were fatal. One case of Kawasaki-like syndrome, which included hepatic function changes, was also reported.

DRUG ABUSE AND DEPENDENCY

Abuse: None reported.

Dependence: Drug dependence has not been reported with chronic administration of olsalazine.

OVERDOSAGE

No overdosage has been reported in humans. Maximum single oral doses of 5 g/kg in mice and rats and 2 g/kg in dogs were not lethal. Symptoms of acute toxicity were decreased motor activity and diarrhea in all species tested and in addition, vomiting in dogs.

DOSAGE AND ADMINISTRATION

The usual dosage in adults for maintenance of remission is 1.0 g/day in two divided doses.

HOW SUPPLIED

Beige colored capsules, containing 250 mg olsalazine sodium imprinted with "DIPENTUM® 250 mg" on the capsule shell. Packaged in bottles of 100 (NDC 53014-726-71) and 300 (NDC 53014-726-82).

Storage: Store at 25°C (77°F). Excursions permitted to 15° to 30°C (59° to 86°F) [see USP Controlled Room Temperature].

Rx only

Marketed by:
Celltech Pharmaceuticals, Inc.
Rochester, NY 14623 USA
Manufactured by: Pharmacia AB, Stockholm, Sweden
LR244 Revised: 9/02

GASTROCROM® ℞

[gas-tro-crŏm]
(cromolyn sodium, USP)
Oral Concentrate
℞ Only

Rev 4/02
R535A

For Oral Use Only – Not for Inhalation or Injection.

DESCRIPTION

Each 5 mL ampule of GASTROCROM contains 100 mg cromolyn sodium, USP, in purified water. Cromolyn sodium is a hygroscopic, white powder having little odor. It may leave a slightly bitter aftertaste. GASTROCROM (cromolyn sodium, USP) Oral Concentrate is clear, colorless, and sterile. It is intended for oral use.

Chemically, cromolyn sodium is disodium 5,5'-[(2- hydroxytrimethylene)dioxy]bis[4-oxo-*4H*-1-benzopyran-2- carboxylate]. The empirical formula is $C_{23}H_{14}Na_2O_{11}$; the molecular weight is 512.34. Its chemical structure is:

NaOOC ... OH ... OCH_2CHCH_2O ... COONa

Pharmacologic Category: Mast cell stabilizer
Therapeutic Category: Antiallergic

CLINICAL PHARMACOLOGY

In vitro and *in vivo* animal studies have shown that cromolyn sodium inhibits the release of mediators from sensitized mast cells. Cromolyn sodium acts by inhibiting the release of histamine and leukotrienes (SRS-A) from the mast cell.

Cromolyn sodium has no intrinsic vasoconstrictor, antihistamine, or glucocorticoid activity.

Cromolyn sodium is poorly absorbed from the gastrointestinal tract. No more than 1% of an administered dose is absorbed by humans after oral administration, the remainder being excreted in the feces. Very little absorption of cromolyn sodium was seen after oral administration of 500 mg by mouth to each of 12 volunteers. From 0.28 to 0.50% of the administered dose was recovered in the first 24 hours of urinary excretion in 3 subjects. The mean urinary excretion of an administered dose over 24 hours in the remaining 9 subjects was 0.45%.

CLINICAL STUDIES

Four randomized, controlled clinical trials were conducted with GASTROCROM in patients with either cutaneous or systemic mastocytosis; two of which utilized a placebo-controlled crossover design, one utilized an active-controlled (chlorpheniramine plus cimetidine) crossover design, and one utilized a placebo-controlled parallel group design. Due to the rare nature of this disease, only 36 patients qualified for study entry, of whom 32 were considered evaluable. Consequently, formal statistical analyses were not performed. Clinically significant improvement in gastrointestinal symptoms (diarrhea, abdominal pain) were seen in the majority of patients with some improvement also seen for cutaneous manifestations (urticaria, pruritus, flushing) and cognitive function. The benefit seen with GASTROCROM 200 mg QID was similar to chlorpheniramine (4 mg QID) plus cimetidine (300 mg QID) for both cutaneous and systemic symptoms of mastocytosis.

Clinical improvement occurred within 2–6 weeks of treatment initiation and persisted for 2–3 weeks after treatment withdrawal. GASTROCROM did not affect urinary histamine levels or peripheral eosinophilia, although neither of these variables appeared to correlate with disease severity. Positive clinical benefits were also reported for 37 of 51 patients who received GASTROCROM in United States and foreign humanitarian programs.

INDICATIONS AND USAGE

GASTROCROM is indicated in the management of patients with mastocytosis. Use of this product has been associated with improvement in diarrhea, flushing, headaches, vomiting, urticaria, abdominal pain, nausea, and itching in some patients.

CONTRAINDICATIONS

GASTROCROM is contraindicated in those patients who have shown hypersensitivity to cromolyn sodium.

WARNINGS

The recommended dosage should be decreased in patients with decreased renal or hepatic function. Severe anaphylactic reactions may occur rarely in association with cromolyn sodium administration.

PRECAUTIONS

In view of the biliary and renal routes of excretion of GASTROCROM, consideration should be given to decreasing the dosage of the drug in patients with impaired renal or hepatic function.

Carcinogenesis, Mutagenesis, and Impairment of Fertility: In carcinogenicity studies in mice, hamsters, and rats, cromolyn sodium had no neoplastic effects at intraperitoneal doses up to 150 mg/kg three days per week for 12 months in mice, at intraperitoneal doses up to 53 mg/kg three days per week for 15 weeks followed by 17.5 mg/kg three days per week for 37 weeks in hamsters, and at subcutaneous doses up to 75 mg/kg six days per week for 18 months in rats. These doses in mice, hamsters, and rats are less than the maximum recommended daily oral dose in adults and children on a mg/m^2 basis.

Cromolyn sodium showed no mutagenic potential in Ames Salmonella/microsome plate assays, mitotic gene conversion in *Saccharomyces cerevisiae* and in an *in vitro* cytogenetic study in human peripheral lymphocytes.

In rats, cromolyn sodium showed no evidence of impaired fertility at subcutaneous doses up to 175 mg/kg in males (approximately equal to the maximum recommended daily oral dose in adults on a mg/m^2 basis) and 100 mg/kg in females (less than the maximum recommended daily oral dose in adults on a mg/m^2 basis).

Pregnancy: Pregnancy Category B. In reproductive studies in pregnant mice, rats, and rabbits, cromolyn sodium produced no evidence of fetal malformations at subcutaneous doses up to 540 mg/kg in mice (approximately equal to the maximum recommended daily oral dose in adults on a mg/m^2 basis) and 164 mg/kg in rats (less than the maximum recommended daily oral dose in adults on a mg/m^2 basis) or at intravenous doses up to 485 mg/kg in rabbits (approximately 4 times the maximum recommended daily oral dose in adults on a mg/m^2 basis). There are, however, no adequate and well controlled studies in pregnant women.

Because animal reproduction studies are not always predictive of human response, this drug should be used during pregnancy only if clearly needed.

Drug Interaction During Pregnancy: In pregnant mice, cromolyn sodium alone did not cause significant increases in resorptions or major malformations at subcutaneous doses up to 540 mg/kg (approximately equal to the maximum recommended daily oral dose in adults on a mg/m^2 basis). Isoproterenol alone increased both resorptions and major malformations (primarily cleft palate) at a subcutaneous dose of 2.7 mg/kg (approximately 7 times the maximum recommended daily inhalation dose in adults on a mg/m^2 basis). The incidence of major malformations increased further when cromolyn sodium at a subcutaneous dose of 540 mg/kg was added to isoproterenol at a subcutaneous dose of 2.7 mg/kg. No such interaction was observed in rats or rabbits.

Nursing Mothers: It is not known whether this drug is excreted in human milk. Because many drugs are excreted in human milk, caution should be exercised when GASTROCROM is administered to a nursing woman.

Pediatric Use: In adult rats no adverse effects of cromolyn sodium were observed at oral doses up to 6144 mg/kg (approximately 25 times the maximum recommended daily oral dose in adults on a mg/m^2 basis). In neonatal rats, cromolyn sodium increased mortality at oral doses of 1000 mg/kg or greater (approximately 9 times the maximum recommended daily oral dose in infants on a mg/m^2 basis) but not at doses of 300 mg/kg or less (approximately 3 times the maximum recommended daily oral dose in infants on a mg/m^2 basis). Plasma and kidney concentrations of cromolyn after oral administration to neonatal rats were up to 20 times greater than those in older rats. In term infants up to six months of age, available clinical data suggest that the dose should not exceed 20 mg/kg/day. The use of this product in pediatric patients less than two years of age should be reserved for patients with severe disease in which the potential benefits clearly outweigh the risks.

Geriatric Use: Clinical studies of GASTROCROM did not include sufficient numbers of subjects aged 65 and over to determine whether they respond differently from younger subjects. Other reported clinical experience has not identified differences in responses between the elderly and younger patients. In general, dose selection for an elderly patient should be cautious, usually starting as the low end of the dosing range, reflecting the greater frequency of decreased hepatic, renal, or cardiac function, and of concomitant disease or other drug therapy.

ADVERSE REACTIONS

Most of the adverse events reported in mastocytosis patients have been transient and could represent symptoms of the disease. The most frequently reported adverse events in mastocytosis patients who have received GASTROCROM during clinical studies were headache and diarrhea, each of which occurred in 4 of the 87 patients. Pruritus, nausea, and myalgia were each reported in 3 patients and abdominal pain, rash, and irritability in 2 patients each. One report of malaise was also recorded.

Other Adverse Events: Additional adverse events have been reported during studies in other clinical conditions and from worldwide postmarketing experience. In most cases the available information is incomplete and attribution to the drug cannot be determined. The majority of these reports involve the gastrointestinal system and include: diarrhea, nausea, abdominal pain, constipation, dyspepsia, flatulence, glossitis, stomatitis, vomiting, dysphagia, esophagospasm.

Other less commonly reported events (the majority representing only a single report) include the following:

Skin:	pruritus, rash, urticaria/angioedema, erythema/burning, photosensitivity
Musculoskeletal:	arthralgia, myalgia, stiffness/weakness of legs
Neurologic:	headache, dizziness, hypoesthesia, paresthesia, migraine, convulsions, flushing
Psychiatric:	psychosis, anxiety, depression, hallucinations, behavior change, insomnia, nervousness
Heart Rate:	tachycardia, premature ventricular contractions (PVCs), palpitations
Respiratory:	pharyngitis, dyspnea
Miscellaneous:	fatigue, edema, unpleasant taste, chest pain, postprandial lightheadedness and lethargy, dysuria, urinary frequency, purpura, hepatic function test abnormal, polycythemia, neutropenia, pancytopenia, tinnitus, lupus erythematosus (LE) syndrome

DOSAGE AND ADMINISTRATION

NOT FOR INHALATION OR INJECTION. SEE DIRECTIONS FOR USE.

The usual starting dose is as follows:

Adults and Adolescents (13 Years and Older): Two ampules four times daily, taken one-half hour before meals and at bedtime.

Children 2–12 Years: One ampule four times daily, taken one-half hour before meals and at bedtime.

Pediatric Patients Under 2 Years: Not recommended.

If satisfactory control of symptoms is not achieved within two to three weeks, the dosage may be increased but should not exceed 40 mg/kg/day.

Patients should be advised that the effect of GASTROCROM therapy is dependent upon its administration at regular intervals, as directed.

Maintenance Dose: Once a therapeutic response has been achieved, the dose may be reduced to the minimum required to maintain the patient with a lower degree of symptomatology. To prevent relapses, the dosage should be maintained.

Administration: GASTROCROM should be administered as a solution at least 1/2 hour before meals and at bedtime after preparation according to the following directions:

1. Break open ampule(s) and squeeze liquid contents of ampule(s) into a glass of water.
2. Stir solution.
3. Drink all of the liquid.

HOW SUPPLIED

GASTROCROM Oral Concentrate is an unpreserved, colorless solution supplied in a low density polyethylene plastic unit dose ampule with 8 ampules per foil pouch. Each 5 mL ampule contains 100 mg cromolyn sodium, USP, in purified water.

NDC 53014-678-70 96 ampules × 5 mL

GASTROCROM Oral Concentrate should be stored between 15°–30°C (59°–86°F) and protected from light. Do not use if it contains a precipitate or becomes discolored. Keep out of the reach of children.

Store ampules in foil pouch until ready for use.

Marketed by:
Celltech Pharmaceuticals, Inc.
Rochester, NY 14623 USA
Manufactured by:
Automatic Liquid Packaging, Inc.
Woodstock, IL 60098 USA
® Celltech Manufacturing, Inc. Rev. 4/02
© 2002, Celltech Pharmaceuticals, Inc.
R535A

Patient Instructions

GASTROCROM®
(cromolyn sodium, USP)
Oral Concentrate

For Oral Use Only – Not for Inhalation or Injection.

How to Use GASTROCROM:

As with all prescription drugs, follow the directions for dosage that your physician recommends.

The effect of GASTROCROM therapy is dependent upon its administration at REGULAR intervals, for as long as recommended by your physician.

Usual Starting Dose:

Adults and Adolescents (13 Years and Older):

Two ampules four times daily, taken one-half hour before meals and at bedtime.

Children 2–12 Years:

One ampule four times daily, taken one-half hour before meals and at bedtime.

Note:

Your physician may decide to increase OR decrease your dosage to achieve optimum results with GASTROCROM. However, do not change your dose or stop taking GASTROCROM without first consulting your physician.

Care & Storage:

GASTROCROM Oral Concentrate should be stored between 15°–30°C (59°–86°F) and protected from light. Do not use if it contains a precipitate (particles or cloudiness) or becomes discolored. Keep out of the reach of children.

Store ampules in foil pouch until ready for use.

Recycling Information: GASTROCROM Oral Concentrate ampules are made with a low density polyethylene plastic (recycling material code: ♺4 LDPE).

Directions for Use:

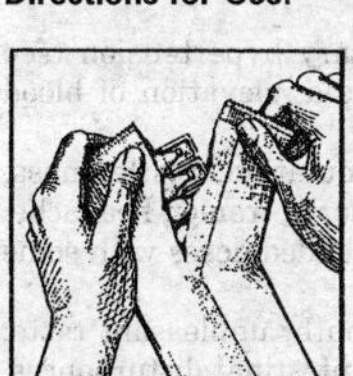

1. Open foil pouch by tearing at serrated edge as shown.

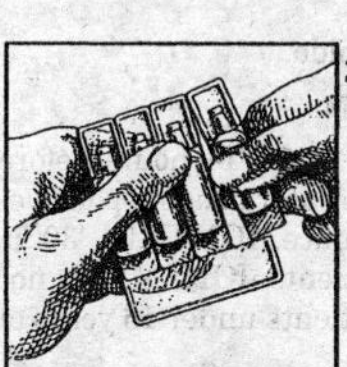

2. Remove ampule(s) from the strip.

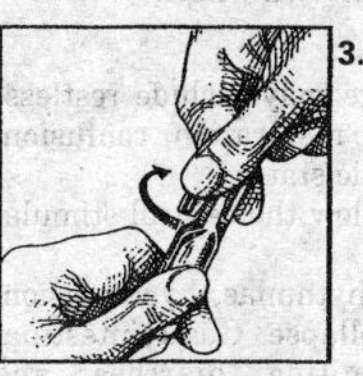

3. Open the ampule by twisting off the tabbed top section.

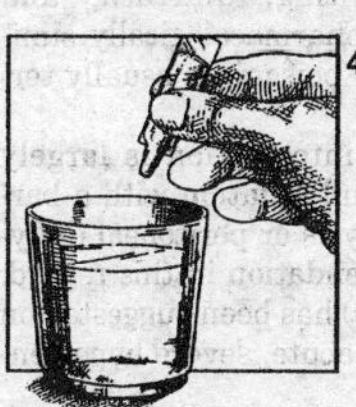

4. Squeeze liquid contents into a glass of water. Stir solution. Drink all of the liquid. Discard the empty ampule.

Marketed by:
Celltech Pharmaceuticals, Inc.
Rochester, NY 14623 USA

Manufactured by:
Automatic Liquid Packaging, Inc., Woodstock, IL 60098 USA
® Celltech Manufacturing, Inc. Rev. 4/02
© 2002, Celltech Pharmaceuticals, Inc. R535A

IONAMIN® CAPSULES ©IV ℞

(phentermine resin)
℞ Only

R523A
Rev. 3/03

DESCRIPTION

IONAMIN '15' and IONAMIN '30' contain 15 mg and 30 mg respectively of phentermine as the cationic exchange resin complex. Phentermine is α, α-dimethyl phenethylamine (phenyl-tertiary-butylamine).

Inactive Ingredients: D&C Yellow No. 10, dibasic calcium phosphate, FD&C Yellow No. 6, gelatin, iron oxides (15 mg capsules only), lactose, magnesium stearate, titanium dioxide.

ACTIONS

IONAMIN is a sympathomimetic amine with pharmacologic activity similar to the prototype drug of this class used in obesity, amphetamine (d- and dℓ-amphetamine). Actions include central nervous system stimulation and elevation of blood pressure. Tachyphylaxis and tolerance have been demonstrated with all drugs of this class in which these phenomena have been looked for.

Drugs of this class used in obesity are commonly known as "anorectics" or "anorexigenics." It has not been established, however, that the action of such drugs in treating obesity is primarily one of appetite suppression. Other central nervous system actions, or metabolic effects may be involved.

Adult obese subjects instructed in dietary management and treated with "anorectic" drugs, lose more weight on the average than those treated with placebo and diet, as determined in relatively short-term clinical trials.

The magnitude of increased weight loss of drug-treated patients over placebo-treated patients is only a fraction of a pound a week. The rate of weight loss is greatest in the first weeks of therapy for both drug and placebo subjects and tends to decrease in succeeding weeks. The possible origins of the increased weight loss due to the various drug effects are not established. The amount of weight loss associated with the use of an "anorectic" drug varies from trial to trial, and the increased weight loss appears to be related in part to variables other than the drugs prescribed, such as the physician-investigator, the population treated, and the diet prescribed. Studies do not permit conclusions as to the relative importance of the drug and non-drug factors on weight loss.

The natural history of obesity is measured in years, whereas the studies cited are restricted to a few weeks' or months' duration; thus, the total impact of drug-induced weight loss over that of diet alone must be considered clinically limited.

The bioavailability of IONAMIN has been studied in humans in which blood levels of phentermine were measured by a gas chromatography method. Blood levels obtained with the 15 mg and 30 mg resin complex formulations indicated slower absorption with a reduced but prolonged peak concentration and without a significant difference in prolongation of blood levels when compared with the same doses of phentermine hydrochloride. The clinical significance of these differences is not known. In clinical trials establishing the efficacy of IONAMIN, a single daily dose produced an effect comparable to that produced by other regimens of "anorectic" drug therapy.

INDICATION

IONAMIN Capsules are indicated as a short-term (a few weeks) adjunct in a regimen of weight reduction based on exercise, behavioral modification, and caloric restriction in the management of exogenous obesity for patients with an initial body mass index ≥30 kg/m^2, or ≥27 kg/m^2 in the presence of other risk factors (e.g., hypertension, diabetes, hyperlipidemia).

Below is a chart of Body Mass Index (BMI) based on various heights and weights.

BMI is calculated by taking the patient's weight, in kilograms (kg), divided by the patient's height, in meters (m), squared. Metric conversions are as follows: pounds ÷ 2.2 = kg; inches × 0.0254 = meters.

[See table at top of next page]

The limited usefulness of agents of this class (see ACTIONS) should be measured against possible risk factors inherent in their use such as those described below.

Continued on next page

Information on the Celltech Pharmaceuticals, Inc. products listed on these pages contains the full prescribing information from product circulars in use as of July 2004. For further information, please consult the package insert currently accompanying the product.

Weight (pounds)	BODY MASS INDEX (BMI), kg/m² Height (feet, inches) 5'0"	5'3"	5'6"	5'9"	6'0"	6'3"
140	27	25	23	21	19	18
150	29	27	24	22	20	19
160	31	28	26	24	22	20
170	33	30	28	25	23	21
180	35	32	29	27	25	23
190	37	34	31	28	26	24
200	39	36	32	30	27	25
210	41	37	34	31	29	26
220	43	39	36	33	30	28
230	45	41	37	34	31	29
240	47	43	39	36	33	30
250	49	44	40	37	34	31

Ionamin—Cont.

CONTRAINDICATIONS

Advanced arteriosclerosis, cardiovascular disease, moderate to severe hypertension, hyperthyroidism, known hypersensitivity, or idiosyncrasy to the sympathomimetic amines, glaucoma.
Agitated states.
Patients with a history of drug abuse.
During or within 14 days following the administration of monoamine oxidase inhibitors (hypertensive crises may result).

WARNINGS

IONAMIN Capsules are indicated only as short-term monotherapy for the management of exogenous obesity. The safety and efficacy of combination therapy with phentermine and any other drug products for weight loss, including selective serotonin reuptake inhibitors (e.g., fluoxetine, sertraline, fluvoxamine, paroxetine), have not been established. Therefore, the coadministration of these drug products for weight loss is not recommended.
Primary Pulmonary Hypertension (PPH)—a rare, frequently fatal disease of the lungs—has been reported to occur in patients receiving a combination of phentermine with fenfluramine or dexfenfluramine. The possibility of an association between PPH and the use of phentermine alone cannot be ruled out. The initial symptom of PPH is usually dyspnea. Other initial symptoms include: angina pectoris, syncope, or lower extremity edema. Patients should be advised to report immediately any deterioration in exercise tolerance. Treatment should be discontinued in patients who develop new, unexplained symptoms of dyspnea, angina pectoris, syncope, or lower extremity edema.
Valvular Heart Disease: Serious regurgitant cardiac valvular disease, primarily affecting the mitral, aortic and/or tricuspid valves, has been reported in otherwise healthy persons who had taken a combination of phentermine with fenfluramine or dexfenfluramine for weight loss. The etiology of these valvulopathies has not been established and their course in individuals after the drugs are stopped is not known.
If tolerance to the "anorectic" effect develops, the recommended dose should not be exceeded in an attempt to increase the effect: rather, the drug should be discontinued.
IONAMIN may impair the ability of the patient to engage in potentially hazardous activities such as operating machinery or driving a motor vehicle; the patient should therefore be cautioned accordingly.
When using CNS active agents, consideration must always be given to the possibility of adverse interactions with alcohol.
Drug Dependence: IONAMIN is related chemically and pharmacologically to amphetamine (d- and dℓ-amphetamine) and other stimulant drugs that have been extensively abused. The possibility of abuse of IONAMIN should be kept in mind when evaluating the desirability of including a drug as part of a weight reduction program. Abuse of amphetamine (d- and dℓ-amphetamine) and related drugs may be associated with intense psychological dependence and severe social dysfunction. There are reports of patients who have increased the dosage of some of these drugs to many times that recommended. Abrupt cessation following prolonged high dosage administration results in extreme fatigue and mental depression; changes are also noted on the sleep EEG. Manifestations of chronic intoxication with anorectic drugs include severe dermatoses, marked insomnia, irritability, hyperactivity, and personality changes. The most severe manifestation of chronic intoxications is psychosis, often clinically indistinguishable from schizophrenia.
Usage in Pregnancy: Safe use in pregnancy has not been established. Use of IONAMIN by women who are or may become pregnant requires that the potential benefit be weighed against the possible hazard to mother and infant.
Pediatric Use: IONAMIN® Capsules (phentermine resin) are not recommended for use in pediatric patients under 16 years of age.

PRECAUTIONS

Caution is to be exercised in prescribing IONAMIN for patients with even mild hypertension. Insulin requirements in diabetes mellitus may be altered in association with the use of IONAMIN and the concomitant dietary regimen.
IONAMIN may decrease the hypotensive effect of adrenergic neuron blocking drugs.
The least amount feasible should be prescribed or dispensed at one time in order to minimize the possibility of overdosage.
Geriatric Use: Clinical studies of IONAMIN did not include sufficient numbers of subjects aged 65 or over to determine whether they respond differently from younger subjects. Other reported clinical experience has not identified differences in responses between the elderly and younger patients. In general, dose selection for an elderly patient should be cautious, usually starting at the low end of the dosing range, reflecting the greater frequency of decreased hepatic, renal, or cardiac function, and of concomitant disease or other drug therapy.
This drug is known to be substantially excreted by the kidney, and the risk of toxic reactions to this drug may be greater in patients with impaired renal function. Because elderly patients are more likely to have decreased renal function, care should be taken in dose selection, and it may be useful to monitor renal function.

ADVERSE REACTIONS

Cardiovascular: Primary pulmonary hypertension (see WARNINGS), palpitation, tachycardia, elevation of blood pressure.
Central Nervous System: Overstimulation, restlessness, dizziness, insomnia, euphoria, dysphoria, tremor, headache; rarely psychotic episodes at recommended doses with some drugs in this class.
Gastrointestinal: Dryness of the mouth, unpleasant taste, diarrhea, constipation, other gastrointestinal disturbances.
Allergic: Urticaria.
Endocrine: Impotence, changes in libido.

DOSAGE AND ADMINISTRATION

One capsule daily, before breakfast or 10–14 hours before retiring. For individuals exhibiting greater drug responsiveness, IONAMIN '15' will usually suffice. IONAMIN '30' is recommended for less responsive patients. IONAMIN is not recommended for use in pediatric patients under 16 years of age.
IONAMIN Capsules should be swallowed whole.

OVERDOSAGE

Manifestations of acute overdosage may include restlessness, tremor, hyperreflexia, rapid respiration, confusion, assaultiveness, hallucinations, panic states.
Fatigue and depression usually follow the central stimulation.
Cardiovascular effects include arrhythmias, hypertension, or hypotension and circulatory collapse. Gastrointestinal symptoms include nausea, vomiting, diarrhea, and abdominal cramps. Overdosage of pharmacologically similar compounds has resulted in fatal poisoning, usually terminating in convulsions and coma.
Management of acute IONAMIN intoxication is largely symptomatic and includes lavage and sedation with a barbiturate. Experience with hemodialysis or peritoneal dialysis is inadequate to permit recommendation in this regard. Intravenous phentolamine (Regitine) has been suggested on pharmacologic grounds for possible acute, severe hypertension, if this complicates overdosage.

HOW SUPPLIED

IONAMIN Capsules (phentermine resin) are available in two strengths:
15 mg, yellow/grey capsules, imprinted with "IONAMIN 15."
NDC 53014-903-71 Bottle of 100's
NDC 53014-903-84 Bottle of 400's
30 mg, yellow/yellow capsules, imprinted with "IONAMIN 30."
NDC 53014-904-71 Bottle of 100's
NDC 53014-904-84 Bottle of 400's
Dispense in a tight container. Store at 25°C (77°F); excursions permitted to 15°–30°C (59°–86°F) [See USP Controlled Room Temperature].
Keep out of the reach of children.
Celltech Pharmaceuticals, Inc.
Rochester, NY 14623 USA

® Celltech Manufacturing, Inc.
Rev. 3/03
R523A

METADATE® CD Ⓒ℞

Once-daily
[*mĕt-ă-dāt*]
(methylphenidate HCl, USP)
Extended-Release Capsules
℞ Only **R312E**
Rev. 7/03

DESCRIPTION

METADATE CD is a central nervous system (CNS) stimulant. The extended-release capsules comprise both immediate-release (IR) and extended-release (ER) beads such that 30% of the dose is provided by the IR component and 70% of the dose is provided by the ER component. METADATE CD is available in three capsule strengths containing 10 mg (3mg IR; 7 mg ER), 20 mg (6 mg IR; 14 mg ER), or 30 mg (9 mg IR; 21 mg ER) of methylphenidate hydrochloride for oral administration.
Chemically, methylphenidate HCl is *d,l* (racemic)-*threo*-methyl α-phenyl-2-piperidineacetate hydrochloride. Its empirical formula is $C_{14}H_{19}NO_2 \cdot HCl$. Its structural formula is:

O OCH₃ H N •HCl

Methylphenidate HCl USP is a white, odorless, crystalline powder. Its solutions are acid to litmus. It is freely soluble in water and in methanol, soluble in alcohol, and slightly soluble in chloroform and in acetone. Its molecular weight is 269.77
METADATE CD also contains the following inert ingredients: Sugar spheres, povidone, hydroxypropylmethylcellulose and polyethylene glycol, ethylcellulose aqueous dispersion, dibutyl sebacate, gelatin, titanium dioxide, FD&C Blue No. 2.

CLINICAL PHARMACOLOGY

Pharmacodynamics: Methylphenidate HCl is a central nervous system (CNS) stimulant. The mode of therapeutic action in Attention Deficit Hyperactivity Disorder (ADHD) is not known. Methylphenidate is thought to block the reuptake of norepinephrine and dopamine into the presynaptic neuron and increase the release of these monoamines into the extraneuronal space. Methylphenidate is a racemic mixture comprised of the *d*- and *l-threo* enantiomers. The *d-threo* enantiomer is more pharmacologically active than the *l-threo* enantiomer.
Pharmacokinetics: The pharmacokinetics of the METADATE CD methylphenidate hydrochloride formulation have been studied in healthy adult volunteers and in children with Attention Deficit Hyperactivity disorder (ADHD).
Absorption and Distribution: Methylphenidate is readily absorbed. METADATE CD has a plasma/time concentration profile showing two phases of drug release with a sharp, initial slope similar to a methylphenidate immediate-release tablet, and a second rising portion approximately three hours later, followed by a gradual decline. (See Figure 1 below.)
Comparison of Immediate Release (IR) and METADATE CD Formulations After Repeated Doses of Methylphenidate HCl in Children with ADHD: METADATE CD was administered as repeated once-daily doses of 20 mg or 40 mg to children aged 7-12 years with ADHD for one week. After a dose of 20 mg, the mean (±SD) early C_{max} was 8.6 (±2.2) ng/mL, the later C_{max} was 10.9 (±3.9)* ng/mL and $AUC_{0\text{-}9h}$ was 63.0 (±16.8) ng•h/mL. The corresponding values after a 40 mg dose were 16.8 (±5.1) ng/mL, 15.1 (±5.8)* ng/mL and 120 (±39.6) ng•h/mL, respectively. The early peak concentrations (median) were reached about 1.5 hours after

dose intake, and the second peak concentrations (median) were reached about 4.5 hours after dose intake. The means for C_{max} and AUC following a dose of 20 mg were slightly lower than those seen with 10 mg of the immediate-release formulation, dosed at 0 and 4 hours.

*25-30% of the subjects had only one observed peak (C_{max}) concentration of methylphenidate.

FIGURE 1

Comparison of Immediate Release (IR) and METADATE CD Formulations After Repeated Doses of Methylphenidate HCl in Children with ADHD

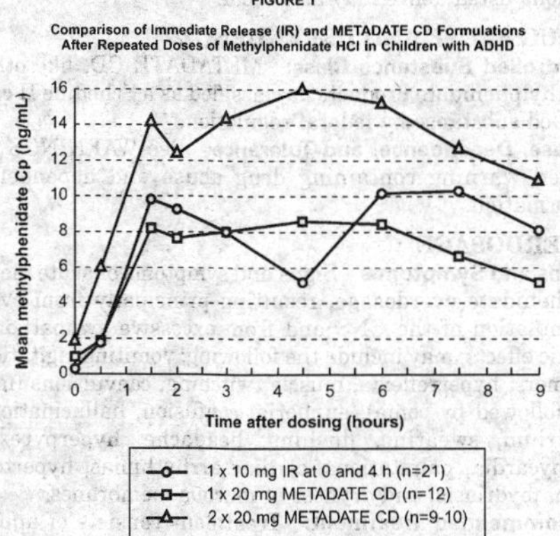

Dose Proportionality: Following single oral doses of 10-60 mg methylphenidate free base as a solution given to ten healthy male volunteers, C_{max} and AUC increased proportionally with increasing doses. After the 60 mg dose, t_{max} was reached 1.5 hours post-dose, with a mean C_{max} of 31.8 ng/mL (range 24.7-40.9 ng/mL).

Following one week of repeated once-daily doses of 20 mg or 40 mg METADATE CD to children aged 7-12 years with ADHD, C_{max} and AUC were proportional to the administered dose.

Food Effects: In a study in adult volunteers to investigate the effects of a high-fat meal on the bioavailability of a dose of 40 mg, the presence of food delayed the early peak by approximately 1 hour (range −2 to 5 hours delay). The plasma levels rose rapidly following the food-induced delay in absorption. Overall, a high-fat meal increased the C_{max} of METADATE CD by about 30% and AUC by about 17%, on average (see DOSAGE and ADMINISTRATION).

After a single dose, the bioavailability (C_{max} and AUC) of methylphenidate in 26 healthy adults was unaffected by sprinkling the capsule contents on applesauce as compared to the intact capsule. This finding demonstrates that a 20 mg METADATE CD Capsule, when opened and sprinkled on one tablespoon of applesauce, is bioequivalent to the intact capsule.

Metabolism and Excretion: In humans, methylphenidate is metabolized primarily via deesterification to alpha-phenyl-piperidine acetic acid (ritalinic acid). The metabolite has little or no pharmacologic activity.

In vitro studies showed that methylphenidate was not metabolized by cytochrome P450 isoenzymes, and did not inhibit cytochrome P450 isoenzymes at clinically observed plasma drug concentrations.

The mean terminal half-life ($t_{½}$) of methylphenidate following administration of METADATE CD ($t_{½}$=6.8h) is longer than the mean terminal $t_{½}$ following administration of methylphenidate hydrochloride immediate-release tablets ($t_{½}$=2.9h) and methylphenidate hydrochloride sustained-release tablets ($t_{½}$=3.4h) in healthy adult volunteers. This suggests that the elimination process observed for METADATE CD is controlled by the release rate of methylphenidate from the extended-release formulation, and that the drug absorption is the rate-limiting process.

Special Populations: *Gender:* The pharmacokinetics of methylphenidate after a single dose of METADATE CD were similar between adult men and women.

Race: The influence of race on the pharmacokinetics of methylphenidate after METADATE CD administration has not been studied.

Age: The pharmacokinetics of methylphenidate after METADATE CD administration have not been studied in children less than 6 years of age.

Renal Insufficiency: There is no experience with the use of METADATE CD in patients with renal insufficiency. After oral administration of radiolabeled methylphenidate in humans, methylphenidate was extensively metabolized and approximately 80% of the radioactivity was excreted in the urine in the form of ritalinic acid. Since renal clearance is not an important route of methylphenidate clearance, renal insufficiency is expected to have little effect on the pharmacokinetics of METADATE CD.

Hepatic Insufficiency: There is no experience with the use of METADATE CD in patients with hepatic insufficiency.

CLINICAL STUDIES

METADATE CD was evaluated in a double-blind, parallel-group, placebo-controlled trial in which 321 untreated or previously treated pediatric patients with a DSM-IV diagnosis of attention deficit hyperactivity disorder (ADHD), 6 to 15 years of age, received a single morning dose for up to 3 weeks. Patients were required to have the combined or predominantly hyperactive-impulsive subtype of ADHD; patients with the predominantly inattentive subtype were excluded. Patients randomized to the METADATE CD group received 20 mg daily for the first week. Their dosage could be increased weekly to a maximum of 60 mg by the third week, depending on individual response to treatment.

The patient's regular school teacher completed the teachers' version of the Conners' Global Index Scale (TCGIS), a scale for assessing ADHD symptoms, in the morning and again in the afternoon on three alternate days of each treatment week. The change from baseline of the overall average (i.e., an average of morning and afternoon scores over 3 days) of the total TCGIS scores during the last week of treatment was analyzed as the primary efficacy parameter. Patients treated with METADATE CD showed a statistically significant improvement in symptom scores from baseline over patients who received placebo. (See Figure 2.) Separate analyses of TCGIS scores in the morning and afternoon revealed superiority in improvement with METADATE CD over placebo during both time periods. (See Figure 3.) This demonstrates that a single morning dose of METADATE CD exerts a treatment effect in both the morning and the afternoon.

FIGURE 2

Least Squares Mean Change from Baseline in TCGIS Scores*

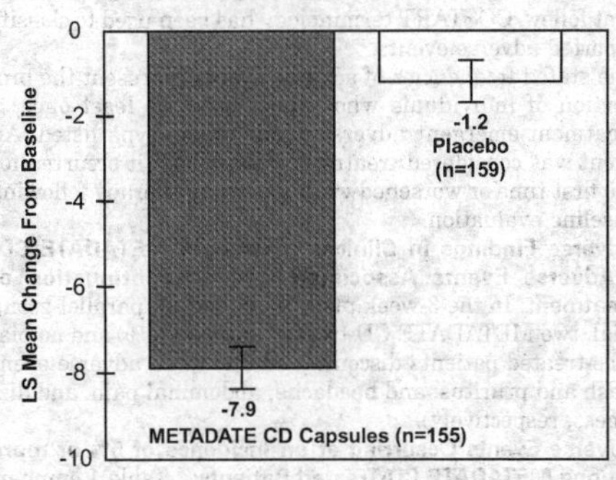

FIGURE 3

Least Squares Mean Change from Baseline in TCGIS Scores, Morning/Afternoon Groups*

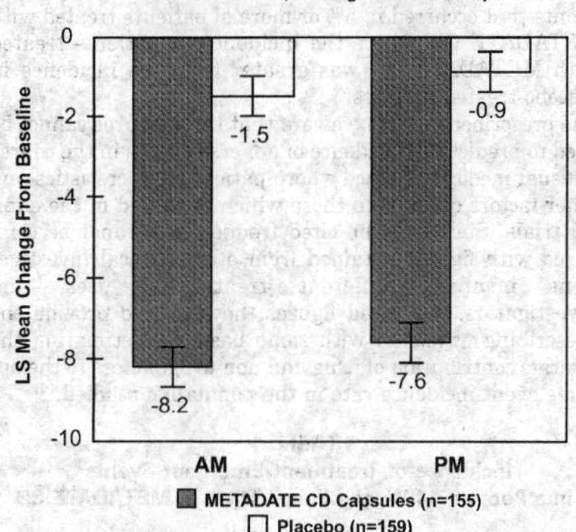

***FIGURES 2 & 3:** Last observation carried forward analysis at week 3.

Error bars represent the standard error of the mean.

INDICATION AND USAGE

Attention Deficit Hyperactivity Disorder (ADHD): METADATE® CD (methylphenidate HCl, USP) Extended-Release Capsules are indicated for the treatment of Attention Deficit Hyperactivity Disorder (ADHD).

The efficacy of METADATE CD in the treatment of ADHD was established in one controlled trial of children aged 6 to 15 who met DSM-IV criteria for ADHD (see CLINICAL PHARMACOLOGY).

A diagnosis of Attention Deficit Hyperactivity Disorder (ADHD; DSM-IV) implies the presence of hyperactive-impulsive or inattentive symptoms that caused impairment and were present before age 7 years. The symptoms must cause clinically significant impairment, e.g., in social, academic, or occupational functioning, and be present in two or more settings, e.g., school (or work) and at home. The symptoms must not be better accounted for by another mental disorder. For the Inattentive Type, at least six of the following symptoms must have persisted for at least 6 months: lack of attention to details/careless mistakes; lack of sustained attention; poor listener; failure to follow through on tasks; poor organization; avoids tasks requiring sustained mental effort; loses things; easily distracted; forgetful. For the Hyperactive-Impulsive Type, at least six of the following symptoms must have persisted for at least 6 months: fidgeting/squirming; leaving seat; inappropriate running/climbing; difficulty with quiet activities; "on the go;" excessive talking; blurting answers; can't wait turn; intrusive. The Combined Types requires both inattentive and hyperactive-impulsive criteria to be met.

Special Diagnostic Considerations: Specific etiology of this syndrome is unknown, and there is no single diagnostic test. Adequate diagnosis requires the use not only of medical but of special psychological, educational, and social resources. Learning may or may not be impaired. The diagnosis must be based upon a complete history and evaluation of the child and not solely on the presence of the required number of DSM-IV characteristics.

Need for Comprehensive Treatment Program: METADATE CD is indicated as an integral part of a total treatment program for ADHD that may include other measures (psychological, educational, social) for patients with this syndrome. Drug treatment may not be indicated for all children with this syndrome. Stimulants are not intended for use in the child who exhibits symptoms secondary to environmental factors and/or other primary psychiatric disorders, including psychosis. Appropriate educational placement is essential and psychosocial intervention is often helpful. When remedial measures alone are insufficient, the decision to prescribe stimulant medication will depend upon the physician's assessment of the chronicity and severity of the child's symptoms.

Long-Term Use: The effectiveness of METADATE CD for long-term use, i.e., for more than 3 weeks, has not been systematically evaluated in controlled trials. Therefore, the physician who elects to use METADATE CD for extended periods should periodically re-evaluate the long-term usefulness of the drug for the individual patient (see DOSAGE and ADMINISTRATION).

CONTRAINDICATIONS

Agitation: METADATE CD is contraindicated in patients with marked anxiety, tension and agitation, since the drug may aggravate these symptoms.

Hypersensitivity to Methylphenidate: METADATE CD is contraindicated in patients known to be hypersensitive to methylphenidate or other components of the product.

Glaucoma: METADATE CD is contraindicated in patients with glaucoma.

Tics: METADATE CD is contraindicated in patients with motor tics or with a family history or diagnosis of Tourette's syndrome. (see ADVERSE REACTIONS).

Monoamine Oxidase Inhibitors: METADATE CD is contraindicated during treatment with monoamine oxidase inhibitors, and also within a minimum of 14 days following discontinuation of a monoamine oxidase inhibitor (hypertensive crises may result).

WARNINGS

Depression: METADATE CD should not be used to treat severe depression.

Fatigue: METADATE CD should not be used for the prevention or treatment of normal fatigue states.

Long-Term Suppression of Growth: Sufficient data on the safety of long-term use of methylphenidate in children are not yet available. Although a causal relationship has not been established, suppression of growth (i.e., weight gain, and/or height) has been reported with the long-term use of stimulants in children. Therefore, patients requiring long-term therapy should be carefully monitored. Patients who are not growing or gaining weight as expected should have their treatment interrupted.

Psychosis: Clinical experience suggests that in psychotic patients, administration of methylphenidate may exacerbate symptoms of behavior disturbance and thought disorder.

Seizures: There is some clinical evidence that methylphenidate may lower the convulsive threshold in patients with prior history of seizures, in patients with prior EEG abnormalities in absence of seizures, and, very rarely, in absence of history of seizures and no prior EEG evidence of seizures. In the presence of seizures, the drug should be discontinued.

Hypertension and other Cardiovascular Conditions: Use cautiously in patients with hypertension. Blood pressure should be monitored at appropriate intervals in patients taking METADATE CD, especially patients with hypertension. Studies of methylphenidate have shown modest increases of resting pulse and systolic and diastolic blood pressure. Therefore, caution is indicated in treating patients whose underlying medical conditions might be compromised by increases in blood pressure or heart rate, e.g., those with pre-existing hypertension, heart failure, recent myocardial infarction, or hyperthyroidism.

Visual Disturbance: Symptoms of visual disturbances have been encountered in rare cases. Difficulties with accommodation and blurring of vision have been reported.

Use in Children Under Six Years of Age: METADATE® CD (methylphenidate HCl, USP) Extended-Release Capsules should not be used in children under six years, since safety and efficacy in this age group have not been established.

DRUG DEPENDENCE: METADATE CD should be given cautiously to patients with a history of drug dependence or alcoholism. Chronic abusive use can lead to marked tolerance and psychological dependence with varying degrees of abnormal behavior. Frank psychotic episodes can occur, especially with parenteral abuse. Careful supervision is required during withdrawal from

Continued on next page

Information on the Celltech Pharmaceuticals, Inc. products listed on these pages contains the full prescribing information from product circulars in use as of July 2004. For further information, please consult the package insert currently accompanying the product.

Metadate CD—Cont.

abusive use since severe depression may occur. Withdrawal following chronic therapeutic use may unmask symptoms of the underlying disorder that may require follow-up.

PRECAUTIONS

Hematologic Monitoring: Periodic CBC, differential, and platelet counts are advised during prolonged therapy.

Information for Patients: Patients should be instructed to take one dose in the morning before breakfast. The patients should be instructed that the capsule may be swallowed whole, or alternatively, the capsule may be opened and the capsule contents sprinkled onto a small amount (tablespoon) of applesauce and given immediately, and not stored for future use. The capsules and the capsule contents must not be crushed or chewed.

Patient information is printed along with this insert. To assure safe and effective use of METADATE CD, the information and instructions provided in the patient information section should be discussed with patients.

Drug Interactions: Because of possible effects on blood pressure, METADATE CD should be used cautiously with pressor agents.

Human pharmacologic studies have shown that methylphenidate may inhibit the metabolism of coumarin anticoagulants, anticonvulsants (e.g., phenobarbital, phenytoin, primidone), and some antidepressants (tricyclics and selective serotonin reuptake inhibitors). Downward dose adjustment of these drugs may be required when given concomitantly with methylphenidate. It may be necessary to adjust the dosage and monitor plasma drug concentrations (or, in the case of coumarin, coagulation times), when initiating or discontinuing concomitant methylphenidate.

Serious adverse events have been reported in concomitant use with clonidine, although no causality for the combination has been established. The safety of using methylphenidate in combination with clonidine or other centrally acting alpha-2 agonists has not been systematically evaluated.

Carcinogenesis, Mutagenesis, and Impairment of Fertility: In a lifetime carcinogenicity study carried out in B6C3F1 mice, methylphenidate caused an increase in hepatocellular adenomas and, in males only, an increase in hepatoblastomas, at a daily dose of approximately 60 mg/kg/day. This dose is approximately 30 times and 4 times the maximum recommended human dose of METADATE CD on a mg/kg and mg/m^2 basis, respectively. Hepatoblastoma is a relatively rare rodent malignant tumor type. There was no increase in total malignant hepatic tumors. The mouse strain used is sensitive to the development of hepatic tumors, and the significance of these results to humans is unknown.

Methylphenidate did not cause any increases in tumors in a lifetime carcinogenicity study carried out in F344 rats; the highest dose used was approximately 45 mg/kg/day, which is approximately 22 times and 5 times the maximum recommended human dose of METADATE CD on a mg/kg and mg/m^2 basis, respectively.

In a 24-week carcinogenicity study in the transgenic mouse strain p53+/−, which is sensitive to genotoxic carcinogens, there was no evidence of carcinogenicity. Male and female mice were fed diets containing the same concentration of methylphenidate as in the lifetime carcinogenicity study; the high-dose groups were exposed to 60 to 74 mg/kg/day of methylphenidate.

Methylphenidate was not mutagenic in the *in vitro* Ames reverse mutation assay or in the *in vitro* mouse lymphoma cell forward mutation assay. Sister chromatid exchanges and chromosome aberrations were increased, indicative of a weak clastogenic response, in an *in vitro* assay in cultured Chinese Hamster Ovary cells. Methylphenidate was negative *in vivo* in males and females in the mouse bone marrow micronucleus assay.

Methylphenidate did not impair fertility in male or female mice that were fed diets containing the drug in an 18-week Continuous Breeding study. The study was conducted at doses up to 160 mg/kg/day, approximately 80-fold and 8-fold the highest recommended human dose of METADATE CD on a mg/kg and mg/m^2 basis, respectively.

Pregnancy: Teratogenic Effects: Pregnancy Category C. Methylphenidate has been shown to have teratogenic effects in rabbits when given in doses of 200 mg/kg/day, which is approximately 100 times and 40 times the maximum recommended human dose on a mg/kg and mg/m^2 basis, respectively.

A reproduction study in rats revealed no evidence of teratogenicity at an oral dose of 58 mg/kg/day. However, this dose, which caused some maternal toxicity, resulted in decreased postnatal pup weights and survival when given to the dams from day one of gestation through the lactation period. This dose is approximately 30 fold and 6 fold the maximum recommended human dose of METADATE CD on a mg/kg and mg/m^2 basis, respectively.

There are no adequate and well-controlled studies in pregnant women. METADATE CD should be used during pregnancy only if the potential benefit justifies the potential risk to the fetus.

Nursing Mothers: It is not known whether methylphenidate is excreted in human milk. Because many drugs are excreted in human milk, caution should be exercised if METADATE CD is administered to a nursing woman.

Pediatric Use: The safety and efficacy of METADATE CD in children under 6 years old have not been established. Long-term effects of methylphenidate in children have not been well established (see WARNINGS).

ADVERSE REACTIONS

The premarketing development program for METADATE CD included exposures in a total of 228 participants in clinical trials (188 pediatric patients with ADHD, 40 healthy adult subjects). These participants received METADATE CD 20, 40, and/or 60 mg/day. The 188 patients (ages 6 to 15) were evaluated in one controlled clinical study, one controlled, crossover clinical study, and one uncontrolled clinical study. Safety data on all patients are included in the discussion that follows. Adverse reactions were assessed by collecting adverse events, results of physical examinations, vital signs, weights, laboratory analyses, and ECGs.

Adverse events during exposure were obtained primarily by general inquiry and recorded by clinical investigators using terminology of their own choosing. Consequently, it is not possible to provide a meaningful estimate of the proportion of individuals experiencing adverse events without first grouping similar types of events into a smaller number of standardized event categories. In the tables and listings that follow, COSTART terminology has been used to classify reported adverse events.

The stated frequencies of adverse events represent the proportion of individuals who experienced, at least once, a treatment-emergent adverse event of the type listed. An event was considered treatment emergent if it occurred for the first time or worsened while receiving therapy following baseline evaluation.

Adverse Findings in Clinical Trials with METADATE CD:

Adverse Events Associated with Discontinuation of Treatment: In the 3-week placebo-controlled, parallel-group trial, two METADATE CD-treated patients (1%) and no placebo-treated patients discontinued due to an adverse event (rash and pruritus; and headache, abdominal pain, and dizziness, respectively).

Adverse Events Occurring at an Incidence of 5% or more Among METADATE CD-Treated Patients: Table 1 enumerates, for a pool of the three studies in pediatric patients with ADHD, at METADATE CD doses of 20, 40, or 60 mg/day, the incidence of treatment-emergent adverse events. One study was a 3-week placebo-controlled, parallel-group trial, one study was a controlled, crossover trial, and the third study was an open titration trial. The table includes only those events that occurred in 5% or more of patients treated with METADATE CD where the incidence in patients treated with METADATE CD was greater than the incidence in placebo-treated patients.

The prescriber should be aware that these figures cannot be used to predict the incidence of adverse events in the course of usual medical practice where patient characteristics and other factors differ from those which prevailed in the clinical trials. Similarly, the cited frequencies cannot be compared with figures obtained from other clinical investigations involving different treatments, uses, and investigators. The cited figures, however, do provide the prescribing physician with some basis for estimating the relative contribution of drug and non-drug factors to the adverse event incidence rate in the population studied.

TABLE 1
Incidence of Treatment-Emergent Events[1] in a Pool of 3-4 Week Clinical Trials of METADATE CD

Body System	Preferred Term	METADATE CD (n=188)	Placebo (n=190)
General	Headache	12%	8%
	Abdominal pain (stomach ache)	7%	4%
Digestive System	Anorexia (loss of appetite)	9%	2%
Nervous System	Insomnia	5%	2%

[1]: Events, regardless of causality, for which the incidence for patients treated with METADATE CD was at least 5% and greater than the incidence among placebo-treated patients. Incidence has been rounded to the nearest whole number.

Adverse Events with Other Methylphenidate HCl Products: Nervousness and insomnia are the most common adverse reactions reported with other methylphenidate products. Other reactions include hypersensitivity (including skin rash, urticaria, fever, arthralgia, exfoliative dermatitis, erythema multiforme with histopathological findings of necrotizing vasculitis, and thrombocytopenic purpura); anorexia; nausea; dizziness; palpitations; headache; dyskinesia; drowsiness; blood pressure and pulse changes, both up and down; tachycardia; angina; cardiac arrhythmia; abdominal pain; weight loss during prolonged therapy. There have been rare reports of Tourette's Syndrome. Toxic psychosis has been reported. Although a definite causal relationship has not been established, the following have been reported in patients taking this drug: instances of abnormal liver function, ranging from transaminase elevation to hepatic coma; isolated cases of cerebral arteritis and/or occlusion; leukopenia and/or anemia; transient depressed mood; a few instances of scalp hair loss. Very rare reports of neuroleptic malignant syndrome (NMS) have been reported, and, in most of these, patients were concurrently receiving therapies associated with NMS. In a single report, a ten year old boy who had been taking methylphenidate for approximately 18 months experienced an NMS-like event within 45 minutes of ingesting his first dose of venlafaxine. It is uncertain whether this case represented a drug-drug interaction, a response to either drug alone, or some other cause.

In children, loss of appetite, abdominal pain, weight loss during prolonged therapy, insomnia and tachycardia may occur more frequently; however, any of the other adverse reactions listed above may also occur.

DRUG ABUSE AND DEPENDENCE

Controlled Substance Class: METADATE CD, like other methylphenidate products, is classified as a Schedule II controlled substance by federal regulation.

Abuse, Dependence, and Tolerance: See WARNINGS for boxed warning containing drug abuse and dependence information.

OVERDOSAGE

Signs and Symptoms: Signs and symptoms of acute methylphenidate overdosage, resulting principally from overstimulation of the CNS and from excessive sympathomimetic effects, may include the following: vomiting, agitation, tremors, hyperreflexia, muscle twitching, convulsions (may be followed by coma), euphoria, confusion, hallucinations, delirium, sweating, flushing, headache, hyperpyrexia, tachycardia, palpitations, cardiac arrhythmias, hypertension, mydriasis, and dryness of mucous membranes.

Recommended Treatment: Treatment consists of appropriate supportive measures. The patient must be protected against self-injury and against external stimuli that would aggravate overstimulation already present. Gastric contents may be evacuated by gastric lavage as indicated. Before performing gastric lavage, control agitation and seizures if present and protect the airway. Other measures to detoxify the gut include administration of activated charcoal and a cathartic. Intensive care must be provided to maintain adequate circulation and respiratory exchange; external cooling procedures may be required for hyperpyrexia.

Efficacy of peritoneal dialysis or extracorporeal hemodialysis for METADATE CD overdosage has not been established.

The prolonged release of methylphenidate from METADATE CD should be considered when treating patients with overdose.

Poison Control Center: As with the management of all overdosage, the possibility of multiple drug ingestion should be considered. The physician may wish to consider contacting a poison control center for up-to-date information on the management of overdosage with methylphenidate.

DOSAGE AND ADMINISTRATION

METADATE CD is administered once daily in the morning, before breakfast.

METADATE CD may be swallowed whole with the aid of liquids, or alternatively, the capsule may be opened and the capsule contents sprinkled onto a small amount (tablespoon) of applesauce and given immediately, and not stored for future use. Drinking some fluids, e.g. water, should follow the intake of the sprinkles with applesauce. The capsules and the capsule contents must not be crushed or chewed. (See PRECAUTIONS: Information for Patients.)

Dosage should be individualized according to the needs and responses of the patient.

Initial Treatment: The recommended starting dose of METADATE CD is 20 mg once daily. Dosage may be adjusted in weekly 10-20 mg increments to a maximum of 60 mg/day taken once daily in the morning, depending upon tolerability and degree of efficacy observed. Daily dosage above 60 mg is not recommended.

Maintenance/Extended Treatment: There is no body of evidence available from controlled trials to indicate how long the patient with ADHD should be treated with METADATE CD. It is generally agreed, however, that pharmacological treatment of ADHD may be needed for extended periods. Nevertheless, the physician who elects to use METADATE CD for extended periods in patients with ADHD should periodically re-evaluate the long-term usefulness of the drug for the individual patient with trials off medication to assess the patient's functioning without pharmacotherapy. Improvement may be sustained when the drug is either temporarily or permanently discontinued.

Dose Reduction and Discontinuation: If paradoxical aggravation of symptoms or other adverse events occur, the dosage should be reduced, or, if necessary, the drug should be discontinued.

If improvement is not observed after appropriate dosage adjustment over a one-month period, the drug should be discontinued.

HOW SUPPLIED

METADATE CD (methylphenidate HCl, USP) Extended-Release Capsules are available in three strengths:

10 mg, green/white capsules, imprinted with "CELLTECH 574" in white letters on the green cap, and "10 mg" in black letters on the white body of the capsule.

NDC 53014-574-07 Bottle of 100 Capsules

20 mg, blue/white capsules, imprinted with "CELLTECH 575" in white letters on the blue cap, and "20 mg" in black letters on the white body of the capsule.

NDC 53014-575-07 Bottle of 100 Capsules
NDC 53014-575-72 Carton of 100 Capsules, Unit Dose
NDC 53014-575-30 Dose Pack of 30 Capsules*

30 mg, reddish-brown/white capsules, imprinted with "CELLTECH 576" in white letters on the reddish-brown cap, and "30 mg" in black letters on the white body of the capsule.

NDC 53014-576-07 Bottle of 100 Capsules

*PHARMACIST: Dispense only in current dose pack.

Store at 25°C (77°F): excursions permitted to 15°-30°C (59°-86°F) [See USP Controlled Room Temperature].

Keep out of the reach of children.

Reference: American Psychiatric Association. *Diagnostic and Statistical Manual of Mental Disorders.* 4th ed. Washington D.C.: American Psychiatric Association 1994.

For more information call 1-888-METADATE (1-888-638-2328) or visit www.metadate-cd.com

Celltech Pharmaceuticals, Inc.
Rochester, NY 14623 USA
® Celltech Pharma Limited

Metadate® CD Extended-Release Capsules: US Patent No. 6,344,215.

Rev. 7/03 R312E

INFORMATION FOR PATIENTS TAKING METADATE® CD OR THEIR PARENTS OR CAREGIVERS

Once daily

METADATE® CD Ⓒ

(methylphenidate HCl, USP)

Extended-Release Capsules

This information is for patients or their parents or caregivers taking METADATE CD Capsules for the treatment of Attention Deficit Hyperactivity Disorder.

Please read this before you start taking METADATE CD. Remember, this information does not take the place of your doctor's instructions. If you have any questions about this information or about METADATE CD, talk to your doctor or pharmacist.

What is METADATE® CD?

METADATE CD is a once-a-day treatment for Attention Deficit Hyperactivity Disorder, or ADHD. METADATE CD contains the drug methylphenidate, a central nervous system stimulant that has been used to treat ADHD for more than 30 years. METADATE CD is taken by mouth, once each day in the morning, before breakfast.

What is Attention Deficit Hyperactivity Disorder?

ADHD has three main types of symptoms: inattention, hyperactivity, and impulsiveness. Symptoms of inattention include not paying attention, making careless mistakes, not listening, not finishing tasks, not following directions, and being easily distracted. Symptoms of hyperactivity and impulsiveness include fidgeting, talking excessively, running around at inappropriate times, and interrupting others. Some patients have more symptoms of hyperactivity and impulsiveness while others have more symptoms of inattentiveness. Some patients have all three types of symptoms. Many people have symptoms like these from time to time, but patients with ADHD have these symptoms more than others their age. Symptoms must be present for at least 6 months to be certain of the diagnosis.

How does METADATE® CD work?

The METADATE CD capsule dissolves right after you swallow it in the morning, giving you an initial dose of methylphenidate. The remaining drug is slowly released during the day to continue to help lessen the symptoms of ADHD. Methylphenidate, the active ingredient in METADATE CD, helps increase attention and decrease impulsiveness and hyperactivity in patients with ADHD.

Who should NOT take METADATE® CD?

You should NOT take METADATE CD if:

- You have significant anxiety, tension, or agitation since METADATE CD may make these conditions worse.
- You are allergic to methylphenidate or any of the other ingredients in METADATE CD.
- You have glaucoma, an eye disease.
- You have tics or Tourette's Syndrome, or a family history of Tourette's Syndrome.

Talk to your doctor if you believe any of these conditions apply to you.

How should I take METADATE® CD?

Do not chew or crush the capsules or the beads inside the capsule. Swallow the METADATE CD Capsules whole with the help of water or other liquids, such as milk or juice. Alternatively, the capsule may be opened and the capsule contents sprinkled onto a small amount (tablespoon) of applesauce and taken immediately (do not store for future use) without chewing. Take a drink of water after the sprinkles with applesauce have been swallowed.

Take METADATE CD once each day in the morning, before breakfast.

Take the dose prescribed by your doctor. Your doctor may adjust the amount of drug you take until it is right for you. From time to time, your doctor may interrupt your treatment to check your symptoms while you are not taking the drug.

What are the possible side effects of METADATE® CD?

In the clinical studies with patients using METADATE CD, the most common side effects were headache, stomach pain, sleeplessness, and decreased appetite. Other side effects seen with methylphenidate, the active ingredient in METADATE CD, include nausea, vomiting, dizziness, nervousness, tics, allergic reactions, increased blood pressure and psychosis (abnormal thinking or hallucinations).

This is not a complete list of possible side effects. Ask your doctor about other side effects. If you develop any side effect, talk to your doctor.

What must I discuss with my doctor before taking METADATE® CD (methylphenidate HCl, USP) Extended-Release Capsules?

Talk to your doctor ***before*** taking METADATE CD if you:

- Are being treated for depression or have symptoms of depression such as feelings of sadness, worthlessness, and hopelessness.
- Have motion tics (hard-to-control, repeated twitching of any parts of your body) or verbal tics (hard-to-control repeating of sounds or words).
- Have someone in your family with motion tics, verbal tics, or Tourette's Syndrome.
- Have abnormal thoughts or visions, hear abnormal sounds, or have been diagnosed with psychosis.
- Have had seizures (convulsions, epilepsy) or abnormal EEGs (electroencephalograms).
- Have high blood pressure.

Tell your doctor ***immediately*** if you develop any of the above conditions or symptoms while taking METADATE CD.

Can I take METADATE® CD with other medicines?

Tell your doctor about ***all*** medicines that you are taking or intend to take. Your doctor should decide whether you can take METADATE CD with other medicines. These include:

- Other medicines that a doctor has prescribed.
- All medicines that you buy yourself without a prescription.
- Any herbal remedies that you may be taking.

You should not take METADATE CD with monoamine oxidase (MAO) inhibitors.

While on METADATE CD, do not start taking a new medicine or herbal remedy before checking with your doctor.

METADATE CD may change the way your body reacts to certain medicines. These include medicines used to treat depression, prevent seizures, or prevent blood clots (commonly called "blood thinners"). Your doctor may need to change your dose of these medicines if you are taking them with METADATE CD.

Other Important Safety Information:

Abuse of methylphenidate can lead to dependence.

Tell your doctor if you have ever abused or been dependent on alcohol or drugs, or if you are now abusing or dependent on alcohol or drugs.

Before taking METADATE CD, tell your doctor if you are pregnant or plan on becoming pregnant. If you take methylphenidate, it may be in your breast milk. Tell your doctor if you are nursing a baby.

Tell your doctor if you have blurred vision when taking METADATE CD.

Slower growth (weight gain and/or height) has been reported with long-term use of methylphenidate in children. Your doctor will be carefully watching your height and weight. If you are not growing or gaining weight as your doctor expects, your doctor may stop your METADATE CD treatment.

Call your doctor ***immediately*** if you take more than the amount of METADATE CD prescribed by your doctor.

What else should I know about METADATE® CD?

METADATE CD has not been studied in children under 6 years of age.

METADATE CD may be a part of your overall treatment for ADHD. Your doctor may also recommend that you have counseling or other therapy.

As with all medicines, never share METADATE CD with anyone else and take only the number of METADATE CD Capsules prescribed by your doctor.

METADATE CD should be stored in a safe place at room temperature (between 59°-86°F).

Keep out of the reach of children.

For more information call 1-888-METADATE
(1-888-638-2328) or visit www.metadate-cd.com

Celltech Pharmaceuticals, Inc.
Rochester, NY 14623 USA
® Celltech Pharma Limited

Metadate® CD Extended-Release Capsules: US Patent No. 6,344,215.

Rev. 7/03 R312E

METADATE® ER TABLETS Ⓒ ℞

[mĕt ə dāte]

(methylphenidate hydrochloride extended-release tablets, USP)

℞ only R533A 6/02

DESCRIPTION

METADATE ER Tablets (methylphenidate hydrochloride extended-release tablets, USP) are a mild central nervous system (CNS) stimulant. METADATE ER is available as extended-release tablets of 10 and 20 mg for oral administration.

Methylphenidate hydrochloride is methyl α-phenyl-2-piperidineacetate hydrochloride, and its structural formula is: [See chemical structure at top of next column]

Methylphenidate hydrochloride is a white, odorless, fine crystalline powder. Its solutions are acid to litmus. It is freely soluble in water and in methanol, soluble in alcohol, and slightly soluble in chloroform and in acetone. Its chemical formula is $C_{14}H_{19}NO_2 \cdot HCl$, and its molecular weight is 269.77.

Inactive Ingredients: Cetyl alcohol, ethylcellulose, anhydrous lactose and magnesium stearate.

CLINICAL PHARMACOLOGY

METADATE ER is a mild central nervous system stimulant.

The mode of action in man is not completely understood, but methylphenidate presumably activates the brain stem arousal system and cortex to produce its stimulant effect.

There is neither specific evidence which clearly establishes the mechanism whereby methylphenidate produces its mental and behavioral effects in children, nor conclusive evidence regarding how these effects relate to the condition of the central nervous system.

METADATE ER in extended-release tablets is more slowly but as extensively absorbed as in the regular tablets. Bioavailability of METADATE 20 mg Extended-Release Tablets was compared to a sustained-release reference product and an immediate-release product. The extent of absorption for the three products was similar, and the rate of absorption of the two sustained-release products was not statistically different.

In another reported study with a brand of Methylphenidate HCl sustained-release, the time to peak rate in children was reported as 4.7 hours (1.3–8.2 hours) for the sustained-release tablet dosage form and 1.9 hours (0.3–4.4 hours) for immediate release tablets. An average of 67% of a sustained-release tablet dosage form was excreted in children compared to 86% in adults.

Based on rate of bioavailability ($AUC_{0\to\infty}$, T_{max}, and C_{max}), no significant statistical difference was found following single dose administration, in fasting and fed adults, of two METADATE 10 mg Extended-Release Tablets, or one methylphenidate hydrochloride, USP sustained-release 20 mg tablet. The administration of the extended-release methylphenidate HCl, USP, tablets with food, resulted in a greater C_{max} and $AUC_{0\to\infty}$, than when administered in a fasting condition.

Pharmacokinetic and statistical analyses for a multiple dose study demonstrated that 3 times daily administration of two METADATE 10 mg Extended-Release Tablets met the requirements for bioequivalence to one methylphenidate hydrochloride, USP sustained-release 20 mg tablet when administered every eight hours. Pharmacokinetic parameters (i.e., $AUC_{0\to\infty}$, T_{max}, C_{max}, C_{min}, and C_{av}) demonstrated achievement of steady state following 3 times daily administration of two METADATE 10 mg Extended-Release Tablets was confirmed.

In a clinical study involving adult subjects who received Extended-release (ER) tablets, plasma concentrations of methylphenidate hydrochloride's major metabolite appeared to be greater in females than in males. No gender differences were observed for methylphenidate hydrochloride's plasma concentration in the same subjects.

INDICATIONS AND USAGE

Attention Deficit Disorders, Narcolepsy: *Attention Deficit Disorders* (previously known as Minimal Brain Dysfunction in Children). Other terms being used to describe the behavioral syndrome below include: Hyperkinetic Child Syndrome, Minimal Brain Damage, Minimal Cerebral Dysfunction, Minor Cerebral Dysfunction.

METADATE ER is indicated as an integral part of a total treatment program which typically includes other remedial measures (psychological, educational, social) for a stabilizing effect in children with a behavioral syndrome characterized by the following group of developmentally inappropriate symptoms: moderate-to-severe distractibility, short attention span, hyperactivity, emotional lability, and impulsivity. The diagnosis of this syndrome should not be made with finality when these symptoms are only of comparatively recent origin. Nonlocalizing (soft) neurological signs, learning disability, and abnormal EEG may or may not be present, and a diagnosis of central nervous system dysfunction may or may not be warranted.

Special Diagnostic Considerations: Specific etiology of this syndrome is unknown, and there is no single diagnostic test. Adequate diagnosis requires the use not only of medical but of special psychological, educational, and social resources.

Characteristics commonly reported include: chronic history of short attention span, distractibility, emotional lability, impulsivity, and moderate-to-severe hyperactivity; minor neurological signs and abnormal EEG. Learning may or may not be impaired. The diagnosis must be based upon a complete history and evaluation of the child and not solely on the presence of one or more of these characteristics.

Continued on next page

Information on the Celltech Pharmaceuticals, Inc. products listed on these pages contains the full prescribing information from product circulars in use as of July 2004. For further information, please consult the package insert currently accompanying the product.

Metadate ER—Cont.

Drug treatment is not indicated for all children with this syndrome. Stimulants are not intended for use in the child who exhibits symptoms secondary to environmental factors and/or primary psychiatric disorders, including psychosis. Appropriate educational placement is essential and psychosocial intervention is generally necessary. When remedial measures alone are insufficient, the decision to prescribe stimulant medication will depend upon the physician's assessment of the chronicity and severity of the child's symptoms.

CONTRAINDICATIONS

Marked anxiety, tension and agitation are contraindications to METADATE ER, since the drug may aggravate these symptoms. METADATE ER is contraindicated also in patients known to be hypersensitive to the drug, in patients with glaucoma, and in patients with motor tics or with a family history or diagnosis of Tourette's syndrome.

METADATE ER is contraindicated during treatment with monoamine oxidase inhibitors, and also within a minimum of 14 days following discontinuation of a monoamine oxidase inhibitor (hypertensive crises may result).

WARNINGS

METADATE ER should not be used in children under six years, since safety and efficacy in this age group have not been established.

Sufficient data on safety and efficacy of long-term use of methylphenidate in children are not yet available. Although a causal relationship has not been established, suppression of growth (i.e. weight gain, and/or height) has been reported with the long-term use of stimulants in children. Therefore, patients requiring long-term therapy should be carefully monitored.

METADATE ER should not be used for severe depression of either exogenous or endogenous origin. Clinical experience suggests that in psychotic children, administration of methylphenidate may exacerbate symptoms of behavior disturbance and thought disorder.

METADATE ER should not be used for the prevention or treatment of normal fatigue states.

There is some clinical evidence that methylphenidate may lower the convulsive threshold in patients with prior history of seizures, with prior EEG abnormalities in absence of seizures, and, very rarely, in absence of history of seizures and no prior EEG evidence of seizures. Safe concomitant use of anticonvulsants and METADATE ER has not been established. In the presence of seizures, the drug should be discontinued.

Use cautiously in patients with hypertension. Blood pressure should be monitored at appropriate intervals in all patients taking METADATE ER, especially those with hypertension.

Symptoms of visual disturbances have been encountered in rare cases. Difficulties with accommodation and blurring of vision have been reported.

Drug Interactions: METADATE ER may decrease the hypotensive effect of guanethidine. Use cautiously with pressor agents.

Human pharmacologic studies have shown that methylphenidate may inhibit the metabolism of coumarin anticoagulants, anticonvulsants (phenobarbital, phenytoin, primidone), phenylbutazone, and tricyclic drugs (imipramine, clomipramine, desipramine). Downward dosage adjustments of these drugs may be required when given concomitantly with METADATE ER.

Serious adverse events have been reported in concomitant use with clonidine, although no causality for the combination has been established. The safety of using methylphenidate in combination with clonidine or other centrally acting alpha-2-agonists has not been systematically evaluated.

Usage in Pregnancy: Adequate animal reproduction studies to establish safe use of methylphenidate during pregnancy have not been conducted. Therefore, until more information is available, METADATE ER should not be prescribed for women of childbearing age unless, in the opinion of the physician, the potential benefits outweigh the possible risks.

> **Drug Dependence:** METADATE® ER Tablets (methylphenidate hydrochloride extended-release tablets, USP) should be given cautiously to emotionally unstable patients, such as those with a history of drug dependence or alcoholism, because such patients may increase dosage on their own initiative.
>
> Chronically abusive use can lead to marked tolerance and psychic dependence with varying degrees of abnormal behavior. Frank psychotic episodes can occur, especially with parenteral abuse. Careful supervision is required during drug withdrawal, since severe depression as well as the effects of chronic overactivity can be unmasked. Long-term follow-up may be required because of the patient's basic personality disturbances.

PRECAUTIONS

Patients with an element of agitation may react adversely; discontinue therapy if necessary.

Periodic CBC, differential, and platelet counts are advised during prolonged therapy.

Drug treatment is not indicated in all cases of this behavioral syndrome and should be considered only in light of the complete history and evaluation of the child. The decision to prescribe METADATE® ER Tablets (methylphenidate hydrochloride extended-release tablets, USP) should depend on the physician's assessment of the chronicity and severity of the child's symptoms and their appropriateness for his/her age. Prescription should not depend solely on the presence of one or more of the behavioral characteristics.

When these symptoms are associated with acute stress reactions, treatment with methylphenidate is usually not indicated.

Long-term effects of methylphenidate in children have not been well established.

Carcinogenesis, Mutagenesis, Impairment of Fertility: In a lifetime carcinogenicity study carried out in B6C3F1 mice, methylphenidate caused an increase in hepatocellular adenomas and, in males only, an increase in hepatoblastomas, at a daily dose of approximately 60 mg/kg/day. This dose is approximately 30 times and 2.5 times the maximum recommended human dose on a mg/kg and mg/m^2 basis respectively.

Hepatoblastoma is a relatively rare rodent malignant tumor type. There was no increase in total malignant hepatic tumors. The mouse strain used is sensitive to the development of hepatic tumors, and the significance of these results to humans is unknown.

Methylphenidate did not cause any increases in tumors in a lifetime carcinogenicity study carried out in F344 rats; the highest dose used was approximately 45 mg/kg/day, which is approximately 22 times and 4 times the maximum recommended human dose on a mg/kg and mg/m^2 basis, respectively.

Methylphenidate was not mutagenic in the *in vitro* Ames reverse mutation assay or in the *in vitro* mouse lymphoma cell forward mutation assay. Sister chromatid exchanges and chromosome aberrations were increased, indicative of a weak clastogenic response, in an *in vitro* assay in cultured Chinese Hamster Ovary (CHO) cells. The genotoxic potential of methylphenidate has not been evaluated in an *in vivo* assay.

ADVERSE REACTIONS

Nervousness and insomnia are the most common adverse reactions but are usually controlled by reducing dosage and omitting the drug in the afternoon or evening. Other reactions include hypersensitivity (including skin rash, urticaria, fever, arthralgia, exfoliative dermatitis, erythema multiforme with histopathological findings of necrotizing vasculitis, and thrombocytopenic purpura); anorexia; nausea; dizziness; palpitations; headache; dyskinesia; drowsiness; blood pressure and pulse changes, both up and down; tachycardia; angina; cardiac arrhythmia; abdominal pain; weight loss during prolonged therapy. There have been rare reports of Tourette's syndrome. Toxic psychosis has been reported. Although a definite causal relationship has not been established, the following have been reported in patients taking this drug: instances of abnormal liver function, ranging from transaminase elevation to hepatic coma; isolated cases of cerebral arteritis and/or occlusion; leukopenia and/or anemia; transient depressed mood; a few instances of scalp hair loss. Very rare reports of neuroleptic malignant syndrome (NMS) have been received, and, in most of these, patients were concurrently receiving therapies associated with NMS. In a single report, a ten year old boy who had been taking methylphenidate for approximately 18 months experienced an NMS-like event within 45 minutes of ingesting his first dose of venlafaxine. It is uncertain whether this case represented a drug-drug interaction, a response to either drug alone, or some other cause.

In children, loss of appetite, abdominal pain, weight loss during prolonged therapy, insomina, and tachycardia may occur more frequently; however, any of the other adverse reactions listed above may also occur.

OVERDOSAGE

Signs and symptoms of acute overdosage, resulting principally from overstimulation of the central nervous system and from excessive sympathomimetic effects, may include the following: vomiting, agitation, tremors, hyperreflexia, muscle twitching, convulsions (may be followed by coma), euphoria, confusion, hallucinations, delirium, sweating, flushing, headache, hyperpyrexia, tachycardia, palpitations, cardiac arrhythmias, hypertension, mydriasis, and dryness of mucous membranes.

Consult with a Certified Poison Control Center regarding treatment for up-to-date guidance and advice.

Treatment consists of appropriate supportive measures. The patient must be protected against self-injury and against external stimuli that would aggravate overstimulation already present. Gastric contents may be evacuated by gastric lavage. In the presence of severe intoxication, use a carefully titrated dosage of a *short-acting* barbiturate *before* performing gastric lavage.

Other measures to detoxify the gut include administration of activated charcoal and a cathartic.

Intensive care must be provided to maintain adequate circulation and respiratory exchange; external cooling procedures may be required for hyperpyrexia.

Efficacy of peritoneal dialysis or extracorporeal hemodialysis for methylphenidate overdosage has not been established.

DOSAGE AND ADMINISTRATION

Dosage should be individualized according to the needs and responses of the patient.

Adults: *Methylphenidate Hydrochloride, USP Immediate-Release Tablets:* Administer in divided doses 2 or 3 times daily, preferably 30 to 45 minutes before meals. Average dosage is 20 to 30 mg daily. Some patients may require 40 to 60 mg daily. In others, 10 to 15 mg daily will be adequate. Patients who are unable to sleep if medication is taken late in the day should take the last dose before 6 p.m.

Extended-Release Tablets: METADATE ER Tablets have a duration of action of approximately 8 hours. Therefore, the extended-release tablets may be used in place of the immediate-release tablets when the 8-hour dosage of METADATE ER Tablets corresponds to the titrated 8-hour dosage of the immediate-release tablets. METADATE ER Tablets must be swallowed whole and never crushed or chewed.

Children (6 years and over): Methylphenidate hydrochloride tablets should be initiated in small doses, with gradual weekly increments. Daily dosage above 60 mg is not recommended.

If improvement is not observed after appropriate dosage adjustment over a one-month period, the drug should be discontinued.

Methylphenidate Hydrochloride, USP Immediate-Release Tablets: Start with 5 mg twice daily (before breakfast and lunch) with gradual increments of 5 to 10 mg weekly.

Extended-Release Tablets: METADATE ER Tablets have a duration of action of approximately 8 hours. Therefore, the extended-release tablets may be used in place of the immediate-release tablets when the 8-hour dosage of METADATE ER Tablets corresponds to the titrated 8-hour dosage of the immediate-release tablets. METADATE ER Tablets must be swallowed whole and never crushed or chewed.

If paradoxical aggravation of symptoms or other adverse effects occur, reduce dosage, or, if necessary, discontinue the drug.

METADATE ER should be periodically discontinued to assess the child's condition. Improvement may be sustained when the drug is either temporarily or permanently discontinued.

Drug treatment should not and need not be indefinite and usually may be discontinued after puberty.

HOW SUPPLIED

METADATE ER Tablets (methylphenidate hydrochloride extended-release tablets, USP) are available as follows:

10 mg: Oval, white, uncoated, unscored, debossed "561 MD".
NDC 53014-593-07 Bottle of 100's

20 mg: Round, white, uncoated, unscored, debossed "562 MD".
NDC 53014-594-07 Bottle of 100's

NOTE: METADATE ER Tablets are color-additive free.

PHARMACIST: Dispense in a tight, light-resistant container as defined in the USP with a child-resistant closure. Store at controlled room temperature 15°–30°C (59°–86°F). [See USP.] Protect from moisture.

Celltech Pharmaceuticals, Inc.
Rochester, NY 14623 USA
®Celltech Pharma Limited.

Rev. 6/02
R533A

PEDIAPRED® ℞

(prednisolone sodium phosphate, USP)
Oral Solution
℞ Only

R529
Rev. 7/01

DESCRIPTION

PEDIAPRED (prednisolone sodium phosphate, USP) Oral Solution is a dye free, colorless to light straw colored, raspberry flavored solution. Each 5 mL (teaspoonful) of PEDIAPRED contains 6.7 mg prednisolone sodium phosphate (5 mg prednisolone base) in a palatable, aqueous vehicle.

PEDIAPRED also contains dibasic sodium phosphate, edetate disodium, methylparaben, purified water, sodium biphosphate, sorbitol, natural and artificial raspberry flavor.

Prednisolone sodium phosphate occurs as white or slightly yellow, friable granules or powder. It is freely soluble in water; soluble in methanol; slightly soluble in alcohol and in chloroform; and very slightly soluble in acetone and in dioxane. The chemical name of prednisolone sodium phosphate is pregna -1,4- diene-3,20-dione,11,17-dihydroxy -21-(phosphonooxy)-, disodium salt, (11β)-. The empirical formula is $C_{21}H_{27}Na_2O_8P$; the molecular weight is 484.39. Its chemical structure is:

Pharmacological Category: Glucocorticoid

CLINICAL PHARMACOLOGY

Naturally occurring glucocorticoids (hydrocortisone), which also have salt-retaining properties, are used as replacement therapy in adrenocortical deficiency states. Their synthetic analogs are primarily used for their potent anti-inflammatory effects in disorders of many organ systems.

Prednisolone is a synthetic adrenocortical steroid drug with predominantly glucocorticoid properties. Some of these properties reproduce the physiological actions of endogenous glucocorticosteroids, but others do not necessarily reflect any of the adrenal hormones' normal functions; they are seen only after administration of large therapeutic doses of the drug. The pharmacological effects of prednisolone which are due to its glucocorticoid properties include: promotion of gluconeogenesis; increased deposition of glycogen in the liver; inhibition of the utilization of glucose; anti-insulin activity; increased catabolism of protein; increased lipolysis; stimulation of fat synthesis and storage; increased glomerular filtration rate and resulting increase in urinary excretion of urate (creatinine excretion remains unchanged); and increased calcium excretion.

Depressed production of eosinophils and lymphocytes occurs, but erythropoiesis and production of polymorphonuclear leukocytes are stimulated. Inflammatory processes (edema, fibrin deposition, capillary dilatation, migration of leukocytes and phagocytosis) and the later stages of wound healing (capillary proliferation, deposition of collagen, cicatrization) are inhibited.

Prednisolone can stimulate secretion of various components of gastric juice. Suppression of the production of corticotropin may lead to suppression of endogenous corticosteroids. Prednisolone has slight mineralocorticoid activity, whereby entry of sodium into cells and loss of intracellular potassium is stimulated. This is particularly evident in the kidney, where rapid ion exchange leads to sodium retention and hypertension.

Prednisolone is rapidly and well absorbed from the gastrointestinal tract following oral administration. PEDIAPRED Oral Solution produces a 14% higher peak plasma level of prednisolone which occurs 20% faster than that seen with tablets. Prednisolone is 70–90% protein-bound in the plasma and it is eliminated from the plasma with a half-life of 2 to 4 hours. It is metabolized mainly in the liver and excreted in the urine as sulfate and glucuronide conjugates.

INDICATIONS AND USAGE

PEDIAPRED Oral Solution is indicated in the following conditions:

1. ***Endocrine Disorders***
Primary or secondary adrenocortical insufficiency (hydrocortisone or cortisone is the first choice; synthetic analogs may be used in conjunction with mineralocorticoids where applicable; in infancy mineralocorticoid supplementation is of particular importance); congenital adrenal hyperplasia; hypercalcemia associated with cancer; nonsuppurative thyroiditis.
2. ***Rheumatic Disorders***
As adjunctive therapy for short term administration (to tide the patient over an acute episode or exacerbation) in: psoriatic arthritis; rheumatoid arthritis, including juvenile rheumatoid arthritis (selected cases may require low dose maintenance therapy); ankylosing spondylitis; acute and subacute bursitis; acute nonspecific tenosynovitis; acute gouty arthritis; epicondylitis. For the treatment of systemic lupus erythematosus, dermatomyositis (polymyositis), polymyalgia rheumatica, Sjogren's syndrome, relapsing polychondritis, and certain cases of vasculitis.
3. ***Dermatologic Diseases***
Pemphigus; bullous dermatitis herpetiformis; severe erythema multiforme (Stevens-Johnson syndrome); exfoliative erythroderma; mycosis fungoides.
4. ***Allergic States***
Control of severe or incapacitating allergic conditions intractable to adequate trials of conventional treatment in adult and pediatric populations with: seasonal or perennial allergic rhinitis; asthma; contact dermatitis; atopic dermatitis; serum sickness; drug hypersensitivity reactions.
5. ***Ophthalmic Diseases***
Uveitis and ocular inflammatory conditions unresponsive to topical corticosteroids; temporal arteritis; sympathetic ophthalmia.
6. ***Respiratory Diseases***
Symptomatic sarcoidosis; idiopathic eosinophilic pneumonias; fulminating or disseminated pulmonary tuberculosis when used concurrently with appropriate antituberculous chemotherapy; asthma (as distinct from allergic asthma listed above under "Allergic States"), hypersensitivity pneumonitis, idiopathic pulmonary fibrosis, acute exacerbations of chronic obstructive pulmonary disease (COPD), and Pneumocystis carinii pneumonia (PCP) associated with hypoxemia occurring in an HIV (+) individual who is also under treatment with appropriate anti-PCP antibiotics. Studies support the efficacy of systemic corticosteroids for the treatment of these conditions: allergic bronchopulmonary aspergillosis, idiopathic bronchiolitis obliterans with organizing pneumonia.
7. ***Hematologic Disorders***
Idiopathic thrombocytopenic purpura in adults; selected cases of secondary thrombocytopenia; acquired (autoimmune) hemolytic anemia; pure red cell aplasia; Diamond-Blackfan anemia.
8. ***Neoplastic Diseases***
For the treatment of acute leukemia and aggressive lymphomas in adults and children.
9. ***Edematous States***
To induce diuresis or remission of proteinuria in nephrotic syndrome in adults with lupus erythematosus and in adults and pediatric populations, with idiopathic nephrotic syndrome, without uremia.
10. ***Gastrointestinal Diseases***
To tide the patient over a critical period of the disease in: ulcerative colitis; regional enteritis.
11. ***Nervous System***
Acute exacerbations of multiple sclerosis.
12. ***Miscellaneous***
Tuberculous meningitis with subarachnoid block or impending block, tuberculosis with enlarged mediastinal lymph nodes causing respiratory difficulty, and tuberculosis with pleural or pericardial effusion (appropriate antituberculous chemotherapy must be used concurrently when treating any tuberculosis complications); Trichinosis with neurologic or myocardial involvement; acute or chronic solid organ rejection (with or without other agents).

CONTRAINDICATIONS

Systemic fungal infections.
Hypersensitivity to the drug or any of its components.

WARNINGS

General: In patients on corticosteroid therapy subjected to unusual stress, increased dosage of rapidly acting corticosteroids before, during and after the stressful situation is indicated.

Endocrine: Corticosteroids can produce reversible hypothalamic-pituitary adrenal (HPA) axis suppression with the potential for glucocorticosteroid insufficiency after withdrawal of treatment.

Metabolic clearance of corticosteroids is decreased in hypothyroid patients and increased in hyperthyroid patients. Changes in thyroid status of the patient may necessitate adjustment in dosage.

Infections (General): Persons who are on drugs which suppress the immune system are more susceptible to infections than healthy individuals. There may be decreased resistance and inability to localize infection when corticosteroids are used. Infection with any pathogen including viral, bacterial, fungal, protozoan or helminthic infection, in any location of the body, may be associated with the use of corticosteroids alone or in combination with other immunosuppressive agents that affect humoral or cellular immunity, or neutrophil function. These infections may be mild to severe, and, with increasing doses of corticosteroids, the rate of occurrence of infectious complications increases. Corticosteroids may also mask some signs of infection after it has already started.

Viral Infections: Chicken pox and measles, for example, can have a more serious or even fatal course in non-immune children or adults on corticosteroids. In such children or adults who have not had these diseases, particular care should be taken to avoid exposure. How the dose, route and duration of corticosteroid administration affect the risk of developing a disseminated infection is not known. The contribution of the underlying disease and/or prior corticosteroid treatment to the risk is also not known. If exposed to chicken pox, prophylaxis with varicella zoster immune globulin (VZIG) may be indicated. If exposed to measles, prophylaxis with immunoglobulin (IG) may be indicated. (See the respective package inserts for complete VZIG and IG prescribing information). If chicken pox develops, treatment with antiviral agents should be considered.

Special Pathogens: Latent disease may be activated or there may be an exacerbation of intercurrent infections due to pathogens, including those caused by Candida, Mycobacterium, Ameba, Toxoplasma, Pneumocystis, Cryptococus, Nocardia, etc.

Corticosteroids may activate latent amebiasis. Therefore, it is recommended that latent or active amebiasis be ruled out before initiating corticosteroid therapy in any patient who has spent time in the tropics or in any patient with unexplained diarrhea.

Similarly, corticosteroids should be used with great care in patients with known or suspected Strongyloides (threadworm) infestation. In such patients, corticosteroid-induced immunosuppression may lead to Strongyloides hyperinfection and dissemination with widespread larval migration, often accompanied by severe enterocolitis and potentially fatal gram-negative septicemia.

Corticosteroids should not be used in cerebral malaria.

Tuberculosis: The use of prednisolone in active tuberculosis should be restricted to those cases of fulminating or disseminated tuberculosis in which the corticosteroid is used for the management of the disease in conjunction with an appropriate antituberculous regimen.

If corticosteroids are indicated in patients with latent tuberculosis or tuberculin reactivity, close observation is necessary as reactivation of the disease may occur. During prolonged corticosteroid therapy these patients should receive chemoprophylaxis.

Vaccination: **Administration of live or live, attenuated vaccines is contraindicated in patients receiving immunosuppressive doses of corticosteroids. Killed or inactivated vaccines may be administered, however, the response to such vaccines can not be predicted.** Immunization procedures may be undertaken in patients who are receiving corticosteroids as replacement therapy, e.g., for Addison's disease.

Ophthalmic: Use of corticosteroids may produce posterior subcapsular cataracts, glaucoma with possible damage to the optic nerves, and may enhance the establishment of secondary ocular infections due to bacteria, fungi, or viruses. The use of oral corticosteroids is not recommended in the treatment of optic neuritis and may led to an increase in the risk of new episodes. Corticosteroids should not be used in active ocular herpes simplex.

Cardio-renal: Average and large doses of hydrocortisone or cortisone can cause elevation of blood pressure, salt and water retention, and increased excretion of potassium. These effects are less likely to occur with the synthetic derivatives except when used in large doses. Dietary salt restriction and potassium supplementation may be necessary. All corticosteroids increase calcium excretion.

PRECAUTIONS

General: The lowest possible dose of corticosteroid should be used to control the condition under treatment, and when reduction in dosage is possible, the reduction should be gradual.

Since complications of treatment with glucocorticoids are dependent on the size of the dose and the duration of treatment, a risk/benefit decision must be made in each individual case as to dose and duration of treatment and as to whether daily or intermittent therapy should be used.

There is an enhanced effect of corticosteroids in patients with hypothyroidism and in those with cirrhosis.

Kaposi's sarcoma has been reported to occur in patients receiving corticosteroid therapy, most often for chronic conditions. Discontinuation of corticosteroids may result in clinical improvement.

Endocrine: Drug-induced secondary adrenocortical insufficiency may be minimized by gradual reduction of dosage. This type of relative insufficiency may persist for months after discontinuation of therapy; therefore, in any situation of stress occurring during that period, hormone therapy should be reinstituted. Since mineralocorticoid secretion may be impaired, salt and/or a mineralocorticoid should be administered concurrently.

Ophthalmic: Intraocular pressure may become elevated in some individuals. If steroid therapy is continued for more than 6 weeks, intraocular pressure should be monitored.

Neuro-psychiatric: Although controlled clinical trials have shown corticosteroids to be effective in speeding the resolution of acute exacerbations of multiple sclerosis, they do not show that they affect the ultimate outcome or natural history of the disease. The studies do show that relatively high doses of corticosteroids are necessary to demonstrate a significant effect. (See DOSAGE AND ADMINSTRATION).

An acute myopathy has been observed with the use of high doses of corticosteroids, most often occurring in patients with disorders of neuromuscular transmission (e.g., myasthenia gravis), or in patients receiving concomitant therapy with neuromuscular blocking drugs (e.g., pancuronium). This acute myopathy is generalized, may involve ocular and respiratory muscles, and may result in quadriparesis. Elevation of creatinine kinase may occur. Clinical improvement or recovery after stopping corticosteroids may require weeks to years.

Psychic derangements may appear when corticosteroids are used, ranging from euphoria, insomnia, mood swings, personality changes, and severe depression, to frank psychotic manifestations. Also, existing emotional instability or psychotic tendencies may be aggravated by corticosteroids.

Gastrointestinal: Steroids should be used with caution in nonspecific ulcerative colitis, if there is a probability of impending perforation, abscess or other pyogenic infection; diverticulitis; fresh intestinal anastomoses; active or latent peptic ulcer.

Signs of peritoneal irritation following gastrointestinal perforation in patients receiving corticosteroids may be minimal or absent.

Cardio-renal: As sodium retention with resultant edema and potassium loss may occur in patients receiving corticosteroids, these agents should be used with caution in patients with hypertension, congestive heart failure, or renal insufficiency.

Musculoskeletal: Corticosteroids decrease bone formation and increase bone resorption both through their effect on calcium regulation (i.e. decreasing absorption and increasing excretion) and inhibition of osteoblast function. This, together with a decrease in the protein matrix of the bone secondary to an increase in protein catabolism, and reduced sex hormone production, may lead to inhibition of bone growth in children and adolescents and the development of osteoporosis at any age. Special consideration should be given to patients at increased risk of osteoporosis (i.e., postmenopausal women) before initiating corticosteroid therapy.

Information for Patients: Patients should be warned not to discontinue the use of PEDIAPRED® (prednisolone sodium phosphate, USP) Oral Solution abruptly or without medical supervision, to advise any medical attendants that they are

Continued on next page

Information on the Celltech Pharmaceuticals, Inc. products listed on these pages contains the full prescribing information from product circulars in use as of July 2004. For further information, please consult the package insert currently accompanying the product.

Pediapred—Cont.

taking PEDIAPRED and to seek medical advice at once should they develop fever or other signs of infection.

Persons who are on immunosuppressant doses of corticosteroids should be warned to avoid exposure to chicken pox or measles. Patients should also be advised that if they are exposed, medical advice should be sought without delay.

Drug Interactions: Drugs such as barbiturates, phenytoin, ephedrine, and rifampin, which induce hepatic microsomal drug metabolizing enzyme activity may enhance metabolism of prednisolone and require that the dosage of PEDIAPRED be increased.

Increased activity of both cyclosporin and corticosteroids may occur when the two are used concurrently. Convulsions have been reported with this concurrent use.

Estrogens may decrease the hepatic metabolism of certain corticosteroids thereby increasing their effect.

Ketoconazole has been reported to decrease the metabolism of certain corticosteroids by up to 60% leading to an increased risk of corticosteroid side effects.

Coadministration of corticosteroids and warfarin usually results in inhibition of response to warfarin, although there have been some conflicting reports. Therefore, coagulation indices should be monitored frequently to maintain the desired anticoagulant effect.

Concomitant use of aspirin (or other non-steroidal anti-inflammatory agents) and corticosteroids increases the risk of gastrointestinal side effects. Aspirin should be used cautiously in conjunction with corticosteroids in hypoprothrombinemia. The clearance of salicylates may be increased with concurrent use of corticosteroids.

When corticosteroids are administered concomitantly with potassium-depleting agents (i.e., diuretics, amphotericin-B), patients should be observed closely for development of hypokalemia. Patients on digitalis glycosides may be at increased risk of arrhythmias due to hypokalemia.

Concomitant use of anticholinesterase agents and corticosteroids may produce severe weakness in patients with myasthenia gravis. If possible, anticholinesterase agents should be withdrawn at least 24 hours before initiating corticosteroid therapy.

Due to inhibition of antibody response, patients on prolonged corticosteroid therapy may exhibit a diminished response to toxoids and live or inactivated vaccines. Corticosteroids may also potentiate the replication of some organisms contained in live attenuated vaccines. If possible, routine administration of vaccines or toxoids should be deferred until corticosteroid therapy is discontinued.

Because corticosteroids may increase blood glucose concentrations, dosage adjustments of antidiabetic agents may be required.

Corticosteroids may suppress reactions to skin tests.

***Pregnancy:* Teratogenic Effects: Pregnancy Category C.** Prednisolone has been shown to be teratogenic in many species when given in doses equivalent to the human dose. Animal studies in which prednisolone has been given to pregnant mice, rats, and rabbits have yielded an increased incidence of cleft palate in the offspring. There are no adequate and well controlled studies in pregnant women. PEDIAPRED should be used during pregnancy only if the potential benefit justifies the potential risk to the fetus. Infants born to mothers who have received corticosteroids during pregnancy should be carefully observed for signs of hypoadrenalism.

Nursing Mothers: Systemically administered corticosteroids appear in human milk and could suppress growth, interfere with endogenous corticosteroid production, or cause other untoward effects. Caution should be exercised when PEDIAPRED is administered to a nursing woman.

Pediatric Use: The efficacy and safety of prednisolone in the pediatric population are based on the well-established course of effect of corticosteroids which is similar in pediatric and adult populations. Published studies provide evidence of efficacy and safety in pediatric patients for the treatment of nephrotic syndrome (>2 years of age), and aggressive lymphomas and leukemias (> 1 month of age). However, some of these conclusions and other indications for pediatric use of corticosteroid, e.g., severe asthma and wheezing, are based on adequate and well-controlled trials conducted in adults, on the premises that the course of the diseases and their pathophysiology are considered to be substantially similar in both populations.

The adverse effects of prednisolone in pediatric patients are similar to those in adults (see ADVERSE REACTIONS). Like adults, pediatric patients should be carefully observed with frequent measurements of blood pressure, weight, height, intraocular pressure, and clinical evaluation for the presence of infection, psychosocial disturbances, thromboembolism, peptic ulcers, cataracts, and osteoporosis. Children who are treated with corticosteroids by any route, including systemically administered corticosteroids, may experience a decrease in their growth velocity. This negative impact of corticosteroids on growth has been observed at low systemic doses and in the absence of laboratory evidence of HPA axis suppression (i.e., cosyntropin stimulation and basal cortisol plasma levels). Growth velocity may therefore be a more sensitive indicator of systemic corticosteroid exposure in children than some commonly used tests of HPA axis function. The linear growth of children treated with corticosteroids by any route should be monitored, and the potential growth effects of prolonged treatment should be weighed against clinical benefits obtained and the availability of other treatment alternatives. In order to minimize the potential growth effects of corticosteroids, children should be titrated to the lowest effective dose.

ADVERSE REACTIONS

(listed alphabetically under each subsection): Fluid and Electrolyte Disturbances: Congestive heart failure in susceptible patients; fluid retention; hypertension; hypokalemic alkalosis; potassium loss; sodium retention.

Cardiovascular: Hypertrophic cardiomyopathy in premature infants.

Musculoskeletal: Aseptic necrosis of femoral and humeral heads; loss of muscle mass; muscle weakness; osteoporosis; pathologic fracture of long bones; steroid myopathy; tendon rupture; vertebral compression fractures.

Gastrointestinal: Abdominal distention; elevation in serum liver enzyme levels (usually reversible upon discontinuation); pancreatitis; peptic ulcer with possible perforation and hemorrhage; ulcerative esophagitis.

Dermatologic: Facial erythema; increased sweating; impaired wound healing; may suppress reactions to skin tests; petechiae and ecchymoses; thin fragile skin; urticaria; edema.

Metabolic: Negative nitrogen balance due to protein catabolism.

Neurological: Convulsions; headache; increased intracranial pressure with papilledema (pseudotumor cerebri) usually following discontinuation of treatment; psychic disorders; vertigo.

Endocrine: Decreased carbohydrate tolerance; development of cushingoid state; hirsutism; increased requirements for insulin or oral hypoglycemic agents in diabetic patients; manifestations of latent diabetes mellitus; menstrual irregularities; secondary adrenocortical and pituitary unresponsiveness, particularly in times of stress, as in trauma, surgery or illness; suppression of growth in children.

Ophthalmic: Exophthalmos; glaucoma; increased intraocular pressure; posterior subcapsular cataracts.

Other: Increased appetite; malaise; nausea; weight gain.

OVERDOSAGE

The effects of accidental ingestion of large quantities of prednisolone over a very short period of time have not been reported, but prolonged use of the drug can produce mental symptoms, moon face, abnormal fat deposits, fluid retention, excessive appetite, weight gain, hypertrichosis, acne, striae, ecchymosis, increased sweating, pigmentation, dry scaly skin, thinning scalp hair, increased blood pressure, tachycardia, thrombophlebitis, decreased resistance to infection, negative nitrogen balance with delayed bone and wound healing, headache, weakness, menstrual disorders, accentuated menopausal symptoms, neuropathy, fractures, osteoporosis, peptic ulcer, decreased glucose tolerance, hypokalemia, and adrenal insufficiency. Hepatomegaly and abdominal distention have been observed in children.

Treatment of acute overdosage is by immediate gastric lavage or emesis followed by supportive and symptomatic therapy. For chronic overdosage in the face of severe disease requiring continuous steroid therapy the dosage of prednisolone may be reduced only temporarily, or alternate day treatment may be introduced.

DOSAGE AND ADMINISTRATION

The initial dosage of PEDIAPRED may vary from 5 mL to 60 mL (5 to 60 mg prednisolone base) per day depending on the specific disease entity being treated. In situations of less severity, lower doses will generally suffice while in selected patients higher initial doses may be required. The initial dosage should be maintained or adjusted until a satisfactory response is noted. If after a reasonable period of time, there is a lack of satisfactory clinical response, PEDIAPRED should be discontinued and the patient placed on other appropriate therapy. **IT SHOULD BE EMPHASIZED THAT DOSAGE REQUIREMENTS ARE VARIABLE AND MUST BE INDIVIDUALIZED ON THE BASIS OF THE DISEASE UNDER TREATMENT AND THE RESPONSE OF THE PATIENT.** After a favorable response is noted, the proper maintenance dosage should be determined by decreasing the initial drug dosage in small decrements at appropriate time intervals until the lowest dosage which will maintain an adequate clinical response is reached. It should be kept in mind that constant monitoring is needed in regard to drug dosage. Included in the situations which may make dosage adjustments necessary are changes in clinical status secondary to remissions or exacerbations in the disease process, the patient's individual drug responsiveness, and the effect of patient exposure to stressful situations not directly related to the disease entity under treatment; in this latter situation it may be necessary to increase the dosage of PEDIAPRED for a period of time consistent with the patient's condition. If after long term therapy the drug is to be stopped, it is recommended that it be withdrawn gradually rather than abruptly.

In the treatment of acute exacerbations of multiple sclerosis, daily doses of 200 mg of prednisolone for a week followed by 80 mg every other day or 4 to 8 mg dexamethasone every other day for one month have been shown to be effective.

In pediatric patients, the initial dose of PEDIAPRED may vary depending on the specific disease entity being treated. The range of initial doses is 0.14 to 2 mg/kg/day in three or four divided doses (4 to 60 mg/m^{2}bsa/day).

The standard regimen used to treat nephrotic syndrome in pediatric patients is 60 mg/m^2/day given in three divided doses for 4 weeks, followed by 4 weeks of single dose alternate-day therapy at 40 mg/m^2/day.

The National Heart, Lung, and Blood Institute (NHLBI) recommended dosing for systemic prednisone, prednisolone or methylprednisolone in children whose asthma is uncontrolled by inhaled corticosteroids and long-acting bronchodilators is 1–2 mg/kg/day in single or divided doses. It is further recommended that short course, or "burst" therapy, be continued until a child achieves a peak expiratory flow rate of 80% of his or her personal best or symptoms resolve. This usually requires 3 to 10 days of treatment, although it can take longer. There is no evidence that tapering the dose after improvement will prevent a relapse.

For the purpose of comparison, the following is the equivalent milligram dosage of the various glucocorticoids:

Cortisone, 25	Triamcinolone, 4
Hydrocortisone, 20	Paramethasone, 2
Prednisolone, 5	Betamethasone, 0.75
Prednisone, 5	Dexamethasone, 0.75
Methylprednisolone, 4	

These dose relationships apply only to oral or intravenous administration of these compounds. When these substances or their derivatives are injected intramuscularly or into joint spaces, their relative properties may be greatly altered.

HOW SUPPLIED

PEDIAPRED (prednisolone sodium phosphate, USP) Oral Solution is a colorless to light straw colored solution containing 6.7 mg prednisolone sodium phosphate (5 mg prednisolone base) per 5 mL (teaspoonful).

NDC 53014-250-01 120 mL bottle

Store at 4°–25°C (39°–77°F). May be refrigerated. Keep tightly closed and out of the reach of children.

Celltech Pharmaceuticals, Inc.
Rochester, NY 14623 USA

SEMPREX®-D CAPSULES ℞

[*sĕm-prĕx*]
(acrivastine and pseudoephedrine hydrochloride)
℞ only

R532B
Rev. 4/04
000281

DESCRIPTION

SEMPREX-D Capsules (acrivastine and pseudoephedrine hydrochloride) are a fixed combination product formulated for oral administration. Acrivastine is an antihistamine and pseudoephedrine is a decongestant. Each capsule contains 8 mg acrivastine and 60 mg pseudoephedrine hydrochloride and the inactive ingredients: lactose, magnesium stearate and sodium starch glycolate. The green and white capsule shell consists of gelatin, D&C Yellow No. 10, FD&C Green No. 3, and titanium dioxide. The yellow band around the capsule consists of gelatin and D&C Yellow No. 10. The capsules may contain one or more parabens and are printed with edible black and white inks.

The chemical name of acrivastine is (*E,E*)-3-[6-[1-(4-methylphenyl)-3-(1-pyrrolidinyl)-1-propenyl]-2-pyridinyl]-2-propenoic acid; the molecular formula is $C_{22}H_{24}N_2O_2$. As an analog of triprolidine hydrochloride, acrivastine is classified as an alkylamine antihistamine. Acrivastine is an odorless, white to pale cream crystalline powder that is soluble in chloroform and alcohol and slightly soluble in water.

The chemical name of pseudoephedrine hydrochloride is [*S*-(*R**,*R**)]-α-[1-(methylamino)ethyl]benzenemethanol hydrochloride; the molecular formula is $C_{10}H_{15}NO \cdot HCl$. Pseudoephedrine is one of the naturally occurring dextrorotatory diastereoisomers of ephedrine and is classified as an indirect sympathomimetic amine. Pseudoephedrine hydrochloride occurs as odorless, fine white to off-white crystals or powder; the drug is soluble in water, alcohol and chloroform.

Structural formulae for the active ingredients of SEMPREX-D Capsules are as follows:

(a) Acrivastine
(Molecular Weight = 348.44)

[See chemical structure at top of next column]

(b) Pseudoephedrine hydrochloride
(Molecular Weight = 201.70)

CLINICAL PHARMACOLOGY

Acrivastine, a structural analog of triprolidine hydrochloride, exhibits H_1-antihistaminic activity in isolated tissues,

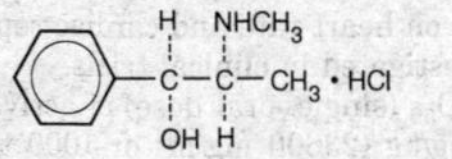

animals, and humans, and has sedative effects in humans (see PRECAUTIONS). The propionic acid derivative of acrivastine is a metabolite in several animal species (as well as in man) and also exhibits H_1-antihistaminic activity.
Pseudoephedrine hydrochloride is an indirect sympathomimetic agent; that is, it releases norepinephrine from adrenergic nerves.
In vitro tests and *in vivo* studies in animals of acrivastine and pseudoephedrine in combination failed to demonstrate evidence of any beneficial or deleterious pharmacologic interaction between the two agents.

Pharmacokinetics and Metabolism
Acrivastine was absorbed rapidly from the combination capsule following oral administration and was as bioavailable as a solution of acrivastine. After administration of SEMPREX-D Capsules, maximum plasma acrivastine concentrations were achieved at 1.14 ± 0.23 hours. A mass balance study in 7 healthy volunteers showed that acrivastine is primarily eliminated by the kidneys. Over a 72-hour collection period, about 84% of the administered total radioactivity was recovered in urine and about 13% in feces, for a combined recovery of about 97%. Further, 67% of the administered radioactive dose was recovered in urine as the unchanged drug, 11% as the propionic acid metabolite, and 6% as other unknown metabolites.
Acrivastine exhibits linear kinetics over dosages ranging from 2 to 32 mg t.i.d. The mean ± SD terminal half-life for acrivastine was 1.9 ± 0.3 hours following single oral doses and increased to 3.5 ± 1.9 hours at steady state. The terminal half-life for the propionic acid metabolite was 3.8 ± 1.4 hours. Because of the short half-lives of both acrivastine and its metabolites, accumulation in the plasma following multiple dosing is not expected.
The steady-state maximum acrivastine plasma concentration was 227 ± 47 ng/mL. The oral clearance, and apparent volume of distribution were 2.9 ± 0.7 mL/min/kg and 0.46 ± 0.05 L/kg, respectively, following a single oral dose; oral clearance did not change at steady state (2.86 ± 0.75 mL/min/kg). The apparent volume of distribution increased to 0.82 ± 0.6 L/kg to parallel the increase in the elimination half-life of the drug.
Acrivastine binding to human plasma proteins was 50 ± 2.0% and was concentration-independent over the range of 5 to 1000 ng/mL. The main binding protein was serum albumin although the drug was slightly bound to α-1-acid glycoprotein. No displacement interaction was observed between acrivastine and either phenytoin or theophylline. The binding of acrivastine was not affected by the presence of pseudoephedrine.
Pseudoephedrine hydrochloride was also rapidly absorbed from the combination capsule, and the capsule was as bioavailable as a solution of pseudoephedrine. Steady state maximum plasma concentration for pseudoephedrine was 498 ± 129 ng/mL. The terminal half-life, oral clearance and apparent volume of distribution were 6.2 ± 1.8 hours, 5.9 ± 1.7 mL/min/kg, and 3.0 ± 0.4 L/kg, respectively. Elimination of pseudoephedrine is primarily through the renal route as 55 to 75% of an administered dose appears unchanged in the urine. Pseudoephedrine elimination, however, is highly dependent upon urine pH; the plasma half-life decreased to about 4 hours at pH 5 and increased to 13 hours at pH 8.
Pseudoephedrine did not bind to human plasma proteins over the concentration range of 50 to 2000 ng/mL.
Acrivastine and pseudoephedrine do not influence the pharmacokinetics of the other drug when administered concomitantly.

Special Populations
A single dose pharmacokinetic study showed that the elimination half-lives of acrivastine, the propionic acid metabolite of acrivastine, and pseudoephedrine were prolonged in patients with chronic renal insufficiency. Compared to normal volunteers, the elimination half-life of acrivastine was about 50% increased in patients with mild renal insufficiency (creatinine clearance = 26 to 48 mL/min) and was increased by about 130% in patients with moderate (creatinine clearance = 12 to 17 mL/min) or severe (creatinine clearance 6 to 10 mL/min) renal insufficiency. Oral clearance of acrivastine was diminished by the same magnitude as the half-life was prolonged in each of the three renally impaired groups. The elimination half-life of the propionic acid metabolite of acrivastine was about 140% increased in patients with mild renal insufficiency and about 5 times increased in patients with moderate or severe renal insufficiency.
Compared to normal volunteers, the elimination half-life of pseudoephedrine was about 3 times increased in patients with mild renal insufficiency, about 7 times increased in patients with moderate renal insufficiency, and about 10 times increased in patients with severe renal insufficiency. Oral clearance of pseudoephedrine was diminished by about the same magnitude as the half-life was prolonged in each of the three renally impaired groups (see PRECAUTIONS: Use in Patients with Diminished Renal Function).
The total body load removed by dialysis is approximately 20%, 27%, and 38% for acrivastine, the propionic acid metabolite of acrivastine, and pseudoephedrine, respectively, and therefore, a supplemental dose after a dialysis session is not required.
Based on a multiple dose cross study comparison, the apparent volume of distribution for acrivastine was 44% lower in elderly (n = 36, 65–75 yr) than in young volunteers (n = 16, 19–33 yr). This difference could be attributed to the decrease in total body water that occurs with aging. Despite this difference, no appreciable differences in plasma acrivastine concentrations were seen in the elderly compared to the young, and no appreciable accumulation of acrivastine occurred in plasma at steady-state. The elimination half-life for pseudoephedrine was 18% longer in elderly (7.9 hours) than in younger subjects (6.7 hours), presumably due to the decline in average renal function that occurs with aging. Despite this difference, clearance of pseudoephedrine was not appreciably different in elderly and younger subjects. Elderly patients can therefore be given the same dosage as younger patients. SEMPREX-D Capsules are not recommended, however, in patients with renal impairment (see PRECAUTIONS: Use in Patients with Diminished Renal Function and Geriatric Use).
The effect of age and sex on the pharmacokinetic parameters of acrivastine and pseudoephedrine was determined in 93 healthy volunteers who participated in various studies. All of the 93 volunteers were Caucasian (81 males and 12 females); 57 were between the ages of 18 and 38 years and 36 were between the ages of 65 and 75 years. There were no age- or sex-related differences in the pharmacokinetic parameters of either acrivastine or pseudoephedrine.
The effect of race on acrivastine and pseudoephedrine pharmacokinetics was examined by screening data obtained from 1035 patients, age 12 to 71 years, who participated in the eight safety and efficacy studies. No race-related differences were observed in the pharmacokinetics of either acrivastine or pseudoephedrine.

Clinical Studies
In healthy volunteers, histamine-induced wheal and flare areas were significantly reduced relative to placebo at 30 minutes after administration of a single dose of acrivastine 8 mg. Maximum reductions of wheal and flare occurred by 1 to 2 hours and significant reductions relative to placebo persisted for up to 6 hours after a single oral dose of acrivastine 8 mg. No additional reductions of wheal and flare were observed following single doses of acrivastine up to 24 mg. The exact correlation between responses on skin testing and clinical efficacy is not established.
Five randomized, placebo- and/or active-controlled trials compared SEMPREX-D with its acrivastine and pseudoephedrine components for the symptomatic relief of seasonal allergic rhinitis. In these studies, 696 patients received four daily doses of acrivastine 8 mg plus pseudoephedrine hydrochloride 60 mg (i.e., SEMPREX-D Capsules or bioequivalent formulations administered concurrently) or the same doses of the components for 14 days. The combination reduced the intensity of sneezing, rhinorrhea, pruritus, and lacrimation more than pseudoephedrine and reduced the intensity of nasal congestion more than acrivastine, demonstrating a contribution of each of the components. The onset of antihistaminic and nasal decongestant actions occurred within one or two hours after the first dose of SEMPREX-D Capsules. Somnolence occurred in about 12% of patients given SEMPREX-D compared with about 6% on placebo.

INDICATIONS AND USAGE
SEMPREX-D Capsules are indicated for relief of symptoms associated with seasonal allergic rhinitis such as sneezing, rhinorrhea, pruritus, lacrimation, and nasal congestion. SEMPREX-D Capsules should be administered when both the antihistaminic activity of acrivastine and the nasal decongestant activity of pseudoephedrine are desired (see CLINICAL PHARMACOLOGY). The efficacy of SEMPREX-D Capsules beyond 14 days of continuous treatment in patients with seasonal allergic rhinitis has not been adequately investigated in clinical trials.
SEMPREX-D Capsules have not been adequately studied for effectiveness in relieving the symptoms of the common cold.

CONTRAINDICATIONS
SEMPREX-D Capsules are contraindicated in patients with a known sensitivity to acrivastine, other alkylamine antihistamines (e.g., triprolidine), pseudoephedrine, other sympathomimetic amines (e.g., phenylpropanolamine), or to any other components of the formulation. SEMPREX-D Capsules are contraindicated in patients with severe hypertension or severe coronary artery disease. SEMPREX-D Capsules are contraindicated in patients taking monoamine oxidase (MAO) inhibitors and for 14 days after stopping use of an MAO inhibitor (see Drug Interactions).

WARNINGS
SEMPREX-D Capsules should be used with caution in patients with hypertension, diabetes mellitus, ischemic heart disease, increased intraocular pressure, hyperthyroidism, prostatic hypertrophy, stenosing peptic ulcer, or pyloroduodenal obstruction. Overdose of sympathomimetic amines may produce CNS stimulation with convulsions or cardiovascular collapse with accompanying hypotension. The elderly are more likely to have adverse reactions to sympathomimetic amines.

PRECAUTIONS
General: Acrivastine is sedating in some patients. In controlled clinical trials, somnolence (i.e., drowsiness, sedation, sleepiness) was more common with SEMPREX-D Capsules (by an average of 6%) than with placebo (see ADVERSE EXPERIENCES).
Patients should be advised to assess their individual responses to SEMPREX-D Capsules before engaging in any activity requiring mental alertness, such as driving a motor vehicle or operating machinery. Concurrent use of SEMPREX-D Capsules with alcohol or other CNS depressants may cause additional reductions in alertness and impairment of CNS performance and should be avoided (see Drug Interactions).
Use in Patients with Diminished Renal Function: Acrivastine and pseudoephedrine are excreted primarily through the kidney. Both compounds therefore accumulate in patients with impaired renal function. Due to the differential effects of renal failure on the serum half-life and clearance of acrivastine and pseudoephedrine, use of SEMPREX-D Capsules, a fixed combination product, in patients with renal impairment (creatinine clearance ≤ 48 mL/min) is not recommended (see OVERDOSAGE and CLINICAL PHARMACOLOGY).
Information to Patients: Patients taking SEMPREX®-D Capsules (acrivastine and pseudoephedrine hydrochloride) should receive the following information. SEMPREX-D Capsules are prescribed to reduce symptoms associated with seasonal allergic rhinitis. Patients should be instructed to take SEMPREX-D Capsules only as prescribed and not to exceed the prescribed dose. Patients should be advised against the concurrent use of SEMPREX-D with over-the-counter antihistamines and decongestants. Patients who are or may become pregnant should be told that this product should be used in pregnancy or during lactation only if the potential benefit justifies the potential risks to the fetus or nursing infant. Due to the risk of hypertensive crisis, patients should be instructed not to take SEMPREX-D Capsules if they are presently taking a monoamine oxidase inhibitor or for 14 days after stopping use of an MAO inhibitor. Patients should be advised to assess their individual responses to SEMPREX-D Capsules before engaging in any activity requiring mental alertness, such as driving a car or operating machinery. Patients should be advised that the concurrent use of SEMPREX-D Capsules with alcohol and other CNS depressants may lead to additional reductions in alertness and impairment of CNS performance and should be avoided.
Drug Interactions: MAO inhibitors and beta-adrenergic agonists increase the effects of sympathomimetic amines. Concomitant use of sympathomimetic amines with MAO inhibitors can result in a hypertensive crisis (see CONTRAINDICATIONS). Because MAO inhibitors are long-acting, SEMPREX-D Capsules should not be taken with an MAO inhibitor or for 14 days after stopping use of an MAO inhibitor.
Because of their pseudoephedrine content, SEMPREX-D Capsules may reduce the antihypertensive effects of drugs that interfere with sympathetic activity. Care should be taken in the administration of SEMPREX-D Capsules concomitantly with other sympathomimetic amines because the combined effects on the cardiovascular system may be harmful to the patient.
Concomitant administration of SEMPREX-D Capsules with alcohol and other CNS depressants may result in additional reductions in alertness and impairment of CNS performance and should be avoided.
No formal drug interaction studies between SEMPREX-D Capsules and other possibly co-administered drugs have been performed.
Carcinogenesis, Mutagenesis, and Impairment of Fertility: Carcinogenicity studies with the combination of acrivastine and pseudoephedrine have not been performed. Oral doses of acrivastine alone at levels up to 40 mg/kg/day (236 mg/m^2/day or 10 times the recommended human daily dose) for 20 to 22 months in rats and up to 250 mg/kg/day (750 mg/m^2/day or 32 times the recommended human daily dose) for 20 to 24 months in mice revealed no evidence of carcinogenic potential. No evidence of mutagenicity (with or without metabolic activation) was observed in the Ames Salmonella mutagenicity assay or in the L5178Y/tk+/− mouse lymphoma assay. In an *in vitro* cytogenetic study performed in cultured human lymphocytes, acrivastine induced structural chromosomal abnormalities in the absence of metabolic activation, but not in its presence. In an *in vivo* cytogenetic study in rats given single oral doses of acrivastine up to 1000 mg/kg (5900 mg/m^2 or 249 times the recommended human daily dose) there were no structural chromosomal alterations.
Reproduction-fertility studies in rats given acrivastine alone at levels up to 200 mg/kg/day (1180 mg/m^2/day or 50 times the recommended human daily dose) had no effect on male or female fertility. Similarly, no effect on fertility was seen in male rats given acrivastine 20 mg/kg/day and pseudoephedrine 100 mg/kg/day (118 and 590 mg/m^2/day or 5 and 3 times the recommended human daily doses, respectively) or in female rats given acrivastine 4 mg/kg/day and pseudoephedrine 20 mg/kg/day (23.6 and 118 mg/m^2/day or 1 and 0.7 times the recommended human daily doses, respectively).

Continued on next page

Information on the Celltech Pharmaceuticals, Inc. products listed on these pages contains the full prescribing information from product circulars in use as of July 2004. For further information, please consult the package insert currently accompanying the product.

Semprex-D—Cont.

Pregnancy: Pregnancy Category B:
Teratogenic Effects: No evidence of teratogenicity was seen in rats and rabbits given acrivastine 1000 and 400 mg/kg/day, respectively (5900 and 4720 mg/m^2/day or 249 and 200 times the recommended human daily dose). No evidence of teratogenicity was seen in rats given a combination of acrivastine 30 mg/kg/day and pseudoephedrine 150 mg/kg/day (177 and 885 mg/m^2/day or 8 and 5 times the recommended human daily dose, respectively). Similarly, no evidence of teratogenicity was observed in rabbits given acrivastine 20 mg/kg/day and pseudoephedrine 100 mg/kg/day (236 and 1180 mg/m^2/day or 10 and 7 times the recommended human daily doses, respectively). There are, however, no adequate and well-controlled studies in pregnant women. Because animal teratology studies are not always predictive of human responses, SEMPREX-D Capsules should be used during pregnancy only if the potential benefit justifies the potential risks to the fetus.
Nonteratogenic Effects: In a perinatal-postnatal study in rats, acrivastine given alone at levels up to 500 mg/kg/day (2950 mg/m^2/day or 124 times the recommended human daily dose) was associated with maternal and neonatal mortality at the maximum dose level. Neonatal survival was decreased in rats given a combination of acrivastine 20 mg/kg/day and pseudoephedrine 100 mg/kg/day (118 and 590 mg/m^2/day or 5 and 3 times the human dose, respectively).
Nursing Mothers: It is not known whether acrivastine is excreted in human milk; pseudoephedrine is excreted in human milk. SEMPREX-D Capsules should only be used in nursing mothers when the potential benefit justifies the potential risks to the nursing infant.
Pediatric Use: Safety and effectiveness of SEMPREX-D Capsules in pediatric patients under the age of 12 years have not been established.
Geriatric Use: Of the total number of subjects in clinical studies of SEMPREX-D, 349 were 60 years of age or older and 53 were 70 years of age and older. No overall differences in safety or effectiveness were observed between these subjects and younger subjects, and other reported clinical experience has not identified differences in responses between the elderly and younger patients, but greater sensitivity of some older individuals cannot be ruled out. Antihistamines, however, as a pharmaceutical class, are more likely to cause dizziness, sedation, bladder-neck obstruction, and hypotension in elderly patients. The elderly are also more likely to have adverse reactions to sympathomimetics such as pseudoephedrine (see CLINICAL PHARMACOLOGY and WARNINGS).
This drug is known to be substantially excreted by the kidney, and the risk of toxic reactions to this drug may be greater in patients with impaired renal function. Because elderly patients are more likely to have decreased renal function, care should be taken in dose selection, and it may be useful to monitor renal function. Use of SEMPREX-D in patients with renal impairment (creatinine clearance ≤ 48 mL/min) is not recommended (see PRECAUTIONS: Use in Patients with Diminished Renal Function).

ADVERSE EXPERIENCES

Information on the incidence of adverse events in clinical investigations conducted in the U.S. was obtained from 33 controlled and 15 uncontrolled clinical studies in which 2499 patients received acrivastine and 2631 patients received acrivastine plus pseudoephedrine hydrochloride for treatment periods ranging from one day to one year. The majority of patients in clinical trials were exposed to acrivastine or acrivastine plus pseudoephedrine for less than 90 days. Acrivastine dosage ranged from 3 to 96 mg/day; 1336 patients received dosages equal to or greater than acrivastine 24 mg/day. Acrivastine plus pseudoephedrine hydrochloride dosages ranged from acrivastine 8 to 48 mg/day plus pseudoephedrine hydrochloride 60 to 240 mg/day. A total of 2335 patients received three or four daily doses of acrivastine 8 mg plus pseudoephedrine hydrochloride 60 mg. In controlled clinical trials, only 12 spontaneously elicited adverse events were reported with frequencies greater than 1% in the acrivastine plus pseudoephedrine hydrochloride treatment group (see table).
[See table below]
The nature and overall frequencies of adverse events from international clinical trials (35 studies involving approximately 1600 patients) were similar to the results obtained in the U.S. studies.
Post-marketing clinical experience reports with acrivastine and acrivastine plus pseudoephedrine have included rare serious hypersensitivity reactions manifested by anaphylaxis, angioedema, bronchospasm, and erythema multiforme. No deaths associated with use of acrivastine or acrivastine plus pseudoephedrine have been reported.
Pseudoephedrine may cause ephedrine-like reactions such as tachycardia, palpitations, headache, dizziness, or nausea (see WARNINGS and OVERDOSAGE).

OVERDOSAGE

There have been no reports of overdosage with Semprex-D Capsules. In the clinical trial program and in international post-marketing experience, there have been two reported overdoses with acrivastine. Doses were 72 mg and 322 mg. Both patients recovered without sequelae. Adverse events included trembling, stridor, loss of consciousness and possible convulsions in the first patient and somnolence in the second.
Since acrivastine and pseudoephedrine have pharmacologically different actions, it is difficult to predict how an individual will respond to overdosage with SEMPREX-D Capsules. However, acute overdosage with SEMPREX-D Capsules may produce clinical signs of either CNS stimulation or depression. Overdosage of sympathomimetics has been associated with the following events: fear, anxiety, tenseness, restlessness, tremor, weakness, pallor, respiratory difficulty, dysuria, insomnia, hallucinations, convulsions, CNS depression, arrhythmias, and cardiovascular collapse with hypotension. Treatment for overdosage with SEMPREX-D Capsules should follow general symptomatic and supportive principles.
In a placebo-controlled, double-blind clinical trial in 18 healthy male subjects, single doses of acrivastine up to 400 mg (50 times the recommended antihistaminic dose) produced only a weak vagolytic effect, manifested as an increase in heart rate, and did not cause cardiac repolarization delays (i.e., increased QTc). Daily doses of acrivastine up to 2400 mg (75 times the recommended antihistamine dose) in an uncontrolled study in 38 cancer patients produced a 15–beats-per-minute increase in mean heart rate and occasional episodes of nausea and vomiting. The effects of acrivastine plus pseudoephedrine at single or multiple doses higher than the recommended daily dose of SEMPREX-D Capsules (i.e., 32 mg acrivastine plus 240 mg pseudoephedrine) on heart rate and cardiac repolarization have not been investigated in clinical trials.
The mean LD_{50} (single, oral dose) of acrivastine is greater than 4000 mg/kg (23600 mg/m^2 or 1000 times the recommended human daily dose) in rats and greater than 1200 mg/kg (3600 mg/m^2 or 153 times the recommended human daily dose) in mice. The mean LD_{50} (single, oral dose) of pseudoephedrine hydrochloride is 2206 mg/kg (13015 mg/m^2 or 73 times the recommended human daily dose) in rats and 726 mg/kg (2178 mg/m^2 or 12 times the recommended human daily dose) in mice. The toxic and lethal concentrations of acrivastine and pseudoephedrine in human biologic fluids are not known. Based upon pharmacokinetic screening data from clinical trials, the maximum plasma acrivastine concentration after dosing with acrivastine 8 mg was 393 ng/mL and the maximum plasma pseudoephedrine concentration after dosing with pseudoephedrine hydrochloride 60 mg was 1308 ng/mL.

DOSAGE AND ADMINISTRATION

The recommended dosage for adults and adolescents 12 years and older is one capsule administered orally, every 4 to 6 hours four times a day.

HOW SUPPLIED

SEMPREX-D Capsules (dark green opaque cap and white opaque body with a yellow band) contain acrivastine 8 mg and pseudoephedrine hydrochloride 60 mg. The cap is printed with "404" in white ink, and the body is printed with "SEMPREX-D" in black ink.
NDC 53014-404-10 Bottle of 100's.
Store at 15° to 25°C (59° to 77°F) in a dry place and protected from light. Keep out of the reach of children.
Marketed by:
Celltech Pharmaceuticals, Inc.
Rochester, NY 14623 USA
Manufactured by:
DSM Pharmaceuticals, Inc.
Greenville, NC 27834 USA
U.S. Patent No. 4650807.
® Celltech Manufacturing, CA Inc.

Rev. 4/04
R532B
000281

ADVERSE EVENTS REPORTED IN CLINICAL TRIALS* (PERCENT OF PATIENTS REPORTING)†

	Controlled Studies			
	Placebo (n = 1767)	Acrivastine (n = 1935)	Pseudoephedrine (n = 887)	Acrivastine plus Pseudoephedrine (n = 1650)
CNS				
Somnolence‡	6	12	8	12
Headache	18	19	19	19
Dizziness	2	3	3	3
Nervousness‡	1	2	4	3
Insomnia‡	1	1	6	4
MISCELLANEOUS				
Nausea	2	3	3	2
Dry Mouth‡	2	3	5	7
Asthenia	2	3	2	2
Dyspepsia	1	1	2	2
Pharyngitis	2	1	1	3
Cough Increase	1	2	1	2
Dysmenorrhea	1	2	3	2

* Includes all events regardless of causal relationship to treatment.
† Includes all adverse events with a reported frequency of >1% for the acrivastine plus pseudoephedrine treatment group.
‡ SEMPREX-D demonstrates a statistically higher frequency of events than placebo, p ≤0.05.

TUSSIONEX® PENNKINETIC®

Ⓒⅲ ℞

[tu-sē-ō-nĕks]
[pĕn-kī-nĕ-tĭk]
(hydrocodone polistirex and chlorpheniramine polistirex)
Extended-Release Suspension **LR 242A**
℞ Only **Rev. 12/02**

DESCRIPTION

Each teaspoonful (5 mL) of TUSSIONEX Pennkinetic Extended-Release Suspension contains hydrocodone polistirex equivalent to 10 mg of hydrocodone bitartrate and chlorpheniramine polistirex equivalent to 8 mg of chlorpheniramine maleate. TUSSIONEX Pennkinetic Extended-Release Suspension provides up to 12-hour relief per dose. Hydrocodone is a centrally-acting narcotic antitussive. Chlorpheniramine is an antihistamine. TUSSIONEX Pennkinetic Extended-Release Suspension is for oral use only.
Hydrocodone Polistirex: sulfonated styrene-divinylbenzene copolymer complex with 4,5α-epoxy-3-methoxy-17-methylmorphinan-6-one.

Chlorpheniramine Polistirex: sulfonated styrene-divinylbenzene copolymer complex with 2-[p-chloro-α-[2-(dimethylamino)ethyl]-benzyl]pyridine.

Inactive Ingredients: Ascorbic acid, D&C Yellow No. 10, ethylcellulose, FD&C Yellow No. 6, flavor, high fructose corn syrup, methylparaben, polyethylene glycol 3350, polysorbate 80, pregelatinized starch, propylene glycol, propylparaben, purified water, sucrose, vegetable oil, xanthan gum.

CLINICAL PHARMACOLOGY

Hydrocodone is a semisynthetic narcotic antitussive and analgesic with multiple actions qualitatively similar to those of codeine. The precise mechanism of action of hydrocodone and other opiates is not known; however, hydrocodone is believed to act directly on the cough center. In excessive doses, hydrocodone, like other opium derivatives, will depress respiration. The effects of hydrocodone in therapeutic doses on the cardiovascular system are insignificant. Hydrocodone can produce miosis, euphoria, physical and psychological dependence.

Chlorpheniramine is an antihistamine drug (H_1 receptor antagonist) that also possesses anticholinergic and sedative activity. It prevents released histamine from dilating capillaries and causing edema of the respiratory mucosa.

Hydrocodone release from TUSSIONEX Pennkinetic Extended-Release Suspension is controlled by the Pennkinetic System, an extended-release drug delivery system which combines an ion-exchange polymer matrix with a diffusion rate-limiting permeable coating. Chlorpheniramine release is prolonged by use of an ion-exchange polymer system.

Following multiple dosing with TUSSIONEX Pennkinetic Extended-Release Suspension, hydrocodone mean (S.D.) peak plasma concentrations of 22.8 (5.9) ng/mL occurred at 3.4 hours. Chlorpheniramine mean (S.D.) peak plasma concentrations of 58.4 (14.7) ng/mL occurred at 6.3 hours following multiple dosing. Peak plasma levels obtained with an immediate-release syrup occurred at approximately 1.5 hours for hydrocodone and 2.8 hours for chlorpheniramine. The plasma half-lives of hydrocodone and chlorpheniramine have been reported to be approximately 4 and 16 hours, respectively.

INDICATIONS AND USAGE

TUSSIONEX Pennkinetic Extended-Release Suspension is indicated for relief of cough and upper respiratory symptoms associated with allergy or a cold.

CONTRAINDICATIONS

Known allergy or sensitivity to hydrocodone or chlorpheniramine.

WARNINGS

Respiratory Depression: As with all narcotics, TUSSIONEX Pennkinetic Extended-Release Suspension produces dose-related respiratory depression by directly acting on brain stem respiratory centers. Hydrocodone affects the center that controls respiratory rhythm, and may produce irregular and periodic breathing. Caution should be exercised when TUSSIONEX Pennkinetic Extended-Release Suspension is used postoperatively and in patients with pulmonary disease or whenever ventilatory function is depressed. If respiratory depression occurs, it may be antagonized by the use of naloxone hydrochloride and other supportive measures when indicated (see OVERDOSAGE).

Head Injury and Increased Intracranial Pressure: The respiratory depressant effects of narcotics and their capacity to elevate cerebrospinal fluid pressure may be markedly exaggerated in the presence of head injury, other intracranial lesions or a pre-existing increase in intracranial pressure. Furthermore, narcotics produce adverse reactions which may obscure the clinical course of patients with head injuries.

Acute Abdominal Conditions: The administration of narcotics may obscure the diagnosis or clinical course of patients with acute abdominal conditions.

Obstructive Bowel Disease: Chronic use of narcotics may result in obstructive bowel disease especially in patients with underlying intestinal motility disorder.

Pediatric Use: In pediatric patients, as well as adults, the respiratory center is sensitive to the depressant action of narcotic cough suppressants in a dose-dependent manner. Benefit to risk ratio should be carefully considered especially in pediatric patients with respiratory embarrassment (e.g., croup) (see PRECAUTIONS).

PRECAUTIONS

General: Caution is advised when prescribing this drug to patients with narrow-angle glaucoma, asthma or prostatic hypertrophy.

Special Risk Patients: As with any narcotic agent, TUSSIONEX Pennkinetic Extended-Release Suspension should be used with caution in elderly or debilitated patients and those with severe impairment of hepatic or renal function, hypothyroidism, Addison's disease, prostatic hypertrophy or urethral stricture. The usual precautions should be observed and the possibility of respiratory depression should be kept in mind.

Information for Patients: As with all narcotics, TUSSIONEX Pennkinetic Extended-Release Suspension may produce marked drowsiness and impair the mental and/or physical abilities required for the performance of potentially hazardous tasks such as driving a car or operating machinery; patients should be cautioned accordingly. TUSSIONEX Pennkinetic Extended-Release Suspension must not be diluted with fluids or mixed with other drugs as this may alter the resin-binding and change the absorption rate, possibly increasing the toxicity. Keep out of the reach of children.

Cough Reflex: Hydrocodone suppresses the cough reflex; as with all narcotics, caution should be exercised when TUSSIONEX Pennkinetic Extended-Release Suspension is used postoperatively, and in patients with pulmonary disease.

Drug Interactions: Patients receiving narcotics, antihistaminics, antipsychotics, antianxiety agents or other CNS depressants (including alcohol) concomitantly with TUSSIONEX Pennkinetic Extended-Release Suspension may exhibit an additive CNS depression. When combined therapy is contemplated, the dose of one or both agents should be reduced.

The use of MAO inhibitors or tricyclic antidepressants with hydrocodone preparations may increase the effect of either the antidepressant or hydrocodone.

The concurrent use of other anticholinergics with hydrocodone may produce paralytic ileus.

Carcinogenesis, Mutagenesis, Impairment of Fertility: Carcinogenicity, mutagenicity and reproductive studies have not been conducted with TUSSIONEX® Pennkinetic® (hydrocodone polistirex and chlorpheniramine polistirex) Extended-Release Suspension.

Pregnancy: Teratogenic Effects – Pregnancy Category C. Hydrocodone has been shown to be teratogenic in hamsters when given in doses 700 times the human dose. There are no adequate and well-controlled studies in pregnant women. TUSSIONEX Pennkinetic Extended-Release Suspension should be used during pregnancy only if the potential benefit justifies the potential risk to the fetus.

Nonteratogenic Effects: Babies born to mothers who have been taking opioids regularly prior to delivery will be physically dependent. The withdrawal signs include irritability and excessive crying, tremors, hyperactive reflexes, increased respiratory rate, increased stools, sneezing, yawning, vomiting and fever. The intensity of the syndrome does not always correlate with the duration of maternal opioid use or dose.

Labor and Delivery: As with all narcotics, administration of TUSSIONEX Pennkinetic Extended-Release Suspension to the mother shortly before delivery may result in some degree of respiratory depression in the newborn, especially if higher doses are used.

Nursing Mothers: It is not known whether this drug is excreted in human milk. Because many drugs are excreted in human milk and because of the potential for serious adverse reactions in nursing infants from TUSSIONEX Pennkinetic Extended-Release Suspension, a decision should be made whether to discontinue nursing or to discontinue the drug, taking into account the importance of the drug to the mother.

Pediatric Use: Safety and effectiveness of TUSSIONEX Pennkinetic Extended-Release Suspension in pediatric patients under six have not been established (see WARNINGS).

Geriatric Use: Clinical studies of TUSSIONEX did not include sufficient numbers of subjects aged 65 and over to determine whether they respond differently from younger subjects. Other reported clinical experience has not identified differences in responses between the elderly and younger patients. In general, dose selection for an elderly patient should be cautious, usually starting at the low end of the dosing range, reflecting the greater frequency of decreased hepatic, renal, or cardiac function, and of concomitant disease or other drug therapy.

This drug is known to be substantially excreted by the kidney, and the risk of toxic reactions to this drug may be greater in patients with impaired renal function. Because elderly patients are more likely to have decreased renal function, care should be taken in dose selection, and it may be useful to monitor renal function.

ADVERSE REACTIONS

Central Nervous System: Sedation, drowsiness, mental clouding, lethargy, impairment of mental and physical performance, anxiety, fear, dysphoria, euphoria, dizziness, psychic dependence, mood changes.

Dermatologic System: Rash, pruritus.

Gastrointestinal System: Nausea and vomiting may occur; they are more frequent in ambulatory than in recumbent patients. Prolonged administration of TUSSIONEX Pennkinetic Extended-Release Suspension may produce constipation.

Genitourinary System: Ureteral spasm, spasm of vesicle sphincters and urinary retention have been reported with opiates.

Respiratory Depression: TUSSIONEX Pennkinetic Extended-Release Suspension may produce dose-related respiratory depression by acting directly on brain stem respiratory centers (see OVERDOSAGE).

Respiratory System: Dryness of the pharynx, occasional tightness of the chest.

DRUG ABUSE AND DEPENDENCE

TUSSIONEX Pennkinetic Extended-Release Suspension is a Schedule III narcotic. Psychic dependence, physical dependence and tolerance may develop upon repeated administration of narcotics; therefore, TUSSIONEX Pennkinetic Extended-Release Suspension should be prescribed and administered with caution. However, psychic dependence is unlikely to develop when TUSSIONEX Pennkinetic Extended-Release Suspension is used for a short time for the treatment of cough. Physical dependence, the condition in which continued administration of the drug is required to prevent the appearance of a withdrawal syndrome, assumes clinically significant proportions only after several weeks of continued oral narcotic use, although some mild degree of physical dependence may develop after a few days of narcotic therapy.

OVERDOSAGE

Signs and Symptoms: Serious overdosage with hydrocodone is characterized by respiratory depression (a decrease in respiratory rate and/or tidal volume, Cheyne-Stokes respiration, cyanosis), extreme somnolence progressing to stupor or coma, skeletal muscle flaccidity, cold and clammy skin, and sometimes bradycardia and hypotension. Although miosis is characteristic of narcotic overdose, mydriasis may occur in terminal narcosis or severe hypoxia. In severe overdosage apnea, circulatory collapse, cardiac arrest and death may occur. The manifestations of chlorpheniramine overdosage may vary from central nervous system depression to stimulation.

Treatment: Primary attention should be given to the reestablishment of adequate respiratory exchange through provision of a patent airway and the institution of assisted or controlled ventilation. The narcotic antagonist naloxone hydrochloride is a specific antidote for respiratory depression which may result from overdosage or unusual sensitivity to narcotics including hydrocodone. Therefore, an appropriate dose of naloxone hydrochloride should be administered, preferably by the intravenous route, simultaneously with efforts at respiratory resuscitation. Since the duration of action of hydrocodone in this formulation may exceed that of the antagonist, the patient should be kept under continued surveillance and repeated doses of the antagonist should be administered as needed to maintain adequate respiration. For further information, see full prescribing information for naloxone hydrochloride. An antagonist should not be administered in the absence of clinically significant respiratory depression. Oxygen, intravenous fluids, vasopressors and other supportive measures should be employed as indicated. Gastric emptying may be useful in removing unabsorbed drug.

DOSAGE AND ADMINISTRATION

Shake well before using.

Adults: 1 teaspoonful (5 mL) every 12 hours; do not exceed 2 teaspoonfuls in 24 hours.

Children 6-12: 1/2 teaspoonful every 12 hours; **do not exceed 1 teaspoonful in 24 hours.**

Not recommended for children under 6 years of age (see PRECAUTIONS).

HOW SUPPLIED

TUSSIONEX Pennkinetic (hydrocodone polistirex and chlorpheniramine polistirex) Extended-Release Suspension is a gold-colored suspension.

NDC 53014-548-67 473 mL bottle

Shake well. Dispense in a well-closed container. Store at 59°-86°F (15°-30°C).

Celltech Pharmaceuticals, Inc.
Rochester, NY 14623 USA

® Celltech Manufacturing, Inc.
Tussionex® Pennkinetic® Extended-Release Suspension: US Patent No. 4,762,709.2
Rev. 12/02
LR242A

ZAROXOLYN® TABLETS ℞

[*zar-″ox ′uh-lin*]
(metolazone tablets, USP) **R522B**
℞ Only **Rev. 2/03**

DO NOT INTERCHANGE: DO NOT INTERCHANGE ZAROXOLYN TABLETS AND OTHER FORMULATIONS OF METOLAZONE THAT SHARE ITS SLOW AND INCOMPLETE BIOAVAILABILITY AND ARE NOT THERAPEUTICALLY EQUIVALENT AT THE SAME DOSES TO MYKROX® TABLETS, A MORE RAPIDLY AVAILABLE AND COMPLETELY BIOAVAILABLE METOLAZONE PRODUCT. FORMULATIONS BIOEQUIVALENT TO ZAROXOLYN AND FORMULATIONS BIOEQUIVALENT TO MYKROX SHOULD NOT BE INTERCHANGED FOR ONE ANOTHER.

DESCRIPTION

ZAROXOLYN Tablets (metolazone tablets, USP) for oral administration contain 2½, 5, or 10 mg of metolazone, USP, a diuretic/saluretic/antihypertensive drug of the quinazoline class.

Metolazone has the molecular formula $C_{16}H_{16}ClN_3O_3S$, the chemical name 7-chloro-1, 2, 3, 4-tetrahydro-2-methyl-3-(2-methylphenyl)-4-oxo-6-quinazolinesulfonamide, and a molecular weight of 365.83. The structural formula is:

Cl H CH3 N N H2NSO2 O CH3

Metolazone is only sparingly soluble in water, but more soluble in plasma, blood, alkali, and organic solvents.

Inactive Ingredients: Magnesium stearate, microcrystalline cellulose and dye: 2½ mg-D&C Red No. 33; 5 mg-FD&C Blue No. 2; 10 mg-D&C Yellow No. 10 and FD&C Yellow No. 6.

Continued on next page

Information on the Celltech Pharmaceuticals, Inc. products listed on these pages contains the full prescribing information from product circulars in use as of July 2004. For further information, please consult the package insert currently accompanying the product.

Zaroxolyn—Cont.

CLINICAL PHARMACOLOGY

ZAROXOLYN (metolazone) is a quinazoline diuretic, with properties generally similar to the thiazide diuretics. The actions of ZAROXOLYN result from interference with the renal tubular mechanism of electrolyte reabsorption. ZAROXOLYN acts primarily to inhibit sodium reabsorption at the cortical diluting site and to a lesser extent in the proximal convoluted tubule. Sodium and chloride ions are excreted in approximately equivalent amounts. The increased delivery of sodium to the distal tubular exchange site results in increased potassium excretion. ZAROXOLYN does not inhibit carbonic anhydrase. A proximal action of metolazone has been shown in humans by increased excretion of phosphate and magnesium ions and by a markedly increased fractional excretion of sodium in patients with severely compromised glomerular filtration. This action has been demonstrated in animals by micropuncture studies.

When ZAROXOLYN Tablets are given, diuresis and saluresis usually begin within one hour and may persist for 24 hours or more. For most patients, the duration of effect can be varied by adjusting the daily dose. High doses may prolong the effect. A single daily dose is recommended. When a desired therapeutic effect has been obtained, it may be possible to reduce dosage to a lower maintenance level.

The diuretic potency of ZAROXOLYN at maximum therapeutic dosage is approximately equal to thiazide diuretics. However, unlike thiazides, ZAROXOLYN may produce diuresis in patients with glomerular filtration rates below 20 mL/min.

ZAROXOLYN and furosemide administered concurrently have produced marked diuresis in some patients where edema or ascites was refractory to treatment with maximum recommended doses of these or other diuretics administered alone. The mechanism of this interaction is unknown (see WARNINGS and PRECAUTIONS, Drug Interactions).

Maximum blood levels of metolazone are found approximately eight hours after dosing. A small fraction of metolazone is metabolized. Most of the drug is excreted in the unconverted form in the urine.

INDICATIONS AND USAGE

ZAROXOLYN is indicated for the treatment of salt and water retention including:

- edema accompanying congestive heart failure;
- edema accompanying renal diseases, including the nephrotic syndrome and states of diminished renal function.

ZAROXOLYN is also indicated for the treatment of hypertension, alone or in combination with other antihypertensive drugs of a different class. MYKROX Tablets, a more rapidly available form of metolazone, are intended for the treatment of new patients with mild to moderate hypertension. A dose titration is necessary if MYKROX Tablets are to be substituted for ZAROXOLYN in the treatment of hypertension. See package circular for MYKROX Tablets (Celltech).

Usage in Pregnancy: The routine use of diuretics in an otherwise healthy woman is inappropriate and exposes mother and fetus to unnecessary hazard. Diuretics do not prevent development of toxemia of pregnancy, and there is no evidence that they are useful in the treatment of developed toxemia.

Edema during pregnancy may arise from pathologic causes or from the physiologic and mechanical consequences of pregnancy. ZAROXOLYN is indicated in pregnancy when edema is due to pathologic causes, just as it is in the absence of pregnancy (see PRECAUTIONS). Dependent edema in pregnancy resulting from restriction of venous return by the expanded uterus is properly treated through elevation of the lower extremities and use of support hose; use of diuretics to lower intravascular volume in this case is illogical and unnecessary. There is hypervolemia during normal pregnancy which is harmful to neither the fetus nor the mother (in the absence of cardiovascular disease), but which is associated with edema, including generalized edema, in the majority of pregnant women. If this edema produces discomfort, increased recumbency will often provide relief. In rare instances, this edema may cause extreme discomfort which is not relieved by rest. In these cases, a short course of diuretics may be appropriate.

CONTRAINDICATIONS

Anuria, hepatic coma or precoma, known allergy or hypersensitivity to metolazone.

WARNINGS

Rapid Onset Hyponatremia and/or Hypokalemia: Rarely, the rapid onset of severe hyponatremia and/or hypokalemia has been reported following initial doses of thiazide and non-thiazide diuretics. When symptoms consistent with severe electrolyte imbalance appear rapidly, drug should be discontinued and supportive measures should be initiated immediately. Parenteral electrolytes may be required. Appropriateness of therapy with this class of drugs should be carefully reevaluated.

Hypokalemia: Hypokalemia may occur with consequent weakness, cramps, and cardiac dysrhythmias. Serum potassium should be determined at regular and appropriate intervals, and dose reduction, potassium supplementation or addition of a potassium-sparing diuretic instituted whenever indicated. Hypokalemia is a particular hazard in patients who are digitalized or who have or have had a ventricular arrhythmia; dangerous or fatal arrhythmias may be precipitated. Hypokalemia is dose related.

Concomitant Therapy: Lithium: In general, diuretics should not be given concomitantly with lithium because they reduce its renal clearance and add a high risk of lithium toxicity. Read prescribing information for lithium preparations before use of such concomitant therapy.

Furosemide: Unusually large or prolonged losses of fluids and electrolytes may result when ZAROXOLYN is administered concomitantly to patients receiving furosemide (see PRECAUTIONS, Drug Interactions).

Other Antihypertensive Drugs: When ZAROXOLYN is used with other antihypertensive drugs, particular care must be taken to avoid excessive reduction of blood pressure, especially during initial therapy.

Cross-Allergy: Cross-allergy may occur when Zaroxolyn is given to patients known to be allergic to sulfonamide-derived drugs, thiazides or quinethazone.

Sensitivity Reactions: Sensitivity reactions (e.g., angioedema, bronchospasm) may occur with or without a history of allergy or bronchial asthma and may occur with the first dose of ZAROXOLYN.

PRECAUTIONS

DO NOT INTERCHANGE

DO NOT INTERCHANGE ZAROXOLYN TABLETS AND OTHER FORMULATIONS OF METOLAZONE THAT SHARE ITS SLOW AND INCOMPLETE BIOAVAILABILITY AND ARE NOT THERAPEUTICALLY EQUIVALENT AT THE SAME DOSES TO MYKROX TABLETS, A MORE RAPIDLY AVAILABLE AND COMPLETELY BIOAVAILABLE METOLAZONE PRODUCT. FORMULATIONS BIOEQUIVALENT TO ZAROXOLYN AND FORMULATIONS BIOEQUIVALENT TO MYKROX SHOULD NOT BE INTERCHANGED FOR ONE ANOTHER.

General: *Fluid and Electrolytes:* All patients receiving therapy with ZAROXOLYN Tablets should have serum electrolyte measurements done at appropriate intervals and be observed for clinical signs of fluid and/or electrolyte imbalance: namely, hyponatremia, hypochloremic alkalosis, and hypokalemia. In patients with severe edema accompanying cardiac failure or renal disease, a low-salt syndrome may be produced, especially with hot weather and a low-salt diet. Serum and urine electrolyte determinations are particularly important when the patient has protracted vomiting, severe diarrhea, or is receiving parenteral fluids. Warning signs of imbalance are: dryness of mouth, thirst, weakness, lethargy, drowsiness, restlessness, muscle pains or cramps, muscle fatigue, hypotension, oliguria, tachycardia, and gastrointestinal disturbances such as nausea and vomiting. Hyponatremia may occur at any time during long term therapy and, on rare occasions, may be life threatening.

The risk of hypokalemia is increased when larger doses are used, when diuresis is rapid, when severe liver disease is present, when corticosteroids are given concomitantly, when oral intake is inadequate or when excess potassium is being lost extrarenally, such as with vomiting or diarrhea.

Thiazide-like diuretics have been shown to increase the urinary excretion of magnesium; this may result in hypomagnesemia.

Glucose Tolerance: Metolazone may raise blood glucose concentrations possibly causing hyperglycemia and glycosuria in patients with diabetes or latent diabetes.

Hyperuricemia: ZAROXOLYN regularly causes an increase in serum uric acid and can occasionally precipitate gouty attacks even in patients without a prior history of them.

Azotemia: Azotemia, presumably prerenal azotemia, may be precipitated during the administration of ZAROXOLYN. If azotemia and oliguria worsen during treatment of patients with severe renal disease, ZAROXOLYN should be discontinued.

Renal Impairment: Use caution when administering ZAROXOLYN Tablets to patients with severely impaired renal function. As most of the drug is excreted by the renal route, accumulation may occur.

Orthostatic Hypotension: Orthostatic hypotension may occur; this may be potentiated by alcohol, barbiturates, narcotics, or concurrent therapy with other antihypertensive drugs.

Hypercalcemia: Hypercalcemia may infrequently occur with metolazone, especially in patients taking high doses of vitamin D or with high bone turnover states, and may signify hidden hyperparathyroidism. Metolazone should be discontinued before tests for parathyroid function are performed.

Systemic Lupus Erythematosus: Thiazide diuretics have exacerbated or activated systemic lupus erythematosus and this possibility should be considered with ZAROXOLYN Tablets.

Information for Patients: Patients should be informed of possible adverse effects, advised to take the medication as directed, and promptly report any possible adverse reactions to the treating physician.

Drug Interactions: *Diuretics:* Furosemide and probably other loop diuretics given concomitantly with metolazone can cause unusually large or prolonged losses of fluid and electrolytes (see WARNINGS).

Other Antihypertensives: When ZAROXOLYN Tablets are used with other antihypertensive drugs, care must be taken, especially during initial therapy. Dosage adjustments of other antihypertensives may be necessary.

Alcohol, Barbiturates, and Narcotics: The hypotensive effects of these drugs may be potentiated by the volume contraction that may be associated with metolazone therapy.

Digitalis Glycosides: Diuretic-induced hypokalemia can increase the sensitivity of the myocardium to digitalis. Serious arrhythmias can result.

Corticosteroids or ACTH: May increase the risk of hypokalemia and increase salt and water retention.

Lithium: Serum lithium levels may increase (see WARNINGS).

Curariform Drugs: Diuretic-induced hypokalemia may enhance neuromuscular blocking effects of curariform drugs (such as tubocurarine) – the most serious effect would be respiratory depression which could proceed to apnea. Accordingly, it may be advisable to discontinue ZAROXOLYN® Tablets (metolazone tablets, USP) three days before elective surgery.

Salicylates and Other Non-Steroidal Anti-Inflammatory Drugs: May decrease the antihypertensive effects of ZAROXOLYN Tablets.

Sympathomimetics: Metolazone may decrease arterial responsiveness to norepinephrine, but this diminution is not sufficient to preclude effectiveness of the pressor agent for therapeutic use.

Insulin and Oral Antidiabetic Agents: See Glucose Tolerance under PRECAUTIONS, General.

Methenamine: Efficacy may be decreased due to urinary alkalizing effect of metolazone.

Anticoagulants: Metolazone, as well as other thiazide-like diuretics, may affect the hypoprothrombinemic response to anticoagulants; dosage adjustments may be necessary.

Drug/Laboratory Test Interactions: None reported.

Carcinogenesis, Mutagenesis, Impairment of Fertility: Mice and rats administered metolazone 5 days/week for up to 18 and 24 months, respectively, at daily doses of 2, 10, and 50 mg/kg, exhibited no evidence of a tumorigenic effect of the drug. The small number of animals examined histologically and poor survival in the mice limit the conclusions that can be reached from these studies.

Metolazone was not mutagenic *in vitro* in the Ames Test using Salmonella typhimurium strains TA-97, TA-98, TA-100, TA-102, and TA-1535.

Reproductive performance has been evaluated in mice and rats. There is no evidence that metolazone possesses the potential for altering reproductive capacity in mice. In a rat study, in which males were treated orally with metolazone at doses of 2, 10, and 50 mg/kg for 127 days prior to mating with untreated females, an increased number of resorption sites was observed in dams mated with males from the 50 mg/kg group. In addition, the birth weight of offspring was decreased and the pregnancy rate was reduced in dams mated with males from the 10 and 50 mg/kg groups.

Pregnancy: Teratogenic Effects—Pregnancy Category B. Reproduction studies performed in mice, rabbits, and rats treated during the appropriate period of gestation at doses up to 50 mg/kg/day have revealed no evidence of harm to the fetus due to metolazone. There are, however, no adequate and well-controlled studies in pregnant women. Because animal reproduction studies are not always predictive of human response, ZAROXOLYN Tablets should be used during pregnancy only if clearly needed. Metolazone crosses the placental barrier and appears in cord blood.

Non-Teratogenic Effects: The use of ZAROXOLYN Tablets in pregnant women requires that the anticipated benefit be weighed against possible hazards to the fetus. These hazards include fetal or neonatal jaundice, thrombocytopenia, and possibly other adverse reactions which have occurred in the adult. It is not known what effect the use of the drug during pregnancy has on the later growth, development, and functional maturation of the child. No such effects have been reported with metolazone.

Labor and Delivery: Based on clinical studies in which women received metolazone in late pregnancy until the time of delivery, there is no evidence that the drug has any adverse effects on the normal course of labor or delivery.

Nursing Mothers: Metolazone appears in breast milk. Because of the potential for serious adverse reactions in nursing infants from metolazone, a decision should be made whether to discontinue nursing or to discontinue the drug, taking into account the importance of the drug to the mother.

Pediatric Use: Safety and effectiveness in pediatric patients have not been established in controlled clinical trials. There is limited experience with the use of ZAROXOLYN in pediatric patients with congestive heart failure, hypertension, bronchopulmonary dysplasia, nephrotic syndrome and nephrogenic diabetes insipidus. Doses used generally ranged from 0.05 to 0.1 mg/kg administered once daily and usually resulted in a 1 to 2.8 kg weight loss and 150 to 300 cc increase in urine output. Not all patients responded and some gained weight. Those patients who did respond did so in the first few days of treatment. Prolonged use (beyond a few days) was generally associated with no further beneficial effect or a return to baseline status and is not recommended.

There is limited experience with the combination of ZAROXOLYN and furosemide in pediatric patients with furosemide-resistant edema. Some benefited while others did not or had an exaggerated response with hypovolemia, tachycardia, and orthostatic hypotension requiring fluid replacement. Severe hypokalemia was reported and there was a tendency for diuresis to persist for up to 24 hours after ZAROXOLYN was discontinued. Hyperbilirubinemia has been reported in 1 neonate. Close clinical and laboratory monitoring of all children treated with diuretics is indicated. See CONTRAINDICATIONS, WARNINGS, PRECAUTIONS.

Geriatric Use: Clinical studies of ZAROXOLYN did not include sufficient numbers of subjects aged 65 and over to determine whether they respond differently from younger subjects. Other reported clinical experience has not identified differences in responses between the elderly and younger patients. In general, dose selection for an elderly patient should be cautious, usually starting at the low end of the dosing range, reflecting the greater frequency of decreased hepatic, renal, or cardiac function, and of concomitant disease or other drug therapy. This drug is known to be substantially excreted by the kidney, and the risk of toxic reactions to this drug may be greater in patients with impaired renal function. Because elderly patients are more likely to have decreased renal function, care should be taken in dose selection, and it may be useful to monitor renal function.

ADVERSE REACTIONS

ZAROXOLYN is usually well tolerated, and most reported adverse reactions have been mild and transient. Many ZAROXOLYN related adverse reactions represent extensions of its expected pharmacologic activity and can be attributed to either its antihypertensive action or its renal/metabolic actions. The following adverse reactions have been reported. Several are single or comparably rare occurrences. Adverse reactions are listed in decreasing order of severity within body systems.

Cardiovascular: Chest pain/discomfort, orthostatic hypotension, excessive volume depletion, hemoconcentration, venous thrombosis, palpitations.

Central and Peripheral Nervous System: Syncope, neuropathy, vertigo, paresthesias, psychotic depression, impotence, dizziness/lightheadedness, drowsiness, fatigue, weakness, restlessness (sometimes resulting in insomnia), headache.

Dermatologic/Hypersensitivity: Toxic epidermal necrolysis (TEN), Stevens-Johnson Syndrome, necrotizing angiitis (cutaneous vasculitis), skin necrosis, purpura, petechiae, dermatitis (photosensitivity), urticaria, pruritus, skin rashes.

Gastrointestinal: Hepatitis, intrahepatic cholestatic jaundice, pancreatitis, vomiting, nausea, epigastric distress, diarrhea, constipation, anorexia, abdominal bloating, abdominal pain.

Hematologic: Aplastic/hypoplastic anemia, agranulocytosis, leukopenia, thrombocytopenia.

Metabolic: Hypokalemia, hyponatremia, hyperuricemia, hypochloremia, hypochloremic alkalosis, hyperglycemia, glycosuria, increase in serum urea nitrogen (BUN) or creatinine, hypophosphatemia, hypomagnesemia, hypercalcemia.

Musculoskeletal: Joint pain, acute gouty attacks, muscle cramps or spasm.

Other: Transient blurred vision, chills, dry mouth.

In addition, adverse reactions reported with similar antihypertensive-diuretics, but which have not been reported to date for ZAROXOLYN include: bitter taste, sialadenitis, xanthopsia, respiratory distress (including pneumonitis), and anaphylactic reactions. These reactions should be considered as possible occurrences with clinical usage of ZAROXOLYN.

Whenever adverse reactions are moderate or severe, ZAROXOLYN dosage should be reduced or therapy withdrawn.

OVERDOSAGE

Intentional overdosage has been reported rarely with metolazone and similar diuretic drugs.

Signs and Symptoms: Orthostatic hypotension, dizziness, drowsiness, syncope, electrolyte abnormalities, hemoconcentration and hemodynamic changes due to plasma volume depletion may occur. In some instances depressed respiration may be observed. At high doses, lethargy of varying degree may progress to coma within a few hours. The mechanism of CNS depression with thiazide overdosage is unknown. Also, GI irritation and hypermotility may occur. Temporary elevation of BUN has been reported, especially in patients with impairment of renal function. Serum electrolyte changes and cardiovascular and renal function should be closely monitored.

Treatment: There is no specific antidote available but immediate evacuation of stomach contents is advised. Dialysis is not likely to be effective. Care should be taken when evacuating the gastric contents to prevent aspiration, especially in the stuporous or comatose patient. Supportive measures should be initiated as required to maintain hydration, electrolyte balance, respiration, and cardiovascular and renal function.

DOSAGE AND ADMINISTRATION

Effective dosage of ZAROXOLYN should be individualized according to indication and patient response. A single daily dose is recommended. Therapy with ZAROXOLYN should be titrated to gain an initial therapeutic response and to determine the minimal dose possible to maintain the desired therapeutic response.

Usual Single Daily Dosage Schedules: Suitable initial dosages will usually fall in the ranges given.

Edema of cardiac failure:
ZAROXOLYN 5 to 20 mg once daily.
Edema of renal disease:
ZAROXOLYN 5 to 20 mg once daily.
Mild to moderate essential hypertension:
ZAROXOLYN 2½ to 5 mg once daily.

New patients—MYKROX® Tablets (metolazone tablets, USP) (see MYKROX package circular). If considered desirable to switch patients currently on ZAROXOLYN to MYKROX, the dose should be determined by titration starting at one tablet (½ mg) once daily and increasing to two tablets (1 mg) once daily if needed.

Treatment of Edematous States: The time interval required for the initial dosage to produce an effect may vary. Diuresis and saluresis usually begin within one hour and persist for 24 hours or longer. When a desired therapeutic effect has been obtained, it may be advisable to reduce the dose if possible. The daily dose depends on the severity of the patient's condition, sodium intake, and responsiveness. A decision to change the daily dose should be based on the results of thorough clinical and laboratory evaluations. If antihypertensive drugs or diuretics are given concurrently with ZAROXOLYN, more careful dosage adjustment may be necessary. For patients who tend to experience paroxysmal nocturnal dyspnea, it may be advisable to employ a larger dose to ensure prolongation of diuresis and saluresis for a full 24-hour period.

Treatment of Hypertension: The time interval required for the initial dosage regimen to show effect may vary from three or four days to three to six weeks in the treatment of elevated blood pressure. Doses should be adjusted at appropriate intervals to achieve maximum therapeutic effect.

HOW SUPPLIED

ZAROXOLYN Tablets (metolazone tablets, USP) are shallow biconvex, round tablets, and are available in three strengths:

2½ mg, pink, debossed "ZAROXOLYN" on one side, and "2½" on reverse side.

NDC 53014-975-71	Bottle of 100's
NDC 53014-975-90	Bottle of 1000's
NDC 53014-975-72	Carton of 100's, unit dose

5 mg, blue, debossed "ZAROXOLYN" on one side, and "5" on reverse side.

NDC 53014-850-71	Bottle of 100's
NDC 53014-850-90	Bottle of 1000's
NDC 53014-850-72	Carton of 100's, unit dose

10 mg, yellow, debossed "ZAROXOLYN" on one side, and "10" on reverse side.

NDC 53014-835-71	Bottle of 100's
NDC 53014-835-90	Bottle of 1000's
NDC 53014-835-72	Carton of 100's, unit dose

Store at 25°C (77°F); excursions permitted to 15°-30°C (59°-86°F) [See USP Controlled Room Temperature]. Protect from light. Keep out of the reach of children.

Celltech Pharmaceuticals, Inc.
Rochester, NY 14623 USA

EDUCATIONAL MATERIAL

For educational information, please write to Celltech Pharmaceuticals, Inc., PO Box 31766, Rochester, NY 14603.

Centocor, Inc.

200 GREAT VALLEY PARKWAY
MALVERN, PA 19355
USA

Direct General Inquiries to:
Ph: (610) 651-6000
(888) 874-3083
Fax: (610) 651-6100

Medical Emergency Contact:
Ph: 1-(800)-457-6399

For Medical Information/Adverse Experience Reporting Contact:
Medical Information
Ph: (800) 457-6399

REMICADE® ℞
[*rĕm-ĭ-kād*]
(infliximab)
for IV Injection

> **WARNING**
> **RISK OF INFECTIONS**
> **TUBERCULOSIS (FREQUENTLY DISSEMINATED OR EXTRAPULMONARY AT CLINICAL PRESENTATION), INVASIVE FUNGAL INFECTIONS, AND OTHER OPPORTUNISTIC INFECTIONS, HAVE BEEN OBSERVED IN PATIENTS RECEIVING REMICADE. SOME OF THESE INFECTIONS HAVE BEEN FATAL (SEE WARNINGS).**
> **PATIENTS SHOULD BE EVALUATED FOR LATENT TUBERCULOSIS INFECTION WITH A TUBERCULIN SKIN TEST.[1] TREATMENT OF LATENT TUBERCULOSIS INFECTION SHOULD BE INITIATED PRIOR TO THERAPY WITH REMICADE.**

DESCRIPTION

REMICADE® is a chimeric IgG1κ monoclonal antibody with an approximate molecular weight of 149,100 daltons. It is composed of human constant and murine variable regions. Infliximab binds specifically to human tumor necrosis factor alpha (TNFα) with an association constant of 10^{10} M^{-1}. Infliximab is produced by a recombinant cell line cultured by continuous perfusion and is purified by a series of steps that includes measures to inactivate and remove viruses.

REMICADE is supplied as a sterile, white, lyophilized powder for intravenous infusion. Following reconstitution with 10 mL of Sterile Water for Injection, USP, the resulting pH is approximately 7.2. Each single-use vial contains 100 mg infliximab, 500 mg sucrose, 0.5 mg polysorbate 80, 2.2 mg monobasic sodium phosphate, monohydrate, and 6.1 mg dibasic sodium phosphate, dihydrate. No preservatives are present.

CLINICAL PHARMACOLOGY

General

Infliximab neutralizes the biological activity of TNFα by binding with high affinity to the soluble and transmembrane forms of TNFα and inhibits binding of TNFα with its receptors.[2,3] Infliximab does not neutralize TNFβ (lymphotoxin α), a related cytokine that utilizes the same receptors as TNFα. Biological activities attributed to TNFα include: induction of pro-inflammatory cytokines such as interleukins (IL) 1 and 6, enhancement of leukocyte migration by increasing endothelial layer permeability and expression of adhesion molecules by endothelial cells and leukocytes, activation of neutrophil and eosinophil functional activity, induction of acute phase reactants and other liver proteins, as well as tissue degrading enzymes produced by synoviocytes and/or chondrocytes. Cells expressing transmembrane TNFα bound by infliximab can be lysed *in vitro*[3] or *in vivo*.[4] Infliximab inhibits the functional activity of TNFα in a wide variety of *in vitro* bioassays utilizing human fibroblasts, endothelial cells, neutrophils, B and T lymphocytes and epithelial cells. Anti-TNFα antibodies reduce disease activity in the cotton-top tamarin colitis model, and decrease synovitis and joint erosions in a murine model of collagen-induced arthritis. Infliximab prevents disease in transgenic mice that develop polyarthritis as a result of constitutive expression of human TNFα, and when administered after disease onset, allows eroded joints to heal.

Pharmacodynamics

Elevated concentrations of TNFα have been found in the joints of rheumatoid arthritis patients and the stools of Crohn's disease patients and correlate with elevated disease activity. In rheumatoid arthritis, treatment with REMICADE reduced infiltration of inflammatory cells into inflamed areas of the joint as well as expression of molecules mediating cellular adhesion [E-selectin, intercellular adhesion molecule-1 (ICAM-1) and vascular cell adhesion molecule-1 (VCAM-1)], chemoattraction [IL-8 and monocyte chemotactic protein (MCP-1)] and tissue degradation [matrix metalloproteinase (MMP) 1 and 3]. In Crohn's disease, treatment with REMICADE reduced infiltration of inflammatory cells and TNFα production in inflamed areas of the intestine, and reduced the proportion of mononuclear cells from the lamina propria able to express TNFα and interferon. After treatment with REMICADE, patients with rheumatoid arthritis or Crohn's disease exhibited decreased levels of serum IL-6 and C-reactive protein (CRP) compared to baseline. Peripheral blood lymphocytes from REMICADE-treated patients showed no significant decrease in number or in proliferative responses to *in vitro* mitogenic stimulation when compared to cells from untreated patients.

Pharmacokinetics

Single intravenous (IV) infusions of 3 mg/kg to 20 mg/kg showed a linear relationship between the dose administered and the maximum serum concentration. The volume of distribution at steady state was independent of dose and indicated that infliximab was distributed primarily within the vascular compartment. Median pharmacokinetic results for doses of 3 mg/kg to 10 mg/kg in rheumatoid arthritis and 5 mg/kg in Crohn's disease indicate that the terminal half-life of infliximab is 8.0 to 9.5 days.

Following an initial dose of REMICADE, repeated infusions at 2 and 6 weeks resulted in predictable concentration-time profiles following each treatment. No systemic accumulation of infliximab occurred upon continued repeated treatment with 3 mg/kg or 10 mg/kg at 4- or 8-week intervals. No major differences in clearance or volume of distribution were observed in patient subgroups defined by age, weight, or gender. It is not known if there are differences in clearance or volume of distribution in patients with marked impairment of hepatic or renal function.

A pediatric Crohn's disease pharmacokinetic study was conducted in 21 patients aged 11 to 17 years old. No notable differences in single-dose pharmacokinetic parameters were observed between pediatric and adult Crohn's disease patients (see PRECAUTIONS, Pediatric Use).

CLINICAL STUDIES

Rheumatoid Arthritis

The safety and efficacy of REMICADE when given in conjunction with methotrexate (MTX) were assessed in a mul-

Continued on next page

Remicade—Cont.

ticenter, randomized, double-blind, placebo-controlled study of 428 patients with active rheumatoid arthritis despite treatment with MTX (the Anti-TNF Trial in Rheumatoid Arthritis with Concomitant Therapy or ATTRACT). Patients enrolled had a median age of 54 years, median disease duration of 8.4 years, median swollen and tender joint count of 20 and 31 respectively, and were on a median dose of 15 mg/wk of MTX. Patients received either placebo + MTX or one of 4 doses/schedules of REMICADE + MTX: 3 mg/kg or 10 mg/kg of REMICADE by IV infusion at weeks 0, 2 and 6 followed by additional infusions every 4 or 8 weeks in combination with MTX. Concurrent use of stable doses of folic acid, oral corticosteroids (≤10 mg/day) and/or nonsteroidal anti-inflammatory drugs was also permitted.

Data on use of REMICADE without concurrent MTX are limited (see ADVERSE REACTIONS, Immunogenicity).[5,6]

Clinical response

All doses/schedules of REMICADE + MTX resulted in improvement in signs and symptoms as measured by the American College of Rheumatology response criteria (ACR 20) with a higher percentage of patients achieving an ACR 20, 50 and 70 compared to placebo + MTX (Table 1). This improvement was observed at week 2 and maintained through week 102. Greater effects on each component of the ACR 20 were observed in all patients treated with REMICADE + MTX compared to placebo + MTX (Table 2). Approximately 10% of patients treated with REMICADE achieved a major clinical response, defined as maintenance of an ACR 70 response over a 6-month period compared to 0% of placebo-treated patients (p≤0.018).

[See table 1 at right]

[See table 2 at right]

Radiographic response

Structural damage in both hands and feet was assessed radiographically at week 54 by the change from baseline in the van der Heijde-modified Sharp score, a composite score of structural damage that measures the number and size of joint erosions and the degree of joint space narrowing in hands/wrists and feet.[7] Approximately 80% of patients had paired x-ray data at 54 weeks and approximately 70% at 102 weeks. The inhibition of progression of structural damage was observed at 54 weeks (Table 3) and maintained through 102 weeks.

[See table 3 at right]

Physical function response

Physical function and disability were assessed using the Health Assessment Questionnaire (HAQ) and the general health-related quality of life questionnaire SF-36. All doses/schedules of REMICADE + MTX showed significantly greater improvement from baseline in HAQ and SF-36 physical component summary score averaged over time through week 54 compared to placebo + MTX, and no worsening in the SF-36 mental component summary score.

The median (interquartile range) improvement from baseline to week 54 in HAQ was 0.1 (−0.1, 0.5) for the placebo + MTX group and 0.4 (0.1, 0.9) for REMICADE + MTX (p<0.001). Both HAQ and SF-36 effects were maintained through week 102. Approximately 80% of patients in all doses/schedules of REMICADE + MTX remained in the trial through 102 weeks.

Active Crohn's Disease

The safety and efficacy of single and multiple doses of REMICADE were assessed in two randomized, double-blind, placebo-controlled clinical studies in 653 patients with moderate to severely active Crohn's disease [Crohn's Disease Activity Index (CDAI) ≥220 and ≤400] with an inadequate response to prior conventional therapies. Concomitant stable doses of aminosalicylates, corticosteroids and/or immunomodulatory agents were permitted and 92% of patients continued to receive at least one of these medications.

In the single-dose trial[8] of 108 patients, 16% (4/25) of placebo patients achieved a clinical response (decrease in CDAI ≥70 points) at week 4 vs. 81% (22/27) of patients receiving 5 mg/kg REMICADE (p<0.001, two-sided, Fisher's Exact test). Additionally, 4% (1/25) of placebo patients and 48% (13/27) of patients receiving 5 mg/kg REMICADE achieved clinical remission (CDAI<150) at week 4.

In a multidose trial (ACCENT I)[9], 545 patients received 5 mg/kg at week 0 and were then randomized to one of three treatment groups; the placebo maintenance group received placebo at weeks 2 and 6, and then every 8 weeks; the 5 mg/kg maintenance group received 5 mg/kg at weeks 2 and 6, and then every 8 weeks; and the 10 mg/kg maintenance group received 5 mg/kg at weeks 2 and 6, and then 10 mg/kg every 8 weeks. Patients in response at week 2 were randomized and analyzed separately from those not in response at week 2. Corticosteroid taper was permitted after week 6.

At week 2, 57% (311/545) of patients were in clinical response. At week 30, a significantly greater proportion of these patients in the 5 mg/kg and 10 mg/kg maintenance groups achieved clinical remission compared to patients in the placebo maintenance group (Table 4).

Additionally, a significantly greater proportion of patients in the 5 mg/kg and 10 mg/kg infliximab maintenance groups were in clinical remission and were able to discontinue corticosteroid use compared to patients in the placebo maintenance group at week 54 (Table 4).

[See table 4 at right]

Table 1
PERCENTAGE OF PATIENTS WHO ACHIEVED AN ACR RESPONSE AT WEEKS 30 AND 54

		REMICADE + MTX			
		3 mg/kg[a]		10 mg/kg[a]	
Response	Placebo + MTX (n=88)	q 8 wks (n=86)	q 4 wks (n=86)	q 8 wks (n=87)	q 4 wks (n=81)
ACR 20					
Week 30	20%	50%	50%	52%	58%
Week 54	17%	42%	48%	59%	59%
ACR 50					
Week 30	5%	27%	29%	31%	26%
Week 54	9%	21%	34%	40%	38%
ACR 70					
Week 30	0%	8%	11%	18%	11%
Week 54	2%	11%	18%	26%	19%

[a] p<0.05 for each outcome compared to placebo

Table 2
COMPONENTS OF ACR 20 AT BASELINE AND 54 WEEKS

	Placebo + MTX (n=88)		REMICADE + MTX[a] (n=340)	
Parameter (medians)	Baseline	Week 54	Baseline	Week 54
No. of Tender Joints	24	16	32	8
No. of Swollen Joints	19	13	20	7
Pain[b]	6.7	6.1	6.8	3.3
Physician's Global Assessment[b]	6.5	5.2	6.2	2.1
Patient's Global Assessment[b]	6.2	6.2	6.3	3.2
Disability Index (HAQ)[c]	1.8	1.5	1.8	1.3
CRP (mg/dL)	3.0	2.3	2.4	0.6

[a] All doses/schedules of REMICADE + MTX

[b] Visual Analog Scale (0=best, 10=worst)

[c] Health Assessment Questionnaire, measurement of 8 categories: dressing and grooming, arising, eating, walking, hygiene, reach, grip, and activities (0=best, 3=worst)

Table 3
RADIOGRAPHIC CHANGE FROM BASELINE TO WEEK 54

		REMICADE + MTX				
		3 mg/kg		10 mg/kg		
Median (10, 90 percentiles)	Placebo + MTX (n=64)	q 8 wks (n=71)	q 4 wks (n=71)	q 8 wks (n=77)	q 4 wks (n=66)	p-value[a]
Total Score						
Baseline	55 (14, 188)	57 (15, 187)	45 (8, 162)	56 (6, 143)	43 (7, 178)	
Change from baseline	4.0 (−1.0, 19.0)	0.5 (−3.0, 5.5)	0.1 (−5.2, 9.0)	0.5 (−4.8, 5.0)	−0.5 (−5.7, 4.0)	p<0.001
Erosion Score						
Baseline	25 (8, 110)	29 (9, 100)	22 (3, 91)	22 (3, 80)	26 (4, 104)	
Change from baseline	2.0 (−1.0, 9.7)	0.0 (−3.0, 4.3)	−0.3 (−3.1, 2.5)	0.5 (−3.0, 2.5)	−0.5 (−2.7, 2.5)	p<0.001
JSN Score						
Baseline	26 (3, 88)	29 (4, 80)	20 (3, 83)	24 (1, 79)	25 (3, 77)	
Change from baseline	1.5 (−0.8, 8.0)	0.0 (−2.5, 4.5)	0.0 (−3.4, 5.0)	0.0 (−3.0, 2.5)	0.0 (−3.0, 3.5)	p<0.001

[a] For comparisons of each dose against placebo

Table 4
CLINICAL REMISSION AND STEROID WITHDRAWAL

	Single 5 mg/kg Dose[a] Placebo Maintenance	Three Dose Induction[b] Infliximab Maintenance q 8 wks	
		5 mg/kg	10 mg/kg
Week 30	25/102	41/104	48/105
Clinical remission	25%	39%	46%
p-value[c]		0.022	0.001
Week 54			
Patients in remission able to discontinue corticosteroid use[d]	6/54 11%	14/56 25%	18/53 34%
p-value[c]		0.059	0.005

[a] REMICADE at week 0

[b] REMICADE 5 mg/kg administered at weeks 0, 2 and 6

[c] p-values represent pairwise comparisons to placebo

[d] Of those receiving corticosteroids at baseline

Patients in the infliximab maintenance groups (5 mg/kg and 10 mg/kg) had a longer time to loss of response than patients in the placebo maintenance group (Figure 1). At weeks 30 and 54, significant improvement from baseline was seen among the 5 mg/kg and 10 mg/kg infliximab-treated groups compared to the placebo group in the disease specific inflammatory bowel disease questionnaire (IBDQ), particularly the bowel and systemic components, and in the physical component summary score of the general health-related quality of life questionnaire SF-36.

[See figure 1 at top of next page]

In a subset of 78 patients who had mucosal ulceration at baseline and who participated in an endoscopic substudy, 13 of 43 patients in the infliximab maintenance group had endoscopic evidence of mucosal healing compared to 1 of 28 patients in the placebo group at week 10. Of the infliximab-treated patients showing mucosal healing at week 10, 9 of 12 patients also showed mucosal healing at week 54.

Patients who achieved a response and subsequently lost response were eligible to receive infliximab on an episodic basis at a dose that was 5 mg/kg higher than the dose to which they were randomized. The majority of such patients responded to the higher dose. Among patients who were not in response at week 2, 59% (92/157) of infliximab maintenance patients responded by week 14 compared to 51% (39/77) of placebo maintenance patients. Among patients who did not

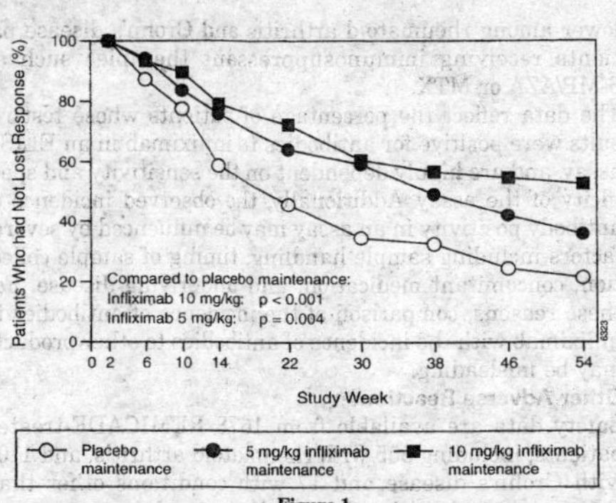

Figure 1
Kaplan-Meier estimate of the proportion of patients who had not lost response through week 54

respond by week 14, additional therapy did not result in significantly more responses (see DOSAGE AND ADMINISTRATION).

Fistulizing Crohn's Disease

The safety and efficacy of REMICADE were assessed in 2 randomized, double-blind, placebo-controlled studies in patients with fistulizing Crohn's disease with fistula(s) that were of at least 3 months duration. Concurrent use of stable doses of corticosteroids, 5-aminosalicylates, antibiotics, MTX, 6-mercaptopurine (6-MP) and/or azathioprine (AZA) was permitted.

In the first trial,[10] 94 patients received three doses of either placebo or REMICADE at weeks 0, 2 and 6. Fistula response (≥50% reduction in number of enterocutaneous fistulas draining upon gentle compression on at least two consecutive visits without an increase in medication or surgery for Crohn's disease) was seen in 68% (21/31) of patients in the 5 mg/kg REMICADE group (p=0.002) and 56% (18/32) of patients in the 10 mg/kg REMICADE group (p=0.021) vs. 26% (8/31) of patients in the placebo arm. The median time to onset of response and median duration of response in REMICADE-treated patients was 2 and 12 weeks, respectively. Closure of all fistula was achieved in 52% of REMICADE-treated patients compared with 13% of placebo-treated patients (p<0.001).

In the second trial (ACCENT II), patients who were enrolled had to have at least one draining enterocutaneous (perianal, abdominal) fistula. All patients received 5 mg/kg REMICADE at weeks 0, 2 and 6. Patients were randomized to placebo or 5 mg/kg REMICADE maintenance at week 14. Patients received maintenance doses at week 14 and then every eight weeks through week 46. Patients who were in fistula response (fistula response was defined the same as in the first trial) at both weeks 10 and 14 were randomized separately from those not in response. The primary endpoint was time from randomization to loss of response among those patients who were in fistula response.

Among the randomized patients (273 of the 296 initially enrolled), 87% had perianal fistulas and 14% had abdominal fistulas. Eight percent also had rectovaginal fistulas. Greater than 90% of the patients had received previous immunosuppressive and antibiotic therapy.

At week 14, 65% (177/273) of patients were in fistula response. Patients randomized to REMICADE maintenance had a longer time to loss of fistula response compared to the placebo maintenance group (Figure 2). At week 54, 38% (33/87) of REMICADE-treated patients had no draining fistulas compared with 22% (20/90) of placebo-treated patients (p=0.02). Compared to placebo maintenance, patients on REMICADE maintenance had a trend toward fewer hospitalizations.

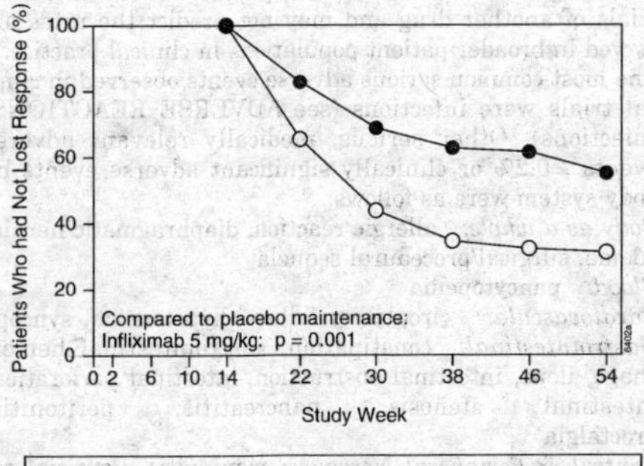

Figure 2
Life table estimates of the proportion of patients who had not lost fistula response through week 54

Patients who achieved a fistula response and subsequently lost response were eligible to receive REMICADE maintenance therapy at a dose that was 5 mg/kg higher than the dose to which they were randomized. Of the placebo maintenance patients, 66% (25/38) responded to 5 mg/kg REMICADE, and 57% (12/21) of REMICADE maintenance patients responded to 10 mg/kg.

Patients who had not achieved a response by week 14 were unlikely to respond to additional doses of REMICADE.

Similar proportions of patients in either group developed new fistulas (17% overall) and similar numbers developed abscesses (15% overall).

INDICATIONS AND USAGE

Rheumatoid Arthritis

REMICADE, in combination with methotrexate, is indicated for reducing signs and symptoms, inhibiting the progression of structural damage and improving physical function in patients with moderately to severely active rheumatoid arthritis who have had an inadequate response to methotrexate.

Crohn's Disease

REMICADE is indicated for reducing signs and symptoms and inducing and maintaining clinical remission in patients with moderately to severely active Crohn's disease who have had an inadequate response to conventional therapy.

REMICADE is indicated for reducing the number of draining enterocutaneous and rectovaginal fistulas and maintaining fistula closure in patients with fistulizing Crohn's disease.

CONTRAINDICATIONS

REMICADE at doses >5 mg/kg should not be administered to patients with moderate to severe heart failure. In a randomized study evaluating REMICADE in patients with moderate to severe heart failure (New York Heart Association [NYHA] Functional Class III/IV), REMICADE treatment at 10 mg/kg was associated with an increased incidence of death and hospitalization due to worsening heart failure (see WARNINGS and ADVERSE REACTIONS, Patients with Heart Failure).

REMICADE should not be administered to patients with known hypersensitivity to any murine proteins or other component of the product.

WARNINGS

RISK OF INFECTIONS
(See boxed WARNING)

SERIOUS INFECTIONS, INCLUDING SEPSIS HAVE BEEN REPORTED IN PATIENTS RECEIVING TNF-BLOCKING AGENTS. SOME OF THESE INFECTIONS HAVE BEEN FATAL. MANY OF THE SERIOUS INFECTIONS IN PATIENTS TREATED WITH REMICADE HAVE OCCURRED IN PATIENTS ON CONCOMITANT IMMUNOSUPPRESSIVE THERAPY THAT, IN ADDITION TO THEIR CROHN'S DISEASE OR RHEUMATOID ARTHRITIS, COULD PREDISPOSE THEM TO INFECTIONS.

REMICADE SHOULD NOT BE GIVEN TO PATIENTS WITH A CLINICALLY IMPORTANT, ACTIVE INFECTION. CAUTION SHOULD BE EXERCISED WHEN CONSIDERING THE USE OF REMICADE IN PATIENTS WITH A CHRONIC INFECTION OR A HISTORY OF RECURRENT INFECTION. PATIENTS SHOULD BE MONITORED FOR SIGNS AND SYMPTOMS OF INFECTION WHILE ON OR AFTER TREATMENT WITH REMICADE. NEW INFECTIONS SHOULD BE CLOSELY MONITORED. IF A PATIENT DEVELOPS A SERIOUS INFECTION, REMICADE THERAPY SHOULD BE DISCONTINUED (see ADVERSE REACTIONS, Infections).

CASES OF HISTOPLASMOSIS, COCCIDIOIDOMYCOSIS, LISTERIOSIS, PNEUMOCYSTOSIS, TUBERCULOSIS, OTHER BACTERIAL, MYCOBACTERIAL AND FUNGAL INFECTIONS HAVE BEEN OBSERVED IN PATIENTS RECEIVING REMICADE. FOR PATIENTS WHO HAVE RESIDED IN REGIONS WHERE HISTOPLASMOSIS OR COCCIDIOIDOMYCOSIS IS ENDEMIC, THE BENEFITS AND RISKS OF REMICADE TREATMENT SHOULD BE CAREFULLY CONSIDERED BEFORE INITIATION OF REMICADE THERAPY.

SERIOUS INFECTIONS WERE SEEN IN CLINICAL STUDIES WITH CONCURRENT USE OF ANAKINRA AND ANOTHER TNFα-BLOCKING AGENT, ETANERCEPT, WITH NO ADDED CLINICAL BENEFIT COMPARED TO ETANERCEPT ALONE. BECAUSE OF THE NATURE OF THE ADVERSE EVENTS SEEN WITH COMBINATION OF ETANERCEPT AND ANAKINRA THERAPY, SIMILAR TOXICITIES MAY ALSO RESULT FROM THE COMBINATION OF ANAKINRA AND OTHER TNFα-BLOCKING AGENTS. THEREFORE, THE COMBINATION OF REMICADE AND ANAKINRA IS NOT RECOMMENDED.

Patients with Heart Failure

REMICADE has been associated with adverse outcomes in patients with heart failure, and should be used in patients with heart failure only after consideration of other treatment options. The results of a randomized study evaluating the use of REMICADE in patients with heart failure (NYHA Functional Class III/IV) suggested higher mortality in patients who received 10 mg/kg REMICADE, and higher rates of cardiovascular adverse events at doses of 5 mg/kg and 10 mg/kg. There have been post-marketing reports of worsening heart failure, with and without identifiable precipitating factors, in patients taking REMICADE. There have also been rare post-marketing reports of new onset heart failure, including heart failure in patients without known pre-existing cardiovascular disease. Some of these patients have been under 50 years of age. If a decision is made to administer REMICADE to patients with heart failure, they should be closely monitored during therapy, and REMICADE should be discontinued if new or worsening symptoms of heart failure appear. (See CONTRAINDICATIONS and ADVERSE REACTIONS, Patients with Heart Failure.)

Hematologic Events

Cases of leukopenia, neutropenia, thrombocytopenia, and pancytopenia, some with a fatal outcome, have been reported in patients receiving REMICADE. The causal relationship to REMICADE therapy remains unclear. Although no high-risk group(s) has been identified, caution should be exercised in patients being treated with REMICADE who have ongoing or a history of significant hematologic abnormalities. All patients should be advised to seek immediate medical attention if they develop signs and symptoms suggestive of blood dyscrasias or infection (e.g., persistent fever) while on REMICADE. Discontinuation of REMICADE therapy should be considered in patients who develop significant hematologic abnormalities.

Hypersensitivity

REMICADE has been associated with hypersensitivity reactions that vary in their time of onset and required hospitalization in some cases. Most hypersensitivity reactions, which include urticaria, dyspnea, and/or hypotension, have occurred during or within 2 hours of REMICADE infusion. However, in some cases, serum sickness-like reactions have been observed in Crohn's disease patients 3 to 12 days after REMICADE therapy was reinstituted following an extended period without REMICADE treatment. Symptoms associated with these reactions include fever, rash, headache, sore throat, myalgias, polyarthralgias, hand and facial edema and/or dysphagia. These reactions were associated with marked increase in antibodies to infliximab, loss of detectable serum concentrations of infliximab, and possible loss of drug efficacy. REMICADE should be discontinued for severe reactions. Medications for the treatment of hypersensitivity reactions (e.g., acetaminophen, antihistamines, corticosteroids and/or epinephrine) should be available for immediate use in the event of a reaction (see ADVERSE REACTIONS, Infusion-related Reactions).

Neurologic Events

Infliximab and other agents that inhibit TNF have been associated in rare cases with optic neuritis, seizure and new onset or exacerbation of clinical symptoms and/or radiographic evidence of central nervous system demyelinating disorders, including multiple sclerosis, and CNS manifestation of systemic vasculitis. Prescribers should exercise caution in considering the use of REMICADE in patients with pre-existing or recent onset of central nervous system demyelinating or seizure disorders. Discontinuation of REMICADE should be considered in patients who develop significant central nervous system adverse reactions.

PRECAUTIONS

Autoimmunity

Treatment with REMICADE may result in the formation of autoantibodies and, rarely, in the development of a lupus-like syndrome. If a patient develops symptoms suggestive of a lupus-like syndrome following treatment with REMICADE, treatment should be discontinued (see ADVERSE REACTIONS, Autoantibodies/Lupus-like Syndrome).

Malignancy

Patients with long duration of Crohn's disease or rheumatoid arthritis and chronic exposure to immunosuppressant therapies are more prone to develop lymphomas (see ADVERSE REACTIONS, Malignancies/Lymphoproliferative Disease). The impact of treatment with REMICADE on these phenomena is unknown.

Vaccinations

No data are available on the response to vaccination or on the secondary transmission of infection by live vaccines in patients receiving anti-TNF therapy. It is recommended that live vaccines not be given concurrently.

Information for Patients

Patients should be provided the REMICADE Patient Information Sheet and provided an opportunity to read it prior to each treatment infusion session. Because caution should be exercised in administering REMICADE to patients with clinically important active infections, it is important that the patient's overall health be assessed at each treatment visit and any questions resulting from the patient's reading of the Patient Information Sheet be discussed.

Drug Interactions

Concurrent administration of etanercept (another TNFα-blocking agent) and anakinra (an interleukin-1 antagonist) has been associated with an increased risk of serious infections, and increased risk of neutropenia and no additional benefit compared to these medicinal products alone. Other TNFα-blocking agents (including REMICADE) used in combination with anakinra may also result in similar toxicities (see WARNINGS, RISK OF INFECTIONS).

Specific drug interaction studies, including interactions with MTX, have not been conducted. The majority of patients in rheumatoid arthritis or Crohn's disease clinical studies received one or more concomitant medications. In rheumatoid arthritis, concomitant medications besides MTX were nonsteroidal anti-inflammatory agents, folic acid, corticosteroids and/or narcotics. Concomitant Crohn's disease medications were antibiotics, antivirals, corticosteroids, 6-MP/AZA and aminosalicylates. Patients with Crohn's disease who received immunosuppressants tended to experience fewer infusion reactions compared to patients on no immunosuppressants (see ADVERSE REACTIONS, Immunogenicity and Infusion-related Reactions).

Serum infliximab concentrations appeared to be unaffected by baseline use of medications for the treatment of Crohn's disease including corticosteroids, antibiotics (metronidazole or ciprofloxacin) and aminosalicylates.

Carcinogenesis, Mutagenesis and Impairment of Fertility

A repeat dose toxicity study was conducted with mice given cV1q anti-mouse TNFα to evaluate tumorigenicity. CV1q is

Continued on next page

Remicade—Cont.

an analogous antibody that inhibits the function of TNFα in mice. Animals were assigned to 1 of 3 dose groups: control, 10 mg/kg or 40 mg/kg cV1q given weekly for 6 months. The weekly doses of 10 mg/kg and 40 mg/kg are 2 and 8 times, respectively, the human dose of 5 mg/kg for Crohn's disease. Results indicated that cV1q did not cause tumorigenicity in mice. No clastogenic or mutagenic effects of infliximab were observed in the *in vivo* mouse micronucleus test or the *Salmonella-Escherichia coli* (Ames) assay, respectively. Chromosomal aberrations were not observed in an assay performed using human lymphocytes. The significance of these findings for human risk is unknown. It is not known whether infliximab can impair fertility in humans. No impairment of fertility was observed in a fertility and general reproduction toxicity study with the analogous mouse antibody used in the 6-month chronic toxicity study.

Pregnancy Category B

Since infliximab does not cross-react with TNFα in species other than humans and chimpanzees, animal reproduction studies have not been conducted with REMICADE. No evidence of maternal toxicity, embryotoxicity or teratogenicity was observed in a developmental toxicity study conducted in mice using an analogous antibody that selectively inhibits the functional activity of mouse TNFα. Doses of 10 to 15 mg/kg in pharmacodynamic animal models with the anti-TNF analogous antibody produced maximal pharmacologic effectiveness. Doses up to 40 mg/kg were shown to produce no adverse effects in animal reproduction studies. It is not known whether REMICADE can cause fetal harm when administered to a pregnant woman or can affect reproduction capacity. REMICADE should be given to a pregnant woman only if clearly needed.

Nursing Mothers

It is not known whether infliximab is excreted in human milk or absorbed systemically after ingestion. Because many drugs and immunoglobulins are excreted in human milk, and because of the potential for adverse reactions in nursing infants from REMICADE, a decision should be made whether to discontinue nursing or to discontinue the drug, taking into account the importance of the drug to the mother.

Pediatric Use

Safety and effectiveness of REMICADE in patients with juvenile rheumatoid arthritis and in pediatric patients with Crohn's disease have not been established.

Geriatric Use

In the ATTRACT study, no overall differences were observed in effectiveness or safety in 72 patients aged 65 or older compared to younger patients. In Crohn's disease studies, there were insufficient numbers of patients aged 65 and over to determine whether they respond differently from patients aged 18 to 65. Because there is a higher incidence of infections in the elderly population in general, caution should be used in treating the elderly (see ADVERSE REACTIONS, Infections).

ADVERSE REACTIONS

The data described herein reflect exposure to REMICADE in 1678 patients, including 842 patients exposed beyond 30 weeks and 295 exposed beyond one year. The most common reason for discontinuation of treatment was infusion-related reactions (e.g. dyspnea, flushing, headache and rash). Adverse events have been reported in a higher proportion of rheumatoid arthritis patients receiving the 10 mg/kg dose than the 3 mg/kg dose, however, no differences were observed in the frequency of adverse events between the 5 mg/kg dose and 10 mg/kg dose in patients with Crohn's disease.

Infusion-related Reactions

Acute infusion reactions

An infusion reaction was defined in clinical trials as any adverse event occurring during an infusion or within 1 to 2 hours after an infusion. Approximately 20% of REMICADE-treated patients in all clinical studies experienced an infusion reaction compared to approximately 10% of placebo-treated patients. Among all REMICADE infusions, 3% were accompanied by nonspecific symptoms such as fever or chills, 1% were accompanied by cardiopulmonary reactions (primarily chest pain, hypotension, hypertension or dyspnea), and <1% were accompanied by pruritus, urticaria, or the combined symptoms of pruritus/urticaria and cardiopulmonary reactions. Serious infusion reactions occurred in <1% of patients and included anaphylaxis, convulsions, erythematous rash and hypotension. Approximately 3% of patients discontinued REMICADE because of infusion reactions, and all patients recovered with treatment and/or discontinuation of the infusion. REMICADE infusions beyond the initial infusion were not associated with a higher incidence of reactions.

Patients who became positive for antibodies to infliximab were more likely (approximately 2- to 3-fold) to have an infusion reaction than were those who were negative. Use of concomitant immunosuppressant agents appeared to reduce the frequency of antibodies to infliximab and infusion reactions (see ADVERSE REACTIONS, Immunogenicity and PRECAUTIONS, Drug Interactions).

In post-marketing experience, cases of anaphylactic-like reactions, including laryngeal/pharyngeal edema and severe bronchospasm, and seizure have been associated with REMICADE administration.

Reactions following readministration

In a study where 37 of 41 patients with Crohn's disease were retreated with infliximab following a 2 to 4 year period without infliximab treatment, 10 patients experienced adverse events manifesting 3 to 12 days following infusion of which 6 were considered serious. Signs and symptoms included myalgia and/or arthralgia with fever and/or rash, with some patients also experiencing pruritus, facial, hand or lip edema, dysphagia, urticaria, sore throat, and headache. Patients experiencing these adverse events had not experienced infusion-related adverse events associated with their initial infliximab therapy. These adverse events occurred in 39% (9/23) of patients who had received liquid formulation which is no longer in use and 7% (1/14) of patients who received lyophilized formulation. The clinical data are not adequate to determine if occurrence of these reactions is due to differences in formulation. Patients' signs and symptoms improved substantially or resolved with treatment in all cases. There are insufficient data on the incidence of these events after drug-free intervals of 1 to 2 years. These events have been observed only infrequently in clinical studies and post-marketing surveillance with retreatment intervals up to 1 year.

Infections

In REMICADE clinical studies, treated infections were reported in 35% of REMICADE-treated patients (average of 53 weeks of follow-up) and in 26% of placebo-treated patients (average of 41 weeks of follow-up). When longer observation of patients on REMICADE was accounted for, the event rate was similar for both groups. The infections most frequently reported were respiratory tract infections (including sinusitis, pharyngitis, and bronchitis) and urinary tract infections. No increased risk of serious infections or sepsis was observed with REMICADE compared with placebo in clinical studies. Among REMICADE-treated patients, serious infections included pneumonia, cellulitis, abscess, skin ulceration, sepsis, and bacterial infection. Three opportunistic infections were reported; coccidioidomycosis (which resulted in death), nocardiosis and cytomegalovirus. Tuberculosis was reported in two patients, one of whom died due to miliary tuberculosis. Other cases of tuberculosis, including disseminated tuberculosis, also have been reported post-marketing. Most of the cases of tuberculosis occurred within the first two months after initiation of therapy with infliximab and may reflect recrudescence of latent disease (see WARNINGS, RISK OF INFECTIONS). During the 54 week ACCENT II trial, 15% of patients with fistulizing Crohn's disease developed a new fistula-related abscess.

In post-marketing experience, infections have been observed with various pathogens including viral, bacterial, fungal, and protozoal organisms. Infections have been noted in all organ systems and have been reported in patients receiving REMICADE alone or in combination with immunosuppressive agents.

Autoantibodies/Lupus-like Syndrome

Approximately 52% of 1261 infliximab-treated patients in clinical trials who were antinuclear antibody (ANA) negative at baseline developed a positive ANA during the trial compared with approximately 19% of 129 placebo-treated patients. Anti-dsDNA antibodies were newly detected in approximately 17% of 1507 infliximab-treated patients compared with 0% of 162 placebo-treated patients. Reports of lupus and lupus-like syndromes, however, remain uncommon.

Malignancies/Lymphoproliferative Disease

In completed clinical studies of REMICADE for up to 102 weeks, 18 of 1678 patients developed 19 new or recurrent malignancies of various types, such as non-Hodgkin's B-cell lymphoma, breast, melanoma, squamous, rectal and basal cell. There are insufficient data to determine whether REMICADE contributed to the development of these malignancies. The observed rates and incidences were similar to those expected for the populations studied[11,12] (see PRECAUTIONS, Malignancy).

Patients with Heart Failure

In a randomized study evaluating REMICADE in moderate to severe heart failure (NYHA Class III/IV; left ventricular ejection fraction ≤35%), 150 patients were randomized to receive treatment with 3 infusions of REMICADE 10 mg/kg, 5 mg/kg, or placebo, at 0, 2, and 6 weeks. Higher incidences of mortality and hospitalization due to worsening heart failure were observed in patients receiving the 10 mg/kg REMICADE dose. At 1 year, 8 patients in the 10 mg/kg REMICADE group had died compared with 4 deaths each in the 5 mg/kg REMICADE and the placebo groups. There were trends towards increased dyspnea, hypotension, angina, and dizziness in both the 10 mg/kg and 5 mg/kg REMICADE treatment groups, versus placebo. REMICADE has not been studied in patients with mild heart failure (NYHA Class I/II). (See CONTRAINDICATIONS and WARNINGS, Patients with Heart Failure.)

Immunogenicity

Treatment with REMICADE can be associated with the development of antibodies to infliximab. The incidence of antibodies to infliximab in patients given a 3-dose induction regimen followed by maintenance dosing was approximately 10% as assessed through one to two years of REMICADE treatment. A higher incidence of antibodies to infliximab was observed in Crohn's disease patients receiving REMICADE after drug free intervals >16 weeks. The majority of antibody-positive patients had low titers. Patients who were antibody-positive were more likely to experience an infusion reaction (see ADVERSE REACTIONS, Infusion-related Reactions). Antibody development was lower among rheumatoid arthritis and Crohn's disease patients receiving immunosuppressant therapies such as 6-MP/AZA or MTX.

The data reflect the percentage of patients whose test results were positive for antibodies to infliximab in an ELISA assay, and are highly dependent on the sensitivity and specificity of the assay. Additionally, the observed incidence of antibody positivity in an assay may be influenced by several factors including sample handling, timing of sample collection, concomitant medication, and underlying disease. For these reasons, comparison of the incidence of antibodies to infliximab with the incidence of antibodies to other products may be misleading.

Other Adverse Reactions

Safety data are available from 1678 REMICADE-treated patients, including 555 with rheumatoid arthritis, and 1106 with Crohn's disease and 17 with conditions other than rheumatoid arthritis or Crohn's disease. Adverse events reported in ≥5% of all patients with rheumatoid arthritis receiving 4 or more infusions are in Table 5. The types and frequencies of adverse reactions observed were similar in REMICADE-treated rheumatoid arthritis and Crohn's disease patients except for abdominal pain which occurred in 26% of REMICADE-treated patients with Crohn's disease. In the Crohn's disease studies, there were insufficient numbers and duration of follow-up for patients who never received REMICADE to provide meaningful comparisons.

Table 5
ADVERSE EVENTS OCCURRING IN 5% OR MORE OF PATIENTS RECEIVING 4 OR MORE INFUSIONS FOR RHEUMATOID ARTHRITIS

	Placebo (n=81)	REMICADE (n=430)
Average weeks of follow-up	73	82
Gastrointestinal		
Abdominal pain	12%	17%
Nausea	23%	24%
Diarrhea	19%	19%
Dyspepsia	9%	10%
Respiratory		
Upper respiratory tract infection	35%	40%
Pharyngitis	12%	17%
Sinusitis	7%	20%
Coughing	9%	18%
Rhinitis	14%	14%
Dyspnea	2%	6%
Skin and appendages disorders		
Rash	7%	18%
Pruritis	2%	9%
Body as a whole–general disorders		
Fatigue	9%	13%
Chest pain	6%	7%
Resistance mechanism disorders		
Fever	11%	13%
Abscess	5%	6%
Moniliasis	2%	8%
Central and peripheral nervous system disorders		
Headache	21%	29%
Musculoskeletal system disorders		
Arthralgia	7%	13%
Back pain	5%	13%
Psychiatric disorders		
Insomnia	4%	6%
Depression	2%	8%
Urinary system disorders		
Urinary tract infection	12%	14%
Cardiovascular disorders, general		
Hypertension	6%	10%

Because clinical trials are conducted under widely varying conditions, adverse reaction rates observed in clinical trials of a drug cannot be directly compared to rates in clinical trials of another drug and may not predict the rates observed in broader patient populations in clinical practice.

The most common serious adverse events observed in clinical trials were infections (see ADVERSE REACTIONS, Infections). Other serious, medically relevant adverse events ≥0.2% or clinically significant adverse events by body system were as follows:

Body as a whole: allergic reaction, diaphragmatic hernia, edema, surgical/procedural sequela

Blood: pancytopenia

Cardiovascular: circulatory failure, hypotension, syncope

Gastrointestinal: constipation, gastrointestinal hemorrhage, ileus, intestinal obstruction, intestinal perforation, intestinal stenosis, pancreatitis, peritonitis, proctalgia

Central & Peripheral Nervous: meningitis, neuritis, peripheral neuropathy, dizziness

Heart Rate and Rhythm: arrhythmia, bradycardia, cardiac arrest, tachycardia

Liver and Biliary: biliary pain, cholecystitis, cholelithiasis, hepatitis

Metabolic and Nutritional: dehydration

Musculoskeletal: intervertebral disk herniation, tendon disorder

Myo-, Endo-, Pericardial and Coronary Valve: myocardial infarction

Platelet, Bleeding and Clotting: thrombocytopenia

Neoplasms: basal cell, breast, lymphoma

Psychiatric: confusion, suicide attempt

Red Blood Cell: anemia, hemolytic anemia

Reproductive: menstrual irregularity
Resistance Mechanism: cellulitis, sepsis, serum sickness
Respiratory: adult respiratory distress syndrome, lower respiratory tract infection, pleural effusion, pleurisy, pulmonary edema, respiratory insufficiency
Skin and Appendages: increased sweating, ulceration
Urinary: renal calculus, renal failure
Vascular (Extracardiac): brain infarction, pulmonary embolism, thrombophlebitis
White Cell and Reticuloendothelial: leukopenia, lymphadenopathy

A greater proportion of patients enrolled into the ATTRACT study who received REMICADE + MTX experienced transient mild (<2 times the upper limit of normal) or moderate (≥2 but <3 times the upper limit of normal) elevations in AST or ALT (49% and 47%, respectively) compared to patients treated with placebo + MTX (27% and 35%, respectively). Six (1.8%) patients treated with REMICADE + MTX experienced more prolonged elevations in their ALT.

The following adverse events have been reported during post-approval use of REMICADE: neutropenia (see WARNINGS, Hematologic Events), interstitial pneumonitis/fibrosis, idiopathic thrombocytopenic purpura, thrombotic thrombocytopenic purpura, pericardial effusion, systemic and cutaneous vasculitis, Guillain-Barré syndrome, transverse myelitis, and neuropathies (additional neurologic events have also been observed, see WARNINGS, Neurologic Events). Because these events are reported voluntarily from a population of uncertain size, it is not always possible to reliably estimate their frequency or establish a causal relationship to REMICADE exposure.

OVERDOSAGE

Single doses up to 20 mg/kg have been administered without any direct toxic effect. In case of overdosage, it is recommended that the patient be monitored for any signs or symptoms of adverse reactions or effects and appropriate symptomatic treatment instituted immediately.

DOSAGE AND ADMINISTRATION

Rheumatoid Arthritis

The recommended dose of REMICADE is 3 mg/kg given as an intravenous infusion followed with additional similar doses at 2 and 6 weeks after the first infusion then every 8 weeks thereafter. REMICADE should be given in combination with methotrexate. For patients who have an incomplete response, consideration may be given to adjusting the dose up to 10 mg/kg or treating as often as every 4 weeks.

Crohn's Disease or Fistulizing Crohn's Disease

The recommended dose of REMICADE is 5 mg/kg given as an induction regimen at 0, 2 and 6 weeks followed by a maintenance regimen of 5 mg/kg every 8 weeks thereafter for the treatment of moderately to severely active Crohn's disease or fistulizing disease. For patients who respond and then lose their response, consideration may be given to treatment with 10 mg/kg. Patients who do not respond by week 14 are unlikely to respond with continued dosing and consideration should be given to discontinue REMICADE in these patients.

Preparation and Administration Instructions

Use aseptic technique.

REMICADE vials do not contain antibacterial preservatives. Therefore, the vials after reconstitution should be used immediately, not re-entered or stored. The diluent to be used for reconstitution is 10 mL of Sterile Water for Injection, USP. The total dose of the reconstituted product must be further diluted to 250 mL with 0.9% Sodium Chloride Injection, USP. The infusion concentration should range between 0.4 mg/mL and 4 mg/mL. The REMICADE infusion should begin within 3 hours of preparation.

1. Calculate the dose and the number of REMICADE vials needed. Each REMICADE vial contains 100 mg of infliximab. Calculate the total volume of reconstituted REMICADE solution required.
2. Reconstitute each REMICADE vial with 10 mL of Sterile Water for Injection, USP, using a syringe equipped with a 21-gauge or smaller needle. Remove the flip-top from the vial and wipe the top with an alcohol swab. Insert the syringe needle into the vial through the center of the rubber stopper and direct the stream of Sterile Water for Injection, USP, to the glass wall of the vial. Do not use the vial if the vacuum is not present. Gently swirl the solution by rotating the vial to dissolve the lyophilized powder. Avoid prolonged or vigorous agitation. DO NOT SHAKE. Foaming of the solution on reconstitution is not unusual. Allow the reconstituted solution to stand for 5 minutes. The solution should be colorless to light yellow and opalescent, and the solution may develop a few translucent particles as infliximab is a protein. Do not use if opaque particles, discoloration, or other foreign particles are present.
3. Dilute the total volume of the reconstituted REMICADE solution dose to 250 mL with 0.9% Sodium Chloride Injection, USP, by withdrawing a volume of 0.9% Sodium Chloride Injection, USP, equal to the volume of reconstituted REMICADE from the 0.9% Sodium Chloride Injection, USP, 250 mL bottle or bag. Slowly add the total volume of reconstituted REMICADE solution to the 250 mL infusion bottle or bag. Gently mix.
4. The infusion solution must be administered over a period of not less than 2 hours and must use an infusion set with an in-line, sterile, non-pyrogenic, low-protein-binding filter (pore size of 1.2 µm or less). Any unused portion of the infusion solution should not be stored for reuse.
5. No physical biochemical compatibility studies have been conducted to evaluate the co-administration of REMICADE with other agents. REMICADE should not be infused concomitantly in the same intravenous line with other agents.
6. Parenteral drug products should be inspected visually for particulate matter and discoloration prior to administration, whenever solution and container permit. If visibly opaque particles, discoloration or other foreign particulates are observed, the solution should not be used.

Storage

Store the lyophilized product under refrigeration at 2°C to 8°C (36°F to 46°F). Do not freeze. Do not use beyond the expiration date. This product contains no preservative.

HOW SUPPLIED

REMICADE lyophilized concentrate for IV injection is supplied in individually-boxed single-use vials in the following strength:

NDC 57894-030-01 100 mg infliximab in a 20 mL vial

REFERENCES

1. American Thoracic Society, Centers for Disease Control and Prevention. Targeted tuberculin testing and treatment of latent tuberculosis infection. *Am J Respir Crit Care Med* 2000;161:S221-S247.
2. Knight DM, Trinh H, Le J, et al. Construction and initial characterization of a mouse-human chimeric anti-TNF antibody. *Molec Immunol* 1993;30:1443-1453.
3. Scallon BJ, Moore MA, Trinh H, et al. Chimeric anti-TNFα monoclonal antibody cA2 binds recombinant transmembrane TNFα and activates immune effector functions. *Cytokine* 1995;7:251-259.
4. ten Hove T, van Montfrans C, Peppelenbosch MP, et al. Infliximab treatment induces apoptosis of lamina propria T lymphocytes in Crohn's disease. *Gut* 2002;50:206-211.
5. Maini RN, Breedveld FC, Kalden JR, et al. Therapeutic efficacy of multiple intravenous infusions of anti-tumor necrosis factor α monoclonal antibody combined with low-dose weekly methotrexate in rheumatoid arthritis. *Arthritis Rheum* 1998;41(9):1552-1563.
6. Elliott MJ, Maini RN, Feldmann M, et al. Randomised double-blind comparison of chimeric monoclonal antibody to tumour necrosis factor alpha (cA2) vs. placebo in rheumatoid arthritis. *Lancet* 1994;344(8930):1105-1110.
7. Van der Heijde DM, van Leeuwen MA, van Riel PL, et al. Biannual radiographic assessments of hands and feet in a three-year prospective follow-up of patients with early rheumatoid arthritis. *Arthritis Rheum* 1992; 35(1):26-34.
8. Targan SR, Hanauer SR, van Deventer SJH, et al. A short-term study of chimeric monoclonal antibody cA2 to tumor necrosis factor α for Crohn's disease. *N Engl J Med* 1997;337(15):1029-1035.
9. Hanauer SB, Feagan BG, Lichtenstein GR, et al. Maintenance infliximab for Crohn's disease: the ACCENT I randomized trial. *Lancet* 2002; 359:1541-1549.
10. Present DH, Rutgeerts P, Targan S, et al. Infliximab for the treatment of fistulas in patients with Crohn's disease. *N Engl J Med* 1999;340:1398-1405.
11. Bernstein C, Blanchard JF, Kliewer E, et al. Cancer risk in patients with inflammatory bowel disease. *Cancer* 2001;91:854-862.
12. Jones M, Symmons D, Finn J, et al. Does exposure to immunosuppressive therapy increase the 10 year malignancy and mortality risks in rheumatoid arthritis? A matched cohort study. *Br J Rheum.* 1996;35:738-745.

Malvern, PA 19355, USA License #1242
1-800-457-6399 Revised July 2004
Rx Only

REMICADE® (infliximab)
Patient Information Sheet

You should read this information sheet before you start using REMICADE® (pronounced rem-eh-kaid) and before each time you are scheduled to receive REMICADE. This information sheet does not take the place of talking with your doctor. You and your doctor should talk about your health and how you are feeling before you start taking REMICADE, while you are taking it and at regular checkups. If you do not understand any of the information in this sheet, you should ask your doctor to explain what it means.

What is REMICADE?

REMICADE is a medicine that is used to treat adults with moderate to severely active rheumatoid arthritis and Crohn's disease. Your doctor has decided to treat you with REMICADE because your disease is still active even though you have tried other treatments.

How does REMICADE work?

The medicine REMICADE is a type of protein that recognizes, attaches to and blocks the action of a substance in your body called tumor necrosis factor. Tumor necrosis factor (TNF) is made by certain blood cells in your body. REMICADE will not cure rheumatoid arthritis or Crohn's disease, but blocking TNF with REMICADE may reduce the inflammation caused by too much TNF in your body. You should also know that REMICADE may help you feel better but can also cause serious side effects and can reduce your body's ability to fight infections (see below).

What should I know about the immune system, and taking REMICADE for Rheumatoid Arthritis or Crohn's Disease?

The immune system protects the body by responding to "invaders" like bacteria, viruses and other foreign matter that enter your body by producing antibodies and putting them into action to fight off the "invaders." In diseases like rheumatoid arthritis and Crohn's disease, your body's immune system produces too much TNF. Too much TNF can cause your immune system to attack healthy tissues in your body and cause inflammation. If this condition is left untreated, it can cause permanent damage to the body's bones, cartilage and tissue.

While taking REMICADE can block the TNF that causes inflammation, it can also lower your body's ability to fight infections. So, taking REMICADE can make you more prone to getting infections or it can make an infection that you already have worse. You should call your doctor right away if you think you have an infection.

What important information should I know about treatment with REMICADE?

REMICADE, like other medicines that affect your immune system, is a strong medicine that can cause serious side effects. Possible serious side effects include:

Serious Infections:

- Some patients have had serious infections while receiving REMICADE. Some of the patients have died from these infections. Serious infections include TB (tuberculosis), and infections caused by viruses, fungi or bacteria that have spread throughout the body. If you develop a fever, feel very tired, have a cough, or have flu-like symptoms, these could be signs that you may be getting an infection. If you have any of these symptoms while you are taking or after you have taken REMICADE, you should tell your doctor right away.

Heart Failure:

- If you have been told that you have a heart problem called congestive heart failure and you are currently being treated with REMICADE, you will need to be closely monitored by your doctor. If you develop new or worse symptoms that are related to your heart condition, such as shortness of breath or swelling of your ankles or feet, you must contact your doctor immediately.

Blood Problems:

- In some patients the body may fail to produce enough of the blood cells that help your body fight infections or help you stop bleeding. Some of the patients have died from this failure to produce blood cells. If you develop a fever that doesn't go away, bruise or bleed very easily or look very pale, call your doctor right away. Your doctor may decide to stop your treatment.

Allergic Reactions:

- Some patients have had severe allergic reactions to REMICADE. These reactions can happen while you are getting your REMICADE infusion or shortly afterwards. The symptoms of an allergic reaction may include hives (red, raised, itchy patches of skin), difficulty breathing, chest pain and high or low blood pressure. Your doctor may decide to stop REMICADE treatment and give you medicines to treat the allergic reaction.
- Some patients who have been taking REMICADE for Crohn's disease have had allergic reactions 3 to 12 days after receiving their REMICADE treatment. The symptoms of this type of delayed reaction may include fever, rash, headache and muscle or joint pain. Call your doctor right away if you develop any of these symptoms or any other unusual symptoms such as difficulty swallowing.

Nervous System Disorders:

- There have been rare cases where people taking REMICADE or other TNF blockers have developed disorders that affected their nervous system. Signs that you could be having a problem include: changes in your vision, weakness in your arms and/or legs, and numbness or tingling in any part of your body.

Other Important Information

People who have been treated for rheumatoid arthritis or Crohn's disease for a long time tend to be more prone to a type of blood cancer called lymphoma. There have been some patients that while taking REMICADE developed other types of cancer, but, the number of people taking REMICADE that developed cancer does not seem to be much different from what you would expect to see in people who are not taking REMICADE.

Some patients have developed symptoms that can resemble a disease called lupus. Lupus-like symptoms may include chest discomfort or pain that doesn't go away, shortness of breath, joint pain, or a rash on the cheeks or arms that gets worse in the sun. If you develop any of these symptoms your doctor may decide to stop your treatment with REMICADE.

What are the more common side effects of REMICADE?

The more common side effects with REMICADE are respiratory infections (that may include sinus infections and sore throat), coughing and stomach pain.

Who should not take REMICADE?

YOU SHOULD NOT take REMICADE if you have:

- Heart failure, unless your doctor has talked to you and decided that you are able to take REMICADE.
- Had an allergic reaction to REMICADE or any other product that was made with murine (mouse) proteins.

What health concerns should I talk to my doctor about?

Before receiving your first treatment with REMICADE you should tell your doctor if you:

- Have or think you may have any kind of infection. The infection could be in only one place in your body (such as an open cut or sore), or an infection that affects your whole body (such as the flu). Having an infection could put you at risk for serious side effects from REMICADE.

Continued on next page

Remicade—Cont.

- Have an infection that won't go away or a history of infection that keeps coming back.
- Have had TB (tuberculosis), or if you have recently been with anyone who might have TB. Your doctor will examine you for TB and perform a skin test. If your doctor feels that you are at risk for TB, he or she may start treating you for TB before you begin REMICADE therapy.
- Have lived in or visited an area of the country where an infection called histoplasmosis or coccidioidomycosis (an infection caused by a fungus that affects the lungs) is common. If you don't know if the area you live in is one where histoplasmosis or coccidioidomycosis is common, ask your doctor.
- Have or have previously had heart failure or other heart conditions.
- Have or have had a condition that affects your nervous system, like multiple sclerosis, or Guillain-Barré syndrome, or if you experience any numbness, or tingling, or have had a seizure.
- Are pregnant or nursing.
- Have recently received or are scheduled to receive a vaccine.

Can I take REMICADE while I am on other medicines?
Tell your doctor if you are taking any other medicines including over the counter medicines, supplements or herbal products before you are treated with REMICADE. If you start taking or plan to start taking any new medicine while you are taking REMICADE, tell your doctor.
REMICADE and KINERET should not be taken together.

How will REMICADE be given to me?
REMICADE will be given to you by a healthcare professional. REMICADE will be given to you by an IV. This means that the medicine will be given to you through a needle placed in a vein in your arm. It will take about 2 hours to give you the full dose of medicine. During that time and for a period after you receive REMICADE, you will be monitored by a healthcare professional. Your doctor may ask you to take other medicines along with REMICADE.
Only a health care professional should prepare the medicine and administer it to you.

How often will I receive REMICADE?
Rheumatoid Arthritis
If you are receiving REMICADE for rheumatoid arthritis you will receive your first dose followed by additional doses at 2 and 6 weeks after the first dose. You will then receive a dose every 8 weeks. Your doctor will monitor your response to REMICADE and may change your dose or dose you more frequently (as often as every 4 weeks).
Crohn's Disease or Fistulizing Crohn's Disease
If you are receiving REMICADE for active Crohn's disease or fistulizing Crohn's disease, you will receive your first dose followed by additional doses at 2 and 6 weeks after the first dose. You will then receive a dose every 8 weeks. Your doctor will monitor your response to REMICADE and may change your dose.

What if I still have questions?
If you have any questions, or problems, always talk first with your doctor. You can also visit the REMICADE internet site at www.remicade.com.
Product developed and manufactured by:
Centocor, Inc.
200 Great Valley Parkway
Malvern, PA 19355
Revised July 2004
IN04240

Shown in Product Identification Guide, page 310

Cephalon, Inc.
145 BRANDYWINE PARKWAY
WEST CHESTER, PA 19380

For Medical Information and Adverse Drug Experience/Product Complaint Reporting Contact:
(800) 896-5855
Fax 610-738-6669

ACTIQ® Ⓒ℞
[āk' tĕk]
(oral transmucosal fentanyl citrate)

PHYSICIANS AND OTHER HEALTHCARE PROVIDERS MUST BECOME FAMILIAR WITH THE IMPORTANT WARNINGS IN THIS LABEL.
***Actiq* is indicated only for the management of breakthrough cancer pain in patients with malignancies who are already receiving and who are tolerant to opioid therapy for their underlying persistent cancer pain.**
Patients considered opioid tolerant are those who are taking at least 60 mg morphine/day, 50 mcg transdermal fentanyl/hour, or an equianalgesic dose of another opioid for a week or longer.
Because life-threatening hypoventilation could occur at any dose in patients not taking chronic opiates, *Actiq* is contraindicated in the management of acute or postoperative pain. This product **must not** be used in opioid non-tolerant patients.
Actiq is intended to be used only in the care of cancer patients and only by oncologists and pain specialists who are knowledgeable of and skilled in the use of Schedule II opioids to treat cancer pain.
Patients and their caregivers must be instructed that *Actiq* contains a medicine in an amount which can be fatal to a child. Patients and their caregivers must be instructed to keep all units out of the reach of children and to discard opened units properly. (See Information for Patients and Their Caregivers for disposal instructions.)

WARNING: May be habit forming

DESCRIPTION
Actiq (oral transmucosal fentanyl citrate) is a solid formulation of fentanyl citrate, a potent opioid analgesic, intended for oral transmucosal administration. *Actiq* is formulated as a white to off-white solid drug matrix on a handle that is radiopaque and is fracture resistant (ABS plastic) under normal conditions when used as directed.
Actiq is designed to be dissolved slowly in the mouth in a manner to facilitate transmucosal absorption. The handle allows the *Actiq* unit to be removed from the mouth if signs of excessive opioid effects appear during administration.
Active Ingredient: Fentanyl citrate, USP is N-(1-Phenethyl-4-piperidyl) propionanilide citrate (1:1). Fentanyl is a highly lipophilic compound (octanol-water partition coefficient at pH 7.4 is 816:1) that is freely soluble in organic solvents and sparingly soluble in water (1:40). The molecular weight of the free base is 336.5 (the citrate salt is 528.6). The pKa of the tertiary nitrogens are 7.3 and 8.4. The compound has the following structural formula:

CH_3CH_2CON–(piperidine)–$N\text{-}CH_2CH_2$–(phenyl) • $HO\text{-}C\text{-}COOH$ (CH_2COOH, CH_2COOH)

Actiq is available in six strengths equivalent to 200, 400, 600, 800, 1200, or 1600 mcg fentanyl base that is identified by the text on the solid drug matrix, the dosage unit handle tag, the blister package, and the shelf carton.
Inactive Ingredients: Hydrated dextrates, citric acid, dibasic sodium phosphate, artificial berry flavor, magnesium stearate, modified food starch, and confectioner's sugar.

CLINICAL PHARMACOLOGY AND PHARMACOKINETICS
Pharmacology:
Fentanyl, a pure opioid agonist, acts primarily through interaction with opioid mu-receptors located in the brain, spinal cord and smooth muscle. The primary site of therapeutic action is the central nervous system (CNS). The most clinically useful pharmacologic effects of the interaction of fentanyl with mu-receptors are analgesia and sedation.
Other opioid effects may include somnolence, hypoventilation, bradycardia, postural hypotension, pruritus, dizziness, nausea, diaphoresis, flushing, euphoria and confusion or difficulty in concentrating at clinically relevant doses.

Clinical Pharmacology
Analgesia:
The analgesic effects of fentanyl are related to the blood level of the drug, if proper allowance is made for the delay into and out of the CNS (a process with a 3-to-5-minute half-life). In opioid non-tolerant individuals, fentanyl provides effects ranging from analgesia at blood levels of 1 to 2 ng/mL, all the way to surgical anesthesia and profound respiratory depression at levels of 10-20 ng/mL.
In general, the minimum effective concentration and the concentration at which toxicity occurs rise with increasing tolerance to any and all opioids. The rate of development of tolerance varies widely among individuals. As a result, the dose of *Actiq* should be individually titrated to achieve the desired effect (see **DOSAGE AND ADMINISTRATION**).
Gastrointestinal (GI) Tract and Other Smooth Muscle:
Opioids increase the tone and decrease contractions of the smooth muscle of the gastrointestinal (GI) tract. This results in prolongation in GI transit time and may be responsible for the constipating effect of opioids. Because opioids may increase biliary tract pressure, some patients with biliary colic may experience worsening of pain.
While opioids generally increase the tone of urinary tract smooth muscle, the overall effect tends to vary, in some cases producing urinary urgency, in others, difficulty in urination.
Respiratory System:
All opioid mu-receptor agonists, including fentanyl, produce dose dependent respiratory depression. The risk of respiratory depression is less in patients receiving chronic opioid therapy who develop tolerance to respiratory depression and other opioid effects. During the titration phase of the clinical trials, somnolence, which may be a precursor to respiratory depression, did increase in patients who were treated with higher doses of *Actiq*. In studies of opioid non-tolerant subjects, respiratory rate and oxygen saturation typically decrease as fentanyl blood concentration increases. Typically, peak respiratory depressive effects (decrease in respiratory rate) are seen 15 to 30 minutes from the start of oral transmucosal fentanyl citrate (OTFC®) administration and may persist for several hours.
Serious or fatal respiratory depression can occur, even at recommended doses, in vulnerable individuals. As with other potent opioids, fentanyl has been associated with cases of serious and fatal respiratory depression in opioid non-tolerant individuals.
Fentanyl depresses the cough reflex as a result of its CNS activity. Although not observed with *Actiq* in clinical trials, fentanyl given rapidly by intravenous injection in large doses may interfere with respiration by causing rigidity in the muscles of respiration. Therefore, physicians and other healthcare providers should be aware of this potential complication. **(See BOX WARNING, CONTRAINDICATIONS, WARNINGS, PRECAUTIONS, ADVERSE REACTIONS, and OVERDOSAGE for additional information on hypoventilation.)**
Pharmacokinetics
Absorption:
The absorption pharmacokinetics of fentanyl from the oral transmucosal dosage form is a combination of an initial rapid absorption from the buccal mucosa and a more prolonged absorption of swallowed fentanyl from the GI tract. Both the blood fentanyl profile and the bioavailability of fentanyl will vary depending on the fraction of the dose that is absorbed through the oral mucosa and the fraction swallowed.
Absolute bioavailability, as determined by area under the concentration-time curve, of 15 mcg/kg in 12 adult males was 50% compared to intravenous fentanyl.
Normally, approximately 25% of the total dose of *Actiq* is rapidly absorbed from the buccal mucosa and becomes systemically available. The remaining 75% of the total dose is swallowed with the saliva and then is slowly absorbed from the GI tract. About 1/3 of this amount (25% of the total dose) escapes hepatic and intestinal first-pass elimination and becomes systemically available. Thus, the generally observed 50% bioavailability of *Actiq* is divided equally between rapid transmucosal and slower GI absorption. Therefore, a unit dose of *Actiq*, if chewed and swallowed, might result in lower peak concentrations and lower bioavailability than when consumed as directed.
Dose proportionality among four of the available strengths of *Actiq* (200, 400, 800, and 1600 mcg) has been demonstrated in a balanced crossover design in adult subjects. Mean serum fentanyl levels following these four doses of *Actiq* are shown in Figure 1. The curves for each dose level are similar in shape with increasing dose levels producing increasing serum fentanyl levels. C_{max} and $AUC_{0\rightarrow\infty}$ increased in a dose-dependent manner that is approximately proportional to the *Actiq* administered.

Figure 1.
Mean Serum Fentanyl Concentration (ng/mL) in Adult Subjects Comparing 4 Doses of *Actiq*

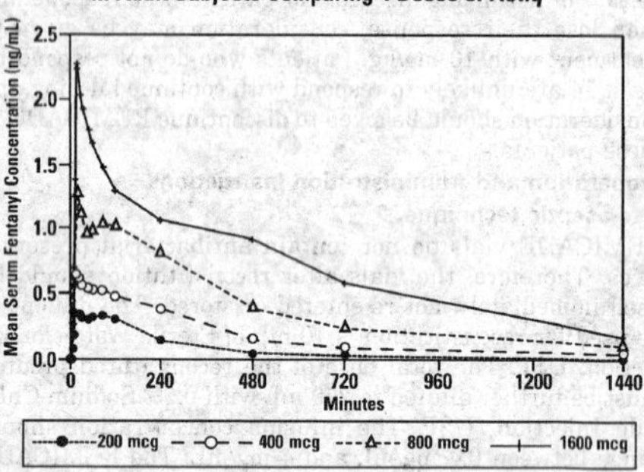

The pharmacokinetic parameters of the four strengths of *Actiq* tested in the dose-proportionality study are shown in Table 1. The mean C_{max} ranged from 0.39–2.51 ng/mL. The median time of maximum plasma concentration (T_{max}) across these four doses of *Actiq* varied from 20-40 minutes (range of 20-480 minutes) as measured after the start of administration.
[See table 1 at top of next page]
Distribution:
Fentanyl is highly lipophilic. Animal data showed that following absorption, fentanyl is rapidly distributed to the brain, heart, lungs, kidneys and spleen followed by a slower redistribution to muscles and fat. The plasma protein binding of fentanyl is 80-85%. The main binding protein is alpha-1-acid glycoprotein, but both albumin and lipoproteins contribute to some extent. The free fraction of fentanyl increases with acidosis. The mean volume of distribution at steady state (Vss) was 4 L/kg.
Metabolism:
Fentanyl is metabolized in the liver and in the intestinal mucosa to norfentanyl by cytochrome P450 3A4 isoform. Norfentanyl was not found to be pharmacologically active in animal studies (see **PRECAUTIONS: Drug Interactions** for additional information).
Elimination:
Fentanyl is primarily (more than 90%) eliminated by biotransformation to N-dealkylated and hydroxylated inactive metabolites. Less than 7% of the dose is excreted unchanged in the urine, and only about 1% is excreted unchanged in the feces. The metabolites are mainly excreted in the urine, while fecal excretion is less important. The total plasma clearance of fentanyl was 0.5 L/hr/kg (range 0.3–0.7 L/hr/kg). The terminal elimination half-life after OTFC administration is about 7 hours.

Special Populations:

Elderly Patients:

Elderly patients have been shown to be twice as sensitive to the effects of fentanyl when administered intravenously, compared with the younger population. While a formal study evaluating the safety profile of *Actiq* in the elderly population has not been performed, in the 257 opioid tolerant cancer patients studied with *Actiq*, approximately 20% were over age 65 years. No difference was noted in the safety profile in this group compared to those aged less than 65 years, though they did titrate to lower doses than younger patients (see **PRECAUTIONS**).

Patients with Renal or Hepatic Impairment:

Actiq should be administered with caution to patients with liver or kidney dysfunction because of the importance of these organs in the metabolism and excretion of drugs and effects on plasma-binding proteins (see **PRECAUTIONS**). Although fentanyl kinetics are known to be altered in both hepatic and renal disease due to alterations in metabolic clearance and plasma proteins, individualized doses of *Actiq* have been used successfully for breakthrough cancer pain in patients with hepatic and renal disorders. The duration of effect for the initial dose of fentanyl is determined by redistribution of the drug, such that diminished metabolic clearance may only become significant with repeated dosing or with excessively large single doses. For these reasons, while doses titrated to clinical effect are recommended for all patients, special care should be taken in patients with severe hepatic or renal disease.

Gender

Both male and female opioid-tolerant cancer patients were studied for the treatment of breakthrough cancer pain. No clinically relevant gender differences were noted either in dosage requirement or in observed adverse events.

CLINICAL TRIALS

Breakthrough Cancer Pain:

Actiq was investigated in clinical trials involving 257 opioid tolerant adult cancer patients experiencing breakthrough cancer pain. Breakthrough cancer pain was defined as a transient flare of moderate-to-severe pain occurring in cancer patients experiencing persistent cancer pain otherwise controlled with maintenance doses of opioid medications including at least 60 mg morphine/day, 50 mcg transdermal fentanyl/hour, or an equianalgesic dose of another opioid for a week or longer.

In two dose titration studies 95 of 127 patients (75%) who were on stable doses of either long-acting oral opioids or transdermal fentanyl for their persistent cancer pain titrated to a successful dose of *Actiq* to treat their breakthrough cancer pain within the dose range offered (200, 400, 600, 800, 1200 and 1600 mcg). In these studies 11% of patients withdrew due to adverse events and 14% withdrew due to other reasons. A "successful" dose was defined as a dose where one unit of *Actiq* could be used consistently for at least two consecutive days to treat breakthrough cancer pain without unacceptable side effects.

The successful dose of *Actiq* for breakthrough cancer pain was not predicted from the daily maintenance dose of opioid used to manage the persistent cancer pain and is thus best determined by dose titration.

A double-blind placebo controlled crossover study was performed in cancer patients to evaluate the effectiveness of *Actiq* for the treatment of breakthrough cancer pain. Of 130 patients who entered the study 92 patients (71%) achieved a successful dose during the titration phase. The distribution of successful doses is shown in Table 2.

Table 2.
Successful Dose of *Actiq* Following Initial Titration

Actiq Dose	Total No (%) (N=92)
200 mcg	13 (14)
400 mcg	19 (21)
600 mcg	14 (15)
800 mcg	18 (20)
1200 mcg	13 (14)
1600 mcg	15 (16)
Mean±SD	789±468 mcg

On average, patients over 65 years of age titrated to a mean dose that was about 200 mcg less than the mean dose to which younger adult patients were titrated.

Actiq produced statistically significantly more pain relief compared with placebo at 15, 30, 45 and 60 minutes following administration (see Figure 2).

[See figure 2 at top of next column]

In this same study patients also rated the performance of medication to treat their breakthrough cancer pain using a different scale ranging from "poor" to "excellent." On average, placebo was rated "fair" and *Actiq* was rated "good."

INDICATIONS AND USAGE

(See BOX WARNING and CONTRAINDICATIONS)

Actiq is indicated only for the management of breakthrough cancer pain in patients with malignancies who are **already receiving and who are tolerant to opioid therapy for their underlying persistent cancer pain.** Patients considered opioid tolerant are those who are taking at least 60 mg morphine/day, 50 mcg transdermal fentanyl/hour, or an equianalgesic dose of another opioid for a week or longer.

Because life-threatening hypoventilation could occur at any dose in patients not taking chronic opiates, *Actiq* is contraindicated in the management of acute or postoperative pain. This product **must not** be used in opioid non-tolerant patients.

Table 1.
Pharmacokinetic Parameters in Adult Subjects Receiving 200, 400, 800, and 1600 mcg Units of *Actiq*

Pharmacokinetic Parameter	200 mcg	400 mcg	800 mcg	1600 mcg
T_{max}, minute median (range)	40 (20-120)	25 (20-240)	25 (20-120)	20 (20-480)
C_{max}, ng/mL mean (% CV)	0.39 (23)	0.75 (33)	1.55 (30)	2.51 (23)
AUC_{0-1440}, ng/mL minute mean (% CV)	102 (65)	243 (67)	573 (64)	1026 (67)
$t_{½}$, minute mean (% CV)	193 (48)	386 (115)	381 (55)	358 (45)

Figure 2
Pain Relief (PR) Scores (Mean±SD) During the Double-Blind Phase-All Patients with Evaluable Episodes on Both *Actiq* and Placebo (N=86)

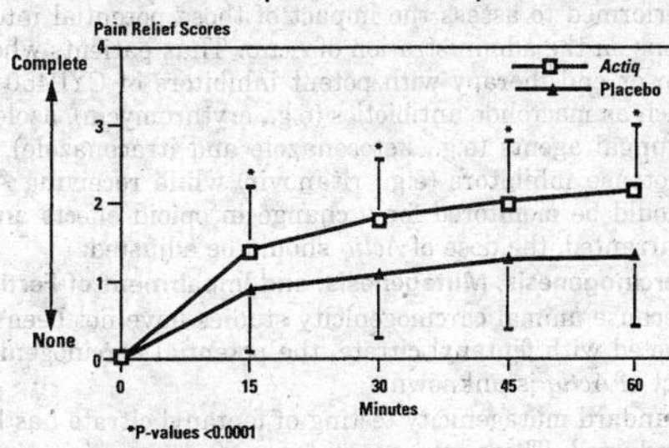

Actiq is intended to be used only in the care of cancer patients and only by oncologists and pain specialists who are knowledgeable of and skilled in the use of Schedule II opioids to treat cancer pain.

Actiq should be individually titrated to a dose that provides adequate analgesia and minimizes side effects. If signs of excessive opioid effects appear before the unit is consumed, the dosage unit should be removed from the patient's mouth immediately, disposed of properly, and subsequent doses should be decreased (see **DOSAGE AND ADMINISTRATION**).

Patients and their caregivers must be instructed that *Actiq* contains a medicine in an amount that can be fatal to a child. Patients and their caregivers must be instructed to keep all units out of the reach of children and to discard opened units properly in a secured container.

CONTRAINDICATIONS

Because life-threatening hypoventilation could occur at any dose in patients not taking chronic opiates, *Actiq* is contraindicated in the management of acute or postoperative pain. The risk of respiratory depression begins to increase with fentanyl plasma levels of 2.0 ng/mL in opioid non-tolerant individuals (see **Pharmacokinetics**). This product **must not** be used in opioid non-tolerant patients.

Patients considered opioid tolerant are those who are taking at least 60 mg morphine/day, 50 mcg transdermal fentanyl/hour, or an equianalgesic dose of another opioid for a week or longer.

Actiq is contraindicated in patients with known intolerance or hypersensitivity to any of its components or the drug fentanyl.

WARNINGS

See BOX WARNING.)

The concomitant use of other CNS depressants, including other opioids, sedatives or hypnotics, general anesthetics, phenothiazines, tranquilizers, skeletal muscle relaxants, sedating antihistamines, potent inhibitors of cytochrome P450 3A4 isoform (e.g., erythromycin, ketoconazole, and certain protease inhibitors), and alcoholic beverages may produce increased depressant effects. Hypoventilation, hypotension, and profound sedation may occur.

Actiq is not recommended for use in patients who have received MAO inhibitors within 14 days, because severe and unpredictable potentiation by MAO inhibitors has been reported with opioid analgesics.

Pediatric Use: The appropriate dosing and safety of *Actiq* in opioid tolerant children with breakthrough cancer pain have not been established below the age of 16 years.

Patients and their caregivers must be instructed that *Actiq* contains a medicine in an amount which can be fatal to a child. Patients and their caregivers must be instructed to keep both used and unused dosage units out of the reach of children. While all units should be disposed of immediately after use, partially consumed units represent a special risk to children. In the event that a unit is not completely consumed it must be properly disposed as soon as possible. (See **SAFETY AND HANDLING, PRECAUTIONS,** and **PATIENT LEAFLET** for specific patient instructions.)

Physicians and dispensing pharmacists must specifically question patients or caregivers about the presence of children in the home on a full time or visiting basis and counsel them regarding the dangers to children from inadvertent exposure.

PRECAUTIONS

General

The initial dose of *Actiq* to treat episodes of breakthrough cancer pain should be 200 mcg. Each patient should be individually titrated to provide adequate analgesia while minimizing side effects.

Opioid analgesics impair the mental and/or physical ability required for the performance of potentially dangerous tasks (e.g., driving a car or operating machinery). Patients taking *Actiq* should be warned of these dangers and should be counseled accordingly.

The use of concomitant CNS active drugs requires special patient care and observation. (See **WARNINGS.**)

Hypoventilation (Respiratory Depression)

As with all opioids, there is a risk of clinically significant hypoventilation in patients using *Actiq*. Accordingly, all patients should be followed for symptoms of respiratory depression. Hypoventilation may occur more readily when opioids are given in conjunction with other agents that depress respiration.

Chronic Pulmonary Disease

Because potent opioids can cause hypoventilation, *Actiq* should be titrated with caution in patients with chronic obstructive pulmonary disease or pre-existing medical conditions predisposing them to hypoventilation. In such patients, even normal therapeutic doses of *Actiq* may further decrease respiratory drive to the point of respiratory failure.

HEAD INJURIES AND INCREASED INTRACRANIAL PRESSURE

Actiq should only be administered with extreme caution in patients who may be particularly susceptible to the intracranial effects of CO_2 retention such as those with evidence of increased intracranial pressure or impaired consciousness. Opioids may obscure the clinical course of a patient with a head injury and should be used only if clinically warranted.

Cardiac Disease

Intravenous fentanyl may produce bradycardia. Therefore, *Actiq* should be used with caution in patients with bradyarrhythmias.

Hepatic or Renal Disease

Actiq should be administered with caution to patients with liver or kidney dysfunction because of the importance of these organs in the metabolism and excretion of drugs and effects on plasma binding proteins (see **PHARMACOKINETICS**).

Information for Patients and Their Caregivers

Patients and their caregivers must be instructed that *Actiq* contains medicine in an amount that could be fatal to a child. Patients and their caregivers must be instructed to keep both used and unused dosage units out of the reach of children. Partially consumed units represent a special risk to children. In the event that a unit is not completely consumed it must be properly disposed as soon as possible. (See **SAFETY AND HANDLING, WARNINGS,** and **PATIENT LEAFLET** for specific patient instructions.)

Frequent consumption of sugar-containing products may increase the risk of dental caries (each *Actiq* unit contains approximately 2 grams of sugar [hydrated dextrates]). The occurrence of dry mouth associated with the use of opioid medications (such as fentanyl) may add to this risk.

Post-marketing reports of dental decay have been received in patients taking *Actiq* (see **ADVERSE REACTIONS** — Post Marketing Experience). In some of these patients, dental decay occurred despite reported oral hygiene. Therefore, patients using *Actiq* should consult their dentist to ensure appropriate oral hygiene.

Diabetic patients should be advised that *Actiq* contains approximately 2 grams of sugar per unit.

Patients and their caregivers should be provided with an *Actiq* Welcome Kit, which contains educational materials and safe storage containers to help patients store *Actiq* and other medicines out of the reach of children. Patients and their caregivers should also have an opportunity to watch the patient safety video, which provides proper product use, storage, handling and disposal directions. Patients should also have an opportunity to discuss the video with their health care providers. Health care professionals should call 1-800-896-5855 to obtain a supply of welcome kits or videos for patient viewing.

Disposal of Used *Actiq* Units

Patients must be instructed to dispose of completely used and partially used *Actiq* units.

1) After consumption of the unit is complete and the matrix is totally dissolved, throw away the handle in a trash container that is out of the reach of children.
2) If any of the drug matrix remains on the handle, place the handle under hot running tap water until all of the drug matrix is dissolved, and then dispose of the handle in a place that is out of the reach of children.
3) Handles in the child-resistant container should be disposed of (as described in steps 1 and 2) at least once a day.

Continued on next page

Actiq—Cont.

If the patient does not entirely consume the unit and the remaining drug cannot be immediately dissolved under hot running water, the patient or caregiver must temporarily store the *Actiq* unit in the specially provided child-resistant container out of the reach of children until proper disposal is possible.

Disposal of Unopened *Actiq* Units When No Longer Needed

Patients and members of their household must be advised to dispose of any unopened units remaining from a prescription as soon as they are no longer needed.

To dispose of the unused *Actiq* units:

1) Remove the *Actiq* unit from its blister package using scissors, and hold the *Actiq* by its handle over the toilet bowl.
2) Using wire-cutting pliers cut off the drug matrix end so that it falls into the toilet.
3) Dispose of the handle in a place that is out of the reach of children.
4) Repeat steps 1, 2, and 3 for each *Actiq* unit. Flush the toilet twice after 5 units have been cut and deposited into the toilet.

Do not flush the entire *Actiq* units, *Actiq* handles, blister packages, or cartons down the toilet. The handle should be disposed of where children cannot reach it (see **SAFETY AND HANDLING**).

Detailed instructions for the proper storage, administration, disposal, and important instructions for managing an overdose of *Actiq* are provided in the *Actiq* Patient Leaflet. Patients should be encouraged to read this information in its entirety and be given an opportunity to have their questions answered.

In the event that a caregiver requires additional assistance in disposing of excess unusable units that remain in the home after a patient has expired, they should be instructed to call the toll-free number (1-800-896-5855) or seek assistance from their local DEA office.

Laboratory Tests

The effects of *Actiq* on laboratory tests have not been evaluated.

Drug Interactions

See **WARNINGS**.

Fentanyl is metabolized in the liver and intestinal mucosa to norfentanyl by the cytochrome P450 3A4 isoform. Drugs that inhibit P450 3A4 activity may increase the bioavailability of swallowed fentanyl (by decreasing intestinal and hepatic first pass metabolism) and may decrease the systemic clearance of fentanyl. The expected clinical results would be increased or prolonged opioid effects. Drugs that induce cytochrome P450 3A4 activity may have the opposite effects. However, no *in vitro* or *in vivo* studies have been performed to assess the impact of those potential interactions on the administration of *Actiq*. Thus patients who begin or end therapy with potent inhibitors of CYP450 3A4 such as macrolide antibiotics (e.g., erythromycin), azole antifungal agents (e.g., ketoconazole and itraconazole), and protease inhibitors (e.g., ritanovir) while receiving *Actiq* should be monitored for a change in opioid effects and, if warranted, the dose of *Actiq* should be adjusted.

Carcinogenesis, Mutagenesis, and Impairment of Fertility

Because animal carcinogenicity studies have not been conducted with fentanyl citrate, the potential carcinogenic effect of *Actiq* is unknown.

Standard mutagenicity testing of fentanyl citrate has been conducted. There was no evidence of mutagenicity in the Ames *Salmonella* or *Escherichia* mutagenicity assay, the *in-vitro* mouse lymphoma mutagenesis assay, and the *in-vivo* micronucleus cytogenetic assay in the mouse.

Reproduction studies in rats revealed a significant decrease in the pregnancy rate of all experimental groups. This decrease was most pronounced in the high dose group (1.25 mg/kg subcutaneously) in which one of twenty animals became pregnant.

Pregnancy—Category C

Fentanyl has been shown to impair fertility and to have an embryocidal effect with an increase in resorptions in rats when given for a period of 12 to 21 days in doses of 30 mcg/kg IV or 160 mcg/kg subcutaneously.

No evidence of teratogenic effects has been observed after administration of fentanyl citrate to rats. There are no adequate and well-controlled studies in pregnant women. *Actiq* should be used during pregnancy only if the potential benefit justifies the potential risk to the fetus.

Labor and Delivery

Actiq is not indicated for use in labor and delivery.

Nursing Mothers

Fentanyl is excreted in human milk; therefore *Actiq* should not be used in nursing women because of the possibility of sedation and/or respiratory depression in their infants.

Pediatric Use

See **WARNINGS**

Geriatric Use

Of the 257 patients in clinical studies of *Actiq* in breakthrough cancer pain, 61 (24%) were 65 and over, while 15 (6%) were 75 and over.

Those patients over the age of 65 titrated to a mean dose that was about 200 mcg less than the mean dose titrated to by younger patients. Previous studies with intravenous fentanyl showed that elderly patients are twice as sensitive to the effects of fentanyl as the younger population.

No difference was noted in the safety profile of the group over 65 as compared to younger patients in *Actiq* clinical trials. However, greater sensitivity in older individuals cannot be ruled out. Therefore, caution should be exercised in individually titrating *Actiq* in elderly patients to provide adequate efficacy while minimizing risk.

ADVERSE REACTIONS

Pre-Marketing Clinical Trial Experience

The safety of *Actiq* has been evaluated in 257 opioid tolerant chronic cancer pain patients. The duration of *Actiq* use varied during the open-label study. Some patients were followed for over 21 months. The average duration of therapy in the open-label study was 129 days.

The adverse events seen with *Actiq* are typical opioid side effects. Frequently, these adverse events will cease or decrease in intensity with continued use of *Actiq,* as the patient is titrated to the proper dose. Opioid side effects should be expected and managed accordingly.

The most serious adverse effects associated with all opioids are respiratory depression (potentially leading to apnea or respiratory arrest), circulatory depression, hypotension, and shock. All patients should be followed for symptoms of respiratory depression.

Because the clinical trials of *Actiq* were designed to evaluate safety and efficacy in treating breakthrough cancer pain, all patients were also taking concomitant opioids, such as sustained-release morphine or transdermal fentanyl, for their persistent cancer pain. The adverse event data presented here reflect the actual percentage of patients experiencing each adverse effect among patients who received *Actiq* for breakthrough cancer pain along with a concomitant opioid for persistent cancer pain. There has been no attempt to correct for concomitant use of other opioids, duration of *Actiq* therapy, or cancer-related symptoms. Adverse events are included regardless of causality or severity.

Three short-term clinical trials with similar titration schemes were conducted in 257 patients with malignancy and breakthrough cancer pain. Data are available for 254 of these patients. The goal of titration in these trials was to find the dose of *Actiq* that provided adequate analgesia with acceptable side effects (successful dose). Patients were titrated from a low dose to a successful dose in a manner similar to current titration dosing guidelines. Table 3 lists by dose groups, adverse events with an overall frequency of 1% or greater that occurred during titration and are commonly associated with opioid administration or are of particular clinical interest. The ability to assign a dose-response relationship to these adverse events is limited by the titration schemes used in these studies. Adverse events are listed in descending order of frequency within each body system.

[See table 3 at left]

Table 3.
Percent of Patients with Specific Adverse Events Commonly Associated with Opioid Administration or of Particular Clinical Interest Which Occurred During Titration (Events in 1% or More of Patients)

Dose Group	200-600 mcg	800-1400 mcg	1600 mcg	>1600 mcg	Any
Number of Patients	**230**	**138**	**54**	**41**	**254**
Body As A Whole					
Asthenia	6	4	0	7	9
Headache	3	4	6	5	6
Accidental Injury	1	1	4	0	2
Digestive					
Nausea	14	15	11	22	23
Vomiting	7	6	6	15	12
Constipation	1	4	2	0	4
Nervous					
Dizziness	10	16	6	15	17
Somnolence	9	9	11	20	17
Confusion	1	6	2	0	4
Anxiety	3	0	2	0	3
Abnormal Gait	0	1	4	0	2
Dry Mouth	1	1	2	0	2
Nervousness	1	1	0	0	2
Vasodilatation	2	0	2	0	2
Hallucinations	0	1	2	2	1
Insomnia	0	1	2	0	1
Thinking Abnormal	0	1	2	0	1
Vertigo	1	0	0	0	1
Respiratory					
Dyspnea	2	3	6	5	4
Skin					
Pruritus	1	0	0	5	2
Rash	1	1	0	2	2
Sweating	1	1	2	2	2
Special Senses					
Abnormal Vision	1	0	2	0	2

The following adverse events not reflected in Table 3 occurred during titration with an overall frequency of 1% or greater and are listed in descending order of frequency within each body system.

Body as a Whole: Pain, fever, abdominal pain, chills, back pain, chest pain, infection
Cardiovascular: Migraine
Digestive: Diarrhea, dyspepsia, flatulence
Metabolic and Nutritional: Peripheral edema, dehydration
Nervous: Hypesthesia
Respiratory: Pharyngitis, cough increased

The following events occurred during titration with an overall frequency of less than 1% and are listed in descending order of frequency within each body system.

Body as a Whole: Flu syndrome, abscess, bone pain
Cardiovascular: Deep thrombophlebitis, hypertension, hypotension
Digestive: Anorexia, eructation, esophageal stenosis, fecal impaction, gum hemorrhage, mouth ulceration, oral moniliasis
Hemic and Lymphatic: Anemia, leukopenia

Metabolic and Nutritional: Edema, hypercalcemia, weight loss
Musculoskeletal: Myalgia, pathological fracture, myasthenia
Nervous: Abnormal dreams, urinary retention, agitation, amnesia, emotional lability, euphoria, incoordination, libido decreased, neuropathy, paresthesia, speech disorder
Respiratory: Hemoptysis, pleural effusion, rhinitis, asthma, hiccup, pneumonia, respiratory insufficiency, sputum increased
Skin and Appendages: Alopecia, exfoliative dermatitis
Special Senses: Taste perversion
Urogenital: Vaginal hemorrhage, dysuria, hematuria, urinary incontinence, urinary tract infection

A long-term extension study was conducted in 156 patients with malignancy and breakthrough cancer pain who were treated for an average of 129 days. Data are available for 152 of these patients. Table 4 lists by dose groups, adverse events with an overall frequency of 1% or greater that occurred during the long-term extension study and are commonly associated with opioid administration or are of particular clinical interest. Adverse events are listed in descending order of frequency within each body system.

[See table 4 at right]

The following events not reflected in Table 4 occurred with an overall frequency of 1% or greater in the long-term extension study and are listed in descending order of frequency within each body system.

Body as a Whole: Pain, fever, back pain, abdominal pain, chest pain, flu syndrome, chills, infection, abdomen enlarged, bone pain, ascites, sepsis, neck pain, viral infection, fungal infection, cachexia, cellulitis, malaise, pelvic pain
Cardiovascular: Deep thrombophlebitis, migraine, palpitation, vascular disorder
Digestive: Diarrhea, anorexia, dyspepsia, dysphagia, oral moniliasis, mouth ulceration, rectal disorder, stomatitis, flatulence, gastrointestinal hemorrhage, gingivitis, jaundice, periodontal abscess, eructation, glossitis, rectal hemorrhage
Hemic and Lymphatic: Anemia, leukopenia, thrombocytopenia, ecchymosis, lymphadenopathy, lymphedema, pancytopenia
Metabolic and Nutritional: Peripheral edema, edema, dehydration, weight loss, hyperglycemia, hypokalemia, hypercalcemia, hypomagnesemia
Musculoskeletal: Myalgia, pathological fracture, joint disorder, leg cramps, arthralgia, bone disorder
Nervous: Hypesthesia, paresthesia, hypokinesia, neuropathy, speech disorder
Respiratory: Cough increased, pharyngitis, pneumonia, rhinitis, sinusitis, bronchitis, epistaxis, asthma, hemoptysis, sputum increased
Skin and Appendages: Skin ulcer, alopecia
Special Senses: Tinnitus, conjunctivitis, ear disorder, taste perversion
Urogenital: Urinary tract infection, urinary incontinence, breast pain, dysuria, hematuria, scrotal edema, hydronephrosis, kidney failure, urinary urgency, urination impaired, breast neoplasm, vaginal hemorrhage, vaginitis

The following events occurred with a frequency of less than 1% in the long-term extension study and are listed in descending order of frequency within each body system.

Body as a Whole: Allergic reaction, cyst, face edema, flank pain, granuloma, bacterial infection, injection site pain, mucous membrane disorder, neck rigidity
Cardiovascular: Angina pectoris, hemorrhage, hypotension, peripheral vascular disorder, postural hypotension, tachycardia
Digestive: Cheilitis, esophagitis, fecal incontinence, gastroenteritis, gastrointestinal disorder, gum hemorrhage, hemorrhage of colon, hepatorenal syndrome, liver tenderness, tooth caries, tooth disorder
Hemic and Lymphatic: Bleeding time increased
Metabolic and Nutritional: Acidosis, generalized edema, hypocalcemia, hypoglycemia, hyponatremia, hypoproteinemia, thirst
Musculoskeletal: Arthritis, muscle atrophy, myopathy, synovitis, tendon disorder
Nervous: Acute brain syndrome, agitation, cerebral ischemia, facial paralysis, foot drop, hallucinations, hemiplegia, miosis, subdural hematoma
Respiratory: Hiccup, hyperventilation, lung disorder, pneumothorax, respiratory failure, voice alteration
Skin and Appendages: Herpes zoster, maculopapular rash, skin discoloration, urticaria, vesiculobullous rash
Special Senses: Ear pain, eye hemorrhage, lacrimation disorder, partial permanent deafness, partial transitory deafness
Urogenital: Kidney pain, nocturia, oliguria, polyuria, pyelonephritis

Post-Marketing Experience

The following adverse reactions have been identified during postapproval use of *Actiq*. Because these reactions are reported voluntarily from a population of uncertain size, it is not always possible to reliably estimate their frequency or establish a causal relationship to drug exposure. Decisions to include these reactions in labeling are typically based on one or more of the following factors: (1) seriousness of the reaction, (2) frequency of the reporting, or (3) strength of causal connection to *Actiq*.
Digestive: Dental decay of varying severity including dental caries, tooth loss, and gum line erosion

Table 4.
Percent of Patients with Adverse Events Commonly Associated with Opioid Administration or of Particular Clinical Interest Which Occurred During Long-Term Treatment (Events in 1% or More of Patients)

Dose Group	200-600 mcg	800-1400 mcg	1600 mcg	>1600 mcg	Any
Number of Patients	**98**	**83**	**53**	**27**	**152**
Body As A Whole					
Asthenia	25	30	17	15	38
Headache	12	17	13	4	20
Accidental Injury	4	6	4	7	9
Hypertonia	2	2	2	0	3
Digestive					
Nausea	31	36	25	26	45
Vomiting	21	28	15	7	31
Constipation	14	11	13	4	20
Intestinal Obstruction	0	2	4	0	3
Cardiovascular					
Hypertension	1	1	0	0	1
Nervous					
Dizziness	12	10	9	0	16
Anxiety	9	8	8	7	15
Somnolence	8	13	8	7	15
Confusion	2	5	13	7	10
Depression	9	4	2	7	9
Insomnia	5	1	8	4	7
Abnormal Gait	5	1	0	0	4
Dry Mouth	3	1	2	4	4
Nervousness	2	2	0	4	3
Stupor	4	1	0	0	3
Vasodilatation	1	1	4	0	3
Thinking Abnormal	2	1	0	0	2
Abnormal Dreams	1	1	0	0	1
Convulsion	0	1	2	0	1
Myoclonus	0	0	4	0	1
Tremor	0	1	2	0	1
Vertigo	0	0	4	0	1
Respiratory					
Dyspnea	15	16	8	7	22
Skin					
Rash	3	5	8	4	8
Sweating	3	2	2	0	4
Pruritus	2	0	2	0	2
Special Senses					
Abnormal Vision	2	2	0	0	3
Urogenital					
Urinary Retention	1	2	0	0	2

DRUG ABUSE AND DEPENDENCE

Fentanyl is a mu-opioid agonist and a Schedule II controlled substance that can produce drug dependence of the morphine type. *Actiq* may be subject to misuse, abuse and addiction.

The administration of *Actiq* should be guided by the response of the patient. Physical dependence, per se, is not ordinarily a concern when one is treating a patient with chronic cancer pain, and fear of tolerance and physical dependence should not deter using doses that adequately relieve the pain.

Opioid analgesics may cause physical dependence. Physical dependence results in withdrawal symptoms in patients who abruptly discontinue the drug. Withdrawal also may be precipitated through the administration of drugs with opioid antagonist activity, e.g., naloxone, nalmefene, or mixed agonist/antagonist analgesics (pentazocine, butorphanol, buprenorphine, nalbuphine).

Physical dependence usually does not occur to a clinically significant degree until after several weeks of continued opioid usage. Tolerance, in which increasingly larger doses are required in order to produce the same degree of analgesia, is initially manifested by a shortened duration of analgesic effect, and subsequently, by decreases in the intensity of analgesia.

The handling of *Actiq* should be managed to minimize the risk of diversion, including restriction of access and accounting procedures as appropriate to the clinical setting and as required by law (see **SAFETY AND HANDLING**).

OVERDOSAGE

Clinical Presentation

The manifestations of *Actiq* overdosage are expected to be similar in nature to intravenous fentanyl and other opioids,

Continued on next page

Actiq—Cont.

and are an extension of its pharmacological actions with the most serious significant effect being hypoventilation (see **CLINICAL PHARMACOLOGY**).

General

Immediate management of opioid overdose includes removal of the *Actiq* unit, if still in the mouth, ensuring a patent airway, physical and verbal stimulation of the patient, and assessment of level of consciousness, ventilatory and circulatory status.

Treatment of Overdosage (Accidental Ingestion) in the Opioid NON-Tolerant Person

Ventilatory support should be provided, intravenous access obtained, and naloxone or other opioid antagonists should be employed as clinically indicated. The duration of respiratory depression following overdose may be longer than the effects of the opioid antagonist's action (e.g., the half-life of naloxone ranges from 30 to 81 minutes) and repeated administration may be necessary. Consult the package insert of the individual opioid antagonist for details about such use.

Treatment of Overdose in Opioid-Tolerant Patients

Ventilatory support should be provided and intravenous access obtained as clinically indicated. Judicious use of naloxone or another opioid antagonist may be warranted in some instances, but it is associated with the risk of precipitating an acute withdrawal syndrome.

General Considerations for Overdose

Management of severe *Actiq* overdose includes: securing a patent airway, assisting or controlling ventilation, establishing intravenous access, and GI decontamination by lavage and/or activated charcoal, once the patient's airway is secure. In the presence of hypoventilation or apnea, ventilation should be assisted or controlled and oxygen administered as indicated.

Patients with overdose should be carefully observed and appropriately managed until their clinical condition is well controlled.

Although muscle rigidity interfering with respiration has not been seen following the use of *Actiq*, this is possible with fentanyl and other opioids. If it occurs, it should be managed by the use of assisted or controlled ventilation, by an opioid antagonist, and as a final alternative, by a neuromuscular blocking agent.

DOSAGE AND ADMINISTRATION

***Actiq* is contraindicated in non-opioid tolerant individuals.** *Actiq* should be individually titrated to a dose that provides adequate analgesia and minimizes side effects (see **Dose Titration**).

As with all opioids, the safety of patients using such products is dependent on health care professionals prescribing them in strict conformity with their approved labeling with respect to patient selection, dosing, and proper conditions for use.

Physicians and dispensing pharmacists must specifically question patients and caregivers about the presence of children in the home on a full time or visiting basis and counsel accordingly regarding the dangers to children of inadvertent exposure to *Actiq*.

Administration of *Actiq*

The blister package should be opened with scissors immediately prior to product use. The patient should place the *Actiq* unit in his or her mouth between the cheek and lower gum, occasionally moving the drug matrix from one side to the other using the handle. The *Actiq* unit should be sucked, not chewed. A unit dose of *Actiq*, if chewed and swallowed, might result in lower peak concentrations and lower bioavailability than when consumed as directed.

The *Actiq* unit should be consumed over a 15-minute period. Longer or shorter consumption times may produce less efficacy than reported in *Actiq* clinical trials. If signs of excessive opioid effects appear before the unit is consumed, the drug matrix should be removed from the patient's mouth immediately and future doses should be decreased.

Patients and caregivers must be instructed that *Actiq* contains medicine in an amount that could be fatal to a child. While all units should be disposed of immediately after use, partially used units represent a special risk and must be disposed of as soon as they are consumed and/or no longer needed. Patients and caregivers should be advised to dispose of any units remaining from a prescription as soon as they are no longer needed (see **Disposal Instructions**).

Dose Titration

Starting Dose: *The initial dose of Actiq to treat episodes of breakthrough cancer pain should be 200 mcg.* Patients should be prescribed an initial titration supply of six 200 mcg *Actiq* units, thus limiting the number of units in the home during titration. Patients should use up all units before increasing to a higher dose.

From this initial dose, patients should be closely followed and the dosage level changed until the patient reaches a dose that provides adequate analgesia using a single *Actiq* dosage unit per breakthrough cancer pain episode.

Patients should record their use of *Actiq* over several episodes of breakthrough cancer pain and review their experience with their physicians to determine if a dosage adjustment is warranted.

Redosing Within a Single Episode: Until the appropriate dose is reached, patients may find it necessary to use an additional *Actiq* unit during a single episode. Redosing may start 15 minutes after the previous unit has been completed (30 minutes after the start of the previous unit). While patients are in the titration phase and consuming units which individually may be subtherapeutic, no more than two units should be taken for each individual breakthrough cancer pain episode.

Increasing the Dose: If treatment of several consecutive breakthrough cancer pain episodes requires more than one *Actiq* per episode, an increase in dose to the next higher available strength should be considered. At each new dose of *Actiq* during titration, it is recommended that six units of the titration dose be prescribed. Each new dose of *Actiq* used in the titration period should be evaluated over several episodes of breakthrough cancer pain (generally 1–2 days) to determine whether it provides adequate efficacy with acceptable side effects. The incidence of side effects is likely to be greater during this initial titration period compared to later, after the effective dose is determined.

Daily Limit: Once a successful dose has been found (i.e., an average episode is treated with a single unit), patients should limit consumption to four or fewer units per day. If consumption increases above four units/day, the dose of the long-acting opioid used for persistent cancer pain should be re-evaluated.

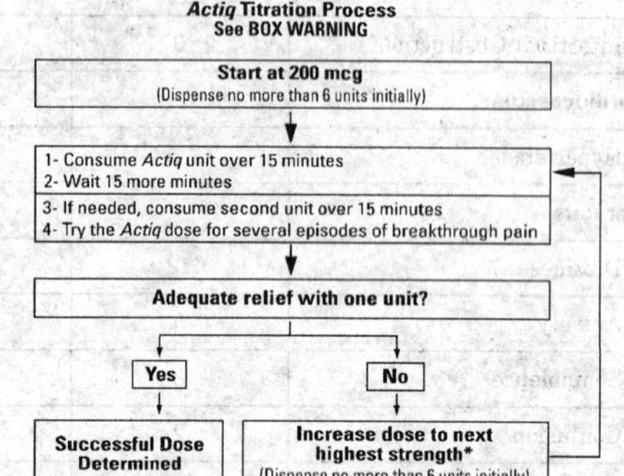

Actiq Titration Process
See BOX WARNING
Start at 200 mcg
(Dispense no more than 6 units initially)
1- Consume *Actiq* unit over 15 minutes
2- Wait 15 more minutes
3- If needed, consume second unit over 15 minutes
4- Try the *Actiq* dose for several episodes of breakthrough pain
Adequate relief with one unit?
Yes
No
Successful Dose Determined
Increase dose to next highest strength*
(Dispense no more than 6 units initially)
*Available dosage strengths include: 200, 400, 600, 800, 1200, and 1600 mcg.

Dosage Adjustment

Experience in a long-term study of *Actiq* used in the treatment of breakthrough cancer pain suggests that dosage adjustment of both *Actiq* and the maintenance (around-the-clock) opioid analgesic may be required in some patients to continue to provide adequate relief of breakthrough cancer pain.

Generally, the *Actiq* dose should be increased when patients require more than one dosage unit per breakthrough cancer pain episode for several consecutive episodes. When titrating to an appropriate dose, small quantities (six units) should be prescribed at each titration step. Physicians should consider increasing the around-the-clock opioid dose used for persistent cancer pain in patients experiencing more than four breakthrough cancer pain episodes daily.

Discontinuation of *Actiq*

For patients requiring discontinuation of opioids, a gradual downward titration is recommended because it is not known at what dose level the opioid may be discontinued without producing the signs and symptoms of abrupt withdrawal.

SAFETY AND HANDLING

Actiq is supplied in individually sealed child-resistant blister packages. The amount of fentanyl contained in *Actiq* can be fatal to a child. Patients and their caregivers must be instructed to keep *Actiq* out of the reach of children (see **BOX WARNING, WARNINGS, PRECAUTIONS,** and **PATIENT LEAFLET**).

Store at 20°–25°C with excursions permitted between 15° and 30°C (59° to 86°F) until ready to use. (See USP Controlled Room Temperature.)

Actiq should be protected from freezing and moisture. Do not use if the blister package has been opened.

DISPOSAL OF ACTIQ

Patients must be advised to dispose of any units remaining from a prescription as soon as they are no longer needed. While all units should be disposed of immediately after use, partially consumed units represent a special risk because they are no longer protected by the child-resistant blister package, yet may contain enough medicine to be fatal to a child (see **Information for Patients**).

A temporary storage bottle is provided as part of the *Actiq* Welcome Kit (see **Information for Patients and Their Caregivers**). This container is to be used by patients or their caregivers in the event that a partially consumed unit cannot be disposed of promptly. Instructions for usage of this container are included in the patient leaflet.

Patients and members of their household must be advised to dispose of any units remaining from a prescription as soon as they are no longer needed. Instructions are included in **Information for Patients and Their Caregivers** and in the patient leaflet. If additional assistance is required, referral to the *Actiq* 800# (1-800-896-5855) should be made.

HOW SUPPLIED

Actiq is supplied in six dosage strengths. Each unit is individually wrapped in a child-resistant, protective blister package. These blister packages are packed 30 per shelf carton for use when patients have been titrated to the appropriate dose.

Patients should be prescribed an initial titration supply of six 200 mcg *Actiq* units. At each new dose of *Actiq* during titration, it is recommended that only six units of the next higher dose be prescribed.

Each dosage unit has a white to off-white color. The dosage strength of each unit is marked on the solid drug matrix, the handle tag, the blister package and the carton. See blister package and carton for product information.

Dosage Strength (fentanyl base)	*Carton/Blister* Package Color	NDC Number
200 mcg	Gray	NDC 63459-502-30
400 mcg	Blue	NDC 63459-504-30
600 mcg	Orange	NDC 63459-506-30
800 mcg	Purple	NDC 63459-508-30
1200 mcg	Green	NDC 63459-512-30
1600 mcg	Burgundy	NDC 63459-516-30

Note: Colors are a secondary aid in product identification. Please be sure to confirm the printed dosage before dispensing.

℞ only.

DEA order form required. A Schedule C-II narcotic.

Manufactured by:
Cephalon, Inc., Salt Lake City, UT 84116, USA
U. S. Patent No. 4,671,953
#1598.01

Shown in Product Identification Guide, page 310

GABITRIL® ℞

[*găb-ĭ-trĭl*]
(tiagabine hydrochloride)
Tablets
℞ only

DESCRIPTION

GABITRIL (tiagabine HCl) is an antiepilepsy drug available as 2 mg, 4 mg, 12 mg, 16 mg tablets for oral administration. Its chemical name is (-)-(R)-1-[4,4-Bis(3-methyl-2-thienyl)-3-butenyl]nipecotic acid hydrochloride, its molecular formula is $C_{20}H_{25}NO_2S_2$ HCl, and its molecular weight is 412.0. Tiagabine HCl is a white to off-white, odorless, crystalline powder. It is insoluble in heptane, sparingly soluble in water, and soluble in aqueous base. The structural formula is:

Inactive Ingredients

GABITRIL tablets contain the following inactive ingredients: Ascorbic acid, colloidal silicon dioxide, crospovidone, hydrogenated vegetable oil wax, hydroxypropyl cellulose, hypromellose, lactose, magnesium stearate, microcrystalline cellulose, pregelatinized starch, stearic acid, and titanium dioxide.

In addition, individual tablets contain:
- 2 mg tablets: FD&C Yellow No. 6.
- 4 mg tablets: D&C Yellow No. 10.
- 12 mg tablets: D&C Yellow No. 10 and FD&C Blue No. 1.
- 16 mg tablets: FD&C Blue No. 2.

CLINICAL PHARMACOLOGY

Mechanism of Action

The precise mechanism by which tiagabine exerts its antiseizure effect is unknown, although it is believed to be related to its ability, documented in *in vitro* experiments, to enhance the activity of gamma aminobutyric acid (GABA), the major inhibitory neurotransmitter in the central nervous system. These experiments have shown that tiagabine binds to recognition sites associated with the GABA uptake carrier. It is thought that, by this action, tiagabine blocks GABA uptake into presynaptic neurons, permitting more GABA to be available for receptor binding on the surfaces of post-synaptic cells. Inhibition of GABA uptake has been shown for synaptosomes, neuronal cell cultures, and glial cell cultures. In rat-derived hippocampal slices, tiagabine has been shown to prolong GABA-mediated inhibitory post-synaptic potentials. Tiagabine increases the amount of GABA available in the extracellular space of the globus pallidus, ventral palladum, and substantia nigra in rats at the ED_{50} and ED_{85} doses for inhibition of pentylenetetrazol (PTZ)-induced tonic seizures. This suggests that tiagabine prevents the propagation of neural impulses that contribute to seizures by a GABA-ergic action.

Tiagabine has shown efficacy in several animal models of seizures. It is effective against the tonic phase of subcutaneous PTZ-induced seizures in mice and rats, seizures induced by the proconvulsant DMCM in mice, audiogenic seizures in genetically epilepsy-prone rats (GEPR), and amygdala-kindled seizures in rats. Tiagabine has little efficacy against maximal electroshock seizures in rats and is only partially effective against subcutaneous PTZ-induced clonic seizures in mice, picrotoxin-induced tonic seizures in the mouse, bicuculline-induced seizures in the rat, and photic seizures in photosensitive baboons. Tiagabine produces a biphasic dose-response curve against PTZ- and DMCM-induced convulsions, with attenuated effectiveness at higher doses.

Based on *in vitro* binding studies, tiagabine does not significantly inhibit the uptake of dopamine, norepinephrine, serotonin, glutamate, or choline and shows little or no binding to dopamine D1 and D2, muscarinic, serotonin $5HT_{1A}$, $5HT_2$, and $5HT_3$, beta-1 and 2 adrenergic, alpha-1 and alpha-2 adrenergic, histamine H2 and H3, adenosine A_1 and A_2, opiate μ and K_1, NMDA glutamate, and $GABA_A$ receptors at 100 μM. It also lacks significant affinity for sodium or calcium channels. Tiagabine binds to histamine H1, serotonin $5HT_{1B}$, benzodiazepine, and chloride channel receptors at concentrations 20 to 400 times those inhibiting the uptake of GABA.

PHARMACOKINETICS

Tiagabine is well absorbed, with food slowing absorption rate but not altering the extent of absorption. Although its elimination half-life is 7 to 9 hours in normal volunteers, it is only 4 to 7 hours in patients receiving hepatic enzyme-inducing drugs (carbamazepine, phenytoin, primidone, and phenobarbital). In clinical trials, most patients were induced.

Absorption and Distribution: Absorption of tiagabine is rapid, with peak plasma concentrations occurring at approximately 45 minutes following an oral dose in the fasting state. Tiagabine is nearly completely absorbed (>95%), with an absolute oral bioavailability of about 90%. A high fat meal decreases the rate (mean T_{max} was prolonged to 2.5 hours, and mean C_{max} was reduced by about 40%) but not the extent (AUC) of tiagabine absorption. In all clinical trials, tiagabine was given with meals.

The pharmacokinetics of tiagabine are linear over the single dose range of 2 to 24 mg. Following multiple dosing, steady state is achieved within 2 days.

Tiagabine is 96% bound to human plasma proteins, mainly to serum albumin and α1-acid glycoprotein over the concentration range of 10 ng/mL to 10,000 ng/mL. While the relationship between tiagabine plasma concentrations and clinical response is not currently understood, trough plasma concentrations observed in controlled clinical trials at doses from 30 to 56 mg/day ranged from <1 ng/mL to 234 ng/mL.

Metabolism and Elimination: Although the metabolism of tiagabine has not been fully elucidated, *in vivo* and *in vitro* studies suggest that at least two metabolic pathways for tiagabine have been identified in humans: 1) thiophene ring oxidation leading to the formation of 5-oxo-tiagabine; and 2) glucuronidation. The 5-oxo-tiagabine metabolite does not contribute to the pharmacologic activity of tiagabine.

Based on *in vitro* data, tiagabine is likely to be metabolized primarily by the 3A isoform subfamily of hepatic cytochrome P450 (CYP 3A), although contributions to the metabolism of tiagabine from CYP 1A2, CYP 2D6 or CYP 2C19 have not been excluded.

Approximately 2% of an oral dose of tiagabine is excreted unchanged, with 25% and 63% of the remaining dose excreted into the urine and feces, respectively, primarily as metabolites, at least 2 of which have not been identified. The mean systemic plasma clearance is 109 mL/min (CV = 23%) and the average elimination half-life for tiagabine in healthy subjects ranged from 7 to 9 hours. The elimination half-life decreased by 50 to 65% in hepatic enzyme-induced patients with epilepsy compared to uninduced patients with epilepsy.

A diurnal effect on the pharmacokinetics of tiagabine was observed. Mean steady-state C_{min} values were 40% lower in the evening than in the morning. Tiagabine steady-state AUC values were also found to be 15% lower following the evening tiagabine dose compared to the AUC following the morning dose.

SPECIAL POPULATIONS

Renal Insufficiency: The pharmacokinetics of total and unbound tiagabine were similar in subjects with normal renal function (creatinine clearance >80 mL/min) and in subjects with mild (creatinine clearance 40 to 80 mL/min), moderate (creatinine clearance 20 to 39 mL/min), or severe (creatinine clearance 5 to 19 mL/min) renal impairment. The pharmacokinetics of total and unbound tiagabine were also unaffected in subjects with renal failure requiring hemodialysis.

Hepatic Insufficiency: In patients with moderate hepatic impairment (Child-Pugh Class B), clearance of unbound tiagabine was reduced by about 60%. Patients with impaired liver function may require reduced initial and maintenance doses of tiagabine and/or longer dosing intervals compared to patients with normal hepatic function (see **PRECAUTIONS**).

Geriatric: The pharmacokinetic profile of tiagabine was similar in healthy elderly and healthy young adults.

Pediatric: Tiagabine has not been investigated in adequate and well-controlled clinical trials in patients below the age of 12. The apparent clearance and volume of distribution of tiagabine per unit body surface area or per kg were fairly similar in 25 children (age: 3 to 10 years) and in adults taking enzyme-inducing antiepilepsy drugs ([AEDs] e.g., carbamazepine or phenytoin). In children who were taking a non-inducing AED (e.g., valproate), the clearance of tiagabine based upon body weight and body surface area was 2 and 1.5-fold higher, respectively, than in uninduced adults with epilepsy.

Table 1
Median Reduction and Median Percent Reduction from Baseline in 4-Week Seizure Rates in Study 1

		Placebo (N=91)	GABITRIL 16 mg/day (N=61)	GABITRIL 32 mg/day (N=87)	GABITRIL 56 mg/day (N=56)	Combined 32 + 56 mg/day (N=143)
Complex Partial	Median Reduction	0.6	0.8	2.2*	2.9*	2.6*
	Median % Reduction†	9%	13%	25%	32%	29%
All Partial	Median Reduction	0.2	1.2	2.7*	3.5*	2.9*
	Median % Reduction†	3%	12%	24%	36%	27%

* p<0.05
† Statistical significance was not assessed for median % reduction.

Table 2
Median Reduction and Median Percent Reduction from Baseline in 4-Week Seizure Rates in Study 2

		Placebo (N=107)	GABITRIL 16 mg BID (N=106)	GABITRIL 8 mg QID (N=104)
Complex Partial	Median Reduction	0.3	1.6	1.3*
	Median % Reduction†	4%	22%	15%
All Partial	Median Reduction	0.5	1.6	1.3
	Median % Reduction†	5%	19%	13%

* p < 0.027, necessary for statistical significance due to multiple comparisons.
† Statistical significance was not assessed for median % reduction.

Gender, Race and Cigarette Smoking: No specific pharmacokinetic studies were conducted to investigate the effect of gender, race and cigarette smoking on the disposition of tiagabine. Retrospective pharmacokinetic analyses, however, suggest that there is no clinically important difference between the clearance of tiagabine in males and females, when adjusted for body weight. Population pharmacokinetic analyses indicated that tiagabine clearance values were not significantly different in Caucasian (N=463), Black (N=23), or Hispanic (N=17) patients with epilepsy, and that tiagabine clearance values were not significantly affected by tobacco use.

Interactions with other Antiepilepsy Drugs: The clearance of tiagabine is affected by the co-administration of hepatic enzyme-inducing antiepilepsy drugs. Tiagabine is eliminated more rapidly in patients who have been taking hepatic enzyme-inducing drugs, e.g. carbamazepine, phenytoin, primidone and phenobarbital than in patients not receiving such treatment (see **PRECAUTIONS, Drug Interactions**).

Interactions with Other Drugs: See **PRECAUTIONS, Drug Interactions.**

CLINICAL STUDIES

The effectiveness of GABITRIL as adjunctive therapy (added to other antiepilepsy drugs) was examined in three multi-center, double-blind, placebo-controlled, parallel-group, clinical trials in 769 patients with refractory partial seizures who were taking at least one hepatic enzyme-inducing antiepilepsy drug (AED), and two placebo-controlled cross-over studies in 90 patients. In the parallel-group trials, patients had a history of at least six complex partial seizures (Study 1 and Study 2, U.S. studies), or six partial seizures of any type (Study 3, European study), occurring alone or in combination with any other seizure type within the 8-week period preceding the first study visit in spite of receiving one or more AEDs at therapeutic concentrations.

In the first two studies, the primary protocol-specified outcome measure was the median reduction from baseline in the 4-week complex partial seizure (CPS) rates during treatment. In the third study, the protocol-specified primary outcome measure was the proportion of patients achieving a 50% or greater reduction from baseline in the 4-week seizure rate of all partial seizures during treatment. The results given below include data for complex partial seizures and all partial seizures for the intent-to-treat population (all patients who received at least one dose of treatment and at least one seizure evaluation) in each study.

Study 1 was a double-blind, placebo-controlled, parallel-group trial comparing GABITRIL 16 mg/day, GABITRIL 32 mg/day, GABITRIL 56 mg/day, and placebo. Study drug was given as a four times a day regimen. After a prospective Baseline Phase of 12 weeks, patients were randomized to one of the four treatment groups described above. The 16-week Treatment Phase consisted of a 4-week Titration Period, followed by a 12-week Fixed-Dose Period, during which concomitant AED doses were held constant. The primary outcome was assessed for the combined 32 and 56 mg/day groups compared to placebo.

Study 2 was a double-blind, placebo-controlled, parallel-group trial consisting of an 8-week Baseline Phase and a 12-week Treatment Phase, the first 4 weeks of which constituted a Titration Period and the last 8 weeks a Fixed-Dose Period. This study compared GABITRIL 16 mg BID and 8 mg QID to placebo. The protocol-specified primary outcome measure was assessed separately for each group treated with GABITRIL.

The following tables display the results of the analyses of these two trials.

[See table 1 above]

[See table 2 above]

Figures 1 to 4 present the proportion of patients (X-axis) whose percent reduction from baseline in the all partial seizure rate was at least as great as that indicated on the Y axis in the three placebo-controlled adjunctive studies (Studies 1, 2, and 3). A positive value on the Y axis indicates an improvement from baseline (i.e., a decrease in seizure rate), while a negative value indicates a worsening from baseline (i.e., an increase in seizure rate). Thus, in a display of this type, the curve for an effective treatment is shifted to the left of the curve for placebo.

Figure 1 indicates that the proportion of patients achieving any particular level of reduction in seizure rate was consistently higher for the combined GABITRIL 32 mg and 56 mg groups compared to the placebo group in Study 1. For example, Figure 1 indicates that approximately 24% of patients treated with GABITRIL experienced a 50% or greater reduction, compared to 4% in the placebo group.

Figure 1
Study 1

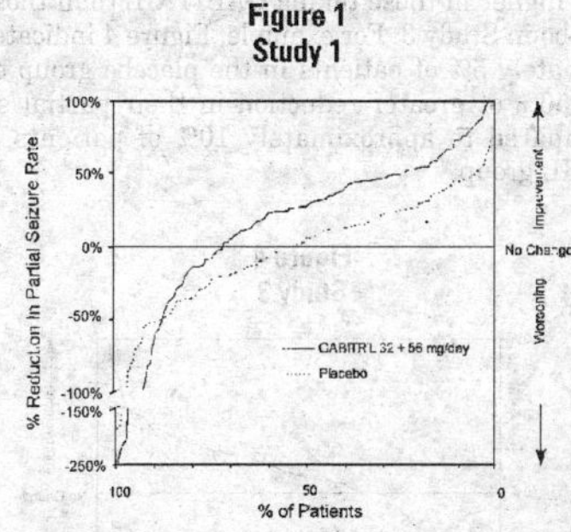

Figure 2 also displays the results for Study 1, which was a dose-response study, by treatment group, without combining GABITRIL dosage groups. Figure 2 indicates a dose-response relationship across the three GABITRIL groups. The proportion of patients achieving any particular level of reduction in all partial seizure rates was consistently higher as the dose of GABITRIL was increased. For example, Figure 2 indicates that approximately 4% of patients in the placebo group experienced a 50% or greater reduction in all partial seizure rate, compared to approximately 10% of the GABITRIL 16 mg/day group, 21% of the GABITRIL 32 mg/day group, and 30% of the GABITRIL 56 mg/day group.

[See figure 2 at top of next column]

Figure 3 indicates that the proportion of patients achieving any particular level of reduction in partial seizure rate was consistently greater in patients taking GABITRIL than in those taking placebo in Study 2. (Study 2 compared placebo to GABITRIL 32 mg/day; one of the GABITRIL groups received 8 mg QID, while the other GABITRIL group received 16 mg BID). For example, Figure 3 indicates that approximately 7% of patients in the placebo group experienced a

Continued on next page

Gabitril—Cont.

Figure 2
Study 1

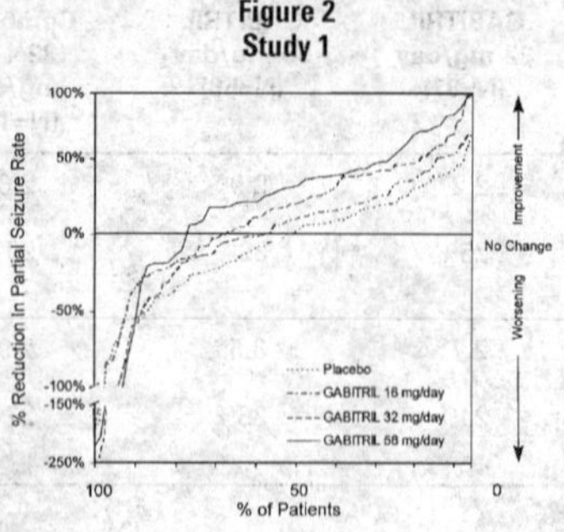

50% or greater reduction in their partial seizure rate, compared to approximately 23% of patients in the GABITRIL 8 mg QID group and 28% of patients in the GABITRIL 16 mg BID group.

Figure 3
Study 2

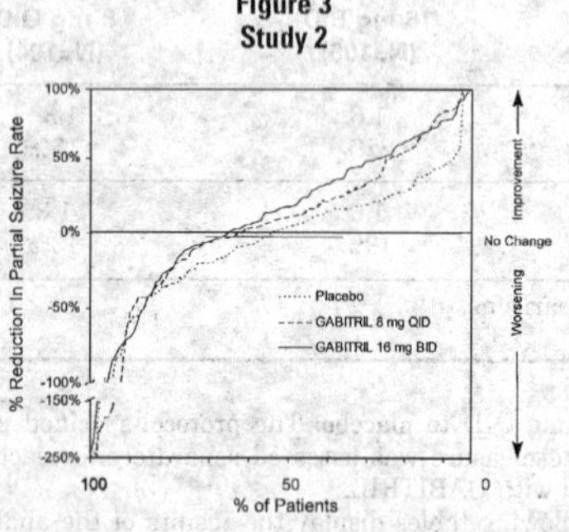

Study 3 was a double-blind, placebo-controlled, parallel-group trial that compared GABITRIL 10 mg TID (N=77) with placebo (N=77). In this trial, patients were followed prospectively during a 12-week Baseline Phase and then randomized to receive study drug during an 18-week Treatment Phase. During the first 6 weeks of treatment (Titration Period), patients were titrated to 30 mg/day, after which they were maintained on this dose during the 12-week Fixed-Dose Period. The protocol-specified primary outcome measure (proportion of patients who achieved at least a 50% reduction from baseline in partial seizure rate) did not reach statistical significance. However, analyses of the median reduction from baseline in 4-week partial seizure rate (the analyses presented above for Study 1 and Study 2) were performed and showed a statistically significant improvement compared to placebo in all partial and complex partial seizure rates (Table 3):

[See table 3 above]

Figure 4 indicates that the proportion of patients achieving any particular level of reduction in seizure activity was consistently higher in those taking GABITRIL than those taking placebo in Study 3. For example, Figure 4 indicates that approximately 5% of patients in the placebo group experienced a 50% or greater reduction in their partial seizure rate compared to approximately 10% of patients in the GABITRIL group.

Figure 4
Study 3

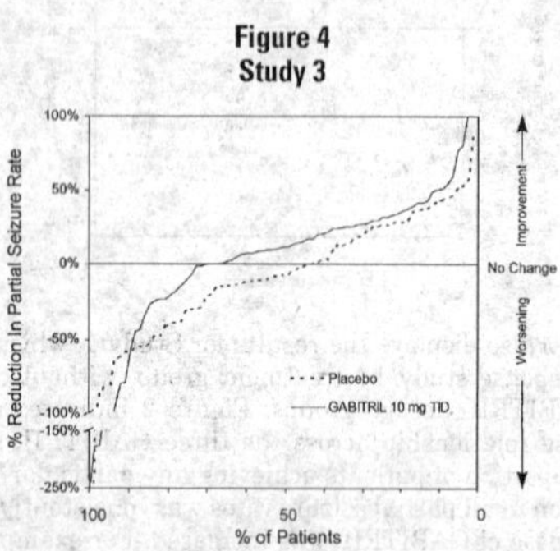

The two other placebo-controlled trials that examined the effectiveness of GABITRIL were small cross-over trials (N=46 and 44). Both trials included an open Screening Phase during which patients were titrated to an optimal dose and then treated with this dose for an additional 4 weeks. After this Open Phase, patients were randomized to one of two blinded treatment sequences (GABITRIL followed by placebo or placebo followed by GABITRIL). The Double-Blind Phase consisted of two Treatment Periods, each lasting 7 weeks (with a 3 week washout between periods). The outcome measures were median with-in patient differences between placebo and GABITRIL Treatment Periods in 4-week complex partial and all partial seizure rates. The reductions in seizure rates were statistically significant in both studies.

Table 3
Median Reduction and Median Percent Reduction from Baseline in 4-Week Seizure Rates in Study 3

		Placebo (N=77)	GABITRIL 30 mg/day (N=77)
Complex Partial‡	Median Reduction	−0.1	1.3*
	Median % Reduction†	−1%	14%
All Partial	Median Reduction	−0.5	1.1*
	Median % Reduction†	−7%	11%

* $p < 0.05$
† Statistical significance was not assessed for median % reduction.
‡ N=72 and 75 for placebo and GABITRIL, respectively.

INDICATIONS AND USAGE

GABITRIL (tiagabine hydrochloride) is indicated as adjunctive therapy in adults and children 12 years and older in the treatment of partial seizures.

CONTRAINDICATIONS

GABITRIL is contraindicated in patients who have demonstrated hypersensitivity to the drug or its ingredients.

WARNINGS

Withdrawal Seizures: As a rule, antiepilepsy drugs should not be abruptly discontinued because of the possibility of increasing seizure frequency. In a placebo-controlled, double-blind, dose-response study (Study 1 described in **CLINICAL STUDIES**) designed, in part, to investigate the capacity of GABITRIL to induce withdrawal seizures, study drug was tapered over a 4-week period after 16 weeks of treatment. Patients' seizure frequency during this 4-week withdrawal period was compared to their baseline seizure frequency (before study drug). For each partial seizure type, for all partial seizure types combined, and for secondarily generalized tonic-clonic seizures, more patients experienced increases in their seizure frequencies during the withdrawal period in the three GABITRIL groups than in the placebo group. The increase in seizure frequency was not affected by dose. GABITRIL should be withdrawn gradually to minimize the potential of increased seizure frequency, unless safety concerns require a more rapid withdrawal.

Cognitive/Neuropsychiatric Adverse Events: Adverse events most often associated with the use of GABITRIL were related to the central nervous system. The most significant of these can be classified into 2 general categories: 1) impaired concentration, speech or language problems, and confusion (effects on thought processes); and 2) somnolence and fatigue (effects on level of consciousness). The majority of these events were mild to moderate. In controlled clinical trials, these events led to discontinuation of treatment with GABITRIL in 6% (31 of 494) of patients compared to 2% (5 of 275) of the placebo-treated patients. A total of 1.6% (8 of 494) of the GABITRIL treated patients in the controlled trials were hospitalized secondary to the occurrence of these events compared to 0% of the placebo treated patients. Some of these events were dose related and usually began during initial titration.

Patients with a history of spike and wave discharges on EEG have been reported to have exacerbations of their EEG abnormalities associated with these cognitive/neuropsychiatric events. This raises the possibility that these clinical events may, in some cases, be a manifestation of underlying seizure activity (see **PRECAUTIONS, EEG**). In the documented cases of spike and wave discharges on EEG with cognitive/neuropsychiatric events, patients usually continued tiagabine, but required dosage adjustment.

Additionally, there have been postmarketing reports of patients who have experienced cognitive/neuropsychiatric symptoms, some accompanied by EEG abnormalities such as generalized spike and wave activity, that have been reported as nonconvulsant status epilepticus. Some reports describe recovery following reduction of dose or discontinuation of GABITRIL.

Status Epilepticus: In the three double-blind, placebo-controlled, parallel-group studies (Studies 1, 2, and 3), the incidence of any type of status epilepticus (simple, complex, or generalized tonic-clonic) in patients receiving GABITRIL was 0.8% (4 of 494 patients) versus 0.7% (2 of 275 patients) receiving placebo. Among the patients treated with GABITRIL across all epilepsy studies (controlled and uncontrolled), 5% had some form of status epilepticus. Of the 5%, 57% of patients experienced complex partial status epilepticus. A critical risk factor for status epilepticus was the presence of a previous history; 33% of patients with a history of status epilepticus had recurrence during GABITRIL treatment. Because adequate information about the incidence of status epilepticus in a similar population of patients with epilepsy who have not received treatment with GABITRIL is not available, it is impossible to state whether or not treatment with GABITRIL is associated with a higher or lower rate of status epilepticus than would be expected to occur in a similar population not treated with GABITRIL.

Sudden Unexpected Death In Epilepsy (SUDEP): There have been as many as 10 cases of sudden unexpected deaths during the clinical development of tiagabine among 2531 patients with epilepsy (3831 patient-years of exposure). This represents an estimated incidence of 0.0026 deaths per patient-year. This rate is within the range of estimates for the incidence of sudden and unexpected deaths in patients with epilepsy not receiving GABITRIL (ranging from 0.0005 for the general population with epilepsy, 0.003 to 0.004 for clinical trial populations similar to that in the clinical development program for GABITRIL, to 0.005 for patients with refractory epilepsy). The estimated SUDEP rates in patients receiving GABITRIL are also similar to those observed in patients receiving other antiepilepsy drugs, chemically unrelated to GABITRIL, that underwent clinical testing in similar populations at about the same time. This evidence suggests that the SUDEP rates reflect population rates, not a drug effect.

PRECAUTIONS

General

Use in Non-Induced Patients: Virtually all experience with GABITRIL has been obtained in patients receiving at least one concomitant enzyme-inducing antiepilepsy drug (AED). Use in non-induced patients (e.g., patients receiving valproate monotherapy) may require lower doses or a slower dose titration of GABITRIL for clinical response. Patients taking a combination of inducing and non-inducing drugs (e.g., carbamazepine and valproate) should be considered to be induced.

Seizures: In post-approval use of GABITRIL, seizures have been reported in patients without a history of seizures. Confounding factors that may have contributed to development of seizures include underlying medical conditions or concomitant medications that can reduce seizure threshold, reported overdose, and manner of dose administration (e.g., high dosage, fast titration rate).

Generalized Weakness: Moderately severe to incapacitating generalized weakness has been reported following administration of GABITRIL in 28 of 2531 (approximately 1%) patients with epilepsy. The weakness resolved in all cases after a reduction in dose or discontinuation of GABITRIL.

Binding in the Eye and Other Melanin-Containing Tissues: When dogs received a single dose of radiolabeled tiagabine, there was evidence of residual binding in the retina and uvea after 3 weeks (the latest time point measured). Although not directly measured, melanin binding is suggested. The ability of available tests to detect potentially adverse consequences, if any, of the binding of tiagabine to melanin-containing tissue is unknown and there was no systematic monitoring for relevant ophthalmological changes during the clinical development of GABITRIL. However, long term (up to one year) toxicological studies of tiagabine in dogs showed no treatment-related ophthalmoscopic changes and macro- and microscopic examinations of the eye were unremarkable. Accordingly, although there are no specific recommendations for periodic ophthalmologic monitoring, prescribers should be aware of the possibility of long-term ophthalmologic effects.

Use in Hepatically-Impaired Patients: Because the clearance of tiagabine is reduced in patients with liver disease, dosage reduction may be necessary in these patients.

Serious Rash: Four patients treated with tiagabine during the product's premarketing clinical testing developed what were considered to be serious rashes. In two patients, the rash was described as maculopapular; in one it was described as vesiculobullous; and in the 4th case, a diagnosis of Stevens Johnson Syndrome was made. In none of the 4 cases is it certain that tiagabine was the primary, or even a contributory, cause of the rash. Nevertheless, drug associated rash can, if extensive and serious, cause irreversible morbidity, even death.

Information for Patients: Patients should be instructed to take GABITRIL only as prescribed.

Patients should be advised that GABITRIL may cause dizziness, somnolence, and other symptoms and signs of CNS depression. Accordingly, they should be advised neither to drive nor to operate other complex machinery until they have gained sufficient experience on GABITRIL to gauge whether or not it affects their mental and/or motor performance adversely. Because of the possible additive depressive effects, caution should also be used when patients are taking other CNS depressants in combination with GABITRIL.

Because teratogenic effects were seen in the offspring of rats exposed to maternally toxic doses of tiagabine and because experience in humans is limited, patients should be advised to notify their physicians if they become pregnant or intend to become pregnant during therapy.

Because of the possibility that tiagabine may be excreted in breast milk, patients should be advised to notify those providing care to themselves and their children if they intend to breast-feed or are breast-feeding an infant.

Laboratory Tests

Therapeutic Monitoring of Plasma Concentrations of Tiagabine: A therapeutic range for tiagabine plasma concentrations has not been established. In controlled trials, trough plasma concentrations observed among patients randomized to doses of tiagabine that were statistically significantly more effective than placebo ranged from <1 ng/mL to 234 ng/mL (median, 10th and 90th percentiles are 23.7 ng/mL, 5.4 ng/mL, and 69.8 ng/mL, respectively). Because of the potential for pharmacokinetic interactions between GABITRIL and drugs that induce or inhibit hepatic metabolizing enzymes, it may be useful to obtain plasma levels of tiagabine before and after changes are made in the therapeutic regimen.

Clinical Chemistry and Hematology: During the development of GABITRIL, no systematic abnormalities on routine laboratory testing were noted. Therefore, no specific guidance is offered regarding routine monitoring; the practitioner retains responsibility for determining how best to monitor the patient in his/her care.

EEG: Patients with a history of spike and wave discharges on EEG have been reported to have exacerbations of their EEG abnormalities associated with cognitive/neuropsychiatric events. This raises the possibility that these clinical events may, in some cases, be a manifestation of underlying seizure activity (see **WARNINGS, Cognitive/Neuropsychiatric Adverse Events**). In the documented cases of spike and wave discharges on EEG with cognitive/neuropsychiatric events, patients usually continued tiagabine, but required dosage adjustment.

Drug Interactions

In evaluating the potential for interactions among co-administered antiepilepsy drugs (AEDs), whether or not an AED induces or does not induce metabolic enzymes is an important consideration. Phenytoin, phenobarbital and carbamazepine are generally classified as enzyme inducers; valproate and gabapentin are not. GABITRIL is considered to be a non-enzyme inducing AED.

The drug interaction data described in this section were obtained from studies involving either healthy subjects or patients with epilepsy.

Effects of GABITRIL on other Antiepilepsy Drugs (AEDs):

Phenytoin: Tiagabine had no effect on the steady-state plasma concentrations of phenytoin in patients with epilepsy.

Carbamazepine: Tiagabine had no effect on the steady-state plasma concentrations of carbamazepine or its epoxide metabolite in patients with epilepsy.

Valproate: Tiagabine causes a slight decrease (about 10%) in steady-state valproate concentrations.

Phenobarbital or Primidone: No formal pharmacokinetic studies have been performed examining the addition of tiagabine to regimens containing phenobarbital or primidone. The addition of tiagabine in a limited number of patients in three well-controlled studies caused no systematic changes in phenobarbital or primidone concentrations when compared to placebo.

Effects of other Antiepilepsy Drugs (AEDs) on GABITRIL:

Carbamazepine: Population pharmacokinetic analyses indicate that tiagabine clearance is 60% greater in patients taking carbamazepine with or without other enzyme-inducing AEDs.

Phenytoin: Population pharmacokinetic analyses indicate that tiagabine clearance is 60% greater in patients taking phenytoin with or without other enzyme-inducing AEDs.

Phenobarbital (Primidone): Population pharmacokinetic analyses indicate that tiagabine clearance is 60% greater in patients taking phenobarbital (primidone) with or without other enzyme-inducing AEDs.

Valproate: The addition of tiagabine to patients taking valproate chronically had no effect on tiagabine pharmacokinetics, but valproate significantly decreased tiagabine binding *in vitro* from 96.3 to 94.8%, which resulted in an increase of approximately 40% in the free tiagabine concentration. The clinical relevance of this *in vitro* finding is unknown.

Interaction of GABITRIL with Other Drugs:

Cimetidine: Co-administration of cimetidine (800 mg/day) to patients taking tiagabine chronically had no effect on tiagabine pharmacokinetics.

Theophylline: A single 10 mg dose of tiagabine did not affect the pharmacokinetics of theophylline at steady state.

Warfarin: No significant differences were observed in the steady-state pharmacokinetics of R-warfarin or S-warfarin with the addition of tiagabine given as a single dose. Prothrombin times were not affected by tiagabine.

Digoxin: Concomitant administration of tiagabine did not affect the steady-state pharmacokinetics of digoxin or the mean daily trough serum level of digoxin.

Ethanol or Triazolam: No significant differences were observed in the pharmacokinetics of triazolam (0.125 mg) and tiagabine (10 mg) when given together as a single dose. The pharmacokinetics of ethanol were not affected by multiple-dose administration of tiagabine. Tiagabine has shown no clinically important potentiation of the pharmacodynamic effects of triazolam or alcohol. Because of the possible additive effects of drugs that may depress the nervous system, ethanol or triazolam should be used cautiously in combination with tiagabine.

Oral Contraceptives: Multiple dose administration of tiagabine (8 mg/day monotherapy) did not alter the pharmacokinetics of oral contraceptives in healthy women of child-bearing age.

Table 4
Treatment-Emergent Adverse Event[1] Incidence in Parallel-Group, Placebo-Controlled, Add-On Trials (events in at least 1% of patients treated with GABITRIL and numerically more frequent than in the placebo group)

Body System/ COSTART	GABITRIL N=494 %	Placebo N=275 %
Body as a Whole		
Abdominal Pain	7	3
Pain (unspecified)	5	3
Cardiovascular		
Vasodilation	2	1
Digestive		
Nausea	11	9
Diarrhea	7	3
Vomiting	7	4
Increased Appetite	2	0
Mouth Ulceration	1	0
Musculoskeletal		
Myasthenia	1	0
Nervous System		
Dizziness	27	15
Asthenia	20	14
Somnolence	18	15
Nervousness	10	3
Tremor	9	3
Difficulty With Concentration/ Attention*	6	2
Insomnia	6	4
Ataxia	5	3
Confusion	5	3
Speech Disorder	4	2
Difficulty With Memory*	4	3
Paresthesia	4	2
Depression	3	1
Emotional Lability	3	2
Abnormal Gait	3	2
Hostility	2	1
Nystagmus	2	1
Language Problems*	2	0
Agitation	1	0
Respiratory System		
Pharyngitis	7	4
Cough Increased	4	3
Skin and Appendages		
Rash	5	4
Pruritus	2	0

[1] Patients in these add-on studies were receiving one to three concomitant enzyme-inducing antiepilepsy drugs in addition to GABITRIL or placebo. Patients may have reported multiple adverse experiences; thus, patients may be included in more than one category.

* COSTART term substituted with a more clinically descriptive term.

Antipyrine: Antipyrine pharmacokinetics were not significantly different before and after tiagabine multiple-dose regimens. This indicates that tiagabine does not cause induction or inhibition of the hepatic microsomal enzyme systems responsible for the metabolism of antipyrine.

Carcinogenesis: In rats, a study of the potential carcinogenicity associated with tiagabine HCl administration showed that 200 mg/kg/day (plasma exposure [AUC] 36 to 100 times that at the maximum recommended human dosage [MRHD] of 56 mg/day) for 2 years resulted in small, but statistically significant increases in the incidences of hepatocellular adenomas in females and Leydig cell tumors of the testis in males. The significance of these findings relative to the use of GABITRIL in humans is unknown. The no effect dosage for induction of tumors in this study was 100 mg/kg/day (17 to 50 times the exposure at the MRHD). No statistically significant increases in tumor formation were noted in mice at dosages up to 250 mg/kg/day (20 times the MRHD on a mg/m^2 basis).

Mutagenesis: Tiagabine produced an increase in structural chromosome aberration frequency in human lymphocytes *in vitro* in the absence of metabolic activation. No increase in chromosomal aberration frequencies was demonstrated in this assay in the presence of metabolic activation. No evidence of genetic toxicity was found in the *in vitro* bacterial gene mutation assays, the *in vitro* HGPRT forward mutation assay in Chinese hamster lung cells, the *in vivo* mouse micronucleus test, or an unscheduled DNA synthesis assay.

Impairment of Fertility: Studies of male and female rats administered dosages of tiagabine HCl prior to and during mating, gestation, and lactation have shown no impairment of fertility at doses up to 100 mg/kg/day. This dose represents approximately 16 times the maximum recommended human dose (MRHD) of 56 mg/day, based on body surface area (mg/m^2). Lowered maternal weight gain and decreased viability and growth in the rat pups were found at 100 mg/kg, but not at 20 mg/kg/day (3 times the MRHD on a mg/m^2 basis).

Pregnancy: Pregnancy Category C: Tiagabine has been shown to have adverse effects on embryo-fetal development, including teratogenic effects, when administered to pregnant rats and rabbits at doses greater than the human therapeutic dose.

An increased incidence of malformed fetuses (various craniofacial, appendicular, and visceral defects) and decreased fetal weights were observed following oral administration of 100 mg/kg/day to pregnant rats during the period of organogenesis. This dose is approximately 16 times the maximum recommended human dose (MRHD) of 56 mg/day, based on body surface area (mg/m^2). Maternal toxicity (transient weight loss/reduced maternal weight gain during gestation) was associated with this dose, but there is no evidence to suggest that the teratogenic effects were secondary to the maternal effects. No adverse maternal or embryo-fetal effects were seen at a dose of 20 mg/kg/day (3 times the MRHD on a mg/m^2 basis).

Decreased maternal weight gain, increased resorption of embryos and increased incidences of fetal variations, but not malformations, were observed when pregnant rabbits were given 25 mg/kg/day (8 times the MRHD on a mg/m^2 basis) during organogenesis. The no effect level for maternal and embryo-fetal toxicity in rabbits was 5 mg/kg/day (equivalent to the MRHD on a mg/m^2 basis).

When female rats were given tiagabine 100 mg/kg/day during late gestation and throughout parturition and lactation, decreased maternal weight gain during gestation, an increase in stillbirths, and decreased postnatal offspring viability and growth were found. There are no adequate and well-controlled studies in pregnant women. Tiagabine should be used during pregnancy only if clearly needed.

Use in Nursing Mothers: Studies in rats have shown that tiagabine HCl and/or its metabolites are excreted in the milk of that species. Levels of excretion of tiagabine and/or its metabolites in human milk have not been determined and effects on the nursing infant are unknown. GABITRIL should be used in women who are nursing only if the benefits clearly outweigh the risks.

Pediatric Use: Safety and effectiveness in pediatric patients below the age of 12 have not been established. The pharmacokinetics of tiagabine were evaluated in pediatric patients age 3 to 10 years (see **CLINICAL PHARMACOLOGY**—Pediatric).

Geriatric Use: Because few patients over the age of 65 (approximately 20) were exposed to GABITRIL during its clinical evaluation, no specific statements about the safety or effectiveness of GABITRIL in this age group could be made.

ADVERSE REACTIONS

The most commonly observed adverse events in placebo-controlled, parallel-group, add-on epilepsy trials associated with the use of GABITRIL in combination with other antiepilepsy drugs not seen at an equivalent frequency among placebo-treated patients were dizziness/light-headedness, asthenia/lack of energy, somnolence, nausea, nervousness/irritability, tremor, abdominal pain, and thinking abnormal/difficulty with concentration or attention.

Approximately 21% of the 2531 patients who received GABITRIL in clinical trials of epilepsy discontinued treat-

Continued on next page

Gabitril—Cont.

ment because of an adverse event. The adverse events most commonly associated with discontinuation were dizziness (1.7%), somnolence (1.6%), depression (1.3%), confusion (1.1%), and asthenia (1.1%).

In Studies 1 and 2 (U.S. studies), the double-blind, placebo-controlled, parallel-group, add-on studies, the proportion of patients who discontinued treatment because of adverse events was 11% for the group treated with GABITRIL and 6% for the placebo group. The most common adverse events considered the primary reason for discontinuation were confusion (1.2%), somnolence (1.0%), and ataxia (1.0%).

Adverse Event Incidence in Controlled Clinical Trials: Table 4 lists treatment-emergent signs and symptoms that occurred in at least 1% of patients treated with GABITRIL for epilepsy participating in parallel-group, placebo-controlled trials and were numerically more common in the GABITRIL group. In these studies, either GABITRIL or placebo was added to the patient's current antiepilepsy drug therapy. Adverse events were usually mild or moderate in intensity.

The prescriber should be aware that these figures, obtained when GABITRIL was added to concurrent antiepilepsy drug therapy, cannot be used to predict the frequency of adverse events in the course of usual medical practice when patient characteristics and other factors may differ from those prevailing during clinical studies. Similarly, the cited frequencies cannot be directly compared with figures obtained from other clinical investigations involving different treatments, uses, or investigators. An inspection of these frequencies, however, does provide the prescribing physician with one basis to estimate the relative contribution of drug and non-drug factors to the adverse event incidences in the population studied.

[See table 4 at top of previous page]

Other events reported by 1% or more of patients treated with GABITRIL but equally or more frequent in the placebo group were: accidental injury, chest pain, constipation, flu syndrome, rhinitis, anorexia, back pain, dry mouth, flatulence, ecchymosis, twitching, fever, amblyopia, conjunctivitis, urinary tract infection, urinary frequency, infection, dyspepsia, gastroenteritis, nausea and vomiting, myalgia, diplopia, headache, anxiety, acne, sinusitis, and incoordination.

Study 1 was a dose-response study including doses of 32 mg and 56 mg. Table 5 shows adverse events reported at a rate of ≥ 5% in at least one GABITRIL group and more frequent than in the placebo group. Among these events, tremor, difficulty with concentration/attention, and perhaps asthenia exhibited a positive relationship to dose.

[See table 5 at right]

The effects of GABITRIL in relation to those of placebo on the incidence of adverse events and the types of adverse events reported were independent of age, weight, and gender. Because only 10% of patients were non-Caucasian in parallel-group, placebo-controlled trials, there is insufficient data to support a statement regarding the distribution of adverse experience reports by race.

Other Adverse Events Observed During All Clinical Trials: GABITRIL has been administered to 2531 patients during all phase 2/3 clinical trials, only some of which were placebo-controlled. During these trials, all adverse events were recorded by the clinical investigators using terminology of their own choosing. To provide a meaningful estimate of the proportion of individuals having adverse events, similar types of events were grouped into a smaller number of standardized categories using modified COSTART dictionary terminology. These categories are used in the listing below. The frequencies presented represent the proportion of the 2531 patients exposed to GABITRIL who experienced events of the type cited on at least one occasion while receiving GABITRIL. All reported events are included except those already listed above, events seen only three times or fewer (unless potentially important), events very unlikely to be drug-related, and those too general to be informative. Events are included without regard to determination of a causal relationship to tiagabine.

Events are further classified within body system categories and enumerated in order of decreasing frequency using the following definitions: frequent adverse events are defined as those occurring in at least 1/100 patients; infrequent adverse events are those occurring in 1/100 to 1/1000 patients; rare events are those occurring in fewer than 1/1000 patients.

Body as a Whole: *Frequent:* Allergic reaction, chest pain, chills, cyst, neck pain, and malaise. *Infrequent:* Abscess, cellulitis, facial edema, halitosis, hernia, neck rigidity, neoplasm, pelvic pain, photosensitivity reaction, sepsis, sudden death, and suicide attempt.

Cardiovascular System: *Frequent:* Hypertension, palpitation, syncope, and tachycardia. *Infrequent:* Angina pectoris, cerebral ischemia, electrocardiogram abnormal, hemorrhage, hypotension, myocardial infarct, pallor, peripheral vascular disorder, phlebitis, postural hypotension, and thrombophlebitis.

Digestive System: *Frequent:* Gingivitis and stomatitis. *Infrequent:* Abnormal stools, cholecystitis, cholelithiasis, dysphagia, eructation, esophagitis, fecal incontinence, gastritis, gastrointestinal hemorrhage, glossitis, gum hyperplasia, hepatomegaly, increased salivation, liver function tests abnormal, melena, periodontal abscess, rectal hemorrhage, thirst, tooth caries, and ulcerative stomatitis.

Table 5
Treatment-Emergent Adverse Event Incidence in Study 1†
(events in at least 5% of patients treated with GABITRIL 32 or 56 mg and numerically more frequent than in the placebo group)

Body System/ COSTART Term	GABITRIL 56 mg (N=57) %	GABITRIL 32 mg (N=88) %	Placebo (N=91) %
Body as a Whole			
Accidental Injury	21	15	20
Infection	19	10	12
Flu Syndrome	9	6	3
Pain	7	2	3
Abdominal Pain	5	7	4
Digestive System			
Diarrhea	2	10	6
Hemic and Lymphatic System			
Ecchymosis	0	6	1
Musculoskeletal System			
Myalgia	5	2	3
Nervous System			
Dizziness	28	31	12
Asthenia	23	18	15
Tremor	21	14	1
Somnolence	19	21	17
Nervousness	14	11	6
Difficulty With Concentration/Attention*	14	7	3
Ataxia	9	6	6
Depression	7	1	0
Insomnia	5	6	3
Abnormal Gait	5	5	3
Hostility	5	5	2
Respiratory System			
Pharyngitis	7	8	6
Special Senses			
Amblyopia	4	9	8
Urogenital System			
Urinary Tract Infection	5	0	2

† Patients in this study were receiving one to three concomitant enzyme-inducing antiepilepsy drugs in addition to GABITRIL or placebo. Patients may have reported multiple adverse experiences; thus, patients may be included in more than one category.
* COSTART term substituted with a more clinically descriptive term.

Table 6
Typical Dosing Titration Regimen for Patients Taking Enzyme-Inducing AEDs

	Initiation and Titration Schedule	Total Daily Dose
Week 1	Initiate at 4 mg once daily	4 mg/day
Week 2	Increase total daily dose by 4 mg	8 mg/day (in two divided doses)
Week 3	Increase total daily dose by 4 mg	12 mg/day (in three divided doses)
Week 4	Increase total daily dose by 4 mg	16 mg/day (in two to four divided doses)
Week 5	Increase total daily dose by 4 to 8 mg	20 to 24 mg/day (in two to four divided doses)
Week 6	Increase total daily dose by 4 to 8 mg	24 to 32 mg/day (in two to four divided doses)
Usual Adult Maintenance Dose:	32 to 56 mg/day in two to four divided doses	

Endocrine System: *Infrequent:* Goiter and hypothyroidism.

Hemic and Lymphatic System: *Frequent:* Lymphadenopathy. *Infrequent:* Anemia, erythrocytes abnormal, leukopenia, petechia, and thrombocytopenia.

Metabolic and Nutritional: *Frequent:* Edema, peripheral edema, weight gain, and weight loss. *Infrequent:* Dehydration, hypercholesteremia, hyperglycemia, hyperlipemia, hypoglycemia, hypokalemia, and hyponatremia.

Musculoskeletal System: *Frequent:* Arthralgia. *Infrequent:* Arthritis, arthrosis, bursitis, generalized spasm, and tendinous contracture.

Nervous System: *Frequent:* Depersonalization, dysarthria, euphoria, hallucination, hyperkinesia, hypertonia, hypesthesia, hypokinesia, hypotonia, migraine, myoclonus, paranoid reaction, personality disorder, reflexes decreased, stupor, twitching, and vertigo. *Infrequent:* Abnormal dreams, apathy, choreoathetosis, circumoral paresthesia, CNS neoplasm, coma, delusions, dry mouth, dystonia, encephalopathy, hemiplegia, leg cramps, libido increased, libido decreased, movement disorder, neuritis, neurosis, paralysis, peripheral neuritis, psychosis, reflexes increased, and urinary retention.

Respiratory System: *Frequent:* Bronchitis, dyspnea, epistaxis, and pneumonia. *Infrequent:* Apnea, asthma, hemoptysis, hiccups, hyperventilation, laryngitis, respiratory disorder, and voice alteration.

Skin and Appendages: *Frequent:* Alopecia, dry skin, and sweating. *Infrequent:* Contact dermatitis, eczema, exfoliative dermatitis, furunculosis, herpes simplex, herpes zoster, hirsutism, maculopapular rash, psoriasis, skin benign neoplasm, skin carcinoma, skin discolorations, skin nodules, skin ulcer, subcutaneous nodule, urticaria, and vesiculobullous rash.

Special Senses: *Frequent:* Abnormal vision, ear pain, otitis media, and tinnitus. *Infrequent:* Blepharitis, blindness, deafness, eye pain, hyperacusis, keratoconjunctivitis, otitis externa, parosmia, photophobia, taste loss, taste perversion, and visual field defect.

Urogenital System: *Frequent:* Dysmenorrhea, dysuria, metrorrhagia, urinary incontinence, and vaginitis. *Infrequent:* Abortion, amenorrhea, breast enlargement, breast pain, cystitis, fibrocystic breast, hematuria, impotence, kidney failure, menorrhagia, nocturia, papanicolaou smear suspicious, polyuria, pyelonephritis, salpingitis, urethritis, urinary urgency, and vaginal hemorrhage.

Post-marketing Reports: The following adverse reactions have been identified during post-approval use of GABITRIL. Because these reactions are reported voluntarily from a population of uncertain size, it is not always possible to reliably estimate their frequency or establish a causal relationship to drug exposure. Decisions to include these reactions in labeling are typically based on one or more of the following factors: (1) seriousness of the reaction, (2) frequency of the reporting, or (3) strength of causal connection to GABITRIL.

Nervous System: Seizures including status epilepticus.

DRUG ABUSE AND DEPENDENCE

The abuse and dependence potential of GABITRIL have not been evaluated in human studies.

OVERDOSAGE

Human Overdose Experience: Human experience of acute overdose with GABITRIL is limited. Eleven patients in clinical trials took single doses of GABITRIL up to 800 mg. All patients fully recovered, usually within one day. The most common symptoms reported after overdose included somnolence, impaired consciousness, agitation, confusion, speech difficulty, hostility, depression, weakness, and myoclonus. One patient who ingested a single dose of 400 mg experienced generalized tonic-clonic status epilepticus, which responded to intravenous phenobarbital.

From post-marketing experience, there have been no reports of fatal overdoses involving GABITRIL alone (doses up to 720 mg) or in combination with other drugs. Symptoms most often accompanying GABITRIL overdose, alone or in combination with other drugs, have included: seizures including status epilecticus in patients with and without underlying seizure disorders, nonconvulsive status epilepticus, coma, ataxia, confusion, somnolence, drowsiness, impaired speech, agitation, lethargy, myoclonus, spike wave stupor, tremors, disorientation, vomiting, hostility, and temporary paralysis. All individuals recovered with supportive care, usually within one day.

Cases of accidental ingestion/overdose have been reported in children as young as 1 year-old. The symptoms associated with overdose in children less than 16 years-old were similar to those observed in adults with the exception of respiratory depression that occurred in 2 brothers ages 2 and 3 years-old who also experienced seizures and may therefore have represented an ictal phenomenon.

Management of Overdose: There is no specific antidote for overdose with GABITRIL. If indicated, elimination of unabsorbed drug should be achieved by emesis or gastric lavage; usual precautions should be observed to maintain the airway. General supportive care of the patient is indicated including monitoring of vital signs and observation of clinical status of the patient. Since tiagabine is mostly metabolized by the liver and is highly protein bound, dialysis is unlikely to be beneficial. A Certified Poison Control Center should be consulted for up to date information on the management of overdose with GABITRIL.

DOSAGE AND ADMINISTRATION

GABITRIL (tiagabine HCl) is recommended as adjunctive therapy in patients 12 years and older. GABITRIL is given orally and should be taken with food.

Adequate and controlled clinical studies with GABITRIL were conducted in patients taking enzyme-inducing AEDs (e.g., phenytoin, carbamazepine, and barbiturates). Patients taking only non-enzyme-inducing AEDs (e.g., valproate, gabapentin, and lamotrigine) may require lower doses or a slower titration of GABITRIL for clinical response.

Adults and Adolescents 12 Years or Older: In adolescents 12 to 18 years old, GABITRIL should be initiated at 4 mg once daily. Modification of concomitant antiepilepsy drugs is not necessary, unless clinically indicated. The total daily dose of GABITRIL may be increased by 4 mg at the beginning of Week 2. Thereafter, the total daily dose may be increased by 4 to 8 mg at weekly intervals until clinical response is achieved or up to 32 mg/day. The total daily dose should be given in divided doses two to four times daily. Doses above 32 mg/day have been tolerated in a small number of adolescent patients for a relatively short duration.

In adults, GABITRIL should be initiated at 4 mg once daily. Modification of concomitant antiepilepsy drugs is not necessary, unless clinically indicated. The total daily dose of GABITRIL may be increased by 4 to 8 mg at weekly intervals until clinical response is achieved or, up to 56 mg/day. The total daily dose should be given in divided doses two to four times daily. Doses above 56 mg/day have not been systematically evaluated in adequate well-controlled trials.

Experience is limited in patients taking total daily doses above 32 mg/day using twice daily dosing. A typical dosing titration regimen for patients taking enzyme-inducing AEDs is provided in Table 6.

[See table 6 on previous page]

HOW SUPPLIED

GABITRIL tablets are available in five dosage strengths.

2 mg orange-peach, round tablets, debossed with [C] on one side and 402 on the opposite side, are available in bottles of 100 (**NDC** 63459-402-01).

4 mg yellow, round tablets, debossed with [C] on one side and 404 on the opposite side, are available in bottles of 100 (**NDC** 63459-404-01).

12 mg green, ovaloid tablets, debossed with [C] on one side and 412 on the opposite side, are available in bottles of 100 (**NDC** 63459-412-01).

16 mg blue, ovaloid tablets, debossed with [C] on one side and 416 on the opposite side, are available in bottles of 100 (**NDC** 63459-416-01).

Recommended Storage: Store tablets at controlled room temperature, between 20-25°C (68-77°F). See USP. Protect from light and moisture.

ANIMAL TOXICOLOGY

In repeat dose toxicology studies, dogs receiving daily oral doses of 5 mg/kg/day or greater experienced unexpected CNS effects throughout the study. These effects occurred acutely and included marked sedation and apparent visual impairment which was characterized by a lack of awareness of objects, failure to fix on and follow moving objects, and absence of a blink reaction. Plasma exposures (AUCs) at 5 mg/kg/day were equal to those in humans receiving the maximum recommended daily human dose of 56 mg/day. The effects were reversible upon cessation of treatment and were not associated with any observed structural abnormality. The implications of these findings for humans are unknown.

Revised: July, 2004

Ref. 03-4957-R5

Manufactured for Cephalon, Inc., West Chester, PA 19380

GAB 014/A JAN 2004 MASTER

Shown in Product Identification Guide, page 310

PROVIGIL® ℞

[pro-vij-el]

(modafinil) Tablets [C-IV]

Rx Only

DESCRIPTION

PROVIGIL (modafinil) is a wakefulness-promoting agent for oral administration. Modafinil is a racemic compound. The chemical name for modafinil is 2-[(diphenylmethyl) sulfinyl]acetamide. The molecular formula is $C_{15}H_{15}NO_2S$ and the molecular weight is 273.36.

The chemical structure is:

Modafinil is a white to off-white, crystalline powder that is practically insoluble in water and cyclohexane. It is sparingly to slightly soluble in methanol and acetone. PROVIGIL tablets contain 100 mg or 200 mg of modafinil and the following inactive ingredients: lactose, microcrystalline cellulose, pregelatinized starch, croscarmellose sodium, povidone, and magnesium stearate.

CLINICAL PHARMACOLOGY

Mechanism of Action and Pharmacology

The precise mechanism(s) through which modafinil promotes wakefulness is unknown. Modafinil has wake-promoting actions like sympathomimetic agents including amphetamine and methylphenidate, although the pharmacologic profile is not identical to that of sympathomimetic amines.

At pharmacologically relevant concentrations, modafinil does not bind to most potentially relevant receptors for sleep/wake regulation, including those for norepinephrine, serotonin, dopamine, GABA, adenosine, histamine-3, melatonin, or benzodiazepines. Modafinil also does not inhibit the activities of MAO-B or phosphodiesterases II-V.

Modafinil is not a direct- or indirect-acting dopamine receptor agonist and is inactive in several *in vivo* preclinical models capable of detecting enhanced dopaminergic activity. *In vitro*, modafinil binds to the dopamine reuptake site and causes an increase in extracellular dopamine, but no increase in dopamine release. In a preclinical model, the wakefulness induced by amphetamine, but not modafinil, is antagonized by the dopamine receptor antagonist haloperidol.

Modafinil does not appear to be a direct or indirect α_1-adrenergic agonist. Although modafinil-induced wakefulness can be attenuated by the α_1-adrenergic receptor antagonist, prazosin, in assay systems known to be responsive to α-adrenergic agonists, modafinil has no activity. Modafinil does not display sympathomimetic activity in the rat vas deferens preparations (agonist-stimulated or electrically stimulated) nor does it increase the formation of the adrenergic receptor-mediated second messenger phosphatidyl inositol in *in vitro* models. Unlike sympathomimetic agents, modafinil does not reduce cataplexy in narcoleptic canines and has minimal effects on cardiovascular and hemodynamic parameters.

In the cat, equal wakefulness-promoting doses of methylphenidate and amphetamine increased neuronal activation throughout the brain. Modafinil at an equivalent wakefulness-promoting dose selectively and prominently increased neuronal activation in more discrete regions of the brain. The relationship of this finding in cats to the effects of modafinil in humans is unknown.

In addition to its wakefulness-promoting effects and increased locomotor activity in animals, in humans, PROVIGIL produces psychoactive and euphoric effects, alterations in mood, perception, thinking, and feelings typical of other CNS stimulants. Modafinil is reinforcing, as evidenced by its self-administration in monkeys previously trained to self-administer cocaine, modafinil was also partially discriminated as stimulant-like.

The optical enantiomers of modafinil have similar pharmacological actions in animals. Two major metabolites of modafinil, modafinil acid and modafinil sulfone, do not appear to contribute to the CNS-activating properties of modafinil.

Pharmacokinetics

Modafinil is a racemic compound, whose enantiomers have different pharmacokinetics (e.g., the half-life of the *l*-isomer is approximately three times that of the *d*-isomer in humans). The enantiomers do not interconvert. At steady state, total exposure to the *l*-isomer is approximately three times that for the *d*-isomer. The trough concentration (C_{minss}) of circulating modafinil after once daily dosing consists of 90% of the *l*-isomer and 10% of the *d*-isomer. The effective elimination half-life of modafinil after multiple doses is about 15 hours. The enantiomers of modafinil exhibit linear kinetics upon multiple dosing of 200-600 mg/day once daily in healthy volunteers. Apparent steady states of total modafinil and *l*-(-)-modafinil are reached after 2-4 days of dosing.

Absorption and Distribution

Absorption of PROVIGIL tablets is rapid, with peak plasma concentrations occurring at 2-4 hours. The bioavailability of PROVIGIL tablets is approximately equal to that of an aqueous suspension. The absolute oral bioavailability was not determined due to the aqueous insolubility (<1 mg/mL) of modafinil, which precluded intravenous administration. Food has no effect on overall PROVIGIL bioavailability; however, its absorption (t_{max}) may be delayed by approximately one hour if taken with food.

Modafinil is well distributed in body tissue with an apparent volume of distribution (~0.9 L/kg) larger than the volume of total body water (0.6 L/kg). In human plasma, *in vitro*, modafinil is moderately bound to plasma protein (~60%, mainly to albumin). At serum concentrations obtained at steady state after doses of 200 mg/day, modafinil exhibits no displacement of protein binding of warfarin, diazepam, or propranolol. Even at much larger concentrations (1000µM; >25 times the C_{max} of 40µM at steady state at 400 mg/day), modafinil has no effect on warfarin binding. Modafinil acid at concentrations >500µM decreases the extent of warfarin binding, but these concentrations are >35 times those achieved therapeutically.

Metabolism and Elimination

The major route of elimination (~90%) is metabolism, primarily by the liver, with subsequent renal elimination of the metabolites. Urine alkalinization has no effect on the elimination of modafinil.

Metabolism occurs through hydrolytic deamidation, S-oxidation, aromatic ring hydroxylation, and glucuronide conjugation. Less than 10% of an administered dose is excreted as the parent compound. In a clinical study using radiolabeled modafinil, a total of 81% of the administered radioactivity was recovered in 11 days post-dose, predominantly in the urine (80% vs. 1.0% in the feces). The largest fraction of the drug in urine was modafinil acid, but at least six other metabolites were present in lower concentrations. Only two metabolites reach appreciable concentrations in plasma, i.e., modafinil acid and modafinil sulfone. In preclinical models, modafinil acid, modafinil sulfone, 2-[(diphenylmethyl)-sulfonyl]acetic acid and 4-hydroxy modafinil, were inactive or did not appear to mediate the arousal effects of modafinil.

In humans, decreases in trough levels of modafinil have sometimes been observed after multiple weeks of dosing, suggesting auto-induction, but the magnitude of the decreases and the inconsistency of their occurrence suggest that their clinical significance is minimal. Significant accumulation of modafinil sulfone has been observed after multiple doses due to its long elimination half-life of 40 hours. Induction of metabolizing enzymes, most importantly cytochrome P-450 (CYP) 3A4, has also been observed *in vitro* after incubation of primary cultures of human hepatocytes with modafinil and *in vivo* after extended administration of modafinil at 400 mg/day. (For further discussion of the effects of modafinil on CYP enzyme activities see **PRECAUTIONS, Drug Interactions**).

Drug-Drug Interactions: Because modafinil and modafinil sulfone are reversible inhibitors of the drug-metabolizing enzyme CYP2C19, co-administration of modafinil with drugs such as diazepam, phenytoin and propranolol, which are largely eliminated via that pathway, may increase the circulating levels of those compounds. In addition, in individuals deficient in the enzyme CYP2D6 (i.e., 7-10% of the Caucasian population; similar or lower in other populations), the levels of CYP2D6 substrates such as tricyclic antidepressants and selective serotonin reuptake inhibitors, which have ancillary routes of elimination through CYP2C19, may be increased by co-administration of modafinil. Dose adjustments may be necessary for patients being treated with these and similar medications (See **PRECAUTIONS, Drug Interactions**).

Coadministration of modafinil with other CNS active drugs such as methylphenidate and dextroamphetamine did not significantly alter the pharmacokinetics of either drug.

Chronic administration of modafinil 400 mg was found to decrease the systemic exposure to two CYP3A4 substrates, ethinyl estradiol and triazolam, after oral administration suggesting that CYP3A4 had been induced. Chronic administration of modafinil can increase the elimination of substrates of CYP3A4. Dose adjustments may be necessary for patients being treated with these and similar medications (See **PRECAUTIONS, Drug Interactions**).

An apparent concentration-related suppression of CYP2C9 activity was observed in human hepatocytes after exposure to modafinil *in vitro* suggesting that there is a potential for a metabolic interaction between modafinil and the substrates of this enzyme (e.g., S-warfarin, phenytoin). However, in an interaction study in healthy volunteers, chronic modafinil treatment did not show a significant effect on the pharmacokinetics of warfarin when compared to placebo. (See **PRECAUTIONS, Drug Interactions,** *Other Drugs*, Warfarin).

Continued on next page

Provigil—Cont.

Special Populations
Gender Effect: The pharmacokinetics of modafinil are not affected by gender.
Age Effect: A slight decrease (~20%) in the oral clearance (CL/F) of modafinil was observed in a single dose study at 200 mg in 12 subjects with a mean age of 63 years (range 53 - 72 years), but the change was considered not likely to be clinically significant. In a multiple dose study (300 mg/day) in 12 patients with a mean age of 82 years (range 67 - 87 years), the mean levels of modafinil in plasma were approximately two times those historically obtained in matched younger subjects. Due to potential effects from the multiple concomitant medications with which most of the patients were being treated, the apparent difference in modafinil pharmacokinetics may not be attributable solely to the effects of aging. However, the results suggest that the clearance of modafinil may be reduced in the elderly (See **DOSAGE AND ADMINISTRATION**).
Race Effect: The influence of race on the pharmacokinetics of modafinil has not been studied.
Renal Impairment: In a single dose 200 mg modafinil study, severe chronic renal failure (creatinine clearance ≤20 mL/min) did not significantly influence the pharmacokinetics of modafinil, but exposure to modafinil acid (an inactive metabolite) was increased 9 fold (See **PRECAUTIONS**).
Hepatic Impairment: Pharmacokinetics and metabolism were examined in patients with cirrhosis of the liver (6 M and 3 F). Three patients had stage B or B+ cirrhosis (per the Child criteria) and 6 patients had stage C or C+ cirrhosis. Clinically 8 of 9 patients were icteric and all had ascites. In these patients, the oral clearance of modafinil was decreased by about 60% and the steady state concentration was doubled compared to normal patients. The dose of PROVIGIL should be reduced in patients with severe hepatic impairment (See **PRECAUTIONS** and **DOSAGE AND ADMINISTRATION**).

CLINICAL TRIALS

The effectiveness of PROVIGIL in reducing excessive sleepiness has been established in the following sleep disorders: narcolepsy, obstructive sleep apnea/hypopnea syndrome (OSAHS), and shift work sleep disorder (SWSD).
Narcolepsy
The effectiveness of PROVIGIL in reducing the excessive sleepiness (ES) associated with narcolepsy was established in two US 9-week, multicenter, placebo-controlled, two-dose (200 mg per day and 400 mg per day) parallel-group, double-blind studies of outpatients who met the ICD-9 and American Sleep Disorders Association criteria for narcolepsy (which are also consistent with the American Psychiatric Association DSM-IV criteria). These criteria include either 1) recurrent daytime naps or lapses into sleep that occur almost daily for at least three months, plus sudden bilateral loss of postural muscle tone in association with intense emotion (cataplexy) or 2) a complaint of excessive sleepiness or sudden muscle weakness with associated features: sleep paralysis, hypnagogic hallucinations, automatic behaviors, disrupted major sleep episode; and polysomnography demonstrating one of the following: sleep latency less than 10 minutes or rapid eye movement (REM) sleep latency less than 20 minutes. In addition, for entry into these studies, all patients were required to have objectively documented excessive daytime sleepiness, a Multiple Sleep Latency Test (MSLT) with two or more sleep onset REM periods, and the absence of any other clinically significant active medical or psychiatric disorder. The MSLT, an objective daytime polysomnographic assessment of the patient's ability to fall asleep in an unstimulating environment, measures latency (in minutes) to sleep onset averaged over 4 test sessions at 2-hour intervals following nocturnal polysomnography. For each test session, the subject was told to lie quietly and attempt to sleep. Each test session was terminated after 20 minutes if no sleep occurred or 15 minutes after sleep onset.
In both studies, the primary measures of effectiveness were 1) sleep latency, as assessed by the Maintenance of Wakefulness Test (MWT) and 2) the change in the patient's overall disease status, as measured by the Clinical Global Impression of Change (CGI-C). For a successful trial, both measures had to show significant improvement.
The MWT measures latency (in minutes) to sleep onset averaged over 4 test sessions at 2 hour intervals following nocturnal polysomnography. For each test session, the subject was asked to attempt to remain awake without using extraordinary measures. Each test session was terminated after 20 minutes if no sleep occurred or 10 minutes after sleep onset. The CGI-C is a 7-point scale, centered at *No Change*, and ranging from *Very Much Worse* to *Very Much Improved*. Patients were rated by evaluators who had no access to any data about the patients other than a measure of their baseline severity. Evaluators were not given any specific guidance about the criteria they were to apply when rating patients.
Other assessments of effect included the Multiple Sleep Latency Test (MSLT), Epworth Sleepiness Scale (ESS; a series of questions designed to assess the degree of sleepiness in everyday situations) the Steer Clear Performance Test (SCPT; a computer-based evaluation of a patient's ability to avoid hitting obstacles in a simulated driving situation), standard nocturnal polysomnography, and patient's daily sleep log. Patients were also assessed with the Quality of Life in Narcolepsy (QOLIN) scale, which contains the validated SF-36 health questionnaire.
Both studies demonstrated improvement in objective and subjective measures of excessive daytime sleepiness for both the 200 mg and 400 mg doses compared to placebo. Patients treated with either dose of PROVIGIL showed a statistically significantly enhanced ability to remain awake on the MWT (all p values <0.001) at weeks 3, 6, 9, and final visit compared to placebo and a statistically significantly greater global improvement, as rated on the CGI-C scale (all p values <0.05).
The average sleep latencies (in minutes) on the MWT at baseline for the 2 controlled trials are shown in Table 1 below, along with the average change from baseline on the MWT at final visit.
The percentages of patients who showed any degree of improvement on the CGI-C in the two clinical trials are shown in Table 2 below.
Similar statistically significant treatment-related improvements were seen on other measures of impairment in narcolepsy, including a patient assessed level of daytime sleepiness on the ESS (p<0.001 for each dose in comparison to placebo).
Although PROVIGIL tended to be numerically superior to placebo on several of the other outcome measures, there were no consistent statistically significant differences between drug and placebo on these measures.
Nighttime sleep measured with polysomnography was not affected by the use of PROVIGIL.
The effectiveness of modafinil in long-term use (greater than 9 weeks) has not been systematically evaluated in placebo-controlled trials. The physician who elects to prescribe PROVIGIL tablets for an extended time in patients with narcolepsy should periodically re-evaluate long-term usefulness for the individual patient.
Obstructive Sleep Apnea/Hypopnea Syndrome (OSAHS)
The effectiveness of PROVIGIL in reducing the excessive sleepiness associated with OSAHS was established in two clinical trials. In both studies, patients were enrolled who met the International Classification of Sleep Disorders (ICSD) criteria for OSAHS (which are also consistent with the American Psychiatric Association DSM-IV criteria). These criteria include either, 1) excessive sleepiness or insomnia, plus frequent episodes of impaired breathing during sleep, and associated features such as loud snoring, morning headaches and dry mouth upon awakening; or 2) excessive sleepiness or insomnia and polysomnography demonstrating one of the following: more than five obstructive apneas, each greater than 10 seconds in duration, per hour of sleep and one or more of the following: frequent arousals from sleep associated with the apneas, bradytachycardia, and arterial oxygen desaturation in association with the apneas. In addition, for entry into these studies, all patients were required to have excessive sleepiness as demonstrated by a score ≥10 on the Epworth Sleepiness Scale, despite treatment with continuous positive airway pressure (CPAP). Evidence that CPAP was effective in reducing episodes of apnea/hypopnea was required along with documentation of CPAP use.
In the first study, a 12-week multicenter placebo-controlled trial, a total of 327 patients were randomized to receive PROVIGIL 200mg/day, PROVIGIL 400mg/day, or matching placebo. The majority of patients (80%) were fully compliant with CPAP, defined as CPAP use >4 hours/night on >70% nights. The remainder were partially CPAP compliant, defined as CPAP use <4 hours/night on >30% nights. CPAP use continued throughout the study. The primary measures of effectiveness were 1) sleep latency, as assessed by the Maintenance of Wakefulness Test (MWT) and 2) the change in the patient's overall disease status, as measured by the Clinical Global Impression of Change (CGI-C) at week 12 or the final visit. (See **CLINICAL TRIALS**, Narcolepsy section above for a description of these tests.)
Patients treated with PROVIGIL showed a statistically significant improvement in the ability to remain awake compared to placebo-treated patients as measured by the MWT (p<0.001) at endpoint [Table 1]. PROVIGIL-treated patients also showed a statistically significant improvement in clinical condition as rated by the CGI-C scale (p<0.001) [Table 2]. The two doses of PROVIGIL performed similarly.
In the second study, a 4-week multicenter placebo-controlled trial, 157 patients were randomized to either PROVIGIL 400 mg/day or placebo. Documentation of regular CPAP use (at least 4 hours/night on 70% of nights) was required for all patients.
The primary outcome measure was the change from baseline on the ESS at week 4 or final visit. The baseline ESS scores for the PROVIGIL and placebo groups were 14.2 and 14.4, respectively. At week 4, the ESS was reduced by 4.6 in the PROVIGIL group and by 2.0 in the placebo group, a difference that was statistically significant (p<0.0001).
Nighttime sleep measured with polysomnography was not affected by the use of PROVIGIL.
The effectiveness of modafinil in long-term use (greater than 12 weeks) has not been systematically evaluated in placebo-controlled trials. The physician who elects to prescribe PROVIGIL tablets for an extended time in patients with OSAHS should periodically reevaluate long-term usefulness for the individual patient.
Shift Work Sleep Disorder (SWSD)
The effectiveness of PROVIGIL for the excessive sleepiness associated with SWSD was demonstrated in a 12-week placebo-controlled clinical trial. A total of 209 patients with chronic SWSD were randomized to receive PROVIGIL 200mg/day or placebo. All patients met the International Classification of Sleep Disorders (ICSD-10) criteria for chronic SWSD (which are consistent with the American Psychiatric Association DSM-IV criteria for Circadian Rhythm Sleep Disorder: Shift Work Type). These criteria include 1) either: a) a primary complaint of excessive sleepiness or insomnia which is temporally associated with a work period (usually night work) that occurs during the habitual sleep phase, or b) polysomnography and the MSLT demonstrate loss of a normal sleep-wake pattern (i.e., disturbed chronobiological rhythmicity); and 2) no other medical or mental disorder accounts for the symptoms, and 3) the symptoms do not meet criteria for any other sleep disorder producing insomnia or excessive sleepiness (e.g., time zone change [jet lag] syndrome).
It should be noted that not all patients with a complaint of sleepiness who are also engaged in shift work meet the criteria for the diagnosis of SWSD. In the clinical trial, only patients who were symptomatic for at least 3 months were enrolled.
Enrolled patients were also required to work a minimum of 5 night shifts per month, have excessive sleepiness at the time of their night shifts (MSLT score < 6 minutes), and have daytime insomnia documented by a daytime polysomnogram (PSG).
The primary measures of effectiveness were 1) sleep latency, as assessed by the Multiple Sleep Latency Test (MSLT) performed during a simulated night shift at week 12 or the final visit and 2) the change in the patient's overall disease status, as measured by the Clinical Global Impression of Change (CGI-C) at week 12 or the final visit. Patients treated with PROVIGIL showed a statistically significant prolongation in the time to sleep onset compared to placebo-treated patients, as measured by the nighttime MSLT [Table 1] (p<0.05). Improvement on the CGI-C was also observed to be statistically significant (p<0.001).
Daytime sleep measured with polysomnography was not affected by the use of PROVIGIL.
The effectiveness of modafinil in long-term use (greater than 12 weeks) has not been systematically evaluated in placebo-controlled trials. The physician who elects to prescribe PROVIGIL for an extended time in patients with SWSD should periodically reevaluate long-term usefulness for the individual patient.
[See table 1 at left]

Table 1. Average Baseline Sleep Latency and Change from Baseline at Final Visit (MWT and MSLT in minutes)

Disorder	Measure	PROVIGIL 200 mg*		PROVIGIL 400 mg*		Placebo	
		Baseline	Change from baseline	Baseline	Change from baseline	Baseline	Change from baseline
Narcolepsy I	MWT	5.8	2.3	6.6	2.3	5.8	-0.7
Narcolepsy II	MWT	6.1	2.2	5.9	2.0	6.0	-0.7
OSAHS	MWT	13.1	1.6	13.6	1.5	13.8	-1.1
SWSD	MSLT	2.1	1.7	–	–	2.0	0.3

*Significantly different than placebo for all trials (p<0.01) for all trials but SWSD, which was p<0.05)

Table 2. Clinical Global Impression of Change (CGI-C) (Percent of Patients Who Improved at Final Visit)

Disorder	PROVIGIL 200 mg*	PROVIGIL 400 mg*	Placebo
Narcolepsy I	64%	72%	37%
Narcolepsy II	58%	60%	38%
OSAHS	61%	68%	37%
SWSD	74%	—	36%

*Significantly different than placebo for all trials (p<0.01)

INDICATIONS AND USAGE

PROVIGIL is indicated to improve wakefulness in patients with excessive sleepiness associated with narcolepsy, obstructive sleep apnea/hypopnea syndrome, and shift work sleep disorder.
In OSAHS, PROVIGIL is indicated as an adjunct to standard treatment(s) for the underlying obstruction. If contin-

uous positive airway pressure (CPAP) is the treatment of choice for a patient, a maximal effort to treat with CPAP for an adequate period of time should be made prior to initiating PROVIGIL. If PROVIGIL is used adjunctively with CPAP, the encouragement of and periodic assessment of CPAP compliance is necessary.

In all cases, careful attention to the diagnosis and treatment of the underlying sleep disorder(s) is of utmost importance. Prescribers should be aware that some patients may have more than one sleep disorder contributing to their excessive sleepiness.

CONTRAINDICATIONS

PROVIGIL is contraindicated in patients with known hypersensitivity to modafinil or its inactive ingredients.

WARNINGS

Patients with abnormal levels of sleepiness who take PROVIGIL should be advised that their level of wakefulness may not return to normal. Patients with excessive sleepiness, including those taking PROVIGIL, should be frequently reassessed for their degree of sleepiness and, if appropriate, advised to avoid driving or any other potentially dangerous activity. Prescribers should also be aware that patients may not acknowledge sleepiness or drowsiness until directly questioned about drowsiness or sleepiness during specific activities.

PRECAUTIONS

Diagnosis of Sleep Disorders

PROVIGIL should be used only in patients who have had a complete evaluation of their excessive sleepiness, and in whom a diagnosis of either narcolepsy, OSAHS, and/or SWSD has been made in accordance with ICSD or DSM diagnostic criteria (See **CLINICAL TRIALS** Section). Such an evaluation usually consists of a complete history and physical examination, and it may be supplemented with testing in a laboratory setting. Some patients may have more than one sleep disorder contributing to their excessive sleepiness (e.g., OSAHS and SWSD coincident in the same patient).

CPAP Use in Patients with OSAHS

In OSAHS, PROVIGIL is indicated as an adjunct to standard treatment(s) for the underlying obstruction. If continuous positive airway pressure (CPAP) is the treatment of choice for a patient, a maximal effort to treat with CPAP for an adequate period of time should be made prior to initiating PROVIGIL. If PROVIGIL is used adjunctively with CPAP, the encouragement of and periodic assessment of CPAP compliance is necessary.

General

Although modafinil has not been shown to produce functional impairment, any drug affecting the CNS may alter judgment, thinking or motor skills. Patients should be cautioned about operating an automobile or other hazardous machinery until they are reasonably certain that PROVIGIL therapy will not adversely affect their ability to engage in such activities.

Patients Using Contraceptives

The effectiveness of steroidal contraceptives may be reduced when used with PROVIGIL tablets and for one month after discontinuation of therapy (See **Drug Interactions**). Alternative or concomitant methods of contraception are recommended for patients treated with PROVIGIL tablets, and for one month after discontinuation of PROVIGIL.

Cardiovascular System

In clinical studies of PROVIGIL, signs and symptoms including chest pain, palpitations, dyspnea and transient ischemic T-wave changes on ECG were observed in three subjects in association with mitral valve prolapse or left ventricular hypertrophy. It is recommended that PROVIGIL tablets not be used in patients with a history of left ventricular hypertrophy or in patients with mitral valve prolapse who have experienced the mitral valve prolapse syndrome when previously receiving CNS stimulants. Such signs may include but are not limited to ischemic ECG changes, chest pain, or arrhythmia.

Modafinil has not been evaluated or used to any appreciable extent in patients with a recent history of myocardial infarction or unstable angina, and such patients should be treated with caution.

Blood pressure monitoring in short-term (<3 months) controlled trials showed no clinically significant changes in mean systolic and diastolic blood pressure in patients receiving PROVIGIL as compared to placebo. However, a retrospective analysis of the use of antihypertensive medication in these studies showed that a greater proportion of patients on PROVIGIL required new or increased use of antihypertensive medications (2.4%) compared to patients on placebo (0.7%). The differential use was slightly larger when only studies in OSAHS were included, with 3.4% of patients on PROVIGIL and 1.1% of patients on placebo requiring such alterations in the use of antihypertensive medication. Increased monitoring of blood pressure may be appropriate in patients on PROVIGIL.

Central Nervous System

There have been reports of psychotic episodes associated with PROVIGIL use. One healthy male volunteer developed ideas of reference, paranoid delusions, and auditory hallucinations in association with multiple daily 600 mg doses of PROVIGIL and sleep deprivation. There was no evidence of psychosis 36 hours after drug discontinuation. Caution should be exercised when PROVIGIL is given to patients with a history of psychosis.

Patients with Severe Renal Impairment

In patients with severe renal impairment (mean creatinine clearance = 16.6 mL/min), a 200 mg single dose of modafinil did not lead to increased exposure to modafinil but resulted in much higher exposure to the inactive metabolite, modafinil acid, than is seen in subjects with normal renal function. There is little information available about the safety of such levels of this metabolite (See **CLINICAL PHARMACOLOGY**).

Patients with Severe Hepatic Impairment

In patients with severe hepatic impairment, with or without cirrhosis (See **CLINICAL PHARMACOLOGY**), PROVIGIL should be administered at a reduced dose as the clearance of modafinil was decreased compared to that in normal subjects (See **DOSAGE AND ADMINISTRATION**).

Elderly Patients

To the extent that elderly patients may have diminished renal and/or hepatic function, dosage reductions should be considered (See **DOSAGE AND ADMINISTRATION**).

Information for Patients

Physicians are advised to discuss the following issues with patients for whom they prescribe PROVIGIL.

PROVIGIL is indicated for patients who have abnormal levels of sleepiness. PROVIGIL has been shown to improve, but not eliminate this abnormal tendency to fall asleep. Therefore, patients should not alter their previous behavior with regard to potentially dangerous activities (e.g., driving, operating machinery) or other activities requiring appropriate levels of wakefulness, until and unless treatment with PROVIGIL has been shown to produce levels of wakefulness that permit such activities. Patients should be advised that PROVIGIL is not a replacement for sleep.

Patients should be informed that it may be critical that they continue to take their previously prescribed treatments (e.g., patients with OSAHS receiving CPAP should continue to do so).

Patients should be informed of the availability of a patient information leaflet, and they should be instructed to read the leaflet prior to taking PROVIGIL. See Patient Information at the end of this labeling for the text of the leaflet provided for patients.

Pregnancy

Patients should be advised to notify their physician if they become pregnant or intend to become pregnant during therapy. Patients should be cautioned regarding the potential increased risk of pregnancy when using steroidal contraceptives (including depot or implantable contraceptives) with PROVIGIL and for one month after discontinuation of therapy (See *Impairment of Fertility* and **Pregnancy**).

Nursing

Patients should be advised to notify their physician if they are breast feeding an infant.

Concomitant Medication

Patients should be advised to inform their physician if they are taking, or plan to take, any prescription or over-the-counter drugs, because of the potential for interactions between PROVIGIL and other drugs.

Alcohol

Patients should be advised that the use of PROVIGIL in combination with alcohol has not been studied. Patients should be advised that it is prudent to avoid alcohol while taking PROVIGIL.

Allergic Reactions

Patients should be advised to notify their physician if they develop a rash, hives, or a related allergic phenomenon.

Drug Interactions

CNS Active Drugs

Methylphenidate - In a single-dose study in healthy volunteers, simultaneous administration of modafinil (200 mg) with methylphenidate (40 mg) did not cause any significant alterations in the pharmacokinetics of either drug. However, the absorption of PROVIGIL may be delayed by approximately one hour when coadministered with methylphenidate.

Dextroamphetamine - In a single dose study in healthy volunteers, simultaneous administration of modafinil (200 mg) with dextroamphetamine (10 mg) did not cause any significant alterations in the pharmacokinetics of either drug. However, the absorption of PROVIGIL may be delayed by approximately one hour when coadministered with dextroamphetamine.

Clomipramine - The coadministration of a single dose of clomipramine (50 mg) on the first of three days of treatment with modafinil (200 mg/day) in healthy volunteers did not show an effect on the pharmacokinetics of either drug. However, one incident of increased levels of clomipramine and its active metabolite desmethylclomipramine has been reported in a patient with narcolepsy during treatment with modafinil.

Triazolam - In the drug interaction study between PROVIGIL and ethinyl estradiol (EE_2), on the same days as those for the plasma sampling for EE_2 pharmacokinetics, a single dose of triazolam (0.125 mg) was also administered. Mean C_{max} and $AUC_{0-\infty}$ of triazolam were decreased by 42% and 59%, respectively, and its elimination half-life was decreased by approximately an hour after the modafinil treatment.

Monoamine Oxidase (MAO) Inhibitors - Interaction studies with monoamine oxidase inhibitors have not been performed. Therefore, caution should be used when concomitantly administering MAO inhibitors and modafinil.

Other Drugs

Warfarin - There were no significant changes in the pharmacokinetic profiles of R- and S-warfarin in healthy subjects given a single dose of racemic warfarin (5 mg) following chronic administration of modafinil (200 mg/day for 7 days followed by 400 mg/day for 27 days) relative to the profiles in subjects given placebo. However, more frequent monitoring of prothrombin times/INR is advisable whenever PROVIGIL is coadministered with warfarin (See **CLINICAL PHARMACOLOGY, Pharmacokinetics,** Drug-Drug Interactions).

Ethinyl Estradiol - Administration of modafinil to female volunteers once daily at 200 mg/day for 7 days followed by 400 mg/day for 21 days resulted in a mean 11% decrease in C_{max} and 18% decrease in AUC_{0-24} of ethinyl estradiol (EE_2; 0.035 mg; administered orally with norgestimate). There was no apparent change in the elimination rate of ethinyl estradiol.

Cyclosporine - One case of an interaction between modafinil and cyclosporine, a substrate of CYP3A4, has been reported in a 41 year old woman who had undergone an organ transplant. After one month of administration of 200 mg/day of modafinil, cyclosporine blood levels were decreased by 50%. The interaction was postulated to be due to the increased metabolism of cyclosporine, since no other factor expected to affect the disposition of the drug had changed. Dosage adjustment for cyclosporine may be needed.

Potential Interactions with Drugs That Inhibit, Induce, or are Metabolized by Cytochrome P-450 Isoenzymes and Other Hepatic Enzymes

In *in vitro* studies using primary human hepatocyte cultures, modafinil was shown to slightly induce CYP1A2, CYP2B6 and CYP3A4 in a concentration-dependent manner. Although induction results based on *in vitro* experiments are not necessarily predictive of response *in vivo*, caution needs to be exercised when PROVIGIL is coadministered with drugs that depend on these three enzymes for their clearance. Specifically, lower blood levels of such drugs could result (See *Other Drugs*, Cyclosporine above).

The exposure of human hepatocytes to modafinil *in vitro* produced an apparent concentration-related suppression of expression of CYP2C9 activity suggesting that there is a potential for a metabolic interaction between modafinil and the substrates of this enzyme (e.g., S-warfarin and phenytoin). In a subsequent clinical study in healthy volunteers, chronic modafinil treatment did not show a significant effect on the single-dose pharmacokinetics of warfarin when compared to placebo (See **PRECAUTIONS, Drug Interactions,** Warfarin).

In vitro studies using human liver microsomes showed that modafinil reversibly inhibited CYP2C19 at pharmacologically relevant concentrations of modafinil. CYP2C19 is also reversibly inhibited, with similar potency, by a circulating metabolite, modafinil sulfone. Although the maximum plasma concentrations of modafinil sulfone are much lower than those of parent modafinil, the combined effect of both compounds could produce sustained partial inhibition of the enzyme. Drugs that are largely eliminated via CYP2C19 metabolism, such as diazepam, propranolol, phenytoin (also via CYP2C9) or S-mephenytoin may have prolonged elimination upon coadministration with PROVIGIL and may require dosage reduction and monitoring for toxicity.

Tricyclic antidepressants - CYP2C19 also provides an ancillary pathway for the metabolism of certain tricyclic antidepressants (e.g., clomipramine and desipramine) that are primarily metabolized by CYP2D6. In tricyclic-treated patients deficient in CYP2D6 (i.e., those who are poor metabolizers of debrisoquine; 7–10% of the Caucasian population; similar or lower in other populations), the amount of metabolism by CYP2C19 may be substantially increased. PROVIGIL may cause elevation of the levels of the tricyclics in this subset of patients. Physicians should be aware that a reduction in the dose of tricyclic agents might be needed in these patients.

In addition, due to the partial involvement of CYP3A4 in the metabolic elimination of modafinil, coadministration of potent inducers of CYP3A4 (e.g., carbamazepine, phenobarbital, rifampin) or inhibitors of CYP3A4 (e.g., ketoconazole, itraconazole) could alter the plasma levels of modafinil.

Carcinogenesis, Mutagenesis, Impairment of Fertility

Carcinogenesis

Carcinogenicity studies were conducted in which modafinil was administered in the diet to mice for 78 weeks and to rats for 104 weeks at doses of 6, 30 and 60 mg/kg/day. The highest dose studied represents 1.5 times (mouse) or 3 times (rat) greater than the recommended human daily dose of 200 mg on a mg/m^2 basis. There was no evidence of tumorigenesis associated with modafinil administration in these studies, but because the mouse study used an inadequate high dose that was not representative of a maximum tolerated dose, the carcinogenic potential of modafinil has not been fully evaluated.

Mutagenesis

There was no evidence of mutagenic or clastogenic potential of modafinil in a series of assays. It was not mutagenic in the *in vitro* Ames bacterial reverse mutation test, the *in vitro* mouse lymphoma/TK locus assay in the presence or absence of metabolic activation; and it was not clastogenic in the *in vitro* human lymphocyte chromosomal aberration assay in the presence or absence of metabolic activation, or in two *in vivo* mouse bone marrow micronucleus assays.

Continued on next page

Provigil—Cont.

Modafinil did not increase unscheduled DNA synthesis in rat hepatocytes. In a cell transformation assay in BALB/3T3 mouse embryo cells, modafinil did not cause an increase in the frequency of transformed foci in the presence or absence of metabolic activation.

Impairment of Fertility

Oral administration of modafinil to male and female rats had no effects on fertility when administered prior to and throughout mating, and continued in females through day 7 of gestation, at doses up to 480 mg/kg/day (23 times the recommended human dose of 200 mg/day on a mg/m^2 basis).

Pregnancy

Pregnancy Category C: Modafinil administered orally to pregnant rats throughout the period of organogenesis caused, in the absence of maternal toxicity, an increase in resorptions and an increased incidence of hydronephrosis and skeletal variations in the offspring at a dose of 200 mg/kg/day (10 times the recommended human dose of 200 mg/day on a mg/m^2 basis) but not at 100 mg/kg/day. However, in a subsequent study of up to 480 mg/kg/day (23 times the recommended human dose on a mg/m^2 basis), which included maternally toxic doses, no adverse effects on embryofetal development were seen.

Modafinil administered orally to pregnant rabbits throughout the period of organogenesis at doses up to 100 mg/kg/day (10 times the recommended human dose on a mg/m^2 basis) had no effects on embryofetal development.

However, in a subsequent study in pregnant rabbits, increased resorptions, and increased alterations in fetuses from a single litter (open eye lids, fused digits, rotated limbs), were observed at 180 mg/kg/day (17 times the recommended human dose on a mg/m^2 basis), a dose that was also maternally toxic.

Modafinil administered orally to rats throughout gestation and lactation at doses up to 200 mg/kg/day (5 times the recommended human dose on a mg/m^2 basis), had no effects on the postnatal development of the offspring.

There are no adequate and well-controlled studies in pregnant women. Modafinil should be used during pregnancy only if the potential benefit justifies the potential risk to the fetus.

Labor and Delivery

The effect of modafinil on labor and delivery in humans has not been systematically investigated. Seven normal births occurred in patients who had received modafinil during pregnancy. One patient gave birth 3 weeks earlier than the expected range of delivery dates (estimated using ultrasound) to a healthy male infant. One woman with a history of spontaneous abortions suffered a spontaneous abortion while being treated with modafinil.

Nursing Mothers

It is not known whether modafinil or its metabolites are excreted in human milk. Because many drugs are excreted in human milk, caution should be exercised when PROVIGIL tablets are administered to a nursing woman.

PEDIATRIC USE

Safety and effectiveness in individuals below 16 years of age have not been established. Leukopenia has been reported in pediatric patients taking PROVIGIL.

GERIATRIC USE

Safety and effectiveness in individuals above 65 years of age have not been established. Experience in a limited number of patients who were greater than 65 years of age in clinical trials showed an incidence of adverse experiences similar to other age groups.

Table 3. Incidence Of Treatment-Emergent Adverse Experiences In Parallel-Group, Placebo-Controlled Clinical Trials[1] In Narcolepsy, OSAHS, and SWSD With PROVIGIL (200 mg, 300 mg and 400 mg)*

Body System	Preferred Term	Modafinil (n = 934)	Placebo (n = 567)
Body as a Whole	Headache	34%	23%
	Back pain	6%	5%
	Flu Syndrome	4%	3%
	Chest Pain	3%	1%
	Chills	1%	0%
	Neck Rigidity	1%	0%
Cardiovascular	Hypertension	3%	1%
	Tachycardia	2%	1%
	Palpitation	2%	1%
	Vasodilatation	2%	0%
Digestive	Nausea	11%	3%
	Diarrhea	6%	5%
	Dyspepsia	5%	4%
	Dry Mouth	4%	2%
	Anorexia	4%	1%
	Constipation	2%	1%
	Abnormal liver function[2]	2%	1%
	Flatulence	1%	0%
	Mouth Ulceration	1%	0%
	Thirst	1%	0%
Hemic/Lymphatic	Eosinophilia	1%	0%
Metabolic/Nutritional	Edema	1%	0%
Nervous	Nervousness	7%	3%
	Insomnia	5%	1%
	Anxiety	5%	1%
	Dizziness	5%	4%
	Depression	2%	1%
	Paresthesia	2%	0%
	Somnolence	2%	1%
	Hypertonia	1%	0%
	Dyskinesia[3]	1%	0%
	Hyperkinesia	1%	0%
	Agitation	1%	0%
	Confusion	1%	0%
	Tremor	1%	0%
	Emotional Lability	1%	0%
	Vertigo	1%	0%
Respiratory	Rhinitis	7%	6%
	Pharyngitis	4%	2%
	Lung Disorder	2%	1%
	Epistaxis	1%	0%
	Asthma	1%	0%
Skin/Appendages	Sweating	1%	0%
	Herpes Simplex	1%	0%
Special Senses	Amblyopia	1%	0%
	Abnormal Vision	1%	0%
	Taste Perversion	1%	0%
	Eye Pain	1%	0%
Urgoenital	Urine Abnormality	1%	0%
	Hematuria	1%	0%
	Pyuria	1%	0%

* Six double-blind, placebo controlled clinical studies in narcolepsy, OSAHS, and SWSD.

[1] Events reported by at least 1% of patients treated with PROVIGIL that were more frequent than in the placebo group are included; incidence is rounded to the nearest 1%. The adverse experience terminology is coded using a standard modified COSTART Dictionary.

Events for which the PROVIGIL incidence was at least 1%, but equal to or less than placebo are not listed in the table. These events included the following: infection, pain, accidental injury, abdominal pain, hypothermia, allergic reaction, asthenia, fever, viral infection, neck pain, migraine, abnormal electrocardiogram, hypotension, tooth disorder, vomiting, periodontal abscess, increased appetite, ecchymosis, hyperglycemia, peripheral edema, weight loss, weight gain, myalgia, leg cramps, arthritis, cataplexy, thinking abnormality, sleep disorder, increased cough, sinusitis, dyspnea, bronchitis, rash, conjunctivitis, ear pain, dysmenorrhea[4], urinary tract infection.

[2] Elevated liver enzymes.

[3] Oro-facial dyskinesias.

[4] Incidence adjusted for gender.

ADVERSE REACTIONS

Modafinil has been evaluated for safety in over 3500 patients, of whom more than 2000 patients with excessive sleepiness associated with primary disorders of sleep and wakefulness were given at least one dose of modafinil. In clinical trials, modafinil has been found to be generally well tolerated and most adverse experiences were mild to moderate.

The most commonly observed adverse events (≥5%) associated with the use of PROVIGIL more frequently than placebo-treated patients in the placebo-controlled clinical studies in primary disorders of sleep and wakefulness were headache, nausea, nervousness, rhinitis, diarrhea, back pain, anxiety, insomnia, dizziness, and dyspepsia. The adverse event profile was similar across these studies.

In the placebo-controlled clinical trials, 74 of the 934 patients (8%) who received PROVIGIL discontinued due to an adverse experience compared to 3% of patients that received placebo. The most frequent reasons for discontinuation that occurred at a higher rate for PROVIGIL than placebo patients were headache (2%), nausea, anxiety, dizziness, insomnia, chest pain and nervousness (each <1%). In a Canadian clinical trial, a 35 year old obese narcoleptic male with a prior history of syncopal episodes experienced a 9-second episode of asystole after 27 days of modafinil treatment (300 mg/day in divided doses).

Incidence in Controlled Trials

The following table (Table 3) presents the adverse experiences that occurred at a rate of 1% or more and were more frequent in patients treated with PROVIGIL than in placebo patients in the principal, placebo-controlled clinical trials.

The prescriber should be aware that the figures provided below cannot be used to predict the frequency of adverse experiences in the course of usual medical practice, where patient characteristics and other factors may differ from those occurring during clinical studies. Similarly, the cited frequencies cannot be directly compared with figures obtained from other clinical investigations involving different treatments, uses, or investigators. Review of these frequencies, however, provides prescribers with a basis to estimate the relative contribution of drug and non-drug factors to the incidence of adverse events in the population studied.

[See table 3 at left]

Dose Dependency of Adverse Events

In the placebo-controlled clinical trials which compared doses of 200, 300, and 400 mg/day of PROVIGIL and placebo, the only adverse events that were clearly dose related were headache and anxiety.

Vital Sign Changes

While there was no consistent change in mean values of heart rate or systolic and diastolic blood pressure, the requirement for antihypertensive medication was slightly greater in patients on PROVIGIL compared to placebo (See **PRECAUTIONS**).

Weight Changes

There were no clinically significant differences in body weight change in patients treated with PROVIGIL compared to placebo-treated patients in the placebo-controlled clinical trials.

Laboratory Changes

Clinical chemistry, hematology, and urinalysis parameters were monitored in Phase 1, 2, and 3 studies. In these studies, mean plasma levels of gamma glutamyltransferase (GGT) and alkaline phosphatase (AP) were found to be higher following administration of PROVIGIL, but not placebo. Few subjects, however, had GGT or AP elevations outside of the normal range. Shifts to higher, but not clinically significantly abnormal, GGT and AP values appeared to increase with time in the population treated with PROVIGIL in the Phase 3 clinical trials. No differences were apparent in alanine aminotransferase, aspartate aminotransferase, total protein, albumin, or total bilirubin.

ECG Changes

No treatment-emergent pattern of ECG abnormalities was found in placebo-controlled clinical trials following administration of PROVIGIL.

Postmarketing Reports

In addition to the adverse events observed during clinical trials, the following adverse events have been identified during post-approval use of PROVIGIL in clinical practice.

Because these adverse events are reported voluntarily from a population of uncertain size, reliable estimates of their frequency cannot be made.

Hematologic: agranulocytosis

Central Nervous System: symptoms of psychosis, symptoms of mania

Hypersensitivity: urticaria (hives), angioedema

DRUG ABUSE AND DEPENDENCE

Controlled Substance Class

Modafinil (PROVIGIL) is listed in Schedule IV of the Controlled Substances Act.

Abuse Potential and Dependence

In addition to its wakefulness-promoting effect and increased locomotor activity in animals, in humans, PROVIGIL produces psychoactive and euphoric effects, alterations in mood, perception, thinking and feelings typical of other CNS stimulants. In *in vitro* binding studies, modafinil binds to the dopamine reuptake site and causes an increase in extracellular dopamine, but no increase in dopamine release. Modafinil is reinforcing, as evidenced by its self-administration in monkeys previously trained to self-administer cocaine. In some studies, modafinil was also partially discriminated as stimulant-like. Physicians should follow patients closely, especially those with a history of drug and/or stimulant (e.g., methylphenidate, amphetamine, or cocaine) abuse. Patients should be observed for signs of misuse or abuse (e.g., incrementation of doses or drug-seeking behavior).

The abuse potential of modafinil (200, 400, and 800 mg) was assessed relative to methylphenidate (45 and 90 mg) in an inpatient study in individuals experienced with drugs of abuse. Results from this clinical study demonstrated that modafinil produced psychoactive and euphoric effects and feelings consistent with other scheduled CNS stimulants (methylphenidate).

Withdrawal

The effects of modafinil withdrawal were monitored following 9 weeks of modafinil use in one US Phase 3 controlled clinical trial. No specific symptoms of withdrawal were observed during 14 days of observation, although sleepiness returned in narcoleptic patients.

OVERDOSAGE

Human Experience

In clinical trials, a total of 151 protocol-specified doses ranging from 1000 to 1600 mg/day (5 to 8 times the recommended daily dose of 200 mg) have been administered to 32 subjects, including 13 subjects who received doses of 1000 or 1200 mg/day for 7 to 21 consecutive days. In addition, several intentional acute overdoses occurred; the two largest being 4500 mg and 4000 mg taken by two subjects participating in foreign depression studies. None of these study subjects experienced any unexpected or life-threatening effects. Adverse experiences that were reported at these doses included excitation or agitation, insomnia, and slight or moderate elevations in hemodynamic parameters. Other observed high-dose effects in clinical studies have included anxiety, irritability, aggressiveness, confusion, nervousness, tremor, palpitations, sleep disturbances, nausea, diarrhea and decreased prothrombin time.

From post-marketing experience, there have been no reports of fatal overdoses involving modafinil alone (doses up to 12 grams). Overdoses involving multiple drugs, including modafinil, have resulted in fatal outcomes. Symptoms most often accompanying modafinil overdose, alone or in combination with other drugs have included: insomnia; central nervous system symptoms such as restlessness, disorientation, confusion, excitation and hallucination; digestive changes such as nausea and diarrhea; and cardiovascular changes such as tachycardia, bradycardia, hypertension and chest pain.

Cases of accidental ingestion/overdose have been reported in children as young as 11 months of age. The highest reported accidental ingestion on a mg/kg basis occurred in a three-year-old boy who ingested 800-1000 mg (50-63 mg/kg) of modafinil. The child remained stable. The symptoms associated with overdose in children were similar to those observed in adults.

Overdose Management

No specific antidote to the toxic effects of modafinil overdose has been identified to date. Such overdoses should be managed with primarily supportive care, including cardiovascular monitoring. If there are no contraindications, induced emesis or gastric lavage should be considered. There are no data to suggest the utility of dialysis or urinary acidification or alkalinization in enhancing drug elimination. The physician should consider contacting a poison-control center on the treatment of any overdose.

DOSAGE AND ADMINISTRATION

The recommended dose of PROVIGIL is 200 mg given once a day.

For patients with narcolepsy and OSAHS, PROVIGIL should be taken as a single dose in the morning.

For patients with SWSD, PROVIGIL should be taken approximately 1 hour prior to the start of their work shift.

Doses up to 400 mg/day, given as a single dose, have been well tolerated, but there is no consistent evidence that this dose confers additional benefit beyond that of the 200 mg dose (See **CLINICAL PHARMACOLOGY** and **CLINICAL TRIALS**).

Dosage adjustment should be considered for concomitant medications that are substrates for CYP3A4, such as triazolam and cyclosporine (See **PRECAUTIONS, Drug Interactions**).

Drugs that are largely eliminated via CYP2C19 metabolism, such as diazepam, propranolol, phenytoin (also via CYP2C9) or S-mephenytoin may have prolonged elimination upon coadministration with PROVIGIL and may require dosage reduction and monitoring for toxicity.

In patients with severe hepatic impairment, the dose of PROVIGIL should be reduced to one-half of that recommended for patients with normal hepatic function (See **CLINICAL PHARMACOLOGY** and **PRECAUTIONS**).

There is inadequate information to determine safety and efficacy of dosing in patients with severe renal impairment (See **CLINICAL PHARMACOLOGY** and **PRECAUTIONS**).

In elderly patients, elimination of PROVIGIL and its metabolites may be reduced as a consequence of aging. Therefore, consideration should be given to the use of lower doses in this population (See **CLINICAL PHARMACOLOGY** and **PRECAUTIONS**).

HOW SUPPLIED

PROVIGIL® (modafinil) Tablets

100 mg Each capsule-shaped, white, uncoated tablet is debossed with "PROVIGIL" on one side and "100 MG" on the other.

NDC 63459-101-01 - Bottles of 100

200 mg Each capsule-shaped, white, scored, uncoated tablet is debossed with "PROVIGIL" on one side and "200 MG" on the other.

NDC 63459-201-01 - Bottles of 100

Store at 20°-25° C (68°-77° F).

Manufactured for: **Cephalon, Inc.**
West Chester, PA 19380

U.S. Patent Nos. RE37,516 / 6,462,089

April 2004

PROV-007

PATIENT INFORMATION

PROVIGIL® (pro-vij-el) Tablets [C-IV]

Generic name: modafinil

Read the Patient Information that comes with PROVIGIL before you start taking it and each time you get a refill. There may be new information. This leaflet does not take the place of talking with your doctor about your condition or treatment.

What is the most important information I should know about PROVIGIL?

PROVIGIL may help treat the excessive sleepiness caused by certain sleep disorders, but it may not stop all your sleepiness. Regardless of how improved you may feel, do not change your daily habits until your doctor tells you it is okay. Discuss your level of sleepiness with your doctor at each visit. People with sleep disorders should always be careful about doing things that could be dangerous, including driving a car.

What is PROVIGIL?

PROVIGIL is a medicine to treat unusually sleepy people who have one of the following diagnosed sleep disorders:

- narcolepsy
- obstructive sleep apnea/hypopnea syndrome (OSAHS). PROVIGIL is used along with other medical treatments for OSAHS.
- shift work sleep disorder (SWSD)

You should be diagnosed with one of these sleep disorders before taking PROVIGIL, as sleepiness can be a symptom of other medical conditions that need to be treated.

PROVIGIL will not cure the above sleep disorders. PROVIGIL may help the sleepiness caused by these conditions, but it may not stop all your sleepiness. PROVIGIL is not meant to be used in place of getting enough sleep. You should follow your doctor's advice about good sleep habits and using other treatments.

PROVIGIL is a controlled substance [C-IV]. This means that PROVIGIL may be a target for people who abuse medicines or street drugs. Keep your PROVIGIL in a safe place. Giving away PROVIGIL is against the law.

Who should not take PROVIGIL?

Do not take PROVIGIL if you are allergic to any of its ingredients. The active ingredient is modafinil. See the end of this leaflet for a complete list of ingredients.

It is not known if PROVIGIL is right for children under the age of 16. Low levels of white blood cells (cells that fight infections) have happened in some children who have taken PROVIGIL.

Before starting PROVIGIL tell your doctor

- about all your medical conditions, including if you:
  - are pregnant, are planning to become pregnant, or are breastfeeding. It is not known if PROVIGIL may harm your unborn baby, or if PROVIGIL passes into your milk and if it can harm your baby.
  - have high blood pressure or heart problems.
  - have liver or kidney problems.
  - have abused medicines called "stimulants" or street drugs.
  - have or had a mental problem called psychosis.
- about all the medicines you take, including prescription and non-prescription medicines, vitamins, and herbal supplements. PROVIGIL and many other medicines can interact with each other causing side effects. PROVIGIL may affect the way other medicines work, and other medicines may affect how PROVIGIL works. Keep a list of all the medicines you take. Your doctor or pharmacist will tell you if it is safe to take PROVIGIL and other medicines together. Do not take other medicines with PROVIGIL unless your doctor has told you it is okay.

PROVIGIL can affect hormonal birth control methods (contraceptives). Women who use hormonal contraceptives such as birth control pills, shots, implants, intrauterine devices (IUDs), or patches, may have a higher chance for getting pregnant while taking PROVIGIL, and for one month after stopping PROVIGIL. Talk to your doctor about birth control methods that are right for you while using PROVIGIL.

How should I take PROVIGIL?

- Take PROVIGIL exactly as prescribed by your doctor. Your doctor will prescribe the dose of PROVIGIL that is right for you. Do not change your dose of PROVIGIL without talking to your doctor. Do not take more PROVIGIL than prescribed.
- Your doctor will tell you the right time of day to take PROVIGIL. Patients with narcolepsy or OSAHS usually take one dose of PROVIGIL every day in the morning. PROVIGIL may help you stay awake during the day but it should not affect nighttime sleep. Patients with SWSD usually take PROVIGIL about 1 hour before their work shift. Do not change the time of day you take PROVIGIL unless you have talked to your doctor.
- You can take PROVIGIL with or without food.
- If you take more than your prescribed dose, or take PROVIGIL too late in your waking day, you may find it harder to go to sleep. Call your doctor if you have any concerns.

What should I avoid while taking PROVIGIL?

- People with sleep disorders should always be careful about doing things that could be dangerous, including driving a car. Discuss your level of sleepiness with your doctor at each visit. Do not change your daily habits until your doctor tells you it is okay.
- Do not take other medicines including prescription and non-prescription medicines, vitamins or herbal supplements unless your doctor has told you it is okay.
- You should avoid drinking alcohol.

What are the possible side effects of PROVIGIL?

The most common side effects of PROVIGIL are headache, nausea, nervousness, stuffy nose, diarrhea, back pain, anxiety, trouble sleeping, dizziness, and upset stomach.

PROVIGIL may cause the following infrequent serious side effects. Call your doctor or get emergency help if you have any of these or any other serious side effects while taking PROVIGIL:

- chest pain.
- mental problems.
- allergic reactions, such as a rash, hives or other allergic reaction.

Some effects of PROVIGIL on the brain are similar to other medications called "stimulants". If you have a history of drug and/or stimulant use or abuse you should discuss this with your doctor before starting PROVIGIL.

Tell your doctor if you get any side effects while taking PROVIGIL.

These are not all the side effects of PROVIGIL. For more information, ask your doctor or pharmacist.

How should I store PROVIGIL?

- Store PROVIGIL at room temperature, 68° to 77° F (20° to 25° C).
- Store PROVIGIL in a safe place.
- Keep PROVIGIL and all medicines out of the reach of children.

General information about PROVIGIL

Medicines are sometimes prescribed for conditions that are not listed in patient information leaflets. Do not use PROVIGIL for a condition for which it was not prescribed. This medication is for your use only. Do not share this medication with others.

This leaflet summarizes the most important information about PROVIGIL. If you would like more information, talk with your doctor. You can ask your doctor or pharmacist for information about PROVIGIL that is written for health professionals. For more information, please call 1-800-896-5855, or go to www.provigil.com.

What are the ingredients in PROVIGIL?

Active Ingredient: modafinil

Inactive Ingredients: lactose, microcrystalline cellulose, pregelatinized starch, croscarmellose sodium, povidone, and magnesium stearate.

Rx Only

April 2004

Cephalon, Inc. West Chester, PA 19380.

This Patient Information Leaflet has been approved by the U.S. Food and Drug Administration.

Shown in Product Identification Guide, page 311

For information on over-the-counter drugs, consult **PDR For Nonprescription Drugs and Dietary Supplements.**

Cetylite Industries, Inc.

9051 RIVER ROAD
P.O. BOX 90006
PENNSAUKEN, NJ 08110-0700

Direct Inquiries to:
Mr. Stanley L. Wachman, President
(856) 665-6111
(800) 257-7740
FAX: (856) 665-5408

CETACAINE® ℞

[set'a-cane"]
TOPICAL ANESTHETIC

ACTIVE INGREDIENTS

Benzocaine	14.0%
Butyl Aminobenzoate	2.0%
Tetracaine Hydrochloride	2.0%

CONTAINS

Benzalkonium Chloride	0.5%
Cetyl Dimethyl Ethyl Ammonium Bromide	0.005%

In bland, water-soluble base.

ACTION

The onset of Cetacaine produced anesthesia is rapid (approximately 30 seconds) and the duration of anesthesia is typically 30–60 minutes, when used as directed. This effect is due to the rapid onset, but short duration of action of Benzocaine coupled with the slow onset, but extended duration of Tetracaine HCl and bridged by the intermediate action of Butamben.

It is believed that all of these agents act by reversibly blocking nerve conduction. Speed and duration of action is determined by the ability of the agent to be absorbed by the mucous membrane and nerve sheath and then to diffuse out, and ultimately be metabolized (primarily by plasma cholinesterases) to inert metabolites which are excreted in the urine.

INDICATIONS

Cetacaine is a topical anesthetic indicated for the production of anesthesia of all accessible mucous membrane except the eyes. Cetacaine Spray is indicated for use to control pain or gagging. Cetacaine in all forms is indicated to control pain and for use for surgical or endoscopic or other procedures in the ear, nose, mouth, pharynx, larynx, trachea, bronchi, and esophagus. It may also be used for vaginal or rectal procedures when feasible.

DOSAGE AND ADMINISTRATION

Cetacaine Spray should be applied for approximately one second or less for normal anesthesia. Only a limited quantity of Cetacaine is required for anesthesia. Spray in excess of two seconds is contraindicated. Average expulsion rate of residue from spray, at normal temperatures, is 200 mg per second.

Tissue need not be dried prior to application of Cetacaine. Cetacaine should be applied directly to the site where pain control is required. Cetacaine Liquid may be applied with a cotton applicator or directly to tissue. The cotton applicator should not be held in position for extended periods of time, since local reactions to benzoate topical anesthetics are related to the length of time of application.

ADVERSE REACTIONS

Hypersensitivity Reactions: Unpredictable adverse reactions (ie, hypersensitivity, including anaphylaxis) are extremely rare.

Localized allergic reactions may occur after prolonged or repeated use of any aminobenzoate anesthetic. The most common adverse reaction caused by local anesthetics is contact dermatitis charaterized by erythema and pruritus that may progress to vesiculation and oozing. This occurs most commonly in patients following prolonged self-medication, which is contraindicated. If rash, urticaria, edema, or other manifestations of allergy develop during use, the drug should be discontinued. To minimize the possibility of a serious allergic reaction, Cetacaine preparations should not be applied for prolonged periods except under continual supervision. Dehydration of the epithelium or an escharotic effect may also result from prolonged contact.

PRECAUTION

On rare occasions, methemoglobinemia has been reported in connection with the use of benzocaine-containing products. Care should be used not to exceed a two second spray. If a patient becomes cyanotic, treat appropriately to counteract (such as with methylene blue, if medically indicated).

USE IN PREGNANCY

Safe use of Cetacaine has not been established with respect to possible adverse effects upon fetal development. Therefore, Cetacaine should not be used during early pregnancy, unless in the judgement of a physician, the potential benefits outweigh the unknown hazards. Routine precaution for the use of any topical anesthetic should be observed when Cetacaine is used.

Appropriate pediatric dosage has not been established for this product.

CONTRAINDICATIONS

Cetacaine is not suitable and should never be used for injection. Do not use on the eyes. To avoid excessive systemic absorption, Cetacaine should not be applied to large areas of denuded or inflamed tissue. Cetacaine should not be administered to patients who are hypersensitive to any of its ingredients or to patients known to have cholinesterase deficiencies. Tolerance may vary with the status of the patient. Dosage should be reduced in the debilitated elderly, acutely ill, and very young patients.

Individual dosage of tetracaine hydrochloride in excess of 20 mg is contraindicated. Cetacaine should not be used under dentures or cotton rolls, as retention of the active ingredients under a denture or cotton roll could possibly cause an escharotic effect. Routine precaution for the use of any topical anesthetic should be observed when using Cetacaine.

Jetco® Cannula for Cetacaine Spray

- The supplied 4" stainless steel Jetco® cannula (J-4) for Cetacaine Spray is especially designed for accessibility and application of Cetacaine, at the required site of pain control.
- The Jetco cannula is also available in 6", (J-6) and 8" curved configuration, (J-8).
- Replacement Jetco cannulas are available.
- The Jetco cannula is inserted firmly into the protruding plastic stem on each bottle of Cetacaine Spray.
- The Jetco cannula may be removed and reinserted as many times as required for cleansing or sterilization, and is autoclavable.

PACKAGING AVAILABLE

Cetacaine Spray 56 g. including propellant.
Cetacaine Liquid 56 g.
Cetacaine Hospital Gel 29 g. Tube.

CAUTION

Federal law prohibits dispensing Cetacaine without prescription.

CETYLITE
INDUSTRIES, INC.
9051 River Road
Pennsauken, NJ 08110-3293
1-800-257-7740
www.cetylite.com
Made in U.S.A. Rev. 11/99

Shown in Product Identification Guide, page 311

Chiron Corporation

4560 HORTON STREET
EMERYVILLE, CA 94608-2916

For Medical Information Contact:
Generally:
Drug Information Services:
(800) CHIRON-8 selection #2
(800) 244-7668 selection #2
FAX: (510) 923-3435
e-mail: drug_info@chiron.com
Adverse Event Reporting:
(800) CHIRON-8 selection #3
(800) 244-7668 selection #3
After Hours and Weekends:
(415) 487-8335
Sales and Ordering:
(800) CHIRON-8 selection #1
(800) 244-7668 selection #1
FAX: (510) 923-3434

PROLEUKIN® ℞

[prō-lū´-kin]
Aldesleukin For Injection
Rx Only

WARNINGS

Therapy with PROLEUKIN® (aldesleukin) for injection should be restricted to patients with normal cardiac and pulmonary functions as defined by thallium stress testing and formal pulmonary function testing. Extreme caution should be used in patients with a normal thallium stress test and a normal pulmonary function test who have a history of cardiac or pulmonary disease.

PROLEUKIN should be administered in a hospital setting under the supervision of a qualified physician experienced in the use of anticancer agents. An intensive care facility and specialists skilled in cardiopulmonary or intensive care medicine must be available.

PROLEUKIN administration has been associated with capillary leak syndrome (CLS) which is characterized by a loss of vascular tone and extravasation of plasma proteins and fluid into the extravascular space. CLS results in hypotension and reduced organ perfusion which may be severe and can result in death. CLS may be associated with cardiac arrhythmias (supraventricular and ventricular), angina, myocardial infarction, respiratory insufficiency requiring intubation, gastrointestinal bleeding or infarction, renal insufficiency, edema, and mental status changes.

PROLEUKIN treatment is associated with impaired neutrophil function (reduced chemotaxis) and with an increased risk of disseminated infection, including sepsis and bacterial endocarditis. Consequently, preexisting bacterial infections should be adequately treated prior to initiation of PROLEUKIN therapy. Patients with indwelling central lines are particularly at risk for infection with gram positive microorganisms. Antibiotic prophylaxis with oxacillin, nafcillin, ciprofloxacin, or vancomycin has been associated with a reduced incidence of staphylococcal infections.

PROLEUKIN administration should be withheld in patients developing moderate to severe lethargy or somnolence; continued administration may result in coma.

DESCRIPTION

PROLEUKIN® (aldesleukin) for injection, a human recombinant interleukin-2 product, is a highly purified protein with a molecular weight of approximately 15,300 daltons. The chemical name is des-alanyl-1, serine-125 human interleukin-2. PROLEUKIN, a lymphokine, is produced by recombinant DNA technology using a genetically engineered *E. coli* strain containing an analog of the human interleukin-2 gene. Genetic engineering techniques were used to modify the human IL-2 gene, and the resulting expression clone encodes a modified human interleukin-2. This recombinant form differs from native interleukin-2 in the following ways: a) PROLEUKIN is not glycosylated because it is derived from *E. coli*; b) the molecule has no N-terminal alanine; the codon for this amino acid was deleted during the genetic engineering procedure; c) the molecule has serine substituted for cysteine at amino acid position 125; this was accomplished by site specific manipulation during the genetic engineering procedure; and d) the aggregation state of PROLEUKIN is likely to be different from that of native interleukin-2.

The *in vitro* biological activities of the native nonrecombinant molecule have been reproduced with PROLEUKIN.[1,2]

PROLEUKIN is supplied as a sterile, white to off-white, lyophilized cake in single-use vials intended for intravenous (IV) administration. When reconstituted with 1.2 mL Sterile Water for Injection, USP, each mL contains 18 million IU (1.1 mg) PROLEUKIN, 50 mg mannitol, and 0.18 mg sodium dodecyl sulfate, buffered with approximately 0.17 mg monobasic and 0.89 mg dibasic sodium phosphate to a pH of 7.5 (range 7.2 to 7.8). The manufacturing process for PROLEUKIN involves fermentation in a defined medium containing tetracycline hydrochloride. The presence of the antibiotic is not detectable in the final product. PROLEUKIN contains no preservatives in the final product.

PROLEUKIN biological potency is determined by a lymphocyte proliferation bioassay and is expressed in International Units (IU) as established by the World Health Organization 1st International Standard for Interleukin-2 (human). The relationship between potency and protein mass is as follows:

18 million (18 X 10^6) IU PROLEUKIN = 1.1 mg protein

CLINICAL PHARMACOLOGY

PROLEUKIN® (aldesleukin) has been shown to possess the biological activities of human native interleukin-2.[1,2]

In vitro studies performed on human cell lines demonstrate the immunoregulatory properties of PROLEUKIN, including: a) enhancement of lymphocyte mitogenesis and stimulation of long-term growth of human interleukin-2 dependent cell lines; b) enhancement of lymphocyte cytotoxicity; c) induction of killer cell (lymphokine-activated (LAK) and natural (NK)) activity; and d) induction of interferon-gamma production.

The *in vivo* administration of PROLEUKIN in animals and humans produces multiple immunological effects in a dose dependent manner. These effects include activation of cellular immunity with profound lymphocytosis, eosinophilia, and thrombocytopenia, and the production of cytokines including tumor necrosis factor, IL-1 and gamma interferon.[3]

In vivo experiments in murine tumor models have shown inhibition of tumor growth.[4] The exact mechanism by which PROLEUKIN mediates its antitumor activity in animals and humans is unknown.

Pharmacokinetics: PROLEUKIN exists as biologically active, non-covalently bound microaggregates with an average size of 27 recombinant interleukin-2 molecules. The solubilizing agent, sodium dodecyl sulfate, may have an effect on the kinetic properties of this product.

The pharmacokinetic profile of PROLEUKIN is characterized by high plasma concentrations following a short IV infusion, rapid distribution into the extravascular space and elimination from the body by metabolism in the kidneys with little or no bioactive protein excreted in the urine. Studies of IV PROLEUKIN in sheep and humans indicate that upon completion of infusion, approximately 30% of the administered dose is detectable in plasma. This finding is consistent with studies in rats using radiolabeled PROLEUKIN, which demonstrate a rapid (<1 min) uptake of the majority of the label into the lungs, liver, kidney, and spleen.

The serum half-life (T 1/2) curves of PROLEUKIN remaining in the plasma are derived from studies done in 52 cancer patients following a 5-minute IV infusion. These patients were shown to have a distribution and elimination T 1/2 of 13 and 85 minutes, respectively.

Following the initial rapid organ distribution, the primary route of clearance of circulating PROLEUKIN is the kidney. In humans and animals, PROLEUKIN is cleared from the circulation by both glomerular filtration and peritubular extraction in the kidney.[5–8] This dual mechanism for delivery of PROLEUKIN to the proximal tubule may account for the preservation of clearance in patients with rising serum creatinine values. Greater than 80% of the amount of PROLEUKIN distributed to plasma, cleared from the circulation and presented to the kidney is metabolized to amino acids in the cells lining the proximal convoluted tubules. In humans, the mean clearance rate in cancer patients is 268 mL/min.

The relatively rapid clearance of PROLEUKIN has led to dosage schedules characterized by frequent, short infusions. Observed serum levels are proportional to the dose of PROLEUKIN.

Immunogenicity: Fifty-seven of 77 (74%) metastatic renal cell carcinoma patients treated with an every 8-hour PROLEUKIN regimen and 33 of 50 (66%) metastatic melanoma patients treated with a variety of IV regimens developed low titers of non-neutralizing anti-PROLEUKIN antibodies. Neutralizing antibodies were not detected in this group of patients, but have been detected in 1/106 (<1%) patients treated with IV PROLEUKIN using a wide variety of schedules and doses. The clinical significance of anti-PROLEUKIN antibodies is unknown.

Clinical Experience: Two hundred fifty-five patients with metastatic renal cell cancer (metastatic RCC) were treated with single agent PROLEUKIN in 7 clinical studies conducted at 21 institutions. Two hundred seventy patients with metastatic melanoma were treated with single agent PROLEUKIN in 8 clinical studies conducted at 22 institutions. Patients enrolled in trials of single agent PROLEUKIN were required to have an Eastern Cooperative Oncology Group (ECOG) Performance Status (PS) of 0 or 1 and normal organ function as determined by cardiac stress test, pulmonary function tests, and creatinine ≤1.5 mg/dL. Patients with brain metastases, active infections, organ allografts and diseases requiring steroid treatment were excluded.

PROLEUKIN was given by 15 min IV infusion every 8 hours for up to 5 days (maximum of 14 doses). No treatment was given on days 6 to 14 and then dosing was repeated for up to 5 days on days 15 to 19 (maximum of 14 doses). These 2 cycles constituted 1 course of therapy. Patients could receive a maximum of 28 doses during a course of therapy. In practice >90% of patients had doses withheld. Metastatic RCC patients received a median of 20 of 28 scheduled doses of PROLEUKIN. Metastatic melanoma patients received a median of 18 of 28 scheduled doses of PROLEUKIN during the first course of therapy. Doses were withheld for specific toxicities (See "**DOSAGE AND ADMINISTRATION**" section, "**Dose Modifications**" subsection and "**ADVERSE REACTIONS**" section).

In the renal cell cancer studies (n=255), objective response was seen in 37 (15%) patients, with 17 (7%) complete and 20 (8%) partial responders (See Table l). The 95% confidence interval for objective response was 11% to 20%. Onset of tumor regression was observed as early as 4 weeks after completion of the first course of treatment, and in some cases, tumor regression continued for up to 12 months after the start of treatment. Responses were observed in both lung and non-lung sites (e.g., liver, lymph node, renal bed occurrences, soft tissue). Responses were also observed in patients with individual bulky lesions and high tumor burden.

In the metastatic melanoma studies (n=270), objective response was seen in 43 (16%) patients, with 17 (6%) complete and 26 (10%) partial responders (See Table l). The 95% confidence interval for objective response was 12% to 21%. Responses in metastatic melanoma patients were observed in both visceral and non-visceral sites (e.g., lung, liver, lymph node, soft tissue, adrenal, subcutaneous). Responses were also observed in patients with individual bulky lesions and large cumulative tumor burden.

TABLE I: PROLEUKIN CLINICAL RESPONSE DATA

	METASTATIC RCC		METASTATIC MELANOMA	
	Number of Responding Patients (response rate)	Median Response Duration in Months (range)	Number of Responding Patients (response rate)	Median Response Duration in Months (range)
CR's	17 (7%)	80+* (7 to 131+)	17 (6%)	59+* (3 to 122+)
PR's	20 (8%)	20 (3 to 126+)	26 (10%)	6 (1 to 111+)
PR's + CR's	37 (15%)	54 (3 to 131+)	43 (16%)	9 (1 to 122+)

(+) sign means ongoing

* Median duration not yet observed; a conservative value is presented which represents the minimum median duration of response.

An analysis of prognostic factors showed that a better ECOG performance status (see Table ll) was significantly associated with response.

TABLE II: PROLEUKIN CLINICAL RESPONSE BY ECOG PERFORMANCE STATUS (PS)

Pre Treatment	METASTATIC RCC		METASTATIC MELANOMA	
ECOG PS	CR	PR	CR	PR
0	14/166 (8%)	16/166 (10%)	14/191 (7%)	22/191 (12%)
≥1	3/89 (3%)	4/89 (4%)	3/79 (4%)	4/79 (5%)

INDICATIONS AND USAGE

PROLEUKIN® (aldesleukin) is indicated for the treatment of adults with metastatic renal cell carcinoma (metastatic RCC).

PROLEUKIN is indicated for the treatment of adults with metastatic melanoma.

Careful patient selection is mandatory prior to the administration of PROLEUKIN. See "**CONTRAINDICATIONS**", "**WARNINGS**" and "**PRECAUTIONS**" sections regarding patient screening, including recommended cardiac and pulmonary function tests and laboratory tests.

Evaluation of clinical studies to date reveals that patients with more favorable ECOG performance status (ECOG PS O) at treatment initiation respond better to PROLEUKIN, with a higher response rate and lower toxicity (See "**CLINICAL PHARMACOLOGY**" section, "**Clinical Experience**" subsection and "**ADVERSE REACTIONS**" section). Therefore, selection of patients for treatment should include assessment of performance status.

Experience in patients with ECOG PS >1 is extremely limited.

CONTRAINDICATIONS

PROLEUKIN® (aldesleukin) is contraindicated in patients with a known history of hypersensitivity to interleukin-2 or any component of the PROLEUKIN formulation.

PROLEUKIN is contraindicated in patients with an abnormal thallium stress test or abnormal pulmonary function tests and those with organ allografts. Retreatment with PROLEUKIN is contraindicated in patients who have experienced the following drug-related toxicities while receiving an earlier course of therapy:

- Sustained ventricular tachycardia (≥5 beats)
- Cardiac arrhythmias not controlled or unresponsive to management
- Chest pain with ECG changes, consistent with angina or myocardial infarction
- Cardiac tamponade
- Intubation for >72 hours
- Renal failure requiring dialysis >72 hours
- Coma or toxic psychosis lasting >48 hours
- Repetitive or difficult to control seizures
- Bowel ischemia/perforation
- GI bleeding requiring surgery

WARNINGS

See boxed "**WARNINGS**"

Because of the severe adverse events which generally accompany PROLEUKIN® (aldesleukin) therapy at the recommended dosages, thorough clinical evaluation should be performed to identify patients with significant cardiac, pulmonary, renal, hepatic, or CNS impairment in whom PROLEUKIN is contraindicated. Patients with normal cardiovascular, pulmonary, hepatic, and CNS function may experience serious, life threatening or fatal adverse events. Adverse events are frequent, often serious, and sometimes fatal.

Should adverse events, which require dose modification occur, dosage should be withheld rather than reduced (See "**DOSAGE AND ADMINISTRATION**" section, "**Dose Modifications**" subsection).

PROLEUKIN has been associated with exacerbation of preexisting or initial presentation of autoimmune disease and inflammatory disorders. Exacerbation of Crohn's disease, scleroderma, thyroiditis, inflammatory arthritis, diabetes mellitus, oculo-bulbar myasthenia gravis, crescentic IgA glomerulonephritis, cholecystitis, cerebral vasculitis, Stevens-Johnson syndrome and bullous pemphigoid, has been reported following treatment with IL-2.

All patients should have thorough evaluation and treatment of CNS metastases and have a negative scan prior to receiving PROLEUKIN therapy. New neurologic signs, symptoms, and anatomic lesions following PROLEUKIN therapy have been reported in patients without evidence of CNS metastases. Clinical manifestations included changes in mental status, speech difficulties, cortical blindness, limb or gait ataxia, hallucinations, agitation, obtundation, and coma. Radiological findings included multiple and, less commonly, single cortical lesions on MRI and evidence of demyelination. Neurologic signs and symptoms associated with PROLEUKIN therapy usually improve after discontinuation of PROLEUKIN therapy; however, there are reports of permanent neurologic defects. One case of possible cerebral vasculitis, responsive to dexamethasone, has been reported. In patients with known seizure disorders, extreme caution should be exercised as PROLEUKIN may cause seizures.

PRECAUTIONS

General: Patients should have normal cardiac, pulmonary, hepatic, and CNS function at the start of therapy. (See "**PRECAUTIONS**" section, "**Laboratory Tests**" subsection).

Capillary leak syndrome (CLS) begins immediately after PROLEUKIN® (aldesleukin) treatment starts and is marked by increased capillary permeability to protein and fluids and reduced vascular tone. In most patients, this results in a concomitant drop in mean arterial blood pressure within 2 to 12 hours after the start of treatment. With continued therapy, clinically significant hypotension (defined as systolic blood pressure below 90 mm Hg or a 20 mm Hg drop from baseline systolic pressure) and hypoperfusion will occur. In addition, extravasation of protein and fluids into the extravascular space will lead to the formation of edema and creation of new effusions.

Medical management of CLS begins with careful monitoring of the patient's fluid and organ perfusion status. This is achieved by frequent determination of blood pressure and pulse, and by monitoring organ function, which includes assessment of mental status and urine output. Hypovolemia is assessed by catheterization and central pressure monitoring.

Flexibility in fluid and pressor management is essential for maintaining organ perfusion and blood pressure. Consequently, extreme caution should be used in treating patients with fixed requirements for large volumes of fluid (e.g., patients with hypercalcemia). Administration of IV fluids, either colloids or crystalloids is recommended for treatment of hypovolemia. Correction of hypovolemia may require large volumes of IV fluids but caution is required because unrestrained fluid administration may exacerbate problems associated with edema formation or effusions. With extravascular fluid accumulation, edema is common and ascites, pleural or pericardial effusions may develop. Management of these events depends on a careful balancing of the effects of fluid shifts so that neither the consequences of hypovolemia (e.g., impaired organ perfusion) nor the consequences of fluid accumulations (e.g., pulmonary edema) exceed the patient's tolerance.

Clinical experience has shown that early administration of dopamine (1 to 5 μg/kg/min) to patients manifesting capillary leak syndrome, before the onset of hypotension, can help to maintain organ perfusion particularly to the kidney and thus preserve urine output. Weight and urine output should be carefully monitored. If organ perfusion and blood pressure are not sustained by dopamine therapy, clinical investigators have increased the dose of dopamine to 6 to 10 μg/kg/min or have added phenylephrine hydrochloride (1 to 5 μg/kg/min) to low dose dopamine (See "**ADVERSE REACTIONS**" section). Prolonged use of pressors, either in combination or as individual agents, at relatively high doses, may be associated with cardiac rhythm disturbances. If there has been excessive weight gain or edema formation, particularly if associated with shortness of breath from pulmonary congestion, use of diuretics, once blood pressure has normalized, has been shown to hasten recovery. **NOTE: Prior to the use of any product mentioned, the physician should refer to the package insert for the respective product.**

PROLEUKIN® (aldesleukin) treatment should be withheld for failure to maintain organ perfusion as demonstrated by altered mental status, reduced urine output, a fall in the systolic blood pressure below 90 mm Hg or onset of cardiac arrhythmias (See "**DOSAGE AND ADMINISTRATION**" section, "**Dose Modifications**" subsection). Recovery from CLS begins soon after cessation of PROLEUKIN therapy. Usually, within a few hours, the blood pressure rises, organ perfusion is restored and reabsorption of extravasated fluid and protein begins.

Kidney and liver function are impaired during PROLEUKIN treatment. Use of concomitant nephrotoxic or hepatotoxic medications may further increase toxicity to the kidney or liver.

Mental status changes including irritability, confusion, or depression which occur while receiving PROLEUKIN may be indicators of bacteremia or early bacterial sepsis, hypoperfusion, occult CNS malignancy, or direct PROLEUKIN-induced CNS toxicity. Alterations in mental status due solely to PROLEUKIN therapy may progress for several days before recovery begins. Rarely, patients have sustained permanent neurologic deficits (See "**PRECAUTIONS**" section "**Drug Interactions**" subsection).

Exacerbation of preexisting autoimmune disease or initial presentation of autoimmune and inflammatory disorders has been reported following PROLEUKIN alone or in combination with interferon (See "**PRECAUTIONS**" section "**Drug Interactions**" subsection and "**ADVERSE REACTIONS**" section). Hypothyroidism, sometimes preceded by hyperthyroidism, has been reported following PROLEUKIN treatment. Some of these patients required thyroid replacement therapy. Changes in thyroid function may be a manifestation of autoimmunity. Onset of symptomatic hyperglycemia and/or diabetes mellitus has been reported during PROLEUKIN therapy.

Continued on next page

Proleukin—Cont.

PROLEUKIN enhancement of cellular immune function may increase the risk of allograft rejection in transplant patients.

Laboratory Tests: The following clinical evaluations are recommended for all patients, prior to beginning treatment and then daily during drug administration.

- Standard hematologic tests-including CBC, differential and platelet counts
- Blood chemistries-including electrolytes, renal and hepatic function tests
- Chest x-rays

Serum creatinine should be ≤1.5 mg/dL prior to initiation of PROLEUKIN treatment.

All patients should have baseline pulmonary function tests with arterial blood gases. Adequate pulmonary function should be documented (FEV_1 >2 liters or ≥75% of predicted for height and age) prior to initiating therapy.

All patients should be screened with a stress thallium study. Normal ejection fraction and unimpaired wall motion should be documented. If a thallium stress test suggests minor wall motion abnormalities further testing is suggested to exclude significant coronary artery disease.

Daily monitoring during therapy with PROLEUKIN should include vital signs (temperature, pulse, blood pressure, and respiration rate), weight, and fluid intake and output. In a patient with a decreased systolic blood pressure, especially less than 90 mm Hg, constant cardiac rhythm monitoring should be conducted. If an abnormal complex or rhythm is seen, an ECG should be performed. Vital signs in these hypotensive patients should be taken hourly.

During treatment, pulmonary function should be monitored on a regular basis by clinical examination, assessment of vital signs and pulse oximetry. Patients with dyspnea or clinical signs of respiratory impairment (tachypnea or rales) should be further assessed with arterial blood gas determination. These tests are to be repeated as often as clinically indicated.

Cardiac function should be assessed daily by clinical examination and assessment of vital signs. Patients with signs or symptoms of chest pain, murmurs, gallops, irregular rhythm or palpitations should be further assessed with an ECG examination and cardiac enzyme evaluation. Evidence of myocardial injury, including findings compatible with myocardial infarction or myocarditis, has been reported. Ventricular hypokinesia due to myocarditis may be persistent for several months. If there is evidence of cardiac ischemia or congestive heart failure, PROLEUKIN therapy should be held, and a repeat thallium study should be done.

Drug Interactions: PROLEUKIN may affect central nervous function. Therefore, interactions could occur following concomitant administration of psychotropic drugs (e.g., narcotics, analgesics, antiemetics, sedatives, tranquilizers).

Concurrent administration of drugs possessing nephrotoxic (e.g., aminoglycosides, indomethacin), myelotoxic (e.g., cytotoxic chemotherapy), cardiotoxic (e.g., doxorubicin) or hepatotoxic (e.g., methotrexate, asparaginase) effects with PROLEUKIN may increase toxicity in these organ systems. The safety and efficacy of PROLEUKIN in combination with any antineoplastic agents have not been established.

In addition, reduced kidney and liver function secondary to PROLEUKIN treatment may delay elimination of concomitant medications and increase the risk of adverse events from those drugs.

Hypersensitivity reactions have been reported in patients receiving combination regimens containing sequential high dose PROLEUKIN and antineoplastic agents, specifically, dacarbazine, cis-platinum, tamoxifen and interferon-alfa. These reactions consisted of erythema, pruritus, and hypotension and occurred within hours of administration of chemotherapy. These events required medical intervention in some patients.

Myocardial injury, including myocardial infarction, myocarditis, ventricular hypokinesia, and severe rhabdomyolysis appear to be increased in patients receiving PROLEUKIN and interferon-alfa concurrently.

Exacerbation or the initial presentation of a number of autoimmune and inflammatory disorders has been observed following concurrent use of interferon-alfa and PROLEUKIN, including crescentic IgA glomerulonephritis, oculobulbar myasthenia gravis, inflammatory arthritis, thyroiditis, bullous pemphigoid, and Stevens-Johnson syndrome.

Although glucocorticoids have been shown to reduce PROLEUKIN-induced side effects including fever, renal insufficiency, hyperbilirubinemia, confusion, and dyspnea, concomitant administration of these agents with PROLEUKIN may reduce the antitumor effectiveness of PROLEUKIN and thus should be avoided.[12]

Beta-blockers and other antihypertensives may potentiate the hypotension seen with PROLEUKIN.

Delayed Adverse Reactions to Iodinated Contrast Media: A review of the literature revealed that 12.6% (range 11–28%) of 501 patients treated with various interleukin-2 containing regimens who were subsequently administered radiographic iodinated contrast media experienced acute, atypical adverse reactions. The onset of symptoms usually occurred within hours (most commonly 1 to 4 hours) following the administration of contrast media. These reactions include fever, chills, nausea, vomiting, pruritus, rash, diarrhea, hypotension, edema, and oliguria. Some clinicians have noted that these reactions resemble the immediate side effects caused by interleukin-2 administration, however the cause of contrast reactions after interleukin-2 therapy is unknown. Most events were reported to occur when contrast media was given within 4 weeks after the last dose of interleukin-2. These events were also reported to occur when contrast media was given several months after interleukin-2 treatment.[13]

Carcinogenesis, Mutagenesis, Impairment of Fertility: There have been no studies conducted assessing the carcinogenic or mutagenic potential of PROLEUKIN.

There have been no studies conducted assessing the effect of PROLEUKIN on fertility. It is recommended that this drug not be administered to fertile persons of either gender not practicing effective contraception.

Pregnancy: *Pregnancy Category C.* PROLEUKIN has been shown to have embryolethal effects in rats when given in doses at 27 to 36 times the human dose (scaled by body weight). Significant maternal toxicities were observed in pregnant rats administered PROLEUKIN by IV injection at doses 2.1 to 36 times higher than the human dose during critical period of organogenesis. No evidence of teratogenicity was observed other than that attributed to maternal toxicity. There are no adequate well-controlled studies of PROLEUKIN in pregnant women. PROLEUKIN should be used during pregnancy only if the potential benefit justifies the potential risk to the fetus.

Nursing Mothers: It is not known whether this drug is excreted in human milk. Because many drugs are excreted in human milk and because of the potential for serious adverse reactions in nursing infants from PROLEUKIN, a decision should be made whether to discontinue nursing or to discontinue the drug, taking into account the importance of the drug to the mother.

Pediatric Use: Safety and effectiveness in children under 18 years of age have not been established.

Geriatric Use: There were a small number of patients aged 65 and over in clinical trials of PROLEUKIN; experience is limited to 27 patients, eight with metastatic melanoma and nineteen with metastatic renal cell carcinoma. The response rates were similar in patients 65 years and over as compared to those less than 65 years of age. The median number of courses and the median number of doses per course were similar between older and younger patients.

PROLEUKIN is known to be substantially excreted by the kidney, and the risk of toxic reactions to this drug may be greater in patients with impaired renal function. The pattern of organ system toxicity and the proportion of patients with severe toxicities by organ system were generally similar in patients 65 and older and younger patients. There was a trend, however, towards an increased incidence of severe urogenital toxicities and dyspnea in the older patients.

TABLE III: ADVERSE EVENTS OCCURRING IN ≥10% OF PATIENTS (n=525)

Body System	% Patients	Body System	% Patients
Body as a Whole		Metabolic and Nutritional Disorders	
Chills	52	Bilirubinemia	40
Fever	29	Creatinine increase	33
Malaise	27	Peripheral edema	28
Asthenia	23	SGOT increase	23
Infection	13	Weight gain	16
Pain	12	Edema	15
Abdominal pain	11	Acidosis	12
Abdomen enlarged	10	Hypomagnesium	12
Cardiovascular		Hypocalcemia	11
Hypotension	71	Alkaline phosphatase increase	10
Tachycardia	23	Nervous	
Vasodilation	13	Confusion	34
Supraventricular tachycardia	12	Somnolence	22
Cardiovascular disorder[a]	11	Anxiety	12
Arrhythmia	10	Dizziness	11
Digestive		Respiratory	
Diarrhea	67	Dyspnea	43
Vomiting	50	Lung disorder[b]	24
Nausea	35	Respiratory disorder[c]	11
Stomatitis	22	Cough increase	11
Anorexia	20	Rhinitis	10
Nausea and vomiting	19	Skin and Appendages	
Hemic and Lymphatic		Rash	42
Thrombocytopenia	37	Pruritus	24
Anemia	29	Exfoliative dermatitis	18
Leukopenia	16	Urogenital	
		Oliguria	63

[a] Cardiovascular disorder: fluctuations in blood pressure, asymptomatic ECG changes, CHF.
[b] Lung disorder: physical findings associated with pulmonary congestion, rales, rhonchi.
[c] Respiratory disorder: ARDS, CXR infiltrates, unspecified pulmonary changes.

TABLE IV: LIFE-THREATENING (GRADE 4) ADVERSE EVENTS (n=525)

Body System	# (%) Patients	Body System	# (%) Patients
Body as a Whole		Metabolic and Nutritional Disorders	
Fever	5 (1%)	Bilirubinemia	13 (2%)
Infection	7 (1%)	Creatinine increase	5 (1%)
Sepsis	6 (1%)	SGOT increase	3 (1%)
Cardiovascular		Acidosis	4 (1%)
Hypotension	15 (3%)	Nervous	
Supraventricular tachycardia	3 (1%)	Confusion	5 (1%)
Cardiovascular disorder[a]	7 (1%)	Stupor	3 (1%)
Myocardial infarct	7 (1%)	Coma	8 (2%)
Ventricular tachycardia	5 (1%)	Psychosis	7 (1%)
Heart arrest	4 (1%)	Respiratory	
Digestive		Dyspnea	5 (1%)
Diarrhea	10 (2%)	Respiratory disorder[c]	14 (3%)
Vomiting	7 (1%)	Apnea	5 (1%)
Hemic and Lymphatic		Urogenital	
Thrombocytopenia	5 (1%)	Oliguria	33 (6%)
Coagulation disorder[b]	4 (1%)	Anuria	25 (5%)
		Acute kidney failure	3 (1%)

[a] Cardiovascular disorder: fluctuations in blood pressure.
[b] Coagulation disorder: intravascular coagulopathy.
[c] Respiratory disorder: ARDS, respiratory failure, intubation.

ADVERSE REACTIONS

The rate of drug-related deaths in the 255 metastatic RCC patients who received single-agent PROLEUKIN® (aldesleukin) was 4% (11/255); the rate of drug-related deaths in the 270 metastatic melanoma patients who received single-agent PROLEUKIN was 2% (6/270).

The following data on common adverse events (reported in greater than 10% of patients, any grade), presented by body system, decreasing frequency and by preferred term (COSTART) are based on 525 patients (255 with renal cell cancer and 270 with metastatic melanoma) treated with the recommended infusion dosing regimen.

[See table III above]

The following data on life-threatening adverse events (reported in greater than 1% of patients, grade 4), presented by body system, and by preferred term (COSTART) are based on 525 patients (255 with renal cell cancer and 270 with metastatic melanoma) treated with the recommended infusion dosing regimen.

[See table IV above]

The following life-threatening (grade 4) events were reported by <1% of the 525 patients: hypothermia; shock; bradycardia; ventricular extrasystoles; myocardial ischemia; syncope; hemorrhage; atrial arrhythmia; phlebitis; AV block second degree; endocarditis; pericardial effusion; peripheral gangrene; thrombosis; coronary artery disorder; stomatitis; nausea and vomiting; liver function tests abnormal; gastrointestinal hemorrhage; hematemesis; bloody diarrhea; gastrointestinal disorder; intestinal perforation; pancreatitis; anemia; leukopenia; leukocytosis; hypocalcemia; alkaline phosphatase increase; BUN increase; hyperuricemia; NPN increase; respiratory acidosis; somnolence; agitation; neuropathy; paranoid reaction; convulsion; grand mal convulsion; delirium; asthma, lung edema; hyperventilation; hypoxia; hemoptysis; hypoventilation; pneumothorax; mydriasis; pupillary disorder; kidney function abnormal; kidney failure; acute tubular necrosis.

In an additional population of greater than 1,800 patients treated with PROLEUKIN-based regimens using a variety of doses and schedules (e.g., subcutaneous, continuous infusion, administration with LAK cells) the following serious adverse events were reported: duodenal ulceration; bowel necrosis; myocarditis; supraventricular tachycardia; permanent or transient blindness secondary to optic neuritis; transient ischemic attacks; meningitis; cerebral edema; pericarditis; allergic interstitial nephritis; tracheo-esophageal fistula.

In the same clinical population, the following fatal events each occurred with a frequency of <1%: malignant hyperthermia; cardiac arrest; myocardial infarction; pulmonary emboli; stroke; intestinal perforation; liver or renal failure; severe depression leading to suicide; pulmonary edema; respiratory arrest; respiratory failure.

In patients with both metastatic RCC and metastatic melanoma, those with ECOG PS of 1 or higher had a higher treatment-related mortality, and serious adverse events.

Most adverse reactions are self-limiting and, usually, but not invariably, reverse or improve within 2 or 3 days of discontinuation of therapy. Examples of adverse reactions with permanent sequelae include: myocardial infarction, bowel perforation/infarction, and gangrene.

In post marketing experience, the following serious adverse events have been reported in a variety of treatment regimens that include interleukin-2: anaphylaxis; cellulitis; injection site necrosis; retroperitoneal hemorrhage; cardiomyopathy; cerebral hemorrhage; fatal endocarditis; hypertension; cholecystitis; colitis; gastritis; hepatitis; hepatosplenomegaly; intestinal obstruction; hyperthyroidism, neutropenia; myopathy; myositis; rhabdomyolysis; cerebral lesions; encephalopathy; extrapyramidal syndrome; insomnia; neuralgia; neuritis; neuropathy (demyelination); urticaria; pneumonia (bacterial, fungal, viral).

Exacerbation or initial presentation of a number of autoimmune and inflammatory disorders have been reported (See **"WARNINGS"** section, **"PRECAUTIONS"** section, **"Drug Interactions"** subsection). Persistent but nonprogressive vitiligo has been observed in malignant melanoma patients treated with interleukin-2. Synergistic, additive and novel toxicities have been reported with PROLEUKIN used in combination with other drugs. Novel toxicities include delayed adverse reactions to iodinated contrast media and hypersensitivity reactions to antineoplastic agents (See **"PRECAUTIONS"** section, **"Drug Interactions"** subsection).

Experience has shown the following concomitant medications to be useful in the management of patients on PROLEUKIN therapy: a) standard antipyretic therapy, including nonsteroidal anti-inflammatories (NSAIDs), started immediately prior to PROLEUKIN to reduce fever. Renal function should be monitored as some NSAIDs may cause synergistic nephrotoxicity; b) meperidine used to control the rigors associated with fever; c) H_2 antagonists given for prophylaxis of gastrointestinal irritation and bleeding; d) antiemetics and antidiarrheals used as needed to treat other gastrointestinal side effects. Generally these medications were discontinued 12 hours after the last dose of PROLEUKIN.

Patients with indwelling central lines have a higher risk of infection with gram positive organisms.[9–11] A reduced incidence of staphylococcal infections in PROLEUKIN studies has been associated with the use of antibiotic prophylaxis which includes the use of oxacillin, nafcillin, ciprofloxacin, or vancomycin. Hydroxyzine or diphenhydramine has been used to control symptoms from pruritic rashes and continued until resolution of pruritus. Topical creams and ointments should be applied as needed for skin manifestations. Preparations containing a steroid (e.g., hydrocortisone) should be avoided. **NOTE: Prior to the use of any product mentioned, the physician should refer to the package insert for the respective product.**

OVERDOSAGE

Side effects following the use of PROLEUKIN® (aldesleukin) appear to be dose-related. Exceeding the recommended dose has been associated with a more rapid onset of expected dose-limiting toxicities. Symptoms which persist after cessation of PROLEUKIN should be monitored and treated supportively. Life-threatening toxicities may be ameliorated by the intravenous administration of dexamethasone, which may also result in loss of the therapeutic effects of PROLEUKIN.[12] **NOTE: Prior to the use of dexamethasone, the physician should refer to the package insert for this product.**

DOSAGE AND ADMINISTRATION

The recommended PROLEUKIN® (aldesleukin) for injection treatment regimen is administered by a 15-minute IV infusion every 8 hours. Before initiating treatment, carefully review the **"INDICATIONS AND USAGE"**, **"CONTRAINDICATIONS"**, **"WARNINGS"**, **"PRECAUTIONS"**, and **"ADVERSE REACTIONS"** sections, particularly regarding patient selection, possible serious adverse events, patient monitoring and withholding dosage. The following schedule has been used to treat adult patients with metastatic renal cell carcinoma (metastatic RCC) or metastatic melanoma. Each course of treatment consists of two 5-day treatment cycles separated by a rest period.

600,000 IU/kg (0.037 mg/kg) dose administered every 8 hours by a 15-minute IV infusion for a maximum of 14 doses. Following 9 days of rest, the schedule is repeated for another 14 doses, for a maximum of 28 doses per course, as tolerated. During clinical trials, doses were frequently withheld for toxicity (See **"Clinical Experience"** and **"Dose Modifications"** subsections). Metastatic RCC patients treated with this schedule received a median of 20 of the 28 doses during the first course of therapy. Metastatic melanoma patients received a median of 18 doses during the first course of therapy.

Retreatment: Patients should be evaluated for response approximately 4 weeks after completion of a course of therapy and again immediately prior to the scheduled start of the next treatment course. Additional courses of treatment should be given to patients only if there is some tumor shrinkage following the last course and retreatment is not contraindicated (See **"CONTRAINDICATIONS"** section). Each treatment course should be separated by a rest period of at least 7 weeks from the date of hospital discharge.

Dose Modifications: Dose modification for toxicity should be accomplished by withholding or interrupting a dose rather than reducing the dose to be given. Decisions to stop, hold, or restart PROLEUKIN therapy must be made after a global assessment of the patient. With this in mind, the following guidelines should be used:

[See first table above]

[See second table above]

Retreatment with PROLEUKIN is contraindicated in patients who have experienced the following toxicities:

Body System	
Cardiovascular	Sustained ventricular tachycardia (≥5 beats)
	Cardiac rhythm disturbances not controlled or unresponsive to management
	Chest pain with ECG changes, consistent with angina or myocardial infarction
	Cardiac tamponade
Respiratory	Intubation for >72 hours
Urogenital	Renal failure requiring dialysis >72 hours
Nervous	Coma or toxic psychosis lasting >48 hours
	Repetitive or difficult to control seizures
Digestive	Bowel ischemia/perforation
	GI bleeding requiring surgery

Doses should be held and restarted according to the following:

Body System	Hold dose for	Subsequent doses may be given if
Cardiovascular	Atrial fibrillation, supraventricular tachycardia, or bradycardia that requires treatment or is recurrent or persistent	Patient is asymptomatic with full recovery to normal sinus rhythm
	Systolic bp <90 mm Hg with increasing requirements for pressors	Systolic bp ≥90 mmHg and stable or improving requirements for pressors
	Any ECG change consistent with MI, ischemia or myocarditis with or without chest pain; suspicion of cardiac ischemia	Patient is asymptomatic, MI and myocarditis have been ruled out, clinical suspicion of angina is low; there is no evidence of ventricular hypokinesia
Respiratory	O_2 saturation <90%	O_2 saturation >90%
Nervous	Mental status changes, including moderate confusion or agitation	Mental status changes completely resolved
Body as a Whole	Sepsis syndrome, patient is clinically unstable	Sepsis syndrome has resolved, patient is clinically stable, infection is under treatment
Urogenital	Serum creatinine > 4.5 mg/dL or a serum creatinine of ≥4 mg/dL in the presence of severe volume overload, acidosis, or hyperkalemia	Serum creatinine <4 mg/dL and fluid and electrolyte status is stable
	Persistent oliguria, urine output of <10 mL/hour for 16 to 24 hours with rising serum creatinine	Urine output >10 mL/hour with a decrease of serum creatinine >1.5 mg/dL or normalization of serum creatinine
Digestive	Signs of hepatic failure including encephalopathy, increasing ascites, liver pain, hypoglycemia	All signs of hepatic failure have resolved*
	Stool guaiac repeatedly >3-4+	Stool guaiac negative
Skin	Bullous dermatitis or marked worsening of pre-existing skin condition, avoid topical steroid therapy	Resolution of all signs of bullous dermatitis

* Discontinue all further treatment for that course. A new course of treatment, if warranted, should be initiated no sooner than 7 weeks after cessation of adverse event and hospital discharge.

Reconstitution and Dilution Directions: Reconstitution and dilution procedures other than those recommended may alter the delivery and/or pharmacology of PROLEUKIN and thus should be avoided.

1. PROLEUKIN® (aldesleukin) is a sterile, white to off-white, preservative-free, lyophilized powder suitable for IV infusion upon reconstitution and dilution. **EACH VIAL CONTAINS 22 MILLION IU (1.3 MG) OF PROLEUKIN AND SHOULD BE RECONSTITUTED ASEPTICALLY WITH 1.2 ML OF STERILE WATER FOR INJECTION, USP. WHEN RECONSTITUTED AS DIRECTED, EACH ML CONTAINS 18 MILLION IU (1.1 MG) PROLEUKIN.** The resulting solution should be a clear, colorless to slightly yellow liquid. The vial is for single-use only and any unused portion should be discarded.
2. During reconstitution, the Sterile Water for Injection, USP should be directed at the side of the vial and the contents gently swirled to avoid excess foaming. DO NOT SHAKE.
3. The dose of PROLEUKIN, reconstituted with Sterile Water for Injection, USP (without preservative) should be diluted aseptically in 50 mL of 5% Dextrose Injection, USP (D5W) and infused over a 15-minute period.
   In cases where the total dose of PROLEUKIN is 1.5 mg or less (e.g., a patient with a body weight of less than 40 kilograms), the dose of PROLEUKIN should be diluted in a smaller volume of D5W. Concentrations of PROLEUKIN below 30 µg/mL and above 70 µg/mL have shown increased variability in drug delivery. Dilution and delivery of PROLEUKIN outside of this concentration range should be avoided.
4. Glass bottles and plastic (polyvinyl chloride) bags have been used in clinical trials with comparable results. It is recommended that plastic bags be used as the dilution container since experimental studies suggest that use of plastic containers results in more consistent drug delivery. **In-line filters should not be used when administering PROLEUKIN.**
5. Before and after reconstitution and dilution, store in a refrigerator at 2° to 8°C (36° to 46°F). Do not freeze. Administer PROLEUKIN within 48 hours of reconstitution. The solution should be brought to room temperature prior to infusion in the patient.
6. Reconstitution or dilution with Bacteriostatic Water for Injection, USP, or 0.9% Sodium Chloride Injection, USP should be avoided because of increased aggregation. PROLEUKIN should not be coadministered with other drugs in the same container.

Continued on next page

Proleukin—Cont.

7. Parenteral drug products should be inspected visually for particulate matter and discoloration prior to administration, whenever solution and container permit.

HOW SUPPLIED

PROLEUKIN® (aldesleukin) for injection is supplied in individually boxed single-use vials. Each vial contains 22 × 10^6 IU of PROLEUKIN. Discard unused portion.

NDC 53905-991-01 Individually boxed single-use vial

Store vials of lyophilized PROLEUKIN in a refrigerator at 2° to 8°C (36° to 46°F). PROTECT FROM LIGHT. Store in carton until time of use.

Reconstituted or diluted PROLEUKIN is stable for up to 48 hours at refrigerated and room temperatures, 2° to 25°C (36° to 77°F). However, since this product contains no preservative, the reconstituted and diluted solutions should be stored in the refrigerator.

Do not use beyond the expiration date printed on the vial.

NOTE: This product contains no preservative.

Rx Only

REFERENCES

1. Doyle MV, Lee MT, Fong S. Comparison of the biological activities of human recombinant interleukin-2^{125} and native interleukin-2. *J Biol Response Mod* 1985; **4**:96-109.
2. Ralph P, Nakoinz I, Doyle M, et al. Human B and T lymphocyte stimulating properties of interleukin-2 (IL-2) muteins. In: *Immune Regulation by Characterized Polypeptides.* Alan R. Liss, Inc. 1987; 453-62.
3. Winkelhake JL and Gauny SS. Human recombinant interleukin-2 as an experimental therapeutic. *Pharmacol Rev* 1990; **42**:1-28.
4. Rosenberg SA, Mule JJ, Spiess PJ, et al. Regression of established pulmonary metastases and subcutaneous tumor mediated by the systemic administration of high-dose recombinant interleukin-2. *J Exp Med* 1985; **161**: 1169-88.
5. Konrad MW, Hemstreet G, Hersh EM, et al. Pharmacokinetics of recombinant interleukin-2 in humans. *Cancer Res* 1990; **50**:2009-17.
6. Donohue JH and Rosenberg SA. The fate of interleukin-2 after *in vivo* administration. *J Immunol* 1983; **130**: 2203-8.
7. Koths K, Halenbeck R. Pharmacokinetic studies on ^{35}S-labeled recombinant interleukin-2 in mice. In: Sorg C and Schimpl A, eds. *Cellular And Molecular Biology Of Lymphokines.* Academic Press: Orlando, FL, 1985;779.
8. Gibbons JA, Luo ZP, Hansen ER et al. Quantitation of the renal clearance of interleukin-2 using nephrectomized and ureter ligated rats. *J Pharmacol Exp Ther* 1995; **272**: 119-125.
9. Bock SN, Lee RE, Fisher B, et al. A prospective randomized trial evaluating prophylactic antibiotics to prevent triple-lumen catheter-related sepsis in patients treated with immunotherapy. *J Clin Oncol* 1990; **8**:161-69.
10. Hartman LC, Urba WJ, Steis RG, et al. Use of prophylactic antibiotics for prevention of intravascular catheter-related infections in interleukin-2-treated patients. *J Natl Cancer Inst* 1989; **81**:1190-93.
11. Snydman DR, Sullivan B, Gill M, et al. Nosocomial sepsis associated with interleukin-2. *Ann Intern Med* 1990; **112**:102-07.
12. Mier JW, Vachino G, Klempner MS, et al. Inhibition of interleukin-2-induced tumor necrosis factor release by dexamethasone: Prevention of an acquired neutrophil chemotaxis defect and differential suppression of interleukin-2 associated side effects. *Blood* 1990; **76**:1933-40.
13. Choyke PL, Miller DL, Lotze MT, et al. Delayed reactions to contrast media after interleukin-2-immunotherapy. *Radiology* 1992; **183**:111-114.

Manufactured by:
Chiron Corporation
Emeryville, CA 94608
U.S. License No. 1106
Distributed by:
Chiron Corporation
Emeryville, CA 94608
For additional information, contact Chiron Corporations Professional Services 1-800-244-7668, selection 2.
U.S. Patent Nos. RE 33653; 4,530,787; 4,569,790; 4,604,377; 4,748,234; 4,572,798; 4,853,332; 4,959,314; 5,464,939

10000340 Revised September 2000

RABAVERT® ℞

[*rāb-Ā-vərt*]

Rabies Vaccine

Rabies Vaccine for Human Use

DESCRIPTION

RabAvert® Rabies Vaccine produced by Chiron Behring GmbH & Co KG is a sterile freeze-dried vaccine obtained by growing the fixed-virus strain Flury LEP in primary cultures of chicken fibroblasts. The strain Flury LEP was obtained from American Type Culture Collection as the 59th egg passage. The growth medium for propagation of the virus is a synthetic cell culture medium with the addition of human albumin, polygeline (processed bovine gelatin) and antibiotics. The virus is inactivated with β-propiolactone, and further processed by zonal centrifugation in a sucrose density-gradient. The vaccine is lyophilized after addition of a stabilizer solution which consists of buffered polygeline and potassium glutamate. One dose of reconstituted vaccine contains less than 12 mg polygeline (processed bovine gelatin), less than 0.3 mg human serum albumin, 1 mg potassium glutamate and 0.3 mg sodium EDTA. Small quantities of bovine serum are used in the cell culture process. Bovine components originate only from source countries known to be free of bovine spongiform encephalopathy. Minimal amounts of chicken protein may be present in the final product; ovalbumin content is less than 3 ng/dose (1 mL), based on ELISA. Antibiotics (neomycin, chlortetracycline, amphotericin B) added during cell and virus propagation are largely removed during subsequent steps in the manufacturing process. In the final vaccine, neomycin is present at < 1 µg, chlortetracycline at ≤ 20 ng, and amphotericin B at ≤ 2 ng per dose. RabAvert® is intended for intramuscular (IM) injection. The vaccine contains no preservative and should be used immediately after reconstitution with the supplied Sterile Diluent for RabAvert® (Water For Injection). The potency of the final product is determined by the NIH mouse potency test using the US reference standard. The potency of one dose (1.0 mL) RabAvert® is at least 2.5 IU of rabies antigen. RabAvert® is a white, freeze-dried vaccine for reconstitution with the diluent prior to use; the reconstituted vaccine is a clear to slightly opaque, colorless suspension.

CLINICAL PHARMACOLOGY

Rabies in the United States

Over the last 100 years, the epidemiology of rabies in animals in the United States has changed dramatically. More than 90% of all animal rabies cases reported annually to the Centers for Disease Control and Prevention (CDC) now occur in wildlife, whereas before 1960 the majority were in domestic animals. The principal rabies hosts today are wild terrestrial carnivores and bats. Annual human deaths have fallen from more than a hundred at the turn of the century to one to two per year despite major epizootics of animal rabies in several geographic areas. Within the United States, only Hawaii has remained rabies free. Although rabies among humans is rare in the United States, every year tens of thousands of people receive rabies vaccine for postexposure prophylaxis.

Rabies is a viral infection transmitted via the saliva of infected mammals. The virus enters the central nervous system of the host, causing an encephalomyelitis that is almost invariably fatal. The incubation period varies between 5 days and several years, but is usually between 20 and 60 days. Clinical rabies presents either in a furious or in a paralytic form. Clinical illness most often starts with prodromal complaints of malaise, anorexia, fatigue, headache, and fever followed by pain or paresthesia at the site of exposure. Anxiety, agitation, irritability may be prominent during this period, followed by hyperactivity, disorientation, seizures, aero- and hydrophobia, hypersalivation, and eventually paralysis, coma and death.

Modern day prophylaxis has proven nearly 100% successful; most human fatalities now occur in people who fail to seek medical treatment, usually because they do not recognize a risk in the animal contact leading to the infection. Inappropriate postexposure prophylaxis may also result in clinical rabies. Survival after clinical rabies is extremely rare, and is associated with severe brain damage and permanent disability.

RabAvert® (in combination with passive immunization with Human Rabies Immune Globulin [HRIG] and local wound treatment) in postexposure treatment against rabies has been shown to protect patients of all age groups from rabies, when the vaccine was administered according to the CDC's Advisory Committee on Immunization Practices (ACIP) or World Health Organization (WHO) guidelines and as soon as possible after rabid animal contact. Anti-rabies antibody titers after immunization have been shown to reach levels well above the minimum antibody titer accepted as seroconversion (protective titer) within 14 days after initiating the postexposure treatment series. The minimum antibody titer accepted as seroconversion is a 1:5 titer (complete inhibition in the rapid fluorescent focus inhibition test [RFFIT] at 1:5 dilution) as specified by the CDC (1), or ≥ 0.5 IU per milliliter (mL) as specified by the WHO (2,3).

Clinical Studies

Preexposure Vaccination

The immunogenicity of RabAvert® has been demonstrated in clinical trials conducted in different countries such as the USA (4,5), UK (6), Croatia (7), and Thailand (8-10). When administered according to the recommended immunization schedule (days 0, 7, 21 or 0, 7, 28), 100% of subjects attained a protective titer. In two studies carried out in the USA in 101 subjects, antibody titers > 0.5 IU/mL were obtained by day 28 in all subjects. In studies carried out in Thailand in 22 subjects, and in Croatia in 25 subjects, antibody titers of > 0.5 IU/mL were obtained by day 14 (injections on days 0, 7, 21) in all subjects.

The ability of RabAvert® to boost previously immunized subjects was evaluated in three clinical trials. In the Thailand study, preexposure booster doses were administered to 10 individuals. Antibody titers of > 0.5 IU/mL were present at baseline on day 0 in all subjects (9). Titers after a booster dose were enhanced from geometric mean titers (GMT) of 1.91 IU/mL to 23.66 IU/mL on day 30. In an additional booster study, individuals known to have been immunized with Human Diploid Cell Vaccine (HDCV) were boosted with RabAvert®. In this study, a booster response was observed on day 14 for all (22/22) individuals (11). In a trial carried out in the USA (4), a RabAvert® IM booster dose resulted in a significant increase in titers in all (35/35) subjects, regardless of whether they had received RabAvert® or HDCV as the primary vaccine.

Persistence of antibody after immunization with RabAvert® has been evaluated. In a trial performed in the UK, neutralizing antibody titers > 0.5 IU/mL were present 2 years after immunization in all sera (6/6) tested.

Preexposure Vaccination in Children

Preexposure administration of RabAvert® in 11 Thai children from the age of 2 years and older resulted in antibody levels higher than 0.5 IU/mL on day 14 in all children (12).

Postexposure Treatment

RabAvert®, when used in the recommended postexposure WHO program of 5 to 6 IM injections of 1 mL (days 0, 3, 7, 14, 30, and one optionally on day 90) provided protective titers of neutralizing antibody (> 0.5 IU/mL) in 158/160 patients (8, 9, 13-16) within 14 days and in 215/216 patients by day 28-38.

Of these, 203 were followed for at least 10 months. No case of rabies was observed (8, 9, 13-20). Some patients received Human Rabies Immune Globulin (HRIG), 20–30 IU per kg body weight, or Equine Rabies Immune Globulin (ERIG), 40 IU per kg body weight, at the time of the first dose. In most studies (8, 9, 13, 17), the addition of either HRIG or ERIG caused a slight decrease in GMTs which was neither clinically relevant nor statistically significant. In one study (16), patients receiving HRIG had significantly lower ($p < 0.05$) GMTs on day 14; however, again this was not clinically relevant. After day 14 there was no statistical significance.

The results of several studies of normal volunteers receiving the postexposure WHO regimen, i.e., "simulated" postexposure, show that with sampling by day 28-30, 205/208 vaccinees had protective titers > 0.5 IU/mL.

No postexposure vaccine failures have occurred in the United States since cell culture vaccines have been routinely used (1). Failures have occurred abroad, almost always after deviation from the recommended postexposure treatment protocol (21-24). In two cases with bites to the face, treatment failed although no deviation from the recommended postexposure treatment protocol appeared to have occurred (25).

Postexposure Treatment in Children

In a 10-year serosurveillance study, RabAvert® has been administered to 91 children aged 1 to 5 years and 436 children and adolescents aged 6 to 20 years (19). The vaccine was effective in both age groups. None of these patients developed rabies.

One newborn has received RabAvert® on an immunization schedule of days 0, 3, 7, 14 and 30; the antibody concentration on day 37 was 2.34 IU/mL. There were no clinically significant adverse events (26).

INDICATIONS AND USAGE

RabAvert® is indicated for preexposure vaccination, in both primary series and booster dose, and for postexposure prophylaxis against rabies in all age groups.

Usually, an immunization series is initiated and completed with one vaccine product. No clinical studies have been conducted that document a change in efficacy or the frequency of adverse reactions when the series is completed with a second vaccine product. However, for booster immunization, RabAvert® was shown to elicit protective antibody level responses in persons tested who received a primary series with HDCV (4,11).

A. Preexposure Vaccination—See Table 1

(see also **DOSAGE AND ADMINISTRATION** section below)

Preexposure vaccination consists of three doses of RabAvert® 1.0 mL, intramuscularly (deltoid region), one each on days 0, 7, and 21 or 28 (1) (see also Table 1 for criteria for preexposure vaccination).

Preexposure vaccination does not eliminate the need for additional therapy after a known rabies exposure (see also **DOSAGE AND ADMINISTRATION** section, subsection C).

Preexposure vaccination should be offered to persons in high-risk groups, such as veterinarians, animal handlers, wildlife officers in areas where animal rabies is enzootic, certain laboratory workers, and persons spending time in foreign countries where rabies is endemic. Persons whose activities bring them into contact with potentially rabid dogs, cats, foxes, skunks, bats, or other species at risk of having rabies should also be considered for preexposure vaccination. International travelers might be candidates for preexposure vaccination if they are likely to come in contact with animals in areas where dog rabies is enzootic and immediate access to appropriate medical care, including biologics, might be limited (27, 28).

Preexposure vaccination is given for several reasons. First, it may provide protection to persons with inapparent exposure to rabies. Second, it may protect persons whose postexposure therapy might be expected to be delayed. Finally, although it does not eliminate the need for prompt therapy after a rabies exposure, it simplifies therapy by eliminating the need for globulin and decreasing the number of doses of vaccine needed. This is of particular importance for persons at high risk of being exposed in countries where the available rabies immunizing products may carry a higher risk of adverse reactions.

In some instances, booster doses of vaccine should be administered to maintain a serum titer corresponding to at least complete neutralization at a 1:5 serum dilution by the RFFIT (see Table 1); each booster immunization consists of a single dose. See **CLINICAL PHARMACOLOGY**. Serum antibody determinations to decide upon the need for a booster dose is suggested by the ACIP and is considered cost-effective.
[See table 1 at right]

B. Postexposure Treatment—See Table 2
(see also **DOSAGE AND ADMINISTRATION** section below)
The following recommendations are only a guide. In applying them, take into account the animal species involved, the circumstances of the bite or other exposure, the immunization status of the animal, and presence of rabies in the region (as outlined below). Local or state public health officials should be consulted if questions arise about the need for rabies prophylaxis (1).
[See table 2 at right]
In the United States, the following factors should be considered before antirabies treatment is initiated.

Species of Biting Animal
Wild terrestrial animals (especially skunks, raccoons, foxes and coyotes) and bats are the animals most commonly infected with rabies and are the most important potential source of infection for both humans and domestic animals. Unless a wild animal is tested and shown not to be rabid, postexposure prophylaxis should be initiated upon bite or nonbite exposure to the animals (see definition in "Type of Exposure" below). If treatment has been initiated and subsequent testing in a qualified laboratory shows the exposing animal is not rabid, postexposure prophylaxis can be discontinued (1).
The likelihood of rabies in a domestic animal varies from region to region; hence the need for postexposure prophylaxis also varies (1).
Small rodents (such as squirrels, hamsters, guinea pigs, gerbils, chipmunks, rats, and mice) and lagomorphs (including rabbits and hares) are almost never found to be infected with rabies and have not been known to transmit rabies to humans in the United States. Bites from large rodents such as woodchucks (including groundhogs) and beavers, should be considered as possible rabies exposures, especially in regions where rabies is enzootic in raccoons (30). In all cases involving rodents, the state or local health department should be consulted before a decision is made to initiate antirabies postexposure prophylaxis (1).

Circumstances of Biting Incident
An UNPROVOKED attack is more likely than a provoked attack to indicate the animal is rabid. Bites inflicted on a person attempting to feed or handle an apparently healthy animal should generally be regarded as PROVOKED. A currently vaccinated dog, cat or ferret is unlikely to become infected with rabies (1).

Type of Exposure
Rabies is transmitted by introducing the virus into open cuts or wounds in skin or via mucous membranes. The likelihood of rabies infection varies with the nature and extent of exposure. Two categories of exposure should be considered:
Bite: Any penetration of the skin by teeth. Bites to highly innervated areas such as the face and hands carry the highest risk, but the site of the bite should not influence the decision to begin treatment. Recent epidemiologic data suggest that even the very limited injury inflicted by a bat bite (compared to lesions caused by terrestrial carnivores) should prompt consideration of postexposure prophylaxis unless the bat is available for testing and is negative for evidence of rabies (1).
Nonbite: The contamination of open wounds, abrasions, mucous membranes, or theoretically, scratches, with saliva or other potentially infectious material (such as neural tissue) from a rabid animal constitutes a nonbite exposure. In all instances of potential human exposures involving bats, and the bat is not available for testing, postexposure prophylaxis might be appropriate even if a bite, scratch or mucous membrane exposure is not apparent when there is reasonable probability that such exposure might have occurred. Postexposure prophylaxis can be considered for persons who were in the same room as the bat and who might be unaware that a bite or direct contact had occurred (e.g., a sleeping person awakens to find a bat in the room or an adult witnesses a bat in the room with a previously unattended child, mentally disabled person, or intoxicated person) and rabies cannot be ruled out by testing the bat. Other contact by itself, such as petting a rabid animal and contact with blood, urine, or feces (e.g., guano) of a rabid animal, does not constitute an exposure and is not an indication for prophylaxis. Because the rabies virus is inactivated by desiccation and ultraviolet irradiation, in general, if the material containing the virus is dry, the virus can be considered noninfectious. Two cases of rabies have been attributed to probable aerosol exposures in laboratories, and two cases of rabies in Texas could possibly have been due to airborne exposures in caves containing millions of bats (1).
The only documented cases for rabies from human-to-human transmission occurred in eight patients, including two in the USA, who received corneas transplanted from persons who died of rabies undiagnosed at the time of death (1). Stringent guidelines for acceptance of donor corneas have been implemented to reduce this risk.
Bite and nonbite exposure from humans with rabies theoretically could transmit rabies, but no laboratory-diagnosed

TABLE 1: RABIES PREEXPOSURE PROPHYLAXIS GUIDE – UNITED STATES, 1999

Risk Category and Nature of Risk	Typical Populations	Preexposure Recommendations
Continuous. Virus present continuously, often in high concentrations. Specific exposures likely to go unrecognized. Bite, nonbite or aerosol exposure.	Rabies research lab workers,* rabies biologics production workers.	Primary course. Serologic testing every 6 months; booster vaccination if antibody titer is below acceptable level.*
Frequent. Exposure usually episodic, with source recognized, but exposure might be unrecognized. Bite, nonbite or aerosol exposure.	Rabies diagnostic lab workers,* spelunkers, veterinarians and staff, and animal-control and wildlife workers in rabies enzootic areas.	Primary course. Serologic testing every 2 years; booster vaccination if antibody titer is below acceptable level.**
Infrequent (greater than population-at-large). Exposure nearly always episodic with source recognized. Bite or nonbite exposure.	Veterinarians and animal-control and wildlife workers in areas with low rabies rates. Veterinary students. Travelers visiting areas where rabies in enzootic and immediate access to appropriate medical care including biologics is limited.	Primary course. No serologic testing or booster vaccination.**
Rare (population-at-large). Exposures always episodic. with source recognized. Bite or nonbite exposure.	US population-at-large, including persons in rabies- epizootic areas.	No vaccination necessary.

Adapted from the Recommendations of the Advisory Committee on Immunization Practices: Human Rabies Prevention – United States, 1999. (1)
* Judgment of relative risk and extra monitoring of vaccination status of laboratory workers is the responsibility of the laboratory supervisor (29).
**Minimum acceptable antibody level is complete virus neutralization at a 1:5 serum dilution by RFFIT. A booster dose should be administered if the titer falls below this level.

TABLE 2: RABIES POSTEXPOSURE PROPHYLAXIS GUIDE – UNITED STATES, 1999

Animal type	Evaluation and disposition of animal	Postexposure prophylaxis recommendations
Dogs, cats and ferrets	Healthy and available for 10 days observation Rabid or suspected rabid Unknown (e.g., escaped)	Should not begin prophylaxis unless animal develops clinical signs of rabies* Immediately vaccinate Consult public health officials
Skunks, raccoons, bats, foxes, and most other carnivores	Regarded as rabid unless animal proven negative by laboratory tests**	Consider immediate vaccination
Livestock, small rodents, lagomorphs (rabbits and hares), large rodents (woodchucks and beavers), and other mammals	Consider individually	Consult public health officials. Bites of squirrels, hamsters, guinea pigs, gerbils, chipmunks, rats, mice, other small rodents, rabbits, and hares almost never require antirabies postexposure prophylaxis

Adapted from the Recommendations of the Advisory Committee on Immunization Practices: Human Rabies Prevention – United States, 1999. (1)
* During the 10-day observation period, begin postexposure prophylaxis at the first sign of rabies in a dog, cat or ferret that has bitten someone. If the animal exhibits clinical signs of rabies, it should be euthanized immediately and tested.
**The animal should be euthanized and tested as soon as possible. Holding for observation is not recommended. Discontinue vaccine if immunofluorescence test results of the animal are negative.

cases occurring under such situations have been documented. Each potential exposure to human rabies should be carefully evaluated to minimize unnecessary rabies prophylaxis (1).

Postexposure Treatment Schedule
(see also **DOSAGE AND ADMINISTRATION** section below)
The essential components of rabies postexposure prophylaxis are prompt local treatment of wounds and administration of both Human Rabies Immune Globulin (HRIG) and vaccine.
A complete course of postexposure treatment for previously unvaccinated adults and children consists of a total of 5 doses of vaccine, each 1.0 mL: one IM injection (deltoid) on each of days 0, 3, 7, 14 and 28. For previously immunized adults and children, a total of 2 doses of vaccine, each 1.0 mL: one IM injection (deltoid) on each of days 0 and 3. No HRIG should be administered to previously vaccinated persons as it may blunt their rapid memory response to rabies antigen.

1. Local Treatment of Wounds
Immediate and thorough washing of all bite wounds and scratches with soap and water is an important measure for preventing rabies. In animal studies, thorough local wound cleansing alone has been shown to reduce markedly the likelihood of rabies. Whenever possible, bite injuries should not be sutured to avoid further and/or deeper contamination. Tetanus prophylaxis and measures to control bacterial infection should be given as indicated (1).

2. Postexposure Prophylaxis of Rabies
The regimen for postexposure prophylaxis depends on whether or not the patient has been previously immunized against rabies (see below). For persons who have not previously been immunized against rabies, the schedule consists of an initial injection IM of HRIG exactly 20 IU per kilogram body weight in total. If anatomically feasible, the FULL DOSE of HRIG should be thoroughly infiltrated in the area around and into the wounds. Any remaining volume of HRIG should be injected IM at a site distant from rabies vaccine administration. HRIG should never be administered in the same syringe or in the same anatomical site as the rabies vaccine. HRIG is administered only once (for specific instructions for HRIG use, see the product package insert). The HRIG injection is followed by a series of 5 individual injections of RabAvert® (1.0 mL each) given IM on days 0, 3, 7, 14 and 28. Postexposure rabies prophylaxis should begin the same day exposure occurred or as soon after exposure as possible. The combined use of HRIG and RabAvert® is recommended by the CDC for both bite and non-bite exposures, regardless of the interval between exposure and initiation of treatment.
In the event that HRIG is not readily available for the initiation of treatment, it can be given through the seventh day after administration of the first dose of vaccine. HRIG is not indicated beyond the seventh day because an antibody response to RabAvert® is presumed to have begun by that time (1).
The sooner treatment is begun after exposure, the better. However, there have been instances in which the decision to begin treatment was made as late as 6 months or longer after exposure due to delay in recognition that an exposure had occurred. Postexposure antirabies treatment should always include administration of both passive antibody (HRIG) and immunization, with the exception of persons who have previously received complete immunization regimens (preexposure or postexposure) with a cell culture vaccine, or persons who have been immunized with other types of vaccines and have had documented rabies antibody titers. Persons who have previously received rabies immunization should receive 2 IM doses of RabAvert®: 1 on day 0 and another on day 3. They should not be given HRIG as this may blunt their rapid memory response to rabies antigen.

3. Postexposure Prophylaxis Outside the United States
If postexposure treatment is begun outside the United States with regimens or biologics that are not used in the United States, it may be prudent to provide additional treatment when the patient reaches the USA. State or local health departments should be contacted for specific advice in such cases (1).

CONTRAINDICATIONS

In view of the almost invariably fatal outcome of rabies, there is no contraindication to postexposure prophylaxis, including pregnancy (1).
Hypersensitivity
History of anaphylaxis to the vaccine or any of the vaccine components constitutes a contraindication to preexposure vaccination with this vaccine.

Continued on next page

RabAvert—Cont.

In the case of postexposure prophylaxis, if an alternative product is not available, the patient should be vaccinated with caution with the necessary medical equipment and emergency supplies available and observed carefully after vaccination. A patient's risk of acquiring rabies must be carefully considered before deciding to discontinue vaccination. Advice and assistance on the management of serious adverse reactions for persons receiving rabies vaccines may be sought from the state health department or CDC.

WARNINGS

Anaphylaxis, encephalitis including death, meningitis, neuroparalytic events such as encephalitis, transient paralysis, Guillain-Barre Syndrome, myelitis, and retrobulbar neuritis; and multiple sclerosis have been reported to be temporally associated with the use of RabAvert®. See **PRECAUTIONS** and **ADVERSE EVENTS** sections. A patient's risk of developing rabies must be carefully considered, however, before deciding to discontinue immunization.

RABAVERT® MUST NOT BE USED SUBCUTANEOUSLY OR INTRADERMALLY.

RabAvert® must be injected intramuscularly. For adults, the deltoid area is the preferred site of immunization; for small children and infants, administration into the anterolateral zone of the thigh is preferred. The use of the gluteal region should be avoided, since administration in this area may result in lower neutralizing antibody titers (1).

DO NOT INJECT INTRAVASCULARLY.

Unintentional intravascular injection may result in systemic reactions, including shock. Immediate measures include catecholamines, volume replacement, high doses of corticosteroids, and oxygen.

Development of active immunity after vaccination may be impaired in immune-compromised individuals. Please refer to **Drug Interactions**, under **PRECAUTIONS**.

This product contains albumin, a derivative of human blood. It is present in RabAvert® at concentrations of less than 0.3 mg/dose. Based on effective donor screening and product manufacturing processes, it carries an extremely remote risk for transmission of viral diseases. A theoretical risk for transmission of Creutzfeld-Jakob disease (CJD) also is considered extremely remote. No cases of transmission of viral diseases or CJD have ever been identified for albumin.

PRECAUTIONS

General

Care is to be taken by the health care provider for the safe and effective use of the product. The health care provider should also question the patient, parent or guardian about 1) the current health status of the vaccinee; and 2) reactions to a previous dose of RabAvert®, or a similar product. Preexposure vaccination should be postponed in the case of sick and convalescent persons, and those considered to be in the incubation stage of an infectious disease. A separate, sterile syringe and needle or a sterile disposable unit should be used for each patient to prevent transmission of hepatitis and other infectious agents from person to person. Needles should not be recapped and should be properly disposed of. As with any rabies vaccine, vaccination with RabAvert® may not protect 100% of susceptible individuals.

Hypersensitivity

At present there is no evidence that persons are at increased risk if they have egg hypersensitivities that are not anaphylactic or anaphylactoid in nature. Although there is no safety data regarding the use of RabAvert® in patients with egg allergies, experience with other vaccines derived from primary cultures of chick embryo fibroblasts demonstrates that documented egg hypersensitivity does not necessarily predict an increased likelihood of adverse reactions. There is no evidence to indicate that persons with allergies to chickens or feathers are at increased risk of reaction to vaccines produced in primary cultures of chick embryo fibroblasts.

Since reconstituted RabAvert® contains processed bovine gelatin and trace amounts of chicken protein, neomycin, chlortetracycline and amphotericin B, the possibility of allergic reactions in individuals hypersensitive to these substances should be considered when administering the vaccine.

Epinephrine injection (1:1000) must be immediately available should anaphylactic or other allergic reactions occur.

When a person with a history of hypersensitivity must be given RabAvert®, antihistamines may be given; epinephrine (1:1000), volume replacement, corticosteroids and oxygen should be readily available to counteract anaphylactic reactions.

Drug Interactions

Radiation therapy, antimalarials, corticosteroids, other immunosuppressive agents and immunosuppressive illnesses can interfere with the development of active immunity after vaccination, and may diminish the protective efficacy of the vaccine. Preexposure vaccination should be administered to such persons with the awareness that the immune response may be inadequate. Immunosuppressive agents should not be administered during postexposure therapy unless essential for the treatment of other conditions. When rabies postexposure prophylaxis is administered to persons receiving corticosteroids or other immunosuppressive therapy, or who are immunosuppressed, it is important that a serum sample on day 14 (the day of the fourth vaccination) be tested for rabies antibody to ensure that an acceptable antibody response has been induced (1).

HRIG must not be administered at more than the recommended dose, since active immunization to the vaccine may be impaired.

No data are available regarding the concurrent administration of RabAvert® with other vaccines.

Carcinogenesis, Mutagenesis, Impairment of Fertility

Long-term studies with RabAvert® have not been conducted to assess the potential for carcinogenesis, mutagenesis, or impairment of fertility.

Use in Pregnancy

Pregnancy Category C. Animal reproductive studies have not been conducted with RabAvert®. It is also not known whether RabAvert® can cause fetal harm when administered to a pregnant woman or can affect reproduction capacity. RabAvert® should be given to a pregnant woman only if clearly needed. The ACIP has issued recommendations for use of rabies vaccine in pregnant women (1).

Use in Nursing Mothers

It is not known whether RabAvert® is excreted in animal or human milk, but many drugs are excreted in human milk. Although there are no data, because of the potential consequences of inadequately treated rabies exposure, nursing is not considered a contraindication to postexposure prophylaxis. If the risk of exposure to rabies is substantial, preexposure vaccination might also be indicated during nursing.

Pediatric Use

Children and infants receive the same dose of 1 mL, given IM, as do adults.

Only limited data on the safety and efficacy of RabAvert® in the pediatric age group are available. However, in three studies some preexposure and postexposure experience has been gained (12, 19, 26; see also **Clinical Studies in CLINICAL PHARMACOLOGY** section).

Geriatric Use

Clinical studies of RabAvert® did not include sufficient numbers of subjects aged 65 and over to determine whether they respond differently from younger subjects. Other reported clinical experience has not identified differences in responses between the elderly and younger patients.

ADVERSE REACTIONS

In very rare cases, neurological and neuroparalytical events have been reported in temporal association with administration of RabAvert® (see also **WARNINGS** section). These include cases of hypersensitivity (see **CONTRAINDICATIONS, WARNINGS, and PRECAUTIONS** sections).

The most commonly occurring adverse reactions are injection site reactions, such as injection site erythema, induration and pain; flu-like symptoms, such as asthenia, fatigue, fever, headache, myalgia and malaise; arthralgia, dizziness, lymphadenopathy, nausea, and rash.

A patient's risk of acquiring rabies must be carefully considered before deciding to discontinue vaccination. Advice and assistance on the management of serious adverse reactions for persons receiving rabies vaccines may be sought from the state health department or CDC (see also **CONTRAINDICATIONS** section).

Local reactions such as induration, swelling and reddening have been reported more often than systemic reactions. In a comparative trial in normal volunteers, Dreesen *et al.* (4) described their experience with RabAvert® compared to a HDCV rabies vaccine. Nineteen subjects received RabAvert® and 20 received HDCV. The most commonly reported adverse reaction was pain at the injection site, reported in 45% of the HDCV group, and 34% of the RabAvert® group. Localized lymphadenopathy was reported in about 15% of each group. The most common systemic reactions were malaise (15 % RabAvert® group vs. 25 % HDCV group), headache (10 % RabAvert® group vs. 20 % HDCV group), and dizziness (15 % RabAvert® group vs. 10 % HDCV group). In a recent study in the USA (5), 83 subjects received RabAvert® and 82 received HDCV. Again, the most common adverse reaction was pain at the injection site in 80% in the HDCV group and 84% in the RabAvert® group. The most common systemic reactions were headache (52% RabAvert® group vs. 45% HDCV group), myalgia (53% RabAvert® group vs. 38% HDCV group) and malaise (20% RabAvert® group vs. 17% HDCV group). None of the adverse events were serious, almost all adverse events were of mild or moderate intensity. Statistically significant differences between vaccination groups were not found. Both vaccines were generally well tolerated.

Uncommonly observed adverse events include temperatures above 38°C (100°F), swollen lymph nodes, pain in limbs and gastrointestinal complaints. In rare cases, patients have experienced severe headache, fatigue, circulatory reactions, sweating, chills, monoarthritis and allergic reactions; transient paresthesias and one case of suspected urticaria pigmentosa have also been reported.

Observed During Clinical Practice (See **WARNINGS** and **PRECAUTIONS**)

The following adverse reactions have been identified during post approval use of RabAvert®. Because these reactions are reported voluntarily from a population of uncertain size, estimates of frequency cannot be made. These events have been chosen for inclusion due to their seriousness, frequency of reporting, causal connection to RabAvert®, or a combination of these factors:

Allergic: Anaphylaxis, Type III hypersensitivity-like reactions, bronchospasm, urticaria, pruritis, edema

CNS: Neuroparalysis, encephalitis, meningitis, transient paralysis, Guillain-Barre Syndrome, myelitis, retrobulbar neuritis, multiple sclerosis, vertigo, visual disturbance

Cardiac: Palpitations, hot flush

Local: Extensive limb swelling

The use of corticosteroids to treat life-threatening neuroparalytic reactions may inhibit the development of immunity to rabies (see **PRECAUTIONS**, *Drug Interactions*).

Once initiated, rabies prophylaxis should not be interrupted or discontinued because of local or mild systemic adverse reactions to rabies vaccine. Usually such reactions can be successfully managed with anti-inflammatory and antipyretic agents.

Reporting of Adverse Events

Adverse events should be reported by the health care provider or patient to the US Department of Health and Human Services (DHHS) Vaccine Adverse Event Reporting System (VAERS). Report forms and information about reporting requirements or completion of the form can be obtained from VAERS by calling the toll-free number 1-800-822-7967 (1). In the USA, such events can be reported to the Professional Services department, Chiron Corporation: phone: 1-800-CHIRON-8.

DOSAGE AND ADMINISTRATION

The individual dose for adults, children, and infants is 1 mL, given intramuscularly.

In adults, administer vaccine by IM injection into the deltoid muscle. In small children and infants, administer vaccine into the anterolateral zone of the thigh. The gluteal area should be avoided for vaccine injections, since administration in this area may result in lower neutralizing antibody titers. Care should be taken to avoid injection into or near blood vessels and nerves. After aspiration, if blood or any suspicious discoloration appears in the syringe, do not inject but discard contents and repeat procedure using a new dose of vaccine, at a different site.

A. Preexposure Dosage

1. Primary Immunization

In the United States, the Advisory Committee on Immunization Practices (ACIP) recommends three injections of 1.0 mL each: one injection on day 0 and one on day 7, and one either on day 21 or 28 (for criteria for preexposure vaccination, see Table 1).

2. Booster Immunization

The individual booster dose is 1 mL, given intramuscularly. Booster immunization is given to persons who have received previous rabies immunization and remain at increased risk of rabies exposure by reasons of occupation or avocation.

Persons who work with live rabies virus in research laboratories or vaccine production facilities (continuous-risk category: see Table 1) should have a serum sample tested for rabies antibodies every 6 months. The minimum acceptable antibody level is complete virus neutralization at a 1:5 serum dilution by the rapid fluorescent focus inhibition test (RFFIT). A booster dose should be administered if the titer falls below this level.

The frequent-risk category includes other laboratory workers such as those doing rabies diagnostic testing, spelunkers, veterinarians and staff, animal-control and wildlife officers in areas where rabies is epizootic. Persons in the frequent-risk category should have a serum sample tested for rabies antibodies every 2 years and, if the titer is less than complete neutralization at a 1:5 serum dilution by RFFIT, should have a booster dose of vaccine. Alternatively, a booster can be administered in the absence of a titer determination.

The infrequent-risk category, including veterinarians, animal-control and wildlife officers working in areas of low rabies enzooticity (infrequent-exposure group) and international travelers to rabies enzootic areas do not require routine preexposure booster doses of RabAvert® after completion of a full primary preexposure vaccination scheme (Table 1).

B. Postexposure Dosage

Immunization should begin as soon as possible after exposure. A complete course of immunization consists of a total of 5 injections of 1 mL each: one injection on each of days 0, 3, 7, 14 and 28 in conjunction with the administration of HRIG on day 0. For children, see **Pediatric Use** section under **PRECAUTIONS**.

Begin with the administration of HRIG. Give 20 IU/kg body weight.

This formula is applicable to all age groups, including infants and children. The recommended dosage of HRIG should not exceed 20 IU/kg body weight because it may otherwise interfere with active antibody production. Since vaccine-induced antibody appears within 1 week, HRIG is not indicated more than 7 days after initiating postexposure prophylaxis with RabAvert®. If anatomically feasible, the FULL DOSE of HRIG should be thoroughly infiltrated in the area around and into the wounds. Any remaining volume of HRIG should be injected IM at a site distant from rabies vaccine administration. HRIG should never be administered in the same syringe or in the same anatomical site as the rabies vaccine.

Because the antibody response following the recommended immunization regimen with RabAvert® has been satisfactory, routine post-immunization serologic testing is not recommended. Serologic testing is indicated in unusual circumstances, as when the patient is known to be immunosuppressed. Contact the appropriate state health department or the CDC for recommendations.

C. Postexposure Prophylaxis of Previously Immunized Persons

When rabies exposure occurs in a previously vaccinated person, then that person should receive two IM (deltoid) doses (1.0 mL each) of RabAvert®: one immediately and one 3 days later. HRIG should not be given in these cases. Persons considered to have been immunized previously are those who received a complete preexposure vaccination or postexposure prophylaxis with RabAvert® or other tissue culture vaccines or have been documented to have had a protective antibody response to another rabies vaccine. If the immune status of a previously vaccinated person is not known, full postexposure antirabies treatment (HRIG plus 5 doses of vaccine) is recommended. In such cases, if a protective titer can be demonstrated in a serum sample collected before vaccine is given, treatment can be discontinued after at least two doses of vaccine.

Instructions for Reconstituting RabAvert®

Using the longer of the 2 needles supplied, withdraw the entire contents of the Sterile Diluent for RabAvert® into the syringe. Insert the needle at a 45° angle and slowly inject the entire contents of the diluent vial into the vaccine vial. Mix gently to avoid foaming. The white, freeze-dried vaccine dissolves to give a clear or slightly opaque suspension. Withdraw the total amount of dissolved vaccine into the syringe and replace the long needle with the smaller needle for IM injection. The reconstituted vaccine should be used immediately.

Parenteral drug products should be inspected visually for particulate matter and discoloration prior to administration. If either of these conditions exists, the vaccine should not be administered. A separate, sterile syringe and needle or a sterile disposable unit should be used for each patient to prevent transmission of hepatitis and other infectious agents from person to person. Needles should not be recapped and should be properly disposed of.

The lyophilization of the vaccine is performed under reduced pressure and the subsequent closure of the vials needs to be done under vacuum. Additionally, if there is no negative pressure in the vial, injection of Sterile Diluent for RabAvert® would lead to an excess positive pressure in the vial. After reconstitution of the vaccine, it is recommended to unscrew the syringe from the needle to eliminate the negative pressure. After that, the vaccine can be easily withdrawn from the vial. It is not recommended to induce excess pressure, since over-pressurization will create the problems in withdrawing the proper amount of the vaccine.

HOW SUPPLIED

Package with:
1 vial of freeze-dried vaccine containing a single dose
1 vial of Sterile Diluent for RabAvert® (1 mL)
1 disposable syringe
1 smaller needle for injection, 25 gauge × 1″
1 longer needle for reconstitution, 21 gauge × 1.5″
N.D.C.# 53905-501-01
CAUTION: Federal law prohibits dispensing without a prescription

Storage

RabAvert® should be stored protected from light at 2°C to 8°C (36°F to 46°F). After reconstitution the vaccine is to be used immediately. The vaccine may not be used after the expiration date given on package and container.

REFERENCES

1. CDC. Recommendations of the Advisory Committee on Immunization Practices (ACIP). Human Rabies Prevention – United States, 1999. Morbidity and Mortality Weekly Report Recommendations and Report, January 8, 1999, Vol.48, RR-1, pg1.1-21.
2. Smith JS, Yager, PA & Baer, GM. A rapid reproducible test for determining rabies neutralizing antibody. Bull WHO. 1973; 48: 535-541.
3. Eighth Report of the WHO Expert Committee on Rabies. WHO Technical Report Series, no. 824; 1992.
4. Dreesen DW, et al. Two-year comparative trial on the immunogenicity and adverse effects of purified chick embryo cell rabies vaccine for preexposure immunization. Vaccine. 1989; 7: 397-400.
5. Dreesen, DW. Investigation of antibody response to purified chick embryo cell tissue culture vaccine (PCECV) or human diploid cell culture vaccine (HDCV) in healthy volunteers. Study synopsis 7USA401RA, September 1996 – December 1996 (unpublished).
6. Nicholson KG, et al. Preexposure studies with purified chick embryo cell culture rabies vaccine and human diploid cell vaccine: serological and clinical responses in man. Vaccine. 1987; 5: 208-210.
7. Vodopija I, et al. An evaluation of second generation tissue culture rabies vaccines for use in man: a four-vaccine comparative immunogenicity study using a preexposure vaccination schedule and an abbreviated 2-1-1 postexposure schedule. Vaccine. 1986; 4: 245-248.
8. Wasi C, et al. Purified chick embryo cell rabies vaccine (letter). Lancet. 1986; 1: 40.
9. Wasi C. Rabies prophylaxis with purified chick embryo (PCEC) rabies vaccine. Protocol 8T-201RA, 1983 - 1984 (unpublished).
10. Wasi C. Personal communication to Behringwerke AG, 1990.
11. Bijok U, et al. Clinical trials in healthy volunteers with the new purified chick embryo cell rabies vaccine for man. J Commun Dis. 1984; 16: 61-69.
12. Lumbiganon P, et al. Preexposure vaccination with purified chick embryo cell rabies vaccines in children. Asian Pacific J Allergy Immunol 1989; 7: 99-101.
13. Vodopija I. Post-exposure rabies prophylaxis with purified chick embryo cell (PCEC) rabies vaccine. Protocol 7YU-201RA, 1983-1985 (unpublished).
14. John J. Evaluation of purified chick embryo cell culture (PCEC) rabies vaccine, 1987 (unpublished).
15. Tanphaichitra D, Siristonpun Y. Study of the efficacy of a purified chick embryo cell vaccine in patients bitten by rabid animals. Intern Med. 1987; 3: 158-160.
16. Thongcharoen P, et al. Effectiveness of new economical schedule of rabies postexposure prophylaxis using purified chick embryo cell tissue culture rabies vaccine. Protocol 7T—301IP, 1993 (unpublished).
17. Ljubicic M, et al. Efficacy of PCEC vaccines in postexposure rabies prophylaxis. In: Vodopija, Nicholson, Smerdel & Bijok (eds.): Improvements in rabies postexposure treatment (Proceedings of a meeting in Dubrovnik, Yogoslavia). Zagreb Institute of Public Health 1985.17.
18. Madhusudana SN, Tripathi KK. Post exposure studies with human diploid cell rabies vaccine and purified chick embryo cell vaccine: Comparative Serological Responses in Man. Zbl Bakt 1989; 271: 345-350.
19. Sehgal S, et al. Ten year longitudinal study of efficacy and safety of purified chick embryo cell vaccine for preand postexposure prophylaxis of rabies in Indian population. J Commun Dis. 1995; 27: 36-43.
20. Sehgal S, et al. Clinical evaluation of purified chick embryo cell antirabies vaccine for postexposure treatment. J Commun Dis. 1988; 20: 293-300.
21. Fishbein DB, et al. Administration of human diploid-cell rabies vaccine in the gluteal area. N Engl J Med 1988; 318: 124-125.
22. Shill M, et al. Fatal rabies encephalitis despite appropriate postexposure prophylaxis. A case report. N Engl J Med 1987; 316: 1257-1258.
23. Wilde H, et al. Failure of rabies postexposure treatment in Thailand. Vaccine 1989; 7: 49–52.
24. Kuwert EK, et al. postexposure use of human diploid cell culture rabies vaccine. Dev Biol Stand 1977; 37: 273-286.
25. Hemachudha T, et al. Additional reports of failure to respond to treatment after rabies exposure in Thailand. Clin Infect Dis 1999; 28: 143-144.
26. Lumbiganon P, Wasi C. Survival after rabies immunisation in newborn infant of affected mother. Lancet 1990; 336: 319-320.
27. Centers for Disease Control and Prevention. Health Information for International Travel, 2003–2004 (The Yellow Book). Atlanta: US Department of Health and Human Services, Public Health Service, 2003. Internet version at: http://www.cdc.gov/travel/yb
28. World Health Organization. International Travel and Health, 2002. Geneva, Switzerland. Internet version at: http://www.who.int/ith
29. CDC and NIH. Biosafety in microbiological and biomedical laboratories. 3rd. ed. Washington, D.C. HHS Publication no. (CDC) 93-8395, Washington, DC: US Department of Health and Human Services, 1993.
30. Krebs JW, et al. Rabies surveillance in the United States in 2001. J Am Vet Med Assoc. 2002; 221: 1690-1701.

Manufactured by:
Chiron Behring GmbH & Co KG
D-35006 Marburg, Germany
US License No. 1222
Distributed by:
Chiron Corporation
Emeryville, CA. 94608, USA
Rev. 04/04

Shown in Product Identification Guide, page 311

TOBI® ℞

Tobramycin Solution for Inhalation
Nebulizer Solution—For Inhalation Use Only

PRESCRIBING INFORMATION

DESCRIPTION

TOBI® is a tobramycin solution for inhalation. It is a sterile, clear, slightly yellow, non-pyrogenic, aqueous solution with the pH and salinity adjusted specifically for administration by a compressed air driven reusable nebulizer. The chemical formula for tobramycin is $C_{18}H_{37}N_5O_9$ and the molecular weight is 467.52. Tobramycin is *O*-3-amino-3-deoxy-α-D-glucopyranosyl-(1→4)-*O*-[2,6-diamino-2,3,6-trideoxy-α-D-*ribo*-hexopyranosyl-(1→6)]-2-deoxy-L-streptamine. The structural formula for tobramycin is:

Each single-use 5 mL ampule contains 300 mg tobramycin and 11.25 mg sodium chloride in sterile water for injection. Sulfuric acid and sodium hydroxide are added to adjust the pH to 6.0. Nitrogen is used for sparging. All ingredients meet USP requirements. The formulation contains no preservatives.

CLINICAL PHARMACOLOGY

TOBI is specifically formulated for administration by inhalation. When inhaled, tobramycin is concentrated in the airways.

Pharmacokinetics

TOBI contains tobramycin, a cationic polar molecule that does not readily cross epithelial membranes.[1] The bioavailability of TOBI may vary because of individual differences in nebulizer performance and airway pathology.[2] Following administration of TOBI, tobramycin remains concentrated primarily in the airways.

Sputum Concentrations: Ten minutes after inhalation of the first 300 mg dose of TOBI, the average concentration of tobramycin was 1237 μg/g (ranging from 35 to 7414 μg/g) in sputum. Tobramycin does not accumulate in sputum; after 20 weeks of therapy with the TOBI regimen, the average concentration of tobramycin at ten minutes after inhalation was 1154 μg/g (ranging from 39 to 8085 μg/g) in sputum. High variability of tobramycin concentration in sputum was observed. Two hours after inhalation, sputum concentrations declined to approximately 14% of tobramycin levels at ten minutes after inhalation.

Serum Concentrations: The average serum concentration of tobramycin one hour after inhalation of a single 300 mg dose of TOBI by cystic fibrosis patients was 0.95 μg/mL. After 20 weeks of therapy on the TOBI regimen, the average serum tobramycin concentration one hour after dosing was 1.05 μg/mL.

Elimination: The elimination half-life of tobramycin from serum is approximately 2 hours after intravenous (IV) administration. Assuming tobramycin absorbed following inhalation behaves similarly to tobramycin following IV administration, systemically absorbed tobramycin is eliminated principally by glomerular filtration. Unabsorbed tobramycin, following TOBI administration, is probably eliminated primarily in expectorated sputum.

Microbiology

Tobramycin is an aminoglycoside antibiotic produced by *Streptomyces tenebrarius.*[1] It acts primarily by disrupting protein synthesis, leading to altered cell membrane permeability, progressive disruption of the cell envelope, and eventual cell death.[3]

Tobramycin has *in vitro* activity against a wide range of gram-negative organisms including *Pseudomonas aeruginosa*. It is bactericidal at concentrations equal to or slightly greater than inhibitory concentrations.

Susceptibility Testing

A single sputum sample from a cystic fibrosis patient may contain multiple morphotypes of *Pseudomonas aeruginosa* and each morphotype may have a different level of *in vitro* susceptibility to tobramycin. Treatment for 6 months with TOBI in two clinical studies did not affect the susceptibility of the majority of *P. aeruginosa* isolates tested; however, increased minimum inhibitory concentrations (MICs) were noted in some patients. The clinical significance of this information has not been clearly established in the treatment of *P. aeruginosa* in cystic fibrosis patients. For additional information regarding the effects of TOBI on *P. aeruginosa* MIC values and bacterial sputum density, please refer to the **CLINICAL STUDIES** section.

The *in vitro* antimicrobial susceptibility test methods used for parenteral tobramycin therapy can be used to monitor the susceptibility of *P. aeruginosa* isolated from cystic fibrosis patients. If decreased susceptibility is noted, the results should be reported to the clinician.

Susceptibility breakpoints established for parenteral administration of tobramycin do not apply to aerosolized administration of TOBI. The relationship between *in vitro* susceptibility test results and clinical outcome with TOBI therapy is not clear.

INDICATIONS AND USAGE

TOBI is indicated for the management of cystic fibrosis patients with *P. aeruginosa.*

Safety and efficacy have not been demonstrated in patients under the age of 6 years, patients with FEV_1 <25% or >75% predicted, or patients colonized with *Burkholderia cepacia* (see **CLINICAL STUDIES**).

CONTRAINDICATIONS

TOBI is contraindicated in patients with a known hypersensitivity to any aminoglycoside.

WARNINGS

Caution should be exercised when prescribing TOBI to patients with known or suspected renal, auditory, vestibular, or neuromuscular dysfunction. Patients receiving concomitant parenteral aminoglycoside therapy should be monitored as clinically appropriate.

Aminoglycosides can cause fetal harm when administered to a pregnant woman. Aminoglycosides cross the placenta, and streptomycin has been associated with several reports of total, irreversible, bilateral congenital deafness in pediatric patients exposed *in utero*. Patients who use TOBI during pregnancy, or become pregnant while taking TOBI should be apprised of the potential hazard to the fetus.

Ototoxicity

Ototoxicity, as measured by complaints of hearing loss or by audiometric evaluations, did not occur with TOBI therapy during clinical studies. However, transient tinnitus occurred in eight TOBI-treated patients versus no placebo patients in the clinical studies. Tinnitus may be a sentinel symptom of ototoxicity, and therefore the onset of this symp-

Continued on next page

TOBI—Cont.

tom warrants caution (see **ADVERSE REACTIONS**). Ototoxicity, manifested as both auditory and vestibular toxicity, has been reported with parenteral aminoglycosides. Vestibular toxicity may be manifested by vertigo, ataxia or dizziness. **In postmarketing experience, patients receiving TOBI have reported hearing loss.** Some of these reports occurred in patients with previous or concomitant treatment with systemic aminoglycosides. Patients with hearing loss frequently reported tinnitus.

Nephrotoxicity

Nephrotoxicity was not seen during TOBI clinical studies but has been associated with aminoglycosides as a class. If nephrotoxicity occurs in a patient receiving TOBI, tobramycin therapy should be discontinued until serum concentrations fall below 2 µg/mL.

Muscular Disorders

TOBI should be used cautiously in patients with muscular disorders, such as myasthenia gravis or Parkinson's disease, since aminoglycosides may aggravate muscle weakness because of a potential curare-like effect on neuromuscular function.

Bronchospasm

Bronchospasm can occur with inhalation of TOBI. In clinical studies of TOBI, changes in FEV_1 measured after the inhaled dose were similar in the TOBI and placebo groups. Bronchospasm should be treated as medically appropriate.

PRECAUTIONS

Information for Patients

NOTE: In addition to information provided below, a Patient Medication Guide providing instructions for proper use of TOBI is contained inside the package.

Safety Information

TOBI is in a class of antibiotics that have caused hearing loss, dizziness, kidney damage, and harm to a fetus. Ringing in the ears and hoarseness were two symptoms that were seen in more patients taking TOBI than placebo in research studies. Patients with cystic fibrosis can have many symptoms. Some of these symptoms may be related to your medications. If you have new or worsening symptoms, you should tell your doctor.

Hearing: You should tell your doctor if you have ringing in the ears, dizziness, or any changes in hearing.

Kidney Damage: Inform your doctor if you have any history of kidney problems.

Pregnancy: If you want to become pregnant or are pregnant while on TOBI, you should talk with your doctor about the possibility of TOBI causing any harm.

Nursing Mothers: If you are nursing a baby, you should talk with your doctor before using TOBI.

TOBI Packaging

TOBI comes in a single dose, ready-to-use ampule containing 300 mg tobramycin. Each box of TOBI contains a 28-day supply - 56 ampules packaged in 14 foil pouches. Each foil pouch contains four ampules, for two days of TOBI therapy.

Dosage

The 300 mg dose of TOBI is the same for patients regardless of age or weight. TOBI has not been studied in patients less than six years old. Doses should be inhaled as close to 12 hours apart as possible and not less than six hours apart.

You should not mix TOBI with dornase alfa (PULMOZYME®, Genentech) in the nebulizer.

If you are taking several medications the recommended order is as follows: bronchodilator first, followed by chest physiotherapy, then other inhaled medications and, finally, TOBI.

Treatment Schedule

You should take TOBI in repeated cycles of 28 days on drug followed by 28 days off drug. You should take TOBI twice a day during the 28 day period on drug.

How to Administer TOBI

THIS INFORMATION IS NOT INTENDED TO REPLACE CONSULTATION WITH YOUR PHYSICIAN AND CF CARE TEAM ABOUT PROPERLY TAKING MEDICATION OR USING INHALATION EQUIPMENT.

TOBI is specially formulated for inhalation using a PARI LC PLUS™ Reusable Nebulizer and a DeVilbiss Pulmo-Aide® air compressor. TOBI can be taken at home, school, or at work. The following are instructions on how to use the DeVilbiss Pulmo-Aide air-compressor and PARI LC PLUS Reusable Nebulizer to administer TOBI.

You will need the following supplies:

- TOBI plastic ampule (vial)
- DeVilbiss Pulmo-Aide air compressor
- PARI LC PLUS Reusable Nebulizer
- Tubing to connect the nebulizer and compressor
- Clean paper or cloth towels
- Nose clips (optional)

It is important that your nebulizer and compressor function properly before starting your TOBI therapy.

Note: Please refer to the manufacturers' care and use instructions for important information.

Preparing Your TOBI for Inhalation

1. Wash your hands thoroughly with soap and water.

2a. TOBI is packaged with four ampules per foil pouch

2b. Separate one ampule by gently pulling apart at the bottom tabs. Store all remaining ampules in the refrigerator as directed.

3. Lay out the contents of a PARI LC PLUS Reusable Nebulizer package on a clean, dry paper or cloth towel. You should have the following parts:

- Nebulizer Top and Bottom (Nebulizer Cup) Assembly
- Inspiratory Valve Cap
- Mouthpiece with Valve
- Tubing

4. Remove the Nebulizer Top from the Nebulizer Cup by twisting the Nebulizer Top counter-clock-wise, and then lifting. Place the Nebulizer Top on the clean paper or cloth towel. Stand the Nebulizer Cup upright on the towel.
5. Connect one end of the tubing to the compressor air outlet. The tubing should fit snugly. Plug in your compressor to an electrical outlet.
6. Open the TOBI ampule by holding the bottom tab with one hand and twisting off the top of the ampule with the other hand. Be careful not to squeeze the ampule until you are ready to empty its contents into the Nebulizer Cup.
7. Squeeze **all** the contents of the ampule into the Nebulizer Cup.
8. Replace the Nebulizer Top. Note: In order to insert the Nebulizer Top into the Nebulizer Cup, the semi-circle halfway down the stem of the Nebulizer Top should face the Nebulizer Outlet.
9. Attach the Mouthpiece to the Nebulizer Outlet. Then firmly push the Inspiratory Valve Cap in place on the Nebulizer Top. Note: the Inspiratory Valve Cap will fit snugly.
10. Connect the free end of the tubing to the Air Intake on the bottom of the nebulizer, making sure to keep the nebulizer upright. Press the tubing on the Air Intake firmly.

TOBI Treatment

1. Turn on the compressor.
2. Check for a steady mist from the Mouthpiece. If there is no mist, check all tubing connections and confirm that the compressor is working properly.
3. Sit or stand in an upright position that will allow you to breathe normally.
4. Place Mouthpiece between your teeth and on top of your tongue and breathe normally only through your mouth. Nose clips may help you breathe through your mouth and not through your nose. Do not block airflow with your tongue.
5. Continue treatment until all your TOBI is gone, and there is no longer any mist being produced. You may hear a sputtering sound when the Nebulizer Cup is empty. The entire TOBI treatment should take approximately 15 minutes to complete. Note: if you are interrupted, need to cough or rest during your TOBI treatment, turn off the compressor to save your medication. Turn the compressor back on when you are ready to resume your therapy.
6. Follow the nebulizer cleaning and disinfecting instructions after completing therapy.

Cleaning Your Nebulizer

To reduce the risk of infection, illness or injury from contamination, you must thoroughly clean all parts of the nebulizer as instructed after each treatment. Never use a nebulizer with a clogged nozzle. If the nozzle is clogged, no aerosol mist is produced, which will alter the effectiveness of the treatment. Replace the nebulizer if clogging occurs.

1. Remove tubing from nebulizer and disassemble nebulizer parts.
2. Wash all parts (except tubing) with warm water and liquid dish soap.
3. Rinse thoroughly with warm water and shake out water.
4. Air dry or hand dry nebulizer parts on a clean, lint-free cloth. Reassemble nebulizer when dry, and store.
5. You can also wash all parts of the nebulizer in a dishwasher (except tubing). Place the nebulizer parts in a dishwasher basket, then place on the top rack of the dishwasher. Remove and dry the parts when the cycle is complete.

Disinfecting Your Nebulizer

Your nebulizer is for your use only—Do not share your nebulizer with other people. You must regularly disinfect the nebulizer. Failure to do so could lead to serious or fatal illness.

1. Clean the nebulizer as described above. Every other treatment day, soak all parts of the nebulizer (except tubing) in a solution of 1 part distilled white vinegar and 3 parts hot tap water for 1 hour. You can substitute respiratory equipment disinfectants (such as Control III®) for distilled white vinegar (follow manufacturer's instructions for mixing). Rinse all parts of the nebulizer thoroughly with warm tap water and dry with a clean, lint-free cloth. Discard the vinegar solution when disinfection is complete.
2. The nebulizer parts (except tubing) may also be disinfected by boiling them in water for a full 10 minutes. Dry parts on a clean, lint-free cloth.

Care and Use of Your Pulmo-Aide Compressor

Follow the manufacturer's instructions for care and use of your compressor.

Filter Change:

1. DeVilbiss Compressor filters should be changed every six months or sooner if filter turns completely gray in color.

Compressor Cleaning:

1. With power switch in the "Off" position, unplug power cord from wall outlet.
2. Wipe outside of the compressor cabinet with a clean, damp cloth every few days to keep dust free.

Caution: Do not submerge in water: doing so will result in compressor damage.

Storage Instructions

You should store TOBI ampules in a refrigerator (2–8°C or 36–46°F). However, when you don't have a refrigerator available (e.g., transporting your TOBI), you may store the foil pouches (opened or unopened) at room temperature (up to 25°C/77°F) for up to 28 days.

Avoid exposing TOBI ampules to intense light.

Unrefrigerated TOBI, which is normally slightly yellow, may darken with age; however, the color change does not indicate any change in the quality of the product.

You should not use TOBI if it is cloudy, if there are particles in the solution, or if it has been stored at room temperature for more than 28 days. You should not use TOBI beyond the expiration date stamped on the ampule.

Additional Information

Nebulizer: 1-800-327-8632
Compressor: 1-800-333-4000
TOBI: 1-800-CHIRON8

Laboratory Tests

Audiograms

Clinical studies of TOBI did not identify hearing loss using audiometric tests which evaluated hearing up to 8000 Hz. **Physicians should consider an audiogram for patients who show any evidence of auditory dysfunction, or who are at increased risk for auditory dysfunction.** Tinnitus may be a sentinel symptom of ototoxicity, and therefore the onset of this symptom warrents caution.

Serum Concentrations

In patients with normal renal function treated with TOBI, serum tobramycin concentrations are approximately 1 µg/mL one hour after dose administration and do not require routine monitoring. Serum concentrations of tobramycin in patients with renal dysfunction or patients treated with concomitant parenteral tobramycin should be monitored at the discretion of the treating physician.

Renal Function

The clinical studies of TOBI did not reveal any imbalance in the percentage of patients in the TOBI and placebo groups who experienced at least a 50% rise in serum creatinine from baseline (see **ADVERSE REACTIONS**). Laboratory tests of urine and renal function should be conducted at the discretion of the treating physician.

Drug Interactions

In clinical studies of TOBI, patients taking TOBI concomitantly with dornase alfa (PULMOZYME®, Genentech), β-agonists, inhaled corticosteroids, other anti-pseudomonal antibiotics, or parenteral aminoglycosides demonstrated adverse experience profiles similar to the study population as a whole.

Concurrent and/or sequential use of TOBI with other drugs with neurotoxic or ototoxic potential should be avoided. Some diuretics can enhance aminoglycoside toxicity by altering antibiotic concentrations in serum and tissue. TOBI should not be administered concomitantly with ethacrynic acid, furosemide, urea, or mannitol.

Carcinogenesis, Mutagenesis, Impairment of Fertility

A two-year rat inhalation toxicology study to assess carcinogenic potential of TOBI is in progress.

TOBI has been evaluated for genotoxicity in a battery of *in vitro* and *in vivo* tests. The Ames bacterial reversion test, conducted with five tester strains, failed to show a significant increase in revertants with or without metabolic activation in all strains. Tobramycin was negative in the mouse lymphoma forward mutation assay, did not induce chromosomal aberrations in Chinese hamster ovary cells, and was negative in the mouse micronucleus test.

Subcutaneous administration of up to 100 mg/kg of tobramycin did not affect mating behavior or cause impairment of fertility in male or female rats.

Pregnancy

Teratogenic Effects—Pregnancy Category D

(See **WARNINGS**).

No reproduction toxicology studies have been conducted with TOBI. However, subcutaneous administration of tobramycin at doses of 100 or 20 mg/kg/day during organogenesis was not teratogenic in rats or rabbits, respectively. Doses of tobramycin ≥40 mg/kg/day were severely maternally toxic to rabbits and precluded the evaluation of teratogenicity. Aminoglycosides can cause fetal harm (e.g., congenital deafness) when administered to a pregnant woman. Ototoxicity was not evaluated in offspring during nonclinical reproduction toxicity studies with tobramycin. If TOBI is used during pregnancy, or if the patient becomes pregnant while taking TOBI, the patient should be apprised of the potential hazard to the fetus.

Nursing Mothers

It is not known if TOBI will reach sufficient concentrations after administration by inhalation to be excreted in human breast milk. Because of the potential for ototoxicity and nephrotoxicity in infants, a decision should be made whether to terminate nursing or discontinue TOBI.

Pediatric Use

The safety and efficacy of TOBI have not been studied in pediatric patients under 6 years of age.

ADVERSE REACTIONS

TOBI was generally well tolerated during two clinical studies in 258 cystic fibrosis patients ranging in age from 6 to 48 years. Patients received TOBI in alternating periods of 28 days on and 28 days off drug in addition to their standard cystic fibrosis therapy for a total of 24 weeks.

Voice alteration and tinnitus were the only adverse experiences reported by significantly more TOBI-treated patients. Thirty-three patients (13%) treated with TOBI complained of voice alteration compared to 17 (7%) placebo patients. Voice alteration was more common in the on-drug periods.

Eight patients from the TOBI group (3%) reported tinnitus compared to no placebo patients. All episodes were transient, resolved without discontinuation of the TOBI treatment regimen, and were not associated with loss of hearing in audiograms. Tinnitus is one of the sentinel symptoms of cochlear toxicity, and patients with this symptom should be carefully monitored for high frequency hearing loss. The numbers of patients reporting vestibular adverse experiences such as dizziness were similar in the TOBI and placebo groups.

Nine (3%) patients in the TOBI group and nine (3%) patients in the placebo group had increases in serum creatinine of at least 50% over baseline. In all nine patients in the TOBI group, creatinine decreased at the next visit.

Table 1 lists the percent of patients with treatment-emergent adverse experiences (spontaneously reported and solicited) that occurred in >5% of TOBI patients during the two Phase III studies.

Table 1: Percent of Patients With Treatment Emergent Adverse Experiences Occurring in >5% of TOBI Patients

Adverse Event	TOBI (n=258) %	Placebo (n=262) %
Cough increased	46.1	47.3
Pharyngitis	38.0	39.3
Sputum increased	37.6	39.7
Asthenia	35.7	39.3
Rhinitis	34.5	33.6
Dyspnea	33.7	38.5
Fever[1]	32.9	43.5
Lung Disorder	31.4	31.3
Headache	26.7	32.1
Chest pain	26.0	29.8
Sputum discoloration	21.3	19.8
Hemoptysis	19.4	23.7
Anorexia	18.6	27.9
Lung Function decreased[2]	16.3	15.3
Asthma	15.9	20.2
Vomiting	14.0	22.1
Abdominal pain	12.8	23.7
Voice alteration	12.8	6.5
Nausea	11.2	16.0
Weight loss	10.1	15.3
Pain	8.1	12.6
Sinusitis	8.1	9.2
Ear pain	7.4	8.8
Back pain	7.0	8.0
Epistaxis	7.0	6.5
Taste perversion	6.6	6.9
Diarrhea	6.2	10.3
Malaise	6.2	5.3
Lower Resp. Tract Infection	5.8	8.0
Dizziness	5.8	7.6
Hyperventilation	5.4	9.9
Rash	5.4	6.1

[1] Includes subjective complaints of fever.
[2] Includes reported decreases in pulmonary function tests or decreased lung volume on chest radiograph associated with intercurrent illness or study drug administration.

OVERDOSAGE

Signs and symptoms of acute toxicity from overdosage of IV tobramycin might include dizziness, tinnitus, vertigo, loss of high-tone hearing acuity, respiratory failure, and neuromuscular blockade. Administration by inhalation results in low systemic bioavailability of tobramycin. Tobramycin is not significantly absorbed following oral administration. Tobramycin serum concentrations may be helpful in monitoring overdosage.

In all cases of suspected overdosage, physicians should contact the Regional Poison Control Center for information about effective treatment. In the case of any overdosage, the possibility of drug interactions with alterations in drug disposition should be considered.

DOSAGE AND ADMINISTRATION

The recommended dosage for both adults and pediatric patients 6 years of age and older is one single-use ampule (300 mg) administered BID for 28 days. Dosage is not adjusted by weight. All patients should be administered 300 mg BID. The doses should be taken as close to 12 hours apart as possible; they should not be taken less than six hours apart.

TOBI is inhaled while the patient is sitting or standing upright and breathing normally through the mouthpiece of the nebulizer. Nose clips may help the patient breathe through the mouth.

TOBI is administered BID in alternating periods of 28 days. After 28 days of therapy, patients should stop TOBI therapy for the next 28 days, and then resume therapy for the next 28 day on/28 day off cycle.

TOBI is supplied as a single-use ampule and is administered by inhalation, using a hand-held PARI LC PLUS Reusable Nebulizer with a DeVilbiss Pulmo-Aide compressor. TOBI is not for subcutaneous, intravenous or intrathecal administration.

Usage

TOBI is administered by inhalation over an approximately 15 minute period, using a hand-held PARI LC PLUS Reusable Nebulizer with a DeVilbiss Pulmo-Aide compressor. TOBI should not be diluted or mixed with dornase alfa (PULMOZYME®, Genentech) in the nebulizer.

During clinical studies, patients on multiple therapies were instructed to take them first, followed by TOBI.

HOW SUPPLIED

TOBI is supplied in single-use, low-density polyethylene plastic 5 mL ampules. TOBI is packaged in boxes of 56 ampules (14 flexible, laminated foil over-pouches, each containing 4 ampules).

NDC 53905-065-01

Storage

TOBI should be stored under refrigeration at 2–8°C/36–46°F. Upon removal from the refrigerator, or if refrigeration is unavailable, TOBI pouches (opened or unopened) may be stored at room temperature (up to 25°C/77°F) for up to 28 days. TOBI should not be used beyond the expiration date stamped on the ampule when stored under refrigeration (2–8°C/36–46°F) or beyond 28 days when stored at room temperature (25°C/77°F).

TOBI ampules should not be exposed to intense light. The solution in the ampule is slightly yellow, but may darken with age if not stored in the refrigerator; however, the color change does not indicate any change in the quality of the product as long as it is stored within the recommended storage conditions.

CLINICAL STUDIES

Two identically designed, double-blind, randomized, placebo-controlled, parallel group, 24-week clinical studies (Study 1 and Study 2) at a total of 69 cystic fibrosis centers in the United States were conducted in cystic fibrosis patients with *P. aeruginosa*. Subjects who were less than six years of age, had a baseline creatinine of > 2 mg/dL, or had *Burkholderia cepacia* isolated from sputum were excluded. All subjects had baseline FEV_1 % predicted between 25% and 75%. In these clinical studies, 258 patients received TOBI therapy on an outpatient basis (see Table 2) using a hand-held PARI LC PLUS Reusable Nebulizer with a DeVilbiss Pulmo-Aide compressor.

[See table 2 above]

Table 2: Dosing Regimens in Clinical Studies

	Cycle 1		Cycle 2		Cycle 3	
	28 days	28 days	28 days	28 days	28 days	28 days
TOBI regimen n=258	TOBI 300 mg BID	no drug	TOBI 300 mg BID	no drug	TOBI 300 mg BID	no drug
Placebo regimen n=262	placebo BID	no drug	placebo BID	no drug	placebo BID	no drug

All patients received either TOBI or placebo (saline with 1.25 mg quinine for flavoring) in addition to standard treatment recommended for cystic fibrosis patients, which included oral and parenteral anti-pseudomonal therapy, β_2-agonists, cromolyn, inhaled steroids, and airway clearance techniques. In addition, approximately 77% of patients were concurrently treated with dornase alfa (PULMOZYME®, Genentech).

In each study, TOBI-treated patients experienced significant improvement in pulmonary function. Improvement was demonstrated in the TOBI group in Study 1 by an average increase in FEV_1% predicted of about 11% relative to baseline (Week 0) during 24 weeks compared to no average change in placebo patients. In Study 2, TOBI treated patients had an average increase of about 7% compared to an average decrease of about 1% in placebo patients. Figure 1 shows the average relative change in FEV_1% predicted over 24 weeks for both studies.

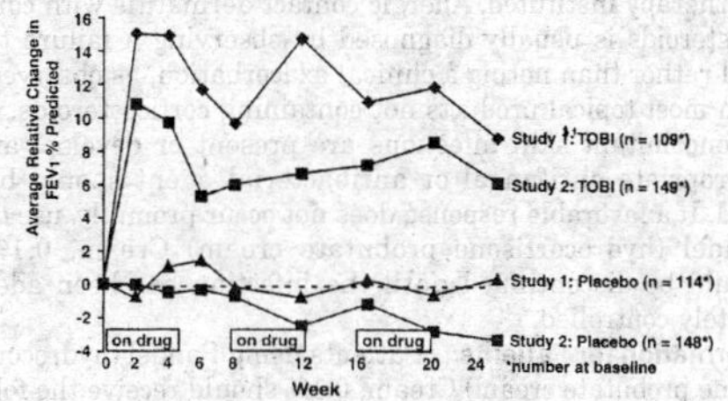

Figure 1: Relative Change From Baseline in FEV_1% Predicted

In each study, TOBI therapy resulted in a significant reduction in the number of *P. aeruginosa* colony forming units (CFUs) in sputum during the on-drug periods. Sputum bacterial density returned to baseline during the off-drug periods. Reductions in sputum bacterial density were smaller in each successive cycle (see Figure 2).

[See figure 2 at top of next column]

Patients treated with TOBI were hospitalized for an average of 5.1 days compared to 8.1 days for placebo patients. Patients treated with TOBI required an average of 9.6 days of parenteral anti-pseudomonal antibiotic treatment compared to 14.1 days for placebo patients. During the six

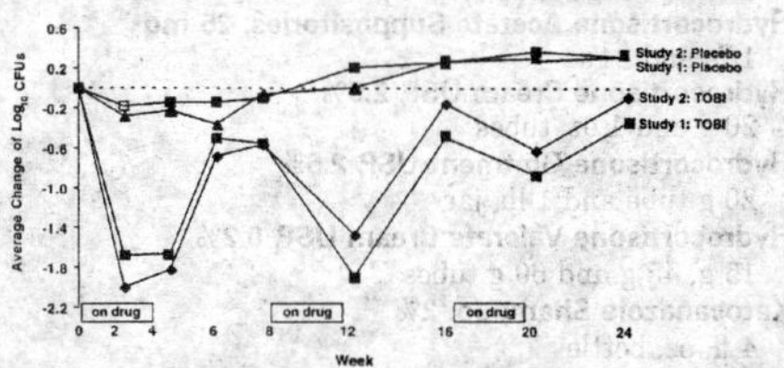

Figure 2: Absolute Change From Baseline in Log_{10} CFUs

months of treatment, 40% of TOBI patients and 53% of placebo patients were treated with parenteral anti-pseudomonal antibiotics.

The relationship between *in vitro* susceptibility test results and clinical outcome with TOBI therapy is not clear. However, four TOBI patients who began the clinical trial with *P. aeruginosa* isolates having MIC values ≥128 µg/mL did not experience an improvement in FEV_1 or a decrease in sputum bacterial density.

Treatment with TOBI did not affect the susceptibility of the majority of *P. aeruginosa* isolates during the six month studies. However, some *P. aeruginosa* isolates did exhibit increased tobramycin MICs. The percentage of patients with *P. aeruginosa* isolates with tobramycin MICs ≥ 16 µg/mL was 13% at the beginning, and 23% at the end of six months of the TOBI regimen.

REFERENCES

1. Neu HC. Tobramycin: an overview. [Review]. J Infect Dis 1976; Suppl 134:S3-19.
2. Weber A, Smith A, Williams-Warren J et al. Nebulizer delivery of tobramycin to the lower respiratory tract. Pediatr Pulmonol 1994; 17 (5):331-9.
3. Bryan LE. Aminoglycoside resistance. Bryan LE, Ed. Antimicrobial drug resistance. Orlando, FL: Academic Press, 1984: 241-77.

Rx Only

Manufactured for
CHIRON Corporation
Emeryville, CA 94608
by Automatic Liquid Packaging, Inc.,
Woodstock, IL 60098
Packaged by Packaging Coordinators Inc.,
Philadelphia, PA 19114-1123

DATE OF ISSUANCE 4/2001

Shown in Product Identification Guide, page 311

Clay-Park Labs, Inc.

1700 BATHGATE AVENUE
BRONX, NY 10457

Direct Inquiries to:
1-800-933-5550

Products:

Name/Product Description
How Supplied

Ammonium Lactate Cream, 12%
385 g pump bottle and 280 g carton (2–140 g tubes)
Ammonium Lactate Lotion, 12%
225 g and 400 g bottles
Antipyrine/Benzocaine Otic Drops
15 ml
Betametasone Dipropionate Cream USP (Augmented), 0.05% (base)
15 g and 50 g tubes
Betamethasone Dipropionate Lotion USP, 0.05%
20 ml and 60 ml bottles
Clindamycin Phosphate Pledgets, 1%
60's and 69's
Desonide Cream 0.05%
15 g and 60 g tubes
Desonide Ointment 0.05%
15 g and 60 g tubes

Continued on next page

Desoximetasone Cream USP, 0.25%
15 g and 60 g tubes
Econazole Nitrate Cream, 1%
15 g, 30 g and 85 g tubes
Erythromycin-Benzoyl Peroxide Topical Gel
23.3 g and 46.6 g jars
Erythromycin Topical Solution USP, 2%
60 ml bottle
Fluticasone Propionate Cream, 0.05%
15 g, 30 g and 60 g tubes
Fluticasone Propionate Ointment, 0.005%
15 g, 30 g and 60 g tubes
Gentamicin Sulfate Cream, USP
15g and 30g tubes
Gentamicin Sulfate Ointment, USP
15g and 30g tubes
Hydrocortisone Acetate Suppositories, 25 mg
12's and 24's
Hydrocortisone Cream USP, 2.5%
20 g and 1 oz. tubes
Hydrocortisone Ointment USP, 2.5%
20 g tube and 1 lb. jar
Hydrocortisone Valerate Cream USP, 0.2%
15 g, 45 g and 60 g tubes
Ketocanazole Shampoo, 2%
4 fl. oz. bottle
Mometasone Furoate Ointment USP, 0.1%
15 g and 45 g tubes
Mupirocin Ointment USP, 2%
15 g, 22 g and 30 g tubes
Nystatin Cream, USP
15 g and 30 g tubes
Nystatin Ointment, USP
15 g and 30 g tubes
Permethrin Cream, 5%
60 g tube
Promethazine Hydrochloride Suppositories USP, 12.5 mg
12's
Promethazine Hydrochloride Suppositories USP, 25 mg
12's
Selenium Sulfide Lotion USP, 2.5%
4 oz. bottle
Trimethobenzamide Suppositories, 100 mg
10's and 50's
Trimethobenzamide Suppositories, 200 mg
10's and 50's
Triamcinolone Acetonide Cream USP, 0.025%
15 g and 80 g tubes; 1 lb. jar
Triamcinolone Acetonide Cream USP, 0.1%
15 g and 80 g tubes; 1 lb. and 5 lb. jars
Triamcinolone Acetonide Cream USP, 0.5%
15 g tube
Triamcinolone Acetonide Ointment USP, 0.025%
15 g and 80 g tubes; 1 lb. jar
Triamcinolone Acetonide Ointment USP, 0.1%
15 g and 80 g tubes; 1 lb. jar
Triamcinolone Acetonide Ointment USP, 0.5%
15 g tube
Tridesilon® (desonide) Cream 0.05%
15 g and 60 g tubes
Tridesilon® (desonide) Ointment 0.05%
15 g and 60 g tubes

CollaGenex Pharmaceuticals, Inc.

41 UNIVERSITY DRIVE, STE. 200
NEWTOWN, PA 18940

Direct inquiries to:
888-339-5678

PANDEL® ℞

[*păn-děl*]
(hydrocortisone probutate cream)
Cream, 0.1%
℞ only
For Dermatologic Use Only
Not for Ophthalmic Use

DESCRIPTION

Pandel Cream contains hydrocortisone probutate, a synthetic adrenocorticosteroid, for dermatologic use. The topical corticosteroids constitute a class of primarily synthetic steroids used as anti-inflammatory and anti-pruritic agents.

Hydrocortisone probutate is a tasteless and odorless white crystalline powder practically insoluble in hexane or water, slightly soluble in ether, and very soluble in dichloromethane, methanol and acetone. Chemically, it is 11β,17,21-trihydroxypregn-4-ene-3,20-dione 17-butyrate 21-propionate. The structural formula is:

[See chemical structure at top of next column]

Each gram of Pandel (hydrocortisone probutate cream) Cream, 0.1% contains: 1 mg of hydrocortisone probutate in a cream base of propylene glycol, white petrolatum, light mineral oil, stearyl alcohol, polysorbate 60, sorbitan monostearate, glyceryl monostearate, PEG-20 stearate, glyceryl stearate SE, methylparaben, butylparaben, citric acid, sodium citrate anhydrous, and purified water.

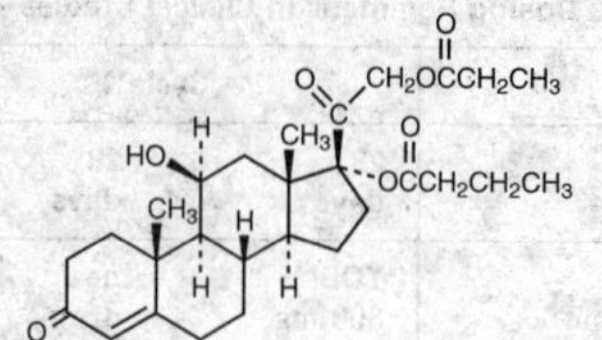

Molecular Formula: $C_{28}H_{40}O_7$ Molecular Weight: 488.62

CLINICAL PHARMACOLOGY

Topical corticosteroids share anti-inflammatory, antipruritic and vasoconstrictive actions. The mechanism of anti-inflammatory activity of the topical corticosteroids is unclear. However, corticosteroids are thought to act by the induction of phospholipase A_2 inhibitory proteins, collectively called lipocortins. It is postulated that these proteins control the biosynthesis of potent mediators of inflammation such as prostaglandins and leukotrienes by inhibiting the release of their common precursor arachidonic acid. Arachidonic acid is released from membrane phospholipids by phospholipase A_2.

Pharmacokinetics: The extent of percutaneous absorption of topical corticosteroids is determined by many factors, including the vehicle and the integrity of the epidermal barrier. Use of occlusive dressings with hydrocortisone for up to 24 hours has not been shown to increase penetration; however, occlusion of hydrocortisone for 96 hours does markedly enhance penetration. Topical corticosteroids can be absorbed from normal intact skin. Inflammation and/or other disease processes in the skin increase percutaneous absorption.

Studies performed with Pandel (hydrocortisone probutate cream) Cream, 0.1% indicate that it is in the medium range of potency compared with other topical corticosteroids.

INDICATIONS AND USAGE

Pandel (hydrocortisone probutate cream) Cream, 0.1% is a medium potency corticosteroid indicated for the relief of the inflammatory and pruritic manifestations of corticosteroid-responsive dermatoses in patients 18 years of age or older.

CONTRAINDICATIONS

Pandel (hydrocortisone probutate cream) Cream, 0.1% is contraindicated in those patients who are hypersensitive to hydrocortisone probutate or to any of the components of the preparation.

PRECAUTIONS

General: Systemic absorption of topical corticosteroids can produce reversible hypothalamic-pituitary-adrenal (HPA) axis suppression with the potential for glucocorticosteroid insufficiency after withdrawal of treatment. Manifestations of Cushing's syndrome, hyperglycemia, and glucosuria can also be produced in some patients by systemic absorption of topical corticosteroids while on treatment.

Patients applying a topical steroid to a large surface area or to areas under occlusion should be evaluated periodically for evidence of HPA-axis suppression. This may be done by using the ACTH stimulation, A.M. plasma cortisol or urinary free cortisol tests.

If HPA axis suppression is noted, an attempt should be made to withdraw the drug, to reduce the frequency of application, or to substitute a less potent steroid. Recovery of HPA axis function is generally prompt and complete upon discontinuation of the drug. Infrequently, signs and symptoms of steroid withdrawal may occur, requiring supplemental systemic corticosteroids. For information on systemic supplementation, see prescribing information for those products.

Pediatric patients may be more susceptible to systemic toxicity from equivalent doses due to their larger skin surface to body mass ratios. (See **PRECAUTIONS–Pediatric Use**).

If irritation develops, Pandel (hydrocortisone probutate cream) Cream, 0.1% should be discontinued and appropriate therapy instituted. Allergic contact dermatitis with corticosteroids is usually diagnosed by observing a failure to heal rather than noting a clinical exacerbation, as observed with most topical products not containing corticosteroids.

If concomitant skin infections are present or develop, an appropriate antifungal or antibacterial agent should be used. If a favorable response does not occur promptly, use of Pandel (hydrocortisone probutate cream) Cream, 0.1% should be discontinued until the infection has been adequately controlled.

Information for Patients: Patients using Pandel (hydrocortisone probutate cream) Cream, 0.1% should receive the following information and instructions:

1. This medication is to be used as directed by the physician. It is for external use only. Avoid contact with the eyes.
2. This medication should not be used for any disorder other than that for which it was prescribed.
3. The treated skin area should not be bandaged or otherwise covered or wrapped so as to be occlusive, unless directed by the physician.
4. Patients should report to their physician any signs of local adverse reactions.
5. Parents of pediatric patients should be advised not to use Pandel (hydrocortisone probutate cream) Cream, 0.1% in the treatment of diaper dermatitis. Pandel (hydrocortisone probutate cream) Cream, 0.1% should not be applied in the diaper area as diapers or plastic pants may constitute occlusive dressings (See **DOSAGE AND ADMINISTRATION**).
6. This medication should not be used on the face, underarms, or groin areas unless directed by the physician.
7. As with other corticosteroids, therapy should be discontinued when control is achieved. If no improvement is seen within two weeks, contact the physician.

Laboratory Tests: The following tests may be helpful in evaluating if HPA axis suppression does occur:
ACTH stimulation test
A.M. plasma cortisol test
Urinary free cortisol test

Carcinogenesis, Mutagenesis and Impairment of Fertility: Long-term animal studies have not been performed to evaluate the carcinogenic potential or the effect on fertility of topical corticosteroids.

In two mutagenicity experiments using hydrocortisone probutate, negative responses were observed in the occurrence of micronuclei in the bone marrow of mice and in the Ames reverse mutation test bacterial assay - with and without metabolic activation.

Pregnancy: Teratogenic Effects – *Pregnancy Category C.* Corticosteroids have been shown to be teratogenic in laboratory animals when administered systemically at relatively low dosage levels. Some corticosteroids have been shown to be teratogenic after dermal application to laboratory animals.

Hydrocortisone probutate has not been tested for teratogenicity when applied topically; however, it is absorbed percutaneously, and studies in Wistar rats using the subcutaneous route resulted in teratogenicity at dose levels equal to or greater than 1 mg/kg. This dose is approximately 12 times the human average topical dose of Pandel Cream, 0.1% assuming 3% absorption and an application of 30 g/day on a 70 kg individual. Abnormalities seen included delayed ossification of the caudal vertebrae and other skeletal variations, cleft palate, umbilical hernia, edema, and exencephalia.

In rabbits, hydrocortisone probutate given by the subcutaneous route was teratogenic at doses equal to or greater than 0.1 mg/kg. This dose is approximately 2 times the human average topical dose of Pandel Cream, 0.1% assuming 3% absorption and an application of 30 g/day on a 70 kg individual. Abnormalities seen included delayed ossification of the caudal vertebrae and other skeletal abnormalities, cleft palate and increased fetal mortality.

The differences between the doses used in animal studies and the proposed human dose may not fully predict the human outcome. The animals received a bolus subcutaneous dose, whereas humans receive a dermal application, where absorption is lower and highly dependent on various factors (e.g., vehicle, integrity of epidermal barrier, occlusion).

There are no adequate and well-controlled studies of the teratogenic potential of hydrocortisone probutate in pregnant women. Although human epidemiological studies do not indicate an increased incidence of teratogenicity with the use of topical corticosteroids, Pandel Cream should be used during pregnancy only if the potential benefit justifies the potential risk to the fetus.

Nursing Mothers: Systemically administered corticosteroids appear in human milk and could suppress growth, interfere with endogenous corticosteroid production, or cause other untoward effects. It is not known whether topical administration of corticosteroids could result in sufficient systemic absorption to produce detectable quantities in human milk. Because many drugs are excreted in human milk, caution should be exercised when Pandel (hydrocortisone probutate cream) Cream, 0.1% is administered to a nursing woman.

Pediatric Use: Safety and effectiveness in pediatric patients have not been established. Because of a higher ratio of skin surface area to body mass, pediatric patients are at a greater risk than adults of HPA axis suppression and Cushing's syndrome when they are treated with topical corticosteroids. They are therefore also at a greater risk of adrenal insufficiency during and/or after withdrawal of treatment. Adverse effects including striae have been reported with inappropriate use of topical corticosteroids in infants and children.

Hypothalamic-pituitary-adrenal (HPA) axis suppression, Cushing's syndrome, linear growth retardation, delayed weight gain, and intracranial hypertension have been reported in children receiving topical corticosteroids. Manifestations of adrenal suppression in children include low plasma cortisol levels and an absence of response to ACTH stimulation. Manifestations of intracranial hypertension include bulging fontanelles, headaches, and bilateral papilledema.

ADVERSE REACTIONS

The most frequent adverse reactions reported for Pandel (hydrocortisone probutate cream) Cream, 0.1% have included burning in 4, stinging in 2, and moderate paresthesia in 1 out of 226 patients.

The following local adverse reactions are reported with topical corticosteroids, and they may occur more frequently with the use of occlusive dressings. These reactions are listed in an approximate decreasing order of occurrence: burning, itching, irritation, dryness, folliculitis, hypertrichosis, acneiform eruptions, hypopigmentation, perioral dermatitis, allergic contact dermatitis, secondary infections, skin atrophy, striae, miliaria.

OVERDOSAGE

Topically applied corticosteroids can be absorbed in sufficient amounts to produce systemic effects. (See **PRECAUTIONS**).

DOSAGE AND ADMINISTRATION

Apply a thin film of Pandel (hydrocortisone probutate cream) Cream, 0.1% to the affected area once or twice a day depending on the severity of the condition. Massage gently until the medication disappears.

Occlusive dressings may be used for the management of refractory lesions of psoriasis and other deep-seated dermatoses, such as localized neurodermatitis (lichen simplex chronicus).

As with other corticosteroids, therapy should be discontinued when control is achieved. If no improvement is seen within 2 weeks, reassessment of the diagnosis may be necessary.

Pandel (hydrocortisone probutate cream) Cream, 0.1% should not be used with occlusive dressings unless directed by the physician. Pandel (hydrocortisone probutate cream) Cream, 0.1% should not be applied in the diaper area, as diapers or plastic pants may constitute occlusive dressings.

HOW SUPPLIED

Pandel (hydrocortisone probutate cream) Cream, 0.1%, a white to off-white opaque cream is supplied as follows:
15 g tubes NDC 64682-200-15
45 g tubes NDC 64682-200-45
80 g tubes NDC 64682-200-80
Store at controlled room temperature 15°-30°C (59°-86°F).
Manufactured for CollaGenex Pharmaceuticals, Inc.
Newtown, PA 18940
by Altana Inc., Melville, New York 11747

PERIOSTAT® ℞

[pĕrĭo-stat]
(doxycycline hyclate tablets) 20 mg

1841–00
Rev. 10/03

DESCRIPTION

Periostat® is available as a 20 mg tablet formulation of doxycycline for oral administration.

The structural formula of doxycycline hyclate is:

with an empirical formula of $(C_{22}H_{24}N_2O_8 \cdot HCl)_2 \cdot C_2H_6O \cdot H_2O$ and a molecular weight of 1025.89. The chemical designation for doxycycline is 4-(dimethylamino)-1,4,4a,5,5a,6,11,12a-octahydro-3,5,10,12,12a-pentahydroxy-6-methyl-1,11-dioxo-2-naphthacenecarboxamide monohydrochloride, compound with ethyl alcohol (2:1), monohydrate.

Doxycycline hyclate is a yellow to light-yellow crystalline powder which is soluble in water.

Inert ingredients in the formulation are: hydroxypropyl methylcellulose, lactose, magnesium stearate, microcrystalline cellulose, titanium dioxide, and triacetin. Each tablet contains 23 mg of doxycycline hyclate equivalent to 20 mg of doxycycline.

CLINICAL PHARMACOLOGY

After oral administration, doxycycline hyclate is rapidly and nearly completely absorbed from the gastrointestinal tract. Doxycycline is eliminated with a half-life of approximately 18 hours by renal and fecal excretion of unchanged drug.

Mechanism of Action: Doxycycline has been shown to inhibit collagenase activity in vitro.[1] Additional studies have shown that doxycycline reduces the elevated collagenase activity in the gingival crevicular fluid of patients with adult periodontitis.[2,3] The clinical significance of these findings is not known.

Microbiology: Doxycycline is a member of the tetracycline class of antibiotics. The dosage of doxycycline achieved with this product during administration is well below the concentration required to inhibit microorganisms commonly associated with adult periodontitis. Clinical studies with this product demonstrated no effect on total anaerobic and facultative bacteria in plaque samples from patients administered this dose regimen for 9 to 18 months. This product **should not** be used for reducing the numbers of or eliminating those microorganisms associated with periodontitis.

Pharmacokinetics

The pharmacokinetics of doxycycline following oral administration of Periostat® were investigated in 4 volunteer studies involving 107 adults. Additionally, doxycycline pharmacokinetics have been characterized in numerous scientific publications.[4] Pharmacokinetic parameters for Periostat® following single oral doses and at steady-state in healthy subjects are presented as follows:
[See first table above]

Absorption: Doxycycline is well absorbed after oral administration. In a single-dose study, concomitant administration of Periostat® with a 1000 calorie, high-fat, high-protein meal which included dairy products, in healthy volunteers, resulted in a decrease in the rate and extent of absorption and delay in the time to maximum concentration.

Pharmacokinetic Parameters for Periostat®

	n	Cmax* (ng/mL)	Tmax** (hr)	Cl/F* (L/hr)	$t_{1/2}$* (hr)
Single dose 20 mg (tablet)	20	362 ± 101	1.4 (1.0–2.5)	3.85 ± 1.3	18.1 ± 4.85
Steady-State 20 mg BID***	30	790 ± 285	2 (0.98–12.0)	3.76 ± 1.06	Not Determined

* Mean ± SD
** Mean and range
***Steady-State data were obtained from normal volunteers administered a bioequivalent formulation.

Clinical Results at Nine Months of Doxycycline Hyclate Capsules, 20 mg, as an Adjunct to SRP (Bioequivalent to Doxycycline Hyclate Tablets, 20 mg)

Parameter	Baseline Pocket Depth 0–3 mm	4–6 mm	≥ 7 mm
Number of Patients (Periostat® 20mg BID)	90	90	79
Number of Patients (Placebo)	93	93	78
Mean Gain (SD//) in ALv✓			
Periostat® 20 mg BID	0.25 (0.29) mm	1.03 (0.47) mm*	1.55 (1.16) mm*
Placebo	0.20 (0.29) mm	0.86 (0.48) mm	1.17 (1.15) mm
Mean Decrease (SD//) in PD✓✓			
Periostat® 20 mg BID	0.16 (0.19) mm**	0.95 (0.47) mm**	1.68 (1.07) mm**
Placebo	0.05 (0.19) mm	0.69 (0.48) mm	1.20 (1.06) mm
% of Sites (SD//) with loss of ALv✓ ≥2 mm			
Periostat® 20 mg BID	1.9 (4.2)%	1.3 (4.5)%	0.3 (9.4)%*
Placebo	2.2 (4.1)%	2.4 (4.4)%	3.6 (9.4)%
% of Sites (SD//) with BOP/			
Periostat® 20 mg BID	39 (19)%**	64 (18)%*	75 (29)%
Placebo	46 (19)%	70 (18)%	80 (29)%

* $p<0.050$ vs. the placebo control group.
** $p<0.010$ vs. the placebo control group.
✓ Alv = Clinical Attachment Level
✓✓ PD = Pocket Depth
/ BOP = Bleeding on Probing
// SD = Standard Deviation

Distribution: Doxycycline is greater than 90% bound to plasma proteins. Its apparent volume of distribution is variously reported as between 52.6 and 134 L.[4,6]

Metabolism: Major metabolites of doxycycline have not been identified. However, enzyme inducers such as barbiturates, carbamazepine, and phenytoin decrease the half-life of doxycycline.

Excretion: Doxycycline is excreted in the urine and feces as unchanged drug. It is variously reported that between 29% and 55.4% of an administered dose can be accounted for in the urine by 72 hours.[5,6] Half-life averaged 18 hours in subjects receiving a single 20 mg doxycycline dose.

Special Populations

Geriatric: Doxycycline pharmacokinetics have not been evaluated in geriatric patients.

Pediatric: Doxycycline pharmacokinetics have not been evaluated in pediatric patients. (See **WARNINGS** section).

Gender: Doxycycline pharmacokinetics were compared in 9 men and 11 women under fed and fasted conditions. While female subjects had a higher rate (Cmax) and extent of absorption (AUC), these differences are thought to be due to differences in body weight/lean body mass. Differences in other pharmacokinetic parameters were not significant.

Race: Differences in doxycycline pharmacokinetics among racial groups have not been evaluated.

Renal Insufficiency: Studies have shown no significant difference in serum half-life of doxycycline in patients with normal and severely impaired renal function. Hemodialysis does not alter the half-life of doxycycline.

Hepatic Insufficiency: Doxycycline pharmacokinetics have not been evaluated in patients with hepatic insufficiency.

Drug Interactions: (See **PRECAUTIONS** section)

Clinical Study

In a randomized, multi-centered, double-blind, 9-month Phase 3 study involving 190 adult patients with periodontal disease [at least two probing sites per quadrant of between 5 and 9 mm pocket depth (PD) and attachment level (ALv)], the effects of oral administration of 20 mg twice a day of doxycycline hyclate (using a bioequivalent capsule formulation) plus scaling and root planing (SRP) were compared to placebo control plus SRP. Both treatment groups were administered a course of scaling and root planing in 2 quadrants at Baseline. Measurements of ALv, PD and bleeding-on-probing (BOP) were obtained at Baseline, 3, 6, and 9 months from each site about each tooth in the two quadrants that received SRP using the UNC-15 manual probe. Each tooth site was categorized into one of three strata based on Baseline PD: 0–3 mm (no disease), 4–6 mm (mild/moderate disease), ≥ 7 mm (severe disease). For each stratum and treatment group, the following were calculated at month 3, 6, and 9: mean change in ALv from baseline, mean change in PD from baseline, mean percentage of tooth sites per patient exhibiting attachment loss of ≥ 2 mm from baseline, and percentage of tooth sites with bleeding on probing. The results are summarized in the following table.
[See second table above]

INDICATIONS AND USAGE

Periostat® is indicated for use as an adjunct to scaling and root planing to promote attachment level gain and to reduce pocket depth in patients with adult periodontitis.

CONTRAINDICATIONS

This drug is contraindicated in persons who have shown hypersensitivity to doxycycline or any of the other tetracyclines.

WARNINGS

THE USE OF DRUGS OF THE TETRACYCLINE CLASS DURING TOOTH DEVELOPMENT (LAST HALF OF PREGNANCY, INFANCY AND CHILDHOOD TO THE AGE OF 8 YEARS) MAY CAUSE PERMANENT DISCOLORATION OF THE TEETH (YELLOW-GRAY-BROWN). This adverse reaction is more common during long-term use of the drugs but has been observed following repeated short-term courses. Enamel hypoplasia has also been reported. TETRACYCLINE DRUGS, THEREFORE, SHOULD NOT BE USED IN THIS AGE GROUP AND IN PREGNANT OR NURSING MOTHERS UNLESS THE POTENTIAL BENEFITS MAY BE ACCEPTABLE DESPITE THE POTENTIAL RISKS.

All tetracyclines form a stable calcium complex in any bone forming tissue. A decrease in fibula growth rate has been observed in premature infants given oral tetracyclines in doses of 25 mg/kg every 6 hours. This reaction was shown to be reversible when the drug was discontinued.

Doxycycline can cause fetal harm when administered to a pregnant woman. Results of animal studies indicate that tetracyclines cross the placenta, are found in fetal tissues, and can have toxic effects on the developing fetus (often related to retardation of skeletal development). Evidence of embryotoxicity has also been noted in animals treated early in pregnancy. If any tetracyclines are used during pregnancy, or if the patient becomes pregnant while taking this drug, the patient should be apprised of the potential hazard to the fetus.

The catabolic action of the tetracyclines may cause an increase in BUN. Previous studies have not observed an increase in BUN with the use of doxycycline in patients with impaired renal function.

Photosensitivity manifested by an exaggerated sunburn reaction has been observed in some individuals taking tetracyclines. Patients apt to be exposed to direct sunlight or ul-

Continued on next page

Periostat—Cont.

traviolet light should be advised that this reaction can occur with tetracycline drugs, and treatment should be discontinued at the first evidence of skin erythema.

PRECAUTIONS

While no overgrowth by opportunistic microorganisms such as yeast were noted during clinical studies, as with other antimicrobials, Periostat® therapy may result in overgrowth of nonsusceptible microorganisms including fungi.
The use of tetracyclines may increase the incidence of vaginal candidiasis.
Periostat® should be used with caution in patients with a history or predisposition to oral candidiasis. The safety and effectiveness of Periostat® has not been established for the treatment of periodontitis in patients with coexistant oral candidiasis.
If superinfection is suspected, appropriate measures should be taken.

Laboratory Tests: In long term therapy, periodic laboratory evaluations of organ systems, including hematopoietic, renal, and hepatic studies should be performed.

Drug Interactions: Because tetracyclines have been shown to depress plasma prothrombin activity, patients who are on anticoagulant therapy may require downward adjustment of their anticoagulant dosage.
Since bacterial antibiotics, such as the tetracycline class of antibiotics, may interfere with the bactericidal action of members of the -lactam (e.g. penicillin) class of antibiotics, it is not advisable to administer these antibiotics concomitantly.
Absorption of tetracyclines is impaired by antacids containing aluminum, calcium, or magnesium, and iron-containing preparations, and by bismuth subsalicylate.
Barbiturates, carbamazepine, and phenytoin decrease the half-life of doxycycline.
The concurrent use of tetracycline and methoxyflurane has been reported to result in fatal renal toxicity.
Concurrent use of tetracyclines may render oral contraceptives less effective.

Drug/Laboratory Test Interactions: False elevations of urinary catecholamine levels may occur due to interference with the fluorescence test.

Carcinogenesis, Mutagenesis, Impairment of Fertility: Doxycycline hyclate was assessed for potential to induce carcinogenesis in a study in which the compound was administered to Sprague-Dawley rats by gavage at dosages of 20, 75, and 200 mg/kg/day for two years. An increased incidence of uterine polyps was observed in female rats that received 200 mg/kg/day, a dosage that resulted in a systemic exposure to doxycycline approximately nine times that observed in female humans that used Periostat (exposure comparison based upon AUC values). No impact upon tumor incidence was observed in male rats at 200 mg/kg/day, or in either gender at the other dosages studied. Evidence of oncogenic activity was obtained in studies with related compounds, i.e., oxytetracycline (adrenal and pituitary tumors), and minocycline (thyroid tumors).
Doxycycline hyclate demonstrated no potential to cause genetic toxicity in an *in vitro* point mutation study with mammalian cells (CHO/HGPRT forward mutation assay) or in an *in vivo* micronucleus assay conducted in CD-1 mice. However, data from an *in vitro* assay with CHO cells for potential to cause chromosomal aberrations suggest that doxycycline hyclate is a weak clastogen.
Oral administration of doxycycline hyclate to male and female Sprague-Dawley rats adversely affected fertility and reproductive performance, as evidenced by increased time for mating to occur, reduced sperm motility, velocity, and concentration, abnormal sperm morphology, and increased pre-and post-implantation losses. Doxycycline hyclate induced reproductive toxicity at all dosages that were examined in this study, as even the lowest dosage tested (50 mg/kg/day) induced a statistically significant reduction in sperm velocity. Note that 50 mg/kg/day is approximately 10 times the amount of doxycycline hyclate contained in the recommended daily dose of Periostat® for a 60 kg human when compared on the basis of body surface area estimates (mg/m^2). Although doxycycline impairs the fertility of rats when administered at sufficient dosage, the effect of Periostat® on human fertility is unknown.

Pregnancy: ***Teratogenic Effects:*** Pregnancy Category D. (See **WARNINGS** Section). Results from animal studies indicate that doxycycline crosses the placenta and is found in fetal tissues.

Nonteratogenic effects: (See **WARNINGS** Section).

Labor and Delivery: The effect of tetracyclines on labor and delivery is unknown.

Nursing Mothers: Tetracyclines are excreted in human milk. Because of the potential for serious adverse reactions in nursing infants from doxycycline, the use of Periostat® in nursing mothers is contraindicated. (See **WARNINGS** Section).

Pediatric Use: The use of Periostat® in infancy and childhood is contraindicated. (See **WARNINGS** section.)

ADVERSE REACTIONS

Adverse Reactions in Clinical Trials of a bioequivalent form of doxycycline hyclate capsules: In clinical trials of adult patients with periodontal disease 213 patients received 20 mg BID over a 9–12 month period. The most frequent adverse reactions occurring in studies involving treatment with a bioequivalent form of doxycycline hyclate capsules or placebo are listed below:

Incidence (%) of Adverse Reactions in Clinical Trials of Doxycycline Hyclate Capsules, 20mg (Bioequivalent to Doxycycline Hyclate Tablets, 20mg) vs. Placebo

Adverse Reaction	Doxycycline Hyclate Capsules 20 mg BID (n=213)	Placebo (n=215)
Headache	55 (26%)	56 (26%)
Common Cold	47 (22%)	46 (21%)
Flu Symptoms	24 (11%)	40 (19%)
Tooth Ache	14 (7%)	28 (13%)
Periodontal Abscess	8 (4%)	21 (10%)
Tooth Disorder	13 (6%)	19 (9%)
Nausea	17 (8%)	12 (6%)
Sinusitis	7 (3%)	18 (8%)
Injury	11 (5%)	18 (8%)
Dyspepsia	13 (6%)	5 (2%)
Sore Throat	11 (5%)	13 (6%)
Joint Pain	12 (6%)	8 (4%)
Diarrhea	12 (6%)	8 (4%)
Sinus Congestion	11 (5%)	11 (5%)
Coughing	9 (4%)	11 (5%)
Sinus Headache	8 (4%)	8 (4%)
Rash	8 (4%)	6 (3%)
Back Pain	7 (3%)	8 (4%)
Back Ache	4 (2%)	9 (4%)
Menstrual Cramp	9 (4%)	5 (2%)
Acid Indigestion	8 (4%)	7 (3%)
Pain	8 (4%)	5 (2%)
Infection	4 (2%)	6 (3%)
Gum Pain	1 (<1%)	6 (3%)
Bronchitis	7 (3%)	5 (2%)
Muscle Pain	2 (1%)	6 (3%)

Note: Percentages are based on total number of study participants in each treatment group.

Adverse Reactions for Tetracyclines: The following adverse reactions have been observed in patients receiving tetracyclines:
Gastrointestinal: anorexia, nausea, vomiting, diarrhea, glossitis, dysphagia, enterocolitis, and inflammatory lesions (with vaginal candidiasis) in the anogenital region. Hepatotoxicity has been reported rarely. Rare instances of esophagitis and esophageal ulcerations have been reported in patients receiving the capsule forms of the drugs in the tetracycline class. Most of these patients took medications immediately before going to bed. (See **DOSAGE AND ADMINISTRATION** Section).
Skin: maculopapular and erythematous rashes. Exfoliative dermatitis has been reported but is uncommon. Photosensitivity is discussed above. (See **WARNINGS** Section).
Renal toxicity: Rise in BUN has been reported and is apparently dose related. (See **WARNINGS** Section).
Hypersensitivity reactions: urticaria, angioneurotic edema, anaphylaxis, anaphylactoid purpura, serum sickness, pericarditis, and exacerbation of systemic lupus erythematosus.
Blood: Hemolytic anemia, thrombocytopenia, neutropenia, and eosinophilia have been reported.

OVERDOSAGE

In case of overdosage, discontinue medication, treat symptomatically and institute supportive measures. Dialysis does not alter serum half-life and thus would not be of benefit in treating cases of overdose.

DOSAGE AND ADMINISTRATION

THE DOSAGE OF PERIOSTAT® DIFFERS FROM THAT OF DOXYCYCLINE USED TO TREAT INFECTIONS. EXCEEDING THE RECOMMENDED DOSAGE MAY RESULT IN AN INCREASED INCIDENCE OF SIDE EFFECTS INCLUDING THE DEVELOPMENT OF RESISTANT MICROORGANISMS.
Periostat® 20 mg twice daily as an adjunct following scaling and root planing may be administered for up to 9 months. Periostat® should be taken twice daily at 12 hour intervals, usually in the morning and evening. It is recommended that if Periostat® is taken close to meal times, allow at least one hour prior to or two hours after meals. Safety beyond 12 months and efficacy beyond 9 months have not been established.
Administration of adequate amounts of fluid along with the tablets is recommended to wash down the drug and reduce the risk of esophageal irritation and ulceration. (See **ADVERSE REACTIONS** Section).

HOW SUPPLIED

Periostat® (white tablet imprinted with a PS20) containing doxycycline hyclate equivalent to 20 mg doxycycline. Bottle of 60 (NDC 64682-008-01), Bottle of 100 (NDC 64682-008-02) and Bottle of 1000 (NDC 64682-008-03).

Storage: All products are to be stored at controlled room temperatures of 15°C–30°C (59°F–86°F) and dispensed in tight, light-resistant containers (USP).

Rx Only

PERIOSTAT® is a trademark of CollaGenex Pharmaceuticals, Inc., Newtown, PA, 18940
Manufactured by:
Pharmaceutical Manufacturing Research Services, Inc.
Horsham, PA 19044
Marketed by:
CollaGenex Pharmaceuticals, Inc.
Newtown, PA, 18940

REFERENCES

1. Golub L.M., Sorsa T., Lee H-M, Ciancio S., Sorbi D., Ramamurthy N.S., Gruber B., Salo T., Konttinen Y.T.: Doxycycline Inhibits Neutrophil (PMN)-type Matrix Metalloproteinases in Human Adult Periodontitis Gingiva. J. Clin. Periodontol 1995; 22: 100–109.
2. Golub L.M., Ciancio S., Ramamurthy N.S., Leung M., McNamara T.F.: Low-dose Doxycycline Therapy: Effect on Gingival and Crevicular Fluid Collagenase Activity in Humans. J. Periodont Res 1990; 25: 321–330.
3. Golub L.M., Lee H.M., Greenwald R.A., Ryan M.E., Salo T., Giannobile W.V.: A Matrix Metalloproteinase Inhibitor Reduces Bone-type Collagen Degradation Fragments and Specific Collegenases in Gingival Crevicular Fluid During Adult Periodontitis. Inflammation Research 1997; 46: 310–319.
4. Saivain S., Houin G.: Clinical Pharmacokinetics of Doxycycline and Minocycline. Clin. Pharmacokinetics 1988; 15; 355–366.
5. Schach von Wittenau M., Twomey T.: The Disposition of Doxycycline by Man and Dog. Chemotherapy 1971; 16: 217–228.
6. Campistron G., Coulais Y., Caillard C., Mosser J., Pontagnier H., Houin G.: Pharmacokinetics and Bioavailability of Doxycycline in Humans. Arzneimittel Forschung 1986; 36: 1705–1707.

Columbia Laboratories, Inc.

354 EISENHOWER PARKWAY
SECOND FLOOR – PLAZA I
LIVINGSTON, NJ 07039

Direct Inquiries To:
(973) 994-3999
Fax: (973) 994-3001
(973) 994-2771

PROCHIEVE® 4% ℞
PROCHIEVE® 8% ℞
[*prō'chēv*]
(progesterone gel)

DESCRIPTION

Prochieve® (progesterone gel) is a bioadhesive vaginal gel containing micronized progesterone in an emulsion system, which is contained in single use, one piece polyethylene vaginal applicators. The carrier vehicle is an oil in water emulsion containing the water swellable, but insoluble polymer, polycarbophil. The progesterone is partially soluble in both the oil and water phase of the vehicle, with the majority of the progesterone existing as a suspension. Physically, Prochieve® has the appearance of a soft, white to off-white gel.
The active ingredient, progesterone, is present in either a 4% or an 8% concentration (w/w). The chemical name for progesterone is pregn-4-ene-3,20-dione. It has an empirical formula of $C_{21}H_{30}O_2$ and a molecular weight of 314.5. The structural formula is:

Progesterone exists in two polymorphic forms. Form 1, which is the form used in Prochieve®, exists as white orthorhombic prisms with a melting point of 127-131°C.

Each applicator delivers 1.125 grams of Prochieve® gel containing either 45 mg (4% gel) or 90 mg (8% gel) of progesterone in a base containing glycerin, mineral oil, polycarbophil, carbomer 934P, hydrogenated palm oil glyceride, sorbic acid, sodium hydroxide and purified water.

CLINICAL PHARMACOLOGY

Progesterone is a naturally occurring steroid that is secreted by the ovary, placenta, and adrenal gland. In the presence of adequate estrogen, progesterone transforms a proliferative endometrium into a secretory endometrium. Progesterone is essential for the development of decidual tissue, and the effect of progesterone on the differentiation of glandular epithelia and stroma has been extensively studied. Progesterone is necessary to increase endometrial receptivity for implantation of an embryo. Once an embryo is implanted, progesterone acts to maintain the pregnancy. Normal or near-normal endometrial responses to oral estradiol and intramuscular progesterone have been noted in functionally agonadal women through the sixth decade of life. Progesterone administration decreases the circulatory levels of gonadotropins.

Pharmacokinetics

Absorption

Due to the sustained release properties of Prochieve®, progesterone absorption is prolonged with an absorption half-life of approximately 25-50 hours, and an elimination half-life of 5-20 minutes. Therefore, the pharmacokinetics of Prochieve® are rate-limited by absorption rather than by elimination.

The bioavailability of progesterone in Prochieve® was determined relative to progesterone administered intramuscularly. In a single dose crossover study, 20 healthy, estrogenized postmenopausal women received 45 mg or 90 mg progesterone vaginally in Prochieve® 4% or Prochieve® 8%, or 45 mg or 90 mg progesterone intramuscularly. The pharmacokinetic parameters (mean ± standard deviation) are shown in Table 1.

[See table 1 above]

The multiple dose pharmacokinetics of Prochieve® 4% and Prochieve® 8% administered every other day and Prochieve® 8% administered daily or twice daily for 12 days were studied in 10 healthy, estrogenized postmenopausal women in two separate studies. Steady state was achieved within the first 24 hours after initiation of treatment. The pharmacokinetic parameters (mean ± standard deviation) after the last administration of Prochieve® 4% or 8% derived from these studies are shown in Table 2.

[See table 2 at right]

TABLE 1
Single Dose Relative Bioavailability

	PROCHIEVE® 4%	45 mg Intramuscular Progesterone	PROCHIEVE® 8%	90 mg Intramuscular Progesterone
C_{max} (ng/mL)	13.15±6.49	39.06±13.68	14.87±6.32	53.76±14.9
$C_{avg\ 0-24}$ (ng/mL)	6.94±4.24	22.41±4.92	6.98±3.21	28.98±8.75
AUC_{0-96} (ng•hr/mL)	288.63±273.72	806.26±102.75	296.78±129.90	1378.91±176.39
T_{max} (hr)	5.6±1.84	8.2±6.43	6.8±3.3	9.2±2.7
$t_{1/2}$ (hr)	55.13±28.04	28.05±16.87	34.8±11.3	19.6±6.0
F (%)	27.6		19.8	

C_{max} - maximum progesterone serum concentration
$C_{avg\ 0-24}$ - average progesterone serum concentration over 24 hours
AUC_{0-96} - area under the drug concentration versus time curve from 0-96 hours post dose
T_{max} - time to maximum progesterone concentration
$t_{1/2}$ - elimination half-life
F - relative bioavailability

TABLE 2
Multiple Dose Pharmacokinetics

	Assisted Reproductive Technology		Secondary Amenorrhea	
	Daily Dosing 8%	Twice Daily Dosing 8%	Every Other Day Dosing 4%	Every Other Day Dosing 8%
C_{max} (ng/mL)	15.97 ± 5.05	14.57 ± 4.49	13.21 ± 9.46	13.67 ± 3.58
C_{avg} (ng/mL)	8.99 ± 3.53	11.6 ± 3.47	4.05 ± 2.85	6.75 ± 2.83
T_{max} (hr)	5.40 ± 0.97	3.55 ± 2.48	6.67 ± 3.16	7.00 ± 2.88
AUC_{0-t} (ng•hr/mL)	391.98 ± 153.28	138.72 ± 41.58	242.15 ± 167.88	438.36 ± 223.36
$t_{1/2}$ (hr)	45.00 ± 34.70	25.91 ± 6.15	49.87 ± 31.20	39.08 ± 12.88

Distribution

Progesterone is extensively bound to serum proteins (~96-99%), primarily to serum albumin and corticosteroid binding globulin.

Metabolism

The major urinary metabolite of oral progesterone is 5β-pregnan-3α, 20α-diol glucuronide which is present in plasma in the conjugated form only. Plasma metabolites also include 5β-pregnan-3α-ol-20-one (5β-pregnanolone) and 5α-pregnan-3α-ol-20-one (5α-pregnanolone).

Excretion

Progesterone undergoes both biliary and renal elimination. Following an injection of labeled progesterone, 50-60% of the excretion of progesterone metabolites occurs via the kidney; approximately 10% occurs via the bile and feces, the second major excretory pathway. Overall recovery of labeled material accounts for 70% of an administered dose, with the remainder of the dose not characterized with respect to elimination. Only a small portion of unchanged progesterone is excreted in the bile.

Clinical Studies

Assisted Reproductive Technology

In a single-center, open-label study (COL1620-007US), 99 women (aged 28-47 years) with either partial (n=84) or premature ovarian failure (n=15) who were candidates to receive a donor oocyte transfer as an Assisted Reproductive Technology ("ART") procedure were randomized to receive either Prochieve® 8% twice daily (n=68) or intramuscular progesterone 100 mg daily (n=31). The study was divided into three phases (Pilot, Donor Egg and Treatment). The first phase of the study consisted of a test Pilot Cycle to ensure that the administration of transdermal estradiol and progesterone would adequately prime the endometrium to receive the donor egg. The second phase was the Donor Egg Cycle during which a fertilized oocyte was implanted. Prochieve® 8% was administered beginning the evening of Day 14 of the Pilot and Donor Egg cycles. Subjects with partial ovarian function also underwent a Pre-Pilot Cycle and a Pre-Donor Egg Cycle during which time they were administered only leuprolide acetate to suppress remaining ovarian function. The Pre-Pilot Cycle, Pilot Cycle, Pre-Donor Egg Cycle, and Donor Egg Cycle each lasted approximately 34 days. The third phase of the study consisted of a 10-week treatment period to maintain a pregnancy until placental autonomy was achieved.

Sixty-one women received Prochieve® 8% as part of the Pilot Cycle to determine their endometrial response. Of the 55 evaluable endometrial biopsies in the Prochieve® 8% group performed on Day 25-27, all were histologically "in-phase", consistent with luteal phase biopsy specimens of menstruating women at comparable time intervals. Fifty-four women who received Prochieve® 8% and had a histologically "in-phase" biopsy received a donor oocyte transfer. Among these 54 Prochieve®-treated women, clinical pregnancies (assessed about week 10 after transfer by clinical examination, ultrasound and/or β-hCG levels) occurred in 26 women (48%). In these 26 women, 17 women (31%) delivered a total of 25 newborns, seven women (13%) had spontaneous abortions and two women (4%) had elective abortions.

In a second study (COL1620-F01), Prochieve® 8% was used in luteal phase support of women with tubal or idiopathic infertility due to endometriosis and normal ovulatory cycles, undergoing *in vitro* fertilization ("IVF") procedures. All women received a GnRH analog to suppress endogenous progesterone, human menopausal gonadotropins, and human chorionic gonadotropin. In this multi-center, open-label study, 139 women (aged 22-38 years) received Prochieve® 8% once daily beginning within 24 hours of embryo transfer and continuing through Day 30 post-transfer. Clinical pregnancies assessed at Day 90 post-transfer were seen in 36 (26%) of women. Thirty-two women (23%) delivered newborns and four women (3%) had spontaneous abortions. (See **PRECAUTIONS**, subsection **Pregnancy**)

Secondary Amenorrhea

In three parallel, open-label studies (COL1620-004US, COL1620-005US, COL1620-009US), 127 women (aged 18-44) with hypothalamic amenorrhea or premature ovarian failure were randomized to receive either Prochieve® 4% (n=62) or Prochieve® 8% (n=65). All women were treated with either conjugated estrogens 0.625 mg daily (n=100) or transdermal estradiol (delivering 50 mcg/day) twice weekly (n=27).

Estrogen therapy was continuous for the entire three 28-day cycle studies. At Day 15 of the second cycle (six weeks after initiating estrogen replacement), women who demonstrated adequate response to estrogen therapy (by ultrasound) and who continued to be amenorrheic received Prochieve® every other day for six doses (Day 15 through Day 25 of the cycle).

In cycle 2, Prochieve® 4% induced bleeding in 79% of women and Prochieve® 8% induced bleeding in 77% of women. In the third cycle, estrogen was continued and Prochieve® was administered every other day beginning on Day 15 for six doses. On Day 24 an endometrial biopsy was performed. In 53 women who received Prochieve® 4%, biopsy results were as follows: 7% proliferative, 40% late secretory, 19% mid secretory, 13% early secretory, 7% atrophic, 6% menstrual endometrium, 6% inactive endometrium and 2% negative endometrium. In 54 women who received Prochieve® 8%, biopsy results were as follows: 44% late secretory, 19% mid secretory, 11% early secretory, 19% atrophic, 5% menstrual endometrium and 2% "oral contraceptive like" endometrium.

INDICATIONS AND USAGE

Assisted Reproductive Technology

Prochieve® 8% is indicated for progesterone supplementation or replacement as part of an Assisted Reproductive Technology ("ART") treatment for infertile women with progesterone deficiency.

Secondary Amenorrhea

Prochieve® 4% is indicated for the treatment of secondary amenorrhea. Prochieve® 8% is indicated for use in women who have failed to respond to treatment with Prochieve® 4%.

CONTRAINDICATIONS

Prochieve® should not be used in individuals with any of the following conditions:

1. Known sensitivity to Prochieve® (progesterone or any of the other ingredients)
2. Undiagnosed vaginal bleeding
3. Liver dysfunction or disease
4. Known or suspected malignancy of the breast or genital organs
5. Missed abortion
6. Active thrombophlebitis or thromboembolic disorders, or a history of hormone-associated thrombophlebitis or thromboembolic disorders

WARNINGS

The physician should be alert to the earliest manifestations of thrombotic disorders (thrombophlebitis, cerebrovascular disorders, pulmonary embolism, and retinal thrombosis). Should any of these occur or be suspected, the drug should be discontinued immediately.

Progesterone and progestins have been used to prevent miscarriage in women with a history of recurrent spontaneous pregnancy losses. No adequate evidence is available to show that they are effective for this purpose.

PRECAUTIONS

General

1. The pretreatment physical examination should include special reference to breast and pelvic organs, as well as Papanicolaou smear.
2. In cases of breakthrough bleeding, as in all cases of irregular vaginal bleeding, nonfunctional causes should be considered. In cases of undiagnosed vaginal bleeding, adequate diagnostic measures should be undertaken.
3. Because progestogens may cause some degree of fluid retention, conditions which might be influenced by this factor (e.g., epilepsy, migraine, asthma, cardiac or renal dysfunction) require careful observation.
4. The pathologist should be advised of progesterone therapy when relevant specimens are submitted.
5. Patients who have a history of psychic depression should be carefully observed and the drug discontinued if the depression recurs to a serious degree.
6. A decrease in glucose tolerance has been observed in a small percentage of patients on estrogen-progestin combination drugs. The mechanism of this decrease is not known. For this reason, diabetic patients should be carefully observed while receiving progestin therapy.

Information for Patients

The product should not be used concurrently with other local intravaginal therapy. If other local intravaginal therapy is to be used concurrently, there should be at least a 6-hour period before or after Prochieve® administration. Small, white globules may appear as a vaginal discharge possibly due to gel accumulation, even several days after usage.

Drug Interactions

No drug interactions have been assessed with Prochieve®.

Carcinogenesis, Mutagenesis, Impairment of Fertility

Nonclinical toxicity studies to determine the potential of Prochieve® to cause carcinogenicity or mutagenicity have not been performed. The effect of Prochieve® on fertility has not been evaluated in animals.

Continued on next page

Prochieve—Cont.

Pregnancy (See **CLINICAL PHARMACOLOGY**, subsection **Clinical Studies)**
Prochieve® 8% has been used to support embryo implantation and maintain pregnancies through its use as part of ART treatment regimens in two clinical studies (studies COL1620-007US and COL1620-F01). In the first study (COL1620-007US), 54 Prochieve®-treated women had donor oocyte transfer procedures, and clinical pregnancies occurred in 26 women (48%). The outcomes of these 26 pregnancies were as follows: one woman had an elective termination of pregnancy at 19 weeks due to congenital malformations (omphalocele) associated with a chromosomal abnormality; one woman pregnant with triplets had an elective termination of her pregnancy; seven women had spontaneous abortions; and 17 women delivered 25 apparently normal newborns.
In the second study (COL1620-F01), Prochieve® 8% was used in the luteal phase support of women undergoing *in vitro* fertilization ("IVF") procedures. In this multi-center, open-label study, 139 women received Prochieve® 8% once daily beginning within 24 hours of embryo transfer and continuing through Day 30 post-transfer.
Clinical pregnancies assessed at Day 90 post-transfer were seen in 36 (26%) of women. Thirty-two women (23%) delivered newborns and four women (3%) had spontaneous abortions. Of the 47 newborns delivered, one had a teratoma associated with a cleft palate; one had respiratory distress syndrome; 44 were apparently normal and one was lost to follow-up.
Geriatric Use
The safety and effectiveness in geriatric patients (over age 65) have not been established.
Pediatric Use
Safety and effectiveness in pediatric patients have not been established.
Nursing Mothers
Detectable amounts of progestins have been identified in the milk of mothers receiving them. The effect of this on the nursing infant has not been determined.

ADVERSE REACTIONS

Assisted Reproductive Technology
In a study of 61 women with ovarian failure undergoing a donor oocyte transfer procedure receiving Prochieve® 8% twice daily, treatment-emergent adverse events occurring in 5% or more of the women are shown in Table 3.

TABLE 3
Treatment-Emergent Adverse Events in ≥5% of Women Receiving Prochieve® 8% Twice Daily
Study COL1620-007US (n=61)

Body as a Whole	
Bloating	7%
Cramps NOS	15%
Pain	8%
Central and Peripheral Nervous System	
Dizziness	5%
Headache	13%
Gastro-Intestinal System	
Nausea	7%
Reproductive, Female	
Breast Pain	13%
Moniliasis Genital	5%
Vaginal Discharge	7%
Skin and Appendages	
Pruritus Genital	5%

In a second clinical study of 139 women using Prochieve® 8% once daily for luteal phase support while undergoing an *in vitro* fertilization procedure, treatment-emergent adverse events reported in ≥5% of the women are shown in Table 4.

TABLE 4
Treatment-Emergent Adverse Events in ≥5% of Women Receiving Prochieve® 8% Once Daily
Study COL1620-F01 (n=139)

Body as a Whole	
Abdominal Pain	12%
Perineal Pain Female	17%
Central and Peripheral Nervous System	
Headache	17%
Gastro-Intestinal System	
Constipation	27%
Diarrhea	8%
Nausea	22%
Vomiting	5%
Musculo-Skeletal System	
Arthralgia	8%
Psychiatric	
Depression	11%
Libido Decreased	10%
Nervousness	16%
Somnolence	27%
Reproductive, Female	
Breast Enlargement	40%
Dyspareunia	6%
Urinary System	
Nocturia	13%

Secondary Amenorrhea
In three studies, 127 women with secondary amenorrhea received estrogen replacement therapy and Prochieve® 4% or 8% every other day for six doses. Treatment emergent adverse events during estrogen and Prochieve® treatment that occurred in 5% or more of women are shown in Table 5.

TABLE 5
Treatment-Emergent Adverse Events in ≥5% of Women Receiving Estrogen Treatment and Prochieve® Every Other Day
Studies COL1620-004US, COL1620-005US, COL1620-009US

	Estrogen +Prochieve® 4% n=65	Estrogen +Prochieve® 8% n=62
Body as a Whole		
Abdominal Pain	3 (5%)	6 (9%)
Appetite Increased	3 (5%)	5 (8%)
Bloating	8 (13%)	8 (12%)
Cramps NOS	12 (19%)	17 (26%)
Fatigue	13 (21%)	14 (22%)
Central and Peripheral Nervous System		
Headache	12 (19%)	10 (15%)
Gastro-Intestinal System		
Nausea	5 (8%)	4 (6%)
Musculo-Skeletal System		
Back Pain	5 (8%)	2 (3%)
Myalgia	5 (8%)	0 (0%)
Psychiatric		
Depression	12 (19%)	10 (15%)
Emotional Lability	14 (23%)	14 (22%)
Sleep Disorder	11 (18%)	12 (18%)
Reproductive, Female		
Vaginal Discharge	7 (11%)	2 (3%)
Resistance Mechanism		
Upper Respiratory Tract Infection	3 (5%)	5 (8%)
Skin and Appendages		
Pruritus genital	1 (2%)	4 (6%)

Additional adverse events reported in women at a frequency <5% in Prochieve® ART and secondary amenorrhea studies and not listed in the tables above include:
Autonomic Nervous System—mouth dry, sweating increased
Body as a Whole—abnormal crying, allergic reaction, allergy, appetite decreased, asthenia, edema, face edema, fever, hot flushes, influenzalike symptoms, water retention, xerophthalmia
Cardiovascular, General—syncope
Central and Peripheral Nervous System—migraine, tremor
Gastro-Intestinal—dyspepsia, eructation, flatulence, gastritis, toothache
Metabolic and Nutritional—thirst
Musculo-Skeletal System—cramps legs, leg pain, skeletal pain
Neoplasm—benign cyst
Platelet, Bleeding & Clotting—purpura
Psychiatric—aggressive reactions, forgetfulness, insomnia
Red Blood Cell—anemia
Reproductive, Female—dysmenorrhea, premenstrual tension, vaginal dryness
Resistance Mechanism—infection, pharyngitis, sinusitis, urinary tract infection
Respiratory System—asthma, dyspnea, hyperventilation, rhinitis
Skin and Appendages—acne, pruritis, rash, seborrhea, skin discoloration, skin disorder, urticaria
Urinary System—cystitis, dysuria, micturition frequency
Vision Disorders—conjunctivitis

OVERDOSAGE

There have been no reports of overdosage with Prochieve®. In the case of overdosage, however, discontinue Prochieve®, treat the patient symptomatically, and institute supportive measures.
As with all prescription drugs, this medicine should be kept out of the reach of children.

DOSAGE AND ADMINISTRATION

Assisted Reproductive Technology
Prochieve® 8% is administered vaginally at a dose of 90 mg once daily in women who require progesterone supplementation. Prochieve® 8% is administered vaginally at a dose of 90 mg twice daily in women with partial or complete ovarian failure who require progesterone replacement. If pregnancy occurs, treatment may be continued until placental autonomy is achieved, up to 10-12 weeks.
Secondary Amenorrhea
Prochieve® 4% is administered vaginally every other day up to a total of six doses. For women who fail to respond, a trial of Prochieve® 8% every other day up to a total of six doses may be instituted.
It is important to note that a dosage increase from the 4% gel can only be accomplished by using the 8% gel. Increasing the volume of gel administered does not increase the amount of progesterone absorbed.
SEE Prochieve® PATIENT INFORMATION SHEET - HOW TO USE Prochieve®. Note: The PATIENT INFORMATION SHEET contains special instructions for using the applicator at altitudes above 2500 feet in order to avoid a partial release of Prochieve® before vaginal insertion.

HOW SUPPLIED

Prochieve® is available in the following strengths:
4% gel (45 mg) in a single use, one piece, disposable, white polyethylene vaginal applicator with a twist-off top. Each applicator contains 1.45 g of gel and delivers 1.125 g of gel.
NDC-55056-0406-1 - 6 Single-use prefilled applicators.
8% gel (90 mg) in a single use, one piece, disposable, white polyethylene vaginal applicator with a twist-off top. Each applicator contains 1.45 g of gel and delivers 1.125 g of gel.
NDC-55056-0806-1 - 6 Single-use prefilled applicators.
NDC-55056-0818-1 - 18 Single-use prefilled applicators
Each applicator is wrapped and sealed in a foil overwrap.
Store at 25°C (77°F); excursions permitted to 15-30°C (59-86°F).
Rx only.
U.S. Patent Numbers 4,615,697 and 5,543,150.
Manufactured for: Columbia Laboratories, Inc. Livingston, NJ 07039
Manufactured by: Fleet Laboratories Ltd., Watford, United Kingdom
40905010002 Revised February 2004
Shown in Product Identification Guide, page 311

STRIANT® Ⓒ℞

[*strī'ănt*]
(testosterone buccal system)
mucoadhesive

DESCRIPTION

Striant® (testosterone buccal system) is designed to adhere to the gum or inner cheek. It provides a controlled and sustained release of testosterone through the buccal mucosa as the buccal system gradually hydrates. Insertion of Striant® twice a day, in the morning and in the evening, provides continuous systemic delivery of testosterone.
Striant® is a white to off-white colored, monoconvex, tablet-like, mucoadhesive buccal system. Striant® adheres to the gum tissue above the incisors, with the flat surface facing the cheek mucosa.
The active ingredient in Striant® is testosterone. Each buccal system contains 30 mg of testosterone. Testosterone USP is practically white crystalline powder chemically described as 17-beta hydroxyandrost-4-en-3one.

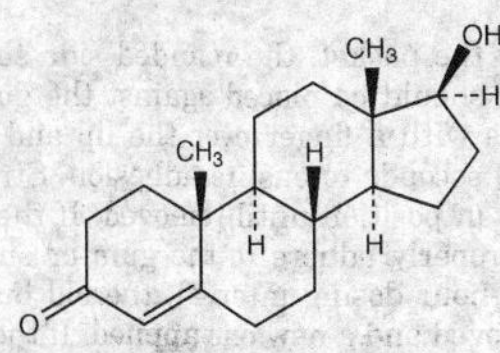

$C_{19}H_{28}O_2$ M.W.: 288.42

Other pharmacologically inactive ingredients in Striant® are anhydrous lactose NF, carbomer 934P, hypromellose USP, magnesium stearate NF, lactose monohydrate NF, polycarbophil USP, colloidal silicon dioxide NF, starch NF and talc USP.

CLINICAL PHARMACOLOGY

Striant® delivers physiologic amounts of testosterone to the systemic circulation, thereby producing circulating testosterone concentrations in hypogonadal males that approximate physiologic levels seen in healthy young men (300 – 1050 ng/dL).

Testosterone – General Androgen Effects:

Endogenous androgens, including testosterone and dihydrotestosterone (DHT) are responsible for the normal growth and development of the male sex organs and for maintenance of secondary sex characteristics. These effects include the growth and maturation of prostate, seminal vesicles, penis, and scrotum; the development of male hair distribution, such as facial, pubic, chest, and axillary hair; laryngeal enlargement, vocal chord thickening, and alterations in body musculature and fat distribution. Testosterone and DHT are necessary for the normal development of secondary sex characteristics.

Male hypogonadism results from insufficient production of testosterone and is characterized by low serum testosterone concentrations. Symptoms associated with male hypogonadism include impotence and decreased sexual desire, fatigue and loss of energy, mood depression, regression of secondary sexual characteristics and osteoporosis. Hypogonadism is a risk factor for osteoporosis in men.

Drugs in the androgen class also promote retention of nitrogen, sodium, potassium, phosphorus, and decreased urinary excretion of calcium. Androgens have been reported to increase protein anabolism and decrease protein catabolism. Nitrogen balance is improved only when there is sufficient intake of calories and protein.

Androgens are responsible for the growth spurt of adolescence and for the eventual termination of linear growth brought about by fusion of the epiphyseal growth centers. In children, exogenous androgens accelerate linear growth rates but may cause a disproportionate advancement in bone maturation. Use by children and adolescents over long periods may result in fusion of the epiphyseal growth centers and termination of the growth process. Androgens have been reported to stimulate the production of red blood cells by enhancing the production of erythropoietin.

During exogenous administration of androgens, endogenous testosterone release may be inhibited through feedback inhibition of pituitary luteinizing hormone (LH). At large doses of exogenous androgens, spermatogenesis may also be suppressed through feedback inhibition of pituitary follicle-stimulating hormone (FSH).

Pharmacokinetics

Absorption

When applied to the buccal mucosa, Striant® slowly releases testosterone, allowing for absorption of testosterone through gum and cheek surfaces that are in contact with the buccal system. Since venous drainage from the mouth is to the superior vena cava, trans-buccal delivery of testosterone circumvents first-pass (hepatic) metabolism.

Following the initial application of Striant®, the serum testosterone concentration rises to a maximum within 10-12 hours. The mean maximum (C_{max}) and mean average serum total testosterone concentrations for the 12 hour dosing period ($C_{avg(0-12)}$) are within the normal physiologic range.

Striant® is intended for twice daily dosing. Serum concentrations of testosterone reach steady-state levels after the second dose of twice daily Striant® dosing. Following removal of Striant®, the serum testosterone concentration decreases to a level below the normal range within 2-4 hours. With twice-daily repeated dosing, mean pharmacokinetic parameters at steady-state for total testosterone serum concentration were very similar between studies of 7-day and 12-week dosing durations. Mean $C_{avg(0-24)}$ across the studies ranged from 520 to 550 ng/dL and these mean values were within the physiologic range (see Table 1).

Table 1. Mean (±SD) Steady-State Serum Total Testosterone Concentrations During Treatment with Striant® (on Final Day of Treatment)

	Study 1	Study 2
	12-weeks (N=82)	7-days (N=29)
$C_{avg(0-24)}$ (ng/dL)	520 (±205)	550 (±169)
$C_{max(0-24)}$ (ng/dL)	970 (±442)	910 (±319)
$C_{min(0-24)}$ (ng/dL)	290 (±130)	320 (±131)

Although no specific food effect study was conducted, pivotal Phase 3 study results showed that consumption of food and beverage did not significantly affect the absorption of testosterone from Striant®.

The effects of toothbrushing, mouthwashing, chewing gum and alcoholic beverages on the use and absorption of Striant® were not investigated in controlled studies, however, Phase 3 clinical studies permitted patients to do these activities indicating the use of Striant® was not significantly affected by these activities.

Distribution

Circulating testosterone is chiefly bound in the serum to sex hormone-binding globulin (SHBG) and albumin. The albumin-bound fraction of testosterone easily dissociates from albumin and is presumed to be bioactive. The portion of testosterone bound to SHBG is not considered biologically active. The amount of SHBG in the serum and the total testosterone level will determine the distribution of bioactive and nonbioactive androgen. SHBG-binding capacity is high in prepubertal children, declines during puberty and adulthood, and increases again during the later decades of life. Approximately 40% of testosterone in plasma is bound to SHBG, 2% remains unbound (free) and the rest is bound to albumin and other proteins.

Metabolism

There is considerable variation in the half-life of testosterone as reported in the literature, ranging from ten to 100 minutes. Testosterone is metabolized to various 17-keto steroids through two different pathways, and the major active metabolites are estradiol and dihydrotestosterone (DHT). DHT binds with greater affinity to SHBG than does testosterone. In many tissues the activity of testosterone appears to depend on reduction to DHT, which binds to cytosol receptor proteins. The steroid-receptor complex is transported to the nucleus where it initiates transcription and cellular changes related to androgen action. In reproductive tissues, DHT is further metabolized to 3-alpha and 3-beta androstanediol.

Mean DHT concentrations increase in parallel with testosterone concentrations during Striant® treatment. After 24 hours of treatment, mean DHT serum concentrations are within normal range. The mean steady-state T/DHT ratio during treatment with Striant® remained within normal limits as determined by the analytical laboratory involved with the clinical trials. These ratios ranged from approximately 9-12.

Excretion

About 90% of a dose of testosterone given intramuscularly is excreted in the urine as glucuronic and sulfuric acid conjugates of testosterone and its metabolites; about 6% of a dose is excreted in the feces, mostly in the unconjugated form. Inactivation of testosterone occurs primarily in the liver.

Special Populations

No formal studies were conducted comparing the pharmacokinetics of testosterone in different racial groups or in compromised patients with renal or hepatic insufficiencies.

Clinical Studies

Striant® was evaluated in a multicenter, open-label, single arm, Phase 3 trial in 98 hypogonadal men (Study 1). In this study, Striant® was administered twice daily for 12 weeks. The mean age was 53.6 years (range 20 to 75 years). Overall, 68 (69.4%) patients were Caucasian, 9 (9.2%) were African-American, 15 (15.3%) were Hispanic, 4 (4.1%) were Asian, and 2 (2.0%) were of another ethnic origin. At baseline, ten patients (10.2%) reported current use of tobacco and forty-one (41.8%) drank alcohol. Of 82 patients who completed the trial and had sufficient data for full analysis, 86.6% had mean serum testosterone concentration ($C_{avg(0-24)}$) values within the physiologic range.

The mean (±SD) time-averaged steady-state daily testosterone concentration ($C_{avg(0-24)}$) at Week 12 was 520 (±205) ng/dL compared with a mean of 149 (±99) ng/dL at Baseline. At Week 12, the mean percentage of time over the 24-hour sampling period that total testosterone concentrations remained within the normal range of 300 - 1050 ng/dL was 76%. Table 1 above provides the steady-state serum testosterone concentrations in greater detail.

Striant® was also evaluated in a 7-day multicenter, open-label, parallel study comparing Striant® and an approved testosterone transdermal system (Study 2). In this study, Striant® was again administered twice daily. On Day 7, the mean $C_{avg(0-24)}$ for the 29 patients who received Striant® was 550 (±169) ng/dL compared with a mean of 119 (±78) ng/dL at Baseline. At Day 7, the mean percentage of time for Striant® over the 24-hour sampling period that testosterone concentrations remained within the physiologic range of 300-1050 ng/dL was 84%. Additional pharmacokinetic data for this study are presented in Table 1 above.

Figure 1 below shows the mean total testosterone serum concentration versus time at steady-state for two representative consecutive dosing intervals from both the 7-day and 12 week studies. The figure shows that the concentration-time curves for the different duration studies are consistent. [See figure 1 at top of next column]

In both clinical trials, mean DHT concentrations increased in parallel with testosterone concentrations, with the total testosterone/DHT ratio (9 - 12) indicating no alteration in metabolism of testosterone to DHT in testosterone deficient men treated with Striant® as compared with young, healthy eugonadal men.

During continuous treatment there was no accumulation of testosterone, and mean total testosterone, free testosterone, and DHT were maintained within their physiologic ranges.

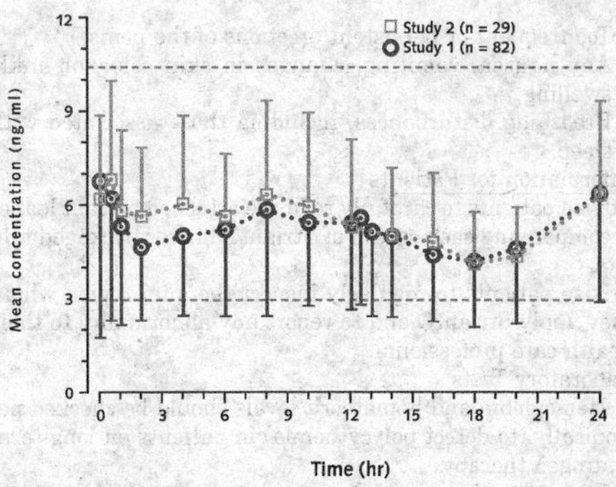

Figure 1: Mean (SD) total testosterone concentration-time curves for two consecutive dosing intervals at steady-state for both the 12- week study (Study 1) and the 7-day study (Study 2) of Striant®. (The horizontal dotted lines represent the upper and lower limit of normal for the normal physiologic range in healthy adult males).

INDICATIONS AND USAGE

Striant® is indicated for replacement therapy in males for conditions associated with a deficiency or absence of endogenous testosterone:

Primary hypogonadism (congenital or acquired) – testicular failure due to cryptorchidism, bilateral torsion, orchitis, vanishing testis syndrome, orchidectomy, Klinefelter's syndrome, chemotherapy, or toxic damage from alcohol or heavy metals. These men usually have low serum testosterone levels and gonadotropins (FSH, LH) above the normal range.

Hypogonadotropic hypogonadism (congenital or acquired) — idiopathic gonadotropin or LHRH deficiency, or pituitary hypothalamic injury from tumors, trauma, or radiation. These patients have low serum testosterone levels but have gonadotropins in the normal or low range.

CONTRAINDICATIONS

Androgens are contraindicated in men with carcinoma of the breast or known or suspected carcinoma of the prostate. Striant® is not indicated for use in women, and must not be used in women. Testosterone supplements may cause fetal harm.

Striant® should not be used in patients with known hypersensitivity to any of its ingredients, including testosterone USP that is chemically synthesized from soy.

WARNINGS

1. Prolonged use of high doses of orally active 17-alpha-alkyl androgens (e.g., methyltestosterone) have been associated with serious hepatic adverse effects (peliosis hepatis, hepatic neoplasms, cholestatic hepatitis, and jaundice). Peliosis hepatis can be a life-threatening or fatal complication. Long-term therapy with testosterone enanthate, which elevates blood levels for prolonged periods, has produced multiple hepatic adenomas. Testosterone is not known to produce these adverse effects.

2. Geriatric patients treated with androgens may be at an increased risk for the development of prostatic hyperplasia and prostatic carcinoma.

3. Geriatric patients and other patients with clinical or demographic characteristics that are recognized to be associated with an increased risk of prostate cancer should be evaluated for the presence of prostate cancer prior to initiation of testosterone replacement therapy. In men receiving testosterone replacement therapy, surveillance for prostate cancer should be consistent with current practices for eugonadal men (see PRECAUTIONS: Carcinogenesis, Mutagenesis, Impairment of Fertility and Laboratory Tests).

4. Edema with or without congestive heart failure may be a serious complication in patients with preexisting cardiac, renal, or hepatic disease. In addition to discontinuation of the drug, diuretic therapy may be required.

5. Gynecomastia frequently develops and occasionally persists in patients being treated for hypogonadism.

6. The treatment of hypogonadal men with testosterone esters may potentiate sleep apnea in some patients especially those with risk factors such as obesity or chronic lung diseases.

PRECAUTIONS

Striant® is applied to the upper gum just above the incisor tooth on either side of the mouth. Long-term data on gum safety is available for 117 patients and 51 patients with at least 6 months and 1 year of exposure, respectively. While the available data supports the overall oral safety of Striant®, longer-term data is not currently available and studies continue. Until such longer-term data become available, it is recommended that patients regularly inspect their own gum region where Striant® is applied. Any abnormal finding should be brought promptly to the attention of the patient's physician. In such circumstances, dental consultation may be appropriate.

General

The physician should instruct patients to report any of the following:

Continued on next page

Striant—Cont.

- Too frequent or persistent erections of the penis.
- Any nausea, vomiting, changes in skin color, or ankle swelling.
- Breathing disturbances, including those associated with sleep.

Information for Patients
Advise patients to carefully read the attached patient leaflet accompanying each carton of Striant® blister packaged tablets.
Advise patients to regularly inspect the gum region where they apply Striant® and to report any abnormality to their health care professional.
Laboratory Tests
1. Hemoglobin and hematocrit levels should be checked periodically (to detect polycythemia) in patients on long-term androgen therapy.
2. Liver function, prostate specific antigen (PSA), cholesterol and high-density lipoprotein should be checked periodically.
3. Serum total testosterone concentrations may be checked four to twelve weeks after initiating treatment with Striant®. To capture the maximum serum concentration, an early morning sample (just prior to applying the A.M. dose) is recommended. In the infrequent circumstance where the total testosterone concentration in this sample is excessive, therapy with Striant® should be discontinued and an alternative treatment considered.
Drug interactions
Oxyphenbutazone: Concurrent administration of oxyphenbutazone and androgens may result in elevated serum levels of oxyphenbutazone.
Insulin: In diabetic patients, the metabolic effects of androgens may decrease blood glucose and therefore, insulin requirements.
Corticosteroids: Concurrent administration of testosterone with ACTH or corticosteroids may enhance edema formation and should be administered cautiously, particularly in patients with cardiac or hepatic disease.
Drug/Laboratory Test Interactions
Androgens may decrease levels of thyroxin-binding globulin, resulting in decreased total T4 serum levels and increased resin uptake of T3 and T4. Free thyroid hormone levels remain unchanged, however, and there is no clinical evidence of thyroid dysfunction.
Carcinogenesis, mutagenesis, impairment of fertility
Animal data: Testosterone has been tested by subcutaneous injection and implantation in mice and rats. In mice, the implant induced cervical-uterine tumors, which metastasized in some cases. There is suggestive evidence that injection of testosterone into some strains of female mice increases their susceptibility to hepatoma. Testosterone is also known to increase the number of tumors and decrease the degree of differentiation of chemically induced carcinomas of the liver in rats.
Human data: There were rare reports of hepatocellular carcinoma in patients receiving long-term therapy with androgens in high doses. Withdrawal of the drugs did not lead to regression of the tumors in all cases.
Striant® has been evaluated in patients for 1 year without reports of cancer related to the product. However, safety in patients beyond 1 year has not been established.
Geriatric patients treated with androgens may be at an increased risk for the development of prostatic hyperplasia and prostatic carcinoma.
Geriatric patients and other patients with clinical or demographic characteristics that are recognized to be associated with an increased risk of prostate cancer should be evaluated for the presence of prostate cancer prior to initiation of testosterone replacement therapy.
In men receiving testosterone replacement therapy, surveillance for prostate cancer should be consistent with current practices for eugonadal men.
Pregnancy Category X (see CONTRAINDICATIONS) – Teratogenic Effects: Striant® is not indicated for women and must not be used in women.
Labor and Delivery: Striant® is not indicated for women and must not be used in women.
Nursing Mothers: Striant® is not indicated for women and must not be used in women.
Pediatric Use: Safety and effectiveness in pediatric male patients below the age of 18 have not yet been established
Geriatric Use: Of the total number of subjects in clinical studies of Striant®, 51 patients (16.5 percent) were 65 and over. No overall differences in safety or effectiveness were observed between these subjects and younger subjects. However, in Study 1, in patients 65 years of age and older, the total testosterone $C_{avg(0-24)}$ value was higher by 12.7% compared to patients less than 65 years of age. In addition, the total T to DHT area-under-the curve ratio was lower in the older population compared to the younger population by 15.6%. These differences may not be clinically significant.

ADVERSE REACTIONS

In all clinical studies combined, a total of 308 patients were treated with Striant® for up to 12 months
Twelve Week Trials
In the pivotal, Phase 3, open-label controlled study (Study 1), 98 patients received Striant® for up to 12 weeks. Adverse events judged possibly, probably, or definitely related to the use of Striant® and reported by ≥ 1% of patients in Study 1 are listed in Table 2.

Table 2. Incidences of Adverse Events Possibly, Probably or Definitely Related to Use of Striant® in Study 1

Adverse Event	Striant® (n=98)
Gum or Mouth Irritation	9.2%
Taste Bitter	4.1%
Gum Pain	3.1%
Gum Tenderness	3.1%
Headache	3.1%
Gum Edema	2.0%
Taste Perversion	2.0%

Please see "Gum-related adverse events and gum examinations" subsection for further information. The majority of gum-related adverse events were transient. Gum irritation generally resolved in 1 to 8 days. Gum tenderness resolved in 1 to 14 days.
The following adverse events judged possibly, probably or definitely related to the use of Striant® occurred in 1 patient each in Study 1: abdominal cramp, acne, anxiety, asthma (acute), breast enlargement, breast pain, buccal mucosal roughening, difficulty in micturition, fatigue, gingivitis, gum blister, gustatory sense diminished, hematocrit increased, lipids serum increased, liver function tests abnormal, nose edema, stinging of lips, and toothache.
There was one additional 12-week study in 12 patients. In this study, additional adverse events judged at least possibly related to Striant® and reported by 1 patient each included emotional lability and hypertension.
Long-Term Extension Trials
In two long-term extension trials, a total of 117 and 51 patients received Striant® for at least 6 months and 1 year, respectively.
Of 117 patients treated for at least 6 months, adverse events judged possibly, probably, or definitely related to treatment and reported by 1 patient each included: anxiety, buccal inflammation, depression, dry mouth, gastrointestinal disorder, gum redness, hypertension, infection, medication error, nausea, pruritis, renal function abnormal, stomatitis, taste bitter, taste perversion, and toothache. Polycythemia and increased serum prostate specific antigen (PSA) were reported in three and two patients, respectively.
Adverse events reported in the 51 patients treated for at least one year were similar to those reported after 6 months of treatment and lower in incidence.
Gum-related adverse events and gum examinations
In the pivotal controlled study (Study 1), all reported gum-related adverse events were collected and gum examinations were conducted at Baseline and every month thereafter.
In Study 1, a total of 16 patients reported 19 gum-related adverse events. Of these, ten patients (10.2%) reported 12 events of mild intensity, four patients (4.1%) reported 5 events of moderate intensity, and two patients (2.0%) reported 2 events of severe intensity. Most of these events were judged probably or definitely related to treatment with Striant®. Four patients (4.1%) discontinued treatment with Striant® due to gum or mouth-related adverse events including two with severe gum irritation, one with mouth irritation, and one with "bad taste in mouth". The majority of gum-related adverse events were transient. Gum irritation generally resolved in 1 to 8 days. Gum tenderness resolved in 1 to 14 days.
In Study 1, monthly gum examinations were conducted to assess for gingivitis, gum edema, oral lesions, ulcerations or leukoplakia. No cases of ulceration or leukoplakia were observed. No new oral lesions were observed. Gingivitis was common at Baseline (32.6%), and was reduced at Week 4 (10.2%), Week 8 (10.2%) and Week 12 (11.2%). Similar findings were seen for gum edema.
In the two long-term extension trials, gum examinations were conducted every 3 months while on treatment. In one of these trials, no patient had a gum abnormality, and in the other trial, moderate gingivitis and mild gum edema were reported by 1 patient each.

DRUG ABUSE AND DEPENDENCE

Striant® contains testosterone, a Schedule III controlled substance as defined by the Anabolic Steroids Control Act.

OVERDOSAGE

There is one report of acute overdosage with testosterone enanthate injection: testosterone levels of up to 11,400 ng/dL were implicated in a cerebrovascular accident. Oral ingestion of Striant® is not expected to result in clinically significant serum testosterone concentrations due to extensive first-pass (hepatic) metabolism.

DOSAGE AND ADMINISTRATION

The recommended dosing schedule for Striant® is the application of one buccal system (30 mg) to the gum region twice daily; morning and evening (about 12 hours apart). Striant® should be placed in a comfortable position just above the incisor tooth (on either side of the mouth). With each application, Striant® should be rotated to alternate sides of the mouth.
Upon opening the packet, the rounded side surface of the buccal system should be placed against the gum and held firmly in place with a finger over the lip and against the product for 30 seconds to ensure adhesion. Striant® is designed to stay in position until removed. If the buccal system fails to properly adhere to the gum or should fall off during the 12-hour dosing interval, the old buccal system should be removed and a new one applied. If the buccal system falls out of position within 4 hours prior to the next dose, a new buccal system should be applied and it may remain in place until the time of next regularly scheduled dosing.
Patients should take care to avoid dislodging the buccal system. Patients should check to see if Striant® is in place following toothbrushing, use of mouthwash and consumption of food or alcoholic/non-alcoholic beverages. Striant® should not be chewed or swallowed. To remove Striant®, gently slide it downwards from the gum towards the tooth to avoid scratching the gum.

HOW SUPPLIED

Striant® (testosterone buccal system) is for buccal administration only. It contains testosterone, a Schedule III controlled substance as defined by the Anabolic Steroids Control Act.
Striant® is supplied in transparent blister packs containing 10 doses. It is white to off- white colored with a flat edge on one side and a convex surface on the other.
Striant® is debossed on its flat side, as shown below:

Each Striant® buccal system contains 30 mg of testosterone and is supplied as follows:

NDC Number	Strength	Package Size
55056-3060-1	30 mg	6 blister packs, 10 buccal systems per blister: 30 mg per buccal system

Storage and Disposal. Store at 20–25°C (68-77°F) [see USP Controlled Room temperature]. Protect from heat and moisture. Damaged blister packages should not be used. Discarded Striant® buccal systems should be disposed of in household trash in a manner that prevents accidental application or ingestion by children or pets.
Rx Only
Manufactured by: Mipharm S.p.A. Milan, Italy
Manufactured for:
Columbia Laboratories, Inc. Livingston, NJ 07039
US Patent Numbers: 6,248,358
others pending
PHYSTN002/41005010002

Patient Information

STRIANT® CIII
(testosterone buccal system)
mucoadhesive
Read the Patient Information that comes with Striant® [STRI' ant] before you start using it and each time you get a refill. There may be new information. This information does not take the place of information from your healthcare provider about your medical condition or your treatment.
What is Striant®?
Striant® is a hormone medicine that contains testosterone. It is used to treat adult men when their bodies do not make any testosterone or not enough testosterone (hypogonadism). Striant® is a white to off-white tablet-like buccal system that is applied to the upper gum area of the mouth.
Striant® is not to be chewed or swallowed.
Striant® is a controlled substance (**CIII**) because it contains testosterone. Therefore, you should keep your Striant® in a secure place. Do not share or sell your Striant®.
Who should not use Striant®?
Do not use Striant® if you:
- have breast cancer (rare in men).
- have prostate cancer.
- are a woman (especially if you are pregnant or breast-feeding). Striant may harm the babies of pregnant and breast-feeding women.
- are allergic to Striant®. The active ingredient in Striant® is testosterone USP. See the end of this leaflet for a list of all ingredients in Striant®.

Tell your doctor if you have or had:
- problems urinating due to an enlarged prostate.
- liver problems.
- kidney problems.
- heart problems.
- lung problems.
- diabetes.
- weight problems (obesity).

Tell your doctor about all the medicines you take, including prescription and non- prescription medicines, vitamins, and herbal supplements. Some medicines may cause serious side effects if taken while you also take Striant®. Some medicines may affect how Striant® works, or Striant® may affect how your other medicines work. Be sure to tell your doctor if you use insulin for diabetes. Your dose of insulin may need to be adjusted if you use Striant®.

How should I use Striant®?
Use Striant® twice a day, once in the morning and once at night (about 12 hours apart). You may find it convenient to apply morning dose after brushing your teeth following breakfast and evening dose following your evening meal. Striant® should be applied as follows:

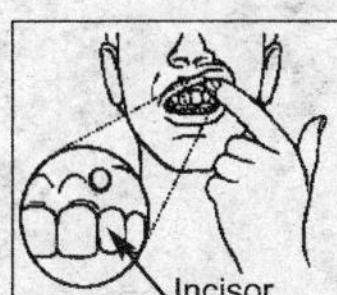

• Tear off individual unit then start at the corner tab and peel off paper backing. Push buccal system through foil from the front. You will notice that Striant® is curved on one side and flat on the other side. The flat side has a marking on it (company logo).

• Before you apply Striant®, locate the area on your upper gum, just above either the left or right incisor (see picture). The incisor is the tooth just to the right or left of your two front teeth.

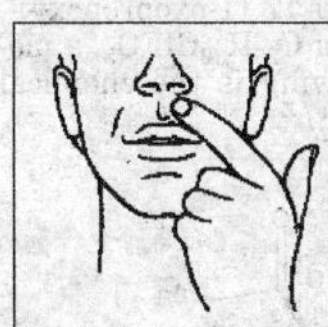

• Place the flat side of the Striant® system on your fingertip. Gently push the curved side of Striant® against your upper gum in the area shown. Push the Striant® system up as high as it will go on the gum. If you have applied Striant® correctly, the flat side will be facing your cheek.

• Using your finger on the outside of your upper lip, hold the Striant® buccal system in place for 30 seconds (see picture). This will make the buccal system stick to your gum or cheek.

• As the Striant® buccal system absorbs moisture from your mouth, it will begin to soften and will mold to the shape of your gum. You should be aware that Striant® does not dissolve completely, but will remain in place for 12 hours. Striant® is made to stay in place until you remove it.

• Remove Striant® by gently sliding it to the front or back of your mouth to loosen it. Then slide it downwards from your gum to your tooth. This will avoid scratching the gum.

• **With each application, you should rotate Striant® to alternate sides of your mouth.**

• If Striant® does not stick or falls off within the first 8 hours, remove the original system and apply a new one. This counts as replacing the first dose. Apply the next system about 12 hours after the original buccal system was applied.

• If Striant® falls off after 8 hours but before 12 hours, replace the original buccal system. This replacement can serve as the second dose for that day.

• If Striant® sticks to your cheek and not your gum, this is acceptable. Do not replace the buccal system if this should happen.

• Check to see if Striant® is in place following toothbrushing, use of mouthwash and consumption of food or alcoholic/nonalcoholic beverages. If Striant® does not stick or falls off, follow the above mentioned directions to replace with a new system.

What are the possible side effects of testosterone replacement therapy?
Inform your doctor immediately if any of the following symptoms appear while using Striant®.

• **Liver problems.** Tell your doctor if:
  • Your skin or white part of your eyes turns yellow (jaundice).
  • Your urine turns dark.
  • Your bowel movements (stool) turns light in color.
  • You don't feel like eating for several days or longer.
  • You feel sick to your stomach (nausea).
  • You have lower abdominal pain (stomach).
• **Problems urinating.** Tell your doctor if you develop problems urinating while using Striant®. Older patients who use testosterone replacement therapies may have an increased chance of developing prostate enlargement or prostate cancer.
• **Extra fluid in the body (edema).** Edema can be dangerous if you have heart, kidney or liver problems. Tell your doctor if your ankles and legs swell or if you put on weight quickly.
• **Breathing problems, including a sleep problem called "sleep apnea".** Sleep apnea is when you stop breathing for short times while you are sleeping. This happens more in patients who are overweight or who have lung disease. Tell your doctor if you have breathing problems or if you or your partner notice changes in your breathing when you are sleeping.
• **Penile erections** that are painful, that occur too frequently, or that last for too long a duration.
• **Breast enlargement** – which sometimes does not go away.
• **Emotional changes** – such as depression.

Your doctor may do blood tests to check your red blood cells, liver function, cholesterol levels, testosterone levels and prostate (PSA) while you are using Striant®, to see how Striant® is affecting your body.
Striant® may also cause these side effects:
• redness, irritation, swelling and pain at the gum application site.
• gum infection (gingivitis)-gum side effects are usually temporary, and should resolve within several days. However, some gum side effects may last up to two weeks. If you should have gum side effects, they usually resolve while taking Striant®. Any abnormal finding should be brought to the attention of your physician.
• a change in how food tastes to you, a bitter taste in your mouth, or an unusual taste in your mouth.
• headache.

These are not all the possible side effects of Striant®. For more information, ask your doctor or pharmacist.
You should regularly examine your gums where Striant® is applied. Any abnormal finding should be brought to the attention of your physician.

How should Striant® be stored?
Keep Striant® at a temperature between 68° and 77° F (20-25° C). Protect from heat and moisture. Do not use a damaged blister package. **Keep Striant® and all medicines out of the reach of children.** Discarded Striant® buccal systems should be thrown away in a household trash can in a way that prevents children or pets from accidentally using or taking them.

General information about the safe and effective use of Striant®. Medicines are sometimes prescribed for conditions that are not mentioned in patient information leaflets. Do not use Striant® for a condition for which it was not prescribed. Do not give Striant® to other people, even if they have the same symptoms you have. It may harm them, and you should be aware that Striant® is a controlled substance.
This leaflet summarizes the most important information about Striant®. If you would like more information, talk with your doctor. You can ask your doctor or pharmacist for information about Striant® that is written for health professionals.

What are the ingredients of Striant®?
Active Ingredient: Testosterone USP (30 mg in each buccal system)
Inactive Ingredients: anhydrous lactose NF, carbomer 934P, hypromellose USP, magnesium stearate NF, lactose monohydrate NF, polycarbophil USP, colloidal silicon dioxide NF, starch NF, and talc USP.

How is Striant® supplied?
Striant® is supplied in a transparent blister in a white card. Each card contains 10 buccal systems. There are a total of 6 blister cards (60 buccal systems) in each carton.

Rx Only
Manufactured by:
Mipharm S.p.A, Milan, Italy
Manufactured for:
Columbia Laboratories, Inc.,
Livingston, NJ 07039
US Patent Numbers: 6,248,358
others pending

PATSTN002/41005010002 USA/930874/0

Shown in Product Identification Guide, page 311

Connetics Corporation
3290 WEST BAYSHORE ROAD
PALO ALTO, CA 94303

Direct Inquiries to:
(650) 843-2800
FAX: (650) 843-2899
www.connetics.com

For Medical Information Contact:
Medical Information Department
(877) 821-5337
FAX: (510) 595-8183
E-mail: medicalaffairs@connetics.com

LUXÍQ® ℞
[*lŭk-sēk*]
(betamethasone valerate) Foam, 0.12%
℞ Only
For Dermatologic Use Only
Not for Ophthalmic Use

DESCRIPTION
Luxíq contains betamethasone valerate, USP, a synthetic corticosteroid, for topical dermatologic use. The corticosteroids constitute a class of primarily synthetic steroids used topically as anti-inflammatory agents.
Chemically, betamethasone valerate is 9-fluoro-11β,17,21-trihydroxy-16β-methylpregna-1, 4-diene-3, 20-dione 17-valerate, with the empirical formula $C_{27}H_{37}FO_6$, a molecular weight of 476.58 (CAS Registry Number 2152-44-5) and the following structural formula:

Betamethasone 17-valerate

Betamethasone valerate is a white to practically white, odorless crystalline powder, and is practically insoluble in water, freely soluble in acetone and in chloroform, soluble in alcohol, and slightly soluble in benzene and in ether.
Each gram of Luxíq contains 1.2 mg betamethasone valerate, USP, in a hydroalcoholic, thermolabile foam. The foam also contains cetyl alcohol, citric acid, ethanol (60.4%), polysorbate 60, potassium citrate, propylene glycol, purified water, and stearyl alcohol, and is dispensed from an aluminum can pressurized with a hydrocarbon propellant (propane/butane).

CLINICAL PHARMACOLOGY
Like other topical corticosteroids, betamethasone valerate foam has anti-inflammatory, antipruritic, and vasoconstrictive properties. The mechanism of the anti-inflammatory activity of the topical steroids, in general, is unclear. However, corticosteroids are thought to act by the induction of phospholipase A_2 inhibitory proteins, collectively called lipocortins. It is postulated that these proteins control the biosynthesis of potent mediators of inflammation such as prostaglandins and leukotrienes by inhibiting the release of their common precursor arachidonic acid. Arachidonic acid is released from membrane phospholipids by phospholipase A_2.

Pharmacokinetics:
Topical corticosteroids can be absorbed from intact healthy skin. The extent of percutaneous absorption of topical corticosteroids is determined by many factors, including the vehicle and the integrity of the epidermal barrier. Occlusion, inflammation and/or other disease processes in the skin may also increase percutaneous absorption.
The use of pharmacodynamic endpoints for assessing the systemic exposure of topical corticosteroids is necessary due to the fact that circulating levels are well below the level of detection. Once absorbed through the skin, topical corticosteroids are handled through pharmacokinetic pathways similar to systemically administered corticosteroids. They are metabolized, primarily in the liver, and are then excreted by the kidneys. In addition, some corticosteroids and their metabolites are also excreted in the bile.

CLINICAL STUDIES
The safety and efficacy of Luxíq has been demonstrated in a four-week trial. An adequate and well-controlled clinical trial was conducted in 190 patients with moderate to severe scalp psoriasis. Patients were treated twice daily for four weeks with Luxíq Foam, Placebo foam, a commercially available betamethasone valerate lotion 0.12% (formerly expressed as 0.1% betamethasone), or Placebo lotion. At four weeks of treatment, study results of 159 patients demonstrated that the efficacy of Luxíq Foam in treating scalp psoriasis is superior to that of Placebo foam, and is comparable to that of a currently marketed BMV lotion (see Table below).
[See table below]

Subjects with Target Lesion Parameter Clear at Endpoint	Luxíq Foam n (%)	BMV lotion n (%)	Placebo foam n (%)
Scaling	30 (47%)	22 (35%)	2 (6%)
Erythema	26 (41%)	16 (25%)	2 (6%)
Plaque Thickness	42 (66%)	25 (40%)	5 (16%)
Investigator's Global: Subjects Completely Clear or Almost Clear at Endpoint	43 (67%)	29 (46%)	6 (19%)

INDICATIONS AND USAGE
Luxíq is a medium potency topical corticosteroid indicated for relief of the inflammatory and pruritic manifestations of corticosteroid-responsive dermatoses of the scalp.

CONTRAINDICATIONS
Luxíq is contraindicated in patients who are hypersensitive to betamethasone valerate, to other corticosteroids, or to any ingredient in this preparation.

PRECAUTIONS
General: Systemic absorption of topical corticosteroids has caused reversible hypothalamic-pituitary-adrenal (HPA) axis suppression with the potential for glucocorticosteroid insufficiency after withdrawal of treatment. Manifestations of Cushing's syndrome, hyperglycemia, and glucosuria can also be produced in some patients by systemic absorption of topical corticosteroids while on treatment.
Conditions which augment systemic absorption include the application of the more potent steroids, use over large surface areas, prolonged use, and the addition of occlusive dressings.

Continued on next page

Incidence and severity of burning/itching/stinging

Product	Total incidence	Maximum severity		
		Mild	Moderate	Severe
Luxíq Foam n=63	34 (54%)	28 (44%)	5 (8%)	1 (2%)
Betamethasone valerate lotion n=63	33 (52%)	26 (41%)	6 (10%)	1 (2%)
Placebo Foam n=32	24 (75%)	13 (41%)	7 (22%)	4 (12%)
Placebo Lotion n=30	20 (67%)	12 (40%)	5 (17%)	3 (10%)

Luxíq—Cont.

Therefore, patients applying a topical steroid to a large surface area or to areas under occlusion should be evaluated periodically for evidence of HPA axis suppression. If HPA axis suppression is noted, an attempt should be made to withdraw the drug, to reduce the frequency of application, or to substitute a less potent steroid.
Recovery of HPA axis function is generally prompt upon discontinuation of topical corticosteroids. Infrequently, signs and symptoms of glucocorticosteroid insufficiency may occur requiring supplemental systemic corticosteroids. For information on systemic supplementation, see prescribing information for those products.
Pediatric patients may be more susceptible to systemic toxicity from equivalent doses due to their larger skin surface to body mass ratios. (See **PRECAUTIONS-Pediatric Use.**)
If irritation develops, Luxíq should be discontinued and appropriate therapy instituted. Allergic contact dermatitis with corticosteroids is usually diagnosed by observing a failure to heal rather than noting a clinical exacerbation, as with most topical products not containing corticosteroids. Such an observation should be corroborated with appropriate diagnostic patch testing.
In the presence of dermatological infections, the use of an appropriate antifungal or antibacterial agent should be instituted. If a favorable response does not occur promptly, use of Luxíq should be discontinued until the infection has been adequately controlled.
Information for Patients: Patients using topical corticosteroids should receive the following information and instructions:

1. This medication is to be used as directed by the physician. It is for external use only. Avoid contact with the eyes.
2. This medication should not be used for any disorder other than that for which it was prescribed.
3. The treated scalp area should not be bandaged or otherwise covered or wrapped so as to be occlusive unless directed by the physician.
4. Patients should report to their physician any signs of local adverse reactions.
5. As with other corticosteroids, therapy should be discontinued when control is achieved. If no improvement is seen within 2 weeks, contact the physician.

Laboratory Tests: The following tests may be helpful in evaluating patients for HPA axis suppression:
ACTH stimulation test
A.M. plasma cortisol test
Urinary free cortisol test
Carcinogenesis, Mutagenesis, and Impairment of Fertility: Long-term animal studies have not been performed to evaluate the carcinogenic potential or the effect on fertility of betamethasone valerate.
Betamethasone was genotoxic in the *in vitro* human peripheral blood lymphocyte chromosome aberration assay with metabolic activation and in the *in vivo* mouse bone marrow micronucleus assay.
Pregnancy Category C: Corticosteroids have been shown to be teratogenic in laboratory animals when administered systemically at relatively low dosage levels. Some corticosteroids have been shown to be teratogenic after dermal application in laboratory animals. There are no adequate and well-controlled studies in pregnant women. Therefore, Luxíq should be used during pregnancy only if the potential benefit justifies the potential risk to the fetus.
Drugs of this class should not be used extensively on pregnant patients, in large amounts, or for prolonged periods of time.
Nursing Mothers: Systemically administered corticosteroids appear in human milk and could suppress growth, interfere with endogenous corticosteroid production, or cause other untoward effects. It is not known whether topical administration of corticosteroids could result in sufficient systemic absorption to produce detectable quantities in breast milk. Because many drugs are excreted in human milk, caution should be exercised when Luxíq is administered to a nursing woman.
Pediatric Use: Safety and effectiveness in pediatric patients have not been established. Because of a higher ratio of skin surface area to body mass, pediatric patients are at a greater risk than adults of HPA axis suppression and Cushing's syndrome when they are treated with topical corticosteroids. They are therefore also at greater risk of adrenal insufficiency during and/or after withdrawal of treatment. Adverse effects including striae have been reported with inappropriate use of topical corticosteroids in infants and children.
Hypothalamic-pituitary-adrenal (HPA) axis suppression, Cushing's syndrome, linear growth retardation, delayed weight gain, and intracranial hypertension have been reported in children receiving topical corticosteroids. Manifestations of adrenal suppression in children include low plasma cortisol levels and an absence of response to ACTH stimulation. Manifestations of intracranial hypertension include bulging fontanelles, headaches, and bilateral papilledema.
Administration of topical corticosteroids to children should be limited to the least amount compatible with an effective therapeutic regimen. Chronic corticosteroid therapy may interfere with the growth and development of children.

ADVERSE REACTIONS

The most frequent adverse event was burning/itching/stinging at the application site; the incidence and severity of this event were as follows:
[See table above]
Other adverse events which were considered to be possibly, probably, or definitely related to Luxíq occurred in 1 patient each; these were paresthesia, pruritus, acne, alopecia, and conjunctivitis.
The following additional local adverse reactions have been reported with topical corticosteroids, and they may occur more frequently with the use of occlusive dressings. These reactions are listed in an approximately decreasing order of occurrence: irritation; dryness; folliculitis; acneiform eruptions; hypopigmentation; perioral dermatitis; allergic contact dermatitis; secondary infection; skin atrophy; striae; and miliaria.
Systemic absorption of topical corticosteroids has produced reversible hypothalamic-pituitary-adrenal (HPA) axis suppression, manifestations of Cushing's syndrome, hyperglycemia, and glucosuria in some patients.

OVERDOSAGE

Topically applied Luxíq can be absorbed in sufficient amounts to produce systemic effects. (See **PRECAUTIONS**)

DOSAGE AND ADMINISTRATION

Note: For proper dispensing of foam, can must be inverted. For application to the scalp invert can and dispense a small amount of Luxíq onto a saucer or other cool surface. Do not dispense directly onto hands as foam will begin to melt immediately upon contact with warm skin. Pick up small amounts of foam with fingers and gently massage into affected area until foam disappears. Repeat until entire affected scalp area is treated. Apply twice daily, once in the morning and once at night.
As with other corticosteroids, therapy should be discontinued when control is achieved. If no improvement is seen within 2 weeks, reassessment of the diagnosis may be necessary.
Luxíq should not be used with occlusive dressings unless directed by a physician.

HOW SUPPLIED

Luxíq is supplied in 100 gram (NDC 63032-021-00) and 50 gram (NDC 63032-021-50) aluminum cans.
Store at controlled room temperature 68–77°F (20–25°C).

WARNING

FLAMMABLE. AVOID FIRE, FLAME OR SMOKING DURING AND IMMEDIATELY FOLLOWING APPLICATION. Keep out of reach of children. Contents under pressure. Do not puncture or incinerate container. Do not expose to heat or store at temperatures above 120°F (49°C).
Manufactured for
Connetics Corporation
Palo Alto, CA 94303
USA
Printed in: USA
May 2003
For additional information:
1-877-821-5337 or visit
www.luxiq.com
AW NO.: AW-0182 P/N: 181484ZZ
Connetics®
Delivered in VersaFoam™

OLUX® Foam, 0.05% ℞

[*ō-lŭks*]
(clobetasol propionate)
℞ Only
For Dermatologic Use Only
Not for Ophthalmic Use

DESCRIPTION

OLUX Foam contains clobetasol propionate, USP, a synthetic corticosteroid, for topical dermatologic use. Clobetasol, an analog of prednisolone, has a high degree of glucocorticoid activity and a slight degree of mineralocorticoid activity.
Clobetasol propionate is pregna-1,4-diene-3,20-dione, 21-chloro-9-fluoro-11-hydroxy-16-methyl-17 (1-oxopropoxy)-, (11β,16β)-, with the empirical formula $C_{25}H_{32}ClFO_5$, a molecular weight of 466.97. The following is the chemical structure:

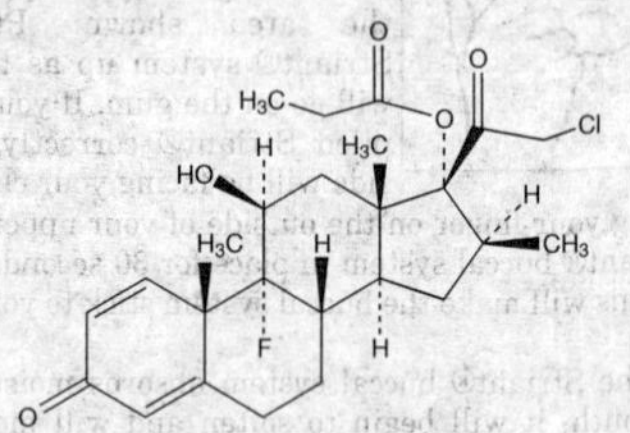

clobetasol propionate

Clobetasol propionate is a white or almost white, odorless, crystalline powder and is insoluble in water.
Each gram of OLUX Foam contains 0.5 mg clobetasol propionate, USP, in a thermolabile foam which consists of cetyl alcohol, citric acid, ethanol (60%), polysorbate 60, potassium citrate, propylene glycol, purified water, and stearyl alcohol. OLUX Foam is dispensed from an aluminum can pressurized with a hydrocarbon propellant (propane/butane).

CLINICAL PHARMACOLOGY

Like other topical corticosteroids, clobetasol propionate foam has anti-inflammatory, antipruritic, and vasoconstrictive properties. The precise mechanism of the anti-inflammatory activity of topical steroids in the treatment of steroid-responsive dermatoses, in general, is uncertain. However, corticosteroids are thought to act by the induction of phospholipase A_2 inhibitory proteins, collectively called lipocortins. It is postulated that these proteins control the biosynthesis of potent mediators of inflammation such as prostaglandins and leukotrienes by inhibiting the release of their common precursor arachidonic acid. Arachidonic acid is released from membrane phospholipids by phospholipase A_2.
Pharmacokinetics:
Topical corticosteroids can be absorbed from intact healthy skin. The extent of percutaneous absorption of topical corticosteroids is determined by many factors, including the vehicle and the integrity of the epidermal barrier. Occlusion, inflammation and/or other disease processes in the skin may also increase percutaneous absorption.
Once absorbed through the skin, topical corticosteroids are handled through pharmacokinetic pathways similar to systemically administered corticosteroids. Due to the fact that circulating levels are well below the level of detection, the use of pharmacodynamic endpoints for assessing the systemic exposure of topical corticosteroids is necessary. They are metabolized, primarily in the liver, and are then excreted by the kidneys. In addition, some corticosteroids and their metabolites are also excreted in the bile.

CLINICAL STUDIES

A well-controlled clinical study evaluated 188 subjects with moderate to severe scalp psoriasis. Subjects were treated twice daily for 2 weeks with one of four treatments: OLUX Foam, Vehicle foam, a commercially available clobetasol propionate solution (Temovate® Scalp Application), or Vehicle solution. The efficacy of OLUX Foam in treating scalp psoriasis at the end of the 2 weeks' treatment was superior to that of Vehicle (foam and solution), and was comparable to that of Temovate Scalp Application. *See Table 1 below.*

Table 1: Efficacy results from a controlled clinical trial in scalp psoriasis

	OLUX Foam n (%)	Vehicle Foam n (%)
Total number of subjects	62	31
Subjects with Treatment Success*	39 (63)	1 (3)
Subjects with Parameter Clear at Endpoint (Scalp Psoriasis)		
Scaling - Clear at Endpoint	42 (68)	3 (10)

Erythema - Clear at Endpoint	27 (44)	2 (6)
Plaque Thickness - Clear at Endpoint	41 (66)	3 (10)

*Defined as a composite of an Investigator's Global Assessment of "completely clear" or "almost clear," a plaque thickness score of 0, an erythema score of 0 or 1, and a scaling score of 0 or 1 at Endpoint, scored on a severity scale of 0-4.

Another well-controlled clinical study evaluated 279 subjects with mild to moderate plaque-type psoriasis (mean Body Surface Area at baseline was 6.7% with a range from 1% to 20%) of non-scalp regions. Subjects were treated twice daily for 2 weeks with OLUX Foam or Vehicle foam. The face and intertriginous areas were excluded from treatment. The efficacy of OLUX Foam in treating non-scalp psoriasis at the end of the 2 weeks' treatment was superior to that of Vehicle foam. *See Table 2 below.*

Table 2: Efficacy results from a controlled clinical trial in non-scalp psoriasis

	OLUX Foam n (%)	Vehicle Foam n (%)
Total number of subjects	139	140
Subjects with Treatment Success*	39 (28)	4 (3)
Physician's Static Global Assessment - Clear or Almost Clear at Endpoint	94 (68)	30 (21)
Scaling - Clear or Almost Clear at Endpoint	101 (73)	42 (30)
Erythema - Clear or Almost Clear at Endpoint	88 (63)	35 (25)
Plaque Thickness - Clear at Endpoint	44 (32)	5 (4)

*Defined as a composite of a Physician's Static Global Assessment score of 0 or 1, scaling score of 0 or 1, an erythema score of 0 or 1 and a plaque thickness score of 0, based on a severity scale of 0-5 at Endpoint.

INDICATIONS AND USAGE

OLUX Foam is a super-potent topical corticosteroid indicated for short-term topical treatment of the inflammatory and pruritic manifestations of moderate to severe corticosteroid-responsive dermatoses of the scalp, and for short-term topical treatment of mild to moderate plaque-type psoriasis of non-scalp regions excluding the face and intertriginous areas.

Treatment beyond 2 consecutive weeks is not recommended and the total dosage should not exceed 50 g per week because of the potential for the drug to suppress the hypothalamic-pituitary-adrenal (HPA) axis. In a controlled pharmacokinetic study, some subjects experienced reversible suppression of the adrenals following 14 days of OLUX Foam therapy (See ADVERSE REACTIONS).

Use in children under 12 years of age is not recommended.

CONTRAINDICATIONS

OLUX Foam is contraindicated in patients who are hypersensitive to clobetasol propionate, to other corticosteroids, or to any ingredient in this preparation.

PRECAUTIONS

General: Clobetasol propionate is a super-potent topical corticosteroid that has been shown to suppress the adrenals at 7.0 g of OLUX Foam per day. Lesser amounts of OLUX Foam were not studied. Systemic absorption of topical corticosteroids has caused reversible adrenal suppression with the potential for glucocorticosteroid insufficiency after withdrawal of treatment. Manifestations of Cushing's syndrome, hyperglycemia, and glucosuria can also be produced in some patients by systemic absorption of topical corticosteroids while on treatment.

Conditions which augment systemic absorption include the application of more potent steroids, use over large surface areas, prolonged use, and the addition of occlusive dressings.

Patients applying a topical steroid to a large surface area or to areas under occlusion should be evaluated periodically for evidence of adrenal suppression. If adrenal suppression is noted, an attempt should be made to withdraw the drug, to reduce the frequency of application, or to substitute a less potent steroid.

Recovery of HPA axis function is generally prompt upon discontinuation of topical corticosteroids. Infrequently, signs and symptoms of glucocorticosteroid insufficiency may occur requiring supplemental systemic corticosteroids. For information on systemic supplementation, see prescribing information for those products.

Pediatric patients may be more susceptible to systemic toxicity from equivalent doses due to their larger skin surface to body mass ratios. See ***PRECAUTIONS-Pediatric Use.***

If irritation develops, OLUX Foam should be discontinued and appropriate therapy instituted. Allergic contact dermatitis with corticosteroids is usually diagnosed by observing a failure to heal rather than by noting a clinical exacerbation, as with most topical products not containing corticosteroids. Such an observation should be corroborated with appropriate diagnostic patch testing.

In the presence of dermatological infections, the use of an appropriate antifungal or antibacterial agent should be instituted. If a favorable response does not occur promptly, use of OLUX Foam should be discontinued until the infection has been adequately controlled.

Information for Patients: Patients using topical corticosteroids should receive the following information and instructions:

1. This medication is to be used as directed by the physician and should not be used longer than the prescribed time period. It is for external use only. Avoid contact with the eyes.
2. This medication should not be used for any disorder other than that for which it was prescribed.
3. The treated area should not be bandaged or otherwise covered or wrapped so as to be occlusive unless directed by the physician.
4. Patients should report to their physician any signs of local adverse reactions.

Laboratory Tests: The following tests may be helpful in evaluating patients for adrenal suppression:

ACTH stimulation test
A.M. plasma cortisol test
Urinary free cortisol test

Carcinogenesis, Mutagenesis, and Impairment of Fertility: Long-term animal studies have not been performed to evaluate the carcinogenic potential of clobetasol propionate.

Clobetasol propionate was non-mutagenic in three different test systems: the Ames test, the *Saccharomyces cerevisiae* gene conversion assay, and the *E. coli* B WP2 fluctuation test.

Studies in the rat following subcutaneous administration of clobetasol propionate at dosage levels up to 0.05 mg/kg per day revealed that the females exhibited an increase in the number of resorbed embryos and a decrease in the number of living fetuses at the highest dose.

Pregnancy: *Teratogenic Effects: Pregnancy Category C:* Corticosteroids have been shown to be teratogenic in laboratory animals when administered systemically at relatively low dosage levels. Some corticosteroids have been shown to be teratogenic after dermal application to laboratory animals.

Clobetasol propionate has not been tested for teratogenicity by the topical route; however, it is absorbed percutaneously, and when administered subcutaneously, it was a significant teratogen in both the rabbit and the mouse. Clobetasol propionate has greater teratogenic potential than steroids that are less potent.

Teratogenicity studies in mice using the subcutaneous route resulted in fetotoxicity at the highest dose tested (1 mg/kg) and teratogenicity at all dose levels tested down to 0.03 mg/kg. These doses are approximately 1.4 and 0.04 times, respectively, the human topical dose of OLUX based on body surface area comparisons. Abnormalities seen included cleft palate and skeletal abnormalities.

In rabbits, clobetasol propionate was teratogenic at doses of 0.003 and 0.01 mg/kg. These doses are approximately 0.02 and 0.05 times, respectively, the human topical dose of OLUX based on body surface area comparisons. Abnormalities seen included cleft palate, cranioschisis, and other skeletal abnormalities.

There are no adequate and well-controlled studies of the teratogenic potential of clobetasol propionate in pregnant women. OLUX Foam should be used during pregnancy only if the potential benefit justifies the potential risk to the fetus.

Drugs of this class should not be used extensively on pregnant patients, in large amounts, or for prolonged periods of time.

Nursing Mothers: Systemically administered corticosteroids appear in human milk and could suppress growth, interfere with endogenous corticosteroid production, or cause other untoward effects. It is not known whether topical administration of corticosteroids could result in sufficient systemic absorption to produce detectable quantities in breast milk. Because many drugs are excreted in human milk, caution should be exercised when OLUX Foam is administered to a nursing woman.

Pediatric Use: Safety and effectiveness of OLUX Foam in pediatric patients have not been established; therefore, use in children under 12 years of age is not recommended. Because of a higher ratio of skin surface area to body mass, pediatric patients are at a greater risk than adults of adrenal suppression and Cushing's syndrome when they are treated with topical corticosteroids. Pediatric patients are therefore at greater risk of adrenal insufficiency during and/or after withdrawal of treatment. Adverse effects including striae have been reported with inappropriate use of topical corticosteroids in infants and children.

Adrenal suppression, Cushing's syndrome, linear growth retardation, delayed weight gain, and intracranial hypertension have been reported in children receiving topical corticosteroids. Manifestations of adrenal suppression in children include low plasma cortisol levels and an absence of response to ACTH stimulation. Manifestations of intracranial hypertension include bulging fontanelles, headaches, and bilateral papilledema.

Geriatric Use: Clinical studies of OLUX Foam did not include sufficient numbers of subjects aged 65 and over to determine whether they respond differently from younger subjects. Other reported clinical experience has not identified differences in responses between the elderly and younger patients. In general, dose selection for an elderly patient should be cautious, usually starting at the low end of the dosing range, reflecting the greater frequency of decreased hepatic, renal, or cardiac function, and of concomitant disease or other drug therapy.

ADVERSE REACTIONS

In a controlled pharmacokinetic study, 5 of 13 subjects experienced reversible suppression of the adrenals at any time during the 14 days of OLUX Foam therapy to at least 20% of the body surface area. Of the 13 subjects studied, 1 of 9 with psoriasis were suppressed after 14 days and all 4 of the subjects with atopic dermatitis had abnormal cortisol levels indicative of adrenal suppression at some time after starting therapy with OLUX Foam. (See Table 3 below.)

Table 3: Subjects with reversible HPA axis suppression at any time during treatment

Dermatosis	OLUX Foam
Psoriasis	1 of 9
Atopic Dermatitis*	4 of 4

*OLUX Foam is not indicated for non-scalp atopic dermatitis, as the safety and efficacy of OLUX Foam in non-scalp atopic dermatitis has not been established. Use in children under 12 years of age is not recommended.

Systemic absorption of topical corticosteroids has produced reversible adrenal suppression, manifestations of Cushing's syndrome, hyperglycemia, and glucosuria in some patients (see PRECAUTIONS).

In a controlled clinical trial (188 subjects) with OLUX Foam in subjects with psoriasis of the scalp, there were no localized scalp adverse reactions reported in the OLUX Foam treated subjects. In two controlled clinical trials (360 subjects) with OLUX Foam in subjects with psoriasis of non-scalp regions, localized adverse events that occurred in the OLUX Foam treated subjects included application site burning (10%), application site dryness (<1%), and other application site reactions (4%).

In larger controlled trials with other clobetasol propionate formulations, the most frequently reported local adverse reactions have included burning, stinging, irritation, pruritus, erythema, folliculitis, cracking and fissuring of the skin, numbness of the fingers, skin atrophy, and telangiectasia (all less than 2%).

The following additional local adverse reactions have been reported with topical corticosteroids, but they may occur more frequently with the use of occlusive dressings and higher potency corticosteroids such as OLUX Foam. These reactions are listed in an approximate decreasing order of occurrence: dryness, hypertrichosis, acneiform eruptions, hypopigmentation, perioral dermatitis, allergic contact dermatitis, maceration of the skin, secondary infection, striae, and miliaria.

OVERDOSAGE

Topically applied OLUX Foam can be absorbed in sufficient amounts to produce systemic effects. See PRECAUTIONS.

DOSAGE AND ADMINISTRATION

Note: For proper dispensing of foam, hold the can upside down and depress the actuator.

OLUX Foam should be applied to the affected area twice daily, once in the morning and once at night. Invert the can and dispense a small amount of OLUX Foam (up to a maximum of a golf-ball-size dollop or one and a half capfuls) into the cap of the can, onto a saucer or other cool surface, or to the lesion, taking care to avoid contact with the eyes. Dispensing directly onto hands is not recommended (unless the hands are the affected area), as the foam will begin to melt immediately upon contact with warm skin. When applying OLUX Foam to a hair-bearing area, move the hair away from the affected area so that the foam can be applied to each affected area. Pick up small amounts with fingertips and gently massage into affected area until the foam disappears. Repeat until entire affected area is treated.

Apply the smallest amount possible that sufficiently covers the affected area(s). No more than one and a half capfuls of foam should be used at each application. Do not apply to face or intertriginous areas.

OLUX Foam is a super-high-potency topical corticosteroid; therefore, treatment should be limited to 2 consecutive weeks and amounts greater than 50 g/week should not be used. Use in pediatric patients under 12 years of age is not recommended.

Unless directed by a physician, OLUX Foam should not be used with occlusive dressings.

Instructions for applying OLUX Foam

Apply OLUX Foam twice a day, once in the morning and once at night. Apply only enough to cover the affected areas. OLUX Foam should not be applied to the groin, armpits, or other skin fold areas.

Continued on next page

Olux—Cont.

To use OLUX Foam:

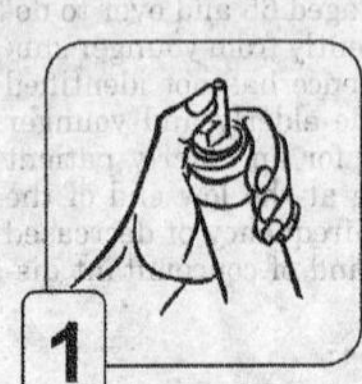

Before applying OLUX Foam for the first time, break the tiny plastic piece at the base of the can's rim by gently pushing back (away from the piece) on the nozzle.

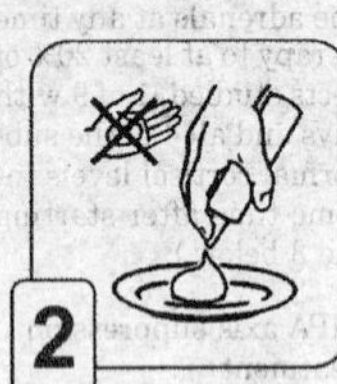

Turn the can upside down.
Push the button to squirt a small amount of OLUX Foam into the cap of the can, onto a saucer or other cool surface, or your affected skin area. This amount should be no more than 1 1/2 capfuls, about the size of a golf ball. **Do not** squirt OLUX Foam directly onto your hands (unless your hands are the affected areas), because the foam will begin to melt right away on contact with your warm skin.
If your fingers are warm, rinse them in cold water first. (Be sure to dry them thoroughly before handling the foam.)
If the can seems warm or the foam seems runny, run the can under cold water.

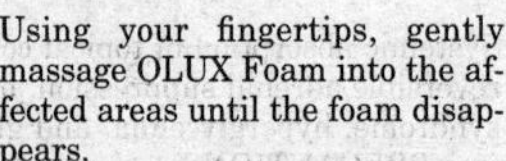

Using your fingertips, gently massage OLUX Foam into the affected areas until the foam disappears.
If you are treating areas with hair such as the scalp, move any hair away so that the foam can be applied directly to the affected areas.
Repeat the process until the affected areas are treated.
Keep the foam away from your eyes, as it will sting and may cause eye problems if there is frequent contact with your eyes. If the foam gets in your eyes, rinse them well with cold water right away. If the stinging continues, contact your doctor right away.

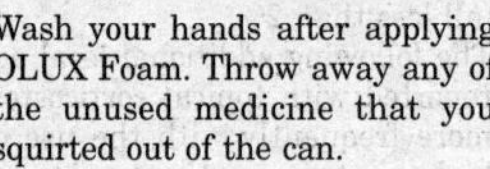

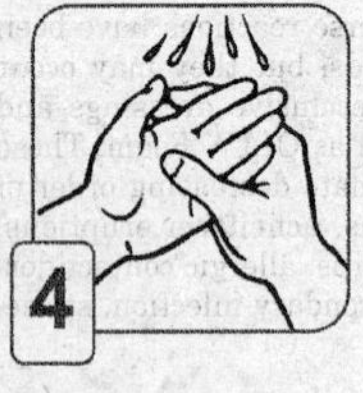

Wash your hands after applying OLUX Foam. Throw away any of the unused medicine that you squirted out of the can.

HOW SUPPLIED

OLUX Foam is supplied in 100 g (NDC 63032-031-00) and 50 g (NDC 63032-031-50) aluminum cans.
Store at controlled room temperature 68-77°F (20-25°C).

WARNING

FLAMMABLE. AVOID FIRE, FLAME OR SMOKING DURING AND IMMEDIATELY FOLLOWING APPLICATION. Keep out of reach of children. Contents under pressure. Do not puncture or incinerate container. Do not expose to heat or store at temperatures above 120°F (49°C).
Manufactured for:
Connetics Corporation
Palo Alto, CA 94303
USA
Printed in USA
January 2004
For additional information:
1-877-821-5337 or visit
www.olux.com
Connetics®
AW No: AW-0183-r2 P/N: PRM-OLU1-073
Delivered in VersaFoam™
VersaFoam is a trademark, and OLUX and Connetics are registered trademarks, of Connetics Corporation.

SORIATANE® ℞

[sōr-ĭ-ă-tēn]
(acitretin)
CAPSULES
[See figure at top of next column]

CONTRAINDICATIONS AND WARNINGS:
Soriatane must not be used by females who are

CAUSES BIRTH DEFECTS

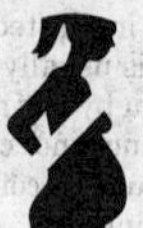

DO NOT GET PREGNANT

pregnant, or who intend to become pregnant during therapy or at any time for at least 3 years following discontinuation of therapy. Soriatane also must not be used by females who may not use reliable contraception while undergoing treatment and for at least 3 years following discontinuation of treatment. Acitretin is a metabolite of etretinate (Tegison®), and major human fetal abnormalities have been reported with the administration of acitretin and etretinate. Potentially, any fetus exposed can be affected.

Clinical evidence has shown that concurrent ingestion of acitretin and ethanol has been associated with the formation of etretinate, which has a significantly longer elimination half-life than acitretin. Because the longer elimination half-life of etretinate would increase the duration of teratogenic potential for female patients, ethanol must not be ingested by female patients either during treatment with Soriatane or for 2 months after cessation of therapy. This allows for elimination of acitretin, thus removing the substrate for transesterification to etretinate. The mechanism of the metabolic process for conversion of acitretin to etretinate has not been fully defined. It is not known whether substances other than ethanol are associated with transesterification.

Acitretin has been shown to be embryotoxic and/or teratogenic in rabbits, mice, and rats at oral doses of 0.6, 3 and 15 mg/kg, respectively. These doses are approximately 0.2, 0.3 and 3 times the maximum recommended therapeutic dose, respectively, based on a mg/m² comparison.

Major human fetal abnormalities associated with acitretin and/or etretinate administration have been reported including meningomyelocele, meningoencephalocele, multiple synostoses, facial dysmorphia, syndactyly, absence of terminal phalanges, malformations of hip, ankle and forearm, low-set ears, high palate, decreased cranial volume, cardiovascular malformation and alterations of the skull and cervical vertebrae.

Soriatane should be prescribed only by those who have special competence in the diagnosis and treatment of severe psoriasis, are experienced in the use of systemic retinoids, and understand the risk of teratogenicity.

Important Information for Women of Childbearing Potential:

Soriatane should be considered only for women with severe psoriasis unresponsive to other therapies or whose clinical condition contraindicates the use of other treatments.

Females of reproductive potential must not be given a prescription for Soriatane until pregnancy is excluded. Soriatane is contraindicated in females of reproductive potential unless the patient meets ALL of the following conditions:

- **Must have had 2 negative urine or serum pregnancy tests with a sensitivity of at least 25 mIU/mL before receiving the initial Soriatane prescription. The first test (a screening test) is obtained by the prescriber when the decision is made to pursue Soriatane therapy. The second pregnancy test (a confirmation test) should be done during the first 5 days of the menstrual period immediately preceding the beginning of Soriatane therapy. For patients with amenorrhea, the second test should be done at least 11 days after the last act of unprotected sexual intercourse (without using 2 effective forms of contraception [birth control] simultaneously). Timing of pregnancy testing throughout the treatment course should be monthly or individualized based on the prescriber's clinical judgment.**
- **Must have selected and have committed to use 2 effective forms of contraception (birth control) simultaneously, at least 1 of which must be a primary form, unless absolute abstinence is the chosen method, or the patient has undergone a hysterectomy or is clearly postmenopausal.**
- **Patients must use 2 effective forms of contraception (birth control) simultaneously for at least 1 month prior to initiation of Soriatane therapy, during Soriatane therapy, and for at least 3 years after discontinuing Soriatane therapy. A Soriatane Patient Referral Form is available so that patients can receive an initial free contraceptive counseling session and pregnancy testing. Counseling about contraception and behaviors associated with an increased risk of pregnancy must be repeated on a regular basis by the prescriber. To encourage compliance with this recommendation, a limited supply of the drug should be prescribed.**

Effective forms of contraception include both primary and secondary forms of contraception. Primary forms of contraception include: tubal ligation, partner's vasectomy, intrauterine devices, birth control pills, and injectable/implantable/insertable/topical hormonal birth control products. Secondary forms of contraception include diaphragms, latex condoms, and cervical caps; each secondary form must be used with a spermicide.

Any birth control method can fail. Therefore, it is critically important that women of childbearing potential use 2 effective forms of contraception (birth control) simultaneously. It has not been established if there is a pharmacokinetic interaction between acitretin and combined oral contraceptives. However, it *has been* established that acitretin interferes with the contraceptive effect of microdosed progestin preparations.[1] Microdosed "minipill" progestin preparations are *not* recommended for use with Soriatane. *It is not known whether other progestational contraceptives, such as implants and injectables, are adequate methods of contraception during acitretin therapy.*

Prescribers are advised to consult the package insert of any medication administered concomitantly with hormonal contraceptives, since some medications may decrease the effectiveness of these birth control products. Patients should be prospectively cautioned not to self-medicate with the herbal supplement St. John's Wort because a possible interaction has been suggested with hormonal contraceptives based on reports of breakthrough bleeding on oral contraceptives shortly after starting St. John's Wort. Pregnancies have been reported by users of combined hormonal contraceptives who also used some form of St. John's Wort (see PRECAUTIONS).

- **Must have signed a Patient Agreement/Informed Consent for Female Patients that contains warnings about the risk of potential birth defects if the fetus is exposed to Soriatane, about contraceptive failure, and about the fact that they must not ingest beverages or products containing ethanol while taking Soriatane and for 2 months after Soriatane treatment has been discontinued.**

If pregnancy does occur during Soriatane therapy or at any time for at least 3 years following discontinuation of Soriatane therapy, the prescriber and patient should discuss the possible effects on the pregnancy. The available information is as follows:

Acitretin, the active metabolite of etretinate, is teratogenic and is contraindicated during pregnancy. The risk of severe fetal malformations is well established when systemic retinoids are taken during pregnancy. Pregnancy must also be prevented after stopping acitretin therapy, while the drug is being eliminated to below a threshold blood concentration that would be associated with an increased incidence of birth defects. Because this threshold has not been established for acitretin in humans and because elimination rates vary among patients, the duration of posttherapy contraception to achieve adequate elimination cannot be calculated precisely. It is strongly recommended that contraception be continued for at least 3 years after stopping treatment with acitretin, based on the following considerations:

- **In the absence of transesterification to form etretinate, greater than 98% of the acitretin would be eliminated within 2 months, assuming a mean elimination half-life of 49 hours.**
- **In cases where etretinate is formed, as has been demonstrated with concomitant administration of acitretin and ethanol,**
  - ◆**greater than 98% of the etretinate formed would be eliminated in 2 years, assuming a mean elimination half-life of 120 days.**
  - ◆**greater than 98% of the etretinate formed would be eliminated in 3 years, based on the longest demonstrated elimination half-life of 168 days.**

  However, etretinate was found in plasma and subcutaneous fat in one patient reported to have had sporadic alcohol intake, 52 months after she stopped acitretin therapy.[2]
- **Severe birth defects have been reported where conception occurred during the time interval when the patient was being treated with acitretin and/or etretinate. In addition, severe birth defects have also been reported when conception occurred *after* the mother completed therapy. These cases have been reported both prospectively (before the outcome was known) and retrospectively (after the outcome was known). The events below are listed without distinction as to whether the reported birth defects are consistent with retinoid-induced embryopathy or not.**
  - ◆**There have been 318 prospectively reported cases involving pregnancies and the use of etretinate, acitretin or both. In 238 of these cases, the conception occurred *after* the last dose of etretinate (103 cases), acitretin (126) or both (9). Fetal outcome remained unknown in approximately one-half of these cases, of which 62 were terminated and 14 were spontaneous abortions. Fetal outcome is known for the other 118 cases and 15 of the outcomes were abnormal (including cases of absent**

hand/wrist, clubfoot, GI malformation, hypocalcemia, hypotonia, limb malformation, neonatal apnea/anemia, neonatal ichthyosis, placental disorder/death, undescended testicle and 5 cases of premature birth). In the 126 prospectively reported cases where conception occurred after the last dose of acitretin only, 43 cases involved conception at least 1 year but less than 2 years after the last dose. There were 3 reports of abnormal outcomes out of these 43 cases (involving limb malformation, GI tract malformations and premature birth). There were only 4 cases where conception occurred at least 2 years after the last dose but there were no reports of birth defects in these cases.

- ◆There is also a total of 35 retrospectively reported cases where conception occurred at least one year after the last dose of etretinate, acitretin or both. From these cases there are 3 reports of birth defects when the conception occurred at least 1 year but less than 2 years after the last dose of acitretin (including heart malformations, Turner's Syndrome, and unspecified congenital malformations) and 4 reports of birth defects when conception occurred 2 or more years after the last dose of acitretin (including foot malformation, cardiac malformations [2 cases] and unspecified neonatal and infancy disorder). There were 3 additional abnormal outcomes in cases where conception occurred 2 or more years after the last dose of etretinate (including chromosome disorder, forearm aplasia, and stillbirth).
- ◆Females who have taken Tegison (etretinate) must continue to follow the contraceptive recommendations for Tegison. Tegison is no longer marketed in the US; for information, call Connetics at 1-888-500-DERM (3376).
- ◆Patients should not donate blood during and for at least 3 years following the completion of Soriatane therapy because women of childbearing potential must not receive blood from patients being treated with Soriatane.

Important Information For Males Taking Soriatane:

- Patients should not donate blood during and for at least 3 years following Soriatane therapy because women of childbearing potential must not receive blood from patients being treated with Soriatane.
- Samples of seminal fluid from 3 male patients treated with acitretin and 6 male patients treated with etretinate have been assayed for the presence of acitretin. The maximum concentration of acitretin observed in the seminal fluid of these men was 12.5 ng/mL. Assuming an ejaculate volume of 10 mL, the amount of drug transferred in semen would be 125 ng, which is 1/200,000 of a single 25 mg capsule. Thus, although it appears that residual acitretin in seminal fluid poses little, if any, risk to a fetus while a male patient is taking the drug or after it is discontinued, the no-effect limit for teratogenicity is unknown and there is no registry for birth defects associated with acitretin. The available data are as follows:

  There have been 25 cases of reported conception when the male partner was taking acitretin. The pregnancy outcome is known in 13 of these 25 cases. Of these, 9 reports were retrospective and 4 were prospective (meaning the pregnancy was reported prior to knowledge of the outcome) [3].

For All Patients: **A SORIATANE MEDICATION GUIDE MUST BE GIVEN TO THE PATIENT EACH TIME SORIATANE IS DISPENSED, AS REQUIRED BY LAW.**

Timing of Paternal Acitretin Treatment Relative to Conception	Delivery of Healthy Neonate	Spontaneous Abortion	Induced Abortion	Total
At time of conception	5*	5	1	11
Discontinued ~4 weeks prior	0	0	1**	1
Discontinued ~6 to 8 months prior	0	1	0	1

*Four of 5 cases were prospective.
**With malformation pattern not typical of retinoid embryopathy (bilateral cystic hygromas of neck, hypoplasia of lungs bilateral, pulmonary atresia, VSD with overriding truncus arteriosus).

[See table above]

DESCRIPTION

Soriatane (acitretin), a retinoid, is available in 10 mg and 25 mg gelatin capsules for oral administration. Chemically, acitretin is all-*trans*-9-(4-methoxy-2,3,6-trimethylphenyl)-3,7-dimethyl-2,4,6,8-nonatetraenoic acid. It is a metabolite of etretinate and is related to both retinoic acid and retinol (vitamin A). It is a yellow to greenish-yellow powder with a molecular weight of 326.44. The structural formula is:

CH_3 CH_3 CH_3 H_3C COOH CH_3O CH_3

Each capsule contains acitretin, microcrystalline cellulose, sodium ascorbate, gelatin, black monogramming ink and maltodextrin (a mixture of polysaccharides).

Gelatin capsule shells contain gelatin, iron oxide (yellow, black, and red), and titanium dioxide. They may also contain benzyl alcohol, carboxymethylcellulose sodium, edetate calcium disodium.

CLINICAL PHARMACOLOGY

The mechanism of action of Soriatane is unknown.

Pharmacokinetics: *Absorption:* Oral absorption of acitretin is optimal when given with food. For this reason, acitretin was given with food in all of the following studies. After administration of a single 50 mg oral dose of acitretin to 18 healthy subjects, maximum plasma concentrations ranged from 196 to 728 ng/mL (mean 416 ng/mL) and were achieved in 2 to 5 hours (mean 2.7 hours). The oral absorption of acitretin is linear and proportional with increasing doses from 25 to 100 mg. Approximately 72% (range 47% to 109%) of the administered dose was absorbed after a single 50 mg dose of acitretin was given to 12 healthy subjects.

Distribution: Acitretin is more than 99.9% bound to plasma proteins, primarily albumin.

Metabolism (see *Pharmacokinetic Drug Interactions: Ethanol*): Following oral absorption, acitretin undergoes extensive metabolism and interconversion by simple isomerization to its 13-*cis* form (*cis*-acitretin). The formation of *cis*-acitretin relative to parent compound is not altered by dose or fed/fast conditions of oral administration of acitretin. Both parent compound and isomer are further metabolized into chain-shortened breakdown products and conjugates, which are excreted. Following multiple-dose administration of acitretin, steady-state concentrations of acitretin and *cis*-acitretin in plasma are achieved within approximately 3 weeks.

Elimination: The chain-shortened metabolites and conjugates of acitretin and *cis*-acitretin are ultimately excreted in the feces (34% to 54%) and urine (16% to 53%). The terminal elimination half-life of acitretin following multiple-dose administration is 49 hours (range 33 to 96 hours), and that of *cis*-acitretin under the same conditions is 63 hours (range 28 to 157 hours). The accumulation ratio of the parent compound is 1.2; that of *cis*-acitretin is 6.6.

Special Populations: *Psoriasis:* In an 8-week study of acitretin pharmacokinetics in patients with psoriasis, mean steady-state trough concentrations of acitretin increased in a dose proportional manner with dosages ranging from 10 to 50 mg daily. Acitretin plasma concentrations were nonmeasurable (<4 ng/mL) in all patients 3 weeks after cessation of therapy.

Elderly: In a multiple-dose study in healthy young (n=6) and elderly (n=8) subjects, a two-fold increase in acitretin plasma concentrations were seen in elderly subjects, although the elimination half-life did not change.

Renal Failure: Plasma concentrations of acitretin were significantly (59.3%) lower in end-stage renal failure subjects (n=6) when compared to age-matched controls, following single 50 mg oral doses. Acitretin was not removed by hemodialysis in these subjects.

Pharmacokinetic Drug Interactions (see also boxed CONTRAINDICATIONS AND WARNINGS and PRECAUTIONS: *Drug Interactions*): In studies of in vivo pharmacokinetic drug interactions, no interaction was seen between acitretin and cimetidine, digoxin, phenprocoumon or glyburide.

Ethanol: Clinical evidence has shown that etretinate (a retinoid with a much longer half-life, see below) can be formed with concurrent ingestion of acitretin and ethanol. In a two-way crossover study, all 10 subjects formed etretinate with concurrent ingestion of a single 100 mg oral dose of acitretin during a 3-hour period of ethanol ingestion (total ethanol, approximately 1.4 g/kg body weight). A mean peak etretinate concentration of 59 ng/mL (range 22 to 105 ng/mL) was observed, and extrapolation of AUC values indicated that the formation of etretinate in this study was comparable to a single 5 mg oral dose of etretinate. There was no detectable formation of etretinate when a single 100 mg oral dose of acitretin was administered without concurrent ethanol ingestion, although the formation of etretinate without concurrent ethanol ingestion cannot be excluded (see boxed CONTRAINDICATIONS AND WARNINGS). Of 93 evaluable psoriatic patients on acitretin therapy in several foreign studies (10 to 80 mg/day), 16% had measurable etretinate levels (>5 ng/mL). Etretinate has a much longer elimination half-life compared to that of acitretin. In one study the apparent mean terminal half-life after 6 months of therapy was approximately 120 days (range 84 to 168 days). In another study of 47 patients treated chronically with etretinate, 5 had detectable serum drug levels (in the range of 0.5 to 12 ng/mL) 2.1 to 2.9 years after therapy was discontinued. The long half-life appears to be due to storage of etretinate in adipose tissue.

Progestin-only Contraceptives: It has not been established if there is a pharmacokinetic interaction between acitretin and combined oral contraceptives. However, it *has been* established that acitretin interferes with the contraceptive effect of microdosed progestin preparations.[1] Microdosed "minipill" progestin preparations are *not* recommended for use with Soriatane. *It is not known whether other progestational contraceptives, such as implants and injectables, are adequate methods of contraception during acitretin therapy.*

CLINICAL STUDIES

In two double-blind placebo controlled studies, Soriatane was administered once daily to patients with severe psoriasis (ie, covering at least 10% to 20% of the body surface area). At 8 weeks (see Table 1) patients treated in Study A with 50 mg Soriatane per day showed significant improvements ($p \leq 0.05$) relative to baseline and to placebo in the physician's global evaluation and in the mean ratings of severity of psoriasis (scaling, thickness, and erythema). In study B, differences from baseline and from placebo were statistically significant ($p \leq 0.05$) for all variables at both the 25 mg and 50 mg doses; it should be noted for Study B that no statistical adjustment for multiplicity was carried out.

Table 1. Summary of the Soriatane Efficacy Results of the 8-Week Double-Blind Phase of Studies A and B

	Study A		Study B		
	Total daily dose		Total daily dose		
Efficacy Variables	**Placebo (N=29)**	**50 mg (N=29)**	**Placebo (N=72)**	**25 mg (N=74)**	**50 mg (N=71)**
Physician's Global Evaluation					
Baseline	4.62	4.55	4.43	4.37	4.49
Mean Change After 8 Weeks	-0.29	-2.00*	-0.06	-1.06*	-1.57*
Scaling					
Baseline	4.10	3.76	3.97	4.11	4.10
Mean Change After 8 Weeks	-0.22	-1.62*	-0.21	-1.50*	-1.78*
Thickness					
Baseline	4.10	4.10	4.03	4.11	4.20
Mean Change After 8 Weeks	-0.39	-2.10*	-0.18	-1.43*	-2.11*
Erythema					
Baseline	4.21	4.59	4.42	4.24	4.45
Mean Change After 8 Weeks	-0.33	-2.10*	-0.37	-1.12*	-1.65*

*Values were statistically significantly different from placebo and from baseline ($p \leq 0.05$). No adjustment for multiplicity was done for Study B.

The efficacy variables consisted of: the mean severity rating of scale, lesion thickness, erythema, and the physician's global evaluation of the current status of the disease. Ratings of scaling, erythema, and lesion thickness, and the ratings of the global assessments were made using a seven-point scale (0=none, 1=trace, 2=mild, 3=mild-moderate, 4=moderate, 5=moderate-severe, 6=severe).

A subset of 141 patients from both pivotal studies A and B continued to receive Soriatane in an open fashion for up to 24 weeks. At the end of the treatment period, all efficacy variables, as indicated in Table 2, were significantly improved ($p \leq 0.01$) from baseline, including extent of psoriasis, mean ratings of psoriasis severity and physician's global evaluation.

Table 2. Summary of the First Course of Soriatane Therapy (24 Weeks)

Variables	Study A	Study B
Mean Total Daily Soriatane Dose (mg)	43.1	43.1
Mean Duration of Therapy (Weeks)	21.1	22.6
Physician's Global Evaluation	**N=39**	**N=98**
Baseline	4.51	4.43
Mean Change From Baseline	-2.26*	-2.60*
Scaling	**N=59**	**N=132**
Baseline	3.97	4.07
Mean Change From Baseline	-2.15*	-2.42*
Thickness	**N=59**	**N=132**
Baseline	4.00	4.12
Mean Change From Baseline	-2.44*	-2.66*
Erythema	**N=59**	**N=132**
Baseline	4.35	4.33
Mean Change From Baseline	-2.31*	-2.29*

Continued on next page

Soriatane—Cont.

*Indicates that the difference from baseline was statistically significant ($p \leq 0.01$).

The efficacy variables consisted of: the mean severity rating of scale, lesion thickness, erythema, and the physician's global evaluation of the current status of the disease. Ratings of scaling, erythema, and lesion thickness, and the ratings of the global assessments were made using a seven-point scale (0=none, 1=trace, 2=mild, 3=mild-moderate, 4=moderate, 5=moderate-severe, 6=severe).

All efficacy variables improved significantly in a subset of 55 patients from Study A treated for a second, 6-month maintenance course of therapy (for a total of 12 months of treatment); a small subset of patients (n=4) from Study A continued to improve after a third 6-month course of therapy (for a total of 18 months of treatment).

INDICATIONS AND USAGE

Soriatane is indicated for the treatment of severe psoriasis in adults. Because of significant adverse effects associated with its use, Soriatane should be prescribed only by those knowledgeable in the systemic use of retinoids. In females of reproductive potential, Soriatane should be reserved for non-pregnant patients who are unresponsive to other therapies or whose clinical condition contraindicates the use of other treatments (see boxed CONTRAINDICATIONS AND WARNINGS — Soriatane can cause severe birth defects).

Most patients experience relapse of psoriasis after discontinuing therapy. Subsequent courses, when clinically indicated, have produced efficacy results similar to the initial course of therapy.

CONTRAINDICATIONS

Pregnancy Category X (see boxed CONTRAINDICATIONS AND WARNINGS).

Soriatane is contraindicated in patients with severely impaired liver or kidney function and in patients with chronic abnormally elevated blood lipid values (see boxed WARNINGS: *Hepatotoxicity*, WARNINGS: *Lipids and Possible Cardiovascular Effects*, and PRECAUTIONS).

An increased risk of hepatitis has been reported to result from combined use of methotrexate and etretinate. Consequently, the combination of methotrexate with Soriatane is also contraindicated (see PRECAUTIONS: *Drug Interactions*).

Since both Soriatane and tetracyclines can cause increased intracranial pressure, their combined use is contraindicated (see WARNINGS: *Pseudotumor Cerebri*).

Soriatane is contraindicated in cases of hypersensitivity to the preparation (acitretin or excipients) or to other retinoids.

WARNINGS

(see also boxed CONTRAINDICATIONS AND WARNINGS)

Hepatotoxicity: **Of the 525 patients treated in US clinical trials, 2 had clinical jaundice with elevated serum bilirubin and transaminases considered related to Soriatane treatment. Liver function test results in these patients returned to normal after Soriatane was discontinued. Two of the 1289 patients treated in European clinical trials developed biopsy-confirmed toxic hepatitis. A second biopsy in one of these patients revealed nodule formation suggestive of cirrhosis. One patient in a Canadian clinical trial of 63 patients developed a three-fold increase of transaminases. A liver biopsy of this patient showed mild lobular disarray, multifocal hepatocyte loss and mild triaditis of the portal tracts compatible with acute reversible hepatic injury. The patient's transaminase levels returned to normal 2 months after Soriatane was discontinued.**

The potential of Soriatane therapy to induce hepatotoxicity was prospectively evaluated using liver biopsies in an open-label study of 128 patients. Pretreatment and posttreatment biopsies were available for 87 patients. A comparison of liver biopsy findings before and after therapy revealed 49 (58%) patients showed no change, 21 (25%) improved and 14 (17%) patients had a worsening of their liver biopsy status. For 6 patients, the classification changed from class 0 (no pathology) to class I (normal fatty infiltration; nuclear variability and portal inflammation; both mild); for 7 patients, the change was from class I to class II (fatty infiltration, nuclear variability, portal inflammation and focal necrosis; all moderate to severe); and for 1 patient, the change was from class II to class IIIb (fibrosis, moderate to severe). No correlation could be found between liver function test result abnormalities and the change in liver biopsy status, and no cumulative dose relationship was found.

Elevations of AST (SGOT), ALT (SGPT), GGT (GGTP) or LDH have occurred in approximately 1 in 3 patients treated with Soriatane. Of the 525 patients treated in clinical trials in the US, treatment was discontinued in 20 (3.8%) due to elevated liver function test results. If hepatotoxicity is suspected during treatment with Soriatane, the drug should be discontinued and the etiology further investigated.

Ten of 652 patients treated in US clinical trials of etretinate, of which acitretin is the active metabolite, had clinical or histologic hepatitis considered to be possibly or probably related to etretinate treatment. There have been reports of hepatitis-related deaths worldwide; a few of these patients had received etretinate for a month or less before presenting with hepatic symptoms or signs.

Table 3. Adverse Events Frequently Reported During Clinical Trials Percent of Patients Reporting (N=525)

BODY SYSTEM	>75%	50% to 75%	25% to 50%	10% to 25%
CNS				Rigors
Eye Disorders				Xerophthalmia
Mucous Membranes	Cheilitis		Rhinitis	Dry mouth Epistaxis
Musculoskeletal				Arthralgia Spinal hyperostosis (progression of existing lesions)
Skin and Appendages		Alopecia Skin peeling	Dry skin Nail disorder Pruritus	Erythematous rash Hyperesthesia Paresthesia Paronychia Skin atrophy Sticky skin

Hyperostosis: In adults receiving long-term treatment with Soriatane, appropriate examinations should be periodically performed in view of possible ossification abnormalities (see ADVERSE REACTIONS). Because the frequency and severity of iatrogenic bony abnormality in adults is low, periodic radiography is only warranted in the presence of symptoms or long-term use of Soriatane. If such disorders arise, the continuation of therapy should be discussed with the patient on the basis of a careful risk/benefit analysis. In clinical trials with Soriatane, patients were prospectively evaluated for evidence of development or change in bony abnormalities of the vertebral column, knees and ankles.

Vertebral Results: Of 380 patients treated with Soriatane, 15% had preexisting abnormalities of the spine which showed new changes or progression of preexisting findings. Changes included degenerative spurs, anterior bridging of spinal vertebrae, diffuse idiopathic skeletal hyperostosis, ligament calcification and narrowing and destruction of a cervical disc space. De novo changes (formation of small spurs) were seen in 3 patients after 1½ to 2½ years.

Skeletal Appendicular Results: Six of 128 patients treated with Soriatane showed abnormalities in the knees and ankles before treatment that progressed during treatment. In 5, these changes involved the formation of additional spurs or enlargement of existing spurs. The sixth patient had degenerative joint disease which worsened. No patients developed spurs de novo. Clinical complaints did not predict radiographic changes.

Lipids and Possible Cardiovascular Effects: Blood lipid determinations should be performed before Soriatane is administered and again at intervals of 1 to 2 weeks until the lipid response to the drug is established, usually within 4 to 8 weeks. In patients receiving Soriatane during clinical trials, 66% and 33% experienced elevation in triglycerides and cholesterol, respectively. Decreased high density lipoproteins (HDL) occurred in 40% of patients. These effects of Soriatane were generally reversible upon cessation of therapy.

Patients with an increased tendency to develop hypertriglyceridemia included those with disturbances of lipid metabolism, diabetes mellitus, obesity, increased alcohol intake or a familial history of these conditions. Because of the risk of hypertriglyceridemia, serum lipids must be more closely monitored in high-risk patients and during long-term treatment.

Hypertriglyceridemia and lowered HDL may increase a patient's cardiovascular risk status. Although no causal relationship has been established, there have been post-marketing reports of acute myocardial infarction or thromboembolic events in patients on Soriatane therapy. In addition, elevation of serum triglycerides to greater than 800 mg/dL has been associated with fatal fulminant pancreatitis. Therefore, dietary modifications, reduction in Soriatane dose, or drug therapy should be employed to control significant elevations of triglycerides. If, despite these measures, hypertriglyceridemia and low HDL levels persist, the discontinuation of Soriatane should be considered.

Ophthalmologic Effects: The eyes and vision of 329 patients treated with Soriatane were examined by ophthalmologists. The findings included dry eyes (23%), irritation of eyes (9%) and brow and lash loss (5%). The following were reported in less than 5% of patients: Bell's Palsy, blepharitis and/or crusting of lids, blurred vision, conjunctivitis, corneal epithelial abnormality, cortical cataract, decreased night vision, diplopia, itchy eyes or eyelids, nuclear cataract, pannus, papilledema, photophobia, posterior subcapsular cataract, recurrent sties and subepithelial corneal lesions.

Any patient treated with Soriatane who is experiencing visual difficulties should discontinue the drug and undergo ophthalmologic evaluation.

Pancreatitis: Lipid elevations occur in 25% to 50% of patients treated with Soriatane. Triglyceride increases sufficient to be associated with pancreatitis are much less common, although fatal fulminant pancreatitis has been reported. There have been rare reports of pancreatitis during Soriatane therapy in the absence of hypertriglyceridemia.

Pseudotumor Cerebri: Soriatane and other retinoids administered orally have been associated with cases of pseudotumor cerebri (benign intracranial hypertension). Some of these events involved concomitant use of isotretinoin and tetracyclines. However, the event seen in a single Soriatane patient was not associated with tetracyline use. Early signs and symptoms include papilledema, headache, nausea and vomiting and visual disturbances. Patients with these signs and symptoms should be examined for papilledema and, if present, should discontinue Soriatane immediately and be referred for neurological evaluation and care. Since both Soriatane and tetracyclines can cause increased intracranial pressure, their combined use is contraindicated (see CONTRAINDICATIONS).

PRECAUTIONS

Information for Patients **(see Medication Guide for all patients and Patient Agreement/Informed Consent for Female Patients at end of professional labeling):**

Patients should be instructed to read the Medication Guide supplied as required by law when Soriatane is dispensed.

Females of reproductive potential: **Soriatane can cause severe birth defects.** Female patients must not be pregnant when Soriatane therapy is initiated, they must not become pregnant while taking Soriatane, and for at least 3 years after stopping Soriatane, so that the drug can be eliminated to below a blood concentration that would be associated with an increased incidence of birth defects. Because this threshold has not been established for acitretin in humans and because elimination rates vary among patients, the duration of posttherapy contraception to achieve adequate elimination cannot be calculated precisely (see boxed CONTRAINDICATIONS AND WARNINGS).

Females of reproductive potential should also be advised that they must not ingest beverages or products containing ethanol while taking Soriatane and for 2 months after Soriatane treatment has been discontinued. This allows for elimination of the acitretin which can be converted to etretinate in the presence of alcohol.

Female patients should be advised that any method of birth control can fail, including tubal ligation, and that micro-dosed progestin "minipill" preparations are not recommended for use with Soriatane (see CLINICAL PHARMACOLOGY: *Pharmacokinetic Drug Interactions*). Data from one patient who received a very low-dosed progestin contraceptive (levonorgestrel 0.03 mg) had a significant increase of the progesterone level after three menstrual cycles during acitretin treatment.[2]

Female patients should sign a consent form prior to beginning Soriatane therapy (see boxed CONTRAINDICATIONS AND WARNINGS).

Nursing Mothers: Studies on lactating rats have shown that etretinate is excreted in the milk. There is one prospective case report where acitretin is reported to be excreted in human milk. Therefore, nursing mothers should not receive Soriatane prior to or during nursing because of the potential for serious adverse reactions in nursing infants.

All Patients:

Depression and/or other psychiatric symptoms such as aggressive feelings or thoughts of self-harm have been reported. These events, including self-injurious behavior, have been reported in patients taking other systemically administered retinoids, as well as in patients taking Soriatane. Since other factors may have contributed to these events, it is not known if they are related to Soriatane. Patients should be counseled to stop taking Soriatane and notify their prescriber immediately if they experience psychiatric symptoms.

Patients should be advised that a transient worsening of psoriasis is sometimes seen during the initial treatment period. Patients should be advised that they may have to wait 2 to 3 months before they get the full benefit of Soriatane, although some patients may achieve significant improvements within the first 8 weeks of treatment as demonstrated in clinical trials.

Decreased night vision has been reported with Soriatane therapy. Patients should be advised of this potential problem and warned to be cautious when driving or operating any vehicle at night. Visual problems should be carefully monitored (see WARNINGS and ADVERSE REACTIONS). Patients should be advised that they may experience decreased tolerance to contact lenses during the treatment period and sometimes after treatment has stopped.

Patients should not donate blood during and for at least 3 years following therapy because Soriatane can cause birth defects and women of childbearing potential must not receive blood from patients being treated with Soriatane.

Because of the relationship of Soriatane to vitamin A, patients should be advised against taking vitamin A supplements in excess of minimum recommended daily allowances to avoid possible additive toxic effects.

Patients should avoid the use of sun lamps and excessive exposure to sunlight (non-medical UV exposure) because the effects of UV light are enhanced by retinoids.

Patients should be advised that they must not give their Soriatane capsules to any other person.

For Prescribers:

Phototherapy: Significantly lower doses of phototherapy are required when Soriatane is used because Soriatane-induced effects on the stratum corneum can increase the risk of erythema (burning) (see DOSAGE AND ADMINISTRATION).

Drug Interactions:

Ethanol: Clinical evidence has shown that etretinate can be formed with concurrent ingestion of acitretin and ethanol (see boxed CONTRAINDICATIONS AND WARNINGS and CLINICAL PHARMACOLOGY: *Pharmacokinetics*).

Glibenclamide: In a study of 7 healthy male volunteers, acitretin treatment potentiated the blood glucose lowering effect of glibenclamide (a sulfonylurea similar to chlorpropamide) in 3 of the 7 subjects. Repeating the study with 6 healthy male volunteers in the absence of glibenclamide did not detect an effect of acitretin on glucose tolerance. Careful supervision of diabetic patients under treatment with Soriatane is recommended (see CLINICAL PHARMACOLOGY: *Pharmacokinetics* and DOSAGE AND ADMINISTRATION).

Hormonal Contraceptives: It has not been established if there is a pharmacokinetic interaction between acitretin and combined oral contraceptives. However, it *has been* established that acitretin interferes with the contraceptive effect of microdosed progestin "minipill" preparations. Microdosed "minipill" progestin preparations are *not* recommended for use with Soriatane (see CLINICAL PHARMACOLOGY: *Pharmacokinetic Drug Interactions*). *It is not known whether other progestational contraceptives, such as implants and injectables, are adequate methods of contraception during acitretin therapy.*

Methotrexate: An increased risk of hepatitis has been reported to result from combined use of methotrexate and etretinate. Consequently, the combination of methotrexate with acitretin is also contraindicated (see CONTRAINDICATIONS).

Phenytoin: If acitretin is given concurrently with phenytoin, the protein binding of phenytoin may be reduced.

Tetracyclines: Since both acitretin and tetracyclines can cause increased intracranial pressure, their combined use is contraindicated (see CONTRAINDICATIONS and WARNINGS: *Pseudotumor Cerebri*).

Vitamin A and oral retinoids: Concomitant administration of vitamin A and/or other oral retinoids with acitretin must be avoided because of the risk of hypervitaminosis A.

Other: There appears to be no pharmacokinetic interaction between acitretin and cimetidine, digoxin, or glyburide. Investigations into the effect of acitretin on the protein binding of anticoagulants of the coumarin type (warfarin) revealed no interaction.

Laboratory Tests: If significant abnormal laboratory results are obtained, either dosage reduction with careful monitoring or treatment discontinuation is recommended, depending on clinical judgement.

Blood Sugar: Some patients receiving retinoids have experienced problems with blood sugar control. In addition, new cases of diabetes have been diagnosed during retinoid therapy, including diabetic ketoacidosis. In diabetics, blood-sugar levels should be monitored very carefully.

Lipids: In clinical studies, the incidence of hypertriglyceridemia was 66%, hypercholesterolemia was 33% and that of decreased HDL was 40%. Pretreatment and follow-up measurements should be obtained under fasting conditions. It is recommended that these tests be performed weekly or every other week until the lipid response to Soriatane has stabilized (see WARNINGS).

Liver Function Tests: Elevations of AST (SGOT), ALT (SGPT) or LDH were experienced by approximately 1 in 3 patients treated with Soriatane. It is recommended that these tests be performed prior to initiation of Soriatane therapy, at 1- to 2-week intervals until stable and thereafter at intervals as clinically indicated (see CONTRAINDICATIONS and boxed WARNINGS).

Carcinogenesis, Mutagenesis and Impairment of Fertility:

Carcinogenesis: A carcinogenesis study of acitretin in Wistar rats, at doses up to 2 mg/kg/day administered 7 days/week for 104 weeks, has been completed. There were no neoplastic lesions observed that were considered to have been related to treatment with acitretin. An 80-week carcinogenesis study in mice has been completed with etretinate, the ethyl ester of acitretin. Blood level data obtained during this study demonstrated that etretinate was metabolized to acitretin and that blood levels of acitretin exceeded those of etretinate at all times studied. In the etretinate study, an increased incidence of blood vessel tumors (hemangiomas and hemangiosarcomas at several different sites) was noted

Table 4. Adverse Events Less Frequently Reported During Clinical Trials (Some of Which May Bear No Relationship to Therapy) Percent of Patients Reporting (N=525)

BODY SYSTEM	1% to 10%		<1%	
Body as a Whole	Anorexia Edema Fatigue Hot flashes Increased appetite		Alcohol intolerance Dizziness Fever Influenza-like symptoms	Malaise Moniliasis Muscle weakness Weight increase
Cardiovascular	Flushing		Chest pain Cyanosis Increased bleeding time	Intermittent claudication Peripheral ischemia
CNS (also see Psychiatric)	Headache Pain		Abnormal gait Migraine Neuritis	Pseudotumor cerebri (intracranial hypertension)
Eye Disorders	Abnormal/blurred vision Blepharitis Conjunctivitis/ irritation Corneal epithelial abnormality	Decreased night vision/night blindness Eye abnormality Eye pain Photophobia	Abnormal lacrimation Chalazion Conjunctival hemorrhage Corneal ulceration Diplopia Ectropion	Itchy eyes and lids Papilledema Recurrent sties Subepithelial corneal lesions
Gastrointestinal	Abdominal pain Diarrhea Nausea Tongue disorder		Constipation Dyspepsia Esophagitis Gastritis Gastroenteritis	Glossitis Hemorrhoids Melena Tenesmus Tongue ulceration
Liver and Biliary			Hepatic function abnormal Hepatitis Jaundice	
Mucous Membranes	Gingival bleeding Gingivitis Increased saliva	Stomatitis Thirst Ulcerative stomatitis	Altered saliva Anal disorder Gum hyperplasia	Hemorrhage Pharyngitis
Musculoskeletal	Arthritis Arthrosis Back pain Hypertonia Myalgia	Osteodynia Peripheral joint hyperostosis (progression of existing lesions)	Bone disorder Olecranon bursitis Spinal hyperostosis (new lesions) Tendonitis	
Psychiatric	Depression Insomnia Somnolence		Anxiety Dysphonia Libido decreased Nervousness	
Reproductive				Atrophic vaginitis Leukorrhea
Respiratory	Sinusitis		Coughing Increased sputum Laryngitis	
Skin and Appendages	Abnormal skin odor Abnormal hair texture Bullous eruption Cold/clammy skin Dermatitis Increased sweating Infection	Psoriasiform rash Purpura Pyogenic granuloma Rash Seborrhea Skin fissures Skin ulceration Sunburn	Acne Breast pain Cyst Eczema Fungal infection Furunculosis Hair discoloration Herpes simplex Hyperkeratosis Hypertrichosis Hypoesthesia Impaired healing Otitis media Otitis externa	Photosensitivity reaction Psoriasis aggravated Scleroderma Skin nodule Skin hypertrophy Skin disorder Skin irritation Sweat gland disorder Urticaria Verrucae
Special Senses / Other	Earache Taste perversion Tinnitus		Ceruminosis Deafness Taste loss	
Urinary			Abnormal urine Dysuria Penis disorder	

in male, but not female, mice at doses approximately one-half the maximum recommended human therapeutic dose based on a mg/m^2 comparison.

Mutagenesis: Acitretin was evaluated for mutagenic potential in the Ames test, in the Chinese hamster (V79/HGPRT) assay, in unscheduled DNA synthesis assays using rat hepatocytes and human fibroblasts and in an in vivo mouse micronucleus assay. No evidence of mutagenicity of acitretin was demonstrated in any of these assays.

Impairment of Fertility: In a fertility study in rats, the fertility of treated animals was not impaired at the highest dosage of acitretin tested, 3 mg/kg/day (approximately one-half the maximum recommended therapeutic dose based on a mg/m^2 comparison). Chronic toxicity studies in dogs revealed testicular changes (reversible mild to moderate spermatogenic arrest and appearance of multinucleated giant cells) in the highest dosage group (50 then 30 mg/kg/day).

No decreases in sperm count or concentration and no changes in sperm motility or morphology were noted in 31 men (17 psoriatic patients, 8 patients with disorders of keratinization and 6 healthy volunteers) given 30 to 50 mg/day of acitretin for at least 12 weeks. In these studies, no deleterious effects were seen on either testosterone production, LH or FSH in any of the 31 men.[4–6] No deleterious effects were seen on the hypothalamic-pituitary axis in any of the 18 men where it was measured.[4,5]

Pregnancy: *Teratogenic Effects:* **Pregnancy Category X (see boxed CONTRAINDICATIONS AND WARNINGS).**

In a study in which acitretin was administered to male rats only at a dosage of 5 mg/kg/day for 10 weeks (approximate duration of one spermatogenic cycle) prior to and during mating with untreated female rats, no teratogenic effects were observed in the progeny (see boxed CONTRAINDICATIONS AND WARNINGS for information about male use of Soriatane).

Nonteratogenic Effects: In rats dosed at 3 mg/kg/day (approximately one-half the maximum recommended therapeutic dose based on a mg/m^2 comparison), slightly de-

Continued on next page

Soriatane—Cont.

creased pup survival and delayed incisor eruption were noted. At the next lowest dose tested, 1 mg/kg/day, no treatment-related adverse effects were observed.

Pediatric Use: Safety and effectiveness in pediatric patients have not been established. No clinical studies have been conducted in pediatric patients. Ossification of interosseous ligaments and tendons of the extremities, skeletal hyperostoses, decreases in bone mineral density, and premature epiphyseal closure have been reported in children taking other systemic retinoids, including etretinate, a metabolite of Soriatane. A causal relationship between these effects and Soriatane has not been established. While it is not known that these occurrences are more severe or more frequent in children, there is special concern in pediatric patients because of the implications for growth potential (see WARNINGS: *Hyperostosis*).

Geriatric Use: Clinical studies of Soriatane did not include sufficient numbers of subjects aged 65 and over to determine whether they respond differently than younger subjects. Other reported clinical experience has not identified differences in responses between the elderly and younger patients. In general, dose selection for an elderly patient should be cautious, usually starting at the low end of the dosing range, reflecting the greater frequency of decreased hepatic, renal, or cardiac function, and of concomitant disease or other drug therapy. A twofold increase in acitretin plasma concentrations was seen in healthy elderly subjects compared with young subjects, although the elimination half-life did not change (see CLINICAL PHARMACOLOGY: *Special Populations*).

ADVERSE REACTIONS

Hypervitaminosis A produces a wide spectrum of signs and symptoms primarily of the mucocutaneous, musculoskeletal, hepatic, neuropsychiatric, and central nervous systems. Many of the clinical adverse reactions reported to date with Soriatane administration resemble those of the hypervitaminosis A syndrome.

Adverse Events/Postmarketing Reports: In addition to the events listed in the tables for the clinical trials, the following adverse events have been identified during postapproval use of Soriatane. Because these events are reported voluntarily from a population of uncertain size, it is not always possible to reliably estimate their frequency or establish a causal relationship to drug exposure.

Cardiovascular: Acute myocardial infarction, thromboembolism (see WARNINGS), stroke

Nervous System: Myopathy with peripheral neuropathy has been reported during Soriatane therapy. Both conditions improved with discontinuation of the drug.

Psychiatric: Aggressive feelings and/or suicidal thoughts have been reported. These events, including self-injurious behavior, have been reported in patients taking other systemically administered retinoids, as well as in patients taking Soriatane. Since other factors may have contributed to these events, it is not known if they are related to Soriatane (see PRECAUTIONS).

Reproductive: Vulvo-vaginitis due to *Candida albicans*

Skin and Appendages: Thinning of the skin, skin fragility and scaling may occur all over the body, particularly on the palms and soles; nail fragility is frequently observed.

Clinical Trials: During clinical trials with Soriatane, 513/525 (98%) of patients reported a total of 3545 adverse events. One-hundred sixteen patients (22%) left studies prematurely, primarily because of adverse experiences involving the mucous membranes and skin. Three patients died. Two of the deaths were not drug related (pancreatic adenocarcinoma and lung cancer); the other patient died of an acute myocardial infarction, considered remotely related to drug therapy. In clinical trials, Soriatane was associated with elevations in liver function test results or triglyceride levels and hepatitis.

The tables below list by body system and frequency the adverse events reported during clinical trials of 525 patients with psoriasis.

[See table 3 at top of page 1158]

[See table 4 at top of previous page]

Laboratory: Soriatane therapy induces changes in liver function tests in a significant number of patients. Elevations of AST (SGOT), ALT (SGPT) or LDH were experienced by approximately 1 in 3 patients treated with Soriatane. In most patients, elevations were slight to moderate and returned to normal either during continuation of therapy or after cessation of treatment. In patients receiving Soriatane during clinical trials, 66% and 33% experienced elevation in triglycerides and cholesterol, respectively. Decreased high density lipoproteins (HDL) occurred in 40% (see WARNINGS). Transient, usually reversible elevations of alkaline phosphatase have been observed.

Table 5 lists the laboratory abnormalities reported during clinical trials.

[See table 5 below]

OVERDOSAGE

In the event of acute overdosage, Soriatane must be withdrawn at once. Symptoms of overdose are identical to acute hypervitaminosis A, ie, headache and vertigo. The acute oral toxicity (LD_{50}) of acitretin in both mice and rats was greater than 4000 mg/kg.

In one reported case of overdose, a 32-year-old male with Darier's disease took 21 × 25 mg capsules (525 mg single dose). He vomited several hours later but experienced no other ill effects.

All female patients of childbearing potential who have taken an overdose of Soriatane must: 1) Have a pregnancy test at the time of overdose; 2) Be counseled as per the boxed CONTRAINDICATIONS AND WARNINGS and PRECAUTIONS sections regarding birth defects and contraceptive use for at least 3 years' duration after the overdose.

DOSAGE AND ADMINISTRATION

There is intersubject variation in the pharmacokinetics, clinical efficacy and incidence of side effects with Soriatane. A number of the more common side effects are dose related. Individualization of dosage is required to achieve sufficient therapeutic response while minimizing side effects. Soriatane therapy should be initiated at 25 to 50 mg per day, given as a single dose with the main meal. Maintenance doses of 25 to 50 mg per day may be given dependent upon an individual patient's response to initial treatment. Relapses may be treated as outlined for initial therapy.

When Soriatane is used with phototherapy, the prescriber should decrease the phototherapy dose, dependent on the patient's individual response (see PRECAUTIONS: General).

Females who have taken Tegison (etretinate) must continue to follow the contraceptive recommendations for Tegison.

Information for Pharmacists: A Soriatane Medication Guide must be given to the patient each time Soriatane is dispensed, as required by law.

HOW SUPPLIED

Brown and white capsules, 10 mg, imprinted SORIATANE 10; bottles of 30 (NDC 0004-0288-57).

Brown and yellow capsules, 25 mg, imprinted SORIATANE 25; bottles of 30 (NDC 0004-0289-57).

Store between 15° and 25°C (59° and 77°F). Protect from light. Avoid exposure to high temperatures and humidity after the bottle is opened.

REFERENCES

1. Berbis Ph, et al.: *Arch Dermatol Res* (1988) 280:388-389. **2.** Maier H, Honigsmann H: Concentration of etretinate in plasma and subcutaneous fat after long-term acitretin. *Lancet* 348:1107, 1996. **3.** Geiger JM, Walker M: Is there a reproductive safety risk in male patients treated with acitretin (Neotigason®/Soriatane®)? *Dermatology* 205: 105-107, 2002. **4.** Sigg C, et al.: Andrological investigations in patients treated with etretin. *Dermatologica* 175:48-49, 1987. **5.** Parsch EM, et al.: Andrological investigation in men treated with acitretin (Ro 10-1670). *Andrologia* 22: 479-482, 1990. **6.** Kadar L, et al.: Spermatological investigations in psoriatic patients treated with acitretin. In: Pharmacology of Retinoids in the Skin; Reichert U. et al., ed, KARGER, Basel, vol. 3, pp 253-254, 1988.

PATIENT AGREEMENT/INFORMED CONSENT for FEMALE Patients

To be completed by the patient, her parent/guardian* and signed by her prescriber.

Read each item below and initial in the space provided to show that you understand each item and agree to follow your prescriber's instructions. **Do not sign this consent and do not take Soriatane if there is anything that you do not understand.**

*A parent or guardian of a minor patient (under age 18) must also read and initial each item before signing the consent.

(Patient's Name)

1. I understand that there is a very high risk that my unborn baby could have severe birth defects if I am pregnant or become pregnant while taking Soriatane in any amount even for short periods of time. Birth defects have also happened in babies of women who became pregnant after stopping Soriatane treatment. INITIAL: ______
2. I understand that I must not take Soriatane if I am pregnant. INITIAL: ______
3. I understand that I must not become pregnant while taking Soriatane and for at least 3 years after the end of my treatment with Soriatane. INITIAL: ______
4. I know that I must avoid drinks, food, and medicines, including over-the-counter products, that contain alcohol. This is extremely important, because alcohol changes Soriatane in the blood into a drug that takes even longer to leave the body. This means the risk of birth defects may last longer than 3 years if I swallow any form of alcohol during Soriatane therapy or for 2 months after I stop taking Soriatane. INITIAL: ______
5. I understand that I must avoid sexual intercourse completely, or I must use 2 separate effective forms of birth control (contraception) **at the same time.** The only ex-

Table 5. Abnormal Laboratory Test Results Reported During Clinical Trials
Percent of Patients Reporting

BODY SYSTEM	50% to 75%	25% to 50%	10% to 25%	1% to 10%
Electrolytes			Increased: – Phosphorus – Potassium – Sodium Increased and decreased: –Magnesium	Decreased: – Phosphorus – Potassium – Sodium Increased and decreased: – Calcium – Chloride
Hematologic		Increased: – Reticulocytes	Decreased: – Hematocrit – Hemoglobin – WBC Increased: – Haptoglobin – Neutrophils – WBC	Increased: – Bands – Basophils – Eosinophils – Hematocrit – Hemoglobin – Lymphocytes – Monocytes Decreased: – Haptoglobin – Lymphocytes – Neutrophils – Reticulocytes Increased or decreased: – Platelets – RBC
Hepatic		Increased: – Cholesterol – LDH – SGOT – SGPT Decreased: – HDL cholesterol	Increased: – Alkaline phosphatase – Direct bilirubin – GGTP	Increased: – Globulin – Total bilirubin – Total protein Increased and decreased: – Serum albumin
Miscellaneous	Increased – Triglycerides	Increased: – CPK – Fasting blood sugar	Decreased: – Fasting blood sugar – High occult blood	Increased and decreased: – Iron
Renal			Increased: – Uric acid	Increased: – BUN – Creatinine
Urinary		WBC in urine	Acetonuria Hematuria RBC in urine	Glycosuria Proteinuria

ception is if I have had surgery to remove the womb (a hysterectomy) or my prescriber has told me I have gone completely through menopause.

INITIAL: ________

6. I have been told by my prescriber that 2 effective forms of birth control (contraception) must be used at the same time for at least 1 month before starting Soriatane, for the entire time of Soriatane therapy, and for at least 3 years after Soriatane treatment has stopped.

INITIAL: ________

7. I understand that birth control pills and injectable/implantable/insertable/topical (patch) hormonal birth control products are among the most effective forms of birth control. However, any form of birth control can fail. Therefore, I must use 2 different methods at the same time, every time I have sexual intercourse, even if 1 of the methods I choose is birth control pills, injections, or tubal ligation (tube-tying).

INITIAL: ________

8. I understand that the following are considered effective forms of birth control: Primary: Tubal ligation (tying my tubes), partner's vasectomy, birth control pills, injectable/implantable/insertable/topical (patch) hormonal birth control products, and an IUD (intrauterine device).
Secondary: Diaphragms, latex condoms, and cervical caps. Each must be used with a spermicide, which is a special cream or jelly that kills sperm.
I understand that at least 1 of my 2 methods of birth control must be a primary method.

INITIAL: ________

9. I will talk with my prescriber about any medicines or dietary supplements I plan to take during my Soriatane treatment because hormonal birth control methods (for example, birth control pills) may not work if I am taking certain medicines or herbal products (for example, St. John's Wort).

INITIAL: ________

10. I understand that if I have taken Tegison (etretinate), I must continue to follow the birth control (contraception) recommendations for Tegison.

INITIAL: ________

11. Unless I have had a hysterectomy or my prescriber says I have gone completely through menopause, I understand that I must have 2 negative pregnancy test results before I can get a prescription for Soriatane. The first pregnancy test should be done when my prescriber decides to prescribe Soriatane. The second pregnancy test should be done during the first 5 days of my menstrual period right before starting Soriatane therapy, or as instructed by my prescriber. I will then have pregnancy tests on a regular basis as instructed by my prescriber during my Soriatane therapy.

INITIAL: ________

12. I understand that I should not start taking Soriatane until I am *sure* that I am not pregnant and have negative results from 2 pregnancy tests.

INITIAL: ________

13. I have read and understand the materials my prescriber has given to me, including the Soriatane Pregnancy Prevention Program. My prescriber gave me and asked me to watch the video about contraception (birth control). I was told about a confidential counseling line that I may call at Connetics for more information about birth control(1-888-500-DERM (3376)).

INITIAL: ________

14. I have received information on emergency contraception (birth control).

INITIAL: ________

15. I understand that I may receive a free contraceptive (birth control) counseling session and pregnancy testing. My prescriber can give me a Soriatane Patient Referral Form for this free consultation.

INITIAL: ________

16. I understand that I should receive counseling from my prescriber, repeated on a regular basis, about contraception (birth control) and behaviors associated with an increased risk of pregnancy.

INITIAL: ________

17. I understand that I must stop taking Soriatane right away and call my prescriber if I get pregnant, miss my menstrual period, stop using birth control, or have sexual intercourse without using my 2 birth control methods during and at least 3 years after stopping Soriatane treatment.

INITIAL: ________

18. If I do become pregnant while on Soriatane or at any time within 3 years of stopping Soriatane, I understand that I should report my pregnancy to Connetics at 1-888-500-DERM (3376) or to the Food and Drug Administration (FDA) MedWatch program at 1-800-FDA-1088. The information I share will be kept confidential (private) and will help the company and the FDA evaluate the Pregnancy Prevention Program.

INITIAL: ________

My prescriber has answered all my questions about Soriatane. I understand that it is my responsibility not to get pregnant during Soriatane treatment or for at least 3 years after I stop taking Soriatane. I now authorize my prescriber ________ to begin my treatment with Soriatane.

Patient signature: ________ Date: ________

Parent/guardian signature (if under age 18): ________

________ Date: ________

Please print: Patient name and address ________

________ Telephone: ________

I have fully explained to the patient, ________, the nature and purpose of the treatment described above and the risks to females of childbearing potential. I have asked the patient if she has any questions regarding her treatment with Soriatane and have answered those questions to the best of my ability.

Prescriber signature: ________ Date: ________

Medication Guide for Patients:

Read this Medication Guide carefully before you start taking Soriatane and read it each time you get more Soriatane. There may be new information.

The first information in this Guide is about birth defects and how to avoid pregnancy. **After this section there is important safety information about possible effects for any patient taking Soriatane.** ALL patients should read this entire Medication Guide carefully.

This information does not take the place of talking with your prescriber about your medical condition or treatment.

What is the most important information I should know about Soriatane?

Soriatane can cause severe birth defects. If you are a female who can get pregnant, you should use Soriatane only if you are not pregnant now, can avoid becoming pregnant for at least 3 years, and other medicines do not work for your severe psoriasis or you cannot use other psoriasis medicines. Information about effects on unborn babies and about how to avoid pregnancy is found in the next section: "What are the important warnings and instructions for females taking Soriatane?".

CAUSES BIRTH DEFECTS

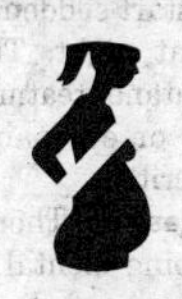

DO NOT GET PREGNANT

What are the important warnings and instructions for females taking Soriatane?

- **Before you receive your Soriatane prescription, you should have discussed and signed a Patient Information/Consent form with your prescriber. This is to help make sure you understand the risk of birth defects and how to avoid getting pregnant. If you did not talk to your prescriber about this and sign the form, contact your prescriber.**
- **You must not take Soriatane if you are pregnant or might become pregnant during treatment or at any time for at least 3 years after you stop treatment because Soriatane can cause severe birth defects.**
- **During Soriatane treatment and for 2 months after you stop Soriatane treatment, you must avoid drinks, foods, and all medicines that contain alcohol. This includes over-the-counter products that contain alcohol.** Avoiding alcohol is very important, because alcohol changes Soriatane into a drug that may take longer than 3 years to leave your body. The chance of birth defects may last longer than 3 years if you swallow any form of alcohol during Soriatane therapy and for 2 months after you stop taking Soriatane.
- **You and your prescriber must be sure you are not pregnant before you start Soriatane therapy. You must** have **negative** results from **2 pregnancy tests.** A negative result shows you are not pregnant. Because it takes a few days after pregnancy begins for a test to show that you are pregnant, the first negative test may not ensure you are not pregnant. Do not take Soriatane until you have negative results from 2 pregnancy tests.
- The **first pregnancy test** will be done at the time you and your prescriber decide if Soriatane might be right for you.
- The **second pregnancy test** will usually be done during the first 5 days of your menstrual period, right before you plan to start Soriatane. Your prescriber may suggest another time.
- **Discuss effective birth control (contraception) with your prescriber. You must use 2 effective forms of birth control (contraception) at the same time during all of the following:**
  - for at least 1 month before beginning Soriatane treatment
  - during treatment with Soriatane
  - for at least 3 years after stopping Soriatane treatment
- **You must use 2 effective forms of birth control (contraception) at the same time even if you think you cannot become pregnant, unless 1 of the following is true for you:**
  - You had your womb (uterus) removed during an operation (a hysterectomy).
  - Your prescriber said you have gone completely through menopause (the "change of life").
  - You choose a method called "abstinence". This means that you are absolutely certain (100% sure) you will not have sex with a male partner for at least 1 month before, during, and for at least 3 years after Soriatane treatment.
- **You can get a free birth control counseling session and pregnancy testing from a prescriber or family planning expert. Your prescriber can give you a Soriatane Patient Referral Form for this free session.**
- **You must use 2 effective forms of birth control (contraception) at the same time every time you repeat Soriatane treatment. You must use birth control for at least 1 month before you start Soriatane, during treatment, and at least 3 years after you stop Soriatane treatment.**
- **The following are considered effective forms of birth control:**

Primary Forms:
- having your tubes tied (tubal ligation)
- partner's vasectomy
- IUD (intrauterine device)
- birth control pills that contain both estrogen and progestin (combination oral contraceptives)
- hormonal birth control products that are injected, implanted, or inserted in your body
- birth control patch

Secondary Forms (use with a Primary Form):
- diaphragms with spermicide
- latex condoms with spermicide
- cervical caps with spermicide

At least 1 of your 2 methods of birth control must be a primary form.

- **If you have sex at any time without using 2 effective forms of birth control (contraception) at the same time, or if you get pregnant or miss your period, stop using Soriatane and call your prescriber right away.**
- **Consider "Emergency Contraception" (EC) if you have sex with a male without correctly using 2 effective forms of birth control (contraception) at the same time.** EC is also called "emergency birth control" or the "morning after" pill. Contact your prescriber **as soon as possible** if you have sex without using 2 effective forms of birth control (contraception) at the same time, because EC works best if it is used within 1 or 2 days after sex. EC is not a replacement for your usual 2 effective forms of birth control (contraception) because it is not as effective as regular birth control methods.
  You can get EC from private doctors or nurse practitioners, women's health centers, or hospital emergency rooms. You can get the name and phone number of EC providers nearest you by calling the free Emergency Contraception Hotline at 1-888-NOT-2-LATE (1-888-668-2528).
- **Stop taking Soriatane right away and contact your prescriber if you get pregnant while taking Soriatane or at any time for at least 3 years after treatment has stopped. You need to discuss the possible effects on the unborn baby with your prescriber.**
- **If you do become pregnant while taking Soriatane or at any time for at least 3 years after stopping Soriatane, you should report your pregnancy to Connetics at 1-888-500-DERM (3376) or directly to the Food and Drug Administration (FDA) MedWatch program (1-800-FDA-1088).** Your name will be kept in private (confidential). The information you share will help the FDA and the manufacturer evaluate the Pregnancy Prevention Program for Soriatane.
- **Do not take Soriatane if you are breast feeding.** Soriatane can pass into your milk and may harm your baby. You will need to choose either to breast feed or take Soriatane, but not both.

What should males know before taking Soriatane?

Small amounts of Soriatane are found in the semen of males taking Soriatane. Based upon available information, it appears that these small amounts of Soriatane in semen pose little, if any, risk to an unborn child while a male patient is taking the drug or after it is discontinued. Discuss any concerns you have about this with your prescriber.

All patients should read the rest of this Medication Guide.

What is Soriatane?

Soriatane is a medicine used to treat severe forms of psoriasis in adults. Psoriasis is a skin disease that causes cells in the outer layer of the skin to grow faster than normal and pile up on the skin's surface. In the most common type of psoriasis, the skin becomes inflamed and produces red, thickened areas, often with silvery scales. **Because Soriatane can have serious side effects,** you should talk with your prescriber about whether Soriatane's possible benefits outweigh its possible risks.

Soriatane may not work right away. You may have to wait 2 to 3 months before you get the full benefit of Soriatane. Psoriasis gets worse for some patients when they first start Soriatane treatment.

Soriatane has not been studied in children.

Who should not take Soriatane?

- **Do NOT take Soriatane if you can get pregnant.** Do not take Soriatane if you are pregnant or might get pregnant during Soriatane treatment or at any time for **at least 3 years** after you stop Soriatane treatment (see "What are the important warnings and instructions for females taking Soriatane?").
- **Do NOT take Soriatane if you are breast feeding.** Soriatane can pass into your milk and may harm your baby. You will need to choose either to breast feed or take Soriatane, but not both.
- **Do NOT take Soriatane if you have severe liver or kidney disease.**

Continued on next page

Soriatane—Cont.

- **Do NOT take Soriatane if you have repeated high blood lipids** (fat in the blood).
- **Do NOT take Soriatane if you take these medicines:**
  - methotrexate
  - tetracyclines

  The use of these medicines with Soriatane may cause **serious** side effects.
- **Do NOT take Soriatane if you are allergic to acitretin,** the active ingredient in Soriatane, to any of the other ingredients (see the end of this Medication Guide for a list of all the ingredients in Soriatane), or to any similar drugs (ask your prescriber or pharmacist whether any drugs you are allergic to are related to Soriatane).

Tell your prescriber if you have or ever had:
- diabetes or high blood sugar
- liver problems
- kidney problems
- high cholesterol or high triglycerides (fat in the blood)
- heart disease
- depression
- alcoholism
- an allergic reaction to a medication

Your prescriber needs this information to decide if Soriatane is right for you and to know what dose is best for you.

Tell your prescriber about all the medicines you take, including prescription and non-prescription medicines, vitamins, and herbal supplements. Some medicines can cause **serious side effects** if taken while you also take Soriatane. Some medicines may affect how Soriatane works, or Soriatane may affect how your other medicines work. **Be especially sure to tell your prescriber if you are taking the following medicines:**
- methotrexate
- tetracyclines
- phenytoin
- vitamin A supplements
- progestin-only oral contraceptives ("minipills")
- Tegison® or Tigason (etretinate). Tell your prescriber if you have ever taken this medicine in the past.
- St. John's Wort herbal supplement

Tell your prescriber if you are getting phototherapy treatment. Your doses of phototherapy may need to be changed to prevent a burn.

How should I take Soriatane?
- Take Soriatane with food.
- Be sure to take your medicine as prescribed by your prescriber. The dose of Soriatane varies from patient to patient. The number of capsules you must take is chosen specially for you by your prescriber. This dose may change during treatment.
- If you miss a dose, do not double the next dose. Skip the missed dose and resume your normal schedule.
- If you take too much Soriatane (overdose), call your local poison control center or emergency room.

You should have **blood tests** for liver function, cholesterol and triglycerides before starting treatment and during treatment to check your body's response to Soriatane. Your prescriber may also do other tests.

Once you stop taking Soriatane, your psoriasis may return. Do *not* treat this new psoriasis with leftover Soriatane. It is important to see your prescriber again for treatment recommendations because your situation may have changed.

What should I avoid while taking Soriatane?
- **Avoid pregnancy.** See "What is the most important information I should know about Soriatane?", and "What are the important warnings and instructions for females taking Soriatane?".
- **Avoid breast feeding.** See "What are the important warnings and instructions for females taking Soriatane?".
- **Avoid alcohol.** Females must avoid drinks, foods, medicines, and over-the-counter products that contain alcohol. The risk of birth defects may continue for longer than 3 years if you swallow any form of alcohol during Soriatane treatment and for 2 months after stopping Soriatane (see "What are the important warnings and instructions for females taking Soriatane?").
- **Avoid giving blood. Do not donate blood** while you are taking Soriatane and **for at least 3 years after stopping** Soriatane treatment. Soriatane in your blood can harm an unborn baby if your blood is given to a pregnant woman. Soriatane does not affect your ability to **receive** a blood transfusion.
- **Avoid progestin-only birth control pills ("minipills").** This type of birth control pill may not work while you take Soriatane. Ask your prescriber if you are not sure what type of pills you are using.
- **Avoid night driving if you develop any sudden vision problems.** Stop taking Soriatane and call your prescriber if this occurs (see "Serious side effects").
- **Avoid non-medical ultraviolet (UV) light.** Soriatane can make your skin more sensitive to UV light. Do not use sunlamps, and avoid sunlight as much as possible. If you are taking light treatment (phototherapy), your prescriber may need to change your light dosages to avoid burns.
- **Avoid dietary supplements containing vitamin A.** Soriatane is related to vitamin A. Therefore, do not take supplements containing vitamin A, because they may add to the unwanted effects of Soriatane. Check with your prescriber or pharmacist if you have any questions about vitamin supplements.
- **DO NOT SHARE Soriatane with anyone else, even if they have the same symptoms.** Your medicine may harm them or their unborn child.

What are the possible side effects of Soriatane?
- **Soriatane can cause birth defects.** See "What is the most important information I should know about Soriatane?" and "What are the important warnings and instructions for females taking Soriatane?"
- Psoriasis gets worse for some patients when they first start Soriatane treatment. Some patients have more redness or itching. If this happens, tell your prescriber. These symptoms usually get better as treatment continues, but your prescriber may need to change the amount of your medicine.

Serious side effects. These do not happen often, but they can lead to permanent harm, or rarely, to death. Stop taking Soriatane and call your prescriber right away if you get the following signs or symptoms:
- **Bad headaches, nausea, vomiting, blurred vision.** These symptoms can be signs of increased brain pressure that can lead to blindness or even death.
- **Decreased vision in the dark** (night blindness). Since this can start suddenly, you should be very careful when driving at night. This problem usually goes away when Soriatane treatment stops. If you develop **any** vision problems or eye pain stop taking Soriatane and call your prescriber.
- **Depression.** There have been some reports of patients developing mental problems including a depressed mood, aggressive feelings, or thoughts of ending their own life (suicide). These events, including suicidal behavior, have been reported in patients taking other drugs similar to Soriatane as well as in patients taking Soriatane. Since other things may have contributed to these problems, it is not known if they are related to Soriatane. It is very important to stop taking Soriatane and call your prescriber right away if you develop such problems.
- **Yellowing of your skin or the whites of your eyes, nausea and vomiting, loss of appetite, or dark urine.** These can be signs of serious liver damage.
- **Aches or pains in your bones, joints, muscles, or back; trouble moving; loss of feeling in your hands or feet.** These can be signs of abnormal changes to your bones or muscles.
- **Frequent urination, great thirst or hunger.** Soriatane can affect blood sugar control, even if you do not already have diabetes. These are some of the signs of high blood sugar.
- **Shortness of breath, dizziness, nausea, chest pain, weakness, trouble speaking, or swelling of a leg. These may be signs of a heart attack, blood clots, or stroke.** Soriatane can cause serious changes in blood fats (lipids). It is possible for these changes to cause blood vessel blockages that lead to heart attacks, strokes, or blood clots.

Common side effects. If you develop any of these side effects or any unusual reaction, check with your prescriber to find out if you need to change the amount of Soriatane you take. These side effects usually get better if the Soriatane dose is reduced or Soriatane is stopped.
- **Chapped lips; peeling fingertips, palms, and soles; itching; scaly skin all over; weak nails; sticky or fragile (weak) skin; runny or dry nose, or nosebleeds.** Your prescriber or pharmacist can recommend a lotion or cream to help treat drying or chapping.
- **Dry mouth**
- **Joint pain**
- **Tight muscles**
- **Hair loss.** Most patients have some hair loss, but this condition varies among patients. No one can tell if you will lose hair, how much hair you may lose or if and when it may grow back.
- **Dry eyes.** Soriatane may dry your eyes. Wearing **contact lenses** may be uncomfortable during and after treatment with Soriatane because of the dry feeling in your eyes. If this happens, remove your contact lenses and call your prescriber. Also read the section about vision under "Serious side effects".
- **Rise in blood fats (lipids).** Soriatane can cause your blood fats (lipids) to rise. Most of the time this is not serious. But sometimes the increase can become a serious problem (see information under "Serious side effects"). You should have blood tests as directed by your prescriber.

These are not all the possible side effects of Soriatane. For more information, ask your prescriber or pharmacist.

How should I store Soriatane?

Keep Soriatane away from sunlight, high temperature, and humidity. **Keep Soriatane away from children.**

What are the ingredients in Soriatane?

Active ingredient: acitretin

Inactive ingredients: microcrystalline cellulose, sodium ascorbate, gelatin, black monogramming ink and maltodextrin (a mixture of polysaccharides). Gelatin capsule shells contain gelatin, iron oxide (yellow, black, and red), and titanium dioxide. They may also contain benzyl alcohol, carboxymethylcellulose sodium, edetate calcium disodium.

General information about the safe and effective use of Soriatane

Medicines are sometimes prescribed for purposes other than those listed in a Medication Guide. Do not use Soriatane for a condition for which it was not prescribed. Do not give Soriatane to other people, even if they have the same symptoms that you have.

This Medication Guide summarizes the most important information about Soriatane. If you would like more information, talk with your prescriber. You can ask your pharmacist or prescriber for information about Soriatane that is written for health professionals.

This Medication Guide has been approved by the U.S. Food and Drug Administration.

Tegison® is a registered trademark of Hoffmann-La Roche Inc.

℞ only

Manufactured for
Connetics Corporation
Palo Alto, CA 94303
27898424
March 2004

connetics®

The interlocking C design is a trademark, and Connetics and Soriatane are registered trademarks of Connetics Corporation.

Shown in Product Identification Guide, page 311

CPH International Corp.

P. O. BOX 11439
OAKLAND, CA 94611

For Medical Information Contact:
Fax: (510) 352-6009

The following products are available for export.

Direct inquiries to
CPH International Corp. P.O. Box 94611 Oakland, CA 94611
Fax: (510) 352-6009

In addition to the labeling of the products listed below, the following products are also available from CPH International Corp.:

PROCIRC/ECOTRAN/GINKO-Q/UBIGIN-Q
MULTIZYME/SUPERZYME CHEWABLE/NEO-PROZYME/ABSORPASE
NT-KINASE 500/FIBRINASE
ACROBIN, CINAPLEX, FENAXIN, PANEMAX, RENIPLY, SNOVAR, TOFIPAN, VASONAMIN, ZIZODAL.

CATASOD®-OCUXTRA/ OPTIGOLD®/MACUTEIN® OTC
Lutein and Zeaxanthin with ocular antioxidants

DESCRIPTION

Lutein and Zeaxanthin are found in the macula of the human retina, as well as the human crystalline lens. They play a role in protection against age-related macular degeneration (ARMD) and cataract formation. The antioxidant properties of lutein and zeaxanthin together with ocular antioxidants (selenium, zinc, copper, vitamin A, C, E, etc.) inhibit free radical damage caused by light and oxygen.

INDICATIONS

CATASOD®-OCUXTRA is formulated to provide antioxidant protection and support for the eye. The formulation contains 5 mg of Lutein/Zeaxanthin and essential ocular antioxidants.

CYNAXIN®/ATK-250/ARTICHIN/SCOKIN OTC
Cynarin from 250 mg leaf extract of Cynara scolymus

DESCRIPTION

Cynarin, lipotropic factors and vitamin B complex are of value for persons who are suffering from liver dysfunction such as hepatitis fatty liver, alcoholism and hepatic intoxication. The pharmacological actions of cynara scolymus (European globe artichoke) leaves are hepatic cell regenerating, choleretic, diuretic and cholesterol lowering, etc..

IMMULEIN® OTC
Hepalein® and hepatonic preparation

DESCRIPTION

IMMULEIN® is a homeopathic formulation of Hepalein® (natural antibody substance processed from bile extract), lipotropic factors, amino acids. serum albumin and vitamins. The formula is of value for persons who are suffering from liver disorders, viral hepatitis and alcoholism.

Cubist Pharmaceuticals, Inc.
65 HAYDEN AVENUE
LEXINGTON, MA 02421

Direct Inquiries to:
1-866-RX-DAPTO
(phone) 866-793-2786
(fax) 866-305-2039

CUBICIN® ℞

[kew-bĭ-sĭn]
(daptomycin for injection)
℞ only

To reduce the development of drug-resistant bacteria and maintain the effectiveness of CUBICIN and other antibacterial drugs, CUBICIN should be used only to treat or prevent infections caused by bacteria.

DESCRIPTION

CUBICIN contains daptomycin, a cyclic lipopeptide antibacterial agent derived from the fermentation of *Streptomyces roseosporus*. The chemical name is *N*-decanoyl-L-tryptophyl-L-asparaginyl-L-aspartyl-L-threonylglycyl-L-ornithyl-L-aspartyl-D-alanyl-L-aspartylglycyl-D-seryl-*threo*-3-methyl-L-glutamyl-3-anthraniloyl-L-alanine ϵ_1-lactone. The chemical structure is:

The empirical formula is $C_{72}H_{101}N_{17}O_{26}$; the molecular weight is 1620.67. CUBICIN is supplied as a sterile, preservative-free, pale yellow to light brown, lyophilized cake containing approximately 900 mg/g of daptomycin for intravenous use following reconstitution with 0.9% sodium chloride injection. The only inactive ingredient is sodium hydroxide, which is used in minimal quantities for pH adjustment. Freshly reconstituted solutions of CUBICIN range in color from pale yellow to light brown.

CLINICAL PHARMACOLOGY

Pharmacokinetics: The mean (SD) pharmacokinetic parameters of daptomycin on Day 7 following the intravenous administration of 4 mg/kg, 6 mg/kg, and 8 mg/kg q24h to healthy young adults (mean age 35.8 years) are summarized in Table 1.

[See table 1 above]

Table 1 Mean (SD) Daptomycin Pharmacokinetic Parameters in Healthy Volunteers on Day 7

Dose mg/kg	C_{max} (μg/mL)	T_{max}* (h)	AUC_{0-24} (μg•h/mL)	$t_{1/2}$ (h)	V_d (L/kg)	CL_T (mL/h/kg)	CL_R (mL/h/kg)	Ae_{24} %
4 (n=6)	57.8 (3.0)	0.8 (0.5,1.0)	494 (75)	8.1 (1.0)	0.096 (0.009)	8.3 (1.3)	4.8 (1.3)	53.0 (10.8)
6 (n=6)	98.6 (12)	0.5 (0.5,1.0)	747 (91)	8.9 (1.3)	0.104 (0.013)	8.1 (1.0)	4.4 (0.3)	47.4 (11.5)
8 (n=6)	133 (13.5)	0.5 (0.5,1.0)	1130 (117)	9.0 (1.2)	0.092 (0.012)	7.2 (0.8)	3.7 (0.5)	52.1 (5.19)

*Median (minimum, maximum)
C_{max} = Maximum plasma concentration; T_{max} = Time to C_{max}; AUC_{0-24} = Area under concentration-time curve from 0 to 24 hours; $t_{1/2}$ = Terminal elimination half-life; V_d = Apparent volume of distribution; CL_T = Systemic clearance; CL_R = Renal clearance; Ae_{24} = Percent of dose recovered in urine over 24 hours as unchanged daptomycin following the first dose.

Daptomycin pharmacokinetics are nearly linear and time-independent at doses up to 6 mg/kg administered once daily for 7 days. Steady-state concentrations are achieved by the third daily dose. The mean (SD) steady-state trough concentrations (Days 4 to 8) attained following administration of 4, 6, and 8 mg/kg q24h are 5.9 (1.6), 9.4 (2.5), and 14.9 (2.9) μg/mL, respectively.

Distribution: Daptomycin is reversibly bound to human plasma proteins, primarily to serum albumin, in a concentration-independent manner. The mean serum protein binding of daptomycin was approximately 92% in healthy adults after the administration of 4 mg/kg or 6 mg/kg. Serum protein binding was not altered as a function of daptomycin concentration, dose, or number of doses received.

In clinical studies, mean serum protein binding in subjects with CL_{CR} ≥30 mL/min was comparable to that observed in healthy subjects with normal renal function. However, there was a trend toward decreasing serum protein binding among subjects with CL_{CR} <30 mL/min (87.6%), including hemodialysis patients (85.9%) and CAPD patients (83.5%). The protein binding of daptomycin in subjects with hepatic impairment (Child-Pugh B) was similar to healthy adult subjects. The apparent volume of distribution of daptomycin at steady-state in healthy adult subjects was approximately 0.09 L/kg.

Metabolism: *In vitro* studies with human hepatocytes indicate that daptomycin does not inhibit or induce the activities of the following human cytochrome (CYP) P450 isoforms: 1A2, 2A6, 2C9, 2C19, 2D6, 2E1, and 3A4. It is unlikely that daptomycin will inhibit or induce the metabolism of drugs metabolized by the CYP P450 system. It is unknown whether daptomycin is a substrate of the CYP P450 system.

In 5 healthy young adults, after infusion of radiolabeled ^{14}C-daptomycin, the plasma total radioactivity was similar to the concentration determined by microbiological assay. Inactive metabolites of daptomycin have been detected in the urine, as determined by the difference in total radiolabeled concentrations and microbiologically active concentrations. The site of metabolism has not been identified.

Excretion: Daptomycin is excreted primarily by the kidney. In a mass balance study of 5 healthy subjects using radiolabeled daptomycin, approximately 78% of the administered dose was recovered from urine based on total radioactivity (approximately 52% of the dose based on microbiologically active concentrations) and 5.7% of the dose was recovered from feces (collected for up to 9 days), based on total radioactivity.

Because renal excretion is the primary route of elimination, dosing adjustment is necessary in patients with severe renal insufficiency (CL_{CR} <30 mL/min) (see **DOSAGE AND ADMINISTRATION**).

SPECIAL POPULATIONS

Renal Insufficiency: Population derived pharmacokinetic parameters were determined for patients with skin and skin structure infections and healthy non-infected subjects with varying degrees of renal function (n=282). Following the administration of a single 4 mg/kg IV dose of daptomycin, the plasma clearance (CL_T) was reduced and the systemic exposure ($AUC_{0-\infty}$) was increased with decreasing renal function (see Table 2). The mean $AUC_{0-\infty}$ was not markedly different for subjects and patients with CL_{CR} 30-80 mL/min as compared to those with normal renal function (CL_{CR} >80 mL/min). The mean $AUC_{0-\infty}$ values for subjects and patients with CL_{CR} <30 mL/min and hemodialysis (dosed post dialysis) / CAPD subjects were approximately 2- and 3-times higher, respectively, than the values in individuals with normal renal function. The mean C_{max} ranged from 59.6 μg/mL to 69.6 μg/mL in subjects with CL_{CR} ≥30 mL/min while those with CL_{CR} <30 mL/min ranged from 41.1 μg/mL to 57.7 μg/mL in 11 non-infected adult subjects undergoing dialysis, approximately 15% and 11% of the administered dose was removed by 4 hours of hemodialysis and 48 hours of CAPD, respectively. The recommended dosing regimens is 4 mg/kg once every 24 hours for patients with CL_{CR} ≥30 mL/min and 4 mg/kg once every 48 hours for CL_{CR} <30 mL/min, including those on hemodialysis and CAPD. Daptomycin should be administered following the completion of hemodialysis on hemodialysis days (see **DOSAGE AND ADMINISTRATION**).

[See table 2 above]

Table 2 Mean (SD) Daptomycin Population Pharmacokinetic Parameters Following a Single 30-Minute Intravenous Infusion of 4 mg/kg to Infected Patients and Non-Infected Subjects with Varying Degrees of Renal Function

Renal Function	$AUC_{0-\infty}$ (μg•h/mL)	$t_{1/2}$ (h)	V_{SS} (L/kg)	CL_T (mL/h/kg)
Normal (CL_{CR} >80 mL/min) (N=165)	417 (155)	9.39 (4.74)	0.13 (0.05)	10.9 (4.0)
Mild Renal Impairment (CL_{CR} 50-80 mL/min) (N=64)	466 (177)	10.75 (8.36)	0.12 (0.05)	9.9 (4.0)
Moderate Renal Impairment (CL_{CR} 30-<50 mL/min) (N=24)	560 (258)	14.70 (10.50)	0.15 (0.06)	8.5 (3.4)
Severe Renal Impairment (CL_{CR} <30 mL/min) (N=8)	925 (467)	27.83 (14.85)	0.20 (0.15)	5.9 (3.9)
Hemodialysis and CAPD (N=21)	1244 (374)	29.81 (6.13)	0.15 (0.04)	3.7 (1.9)

Note: CL_{CR}= Creatinine clearance estimated using the Cockroft-Gault equation with actual body weight.

Hepatic Insufficiency: The pharmacokinetics of daptomycin were evaluated in 10 subjects with moderate hepatic impairment (Child-Pugh Class B) and compared with healthy volunteers (n=9) matched for gender, age, and weight. The pharmacokinetics of daptomycin were not altered in subjects with moderate hepatic impairment. No dosage adjustment is warranted when administering daptomycin to patients with mild to moderate hepatic impairment. The pharmacokinetics of daptomycin in patients with severe hepatic insufficiency have not been evaluated.

Gender: No clinically significant gender-related differences in daptomycin pharmacokinetics have been observed between healthy male and female subjects. No dosage adjustment is warranted based on gender when administering daptomycin.

Geriatric: The pharmacokinetics of daptomycin were evaluated in 12 healthy elderly subjects (≥75 years of age) and 11 healthy young matched controls (18-30 years of age). Following administration of a single intravenous 4 mg/kg dose, the mean total clearance of daptomycin was reduced approximately 35% and the mean $AUC_{0-\infty}$ increased approximately 58% in elderly subjects compared to young healthy subjects. There were no differences in C_{max}. No dosage adjustment is warranted for elderly patients with normal (for age) renal function.

Obesity: The pharmacokinetics of daptomycin were evaluated in six moderately obese (Body Mass Index [BMI] 25-39.9 kg/m^2) and six extremely dose (BMI ≥40 kg/m^2) subjects and controls matched for age, sex, and renal function. Following administration of a single intravenous 4 mg/kg dose based on total body weight, the plasma clearance of daptomycin increased approximately 18% in moderately obese subjects and 46% in extremely obese subjects compared with non-obese controls. The $AUC_{0-\infty}$ of daptomycin increased approximately 30% in moderately obese and 31% in extremely obese subjects compared with non-obese controls. The differences were most likely due to differences in the renal clearance of daptomycin. No dosage adjustment of daptomycin is warranted in obese subjects.

Pediatric: The pharmacokinetics of daptomycin in pediatric populations (<18 years of age) have not been established.

DRUG-DRUG INTERACTIONS

Drug-drug interaction studies were performed with daptomycin and other drugs that are likely to either be co-administered or associated with overlapping toxicity.

Aztreonam: In a study in which 15 healthy adult subjects received a single dose of daptomycin IV 6 mg/kg, aztreonam 1000 mg IV, and both in combination, the C_{max} and $AUC_{0-\infty}$ of daptomycin were not significantly altered by aztreonam; the C_{max} and $AUC_{0-\infty}$ of aztreonam were not significantly altered by daptomycin. No dosage adjustment of either antibiotic is warranted when co-administered.

Tobramycin: In a study in which 6 healthy adult males received a single dose of daptomycin IV 2 mg/kg, tobramycin IV 1 mg/kg, and both in combination, the mean C_{max} and $AUC_{0-\infty}$ of daptomycin increased 12.7% and 8.7%, respectively, when administered with tobramycin. The mean C_{max} and $AUC_{0-\infty}$ of tobramycin decreased 10.7% and 6.6%, respectively, when administered with daptomycin. None of these differences was statistically significant. The interaction between daptomycin and tobramycin with a clinical dose of daptomycin (4 mg/kg) is unknown. Caution is warranted when daptomycin is co-administered with tobramycin.

Warfarin: In 16 healthy subjects, concomitant administration of daptomycin 6 mg/kg once daily for 5 days followed by a single oral dose of warfarin (25 mg) had no significant effect on the pharmacokinetics of either drug and did not significantly alter the INR (International Normalized Ratio) (see **PRECAUTIONS, Drug Interactions**).

Simvastatin: In 20 healthy subjects on a stable daily dose of simvastatin 40 mg, administration of daptomycin IV 4 mg/kg once daily for 14 days (n=10) was not associated with a higher incidence of adverse events than subjects receiving placebo once daily (n=10) (see **PRECAUTIONS, Drug Interactions**).

Probenecid: Concomitant administration of probenecid (500 mg four times daily) and a single dose of daptomycin IV 4 mg/kg did not significantly alter the C_{max} and $AUC_{0-\infty}$ of daptomycin. No dosage adjustment of daptomycin is warranted when daptomycin is co-administered with probenecid.

MICROBIOLOGY

Daptomycin is an antibacterial agent of a new class of antibiotics, the cyclic lipopeptides. Daptomycin is a natural

Continued on next page

Cubicin—Cont.

product which has clinical utility in the treatment of infections caused by aerobic Gram-positive bacteria. The *in vitro* spectrum of activity of daptomycin encompasses most clinically relevant Gram-positive pathogenic bacteria. Daptomycin retains potency against antibiotic-resistant Gram-positive bacteria, including isolates resistant to methicillin, vancomycin, and linezolid.

Daptomycin exhibits rapid, concentration-dependent bactericidal activity against Gram-positive organisms *in vitro*. This has been demonstrated both by time-kill curves and by MBC/MIC ratios using broth dilution methodology.

In vitro studies have demonstrated additive or indifferent interactions of daptomycin with other antibiotics. Antagonism, as determined by kill curve studies, has not been observed. *In vitro* synergistic interactions occurred with aminoglycosides and β-lactam antibiotics against some isolates of staphylococci and enterococci, including some MRSA isolates.

Mechanism of Action: The mechanism of action of daptomycin is distinct from any other antibiotic. Daptomycin binds to bacterial membranes and causes a rapid depolarization of membrane potential. The loss of membrane potential leads to inhibition of protein, DNA, and RNA synthesis, which results in bacterial cell death.

Resistance

Mechanisms of resistance: At this time, no mechanism of resistance to daptomycin has been identified. Currently, there are no known transferable elements that confer resistance to daptomycin.

Cross-resistance: Cross-resistance has not been observed with any other class of antibiotic.

Other: The emergence of resistance to daptomycin occurred in 2 of more than 1000 (<0.2%) infected subjects across the entire set of Phase 2 and 3 clinical trials. In one case, a resistant *S aureus* was isolated from a patient in a Phase 2 study who received daptomycin at less than the protocol-specified dose for the initial 5 days of therapy. In the second case, a resistant *E faecalis* was isolated from a patient with an infected chronic decubitus ulcer enrolled in a salvage trial.

Daptomycin has been shown to be active against most isolates of the following microorganisms both *in vitro* and in clinical infections, as described in the **INDICATIONS AND USAGE** section.

Aerobic and facultative Gram-positive microorganisms

Enterococcus faecalis (vancomycin-susceptible strains only)
Staphylococcus aureus (including methicillin-resistant strains)
Streptococcus agalactiae
Streptococcus dysgalactiae subsp *equisimilis*
Streptococcus pyogenes

The following *in vitro* data are available, but their clinical significance is unknown. Greater than 90% of the following microorganisms demonstrate an *in vitro* MIC less than or equal to the susceptible breakpoint for daptomycin versus the bacterial genus. The efficacy of daptomycin in treating clinical infections due to these microorganisms has not been established in adequate and well-controlled clinical trials.

Aerobic and facultative Gram-positive microorganisms

Corynebacterium jeikeium
Enterococcus faecalis (vancomycin-resistant strains)
Enterococcus faecium (including vancomycin-resistant strains)
Staphylococcus epidermidis (including methicillin-resistant strains)
Staphylococcus haemolyticus

Susceptibility Testing Methods

Susceptibility testing by dilution methods requires the use of daptomycin susceptibility powder. The testing also requires the presence of physiological levels of free calcium ions (50 mg/L calcium chloride) in Mueller-Hinton broth medium and a minimum of 28 mg/L calcium chloride in Mueller-Hinton agar medium.

Dilution technique: Quantitative methods are used to determine antimicrobial MICs. These MICs provide estimates of the susceptibility of bacteria to antimicrobial compounds. The MICs should be determined using a standardized procedure.[2,3] Standardized procedures are based on a dilution method (broth or agar) or equivalent with standardized inoculum concentrations and standardized concentrations of daptomycin powder. The MIC values should be interpreted according to the criteria in Table 3.

Diffusion technique: Quantitative methods that require measurement of zone diameters also provide reproducible estimates of the susceptibility of bacteria to antimicrobial compounds. One such standardized procedure requires the use of standardized inoculum concentrations.[1,3] This procedure uses paper disks impregnated with 30 µg of daptomycin to test the susceptibility of microorganisms to daptomycin. The disk diffusion interpretive criteria are provided in Table 3.

[See table 3 above]

A report of "Susceptible" indicates that the pathogen is likely to be inhibited if the antimicrobial compound in the blood reaches the concentrations usually achievable.

Quality Control: Standardized susceptibility test procedures require the use of quality control microorganisms to control the technical aspects of the procedures. Standard daptomycin powder should provide the range of values noted in Table 4. Quality control microorganisms are specific strains of organisms with intrinsic biological properties relating to resistance mechanisms and their genetic expression within bacteria; the specific strains used for microbiological quality control are not clinically significant.

Table 3 Susceptibility Interpretive Criteria for Daptomycin

Pathogen	Minimal inhibitory concentration (µg/mL)[a]			Disk diffusion zone diameter (mm)[b]		
	S	I	R	S	I	R
Staphylococcus aureus (methicillin-susceptible and methicillin-resistant)	≤1	(c)	(c)	≥16	(c)	(c)
Streptococcus pyogenes, *Streptococcus agalactiae*, and *Streptococcus dysgalactiae* subsp *equisimilis*	≤1	(c)	(c)	≥16	(c)	(c)
Enterococcus faecalis (vancomycin-susceptible only)	≤4	(c)	(c)	≥11	(c)	(c)

a. The MIC interpretive criteria for *S aureus* and *E faecalis* are applicable only to tests performed by broth microdilution using Mueller-Hinton broth adjusted to a calcium content of 50 mg/L; the MIC interpretive criteria for *Streptococcus* spp other than *S pneumoniae* are applicable only to tests performed by broth microdilution using Mueller-Hinton broth adjusted to a calcium content of 50 mg/L, supplemented with 2–5% lysed horse blood inoculated with a direct colony suspension and incubated in ambient air at 35°C for 20 to 24 hours.
b. The zone diameter interpretive criteria for *Streptococcus* spp other than *S pneumoniae* are applicable only to tests performed using Mueller-Hinton agar supplemented with 5% defibrinated sheep blood and incubated in 5% CO_2 at 35°C for 20 to 24 hours.
c. The current absence of data on daptomycin-resistant strains precludes defining any categories other than "Susceptible." Strains yielding test results suggestive of a "non-susceptible" category should be retested, and if the result is confirmed, the isolate should be submitted to a reference laboratory for further testing.

Table 4 Acceptable Quality Control Ranges for Daptomycin to Be Used in Validation of Susceptibility Test Results

QC Strain	Acceptable Quality Control Ranges: Minimum Inhibitory Concentration (MIC in µg/mL)[a]	Disk Diffusion (zone diameters in mm)[b]
Enterococcus faecalis ATCC 29212	1–8	Not applicable
Staphylococcus aureus ATCC 29213	0.25–1	Not applicable
Staphylococcus aureus ATCC 25923	Not applicable	18–23
Streptococcus pneumoniae ATCC 49619[c]	0.06–0.5[d]	19–26[e]

a. Quality control ranges reflect MICs obtained when Mueller-Hinton broth is supplemented with calcium to a final concentration of 50 mg/L.
b. Some lots of Mueller-Hinton agar are deficient in calcium and give small zone diameters.
c. This organism may be used for validation of susceptibility test results when testing *Streptococcus* spp other than *S pneumoniae*.
d. This quality control range for *S pneumoniae* is applicable only to tests performed by broth microdilution using cation adjusted Mueller-Hinton broth with 2–5% lysed horse blood inoculated with a direct colony suspension and incubated in ambient air at 35°C for 20 to 24 hours.
e. This quality control zone diameter range is applicable only to tests performed using Mueller-Hinton agar supplemented with 5% defibrinated sheep blood inoculated with a direct colony suspension and incubated in 5% CO_2 at 35°C for 20 to 24 hours.

INDICATIONS AND USAGE

CUBICIN (daptomycin for injection) is indicated for the treatment of complicated skin and skin structure infections caused by susceptible strains of the following Gram-positive microorganisms (see also **DOSAGE AND ADMINISTRATION**): *Staphylococcus aureus* (including methicillin-resistant strains), *Streptococcus pyogenes, Streptococcus agalactiae, Streptococcus dysgalactiae* subsp. *equisimilis* and *Enterococcus faecalis* (vancomycin-susceptible strains only). Combination therapy may be clinically indicated if the documented or presumed pathogens include Gram-negative or anaerobic organisms (see **CLINICAL STUDIES**).

Daptomycin is not indicated for the treatment of pneumonia.

Appropriate specimens for microbiological examination should be obtained in order to isolate and identify the causative pathogens and to determine their susceptibility to daptomycin. Empiric therapy may be initiated while awaiting test results. Antimicrobial therapy should be adjusted as needed based upon test results.

To reduce the development of drug-resistant bacteria and maintain the effectiveness of CUBICIN and other antibacterial drugs, CUBICIN should be used only to treat or prevent infections that are proven or strongly suspected to be caused by susceptible bacteria. When culture and susceptibility information are available, they should be considered in selecting or modifying antibacterial therapy. In the absence of such data, local epidemiology and susceptibility patterns may contribute to the empiric selection of therapy.

CONTRAINDICATIONS

CUBICIN is contraindicated in patients with known hypersensitivity to daptomycin.

WARNINGS

Pseudomembranous colitis has been reported with nearly all antibacterial agents, including daptomycin, and may range in severity from mild to life-threatening. Therefore, it is important to consider this diagnosis in patients who present with diarrhea subsequent to the administration of any antibacterial agent.

Treatment with antibacterial agents alters the normal flora of the colon and may permit overgrowth of clostridia. Studies indicated that a toxin produced by *Clostridium difficile* is a primary cause of "antibiotic-associated colitis."

If a diagnosis of pseudomembranous colitis has been established, appropriate therapeutic measures should be initiated. Mild cases of pseudomembranous colitis usually respond to drug discontinuation alone. In moderate to severe cases, consideration should be given to management with fluids and electrolytes, protein supplementation, and treatment with an antibacterial agent clinically effective against *C. difficile*.

PRECAUTIONS

General: The use of antibiotics may promote the overgrowth of nonsusceptible organisms. Should superinfection occur during therapy, appropriate measures should be taken.

Prescribing CUBICIN in the absence of a proven or strongly suspected bacterial infection or a prophylactic indication is unlikely to provide benefit to the patient and increases the risk of the development of drug-resistant bacteria.

Skeletal Muscle: In Phase 3 complicated skin and skin structure infection (cSSSI) trials, elevations in serum creatine phosphokinase (CPK) were reported as clinical adverse events in 15/534 (2.8%) daptomycin-treated patients, compared to 10/558 (1.8%) comparator-treated patients. Skeletal muscle effects associated with daptomycin were observed in animals (see **ANIMAL PHARMACOLOGY**).

Patients receiving CUBICIN should be monitored for the development of muscle pain or weakness, particularly of the distal extremities. CPK levels should be monitored weekly in patients who receive CUBICIN. Patients who develop unexplained elevations in CPK while receiving daptomycin should be monitored more frequently. Among patients with abnormal CPK (>500 U/L) at baseline, 2/19 (10.5%) treated with CUBICIN and 4/24 (16.7%) treated with comparator developed further increases in CPK while on therapy. In this same population, no patients developed myopathy. Daptomycin-treated patients with baseline CPK >500 U/L (n=19) did not experience an increased incidence of CPK elevations or myopathy relative to those treated with comparator (n=24).

CUBICIN should be discontinued in patients with unexplained signs and symptoms of myopathy in conjunction with CPK elevation >1000 U/L (~5× ULN), or in patients without reported symptoms who have marked elevations in CPK (≥10× ULN). In addition, consideration should be given to temporarily suspending agents associated with rhabdomyolysis, such as HMG-CoA reductase inhibitors, in patients receiving CUBICIN.

In a small number of patients in Phase 1 and Phase 2 studies, administration of CUBICIN was associated with decreases in nerve conduction velocity and with adverse events (eg, paresthesias, Bell's palsy), possibly reflective of peripheral or cranial neuropathy. Nerve conduction deficits were also detected in a similar number of comparator subjects in these studies.

In Phase 3 cSSSI and CAP studies, 7/989 (0.7%) daptomycin-treated patients and 7/1018 (0.7%) comparator-treated patients experienced paresthesias. New or worsening peripheral neuropathy was not diagnosed in any of these patients. In animals, effects of daptomycin on peripheral nerve were observed (see **ANIMAL PHARMACOL-**

OGY). Therefore, physicians should be alert to the possibility of signs and symptoms of neuropathy in patients receiving CUBICIN.

Drug Interactions: **Warfarin** Concomitant administration of daptomycin (6 mg/kg once every 24 hours for 5 days) and warfarin (25 mg single oral dose) had no significant effect on the pharmacokinetics of either drug, and the INR was not significantly altered. As experience with the concomitant administration of daptomycin and warfarin is limited to volunteer studies, anticoagulant activity in patients receiving daptomycin and warfarin should be monitored for the first several days after initiating therapy with CUBICIN (see **CLINICAL PHARMACOLOGY, Drug-Drug Interactions**).

HMG-CoA Reductase Inhibitors Inhibitors of HMG-CoA reductase may cause myopathy, which is manifested as muscle pain or weakness associated with elevated levels of CPK. There were no reports of skeletal myopathy in a placebo-controlled Phase I trial in which 10 healthy subjects on stable simvastatin therapy were treated concurrently with daptomycin (4 mg/kg once every 24 hours) for 14 days. Experience with co-administration of HMG-CoA reductase inhibitors and CUBICIN in patients is limited, therefore, consideration should be given to temporarily suspending use of HMG-CoA reductase inhibitors in patients receiving CUBICIN.

Drug-Laboratory Test Interactions: There are no reported drug-laboratory test interactions.

Carcinogenesis, Mutagenesis, Impairment of Fertility: Long-term carcinogenicity studies in animals have not been conducted to evaluate the carcinogenic potential of daptomycin. However, neither mutagenic nor clastogenic potential was found in a battery of genotoxicity tests, including the Ames assay, a mammalian cell gene mutation assay, a test for chromosomal aberrations in Chinese hamster ovary cells, an *in vivo* micronucleus assay, an *in vitro* DNA repair assay, and an *in vivo* sister chromatid exchange assay in Chinese hamsters.

Daptomycin did not affect the fertility or reproductive performance of male and female rats when administered intravenously at doses up to 150 mg/kg/day, which is approximately 9 times the estimated human exposure level based upon AUCs.

Pregnancy: **Teratogenic Effects: Pregnancy Category B** Reproductive and teratology studies performed in rats and rabbits at doses of up to 75 mg/kg, 3 and 6 times the human dose, respectively, on a body surface area basis, have revealed no evidence of harm to the fetus due to CUBICIN. There are, however, no adequate and well-controlled studies in pregnant women. Because animal reproduction studies are not always predictive of human response, this drug should be used during pregnancy only if clearly needed.

Nursing Mothers: It is not known if daptomycin is excreted in human milk. Caution should be exercised when CUBICIN is administered to nursing women.

Pediatric Use: Safety and efficacy of CUBICIN in patients under the age of 18 have not been established.

Geriatric Use: Of the 534 patients treated with CUBICIN in Phase 3 controlled clinical trials of complicated skin and skin structure infection, 27.0% were 65 years of age or older and 12.4% were 75 years or older. In the two Phase 3 clinical studies in patients with cSSSI, lower clinical success rates were seen in patients ≥65 years of age compared to those <65 years of age. In addition, treatment-emergent adverse events were more common in patients ≥65 years old than in patients <65 years of age in both cSSSI studies.

ANIMAL PHARMACOLOGY

In animals, daptomycin administration has been associated with effects on skeletal muscle with no changes in cardiac or smooth muscle. Skeletal muscle effects were characterized by degenerative/regenerative changes and variable elevations in CPK. No fibrosis or rhabdomyolysis was evident in repeat dose studies up to the highest doses tested in rats (150 mg/kg/day) and dogs (100 mg/kg/day). The degree of skeletal myopathy showed no increase when treatment was extended from 1 month to up to 6 months. Severity was dose dependent. All muscle effects, including microscopic changes, were fully reversible within 30 days following cessation of dosing.

In adult animals, effects on peripheral nerve (characterized by axonal degeneration and frequently accompanied by significant losses of patellar reflex, gag reflex, and pain perception) were observed at doses higher than those associated with skeletal myopathy. Deficits in the dogs' patellar reflexes were seen within 2 weeks of the start of treatment at 40 mg/kg (3.5 times the human AUC), with some clinical improvement noted within 2 weeks of the cessation of dosing. However, at 75 mg/kg daily for 1 month, 7/8 dogs failed to regain full patellar reflex responses within the duration of a 3 month recovery period. In a separate study in dogs receiving doses of 75 and 100 mg/kg/day for 2 weeks, minimal residual histological changes were noted at 6 months after cessation of dosing. However, recovery of peripheral nerve function was evident.

Tissue distribution studies in rats have shown that daptomycin is retained in the kidney but does not appear to penetrate across the blood-brain barrier following single and multiple doses.

ADVERSE REACTIONS

Because clinical trials are conducted under widely varying conditions, adverse reaction rates observed in the clinical trials of a drug cannot be directly compared to rates in the clinical trials of another drug and may not reflect the rates observed in practice. The adverse reaction information from clinical trials does, however, provide a basis for identifying the adverse events that appear to be related to drug use and for approximating rates.

Clinical studies sponsored by Cubist enrolled 1409 patients treated with daptomycin and 1185 treated with comparator. Most adverse events reported in these clinical studies were described as mild or moderate in intensity. In Phase 3 cSSSI trials, daptomycin was discontinued in 15/534 (2.8%) patients due to an adverse event while comparator was discontinued in 17/558 (3.0%) patients.

The rates of most common adverse events, organized by body system, observed in cSSSI patients are displayed in Table 5.

Table 6 Incidence (%) of Creatine Phosphokinase (CPK) Elevations From Baseline While on Therapy in Either Daptomycin or Comparator Treatment Groups in Phase 3 cSSSI Studies

	All patients				Patients with normal CPK at baseline			
	Daptomycin (N=430)		Comparator (N=459)		Daptomycin (N=374)		Comparator (N=392)	
	%	n	%	n	%	n	%	n
No increase	90.7%	390	91.1%	418	91.2%	341	91.1%	357
Maximum Value >1× ULN*	9.3%	40	8.9%	41	8.8%	33	8.9%	35
>2× ULN	4.9%	21	4.8%	22	3.7%	14	3.1%	12
>4× ULN	1.4%	6	1.5%	7	1.1%	4	1.0%	4
>5× ULN	1.4%	6	0.4%	2	1.1%	4	0.0%	0
>10× ULN	0.5%	2	0.2%	1	0.2%	1	0.0%	0

* ULN (Upper Limit of Normal) is defined as 200 U/L.
Note: Elevations in CPK observed in patients treated with daptomycin or comparator were not clinically or statistically significantly different (P <0.05).

Table 5 Incidence (%) of Adverse Events that Occurred in ≥ 2% of Patients in Either Daptomycin or Comparator Treatment Groups in Phase 3 cSSSI Studies

Adverse Event	Daptomycin (N=534)	Comparator* (N=558)
Gastrointestinal disorders		
Constipation	6.2%	6.8%
Nausea	5.8%	9.5%
Diarrhea	5.2%	4.3%
Vomiting	3.2%	3.8%
Dyspepsia	0.9%	2.5%
General disorders		
Injection site reactions	5.8%	7.7%
Fever	1.9%	2.5%
Nervous system disorders		
Headache	5.4%	5.4%
Insomnia	4.5%	5.4%
Dizziness	2.2%	2.0%
Skin/subcutaneous disorders		
Rash	4.3%	3.8%
Pruritis	2.8%	3.8%
Diagnostic investigations		
Abnormal liver function tests	3.0%	1.6%
Elevated CPK	2.8%	1.8%
Infections		
Fungal infections	2.6%	3.2%
Urinary tract infections	2.4%	0.5%
Vascular disorders		
Hypotension	2.4%	1.4%
Hypertension	1.1%	2.0%
Renal/urinary disorders		
Renal failure	2.2%	2.7%
Blood/lymphatic disorders		
Anemia	2.1%	2.3%
Respiratory disorders		
Dyspnea	2.1%	1.6%
Musculoskeletal disorders		
Limb pain	1.5%	2.0%
Arthralgia	0.9%	2.2%

* Comparators included vancomycin (1 g IV q12h) and semi-synthetic penicillins (ie, nafcillin, oxacillin, cloxacillin, flucloxacillin; 4-12 g/day in divided doses)

In Phase 3 studies of community-acquired pneumonia (CAP), the death rate and rates of serious cardiorespiratory adverse events were higher in daptomycin-treated patients than in comparator-treated patients. These differences were due to lack of therapeutic effectiveness of daptomycin in the treatment of CAP in patients experiencing these adverse events (see **INDICATIONS AND USAGE**). Additional adverse events that occurred in 1-2% of patients in either daptomycin- or comparator-treatment groups in the cSSSI studies are as follows: edema, cellulitis, hypoglycemia, elevated alkaline phosphatase, cough, back pain, abdominal pain, hypokalemia, hyperglycemia, decreased appetite, anxiety, chest pain, sore throat, cardiac failure, confusion, and Candida infections. These events occurred at rates ranging from 0.2-1.7% in daptomycin-treated patients and at rates of 0.4-1.8% in comparator-treated patients.

Additional drug-related adverse events (possibly or probably related) that occurred in <1% of patients receiving daptomycin in cSSSI trials are as follows:

Body as a Whole: fatigue, weakness, rigors, discomfort, jitteriness, flushing, hypersensitivity

Blood/Lymphatic System: leukocytosis, thrombocytopenia, thrombocytosis, eosinophilia, increased international normalized ratio

Cardiovascular System: supraventricular arrhythmia

Dermatologic System: eczema

Digestive System: abdominal distension, flatulence, stomatitis, jaundice, increased serum lactate dehydrogenase

Metabolic/Nutritional System: hypomagnesemia, increased serum bicarbonate, electrolyte disturbance

Musculoskeletal System: myalgia, muscle cramps, muscle weakness, osteomyelitis

Nervous System: vertigo, mental status change, paraesthesia

Special Senses: taste disturbance, eye irritation

Laboratory Changes

[See table 6 above]

In clinical trials, 0.2% of patients treated with CUBICIN had symptoms of muscle pain or weakness associated with CPK elevations to greater than 4 times the upper limit of normal. The symptoms resolved within 3 days and CPK returned to normal within 7-10 days after discontinuing treatment (see **PRECAUTIONS, Skeletal Muscle**). In Phase 3 comparator-controlled trials, there was no clinically or statistically significant difference (P <0.05) in the frequency of CPK elevations between patients treated with CUBICIN and those treated with comparator. CPK elevations in both groups were generally related to medical conditions, for example, skin and skin structure infection, surgical procedures, or intramuscular injections, and were not associated with muscle symptoms.

There were no substantial differences between CUBICIN and the comparators in the frequency or distribution of changes in other laboratory parameters, regardless of drug relationship.

OVERDOSAGE

In the event of overdosage, supportive care is advised with maintenance of glomerular filtration. Daptomycin is slowly cleared from the body by hemodialysis (approximately 15% recovered over 4 hours) or by peritoneal dialysis (approximately 11% recovered over 48 hours).

DOSAGE AND ADMINISTRATION

Complicated Skin and Skin Structure Infections: CUBICIN 4 mg/kg should be administered over a 30-minute period by intravenous infusion in 0.9% sodium chloride injection once every 24 hours for 7-14 days. Doses of CUBICIN higher than 4 mg/kg/day have not been studied in Phase 3 controlled clinical trials. In Phase 1 and 2 clinical studies, CPK elevations appeared to be more frequent when daptomycin was dosed more frequently than once daily. Therefore, CUBICIN should not be dosed more frequently than once a day.

Because daptomycin is eliminated primarily by the kidney, a dosage modification is recommended for patients with creatinine clearance <30 mL/min, including patients receiving hemodialysis or continuous ambulatory peritoneal dialysis (CAPD), as listed in Table 7. The recommended dosing regimen is 4 mg/kg once every 24 hours for patients with CL_{CR} ≥ 30 mL/min and 4 mg/kg once every 48 hours for CL_{CR} <30 mL/min, including those on hemodialysis or CAPD. When possible, CUBICIN should be administered following hemodialysis on hemodialysis days (see **CLINICAL PHARMACOLOGY**).

Continued on next page

Table 8 Investigator's Primary Diagnosis in the Complicated Skin and Skin Structure Infection Studies (Population: ITT)

Parameters	Study 9801 CUBICIN/Comparator[a] N=264/N=266	Study 9901 CUBICIN/Comparator[a] N=270/N=292	Pooled CUBICIN/Comparator[a] N=534/N=558
Wound Infection	99 (37.5%)/116 (43.6%)	102 (37.8%)/108 (37.0%)	201 (37.6%)/224 (40.1%)
Major Abscess	55 (20.8%)/43 (16.2%)	59 (21.9%)/65 (22.3%)	114 (21.3%)/108 (19.4%)
Ulcer Infection	71 (26.9%)/75 (28.2%)	53 (19.6%)/68 (23.3%)	124 (23.2%)/143 (25.6%)
Other Infection[b]	39 (14.8%)/32 (12.0%)	56 (20.7%)/51 (17.5%)	95 (17.8%)/83 (14.9%)

a. Vancomycin or semi-synthetic penicillins
b. The majority of cases were subsequently categorized as complicated cellulitis, major abscesses, or traumatic wound infections.

Table 9 Clinical Success Rates by Infecting Pathogen, Primary Comparative Complicated Skin and Skin Structure Infection Studies (Population: Microbiologically Evaluable)

Pathogen	Success Rate CUBICIN n/N (%)	Comparator[a] n/N (%)
Methicillin-susceptible *Staphylococcus aureus* (MSSA)[b]	170/198 (85.9)	180/207 (87.0)
Methicillin-resistant *Staphylococcus aureus* (MRSA)[b]	21/28 (75.0)	25/36 (69.4)
Streptococcus pyogenes	79/84 (94.0)	80/88 (90.9)
Streptococcus agalactiae	23/27 (85.2)	22/29 (75.9)
Streptococcus dysgalactiae subsp *equisimilis*	8/8 (100.0)	9/11 (81.8)
Enterococcus faecalis (vancomycin-susceptible only)[b]	27/37 (73.0)	40/53 (75.5)

a. Vancomycin or semi-synthetic penicillins
b. As determined by the central laboratory

Cubicin—Cont.

Table 7 Recommended Dosage of CUBICIN (daptomycin for injection) in Adult Patients With Renal Impairment

Creatinine Clearance	Dosage Regimen
≥30 mL/min	4 mg/kg once every 24 hours
<30 mL/min, including hemodialysis or CAPD	4 mg/kg once every 48 hours

Preparation of Daptomycin for Administration: CUBICIN is supplied in single-use vials containing either 250 or 500 mg daptomycin as a sterile, lyophilized powder. The contents of a CUBICIN 250 mg vial should be reconstituted with 5 mL of 0.9% sodium chloride injection. The contents of a CUBICIN 500 mg vial should be reconstituted with 10 mL of 0.9% sodium chloride injection. Reconstituted CUBICIN should be further diluted with 0.9% sodium chloride injection to be administered by intravenous infusion over a period of 30 minutes.
Since no preservative or bacteriostatic agent is present in this product, aseptic technique must be used in preparation of final intravenous solution. Stability studies have shown that the reconstituted solution is stable in the vial for 12 hours at room temperature or up to 48 hours if stored under refrigeration at 2 to 8°C (36 to 46°F). The diluted solution is stable in the infusion bag for 12 hours at room temperature or 48 hours if stored under refrigeration. The combined time (vial and infusion bag) at room temperature should not exceed 12 hours; the combined time (vial and infusion bag) under refrigeration should not exceed 48 hours.
CUBICIN vials are for single-use only.
Parenteral drug products should be inspected visually for particulate matter prior to administration.
Because only limited data are available on the compatibility of CUBICIN with other intravenous substances, additives or other medications should not be added to daptomycin single-use vials or infused simultaneously through the same intravenous line. If the same intravenous line is used for sequential infusion of several different drugs, the line should be flushed with a compatible infusion solution before and after infusion with daptomycin.
Compatible Intravenous Solutions: CUBICIN is compatible with 0.9% sodium chloride injection and lactated Ringer's injection. CUBICIN is not compatible with dextrose-containing diluents.

HOW SUPPLIED

CUBICIN (daptomycin for injection) – Pale yellow to light brown lyophilized cake
Single-use 10 mL capacity vials:
500 mg/vial: Packages of 1 (NDC 67919-011-01)
250 mg/vial: Packages of 1 (NDC 67919-010-01)

STORAGE

Store original packages at refrigerated temperatures 2 to 8°C (36 to 46°F); avoid excessive heat.

CLINICAL STUDIES

Complicated Skin and Skin Structure Infections: Adult patients with clinically documented complicated skin and skin structure infections (Table 8) were enrolled in 2 randomized, multinational, multicenter, investigator-blinded studies comparing CUBICIN (4 mg/kg IV q24h) with either vancomycin (1 g IV q12h) or a semi-synthetic penicillin (ie, nafcillin, oxacillin, cloxacillin, or flucloxacillin; 4-12 g IV per day). Patients known to have bacteremia at baseline were excluded. Patients with creatinine clearance between 30-70 mL/min were to receive a lower dose of CUBICIN as specified in the protocol; however, the majority of patients in this subpopulation did not have the dose of daptomycin adjusted. Patients could switch to oral therapy after a minimum of 4 days of IV treatment if clinical improvement was demonstrated.
One study was conducted primarily in the United States and South Africa (study 9801), and the second (study 9901) was conducted at non–U.S. sites only. Both studies were similar in design but differed in patient characteristics, including history of diabetes and peripheral vascular disease. There were a total of 534 patients treated with CUBICIN and 558 treated with comparator in the 2 studies. The majority (89.7%) of patients received IV medication exclusively.
The efficacy endpoints in both studies were the clinical success rates in the intent-to-treat (ITT) population and in the clinically evaluable (CE) population. In study 9801, clinical success rates in the ITT population were 62.5% (165/264) in patients treated with daptomycin and 60.9% (162/266) in patients treated with comparator drugs. Clinical success rates in the CE population were 76.0% (158/208) in patients treated with daptomycin and 76.7% (158/206) in patients treated with comparator drugs. In study 9901, clinical success rates in the ITT population were 80.4% (217/270) in patients treated with daptomycin and 80.5% (235/292) in patients treated with comparator drugs. Clinical success rates in the CE population were 89.9% (214/238) in patients treated with daptomycin and 90.4% (226/250) in patients treated with comparator drugs.
The success rates by pathogen for microbiologically evaluable patients are presented in Table 9.
[See table 8 above]
[See table 9 above]
℞ **only**
US Patent Nos. 6,468,967; 5,912,226; 4,885,243; 4,874,843
CUBICIN is a trademark of Cubist Pharmaceuticals, Inc.
Manufactured for:
Cubist Pharmaceuticals, Inc.
Lexington, MA 02421
Manufactured by:
Abbott Laboratories
Hospital Products Division
McPherson, KS 67460
For all medical inquiries, call 866-793-2786.

REFERENCES

1. National Committee for Clinical Laboratory Standards. Performance standards for antimicrobial disk susceptibility tests; approved standard–eighth edition. NCCLS document M2-A8, Villanova, (PA). 2003 January.
2. National Committee for Clinical Laboratory Standards. Methods for dilution antimicrobial susceptibility test for bacteria that grow aerobically; approved standard–sixth edition. NCCLS document M7-A6,Villanova, (PA). 2003 January.
3. National Committee for Clinical Laboratory Standards. Performance standards for antimicrobial susceptibility testing; thirteenth informational supplement. NCCLS document M100-S13, Villanova, (PA). 2003 January.
September 2003

Lexington, MA 02421
1109090803
Shown in Product Identification Guide, page 311

Daiichi Pharmaceutical Corp.

11 PHILIPS PARKWAY
MONTVALE, NJ 07645

Direct Inquiries to:
Ph: (877) 324-4244 (877-DAIICHI)
Fax: (888) 727-5666
For Medical Emergencies and Product Information Contact:
Medical Services Department
Ph: (888) 727-2500
Fax: (888) 272-7979

EVOXAC® CAPSULES ℞

(cevimeline hydrochloride)

DESCRIPTION

Cevimeline is cis-2'-methylspiro (1-azabicyclo [2.2.2] octane-3, 5' -[1,3] oxathiolane) hydrochloride, hydrate (2:1). Its empirical formula is $C_{10}H_{17}NOS.HCl.½ H_2O$, and its structural formula is:

[structural formula: • HCl • 1/2 H₂O]

Cevimeline has a molecular weight of 244.79. It is a white to off white crystalline powder with a melting point range of 201 to 203°C. It is freely soluble in alcohol and chloroform, very soluble in water, and virtually insoluble in ether. The pH of a 1% solution ranges from 4.6 to 5.6. Inactive ingredients include lactose monohydrate, hydroxypropyl cellulose, and magesium stearate.

CLINICAL PHARMACOLOGY

Pharmacodynamics
Cevimeline is a cholinergic agonist which binds to muscarinic receptors. Muscarinic agonists in sufficient dosage can increase secretion of exocrine glands, such as salivary and sweat glands and increase tone of the smooth muscle in the gastrointestinal and urinary tracts.
Pharmacokinetics
Absorption: After administration of a single 30 mg capsule, cevimeline was rapidly absorbed with a mean time to peak concentration of 1.5 to 2 hours. No accumulation of active drug or its metabolites was observed following multiple dose administration. When administered with food, there is a decrease in the rate of absorption, with a fasting T_{MAX} of 1.53 hours and a T_{MAX} of 2.86 hours after a meal; the peak concentration is reduced by 17.3%. Single oral doses across the clinical dose range are dose proportional.
Distribution: Cevimeline has a volume of distribution of approximately 6L/kg and is <20% bound to human plasma proteins. This suggests that cevimeline is extensively bound to tissues; however, the specific binding sites are unknown.
Metabolism: Isozymes CYP2D6 and CYP3A3/4 are responsible for the metabolism of cevimeline. After 24 hours, 86.7% of the dose was recovered (16.0% unchanged, 44.5% as cis and trans-sulfoxide, 22.3% of the dose as glucuronic acid conjugate and 4% of the dose as N-oxide of cevimeline). Approximately 8% of the trans-sulfoxide metabolite is then converted into the corresponding glucuronic acid conjugate and eliminated. Cevimeline did not inhibit cytochrome P450 isozymes 1A2, 2A6, 2C9, 2C19, 2D6, 2E1, and 3A4.
Excretion: The mean half-life of cevimeline is 5+/−1 hours. After 24 hours, 84% of a 30 mg dose of cevimeline was excreted in urine. After seven days, 97% of the dose was recovered in the urine and 0.5% was recovered in the feces.
Special Populations: The effects of renal impairment, hepatic impairment, or ethnicity on the pharmacokinetics of cevimeline have not been investigated.
Clinical Studies
Cevimeline has been shown to improve the symptoms of dry mouth in patients with Sjögren's Syndrome.
A 6-week, randomized, double blind, placebo-controlled study was conducted in 75 patients (10 men, 65 women) with a mean age of 53.6 years (range 33–75). The racial distribution was Caucasian 92%, Black 1% and other 7%. The effects of cevimeline at 30 mg tid (90 mg/day) and 60 mg tid (180 mg/day) were compared to those of placebo. Patients were evaluated by a measure called global improvement, which is defined as a response of "better" to the question,

"Please rate the overall condition of your dry mouth now compared with how you felt before starting treatment in this study." Patients also had the option of selecting "worse" or "no change" as answers. Seventy-six percent of the patients in the 30 mg tid group reported a global improvement in their dry mouth symptoms compared to 35% of the patients in the placebo group. This difference was statistically significant at p=0.0043. There was no evidence that patients in the 60 mg tid group had better global evaluation scores than the patients in the 30 mg tid group.

A 12-week, randomized, double-blind, placebo-controlled study was conducted in 197 patients (10 men, 187 women) with a mean age of 54.5 years (range 23–74). The racial distribution was Caucasian 91.4%, Black 3% and other 5.6%. The effects of cevimeline at 15 mg tid (45 mg/day) and 30 mg tid (90 mg/day) were compared to those of placebo. Statistically significant global improvement in the symptoms of dry mouth (p=0.0004) was seen for the 30 mg tid group compared to placebo, but not for the 15 mg group compared to placebo. Salivary flow showed statistically significant increases at both doses of cevimeline during the study compared to placebo.

A second 12-week, randomized, double-blind, placebo-controlled study was conducted in 212 patients (11 men, 201 women) with a mean age of 55.3 years (range 24–75). The racial distribution was Caucasian 88.7%, Black 1.9% and other 9.4%. The effects of cevimeline at 15 mg tid (45 mg/day) and 30 mg tid (90 mg/day) were compared to those of placebo. No statistically significant differences were noted in the patient global evaluations. However, there was a higher placebo response rate in this study compared to the aforementioned studies. The 30 mg tid group showed a statistically significant increase in salivary flow from pre-dose to post-dose compared to placebo (p=0.0017).

INDICATIONS AND USAGE

Cevimeline is indicated for the treatment of symptoms of dry mouth in patients with Sjögren's Syndrome.

CONTRAINDICATIONS

Cevimeline is contraindicated in patients with uncontrolled asthma, known hypersensitivity to cevimeline, and when miosis is undesirable, e.g., in acute iritis and in narrow-angle (angle-closure) glaucoma.

WARNINGS

Cardiovascular Disease:

Cevimeline can potentially alter cardiac conduction and/or heart rate. Patients with significant cardiovascular disease may potentially be unable to compensate for transient changes in hemodynamics or rhythm induced by EVOXAC®. EVOXAC® should be used with caution and under close medical supervision in patients with a history of cardiovascular disease evidenced by angina pectoris or myocardial infarction.

Pulmonary Disease:

Cevimeline can potentially increase airway resistance, bronchial smooth muscle tone, and bronchial secretions. Cevimeline should be administered with caution and with close medical supervision to patients with controlled asthma, chronic bronchitis, or chronic obstructive pulmonary disease.

Ocular:

Ophthalmic formulations of muscarinic agonists have been reported to cause visual blurring which may result in decreased visual acuity, especially at night and in patients with central lens changes, and to cause impairment of depth perception. Caution should be advised while driving at night or performing hazardous activities in reduced lighting.

PRECAUTIONS

General:

Cevimeline toxicity is characterized by an exaggeration of its parasympathomimetic effects. These may include: headache, visual disturbance, lacrimation, sweating, respiratory distress, gastrointestinal spasm, nausea, vomiting, diarrhea, atrioventricular block, tachycardia, bradycardia, hypotension, hypertension, shock, mental confusion, cardiac arrhythmia, and tremors.

Cevimeline should be administered with caution to patients with a history of nephrolithiasis or cholelithiasis. Contractions of the gallbladder or biliary smooth muscle could precipitate complications such as cholecystitis, cholangitis and biliary obstruction. An increase in the ureteral smooth muscle tone could theoretically precipitate renal colic or ureteral reflux in patients with nephrolithiasis.

Information for Patients: Patients should be informed that cevimeline may cause visual disturbances, especially at night, that could impair their ability to drive safely.

If a patient sweats excessively while taking cevimeline, dehydration may develop. The patient should drink extra water and consult a health care provider.

Drug Interactions:

Cevimeline should be administered with caution to patients taking beta adrenergic antagonists, because of the possibility of conduction disturbances. Drugs with parasympathomimetic effects administered concurrently with cevimeline can be expected to have additive effects. Cevimeline might interfere with desirable antimuscarinic effects of drugs used concomitantly.

Drugs which inhibit CYP2D6 and CYP3A3/4 also inhibit the metabolism of cevimeline. Cevimeline should be used with caution in individuals known or suspected to be deficient in CYP2D6 activity, based on previous experience, as they may be at a higher risk of adverse events. In an *in vitro* study, cytochrome P450 isozymes 1A2, 2A6, 2C9, 2C19, 2D6, 2E1, and 3A4 were not inhibited by exposure to cevimeline.

Carcinogenesis, Mutagenesis and Impairment of Fertility:

Lifetime carcinogenicity studies were conducted in CD-1 mice and F-344 rats. A statistically significant increase in the incidence of adenocarcinomas of the uterus was observed in female rats that received cevimeline at a dosage of 100 mg/kg/day (approximately 8 times the maximum human exposure based on comparison of AUC data). No other significant differences in tumor incidence were observed in either mice or rats.

Cevimeline exhibited no evidence of mutagenicity or clastogenicity in a battery of assays that included an Ames test, an *in vitro* chromosomal aberration study in mammalian cells, a mouse lymphoma study in L5178Y cells, or a micronucleus assay conducted *in vivo* in ICR mice.

Cevimeline did not adversely affect the reproductive performance or fertility of male Sprague-Dawley rats when administered for 63 days prior to mating and throughout the period of mating at dosages up to 45 mg/kg/day (approximately 5 times the maximum recommended dose for a 60 kg human following normalization of the data on the basis of body surface area estimates). Females that were treated with cevimeline at dosages up to 45 mg/kg/day from 14 days prior to mating through day seven of gestation exhibited a statistically significantly smaller number of implantations than did control animals.

Pregnancy:

Pregnancy Category C.

Cevimeline was associated with a reduction in the mean number of implantations when given to pregnant Sprague-Dawley rats from 14 days prior to mating through day seven of gestation at a dosage of 45 mg/kg/day (approximately 5 times the maximum recommended dose for a 60 kg human when compared on the basis of body surface area estimates). This effect may have been secondary to maternal toxicity. There are no adequate and well-controlled studies in pregnant women. Cevimeline should be used during pregnancy only if the potential benefit justifies the potential risk to the fetus.

Nursing Mothers:

It is not known whether this drug is secreted in human milk. Because many drugs are excreted in human milk, and because of the potential for serious adverse reactions in nursing infants from EVOXAC®, a decision should be made whether to discontinue nursing or discontinue the drug, taking into account the importance of the drug to the mother.

Pediatric Use:

Safety and effectiveness in pediatric patients have not been established.

Geriatric Use:

Although clinical studies of cevimeline included subjects over the age of 65, the numbers were not sufficient to determine whether they respond differently from younger subjects. Special care should be exercised when cevimeline treatment is initiated in an elderly patient, considering the greater frequency of decreased hepatic, renal, or cardiac function, and of concomitant disease or other drug therapy in the elderly.

ADVERSE REACTIONS

Cevimeline was administered to 1777 patients during clinical trials worldwide, including Sjögren's patients and patients with other conditions. In placebo-controlled Sjögren's studies in the U.S., 320 patients received cevimeline doses ranging from 15 mg tid to 60 mg tid, of whom 93% were women and 7% were men. Demographic distribution was 90% Caucasian, 5% Hispanic, 3% Black and 2% of other origin. In these studies, 14.6% of patients discontinued treatment with cevimeline due to adverse events.

The following adverse events associated with muscarinic agonism were observed in the clinical trials of cevimeline in Sjögren's syndrome patients:

Adverse Event	Cevimeline 30 mg (tid) n*=533	Placebo (tid) n=164
Excessive Sweating	18.7%	2.4%
Nausea	13.8%	7.9%
Rhinitis	11.2%	5.4%
Diarrhea	10.3%	10.3%
Excessive Salivation	2.2%	0.6%
Urinary Frequency	0.9%	1.8%
Asthenia	0.5%	0.0%
Flushing	0.3%	0.6%
Polyuria	0.1%	0.6%

*n is the total number of patients exposed to the dose at any time during the study.

In addition, the following adverse events (≥3% incidence) were reported in the Sjögren's clinical trials:

Adverse Event	Cevimeline 30 mg (tid) n*=533	Placebo (tid) n=164
Headache	14.4%	20.1%
Sinusitis	12.3%	10.9%
Upper Respiratory Tract Infection	11.4%	9.1%
Dyspepsia	7.8%	8.5%
Abdominal Pain	7.6%	6.7%
Urinary Tract Infection	6.1%	3.0%
Coughing	6.1%	3.0%
Pharyngitis	5.2%	5.4%
Vomiting	4.6%	2.4%
Injury	4.5%	2.4%
Back Pain	4.5%	4.2%
Rash	4.3%	6.0%
Conjunctivitis	4.3%	3.6%
Dizziness	4.1%	7.3%
Bronchitis	4.1%	1.2%
Arthralgia	3.7%	1.8%
Surgical Intervention	3.3%	3.0%
Fatigue	3.3%	1.2%
Pain	3.3%	3.0%
Skeletal Pain	2.8%	1.8%
Insomnia	2.4%	1.2%
Hot Flushes	2.4%	0.0%
Rigors	1.3%	1.2%
Anxiety	1.3%	1.2%

*n is the total number of patients exposed to the dose at any time during the study.

The following events were reported in Sjögren's patients at incidences of <3% and ≥1%: constipation, tremor, abnormal vision, hypertonia, peripheral edema, chest pain, myalgia, fever, anorexia, eye pain, earache, dry mouth, vertigo, salivary gland pain, pruritus, influenza-like symptoms, eye infection, post-operative pain, vaginitis, skin disorder, depression, hiccup, hyporeflexia, infection, fungal infection, sialoadenitis, otitis media, erythematous rash, pneumonia, edema, salivary gland enlargement, allergy, gastroesophageal reflux, eye abnormality, migraine, tooth disorder, epistaxis, flatulence, toothache, ulcerative stomatitis, anemia, hypoesthesia, cystitis, leg cramps, abscess, eructation, moniliasis, palpitation, increased amylase, xerophthalmia, allergic reaction.

The following events were reported rarely in treated Sjögren's patients (<1%): Causal relation is unknown:

Body as a Whole Disorders: aggravated allergy, precordial chest pain, abnormal crying, hematoma, leg pain, edema, periorbital edema, activated pain trauma, pallor, changed sensation temperature, weight decrease, weight increase, choking, mouth edema, syncope, malaise, face edema, substernal chest pain

Cardiovascular Disorders: abnormal ECG, heart disorder, heart murmur, aggravated hypertension, hypotension, arrhythmia, extrasystoles, t wave inversion, tachycardia, supraventricular tachycardia, angina pectoris, myocardial infarction, pericarditis, pulmonary embolism, peripheral ischemia, superficial phlebitis, purpura, deep thrombophlebitis, vascular disorder, vasculitis, hypertension

Digestive Disorders: appendicitis, increased appetite, ulcerative colitis, diverticulitis, duodenitis, dysphagia, enterocolitis, gastric ulcer, gastritis, gastroenteritis, gastrointestinal hemorrhage, gingivitis, glossitis, rectum hemorrhage, hemorrhoids, ileus, irritable bowel syndrome, melena, mucositis, esophageal stricture, esophagitis, oral hemorrhage, peptic ulcer, periodontal destruction, rectal disorder, stomatitis, tenesmus, tongue discoloration, tongue disorder, geographic tongue, tongue ulceration, dental caries.

Endocrine Disorders: increased glucocorticoids, goiter, hypothyroidism

Hematologic Disorders: thrombocytopenic purpura, thrombocythemia, thrombocytopenia, hypochromic anemia, eosinophilia, granulocytopenia, leucopenia, leukocytosis, cervical lymphadenopathy, lymphadenopathy

Liver and Biliary System Disorders: cholelithiasis, increased gamma-glutamyl transferase, increased hepatic enzymes, abnormal hepatic function, viral hepatitis, increased serum glutamate oxaloacetic transaminase (SGOT) (also called AST-aspartate aminotransferase), increased serum glutamate pyruvate transaminase (SGPT) (also called ALT-alanine aminotransferase)

Metabolic and Nutritional Disorders: dehydration, diabetes mellitus, hypercalcemia, hypercholesterolemia, hyperglycemia, hyperlipemia, hypertriglyceridemia, hyperuricemia, hypoglycemia, hypokalemia, hyponatremia, thirst

Musculoskeletal Disorders: arthritis, aggravated arthritis, arthropathy, femoral head avascular necrosis, bone disorder, bursitis, costochondritis, plantar fasciitis, muscle weakness, osteomyelitis, osteoporosis, synovitis, tendinitis, tenosynovitis

Neoplasms: basal cell carcinoma, squamous carcinoma

Nervous Disorders: carpal tunnel syndrome, coma, abnormal coordination, dysesthesia, dyskinesia, dysphonia, aggravated multiple sclerosis, involuntary muscle contractions, neuralgia, neuropathy, paresthesia, speech disorder, agitation, confusion, depersonalization, aggravated depression, abnormal dreaming, emotional lability, manic reaction, paroniria, somnolence, abnormal thinking, hyperkinesia, hallucination

Miscellaneous Disorders: fall, food poisoning, heat stroke, joint dislocation, post-operative hemorrhage

Resistance Mechanism Disorders: cellulitis, herpes simplex, herpes zoster, bacterial infection, viral infection, genital moniliasis, sepsis

Continued on next page

Evoxac—Cont.

Respiratory Disorders: asthma, bronchospasm, chronic obstructive airway disease, dyspnea, hemoptysis, laryngitis, nasal ulcer, pleural effusion, pleurisy, pulmonary congestion, pulmonary fibrosis, respiratory disorder
Rheumatologic Disorders: aggravated rheumatoid arthritis, lupus erythematosus rash, lupus erythematosus syndrome
Skin and Appendages Disorders: acne, alopecia, burn, dermatitis, contact dermatitis, lichenoid dermatitis, eczema, furunculosis, hyperkeratosis, lichen planus, nail discoloration, nail disorder, onychia, onychomycosis, paronychia, photosensitivity reaction, rosacea, scleroderma, seborrhea, skin discoloration, dry skin, skin exfoliation, skin hypertrophy, skin ulceration, urticaria, verruca, bullous eruption, cold clammy skin
Special Senses Disorders: deafness, decreased hearing, motion sickness, parosmia, taste perversion, blepharitis, cataract, corneal opacity, corneal ulceration, diplopia, glaucoma, anterior chamber eye hemorrhage, keratitis, keratoconjunctivitis, mydriasis, myopia, photopsia, retinal deposits, retinal disorder, scleritis, vitreous detachment, tinnitus
Urogenital Disorders: epididymitis, prostatic disorder, abnormal sexual function, amenorrhea, female breast neoplasm, malignant female breast neoplasm, female breast pain, positive cervical smear test, dysmenorrhea, endometrial disorder, intermenstrual bleeding, leukorrhea, menorrhagia, menstrual disorder, ovarian cyst, ovarian disorder, genital pruritus, uterine hemorrhage, vaginal hemorrhage, atrophic vaginitis, albuminuria, bladder discomfort, increased blood urea nitrogen, dysuria, hematuria, micturition disorder, nephrosis, nocturia, increased nonprotein nitrogen, pyelonephritis, renal calculus, abnormal renal function, renal pain, strangury, urethral disorder, abnormal urine, urinary incontinence, decreased urine flow, pyuria

In one subject with lupus erythematosus receiving concomitant multiple drug therapy, a highly elevated ALT level was noted after the fourth week of cevimeline therapy. In two other subjects receiving cevimeline in the clinical trials, very high AST levels were noted. The significance of these findings is unknown.

Additional adverse events (relationship unknown) which occurred in other clinical studies (patient population different from Sjögren's patients) are as follows:

cholinergic syndrome, blood pressure fluctuation, cardiomegaly, postural hypotension, aphasia, convulsions, abnormal gait, hyperesthesia, paralysis, abnormal sexual function, enlarged abdomen, change in bowel habits, gum hyperplasia, intestinal obstruction, bundle branch block, increased creatine phosphokinase, electrolyte abnormality, glycosuria, gout, hyperkalemia, hyperproteinemia, increased lactic dehydrogenase (LDH), increased alkaline phosphatase, failure to thrive, abnormal platelets, aggressive reaction, amnesia, apathy, delirium, delusion, dementia, illusion, impotence, neurosis, paranoid reaction, personality disorder, hyperhemoglobinemia, apnea, atelectasis, yawning, oliguria, urinary retention, distended vein, lymphocytosis

MANAGEMENT OF OVERDOSE

Management of the signs and symptoms of acute overdosage should be handled in a manner consistent with that indicated for other muscarinic agonists: general supportive measures should be instituted. If medically indicated, atropine, an anti-cholinergic agent, may be of value as an antidote for emergency use in patients who have had an overdose of cevimeline. If medically indicated, epinephrine may also be of value in the presence of severe cardiovascular depression or bronchoconstriction. It is not known if cevimeline is dialyzable.

DOSAGE AND ADMINISTRATION

The recommended dose of cevimeline hydrochloride is 30 mg taken three times a day. There is insufficient safety information to support doses greater than 30 mg tid. There is also insufficient evidence for additional efficacy of cevimeline hydrochloride at doses greater than 30 mg tid.

HOW SUPPLIED

EVOXAC® is available as white, hard gelatin capsules containing 30 mg of cevimeline hydrochloride. EVOXAC® capsules have a white opaque cap and a white opaque body. The capsules are imprinted with "EVOXAC" on the cap and "30 mg" on the body with a black bar above "30 mg". It is supplied in child resistant bottles of:

100 capsules (**NDC 63395-201-13**)

Store at 25°C (77°F) excursion permitted to 15°–30°C (59°–86°F)

℞ Only

Manufactured by:
YAMANOUCHI PHARMA TECHNOLOGIES, INC.
Norman, OK 73072
Distributed and Marketed by:
Daiichi Pharmaceutical Corporation
Montvale, NJ 07645
EVOXAC is a registered trademark of
Daiichi Pharmaceutical Co., Ltd.
SRT17 Revised 11/2002

Shown in Product Identification Guide, page 311

FLOXIN® OTIC ℞

[flox-in]
(ofloxacin otic) solution 0.3%

DESCRIPTION

FLOXIN® Otic (ofloxacin otic) solution 0.3% is a sterile aqueous anti-infective (anti-bacterial) solution for otic use. Chemically, ofloxacin has three condensed 6-membered rings made up of a fluorinated carboxyquinolone with a benzoxazine ring. The chemical name of ofloxacin is: (±)-9-fluoro-2,3-dihydro-3-methyl-10-(4-methyl-1-piperazinyl)-7-oxo-7*H*-pyrido [1,2,3-*de*]-1,4-benzoxazine-6-carboxylic acid. The empirical formula of ofloxacin is $C_{18}H_{20}FN_3O_4$ and its molecular weight is 361.38. The structural formula is:

FLOXIN® Otic contains 0.3% (3 mg/mL) ofloxacin with benzalkonium chloride (0.0025%), sodium chloride (0.9%), and water for injection. Hydrochloric acid and sodium hydroxide are added to adjust the pH to 6.5±0.5.

CLINICAL PHARMACOLOGY

Pharmacokinetics: Drug concentrations in serum (in subjects with tympanostomy tubes and perforated tympanic membranes), in otorrhea, and in mucosa of the middle ear (in subjects with perforated tympanic membranes) were determined following otic administration of ofloxacin solution. In two single-dose studies, mean ofloxacin serum concentrations were low in adult patients with tympanostomy tubes, with and without otorrhea, after otic administration of a 0.3% solution (4.1 ng/mL (n=3) and 5.4 ng/mL (n=5), respectively). In adults with perforated tympanic membranes, the maximum serum drug level of ofloxacin detected was 10 ng/mL after administration of a 0.3% solution. Ofloxacin was detectable in the middle ear mucosa of some adult subjects with perforated tympanic membranes (11 of 16 subjects). The variability of ofloxacin concentration in middle ear mucosa was high. The concentrations ranged from 1.2 to 602 µg/g after otic administration of a 0.3% solution. Ofloxacin was present in high concentrations in otorrhea (389 - 2850 µg/g, n=13) 30 minutes after otic administration of a 0.3% solution in subjects with chronic suppurative otitis media and perforated tympanic membranes. However, the measurement of ofloxacin in the otorrhea does not necessarily reflect the exposure of the middle ear to ofloxacin.

Microbiology: Ofloxacin has *in vitro* activity against a wide range of gram-negative and gram-positive microorganisms. Ofloxacin exerts its antibacterial activity by inhibiting DNA gyrase, a bacterial topoisomerase. DNA gyrase is an essential enzyme which controls DNA topology and assists in DNA replication, repair, deactivation, and transcription. Cross-resistance has been observed between ofloxacin and other fluoroquinolones. There is generally no cross-resistance between ofloxacin and other classes of antibacterial agents such as beta-lactams or aminoglycosides.

Ofloxacin has been shown to be active against most isolates of the following microorganisms, both *in vitro* and clinically in otic infections as described in the **INDICATIONS AND USAGE** section.

Aerobic and facultative gram-positive microorganisms:
Staphylococcus aureus
Streptococcus pneumoniae

Aerobic and facultative gram-negative microorganisms:
Escherichia coli
Haemophilus influenzae
Moraxella catarrhalis
Proteus mirabilis
Pseudomonas aeruginosa

INDICATIONS AND USAGE

FLOXIN® Otic (ofloxacin otic) solution 0.3% is indicated for the treatment of infections caused by susceptible isolates of the designated microorganisms in the specific conditions listed below:

Otitis Externa in adults and pediatric patients, 6 months and older, due to *Escherichia coli, Pseudomonas aeruginosa,* and *Staphylococcus aureus.*

Chronic Suppurative Otitis Media in patients 12 years and older with perforated tympanic membranes due to *Proteus mirabilis, Pseudomonas aeruginosa,* and *Staphylococcus aureus.*

Acute Otitis Media in pediatric patients one year and older with tympanostomy tubes due to *Haemophilus influenzae, Moraxella catarrhalis, Pseudomonas aeruginosa, Staphylococcus aureus,* and *Streptococcus pneumoniae.*

CONTRAINDICATIONS

FLOXIN® Otic (ofloxacin otic) solution 0.3% is contraindicated in patients with a history of hypersensitivity to ofloxacin, to other quinolones, or to any of the components in this medication.

WARNINGS

NOT FOR OPHTHALMIC USE.
NOT FOR INJECTION.

Serious and occasionally fatal hypersensitivity (anaphylactic) reactions, some following the first dose, have been reported in patients receiving systemic quinolones, including ofloxacin. Some reactions were accompanied by cardiovascular collapse, loss of consciousness, angioedema (including laryngeal, pharyngeal or facial edema), airway obstruction, dyspnea, urticaria, and itching. If an allergic reaction to ofloxacin is suspected, stop the drug. Serious acute hypersensitivity reactions may require immediate emergency treatment. Oxygen and airway management, including intubation, should be administered as clinically indicated.

PRECAUTIONS

General: As with other anti-infective preparations, prolonged use may result in over-growth of nonsusceptible organisms, including fungi. If the infection is not improved after one week, cultures should be obtained to guide further treatment. If otorrhea persists after a full course of therapy, or if two or more episodes of otorrhea occur within six months, further evaluation is recommended to exclude an underlying condition such as cholesteatoma, foreign body, or a tumor.

The systemic administration of quinolones, including ofloxacin at doses much higher than given or absorbed by the otic route, has led to lesions or erosions of the cartilage in weight-bearing joints and other signs of arthropathy in immature animals of various species.

Young growing guinea pigs dosed in the middle ear with 0.3% ofloxacin otic solution showed no systemic effects, lesions or erosions of the cartilage in weight-bearing joints, or other signs of arthropathy. No drug-related structural or functional changes of the cochlea and no lesions in the ossicles were noted in the guinea pig following otic administration of 0.3% ofloxacin for one month.

No signs of local irritation were found when 0.3% ofloxacin was applied topically in the rabbit eye. Ofloxacin was also shown to lack dermal sensitizing potential in the guinea pig maximization study.

Information for Patients: Avoid contaminating the applicator tip with material from the fingers or other sources. This precaution is necessary if the sterility of the drops is to be preserved. Systemic quinolones, including ofloxacin, have been associated with hypersensitivity reactions, even following a single dose. Discontinue use immediately and contact your physician at the first sign of a rash or allergic reaction.

Otitis Externa

Prior to administration of FLOXIN® Otic, the solution should be warmed by holding the bottle in the hand for one or two minutes to avoid dizziness which may result from the instillation of a cold solution. The patient should lie with the affected ear upward, and then the drops should be instilled. This position should be maintained for five minutes to facilitate penetration of the drops into the ear canal. Repeat, if necessary, for the opposite ear (see **DOSAGE AND ADMINISTRATION**).

Acute Otitis Media and Chronic Suppurative Otitis Media

Prior to administration of FLOXIN® Otic, the solution should be warmed by holding the bottle in the hand for one or two minutes to avoid dizziness which may result from the instillation of a cold solution. The patient should lie with the affected ear upward, and then the drops should be instilled. The tragus should then be pumped 4 times by pushing inward to facilitate penetration of the drops into the middle ear. This position should be maintained for five minutes. Repeat, if necessary, for the opposite ear (see **DOSAGE AND ADMINISTRATION**).

Drug Interactions: Specific drug interaction studies have not been conducted with FLOXIN® Otic.

Carcinogenesis, Mutagenesis, Impairment of Fertility

Long-term studies to determine the carcinogenic potential of ofloxacin have not been conducted. Ofloxacin was not mutagenic in the Ames test, the sister chromatid exchange assay (Chinese hamster and human cell lines), the unscheduled DNA synthesis (UDS) assay using human fibroblasts, the dominant lethal assay, or the mouse micronucleus assay. Ofloxacin was positive in the rat hepatocyte UDS assay, and in the mouse lymphoma assay. In rats, ofloxacin did not affect male or female reproductive performance at oral doses up to 360 mg/kg/day. This would be over 1000 times the maximum recommended clinical dose, based upon body surface area, assuming total absorption of ofloxacin from the ear of a patient treated with FLOXIN® Otic twice per day.

Pregnancy

Teratogenic effects: Pregnancy Category C. Ofloxacin has been shown to have an embryocidal effect in rats at a dose of 810 mg/kg/day and in rabbits at 160 mg/kg/day.

These dosages resulted in decreased fetal body weights and increased fetal mortality in rats and rabbits, respectively. Minor fetal skeletal variations were reported in rats receiving doses of 810 mg/kg/day. Ofloxacin has not been shown to be teratogenic at doses as high as 810 mg/kg/day and 160 mg/kg/day when administered to pregnant rats and rabbits, respectively.

Ofloxacin has not been shown to have any adverse effects on the developing embryo or fetus at doses relevant to the amount of ofloxacin that will be delivered ototopically at the recommended clinical doses.

Nonteratogenic Effects: Additional studies in the rat demonstrated that doses up to 360 mg/kg/day during late gestation had no adverse effects on late fetal development, labor, delivery, lactation, neonatal viability, or growth of the newborn. There are, however, no adequate and well-controlled studies in pregnant women. FLOXIN® Otic should be used during pregnancy only if the potential benefit justifies the potential risk to the fetus.

Nursing Mothers: In nursing women, a single 200 mg oral dose resulted in concentrations of ofloxacin in milk which were similar to those found in plasma. It is not known whether ofloxacin is excreted in human milk following topical otic administration. Because of the potential for serious adverse reactions from ofloxacin in nursing infants, a decision should be made whether to discontinue nursing or to discontinue the drug, taking into account the importance of the drug to the mother.

Adverse Event	Incidence Rate		
	Studies 002/003† BID (N=229)	Studies 016/017† QD (N=310)	Study 020† QD (N=489)
Application Site Reaction	3%	16.8%	0.6%
Pruritus	4%	1.2%	1.0%
Earache	1%	0.6%	0.8%
Dizziness	1%	0.0%	0.6%
Headache	0%	0.3%	0.2%
Vertigo	1%	0.0%	0.0%

† Studies 002/003 (BID) and 016/017 (QD) were active-controlled and comparative.
Study 020 (QD) was open and non-comparative.
An unexpected increased incidence of application site reaction was seen in studies 016/017 and was similar for both ofloxacin and the active control drug (neomycin-polymyxin B sulfate-hydrocortisone). This finding is believed to be the result of specific questioning of the subjects regarding the incidence of application site reactions.

Pediatric Use: Safety and efficacy have been demonstrated in pediatric patients of the following ages for the listed indications:

- six months and older: otitis externa with intact tympanic membranes
- one year and older: acute otitis media with tympanostomy tubes
- twelve years and older: chronic suppurative otitis media with perforated tympanic membranes

Safety and efficacy in pediatric patients below these ages have not been established.

Although no data are available on patients less than age 6 months, there are no known safety concerns or differences in the disease process in this population that will preclude use of this product.

No changes in hearing function occurred in 30 pediatric subjects treated with ofloxacin otic and tested for audiometric parameters.

Although quinolones, including ofloxacin, have been shown to cause arthropathy in immature animals after systemic administration, young growing guinea pigs dosed in the middle ear with 0.3% ofloxacin otic solution for one month showed no systemic effects, quinolone-induced lesions, erosions of the cartilage in weight-bearing joints, or other signs of arthropathy.

ADVERSE REACTIONS

Subjects with Otitis Externa

In the phase III clinical trials performed in support of once-daily dosing, 799 subjects with otitis externa and intact tympanic membranes were treated with ofloxacin otic solution. The studies, which served as the basis for approval, were 020 (pediatric, adolescents and adults), 016 (adolescents and adults) and 017 (pediatric). The following treatment-related adverse events occurred in two or more of the subjects.

[See table above]

In once daily dosing studies, there were also single reports of nausea, seborrhea, loss of hearing, tinnitus, otitis externa, otitis media, tremor, hypertension and fungal infection.

In twice daily dosing studies, the following treatment-related adverse events were each reported in a single subject: dermatitis, eczema, erythematous rash, follicular rash, hypoaesthesia, tinnitus, dyspepsia, hot flushes, flushing and otorrhagia.

Subjects with Acute Otitis Media with Tympanostomy Tubes (AOM TT) and Subjects with Chronic Suppurative Otitis Media (CSOM) with Perforated Tympanic Membranes

In phase III clinical trials which formed the basis for approval, the following treatment-related adverse events occurred in 1% or more of the 656 subjects with non-intact tympanic membranes in AOM TT or CSOM treated twice-daily with ofloxacin otic solution:

Adverse Event	Incidence (N = 656)
Taste Perversion	7%
Earache	1%
Pruritus	1%
Paraesthesia	1%
Rash	1%
Dizziness	1%

Other treatment-related adverse reactions reported in subjects with non-intact tympanic membranes included: diarrhea (0.6%), nausea (0.3%), vomiting (0.3%), dry mouth (0.5%), headache (0.3%), vertigo (0.5%), otorrhagia (0.6%), tinnitus (0.3%), fever (0.3%). The following treatment-related adverse events were each reported in a single subject: application site reaction, otitis externa, urticaria, abdominal pain, dysaesthesia, hyperkinesia, halitosis, inflammation, pain, insomnia, coughing, pharyngitis, rhinitis, sinusitis, and tachycardia.

Post-marketing Adverse Events

Cases of uncommon transient neuropsychiatric disturbances have been included in spontaneous post-marketing reports. A causal relationship with ofloxacin otic solution 0.3% is unknown.

DOSAGE AND ADMINISTRATION

Otitis Externa: The recommended dosage regimen for the treatment of otitis externa is:

For pediatric patients (from 6 months to 13 years old): Five drops (0.25 mL, 0.75 mg ofloxacin) instilled into the affected ear once daily for seven days.

For patients 13 years and older: Ten drops (0.5 mL, 1.5 mg ofloxacin) instilled into the affected ear once daily for seven days.

The solution should be warmed by holding the bottle in the hand for one or two minutes to avoid dizziness which may result from the instillation of a cold solution. The patient should lie with the affected ear upward, and then the drops should be instilled. This position should be maintained for five minutes to facilitate penetration of the drops into the ear canal. Repeat, if necessary, for the opposite ear.

Acute Otitis Media in pediatric patients with tympanostomy tubes: The recommended dosage regimen for the treatment of acute otitis media in pediatric patients (from 1 to 12 years old) with tympanostomy tubes is:

Five drops (0.25 mL, 0.75 mg ofloxacin) instilled into the affected ear twice daily for ten days. The solution should be warmed by holding the bottle in the hand for one or two minutes to avoid dizziness which may result from the instillation of a cold solution. The patient should lie with the affected ear upward, and then the drops should be instilled. The tragus should then be pumped 4 times by pushing inward to facilitate penetration of the drops into the middle ear. This position should be maintained for five minutes. Repeat, if necessary, for the opposite ear.

Chronic Suppurative Otitis Media with perforated tympanic membranes: The recommended dosage regimen for the treatment of chronic suppurative otitis media with perforated tympanic membranes in patients 12 years and older is:

Ten drops (0.5 mL, 1.5 mg ofloxacin) instilled into the affected ear twice daily for fourteen days. The solution should be warmed by holding the bottle in the hand for one or two minutes to avoid dizziness which may result from the instillation of a cold solution. The patient should lie with the affected ear upward, before instilling the drops. The tragus should then be pumped 4 times by pushing inward to facilitate penetration into the middle ear. This position should be maintained for five minutes. Repeat, if necessary, for the opposite ear.

HOW SUPPLIED

FLOXIN® Otic (ofloxacin otic) solution 0.3% is supplied in plastic dropper bottles containing 5 mL and 10 mL.

NDC 63395-101-05 FLOXIN® Otic 5 mL
NDC 63395-101-10 FLOXIN® Otic 10 mL

Storage Conditions: Store at 25°C (77°F), excursions permitted to 15-30°C (59-86°F). Protect from light.

℞ Only

Daiichi Pharmaceutical Corporation
Montvale, NJ 07645
Revised May 2004
Covered by U.S. Patent No. 5,401,741

Shown in Product Identification Guide, page 311

FLOXIN® OTIC SINGLES™ ℞

[Flox-in]
(ofloxacin otic) solution 0.3%

DESCRIPTION

FLOXIN® Otic SINGLES™ (ofloxacin otic) solution 0.3% is a sterile aqueous antiinfective (anti-bacterial) solution for otic use. Chemically, ofloxacin has three condensed 6-membered rings made up of a fluorinated carboxyquinolone with a benzoxazine ring. The chemical name of ofloxacin is: (±)-9-fluoro-2,3-dihydro-3-methyl-10-(4-methyl-1-piperazinyl)-7-oxo-7*H*-pyrido [1,2,3-*de*]-1,4-benzoxazine-6-carboxylic acid. The empirical formula of ofloxacin is $C_{18}H_{20}FN_3O_4$ and its molecular weight is 361.38. The structural formula is:

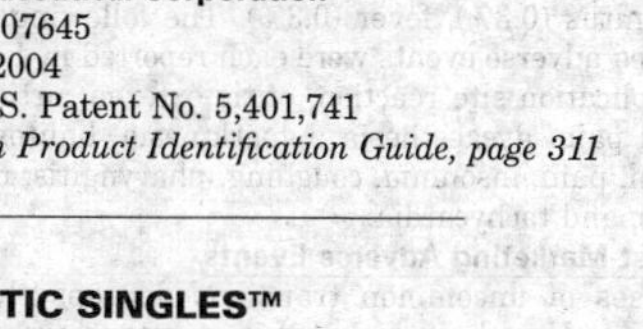

FLOXIN® Otic SINGLES™ contains 0.3% (3 mg/mL) ofloxacin with benzalkonium chloride (0.0025%), sodium chloride (0.9%), and water for injection. Hydrochloric acid and sodium hydroxide are added to adjust the pH to 6.5±0.5.

CLINICAL PHARMACOLOGY

Pharmacokinetics: Drug concentrations in serum (in subjects with tympanostomy tubes and perforated tympanic membranes), in otorrhea, and in mucosa of the middle ear (in subjects with perforated tympanic membranes) were determined following otic administration of ofloxacin solution. In two single-dose studies, mean ofloxacin serum concentrations were low in adult patients with tympanostomy tubes, with and without otorrhea, after otic administration of a 0.3% solution (4.1 ng/mL (n=3) and 5.4 ng/mL (n=5), respectively). In adults with perforated tympanic membranes, the maximum serum drug level of ofloxacin detected was 10 ng/mL after administration of a 0.3% solution. Ofloxacin was detectable in the middle ear mucosa of some adult subjects with perforated tympanic membranes (11 of 16 subjects). The variability of ofloxacin concentration in middle ear mucosa was high. The concentrations ranged from 1.2 to 602 µg/g after otic administration of a 0.3% solution. Ofloxacin was present in high concentrations in otorrhea (389–2850 µg/g, n=13) 30 minutes after otic administration of a 0.3% solution in subjects with chronic suppurative otitis media and perforated tympanic membranes. However, the measurement of ofloxacin in the otorrhea does not necessarily reflect the exposure of the middle ear to ofloxacin.

Microbiology: Ofloxacin has *in vitro* activity against a wide range of gram-negative and gram-positive microorganisms. Ofloxacin exerts its antibacterial activity by inhibiting DNA gyrase, a bacterial topoisomerase. DNA gyrase is an essential enzyme which controls DNA topology and assists in DNA replication, repair, deactivation, and transcription. Cross-resistance has been observed between ofloxacin and other fluoroquinolones. There is generally no cross-resistance between ofloxacin and other classes of antibacterial agents such as beta-lactams or aminoglycosides.

Ofloxacin has been shown to be active against most isolates of the following microorganisms, both *in vitro* and clinically in otic infections as described in the **INDICATIONS AND USAGE** section.

Aerobic and facultative gram-positive microorganisms:
Staphylococcus aureus *Streptococcus pneumoniae*

Aerobic and facultative gram-negative microorganisms:
Escherichia coli *Proteus mirabilis*
Haemophilus influenzae *Pseudomonas aeruginosa*
Moraxella catarrhalis

INDICATIONS AND USAGE

FLOXIN® Otic SINGLES™ (ofloxacin otic) solution 0.3% is indicated for the treatment of infections caused by susceptible isolates of the designated microorganisms in the specific conditions listed below:

Otitis Externa in adults and pediatric patients, 6 months and older, due to *Escherichia coli, Pseudomonas aeruginosa,* and *Staphylococcus aureus.*

Chronic Suppurative Otitis Media in patients 12 years and older with perforated tympanic membranes due to *Proteus mirabilis, Pseudomonas aeruginosa,* and *Staphylococcus aureus.*

Acute Otitis Media in pediatric patients one year and older with tympanostomy tubes due to *Haemophilus influenzae, Moraxella catarrhalis, Pseudomonas aeruginosa, Staphylococcus aureus,* and *Streptococcus pneumoniae.*

CONTRAINDICATIONS

FLOXIN® Otic SINGLES™ (ofloxacin otic) solution 0.3% is contraindicated in patients with a history of hypersensitivity to ofloxacin, to other quinolones, or to any of the components in this medication.

WARNINGS

NOT FOR OPHTHALMIC USE.
NOT FOR INJECTION.

Serious and occasionally fatal hypersensitivity (anaphylactic) reactions, some following the first dose, have been reported in patients receiving systemic quinolones, including ofloxacin. Some reactions were accompanied by cardiovascular collapse, loss of consciousness, angioedema (including laryngeal, pharyngeal or facial edema), airway obstruction, dyspnea, urticaria, and itching. If an allergic reaction to ofloxacin is suspected, stop the drug. Serious acute hypersensitivity reactions may require immediate emergency treatment. Oxygen and airway management, including intubation, should be administered as clinically indicated.

PRECAUTIONS

General: As with other anti-infective preparations, prolonged use may result in over-growth of nonsusceptible organisms, including fungi. If the infection is not improved after one week, cultures should be obtained to guide further treatment. If otorrhea persists after a full course of therapy, or if two or more episodes of otorrhea occur within six months, further evaluation is recommended to exclude an underlying condition such as cholesteatoma, foreign body, or a tumor.

The systemic administration of quinolones, including ofloxacin at doses much higher than given or absorbed by the otic route, has led to lesions or erosions of the cartilage in weight-bearing joints and other signs of arthropathy in immature animals of various species.

Young growing guinea pigs dosed in the middle ear with 0.3% ofloxacin otic solution showed no systemic effects, lesions or erosions of the cartilage in weight-bearing joints, or other signs of arthropathy. No drug-related structural or functional changes of the cochlea and no lesions in the ossicles were noted in the guinea pig following otic administration of 0.3% ofloxacin for one month.

Continued on next page

Floxin Otic Singles—Cont.

No signs of local irritation were found when 0.3% ofloxacin was applied topically in the rabbit eye. Ofloxacin was also shown to lack dermal sensitizing potential in the guinea pig maximization study.

Information for Patients: Avoid contaminating the applicator tip with material from the fingers or other sources. This precaution is necessary if the sterility of the drops is to be preserved. Systemic quinolones, including ofloxacin, have been associated with hypersensitivity reactions, even following a single dose. Discontinue use immediately and contact your physician at the first sign of a rash or allergic reaction.

Otitis Externa

Prior to administration of FLOXIN® Otic SINGLES™, the solution should be warmed by holding the single-dispensing container(s) in the hand for one or two minutes to avoid dizziness which may result from the instillation of a cold solution. The patient should lie with the affected ear upward, and then the drops should be instilled. This position should be maintained for five minutes to facilitate penetration of the drops into the ear canal. Repeat, if necessary, for the opposite ear (see **DOSAGE AND ADMINISTRATION**).

Acute Otitis Media and Chronic Suppurative Otitis Media

Prior to administration of FLOXIN® Otic SINGLES™, the solution should be warmed by holding the single-dispensing container(s) in the hand for one or two minutes to avoid dizziness which may result from the instillation of a cold solution. The patient should lie with the affected ear upward, and then the drops should be instilled. The tragus should then be pumped 4 times by pushing inward to facilitate penetration of the drops into the middle ear. This position should be maintained for five minutes. Repeat, if necessary, for the opposite ear (see **DOSAGE AND ADMINISTRATION**).

Drug Interactions: Specific drug interaction studies have not been conducted with FLOXIN® Otic SINGLES™.

Carcinogenesis, Mutagenesis, Impairment of Fertility

Long-term studies to determine the carcinogenic potential of ofloxacin have not been conducted. Ofloxacin was not mutagenic in the Ames test, the sister chromatid exchange assay (Chinese hamster and human cell lines), the unscheduled DNA synthesis (UDS) assay using human fibroblasts, the dominant lethal assay, or the mouse micronucleus assay. Ofloxacin was positive in the rat hepatocyte UDS assay, and in the mouse lymphoma assay. In rats, ofloxacin did not affect male or female reproductive performance at oral doses up to 360 mg/kg/day. This would be over 1000 times the maximum recommended clinical dose, based upon body surface area, assuming total absorption of ofloxacin from the ear of a patient treated with FLOXIN® Otic twice per day.

Pregnancy

Teratogenic effects: Pregnancy Category C. Ofloxacin has been shown to have an embryocidal effect in rats at a dose of 810 mg/kg/day and in rabbits at 160 mg/kg/day.

These dosages resulted in decreased fetal body weights and increased fetal mortality in rats and rabbits, respectively. Minor fetal skeletal variations were reported in rats receiving doses of 810 mg/kg/day. Ofloxacin has not been shown to be teratogenic at doses as high as 810 mg/kg/day and 160 mg/kg/day when administered to pregnant rats and rabbits, respectively.

Ofloxacin has not been shown to have any adverse effects on the developing embryo or fetus at doses relevant to the amount of ofloxacin that will be delivered ototopically at the recommended clinical doses.

Nonteratogenic Effects: Additional studies in the rat demonstrated that doses up to 360 mg/kg/day during late gestation had no adverse effects on late fetal development, labor, delivery, lactation, neonatal viability, or growth of the newborn. There are, however, no adequate and well-controlled studies in pregnant women. FLOXIN® Otic SINGLES™ should be used during pregnancy only if the potential benefit justifies the potential risk to the fetus.

Nursing Mothers: In nursing women, a single 200 mg oral dose resulted in concentrations of ofloxacin in milk which were similar to those found in plasma. It is not known whether ofloxacin is excreted in human milk following topical otic administration. Because of the potential for serious adverse reactions from ofloxacin in nursing infants, a decision should be made whether to discontinue nursing or to discontinue the drug, taking into account the importance of the drug to the mother.

Pediatric Use: Safety and efficacy have been demonstrated in pediatric patients of the following ages for the listed indications:

- six months and older: otitis externa with intact tympanic membranes
- one year and older: acute otitis media with tympanostomy tubes
- twelve years and older: chronic suppurative otitis media with perforated tympanic membranes

Safety and efficacy in pediatric patients below these ages have not been established.

Although no data are available on patients less than age 6 months, there are no known safety concerns or differences in the disease process in this population that will preclude use of this product.

No changes in hearing function occurred in 30 pediatric subjects treated with ofloxacin otic and tested for audiometric parameters.

Although quinolones, including ofloxacin, have been shown to cause arthropathy in immature animals after systemic administration, young growing guinea pigs dosed in the middle ear with 0.3% ofloxacin otic solution for one month showed no systemic effects, quinolone-induced lesions, erosions of the cartilage in weight-bearing joints, or other signs of arthropathy.

ADVERSE REACTIONS

Subjects with Otitis Externa

In the phase III clinical trials performed in support of once-daily dosing, 799 subjects with otitis externa and intact tympanic membranes were treated with ofloxacin otic solution. The studies, which served as the basis for approval, were 020 (pediatric, adolescents and adults), 016 (adolescents and adults) and 017 (pediatric). The following treatment-related adverse events occurred in two or more of the subjects.

[See table below]

In once daily dosing studies, there were also single reports of nausea, seborrhea, loss of hearing, tinnitus, otitis externa, otitis media, tremor, hypertension and fungal infection.

In twice daily dosing studies, the following treatment-related adverse events were each reported in a single subject: dermatitis, eczema, erythematous rash, follicular rash, hypoaesthesia, tinnitus, dyspepsia, hot flushes, flushing and otorrhagia.

Subjects with Acute Otitis Media with Tympanostomy Tubes (AOM TT) and Subjects with Chronic Suppurative Otitis Media (CSOM) with Perforated Tympanic Membranes

In phase III clinical trials which formed the basis for approval, the following treatment-related adverse events occurred in 1% or more of the 656 subjects with nonintact tympanic membranes in AOM TT or CSOM treated twice-daily with ofloxacin otic solution:

Adverse Event	Incidence (N = 656)
Taste Perversion	7%
Earache	1%
Pruritus	1%
Paraesthesia	1%
Rash	1%
Dizziness	1%

Other treatment-related adverse reactions reported in subjects with non-intact tympanic membranes included: diarrhea (0.6%), nausea (0.3%), vomiting (0.3%), dry mouth (0.5%), headache (0.3%), vertigo (0.5%), otorrhagia (0.6%), tinnitus (0.3%), fever (0.3%). The following treatment-related adverse events were each reported in a single subject: application site reaction, otitis externa, urticaria, abdominal pain, dysaesthesia, hyperkinesia, halitosis, inflammation, pain, insomnia, coughing, pharyngitis, rhinitis, sinusitis, and tachycardia.

Post-Marketing Adverse Events

Cases of uncommon transient neuropsychiatric disturbances have been included in spontaneous post-marketing reports. A causal relationship with ofloxacin otic solution 0.3% is unknown.

DOSAGE AND ADMINISTRATION

Otitis Externa: The recommended dosage regimen for the treatment of otitis externa is:

For pediatric patients (from 6 months to 13 years old): instill the contents of 1 single-dispensing container into the affected ear once daily for seven days.

For patients 13 years and older: instill the contents of 2 single-dispensing containers into the affected ear once daily for seven days.

The solution should be warmed by holding the container in the hand for one or two minutes to avoid dizziness which may result from the instillation of a cold solution. The patient should lie with the affected ear upward, and then the drops should be instilled. This position should be maintained for five minutes to facilitate penetration of the drops into the ear canal. Repeat, if necessary, for the opposite ear.

Acute Otitis Media in pediatric patients with tympanostomy tubes: The recommended dosage regimen for the treatment of acute otitis media in pediatric patients (from 1 to 12 years old) with tympanostomy tubes is:

Instill the contents of 1 single-dispensing container into the affected ear twice daily for ten days. The solution should be warmed by holding the container in the hand for one or two minutes to avoid dizziness which may result from the instillation of a cold solution. The patient should lie with the affected ear upward, and then the medication should be instilled. The tragus should then be pumped 4 times by pushing inward to facilitate penetration of the medication into the middle ear. This position should be maintained for five minutes. Repeat, if necessary, for the opposite ear.

Chronic Suppurative Otitis Media with perforated tympanic membranes: The recommended dosage regimen for the treatment of chronic suppurative otitis media with perforated tympanic membranes in patients 12 years and older is:

Instill the contents of 2 single-dispensing containers into the affected ear twice daily for fourteen days. The solution should be warmed by holding the container in the hand for one or two minutes to avoid dizziness which may result from the instillation of a cold solution. The patient should lie with the affected ear upward, before instilling the medication. The tragus should then be pumped 4 times by pushing inward to facilitate penetration into the middle ear. This position should be maintained for five minutes. Repeat, if necessary, for the opposite ear.

HOW SUPPLIED

FLOXIN® Otic SINGLES™ (ofloxacin otic) solution 0.3% is supplied in plastic single-dispensing containers, 0.25 mL each, packaged 2 per foil pouch.

NDC 63395-101-01 FLOXIN® Otic SINGLES™, 1 foil pouch containing 2 single-dispensing containers, per Physician Sample box.

NDC 63395-101-11 FLOXIN® Otic SINGLES™, 10 foil pouches each containing 2 single-dispensing containers (5 mL net volume), per carton.

Storage Conditions: Store at 25°C (77°F), excursions permitted to 15–30°C (59–86°F). Protect from light.

℞ **Only**

Daiichi Pharmaceutical Corporation
Montvale, NJ 07645
Revised May 2004
Covered by U.S. Patent No. 5,401,741

	Incidence Rate		
Adverse Event	Studies 002/003† BID (N=229)	Studies 016/017† QD (N=310)	Study 020† QD (N=489)
Application Site Reaction	3%	16.8%	0.6%
Pruritus	4%	1.2%	1.0%
Earache	1%	0.6%	0.8%
Dizziness	1%	0.0%	0.6%
Headache	0%	0.3%	0.2%
Vertigo	1%	0.0%	0.0%

† Studies 002/003 (BID) and 016/017 (QD) were active-controlled and comparative. Study 020 (QD) was open and non-comparative.

An unexpected increased incidence of application site reaction was seen in studies 016/017 and was similar for both ofloxacin and the active control drug (neomycin-polymyxin B sulfate-hydrocortisone). This finding is believed to be the result of specific questioning of the subjects regarding the incidence of application site reactions.

Dermik Laboratories

1050 WESTLAKES DRIVE
BERWYN, PA 19312

Direct Inquiries to:
Customer Service
Somerset Corporate Center, Blg 3
300 Somerset Corporate Blvd
Bridgewater, NJ 08807-2854
(800) 207-8049

For Medical Information Contact:
Medical Information Services
Somerset Corporate Center, Blg 3
300 Somerset Corporate Blvd
Bridgewater, NJ 08807-2854
(800) 633-1610
www.dermik.com

BENZACLIN® TOPICAL GEL ℞

(clindamycin–benzoyl peroxide gel)
Topical Gel: clindamycin (1%) as clindamycin phosphate, benzoyl peroxide (5%)
For Dermatological Use Only—Not for Ophthalmic Use
Reconstitute Before Dispensing

DESCRIPTION

BenzaClin® Topical Gel contains clindamycin phosphate, (7(S)-chloro-7-deoxylincomycin-2-phosphate). Clindamycin phosphate is a water soluble ester of the semi-synthetic antibiotic produced by a 7(S)-chloro-substitution of the 7(R)-hydroxyl group of the parent antibiotic lincomycin.

Chemically, clindamycin phosphate is ($C_{18}H_{34}ClN_2O_8PS$). The structural formula for clindamycin is represented below:

[See chemical structure at top of next column]

Clindamycin phosphate has molecular weight of 504.97 and its chemical name is Methyl 7-chloro-6,7,8-trideoxy-6-

(1-methyl-trans-4-propyl-L-2-pyrrolidinecarboxamido)-1-thio-L-threo-alpha-D-galacto-octopyranoside 2-(dihydrogen phosphate).

BenzaClin Topical Gel also contains benzoyl peroxide, for topical use. Chemically, benzoyl peroxide is ($C_{14}H_{10}O_4$). It has the following structural formula:

Benzoyl peroxide has a molecular weight of 242.23.

Each gram of **BenzaClin Topical Gel** contains, as dispensed, 10 mg (1%) clindamycin as phosphate and 50 mg (5%) benzoyl peroxide in a base of carbomer, sodium hydroxide, dioctyl sodium sulfosuccinate, and purified water.

CLINICAL PHARMACOLOGY

An *in vitro* percutaneous penetration study comparing **BenzaClin Topical Gel** and topical 1% clindamycin gel alone, demonstrated there was no statistical difference in penetration between the two drugs. Mean systemic bioavailability of topical clindamycin in **BenzaClin Topical Gel** is suggested to be less than 1%.

Benzoyl peroxide has been shown to be absorbed by the skin where it is converted to benzoic acid. Less than 2% of the dose enters systemic circulation as benzoic acid. It is suggested that the lipophilic nature of benzoyl peroxide acts to concentrate the compound into the lipid-rich sebaceous follicle.

Microbiology:

The clindamycin and benzoyl peroxide components individually have been shown to have *in vitro* activity against *Propionibacterium acnes* an organism which has been associated with acne vulgaris; however, the clinical significance of this activity against *P. acnes* was not examined in clinical trials with this product.

CLINICAL STUDIES

In two adequate and well controlled clinical studies of 758 patients, 214 used BenzaClin, 210 used benzoyl peroxide, 168 used clindamycin, and 166 used vehicle. **BenzaClin** applied twice daily for 10 weeks was significantly more effective than vehicle in the treatment of moderate to moderately severe facial acne vulgaris. Patients were evaluated and acne lesions counted at each clinical visit; weeks, 2, 4, 6, 8 and 10. The primary efficacy measures were the lesion counts and the investigator's global assessment evaluated at week 10. Patients were instructed to wash the face with a mild soap, using only the hands. Fifteen minutes after the face was thoroughly dry, application was made to the entire face. Non-medicated make-up could be applied at one hour after the **BenzaClin** application. If a moisturizer was required, the patients were provided a moisturizer to be used as needed. Patients were instructed to avoid sun exposure.

Percent reductions in lesion counts after treatment for 10 weeks in these two studies are shown below:

[See first table above]

The BenzaClin group showed greater overall improvement than the benzoyl peroxide, clindamycin and vehicle groups as rated by the investigator.

INDICATIONS AND USAGE

BenzaClin Topical Gel is indicated for the topical treatment of acne vulgaris.

CONTRAINDICATIONS

BenzaClin Topical Gel is contraindicated in those individuals who have shown hypersensitivity to any of its components or to lincomycin. It is also contraindicated in those having a history of regional enteritis, ulcerative colitis, or antibiotic-associated colitis.

WARNINGS

ORALLY AND PARENTERALLY ADMINISTERED CLINDAMYCIN HAS BEEN ASSOCIATED WITH SEVERE COLITIS WHICH MAY RESULT IN PATIENT DEATH. USE OF THE TOPICAL FORMULATION OF CLINDAMYCIN RESULTS IN ABSORPTION OF THE ANTIBIOTIC FROM THE SKIN SURFACE. DIARRHEA, BLOODY DIARRHEA, AND COLITIS (INCLUDING PSEUDOMEMBRANOUS COLITIS) HAVE BEEN REPORTED WITH THE USE OF TOPICAL AND SYSTEMIC CLINDAMYCIN. STUDIES INDICATE A TOXIN(S) PRODUCED BY CLOSTRIDIA IS ONE PRIMARY CAUSE OF ANTIBIOTIC-ASSOCIATED COLITIS. THE COLITIS IS USUALLY CHARACTERIZED BY SEVERE PERSISTENT DIARRHEA AND SEVERE ABDOMINAL CRAMPS AND MAY BE ASSOCIATED WITH THE PASSAGE OF BLOOD AND MUCUS. ENDOSCOPIC EXAMINATION MAY REVEAL PSEUDOMEMBRANOUS COLITIS. STOOL CULTURE FOR *Clostridium Difficile* AND STOOL ASSAY FOR *C. Difficile* TOXIN MAY BE HELPFUL DIAGNOSTICALLY. WHEN SIGNIFICANT DIARRHEA OCCURS, THE DRUG SHOULD BE DISCONTINUED. LARGE BOWEL ENDOSCOPY SHOULD BE CONSIDERED TO ESTABLISH A DEFINITIVE DIAGNOSIS IN CASES OF SEVERE DIARRHEA.

Study 1

BenzaClin n=120	Benzoyl peroxide n=120	Clindamycin n=120	Vehicle n=120
Mean percent reduction in inflammatory lesion counts			
46%	32%	16%	+3%
Mean percent reduction in non-inflammatory lesion counts			
22%	22%	9%	+1%
Mean percent reduction in total lesion counts			
36%	28%	15%	0.2%

Study 2

BenzaClin n=95	Benzoyl peroxide n=95	Clindamycin n=49	Vehicle n=48
Mean percent reduction in inflammatory lesion counts			
63%	53%	45%	42%
Mean percent reduction in non-inflammatory lesion counts			
54%	50%	39%	36%
Mean percent reduction in total lesion counts			
58%	52%	42%	39%

Size (Net Weight)	NDC 0066-	Benzoyl Peroxide Gel	Active Clindamycin Powder (in plastic vial)	Purified Water To Be Added to each vial
25 grams	0494-25	19.7g	0.3g (1 vial)*	5 mL
50 grams	0494-50	41.4g	0.6g (2 vials)*	5 mL

*Each vial contains 0.3g Clindamycin Phosphate

ANTIPERISTALTIC AGENTS SUCH AS OPIATES AND DIPHENOXYLATE WITH ATROPINE MAY PROLONG AND/OR WORSEN THE CONDITION. DIARRHEA, COLITIS, AND PSEUDOMEMBRANOUS COLITIS HAVE BEEN OBSERVED TO BEGIN UP TO SEVERAL WEEKS FOLLOWING CESSATION OF ORAL AND PARENTERAL THERAPY WITH CLINDAMYCIN.

Mild cases of pseudomembranous colitis usually respond to drug discontinuation alone. In moderate to severe cases, consideration should be given to management with fluids and electrolytes, protein supplementation and treatment with an antibacterial drug clinically effective against *C. difficile* colitis.

PRECAUTIONS

General: For dermatological use only; not for ophthalmic use. Concomitant topical acne therapy should be used with caution because a possible cumulative irritancy effect may occur, especially with the use of peeling, desquamating, or abrasive agents.

The use of antibiotic agents may be associated with the overgrowth of nonsusceptible organisms including fungi. If this occurs, discontinue use of this medication and take appropriate measures.

Avoid contact with eyes and mucous membranes.

Clindamyin and erythromycin containing products should not be used in combination. *In vitro* studies have shown antagonism between these two antimicrobials. The clinical significance of this *in vitro* antagonism is not known.

Information for Patients: Patients using **BenzaClin Topical Gel** should receive the following information and instructions:

1. **BenzaClin Topical Gel** is to be used as directed by the physician. It is for external use only. Avoid contact with eyes, and inside the nose, mouth, and all mucous membranes, as this product may be irritating.
2. This medication should not be used for any disorder other than that for which it was prescribed.
3. Patients should not use any other topical acne preparation unless otherwise directed by physician.
4. Patients should report any signs of local adverse reactions to their physician.
5. **BenzaClin Topical Gel** may bleach hair or colored fabric.
6. **BenzaClin Topical Gel** can be stored at room temperature up to 25°C (77°F) for 3 months. Do not freeze. Discard any unused product after 3 months.
7. Before applying **BenzaClin Topical Gel** to affected areas wash the skin gently, then rinse with warm water and pat dry.

Carcinogenesis, Mutagenesis, Impairment of Fertility: Benzoyl peroxide has been shown to be a tumor promoter and progression agent in a number of animal studies. The clinical significance of this is unknown.

Benzoyl peroxide in acetone at doses of 5 and 10 mg administered twice per week induced skin tumors in transgenic Tg.AC mice in a study using 20 weeks of topical treatment.

Genotoxicity studies were not conducted with **BenzaClin Topical Gel.** Clindamycin phosphate was not genotoxic in *Salmonella typhimurium* or in a rat micronucleus test. Clindamycin phosphate sulfoxide, an oxidative degradation product of clindamycin phosphate and benzoyl peroxide, was not clastogenic in a mouse micronucleus test. Benzoyl peroxide has been found to cause DNA strand breaks in a variety of mammalian cell types, to be mutagenic in *S. typhimurium* tests by some but not all investigators, and to cause sister chromatid exchanges in Chinese hamster ovary cells. Studies have not been performed with **BenzaClin Topical Gel** or benzoyl peroxide to evaluate the effect on fertility. Fertility studies in rats treated orally with up to 300 mg/kg/day of clindamycin (approximately 120 times the amount of clindamycin in the highest recommended adult human dose of 2.5 g BenzaClin Topical Gel, based on mg/m^2) revealed no effects on fertility or mating ability.

Pregnancy: Teratogenic Effects: Pregnancy Category C: Animal reproductive/developmental toxicity studies have not been conducted with **BenzaClin Topical Gel** or benzoyl peroxide. Developmental toxicity studies performed in rats and mice using oral doses of clindamycin up to 600 mg/kg/day (240 and 120 times amount of clindamycin in the highest recommended adult human dose based on mg/m^2, respectively) or subcutaneous doses of clindamycin up to 250 mg/kg/day (100 and 50 times the amount of clindamycin in the highest recommended adult human dose based on mg/m^2, respectively) revealed no evidence of teratogenicity.

There are no well-controlled trials in pregnant women treated with **BenzaClin Topical Gel**. It also is not known whether **BenzaClin Topical Gel** can cause fetal harm when administered to a pregnant woman.

Nursing Women: It is not known whether **BenzaClin Topical Gel** is excreted in human milk after topical application. However, orally and parenterally administered clindamycin has been reported to appear in breast milk. Because of the potential for serious adverse reactions in nursing infants, a decision should be made whether to discontinue nursing or to discontinue the drug, taking into account the importance of the drug to the mother.

Pediatric Use: Safety and effectiveness of this product in pediatric patients below the age of 12 have not been established.

ADVERSE REACTIONS

During clinical trials, the most frequently reported adverse event in the **BenzaClin** treatment group was dry skin (12%). The Table below lists local adverse events reported by at least 1% of patients in the **BenzaClin** and vehicle groups.

Local Adverse Events - all causalities in >/= 1% of patients

	BenzaClin n = 420	Vehicle n = 168
Application site reaction	13 (3%)	1 (<1%)
Dry skin	50 (12%)	10 (6%)

Continued on next page

Benzaclin—Cont.

Pruritus	8 (2%)	1 (<1%)
Peeling	9 (2%)	-
Erythema	6 (1%)	1 (<1%)
Sunburn	5 (1%)	-

The actual incidence of dry skin might have been greater were it not for the use of a moisturizer in these studies.

DOSAGE AND ADMINISTRATION

BenzaClin Topical Gel should be applied twice daily, morning and evening, or as directed by a physician, to affected areas after the skin is gently washed, rinsed with warm water and patted dry.

HOW SUPPLIED AND COMPOUNDING INSTRUCTIONS

[See second table at top of previous page]

Prior to dispensing, tap each vial until powder flows freely. Add 5 mL of purified water to each vial (to the mark) and immediately shake to completely dissolve clindamycin. If needed, add additional purified water to bring level up to the mark. Add the solution in each vial to the gel and stir until homogenous in appearance (1 to 1½ minutes). **BenzaClin Topical Gel** (as reconstituted) can be stored at room temperature up to 25°C (77°F) for 3 months. Place a 3 month expiration date on the label immediately following mixing.

Store at room temperature up to 25°C (77°F) [see USP].

Do not freeze. Keep tightly closed. Keep out of the reach of children.

US Patents 5,446,028; 5,767,098; 6,013,637

Prescribing Information as of September 2003

Rx Only

DERMIK LABORATORIES

A Division of Aventis Pharmaceuticals Inc.

Berwyn, PA 19312 USA

MICROGEL™ FORMULA ℞
5 Benzagel® & 10 Benzagel®

Acne Gel

(benzoyl peroxide gel)

DESCRIPTION

Each gram of **5 Benzagel®** and **10 Benzagel®** contains 50 mg and 100 mg respectively, of benzoyl peroxide in a gel vehicle of purified water, carbomer 940, 14% alcohol, sodium hydroxide, docusate sodium and fragrances.

Benzoyl peroxide is an antibacterial and keratolytic agent.

The structural formula is:

Hydrous Benzoyl Peroxide

HOW SUPPLIED

5 Benzagel is available in 1.5 oz. (42.5 g) (NDC 0066-0430-15) plastic tubes; **10 Benzagel** is available in 1.5 oz. (42.5 g) (NDC 0066-0431-15) plastic tubes.

5 Benzagel contains 50 mg benzoyl peroxide per gram and **10 Benzagel** contains 100 mg of benzoyl peroxide per gram.

Store at Controlled Room Temperature 20 to 25°C (68 to 77°F) [see USP].

Pat.No 4,387,107

Prescribing Information as of April 2003

Rx Only

Dermik Laboratories

A Division of Aventis Pharmaceuticals Inc

Berwyn, PA 19312 USA

BENZAMYCIN® PAK ℞

(erythromycin 3%-benzoyl peroxide 5% topical gel)

For Dermatological Use Only—Not for Ophthalmic Use

DESCRIPTION

Benzamycin® Pak contains erythromycin [(3R*, 4S*, 5S*, 6R*, 7R*, 9R*, 11R*, 12R*, 13S*, 14R*)-4-[(2,6-dideoxy-3-C-methyl-3-O-methyl-a-L-ribo-hexopyranosyl)-oxy]-14-ethyl-7,12,13-trihydroxy-3,5,7,9,11,13-hexa-methyl-6-[[3,4,6-trideoxy-3-(dimethylamino)-b-D-xylo-hexopyranosyl]oxy]oxacyclotetradecane-2,10-dione]. Erythromycin is a macrolide antibiotic produced from a strain of *Saccharopolyspora erythraea* (formerly *Streptomyces erythreus*). It is a base and readily forms salts with acids.

Chemically, erythromycin is ($C_{37}H_{67}NO_{13}$). It has the following structural formula:

[See chemical structure at top of next column]

Erythromycin has the molecular weight of 733.94. It is a white crystalline powder and has a solubility of approximately 1 mg/mL in water and is soluble in alcohol at 25°C.

Size (Net Weight)	NDC 0066-	Benzoyl Peroxide Gel	Active Erythromycin Powder (In Plastic Vial)	70% Ethyl Alcohol To Be Added
46.6 grams (as dispensed)	0510-46	40 grams	1.6 grams	6 mL

Benzamycin® Pak also contains benzoyl peroxide for topical use. Benzoyl peroxide is an oxidizing agent demonstrating antibacterial activity.

Chemically, benzoyl peroxide is ($C_{14}H_{10}O_4$). It has the following structural formula:

Benzoyl peroxide has the molecular weight of 242.23. It is a white granular powder and is sparingly soluble in water and alcohol and soluble in acetone, chloroform and ether.

Each gram of product, as dispensed, contains 30 mg of erythromycin and 50 mg of benzoyl peroxide in a base of SD Alcohol 40B, purified water, hydroxypropyl cellulose, carbomer 934, sodium hydroxide, dioctyl sodium sulfosuccinate 75%. Each Benzamycin® Pak contains 0.8 grams of product.

HOW SUPPLIED

60 Pouches per carton **NDC 0066-0577-60**

Store at Room Temperature 20 to 25°C (68 to 77°F).

Keep away from heat and any open flame.

Keep out of the reach of children.

Prescribing Information as of July 2002

Rx only

Manufactured for:

Dermik Laboratories

A Division of Aventis Pharmaceuticals Inc.

Berwyn, PA, 19312 USA

by:

DPT Lakewood, Inc

Lakewood, NJ 08701 USA

BENZAMYCIN® Topical Gel ℞

(3% erythromycin, 5% benzoyl peroxide)

Topical Gel: erythromycin (3%), benzoyl peroxide (5%)

For Dermatological Use Only – Not for Ophthalmic Use

Reconstitute Before Dispensing

DESCRIPTION

Benzamycin® Topical Gel contains erythromycin [(3R*, 4S*, 5S*, 6R*, 7R*, 9R*, 11R*, 12R*, 13S*, 14R*)-4-[(2,6-Dideoxy-3-*C*-methyl-3-*O*-methyl-*a*-L-*ribo*-hexopyranosyl)-oxy]-14-ethyl-7,12,13-trihydroxy-3,5,7,9,11,13-hexamethyl-6-[[3,4,6-trideoxy-3-(dimethylamino)-*b*-D-*xylo*-hexopyranosyl]oxy]oxacyclotetradecane-2,10-dione]. Erythromycin is a macrolide antibiotic produced from a strain of *Saccharopolyspora erythraea* (formerly *Streptomyces erythreus*). It is a base and readily forms salts with acids.

Chemically, erythromycin is ($C_{37}H_{67}NO_{13}$). It has the following structural formula:

Erythromycin has the molecular weight of 733.94. It is a white crystalline powder and has a solubility of approximately 1 mg/mL in water and is soluble in alcohol at 25°C.

BENZAMYCIN Topical Gel also contains benzoyl peroxide for topical use. Benzoyl peroxide is an antibacterial and keratolytic agent.

Chemically, benzoyl peroxide is ($C_{14}H_{10}O_4$). It has the following structural formula:

Benzoyl peroxide has the molecular weight of 242.23. It is a white granular powder and is sparingly soluble in water and alcohol and soluble in acetone, chloroform and ether.

Each gram of BENZAMYCIN Topical Gel contains, as dispensed, 30 mg (3%) of erythromycin and 50 mg (5%) of benzoyl peroxide in a base of purified water USP, carbomer, alcohol 20%, sodium hydroxide NF, docusate sodium and fragrance.

HOW SUPPLIED AND COMPOUNDING DIRECTIONS

[See table above]

Prior to dispensing, tap vial until all powder flows freely. Add indicated amount of room temperature 70% ethyl alcohol to vial (to the mark) and immediately shake to completely dissolve erythromycin. Add this solution to gel and stir until homogeneous in appearance (1 to 1 1/2 minutes). BENZAMYCIN Topical Gel should then be stored under refrigeration. Do not freeze. Place a 3-month expiration date on the label.

Note: ***Prior to reconstitution,*** **store at room temperature between 15° and 30°C (59° – 86°F).**

After reconstitution, **store under refrigeration between 2° and 8°C (36° – 46°F).**

Do not freeze. Keep tightly closed. Keep out of the reach of children.

U.S. Patent Nos. 4,387,107 and 4,497,794.

Prescribing Information as of December 2002 (b).

Rx only

Manufactured for

Dermik Laboratories

A Division of Aventis Pharmaceuticals Inc.

Berwyn, PA 19312 USA

by

Aventis Pharmaceuticals Puerto Rico Inc.

Manati, Puerto Rico 00674

CARAC® CREAM 0.5% ℞

(fluorouracil cream)

FOR TOPICAL DERMATOLOGICAL USE ONLY (NOT FOR OPHTHALMIC, ORAL, OR INTRAVAGINAL USE)

℞ Only

DESCRIPTION

Carac® (fluorouracil cream) Cream, 0.5%, contains fluorouracil for topical dermatologic use. Chemically, fluorouracil is 5-fluoro-2,4(1H, 3H)-pyrimidinedione. The molecular formula is $C_4H_3FN_2O_2$. Fluorouracil has a molecular weight of 130.08.

Carac Cream contains 0.5% fluorouracil, with 0.35% being incorporated into a patented porous microsphere (Microsponge®)* composed of methyl methacrylate / glycol dimethacrylate crosspolymer and dimethicone. The cream formulation contains the following other inactive ingredients: carbomer 940, dimethicone, glycerin, methyl gluceth-20, methyl methacrylate / glycol dimethacrylate crosspolymer, methylparaben, octyl hydroxy stearate, polyethylene glycol 400, polysorbate 80, propylene glycol, propylparaben, purified water, sorbitan monooleate, stearic acid, and trolamine.

CLINICAL PHARMACOLOGY

There is evidence that the metabolism of fluorouracil in the anabolic pathway blocks the methylation reaction of deoxyuridylic acid to thymidylic acid. In this manner, fluorouracil interferes with the synthesis of deoxyribonucleic acid (DNA) and to a lesser extent inhibits the formation of ribonucleic acid (RNA). Since DNA and RNA are essential for cell division and growth, the effect of fluorouracil may be to create a thymine deficiency that provokes unbalanced growth and death of the cell. The effects of DNA and RNA deprivation are most marked on those cells that grow more rapidly and take up fluorouracil at a more rapid rate. The contribution to efficacy or safety of individual components of the vehicle has not been established.

Pharmacokinetics: A multiple-dose, randomized, open-label, parallel study was performed in 21 patients with actinic keratoses. Twenty patients had pharmacokinetic samples collected: 10 patients treated with Carac and 10 treated with Efudex®[†] 5% Cream. Patients were treated for a maximum of 28 days with Carac, 1 g once daily in the morning; or Efudex® 5% Cream, 1 g twice daily, in the morning and evening. Steady-state plasma concentrations and the amounts of fluorouracil in urine resulting from the topical application of either product were measured. Three patients who received Carac and nine patients who received Efudex® 5% Cream had measurable plasma fluorouracil levels; however, only one patient receiving Carac and six patients receiving Efudex® 5% Cream had a sufficient number of data points to calculate mean pharmacokinetic parameters.

Plasma Pharmacokinetic Summary

PK Parameter	Carac n=1	Efudex (Mean±SD) n=6
C_{max}	0.77 ng/mL	11.49±8.24 ng/mL
T_{max}	1.00 hr	1.03±0.028 hr
AUC (0–24)	2.80 ng hr/mL	22.39±7.89 ng hr/mL

Five of 10 patients receiving Carac and nine of 10 patients receiving Efudex® 5% Cream had measurable urine fluorouracil levels.

[See first table at right]

Both Carac and Efudex® 5% Cream demonstrated low measurable plasma concentrations for fluorouracil when administered under steady-state conditions. Cumulative urinary excretion of fluorouracil was low for Carac and for Efudex®, corresponding to 0.055% and 0.24% of the applied doses, respectively.

Clinical Trials:

Under the experimental conditions of the topical safety studies, Carac was not observed to cause contact sensitization. However, approximately 95% of subjects in the active arms of the Phase 3 clinical studies experienced facial irritation. Irritation is likely and sensitization is unlikely based on the results of the topical safety and Phase 3 studies.

Two Phase 3 identically designed, multi-center, vehicle-controlled, double-blind studies were conducted to evaluate the clinical safety and efficacy of Carac. Patients with 5 or more actinic keratoses (AKs) on the face or anterior bald scalp were randomly allocated to active or vehicle treatment in a 2:1 ratio. Patients were randomly allocated to treatment durations of 1, 2, or 4 weeks in a 1:1:1 ratio. They applied the study cream once daily to the entire face/anterior bald scalp. Each patient's clinical response was evaluated 4 weeks after the patient's last scheduled application of study cream. No additional post-treatment follow-up efficacy or safety assessments were performed beyond 4 weeks after the last scheduled application. The following graphs show the percentage of patients in whom 100% of treated lesions cleared, and the percentage of patients in whom 75% or more of treated lesions cleared. Treatment with Carac Cream for 1, 2, or 4 weeks is compared to treatment with vehicle cream. Outcomes from 1, 2, and 4 weeks of treatment with vehicle cream are pooled because duration of treatment with vehicle had no substantive effect on clearance. Results from the two Phase 3 studies are shown separately. Although all treatment regimens of Carac studied demonstrated efficacy over vehicle for the treatment of actinic keratosis, continuing treatment up to 4 weeks as tolerated results in further lesion reduction and clearing.

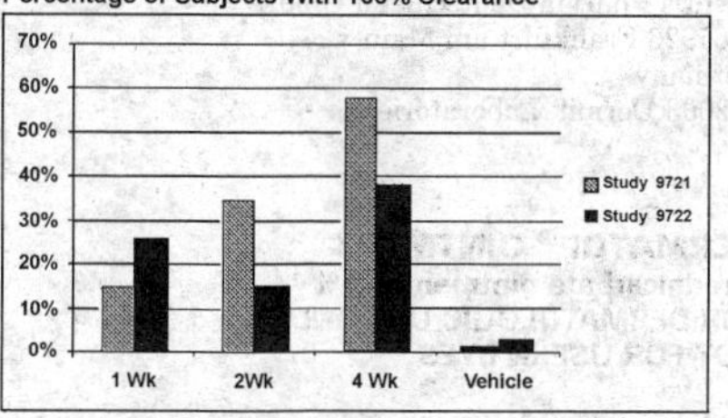

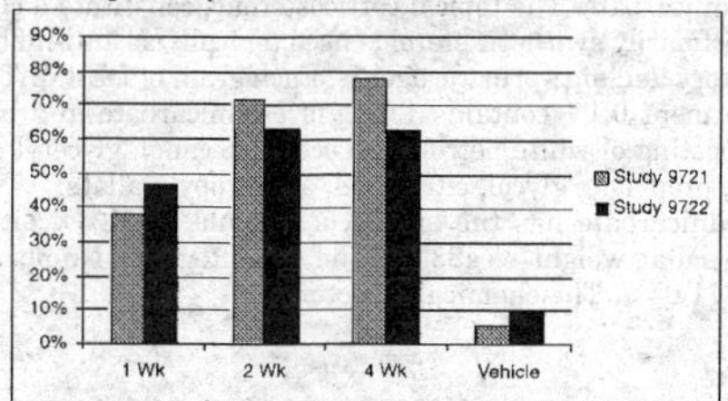

Clinical efficacy and safety in the treatment of AKs on the ears and other sun-exposed areas were not evaluated in the studies.

INDICATIONS AND USAGE

Carac is indicated for the topical treatment of multiple actinic or solar keratoses of the face and anterior scalp.

CONTRAINDICATIONS

Fluorouracil may cause fetal harm when administered to a pregnant woman. Fluorouracil is contraindicated in women who are or may become pregnant. If this drug is used during pregnancy, or if the patient becomes pregnant while taking this drug, the patient should be apprised of the potential hazard to the fetus.

No adequate and well-controlled studies have been conducted in pregnant women with either topical or parenteral forms of fluorouracil. One birth defect (ventricular septal defect) and cases of miscarriage have been reported when fluorouracil was applied to mucous membrane areas. Multiple birth defects have been reported in the fetus of a patient treated with intravenous fluorouracil.

Animal reproduction studies have not been conducted with Carac. Fluorouracil, the active ingredient, has been shown to be teratogenic in mice, rats, and hamsters when administered parenterally at doses greater than or equal to 10, 15, and 33 mg/kg/day, respectively, [4X, 11X, and 20X, respectively, the Maximum Recommended Human Dose (MRHD) based on body surface area (BSA)]. Fluorouracil was administered during the period of organogenesis for each species. Embryolethal effects occurred in monkeys at parenteral doses greater than 40 mg/kg/day (65X the MRHD based on BSA) administered during the period of organogenesis.

Carac should not be used in patients with dihydropyrimidine dehydrogenase (DPD) enzyme deficiency. A large percentage of fluorouracil is catabolized by the enzyme dihydropyrimidine dehydrogenase (DPD). DPD enzyme deficiency can result in shunting of fluorouracil to the anabolic pathway, leading to cytotoxic activity and potential toxicities.

Carac is contraindicated in patients with known hypersensitivity to any of its components.

WARNINGS

The potential for a delayed hypersensitivity reaction to fluorouracil exists. Patch testing to prove hypersensitivity may be inconclusive.

Patients should discontinue therapy with Carac if symptoms of DPD enzyme deficiency develop.

Rarely, unexpected, systemic toxicity (e.g. stomatitis, diarrhea, neutropenia, and neurotoxicity) associated with parenteral administration of fluorouracil has been attributed to deficiency of dihydropyrimidine dehydrogenase "DPD" activity. One case of life threatening systemic toxicity has been reported with the topical use of 5% fluorouracil in a patient with a complete absence of DPD enzyme activity. Symptoms included severe abdominal pain, bloody diarrhea, vomiting, fever, and chills. Physical examination revealed stomatitis, erythematous skin rash, neutropenia, thrombocytopenia, inflammation of the esophagus, stomach, and small bowel. Although this case was observed with 5% fluorouracil cream, it is unknown whether patients with profound DPD enzyme deficiency would develop systemic toxicity with lower concentrations of topically applied fluorouracil.

Applications to mucous membranes should be avoided due to the possibility of local inflammation and ulceration.

PRECAUTIONS

General: There is a possibility of increased absorption through ulcerated or inflamed skin.

Information for the Patient: Patients using Carac should receive the following information and instructions:

1. This medication is to be used as directed.
2. This medication should not be used for any disorder other than that for which it was prescribed.
3. It is for external use only.
4. Avoid contact with the eyes, eyelids, nostrils, and mouth.
5. Cleanse affected area and wait 10 minutes before applying Carac.
6. Wash hands immediately after applying Carac.
7. Avoid prolonged exposure to sunlight or other forms of ultraviolet irradiation during treatment, as the intensity of the reaction may be increased.
8. Most patients using Carac get skin reactions where the medicine is used. These reactions include redness, dryness, burning, pain, erosion (loss of the upper layer of skin), and swelling. Irritation at the application site may persist for two or more weeks after therapy is discontinued. Treated areas may be unsightly during and after therapy.
9. If you develop abdominal pain, bloody diarrhea, vomiting, fever, or chills while on Carac therapy, stop the medication and contact your physician and/or pharmacist.
10. Report any side effects to the physician and/or pharmacist.

Laboratory Tests: To rule out the presence of a frank neoplasm, a biopsy may be considered for those areas failing to respond to treatment or recurring after treatment.

Urine Pharmacokinetic Summary

PK Parameter	Carac (Mean±SD) (Range) n=10	Efudex (Mean±SD) (Range) n=10
Cum Ae‡ (min-max)	2.74±5.22 mcg (0–15.02)	119.83±94.80 mcg (0–329.87)
Max excretion rate (min-max)	0.19±0.52 mcg/hr (0–1.67)	40.27±47.14 mcg/hr (0–164.5)

‡Cumulative urinary excretion

Summary of Facial Irritation Signs and Symptoms—Pooled Phase 3 Studies

Clinical Sign or Symptom	Active One Week N=85	Active Two Week N=87	Active Four Week N=85	ALL Active Treatments N=257	Vehicle Treatments N=127
	n (%)	n (%)	n (%)	n (%)	n (%)
Erythema	76 (89.4)	82 (94.3)	82 (96.5)	240 (93.4)	76 (59.8)
Dryness	59 (69.4)	76 (87.4)	79 (92.9)	214 (83.3)	60 (47.2)
Burning	51 (60.0)	70 (80.5)	71 (83.5)	192 (74.7)	28 (22.0)
Erosion	21 (24.7)	38 (43.7)	54 (63.5)	113 (44.0)	17 (13.4)
Pain	26 (30.6)	34 (39.1)	52 (61.2)	112 (43.6)	7 (5.5)
Edema	12 (14.1)	28 (32.2)	51 (60.0)	91 (35.4)	6 (4.7)

Carcinogenesis, Mutagenesis, and Impairment of Fertility: Adequate long-term studies in animals to evaluate carcinogenic potential have not been conducted with fluorouracil. Studies with the active ingredient of Carac, fluorouracil, have shown positive effects in *in vitro* and *in vivo* tests for mutagenicity and on impairment of fertility in *in vivo* animal studies.

Fluorouracil produced morphological transformation of cells in *in vitro* cell transformation assays. Morphological transformation was also produced in an *in vitro* assay by a metabolite of fluorouracil, and the transformed cells produced malignant tumors when injected into immunosuppressed syngeneic mice. Fluorouracil has been shown to exert mutagenic activity in yeast cells, *Bacillus subtilis*, and *Drosophila* assays. In addition, fluorouracil has produced chromosome damage at concentrations of 1.0 and 2.0 mcg/mL in an *in vitro* hamster fibroblast assay, was positive in a microwell mouse lymphoma assay, and was positive in *in vivo* micronucleus assays in rats and mice following intraperitoneal administration. Some patients receiving cumulative doses of 0.24 to 1.0 g of fluorouracil parenterally have shown an increase in numerical and structural chromosome aberrations in peripheral blood lymphocytes.

Fluorouracil has been shown to impair fertility after parenteral administration in rats. Fluorouracil administered at intraperitoneal doses of 125 and 250 mg/kg has been shown to induce chromosomal aberrations and changes in chromosome organization of spermatogonia in rats. In mice, single-dose intravenous and intraperitoneal injections of fluorouracil have been reported to kill differentiated spermatogonia and spermatocytes at a dose of 500 mg/kg and produce abnormalities in spermatids at 50 mg/kg.

Pediatric Use: Actinic keratosis is not a condition seen within the pediatric population, except in association with rare genetic diseases. Carac should not be used in children. The safety and effectiveness of Carac have not been established in patients less than 18 years old.

Geriatric Use: No significant differences in safety and efficacy measures were demonstrated in patients age 65 and older compared to all other patients.

Pregnancy: Teratogenic Effects: Pregnancy Category X: See **CONTRAINDICATIONS.**

Nursing Women: It is not known whether fluorouracil is excreted in human milk. Because many drugs are excreted in human milk and because of the potential for serious adverse reactions in nursing infants from fluorouracil, a decision should be made whether to discontinue nursing or to discontinue the drug, taking into account the importance of the drug to the mother.

ADVERSE REACTIONS

The following were adverse events considered to be drug-related and occurring with a frequency of ≥1% with Carac: application site reaction (94.6%) and eye irritation (5.4%). The signs and symptoms of facial irritation (application site reaction) are presented below.

[See second table above]

During clinical trials, irritation generally began on day 4 and persisted for the remainder of treatment. Severity of facial irritation at the last treatment visit was slightly below baseline for the vehicle group, mild to moderate for the 1 week active treatment group, and moderate for the 2 and 4 week active treatment groups. Mean severity declined rapidly for each active group after completion of treatment and was below baseline for each group at the week 2 post-treatment follow-up visit.

Thirty-one patients (12% of those treated with Carac in the Phase 3 clinical studies) discontinued study treatment early due to facial irritation. Except for three patients, discontinuation of treatment occurred on or after day 11 of treatment.

Eye irritation adverse events, described as mild to moderate in intensity, were characterized as burning, watering, sen-

Continued on next page

Summary of All Adverse Events Reported in ≥1% of Patients in the Combined Active Treatment and Vehicle Groups—Pooled Phase 3 Studies

Adverse Event	9721 and 9722 Combined Active One Week N=85	Active Two Week N=87	Active Four Week N=85	ALL Active Treatments N=257	Vehicle Treatments N=127
	n (%)	n (%)	n (%)	n (%)	n (%)
Body as a whole	7 (8.2)	6 (6.9)	12 (14.1)	25 (9.7)	15 (11.8)
Headache	3 (3.5)	2 (2.3)	3 (3.5)	8 (3.1)	3 (2.4)
Common Cold	4 (4.7)	0	2 (2.4)	6 (2.3)	3 (2.4)
Allergy	0	2 (2.3)	1 (1.2)	3 (1.2)	2 (1.6)
Infection Upper Respiratory	0	0	0	0	2 (1.6)
Musculoskeletal	1 (1.2)	1 (1.1)	1 (1.2)	3 (1.2)	5 (3.9)
Muscle Soreness	0	0	0	0	2 (1.6)
Respiratory	5 (5.9)	0	1 (1.2)	6 (2.3)	6 (4.7)
Sinusitis	4 (4.7)	0	0	4 (1.6)	2 (1.6)
Skin & Appendages	78 (91.8)	83 (95.4)	82 (96.5)	243 (94.6)	85 (66.9)
Application Site Reaction	78 (91.8)	83 (95.4)	82 (96.5)	243 (94.6)	83 (65.4)
Irritation Skin	1 (1.2)	0	2 (2.4)	3 (1.2)	0
Special Senses	6 (7.1)	4 (4.6)	6 (7.1)	16 (6.2)	6 (4.7)
Eye Irritation	5 (5.9)	3 (3.4)	6 (7.1)	14 (5.4)	3 (2.4)

Carac—Cont.

sitivity, stinging and itching. These adverse events occurred across all treatment arms in one of the two Phase 3 studies. [See table above]

Adverse Experiences Reported by Body System:

In the Phase 3 studies, no serious adverse event was considered related to study drug. A total of five patients, three in the active treatment groups and two in the vehicle group, experienced at least one serious adverse event. Three patients died as a result of adverse event(s) considered unrelated to study drug (stomach cancer, myocardial infarction, and cardiac failure).

Post-treatment clinical laboratory tests other than pregnancy tests were not performed during the Phase 3 clinical studies. Clinical laboratory tests were performed during conduct of a Phase 2 study of 104 patients and 21 patients in a Phase 1 study. No abnormal serum chemistry, hematology, or urinalysis results in these studies were considered clinically significant.

DOSAGE AND ADMINISTRATION

Carac Cream should be applied once a day to the skin where actinic keratosis lesions appear, using enough to cover the entire area with a thin film. Carac Cream should not be applied near the eyes, nostrils, or mouth. Carac Cream should be applied ten minutes after thoroughly washing, rinsing, and drying the entire area. Carac Cream may be applied using the fingertips. Immediately after application, the hands should be thoroughly washed. Carac should be applied up to 4 weeks as tolerated. Continued treatment up to 4 weeks results in greater lesion reduction. Local irritation is not markedly increased by extending treatment from 2 to 4 weeks, and is generally resolved within 2 weeks of cessation of treatment.

OVERDOSE

Ordinarily, topical overdosage will not cause acute problems. If Carac is accidentally ingested, induce emesis and gastric lavage. Administer symptomatic and supportive care as needed. If contact is made with the eye, flush with copious amounts of water.

HOW SUPPLIED

Cream—30 gram tube NDC 0066-7150-30

Store at Controlled Room Temperature 20 to 25°C (68 to 77°F) [see USP].

Prescribing Information as of December 2003(a)

Keep out of the reach of children.

Rx only

Manufactured for:
Dermik Laboratories
A division of Aventis Pharmaceuticals Inc
Berwyn, PA 19312 USA
Manufactured by:
Pharmaceutical Manufacturing Research Services, Inc
Horsham, PA 19044 USA

*Microsponge® is a registered trademark of Cardinal Health, Inc. or one of its subsidiaries.

†Efudex® is a registered trademark of ICN Pharmaceuticals, Inc.

PATIENT INFORMATION

Carac® Cream, 0.5%
(fluorouracil cream)

Read this leaflet carefully before you start to use your medicine. Read the information you get every time you get more medicine. There may be new information about the drug. This leaflet does not take the place of talks with your doctor. If you have any questions or are not sure about something, ask your doctor or pharmacist.

What is Carac?

Carac (Care ack) is a cream used by adults to treat skin conditions on the face and front part of the scalp called solar keratosis or actinic keratosis.

Who should not use Carac?

Do not use Carac

- if you are pregnant or might become pregnant. Carac may harm your unborn child.
- if you are nursing a baby. We do not know if Carac can pass to the baby through the milk.
- if you have dihydropyrimidine dehydrogenase (DPD) enzyme deficiency. The active ingredient in Carac, fluorouracil, can cause serious side effects in patients who are DPD enzyme deficient. If you have DPD enzyme deficiency and use medications containing fluorouracil, you may develop serious side effects such as stomach pain, bloody diarrhea, vomiting, fever, or chills.
- if you are allergic to the ingredients in Carac. Ask your doctor or pharmacist about the inactive ingredients.
- if under 18 years of age. Carac should not be used in children.

Tell your doctor if you are able to become pregnant. Your doctor may advise you about birth control to avoid pregnancy.

How should I use Carac?

Use Carac once a day as instructed by your doctor. Use it only on your skin. You should use Carac for up to 4 weeks.

1. Clean the area where you will apply Carac. Rinse well and dry the area with a towel and wait 10 minutes before applying Carac.
2. Put Carac on your face as directed by your physician, using your fingertips. Use enough to cover the affected skin.
3. Avoid contact with your eyes, nostrils, and mouth.
4. Wash your hands as soon as you finish putting the Carac on your skin.
5. A moisturizer/sunscreen may be applied 2 hours after Carac has been applied. Do not use any other skin products including creams, lotions, medications or cosmetics–unless instructed by your doctor.

What should I avoid while using Carac?

Avoid sunlight or other ultraviolet light (such as tanning booths) as much as possible while using Carac. Sunlight may increase your side effects. When exposed to sunlight, wear a hat and use sunscreen.

Do not cover the treated skin with a dressing.

Do not breast feed or become pregnant while using Carac. If you do become pregnant, stop using Carac and tell your doctor right away.

What are the possible side effects of Carac?

Most patients using Carac get skin reactions where the medicine is used. These reactions include redness, dryness, burning, pain, erosion (loss of the upper layer of skin), and swelling. Irritation may continue for two or more weeks after treatment is over. The treated area may become unsightly during therapy.

Some patients get eye irritation. Eye irritation might consist of burning, sensitivity, itching, stinging, and watering. If you are concerned about side effects, talk to your doctor.

A few patients have reported side effects such as stomach pain, diarrhea, vomiting, fever, or chills, possibly due to the lack of a specific enzyme, DPD, in their body. If you experience any of these symptoms, discontinue therapy immediately, and contact your doctor.

Storage information

Keep this medicine at room temperature (68–77°F/ 20–25°C). Throw away unused medicine. Keep this medicine out of the reach of children.

General advice about prescription medicines

Medicines are sometimes prescribed for conditions that are not described in patient information leaflets. Do not use it for a condition for which it was not prescribed. This medicine is for your use only. Never give it to other people. It may harm them even if their skin problem appears to be the same as yours. Do not use **Carac** after the expiration date on the tube.

Prescribing Information as of December 2003(a).

Manufactured for:
Dermik Laboratories
A Division of Aventis Pharmaceuticals Inc.
Berwyn, PA 19312 USA
Manufactured by:
Pharmaceutical Manufacturing Research Services, Inc.
Horsham, PA 19044 USA

DERMATOP® EMOLLIENT CREAM ℞

[*dər-mă-tŏp*]

(prednicarbate emollient cream) 0.1%
FOR DERMATOLOGIC USE ONLY.
NOT FOR USE IN EYES.

DESCRIPTION

DERMATOP® Emollient Cream (prednicarbate emollient cream) 0.1% contains prednicarbate, a synthetic corticosteroid for topical dermatologic use. The chemical name of prednicarbate is 11β, 17, 21-trihydroxypregna-1,4-diene- 3,20-dione 17-(ethyl carbonate) 21-propionate. Prednicarbate has the empirical formula $C_{27}H_{36}O_8$ and a molecular weight of 488.58. Topical corticosteroids constitute a class of primarily synthetic steroids used topically as anti-inflammatory and antipruritic agents.

The CAS Registry Number is 73771–04–7. The chemical structure is:

Prednicarbate is a practically odorless white to yellow-white powder insoluble to practically insoluble in water and freely soluble in ethanol.

Each gram of DERMATOP Emollient Cream 0.1% contains 1.0 mg of prednicarbate in a base consisting of white petrolatum USP, purified water USP, isopropyl myristate NF, lanolin alcohols NF, mineral oil USP, cetostearyl alcohol NF, aluminum stearate, edetate disodium USP, lactic acid USP, and magnesium stearate DAB 9.

HOW SUPPLIED

DERMATOP Emollient Cream (prednicarbate emollient cream) 0.1% is supplied in 15 g (NDC 0066-0507-15) and 60 g (NDC 0066-0507-60) tubes.

Store between 41 and 77°F (5 and 25°C).

Prescribing Information as of May 2003.

℞ Only

U.S. Patent 4,242,334

Manufactured for:
Dermik Laboratories
A Division of Aventis Pharmaceuticals Inc.
Berwyn, PA 19312 USA
by:
Aventis Pharma Deutschland GmbH
D-65926 Frankfurt am Main
Germany

DERMATOP® OINTMENT ℞

(prednicarbate ointment) 0.1%
FOR DERMATOLOGIC USE ONLY.
NOT FOR USE IN EYES.

DESCRIPTION

DERMATOP® Ointment (prednicarbate ointment) 0.1% contains the non-halogenated prednisolone derivative prednicarbate. The topical corticosteroids constitute a class of primarily synthetic steroids used topically as anti-inflammatory and anti-pruritic agents. Each gram of DERMATOP Ointment 0.1% contains 1.0mg of prednicarbate in a base consisting of white petrolatum octyldodecanol, glyceryl oleate, propylene glycol, citric acid, and propyl gallate.

Prednicarbate has the empirical formula $C_{27}H_{36}O_8$ and a molecular weight of 488.58. The CAS Registry Number is 73771-04-7. The chemical structure is:

HOW SUPPLIED

DERMATOP Ointment (prednicarbate ointment) 0.1% is supplied in 15 gram (NDC 0066-0508-15) and 60 gram (NDC 0066-0508-60) tubes.

Store at controlled room temperature (59 to 86°F or 15 to 30°C).

℞ Only.

Prescribing information as of February 2004(a).

US Patent 4,242,334 has been extended.

Manufactured for:
Dermik Laboratories
A Division of Aventis Pharmaceuticals Inc.
Berwyn, PA 19312 USA
by:
Aventis Pharma Deutschland GmbH
D-65926 Frankfurt am Main
Germany

KLARON® ℞

(sodium sulfacetamide lotion)
Lotion, 10%

DESCRIPTION

Each mL of **Klaron®** (sodium sulfacetamide lotion) **Lotion, 10%** contains 100 mg of sodium sulfacetamide in a vehicle consisting of purified water; propylene glycol; lauramide DEA (and) diethanolamine; polyethylene glycol 400, monolaurate; hydroxyethyl cellulose; sodium chloride; sodium metabisulfite; methylparaben; xanthan gum; EDTA and simethicone.
Sodium sulfacetamide is a sulfonamide with antibacterial activity. Chemically, sodium sulfacetamide is N′ -[(4-aminophenyl) sulfonyl] - acetamide, monosodium salt, monohydrate. The structural formula is:

Na
NH_2— —$SO_2NCOCH_3 \cdot H_2O$

CLINICAL PHARMACOLOGY

The most widely accepted mechanism of action of sulfonamides is the Woods-Fildes theory, based on sulfonamides acting as a competitive inhibitor of para-aminobenzoic acid (PABA) utilization, an essential component for bacterial growth. While absorption through intact skin in humans has not been determined, *in vitro* studies with human cadaver skin indicated a percutaneous absorption of about 4%. Sodium sulfacetamide is readily absorbed from the gastrointestinal tract when taken orally and excreted in the urine largely unchanged. The biological half-life has been reported to be between 7 to 13 hours.

INDICATIONS

Klaron Lotion is indicated in the topical treatment of *acne vulgaris.*

CONTRAINDICATIONS

Klaron Lotion is contraindicated for use by patients having known hypersensitivity to sulfonamides or any other component of this preparation (see **WARNINGS** section).

WARNINGS

Fatalities have occurred, although rarely, due to severe reactions to sulfonamides including Stevens-Johnson syndrome, toxic epidermal necrolysis, fulminant hepatic necrosis, agranulocytosis, aplastic anemia, and other blood dyscrasias. Hypersensitivity reactions may occur when a sulfonamide is readministered, irrespective of the route of administration. Sensitivity reactions have been reported in individuals with no prior history of sulfonamide hypersensitivity. At the first sign of hypersensitivity, skin rash or other reactions, discontinue use of this preparation (see **ADVERSE REACTIONS** section).
Klaron Lotion contains sodium metabisulfite, a sulfite that may cause allergic-type reactions including anaphylactic symptoms and life-threatening or less severe asthmatic episodes in certain susceptible people. The overall prevalence of sulfite sensitivity in the general population is unknown and probably low. Sulfite sensitivity is seen more frequently in asthmatic than in non-asthmatic people (see **CONTRAINDICATIONS** section).

PRECAUTIONS

General: For external use only. Keep away from eyes. If irritation develops, use of the product should be discontinued and appropriate therapy instituted. Patients should be carefully observed for possible local irritation or sensitization during long-term therapy. Hypersensitivity reactions may occur when a sulfonamide is readministered irrespective of the route of administration, and cross-sensitivity between different sulfonamides may occur. Sodium sulfacetamide can cause reddening and scaling of the skin. Particular caution should be employed if areas of involved skin to be treated are denuded or abraded.

Keep out of reach of children.

Carcinogenesis, Mutagenesis and Impairment of Fertility: Long-term studies in animals have not been performed to evaluate carcinogenic potential.
Pregnancy - Category C: Animal reproduction studies have not been conducted with **Klaron Lotion**. It is also not known whether **Klaron Lotion** can cause fetal harm when administered to a pregnant woman or can affect reproduction capacity. **Klaron Lotion** should be given to a pregnant woman only if clearly needed.
Kernicterus may occur in the newborn as a result of treatment of a pregnant woman at term with orally administered sulfonamide. There are no adequate and well controlled studies of **Klaron Lotion** in pregnant women, and it is not known whether topically applied sulfonamides can cause fetal harm when administered to a pregnant woman.
Nursing Mothers: It is not known whether sodium sulfacetamide is excreted in the human milk following topical use of **Klaron Lotion**. Systemically administered sulfonamides are capable of producing kernicterus in the infants of lactating women. Small amounts of orally administered sulfonamides have been reported to be eliminated in human milk. Because many drugs are excreted in human milk, caution should be exercised in prescribing for nursing women.
Pediatric Use: Safety and effectiveness in pediatric patients under the age of 12 have not been established.

ADVERSE REACTIONS

In controlled clinical trials for the management of *acne vulgaris*, the occurrence of adverse reactions associated with the use of **Klaron Lotion** was infrequent and restricted to local events. The total incidence of adverse reactions reported in these studies was less than 2%. Only one of 105 patients treated with **Klaron Lotion** had adverse reactions of erythema, itching and edema. It has been reported that sodium sulfacetamide may cause local irritation, stinging and burning. While the irritation may be transient, occasionally, the use of medication has to be discontinued.

DOSAGE AND ADMINISTRATION

Apply a thin film to affected areas twice daily.

HOW SUPPLIED

2 FL OZ (59 mL) bottles (**NDC** 0066-7500-02).
4 FL OZ (118 mL) bottles (**NDC** 0066-7500-04)
Store at Controlled Room Temperature 20° to 25°C (68° to 77°F) (See USP).
Shake well before using. Keep tightly closed.
Rx only
Prescribing Information as of July 2002
Manufactured for:
Dermik Laboratories
A Division of Aventis Pharmaceuticals Inc
Berwyn, PA 19312
by:
DPT Lakewood, Inc.
Lakewood, NJ 08701 USA

NORITATE® ℞

(metronidazole cream)
Cream, 1%
FOR TOPICAL USE ONLY
(NOT FOR OPHTHALMIC USE)

DESCRIPTION

NORITATE® (metronidazole cream) **Cream, 1%,** contains metronidazole, USP. Chemically, metronidazole is 2-methyl-5-nitro-1*H*-imidazole-1-ethanol. The molecular formula for metronidazole is $C_6H_9N_3O_3$. It has the following structural formula:

OH
O_2N N CH_3
N

Metronidazole has a molecular weight of 171.16. It is a white to pale yellow crystalline powder. It is slightly soluble in alcohol and has a solubility in water of 10 mg/mL at 20°C. Metronidazole is a member of the imidazole class of antibacterial agents and is classified as an antiprotozoal and anti-bacterial agent.
NORITATE is an emollient cream; each gram contains 10 mg micronized metronidazole USP, in a base of purified water USP, stearic acid NF, glyceryl monostearate NF, glycerin USP, methylparaben NF, trolamine NF and propylparaben NF.

CLINICAL PHARMACOLOGY

Pharmacokinetics: When one gram dose of **NORITATE** cream, 1%, was applied in a single application to the face of 16 healthy volunteers, low concentrations of metronidazole were detected in the plasma of 7 of the volunteers. The mean ± SD C_{max} of metronidazole was 27.6 ± 7.3 ng/mL, which is about 1% of the value reported for a single 250 mg oral dose of metronidazole. The time to maximum plasma concentration (T_{max}) in the volunteers with detectable metronidazole was 8–12 hours after topical application.
Pharmacodynamics: The mechanisms by which metronidazole acts in reducing inflammatory lesions of rosacea are unknown.
Clinical Studies: Safety and efficacy of **NORITATE** were evaluated in two randomized vehicle-controlled clinical studies for the treatment of rosacea, which excluded patients who had nodules, moderate or severe rhinophyma, dense telangiectases, plaque-like facial edema or ocular involvement and those who had a history of not responding to metronidazole therapy for rosacea. Of the patients included in the efficacy database (n=416), there were 142 men and 274 women. Endpoint efficacy data comparisons for patients treated with daily **NORITATE** or vehicle applications are listed below.
[See table below]
Safety Studies: Studies of contact sensitization (n=258), phototoxicity (n=21), and photocontact sensitization (n=29) of **NORITATE** were conducted. No evidence of sensitization or phototoxicity was seen in these studies.

INDICATIONS AND USAGE

NORITATE is indicated for the topical treatment of inflammatory lesions and erythema of rosacea.

CONTRAINDICATIONS

NORITATE is contraindicated in those patients with a history of hypersensitivity to metronidazole or to any other ingredient in this formulation.

PRECAUTIONS

General: If a reaction suggesting local skin irritation occurs, patients should be directed to discontinue use of the medication. Conjunctivitis associated with topical use of metronidazole on the face has been reported. Contact with the eyes should be avoided. Metronidazole is a nitroimidazole and should be used with care in patients with evidence of, or history of, blood dyscrasia.
Information for Patients: Patients using **NORITATE** should receive the following information and instructions:

1. This medication is to be used as directed.
2. It is for external use only.
3. Avoid contact with the eyes.
4. Cleanse affected area(s) before applying **NORITATE**.
5. This medication should not be used for any disorder other than that for which it is prescribed.
6. Patients should report any adverse reaction to their physician.

Drug Interactions: Oral metronidazole has been reported to potentiate the anticoagulant effect of coumarin and warfarin resulting in a prolongation of prothrombin time. Drug interactions should be kept in mind when **NORITATE** is prescribed for patients who are receiving anticoagulant treatment, although they are less likely to occur with topical metronidazole administration because of low absorption. (See **CLINICAL PHARMACOLOGY**, **Pharmacokinetics** section)
Carcinogenesis, Mutagenesis and Impairment of Fertility: Metronidazole has shown evidence of carcinogenic activity in a number of studies involving chronic, oral administration in mice and rats but not in studies involving hamsters. In several long term studies in mice, oral doses of approximately 225 mg/m^2/day or greater (approximately 37 times the human topical dose on a mg/m^2 basis) were associated with an increase in pulmonary tumors and lymphomas. Several long term oral studies in the rat have shown statistically significant increases in mammary and hepatic tumors at doses >885 mg/m^2/day (144 times the topical human dose).
Metronidazole has shown evidence of mutagenic activity in several *in vitro* bacterial assay systems. In addition, a dose-related increase in the frequency of micronuclei was observed in mice after intraperitoneal injections. An increase in chromosomal aberrations in peripheral blood lymphocytes was reported in patients with Crohn's disease who were treated with 200 to 1200 mg/day of metronidazole for 1 to 24 months. However, in another study, no increase in chromosomal aberrations in circulating lymphocytes was observed in patients with Crohn's disease treated with the drug for 8 months.
In one published study, using albino hairless mice, intraperitoneal administration of metronidazole at a dose of 45 mg/m^2/day (approximately 7 times the human topical dose on a mg/m^2 basis) was associated with an increase in ultraviolet radiation-induced skin carcinogenesis. Neither dermal carcinogenicity nor photocarcinogenicity studies have been performed with **NORITATE** or any marketed metronidazole formulations.
Pregnancy: *Teratogenic Effects:* Pregnancy Category B. There are no adequate and well controlled studies with the use of **NORITATE** in pregnant women.

Continued on next page

Inflammatory Lesion Counts and Erythema Severity Scores in Two Clinical Trials for Rosacea

	Noritate				Vehicle			
	Study 1		Study 2		Study 1		Study 2	
	N	Result	N	Result	N	Result	N	Result
Papules + Pustules Count								
Baseline	89	15	92	19	50	18	49	17
Week-10	80	7*	82	8	45	15	41	12
Reduction		49%*		58%*		17%		30%
Papules Count								
Baseline	89	13	92	17	50	15	49	15
Week-10	80	7*	82	7	45	12	41	11
Reduction		41%*		55%*		14%		28%
Erythema Score								
Baseline	89	2.2	92	2.3	50	2.2	49	2.2
Week-10	80	1.3*	82	1.4*	45	1.7	40	1.8
Reduction		42%*		40%*		25%		19%

* Statistically significant differences between **NORITATE** and vehicle groups with p≤0.05. Erythema scores: 0=none, 1=mild, 2=moderate and 3=severe.

Noritate—Cont.

Metronidazole crosses the placental barrier and enters the fetal circulation rapidly. No fetotoxicity was observed after oral administration of metronidazole to rats or mice at 200 and 20 times, respectively, the expected clinical dose. However, oral metronidazole has shown carcinogenic activity in rodents. Because animal reproduction studies are not always predictive of human response, **NORITATE** should be used during pregnancy only if clearly needed.

Nursing Mothers: After oral administration, metronidazole is secreted in breast milk in concentrations similar to those found in the plasma. Even though blood levels taken after topical metronidazole application are significantly lower than those achieved after oral metronidazole, a decision should be made whether to discontinue nursing or to discontinue the drug, taking into account the importance of the drug to the mother and the risk to the infant.

Pediatric Use: Safety and effectiveness in pediatric patients have not been established.

ADVERSE REACTIONS

Safety data from 302 patients who used **NORITATE** (n=200) or vehicle control (n=102) once daily in clinical trials and experienced an adverse event considered to be treatment-related include: application site reaction (**NORITATE** 1, vehicle 1), condition aggravated (**NORITATE** 1, vehicle 0), paresthesia (**NORITATE** 0, vehicle 1), acne (**NORITATE** 1, vehicle 0), dry skin (**NORITATE** 0, vehicle 2). The majority of adverse reactions were mild to moderate in severity.

Two patients treated with **NORITATE** once daily discontinued treatment because of adverse events: one for a severe flare of comedonal acne and one for rosacea aggravated.

Additional clinical adverse effects reported spontaneously since the drug was marketed are uncommon & include tingling or numbness of extremities, allergic reactions, skin & eye irritation, rash, headache, nausea and dry mouth.

DOSAGE AND ADMINISTRATION

Areas to be treated should be cleansed before application of **NORITATE**. Apply and rub in a thin film of **NORITATE** once daily to entire affected area(s). Patients may use cosmetics after application of **NORITATE**.

HOW SUPPLIED

Cream—30 gram aluminum tube NDC 0066-9850-30 and 60 gram aluminum tube NDC 0066-9850-60.

Keep out of the reach of children.

Storage Conditions: Store at controlled room temperature: 20 to 25°C (68 to 77°F).

Prescribing Information as of September 2003

Rx Only

Marketed by
Dermik Laboratories
A Division of Aventis Pharmaceuticals Inc.
Berwyn, PA 19312 USA

Manufactured by
Aventis Pharma Inc
2150 St. Elzéar Blvd, West
Laval, Quebec, Canada
H7L 4A8
Made in Canada
© 2003 Dermik Laboratories

PENLAC® NAIL LACQUER ℞
(ciclopirox) Topical Solution, 8%

FOR USE ON FINGERNAILS AND TOENAILS AND IMMEDIATELY ADJACENT SKIN ONLY
NOT FOR USE IN EYES

DESCRIPTION

PENLAC® NAIL LACQUER (ciclopirox) Topical Solution, 8%, contains a synthetic antifungal agent, ciclopirox. It is intended for topical use on fingernails and toenails and immediately adjacent skin.

Each gram of PENLAC® NAIL LACQUER (ciclopirox) Topical Solution, 8%, contains 80 mg ciclopirox in a solution base consisting of ethyl acetate, NF; isopropyl alcohol, USP; and butyl monoester of poly[methylvinyl ether/maleic acid] in isopropyl alcohol. Ethyl acetate and isopropyl alcohol are solvents that vaporize after application.

PENLAC® NAIL LACQUER (ciclopirox) Topical Solution, 8%, is a clear, colorless to slightly yellowish solution.

The chemical name for ciclopirox is 6-cyclohexyl-1-hydroxy-4-methyl-2(1H)-pyridone, with the empirical formula $C_{12}H_{17}NO_2$ and a molecular weight of 207.27. The CAS Registry Number is [29342-05-0]. The chemical structure is:

CLINICAL PHARMACOLOGY

Microbiology

Mechanism of Action

The mechanism of action of ciclopirox has been investigated using various *in vitro* and *in vivo* infection models. One *in vitro* study suggested that ciclopirox acts by chelation of polyvalent cations (Fe^{+3} or Al^{+3}) resulting in the inhibition of the metal-dependent enzymes that are responsible for the degradation of peroxides within the fungal cell. The clinical significance of this observation is not known.

At Week 48 (plus Last Observation Carried Forward) for the Intent-to-Treat (ITT) Population

	Study 312		Study 313	
	Active	Vehicle	Active	Vehicle
Complete Cure*	6/110 (5.5%)	1/109 (0.9%)	10/118 (8.5%)	0/117 (0%)
Almost Clear**	7/107 (6.5%)	1/108 (0.9%)	14/116 (12%)	1/115 (0.9%)
Negative Mycology Alone***	30/105 (29%)	12/106 (11%)	41/115 (36%)	10/114 (9%)

*Clear nail and negative mycology
**≤10% nail involvement and negative mycology
***Negative KOH and negative culture

Activity *in vitro* and *ex vivo*

In vitro methodologies employing various broth or solid media with and without additional nutrients have been utilized to determine ciclopirox minimum inhibitory concentration (MIC) values for the dermatophytic molds.[1–2] As a consequence, a broad range of MIC values, 1–20 µg/mL, were obtained for *Trichophyton rubrum* and *Trichophyton mentagrophytes* species. Correlation between *in vitro* MIC results and clinical outcome has yet to be established for ciclopirox.

One *ex vivo* study was conducted evaluating 8% ciclopirox against new and established *Trichophyton rubrum* and *Trichophyton mentagrophytes* infections in ovine hoof material.[3] After 10 days of treatment the growth of *T. rubrum* and *T. mentagrophytes* in the established infection model was very minimally affected. Elimination of the molds from hoof material was not achieved in either the new or established infection models.

Susceptibility testing for *Trichophyton rubrum* species

In vitro susceptibility testing methods for determining ciclopirox MIC values against the dermatophytic molds, including *Trichophyton rubrum* species, have not been standardized or validated. Ciclopirox MIC values will vary depending on the susceptibility testing method employed, composition and pH of media and the utilization of nutritional supplements. Breakpoints to determine whether clinical isolates of *Trichophyton rubrum* are susceptible or resistant to ciclopirox have not been established.

Resistance

Studies have not been conducted to evaluate drug resistance development in *T. rubrum* species exposed to 8% ciclopirox topical solution. Studies assessing cross-resistance to ciclopirox and other known antifungal agents have not been performed.

Antifungal Drug Interactions

No studies have been conducted to determine whether ciclopirox might reduce the effectiveness of systemic antifungal agents for onychomycosis. Therefore, the concomitant use of 8% ciclopirox topical solution and systemic antifungal agents for onychomycosis is not recommended.

Pharmacokinetics

As demonstrated in pharmacokinetic studies in animals and man, ciclopirox olamine is rapidly absorbed after oral administration and completely eliminated in all species via feces and urine. Most of the compound is excreted either unchanged or as glucuronide. After oral administration of 10 mg of radiolabeled drug (14C-ciclopirox) to healthy volunteers, approximately 96% of the radioactivity was excreted renally within 12 hours of administration. Ninety-four percent of the renally excreted radioactivity was in the form of glucuronides. Thus, glucuronidation is the main metabolic pathway of this compound.

Systemic absorption of ciclopirox was determined in 5 patients with dermatophytic onychomycoses, after application of PENLAC® NAIL LACQUER (ciclopirox) Topical Solution, 8%, to all 20 digits and adjacent 5 mm of skin once daily for six months. Random serum concentrations and 24 hour urinary excretion of ciclopirox were determined at two weeks and at 1, 2, 4 and 6 months after initiation of treatment and 4 weeks post-treatment. In this study, ciclopirox serum levels ranged from 12–80 ng/mL. Based on urinary data, mean absorption of ciclopirox from the dosage form was <5% of the applied dose. One month after cessation of treatment, serum and urine levels of ciclopirox were below the limit of detection.

In two vehicle-controlled trials, patients applied PENLAC® NAIL LACQUER (ciclopirox) Topical Solution, 8%, to all toenails and affected fingernails. Out of a total of 66 randomly selected patients on active treatment, 24 had detectable serum ciclopirox concentrations at some point during the dosing interval (range 10.0–24.6 ng/mL). It should be noted that eleven of these 24 patients took concomitant medication containing ciclopirox as ciclopirox olamine (Loprox® Cream, 0.77%).

The penetration of the PENLAC® NAIL LACQUER (ciclopirox) Topical Solution, 8%, was evaluated in an *in vitro* investigation. Radiolabeled ciclopirox applied once to onychomycotic toenails that were avulsed demonstrated penetration up to a depth of approximately 0.4 mm. As expected, nail plate concentrations decreased as a function of nail depth. The clinical significance of these findings in nail plates is unknown. Nail bed concentrations were not determined.

INDICATIONS AND USAGE

(To understand fully the indication for this product, please read the entire INDICATION AND USAGE section of the labeling.)

PENLAC® NAIL LACQUER (ciclopirox) Topical Solution, 8%, as a component of a comprehensive management program, is indicated as topical treatment in immunocompetent patients with mild to moderate onychomycosis of fingernails and toenails without lunula involvement, due to *Trichophyton rubrum*. The comprehensive management program includes removal of the unattached, infected nails as frequently as monthly, by a health care professional who has special competence in the diagnosis and treatment of nail disorders, including minor nail procedures.

- No studies have been conducted to determine whether ciclopirox might reduce the effectiveness of systemic antifungal agents for onychomycosis. Therefore, the concomitant use of 8% ciclopirox topical solution and systemic antifungal agents for onychomycosis, is not recommended.
- PENLAC® NAIL LACQUER (ciclopirox) Topical Solution, 8%, should be used only under medical supervision as described above.
- The effectiveness and safety of PENLAC® NAIL LACQUER (ciclopirox) Topical Solution, 8%, in the following populations has not been studied. The clinical trials with use of PENLAC® NAIL LACQUER (ciclopirox) Topical Solution, 8%, excluded patients who: were pregnant or nursing, planned to become pregnant, had a history of immunosuppression (e.g., extensive, persistent, or unusual distribution of dermatomycoses, extensive seborrheic dermatitis, recent or recurring herpes zoster, or persistent herpes simplex), were HIV seropositive, received organ transplant, required medication to control epilepsy, were insulin dependent diabetics or had diabetic neuropathy. Patients with severe plantar (moccasin) tinea pedis were also excluded.
- The safety and efficacy of using PENLAC® NAIL LACQUER (ciclopirox) Topical Solution, 8%, daily for greater than 48 weeks have not been established.

Clinical Trials Data

The results of use of PENLAC® NAIL LACQUER (ciclopirox) Topical Solution, 8%, in treatment of onychomycosis of the toenail without lunula involvement were obtained from two double-blind, placebo-controlled studies conducted in the US. In these studies, patients with onychomycosis of the great toenails without lunula involvement were treated with ciclopirox topical solution, 8%, in conjunction with monthly removal of the unattached, infected toenail by the investigator. PENLAC® NAIL LACQUER (ciclopirox) Topical Solution, 8%, was applied for 48 weeks. At baseline, patients had 20–65% involvement of the target great toenail plate. Statistical significance was demonstrated in one of two studies for the endpoint "complete cure" (clear nail and negative mycology) and in two studies for the endpoint "almost clear" (≤10% nail involvement and negative mycology) at the end of study. These results are presented below.

[See table above]

The summary of reported patient outcomes for the ITT population at 12 weeks following the end of treatment are presented below. Note that post-treatment efficacy assessments were scheduled only for patients who achieved a complete cure.

[See table at top of next page]

CONTRAINDICATIONS

PENLAC® NAIL LACQUER (ciclopirox) Topical Solution, 8%, is contraindicated in individuals who have shown hypersensitivity to any of its components.

WARNINGS

PENLAC® NAIL LACQUER (ciclopirox) Topical Solution, 8%, is not for ophthalmic, oral, or intravaginal use. For use on nails and immediately adjacent skin only.

PRECAUTIONS

If a reaction suggesting sensitivity or chemical irritation should occur with the use of PENLAC® NAIL LACQUER (ciclopirox) Topical Solution, 8%, treatment should be discontinued and appropriate therapy instituted.

So far there is no relevant clinical experience with patients with insulin dependent diabetes or who have diabetic neuropathy. The risk of removal of the unattached, infected nail, by the health care professional and trimming by the patient, should be carefully considered before prescribing to patients with a history of insulin dependent diabetes mellitus or diabetic neuropathy.

Information for Patients

Patients should have detailed instructions regarding the use of PENLAC® NAIL LACQUER (ciclopirox) Topical Solution, 8%, as a component of a comprehensive management program for onychomycosis in order to achieve maximum benefit with the use of this product.

The patient should be told to:

1. Use PENLAC® NAIL LACQUER (ciclopirox) Topical Solution, 8%, as directed by a health care professional. Avoid contact with the eyes and mucous membranes. Contact with skin other than skin immediately surrounding the treated nail(s) should be avoided. PENLAC® NAIL LACQUER (ciclopirox) Topical Solution, 8%, is for external use only.
2. PENLAC® NAIL LACQUER (ciclopirox) Topical Solution, 8%, should be applied evenly over the entire nail plate and 5 mm of surrounding skin. If possible, PENLAC® NAIL LACQUER (ciclopirox) Topical Solution, 8%, should be applied to the nail bed, hyponychium, and the under surface of the nail plate when it is free of the nail bed (e.g., onycholysis). Contact with the surrounding skin may produce mild, transient irritation (redness).
3. Removal of the unattached, infected nail, as frequently as monthly, by a health care professional is needed with use of this medication. Inform a health care professional if they have diabetes or problems with numbness in your toes or fingers for consideration of the appropriate nail management program.
4. Inform a health care professional if the area of application shows signs of increased irritation (redness, itching, burning, blistering, swelling, oozing).
5. Up to 48 weeks of daily applications with PENLAC® NAIL LACQUER (ciclopirox) Topical Solution, 8%, and professional removal of the unattached, infected nail, as frequently as monthly, are considered the full treatment needed to achieve a clear or almost clear nail (defined as 10% or less residual nail involvement).
6. Six months of therapy with professional removal of the unattached, infected nail may be required before initial improvement of symptoms is noticed.
7. A completely clear nail may not be achieved with use of this medication. In clinical studies less than 12% of patients were able to achieve either a completely clear or almost clear toenail.
8. Do not use the medication for any disorder other than that for which it is prescribed.
9. Do not use nail polish or other nail cosmetic products on the treated nails.
10. Avoid use near heat or open flame, because product is flammable.

Carcinogenesis, Mutagenesis, Impairment of Fertility:

No carcinogenicity study was conducted with PENLAC® NAIL LACQUER (ciclopirox) Topical Solution, 8%, formulation. A carcinogenicity study of ciclopirox (1% and 5% solutions in polyethylene glycol 400) in female mice dosed topically twice per week for 50 weeks followed by a 6-month drug-free observation period prior to necropsy revealed no evidence of tumors at the application sites.

In human systemic tolerability studies following daily application (~340 mg of PENLAC® NAIL LACQUER (ciclopirox) Topical Solution, 8%) in subjects with distal subungual onychomycosis, the average maximal serum level of ciclopirox was 31±28 ng/mL after two months of once daily applications. This level was 159 times lower than the lowest toxic dose and 115 times lower than the highest nontoxic dose in rats and dogs fed 7.7 and 23.1 mg ciclopirox (as ciclopirox olamine)/kg/day.

The following *in vitro* genotoxicity tests have been conducted with ciclopirox: evaluation of gene mutation in Ames *Salmonella* and *E. coli* assays (negative); chromosome aberration assays in V79 Chinese hamster lung fibroblasts, with and without metabolic activation (positive); gene mutation assay in the HGPRT-test with V79 Chinese hamster lung fibroblasts (negative); unscheduled DNA synthesis in human A549 cells (negative); and BALB/c3T3 cell transformation assay (negative). In an *in vivo* Chinese hamster bone marrow cytogenetic assay, ciclopirox was negative for chromosome aberrations at 5,000 mg/kg.

The following *in vitro* genotoxicity tests were conducted with PENLAC® NAIL LACQUER (ciclopirox) Topical Solution, 8%: Ames *Salmonella* test (negative); unscheduled DNA synthesis in the rat hepatocytes (negative); cell transformation assay in BALB/c3T3 cell assay (positive). The positive response of the lacquer formulation in the BALB/c3T3 assay was attributed to its butyl monoester of poly-[methylvinyl ether/maleic acid] resin component (Gantrez® ES-435), which also tested positive in this test. The cell transformation assay may have been confounded because of the film-forming nature of the resin. Gantrez® ES-435 tested nonmutagenic in both the *in vitro* mouse lymphoma forward mutation assay with or without activation and unscheduled DNA synthesis assay in rat hepatocytes.

Oral reproduction studies in rats at doses up to 3.85 mg ciclopirox (as ciclopirox olamine)/kg/day [equivalent to approximately 1.4 times the potential exposure at the maximum recommended human topical dose (MRHTD)] did not reveal any specific effects on fertility or other reproductive parameters. MRHTD (mg/m^2) is based on the assumption of 100% systemic absorption of 27.12 mg ciclopirox (~340 mg PENLAC® NAIL LACQUER (ciclopirox) Topical Solution, 8%) that will cover all the fingernails and toenails including 5 mm proximal and lateral fold area plus onycholysis to a maximal extent of 50%.

Post-treatment Week 12 Data for Patients Who Achieved Complete Cure at Week 48

	Study 312		Study 313	
	Active	Vehicle	Active	Vehicle
Number of Treated Patients	112	111	119	118
Complete Cure at Week 48	6	1	10	0
Post-treatment Week 12 Outcomes:				
Patients Missing All Week 12 Assessments	2	0	2	0
Patients with Week 12 Assessments	4	1	8	0
Complete Cure	3	1	4	0
Almost Clear	2*	1	1*	0
Negative Mycology	3	1	5	0

*Four patients (from studies 312 and 313) who were completely cured did not have post-treatment Week 12 planimetry data.

Pregnancy

Teratogenic effects: Pregnancy Category B

Teratology studies in mice, rats, rabbits, and monkeys at oral doses of up to 77, 23, 23, or 38.5 mg, respectively, of ciclopirox as ciclopirox olamine/kg/day (14, 8, 17, and 28 times MRHTD), or in rats and rabbits receiving topical doses of up to 92.4 and 77 mg/kg/day, respectively (33 and 55 times MRHTD), did not indicate any significant fetal malformations.

There are no adequate or well-controlled studies of topically applied ciclopirox in pregnant women. PENLAC® NAIL LACQUER (ciclopirox) Topical Solution, 8%, should be used during pregnancy only if the potential benefit justifies the potential risk to the fetus.

Nursing Mothers

It is not known whether this drug is excreted in human milk. Since many drugs are excreted in human milk, caution should be exercised when PENLAC® NAIL LACQUER (ciclopirox) Topical Solution, 8%, is administered to a nursing woman.

Pediatric Use

Based on the safety profile in adults, PENLAC® NAIL LACQUER (ciclopirox) Topical Solution, 8% is considered safe for use in children twelve years and older. No clinical trials have been conducted in the pediatric population.

Geriatric Use

Clinical studies of PENLAC® NAIL LACQUER (ciclopirox) Topical Solution, 8%, did not include sufficient numbers of subjects aged 65 and over to determine whether they respond differently from younger subjects. Other reported clinical experience has not identified differences in responses between elderly and younger patients.

ADVERSE REACTIONS

In the vehicle-controlled clinical trials conducted in the US, 9% (30/327) of patients treated with PENLAC® NAIL LACQUER (ciclopirox) Topical Solution, 8% and 7% (23/328) of patients treated with vehicle reported treatment-emergent adverse events (TEAE) considered by the investigator to be causally related to the test material.

The incidence of these adverse events, within each body system, was similar between the treatment groups except for Skin and Appendages: 8% (27/327) and 4% (14/328) of subjects in the ciclopirox and vehicle groups reported at least one adverse event, respectively. The most common were rash-related adverse events: periungual erythema and erythema of the proximal nail fold were reported more frequently in patients treated with PENLAC® NAIL LACQUER (ciclopirox) Topical Solution, 8%, (5% [16/327]) than in patients treated with vehicle (1% [3/328]). Other TEAEs thought to be causally related included nail disorders such as shape change, irritation, ingrown toenail, and discoloration.

The incidence of nail disorders was similar between the treatment groups (2% [6/327] in the PENLAC® NAIL LACQUER (ciclopirox) Topical Solution, 8%, group and 2% [7/328] in the vehicle group). Moreover, application site reactions and/or burning of the skin occurred in 1% of patients treated with PENLAC® NAIL LACQUER (ciclopirox) Topical Solution, 8%, (3/327) and vehicle (4/328).

A 21-Day Cumulative Irritancy study was conducted under conditions of semi-occlusion. Mild reactions were seen in 46% of patients with the PENLAC® NAIL LACQUER (ciclopirox) Topical Solution, 8%, 32% with the vehicle and 2% with the negative control, but all were reactions of mild transient erythema. There was no evidence of allergic contact sensitization for either the PENLAC® NAIL LACQUER (ciclopirox) Topical Solution, 8%, or the vehicle base. In the vehicle-controlled studies, one patient treated with PENLAC® NAIL LACQUER (ciclopirox) Topical Solution, 8%, discontinued treatment due to a rash, localized to the palm (causal relation to test material undetermined).

Use of PENLAC® NAIL LACQUER (ciclopirox) Topical Solution, 8%, for 48 additional weeks was evaluated in an open-label extension study conducted in patients previously treated in the vehicle-controlled studies. Three percent (9/281) of subjects treated with PENLAC® NAIL LACQUER (ciclopirox) Topical Solution, 8%, experienced at least one TEAE that the investigator thought was causally related to the test material. Mild rash in the form of periungual erythema (1% [2/281]) and nail disorders (1% [4/281]) were the most frequently reported. Four patients discontinued because of TEAEs. Two of the four had events considered to be related to test material: one patient's great toenail "broke away" and another had an elevated creatine phosphokinase level on Day 1 (after 48 weeks of treatment with vehicle in the previous vehicle-controlled study).

DOSAGE AND ADMINISTRATION

PENLAC® NAIL LACQUER (ciclopirox) Topical Solution, 8%, should be used as a component of a comprehensive management program for onychomycosis. Removal of the unattached, infected nail, as frequently as monthly, by a health care professional, weekly trimming by the patient, and daily application of the medication are all integral parts of this therapy. Careful consideration of the appropriate nail management program should be given to patients with diabetes (see PRECAUTIONS)

Nail Care By Health Care Professionals

Removal of the unattached, infected nail, as frequently as monthly, trimming of onycholytic nail, and filing of excess horny material should be performed by professionals trained in treatment of nail disorders.

Nail Care By Patient

Patients should file away (with emery board) loose nail material and trim nails, as required, or as directed by the health care professional, every seven days after PENLAC® NAIL LACQUER (ciclopirox) Topical Solution, 8%, is removed with alcohol.

PENLAC® NAIL LACQUER (ciclopirox) Topical Solution, 8%, should be applied once daily (preferably at bedtime or eight hours before washing) to all affected nails with the applicator brush provided. The PENLAC® NAIL LACQUER (ciclopirox) Topical Solution, 8%, should be applied evenly over the entire nail plate.

If possible, PENLAC® NAIL LACQUER (ciclopirox) Topical Solution, 8%, should be applied to the nail bed, hyponychium, and the under surface of the nail plate when it is free of the nail bed (e.g., onycholysis).

The PENLAC® NAIL LACQUER (ciclopirox) Topical Solution, 8%, should not be removed on a daily basis. Daily applications should be made over the previous coat and removed with alcohol every seven days. This cycle should be repeated throughout the duration of therapy.

HOW SUPPLIED

PENLAC® NAIL LACQUER (ciclopirox) Topical Solution, 8%, is supplied in 3.3 mL (NDC 0066-8008-01) and 6.6 mL (NDC 0066-8008-02) glass bottles with screw caps which are fitted with brushes.

Protect from light (e.g., store the bottle in the carton after every use).

PENLAC® NAIL LACQUER (ciclopirox) Topical Solution, 8%, should be stored at room temperature between 59° and 86°F (15° and 30°C).

CAUTION: Flammable. Keep away from heat and flame.

Rx ONLY.

Prescribing Information as of December 2003

Manufactured for:
Dermik Laboratories
A Division of Aventis Pharmaceuticals Inc
Berwyn, PA 19312 USA
by:
Aventis Pharma Deutschland GmbH
D-65926 Frankfurt am Main
Germany

REFERENCES:

1. Dittmar W., Lohaus G. 1973. HOE296, A new antimycotic compound with a broad antimicrobial spectrum. *Arzneim-Forsch. / Drug Res.* 23:670–674.
2. Niewerth et. al., 1998. Antimicrobial susceptibility testing of dermatophytes: Comparison of the agar macrodilution and broth micro dilution tests. *Chemotherapy.* 44:31–35.
3. Yang et. al. 1997. A new simulation model for studying in vitro topical penetration of antifungal drugs into hard keratin. *J. Mycol. Med.* 7:195–98.

Gantrez is a registered trademark of GAF Corporation

PENLAC® NAIL LACQUER (ciclopirox)
Topical Solution, 8%

Patient Information and Instructions

Patients should have detailed instructions regarding the use of PENLAC® NAIL LACQUER (ciclopirox) Topical Solution, 8%, as a component of a comprehensive management program for onychomycosis in order to achieve maxi-

Continued on next page

Penlac—Cont.

mum benefit with the use of this product. Discuss your treatment plan with your health care professional for regular removal of the unattached, infected nail.

Before using this medication, tell your doctor if you:

- Are pregnant or nursing
- Are an insulin dependent diabetic or have diabetic neuropathy
- Have a history of immunosuppression
- Are immunocompromised (e.g., received an organ transplant, etc.)
- Require medication to control epilepsy
- Use or require topical corticosteroids on a repeated monthly basis
- Use steroid inhalers on a regular basis

Patient Information:

- Use PENLAC® NAIL LACQUER (ciclopirox) Topical Solution, 8%, as directed by your health care professional.
- PENLAC® NAIL LACQUER (ciclopirox) Topical Solution, 8%, is for external use only.
- Contact with skin other than skin immediately surrounding the treated nail(s) should be avoided.
- Avoid contact with the eyes and mucous membranes.
- Removal of the unattached, infected nail, as frequently as monthly, by your health care professional is needed with use of this medication to obtain maximal benefit with use of this product. If you have diabetes or problems with numbness in your toes or fingers, talk to your health care provider before trimming your nails or removing any nail material.
- Inform your health care professional if the area of application shows signs of increased irritation (redness, itching, burning, blistering, swelling, oozing).
- Up to 48 weeks of daily applications with PENLAC® NAIL LACQUER (ciclopirox) Topical Solution, 8%, and professional removal, as frequently as monthly, of the unattached, infected nail are considered the full treatment time to achieve a clear or almost clear nail (defined as 10% or less residual nail involvement). Six months of therapy with professional removal of the unattached, infected nail may be required before initial improvement of symptoms is noticed.
- A completely clear nail may not be achieved with use of this medication. In clinical studies less than 12% of patients were able to achieve either a clear or almost clear toenail.
- Do not use nail polish or other nail cosmetic products on the treated nails.
- Avoid use near heat or open flame, because product is flammable.

Patient Instructions

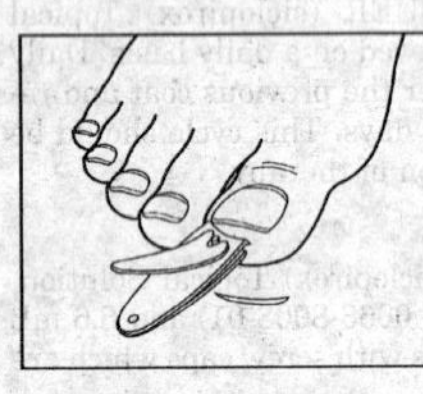

1. Before starting treatment, remove any loose nail or nail material using nail clippers or nail files. If you have diabetes or problems with numbness in your toes or fingers, talk to your health care provider before trimming your nails or removing any nail material.

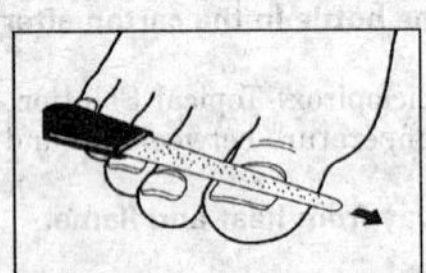

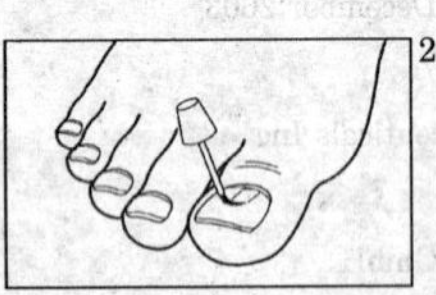

2. Apply PENLAC® NAIL LACQUER (ciclopirox) Topical Solution, 8%, once daily (preferably at bedtime) to all affected nails with the applicator brush provided. Apply the lacquer evenly over the entire nail. Where possible, nail lacquer should also be applied to the underside of the nail and to the skin beneath it. Allow lacquer to dry (approximately 30 seconds) before putting on socks or stockings. After applying medication, wait 8 hours before taking a bath or shower.

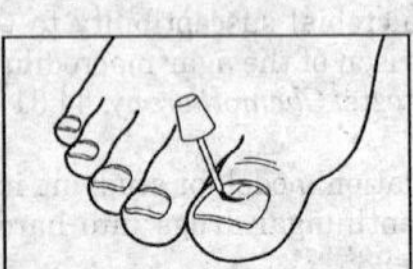

3. Apply PENLAC® NAIL LACQUER (ciclopirox) Topical Solution, 8%, daily over the previous coat.

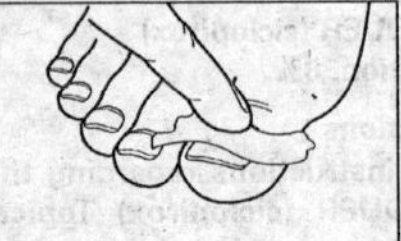

4. Once a week, remove the PENLAC® NAIL LACQUER (ciclopirox) Topical Solution, 8%, with alcohol. Remove as much as possible of the damaged nail using scissors, nail clippers, or nail files.
5. Repeat process (steps 2 through 4).

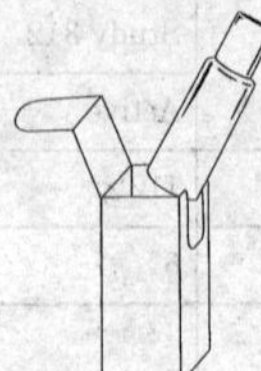

Please Note:

1. To prevent screw cap from sticking to the bottle, do not allow solution to get into the bottle threads.
2. To prevent the solution from drying out, bottle should be closed tightly after every use.
3. To protect from light, replace bottle into carton after each use.

Prescribing Information as of December 2003
Manufactured for:
Dermik Laboratories
A Division of Aventis Pharmaceuticals Inc
Berwyn, PA 19312 USA
by:
Aventis Pharma Deutschland GmbH
D-65926 Frankfurt am Main
Germany

PSORCON® E Emollient Cream ℞

(diflorasone diacetate cream) 0.05%
Not For Ophthalmic Use

Prescribing information as of December 2001

DESCRIPTION

Each gram of **Psorcon E** Emollient Cream contains 0.5 mg diflorasone diacetate in a cream base. Chemically, diflorasone diacetate is: 6α,9-difluoro - 11β,17,21 - trihydroxy - 16β - methyl-pregna 1,4 - diene - 3,20 - dione 17,21 - diacetate. The structural formula is represented below:

Each gram of **Psorcon E** Emollient Cream contains 0.5 mg diflorasone diacetate in a hydrophilic vanishing cream base of propylene glycol, stearyl alcohol, cetyl alcohol, sorbitan monostearate, polysorbate 60, mineral oil and purified water.

HOW SUPPLIED

Psorcon E Emollient Cream is available in the following size tubes:

15 gram	NDC 0066-0272-17
30 gram	NDC 0066-0272-31
60 gram	NDC 0066-0272-60

Store at controlled room temperature, 20° to 25° C (68° to 77°F) [see USP].
Rx only
Prescribing Information as of December 2001
Manufactured for
Dermik Laboratories, Inc.
Berwyn, PA 19312
By Pharmacia & Upjohn Company
A Subsidiary of Pharmacia Corporation
Kalamazoo, MI, USA 49001

Revised December 2001

PSORCON® E Emollient Ointment ℞

(diflorasone diacetate ointment) 0.05%
Not For Ophthalmic Use

Prescribing Information as of December 2001

DESCRIPTION

Each gram of **Psorcon E** Emollient Ointment contains 0.5 mg diflorasone diacetate in an ointment base. Chemically, diflorasone diacetate is: 6α,9-difluoro - 11β, 17,21 - trihydroxy - 16β- methyl-pregna - 1,4-diene - 3,20 - dione 17,21 - diacetate. The structural formula is represented below:

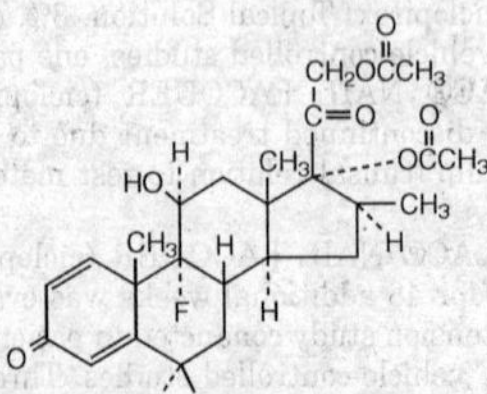

Psorcon E Emollient Ointment contains diflorasone diacetate in an emollient, occlusive base consisting of polyoxypropylene 15-stearyl ether, stearic acid, lanolin alcohol and white petrolatum.

HOW SUPPLIED

Psorcon E Emollient Ointment is available as follows:

15 gram tube	NDC 0066-0275-17
30 gram tube	NDC 0066-0275-31
60 gram tube	NDC 0066-0275-60

Store at controlled room temperature, 20° to 25° C (68° to 77° F) [see USP].
Prescribing Information as of December 2001
Rx only
Manufactured for
Dermik Laboratories, Inc.
Berwyn, PA 19312
By Pharmacia & Upjohn Company
A Subsidiary of Pharmacia Corporation
Kalamazoo, MI, USA 49001

SULFACET-R® LOTION ℞

(Sodium Sulfacetamide 10% and Sulfur 5%)

DESCRIPTION

Each mL of **Sulfacet-R® Lotion** (sodium sulfacetamide 10% and sulfur 5%) as dispensed contains 100 mg of sodium sulfacetamide and 50 mg of sulfur in a tinted lotion of 2-bromo-2-nitropropane-1, 3 diol, attapulgite, butylparaben, hydroxyethyl cellulose, iron oxides, lauramide DEA (and) diethanolamine, methylparaben, polyethylene glycol 400 monolaurate, propylene glycol, purified water, silicone emulsion, sodium chloride, sodium metabisulfite, sodium polynaphthalenesulfonate, talc, xanthan gum, and zinc oxide. Color Blender contains an additional inactive ingredient, polyethylene glycol 400, NF.
Sodium sulfacetamide is a sulfonamide with antibacterial activity while sulfur acts as a keratolytic agent. Chemically sodium sulfacetamide is N'-[(4-aminophenyl) sulfonyl]-acetamide, monosodium salt, monohydrate.
The structural formula is:
Sulfacetamide Sodium

HOW SUPPLIED

25 g bottles (NDC 0066-0028-25).
Store at room temperature. Keep tightly closed.
Prescribing Information as of April 2003.
Rx Only
Dermik Laboratories
A Division of Aventis Pharmaceuticals Inc
Berwyn, PA 19312 USA

SULFACET-R® TINT FREE LOTION ℞

(Sodium Sulfacetamide 10% and Sulfur 5%)

DESCRIPTION

Each mL of **Sulfacet-R® Tint Free Lotion** (sodium sulfacetamide 10% and sulfur 5%) as dispensed contains 100 mg of sodium sulfacetamide and 50 mg of sulfur in a lotion of 2-bromo-2-nitropropane-1, 3 diol, attapulgite, butylparaben, hydroxyethyl cellulose, iron oxides, lauramide DEA (and) diethanolamine, methylparaben, polyethylene glycol 400 monolaurate, propylene glycol, purified water, silicone emulsion, sodium chloride, sodium metabisulfite, sodium polynaphthalenesulfonate, talc, xanthan gum, and zinc oxide.
Sodium sulfacetamide is a sulfonamide with antibacterial activity while sulfur acts as a keratolytic agent. Chemically sodium sulfacetamide is N'-[(4-aminophenyl) sulfonyl]-acetamide, monosodium salt, monohydrate. The structural formula is:
Sulfacetamide Sodium

HOW SUPPLIED

25 g bottles (NDC 0066-9028-25).
Store at room temperature. Keep tightly closed.
Prescribing Information as of February 2001.
Rx ONLY
Dermik Laboratories, Inc.
Berwyn, PA USA 19312

VANAMIDE™ ℞

[vă'nă-mīd]
urea cream, 40%
For topical use only. Not for ophthalmic use.

DESCRIPTION

Vanamide™ is a keratolytic, emollient cream which is a potent tissue softener for skin or nails. Each gram of **Vanamide** contains urea (40%), purified water, light mineral oil, glyceryl stearate, cetyl alcohol, petrolatum, gluconolactone, triethanolamine, xanthan gum and propylene glycol.

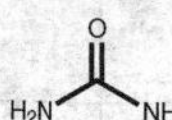

HOW SUPPLIED

Vanamide *urea cream, 40%* is supplied in:
85 gram tube, NDC 0066-0603-03 and 199 gram tube, NDC 0066-0603-07.
Store at controlled room temperature 15–30°C (59–86°F).
Protect from freezing.
℞ **Only.**
Prescribing Information as of September 2002.

How to properly use Vanamide™
urea cream, 40%

Potent tissue-softener for skin or nails. Easy steps to help thin and soften thick, severely rough or dry skin, calluses and nail tissue, including ingrown nails.

1. Apply **Vanamide** to affected areas. Protect surrounding skin.
2. Smooth over affected skin area(s) until cream is absorbed. If desired, cover with adhesive bandage or gauze, secured with adhesive tape. When applying to diseased or damaged nail surfaces, use an ample amount. Cover as above. It is then advisable to remove the "finger" from a plastic or vinyl glove and slip over the bandage covered site. Secure glove finger with additional adhesive tape. Keep dry and occlusive for 3–7 days.
3. Use soap and water to wash off any excess product on unaffected skin areas, including hands. Avoid contact with eyes.

Manufactured for:
Dermik Laboratories
A Division of Aventis Pharmaceuticals Inc.
Berwyn, PA 19312 USA
by:
DPT Lakewood, Inc.
Lakewood, NJ 08701 USA

VYTONE® Cream 1% ℞
(hydrocortisone-iodoquinol)

DESCRIPTION

Each gram of Vytone® Cream 1% contains 10 mg of hydrocortisone and 10 mg of iodoquinol in a greaseless base of purified water, propylene glycol, glyceryl monostearate SE, cholesterol and related sterols, isopropyl myristate, polysorbate 60, cetyl alcohol, sorbitan monostearate, polyoxyl 40 stearate, sorbic acid, and polysorbate 20.

Chemically, hydrocortisone is [Pregn-4-ene-3,20-dione, 11, 17, 21- trihydroxy-, (11β)-] with the molecular formula ($C_{21}H_{30}O_5$) and is represented by the following structural formula:

and iodoquinol, 5,7-diiodo-8-quinolinol ($C_9H_5I_2NO$) is represented by the following structure:

Hydrocortisone is an anti-inflammatory and antipruritic agent, while iodoquinol is an antifungal and antibacterial agent.

HOW SUPPLIED

1%–Tube 1 oz NDC 0066-0051-01
Store at room temperature. Keep tightly closed.
Prescribing Information as of June 2001(a).
Rx ONLY
Dermik Laboratories, Inc.
Berwyn, PA 19312 USA

For information on over-the-counter drugs, consult **PDR For Nonprescription Drugs and Dietary Supplements.**

DEY, L.P.
2751 NAPA VALLEY CORPORATE DRIVE
NAPA, CA 94558

Direct Inquiries to:
DEY, L.P.
(800) 755-5560
FAX: (707) 224-8918
www.dey.com

For Medical Information Contact:
Gerald L. Klein, M.D.
Vice President
Medical Affairs & Clinical Research
800-429-7751
Fax: 510-595-8183

Brand Name or Generic Name	Concentration Or Size	NDC or Product #
AccuNeb® (albuterol sulfate) Inhalation Solution (℞)	Twenty-Five 3 mL Vials 1.25 mg (*Potency expressed as albuterol, equivalent to 1.5 mg albuterol sulfate)	49502-693-03
	Twenty-Five 3 mL Vials 0.63 mg (*Potency expressed as albuterol, equivalent to 0.75 albuterol sulfate)	49502-692-03
Shown in Product Identification Guide, page 310		
Albuterol Sulfate Inhalation Solution (℞)	Twenty-Five 3 mL Vials 0.083% (expressed as Albuterol)	49502-697-24
	Thirty 3 mL Vials 0.083% (expressed as Albuterol)	49502-697-29
		49502-697-61
	Thirty 3 mL Vials 0.083% (expressed as Albuterol) (Individually wrapped)	49502-697-30
	Sixty 3 mL Vials 0.083% (expressed as Albuterol)	49502-697-61
Shown in Product Identification Guide, page 310		
Curosurf® (℞) (poractant alfa) Intratracheal Suspension	One 1.5 mL Vial (120 mg)	49502-180-01
	One 3 mL Vial (240 mg)	49502-180-03
DuoNeb® (ipratropium bromide and albuterol sulfate) Inhalation Solution (℞)	Thirty 3 mL Vials Ipratropium bromide 0.5 mg/Albuterol sulfate 3.0 mg* (*Equivalent to 2.5 mg albuterol base)	49502-672-30
	Thirty 3 mL Vials Ipratropium bromide 0.5 mg/Albuterol sulfate 3.0 mg* (*Equivalent to 2.5 mg albuterol base) (Individually wrapped)	49502-672-31
	Sixty 3 mL Vials Ipratropium bromide 0.5 mg/Albuterol sulfate 3.0 mg* (*Equivalent to 2.5 mg albuterol base)	49502-672-60
Shown in Product Identification Guide, page 310		
EpiPen® epinephrine Auto-Injector (℞)	0.3 mg	49502-500-01
EpiPen® Jr epinephrine Auto-Injector (℞)	0.15 mg	49502-501-01
EpiPen 2-Pak® (℞)	Two Epinephrine Auto-Injectors with trainer 0.3 mg	49502-500-02
EpiPen Jr 2-Pak® (℞)	Two Epinephrine Auto-injectors with trainer 0.15 mg	49502-501-02
Shown in Product Identification Guide, page 310		
Cromolyn Sodium Inhalation Solution USP (℞)	Sixty 2 mL Vials 20 mg/mL	49502-689-61
Ipratropium Bromide Inhalation Solution (℞)	Twenty-five 2.5 mL Vials (0.5 mg/2.5 mL)	49502-685-24
	Thirty 2.5 ml Vials (0.5/2.5 mL)	49502-685-29
	Thirty 2.5 mL Vials (0.5/2.5 mL) (Individually wrapped)	49502-685-30
	Sixty 2.5 mL Vials (0.5/2.5 mL)	49502-685-61
Shown in Product Identification Guide, page 310		
Metaproterenol Sulfate Inhalation Solution USP (℞)	Twenty-five 2.5 mL Vials 0.4%	49502-678-24
	Twenty-five 2.5 mL Vials 0.6%	49502-676-24
Sodium Chloride Inhalation Solution USP (OTC)	One Hundred 3 mL Vials 0.45%	49502-820-03
	One Hundred 5 mL Vials 0.45%	49502-820-05
	One Hundred 3 mL Vials 0.9%	49502-830-03
	One Hundred 5 mL Vials 0.9%	49502-830-05
	Fifty 15 mL Vials 0.9%	49502-830-50
Sodium Chloride Solution (℞)	Fifty 15 mL Vials 3%	49502-640-15
	Fifty 15 mL Vials 10%	49502-641-15

ACCUNEB® ℞
(albuterol sulfate)
Inhalation Solution
1.25 mg*/3 mL and 0.63 mg*/3 mL
(*Potency expressed as albuterol, equivalent to 1.5 mg and 0.75 mg albuterol sulfate)

PRESCRIBING INFORMATION

DESCRIPTION

AccuNeb® (albuterol sulfate) inhalation solution is a sterile, clear, colorless solution of the sulfate salt of racemic albuterol, albuterol sulfate. Albuterol sulfate is a relatively selective beta$_2$-adrenergic bronchodilator (see CLINICAL PHARMACOLOGY). The chemical name for albuterol sulfate is α_1 [(tert-butylamino) methyl]-4-hydroxy-m-xylene-α, α′-diol sulfate (2:1) (salt), and its established chemical structure is as follows:

The molecular weight of albuterol sulfate is 576.7 and the empirical formula is $(C_{13}H_{21}NO_3)_2 \bullet H_2SO_4$. Albuterol sulfate is a white crystalline powder, soluble in water and slightly soluble in ethanol. The World Health Organization recommended name for albuterol is salbutamol.

AccuNeb (albuterol sulfate) Inhalation Solution is supplied in two strengths in unit dose vials. Each unit dose vial contains either 0.75 mg of albuterol sulfate (equivalent to 0.63 mg of albuterol) or 1.50 mg of albuterol sulfate (equivalent to 1.25 mg of albuterol) with sodium chloride and sulfuric acid in a 3-mL isotonic, sterile, aqueous solution. Sodium chloride is added to adjust isotonicity of the solution and sulfuric acid is added to adjust pH of the solution to 3.5 (see HOW SUPPLIED).

AccuNeb (albuterol sulfate) Inhalation Solution does not require dilution prior to administration by nebulization. For AccuNeb, like all other nebulized treatments, the amount delivered to the lungs will depend on patient factors, the jet nebulizer utilized, and compressor performance. Using the Pari LC Plus™ nebulizer (with face mask or mouthpiece) connected to a Pari PRONEB™ compressor, under in vitro conditions, the mean delivered dose from the mouth piece (% nominal dose) was approximately 43% of albuterol (1.25 mg strength) and 39% of albuterol (0.63 mg strength) at a mean flow rate of 3.6 L/min. The mean nebulization time was 15 minutes or less. AccuNeb should be administered from a jet nebulizer at an adequate flow rate, via a mouthpiece or face mask (see DOSAGE AND ADMINISTRATION).

CLINICAL PHARMACOLOGY

The prime action of beta-adrenergic drugs is to stimulate adenyl cyclase, the enzyme which catalyzes the formation of cyclic-3′,5′-adenosine monophosphate (cyclic AMP) from adenosine triphosphate (ATP). The cyclic AMP thus formed mediates the cellular responses. In vitro studies and in vivo pharmacologic studies have demonstrated that albuterol has a preferential effect on beta$_2$-adrenergic receptors compared with isoproterenol. While it is recognized that beta$_2$-adrenergic receptors are the predominant receptors in bronchial smooth muscle, recent data indicate that 10% to 50% of the beta-receptors in the human heart may be beta$_2$-receptors. The precise function of these receptors, however, is not yet established. Controlled clinical studies and other

Continued on next page

Accuneb—Cont.

clinical experience have shown that inhaled albuterol, like other beta-adrenergic drugs, can produce a significant cardiovascular effect in some patients, as measured by pulse rate, blood pressure, symptoms, and/or electrocardiographic changes. Albuterol is longer acting than isoproterenol in most patients by any route of administration because it is not a substrate for the cellular uptake processes for catecholamines nor for catechol-*O*-methyl transferase.

Pharmacokinetics: Studies in asthmatic patients have shown that less than 20% of a single albuterol dose was absorbed following either intermittent positive-pressure breathing (IPPB) or nebulizer administration; the remaining amount was recovered from the nebulizer and apparatus, and expired air. Most of the absorbed dose was recovered in urine collected during the 24 hours after drug administration. Following oral administration of 4 mg albuterol, the elimination half-life was five to six hours. Following a 3 mg dose of nebulized albuterol in adults, the mean maximum albuterol plasma level at 0.5 hours was 2.1 ng/mL (range, 1.4 to 3.2 ng/mL). The pharmacokinetics of albuterol following administration of 0.63 mg or 1.25 mg albuterol sulfate inhalation solution by nebulization have not been determined in children 2 to 12 years old.

Animal Pharmacology/Toxicology: Intravenous studies in rats with albuterol sulfate have demonstrated that albuterol crosses the blood-brain barrier and reaches brain concentrations amounting to approximately 5% of plasma concentrations. In structures outside the blood-brain barrier (pineal and pituitary glands), albuterol concentrations were found to be 100 times those found in whole brain.

Studies in laboratory animals (minipigs, rodents, and dogs) have demonstrated the occurrence of cardiac arrhythmias and sudden death (with histologic evidence of myocardial necrosis) when beta-agonists and methylxanthines are administered concurrently. The clinical significance of these findings is unknown.

Clinical Trials: The safety and efficacy of AccuNeb was evaluated in a 4-week, multi-center, randomized, double-blind, placebo-controlled, parallel group study in 349 children 6 to 12 years of age with mild-to-moderate asthma (mean baseline FEV_1 60% to 70% of predicted). Approximately half of the patients were also receiving inhaled corticosteroids. Patients were randomized to receive AccuNeb 0.63 mg, AccuNeb 1.25 mg, or placebo three times a day administered via a Pari LC Plus™ nebulizer and a Pari PRONEB™ compressor. Racemic albuterol, delivered by a chlorofluorocarbon (CFC) metered dose inhaler (MDI) or nebulized, was used on an as-needed basis as the rescue medication.

Efficacy, as measured by the mean percent change from baseline in the area under the 6-hour curve for FEV_1, was demonstrated for both active treatment regimens (n=112 [1.25 mg group] and n=110 [0.63 mg group]) compared with placebo (n=110) on day 1 and day 28. Figures 1 and 2 illustrate the mean percentage change from pre-dose FEV_1 on day 1 and day 28, respectively. The mean baseline FEV_1 for all patients was 1.49 L.

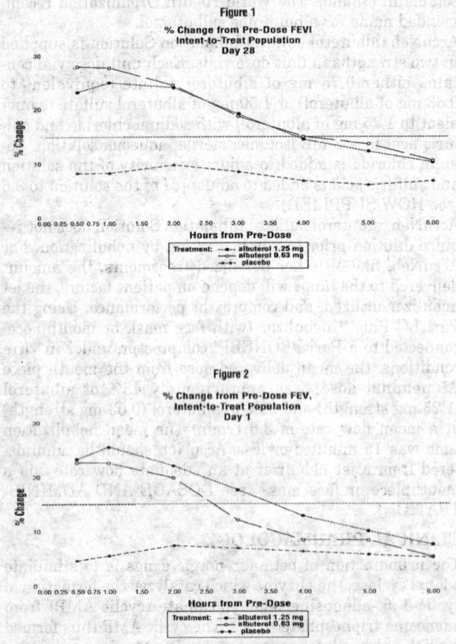

The onset of a 15% increase in FEV_1 over baseline for both doses of AccuNeb was seen at 30 minutes (the first post-dose assessment). The mean time to peak effect was approximately 30 to 60 minutes for both doses on day 1 and after 4 weeks of treatment. The mean duration of effect, as measured by a >15% increase from baseline in FEV_1, was approximately 2.5 hours for both doses on day 1 and approximately 2 hours for both doses after 4 weeks of treatment. In some patients, the duration of effect was as long as 6 hours.

Table 1: Adverse Events with an Incidence of >1% of Patients Receiving AccuNeb and Greater than Placebo (expressed as % of treatment group)

	1.25 mg AccuNeb (N=115)	0.63 mg AccuNeb (N=117)	Placebo (N=117)
Asthma Exacerbation	13	11.1	8.5
Otitis Media	4.3	0.9	0
Allergic Reaction	0.9	3.4	1.7
Gastroenteritis	0.9	3.4	0.9
Cold Symptoms	0	3.4	1.7
Flu Syndrome	2.6	2.6	1.7
Lymphadenopathy	2.6	0.9	1.7
Skin/Appendage Infection	1.7	0	0
Urticaria	1.7	0.9	0
Migraine	0.9	1.7	0
Chest Pain	0.9	1.7	0
Bronchitis	0.9	1.7	0.9
Nausea	1.7	0.9	0.9

INDICATIONS AND USAGE

AccuNeb is indicated for the relief of bronchospasm in patients 2 to 12 years of age with asthma (reversible obstructive airway disease).

CONTRAINDICATIONS

AccuNeb is contraindicated in patients with a history of hypersensitivity to any of its components.

WARNINGS

Paradoxical Bronchospasm: As with other inhaled beta-adrenergic agonists, AccuNeb can produce paradoxical bronchospasm, which may be life threatening. If paradoxical bronchospasm occurs, AccuNeb should be discontinued immediately and alternative therapy instituted. It should be noted that paradoxical bronchospasm, when associated with inhaled formulations, frequently occurs with the first use of a new canister or vial.

Use of Anti-Inflammatory Agents: The use of beta-adrenergic bronchodilators alone may not be adequate to control asthma in many patients. Early consideration should be given to adding anti-inflammatory agents (e.g., corticosteroids).

Deterioration of Asthma: Asthma may deteriorate acutely over a period of hours or chronically over several days or longer. If the patient needs more doses of AccuNeb than usual, this may be a marker of destabilization of asthma and requires reevaluation of the patient and the treatment regimen, giving special consideration of the possible need for anti-inflammatory treatment (e.g., corticosteroids).

Fatalities have been reported in association with excessive use of inhaled sympathomimetic drugs and with the home use of nebulizers. It is, therefore, essential that the physician instruct the patient in the need for further evaluation, if his/her asthma becomes worse.

Cardiovascular Effects: AccuNeb, like other beta-adrenergic agonists, can produce a clinically significant cardiovascular effect in some patients as measured by pulse rate, blood pressure, and/or symptoms. Although such effects are uncommon for AccuNeb at recommended doses, if they occur, the drug may need to be discontinued. In addition, beta-agonists have been reported to produce ECG changes, such as flattening of the T-wave, prolongation of the QTc interval, and ST segment depression. The clinical significance of these findings is unknown. Therefore, AccuNeb like all other sympathomimetic amines, should be used with caution in patients with cardiovascular disorders, especially coronary insufficiency, cardiac arrhythmias, and hypertension.

Immediate Hypersensitivity Reactions: Immediate hypersensitivity reactions may occur after administration of albuterol as demonstrated by rare cases of urticaria, angioedema, rash, bronchospasm, and oropharyngeal edema.

PRECAUTIONS

General: Large doses of intravenous albuterol have been reported to aggravate pre-existing diabetes mellitus and ketoacidosis. As with other beta-agonists, inhaled and intravenous albuterol may produce a significant hypokalemia in some patients, possibly through intracellular shunting, which has the potential to produce adverse cardiovascular effects. The decrease is usually transient, not requiring potassium supplementation.

Information for Patients: The action of AccuNeb may last up to six hours, and therefore it should not be used more frequently than recommended. Do not increase the dose or frequency of medication without consulting your physician. If you find that treatment with AccuNeb becomes less effective for symptomatic relief, your symptoms become worse, and/or you need to use the product more frequently than usual, you should seek medical attention immediately. All asthma medication should only be used under the supervision and direction of a physician. Common effects with medications such as AccuNeb include palpitations, chest pain, rapid heart rate, tremor, or nervousness.

If you are pregnant or nursing, contact your physician about the use of AccuNeb. Effective and safe use of AccuNeb includes an understanding of the way it should be administered.

If the solution in the vial changes color or becomes cloudy, you should not use it.

The drug compatibility (physical and chemical), clinical efficacy, and safety of AccuNeb solution, when mixed with other drugs in a nebulizer, has not been established.

See illustrated Patient's Instructions for Use.

Drug Interactions: Other short-acting sympathomimetic aerosol bronchodilators or epinephrine should not be used concomitantly with AccuNeb.

AccuNeb should be administered with extreme caution to patients being treated with monoamine oxidase inhibitors or tricyclic anti-depressants or within 2 weeks of discontinuation of such agents, since the action of albuterol on the vascular system may be potentiated.

Beta-receptor blocking agents not only block the pulmonary effect of beta-agonists, such as AccuNeb, but may produce severe bronchospasm in asthmatic patients. Therefore, patients with asthma should not normally be treated with beta-blockers. However, under certain circumstances (e.g., prophylaxis after myocardial infarction), there may be no acceptable alternatives to the use of beta-adrenergic blocking agents in patients with asthma. In this setting, cardioselective beta-blockers should be considered, although they should be administered with caution.

The ECG changes and/or hypokalemia that may result from the administration of non-potassium sparing diuretics (such as loop or thiazide diuretics) can be acutely worsened by beta-agonists, especially when the dose of the beta-agonist is exceeded. Although the clinical significance of these effects is unknown, caution is advised in the co-administration of beta-agonists with non-potassium sparing diuretics.

Mean decreases of 16% to 22% in serum digoxin levels were demonstrated after single dose intravenous and oral administration of albuterol, respectively, to normal volunteers who had received digoxin for 10 days. The clinical significance of these findings for patients with obstructive airway disease who are receiving albuterol and digoxin on a chronic basis is unclear. Nevertheless, it would be prudent to carefully evaluate the serum digoxin levels in patients who are currently receiving digoxin and albuterol.

Carcinogenesis, Mutagenesis, and Impairment of Fertility: In a 2-year study in Sprague-Dawley rats, albuterol sulfate caused a significant dose-related increase in the incidence of benign leiomyomas of the mesovarium and above dietary doses of 2 mg/kg (approximately equivalent to the maximum recommended daily inhalation dose for AccuNeb on a mg/m^2 basis). In another study, this effect was blocked by the co-administration of propranolol, a non-selective beta-adrenergic antagonist.

In an 18-month study in CD-1 mice, albuterol sulfate showed no evidence of tumorigenicity at dietary doses up to 500 mg/kg (approximately 140 times the maximum recommended daily inhalation dose of AccuNeb on a mg/m^2 basis). In a 22-month study in Golden hamsters, albuterol sulfate showed no evidence of tumorigenicity at dietary doses up to 50 mg/kg (approximately 20 times the maximum recommended daily inhalation dose of AccuNeb on a mg/m^2 basis).

Albuterol sulfate was not mutagenic in the Ames test or a mutation test in yeast. Albuterol sulfate was not clastogenic in a human peripheral lymphocyte assay or in an AH_1 strain mouse micronucleus assay.

Reproduction studies in rats demonstrated no evidence of impaired fertility at oral doses of albuterol sulfate up to 50 mg/kg (approximately 30 times the maximum recommended daily inhalation dose of AccuNeb on a mg/m^2 basis).

Pregnancy: Teratogenic Effects: Pregnancy Category C: Albuterol has been shown to be teratogenic in mice. A study in CD-1 mice given albuterol subcutaneously showed cleft palate formation in 5 of 111 (4.5%) fetuses at 0.25 mg/kg (less than the maximum recommended daily inhalation dose of AccuNeb on a mg/m^2 basis) and cleft palate formation in 10 of 108 (9.3%) fetuses at 2.5 mg/kg (approximately equal to the maximum recommended daily inhalation dose of AccuNeb on a mg/m^2 basis). The drug did not induce cleft palate formation when administered subcutaneously at a dose of 0.025 mg/kg (less than the maximum recommended daily inhalation dose of AccuNeb on a mg/m^2 basis). Cleft palate formation also occurred in 23 of 72 (30.5%) fetuses from females treated subcutaneously with 2.5 mg/kg isoproterenol (positive control). A reproduction study in Stride rabbits revealed cranioschisis in 7 of 19 (37%) fetuses when albuterol sulfate was administered orally at 50 mg/kg (approximately 60 times the maximum recommended daily inhalation dose of AccuNeb on a mg/m^2 basis).

A study in which pregnant rats were dosed with radiolabelled albuterol sulfate demonstrated that drug-related material was transferred from the maternal circulation to the fetus.

There are no adequate and well-controlled studies of the use of albuterol sulfate in pregnant women. Albuterol should be used during pregnancy only if the potential benefit justifies the potential risk to the fetus.

During worldwide marketing experience, various congenital anomalies, including cleft palate and limb defects, have been reported in the offspring of patients being treated with albuterol. Some of the mothers were taking multiple medications during their pregnancies. Because no consistent pattern of defects can be discerned, a relationship between albuterol use and congenital anomalies has not been established.

Labor and Delivery: Oral albuterol has been shown to delay pre-term labor in some reports. There are presently no well-controlled studies that demonstrate that it will stop pre-term labor or prevent labor at term. Because of the potential for beta agonist interference with uterine contractility, use of AccuNeb for relief of bronchospasm during labor should be restricted to those patients in whom the benefits clearly outweigh the risk.

Albuterol has not been approved for the management of preterm labor. The benefit:risk ratio when albuterol is administered for tocolysis has not been established. Serious adverse reactions, including pulmonary edema, have been reported following administration of albuterol to women in labor.

Nursing Mothers: It is not known whether this drug is excreted in human milk. Because of the potential for tumorigenicity shown for albuterol in some animal studies, a decision should be made whether to discontinue nursing or to discontinue the drug, taking into account the importance of the drug to the mother.

Pediatric Use: Safety and effectiveness of AccuNeb 1.25 mg and 0.63 mg have been established in pediatric patients between the ages of 2 and 12 years. The use of AccuNeb in these age groups is supported by evidence from adequate and well-controlled studies of AccuNeb in children age 6 to 12 years and published reports of albuterol sulfate trials in pediatric patients 3 years of age and older. The safety and effectiveness of AccuNeb in children below 2 years of age have not been established.

ADVERSE REACTIONS

Adverse events reported in >1% of patients receiving AccuNeb and more frequently than in patients receiving placebo in a four-week double-blind study are listed in the following table.

[See table 1 at top of previous page]

There was one case of ST segment depression in the 1.25 mg AccuNeb treatment group.

No clinically relevant laboratory abnormalities related to AccuNeb administration were seen in this study.

OVERDOSAGE

The expected symptoms with overdosage are those of excessive beta-adrenergic stimulation and/or occurrence or exaggeration of symptoms such as seizures, angina, hypertension or hypotension, tachycardia with rates up to 200 beats per minute, arrhythmias, nervousness, headache, tremor, dry mouth, palpitation, nausea, dizziness, fatigue, malaise, insomnia, and exaggeration of the pharmacological effects listed in ADVERSE REACTIONS. Hypokalemia may also occur. As with all sympathomimetic aerosol medications, cardiac arrest and even death may be associated with abuse of AccuNeb. Treatment consists of discontinuation of AccuNeb together with appropriate symptomatic therapy. The judicious use of a cardioselective beta-receptor blocker may be considered, bearing in mind that such medication can produce bronchospasm. There is insufficient evidence to determine if dialysis is beneficial for overdosage of AccuNeb. The oral median lethal dose of albuterol sulfate in mice is greater than 2000 mg/kg (approximately 580 times the maximum recommended daily inhalation dose of AccuNeb on a mg/m^2 basis). The subcutaneous median lethal dose of albuterol sulfate in mature rats and small young rats is approximately 450 mg/kg and 2000 mg/kg, respectively (approximately 260 and 1200 times the maximum recommended daily inhalation dose of AccuNeb on a mg/m^2 basis). The inhalation median lethal dose has not been determined in animals.

DOSAGE AND ADMINISTRATION

The usual starting dosage for patients 2 to 12 years of age is 1.25 mg or 0.63 mg of AccuNeb administered 3 or 4 times daily, as needed, by nebulization. More frequent administration is not recommended.

To administer 1.25 mg or 0.63 mg of albuterol, use the entire contents of one unit-dose vial (3 mL of 1.25 mg or 0.63 mg inhalation solution) by nebulization. Adjust nebulizer flow rate to deliver AccuNeb over 5 to 15 minutes.

The use of AccuNeb can be continued as medically indicated to control recurring bouts of bronchospasm. During this time most patients gain optimum benefit from regular use of the inhalation solution.

Patients 6 to 12 years of age with more severe asthma (baseline FEV_1 less than 60% predicted), weight >40 kg, or patients 11 to 12 years of age may achieve a better initial response with the 1.25 mg dose.

AccuNeb has not been studied in the setting of acute attacks of bronchospasm. A 2.5 mg dose of albuterol provided by a higher concentration product (2.5 mg albuterol per 3 mL) may be more appropriate for treating acute exacerbations, particularly in children 6 years old and above.

If a previously effective dosage regimen fails to provide the usual relief, medical advice should be sought immediately, as this is often a sign of seriously worsening asthma which would require reassessment of therapy.

The drug compatibility (physical and chemical), clinical efficacy and safety of AccuNeb solution, when mixed with other drugs in a nebulizer have not been established.

The safety and efficacy of AccuNeb have been established in clinical trials when administered using the Pari LC Plus™ nebulizer and Pari PRONEB™ compressor. The safety and efficacy of AccuNeb when administered with other nebulizer systems have not been established.

AccuNeb should be administered via jet nebulizer connected to an air compressor with adequate air flow, equipped with a mouthpiece or suitable face mask.

HOW SUPPLIED

AccuNeb (albuterol sulfate) Inhalation Solution is supplied as a 3 mL, clear, colorless, sterile, preservative-free, aqueous solution in two different strengths, 0.63 mg and 1.25 mg, of albuterol (equivalent to 0.75 mg of albuterol sulfate or 1.5 mg of albuterol sulfate per 3 mL) in unit-dose low-density polyethylene (LDPE) vials. Each unit-dose LDPE vial is protected in a foil-pouch, and each foil pouch contains 5 unit-dose LDPE vials. Each strength of AccuNeb (albuterol sulfate) Inhalation Solution is available in a shelf carton containing multiple foil pouches.

AccuNeb® (albuterol sulfate) Inhalation Solution, 0.63 mg (potency expressed as albuterol) contains 0.75 mg albuterol sulfate per 3 mL in unit-dose vials and is available in the following packaging configuration.

NDC 49502-692-03 5 foil pouches, each containing 5 vials, total 25 vials per carton

AccuNeb® (albuterol sulfate) Inhalation Solution, 1.25 mg (potency expressed as albuterol) contains 1.50 mg albuterol sulfate per 3 mL in unit-dose vials and is available in the following packaging configuration.

NDC 49502-693-03 5 foil pouches, each containing 5 vials, total 25 vials per carton

Rx Only.

STORAGE

Store between 2°C and 25°C (36°F–77°F). Protect from light and excessive heat.

Store unit-dose vials in protective foil pouch at all times. Once removed from the foil pouch, use vial(s) within one week. Discard the vial if the solution is not colorless.

Keep out of the reach of children.

DEY, Napa, CA 94558

03-492-21A September 2001

AccuNeb®

(albuterol sulfate)

Inhalation Solution

1.25 mg*/3 mL and 0.63 mg*/3 mL

(*Potency expressed as albuterol, equivalent to 1.5 mg and 0.75 mg albuterol sulfate)

PATIENT'S INSTRUCTIONS FOR USE

Read this patient information completely every time your prescription is filled as information may have changed. Keep these instructions with your medication, as you may want to read them again.

AccuNeb should only be used under the direction of a physician. Your physician and pharmacist have more information about AccuNeb and the condition for which it has been prescribed. Contact them if you have additional questions.

Storing your Medicine

Store AccuNeb between 2° and 25° C (36° and 77° F). Vials should be protected from light before use, therefore, keep unused vials in the foil pouch. Do not use after the expiration (EXP) date printed on the vial.

Dose

AccuNeb is supplied as a single-dose, ready-to-use vial containing 3 mL of solution. No mixing or dilution is needed. Use one new vial with each nebulizer treatment.

Instructions for Use

1. Remove one vial from the foil pouch. Place remaining vials back into foil pouch for storage.
2. Twist the cap completely off the vial and squeeze the contents into the nebulizer reservoir (Figure 1).

Figure 1

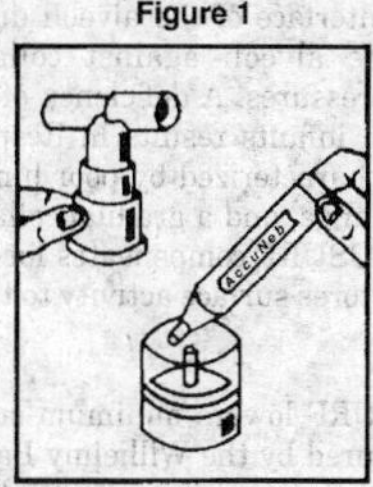

3. Connect the nebulizer to the mouthpiece or face mask (Figure 2).

Figure 2

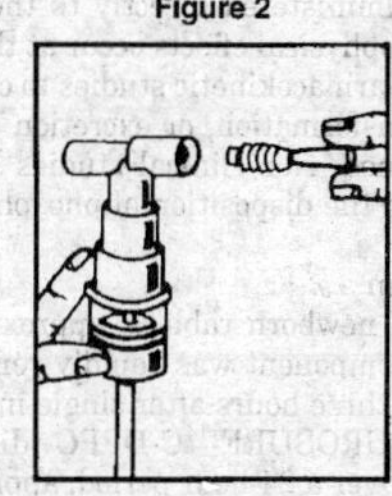

4. Connect the nebulizer to the compressor.
5. Sit in a comfortable, upright position; place the mouthpiece in your mouth (Figure 3) or put on the face mask (Figure 4); and turn on the compressor.

Figure 3

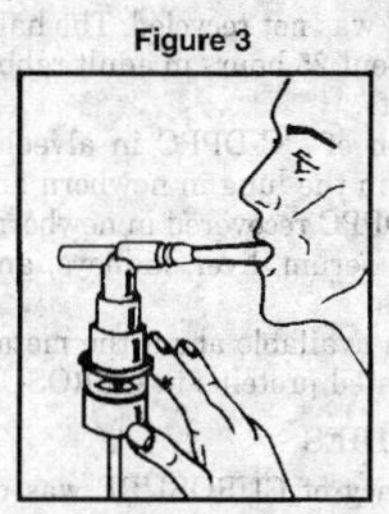

Figure 4

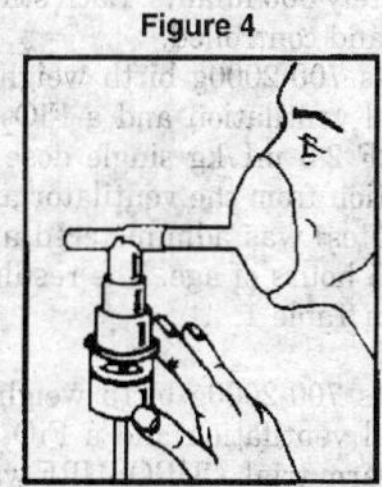

6. Breathe as calmly, deeply and evenly as possible through your mouth until no more mist is formed in the nebulizer chamber (about 5–15 minutes). At this point, the treatment is finished.
7. Clean the nebulizer (see manufacturer's instructions).

DEY, Napa, CA 94558

03-492-21A September 2001

Shown in Product Identification Guide, page 311

CUROSURF® ℞

[kər'ō-sîrf]

(poractant alfa)

Intratracheal Suspension

DESCRIPTION

CUROSURF® (poractant alfa) Intratracheal Suspension is a sterile, non-pyrogenic pulmonary surfactant intended for intratracheal use only. It is an extract of natural porcine lung surfactant consisting of 99% polar lipids (mainly phospholipids) and 1% hydrophobic low molecular weight proteins (surfactant associated proteins SP-B and SP-C). It is suspended in 0.9% sodium chloride solution. The pH is adjusted as required with sodium bicarbonate to a pH of 6.2 (5.5-6.5). CUROSURF contains no preservatives.

CUROSURF is a white to creamy white suspension of poractant alfa. Each milliliter of surfactant mixture contains 80 mg of surfactant (extract) that includes 76 mg of phospholipids and 1 mg of protein of which 0.2 mg is SP-B. The amount of phospholipids is calculated from the content of phosphorus and contains 55 mg of phosphotidylcholine of which 30 mg is dipalmitoylphosphatidylcholine.

Continued on next page

Curosurf—Cont.

CLINICAL PHARMACOLOGY

Mechanism of Action

Endogenous pulmonary surfactant reduces surface tension at the air-liquid interface of the alveoli during ventilation and stabilizes the alveoli against collapse at resting transpulmonary pressures. A deficiency of pulmonary surfactant in preterm infants results in Respiratory Distress Syndrome (RDS) characterized by poor lung expansion, inadequate gas exchange, and a gradual collapse of the lungs (atelectasis). CUROSURF compensates for the deficiency of surfactant and restores surface activity to the lungs of these infants.

Activity

In vitro—CUROSURF lowers minimum surface tension to ≤4mN/m as measured by the Wilhelmy Balance System.
In vivo—In several pharmacodynamic studies, CUROSURF improved lung compliance, pulmonary gas exchange, or survival in premature rabbits.

Pharmacokinetics

CUROSURF is administered directly to the target organ, the lung, where biophysical effects occur at the alveolar surface. No human pharmacokinetic studies to characterize the absorption, biotransformation, or excretion of CUROSURF have been performed. Non-clinical studies have been performed to evaluate the disposition of phospholipids present in CUROSURF.

Animal Metabolism

In both adult and newborn rabbits, approximately 50% of the radiolabeled component was rapidly removed from the alveoli in the first three hours after single intratracheal administration of CUROSURF-^{14}C-DPPC (dipalmitoylphosphatidylcholine). Over a 24-hour period, approximately 45% of the labeled DPPC was cleared from the lungs of adult rabbits compared to approximately 20% in newborn rabbits. In newborn rabbits, CUROSURF-^{14}C-DPPC passed from the alveolar space into the lung parenchyma and then was secreted again into the alveoli, whereas in adult rabbits, most of the DPPC was not recycled. The half-life in the lung appeared to be about 25 hours in adult rabbits and 67 hours in newborn rabbits.
The concentration of ^{14}C-DPPC in alveolar macrophages was ≤2% of that in the lung in newborn and adult rabbits. Of the total ^{14}C-DPPC recovered in newborn rabbits, <0.6% was found in the serum, liver, kidneys, and brain, respectively, at 48 hours.
No information is available about the metabolic rate of the surfactant-associated proteins in CUROSURF.

CLINICAL STUDIES

The clinical efficacy of CUROSURF was demonstrated in one single-dose study (Study 1) and one multiple-dose study (Study 2) in the treatment of established neonatal RDS involving approximately 500 infants. Each study was randomized, multicenter, and controlled.
In Study 1, infants 700-2000g birth weight with RDS requiring mechanical ventilation and a $FiO_2 \geq 0.60$ were enrolled. CUROSURF 2.5 mL/kg single dose (200 mg/kg) or control (disconnection from the ventilator and manual ventilation for 2 minutes) was administered after RDS developed and before 15 hours of age. The results from Study 1 are shown below in Table 1.
[See table 1 above]

TABLE 1

EFFICACY PARAMETER	SINGLE DOSE CUROSURF n=78 %	CONTROL n=67 %	P-VALUE
MORTALITY at 28 DAYS (ALL CAUSES)	31	48	≤0.05
BRONCHOPULMONARY DYSPLASIA*	18	22	N.S.
PNEUMOTHORAX	21	36	≤0.05
PULMONARY INTERSTITIAL EMPHYSEMA	21	38	≤0.05

*Bronchopulmonary dysplasia (BPD) diagnosed by positive x-ray and supplemental oxygen dependence at 28 days of life.
N.S.: not statistically significant

In Study 2, infants 700-2000g birth weight with RDS requiring mechanical ventilation and a $FiO_2 \geq 0.60$ were enrolled. In this two-arm trial, CUROSURF was administered after RDS developed and before 15 hours of age, as a single-dose or as multiple doses. In the single-dose arm, infants received CUROSURF 2.5mL/kg (200mg/kg). In the multiple-dose arm, the initial dose of CUROSURF was 2.5mL/kg (200mg/kg) and subsequent doses of CUROSURF were 1.25mL/kg (100mg/kg). The results from Study 2 are shown below in Table 2.
[See table 2 above]

TABLE 2

EFFICACY PARAMETER	SINGLE-DOSE CUROSURF n=184 %	MULTIPLE-DOSE CUROSURF n=173 %	P-VALUE
MORTALITY at 28 DAYS (ALL CAUSES)	21	13	0.048
BRONCHOPULMONARY DYSPLASIA	18	18	N.S.
PNEUMOTHORAX	17	9	0.03
PULMONARY INTERSTITIAL EMPHYSEMA	27	22	N.S.

N.S.: not statistically significant

ACUTE CLINICAL EFFECTS

As with other surfactants, marked improvements in oxygenation may occur within minutes of the administration of CUROSURF.

INDICATION AND USAGE

CUROSURF is indicated for the treatment (rescue) of Respiratory Distress Syndrome (RDS) in premature infants. CUROSURF reduces mortality and pneumothoraces associated with RDS.

WARNINGS

CUROSURF is intended for intratracheal use only.
THE ADMINISTRATION OF EXOGENOUS SURFACTANTS, INCLUDING CUROSURF, CAN RAPIDLY AFFECT OXYGENATION AND LUNG COMPLIANCE. Therefore, infants receiving CUROSURF should receive frequent clinical and laboratory assessments so that oxygen and ventilatory support can be modified to respond to respiratory changes. CUROSURF should only be administered by those trained and experienced in the care, resuscitation, and stabilization of pre-term infants.
TRANSIENT ADVERSE EFFECTS SEEN WITH THE ADMINISTRATION OF CUROSURF INCLUDE BRADYCARDIA, HYPOTENSION, ENDOTRACHEAL TUBE BLOCKAGE, AND OXYGEN DESATURATION. These events require stopping Curosurf administration and taking appropriate measures to alleviate the condition. After the patient is stable, dosing may proceed with appropriate monitoring.

TABLE 3

COMPLICATIONS OF PREMATURITY	CUROSURF 2.5 mL/kg (200 mg/kg) n=78 %	CONTROL* n=66 %
Acquired Pneumonia	17	21
Acquired Septicemia	14	18
Bronchopulmonary Dysplasia	18	22
Intracranial Hemorrhage	51	64
Patent Ductus Arteriosus	60	48
Pneumothorax	21	36
Pulmonary Interstitial Emphysema	21	38

*Control patients were disconnected from the ventilator and manually ventilated for 2 minutes. No surfactant was instilled.

PRECAUTIONS

General

Correction of acidosis, hypotension, anemia, hypoglycemia, and hypothermia is recommended prior to CUROSURF administration.
Surfactant administration can be expected to reduce the severity of RDS but will not eliminate the mortality and morbidity associated with other complications of prematurity.
Sufficient information is not available on the effects of administering initial doses of CUROSURF other than 2.5 mL/kg (200 mg/kg), subsequent doses other than 1.25 mL/kg (100 mg/kg), administration of more than three total doses, dosing more frequently than every 12 hours, or initiating therapy with CUROSURF more than 15 hours after diagnosing RDS. Adequate data are not available on the use of CUROSURF in conjunction with experimental therapies of RDS, e.g., high-frequency ventilation.

Carcinogenesis, Mutagenesis, Impairment of Fertility

Studies to assess potential carcinogenic and reproductive effects of CUROSURF, or other surfactants, have not been conducted.
Mutagenicity studies of CUROSURF, which included the Ames test, gene mutation assay in Chinese hamster V79 cells, chromosomal aberration assay in Chinese hamster ovarian cells, unscheduled DNA synthesis in HELA S3 cells, and *in vivo* mouse nuclear test, were negative.

ADVERSE REACTIONS

Transient adverse effects seen with the administration of CUROSURF include bradycardia, hypotension, endotracheal tube blockage, and oxygen desaturation.
The rates of common complications of prematurity observed in Study 1 are shown below in Table 3.
[See table 3 above]
Immunological studies have not demonstrated differences in levels of surfactant-anti-surfactant immune complexes and anti-CUROSURF antibodies between patients treated with CUROSURF and patients who received control treatment.

FOLLOW-UP EVALUATIONS

Seventy-six infants (45 treated with CUROSURF) were evaluated at 1 year of age and 73 infants (44 treated with CUROSURF) at 2 years of age. Data from follow-up evaluations for weight and length, persistent respiratory symptoms, incidence of cerebral palsy, visual impairment, or auditory impairment was similar between treatment groups. In 16 patients (10 treated with CUROSURF and 6 controls) evaluated at 5.5 years of age, the developmental quotient, derived using the Griffiths Mental Developmental Scales, was similar between groups.

OVERDOSAGE

There have been no reports of overdosage following the administration of CUROSURF.
In the event of accidental overdosage, and only if there are clear clinical effects on the infant's respiration, ventilation, or oxygenation, as much of the suspension as possible should be aspirated and the infant should be managed with supportive treatment, with particular attention to fluid and electrolyte balance.

DOSAGE AND ADMINISTRATION

FOR INTRATRACHEAL ADMINISTRATION ONLY.

General

CUROSURF is administered intratracheally by instillation through a 5 French end-hole catheter, and briefly disconnecting the endotracheal tube from the ventilator. Alternatively, CUROSURF may be administered through the secondary lumen of a dual lumen endotracheal tube without interrupting mechanical ventilation.
Before administering CUROSURF, assure proper placement and patency of the endotracheal tube. At the discretion of the clinician, the endotracheal tube may be suctioned before administering Curosurf. The infant should be allowed to stabilize before proceeding with dosing.

Initial Dose

The initial recommended dose of CUROSURF is 2.5 mL/kg birth weight. This dose may be determined from the CUROSURF dosing chart below.

For endotracheal tube instillation using a 5 French end-hole catheter

Slowly withdraw the entire contents of the vial of CUROSURF into a 3 or 5 mL plastic syringe through a large-gauge needle (e.g., at least 20 gauge). Attach the precut 8-cm 5 end-hole French catheter to the syringe. Fill the catheter with CUROSURF. Discard excess CUROSURF through the catheter so that only the total dose to be given remains in the syringe.
Immediately before CUROSURF administration, the infant's ventilator settings should be changed to a rate of

TABLE 4

CUROSURF DOSING CHART

WEIGHT (grams)	INITIAL DOSE 2.5mL/kg	REPEAT DOSE 1.25 mL/kg	WEIGHT (grams)	INITIAL DOSE 2.5mL/kg	REPEAT DOSE 1.25 mL/kg
	EACH DOSE (mL)			EACH DOSE (mL)	
600-650	1.60	0.80	1301-1350	3.30	1.65
651-700	1.70	0.85	1351-1400	3.50	1.75
701-750	1.80	0.90	1401-1450	3.60	1.80
751-800	2.00	1.00	1451-1500	3.70	1.85
801-850	2.10	1.05	1501-1550	3.80	1.90
851-900	2.20	1.10	1551-1600	4.00	2.00
901-950	2.30	1.15	1601-1650	4.10	2.05
951-1000	2.50	1.25	1651-1700	4.20	2.10
1001-1050	2.60	1.30	1701-1750	4.30	2.15
1051-1100	2.70	1.35	1751-1800	4.50	2.25
1101-1150	2.80	1.40	1801-1850	4.60	2.30
1151-1200	3.00	1.50	1851-1900	4.70	2.35
1201-1250	3.10	1.55	1901-1950	4.80	2.40
1251-1300	3.20	1.60	1951-2000	5.00	2.50

40-60 breaths/minute, inspiratory time 0.5 second, and supplemental oxygen sufficient to maintain SaO_2>92%. Keep the infant in a neutral position (head and body in alignment without inclination). Briefly disconnect the endotracheal tube from the ventilator. Insert the pre-cut 5 French catheter into the endotracheal tube and instill the first aliquot (1.25 mL/kg birth weight) of CUROSURF. The infant should be positioned such that either the right or left side is dependent for this aliquot. After the first aliquot is instilled, remove the catheter from the endotracheal tube and manually ventilate the infant with 100% oxygen at a rate of 40-60 breaths/minute for one minute. When the infant is stable, reposition the infant such that the other side is dependant and administer the remaining aliquot using the same procedures. Do not suction airways for 1 hour after surfactant instillation unless signs of significant airway obstruction occur.

After completion of the dosing procedure, resume usual ventilator management and clinical care. In the clinical trials, ventilator management was modified to maintain a PaO_2 of about 55 mmHg, $PaCO_2$ of 35-45, and pH >7.3.

For endotracheal instillation using the secondary lumen of a dual lumen endotracheal tube

Slowly withdraw the entire contents of the vial of CUROSURF into a 3 or 5 mL plastic syringe through a large-gauge needle (e.g., at least 20 gauge). Do not attach 5 French end-hole catheter. Keep the infant in a neutral position (head and body in alignment without inclination). Administer CUROSURF through the proximal end of the secondary lumen of the endotracheal tube as a single dose, given over 1 minute, and without interrupting mechanical ventilation. After completion of this dosing procedure, ventilatory management may require transient increases in FiO_2, ventilatory rate, or PIP.

Repeat doses

Up to two repeat doses of 1.25 mL/kg birth weight each may be administered, using the same techniques described for the initial dose. Repeat doses should be administered, at approximately 12-hour intervals, in infants who remain intubated and in whom RDS is considered responsible for their persisting or deteriorating respiratory status. The maximum recommended total dose (sum of the initial and up to two repeat doses) is 5 mL/kg.

[See table above]

Directions for Use

CUROSURF should be inspected visually for discoloration prior to administration. The color of CUROSURF is white to creamy white. CUROSURF should be stored in a refrigerator at +2 to +8°C (36-46°F). Before use, the vial should be slowly warmed to room temperature and gently turned upside-down, in order to obtain a uniform suspension. DO NOT SHAKE.

Unopened, unused vials of CUROSURF that have warmed to room temperature can be returned to refrigerated storage within 24 hours for future use. Do not warm to room temperature and return to refrigerated storage more than once. Protect from light. Each single-use vial should be entered only once and the vial with any unused material should be discarded after the initial entry.

Dosing Precautions

Transient episodes of bradycardia, decreased oxygen saturation, reflux of the surfactant into the endotracheal tube, and airway obstruction have occurred during the dosing procedure of CUROSURF. These events require interrupting the administration of CUROSURF and taking the appropriate measures to alleviate the condition. After stabilization, dosing may resume with appropriate monitoring.

HOW SUPPLIED

CUROSURF® (poractant alfa) Intratracheal Suspension (NDC Numbers: 49502-180-01 [1.5 mL]; 49502-180-03 [3 mL]) is available in sterile, ready-to-use rubber-stoppered clear glass vials containing 1.5 mL [120 mg phospholipids (extract)] or 3 mL [240 mg phospholipids (extract)] of suspension. One vial per carton.

Store CUROSURF Intratracheal Suspension in a refrigerator at +2 to +8°C (36-46°F). Unopened vials of CUROSURF may be warmed to room temperature for up to 24 hours prior to use. CUROSURF should not be warmed to room temperature and returned to the refrigerator more than once. PROTECT FROM LIGHT. Do not shake. Vials are for single use only. After opening the vial discard the unused portion of the drug.

Rx only.

DEY

Manufactured for:
DEY, Napa, CA 94558
Manufactured by and licensed from:
chiesi
Chiesi Farmaceutici, S.p.A.
Parma, Italy 43100
05/2004 03-572-03A
82W03.04/01

Shown in Product Identification Guide, page 311

DUONEB® ℞

[*dew'ō-nĕb*]

(Ipratropium Bromide 0.5 mg/Albuterol Sulfate 3.0 mg*)
Inhalation Solution
***Equivalent to 2.5 mg albuterol base**

DESCRIPTION

The active components in DuoNeb® are albuterol sulfate and ipratropium bromide.

Albuterol sulfate, is a salt of racemic albuterol and a relatively selective β_2-adrenergic bronchodilator chemically described as α^1-[(tert-butylamino)methyl]-4-hydroxy-m-xylene-α, α'-diol sulfate (2:1) (salt). It has a molecular weight of 576.7 and the empirical formula is $(C_{13}H_{21}NO_3)_2 \bullet H_2SO_4$. It is a white crystalline powder, soluble in water and slightly soluble in ethanol. The World Health Organization recommended name for albuterol base is salbutamol.

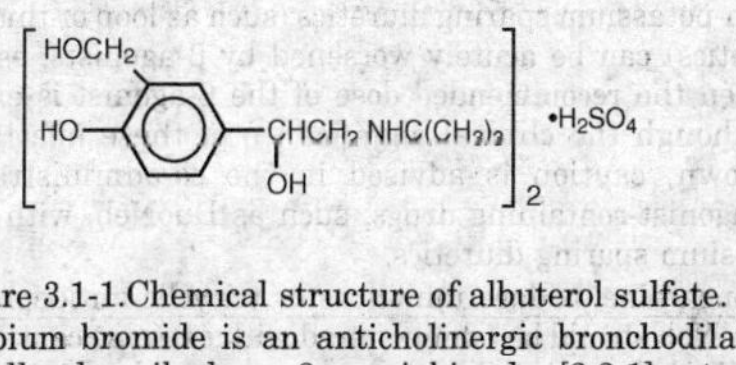

Figure 3.1-1.Chemical structure of albuterol sulfate.

Ipratropium bromide is an anticholinergic bronchodilator chemically described as 8-azoniabicyclo [3.2.1]-octane, 3-(3-hydroxy-1-oxo-2-phenylpropoxy)-8methyl-8-(1-methylethyl)-, bromide, monohydrate (endo, syn)-, (±)-; a synthetic quaternary ammonium compound, chemically related to atropine. It has a molecular weight of 430.4 and the empirical formula is $C_{20}H_{30}BrNO_3 \bullet H_2O$. It is a white crystalline substance, freely soluble in water and lower alcohols, and insoluble in lipophilic solvents such as ether, chloroform, and fluorocarbons.

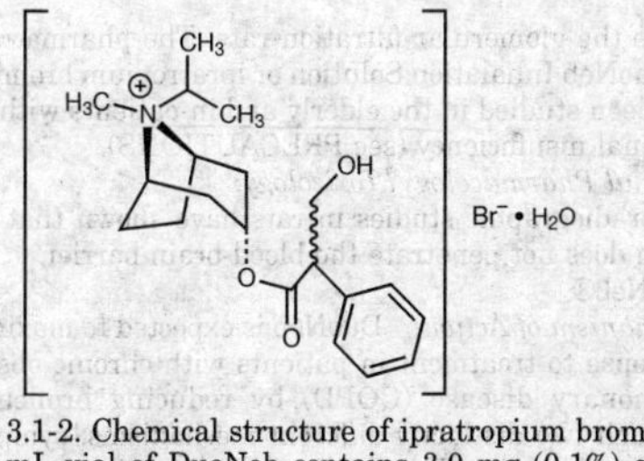

Figure 3.1-2. Chemical structure of ipratropium bromide.

Each 3 mL vial of DuoNeb contains 3.0 mg (0.1%) of albuterol sulfate (equivalent to 2.5 mg (0.083%) of albuterol base) and 0.5 mg (0.017%) of ipratropium bromide in an isotonic, sterile, aqueous solution containing sodium chloride, hydrochloric acid to adjust to pH 4, and edetate disodium, USP (a chelating agent).

DuoNeb is a clear, colorless solution. It does not require dilution prior to administration by nebulization. For DuoNeb Inhalation Solution, like all other nebulized treatments, the amount delivered to the lungs will depend on patient factors, the jet nebulizer utilized, and compressor performance. Using the Pari-LC-Plus™ nebulizer (with face mask or mouthpiece) connected to a PRONEB™ compressor system, under in vitro conditions, the mean delivered dose from the mouth piece (% nominal dose) was approximately 46% of albuterol and 42% of ipratropium bromide at a mean flow rate of 3.6 L/min. The mean nebulization time was 15 minutes or less. DuoNeb should be administered from jet nebulizers at adequate flow rates, via face masks or mouthpieces (see DOSAGE AND ADMINISTRATION).

CLINICAL PHARMACOLOGY

DuoNeb Inhalation Solution is a combination of the β_2-adrenergic bronchodilator, albuterol sulfate, and the cholinergic bronchodilator, ipratropium bromide.

Albuterol sulfate

Mechanism of Action. The prime action of β-adrenergic drugs is to stimulate adenyl cyclase, the enzyme that catalyzes the formation of cyclic-3',5'-adenosine monophosphate (cAMP) from adenosine triphosphate (ATP). The cAMP thus formed mediates the cellular responses. In vitro studies and in vivo pharmacologic studies have demonstrated that albuterol has a preferential effect on β_2-adrenergic receptors compared with isoproterenol. While it is recognized that β_2-adrenergic receptors are the predominant receptors in bronchial smooth muscle, recent data indicated that 10% to 50% of the β-receptors in the human heart may be β_2-receptors. The precise function of these receptors, however, is not yet established. Albuterol has been shown in most controlled clinical trials to have more effect on the respiratory tract, in the form of bronchial smooth muscle relaxation, than isoproterenol at comparable doses while producing fewer cardiovascular effects. Controlled clinical studies and other clinical experience have shown that inhaled albuterol, like other β-adrenergic agonist drugs, can produce a significant cardiovascular effect in some patients.

Pharmacokinetics: Albuterol sulfate is longer acting than isoproterenol in most patients by any route of administration, because it is not a substrate for the cellular uptake processes for catecholamine nor for the metabolism of catechol-O-methyl transferase. Instead the drug is conjugatively metabolized to albuterol 4'-O-sulfate.

Animal Pharmacology / Toxicology: Intravenous studies in rats with albuterol sulfate have demonstrated that albuterol crosses the blood-brain barrier and reaches brain concentrations amounting to approximately 5% of plasma concentrations. In structures outside of the blood-brain barrier (pineal and pituitary glands), albuterol concentrations were found to be 100 times those found in whole brain.

Studies in laboratory animals (minipigs, rodents, and dogs) have demonstrated the occurrence of cardiac arrythmias and sudden death (with histological evidence of myocardial necrosis) when beta-agonists and methyl-xanthines are administered concurrently. The clinical significance of these findings is unknown.

Ipratropium bromide

Mechanism of Action: Ipratropium bromide is an anticholinergic (parasympatholytic) agent, which blocks the muscarinic receptors of acetylcholine, and, based on animal studies, appears to inhibit vagally mediated reflexes by antagonizing the action of acetylcholine, the transmitter agent released from the vagus nerve. Anticholinergics prevent the increases in intracellular concentration of cyclic guanosine monophosphate (cGMP), resulting from the interaction of acetylcholine with the muscarinic receptors of bronchial smooth muscle.

Pharmacokinetics: The bronchodilation following inhalation of ipratropium is primarily a local, site-specific effect, not a systemic one. Much of an inhaled dose is swallowed as shown by fecal excretion studies. Following nebulization of a 1-mg dose to healthy volunteers, a mean of 4% of the dose was excreted unchanged in the urine.

Ipratropium bromide is minimally (0% to 9% in vitro) bound to plasma albumin and α_1-acid glycoproteins. It is partially metabolized to inactive ester hydrolysis products. Following intravenous administration, approximately one-half is excreted unchanged in the urine. The half-life of elimination is about 1.6 hours after intravenous administration. Ipratropium bromide that reaches the systemic circulation is reportedly removed by the kidneys rapidly at a rate that ex-

Continued on next page

Duoneb—Cont.

ceeds the glomerular filtration rate. The pharmacokinetics of DuoNeb Inhalation Solution or ipratropium bromide have not been studied in the elderly and in patients with hepatic or renal insufficiency (see PRECAUTIONS).

Animal Pharmacology / Toxicology:

Autoradiographic studies in rats have shown that ipratropium does not penetrate the blood-brain barrier.

DuoNeb®

Mechanism of Action: DuoNeb is expected to maximize the response to treatment in patients with chronic obstructive pulmonary disease (COPD) by reducing bronchospasm through two distinctly different mechanisms: sympathomimetic (albuterol sulfate) and anticholinergic/parasympatholytic (ipratropium bromide). Simultaneous administration of both an anticholinergic and a β_2-sympathomimetic is designed to produce greater bronchodilation effects than when either drug is utilized alone at its recommended dosage.

Animal Pharmacology / Toxicology:

In 30-day studies in Sprague-Dawley rats and Beagle dogs, subcutaneous doses of up to 205.5 mcg/kg of ipratropium administered with up to 1000 mcg/kg albuterol in rats and 3.16 mcg/kg ipratropium and 15 mcg/kg albuterol in dogs (less than the maximum recommended daily inhalation dose for adults on a mg/m^2 basis) did not cause death or potentiation of the cardiotoxicity induced by albuterol administered alone.

Pharmacokinetics:

In a double blind, double period, crossover study, 15 male and female subjects were administered single doses of DuoNeb or albuterol sulfate inhalation solution at two times the recommended single doses as two inhalations separated by 15 minutes. The total nebulized dose of albuterol sulfate from both treatments was 6.0 mg and the total dose of ipratropium bromide from DuoNeb was 1.0 mg. Peak albuterol plasma concentrations occurred at 0.8 hours after dosing for both treatments. The mean peak albuterol concentration following administration of albuterol sulfate alone was 4.86 (± 2.65) mg/mL and it was 4.65 (± 2.92) mg/mL for DuoNeb. Mean AUC values for the two treatments were 26.6 (± 15.2) ng•hr/mL (albuterol sulfate alone) versus 24.2 (± 14.5) ng•hr/mL (DuoNeb). The mean $t_{1/2}$ values were 7.2 (± 1.3) hours (albuterol sulfate alone) and 6.7 (± 1.7) hours (DuoNeb). A mean of 8.4 (± 8.9)% of the albuterol dose was excreted unchanged in urine following administration of two vials of DuoNeb which is similar to 8.8 (± 7.3)% that was obtained from albuterol sulfate inhalation solution. There were no statistically significant differences in the pharmacokinetics of albuterol between the two treatments. For ipratropium, a mean of 3.9 (± 5.1)% of the ipratropium bromide dose was excreted unchanged in urine following two vials of DuoNeb Inhalation Solution, which is comparable with previously reported data.

Clinical Trials: In a 12 week, randomized, double-blind, positive-control, crossover study of albuterol sulfate, ipratropium bromide, and DuoNeb, 863 COPD patients were evaluated for bronchodilator efficacy comparing DuoNeb with albuterol sulfate and ipratropium bromide alone.

DuoNeb demonstrated significantly better changes in FEV$_1$, as measured from baseline to peak response, when compared with either albuterol sulfate or ipratropium bromide. DuoNeb was also shown to have the rapid onset associated with albuterol sulfate, with a mean time to peak FEV$_1$ of 1.5 hours, and the extended duration associated with ipratropium bromide with a duration of 15% response in FEV$_1$ of 4.3 hours.

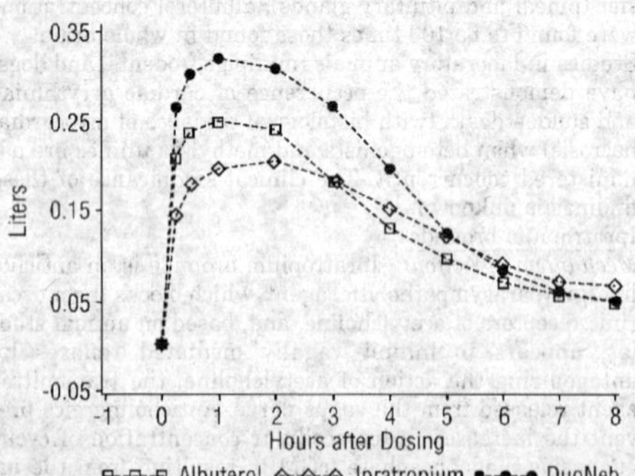

Figure 3.1-3. Mean Change in FEV$_1$ — Measured on Day 14

This study demonstrated that each component of DuoNeb contributed to the improvement in pulmonary function, especially during the first 4 to 5 hours after dosing, and that DuoNeb was significantly more effective than albuterol sulfate or ipratropium bromide alone.

INDICATIONS AND USAGE

DuoNeb is indicated for the treatment of bronchospasm associated with COPD in patients requiring more than one bronchodilator.

CONTRAINDICATIONS

DuoNeb is contraindicated in patients with a history of hypersensitivity to any of its components, or to atropine and its derivatives.

WARNINGS

Paradoxical Bronchospasm: In the clinical study of DuoNeb, paradoxical bronchospasm was not observed. However, paradoxical bronchospasm has been observed with both inhaled ipratropium bromide and albuterol products and can be life-threatening. If this occurs, DuoNeb should be discontinued immediately and alternative therapy instituted.

Do Not Exceed Recommended Dose: Fatalities have been reported in association with excessive use of inhaled products containing sympathomimetic amines and with the home use of nebulizers.

Cardiovascular Effect: DuoNeb, like other beta adrenergic agonists, can produce a clinically significant cardiovascular effect in some patients as measured by pulse rate, blood pressure, and/or symptoms. Although such effects are uncommon for DuoNeb at recommended doses, if they occur, the drug may need to be discontinued. In addition, beta agonists have been reported to produce ECG changes, such as flattening of the T-wave, prolongation of the QTc interval, and ST segment depression. The clinical significance of these findings is unknown. Therefore, DuoNeb, like other sympathomimetic amines, should be used with caution in patients with cardiovascular disorders, especially coronary insufficiency, cardiac arrhythmias, and hypertension.

Immediate Hypersensitivity Reactions: Immediate hypersensitivity reactions to albuterol and/or ipratropium bromide may occur after the administration of DuoNeb as demonstrated by rare cases of urticaria, angioedema, rash, pruritus, oropharyngeal edema, bronchospasm, and anaphylaxis.

PRECAUTIONS

General

1. Effects Seen with Sympathomimetic Drugs: As with all products containing sympathomimetic amines, DuoNeb should be used with caution in patients with cardiovascular disorders, especially coronary insufficiency, cardiac arrhythmias, and hypertension; in patients with convulsive disorders, hyperthyroidism, or diabetes mellitus; and in patients who are unusually responsive to sympathomimetic amines. Large doses of intravenous albuterol have been reported to aggravate pre-existing diabetes mellitus and ketoacidosis. Additionally, β-agonists may cause a decrease in serum potassium in some patients, possibly through intracellular shunting. The decrease is usually transient, not requiring supplementation.

2. Effects Seen with Anticholinergic Drugs: Due to the presence of ipratropium bromide in DuoNeb, it should be used with caution in patients with narrow-angle glaucoma, prostatic hypertrophy, or bladder-neck obstruction.

3. Use in Hepatic or Renal Diseases: DuoNeb has not been studied in patients with hepatic or renal insufficiency. It should be used with caution in these patient populations.

Information for Patients

The action of DuoNeb should last up to 5 hours. DuoNeb should not be used more frequently than recommended. Patients should be instructed not to increase the dose or frequency of DuoNeb without consulting their healthcare provider. If symptoms worsen, patients should be instructed to seek medical consultation.

Patients must avoid exposing their eyes to this product as temporary papillary dilation, blurred vision, eye pain, or precipitation or worsening of narrow-angle glaucoma may occur, and therefore proper nebulizer technique should be assured, particularly if a mask is used.

If a patient becomes pregnant or begins nursing while on DuoNeb, they should contact their healthcare provider about use of DuoNeb.

See the illustrated Patient's Instruction for Use in the product package insert.

Drug Interactions

Anticholinergic agents: Although ipratropium bromide is minimally absorbed into the systemic circulation, there is some potential for an additive interaction with concomitantly used anticholinergic medications. Caution is, therefore, advised in the co-administration of DuoNeb with other drugs having anticholinergic properties.

β-adrenergic agents: Caution is advised in the co-administration of DuoNeb and other sympathomimetic agents due to the increased risk of adverse cardiovascular effects.

β-receptor blocking agents: These agents and albuterol sulfate inhibit the effect of each other. β-receptor blocking agents should be used with caution in patients with hyperreactive airways, and if used, relatively selective β_1 selective agents are recommended.

Diuretics: The electrocardiogram (ECG) changes and/or hypokalemia that may result from the administration of non-potassium sparing diuretics (such as loop or thiazide diuretics) can be acutely worsened by β-agonists, especially when the recommended dose of the β-agonist is exceeded. Although the clinical significance of these effects is not known, caution is advised in the co-administration of β-agonist-containing drugs, such as DuoNeb, with non-potassium sparing diuretics.

Monoamine oxidase inhibitors or tricyclic antidepressants: DuoNeb should be administered with extreme caution to patients being treated with monoamine oxidase inhibitors or tricyclic antidepressants, or within 2 weeks of discontinuation of such agents because the action of albuterol sulfate on the cardiovascular system may be potentiated.

Carcinogenesis, Mutagenesis, Impairment of Fertility

Albuterol Sulfate: In a 2-year study in Sprague-Dawley rats, albuterol sulfate caused a significant dose-related increase in the incidence of benign leiomyomas of the mesovarium at and above dietary doses of 2 mg/kg (approximately equal to the maximum recommended daily inhalation dose for adults on a mg/m^2 basis). In another study, this effect was blocked by the coadministration of propranolol, a non-selective beta-adrenergic antagonist.

In an 18-month study in CD-1 mice, albuterol sulfate showed no evidence of tumorigenicity at dietary doses up to 500 mg/kg (approximately 140 times the maximum recommended daily inhalation dose for adults on a mg/m^2 basis). In a 22-month study in Golden hamsters, albuterol sulfate showed no evidence of tumorigenicity at dietary doses up to 50 mg/kg (approximately 20 times the maximum recommended daily inhalation dose for adults on a mg/m^2 basis). Albuterol sulfate was not mutagenic in the Ames test or a mutation test in yeast. Albuterol sulfate was not clastogenic in a human peripheral lymphocyte assay or in an AH1 strain mouse micronucleous assay.

Reproduction studies in rats demonstrated no evidence of impaired fertility at oral doses of albuterol sulfate up to 50 mg/kg (approximately 25 times the maximum recommended daily inhalation dose for adults on a mg/m^2 basis).

Ipratropium bromide: In 2-year studies in Sprague-Dawley rats and CD-1 mice, ipratropium bromide showed no evidence of tumorigenicity at oral doses up to 6 mg/kg (approximately 15 times and 8 times the maximum recommended daily inhalation dose for adults in rats and mice respectively, on a mg/m^2 basis).

Ipratropium bromide was not mutagenic in the Ames test and mouse dominant lethal test. Ipratropium bromide was not clastogenic in a mouse micronucleous assay.

A reproduction study in rats demonstrated decreased conception and increased resorptions when ipratropium bromide was administered orally at a dose of 90 mg/kg (approximately 240 times the maximum recommended daily inhalation dose for adults on a mg/m^2 basis). These effects were not seen with a dose of 50 mg/kg (approximately 140 times the maximum recommended daily inhalation dose for adults on a mg/m^2 basis).

Pregnancy

TERATOGENIC EFFECTS: Pregnancy Category C

Albuterol sulfate: *Pregnancy Category C.* Albuterol sulfate has been shown to be teratogenic in mice. A study in CD-1 mice given albuterol sulfate subcutaneously showed cleft palate formation in 5 of 111 (4.5%) fetuses at 0.25 mg/kg (less than the maximum recommended daily inhalation dose for adults on a mg/m^2 basis) and in 10 of 108 (9.3%) fetuses at 2.5 mg/kg (approximately equal to the maximum recommended daily inhalation dose for adults on a mg/m^2 basis). The drug did not induce cleft palate formation when administered subcutaneously at a dose of 0.025 mg/kg (less than the maximum recommended daily inhalation dose for adults on a mg/m^2 basis). Cleft palate formation also occurred in 22 of 72 (30.5%) fetuses from females treated subcutaneously with 2.5 mg/kg isoproterenol (positive control).

A reproduction study in Stride rabbits revealed cranioschisis in 7 of 19 (37%) fetuses when albuterol was administered orally at a dose of 50 mg/kg (approximately 55 times the maximum recommended daily inhalation dose for adults on a mg/m^2 basis).

A study in which pregnant rats were dosed with radiolabeled albuterol sulfate demonstrated that drug-related material is transferred from the maternal circulation to the fetus.

During worldwide marketing experience, various congenital anomalies, including cleft palate and limb defects, have been reported in the offspring of patients being treated with albuterol. Some of the mothers were taking multiple medications during their pregnancies. Because no consistent pattern of defects can be discerned, a relationship between albuterol use and congenital anomalies has not been established.

Ipratropium bromide: *Pregnancy Category B.* Reproduction studies in CD-1 mice, Sprague-Dawley rats and New Zealand rabbits demonstrated no evidence of teratogenicity at oral doses up to 10, 100, and 125 mg/kg, respectively (approximately 15, 270, and 680 times the maximum recommended daily inhalation dose for adults on a mg/m^2 basis). Reproduction studies in rats and rabbits demonstrated no evidence of teratogenicity at inhalation doses up to 1.5 and 1.8 mg/kg, respectively (approximately 4 and 10 times the maximum recommended daily inhalation dose for adults on a mg/m^2 basis). There are no adequate and well-controlled studies of the use of DuoNeb, albuterol sulfate, or ipratropium bromide in pregnant women. DuoNeb should be used during pregnancy only if the potential benefit justifies the potential risk to the fetus.

Labor and Delivery

Oral albuterol sulfate has been shown to delay preterm labor in some reports. Because of the potential of albuterol to interfere with uterine contractility, use of DuoNeb during labor should be restricted to those patients in whom the benefits clearly outweigh the risks.

Nursing Mothers

It is not known whether the components of DuoNeb are excreted in human milk. Although lipid-insoluble quaternary bases pass into breast milk, it is unlikely that ipratropium bromide would reach the infant to an important extent, especially when taken as a nebulized solution. Because of the potential for tumorigenicity shown for albuterol sulfate in some animals, a decision should be made whether to discontinue nursing or discontinue DuoNeb, taking into account the importance of the drug to the mother.

ADVERSE EVENTS OCCURRING IN ≥ 1% OF ≥ 1 TREATMENT GROUP(S) AND WHERE THE COMBINATION TREATMENT SHOWED THE HIGHEST PERCENTAGE

Body System COSTART Term	Albuterol n (%)	Ipratropium n (%)	DuoNeb n (%)
NUMBER OF PATIENTS	761	754	765
N (%) Patients with AE	327 (43.0)	329 (43.6)	367 (48.0)
BODY AS A WHOLE			
Pain	8 (1.1)	4 (0.5)	10 (1.3)
Pain chest	11 (1.4)	14 (1.9)	20 (2.6)
DIGESTIVE			
Diarrhea	5 (0.7)	9 (1.2)	14 (1.8)
Dyspepsia	7 (0.9)	8 (1.1)	10 (1.3)
Nausea	7 (0.9)	6 (0.8)	11 (1.4)
MUSCULO-SKELETAL			
Cramps leg	8 (1.1)	6 (0.8)	11 (1.4)
RESPIRATORY			
Bronchitis	11 (1.4)	13 (1.7)	13 (1.7)
Lung Disease	36 (4.7)	34 (4.5)	49 (6.4)
Pharyngitis	27 (3.5)	27 (3.6)	34 (4.4)
Pneumonia	7 (0.9)	8 (1.1)	10 (1.3)
UROGENITAL			
Infection urinary tract	3 (0.4)	9 (1.2)	12 (1.6)

Pediatric Use
The safety and effectiveness of DuoNeb in patients below 18 years of age have not been established.

Geriatric Use
Of the total number of subjects in clinical studies of DuoNeb, 62 percent were 65 and over, while 19 percent were 75 and over. No overall differences in safety or effectiveness were observed between these subjects and younger subjects, and other reported clinical experience has not identified differences in responses between the elderly and younger patients, but greater sensitivity of some older individuals cannot be ruled out.

ADVERSE REACTIONS

Adverse reaction information concerning DuoNeb was derived from the 12-week controlled clinical trial.
[See table above]
Additional adverse reactions reported in more than 1% of patients treated with DuoNeb included constipation and voice alterations.
In the clinical trial, there was a 0.3% incidence of possible allergic-type reactions, including skin rash, pruritus, and urticaria.
Additional information derived from the published literature on the use of albuterol sulfate and ipratropium bromide singly or in combination includes precipitation or worsening of narrow-angle glaucoma, acute eye pain, blurred vision, paradoxical bronchospasm, wheezing, exacerbation of COPD symptoms, drowsiness, aching, flushing, upper respiratory tract infection, palpitations, taste perversion, elevated heart rate, sinusitis, back pain and sore throat.

OVERDOSAGE

The effects of overdosage with DuoNeb are expected to be related primarily to albuterol sulfate, since ipratropium bromide is not well-absorbed systemically after oral or aerosol administration. The expected symptoms with overdosage are those of excessive beta-adrenergic stimulation and/or occurrence or exaggeration of symptoms such as seizures, angina, hypertension or hypotension, tachycardia with rates up to 200 beats per minute, arrhythmia, nervousness, headache, tremor, dry mouth, palpitation, nausea, dizziness, fatigue, malaise, insomnia, and exaggeration of pharmacological effects listed in ADVERSE REACTIONS. Hypokalemia may also occur. As with all sympathomimetic aerosol medications, cardiac arrest and even death may be associated with abuse of DuoNeb. Treatment consists of discontinuation of DuoNeb together with appropriate symptomatic therapy. The judicious use of a cardioselective beta-receptor blocker may be considered, bearing in mind that such medication can produce bronchospasm. There is insufficient evidence to determine if dialysis is beneficial for overdosage of DuoNeb.
The oral median lethal dose of albuterol sulfate in mice is greater than 2000 mg/kg (approximately 540 times the maximum recommended daily inhalation dose of DuoNeb on a mg/m^2 basis). The subcutaneous median lethal dose of albuterol sulfate in mature rats and small young rats is approximately 450 and 2000 mg/kg respectively (approximately 240 and 1100 times the maximum recommended daily inhalation dose of DuoNeb on a mg/m^2 basis, respectively). The inhalation median lethal dose has not been determined in animals. The oral median lethal dose of ipratropium bromide in mice, rats and dogs is greater than 1000 mg/kg, approximately 1700 mg/kg and approximately 400 mg/kg, respectively (approximately 1400, 4600, and 3600 times the maximum recommended daily inhalation dose in adults on a mg/m^2 basis, respectively).

DOSAGE AND ADMINISTRATION

The recommended dose of DuoNeb is one 3 mL vial administered 4 times per day via nebulization with up to 2 additional 3 mL doses allowed per day, if needed. Safety and efficacy of additional doses or increased frequency of administration of DuoNeb beyond these guidelines has not been studied and the safety and efficacy of extra doses of albuterol sulfate or ipratropium bromide in addition to the recommended doses of DuoNeb have not been studied.
The use of DuoNeb can be continued as medically indicated to control recurring bouts of bronchospasm. If a previously effective regimen fails to provide the usual relief, medical advice should be sought immediately, as this is often a sign of worsening COPD, which would require reassessment of therapy.
A Pari-LC-Plus™ nebulizer (with face mask or mouthpiece) connected to a PRONEB™ compressor was used to deliver DuoNeb to each patient in one U.S. clinical study. The safety and efficacy of DuoNeb delivered by other nebulizers and compressors have not been established.
DuoNeb should be administered via jet nebulizer connected to an air compressor with an adequate air flow, equipped with a mouthpiece or suitable face mask.

HOW SUPPLIED

DuoNeb is supplied as a 3-mL sterile solution for nebulization in sterile low-density polyethylene unit-dose vials. Store in pouch untill time of use. Supplied in cartons as listed below.

NDC 49502-672-30	30 vials per carton/5 vials per foil pouch
NDC 49502-672-60	60 vials per carton/5 vials per foil pouch
NDC 49502-672-31	30 vials per carton/1 vial per foil pouch

Store between 2°C and 25°C (36°F and 77°F). Protect from light.

DEY
DEY, Napa, CA 94558

03-485-22 May 2003

DuoNeb®
(Ipratropium Bromide 0.5 mg/Albuterol Sulfate 3.0 mg*) Inhalation Solution
***Equivalent to 2.5 mg albuterol base**

Patient's Instructions for Use

Read this patient information completely every time your prescription is filled as information may have changed. Keep these instructions with your medication as you may want to read them again.
DuoNeb should only be used under the direction of a physician. Your physician and pharmacist have more information about DuoNeb and the condition for which it has been prescribed. Contact them if you have additional questions.

Storing your Medicine
Store DuoNeb between 2°C and 25°C (36°F and 77°F). Vials should be protected from light before use, therefore, keep unused vials in the foil pouch or carton. Do not use after the expiration (EXP) date printed on the carton.

Dose
DuoNeb is supplied as a single-dose, ready-to-use vial containing 3 mL of solution. No mixing or dilution is needed. Use one new vial for each nebulizer treatment.
FOLLOW THESE DIRECTIONS FOR USE OF YOUR NEBULIZER/COMPRESSOR OR THE DIRECTIONS GIVEN BY YOUR HEALTHCARE PROVIDER. A TYPICAL EXAMPLE IS SHOWN BELOW.

Instructions for Use
1. Remove one vial from the foil pouch. Place remaining vials back into pouch for storage.
2. Twist the cap completely off the vial and squeeze the contents into the nebulizer reservoir (Figure 1).

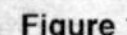
Figure 1

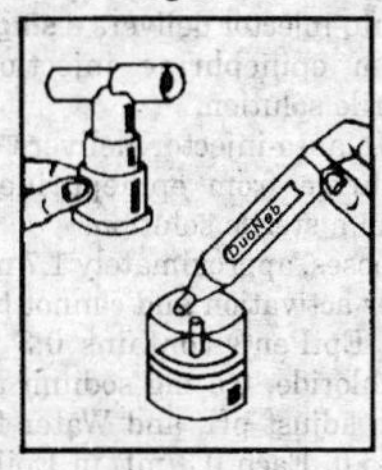

3. Connect the nebulizer to the mouthpiece or face mask (Figure 2).

Figure 2

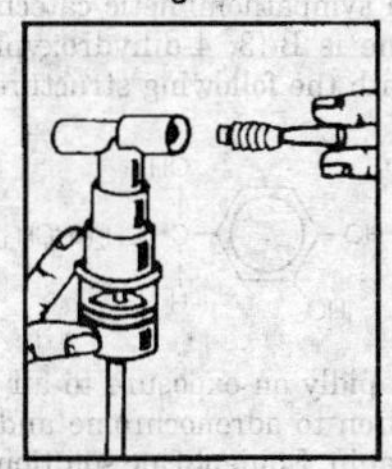

4. Connect the nebulizer to the compressor.
5. Sit in a comfortable, upright position; place the mouthpiece in your mouth (Figure 3) or put on the face mask (Figure 4); and turn on the compressor.

Figure 3

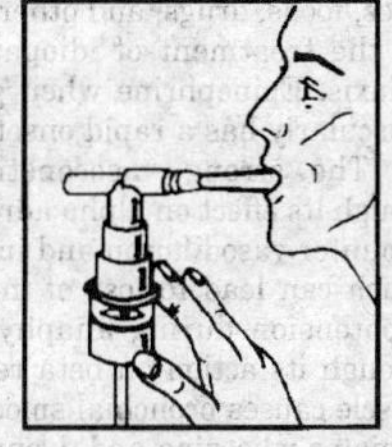

Figure 4

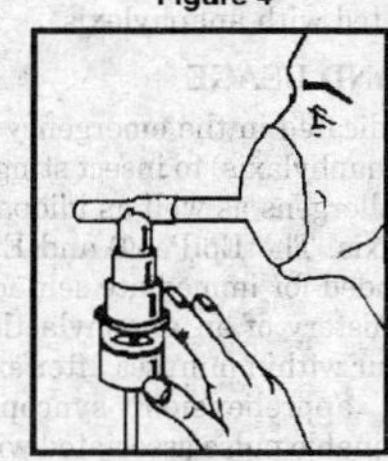

6. Breathe as calmly, deeply and evenly as possible through your mouth until no more mist is formed in the nebulizer chamber (about 5-15 minutes). At this point, the treatment is finished.
7. Clean the nebulizer (see manufacturer's instructions).

DEY
DEY, Napa, CA 94558

03-485-22A May 2003
Shown in Product Identification Guide, page 311

EPIPEN® 0.3 mg
EPINEPHRINE AUTO-INJECTOR ℞
Auto-Injector for Intramuscular Injection of Epinephrine For the Emergency Treatment of Allergic Reactions (Anaphylaxis)
Delivers a single 0.3 mg intramuscular dose of epinephrine from epinephrine injection, USP, 1:1000 (0.3 mL).

EPIPEN® JR 0.15 mg EPINEPHRINE AUTO-INJECTOR ℞
Auto-Injector for Intramuscular Injection of Epinephrine For the Emergency Treatment of Allergic Reactions (Anaphylaxis)
Delivers a single 0.15 mg intramuscular dose of epinephrine from epinephrine injection, USP, 1:2000 (0.3 mL).

Continued on next page

EpiPen/EpiPen Jr—Cont.

IMPORTANT INFORMATION

- **DO NOT REMOVE ACTIVATION CAP UNTIL READY FOR USE.**
- **A SINGLE DOSE OF 0.3 ML OF SOLUTION IS DISPENSED. THE MAJORITY OF THE DRUG PRODUCT, 1.7 ML, REMAINS IN THE AUTO-INJECTOR AFTER ACTIVATION AND CANNOT BE USED.**
- **THE UNIT CONTAINS NO LATEX.**

DESCRIPTION

The EpiPen® and EpiPen® Jr auto-injectors contain 2 mL epinephrine injection for emergency intramuscular use.
Each EpiPen® auto-injector delivers **a single dose** of 0.3 mg epinephrine from epinephrine injection, USP, 1:1000 (0.3 mL) in a sterile solution.
Each EpiPen® Jr auto-injector delivers **a single dose** of 0.15 mg epinephrine from epinephrine injection, USP, 1:2000 (0.3 mL) in a sterile solution.
For stability purposes, approximately 1.7 mL remains in the auto-injector after activation and cannot be used.
Each 0.3 mL in EpiPen® contains 0.3 mg epinephrine, 1.8 mg sodium chloride, 0.5 mg sodium metabisulfite, hydrochloric acid to adjust pH, and Water for Injection. The pH range is 2.2–5.0. Each 0.3 mL in EpiPen® Jr contains 0.15 mg epinephrine, 1.8 mg sodium chloride, 0.5 mg sodium metabisulfite, hydrochloric acid to adjust pH, and Water for Injection. The pH range is 2.2–5.0.
Epinephrine is a sympathomimetic catecholamine. Chemically, epinephrine is B-(3, 4-dihydroxyphenyl)-a-methylaminoethanol, with the following structure:

It deteriorates rapidly on exposure to air or light, turning pink from oxidation to adrenochrome and brown from the formation of melanin. Epinephrine solutions which show evidence of discoloration should be replaced.

CLINICAL PHARMACOLOGY

Epinephrine is a sympathomimetic drug, acting on both alpha and beta receptors. It is the drug of choice for the emergency treatment of severe allergic reactions (Type I) to insect stings or bites, foods, drugs, and other allergens. It can also be used in the treatment of idiopathic or exercise-induced anaphylaxis. Epinephrine when given subcutaneously or intramuscularly has a rapid onset and short duration of action. The strong vasoconstrictor action of epinephrine through its effect on alpha adrenergic receptors acts quickly to counter vasodilation and increased vascular permeability which can lead to loss of intravascular fluid volume and hypotension during anaphylactic reactions. Epinephrine through its action on beta receptors on bronchial smooth muscle causes bronchial smooth muscle relaxation which alleviates wheezing and dyspnea. Epinephrine also alleviates pruritis, urticaria, and angioedema and may be effective in relieving gastrointestinal and genitourinary symptoms associated with anaphylaxis.

INDICATIONS AND USAGE

Epinephrine is indicated in the emergency treatment of allergic reactions (anaphylaxis) to insect stings or bites, foods, drugs and other allergens as well as idiopathic or exercise-induced anaphylaxis. The EpiPen® and EpiPen® Jr auto-injectors are intended for immediate self-administration by a person with a history of an anaphylactic reaction. Such reactions may occur within minutes after exposure and consist of flushing, apprehension, syncope, tachycardia, thready or unobtainable pulse associated with a fall in blood pressure, convulsions, vomiting, diarrhea and abdominal cramps, involuntary voiding, wheezing, dyspnea due to laryngeal spasm, pruritis, rashes, uticaria or angioedema. The EpiPen® and EpiPen® Jr are designed as emergency supportive therapy only and are not a replacement or substitute for immediate medical or hospital care.

CONTRAINDICATIONS

There are no absolute contraindications to the use of epinephrine in a life-threatening situation.

WARNINGS

Epinephrine is light sensitive and should be stored in the tube provided. Store at room temperature (15°–30°C/59°–86°F). Do not refrigerate. Before using, check to make sure the solution in the auto-injector is not discolored. Replace the auto-injector if the solution is discolored or contains a precipitate. Avoid possible inadvertent intravascular administration. EpiPen® and EpiPen® Jr should **only** be injected into the anterolateral aspect of the thigh. DO NOT INJECT INTO BUTTOCK.
Large doses or accidental intravenous injection of epinephrine may result in cerebral hemorrhage due to sharp rise in blood pressure. DO NOT INJECT INTRAVENOUSLY. Rapidly acting vasodilators can counteract the marked pressor effects of epinephrine.
Epinephrine is the preferred treatment for serious allergic or other emergency situations even though this product contains sodium metabisulfite, a sulfite that may in other products cause allergic-type reactions including anaphylactic symptoms or life-threatening or less severe asthmatic episodes in certain susceptible persons. The alternatives to using epinephrine in a life-threatening situation may not be satisfactory. The presence of a sulfite in this product should not deter administration of the drug for treatment of serious allergic or other emergency situations.
Accidental injection into the hands or feet may result in loss of blood flow to the affected area and should be avoided. If there is an accidental injection into these areas, advise the patient to go immediately to the nearest emergency room for treatment. EpiPen® and EpiPen® Jr. should **only** be injected into the anterolateral aspect of the thigh.

PRECAUTIONS

Epinephrine is essential for the treatment of anaphylaxis. Patients with a history of severe allergic reactions (anaphylaxis) to insect stings or bites, foods, drugs, and other allergens as well as idiopathic and exercise-induced anaphylaxis should be carefully instructed about the circumstances under which this life-saving medication should be used. It must be clearly determined that the patient is at risk of future anaphylaxis, since the following risks may be associated with epinephrine administration (see Dosage and Administration).
Epinephrine is ordinarily administered with extreme caution in patients who have heart disease. Use of epinephrine with drugs that may sensitize the heart to arrhythmias, e.g., digitalis, mercurial diuretics, or quinidine, ordinarily is not recommended. Anginal pain may be induced by epinephrine in patients with coronary insufficiency.
The effects of epinephrine may be potentiated by tricyclic antidepressants and monoamine oxidase inhibitors.
Some patients may be at greater risk of developing adverse reactions after epinephrine administration. These include: hyperthyroid individuals, individuals with cardiovascular disease, hypertension, or diabetes, elderly individuals, pregnant women, pediatric patients under 30 kg (66 lbs.) body weight using EpiPen®, and pediatric patients under 15 kg (33 lbs.) body weight using EpiPen® Jr.
Despite these concerns, epinephrine is essential for the treatment of anaphylaxis. Therefore, patients with these conditions, and/or any other person who might be in a position to administer EpiPen® or EpiPen® Jr to a patient experiencing anaphylaxis should be carefully instructed in regard to the circumstances under which this life-saving medication should be used.

CARCINOGENESIS, MUTAGENESIS, IMPAIRMENT OF FERTILITY

Studies of epinephrine in animals to evaluate the carcinogenic and mutagenic potential or the effect on fertility have not been conducted. This should not prevent the use of this life-saving medication under the conditions noted under INDICATIONS AND USAGE and as indicated under PRECAUTIONS above.

USAGE IN PREGNANCY

Pregnancy Category C: Epinephrine has been shown to be teratogenic in rats when given in doses about 25 times the human dose. There are no adequate and well-controlled studies in pregnant women. Epinephrine should be used during pregnancy only if the potential benefit justifies the potential risk to the fetus.

PEDIATRIC USE

Epinephrine may be given safely to pediatric patients at a dosage appropriate to body weight (see Dosage and Administration).

ADVERSE REACTIONS

Side effects of epinephrine may include palpitations, tachycardia, sweating, nausea and vomiting, respiratory difficulty, pallor, dizziness, weakness, tremor, headache, apprehension, nervousness and anxiety.
Cardiac arrhythmias may follow administration of epinephrine.

OVERDOSAGE

Overdosage or inadvertent intravascular injection of epinephrine may cause cerebral hemorrhage resulting from a sharp rise in blood pressure. Fatalities may also result from pulmonary edema because of peripheral vascular constriction together with cardiac stimulation.

DOSAGE AND ADMINISTRATION

A physician who prescribes EpiPen® or EpiPen® Jr should take appropriate steps to insure that the patient (or parent) understands the indications and use of this device thoroughly. The physician should review with the patient or any other person who might be in a position to administer EpiPen® or EpiPen® Jr to a patient experiencing anaphylaxis, in detail, the patient instructions and operation of the EpiPen® or EpiPen® Jr auto-injector. Inject the delivered dose of the EpiPen® auto-injector (0.3 mL epinephrine injection, USP, 1:1000) or the EpiPen® Jr auto injector (0.3mL epinephrine injection, USP, 1:2000) intramuscularly into the anterolateral aspect of the thigh, through clothing if necessary. See detailed Directions for Use on the accompanying Patient Instructions.
Usual epinephrine adult dose for allergic emergencies is 0.3 mg. For pediatric use, the appropriate dosage may be 0.15 or 0.30 mg depending upon the body weight of the patient. A dosage of 0.01 mg/kg body weight is recommended. EpiPen® Jr, which provides a dosage of 0.15 mg, may be more appropriate for patients weighing less than 30 kg. However, the prescribing physician has the option of prescribing more or less than these amounts, based on careful assessment of each individual patient and recognizing the life-threatening nature of the reactions for which this drug is being prescribed. The physician should consider using other forms of injectable epinephrine if doses lower than 0.15 mg are felt to be necessary.
Each EpiPen® or EpiPen® Jr contains a single dose of epinephrine. With severe persistent anaphylaxis, repeat injections with an additional EpiPen® may be necessary.
Parenteral drug products should be periodically inspected visually by the patient for particulate matter or discoloration and should be replaced if these are present.

HOW SUPPLIED

EpiPen® auto-injectors (epinephrine injection, USP, 1:1000, 0.3 mL) are available in individual cartons, NDC 49502-500-01, and as EpiPen 2-Pak®, a pack that contains two EpiPen® auto-injectors (epinephrine injections, USP, 1:1000, 0.3 mL) and one EpiPen® trainer device, NDC 49502-500-02.
EpiPen® Jr auto-injectors (epinephrine injection, USP, 1:2000, 0.3 mL) are available in individual cartons, NDC 49502-501-01, and as EpiPen Jr 2-Pak®, a pack that contains two EpiPen® Jr auto-injectors (epinephrine injections, USP, 1:2000, 0.3 mL) and one EpiPen® trainer device, NDC 49502-501-02.
Store in a dark place at room temperature (15°–30°C/59°–86°F). Do not refrigerate. Contains no latex.
Rx only.

MANUFACTURED FOR DEY, NAPA, CALIFORNIA, 94558, U.S.A

by Meridian Medical Technologies, Inc., Columbia, MD 21046, U.S.A.

12/02 03-500-02A

Shown in Product Identification Guide, page 313

Duramed Pharmaceuticals, Inc. Subsidiary of Barr Pharmaceuticals, Inc.

2 QUAKER RD.
POMONA, NY 10970

Direct Inquiries to:
877-405-0369

AYGESTIN® ℞

[*ā'jĕs-tĭn*]
(norethindrone acetate tablets, USP)
℞ only

DESCRIPTION

Aygestin (norethindrone acetate tablets, USP) — 5 mg oral tablets. Aygestin, (17-hydroxy-19-nor-17α-pregn-4-en-20-yn-3-one acetate), a synthetic, orally active progestin, is the acetic acid ester of norethindrone. It is a white, or creamy white, crystalline powder.

Aygestin Tablets contain the following inactive ingredients: lactose, magnesium stearate, and microcrystalline cellulose.

CLINICAL PHARMACOLOGY

Norethindrone acetate induces secretory changes in an estrogen-primed endometrium. It acts to inhibit the secretion of pituitary gonadotropins which, in turn, prevent follicular maturation and ovulation. On a weight basis, it is twice as potent as norethindrone.

INDICATIONS AND USAGE

Aygestin is indicated for the treatment of secondary amenorrhea, endometriosis, and abnormal uterine bleeding due to hormonal imbalance in the absence of organic pathology, such as submucous fibroids or uterine cancer.

CONTRAINDICATIONS

Known or suspected pregnancy.
Thrombophlebitis, thromboembolic disorders, cerebral apoplexy, or a past history of these conditions.
Markedly impaired liver function or liver disease.
Known or suspected carcinoma of the breast.
Undiagnosed vaginal bleeding.
Missed abortion.
As a diagnostic test for pregnancy.
Hypersensitivity to norethindrone acetate tablets.

WARNINGS

1. Discontinue medication pending examination if there is a sudden partial or complete loss of vision or if there is sudden onset of proptosis, diplopia, or migraine. If examination reveals papilledema or retinal vascular lesions, medication should be withdrawn. There have been reports of retinal vascular thrombosis coincident with the use of progestins.

2. Because of the occasional occurrence of thrombophlebitis and pulmonary embolism in patients taking progestogens, the physician should be alert to the earliest manifestations of the disease. Care should be used when prescribing progestins to a population that may be predisposed to thrombotic disorders (e.g., past history of thrombotic events, thrombophilia, obesity, cardiovascular disease, prolonged immobilization).
3. Several reports suggest an association between intrauterine exposure to progestational drugs in the first trimester of pregnancy and genital abnormalities in male and female fetuses. The risk of hypospadias, 5 to 8 per 1,000 male births in the general population, may be approximately doubled with exposure to these drugs. There are insufficient data to quantify the risk to exposed female fetuses, but insofar as some of these drugs induce mild virilization of the external genitalia of the female fetus, and because of the increased association of hypospadias in the male fetus, it is prudent to avoid the use of these drugs during the first trimester of pregnancy.

PRECAUTIONS

General Precautions:

1. The pretreatment physical examination should include special reference to breasts and pelvic organs, as well as a Papanicolaou smear.
2. Because this drug may cause some degree of fluid retention, conditions which might be influenced by this factor, such as epilepsy, migraine, asthma, cardiac or renal dysfunctions, require careful observation.
3. In cases of breakthrough bleeding, as in all cases of irregular bleeding per vagina, nonfunctional causes should be borne in mind. In cases of undiagnosed vaginal bleeding, adequate diagnostic measures are indicated.
4. Patients who have a history of psychic depression should be carefully observed and the drug discontinued if the depression recurs to a serious degree.
5. Any possible influence of prolonged progestogen therapy on pituitary, ovarian, adrenal, hepatic, or uterine functions awaits further study.
6. Data suggest that progestin therapy may have adverse effects on lipid and carbohydrate metabolism. The choice of progestin, its dose, and its regimen may be important in minimizing these adverse effects, but these issues will require further study before they are clarified. Women with hyperlipidemias and/or diabetes should be monitored closely during progestin therapy.
7. The age of the patient constitutes no absolute limiting factor, although treatment with progestogens may mask the onset of the climacteric.
8. The pathologist should be advised of progestogen therapy when relevant specimens are submitted.

Information for the Patient:
See text which appears at the end of this insert.

Carcinogenesis, Mutagenesis, and Impairment of Fertility:
Some beagle dogs treated with medroxyprogesterone acetate developed mammary nodules. Although nodules occasionally appeared in control animals, they were intermittent in nature, whereas nodules in treated animals were larger and more numerous, and persisted. There is no general agreement as to whether the nodules are benign or malignant. Their significance with respect to humans has not been established.

Pregnancy Category X:
Norethindrone acetate is contraindicated during pregnancy as it may cause fetal harm when administered to pregnant women. Several reports suggest an association between intrauterine exposure to progestational drugs in the first trimester of pregnancy and genital abnormalities in male and female fetuses. Hypospadias occurs in about 5 to 8 per 1,000 male births and is about doubled with exposure to these drugs. Some progestational drugs induce mild virilization of the external genitalia of female fetuses.

Nursing Mothers:
Detectable amounts of progestogens have been identified in the milk of mothers receiving them. The effect of this on the nursing infant has not been determined.

Pediatric Use:
Safety and effectiveness in pediatric patients have not been established.

ADVERSE REACTIONS

See "**WARNINGS**" for further information on Retinal vascular thrombosis, Thrombotic and thromboembolic events, and Use in pregnancy. The following adverse reactions have been observed in women taking progestins:
Breakthrough bleeding.
Spotting.
Change in menstrual flow.
Amenorrhea.
Edema.
Changes in weight (decreases, increases).
Changes in cervical erosion and cervical secretions.
Cholestatic jaundice.
Rash (allergic) with and without pruritus.
Melasma or chloasma.
Mental depression.
Acne.
Breast enlargement/tenderness.
Headache/migraine.
Urticaria.
Abnormalities of liver tests (i.e., AST, ALT, Bilirubin).
Mood swings.
Nausea.
Insomnia.
Anaphylactic/anaphylactoid reactions.
Thrombotic and thromboembolic events (e.g., deep vein thrombosis, pulmonary embolism, retinal vascular thrombosis, cerebral thrombosis and embolism).
Optic neuritis (which may lead to partial or complete loss of vision).
Progestins may alter the result of pregnanediol determinations. The following laboratory results may be altered by the concomitant use of estrogens with progestins:
Hepatic function.
Coagulation tests — increase in prothrombin, factors VII, VIII, IX, and X.
Increase in PBI, BEI, and a decrease in T^3 uptake.
Reduced response to metyrapone test.
The following adverse reactions have been observed in patients receiving estrogen-progestogen combination drugs:

1. Rise in blood pressure in susceptible individuals.
2. Premenstrual-like syndrome.
3. Changes in libido.
4. Changes in appetite.
5. Cystitis-like syndrome.
6. Headache.
7. Nervousness.
8. Dizziness.
9. Fatigue.
10. Backache.
11. Hirsutism.
12. Loss of scalp hair.
13. Erythema multiforme.
14. Erythema nodosum.
15. Hemorrhagic eruption.
16. Itching.

In view of these observations, patients on progestogen therapy should be carefully observed.

DOSAGE AND ADMINISTRATION

Therapy with Aygestin® (norethindrone acetate tablets, USP) must be adapted to the specific indications and therapeutic response of the individual patient. This dosage schedule assumes the interval between menses to be 28 days.

Secondary amenorrhea, abnormal uterine bleeding due to hormonal imbalance in the absence of organic pathology: 2.5 to 10 mg Aygestin may be given daily for 5 to 10 days during the second half of the theoretical menstrual cycle to produce an optimum secretory transformation of an endometrium that has been adequately primed with either endogenous or exogenous estrogen.

Progestin withdrawal bleeding usually occurs within three to seven days after discontinuing Aygestin therapy. Patients with a past history of recurrent episodes of abnormal uterine bleeding may benefit from planned menstrual cycling with Aygestin.

Endometriosis: Initial daily dosage of 5 mg Aygestin for two weeks. Dosage should be increased by 2.5 mg per day every two weeks until 15 mg per day of Aygestin is reached. Therapy may be held at this level for six to nine months or until annoying breakthrough bleeding demands temporary termination.

HOW SUPPLIED

Aygestin® (norethindrone acetate tablets, USP) are available as:

5 mg: White, oval, flat-faced, beveled edge biconvex tablet scored on one side. Debossed with **5 Aygestin** on the unscored side and **b/424** on the scored side.
Available in bottle of:
50 NDC 51285-424-10

Store at controlled room temperature 20° to 25°C (68° to 77°F); with excursions permitted between 15° to 30°C (59° to 86°F) [See USP].
Dispense in a well-closed container.

INFORMATION FOR THE PATIENT

Your doctor has prescribed Aygestin (norethindrone acetate tablets, USP), a progestin, for you. Aygestin is similar to the progesterone hormones naturally produced by the body. Progestins are used to treat menstrual disorders and to test if the body is producing certain hormones.

WARNINGS

AYGESTIN TABLETS SHOULD NOT BE USED IN WOMEN WITH THE FOLLOWING CONDITIONS:
— Known or suspected pregnancy.
— History of blood clots in the legs, lungs, eyes, brain, or elsewhere, or a past history of these conditions.
— Liver impairment or disease.
— Known or suspected cancer of the breast.
— Undiagnosed vaginal bleeding.
— Hypersensitivity to Aygestin tablets.

The information below relates only to the risk to the unborn child associated with use of progestin during pregnancy, abnormal blood clotting, and eye abnormalities.

Risk to the Fetus:
Aygestin tablets should not be used if you are pregnant. Norethindrone acetate is contraindicated during pregnancy as it may cause fetal harm when administered to pregnant women. There is an increased risk of minor birth defects in children whose mothers take this drug during the first 4 months of pregnancy. Several reports suggest an association between mothers who take these drugs in the first trimester of pregnancy and genital abnormalities in male and female babies. The risk to the male baby is the possibility of being born with a condition in which the opening of the penis is on the underside rather than the tip of the penis (hypospadias). Hypospadias occurs in about 5 to 8 per 1,000 male births and is about doubled with exposure to these drugs. There is not enough information to quantify the risk to exposed female fetuses, but enlargement of the clitoris and fusion of the labia may occur, although rarely. Therefore, avoid using the drug during the first trimester of pregnancy. If you take Aygestin (norethindrone acetate tablets, USP) and later find you were pregnant when you took it, be sure to discuss this with your doctor as soon as possible.

Abnormal Blood Clotting:
Use of progestational drugs has been associated with changes in the blood-clotting system. These changes allow the blood to clot more easily, possibly allowing clots to form in the bloodstream. If blood clots do form in your bloodstream, they can cut off the blood supply to vital organs, causing serious problems. These problems may include a stroke (by cutting off blood to part of the brain), a heart attack (by cutting off blood to part of the heart), a pulmonary embolus (by cutting off blood to part of the lungs), visual loss or blindness (by cutting off blood vessels in the eye), or other problems. Any of these conditions may cause death or serious long-term disability. Call your doctor immediately if you suspect you have any of these conditions. He or she may advise you to stop using the drug.

Eye Abnormalities:
Discontinue medication and call your physician immediately if you experience sudden partial or complete loss of vision, blurred vision, or sudden onset of bulging eyes, double vision, or migraine.

OTHER INFORMATION

For further information on the use, side effects and other risks associated with this product, ask your doctor. If you want more information, ask your doctor to show you the professional labeling. The professional labeling is also published in a book called the *Physicians' Desk Reference*, which is available in bookstores and public libraries.

DURAMED PHARMACEUTICALS, INC.
A subsidiary of Barr Laboratories, Inc.
Pomona, NY 10970
Revised JULY 2003
BR-424

Shown in Product Identification Guide, page 311

CENESTIN® ℞
[*sĕ′nĕ″stĭn*]
(synthetic conjugated estrogens, A)
Tablets
℞ only

ESTROGENS INCREASE THE RISK OF ENDOMETRIAL CANCER

Close clinical surveillance of all women taking estrogens is important. Adequate diagnostic measures, including endometrial sampling when indicated, should be undertaken to rule out malignancy in all cases of undiagnosed persistent or recurring abnormal vaginal bleeding. There is no evidence that the use of "natural" estrogens results in a different endometrial risk profile than synthetic estrogens at equivalent estrogen doses. (See **WARNINGS, Malignant neoplasms,** *Endometrial cancer.)*

CARDIOVASCULAR AND OTHER RISKS

Estrogens with and without progestins should not be used for the prevention of cardiovascular disease. (See **WARNINGS, Cardiovascular disorders.**)

The Women's Health Initiative (WHI) study reported increased risks of myocardial infarction, stroke, invasive breast cancer, pulmonary emboli, and deep vein thrombosis in postmenopausal women (50 to 79 years of age) during 5 years of treatment with oral conjugated equine estrogens (CE 0.625 mg) combined with medroxyprogesterone acetate (MPA 2.5 mg) relative to placebo. (See **CLINICAL PHARMACOLOGY, Clinical Studies.**)

Other doses of oral conjugated estrogens with medroxyprogesterone, and other combinations and dosage forms of estrogens and progestins were not studied in the WHI clinical trials and, in the absence of comparable data, these risks should be assumed to be similar. Because of these risks, estrogens with or without progestins should be prescribed at the lowest effective doses and for the shortest duration consistent with treatment goals and risks for the individual woman.

DESCRIPTION

Synthetic conjugated estrogens, A tablets contain a blend of nine (9) synthetic estrogenic substances. The estrogenic substances are sodium estrone sulfate, sodium equilin sulfate, sodium 17α-dihydroequilin sulfate, sodium 17α-estradiol sulfate, sodium 17β-dihydroequilin sulfate, sodium 17α-dihydroequilenin sulfate, sodium 17β-dihy-

Continued on next page

Cenestin—Cont.

droequilenin sulfate, sodium equilenin sulfate and sodium 17β-estradiol sulfate.
The structural formulae for these estrogens are:

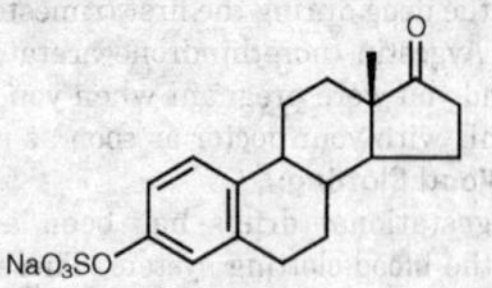

$C_{18}H_{21}NaO_5S$
372.42
Sodium Estrone Sulfate

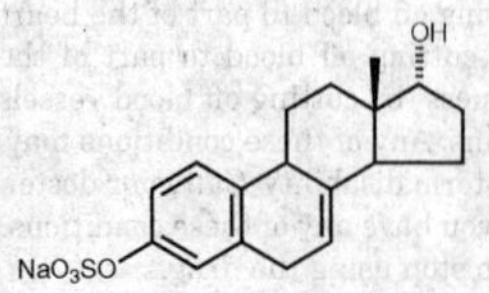

$C_{18}H_{21}NaO_5S$
372.42
Sodium 17α-Dihydroequilin Sulfate

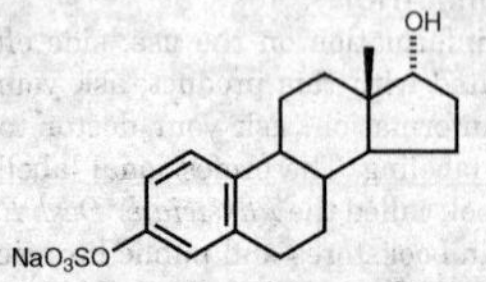

$C_{18}H_{23}NaO_5S$
374.44
Sodium 17α-Estradiol Sulfate

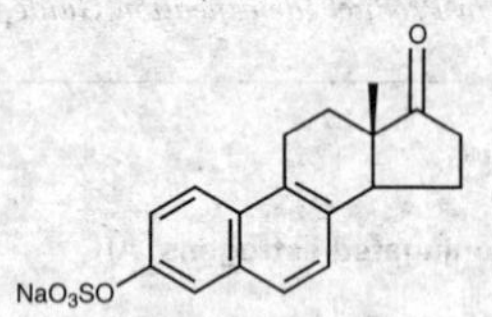

$C_{18}H_{17}NaO_5S$
368.39
Sodium Equilenin Sulfate

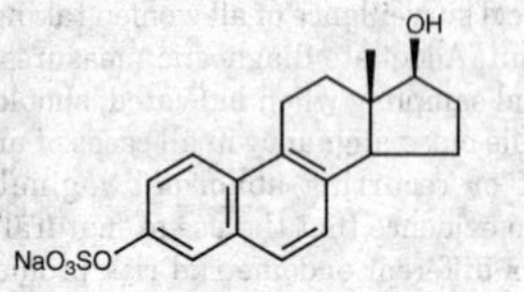

$C_{18}H_{19}NaO_5S$
370.41
Sodium 17β-Dihydroequilenin Sulfate

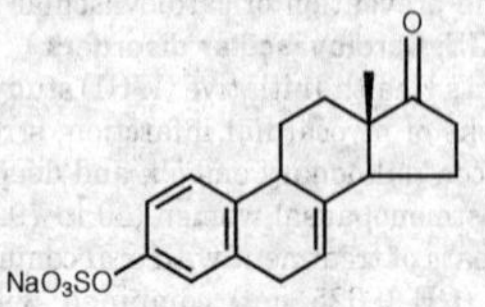

$C_{18}H_{19}NaO_5S$
370.41
Sodium Equilin Sulfate

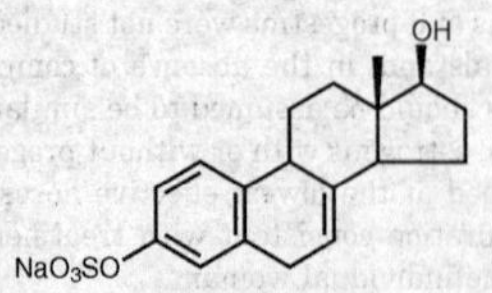

$C_{18}H_{21}NaO_5S$
372.42
Sodium 17β-Dihydroequilin Sulfate

[See first chemical structure at top of next column]
[See second chemical structure at top of next column]
Tablets for oral administration, are available in 0.3 mg, 0.45 mg, 0.625 mg, 0.9 mg and 1.25 mg strengths of synthetic conjugated estrogens, A. Tablets also contain the following inactive ingredients: ethylcellulose, hypromellose,

Table 1
PHARMACOKINETIC PARAMETERS FOR UNCONJUGATED AND CONJUGATED ESTROGENS IN HEALTHY POSTMENOPAUSAL WOMEN UNDER FASTING CONDITIONS

Pharmacokinetic Parameters of Unconjugated Estrogens Following a Dose of 2 × 0.625 mg Cenestin

Drug	C_{max} (pg/mL) CV%	t_{max} (h) CV%	AUC_{0-72h} (pg•hr/mL) CV%
Baseline-corrected estrone	84.5 (41.7)	8.25 (35.6)	1749 (43.8)
Equilin	45.6 (47.3)	7.78 (28.8)	723 (67.9)

Pharmacokinetic Parameters of Conjugated Estrogens Following a Dose of 2 × 0.625 mg Cenestin

Drug	C_{max} (ng/mL) CV%	t_{max} (h) CV%	$t_{1/2}$ (h) CV%	AUC_{0-72h} (ng•hr/mL) CV%
Baseline-corrected estrone	4.43 (40.4)	7.7 (30.3)	10.6 (25.4)	69.89 (39.2)
Equilin	3.27 (43.5)	5.8 (31.1)	9.7 (23.0)	46.46 (47.5)

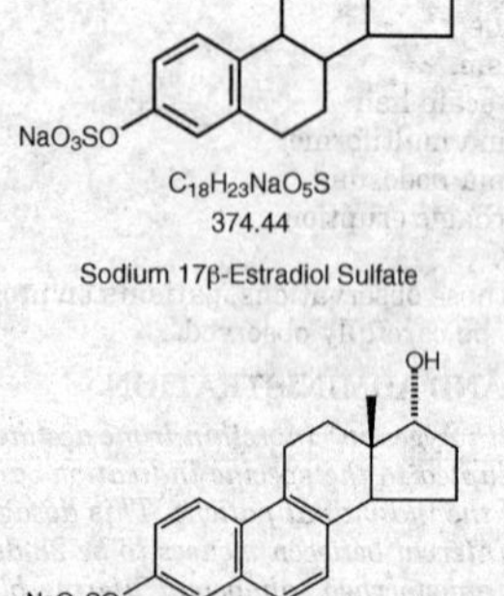
$C_{18}H_{23}NaO_5S$
374.44
Sodium 17β-Estradiol Sulfate

$C_{18}H_{19}NaO_5S$
370.41
Sodium 17α–Dihydroequilenin Sulfate

lactose monohydrate, magnesium stearate, polyethylene glycol, polysorbate 80, pregelatinized starch, titanium dioxide, and triethyl citrate.
-0.3 mg tablets also contain FD&C Blue No. 2 aluminum lake and D&C Yellow No. 10 aluminum lake.
-0.45 mg tablets also contain FD&C Yellow No. 6/Sunset Yellow FCF lake.
-0.625 mg tablets also contain FD&C Red No. 40 aluminum lake.
-0.9 mg tablets do not contain additional color additives.
-1.25 mg tablets also contain FD&C Blue No. 2 aluminum lake.

CLINICAL PHARMACOLOGY

Endogenous estrogens are largely responsible for the development and maintenance of the female reproductive system and secondary sexual characteristics. Although circulating estrogens exist in a dynamic equilibrium of metabolic interconversions, estradiol is the principal intracellular human estrogen and is substantially more potent than its metabolites, estrone and estriol at the receptor level.

The primary source of estrogen in normally cycling adult women is the ovarian follicle, which secretes 70 to 500 mcg of estradiol daily, depending on the phase of the menstrual cycle. After menopause, most endogenous estrogen is produced by conversion of androstenedione, secreted by the adrenal cortex, to estrone by peripheral tissues. Thus, estrone and the sulfate-conjugated form, estrone sulfate, are the most abundant circulating estrogens in postmenopausal women.

Estrogens act through binding to nuclear receptors in estrogen-responsive tissues. To date, two estrogen receptors have been identified. These vary in proportion from tissue to tissue.

Circulating estrogens modulate the pituitary secretion of the gonadotropins, luteinizing hormone (LH) and follicle stimulating hormone (FSH) through a negative feedback mechanism. Estrogens act to reduce the elevated levels of these hormones seen in postmenopausal women.

Pharmacokinetics

Absorption

Synthetic conjugated estrogens, A are soluble in water and are well absorbed from the gastrointestinal tract after release from the drug formulation. The Cenestin tablet releases the synthetic conjugated estrogens, A slowly over a period of several hours. The effect of food on the bioavailability of synthetic conjugated estrogens, A from Cenestin has not been studied.
[See table 1 above]
[See figure 1 at top of next column]

Distribution

The distribution of exogenous estrogens is similar to that of endogenous estrogens. Estrogens are widely distributed in the body and are generally found in higher concentrations in the sex hormone target organs. Estrogens circulate in the blood largely bound to sex hormone binding globulin (SHBG) and albumin.

Figure 1

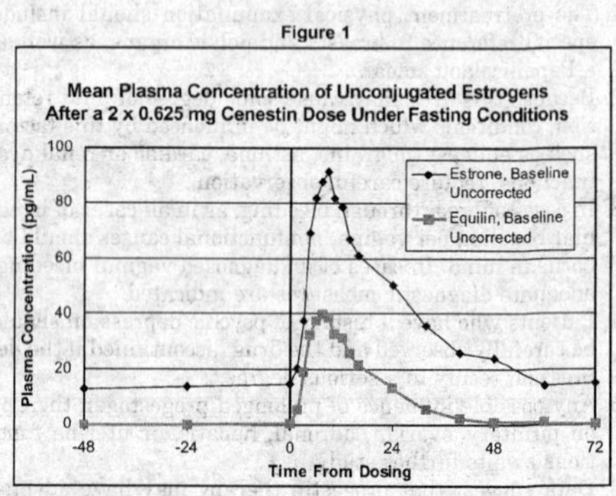

Metabolism

Exogenous estrogens are metabolized in the same manner as endogenous estrogens. Circulating estrogens exist in a dynamic equilibrium of metabolic interconversions. These transformations take place mainly in the liver. Estradiol is converted reversibly to estrone, and both can be converted to estriol, which is the major urinary metabolite. Estrogens also undergo enterohepatic recirculation via sulfate and glucuronide conjugation in the liver, biliary secretion of conjugates into the intestine, and hydrolysis in the gut followed by reabsorption. In postmenopausal women a significant portion of the circulating estrogens exist as sulfate conjugates, especially estrone sulfate, which serves as a circulating reservoir for the formation of more active estrogens.

Excretion

Estradiol, estrone, and estriol are excreted in the urine along with glucuronide and sulfate conjugates.

Special Populations

Cenestin was investigated in postmenopausal women. No pharmacokinetic studies were conducted in special populations, including patients with renal or hepatic impairment.

Drug Interactions

In vitro and *in vivo* studies have shown that estrogens are metabolized partially by cytochrome P450 3A4 (CYP3A4). Therefore, inducers and inhibitors of CYP3A4 may affect estrogen drug metabolism. Inducers of CYP3A4 such as St. John's Wort preparations (Hypericum perforatum), phenobarbital, carbamazepine, and rifampin may reduce plasma concentrations of estrogens, possibly resulting in a decrease in therapeutic effects and/or changes in the uterine bleeding profile. Inhibitors of CYP3A4 such as erythromycin, clarithromycin, ketoconazole, itraconazole, ritonavir and grapefruit juice may increase plasma concentrations of estrogens and may result in side effects.

Clinical Studies

Effects on vasomotor symptoms

A randomized, placebo-controlled multicenter clinical study was conducted evaluating the effectiveness of Cenestin for the treatment of moderate to severe vasomotor symptoms in 120 postmenopausal women between 38 and 66 years of age (68% were Caucasian). Patients were randomized to receive either placebo or 0.625 mg Cenestin daily for 12 weeks. Dose titration was allowed after one week of treatment. The starting dose was either doubled (2 × 0.625 mg Cenestin or placebo taken daily) or reduced (0.3 mg Cenestin or placebo taken daily), if necessary. Efficacy was assessed at 4 and 12 weeks of treatment. By week 12, 10% of the study participants remained on a single 0.625 mg Cenestin tablet daily while 77% required two (0.625 mg) tablets daily. The results in Table 2 indicate that compared to placebo, Cenestin produced a reduction in moderate to severe vasomotor symptoms at weeks 4 and 12.

A second randomized, placebo-controlled multicenter clinical study was conducted evaluating the effectiveness of 0.45 mg Cenestin tablets, for the treatment of moderate to severe vasomotor symptoms in 104 menopausal women between 52 and 74 years of age (76% were Caucasian). Patients were randomized to receive either placebo or 0.45 mg Cenestin daily for 12 weeks. Efficacy was assessed at 4 and 12 weeks of treatment. The mean change in the number of moderate to severe hot flushes per week shown in Table 3 indicate that compared to placebo, 0.45 mg Cenestin produced a reduction in moderate to severe vasomotor symptoms at weeks 4 and 12. A corresponding reduction in the severity of hot flushes was demonstrated at weeks 5 and 12.

Table 2
Clinical Response[a]
Mean Change in the Number of Moderate to Severe Hot Flushes Per Week, 0.625 mg and 2 × 0.625 mg Cenestin, ITT Population

	Cenestin[b] 0.625 mg and 2 × 0.625 mg (n=70)	Placebo (n=47)
Baseline		
Mean # (SD)	96.8 (42.6)	94.1 (33.9)
Week 4		
Mean # (SD)	28.7 (28.8)	45.7 (36.8)
Mean Change from Baseline (SD)	-68.1 (43.9)	-48.4 (46.2)
P-value vs. Placebo	p=.022	
Week 12		
Mean # (SD)	16.5 (25.7)	37.8 (38.7)
Mean Change from Baseline (SD)	-80.3 (50.3)	-56.3 (48.0)
P-value vs. Placebo	p=.010	

Mean = Arithmetic Mean, SD = Standard Deviation
[a]Intent-to-treat population = 117
[b]: Combined results for 0.625 mg and 0.625 mg Cenestin tablets.

Table 3
Clinical Response*
Mean Change in the Number of Moderate to Severe Hot Flushes Per Week, 0.45 mg Cenestin, ITT Population

	Cenestin 0.45 mg (n=53)	Placebo (n=51)
Baseline		
Mean # (SD)	95.9 (37.0)	95.9 (41.6)
Week 4		
Mean # (SD)	45.7 (45.9)	59.4 (46.2)
Mean Change from Baseline (SD)	-50.3 (35.4)	-36.5 (42.9)
P-value vs. Placebo	p=.014	
Week 12		
Mean # (SD)	26.1 (43.0)	50.5 (48.4)
Mean Change from Baseline (SD)	-69.9 (38.1)	-45.4 (44.7)
P-value vs. Placebo	p<.001	

Mean = Arithmetic Mean, SD = Standard Deviation
*Intent-to-treat population = 104

Effects on vulvar and vaginal atrophy

The effects of 0.3 mg Cenestin on moderate to severe symptoms of vulvar and vaginal atrophy were confirmed in a 16-week, randomized, placebo-controlled, multicenter clinical study in 72 postmenopausal women between 30 and 77 years of age (53% were Caucasian). Patients were randomized to receive either placebo or 0.3 mg Cenestin daily for 16 weeks. Efficacy was assessed at weeks 12 and 16 for vaginal wall cytology and week 16 for vaginal pH. Results for percent of superficial cells from a maturation index of the vaginal mucosa are shown in Figure 2. Mean vaginal pH decreased from a baseline of 6.20 to 5.14 for Cenestin and increased to 6.15 from a baseline of 6.03 for placebo.

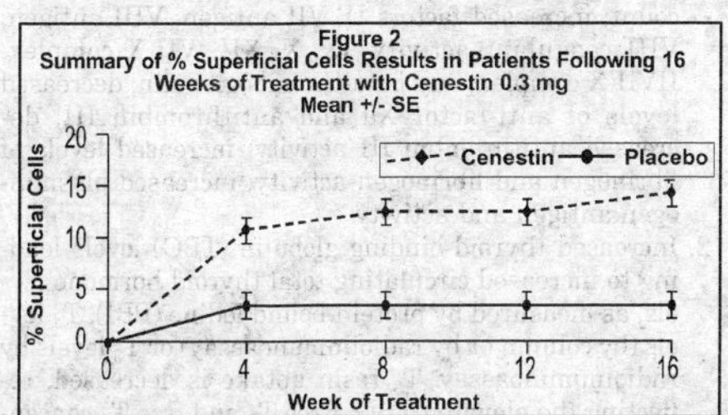

Women's Health Initiative Studies.

The Women's Health Initiative (WHI) enrolled a total of 27,000 predominantly healthy postmenopausal women to assess the risks and benefits of either the use of oral 0.625 mg conjugated equine estrogens (CE) per day alone or the use of oral 0.625 mg conjugated estrogens plus 2.5 mg medroxyprogesterone acetate (MPA) per day compared to placebo in prevention of certain chronic diseases. The primary endpoint was the incidence of coronary heart disease (CHD) (nonfatal myocardial infarction and CHD death), with invasive breast cancer as the primary adverse outcome studied. A "global index" included the earliest occurrence of CHD, invasive breast cancer, stroke, pulmonary embolism (PE), endometrial cancer, colorectal cancer, hip fracture, or death due to other cause. The study did not evaluate the effects of CE or CE/MPA on menopausal symptoms.

The CE-only substudy is continuing and results have not been reported. The CE/MPA substudy was stopped early because, according to the predefined stopping rule, the increased risk of breast cancer and cardiovascular events exceeded the specified benefits included in the "global index." Results of the CE/MPA substudy, which included 16,608 women (average age of 63 years range 50 to 79; 83.9% White, 6.5% Black, 5.5% Hispanic), after an average follow-up of 5.2 years are presented in Table 4 below:

Table 4
Relative and Absolute Risk Seen in the Estrogen/Progestin Substudy of the WHI[a]

Event[c]	Relative Risk Conjugated Equine Estrogens/ Medroxyprogesterone Acetate vs Placebo at 5.2 years (95% CI*)	Placebo n = 8102	CEE/MPA n = 8506
		Absolute Risk per 10,000 Person-years	
CHD events	1.29 (1.02-1.63)	30	37
Non-fatal MI	*1.32 (1.02-1.72)*	*23*	*30*
CHD death	*1.18 (0.70-1.97)*	*6*	*7*
Invasive breast cancer[b]	1.26 (1.00-1.59)	30	38
Stroke	1.41 (1.07-1.85)	21	29
Pulmonary embolism	2.13 (1.39-3.25)	8	16
Colorectal cancer	0.63 (0.43-0.92)	16	10
Endometrial cancer	0.83 (0.47-1.47)	6	5
Hip fracture	0.66 (0.45-0.98)	15	10
Death due to causes other than the events above	0.92 (0.74-1.14)	40	37
Global index[c]	1.15 (1.03-1.28)	151	170
Deep vein thrombosis[d]	2.07 (1.49-2.87)	13	26
Vertebral fractures[d]	0.66 (0.44-0.98)	15	9
Other osteoporotic fractures[d]	0.77 (0.69-0.86)	170	131

[a] adapted from JAMA, 2002; 288:321-333.
[b] Includes metastatic and non-metastatic breast cancer with the exception of in situ breast cancer.
[c] a subset of the events was combined in a "global index," defined as the earliest occurrence of CHD events, invasive breast cancer, stroke, pulmonary embolism, endometrial cancer, colorectal cancer, hip fracture, or death due to other causes.
[d] not included in Global Index.
*nominal confidence intervals unadjusted for multiple looks and multiple comparisons.

[See table 4 above]

For those outcomes included in the "global index," absolute excess risks per 10,000 women-years in the group treated with CE/MPA were 7 more CHD events, 8 more strokes, 8 more PEs, and 8 more invasive breast cancers, while absolute risk reductions per 10,000 women-years were 6 fewer colorectal cancers and 5 fewer hip fractures. The absolute excess risk of events included in the "global index" was 19 per 10,000 women-years. There was no difference between the groups in terms of all-cause mortality. (See **BOXED WARNINGS, WARNINGS,** and **PRECAUTIONS.**)

INDICATIONS AND USAGE

Cenestin therapy is indicated for the:

1. Treatment of moderate-to-severe vasomotor symptoms associated with the menopause.
   - 0.45 mg Cenestin
   - 0.625 mg Cenestin
   - 0.9 mg Cenestin
   - 1.25 mg Cenestin
2. Treatment of moderate to severe symptoms of vulvar and vaginal atrophy associated with the menopause. When prescribing solely for the treatment of symptoms of vulvar and vaginal atrophy, topical vaginal products should be considered.
   - 0.3 mg Cenestin

CONTRAINDICATIONS

Cenestin should not be used in individuals with any of the following conditions:

1. Undiagnosed abnormal genital bleeding.
2. Known, suspected, or history of cancer of the breast.
3. Known or suspected estrogen-dependent neoplasia.
4. Active deep vein thrombosis, pulmonary embolism or a history of these conditions.
5. Active or recent (e.g., within the past year) arterial thromboembolic disease (e.g., stroke, myocardial infarction).
6. Liver dysfunction or disease.
7. Cenestin therapy should not be used in patients with known hypersensitivity to its ingredients.
8. Known or suspected pregnancy. There is no indication for Cenestin in pregnancy. There appears to be little or no increased risk of birth defects in children born to women who have used estrogens and progestins from oral contraceptives inadvertently during early pregnancy. (See **PRECAUTIONS.**)

WARNINGS

See **BOXED WARNINGS.**

1. Cardiovascular disorders.

Estrogen and estrogen/progestin therapy have been associated with an increased risk of cardiovascular events such as myocardial infarction and stroke, as well as venous thrombosis and pulmonary embolism (venous thromboembolism or VTE). Should any of these occur or be suspected, estrogens should be discontinued immediately.

Risk factors for arterial vascular disease (e.g., hypertension, diabetes mellitus, tobacco use, hypercholesterolemia, and obesity) and/or venous thromboembolism (e.g., personal history or family history of VTE, obesity, and systemic lupus erythematosus) should be managed appropriately.

a. Coronary heart disease and stroke. In the Women's Health Initiative (WHI) study, an increase in the number of myocardial infarctions and strokes has been observed in women receiving CE compared to placebo. These observations are preliminary, and the study is continuing. (See **CLINICAL PHARMACOLOGY, Clinical Studies.**)

In the CE/MPA substudy of WHI, an increased risk of coronary heart disease (CHD) events (defined as non-fatal myocardial infarction and CHD death) was observed in women receiving CE/MPA compared to women receiving placebo (37 vs 30 per 10,000 women-years). The increase in risk was observed in year one and persisted.

In the same substudy of WHI, an increased risk of stroke was observed in women receiving CE/MPA compared to women receiving placebo (29 vs 21 per 10,000 women-years). The increase in risk was observed after the first year and persisted.

In postmenopausal women with documented heart disease (n = 2,763, average age 66.7 years) a controlled clinical trial of secondary prevention of cardiovascular disease (Heart and Estrogen/Progestin Replacement Study; HERS) treatment with CE/MPA (0.625 mg/2.5 mg per day) demonstrated no cardiovascular benefit. During an average follow-up of 4.1 years, treatment with CE/MPA did not reduce the overall rate of CHD events in postmenopausal women with established coronary heart disease. There were more CHD events in the CE/MPA-treated group than in the placebo group in year 1, but not during the subsequent years. Two thousand three hundred and twenty one women from the original HERS trial agreed to participate in an open label extension of HERS, HERS II. Average follow-up in HERS II was an additional 2.7 years, for a total of 6.8 years overall. Rates of CHD events were comparable among women in the CE/MPA group and the placebo group in HERS, HERS II, and overall.

Large doses of estrogen (5 mg conjugated estrogens per day), comparable to those used to treat cancer of the prostate and breast, have been shown in a large prospective clinical trial in men to increase the risks of nonfatal myocardial infarction, pulmonary embolism, and thrombophlebitis.

b. Venous thromboembolism (VTE). In the Women's Health Initiative (WHI) study, an increase in VTE has been observed in women receiving CE compared to placebo. These observations are preliminary, and the study is continuing. (See **CLINICAL PHARMACOLOGY, Clinical Studies.**)

In the CE/MPA substudy of WHI, a 2-fold greater rate of VTE, including deep venous thrombosis and pulmonary embolism, was observed in women receiving CE/MPA compared to women receiving placebo. The rate of VTE was 34 per 10,000 women-years in the CE/MPA group compared to 16 per 10,000 women-years in the placebo group. The increase in VTE risk was observed during the first year and persisted.

If feasible, estrogens should be discontinued at least 4 to 6 weeks before surgery of the type associated with an increased risk of thromboembolism, or during periods of prolonged immobilization.

Continued on next page

Cenestin—Cont.

2. Malignant neoplasms.

a. Endometrial cancer. The use of unopposed estrogens in women with intact uteri has been associated with an increased risk of endometrial cancer. The reported endometrial cancer risk among unopposed estrogen users is about 2- to 12-fold greater than in non-users, and appears dependent on duration of treatment and on estrogen dose. Most studies show no significant increased risk associated with use of estrogens for less than one year. The greatest risk appears associated with prolonged use, with increased risks of 15- to 24-fold for five to ten years or more and this risk has been shown to persist for at least 8 to 15 years after estrogen therapy is discontinued.

Clinical surveillance of all women taking estrogen/progestin combinations is important. Adequate diagnostic measures, including endometrial sampling when indicated, should be undertaken to rule out malignancy in all cases of undiagnosed persistent or recurring abnormal vaginal bleeding. There is no evidence that the use of natural estrogens results in a different endometrial risk profile than synthetic estrogens of equivalent estrogen dose. Adding a progestin to estrogen therapy has been shown to reduce the risk of endometrial hyperplasia, which may be a precursor to endometrial cancer.

b. Breast cancer. Estrogen and estrogen/progestin therapy in postmenopausal women has been associated with an increased risk of breast cancer. In the CE/MPA substudy of the Women's Health Initiative (WHI) study, a 26% increase of invasive breast cancer (38 vs 30 per 10,000 women-years) after an average of 5.2 years of treatment was observed in women receiving CE/MPA compared to women receiving placebo. The increased risk of breast cancer became apparent after 4 years on CE/MPA. The women reporting prior postmenopausal use of estrogen and/or estrogen with progestin had a higher relative risk for breast cancer associated with CE/MPA than those who had never used these hormones. (See **CLINICAL PHARMACOLOGY, Clinical Studies.**)

In the WHI, no increased risk of breast cancer in CE-treated women compared to placebo was reported after an average of 5.2 years of therapy. These data are preliminary and that substudy of WHI is continuing.

Epidemiologic studies have reported an increased risk of breast cancer in association with increasing duration of postmenopausal treatment with estrogens with or without a progestin. This association was reanalyzed in original data from 51 studies that involved various doses and types of estrogens, with and without progestins. In the reanalysis, an increased risk of having breast cancer diagnosed became apparent after about 5 years of continued treatment, and subsided after treatment had been discontinued for 5 years or longer. Some later studies have suggested that postmenopausal treatment with estrogen and progestin increases the risk of breast cancer more than treatment with estrogen alone.

A postmenopausal woman without a uterus who requires estrogen should receive estrogen-alone therapy, and should not be exposed unnecessarily to progestins. All postmenopausal women should receive yearly breast exams by a healthcare provider and perform monthly self-examinations. In addition, mammography examinations should be scheduled based on patient age and risk factors.

3. Gallbladder disease

A 2 to 4-fold increase in the risk of gallbladder disease requiring surgery in postmenopausal women receiving estrogens has been reported.

4. Hypercalcemia

Estrogen administration may lead to severe hypercalcemia in patients with breast cancer and bone metastases. If hypercalcemia occurs, use of the drug should be stopped and appropriate measures taken to reduce the serum calcium level.

5. Visual abnormalities

Retinal vascular thrombosis has been reported in patients receiving estrogens. Discontinue medication pending examination if there is sudden partial or complete loss of vision, or a sudden onset of proptosis, diplopia, or migraine. If examination reveals papilledema or renal vascular lesions, estrogens should be permanently discontinued.

PRECAUTIONS

A. General

1. ***Addition of a progestin when a woman has not had a hysterectomy.*** Studies of the addition of a progestin for 10 or more days of a cycle of estrogen administration, or daily with estrogen in a continuous regimen, have reported a lowered incidence of endometrial hyperplasia than would be induced by estrogen treatment alone. Endometrial hyperplasia may be a precursor to endometrial cancer. There are, however, possible risks that may be associated with the use of progestins in estrogen replacement regimens. These include:
   a. A possible increased risk of breast cancer.
   b. Adverse effects on lipoprotein metabolism (e.g., lowering HDL, raising LDL).
   c. Impairment of glucose tolerance.
2. ***Elevated blood pressure.*** In a small number of case reports, substantial increases in blood pressure have been attributed to idiosyncratic reactions to estrogens. In a large, randomized, placebo controlled clinical trial, a generalized effect of estrogen therapy on blood pressure was not seen. Blood pressure should be monitored at regular intervals with estrogen use.

Table 5
Number (%) of Patients with Adverse Events With ≥5% Occurrence Rate By Body System and Treatment Group

Body System Adverse Event	Cenestin* 0.625 mg and 2 × 0.625 mg n (%)	Placebo n (%)	Total n (%)
Number of Patients Who Received Medication	72 (100)	48 (100)	120 (100)
Number of Patients With Adverse Events	68 (94)	43 (90)	111 (93)
Number of Patients Without Any Adverse Events	4 (6)	5 (10)	9 (8)
Body As A Whole			
Abdominal Pain	20 (28)	11 (23)	31 (26)
Asthenia	24 (33)	20 (42)	44 (37)
Back Pain	10 (14)	6 (13)	16 (13)
Fever	1 (1)	3 (6)	4 (3)
Headache	49 (68)	32 (67)	81 (68)
Infection	10 (14)	5 (10)	15 (13)
Pain	8 (11)	9 (19)	17 (14)
Cardiovascular System			
Palpitation	15 (21)	13 (27)	28 (23)
Digestive System			
Constipation	4 (6)	2 (4)	6 (5)
Diarrhea	4 (6)	0 (0)	4 (3)
Dyspepsia	7 (10)	3 (6)	10 (8)
Flatulence	21 (29)	14 (29)	35 (29)
Nausea	13 (18)	9 (19)	22 (18)
Vomiting	5 (7)	1 (2)	6 (5)
Metabolic and Nutritional			
Peripheral Edema	7 (10)	6 (13)	13 (11)
Musculoskeletal System			
Arthralgia	18 (25)	13 (27)	31 (26)
Myalgia	20 (28)	15 (31)	35 (29)
Nervous System			
Depression	20 (28)	18 (38)	38 (32)
Dizziness	8 (11)	5 (10)	13 (11)
Hypertonia	4 (6)	0 (0)	4 (3)
Insomnia	30 (42)	23 (48)	53 (44)
Leg Cramps	7 (10)	3 (6)	10 (8)
Nervousness	20 (28)	20 (42)	40 (33)
Paresthesia	24 (33)	15 (31)	39 (33)
Vertigo	12 (17)	12 (25)	24 (20)
Respiratory System			
Cough Increased	4 (6)	1 (2)	5 (4)
Pharyngitis	6 (8)	4 (8)	10 (8)
Rhinitis	6 (8)	7 (15)	13 (11)
Skin and Appendages			
Rash	3 (4)	3 (6)	6 (5)
Urogenital System			
Breast Pain	21 (29)	7 (15)	28 (23)
Dysmenorrhea	4 (6)	3 (6)	7 (6)
Metrorrhagia	10 (14)	3 (6)	13 (11)

*Combined results for 0.625 mg and 2 × 0.625 mg Cenestin Tablets

3. ***Hypertriglyceridemia.*** In patients with pre-existing hypertriglyceridemia, estrogen therapy may be associated with elevations of plasma triglycerides leading to pancreatitis and other complications.
4. ***Impaired liver function and past history of cholestatic jaundice.*** Estrogens may be poorly metabolized in patients with impaired liver function. For patients with a history of cholestatic jaundice associated with past estrogen use or with pregnancy, caution should be exercised and in the case of recurrence, medication should be discontinued.
5. ***Hypothyroidism.*** Estrogen administration leads to increased thyroid-binding globulin (TBG) levels. Patients with normal thyroid function can compensate for the increased TBG by making more thyroid hormone, thus maintaining free T_4 and T_3 serum concentrations in the normal range. Patients dependent on thyroid hormone replacement therapy who are also receiving estrogens may require increased doses of their thyroid replacement therapy. These patients should have their thyroid function monitored in order to maintain their free thyroid hormone levels in an acceptable range.
6. ***Fluid retention.*** Because estrogens may cause some degree of fluid retention, patients with conditions that might be influenced by this factor, such as a cardiac or renal dysfunction, warrant careful observation when estrogens are prescribed.
7. ***Hypocalcemia.*** Estrogens should be used with caution in individuals with severe hypocalcemia.
8. ***Ovarian cancer.*** Use of estrogen-only products, in particular for ten or more years, has been associated with an increased risk of ovarian cancer in some epidemiological studies. Other studies did not show a significant association. Data are insufficient to determine whether there is an increased risk with estrogen/progestin combination therapy in postmenopausal women.
9. ***Exacerbation of endometriosis.*** Endometriosis may be exacerbated with administration of estrogen therapy. A few cases of malignant transformation of residual endometrial implants have been reported in women treated post-hysterectomy with estrogen alone therapy. For patients known to have residual endometriosis post-hysterectomy, the addition of progestin should be considered.
10. ***Exacerbation of other conditions.*** Estrogens may cause an exacerbation of asthma, diabetes mellitus, epilepsy, migraine, porphyria, systemic lupus erythematosus, and hepatic hemangiomas and should be used with caution in women with these conditions.

B. Patient Information

Physicians are advised to discuss the PATIENT INFORMATION leaflet with patients for whom they prescribe Cenestin.

C. Laboratory Tests

Estrogen administration should be initiated at the lowest dose for the approved indication and then guided by clinical response, rather than by serum hormone levels (e.g., estradiol, FSH).

D. Drug/Laboratory Test Interactions

1. Accelerated prothrombin time, partial thromboplastin time, and platelet aggregation time; increased platelet count; increased factors II, VII antigen, VIII antigen, VIII coagulant activity, IX, X, XII, VII-X complex, IIVII-X complex, and beta-thromboglobulin; decreased levels of anti-factor Xa and antithrombin III, decreased antithrombin III activity; increased levels of fibrinogen and fibrinogen activity; increased plasminogen antigen and activity.
2. Increased thyroid-binding globulin (TBG) levels leading to increased circulating total thyroid hormone levels, as measured by protein-bound iodine (PBI), T_4 levels (by column or by radioimmunoassay) or T_3 levels by radioimmunoassay. T_3 resin uptake is decreased, reflecting the elevated TBG. Free T_4 and free T_3 concentrations are unaltered. Patients on thyroid replacement therapy may require higher doses of thyroid hormone.
3. Other binding proteins may be elevated in serum (i.e., corticosteroid binding globulin (CBG), sex hormone-binding globulin (SHBG)) leading to increased total circulating corticosteroids and sex steroids, respectively. Free hormone concentrations may be decreased. Other plasma proteins may be increased (angiotensinogen/renin substrate, alpha-1-antitrypsin, ceruloplasmin).
4. Increased plasma HDL and HDL_2 cholesterol subfraction concentrations, reduced LDL cholesterol concentration, increased triglyceride levels.
5. Impaired glucose tolerance.
6. Reduced response to metyrapone test.

E. Carcinogenesis, Mutagenesis, Impairment of Fertility

Long-term continuous administration of estrogen, with and without progestin, in women, with and without a uterus, has shown an increased risk of endometrial cancer, breast cancer, and ovarian cancer. (See **BOXED WARNINGS**, **WARNINGS** and **PRECAUTIONS**.)

Long-term continuous administration of natural and synthetic estrogens in certain animal species increases the frequency of carcinomas of the breast, uterus, cervix, vagina, testis, and liver.

F. Pregnancy

Cenestin should not be used in pregnancy. (See **CONTRAINDICATIONS**.)

G. Nursing Mothers

Estrogen administration to nursing mothers has been shown to decrease the quantity and quality of the milk. Detectable amounts of estrogens have been identified in the milk of mothers receiving this drug. Caution should be exercised when Cenestin is administered to a nursing woman.

H. Pediatric Use

Cenestin is not indicated in children.

I. Geriatric Use

There have not been sufficient numbers of geriatric patients involved in studies utilizing Cenestin to determine whether those over 65 years of age differ from younger subjects in their response to Cenestin.

ADVERSE REACTIONS

See **BOXED WARNINGS**, **WARNINGS** and **PRECAUTIONS**.

Because clinical trials are conducted under widely varying conditions, adverse reaction rates observed in the clinical trials of a drug cannot be directly compared to rates in the clinical trials of another drug and may not reflect the rates observed in practice. The adverse reaction information from clinical trials does, however, provide a basis for identifying the adverse events that appear to be related to drug use and for approximating rates.

In a 12-week clinical trial that included 72 women treated with 0.625 mg and 2 x 0.625 mg Cenestin and 48 women treated with placebo, adverse events that occurred at a rate of ≥ 5% are summarized in Table 5.

[See table 5 at top of previous page]

In a second 12-week clinical trial that included 52 women treated with 0.45 mg Cenestin and 51 women treated with placebo, adverse events that occurred at a rate of >5% are summarized in Table 6

[See table 6 at right]

The following additional adverse reactions have been reported with estrogen and/or progestin therapy:

1. Genitourinary system.

Changes in vaginal bleeding pattern and abnormal withdrawal bleeding or flow; breakthrough bleeding; spotting; dysmenorrhea, increase in size of uterine leiomyomata; vaginitis, including vaginal candidiasis; change in amount of cervical secretion; changes in cervical ectropion; ovarian cancer; endometrial hyperplasia; endometrial cancer.

2. Breasts.

Tenderness, enlargement, pain, nipple discharge, galactorrhea; fibrocystic breast changes; breast cancer.

3. Cardiovascular.

Deep and superficial venous thrombosis; pulmonary embolism; thrombophlebitis; myocardial infarction; stroke; increase in blood pressure.

4. Gastrointestinal.

Nausea, vomiting; abdominal cramps, bloating; cholestatic jaundice; increased incidence of gallbladder disease; pancreatitis, enlargement of hepatic hemangiomas.

5. Skin.

Chloasma or melasma, which may persist when drug is discontinued; erythema multiforme; erythema nodosum; hemorrhagic eruption; loss of scalp hair; hirsutism; pruritus, rash.

6. Eyes.

Retinal vascular thrombosis; intolerance to contact lenses.

7. Central nervous system.

Headache; migraine; dizziness; mental depression; chorea; nervousness; mood disturbances; irritability; exacerbation of epilepsy.

8. Miscellaneous.

Increase or decrease in weight; reduced carbohydrate tolerance; aggravation of porphyria; edema; arthalgias; leg cramps; changes in libido; anaphylactoid/anaphylactic reactions including urticaria and angioedema; hypocalcemia; exacerbation of asthma; increased triglycerides.

OVERDOSAGE

Serious ill effects have not been reported following acute ingestion of large doses of estrogen containing drug products by young children. Overdosage of estrogen may cause nausea and vomiting, and withdrawal bleeding may occur in females.

DOSAGE AND ADMINISTRATION

When estrogen is prescribed for a postmenopausal woman with a uterus, progestin should also be initiated to reduce the risk of endometrial cancer. A woman without a uterus does not need progestin. Use of estrogen, alone or in combination with a progestin, should be with the lowest effective dose and for the shortest duration consistent with treatment goals and risks for the individual woman. Patients should be reevaluated periodically as clinically appropriate (e.g., 3-month to 6-month intervals) to determine if treatment is still necessary (see **BOXED WARNINGS** and **WARNINGS**). For women who have a uterus, adequate diagnostic measures, such as endometrial sampling, when indicated, should be undertaken to rule out malignancy in cases of undiagnosed persistent or recurring abnormal vaginal bleeding.

Table 6
Number (%) of Patients with a ≥5% Occurrence Rate By Body System and Treatment Group

Body System and Term	Cenestin 0.45 mg	Control	p-value
Any Adverse Event %	40 (75.5%)	39 (76.5%)	1.0000
Body As A Whole	20 (37.7%)	24 (47.1%)	0.4275
Asthenia	6 (11.3%)	7 (13.7%)	0.7731
Headache	6 (11.3%)	8 (15.7%)	0.5748
Infection	1 (1.9%)	6 (11.8%)	0.0576
Pain	6 (11.3%)	1 (2.0%)	0.1128
Pain abdominal	5 (9.4%)	3 (5.9%)	0.7159
Cardiovascular	5 (9.4%)	10 (19.6%)	0.1695
Palpitations	3 (5.7%)	3 (5.9%)	1.0000
Vasodilations	2 (3.8%)	4 (7.8%)	0.4324
Digestive	8 (15.1%)	7 (13.7%)	1.0000
Nausea	5 (9.4%)	2 (3.9%)	0.4374
Metabolic and Nutritional	5 (9.4%)	3 (5.9%)	0.7159
Weight increase	3 (5.7%)	2 (3.9%)	1.0000
Musculoskeletal	5 (9.4%)	6 (11.8%)	0.7582
Arthralgia	5 (9.4%)	5 (9.8%)	1.0000
Myalgia	2 (3.8%)	6 (11.8%)	0.1566
Neurological	15 (28.3%)	19 (37.3%)	0.4044
Anxiety	3 (5.7%)	1 (2.0%)	0.6179
Depression	2 (3.8%)	7 (13.7%)	0.0895
Insomnia	3 (5.7%)	5 (9.8%)	0.4839
Nervousness	2 (3.8%)	7 (13.7%)	0.0895
Paresthesia	4 (7.5%)	3 (5.9%)	1.0000
Vertigo	3 (5.7%)	3 (5.9%)	1.0000
Respiratory	10 (18.9%)	6 (11.8%)	0.4173
Upper Respiratory Tract Infection	7 (13.2%)	1 (2.0%)	0.0603
Rhinitis	3 (5.7%)	2 (3.9%)	1.0000
Pharyngitis	1 (1.9%)	3 (5.9%)	0.3581
Urogenital	19 (35.8%)	7 (13.7%)	0.0124
Endometrial thickening	10 (18.9%)	4 (7.8%)	0.1503
Vaginitis	4 (7.5%)	1 (2.0%)	0.3632

P-value by Fisher's Exact (2-tail) Test
If a subject experiences the same event more than once, the first occurrence is tabulated.

1. For treatment of moderate to severe vasomotor symptoms associated with the menopause.
   - Cenestin 0.45 mg
   - Cenestin 0.625 mg
   - Cenestin 0.9 mg
   - Cenestin 1.25 mg

   Patients should be started at Cenestin 0.45 mg daily. Subsequent dosage adjustment may be made based upon the individual patient response.This dose should be periodically reassessed by the healthcare provider. The lowest effective dose of Cenestin for the treatment of moderate to severe vasomotor symptoms has not been determined.
2. For treatment of moderate to severe symptoms of vulvar and vaginal atrophy associated with the menopause. When prescribing solely for the treatment of symptoms of vulvar and vaginal atrophy, topical vaginal products should be considered.
   - Cenestin 0.3 mg daily

HOW SUPPLIED

Cenestin (synthetic conjugated estrogens, A) Tablets are available as:

0.3 mg: Round, green, film-coated, and are debossed with letters, **dp**, and number, 41.
Available in bottles of:
30 NDC 51285-441-30
100 NDC 51285-441-02
1000 NDC 51285-441-05

0.45 mg: Round, orange, film-coated, and are debossed with letters, **dp**, and number, 46.
Available in bottles of:
30 NDC 51285-446-30
100 NDC 51285-446-02
1000 NDC 51285-446-05

0.625 mg: Round, red, film-coated, and are debossed with letters, **dp**, and number, 42.
Available in bottles of:
30 NDC 51285-442-30
100 NDC 51285-442-02
1000 NDC 51285-442-05

0.9 mg: Round, white, film-coated, and are debossed with letters, **dp**, and number, 43.
Available in bottles of:
30 NDC 51285-443-30
100 NDC 51285-443-02
1000 NDC 51285-443-05

1.25 mg: Round, blue, film-coated, and are debossed with letters, **dp**, and number, 44.
Available in bottles of:
30 NDC 51285-444-30
100 NDC 51285-444-02
1000 NDC 51285-444-05

Store at 20-25°C (68-77°F); excursions are permitted to 15-30°C (59-86°F) [See USP Controlled Room Temperature].
Dispense in tight container.
Dispense in child-resistant packaging.
Pharmacist: Include one "Information for the patient" leaflet with each package dispensed.

PATIENT INFORMATION

Revised FEBRUARY 2004
Cenestin®
(synthetic conjugated estrogens, A) Tablets

Read this PATIENT INFORMATION before you start taking Cenestin and read what you get each time you refill Cenestin. There may be new information. This information does not take the place of talking to your healthcare provider about your medical condition or your treatment.

What is the most important information I should know about Cenestin (synthetic estrogen mixture)?

- Estrogens increase the chances of getting cancer of the uterus.

Report any unusual vaginal bleeding right away while you are taking estrogens. Vaginal bleeding after menopause may be a warning sign of cancer of the uterus (womb). Your healthcare provider should check any unusual vaginal bleeding to find out the cause.

- Do not use estrogens with or without progestins to prevent heart disease, heart attacks, or strokes.

Using estrogens with or without progestins may increase your chances of getting heart attack, strokes, breast cancer, and blood clots. You and your healthcare provider should talk regularly about whether you still need treatment with Cenestin.

What is Cenestin?

Cenestin is a medicine that contains a mixture of synthetic estrogens made from a plant source.

What is Cenestin used for?

Cenestin is used after menopause to:

- **reduce moderate or severe hot flashes.**
  Estrogens are hormones made by a woman's ovaries. The ovaries normally stop making estrogens when a woman is between 45 to 55 years old. This drop in body estrogen levels causes the "change of life" or menopause (the end of monthly menstrual periods). Sometimes, both ovaries are removed during an operation before natural menopause takes place. The sudden drop in estrogen levels causes "surgical menopause."
  When estrogen levels begin dropping, some women develop very uncomfortable symptoms, such as feelings of warmth in the face, neck, and chest, or sudden strong feelings of heat and sweating ("hot flashes" or "hot flushes"). In some women, the symptoms are mild, and they will not need estrogens. In other women, symptoms can be more severe.You and your healthcare provider should talk regularly about whether you still need treatment with Cenestin.
- **treat moderate to severe dryness, itching, and burning in and around the vagina.** You and your healthcare provider should talk regularly about whether you still need treatment with Cenestin to control these problems. If you use Cenestin only to treat your dryness, itching, and burning in and around your vagina, talk with your healthcare provider about whether a topical vaginal product would be better for you.

Continued on next page

Cenestin—Cont.

Who Should Not Take Cenestin?
Do not start taking Cenestin if you:
- **have unusual vaginal bleeding.**
- **currently have or have had certain cancers.** Estrogens may increase the risk of certain types of cancers, including cancer of the breast or uterus. If you have or had cancer, talk with your healthcare provider about whether you should take Cenestin.
- **had a stroke or heart attack in the past year.**
- **currently have or have had blood clots.**
- **currently have or have had liver problems.**
- **are allergic to Cenestin or any of its ingredients.** See the end of this leaflet for a list of ingredients in Cenestin.
- **think you may be pregnant.**

TELL YOUR HEALTHCARE PROVIDER:
- **if you are breastfeeding.** The synthetic estrogen hormones in Cenestin can pass into your milk.
- **about all of your medical problems.** Your healthcare provider may need to check you more carefully if you have certain conditions, such as asthma (wheezing), epilepsy (seizures), migraine, endometriosis, lupus, or problems with your heart, liver, thyroid, kidneys, or have high calcium levels in your blood.
- **about all the medicines you take,** including prescription and nonprescription medicines, vitamins, and herbal supplements. Some medicines may affect how Cenestin works. Cenestin may also affect how your other medicines work.
- **if you are going to have surgery or will be on bed rest.** You may need to stop taking estrogens.

How Should I Take Cenestin?
Take one Cenestin tablet each day at about the same time. If you miss a dose, take it as soon as possible. If it is almost time for your next dose, skip the missed dose and go back to your normal schedule. Do not take 2 doses at the same time. Start at the lowest dose and talk to your healthcare provider about how well that dose is working for you. Estrogens should be used only as long as needed. You and your healthcare provider should talk regularly (for example every 3 to 6 months) about whether you still need treatment with Cenestin.

What are the possible risks and side effects of estrogens?
Less common but serious side effects include:
- Breast cancer
- Cancer of the uterus
- Stroke
- Heart attack
- Blood clots
- Gallbladder disease
- Ovarian cancer

These are some of the warning signs of serious side effects:
- Breast lumps
- Unusual vaginal bleeding
- Dizziness and faintness
- Changes in speech
- Severe headaches
- Chest pain
- Shortness of breath
- Pains in your legs
- Changes in vision
- Vomiting

Call your healthcare provider right away if you get any of these warning signs, or any other unusual symptom that concerns you.

Common side effects include:
- Headache
- Breast pain
- Irregular vaginal bleeding or spotting
- Stomach/abdominal cramps, bloating
- Nausea and vomiting
- Hair loss

Other side effects include:
- High blood pressure
- Liver problems
- High blood sugar
- Fluid retention
- Enlargement of benign tumors of the uterus ("fibroids")
- Vaginal yeast infection

These are not all the possible side effects of Cenestin. For more information, ask your healthcare provider or pharmacist.

What can I do to lower my chances of getting a serious side effect with Cenestin?
- Talk with your healthcare provider regularly about whether you should continue taking Cenestin.
- If you have a uterus, talk to your healthcare provider about whether the addition of a progestin is right for you.
- See your healthcare provider right away if you get vaginal bleeding while taking Cenestin.
- Have a breast exam and mammogram (breast X-ray) every year unless your healthcare provider tells you something else. If members of your family have had breast cancer or if you have ever had breast lumps or an abnormal mammogram, you may need to have breast exams more often.
- If you have high blood pressure, high cholesterol (fat in the blood), diabetes, are overweight, or if you use tobacco, you may have higher chances for getting heart disease. Ask your healthcare provider for ways to lower your chances for getting heart disease.

General information about safe and effective use of Cenestin.
Medicines are sometimes prescribed for conditions that are not mentioned in patient information leaflets. Do not take Cenestin for conditions for which it was not prescribed. Do not give Cenestin to other people, even if they have the same symptoms you have. It may harm them.

Keep Cenestin out of the reach of children.
This leaflet provides a summary of the most important information about Cenestin. If you would like more information, talk with your healthcare provider or pharmacist. You can ask for information about Cenestin that is written for health professionals. You can get more information by calling the toll free number 877-405-0369.

What are the ingredients in Cenestin?
Tablets for oral administration, are available in 0.3 mg, 0.45 mg, 0.625 mg, 0.9 mg and 1.25 mg strengths of synthetic conjugated estrogens, A. Tablets also contain the following inactive ingredients: ethylcellulose, hypromellose, lactose monohydrate, magnesium stearate, polyethylene glycol, polysorbate 80, pregelatinized starch, titanium dioxide, and triethyl citrate.
-0.3 mg tablets also contain FD&C Blue No. 2 aluminum lake and D&C Yellow No. 10 aluminum lake.
-0.45 mg tablets also contain FD&C Yellow No. 6/Sunset Yellow FCF lake.
-0.625 mg tablets also contain FD&C Red No. 40 aluminum lake.
-0.9 mg tablets do not contain any additional color additives.
-1.25 mg tablets also contain FD&C Blue No. 2 aluminum lake.

Manufactured By:
Duramed Pharmaceuticals, Inc.
Subsidiary of Barr Pharmaceuticals, Inc.
Pomona, New York 10970
Revised FEBRUARY 2004
BR - 41, 46, 42, 43, 44

Shown in Product Identification Guide, page 311

ECR Pharmaceuticals

Distributor of ECR &
Wm. P. Poythress Products
3969 DEEP ROCK ROAD
P. O. BOX 71600
RICHMOND, VA 23255

Direct Inquiries to:
Professional Services Department
(804) 527-1950
FAX: (804) 527-1959

For Medical Information Contact:
In Emergencies:
Professional Services Department
(804) 527-1950
FAX: (804) 527-1959

NDC 00095	Product	
—0131	**Anaplex DM Cough Syrup** Each teaspoon (5 ml) contains: Dextromethrophan Hydrobromide, 30 mg. Brompheniramine Maleate, 4 mg. Pseudoephedrine HCl, 60 mg. Sugar Free, Alcohol Free, Dye Free	℞
—0130	**Anaplex HD Cough Syrup** Each teaspoon (5 ml) contains: Hydrocodone Bitartrate, 1.7 mg; Pseudoephedrine HCl, 30 mg. Brompheniramine Maleate, 2 mg. Sugar Free. Alcohol Free, Dye Free	℞ CIII
—0240	**Bupap Tablets** (Butalbital, 50 mg; Acetaminophen, 650 mg)	℞
—0086	**DEXPAK Taperpak** Weighted, tapered, oral Corticosteroid Therapy. Each package contains 51 tablets, dexamethasone, USP 1.5 mg	℞
—6004	**Lodrane Liquid** Each teaspoon (5 ml) contains: Brompheniramine Maleate, 4 mg; Pseudoephedrine HCl, 60 mg. Sugar Free. Alcohol Free. Dye Free.	℞
—0006	**Lodrane 12 Hour Extended Release Tablets** (Brompheniramine Maleate, 6 mg.) Sustained Release, Dye Free	℞
—0645	**Lodrane 12 D Extended Release Tablets** (Brompheniramine Maleate, 6 mg; Pseudoephedrine HCl, 45 mg) Sustained Release, Dye Free	℞
—1200	**Lodrane 24 Extended Release Capsules** (Brompheniramine maleate, 12 mg) Once a Day Dosage. Dye Free.	℞
—1290	**Lodrane 24 D Extended Release Capsules** (Brompheniramine maleate, 12 mg; Pseudoephedrine HCl, 90 mg) Once a Day Dosage. Dye Free.	℞
—0008	**Lodrane Sustained Release Liquid** Each teaspoon (5 ml) contains: Brompheniramine tannate, 8 mg	℞
—9008	**Lodrane D Sustained Release Liquid** Each teaspoon (5 ml) contains: Brompheniramine tannate, 8 mg; Pseudoephedrine tannate, 90 mg	℞
—0225	**Nasatab LA Tablets** (Guaifenesin, 500 mg; Pseudoephedrine HCl, 120 mg) Sustained Release, Dye Free	℞
—0021	**Panalgesic Gold Cream** (Methyl Salicylate, 35%; Menthol, 4%)	OTC
—0120	**Panalgesic Gold Liniment** (Methyl Salicylate, 55%; Camphor, 3%; Menthol, 1%)	OTC
—0066	**Pneumotussin Tablets** (Guaifenesin, 300 mg; Hydrocodone Bitartrate, 2.5 mg)	℞ CIII
—0067	**Pneumotussin 2.5 Cough Syrup** Each teaspoon (5 ml) contains: (Guaifenesin, 200 mg; Hydrocodone Bitartrate, 2.5 mg)	℞ CIII

Eisai Inc.

500 FRANK W. BURR BOULEVARD
TEANECK, NJ 07666

Direct Inquiries to:
Eisai Medical Services
1 (888) 422-4743 (888) 4Aciphe(x)
FAX: (201) 287-9744

Medical Emergency Contact:
Medical Emergencies:
24 hours/day, 7 days/week
1 (888) 422-4743 (888) 4Aciphe(x)

ACIPHEX® ℞
[*'a-se-feks*]
(rabeprazole sodium)
Delayed-Release Tablets

DESCRIPTION
The active ingredient in ACIPHEX® Delayed-Release Tablets is rabeprazole sodium, a substituted benzimidazole that inhibits gastric acid secretion. Rabeprazole sodium is known chemically as 2-[[[4-(3-methoxypropoxy)-3-methyl-2-pyridinyl]-methyl]sulfinyl]-1*H*–benzimidazole sodium salt. It has an empirical formula of $C_{18}H_{20}N_3NaO_3S$ and a molecular weight of 381.43. Rabeprazole sodium is a white to slightly yellowish-white solid. It is very soluble in water and methanol, freely soluble in ethanol, chloroform and ethyl acetate and insoluble in ether and n-hexane. The stability of rabeprazole sodium is a function of pH; it is rapidly degraded in acid media, and is more stable under alkaline conditions. The structural formula is:

RABEPRAZOLE SODIUM

ACIPHEX® is available for oral administration as delayed-release, enteric-coated tablets containing 20 mg of rabeprazole sodium. Inactive ingredients are carnauba wax, crospovidone, diacetylated monoglycerides, ethylcellulose, hydroxypropyl cellulose, hypromellose phthalate, magnesium stearate, mannitol, sodium hydroxide, sodium stearyl fumarate, talc, titanium dioxide, and yellow ferric oxide as a coloring agent.

CLINICAL PHARMACOLOGY

Pharmacokinetics and Metabolism

ACIPHEX® delayed-release tablets are enteric-coated to allow rabeprazole sodium, which is acid labile, to pass through the stomach relatively intact. After oral administration of 20 mg ACIPHEX®, peak plasma concentrations (C_{max}) of rabeprazole occur over a range of 2.0 to 5.0 hours (T_{max}). The rabeprazole C_{max} and AUC are linear over an oral dose range of 10 mg to 40 mg. There is no appreciable accumulation when doses of 10 mg to 40 mg are administered every 24 hours; the pharmacokinetics of rabeprazole are not altered by multiple dosing. The plasma half-life ranges from 1 to 2 hours.

Absorption: Absolute bioavailability for a 20 mg oral tablet of rabeprazole (compared to intravenous administration) is approximately 52%. When rabeprazole is administered with a high fat meal, its T_{max} is variable and may delay its absorption up to 4 hours or longer, however, the C_{max} and the extent of rabeprazole absorption (AUC) are not significantly altered. Thus rabeprazole may be taken without regard to timing of meals.

Distribution: Rabeprazole is 96.3% bound to human plasma proteins.

Metabolism: Rabeprazole is extensively metabolized. The thioether and sulphone are the primary metabolites measured in human plasma. These metabolites were not observed to have significant antisecretory activity. *In vitro* studies have demonstrated that rabeprazole is metabolized in the liver primarily by cytochromes P450 3A (CYP3A) to a sulphone metabolite and cytochromes P450 2C19 (CYP2C19) to desmethyl rabeprazole. The thioether metabolite is formed non-enzymatically by reduction of rabeprazole. CYP2C19 exhibits a known genetic polymorphism due to its deficiency in some sub-populations (e.g. 3 to 5% of Caucasians and 17 to 20% of Asians). Rabeprazole metabolism is slow in these sub-populations, therefore, they are referred to as poor metabolizers of the drug.

Elimination: Following a single 20 mg oral dose of ^{14}C-labeled rabeprazole, approximately 90% of the drug was eliminated in the urine, primarily as thioether carboxylic acid; its glucuronide, and mercapturic acid metabolites. The remainder of the dose was recovered in the feces. Total recovery of radioactivity was 99.8%. No unchanged rabeprazole was recovered in the urine or feces.

Special Populations

Geriatric: In 20 healthy elderly subjects administered 20 mg rabeprazole once daily for seven days, AUC values approximately doubled and the C_{max} increased by 60% compared to values in a parallel younger control group. There was no evidence of drug accumulation after once daily administration. (see PRECAUTIONS).

Pediatric: The pharmacokinetics of rabeprazole in pediatric patients under the age of 18 years have not been studied.

Gender and Race: In analyses adjusted for body mass and height, rabeprazole pharmacokinetics showed no clinically significant differences between male and female subjects. In studies that used different formulations of rabeprazole, $AUC_{0-\infty}$ values for healthy Japanese men were approximately 50–60% greater than values derived from pooled data from healthy men in the United States.

Renal Disease: In 10 patients with stable end-stage renal disease requiring maintenance hemodialysis (creatinine clearance ≤5 mL/min/1.73 m^2), no clinically significant differences were observed in the pharmacokinetics of rabeprazole after a single 20 mg oral dose when compared to 10 healthy volunteers.

Hepatic Disease: In a single dose study of 10 patients with chronic mild to moderate compensated cirrhosis of the liver who were administered a 20 mg dose of rabeprazole, AUC_{0-24} was approximately doubled, the elimination half-life was 2- to 3-fold higher, and total body clearance was decreased to less than half compared to values in healthy men.

In a multiple dose study of 12 patients with mild to moderate hepatic impairment administered 20 mg rabeprazole once daily for eight days, $AUC_{0-\infty}$ and C_{max} values increased approximately 20% compared to values in healthy age- and gender-matched subjects. These increases were not statistically significant.

No information exists on rabeprazole disposition in patients with severe hepatic impairment. Please refer to the DOSAGE AND ADMINISTRATION section for information on dosage adjustment in patients with hepatic impairment.

Combined Administration with Antimicrobials: Sixteen healthy volunteers genotyped as extensive metabolizers with respect to CYP2C19 were given 20 mg rabeprazole sodium, 1000 mg amoxicillin, 500 mg clarithromycin, or all 3 drugs in a four-way crossover study. Each of the four regimens was administered twice daily for 6 days. The AUC and C_{max} for clarithromycin and amoxicillin were not different following combined administration compared to values following single administration. However, the rabeprazole AUC and C_{max} increased by 11% and 34%, respectively, following combined administration. The AUC and C_{max} for 14-hydroxyclarithromycin (active metabolite of clarithromycin) also increased by 42% and 46%, respectively. This increase in exposure to rabeprazole and 14-hydroxyclarithromycin is not expected to produce safety concerns.

PHARMACODYNAMICS

Mechanism of Action

Rabeprazole belongs to a class of antisecretory compounds (substituted benzimidazole proton-pump inhibitors) that do not exhibit anticholinergic or histamine H_2-receptor antagonist properties, but suppress gastric acid secretion by inhibiting the gastric H^+, K^+ATPase at the secretory surface of the gastric parietal cell. Because this enzyme is regarded as the acid (proton) pump within the parietal cell, rabeprazole has been characterized as a gastric proton-pump inhibitor. Rabeprazole blocks the final step of gastric acid secretion.

In gastric parietal cells, rabeprazole is protonated, accumulates, and is transformed to an active sulfenamide. When studied *in vitro*, rabeprazole is chemically activated at pH 1.2 with a half-life of 78 seconds. It inhibits acid transport in porcine gastric vesicles with a half-life of 90 seconds.

AUC Acidity (mmol·hr/L)
ACIPHEX® Versus Placebo on Day 7
of Once Daily Dosing (mean ± SD)

	Treatment			
AUC interval (hrs)	10 mg RBP (N=24)	20 mg RBP (N=24)	40 mg RBP (N=24)	Placebo (N=24)
08:00 – 13:00	19.6±21.5*	12.9±23*	7.6±14.7*	91.1±39.7
13:00 – 19:00	5.6±9.7*	8.3±29.8*	1.3±5.2*	95.5±48.7
19:00 – 22:00	0.1±0.1*	0.1±0.06*	0.0±0.02*	11.9±12.5
22:00 – 08:00	129.2±84*	109.6±67.2*	76.9±58.4*	479.9±165
AUC 0–24 hours	155.5±90.6*	130.9±81*	85.8±64.3*	678.5±216

*(p<0.001 versus placebo)

Gastric Acid Parameters
ACIPHEX® Once Daily Dosing Versus Placebo on Day 1 and Day 8

	ACIPHEX® 20 mg QD		Placebo	
Parameter	Day 1	Day 8	Day 1	Day 8
Mean AUC_{0-24} Acidity	340.8*	176.9*	925.5	862.4
Median trough pH (23-hr)[a]	3.77	3.51	1.27	1.38
% Time Gastric pH>3[b]	54.6*	68.7*	19.1	21.7
% Time Gastric pH>4[b]	44.1*	60.3*	7.6	11.0

[a] No inferential statistics conducted for this parameter.
* (p<0.001 versus placebo)
[b] Gastric pH was measured every hour over a 24-hour period.

Antisecretory Activity

The anti-secretory effect begins within one hour after oral administration of 20 mg ACIPHEX®. The median inhibitory effect of ACIPHEX® on 24 hour gastric acidity is 88% of maximal after the first dose. ACIPHEX® 20 mg inhibits basal and peptone mealstimulated acid secretion versus placebo by 86% and 95%, respectively, and increases the percent of a 24-hour period that the gastric pH>3 from 10% to 65% (see table below). This relatively prolonged pharmacodynamic action compared to the short pharmacokinetic half-life (1–2 hours) reflects the sustained inactivation of the H^+, K^+ATPase.

Gastric Acid Parameters
ACIPHEX® Versus Placebo After 7 Days of Once Daily Dosing

Parameter	ACIPHEX® (20 mg QD)	Placebo
Basal Acid Output (mmol/hr)	0.4*	2.8
Stimulated Acid Output (mmol/hr)	0.6*	13.3
% Time Gastric pH>3	65*	10

*(p<0.01 versus placebo)

Compared to placebo, ACIPHEX®, 10 mg, 20 mg, and 40 mg, administered once daily for 7 days significantly decreased intragastric acidity with all doses for each of four meal-related intervals and the 24-hour time period overall. In this study, there were no statistically significant differences between doses; however, there was a significant dose-related decrease in intragastric acidity. The ability of rabeprazole to cause a dose-related decrease in mean intragastric acidity is illustrated below.

[See first table above]

After administration of 20 mg ACIPHEX® once daily for eight days, the mean percent of time that gastric pH>3 or gastric pH>4 after a single dose (Day 1) and multiple doses (Day 8) was significantly greater than placebo (see table below). The decrease in gastric acidity and the increase in gastric pH observed with 20 mg ACIPHEX® administered once daily for eight days were compared to the same parameters for placebo, as illustrated below:

[See second table above]

Effects on Esophageal Acid Exposure

In patients with gastroesophageal reflux disease (GERD) and moderate to severe esophageal acid exposure, ACIPHEX® 20 mg and 40 mg per day decreased 24-hour esophageal acid exposure. After seven days of treatment, the percentage of time that esophageal pH<4 decreased from baselines of 24.7% for 20 mg and 23.7% for 40 mg, to 5.1% and 2.0%, respectively. Normalization of 24-hour intraesophageal acid exposure was correlated to gastric pH>4 for at least 35% of the 24-hour period; this level was achieved in 90% of subjects receiving ACIPHEX® 20 mg and in 100% of subjects receiving ACIPHEX® 40 mg. With ACIPHEX® 20 mg and 40 mg per day, significant effects on gastric and esophageal pH were noted after one day of treatment, and more pronounced after seven days of treatment.

Effects on Serum Gastrin

In patients given daily doses of ACIPHEX® for up to eight weeks to treat ulcerative or erosive esophagitis and in patients treated for up to 52 weeks to prevent recurrence of disease the median fasting gastrin level increased in a dose-related manner. The group median values stayed within the normal range.

In a group of subjects treated daily with ACIPHEX® 20 mg for 4 weeks a doubling of mean serum gastrin concentrations were observed. Approximately 35% of these treated subjects developed serum gastrin concentrations above the upper limit of normal. In a study of CYP2C19 genotyped subjects in Japan, poor metabolizers developed statistically significantly higher serum gastrin concentrations than extensive metabolizers.

Effects on Enterochromaffin-like (ECL) Cells

Increased serum gastrin secondary to antisecretory agents stimulates proliferation of gastric ECL cells which, over time, may result in ECL cell hyperplasia in rats and mice and gastric carcinoids in rats, especially in females (see Carcinogenesis, Mutagenesis, Impairment of Fertility).

In over 400 patients treated with ACIPHEX® (10 or 20 mg/day) for up to one year, the incidence of ECL cell hyperplasia increased with time and dose, which is consistent with the pharmacological action of the proton-pump inhibitor. No patient developed the adenomatoid, dysplastic or neoplastic changes of ECL cells in the gastric mucosa. No patient developed the carcinoid tumors observed in rats.

Endocrine Effects

Studies in humans for up to one year have not revealed clinically significant effects on the endocrine system. In healthy male volunteers treated with ACIPHEX® for 13 days, no clinically relevant changes have been detected in the following endocrine parameters examined: 17 β-estradiol, thyroid stimulating hormone, tri-iodothyronine, thyroxine, thyroxine-binding protein, parathyroid hormone, insulin, glucagon, renin, aldosterone, follicle-stimulating hormone, luteotrophic hormone, prolactin, somatotrophic hormone, dehydroepiandrosterone, cortisol-binding globulin, and urinary 6β-hydroxycortisol, serum testosterone and circadian cortisol profile.

Other Effects

In humans treated with ACIPHEX® for up to one year, no systemic effects have been observed on the central nervous, lymphoid, hematopoietic, renal, hepatic, cardiovascular, or respiratory systems. No data are available on long-term treatment with ACIPHEX® and ocular effects.

Microbiology

Rabeprazole sodium, amoxicillin and clarithromycin as a three drug regimen has been shown to be active against most strains of *Helicobacter pylori* in vitro and in clinical infections as described in the **CLINICAL STUDIES** and **INDICATIONS AND USAGE** sections.

Helicobacter pylori

Susceptibility testing of *H. pylori* isolates was performed for amoxicillin and clarithromycin using agar dilution methodology[1], and minimum inhibitory concentrations (MICs) were determined. The clarithromycin and amoxicillin MIC values should be interpreted according to the following criteria:

Continued on next page

Aciphex—Cont.

Clarithromycin MIC (µg/mL)[a]	Interpretation
≤ 0.25	Susceptible (S)
0.5	Intermediate (I)
≥ 1.0	Resistant (R)

Amoxicillin MIC (µg/mL)[a,b]	Interpretation
≤ 0.25	Susceptible (S)

[a] These are breakpoints for the agar dilution methodology and they should not be used to interpret results using alternative methods.
[b] There were not enough organisms with MICs > 0.25 µg/mL to determine a resistance breakpoint.

Standardized susceptibility test procedures require the use of laboratory control microorganisms to control the technical aspects of the laboratory procedures. Standard clarithromycin and amoxicillin powders should provide the following MIC values:

Microorganism	Antimicrobial Agent	MIC (µg/mL)[a]
H. pylori ATCC 43504	Clarithromycin	0.015–0.12 µg/mL
H. pylori ATCC 43504	Amoxicillin	0.015–0.12 µg/mL

[a] These are quality control ranges for the agar dilution methodology and they should not be used to control test results obtained using alternative methods.

Incidence of Antibiotic-Resistant Organisms Among Clinical Isolates

Pretreatment Resistance: Clarithromycin pretreatment resistance rate (MIC ≥ 1 µg/mL) to *H. pylori* was 9% (51/560) at baseline in all treatment groups combined. A total of > 99% (558/560) of patients had *H. pylori* isolates which were considered to be susceptible (MIC ≤ 0.25 µg/mL) to amoxicillin at baseline. Two patients had baseline *H. pylori* isolates with an amoxicillin MIC of 0.5 µg/mL.

Clarithromycin Susceptibility Test Results and Clinical/Bacteriologic Outcomes: For the U.S. multicenter study, the baseline *H. pylori* clarithromycin susceptibility results and the *H. pylori* eradication results post-treatment are shown in the table below:

[See first table above]

Patients with persistent *H. pylori* infection following rabeprazole, amoxicillin, and clarithromycin therapy will likely have clarithromycin resistant clinical isolates. Therefore, clarithromycin susceptibility testing should be done when possible. If resistance to clarithromycin is demonstrated or susceptibility testing is not possible, alternative antimicrobial therapy should be instituted.

Amoxicillin Susceptibility Test Results and Clinical/Bacteriological Outcomes: In the U.S. multicenter study, a total of >99% (558/560) of patients had *H. pylori* isolates which were considered to be susceptible (MIC ≤ 0.25 µg/mL) to amoxicillin at baseline. The other 2 patients had baseline *H. pylori* isolates with an amoxicillin MIC of 0.5 µg/mL, and both isolates were clarithromycin-resistant at baseline; in one case the *H. pylori* was eradicated. In the 7- and 10-day treatment groups 75% (107/145) and 79% (112/142), respectively, of the patients who had pretreatment amoxicillin susceptible MICs (≤ 0.25 µg/mL) were eradicated of *H. pylori*. No patients developed amoxicillin-resistant *H. pylori* during therapy.

CLINICAL STUDIES

Healing of Erosive or Ulcerative Gastroesophageal Reflux Disease (GERD)

In a U.S., multicenter, randomized, double-blind, placebo-controlled study, 103 patients were treated for up to eight weeks with placebo, 10 mg, 20 mg or 40 mg ACIPHEX® QD. For this and all studies of GERD healing, only patients with GERD symptoms and at least grade 2 esophagitis (modified Hetzel-Dent grading scale) were eligible for entry. Endoscopic healing was defined as grade 0 or 1. Each rabeprazole dose was significantly superior to placebo in producing endoscopic healing after four and eight weeks of treatment. The percentage of patients demonstrating endoscopic healing was as follows:

[See second table above]

In addition, there was a statistically significant difference in favor of the ACIPHEX® 10 mg, 20 mg, and 40 mg doses compared to placebo at Weeks 4 and 8 regarding complete resolution of GERD heartburn frequency (p≤0.026). All ACIPHEX® groups reported significantly greater rates of complete resolution of GERD daytime heartburn severity compared to placebo at Weeks 4 and 8 (p≤0.036). Mean reductions from baseline in daily antacid dose were statistically significant for all ACIPHEX® groups when compared to placebo at both Weeks 4 and 8 (p≤0.007).

In a North American multicenter, randomized, double-blind, active-controlled study of 336 patients, ACIPHEX® was statistically superior to ranitidine with respect to the percentage of patients healed at endoscopy after four and eight weeks of treatment (see table below):

Clarithromycin Susceptibility Test Results and Clinical/Bacteriologic Outcomes[a] for a Three Drug Regimen (Rabeprazole 20 mg twice daily, amoxicillin 1000 mg twice daily, and clarithromycin 500 mg twice daily for 7 or 10 days)

Days of RAC Therapy	Clarithromycin Pretreatment Results	Total Number	*H. pylori* Negative (Eradicated)	*H. pylori* Positive (Persistent) Post-Treatment Susceptibility Results			
				S[b]	I[b]	R[b]	No MIC
7	Susceptible[b]	129	103	2	0	1	23
7	Intermediate[b]	0	0	0	0	0	0
7	Resistant[b]	16	5	2	1	4	4
10	Susceptible[b]	133	111	3	1	2	16
10	Intermediate[b]	0	0	0	0	0	0
10	Resistant[b]	9	1	0	0	5	3

[a] Includes only patients with pretreatment and post-treatment clarithromycin susceptibility test results.
[b] Susceptible (S) MIC ≤ 0.25 µg/mL, Intermediate (I) MIC = 0.5 µg/mL, Resistant (R) MIC ≥ 1 µg/mL

Healing of Erosive or Ulcerative Gastroesophageal Reflux Disease (GERD) Percentage of Patients Healed

Week	10 mg ACIPHEX® QD N=27	20 mg ACIPHEX® QD N=25	40 mg ACIPHEX® QD N=26	Placebo N=25
4	63%*	56%*	54%*	0%
8	93%*	84%*	85%*	12%

*(p<0.001 versus placebo)

Long-term Maintenance of Healing of Erosive or Ulcerative Gastroesophageal Reflux Disease (GERD Maintenance) Percent of Patients in Endoscopic Remission

	ACIPHEX® 10 mg	ACIPHEX® 20 mg	Placebo
Study 1	N=66	N=67	N=70
Week 4	83%*	96%*	44%
Week 13	79%*	93%*	39%
Week 26	77%*	93%*	31%
Week 39	76%*	91%*	30%
Week 52	73%*	90%*	29%
Study 2	N=93	N=93	N=99
Week 4	89%*	94%*	40%
Week 13	86%*	91%*	33%
Week 26	85%*	89%*	30%
Week 39	84%*	88%*	29%
Week 52	77%*	86%*	29%
COMBINED STUDIES	N=159	N=160	N=169
Week 4	87%*	94%*	42%
Week 13	83%*	92%*	36%
Week 26	82%*	91%*	31%
Week 39	81%*	89%*	30%
Week 52	75%*	87%*	29%

*(p<0.001 versus placebo)

Healing of Erosive or Ulcerative Gastroesophageal Reflux Disease (GERD) Percentage of Patients Healed

Week	ACIPHEX® 20 mg QD N=167	Ranitidine 150 mg QID N=169
4	59%*	36%
8	87%*	66%

*(p<0.001 versus ranitidine)

ACIPHEX® 20 mg once daily was significantly more effective than ranitidine 150 mg QID in the percentage of patients with complete resolution of heartburn at Weeks 4 and 8 (p<0.001). ACIPHEX® 20 mg once daily was also more effective in complete resolution of daytime heartburn (p≤0.025), and night time heartburn (p≤0.012) at both Weeks 4 and 8, with significant differences by the end of the first week of the study.

Long-term Maintenance of Healing of Erosive or Ulcerative Gastroesophageal Reflux Disease (GERD Maintenance)

The long-term maintenance of healing in patients with erosive or ulcerative GERD previously healed with gastric antisecretory therapy was assessed in two U.S., multicenter, randomized, double-blind, placebo-controlled studies of identical design of 52 weeks duration. The two studies randomized 209 and 285 patients, respectively, to receive either 10 mg or 20 mg of ACIPHEX® QD or placebo. As demonstrated in the tables below, ACIPHEX® was significantly superior to placebo in both studies with respect to the maintenance of healing of GERD and the proportions of patients remaining free of heartburn symptoms at 52 weeks:

[See third table above]

[See first table at top of next page]

Symptomatic Gastroesophageal Reflux Disease (GERD)

Two U.S., multicenter, double-blind, placebo controlled studies were conducted in 316 patients with daytime and nighttime heartburn. Patients reported 5 or more periods of moderate to very severe heartburn during the placebo treatment phase the week prior to randomization. Patients were confirmed by endoscopy to have no esophageal erosions.

The percentage of heartburn free daytime and/or nighttime periods was greater with ACIPHEX® 20 mg compared to placebo over the 4 weeks of study in Study RAB-USA-2 (47% vs. 23%) and Study RAB-USA-3 (52% vs. 28%). The mean decreases from baseline in average daytime and nighttime heartburn scores were significantly greater for ACIPHEX® 20 mg as compared to placebo at week 4.

Graphical displays depicting the daily mean daytime and nighttime scores are provided in Figures 1 to 4.

Figure 1: Mean Daytime heartburn scores RAB - USA - 2

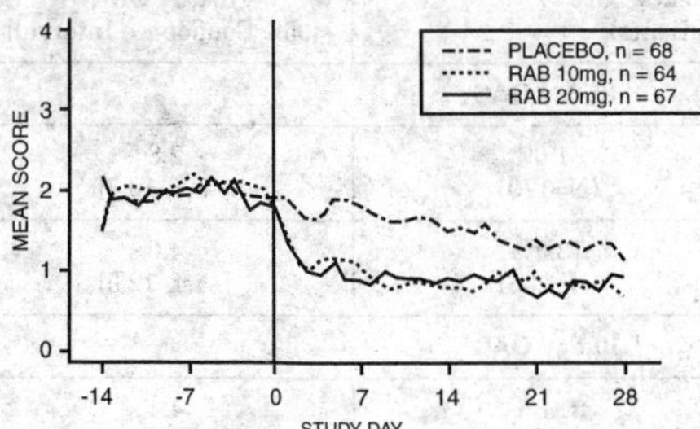

Figure 2: Mean Nighttime heartburn scores RAB - USA - 2

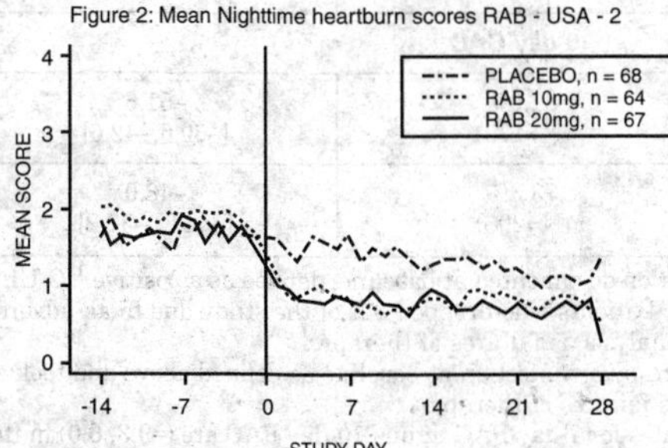

Figure 3: Mean Daytime heartburn scores RAB - USA - 3

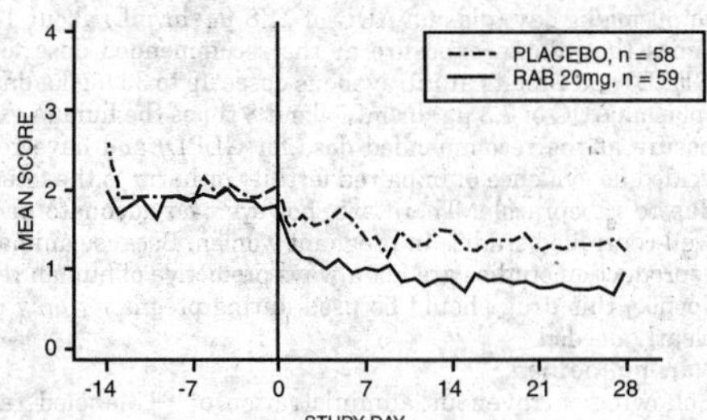

Figure 4: Mean Nighttime heartburn scores RAB - USA - 3

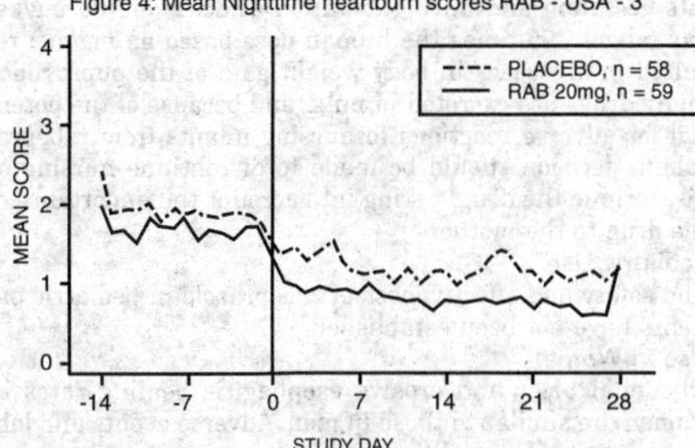

ACIPHEX® 20 mg also significantly reduced daily antacid consumption versus placebo over 4 weeks ($p<0.001$).

Healing of Duodenal Ulcers

In a U.S., randomized, double-blind, multicenter study assessing the effectiveness of 20 mg and 40 mg of ACIPHEX® QD versus placebo for healing endoscopically defined duodenal ulcers, 100 patients were treated for up to four weeks. ACIPHEX® was significantly superior to placebo in producing healing of duodenal ulcers. The percentages of patients with endoscopic healing are presented below:

Healing of Duodenal Ulcers
Percentage of Patients Healed

Week	ACIPHEX® 20 mg QD N=34	ACIPHEX® 40 mg QD N=33	Placebo N=33
2	44%	42%	21%
4	79%*	91%*	39%

* $p\leq0.001$ versus placebo

At Weeks 2 and 4, significantly more patients in the ACIPHEX® 20 and 40 mg groups reported complete resolution of ulcer pain frequency ($p\leq0.018$), daytime pain severity ($p\leq0.023$), and nighttime pain severity ($p\leq0.035$) compared with placebo patients. The only exception was the ACIPHEX® 40 mg group versus placebo at Week 2 for duodenal ulcer pain frequency ($p=0.094$). Significant differences in resolution of daytime and nighttime pain were noted in both ACIPHEX® groups relative to placebo by the end of the first week of the study. Significant reductions in daily antacid use were also noted in both ACIPHEX® groups compared to placebo at Weeks 2 and 4 ($p<0.001$).

Long-term Maintenance of Healing of Erosive or Ulcerative Gastroesophageal Reflux Disease (GERD Maintenance): Percent of Patients Without Relapse in Heartburn Frequency and Daytime and Nighttime Heartburn Severity at Week 52

	ACIPHEX® 10 mg	ACIPHEX® 20 mg	Placebo
Heartburn Frequency			
Study 1	46/55 (84%)*	48/52 (92%)*	17/45 (38%)
Study 2	50/72 (69%)*	57/72 (79%)*	22/79 (28%)
Daytime Heartburn Severity			
Study 1	61/64 (95%)*	60/62 (97%)*	42/61 (69%)
Study 2	73/84 (87%)†	82/87 (94%)*	67/90 (74%)
Nighttime Heartburn Severity			
Study 1	57/61 (93%)*	60/61 (98%)*	37/56 (66%)
Study 2	67/80 (84%)	79/87 (91%)†	64/87 (74%)

* $p\leq0.001$ versus placebo
† $0.001<p<0.05$ versus placebo

Healing of Duodenal Ulcers
Percentage of Patients Healed

Week	ACIPHEX® 20 mg QD N=102	Omeprazole 20 mg QD N=103	95% Confidence Interval for the Treatment Difference (ACIPHEX® - Omeprazole)
2	69%	61%	(−6%, 22%)
4	98%	93%	(−3%, 15%)

An international randomized, double-blind, active-controlled trial was conducted in 205 patients comparing 20 mg ACIPHEX® QD with 20 mg omeprazole QD. The study was designed to provide at least 80% power to exclude a difference of at least 10% between ACIPHEX® and omeprazole, assuming four-week healing response rates of 93% for both groups. In patients with endoscopically defined duodenal ulcers treated for up to four weeks, ACIPHEX® was comparable to omeprazole in producing healing of duodenal ulcers. The percentages of patients with endoscopic healing at two and four weeks are presented below:

[See second table above]

ACIPHEX® and omeprazole were comparable in providing complete resolution of symptoms.

***Helicobacter pylori* Eradication in Patients with Peptic Ulcer Disease or Symptomatic Non-Ulcer Disease**

The U.S. multicenter study was a double blind, parallel group comparison of rabeprazole, amoxicillin, and clarithromycin for 3, 7, or 10 days vs. omeprazole, amoxicillin and clarithromycin for 10 days. Therapy consisted of rabeprazole 20 mg twice daily, amoxicillin 1000 mg twice daily, and clarithromycin 500 mg twice daily (RAC) or omeprazole 20 mg twice daily, amoxicillin 1000 mg twice daily, and clarithromycin 500 mg twice daily (OAC). Patients with *H. pylori* infection were stratified in a 1:1 ratio for those with peptic ulcer disease (active or a history of ulcer in the past five years) [PUD] and those who were symptomatic but without peptic ulcer disease [NPUD], as determined by upper gastrointestinal endoscopy. The overall *H. pylori* eradication rates, defined as negative ^{13}C-UBT for *H. pylori* $\geq$ 6 weeks from the end of the treatment are shown in the following table. The eradication rates in the 7-day and 10-day RAC regimens were found to be similar to 10-day OAC regimen using either the Intent-to-Treat (ITT) or Per-Protocol (PP) populations. Eradication rates in the RAC 3-day regimen were inferior to the other regimens.

[See table at top of next page]

Pathological Hypersecretory Conditions Including Zollinger-Ellison Syndrome

Twelve patients with idiopathic gastric hypersecretion or Zollinger-Ellison syndrome have been treated successfully with ACIPHEX® at doses from 20 to 120 mg for up to 12 months. ACIPHEX® produced satisfactory inhibition of gastric acid secretion in all patients and complete resolution of signs and symptoms of acid-peptic disease where present. ACIPHEX® also prevented recurrence of gastric hypersecretion and manifestations of acid-peptic disease in all patients. The high doses of ACIPHEX® used to treat this small cohort of patients with gastric hypersecretion were well tolerated.

INDICATIONS AND USAGE

Healing of Erosive or Ulcerative Gastroesophageal Reflux Disease (GERD)

ACIPHEX® is indicated for short-term (4 to 8 weeks) treatment in the healing and symptomatic relief of erosive or ulcerative gastroesophageal reflux disease (GERD). For those patients who have not healed after 8 weeks of treatment, an additional 8-week course of ACIPHEX® may be considered.

Maintenance of Healing of Erosive or Ulcerative Gastroesophageal Reflux Disease (GERD)

ACIPHEX® is indicated for maintaining healing and reduction in relapse rates of heartburn symptoms in patients with erosive or ulcerative gastroesophageal reflux disease (GERD Maintenance). Controlled studies do not extend beyond 12 months.

Treatment of Symptomatic Gastroesophageal Reflux Disease (GERD)

ACIPHEX® is indicated for the treatment of daytime and nighttime heartburn and other symptoms associated with GERD.

Healing of Duodenal Ulcers

ACIPHEX® is indicated for short-term (up to four weeks) treatment in the healing and symptomatic relief of duodenal ulcers. Most patients heal within four weeks.

***Helicobacter pylori* Eradication to Reduce the Risk of Duodenal Ulcer Recurrence**

ACIPHEX® in combination with amoxicillin and clarithromycin as a three drug regimen, is indicated for the treatment of patients with *H. pylori* infection and duodenal ulcer disease (active or history within the past 5 years) to eradicate *H. pylori*. Eradication of *H. pylori* has been shown to reduce the risk of duodenal ulcer recurrence. (See **CLINICAL STUDIES** and **DOSAGE AND ADMINISTRATION**.)

In patients who fail therapy, susceptibility testing should be done. If resistance to clarithromycin is demonstrated or susceptibility testing is not possible, alternative antimicrobial therapy should be instituted. (See **CLINICAL PHARMACOLOGY, Microbiology** and the clarithromycin package insert, **CLINICAL PHARMACOLOGY, Microbiology**.)

Treatment of Pathological Hypersecretory Conditions, Including Zollinger-Ellison Syndrome

ACIPHEX® is indicated for the long-term treatment of pathological hypersecretory conditions, including Zollinger-Ellison syndrome.

CONTRAINDICATIONS

Rabeprazole is contraindicated in patients with known hypersensitivity to rabeprazole, substituted benzimidazoles or to any component of the formulation.

Clarithromycin is contraindicated in patients with known hypersensitivity to any macrolide antibiotic.

Concomitant administration of clarithromycin with pimozide and cisapride is contraindicated. There have been postmarketing reports of drug interactions when clarithromycin and/or erythromycin are co-administered with pimozide resulting in cardiac arrhythmias (QT prolongation, ventricular tachycardia, ventricular fibrillation, and torsade de pointes) most likely due to inhibition of hepatic metabolism of pimozide by erythromycin and clarithromycin. Fatalities have been reported. (Please refer to full prescribing information for clarithromycin.)

Amoxicillin is contraindicated in patients with a known hypersensitivity to any penicillin. (Please refer to full prescribing information for amoxicillin.)

WARNINGS

CLARITHROMYCIN SHOULD NOT BE USED IN PREGNANT WOMEN EXCEPT IN CLINICAL CIRCUMSTANCES WHERE NO ALTERNATIVE THERAPY IS APPROPRIATE. If pregnancy

Continued on next page

Aciphex—Cont.

occurs while taking clarithromycin, the patient should be apprised of the potential hazard to the fetus. (See **WARNINGS** in prescribing information for clarithromycin.)

Amoxicillin: Serious and occasionally fatal hypersensitivity (anaphylactic) reactions have been reported in patients on penicillin therapy. These reactions are more likely to occur in individuals with a history of penicillin hypersensitivity and/or a history of sensitivity to multiple allergens.

There have been well-documented reports of individuals with a history of penicillin hypersensitivity reactions who have experienced severe hypersensitivity reactions when treated with a cephalosporin. Before initiating therapy with any penicillin, careful inquiry should be made concerning previous hypersensitivity reactions to penicillin, cephalosporin, and other allergens. If an allergic reaction occurs, amoxicillin should be discontinued and the appropriate therapy instituted. (See **WARNINGS** in prescribing information for amoxicillin.)

SERIOUS ANAPHYLACTIC REACTIONS REQUIRE IMMEDIATE EMERGENCY TREATMENT WITH EPINEPHRINE. OXYGEN, INTRAVENOUS STEROIDS, AND AIRWAY MANAGEMENT, INCLUDING INTUBATION, SHOULD ALSO BE ADMINISTERED AS INDICATED.

Pseudomembranous colitis has been reported with nearly all antibacterial agents, including clarithromycin and amoxicillin, and may range in severity from mild to life threatening. Therefore, it is important to consider this diagnosis in patients who present with diarrhea subsequent to the administration of antibacterial agents.

Treatment with antibacterial agents alters the normal flora of the colon and may permit overgrowth of clostridia. Studies indicate that a toxin produced by *Clostridium difficile* is a primary cause of "antibiotic-associated colitis".

After the diagnosis of pseudomembranous colitis has been established, therapeutic measures should be initiated. Mild cases of pseudomembranous colitis usually respond to discontinuation of the drug alone. In moderate to severe cases, consideration should be given to management with fluid and electrolytes, protein supplementation, and treatment with an antibacterial drug clinically effective against *Clostridium difficile colitis.*

Helicobater pylori Eradication at ≥ 6 Weeks After The End of Treatment

	Treatment Group Percent (%) of Patients Cured (Number of Patients)		Difference (RAC – OAC) [95% Confidence Interval]
	7-day RAC*	**10-day OAC**	
Per Protocol[a]	84.3% (N=166)	81.6% (N=179)	2.8 [–5.2, 10.7]
Intent-to-Treat[b]	77.3% (N=194)	73.3% (N=206)	4.0 [–4.4, 12.5]
	10-day RAC*	**10-day OAC**	
Per Protocol[a]	86.0% (N=171)	81.6% (N=179)	4.4 [–3.3, 12.1]
Intent-to-Treat[b]	78.1% (N=196)	73.3% (N=206)	4.8 [–3.6, 13.2]
	3-day RAC	**10-day OAC**	
Per Protocol[a]	29.9% (N=167)	81.6% (N=179)	–51.6 [–60.6,–42.6]
Intent-to-Treat[b]	27.3% (N=187)	73.3% (N=206)	–46.0 [–54.8, –37.2]

[a] Patients were included in the analysis if they had *H. pylori* infection documented at baseline, defined as a positive ^{13}C-UBT plus rapid urease test or culture and were not protocol violators. Patients who dropped out of the study due to an adverse event related to the study drug were included in the evaluable analysis as failures of therapy.
[b] Patients were included in the analysis if they had documented *H. pylori* infection at baseline as defined above and took at least one dose of study medication. All dropouts were included as failures of therapy.
* The 95% confidence intervals for the difference in eradication rates for 7-day RAC minus 10-day RAC are (–9.3, 6.0) in the PP population and (–9.0, 7.5) in the ITT population.

PRECAUTIONS

General

Symptomatic response to therapy with rabeprazole does not preclude the presence of gastric malignancy.

Patients with healed GERD were treated for up to 40 months with rabeprazole and monitored with serial gastric biopsies. Patients without *H. pylori* infection (221 of 326 patients) had no clinically important pathologic changes in the gastric mucosa. Patients with *H. pylori* infection at baseline (105 of 326 patients) had mild or moderate inflammation in the gastric body or mild inflammation in the gastric antrum. Patients with mild grades of infection or inflammation in the gastric body tended to change to moderate, whereas those graded moderate at baseline tended to remain stable. Patients with mild grades of infection or inflammation in the gastric antrum tended to remain stable. At baseline 8% of patients had atrophy of glands in the gastric body and 15% had atrophy in the gastric antrum. At endpoint, 15% of patients had atrophy of glands in the gastric body and 11% had atrophy in the gastric antrum. Approximately 4% of patients had intestinal metaplasia at some point during follow-up, but no consistent changes were seen.

Steady state interactions of rabeprazole and warfarin have not been adequately evaluated in patients. There have been reports of increased INR and prothrombin time in patients receiving a proton pump inhibitor and warfarin concomitantly. Increases in INR and prothrombin time may lead to abnormal bleeding and even death. Patients treated with a proton pump inhibitor and warfarin concomitantly may need to be monitored for increases in INR and prothrombin time.

Information for Patients

Patients should be cautioned that ACIPHEX® delayed-release tablets should be swallowed whole. The tablets should not be chewed, crushed, or split. ACIPHEX® can be taken with or without food.

Drug Interactions

Rabeprazole is metabolized by the cytochrome P450 (CYP450) drug metabolizing enzyme system. Studies in healthy subjects have shown that rabeprazole does not have clinically significant interactions with other drugs metabolized by the CYP450 system, such as warfarin and theophylline given as single oral doses, diazepam as a single intravenous dose, and phenytoin given as a single intravenous dose (with supplemental oral dosing). Steady state interactions of rabeprazole and other drugs metabolized by this enzyme system have not been studied in patients. There have been reports of increased INR and prothrombin time in patients receiving proton pump inhibitors, including rabeprazole, and warfarin concomitantly. Increases in INR and prothrombin time may lead to abnormal bleeding and even death.

In vitro incubations employing human liver microsomes indicated that rabeprazole inhibited cyclosporine metabolism with an IC_{50} of 62 micromolar, a concentration that is over 50 times higher than the C_{max} in healthy volunteers following 14 days of dosing with 20 mg of rabeprazole. This degree of inhibition is similar to that by omeprazole at equivalent concentrations.

Rabeprazole produces sustained inhibition of gastric acid secretion. An interaction with compounds which are dependent on gastric pH for absorption may occur due to the magnitude of acid suppression observed with rabeprazole. For example, in normal subjects, co-administration of rabeprazole 20 mg QD resulted in an approximately 30% decrease in the bioavailability of ketoconazole and increases in the AUC and C_{max} for digoxin of 19% and 29%, respectively. Therefore, patients may need to be monitored when such drugs are taken concomitantly with rabeprazole. Co-administration of rabeprazole and antacids produced no clinically relevant changes in plasma rabeprazole concentrations.

In a clinical study in Japan evaluating rabeprazole in patients categorized by CYP2C19 genotype (n=6 per genotype category), gastric acid suppression was higher in poor metabolizers as compared to extensive metabolizers. This could be due to higher rabeprazole plasma levels in poor metabolizers. Whether or not interactions of rabeprazole sodium with other drugs metabolized by CYP2C19 would be different between extensive metabolizers and poor metabolizers has not been studied.

Combined Administration with Clarithromycin

Combined administration consisting of rabeprazole, amoxicillin, and clarithromycin resulted in increases in plasma concentrations of rabeprazole and 14-hydroxyclarithromycin. (See **CLINICAL PHARMACOLOGY, Combination Therapy with Antimicrobials.**)

Concomitant administration of clarithromycin with pimozide and cisapride is contraindicated. (See **PRECAUTIONS** in prescribing information for clarithromycin.) (See **PRECAUTIONS** in prescribing information for amoxicillin.)

Carcinogenesis, Mutagenesis, Impairment of Fertility

In a 88/104-week carcinogenicity study in CD-1 mice, rabeprazole at oral doses up to 100 mg/kg/day did not produce any increased tumor occurrence. The highest tested dose produced a systemic exposure to rabeprazole (AUC) of 1.40 µg•hr/mL which is 1.6 times the human exposure (plasma $AUC_{0-\infty}$ = 0.88 µg•hr/mL) at the recommended dose for GERD (20 mg/day). In a 104-week carcinogenicity study in Sprague-Dawley rats, males were treated with oral doses of 5, 15, 30 and 60 mg/kg/day and females with 5, 15, 30, 60 and 120 mg/kg/day. Rabeprazole produced gastric enterochromaffin-like (ECL) cell hyperplasia in male and female rats and ECL cell carcinoid tumors in female rats at all doses including the lowest tested dose. The lowest dose (5 mg/kg/day) produced a systemic exposure to rabeprazole (AUC) of about 0.1 µg•hr/mL which is about 0.1 times the human exposure at the recommended dose for GERD. In male rats, no treatment related tumors were observed at doses up to 60 mg/kg/day producing a rabeprazole plasma exposure (AUC) of about 0.2 µg•hr/mL (0.2 times the human exposure at the recommended dose for GERD).

Rabeprazole was positive in the Ames test, the Chinese hamster ovary cell (CHO/HGPRT) forward gene mutation test and the mouse lymphoma cell (L5178Y/TK+/–) forward gene mutation test. Its demethylated-metabolite was also positive in the Ames test. Rabeprazole was negative in the *in vitro* Chinese hamster lung cell chromosome aberration test, the *in vivo* mouse micronucleus test, and the *in vivo* and *ex vivo* rat hepatocyte unscheduled DNA synthesis (UDS) tests.

Rabeprazole at intravenous doses up to 30 mg/kg/day (plasma AUC of 8.8 µg•hr/mL, about 10 times the human exposure at the recommended dose for GERD) was found to have no effect on fertility and reproductive performance of male and female rats.

Pregnancy

Teratogenic Effects. Pregnancy Category B: Teratology studies have been performed in rats at intravenous doses up to 50 mg/kg/day (plasma AUC of 11.8 µg•hr/mL, about 13 times the human exposure at the recommended dose for GERD) and rabbits at intravenous doses up to 30 mg/kg/day (plasma AUC of 7.3 µg•hr/mL, about 8 times the human exposure at the recommended dose for GERD) and have revealed no evidence of impaired fertility or harm to the fetus due to rabeprazole. There are, however, no adequate and well-controlled studies in pregnant women. Because animal reproduction studies are not always predictive of human response, this drug should be used during pregnancy only if clearly needed.

Nursing Mothers

Following intravenous administration of ^{14}C-labeled rabeprazole to lactating rats, radioactivity in milk reached levels that were 2- to 7-fold higher than levels in the blood. It is not known if unmetabolized rabeprazole is excreted in human breast milk. Administration of rabeprazole to rats in late gestation and during lactation at doses of 400 mg/kg/day (about 195-times the human dose based on mg/m^2) resulted in decreases in body weight gain of the pups. Since many drugs are excreted in milk, and because of the potential for adverse reactions to nursing infants from rabeprazole, a decision should be made to discontinue nursing or discontinue the drug, taking into account the importance of the drug to the mother.

Pediatric Use

The safety and effectiveness of rabeprazole in pediatric patients have not been established.

Use in Women

Duodenal ulcer and erosive esophagitis healing rates in women are similar to those in men. Adverse events and laboratory test abnormalities in women occurred at rates similar to those in men.

Geriatric Use

Of the total number of subjects in clinical studies of ACIPHEX®, 19% were 65 years and over, while 4% were 75 years and over. No overall differences in safety or effectiveness were observed between these subjects and younger subjects, and other reported clinical experience has not identified differences in responses between the elderly and younger patients, but greater sensitivity of some older individuals cannot be ruled out.

ADVERSE REACTIONS

Worldwide, over 2900 patients have been treated with rabeprazole in Phase II-III clinical trials involving various dosages and durations of treatment. In general, rabeprazole treatment has been well-tolerated in both short-term and long-term trials. The adverse events rates were generally similar between the 10 and 20 mg doses.

Incidence in Controlled North American and European Clinical Trials

In an analysis of adverse events assessed as possibly or probably related to treatment appearing in greater than 1% of ACIPHEX® patients and appearing with greater frequency than placebo in controlled North American and European trials, the incidence of headache was 2.4% (n=1552) for ACIPHEX® versus 1.6% (n=258) for placebo.

In short and long-term studies, the following adverse events, regardless of causality, were reported in ACIPHEX®-treated patients. Rare events are those reported in ≤1/1000 patients.

Body as a Whole: asthenia, fever, allergic reaction, chills, malaise, chest pain substernal, neck rigidity, photosensitivity reaction. Rare: abdomen enlarged, face edema, hangover effect. *Cardiovascular System:* hypertension, myocardial infarct, electrocardiogram abnormal, migraine, syncope, angina pectoris, bundle branch block, palpitation, sinus bradycardia, tachycardia. Rare: bradycardia, pulmonary embolus, supraventricular tachycardia, thrombophlebitis, vasodilation, QTC prolongation and ventricular tachycardia. *Digestive System:* diarrhea, nausea, abdominal pain, vomiting, dyspepsia, flatulence, constipation, dry mouth, eructation, gastroenteritis, rectal hemorrhage, melena, anorexia, cholelithiasis, mouth ulceration, stomatitis, dysphagia, gingivitis, cholecystitis, increased appetite, abnormal stools, colitis, esophagitis, glossitis, pancreatitis, proctitis. Rare: bloody diarrhea, cholangitis, duodenitis, gastrointestinal hemorrhage, hepatic encephalopathy, hepatitis, hepatoma, liver fatty deposit, salivary gland enlargement, thirst. *Endocrine System:* hyperthyroidism, hypothyroidism. *Hemic & Lymphatic System:* anemia, ecchymosis, lymphadenopathy, hypochromic anemia. *Metabolic & Nutritional Disorders:* peripheral edema, edema, weight gain, gout, dehydration, weight loss. *Musculo-Skeletal System:* myalgia, arthritis, leg cramps, bone pain, arthrosis, bursitis. Rare: twitching. *Nervous System:* insomnia, anxiety, dizziness, depression, nervousness, somnolence, hypertonia, neuralgia, vertigo, convulsion, abnormal dreams, libido decreased, neuropathy, paresthesia, tremor. Rare: agitation, amnesia, confusion, extrapyramidal syndrome, hyperkinesia. *Respiratory System:* dyspnea, asthma, epistaxis, laryngitis, hiccup, hyperventilation. Rare: apnea, hypoventilation. *Skin and Appendages:* rash, pruritus, sweating, urticaria, alopecia. Rare: dry skin, herpes zoster, psoriasis, skin discoloration. *Special Senses:* cataract, amblyopia, glaucoma, dry eyes, abnormal vision, tinnitus, otitis media. Rare: corneal opacity, blurry vision, diplopia, deafness, eye pain, retinal degeneration, strabismus. *Urogenital System:* cystitis, urinary frequency, dysmenorrhea, dysuria, kidney calculus, metrorrhagia, polyuria. Rare: breast enlargement, hematuria, impotence, leukorrhea, menorrhagia, orchitis, urinary incontinence.

Laboratory Values: The following changes in laboratory parameters were reported as adverse events: abnormal platelets, albuminuria, creatine phosphokinase increased, erythrocytes abnormal, hypercholesteremia, hyperglycemia, hyperlipemia, hypokalemia, hyponatremia, leukocytosis, leukorrhea, liver function tests abnormal, prostatic specific antigen increase, SGPT increased, urine abnormality, WBC abnormal.

In controlled clinical studies, 3/1456 (0.2%) patients treated with rabeprazole and 2/237 (0.8%) patients treated with placebo developed treatment-emergent abnormalities (which were either new on study or present at study entry with an increase of 1.25 × baseline value) in SGOT (AST), SGPT (ALT), or both. None of the three rabeprazole patients experienced chills, fever, right upper quadrant pain, nausea or jaundice.

Combination Treatment with Amoxicillin and Clarithromycin: In clinical trials using combination therapy with rabeprazole plus amoxicillin and clarithromycin (RAC), no adverse events unique to this drug combination were observed. In the U.S. multicenter study, the most frequently reported drug related adverse events for patients who received RAC therapy for 7 or 10 days were diarrhea (8% and 7%) and taste perversion (6% and 10%), respectively.

No clinically significant laboratory abnormalities particular to the drug combinations were observed.

For more information on adverse events or laboratory changes with amoxicillin or clarithromycin, refer to their respective package prescribing information, **ADVERSE REACTIONS** section.

Post-Marketing Adverse Events: Additional adverse events reported from worldwide marketing experience with rabeprazole sodium are: sudden death; coma and hyperammonemia; jaundice; rhabdomyolysis; disorientation and delirium; anaphylaxis; angioedema; bullous and other drug eruptions of the skin; severe dermatologic reactions, including toxic epidermal necrolysis (some fatal), Stevens-Johnson syndrome, and erythema multiforme; interstitial pneumonia; interstitial nephritis; and TSH elevations. In most instances, the relationship to rabeprazole sodium was unclear. In addition, agranulocytosis, hemolytic anemia, leukopenia, pancytopenia, and thrombocytopenia have been reported. Increases in prothrombin time/INR in patients treated with concomitant warfarin have been reported.

OVERDOSAGE

Because strategies for the management of overdose are continually evolving, it is advisable to contact a Poison Control Center to determine the latest recommendations for the management of an overdose of any drug. There has been no experience with large overdoses with rabeprazole. Seven reports of accidental overdosage with rabeprazole have been received. The maximum reported overdose was 80 mg. There were no clinical signs or symptoms associated with any reported overdose. Patients with Zollinger-Ellison syndrome have been treated with up to 120 mg rabeprazole QD. No specific antidote for rabeprazole is known. Rabeprazole is extensively protein bound and is not readily dialyzable. In the event of overdosage, treatment should be symptomatic and supportive.

Single oral doses of rabeprazole at 786 mg/kg and 1024 mg/kg were lethal to mice and rats, respectively. The single oral dose of 2000 mg/kg was not lethal to dogs. The major symptoms of acute toxicity were hypoactivity, labored respiration, lateral or prone position and convulsion in mice and rats and watery diarrhea, tremor, convulsion and coma in dogs.

DOSAGE AND ADMINISTRATION

Healing of Erosive or Ulcerative Gastroesophageal Reflux Disease (GERD)

The recommended adult oral dose is one ACIPHEX® 20 mg delayed-release tablet to be taken once daily for four to eight weeks. (See **INDICATIONS AND USAGE**). For those patients who have not healed after 8 weeks of treatment, an additional 8-week course of ACIPHEX® may be considered.

Maintenance of Healing of Erosive or Ulcerative Gastroesophageal Reflux Disease (GERD Maintenance)

The recommended adult oral dose is one ACIPHEX® 20 mg delayed-release tablet to be taken once daily. (See **INDICATIONS AND USAGE**).

Treatment of Symptomatic Gastroesophageal Reflux Disease (GERD)

The recommended adult oral dose is one ACIPHEX® 20 mg delayed-release tablet to be taken once daily for 4 weeks. (See **INDICATIONS AND USAGE**). If symptoms do not resolve completely after 4 weeks, an additional course of treatment may be considered.

Healing of Duodenal Ulcers

The recommended adult oral dose is one ACIPHEX® 20 mg delayed-release tablet to be taken once daily after the morning meal for a period up to four weeks. (See **INDICATIONS AND USAGE**). Most patients with duodenal ulcer heal within four weeks. A few patients may require additional therapy to achieve healing.

***Helicobacter pylori* Eradication to Reduce the Risk of Duodenal Ulcer Recurrence**

Three Drug Regimen[a]:

Aciphex	20 mg	Twice Daily for 7 Days
Amoxicillin	1000 mg	Twice Daily for 7 Days
Clarithromycin	500 mg	Twice Daily for 7 Days

All three medications should be taken twice daily with the morning and evening meals.

[a] It is important that patients comply with the full 7-day regimen. (See **CLINICAL STUDIES** section.)

Treatment of Pathological Hypersecretory Conditions Including Zollinger-Ellison Syndrome

The dosage of ACIPHEX® in patients with pathologic hypersecretory conditions varies with the individual patient. The recommended adult oral starting dose is 60 mg once a day. Doses should be adjusted to individual patient needs and should continue for as long as clinically indicated. Some patients may require divided doses. Doses up to 100 mg QD and 60 mg BID have been administered. Some patients with Zollinger-Ellison syndrome have been treated continuously with ACIPHEX® for up to one year.

No dosage adjustment is necessary in elderly patients, in patients with renal disease or in patients with mild to moderate hepatic impairment. Administration of rabeprazole to patients with mild to moderate liver impairment resulted in increased exposure and decreased elimination. Due to the lack of clinical data on rabeprazole in patients with severe hepatic impairment, caution should be exercised in those patients.

ACIPHEX® tablets should be swallowed whole. The tablets should not be chewed, crushed, or split. ACIPHEX® can be taken with or without food.

HOW SUPPLIED

ACIPHEX® 20 mg is supplied as delayed-release light yellow enteric-coated tablets. The name and strength, in mg, (ACIPHEX 20) is imprinted on one side.

Bottles of 30 (NDC#62856-243-30)

Bottles of 90 (NDC#62856-243-90)

Unit Dose Blisters Package of 100 (10 × 10) (NDC#62856-243-41)

Store at 25°C (77°F); excursions permitted to 15–30°C (59–86°F). Protect from moisture.

REFERENCES

1. National Committee for Clinical Laboratory Standards. *Methods for Dilution Antimicrobial Susceptibility Tests for Bacteria That Grow Aerobically*—Fifth Edition. Approved Standard NCCLS Document M7-A5, Vol. 20, No. 2, NCCLS, Wayne, PA, January 2000.

Rx only.

ACIPHEX® is a registered trademark of Eisai Co., Ltd., Tokyo, Japan.

Manufactured and Marketed by Eisai Inc., Teaneck, NJ 07666

Marketed by Janssen Pharmaceutica Inc., Titusville, NJ 08560

Revised August 2003

200298

Shown in Product Identification Guide, page 311

ARICEPT® ℞

[ă-rĭ-sĕpt]

(Donepezil Hydrochloride Tablets)

DESCRIPTION

ARICEPT® (donepezil hydrochloride) is a reversible inhibitor of the enzyme acetylcholinesterase, known chemically as (±)-2,3-dihydro-5,6-dimethoxy-2-[[1-(phenylmethyl)-4-piperidinyl]methyl]-1*H*-inden-1-one hydrochloride. Donepezil hydrochloride is commonly referred to in the pharmacological literature as E2020. It has an empirical formula of $C_{24}H_{29}NO_3HCl$ and a molecular weight of 415.96. Donepezil hydrochloride is a white crystalline powder and is freely soluble in chloroform, soluble in water and in glacial acetic acid, slightly soluble in ethanol and in acetonitrile and practically insoluble in ethyl acetate and in n-hexane.

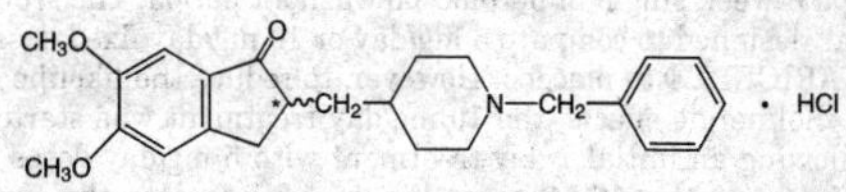

ARICEPT® is available for oral administration in film-coated tablets containing 5 or 10 mg of donepezil hydrochloride. Inactive ingredients are lactose monohydrate, corn starch, microcrystalline cellulose, hydroxypropyl cellulose, and magnesium stearate. The film coating contains talc, polyethylene glycol, hypromellose and titanium dioxide. Additionally, the 10 mg tablet contains yellow iron oxide (synthetic) as a coloring agent.

CLINICAL PHARMACOLOGY

Current theories on the pathogenesis of the cognitive signs and symptoms of Alzheimer's Disease attribute some of them to a deficiency of cholinergic neurotransmission.

Donepezil hydrochloride is postulated to exert its therapeutic effect by enhancing cholinergic function. This is accomplished by increasing the concentration of acetylcholine through reversible inhibition of its hydrolysis by acetylcholinesterase. If this proposed mechanism of action is correct, donepezil's effect may lessen as the disease process advances and fewer cholinergic neurons remain functionally intact. There is no evidence that donepezil alters the course of the underlying dementing process.

Clinical Trial Data

The effectiveness of ARICEPT® as a treatment for Alzheimer's Disease is demonstrated by the results of two randomized, double-blind, placebo-controlled clinical investigations in patients with Alzheimer's Disease (diagnosed by NINCDS and DSM III-R criteria, Mini-Mental State Examination ≥ 10 and ≤ 26 and Clinical Dementia Rating of 1 or 2). The mean age of patients participating in ARICEPT® trials was 73 years with a range of 50 to 94. Approximately 62% of patients were women and 38% were men. The racial distribution was white 95%, black 3% and other races 2%.

Study Outcome Measures: In each study, the effectiveness of treatment with ARICEPT® was evaluated using a dual outcome assessment strategy.

The ability of ARICEPT® to improve cognitive performance was assessed with the cognitive subscale of the Alzheimer's Disease Assessment Scale (ADAS-cog), a multi-item instrument that has been extensively validated in longitudinal cohorts of Alzheimer's Disease patients. The ADAS-cog examines selected aspects of cognitive performance including elements of memory, orientation, attention, reasoning, language and praxis. The ADAS-cog scoring range is from 0 to 70, with higher scores indicating greater cognitive impairment. Elderly normal adults may score as low as 0 or 1, but it is not unusual for non-demented adults to score slightly higher.

The patients recruited as participants in each study had mean scores on the Alzheimer's Disease Assessment Scale (ADAS-cog) of approximately 26 units, with a range from 4 to 61. Experience gained in longitudinal studies of ambulatory patients with mild to moderate Alzheimer's Disease suggest that they gain 6 to 12 units a year on the ADAS-cog. However, lesser degrees of change are seen in patients with very mild or very advanced disease because the ADAS-cog is not uniformly sensitive to change over the course of the disease. The annualized rate of decline in the placebo patients participating in ARICEPT® trials was approximately 2 to 4 units per year.

The ability of ARICEPT® to produce an overall clinical effect was assessed using a Clinician's Interview Based Impression of Change that required the use of caregiver information, the CIBIC plus. The CIBIC plus is not a single instrument and is not a standardized instrument like the ADAS-cog. Clinical trials for investigational drugs have used a variety of CIBIC formats, each different in terms of depth and structure. As such, results from a CIBIC plus reflect clinical experience from the trial or trials in which it was used and cannot be compared directly with the results of CIBIC plus evaluations from other clinical trials. The CIBIC plus used in ARICEPT® trials was a semi-structured instrument that was intended to examine four major areas of patient function: General, Cognitive, Behavioral and Activities of Daily Living. It represents the assessment of a skilled clinician based upon his/her observations at an interview with the patient, in combination with information supplied by a caregiver familiar with the behavior of the patient over the interval rated. The CIBIC plus is scored as a seven point categorical rating, ranging from a score of 1, indicating "markedly improved," to a score of 4, indicating "no change" to a score of 7, indicating "markedly worse." The

Continued on next page

Aricept—Cont.

CIBIC plus has not been systematically compared directly to assessments not using information from caregivers (CIBIC) or other global methods.

Thirty-Week Study

In a study of 30 weeks duration, 473 patients were randomized to receive single daily doses of placebo, 5 mg/day or 10 mg/day of ARICEPT®. The 30-week study was divided into a 24-week double-blind active treatment phase followed by a 6-week single-blind placebo washout period. The study was designed to compare 5 mg/day or 10 mg/day fixed doses of ARICEPT® to placebo. However, to reduce the likelihood of cholinergic effects, the 10 mg/day treatment was started following an initial 7-day treatment with 5 mg/day doses.

Effects on the ADAS-cog: Figure 1 illustrates the time course for the change from baseline in ADAS-cog scores for all three dose groups over the 30 weeks of the study. After 24 weeks of treatment, the mean differences in the ADAS-cog change scores for ARICEPT® treated patients compared to the patients on placebo were 2.8 and 3.1 units for the 5 mg/day and 10 mg/day treatments, respectively. These differences were statistically significant. While the treatment effect size may appear to be slightly greater for the 10 mg/day treatment, there was no statistically significant difference between the two active treatments.

Following 6 weeks of placebo washout, scores on the ADAS-cog for both the ARICEPT® treatment groups were indistinguishable from those patients who had received only placebo for 30 weeks. This suggests that the beneficial effects of ARICEPT® abate over 6 weeks following discontinuation of treatment and do not represent a change in the underlying disease. There was no evidence of a rebound effect 6 weeks after abrupt discontinuation of therapy.

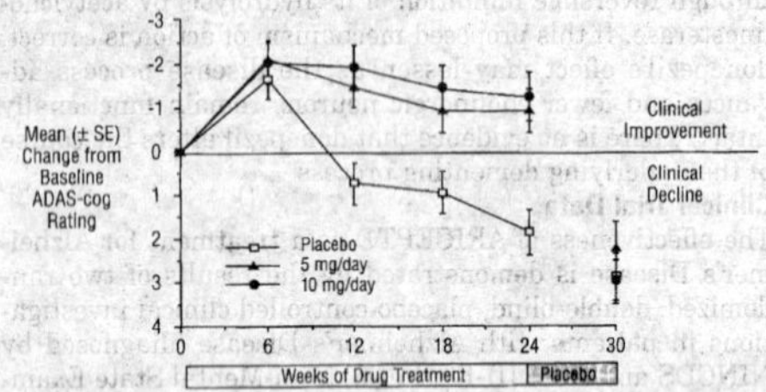

Figure 1. Time-course of the Change from Baseline in ADAS-cog Score for Patients Completing 24 Weeks of Treatment.

Figure 2 illustrates the cumulative percentages of patients from each of the three treatment groups who had attained the measure of improvement in ADAS-cog score shown on the X axis. Three change scores, (7-point and 4-point reductions from baseline or no change in score) have been identified for illustrative purposes and the percent of patients in each group achieving that result is shown in the inset table. The curves demonstrate that both patients assigned to placebo and ARICEPT® have a wide range of responses, but that the active treatment groups are more likely to show the greater improvements. A curve for an effective treatment would be shifted to the left of the curve for placebo, while an ineffective or deleterious treatment would be superimposed upon or shifted to the right of the curve for placebo, respectively.

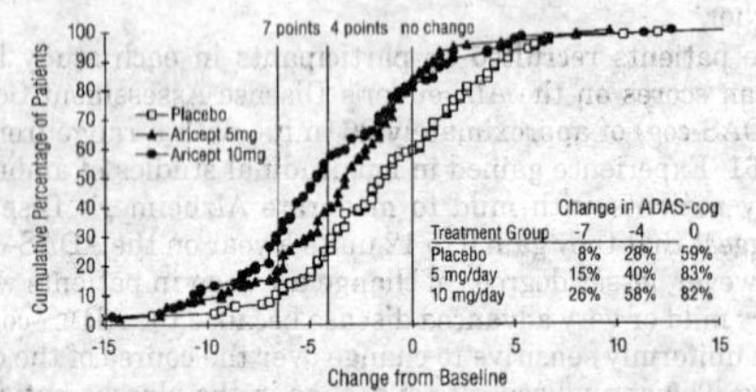

Figure 2. Cumulative Percentage of Patients Completing 24 Weeks of Double-blind Treatment with Specified Changes from Baseline ADAS-cog Scores. The Percentages of Randomized Patients who Completed the Study were: Placebo 80%, 5 mg/day 85% and 10 mg/day 68%.

Effects on the CIBIC plus: Figure 3 is a histogram of the frequency distribution of CIBIC plus scores attained by patients assigned to each of the three treatment groups who completed 24 weeks of treatment. The mean drug-placebo differences for these groups of patients were 0.35 units and 0.39 units for 5 mg/day and 10 mg/day of ARICEPT®, respectively. These differences were statistically significant. There was no statistically significant difference between the two active treatments.

[See figure at top of next column]

Fifteen-Week Study

In a study of 15 weeks duration, patients were randomized to receive single daily doses of placebo or either 5 mg/day or 10 mg/day of ARICEPT® for 12 weeks, followed by a 3-week placebo washout period. As in the 30-week study, to avoid acute cholinergic effects, the 10 mg/day treatment followed an initial 7-day treatment with 5 mg/day doses.

Effects on the ADAS-Cog: Figure 4 illustrates the time course of the change from baseline in ADAS-cog scores for all three dose groups over the 15 weeks of the study. After 12 weeks of treatment, the differences in mean ADAS-cog change scores for the ARICEPT® treated patients compared to the patients on placebo were 2.7 and 3.0 units each, for

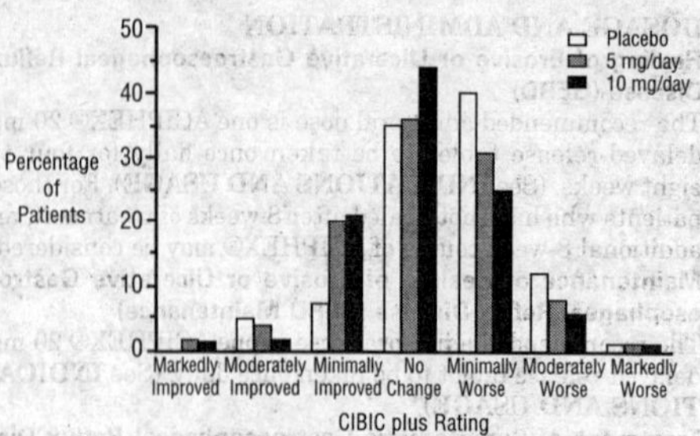

Figure 3. Frequency Distribution of CIBIC plus Scores at Week 24

the 5 and 10 mg/day ARICEPT® treatment groups respectively. These differences were statistically significant. The effect size for the 10 mg/day group may appear to be slightly larger than that for 5 mg/day. However, the differences between active treatments were not statistically significant.

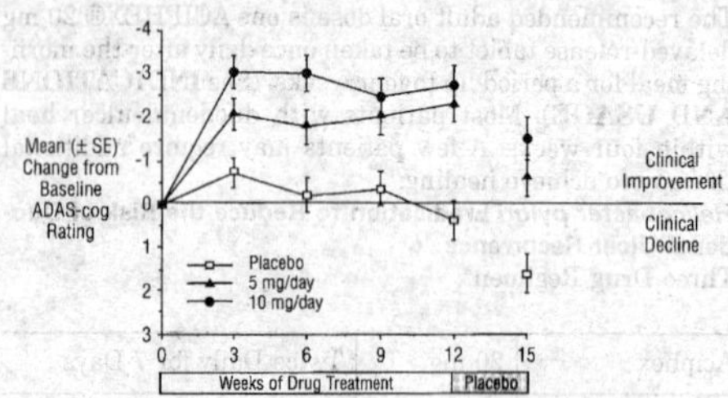

Figure 4. Time-course of the Change from Baseline in ADAS-cog Score for Patients Completing the 15-week Study.

Following 3 weeks of placebo washout, scores on the ADAS-cog for both the ARICEPT® treatment groups increased, indicating that discontinuation of ARICEPT® resulted in a loss of its treatment effect. The duration of this placebo washout period was not sufficient to characterize the rate of loss of the treatment effect, but, the 30-week study (see above) demonstrated that treatment effects associated with the use of ARICEPT® abate within 6 weeks of treatment discontinuation.

Figure 5 illustrates the cumulative percentages of patients from each of the three treatment groups who attained the measure of improvement in ADAS-cog score shown on the X axis. The same three change scores, (7-point and 4-point reductions from baseline or no change in score) as selected for the 30-week study have been used for this illustration. The percentages of patients achieving those results are shown in the inset table.

As observed in the 30-week study, the curves demonstrate that patients assigned to either placebo or to ARICEPT® have a wide range of responses, but that the ARICEPT® treated patients are more likely to show the greater improvements in cognitive performance.

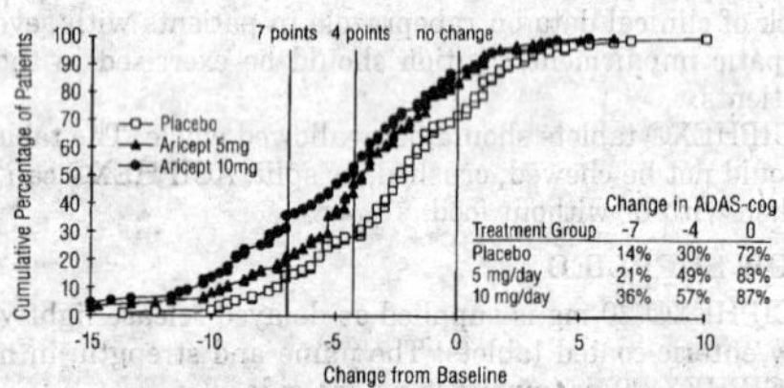

Figure 5. Cumulative Percentage of Patients with Specified Changes from Baseline ADAS-cog Scores. The Percentages of Randomized Patients Within Each Treatment Group Who Completed the Study Were: Placebo 93%, 5 mg/day 90% and 10 mg/day 82%.

Effects on the CIBIC plus: Figure 6 is a histogram of the frequency distribution of CIBIC plus scores attained by patients assigned to each of the three treatment groups who completed 12 weeks of treatment. The differences in mean scores for ARICEPT® treated patients compared to the patients on placebo at Week 12 were 0.36 and 0.38 units for the 5 mg/day and 10 mg/day treatment groups, respectively. These differences were statistically significant.

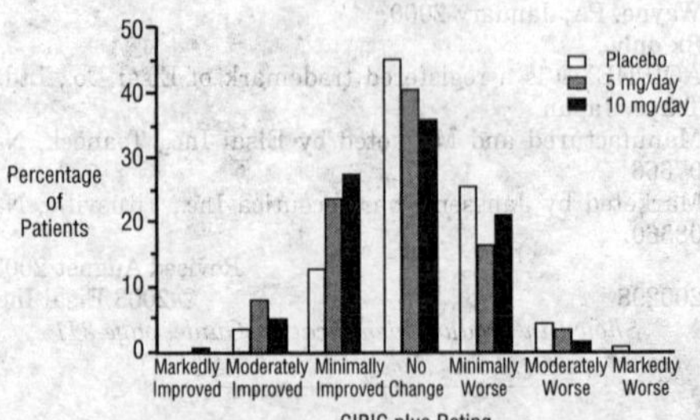

Figure 6. Frequency Distribution of CIBIC plus Scores at Week 12

In both studies, patient age, sex and race were not found to predict the clinical outcome of ARICEPT® treatment.

Clinical Pharmacokinetics

Donepezil is well absorbed with a relative oral bioavailability of 100% and reaches peak plasma concentrations in 3 to 4 hours. Pharmacokinetics are linear over a dose range of 1-10 mg given once daily. Neither food nor time of administration (morning vs. evening dose) influences the rate or extent of absorption. The elimination half life of donepezil is about 70 hours and the mean apparent plasma clearance (Cl/F) is 0.13 L/hr/kg. Following multiple dose administration, donepezil accumulates in plasma by 4-7 fold and steady state is reached within 15 days. The steady state volume of distribution is 12 L/kg. Donepezil is approximately 96% bound to human plasma proteins, mainly to albumins (about 75%) and alpha$_1$ - acid glycoprotein (about 21%) over the concentration range of 2-1000 ng/mL.

Donepezil is both excreted in the urine intact and extensively metabolized to four major metabolites, two of which are known to be active, and a number of minor metabolites, not all of which have been identified. Donepezil is metabolized by CYP 450 isoenzymes 2D6 and 3A4 and undergoes glucuronidation. Following administration of ^{14}C-labeled donepezil, plasma radioactivity, expressed as a percent of the administered dose, was present primarily as intact donepezil (53%) and as 6-O-desmethyl donepezil (11%), which has been reported to inhibit AChE to the same extent as donepezil *in vitro* and was found in plasma at concentrations equal to about 20% of donepezil. Approximately 57% and 15% of the total radioactivity was recovered in urine and feces, respectively, over a period of 10 days, while 28% remained unrecovered, with about 17% of the donepezil dose recovered in the urine as unchanged drug.

Special Populations:

Hepatic Disease: In a study of 10 patients with stable alcoholic cirrhosis, the clearance of ARICEPT® was decreased by 20% relative to 10 healthy age and sex matched subjects.

Renal Disease: In a study of 11 patients with moderate to severe renal impairment ($Cl_{Cr} < 18$ mL/min/1.73 m^2) the clearance of ARICEPT® did not differ from 11 age and sex matched healthy subjects.

Age: No formal pharmacokinetic study was conducted to examine age related differences in the pharmacokinetics of ARICEPT®. However, mean plasma ARICEPT® concentrations measured during therapeutic drug monitoring of elderly patients with Alzheimer's Disease are comparable to those observed in young healthy volunteers.

Gender and Race: No specific pharmacokinetic study was conducted to investigate the effects of gender and race on the disposition of ARICEPT®. However, retrospective pharmacokinetic analysis indicates that gender and race (Japanese and Caucasians) did not affect the clearance of ARICEPT®.

Drug-Drug Interactions

Drugs Highly Bound to Plasma Proteins: Drug displacement studies have been performed *in vitro* between this highly bound drug (96%) and other drugs such as furosemide, digoxin, and warfarin. ARICEPT® at concentrations of 0.3-10 µg/mL did not affect the binding of furosemide (5 µg/mL), digoxin (2 ng/mL), and warfarin (3 µg/mL) to human albumin. Similarly, the binding of ARICEPT® to human albumin was not affected by furosemide, digoxin and warfarin.

Effect of ARICEPT® on the Metabolism of Other Drugs: No *in vivo* clinical trials have investigated the effect of ARICEPT® on the clearance of drugs metabolized by CYP 3A4 (e.g. cisapride, terfenadine) or by CYP 2D6 (e.g. imipramine). However, *in vitro* studies show a low rate of binding to these enzymes (mean K_i about 50-130 µM), that, given the therapeutic plasma concentrations of donepezil (164 nM), indicates little likelihood of interference.

Whether ARICEPT® has any potential for enzyme induction is not known.

Formal pharmacokinetic studies evaluated the potential of ARICEPT® for interaction with theophylline, cimetidine, warfarin, digoxin and ketoconazole. No effects of ARICEPT® on the pharmacokinetics of these drugs were observed.

Effect of Other Drugs on the Metabolism of ARICEPT®: Ketoconazole and quinidine, inhibitors of CYP450, 3A4 and 2D6, respectively, inhibit donepezil metabolism *in vitro*. Whether there is a clinical effect of quinidine is not known. In a 7-day crossover study in 18 healthy volunteers, ketoconazole (200mg q.d.) increased mean donepezil (5mg q.d.) concentrations ($AUC_{0\text{-}24}$ and C_{max}) by 36%. The clinical relevance of this increase in concentration is unknown.

Inducers of CYP 2D6 and CYP 3A4 (e.g., phenytoin, carbamazepine, dexamethasone, rifampin, and phenobarbital) could increase the rate of elimination of ARICEPT®.

Formal pharmacokinetic studies demonstrated that the metabolism of ARICEPT® is not significantly affected by concurrent administration of digoxin or cimetidine.

INDICATIONS AND USAGE

ARICEPT® is indicated for the treatment of mild to moderate dementia of the Alzheimer's type.

CONTRAINDICATIONS

ARICEPT® is contraindicated in patients with known hypersensitivity to donepezil hydrochloride or to piperidine derivatives.

WARNINGS

Anesthesia: ARICEPT®, as a cholinesterase inhibitor, is likely to exaggerate succinylcholine-type muscle relaxation during anesthesia.

Cardiovascular Conditions: Because of their pharmacological action, cholinesterase inhibitors may have vagotonic effects on the sinoatrial and atrioventricular nodes. This effect may manifest as bradycardia or heart block in patients both with and without known underlying cardiac conduction abnormalities. Syncopal episodes have been reported in association with the use of ARICEPT®.

Gastrointestinal Conditions: Through their primary action, cholinesterase inhibitors may be expected to increase gastric acid secretion due to increased cholinergic activity. Therefore, patients should be monitored closely for symptoms of active or occult gastrointestinal bleeding, especially those at increased risk for developing ulcers, e.g., those with a history of ulcer disease or those receiving concurrent nonsteroidal anti-inflammatory drugs (NSAIDS). Clinical studies of ARICEPT® have shown no increase, relative to placebo, in the incidence of either peptic ulcer disease or gastrointestinal bleeding.

ARICEPT®, as a predictable consequence of its pharmacological properties, has been shown to produce diarrhea, nausea and vomiting. These effects, when they occur, appear more frequently with the 10 mg/day dose than with the 5 mg/day dose. In most cases, these effects have been mild and transient, sometimes lasting one to three weeks, and have resolved during continued use of ARICEPT®.

Genitourinary: Although not observed in clinical trials of ARICEPT®, cholinomimetics may cause bladder outflow obstruction.

Neurological Conditions: Seizures: Cholinomimetics are believed to have some potential to cause generalized convulsions. However, seizure activity also may be a manifestation of Alzheimer's Disease.

Pulmonary Conditions: Because of their cholinomimetic actions, cholinesterase inhibitors should be prescribed with care to patients with a history of asthma or obstructive pulmonary disease.

PRECAUTIONS

Drug-Drug Interactions (see Clinical Pharmacology: Clinical Pharmacokinetics: Drug-drug Interactions)

Effect of ARICEPT® on the Metabolism of Other Drugs: No *in vivo* clinical trials have investigated the effect of ARICEPT® on the clearance of drugs metabolized by CYP 3A4 (e.g. cisapride, terfenadine) or by CYP 2D6 (e.g. imipramine). However, *in vitro* studies show a low rate of binding to these enzymes (mean K_i about 50-130 μM), that, given the therapeutic plasma concentrations of donepezil (164 nM), indicates little likelihood of interference.

Whether ARICEPT® has any potential for enzyme induction is not known.

Formal pharmacokinetic studies evaluated the potential of ARICEPT® for interaction with theophylline, cimetidine, warfarin, digoxin and ketoconazole. No effects of ARICEPT® on the pharmacokinetics of these drugs were observed.

Effect of Other Drugs on the Metabolism of ARICEPT®: Ketoconazole and quinidine, inhibitors of CYP450, 3A4 and 2D6, respectively, inhibit donepezil metabolism *in vitro*. Whether there is a clinical effect of quinidine is not known. In a 7-day crossover study in 18 healthy volunteers, ketoconazole (200mg q.d.) increased mean donepezil (5mg q.d.) concentrations (AUC_{0-24} and C_{max}) by 36%. The clinical relevance of this increase in concentration is unknown.

Inducers of CYP 2D6 and CYP 3A4 (e.g., phenytoin, carbamazepine, dexamethasone, rifampin, and phenobarbital) could increase the rate of elimination of ARICEPT®.

Formal pharmacokinetic studies demonstrated that the metabolism of ARICEPT® is not significantly affected by concurrent administration of digoxin or cimetidine.

Use with Anticholinergics: Because of their mechanism of action, cholinesterase inhibitors have the potential to interfere with the activity of anticholinergic medications.

Use with Cholinomimetics and Other Cholinesterase Inhibitors: A synergistic effect may be expected when cholinesterase inhibitors are given concurrently with succinylcholine, similar neuromuscular blocking agents or cholinergic agonists such as bethanechol.

Carcinogenesis, Mutagenesis, Impairment of Fertility

No evidence of a carcinogenic potential was obtained in an 88-week carcinogenicity study of donepezil hydrochloride conducted in CD-1 mice at doses up to 180 mg/kg/day (approximately 90 times the maximum recommended human dose on a mg/m^2 basis), or in a 104-week carcinogenicity study in Sprague-Dawley rats at doses up to 30mg/kg/day (approximately 30 times the maximum recommended human dose on a mg/m^2 basis).

Donepezil was not mutagenic in the Ames reverse mutation assay in bacteria, or in a mouse lymphoma forward mutation assay *in vitro*. In the chromosome aberration test in cultures of Chinese hamster lung (CHL) cells, some clastogenic effects were observed. Donepezil was not clastogenic in the *in vivo* mouse micronucleus test and was not genotoxic in an *in vivo* unscheduled DNA synthesis assay in rats. Donepezil had no effect on fertility in rats at doses up to 10 mg/kg/day (approximately 8 times the maximum recommended human dose on a mg/m^2 basis).

Pregnancy

Pregnancy Category C: Teratology studies conducted in pregnant rats at doses up to 16 mg/kg/day (approximately 13 times the maximum recommended human dose on a mg/m^2 basis) and in pregnant rabbits at doses up to 10 mg/kg/day (approximately 16 times the maximum recommended human dose on a mg/m^2 basis) did not disclose any evidence for a teratogenic potential of donepezil. However, in a study in which pregnant rats were given up to 10 mg/kg/day (approximately 8 times the maximum recommended human dose on a mg/m^2 basis) from day 17 of gestation through day 20 postpartum, there was a slight increase in still births and a slight decrease in pup survival through day 4 postpartum at this dose; the next lower dose tested was 3 mg/kg/day. There are no adequate or well-controlled studies in pregnant women. ARICEPT® should be used during pregnancy only if the potential benefit justifies the potential risk to the fetus.

Nursing Mothers

It is not known whether donepezil is excreted in human breast milk. ARICEPT® has no indication for use in nursing mothers.

Pediatric Use

There are no adequate and well-controlled trials to document the safety and efficacy of ARICEPT® in any illness occurring in children.

Geriatric Use

Alzheimer's disease is a disorder occurring primarily in individuals over 55 years of age. The mean age of patients enrolled in the clinical studies with ARICEPT® was 73 years; 80% of these patients were between 65 and 84 years old and 49% of patients were at or above the age of 75. The efficacy and safety data presented in the clinical trials section were obtained from these patients. There were no clinically significant differences in most adverse events reported by patient groups ≥ 65 years old and < 65 years old.

ADVERSE REACTIONS

Adverse Events Leading to Discontinuation

The rates of discontinuation from controlled clinical trials of ARICEPT® due to adverse events for the ARICEPT® 5 mg/day treatment groups were comparable to those of placebo-treatment groups at approximately 5%. The rate of discontinuation of patients who received 7-day escalations from 5 mg/day to 10 mg/day, was higher at 13%.

The most common adverse events leading to discontinuation, defined as those occurring in at least 2% of patients and at twice the incidence seen in placebo patients, are shown in Table 1.

Table 1. Most Frequent Adverse Events Leading to Withdrawal from Controlled Clinical Trials by Dose Group

Dose Group	Placebo	5 mg/day ARICEPT®	10 mg/day ARICEPT®
Patients Randomized	355	350	315
Event/% Discontinuing			
Nausea	1%	1%	3%
Diarrhea	0%	<1%	3%
Vomiting	<1%	<1%	2%

Most Frequent Adverse Clinical Events Seen in Association with the Use of ARICEPT®

The most common adverse events, defined as those occurring at a frequency of at least 5% in patients receiving 10 mg/day and twice the placebo rate, are largely predicted by ARICEPT®'s cholinomimetic effects. These include nausea, diarrhea, insomnia, vomiting, muscle cramp, fatigue and anorexia. These adverse events were often of mild intensity and transient, resolving during continued ARICEPT® treatment without the need for dose modification.

There is evidence to suggest that the frequency of these common adverse events may be affected by the rate of titration. An open-label study was conducted with 269 patients who received placebo in the 15 and 30-week studies. These patients were titrated to a dose of 10 mg/day over a 6-week period. The rates of common adverse events were lower than those seen in patients titrated to 10 mg/day over one week in the controlled clinical trials and were comparable to those seen in patients on 5 mg/day.

See Table 2 for a comparison of the most common adverse events following one and six week titration regimens.

Table 2. Comparison of rates of adverse events in patients titrated to 10 mg/day over 1 and 6 weeks

	No titration		One week titration	Six week titration
Adverse Event	Placebo (n=315)	5 mg/day (n=311)	10 mg/day (n=315)	10 mg/day (n=269)
Nausea	6%	5%	19%	6%
Diarrhea	5%	8%	15%	9%
Insomnia	6%	6%	14%	6%
Fatigue	3%	4%	8%	3%
Vomiting	3%	3%	8%	5%
Muscle cramps	2%	6%	8%	3%
Anorexia	2%	3%	7%	3%

Adverse Events Reported in Controlled Trials

The events cited reflect experience gained under closely monitored conditions of clinical trials in a highly selected patient population. In actual clinical practice or in other clinical trials, these frequency estimates may not apply, as the conditions of use, reporting behavior, and the kinds of patients treated may differ. Table 3 lists treatment emergent signs and symptoms that were reported in at least 2% of patients in placebo-controlled trials who received ARICEPT® and for which the rate of occurrence was greater for ARICEPT® assigned than placebo assigned patients. In general, adverse events occurred more frequently in female patients and with advancing age.

Table 3. Adverse Events Reported in Controlled Clinical Trials in at Least 2% of Patients Receiving ARICEPT® and at a Higher Frequency than Placebo-treated Patients

Body System/Adverse Event	Placebo (n=355)	ARICEPT® (n=747)
Percent of Patients with any Adverse Event	72	74
Body as a Whole		
Headache	9	10
Pain, various locations	8	9
Accident	6	7
Fatigue	3	5
Cardiovascular System		
Syncope	1	2
Digestive System		
Nausea	6	11
Diarrhea	5	10
Vomiting	3	5
Anorexia	2	4
Hemic and Lymphatic System		
Ecchymosis	3	4
Metabolic and Nutritional Systems		
Weight Decrease	1	3
Musculoskeletal System		
Muscle Cramps	2	6
Arthritis	1	2
Nervous System		
Insomnia	6	9
Dizziness	6	8
Depression	<1	3
Abnormal Dreams	0	3
Somnolence	<1	2
Urogenital System		
Frequent Urination	1	2

Other Adverse Events Observed During Clinical Trials

ARICEPT® has been administered to over 1700 individuals during clinical trials worldwide. Approximately 1200 of these patients have been treated for at least 3 months and more than 1000 patients have been treated for at least 6 months. Controlled and uncontrolled trials in the United States included approximately 900 patients. In regards to the highest dose of 10 mg/day, this population includes 650 patients treated for 3 months, 475 patients treated for 6 months and 116 patients treated for over 1 year. The range of patient exposure is from 1 to 1214 days.

Treatment emergent signs and symptoms that occurred during 3 controlled clinical trials and two open-label trials in the United States were recorded as adverse events by the clinical investigators using terminology of their own choosing. To provide an overall estimate of the proportion of individuals having similar types of events, the events were grouped into a smaller number of standardized categories using a modified COSTART dictionary and event frequencies were calculated across all studies. These categories are used in the listing below. The frequencies represent the proportion of 900 patients from these trials who experienced that event while receiving ARICEPT®. All adverse events occurring at least twice are included, except for those al-

Continued on next page

Aricept—Cont.

ready listed in Tables 2 or 3, COSTART terms too general to be informative, or events less likely to be drug caused. Events are classified by body system and listed using the following definitions: *frequent adverse events* - those occurring in at least 1/100 patients; *infrequent adverse events* - those occurring in 1/100 to 1/1000 patients. These adverse events are not necessarily related to ARICEPT® treatment and in most cases were observed at a similar frequency in placebo-treated patients in the controlled studies. No important additional adverse events were seen in studies conducted outside the United States.

Body as a Whole: *Frequent:* influenza, chest pain, toothache; *Infrequent:* fever, edema face, periorbital edema, hernia hiatal, abscess, cellulitis, chills, generalized coldness, head fullness, listlessness.

Cardiovascular System: *Frequent:* hypertension, vasodilation, atrial fibrillation, hot flashes, hypotension; *Infrequent:* angina pectoris, postural hypotension, myocardial infarction, AV block (first degree), congestive heart failure, arteritis, bradycardia, peripheral vascular disease, supraventricular tachycardia, deep vein thrombosis.

Digestive System: *Frequent:* fecal incontinence, gastrointestinal bleeding, bloating, epigastric pain; *Infrequent:* eructation, gingivitis, increased appetite, flatulence, periodontal abscess, cholelithiasis, diverticulitis, drooling, dry mouth, fever sore, gastritis, irritable colon, tongue edema, epigastric distress, gastroenteritis, increased transaminases, hemorrhoids, ileus, increased thirst, jaundice, melena, polydipsia, duodenal ulcer, stomach ulcer.

Endocrine System: *Infrequent:* diabetes mellitus, goiter.

Hemic and Lymphatic System: *Infrequent:* anemia, thrombocythemia, thrombocytopenia, eosinophilia, erythrocytopenia.

Metabolic and Nutritional Disorders: *Frequent:* dehydration; *Infrequent:* gout, hypokalemia, increased creatine kinase, hyperglycemia, weight increase, increased lactate dehydrogenase.

Musculoskeletal System: *Frequent:* bone fracture; *Infrequent:* muscle weakness, muscle fasciculation.

Nervous System: *Frequent:* delusions, tremor, irritability, paresthesia, aggression, vertigo, ataxia, increased libido, restlessness, abnormal crying, nervousness, aphasia; *Infrequent:* cerebrovascular accident, intracranial hemorrhage, transient ischemic attack, emotional lability, neuralgia, coldness (localized), muscle spasm, dysphoria, gait abnormality, hypertonia, hypokinesia, neurodermatitis, numbness (localized), paranoia, dysarthria, dysphasia, hostility, decreased libido, melancholia, emotional withdrawal, nystagmus, pacing.

Respiratory System: *Frequent:* dyspnea, sore throat, bronchitis; *Infrequent:* epistaxis, post nasal drip, pneumonia, hyperventilation, pulmonary congestion, wheezing, hypoxia, pharyngitis, pleurisy, pulmonary collapse, sleep apnea, snoring.

Skin and Appendages: *Frequent:* pruritus, diaphoresis, urticaria; *Infrequent:* dermatitis, erythema, skin discoloration, hyperkeratosis, alopecia, fungal dermatitis, herpes zoster, hirsutism, skin striae, night sweats, skin ulcer.

Special Senses: *Frequent:* cataract, eye irritation, vision blurred; *Infrequent:* dry eyes, glaucoma, earache, tinnitus, blepharitis, decreased hearing, retinal hemorrhage, otitis externa, otitis media, bad taste, conjunctival hemorrhage, ear buzzing, motion sickness, spots before eyes.

Urogenital System: *Frequent:* urinary incontinence, nocturia; *Infrequent:* dysuria, hematuria, urinary urgency, metrorrhagia, cystitis, enuresis, prostate hypertrophy, pyelonephritis, inability to empty bladder, breast fibroadenosis, fibrocystic breast, mastitis, pyuria, renal failure, vaginitis.

Postintroduction Reports

Voluntary reports of adverse events temporally associated with ARICEPT® that have been received since market introduction that are not listed above, and that there is inadequate data to determine the causal relationship with the drug include the following: abdominal pain, agitation, cholecystitis, confusion, convulsions, hallucinations, heart block (all types), hemolytic anemia, hepatitis, hyponatremia, neuroleptic malignant syndrome, pancreatitis, and rash.

OVERDOSAGE

Because strategies for the management of overdose are continually evolving, it is advisable to contact a Poison Control Center to determine the latest recommendations for the management of an overdose of any drug.

As in any case of overdose, general supportive measures should be utilized. Overdosage with cholinesterase inhibitors can result in cholinergic crisis characterized by severe nausea, vomiting, salivation, sweating, bradycardia, hypotension, respiratory depression, collapse and convulsions. Increasing muscle weakness is a possibility and may result in death if respiratory muscles are involved. Tertiary anticholinergics such as atropine may be used as an antidote for ARICEPT® overdosage. Intravenous atropine sulfate titrated to effect is recommended: an initial dose of 1.0 to 2.0 mg IV with subsequent doses based upon clinical response. Atypical responses in blood pressure and heart rate have been reported with other cholinomimetics when coadministered with quaternary anticholinergics such as glycopyrrolate. It is not known whether ARICEPT® and/or its metabolites can be removed by dialysis (hemodialysis, peritoneal dialysis, or hemofiltration).

Dose-related signs of toxicity in animals included reduced spontaneous movement, prone position, staggering gait, lacrimation, clonic convulsions, depressed respiration, salivation, miosis, tremors, fasciculation and lower body surface temperature.

DOSAGE AND ADMINISTRATION

The dosages of ARICEPT® shown to be effective in controlled clinical trials are 5 mg and 10 mg administered once per day.

The higher dose of 10 mg did not provide a statistically significantly greater clinical benefit than 5 mg. There is a suggestion, however, based upon order of group mean scores and dose trend analyses of data from these clinical trials, that a daily dose of 10 mg of ARICEPT® might provide additional benefit for some patients. Accordingly, whether or not to employ a dose of 10 mg is a matter of prescriber and patient preference.

Evidence from the controlled trials indicates that the 10 mg dose, with a one week titration, is likely to be associated with a higher incidence of cholinergic adverse events than the 5 mg dose. In open label trials using a 6 week titration, the frequency of these same adverse events was similar between the 5 mg and 10 mg dose groups. Therefore, because steady state is not achieved for 15 days and because the incidence of untoward effects may be influenced by the rate of dose escalation, treatment with a dose of 10 mg should not be contemplated until patients have been on a daily dose of 5 mg for 4 to 6 weeks.

ARICEPT® should be taken in the evening, just prior to retiring. ARICEPT® can be taken with or without food.

HOW SUPPLIED

ARICEPT® is supplied as film-coated, round tablets containing either 5 mg or 10 mg of donepezil hydrochloride.

The 5 mg tablets are white. The strength, in mg (5), is debossed on one side and ARICEPT is debossed on the other side.

The 10 mg tablets are yellow. The strength, in mg (10), is debossed on one side and ARICEPT is debossed on the other side.

5 mg (White)	Bottles of 30 (NDC# 62856-245-30)
	Bottles of 90 (NDC# 62856-245-90)
	Unit Dose Blister Package 100 (10x10) (NDC# 62856-245-41)
10 mg (Yellow)	Bottles of 30 (NDC# 62856-246-30)
	Bottles of 90 (NDC# 62856-246-90)
	Unit Dose Blister Package 100 (10x10) (NDC# 62856-246-41)

Storage: Store at controlled room temperature, 15°C to 30°C (59°F to 86°F).

℞ only

ARICEPT® is a registered trademark of Eisai Co., Ltd.

Manufactured and Marketed by Eisai Inc., Teaneck, NJ 07666

Marketed by Pfizer Inc, New York, NY 10017

Printed in U.S.A.

200336 Revised April 2004

Shown in Product Identification Guide, page 311

ZONEGRAN® ℞

[*zōn'ə-grăn*]

(zonisamide)

Capsules

℞ only

DESCRIPTION

ZONEGRAN® (zonisamide) is an antiseizure drug chemically classified as a sulfonamide and unrelated to other antiseizure agents. The active ingredient is zonisamide, 1,2-benzisoxazole-3-methanesulfonamide. The empirical formula is $C_8H_8N_2O_3S$ with a molecular weight of 212.23. Zonisamide is a white powder, pKa = 10.2, and is moderately soluble in water (0.80 mg/mL) and 0.1 N HCl (0.50 mg/mL). The chemical structure is:

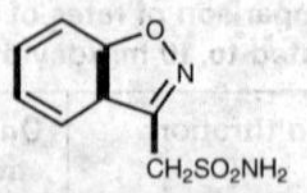

$CH_2SO_2NH_2$

ZONEGRAN is supplied for oral administration as capsules containing 25 mg, 50 mg or 100 mg zonisamide. Each capsule contains the labeled amount of zonisamide plus the following inactive ingredients: microcrystalline cellulose, hydrogenated vegetable oil, sodium lauryl sulfate, gelatin, and colorants.

CLINICAL PHARMACOLOGY

Mechanism of Action: The precise mechanism(s) by which zonisamide exerts its antiseizure effect is unknown. Zonisamide demonstrated anticonvulsant activity in several experimental models. In animals, zonisamide was effective against tonic extension seizures induced by maximal electroshock but ineffective against clonic seizures induced by subcutaneous pentylenetetrazol. Zonisamide raised the threshold for generalized seizures in the kindled rat model and reduced the duration of cortical focal seizures induced by electrical stimulation of the visual cortex in cats. Furthermore, zonisamide suppressed both interictal spikes and the secondarily generalized seizures produced by cortical application of tungstic acid gel in rats or by cortical freezing in cats. The relevance of these models to human epilepsy is unknown.

Zonisamide may produce these effects through action at sodium and calcium channels. *In vitro* pharmacological studies suggest that zonisamide blocks sodium channels and reduces voltage-dependent, transient inward currents (T-type Ca^{2+} currents), consequently stabilizing neuronal membranes and suppressing neuronal hypersynchronization. *In vitro* binding studies have demonstrated that zonisamide binds to the GABA/benzodiazepine receptor ionophore complex in an allosteric fashion which does not produce changes in chloride flux. Other *in vitro* studies have demonstrated that zonisamide (10–30 µg/mL) suppresses synaptically-driven electrical activity without affecting postsynaptic GABA or glutamate responses (cultured mouse spinal cord neurons) or neuronal or glial uptake of [^{3}H]-GABA (rat hippocampal slices). Thus, zonisamide does not appear to potentiate the synaptic activity of GABA. *In vivo* microdialysis studies demonstrated that zonisamide facilitates both dopaminergic and serotonergic neurotransmission. Zonisamide also has weak carbonic anhydrase inhibiting activity, but this pharmacologic effect is not thought to be a major contributing factor in the antiseizure activity of zonisamide.

Pharmacokinetics: Following a 200–400 mg oral zonisamide dose, peak plasma concentrations (range: 2–5 µg/mL) in normal volunteers occur within 2–6 hours. In the presence of food, the time to maximum concentration is delayed, occurring at 4–6 hours, but food has no effect on the bioavailability of zonisamide. Zonisamide extensively binds to erythrocytes, resulting in an eight-fold higher concentration of zonisamide in red blood cells (RBC) than in plasma. The pharmacokinetics of zonisamide are dose proportional in the range of 200–400 mg, but the C_{max} and AUC increase disproportionately at 800 mg, perhaps due to saturable binding of zonisamide to RBC. Once a stable dose is reached, steady state is achieved within 14 days. The elimination half-life of zonisamide in plasma is about 63 hours. The elimination half-life of zonisamide in RBC is approximately 105 hours.

The apparent volume of distribution (V/F) of zonisamide is about 1.45 L/kg following a 400 mg oral dose. Zonisamide, at concentrations of 1.0–7.0 µg/mL, is approximately 40% bound to human plasma proteins. Protein binding of zonisamide is unaffected in the presence of therapeutic concentrations of phenytoin, phenobarbital or carbamazepine.

Metabolism and Excretion: Following oral administration of ^{14}C-zonisamide to healthy volunteers, only zonisamide was detected in plasma. Zonisamide is excreted primarily in urine as parent drug and as the glucuronide of a metabolite. Following multiple dosing, 62% of the ^{14}C dose was recovered in the urine, with 3% in the feces by day 10. Zonisamide undergoes acetylation to form N-acetyl zonisamide and reduction to form the open ring metabolite, 2-sulfamoylacetyl phenol (SMAP). Of the excreted dose, 35% was recovered as zonisamide, 15% as N-acetyl zonisamide, and 50% as the glucuronide of SMAP. Reduction of zonisamide to SMAP is mediated by cytochrome P450 isozyme 3A4 (CYP3A4). Zonisamide does not induce its own metabolism. Plasma clearance of zonisamide is approximately 0.30–0.35 mL/min/kg in patients not receiving enzyme-inducing antiepilepsy drugs (AEDs). The clearance of zonisamide is increased to 0.5 mL/min/kg in patients concurrently on enzyme-inducing AEDs.

Renal clearance is about 3.5 mL/min. The clearance of an oral dose of zonisamide from RBC is 2 mL/min.

Special Populations:

Renal Insufficiency: Single 300 mg zonisamide doses were administered to three groups of volunteers. Group 1 was a healthy group with a creatinine clearance ranging from 70–152 mL/min. Group 2 and Group 3 had creatinine clearances ranging from 14.5–59 mL/min and 10–20 mL/min, respectively. Zonisamide renal clearance decreased with decreasing renal function (3.42, 2.50, 2.23 mL/min, respectively). Marked renal impairment (creatinine clearance < 20 mL/min) was associated with an increase in zonisamide AUC of 35% (see **DOSAGE AND ADMINISTRATION** section).

Hepatic Disease: The pharmacokinetics of zonisamide in patients with impaired liver function have not been studied (see **DOSAGE AND ADMINISTRATION** section).

Age: The pharmacokinetics of a 300 mg single dose of zonisamide was similar in young (mean age 28 years) and elderly subjects (mean age 69 years).

Gender and Race: Information on the effect of gender and race on the pharmacokinetics of zonisamide is not available.

Interactions of Zonisamide with Other Antiepilepsy Drugs (AEDs): Concurrent medication with drugs that either induce or inhibit CYP3A4 may alter serum concentrations of zonisamide. Concomitant administration of phenytoin and carbamazepine increases zonisamide plasma clearance from 0.30–0.35 mL/min/kg to 0.35–0.5 mL/min/kg. The half-life of zonisamide is decreased to 27 hours by phenytoin, to 38 hours by phenobarbital and carbamazepine, and to 46 hours by valproate. Plasma protein binding of phenytoin and carbamazepine was not affected by zonisamide administration (see **PRECAUTIONS, Drug Interactions** subsection).

Clinical Studies: The effectiveness of ZONEGRAN as adjunctive therapy (added to other antiepilepsy drugs) has been established in three multicenter, placebo-controlled, double blind, 3-month clinical trials (two domestic, one European) in 499 patients with refractory partial onset seizures with or without secondary generalization. Each patient had a history of at least four partial onset seizures per month in spite of receiving one or two antiepilepsy drugs at therapeutic concentrations. The 499 patients (209 women, 290 men) ranged in age from 13–68 years with a mean age of about 35 years. In the two US studies, over 80% of patients were Caucasian; 100% of patients in the European study were Caucasian. ZONEGRAN or placebo was added to the existing therapy. The primary measure of effectiveness was median percent reduction from baseline in partial seizure frequency. The secondary measure was proportion of patients achieving a 50% or greater seizure reduction from baseline (responders). The results described below are for all partial seizures in the intent-to-treat populations.

In the first study (n = 203), all patients had a 1-month baseline observation period, then received placebo or ZONEGRAN in one of two dose escalation regimens; either 1) 100 mg/day for five weeks, 200 mg/day for one week, 300 mg/day for one week, and then 400 mg/day for five weeks; or 2) 100 mg/day for one week, followed by 200 mg/day for five weeks, then 300 mg/day for one week, then 400 mg/day for five weeks. This design allowed a 100 mg vs. placebo comparison over weeks 1–5, and a 200 mg vs. placebo comparison over weeks 2–6; the primary comparison was 400 mg (both escalation groups combined) vs. placebo over weeks 8–12. The total daily dose was given as twice a day dosing. Statistically significant treatment differences favoring ZONEGRAN were seen for doses of 100, 200, and 400 mg/day.

In the second (n = 152) and third (n = 138) studies, patients had a 2–3 month baseline, then were randomly assigned to placebo or ZONEGRAN for three months. ZONEGRAN was introduced by administering 100 mg/day for the first week, 200 mg/day the second week, then 400 mg/day for two weeks, after which the dose (ZONEGRAN or placebo) could be adjusted as necessary to a maximum dose of 20 mg/kg/day or a maximum plasma level of 40 μg/mL. In the second study, the total daily dose was given as twice a day dosing; in the third study, it was given as a single daily dose. The average final maintenance doses received in the studies were 530 and 430 mg/day in the second and third studies, respectively. Both studies demonstrated statistically significant differences favoring ZONEGRAN for doses of 400–600 mg/day, and there was no apparent difference between once daily and twice daily dosing (in different studies). Analysis of the data (first 4 weeks) during titration demonstrated statistically significant differences favoring ZONEGRAN at doses between 100 and 400 mg/day. The primary comparison in both trials was for any dose over Weeks 5–12.

[See table 1 above]

[See table 2 above]

Figure 1 presents the proportion of patients (X-axis) whose percentage reduction from baseline in the all partial seizure rate was at least as great as that indicated on the Y-axis in the second and third placebo-controlled trials. A positive value on the Y-axis indicates an improvement from baseline (i.e., a decrease in seizure rate), while a negative value indicates a worsening from baseline (i.e., an increase in seizure rate). Thus, in a display of this type, the curve for an effective treatment is shifted to the left of the curve for placebo. The proportion of patients achieving any particular level of reduction in seizure rate was consistently higher for the ZONEGRAN groups compared to the placebo groups. For example, Figure 1 indicates that approximately 27% of patients treated with ZONEGRAN experienced a 75% or greater reduction, compared to approximately 12% in the placebo groups.

Figure 1 Proportion of Patients Achieving Differing Levels of Seizure Reduction in ZONEGRAN and Placebo Groups in Studies 2 and 3

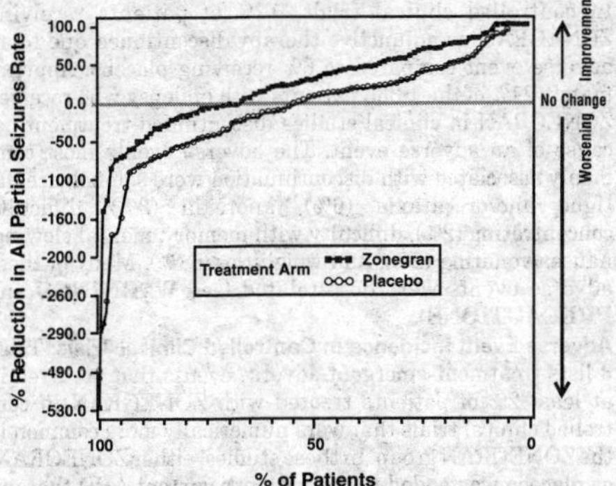

No differences in efficacy based on age, sex or race, as measured by a change in seizure frequency from baseline, were detected.

INDICATIONS AND USAGE

ZONEGRAN is indicated as adjunctive therapy in the treatment of partial seizures in adults with epilepsy.

Table 1. Median % Reduction in All Partial Seizures and % Responders in Primary Efficacy Analyses: Intent-To-Treat Analysis

Study	Median % reduction in partial seizures ZONEGRAN	Placebo	% Responders ZONEGRAN	Placebo
Study 1:	n=98	n=72	n=98	n=72
Weeks 8–12:	40.5%*	9.0%	41.8%*	22.2%
Study 2:	n=69	n=72	n=69	n=72
Weeks 5–12:	29.6%*	-3.2%	29.0%	15.0%
Study 3:	n=67	n=66	n=67	n=66
Weeks 5–12:	27.2%*	-1.1%	28.0%*	12.0%

*p<0.05 compared to placebo

Table 2. Median % Reduction in All Partial Seizures and % Responders for Dose Analyses in Study 1: Intent-To-Treat Analysis

Dose Group	Median % reduction in partial seizures ZONEGRAN	Placebo	% Responders ZONEGRAN	Placebo
100–400 mg/day:	n=112	n=83	n=112	n=83
Weeks 1–12:	32.3%*	5.6%	32.1%*	9.6%
100 mg/day:	n=56	n=80	n=56	n=80
Weeks 1–5:	24.7%*	8.3%	25.0%*	11.3%
200 mg/day:	n=55	n=82	n=55	n=82
Weeks 2–6:	20.4%*	4.0%	25.5%*	9.8%

*p<0.05 compared to placebo

CONTRAINDICATIONS

ZONEGRAN is contraindicated in patients who have demonstrated hypersensitivity to sulfonamides or zonisamide.

WARNINGS

Potentially Fatal Reactions to Sulfonamides: Fatalities have occurred, although rarely, as a result of severe reactions to sulfonamides (zonisamide is a sulfonamide) including Stevens-Johnson syndrome, toxic epidermal necrolysis, fulminant hepatic necrosis, agranulocytosis, aplastic anemia, and other blood dyscrasias. Such reactions may occur when a sulfonamide is readministered irrespective of the route of administration. If signs of hypersensitivity or other serious reactions occur, discontinue zonisamide immediately. Specific experience with sulfonamide-type adverse reaction to zonisamide is described below.

Serious Skin Reactions: Consideration should be given to discontinuing ZONEGRAN in patients who develop an otherwise unexplained rash. If the drug is not discontinued, patients should be observed frequently. Seven deaths from severe rash [i.e. Stevens-Johnson syndrome (SJS) and toxic epidermal necrolysis (TEN)] were reported in the first 11 years of marketing in Japan. All of the patients were receiving other drugs in addition to zonisamide. In post-marketing experience from Japan, a total of 49 cases of SJS or TEN have been reported, a reporting rate of 46 per million patient-years of exposure. Although this rate is greater than background, it is probably an underestimate of the true incidence because of under-reporting. There were no confirmed cases of SJS or TEN in the US, European, or Japanese development programs.

In the US and European randomized controlled trials, 6 of 269 (2.2%) zonisamide patients discontinued treatment because of rash compared to none on placebo. Across all trials during the US and European development, rash that led to discontinuation of zonisamide was reported in 1.4% of patients (12.0 events per 1000 patient-years of exposure). During Japanese development, serious rash or rash that led to study drug discontinuation was reported in 2.0% of patients (27.8 events per 1000 patient years). Rash usually occurred early in treatment, with 85% reported within 16 weeks in the US and European studies and 90% reported within two weeks in the Japanese studies. There was no apparent relationship of dose to the occurrence of rash.

Serious Hematologic Events: Two confirmed cases of aplastic anemia and one confirmed case of agranulocytosis were reported in the first 11 years of marketing in Japan, rates greater than generally accepted background rates. There were no cases of aplastic anemia and two confirmed cases of agranulocytosis in the US, European, or Japanese development programs. There is inadequate information to assess the relationship, if any, between dose and duration of treatment and these events.

Oligohidrosis and Hyperthermia in Pediatric Patients: Oligohidrosis, sometimes resulting in heat stroke and hospitalization, is seen in association with zonisamide in pediatric patients.

During the pre-approval development program in Japan, one case of oligohidrosis was reported in 403 pediatric patients, an incidence of 1 case per 285 patient-years of exposure. While there were no cases reported in the US or European development programs, fewer than 100 pediatric patients participated in these trials.

In the first 11 years of marketing in Japan, 38 cases were reported, an estimated reporting rate of about 1 case per 10,000 patient-years of exposure. In the first year of marketing in the US, 2 cases were reported, an estimated reporting rate of about 12 cases per 10,000 patient-years of exposure. These rates are underestimates of the true incidence because of under-reporting. There has also been one report of heat stroke in an 18-year-old patient in the US. Decreased sweating and an elevation in body temperature above normal characterized these cases. Many cases were reported after exposure to elevated environmental temperatures. Heat stroke, requiring hospitalization, was diagnosed in some cases. There have been no reported deaths. Pediatric patients appear to be at an increased risk for zonisamide-associated oligohidrosis and hyperthermia. Patients, especially pediatric patients, treated with Zonegran should be monitored closely for evidence of decreased sweating and increased body temperature, especially in warm or hot weather. Caution should be used when zonisamide is prescribed with other drugs that predispose patients to heat-related disorders; these drugs include, but are not limited to, carbonic anhydrase inhibitors and drugs with anticholinergic activity.

The practitioner should be aware that the safety and effectiveness of zonisamide in pediatric patients have not been established, and that zonisamide is not approved for use in pediatric patients.

Seizures on Withdrawal: As with other AEDs, abrupt withdrawal of ZONEGRAN in patients with epilepsy may precipitate increased seizure frequency or status epilepticus. Dose reduction or discontinuation of zonisamide should be done gradually.

Teratogenicity: Women of child bearing potential who are given zonisamide should be advised to use effective contraception. Zonisamide was teratogenic in mice, rats, and dogs and embryolethal in monkeys when administered during the period of organogenesis. A variety of fetal abnormalities, including cardiovascular defects, and embryo-fetal deaths occurred at maternal plasma levels similar to or lower than therapeutic levels in humans. These findings suggest that the use of ZONEGRAN during pregnancy in humans may present a significant risk to the fetus (see **PRECAUTIONS, Pregnancy** subsection). It cannot be said with any confidence, however, that even mild seizures do not pose some hazards to the developing fetus. Zonisamide should be used during pregnancy only if the potential benefit justifies the potential risk to the fetus.

Cognitive/Neuropsychiatric Adverse Events: Use of ZONEGRAN was frequently associated with central nervous system-related adverse events. The most significant of these can be classified into three general categories: 1) psychiatric symptoms, including depression and psychosis, 2) psychomotor slowing, difficulty with concentration, and speech or language problems, in particular, word-finding difficulties, and 3) somnolence or fatigue.

In placebo-controlled trials, 2.2% of patients discontinued ZONEGRAN or were hospitalized for depression compared to 0.4% of placebo patients, while 1.1% of ZONEGRAN and 0.4% of placebo patients attempted suicide. Among all epilepsy patients treated with ZONEGRAN, 1.4% were discontinued and 1.0% were hospitalized because of reported depression or suicide attempts. In placebo-controlled trials, 2.2% of patients discontinued ZONEGRAN or were hospitalized due to psychosis or psychosis-related symptoms compared to none of the placebo patients. Among all epilepsy patients treated with ZONEGRAN, 0.9% were discontinued and 1.4% were hospitalized because of reported psychosis or related symptoms.

Psychomotor slowing and difficulty with concentration occurred in the first month of treatment and were associated with doses above 300 mg/day. Speech and language problems tended to occur after 6–10 weeks of treatment and at doses above 300 mg/day. Although in most cases these events were of mild to moderate severity, they at times led to withdrawal from treatment.

Somnolence and fatigue were frequently reported CNS adverse events during clinical trials with ZONEGRAN. Although in most cases these events were of mild to moderate severity, they led to withdrawal from treatment in 0.2% of the patients enrolled in controlled trials. Somnolence and

Continued on next page

Zonegran—Cont.

fatigue tended to occur within the first month of treatment. Somnolence and fatigue occurred most frequently at doses of 300–500 mg/day. **Patients should be cautioned about this possibility and special care should be taken by patients if they drive, operate machinery, or perform any hazardous task.**

PRECAUTIONS

General: Somnolence is commonly reported, especially at higher doses of ZONEGRAN (see **WARNINGS: Cognitive/Neuropsychiatric Adverse Events** subsection). Zonisamide is metabolized by the liver and eliminated by the kidneys; caution should therefore be exercised when administering ZONEGRAN to patients with hepatic and renal dysfunction (see **CLINICAL PHARMACOLOGY, Special Populations** subsection).

Kidney Stones: Among 991 patients treated during the development of ZONEGRAN, 40 patients (4.0%) with epilepsy receiving ZONEGRAN developed clinically possible or confirmed kidney stones (e.g. clinical symptomatology, sonography, etc.), a rate of 34 per 1000 patient-years of exposure (40 patients with 1168 years of exposure). Of these, 12 were symptomatic, and 28 were described as possible kidney stones based on sonographic detection. In nine patients, the diagnosis was confirmed by a passage of a stone or by a definitive sonographic finding. The rate of occurrence of kidney stones was 28.7 per 1000 patient-years of exposure in the first six months, 62.6 per 1000 patient-years of exposure between 6 and 12 months, and 24.3 per 1000 patient-years of exposure after 12 months of use. There are no normative sonographic data available for either the general population or patients with epilepsy. The clinical significance of the sonographic finding is unknown. The analyzed stones were composed of calcium or urate salts. In general, increasing fluid intake and urine output can help reduce the risk of stone formation, particularly in those with predisposing risk factors. It is unknown, however, whether these measures will reduce the risk of stone formation in patients treated with ZONEGRAN.

Effect on Renal Function: In several clinical studies, zonisamide was associated with a statistically significant 8% mean increase from baseline of serum creatinine and blood urea nitrogen (BUN) compared to essentially no change in the placebo patients. The increase appeared to persist over time but was not progressive; this has been interpreted as an effect on glomerular filtration rate (GFR). There were no episodes of unexplained acute renal failure in clinical development in the US, Europe, or Japan. The decrease in GFR appeared within the first 4 weeks of treatment. In a 30-day study, the GFR returned to baseline within 2–3 weeks of drug discontinuation. There is no information about reversibility, after drug discontinuation, of the effects on GFR after long-term use. ZONEGRAN should be discontinued in patients who develop acute renal failure or a clinically significant sustained increase in the creatinine/BUN concentration. ZONEGRAN should not be used in patients with renal failure (estimated GFR <50 mL/min) as there has been insufficient experience concerning drug dosing and toxicity.

Sudden Unexplained Death in Epilepsy: During the development of ZONEGRAN, nine sudden unexplained deaths occurred among 991 patients with epilepsy receiving ZONEGRAN for whom accurate exposure data are available. This represents an incidence of 7.7 deaths per 1000 patient years. Although this rate exceeds that expected in a healthy population, it is within the range of estimates for the incidence of sudden unexplained deaths in patients with refractory epilepsy not receiving ZONEGRAN (ranging from 0.5 per 1000 patient-years for the general population of patients with epilepsy, to 2–5 per 1000 patient-years for patients with refractory epilepsy; higher incidences range from 9–15 per 1000 patient-years among surgical candidates and surgical failures). Some of the deaths could represent seizure-related deaths in which the seizure was not observed.

Status Epilepticus: Estimates of the incidence of treatment emergent status epilepticus in ZONEGRAN-treated patients are difficult because a standard definition was not employed. Nonetheless, in controlled trials, 1.1% of patients treated with ZONEGRAN had an event labeled as status epilepticus compared to none of the patients treated with placebo. Among patients treated with ZONEGRAN across all epilepsy studies (controlled and uncontrolled), 1.0% of patients had an event reported as status epilepticus.

Creatine Phosphokinase (CPK) Elevation and Pancreatitis: In the post-market setting, the following rare adverse events have been observed (<1:1000):

If patients taking zonisamide develop severe muscle pain and/or weakness, either in the presence or absence of a fever, markers of muscle damage should be assessed, including serum CPK and aldolase levels. If elevated, in the absence of another obvious cause such as trauma, grand mal seizures, etc., tapering and/or discontinuance of zonisamide should be considered and appropriate treatment initiated.

Patients taking zonisamide that manifest clinical signs and symptoms of pancreatitis should have pancreatic lipase and amylase levels monitored. If pancreatitis is evident, in the absence of another obvious cause, tapering and/or discontinuation of zonisamide should be considered and appropriate treatment initiated.

Information for Patients: Patients should be advised as follows:

1. **ZONEGRAN may produce drowsiness, especially at higher doses. Patients should be advised not to drive a car or operate other complex machinery until they have gained experience on ZONEGRAN sufficient to determine whether it affects their performance.**
2. Patients should contact their physician immediately if a skin rash develops or seizures worsen.
3. Patients should contact their physician immediately if they develop signs or symptoms, such as sudden back pain, abdominal pain, and/or blood in the urine, that could indicate a kidney stone. Increasing fluid intake and urine output may reduce the risk of stone formation, particularly in those with predisposing risk factors for stones.
4. Patients should contact their physician immediately if a child has been taking ZONEGRAN and is not sweating as usual with or without a fever.
5. Because zonisamide can cause hematological complications, patients should contact their physician immediately if they develop a fever, sore throat, oral ulcers, or easy bruising.
6. As with other AEDs, patients should contact their physician if they intend to become pregnant or are pregnant during ZONEGRAN therapy. Patients should notify their physician if they intend to breast-feed or are breast-feeding an infant.
7. Patients should contact their physician immediately if they develop severe muscle pain and/or weakness.

Laboratory Tests: In several clinical studies, zonisamide was associated with a mean increase in the concentration of serum creatinine and blood urea nitrogen (BUN) of approximately 8% over the baseline measurement. Consideration should be given to monitoring renal function periodically (see **PRECAUTIONS, Effect on Renal Function** subsection).

Zonisamide was associated with an increase in serum alkaline phosphatase. In the randomized, controlled trials, a mean increase of approximately 7% over baseline was associated with zonisamide compared to a 3% mean increase in placebo-treated patients. These changes were not statistically significant. The clinical relevance of these changes is unknown.

Drug Interactions: *Effects of ZONEGRAN on the pharmacokinetics of other antiepilepsy drugs (AEDs):* Zonisamide had no appreciable effect on the steady state plasma concentrations of phenytoin, carbamazepine, or valproate during clinical trials. Zonisamide did not inhibit mixed-function liver oxidase enzymes (cytochrome P450), as measured in human liver microsomal preparations, *in vitro*. Zonisamide is not expected to interfere with the metabolism of other drugs that are metabolized by cytochrome P450 isozymes.

Effects of other drugs on ZONEGRAN pharmacokinetics: Drugs that induce liver enzymes increase the metabolism and clearance of zonisamide and decrease its half-life. The half-life of zonisamide following a 400 mg dose in patients concurrently on enzyme-inducing AEDs such as phenytoin, carbamazepine, or phenobarbital was between 27–38 hours; the half-life of zonisamide in patients concurrently on the non-enzyme inducing AED, valproate, was 46 hours. Concurrent medication with drugs that either induce or inhibit CYP3A4 would be expected to alter serum concentrations of zonisamide.

Interaction with cimetidine: Zonisamide single dose pharmacokinetic parameters were not affected by cimetidine (300 mg four times a day for 12 days).

Carcinogenicity, Mutagenesis, Impairment of Fertility: No evidence of carcinogenicity was found in mice or rats following dietary administration of zonisamide for two years at doses of up to 80 mg/kg/day. In mice, this dose is approximately equivalent to the maximum recommended human dose (MRHD) of 400 mg/day on a mg/m^2 basis. In rats, this dose is 1–2 times the MRHD on a mg/m^2 basis.

Zonisamide increased mutation frequency in Chinese hamster lung cells in the absence of metabolic activation. Zonisamide was not mutagenic or clastogenic in the Ames test, mouse lymphoma assay, sister chromatid exchange test, and human lymphocyte cytogenetics assay *in vitro*, and the rat bone marrow cytogenetics assay *in vivo*.

Rats treated with zonisamide (20, 60, or 200 mg/kg) before mating and during the initial gestation phase showed signs of reproductive toxicity (decreased corpora lutea, implantations, and live fetuses) at all doses. The low dose in this study is approximately 0.5 times the maximum recommended human dose (MRHD) on a mg/m^2 basis. The effect of zonisamide on human fertility is unknown.

Pregnancy: Pregnancy Category C (see **WARNINGS, Teratogenicity** subsection): Zonisamide was teratogenic in mice, rats, and dogs and embryolethal in monkeys when administered during the period of organogenesis. Fetal abnormalities or embryo-fetal deaths occurred in these species at zonisamide dosage and maternal plasma levels similar to or lower than therapeutic levels in humans, indicating that use of this drug in pregnancy entails a significant risk to the fetus. A variety of external, visceral, and skeletal malformations was produced in animals by prenatal exposure to zonisamide. Cardiovascular defects were prominent in both rats and dogs.

Following administration of zonisamide (10, 30, or 60 mg/kg/day) to pregnant dogs during organogenesis, increased incidences of fetal cardiovascular malformations (ventricular septal defects, cardiomegaly, various valvular and arterial anomalies) were found at doses of 30 mg/kg/day or greater. The low effect dose for malformations produced peak maternal plasma zonisamide levels (25 µg/mL) about 0.5 times the highest plasma levels measured in patients receiving the maximum recommended human dose (MRHD) of 400 mg/day. In dogs, cardiovascular malformations were found in approximately 50% of all fetuses exposed to the high dose, which was associated with maternal plasma levels (44 µg/mL) approximately equal to the highest levels measured in humans receiving the MRHD. Incidences of skeletal malformations were also increased at the high dose, and fetal growth retardation and increased frequencies of skeletal variations were seen at all doses in this study. The low dose produced maternal plasma levels (12 µg/mL) about 0.25 times the highest human levels.

In cynomolgus monkeys, administration of zonisamide (10 or 20 mg/kg/day) to pregnant animals during organogenesis resulted in embryo-fetal deaths at both doses. The possibility that these deaths were due to malformations cannot be ruled out. The lowest embryolethal dose in monkeys was associated with peak maternal plasma zonisamide levels (5 µg/mL) approximately 0.1 times the highest levels measured in patients at the MRHD.

In a mouse embryo-fetal development study, treatment of pregnant animals with zonisamide (125, 250, or 500 mg/kg/day) during the period of organogenesis resulted in increased incidences of fetal malformations (skeletal and/or craniofacial defects) at all doses tested. The low dose in this study is approximately 1.5 times the MRHD on a mg/m^2 basis. In rats, increased frequencies of malformations (cardiovascular defects) and variations (persistent cords of thymic tissue, decreased skeletal ossification) were observed among the offspring of dams treated with zonisamide (20, 60, or 200 mg/kg/day) throughout organogenesis at all doses. The low effect dose is approximately 0.5 times the MRHD on a mg/m^2 basis.

Perinatal death was increased among the offspring of rats treated with zonisamide (10, 30, or 60 mg/kg/day) from the latter part of gestation up to weaning at the high dose, or approximately 1.4 times the MRHD on a mg/m^2 basis. The no effect level of 30 mg/kg/day is approximately 0.7 times the MRHD on a mg/m^2 basis.

There are no adequate and well-controlled studies in pregnant women. ZONEGRAN should be used during pregnancy only if the potential benefit justifies the potential risk to the fetus.

Labor and Delivery: The effect of ZONEGRAN on labor and delivery in humans is not known.

Use in Nursing Mothers: It is not known whether zonisamide is excreted in human milk. Because many drugs are excreted in human milk and because of the potential for serious adverse reactions in nursing infants from zonisamide, a decision should be made whether to discontinue nursing or to discontinue drug, taking into account the importance of the drug to the mother. ZONEGRAN should be used in nursing mothers only if the benefits outweigh the risks.

Pediatric Use: The safety and effectiveness of ZONEGRAN in children under age 16 have not been established. Cases of oligohidrosis and hyperpyrexia have been reported (see **WARNINGS, Oligohidrosis and Hyperthermia in Pediatric Patients** subsection).

Geriatric Use: Single dose pharmacokinetic parameters are similar in elderly and young healthy volunteers (see **CLINICAL PHARMACOLOGY, Special Populations** subsection). Clinical studies of zonisamide did not include sufficient numbers of subjects aged 65 and over to determine whether they respond differently from younger subjects. Other reported clinical experience has not identified differences in responses between the elderly and younger patients. In general, dose selection for an elderly patient should be cautious, usually starting at the low end of the dosing range, reflecting the greater frequency of decreased hepatic, renal, or cardiac function, and of concomitant disease or other drug therapy.

ADVERSE REACTIONS

The most commonly observed adverse events associated with the use of ZONEGRAN in controlled clinical trials that were not seen at an equivalent frequency among placebo-treated patients were somnolence, anorexia, dizziness, headache, nausea, and agitation/irritability.

In controlled clinical trials, 12% of patients receiving ZONEGRAN as adjunctive therapy discontinued due to an adverse event compared to 6% receiving placebo. Approximately 21% of the 1,336 patients with epilepsy who received ZONEGRAN in clinical studies discontinued treatment because of an adverse event. The adverse events most commonly associated with discontinuation were somnolence, fatigue and/or ataxia (6%), anorexia (3%), difficulty concentrating (2%), difficulty with memory, mental slowing, nausea/vomiting (2%), and weight loss (1%). Many of these adverse events were dose-related (see **WARNINGS** and **PRECAUTIONS**).

Adverse Event Incidence in Controlled Clinical Trials: Table 3 lists treatment-emergent adverse events that occurred in at least 2% of patients treated with ZONEGRAN in controlled clinical trials that were numerically more common in the ZONEGRAN group. In these studies, either ZONEGRAN or placebo was added to the patient's current AED therapy. Adverse events were usually mild or moderate in intensity. The prescriber should be aware that these figures, obtained when ZONEGRAN was added to concurrent AED therapy, cannot be used to predict the frequency of adverse events in the course of usual medical practice when patient characteristics and other factors may differ from those prevailing during clinical studies. Similarly, the cited frequencies cannot be directly compared with figures obtained from other clinical investigations involving different treatments, uses, or investigators. An inspection of these frequencies, however, does provide the prescriber with one basis by which to estimate the relative contribution of drug and non-drug factors to the adverse event incidences in the population studied.

TABLE 3: Incidence (%) of Treatment-Emergent Adverse Events in Placebo-Controlled, Add-On Trials (Events that occurred in at least 2% of ZONEGRAN-treated patients and occurred more frequently in ZONEGRAN-treated than placebo-treated patients)

BODY SYSTEM/ PREFERRED TERM	ZONEGRAN (n=269) %	PLACEBO (n=230) %
BODY AS A WHOLE		
Headache	10	8
Abdominal Pain	6	3
Flu Syndrome	4	3
DIGESTIVE		
Anorexia	13	6
Nausea	9	6
Diarrhea	5	2
Dyspepsia	3	1
Constipation	2	1
Dry Mouth	2	1
HEMATOLOGIC AND LYMPHATIC		
Ecchymosis	2	1
METABOLIC AND NUTRITIONAL		
Weight Loss	3	2
NERVOUS SYSTEM		
Dizziness	13	7
Ataxia	6	1
Nystagmus	4	2
Paresthesia	4	1
NEUROPSYCHIATRIC AND COGNITIVE DYSFUNCTION-ALTERED COGNITIVE FUNCTION		
Confusion	6	3
Difficulty Concentrating	6	2
Difficulty with Memory	6	2
Mental Slowing	4	2
NEUROPSYCHIATRIC AND COGNITIVE DYSFUNCTION-BEHAVIORAL ABNORMALITIES (NON-PSYCHOSIS-RELATED)		
Agitation/Irritability	9	4
Depression	6	3
Insomnia	6	3
Anxiety	3	2
Nervousness	2	1
NEUROPSYCHIATRIC AND COGNITIVE DYSFUNCTION-BEHAVIORAL ABNORMALITIES (PSYCHOSIS-RELATED)		
Schizophrenic/ Schizophreniform Behavior	2	0
NEUROPSYCHIATRIC AND COGNITIVE DYSFUNCTION-CNS DEPRESSION		
Somnolence	17	7
Fatigue	8	6
Tiredness	7	5
NEUROPSYCHIATRIC AND COGNITIVE DYSFUNCTION-SPEECH AND LANGUAGE ABNORMALITIES		
Speech Abnormalities	5	2
Difficulties in Verbal Expression	2	<1
RESPIRATORY		
Rhinitis	2	1
SKIN AND APPENDAGES		
Rash	3	2
SPECIAL SENSES		
Diplopia	6	3
Taste Perversion	2	0

Other Adverse Events Observed During Clinical Trials: ZONEGRAN has been administered to 1,598 individuals during all clinical trials, only some of which were placebo-controlled. During these trials, all events were recorded by the investigators using their own terms. To provide a useful estimate of the proportion of individuals having adverse events, similar events have been grouped into a smaller number of standardized categories using a modified COSTART dictionary. The frequencies represent the proportion of the 1,598 individuals exposed to ZONEGRAN who experienced an event on at least one occasion. All events are included except those already listed in the previous table or discussed in **WARNINGS** or **PRECAUTIONS**, trivial events, those too general to be informative, and those not reasonably associated with ZONEGRAN.

Events are further classified within each category and listed in order of decreasing frequency as follows: frequent occurring in at least 1:100 patient; infrequent occurring in 1:100 to 1:1000 patients; rare occurring in fewer than 1:1000 patients.

Body as a Whole: *Frequent:* Accidental injury, asthenia. *Infrequent:* Chest pain, flank pain, malaise, allergic reaction, face edema, neck rigidity. *Rare:* Lupus erythematosus.

Cardiovascular: *Infrequent:* Palpitation, tachycardia, vascular insufficiency, hypotension, hypertension, thrombophlebitis, syncope, bradycardia. *Rare:* Atrial fibrillation, heart failure, pulmonary embolus, ventricular extrasystoles.

Digestive: *Frequent:* Vomiting. *Infrequent:* Flatulence, gingivitis, gum hyperplasia, gastritis, gastroenteritis, stomatitis, cholelithiasis, glossitis, melena, rectal hemorrhage, ulcerative stomatitis, gastro-duodenal ulcer, dysphagia, gum hemorrhage. *Rare:* Cholangitis, hematemesis, cholecystitis, cholestatic jaundice, colitis, duodenitis, esophagitis, fecal incontinence, mouth ulceration.

Hematologic and Lymphatic: *Infrequent:* Leukopenia, anemia, immunodeficiency, lymphadenopathy. *Rare:* Thrombocytopenia, microcytic anemia, petechia.

Metabolic and Nutritional: *Infrequent:* Peripheral edema, weight gain, edema, thirst, dehydration. *Rare:* Hypoglycemia, hyponatremia, lactic dehydrogenase increased, SGOT increased, SGPT increased.

Musculoskeletal: *Infrequent:* Leg cramps, myalgia, myasthenia, arthralgia, arthritis.

Nervous System: *Frequent:* Tremor, convulsion, abnormal gait, hyperesthesia, incoordination. *Infrequent:* Hypertonia, twitching, abnormal dreams, vertigo, libido decreased, neuropathy, hyperkinesia, movement disorder, dysarthria, cerebrovascular accident, hypotonia, peripheral neuritis, paresthesia, reflexes increased. *Rare:* Circumoral paresthesia, dyskinesia, dystonia, encephalopathy, facial paralysis, hypokinesia, hyperesthesia, myoclonus, oculogyric crisis.

Behavioral Abnormalities—Non-Psychosis-Related: *Infrequent:* Euphoria.

Respiratory: *Frequent:* Pharyngitis, cough increased. Infrequent: Dyspnea. *Rare:* Apnea, hemoptysis.

Skin and Appendages: *Frequent:* Pruritus. *Infrequent:* Maculopapular rash, acne, alopecia, dry skin, sweating, eczema, urticaria, hirsutism, pustular rash, vesiculobullous rash.

Special Senses: *Frequent:* Amblyopia, tinnitus. *Infrequent:* Conjunctivitis, parosmia, deafness, visual field defect, glaucoma. *Rare:* Photophobia, iritis.

Urogenital: *Infrequent:* Urinary frequency, dysuria, urinary incontinence, hematuria, impotence, urinary retention, urinary urgency, amenorrhea, polyuria, nocturia. *Rare:* Albuminuria, enuresis, bladder pain, bladder calculus, gynecomastia, mastitis, menorrhagia.

DRUG ABUSE AND DEPENDENCE

The abuse and dependence potential of ZONEGRAN has not been evaluated in human studies (see **WARNINGS, Cognitive/Neuropsychiatric Adverse Events** subsection). In a series of animal studies, zonisamide did not demonstrate abuse liability and dependence potential. Monkeys did not self-administer zonisamide in a standard reinforcing paradigm. Rats exposed to zonisamide did not exhibit signs of physical dependence of the CNS-depressant type. Rats did not generalize the effects of diazepam to zonisamide in a standard discrimination paradigm after training, suggesting that zonisamide does not have abuse potential of the benzodiazepine-CNS depressant type.

OVERDOSAGE

Human Experience: Experience with ZONEGRAN daily doses over 800 mg/day is limited. During ZONEGRAN clinical development, three patients ingested unknown amounts of ZONEGRAN as suicide attempts, and all three were hospitalized with CNS symptoms. One patient became comatose and developed bradycardia, hypotension, and respiratory depression; the zonisamide plasma level was 100.1 μg/mL measured 31 hours post-ingestion. Zonisamide plasma levels fell with a half-life of 57 hours, and the patient became alert five days later.

Management: No specific antidotes for ZONEGRAN overdosage are available. Following a suspected recent overdose, emesis should be induced or gastric lavage performed with the usual precautions to protect the airway. General supportive care is indicated, including frequent monitoring of vital signs and close observation.

Zonisamide has a long half-life (see **CLINICAL PHARMACOLOGY** section). Due to the low protein binding of zonisamide (40%), renal dialysis may not be effective. A poison control center should be contacted for information on the management of ZONEGRAN overdosage.

DOSAGE AND ADMINISTRATION

ZONEGRAN (zonisamide) is recommended as adjunctive therapy for the treatment of partial seizures in adults. Safety and efficacy in pediatric patients below the age of 16 have not been established. ZONEGRAN should be administered once or twice daily, using 25 mg, 50 mg or 100 mg capsules. ZONEGRAN is given orally and can be taken with or without food. Capsules should be swallowed whole.

Adults over Age 16: The prescriber should be aware that, because of the long half-life of zonisamide, up to two weeks may be required to achieve steady state levels upon reaching a stable dose or following dosage adjustment. Although the regimen described below is one that has been shown to be tolerated, the prescriber may wish to prolong the duration of treatment at the lower doses in order to fully assess the effects of zonisamide at steady state, noting that many of the side effects of zonisamide are more frequent at doses of 300 mg per day and above. Although there is some evidence of greater response at doses above 100–200 mg/day, the increase appears small and formal dose-response studies have not been conducted.

The initial dose of ZONEGRAN should be 100 mg daily. After two weeks, the dose may be increased to 200 mg/day for at least two weeks. It can be increased to 300 mg/day and 400 mg/day, with the dose stable for at least two weeks to achieve steady state at each level. Evidence from controlled trials suggests that ZONEGRAN doses of 100–600 mg/day are effective, but there is no suggestion of increasing response above 400 mg/day (see **CLINICAL PHARMACOLOGY, Clinical Studies** subsection). There is little experience with doses greater than 600 mg/day.

Patients with Renal or Hepatic Disease: Because zonisamide is metabolized in the liver and excreted by the kidneys, patients with renal or hepatic disease should be treated with caution, and might require slower titration and more frequent monitoring (see **CLINICAL PHARMACOLOGY** and **PRECAUTIONS**).

HOW SUPPLIED

ZONEGRAN is available as 25 mg, 50 mg and 100 mg two-piece hard gelatin capsules. The capsules are printed in black with a stylized E and "ZONEGRAN 25," "ZONEGRAN 50," or "ZONEGRAN 100," respectively. ZONEGRAN is available in bottles of 100 with strengths and colors as follows:

Dosage Strength	Capsule Colors	NDC #
25 mg	White opaque body with white opaque cap.	62856-681-10
50 mg	White opaque body with gray opaque cap.	62856-682-10
100 mg	White opaque body with red opaque cap.	62856-680-10

Store at 25°C (77°F), excursions permitted to 15–30° C (59–86°F) [see USP Controlled Room Temperature], in a dry place and protected from light.

US Patent #6,342,515

ANIMAL TOXICOLOGY

In dogs treated with zonisamide (10, 30, or 75 mg/kg/day) for 1 year, dark brown discoloration of the liver and concentric lamellar bodies in the cytoplasm of hepatocytes were observed in association with clinical chemistry changes indicative of liver damage (elevated alkaline phosphatase, gamma glutamyl transferase, and alanine amino transferase; decreased albumin) and altered drug metabolism at the highest dose, which is approximately 6 times the maximum recommended human dose (MRHD) of 400 mg/day on a mg/m^2 basis. Gross liver changes not clearly accompanied by biochemical evidence of hepatotoxicity were noted at 30 mg/kg/day, or approximately 2.4 times the MRHD on mg/m^2 basis. The no effect dose of 10 mg/kg/day is slightly less than the MRHD on mg/m^2 basis. The significance of these findings for humans is not known.

Manufactured by:
Elan Pharma International Ltd.
Distributed by:
Eisai Inc., Teaneck, NJ 07666
ZONEGRAN® is a registered trademark of Dainippon Pharmaceutical Co. Ltd. and licensed exclusively to Eisai Inc.

Eisai
200342
Revised May 2004
Printed in the USA

PATIENT INFORMATION LEAFLET

Questions and Answers about ZONEGRAN® (zonisamide) capsules

What is the most important information I should know about ZONEGRAN?

Some people taking ZONEGRAN (ZON-uh-gran) can get serious reactions. **If you get any of the following symptoms, call your doctor right away:**

- Rash (may be a sign of a dangerous condition)
- Fever, sore throat, sores in your mouth, or bruising easily (may be signs of a blood problem)
- Sudden back pain, abdominal (stomach area) pain, pain when urinating, bloody or dark urine (may be signs of a kidney stone)
- Decreased sweating or a rise in body temperature (especially in patients under 17 years old)
- Depression
- Thoughts that are unusual for you
- Speech or language problems
- Severe muscle pain and/or weakness

ZONEGRAN can cause drowsiness and coordination problems. **Do not drive or operate dangerous machinery until you know how ZONEGRAN affects you.**

What is ZONEGRAN?

ZONEGRAN is a medicine to treat partial seizures in adults. It is taken with other seizure medicines to help control your seizures.

Continued on next page

Zonegran—Cont.

Who should not take ZONEGRAN?

Talk to your doctor first before stopping ZONEGRAN.

Tell your doctor if you are allergic to sulfa drugs. Do not take ZONEGRAN if you are allergic to any sulfa drugs (for example, Bactrim™ or Septra®) or ZONEGRAN.

How should I take ZONEGRAN?

Be sure to follow your doctor's directions. Starting a new medicine can be confusing. If you have any questions, call your doctor.

ZONEGRAN is available as 25 mg, 50 mg, and 100 mg capsules. The usual recommended starting dose of ZONEGRAN is 100 mg each day. After a week or so, your doctor may increase your dose of ZONEGRAN. This may occur more than once. It is done to get the best control for your seizures. Take only the number of ZONEGRAN capsules you were told to take.

It is important to swallow ZONEGRAN capsules whole. Do not bite into or break the capsules. You may take ZONEGRAN with or without food.

Talk to your doctor about what to do if you miss a dose.

If you think you have overdosed on your medicine, call your local poison control center or emergency room right away.

Drink 6–8 glasses of water a day. This may help prevent kidney stones.

Talk to your doctor before stopping ZONEGRAN or any other seizure medicine. Stopping a seizure medicine all at once can cause status epilepticus, a serious problem.

What should I avoid while taking ZONEGRAN?

ZONEGRAN may make you drowsy. Do not drive a car or operate complex machinery until you know how ZONEGRAN may affect you.

Tell your doctor about any other medicines you may be taking, including non-prescription medicines.

Tell your doctor right away if you are pregnant or plan to become pregnant. You and your doctor can decide if the benefits of taking ZONEGRAN outweigh the risks. ZONEGRAN may cause birth defects.

It is not known whether ZONEGRAN is passed through breast milk to the baby. Before taking ZONEGRAN, tell your doctor if you are nursing or planning to nurse your baby.

What are the possible or reasonably likely side effects of ZONEGRAN?

The most common side effects are drowsiness, loss of appetite, dizziness, headache, nausea, agitation, and irritability. These side effects could occur at any time, but most often occur in the first 4 weeks.

Contact your doctor right away if:

- you develop skin rash
- your seizures worsen
- you develop signs of kidney stones (sudden back pain, abdominal pain, blood in your urine)
- you develop signs of a blood problem (fever, sore throat, sores in your mouth, or bruising easily)
- you get depressed
- you start having thoughts that are unusual for you
- you are very drowsy, have difficulty concentrating, or have coordination problems
- you develop speech or language problems

Other information about ZONEGRAN:

Medicines are sometimes prescribed for purposes other than those listed in a patient leaflet. Use ZONEGRAN only for the reason your doctor told you. Do not use it for another reason. Do not share your ZONEGRAN with others.

This is a summary of information about ZONEGRAN. Call your healthcare professional with any questions. Your doctor or pharmacist can give you the complete information about ZONEGRAN that is written for health professionals. You can also get information about ZONEGRAN at www.eisai.com. You can get information and help from the Epilepsy Foundation at 800-EFA-1000 or www.efa.org.

Eisai

Manufactured by:
Elan Pharma International Ltd.
Distributed by:
Eisai Inc., Teaneck, NJ 07666

ZONEGRAN® is a registered trademark of Dainippon Pharmaceutical Co. Ltd. and licensed exclusively to Eisai Inc.

All other product names may be trademarks of the respective companies with which they are associated.

Shown in Product Identification Guide, page 311

Available to physicians through Eisai Medical Sales Specialists and Representatives, free of charge.

Griest Screener/Aricept Memory Checklist
(also available in Spanish)
(Above are disease specific brochures)
How Aricept Can Help (for patients on Aricept)
(also available in Spanish)
Aricept Weekly Diary
(also available in Spanish)

Elan Pharmaceuticals

7475 LUSK BLVD.
SAN DIEGO, CA 92121

For Medical Information Contact:
(888) NEURO-05
(888) 638-7605
To Report Adverse Events Contact:
(877) ELAN GSS
(877) 352–6477

The products below are distributed by Elan Pharmaceuticals

AZACTAM® ℞

[*ăz-ăk-tăm*]
(aztreonam for injection, USP)
Rx only

To reduce the development of drug-resistant bacteria and maintain the effectiveness of AZACTAM® and other antibacterial drugs, AZACTAM should be used only to treat or prevent infections that are proven or strongly suspected to be caused by bacteria.

DESCRIPTION

AZACTAM® (aztreonam for injection, USP) contains the active ingredient aztreonam, a monobactam. It was originally isolated from *Chromobacterium violaceum*. It is a synthetic bactericidal antibiotic.

The monobactams, having a unique monocyclic beta-lactam nucleus, are structurally different from other beta-lactam antibiotics (e.g., penicillins, cephalosporins, cephamycins). The sulfonic acid substituent in the 1-position of the ring activates the beta-lactam moiety; an aminothiazolyl oxime side chain in the 3-position and a methyl group in the 4-position confer the specific antibacterial spectrum and beta-lactamase stability.

Aztreonam is designated chemically as (Z)-2-[[[(2-amino-4-thiazolyl) [[(2S,3S)-2-methyl-4-oxo-1-sulfo-3-azetidinyl]carbamoyl]methylene]amino]oxy]-2-methylpropionic acid. Structural formula:

$C_{13}H_{17}N_5O_8S_2$ MW 435.44

AZACTAM is a sterile, nonpyrogenic, sodium-free, white powder containing approximately 780 mg arginine per gram of aztreonam. Following constitution, the product is for intramuscular or intravenous use. Aqueous solutions of the product have a pH in the range of 4.5 to 7.5.

CLINICAL PHARMACOLOGY

Single 30-minute intravenous infusions of 500-mg, 1-g and 2-g doses of AZACTAM (aztreonam for injection, USP) in healthy subjects produced aztreonam peak serum levels of 54, 90 and 204 µg/mL, respectively, immediately after administration; at eight hours, serum levels were 1, 3 and 6 µg/mL, respectively (Figure 1). Single 3-minute intravenous injections of the same doses resulted in serum levels of 58, 125 and 242 µg/mL at five minutes following completion of injection.

Serum concentrations of aztreonam in healthy subjects following completion of single intramuscular injections of 500-mg and 1-g doses are depicted in Figure 1; maximum serum concentrations occur at about one hour. After identical single intravenous or intramuscular doses of AZACTAM, the serum concentrations of aztreonam are comparable at one hour (1.5 hours from start of intravenous infusion) with similar slopes of serum concentrations thereafter.

FIGURE 1

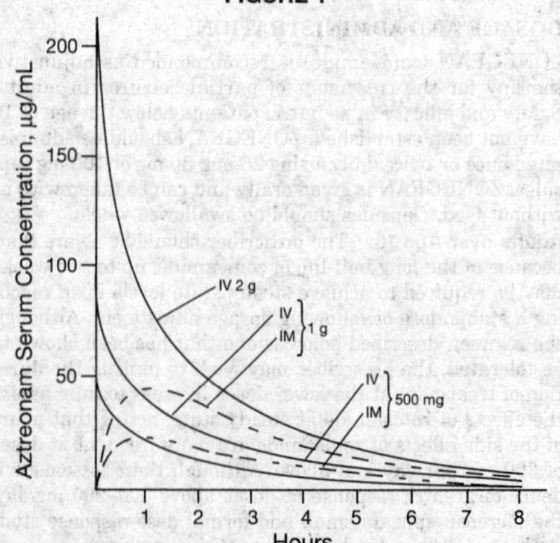

The serum levels of aztreonam following single 500-mg or 1-g (intramuscular or intravenous) or 2-g (intravenous) doses of AZACTAM exceed the MIC_{90} for *Neisseria* sp., *Haemophilus influenzae* and most genera of the Enterobacteriaceae for eight hours (for *Enterobacter* sp., the eight-hour serum levels exceed the MIC for 80 percent of strains). For *Pseudomonas aeruginosa*, a single 2-g intravenous dose produces serum levels that exceed the MIC_{90} for approximately four to six hours. All of the above doses of AZACTAM result in average urine levels of aztreonam that exceed the MIC_{90} for the same pathogens for up to 12 hours.

When aztreonam pharmacokinetics were assessed for adult and pediatric patients, they were found to be comparable (down to 9-months old). The serum half-life of aztreonam averaged 1.7 hours (1.5 to 2.0) in subjects with normal renal function, independent of the dose and route of administration. In healthy subjects, based on a 70 kg person, the serum clearance was 91 mL/min and renal clearance was 56 mL/min; the apparent mean volume of distribution at steady-state averaged 12.6 liters, approximately equivalent to extracellular fluid volume.

In elderly patients, the mean serum half-life of aztreonam increased and the renal clearance decreased, consistent with the age-related decrease in creatinine clearance.[1–4] The dosage of AZACTAM should be adjusted accordingly (See **DOSAGE AND ADMINISTRATION: Renal Impairment in Adult Patients.**)

In patients with impaired renal function, the serum half-life of aztreonam is prolonged (See **DOSAGE AND ADMINISTRATION: Renal Impairment in Adult Patients.**) The serum half-life of aztreonam is only slightly prolonged in patients with hepatic impairment since the liver is a minor pathway of excretion.

Average urine concentrations of aztreonam were approximately 1100, 3500 and 6600 µg/mL within the first two hours following single 500-mg, 1-g and 2-g intravenous doses of AZACTAM (30-minute infusions), respectively. The range of average concentrations for aztreonam in the 8- to 12-hour urine specimens in these studies was 25 to 120 µg/mL. After intramuscular injection of single 500 mg and 1 g doses of AZACTAM, urinary levels were approximately 500 and 1200 µg/mL, respectively, within the first two hours, declining to 180 and 470 µg/mL in the six to eight hour specimens. In healthy subjects, aztreonam is excreted in the urine about equally by active tubular secretion and glomerular filtration. Approximately 60 to 70 percent of an intravenous or intramuscular dose was recovered in the urine by eight hours. Urinary excretion of a single parenteral dose was essentially complete by 12 hours after injection. About 12 percent of a single intravenous radiolabeled dose was recovered in the feces. Unchanged aztreonam and the inactive beta-lactam ring hydrolysis product of aztreonam were present in feces and urine.

Intravenous or intramuscular administration of a single 500-mg or 1-g dose of AZACTAM every eight hours for seven days to healthy subjects produced no apparent accumulation of aztreonam or modification of its disposition characteristics; serum protein binding averaged 56 percent and was independent of dose. An average of about 6 percent of a 1 g intramuscular dose was excreted as a microbiologically inactive open beta-lactam ring hydrolysis product (serum half-life approximately 26 hours) of aztreonam in the zero to eight hour urine collection on the last day of multiple dosing.

Renal function was monitored in healthy subjects given aztreonam; standard tests (serum creatinine, creatinine clearance, BUN, urinalysis and total urinary protein excretion) as well as special tests (excretion of N-acetyl-β-glucosaminidase, alanine aminopeptidase and β_2-microglobulin) were used. No abnormal results were obtained.

Aztreonam achieves measurable concentrations in the following body fluids and tissues:

[See table at top of next page]

The concentration of aztreonam in saliva at 30 minutes after a single 1-g intravenous dose (9 patients) was 0.2 µg/mL; in human milk at two hours after a single 1-g intravenous dose (6 patients), 0.2 µg/mL, and at six hours after a single 1-g intramuscular dose (6 patients), 0.3 µg/mL; in amniotic fluid at six to eight hours after a single 1-g intravenous dose (5 patients), 2 µg/mL. The concentration of aztreonam in peritoneal fluid obtained one to six hours after multiple 2-g intravenous doses ranged between 12 and 90 µg/mL in 7 of 8 patients studied.

Aztreonam given intravenously rapidly reaches therapeutic concentrations in peritoneal dialysis fluid; conversely, aztreonam given intraperitoneally in dialysis fluid rapidly produces therapeutic serum levels.

Concomitant administration of probenecid or furosemide and AZACTAM (aztreonam for injection, USP) causes clinically insignificant increases in the serum levels of aztreonam. Single-dose intravenous pharmacokinetic studies have not shown any significant interaction between aztreonam and concomitantly administered gentamicin, nafcillin sodium, cephradine, clindamycin or metronidazole. No reports of disulfiram-like reactions with alcohol ingestion have been noted; this is not unexpected since aztreonam does not contain a methyl-tetrazole side chain.

Microbiology

Aztreonam exhibits potent and specific activity *in vitro* against a wide spectrum of gram-negative aerobic pathogens including *Pseudomonas aeruginosa*. The bactericidal action of aztreonam results from the inhibition of bacterial cell wall synthesis due to a high affinity of aztreonam for penicillin binding protein 3 (PBP3). Aztreonam, unlike the majority of beta-lactam antibiotics, does not induce beta-lactamase activity and its molecular structure confers a high degree of resistance to hydrolysis by beta-lactamases (i.e., penicillinases and cephalosporinases) produced by most gram-negative and gram-positive pathogens; it is, therefore, usually active against gram-negative aerobic microorganisms that are resistant to antibiotics hydrolyzed by beta-lactamases. It is active against many strains that are multiply-resistant to other antibiotics, such as certain cephalosporins, penicillin, and aminoglycosides. Aztreonam maintains its antimicrobial activity over a pH range of 6 to 8 *in vitro*, as well as in the presence of human serum and under anaerobic conditions.

Aztreonam has been shown to be active against most strains of the following microorganisms, both *in vitro* and in clinical infections as described in the **INDICATIONS AND USAGE** section.

Aerobic gram-negative microorganisms:

Citrobacter species, including *C. freundii*
Enterobacter species, including *E. cloacae*
Escherichia coli
Haemophilus influenzae (including ampicillin-resistant and other penicillinase-producing strains)
Klebsiella oxytoca
Klebsiella pneumoniae
Proteus mirabilis
Pseudomonas aeruginosa
Serratia species, including *S. marcescens*

The following *in vitro* data are available, **but their clinical significance is unknown.**

Aztreonam exhibits *in vitro* minimal inhibitory concentrations (MICs) of 8 µg/mL or less against most (≥90%) strains of the following microorganisms; however, the safety and effectiveness of aztreonam in treating clinical infections due to these microorganisms have not been established in adequate and well-controlled clinical trials.

Aerobic gram-negative microorganisms:

Aeromonas hydrophila
Morganella morganii
Neisseria gonorrhoeae (including penicillinase-producing strains)
Pasteurella multocida
Proteus vulgaris
Providencia stuartii
Providencia rettgeri
Yersinia enterocolitica

Aztreonam and aminoglycosides have been shown to be synergistic *in vitro* against most strains of *P. aeruginosa*, many strains of Enterobacteriaceae, and other gram-negative aerobic bacilli.

Alterations of the anaerobic intestinal flora by broad spectrum antibiotics may decrease colonization resistance, thus permitting overgrowth of potential pathogens, e.g., *Candida* and *Clostrium* species. Aztreonam has little effect on the anaerobic intestinal microflora in *in vitro* studies. *Clostridium difficile* and its cytotoxin were not found in animal models following administration of aztreonam. (See **ADVERSE REACTIONS**: ***Gastrointestinal.***)

Susceptibility Testing

Dilution Techniques: Quantitative methods are used to determine antimicrobial minimal inhibitory concentrations (MICs). These MICs provide estimates of the susceptibility of bacteria to antimicrobial compounds. The MICs should be determined using a standardized procedure. Standardized procedures are based on a dilution method[5] (broth or agar) or equivalent with standardized inoculum concentrations and standardized concentrations of aztreonam powder. The MIC values should be interpreted according to the following criteria:

For testing aerobic microorganisms other than *Haemophilus influenzae*:

MIC (µg/mL)	Interpretation
≤8	Susceptible (S)
16	Intermediate (I)
≥32	Resistant (R)

When testing *Haemophilus influenzae*[a]:

MIC (µg/mL)	Interpretation[b]
≤2	Susceptible (S)

a. Interpretative criteria applicable only to tests performed by broth microdilution method using *Haemophilus* Test Medium (HTM).[5]

b. The current absence of data on resistant strains precludes defining any categories other than "Susceptible". Strains yielding MIC results suggestive of a "nonsusceptible" category should be submitted to a reference laboratory for further testing.

A report of "Susceptible" indicates that the pathogen is likely to be inhibited if the antimicrobial compound in the blood reaches the concentrations usually achievable. A report of "Intermediate" indicates that the result should be considered equivocal, and, if the microorganism is not fully susceptible to alternative, clinically feasible drugs, the test should be repeated. This category implies possible clinical applicability in body sites where the drug is physiologically concentrated or in situations where high dosage of drug can be used. This category also provides a buffer zone which prevents small uncontrolled technical factors from causing major discrepancies in interpretation. A report of "Resistant" indicates that the pathogen is not likely to be inhibited if

EXTRAVASCULAR CONCENTRATIONS OF AZTREONAM AFTER A SINGLE PARENTERAL DOSE*

Fluid or Tissue	Dose (g)	Route	Hours Post-injection	Number of Patients	Mean Concentration (µg/mL or µg/g)
Fluids					
bile	1	IV	2	10	39
blister fluid	1	IV	1	6	20
bronchial secretion	2	IV	4	7	5
cerebrospinal fluid (inflamed meninges)	2	IV	0.9–4.3	16	3
pericardial fluid	2	IV	1	6	33
pleural fluid	2	IV	1.1–3.0	3	51
synovial fluid	2	IV	0.8–1.9	11	83
Tissues					
atrial appendage	2	IV	0.9–1.6	12	22
endometrium	2	IV	0.7–1.9	4	9
fallopian tube	2	IV	0.7–1.9	8	12
fat	2	IV	1.3–2.0	10	5
femur	2	IV	1.0–2.1	15	16
gallbladder	2	IV	0.8–1.3	4	23
kidney	2	IV	2.4–5.6	5	67
large intestine	2	IV	0.8–1.9	9	12
liver	2	IV	0.9–2.0	6	47
lung	2	IV	1.2–2.1	6	22
myometrium	2	IV	0.7–1.9	9	11
ovary	2	IV	0.7–1.9	7	13
prostate	1	IM	0.8–3.0	8	8
skeletal muscle	2	IV	0.3–0.7	6	16
skin	2	IV	0.0–1.0	8	25
sternum	2	IV	1	6	6

*Tissue penetration is regarded as essential to therapeutic efficacy, but specific tissue levels have not been correlated with specific therapeutic effects.

the antimicrobial compound in the blood reaches the concentrations usually achievable; other therapy should be selected.

Standardized susceptibility test procedures require the use of laboratory control microorganisms to control the technical aspects of the laboratory procedures. Standard aztreonam powder should provide the following MIC values:

Microorganism	MIC (µg/mL)
Escherichia coli ATCC 25922	0.06–0.25
Haemophilus influenzae[a] ATCC 49247	0.12–0.5
Pseudomonas aeruginosa ATCC 27853	2.0–8.0

a. Range applicable only to tests performed by broth microdilution method using *Haemophilus* Test Medium (HTM).[5]

Diffusion Techniques: Quantitative methods that require measurement of zone diameters also provide reproducible estimates of the susceptibility of bacteria to antimicrobial compounds. One such standardized procedure[6] requires the use of standardized inoculum concentrations. This procedure uses paper disks impregnated with 30-µg aztreonam to test the susceptibility of microorganisms to aztreonam.

Reports from the laboratory providing results of the standard single-disk susceptibility test with a 30-µg aztreonam disk should be interpreted according to the following criteria:

For testing aerobic microorganisms other than *Haemophilus influenzae*:

Zone Diameter	Interpretation
≥22	Susceptible (S)
16–21	Intermediate (I)
≤15	Resistant (R)

When testing *Haemophilus influenzae*[a]:

Zone Diameter	Interpretation[b]
≥26	Susceptible (S)

a. Interpretative criteria applicable only to tests performed by disk diffusion method using *Haemophilus* Test Medium (HTM).[6]

b. The current absence of data on resistant strains precludes defining any categories other than "Susceptible". Strains yielding zone diameter results suggestive of a "nonsusceptible" category should be submitted to a reference laboratory for further testing.

Interpretation should be as stated above for results using dilution techniques. Interpretation involves correlation of the diameter obtained in the disk test with the MIC for aztreonam.

As with standardized dilution techniques, diffusion methods require the use of laboratory control microorganisms that are used to control the technical aspects of the laboratory procedures. For the diffusion technique, the 30-µg aztreonam disk should provide the following zone diameters in these laboratory test quality control strains.

Microorganism	Zone Diameter (mm)
Escherichia coli ATCC 25922	28–36 mm
Haemophilus influenzae[a] ATCC 49247	30–38 mm
Pseudomonas aeruginosa ATCC 27853	23–29 mm

a. Range applicable to tests performed by disk diffusion method using *Haemophilus* Test Medium (HTM).[6]

INDICATIONS AND USAGE

To reduce the development of drug-resistant bacteria and maintain the effectiveness of AZACTAM® (aztreonam for injection, USP) and other anti-bacterial drugs, AZACTAM should be used only to treat or prevent infections that are proven or strongly suspected to be caused by susceptible bacteria. When culture and susceptibility information are available, they should be considered in selecting or modifying antibacterial therapy. In the absence of such data, local epidemiology and susceptibility patterns may contribute to the empiric selection of therapy.

AZACTAM (aztreonam for injection, USP) is indicated for the treatment of the following infections caused by susceptible gram-negative microorganisms:

Urinary Tract Infections (complicated and uncomplicated), including pyelonephritis and cystitis (initial and recurrent) caused by *Escherichia coli, Klebsiella pneumoniae, Proteus mirabilis, Pseudomonas aeruginosa, Enterobacter cloacae, Klebsiella oxytoca**, *Citrobacter* species* and *Serratia marcescens**.

Lower Respiratory Tract Infections, including pneumonia and bronchitis caused by *Escherichia coli, Klebsiella pneumoniae, Pseudomonas aeruginosa, Haemophilus influenzae, Proteus mirabilis, Enterobacter* species and *Serratia marcescens**.

Septicemia caused by *Escherichia coli, Klebsiella pneumoniae, Pseudomonas aeruginosa, Proteus mirabilis**, *Serratia marcescens** and *Enterobacter* species.

Skin and Skin-Structure Infections, including those associated with postoperative wounds, ulcers and burns caused by *Escherichia coli, Proteus mirabilis, Serratia marcescens, Enterobacter* species, *Pseudomonas aeruginosa, Klebsiella pneumoniae* and *Citrobacter* species*.

Intra-abdominal Infections, including peritonitis caused by *Escherichia coli, Klebsiella* species including *K. pneumoniae, Enterobacter* species including *E. cloacae**, *Pseudomonas aeruginosa, Citrobacter* species* including *C. freundii** and *Serratia* species* including *S. marcescens**.

Gynecologic Infections, including endometritis and pelvic cellulitis caused by *Escherichia coli, Klebsiella pneumoniae**, *Enterobacter* species* including *E. cloacae** and *Proteus mirabilis**.

*Efficacy for this organism in this organ system was studied in fewer than ten infections.

AZACTAM is indicated for adjunctive therapy to surgery in the management of infections caused by susceptible organisms, including abscesses, infections complicating hollow viscus perforations, cutaneous infections and infections of serous surfaces. AZACTAM is effective against most of the commonly encountered gram-negative aerobic pathogens seen in general surgery.

Concurrent Therapy

Concurrent initial therapy with other antimicrobial agents and AZACTAM® (aztreonam for injection, USP) is recommended before the causative organism(s) is known in seriously ill patients who are also at risk of having an infection due to gram-positive aerobic pathogens. If anaerobic organisms are also suspected as etiologic agents, therapy should be initiated using an anti-anaerobic agent concurrently with AZACTAM (see **DOSAGE AND ADMINISTRATION**). Certain antibiotics (e.g., cefoxitin, imipenem) may induce high levels of beta-lactamase in vitro in some gram-negative aerobes such as Enterobacter and Pseudomonas species, resulting in antagonism to many beta-lactam antibiotics including aztreonam. These *in vitro* findings suggest that such beta-lactamase inducing antibiotics not be used concurrently with aztreonam. Following identification and

Continued on next page

Azactam—Cont.

susceptibility testing of the causative organism(s), appropriate antibiotic therapy should be continued.

CONTRAINDICATIONS

This preparation is contraindicated in patients with known hypersensitivity to aztreonam or any other component in the formulation.

WARNINGS

Both animal and human data suggest that AZACTAM is rarely cross-reactive with other beta-lactam antibiotics and weakly immunogenic. Treatment with aztreonam can result in hypersensitivity reactions in patients with or without prior exposure. (See **CONTRAINDICATIONS**.)

Careful inquiry should be made to determine whether the patient has any history of hypersensitivity reactions to any allergens.

While cross-reactivity of aztreonam with other beta-lactam antibiotics is rare, this drug should be administered with caution to any patient with a history of hypersensitivity to beta-lactams (e.g., penicillins, cephalosporins, and/or carbapenems). Treatment with aztreonam can result in hypersensitivity reactions in patients with or without prior exposure to aztreonam. If an allergic reaction to aztreonam occurs, discontinue the drug and institute supportive treatment as appropriate (e.g., maintenance of ventilation, pressor amines, antihistamines, corticosteroids). Serious hypersensitivity reactions may require epinephrine and other emergency measures. (See **ADVERSE REACTIONS**.)

Pseudomembranous colitis has been reported with nearly all antibacterial agents, including aztreonam, and may range in severity from mild to life-threatening. Therefore, it is important to consider this diagnosis in patients who present with diarrhea subsequent to the administration of antibacterial agents.

Treatment with antibacterial agents alters the normal flora of the colon and may permit overgrowth of clostridia. Studies indicate that a toxin produced by *Clostridium difficile* is one primary cause of "antibiotic-associated colitis."

After the diagnosis of pseudomembranous colitis has been established, therapeutic measures should be initiated. Mild cases of pseudomembranous colitis usually respond to drug discontinuation alone. In moderate to severe cases, consideration should be given to management with fluids and electrolytes, protein supplementation, and treatment with an antibacterial drug clinically effective against *C. difficile* colitis.

Rare cases of toxic epidermal necrolysis have been reported in association with aztreonam in patients undergoing bone marrow transplant with multiple risk factors including sepsis, radiation therapy and other concomitantly administered drugs associated with toxic epidermal necrolysis.

PRECAUTIONS

General

Prescribing AZACTAM in the absence of a proven or strongly suspected bacterial infection or a prophylactic indication is unlikely to provide benefit to the patient and increases the risk of the development of drug-resistant bacteria.

In patients with impaired hepatic or renal function, appropriate monitoring is recommended during therapy.

If an aminoglycoside is used concurrently with aztreonam, especially if high dosages of the former are used or if therapy is prolonged, renal function should be monitored because of the potential nephrotoxicity and ototoxicity of aminoglycoside antibiotics.

The use of antibiotics may promote the overgrowth of nonsusceptible organisms, including gram-positive organisms (*Staphylococcus aureus* and *Streptococcus faecalis*) and fungi. Should superinfection occur during therapy, appropriate measures should be taken.

Information for Patients

Patients should be counseled that antibacterial drugs including AZACTAM should only be used to treat bacterial infections. They do not treat viral infections (e.g., the common cold). When AZACTAM is prescribed to treat a bacterial infection, patients should be told that although it is common to feel better early in the course of therapy, the medication should be taken exactly as directed. Skipping doses or not completing the full course of therapy may (1) decrease the effectiveness of the immediate treatment and (2) increase the likelihood that bacteria will develop resistance and will not be treatable by AZACTAM or other antibacterial drugs in the future.

Carcinogenesis, Mutagenesis, Impairment of Fertility

Carcinogenicity studies in animals have not been performed.

Genetic toxicology studies performed *in vivo* and *in vitro* with aztreonam in several standard laboratory models revealed no evidence of mutagenic potential at the chromosomal or gene level.

Two-generation reproduction studies in rats at daily doses up to 20 times the maximum recommended human dose, prior to and during gestation and lactation, revealed no evidence of impaired fertility. There was a slightly reduced survival rate during the lactation period in the offspring of rats that received the highest dosage, but not in offspring of rats that received five times the maximum recommended human dose.

Pregnancy

Pregnancy Category B

Aztreonam crosses the placenta and enters the fetal circulation.

Studies in pregnant rats and rabbits, with daily doses up to 15 and 5 times, respectively, the maximum recommended human dose, revealed no evidence of embryo- or fetotoxicity or teratogenicity. No drug induced changes were seen in any of the maternal, fetal, or neonatal parameters that were monitored in rats receiving 15 times the maximum recommended human dose of aztreonam during late gestation and lactation.

There are no adequate and well-controlled studies in pregnant women. Because animal reproduction studies are not always predictive of human response, aztreonam should be used during pregnancy only if clearly needed.

Nursing Mothers

Aztreonam is excreted in human milk in concentrations that are less than 1 percent of concentrations determined in simultaneously obtained maternal serum; consideration should be given to temporary discontinuation of nursing and use of formula feedings.

Pediatric Use

The safety and effectiveness of intravenous AZACTAM (aztreonam for injection, USP) have been established in the age groups 9 months to 16 years. Use of AZACTAM in these age groups is supported by evidence from adequate and well-controlled studies of AZACTAM in adults with additional efficacy, safety, and pharmacokinetic data from noncomparative clinical studies in pediatric patients. Sufficient data are not available for pediatric patients under 9 months of age or for the following treatment indications/pathogens: septicemia and skin and skin-structure infections (where the skin infection is believed or known to be due to *H. influenzae* type b). In pediatric patients with cystic fibrosis, higher doses of AZACTAM may be warranted. (See **CLINICAL PHARMACOLOGY, DOSAGE AND ADMINISTRATION**, and **CLINICAL STUDIES**.)

Geriatric Use

Clinical studies of AZACTAM did not include sufficient numbers of subjects aged 65 years and older to determine whether they respond differently from younger subjects. Other reported clinical experience has not identified differences in responses between the elderly and younger patients.[7–10] In general, dose selection for an elderly patient should be cautious, reflecting the greater frequency of decreased hepatic, renal, or cardiac function, and of concomitant disease or other drug therapy.

In elderly patients, the mean serum half-life of aztreonam increased and the renal clearance decreased, consistent with the age-related decrease in creatinine clearance.[1–4]

Since aztreonam is known to be substantially excreted by the kidney, the risk of toxic reactions to this drug may be greater in patients with impaired renal function. Because elderly patients are more likely to have decreased renal function, renal function should be monitored and dosage adjustments made accordingly (See **DOSAGE AND ADMINISTRATION: Renal Impairment in Adult Patients** and **Dosage in the Elderly**).

AZACTAM contains no sodium.

ADVERSE REACTIONS

Local reactions such as phlebitis/thrombophlebitis following IV administration, and discomfort/swelling at the injection site following IM administration occurred at rates of approximately 1.9 percent and 2.4 percent, respectively.

Systemic reactions (considered to be related to therapy or of uncertain etiology) occurring at an incidence of 1 to 1.3 percent include diarrhea, nausea and/or vomiting, and rash. Reactions occurring at an incidence of less than 1 percent are listed within each body system in order of decreasing severity:

Hypersensitivity—anaphylaxis, angioedema, bronchospasm

Hematologic—pancytopenia, neutropenia, thrombocytopenia, anemia, eosinophilia, leukocytosis, thrombocytosis

Gastrointestinal—abdominal cramps; rare cases of *C. difficile*-associated diarrhea, including pseudomembranous colitis, or gastrointestinal bleeding have been reported. Onset of pseudomembranous colitis symptoms may occur during or after antibiotic treatment. (See **WARNINGS**.)

Dermatologic—toxic epidermal necrolysis (see **WARNINGS**), purpura, erythema multiforme, exfoliative dermatitis, urticaria, petechiae, pruritus, diaphoresis

Cardiovascular—hypotension, transient ECG changes (ventricular bigeminy and PVC), flushing

Respiratory—wheezing, dyspnea, chest pain

Hepatobiliary—hepatitis, jaundice

Nervous System—seizure, confusion, vertigo, paresthesia, insomnia, dizziness

Musculoskeletal—muscular aches

Special Senses—tinnitus, diplopia, mouth ulcer, altered taste, numb tongue, sneezing, nasal congestion, halitosis

Other—vaginal candidiasis, vaginitis, breast tenderness

Body as a Whole—weakness, headache, fever, malaise

Pediatric Adverse Reactions

Of the 612 pediatric patients who were treated with AZACTAM in clinical trials, less than 1% required discontinuation of therapy due to adverse events. The following systemic adverse events, regardless of drug relationship, occurred in at least 1% of treated patients in domestic clinical trials: rash (4.3%), diarrhea (1.4%), and fever (1.0%). These adverse events were comparable to those observed in adult clinical trials.

In 343 pediatric patients receiving intravenous therapy, the following local reactions were noted: pain (12%), erythema (2.9%), induration (0.9%), and phlebitis (2.1%). In the US patient population, pain occurred in 1.5% of patients, while each of the remaining three local reactions had an incidence of 0.5%.

The following laboratory adverse events, regardless of drug relationship, occurred in at least 1% of treated patients: increased eosinophils (6.3%), increased platelets (3.6%), neutropenia (3.2%), increased AST (3.8%), increased ALT (6.5%), and increased serum creatinine (5.8%).

In US pediatric clinical trials, neutropenia (absolute neutrophil count less than 1000/mm^3) occurred in 11.3% of patients (8/71) younger than 2 years receiving 30 mg/kg q6h. AST and ALT elevations to greater than 3 times the upper limit of normal were noted in 15–20% of patients aged 2 years or above receiving 50 mg/kg q6h. The increased frequency of these reported laboratory adverse events may be due to either increased severity of illness treated or higher doses of AZACTAM administered.

Adverse Laboratory Changes

Adverse laboratory changes without regard to drug relationship that were reported during clinical trials were:

Hepatic—elevations of AST (SGOT), ALT (SGPT), and alkaline phosphatase; signs or symptoms of hepatobiliary dysfunction occurred in less than 1 percent of recipients (see above).

Hematologic—increases in prothrombin and partial thromboplastin times, positive Coombs' test.

Renal—increases in serum creatinine.

OVERDOSAGE

If necessary, aztreonam may be cleared from the serum by hemodialysis and/or peritoneal dialysis.

DOSAGE AND ADMINISTRATION

Dosage in Adult Patients

AZACTAM may be administered intravenously or by intramuscular injection. Dosage and route of administration should be determined by susceptibility of the causative organisms, severity and site of infection, and the condition of the patient.

The intravenous route is recommended for patients requiring single doses greater than 1 g or those with bacterial septicemia, localized parenchymal abscess (e.g., intra-abdominal abscess), peritonitis or other severe systemic or life-threatening infections.

The duration of therapy depends on the severity of infection. Generally, AZACTAM should be continued for at least 48 hours after the patient becomes asymptomatic or evidence of bacterial eradication has been obtained. Persistent infections may require treatment for several weeks. Doses smaller than those indicated should not be used.

Renal Impairment in Adult Patients

Prolonged serum levels of aztreonam may occur in patients with transient or persistent renal insufficiency. Therefore, the dosage of AZACTAM should be halved in patients with estimated creatinine clearances between 10 and 30 mL/min/1.73 m^2 after an initial loading dose of 1 g or 2 g.

When only the serum creatinine concentration is available, the following formula (based on sex, weight, and age of the patient) may be used to approximate the creatinine clearance (Clcr). The serum creatinine should represent a steady state of renal function.

[See table below]

In patients with severe renal failure (creatinine clearance less than 10 mL/min/1.73 m^2), such as those supported by hemodialysis, the usual dose of 500 mg, 1 g or 2 g should be given initially. The maintenance dose should be one-fourth of the usual initial dose given at the usual fixed interval of 6, 8 or 12 hours. For serious or life-threatening infections, in addition to the maintenance doses, one-eighth of the initial dose should be given after each hemodialysis session.

Dosage in The Elderly

Renal status is a major determinant of dosage in the elderly; these patients in particular may have diminished renal function. Serum creatinine may not be an accurate determinant of renal status. Therefore, as with all antibiotics eliminated by the kidneys, estimates of creatinine clearance should be obtained, and appropriate dosage modifications made if necessary.

Dosage in Pediatric Patients

AZACTAM (aztreonam for injection, USP) should be administered intravenously to pediatric patients with normal renal function. There are insufficient data regarding intramuscular administration to pediatric patients or dosing in pediatric patients with renal impairment. (See **PRECAUTIONS: Pediatric Use**.)

$$\text{Males: Clcr} = \frac{\text{weight (kg)} \times (140\text{-age})}{72 \times \text{serum creatinine (mg/dL)}}$$

Females: 0.85 × above value

AZACTAM DOSAGE GUIDELINES

Type of Infection	Dose	Frequency (hours)
ADULTS*		
Urinary tract infections	500 mg or 1 g	8 or 12
Moderately severe systemic infections	1 g or 2 g	8 or 12
Severe systemic or life-threatening infections	2g	6 or 8
*Maximum recommended dose is 8 g per day.		
PEDIATRIC PATIENTS**		
Mild to moderate infections	30 mg/kg	8
Moderate to severe infections	30 mg/kg	6 or 8
**Maximum recommended dose is 120 mg/kg/day.		

Because of the serious nature of infections due to *Pseudomonas aeruginosa*, dosage of 2 g every six or eight hours is recommended, at least upon initiation of therapy, in systemic infections caused by this organism in adults.

CLINICAL STUDIES

A total of 612 pediatric patients aged 1 month to 12 years were enrolled in uncontrolled clinical trials of aztreonam in the treatment of serious gram-negative infections, including urinary tract, lower respiratory tract, skin and skin-structure, and intra-abdominal infections.

Preparation Of Parenteral Solutions

General

Upon the addition of the diluent to the container, contents should be shaken **immediately** and **vigorously**. Constituted solutions are not for multiple-dose use; should the entire volume in the container not be used for a single-dose, the unused solution must be discarded.

Depending upon the concentration of aztreonam and diluent used, constituted AZACTAM yields a colorless to light straw yellow solution which may develop a slight pink tint on standing (potency is not affected). Parenteral drug products should be inspected visually for particulate matter and discoloration whenever solution and container permit.

Admixtures With Other Antibiotics

Intravenous infusion solutions of AZACTAM not exceeding 2% w/v prepared with Sodium Chloride Injection USP 0.9% or Dextrose Injection USP 5%, to which clindamycin phosphate, gentamicin sulfate, tobramycin sulfate, or cefazolin sodium have been added at concentrations usually used clinically, are stable for up to 48 hours at room temperature or seven days under refrigeration. Ampicillin sodium admixtures with aztreonam in Sodium Chloride Injection USP 0.9% are stable for 24 hours at room temperature and 48 hours under refrigeration; stability in Dextrose Injection USP 5% is two hours at room temperature and eight hours under refrigeration.

Aztreonam-cloxacillin sodium and aztreonam-vancomycin hydrochloride admixtures are stable in Dianeal® 137 (Peritoneal Dialysis Solution) with 4.25% Dextrose for up to 24 hours at room temperature.

Aztreonam is incompatible with nafcillin sodium, cephradine, and metronidazole.

Other admixtures are not recommended since compatibility data are not available.

Intravenous (IV) Solutions

For Bolus Injection: The contents of an AZACTAM (aztreonam for injection, USP) 15 mL capacity vial should be constituted with 6 to 10 mL Sterile Water for Injection USP. *For Infusion:* Contents of the 100 mL capacity bottle should be constituted to a final concentration not exceeding 2% w/v (at least 50 mL of any appropriate infusion solution listed below per gram aztreonam). These solutions may be frozen immediately after constitution in the original container. (See **Stability** below.)

If the contents of a 15 mL capacity vial are to be transferred to an appropriate infusion solution, each gram of aztreonam should be initially constituted with at least 3 mL Sterile Water for Injection USP. Further dilution may be obtained with one of the following intravenous infusion solutions:

- Sodium Chloride Injection USP, 0.9%
- Ringer's Injection USP
- Lactated Ringer's Injection USP
- Dextrose Injection USP, 5% or 10%
- Dextrose and Sodium Chloride Injection USP, 5%:0.9%, 5%:0.45% or 5%:0.2%
- Sodium Lactate Injection USP (M/6 Sodium Lactate)
- Ionosol® B and 5% Dextrose
- Isolyte® E
- Isolyte® E with 5% Dextrose
- Isolyte® M with 5% Dextrose
- Normosol®-R
- Normosol®-R and 5% Dextrose
- Normosol®-M and 5% Dextrose
- Mannitol Injection USP, 5% or 10%
- Lactated Ringer's and 5% Dextrose Injection
- Plasma-Lyte® M and 5% Dextrose
- 10% Travert® Injection
- 10% Travert® and Electrolyte No. 1 Injection
- 10% Travert® and Electrolyte No. 2 Injection
- 10% Travert® and Electrolyte No. 3 Injection

Intramuscular (IM) Solutions

The contents of an AZACTAM 15 mL capacity vial should be constituted with at least 3 mL of an appropriate diluent per gram aztreonam. The following diluents may be used:

- Sterile Water for Injection USP
- Sterile Bacteriostatic Water for Injection, USP (with benzyl alcohol or with methyl- and propylparabens)
- Sodium Chloride Injection USP, 0.9%
- Bacteriostatic Sodium Chloride Injection USP (with benzyl alcohol)

Stability Of IV And IM Solutions

AZACTAM solutions for IV infusion at concentrations not exceeding 2% w/v must be used within 48 hours following constitution if kept at controlled room temperature (59°– 86° F/15°– 30° C) or within seven days if refrigerated (36°– 46° F/2°– 8° C).

Frozen aztreonam infusion solutions may be stored for up to three months at -4° F/-20° C; frozen solutions may be thawed at controlled room temperature or by overnight refrigeration. Solutions that have been thawed and maintained at controlled room temperature or under refrigeration should be used within 24 or 72 hours after removal from the freezer, respectively. Solutions should not be refrozen.

AZACTAM solutions at concentrations exceeding 2% w/v, except those prepared with Sterile Water for Injection USP or Sodium Chloride Injection USP, should be used promptly after preparation; the two excepted solutions must be used within 48 hours if stored at controlled room temperature or within seven days if refrigerated.

Intravenous Administration

Bolus Injection: A bolus injection may be used to initiate therapy. The dose should be **slowly** injected directly into a vein, or the tubing of a suitable administration set, over a period of three to five minutes (see next paragraph regarding flushing of tubing).

Infusion: With any intermittent infusion of aztreonam and another drug with which it is not pharmaceutically compatible, the common delivery tube should be flushed before and after delivery of aztreonam with any appropriate infusion solution compatible with both drug solutions; the drugs should not be delivered simultaneously. Any AZACTAM (aztreonam for injection, USP) infusion should be completed within a 20 to 60 minute period. With use of a *Y-type administration set*, careful attention should be given to the calculated volume of aztreonam solution required so that the entire dose will be infused. A volume control administration set may be used to deliver an initial dilution of AZACTAM (see **Preparation Of Parenteral Solutions, For Infusion**) into a compatible infusion solution during administration; in this case, the final dilution of aztreonam should provide a concentration not exceeding 2% w/v.

Intramuscular Administration

The dose should be given by deep injection into a large muscle mass (such as the upper outer quadrant of the gluteus maximus or lateral part of the thigh). Aztreonam is well tolerated and should not be admixed with any local anesthetic agent.

HOW SUPPLIED

AZACTAM® (aztreonam for injection, USP)—Lyophilized

Single-dose 15 mL capacity vials:

500 mg/vial: Packages of 10 NDC 51479-040-05
1 g/vial: Packages of 10 NDC 51479-041-15
2 g/vial: Packages of 10 NDC 51479-042-15

Single-dose 100 mL capacity intravenous infusion bottles with bail bands:

1 g/bottle: Packages of 10 NDC 51479-041-10
2 g/bottle: Packages of 10 NDC 51479-042-10

Storage

Store original packages at room temperature; avoid excessive heat.

ALSO SUPPLIED AS:

AZACTAM® (aztreonam injection) in Galaxy® plastic container (PL 2040) as a frozen, 50 mL single-dose intravenous solution as follows:

1 g aztreonam/50 mL container: Packages of 24 NDC 51479-048-01

2 g aztreonam/50 mL container: Packages of 24 NDC 51479-049-01

REFERENCES

1. Naber KG, Dette GA, Kees F, Knothe H, Grobecker H. Pharmacokinetics, *in vitro* activity, therapeutic efficacy, and clinical safety of aztreonam vs. cefotaxime in the treatment of complicated urinary tract infections. *J Antimicrob Chemother* 1986; 17:517–527.
2. Creasey WA, Platt TB, Frantz M, Sugerman AA. Pharmacokinetics of aztreonam in elderly male volunteers. *Br J Clin Pharmacol* 1985; 19:233–237.
3. Meyers BR, Wilkinson P, Mendelson MH, *et al.* Pharmacokinetics of aztreonam in healthy elderly and young adult volunteers. *J Clin Pharmacol* 1993; 33:470–474.
4. Sattler FR, Schramm M, Swabb EA. Safety of aztreonam and SQ 26,992 in elderly patients with renal insufficiency. *Rev Infect Dis* 1985; 7 (suppl 4):S622-S627.
5. National Committee for Clinical Laboratory Standards. *Methods for Dilution Antimicrobial Susceptibility Tests for Bacteria that Grow Aerobically* — Fifth Edition. Approved Standard NCCLS Document M7-A5, Vol. 20, No. 2, NCCLS, Wayne PA, January 2000.
6. National Committee for Clinical Laboratory Standards. *Performance Standards for Antimicrobial Disk Susceptibility Tests* — Seventh Edition. Approved Standard NCCLS Document M2-A7, Vol. 20, No. 1, NCCLS, Wayne, PA, January 2000.
7. Deger F, Douchamps J, Freschi E, *et al.* Aztreonam in the treatment of serious gram-negative infections in the elderly. *Int J Clin Pharmacol Ther and Toxicol* 1988; 26: 22–26.
8. Knockaert DC, Dejaeger E, Nestor L, *et al.* Aztreonam-flucloxacilin double beta-lactam treatment as empirical therapy of serious infections in very elderly patients. *Age and Aging* 1981; 20:135–139.
9. Roelandts F. Clinical use of aztreonam in a psychogeriatric population. *Acta Clin Belg* 1992; 47:251–255.
10. Andrews R, Fasoli R, Scoggins WG, *et al.* Combined aztreonam and gentamicin therapy for pseudomonal lower respiratory tract infections. *Clin Therap* 1994; 16:236–252.
11. National Committee for Clinical Laboratory Standards. *Performance Standards for Antimicrobial Susceptibility Testing* — Eleventh Informational Supplement, NCCLS Document M100-S11, Vol. 21, No. 1, NCCLS, Wayne, PA, January 2001.

AZACTAM® (aztreonam for injection, USP) is a registered trademark of Bristol-Myers Squibb Company licensed exclusively in the US to EPI. Galaxy®, Dianeal®, Plasma-Lyte®, and Travert® are registered trademarks of Baxter International, Inc. Ionosol® and Normosol® are registered trademarks of Abbott Laboratories Corporation. Isolyte® is a registered trademark of McGraw Inc.

Manufactured by
Bristol-Myers Squibb Company
Princeton, NJ 08543 U.S.A.
Distributed by
Elan Biopharmaceuticals, a business unit of Elan Pharmaceuticals, Inc. (EPI),
a member of the Elan Group,
San Diego, CA 92121 USA
Made in Italy

AZL 1120404/6000849-A Revised January 2004

MAXIPIME® ℞

[*măk'sĭ-pīm*]

(Cefepime Hydrochloride, USP) for Injection
For Intravenous or Intramuscular Use
Rx only

To reduce the development of drug-resistant bacteria and maintain the effectiveness of MAXIPIME® and other antibacterial drugs, MAXIPIME should be used only to treat or prevent infections that are proven or strongly suspected to be caused by bacteria.

DESCRIPTION

MAXIPIME (cefepime hydrochloride, USP) is a semi-synthetic, broad spectrum, cephalosporin antibiotic for parenteral administration. The chemical name is 1-[[(6R,7R)-7-[2-(2-amino-4-thiazolyl)-glyoxylamido]-2-carboxy-8-oxo-5-thia-1-azabicyclo[4.2.0] oct-2-en-3-yl]methyl]-1-methylpyrrolidinium chloride, 7^2-(Z)-(O-methyloxime), monohydrochloride, monohydrate, which corresponds to the following structural formula:

OCH₃ · HCl • H₂N · Cl⁻ · • H₂O · COOH · CH₃

Cefepime hydrochloride is a white to pale yellow powder. Cefepime hydrochloride contains the equivalent of not less than 825 µg and not more than 911 µg of cefepime ($C_{19}H_{24}N_6O_5S_2$) per mg, calculated on an anhydrous basis. It is highly soluble in water.

MAXIPIME for Injection is supplied for intramuscular or intravenous administration in strengths equivalent to 500 mg, 1 g, and 2 g of cefepime. (See **DOSAGE AND ADMINISTRATION.**) MAXIPIME is a sterile, dry mixture of cefepime hydrochloride and L-arginine. It contains the equivalent of not less than 90.0 percent and not more than 115.0 percent of the labeled amount of cefepime ($C_{19}H_{24}N_6O_5S_2$). The L-arginine, at an approximate concentration of 725 mg/g of cefepime, is added to control the pH of the constituted solution at 4.0–6.0. Freshly constituted solutions of MAXIPIME will range in color from colorless to amber.

CLINICAL PHARMACOLOGY

Pharmacokinetics

The average plasma concentrations of cefepime observed in healthy adult male volunteers (n=9) at various times following single 30-minute infusions (IV) of cefepime 500 mg, 1 g, and 2 g are summarized in Table 1. Elimination of cefepime is principally via renal excretion with an average (±SD) half-life of 2.0 (±0.3) hours and total body clearance of 120.0 (±8.0) mL/min in healthy volunteers. Cefepime pharmacokinetics are linear over the range 250 mg to 2 g. There is no

Continued on next page

Maxipime—Cont.

evidence of accumulation in healthy adult male volunteers (n=7) receiving clinically relevant doses for a period of 9 days.

Absorption

The average plasma concentrations of cefepime and its derived pharmacokinetic parameters after intravenous administration are portrayed in Table 1.

[See table 1 at right]

Following intramuscular (IM) administration, cefepime is completely absorbed. The average plasma concentrations of cefepime at various times following a single IM injection are summarized in Table 2. The pharmacokinetics of cefepime are linear over the range of 500 mg to 2 g IM and do not vary with respect to treatment duration.

[See table 2 at right]

Distribution

The average steady-state volume of distribution of cefepime is 18.0 (±2.0) L. The serum protein binding of cefepime is approximately 20% and is independent of its concentration in serum.

Cefepime is excreted in human milk. A nursing infant consuming approximately 1000 mL of human milk per day would receive approximately 0.5 mg of cefepime per day. (See **PRECAUTIONS: Nursing Mothers.**)

Concentrations of cefepime achieved in specific tissues and body fluids are listed in Table 3.

[See table 3 at right]

Data suggest that cefepime does cross the inflamed blood-brain barrier. **The clinical relevance of these data are uncertain at this time.**

Metabolism and Excretion

Cefepime is metabolized to N-methylpyrrolidine (NMP) which is rapidly converted to the N-oxide (NMP-N-oxide). Urinary recovery of unchanged cefepime accounts for approximately 85% of the administered dose. Less than 1% of the administered dose is recovered from urine as NMP, 6.8% as NMP-N-oxide, and 2.5% as an epimer of cefepime. Because renal excretion is a significant pathway of elimination, patients with renal dysfunction and patients undergoing hemodialysis require dosage adjustment. (See **DOSAGE AND ADMINISTRATION.**)

Special Populations

Pediatric patients: Cefepime pharmacokinetics have been evaluated in pediatric patients from 2 months to 11 years of age following single and multiple doses on q8h (n=29) and q12h (n=13) schedules. Following a single IV dose, total body clearance and the steady-state volume of distribution averaged 3.3 (±1.0) mL/min/kg and 0.3 (±0.1) L/kg, respectively. The urinary recovery of unchanged cefepime was 60.4 (±30.4)% of the administered dose, and the average renal clearance was 2.0 (±1.1) mL/min/kg. There were no significant effects of age or gender (25 male vs 17 female) on total body clearance or volume of distribution, corrected for body weight. No accumulation was seen when cefepime was given at 50 mg/kg q12h (n=13), while C_{max}, AUC, and $t_{1/2}$ were increased about 15% at steady state after 50 mg/kg q8h. The exposure to cefepime following a 50 mg/kg IV dose in a pediatric patient is comparable to that in an adult treated with a 2 g IV dose. The absolute bioavailability of cefepime after an IM dose of 50 mg/kg was 82.3 (±15)% in eight patients.

Geriatric patients: Cefepime pharmacokinetics have been investigated in elderly (65 years of age and older) men (n=12) and women (n=12) whose mean (SD) creatinine clearance was 74.0 (±15.0) mL/min. There appeared to be a decrease in cefepime total body clearance as a function of creatinine clearance. Therefore, dosage administration of cefepime in the elderly should be adjusted as appropriate if the patient's creatinine clearance is 60 mL/min or less. (See **DOSAGE AND ADMINISTRATION.**)

Renal insufficiency: Cefepime pharmacokinetics have been investigated in patients with various degrees of renal insufficiency (n=30). The average half-life in patients requiring hemodialysis was 13.5 (±2.7) hours and in patients requiring continuous peritoneal dialysis was 19.0 (±2.0) hours. Cefepime total body clearance decreased proportionally with creatinine clearance in patients with abnormal renal function, which serves as the basis for dosage adjustment recommendations in this group of patients. (See **DOSAGE AND ADMINISTRATION.**)

Hepatic insufficiency: The pharmacokinetics of cefepime were unaltered in patients with impaired hepatic function who received a single 1 g dose (n=11).

Microbiology

Cefepime is a bactericidal agent that acts by inhibition of bacterial cell wall synthesis. Cefepime has a broad spectrum of *in vitro* activity that encompasses a wide range of gram-positive and gram-negative bacteria. Cefepime has a low affinity for chromosomally-encoded beta-lactamases. Cefepime is highly resistant to hydrolysis by most beta-lactamases and exhibits rapid penetration into gram-negative bacterial cells. Within bacterial cells, the molecular targets of cefepime are the penicillin binding proteins (PBP).

Cefepime has been shown to be active against most strains of the following microorganisms, both *in vitro* and in clinical infections as described in the **INDICATIONS AND USAGE** section.

Aerobic Gram-Negative Microorganisms:
- *Enterobacter*
- *Escherichia coli*
- *Klebsiella pneumoniae*
- *Proteus mirabilis*
- *Pseudomonas aeruginosa*

Aerobic Gram-Positive Microorganisms:
- *Staphylococcus aureus (methicillin-susceptible strains only)*
- *Streptococcus pneumoniae*
- *Streptococcus pyogenes (Lancefield's Group A streptococci)*
- Viridans group streptococci

The following *in vitro* data are available, **but their clinical significance is unknown**. Cefepime has been shown to have *in vitro* activity against most strains of the following microorganisms; however, the safety and effectiveness of cefepime in treating clinical infections due to these microorganisms have not been established in adequate and well-controlled trials.

Aerobic Gram-Positive Microorganisms:
- *Staphylococcus epidermidis (methicillin-susceptible strains only)*
- *Staphylococcus saprophyticus*
- *Streptococcus agalactiae (Lancefield's Group B streptococci)*

NOTE: Most strains of enterococci, eg, *Enterococcus faecalis*, and methicillin-resistant staphylococci are resistant to cefepime.

Aerobic Gram-Negative Microorganisms:
- *Acinetobacter calcoaceticus subsp. lwoffi*
- *Citrobacter diversus*
- *Citrobacter freundii*
- *Enterobacter agglomerans*
- *Haemophilus influenzae (including beta-lactamase producing strains)*
- *Hafnia alvei*
- *Klebsiella oxytoca*
- *Moraxella catarrhalis (including beta-lactamase producing strains)*
- *Morganella morganii*
- *Proteus vulgaris*
- *Providencia rettgeri*

TABLE 1
Average Plasma Concentrations in μg/mL of Cefepime and Derived Pharmacokinetic Parameters (±SD), Intravenous Administration

Parameter	MAXIPIME 500 mg IV	MAXIPIME 1 g IV	MAXIPIME 2 g IV
0.5 h	38.2	78.7	163.1
1.0 h	21.6	44.5	85.8
2.0 h	11.6	24.3	44.8
4.0 h	5.0	10.5	19.2
8.0 h	1.4	2.4	3.9
12.0 h	0.2	0.6	1.1
C_{max}, μg/mL	39.1 (3.5)	81.7 (5.1)	163.9 (25.3)
AUC, h•μg/mL	70.8 (6.7)	148.5 (15.1)	284.8 (30.6)
Number of subjects (male)	9	9	9

TABLE 2
Average Plasma Concentrations in μg/mL of Cefepime and Derived Pharmacokinetic Parameters (±SD), Intramuscular Administration

Parameter	MAXIPIME 500 mg IM	MAXIPIME 1 g IM	MAXIPIME 2 g IM
0.5 h	8.2	14.8	36.1
1.0 h	12.5	25.9	49.9
2.0 h	12.0	26.3	51.3
4.0 h	6.9	16.0	31.5
8.0 h	1.9	4.5	8.7
12.0 h	0.7	1.4	2.3
C_{max}, μg/mL	13.9 (3.4)	29.6 (4.4)	57.5 (9.5)
T_{max}, h	1.4 (0.9)	1.6 (0.4)	1.5 (0.4)
AUC, h•μg/mL	60.0 (8.0)	137.0 (11.0)	262.0 (23.0)
Number of subjects (male)	6	6	12

TABLE 3
Average Concentrations of Cefepime in Specific Body Fluids (μg/mL) or Tissues (μg/g)

Tissue or Fluid	Dose/Route	# of Patients	Average Time of Sample Post-Dose (h)	Average Concentration
Blister Fluid	2 g IV	6	1.5	81.4 μg/mL
Bronchial Mucosa	2 g IV	20	4.8	24.1 μg/g
Sputum	2 g IV	5	4.0	7.4 μg/mL
Urine	500 mg IV	8	0–4	292.0 μg/mL
	1 g IV	12	0–4	926.0 μg/mL
	2 g IV	12	0–4	3120.0 μg/mL
Bile	2 g IV	26	9.4	17.8 μg/mL
Peritoneal Fluid	2 g IV	19	4.4	18.3 μg/mL
Appendix	2 g IV	31	5.7	5.2 μg/g
Gallbladder	2 g IV	38	8.9	11.9 μg/g
Prostate	2 g IV	5	1.0	31.5 μg/g

Providencia stuartii
Serratia marcescens
NOTE: Cefepime is inactive against many strains of *Stenotrophomonas* (formerly *Xanthomonas maltophilia* and *Pseudomonas maltophilia*).
Anaerobic Microorganisms:
NOTE: Cefepime is inactive against most strains of *Clostridium difficile*.

Susceptibility Tests

Dilution Techniques: Quantitative methods are used to determine antimicrobial minimum inhibitory concentrations (MICs). These MICs provide estimates of the susceptibility of bacteria to antimicrobial compounds. The MICs should be determined using a standardized procedure. Standardized procedures are based on a dilution method[1] (broth or agar) or equivalent with standardized inoculum concentrations and standardized concentrations of cefepime powder. The MIC values should be interpreted according to the following criteria:
[See table 4 at right]

TABLE 4

Microorganism	MIC (μg/mL) Susceptible (S)	Intermediate (I)	Resistant (R)
Microorganisms other than *Haemophilus* spp.* and *S. pneumoniae*	≤8	16	≥32
Haemophilus spp.*	≤2	—*	—*
*Streptococcus pneumoniae**	≤0.5	1	≥2

*NOTE: Isolates from these species should be tested for susceptibility using specialized dilution testing methods.[1] Also, strains of *Haemophilus* spp. with MICs greater than 2 μg/mL should be considered equivocal and should be further evaluated.

A report of "Susceptible" indicates that the pathogen is likely to be inhibited if the antimicrobial compound in the blood reaches the concentrations usually achievable. A report of "Intermediate" indicates that the result should be considered equivocal, and, if the microorganism is not fully susceptible to alternative, clinically feasible drugs, the test should be repeated. This category implies possible clinical applicability in body sites where the drug is physiologically concentrated or in situations where high dosage of drug can be used. This category also provides a buffer zone which prevents small uncontrolled technical factors from causing major discrepancies in interpretation. A report of "Resistant" indicates that the pathogen is not likely to be inhibited if the antimicrobial compound in the blood reaches the concentrations usually achievable; other therapy should be selected.

Standardized susceptibility test procedures require the use of laboratory control microorganisms to control the technical aspects of the laboratory procedures. Laboratory control microorganisms are specific strains of microbiological assay organisms with intrinsic biological properties relating to resistance mechanisms and their genetic expression within bacteria; the specific strains are not clinically significant in their current microbiological status. Standard cefepime powder should provide the following MIC values (Table 5) when tested against the designated quality control strains:
[See table 5 at right]

Table 5

Microorganism	ATCC	MIC (μg/mL)
Escherichia coli	25922	0.016–0.12
Staphylococcus aureus	29213	1–4
Pseudomonas aeruginosa	27853	1–4
Haemophilus influenzae	49247	0.5–2
Streptococcus pneumoniae	49619	0.06–0.25

Diffusion Techniques: Quantitative methods that require measurement of zone diameters also provide reproducible estimates of the susceptibility of bacteria to antimicrobial compounds. One such standardized procedure[2] requires the use of standardized inoculum concentrations. This procedure uses paper disks impregnated with 30 μg of cefepime to test the susceptibility of microorganisms to cefepime. Interpretation is identical to that stated above for results using dilution techniques.

Reports from the laboratory providing results of the standard single-disk susceptibility test with a 30-μg cefepime disk should be interpreted according to the following criteria:
[See table 6 at right]

TABLE 6

Microorganism	Zone Diameter (mm) Susceptible (S)	Intermediate (I)	Resistant (R)
Microorganisms other than *Haemophilus* spp.* and *S. pneumoniae**	≥18	15–17	≤14
Haemophilus spp.*	≥26	—*	—*

*NOTE: Isolates from these species should be tested for susceptibility using specialized diffusion testing methods[2]. Isolates of *Haemophilus* spp. with zones smaller than 26 mm should be considered equivocal and should be further evaluated. Isolates of *S. pneumoniae* should be tested against a 1-μg oxacillin disk; isolates with oxacillin zone sizes larger than or equal to 20 mm may be considered susceptible to cefepime.

As with standardized dilution techniques, diffusion methods require the use of laboratory control microorganisms to control the technical aspects of the laboratory procedures. Laboratory control microorganisms are specific strains of microbiological assay organisms with intrinsic biological properties relating to resistance mechanisms and their genetic expression within bacteria; the specific strains are not clinically significant in their current microbiological status. For the diffusion technique, the 30-μg cefepime disk should provide the following zone diameters in these laboratory test quality control strains (Table 7):
[See table 7 at right]

TABLE 7

Microorganism	ATCC	Zone Size Range (mm)
Escherichia coli	25922	29–35
Staphylococcus aureus	25923	23–29
Pseudomonas aeruginosa	27853	24–30
Haemophilus influenzae	49247	25–31

INDICATIONS AND USAGE

MAXIPIME is indicated in the treatment of the following infections caused by susceptible strains of the designated microorganisms (see also **PRECAUTIONS: Pediatric Use** and **DOSAGE AND ADMINISTRATION**):

Pneumonia (moderate to severe) caused by *Streptococcus pneumoniae*, including cases associated with concurrent bacteremia, *Pseudomonas aeruginosa, Klebsiella pneumoniae*, or *Enterobacter* species.

Empiric Therapy for Febrile Neutropenic Patients. Cefepime as monotherapy is indicated for empiric treatment of febrile neutropenic patients. In patients at high risk for severe infection (including patients with a history of recent bone marrow transplantation, with hypotension at presentation, with an underlying hematologic malignancy, or with severe or prolonged neutropenia), antimicrobial monotherapy may not be appropriate. Insufficient data exist to support the efficacy of cefepime monotherapy in such patients. (See **CLINICAL STUDIES**.)

Uncomplicated and Complicated Urinary Tract Infections (including pyelonephritis) caused by *Escherichia coli* or *Klebsiella pneumoniae*, when the infection is severe, or caused by *Escherichia coli, Klebsiella pneumoniae*, or *Proteus mirabilis*, when the infection is mild to moderate, including cases associated with concurrent bacteremia with these microorganisms.

Uncomplicated Skin and Skin Structure Infections caused by *Staphylococcus aureus* (methicillin-susceptible strains only) or *Streptococcus pyogenes*.

Complicated Intra-abdominal Infections (used in combination with metronidazole) caused by *Escherichia coli*, viridans group streptococci, *Pseudomonas aeruginosa, Klebsiella pneumoniae, Enterobacter* species, or *Bacteroides fragilis*. (See **CLINICAL STUDIES**.)

To reduce the development of drug-resistant bacteria and maintain the effectiveness of MAXIPIME and other antibacterial drugs, MAXIPIME should be used only to treat or prevent infections that are proven or strongly suspected to be caused by susceptible bacteria. When culture and susceptibility information are available, they should be considered in selecting or modifying antibacterial therapy. In the absence of such data, local epidemiology and susceptibility patterns may contribute to the empiric selection of therapy.

CLINICAL STUDIES

Febrile Neutropenic Patients

The safety and efficacy of empiric cefepime monotherapy of febrile neutropenic patients have been assessed in two multicenter, randomized trials, comparing cefepime monotherapy (at a dose of 2 g IV q8h) to ceftazidime monotherapy (at a dose of 2 g IV q8h). These studies comprised 317 evaluable patients. Table 8 describes the characteristics of the evaluable patient population.
[See table 8 above]

TABLE 8
Demographics of Evaluable Patients (First Episodes Only)

	Cefepime	Ceftazidime
Total	164	153
Median age (yr)	56.0 (range, 18–82)	55.0 (range, 16–84)
Male	86 (52%)	85 (56%)
Female	78 (48%)	68 (44%)
Leukemia	65 (40%)	52 (34%)
Other hematologic malignancies	43 (26%)	36 (24%)
Solid tumor	54 (33%)	56 (37%)
Median ANC nadir (cells/μL)	20.0 (range, 0–500)	20.0 (range, 0–500)
Median duration of neutropenia (days)	6.0 (range, 0–39)	6.0 (range, 0–32)
Indwelling venous catheter	97 (59%)	86 (56%)
Prophylactic antibiotics	62 (38%)	64 (42%)
Bone marrow graft	9 (5%)	7 (5%)
SBP <90 mm Hg at entry	7 (4%)	2 (1%)

ANC = absolute neutrophil count; SBP = systolic blood pressure.

Table 9 describes the clinical response rates observed. For all outcome measures, cefepime was therapeutically equivalent to ceftazidime.
[See table 9 at top of next page]

Insufficient data exist to support the efficacy of cefepime monotherapy in patients at high risk for severe infection (including patients with a history of recent bone marrow transplantation, with hypotension at presentation, with an underlying hematologic malignancy, or with severe or prolonged neutropenia). No data are available in patients with septic shock.

Complicated Intra-abdominal Infections

Patients hospitalized with complicated intra-abdominal infections participated in a randomized, double-blind, multi-

Continued on next page

Maxipime—Cont.

center trial comparing the combination of cefepime (2 g q12h) plus intravenous metronidazole (500 mg q6h) versus imipenem/cilastatin (500 mg q6h) for a maximum duration of 14 days of therapy. The study was designed to demonstrate equivalence of the two therapies. The primary analyses were conducted on the protocol-valid population, which consisted of those with a surgically confirmed complicated infection, at least one pathogen isolated pretreatment, at least 5 days of treatment, and a 4 to 6 week follow-up assessment for cured patients. Subjects in the imipenem/cilastatin arm had higher APACHE II scores at baseline. The treatment groups were otherwise generally comparable with regard to their pretreatment characteristics. The overall clinical cure rate among the protocol-valid patients was 81% (51 cured/63 evaluable patients) in the cefepime plus metronidazole group and 66% (62/94) in the imipenem/cilastatin group. The observed differences in efficacy may have been due to a greater proportion of patients with high APACHE II scores in the imipenem/cilastatin group.

TABLE 9
Pooled Response Rates for Empiric Therapy of Febrile Neutropenic Patients

Outcome Measures	% Response Cefepime (n=164)	Ceftazidime (n=153)
Primary episode resolved with no treatment modification, no new febrile episodes or infection, and oral antibiotics allowed for completion of treatment	**51**	**55**
Primary episode resolved with no treatment modification, no new febrile episodes or infection, and no post-treatment oral antibiotics	**34**	**39**
Survival, any treatment modification allowed	93	97
Primary episode resolved with no treatment modification and oral antibiotics allowed for completion of treatment	62	67
Primary episode resolved with no treatment modification and no post-treatment oral antibiotics	46	51

TABLE 10
Adverse Clinical Reactions
Cefepime Multiple-Dose Dosing Regimens
Clinical Trials—North America

INCIDENCE EQUAL TO OR GREATER THAN 1%	Local reactions (3.0%), including phlebitis (1.3%), pain and/or inflammation (0.6%)*; rash (1.1%)
INCIDENCE LESS THAN 1% BUT GREATER THAN 0.1%	Colitis (including pseudomembranous colitis), diarrhea, fever, headache, nausea, oral moniliasis, pruritus, urticaria, vaginitis, vomiting

*Local reactions, irrespective of relationship to cefepime in those patients who received intravenous infusion (n=3048).

CONTRAINDICATIONS

MAXIPIME is contraindicated in patients who have shown immediate hypersensitivity reactions to cefepime or the cephalosporin class of antibiotics, penicillins or other beta-lactam antibiotics.

WARNINGS

BEFORE THERAPY WITH MAXIPIME (CEFEPIME HYDROCHLORIDE) FOR INJECTION IS INSTITUTED, CAREFUL INQUIRY SHOULD BE MADE TO DETERMINE WHETHER THE PATIENT HAS HAD PREVIOUS IMMEDIATE HYPERSENSITIVITY REACTIONS TO CEFEPIME, CEPHALOSPORINS, PENICILLINS, OR OTHER DRUGS. IF THIS PRODUCT IS TO BE GIVEN TO PENICILLIN-SENSITIVE PATIENTS, CAUTION SHOULD BE EXERCISED BECAUSE CROSS-HYPERSENSITIVITY AMONG BETA-LACTAM ANTIBIOTICS HAS BEEN CLEARLY DOCUMENTED AND MAY OCCUR IN UP TO 10% OF PATIENTS WITH A HISTORY OF PENICILLIN ALLERGY. IF AN ALLERGIC REACTION TO MAXIPIME OCCURS, DISCONTINUE THE DRUG. SERIOUS ACUTE HYPERSENSITIVITY REACTIONS MAY REQUIRE TREATMENT WITH EPINEPHRINE AND OTHER EMERGENCY MEASURES INCLUDING OXYGEN, CORTICOSTEROIDS, INTRAVENOUS FLUIDS, INTRAVENOUS ANTIHISTAMINES, PRESSOR AMINES, AND AIRWAY MANAGEMENT, AS CLINICALLY INDICATED.

In patients with impaired renal function (creatinine clearance ≤ 60 mL/min), the dose of MAXIPIME should be adjusted to compensate for the slower rate of renal elimination. Because high and prolonged serum antibiotic concentrations can occur from usual dosages in patients with renal insufficiency or other conditions that may compromise renal function, the maintenance dosage should be reduced when cefepime is administered to such patients. Continued dosage should be determined by degree of renal impairment, severity of infection, and susceptibility of the causative organisms. (See specific recommendations for dosing adjustment in **DOSAGE AND ADMINISTRATION**.)

During postmarketing surveillance, serious adverse events have been reported including life-threatening or fatal occurrences of the following: encephalopathy (disturbance of consciousness including confusion, hallucinations, stupor, and coma), myoclonus, and seizures (see **ADVERSE REACTIONS: Postmarketing Experience**). Most cases occurred in patients with renal impairment who received doses of cefepime that exceeded the recommended dosage schedules. However, some cases of encephalopathy occurred in patients receiving a dosage adjustment for their renal function. In the majority of cases, symptoms of neurotoxicity were reversible and resolved after discontinuation of cefepime and/or after hemodialysis.

Pseudomembranous colitis has been reported with nearly all antibacterial agents, including MAXIPIME, and may range in severity from mild to life-threatening. Therefore, it is important to consider this diagnosis in patients who present with diarrhea subsequent to the administration of antibacterial agents.

Treatment with antibacterial agents alters the normal flora of the colon and may permit overgrowth of clostridia. Studies indicate that a toxin produced by *Clostridium difficile* is a primary cause of "antibiotic-associated colitis".

After the diagnosis of pseudomembranous colitis has been established, therapeutic measures should be initiated. Mild cases of pseudomembranous colitis usually respond to drug discontinuation alone. In moderate-to-severe cases, consideration should be given to management with fluids and electrolytes, protein supplementation, and treatment with an antibacterial drug clinically effective against *Clostridium difficile* colitis.

PRECAUTIONS

General

Prescribing MAXIPIME in the absence of proven or strongly suspected bacterial infection or a prophylactic indication is unlikely to provide benefit to the patient and increases the risk of the development of drug-resistant bacteria.

As with other antimicrobials, prolonged use of MAXIPIME may result in overgrowth of nonsusceptible microorganisms. Repeated evaluation of the patient's condition is essential. Should superinfection occur during therapy, appropriate measures should be taken.

Many cephalosporins, including cefepime, have been associated with a fall in prothrombin activity. Those at risk include patients with renal or hepatic impairment, or poor nutritional state, as well as patients receiving a protracted course of antimicrobial therapy. Prothrombin time should be monitored in patients at risk, and exogenous vitamin K administered as indicated.

Positive direct Coombs' tests have been reported during treatment with MAXIPIME. In hematologic studies or in transfusion cross-matching procedures when antiglobulin tests are performed on the minor side or in Coombs' testing of newborns whose mothers have received cephalosporin antibiotics before parturition, it should be recognized that a positive Coombs' test may be due to the drug.

MAXIPIME (cefepime hydrochloride) should be prescribed with caution in individuals with a history of gastrointestinal disease, particularly colitis.

Arginine has been shown to alter glucose metabolism and elevate serum potassium transiently when administered at 33 times the amount provided by the maximum recommended human dose of MAXIPIME. The effect of lower doses is not presently known.

Information for Patients

Patients should be counseled that antibacterial drugs including MAXIPIME should only be used to treat bacterial infections. They do not treat viral infections (eg, the common cold). When MAXIPIME is prescribed to treat a bacterial infection, patients should be told that although it is common to feel better early in the course of therapy, the medication should be taken exactly as directed. Skipping doses or not completing the full course of therapy may (1) decrease the effectiveness of the immediate treatment and (2) increase the likelihood that bacteria will develop resistance and will not be treatable by MAXIPIME or other antibacterial drugs in the future.

Drug Interactions

Renal function should be monitored carefully if high doses of aminoglycosides are to be administered with MAXIPIME because of the increased potential of nephrotoxicity and ototoxicity of aminoglycoside antibiotics. Nephrotoxicity has been reported following concomitant administration of other cephalosporins with potent diuretics such as furosemide.

Drug/Laboratory Test Interactions

The administration of cefepime may result in a false-positive reaction for glucose in the urine when using Clinitest® tablets. It is recommended that glucose tests based on enzymatic glucose oxidase reactions (such as Clinistix®) be used.

Carcinogenesis, Mutagenesis, and Impairment of Fertility

No long-term animal carcinogenicity studies have been conducted with cefepime. A battery of *in vivo* and *in vitro* genetic toxicity tests, including the Ames Salmonella reverse mutation assay, CHO/HGPRT mammalian cell forward gene mutation assay, chromosomal aberration and sister chromatid exchange assays in human lymphocytes, CHO fibroblast clastogenesis assay, and cytogenetic and micronucleus assays in mice were conducted. The overall conclusion of these tests indicated no definitive evidence of genotoxic potential. No untoward effects on fertility or reproduction have been observed in rats, mice, and rabbits when cefepime is administered subcutaneously at 1 to 4 times the recommended maximum human dose calculated on a mg/m^2 basis.

Usage in Pregnancy—Teratogenic effects—Pregnancy Category B

Cefepime was not teratogenic or embryocidal when administered during the period of organogenesis to rats at doses up to 1000 mg/kg/day (4 times the recommended maximum human dose calculated on a mg/m^2 basis) or to mice at doses up to 1200 mg/kg (2 times the recommended maximum human dose calculated on a mg/m^2 basis) or to rabbits at a dose level of 100 mg/kg (approximately equal to the recommended maximum human dose calculated on a mg/m^2 basis).

There are, however, no adequate and well-controlled studies of cefepime use in pregnant women. Because animal reproduction studies are not always predictive of human response, this drug should be used during pregnancy only if clearly needed.

Nursing Mothers

Cefepime is excreted in human breast milk in very low concentrations (0.5 µg/mL). Caution should be exercised when cefepime is administered to a nursing woman.

Labor and Delivery

Cefepime has not been studied for use during labor and delivery. Treatment should only be given if clearly indicated.

Pediatric Use

The safety and effectiveness of cefepime in the treatment of uncomplicated and complicated urinary tract infections (including pyelonephritis), uncomplicated skin and skin structure infections, pneumonia, and as empiric therapy for febrile neutropenic patients have been established in the age groups 2 months up to 16 years. Use of MAXIPIME in these age groups is supported by evidence from adequate and well-controlled studies of cefepime in adults with additional pharmacokinetic and safety data from pediatric trials (see **CLINICAL PHARMACOLOGY**).

Safety and effectiveness in pediatric patients below the age of 2 months have not been established. There are insufficient clinical data to support the use of MAXIPIME in pediatric patients under 2 months of age or for the treatment of serious infections in the pediatric population where the suspected or proven pathogen is *Haemophilus influenzae* type b.

IN THOSE PATIENTS IN WHOM MENINGEAL SEEDING FROM A DISTANT INFECTION SITE OR IN WHOM MENINGITIS IS SUSPECTED OR DOCUMENTED, AN ALTERNATE AGENT WITH DEMONSTRATED CLINICAL EFFICACY IN THIS SETTING SHOULD BE USED.

Geriatric Use

Of the more than 6400 adults treated with MAXIPIME in clinical studies, 35% were 65 years or older while 16% were 75 years or older. When geriatric patients received the usual recommended adult dose, clinical efficacy and safety were comparable to clinical efficacy and safety in nongeriatric adult patients.

Serious adverse events have occurred in geriatric patients with renal insufficiency given unadjusted doses of cefepime, including life-threatening or fatal occurrences of the following: encephalopathy, myoclonus, and seizures. (See **WARNINGS** and **ADVERSE REACTIONS**.)

This drug is known to be substantially excreted by the kidney, and the risk of toxic reactions to this drug may be greater in patients with impaired renal function. Because elderly patients are more likely to have decreased renal function, care should be taken in dose selection, and renal function should be monitored. (See **CLINICAL PHARMACOLOGY: Special Populations**, **WARNINGS**; and **DOSAGE AND ADMINISTRATION**.)

ADVERSE REACTIONS

Clinical Trials

In clinical trials using multiple doses of cefepime, 4137 patients were treated with the recommended dosages of cefepime (500 mg to 2 g IV q12h). There were no deaths or permanent disabilities thought related to drug toxicity. Sixty-four (1.5%) patients discontinued medication due to adverse events thought by the investigators to be possibly, probably, or almost certainly related to drug toxicity. Thirty-three (51%) of these 64 patients who discontinued therapy did so because of rash. The percentage of cefepime-treated patients who discontinued study drug because of drug-related adverse events was very similar at daily doses of 500 mg, 1 g, and 2 g q12h (0.8%, 1.1%, and 2.0%, respectively). However, the incidence of discontinuation due to rash increased with the higher recommended doses.

The following adverse events were thought to be probably related to cefepime during evaluation of the drug in clinical trials conducted in North America (n=3125 cefepime-treated patients).

[See table 10 on previous page]

At the higher dose of 2 g q8h, the incidence of probably-related adverse events was higher among the 795 patients who received this dose of cefepime. They consisted of rash (4%), diarrhea (3%), nausea (2%), vomiting (1%), pruritus (1%), fever (1%), and headache (1%).

The following adverse laboratory changes, irrespective of relationship to therapy with cefepime, were seen during clinical trials conducted in North America.

[See table 11 at right]

A similar safety profile was seen in clinical trials of pediatric patients (see **PRECAUTIONS: Pediatric Use**).

Postmarketing Experience

In addition to the events reported during North American clinical trials with cefepime, the following adverse experiences have been reported during worldwide postmarketing experience.

As with some other drugs in this class, encephalopathy (disturbance of consciousness including confusion, hallucinations, stupor, and coma), myoclonus, and seizures have been reported. Although most cases occurred in patients with renal impairment who received doses of cefepime that exceeded recommended dosage schedules, some cases of encephalopathy occurred in patients receiving a dosage adjustment for their renal function. (See also **WARNINGS.**) If seizures associated with drug therapy occur, the drug should be discontinued. Anticonvulsant therapy can be given if clinically indicated. Precautions should be taken to adjust daily dosage in patients with renal insufficiency or other conditions that may compromise renal function to reduce antibiotic concentrations that can lead or contribute to these and other serious adverse events, including renal failure.

As with other cephalosporins, anaphylaxis including anaphylactic shock, transient leukopenia, neutropenia, agranulocytosis, and thrombocytopenia have been reported.

Cephalosporin-class Adverse Reactions

In addition to the adverse reactions listed above that have been observed in patients treated with cefepime, the following adverse reactions and altered laboratory tests have been reported for cephalosporin-class antibiotics:

Stevens-Johnson syndrome, erythema multiforme, toxic epidermal necrolysis, renal dysfunction, toxic nephropathy, aplastic anemia, hemolytic anemia, hemorrhage, hepatic dysfunction including cholestasis, and pancytopenia.

OVERDOSAGE

Patients who receive an overdose should be carefully observed and given supportive treatment. In the presence of renal insufficiency, hemodialysis, not peritoneal dialysis, is recommended to aid in the removal of cefepime from the body. Accidental overdosing has occurred when large doses were given to patients with impaired renal function. Symptoms of overdose include encephalopathy (disturbance of consciousness including confusion, hallucinations, stupor, and coma), myoclonus, seizures, and neuromuscular excitability. (See **WARNINGS**, **ADVERSE REACTIONS**, and **DOSAGE AND ADMINISTRATION**.)

DOSAGE AND ADMINISTRATION

The recommended adult and pediatric dosages and routes of administration are outlined in the following table. MAXIPIME should be administered intravenously over approximately 30 minutes.

[See table 12 at right]

Impaired Hepatic Function—No adjustment is necessary for patients with impaired hepatic function.

Impaired Renal Function—In patients with impaired renal function (creatinine clearance ≤ 60 mL/min), the dose of MAXIPIME should be adjusted to compensate for the slower rate of renal elimination. The recommended initial dose of MAXIPIME should be the same as in patients with normal renal function except in patients undergoing hemodialysis. The recommended doses of MAXIPIME in patients with renal insufficiency are presented in Table 13.

When only serum creatinine is available, the following formula (Cockcroft and Gault equation)[3] may be used to estimate creatinine clearance. The serum creatinine should represent a steady state of renal function:

[See third table at right]
[See table 13 at right]

In patients undergoing continuous ambulatory peritoneal dialysis, MAXIPIME may be administered at normally recommended doses at a dosage interval of every 48 hours (see Table 13).

In patients undergoing hemodialysis, approximately 68% of the total amount of cefepime present in the body at the start of dialysis will be removed during a 3-hour dialysis period.

TABLE 11
Adverse Laboratory Changes
Cefepime Multiple-Dose Dosing Regimens
Clinical Trials—North America

INCIDENCE EQUAL TO OR GREATER THAN 1%	Positive Coombs' test (without hemolysis) (16.2%); decreased phosphorus (2.8%); increased ALT/SGPT (2.8%), AST/SGOT (2.4%), eosinophils (1.7%); abnormal PTT (1.6%), PT (1.4%)
INCIDENCE LESS THAN 1% BUT GREATER THAN 0.1%	Increased alkaline phosphatase, BUN, calcium, creatinine, phosphorus, potassium, total bilirubin; decreased calcium,* hematocrit, neutrophils, platelets, WBC

* Hypocalcemia was more common among elderly patients. Clinical consequences from changes in either calcium or phosphorus were not reported.

Table 12
Recommended Dosage Schedule for MAXIPIME in Patients with CrCL >60 mL/min

Site and Type of Infection	Dose	Frequency	Duration (days)
Adults			
Moderate to Severe Pneumonia due to *S. pneumoniae*,* *P. aeruginosa*, *K. pneumoniae*, or *Enterobacter* species	1-2 g IV	q12h	10
Empiric therapy for febrile neutropenic patients (See **INDICATIONS AND USAGE** and **CLINICAL STUDIES**.)	2 g IV	q8h	7**
Mild to Moderate Uncomplicated or Complicated Urinary Tract Infections, including pyelonephritis, due to *E. coli*, *K. pneumoniae*, or *P. mirabilis**	0.5-1 g IV/IM***	q12h	7-10
Severe Uncomplicated or Complicated Urinary Tract Infections, including pyelonephritis, due to *E. coli* or *K. pneumoniae**	2 g IV	q12h	10
Moderate to Severe Uncomplicated Skin and Skin Structure Infections due to *S. aureus* or *S. pyogenes*	2 g IV	q12h	10
Complicated Intra-abdominal Infections (used in combination with metronidazole) caused by *E. coli*, viridans group streptococci, *P. aeruginosa*, *K. pneumoniae*, *Enterobacter* species, or *B. fragilis*. (See **CLINICAL STUDIES**.)	2 g IV	q12h	7-10

Pediatric Patients (2 months up to 16 years)
The maximum dose for pediatric patients should not exceed the recommended adult dose. The usual recommended dosage in pediatric patients up to 40 kg in weight for uncomplicated and complicated urinary tract infections (including pyelonephritis), uncomplicated skin and skin structure infections, and pneumonia is 50 mg/kg/dose, administered q12h (50 mg/kg/dose, q8h for febrile neutropenic patients), for durations as given above.

* including cases associated with concurrent bacteremia.
** or until resolution of neutropenia. In patients whose fever resolves but who remain neutropenic for more than 7 days, the need for continued antimicrobial therapy should be re-evaluated frequently.
*** IM route of administration is indicated only for mild to moderate, uncomplicated or complicated UTIs due to *E. coli* when the IM route is considered to be a more appropriate route of drug administration.

$$\text{Males: Creatinine Clearance (mL/min)} = \frac{\text{Weight (kg)} \times (140\text{–age})}{72 \times \text{serum creatinine (mg/dL)}}$$

Females: 0.85 × above value

TABLE 13
Recommended Dosing Schedule for MAXIPIME in Adult Patients (Normal Renal Function, Renal Insufficiency, and Hemodialysis)

Creatinine Clearance (mL/min)	Recommended Maintenance Schedule			
>60 Normal recommended dosing schedule	500 mg q12h	1 g q12h	2 g q12h	2 g q8h
30–60	500 mg q24h	1 g q24h	2 g q24h	2 g q12h
11–29	500 mg q24h	500 mg q24h	1 g q24h	2 g q24h
<11	250 mg q24h	250 mg q24h	500 mg q24h	1 g q24h
CAPD	500 mg q48h	1 g q48h	2 g q48h	2 g q48h
Hemodialysis*	1 g on day 1, then 500 mg q24h thereafter			1 g q24h

* On hemodialysis days, cefepime should be administered following hemodialysis. Whenever possible, cefepime should be administered at the same time each day.

The dosage of MAXIPIME for hemodialysis patients is 1 g on Day 1 followed by 500 mg q24h for the treatment of all infections except febrile neutropenia, which is 1 g q24h. MAXIPIME should be administered at the same time each day following the completion of hemodialysis on hemodialysis days (see Table 13).

Data in pediatric patients with impaired renal function are not available; however, since cefepime pharmacokinetics are similar in adults and pediatric patients (see **CLINICAL PHARMACOLOGY**), changes in the dosing regimen proportional to those in adults (see Tables 12 and 13) are recommended for pediatric patients.

Administration:

For Intravenous Infusion, constitute the 1 g or 2 g piggyback (100 mL) bottle with 50 or 100 mL of a compatible IV fluid listed in the **Compatibility and Stability** subsection. Alternatively, constitute the 500 mg, 1 g, or 2 g vial, and add an appropriate quantity of the resulting solution to an IV container with one of the compatible IV fluids. **THE RESULTING SOLUTION SHOULD BE ADMINISTERED OVER APPROXIMATELY 30 MINUTES.**

Intermittent IV infusion with a Y-type administration set can be accomplished with compatible solutions. However, during infusion of a solution containing cefepime, it is desirable to discontinue the other solution.

ADD-Vantage® vials are to be constituted only with 50 or 100 mL of 5% Dextrose Injection or 0.9% Sodium Chloride Injection in Abbott ADD-Vantage® flexible diluent containers. (See ADD-Vantage® Vial Instructions for Use.)

Intramuscular Administration: For IM administration, MAXIPIME (cefepime hydrochloride) should be constituted with one of the following diluents: Sterile Water for Injection, 0.9% Sodium Chloride, 5% Dextrose Injection, 0.5% or 1.0% Lidocaine Hydrochloride, or Sterile Bacteriostatic Wa-

Continued on next page

TABLE 14
Preparation of Solutions of MAXIPIME

Single-Dose Vials for Intravenous/Intramuscular Administration	Amount of Diluent to be added (mL)	Approximate Available Volume (mL)	Approximate Cefepime Concentration (mg/mL)
cefepime vial content			
500 mg (IV)	5.0	5.6	100
500 mg (IM)	1.3	1.8	280
1 g (IV)	10.0	11.3	100
1 g (IM)	2.4	3.6	280
2 g (IV)	10.0	12.5	160
Piggyback (100 mL)			
1 g bottle	50	50	20
1 g bottle	100	100	10
2 g bottle	50	50	40
2 g bottle	100	100	20
ADD-Vantage®			
1 g vial	50	50	20
1 g vial	100	100	10
2 g vial	50	50	40
2 g vial	100	100	20

Table 15
Cefepime Admixture Stability

MAXIPIME Concentration	Admixture and Concentration	IV Infusion Solutions	Stability Time for RT/L (20°–25° C)	Stability Time for Refrigeration (2°–8° C)
40 mg/mL	Amikacin 6 mg/mL	NS or D5W	24 hours	7 days
40 mg/mL	Ampicillin 1 mg/mL	D5W	8 hours	8 hours
40 mg/mL	Ampicillin 10 mg/mL	D5W	2 hours	8 hours
40 mg/mL	Ampicillin 1 mg/mL	NS	24 hours	48 hours
40 mg/mL	Ampicillin 10 mg/mL	NS	8 hours	48 hours
4 mg/mL	Ampicillin 40 mg/mL	NS	8 hours	8 hours
4–40 mg/mL	Clindamycin Phosphate 0.25–6 mg/mL	NS or D5W	24 hours	7 days
4 mg/mL	Heparin 10–50 units/mL	NS or D5W	24 hours	7 days
4 mg/mL	Potassium Chloride 10–40 mEq/L	NS or D5W	24 hours	7 days
4 mg/mL	Theophylline 0.8 mg/mL	D5W	24 hours	7 days
1–4 mg/mL	na	Aminosyn® II 4.25% with electrolytes and calcium	8 hours	3 days
0.125–0.25 mg/mL	na	Inpersol™ with 4.25% dextrose	24 hours	7 days

NS = 0.9% Sodium Chloride Injection.
D5W = 5% Dextrose Injection.
na = not applicable.
RT/L = Ambient room temperature and light.

500 mg*	15 mL vial (tray of 10)	NDC 51479-053-10
1 g*	Piggyback bottle 100 mL (tray of 10)	NDC 51479-054-10
1 g*	ADD-Vantage® vial (tray of 10)	NDC 51479-054-20
1 g*	15 mL vial (tray of 10)	NDC 51479-054-30
2 g*	Piggyback bottle 100 mL (tray of 10)	NDC 51479-055-20
2 g*	ADD-Vantage® vial (tray of 10)	NDC 51479-055-10
2 g*	20 mL vial (tray of 10)	NDC 51479-055-30

*Based on cefepime activity

Maxipime—Cont.

ter for Injection with Parabens or Benzyl Alcohol (refer to Table 14).
Preparation of MAXIPIME solutions is summarized in Table 14.
[See table 14 above]
Compatibility and Stability:
Intravenous: MAXIPIME is compatible at concentrations between 1 and 40 mg/mL with the following IV infusion fluids: 0.9% Sodium Chloride Injection, 5% and 10% Dextrose Injection, M/6 Sodium Lactate Injection, 5% Dextrose and 0.9% Sodium Chloride Injection, Lactated Ringers and 5% Dextrose Injection, Normosol-R™, and Normosol-M™ in 5% Dextrose Injection. These solutions may be stored up to 24 hours at controlled room temperature 20°–25° C (68°–77° F) or 7 days in a refrigerator 2°–8° C (36°–46° F). MAXIPIME in ADD-Vantage® vials is stable at concentrations of 10–40 mg/mL in 5% Dextrose Injection or 0.9% Sodium Chloride Injection for 24 hours at controlled room temperature 20°–25° C or 7 days in a refrigerator 2°–8° C. MAXIPIME admixture compatibility information is summarized in Table 15.
[See table 15 at left]
Solutions of MAXIPIME, like those of most beta-lactam antibiotics, should not be added to solutions of ampicillin at a concentration greater than 40 mg/mL, and should not be added to metronidazole, vancomycin, gentamicin, tobramycin, netilmicin sulfate or aminophylline because of potential interaction. However, if concurrent therapy with MAXIPIME is indicated, each of these antibiotics can be administered separately.
Intramuscular: MAXIPIME (cefepime hydrochloride) constituted as directed is stable for 24 hours at controlled room temperature 20°–25° C (68°–77° F) or for 7 days in a refrigerator 2°–8° C (36°–46° F) with the following diluents: Sterile Water for Injection, 0.9% Sodium Chloride Injection, 5% Dextrose Injection, Sterile Bacteriostatic Water for Injection with Parabens or Benzyl Alcohol, or 0.5% or 1% Lidocaine Hydrochloride.
NOTE: PARENTERAL DRUGS SHOULD BE INSPECTED VISUALLY FOR PARTICULATE MATTER BEFORE ADMINISTRATION.
As with other cephalosporins, the color of MAXIPIME powder, as well as its solutions, tends to darken depending on storage conditions; however, when stored as recommended, the product potency is not adversely affected.

HOW SUPPLIED

MAXIPIME® (cefepime hydrochloride, USP) for Injection is supplied as follows:
[See third table at left]
Storage
MAXIPIME IN THE DRY STATE SHOULD BE STORED BETWEEN 2°–25° C (36°–77° F) AND PROTECTED FROM LIGHT.
US Patent Nos. 4,406,899, 4,994,451, and 5,244,891

REFERENCES

(1) National Committee for Clinical Laboratory Standards. *Methods for Dilution Antimicrobial Susceptibility Tests for Bacteria that Grow Aerobically*—Third Edition. Approved Standard NCCLS Document M7-A3, Vol. 13, No. 25, NCCLS, Villanova, PA, December 1993.
(2) National Committee for Clinical Laboratory Standards. *Performance Standards for Antimicrobial Disk Susceptibility Tests*—Fifth Edition. Approved Standard NCCLS Document M2-A5, Vol. 13, No. 24, NCCLS, Villanova, PA, December 1993.
(3) Cockcroft DW, Gault MH. Prediction of creatinine clearance from serum creatinine. *Nephron*. 1976; 16:31-41.

MAXIPIME® is a registered trademark of Bristol-Myers Squibb Company licensed exclusively in the US to EPI.
ADD-Vantage® is a registered trademark of Abbott Laboratories.
Normosol-R™ and Normosol-M™ are trademarks of Abbott Laboratories.
Aminosyn® is a registered trademark of Abbott Laboratories.
Inpersol™ is a trademark of Abbott Laboratories.
Clinitest® and Clinistix® are registered trademarks of Bayer HealthCare LLC.
Manufactured by
Bristol-Myers Squibb Company
Princeton, NJ 08543 USA
Distributed by
Elan Biopharmaceuticals, a business unit of Elan Pharmaceuticals, Inc. (EPI),
a member of the Elan Group, San Diego, CA 92121 USA
MAX3630304 6001123-A Revised December 2003

ENDO PHARMACEUTICALS

100 Painters Drive
Chadds Ford, PA 19317
Endo Generic Products

Direct Inquiries to:
Customer Service:
(800) 462-3636
Fax: 877-329-3636

For Medical Information/Adverse Drug Experience Reporting Contact:
(800) 462-3636

Other Specialty Products Available:
Carbidopa and Levodopa Tablets, USP
Endocet® Tablets CII, USP
Endodan® Tablets CII, USP
Morphine Sulfate Extended-Release Tablets, CII

ANTITUSSIVE HYCODAN®

Ⓒ℞

[hī-kō-dan]
(hydrocodone bitartrate and homatropine methylbromide)
TABLETS AND SYRUP

DESCRIPTION

HYCODAN contains hydrocodone (dihydrocodeinone) bitartrate, a semisynthetic centrally-acting opioid antitussive. Homatropine methylbromide is included in a subtherapeutic amount to discourage deliberate overdosage.

Each HYCODAN tablet or teaspoonful (5 mL) contains:
Hydrocodone Bitartrate, USP 5 mg
Homatropine Methylbromide, USP 1.5 mg
HYCODAN tablets also contain: calcium phosphate dibasic, colloidal silicon dioxide, lactose, magnesium stearate, starch and stearic acid.
HYCODAN syrup also contains: caramel coloring, FD&C Red 40, liquid sugar, methylparaben, propylparaben, sorbitol solution and wild cherry imitation flavor.
The hydrocodone component is 4,5α-epoxy-3-methoxy-17-methylmorphinan-6-one tartrate (1:1) hydrate (2:5), a fine white crystal or crystalline powder, which is derived from the opium alkaloid, thebaine, has a molecular weight of (494.50), and may be represented by the following structural formula:

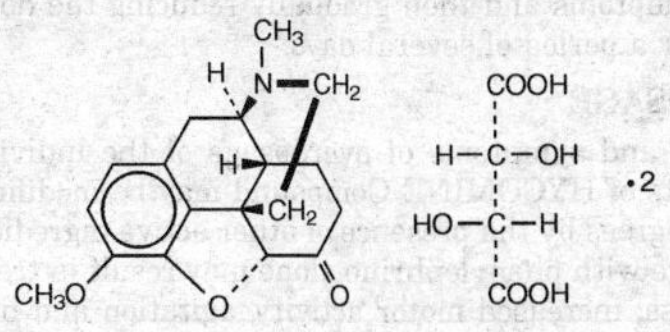

$C_{18}H_{21}NO_3 \cdot C_4H_6O_6 \cdot 2\ ^1/_2H_2O$
HYDROCODONE BITARTRATE

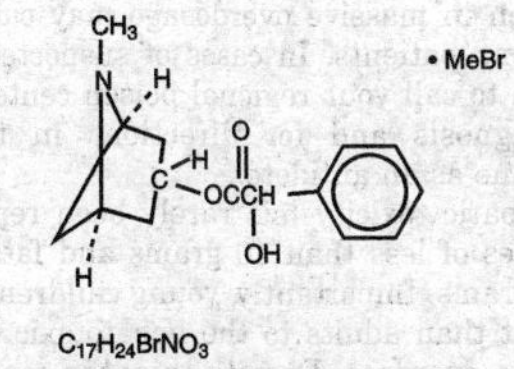

$C_{17}H_{24}BrNO_3$
HOMATROPINE METHYLBROMIDE

Homatropine methylbromide is 8-Azoniabicyclo [3.2.1] octane,3-[(hydroxyphenylacetyl)oxy]-8,8-dimethyl-,bromide, endo-; a white crystal or fine white crystalline powder, with a molecular weight of (370.29).

CLINICAL PHARMACOLOGY

Hydrocodone is a semisynthetic opioid antitussive and analgesic with multiple actions qualitatively similar to those of codeine. The precise mechanism of action of hydrocodone and other opiates is not known; however, hydrocodone is believed to act directly on the cough center. In excessive doses, hydrocodone, like other opium derivatives, will depress respiration. The effects of hydrocodone in therapeutic doses on the cardiovascular system are insignificant. Hydrocodone can produce miosis, euphoria, physical and physiological dependence.
Following a 10 mg oral dose of hydrocodone administered to five adult male subjects, the mean peak concentration was 23.6 ± 5.2 ng/mL. Maximum serum levels were achieved at 1.3 ± 0.3 hours and the half-life was determined to be 3.8 ± 0.3 hours. Hydrocodone exhibits a complex pattern of metabolism including O-demethylation, N-demethylation and 6-keto reduction to the corresponding 6-α- and 6-β-hydroxymetabolites.

INDICATIONS AND USAGE

HYCODAN (hydrocodone bitartrate and homatropine methylbromide) is indicated for the symptomatic relief of cough.

CONTRAINDICATIONS

HYCODAN should not be administered to patients who are hypersensitive to hydrocodone or homatropine methylbromide.

WARNINGS

Hydrocodone can produce drug dependence of the morphine type and, therefore, has the potential for being abused. Psychic dependence, physical dependence and tolerance may develop upon repeated administration of HYCODAN and it should be prescribed and administered with the same degree of caution appropriate to the use of other opioid drugs (see **DRUG ABUSE AND DEPENDENCE**).

Respiratory Depression

HYCODAN produces dose-related respiratory depression by directly acting on brain stem respiratory centers. If respiratory depression occurs, it may be antagonized by the use of naloxone hydrochloride and other supportive measures when indicated.

Head Injury and Increased Intracranial Pressure

The respiratory depression properties of opioids and their capacity to elevate cerebrospinal fluid pressure may be markedly exaggerated in the presence of head injury, other intracranial lesions or a pre-existing increase in intracranial pressure. Furthermore, opioids produce adverse reactions which may obscure the clinical course of patients with head injuries.

Acute Abdominal Conditions

The administration of HYCODAN or other opioids may obscure the diagnosis or clinical course of patients with acute abdominal conditions.

Pediatric Use

In young pediatric patients, as well as adults, the respiratory center is sensitive to the depressant action of opioid cough suppressants in a dose-dependent manner. Benefit to risk ratio should be carefully considered especially in the pediatric population with respiratory embarrassment (e.g., croup).

PRECAUTIONS

General

Before prescribing medication to suppress or modify cough, it is important to ascertain that the underlying cause of cough is identified, that modification of cough does not increase the risk of clinical or physiological complications, and that appropriate therapy for the primary disease is provided.

Special Risk Patients

HYCODAN (hydrocodone bitartrate and homatropine methylbromide) should be given with caution to certain patients such as the elderly or debilitated, and those with severe impairment of hepatic or renal functions, hypothyroidism, Addison's disease, prostatic hypertrophy or urethral stricture, asthma, and narrow-angle glaucoma.

Information for Patients

Hydrocodone may impair the mental and/or physical abilities required for the performance of potentially hazardous tasks such as driving a car or operating machinery. The patient using HYCODAN should be cautioned accordingly.

Drug Interactions

Patients receiving opioids, antihistamines, antipsychotics, antianxiety agents or other CNS depressants (including alcohol) concomitantly with HYCODAN may exhibit an additive CNS depression. When combined therapy is contemplated, the dose of one or both agents should be reduced. The use of MAO inhibitors or tricyclic antidepressants with hydrocodone preparations may increase the effect of either the antidepressant or hydrocodone.

Carcinogenesis, Mutagenesis, Impairment of Fertility

Studies of HYCODAN in animals to evaluate the carcinogenic and mutagenic potential and the effect on fertility have not been conducted.

Pregnancy

Teratogenic Effects: Pregnancy Category C: Animal reproduction studies have not been conducted with HYCODAN. It is also not known whether HYCODAN can cause fetal harm when administered to a pregnant woman or can affect reproduction capacity. HYCODAN should be given to a pregnant woman only if clearly needed.
Nonteratogenic Effects: Babies born to mothers who have been taking opioids regularly prior to delivery will be physically dependent. The withdrawal signs include irritability and excessive crying, tremors, hyperactive reflexes, increased respiratory rate, increased stools, sneezing, yawning, vomiting and fever. The intensity of the syndrome does not always correlate with the duration of maternal opioid use or dose.

Labor and Delivery

As with all opioids, administration of HYCODAN to the mother shortly before delivery may result in some degree of respiratory depression in the newborn, especially if higher doses are used.

Nursing Mothers

It is not known whether this drug is excreted in human milk. Because many drugs are excreted in human milk and because of the potential for serious adverse reactions in nursing infants from HYCODAN, a decision should be made whether to discontinue nursing or to discontinue the drug, taking into account the importance of the drug to the mother.

Pediatric Use

Safety and effectiveness of HYCODAN in pediatric patients under six have not been established.

ADVERSE REACTIONS

Central Nervous System

Sedation, drowsiness, mental clouding, lethargy, impairment of mental and physical performance, anxiety, fear, dysphoria, dizziness, psychic dependence, mood changes.

Gastrointestinal System

Nausea and vomiting may occur; they are more frequent in ambulatory than in recumbent patients. Prolonged administration of HYCODAN may produce constipation.

Genitourinary System

Ureteral spasm, spasm of vesicle sphincters and urinary retention have been reported with opiates.

Respiratory Depression

HYCODAN may produce dose-related respiratory depression by acting directly on brain stem respiratory centers (see **OVERDOSAGE**).

Dermatological

Skin rash, pruritus.

DRUG ABUSE AND DEPENDENCE

HYCODAN (hydrocodone bitartrate and homatropine methylbromide) is a Schedule III opioid. Psychic dependence, physical dependence and tolerance may develop upon repeated administration of opioids; therefore, HYCODAN should be prescribed and administered with caution. However, psychic dependence is unlikely to develop when HYCODAN is used for a short time for the treatment of cough. Physical dependence, the condition in which continued administration of the drug is required to prevent the appearance of a withdrawal syndrome, assumes clinically significant proportions only after several weeks of continued oral opioid use, although some mild degree of physical dependence may develop after a few days of opioid therapy.

OVERDOSAGE

Signs and Symptoms

Serious overdosage with hydrocodone is characterized by respiratory depression (a decrease in respiratory rate and/or tidal volume, Cheyne-Stokes respiration, cyanosis), extreme somnolence progressing to stupor or coma, skeletal muscle flaccidity, cold and clammy skin, and sometimes bradycardia and hypotension. In severe overdosage, apnea, circulatory collapse, cardiac arrest and death may occur. The ingestion of very large amounts of HYCODAN may, in addition, result in acute homatropine intoxication.

Treatment

Primary attention should be given to the reestablishment of adequate respiratory exchange through provision of a patent airway and the institution of assisted or controlled ventilation. The opioid antagonist naloxone hydrochloride is a specific antidote for respiratory depression which may result from overdosage or unusual sensitivity to opioids including hydrocodone. Therefore, an appropriate dose of naloxone hydrochloride should be administered, preferably by the intravenous route, simultaneously with efforts at respiratory resuscitation. For further information, see full prescribing information for naloxone hydrochloride. An antagonist should not be administered in the absence of clinically significant respiratory depression. Oxygen, intravenous fluids, vasopressors and other supportive measures should be employed as indicated. Gastric emptying may be useful in removing unabsorbed drug.

DOSAGE AND ADMINISTRATION

Adults

One (1) tablet or one (1) teaspoonful (5 mL) of the syrup every 4 to 6 hours as needed; do not exceed six (6) tablets or six (6) teaspoonfuls in 24 hours.

Children 6 to 12 Years of Age

One-half ($^1/_2$) tablet or one-half ($^1/_2$) teaspoonful (2.5 mL) of the syrup every 4 to 6 hours as needed; do not exceed three (3) tablets or three (3) teaspoonfuls in 24 hours.

HOW SUPPLIED

HYCODAN is supplied as a white, biconvex tablet, one face bisected and debossed with "HYCODAN", and the other face plain, available in:
Bottles of 100 NDC 63481-042-70
Bottles of 500 NDC 63481-042-85
Store tablets at 25°C (77°F); excursions permitted to 15°–30°C (59°–86°F). [See USP Controlled Room Temperature.]
Dispense in a tight, light-resistant container, as defined in the USP, with a child-resistant closure (as required).
HYCODAN is also available as a clear red colored, wild cherry flavored syrup in:
Bottles of one pint NDC 63481-234-16
Store syrup at 25°C (77°F); excursions permitted to 15°–30°C (59°–86°F). [See USP Controlled Room Temperature].
Oral prescription where permitted by State law.
HYCODAN® is a Registered Trademark of Endo Pharmaceuticals Inc.

6479-04/Rev. February, 2003
Shown in Product Identification Guide, page 311

HYCOMINE® COMPOUND CIII ℞

DESCRIPTION

HYCOMINE Compound tablets contain hydrocodone (dihydrocodeinone) bitartrate, a semi-synthetic centrally-acting opioid antitussive; chlorpheniramine maleate, an antihistamine; phenylephrine hydrochloride, a sympathomimetic amine decongestant; acetaminophen, an analgesic/antipyretic; and caffeine, a centrally-acting stimulant, for oral administration.

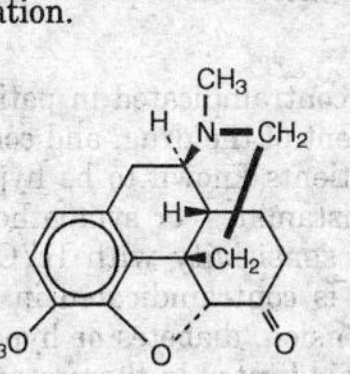

HYDROCODONE BITARTRATE

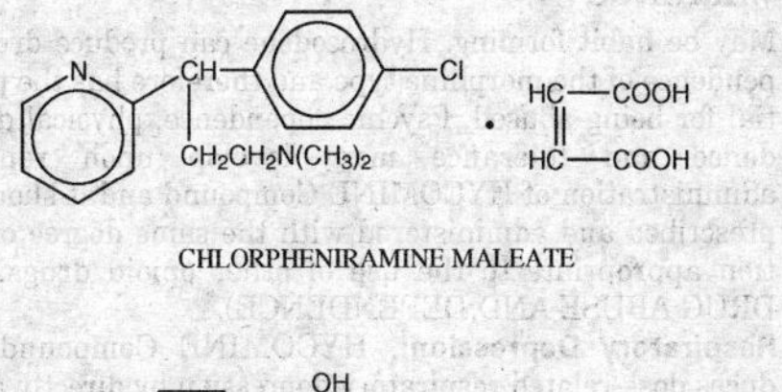

CHLORPHENIRAMINE MALEATE

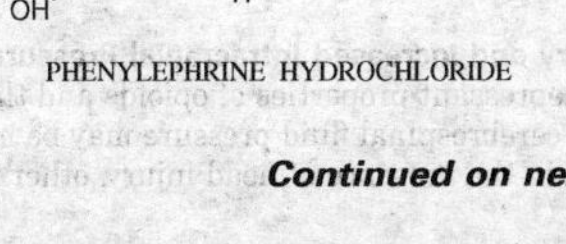

PHENYLEPHRINE HYDROCHLORIDE

Continued on next page

Hycomine—Cont.

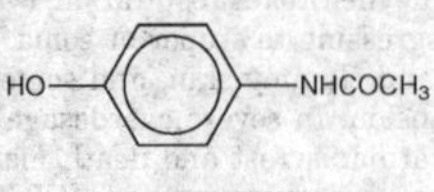

ACETAMINOPHEN

CAFFEINE

Each HYCOMINE Compound tablet contains:

Hydrocodone Bitartrate, USP	5 mg
Chlorpheniramine Maleate, USP	2 mg
Phenylephrine Hydrochloride, USP	10 mg
Acetaminophen, USP	250 mg
Caffeine, Anhydrous, USP	30 mg

HYCOMINE Compound tablets also contain: cherry flavor, colloidal silicon dioxide, FD&C Red 40, magnesium stearate, microcrystalline cellulose, povidone and starch.

CLINICAL PHARMACOLOGY

Clinical trials have proven hydrocodone bitartrate to be an effective antitussive agent which is pharmacologically 2 to 8 times as potent as codeine. At equi-effective doses, its sedative action is greater than codeine. The precise mechanism of action of hydrocodone and other opiates is not known, however, hydrocodone is believed to act by directly depressing the cough center. In excessive doses hydrocodone, like other opium derivatives, will depress respiration. The effects of hydrocodone in therapeutic doses on the cardiovascular system is insignificant. The constipation effects of hydrocodone are much weaker than that of morphine and no stronger than that of codeine. Hydrocodone can produce miosis, euphoria, physical and psychological dependence. At therapeutic antitussive doses, it does exert analgesic effects.
Following a 10 mg oral dose of hydrocodone administered to five adult male human subjects, the mean peak concentration was 23.6 ± 5.2 ng/mL. Maximum serum levels were achieved at 1.3 ± 0.3 hours and the half-life was determined to be 3.8 ± 0.3 hours. Hydrocodone exhibits a complex pattern of metabolism including O-demethylation, N-demethylation and 6-keto reduction to the corresponding 6–α– and 6–β–hydroxymetabolites.
Chlorpheniramine maleate is a competitive H_1-receptor histamine blocking drug, thereby counteracting the effects of histamine release associated with allergic manifestations of upper respiratory tract inflammatory disorders. H_1-blocking drugs inhibit the actions of histamine on smooth muscle, capillary permeability, and can both stimulate and depress the central nervous system. Phenylephrine hydrochloride effects its vasoconstrictor activity by releasing noradrenaline from sympathetic nerve endings, and from direct stimulation of α-adrenoreceptors in blood vessels. Acetaminophen is an antipyretic and peripherally acting analgesic. Caffeine is a central nervous system stimulant.

INDICATIONS AND USAGE

HYCOMINE Compound is indicated for the symptomatic relief of cough, nasal congestion, and discomfort associated with upper respiratory tract infections.

CONTRAINDICATIONS

HYCOMINE Compound is contraindicated in patients hypersensitive to any component of the drug, and concurrent MAO inhibitor therapy. Patients known to be hypersensitive to other opioids, antihistamines, or sympathomimetic amines may exhibit cross sensitivity with HYCOMINE Compound. Phenylephrine is contraindicated in patients with heart disease, hypertension, diabetes or hyperthyroidism. Hydrocodone is contraindicated in the presence of an intracranial lesion associated with increased intracranial pressure, and whenever ventilatory function is depressed.

WARNINGS

May be habit forming. Hydrocodone can produce drug dependence of the morphine type and therefore has the potential for being abused. Psychic dependence, physical dependence and tolerance may develop upon repeated administration of HYCOMINE Compound and it should be prescribed and administered with the same degree of caution appropriate to the use of other opioid drugs. (See DRUG ABUSE AND DEPENDENCE).
Respiratory Depression: HYCOMINE Compound produces dose-related respiratory depression by directly acting on brain stem respiratory centers. If respiratory depression occurs, it may be antagonized by the use of NARCAN® (naloxone hydrochloride) and other supportive measures when indicated.
Head Injury and Increased Intracranial Pressure: The respiratory depressant properties of opioids and their capacity to elevate cerebrospinal fluid pressure may be markedly exaggerated in the presence of head injury, other intracranial lesions or a pre-existing increase in intracranial pressure. Furthermore, opioids produce adverse reactions which may obscure the clinical course of patients with head injuries.
Acute Abdominal Conditions: The administration of HYCOMINE Compound or other opioids may obscure the diagnosis or clinical course of patients with acute abdominal conditions.
Phenylephrine: Hypertensive crises can occur with concurrent use of phenylephrine and monoamine oxidase (MAO) inhibitors, indomethacin or with beta-blockers and methyldopa.
If a hypertensive crisis occurs these drugs should be discontinued immediately and therapy to lower blood pressure should be instituted immediately. Fever should be managed by means of external cooling.
Chlorpheniramine: Antihistamines may produce drowsiness or excitation, particularly in children and elderly patients.

PRECAUTIONS

Before prescribing medication to suppress or modify cough, it is important to ascertain that the underlying cause of cough is identified, that modification of cough does not increase the risk of clinical or physiologic complications, and that appropriate therapy for the primary disease is provided.
Usage in Ambulatory Patients: Hydrocodone, like all opioids, and antihistamines such as chlorpheniramine maleate, may impair the mental and/or physical abilities required for the performance of potentially hazardous tasks such as driving a car or operating machinery; phenylephrine may produce a rapid pulse, dizziness or palpitations; patients should be cautioned accordingly.
Drug Interactions: Patients receiving other opioid analgesics, general anesthetics, phenothiazines, other tranquilizers, sedative-hypnotics or other CNS depressants (including alcohol) concomitantly with hydrocodone may exhibit an additive CNS depression. When such combined therapy is contemplated, the dose of one or both agents should be reduced. The use of phenylephrine with other sympathomimetic amines and MAO inhibitors may produce an additive elevation of blood pressure. MAO inhibitors may prolong the anticholinergic effects of antihistamines. (See WARNINGS).
Carcinogenesis, Mutagenesis, Impairment of Fertility: Carcinogenicity, mutagenicity, and reproduction studies have not been conducted with HYCOMINE Compound.
Usage in Pregnancy: Pregnancy Category C. Animal reproduction studies have not been conducted with HYCOMINE Compound. It is also not known whether HYCOMINE Compound can cause fetal harm when administered to a pregnant woman or can affect reproductive capacity. HYCOMINE Compound should be given to a pregnant woman only if clearly needed.
Nonteratogenic Effects: Babies born to mothers who have been taking opioids regularly prior to delivery will be physically dependent. The withdrawal signs include irritability and excessive crying, tremors, hyperactive reflexes, increased respiratory rate, increased stools, sneezing, yawning, vomiting and fever. The intensity of the syndrome does not always correlate with the duration of maternal opioid use or dose. Chlorpromazine 0.7–1.0 mg/kg q 6 h, phenobarbital 2 mg/kg q 6 h, and paregoric 2–4 drops/kg q 4 h, have been used to treat withdrawal symptoms in infants. The duration of therapy is 4 to 28 days, with dosages decreased as tolerated.
Nursing Mothers: It is not known whether this drug is excreted in human milk. Because many drugs are excreted in human milk and because of the potential for serious adverse reactions in nursing infants from HYCOMINE Compound, a decision should be made whether to discontinue nursing or discontinue the drug, taking into account the importance of the drug to the mother.
Pediatric Use: Safety and effectiveness in pediatric patients below the age of 2 years have not been established.

ADVERSE REACTIONS

Respiratory System: Hydrocodone produces dose-related respiratory depression by acting directly on brain stem respiratory centers.
Cardiovascular System: Hypertension, postural hypotension, tachycardia and palpitations.
Genitourinary System: Ureteral spasm, spasm of vesical sphincters and urinary retention have been reported with opiates.
Central Nervous System: Sedation, drowsiness, mental clouding, lethargy, impairment of mental and physical performance, anxiety, fear, dysphoria, dizziness, psychic dependence, mood changes, and blurred vision.
Gastrointestinal System: Nausea and vomiting occur more frequently in ambulatory than in recumbent patients.

DRUG ABUSE AND DEPENDENCE

Special care should be exercised in prescribing hydrocodone for emotionally unstable patients and for those with a history of drug misuse. Such patients should be closely supervised when long-term therapy is contemplated.
HYCOMINE Compound is a Schedule III opioid. Psychic dependence, physical dependence, and tolerance may develop upon repeated administration of opioids; therefore, HYCOMINE Compound should always be prescribed and administered with caution. Physical dependence is the condition in which continued administration of the drug is required to prevent the appearance of a withdrawal syndrome.
Patients physically dependent on opioids will develop an abstinence syndrome upon abrupt discontinuation of the opioid or following the administration of a opioid antagonist. The character and severity of the withdrawal symptoms are related to the degree of physical dependence. Manifestations of opioid withdrawal are similar to but milder than that of morphine and include lacrimation, rhinorrhea, yawning, sweating, restlessness, dilated pupils, anorexia, gooseflesh, irritability and tremor. In more severe forms, nausea, vomiting, intestinal spasm and diarrhea, increased heart rate and blood pressure, chills, and pains in bones and muscles of the back and extremities may occur. Peak effects will usually be apparent at 48 to 72 hours.
Treatment of withdrawal is usually managed by providing sufficient quantities of an opioid to suppress **severe** withdrawal symptoms and then gradually reducing the dose of opioid over a period of several days.

OVERDOSAGE

The signs and symptoms of overdosage of the individual components of HYCOMINE Compound may be modified in varying degrees by the presence of other active ingredients. Overdosage with phenylephrine alone may result in tremor, restlessness, increased motor activity, agitation and hallucinations.

Acetaminophen

Signs and Symptoms: In acute acetaminophen overdosage, dose-dependent, potentially fatal hepatic necrosis is the most serious adverse effect. Renal tubular necrosis, hypoglycemic coma and thrombocytopenia may also occur.
Acetaminophen in massive overdosage may cause hepatic toxicity in some patients. In cases of suspected overdose, you may wish to call your regional poison center for assistance in diagnosis and for directions in the use of N-acetylcysteine as an antidote.
In adults, hepatic toxicity has rarely been reported with acute overdoses of less than 10 grams and fatalities with less than 15 grams. Importantly, young children seem to be more resistant than adults to the hepatotoxic effect of an acetaminophen overdose. Despite this, the measures outlined below should be initiated in any adult or child suspected of having ingested an acetaminophen overdose.
Early symptoms following a potentially hepatotoxic overdose may include nausea, vomiting, diaphoresis and general malaise. Clinical and laboratory evidence of hepatic toxicity may not be apparent until 48 to 72 hours post-ingestion.
Treatment: The stomach should be emptied promptly by lavage or by induction of emesis with syrup of ipecac. Patient's estimates of the quantity of a drug ingested are notoriously unreliable. Therefore, if an acetaminophen overdose is suspected, a serum acetaminophen assay should be obtained as early as possible, but no sooner than four hours following ingestion. Liver function studies should be obtained initially and repeated at 24-hour intervals.
The antidote, N-acetylcysteine should be administered as early as possible, preferably within 16 hours of the overdose ingestions for optimal results, but in any case, within 24 hours. Following recovery, there are no residual structural or functional hepatic abnormalities.

Hydrocodone

Signs and Symptoms: Serious overdosage with hydrocodone is characterized by respiratory depression (a decrease in respiratory rate and/or tidal volume, Cheyne-Stokes respiration, cyanosis), extreme somnolence progressing to stupor or coma, skeletal muscle flaccidity, cold and clammy skin, and sometimes bradycardia and hypotension. In severe overdosage, apnea, circulatory collapse, cardiac arrest and death may occur.
Treatment: Primary attention should be given to the reestablishment of adequate respiratory exchange through provision of a patent airway and the institution of assisted or controlled ventilation. The opioid antagonist naloxone hydrochloride is a specific antidote for respiratory depression which may result from overdosage or unusual sensitivity to opioids including hydrocodone. Therefore, an appropriate dose of naloxone hydrochloride should be administered, preferably by the intravenous route, simultaneously with efforts at respiratory resuscitation. For further information, see full prescribing information for naloxone hydrochloride. An antagonist should not be administered in the absence of clinically significant respiratory depression. Oxygen, intravenous fluids, vasopressors and other supportive measures should be employed as indicated. Gastric emptying may be useful in removing unabsorbed drug. Activated charcoal may be of benefit.

DOSAGE AND ADMINISTRATION

Usual dosage, not less than 4 hours apart:
Adults: 1 tablet 4 times a day
Children: 6 to 12 years: 1/2 tablet 4 times a day
The total daily consumption of acetaminophen should not exceed 4 grams.

HOW SUPPLIED

HYCOMINE® Compound is available as a coral pink, round tablet scored and debossed with "HYCOMINE" on one side and plain on the other, supplied in bottles as follows:
Bottles of 100 NDC 63481-048-70
Bottles of 500 NDC 63481-048-85
Oral prescription where permitted by State law.
Store at 25°C (77°F); excursions permitted to 15°–30°C (59°–86°F). [See USP Controlled Room Temperature.] Dispense in a tight, light-resistant container as defined in the USP, with a child-resistant closure (as required).

HYCOMINE® is a Registered Trademark of Endo Pharmaceuticals Inc.
NARCAN® is a Registered Trademark of Endo Pharmaceuticals Inc.

6491-03/May, 2003

Shown in Product Identification Guide, page 311

HYCOTUSS® Ⓒ℞

[*hī-kō-tus*]
(hydrocodone bitartrate and guaifenesin)
Expectorant Syrup

DESCRIPTION

HYCOTUSS Expectorant Syrup contains hydrocodone (dihydrocodeinone) bitartrate, a semi-synthetic centrally-acting opioid antitussive and guaifenesin, an expectorant for oral administration.

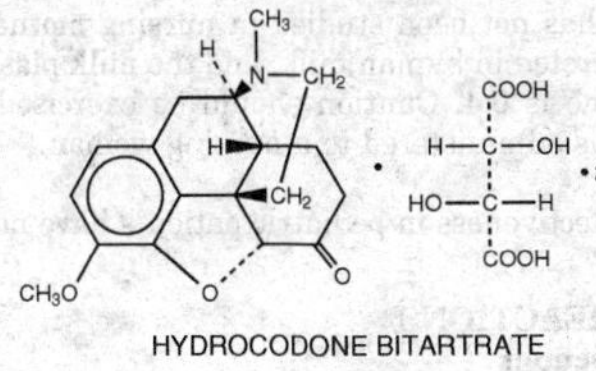

HYDROCODONE BITARTRATE

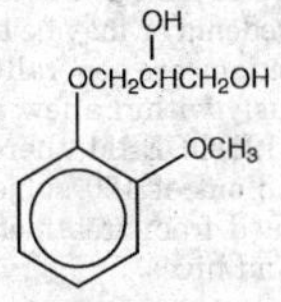

GUAIFENESIN

Each teaspoonful (5 mL) contains:

Hydrocodone bitartrate, USP	5 mg
Guaifenesin, USP	100 mg
Alcohol, USP	10% v/v

HYCOTUSS Expectorant Syrup also contains: artificial butterscotch flavor, FD&C Red 40, FD&C Yellow 6, glycerin, liquid sugar, methylparaben, propylparaben, saccharin sodium, and sorbitol solution.

CLINICAL PHARMACOLOGY

Clinical trials have proven hydrocodone bitartrate to be an effective antitussive agent which is pharmacologically 2 to 8 times as potent as codeine. At equi-effective doses, its sedative action is greater than codeine. The precise mechanism of action of hydrocodone and other opiates is not known, however, hydrocodone is believed to act by directly depressing the cough center. In excessive doses hydrocodone, like other opium derivatives, can depress respiration. The effects of hydrocodone in therapeutic doses on the cardiovascular system is insignificant. The constipation effects of hydrocodone are much weaker than that of morphine and no stronger than that of codeine. Hydrocodone can produce miosis, euphoria, physical and psychological dependence. At therapeutic antitussive doses, it does exert analgesic effects. Following a 10 mg oral dose of hydrocodone administered to five male human subjects, the mean peak concentration was 23.6 ± 5.2 ng/mL. Maximum serum levels were achieved at 1.3 ± 0.3 hours and half-life was determined to be 3.8 ± 0.3 hours. Hydrocodone exhibits a complex pattern of metabolism including O-demethylation, N-demethylation and 6-keto reduction to the corresponding 6-α- and 6-β-hydroxymetabolites.

The exact mechanism of action is not established but guaifenesin is believed to act by stimulating receptors in the gastric mucosa that initiates a reflex secretion of respiratory tract fluid, thereby increasing the volume and decreasing the viscosity of bronchial secretions. Studies with guaifenesin indicate that it is rapidly absorbed from the gastrointestinal tract and has a half-life of one hour.

INDICATIONS AND USAGE

HYCOTUSS (hydrocodone bitartrate and guaifenesin) Expectorant Syrup is indicated for the symptomatic relief of irritating non-productive cough associated with upper and lower respiratory tract congestion.

CONTRAINDICATIONS

HYCOTUSS Expectorant Syrup is contraindicated in patients hypersensitive to hydrocodone or guaifenesin. Patients known to be hypersensitive to other opioids may exhibit cross sensitivity to HYCOTUSS Expectorant Syrup. Hydrocodone is contraindicated in the presence of an intracranial lesion associated with increased intracranial pressure; and whenever ventilatory function is depressed.

WARNINGS

May be habit forming. Hydrocodone can produce drug dependence of the morphine type and therefore has the potential for being abused. Psychic dependence, physical dependence and tolerance may develop upon repeated administration of HYCOTUSS Expectorant Syrup and it should be prescribed and administered with the same degree of caution appropriate to the use of other opioid drugs (See DRUG ABUSE AND DEPENDENCE).

Respiratory Depression: HYCOTUSS Expectorant Syrup produces dose-related respiratory depression by directly acting on the brain stem respiratory centers. If respiratory depression occurs, it may be antagonized by the use of NARCAN® (naloxone hydrochloride) and other supportive measures when indicated.

Head Injury and Increased Intracranial Pressure: The respiratory depressant properties of opioids and their capacity to elevate cerebrospinal fluid pressure may be markedly exaggerated in the presence of head injury, other intracranial lesions or a pre-existing increase in intracranial pressure. Furthermore, narcotics produce adverse reactions which may obscure the clinical course of patients with head injuries.

Acute Abdominal Conditions: The administration of HYCOTUSS Expectorant Syrup or other opioids may obscure the diagnosis or clinical course of patients with acute abdominal conditions.

PRECAUTIONS

Before prescribing medication to suppress or modify cough, it is important to ascertain that the underlying cause of cough is identified, that modification of cough does not increase the risk of clinical or physiologic complications, and that appropriate therapy for the primary disease is provided.

Usage in Ambulatory Patients: Hydrocodone, like all opioids, may impair the mental and/or physical abilities required for the performance of potentially hazardous tasks such as driving a car or operating machinery, and patients should be warned accordingly.

Drug Interactions: Patients receiving other opioids, analgesics, general anesthetics, phenothiazines, other tranquilizers, sedative hypnotics or other CNS depressants (including alcohol) concomitantly with hydrocodone may exhibit an additive CNS depression. When such combined therapy is contemplated, the dose of one or both agents should be reduced (see WARNINGS).

Laboratory Interactions: The metabolite of guaifenesin has been found to produce an apparent increase in urinary 5-hydroxyindoleacetic acid, and guaifenesin therefore may interfere with the interpretation of this test for the diagnosis of carcinoid syndrome. Guaifenesin administration should be discontinued 24 hours prior to the collection of urine specimens for the determination of 5-hydroxyindoleacetic acid.

Carcinogenesis, Mutagenesis, Impairment of Fertility: Carcinogenicity, mutagenicity and reproduction studies have not been conducted with HYCOTUSS (hydrocodone bitartrate and guaifenesin) Expectorant Syrup.

Usage in Pregnancy: Pregnancy Category C. Animal reproduction studies have not been conducted with HYCOTUSS Expectorant Syrup. It is also not known whether HYCOTUSS Expectorant Syrup can cause fetal harm when administered to a pregnant woman or can affect reproductive capacity. HYCOTUSS Expectorant Syrup should be given to a pregnant woman only if clearly needed.

Nonteratogenic Effects: Babies born to mothers who have been taking opioids regularly prior to delivery will be physically dependent. The withdrawal signs include irritability and excessive crying, tremors, hyperactive reflexes, increased respiratory rate, increased stools, sneezing, yawning, vomiting and fever. The intensity of the syndrome does not always correlate with the duration of maternal opioid use or dose. There is no consensus on the best method of managing withdrawal. Chlorpromazine 0.7–1.0 mg/kg q 6 h, phenobarbital 2 mg/kg q 6 h, and paregoric 2–4 drops/kg q 4 h, have been used to treat withdrawal symptoms in infants. The duration of therapy is 4 to 28 days, with the dosages decreased as tolerated.

Nursing Mothers: It is not known whether this drug is excreted in human milk. Because many drugs are excreted in human milk and because of the potential for serious adverse reactions in nursing infants from HYCOTUSS Expectorant Syrup, a decision should be made whether to discontinue nursing or discontinue the drug, taking into account the importance of the drug to the mother.

ADVERSE REACTIONS

Respiratory System: Hydrocodone produces dose-related respiratory depression by acting directly on brain stem respiratory centers.

Cardiovascular System: Hypertension, postural hypotension and palpitations.

Genitourinary System: Ureteral spasm, spasm of vesical sphincters and urinary retention have been reported with opiates.

Central Nervous System: Sedation, drowsiness, mental clouding, lethargy, impairment of mental and physical performance, anxiety, fear, dysphoria, dizziness, psychic dependence, mood changes and blurred vision.

Gastrointestinal System: Nausea and vomiting occur more frequently in ambulatory than in recumbent patients.

DRUG ABUSE AND DEPENDENCE

Special care should be exercised in prescribing hydrocodone for emotionally unstable patients and for those with a history of drug misuse. Such patients should be closely supervised when long-term therapy is contemplated.

HYCOTUSS Expectorant Syrup is a Schedule III opioid. Psychic dependence, physical dependence and tolerance may develop upon repeated administration of opioids; therefore, HYCOTUSS Expectorant Syrup should always be prescribed and administered with caution. Physical dependence is the condition in which continued administration of the drug is required to prevent the appearance of a withdrawal syndrome.

Patients physically dependent on opioids will develop an abstinence syndrome upon abrupt discontinuation of the opioid or following the administration of a opioid antagonist. The character and severity of the withdrawal symptoms are related to the degree of physical dependence. Manifestations of opioid withdrawal are similar to but milder than that of morphine and include lacrimation, rhinorrhea, yawning, sweating, restlessness, dilated pupils, anorexia, gooseflesh, irritability and tremor. In more severe forms, nausea, vomiting, intestinal spasm and diarrhea, increased heart rate and blood pressure, chills, and pains in bones and muscles of the back and extremities may occur. Peak effects will usually be apparent at 48 to 72 hours.

Treatment of withdrawal is usually managed by providing sufficient quantities of an opioid to suppress **severe** withdrawal symptoms and then gradually reducing the dose of opioid over a period of several days.

OVERDOSAGE

Signs and Symptoms: Serious overdosage with HYCOTUSS (hydrocodone bitartrate and guaifenesin) Expectorant Syrup is characterized by respiratory depression (a decrease in respiratory rate and/or tidal volume, Cheyne-Stokes respiration, cyanosis), extreme somnolence progressing to stupor or coma, skeletal muscle flaccidity, cold and clammy skin, and sometimes bradycardia and hypotension. In severe overdosage, apnea, circulatory collapse, cardiac arrest, and death may occur.

Treatment: Primary attention should be given to the reestablishment of adequate respiratory exchange through provision of a patent airway and the institution of assisted or controlled ventilation. The opioid antagonist naloxone hydrochloride is a specific antidote for respiratory depression which may result from overdosage or unusual sensitivity to opioids including hydrocodone. Therefore, an appropriate dose of naloxone hydrochloride should be administered, preferably by the intravenous route, simultaneously with efforts at respiratory resuscitation. For further information, see full prescribing information for naloxone hydrochloride. An antagonist should not be administered in the absence of clinically significant respiratory depression. Oxygen, intravenous fluids, vasopressors, and other supportive measures should be employed as indicated. Gastric emptying may be useful in removing unabsorbed drug. Activated charcoal may be of benefit.

DOSAGE AND ADMINISTRATION

Usual Adult Dose: One teaspoonful (5 mL) after meals and at bedtime, not less than 4 hours apart (not to exceed 6 teaspoonsful in a 24 hour period). Treatment should be initiated with one teaspoonful and subsequent doses, up to a maximum single dose of 3 teaspoonsful, adjusted if required.

Usual Children's Dose:

Over 12 years: Initial dose 1 teaspoonful; maximum single dose, 2 teaspoonsful.

6 to 12 years: Initial dose 1/2 teaspoonful; maximum single dose, 1 teaspoonful.

HOW SUPPLIED

HYCOTUSS Expectorant Syrup is available as an orange-colored, butterscotch flavored syrup in bottles as follows:

480 mL (One pint) NDC 63481-235-16

Store at 25°C (77°F); excursions permitted to 15°–30°C (59°–86°F). [See USP Controlled Room Temperature.]

Dispense in a tight, light-resistant container as defined in the USP, with a child-resistant closure (as required).

Oral prescription where permitted by State Law.

HYCOTUSS® is a Registered Trademark of Endo Pharmaceuticals Inc.

NARCAN® is a Registered Trademark of Endo Pharmaceuticals Inc.

6481-03/April, 2003

LIDODERM® ℞

[*lī-dō-dĕrm*]
(Lidocaine Patch 5%)

DESCRIPTION

LIDODERM (lidocaine patch 5%) is comprised of an adhesive material containing 5% lidocaine, which is applied to a non-woven polyester felt backing and covered with a polyethylene terephthalate (PET) film release liner. The release liner is removed prior to application to the skin. The size of the patch is 10 cm × 14 cm.

Lidocaine is chemically designated as acetamide, 2-(diethylamino)-N-(2,6-dimethylphenyl), has an octanol:water partition ratio of 43 at pH 7.4, and has the following structure:

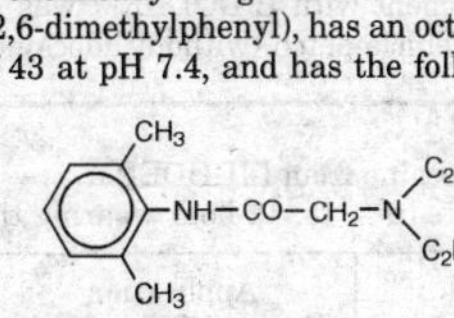

Each adhesive patch contains 700 mg of lidocaine (50 mg per gram adhesive) in an aqueous base. It also contains the

Continued on next page

Lidoderm—Cont.

following inactive ingredients: dihydroxyaluminum aminoacetate, disodium edetate, gelatin, glycerin, kaolin, methylparaben, polyacrylic acid, polyvinyl alcohol, propylene glycol, propylparaben, sodium carboxymethylcellulose, sodium polyacrylate, D-sorbitol, tartaric acid, and urea.

CLINICAL PHARMACOLOGY

Pharmacodynamics

Lidocaine is an amide-type local anesthetic agent and is suggested to stabilize neuronal membranes by inhibiting the ionic fluxes required for the initiation and conduction of impulses.

The penetration of lidocaine into intact skin after application of LIDODERM is sufficient to produce an analgesic effect, but less than the amount necessary to produce a complete sensory block.

Pharmacokinetics

Absorption: The amount of lidocaine systemically absorbed from LIDODERM is directly related to both the duration of application and the surface area over which it is applied. In a pharmacokinetic study, three LIDODERM patches were applied over an area of 420 cm^2 of intact skin on the back of normal volunteers for 12 hours. Blood samples were withdrawn for determination of lidocaine concentration during the application and for 12 hours after removal of patches. The results are summarized in Table 1. [See table 1 below]

When LIDODERM is used according to the recommended dosing instructions, only 3 ± 2% of the dose applied is expected to be absorbed. At least 95% (665 mg) of lidocaine will remain in a used patch. Mean peak blood concentration of lidocaine is about 0.13 μg/mL (about 1/10 of the therapeutic concentration required to treat cardiac arrhythmias). Repeated application of three patches simultaneously for 12 hours (recommended maximum daily dose), once per day for three days, indicated that the lidocaine concentration does not increase with daily use. The mean plasma pharmacokinetic profile for the 15 healthy volunteers is shown in Figure 1.

Figure 1
Mean lidocaine blood concentrations after three consecutive daily applications of three LIDODERM patches simultaneously for 12 hours per day in healthy volunteers (n = 15).

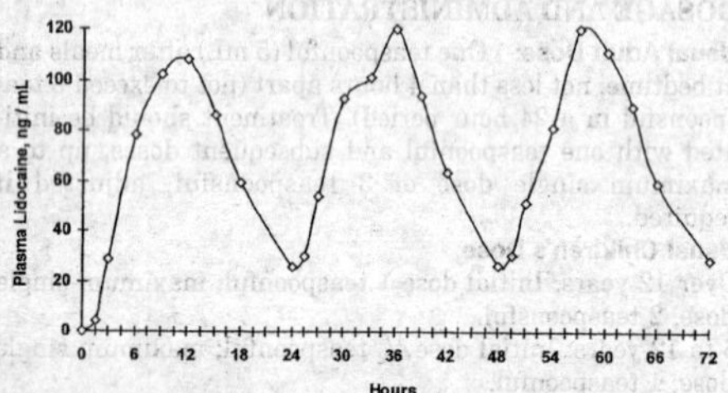

Distribution: When lidocaine is administered intravenously to healthy volunteers, the volume of distribution is 0.7 to 2.7 L/kg (mean 1.5 ± 0.6 SD, n = 15). At concentrations produced by application of LIDODERM, lidocaine is approximately 70% bound to plasma proteins, primarily alpha-1-acid glycoprotein. At much higher plasma concentrations (1 to 4 μg/mL of free base), the plasma protein binding of lidocaine is concentration dependent. Lidocaine crosses the placental and blood brain barriers, presumably by passive diffusion.

Metabolism: It is not known if lidocaine is metabolized in the skin. Lidocaine is metabolized rapidly by the liver to a number of metabolites, including monoethylglycinexylidide (MEGX) and glycinexylidide (GX), both of which have pharmacologic activity similar to, but less potent than that of lidocaine. A minor metabolite, 2,6-xylidine, has unknown pharmacologic activity but is carcinogenic in rats. The blood concentration of this metabolite is negligible following application of LIDODERM (lidocaine patch 5%). Following intravenous administration, MEGX and GX concentrations in serum range from 11 to 36% and from 5 to 11% of lidocaine concentrations, respectively.

Excretion: Lidocaine and its metabolites are excreted by the kidneys. Less than 10% of lidocaine is excreted unchanged. The half-life of lidocaine elimination from the plasma following IV administration is 81 to 149 minutes (mean 107 ± 22 SD, n = 15). The systemic clearance is 0.33 to 0.90 L/min (mean 0.64 ± 0.18 SD, n = 15).

CLINICAL STUDIES

Single-dose treatment with LIDODERM was compared to treatment with vehicle patch (without lidocaine), and to no treatment (observation only) in a double-blind, crossover clinical trial with 35 post-herpetic neuralgia patients. Pain intensity and pain relief scores were evaluated periodically for 12 hours. LIDODERM performed statistically better than vehicle patch in terms of pain intensity from 4 to 12 hours.

Multiple-dose, two-week treatment with LIDODERM was compared to vehicle patch (without lidocaine) in a double-blind, crossover clinical trial of withdrawal-type design conducted in 32 patients, who were considered as responders to the open-label use of LIDODERM prior to the study. The constant type of pain was evaluated but not the pain induced by sensory stimuli (dysesthesia). Statistically significant differences favoring LIDODERM were observed in terms of time to exit from the trial (14 versus 3.8 days at p-value <0.001), daily average pain relief, and patient's preference of treatment. About half of the patients also took oral medication commonly used in the treatment of post-herpetic neuralgia. The extent of use of concomitant medication was similar in the two treatment groups.

INDICATION AND USAGE

LIDODERM is indicated for relief of pain associated with post-herpetic neuralgia. It should be applied only to **intact skin.**

CONTRAINDICATIONS

LIDODERM is contraindicated in patients with a known history of sensitivity to local anesthetics of the amide type, or to any other component of the product.

WARNINGS

Accidental Exposure in Children

Even a *used* LIDODERM patch contains a large amount of lidocaine (at least 665 mg). The potential exists for a small child or a pet to suffer serious adverse effects from chewing or ingesting a new or used LIDODERM patch, although the risk with this formulation has not been evaluated. It is important for patients to **store and dispose of LIDODERM out of the reach of children and pets.**

Excessive Dosing

Excessive dosing by applying LIDODERM to larger areas or for longer than the recommended wearing time could result in increased absorption of lidocaine and high blood concentrations, leading to serious adverse effects (see ADVERSE REACTIONS, Systemic Reactions). Lidocaine toxicity could be expected at lidocaine blood concentrations above 5 μg/mL. The blood concentration of lidocaine is determined by the rate of systemic absorption and elimination. Longer duration of application, application of more than the recommended number of patches, smaller patients, or impaired elimination may all contribute to increasing the blood concentration of lidocaine. With recommended dosing of LIDODERM, the average peak blood concentration is about 0.13 μg/mL, but concentrations higher than 0.25 μg/mL have been observed in some individuals.

PRECAUTIONS

General

Hepatic Disease: Patients with severe hepatic disease are at greater risk of developing toxic blood concentrations of lidocaine, because of their inability to metabolize lidocaine normally.

Allergic Reactions: Patients allergic to para-aminobenzoic acid derivatives (procaine, tetracaine, benzocaine, etc.) have not shown cross sensitivity to lidocaine. However, LIDODERM should be used with caution in patients with a history of drug sensitivities, especially if the etiologic agent is uncertain.

Non-intact Skin: Application to broken or inflamed skin, although not tested, may result in higher blood concentrations of lidocaine from increased absorption. LIDODERM is only recommended for use on intact skin.

Eye Exposure: The contact of LIDODERM with eyes, although not studied, should be avoided based on the findings of severe eye irritation with the use of similar products in animals. If eye contact occurs, immediately wash out the eye with water or saline and protect the eye until sensation returns.

Drug Interactions

Antiarrhythmic Drugs: LIDODERM should be used with caution in patients receiving Class I antiarrhythmic drugs (such as tocainide and mexiletine) since the toxic effects are additive and potentially synergistic.

Local Anesthetics: When LIDODERM is used concomitantly with other products containing local anesthetic agents, the amount absorbed from all formulations must be considered.

Carcinogenesis, Mutagenesis, Impairment of Fertility

Carcinogenesis: A minor metabolite, 2,6-xylidine, has been found to be carcinogenic in rats. The blood concentration of this metabolite is negligible following application of LIDODERM.

Mutagenesis: Lidocaine HCl is not mutagenic in Salmonella/mammalian microsome test nor clastogenic in chromosome aberration assay with human lymphocytes and mouse micronucleus test.

Impairment of Fertility: The effect of LIDODERM on fertility has not been studied.

Pregnancy

Teratogenic Effects: **Pregnancy Category B.** LIDODERM (lidocaine patch 5%) has not been studied in pregnancy. Reproduction studies with lidocaine have been performed in rats at doses up to 30 mg/kg subcutaneously and have revealed no evidence of harm to the fetus due to lidocaine. There are, however, no adequate and well-controlled studies in pregnant women. Because animal reproduction studies are not always predictive of human response, LIDODERM should be used during pregnancy only if clearly needed.

Labor and Delivery

LIDODERM has not been studied in labor and delivery. Lidocaine is not contraindicated in labor and delivery. Should LIDODERM be used concomitantly with other products containing lidocaine, total doses contributed by all formulations must be considered.

Nursing Mothers

LIDODERM has not been studied in nursing mothers. Lidocaine is excreted in human milk, and the milk:plasma ratio of lidocaine is 0.4. Caution should be exercised when LIDODERM is administered to a nursing woman.

Pediatric Use

Safety and effectiveness in pediatric patients have not been established.

ADVERSE REACTIONS

Localized Reactions

During or immediately after treatment with LIDODERM (lidocaine patch 5%), the skin at the site of treatment may develop erythema or edema or may be the locus of abnormal sensation. These reactions are generally mild and transient, resolving spontaneously within a few minutes to hours. In clinical studies with LIDODERM, there were no serious reactions reported. One out of 150 subjects in a three-week study was discontinued from treatment because of a skin reaction (erythema and hives).

Allergic Reactions

Allergic and anaphylactoid reactions associated with lidocaine, although rare, can occur. They are characterized by urticaria, angioedema, bronchospasm, and shock. If they occur, they should be managed by conventional means. The detection of sensitivity by skin testing is of doubtful value.

Systemic (Dose-Related) Reactions

Systemic adverse reactions following appropriate use of LIDODERM are unlikely, due to the small dose absorbed (see CLINICAL PHARMACOLOGY, Pharmacokinetics). Systemic adverse effects of lidocaine are similar in nature to those observed with other amide local anesthetic agents, including CNS excitation and/or depression (light-headedness, nervousness, apprehension, euphoria, confusion, dizziness, drowsiness, tinnitus, blurred or double vision, vomiting, sensations of heat, cold or numbness, twitching, tremors, convulsions, unconsciousness, respiratory depression and arrest). Excitatory CNS reactions may be brief or not occur at all, in which case the first manifestation may be drowsiness merging into unconsciousness. Cardiovascular manifestations may include bradycardia, hypotension and cardiovascular collapse leading to arrest.

OVERDOSAGE

Lidocaine overdose from cutaneous absorption is rare, but could occur. If there is any suspicion of lidocaine overdose (see ADVERSE REACTIONS, Systemic Reactions), drug blood concentration should be checked. The management of overdose includes close monitoring, supportive care, and symptomatic treatment. Dialysis is of negligible value in the treatment of acute overdose with lidocaine.

In the absence of massive topical overdose or oral ingestion, evaluation of symptoms of toxicity should include consideration of other etiologies for the clinical effects, or overdosage from other sources of lidocaine or other local anesthetics.

The oral LD_{50} of lidocaine HCl is 459 (346–773) mg/kg (as the salt) in non-fasted female rats and 214 (159–324) mg/kg (as the salt) in fasted female rats, which are equivalent to roughly 4000 mg and 2000 mg, respectively, in a 60 to 70 kg man based on the equivalent surface area dosage conversion factors between species.

DOSAGE AND ADMINISTRATION

Apply LIDODERM to intact skin to cover the most painful area. Apply up to three patches, only once for up to 12 hours within a 24-hour period. Patches may be cut into smaller sizes with scissors prior to removal of the release liner. Clothing may be worn over the area of application. Smaller areas of treatment are recommended in a debilitated patient, or a patient with impaired elimination.

If irritation or a burning sensation occurs during application, remove the patch(es) and do not reapply until the irritation subsides.

When LIDODERM is used concomitantly with other products containing local anesthetic agents, the amount absorbed from all formulations must be considered.

HANDLING AND DISPOSAL

Hands should be washed after the handling of LIDODERM, and eye contact with LIDODERM should be avoided. The used patch should be immediately disposed of in such a way as to prevent its access by children or pets.

HOW SUPPLIED

LIDODERM (lidocaine patch 5%) is available as the following:

Table 1
Absorption of lidocaine from LIDODERM
Normal volunteers (n = 15, 12-hour wearing time)

LIDODERM Patch	Application Site	Area (cm^2)	Dose Absorbed (mg)	C_{max} (μg/mL)	T_{max} (hr)
3 patches (2100 mg)	Back	420	64 ± 32	0.13 ± 0.06	11 hr

Carton of 30 patches, packaged into individual child-resistant envelopes NDC 63481-687-06.
Store at 25°C (77°F); excursions permitted to 15°–30°C (59°–86°F). [See USP Controlled Room Temperature].
LIDODERM® is a Registered Trademark of Hind Health Care, Inc.

6524-07/March, 2004

Shown in Product Identification Guide, page 311

MOBAN® ℞

[*mō 'ban*]

(Molindone Hydrochloride Tablets, USP)

℞ only

DESCRIPTION

MOBAN (molindone hydrochloride) is a dihydroindolone compound which is not structurally related to the phenothiazines, the butyrophenones or the thioxanthenes.
MOBAN is 3-ethyl-6, 7-dihydro-2-methyl-5-(morpholinomethyl) indol-4 (5*H*)-one hydrochloride. It is a white to off-white crystalline powder, freely soluble in water and alcohol.
MOBAN Tablets contain the following inactive ingredients: Calcium sulfate, lactose, magnesium stearate, microcrystalline cellulose and povidone.

The 5 mg strength also contains alginic acid, colloidal silicon dioxide and FD&C Yellow 6.

The 10 mg strength also contains alginic acid, colloidal silicon dioxide, FD&C Blue 2 and FD&C Red 40.

The 25 mg strength also contains alginic acid, colloidal silicon dioxide, D&C Yellow 10, FD&C Blue 2, and FD&C Yellow 6.

The 50 mg strength also contains FD&C Blue 2 and sodium starch glycolate.

Molindone Hydrochloride is represented by the following structural formula:

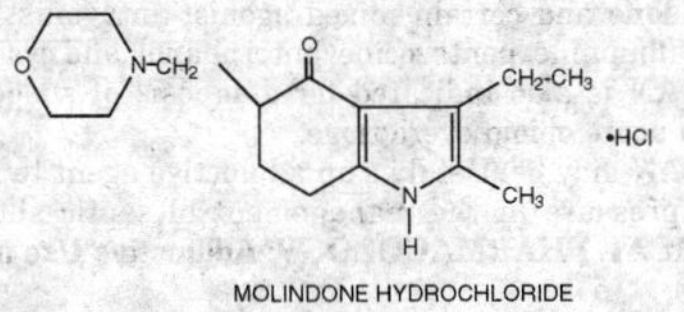

MOLINDONE HYDROCHLORIDE

The empirical formula is $C_{16}H_{24}N_2O_2 \bullet HCl$ representing a molecular weight of 312.83.

CLINICAL PHARMACOLOGY

MOBAN has a pharmacological profile in laboratory animals which predominantly resembles that of other antipsychotic agents causing reduction of spontaneous locomotion and aggressiveness, suppression of a conditioned response and antagonism of the bizarre stereotyped behavior and hyperactivity induced by amphetamines. In addition, MOBAN antagonizes the depression caused by the tranquilizing agent tetrabenazine.
In human clinical studies an antipsychotic effect is achieved in the absence of muscle relaxing or incoordinating effects. Based on EEG studies, MOBAN exerts its effect on the ascending reticular activating system.
Human metabolite studies show MOBAN to be rapidly absorbed and metabolized when given orally. Unmetabolized drug reached a peak level at 1.5 hours. Pharmacological effect from a single oral dose persists for 24-36 hours. There are 36 recognized metabolites with less than 2-3% unmetabolized MOBAN being excreted in urine and feces.

INDICATIONS AND USAGE

MOBAN is indicated for the management of schizophrenia. The efficacy of MOBAN in schizophrenia was established in clinical studies which enrolled newly hospitalized and chronically hospitalized, acutely ill, schizophrenic patients as subjects.

CONTRAINDICATIONS

MOBAN is contraindicated in severe central nervous system depression (alcohol, barbiturates, narcotics, etc.) or comatose states, and in patients with known hypersensitivity to the drug.

WARNINGS

Tardive Dyskinesia

Tardive dyskinesia, a syndrome consisting of potentially irreversible, involuntary, dyskinetic movements may develop in patients treated with antipsychotic drugs. Although the prevalence of the syndrome appears to be highest among the elderly, especially elderly women, it is impossible to rely upon prevalence estimates to predict, at the inception of antipsychotic treatment, which patients are likely to develop the syndrome. Whether antipsychotic drug products differ in their potential to cause tardive dyskinesia is unknown.
Both the risk of developing the syndrome and the likelihood that it will become irreversible are believed to increase as the duration of treatment and the total cumulative dose of antipsychotic drugs administered to the patient increase. However, the syndrome can develop, although much less commonly, after relatively brief treatment periods at low doses.
There is no known treatment for established cases of tardive dyskinesia, although the syndrome may remit, partially or completely, if antipsychotic treatment is withdrawn. Antipsychotic treatment, itself, however, may suppress (or partially suppress) the signs and symptoms of the syndrome and thereby may possibly mask the underlying disease process. The effect that symptomatic suppression has upon the long-term course of the syndrome is unknown.
Given these considerations, antipsychotics should be prescribed in a manner that is most likely to minimize the occurrence of tardive dyskinesia. Chronic antipsychotic treatment should generally be reserved for patients who suffer from a chronic illness that, 1) is known to respond to antipsychotic drugs, and 2) for whom alternative, equally effective, but potentially less harmful treatments are not available or appropriate. In patients who do require chronic treatment, the smallest dose and the shortest duration of treatment producing a satisfactory clinical response should be sought. The need for continued treatment should be reassessed periodically.
If signs and symptoms of tardive dyskinesia appear in a patient on antipsychotics, drug discontinuation should be considered. However, some patients may require treatment despite the presence of the syndrome.
(For further information about the description of tardive dyskinesia and its clinical detection, please refer to the section on Adverse Reactions.)

Neuroleptic Malignant Syndrome (NMS)

A potentially fatal symptom complex sometimes referred to as Neuroleptic Malignant Syndrome (NMS) has been reported in association with antipsychotic drugs. Clinical manifestations of NMS are hyperpyrexia, muscle rigidity, altered mental status and evidence of autonomic instability (irregular pulse or blood pressure, tachycardia, diaphoresis, and cardiac dysrhythmias).
The diagnostic evaluation of patients with this syndrome is complicated. In arriving at a diagnosis, it is important to identify cases where the clinical presentation includes both serious medical illness (e.g., pneumonia, systemic infection, etc.) and untreated or inadequately treated extrapyramidal signs and symptoms (EPS). Other important considerations in the differential diagnosis include central anticholinergic toxicity, heat stroke, drug fever and primary central nervous system (CNS) pathology.
The management of NMS should include, 1) immediate discontinuation of antipsychotic drugs and other drugs not essential to concurrent therapy, 2) intensive symptomatic treatment and medical monitoring, and 3) treatment of any concomitant serious medical problems for which specific treatments are available. There is no general agreement about specific pharmacological treatment regimens for uncomplicated NMS.
If a patient requires antipsychotic drug treatment after recovery from NMS, the potential reintroduction of drug therapy should be carefully considered. The patient should be carefully monitored, since recurrences of NMS have been reported.

PRECAUTIONS

General

Some patients receiving MOBAN (molindone hydrochloride) may note drowsiness initially and they should be advised against activities requiring mental alertness until their response to the drug has been established.
Increased activity has been noted in patients receiving MOBAN. Caution should be exercised where increased activity may be harmful.
MOBAN does not lower the seizure threshold in experimental animals to the degree noted with more sedating antipsychotic drugs. However, in humans convulsive seizures have been reported in a few instances.
The physician should be aware that this tablet preparation contains calcium sulfate as an excipient and that calcium ions may interfere with the absorption of preparations containing phenytoin sodium and tetracyclines.
MOBAN has an antiemetic effect in animals. A similar effect may occur in humans and may obscure signs of intestinal obstruction or brain tumor.
Antipsychotic drugs elevate prolactin levels; the elevation persists during chronic administration. Tissue culture experiments indicate that approximately one-third of human breast cancers are prolactin dependent *in vitro*, a factor of potential importance if the prescription of these drugs is contemplated in a patient with a previously detected breast cancer. Although disturbances such as galactorrhea, amenorrhea, gynecomastia, and impotence have been reported, the clinical significance of elevated serum prolactin levels is unknown for most patients. An increase in mammary neoplasms has been found in rodents after chronic administration of antipsychotic drugs. Neither clinical studies nor epidemiologic studies conducted to date, however, have shown an association between chronic administration of these drugs and mammary tumorigenesis; the available evidence is considered too limited to be conclusive at this time.
MOBAN has not been shown effective in the management of behavioral complications in patients with mental retardation.

Drug Interactions

Potentiation of drugs administered concurrently with MOBAN has not been reported. Additionally, animal studies have not shown increased toxicity when MOBAN is given concurrently with representative members of three classes of drugs (i.e., barbiturates, chloral hydrate and antiparkinson drugs).

Pregnancy

Studies in pregnant patients have not been carried out. Reproduction studies have been performed in the following animals:

Pregnant Rats oral dose—	
no adverse effect	20 mg/kg/day—10 days
no adverse effect	40 mg/kg/day—10 days
Pregnant Mice oral dose—	
slight increase resorptions	20 mg/kg/day—10 days
slight increase resorptions	40 mg/kg/day—10 days
Pregnant Rabbits oral dose—	
no adverse effect	5 mg/kg/day—12 days
no adverse effect	10 mg/kg/day—12 days
no adverse effect	20 mg/kg/day—12 days

Animal reproduction studies have not demonstrated a teratogenic potential. The anticipated benefits must be weighed against the unknown risks to the fetus if used in pregnant patients.

Nursing Mothers

Data are not available on the content of MOBAN (molindone hydrochloride) in the milk of nursing mothers.

Pediatric Use

Use of MOBAN in pediatric patients below the age of twelve years is not recommended because safe and effective conditions for its usage have not been established.

ADVERSE REACTIONS

CNS Effects

The most frequently occurring effect is initial drowsiness that generally subsides with continued usage of the drug or lowering of the dose.
Noted less frequently were depression, hyperactivity and euphoria.

Neurological

Extrapyramidal Reactions

Extrapyramidal reactions noted below may occur in susceptible individuals and are usually reversible with appropriate management.

Akathisia

Motor restlessness may occur early.

Parkinson Syndrome

Akinesia, characterized by rigidity, immobility and reduction of voluntary movements and tremor, have been observed. Occurrence is less frequent than akathisia.

Dystonic Syndrome

Prolonged abnormal contractions of muscle groups occur infrequently. These symptoms may be managed by the addition of a synthetic antiparkinson agent (other than L-dopa), small doses of sedative drugs, and/or reduction in dosage.

Tardive Dyskinesia

Antipsychotic drugs are known to cause a syndrome of dyskinetic movements commonly referred to as tardive dyskinesia. The movements may appear during treatment or upon withdrawal of treatment and may be either reversible or irreversible (i.e., persistent) upon cessation of further antipsychotic administration.
The syndrome is known to have a variable latency for development and the duration of the latency cannot be determined reliably. It is thus wise to assume that any antipsychotic agent has the capacity to induce the syndrome and act accordingly until sufficient data has been collected to settle the issue definitively for a specific drug product. In the case of antipsychotics known to produce the irreversible syndrome, the following has been observed.
Tardive dyskinesia has appeared in some patients on long-term therapy and has also appeared after drug therapy has been discontinued. The risk appears to be greater in elderly patients on high-dose therapy, especially females. The symptoms are persistent and in some patients appear to be irreversible. The syndrome is characterized by rhythmical involuntary movements of the tongue, face, mouth or jaw (e.g., protrusion of tongue, puffing of cheeks, puckering of mouth, chewing movements). There may be involuntary movements of extremities.
There is no known effective treatment of tardive dyskinesia; antiparkinsonism agents usually do not alleviate the symptoms of this syndrome. It is suggested that all antipsychotic agents be discontinued if these symptoms appear. Should it be necessary to reinstitute treatment, or increase the dosage of the agent, or switch to a different antipsychotic agent, the syndrome may be masked. It has been reported that fine vermicular movements of the tongue may be an early sign of the syndrome and if the medication is stopped at that time the syndrome may not develop (See WARNINGS).

Autonomic Nervous System

Occasionally blurring of vision, tachycardia, nausea, dry mouth and salivation have been reported. Urinary retention and constipation may occur particularly if anticholinergic drugs are used to treat extrapyramidal symptoms. One patient being treated with MOBAN experienced priapism which required surgical intervention, apparently resulting in residual impairment of erectile function.

Laboratory Tests

There have been rare reports of leucocytosis. If such reactions occur, treatment with MOBAN may continue if clinical symptoms are absent. Alterations of blood glucose, B.U.N., and red blood cells have not been considered clinically significant.

Metabolic and Endocrine Effects

Alteration of thyroid function has not been significant. Amenorrhea has been reported infrequently. Resumption of

Continued on next page

5 mg	Orange, round, biconvex tablet, one face debossed with "Moban 5", and the other face plain.	NDC 63481-072-70
10 mg	Lavender, round, biconvex tablet, one face debossed with "Moban 10", and the other face plain.	NDC 63481-073-70
25 mg	Green, round, biconvex tablet, one face debossed with "Moban 25", and the other face plain with partial bisect.	NDC 63481-074-70
50 mg	Blue, round, biconvex tablet, one face with partial bisect and debossed with "Moban 50", and the other face plain.	NDC 63481-076-70

Moban—Cont.

menses in previously amenorrheic women has been reported. Initially heavy menses may occur. Galactorrhea and gynecomastia have been reported infrequently. Increase in libido has been noted in some patients. Impotence has not been reported. Although both weight gain and weight loss have been in the direction of normal or ideal weight, excessive weight gain has not occurred with MOBAN.

Hepatic Effects

There have been rare reports of clinically significant alterations in liver function in association with MOBAN use.

Cardiovascular

Rare, transient, non-specific T wave changes have been reported on E.K.G. Association with a clinical syndrome has not been established. Rarely has significant hypotension been reported.

Ophthalmological

Lens opacities and pigmentary retinopathy have not been reported where patients have received MOBAN. In some patients, phenothiazine induced lenticular opacities have resolved following discontinuation of the phenothiazine while continuing therapy with MOBAN.

Skin

Early, non-specific skin rash, probably of allergic origin, has occasionally been reported. Skin pigmentation has not been seen with MOBAN usage alone.

MOBAN has certain pharmacological similarities to other antipsychotic agents. Because adverse reactions are often extensions of the pharmacological activity of a drug, all of the known pharmacological effects associated with other antipsychotic drugs should be kept in mind when MOBAN is used. Upon abrupt withdrawal after prolonged high dosage an abstinence syndrome has not been noted.

OVERDOSAGE

Symptomatic, supportive therapy should be the rule.

Gastric lavage is indicated for the reduction of absorption of MOBAN which is freely soluble in water.

Since the adsorption of MOBAN by activated charcoal has not been determined, the use of this anitdote must be considered of theoretical value.

Emesis in a comatose patient is contraindicated. Additionally, while the emetic effect of apomorphine is blocked by MOBAN in animals, this blocking effect has not been determined in humans.

A significant increase in the rate of removal of unmetabolized MOBAN from the body by forced diuresis, peritoneal or renal dialysis would not be expected. (Only 2% of a single ingested dose of MOBAN is excreted unmetabolized in the urine). However, poor response of the patient may justify use of these procedures.

While the use of laxatives or enemas might be based on general principles, the amount of unmetabolized MOBAN in feces is less than 1%. Extrapyramidal symptoms have responded to the use of Diphenhydramine (Benadryl®)*, Amantadine HCl (Symmetrel®)† and the synthetic anticholinergic antiparkinson agents, (i.e., Artane®‡, Cogentin®§, Akineton®¶).

DOSAGE AND ADMINISTRATION

Initial and maintenance doses of MOBAN should be individualized.

Initial Dosage Schedule

The usual starting dosage is 50-75 mg/day.

— Increase to 100 mg/day in 3 or 4 days.

— Based on severity of symptomatology, dosage may be titrated up or down depending on individual patient response.

— An increase to 225 mg/day may be required in patients with severe symptomatology.

Elderly and debilitated patients should be started on lower dosage.

Maintenance Dosage Schedule

1. Mild-5 mg-15 mg three or four times a day.
2. Moderate-10 mg-25 mg three or four times a day.
3. Severe-225 mg/day may be required.

HOW SUPPLIED

MOBAN (molindone hydrochloride) tablets are supplied in bottles of 100 tablets as follows:

[See table above]

Store at 25°C (77°F); excursions permitted to 15°-30°C (59°-86°F). Dispense in a tight, light-resistant container as defined in the USP, with a child-resistant closure (as required).

KEEP TIGHTLY CLOSED.

*Benadryl is a registered trademark of Warner-Lambert.
†Symmetrel is a registered trademark of Endo Pharmaceuticals Inc.
‡Artane is a registered trademark of Lederle Laboratories.
§Cogentin is a registered trademark of Merck & Co., Inc.
¶Akineton is a registered trademark of Knoll Laboratories.

MOBAN is a registered trademark of Endo Pharmaceuticals Inc.

Manufactured for:
Endo Pharmaceuticals Inc.
Chadds Ford, Pennsylvania 19317

Printed in U.S.A. 6498-04/January, 2003
411842

Shown in Product Identification Guide, page 311

NARCAN® ℞

[*nar'kan*]

(Naloxone Hydrochloride Injection, USP)

Opioid Antagonist

℞ only

DESCRIPTION

NARCAN (naloxone hydrochloride injection, USP), an opioid antagonist, is a synthetic congener of oxymorphone. In structure it differs from oxymorphone in that the methyl group on the nitrogen atom is replaced by an allyl group.

CH₂–CH=CH₂ •HCl
NALOXONE HYDROCHLORIDE
(-)-17-Allyl-4, 5α-epoxy-3, 14 -dihydroxy morphinan-6-one hydrochloride

Naloxone hydrochloride occurs as a white to slightly off-white powder, and is soluble in water, in dilute acids, and in strong alkali; slightly soluble in alcohol; practically insoluble in ether and in chloroform.

NARCAN injection is available as a sterile solution for intravenous, intramuscular and subcutaneous administration in three concentrations: 0.02 mg, 0.4 mg and 1 mg of naloxone hydrochloride per mL.

pH is adjusted to 3.5 ± 0.5 with hydrochloric acid.

The 0.02 mg/mL strength is an unpreserved, paraben-free formulation containing 9 mg/mL sodium chloride.

The 0.4 mg/mL vial contains 8.6 mg/mL of sodium chloride and 2 mg/mL of methylparaben and propylparaben as preservatives in a ratio of 9:1. The 0.4 mg/mL ampul is also available in an unpreserved, paraben-free formulation containing 9 mg/mL of sodium chloride.

The 1 mg/mL vial contains 8.35 mg/mL of sodium chloride and 2 mg/mL of methylparaben and propylparaben as preservatives in a ratio of 9:1. The 1 mg/mL ampul is also available in an unpreserved, paraben-free formulation containing 9 mg/mL of sodium chloride.

CLINICAL PHARMACOLOGY

Complete or Partial Reversal of Opioid Depression

NARCAN prevents or reverses the effects of opioids including respiratory depression, sedation and hypotension. Also, NARCAN can reverse the psychotomimetic and dysphoric effects of agonist-antagonists such as pentazocine.

NARCAN is an essentially pure opioid antagonist, i.e., it does not possess the "agonistic" or morphine-like properties characteristic of other opioid antagonists. When administered in usual doses and in the absence of opioids or agonistic effects of other opioid antagonists, it exhibits essentially no pharmacologic activity.

NARCAN has not been shown to produce tolerance or cause physical or psychological dependence. In the presence of physical dependence on opioids, NARCAN will produce withdrawal symptoms. However, in the presence of opioid dependence, opiate withdrawal symptoms may appear within minutes of NARCAN administration and subside in about 2 hours. The severity and duration of the withdrawal syndrome are related to the dose of NARCAN and to the degree and type of opioid dependence.

While the mechanism of action of NARCAN is not fully understood, *in vitro* evidence suggests that NARCAN antagonizes opioid effects by competing for the μ, κ and σ opiate receptor sites in the CNS, with the greatest affinity for the μ receptor.

When NARCAN is administered intravenously (I.V.), the onset of action is generally apparent within two minutes. The onset of action is slightly less rapid when it is administered subcutaneously (S.C.) or intramuscularly (I.M.). The duration of action is dependent upon the dose and route of administration of NARCAN. Intramuscular administration produces a more prolonged effect than intravenous administration. Since the duration of action of NARCAN may be shorter than that of some opiates, the effects of the opiate may return as the effects of NARCAN dissipates. The requirement for repeat doses of NARCAN will also be dependent upon the amount, type and route of administration of the opioid being antagonized.

Adjunctive Use in Septic Shock

NARCAN has been shown in some cases of septic shock to produce a rise in blood pressure that may last up to several hours; however, this pressor response has not been demonstrated to improve patient survival. In some studies, treatment with NARCAN in the setting of septic shock has been associated with adverse effects, including agitation, nausea and vomiting, pulmonary edema, hypotension, cardiac arrhythmias, and seizures. The decision to use NARCAN in septic shock should be exercised with caution, particularly in patients who may have underlying pain or have previously received opioid therapy and may have developed opioid tolerance.

Because of the limited number of patients who have been treated, optimal dosage and treatment regimens have not been established.

PHARMACOKINETICS

Distribution

Following parenteral administration, NARCAN is rapidly distributed in the body and readily crosses the placenta. Plasma protein binding occurs but is relatively weak. Plasma albumin is the major binding constituent but significant binding of naloxone also occurs to plasma constituents other than albumin. It is not known whether naloxone is excreted into human milk.

Metabolism and Elimination

NARCAN is metabolized in the liver, primarily by glucuronide conjugation with naloxone-3-glucoronide as the major metabolite. In one study the serum half-life in adults ranged from 30 to 81 minutes (mean 64 ± 12 minutes). In a neonatal study the mean plasma half-life was observed to be 3.1 ± 0.5 hours. After an oral or intravenous dose, about 25–40% of the drug is excreted as metabolites in urine within 6 hours, about 50% in 24 hours, and 60–70% in 72 hours.

INDICATIONS AND USAGE

NARCAN is indicated for the complete or partial reversal of opioid depression, including respiratory depression, induced by natural and synthetic opioids, including propoxyphene, methadone and certain mixed agonist-antagonist analgesics: nalbuphine, pentazocine, butorphanol, and cyclazocine. NARCAN is also indicated for diagnosis of suspected or known acute opioid overdosage.

NARCAN may be useful as an adjunctive agent to increase blood pressure in the management of septic shock (see **CLINICAL PHARMACOLOGY; Adjunctive Use in Septic Shock**).

CONTRAINDICATIONS

NARCAN is contraindicated in patients known to be hypersensitive to naloxone hydrochloride or to any of the other ingredients in NARCAN.

WARNINGS

Drug Dependence

NARCAN should be administered cautiously to persons including newborns of mothers who are known or suspected to be physically dependent on opioids. In such cases an abrupt and complete reversal of opioid effects may precipitate an acute withdrawal syndrome.

The signs and symptoms of opioid withdrawal in a patient physically dependent on opioids may include, but are not limited to, the following: body aches, diarrhea, tachycardia, fever, runny nose, sneezing, piloerection, sweating, yawning, nausea or vomiting, nervousness, restlessness or irritability, shivering or trembling, abdominal cramps, weakness, and increased blood pressure. In the neonate, opioid withdrawal may also include: convulsions, excessive crying, and hyperactive reflexes.

Repeat Administration

The patient who has satisfactorily responded to NARCAN should be kept under continued surveillance and repeated doses of NARCAN should be administered, as necessary, since the duration of action of some opioids may exceed that of NARCAN.

Respiratory Depression due to Other Drugs

NARCAN is not effective against respiratory depression due to non-opioid drugs and in the management of acute toxicity caused by levopropoxyphene. Reversal of respiratory depression by partial agonists or mixed agonist/antagonists, such as buprenorphine and pentazocine, may be incomplete or require higher doses of naloxone. If an incomplete response occurs, respirations should be mechanically assisted as clinically indicated.

PRECAUTIONS

General

In addition to NARCAN, other resuscitative measures such as maintenance of a free airway, artificial ventilation, cardiac massage, and vasopressor agents should be available and employed when necessary to counteract acute opioid poisoning.

Abrupt postoperative reversal of opioid depression may result in nausea, vomiting, sweating, tremulousness, tachycardia, increased blood pressure, seizures, ventricular tachycardia and fibrillation, pulmonary edema, and cardiac arrest which may result in death. Excessive doses of NARCAN in postoperative patients may result in significant reversal of analgesia and may cause agitation (see **PRECAUTIONS** and **DOSAGE AND ADMINISTRATION; Usage in Adults-Postoperative Opioid Depression**). Several instances of hypotension, hypertension, ventricular tachycardia and fibrillation, pulmonary edema, and cardiac arrest have been reported in postoperative patients. Death, coma, and encephalopathy have been reported as sequelae of these events. These have occurred in patients most of whom had pre-existing cardiovascular disorders or received other drugs which may have similar adverse cardiovascular effects. Although a direct cause and effect relationship has not been established, NARCAN should be used with caution in patients with pre-existing cardiac disease or patients who have received medications with potential adverse cardiovascular effects, such as hypotension, ventricular tachycardia or fibrillation, and pulmonary edema. It has been suggested that the pathogenesis of pulmonary edema associated with the use of NARCAN is similar to neurogenic pulmonary edema, i.e., a centrally mediated massive catecholamine response leading to a dramatic shift of blood volume into the pulmonary vascular bed resulting in increased hydrostatic pressures.

Drug Interactions

Large doses of naloxone are required to antagonize buprenorphine since the latter has a long duration of action due to its slow rate of binding and subsequent slow dissociation from the opioid receptor. Buprenorphine antagonism is characterized by a gradual onset of the reversal effects and a decreased duration of action of the normally prolonged respiratory depression. The barbiturate methohexital appears to block the acute onset of withdrawal symptoms induced by naloxone in opiate addicts.

Carcinogenesis, Mutagenesis, Impairment of Fertility

Studies in animals to assess the carcinogenic potential of NARCAN have not been conducted. NARCAN was weakly positive in the Ames mutagenicity and in the *in vitro* human lymphocyte chromosome aberration test but was negative in the *in vitro* Chinese hamster V79 cell HGPRT mutagenicity assay and in the *in vivo* rat bone marrow chromosome aberration study. Reproduction studies conducted in mice and rats at doses 4-times and 8-times, respectively, the dose of a 50 kg human given 10 mg/day (when based on surface area or mg/m^2), demonstrated no embryotoxic or teratogenic effects due to NARCAN.

Use in Pregnancy

Teratogenic Effects: Pregnancy Category C: Teratology studies conducted in mice and rats at doses 4-times and 8-times, respectively, the dose of a 50 kg human given 10 mg/day (when based on surface area or mg/m^2), demonstrated no embryotoxic or teratogenic effects due to NARCAN. There are, however, no adequate and well-controlled studies in pregnant women. Because animal reproduction studies are not always predictive of human response, NARCAN should be used during pregnancy only if clearly needed.

Non-teratogenic Effects: Risk-benefit must be considered before NARCAN is administered to a pregnant woman who is known or suspected to be opioid-dependent since maternal dependence may often be accompanied by fetal dependence. Naloxone crosses the placenta, and may precipitate withdrawal in the fetus as well as in the mother. Patients with mild to moderate hypertension who receive naloxone during labor should be carefully monitored as severe hypertension may occur.

Use in Labor and Delivery

It is not known if NARCAN affects the duration of labor and/or delivery. However, published reports indicated that administration of naloxone during labor did not adversely affect maternal or neonatal status.

Nursing Mothers

It is not known whether NARCAN is excreted in human milk. Because many drugs are excreted in human milk, caution should be exercised when NARCAN is administered to a nursing woman.

Pediatric Use

NARCAN (naloxone hydrochloride injection, USP) may be administered intravenously, intramuscularly or subcutaneously in children and neonates to reverse the effects of opiates.The American Academy of Pediatrics, however, does not endorse subcutaneous or intramuscular administration in opiate intoxication since absorption may be erratic or delayed. Although the opiate-intoxicated child responds dramatically to NARCAN, he/she must be carefully monitored for at least 24 hours as a relapse may occur as naloxone is metabolized.

When NARCAN is given to the mother shortly before delivery, the duration of its effect lasts only for the first two hours of neonatal life. It is preferable to administer NARCAN directly to the neonate if needed after delivery. NARCAN has no apparent benefit as an additional method of resuscitation in the newly born infant with intrauterine asphyxia which is not related to opioid use.

Usage in Pediatric Patients and Neonates for Septic Shock: The safety and effectiveness of NARCAN in the treatment of hypotension in pediatric patients and neonates with septic shock have not been established. One study of two neonates in septic shock reported a positive pressor response; however, one patient subsequently died after intractable seizures.

Geriatric Use

Clinical studies of NARCAN did not include sufficient numbers of subjects aged 65 and over to determine whether they respond differently from younger subjects. Other reported clinical experience has not identified differences in responses between the elderly and younger patients. In general, dose selection for an elderly patient should be cautious, usually starting at the low end of the dosing range, reflecting the greater frequency of decreased hepatic, renal, or cardiac function, and of concomitant disease or other drug therapy.

Renal Insufficiency/Failure

The safety and effectiveness of NARCAN in patients with renal insufficiency/failure have not been established in well-controlled clinical trials. Caution should be exercised when NARCAN is administered to this patient population.

Liver Disease

The safety and effectiveness of NARCAN in patients with liver disease have not been established in well-controlled clinical trials. Caution should be exercised when NARCAN is administered to patients with liver disease.

ADVERSE REACTIONS

Postoperative

The following adverse events have been associated with the use of NARCAN in postoperative patients: hypotension, hypertension, ventricular tachycardia and fibrillation, dyspnea, pulmonary edema, and cardiac arrest. Death, coma, and encephalopathy have been reported as sequelae of these events. Excessive doses of NARCAN in postoperative patients may result in significant reversal of analgesia and may cause agitation (see **PRECAUTIONS and DOSAGE AND ADMINISTRATION; Usage in Adults-Postoperative Opioid Depression**).

Opioid Depression

Abrupt reversal of opioid depression may result in nausea, vomiting, sweating, tachycardia, increased blood pressure, tremulousness, seizures, ventricular tachycardia and fibrillation, pulmonary edema, and cardiac arrest which may result in death (see **PRECAUTIONS**).

Opioid Dependence

Abrupt reversal of opioid effects in persons who are physically dependent on opioids may precipitate an acute withdrawal syndrome which may include, but is not limited to, the following signs and symptoms: body aches, fever, sweating, runny nose, sneezing, piloerection, yawning, weakness, shivering or trembling, nervousness, restlessness or irritability, diarrhea, nausea or vomiting, abdominal cramps, increased blood pressure, tachycardia. In the neonate, opioid withdrawal may also include: convulsions; excessive crying; hyperactive reflexes (see **WARNINGS**).

Adverse events associated with the postoperative use of NARCAN are listed by organ system and in decreasing order of frequency as follows:

Cardiac Disorders: pulmonary edema, cardiac arrest or failure, tachycardia, ventricular fibrillation, and ventricular tachycardia. Death, coma, and encephalopathy have been reported as sequelae of these events.

Gastrointestinal Disorders: vomiting, nausea

Nervous System Disorders: convulsions, paraesthesia, grand mal convulsion

Psychiatric Disorders: agitation, hallucination, tremulousness

Respiratory, Thoracic and Mediastinal Disorders: dyspnea, respiratory depression, hypoxia

Skin and Subcutaneous Tissue Disorders: nonspecific injection site reactions, sweating

Vascular Disorders: hypertension, hypotension, hot flushes or flushing.

See also **PRECAUTIONS and DOSAGE AND ADMINISTRATION; Usage in Adults; Postoperative Opioid Depression.**

DRUG ABUSE AND DEPENDENCE

NARCAN is an opioid antagonist. Physical dependence associated with the use of NARCAN has not been reported. Tolerance to the opioid antagonist effect of NARCAN is not known to occur.

OVERDOSAGE

There is limited clinical experience with NARCAN overdosage in humans.

Adult Patients

In one small study, volunteers who received 24 mg/70 kg did not demonstrate toxicity.

In another study, 36 patients with acute stroke received a loading dose of 4 mg/kg (10 mg/m^2/min) of NARCAN followed immediately by 2 mg/kg/hr for 24 hours. Twenty-three patients experienced adverse events associated with naloxone use, and naloxone was discontinued in seven patients because of adverse effects. The most serious adverse events were: seizures (2 patients), severe hypertension (1), and hypotension and/or bradycardia (3).

At doses of 2 mg/kg in normal subjects, cognitive impairment and behavioral symptoms, including irritability, anxiety, tension, suspiciousness, sadness, difficulty concentrating, and lack of appetite have been reported. In addition, somatic symptoms, including dizziness, heaviness, sweating, nausea, and stomachaches were also reported. Although complete information is not available, behavioral symptoms were reported to often persist for 2–3 days.

Pediatric Patients

Up to 11 doses of 0.2 mg of naloxone (2.2 mg) have been administered to children following overdose of diphenoxylate hydrochloride with atropine sulfate. Pediatric reports include a 2-1/2 year-old child who inadvertently received a dose of 20 mg of naloxone for treatment of respiratory depression following overdose with diphenoxylate hydrochloride with atropine sulfate. The child responded well and recovered without adverse sequelae. There is also a report of a 4-1/2 year-old child who received 11 doses during a 12-hour period, with no adverse sequelae.

Patient Management

Patients who experience a NARCAN overdose should be treated symptomatically in a closely supervised environment. Physicians should contact a poison control center for the most up-to-date patient management information.

DOSAGE AND ADMINISTRATION

NARCAN may be administered intravenously, intramuscularly, or subcutaneously. The most rapid onset of action is achieved by intravenous administration, which is recommended in emergency situations.

Since the duration of action of some opioids may exceed that of NARCAN, the patient should be kept under continued surveillance. Repeated doses of NARCAN should be administered, as necessary.

Intravenous Infusion

NARCAN may be diluted for intravenous infusion in normal saline or 5% dextrose solutions. The addition of 2 mg of NARCAN in 500 mL of either solution provides a concentration of 0.004 mg/mL. Mixtures should be used within 24 hours. After 24 hours, the remaining unused mixture must be discarded. The rate of administration should be titrated in accordance with the patient's response.

NARCAN should not be mixed with preparations containing bisulfite, metabisulfite, long-chain or high molecular weight anions, or any solution having an alkaline pH. No drug or chemical agent should be added to NARCAN unless its effect on the chemical and physical stability of the solution has first been established.

General

Parenteral drug products should be inspected visually for particulate matter and discoloration prior to administration whenever solution and container permit.

Usage in Adults

Opioid Overdose–Known or Suspected: An initial dose of 0.4 mg to 2 mg of NARCAN may be administered intravenously. If the desired degree of counteraction and improvement in respiratory functions are not obtained, it may be repeated at two- to three-minute intervals. If no response is observed after 10 mg of NARCAN have been administered, the diagnosis of opioid-induced or partial opioid-induced toxicity should be questioned. Intramuscular or subcutaneous administration may be necessary if the intravenous route is not available.

Postoperative Opioid Depression: For the partial reversal of opioid depression following the use of opioids during surgery, smaller doses of NARCAN are usually sufficient. The dose of NARCAN should be titrated according to the patient's response. For the initial reversal of respiratory depression, NARCAN should be injected in increments of 0.1 to 0.2 mg intravenously at two- to three-minute intervals to the desired degree of reversal i.e., adequate ventilation and alertness without significant pain or discomfort. Larger than necessary dosage of NARCAN may result in significant reversal of analgesia and increase in blood pressure. Similarly, too rapid reversal may induce nausea, vomiting, sweating or circulatory stress.

Repeat doses of NARCAN may be required within one- to two-hour intervals depending upon the amount, type (i.e., short or long acting) and time interval since last administration of an opioid. Supplemental intramuscular doses have been shown to produce a longer lasting effect.

Septic Shock: The optimal dosage of NARCAN or duration of therapy for the treatment of hypotension in septic shock patients has not been established (see **CLINICAL PHARMACOLOGY**).

Usage in Children

Opioid Overdose–Known or Suspected: The usual initial dose in children is 0.01 mg/kg body weight given I.V. If this dose does not result in the desired degree of clinical improvement, a subsequent dose of 0.1 mg/kg body weight may be administered. If an I.V. route of administration is not available, NARCAN may be administered I.M. or S.C. in divided doses. If necessary, NARCAN can be diluted with sterile water for injection.

Postoperative Opioid Depression: Follow the recommendations and cautions under **Adult Postoperative Depression**. For the initial reversal of respiratory depression, NARCAN should be injected in increments of 0.005 mg to 0.01 mg intravenously at two- to three-minute intervals to the desired degree of reversal.

Usage in Neonates

Opioid-induced Depression: The usual initial dose is 0.01 mg/kg body weight administered I.V., I.M. or S.C. This dose may be repeated in accordance with adult administration guidelines for postoperative opioid depression.

HOW SUPPLIED

NARCAN (naloxone hydrochloride injection, USP) for intravenous, intramuscular, and subcutaneous administration is available as:

Multiple Dose Vials

0.4 mg/mL	10 mL multiple dose vial-box of 1, NDC 63481-365-05
1 mg/mL	10 mL multiple dose vial-box of 1, NDC 63481-368-05

Preservative-Free Ampules

0.02 mg/mL	2 mL unit dose ampule-box of 10, NDC 63481-359-10
0.4 mg/mL	1 mL unit dose ampule-box of 10, NDC 63481-358-10
1 mg/mL	2 mL unit dose ampule-box of 10, NDC 63481-377-10

Store at 25°C (77°F); excursions permitted to 15°–30°C (59°–86°F). [See USP Controlled Room Temperature.] Protect from light.

Store in carton until contents have been used.

Continued on next page

Narcan—Cont.

Manufactured for:
Endo Pharmaceuticals Inc.
Chadds Ford, Pennsylvania 19317
NARCAN is a Registered Trademark of Endo Pharmaceuticals Inc.

51-022523-00/July, 2003

NUBAIN® ℞

[nū 'bān]
(Nalbuphine Hydrochloride)
℞ only

DESCRIPTION

NUBAIN (nalbuphine hydrochloride) is a synthetic opioid agonist-antagonist analgesic of the phenanthrene series. It is chemically related to both the widely used opioid antagonist, naloxone, and the potent opioid analgesic, oxymorphone. Chemically nalbuphine hydrochloride is 17-(cyclobutylmethyl)-4,5α-epoxymorphinan-3,6α,14-triol hydrochloride. Nalbuphine hydrochloride molecular weight is 393.91 and is soluble in H_2O (35.5 mg/mL @ 25°C) and ethanol (0.8%); insoluble in $CHCl_3$ and ether. Nalbuphine hydrochloride has pKa values of 8.71 and 9.96. The molecular formula is $C_{21}H_{27}NO_4 \cdot HCl$. The structural formula is:

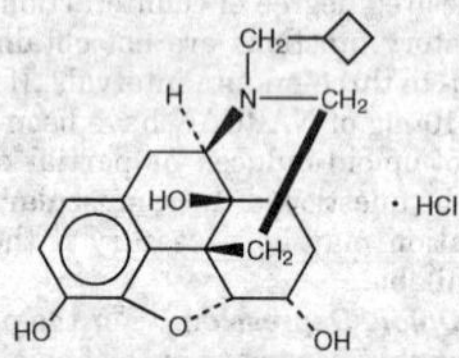

NUBAIN is a sterile solution suitable for subcutaneous, intramuscular, or intravenous injection. NUBAIN is available in two concentrations, 10 mg and 20 mg of nalbuphine hydrochloride per mL. Both strengths in 10 mL vials contain 0.94% sodium citrate hydrous, 1.26% citric acid anhydrous, and 0.2% of a 9:1 mixture of methylparaben and propylparaben as preservatives; pH is adjusted, if necessary, to 3.5 to 3.7 with hydrochloric acid. The 10 mg/mL strength contains 0.2% sodium chloride.

NUBAIN is also available in ampuls in a sterile, paraben-free formulation in two concentrations, 10 mg and 20 mg of nalbuphine hydrochloride per mL. One mL of each strength contains 0.94% sodium citrate hydrous, and 1.26% citric acid anhydrous; pH is adjusted, if necessary, to 3.5 to 3.7 with hydrochloric acid. The 10 mg/mL strength contains 0.2% sodium chloride.

CLINICAL PHARMACOLOGY

NUBAIN is a potent analgesic. Its analgesic potency is essentially equivalent to that of morphine on a milligram basis. Receptor studies show that NUBAIN binds to mu, kappa, and delta receptors, but not to sigma receptors. NUBAIN is primarily a kappa agonist/partial mu antagonist analgesic.

The onset of action of NUBAIN occurs within 2 to 3 minutes after intravenous administration, and in less than 15 minutes following subcutaneous or intramuscular injection. The plasma half-life of nalbuphine is 5 hours, and in clinical studies the duration of analgesic activity has been reported to range from 3 to 6 hours.

The opioid antagonist activity of NUBAIN is one-fourth as potent as nalorphine and 10 times that of pentazocine.

NUBAIN may produce the same degree of respiratory depression as equianalgesic doses of morphine. However, NUBAIN exhibits a ceiling effect such that increases in dose greater than 30 mg do not produce further respiratory depression in the absence of other CNS active medications affecting respiration.

NUBAIN by itself has potent opioid antagonist activity at doses equal to or lower than its analgesic dose. When administered following or concurrent with mu agonist opioid analgesics (e.g., morphine, oxymorphone, fentanyl), NUBAIN may partially reverse or block opioid-induced respiratory depression from the mu agonist analgesic. NUBAIN may precipitate withdrawal in patients dependent on opioid drugs. NUBAIN should be used with caution in patients who have been receiving mu opioid analgesics on a regular basis.

INDICATIONS AND USAGE

NUBAIN is indicated for the relief of moderate to severe pain. NUBAIN can also be used as a supplement to balanced anesthesia, for preoperative and postoperative analgesia, and for obstetrical analgesia during labor and delivery.

CONTRAINDICATIONS

NUBAIN should not be administered to patients who are hypersensitive to nalbuphine hydrochloride, or to any of the other ingredients in NUBAIN.

WARNINGS

NUBAIN should be administered as a supplement to general anesthesia only by persons specifically trained in the use of intravenous anesthetics and management of the respiratory effects of potent opioids.

Naloxone, resuscitative and intubation equipment and oxygen should be readily available.

Drug Abuse

Caution should be observed in prescribing NUBAIN for emotionally unstable patients, or for individuals with a history of opioid abuse. Such patients should be closely supervised when long-term therapy is contemplated (see **DRUG ABUSE AND DEPENDENCE**).

Use in Ambulatory Patients

NUBAIN may impair the mental or physical abilities required for the performance of potentially dangerous tasks such as driving a car or operating machinery. Therefore, NUBAIN should be administered with caution to ambulatory patients who should be warned to avoid such hazards.

Use in Emergency Procedures

Maintain patient under observation until recovered from NUBAIN effects that would affect driving or other potentially dangerous tasks.

Use in Pregnancy (Other Than Labor)

Severe fetal bradycardia has been reported when NUBAIN is administered during labor. Naloxone may reverse these effects. Although there are no reports of fetal bradycardia earlier in pregnancy, it is possible that this may occur. This drug should be used in pregnancy only if clearly needed, if the potential benefit outweighs the risk to the fetus, and if appropriate measures such as fetal monitoring are taken to detect and manage any potential adverse effect on the fetus.

Use During Labor and Delivery

The placental transfer of nalbuphine is high, rapid, and variable with a maternal to fetal ratio ranging from 1:0.37 to 1:6. Fetal and neonatal adverse effects that have been reported following the administration of nalbuphine to the mother during labor include fetal bradycardia, respiratory depression at birth, apnea, cyanosis and hypotonia. Maternal administration of naloxone during labor has normalized these effects in some cases. Severe and prolonged fetal bradycardia has been reported. Permanent neurological damage attributed to fetal bradycardia has occurred. A sinusoidal fetal heart rate pattern associated with the use of nalbuphine has also been reported. NUBAIN should be used during labor and delivery only if clearly indicated and only if the potential benefit outweighs the risk to the infant. Newborns should be monitored for respiratory depression, apnea, bradycardia, and arrhythmias if NUBAIN has been used.

Head Injury and Increased Intracranial Pressure

The possible respiratory depressant effects and the potential of potent analgesics to elevate cerebrospinal fluid pressure (resulting from vasodilation following CO_2 retention) may be markedly exaggerated in the presence of head injury, intracranial lesions or a pre-existing increase in intracranial pressure. Furthermore, potent analgesics can produce effects which may obscure the clinical course of patients with head injuries. Therefore, NUBAIN should be used in these circumstances only when essential, and then should be administered with extreme caution.

Interaction with Other Central Nervous System Depressants

Although NUBAIN possesses opioid antagonist activity, there is evidence that in nondependent patients it will not antagonize an opioid analgesic administered just before, concurrently, or just after an injection of NUBAIN. Therefore, patients receiving an opioid analgesic, general anesthetics, phenothiazines, or other tranquilizers, sedatives, hypnotics, or other CNS depressants (including alcohol) concomitantly with NUBAIN may exhibit an additive effect. When such combined therapy is contemplated, the dose of one or both agents should be reduced.

PRECAUTIONS

General

Impaired Respiration: At the usual adult dose of 10 mg/70 kg, NUBAIN causes some respiratory depression approximately equal to that produced by equal doses of morphine. However, in contrast to morphine, respiratory depression is not appreciably increased with higher doses of NUBAIN. Respiratory depression induced by NUBAIN can be reversed by NARCAN® (naloxone hydrochloride) when indicated. NUBAIN should be administered with caution at low doses to patients with impaired respiration (e.g., from other medication, uremia, bronchial asthma, severe infection, cyanosis, or respiratory obstructions).

Impaired Renal or Hepatic Function: Because NUBAIN is metabolized in the liver and excreted by the kidneys, NUBAIN should be used with caution in patients with renal or liver dysfunction and administered in reduced amounts.

Myocardial Infarction: As with all potent analgesics, NUBAIN should be used with caution in patients with myocardial infarction who have nausea or vomiting.

Biliary Tract Surgery: As with all opioid analgesics, NUBAIN should be used with caution in patients about to undergo surgery of the biliary tract since it may cause spasm of the sphincter of Oddi.

Cardiovascular System: During evaluation of NUBAIN in anesthesia, a higher incidence of bradycardia has been reported in patients who did not receive atropine pre-operatively.

Information for Patients

Patients should be advised of the following information:

— NUBAIN is associated with sedation and may impair mental and physical abilities required for the performance of potentially dangerous tasks such as driving a car or operating machinery.
— NUBAIN is to be used as prescribed by a physician. Dose or frequency should not be increased without first consulting with a physician since NUBAIN may cause psychological or physical dependence.
— The use of NUBAIN with other opioids can cause signs and symptoms of withdrawal.
— Abrupt discontinuation of NUBAIN after prolonged usage may cause signs and symptoms of withdrawal.

Laboratory Tests

NUBAIN may interfere with enzymatic methods for the detection of opioids depending on the specificity/sensitivity of the test. Consult the test manufacturer for specific details.

Carcinogenesis, Mutagenesis, Impairment of Fertility

Carcinogenesis

Long term carcinogenicity studies were performed in rats (24 months) and mice (19 months) by oral administration at doses up to 200 mg/kg (1180 mg/m^2) and 200 mg/kg (600 mg/m^2) per day, respectively. There was no evidence of an increase in tumors in either species related to NUBAIN administration. The maximum recommended human dose (MRHD) in a day is 160 mg subcutaneously, intramuscularly or intravenously, or approximately 100 mg/m^2/day for a 60 kg subject.

Mutagenesis

NUBAIN did not have mutagenic activity in the AMES test with four bacterial strains, in the Chinese Hamster Ovary HGPRT assays or in the Sister Chromatids Exchange Assay. However, NUBAIN induced an increased frequency of mutation in the mouse lymphoma assay. Clastogenic activity was not observed in the mouse micronucleus test of the cytogenicity bone marrow assay in rats.

Impairment of Fertility

A reproduction study was performed in male and female rats at subcutaneous doses up to 56 mg/kg/day or 330 mg/m^2/day. NUBAIN did not affect either male or female fertility rats.

Usage in Pregnancy

Teratogenic Effects: Pregnancy Category B: Reproduction studies have been performed in rats by subcutaneous administration of nalbuphine up to 100 mg/kg/day, or 590 mg/m^2/day which is approximately 6 times the MRHD, and in rabbits by intravenous administration of nalbuphine up to 32 mg/kg/day, or 378 mg/m^2/day which is approximately 4 times the MRHD. The results did not reveal evidence of developmental toxicity, including teratogenicity, or harm to the fetus. There are, however, no adequate and well-controlled studies in pregnant women. Because animal reproduction studies are not always predictive of human response, this drug should be used during pregnancy only if clearly needed.

Non-teratogenic Effects: Neonatal body weight and survival rates were reduced at birth and during lactation when nalbuphine was subcutaneously administered to female and male rats prior to mating and throughout gestation and lactation or to pregnant rats during the last third of gestation and throughout lactation at doses approximately 4 times the maximum recommended human dose.

Use During Labor and Delivery

See **WARNINGS**.

Nursing Mothers

Limited data suggest that NUBAIN is excreted in maternal milk but only in a small amount (less than 1% of the administered dose) and with a clinically insignificant effect. Caution should be exercised when NUBAIN is administered to a nursing woman.

Pediatric Use

Safety and effectiveness in pediatric patients below the age of 18 years have not been established.

ADVERSE REACTIONS

The most frequent adverse reaction in 1066 patients treated in clinical studies with NUBAIN was sedation 381 (36%).

Less frequent reactions were: sweaty/clammy 99 (9%), nausea/vomiting 68 (6%), dizziness/vertigo 58 (5%), dry mouth 44 (4%), and headache 27 (3%).

Other adverse reactions which occurred (reported incidence of 1% or less) were:

CNS Effects: Nervousness, depression, restlessness, crying, euphoria, floating, hostility, unusual dreams, confusion, faintness, hallucinations, dysphoria, feeling of heaviness, numbness, tingling, unreality. The incidence of psychotomimetic effects, such as unreality, depersonalization, delusions, dysphoria and hallucinations has been shown to be less than that which occurs with pentazocine.

Cardiovascular: Hypertension, hypotension, bradycardia, tachycardia.

Gastrointestinal: Cramps, dyspepsia, bitter taste.

Respiratory: Depression, dyspnea, asthma.

Dermatologic: Itching, burning, urticaria.

Miscellaneous: Speech difficulty, urinary urgency, blurred vision, flushing and warmth.

Allergic Reactions: Anaphylactic/anaphylactoid and other serious hypersensitivity reactions have been reported following the use of nalbuphine and may require immediate, supportive medical treatment. These reactions may include shock, respiratory distress, respiratory arrest, bradycardia, cardiac arrest, hypotension, or laryngeal edema. Other allergic-type reactions reported include stridor, bronchospasm, wheezing, edema, rash, pruritus, nausea, vomiting, diaphoresis, weakness, and shakiness.

Post-marketing: Other reports include pulmonary edema, agitation, seizures, and injection site reactions such as pain, swelling, redness, burning, and hot sensations.

DRUG ABUSE AND DEPENDENCE

There have been reports of abuse and dependence associated with NUBAIN among health care providers, patients and bodybuilders. There have been reported instances of psychological and physical dependence and tolerance in patients abusing NUBAIN. Individuals with a prior history of opioid or other substance abuse or dependence may be at greater risk in responding to reinforcing properties of NUBAIN.

Abrupt discontinuation of NUBAIN following prolonged use has been followed by symptoms of opioid withdrawal, i.e., abdominal cramps, nausea and vomiting, rhinorrhea, lacrimation, restlessness, anxiety, elevated temperature and piloerection.

OVERDOSAGE

The immediate intravenous administration of an opiate antagonist such as naloxone or nalmefene is a specific antidote. Oxygen, intravenous fluids, vasopressors and other supportive measures should be used as indicated.

The administration of single doses of 72 mg of NUBAIN subcutaneously to eight normal subjects has been reported to have resulted primarily in symptoms of sleepiness and mild dysphoria.

DOSAGE AND ADMINISTRATION

The usual recommended adult dose is 10 mg for a 70 kg individual, administered subcutaneously, intramuscularly or intravenously; this dose may be repeated every 3 to 6 hours as necessary. Dosage should be adjusted according to the severity of the pain, physical status of the patient, and other medications which the patient may be receiving. (See **Interaction with Other Central Nervous System Depressants** under **WARNINGS**). In non-tolerant individuals, the recommended single maximum dose is 20 mg, with a maximum total daily dose of 160 mg.

The use of NUBAIN as a supplement to balanced anesthesia requires larger doses than those recommended for analgesia. Induction doses of NUBAIN range from 0.3 mg/kg to 3 mg/kg intravenously to be administered over a 10 to 15 minute period with maintenance doses of 0.25 to 0.5 mg/kg in single intravenous administrations as required. The use of NUBAIN may be followed by respiratory depression which can be reversed with the opioid antagonist NARCAN® (naloxone hydrochloride).

NUBAIN is physically incompatible with nafcillin and keterolac.

Patients Dependent on Opioids

Patients who have been taking opioids chronically may experience withdrawal symptoms upon the administration of NUBAIN. If unduly troublesome, opioid withdrawal symptoms can be controlled by the slow intravenous administration of small increments of morphine, until relief occurs. If the previous analgesic was morphine, meperidine, codeine, or other opioid with similar duration of activity, one-fourth of the anticipated dose of NUBAIN can be administered initially and the patient observed for signs of withdrawal, i.e., abdominal cramps, nausea and vomiting, lacrimation, rhinorrhea, anxiety, restlessness, elevation of temperature or piloerection. If untoward symptoms do not occur, progressively larger doses may be tried at appropriate intervals until the desired level of analgesia is obtained with NUBAIN.

Parenteral drug products should be inspected visually for particulate matter and discoloration prior to administration whenever solution and container permit.

HOW SUPPLIED

NUBAIN® (nalbuphine hydrochloride) injection for intramuscular, subcutaneous, or intravenous use is a sterile solution available in:

NDC 63481-508-05	(sulfite-free) 10 mg/mL, 10 mL multiple dose vials (box of 1)
NDC 63481-432-10	(sulfite/paraben-free) 10 mg/mL, 1 mL ampuls (box of 10)
NDC 63481-509-05	(sulfite-free) 20 mg/mL, 10 mL multiple dose vials (box of 1)
NDC 63481-433-10	(sulfite/paraben-free) 20 mg/mL, 1 mL ampuls (box of 10)

Store at 25°C (77°F); excursions permitted to 15°-30°C (59°-86°F). [See USP Controlled Room Temperature]. Protect from excessive light. Store in carton until contents have been used.

Manufactured for:
Endo Pharmaceuticals Inc.
Chadds Ford, Pennsylvania 19317
Manufactured by:
Bristol-Myers Squibb Holdings Pharma, Ltd.
Manati, Puerto Rico 00674 USA
NUBAIN® is a Registered Trademark of Endo Pharmaceuticals Inc.
NARCAN® is a Registered Trademark of Endo Pharmaceuticals Inc.

51-022542-00/May, 2003

NUMORPHAN® Ⓒ℞

[*nū-mor 'fan*]

(Oxymorphone Hydrochloride Injection, USP)
(Oxymorphone Hydrochloride Suppositories, USP)
Opioid Analgesic

DESCRIPTION

NUMORPHAN (oxymorphone hydrochloride, USP), a semi-synthetic opioid substitute for morphine, is a potent analgesic.

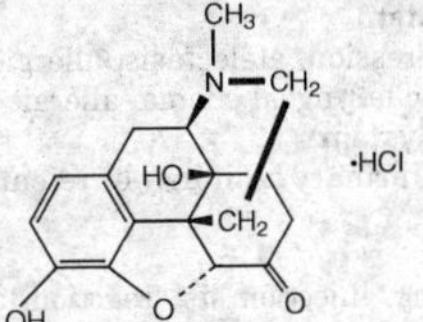

4,5α -Epoxy-3, 14-dihydroxy-17-methylmorphinan-6-one hydrochloride

Oxymorphone hydrochloride is a white or slightly off-white, odorless powder, which is sparingly soluble in alcohol and ether, but freely soluble in water. The molecular weight of oxymorphone hydrochloride is 337.80. The pK_{a1} and pK_{a2} of oxymorphone at 37°C are 8.17 and 9.54, respectively. The octanol/aqueous partition coefficient at 37°C and pH 7.4 is 0.98.

NUMORPHAN Injection is available in two concentrations, 1 mg/mL, 1 mL ampul and 1.5 mg/mL, 10 mL vial of oxymorphone hydrochloride. In addition, each 1 mg/mL ampul contains 8.0 mg/mL sodium chloride. Each 1.5 mg/mL vial contains 8.0 mg/mL sodium chloride, 1.8 mg/mL methylparaben and 0.2 mg/mL propylparaben. pH for both the ampul and vial is adjusted with hydrochloric acid.

The NUMORPHAN Rectal Suppository is available in a concentration of 5 mg of oxymorphone hydrochloride in a base consisting of polyethylene glycol 1000 and polyethylene glycol 3350.

CLINICAL PHARMACOLOGY

NUMORPHAN is a potent opioid analgesic. Administered parenterally, 1 mg of NUMORPHAN is approximately equivalent in analgesic activity to 10 mg of morphine sulfate.

Many of the effects described below are common to the class of opioid analgesics, including NUMORPHAN.

Central Nervous System (CNS)

Opioid analgesics exert their principal pharmacologic effects on the CNS and the gastrointestinal tract. The principal actions of therapeutic value are analgesia and sedation. The precise mechanism of the analgesic action is unknown. However, specific CNS opiate receptors have been identified and likely play a role in the expression of analgesic effects. Opioids produce respiratory depression by direct action on brain stem respiratory centers. The mechanism of respiratory depression involves a reduction in the responsiveness of the brain stem respiratory centers to increases in carbon dioxide tension and to electrical stimulation. Opioids depress the cough reflex by direct action on the cough center in the medulla. Opioids cause miosis. Pinpoint pupils are a common sign of opioid overdose but are not pathognomonic. Marked mydriasis may be seen with worsening hypoxia.

Gastrointestinal Tract and Other Smooth Muscle

Opioids decrease gastric, biliary, and pancreatic secretions. These drugs cause a reduction in motility associated with an increase in tone in the antrum of the stomach and duodenum. Digestion of food in the small intestine is delayed and propulsive contractions are decreased. Propulsive peristaltic waves in the colon are decreased while tone is increased to the point of spasm. The end result is constipation. Opioids can cause a marked increase in biliary tract pressure as a result of spasm of the sphincter of Oddi.

Opioids increase smooth muscle tone in the urinary tract and can induce spasms. Urinary urgency and difficulty with urination may result. These effects, in conjunction with the central effect of these drugs on release of vasopressin, may produce oliguria.

Pharmacokinetics

The onset of action of parenterally administered NUMORPHAN is rapid; initial effects are usually perceived within 5 to 10 minutes. Its duration of action is approximately 3 to 6 hours.

Distribution: After an IV dose, the steady state volume of distribution was 3.08 ± 1.14 L/kg in healthy male and female subjects.

Metabolism: Oxymorphone undergoes extensive hepatic metabolism in humans. After a 10 mg oral dose, 49% was excreted over a five-day period in the urine. Of this, 82% was excreted in the first 24 hours after administration. The recovered drug-related products contained the oxymorphone (1.9%), the conjugate of oxymorphone (44.1%), the 6β-carbinol produced by 6-keto reduction of oxymorphone (0.3%), and the conjugates of 6β-carbinol (2.6%) and 6α-carbinol (0.1%).

Elimination: In healthy subjects, the mean terminal half-life of oxymorphone was 1.3 ± 0.7 hours. The mean systemic clearance was 2.0 ± 0.5 L/min.

INDICATIONS AND USAGE

NUMORPHAN Suppository is indicated for the relief of moderate to severe pain.

NUMORPHAN Injection is indicated for the relief of moderate to severe pain. It is also indicated for preoperative medication, for support of anesthesia, for obstetrical analgesia, and for relief of anxiety in patients with dyspnea associated with pulmonary edema secondary to acute left ventricular dysfunction.

CONTRAINDICATIONS

NUMORPHAN should not be administered to patients who are hypersensitive to oxymorphone hydrochloride or to any of the other ingredients in NUMORPHAN, or hypersensitive to morphine analogs.

NUMORPHAN should not be administered to individuals during an acute asthmatic attack or to patients with severe respiratory depression, upper airway obstruction, or any patient who has or is suspected of having a paralytic ileus. NUMORPHAN should not be used in the treatment of pulmonary edema secondary to a chemical respiratory irritant. Opioid analgesics cause pooling of blood in the extremities by decreasing peripheral vascular resistance. This effect results in decreases in venous return, cardiac work, and pulmonary venous pressure, and blood is shifted from the central to peripheral circulation which would not be beneficial in the treatment of pulmonary edema secondary to a chemical respiratory irritant.

WARNINGS

Interactions with Other Central Nervous System Depressants

Patients receiving other opioid analgesics, general anesthetics, phenothiazines, other tranquilizers, sedatives, hypnotics or other CNS depressants (including alcohol) concomitantly with NUMORPHAN may exhibit an additive CNS depression (See **PRECAUTIONS**; **Drug Interactions**).

Respiratory Depression

NUMORPHAN should be administered with extreme caution to patients with conditions accompanied by hypoxia, hypercapnia or decreased respiratory reserve such as: asthma, chronic obstructive pulmonary disease or cor pulmonale, severe obesity, sleep apnea syndrome, myxedema, kyphoscoliosis, CNS depression or coma.

Head Injury and Increased Intracranial Pressure

The possible respiratory depressant effects of potent analgesics and their potential to elevate cerebrospinal fluid pressure (resulting from vasodilation following CO_2 retention) may be markedly exaggerated in the presence of head injury, intracranial lesions or a preexisting increase in intracranial pressure. Furthermore, potent analgesics can produce effects which may obscure the clinical course of patients with head injuries. Therefore, NUMORPHAN should be used in these circumstances only when essential, and then should be administered with extreme caution.

Acute Abdominal Conditions

The administration of opioids may obscure the diagnosis or clinical course of patients with acute abdominal conditions.

Drug Dependence

NUMORPHAN, as with other opioid drugs, can produce tolerance, psychological dependence, and physical dependence and has the potential for being abused (See **DRUG ABUSE AND DEPENDENCE**).

Pregnancy

Safe use in pregnancy has not been established (relative to possible adverse effects on fetal development). As with other analgesics, the use of NUMORPHAN in pregnancy, in nursing mothers, or in women of child-bearing potential requires that the possible benefits of the drug be weighed against the possible hazards to the mother and the child (See **PRECAUTIONS**).

PRECAUTIONS

General

Special Risk Patients: NUMORPHAN should be used with caution in elderly and debilitated patients and in patients who are known to be sensitive to central nervous system depressants, such as those with cardiovascular, pulmonary, renal or hepatic disease. Caution should also be exercised in patients with hypothyroidism, acute alcoholism, delirium tremens, convulsive disorders, Addison's disease, gallbladder disease or gallstones, prostatic hypertrophy or urethral stricture, recent gastrointestinal or genitourinary tract surgery, inflammatory bowel disease, diarrhea secondary to poisoning until the toxin is eliminated, diarrhea secondary to pseudomembranous colitis, cardiac arrhythmias, increased ocular pressure, and toxic psychosis. Debilitated and elderly patients and those with severe liver disease should receive smaller doses of NUMORPHAN.

Hypotensive Effect: Opioid analgesics may cause severe hypotension in patients whose ability to maintain blood pressure has been compromised by a depleted blood volume or coadministration of drugs such as phenothiazines or general anesthetics. Administer with caution to patients in circulatory shock, since vasodilatation produced by the drug may further reduce cardiac output and blood pressure. Orthostatic hypotension may occur in ambulatory patients.

Information for Patients

Patients should be cautioned regarding the following:

Drowsiness, dizziness, or lightheadedness related to the use of this medication may impair mental and/or physical abilities required for the performance of potentially hazardous tasks, such as driving a car, operating machinery, etc.

This medication, like other opioid analgesics, will add to the effect of alcohol and other CNS depressants [such as antihistamines, sedatives, hypnotics, tranquilizers, general anesthetics, phenothiazines, other opioids, tricyclic antidepressants, and monoamine oxidase (MAO) inhibitors]. Alcohol should not be consumed while taking NUMORPHAN.

Withdrawal side effects may be precipitated by suddenly stopping this drug after prolonged use (regular use for several weeks or more). The medication should be gradually reduced before completely discontinuing use.

Elderly patients are more sensitive to opioid analgesics, especially the respiratory depressant effects and opioid induced urinary retention. Lower doses or longer dosing intervals may be required.

Continued on next page

Numorphan —Cont.

Orthostatic hypotension may occur with the use of this medication, especially in ambulatory patients. Patients should get up slowly from a lying or sitting position.
NUMORPHAN may be habit forming and has the potential for being abused. Tolerance, psychological and physical dependence can occur.
Safe use in pregnancy has not been established. Prolonged use of opioid analgesics during pregnancy may cause fetal-neonatal physical dependence, and neonatal withdrawal may occur.

Laboratory Tests
Opioids may increase biliary tract pressure with resultant increases in plasma amylase or lipase.

Drug Interactions
The concomitant use of other CNS depressants including sedatives, hypnotics, tranquilizers, general anesthetics, phenothiazines, other opioids, tricyclic antidepressants, monoamine oxidase (MAO) inhibitors, and alcohol may produce additive CNS depressant effects. When such combined therapy is contemplated, the dose of one or both agents should be reduced (See **WARNINGS**).
Anticholinergics or other medications with anticholinergic activity when used concurrently with opioid analgesics may result in increased risk of urinary retention and/or severe constipation, which may lead to paralytic ileus.
It has been reported that the incidence of bradycardia was increased when oxymorphone was combined with propofol for induction of anesthesia.
In addition, CNS toxicity has been reported (confusion, disorientation, respiratory depression, apnea, seizures) following coadministration of cimetidine with opioid analgesics; no clear-cut cause and effect relationship was established.

Carcinogenesis, Mutagenesis, Impairment of Fertility
Long-term studies have not been performed in animals to evaluate the carcinogenic potential of NUMORPHAN (oxymorphone hydrochloride, USP). Studies to evaluate the mutagenic potential of NUMORPHAN have not been conducted. There have been no studies to evaluate the effect of NUMORPHAN on fertility.

Usage in Pregnancy
Teratogenic Effects: Pregnancy Category C: NUMORPHAN was reported to produce malformations in offspring of hamsters that received 1,500 times the recommended dose on Day 8 of gestation. There have been no adequate and well-controlled studies of reproductive toxicity in other laboratory animals or in pregnant women. It is not known whether NUMORPHAN can cause fetal harm when administered to a pregnant woman or can affect reproductive capacity. As with other opioid analgesics, the use of NUMORPHAN in pregnancy or in women of child-bearing potential requires that the possible benefits of the drug be weighed against the possible hazards to the mother and the child.
Non-teratogenic Effects: Prolonged use of opioid analgesics during pregnancy may cause fetal-neonatal physical dependence. Neonatal withdrawal may occur. Symptoms usually appear during the first days of life and may include convulsions, irritability, excessive crying, tremors, hyperactive reflexes, fever, vomiting, diarrhea, sneezing, yawning, and increased respiratory rate.

Labor and Delivery
NUMORPHAN should be used with caution during labor. Sinusoidal fetal heart rate patterns may occur with the use of opioid analgesics.
Opioid analgesics in therapeutic doses may prolong labor. Generally, the effect of opioids on the pregnant uterus appears to depend on the time of administration; administration of the drugs during the latent phase of the first stage of labor, or before cervical dilation of 4–5 cm has occurred, may hamper the progress of labor.
Opioid analgesics, including NUMORPHAN, may cause respiratory depression in the newborn. The effect of NUMORPHAN, if any, on the later growth, development, and functional maturation of the child is unknown.

Nursing Mothers
It is not known whether NUMORPHAN is excreted in human milk. Because many drugs, including some opioids, are excreted in human milk, caution should be exercised when NUMORPHAN is administered to a nursing woman.

Pediatric Use
Safety and effectiveness of NUMORPHAN in pediatric patients below the age of 18 years have not been established.

ADVERSE REACTIONS

As with all potent opioid analgesics, possible side effects when using NUMORPHAN include:

Central Nervous System
Drowsiness, sedation, lightheadedness, unusual tiredness or weakness, headache, dysphoria, euphoria, miosis, diplopia, blurred vision, nervousness, restlessness, confusion, mental clouding, trouble sleeping, paradoxical CNS stimulation, hallucinations, mental depression.

Gastrointestinal System
Nausea, vomiting, dry mouth, constipation, biliary tract spasm, cramps or pain, loss of appetite, paralytic ileus or toxic megacolon in patients with inflammatory bowel disease.

Cardiovascular System
Hypotension, orthostatic hypotension particularly in ambulatory patients, tachycardia, bradycardia, palpitations, flushing.

Respiratory System
Respiratory depression, atelectasis, allergic bronchospastic reaction, allergic laryngeal edema, allergic laryngospasm.

Genitourinary System
Ureteral spasm, urinary hesitancy or retention, antidiuretic effect.

Dermatologic
Itching, sweating, injection site reaction, allergic reaction (such as skin rash, hives, and/or itching, swelling of the face).

DRUG ABUSE AND DEPENDENCE

NUMORPHAN is a Schedule II opioid and is subject to the Federal Controlled Substances Act.
NUMORPHAN, as with other opioid drugs, can produce tolerance, psychological dependence, and physical dependence and has the potential for being abused. The addiction potential of the drug appears to be about the same as for morphine.
Withdrawal symptoms may occur when opioids are abruptly discontinued after prolonged use. Withdrawal symptoms may be characterized by some or all of the following: restlessness, lacrimation, rhinorrhea, yawning, perspiration, gooseflesh, restless sleep, and mydriasis during the first 24 hours. These symptoms often increase in severity and over the next 72 hours may be accompanied by increasing irritability, anxiety, weakness, twitching, and spasms of muscles; kicking movements; severe backaches; abdominal and leg pains; abdominal and muscle cramps; hot and cold flashes; insomnia; nausea, anorexia, vomiting, intestinal spasm, diarrhea, coryza, and repetitive sneezing; increase in body temperature, blood pressure, respiratory rate and heart rate. Because of excessive loss of fluids through sweating, vomiting and diarrhea, there is usually marked weight loss, dehydration, ketosis, and disturbances in acid-base balance. Cardiovascular collapse can occur. Without treatment most observable symptoms disappear in 5–14 days; however, there appears to be a phase of secondary or chronic abstinence which may last for 2–6 months characterized by decreasing insomnia, irritability, and muscular aches. In addition, the patient may have miosis and a slight lowering of blood pressure, pulse rate, and body temperature; respiratory centers exhibit a decreased response to the stimulatory effects of carbon dioxide.
The dose of NUMORPHAN should be gradually reduced before discontinuation in those patients who require treatment for physical dependence.
Infants born to mothers physically dependent on opioids will also be physically dependent and may exhibit respiratory difficulties and withdrawal symptoms (See **PRECAUTIONS; Usage in Pregnancy**).

OVERDOSAGE

Signs and Symptons
Serious overdosage with NUMORPHAN is characterized by respiratory depression, (a decrease in respiratory rate and/or tidal volume, Cheyne-Stokes respiration, cyanosis), extreme somnolence progressing to stupor or coma, skeletal muscle flaccidity, cold and clammy skin, and sometimes bradycardia and hypotension. In severe overdosage, apnea, circulatory collapse, cardiac arrest and death may occur.

Treatment
Primary attention should be given to the reestablishment of adequate respiratory exchange through provision of a patent airway and the institution of assisted or controlled ventilation. The opioid antagonist naloxone hydrochloride (NARCAN®) is a specific antidote against respiratory depression which may result from overdosage or unusual sensitivity to opioids including oxymorphone. Therefore, an appropriate dose of naloxone hydrochloride should be administered (usual initial adult dose 0.4 mg–2 mg) preferably by the intravenous route and simultaneously with efforts at respiratory resuscitation. Since the duration of action of oxymorphone may exceed that of the antagonist, the patient should be kept under continued surveillance and repeated doses of the antagonist should be administered as needed to maintain adequate respiration.
Naloxone hydrochloride should not be administered in the absence of clinically significant respiratory or cardiovascular depression. In addition, it should be considered that the use of an opioid antagonist in patients physically dependent on opioids may precipitate an acute withdrawal syndrome that cannot be readily suppressed while the action of the antagonist persists. If respiratory depression is associated with muscular rigidity, administration of a neuromuscular blocking agent may be necessary to facilitate assisted or controlled ventilation. Muscular rigidity may also respond to opioid antagonist therapy.
Oxygen, intravenous fluids, vasopressors and other supportive measures should be employed as indicated.

DOSAGE AND ADMINISTRATION

Smaller doses of NUMORPHAN than those recommended below should be used for debilitated and elderly patients and those with severe liver disease.

Usual Adult Dosage of NUMORPHAN Injection
Subcutaneous or intramuscular administration: initially 1 mg to 1.5 mg, repeated every 4 to 6 hours as needed. Intravenous: 0.5 mg initially. In nondebilitated patients the dose can be cautiously increased until satisfactory pain relief is obtained. For analgesia during labor 0.5 mg to 1 mg intramuscularly is recommended.
Parenteral drug products should be inspected visually for particulate matter and discoloration prior to administration whenever solution and container permit.

Usual Adult Dosage of NUMORPHAN Rectal Suppositories
One suppository, 5 mg, every 4 to 6 hours. In nondebilitated patients the dose can be cautiously increased until satisfactory pain relief is obtained.

HOW SUPPLIED

For Injection
DEA Order Form Required
1 mg/mL 1 mL ampuls (paraben/sodium dithionite-free) (box of 10) NDC 63481-444-10
1.5 mg/mL 10 mL multiple dose vials (sodium dithionite-free) (box of 1) NDC 63481-445-01
Store at 25°C (77°F); excursions permitted to 15°–30°C (59°–86°F). [See USP Controlled Room Temperature].
Protect from light.

For Rectal Suppositories
DEA Order Form Required
5 mg Wrapped in gold foil (box of 6) NDC 63481-761-06
Store under refrigeration 2°–8°C (36°–46°F).

NUMORPHAN® is a Registered Trademark of Endo Pharmaceuticals Inc.
NARCAN® is a Registered Trademark of Endo Pharmaceuticals Inc.

6477-02/January, 2002

PERCOCET® Ⓒ ℞

[*perk' ō-sĕt*]
(Oxycodone and Acetaminophen Tablets, USP)
℞ only

DESCRIPTION

Each tablet, for oral administration, contains oxycodone hydrochloride and acetaminophen in the following strengths:

Oxycodone Hydrochloride 2.5 mg
Acetaminophen, USP 325 mg
2.5 mg oxycodone HCl is equivalent to 2.2409 mg of oxycodone.

Oxycodone Hydrochloride 5 mg
Acetaminophen, USP 325 mg
5 mg oxycodone HCl is equivalent to 4.4815 mg of oxycodone.

Oxycodone Hydrochloride 7.5 mg
Acetaminophen, USP 325 mg
7.5 mg oxycodone HCl is equivalent to 6.7228 mg of oxycodone.

Oxycodone Hydrochloride 7.5 mg
Acetaminophen, USP 500 mg
7.5 mg oxycodone HCl is equivalent to 6.7228 mg of oxycodone.

Oxycodone Hydrochloride 10 mg
Acetaminophen, USP 325 mg
10 mg oxycodone HCl is equivalent to 8.9637 mg of oxycodone.

Oxycodone Hydrochloride 10 mg
Acetaminophen, USP 650 mg
10 mg oxycodone HCl is equivalent to 8.9637 mg of oxycodone.

All strengths of PERCOCET also contain the following inactive ingredients: Colloidal silicon dioxide, croscarmellose sodium, crospovidone, microcrystalline cellulose, povidone, pregelatinized starch, and stearic acid. In addition, the 2.5 mg/325 mg strength contains FD&C Red No. 40 Aluminum Lake and the 5 mg/325 mg strength contains FD&C Blue No. 1 Aluminum Lake. The 7.5 mg/325 mg strength and the 7.5 mg/500 mg strength contains FD&C Yellow No. 6 Aluminum Lake. The 10 mg/325 mg strength and the 10 mg/650 mg strength contains D&C Yellow No. 10 Aluminum Lake.
Acetaminophen, 4′-hydroxyacetanilide, is a non-opiate, non-salicylate analgesic and antipyretic which occurs as a white, odorless, crystalline powder, possessing a slightly bitter taste. The molecular formula for acetaminophen is $C_8H_9NO_2$ and the molecular weight is 151.17. It may be represented by the following structural formula:

CH_3CONH— —OH

Oxycodone, 14-hydroxydihydrocodeinone, is a semisynthetic pure opioid agonist which occurs as a white, odorless, crystalline powder having a saline, bitter taste. The molecular formula for oxycodone hydrochloride is $C_{18}H_{21}NO_4$•HCl and the molecular weight 351.83. It is derived from the opium alkaloid thebaine, and may be represented by the following structural formula:

CH_3 N HO CH_3O O O

CLINICAL PHARMACOLOGY

The principal ingredient, oxycodone, is a semisynthetic opioid analgesic with multiple actions qualitatively similar to those of morphine; the most prominent involves the central nervous system and organs composed of smooth muscle. The principal actions of therapeutic value of the oxycodone in PERCOCET are analgesia and sedation.

Oxycodone is similar to codeine and methadone in that it retains at least one-half of its analgesic activity when administered orally.

Acetaminophen is a non-opiate, non-salicylate analgesic and antipyretic.

INDICATIONS AND USAGE

PERCOCET is indicated for the relief of moderate to moderately severe pain.

CONTRAINDICATIONS

PERCOCET should not be administered to patients who are hypersensitive to oxycodone, acetaminophen, or any other components of this product.

WARNINGS

Drug Dependence

Oxycodone can produce drug dependence of the morphine type and, therefore, has the potential for being abused. Psychic dependence, physical dependence and tolerance may develop upon repeated administration of PERCOCET, and it should be prescribed and administered with the same degree of caution appropriate to the use of other oral opioid-containing medications. Like other opioid-containing medications, PERCOCET is subject to the Federal Controlled Substances Act (Schedule II).

PRECAUTIONS

General

Head Injury and Increased Intracranial Pressure: The respiratory depressant effects of opioids and their capacity to elevate cerebrospinal fluid pressure may be markedly exaggerated in the presence of head injury, other intracranial lesions or a pre-existing increase in intracranial pressure. Furthermore, opioids produce adverse reactions which may obscure the clinical course of patients with head injuries.

Acute Abdominal Conditions: The administration of PERCOCET (Oxycodone and Acetaminophen Tablets, USP) or other opioids may obscure the diagnosis or clinical course in patients with acute abdominal conditions.

Special Risk Patients: PERCOCET should be given with caution to certain patients such as the elderly or debilitated, and those with severe impairment of hepatic or renal function, hypothyroidism, Addison's disease, and prostatic hypertrophy or urethral stricture.

Information for Patients

Oxycodone may impair the mental and/or physical abilities required for the performance of potentially hazardous tasks such as driving a car or operating machinery. The patient using PERCOCET should be cautioned accordingly.

Drug Interactions

Patients receiving other opioid analgesics, general anesthetics, phenothiazines, other tranquilizers, sedative-hypnotics or other CNS depressants (including alcohol) concomitantly with PERCOCET may exhibit an additive CNS depression. When such combined therapy is contemplated, the dose of one or both agents should be reduced.

The concurrent use of anticholinergics with opioids may produce paralytic ileus.

Usage in Pregnancy

Teratogenic Effects; Pregnancy Category C: Animal reproductive studies have not been conducted with PERCOCET. It is also not known whether PERCOCET can cause fetal harm when administered to a pregnant woman or can affect reproductive capacity. PERCOCET should not be given to a pregnant woman unless in the judgment of the physician, the potential benefits outweigh the possible hazards.

Nonteratogenic Effects: Use of opioids during pregnancy may produce physical dependence in the neonate.

Labor and Delivery: As with all opioids, administration of PERCOCET to the mother shortly before delivery may result in some degree of respiratory depression in the newborn and the mother, especially if higher doses are used.

Nursing Mothers

It is not known whether PERCOCET is excreted in human milk. Because many drugs are excreted in human milk, caution should be exercised when PERCOCET is administered to a nursing woman.

Pediatric Use

Safety and effectiveness in pediatric patients have not been established.

ADVERSE REACTIONS

The most frequently observed adverse reactions include lightheadedness, dizziness, sedation, nausea and vomiting. These effects seem to be more prominent in ambulatory than in nonambulatory patients, and some of these adverse reactions may be alleviated if the patient lies down.

Other adverse reactions include euphoria, dysphoria, constipation, skin rash and pruritus. At higher doses, oxycodone has most of the disadvantages of morphine including respiratory depression.

DRUG ABUSE AND DEPENDENCE

PERCOCET (Oxycodone and Acetaminophen Tablets, USP) is a Schedule II controlled substance.

Oxycodone can produce drug dependence and has the potential for being abused (See WARNINGS).

2.5 mg/325 mg Pink oval tablet embossed with "PERCOCET" on one side and "2.5" on the other.	Bottles of 100 Bottles of 500 Unit dose package of 100 tablets	NDC 63481-627-70 NDC 63481-627-85 NDC 63481-627-75
5 mg/325 mg Blue, round, tablet, embossed with "PERCOCET" and "5" on one side and bisect on the other.	Bottles of 100 Bottles of 500 Unit dose package of 100 tablets	NDC 63481-623-70 NDC 63481-623-85 NDC 63481-623-75
7.5 mg/325 mg Peach oval-shaped tablet embossed with "PERCOCET" on one side and "7.5/325" on the other.	Bottles of 100 Bottles of 500 Unit dose package of 100 tablets	NDC 63481-628-70 NDC 63481-628-85 NDC 63481-628-75
7.5 mg/500 mg Peach capsule-shaped tablet embossed with "PERCOCET" on one side and "7.5" on the other.	Bottles of 100	NDC 63481-621-70
10 mg/325 mg Yellow capsule-shaped tablet embossed with "PERCOCET" on one side and "10/325" on the other.	Bottles of 100 Bottles of 500 Unit dose package of 100 tablets	NDC 63481-629-70 NDC 63481-629-85 NDC 63481-629-85
10 mg/650 mg Yellow oval tablet embossed with "PERCOCET" on one side and "10" on the other.	Bottles of 100	NDC 63481-622-70

OVERDOSAGE

Acetaminophen

Signs and Symptoms: In acute acetaminophen overdosage, dose-dependent, potentially fatal hepatic necrosis is the most serious adverse effect. Renal tubular necrosis, hypoglycemic coma and thrombocytopenia may also occur.

In adults, hepatic toxicity has rarely been reported with acute overdoses of less than 10 grams and fatalities with less than 15 grams. Importantly, young children seem to be more resistant than adults to the hepatotoxic effect of an acetaminophen overdose. Despite this, the measures outlined below should be initiated in any adult or child suspected of having ingested an acetaminophen overdose.

Early symptoms following a potentially hepatotoxic overdose may include: nausea, vomiting, diaphoresis and general malaise. Clinical and laboratory evidence of hepatic toxicity may not be apparent until 48 to 72 hours post-ingestion.

Treatment: The stomach should be emptied promptly by lavage or by induction of emesis with syrup of ipecac. Patient's estimates of the quantity of a drug ingested are notoriously unreliable. Therefore, if an acetaminophen overdose is suspected, a serum acetaminophen assay should be obtained as early as possible, but no sooner than four hours following ingestion. Liver function studies should be obtained initially and repeated at 24-hour intervals.

The antidote, N-acetylcysteine, should be administered as early as possible, preferably within 16 hours of the overdose ingestion for optimal results, but in any case, within 24 hours. Following recovery, there are no residual, structural, or functional hepatic abnormalities.

Oxycodone

Signs and Symptoms: Serious overdosage with oxycodone is characterized by respiratory depression (a decrease in respiratory rate and/or tidal volume, Cheyne-Stokes respiration, cyanosis), extreme somnolence progressing to stupor or coma, skeletal muscle flaccidity, cold and clammy skin, and sometimes bradycardia and hypotension. In severe overdosage, apnea, circulatory collapse, cardiac arrest and death may occur.

Treatment: Primary attention should be given to the reestablishment of adequate respiratory exchange through provision of a patent airway and the institution of assisted or controlled ventilation. The opioid antagonist naloxone hydrochloride is a specific antidote against respiratory depression which may result from overdosage or unusual sensitivity to opioids, including oxycodone. Therefore, an appropriate dose of naloxone hydrochloride (usual initial adult dose 0.4 mg to 2 mg) should be administered preferably by the intravenous route, and simultaneously with efforts at respiratory resuscitation (see package insert). Since the duration of action of oxycodone may exceed that of the antagonist, the patient should be kept under continued surveillance and repeated doses of the antagonist should be administered as needed to maintain adequate respiration.

An antagonist should not be administered in the absence of clinically significant respiratory or cardiovascular depression. Oxygen, intravenous fluids, vasopressors and other supportive measures should be employed as indicated.

Gastric emptying may be useful in removing unabsorbed drug.

DOSAGE AND ADMINISTRATION

Dosage should be adjusted according to the severity of the pain and the response of the patient. It may occasionally be necessary to exceed the usual dosage recommended below in cases of more severe pain or in those patients who have become tolerant to the analgesic effect of opioids. PERCOCET (Oxycodone and Acetaminophen Tablets, USP) is given orally.

Percocet 2.5 mg/325 mg

The usual adult dosage is one or two tablets every six hours. The total daily dose of acetaminophen should not exceed 4 grams.

Percocet 5 mg/325 mg; Percocet 7.5 mg/325 mg; Percocet 7.5 mg/500 mg; Percocet 10 mg/325 mg; Percocet 10 mg/650 mg

The usual adult dosage is one tablet every 6 hours as needed for pain. The total daily dose of acetaminophen should not exceed 4 grams.

Strength	Maximal Daily Dose
Percocet 2.5 mg/325 mg	12 Tablets
Percocet 5 mg/325 mg	12 Tablets
Percocet 7.5 mg/325 mg	8 Tablets
Percocet 7.5 mg/500 mg	8 Tablets
Percocet 10 mg/325 mg	6 Tablets
Percocet 10 mg/650 mg	6 Tablets

HOW SUPPLIED

PERCOCET (Oxycodone and Acetaminophen Tablets, USP) are supplied as follows:

[See table above]

Store at 25°C (77°F); excursions permitted to 15°-30°C (59°-86°F). [See USP Controlled Room Temperature.]

Dispense in a tight, light-resistant container as defined in the USP, with a child-resistant closure (as required).

DEA Order Form Required.

Manufactured for:

Endo Pharmaceuticals Inc.

Chadds Ford, Pennsylvania 19317

PERCOCET® is a Registered Trademark of Endo Pharmaceuticals Inc.

Printed in U.S.A. 412842/April, 2003
412942

Shown in Product Identification Guide, page 311

PERCODAN® Ⓒ℞

[perk 'o-dan]

(Oxycodone and Aspirin Tablets, USP)

DESCRIPTION

Each tablet of PERCODAN contains:

Oxycodone Hydrochloride, USP	4.5 mg*
Oxycodone Terephthalate, USP	0.38 mg**
Aspirin, USP	325 mg

*4.5 mg oxycodone HCl is equivalent to 4.0338 mg of oxycodone.

**0.38 mg oxycodone terephthalate is equivalent to 0.3008 mg of oxycodone.

PERCODAN Tablets also contain: D&C Yellow 10, FD&C Yellow 6, microcrystalline cellulose and starch.

The oxycodone component is 14-hydroxydihydrocodeinone, a white odorless crystalline powder which is derived from the opium alkaloid, thebaine, and may be represented by the following structural formula:

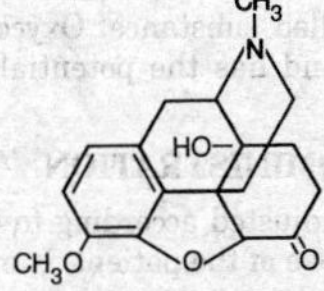

Continued on next page

Percodan—Cont.

CLINICAL PHARMACOLOGY

The principal ingredient, oxycodone, is a semisynthetic opioid analgesic with multiple actions qualitatively similar to those of morphine; the most prominent of these involve the central nervous system and organs composed of smooth muscle. The principal actions of therapeutic value of the oxycodone in PERCODAN are analgesia and sedation.

Oxycodone is similar to codeine and methadone in that it retains at least one-half of its analgesic activity when administered orally.

PERCODAN also contains the non-opioid antipyretic-analgesic, aspirin.

INDICATIONS

For the relief of moderate to moderately severe pain.

CONTRAINDICATIONS

Hypersensitivity to oxycodone or aspirin.

WARNINGS

Drug Dependence

Oxycodone can produce drug dependence of the morphine type and, therefore, has the potential for being abused. Psychic dependence, physical dependence and tolerance may develop upon repeated administration of PERCODAN, and it should be prescribed and administered with the same degree of caution appropriate to the use of other oral opioid-containing medications. Like other opioid-containing medications, PERCODAN is subject to the Federal Controlled Substances Act.

Usage in Ambulatory Patients

Oxycodone may impair the mental and/or physical abilities required for the performance of potentially hazardous tasks such as driving a car or operating machinery. The patient using PERCODAN should be cautioned accordingly.

Interaction with Other Central Nervous System Depressants

Patients receiving other opioid analgesics, general anesthetics, phenothiazines, other tranquilizers, sedative-hypnotics or other CNS depressants (including alcohol) concomitantly with PERCODAN may exhibit an additive CNS depression. When such combined therapy is contemplated, the dose of one or both agents should be reduced.

Usage in Pregnancy

Safe use in pregnancy has not been established relative to possible adverse effects on fetal development. Therefore, PERCODAN should not be used in pregnant women unless, in the judgment of the physician, the potential benefits outweigh the possible hazards.

Pediatric Use

PERCODAN should not be administered to pediatric patients.

Reye Syndrome is a rare but serious disease which can follow flu or chicken pox in children and teenagers. While the cause of Reye Syndrome is unknown, some reports claim aspirin (or salicylates) may increase the risk of developing this disease.

Salicylates should be used with caution in the presence of peptic ulcer or coagulation abnormalities.

PRECAUTIONS

Head Injury and Increased Intracranial Pressure

The respiratory depressant effects of opioids and their capacity to elevate cerebrospinal fluid pressure may be markedly exaggerated in the presence of head injury, other intracranial lesions or a pre-existing increase in intracranial pressure. Furthermore, opioids produce adverse reactions which may obscure the clinical course of patients with head injuries.

Acute Abdominal Conditions

The administration of PERCODAN or other opioids may obscure the diagnosis or clinical course in patients with acute abdominal conditions.

Special Risk Patients

PERCODAN should be given with caution to certain patients such as the elderly or debilitated, and those with severe impairment of hepatic or renal function, hypothyroidism, Addison's disease, and prostatic hypertrophy or urethral stricture.

ADVERSE REACTIONS

The most frequently observed adverse reactions include lightheadedness, dizziness, sedation, nausea and vomiting. These effects seem to be more prominent in ambulatory than in nonambulatory patients, and some of these adverse reactions may be alleviated if the patient lies down.

Other adverse reactions include euphoria, dysphoria, constipation and pruritus.

DRUG ABUSE AND DEPENDENCE

PERCODAN (oxycodone and aspirin tablets, USP) is a Schedule II controlled substance. Oxycodone can produce drug dependence and has the potential for being abused (See **WARNINGS**).

DOSAGE AND ADMINISTRATION

Dosage should be adjusted according to the severity of the pain and the response of the patient. It may occasionally be necessary to exceed the usual dosage recommended below in cases of more severe pain or in those patients who have become tolerant to the analgesic effect of opioids. PERCODAN is given orally. The usual adult dosage is one tablet every 6 hours as needed for pain. The total daily dose of aspirin should not exceed 4 grams or 12 tablets.

DRUG INTERACTIONS

The CNS depressant effects of PERCODAN may be additive with that of other CNS depressants (See **WARNINGS**).

Aspirin may enhance the effect of anticoagulants and inhibit the uricosuric effects of uricosuric agents.

MANAGEMENT OF OVERDOSAGE

Signs and Symptoms

Serious overdose with PERCODAN is characterized by respiratory depression (a decrease in respiratory rate and/or tidal volume, Cheyne-Stokes respiration, cyanosis), extreme somnolence progressing to stupor or coma, skeletal muscle flaccidity, cold and clammy skin, and sometimes bradycardia and hypotension. In severe overdosage, apnea, circulatory collapse, cardiac arrest and death may occur. The ingestion of very large amounts of PERCODAN may, in addition, result in acute salicylate intoxication.

Treatment

Primary attention should be given to the reestablishment of adequate respiratory exchange through provision of a patent airway and the institution of assisted or controlled ventilation. The opioid antagonist naloxone hydrochloride (NARCAN®) is a specific antidote against respiratory depression which may result from overdosage or unusual sensitivity to opioids including oxycodone. Therefore, an appropriate dose of naloxone hydrochloride should be administered (usual initial adult dose 0.4 mg–2 mg) preferably by the intravenous route, simultaneously with efforts at respiratory resuscitation. Since the duration of action of oxycodone may exceed that of the antagonist, the patient should be kept under continued surveillance and repeated doses of the antagonist should be administered as needed to maintain adequate respiration.

Oxygen, intravenous fluids, vasopressors and other supportive measures should be employed as indicated.

Gastric emptying may be useful in removing unabsorbed drug.

HOW SUPPLIED

PERCODAN (oxycodone and aspirin tablets, USP), supplied as a yellow tablet, with one face scored and inscribed "PERCODAN" and plain on the other side is available in:

Bottles of 100 NDC 63481-135-70
Bottles of 500 NDC 63481-135-85

Store at 25°C (77°F); excursions permitted to 15°–30°C (59°–86°F). [See USP Controlled Room Temperature].

Dispense in a tight, light-resistant container as defined in the USP, with a child-resistant closure (as required).

DEA Order Form Required.

PERCODAN® is a Registered Trademark of Endo Pharmaceuticals Inc.

NARCAN® is a Registered Trademark of Endo Pharmaceuticals Inc.

51-022552–00/May, 2003

Shown in Product Identification Guide, page 311

SYMMETREL® ℞

[sim 'e-trel]

(Amantadine Hydrochloride, USP)
Tablets and Syrup
℞ only

DESCRIPTION

SYMMETREL (Amantadine Hydrochloride, USP) is designated generically as amantadine hydrochloride and chemically as 1-adamantanamine hydrochloride.

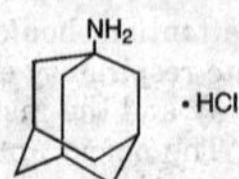

Amantadine hydrochloride is a stable white or nearly white crystalline powder, freely soluble in water and soluble in alcohol and in chloroform.

Amantadine hydrochloride has pharmacological actions as both an anti-Parkinson and an antiviral drug.

SYMMETREL is available in tablets and syrup.

Each tablet intended for oral administration contains 100 mg amantadine hydrochloride and has the following inactive ingredients: hydroxypropyl methylcellulose, magnesium stearate, microcrystalline cellulose, sodium starch glycolate, FD&C Yellow No. 6.

SYMMETREL syrup contains 50 mg of amantadine hydrochloride per 5 mL and has the following inactive ingredients: artificial raspberry flavor, citric acid, methylparaben, propylparaben, and sorbitol solution.

CLINICAL PHARMACOLOGY

Pharmacodynamics

Mechanism of Action: Antiviral The mechanism by which amantadine exerts its antiviral activity is not clearly understood. It appears to mainly prevent the release of infectious viral nucleic acid into the host cell by interfering with the function of the transmembrane domain of the viral M2 protein. In certain cases, amantadine is also known to prevent virus assembly during virus replication. It does not appear to interfere with the immunogenicity of inactivated influenza A virus vaccine.

Antiviral Activity: Amantadine inhibits the replication of influenza A virus isolates from each of the subtypes, i.e., H1N1, H2N2 and H3N2. It has very little or no activity against influenza B virus isolates. A quantitative relationship between the *in vitro* susceptibility of influenza A virus to amantadine and the clinical response to therapy has not been established in man. Sensitivity test results, expressed as the concentration of amantadine required to inhibit by 50% the growth of virus (ED_{50}) in tissue culture vary greatly (from 0.1 μg/mL to 25.0 μg/mL) depending upon the assay protocol used, size of virus inoculum, isolates of influenza A virus strains tested, and the cell type used. Host cells in tissue culture readily tolerated amantadine up to a concentration of 100 μg/mL.

Drug Resistance: Influenza A variants with reduced *in vitro* sensitivity to amantadine have been isolated from epidemic strains in areas where adamantane derivatives are being used. Influenza viruses with reduced *in vitro* sensitivity have been shown to be transmissible and to cause typical influenza illness. The quantitative relationship between the *in vitro* sensitivity of influenza A variants to amantadine and the clinical response to therapy has not been established.

Mechanism of Action: Parkinson's Disease The mechanism of action of amantadine in the treatment of Parkinson's Disease and drug-induced extrapyramidal reactions is not known. Data from earlier animal studies suggest that SYMMETREL may have direct and indirect effects on dopamine neurons. More recent studies have demonstrated that amantadine is a weak, non-competitive NMDA receptor antagonist (K_i = 10μM). Although amantadine has not been shown to possess direct anticholinergic activity in animal studies, clinically, it exhibits anticholinergic-like side effects such as dry mouth, urinary retention, and constipation.

Pharmacokinetics

SYMMETREL is well absorbed orally. Maximum plasma concentrations are directly related to dose for doses up to 200 mg/day. Doses above 200 mg/day may result in a greater than proportional increase in maximum plasma concentrations. It is primarily excreted unchanged in the urine by glomerular filtration and tubular secretion. Eight metabolites of amantadine have been identified in human urine. One metabolite, an N-acetylated compound, was quantified in human urine and accounted for 5-15% of the administered dose. Plasma acetylamantadine accounted for up to 80% of the concurrent amantadine plasma concentration in 5 of 12 healthy volunteers following the ingestion of a 200 mg dose of amantadine. Acetylamantadine was not detected in the plasma of the remaining seven volunteers. The contribution of this metabolite to efficacy or toxicity is not known.

There appears to be a relationship between plasma amantadine concentrations and toxicity. As concentration increases, toxicity seems to be more prevalent, however, absolute values of amantadine concentrations associated with adverse effects have not been fully defined.

Amantadine pharmacokinetics were determined in 24 normal adult male volunteers after the oral administration of a single amantadine hydrochloride 100 mg soft gel capsule. The mean ± SD maximum plasma concentration was 0.22 ± 0.03 μg/mL (range: 0.18 to 0.32 μg/mL). The time to peak concentration was 3.3 ± 1.5 hours (range: 1.5 to 8.0 hours). The apparent oral clearance was 0.28 ± 0.11 L/hr/kg (range: 0.14 to 0.62 L/hr/kg). The half-life was 17 ± 4 hours (range: 10 to 25 hours). Across other studies, amantadine plasma half-life has averaged 16 ± 6 hours (range: 9 to 31 hours) in 19 healthy volunteers.

After oral administration of a single dose of 100 mg amantadine syrup to five healthy volunteers, the mean ± SD maximum plasma concentration C_{max} was 0.24 ± 0.04 μg/mL and ranged from 0.18 to 0.28 μg/mL. After 15 days of amantadine 100 mg b.i.d., the C_{max} was 0.47 ± 0.11 μg/mL in four of the five volunteers. The administration of amantadine tablets as a 200 mg single dose to 6 healthy subjects resulted in a C_{max} of 0.51 ± 0.14 μg/mL. Across studies, the time to C_{max} (T_{max}) averaged about 2 to 4 hours.

Plasma amantadine clearance ranged from 0.2 to 0.3 L/hr/kg after the administration of 5 mg to 25 mg intravenous doses of amantadine to 15 healthy volunteers.

In six healthy volunteers, the ratio of amantadine renal clearance to apparent oral plasma clearance was 0.79 ± 0.17 (mean ± SD).

The volume of distribution determined after the intravenous administration of amantadine to 15 healthy subjects was 3 to 8 L/kg, suggesting tissue binding. Amantadine, after single oral 200 mg doses to 6 healthy young subjects and to 6 healthy elderly subjects has been found in nasal mucus at mean ± SD concentrations of 0.15 ± 0.16, 0.28 ± 0.26, and 0.39 ± 0.34 μg/g at 1, 4, and 8 hours after dosing, respectively. These concentrations represented 31 ± 33%, 59 ± 61%, and 95 ± 86% of the corresponding plasma amantadine concentrations. Amantadine is approximately 67% bound to plasma proteins over a concentration range of 0.1 to 2.0 μg/mL. Following the administration of amantadine 100 mg as a single dose, the mean ± SD red blood cell to plasma ratio ranged from 2.7 ± 0.5 in 6 healthy subjects to 1.4 ± 0.2 in 8 patients with renal insufficiency.

The apparent oral plasma clearance of amantadine is reduced and the plasma half-life and plasma concentrations are increased in healthy elderly individuals age 60 and older. After single dose administration of 25 to 75 mg to 7 healthy, elderly male volunteers, the apparent plasma clearance of amantadine was 0.10 ± 0.04 L/hr/kg (range 0.06 to 0.17 L/hr/kg) and the half-life was 29 ± 7 hours (range 20 to 41 hours). Whether these changes are due to decline in renal function or other age related factors is not known.

In a study of young healthy subjects (n=20), mean renal clearance of amantadine, normalized for body mass index, was 1.5 fold higher in males compared to females ($p<0.032$).

Compared with otherwise healthy adult individuals, the clearance of amantadine is significantly reduced in adult patients with renal insufficiency. The elimination half-life increases two to three fold or greater when creatinine clearance is less than 40 mL/min/1.73m^2 and averages eight days in patients on chronic maintenance hemodialysis. Amantadine is removed in negligible amounts by hemodialysis.

The pH of the urine has been reported to influence the excretion rate of SYMMETREL. Since the excretion rate of SYMMETREL increases rapidly when the urine is acidic, the administration of urine acidifying drugs may increase the elimination of the drug from the body.

INDICATIONS AND USAGE

SYMMETREL is indicated for the prophylaxis and treatment of signs and symptoms of infection caused by various strains of influenza A virus. SYMMETREL is also indicated in the treatment of parkinsonism and drug-induced extrapyramidal reactions.

Influenza A Prophylaxis: SYMMETREL (Amantadine Hydrochloride, USP) is indicated for chemoprophylaxis against signs and symptoms of influenza A virus infection when early vaccination is not feasible or when the vaccine is contraindicated or not available. In the prophylaxis of influenza, early vaccination on an annual basis as recommended by the Centers for Disease Control's Immunization Practices Advisory Committee is the method of choice. Because SYMMETREL does not completely prevent the host immune response to influenza A infection, individuals who take this drug may still develop immune responses to natural disease or vaccination and may be protected when later exposed to antigenically related viruses. Following vaccination during an influenza A outbreak, SYMMETREL prophylaxis should be considered for the 2- to 4-week time period required to develop an antibody response.

Influenza A Treatment: SYMMETREL is also indicated in the treatment of uncomplicated respiratory tract illness caused by influenza A virus strains especially when administered early in the course of illness. There are no well-controlled clinical studies demonstrating that treatment with SYMMETREL will avoid the development of influenza A virus pneumonitis or other complications in high risk patients.

There is no clinical evidence indicating that SYMMETREL is effective in the prophylaxis or treatment of viral respiratory tract illnesses other than those caused by influenza A virus strains.

Parkinson's Disease/Syndrome: SYMMETREL is indicated in the treatment of idiopathic Parkinson's disease (Paralysis Agitans), postencephalitic parkinsonism, and symptomatic parkinsonism which may follow injury to the nervous system by carbon monoxide intoxication. It is indicated in those elderly patients believed to develop parkinsonism in association with cerebral arteriosclerosis. In the treatment of Parkinson's disease, SYMMETREL is less effective than levodopa, (-),-3-(3,4-dihydroxyphenyl)-L-alanine, and its efficacy in comparison with the anticholinergic antiparkinson drugs has not yet been established.

Drug-Induced Extrapyramidal Reactions: SYMMETREL is indicated in the treatment of drug-induced extrapyramidal reactions. Although anticholinergic-type side effects have been noted with SYMMETREL when used in patients with drug-induced extrapyramidal reactions, there is a lower incidence of these side effects than that observed with the anticholinergic antiparkinson drugs.

CONTRAINDICATIONS

SYMMETREL is contraindicated in patients with known hypersensitivity to amantadine hydrochloride or to any of the other ingredients in SYMMETREL.

WARNINGS

Deaths: Deaths have been reported from overdose with SYMMETREL. The lowest reported acute lethal dose was 1 gram. Acute toxicity may be attributable to the anticholinergic effects of amantadine. Drug overdose has resulted in cardiac, respiratory, renal or central nervous system toxicity. Cardiac dysfunction includes arrhythmia, tachycardia and hypertension (see OVERDOSAGE).

Suicide Attempts: Suicide attempts, some of which have been fatal, have been reported in patients treated with SYMMETREL, many of whom received short courses for influenza treatment or prophylaxis. The incidence of suicide attempts is not known and the pathophysiologic mechanism is not understood. Suicide attempts and suicidal ideation have been reported in patients with and without prior history of psychiatric illness. SYMMETREL can exacerbate mental problems in patients with a history of psychiatric disorders or substance abuse. Patients who attempt suicide may exhibit abnormal mental states which include disorientation, confusion, depression, personality changes, agitation, aggressive behavior, hallucinations, paranoia, other psychotic reactions, and somnolence or insomnia. Because of the possibility of serious adverse effects, caution should be observed when prescribing SYMMETREL to patients being treated with drugs having CNS effects, or for whom the potential risks outweigh the benefit of treatment.

CNS Effects: Patients with a history of epilepsy or other "seizures" should be observed closely for possible increased seizure activity.

Patients receiving SYMMETREL who note central nervous system effects or blurring of vision should be cautioned against driving or working in situations where alertness and adequate motor coordination are important.

Other: Patients with a history of congestive heart failure or peripheral edema should be followed closely as there are patients who developed congestive heart failure while receiving SYMMETREL.

Patients with Parkinson's disease improving on SYMMETREL should resume normal activities gradually and cautiously, consistent with other medical considerations, such as the presence of osteoporosis or phlebothrombosis.

Because SYMMETREL has anticholinergic effects and may cause mydriasis, it should not be given to patients with untreated angle closure glaucoma.

PRECAUTIONS

SYMMETREL should not be discontinued abruptly in patients with Parkinson's disease since a few patients have experienced a parkinsonian crisis, i.e., a sudden marked clinical deterioration, when this medication was suddenly stopped. The dose of anticholinergic drugs or of SYMMETREL should be reduced if atropine-like effects appear when these drugs are used concurrently. Abrupt discontinuation may also precipitate delirium, agitation, delusions, hallucinations, paranoid reaction, stupor, anxiety, depression and slurred speech.

Neuroleptic Malignant Syndrome (NMS): Sporadic cases of possible Neuroleptic Malignant Syndrome (NMS) have been reported in association with dose reduction or withdrawal of SYMMETREL therapy. Therefore, patients should be observed carefully when the dosage of SYMMETREL is reduced abruptly or discontinued, especially if the patient is receiving neuroleptics.

NMS is an uncommon but life-threatening syndrome characterized by fever or hyperthermia; neurologic findings including muscle rigidity, involuntary movements, altered consciousness; mental status changes; other disturbances such as autonomic dysfunction, tachycardia, tachypnea, hyper- or hypotension; laboratory findings such as creatine phosphokinase elevation, leukocytosis, myoglobinuria, and increased serum myoglobin.

The early diagnosis of this condition is important for the appropriate management of these patients. Considering NMS as a possible diagnosis and ruling out other acute illnesses (e.g., pneumonia, systemic infection, etc.) is essential. This may be especially complex if the clinical presentation includes both serious medical illness and untreated or inadequately treated extrapyramidal signs and symptoms (EPS). Other important considerations in the differential diagnosis include central anticholinergic toxicity, heat stroke, drug fever and primary central nervous system (CNS) pathology.

The management of NMS should include: 1) intensive symptomatic treatment and medical monitoring, and 2) treatment of any concomitant serious medical problems for which specific treatments are available. Dopamine agonists, such as bromocriptine, and muscle relaxants, such as dantrolene are often used in the treatment of NMS, however, their effectiveness has not been demonstrated in controlled studies.

Renal disease: Because SYMMETREL is mainly excreted in the urine, it accumulates in the plasma and in the body when renal function declines. Thus, the dose of SYMMETREL should be reduced in patients with renal impairment and in individuals who are 65 years of age or older (see DOSAGE AND ADMINISTRATION; Dosage for Impaired Renal Function).

Liver disease: Care should be exercised when administering SYMMETREL to patients with liver disease. Rare instances of reversible elevation of liver enzymes have been reported in patients receiving SYMMETREL, though a specific relationship between the drug and such changes has not been established.

Other: The dose of SYMMETREL may need careful adjustment in patients with congestive heart failure, peripheral edema, or orthostatic hypotension. Care should be exercised when administering SYMMETREL to patients with a history of recurrent eczematoid rash, or to patients with psychosis or severe psychoneurosis not controlled by chemotherapeutic agents.

Serious bacterial infections may begin with influenza-like symptoms or may coexist with or occur as complications during the course of influenza. SYMMETREL has not been shown to prevent such complications.

Information for Patients:

Patients should be advised of the following information:

Blurry vision and/or impaired mental acuity may occur.

Gradually increase physical activity as the symptoms of Parkinson's disease improve.

Avoid excessive alcohol usage, since it may increase the potential for CNS effects such as dizziness, confusion, lightheadedness and orthostatic hypotension.

Avoid getting up suddenly from a sitting or lying position. If dizziness or lightheadedness occurs, notify physician.

Notify physician if mood/mental changes, swelling of extremities, difficulty urinating and/or shortness of breath occur.

Do not take more medication than prescribed because of the risk of overdose. If there is no improvement in a few days, or if medication appears less effective after a few weeks, discuss with a physician.

Consult physician before discontinuing medication.

Seek medical attention immediately if it is suspected that an overdose of medication has been taken.

Drug Interactions: Careful observation is required when SYMMETREL is administered concurrently with central nervous system stimulants.

Agents with anticholinergic properties may potentiate the anticholinergic-like side effects of amantadine.

Coadministration of thioridazine has been reported to worsen the tremor in elderly patients with Parkinson's disease, however, it is not known if other phenothiazines produce a similar response. Coadministration of Dyazide (triamterene/hydrochlorothiazide) resulted in a higher plasma amantadine concentration in a 61-year-old man receiving SYMMETREL (Amantadine Hydrochloride, USP) 100 mg TID for Parkinson's disease.[1] It is not known which of the components of Dyazide contributed to the observation or if related drugs produce a similar response.

Coadministration of quinine or quinidine with amantadine was shown to reduce the renal clearance of amantadine by about 30%.

Carcinogenesis and Mutagenesis: Long-term *in vivo* animal studies designed to evaluate the carcinogenic potential of SYMMETREL have not been performed. In several *in vitro* assays for gene mutation, SYMMETREL did not increase the number of spontaneously observed mutations in four strains of *Salmonella typhimurium* (Ames Test) or in a mammalian cell line (Chinese Hamster Ovary cells) when incubations were performed either with or without a liver metabolic activation extract. Further, there was no evidence of chromosome damage observed in an *in vitro* test using freshly derived and stimulated human peripheral blood lymphocytes (with and without metabolic activation) or in an *in vivo* mouse bone marrow micronucleus test (140-550 mg/kg; estimated human equivalent doses of 11.7-45.8 mg/kg based on body surface area conversion).

Impairment of Fertility: The effect of amantadine on fertility has not been adequately tested, that is, in a study conducted under Good Laboratory Practice (GLP) and according to current recommended methodology. In a three litter, non-GLP, reproduction study in rats, Symmetrel at a dose of 32 mg/kg/day (equal to the maximum recommended human dose on a mg/m^2 basis) administered to both males and females slightly impaired fertility. There were no effects on fertility at a dose level of 10 mg/kg/day (or 0.3 times the maximum recommended human dose on a mg/m^2 basis); intermediate doses were not tested.

Failed fertility has been reported during human *in vitro* fertilization (IVF) when the sperm donor ingested amantadine 2 weeks prior to, and during the IVF cycle.

Pregnancy Category C: The effect of amantadine on embryofetal and peri-postnatal development has not been adequately tested, that is, in studies conducted under Good Laboratory Practice (GLP) and according to current recommended methodology. However, in two non-GLP studies in rats in which females were dosed from 5 days prior to mating to Day 6 of gestation or on Days 7-14 of gestation, Symmetrel produced increases in embryonic death at an oral dose of 100 mg/kg (or 3 times the maximum recommended human dose on a mg/m^2 basis). In the non-GLP rat study in which females were dosed on Days 7-14 of gestation, there was a marked increase in severe visceral and skeletal malformations at oral doses of 50 and 100 mg/kg (or 1.5 and 3 times, respectively, the maximum recommended human dose on a mg/m^2 basis). The no-effect dose for teratogenicity was 37 mg/kg (equal to the maximum recommended human dose on a mg/m^2 basis). The safety margins reported may not accurately reflect the risk considering the questionable quality of the study on which they are based. There are no adequate and well-controlled studies in pregnant women. Human data regarding teratogenicity after maternal use of amantadine is scarce. Tetralogy of Fallot and tibial hemimelia (normal karyotype) occurred in an infant exposed to amantadine during the first trimester of pregnancy (100 mg P.O. for 7 days during the 6th and 7th week of gestation). Cardiovascular maldevelopment (single ventricle with pulmonary atresia) was associated with maternal exposure to amantadine (100 mg/d) administered during the first 2 weeks of pregnancy. SYMMETREL should be used during pregnancy only if the potential benefit justifies the potential risk to the embryo or fetus.

Nursing Mothers: SYMMETREL is excreted in human milk. Use is not recommended in nursing mothers.

Pediatric Use: The safety and efficacy of SYMMETREL in newborn infants and infants below the age of 1 year have not been established.

Usage in the Elderly: Because SYMMETREL is primarily excreted in the urine, it accumulates in the plasma and in the body when renal function declines. Thus, the dose of SYMMETREL should be reduced in patients with renal impairment and in individuals who are 65 years of age or older. The dose of SYMMETREL may need reduction in patients with congestive heart failure, peripheral edema, or orthostatic hypotension (see DOSAGE AND ADMINISTRATION).

ADVERSE REACTIONS

The adverse reactions reported most frequently at the recommended dose of SYMMETREL (5-10%) are: nausea, dizziness (lightheadedness), and insomnia.

Less frequently (1-5%) reported adverse reactions are: depression, anxiety and irritability, hallucinations, confusion,

Continued on next page

Symmetrel —Cont.

anorexia, dry mouth, constipation, ataxia, livedo reticularis, peripheral edema, orthostatic hypotension, headache, somnolence, nervousness, dream abnormality, agitation, dry nose, diarrhea and fatigue.

Infrequently (0.1-1%) occurring adverse reactions are: congestive heart failure, psychosis, urinary retention, dyspnea, skin rash, vomiting, weakness, slurred speech, euphoria, thinking abnormality, amnesia, hyperkinesia, hypertension, decreased libido, and visual disturbance, including punctate subepithelial or other corneal opacity, corneal edema, decreased visual acuity, sensitivity to light, and optic nerve palsy.

Rare (less than 0.1%) occurring adverse reactions are: instances of convulsion, leukopenia, neutropenia, eczematoid dermatitis, oculogyric episodes, suicidal attempt, suicide, and suicidal ideation (see WARNINGS).

Other adverse reactions reported during postmarketing experience with SYMMETREL usage include:

Nervous System/Psychiatric—coma, stupor, delirium, hypokinesia, hypertonia, delusions, aggressive behavior, paranoid reaction, manic reaction, involuntary muscle contractions, gait abnormalities, paresthesia, EEG changes, and tremor. Abrupt discontinuation may also precipitate delirium, agitation, delusions, hallucinations, paranoid reaction, stupor, anxiety, depression and slurred speech;

Cardiovascular—cardiac arrest, arrhythmias including malignant arrhythmias, hypotension, and tachycardia;

Respiratory—acute respiratory failure, pulmonary edema, and tachypnea;

Gastrointestinal—dysphagia;

Hematologic—leukocytosis;

Special Senses—keratitis and mydriasis;

Skin and Appendages—pruritus and diaphoresis;

Miscellaneous—neuroleptic malignant syndrome (see WARNINGS), allergic reactions including anaphylactic reactions, edema, and fever;

Laboratory Test—elevated: CPK, BUN, serum creatiine, alkaline phosphatase, LDH, bilirubin, GGT, SGOT, and SGPT.

OVERDOSAGE

Deaths have been reported from overdose with SYMMETREL. The lowest reported acute lethal dose was 1 gram. Because some patients have attempted suicide by overdosing with amantadine, prescriptions should be written for the smallest quantity consistent with good patient management.

Acute toxicity may be attributable to the anticholinergic effects of amantadine. Drug overdose has resulted in cardiac, respiratory, renal or central nervous system toxicity. Cardiac dysfunction includes arrhythmia, tachycardia and hypertension. Pulmonary edema and respiratory distress (including adult respiratory distress syndrome—ARDS) have been reported; renal dysfunction including increased BUN, decreased creatinine clearance and renal insufficiency can occur. Central nervous system effects that have been reported include insomnia, anxiety, agitation, aggressive behavior, hypertonia, hyperkinesia, ataxia, gait abnormality, tremor, confusion, disorientation, depersonalization, fear, delirium, hallucinations, psychotic reactions, lethargy, somnolence and coma. Seizures may be exacerbated in patients with prior history of seizure disorders. Hyperthermia has also been observed in cases where a drug overdose has occurred.

There is no specific antidote for an overdose of SYMMETREL. However, slowly administered intravenous physostigmine in 1 and 2 mg doses in an adult[2] at 1- to 2-hour intervals and 0.5 mg doses in a child[3] at 5- to 10-minute intervals up to a maximum of 2 mg/hour have been reported to be effective in the control of central nervous system toxicity caused by amantadine hydrochloride. For acute overdosing, general supportive measures should be employed along with immediate gastric lavage or induction of emesis. Fluids should be forced, and if necessary, given intravenously. The pH of the urine has been reported to influence the excretion rate of SYMMETREL. Since the excretion rate of SYMMETREL increases rapidly when the urine is acidic, the administration of urine acidifying drugs may increase the elimination of the drug from the body. The blood pressure, pulse, respiration and temperature should be monitored. The patient should be observed for hyperactivity and convulsions; if required, sedation, and anticonvulsant therapy should be administered. The patient should be observed for the possible development of arrhythmias and hypotension; if required, appropriate antiarrhythmic and antihypotensive therapy should be given. Electrocardiographic monitoring may be required after ingestion, since malignant tachyarrhythmias can appear after overdose.

Care should be exercised when administering adrenergic agents, such as isoproterenol, to patients with a SYMMETREL overdose, since the dopaminergic activity of SYMMETREL has been reported to induce malignant arrhythmias.

The blood electrolytes, urine pH and urinary output should be monitored. If there is no record of recent voiding, catheterization should be done.

DOSAGE AND ADMINISTRATION

The dose of SYMMETREL (Amantadine Hydrochloride, USP) may need reduction in patients with congestive heart failure, peripheral edema, orthostatic hypotension, or impaired renal function (see Dosage for Impaired Renal Function).

Dosage for Prophylaxis and Treatment of Uncomplicated Influenza A Virus Illness:

Adult: The adult daily dosage of SYMMETREL is 200 mg; two 100 mg tablets (or four teaspoonfuls of syrup) as a single daily dose. The daily dosage may be split into one tablet of 100 mg (or two teaspoonfuls of syrup) twice a day. If central nervous system effects develop in once-a-day dosage, a split dosage schedule may reduce such complaints. In persons 65 years of age or older, the daily dosage of SYMMETREL is 100 mg.

A 100 mg daily dose has also been shown in experimental challenge studies to be effective as prophylaxis in healthy adults who are not at high risk for influenza-related complications. However, it has not been demonstrated that a 100 mg daily dose is as effective as a 200 mg daily dose for prophylaxis, nor has the 100 mg daily dose been studied in the treatment of acute influenza illness. In recent clinical trials, the incidence of central nervous system (CNS) side effects associated with the 100 mg daily dose was at or near the level of placebo. The 100 mg dose is recommended for persons who have demonstrated intolerance to 200 mg of SYMMETREL daily because of CNS or other toxicities.

Pediatric Patients: 1 yr.–9 yrs. of age: The total daily dose should be calculated on the basis of 2 to 4 mg/lb/day (4.4 to 8.8 mg/kg/day), but not to exceed 150 mg per day.

9 yrs.–12 yrs. of age: The total daily dose is 200 mg given as one tablet of 100 mg (or two teaspoonfuls of syrup) twice a day. The 100 mg daily dose has not been studied in this pediatric population. Therefore, there are no data which demonstrate that this dose is as effective as or is safer than the 200 mg daily dose in this patient population.

Prophylactic dosing should be started in anticipation of an influenza A outbreak and before or after contact with individuals with influenza A virus respiratory tract illness.

SYMMETREL should be continued daily for at least 10 days following a known exposure. If SYMMETREL is used chemoprophylactically in conjunction with inactivated influenza A virus vaccine until protective antibody responses develop, then it should be administered for 2 to 4 weeks after the vaccine has been given. When inactivated influenza A virus vaccine is unavailable or contraindicated, SYMMETREL should be administered for the duration of known influenza A in the community because of repeated and unknown exposure.

Treatment of influenza A virus illness should be started as soon as possible, preferably within 24 to 48 hours after onset of signs and symptoms, and should be continued for 24 to 48 hours after the disappearance of signs and symptoms.

Dosage for Parkinsonism:

Adult: The usual dose of SYMMETREL is 100 mg twice a day when used alone. SYMMETREL has an onset of action usually within 48 hours.

The initial dose of SYMMETREL is 100 mg daily for patients with serious associated medical illnesses or who are receiving high doses of other antiparkinson drugs. After one to several weeks at 100 mg once daily, the dose may be increased to 100 mg twice daily, if necessary.

Occasionally, patients whose responses are not optimal with SYMMETREL at 200 mg daily may benefit from an increase up to 400 mg daily in divided doses. However, such patients should be supervised closely by their physicians.

Patients initially deriving benefit from SYMMETREL not uncommonly experience a fall-off of effectiveness after a few months. Benefit may be regained by increasing the dose to 300 mg daily. Alternatively, temporary discontinuation of SYMMETREL for several weeks, followed by reinitiation of the drug, may result in regaining benefit in some patients. A decision to use other antiparkinson drugs may be necessary.

Dosage for Concomitant Therapy: Some patients who do not respond to anticholinergic antiparkinson drugs may respond to SYMMETREL. When SYMMETREL or anticholinergic antiparkinson drugs are each used with marginal benefit, concomitant use may produce additional benefit.

When SYMMETREL and levodopa are initiated concurrently, the patient can exhibit rapid therapeutic benefits. SYMMETREL should be held constant at 100 mg daily or twice daily while the daily dose of levodopa is gradually increased to optimal benefit.

When SYMMETREL is added to optimal well-tolerated doses of levodopa, additional benefit may result, including smoothing out the fluctuations in improvement which sometimes occur in patients on levodopa alone. Patients who require a reduction in their usual dose of levodopa because of development of side effects may possibly regain lost benefit with the addition of SYMMETREL.

Dosage for Drug-Induced Extrapyramidal Reactions:

Adult: The usual dose of SYMMETREL is 100 mg twice a day. Occasionally, patients whose responses are not optimal with SYMMETREL at 200 mg daily may benefit from an increase up to 300 mg daily in divided doses.

Dosage for Impaired Renal Function:

Depending upon creatinine clearance, the following dosage adjustments are recommended:

CREATININE CLEARANCE (mL/min/1.73 m^2)	SYMMETREL DOSAGE
30-50	200 mg 1st day and 100 mg each day thereafter
15-29	200 mg 1st day followed by 100 mg on alternate days
<15	200 mg every 7 days

The recommended dosage for patients on hemodialysis is 200 mg every 7 days.

HOW SUPPLIED

SYMMETREL (Amantadine Hydrochloride, USP) is available in light orange, convex curved, triangular shaped 100 mg tablets with "SYMMETREL" debossed on one side and plain on the other side as follows:

Bottles of 100 NDC 63481-108-70

As a clear, colorless syrup [each 5 mL (1 teaspoonful) contains 50 mg amantadine hydrochloride] in:

16 oz. (480 mL) bottles NDC 63481-205-16

Store at 25°C (77°F), excursions permitted to 15°-30°C (59°-86°F). [See USP Controlled Room Temperature].

Dispense in a tight container as defined in the USP, with a child-resistant closure (as required).

REFERENCES

[1] W.W. Wilson and A.H. Rajput, Amantadine-Dyazide Interaction, *Can. Med. Assoc. J.* 129:974-975, 1983.

[2] D.F. Casey, *N. Engl. J. Med.* 298:516, 1978.

[3] C.D. Berkowitz, *J. Pediatr.* 95:144, 1979.

Manufactured for:
Endo Pharmaceuticals Inc.
Chadds Ford, PA 19317
Manufactured by:
Bristol-Myers Squibb Company
Princeton, NJ 08543 USA

Printed in U.S.A. 6486-06/March, 2003

Shown in Product Identification Guide, page 311

ZYDONE® ℂ℞

[*zī ″dōn*]

(Hydrocodone Bitartrate and Acetaminophen Tablets, USP)

DESCRIPTION

ZYDONE (hydrocodone bitartrate and acetaminophen tablets) for oral administration, contain hydrocodone bitartrate and acetaminophen in the following strengths:

Hydrocodone Bitartrate, USP	5 mg
Acetaminophen, USP	400 mg
Hydrocodone Bitartrate, USP	7.5 mg
Acetaminophen, USP	400 mg
Hydrocodone Bitartrate, USP	10 mg
Acetaminophen, USP	400 mg

In addition, each tablet contains the following inactive ingredients: colloidal silicon dioxide, croscarmellose sodium, crospovidone, microcrystalline cellulose, povidone, pregelatinized starch, and stearic acid. The 5 mg/400 mg strength contains FD&C Yellow No. 10; 7.5 mg/400 mg contains FD&C Blue No. 2; and 10 mg/400 mg contains FD&C Red No. 40.

Zydone Tablets meet USP Dissolution Test 1.

Hydrocodone bitartrate is an opioid analgesic and antitussive and occurs as fine, white crystals or as a crystalline powder. It is affected by light. The chemical name is 4,5α-Epoxy-3-methoxy-17-methylmorphinan-6-one tartrate (1:1) hydrate (2:5). It has the following structural formula:

$C_{18}H_{21}NO_3 \cdot C_4H_6O_6 \cdot 2\frac{1}{2} H_2O$ MW = 494.50

Acetaminophen, 4′-Hydroxyacetanilide, a slightly bitter, white, odorless, crystalline powder, is a non-opiate, non-salicylate analgesic and antipyretic. It has the following structural formula:

$C_8H_9NO_2$ MW = 151.17

CLINICAL PHARMACOLOGY

Hydrocodone is a semisynthetic opioid analgesic and antitussive with multiple actions qualitatively similar to those of codeine. Most of these involve the central nervous system and smooth muscle. The precise mechanism of action of hydrocodone and other opiates is not known, although it is believed to relate to the existence of opiate receptors in the central nervous system. In addition to analgesia, opioids may produce drowsiness, changes in mood and mental clouding.

The analgesic action of acetaminophen involves peripheral influences, but the specific mechanism is as yet undetermined. Antipyretic activity is mediated through hypothalamic heat-regulating centers. Acetaminophen inhibits prostaglandin synthetase. Therapeutic doses of acetaminophen have negligible effects on the cardiovascular or respiratory systems; however, toxic doses may cause circulatory failure and rapid, shallow breathing.

Pharmacokinetics

The behavior of the individual components is described below.

Hydrocodone: Following a 10 mg oral dose of hydrocodone administered to five adult male subjects, the mean peak concentration was 23.6 ± 5.2 ng/mL. Maximum serum levels were achieved at 1.3 ± 0.3 hours and the half-life was determined to be 3.8 ± 0.3 hours. Hydrocodone exhibits a complex pattern of metabolism including O-demethylation, N-demethylation and 6-keto reduction to the corresponding 6-α- and 6-β-hydroxymetabolites.

See **OVERDOSAGE** for toxicity information.

Acetaminophen: Acetaminophen is rapidly absorbed from the gastrointestinal tract and is distributed throughout most body tissues. The plasma half-life is 1.25 to 3 hours, but may be increased by liver damage and following overdosage. Elimination of acetaminophen is principally by liver metabolism (conjugation) and subsequent renal excretion of metabolites. Approximately 85% of an oral dose appears in the urine within 24 hours of administration, most as the glucuronide conjugate, with small amounts of other conjugates and unchanged drug.

See **OVERDOSAGE** for toxicity information.

INDICATIONS AND USAGE

ZYDONE (hydrocodone bitartrate and acetaminophen tablets) is indicated for the relief of moderate to moderately severe pain.

CONTRAINDICATIONS

ZYDONE tablets should not be administered to patients who have previously exhibited hypersensitivity to hydrocodone, acetaminophen, or any other component of this product.

Patients known to be hypersensitive to other opioids may exhibit cross-sensitivity to hydrocodone.

WARNINGS

Respiratory Depression

At high doses or in sensitive patients, hydrocodone may produce dose-related respiratory depression by acting directly on the brain stem respiratory center. Hydrocodone also affects the center that controls respiratory rhythm, and may produce irregular and periodic breathing.

Head Injury and Increased Intracranial Pressure

The respiratory depressant effects of opioids and their capacity to elevate cerebrospinal fluid pressure may be markedly exaggerated in the presence of head injury, other intracranial lesions or a preexisting increase in intracranial pressure. Furthermore, opioids produce adverse reactions which may obscure the clinical course of patients with head injuries.

Acute Abdominal Conditions

The administration of opioids may obscure the diagnosis or clinical course of patients with acute abdominal conditions.

PRECAUTIONS

General:

Special Risk Patients: As with any opioid analgesic agent, ZYDONE tablets should be used with caution in elderly or debilitated patients, and those with severe impairment of hepatic or renal function, hypothyroidism, Addison's disease, prostatic hypertrophy or urethral stricture. The usual precautions should be observed and the possibility of respiratory depression should be kept in mind.

Cough Reflex: Hydrocodone suppresses the cough reflex; as with all opioids, caution should be exercised when ZYDONE tablets are used postoperatively and in patients with pulmonary disease.

Information for Patients

Hydrocodone, like all opioids, may impair mental and/or physical abilities required for the performance of potentially hazardous tasks such as driving a car or operating machinery; patients should be cautioned accordingly.

Alcohol and other CNS depressants may produce an additive CNS depression, when taken with this combination product, and should be avoided.

Hydrocodone may be habit-forming. Patients should take the drug only for as long as it is prescribed, in the amounts prescribed, and no more frequently than prescribed.

Laboratory Tests

In patients with severe hepatic or renal disease, effects of therapy should be monitored with serial liver and/or renal function tests.

Drug Interactions

Patients receiving opioids, antihistamines, antipsychotics, antianxiety agents, or other CNS depressants (including alcohol) concomitantly with hydrocodone bitartrate and acetaminophen tablets may exhibit an additive CNS depression. When combined therapy is contemplated, the dose of one or both agents should be reduced.

The use of MAO inhibitors or tricyclic antidepressants with hydrocodone preparations may increase the effect of either the antidepressant or hydrocodone.

Drug/Laboratory Test Interactions

Acetaminophen may produce false-positive test results for urinary 5-hydroxyindoleacetic acid.

5 mg/400 mg Yellow, elongated octagonal, convex tablets debossed with "E" on one side and "5" on the other.	Bottles of 100	NDC 63481-668-70
7.5 mg/400 mg Blue, elongated octagonal, convex tablets debossed with "E" on one side and "7.5" on the other.	Bottles of 100	NDC 63481-669-70
10 mg/400 mg Red, elongated octagonal, convex tablets debossed with "E" on one side and "10" on the other.	Bottles of 100	NDC 63481-698-70

Carcinogenesis, Mutagenesis, Impairment of Fertility

No adequate studies have been conducted in animals to determine whether hydrocodone or acetaminophen have a potential for carcinogenesis, mutagenesis, or impairment of fertility.

Pregnancy

***Teratogenic Effects;* Pregnancy Category C:** There are no adequate and well-controlled studies in pregnant women. ZYDONE tablets should be used during pregnancy only if the potential benefit justifies the potential risk to the fetus.

Nonteratogenic Effects: Babies born to mothers who have been taking opioids regularly prior to delivery will be physically dependent. The withdrawal signs include irritability and excessive crying, tremors, hyperactive reflexes, increased respiratory rate, increased stools, sneezing, yawning, vomiting, and fever. The intensity of the syndrome does not always correlate with the duration of maternal opioid use or dose. There is no consensus on the best method of managing withdrawal.

Labor and Delivery

As with all opioids, administration of this product to the mother shortly before delivery may result in some degree of respiratory depression in the newborn, especially if higher doses are used.

Nursing Mothers

Acetaminophen is excreted in breast milk in small amounts, but the significance of its effects on nursing infants is not known. It is not known whether hydrocodone is excreted in human milk. Because many drugs are excreted in human milk and because of the potential for serious adverse reactions in nursing infants from hydrocodone and acetaminophen, a decision should be made whether to discontinue nursing or to discontinue the drug, taking into account the importance of the drug to the mother.

Pediatric Use

Safety and effectiveness in the pediatric patients have not been established.

ADVERSE REACTIONS

The most frequently reported adverse reactions are lightheadedness, dizziness, sedation, nausea and vomiting. These effects seem to be more prominent in ambulatory than in non-ambulatory patients, and some of these adverse reactions may be alleviated if the patient lies down.

Other adverse reactions include:

Central Nervous System: Drowsiness, mental clouding, lethargy, impairment of mental and physical performance, anxiety, fear, dysphoria, psychic dependence, mood changes.

Gastrointestinal System: Prolonged administration of ZYDONE (hydrocodone bitartrate and acetaminophen tablets) may produce constipation.

Genitourinary System: Ureteral spasm, spasm of vesical sphincters and urinary retention have been reported with opiates.

Respiratory Depression: Hydrocodone bitartrate may produce dose-related respiratory depression by acting directly on brain stem respiratory centers (see **OVERDOSAGE**).

Special Senses: Cases of hearing impairment or permanent loss have been reported predominantly in patients with chronic overdose.

Dermatological: Skin rash, pruritus.

The following adverse drug events may be borne in mind as potential effects of acetaminophen: allergic reactions, rash, thrombocytopenia, agranulocytosis.

Potential effects of high dosage are listed in the **OVERDOSAGE** section.

DRUG ABUSE AND DEPENDENCE

Controlled Substance

ZYDONE tablets are classified as a Schedule III controlled substance.

Abuse and Dependence

Psychic dependence, physical dependence, and tolerance may develop upon repeated administration of opioids; therefore, this product should be prescribed and administered with caution. However, psychic dependence is unlikely to develop when hydrocodone bitartrate and acetaminophen tablets are used for a short time for the treatment of pain. Physical dependence, the condition in which continued administration of the drug is required to prevent the appearance of a withdrawal syndrome, assumes clinically significant proportions only after several weeks of continued opioid use, although some mild degree of physical dependence may develop after a few days of opioid therapy. Tolerance, in which increasingly large doses are required in order to produce the same degree of analgesia, is manifested initially by a shortened duration of analgesic effect, and subsequently by decreases in the intensity of analgesia. The rate of development of tolerance varies among patients.

OVERDOSAGE

Following an acute overdosage, toxicity may result from hydrocodone or acetaminophen.

Signs and Symptoms

Hydrocodone: Serious overdose with hydrocodone is characterized by respiratory depression (a decrease in respiratory rate and/or tidal volume, Cheyne-Stokes respiration, cyanosis) extreme somnolence progressing to stupor or coma, sketetal muscle flaccidity, cold and clammy skin, and sometimes bradycardia and hypotension. In severe overdosage, apnea, circulatory collapse, cardiac arrest and death may occur.

Acetaminophen: In acetaminophen overdosage: dose-dependent, potentially fatal hepatic necrosis is the most serious adverse effect. Renal tubular necrosis, hypoglycemic coma and thrombocytopenia may also occur.

Early symptoms following a potentially hepatotoxic overdose may include: nausea, vomiting, diaphoresis and general malaise. Clinical and laboratory evidence of hepatic toxicity may not be apparent until 48 to 72 hours post-ingestion.

In adults, hepatic toxicity has rarely been reported with acute overdose of less than 10 grams or fatalities with less than 15 grams.

Treatment

A single or multiple overdose with hydrocodone and acetaminophen is a potentially lethal polydrug overdose, and consultation with a regional poison control center is recommended.

Immediate treatment includes support of cardiorespiratory function and measures to reduce drug absorption. Vomiting should be induced mechanically, or with syrup of ipecac, if the patient is alert (adequate pharyngeal and laryngeal reflexes). Oral activated charcoal (1 g/kg) should follow gastric emptying. The first dose should be accompanied by an appropriate cathartic. If repeated doses are used, the cathartic might be included with alternate doses as required. Hypotension is usually hypovolemic and should respond to fluids. Vasopressors and other supportive measures should be employed as indicated. A cuffed endotracheal tube should be inserted before gastric lavage of the unconscious patient and, when necessary, to provide assisted respiration.

Meticulous attention should be given to maintaining adequate pulmonary ventilation. In severe cases of intoxication, peritoneal dialysis, or preferably hemodialysis may be considered. If hypoprothrombinemia occurs due to acetaminophen overdose, vitamin K should be administered intravenously.

Naloxone, an opioid antagonist, can reverse respiratory depression and coma associated with opioid overdose. NARCAN® (naloxone hydrochloride) 0.4 mg to 2 mg is given parenterally. Since the duration of action of hydrocodone may exceed that of naloxone, the patient should be kept under continuous surveillance and repeated doses of the antagonist should be administered as needed to maintain adequate respiration. An opioid antagonist should not be administered in the absence of clinically significant respiratory or cardiovascular depression.

If the dose of acetaminophen may have exceeded 140 mg/kg, acetylcysteine should be administered as early as possible. Serum acetaminophen levels should be obtained, since levels four or more hours following ingestion help predict acetaminophen toxicity. Do not await acetaminophen assay results before initiating treatment. Hepatic enzymes should be obtained initially, and repeated at 24-hour intervals.

Methemoglobinemia over 30% should be treated with methylene blue by slow intravenous administration.

The toxic dose for adults for acetaminophen is 10 grams.

DOSAGE AND ADMINISTRATION

Dosage should be adjusted according to the severity of pain and response of the patient. However, it should be kept in mind that tolerance to hydrocodone can develop with continued use and that the incidence of untoward effects is dose related.

5 mg/400 mg: The usual adult dose is one or two tablets every four to six hours as needed for pain. The total daily dosage should not exceed eight tablets.

Continued on next page

Zydone—Cont.

7.5 mg/400 mg: The usual adult dosage is one tablet every four to six hours as needed for pain. The total daily dosage should not exceed six tablets.
10 mg/400 mg: The usual adult dosage is one tablet every four to six hours as needed for pain. The total daily dosage should not exceed six tablets.

HOW SUPPLIED

ZYDONE (hydrocodone bitartrate and acetaminophen tablets, USP) is supplied as follows:
[See table at top of previous page]
Store at 25°C (77°F); excursions permitted to 15°–30°C (59°–86°F). [See USP Controlled Room Temperature].
Dispense in a tight, light-resistant container as defined in the USP, with a child-resistant closure (as required).
A Schedule III Opioid. Oral prescription where permitted by State law.
ZYDONE® is a Registered Trademark of Endo Pharmaceuticals Inc.
NARCAN® is Registered Trademark of Endo Pharmaceuticals Inc.

6476-04/November, 2002
411242

Shown in Product Identification Guide, page 312

Enzon Pharmaceuticals, Inc.

685 ROUTE 202/206 N
BRIDGEWATER, NJ 08807

Direct Inquiries to:
908-541-8600

ABELCET® ℞

[*ā-bəl″set*]
(Amphotericin B Lipid Complex Injection)

DESCRIPTION

ABELCET® is a sterile, pyrogen-free suspension for intravenous infusion. ABELCET® consists of amphotericin B complexed with two phospholipids in a 1:1 drug-to-lipid molar ratio. The two phospholipids, L-α-dimyristoylphosphatidylcholine (DMPC) and L-α-dimyristoylphosphatidylglycerol (DMPG), are present in a 7:3 molar ratio. ABELCET® is yellow and opaque in appearance, with a pH of 5-7.

NOTE: Liposomal encapsulation or incorporation in a lipid complex can substantially affect a drug's functional properties relative to those of the unencapsulated or nonlipid-associated drug. In addition, different liposomal or lipid-complexed products with a common active ingredient may vary from one another in the chemical composition and physical form of the lipid component. Such differences may affect functional properties of these drug products.

Amphotericin B is a polyene, antifungal antibiotic produced from a strain of *Streptomyces nodosus*. Amphotericin B is designated chemically as [1R-(1R*, 3S*, 5R*, 6R*, 9R*, 11R*, 15S*, 16R*, 17R*, 18S*, 19E, 21E, 23E, 25E, 27E, 29E, 31E, 33R*, 35S*, 36R*, 37S*)]-33-[(3-Amino-3, 6-dideoxy-β-D-mannopyranosyl) oxy]-1,3,5,6,9,11,17,37-octahydroxy-15,16,18-trimethyl-13-oxo-14,39-dioxabicyclo[33.3.1] nonatriaconta-19, 21, 23, 25, 27, 29, 31-heptaene-36-carboxylic acid.

It has a molecular weight of 924.09 and a molecular formula of $C_{47}H_{73}NO_{17}$. The structural formula is:

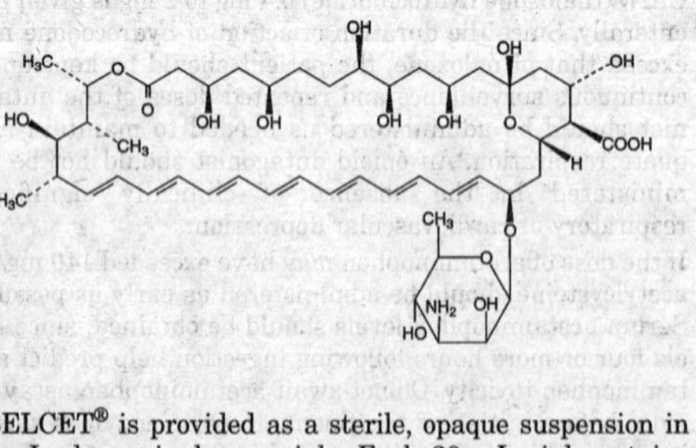

ABELCET® is provided as a sterile, opaque suspension in 20 mL glass, single-use vials. Each 20 mL vial contains 100 mg of amphotericin B (see DOSAGE AND ADMINISTRATION), and each mL of ABELCET® contains:

Amphotericin B USP	5 mg
L-α-dimyristoylphosphatidylcholine (DMPC)	3.4 mg
L-α-dimyristoylphosphatidylglycerol (DMPG)	1.5 mg
Sodium Chloride USP	9 mg
Water for Injection USP, q.s. 1 mL	

MICROBIOLOGY

Mechanism of Action

The active component of ABELCET®, amphotericin B, acts by binding to sterols in the cell membrane of susceptible fungi, with a resultant change in the permeability of the membrane. Mammalian cell membranes also contain sterols, and damage to human cells is believed to occur through the same mechanism of action.

Pharmacokinetic Parameters of Amphotericin B in Whole Blood in Patients Administered Multiple Doses of ABELCET® or Amphotericin B Desoxycholate

Pharmacokinetic Parameter	ABELCET® 5 mg/kg/day for 5–7 days Mean ± SD	Amphotericin B 0.6 mg/kg/day for 42 days[a] Mean ± SD
Peak Concentration (µg/mL	1.7 ± 0.8 (n=10)[b]	1.1 ± 0.2 (n=5)
Concentration at End of Dosing Interval (µg/mL)	0.6 ± 0.3 (n=10)[b]	0.4 ± 0.2 (n=5)
Area Under Blood Concentration-Time Curve (AUC_{0-24}) (µg•h/mL)	14 ± 7 (n=14)[b,c]	17.1 ± 5 (n=5)
Clearance (mL/h•kg)	436 ± 188.5 (n=14)[b,c]	38 ± 15 (n=5)
Apparent Volume of Distribution (Vd_{area}) (L/kg)	131 ± 57.7 (n=8)[c]	5 ± 2.8 (n=5)
Terminal Elimination Half-Life (h)	173.4 ± 78 (n=8)[c]	91.1 ± 40.9 (n=5)
Amount Excreted in Urine Over 24 h After Last Dose (% of dose)[d]	0.9 ± 0.4 (n=8)[c]	9.6 ± 2.5 (n=8)

[a] Data from patients with mucocutaneous leishmaniasis. Infusion rate was 0.25 mg/kg/h.
[b] Data from studies in patients with cytologically proven cancer being treated with chemotherapy or neutropenic patients with presumed or proven fungal infection. Infusion rate was 2.5 mg/kg/h.
[c] Data from patients with mucocutaneous leishmaniasis. Infusion rate was 4 mg/kg/h.
[d] Percentage of dose excreted in 24 hours after last dose.

Activity *in vitro* and *in vivo*

ABELCET® shows *in vitro* activity against *Aspergillus* sp. (n=3) and *Candida* sp. (n=10), with MICs generally <1 µg/mL. Depending upon the species and strain of *Aspergillus* and *Candida* tested, significant *in vitro* differences in susceptibility to amphotericin B have been reported (MICs ranging from 0.1 to >10 µg/mL). However, standardized techniques for susceptibility testing for antifungal agents have not been established, and results of susceptibility studies do not necessarily correlate with clinical outcome.
ABELCET® is active in animal models against *Aspergillus fumigatus, Candida albicans, C. guillermondii, C. stellatoideae,* and *C. tropicalis, Cryptococcus sp., Coccidioidomyces sp., Histoplasma sp., and Blastomyces sp.* in which endpoints were clearance of microorganisms from target organ(s) and/or prolonged survival of infected animals.

Drug Resistance

Fungal species with decreased susceptibility to amphotericin B have been isolated after serial passage in culture media containing the drug, and from some patients receiving prolonged therapy. Although the relevance of drug resistance to clinical outcome has not been established, fungal species which are resistant to amphotericin B may also be resistant to ABELCET®.

CLINICAL PHARMACOLOGY

Pharmacokinetics

The assay used to measure amphotericin B in the blood after the administration of ABELCET® does not distinguish amphotericin B that is complexed with the phospholipids of ABELCET® from amphotericin B that is uncomplexed.
The pharmacokinetics of amphotericin B after the administration of ABELCET® are nonlinear. Volume of distribution and clearance from blood increase with increasing dose of ABELCET®, resulting in less than proportional increases in blood concentrations of amphotericin B over a dose range of 0.6-5 mg/kg/day. The pharmacokinetics of amphotericin B in whole blood after the administration of ABELCET® and amphotericin B desoxycholate are:
[See table above]
The large volume of distribution and high clearance from blood of amphotericin B after the admistration of ABELCET® probably reflect uptake by tissues. The long terminal elimination half-life probably reflects a slow redistribution from tissues. Although amphotericin B is excreted slowly. there is little accumulation in the blood after repeated dosing. AUC of amphotericin B increased approximately 34% from day 1 after the administration of ABELCET® 5 mg/kg/day for 7 days. The effect of gender or ethnicity on the pharmacokinetics of ABELCET® has not been studied.
Tissue concentrations of amphotericin B have been obtained at autopsy from one heart transplant patient who received three doses of ABELCET® at 5.3 mg/kg/day:

Concentration in Human Tissues

Organ	Amphotericin B Tissue Concentration (µg/g)
Spleen	290
Lung	222
Liver	196
Lymph Node	7.6
Kidney	6.9
Heart	5
Brain	1.6

This pattern of distribution is consistent with that observed in preclinical studies in dogs in which greatest concentrations of amphotericin B after ABELCET® administration were observed in the liver, spleen, and lung; however, the relationship of tissue concentrations of amphotericin B to its biological activity when administered as ABELCET® is unknown.

Special Populations

Hepatic Impairment: The effect of hepatic impairment on the disposition of ABELCET® is not known.
Renal Impairment: The effect of renal impairment on the disposition of ABELCET® is not known. The effect of dialysis on the elimination of ABELCET® has not been studied; however, amphotericin B is not removed by hemodialysis when administered as amphotericin B desoxycholate.
Pediatric and Elderly Patients: The pharmacokinetics and pharmacodynamics of pediatric patients (≤16 years of age) and elderly patients (≥65 years of age) have not been studied.

INDICATIONS AND USAGE

ABELCET® indicated for the treatment of invasive fungal infections in patients who are refractory to or intolerant of conventional amphotericin B therapy. This is based on open-label treatment of patients judged by their physicians to be intolerant to or failing conventional amphotericin B therapy (See DESCRIPTION OF CLINICAL STUDIES).

DESCRIPTION OF CLINICAL STUDIES

Fungal infections

Data from 473 patients were pooled from three open-label studies in which ABELCET® was provided for the treatment of patients with invasive fungal infections who were judged by their physicians to be refractory to or intolerant of conventional amphotericin B, or who had preexisting nephrotoxicity. Results of these studies demonstrated effectiveness of ABELCET® in the treatment of invasive fungal infections as a second line therapy.
Patients were defined by their individual physician as being refractory to or falling conventional amphotericin B therapy based on overall clinical judgement after receiving a minimum total dose of 500 mg of amphotericin B. Nephrotoxicity was defined as a serum creatinine that had increased to >2.5 mg/dL in adults and >1.5 mg/dL in pediatric patients, or a creatinine clearance of <25 mL/min while receiving conventional amphotericin B therapy.
Of the 473 patients, four were enrolled more than once; each enrollment contributed separately to the denominator. The median age was 39 years (range of <1 to 93 years); 307 patients were male and 166 female. Patients were Caucasian (381, 81%), African-American (41, 9%), Hispanic (27, 6%), Asian (10, 2%), and various other races (14, 3%). The median baseline neutrophil count was 4,000 PMN/mm^3 of these, 101 (21%) had a baseline neutrophil count $<500/mm^3$.
Two-hundred eighty-two patients of the 473 patients were considered evaluable for response to therapy; the other 191 patients were excluded on the basis of unconfirmed diagnosis, confounding factors, concomitant systemic antifungal therapy, or receiving 4 doses or less of ABELCET®. For evaluable patients, the following fungal infections were treated (n=282): aspergillosis (n=111), candidiasis (n=87), zygomycosis (n=25), cryptococcosis (n=16), and fusariosis (n=11). There were fewer than 10 evaluable patients for each of several other fungal species treated.
For each type of fungal infection listed above there were some patients successfully treated. However, in the absence of controlled studies it is unknown how response would have compared to either continuing conventional amphotericin B therapy or the use of alternative antifungal agents.
Renal Function: Patients with aspergillosis who initiated treatment with ABELCET® when serum creatinine was above 2.5 mg/dL experienced a decline in serum creatinine during treatment (Figure 1). Serum creatinine levels were also lower during treatment with ABELCET® when compared to the serum creatinine levels of patients treated with conventional amphotericin B in a retrospective historical control study. Meaningful statistical testing of the differences between these two groups in precluded since these data were obtained from two separate studies.
[See figure 1 at top of next column]
[See figure 2 at top of next column]
In a randomized study of ABELCET® for the treatment of invasive candidiasis in patients with normal baseline renal function, the incidence of nephrotoxicity was significantly less for ABELCET® at a dose of 5 mg/kg/day than for conventional amphotericin B at a dose of 0.7 mg/kg/day.
Despite generally less nephrotoxicity of ABELCET® observed at a dose of 5 mg/kg/day compared with conventional amphotericin B therapy at a dose range of 0.6-1 mg/kg/day, dose-limiting renal toxicity may still be observed with ABELCET®. Renal toxicity of doses greater than 5 mg/kg/day of ABELCET® has not been formally studied.

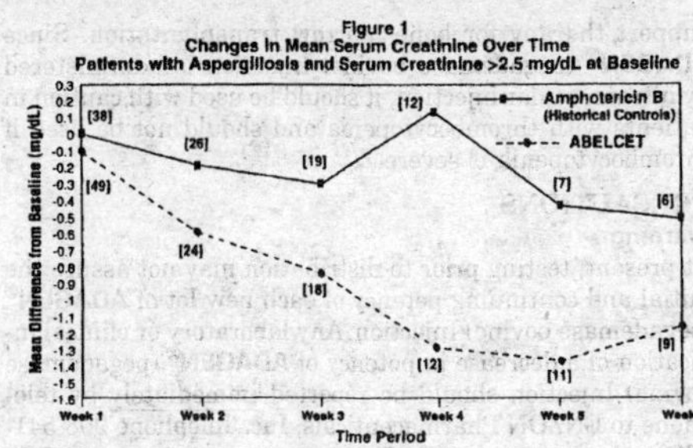

[ ]= Number of patients at each time point.
Note: These curves do not represent the clinical course of a given patient, but that of an open-label cohort of patients.

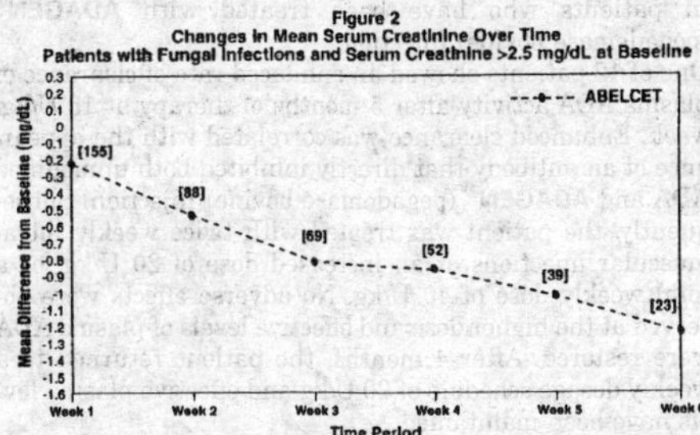

[ ]= Number of patients at each time point.
Note: These curves do not represent the clinical course of a given patient, but that of an open-label cohort of patients.

CONTRAINDICATIONS

ABELCET® is contraindicated in patients who have shown hypersensitivity to amphotericin B or any other component in the formulation.

WARNINGS

Anaphylaxis has been reported with amphotericin B desoxycholate and other amphotericin B-containing drugs. Anaphylaxis has been reported with ABELCET® with an incidence rate of <0.1%. If severe respiratory distress occurs, the infusion should be immediately discontinued. The patient should not receive further infusions of ABELCET®.

PRECAUTIONS

General: As with any amphotericin B-containing product, during the initial dosing of ABELCET®, the drug should be administered under close clinical observation by medically trained personnel.

Acute reactions including fever and chills may occur 1 to 2 hours after starting an intravenous infusion of ABELCET®. These reactions are usually more common with the first few doses of ABELCET® and generally diminish with subsequent doses. Infusion has been rarely associated with hypotension, bronchospasm, arrhythmias, and shock.

Laboratory Tests: Serum creatinine should be monitored frequently during ABELCET® therapy (see ADVERSE REACTIONS). It is also advisable to regularly monitor liver function, serum electrolytes (particularly magnesium and potassium), and complete blood counts.

Drug Interactions: No formal clinical studies of drug interactions have been conducted with ABELCET®. However, when administered concomitantly, the following drugs are known to interact with amphotericin B; therefore, the following drugs may interact with ABELCET®:

Antineoplastic agents: Concurrent use of antineoplastic agents and amphotericin B may enhance the potential for renal toxicity, bronchospasm, and hypotension. Antineoplastic agents should be given concomitantly with ABELCET® with great caution.

Corticosteroids and corticotropin (ACTH): Concurrent use of corticosteroids and corticotropin (ACTH) with amphotericin B may potentiate hypokalemia which could predispose the patient to cardiac dysfunction. If used concomitantly with ABELCET®, serum electrolytes and cardiac function should be closely monitored.

Cyclosporin A: Data from a prospective study of prophylactic ABELCET® in 22 patients undergoing bone marrow transplantation suggested that concurrent initiation of cyclosporin A and ABELCET® within several days of bone marrow ablation may be associated with increased nephrotoxicity.

Digitalis glycosides: Concurrent use of amphotericin B may induce hypokalemia and may potentiate digitalis toxicity. When administered concomitantly with ABELCET®, serum potassium levels should be closely monitored.

Flucytosine: Concurrent use of flucytosine with amphotericin B-containing preparations may increase the toxicity of flucytosine by possibly increasing its cellular uptake and/or impairing its renal excretion. Flucytosine should be given concomitantly with ABELCET® with caution.

Imidazoles (e.g., ketoconazole, miconazole, clotrimazole, fluconazole, etc.): Antagonism between amphotericin B and imidazole derivatives such as miconazole and ketoconazole, which inhibit ergosterol synthesis, has been reported in both *in vitro* and *in vivo* animal studies. The clinical significance of these findings has not been determined.

Leukocyte transfusions: Acute pulmonary toxicity has been reported in patients receiving intravenous amphotericin B and leukocyte transfusions. Leukocyte transfusions and ABELCET® should not be given concurrently.

Other nephrotoxic medications: Concurrent use of amphotericin B and agents such as aminoglcosides and pentamidine may enhance the potential for drug-induced renal toxicity. Aminoglycosides and pentamidine should be used concomitantly with ABELCET® only with great caution. Intensive monitoring of renal function is recommended in patients requiring any combination of nephrotoxic medications.

Skeletal muscle relaxants: Amphotericin B-induced hypokalemia may enhance the curariform effect of skeletal muscle relaxants (e.g., tubocurarine) due to hypokalemia. When administered concomitantly with ABELCET®, serum potassium levels should be closely monitored.

Zidovudine: Increased myelotoxicity and nephrotoxicity were observed in dogs when either ABELCET® (at doses 0.16 or 0.5 times the recommended human dose) or amphotericin B desoxycholate (at 0.5 times the recommended human dose) were administered concomitantly with zidovudine for 30 days. If zidovudine is used concomitantly with ABELCET®, renal and hematologic function should be closely monitored.

Carcinogenesis, Mutagenesis, and Impairment of Fertility: No long-term studies in animals have been performed to evaluate the carcinogenic potential of ABELCET®. The following *in vitro* (with and without metabolic activation) and *in vivo* studies to assess ABELCET® for mutagenic potential were conducted: bacterial reverse mutation assay, mouse lymphoma forward mutation assay, chromosomal aberration assay in CHO cells, and *in vivo* mouse micronucleus assay. ABELCET® was found to be without mutagenic effects in all assay systems. Studies demonstrated that ABELCET® had no impact on fertility in male and female rats at doses up to 0.32 times the recommended human dose (based on body surface area considerations).

Pregnancy: There are no reports of pregnant women having been treated with ABELCET®. Teratogenic Effects. Pregnancy Category B: Reproductive studies in rats and rabbits at doses of ABELCET® up to 0.64 times the human dose revealed no harm to the fetus. Because animal reproductive studies are not always predictive of human response, and adequate and well-controlled studies have not been conducted in pregnant women. ABELCET® should be used during pregnancy only after taking into account the importance of the drug to the mother.

Nursing Mothers: It is not known whether ABELCET® is excreted in human milk. Because many drugs are excreted in human milk, and because of the potential for serious adverse reactions in breast-fed infants from ABELCET®, a decision should be made whether to discontinue nursing or to discontinue the drug, taking into account the importance of the drug to the mother.

Pediatric Use: One hundred eleven children (2 were enrolled twice and counted as separate patients), age 16 years and under, of whom 11 were less than 1 year, have been treated with ABELCET® at 5 mg/kg/day in two open-label studies and one small, prospective, single-arm study. In one single-center study, 5 children with hepatosplenic candidiasis were effectively treated with 2.5 mg/kg/day of ABELCET®. No serious unexpected adverse events have been reported.

Geriatric Use: Forty-nine elderly patients, age 65 years or over, have been treated with ABELCET® at 5 mg/kg/day in two open-label studies and one small, prospective, single-arm study. No serious unexpected adverse events have been reported.

ADVERSE REACTIONS

The total safety data base is composed of 921 patients treated with ABELCET® (5 patients were enrolled twice and counted as separate patients), of whom 775 were treated with 5 mg/kg/day. Of these 775 patients, 194 patients were treated in four comparative studies; 25 were treated in open-label, non-comparative studies; and 556 patients were treated in an open-label, emergency-use program. Most had underlying hematologic neoplasms, and many were receiving multiple concomitant medications. Of the 556 patients treated with ABELCET®, 9% discontinued treatment due to adverse events regardless of presumed relationship to study drug.

In general, the adverse events most commonly reported with ABELCET® were transient chills and/or fever during infusion of the drug.

Adverse Events[a] with an incidence of ≥3% (N=556)

Adverse Event	Percentage (%) of Patients
Chills	18
Fever	14
Increased Serum Creatitine	11
Multiple Organ Failure	11
Nausea	9
Hypotension	8
Respiratory Failure	8
Vomiting	8
Dyspnea	7
Sepsis	7
Diarrhea	6
Headache	6
Heart Arrest	6
Hypertension	5
Hypokalemia	5
Infection	5
Kidney Failure	5
Pain	5
Thrombocytopenia	5
Abdominal Pain	4
Anemia	4
Bilirubinemia	4
Gastrointestinal Hemorrhage	4
Leukopenia	4
Rash	4
Respiratory Disorder	4
Chest Pain	3
Nausea and Vomiting	3

[a] The causal association between these adverse events and ABELCET® is uncertain.

The following adverse events have also been reported in patients using ABELCET® in open-label, uncontrolled clinical studies. The causal association between these adverse events and ABELCET® is uncertain.

Body as a whole: malaise, weight loss, deafness, injection site reaction including inflammation

Allergic bronchospasm, wheezing, asthma, anaphylactoid and other allergic reactions

Cardiopulmonary: cardiac failure, pulmonary edema, shock, myocardial infarction, hemoptysis, tachypnea, thrombophlebitis, pulmonary embolus, cardiomyopathy, pleural effusion, arrhythmias including ventricular fibrillation.

Dermatological: maculopapular rash, pruritus, exfoliative dermatitis, erythema multiforme

Gastrointestinal: acute liver failure, hepatitis, jaundice, melena, anorexia, dyspepsia, cramping, epigastric pain, veno-occlusive liver disease, diarrhea, hepatomegaly, cholangitis, cholecystitis

Hematologic: coagulation defects, leukocytosis, blood dyscrasias including eosinophilia

Musculoskeletal: myasthenia, including bone, muscle, and joint pains

Neurologic: convulsions, tinnitus, visual impairment, hearing loss, peripheral neuropathy, transient vertigo, diplopia, encephalopathy, cerebral vascular accident, extrapyramidal syndrome and other neurologic symptoms

Urogenital: oliguria, decreased renal function, anuria, renal tubular acidosis, impotence, dysuria

Serum electrolyte abnormalities: hypomagnesemia, hyperkalemia, hypocalcemia, hypercalcemia

Liver function test abnormalities: increased AST, ALT, alkaline phosphatase, LDH

Renal function test abnormalities: increased BUN

Other test abnormalities: acidosis, hyperamylasemia, hypoglycemia, hyperglycemia, hyperuricemia, hypophosphatemia

OVERDOSAGE

Amphotericin B desoxycholate overdose has been reported to result in cardio-respiratory arrest. Fifteen patients have been reported to have received one or more doses of ABELCET® between 7-13 mg/kg. None of these patients had a serious acute reaction to ABELCET®. If an overdose is suspected, discontinue therapy, monitor the patient's clinical status, and administer supportive therapy as required. ABELCET® is not hemodialyzable.

DOSAGE AND ADMINISTRATION

The recommended daily dosage for adults and children is 5 mg/kg given as a single infusion. ABELCET® should be administered by intravenous infusion at a rate of 2.5 mg/kg/h. If the infusion time exceeds 2 hours, mix the contents by shaking the infusion bag every 2 hours.

Renal toxicity of ABELCET®, as measured by serum creatinine levels, has been shown to be dose dependent. Decisions about dose adjustments should be made only after taking into account the overall clinical condition of the patient.

Preparation of Admixture for Infusion: Shake the vial gently until there is no evidence of any yellow sediment at the bottom. Withdraw the appropriate dose of ABELCET® from the required number of vials into one or more sterile syringes using an 18-gauge needle. Remove the needle from each syringe filled with ABELCET® and replace with the 5-micron filter needle supplied with each vial. Each filter needle may be used to filter the contents of up to four 100 mg vials. Insert the filter needle of the syringe into an IV bag containing 5% Dextrose Injection USP, and empty the contents of the syringe into the bag. The final infusion concentration should be 1 mg/mL. For pediatric patients and patients with cardiovascular disease the drug may be diluted with 5% Dextrose Injection to a final infusion concentration of 2 mg/mL. Before infusion, shake the bag until the contents are thoroughly mixed. Do not use the admixture after dilution with 5% Dextrose Injection if there is any evidence of foreign matter. Vials are for single use. Unused material should be discarded. Aseptic technique must be strictly observed throughout handling of ABELCET®, since no bacteriostatic agent or preservative is present.

DO NOT DILUTE WITH SALINE SOLUTIONS OR MIX WITH OTHER DRUGS OR ELECTROLYTES as the compatibility of ABELCET® with these materials has not been established. An existing intravenous line should be flushed

Continued on next page

Abelcet—Cont.

with 5% Dextrose Injection before infusion of ABELCET®, or a separate infusion line should be used. DO NOT USE AN IN-LINE FILTER.
The diluted ready-for-use admixture is stable for up to 48 hours at 2° to 8°C (36° to 46°F) and additional 6 hours at room temperature.

HOW SUPPLIED

Single-use vials along with 5-micron filter needles are individually packaged.
100 mg of ABELCET® in 20 mL of suspension NDC 57665-101-41

STORAGE

Prior to admixture, ABELCET® should be stored at 2° to 8°C (36° to 46°F) and protected from exposure to light. Do not freeze. ABELCET® should be retained in the carton until time of use.
The admixed ABELCET® and 5% Dextrose Injection may be stored for up to 48 hours at 2° to 8°C (36° to 46°F) and an additional 6 hours at room temperature. Do not freeze. Any unused material should be discarded.
U.S. Patent Nos. 4,973,465
5,616,334 11/02
I-101-41-US-K

ENZON Pharmaceuticals

Distributed by: ENZON Pharmaceuticals, Piscataway, NJ 08854
ABELCET® is a registered trademark of ENZON Pharmaceuticals.

ADAGEN® ℞

[ădă-jĕn]
(pegademase bovine) Injection

DESCRIPTION

ADAGEN® (pegademase bovine) Injection is a modified enzyme used for enzyme replacement therapy for the treatment of severe combined immunodeficiency disease (SCID) associated with a deficiency of adenosine deaminase.
ADAGEN® (pegademase bovine) Injection is supplied in an isotonic, pyrogen free, sterile solution, pH 7.2–7.4, for intramuscular injection only. The solution is clear and colorless. It is supplied in 1.5 mL single-dose vials.
The chemical name for **ADAGEN®** (pegademase bovine) Injection is (monomethoxypolyethylene glycol succinimidyl)$_{11-17}$-adenosine deaminase. It is a conjugate of numerous strands of monomethoxypolyethylene glycol (PEG), molecular weight 5,000, covalently attached to the enzyme adenosine deaminase (ADA). ADA (adenosine deaminase EC 3.5.4.4) used in the manufacture of **ADAGEN®** (pegademase bovine) Injection is derived from bovine intestine.
The structural formula of **ADAGEN®** (pegademase bovine) Injection is:

$$[CH_3\text{-}(OCH_2CH_2)_x\text{-}O\text{-}\underset{\substack{\|\\ O}}{C}\text{-}CH_2CH_2\text{-}\underset{\substack{\|\\ O}}{C}\text{-}NH]_y\text{-adenosine deaminase}$$

x≈ 114 oxyethylene groups per PEG strand.
y≈ 11-17 primary amino groups of lysine onto which succinyl PEG is attached.

Each milliliter of **ADAGEN®** (pegademase bovine) Injection contains:

Pegademase bovine	250 units*
Monobasic sodium phosphate, USP	1.20 mg
Dibasic sodium phosphate, USP	5.58 mg
Sodium Chloride, USP	8.50 mg
Water for injection, USP	q.s. to 1.0 mL

*One unit of activity is defined as the amount of ADA that converts 1 μM of adenosine to inosine per minute at 25° C and pH 7.3.

CLINICAL PHARMACOLOGY

Severe Combined Immunodeficiency Disease Associated with ADA Deficiency

Severe combined immunodeficiency disease (SCID) associated with a deficiency of ADA is a rare, inherited, and often fatal disease. In the absence of the ADA enzyme, the purine substrates adenosine and 2′-deoxyadenosine accumulate, causing metabolic abnormalities that are directly toxic to lymphocytes.
The immune deficiency can be cured by bone marrow transplantation. When a suitable bone marrow donor is unavailable or when bone marrow transplantation fails, non-selective replacement of the ADA enzyme has been provided by periodic irradiated red blood cell transfusions. However, transmission of viral infections and iron overload are serious risks associated with irradiated red blood cell transfusions, and relatively few ADA deficient patients have benefitted from chronic transfusion therapy.
ADAGEN® (pegademase bovine) Injection provides specific and direct replacement of the deficient enzyme, but will not benefit patients with immunodeficiency due to other causes.
In patients with ADA deficiency, rigorous adherence to a schedule of **ADAGEN®** (pegademase bovine) Injection administration can eliminate the toxic metabolites of ADA deficiency and result in improved immune function. It is imperative that treatment with **ADAGEN®** (pegademase bovine) Injection be carefully monitored by measurement of the level of ADA activity in plasma. Monitoring of the level of deoxyadenosine triphosphate (dATP) in erythrocytes is also helpful in determining that the dose of **ADAGEN®** (pegademase bovine) Injection is adequate.

Actions

ADAGEN® (pegademase bovine) Injection provides specific replacement of the deficient enzyme.
In the absence of the enzyme ADA, the purine substrates adenosine, 2′-deoxyadenosine and their metabolites are toxic to lymphocytes. The direct action of **ADAGEN®** (pegademase bovine) Injection is the correction of these metabolic abnormalities. Improvement in immune function and diminished frequency of opportunistic infections compared with the natural history of combined immunodeficiency due to ADA deficiency only occurs after metabolic abnormalities are corrected. There is a lag between the correction of the metabolic abnormalities and improved immune function. This period of time is variable, and has been reported to be from a few weeks to as long as 6 months. In contrast to the natural history of combined immunodeficiency disease due to ADA deficiency, a trend toward diminished frequency of opportunistic infections and fewer complications of infections has occurred in patients receiving **ADAGEN®** (pegademase bovine) Injection.

Pharmacokinetics

The pharmacokinetics and biochemical of **ADAGEN®** (pegademase bovine) Injection have been studied in six children ranging in age from 6 weeks to 12 years with SCID associated with ADA deficiency.
After the intramuscular Injection of **ADAGEN®** (pegademase bovine) Injection, peak plasma levels of ADA activity were reached 2 to 3 days following administration. The plasma elimination half-life of ADA following the administration of **ADAGEN®** (pegademase bovine) Injection was variable, even for the same child. The range was 3 to > 6 days. Following weekly injections of **ADAGEN®** (pegademase bovine) Injection at 15 U/kg, the average trough level of ADA activity in plasma was between 20 and 25 μmol/hr/mL.

Biochemical Effects

The changes in red blood cell deoxyadenosine nucleotide (dATP) and S-adenosylhomocysteine hydrolase (SAHase) have been evaluated. In patients with ADA deficiency, inadequate elimination of 2′-deoxyadenosine caused a marked elevation in dATP and a decrease in SAHase level in red blood cells. Prior to treatment with **ADAGEN®** (pegademase bovine) Injection, the levels of dATP in the red blood cells ranged from 0.056 to 0.899 μmol/mL of erythrocytes. After 2 months of maintenance treatment with **ADAGEN®** (pegademase bovine) Injection, the levels decreased to 0.007 to 0.015 μmol/mL. The normal value of dATP is below 0.001 μmol/mL. In the same period of time, the levels of SAHase increased from the pretreatment range of 0.09 to 0.22 nmol/hr/mg protein to a range of 2.37 to 5.16 nmol/hr/mg protein. The normal value for SAHase is 4.18± 1.9 nmol/hr/mg protein.
The optimal dosage and schedule of administration of **ADAGEN®** (pegademase bovine) Injection should be established for each patient, based on monitoring of plasma ADA activity levels (trough levels before maintenance injection), biochemical markers of ADA deficiency (primarily red cell dATP content), and parameters of immune function. Since improvement in immune function follows correction of metabolic abnormalities, maintenance dosage in individual patients should be aimed at achieving the following biochemical goals: 1) maintain plasma ADA activity (trough levels) in the range of 15–35 μmol/hr/mL (assayed at 37° C); and 2) decline in erythrocyte dATP to ≤0.005–0.015 μmol/mL packed erythrocytes, or ≤1% of the total erythrocyte adenine nucleotide (ATP + dATP) content, with a normal ATP level, as measured in a pre-injection sample.
In vitro immunologic data (lymphocyte response to mitogens and lymphocyte surface antigens) were obtained, but their clinical significance is unknown. Prior to treatment with **ADAGEN®** (pegademase bovine) Injection, immune status was significantly below normal, as indicated by <10% of normal mitogen responses and circulating mononuclear cells bearing T-cell surface antigens. These parameters improved, though not always to normal, within 2 to 6 months of therapy.

INDICATIONS AND USAGE

ADAGEN® (pegademase bovine) Injection is indicated for enzyme replacement therapy for adenosine deaminase (ADA) deficiency in patients with severe combined immunodeficiency disease (SCID) who are not suitable candidates for – or who have failed – bone marrow transplantation.
ADAGEN® (pegademase bovine) Injection is recommended for use in infants from birth or in children of any age at the time of diagnosis. **ADAGEN®** (pegademase bovine) Injection is not intended as a replacement for HLA identical bone marrow transplant therapy. **ADAGEN®** (pegademase bovine) Injection is also not intended to replace continued close medical supervision and the initiation of appropriate diagnostic tests and therapy (e.g., antibiotics, nutrition, oxygen, gammaglobulin) as indicated for intercurrent illnesses.

CONTRAINDICATIONS

There is no evidence to support the safety and efficacy of **ADAGEN®** (pegademase bovine) Injection as preparatory or support therapy for bone marrow transplantation. Since **ADAGEN®** (pegademase bovine) Injection is administered by intramuscular injection, it should be used with caution in patients with thrombocytopenia and should not be used if thrombocytopenia is severe.

PRECAUTIONS

Warning

At present, testing prior to distribution may not assure the initial and continuing potency of each new lot of **ADAGEN®** (pegademase bovine) Injection. Any laboratory or clinical indication of a decrease in potency of **ADAGEN®** (pegademase bovine) Injection should be reported immediately by telephone to ENZON Pharmaceuticals, Inc. Telephone 908-541-8600.

General

There have been no reports of hypersensitivity reactions in patients who have been treated with **ADAGEN®** (pegademase bovine) Injection.
One of 12 patients showed an enhanced rate of clearance of plasma ADA activity after 5 months of therapy at 15 U/kg/week. Enhanced clearance was correlated with the appearance of an antibody that directly inhibited both unmodified ADA and **ADAGEN®** (pegademase bovine) Injection. Subsequently, the patient was treated with twice weekly intramuscular injections at an increased dose of 20 U/kg, or a total weekly dose of 40 U/kg. No adverse effects were observed at the higher dose and effective levels of plasma ADA were restored. After 4 months, the patient returned to a weekly dosage schedule of 20 U/kg and effective plasma levels have been maintained.
Appropriate care to protect immune deficient patients should be maintained until improvement to immune function has been documented. The degree of immune function improvement may vary from patient to patient and, therefore, each patient will require appropriate care consistent with immunologic status.

Laboratory Tests

The treatment of SCID associated with ADA deficiency with **ADAGEN®** (pegademase bovine) Injection should be monitored by measuring plasma ADA activity and red blood cell dATP levels.
Plasma ADA activity and red cell dATP should be determined prior to treatment. Once treatment with **ADAGEN®** (pegademase bovine) Injection has been initiated, a desirable range of plasma ADA activity (trough level before maintenance injection) should be 15–35 μmol/hr/mL. This minimum trough level will ensure that plasma ADA activity from injection to injection is maintained above the level of total erythrocyte ADA activity in the blood of normal individuals.
Plasma ADA activity (pre-injection) should be determined every 1–2 weeks during the first 8–12 weeks of treatment in order to establish an effective dose of **ADAGEN®** (pegademase bovine) Injection. After two months of maintenance treatment with **ADAGEN®** (pegademase bovine) Injection, red cell dATP levels decrease to a range of ≤0.005 to 0.015 μmol/mL. The normal value of dATP is below 0.001 μmol/mL. Once the level of dATP has fallen adequately, it should be measured 2–4 times a year during the remainder of the first year and 2–3 times a year thereafter, assuming no interruption in therapy.
Between 3 and 9 months, plasma ADA should be determined twice a month, then monthly until after 18–24 months of treatment with **ADAGEN®** (pegademase bovine) Injection.
Patients who have successfully been maintained on therapy for two years should continue to have plasma ADA measured every 2–4 months and red cell dATP measured twice yearly. More frequent monitoring would be necessary if therapy were interrupted or if an enhanced rate of clearance of plasma ADA activity develops.
Once effective ADA plasma levels have been established, should a patient's plasma ADA activity level fall below 10 μmol/hr/mL (which cannot be attributed to improper dosing, sample handling or antibody development) then all patients receiving this lot of **ADAGEN®** (pegademase bovine) Injection will be required to have a blood sample for plasma ADA determination taken prior to their next injection of **ADAGEN®** (pegademase bovine) Injection. The index patient will require re-testing for determination of plasma ADA activity prior to his/her next injection of **ADAGEN®** (pegademase bovine) Injection. If this value, as well as the value from one of the other patients from a different site, is less than 10 μmol/hr/mL then the lot in use will be recalled and replaced with a new clinical lot by ENZON Pharmaceuticals, Inc.
Immune function, including the ability to produce antibodies, generally improves after 2–6 months of therapy, and matures over a longer period. Compared with the natural history of combined immunodeficiency disease due to ADA deficiency, a trend toward diminished frequency of opportunistic infections and fewer complications of infections has occurred in patients receiving **ADAGEN®** (pegademase bovine) Injection. However, the lag between the correction of the metabolic abnormalities and improved immune function with a trend toward diminished frequency of infections and complications of infection is variable, and has ranged from a few weeks to approximately 6 months. Improvement in the general clinical status of the patient may be gradual (as evidenced by improvement in various clinical parameters) but should be apparent by the end of the first year of therapy.
Antibody to **ADAGEN®** (pegademase bovine) Injection may develop in patients and may result in more rapid clearance

of **ADAGEN®** (pegademase bovine) Injection. Antibody to **ADAGEN®** (pegademase bovine) Injection should be suspected if a persistent fall in pre-injection levels of plasma ADA to <10 μmol/hr/mL occurs. If other causes for a decline in plasma ADA levels can be ruled out [such a improper storage of **ADAGEN®** (pegademase bovine) Injection vials (freezing or prolonged storage at temperatures above 8° C), or improper handling of plasma samples (e.g., repeated freezing and thawing during transport to laboratory)], then a specific assay for antibody to ADA and **ADAGEN®** (pegademase bovine) Injection (ELISA, enzyme inhibition) should be performed.

In patients undergoing treatment with **ADAGEN®** (pegademase bovine) Injection, a decline in immune function, with increased risk of opportunistic infections and complications of infection, will result from failure to maintain adequate levels of plasma ADA activity [whether due to the development of antibody to **ADAGEN®** (pegademase bovine) Injection, to improper calculation of **ADAGEN®** (pegademase bovine) Injection dosage, to interruption of treatment or to improper storage of **ADAGEN®** (pegademase bovine) Injection with subsequent loss of activity]. If a persistent decline in plasma ADA activity occurs, immune function and clinical status should be monitored closely and precautions should be taken to minimize the risk of infection. If antibody to ADA or **ADAGEN®** (pegademase bovine) Injection is found to be the cause of a persistent fall in plasma ADA activity, then adjustment in the dosage of **ADAGEN®** (pegademase bovine) Injection and other measures may be taken to induce tolerance and restore adequate ADA activity.

Drug Interactions

There are no known drug interactions with **ADAGEN®** (pegademase bovine) Injection. However, Vidarabine is a substrate for ADA and 2′-deoxycoformycin is a potent inhibitor of ADA. Thus, the activities of these drugs and **ADAGEN®** (pegademase bovine) Injection could be substantially altered if they are used in combination with one another.

Carcinogenesis, Mutagenesis, Impairment of Fertility

Long-term carcinogenic studies in animals have not been performed with **ADAGEN®** (pegademase bovine) Injection nor have studies been performed on impairment of fertility. **ADAGEN®** (pegademase bovine) Injection did not exhibit a mutagenic effect when tested against Salmonella typhimurium strains in the Ames assay.

Pregnancy

Pregnancy Category C. Animal reproduction studies have not been conducted with **ADAGEN®** (pegademase bovine) Injection. It is also not known whether **ADAGEN®** (pegademase bovine) Injection can cause fetal harm when administered to a pregnant woman or can affect reproduction capacity. **ADAGEN®** (pegademase bovine) Injection should be given to a pregnant woman only if clearly needed.

Nursing Mothers

It is not known whether **ADAGEN®** (pegademase bovine) Injection is excreted in human milk. Because many drugs are excreted in human milk, caution should be exercised when **ADAGEN®** (pegademase bovine) Injection is administered to a nursing woman.

ADVERSE REACTIONS

Clinical experience with **ADAGEN®** (pegademase bovine) Injection has been limited. The following adverse reactions have been reported: headache in one patient and pain at the injection site in two patients.

OVERDOSAGE

There is no documented experience with **ADAGEN®** (pegademase bovine) Injection overdosage. An intraperitoneal dose of 50,000 U/kg of **ADAGEN®** (pegademase bovine) Injection in mice resulted in weight loss up to 9%.

DOSAGE AND ADMINISTRATION

Before prescribing **ADAGEN®** (pegademase bovine) Injection the physician should be thoroughly familiar with the details of this prescribing information. For further information concerning the essential monitoring of **ADAGEN®** (pegademase bovine) Injection therapy, the prescribing physician should contact ENZON Pharmaceuticals, Inc., 20 Kingsbridge Road, Piscataway, NJ 08854-3969. Telephone 908-541-8600.

ADAGEN® (pegademase bovine) Injection is recommended for use in infants from birth or in children of any age at the time of diagnosis.

Parenteral drug products should be inspected visually for particulate matter and discoloration prior to administration, whenever solution and container permits.

ADAGEN® (pegademase bovine) Injection should not be diluted nor mixed with any other drug prior to administration.

ADAGEN® (pegademase bovine) Injection should be administered every 7 days as an intramuscular injection. The dosage of **ADAGEN®** (pegademase bovine) Injection should be individualized. The recommended dosing schedule is 10 U/kg for the first dose, 15 U/kg for the second dose, and 20 U/kg for the third dose. The usual maintenance dose is 20 U/kg per week. Further increases of 5 U/kg/week may be necessary, but a maximum single dose of 30 U/kg should not be exceeded. Plasma levels of ADA more than twice the upper limit of 35 μmol/hr/mL have occurred on occasion in several patients, and have been maintained for several weeks in one patient who received twice weekly injections (20 U/kg per dose) of **ADAGEN®** (pegademase bovine) Injection. No adverse effects have been observed at these higher levels; there is no evidence that maintaining per-injection plasma ADA above 35 μmol/hr/mL produces any additional clinical benefits.

Dose proportionality has not been established and patients should be closely monitored when the dosage is increased. **ADAGEN®** (pegademase bovine) Injection is not recommended for intravenous administration.

The optimal dosage and schedule of administration should be established for each patient based on monitoring of plasma ADA activity levels (trough levels before maintenance injection) and biochemical markers of ADA deficiency (primarily red cell dATP content). Since improvement in immune function follows correction of metabolic abnormalities, maintenance dosage in individual patients should be aimed at achieving the following biochemical goals: 1) maintain plasma ADA activity (trough levels before maintenance injection) in the range of 15–35 μmol/hr/mL (assayed at 37° C); and 2) decline in erythrocyte dATP to ≤0.005–0.015 μmol/mL packed erythrocytes, or ≤1% of the total erythrocyte adenine nucleotide (ATP + dATP) content, with a normal ATP level, as measured in a pre-injection sample. In addition, continued monitoring of immune function and clinical status is essential in any patient with a primary immunodeficiency disease and should be continued in patients undergoing treatment with **ADAGEN®** (pegademase bovine) Injection.

HOW SUPPLIED

ADAGEN® (pegademase bovine) Injection is a clear, colorless solution for intramuscular injection. Each vial contains 250 units/mL and is supplied as a 1.5 mL single-use vial, in boxes of 4 vials (NDC-57665-001-01).

Refrigerate. Store between +2° C and +8° C 36° F and 46° F). DO NOT FREEZE. **ADAGEN®** (pegademase bovine) Injection should not be stored at room temperature. This product should not be used if there are any indications that it may have been frozen.

REFERENCES

1. Hershfield MS, Buckley RH, Greenberg ML, et al. Treatment of adenosine deaminase deficiency with polyethylene glycol-modified adenosine deaminase. N Engl J Med 1987; 316:589–96.
2. Levy Y, Hershfield MS, Fernandez-Mejia C, Polmar ST, Scudiery D, Berger M, Sorensen RU. Adenosine deaminase deficiency with late onset of recurrent infections: response to treatment with polyethylene glycol-modified adenosine deaminase. J Pediatr 1988; 113:312–17.
3. Kredich NM, Hershfield MS. Immunodeficiency diseases caused by adenosine deaminase deficiency and purine nucleoside phosphorylase deficiency. 6th ed. In: Scriver CR, Beaudet AL, Sly WS, Valle D, eds. The metabolic basis of inherited disease. New York: McGraw Hill, 1989; 1045–75.
4. Hirschhorn R. Inherited enzyme deficiencies and immunodeficiency: adenosine deaminase (ADA) and purine nucleoside phosphorylase (PNP) deficiencies. Clin Immunol Immunopathol 1986; 40:157–65.
5. Hirschhorn R, Roegner-Maniscalco V, Kuritsky L, Rosen FS. Bone marrow transplantation only partially restores purine metabolites to normal adenosine deaminase-deficient patients. J Clin Invest 1981; 68:1387–93.
6. Polmar AH, Stern RC, Schwartz AL, Wetzler EM, Chase PA, Hirschhorn R. Enzyme replacement therapy for adenosine deaminase deficiency and severe combined immunodeficiency. N Engl J Med 1976; 295:1337–43.
7. Rubinstein A, Hirschhorn R, Sicklick M, Murphy RA. In vivo and in vitro effects of thymosin and adenosine deaminase on adenosine-deaminase-deficient lymphocytes. N Engl J Med 1979; 300:387–92.
8. Hirschhorn R, Papageorgiou PS, Kesarwala HH, Taft LT. Amelioration of neurologic abnormalities after "enzyme replacement" in adenosine deaminase deficiency. N Engl J Med 1980; 303:377–80.
9. Hirschhorn R, Ratech H, Rubinstein A, et al. Increased excretion of modified adenine nucleosides by children with adenosine deaminase deficiency. Pediatr Res 1982; 16:362–9.
10. Polmar SH. Enzyme replacement and other biochemical approaches to the therapy of adenosine deaminase deficiency. In: Elliott K, Whelan J, eds. Enzyme defects and immune dysfunction. Amsterdam: Excerpta Medica, 1979; 213–30.

U.S. Patent 4,179,337 and pat. pending

ENZON Pharmaceuticals, Inc.
20 Kingsbridge Road
Piscataway, NJ 08854-3969

Issued May, 1999 200-029 b

DEPOCYT® ℞

[*dĕ-pō-sīt*]

(cytarabine liposome injection)
For Intrathecal Use Only
50 mg vial

WARNING

DepoCyt® (cytarabine liposome injection) should be administered only under the supervision of a qualified physician experienced in the use of intrathecal cancer chemotherapeutic agents. Appropriate management of complications is possible only when adequate diagnostic and treatment facilities are readily available. In all clinical studies, chemical arachnoiditis, a syndrome manifested primarily by nausea, vomiting, headache and fever, was a common adverse event. If left untreated, chemical arachnoiditis may be fatal. The incidence and severity of chemical arachnoiditis can be reduced by coadministration of dexamethasone (see WARNINGS). Patients receiving DepoCyt should be treated concurrently with dexamethasone to mitigate the symptoms of chemical arachnoiditis (see DOSAGE AND ADMINISTRATION).

DESCRIPTION

DepoCyt® (cytarabine liposome injection) is a sterile, injectable suspension of the antimetabolite cytarabine, encapsulated into multivesicular lipid-based particles. Chemically, cytarabine is 4-amino-1-β-D-arabinofuranosyl-2(1H)-pyrimidinone, also known as cytosine arabinoside ($C_9H_{13}N_3O_5$, molecular weight 243.22).

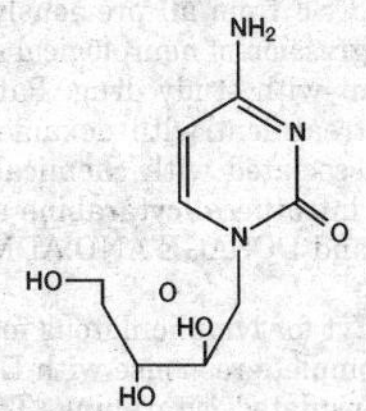

The following is an artist's rendition of a DepoCyt particle:

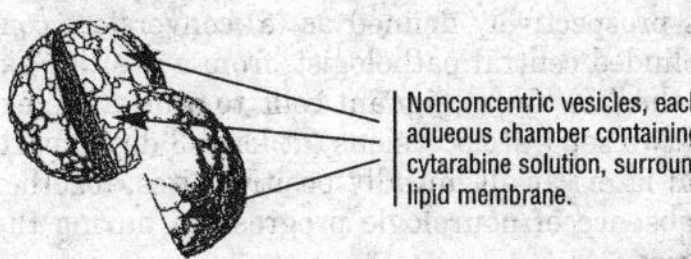

Nonconcentric vesicles, each with an internal, aqueous chamber containing encapsulated cytarabine solution, surrounded by a bilayer lipid membrane.

DepoCyt is available in 5 mL, ready-to-use, single-use vials containing 50 mg of cytarabine. DepoCyt is formulated as a sterile, nonpyrogenic, white to off-white suspension of cytarabine in Sodium Chloride 0.9% w/v in Water for Injection. DepoCyt is preservative-free. Cytarabine, the active ingredient, is present at a concentration of 10 mg/mL and is encapsulated in the particles. Inactive ingredients at their respective approximate concentrations are cholesterol, 4.1 mg/mL; triolein, 1.2 mg/mL; dioleoylphosphatidylcholine (DOPC), 5.7 mg/mL; and dipalmitoylphosphatidylglycerol (DPPG), 1.0 mg/mL. The pH of the product falls within the range from 5.5 to 8.5.

CLINICAL PHARMACOLOGY

Mechanism of Action

DepoCyt® (cytarabine liposome injection) is a sustained-release formulation of the active ingredient cytarabine designed for direct administration into the cerebrospinal fluid (CSF). Cytarabine is a cell cycle phase-specific antineoplastic agent, affecting cells only during the S-phase of cell division. Intracellularly, cytarabine is converted into cytarabine-5′-triphosphate (ara-CTP), which is the active metabolite. The mechanism of action is not completely understood, but it appears that ara-CTP acts primarily through inhibition of DNA polymerase. Incorporation into DNA and RNA may also contribute to cytarabine cytotoxicity. Cytarabine is cytotoxic to a wide variety of proliferating mammalian cells in culture.

Pharmacokinetics

The pharmacokinetics of DepoCyt administered intrathecally to patients at a 50 mg dose every 2 weeks is currently under investigation. However, preliminary analysis of the pharmacokinetic data show that following DepoCyt intrathecal administration in patients, in either the lumbar sac or by intraventricular reservoir, peak levels of free cytarabine were observed within 5 hours in both the ventricle and lumbar sac. These peak levels were followed by a biphasic elimination profile with a terminal phase half-life of 100 to 263 hours over a dose range of 12.5 mg to 75 mg. In contrast, intrathecal administration of 30 mg of free cytarabine showed a biphasic CSF concentration profile with a terminal phase half-life of 3.4 hours. Since the transfer rate of cytarabine from the CSF to plasma is slow and the conversion of cytarabine to ara-U in the plasma is fast, systemic exposure of cytarabine was negligible following intrathecal administration of DepoCyt, 50 mg or 75 mg.

Metabolism and Elimination

The primary route of elimination of cytarabine is metabolism to the inactive compound ara-U (1-β-D-arabinofuranosyluracil or uracilarabinoside), followed by urinary excretion of ara-U. In contrast to systemically administered cytarabine, which is rapidly metabolized to ara-U, conversion to ara-U in the CSF is negligible after intrathecal administration because of the significantly lower cytidine deaminase activity in the CNS tissues and CSF. The CSF clearance rate of cytarabine is similar to the CSF bulk flow rate of 0.24 mL/min.

Drug Interactions

No formal assessments of pharmacokinetic drug-drug interactions between DepoCyt and other agents have been conducted.

Continued on next page

DepoCyt—Cont.

Special Populations
The effects of gender or race on the pharmacokinetics of DepoCyt have not been studied, nor has the effect of renal or hepatic impairment.

CLINICAL STUDIES

DepoCyt® (cytarabine liposome injection) was studied in clinical trials that enrolled patients with neoplastic meningitis due to solid tumors, lymphoma, or leukemia. A randomized multicenter, multi-arm study involving a total of 99 patients compared 50 mg of DepoCyt administered every 2 weeks to standard intrathecal chemotherapy administered twice a week to patients with either solid tumors, lymphoma, or leukemia. For patients with lymphoma, standard therapy consisted of 50 mg of unencapsulated cytarabine given twice a week. Thirty-three lymphoma patients (17 DepoCyt, 16 cytarabine) were enrolled. Patients went off study if they had not achieved a complete response defined as clearing of the CSF from all previously positive sites in the absence of progression of neurological symptoms, after 4 weeks of treatment with study drug. Patients were to receive concurrent treatment with dexamethasone to minimize symptoms associated with chemical arachnoiditis, a known toxicity of intrathecal cytarabine and methotrexate (see WARNINGS and DOSAGE AND ADMINISTRATION).

Lymphoma
Approval of DepoCyt for lymphomatous meningitis is based on an increased complete response with DepoCyt compared to control unencapsulated cytarabine. There has been no demonstration of an improved clinical outcome as a result of the increased response rate. In the controlled trial, complete response was prospectively defined as (a) conversion, confirmed by a blinded central pathologist, from a positive examination of the CSF for malignant cells to a negative examination on two separate occasions (at least 3 days apart, on day 29 and later) at all initially positive sites, together with (b) an absence of neurologic progression during the treatment period.
The complete response rates in the controlled study of lymphoma are shown in Table 1, giving results for all of the 33 lymphoma patients randomized. Although there was a plan for central pathology review of the data, in 4 of the 7 responding patients on the DepoCyt arm this was not accomplished and these cases were considered to have had a complete response based on the reading of an unblinded pathologist. The median overall survival of all treated patients was 99.5 days on the DepoCyt arm and 63 days on the cytarabine arm. In both arms the majority of patients died from progressive systemic disease, not the neoplastic meningitis.

Table 1: Complete Responses in Patients with Lymphomatous Meningitis in the Controlled Study

Intent-to-treat	
DepoCyt®	**Cytarabine**
7/17 (41%)	1/16 (6%)

INDICATIONS

DepoCyt® (cytarabine liposome injection) is indicated for the intrathecal treatment of lymphomatous meningitis. This indication is based on demonstration of increased complete response rate compared to unencapsulated cytarabine. There are no controlled trials that demonstrate a clinical benefit resulting from this treatment, such as improvement in disease-related symptoms, or increased time to disease progression, or increases survival.

CONTRAINDICATIONS

DepoCyt® (cytarabine liposome injection) is contraindicated in patients who are hypersensitive to cytarabine or any component of the formulation, and in patients with active meningeal infection.

WARNINGS (see boxed WARNING)

DepoCyt® (cytarabine liposome injection) should be administered only under the supervision of a qualified physician experienced in the use of cancer chemotherapeutic agents. Appropriate management of complications is possible only when adequate diagnostic and treatment facilities are readily available. Chemical arachnoiditis, a syndrome manifested primarily by nausea, vomiting, headache, and fever has been a common adverse event in all studies. If left untreated, chemical arachnoiditis may be fatal. The incidence and severity of chemical arachnoiditis can be reduced by coadministration of dexamethasone. Patients receiving DepoCyt should be treated concurrently with dexamethasone to mitigate the symptoms of chemical arachnoiditis (see DOSAGE AND ADMINISTRATION).
During the clinical studies, 2 deaths related to DepoCyt were reported. One patient died after developing encephalopathy 36 hours after an intraventricular dose of DepoCyt, 125 mg. This patient was receiving concurrent whole-brain irradiation and had previously received systemic chemotherapy with cyclophosphamide, doxorubicin, and fluorouracil, as well as intraventricular methotrexate. The other patient received DepoCyt, 50 mg by the intraventricular route and developed focal seizures progressing to status epilepticus. This patient died approximately 8 weeks after the last dose of study medication. The death of 1 additional patient was considered "possibly" related to DepoCyt. He was a 63-year-old with extensive lymphoma involving the nasopharynx, brain, and meninges with multiple neurologic deficits who died of apparent disease progression 4 days after his second dose of DepoCyt.

Figure 1: Incidence and Severity of Chemical Arachnoiditis by Cycle in Patients with Lymphomatous Meningitis in the Randomized Study

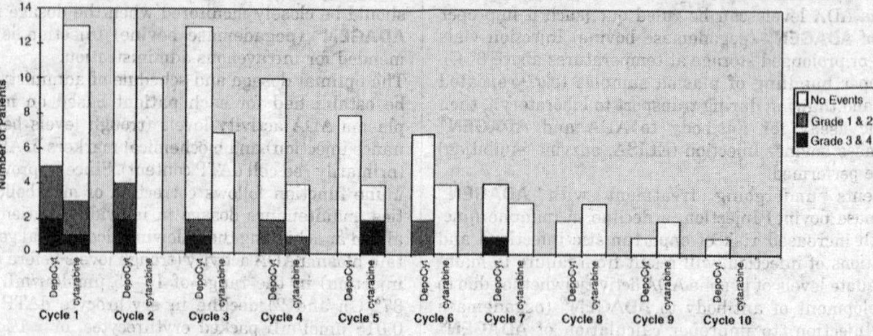

After intrathecal administration of free cytarabine the most frequently reported reactions are nausea, vomiting and fever. Intrathecal administration of free cytarabine may cause myelopathy and other neurologic toxicity and can rarely lead to a permanent neurologic deficit. Administration of intrathecal cytarabine in combination with other chemotherapeutic agents or with cranial/spinal irradiation may increase this risk of neurotoxicity.
Blockage to CSF flow may result in increased free cytarabine concentrations in the CSF and an increased risk of neurotoxicity.

Pregnancy Category D
There are no studies assessing the reproductive toxicity of DepoCyt. Cytarabine, the active component of DepoCyt, can cause fetal harm if a pregnant woman is exposed to the drug systemically. Three anecdotal cases of major limb malformations have been reported in infants after their mothers received intravenous cytarabine, alone or in combination with other agents, during the first trimester. The concern for fetal harm following intrathecal DepoCyt administration is low, however, because systemic exposure to cytarabine is negligible. Cytarabine was teratogenic in mice (cleft palate, phocomelia, deformed appendages, skeletal abnormalities) when doses ≥ 2 mg/kg/day were administered IP during the period of organogenesis (about 0.2 times the recommended human dose on mg/m^2 basis), and in rats (deformed appendages) when 20 mg/kg was administered as a single IP dose on day 12 of gestation (about 4 times the recommended human dose on mg/m^2 basis). Single IP doses of 50 mg/kg in rats (about 10 times the recommended human dose on mg/m^2 basis) on day 14 of gestation also caused reduced prenatal and postnatal brain size and permanent impairment of learning ability. Cytarabine was embryotoxic in mice when administered during the period of organogenesis. Embryotoxicity was characterized by decreased fetal weight at 0.5 mg/kg/day (about 0.05 times the recommended human dose on mg/m^2 basis), and increased early and late resorptions and decreased live litter sizes at 8 mg/kg/day (approximately equal to the recommended human dose on mg/m^2 basis). There are no adequate and well-controlled studies in pregnant women. If this drug is used during pregnancy or if the patient becomes pregnant while taking this drug, the patient should be apprised of the potential harm to the fetus. Despite the low apparent risk for fetal harm, women of childbearing potential should be advised to avoid becoming pregnant.

PRECAUTIONS

General Precautions
DepoCyt® (cytarabine liposome injection) has the potential of producing serious toxicity (see boxed WARNING). All patients receiving DepoCyt should be treated concurrently with dexamethasone to mitigate the symptoms of chemical arachnoiditis (see DOSAGE AND ADMINISTRATION). Toxic effects may be related to a single dose or to cumulative administration. Because toxic effects can occur at any time during therapy (although they are most likely within 5 days of drug administration), patients receiving intrathecal therapy with DepoCyt should be monitored continuously for the development of neurotoxicity. If patients develop neurotoxicity, subsequent doses of DepoCyt should be reduced, and DepoCyt should be discontinued if toxicity persists.
Some patients with neoplastic meningitis receiving treatment with DepoCyt may require concurrent radiation or systemic therapy with other chemotherapeutic agents; this may increase the rate of adverse events.
Anaphylactic reactions following intravenous administration of free cytarabine have been reported.
Although significant systemic exposure to free cytarabine following intrathecal treatment is not expected, some effect on bone marrow function cannot be excluded. Systemic toxicity due to intravenous administration of cytarabine consists primarily of bone marrow suppression with leukopenia, thrombocytopenia, and anemia. Accordingly, careful monitoring of the hematopoietic system is advised.
Transient elevations in CSF protein and white blood cells have been observed in patients following DepoCyt administration and have also been noted after intrathecal treatment with methotrexate or cytarabine.

Information for the Patient
Patients should be informed about the expected adverse events of headache, nausea, vomiting, and fever, and about the early signs and symptoms of neurotoxicity. The importance of concurrent dexamethasone administration should be emphasized at the initiation of each cycle of DepoCyt treatment. Patients should be instructed to seek medical attention if signs or symptoms of neurotoxicity develop, or if oral dexamethasone is not well tolerated (see DOSAGE AND ADMINISTRATION).

Drug Interactions
No formal drug interaction studies of DepoCyt and other drugs were conducted. Concomitant administration of DepoCyt with other antineoplastic agents administered by the intrathecal route has not been studied. With intrathecal cytarabine and other cytotoxic agents administered intrathecally, enhanced neurotoxicity has been associated with coadministration of drugs.

Laboratory Test Interactions
Since DepoCyt particles are similar in size and appearance to white blood cells, care must be taken in interpreting CSF examinations following DepoCyt administration.

Carcinogenesis, Mutagenesis, Impairment of Fertility
No carcinogenicity, mutagenicity, or impairment of fertility studies have been conducted with DepoCyt. The active ingredient of DepoCyt, cytarabine, was mutagenic in *in vitro* tests and was clastogenic *in vitro* (chromosome aberrations and SCE in human leukocytes) and *in vivo* (chromosome aberrations and SCE assay in rodent bone marrow, mouse micronucleus assay). Cytarabine caused the transformation of hamster embryo cells and rat H43 cells *in vitro*. Cytarabine was clastogenic to meiotic cells; a dose-dependent increase in sperm-head abnormalities and chromosomal aberrations occurred in mice given IP cytarabine. Impairment of Fertility: No studies assessing the impact of cytarabine on fertility are available in the literature. Because the systemic exposure to free cytarabine following intrathecal treatment with DepoCyt was negligible, the risk of impaired fertility after intrathecal DepoCyt is likely to be low.

Pregnancy
Pregnancy Category D (see WARNINGS).

Nursing Mothers
It is not known whether cytarabine is excreted in human milk following intrathecal DepoCyt administration. The systemic exposure to free cytarabine following intrathecal treatment with DepoCyt was negligible. Despite the low apparent risk, because many drugs are excreted in human milk and because of the potential for serious adverse reactions in nursing infants, the use of DepoCyt is not recommended in nursing women.

Pediatric Use
The safety and efficacy of DepoCyt in pediatric patients has not been established.

ADVERSE REACTIONS

The toxicity database consists of the observations made during an early uncontrolled study and the controlled multi-arm study described above. In the early study, patients received DepoCyt® (cytarabine liposome injection) at doses ranging from 12.5 mg to 125 mg. In the randomized multi-arm study, DepoCyt was administered at a dose of 50 mg every 2 weeks and was compared to standard intrathecal chemotherapy (cytarabine or methotrexate) in patients with lymphoma, leukemia, and solid tumors; 28 lymphoma patients, 5 leukemia patients, and 59 solid tumor patients received study drug.
Arachnoiditis is an expected and well-documented side effect of both neoplastic meningitis and of intrathecal chemotherapy. For clinical studies of DepoCyt, chemical arachnoiditis was defined as the occurrence of any one of the symptoms of neck rigidity, neck pain, meningism or any two of the symptoms of nausea, vomiting, headache, fever, back pain, or CSF pleocytosis; the grade assigned to an episode of chemical arachnoiditis was the highest severity grade of its component symptoms. Since most of the adverse events reported in the trials were transient episodes associated with drug exposure, the incidence of these events is best expressed by drug cycle. A cycle of treatment for all treatment groups was defined as the 14-day period between DepoCyt doses. The duration of reported symptoms was from 1 to 5 days. Although it was sometimes difficult to distinguish between drug-related chemical arachnoiditis, infectious meningitis, or disease progression, >90% of the chemical arachnoiditis cases reported occurred within 48 hours of the

administration of intrathecal drug, indicating a drug etiology. The incidence and severity of chemical arachnoiditis by cycle in patients with lymphomatous meningitis in the controlled study are shown in Figure 1.

In the early study, chemical arachnoiditis was observed in 100% of cycles without dexamethasone prophylaxis; with concurrent administration of dexamethasone, chemical arachnoiditis was observed in 33% of cycles. Patients receiving DepoCyt should be treated concurrently with dexamethasone to mitigate the symptoms of chemical arachnoiditis (see DOSAGE AND ADMINISTRATION).

[See figure 1 at top of previous page]

Table 2 shows the rate of all adverse events occurring in ≥10 % of patients, as a rate per cycle in the lymphoma randomized study.

Table 2: Comparison of Adverse Events Occurring in ≥ 10% of Patients, by Cycle. Patients with Lymphomatous Meningitis Receiving DepoCyt® or Cytarabine (ara-C) in the Randomized Study

	All Adverse Events %		Grade 3 or 4 Adverse Events %	
Number of Cycles	n=74	n=45	n=74	n=45
Body System/Adverse Event	**DepoCyt®**	**ara-C**	**DepoCyt®**	**ara-C**
Body as a Whole	53	60	18	22
Headache*	28	9	5	2
Asthenia	19	33	5	9
Fever*	11	24	4	0
Back pain*	7	11	0	2
Pain	11	20	3	0
Nervous System	45	53	18	18
Confusion	14	7	4	2
Somnolence	12	11	4	2
Abnormal gait	4	11	1	2
Digestive System	27	44	7	9
Nausea*	11	16	0	4
Vomiting*	12	18	3	2
Constipation	7	11	0	0
Metabolic and Nutritional Disorders	16	24	0	0
Peripheral edema	7	11	0	0
Hemic and Lymphatic System	19	22	11	13
Neutropenia	9	11	8	11
Thrombocytopenia	8	16	5	11
Anemia	1	13	1	4
Urogenital System	11	20	3	2
Urinary incontinence	3	11	0	0
Special Senses	16	18	1	2

*Components of chemical arachnoiditis.

OVERDOSAGE

No overdosages with DepoCyt® (cytarabine liposome injection) have been reported. An overdose with DepoCyt may be associated with severe chemical arachnoiditis including encephalopathy.

In an early uncontrolled study without dexamethasone prophylaxis, single doses up to 125 mg were administered. One patient at the 125 mg dose level died of encephalopathy 36 hours after receiving an intraventricular dose of DepoCyt (see WARNINGS). This patient, however, was also receiving concomitant whole brain irradiation and had previously received intraventricular methotrexate.

There is no antidote for overdose of intrathecal DepoCyt or unencapsulated cytarabine released from DepoCyt. Exchange of CSF with isotonic saline has been carried out in a case of intrathecal overdose of free cytarabine, and such a procedure may be considered in the case of DepoCyt overdose. Management of overdose should be directed at maintaining vital functions.

DOSAGE AND ADMINISTRATION

Preparation of DepoCyt® (cytarabine liposome injection)

DepoCyt is a cytotoxic anticancer drug and, as with other potentially toxic compounds, caution should be used in handling DepoCyt. The use of gloves is recommended. If DepoCyt suspension contacts the skin, wash immediately with soap and water. If it contacts mucous membranes, flush thoroughly with water (see HANDLING AND DISPOSAL). DepoCyt particles are more dense than the diluent and have a tendency to settle with time. Vials of DepoCyt should be allowed to warm to room temperature and gently agitated or inverted to resuspend the particles immediately prior to withdrawal from the vial. Avoid aggressive agitation. No further reconstitution or dilution is required.

DepoCyt Administration

DepoCyt should be withdrawn from the vial immediately before administration. DepoCyt is a single-use vial and does not contain any preservative; DepoCyt should be used within 4 hours of withdrawal from the vial. Unused portions of each vial should be discarded properly (see HANDLING AND DISPOSAL). Do not save any unused portions for later administration. Do not mix DepoCyt with any other medications.

In-line filters must not be used when administering DepoCyt. DepoCyt is administered directly into the CSF via an intraventricular reservoir or by direct injection into the lumbar sac. DepoCyt should be injected slowly over a period of 1–5 minutes. Following drug administration by lumbar puncture, the patient should be instructed to lie flat for 1 hour. Patients should be observed by the physician for immediate toxic reactions.

Patients should be started on dexamethasone 4 mg bid either PO or IV for 5 days beginning on the day of DepoCyt injection.

DepoCyt must only be administered by the intrathecal route.

Further dilution of DepoCyt is not recommended.

Dosing Regimen

For the treatment of lymphomatous meningitis, DepoCyt 50 mg (one vial of DepoCyt) is recommended to be given according to the following schedule:

Induction therapy: DepoCyt, 50 mg, administered intrathecally (intraventricular or lumbar puncture) every 14 days for 2 doses (weeks 1 and 3).

Consolidation therapy: DepoCyt, 50 mg, administered intrathecally (intraventricular or lumbar puncture) every 14 days for 3 doses (weeks 5, 7 and 9) followed by 1 additional dose at week 13.

Maintenance: DepoCyt, 50 mg, administered intrathecally (intraventricular or lumbar puncture) every 28 days for 4 doses (weeks 17, 21, 25 and 29).

If drug-related neurotoxicity develops, the dose should be reduced to 25 mg. If toxicity persists, treatment with DepoCyt should be discontinued.

HANDLING AND DISPOSAL

Procedures for proper handling and disposal of anticancer drugs should be considered. Several guidelines on this subject have been published.[1–7] There is no general agreement that all of the procedures recommended in the guidelines are necessary or appropriate.

HOW SUPPLIED

DepoCyt® (cytarabine liposome injection) is supplied as a sterile, white to off-white suspension in 5 mL glass, single use vials.

Refrigerate at 2° to 8°C (36° to 46°F). Protect from freezing and avoid aggressive agitation.

Available as individual carton containing one ready to use vial. **NDC 57665-331-01.**

Do not use beyond expiration date printed on the label.

REFERENCES

1. *Recommendations for the Safe Handling of Parenteral Antineoplastic Drugs.* Publication NIH 83-2621. For sale by the Superintendent of Documents, U.S. Government Printing Office, Washington, DC 20402.
2. Council on Scientific Affairs. Guidelines for handling parenteral antineoplastics. *JAMA.* 1985; 253:1590-1592.
3. National Study Commission on Cytotoxic Exposure. *Recommendations for handling cytotoxic agents.* Available from Louis P. Jeffrey, ScD, Chairman, National Study Commission on Cytotoxic Exposure, Massachusetts College of Pharmacy and Allied Health Sciences, 179 Longwood Avenue, Boston, Massachusetts 02115.
4. Clinical Oncological Society of Australia. Guidelines and recommendations for safe handling of antineoplastic agents. *Med J Australia.* 1983;1:426-428.
5. Jones RB, et al. Safe handling of chemotherapeutic agents: a report from the Mount Sinai Medical Center. *CA J Clin.* 1983;33:258-263.
6. American Society of Hospital Pharmacists Technical Assistance Bulletin on Handling Cytotoxic and Hazardous Drugs. *Am J Hosp Pharm.* 1990; 47:1033-1049.
7. Controlling Occupational Exposure to Hazardous Drugs (OSHA Work-Practice Guidelines). *Am J Health-Syst Pharm.* 1996;53:1669-1685.

Rx only

For additional information, contact Enzon Professional Services at 866-792-5172.

Manufactured by:
SkyePharma Inc.
San Diego, CA 92121
Distributed by:
ENZON Pharmaceuticals, Inc.
Piscataway, NJ 08854
U.S. Patent Nos. 5,807,572; 5,723,147

ONCASPAR® ℞

[*an'-ca-spar*]
PEGASPARGASE
(PEG-L-asparaginase)

DESCRIPTION

ONCASPAR®, the ENZON trademark for pegaspargase, is a modified version of the enzyme L-asparaginase. It is an oncolytic agent used in combination chemotherapy for the treatment of patients with acute lymphoblastic leukemia who are hypersensitive to native forms of L-asparaginase (as described in **CLINICAL PHARMACOLOGY**).

The generic name of **ONCASPAR®** is **pegaspargase**. The chemical name is monomethoxypolyethylene glycol succinimidyl L-asparaginase. L-asparaginase is modified by covalently conjugating units of monomethoxypolyethylene glycol (PEG), molecular weight of 5,000, to the enzyme, forming the active ingredient PEG-L-asparaginase. The L-asparaginase (L-asparagine amidohydrolase, type EC-2, EC 3.5.1.1) used in the manufacture of **ONCASPAR®** is derived from *Escherichia coli*. ENZON purchases the enzyme L-asparaginase in bulk from Merck, Sharp and Dohme, Division of Merck & Co., Inc., West Point, PA 19486, U.S. License Number 2, Merck & Co., Inc. supplies bulk L-asparaginase as a licensed intermediate for further manufacture by ENZON into PEG-L-asparaginase. Merck & Co., Inc. can only assume responsibility for the bulk intermediate supplied to ENZON.

ONCASPAR® is supplied as an isotonic sterile solution in phosphate buffered saline, pH 7.3, for intramuscular administration only. The solution is clear, colorless and contains no preservatives. It is supplied in 5 mL single-dose vials.

ONCASPAR® activity is expressed in International Units (IU) according to the recommendation of the International Union of Biochemistry. One IU of L-asparaginase is defined as that amount of enzyme required to generate 1 μ mol of ammonia per minute at pH 7.3 and 37°C.

Each milliliter of **ONCASPAR®** contains:

PEG-L-asparaginase	750 IU ± 20 %
Monobasic sodium phosphate, USP	1.20 mg ± 5 %
Dibasic sodium phosphate, USP	5.58 mg ± 5 %
Sodium chloride, USP	8.50 mg ± 5 %
Water for injection, USP	qs to 1.0 mL

The specific activity of **ONCASPAR®** is at least 85 IU per milligram protein.

CLINICAL PHARMACOLOGY

Leukemic cells are unable to synthesize asparagine due to a lack of asparagine synthetase and are dependent on an exogenous source of asparagine for survival. Rapid depletion of asparagine which results from treatment with the enzyme L-asparagine, kills the leukemic cells. Normal cells, however, are less affected by the rapid depletion due to their ability to synthesize asparagine. This is an approach to therapy based on a specific metabolic defect in some leukemic cells which do not produce asparagine synthetase.[1]

In a study in predominately L-asparaginase naive adult patients with leukemia and lymphoma, initial plasma levels of L-asparaginase following intravenous administration were determined. Plasma half-life did not appear to be influenced by dose levels, and it could not be correlated with age, sex, surface area, renal or hepatic function, diagnosis or extent of disease. Apparent volume of distribution was equal to estimated plasma volume. L-asparaginase was measurable for at least 15 days following the initial treatment with **ONCASPAR®**. The enzyme could not be detected in the urine.[2]

In a study of newly diagnosed pediatric patients with acute lymphoblastic leukemia (ALL) who received either a single intramuscular injection of **ONCASPAR®** (2,500 IU/m^2), *E. coli* L-asparaginase (25,000 IU/m^2), or *Erwinia* (25,000 IU/m^2), the plasma half-lives for the three forms of L-asparaginase were:[3]

PLASMA HALF-LIVES OF THREE FORMS OF L-ASPARAGINASE

TREATMENT GROUP	NO. OF PATIENTS	MEAN (DAYS)	STANDARD DEVIATION
ONCASPAR®	10	5.73	3.24
E. coli L-asparaginase	17	1.24	0.17
Erwinia L-asparaginase	10	0.65	0.13

In this same study of newly diagnosed pediatric ALL patients, the *in vivo* early leukemic cell kill after a single intramuscular injection of native *E. coli* L-asparaginase (25,000 IU/m^2), *Erwinia* L-asparaginase (25,000 IU/m^2), and **ONCASPAR®** (2,500 IU/m^2) during a five day "investigational window" was studied.[4] Bone marrow aspirates were taken before and five days after a single dose of one of the three different forms of L-asparaginase. Rhodamine-123 (RH-123), a selectively incorporated fluorescent mitochondrial dye, was used in an *in vitro* assay on the bone marrow aspirates to ascertain cell viability. The percent reduction of viable lymphoblasts at day five for each group is presented in the following table:[4]

RHODAMINE-123 (*IN VIVO* CELL KILL)

TREATMENT GROUP	NO. OF PATIENTS	PERCENT REDUCTION OF VIABLE LYMPHOBLASTS AT DAY 5 MEAN ± S.D.
ONCASPAR®	21	55.7 ± 10.2
E. coli L-asparaginase	28	57.8 ± 10.1
Erwinia L-asparaginase	19	57.9 ± 13.8

In three pharmacokinetic studies, 37 relapsed ALL patients received **ONCASPAR®** at 2,500 IU/m^2 every two weeks. The plasma half-life of **ONCASPAR®** was 3.24 ± 1.83 days in nine patients who were previously hypersensitive to native L-asparaginase and 5.69 ± 3.25 days in 28 non-hypersensitive patients. The area under the curve was 9.50 ± 3.95 IU/mL/day in the previously hypersensitive patients, and 9.83 ± 5.94 IU/mL/day in the non-hypersensitive patients.

Continued on next page

Oncaspar—Cont.

Hypersensitivity Reactions
Hypersensitivity reactions to *E. coli* L-asparaginase have been reported in the literature in 3% to 73% of patients.[1] Patients in **ONCASPAR®** clinical studies were considered to be previously hypersensitive if they experienced a systemic rash, urticaria, bronchospasm, laryngeal edema, or hypotension following administration of any form of native L-asparaginase. Patients were also considered to be previously hypersensitive if they experienced local erythema, urticaria, or swelling, greater than two centimeters, for at least ten minutes following administration of any form of native L-asparaginase. The National Cancer Institute Common Toxicity Criteria (CTC) were used to classify the severity of the hypersensitivity reactions. These are: grade 1 — transient rash (mild); grade 2 — mild bronchospasm (moderate); grade 3 — moderate bronchospasm and/or serum sickness (severe); grade 4 — hypotension and/or anaphylaxis (life-threatening). Additionally, most transient local urticaria were considered grade 2 hypersensitivity reactions, while most sustained urticaria distant from the injection site were considered grade 3 hypersensitivity reactions. In general, the moderate to life-threatening hypersensitivity reactions were considered dose-limiting; that is, they required L-asparaginase treatment to be discontinued.
In separate studies, **ONCASPAR®** was administered intravenously to 48 patients and intramuscularly to 126 patients. The incidence of hypersensitivity reactions when **ONCASPAR®** was administered intramuscularly was 30% in patients who were previously hypersensitive to native L-asparaginase and 11% in non-hypersensitive patients (p-value of 0.007). The incidence of hypersensitivity reactions when **ONCASPAR®** was administered intravenously was 60% in patients who were previously hypersensitive to native L-asparaginase and 12% in non-hypersensitive patients. Since only five previously hypersensitive patients received **ONCASPAR®** intravenously, no meaningful analysis of the incidence of hypersensitivity reactions was possible between either the previously hypersensitive and non-hypersensitive patients, or between the intravenous and intramuscular routes of administration.
The overall incidence of hypersensitivity reactions in 174 patients who received **ONCASPAR®** in five clinical studies is shown in the table below:

INCIDENCE OF ONCASPAR® HYPERSENSITIVITY REACTIONS

PATIENT STATUS	N	CTC GRADE OF HYPERSENSITIVITY REACTION 1	2	3	4	TOTAL
Previously Hypersensitive Patients	62	7	8	4	1	20 (32%)
Non-Hypersensitive Patients	112	5	4	1	1	11 (10%)
Total Patients	174	12	12	5	2	31 (18%)

The probability of previously hypersensitive or non-hypersensitive patients completing 8 doses of **ONCASPAR®** therapy without developing a dose-limiting hypersensitivity reaction was 77% and 95%, respectively.
All of the 62 hypersensitive patients treated with **ONCASPAR®** in five clinical studies had previous hypersensitivity reactions to one or more of the native forms of L-asparaginase. Of the 35 patients who had previous hypersensitivity reactions to *E. coli* L-asparaginase only, 5 (14%) had **ONCASPAR®** dose-limiting hypersensitivity reactions. Of the 27 patients who had hypersensitivity reactions to both *E. coli* and *Erwinia* L-asparaginase, 7 (26%) had **ONCASPAR®** dose-limiting hypersensitivity reactions. The overall incidence of dose-limiting hypersensitivity reactions in 174 patients treated with **ONCASPAR®** was 9% (19% in 62 hypersensitive and 3% in 112 non-hypersensitive patients). Of the total of 9% dose-limiting hypersensitivity reactions, 1% were anaphylactic (CTC grade 4) and the other 8% were ≤ CTC grade 3.
Clinical Activity
ONCASPAR® was evaluated as part of combination therapy in four open label studies comprising 42 multiply-relapsed, previously hypersensitive acute leukemia patients [39 (93%) with ALL] at a dose of 2,000 or 2,500 IU/m^2 administered intramuscularly or intravenously every 14 days during induction combination chemotherapy. The reinduction response rate was 50% (36% complete remissions and 14% partial remissions), with a 95% confidence interval of 35% to 65%. This response rate is comparable to that reported in the literature for relapsed patients treated with native L-asparaginase as part of combination chemotherapy.[1]
ONCASPAR® was also shown to have some activity as a single agent in multiply-relapsed hypersensitive ALL patients, the majority of whom were pediatric. Treatment with **ONCASPAR®** resulted in three responses (one complete remission and two partial remissions) in nine previously hypersensitive patients who would not have been able to receive any further L-asparaginase treatment.
ONCASPAR® was also studied in non-hypersensitive, relapsed ALL patients who were randomized to receive two doses of **ONCASPAR®** at 2,500 IU/m^2 every 14 days or twelve doses of *E. coli* L-asparaginase at 10,000 IU/m^2 three times a week during a 28 day induction combination chemotherapy regimen (which included vincristine and prednisone). Although the enrollment in this study was too small to be conclusive, the data showed that for 20 patients there was no significant difference between the overall response rates of 60% and 50%, respectively, or the complete remission rates of 50% and 50%, respectively.
ONCASPAR® was administered during maintenance therapy regimens to 33 previously hypersensitive patients. The average number of doses received during maintenance therapy was 5.8 (range of 1 to 24) and the average duration of maintenance therapy was 126 (range of 1 to 513) days for this patient population.

INDICATIONS AND USAGE

ONCASPAR® is indicated for patients with acute lymphoblastic leukemia who require L-asparaginase in their treatment regimen, but have developed hypersensitivity to the native forms of L-asparaginase **(SEE CLINICAL PHARMACOLOGY)**. **ONCASPAR®**, like native L-asparginase, is generally used in combination with other chemotherapeutic agents, such as vincristine, methotrexate, cytarabine, daunorubicin, and doxorubicin.[1,5] Use of **ONCASPAR®** as a single agent should only be undertaken when multi-agent chemotherapy is judged to be inappropriate for the patient.

CONTRAINDICATIONS

ONCASPAR® is contraindicated in patients with pancreatitis or a history of pancreatitis. **ONCASPAR®** is contraindicated in patients who have had significant hemorrhagic events associated with prior L-asparaginase therapy. **ONCASPAR®** is also contraindicated in patients who have had previous serious allergic reactions, such as generalized urticaria, bronchospasm, laryngeal edema, hypotension, or other unacceptable adverse reactions to **ONCASPAR®**.

WARNINGS

It is recommended that **ONCASPAR®** be given under the supervision of an individual who is qualified by training and experience to administer cancer chemotherapeutic agents. Especially in patients with known hypersensitivity to the other forms of L-asparaginase, hypersensitivity reactions to **ONCASPAR®**, including life-threatening anaphylaxis, may occur during therapy. As a routine precaution, patients should be kept under observation for one hour with resuscitation equipment and other agents necessary to treat anaphylaxis (epinephrine, oxygen, intravenous steroids, etc.) available.

PRECAUTIONS

General
This drug may be a contact irritant, and the solution must be handled and administered with care. Gloves are recommended. Inhalation of vapors and contact with skin or mucous membranes, especially those of the eyes, must be avoided. In case of contact, wash with copious amounts of water for at least 15 minutes. Anaphylactic reactions require the immediate use of epinephrine, oxygen, intravenous steroids, and antihistamines. Patients taking **ONCASPAR®** are at higher than usual risk for bleeding problems, especially with simultaneous use of other drugs that have anticoagulant properties, such as aspirin, and non-steroidal anti-inflammatories **(SEE DRUG INTERACTIONS)**. **ONCASPAR®** may have immunosuppressive activity. Therefore, it is possible that use of the drug in patients may predispose the patient to infection. Severe hepatic and central nervous system toxicity following multi-agent chemotherapy that includes **ONCASPAR®** may occur. Caution appears warranted when treating patients with **ONCASPAR®** given in combination with hepatotoxic agents, particularly when liver dysfunction is present.
Patients undergoing **ONCASPAR®** therapy must be carefully monitored and the therapeutic regimen adjusted according to response and toxicity. Physicians using a given treatment incorporating **ONCASPAR®** should be thoroughly familiar with its benefits and risks.
Information For Patients
Patients should be informed on the possibility of hypersensitivity reactions, including immediate anaphylaxis, to **ONCASPAR®**. Patients taking **ONCASPAR®** are at higher than usual risk for bleeding problems. Patients should be instructed that the simultaneous use of **ONCASPAR®** with other drugs that may increase the risk of bleeding should be avoided **(SEE DRUG INTERACTIONS)**. **ONCASPAR®** may affect the ability of the liver to function normally in some patients. Therapy with **ONCASPAR®** may increase the toxicity of other medications **(SEE DRUG INTERACTIONS)** **ONCASPAR®** may have immunosuppressive activity. Therefore, it is possible that use of the drug in patients may predispose the patient to infection. Patients should notify their physicians of any adverse reactions that occur.
Laboratory Tests
A fall in circulating lymphoblasts is often noted after initiating therapy. This may be accompanied by a marked rise in serum uric acid. As a guide to the effects of therapy, the patient's peripheral blood count and bone marrow should be monitored.
Frequent serum amylase determinations should be obtained to detect early evidence of pancreatitis **(SEE CONTRAINDICATIONS)**. Blood sugar should be monitored during therapy with **ONCASPAR®** because hyperglycemia may occur. When using **ONCASPAR®** in conjunction with hepatotoxic chemotherapy, patients should be monitored for liver dysfunction.
ONCASPAR® may affect a number of plasma proteins; therefore, monitoring of fibrinogen, PT, and PTT may be indicated.
Drug Interactions
Unfavorable interactions of L-asparaginase with some antitumor agents have been demonstrated.[1] It is recommended, therefore, that **ONCASPAR®** be used in combination regimens only by physicians familiar with the benefits and risks of a given regimen. Depletion of serum protein by **ONCASPAR®** may increase the toxicity of other drugs which are protein bound. Additionally, during the period of its inhibition of protein synthesis and cell replication, **ONCASPAR®** may interfere with the action of drugs such as methotrexate, which require cell replication for their lethal effects. **ONCASPAR®** may interfere with the enzymatic detoxification of other drugs, particularly in the liver. Physicians using a given treatment regimen should be thoroughly familiar with its benefits and risks.
Imbalances in coagulation factors have been noted with the use of **ONCASPAR®** predisposing to bleeding and/or thrombosis. Caution should be used when administering any concurrent anticoagulant therapy, such as coumadin, heparin, dipyridamole, aspirin, or non-steroidal anti-inflammatories.
Carcinogenesis, Mutagenesis, Impairment of Fertility
Long-term carcinogenic studies in animals have not been performed with **ONCASPAR®** nor have studies been performed on impairment of fertility. **ONCASPAR®** did not exhibit a mutagenic effect when tested against *Salmonella typhimurium* strains in the Ames assay.
Pregnancy
Pregnancy Category C. Animal reproduction studies have not been conducted with **ONCASPAR®**. It is also not known whether **ONCASPAR®** can cause fetal harm when administered to a pregnant woman or can affect reproduction capacity. **ONCASPAR®** should be given to a pregnant woman only if clearly needed.
Nursing Mothers
It is not known whether **ONCASPAR®** is excreted in human milk. Because many drugs are excreted in human milk and because of the potential for serious adverse reactions due to **ONCASPAR®** in nursing infants, a decision should be made to discontinue nursing or discontinue the drug, taking into account the importance of the drug to the mother.

ONCASPAR® ADVERSE REACTIONS

Adverse reactions have been reported in adults and pediatric patients. Overall, the adult patients treated with **ONCASPAR®** had a somewhat higher incidence of known L-asparaginase toxicities, except for hypersensitivity reactions, than the pediatric patients treated with **ONCASPAR®**.
Excluding hypersensitivity reactions, the most frequently occurring known L-asparaginase related toxicities and adverse experiences reported for the 174 patients in clinical studies were chemical hepatotoxicities and coagulopathies, the majority of which did not result in any significant clinical events. The incidence of significant clinical events included clinical pancreatitis (1%), hyperglycemia requiring insulin therapy (3%), and thrombosis (4%).
The following adverse reactions related to **ONCASPAR®** were reported for 174 patients in five clinical studies.
The adverse reactions reported most frequently (greater than 5%) were allergic reactions (which may have included rash, erythema, edema, pain, fever chills, urticaria, dyspnea, or bronchospasm), SGT increase, nausea and/or vomiting, fever, and malaise.
The adverse reactions reported occasionally (greater than 1% but less than 5%) were anaphylactic reactions, dyspnea, injection site hypersensitivity, lip edema, rash, urticaria, abdominal pain, chills, pain in the extremities, hypotension, tachycardia, thrombosis, anorexia, diarrhea, jaundice, abnormal liver function test, decreased anticoagulant effect, disseminated intravascular coagulation, decreased fibrinogen, hemolytic anemia, leukopenia, pancytopenia, thrombocytopenia, increased thromboplastin, injection site pain, injection site reaction, bilirubinemia, hyperglycemia, hyperuricemia, hypoglycemia, hypoproteinemia, peripheral edema, increased SGOT, arthralgia, myalgia, convulsion, headache, night sweats, and paresthesia.
The adverse reactions reported rarely (less than 1%) were bronchospasm, petechial rash, face edema, lesional edema, sepsis, septic shock, chest pain, endocarditis, hypertension, constipation, flatulence, gastrointestinal pain, hepatomegaly, increased appetite, liver fatty deposits, coagulation disorder, increased coagulation time, decreased platelet count, purpura, increased amylase, edema, excessive thirst, hyperammonemia, hyponatremia, weight loss, bone pain, joint disorder, confusion, dizziness, emotional lability, somnolence, increased cough, epistaxis, upper respiratory infection, erythema simplex, pruritus, hematuria, increased urinary frequency, and abnormal kidney function.
The following **ONCASPAR®** related reactions have been observed in patients with hematologic malignancies, primarily acute lymphoblastic leukemia (approximately 75%), non-Hodgkins lymphoma (approximately 13%), acute myelogenous leukemia (approximately 3%), and a variety of solid tumors (approximately 9%):
HYPERSENSITIVITY REACTIONS: a variety of hypersensitivity reactions have occurred. These reactions may be acute or delayed, and include acute anaphylaxis, bronchospasm, dyspnea, urticaria, arthralgia, erythema, induration, edema, pain, tenderness, hives, swelling, lip edema, chills, fever, and skin rashes **(SEE WARNINGS AND CONTRAINDICATIONS)**.
PANCREATIC FUNCTION: pancreatitis, sometimes fulminant and fatal, has occurred. Increased serum amylase and lipase have also occurred.

LIVER FUNCTION: a variety of liver function abnormalities have been observed, including elevations of SGOT, SGPT, and bilirubin (direct and indirect). Jaundice, ascites, and hypoalbuminemia, which may be associated with peripheral edema, have been observed. These abnormalities usually are reversible on discontinuance of therapy, and some reversal may occur during the course of therapy. Fatty changes in the liver and liver failure have occurred.
HEMATOLOGIC: hypofibrinogenemia, prolonged prothrombin times, prolonged partial thromboplastin times, and decreased antithrombin III have been observed. Superficial and deep venous, thrombosis, sagittal sinus thrombosis, venous catheter thrombosis, and atrial thrombosis have occurred. Leukopenia, agranulocytosis, pancytopenia, thrombocytopenia, disseminated intravascular coagulation, severe hemolytic anemia, and anemia have been observed. Clinical hemorrhage, which may be fatal; easy bruisability, and ecchymosis have also been observed.
METABOLIC: mild to severe hyperglycemia has been observed in low incidence, and usually responds to discontinuation of **ONCASPAR®** and the judicious use of intravenous fluid and insulin. Hypoglycemia, increased thirst and hyponatremia, uric acid nephropathy, hyperuricemia, hypoproteinemia, and peripheral edema have also been observed. Hypoalbuminemia, proteinuria, weight loss, and metabolic acidosis have occurred. Therapy with **ONCASPAR®** is associated with an increase in blood ammonia during the conversion of L-asparagine to aspartic acid by the enzyme.
NEUROLOGIC: status epilepticus and temporal lobe seizures, somnolence, coma, malaise, mental status changes, dizziness, emotional lability, headache, lip numbness, finger paresthesia, mood changes, night sweats, and a Parkinson-like syndrome have occurred. Mild to severe confusion disorientation, and paresthesia have also occurred. These side effects usually have reversed spontaneously after treatment was stopped.
RENAL: increased BUN, increased creatinine, urinary frequency, hematuria due to thrombopenia, severe hemorrhagic cystitis, renal dysfunction, and renal failure have been observed.
CARDIOVASCULAR: chest pain, subacute bacterial endocarditis, hypertension, severe hypotension, and tachycardia have occurred.
DIGESTIVE: anorexia, constipation, decreased appetite, diarrhea, indigestion, flatulence, gas, gastrointestinal pain, mucositis, hepatomegaly, elevated gamma-glutamyl-transpeptidase, increased appetite, mouth tenderness, severe colitis, and nausea and/or vomiting have been observed.
MUSCULOSKELETAL: diffuse and local musculoskeletal pain, arthralgia, joint stiffness, and cramps have occurred.
RESPIRATORY: cough, epistaxis, severe bronchospasm, and upper respiratory infection have been observed.
SKIN/APPENDAGES: itching, alopecia, fever blister, purpura, hand whiteness and fungal changes, nail whiteness and ridging, erythema simplex, jaundice, and petechial rash have occurred.
GENERAL: localized edema, injection site reactions (including pain, swelling, or redness), malaise, infection, sepsis, fatigue, and septic shock may occur.

OVERDOSAGE

Three patients received 10,000 IU/m^2 of **ONCASPAR®** as an intravenous infusion. One patient experienced a slight increase in liver enzymes. A second patient developed a rash ten minutes after the start of the infusion, which was controlled with the administration of an antihistamine and by slowing down the infusion rate. A third patient did not experience any adverse reactions.

DOSAGE AND ADMINISTRATION

As a component of selected multiple agent regimens, the recommended dose of **ONCASPAR®** is 2,500 IU/m^2 every 14 days by the intramuscular route of administration.
The safety and effectiveness of **ONCASPAR®** have been established in patients with known previous hypersensitivity to L-asparaginase whose ages ranged from 1 to 21 years old. The recommended dose of **ONCASPAR®** for children with a body surface area ≥0.6 m^2 is 2,500 IU/m^2 administered every 14 days. The recommended dose of **ONCASPAR®** for children with a body surface area < 0.6 m^2 is 82.5 IU/kg administered every 14 days.
Do not administer ONCASPAR® if there is any indication that the drug has been frozen. Although there may not be an apparent change in the appearance of the drug, ONCASPAR®'s activity is destroyed after freezing.
When administering **ONCASPAR®** intramuscularly, the volume at a single injection site should be limited to 2 mL. If the volume to be administered is greater than 2 mL, multiple injection sites should be used.
Anaphylactic reactions require the immediate use of antihistamines, epinephrine, oxygen, and intravenous steroids.
Use of **ONCASPAR®** as the sole induction agent should be undertaken only in an unusual situation when a combined regimen, which uses other chemotherapeutic agents such as vincristine, methotrexate, cytarabine, daunorubicin, or doxorubicin, is inappropriate because of toxicity or other specific patient-related factors, or in patients refractory to other therapy. When **ONCASPAR®** is to be used as the sole induction agent, the recommended dosage regimen is also 2,500 IU/m^2 every 14 days.
When a remission is obtained, appropriate maintenance therapy may be instituted. **ONCASPAR®** may be used as part of a maintenance regimen.

Parenteral drug products should be inspected visually for particulate matter, cloudiness or discoloration prior to administration, whenever solution and container permit.

HOW SUPPLIED

Dosage Form
ONCASPAR®: Use only one dose per vial; do not re-enter the vial. Discard unused portions. Do not save unused drug for later administration.
Sterile solution for injection in ready to use single-use vials. Preservative free.
Quantity per Individual Container
5 mL per vial containing 750 IU/mL **ONCASPAR®** in a clear, colorless, phosphate buffered saline solution, pH 7.3. Each vial contains 3,750 IU of **ONCASPAR®**.
Handling and Storage
Avoid excessive agitation. DO NOT SHAKE.
Keep refrigerated at +2°C to +8°C (36°F to 46°F).
Do not use if cloudy of if precipitate is present.
Do not use if stored at room temperature for more than 48 hours.
DO NOT FREEZE. Do not use product if it is known to have been frozen. Freezing destroys activity, which cannot be detected visually.
NDC 57665-002-02
U.S. Patent 4,179,337 and pat pending

20 Kingsbridge Road
Piscataway, NJ 08854-3969 USA

11/5/98 License No. 1171

REFERENCES

1. Capizzi, RL and Holcenberg, JS. Asparaginase. In: Holland and Frei (eds). *Cancer Med* third edition, Lea and Febiger, Phila. PA, 1993.
2. Ho, DH, et al. Clinical pharmacology of polyethylene glycol-L-asparaginase. *Drug Metab Dispos* 14 (3): 349-352, 1986.
3. Asselin, BL, et al. Comparative Pharmacokinetic Studies of Three L-asparaginase Preparations. *J Clin Oncology* (11): 1780-1786, 1993.
4. Data on File at ENZON.
5. Clavell, LA, et al. Four-agent induction and intensive asparaginase therapy for treatment of childhood acute lymphoblastic leukemia. *N Engl J Med* 315 (11): 657-663, 1986.

ENZON Pharmaceuticals, Inc.
20 Kingsbridge Road
Piscataway, NJ 08854 USA PN 200-030A

ESP Pharma

2035 LINCOLN HIGHWAY
SUITE 2150
EDISON, NJ 08817

Direct Inquiries to:
phone: (732) 650-1377

The following list of products is also available from ESP Pharma:
Ismo
Sectal
Tenex
For full prescribing information, please refer to the ESP Pharma website, www.esppharma.com

IV BUSULFEX® ℞

[*bī-sul-fěks*]
(busulfan) Injection
Caution: Must be diluted prior to use.
Rx only

> **WARNING**
> IV BUSULFEX® (busulfan) Injection is a potent cytotoxic drug that causes profound myelosuppression at the recommended dosage. It should be administered under the supervision of a qualified physician who is experienced in allogeneic hematopoietic stem cell transplantation, the use of cancer chemotherapeutic drugs and the management of patients with severe pancytopenia. Appropriate management of therapy and complications is only possible when adequate diagnostic and treatment facilities are readily available. SEE "WARNINGS" SECTION FOR INFORMATION REGARDING BUSULFAN-INDUCED PANCYTOPENIA IN HUMANS.

DESCRIPTION

Busulfan is a bifunctional alkylating agent known chemically as 1,4-butanediol, dimethanesulfonate. BUSULFEX® (busulfan) Injection is intended for intravenous administration. It is supplied as a clear, colorless, sterile, solution in 10 mL single use ampoules.
Each ampoule of BUSULFEX contains 60 mg (6 mg/mL) of busulfan, the active ingredient, a white crystalline powder with a molecular formula of $CH_3SO_2O(CH_2)_4OSO_2CH_3$ and a molecular weight of 246 g/mole. Busulfan is dissolved in N,N-dimethylacetamide (DMA) 33% vol/vol and Polyethylene Glycol 400, 67% vol/vol. The solubility of busulfan in water is 0.1 g/L and the pH of BUSULFEX diluted to approximately 0.5 mg/mL busulfan in 0.9% Sodium Chloride Injection, USP or 5% Dextrose Injection, USP as recommended for infusion reflects the pH of the diluent used and ranges from 3.4 to 3.9.
BUSULFEX is intended for dilution with 0.9% Sodium Chloride Injection, USP or 5% Dextrose Injection, USP prior to intravenous infusion.

CLINICAL PHARMACOLOGY

Mechanism of Action:
Busulfan is a bifunctional alkylating agent in which two labile methanesulfonate groups are attached to opposite ends of a four-carbon alkyl chain. In aqueous media, busulfan hydrolyzes to release the methanesulfonate groups. This produces reactive carbonium ions that can alkylate DNA. DNA damage is thought to be responsible for much of the cytotoxicity of busulfan.
Pharmacokinetics:
The pharmacokinetics of BUSULFEX were studied in 59 patients participating in a prospective trial of a BUSULFEX-cyclophosphamide preparatory regimen prior to allogeneic hematopoietic progenitor stem cell transplantation. Patients received 0.8 mg/kg BUSULFEX every six hours, for a total of 16 doses over four days. Fifty-five of fifty-nine patients (93%) administered BUSULFEX maintained AUC values below the target value (<1500 µM•min).

Table 1: Steady State Pharmacokinetic Parameters Following Busulfex® (busulfan) Infusion (0.8 mg/kg; N=59)

	Mean	CV (%)	Range
C_{max} (ng/mL)	1222	18	496-1684
AUC (µM•min)	1167	20	556-1673
CL (ml/min/kg)*	2.52	25	1.49-4.31

* Clearance normalized to actual body weight for all patients.

BUSULFEX pharmacokinetics showed consistency between dose 9 and dose 13 as demonstrated by reproducibility of steady state C_{max} and a low coefficient of variation for this parameter.
In a pharmacokinetic study of BUSULFEX in 24 pediatric patients, the population pharmacokinetic (PPK) estimates of BUSULFEX for clearance (CL) and volume of distribution (V) were determined. For actual body weight, PPK estimates of CL and V were 4.04 L/hr/20 kg (3.37 ml/min/kg; interpatient variability 23%); and 12.8 L/20 kg (0.64 L/kg; interpatient variability 11%)
Distribution, Metabolism, Excretion:
Studies of distribution, metabolism, and elimination of BUSULFEX have not been done; however, the literature on oral busulfan is relevant. Additionally, for modulating effects on pharmacodynamic parameters see **Drug Interactions.**
Distribution: Busulfan achieves concentrations in the cerebrospinal fluid approximately equal to those in plasma. Irreversible binding to plasma elements, primarily albumin, has been estimated to be 32.4 ± 2.2% which is consistent with the reactive electrophilic properties of busulfan.
Metabolism: Busulfan is predominantly metabolized by conjugation with glutathione, both spontaneously and by glutathione S-transferase (GST) catalysis. This conjugate undergoes further extensive oxidative metabolism in the liver.
Excretion: Following administration of ^{14}C-labeled busulfan to humans, approximately 30% of the radioactivity was excreted into the urine over 48 hours; negligible amounts were recovered in feces. The incomplete recovery of radioactivity may be due to the formation of long-lived metabolites or due to nonspecific alkylation of macromolecules.

CLINICAL STUDIES

Documentation of the safety and efficacy of busulfan as a component of a conditioning regimen prior to allogeneic hematopoietic progenitor cell reconstitution is derived from two sources: i) analysis of a prospective clinical trial of BUSULFEX that involved 61 patients diagnosed with various hematologic malignancies, and ii) the published reports of randomized, controlled trials that employed high-dose oral busulfan as a component of a conditioning regimen for transplantation, which were identified in a literature review of five established commercial databases.
The prospective trial was a single-arm, open-label study in 61 patients who received BUSULFEX as part of a conditioning regimen for allogeneic hematopoietic stem cell transplantation. The study included patients with acute leukemia past first remission (first or subsequent relapse), with high-risk first remission, or with induction failure; chronic myelogenous leukemia (CML) in chronic phase, accelerated phase, or blast crisis; primary refractory or resistant relapsed Hodgkin's disease or non-Hodgkin's lymphoma; and myelodysplastic syndrome. Forty-eight percent of patients (29/61) were heavily pretreated, defined as having at least one of the following: prior radiation, ≥3 prior chemothera-

Continued on next page

Busulfex—Cont.

peutic regimens, or prior hematopoietic stem cell transplant. Seventy-five percent of patients (46/61) were transplanted with active disease.

Patients received 16 BUSULFEX doses of 0.8 mg/kg every 6 hours as a two-hour infusion for 4 days, followed by cyclophosphamide 60 mg/kg once per day for two days (BuCy2 regimen). All patients received 100% of their scheduled BUSULFEX regimen. No dose adjustments were made. After one rest day, allogeneic hematopoietic progenitor cells were infused. The efficacy parameters in this study were myeloablation (defined as one or more of the following: absolute neutrophil count [ANC] less than 0.5×10^9/L, absolute lymphocyte count [ALC] less than 0.1×10^9/L, thrombocytopenia defined as a platelet count less than 20,000/mm^3 or a platelet transfusion requirement) and engraftment (ANC≥0.5×10^9/L).

All patients (61/61) experienced myeloablation. The median time to neutropenia was 4 days. All evaluable patients (60/60) engrafted at a median of 13 days post-transplant (range 9 to 29 days); one patient was considered non-evaluable because he died of a fungal pneumonia 20 days after BMT and before engraftment occurred. All but 13 of the patients were treated with prophylactic G-CSF. Evidence of donor cell engraftment and chimerism was documented in all patients who had a chromosomal sex marker or leukemic marker (43/43), and no patient with chimeric evidence of allogeneic engraftment suffered a later loss of the allogeneic graft. There were no reports of graft failure in the overall study population. The median number of platelet transfusions per patient was 6, and the median number of red blood cell transfusions per patient was 4.

Twenty-three patients (38%) relapsed at a median of 183 days post-transplant (range 36 to 406 days). Sixty-two percent of patients (38/61) were free from disease with a median follow-up of 269 days post-transplant (range 20 to 583 days). Forty-three patients (70%) were alive with a median follow up of 288 days post-transplant (range 51 to 583 days). There were two deaths before BMT Day +28 and six additional patients died by BMT Day +100. Ten patients (16%) died after BMT Day +100, at a median of 199 days post-transplant (range 113 to 275 days).

Oral Busulfan Literature Review. Four publications of randomized, controlled trials that evaluated a high-dose oral busulfan-containing conditioning regimen (busulfan 4 mg/kg/d × 4 days + cyclophosphamide 60 mg/kg/d × 2 days) for allogeneic transplantation in the setting of CML were identified. Two of the studies (Clift and Devergie) had populations confined to CML in chronic phase that were randomized between conditioning with busulfan/cyclophosphamide (BU/CY) and cyclophosphamide/total body irradiation (CY/TBI). A total of 138 patients were treated with BU/CY in these studies. The populations of the two remaining studies (Ringden and Blume) included patients with CML, acute lymphoblastic leukemia (ALL), and acute myelogenous leukemia (AML). In the Nordic BMT Group study published by Ringden, et al., 57 patients had CML, and of those, 30 were treated with BU/CY. Patients with CML in chronic phase, accelerated phase, and blast crisis were eligible for this study. The participants with CML (34/122 patients) in a SWOG study published by Blume, et al., had disease beyond first chronic phase. Twenty of those CML patients were treated with BU/CY, and the TBI comparator arm utilized etoposide instead of cyclophosphamide.

Table 2 below summarizes the efficacy analyses reported from these 4 studies.

[See table 2 below]

INDICATIONS AND USAGE

BUSULFEX® (busulfan) Injection is indicated for use in combination with cyclophosphamide as a conditioning regimen prior to allogeneic hematopoietic progenitor cell transplantation for chronic myelogenous leukemia.

CONTRAINDICATIONS

BUSULFEX is contraindicated in patients with a history of hypersensitivity to any of its components.

WARNINGS

BUSULFEX should be administered under the supervision of a qualified physician experienced in hematopoietic stem cell transplantation. Appropriate management of complications arising from its administration is possible only when adequate diagnostic and treatment facilities are readily available.

The following warnings pertain to different physiologic effects of BUSULFEX in the setting of allogeneic transplantation.

Hematologic: The most frequent serious consequence of treatment with BUSULFEX at the recommended dose and schedule is profound myelosuppression, occurring in all patients. Severe granulocytopenia, thrombocytopenia, anemia, or any combination thereof may develop. Frequent complete blood counts, including white blood cell differentials, and quantitative platelet counts should be monitored during treatment and until recovery is achieved. Absolute neutrophil counts dropped below 0.5×10^9/L at a median of 4 days post-transplant in 100% of patients treated in the BUSULFEX clinical trial. The absolute neutrophil count recovered at a median of 13 days following allogeneic transplantation when prophylactic G-CSF was used in the majority of patients. Thrombocytopenia (<25,000/mm^3 or requiring platelet transfusion) occurred at a median of 5-6 days in 98% of patients. Anemia (hemoglobin <8.0 g/dL) occurred in 69% of patients. Antibiotic therapy and platelet and red blood cell support should be used when medically indicated.

Neurological: Seizures have been reported in patients receiving high-dose oral busulfan at doses producing plasma drug levels similar to those achieved following the recommended dosage of BUSULFEX. Despite prophylactic therapy with phenytoin, one seizure (1/42 patients) was reported during an autologous transplantation clinical trial of BUSULFEX. This episode occurred during the cyclophosphamide portion of the conditioning regimen, 36 hours after the last BUSULFEX dose. Anti-convulsant prophylactic therapy should be initiated prior to BUSULFEX treatment. Caution should be exercised when administering the recommended dose of BUSULFEX to patients with a history of a seizure disorder or head trauma or who are receiving other potentially epileptogenic drugs.

Hepatic: Current literature suggests that high busulfan area under the plasma concentration verses time curve (AUC) values (>1,500 µM•min) may be associated with an increased risk of developing hepatic veno-occlusive disease (HVOD). Patients who have received prior radiation therapy, greater than or equal to three cycles of chemotherapy, or a prior progenitor cell transplant may be at an increased risk of developing HVOD with the recommended BUSULFEX dose and regimen. Based on clinical examination and laboratory findings, hepatic veno-occlusive disease was diagnosed in 8% (5/61) of patients treated with BUSULFEX in the setting of allogeneic transplantation, was fatal in 2/5 cases (40%), and yielded an overall mortality from HVOD in the entire study population of 2/61 (3%). Three of the five patients diagnosed with HVOD were retrospectively found to meet the Jones' criteria. The incidence of HVOD reported in the literature from the randomized, controlled trials (see CLINICAL STUDIES) was 7.7%-12%.

Cardiac: Cardiac tamponade has been reported in pediatric patients with thalassemia (8/400 or 2% in one series) who received high doses of oral busulfan and cyclophosphamide as the preparatory regimen for hematopoietic progenitor cell transplantation. Six of the eight children died and two were saved by rapid pericardiocentesis. Abdominal pain and vomiting preceded the tamponade in most patients. No patients treated in the BUSULFEX (busulfan) Injection clinical trials experienced cardiac tamponade.

Pulmonary: Bronchopulmonary dysplasia with pulmonary fibrosis is a rare but serious complication following chronic busulfan therapy. The average onset of symptoms is 4 years after therapy (range 4 months to 10 years).

Carcinogenicity, Mutagenicity, Impairment of Fertility: Busulfan is a mutagen and a clastogen. In *in vitro* tests it caused mutations in ***Salmonella typhimurium*** and ***Drosophila melanogaster***. Chromosomal aberrations induced by busulfan have been reported *in vivo* (rats, mice, hamsters, and humans) and *in vitro* (rodent and human cells). The intravenous administration of busulfan (48 mg/kg given as biweekly doses of 12 mg/kg, or 30% of the total BUSULFEX dose on a mg/m^2 basis) has been shown to increase the incidence of thymic and ovarian tumors in mice. Four cases of acute leukemia occurred among 19 patients who became pancytopenic in a 243 patient study incorporating busulfan as adjuvant therapy following surgical resection of bronchogenic carcinoma. Clinical appearance of leukemia was observed 5-8 years following oral busulfan treatment. Busulfan is a presumed human carcinogen.

Ovarian suppression and amenorrhea commonly occur in premenopausal women undergoing chronic, low-dose busulfan therapy for chronic myelogenous leukemia. Busulfan depleted oocytes of female rats. Busulfan induced sterility in male rats and hamsters. Sterility, azoospermia and testicular atrophy have been reported in male patients. The solvent DMA may also impair fertility. A DMA daily dose of 0.45 g/kg/d given to rats for nine days (equivalent to 44% of the daily dose of DMA contained in the recommended dose of BUSULFEX on a mg/m^2 basis) significantly decreased spermatogenesis in rats. A single sc dose of 2.2 g/kg (27% of the total DMA dose contained in BUSULFEX on a mg/m^2 basis) four days after insemination terminated pregnancy in 100% of tested hamsters.

Pregnancy: Busulfan may cause fetal harm when administered to a pregnant woman. Busulfan produced teratogenic changes in the offspring of mice, rats and rabbits when given during gestation. Malformations and anomalies included significant alterations in the musculoskeletal system, body weight gain, and size. In pregnant rats, busulfan produced sterility in both male and female offspring due to the absence of germinal cells in the testes and ovaries. The solvent, DMA, may also cause fetal harm when administered to a pregnant woman. In rats, DMA doses of 400 mg/kg/d (about 40% of the daily dose of DMA in the BUSULFEX dose on a mg/m^2 basis) given during organogenesis caused significant developmental anomalies. The most striking abnormalities included anasarca, cleft palate, vertebral anomalies, rib anomalies, and serious anomalies of the vessels of the heart. There are no adequate and well-controlled studies of either busulfan or DMA in pregnant women. If BUSULFEX is used during pregnancy, or if the patient becomes pregnant while receiving BUSULFEX, the patient

Table 2: Summary of efficacy analyses from the randomized, controlled trials utilizing a high dose oral busulfan-containing conditioning regimen identified in a literature review.

Clift, 1994
CML Chronic Phase;

3 year Overall Survival		3 year DFS (p=0.43)		Relapse		Time to Engraftment (ANC ≥500)	
BU/CY	CY/TBI	BU/CY	CY/TBI	BU/CY	CY/TBI	BU/CY	CY/TBI
80%	80%	71%	68%	13%	13%	22.6 days	22.3 days

Devergie, 1995
CML Chronic Phase;

5 year Overall Survival (p=0.5)		5 year DFS (p=0.75)		Relapse (Relative Risk analysis BU/CY:CY/TBI) (p=0.04)		Time to Engraftment (ANC ≥500)	
BU/CY	CY/TBI	BU/CY	CY/TBI	BU/CY	CY/TBI	BU/CY	CY/TBI
60.6% ±11.7%	65.8% ±12.5%	59.1% ±11.8%	51.0% ±14%	4.10 (95% CI = 1.00-20.28)		None Given	None Given

Ringden, 1994
CML, AML, ALL;

3 year Overall Survival (p<0.03)		3 year Relapse Free Survival (p=0.065)		Relapse (p=0.9)		Time to Engraftment (ANC >500)	
BU/CY	CY/TBI	BU/CY	CY/TBI	BU/CY	CY/TBI	BU/CY	CY/TBI
62%	76%	56%	67%	22%	26%	20 days	20 days

Blume, 1993*
CML, AML, ALL; Relative Risk Analysis BU/CY: Etoposide/TBI

RR of Mortality		DFS		RR of Relapse (Relative Risk analysis BU/CY:Eto/TBI)		Time to Engraftment	
BU/CY	Eto/TBI	BU/CY	Eto/TBI	BU/CY	Eto/TBI	BU/CY	Eto/TBI
0.97 (95% CI=0.64-1.48)		Not Given		1.02 (95% CI=0.56-1.86)		Not Given	

* Eto = etoposide. TBI was combined with etoposide in the comparator arm of this study.
BU = Busulfan
CY = Cyclophosphamide
TBI = Total Body Irradiation
DFS = Disease Free Survival
ANC = Absolute Neutrophil Count

should be apprised of the potential hazard to the fetus. Women of childbearing potential should be advised to avoid becoming pregnant.

PRECAUTIONS

Hematologic: At the recommended dosage of BUSULFEX (busulfan) Injection, profound myelosuppression is universal, and can manifest as neutropenia, thrombocytopenia, anemia, or a combination thereof. Patients should be monitored for signs of local or systemic infection or bleeding. Their hematologic status should be evaluated frequently.

Information for Patients: The increased risk of a second malignancy should be explained to the patient.

Laboratory Tests: Patients receiving BUSULFEX should be monitored daily with a complete blood count, including differential count and quantitative platelet count, until engraftment has been demonstrated.

To detect hepatotoxicity, which may herald the onset of hepatic veno-occlusive disease, serum transaminases, alkaline phosphatase, and bilirubin should be evaluated daily through BMT Day +28.

Drug Interactions: Itraconazole decreases busulfan clearance by up to 25%, and may produce an AUC > 1500 µM•min in some patients. Fluconazole, and the 5-HT3 antiemetics odansetron (Zofran®) and granisetron (Kytril®) have all been used with BUSULFEX.

Phenytoin increases the clearance of busulfan by 15% or more, possibly due to the induction of glutathione-S-transferase. Since the pharmacokinetics of BUSULFEX were studied in patients treated with phenytoin, the clearance of BUSULFEX at the recommended dose may be lower and exposure (AUC) higher in patients not treated with phenytoin. Because busulfan is eliminated from the body via conjugation with glutathione, use of acetaminophen prior to (<72 hours) or concurrent with BUSULFEX may result in reduced busulfan clearance based upon the known property of acetaminophen to decrease glutathione levels in the blood and tissues.

Pregnancy: Pregnancy Category D. See **WARNINGS**.

Nursing Mothers: It is not known whether this drug is excreted in human milk. Because many drugs are excreted in human milk and because of the potential for tumorgenicity shown for busulfan in human and animal studies, a decision should be made whether to discontinue nursing or to discontinue the drug, taking into account the importance of the drug to the mother.

Special Populations

Pediatric: The effectiveness of BUSULFEX in the treatment of CML has not been specifically studied in pediatric patients. An open-label, uncontrolled study evaluated the pharmacokinetics of BUSULFEX in 24 pediatric patients receiving BUSULFEX as part of a conditioning regimen administered prior to hematopoietic progenitor cell transplantation for a variety of malignant hematologic (N=15) or non-malignant diseases (N=9). Patients ranged in age from 5 months to 16 years (median 3 years). BUSULFEX dosing was targeted to achieve an area under the plasma concentration curve (AUC) of 900-1350 µM•min with an initial dose of 0.8 mg/kg or 1.0 mg/kg (based on ABW) if the patient was >4 or ≤4 years, respectively. The dose was adjusted based on plasma concentration after completion of dose 1.

Patients received BUSULFEX doses every six hours as a two-hour infusion over four days for a total of 16 doses, followed by cyclophosphamide 50 mg/kg once daily for four days. After one rest day, hematopoietic progenitor cells were infused. All patients received phenytoin as seizure prophylaxis. The target AUC (900-1350 ± 5% µM•min) for BUSULFEX was achieved at dose 1 in 71% (17/24) of patients. Steady state pharmacokinetic testing was performed at dose 9 and 13. BUSULFEX levels were within the target range for 21 of 23 evaluable patients.

All 24 patients experienced neutropenia (absolute neutrophil count $<0.5 \times 10^9$/L) and thrombocytopenia (platelet transfusions or platelet count <20,000/mm^3). Seventy-nine percent (19/24) of patients experienced lymphopenia (absolute lymphocyte count $<0.1 \times 10^9$). In 23 patients, the ANC recovered to $>0.5 \times 10^9$/L (median time to recovery = BMT day +13; range = BMT day +9 to +22). One patient who died on day +20 had not recovered to an ANC $> 0.5 \times 10^9$/L.

Four (17%) patients died during the study. Two patients died within 28 days of transplant; one with pneumonia and capillary leak syndrome, and the other with pneumonia and veno-occlusive disease. Two patients died prior to day 100; one due to progressive disease and one due to multi-organ failure.

Adverse events were reported in all 24 patients during the study period (BMT day -10 through BMT day +28) or post-study surveillance period (day +29 through +100). These included vomiting (100%), nausea (83%), stomatitis (79%), hepatic veno-occlusive disease (HVOD) (21%), graft-versus-host disease (GVHD) (25%), and pneumonia (21%).

Based on the results of this 24-patient clinical trial, a suggested dosing regimen of BUSULFEX in pediatric patients is shown in the following dosing nomogram:

BUSULFEX Dosing Nomogram

Patient's Actual Body Weight (ABW)	BUSULFEX Dosage
≤12 kgs	1.1 (mg/kg)
>12 kgs	0.8 (mg/kg)

Simulations based on a pediatric population pharmacokinetic model indicate that approximately 60% of pediatric patients will achieve a target BUSULFEX exposure (AUC) between 900 to 1350 µM•min with the first dose of BUSULFEX using this dosing nomogram. Therapeutic drug monitoring and dose adjustment following the first dose of BUSULFEX is recommended.

Dose Adjustment Based on Therapeutic Drug Monitoring

Instructions for measuring the AUC of busulfan at dose 1 (see **Blood Sample Collection for AUC Determination**), and the formula for adjustment of subsequent doses to achieve the desired target AUC (1125 µM•min), are provided below.

Adjusted dose (mg) = Actual Dose (mg) × Target AUC (µM•min)/Actual AUC (µM•min)

For example, if a patient received a dose of 11 mg busulfan and if the corresponding AUC measured was 800 µM•min, for a target AUC of 1125 µM•min, the target mg dose would be:

Mg dose = 11 mg × 1125 µM•min / 800 µM•min = 15.5 mg

Busulfex dose adjustment may be made using this formula and instructions below.

Blood Sample Collection for AUC Determination:

Calculate the AUC (µM•min) based on blood samples collected at the following time points:

For dose 1: 2 hr (end of infusion), 4 hr and 6 hr (immediately prior to the next scheduled BUSULFEX administration). Actual sampling times should be recorded.

For doses other than dose 1: Pre-infusion (baseline), 2 hr (end of infusion), 4 hr and 6 hr (immediately prior to the next scheduled BUSULFEX administration).

AUC calculations based on fewer than the three specified samples may result in inaccurate AUC determinations.

For each scheduled blood sample, collect one to three mL of blood into heparinized (Na or Li heparin) Vacutainer® tubes. The blood samples should be placed on wet ice immediately after collection and should be centrifuged (at 4°C) within one hour. The plasma, harvested into appropriate cryovial storage tubes, is to be frozen immediately at -20°C. All plasma samples are to be sent in a frozen state (i.e., on dry ice) to the assay laboratory for the determination of plasma busulfan concentrations.

Calculation of AUC:

BUSULFEX AUC calculations may be made using the following instructions and appropriate standard pharmacokinetic formula:

Dose 1 $AUC_{infinity}$ Calculation: $AUC_{infinity} = AUC_{0\text{-}6hr} + AUC_{extrapolated}$, where $AUC_{0\text{-}6hr}$ is to be estimated using the linear trapezoidal rule and AUC extrapolated can be computed by taking the ratio of the busulfan concentration at Hour 6 and the terminal elimination rate constant, λ_z. The λ_z must be calculated from the terminal elimination phase of the busulfan concentration vs. time curve. A "0" predose busulfan concentration should be assumed, and used in the calculation of AUC.

If the AUC is assessed subsequent to Dose 1, steady-state AUC_{ss} ($AUC_{0\text{-}6hr}$) is to be estimated from the trough, 2 hr, 4 hr and 6 hr concentrations using the linear trapezoidal rule.

Instructions for Drug Administration and Blood Sample Collection for Therapeutic Drug Monitoring:

An administration set with minimal residual hold up (priming) volume (1-3 mL) should be used for drug infusion to ensure accurate delivery of the entire prescribed dose and to ensure accurate collection of blood samples for therapeutic drug monitoring and dose adjustment.

Prime the administration set tubing with drug solution to allow accurate documentation of the start time of BUSULFEX infusion. Collect the blood sample from a peripheral IV line to avoid contamination with infusing drug. If the blood sample is taken directly from the existing central venous catheter (CVC), **DO NOT COLLECT THE BLOOD SAMPLE WHILE THE DRUG IS INFUSING** to ensure that the end of infusion sample is not contaminated with any residual drug. At the end of infusion (2 hr), disconnect the administration tubing and flush the CVC line with 5 cc of normal saline prior to the collection of the end of infusion sample from the CVC port. Collect the blood samples from a different port than that used for the BUSULFEX infusion. When recording the BUSULFEX infusion stop time, do not include the time required to flush the indwelling catheter line. Discard the administration tubing at the end of the two-hour infusion.

See Preparation for Intravenous Administration section for detailed instructions on drug preparation.

Geriatric: Five of sixty-one patients treated in the BUSULFEX clinical trial were over the age of 55 (range 57-64). All achieved myeloablation and engraftment.

Gender, Race: Adjusting BUSULFEX dosage based on gender or race has not been adequately studied.

Renal Insufficiency: BUSULFEX has not been studied in patients with renal impairment.

Hepatic Insufficiency: BUSULFEX has not been administered to patients with hepatic insufficiency.

Other: Busulfan may cause cellular dysplasia in many organs. Cytologic abnormalities characterized by giant, hyperchromatic nuclei have been reported in lymph nodes, pancreas, thyroid, adrenal glands, liver, lungs and bone marrow. This cytologic dysplasia may be severe enough to cause difficulty in the interpretation of exfoliative cytologic examinations of the lungs, bladder, breast and the uterine cervix.

ADVERSE REACTIONS

Dimethylacetamide (DMA), the solvent used in the BUSULFEX formulation, was studied in 1962 as a potential cancer chemotherapy drug. In a Phase 1 trial, the maximum tolerated dose (MTD) was 14.8 g/m^2/d for four days. The daily recommended dose of BUSULFEX contains DMA equivalent to 42% of the MTD on a mg/m^2 basis. The dose-limiting toxicities in the Phase 1 study were hepatotoxicity as evidenced by increased liver transaminase (SGOT) levels and neurological symptoms as evidenced by hallucinations. The hallucinations had a pattern of onset at one day post completion of DMA administration and were associated with EEG changes. The lowest dose at which hallucinations were recognized was equivalent to 1.9 times that delivered in a conditioning regimen utilizing BUSULFEX 0.8 mg/kg every 6 hours × 16 doses. Other neurological toxicities included somnolence, lethargy, and confusion. The relative contribution of DMA and/or other concomitant medications to neurologic and hepatic toxicities observed with BUSULFEX is difficult to ascertain.

Treatment with BUSULFEX at the recommended dose and schedule will result in profound myelosuppression in 100% of patients, including granulocytopenia, thrombocytopenia, anemia, or a combined loss of formed elements of the blood.

Adverse reaction information is primarily derived from the clinical study (N=61) of BUSULFEX and the data obtained for high-dose oral busulfan conditioning in the setting of randomized, controlled trials identified through a literature review.

BUSULFEX Clinical Trials: In the BUSULFEX (busulfan) Injection allogeneic stem cell transplantation clinical trial, all patients were treated with BUSULFEX 0.8 mg/kg as a two-hour infusion every six hours for 16 doses over four days, combined with cyclophosphamide 60 mg/kg × 2 days. Ninety-three percent (93%) of evaluable patients receiving this dose of BUSULFEX maintained an AUC less than 1,500 µM•min for dose 9, which has generally been considered the level that minimizes the risk of HVOD.

Table 3: Summary of the Incidence (20%) of Non-Hematologic Adverse Events through BMT Day +28 in Patients who Received BUSULFEX Prior to Allogeneic Hematopoietic Progenitor Cell Transplantation

Non-Hematological Adverse Events*	Percent Incidence
BODY AS A WHOLE	
Fever	80
Headache	69
Asthenia	51
Chills	46
Pain	44
Edema General	28
Allergic Reaction	26
Chest Pain	26
Inflammation at Inj Site	25
Pain Back	23
CARDIOVASCULAR SYSTEM	
Tachycardia	44
Hypertension	36
Thrombosis	33
Vasodilation	25
DIGESTIVE SYSTEM	
Nausea	98
Stomatitis (Mucositis)	97
Vomiting	95
Anorexia	85
Diarrhea	84
Abdominal Pain	72
Dyspepsia	44
Constipation	38
Dry Mouth	26
Rectal Disorder	25
Abdominal Enlargement	23
METABOLIC AND NUTRITIONAL SYSTEM	
Hypomagnesemia	77
Hyperglycemia	66
Hypokalemia	64
Hypocalcemia	49
Hyperbilirubinemia	49
Edema	36
SGPT Elevation	31
Creatinine Increased	21
NERVOUS SYSTEM	
Insomnia	84
Anxiety	72
Dizziness	30
Depression	23
RESPIRATORY SYSTEM	
Rhinitis	44
Lung Disorder	34
Cough	28
Epistaxis	25
Dyspnea	25

Continued on next page

Busulfex—Cont.

SKIN AND APPENDAGES	
Rash	57
Pruritus	28

* Includes all reported adverse events regardless of severity (toxicity grades 1-4)

The following sections describe clinically significant events occurring in the BUSULFEX clinical trials, regardless of drug attribution. For pediatric information, see Special Populations – Pediatric section.

Hematologic: At the indicated dose and schedule, BUSULFEX produced profound myelosuppression in 100% of patients. Following hematopoietic progenitor cell infusion, recovery of neutrophil counts to ≥500 cells/mm^3 occurred at median day 13 when prophylactic G-CSF was administered to the majority of participants on the study. The median number of platelet transfusions per patient on study was 6, and the median number of red blood cell transfusions on study was 4. Prolonged prothrombin time was reported in one patient (2%).

Gastrointestinal: Gastrointestinal toxicities were frequent and generally considered to be related to the drug. Few were categorized as serious. Mild or moderate nausea occurred in 92% of patients in the allogeneic clinical trial, and mild or moderate vomiting occurred in 95% through BMT Day +28; nausea was severe in 7%. The incidence of vomiting during BUSULFEX administration (BMT Day -7 to -4) was 43% in the allogeneic clinical trial. Grade 3-4 stomatitis developed in 26% of the participants, and grade 3 esophagitis developed in 2%. Grade 3-4 diarrhea was reported in 5% of the allogeneic study participants, while mild or moderate diarrhea occurred in 75%. Mild or moderate constipation occurred in 38% of patients; ileus developed in 8% and was severe in 2%. Forty-four percent (44%) of patients reported mild or moderate dyspepsia. Two percent (2%) of patients experienced mild hematemesis. Pancreatitis developed in 2% of patients. Mild or moderate rectal discomfort occurred in 24% of patients. Severe anorexia occurred in 21% of patients and was mild/moderate in 64%.

Hepatic: Hyperbilirubinemia occurred in 49% of patients in the allogeneic BMT trial. Grade 3/4 hyperbilirubinemia occurred in 30% of patients within 28 days of transplantation and was considered life-threatening in 5% of these patients. Hyperbilirubinemia was associated with graft-versus-host disease in six patients and with hepatic veno-occlusive disease in 5 patients. Grade 3/4 SGPT elevations occurred in 7% of patients. Alkaline phosphatase increases were mild or moderate in 15% of patients. Mild or moderate jaundice developed in 12% of patients, and mild or moderate hepatomegaly developed in 6%.

Hepatic veno-occlusive disease: Hepatic veno-occlusive disease (HVOD) is a recognized potential complication of conditioning therapy prior to transplant. Based on clinical examination and laboratory findings, hepatic veno-occlusive disease was diagnosed in 8% (5/61) of patients treated with BUSULFEX in the setting of allogeneic transplantation, was fatal in 2/5 cases (40%), and yielded an overall mortality from HVOD in the entire study population of 2/61 (3%). Three of the five patients diagnosed with HVOD were retrospectively found to meet the Jones' criteria.

Graft-versus-host disease: Graft-versus-host disease developed in 18% of patients (11/61) receiving allogeneic transplants; it was severe in 3%, and mild or moderate in 15%. There were 3 deaths (5%) attributed to GVHD.

Edema: Patients receiving allogeneic transplant exhibited some form of edema (79%), hypervolemia, or documented weight increase (8%); all events were reported as mild or moderate.

Infection/Fever: Fifty-one percent (51%) of patients experienced one or more episodes of infection. Pneumonia was fatal in one patient (2%) and life-threatening in 3% of patients. Fever was reported in 80% of patients; it was mild or moderate in 78% and severe in 3%. Forty-six percent (46%) of patients experienced chills.

Cardiovascular: Mild or moderate tachycardia was reported in 44% of patients. In 7 patients (11%) it was first reported during BUSULFEX administration. Other rhythm abnormalities, which were all mild or moderate, included arrhythmia (5%), atrial fibrillation (2%), ventricular extrasystoles (2%), and third degree heart block (2%). Mild or moderate thrombosis occurred in 33% of patients, and all episodes were associated with the central venous catheter. Hypertension was reported in 36% of patients and was Grade 3/4 in 7%. Hypotension occurred in 11% of patients and was Grade 3/4 in 3%. Mild vasodilation (flushing and hot flashes) was reported in 25% of patients. Other cardiovascular events included cardiomegaly (5%), mild ECG abnormality (2%), grade 3/4 left-sided heart failure in one patient (2%), and moderate pericardial effusion (2%). These events were reported primarily in the post-cyclophosphamide phase.

Pulmonary: Mild or moderate dyspnea occurred in 25% of patients and was severe in 2%. One patient (2%) experienced severe hyperventilation; and in 2 (3%) additional patients it was mild or moderate. Mild rhinitis and mild or moderate cough were reported in 44% and 28% of patients, respectively. Mild epistaxis events were reported in 25%. Three patients (5%) on the allogeneic study developed documented alveolar hemorrhage. All required mechanical ventilatory support and all died. Non-specific interstitial fibrosis was found on wedge biopsies performed with video assisted thoracoscopy in one patient on the allogeneic study who subsequently died from respiratory failure on BMT Day +98. Other pulmonary events, reported as mild or moderate, included pharyngitis (18%), hiccup (18%), asthma (8%), atelectasis (2%), pleural effusion (3%), hypoxia (2%), hemoptysis (3%), and sinusitis (3%).

Neurologic: The most commonly reported adverse events of the central nervous system were insomnia (84%), anxiety (75%), dizziness (30%), and depression (23%). Severity was mild or moderate except for one patient (1%) who experienced severe insomnia. One patient (1%) developed a life-threatening cerebral hemorrhage and a coma as a terminal event following multi-organ failure after HVOD. Other events considered severe included delirium (2%), agitation (2%), and encephalopathy (2%). The overall incidence of confusion was 11%, and 5% of patients were reported to have experienced hallucinations. The patient who developed delirium and hallucination on the allogeneic study had onset of confusion at the completion of BUSULFEX (busulfan) Injection. The overall incidence of lethargy in the allogeneic BUSULFEX clinical trial was 7%, and somnolence was reported in 2%. One patient (2%) treated in an autologous transplantation study experienced a seizure while receiving cyclophosphamide, despite prophylactic treatment with phenytoin.

Renal: Creatinine was mildly or moderately elevated in 21% of patients. BUN was increased in 3% of patients and to a grade 3/4 level in 2%. Seven percent of patients experienced dysuria, 15% oliguria, and 8% hematuria. There were 4 (7%) Grade 3/4 cases of hemorrhagic cystitis in the allogeneic clinical trial.

Skin: Rash (57%) and pruritus (28%) were reported; both conditions were predominantly mild. Alopecia was mild in 15% of patients and moderate in 2%. Mild vesicular rash was reported in 10% of patients and mild or moderate maculopapular rash in 8%. Vesiculo-bullous rash was reported in 10%, and exfoliative dermatitis in 5%. Erythema nodosum was reported in 2%, acne in 7%, and skin discoloration in 8%.

Metabolic: Hyperglycemia was observed in 67% of patients and Grade 3/4 hyperglycemia was reported in 15%. Hypomagnesemia was mild or moderate in 77% of patients; hypokalemia was mild or moderate in 62% and severe in 2%; hypocalcemia was mild or moderate in 46% and severe in 3%; hypophosphatemia was mild or moderate in 17%; and hyponatremia was reported in 2%.

Other: Other reported events included headache (mild or moderate 64%, severe 5%), abdominal pain (mild or moderate 69%, severe 3%), asthenia (mild or moderate 49%, severe 2%), unspecified pain (mild or moderate 43%, severe 2%), allergic reaction (mild or moderate 24%, severe 2%), injection site inflammation (mild or moderate 25%), injection site pain (mild or moderate 15%), chest pain (mild or moderate 26%), back pain (mild or moderate 23%), myalgia (mild or moderate 16%), arthralgia (mild or moderate 13%), and ear disorder in 3%.

Deaths: There were two deaths through BMT Day +28 in the allogeneic transplant setting. There were an additional six deaths BMT Day +29 through BMT Day +100 in the allogeneic transplant setting.

Oral Busulfan Literature Review. A literature review identified four randomized, controlled trials that evaluated a high-dose oral busulfan-containing conditioning regimen for allogeneic bone marrow transplantation in the setting of CML (see CLINICAL STUDIES). The safety outcomes reported in those trials are summarized in Table 4 below for a mixed population of hematological malignancies (AML, CML, and ALL).

[See table 4 below]

Table 4: Summary of safety analyses from the randomized, controlled trials utilizing a high dose oral busulfan-containing conditioning regimen that were identified in a literature review.

TRM*	VOD**	GVHD***	Pulmonary	Hemorrhagic Cystitis	Seizure
Clift — CML Chronic Phase					
Death ≤100d =4.1% (3/73)	No Report	Acute ≥Grade 2 =35% Chronic =41% (30/73)	1 death from Idiopathic Interstitial Pneumonitis and 1 death from Pulmonary Fibrosis	No Report	No Report
Devergie — CML Chronic Phase					
TRM	VOD	GVHD	Pulmonary	Hemorrhagic Cystitis	Seizure
38%	7.7% (5/65) Deaths=4.6% (3/65)	Acute ≥Grade 2 =41% (24/59 at risk)	Interstitial Pneumonitis= 16.9% (11/65)	10.8% (7/65)	No report
Ringden — CML, AML, ALL					
TRM	VOD	GVHD	Pulmonary	Hemorrhagic Cystitis	Seizure
28%	12%	Acute ≥Grade 2 GVHD=26% Chronic GVHD =45%	Interstitial Pneumonitis =14%	24%	6%
Blume — CML, AML, ALL					
TRM	VOD	GVHD	Pulmonary	Hemorrhagic Cystitis	Seizure
No Report	Deaths =4.9%	Acute ≥Grade 2 GVHD=22% (13/58 at risk) Chronic GVHD =31% (14/45 at risk)	No Report	No Report	No Report

* TRM = Transplantation Related Mortality
** VOD = Veno-Occlusive Disease of the liver
*** GVHD = Graft versus Host Disease

OVERDOSAGE

There is no known antidote to BUSULFEX other than hematopoietic progenitor cell transplantation. In the absence of hematopoietic progenitor cell transplantation, the recommended dosage for BUSULFEX would constitute an overdose of busulfan. The principal toxic effect is profound bone marrow hypoplasia/aplasia and pancytopenia, but the central nervous system, liver, lungs, and gastro intestinal tract may be affected. The hematologic status should be closely monitored and vigorous supportive measures instituted as medically indicated. Survival after a single 140 mg dose of Myleran® Tablets in an 18 kg, 4-year old child has been reported. Inadvertent administration of a greater than normal dose of oral busulfan (2.1 mg/kg; total dose of 23.3 mg/kg) occurred in a 2-year old child prior to a scheduled bone marrow transplant without sequelae. An acute dose of 2.4 g was fatal in a 10-year old boy. There is one report that busulfan is dialyzable, thus dialysis should be considered in the case of overdose. Busulfan is metabolized by conjugation with glutathione, thus administration of glutathione may be considered.

DOSAGE AND ADMINISTRATION

When BUSULFEX (busulfan) Injection is administered as a component of the BuCy conditioning regimen prior to bone marrow or peripheral blood progenitor cell replacement, the recommended doses are as follows:

Adults (BuCy2): The usual adult dose is 0.8 mg/kg of ideal body weight or actual body weight, whichever is lower, administered every six hours for four days (a total of 16 doses). For obese, or severely obese patients, BUSULFEX should be administered based on adjusted ideal body weight. Ideal body weight (IBW) should be calculated as follows (height in cm, and weight in kg): IBW (kg; men)= 50 + 0.91× (height in cm -152); IBW (kg; women)= 45 + 0.91× (height in cm -152). Adjusted ideal body weight (AIBW) should be calculated as follows: AIBW= IBW + 0.25x (actual weight -IBW). Cyclophosphamide is given on each of two days as a one-hour infusion at a dose of 60 mg/kg beginning on BMT day -3, no sooner than six hours following the 16 th dose of BUSULFEX.

BUSULFEX clearance is best predicted when the BUSULFEX dose is administered based on adjusted ideal body weight. Dosing BUSULFEX based on actual body weight, ideal body weight or other factors can produce significant differences in BUSULFEX (busulfan) Injection clearance among lean, normal and obese patients.

BUSULFEX should be administered intravenously via a central venous catheter as a two-hour infusion every six hours for four consecutive days for a total of 16 doses. All patients should be premedicated with phenytoin as busulfan is known to cross the blood brain barrier and induce seizures. Phenytoin reduces busulfan plasma AUC by 15%. Use of other anticonvulsants may result in higher busulfan plasma AUCs, and an increased risk of VOD or seizures. In cases where other anticonvulsants must be used, plasma busulfan exposure should be monitored (See DRUG INTERACTIONS). Antiemetics should be administered prior to the first dose of BUSULFEX and continued on a fixed schedule through administration of BUSULFEX. Where available, pharmacokinetic monitoring may be considered to further optimize therapeutic targeting.

Pediatrics: The effectiveness of BUSULFEX in the treatment of CML has not been specifically studied in pediatric patients. For additional information see Special Populations - Pediatric section.

Preparation and Administration Precautions:

An administration set with minimal residual hold-up volume (2-5 cc) should be used for product administration.

As with other cytotoxic compounds, caution should be exercised in handling and preparing the solution of BUSULFEX. Skin reactions may occur with accidental exposure. The use of gloves is recommended. If BUSULFEX or diluted BUSULFEX solution contacts the skin or mucosa, wash the skin or mucosa thoroughly with water.

BUSULFEX is a clear, colorless solution. Parenteral drug products should be visually inspected for particulate matter and discoloration prior to administration whenever the solution and container permit. If particulate matter is seen in the BUSULFEX ampoule the drug should not be used.

Preparation for Intravenous Administration:

BUSULFEX must be diluted prior to use with either 0.9% Sodium Chloride Injection, USP (normal saline) or 5% Dextrose Injection, USP (D_5W). The diluent quantity should be 10 times the volume of BUSULFEX, so that the final concentration of busulfan is approximately 0.5 mg/mL. Calculation of the dose for a 70 kg patient, would be performed as follows:

(70kg patient) × (0.8 mg/kg) ÷ (6 mg/mL) = 9.3 mL BUSULFEX (56 mg total dose).

To prepare the final solution for infusion, add 9.3 mL of BUSULFEX to 93 mL of diluent (normal saline or D5W) as calculated below:

(9.3 mL BUSULFEX)×(10)=93 mL of either diluent plus the 9.3 mL of BUSULFEX to yield a final concentration of busulfan of 0.54 mg/mL (9.3 mL × 6 mg/mL ÷ 102.3 mL = 0.54 mg/mL).

All transfer procedures require strict adherence to aseptic techniques, preferably employing a vertical laminar flow safety hood while wearing gloves and protective clothing. In accordance with pharmacy practices, filter BUSULFEX using the 5 micron syringe filter provided with each package, using one filter per ampoule. If using the enclosed syringe filter in the forward flow direction, the calculated volume of BUSULFEX should allow for approximately 0.16 ml of residual BUSULFEX that will remain in the filter.

DO NOT put the BUSULFEX into an intravenous bag or large-volume syringe that does not contain normal saline or D_5W. Always add the BUSULFEX to the diluent, not the diluent to the BUSULFEX. Mix thoroughly by inverting several times. USE OF SYRINGE FILTERS OTHER THAN THE SPECIFIC TYPE INCLUDED IN THIS PACKAGE WITH EACH AMPOULE IS NOT RECOMMENDED. DO NOT USE POLYCARBONATE SYRINGES OR POLYCARBONATE FILTER NEEDLES WITH BUSULFEX.

Infusion pumps should be used to administer the diluted BUSULFEX solution. Set the flow rate of the pump to deliver the entire prescribed BUSULFEX dose over two hours. Prior to and following each infusion, flush the indwelling catheter line with approximately 5mL of 0.9% Sodium Chloride Injection, USP or 5% Dextrose Injection, USP. DO NOT infuse concomitantly with another intravenous solution of unknown compatibility. WARNING: RAPID INFUSION OF BUSULFEX HAS NOT BEEN TESTED AND IS NOT RECOMMENDED.

STABILITY

Unopened ampoules of BUSULFEX are stable until the date indicated on the package when stored under refrigeration at 2°-8°C (36°-46°F).

BUSULFEX diluted in 0.9% Sodium Chloride Injection, USP or 5% Dextrose Injection, USP is stable at room temperature (25° C) for up to 8 hours but the infusion must be completed within that time. BUSULFEX diluted in 0.9% Sodium Chloride Injection, USP is stable at refrigerated conditions (2°-8° C) for up to 12 hours but the infusion must be completed within that time.

HOW SUPPLIED

BUSULFEX is supplied as a sterile solution in 10 mL single-use clear glass ampoules each containing 60 mg of busulfan at a concentration of 6 mg/mL for intravenous use.

NDC 67286-0053-8 10mL (6mg/mL) in packages of eight ampoules including eight compatible 5 micron syringe filters.

Unopened ampoules of BUSULFEX must be stored under refrigerated conditions between 2°-8°C (36°-46°F).

HANDLING AND DISPOSAL

Procedures for proper handling and disposal of anticancer drugs should be considered. Several guidelines on this subject have been published.[1,2,3,4,5,6] There is no general agreement that all of the procedures recommended in the guidelines are necessary or appropriate.

Distributed by: ESP Pharma, Inc. Edison, NJ 08817

United States Patent numbers are 5,430,057 and 5,559,148. Canadian Patent number is CA2171738. Patent pending in the European Union.

Revision Date: September 2003 Part No. 4040290

References

1. Recommendations for the safe handling of parenteral antineoplastic drugs. Washington, DC: Division of Safety, National Institutes of Health; 1983. US Department of Health and Human Services, Public Health Service publication NIH 83-2621.
2. AMA Council on Scientific Affairs. Guidelines for handling parenteral antineoplastics. *JAMA* 1985; 253:1590-1591.
3. National Study Commission on Cytotoxic Exposure. Recommendations for handling cytotoxic agents. 1987. Available from Louis P. Jeffrey, Chairman, National Study Commission on Cytotoxic Exposure. Massachusetts College of Pharmacy and Allied Health Sciences, 179 Longhwood Avenue, Boston, MA 02115.
4. Clinical Oncology Society of Australia. Guidelines and recommendations for safe handling of antineoplastic agents. *Med J Australia* 1983; 1:426-428.
5. Jones RB, Frank R, Mass T. Safe handling of chemotherapeutic agents: a report from the Mount Sinai Medical Center. *CA-A Cancer J for Clin* 1983; 33:258-263.
6. American Society of Hospital Pharmacists. ASHP technical assistance bulletin on handling cytotoxic and hazardous drugs. *Am J Hosp Pharm* 1990; 47:1033-1049.

IVBusulfex®
(busulfan) Injection

For questions of a medical nature call 1-866-4ES-PPHARMA

To order IV BUSULFEX call 1-866-4ES-PPHARMA

ESP Pharma
Excellence in Specialty Pharmaceuticals BUS0003-PDR

CARDENE® I.V. ℞
(nicardipine hydrochloride)

℞ only

DESCRIPTION

Cardene (nicardipine HCl) is a calcium ion influx inhibitor (slow channel blocker or calcium channel blocker). Cardene I.V. for intravenous administration contains 2.5 mg/mL of nicardipine hydrochloride. Nicardipine hydrochloride is a dihydropyridine derivative with IUPAC (International Union of Pure and Applied Chemistry) chemical name (±)-2-(benzyl-methyl amino) ethyl methyl 1,4-dihydro-2,6-dimethyl-4-(*m*-nitrophenyl)-3,5-pyridinedicarboxylate monohydrochloride and has the following structure:

$C_{26}H_{29}N_3O_6 \cdot HCl$

Nicardipine hydrochloride is a greenish-yellow, odorless, crystalline powder that melts at about 169° C. It is freely soluble in chloroform, methanol, and glacial acetic acid, sparingly soluble in anhydrous ethanol, slightly soluble in n-butanol, water, 0.01 M potassium dihydrogen phosphate, acetone, and dioxane, very slightly soluble in ethyl acetate, and practically insoluble in benzene, ether, and hexane. It has a molecular weight of 515.99.

Cardene I.V. is available as a sterile, non-pyrogenic, clear, yellow solution in 10 mL ampuls for intravenous infusion after dilution. Each mL contains 2.5 mg nicardipine hydrochloride in Water for Injection, USP with 48.00 mg Sorbitol, NF, buffered to pH 3.5 with 0.525 mg citric acid monohydrate, USP and 0.09 mg sodium hydroxide, NF. Additional citric acid and/or sodium hydroxide may have been added to adjust pH.

CLINICAL PHARMACOLOGY

MECHANISM OF ACTION

Nicardipine inhibits the transmembrane influx of calcium ions into cardiac muscle and smooth muscle without changing serum calcium concentrations. The contractile processes of cardiac muscle and vascular smooth muscle are dependent upon the movement of extracellular calcium ions into these cells through specific ion channels. The effects of nicardipine are more selective to vascular smooth muscle than cardiac muscle. In animal models, nicardipine produced relaxation of coronary vascular smooth muscle at drug levels which cause little or no negative inotropic effect.

PHARMACOKINETICS AND METABOLISM

Following infusion, nicardipine plasma concentrations decline tri-exponentially, with a rapid early distribution phase (α-half-life of 2.7 minutes), an intermediate phase (β-half-life of 44.8 minutes), and a slow terminal phase (γ-half-life of 14.4 hours) that can only be detected after long-term infusions. Total plasma clearance (Cl) is 0.4 L/hr•kg, and the apparent volume of distribution (V_d) using a non-compartment model is 8.3 L/kg. The pharmacokinetics of Cardene I.V. are linear over the dosage range of 0.5 to 40.0 mg/hr.

Rapid dose-related increases in nicardipine plasma concentrations are seen during the first two hours after the start of an infusion of Cardene I.V. Plasma concentrations increase at a much slower rate after the first few hours, and approach steady state at 24 to 48 hours. On termination of the infusion, nicardipine concentrations decrease rapidly, with at least a 50% decrease during the first two hours post-infusion. The effects of nicardipine on blood pressure significantly correlate with plasma concentrations.

Nicardipine is highly protein bound (>95%) in human plasma over a wide concentration range.

Cardene I.V. has been shown to be rapidly and extensively metabolized by the liver. After coadministration of a radioactive intravenous dose of Cardene I.V. with an oral 30 mg dose given every 8 hours, 49% of the radioactivity was recovered in the urine and 43% in the feces within 96 hours. None of the dose was recovered as unchanged nicardipine. Nicardipine does not induce or inhibit its own metabolism and does not induce or inhibit hepatic microsomal enzymes.

The steady-state pharmacokinetics of nicardipine are similar in elderly hypertensive patients (>65 years) and young healthy adults.

HEMODYNAMICS

Cardene I.V. produces significant decreases in systemic vascular resistance. In a study of intra-arterially administered Cardene I.V., the degree of vasodilation and the resultant decrease in blood pressure were more prominent in hypertensive patients than in normotensive volunteers. Administration of Cardene I.V. to normotensive volunteers at dosages of 0.25 to 3.0 mg/hr for eight hours produced changes of <5 mmHg in systolic blood pressure and <3 mmHg in diastolic blood pressure.

An increase in heart rate is a normal response to vasodilation and decrease in blood pressure; in some patients these increases in heart rate may be pronounced. In placebo-controlled trials, the mean increases in heart rate were 7 ± 1 bpm in postoperative patients and 8 ± 1 bpm in patients with severe hypertension at the end of the maintenance period.

Hemodynamic studies following intravenous dosing in patients with coronary artery disease and normal or moderately abnormal left ventricular function have shown significant increases in ejection fraction and cardiac output with no significant change, or a small decrease, in left ventricular end-diastolic pressure (LVEDP). There is evidence that Cardene increases blood flow. Coronary dilatation induced by Cardene I.V. improves perfusion and aerobic metabolism in areas with chronic ischemia, resulting in reduced lactate production and augmented oxygen consumption. In patients with coronary artery disease, Cardene I.V., administered after beta-blockade, significantly improved systolic and diastolic left ventricular function.

In congestive heart failure patients with impaired left ventricular function, Cardene I.V. increased cardiac output both at rest and during exercise. Decreases in left ventricular end-diastolic pressure were also observed. However, in some patients with severe left ventricular dysfunction, it may have a negative inotropic effect and could lead to worsened failure.

"Coronary steal" has not been observed during treatment with Cardene I.V. (Coronary steal is the detrimental redistribution of coronary blood flow in patients with coronary artery disease from underperfused areas toward better perfused areas.) Cardene I.V. has been shown to improve systolic shortening in both normal and hypokinetic segments of myocardial muscle. Radionuclide angiography has confirmed that wall motion remained improved during increased oxygen demand. (Occasional patients have developed increased angina upon receiving Cardene capsules. Whether this represents coronary steal in these patients, or is the result of increased heart rate and decreased diastolic pressure, is not clear.)

In patients with coronary artery disease, Cardene I.V. improves left ventricular diastolic distensibility during the early filing phase, probably due to a faster rate of myocardial relaxation in previously underperfused areas. There is little or no effect on normal myocardium, suggesting the improvement is mainly by indirect mechanisms such as afterload reduction and reduced ischemia. Cardene I.V. has no

Continued on next page

Cardene—Cont.

negative effect on myocardial relaxation at therapeutic doses. The clinical benefits of these properties have not yet been demonstrated.

ELECTROPHYSIOLOGIC EFFECTS

In general, no detrimental effects on the cardiac conduction system have been seen with Cardene I.V. During acute electrophysiologic studies, it increased heart rate and prolonged the corrected QT interval to a minor degree. It did not affect sinus node recovery or SA conduction times. The PA, AH, and HV intervals* or the function and effective refractory periods of the atrium were not prolonged. The relative and effective refractory periods of the His-Purkinje system were slightly shortened.

HEPATIC FUNCTION

Because nicardipine is extensively metabolized by the liver, plasma concentrations are influenced by changes in hepatic function. In a clinical study with Cardene capsules in patients with severe liver disease, plasma concentrations were elevated and the half-life was prolonged (see **"PRECAUTIONS"**). Similar results were obtained in patients with hepatic disease when Cardene I.V. (nicardipine hydrochloride) was adminstered for 24 hours at 0.6 mg/hr.

RENAL FUNCTION

When Cardene I.V. was given to mild to moderate hypertensive patients with moderate degrees of renal impairment, significant reduction in glomerular filtration rate (GFR) and effective renal plasma flow (RPF) was observed. No significant differences in liver blood flow were observed in these patients. A significantly lower systemic clearance and higher area under the curve (AUC) were observed.

When Cardene capsules (20 mg or 30 mg TID) were given to hypertensive patients with impaired renal function, mean plasma concentrations, AUC, and C_{max} were approximately two-fold higher than in healthy controls. There is a transient increase in electrolyte excretion, including sodium (see **"PRECAUTIONS"**).

Acute bolus administration of Cardene I.V. (2.5 mg) in healthy volunteers decreased mean arterial pressure and renal vascular resistance; glomerular filtration rate (GFR), renal plasma flow (RPF), and the filtration fraction were unchanged. In healthy patients undergoing abdominal surgery, Cardene I.V. (10 mg over 20 minutes) increased GFR with no change in RPF when compared with placebo. In hypertensive type II diabetic patients with nephropathy, Cardene capsules (20 mg TID) did not change RPF and GFR, but reduced renal vascular resistance.

PULMONARY FUNCTION

In two well-controlled studies of patients with obstructive airway disease treated with Cardene capsules, no evidence of increased bronchospasm was seen. In one of the studies, Cardene capsules improved forced expiratory volume 1 second (FEV_1) and forced vital capacity (FVC) in comparison with metoprolol. Adverse experiences reported in a limited number of patients with asthma, reactive airway disease, or obstructive airway disease are similar to all patients treated with Cardene capsules.

EFFECTS IN HYPERTENSION

In patients with mild to moderate chronic stable essential hypertension, Cardene I.V. (0.5 to 4.0 mg/hr) produced dose-dependent decreases in blood pressure, although only the decreases at 4.0 mg/hr were statistically different from placebo. At the end of a 48-hour infusion at 4.0 mg/hr, the decreases were 26.0 mmHg (17%) in systolic blood pressure at 20.7 mmHg (20%) in diastolic blood pressure. In other settings (e.g., patients with severe or postoperative hypertension), Cardene I.V. (5 to 15 mg/hr) produced dose-dependent decreases in blood pressure. Higher infusion rates produced therapeutic responses more rapidly. The mean time to therapeutic response for severe hypertension, defined as diastolic blood pressure ≤ 95 mmHg or ≥ 25 mmHg decrease and systolic blood pressure ≤160 mmHg, was 77 ± 5.2 minutes. The average maintenance dose was 8.0 mg/hr. The mean time to therapeutic response for postoperative hypertension, defined as ≥15% reduction in diastolic or systolic blood pressure, was 11.5 ± 0.8 minutes. The average maintenance dose was 3.0 mg/hr.

*PA = conduction time from high to low right atrium; AH = conduction time from low right atrium to His bundle deflection, or AV nodal conduction time; HV = conduction time through the His bundle branch-Purkinje system.

INDICATION AND USAGE

Cardene I.V. is indicated for the short-term treatment of hypertension when oral therapy is not feasible or not desirable.

For prolonged control of blood pressure, patients should be transferred to oral medication as soon as their clinical condition permits (see **"DOSAGE AND ADMINISTRATION"**).

CONTRAINDICATIONS

Cardene I.V. is contraindicated in patients with known hypersensitivity to the drug. Cardene I.V. is also contraindicated in patients with advanced aortic stenosis because part of the effect of Cardene I.V. is secondary to reduced afterload. Reduction of diastolic pressure in these patients may worsen rather than improve myocardial oxygen balance.

WARNINGS

BETA-BLOCKER WITHDRAWAL

Nicardipine is not a beta-blocker and therefore gives no protection against the dangers of abrupt beta-blocker withdrawal; any such withdrawal should be by gradual reduction dose of beta-blocker.

RAPID DECREASES IN BLOOD PRESSURE

No clinical events have been reported suggestive of a too rapid decreases in blood pressure with Cardene I.V. However, as with any antihypertensive agent, blood pressure lowering should be accomplished over as long a time as is compatible with the patient's clinical status.

USE IN PATIENTS WITH ANGINA

Increases in frequency, duration, or severity of angina have been seen in chronic oral therapy with Cardene capsules. Induction or exacerbation of angina has been seen in less than 1% of coronary artery disease patients treated with Cardene I.V. The mechanism of this effect has not been established.

USE IN PATIENTS WITH CONGESTIVE HEART FAILURE

Cardene I.V. reduced afterload without impairing myocardial contractility in preliminary hemodynamic studies of CHF patients. However, *in vitro* and in some patients, a negative inotropic effect has been observed. Therefore, caution should be exercised when using Cardene I.V., particularly in combination with a beta-blocker, in patients with CHF or significant left ventricular dysfunction.

USE IN PATIENTS WITH PHEOCHROMOCYTOMA

Only limited clinical experience exists in use of Cardene I.V. for patients with hypertension associated with pheochromocytoma. Caution should therefore be exercised when using the drug in these patients.

PERIPHERAL VEIN INFUSION SITE

To minimize the risk of peripheral venous irritation, it is recommended that the site of infusion of Cardene I.V., be changed every 12 hours.

PRECAUTIONS

GENERAL

Blood Pressure: Because Cardene I.V. decreases peripheral resistance, monitoring of blood pressure during administration is required. Cardene I.V., like other calcium channel blockers, may occasionally produce symptomatic hypotension. Caution is advised to avoid systemic hypotension when administering the drug to patients who have sustained an acute cerebral infarction or hemorrhage.

Use in Patients with Impaired Hepatic Function: Since nicardipine is metabolized in the liver, the drug should be used with caution in patients with impaired liver function or reduced hepatic blood flow. The use of lower dosages should be considered.

Nicardipine administered intravenously has been reported to increase hepatic venous pressure gradient by 4 mmHg in cirrhotic patients at high doses (5 mg/20 min). Cardene I.V. should therefore be used with caution in patients with portal hypertension.

Use in Patients with Impaired Renal Function: When Cardene I.V. was given to mild to moderate hypertensive patients with moderate renal impairment, a significantly lower systemic clearance and higher AUC was observed. These results are consistent with those seen after oral administration of nicardipine. Careful dose titration is advised when treating renal impaired patients.

DRUG INTERACTIONS

Since Cardene I.V. may be administered to patients already being treated with other medications, including other antihypertensive agents, careful monitoring of these patients is necessary to detect and promptly treat any undesired effects from concomitant administration.

BETA-BLOCKERS

In most patients, Cardene I.V. can safely be used concomitantly with beta-blockers. However, caution should be exercised when using Cardene I.V. in combination with a beta-blocker in congestive heart failure patients (see **"WARNINGS"**).

CIMETIDINE

Cimetidine has been shown to increase nicardipine plasma concentrations with Cardene capsule administration. Patients receiving the two drugs concomitantly should be carefully monitored. Data with other histamine-2 antagonists are not available.

DIGOXIN

Studies have shown that Cardene capsules usually do not alter digoxin plasma concentrations. However, as a precaution, digoxin levels should be evaluated when concomitant therapy with Cardene I.V. is initiated.

FENTANYL ANESTHESIA

Hypotension has been reported during fentanyl anesthesia with concomitant use of a beta-blocker and a calcium channel blocker. Even though such interactions were not seen during clinical studies with Cardene I.V. (nicardipine hydrochloride), an increased volume of circulating fluids might be required if such an interaction were to occur.

CYCLOSPORINE

Concomitant administration of Cardene capsules and cyclosporine results in elevated plasma cyclosporine levels. Plasma concentrations of cyclosporine should therefore be closely monitored during Cardene I.V. administration, and the dose of cyclosporine reduced accordingly.

IN VITRO INTERACTION

The plasma protein binding of nicardipine was not altered when therapeutic concentrations of furosemide, propranolol, dipyridamole, warfarin, quinidine, or naproxen were added to human plasma *in vitro.*

CARCINOGENESIS, MUTAGENESIS, IMPAIRMENT OF FERTILITY

Rats treated with nicardipine in the diet (at concentrations calculated to provide daily dosage levels of 5, 15, or 45 mg/kg/day) for two years showed a dose-dependent increase in thyroid hyperplasia and neoplasia (follicular adenoma/carcinoma). One- and three-month studies in the rat have suggested that these results are linked to a nicardipine-induced reduction in plasma thyroxine (T4) levels with a consequent increase in plasma levels of thyroid stimulating hormone (TSH). Chronic elevation of TSH is known to cause hyperstimulation of the thyroid. In rats on an iodine deficient diet, nicardipine administration for one month was associated with thyroid hyperplasia that was prevented by T4 supplementation. Mice treated with nicardipine in the diet (at concentrations calculated to provide daily dosage levels of up to 100 mg/kg/day) for up to 18 months showed no evidence of neoplasia of any tissue and no evidence of thyroid changes. There was no evidence of thyroid pathology in dogs treated with up to 25 mg nicardipine/kg/day for one year and no evidence of effects of nicardipine on thyroid function (plasma T4 and TSH) in man. There was no evidence of a mutagenic potential of nicardipine in a battery of genotoxicity tests conducted on microbial indicator organisms, in micronucleus tests in mice and hamsters, or in a sister chromatid exchange study in hamsters. No impairment of fertility was seen in male or female rats administered nicardipine at oral doses as high as 100 mg/kg/day (50 times the 40 mg TID maximum recommended dose in man, assuming a patient weight of 60 kg).

Pregnancy Category C: Cardene® I.V. at doses up to 5 mg/kg/day to pregnant rats and up to 0.5 mg/kg/day to pregnant rabbits produced no embryotoxicity or teratogenicity. Embryotoxicity was seen at 10 mg/kg/day in rats and at 1 mg/kg/day in rabbits, but no teratogenicity was observed at these doses.

Nicardipine was embryocidal when administered orally to pregnant Japanese White rabbits, during organogenesis, at 150 mg/kg/day (a dose associated with marked body weight gain suppression in the treated doe), but not at 50 mg/kg/day (25 times the maximum recommended dose in man). No adverse effects on the fetus were observed when New Zealand albino rabbits were treated, during organogenesis, with up to 100 mg nicardipine/kg/day (a dose associated with significant mortality in the treated doe). In pregnant rats administered nicardipine orally at up to 100 mg/kg/day (50 times the maximum recommended human dose) there was no evidence of embryolethality or teratogenicity. However, dystocia, reduced birth weights, reduced neonatal survival, and reduced neonatal weight gain were noted. There are no adequate and well-controlled studies in pregnant women. Cardene should be used during pregnancy only if the potential benefit justifies the potential risk to the fetus.

NURSING MOTHERS

Studies in rats have shown significant concentrations of nicardipine in maternal milk. For this reason, it is recommended that women who wish to breastfeed should not be given this drug.

PEDIATRIC USE

Safety and efficacy in patients under the age of 18 have not been established.

USE IN THE ELDERLY

No significant difference has been observed in the antihypertensive effect of Cardene I.V. in elderly patients (≥ 65 years) compared with other adult patients in clinical studies.

Adverse Experiences

Two hundred forty-four patients participated in two multicenter, double-blind, placebo-controlled trials of Cardene I.V. Adverse experiences were generally not serious and most were expected consequences of vasodilation. Adverse experiences occasionally required dosage adjustment. Therapy was discontinued in approximately 12% of patients, mainly due to hypotension, headache, and tachycardia.

Percent of Patients with Adverse Experiences During the Double-Blind Portion of Controlled Trials

Adverse Experience	Cardene (n=144)	Placebo (n=100)
Body as a Whole		
Headache	14.6	2.0
Asthenia	0.7	0.0
Abdominal pain	0.7	0.0
Chest pain	0.7	0.0
Cardiovascular		
Hypotension	5.6	1.0
Tachycardia	3.5	0.0
ECG abnormality	1.4	0.0
Postural hypotension	1.4	0.0
Ventricular extrasystoles	1.4	0.0
Extrasystoles	0.7	0.0
Hemopericardium	0.7	0.0
Hypertension	0.7	0.0
Supraventricular tachycardia	0.7	0.0
Syncope	0.7	0.0
Vasodilation	0.7	0.0
Ventricular tachycardia	0.7	0.0
Digestive		
Nausea/vomiting	4.9	1.0
Injection Site		
Injection site reaction	1.4	0.0
Injection site pain	0.7	0.0

Metabolic and Nutritional		
Hypokalemia	0.7	0.0
Nervous		
Dizziness	1.4	0.0
Hypesthesia	0.7	0.0
Intracranial hemorrhage	0.7	0.0
Paresthesia	0.7	0.0
Respiratory		
Dyspnea	0.7	0.0
Skin and Appendages		
Sweating	1.4	0.0
Urogenital		
Polyuria	1.4	0.0
Hematuria	0.7	0.0

RARE EVENTS
The following rare events have been reported in clinical trials or in the literature in association with the use of intravenously administered nicardipine.
Body as a Whole: fever, neck pain
Cardiovascular: angina pectoris, atrioventricular block, ST segment depression, inverted T wave, deep-vein thrombophlebitis
Digestive: dyspepsia
Hemic and Lymphatic: thrombocytopenia
Metabolic and Nutritional: hypophosphatemia, peripheral edema
Nervous: confusion, hypertonia
Respiratory: respiratory disorder
Special Senses: conjunctivitis, ear disorder, tinnitus
Urogenital: urinary frequency
Sinus node dysfunction and myocardial infarction, which may be due to disease progression, have been seen in patients on chronic therapy with orally administered nicardipine.

OVERDOSAGE
Several overdosages with orally administered nicardipine have been reported. One adult patient allegedly ingested 600 mg of nicardipine [standard (immediate release) capsules], and another patient, 2160 mg of the sustained release formulation of nicardipine. Symptoms included marked hypotension, bradycardia, palpitations, flushing, drowsiness, confusion and slurred speech. All symptoms resolved without sequelae. An overdosage occurred in a one-year-old child who ingested half of the powder in a 30 mg nicardipine standard capsule. The child remained asymptomatic.
Based on results obtained in laboratory animals, lethal overdose may cause systemic hypotension, bradycardia (following initial tachycardia) and progressive atrioventricular conduction block. Reversible hepatic function abnormalities and sporadic focal hepatic necrosis were noted in some animal species receiving very large doses of nicardipine.
For treatment of overdosage, standard measures including monitoring of cardiac and respiratory functions should be implemented. The patient should be positioned so as to avoid cerebral anoxia.
Frequent blood pressure determinations are essential. Vasopressors are clinically indicated for patients exhibiting profound hypotension. Intravenous calcium gluconate may help reverse the effects of calcium entry blockade.

DOSAGE AND ADMINISTRATION
Cardene I.V. (nicardipine hydrochloride) is intended for intravenous use. DOSAGE MUST BE INDIVIDUALIZED depending upon the severity of hypertension and the response of the patient during dosing. Blood pressure should be monitored both during and after the infusion; too rapid or excessive reduction in either systolic or diastolic blood pressure during parenteral treatment should be avoided.
PREPARATION
WARNING: AMPULS MUST BE DILUTED BEFORE INFUSION
Dilution: Cardene I.V. is administered by slow continuous infusion at a CONCENTRATION OF 0.1 MG/ML. Each ampul (25 mg) should be diluted with 240 mL of compatible intravenous fluid (see below), resulting in 250 mL of solution at a concentration of 0.1 mg/mL.
Cardene I.V. has been found to be compatible and stable in glass or polyvinyl chloride containers for 24 hours at controlled room temperature with:
Dextrose (5%) Injection, USP
Dextrose (5%) and Sodium Chloride (0.45%) Injection, USP
Dextrose (5%) and Sodium Chloride (0.9%) Injection, USP
Dextrose (5%) and 40 mEq Potassium, USP
Sodium Chloride (0.45%) Injection, USP
Sodium Chloride (0.9%) Injection, USP
Cardene I.V. is NOT compatible with Sodium Bicarbonate (5%) Injection, USP or Lactated Ringer's Injection, USP.
THE DILUTED SOLUTION IS STABLE FOR 24 HOURS AT ROOM TEMPERATURE.
Inspection: As with all parenteral drugs, Cardene I.V. should be inspected visually for particulate matter and discoloration prior to administration, whenever solution and container permit. Cardene I.V. is normally light yellow in color.
DOSAGE
As a Substitute for Oral Nicardipine Therapy
The intravenous infusion rate required to produce an average plasma concentration equivalent to a given oral dose at steady state is shown in the following table:

Oral Cardene Dose	Equivalent I.V. Infusion Rate
20 mg q8h	0.5 mg/hr
30 mg q8h	1.2 mg/hr
40 mg q8h	2.2 mg/hr

For Initiation of Therapy in a Drug Free Patient
The time course of blood pressure decrease is dependent on the initial rate of infusion and the frequency of dosage adjustment.
Cardene I.V. is administered by slow continuous infusion at a CONCENTRATION OF 0.1 MG/ML. With constant infusion, blood pressure begins to fall within minutes. It reaches about 50% of its ultimate decrease in about 45 minutes and does not reach final steady state for about 50 hours.
When treating acute hypertensive episodes in patients with chronic hypertension, discontinuation of infusion is followed by a 50% offset of action in 30 ± 7 minutes but plasma levels of drug and gradually decreasing antihypertensive effects exist for about 50 hours.
Titration: For gradual reduction in blood pressure, initiate therapy at 50 mL/hr (5.0 mg/hr). If desired blood pressure reduction is not achieved at this dose, the infusion rate may be increased by 25 mL/hr (2.5 mg/hr) every 15 minutes up to a maximum of 150 mL/hr (15.0 mg/hr), until desired blood pressure reduction is achieved.
For more rapid blood pressure reduction, initiate therapy at 50 mL/hr (5.0 mg/hr). If desired blood pressure reduction is not achieved at this dose, the infusion rate may be increased by 25 mL/hr (2.5 mg/hr) every 5 minutes up to a maximum of 150 mL/hr (15.0 mg/hr), until desired blood pressure reduction is achieved. Following achievement of the blood pressure goal, the infusion rate should be decreased to 30 mL/hr (3 mg/hr).
Maintenance: The rate of infusion should be adjusted as needed to maintain desired response.
CONDITIONS REQUIRING INFUSION ADJUSTMENT
Hypotension or Tachycardia: If there is concern of impending hypotension or tachycardia, the infusion should be discontinued. When blood pressure has stabilized, infusion of Cardene I.V. may be restarted at low doses such as 30 - 50 mL/hr (3.0 - 5.0 mg/hr) and adjusted to maintain desired blood pressure.
Infusion Site Changes: Cardene I.V. should be continued as long as blood pressure control is needed. The infusion site should be changed every 12 hours if administered via peripheral vein.
Impaired Cardiac, Hepatic, or Renal Function: Caution is advised when titrating Cardene I.V. in patients with congestive heart failure or impaired hepatic or renal function (see "**PRECAUTIONS**").
TRANSFER TO ORAL ANTIHYPERTENSIVE AGENTS
If treatment includes transfer to an oral antihypertensive agent other than CARDENE capsules, therapy should generally be initiated upon discontinuation of Cardene I.V.
If Cardene capsules are to be used, the first dose of a TID regimen should be administered 1 hour prior to discontinuation of the infusion.

HOW SUPPLIED
Cardene® I.V. (nicardipine hydrochloride) is available in packages of 10 ampuls of 10 mL as follows:
25 mg (2.5 mg/mL), NDC 67286-0812-3.
Store at controlled room temperature 20° to 25°C (68° to 77°F).
Freezing does not adversely affect the product, but exposure to elevated temperatures should be avoided.
Protect from light. Store ampuls in carton until used.
U S Patent Nos.: 3,985,758; 4,880,823; and 5,164,405
Cardene® is a registered trademark of Roche Palo Alto LLC
Manufactured under license
from Roche Palo Alto LLC by:
Baxter Healthcare Corporation
Deerfield, IL 60015 USA
CI 4806-2
Marketed by:
ESP Pharma, Inc.
Edison, NJ 08817

CIV0021 Revised December 20, 2002

Everett Laboratories, Inc.

29 SPRING STREET
WEST ORANGE, NEW JERSEY 07052

Direct Inquiries to:
Professional Service Department
Phone: (973) 324-0200
Fax: (973) 324-0795
www.everettlabs.com
E mail: evlabs@aol.com

CORTIC®-ND EAR DROPS ℞

NDC# 0642-0012-15
Each 1ml contains:

Hydrocortisone	10 mg
Chloroxylenol	1 mg
Pramoxine HCl	10 mg
Benzalkonium Chloride	0.10 mg

DOSAGE
Children: 3 drops TID for 7 days
Adults: 4–5 drops TID for 7 days

SUPPLIED
In 15ml amber glass bottle with dosage dropper.

RENAX® CAPLET ℞

Vitamin-Mineral formulation to meet the Nutritional Needs of the Renal Patient.
Gluten & Lactose Free

Each caplet contains:

Vitamin E	35 IU
Vitamin C	50 mg
Vitamin B_1 (Thiamine)	3 mg
Vitamin B_2 (Riboflavin)	2 mg
Niacin (as Niacinamide)	20 mg
Folic Acid	2.5 mg
Vitamin B_6	15 mg
Vitamin B_{12}	12 mcg
Biotin	300 mcg
Pantothenic Acid	10 mg
Zinc	20 mg
Selenium	70 mcg

SUPPLIED
Bottles of 90 imprinted EV0300
PATENT PENDING

STROVITE ADVANCE CAPLETS ℞

Antioxidant-Vitamin/Mineral Supplement
IRON FREE, GLUTEN AND LACTOSE-FREE
DYE FREE

Each caplet contains:

Carotenoids (alpha-Carotene, Beta-Carotene, Cryptoxanthin, Lutein and Zeaxanthin)	**3000 IU**
Vitamin E (Succinate)	**100 IU**
Vitamin C (Ascorbic Acid)	**300 mg**
Vitamin D3	**400 IU**
Vitamin B1 (Thiamine HCL)	**20 mg**
Vitamin B2 (Riboflavin)	**5 mg**
Niacin (Niacinamide)	**25 mg**
Vitamin B6 (Pyridoxine HCL)	**25 mg**
Vitamin B12 (Cyanocobalamin)	**50 mcg**
Biotin	**100 mcg**
Pantothenic Acid (Calcium Pantothenate)	**15 mg**
Folic Acid	**1.0 mg**
Alpha Lipoic Acid	**15 mg**
Lutein	**5 mg**
Chromium (Chromic Chloride)	**50 mcg**
Magnesium (Magnesium Oxide)	**50 mg**
Manganese (Manganese Sulfate)	**1.5 mg**
Copper (Cupric Sulfate)	**1.5 mg**
Selenium (Sodium Selenate)	**100 mcg**
Zinc (Zinc Oxide)	**25 mg**

Supplied
Bottles of 100 imprinted EV0208
PATENT # 6,660,293

TRITUSS-A DROPS ℞

Sugar free alcohol free

Each dropperful (1 ml) contains:

Carbinoxamine Maleate	1.0 mg
Phenylephrine HCL	2.0 mg
Dextromethorphan HBr	2.0 mg

DOSAGE
3–6 months - .3 ml to .6 ml 4 ×/day
6–12 months - .6 ml to 1 ml 4×/day
12–24 months - 1 ml to 2 ml 4×/day

Continued on next page

VITAFOL®-OB CAPLETS ℞

NDC# 0642-0079
(Prenatal)
Sugar, sodium & yeast-free
Gluten & lactose-free

Each Caplet Contains:

VITAMINS:	
A (beta carotene)	2700 IU
D (cholecalciferol)	400 IU
C (ascorbic acid)	70 mg
E (as dl-alpha tocopheryl acetate)	30 IU
Folic Acid	1 mg
B1 (thiamine mononitrate)	1.6 mg
B2 (riboflavin)	1.8 mg
B6 (pyridoxine hydrochloride)	2.5 mg
B12 (cyanocobalamin)	12 mcg
Niacin (as niacinamide)	18 mg
MINERALS:	
Calcium (calcium carbonate)	100 mg
Elemental Iron (ferrous fumarate)	65 mg
Magnesium (magnesium oxide)	25 mg
Zinc (zinc oxide)	25 mg
Copper (copper oxide)	2 mg

SUPPLIED

Boxes of (10 × 10) unit dose pack
Imprinted – 0079
USA PATENT PENDING

Faulding Laboratories

for product information, please see Alpharma Branded Products Division

FEI Products LLC

825 WURLITZER DRIVE
NORTH TONAWANDA, NY 14120

For General Information Contact:
1-800-322-4966
For Medical Inquiries/Emergencies Contact:
1-877-601-7163
www.paragard.com

PARAGARD® T 380A ℞

[pă-ră-gard]
(intrauterine copper contraceptive)

PRESCRIBING INFORMATION

Patients should be counseled that this product does not protect against HIV infection (AIDS) and other sexually transmitted diseases.

The ParaGard® T380A should only be inserted, managed, and removed by clinicians that are thoroughly familiar with these procedures.

NOTICE

You have received a Patient Package Insert that Federal Regulations (21 CFR 310.502) require you to furnish to each patient who is considering the use of the ParaGard® T 380A.

The Patient Package Insert contains information on the safety and efficacy of the ParaGard® T 380A. Before inserting the ParaGard® T 380A:

- You should read the physician prescription labeling and be familiar with all the information it contains.
- You should counsel the patient and answer her questions about contraception, the ParaGard® T 380A, and the information in the Patient Package Insert.
- You and the patient should read each section of the Patient Package Insert, and if the patient agrees, she may sign a consent form provided for your convenience.

The Patient Package Insert is also available in Spanish and other foreign languages. Address requests to FEI Products LLC or telephone 1-800-322-4966.

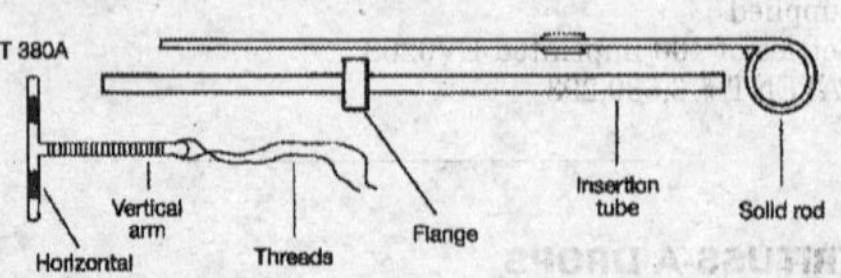

DESCRIPTION

The polyethylene body of the ParaGard® T 380A is wound with approximately 176 mg of copper wire and carries a copper collar of approximately 68.7 mg of copper on each of its transverse arms. The exposed surface areas of copper are 380 ± 23 mm.[2] The dimensions of the ParaGard® T 380A are 36 mm in the vertical direction and 32 mm in the horizontal direction. The tip of the vertical arm of the ParaGard® T 380A is enlarged to form a bulb having a diameter of 3 mm. The ParaGard® T 380A is equipped with a monofilament polyethylene thread which is tied through the bulb, resulting in two threads at the tip to aid in removal of the IUD. The ParaGard® T 380A contains barium sulfate to render it radiopaque.

The ParaGard® T 380A is packaged together with an insertion tube and solid rod in a Tyvek®-polyethylene pouch and then sterilized. The insertion tube is equipped with a movable flange to aid in gauging the depth to which the insertion tube is inserted through the cervical canal and into the uterine cavity.

CLINICAL PHARMACOLOGY

Available data indicate that the contraceptive effectiveness of the ParaGard® T 380A is enhanced by copper being released continuously from the copper coil and sleeves into the uterine cavity. The exact mechanism by which metallic copper enhances the contraceptive effect of an IUD has not been conclusively demonstrated. Various hypotheses have been advanced, including interference with sperm transport, fertilization, and implantation. Clinical studies with copper-bearing IUDs also suggest that fertilization is prevented either due to an altered number or lack of viability of spermatozoa.[1]

INDICATIONS AND USAGE

The ParaGard® T 380A is indicated for intrauterine contraception. ParaGard® T 380A is highly effective. Table II and Table III list an expected pregnancy rate for one year between 0.7 and 0.5, respectively. ParaGard® T 380A should not be kept in place longer than 10 years.

RECOMMENDED PATIENT PROFILE

The ParaGard® T 380A is recommended for women who have had at least one child, are in a stable, mutually monogamous relationship, and have no history of pelvic inflammatory disease.

CONTRAINDICATIONS

The ParaGard® T 380A should not be inserted when one or more of the following conditions exist:

1. Pregnancy or suspicion of pregnancy.
2. Abnormalities of the uterus resulting in distortion of the uterine cavity.
3. Acute pelvic inflammatory disease or a history of pelvic inflammatory disease.
4. Postpartum endometritis or infected abortion in the past 3 months.
5. Known or suspected uterine or cervical malignancy, including unresolved, abnormal "Pap" smear.
6. Genital bleeding of unknown etiology.
7. Untreated acute cervicitis or vaginitis, including bacterial vaginosis, until infection is controlled.
8. Copper-containing IUDs should not be inserted in the presence of diagnosed Wilson's disease.
9. Known allergy to copper.
10. Patient or her partner has multiple sexual partners.
11. Conditions associated with increased susceptibility to infections with microorganisms. Such conditions include, but are not limited to, leukemia, acquired immune deficiency syndrome (AIDS), and I.V. drug abuse.
12. Genital actinomycosis.
13. A previously inserted IUD that has not been removed.

WARNINGS

1. PREGNANCY

Effects on the offspring when pregnancy occurs with the ParaGard® T 380A in place are unknown.

a. Septic Abortion

Reports indicate an increased incidence of septic abortion with septicemia, septic shock, and death in patients becoming pregnant with an IUD in place. Most of these reports have been associated with, but are not limited to, the mid-trimester of pregnancy. In some cases, the initial symptoms have been insidious and not easily recognized. If pregnancy should occur with an IUD *in situ*, the IUD should be removed if the string is visible and removal is easily accomplished. Of course, manipulation may result in spontaneous abortion. If removal proves to be difficult, or if threads are not visible, interruption of the pregnancy should be considered and offered as an option. Rates of mortality with and without contraception are shown in Table I.

b. Continuation of Pregnancy

If the patient elects to maintain the pregnancy and the IUD remains *in situ*, she should be warned that there is an increased risk of spontaneous abortion and sepsis. In addition, she is at increased risk of premature labor and delivery. As a consequence of premature birth, the fetus is at increased risk of damage. She should be followed more closely than the usual obstetrical patient. The patient must be advised to report immediately all abnormal symptoms, such as flu-like syndrome, fever, abdominal cramping or pain, bleeding or vaginal discharge, because generalized symptoms of septicemia may be insidious.

2. ECTOPIC PREGNANCY

a. Patients with a history of ectopic pregnancy are at an increased risk of subsequent pregnancies being ectopic. Although current data indicate that there is no increased risk of ectopic pregnancy in patients using the ParaGard® T 380A and some data suggest there may be a lower risk than the general population using no method of contraception, a pregnancy which occurs with the ParaGard® T 380A in place is more likely to be ectopic than a pregnancy occurring without ParaGard® T 380A.[2-4] Therefore, patients who become pregnant while using the ParaGard® T 380A should be carefully evaluated for the possibility of an ectopic pregnancy.

b. Special attention should be directed to patients with delayed menses, slight metrorrhagia and/or unilateral pelvic pain, and to those patients who wish to terminate a pregnancy because of IUD failure, to determine whether ectopic pregnancy has occurred.

3. PELVIC INFECTION (PELVIC INFLAMMATORY DISEASE, PID)

The ParaGard® T 380A is contraindicated in the presence of PID or in women with a history of PID. Use of all IUDs, including the ParaGard® T 380A, has been associated with an increased incidence of PID. Therefore, a decision to use the ParaGard® T 380A must include consideration of the risks of PID. The highest rate of PID has been reported to occur after insertion and up to four months thereafter. A study suggests that the highest incidence occurs within 20 days postinsertion, then falls, remaining constant thereafter.[5] Administration of prophylactic antibiotics has been reported, although studies do not confirm the utility of this prophylactic measure in reducing PID. PID can necessitate hysterectomy and can also lead to tubo-ovarian abscesses, tubal occlusion and infertility, and tubal damage that can predispose to ectopic pregnancy. PID can result in peritonitis and, infrequently, in death. The effect of PID on fertility is especially important for women who may wish to have children at a later date.

a. Women at special risk of PID

The risk of PID appears to be greater for women who have multiple sexual partners and also for those women whose sexual partners have multiple sexual partners, as PID is most frequently caused by sexually transmitted diseases.

b. PID warning to ParaGard® T 380A users

All women who choose the ParaGard® T 380A must be informed prior to insertion that IUD use has been associated with an increased incidence of PID and that PID can necessitate hysterectomy, can cause tubal damage leading to ectopic pregnancy or infertility or, in infrequent cases, can cause death. Patients must be taught to recognize and report to their physician promptly any symptoms of pelvic inflammatory disease. These symptoms include development of menstrual disorders (prolonged or heavy bleeding), unusual vaginal discharge, abdominal or pelvic pain or tenderness, dyspareunia, chills, and fever.

c. Asymptomatic PID

PID may be asymptomatic but still result in tubal damage and its sequelae.[6,7]

d. Treatment of PID

Following diagnosis of PID, or suspected PID, bacteriologic specimens should be obtained and antibiotic therapy should be initiated promptly. Removal of the ParaGard® T 380A after initiation of antibiotic therapy is usually appropriate. Time should be allowed for therapeutic blood levels to be reached prior to removal. Guidelines for PID treatment are available from the Center for Disease Control (CDC), Atlanta, Georgia. The guidelines were established after deliberation by a group of experts and staff of the CDC, but they should not be construed as rules suitable for use in all patients. Adequate PID treatment requires the application of current standards of therapy prevailing at the time of occurrence of the infection with reference to the prescription labeling of the antibiotic selected.

Genital actinomycosis has been associated primarily with long-term IUD use. If actinomycosis occurs, promptly institute appropriate antibiotic therapy and remove the ParaGard® T 380A.

4. EMBEDMENT

Partial penetration or embedment of the ParaGard® T 380A in the endometrium or myometrium can result in difficult removal. In some cases this can result in breakage of the IUD, necessitating surgical removal.

5. PERFORATION

Partial or total perforation of the uterine wall or cervix may occur with use of the ParaGard® T 380A. The rate of perforation in randomized trials of the ParaGard® T 380A has been 1 in 1,360. Insertions immediately after the expulsion of the placenta are not known to be associated with increased risks of perforation, but insertion later in the first postpartum month, particularly during lactation, has been associated with an increased risk of perforation.[8,9] Thus, unless performed immediately postpartum, insertion should be delayed to the second postpartum month. IUD insertion immediately postabortion in the first trimester is not known to be associated with increased risks of perforation, but insertion after second trimester abortion should be delayed until the second postabortion month.

The possibility of perforation must be kept in mind during insertion and at the time of any subsequent examination. If perforation occurs, the ParaGard® T 380A should be removed as soon as possible. A surgical procedure may be required. Abdominal adhesions, intestinal penetration, intestinal obstruction, and local inflammatory reaction with abscess formation and erosion of adjacent viscera may result if the ParaGard® T 380A is left in the peritoneal cavity. There are reports of migration after insertion.

6. MEDICAL DIATHERMY

The use of medical diathermy (short-wave and microwave) in a patient with a metal-containing IUD may cause heat injury to the surrounding tissue. Therefore, medical diathermy to the abdominal and sacral areas should not be used on patients with a ParaGard® T 380A in place.

7. EFFECTS OF COPPER

Additional amounts of copper available to the body from the ParaGard® T 380A may precipitate symptoms in women with Wilson's disease. The incidence of Wilson's disease is approximately 1 in 200,000. The long term effects of intrauterine copper to a child conceived in the presence of an IUD are unknown.

8. RISKS OF MORTALITY

The available data from a variety of sources have been analyzed to estimate the risk of death associated with various methods of contraception. The estimates of risk of death include the combined risk of the contraceptive method plus the risk of pregnancy or abortion in the event of method failure. The findings of the analysis are shown in Table I.[10]

[See table I at right]

TABLE I – Annual Number of Birth-Related or Method-Related Deaths Associated with Control of Fertility per 100,000 Non-Sterile Women, by Fertility Control Method According to Age

	Age Group					
Methods	**15–19**	**20–24**	**25–29**	**30–34**	**35–39**	**40–44**
No Birth Control Method/Term	4.7	5.4	4.8	6.3	11.7	20.6
No Birth Control Method/AB	2.1	2.0	1.6	1.9	2.8	5.3
IUD	0.2	0.3	0.2	0.1	0.3	0.6
Periodic Abstinence	1.4	1.3	0.7	1.0	1.0	1.9
Withdrawal	0.9	1.7	0.9	1.3	0.8	1.5
Condom	0.6	1.2	0.6	0.9	0.5	1.0
Diaphragm/Cap	0.6	1.1	0.6	0.9	1.6	3.1
Sponge	0.8	1.5	0.8	1.1	2.2	4.1
Spermicides	1.6	1.9	1.4	1.9	1.5	2.7
Oral Contraceptives	0.8	1.3	1.1	1.8	1.0	1.9
Implants/Injectables	0.2	0.6	0.5	0.8	0.5	0.6
Tubal Sterilization	1.3	1.2	1.1	1.1	1.2	1.3
Vasectomy	0.1	0.1	0.1	0.1	0.1	0.2

TABLE II ParaGard® T 380A (Intrauterine Copper Contraceptive) GROSS ANNUAL TERMINATION AND CONTINUATION RATES PER 100* USERS All Copper T 380A IUD Acceptors Combined Population Council and WHO Studies

	YEAR									
Rate of Item	1	2	3	4	5	6	7	8	9	10
Pregnancy	0.7	0.3	0.6	0.2	0.3	0.2	0.0	0.4	0.0	0.0
Expulsion	5.7	2.5	1.6	1.2	0.3	0.0	0.6	1.7	0.2	0.4
Bleeding/Pain	11.9	9.8	7.0	3.5	3.7	2.7	3.0	2.5	2.2	3.7
Other Medical	2.5	2.1	1.6	1.7	0.1	0.3	1.0	0.4	0.7	0.3
Continuation	76.8	78.3	81.2	86.2	89.0	91.9	87.9	88.1	92.0	91.8
No. of Women:										
At Start of Year	4932	3149	2018	1121	872	621	563	483	423	325
At End of Year	3149	2018	1121	872	621	563	483	423	325	230

*Rates were calculated by weighing the annual rates by the number of subjects starting each year for each of the Population Council (3536 acceptors) and the World Health Organization (1396 acceptors) trials.

PRECAUTIONS

Patients should be counseled that this product does not protect against HIV infection (AIDS) and other sexually transmitted diseases.

1. Patient Counseling

Prior to the insertion, the physician, nurse, or other trained health professional must provide the patient with the Patient Package Insert. The patient should be given the opportunity to read the information and discuss fully any questions she may have concerning the ParaGard® T 380A as well as other methods of contraception.

2. Patient Evaluation and Clinical Considerations

a. A complete medical and social history, including that of the partner, should be obtained to determine conditions that might influence the selection of an IUD. A physical examination should include a pelvic examination, a "Pap" smear, and appropriate tests for any other forms of genital disease, such as gonorrhea and chlamydia laboratory evaluations, if indicated. If actinomyces-like organisms are detected on the Pap smear, they should be cultured to determine whether genital actinomyces is present. The physician should determine that the patient is not pregnant.

b. The uterus should be carefully sounded prior to the insertion to determine the degree of patency of the endocervical canal and the internal os, and the direction and depth of the uterine cavity. In occasional cases, severe cervical stenosis may be encountered. Do not use excessive force to overcome this resistance.

c. The uterus should sound to a depth of 6 to 9 centimeters (cm). Insertion of an IUD into a uterine cavity measuring less than 6.0 cm by sounding may increase the incidence of expulsion, bleeding, pain, perforation, and possibly, pregnancy.

d. Clinicians are cautioned that it is imperative for them to become thoroughly familiar with the instructions for use before attempting placement of the ParaGard® T 380A. To reduce the possibility of insertion in the presence of an existing undetermined pregnancy, the optimal time for insertion is the latter part of the menstrual period, or one or two days thereafter. The ParaGard® T 380A should not be inserted postpartum or postabortion until involution of the uterus is complete. The incidence of perforation and expulsion is greater if involution is not complete. Data also suggest that there may be an increased risk of perforation and expulsion if the woman is lactating.[8,9] Other recent studies report no increased incidence of perforation or expulsion in lactating women.[11,12]

The ParaGard® T 380A should be placed at the fundus of the uterine cavity. Proper placement enhances contraceptive effectiveness and helps avoid perforation and partial or complete expulsion that could result in pregnancy.

e. Patients experiencing menorrhagia and/or metrorrhagia following IUD insertion may be at risk for the development of hypochromic microcytic anemia. Careful consideration of this risk must be given before insertion in patients with anemia or a history of menorrhagia or hypermenorrhea. Patients receiving anticoagulants or having a coagulopathy may have a greater risk of menorrhagia or hypermenorrhea.

f. Syncope, bradycardia, or other neurovascular episodes may occur during insertion or removal of IUDs, especially in patients with a previous disposition to these conditions or cervical stenosis.

g. Use of an IUD in patients with cervicitis should be postponed until treatment has eradicated the infection.

h. Patients with valvular or congenital heart disease are more prone to develop subacute bacterial endocarditis than patients who do not have valvular or congenital heart disease. Use of an IUD in these patients may represent a potential source of septic emboli. Patients with known congenital heart disease who may be at increased risk should be treated with appropriate antibiotics at the time of insertion.

i. Patients requiring chronic corticosteroid therapy or insulin for diabetes should be monitored with special care for infection.

j. Since the ParaGard® T 380A may be partially or completely expelled, patients should be reexamined and evaluated shortly after the first postinsertion menses, but no later than 3 months afterwards. Thereafter, annual examination with appropriate evaluation, including a "Pap" smear, should be carried out. The ParaGard® T 380A should be kept in place no longer than 10 years.

k. The patient should be told that some bleeding or cramps may occur during the first few weeks after insertion. If these symptoms continue or are severe she should report them to her physician. She should be instructed on how to check to make certain that the threads still protrude from the cervix and cautioned that there is no contraceptive protection if the ParaGard® T 380A has been expelled. She should check frequently, at least after each menstrual period. She should be cautioned not to dislodge the ParaGard® T 380A by pulling on the thread. If a partial expulsion occurs, removal is indicated.

l. Rarely, a copper-induced urticarial allergic skin reaction may develop in women using a copper-containing IUD. If the symptoms of such an allergic response occur, the patient should be instructed to tell the consulting physician that a copper-containing device is being used.

m. The effect of magnetic resonance imaging of the pelvis was investigated in one study[13] in women with the CU-7® (Intrauterine Copper Contraceptive) and the LIPPES LOOP™ IUD. The CU-7® has a different configuration and contains less copper than the ParaGard® T 380A. The results of the study indicate that neither the CU-7® nor the LIPPES LOOP™ were moved under the influence of the magnetic field nor did they heat during the spin-echo sequences usually employed for pelvic imaging.

3. Insertion Prophylaxis

Observe strict asepsis at insertion; clean the endocervix with an antiseptic solution, because the presence of organisms capable of establishing PID cannot be determined by appearance, and because IUD insertion may be associated with introduction of vaginal bacteria into the uterus. Data do not confirm the utility of prophylactic administration of antibiotics in reducing the incidence of PID, and their use in nursing women is not recommended.

4. Requirements for Continuation and Removal

a. The ParaGard® T 380A must be replaced before the end of the tenth year of use. There is no evidence of decreasing contraceptive efficacy with time before ten years, but the contraceptive effectiveness at longer times has not been established; therefore, the patient should be informed of the known duration of contraceptive efficacy and be advised to return in 10 years for removal and possible insertion of a new ParaGard® T 380A.

b. The ParaGard® T 380A should be removed for the following medical reasons: menorrhagia- and/or metrorrhagia-producing anemia; pelvic infection; genital actinomycosis; intractable pelvic pain; dyspareunia; pregnancy, endometrial or cervical malignancy; uterine or cervical perforation; increase in length of the threads extending from the cervix, or any other indication of partial expulsion. Insertions immediately following placental delivery or first trimester abortion may result in threads becoming slightly longer as the uterus involutes and may not represent expulsion or partial expulsion.

c. If the retrieval threads cannot be visualized, they may have retracted into the uterus or have been broken, or the ParaGard® T 380A may have been broken, or the ParaGard® T 380A may have been expelled. Localization may be made by feeling with a probe, X-ray, or sonography. When the physician elects to recover a ParaGard® T 380A with the threads not visible, the removal instructions should be reviewed.

d. Should the patient's relationship cease to be mutually monogamous, or should her partner become HIV positive, or acquire a sexually transmitted disease, she should be instructed to report this change to her clinician immediately. It may be advisable to recommend the use of a barrier method as a partial protection against acquiring sexually transmitted diseases until the ParaGard® T 380A can be removed.

5. Continuing Care of Patients Using ParaGard® T 380A

a. Any inquiries regarding pain, odorous discharge, bleeding, fever, genital lesions or sores, or a missed period should be promptly responded to and prompt examination is recommended.

b. If examination during visits subsequent to insertion reveals that the length of the threads has visibly or palpably changed from the length at time of insertion, the ParaGard® T 380A should be considered displaced and should be removed. A new ParaGard® T 380A may be inserted at that time or during the next menses if it is certain that conception has not occurred. Under no circumstances should reinsertion with an expelled ParaGard® T 380A be attempted. A new ParaGard® T 380A should be inserted.

c. Since the ParaGard® T 380A may be partially or completely expelled, patients should be reexamined and evaluated shortly after the first postinsertion menses, but no later than 3 months afterwards. Thereafter, at least annual examination with appropriate evaluation, including a "Pap" smear, and if indicated, gonococcal and chlamydial laboratory evaluations, should be carried out. The ParaGard® T 380A should be kept in place no longer than 10 years.

d. In the event a pregnancy is confirmed during ParaGard® T 380A use, the following steps should be taken:

- Determine whether the pregnancy is ectopic and take appropriate measures if it is.
- Inform patient of the risks of leaving an IUD *in situ* or removing it during pregnancy, and of the lack of data on the long term effects of the ParaGard® T 380A on the offspring of women who have had it *in utero* during conception or gestation (see WARNINGS). This information should include the risk of septic spontaneous abortion with the IUD *in situ*.
- If possible, the ParaGard® T 380A should be removed after the patient has been warned of the risks of removal. If removal is difficult, the patient should be counseled about and offered pregnancy termination.
- If the ParaGard® T 380A is left in place, the patient's course should be followed closely.

ADVERSE REACTIONS

These adverse reactions are not listed in any order of frequency or severity.

Reported adverse reactions with intrauterine contraceptives include: endometritis; spontaneous abortion; septic abortion; septicemia; perforation of the uterus and cervix; embedment; fragmentation of the IUD; pelvic infection; tubo-ovarian abscess; tubal damage; vaginitis; leukorrhea; cervical erosion; pregnancy; ectopic pregnancy; fetal damage; difficult removal; complete or partial expulsion of the IUD, particularly in those patients with uteri measuring less than 6.0 cm by sounding; menstrual spotting; prolonga-

Continued on next page

ParaGard T—Cont.

tion of menstrual flow; anemia; amenorrhea or delayed menses; pain and cramping; dysmenorrhea; backaches; dyspareunia; neurovascular episodes, including bradycardia and syncope secondary to insertion. Uterine perforation and IUD displacement into the abdomen have been followed by peritonitis, abdominal adhesions, intestinal penetration, intestinal obstruction, and cystic masses in the pelvis. (Certain of these adverse reactions can lead to loss of fertility, partial or total removal of reproductive organs, hormonal imbalance, or death.) Urticarial allergic skin reaction may occur.

CLINICAL STUDIES

Different event rates have been reported with the use of different intrauterine contraceptives. Inasmuch as these rates are usually derived from separate studies conducted by different investigators in several populations, they cannot be compared with precision. Considerably different rates are likely to be obtained because event rates per unit of time tend to decrease as studies are extended, since more susceptible subjects discontinue due to expulsions, adverse reactions, or pregnancy, leaving the study population richer in less susceptible subjects. In clinical trials conducted by The Population Council[14,15] and WHO, use-effectiveness of the ParaGard® T 380A as calculated by the life table method was determined through ten (10) years of use.

Data suggest a higher pregnancy rate in women under 20.[14,15,17]

[See table II at top of previous page]

TABLE III
GROSS ANNUAL EVENT RATES PER 100 CONTINUING USERS BY YEAR AND PARITY

	1 Year
	Parous
Pregnancy	0.5
Expulsion	2.3
Bleeding/Pain	3.4
Infection	0.3
Other Medical	0.5
Planning Pregnancy	0.6
Other Personal	0.7
Continuation	92.1
No. Completed	1842.0

Rates were calculated by combining the experience on a weighted basis from both an international study by the World Health Organization (2110 women) and a U.S. study by GynoPharma Inc. (230 women).

The lowest expected and typical failure rates during the first year of continuous use of all contraceptive methods are listed in Table IV (Adapted from Reference 16).

[See table IV above]

TABLE IV – Percentage of women experiencing a contraceptive failure during the first year of typical use and the first year of perfect use and the percentage continuing use at the end of the first year, United States.[16]

	% of Women Experiencing an Accidental Pregnancy Within the First Year of Use		% of Women Continuing Use at One Year[3]
Method	Typical Use[1]	Perfect Use[2]	
Chance[4]	85	85	
Spermicides[5]	21	6	43
Periodic Abstinence	20		67
Calendar		9	
Ovulation Method		3	
Sympto-Thermal[6]		2	
Post-Ovulation		1	
Withdrawal Cap[7]	19	4	
Parous Women	36	26	45
Nulliparous Women	18	9	58
Sponge			
Parous Women	36	20	45
Nulliparous Women	18	9	58
Diaphragm[7]	18	6	58
Condom[8]			
Female (Reality)	21	5	56
Male	12	3	63
Pill	3		72
Progestin Only		0.5	
Combined		0.1	
IUD			
Progesterone T	2.0	1.5	81
Copper T 380A (ParaGard® T 380A)	0.8	0.6	78
Depo-Provera®	0.3	0.3	70
Norplant® (6 Capsules)	0.09	0.09	85
Female Sterilization	0.4	0.4	100
Male Sterilization	0.15	0.10	100

Emergency Contraceptive Pills: Treatment initiated within 72 hours after unprotected intercourse reduces the risk of pregnancy by at least 75%.[9]

Lactational Amenorrhea Method: LAM is a highly effective temporary method of contraception.[10]

Footnotes to Table IV:

1. Among *typical* couples who initiate use of a method (not necessarily for the first time), the percentage who experience an accidental pregnancy during the first year if they do not stop use for any other reason.
2. Among couples who initiate use of a method (not necessarily for the first time) and who use it *perfectly* (both consistently and correctly), the percentage who experience an accidental pregnancy during the first year if they do not stop use for any other reason.
3. Among couples attempting to avoid pregnancy, the percentage who continue to use a method for one year.
4. The percentages failing in columns (2) and (3) are based on data from populations where contraception is not used and from women who cease using contraception in order to become pregnant. Among such populations, about 89% become pregnant within one year. This estimate was lowered slightly (to 85%) to represent the percentage who would become pregnant within 1 year among women now relying on reversible methods of contraception if they abandoned contraception altogether.
5. Foams, creams, gels, vaginal suppositories, and vaginal film.
6. Cervical mucous (ovulation) method supplemented by calendar in the pre-ovulatory and basal body temperature in the post-ovulatory phases.
7. With spermicidal cream or jelly.
8. Without spermicides.
9. The treatment schedule is one dose as soon as possible (but no more than 72 hours) after unprotected intercourse, and a second dose 12 hours after the first dose. The hormones that have been studied in the clinical trials of postcoital hormonal contraception are found in Nordette, Levlen, Lo/Ovral (1 dose is 4 pills), Triphasil, Tri-Levlen (1 dose is 4 yellow pills), and Ovral (1 dose is 2 pills).
10. However, to maintain effective protection against pregnancy, another method of contraception must be used as soon as menstruation resumes, the frequency or duration of breastfeeds is reduced, bottle feeds are introduced, or the baby reaches 6 months of age.

HOW SUPPLIED

Available in cartons of one (NDC 50907-0380-6) or five (NDC 50907-0380-7) sterile units. Each ParaGard® T 380A is packaged in a Tyvek®-polyethylene pouch, together with an insertion tube and solid rod.

INSTRUCTIONS FOR USE
ParaGard® T 380A
(Intrauterine Copper Contraceptive)

CLINICIANS SHOULD BE THOROUGHLY FAMILIAR WITH PARAGARD® T 380A INSERTIONS, MANAGEMENT, AND REMOVAL PROCEDURES.

PREVIOUS EDUCATION RE: SURGICAL PROCEDURES WILL REQUIRE VARYING LEVELS OF EXPERIENCE.

The ParaGard® T 380A (Intrauterine Copper Contraceptive) represents a different design in intrauterine contraceptives. Physicians are, therefore, cautioned that they should become thoroughly familiar with instructions for insertion before attempting placement of the ParaGard® T 380A. The insertion technique is different in several respects from that employed with other intrauterine contraceptives and the physician should pay particular attention to the drawings and commentary accompanying these instructions.

A single ParaGard® T 380A is placed at the fundus of the uterine cavity.

The ParaGard® T 380A may be inserted at any time during the cycle. However, it is essential that pregnancy be ruled out before insertion.

The ParaGard® T 380A is indicated for use up to 10 years. Therefore, the ParaGard® T 380A must be removed and a new one inserted on or before 10 years from the date of insertion.

PRELIMINARY PREPARATION AND INSERTION

1. Before insertion, you and the patient will want to review the Patient Package Insert. If the patient agrees, she may sign the Consent Form provided for your records.
2. Take a medical and social history.
3. Refer to CONTRAINDICATIONS, WARNINGS, and PRECAUTIONS.
4. Pelvic examination is to be performed prior to insertion of the ParaGard® T 380A, including a cervical "Pap" smear, and gonococcal and chlamydial evaluations, if indicated, and any other necessary specific tests.
5. If appropriate, commence antibiotic prophylaxis one hour before insertion.
6. Use of aseptic technique during insertion is essential.
7. The endocervix should be cleansed with an antiseptic solution and a tenaculum applied to the cervix with downward traction for correction of the angulation as well as stabilization of the cervix.
8. With a speculum in place, gently insert a sterile sound to determine the depth and direction of the uterine canal. Be sure to determine the position of the uterus before insertion.

CAUTION

Any intrauterine procedure can result in severe pain, bradycardia, and syncope.

It is generally believed that perforations, if they occur, are encountered at the time of insertion, although the perforation may not be detected until some time later. The position of the uterus should be determined during the preinsertion examination. Great care must be exercised during the preinsertion sounding and subsequent insertion. No attempt should be made to force the insertion.

HOW TO LOAD AND INSERT ParaGard® T 380A

STEP 1

To minimize the chance of introducing contamination, do not remove the ParaGard® T 380A from the insertion tube prior to placement in the uterus. Do not bend the arms of the ParaGard® T 380A earlier than 5 minutes before it is to be introduced into the uterus.

In the absence of sterile gloves, this can be accomplished without destroying sterility by folding the arms in the partially opened package. Place the partially opened package on a flat surface and pull the solid rod partially from the package so it will not interfere with assembly. Place thumb and index finger on top of package on ends of the horizontal arms. Push insertion tube against arms of ParaGard® T 380A as indicated by arrow in Fig. 1A to start arms folding.

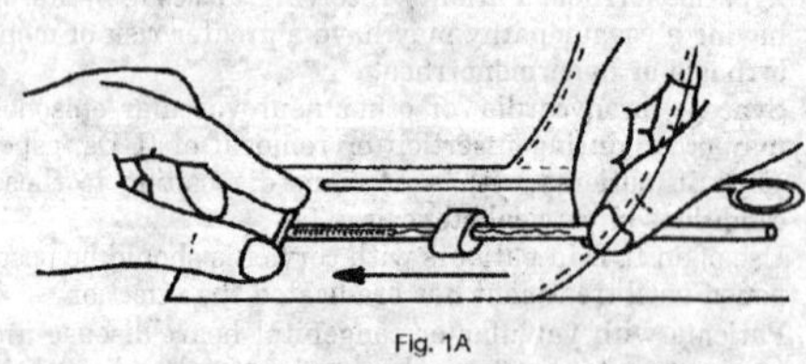

Fig. 1A

Complete the bending by bringing the thumb and index finger together using the other hand to maneuver the insertion tube to pick up the arms of the ParaGard® T 380A (Fig. 1B). Insert no further than necessary to insure retention of the arms. Introduce the solid rod into the insertion tube from the bottom alongside the threads until it touches the bottom of the ParaGard® T 380A.

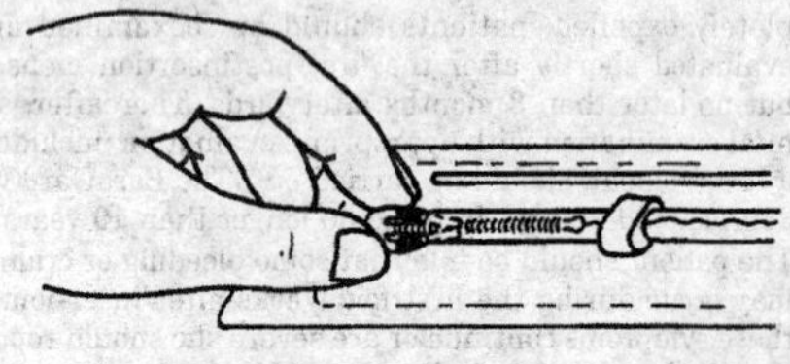

Fig. 1B

STEP 2
Adjust the movable flange so that it indicates the depth to which the ParaGard® T 380A should be inserted and the direction in which the arms of the ParaGard® T 380A will open. At this point, make certain that the horizontal arms of the ParaGard® T 380A and the long axis of the flange lie in the same horizontal plane. Introduce the loaded insertion tube through the cervical canal and upwards until the ParaGard® T 380A lies in contact with the fundus. The movable flange should be at the cervix (Fig. 2).
DO NOT FORCE THE INSERTION.

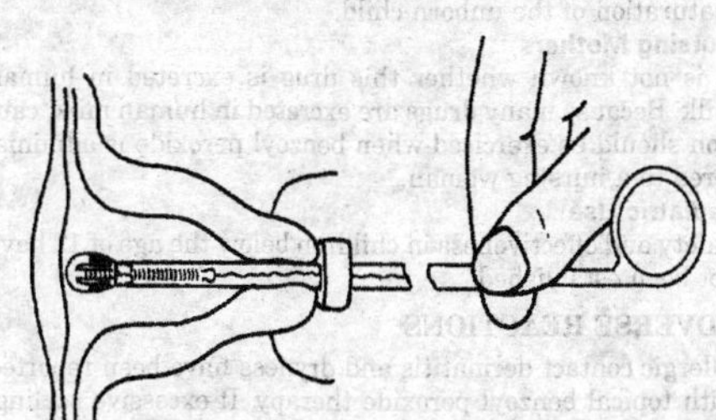
Fig. 2

STEP 3
To release the arms of the ParaGard® T 380A, withdraw the insertion tube not more than ½ inch while the solid rod is not permitted to move. This releases the arms of the ParaGard® T 380A (Fig. 3).

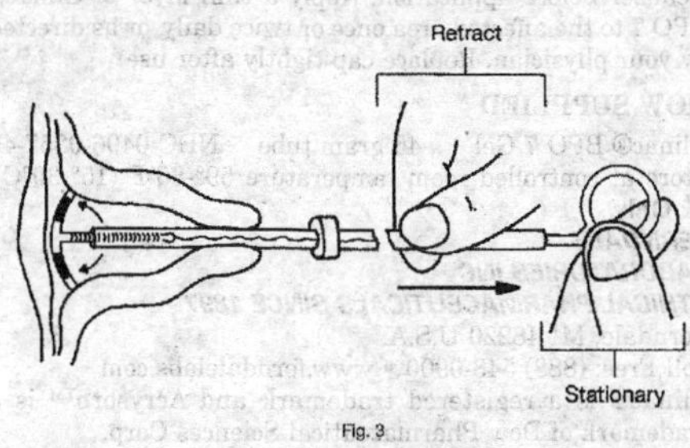

Fig. 3

STEP 4
After the arms are released, the insertion tube should be moved upward gently, until the resistance of the fundus is felt. This will assure placement of the T at the highest possible position within the endometrial cavity (Fig. 4).

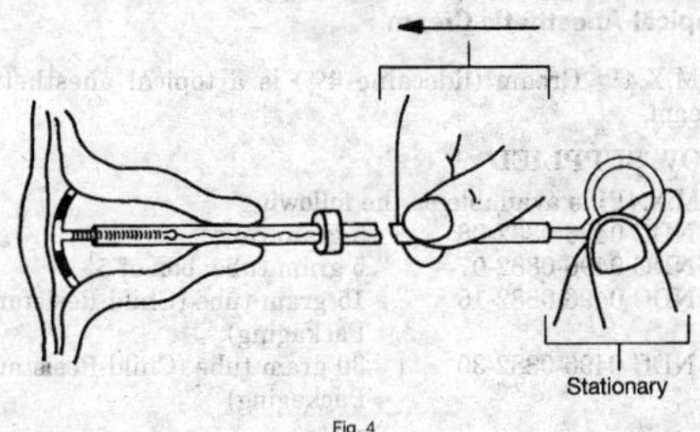

Fig. 4

STEP 5
Withdraw the solid rod while holding the insertion tube stationary (Fig. 5).

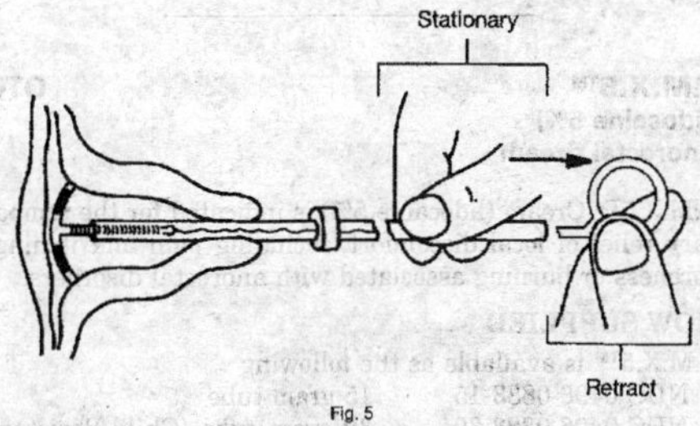

Fig. 5

STEP 6
Withdraw the insertion tube from the cervix. Be sure sufficient length of the threads are visible (approximately 1 in. or 2.5 cm.) to facilitate checking for the presence of the ParaGard® T 380A (Fig. 6). Notation of length of the threads should be made in patient record.
[See figure 6 at top of next column]

HOW TO REMOVE ParaGard® T 380A
To remove the ParaGard® T 380A, pull gently on the exposed threads. The arms of the ParaGard® T 380A will fold upwards as it is withdrawn from the uterus. Even if removal proves difficult, the ParaGard® T 380A should not remain in the uterus after 10 years.

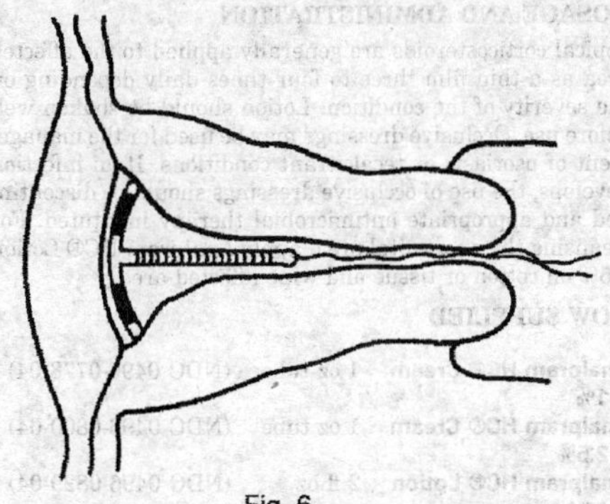
Fig. 6

REFERENCES

1. Alvarez F et al: New insights on the mode of action on intrauterine contraceptives in women. *Fertil Steril* 1988; 49:768–773.
2. World Health Organization's Special Programme of Research, Development and Research Training in Human Reproduction: A multinational case-control study of ectopic pregnancy. *Clin Reprod Fertil* 1985; 3:131–143.
3. Ory HW, Women's Health Study: Ectopic pregnancy and intrauterine contraceptive devices: New perspectives. *Obstet Gynecol* 1981; 57:137–144.
4. Marchbanks PA et al: Risk factors for ectopic pregnancy: A population-based study. *JAMA* 1988; 259:1823–1827.
5. Farley TMM et al: Intrauterine devices and pelvic inflammatory disease: An international perspective. *Lancet* 1992; 339:785–788.
6. Cramer DW et al: Tubal infertility and the intrauterine device. *N Engl J Med* 1985; 312:941–947.
7. Daling JR et al: Primary tubal infertility in relation to the use of an intrauterine device. *N Engl J Med* 1985; 312:937–941.
8. Heartwell SF, Schlesselman S: Risk of uterine perforation among users of intrauterine devices. *Obstet Gynecol* 1983; 61:31–36.
9. Chi I-C, Kelly E: Is lactation a risk factor of IUD and sterilization-related uterine perforations? A hypothesis. *Int J Gynaecol Obstet* 1984; 22:315–317.
10. Harlap S, Kost K, Forrest JD: Preventing pregnancy, protecting health: a new look at birth control choices in the United States. The Alan Guttmacher Institute 1991; 1–129.
11. Chi I-C et al: Performance of the Copper T 380A Intrauterine device in breast feeding women. *Contraception* 1989; 39:603–618.
12. Farr G, Rivera R: Interactions between intrauterine contraceptive device use and breast-feeding status at time of intrauterine contraceptive device insertion. Analysis of TCu-380A acceptors in developing countries. *Am J Obstet Gynecol* 1992; 167:144–151.
13. Mark AS, Hricak H: Intrauterine contraceptive devices: MR imaging. *Radiology* 1987; 311–314.
14. Sivin I, Stern J: Long-acting, more effective Copper T IUDs: A summary of US experience, 1970–1975. *Stud Fam Plann* 1979; 10:263–281.
15. Sivin I, Schmidt F: Effectiveness of IUDs: A review. *Contraception* 1987; 36:55–84.
16. Trussell J: The Essentials of Contraception, in R.A. Hatcher, et al: *Contraceptive Technology*, 16th Revised Ed., New York, Irvington, 1994, p. 113–114.
17. World Health Organization (WHO): Mechanism of action, safety, and efficacy of intrauterine devices. Report of a WHO Scientific Group. Technical Report Series 753. Geneva; World Health Organization, 1987, p. 22.

Manufactured by FEI Products LLC
N. Tonawanda, New York 14120
ECR# 1361
 1017000
Shown in Product Identification Guide, page 312

Ferndale Laboratories, Inc.
780 W. EIGHT MILE ROAD
FERNDALE, MI 48220

Direct Inquiries to:
Dr. Michael Burns
(248) 548-0900
FAX: (248) 548-8427

For Medical Information Contact:
In Emergencies:
Pravin M. Patel
(248) 548-0900
FAX: (248) 548-0708

ANALPRAM HC® CREAM AND LOTION ℞
[*ă'năl-prăm*]
(hydrocortisone acetate and pramoxine hydrochloride)

DESCRIPTION
Analpram HC® Cream is a topical preparation containing hydrocortisone acetate 1% or 2.5% w/w and pramoxine hydrochloride 1% w/w in a hydrophilic cream base containing stearic acid, cetyl alcohol, Aquaphor*, isopropyl palmitate, polyoxyl 40 stearate, propylene glycol, potassium sorbate, sorbic acid, triethanolamine lauryl sulfate, and purified water.
Analpram HC® Lotion is a topical preparation containing hydrocortisone acetate 2.5% w/w and pramoxine hydrochloride 1% w/w in a hydrophilic lotion base containing stearic acid, cetyl alcohol, Forlan-L, glycerin, trolamine, polyoxyl 40 stearate, di-isopropyl adipate, povidone, dimethicone, potassium sorbate, sorbic acid, and purified water.
Topical corticosteroids are anti-inflammatory and antipruritic agents. The structural formulas, the chemical names, molecular formulas and molecular weights for active ingredients are presented below.

hydrocortisone acetate
Pregn-4-ene-3,20-dione, 21-(acetyloxy)-11,
17-dihydroxy-,(11-beta)-
$C_{23}H_{32}O_6$; mol. wt. 404.50

pramoxine hydrochloride
4-(3-(p-butoxyphenoxy)propyl)morpholine hydrochloride
$C_{17}H_{27}NO_3.HCl$; mol. wt: 329.87

CLINICAL PHARMACOLOGY
Topical corticosteroids share anti-inflammatory, antipruritic and vasoconstrictive actions. The mechanism of anti-inflammatory activity of topical corticosteroids is unclear. Various laboratory methods, including vasoconstrictor assays, are used to compare and predict potencies and/or clinical efficacies of the topical corticosteroids. There is some evidence to suggest that a recognizable correlation exists between vasoconstrictor potency and therapeutic efficacy in man.
Pramoxine hydrochloride is a topical anesthetic agent which provides temporary relief from itching and pain. It acts by stabilizing the neuronal membrane of nerve endings with which it comes into contact.
Pharmacokinetics: The extent of percutaneous absorption of topical corticosteroids is determined by many factors including the vehicle, the integrity of the epidermal barrier, and the use of occlusive dressings.
Topical corticosteroids can be absorbed from normal intact skin. Inflammation and/or other disease processes in the skin increase percutaneous absorption. Occlusive dressings substantially increase the percutaneous absorption of topical corticosteroids. Thus, occlusive dressings may be a valuable therapeutic adjunct for treatment of resistant dermatoses. (See DOSAGE AND ADMINISTRATION.)
Once absorbed through the skin, topical corticosteroids are handled through pharmacokinetic pathways similar to systemically administered corticosteroids.
Corticosteroids are bound to plasma proteins in varying degrees. Corticosteroids are metabolized primarily in the liver and are then excreted by the kidneys. Some of the topical corticosteroids and their metabolites are also excreted into the bile.

INDICATIONS AND USAGE
Topical corticosteroids are indicated for the relief of the inflammatory and pruritic manifestations of corticosteroid-responsive dermatoses.

CONTRAINDICATIONS
Topical corticosteroids are contraindicated in those patients with a history of hypersensitivity to any of the components of the preparation.

PRECAUTIONS
General:
Systemic absorption of topical corticosteroids has produced reversible hypothalamic-pituitary-adrenal (HPA) axis suppression, manifestations of Cushing's syndrome, hyperglycemia, and glucosuria in some patients. Conditions which augment systemic absorption include the application of the more potent steroids, use over large surface areas, prolonged use, and the addition of occlusive dressings.
Therefore, patients receiving a large dose of a potent topical steroid applied to a large surface area and under an occlusive dressing should be evaluated periodically for evidence of HPA axis suppression by using the urinary free cortisol and ACTH stimulation tests. If HPA axis suppression is noted, an attempt should be made to withdraw the drug, to reduce the frequency of application, or to substitute a less potent steroid.
Recovery of HPA axis function is generally prompt and complete upon discontinuation of the drug. Infrequently, signs and symptoms of steroid withdrawal may occur, requiring supplemental systemic corticosteroids. Children may absorb

Continued on next page

Analpram HC—Cont.

proportionally larger amounts of topical corticosteroids and thus be more susceptible to systemic toxicity. (See PRECAUTIONS-Pediatric Use.)

If irritation develops, topical corticosteroids should be discontinued and appropriate therapy instituted. In the presence of dermatological infections, the use of an appropriate anti-fungal or antibacterial agent should be instituted. If a favorable response does not occur promptly, the corticosteroid should be discontinued until the infection has been adequately controlled.

Information for the Patient:

Patients using topical corticosteroids should receive the following information and instructions:

1. This medication is to be used as directed by the physician. It is for external use only. Avoid contact with the eyes.
2. Patients should be advised not to use this medication for any disorder other than for which it was prescribed.
3. The treated skin area should not be bandaged or otherwise covered or wrapped as to be occlusive unless directed by the physician.
4. Patients should report any signs of local adverse reactions especially under occlusive dressings.
5. Parents of pediatric patients should be advised not to use tight-fitting diapers or plastic pants on a child being treated in the diaper area, as these garments may constitute occlusive dressings.

Laboratory Tests:

The following tests may be helpful in evaluating the HPA axis suppression:

Urinary free cortisol test
ACTH stimulation test

Carcinogenesis, Mutagenesis, and Impairment of Fertility: Long-term animal studies have not been performed to evaluate the carcinogenic potential or the effect on fertility of topical corticosteroids. Studies to determine mutagenicity with prednisolone and hydrocortisone have revealed negative results.

Pregnancy. Teratogenic Effects. Category C: Corticosteroids are generally teratogenic in laboratory animals when administered systemically at relatively low dosage levels. The more potent corticosteroids have been shown to be teratogenic after dermal application in laboratory animals. There are no adequate and well-controlled studies in pregnant women on teratogenic effects from topically applied corticosteroids. Therefore, topical corticosteroids should be used during pregnancy only if the potential benefit justifies the potential risk to the fetus. Drugs of this class should not be used extensively on pregnant patients, in large amounts, or for prolonged periods of time.

Nursing Mothers:

It is not known whether topical administration of corticosteroids could result in sufficient systemic absorption to produce detectable amounts in breast milk. Systemically administered corticosteroids are secreted into breast milk in quantities NOT likely to have a deleterious effect on the infant. Nevertheless, caution should be exercised when topical corticosteroids are administered to a nursing woman.

Pediatric Use:

Pediatric patients may demonstrate greater susceptibility to topical corticosteroid induced HPA axis suppression and Cushing's syndrome than mature patients because of a larger skin surface area to body weight ratio.

Hypothalamic-pituitary-adrenal (HPA) axis suppression, Cushing's syndrome, and intracranial hypertension have been reported in children receiving topical corticosteroids. Manifestations of adrenal suppression in children include linear growth retardation, delayed weight gain, low plasma cortisol levels, and absence of response to ACTH stimulation. Manifestations of intracranial hypertension include bulging fontanelles, headaches, and bilateral papilledema. Administration of topical corticosteroids to children should be limited to the least amount compatible with an effective therapeutic regimen. Chronic corticosteroid therapy may interfere with the growth and development of children.

ADVERSE REACTIONS

The following local adverse reactions are reported infrequently with topical corticosteroids, but may occur more frequently with the use of occlusive dressings. These reactions are listed in an approximate decreasing order of occurrence:

Burning
Itching
Irritation
Dryness
Folliculitis
Hypertrichosis
Acneiform eruptions
Hypopigmentation
Perioral dermatitis
Allergic contact dermatitis
Maceration of the skin
Secondary infection
Skin atrophy
Striae
Miliaria

OVERDOSAGE

Topically applied corticosteroids can be absorbed in sufficient amounts to produce systemic effects. (See PRECAUTIONS.)

DOSAGE AND ADMINISTRATION

Topical corticosteroids are generally applied to the affected area as a thin film three to four times daily depending on the severity of the condition. Lotion should be shaken well before use. Occlusive dressings may be used for the management of psoriasis or recalcitrant conditions. If an infection develops, the use of occlusive dressings should be discontinued and appropriate antimicrobial therapy instituted. For cleansing the anogenital area, apply Analpram HC® Lotion 2.5% on cotton or tissue and wipe affected area.

HOW SUPPLIED

Analpram HC® Cream 1%	1 oz tube	(NDC 0496-0778-04)
Analpram HC® Cream 2.5%	1 oz tube	(NDC 0496-0800-04)
Analpram HC® Lotion 2.5%	2 fl oz	(NDC 0496-0829-04)

Storage Conditions: Store at controlled room temperature 59°–86°F (15°–30°C).

℞ Only.

FERNDALE LABORATORIES INC.

Ferndale, MI 48220 USA
Toll free (888) 548-0900
www.ferndalelabs.com

*Aquaphor is a trademark of Beiersdorf AG.

Item # AN17
Rev.: 10/02

CLINAC® BPO 7 ℞

[klī'-năk]

(Benzoyl Peroxide Gel USP, 7%)
Acne Control Gel

DESCRIPTION

Clinac® BPO 7 (benzoyl peroxide) is a topical preparation containing 7% benzoyl peroxide as the active ingredient in a gel vehicle containing purified water, propylene glycol, Acrysorb™ (brand of acrylates copolymer), PEG-400, carbomer 940, disodium EDTA, and sodium hydroxide.

The chemical structure for the active ingredient is:

benzoyl peroxide
$C_{14}H_{10}O_4$ (anhydrous) 242.23

CLINICAL PHARMACOLOGY

The exact method of action of benzoyl peroxide in acne vulgaris is not known. Benzoyl peroxide is an antibacterial agent with demonstrated activity against *Propionibacterium acnes*. This action combined with the mild keratolytic effect of benzoyl peroxide is believed to be responsible for its usefulness in acne.

Little is known about the percutaneous penetration, metabolism and excretion of benzoyl peroxide. Benzoyl peroxide is absorbed by the skin where it is metabolized to benzoic acid and excreted as benzoate in the urine. There is no evidence of systemic toxicity caused by benzoyl peroxide in humans.

INDICATIONS AND USAGE

Clinac® BPO 7 is indicated for the topical treatment of mild to moderate acne vulgaris. Clinac® BPO 7 may be used with other acne treatments including retinoic acid products, antibiotics and sulfur/salicylic acid containing preparations.

CONTRAINDICATIONS

Clinac® BPO 7 should not be used in patients who have shown hypersensitivity to benzoyl peroxide or any of the other ingredients in this product.

WARNINGS

FOR EXTERNAL USE ONLY. KEEP OUT OF REACH OF CHILDREN. Avoid contact with eyes, eyelids, lips and mucous membranes. If inadvertent contact occurs, rinse area thoroughly with water. Contact with colored material, including fabric and hair, may result in discoloration. When using Clinac® BPO 7, avoid unnecessary sun exposure and use a sunscreen. In case of accidental ingestion, seek professional assistance or contact a poison control center immediately.

PRECAUTIONS

Information for Patients

- Avoid contact with eyes, eyelids, lips and mucous membranes.
- May discolor hair and fabrics.
- Avoid unnecessary sun exposure and use a sunscreen.
- Use of oil-free make-up recommended.
- If severe irritation develops, discontinue use and consult your physician.

Carcinogenesis, Mutagenesis and Impairment of Fertility

Studies employing a strain of mice that are highly susceptible to developing cancer suggest that benzoyl peroxide acts as a tumor promoter. The clinical significance of these findings to humans is not known. Benzoyl peroxide has not been found to be mutagenic (Ames test) and there are no published data indicating that it impairs fertility.

Pregnancy: Category C

Animal reproductive studies have not been conducted with benzoyl peroxide. It is also not known whether benzoyl peroxide can cause fetal harm when administered to a pregnant woman or can affect reproduction capacity. Benzoyl peroxide should be used by a pregnant woman only if clearly needed. There are no available data on the effect of benzoyl peroxide on the later growth, development and functional maturation of the unborn child.

Nursing Mothers

It is not known whether this drug is excreted in human milk. Because many drugs are excreted in human milk, caution should be exercised when benzoyl peroxide is administered to a nursing woman.

Pediatric Use

Safety and effectiveness in children below the age of 12 have not been established.

ADVERSE REACTIONS

Allergic contact dermatitis and dryness have been reported with topical benzoyl peroxide therapy. If excessive scaling, erythema or edema occurs, the use of Clinac® BPO 7 should be discontinued and appropriate therapy instituted. To hasten resolution of adverse effects, cool compresses may be used. After reaction clears, a reduced dosage schedule may often be resumed if the reaction is judged not to be due to allergenicity.

DOSAGE AND ADMINISTRATION

Wash and dry hands, face and affected areas with a gentle cleanser before application. Apply a thin layer of Clinac® BPO 7 to the affected area once or twice daily, or as directed by your physician. Replace cap tightly after use.

HOW SUPPLIED

Clinac® BPO 7 Gel 45 gram tube NDC 0496-0857-45
Store at controlled room temperature 59°-86°F (15°-30°C).

℞ Only.

FERNDALE LABORATORIES INC
ETHICAL PHARMACEUTICALS SINCE 1897

Ferndale, MI 48220 U.S.A.
Toll Free: (888) 548-0900 • www.ferndalelabs.com

Clinac® is a registered trademark and Acrysorb™ is a trademark of Dow Pharmaceutical Sciences Corp.

MG #14238
Rev: 02/03

L.M.X.4™ OTC

(lidocaine 4%)
Topical Anesthetic Cream

L.M.X.4™ Cream (lidocaine 4%) is a topical anesthetic cream.

HOW SUPPLIED

L.M.X.4™ is available as the following

NDC 0496-0882-08	5 gram tube[1]
NDC 0496-0882-07	5 gram tube, box of 5[1]
NDC 0496-0882-15	15 gram tube (Child-Resistant Packaging)
NDC 0496-0882-30	30 gram tube (Child-Resistant Packaging)

[1] 5 gram formats contain 3M Tegaderm™ bandages for uses where occlusion may be necessary (e.g., pediatrics).

Store between 15° and 30°C (59°–86°F).

L.M.X.4™ is a trademark of Ferndale Laboratories, Inc.

L.M.X.5™ OTC

(lidocaine 5%)
Anorectal Cream

L.M.X.5™ Cream (lidocaine 5%) is indicated for the temporary relief of local discomfort, including pain and itching, soreness or burning associated with anorectal disorders.

HOW SUPPLIED

L.M.X.5™ is available as the following

NDC 0496-0883-15	15 gram tube
NDC 0496-0883-30	30 gram tube (Child-Resistant Packaging)

Store between 15° and 30°C (59°–86°F).

L.M.X.5™ is a trademark of Ferndale Laboratories, Inc.

KRONOFED–A® Kronocaps ℞
KRONOFED–A–JR® Kronocaps ℞

Each sustained release Kronofed A®, white and clear capsule contains:

Pseudoephedrine HCl .... 120 mg
Chlorpheniramine Maleate .... 8 mg

Each sustained release Kronofed-A-Jr®, white and clear capsule contains:

Pseudoephedrine HCl .... 60 mg
Chlorpheniramine Maleate .... 4 mg

HOW SUPPLIED

Kronofed-A® Kronocaps
Bottles of 100 NDC 0496–0382–02
Bottles of 500 NDC 0496–0382–10

Kronofed-A-Jr® Kronocaps
Bottles of 100 NDC 0496–0434–02
Bottles of 500 NDC 0496–0434–10
Kronofed-A is a registered trademark of Ferndale Laboratories, Inc.

LOCOID® ℞

(hydrocortisone butyrate 0.1%)
Cream 0.1%
Ointment 0.1%
Topical Solution 0.1%

For dermatological use only.

DESCRIPTION

LOCOID® cream, ointment and topical solution contain the topical corticosteroid hydrocortisone butyrate, a non-fluorinated hydrocortisone ester. It has the chemical name: pregn-4-ene-3, 20-dione, 11, 21-dihydroxy-17-[(1-oxobutyl) oxy-, (11β)-; the molecular formula: $C_{25}H_{36}O_6$; the molecular weight: 432.54; and the CAS registry number: 13609-67-1. Its structural formula is:

CH₂OH C=O CH₃ HO OCCH₂CH₂CH₃ O CH₃ O

LOCOID® Cream
Each gram of LOCOID® cream contains 1 mg of hydrocortisone butyrate in a hydrophilic base consisting of cetostearyl alcohol, ceteth-20, mineral oil, white petrolatum, citric acid, sodium citrate, propylparaben and butylparaben (preservatives) and purified water.

LOCOID® Ointment
Each gram of LOCOID® ointment contains 1 mg of hydrocortisone butyrate in a base consisting of mineral oil and polyethylene.

LOCOID® Solution
Each mL of LOCOID® solution contains 1 mg of hydrocortisone butyrate in a vehicle consisting of isopropyl alcohol (50%), glycerin, povidone, citric acid, sodium citrate and purified water.

CLINICAL PHARMACOLOGY

Topical corticosteroids share anti-inflammatory, anti-pruritic and vasoconstrictive actions.
The mechanism of anti-inflammatory activity of the topical corticosteroids is unclear. Various laboratory methods, including vasoconstrictor assays, are used to compare and predict potencies and/or clinical efficacies of the topical corticosteroids. There is some evidence to suggest that a recognizable correlation exists between vasoconstrictor potency and therapeutic efficacy in man.

Pharmacokinetics
The extent of percutaneous absorption of topical corticosteroids is determined by many factors including the vehicle, the integrity of the epidermal barrier, and the use of occlusive dressings.
Topical corticosteroids can be absorbed from normal intact skin. Inflammation and/or other disease processes in the skin increase percutaneous absorption. Occlusive dressings substantially increase the percutaneous absorption of topical corticosteroids. Thus, occlusive dressings may be a valuable therapeutic adjunct for treatment of resistant dermatoses. (See DOSAGE AND ADMINISTRATION.)
Once absorbed through the skin, topical corticosteroids are handled through pharmacokinetic pathways similar to systemically administered corticosteroids.
Corticosteroids are bound to plasma proteins in varying degrees. Corticosteroids are metabolized primarily in the liver and are then excreted by the kidneys.
Some of the topical corticosteroids and their metabolites are also excreted into the bile.

INDICATIONS AND USAGE

LOCOID® Cream and Ointment (hydrocortisone butyrate 0.1%) are indicated for the relief of the inflammatory and pruritic manifestations of corticosteroid-responsive dermatoses.
LOCOID® solution (hydrocortisone butyrate 0.1%) is indicated for the relief of the inflammatory and pruritic manifestations of seborrheic dermatitis.

CONTRAINDICATIONS

Topical corticosteroids are contraindicated in those patients with a history of hypersensitivity to any of the components of the preparation.

PRECAUTIONS

General: Systemic absorption of topical corticosteroids has produced reversible hypothalamic-pituitary-adrenal (HPA) axis suppression, manifestations of Cushing's syndrome, hyperglycemia, and glucosuria in some patients. Conditions which augment systemic absorption include the application of the more potent steroids, use over large surface areas, prolonged use, and the addition of occlusive dressings.
Therefore, patients receiving a large dose of a potent topical steroid applied to a large surface area or under an occlusive dressing should be evaluated periodically for evidence of HPA axis suppression by using the urinary free cortisol and ACTH stimulation tests. If HPA axis suppression is noted, an attempt should be made to withdraw the drug, to reduce the frequency of application, or to substitute a less potent steroid.
Recovery of HPA axis function is generally prompt and complete upon discontinuation of the drug. Infrequently, signs and symptoms of steroid withdrawal may occur, requiring supplemental systemic corticosteroids.
Children may absorb proportionally larger amounts of topical corticosteroids and thus be more susceptible to systemic toxicity (See PRECAUTIONS—PEDIATRIC USE.)
If irritation develops, topical corticosteroids should be discontinued and appropriate therapy instituted. In the presence of dermatological infections, the use of an appropriate antifungal or antibacterial agent should be instituted. If a favorable response does not occur promptly, the corticosteroid should be discontinued until the infection has been adequately controlled.

Information for the patient
Patients using topical corticosteroids should receive the following information and instructions:

1. This medication is to be used as directed by the physician. It is for external use only. Avoid contact with the eyes.
2. Patients should be advised not to use this medication for any disorder other than for which it was prescribed.
3. The treated skin area should not be bandaged or otherwise covered or wrapped as to be occlusive unless directed by the physician.
4. Patients should report any signs of local adverse reactions especially under occlusive dressing.
5. Parents of pediatric patients should be advised not to use tight-fitting diapers or plastic pants on a child being treated in the diaper area, as these garments may constitute occlusive dressings.

Laboratory tests
The following tests may be helpful in evaluating the HPA axis suppression:
Urinary free cortisol test
ACTH stimulation test

Carcinogenesis, Mutagenesis, and Impairment of Fertility
Long-term animal studies have not been performed to evaluate the carcinogenic potential or the effect on fertility of topical corticosteroids.
Studies to determine mutagenicity with prednisolone and hydrocortisone have revealed negative results.

Pregnancy Category C
Corticosteroids are generally teratogenic in laboratory animals when administered systemically at relatively low dosage levels. The more potent corticosteroids have been shown to be teratogenic after dermal application in laboratory animals. There are no adequate and well-controlled studies in pregnant women on teratogenic effects from topically applied corticosteroids. Therefore, topical corticosteroids should be used during pregnancy only if the potential benefit justifies the potential risk to the fetus. Drugs of this class should not be used extensively on pregnant patients, in large amounts, or for prolonged periods of time.

Nursing Mothers
It is not known whether topical administration of corticosteroids could result in sufficient systemic absorption to produce detectable quantities in breast milk. Systemically administered corticosteroids are secreted into breast milk, in quantities not likely to have a deleterious effect on the infant. Nevertheless, caution should be exercised when topical corticosteroids are administered to a nursing woman.

Pediatric Use
Pediatric patients may demonstrate greater susceptibility to topical corticosteroid-induced HPA axis suppression and Cushing's syndrome than mature patients because of a larger skin surface area to body weight ratio.
Hypothalamic-pituitary-adrenal (HPA) axis suppression, Cushing's syndrome, and intracranial hypertension have been reported in children receiving topical corticosteroids. Manifestations of adrenal suppression in children include linear growth retardation, delayed weight gain, low plasma cortisol levels, and absence of response to ACTH stimulation. Manifestations of intracranial hypertension include bulging fontanelles, headaches, and bilateral papilledema. Administration of topical corticosteroids to children should be limited to the least amount compatible with an effective therapeutic regimen. Chronic corticosteroid therapy may interfere with the growth and development of children.

ADVERSE REACTIONS

The following local adverse reactions are reported infrequently with topical corticosteroids, but may occur more frequently with the use of occlusive dressings. These reactions are listed in an approximate decreasing order of occurrence: burning, itching, irritation, dryness, folliculitis, hypertrichosis, acneiform eruptions, hypopigmentation, perioral dermatitis, allergic contact dermatitis, maceration of the skin, secondary infection, skin atrophy, striae, miliaria.

OVERDOSAGE

Topically applied corticosteroids can be absorbed in sufficient amounts to produce systemic effects. (See PRECAUTIONS.)

DOSAGE AND ADMINISTRATION

LOCOID® Cream or LOCOID® Ointment (hydrocortisone butyrate 0.1%) should be applied to the affected area as a thin film two to three times daily depending on the severity of the condition.
Occlusive dressings may be used for the management of psoriasis or recalcitrant conditions.
If an infection develops, the use of occlusive dressings should be discontinued and appropriate antimicrobial therapy instituted.
LOCOID® Solution (hydrocortisone butyrate 0.1%) should be applied to the affected area as a thin film from two to three times daily depending on the severity of the condition.

HOW SUPPLIED

LOCOID® Cream (hydrocortisone butyrate 0.1%) is supplied in tubes containing:
15 g NDC 0496-0802-15
45 g NDC 0496-0802-45
LOCOID® Ointment (hydrocortisone butyrate 0.1%) is supplied in tubes containing:
15 g NDC 0496-0803-15
45 g NDC 0496-0803-45
LOCOID® Solution (hydrocortisone butyrate 0.1%) is supplied in polyethylene bottles:
20 mL NDC 0496-0804-20
60 mL NDC 0496-0804-60

STORAGE

LOCOID® Cream: Store between 59° - 77°F (15° - 25°C).
LOCOID® Ointment: Store between 36° - 86°F (2° - 30°C).
LOCOID® Solution: Store between 41° - 77°F (5° - 25°C).

MARKETED BY:
FERNDALE LABORATORIES, INC.
FERNDALE, MICHIGAN 48220
Revised: May 2003

LOCOID LIPOCREAM® ℞

(hydrocortisone butyrate 0.1%)
Cream

For Dermatological Use Only

DESCRIPTION

LOCOID Lipocream® Cream contains the topical corticosteroid hydrocortisone butyrate, a hydrocortisone ester. It has the chemical name: (11β)-11,21-dihydroxy-17-[(1-oxobutyl)oxy]-pregn-4-ene-3,20-dione; the molecular formula: $C_{25}H_{36}O_6$; the molecular weight: 432.54; and the CAS registry number: 13609-67-1. The structural formula is:

CH₂OH C=O CH₃ HO OCCH₂CH₂CH₃ O CH₃ O

LOCOID Lipocream® Cream
Each gram of LOCOID Lipocream® Cream contains 1 mg of hydrocortisone butyrate in a hydrophilic base consisting of cetostearyl alcohol, ceteth-20, mineral oil, white petrolatum, citric acid, sodium citrate, propyl paraben and butyl paraben (preservatives) and purified water.

CLINICAL PHARMACOLOGY

Topical corticosteroids share anti-inflammatory, anti-pruritic and vasoconstrictive actions. The mechanism of anti-inflammatory activity of topical corticosteroids is unclear. Various laboratory methods, including vasoconstrictor assays, are used to compare and predict potencies and/or clinical efficacies of topical corticosteroids. There is some evidence to suggest that a recognizable correlation exists between vasoconstrictor potency and therapeutic efficacy in man.

PHARMACOKINETICS
The extent of percutaneous absorption of topical corticosteroids is determined by many factors including the vehicle, the integrity of the epidermal barrier, and the use of occlusive dressings.
Topical corticosteroids can be absorbed from normal intact skin. Inflammation and/or other disease processes in the skin increase percutaneous absorption. Occlusive dressings or widespread application may increase the possibility of hypothalamic-pituitary-adrenal (HPA) axis suppression.
The vasoconstrictor assay showed that LOCOID Lipocream® Cream had a more pronounced skin blanching effect than LOCOID® Cream, suggesting greater percutaneous absorption from the former. At the present time, no adequate HPA axis suppression studies have been conducted for LOCOID Lipocream® Cream.
Once absorbed through the skin, topical corticosteroids are handled through pharmacokinetic pathways similar to systemically administered corticosteroids.
Corticosteroids are bound to plasma proteins in varying degrees.

Continued on next page

Locoid Lipocream—Cont.

Corticosteroids are metabolized primarily in the liver and are then excreted by the kidneys. Some of the topical corticosteroids and their metabolites are also excreted into the bile.

INDICATIONS AND USAGE

LOCOID Lipocream® (hydrocortisone butyrate 0.1%) Cream is indicated for the relief of the inflammatory and pruritic manifestations of corticosteroid-responsive dermatoses.

CONTRAINDICATIONS

Topical corticosteroids are contraindicated in those patients with a history of hypersensitivity to any of the components of the preparation.

PRECAUTIONS

General

Systemic absorption of topical corticosteroids has produced reversible HPA axis suppression, manifestations of Cushing's syndrome, hyperglycemia, and glucosuria in some patients.

Conditions which increase the risk of systemic toxicity include the application of more potent steroids, use over large surface areas, prolonged use, and the addition of occlusive dressings.

Children may absorb proportionally larger amounts of topical corticosteroids and thus be more susceptible to systemic toxicity. (See PRECAUTIONS — PEDIATRIC USE.)

If irritation develops, topical corticosteroids should be discontinued and appropriate therapy instituted. In the presence of dermatological infections, the use of an appropriate antifungal or antibacterial agent should be instituted. If a favorable response does not occur promptly, the corticosteroid should be discontinued until the infection has been adequately controlled.

Information for the Patient

Patients using topical corticosteroids should receive the following information and instructions:

1. This medication is to be used as directed by the physician. It is for external use only. Avoid contact with the eyes.
2. Patients should be advised not to use this medication for any disorder other than for which it was prescribed.
3. The treated skin area should not be bandaged or otherwise covered or wrapped as to be occlusive.
4. Patients should report any signs of local adverse reactions.
5. Parents of pediatric patients should be advised not to use tight-fitting diapers or plastic pants on a child being treated in the diaper area, as these garments may constitute occlusive dressings.

Laboratory Tests

The following tests may be helpful in evaluating the HPA axis suppression:

Urinary free cortisol test;

ACTH stimulation test;

Carcinogenesis, Mutagenesis, and Impairment of Fertility

Long-term animal studies have not been performed to evaluate the carcinogenic potential or the effect on fertility of topical corticosteroids.

Studies to determine mutagenicity in *Salmonella ryphimurium* strains TA98, TA100, and TA92 with prednisolone and hydrocortisone have revealed negative results.

Pregnancy: Teratogenic Effects: Pregnancy Category C:

Corticosteroids are generally teratogenic in laboratory animals when administered systemically at relatively low dosage levels. Some corticosteroids have been shown to be teratogenic after dermal application in laboratory animals.

In teratogenicity studies, topical administration of 1% or 10% hydrocortisone butyrate in an ointment to pregnant Wistar rats (gestational days 6–15) or New Zealand white rabbits (gestational days 6–18) resulted in no teratogenic findings. However, a dose-dependent increase in fetal resorptions was reported in rabbits, and fetal resorptions were observed in rats treated with 10% hydrocortisone butyrate.

The doses given to rats are approximately 8 to 80 times the human topical dose based on a body surface area comparison (assuming 100% absorption).

For rabbits, the doses given were approximately 0.2 and 2 times the human topical dose. Increased resorptions were also noted in Wistar rats given subcutaneous administrations of hydrocortisone butyrate (9mg/kg/day; 3 times the human topical dose) on gestational days 9 through 15. In CS mice given subcutaneous administrations of 1 mg/kg/day (0.2 times the human topical dose), an increased number of cervical ribs and one fetus with clubbed legs was reported. There are no adequate and well-controlled studies in pregnant women on teratogenic effects from topically applied corticosteroids. Therefore, topical corticosteroids should be used during pregnancy only if the potential benefit justifies the potential risk to the fetus.

LOCOID Lipocream® (hydrocortisone butyrate 0.1%) Cream should not be used extensively on pregnant patients, in large amounts, or for longer than two weeks.

Nursing Mothers

It is not known whether topical administration of corticosteroids could result in sufficient systemic absorption to produce detectable quantities in breast milk.

Systemically administered corticosteroids are secreted into breast milk in quantities not likely to have a deleterious effect on the infant. Nevertheless, caution should be exercised when topical corticosteroids are administered to a nursing woman.

Pediatric Use

Safety and effectiveness in pediatric patients have not been established.

Pediatric patients may demonstrate greater susceptibility to topical corticosteroid-induced HPA axis suppression and Cushing's syndrome than mature patients because of a larger skin surface area to body weight ratio.

HPA axis suppression, Cushing's syndrome, and intracranial hypertension have been reported in children receiving topical corticosteroids.

Manifestations of adrenal suppression in children include linear growth retardation, delayed weight gain, low plasma cortisol levels, and absence of response to ACTH stimulation.

Manifestations of intracranial hypertension include bulging fontanelles, headaches, and bilateral papilledema.

Chronic corticosteroid therapy may interfere with the growth and development of children.

ADVERSE REACTIONS

The following local adverse reactions are reported infrequently with topical corticosteroids but may occur more frequently with the use of occlusive dressings. These reactions are listed in an approximate decreasing order of occurrence: burning, itching, irritation, dryness, folliculitis, hypertrichosis, acneiform eruptions, hypopigmentation, perioral dermatitis, allergic contact dermatitis, maceration of the skin, secondary infection, skin atrophy, striae and miliaria.

OVERDOSAGE

Topically applied corticosteroids can be absorbed in sufficient amounts to produce systemic effects. (See PRECAUTIONS.)

DOSAGE AND ADMINISTRATION

LOCOID Lipocream® (hydrocortisone butyrate 0.1%) Cream should be applied to the affected areas as a thin film two or three times daily (depending on the severity of the condition) and for no longer than two weeks. If an infection develops, appropriate antimicrobial therapy should be instituted.

HOW SUPPLIED

LOCOID Lipocream® (hydrocortisone butyrate 0.1%) Cream is supplied in tubes containing:

15 g NDC 0496-0821-15

45 g NDC 0496-0821-45

STORAGE

Store at controlled temperature between 59° – 77°F (15° – 25°C).

Rx Only.

Marketed by:

FERNDALE LABORATORIES, INC.

Ferndale, Michigan 48220 USA

(888) 548-0900

Revised: May 2004

PRAMOSONE® ℞

CREAM, LOTION AND OINTMENT

(hydrocortisone acetate and pramoxine hydrochloride)

DESCRIPTION

Pramosone® Cream is a topical preparation containing hydrocortisone acetate 1% w/w or 2.5% w/w and pramoxine hydrochloride 1% w/w in a hydrophilic cream base containing stearic acid, cetyl alcohol, aquaphor, isopropyl palmitate, polyoxyl-40-stearate, propylene glycol, potassium sorbate, sorbic acid, triethanolamine lauryl sulfate and purified water.

Pramosone® Lotion is a topical preparation containing hydrocortisone acetate 1% w/w or 2.5% w/w and pramoxine hydrochloride 1% w/w in a hydrophilic lotion base containing stearic acid, cetyl alcohol, forlan-L, glycerin, triethanolamine, polyoxyl-40-stearate, di-isopropyl adipate, povidone, dimethicone, potassium sorbate, sorbic acid, and purified water.

Pramosone® Ointment is a topical preparation containing hydrocortisone acetate 1% w/w or 2.5% w/w and pramoxine hydrochloride 1% w/w in an emollient ointment base containing sorbitan sesquioleate, water, aquaphor and white petrolatum. Topical corticosteroids are anti-inflammatory and anti-pruritic agents. The chemical structural formula for active ingredients is presented below.

hydrocortisone acetate(pregn-4-ene-3,20-dione, 21 - (acetyloxy)-11, 17-dihydroxy-,(11β)-.)

$C_{23}H_{32}O_6$; mol. wt. 404.50

[See chemical structure at top of next column]

CLINICAL PHARMACOLOGY

Topical corticosteroids share anti-inflammatory, antipruritic and vasoconstrictive actions.

$CH_3CH_2CH_2CH_2O$–(C₆H₄)–$OCH_2CH_2CH_2N$(morpholine) O.HCl

The mechanism of anti-inflammatory activity of topical corticosteroids is unclear. Various laboratory methods, including vasoconstrictor assays, are used to compare and predict potencies and/or clinical efficacies of the topical corticosteroids. There is some evidence to suggest that a recognizable correlation exists between vasoconstrictor potency and therapeutic efficacy in man.

Pramoxine hydrochloride is a topical anesthetic agent which provides temporary relief from itching and pain. It acts by stabilizing the neuronal membrane of nerve endings with which it comes into contact.

Pharmacokinetics

The extent of percutaneous absorption of topical corticosteroids is determined by many factors including the vehicle, the integrity of the epidermal barrier, and the use of occlusive dressings.

Topical corticosteroids can be absorbed from normal intact skin. Inflammation and/or other disease processes in the skin increase percutaneous absorption. Occlusive dressings substantially increase the percutaneous absorption of topical corticosteroids. Thus, occlusive dressings may be a valuable therapeutic adjunct for treatment of resistant dermatoses (See DOSAGE AND ADMINISTRATION).

Once absorbed through the skin, topical corticosteroids are handled through pharmacokinetic pathways similar to systemically administered corticosteroids.

Corticosteroids are bound to plasma proteins in varying degrees. Corticosteroids are metabolized primarily in the liver and are then excreted by the kidneys. Some of the topical corticosteroids and their metabolites are also excreted into the bile.

INDICATIONS AND USAGE

Topical corticosteroids are indicated for the relief of the inflammatory and pruritic manifestations of corticosteroid-responsive dermatoses.

CONTRAINDICATIONS

Topical corticosteroids are contraindicated in those patients with a history of hypersensitivity to any of the components of the preparation.

PRECAUTIONS

General: Systemic absorption of topical corticosteroids has produced reversible hypothalamic-pituitary-adrenal (HPA) axis suppression, manifestations of Cushing's syndrome, hyperglycemia, and glucosuria in some patients.

Conditions which augment systemic absorption include the application of the more potent steroids, use over large surface areas, prolonged use, and the addition of occlusive dressings.

Therefore, patients receiving a large dose of a potent topical steroid applied to a large surface area and under an occlusive dressing should be evaluated periodically for evidence of HPA axis suppression by using the urinary free cortisol and ACTH stimulation tests. If HPA axis suppression is noted, an attempt should be made to withdraw the drug, to reduce the frequency of application, or to substitute a less potent steroid.

Recovery of HPA axis function is generally prompt and complete upon discontinuation of the drug. Infrequently, signs and symptoms of steroid withdrawal may occur, requiring supplemental systemic corticosteroids. Children may absorb proportionally larger amounts of topical corticosteroids and thus be more susceptible to systemic toxicity. (See PRECAUTIONS-Pediatric Use). If irritation develops, topical corticosteroids should be discontinued and appropriate therapy instituted. In the presence of dermatological infections, the use of an appropriate anti-fungal or antibacterial agent should be instituted. If a favorable response does not occur promptly, the corticosteroid should be discontinued until the infection has been adequately controlled.

Information for the Patient

Patients using topical corticosteroids should receive the following information and instructions:

1. This medication is to be used as directed by the physician. It is for external use only. Avoid contact with the eyes.
2. Patients should be advised not to use this medication for any disorder other than for which it was prescribed.
3. The treated skin area should not be bandaged or otherwise covered or wrapped as to be occlusive unless directed by the physician.
4. Patients should report any signs of local adverse reactions especially under occlusive dressing.
5. Parents of pediatric patients should be advised not to use tight-fitting diapers or plastic pants on a child being treated in the diaper area, as these garments may constitute occlusive dressings.

Laboratory Tests:

The following tests may be helpful in evaluating the HPA axis suppression:

Urinary free cortisol test

ACTH stimulation test

Carcinogenesis, Mutagenesis, and Impairment of Fertility:

Long-term animal studies have not been performed to evaluate the carcinogenic potential or the effect on fertility of topical corticosteroids.

Studies to determine mutagenicity with prednisolone and hydrocortisone have revealed negative results.

Pregnancy. Teratogenic Effects. Category C:
Corticosteroids are generally teratogenic in laboratory animals when administered systemically at relatively low dosage levels. The more potent corticosteroids have been shown to be teratogenic after dermal application in laboratory animals.
There are no adequate and well-controlled studies in pregnant women on teratogenic effects from topically applied corticosteroids. Therefore, topical corticosteroids should be used during pregnancy only if the potential benefit justifies the potential risk to the fetus. Drugs of this class should not be used extensively on pregnant patients, in large amounts, or for prolonged periods of time.
Nursing Mothers:
It is not known whether topical administration of corticosteroids could result in sufficient systemic absorption to produce detectable amounts in breast milk. Systemically administered corticosteroids are secreted into breast milk in quantities NOT likely to have a deleterious effect on the infant. Nevertheless, caution should be exercised when topical corticosteroids are administered to a nursing woman.
Pediatric Use:
Pediatric patients may demonstrate greater susceptibility to topical corticosteroid-induced HPA axis suppression and Cushing's syndrome than mature patients because of a larger skin surface area to body weight ratio. Hypothalamic-pituitary-adrenal (HPA) axis suppression, Cushing's syndrome, and intracranial hypertension have been reported in children receiving topical corticosteroids. Manifestations of adrenal suppression in children include linear growth retardation, delayed weight gain, low plasma cortisol levels, and absence of response to ACTH stimulation. Manifestations of intracranial hypertension include bulging fontanelles, headaches, and bilateral papilledema.
Administration of topical corticosteroids to children should be limited to the least amount compatible with an effective therapeutic regimen. Chronic corticosteroid therapy may interfere with the growth and development of children.

ADVERSE REACTIONS

The following local adverse reactions are reported infrequently with topical corticosteroids, but may occur more frequently with the use of occlusive dressings. These reactions are listed in an approximate decreasing order of occurrence: Burning, Itching, Irritation, Dryness, Folliculitis, Hypertrichosis, Acneiform eruptions, Hypopigmentation, Perioral dermatitis, Allergic contact dermatitis, Maceration of the skin, Secondary infection, Skin Atrophy, Striae, and Miliaria.

OVERDOSAGE

Topically applied corticosteroids can be absorbed in sufficient amounts to produce systemic effects. (See PRECAUTIONS).

DOSAGE AND ADMINISTRATION

Topical corticosteroids are generally applied to the affected area as a thin film three to four times daily depending on the severity of the condition. Lotion should be shaken well before use. Occlusive dressings may be used for the management of psoriasis or recalcitrant conditions. If an infection develops, the use of occlusive dressings should be discontinued and appropriate antimicrobial therapy instituted.

HOW SUPPLIED

Pramosone® Cream 1%:	Pramosone® Cream 2.5%:
1 oz (NDC 0496-0716-04)	1 oz (NDC 0496-0717-04)
2 oz (NDC 0496-0716-03)	2 oz (NDC 0496-0717-03)
Pramosone® Lotion 1%:	Pramosone® Lotion 2.5%:
2 fl oz (NDC 0496-0729-06)	2 fl oz (NDC 0496-0726-06)
4 fl oz (NDC 0496-0729-04)	4 fl oz (NDC 0496-0726-04)
8 fl oz (NDC 0496-0729-03)	
Pramosone® Ointment 1%:	Pramosone® Ointment 2.5%:
1 oz (NDC 0496-0763-04)	1 oz (NDC 0496-0777-04)

Storage Conditions
Dispense in a tight container as defined in the official compendium. Store at controlled room temperature 59°-86°F (15°-30°C).
℞ **Only.**
FERNDALE LABORATORIES INC
Ferndale, Michigan 48220 USA Rev.: 04/01
Toll Free: (888) 548-0900 #0716I
www.ferndalelabs.com MG #16505

PRAX® LOTION **OTC**
(Pramoxine HCl 1% in an emollient hydrophilic base)

Prax® Lotion provides prompt, temporary relief of dry itching skin and pain due to minor skin irritations.

HOW SUPPLIED
Prax® Lotion is supplied in dispenser bottles containing
15 mL NDC 0496-0748-15
4 fl oz NDC 0496-0748-04
8 fl oz NDC 0496-0748-03
Prax is a registered trademark of Ferndale Laboratories, Inc.

SBR-LIPOCREAM® **OTC**
SBR-Lipocream® is specially designed to help repair and maintain the body's natural skin barrier function. SBR-Lipocream® is for patients with sensitive skin or skin that is predisposed to chronic skin disease and irritation.

HOW SUPPLIED
SBR-Lipocream® is supplied in tubes containing
100 g NDC 0496-0819-01
SBR-Lipocream is a registered trademark of Ferndale Laboratories, Inc.

Ferring Pharmaceuticals Inc.
400 RELLA BOULEVARD
SUITE #300
SUFFERN, NY 10901

Direct Inquiries to:
Ferring Pharmaceuticals Inc.
Customer Service Department
400 Rella Boulevard, Suite #300
Suffern, NY 10901
1-(888)-FERRING (337-7464)

For Medical Information Contact:
In Emergencies:
Ferring Pharmaceuticals Inc.
Professional Services Department
400 Rella Boulevard, Suite #300
Suffern, NY 10901
1-(800)-822-8214

ACTHREL® ℞
(corticorelin ovine triflutate for injection)
For intravenous injection only
DIAGNOSTIC USE ONLY

HOW SUPPLIED
As a 5 mL, amber, single-dose vial (NDC 55566-0302-1). Each vial contains a sterile, nonpyrogenic, lyophilized white cake containing 100 mcg corticorelin ovine (as the trifluroacetate), 0.88 mg ascorbic acid, 10 mg lactose, and 26 mg cysteine hydrochloride monohydrate.
Store refrigerated at 2°C to 8°C (36°F to 46°F) and protect from light.
Please see full prescribing information in the Diagnostic Product Information section.

BRAVELLE™ ℞
[brä-vĕl]
(urofollitropin for injection, purified)
FOR SUBCUTANEOUS OR INTRAMUSCULAR INJECTION

DESCRIPTION
Bravelle™ is a product containing a highly purified preparation of human follicle stimulating hormone (hFSH) extracted from the urine of postmenopausal women. Human FSH consists of two non-covalently linked glycoproteins designated as the α and β subunits. The α subunit has 92 amino acids of which two are modified by attachment of carbohydrates. The β subunit has 111 amino acids of which two are modified by attachment of carbohydrates.
Bravelle™ is a sterile, lyophilized powder intended for subcutaneous (SC) or intramuscular (IM) injection after reconstitution with sterile 0.9% Sodium Chloride Injection, USP. Each vial of Bravelle™ contains 82.5 International Units (IU) of Follicle Stimulating Hormone (FSH) activity, 23 mg Lactose Monohydrate, 0.005 mg Polysorbate 20, and Sodium Phosphate buffer (Sodium Phosphate dibasic, Heptahydrate and Phosphoric acid) for pH adjustments, which, when reconstituted with diluent, will deliver 75 IU of FSH. Bravelle™ contains up to 2% luteinizing hormone (LH) activity based on bioassay. Human Chorionic Gonadotropin (hCG) is not detected in Bravelle™. When stored at 3° to 25°C, up to 40% of the α-subunits may be oxidized.
The in vivo biological activity of urofollitropin for injection, purified is determined by using reference standards calibrated against the First International Standard for follicle-stimulating hormone, (FSH, Urofollitropin), Urinary, Human for Bioassay, National Institute for Biological Standards and Control (NIBSC) at its 46th meeting in 1995. FSH is a glycoprotein that is acidic and water-soluble.
Therapeutic class: Infertility.

CLINICAL PHARMACOLOGY
Bravelle™ administered for 7 to 12 days produces ovarian follicular growth in women who do not have primary ovarian failure. Treatment with Bravelle™ in most instances results only in follicular growth and maturation. When sufficient follicular maturation has occurred, hCG must be given to induce ovulation.
PHARMACOKINETICS
Single doses of 225 IU and multiple daily doses (7 days) of 150 IU of Bravelle™ were administered to healthy volunteer female subjects while their endogenous FSH was suppressed. Sixteen subjects received Bravelle™ SC and 12 received the drug IM. Serum FSH concentrations were determined. Based on the steady state ratio of FSH C_{max} and AUC, SC and IM administration of Bravelle™ were not bioequivalent. Multiple doses of Bravelle™ IM resulted in C_{max} and AUC of 77.7% and 81.8% compared to multiple doses of Bravelle™ SC. The FSH pharmacokinetic parameters for single and multiple dose Bravelle™, administered SC and IM are in Table 1.
[See table 1 below]
Absorption
The maximum plasma concentration of FSH was attained at 20.5 and 17.4 hours following SC and IM single dose administration, respectively. However, following multiple dosing, it was attained at approximately 10 hours following both routes of administration.
Distribution
Human tissue or organ distribution of FSH has not been studied for Bravelle™.
Metabolism
Metabolism of FSH has not been studied for Bravelle™ in humans.
Elimination
The mean elimination half-lives of FSH for SC and IM single dosing are 31.8 and 37 hours, respectively. However, following multiple dosing (× 7 days) they are 20.6 and 15.2 hours for SC and IM, respectively.
Pediatric Populations
Bravelle™ is not indicated in pediatric populations.
Geriatric Populations
Bravelle™ is not indicated in geriatric populations.
Special Populations
The safety and efficacy of Bravelle™ in renal and hepatic insufficiency have not been studied.
Drug Interactions
No drug/drug interaction studies have been conducted for Bravelle™ in humans.

CLINICAL STUDIES
The efficacy of Bravelle™ was established in two randomized, active controlled, multi-center studies, one for in-vitro fertilization [IVF] and one for ovulation induction [OI].
Ovulation Induction
In the randomized, controlled ovulation induction study, patients underwent pituitary suppression with a GnRH agonist before being randomized to Bravelle™ SC, Bravelle™ IM or a commercial recombinant FSH product administered SC. A total of 111 oligo-anovulatory patients were randomized of whom 72 received Bravelle™, starting at a dose of 150 IU daily for 5 days. This was followed by individual titration of the dose from 75 to 450 IU daily based on ultrasound and estradiol (E_2) levels. The total duration of dosing did not exceed 12 days. Results for the Intent-To-Treat Population are summarized in Table 2.

Table 2. Efficacy Outcome by Treatment Groups in Ovulation Induction for Study FPI FSH 99-03 (one cycle of treatment)

	Bravelle™ SC	Bravelle™ IM
Parameter	N=35	N=37
Ovulation (%)	24 (68.6)	26 (70.3)
Received hCG (%)	25 (71.4)	28 (75.7)
Mean Peak Serum E_2 (pg/mL) (SD)	976.5 (680.6)	893.2 (815.2)

Continued on next page

Table 1. FSH Pharmacokinetic Parameters Following Bravelle™ Administration

	Single Dose (225 IU)		Multiple Dose × 7 (150 IU)	
PK Parameters	SC	IM	SC	IM
C_{max} (mIU/mL)	6.0 (1.7)	8.8 (4.5)	14.8 (2.9)	11.5 (2.9)
T_{max} (hrs)	20.5 (7.7)	17.4 (12.2)	9.6 (2.1)	11.3 (8.4)
AUC_{obs} (mIU•hr/mL)	379 (111)	331 (179)	234.7 (77.0)	192.1 (52.3)
$t_{1/2}$ (hrs)	31.8	37	20.6	15.2
Ka (hr^{-1})	0.0500 (0.0231)	0.1408 (0.1227)	0.0905 (0.0383)	0.0358 (0.0108)

Bravelle—Cont.

Chemical Pregnancy (%)	11 (31.4)	8 (21.6)
Clinical Pregnancy (%)	9 (25.7)	7 (18.9)
Continuing Pregnancy (%)	9 (25.7)	7 (18.9)
Pts. w/Live Births (%)	9 (25.7)	6 (16.2)

Assisted Reproductive Technologies [ART]

In the randomized, controlled IVF study FPI FSH 2001-01, patients underwent pituitary suppression with a GnRH agonist before being randomized to Bravelle™ SC or a commercial recombinant FSH product administered SC. A total of 120 patients were randomized of whom 60 received Bravelle™, starting at a dose of 225 IU daily for 5 days. This was followed by individual titration of the dose from 75 to 450 IU daily based on ultrasound and estradiol (E_2) levels. The total duration of dosing did not exceed 12 days. Results are summarized Table 3 for the Intent-To-Treat population.

Table 3. Efficacy Outcome for IVF Study FPI FSH 2001-01 (one cycle of treatment)

	Bravelle™ SC
Parameter	n=60
Mean Total Oocytes Retrieved Per Patient (SD)	11.8 (6.3)
Mean Mature Oocytes Retrieved Per Patient (SD)	9.0 (5.7)
Patients with Oocyte Retrieval (%)	57 (95.0)
Patients with Embryo Transfer (%)	57 (95.0)
Patients with Chemical Pregnancy (%)	28 (46.6)
Patients with Clinical Pregnancy (%)	25 (41.7)
Patients with Continuing Pregnancy (%)	23 (38.3)

INDICATIONS AND USAGE

Ovulation Induction

Bravelle™ administered SC or IM in conjunction with hCG, is indicated for ovulation induction in patients who have previously received pituitary suppression.

Multifollicular Development during ART

Bravelle™ administered SC in conjunction with hCG is indicated for multiple follicular development (controlled ovarian stimulation) during ART cycles in patients who have previously received pituitary suppression.

Selection of Patients

1. Before treatment with Bravelle™ is instituted, a thorough gynecologic and endocrinologic evaluation must be performed. Except for those patients enrolled in an *in vitro* fertilization program, this should include a hysterosalpingography (to rule out uterine and tubal pathology) and documentation of anovulation by means of basal body temperature, serial vaginal smears, examination of cervical mucus, determination of serum (or urine) progesterone, urinary pregnanediol and endometrial biopsy. Patients with tubal pathology should receive Bravelle™ only if enrolled in an *in vitro* fertilization program.
2. Primary ovarian failure should be excluded by the determination of gonadotropin levels.
3. Careful examination should be made to rule out the presence of an early pregnancy.
4. Patients in late reproductive life have a greater predilection to endometrial carcinoma as well as a higher incidence of anovulatory disorders. Cervical dilation and curettage should always be done for diagnosis before starting Bravelle™ therapy in such patients who demonstrate abnormal uterine bleeding or other signs of endometrial abnormalities.
5. Evaluation of the husband's fertility potential should be included in the workup.

CONTRAINDICATIONS

Bravelle™ is contraindicated in women who have:

1. A high FSH level indicating primary ovarian failure.
2. Uncontrolled thyroid and adrenal dysfunction.
3. An organic intracranial lesion such as pituitary tumor.
4. The presence of any cause of infertility other than anovulation.
5. Abnormal bleeding of undetermined origin.
6. Ovarian cysts or enlargement not due to polycystic ovary syndrome.
7. Prior hypersensitivity to urofollitropins, purified.
8. Bravelle™ is contraindicated in women who are pregnant and may cause fetal harm when administered to a pregnant woman. There are limited human data on the effects of Bravelle™ when administered during pregnancy.

WARNINGS

Bravelle™ is a drug that should only be used by physicians who are thoroughly familiar with infertility problems. It is a potent gonadotropic substance capable of causing Ovarian Hyperstimulation Syndrome [OHSS] with or without pulmonary or vascular complications in women. Bravelle™ therapy requires a certain time commitment by physicians and supportive health professionals, and its use requires the availability of appropriate monitoring facilities (see PRECAUTIONS – Laboratory Tests). Bravelle™ should be used with a great deal of care.

Overstimulation of the Ovary During Bravelle™ Therapy

Ovarian Enlargement: Mild to moderate uncomplicated ovarian enlargement which may be accompanied by abdominal distension and/or abdominal pain occurs in approximately 20% of those treated with follitropin and hCG, and generally regresses without treatment within two or three weeks.

In order to minimize the hazard associated with the occasional abnormal ovarian enlargement, which may occur with FSH - hCG therapy, the lowest dose consistent with expectation of good results should be used. Careful monitoring of ovarian response can further minimize the risk of overstimulation.

If the ovaries are abnormally enlarged on the last day of Bravelle™ therapy, hCG should not be administered in the course of therapy; this will reduce the chances of development of the Ovarian Hyperstimulation Syndrome.

OHSS: OHSS is a medical event distinct from uncomplicated ovarian enlargement. OHSS may progress rapidly to become a serious medical event. It is characterized by an apparent dramatic increase in vascular permeability, which can result in a rapid accumulation of fluid in the peritoneal cavity, thorax, and potentially, the pericardium. The early warning signs of development of OHSS are severe pelvic pain, nausea, vomiting, and weight gain. The following symptomatology has been seen with cases of OHSS: abdominal pain, abdominal distension, gastrointestinal symptoms including nausea, vomiting and diarrhea, severe ovarian enlargement, weight gain, dyspnea, and oliguria. Clinical evaluation may reveal hypovolemia, hemoconcentration, electrolyte imbalances, ascites, hemoperitoneum, pleural effusions, hydrothorax, acute pulmonary distress, and thromboembolic events (see "Pulmonary and Vascular Complications" below). Transient liver function test abnormalities suggestive of hepatic dysfunction, which may be accompanied by morphologic changes on liver biopsy, have been reported in association with the Ovarian Hyperstimulation Syndrome (OHSS).

In a clinical study of ovulation induction, 6 of 72 (8.33%) Bravelle™ treated women developed OHSS and two were classified as severe. In a clinical study for multiple follicular development during IVF, 3 of 60 Bravelle™ treated women developed OHSS and 1 was classified as severe. Cases of OHSS are more common, more severe and more protracted if pregnancy occurs. OHSS develops rapidly; therefore patients should be followed for at least two weeks after hCG administration. Most often, OHSS occurs after treatment has been discontinued and reaches its maximum at about 7 to 10 days after treatment. Usually, in cases where OHSS may be developing prior to hCG administration (see PRECAUTIONS – Laboratory Tests), the hCG should be withheld.

If severe OHSS occurs, treatment *must* be stopped and the patient should be hospitalized.

A physician experienced in the management of the syndrome, or who is experienced in the management of fluid and electrolyte imbalances should be consulted.

Pulmonary and Vascular Complications

Serious pulmonary conditions (e.g. atelectasis, acute respiratory distress syndrome) have been reported. In addition, thromboembolic events both in association with, and separate from, the Ovarian Hyperstimulation Syndrome have been reported following FSH therapy. Intravascular thrombosis and embolism, which may originate in venous or arterial vessels, can result in reduced blood flow to critical organs or the extremities. Sequelae of such events have included venous thrombophlebitis, pulmonary embolism, pulmonary infarction, cerebral vascular occlusion (stroke), and arterial occlusion resulting in loss of limb. In rare cases, pulmonary complications and/or thromboembolic events have resulted in death.

Multiple Pregnancies

Multiple pregnancies have occurred following treatment with Bravelle™ SC and IM.

Pregnancy outcomes in a controlled study of 72 patients undergoing ovulation induction with Bravelle™ are shown in Table 4.

Table 4. FPI FSH 99-03 Outcome of Pregnancies

	Bravelle™ SC	Bravelle™ IM
Parameter	N(%)	N(%)
Total Continuing Pregnancies	9 (100)	7 (100)
Singlets	3 (33.3)	5 (71.4)
Total No. with Multiple Pregnancies	6 (66.7)	2 (28.6)
Twins	4	0
Triplets	2	0
Quadruplets	0	1
Quintuplets	0	0
Sextuplets	0	1

The pregnancy outcomes in a controlled study of 60 patients undergoing treatment with Bravelle™ in IVF are shown in Table 5.

Table 5. FPI FSH 2001-01 Outcome of Pregnancies

	Bravelle™ SC
Parameter (%)	N(%)
Total No. of Continuing Pregnancies	23 (100)
Singlets	15 (65.2)
Total No. of Multiple Pregnancies	8 (34.8)
Twins	5
Triplets	3

The patient and her partner should be advised of the potential risk of multiple births before starting treatment.

Hypersensitivity/Anaphylactic Reactions

Hypersensitivity/anaphylactic reactions associated with follitropins for injection, purified administration have been reported in some patients. These reactions presented as generalized urticaria, facial edema, angioneurotic edema, and/or dyspnea suggestive of laryngeal edema. The relationship of these symptoms to uncharacterized urinary proteins is uncertain.

PRECAUTIONS

General

Careful attention should be given to the diagnosis of infertility in the selection of candidates for Bravelle™ therapy (see "**INDICATIONS AND USAGE**-Selection of patients").

Information for Patients

Prior to therapy with Bravelle™, patients should be informed of the duration of treatment and the monitoring of their condition that will be required. Possible adverse reactions (see ADVERSE REACTIONS section) and the risk of multiple births should also be discussed.

Laboratory Tests

The combination of both estradiol levels and ultrasonography are useful for monitoring the growth and development of follicles, timing hCG administration, as well as minimizing the risk of the Ovarian Hyperstimulation Syndrome and multiple gestations.

The clinical confirmation of ovulation, is determined by:

a. A rise in basal body temperature,
b. Increase in serum progesterone, and
c. Menstruation following the shift in basal body temperature.

When used in conjunction with indices of progesterone production, sonographic visualization of the ovaries will assist in determining if ovulation has occurred. Sonographic evidence of ovulation may include the following:

a. Fluid in the cul-de-sac,
b. Ovarian stigmata, and
c. Collapsed follicle.

Because of the subjectivity of the various tests for the determination of follicular maturation and ovulation, it cannot be overemphasized that the physician should choose tests with which he/she is thoroughly familiar.

Carcinogenesis and Mutagenesis

Long-term toxicity studies in animals and in vitro mutagenicity tests have not been performed to evaluate the carcinogenic potential of urofollitropin for injection, purified.

Pregnancy

Pregnancy Category X: See **CONTRAINDICATIONS** section.

Nursing Mothers

It is not known whether this drug is excreted in human milk. Because many drugs are excreted in human milk and because of the potential for serious adverse reactions in the nursing infant from Bravelle™, a decision should be made whether to discontinue nursing or to discontinue the drug, taking into account the importance of the drug to the mother.

Pediatric Patients

Safety and effectiveness in pediatric patients have not been established.

Geriatric Patients

Safety and effectiveness in geriatric patients have not been established.

ADVERSE REACTIONS

The safety of Bravelle™ was examined in four clinical studies that enrolled a total of 222 patients receiving Bravelle™ including 72 for ovulation induction and 150 for IVF.

All adverse events (without regard to causality assessment) occurring ≥ 2% incidence in the clinical study patients receiving Bravelle™ are listed in Table 6, (FPI FSH 99-03 study for ovulation induction) and Table 7 (FPI FSH 99-04, FPI FSH 99-05 and FPI FSH 2001-01 studies for IVF).

Table 6. FPI FSH 99-03 Ovulation Induction Safety Profile

All Patients with Adverse Events ≥2 %

Adverse Events (%)	Bravelle™ SC	Bravelle™ IM
	N=35	N=37
Genitourinary/Reproductive		
OHSS	4 (11.4)	2 (5.4)
Vaginal Hemorrhage	3 (8.6)	0 (0.0)
Ovarian Disorder (Pain, Cyst)	1 (2.9)	3 (8.1)
Urinary tract infection	0	1 (2.7)
Cervix disorder	1 (2.9)	0
Gastrointestinal		
Nausea	2 (5.7)	0 (0.0)
Enlarged Abdomen	1 (2.9)	1 (2.7)
Abdominal Pain	1 (2.9)	2 (5.4)
Vomiting	0	1 (2.7)
Constipation	0	1 (2.7)
Diarrhea	0	1 (2.7)
Metabolic/Nutritional		
Dehydration	0	1 (2.7)
Weight gain	1 (2.9)	0
Skin/Appendages		
Acne	1 (2.9)	0
Exfoliative dermatitis	0	1 (2.7)
Other Body Systems		
Headache	4 (11.4)	3 (8.1)
Pain	2 (5.7)	0 (0.0)
Neck pain	0	1 (2.7)
Respiratory Disorder	2 (5.7)	0 (0.0)
Hot Flashes	2 (5.7)	0 (0.0)
Fever	0	1 (2.7)
Hypertension	0	1 (2.7)
Emotional lability	0	1 (2.7)
Depression	0	1 (2.7)
Accidental injury	0	1 (2.7)

Table 7. Integrated IVF Safety Profile

All Patients with Adverse Events ≥ 2%

Adverse Events (%)	Bravelle ™ SC
	N=150
Genitourinary/Reproductive	
Vaginal hemorrhage	7 (4.7)
Post retrieval pain	12 (8.0)
Pelvic pain/cramps	10 (6.7)
OHSS	9 (6.0)
Uterine spasms	4 (2.7)
Vaginal spotting	4 (2.7)
Urinary tract infection	5 (3.3)
Ovarian disorder	3 (2.0)
Breast tenderness	3 (2.0)
Vaginal Discharge	4 (2.7)
Infection fungal	3 (2.0)
Gastrointestinal	
Abdominal cramps	21 (14.0)
Nausea	13 (8.7)
Abdominal pain	7 (4.7)
Abdominal fullness/enlargement	10 (6.7)
Constipation	3 (2.0)
Other Body Systems	
Headache	19 (12.7)
Pain	8 (5.3)
Rash	4 (2.7)
Respiratory disorder	6 (4.0)
Sinusitis	3 (2.0)
Injection site reaction	6 (4.0)
Hot flash	6 (4.0)
Emotional lability	3 (2.0)

The following medical events have been reported subsequent to pregnancies resulting from gonadotropin therapy in published clinical studies:

1. Spontaneous Abortion
2. Ectopic Pregnancy
3. Premature Labor
4. Postpartum fever
5. Congenital abnormalities

The following adverse reactions have been previously reported during urofollitropin for injection, purified therapy:

1. Pulmonary and vascular complications (see **WARNINGS**),
2. Adnexal torsion (as a complication of ovarian enlargement),
3. Mild to moderate ovarian enlargement,
4. Hemoperitoneum,
5. There have been infrequent reports of ovarian neoplasms, both benign and malignant, in women who have undergone multiple drug regimens for ovulation induction; however, a causal relationship has not been established.

DRUG ABUSE AND DEPENDENCE

There have been no reports of abuse or dependence with follitropins.

OVERDOSAGE

Aside from possible ovarian hyperstimulation (see **WARNINGS**) and multiple gestations (see **WARNINGS**), little is known concerning the consequences of acute overdosage with Bravelle™.

DOSAGE AND ADMINISTRATION

Dosage:

Infertile patients with oligo-anovulation: The dose of Bravelle™ to stimulate development of ovarian follicles must be individualized for each patient. The lowest dose consistent with achieving good results based on clinical experience and reported clinical data should be used.

The recommended initial dose of Bravelle™ for patients who have received GnRH agonist or antagonist pituitary suppression is 150 IU daily administered SC or IM for the first 5 days of treatment. Based on clinical monitoring (including serum estradiol levels and vaginal ultrasound results) subsequent dosing should be adjusted according to individual patient response. Adjustments in dose should not be made more frequently than once every 2 days and should not exceed more than 75 to 150 IU per adjustment. The maximum daily dose of Bravelle™ should not exceed 450 IU and in most cases dosing beyond 12 days is not recommended.

If patient response to Bravelle™ is appropriate, hCG (5000 to 10,000 USP units) should be given 1 day following the last dose of Bravelle™. The hCG should be withheld if the serum estradiol is greater than 2000 pg/mL, if the ovaries are abnormally enlarged or if abdominal pain occurs, and the patient should be advised to refrain from intercourse. These precautions may reduce the risk of Ovarian Hyperstimulation Syndrome and multiple gestations. Patients should be followed closely for at least 2 weeks after hCG administration. If there is inadequate follicle development or ovulation without subsequent pregnancy, the course of treatment with Bravelle™ may be repeated. The couple should be encouraged to have intercourse daily, beginning on the day prior to the administration of hCG until ovulation becomes apparent from the indices employed for the determination of progestational activity. In the light of the foregoing indices and parameters mentioned, it should become obvious that, unless a physician is willing to devote considerable time to these patients and be familiar with and conduct the necessary laboratory studies, he/she should not use Bravelle™.

Assisted Reproductive Technologies: The recommended initial dose of Bravelle™ for patients undergoing IVF and donor egg patients who have received GnRH agonist or antagonist pituitary suppression is 225 IU daily administered SC for the first 5 days of treatment. Based on clinical monitoring (including serum estradiol levels and vaginal ultrasound results) subsequent dosing should be adjusted according to individual patient response. Adjustments in dose should not be made more frequently than once every 2 days and should not exceed more than 75 to 150 IU per adjustment. The maximum daily dose of Bravelle™ given should not exceed 450 IU and in most cases dosing beyond 12 days is not recommended.

Once adequate follicular development is evident, hCG (5000-10,000 USP units) should be administered to induce final follicular maturation in preparation for oocyte retrieval. The administration of hCG must be withheld in cases where the ovaries are abnormally enlarged on the last day of therapy. This should reduce the chance of developing OHSS.

Directions for Using Bravelle™

1) Wash hands thoroughly with soap and water.
2) Before injections, the septum tops of the vials should be wiped with an aseptic solution to prevent contamination of the contents.
3) To prepare the Bravelle™ solution, inject 1 mL of Sterile Saline for Injection, USP into the vial of Bravelle™. **DO NOT SHAKE,** but gently swirl until the solution is clear. Generally, the Bravelle™ dissolves immediately. Check the liquid in the container. If it is not clear or has particles in it, **DO NOT USE IT.**
4) For patients requiring a single injection from multiple vials of Bravelle™, up to 6 vials can be reconstituted with 1 mL of Sterile Saline for Injection, USP. This can be accomplished by reconstituting a single vial as described above (see step 3). Then draw the entire contents of the first vial into a syringe, and inject the contents into a second vial of lyophilized Bravelle™. Gently swirl the second vial, as described above, once again checking to make sure the solution is clear and free of particles. This step can be repeated with 4 additional vials for a total of up to 6 vials of lyophilized Bravelle™ into 1 mL of diluent.
5) Immediately **ADMINISTER** the reconstituted Bravelle™ either **SC** (for ovulation induction or multifollicular development during ART) or **IM** (for ovulation induction). Any unused reconstituted material should be discarded.
6) Draw the reconstituted Bravelle™ into an empty, sterile syringe.
7) Hold the syringe pointing upwards and gently tap the side to force any air bubbles to the top; then squeeze the plunger gently until all the air has been expelled and only Bravelle™ solution is left in the syringe.
8) Bravelle™ works if it is injected **SC** (for ovulation induction or multifollicular development during ART) or **IM** (for ovulation induction). The recommended sites for SC injection are either side of the lower abdomen in alternating fashion with the actual injection site varied a little with each injection. SC injection of Bravelle™ into the thigh is not recommended unless the lower abdomen is not usable because of scarring, surgical deformity or other medical conditions.
   The best site for IM injection of Bravelle™ is the upper outer quadrant of the buttock muscle near the hip. This area contains few blood vessels and major nerves. Stretching the skin helps the needle to go in more easily and pushes the tissue beneath the skin out of the way. This helps the solution disperse correctly.
9) The injection site should be swabbed with a disinfectant to remove any surface bacteria. Clean about two inches around the point where the needle will go in and let the disinfectant dry for at least one minute before proceeding.
10) For **SC** injection, the needle should be inserted at a 90° angle to the skin surface.
    For **IM** injection, the needle should be inserted at a 90° angle to the skin surface. Pushing in with a quick thrust causes the least discomfort.
11) If the needle is correctly positioned, it will be difficult to draw back on the plunger. Any blood drawn into the syringe means the needle tip has penetrated a vein or artery. If this happens, remove the syringe, cover the injection site with a swab containing disinfectant and apply pressure; the site should stop bleeding in a minute or two.
12) Once the needle is properly placed, depress the plunger **slowly** and steadily, so the solution is correctly injected and the skin or muscle tissue is not damaged.
13) Pull the syringe out quickly and apply pressure to the site with a swab containing disinfectant. A gentle massage of the site - while still maintaining pressure - helps disperse the Bravelle™ solution and relieve any discomfort.
14) Use the disposable syringe only once and dispose of it properly.

HOW SUPPLIED

Bravelle™ (urofollitropin for injection, purified) is supplied in a sterile, lyophilized, single dose vial containing 82.5 IU of FSH, to deliver 75 IU FSH after reconstituting with the diluent.

Each vial is available with an accompanying vial of sterile diluent containing 2 mL of 0.9% Sodium Chloride Injection, USP.

75 IU FSH activity, supplied as:

NDC 55566-8505-2: Box of 5 vials + 5 vials diluent.

NDC 55566-8505-3 Box of 100 vials + 100 vials diluent.

Lyophilized powder may be stored refrigerated or at room temperature (3° to 25°C/37° to 77°F). Protect from light. Use immediately after reconstitution. Discard unused material.

Continued on next page

Bravelle—Cont.

℞ only
Vials of sterile diluent of 0.9% Sodium Chloride Injection, USP, manufactured for Ferring Pharmaceuticals Inc.
Manufactured for:
FERRING PHARMACEUTICALS INC.
SUFFERN, NY 10901
By: CARDINAL HEALTH
Albuquerque, New Mexico 87107
6048-03
6-D6048FR-03
12/16/02

DESMOPRESSIN ACETATE ℞
Injection 4 μg/mL

DESCRIPTION

DESMOPRESSIN ACETATE Injection 4 μg/mL is a synthetic analogue of the natural pituitary hormone 8-arginine vasopressin (ADH), an antidiuretic hormone affecting renal water conservation. It is chemically defined as follows:

Mol.Wt. 1183.3
Empirical Formula: $C_{46}H_{64}N_{14}O_{12}S_2 \cdot C_2H_4O_2 \cdot 3H_2O$

$SCH_2CH_2C(=O)$-Tyr-Phe-Gln-Asn-Cys-Pro-D-Arg-Gly-$NH_2 \cdot CH_3COOH \cdot 3H_2O$
(positions 1 2 3 4 5 6 7 8 9)

1-(3-mercaptopropionic acid)-8-D-arginine vasopressin monoacetate (salt) trihydrate.

DESMOPRESSIN ACETATE Injection 4 μg/mL is provided as a sterile, aqueous solution for injection.

Each mL provides:	Desmopressin acetate	4.0 μg
	Sodium chloride	9.0 mg
	Hydrochloric acid to adjust pH to 4	

The 10 mL vial contains chlorobutanol as a preservative (5.0 mg/mL).

CLINICAL PHARMACOLOGY

DESMOPRESSIN ACETATE Injection 4 μg/mL contains as active substance, desmopressin acetate, a synthetic analogue of the natural hormone arginine vasopressin. One mL (4 μg) of DESMOPRESSIN ACETATE solution has an antidiuretic activity of about 16 IU; 1 μg of DESMOPRESSIN ACETATE is equivalent to 4 IU.

DESMOPRESSIN ACETATE has been shown to be more potent than arginine vasopressin in increasing plasma levels of factor VIII activity in patients with hemophilia and von Willebrand's disease Type I.

Dose-response studies were performed in healthy persons, using doses of 0.1 to 0.4 μg/kg body weight, infused over a 10-minute period. Maximal dose response occurred at 0.3 to 0.4 μg/kg. The response to DESMOPRESSIN ACETATE of factor VIII activity and plasminogen activator is dose-related, with maximal plasma levels of 300 to 400 percent of initial concentrations obtained after infusion of 0.4 μg/kg body weight. The increase is rapid and evident within 30 minutes, reaching a maximum at a point ranging from 90 minutes to two hours. The factor VIII related antigen and ristocetin cofactor activity were also increased to a smaller degree, but still are dose-dependent.

1. The biphasic half-lives of DESMOPRESSIN ACETATE were 7.8 and 75.5 minutes for the fast and slow phases, respectively, compared with 2.5 and 14.5 minutes for lysine vasopressin, another form of the hormone. As a result, DESMOPRESSIN ACETATE provides a prompt onset of antidiuretic action with a long duration after each administration.
2. The change in structure of arginine vasopressin to DESMOPRESSIN ACETATE has resulted in a decreased vasopressor action and decreased actions on visceral smooth muscle relative to the enhanced antidiuretic activity, so that clinically effective antidiuretic doses are usually below threshold levels for effects on vascular or visceral smooth muscle.
3. When administered by injection, DESMOPRESSIN ACETATE has an antidiuretic effect about ten times that of an equivalent dose administered intranasally.
4. The bioavailability of the subcutaneous route of administration was determined qualitatively using urine output data. The exact fraction of drug absorbed by that route of administration has not been quantitatively determined.
5. The percentage increase of factor VIII levels in patients with mild hemophilia A and von Willebrand's disease was not significantly different from that observed in normal healthy individuals when treated with 0.3 μg/kg of DESMOPRESSIN ACETATE infused over 10 minutes.
6. Plasminogen activator activity increases rapidly after DESMOPRESSIN ACETATE infusion, but there has been no clinically significant fibrinolysis in patients treated with DESMOPRESSIN ACETATE.
7. The effect of repeated DESMOPRESSIN ACETATE administration when doses were given every 12 to 24 hours has generally shown a gradual diminution of the factor VIII activity increase noted with a single dose. The initial response is reproducible in any particular patient if there are 2 or 3 days between administrations.

INDICATIONS AND USAGE

Hemophilia A: DESMOPRESSIN ACETATE Injection 4 μg/mL is indicated for patients with hemophilia A with factor VIII coagulant activity levels greater than 5%.

DESMOPRESSIN ACETATE will often maintain hemostasis in patients with hemophilia A during surgical procedures and postoperatively when administered 30 minutes prior to scheduled procedure.

DESMOPRESSIN ACETATE will also stop bleeding in hemophilia A patients with episodes of spontaneous or trauma-induced injuries such as hemarthroses, intramuscular hematomas or mucosal bleeding.

DESMOPRESSIN ACETATE is not indicated for the treatment of hemophilia A with factor VIII coagulant activity levels equal to or less than 5%, or for the treatment of hemophilia B, or in patients who have factor VIII antibodies.

In certain clinical situations, it may be justified to try DESMOPRESSIN ACETATE in patients with factor VIII levels between 2% to 5%; however, these patients should be carefully monitored.

von Willebrand's Disease (Type I): DESMOPRESSIN ACETATE Injection 4 μg/mL is indicated for patients with mild to moderate classic von Willebrand's disease (Type I) with factor VIII levels greater than 5%. DESMOPRESSIN ACETATE will often maintain hemostasis in patients with mild to moderate von Willebrand's disease during surgical procedures and postoperatively when administered 30 minutes prior to the scheduled procedure.

DESMOPRESSIN ACETATE will usually stop bleeding in mild to moderate von Willebrand's patients with episodes of spontaneous or trauma-induced injuries such as hemarthroses, intramuscular hematomas or mucosal bleeding.

Those von Willebrand's disease patients who are least likely to respond are those with severe homozygous von Willebrand's disease with factor VIII coagulant activity and factor VIII von Willebrand factor antigen levels less than 1%. Other patients may respond in a variable fashion depending on the type of molecular defect they have. Bleeding time and factor VIII coagulant activity, ristocetin cofactor activity, and von Willebrand factor antigen should be checked during administration of DESMOPRESSIN ACETATE to ensure that adequate levels are being achieved.

DESMOPRESSIN ACETATE is not indicated for the treatment of severe classic von Willebrand's disease (Type I) and when there is evidence of an abnormal molecular form of factor VIII antigen. (See **WARNINGS**.)

Diabetes Insipidus: DESMOPRESSIN ACETATE Injection 4 μg/mL is indicated as antidiuretic replacement therapy in the management of central (cranial) diabetes insipidus and for the management of the temporary polyuria and polydipsia following head trauma or surgery in the pituitary region. DESMOPRESSIN ACETATE is ineffective for the treatment of nephrogenic diabetes insipidus.

DESMOPRESSIN ACETATE is also available as an intranasal preparation. However, this means of delivery can be compromised by a variety of factors that can make nasal insufflation ineffective or inappropriate. These include poor intranasal absorption, nasal congestion and blockage, nasal discharge, atrophy of nasal mucosa, and severe atrophic rhinitis. Intranasal delivery may be inappropriate where there is an impaired level of consciousness. In addition, cranial surgical procedures, such as transsphenoidal hypophysectomy, create situations where an alternative route of administration is needed as in cases of nasal packing or recovery from surgery.

CONTRAINDICATIONS

DESMOPRESSIN ACETATE Injection 4 μg/mL is contraindicated in individuals with known hypersensitivity to desmopressin acetate or to any of the components of **DESMOPRESSIN ACETATE Injection 4 μg/mL.**

WARNINGS

Patients who do not have need of antidiuretic hormone for its antidiuretic effect, in particular those who are young or elderly, should be cautioned to ingest only enough fluid to satisfy thirst, in order to decrease the potential occurrence of water intoxication and hyponatremia.

Fluid intake should be adjusted downward, particularly in very young and elderly patients, in order to decrease the potential occurrence of water intoxication and hyponatremia. Particular attention should be paid to the possibility of the rare occurrence of an extreme decrease in plasma osmolality that may result in seizures which could lead to coma.

DESMOPRESSIN ACETATE should not be used to treat patients with Type IIB von Willebrand's disease since platelet aggregation may be induced.

PRECAUTIONS

General: For injection use only.

DESMOPRESSIN ACETATE Injection 4 μg/mL has infrequently produced changes in blood pressure causing either a slight elevation in blood pressure or a transient fall in blood pressure and a compensatory increase in heart rate. The drug should be used with caution in patients with coronary artery insufficiency and/or hypertensive cardiovascular disease.

DESMOPRESSIN ACETATE should be used with caution in patients with conditions associated with fluid and electrolyte imbalance, such as cystic fibrosis, because these patients are prone to hyponatremia.

There have been rare reports of thrombotic events following **DESMOPRESSIN ACETATE Injection 4 μg/mL** in patients predisposed to thrombus formation. No causality has been determined, however, the drug should be used with caution in these patients.

Severe allergic reactions have been reported rarely. Fatal anaphylaxis has been reported in one patient who received intravenous DESMOPRESSIN ACETATE. It is not known whether antibodies to **DESMOPRESSIN ACETATE Injection 4 μg/mL** are produced after repeated injections.

Hemophilia A: Laboratory tests for assessing patient status include levels of factor VIII coagulant, factor VIII antigen and factor VIII ristocetin cofactor (von Willebrand factor) as well as activated partial thromboplastin time. Factor VIII coagulant activity should be determined before giving DESMOPRESSIN ACETATE for hemostasis. If factor VIII coagulant activity is present at less than 5% of normal, DESMOPRESSIN ACETATE should not be relied on.

von Willebrand's Disease: Laboratory tests for assessing patient status include levels of factor VIII coagulant activity, factor VIII ristocetin cofactor activity, and factor VIII von Willebrand factor antigen. The skin bleeding time may be helpful in following these patients.

Diabetes Insipidus: Laboratory tests for monitoring the patient include urine volume and osmolality. In some cases, plasma osmolality may be required.

Drug Interactions: Although the pressor activity of DESMOPRESSIN ACETATE is very low compared with the antidiuretic activity, use of doses as large as 0.3 μg/kg of DESMOPRESSIN ACETATE with other pressor agents should be done only with careful patient monitoring.

DESMOPRESSIN ACETATE has been used with epsilon aminocaproic acid without adverse effects.

Carcinogenicity, Mutagenicity, Impairment of Fertility: Studies with DESMOPRESSIN ACETATE have not been performed to evaluate carcinogenic potential, mutagenic potential or effects on fertility.

Pregnancy Category B: Fertility studies have not been done. Teratology studies in rats and rabbits at doses from 0.05 to 10 μg/kg/day (approximately 0.1 times the maximum systemic human exposure in rats and up to 38 times the maximum systemic human exposure in rabbits based on surface area, mg/m^2) revealed no harm to the fetus due to DESMOPRESSIN ACETATE. There are, however, no adequate and well controlled studies in pregnant women. Because animal reproduction studies are not always predictive of human response, this drug should be used during pregnancy only if clearly needed.

Several publications of desmopressin acetate's use in the management of diabetes insipidus during pregnancy are available; these include a few anecdotal reports of congenital anomalies and low birth weight babies. However, no causal connection between these events and desmopressin acetate has been established. A fifteen year, Swedish epidemiologic study of the use of desmopressin acetate in pregnant women with diabetes insipidus found the rate of birth defects to be no greater than that in the general population; however the statistical power of this study is low. As opposed to preparations containing natural hormones, desmopressin acetate in antidiuretic doses has no uterotonic action and the physician will have to weigh the therapeutic advantages against the possible risks in each case.

Nursing Mothers: There have been no controlled studies in nursing mothers. A single study in postpartum women demonstrated a marked change in plasma, but little if any change in assayable DESMOPRESSIN ACETATE in breast milk following an intranasal dose of 10 μg. It is not known whether this drug is excreted in human milk. Because many drugs are excreted in human milk, caution should be exercised when DESMOPRESSIN ACETATE is administered to a nursing woman.

Pediatric Use: Use in infants and pediatric patients will require careful fluid intake restriction to prevent possible hyponatremia and water intoxication. **DESMOPRESSIN ACETATE Injection 4 μg/mL** *should not be used in infants less than three months of age* in the treatment of hemophilia A or von Willebrand's disease; safety and effectiveness in pediatric patients under 12 years of age with diabetes insipidus have not been established.

ADVERSE REACTIONS

Infrequently, DESMOPRESSIN ACETATE has produced transient headache, nausea, mild abdominal cramps and vulval pain. These symptoms disappeared with reduction in dosage. Occasionally, injection of DESMOPRESSIN ACETATE has produced local erythema, swelling or burning pain. Occasional facial flushing has been reported with the administration of DESMOPRESSIN ACETATE. **DESMOPRESSIN ACETATE Injection** has infrequently produced changes in blood pressure causing either a slight elevation or a transient fall and a compensatory increase in heart rate. Severe allergic reactions including anaphylaxis have been reported rarely with **DESMOPRESSIN ACETATE Injection.**

See **WARNINGS** for the possibility of water intoxication and hyponatremia.

There have been rare reports of thrombotic events (acute cerebrovascular thrombosis, acute myocardial infarction) following **DESMOPRESSIN ACETATE Injection** in patients predisposed to thrombus formation.

OVERDOSAGE

(See **ADVERSE REACTIONS.**) In case of overdosage, the dosage should be reduced, frequency of administration decreased, or the drug withdrawn according to the severity of the condition.

There is no known specific antidote for desmopressin acetate or **DESMOPRESSIN ACETATE Injection 4 μg/mL.**

An oral LD_{50} has not been established. An intravenous dose of 2 mg/kg in mice demonstrated no effect.

DOSAGE AND ADMINISTRATION

Hemophilia A and von Willebrand's Disease (Type I): DESMOPRESSIN ACETATE Injection 4 µg/mL is administered as an intravenous infusion at a dose of 0.3 µg DESMOPRESSIN ACETATE/kg body weight diluted in sterile physiological saline and infused slowly over 15 to 30 minutes. In adults and children weighing more than 10 kg, 50 mL of diluent is recommended; in children weighing 10 kg or less, 10 mL of diluent is recommended. Blood pressure and pulse should be monitored during infusion. If **DESMOPRESSIN ACETATE Injection 4 µg/mL** is used preoperatively, it should be administered 30 minutes prior to the scheduled procedure.

The necessity for repeat administration of DESMOPRESSIN ACETATE or use of any blood products for hemostasis should be determined by laboratory response as well as the clinical condition of the patient. The tendency toward tachyphylaxis (lessening of response) with repeated administration given more frequently than every 48 hours should be considered in treating each patient.

Diabetes Insipidus: This formulation is administered subcutaneously or by direct intravenous injection. **DESMOPRESSIN ACETATE Injection 4 µg/mL** dosage must be determined for each patient and adjusted according to the pattern of response. Response should be estimated by two parameters: adequate duration of sleep and adequate, not excessive, water turnover.

The usual dosage range in adults is 0.5 mL (2.0 µg) to 1 mL (4.0 µg) daily, administered intravenously or subcutaneously, usually in two divided doses. The morning and evening doses should be separately adjusted for an adequate diurnal rhythm of water turnover. For patients who have been controlled on intranasal DESMOPRESSIN ACETATE and who must be switched to the injection form, either because of poor intranasal absorption or because of the need for surgery, the comparable antidiuretic dose of the injection is about one-tenth the intranasal dose.

Parenteral drug products should be inspected visually for particulate matter and discoloration prior to administration whenever solution and container permit.

HOW SUPPLIED

DESMOPRESSIN ACETATE Injection 4 µg/mL is available as a sterile solution in cartons of ten 1 mL single-dose ampules (NDC 55566-5030-1) and in 10 mL multiple-dose vials (NDC 55566-5040-1), each containing 4.0 µg DESMOPRESSIN ACETATE per mL.

Store refrigerated 2 to 8°C (36 to 46°F).

Rx only

Keep out of the reach of children.

Manufactured for
FERRING PHARMACEUTICALS INC.
SUFFERN, NY 10901
By Ferring Pharmaceuticals, Limhamn, Sweden
Rev. 4/03 6018-02

ADVERSE REACTION	PLACEBO (N=59) %	DESMOPRESSIN ACETATE 20 µg (N=60) %	DESMOPRESSIN ACETATE 40 µg (N=61) %
BODY AS A WHOLE			
Abdominal Pain	0	2	2
Asthenia	0	0	2
Chills	0	0	2
Headache	0	2	5
Throat Pain	2	0	0
NERVOUS SYSTEM			
Depression	2	0	0
Dizziness	0	0	3
RESPIRATORY SYSTEM			
Epistaxis	2	3	0
Nostril Pain	0	2	0
Respiratory Infection	2	0	2
Rhinitis	2	8	3
CARDIOVASCULAR SYSTEM			
Vasodilation	2	0	0
DIGESTIVE SYSTEM			
Gastrointestinal Disorder	0	2	0
Nausea	0	0	2
SKIN & APPENDAGES			
Leg Rash	2	0	0
Rash	2	0	0
SPECIAL SENSES			
Conjunctivitis	0	2	0
Edema Eyes	0	2	0
Lachrymation Disorder	0	0	2

DESMOPRESSIN ACETATE Rhinal Tube ℞

DESCRIPTION

Desmopressin Acetate Rhinal Tube is a synthetic analogue of the natural pituitary hormone 8-arginine vasopressin (ADH), an antidiuretic hormone affecting renal water conservation. It is chemically defined as follows:

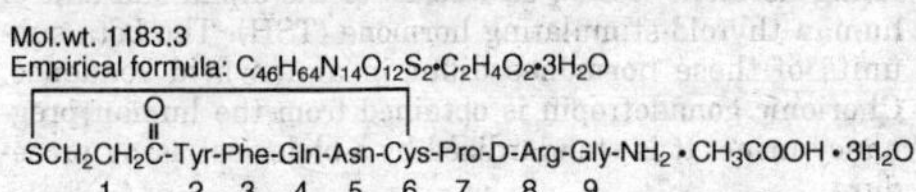

1-(3-mercaptopropionic acid)-8-D-arginine vasopressin monoacetate (salt) trihydrate.

Desmopressin Acetate Rhinal Tube is provided as an aqueous solution for intranasal use.

Each mL contains:

Desmopressin acetate	0.1 mg
Chlorobutanol	5.0 mg
Sodium Chloride	9.0 mg
Hydrochloric acid to adjust pH to approximately 4	

CLINICAL PHARMACOLOGY

Desmopressin Acetate Rhinal Tube contains as active substance desmopressin acetate, a synthetic analogue of the natural hormone arginine vasopressin. One mL (0.1 mg) of intranasal Desmopressin acetate has an antidiuretic activity of about 400 IU; 10 µg of desmopressin acetate is equivalent to 40 IU.

1. The biphasic half-lives for intranasal Desmopressin acetate were 7.8 and 75.5 minutes for the fast and slow phases, compared with 2.5 and 14.5 minutes for lysine vasopressin, another form of the hormone used in this condition. As a result, intranasal Desmopressin acetate provides a prompt onset of antidiuretic action with a long duration after each administration.
2. The change in structure of arginine vasopressin to Desmopressin acetate has resulted in a decreased vasopressor action and decreased actions on visceral smooth muscle relative to the enhanced antidiuretic activity, so that clinically effective antidiuretic doses are usually below threshold levels for effects on vascular or visceral smooth muscle.
3. Desmopressin acetate administered intranasally has an antidiuretic effect about one-tenth that of an equivalent dose administered by injection.

INDICATIONS AND USAGE

Primary Nocturnal Enuresis: Desmopressin Acetate Rhinal Tube is indicated for the management of primary nocturnal enuresis. It may be used alone or adjunctive to behavioral conditioning or other non-pharmacological intervention. It has been shown to be effective in some cases that are refractory to conventional therapies.

Central Cranial Diabetes Insipidus: Desmopressin Acetate Rhinal Tube is indicated as antidiuretic replacement therapy in the management of central cranial diabetes insipidus and for management of the temporary polyuria and polydipsia following head trauma or surgery in the pituitary region. It is ineffective for the treatment of nephrogenic diabetes insipidus.

The use of **Desmopressin Acetate Rhinal Tube** in patients with an established diagnosis will result in a reduction in urinary output with increase in urine osmolality and a decrease in plasma osmolality. This will allow the resumption of a more normal life-style with a decrease in urinary frequency and nocturia.

There are reports of an occasional change in response with time, usually greater than 6 months. Some patients may show a decreased responsiveness, others a shortened duration of effect. There is no evidence this effect is due to the development of binding antibodies but may be due to a local inactivation of the peptide.

Patients are selected for therapy by establishing the diagnosis by means of the water deprivation test, the hypertonic saline infusion test, and/or the response to antidiuretic hormone. Continued response to intranasal Desmopressin acetate can be monitored by urine volume and osmolality.

Desmopressin acetate is also available as a solution for injection when the intranasal route may be compromised. These situations include nasal congestion and blockage, nasal discharge, atrophy of nasal mucosa, and severe atrophic rhinitis. Intranasal delivery may also be inappropriate where there is an impaired level of consciousness. In addition, cranial surgical procedures, such as transsphenoidal hypophysectomy create situations where an alternative route of administration is needed as in cases of nasal packing or recovery from surgery.

CONTRAINDICATIONS

Desmopressin Acetate Rhinal Tube is contraindicated in individuals with known hypersensitivity to desmopressin acetate or to any of the components of **Desmopressin Acetate Rhinal Tube.**

WARNINGS

1. For intranasal use only.
2. In very young and elderly patients in particular, fluid intake should be adjusted downward in order to decrease the potential occurrence of water intoxication and hyponatremia. Particular attention should be paid to the possibility of the rare occurrence of an extreme decrease in plasma osmolality that may result in seizures which could lead to coma.

PRECAUTIONS

General: Intranasal Desmopressin acetate at high dosage has infrequently produced a slight elevation of blood pressure, which disappeared with a reduction in dosage. The drug should be used with caution in patients with coronary artery insufficiency and/or hypertensive cardiovascular disease because of possible rise in blood pressure.

Desmopressin acetate should be used with caution in patients with conditions associated with fluid and electrolyte imbalance, such as cystic fibrosis, because these patients are prone to hyponatremia.

Rare severe allergic reactions have been reported with Desmopressin acetate. Anaphylaxis has been reported with intravenous administration of Desmopressin acetate Injection, but not with Desmopressin Acetate Intranasal.

Central Cranial Diabetes Insipidus: Since **Desmopressin Acetate Rhinal Tube** is used intranasally, changes in the nasal mucosa such as scarring, edema, or other disease may cause erratic, unreliable absorption in which case intranasal Desmopressin acetateshould not be used. For such situations, Desmopressin Acetate Injection should be considered.

Primary Nocturnal Enuresis: If changes in the nasal mucosa have occurred, unreliable absorption may result. **Desmopressin Acetate Rhinal Tube** should be discontinued until the nasal problems resolve.

Laboratory Tests: Laboratory tests for following the patient with central cranial diabetes insipidus or post-surgical or head trauma-related polyuria and polydipsia include urine volume and osmolality. In some cases plasma osmolality measurements may be required. For the healthy patient with primary nocturnal enuresis, serum electrolytes should be checked at least once if therapy is continued beyond 7 days.

Drug Interactions: Although the pressor activity of Desmopressin acetate is very low compared to the antidiuretic activity, use of large doses of intranasal Desmopressin acetate with other pressor agents should only be done with careful patient monitoring.

Carcinogenesis, Mutagenesis, Impairment of Fertility: Studies with Desmopressin acetate have not been performed to evaluate carcinogenic potential, mutagenic potential or effects on fertility.

Pregnancy Category B: Fertility studies have not been done. Teratology studies in rats and rabbits at doses from 0.05 to 10 µg/kg/day (approximately 0.1 times the maximum systemic human exposure in rats and up to 38 times the maximum systemic human exposure in rabbits based on surface area, mg/m²) revealed no harm to the fetus due to Desmopressin acetate. There are, however, no adequate and well controlled studies in pregnant women. Because animal reproduction studies are not always predictive of human response, this drug should be used during pregnancy only if clearly needed.

Several publications of desmopressin acetate's use in the management of diabetes insipidus during pregnancy are available; these include a few anecdotal reports of congenital anomalies and low birth weight babies. However, no causal connection between these events and desmopressin acetate has been established. A fifteen year, Swedish epidemiologic study of the use of desmopressin acetate in pregnant women with diabetes insipidus found the rate of birth defects to be no greater than that in the general population; however the statistical power of this study is low. As opposed to preparations containing natural hormones, desmopressin acetate in antidiuretic doses has no uterotonic action and the physician will have to weigh the therapeutic advantages against the possible risks in each case.

Nursing Mothers: There have been no controlled studies in nursing mothers. A single study in postpartum women demonstrated a marked change in plasma, but little if any change in assayable Desmopressin acetate in breast milk following an intranasal dose of 10 µg. It is not known whether this drug is excreted in human milk. Because many drugs are excreted in human milk, caution should be exer-

Continued on next page

Desmopressin Rhinal—Cont.

cised when Desmopressin acetate is administered to a nursing woman.

Pediatric Use: *Primary Nocturnal Enuresis:* **Desmopressin Acetate Rhinal Tube** has been used in childhood nocturnal enuresis. Short-term (4-8 weeks) **Desmopressin Acetate Rhinal Tube** administration has been shown to be safe and modestly effective in pediatric patients aged 6 years or older with severe childhood nocturnal enuresis. Adequately controlled studies with intranasal Desmopressin acetatein primary nocturnal enuresis have not been conducted beyond 4-8 weeks. The dose should be individually adjusted to achieve the best results.

Central Cranial Diabetes Insipidus: **Desmopressin Acetate Rhinal Tube** has been used in pediatric patients with diabetes insipidus. Use in infants and pediatric patients will require careful fluid intake restriction to prevent possible hyponatremia and water intoxication. The dose must be individually adjusted to the patient with attention in the very young to the danger of an extreme decrease in plasma osmolality with resulting convulsions. Dose should start at 0.05 mL or less.

There are reports of an occasional change in response with time, usually greater than 6 months. Some patients may show a decreased responsiveness, others a shortened duration of effect. There is no evidence this effect is due to the development of binding antibodies but may be due to a local inactivation of the peptide.

ADVERSE REACTIONS

Infrequently, high dosages of intranasal Desmopressin acetate have produced transient headache and nausea. Nasal congestion, rhinitis and flushing have also been reported occasionally along with mild abdominal cramps. These symptoms disappeared with reduction in dosage. Nosebleed, sore throat, cough and upper respiratory infections have also been reported.

The following table lists the percent of patients having adverse experiences without regard to relationship to study drug from the pooled pivotal study data for nocturnal enuresis.

[See table at top of previous page]

See **WARNINGS** for the possibility of water intoxication and hyponatremia.

OVERDOSAGE

(See **ADVERSE REACTIONS**.) In case of overdosage, the dose should be reduced, frequency of administration decreased, or the drug withdrawn according to the severity of the condition. There is no known specific antidote for desmopressin acetate or **Desmopressin Acetate Rhinal Tube**.

An oral LD_{50} has not been established. An intravenous dose of 2 mg/kg in mice demonstrated no effect.

DOSAGE AND ADMINISTRATION

Primary Nocturnal Enuresis: Dosage should be adjusted according to the individual. The recommended initial dose for those 6 years of age and older is 20 µg or 0.2 mL solution intranasally at bedtime. Adjustment up to 40 µg is suggested if the patient does not respond. Some patients may respond to 10 µg and adjustment to that lower dose may be done if the patient has shown a response to 20 µg. It is recommended that one-half of the dose be administered per nostril. Adequately controlled studies with intranasal Desmopressin acetate in primary nocturnal enuresis have not been conducted beyond 4–8 weeks.

Central Cranial Diabetes Insipidus: This drug is administered into the nose through a soft, flexible plastic rhinal tube which has four graduation marks on it that measure 0.2, 0.15, 0.1 and 0.05 mL. **Desmopressin Acetate Rhinal Tube** dosage must be determined for each individual patient and adjusted according to the diurnal pattern of response. Response should be estimated by two parameters: adequate duration of sleep and adequate, not excessive, water turnover. Patients with nasal congestion and blockage have often responded well to intranasal Desmopressin acetate. The usual dosage range in adults is 0.1 to 0.4 mL daily, either as a single dose or divided into two or three doses. Most adults require 0.2 mL daily in two divided doses. The morning and evening doses should be separately adjusted for an adequate diurnal rhythm of water turnover. For children aged 3 months to 12 years, the usual dosage range is 0.05 to 0.3 mL daily, either as a single dose or divided into two doses. About 1/4 to 1/3 of patients can be controlled by a single daily dose of Desmopressin acetate administered intranasally.

HOW SUPPLIED

Desmopressin Acetate Rhinal Tube is available in a 2.5 mL vial, packaged with two rhinal tube applicators per carton (NDC 55566-5020-1). Also available in a shelf packs of 10 × 2.5 mL vials (NDC 55566-5020-2).

Store refrigerated 2 to 8°C (36 to 46°F). When traveling, closed bottles will maintain stability for 3 weeks when stored at controlled room temperature, 20 to 25°C (68 to 77°F).

Rx only

Keep out of the reach of children.

Manufactured for
FERRING PHARMACEUTICALS INC.
SUFFERN, NY 10901
By Ferring Pharmaceuticals, Limhamn, Sweden
Rev. 4/03 6026-02

PATIENT INSTRUCTION GUIDE

DESMOPRESSIN
acetate
RHINAL TUBE

1. Pull plastic tag on neck of bottle.

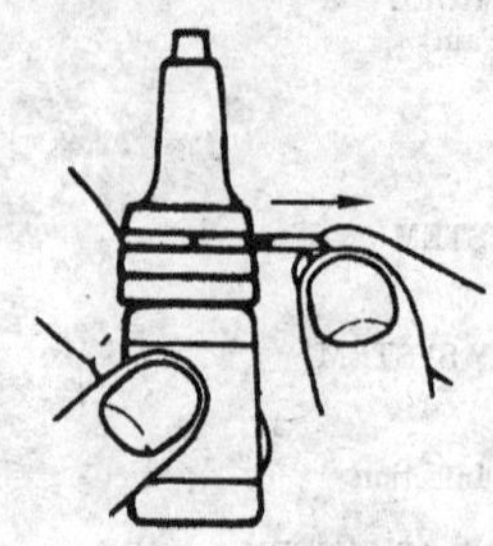

2. Break security seal and remove plastic cap.

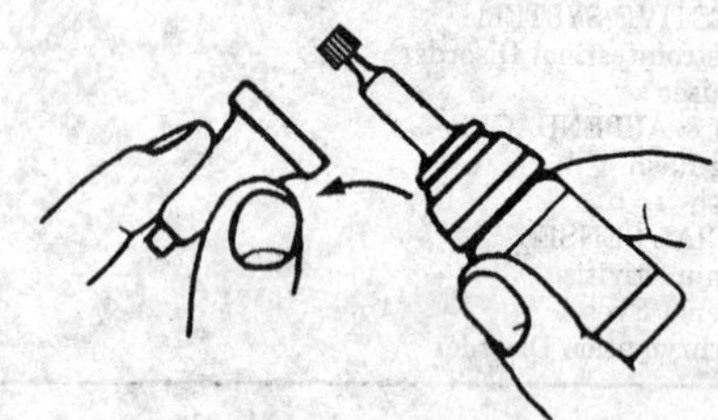

3. Twist off the small knurled seal from the dropper. **Use the same seal reversed to prevent subsequent leakage,** especially if the bottle is not stored upright.

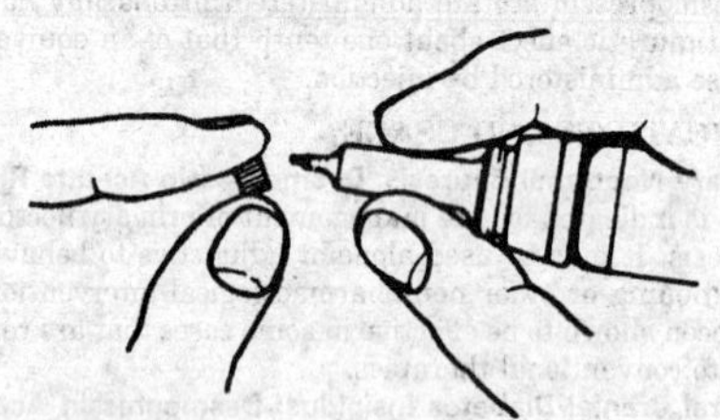

4. The drug is administered by a soft, flexible, plastic rhinal tube which has dose marks at 0.2, 0.15, 0.1 and 0.05 mL. Take the arrow-marked part of the tube in one hand and place the fingers of the other hand around the cylindrical part of the closure. Insert the top of the dropper in a downward position into the arrow-marked end of the tube and squeeze the dropper until the solution has reached the desired calibration mark. The dose is measured from the arrow-marked end of the tube to the appropriate calibration. Disconnect the tube from the bottle by withdrawing the bottle quickly downwards. In order to prevent air bubbles from forming in the tube, maintain constant pressure on the dropper. If difficulty is experienced in filling the tube, a diabetic or tuberculin syringe may be used to draw up the dose and load the tube.

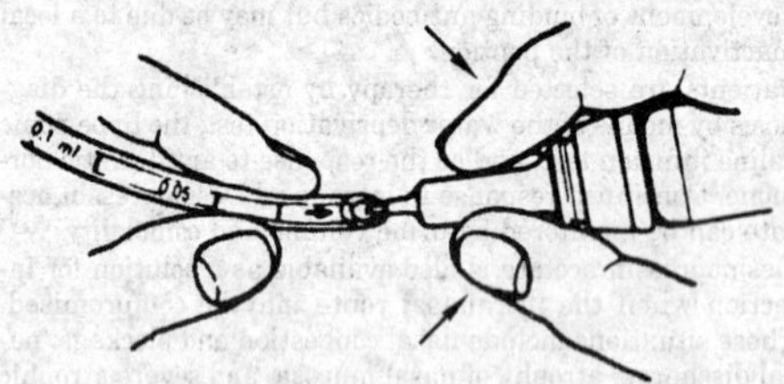

5. Hold the tube with the fingers approximately 3/4 inch from the end and insert into a nostril until the tips of the fingers reach the nostril.

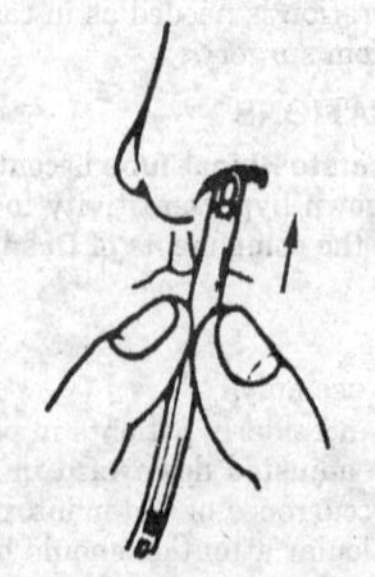

6. Put the other end of the tube into the mouth. Hold the breath, tilt the head back and then blow with a short, strong puff through the tube so that the solution reaches the right place in the nasal cavity. Through this procedure, medication is limited to the nasal cavity and the preparation does not pass down into the throat.
In very young patients, it may be necessary for an adult to blow the solution into the child's nose. In such cases, the tube will not need to be put into the nose as far as in the older child or adult. The tube should be placed in the nose gently just far enough so that the solution does not run out. A baby must be held firmly and securely.

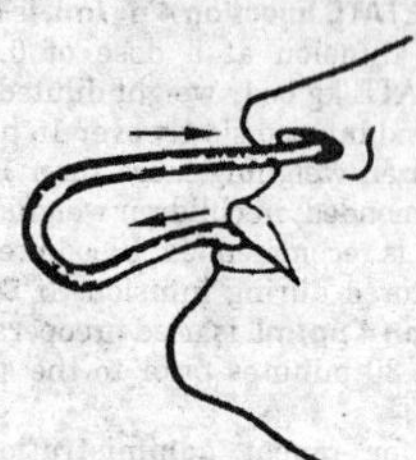

7. **After use, reseal dropper tip and close the bottle with the plastic cap.** Wash the tube in water and shake thoroughly, until no more water is left. The tube can then be used for the next application.

IMPORTANT:
Replace Knurled Seal

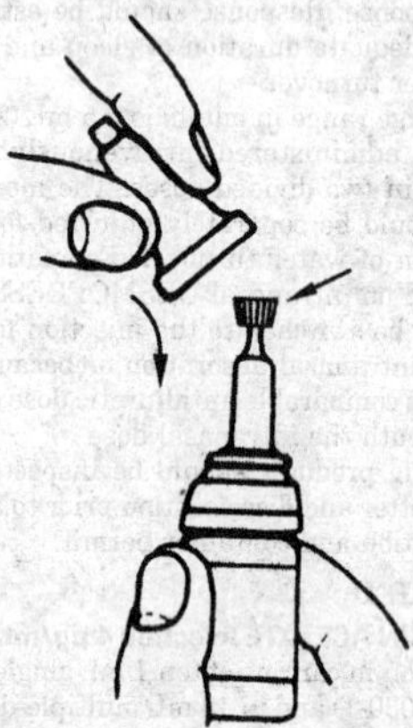

Store refrigerated 2 to 8°C (36 to 46°F). When traveling, closed bottles will maintain stability for 3 weeks when stored at controlled room temperature, 20 to 25°C (68 to 77°F).

Manufactured for
FERRING PHARMACEUTICALS INC.
SUFFERN, NY 10901
By Ferring Pharmaceuticals, Limhamn, Sweden 6026-02

NOVAREL™ ℞
(Chorionic Gonadotropin for Injection, USP)

DESCRIPTION

Human chorionic gonadotropin (HCG), a polypeptide hormone produced by the human placenta, is composed of an alpha and a beta sub-unit. The alpha sub-unit is essentially identical to the alpha sub-units of the human pituitary gonadotropins, luteinizing hormone (LH) and follicle-stimulating hormone (FSH), as well as to the alpha sub-unit of human thyroid-stimulating hormone (TSH). The beta sub-units of these hormones differ in amino acid sequence. Chorionic gonadotropin is obtained from the human pregnancy urine. It is standardized by a biological assay procedure.

Chorionic Gonadotropin for Injection, USP is available in multiple dose vials containing 10,000 USP Units with accompanying Bacteriostatic Water for Injection for reconstitution. When reconstituted with 10 mL of the accompanying diluent each vial contains:

Chorionic gonadotropin	10,000 Units
Mannitol	100 mg
Benzyl alcohol	0.9%
Water for Injection	q.s.

Buffered with dibasic sodium phosphate and monobasic sodium phosphate. Hydrochloric acid and/or sodium hydroxide may have been used for pH adjustment (6.0–8.0). Nitrogen gas is used in the freeze drying process.

CLINICAL PHARMACOLOGY

The action of HCG is virtually identical to that of pituitary LH, although HCG appears to have a small degree of FSH activity as well. It stimulates production of gonadal steroid hormones by stimulating the interstitial cells (Leydig cells) of the testis to produce androgens and the corpus luteum of the ovary to produce progesterone. Androgen stimulation in the male leads to the development of secondary sex characteristics and may stimulate testicular descent when no anatomical impediment to descent is present. This descent is usually reversible when HCG is discontinued. During the normal menstrual cycle, LH participates with FSH in the development and maturation of the normal ovarian follicle, and the mid-cycle LH surge triggers ovulation. HCG can substitute for LH in this function. During a normal pregnancy, HCG secreted by the placenta maintains the corpus luteum after LH secretion decreases, supporting continued secretion of estrogen and progesterone and preventing menstruation. HCG HAS NO KNOWN EFFECT ON FAT MOBILIZATION, APPETITE OR SENSE OF HUNGER, OR BODY FAT DISTRIBUTION.

INDICATIONS AND USAGE

HCG HAS NOT BEEN DEMONSTRATED TO BE EFFECTIVE ADJUNCTIVE THERAPY IN THE TREATMENT OF OBESITY. THERE IS NO SUBSTANTIAL EVIDENCE THAT IT INCREASES WEIGHT LOSS BEYOND THAT RESULTING FROM CALORIC RESTRICTION, THAT IT CAUSES A MORE ATTRACTIVE OR "NORMAL" DISTRIBUTION OF FAT, OR THAT IT DECREASES THE HUNGER AND DISCOMFORT ASSOCIATED WITH CALORIE-RESTRICTED DIETS.

1. Prepubertal cryptorchidism not due to anatomical obstruction. In general, HCG is thought to induce testicular descent in situations when descent would have occurred at puberty. HCG thus may help predict whether or not orchiopexy will be needed in the future. Although, in some cases, descent following HCG administration is permanent, in most cases, the response is temporary. Therapy is usually instituted between the ages four and nine.
2. Selected cases of hypogonadotropic hypogonadism (hypogonadism secondary to a pituitary deficiency) in males.
3. Induction of ovulation and pregnancy in the anovulatory, infertile woman in whom the cause of anovulation is secondary and not due to primary ovarian failure, and who has been appropriately pretreated with human menotropins.

CONTRAINDICATIONS

Precocious puberty, prostatic carcinoma or other androgen-dependent neoplasm, prior allergic reaction to HCG.

WARNINGS

HCG should be used in conjunction with human menopausal gonadotropins only by physicians experienced with infertility problems who are familiar with the criteria for patient selection, contraindications, warnings, precautions and adverse reactions described in the package insert for menotropins. The principal serious adverse reactions are: (1) Ovarian hyperstimulation, a syndrome of sudden ovarian enlargement, ascites with or without pain and/or pleural effusion, (2) Rupture of ovarian cysts with resultant hemoperitoneum, (3) Multiple births and (4) Arterial thromboembolism.

PRECAUTIONS

General

Induction of androgen secretion by HCG may induce precocious puberty in patients treated for cryptorchidism. Therapy should be discontinued if signs of precocious puberty occur.

Since androgens may cause fluid retention, HCG should be used with caution in patients with cardiac or renal disease, epilepsy, migraine or asthma.

Drug/Laboratory Test Interactions

Chorionic gonadotropin may interfere with radioimmunoassay for gonadotropins, particularly luteinizing hormone.

Carcinogenesis, Mutagenesis, Impairment of Fertility

Long-term studies in animals have not been performed to evaluate the carcinogenic or mutagenic potential of chorionic gonadotropin.

Pediatric Use

Safety and effectiveness of chorionic gonadotropin in children below the age of four have not been established.

Pregnancy

Teratogenic Effects: Pregnancy Category C—Chorionic gonadotropin may cause fetal harm when administered to a pregnant woman. Defects of forelimbs and central nervous system and alterations in sex ratio have been reported in mice receiving combined gonadotropin and chorionic gonadotropin therapy in dosages to induce superovulation. Multiple ovulations with resulting plural gestations (mostly twins) have been reported to occur in approximately 20% of pregnancies when conception has followed chorionic gonadotropin therapy.

Nursing Mothers

It is not known whether chorionic gonadotropin is excreted in human milk. Because many drugs are excreted in human milk, caution should be exercised when chorionic gonadotropin is administered to a nursing woman.

ADVERSE REACTIONS

Headache, irritability, restlessness, depression, fatigue, edema, precocious puberty, gynecomastia and pain at the site of injection.

DOSAGE AND ADMINISTRATION

Intramuscular Use Only

The dosage regimen employed in any particular case will depend upon the indication for use, the age and weight of the patient and the physician's preference. The following regimens have been advocated by various authorities.

Prepubertal Cryptorchidism Not Due To Anatomical Obstruction

1. 4,000 USP Units three times weekly for three weeks.
2. 5,000 USP Units every second day for four injections.
3. 15 injections of 500 to 1,000 USP Units over a period of six weeks.
4. 500 USP Units three times weekly for four to six weeks. If this course of treatment is not successful, another is begun one month later giving 1,000 USP Units per injection.

Selected Cases Of Hypogonadotropic Hypogonadism In Males

1. 500 to 1,000 USP Units three times a week for three weeks, followed by the same dose twice a week for three weeks.
2. 4,000 USP Units three times weekly for six to nine months, following which the dosage may be reduced to 2,000 USP Units three times weekly for an additional three months.

Induction of ovulation and pregnancy in the anovulatory, infertile woman in whom the cause of anovulation is secondary and not due to primary ovarian failure and who has been appropriately pretreated with human menotropins (see prescribing information for menotropins for dosage and administration for that drug product). 5,000 to 10,000 USP Units one day following the last dose of menotropins. (A dosage of 10,000 Units is recommended in the labeling for menotropins.)

IMPORTANT: USE COMPLETELY WITHIN 60 DAYS AFTER RECONSTITUTION. REFRIGERATE AFTER RECONSTITUTION.

DIRECTIONS FOR RECONSTITUTION:

Two-Vial Package

Withdraw sterile air from lyophilized vial and inject into diluent vial. Remove 10 mL from diluent vial and add to lyophilized vial; agitate gently until solution is complete.

HOW SUPPLIED

Chorionic Gonadotropin for Injection, USP, lyophilized, is supplied in two-vial packages including Bacteriostatic Water for Injection as diluent as follows:

Product No.	NDC No.	
F25021	55566-1501-1	Chorionic Gonadotropin for Injection, USP, 10,000 USP Units in a 10 mL multiple dose vial with accompanying diluent in packages of 10.

The product is assayed in accord with the USP method and potencies refer to USP Units (International Units) defined in terms of the USP Chorionic Gonadotropin Reference Standard.

Store at controlled room temperature 15°–30°C (59°–86°F).

Rx only

6007-04
NSN 6505-01-145-6377
Manufactured for:
Ferring Pharmaceuticals Inc.
Suffern, NY 10901
By: American Pharmaceutical
Partners, Inc.
Schaumburg, IL 60173
45761C
Revised: September 2002

REPRONEX® ℞
(MENOTROPINS FOR INJECTION, USP) FOR SUBCUTANEOUS INJECTION AND INTRAMUSCULAR INJECTION

DESCRIPTION

Repronex® (menotropins for injection, USP) is a purified preparation of gonadotropins extracted from the urine of postmenopausal women. Each vial of Repronex® contains 75 International Units (IU) or 150 IU of follicle-stimulating hormone (FSH) activity and 75 IU or 150 IU of luteinizing hormone (LH) activity, respectively, plus 20 mg lactose monohydrate in a sterile, lyophilized form. The final product may contain sodium phosphate buffer (sodium phosphate tribasic and phosphoric acid). Repronex® is administered by subcutaneous or intramuscular injection. Human Chorionic Gonadotropin (hCG), a naturally occurring hormone in post-menopausal urine, is detected in Repronex®. Repronex® is biologically standardized for FSH and LH (ICSH) gonadotropin activities in terms of the Second International Reference Preparation for Human Menopausal Gonadotropins established in September, 1964 by the Expert Committee on Biological Standards of the World Health Organization.

Both FSH and LH are glycoproteins that are acidic and water soluble. Therapeutic class: Infertility.

CLINICAL PHARMACOLOGY

Menotropins administered for 7 to 12 days produces ovarian follicular growth in women who do not have primary ovarian failure. Treatment with menotropins in most instances results only in follicular growth and maturation. When sufficient follicular maturation has occurred, hCG must be given to induce ovulation.

PHARMACOKINETICS

Single doses of 300 IU menotropins (Menogon®, Ferring's European formulation) were administered subcutaneously (SC) and intramuscularly (IM) in a 2-period crossover study to 16 healthy female subjects while their endogenous FSH and LH were being suppressed. Serum FSH concentrations were determined. Based on the ratio of FSH C_{max} and $AUC_{0-\infty}$, SC and IM administration of menotropins are not bioequivalent. Compared to IM administration, the SC administration of menotropins results in an increase of FSH C_{max} and $AUC_{0-\infty}$ by 35 and 20%, respectively.

Based on two subjects who received either the highest SC or IM Repronex® dose, FSH pharmacokinetics (PK) appears to be linear up to 450 IU menotropins. The mean accumulation factors for FSH upon six doses of SC or IM 150 to 450 IU/day Repronex® are 1.6 and 1.4, respectively. Upon six doses of SC or IM 150 IU/day Repronex®, the observed serum FSH concentrations range from 1.7 to 15.9 mIU/mL and 0.5 to 10.1 mIU/mL, respectively. The FSH pharmacokinetic parameters from population modeling for these two studies are in Table 1.

[See table 1 below]

Serum LH concentrations upon multiple dose SC or IM Repronex® are low and variable. No recognizable trend in the increase in serum LH concentrations from SC or IM 150 to 450 IU/day Repronex® doses was observed. After the 6th dose of SC or IM 150 IU/day Repronex®, the range of baseline-corrected serum LH concentrations is 0 to 3.2 mIU/mL for both routes of administration.

Absorption

The geometric mean of FSH C_{max} and $AUC_{0-\infty}$ upon single dose SC administration of menotropins is 5.62 mIU/mL and 385.2 mIU•h/mL, respectively; the corresponding geometric median of FSH t_{max} is 12 hours. The geometric mean of FSH C_{max} and $AUC_{0-\infty}$ upon single dose IM administration of menotropins is 4.15 mIU/mL and 320.1 mIU•h/mL, respectively; the corresponding geometric median of FSH t_{max} is 18 hours.

Distribution

Human tissue or organ distribution of FSH and LH have not been studied for Repronex®.

Metabolism

Metabolism of FSH and LH have not been studied for Repronex® in humans.

Excretion

The mean elimination half-lives of FSH upon single dose SC and IM administration of menotropins are 53.7 and 59.2 hours, respectively.

Pediatric Populations

Repronex® is not used in pediatric populations.

Geriatric Populations

Repronex® is not used in geriatric populations.

Special Populations

The safety and efficacy of Repronex® in renal and hepatic insufficiency have not been studied.

Drug Interactions

No drug/drug interaction studies have been conducted for Repronex® in humans.

CLINICAL STUDIES

Efficacy results from a clinical trial in *in vitro* fertilization (IVF) patients and a clinical trial in ovulation induction (OI) in anovulatory and oligovulatory patients are summarized in Tables 2 and 3 respectively. Both studies were multicenter, active control, randomized, parallel group designs. In addition, all patients in both studies underwent pituitary suppression with a GnRH agonist before starting treatment with Repronex® or the control therapy. The IVF study evaluated 186 patients (125 patients received Repronex®). The patients treated with Repronex® received 225 IU Repronex® daily for 5 days. This was followed by individual titration of the dose from 75 to 450 IU daily based on ultrasound and estradiol (E_2) levels. The total duration of dosing did not exceed 12 days. The OI study evaluated 108 patients (72 patients received Repronex®). The patients treated with Repronex® received 150 IU Repronex® daily for 5 days. This was followed by individual titration of the dose from 75 to 450 IU daily based on ultrasound and estradiol (E_2) levels. The total duration of dosing did not exceed 12 days.

[See table 2 at top of next page]
[See table 3 on next page]

Continued on next page

Table 1. FSH Pharmacokinetic Parameters† Upon Menotropins Administration

	Single Dose‡		Multiple Dose¶	
FSH Parameter	SC	IM	SC	IM
$K_a (h^{-1})$	0.128 (42.1)	0.117 (21.3)	0.076 (46.3)	0.064 (63.2)
Cl/F (L/h)	0.770 (17.1)	0.94 (6.9)	1.11 (39.5)	1.44 (43.5)
V/F (L)	39.37 (14.1)	57.68 (11.4)	23.09 (8.3)	23.5 (2.5)

† mean (CV%)
‡ Menogon® (Ferring's European formulation of menotropins)
¶ Repronex®

Repronex—Cont.

INDICATIONS AND USAGE

Repronex®, in conjunction with hCG, is indicated for multiple follicular development (controlled ovarian stimulation) and ovulation induction in patients who have previously received pituitary suppression.

Selection of Patients

1. Before treatment with Repronex® is instituted, a thorough gynecologic and endocrinologic evaluation must be performed. Except for those patients enrolled in an *in vitro* fertilization program, this should include a hysterosalpingogram (to rule out uterine and tubal pathology) and documentation of anovulation by means of basal body temperature, serial vaginal smears, examination of cervical mucus, determination of serum (or urine) progesterone, urinary pregnanediol and endometrial biopsy. Patients with tubal pathology should receive menotropins only if enrolled in an *in vitro* fertilization program.
2. Primary ovarian failure should be excluded by the determination of gonadotropin levels.
3. Careful examination should be made to rule out the presence of an early pregnancy.
4. Patients in late reproductive life have a greater predilection to endometrial carcinoma as well as a higher incidence of anovulatory disorders. Cervical dilation and curettage should always be done for diagnosis before starting Repronex® therapy in such patients who demonstrate abnormal uterine bleeding or other signs of endometrial abnormalities.
5. Evaluation of the husband's fertility potential should be included in the workup.

CONTRAINDICATIONS

Repronex® is contraindicated in women who have:

1. A high FSH level indicating primary ovarian failure.
2. Uncontrolled thyroid and adrenal dysfunction.
3. An organic intracranial lesion such as a pituitary tumor.
4. The presence of any cause of infertility other than anovulation unless they are candidates for *in vitro*-fertilization.
5. Abnormal bleeding of undetermined origin.
6. Ovarian cysts or enlargement not due to polycystic ovary syndrome.
7. Prior hypersensitivity to menotropins.
8. Repronex® is not indicated in women who are pregnant. There are limited human data on the effects of menotropins when administered during pregnancy.

WARNINGS

Repronex® is a drug that should only be used by physicians who are thoroughly familiar with infertility problems. It is a potent gonadotropic substance capable of causing mild to severe adverse reactions in women. Gonadotropin therapy requires a certain time commitment by physicians and supportive health professionals, and its use requires the availability of appropriate monitoring facilities (see **PRECAUTIONS—Laboratory Tests**). In female patients it must be used with a great deal of care.

Overstimulation of the Ovary During Repronex® Therapy

Ovarian Enlargement: Mild to moderate uncomplicated ovarian enlargement which may be accompanied by abdominal distension and/or abdominal pain occurs in approximately 5 to 10% of those treated with Repronex® menotropins and hCG, and generally regresses without treatment within two or three weeks.

In order to minimize the hazard associated with the occasional abnormal ovarian enlargement which may occur with Repronex® hCG therapy, the lowest dose consistent with expectation of good results, should be used. Careful monitoring of ovarian response can further minimize the risk of overstimulation.

If the ovaries are abnormally enlarged on the last day of Repronex® therapy, hCG should not be administered in this course of therapy; this will reduce the chances of development of the Ovarian Hyperstimulation Syndrome.

The Ovarian Hyperstimulation Syndrome (OHSS): OHSS is a medical event distinct from uncomplicated ovarian enlargement. OHSS may progress rapidly to become a serious medical event. It is characterized by an apparent dramatic increase in vascular permeability which can result in a rapid accumulation of fluid in the peritoneal cavity, thorax, and potentially, the pericardium. The early warning signs of development of OHSS are severe pelvic pain, nausea, vomiting, and weight gain. The following symptomatology has been seen with cases of OHSS: abdominal pain, abdominal distension, gastrointestinal symptoms including nausea, vomiting and diarrhea, severe ovarian enlargement, weight gain, dyspnea, and oliguria. Clinical evaluation may reveal hypovolemia, hemoconcentration, electrolyte imbalances, ascites, hemoperitoneum, pleural effusions, hydrothorax, acute pulmonary distress, and thromboembolic events (see "Pulmonary and Vascular Complications" below). Transient liver function test abnormalities suggestive of hepatic dysfunction, which may be accompanied by morphologic changes on liver biopsy, have been reported in association with the Ovarian Hyperstimulation Syndrome (OHSS).

OHSS occured in 3 of 125 (2.4%) Repronex® treated women during ART clinical studies. None of these cases was classified as severe. In Ovulation Induction clinical studies, 4 of 72 (5.5%) Repronex® treated women developed OHSS and of this number one case was classified as severe (1.4%). Cases of OHSS are more common, more severe and more

Table 2. Efficacy Outcomes by Treatment Group for IVF (one cycle of treatment)

Parameter	Repronex® IM	Repronex® SC
	N=65	N=60
Total oocytes Retrieved	13.6	12.7
Mature oocytes Retrieved	9.4	8.6
Pts w/oocyte Retrieval (%)	61(93.8)	55(91.7)
Pts w/Embryo Transfer (%)	58(89.2)	51(85.0)
Pts w/Chemical Pregnancy (%)	31(47.7)	35(58.3)
Pts w/Clinical Pregnancy (%)	25(38.5)	30(50.0)
Pts w/Continuing Pregnancy (%)	24(36.9) [1]	29(48.3) [2]
Pts. w/Live Births (%)	22(33.8) [3]	25(41.7) [4]

1. Continuing pregnancies included 14 single, 7 twins, and 3 triplet pregnancies.
2. Continuing pregnancies included 14 single, 9 twins, 3 triplets, and 3 quadruplet pregnancies.
3. Total of 34 live births. One spontaneous abortion. The follow-up data is not available for one patient.
4. Total of 39 live births. Two spontaneous abortions. The follow-up data is not available for two patients.

Table 3. Efficacy Outcomes by Treatment Groups in Ovulation Induction (one cycle of treatment)

Parameter	Repronex® IM	Repronex® SC
	N=36	N=36
Ovulation (%)	23 (63.9)	25 (69.4)
Received hCG (%)	25 (69.4)	27 (75.0)
Mean Peak Serum E2 (SD)	1158.5 (742.3)	1452.6* (1270.6)
Chemical Pregnancy (%)	4 (11.1)	11 (30.6)
Clinical Pregnancy (%)	4 (11.1)	6 (16.7)
Continuing Pregnancy (%)	4 (11.1) [1]	6 (16.7) [2]
Pts. w/Live Births (%)	4(11.1) [3]	4(11.1) [4]

* Fisher's Exact/Chi-Squared Tests—significant for Repronex® SC vs. Repronex® IM
1. Continuing pregnancies included 2 single and 2 triplet pregnancies.
2. Continuing pregnancies included 3 single, 1 twin and 2 quadruplet pregnancies.
3. Total 6 live births.
4. Total of 6 live births. One spontaneous abortion. The follow-up data is not available for one patient.

protracted if pregnancy occurs. OHSS develops rapidly; therefore patients should be followed for at least two weeks after hCG administration. Most often, OHSS occurs after treatment has been discontinued and reaches its maximum at about seven to ten days following treatment. Usually, OHSS resolves spontaneously with the onset of menses. If there is evidence that OHSS may be developing prior to hCG administration (see **PRECAUTIONS—Laboratory Tests**), the hCG should be withheld.

If OHSS occurs, treatment should be stopped and the patient hospitalized. Treatment is primarily symptomatic, consisting of bed rest, fluid and electrolyte management, and analgesics if needed. The phenomenon of hemoconcentration associated with fluid loss into the peritoneal cavity, pleural cavity, and the pericardial cavity has been seen to occur and should be thoroughly assessed in the following manner: 1) fluid intake and output, 2) weight, 3) hematocrit, 4) serum and urinary electrolytes, 5) urine specific gravity, 6) BUN and creatinine, and 7) abdominal girth. These determinations are to be performed daily or more often if the need arises.

With OHSS there is an increased risk of injury to the ovary. The ascitic, pleural, and pericardial fluid should not be removed unless absolutely necessary to relieve symptoms such as pulmonary distress or cardiac tamponade. Pelvic examination may cause rupture of an ovarian cyst, which may result in hemoperitoneum, and should therefore be avoided. If this does occur, and if bleeding becomes such that surgery is required, the surgical treatment should be designed to control bleeding and to retain as much ovarian tissue as possible. Intercourse should be prohibited in those patients in whom significant ovarian enlargement occurs after ovulation because of the danger of hemoperitoneum resulting from ruptured ovarian cysts.

The management of OHSS may be divided into three phases: the acute, the chronic, and the resolution phases. Because the use of diuretics can accentuate the diminished intravascular volume, diuretics should be avoided except in the late phase of resolution as described below.

Acute Phase: Management during the acute phase should be designed to prevent hemoconcentration due to loss of intravascular volume to the third space and to minimize the risk of thromboembolic phenomena and kidney damage. Treatment is designed to normalize electrolytes while maintaining an acceptable but somewhat reduced intravascular volume. Full correction of the intravascular volume deficit may lead to an unacceptable increase in the amount of third space fluid accumulation. Management includes administration of limited intravenous fluids, electrolytes, and human serum albumin. Monitoring for the development of hyperkalemia is recommended.

Chronic Phase: After stabilizing the patient during the acute phase, excessive fluid accumulation in the third space should be limited by instituting severe potassium, sodium, and fluid restriction.

Resolution Phase: A fall in hematocrit and an increasing urinary output without an increased intake are observed due to the return of third space fluid to the intravascular compartment. Peripheral and/or pulmonary edema may result if the kidneys are unable to excrete third space fluid as rapidly as it is mobilized. Diuretics may be indicated during the resolution phase if necessary to combat pulmonary edema.

Pulmonary and Vascular Complications

Serious pulmonary conditions (e.g., atelectasis, acute respiratory distress syndrome) have been reported. In addition, thromboembolic events both in association with, and separate from, the Ovarian Hyperstimulation Syndrome have been reported following menotropins therapy. Intravascular thrombosis and embolism, which may originate in venous or arterial vessels, can result in reduced blood flow to critical organs or the extremities. Sequelae of such events have included venous thrombophlebitis, pulmonary embolism, pulmonary infarction, cerebral vascular occlusion (stroke), and arterial occlusion resulting in loss of limb. In rare cases, pulmonary complications and/or thromboembolic events have resulted in death.

Multiple Pregnancies

Multiple pregnancies have occurred following treatment with Repronex® IM and SC. In a clinical trial for ovulation induction in which Repronex® IM and Repronex® SC were directly compared, the rates of multiple pregnancies were as follows. Of the four clinical pregnancies with Repronex® IM, two were single and two were multiple pregnancies. Both multiple pregnancies were triplet pregnancies. Of the six clinical pregnancies with Repronex® SC, three were single and three were multiple pregnancies. The three multiple pregnancies included one twin pregnancy and two quadruplet pregnancies.

In a clinical trial of IVF patients in which Repronex® IM and Repronex® SC were directly compared, the rates of multiple pregnancies were as follows. Of the 24 continuing pregnancies on Repronex® IM, 14 were single and 10 were multiple pregnancies. The ten multiple pregnancies included three triplet and seven twin pregnancies. Of the 29 continuing pregnancies on Repronex® SC, 14 were single and 15 were multiple pregnancies. The 15 multiple pregnancies included three quadruplet, three triplet and nine twin pregnancies. The patient and her partner should be advised of the potential risk of multiple births before starting treatment.

Hypersensitivity/Anaphylactic Reactions

Hypersensitivity/anaphylactic reactions associated with menotropins administration have been reported in some patients. These reactions presented as generalized urticaria, facial edema, angioneurotic edema, and/or dyspnea suggestive of laryngeal edema. The relationship of these symptoms to uncharacterized urinary proteins is uncertain.

PRECAUTIONS

General

Careful attention should be given to diagnosis in the selection of candidates for menotropins therapy (see "**INDICATIONS AND USAGE—Selection of Patients**").

Information for Patients

Prior to therapy with Repronex®, patients should be informed of the duration of treatment and the monitoring of their condition that will be required. Possible adverse reactions (see **ADVERSE REACTIONS** section) and the risk of multiple births should also be discussed.

Laboratory Tests

Treatment for Induction of ovulation

The combination of both estradiol levels and ultrasonography are useful for monitoring the growth and development of follicles, timing hCG administration, as well as minimizing the risk of the Ovarian Hyperstimulation Syndrome and multiple gestation.

The clinical confirmation of ovulation, is determined by:

a) A rise in basal body temperature;

b) Increase in serum progesterone; and

c) Menstruation following the shift in basal body temperature.

When used in conjunction with indices of progesterone production, sonographic visualization of the ovaries will assist in determining if ovulation has occurred. Sonographic evidence of ovulation may include the following:

a) Fluid in the cul-de-sac;

b) Ovarian stigmata; and

c) Collapsed follicle.

Because of the subjectivity of the various tests for the determination of follicular maturation and ovulation, it cannot be overemphasized that the physician should choose tests with which he/she is thoroughly familiar.

Carcinogenesis and Mutagenesis

Long-term toxicity studies in animals have not been performed to evaluate the carcinogenic potential of menotropins.

Pregnancy

Pregnancy Category X: See **CONTRAINDICATIONS** section.

Nursing Mothers

It is not known whether this drug is excreted in human milk. Because many drugs are excreted in human milk, caution should be exercised if menotropins are administered to a nursing woman.

Pediatric Patients

Safety and effectiveness in pediatric patients have not been established.

Geriatric Patients

Safety and effectiveness in geriatric patients have not been established.

ADVERSE REACTIONS

The following adverse reactions, reported during menotropins therapy, are listed in decreasing order of potential severity:

1. Pulmonary and vascular complications (see **WARNINGS**)
2. Ovarian Hyperstimulation Syndrome (see **WARNINGS**)
3. Hemoperitoneum
4. Adnexal torsion (as a complication of ovarian enlargement)
5. Mild to moderate ovarian enlargement
6. Ovarian cysts
7. Abdominal pain
8. Sensitivity to menotropins (Febrile reactions suggestive of allergic response have been reported following the administration of menotropins. Reports of flu-like symptoms including fever, chills, musculoskeletal aches, joint pains, nausea, headaches, and malaise have also been reported).
9. Gastrointestinal symptoms (nausea, vomiting, diarrhea, abdominal cramps, bloating)
10. Pain, rash, swelling and/or irritation at the site of injection
11. Body rashes
12. Dizziness, tachycardia, dyspnea, tachypnea

The following medical events have been reported subsequent to pregnancies resulting from menotropins therapy:

1. Ectopic pregnancy
2. Congenital abnormalities

   With menotropin therapy congenital abnormalities have been reported. One infant was shown to have multiple congenital anomalies consisting of aplasia of the sigmoid colon, cecovesicle fistula, bifid scrotum, meningocele, bilateral internal tibial torsion, and right metatarsus adductus. Other reported anomalies include imperforate anus, congenital heart lesions, supernumerary digits, hypospadias, extrophy of the bladder, Down's syndrome and hydrocephalus. The incidence of congenital abnormalities does not exceed that found in the general population.

   There have been infrequent reports of ovarian neoplasms, both benign and malignant, in women who have undergone multiple drug regimens for ovulation induction; however, a causal relationship has not been established.

Adverse events occurring in ≥1% of patients exposed to Repronex® IM or Repronex® SC are described in Table 4.

Table 4. Patients with Adverse Events ≥ 1%

	Repronex® IM (N=101)	Repronex® SC (N=96)
Adverse Events	n (%)	n (%)
INJECTION SITE AEs		
Injection Site Edema	1 (1.0)	8 (8.3)*
Injection Site Reaction	2 (2.0)	8 (8.3)*
GENITOURINARY/REPRODUCTIVE AEs		
OHSS	2 (2.0)	5 (5.2)
Vaginal Hemorrhage	8 (7.9)	3 (3.1)
Ovarian Disease	3 (3.0)	8 (8.3)
Ectopic Pregnancy	1 (1.0)	1 (1.0)
Pelvic Pain	3 (3.0)	1 (1.0)
Breast Tenderness	2 (2.0)	2 (2.1)
GASTROINTESTINAL AEs		
Nausea	4 (4.0)	7(7.3)
Vomiting	0 (0)	3 (3.1)
Diarrhea	0 (0)	2(2.1)
Abdominal Cramping	7(6.9)	5(5.2)
Abdominal Pain	5(5.0)	7(7.3)
Enlarged Abdomen	6(6.0)	2 (2.1)
OTHER BODY SYSTEM AEs		
Headache	6 (6.0)	5 (5.2)
Infection	1(1.0)	0 (0)
Dyspnea	1(1.0)	2(2.1)

* Fisher's Exact/Chi-Squared Tests—significant for Repronex® SC vs. Repronex® IM.

[See table 4 above]

DRUG ABUSE AND DEPENDENCE

There have been no reports of abuse or dependence with menotropins.

OVERDOSAGE

Aside from possible ovarian hyperstimulation (see **WARNINGS**), little is known concerning the consequences of acute overdosage with menotropins.

DOSAGE AND ADMINISTRATION

1. Dosage:

Infertile patients with oligo-anovulation:

The dose of Repronex® to stimulate development of ovarian follicles must be individualized for each patient. The lowest dose consistent with achieving good results based on clinical experience and reported clinical data should be used.

The recommended initial dose of Repronex® for patients who have received GnRH agonist or antagonist pituitary suppression is 150 IU daily for the first 5 days of treatment. Based on clinical monitoring (including serum estradiol levels and vaginal ultrasound results) subsequent dosing should be adjusted according to individual patient response. Adjustments in dose should not be made more frequently than once every 2 days and should not exceed more than 75 to 150 IU per adjustment. The maximum daily dose of Repronex® should not exceed 450 IU and dosing beyond 12 days is not recommended.

If patient response to Repronex® is appropriate, hCG (5000 to 10,000 USP units) should be given 1 day following the last dose of Repronex®. The hCG should be withheld if the serum estradiol is greater than 2000 pg/mL, if the ovaries are abnormally enlarged or if abdominal pain occurs, and the patient should be advised to refrain from intercourse. These precautions may reduce the risk of Ovarian Hyperstimulation Syndrome and multiple gestation. Patients should be followed closely for at least 2 weeks after hCG administration. If there is inadequate follicle development or ovulation without subsequent pregnancy, the course of treatment with Repronex® may be repeated. The couple should be encouraged to have intercourse daily, beginning on the day prior to the administration of hCG until ovulation becomes apparent from the indices employed for the determination of progestational activity. In the light of the foregoing indices and parameters mentioned, it should become obvious that, unless a physician is willing to devote considerable time to these patients and be familiar with and conduct the necessary laboratory studies, he/she should not use Repronex®.

Assisted Reproductive Technologies:

The recommended initial dose of Repronex® for patients who have received GnRH agonist or antagonist pituitary suppression is 225 IU. Based on clinical monitoring (including serum estradiol levels and vaginal ultrasound results) subsequent dosing should be adjusted according to individual patient response. Adjustments in dose should not be made more frequently than once every 2 days and should not exceed more than 75 to 150 IU per adjustment. The maximum daily dose of Repronex® given should not exceed 450 IU and dosing beyond 12 days is not recommended.

Once adequate follicular development is evident, hCG (5000–10,000 USP units) should be administered to induce final follicular maturation in preparation for oocyte retrieval. The administration of hCG must be withheld in cases where the ovaries are abnormally enlarged on the last day of therapy. This should reduce the chance of developing OHSS.

2. Administration:

Dissolve the contents of one to 6 vials of Repronex® in one to two mL of sterile saline and **ADMINISTER SUBCUTANEOUSLY OR INTRAMUSCULARLY** immediately. Any unused reconstituted material should be discarded.

Parenteral drug products should be inspected visually for particulate matter and discoloration prior to administration, whenever solution and container permit.

The lower abdomen (alternating sides) should be used for subcutaneous administration.

HOW SUPPLIED

Repronex® (menotropins for injection, USP) is available in vials as a sterile, lyophilized, white to off-white powder or pellet.

Each vial is available with an accompanying vial of sterile diluent containing 2 mL of 0.9% Sodium Chloride Injection, USP:

75 IU FSH and 75 IU of LH activity, supplied as:

NDC 55566-7185-1—Box of 1 vial + 1 vial diluent.

NDC 55566-7185-2—Box of 5 vials + 5 vials diluent.

150 IU FSH and 150 IU of LH activity, supplied as:

NDC 55566-7125-1—Box of 1 vial + 1 vial diluent.

By biological assay, one IU of LH for the Second International Reference Preparation (2nd-IRP) for hMG is biologically equivalent to approximately 0.5 U of hCG.

Lyophilized powder may be stored refrigerated or at room temperature (3° to 25°C/37° to 77°F). Protect from light. Use immediately after reconstitution. Discard unused material.

℞ only

Vials of sterile diluent of 0.9% Sodium Chloride Injection, USP manufactured for Ferring Pharmaceuticals Inc.

Manufactured for:
FERRING PHARMACEUTICALS INC.
SUFFERN, NY 10901
By: CARDINAL HEALTH
ALBUQUERQUE, NEW MEXICO 87107
6062–02
6–D6062FR-02
3/03

Fielding Pharmaceutical Company

11551 ADIE ROAD
MARYLAND HEIGHTS, MO 63043
(For product information, please see Novavax, Inc.)

First Horizon Pharmaceutical Corporation

6195 SHILOH ROAD
ALPHARETTA, GA 30005

Direct Inquiries to:
Drug Safety Department
800-849-9707
(770) 442-9707
FAX: (770) 442-9594

NITROLINGUAL® PUMPSPRAY ℞

[*nī'trō-lĭn-gwal*]
(nitroglycerin lingual spray)
400 mcg per spray, 60 or 200 Metered Sprays

DESCRIPTION

Nitroglycerin, an organic nitrate, is a vasodilator which has effects on both arteries and veins. The chemical name for nitroglycerin is 1,2,3-propanetriol trinitrate ($C_3H_5N_3O_9$). The compound has a molecular weight of 227.09. The chemical structure is:

CH_2-ONO_2
$CH-ONO_2$
CH_2-ONO_2

Nitrolingual® Pumpspray (nitroglycerin lingual spray 400 mcg) is a metered dose spray containing nitroglycerin. This product delivers nitroglycerin (400 mcg per spray, 60 or 200 metered sprays) in the form of spray droplets onto or under the tongue. Inactive ingredients: medium-chain triglycerides, dehydrated alcohol, medium-chain partial glycerides, peppermint oil.

CLINICAL PHARMACOLOGY

The principal pharmacological action of nitroglycerin is relaxation of vascular smooth muscle, producing a vasodilator effect on both peripheral arteries and veins with more prominent effects on the latter. Dilation of the post-capillary vessels, including large veins, promotes peripheral pooling of blood and decreases venous return to the heart, thereby reducing left ventricular end-diastolic pressure (pre-load). Arteriolar relaxation reduces systemic vascular resistance and arterial pressure (after-load).
The mechanism by which nitroglycerin relieves angina pectoris is not fully understood. Myocardial oxygen consumption or demand (as measured by the pressure-rate product, tension-time index, and stroke-work index) is decreased by both the arterial and venous effects of nitroglycerin and presumably, a more favorable supply-demand ratio is achieved. While the large epicardial coronary arteries are also dilated by nitroglycerin, the extent to which this action contributes to relief of exertional angina is unclear.
Nitroglycerin is rapidly metabolized *in vivo*, with a liver reductase enzyme having primary importance in the formation of glycerol nitrate metabolites and inorganic nitrate. Two active major metabolites, 1,2- and 1,3-dinitroglycerols, the products of hydrolysis, although less potent as vasodilators, have longer plasma half-lives than the parent compound. The dinitrates are further metabolized to mononitrates (considered biologically inactive with respect to cardiovascular effects) and ultimately glycerol and carbon dioxide.
Therapeutic doses of nitroglycerin may reduce systolic, diastolic and mean arterial blood pressure. Effective coronary perfusion pressure is usually maintained, but can be compromised if blood pressure falls excessively or increased heart rate decreases diastolic filling time.
Elevated central venous and pulmonary capillary wedge pressures, pulmonary vascular resistance and systemic vascular resistance are also reduced by nitroglycerin therapy. Heart rate is usually slightly increased, presumably a reflex response to the fall in blood pressure. Cardiac index may be increased, decreased, or unchanged. Patients with elevated left ventricular filling pressure and systemic vascular resistance values in conjunction with a depressed cardiac index are likely to experience an improvement in cardiac index. On the other hand, when filling pressures and cardiac index are normal, cardiac index may be slightly reduced.
In a pharmacokinetic study when a single 0.8 mg dose of Nitrolingual® Pumpspray was administered to healthy volunteers (n = 24), the mean C_{max} and t_{max} were 1,041 pg/mL • min and 7.5 minutes, respectively. Additionally, in these subjects the mean area-under-the-curve (AUC) was 12,769 pg/mL • min.
In a randomized, double-blind single-dose, 5-period cross-over study in 51 patients with exertional angina pectoris significant dose-related increases in exercise tolerance, time to onset of angina and ST-segment depression were seen following doses of 0.2, 0.4, 0.8 and 1.6 mg of nitroglycerin delivered by metered pumpspray as compared to placebo. Additionally the drug was well tolerated as evidenced by a profile of generally mild to moderate adverse events.

INDICATIONS AND USAGE

Nitrolingual® Pumpspray is indicated for acute relief of an attack or prophylaxis of angina pectoris due to coronary artery disease.

CONTRAINDICATIONS

Allergic reactions to organic nitrates are rare. Nitroglycerin is contraindicated in patients who are allergic to it. Nitrolingual® Pumpspray is contraindicated in patients taking certain drugs for erectile dysfunction (phosphodiesterase inhibitors), as their concomitant use can cause severe hypotension. The time course and dose-dependency of this interaction are not known.

WARNINGS

Amplification of the vasodilatory effects of Nitrolingual® Pumpspray by certain drugs (phosphodiesterase inhibitors) used to treat erectile dysfunction can result in severe hypotension. The time course and dose dependence of this interaction have not been studied. Appropriate supportive care has not been studied, but it seems reasonable to treat this as a nitrate overdose, with elevation of the extremities and with central volume expansion. The use of any form of nitroglycerin during the early days of acute myocardial infarction requires particular attention to hemodynamic monitoring and clinical status.

PRECAUTIONS (General)

Severe hypotension, particularly with upright posture, may occur even with small doses of nitroglycerin. The drug, therefore, should be used with caution in subjects who may have volume depletion from diuretic therapy or in patients who have low systolic blood pressure (*e.g.*, below 90 mm Hg). Paradoxical bradycardia and increased angina pectoris may accompany nitroglycerin-induced hypotension.
Nitrate therapy may aggravate the angina caused by hypertrophic cardiomyopathy.
Tolerance to this drug and cross-tolerance to other nitrates and nitrites may occur. Tolerance to the vascular and antianginal effects of nitrates has been demonstrated in clinical trials, experience through occupational exposure, and in isolated tissue experiments in the laboratory.
In industrial workers continuously exposed to nitroglycerin, tolerance clearly occurs. Moreover, physical dependence also occurs since chest pain, acute myocardial infarction, and even sudden death have occurred during temporary withdrawal of nitroglycerin from the workers. In various clinical trials in angina patients, there are reports of anginal attacks being more easily provoked and of rebound in the hemodynamic effects soon after nitrate withdrawal. The relative importance of these observations to the routine, clinical use of nitroglycerin is not known.

PRECAUTIONS (INFORMATION FOR PATIENTS)

Physicians should discuss with patients that Nitrolingual® Pumpspray should not be used with certain drugs taken for erectile dysfunction (phosphodiesterase inhibitors) because of the risk of lowering their blood pressure dangerously.
DRUG INTERACTIONS: Alcohol may enhance sensitivity to the hypotensive effects of nitrates. Nitroglycerin acts directly on vascular muscle. Therefore, any other agents that depend on vascular smooth muscle as the final common path can be expected to have decreased or increased effect depending upon the agent.
Marked symptomatic orthostatic hypotension has been reported when calcium channel blockers and oral controlled-release nitroglycerin were used in combination. Dose adjustments of either class of agents may be necessary.
Concomitant use of nitric oxide donors (like Nitrolingual® Pumpspray) and certain drugs for the treatment of erectile dysfunction (phosphodiesterase inhibitors) can amplify their vasodilatory effects, resulting in severe hypotension. The concomitant use of these drugs is contraindicated (see CONTRAINDICATIONS) and alternative therapies should be used to treat acute angina episodes.
CARCINOGENESIS, MUTAGENESIS, IMPAIRMENT OF FERTILITY: Animal carcinogenesis studies with sublingual nitroglycerin have not been performed.
Rats receiving up to 434 mg/kg/day of dietary nitroglycerin for 2 years developed dose-related fibrotic and neoplastic changes in liver, including carcinomas, and interstitial cell tumors in testes. At high dose, the incidences of hepatocellular carcinomas in both sexes were 52% *vs.* 0% in controls, and incidences of testicular tumors were 52% *vs.* 8% in controls. Lifetime dietary administration of up to 1058 mg/kg/day of nitroglycerin was not tumorigenic in mice.
Nitroglycerin was weakly mutagenic in Ames tests performed in two different laboratories. Nevertheless, there was no evidence of mutagenicity in an *in vivo* dominant lethal assay with male rats treated with doses up to about 363 mg/kg/day, p.o., or in *in vitro* cytogenic tests in rat and dog tissues.
In a three-generation reproduction study, rats received dietary nitroglycerin at doses up to about 434 mg/kg/day for six months prior to mating of the F_0 generation with treatment continuing through successive F_1 and F_2 generations. The high dose was associated with decreased feed intake and body weight gain in both sexes at all matings. No specific effect on the fertility of the F_0 generation was seen. Infertility noted in subsequent generations, however, was attributed to increased interstitial cell tissue and aspermatogenesis in the high-dose males. In this three-generation study there was no clear evidence of teratogenicity.
PREGNANCY: Pregnancy Category C – Animal teratology studies have not been conducted with nitroglycerin-pumpspray. Teratology studies in rats and rabbits, however, were conducted with topically applied nitroglycerin ointment at doses up to 80 mg/kg/day and 240 mg/kg/day, respectively. No toxic effects on dams or fetuses were seen at any dose tested. There are no adequate and well-controlled studies in pregnant women. Nitroglycerin should be given to pregnant women only if clearly needed.
NURSING MOTHERS: It is not known whether nitroglycerin is excreted in human milk. Because many drugs are excreted in human milk, caution should be exercised when Nitrolingual® Pumpspray is administered to a nursing woman.
PEDIATRIC USE: Safety and effectiveness of nitroglycerin in pediatric patients have not been established.

ADVERSE REACTIONS

Adverse reactions to oral nitroglycerin dosage forms, particularly headache and hypotension, are generally dose-related. In clinical trials at various doses of nitroglycerin, the following adverse effects have been observed:
Headache, which may be severe and persistent, is the most commonly reported side effect of nitroglycerin with an incidence on the order of about 50% in some studies. Cutaneous vasodilation with flushing may occur. Transient episodes of dizziness and weakness, as well as other signs of cerebral ischemia associated with postural hypotension, may occasionally develop. Occasionally, an individual may exhibit marked sensitivity to the hypotensive effects of nitrates and severe responses (nausea, vomiting, weakness, restlessness, pallor, perspiration and collapse) may occur even with therapeutic doses. Drug rash and/or exfoliative dermatitis have been reported in patients receiving nitrate therapy. Nausea and vomiting appear to be uncommon.
Nitrolingual® Pumpspray given to 51 chronic stable angina patients in single doses of 0.4, 0.8 and 1.6 mg as part of a double-blind, 5-period single-dose cross-over study exhibited an adverse event profile that was generally mild to moderate. Adverse events occurring at a frequency greater than 2% included: headache, dizziness, and paresthesia. Less frequently reported events in this trial included (≤2%): dyspnea, pharyngitis, rhinitis, vasodilation, peripheral edema, asthenia, and abdominal pain.

OVERDOSAGE

Signs and Symptoms:
Nitrate overdosage may result in: severe hypotension, persistent throbbing headache, vertigo, palpitation, visual disturbance, flushing and perspiring skin (later becoming cold and cyanotic), nausea and vomiting (possibly with colic and even bloody diarrhea), syncope (especially in the upright posture), methemoglobinemia with cyanosis and anorexia, initial hyperpnea, dyspnea and slow breathing, slow pulse (dicrotic and intermittent), heart block, increased intracranial pressure with cerebral symptoms of confusion and moderate fever, paralysis and coma followed by clonic convulsions, and possibly death due to circulatory collapse.
Methemoglobinemia:
Case reports of clinically significant methemoglobinemia are rare at conventional doses of organic nitrates. The formation of methemoglobin is dose-related and in the case of genetic abnormalities of hemoglobin that favor methemoglobin formation, even conventional doses of organic nitrates could produce harmful concentrations of methemoglobin.
Treatment of Overdosage:
Keep the patient recumbent in a shock position and comfortably warm. Passive movement of the extremities may aid venous return. Administer oxygen and artificial ventilation, if necessary. If methemoglobinemia is present, administration of methylene blue (1% solution), 1–2 mg per kilogram of body weight intravenously, may be required. If an excessive quantity of Nitrolingual® Pumpspray has been recently swallowed gastric lavage may be of use.

WARNING

Epinephrine is ineffective in reversing the severe hypotensive events associated with overdosage. It and related compounds are contraindicated in this situation.

DOSAGE AND ADMINISTRATION

At the onset of an attack, one or two metered sprays should be administered onto or under the tongue. No more than three metered sprays are recommended within a 15-minute period. If the chest pain persists, prompt medical attention is recommended. Nitrolingual® Pumpspray may be used prophylactically five to ten minutes prior to engaging in activities which might precipitate an acute attack.
Each metered spray of Nitrolingual® Pumpspray delivers 48 mg of solution containing 400 mcg of nitroglycerin after an initial priming of 1 spray. It will remain adequately primed for 6 weeks. If the product is not used within 6 weeks it can be adequately reprimed with 1 spray. There are 60 or 200 metered sprays per bottle. The total number of available doses is dependent, however, on the number of sprays per use (1 or 2 sprays), and the frequency of repriming.
During application the patient should rest, ideally in the sitting position. The container should be held vertically with the valve head uppermost and the spray orifice as close to the mouth as possible. The dose should preferably be

sprayed onto the tongue by pressing the button firmly and the mouth should be closed immediately after each dose. THE SPRAY SHOULD NOT BE INHALED. The medication should not be expectorated or the mouth rinsed for 5 to 10 minutes following administration. Patients should be instructed to familiarize themselves with the position of the spray orifice, which can be identified by the finger rest on top of the valve, in order to facilitate orientation for administration at night.

HOW SUPPLIED

Each box of Nitrolingual® Pumpspray, contains one clear glass bottle coated with red transparent plastic which assists in containing the glass and medication should the bottle be shattered. Each unit contains 4.9 g (NDC 59630-300-65) or 12 g (NDC 59630-300-20) (Net Content) of nitroglycerin lingual spray which will deliver 60 or 200 metered sprays containing 400 mcgs of nitroglycerin per spray. Store at 25 °C (77 °F); excursions permitted to 15–30 °C (59–86 °F) [see USP Controlled Room Temperature].

Note: Nitrolingual® Pumpspray contains 20% alcohol. Do not forcefully open or burn container after use. Do not spray toward flames.

Rx Only.

Manufactured for FIRST HORIZON PHARMACEUTICAL® CORPORATION, Alpharetta, GA 30005 by G. Pohl-Boskamp GmbH & Co., D-25551 Hohenlockstedt, Germany.

06/04

INFORMATION FOR THE PATIENT

Nitrolingual® Pumpspray
(nitroglycerin lingual spray)
400 mcg per spray, 60 or 200 Metered Sprays

Before using your Nitrolingual® Pumpspray (nitroglycerin lingual spray) 400 mcg per spray, 60 or 200 metered sprays, read carefully the following directions for use.

Nitrolingual® Pumpspray is a metered dose spray which delivers 48 mg of solution containing 400 mcg of nitroglycerin with each spray. Nitroglycerin is absorbed from the tongue and surrounding mucosa producing a prompt therapeutic effect. It is best to use Nitrolingual® Pumpspray in a sitting position.

How to Use Nitrolingual® Pumpspray

1. Remove the plastic cover.
2. **DO NOT SHAKE.**
3. Hold the container upright with forefinger on top of the grooved button.
4. Open the mouth and bring the container as close to it as possible.
5. Press the button firmly with the forefinger to release the spray onto or under the tongue. DO NOT INHALE THE SPRAY.
6. Release button and close mouth. Avoid swallowing immediately after administering the spray. The medication should not be expectorated or the mouth rinsed for 5 to 10 minutes following administration.
7. If you require a second administration to obtain relief, repeat steps 4, 5, and 6.
8. Replace the plastic cover.

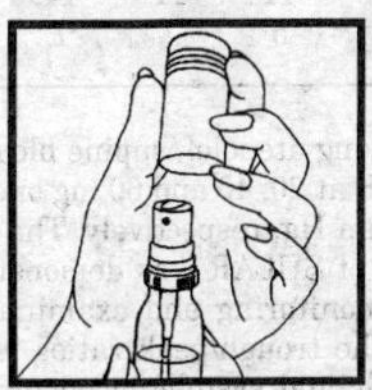

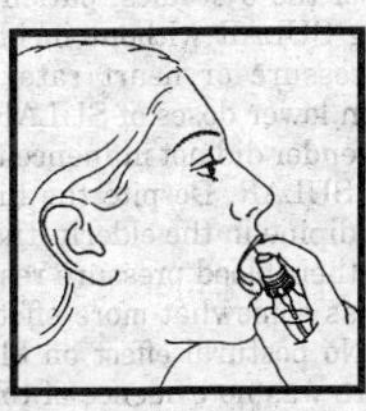

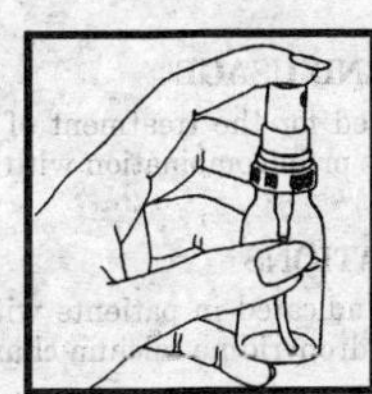

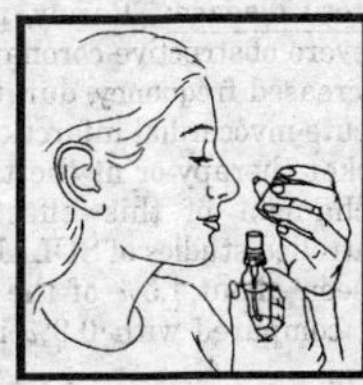

DO NOT SHAKE
HOLD CONTAINER UPRIGHT

NOTE: When using this product for the first time or while priming the container, familiarize yourself with it by actuating the spray into the air (away from yourself and others). Get the feel of your finger resting on the grooved button so that you can use the spray in the dark. **DO NOT SHAKE** the container before use. You may wish to keep additional pumpspray containers handy in convenient locations.

Dosage

During an anginal attack, one or two sprays should be administered into your mouth, preferably onto or under the tongue. Do not inhale spray. The medication should not be expectorated or the mouth rinsed for 5 to 10 minutes following administration. A spray may be repeated approximately every 3–5 minutes as needed. No more than three metered sprays are recommended within a 15-minute period. If chest pain persists, prompt medical attention is recommended. Nitrolingual® Pumpspray may be used 5 to 10 minutes prior to engaging in activities which might provoke an acute attack.

There are approximately 60 or 200 metered sprays of nitroglycerin per Nitrolingual® Pumpspray bottle (including all necessary primes). However, the number of times the medication may be used is dependent on the number of sprays per use (1 or 2 sprays), and frequency of repriming. Each metered spray of Nitrolingual® Pumpspray delivers 400 mcg of nitroglycerin after an initial priming of 1 spray. The container will remain adequately primed for 6 weeks. If the medication is not used within 6 weeks, it can be adequately reprimed with 1 spray.

Precaution

Your physician has determined that this product is likely to help your personal health.

USE THIS PRODUCT AS DIRECTED, BY YOUR PHYSICIAN.

If you have any questions about alternatives, consult with your physician.

Do not share or give your medication to others, particularly those who may appear to be having chest discomfort similar to yours.

Nitrolingual® Pumpspray should be used during an episode of chest pain or may be used 5 to 10 minutes prior to engaging in activities which might provoke an acute attack.

Nitrolingual® Pumpspray is available in a clear glass bottle with a red plastic coating on the exterior. This plastic coating is designed to contain the glass and medication should the bottle be shattered. The transparent container can be used for continuous monitoring of the consumption. The end of the pump should be covered by the fluid level. As with all other sprays, there is a residual volume of fluid at the bottome of the bottle which cannot be used. Nitrolingual® Pumpspray contains 20% alcohol. Do not forcefully open or burn container. Do not spray toward flames. **Keep in a safe place and out of the reach of children.**

Store at 25 °C (77 °F); excursions permitted to 15–30 °C (59–86 °F) [see USP Controlled Room Temperature].

Manufactured for FIRST HORIZON PHARMACEUTICAL® CORPORATION, Alpharetta, GA 30005 by G. Pohl-Boskamp GmbH & Co., D-25551 Hohenlockstedt, Germany.

Shown in Product Identification Guide, page 312

PONSTEL® ℞

[*pŏn 'stĕl"*]
(Mefenamic Acid Capsules)

DESCRIPTION

Ponstel® (mefenamic acid) is a member of the fenamate group of nonsteroidal anti-inflammatory drugs (NSAIDs). Each blue-banded, ivory capsule contains 250 mg of mefenamic acid for oral administration. Mefenamic acid is a white to greyish-white, odorless, microcrystalline powder with a melting point of 230°–231°C and water solubility of 0.004% at pH 7.1. The chemical name is N-2,3-xylylanthranilic acid. The molecular weight is 241.29. Its molecular formula is $C_{15}H_{15}NO_2$ and the structural formula of mefenamic acid is:

COOH, NH, CH_3, CH_3

Each capsule also contains lactose, NF. The capsule shell and/or band contains citric acid, USP; D&C yellow No. 10; FD&C blue No. 1; FD&C red No. 3; FD&C yellow No. 6; gelatin, NF; glycerol monooleate; silicon dioxide, NF; sodium benzoate, NF; sodium lauryl sulfate, NF; titanium dioxide, USP.

HOW SUPPLIED

Ponstel (mefenamic acid) is available as 250 mg blue-banded, ivory capsules, imprinted with "FHPC 400" and "PONSTEL®".

Bottles of 100 NDC 59630-400-10

Storage

Store at 20–25°C (68–77°F) [See USP Controlled Room Temperature].

REFERENCES

1. Neuvonen PJ, Kivisto KT: Enhancement of drug absorption by antacids. An unrecognized drug interaction. *Clin Pharmacokinet.* 27: 120–8, Aug 1994.
2. Tall AR, Mistilits SP: Studies on Ponstan (mefenamic acid): I. Gastro-intestinal blood loss; II. Absorption and excretion of a new formulation. *J Int Med Res* (UK). 1975, 3 (3) p176-82.
3. Winder CV, Kaump DH, Glazko et al: Experimental observations of flufenamic, mefenamic, and meclofenamic acids. *AnnPhys Med* (Eng), Suppl p7–49. 1967.
4. Glazko AJ: Experimental observations of flufenamic, mefenamic, and meclofenamic acids. Part III. Metabolic disposition, in *Fenamates in Medicine.* A Symposium, London, 1966. *Annals of Physical Medicine,* Supplement, pp 23–36, 1967.
5. Data on file, First Horizon (Protocol 356).
6. Budoff PW: Use of mefenamic acid in the treatment of primary dysmenorrhea. *JAMA.* 241:2713–2716, 1979.
7. Buchanan RA, et al. The breast milk excretion of mefenamic acid. *Curr Ther Res.* 10:592, 1968.
8. Corby DG, Decker WJ: Management of acute poisoning with activated charcoal. *Pediatrics.* 54:324, 1974.
9. Champion GD, Graham GG: Pharmacokinetics of nonsteroidal anti-inflammatory agents. *Aust NZ J Med.* 8 (Supp 1): 94–100, Jun 1978.
10. McGurk KA, Remmel RP, Hosagrahara VP, Tosh D, Burchell B: Reactivity of mefenamic acid 1-o- acyl glucuronide with proteins in vitro and ex vivo. *Drug Metab Dispos.* Aug 1996, 24 (8) p842–9.
11. Ito K, Niida Y, Sato J et al: Pharmacokinetics of mefenamic acid in preterm infants with patent ductus arteriosus. *Acta Paediatr JPN.* 36 (4): 387-91, 1994.

Distributed by:
FIRST HORIZON PHARMACEUTICAL CORPORATION
Alpharetta, GA 30005
Revised October 2003
PON-PI-1

PRENATE ELITE™ Tablets ℞

DESCRIPTION

PRENATE ELITE™ is a white oval oil- and water-soluble multivitamin/multimineral film-coated tablet debossed with "PN" on one side.

Each tablet contains:

Elemental Iron (carbonyl iron)	90 mg
Biotin	30 mcg
Pantothenic acid (calcium pantothenate, USP)	6 mg
Calcium (calcium carbonate, USP)	200 mg
Copper (cupric oxide)	2 mg
Zinc (zinc oxide, USP)	15 mg
Folate	1 mg
(L-methylfolate as Metafolin® 600 mcg)	
(folic acid, USP 400 mcg)	
Vitamin D_3 (cholecalciferol)	400 IU
Vitamin E (dl-alpha tocopheryl acetate)	10 IU
Vitamin C (ascorbic acid, USP)	120 mg
Vitamin B_1 (thiamine mononitrate, USP)	3 mg
Vitamin B_2 (riboflavin, USP)	3.4 mg
Vitamin B_6 (pyridoxine HCl)	20 mg
Vitamin B_{12} (cyanocobalamin)	12 mcg
Niacinamide, USP	20 mg
Magnesium (magnesium oxide, USP)	30 mg
Docusate Sodium, USP	50 mg

Other Ingredients: calcium phosphate dibasic, carnauba wax, crospovidone, dextrin, dl-alpha tocopherol, gelatin, hypromellose, lactose, magnesium stearate, mono and diglycerides, polacrilin, pregelatinized starch, propylene glycol, silicon dioxide, sodium benzoate, partially hydrogenated soybean oil, starch, stearic acid, sucrose, titanium dioxide, and other ingredients.

INDICATIONS

PRENATE ELITE™ is a multivitamin/multimineral nutritional supplement indicated for use in improving the nutritional status of women throughout pregnancy and in the postnatal period for both lactating and nonlactating mothers. PRENATE ELITE™ can also be beneficial in improving the nutritional status of women prior to conception.

CONTRAINDICATIONS

This product is contraindicated in patients with a known hypersensitivity to any of the ingredients.

WARNING

Accidental overdose of iron-containing products is a leading cause of fatal poisoning in children under 6. Keep this product out of reach of children. In case of accidental overdose, call a doctor or poison control center immediately.

PRECAUTIONS

Folic acid alone is improper therapy in the treatment of pernicious anemia and other megaloblastic anemias where vitamin B_{12} is deficient. Folic acid in doses above 0.1 mg daily

Continued on next page

Prenate Elite—Cont.

may obscure pernicious anemia in that hematologic remission can occur while neurological manifestations progress.

ADVERSE REACTIONS

Allergic sensitization has been reported following both oral and parenteral administration of folic acid.

DOSAGE AND ADMINISTRATION

One tablet daily or as directed by a physician.

HOW SUPPLIED

Child-resistant unit-dose packs of 90 geltabs
NDC 59630-411-90

KEEP THIS AND ALL DRUGS OUT OF THE REACH OF CHILDREN.

Store at 20°-25°C (68°-77°F). Excursions permitted to 15°-30°C (59°-86°F). [See USP Controlled Room Temperature]

NOTICE: Contact with moisture may produce surface discoloration and/or erosion of the tablet.

FIRST HORIZON PHARMACEUTICAL® CORPORATION
Manufactured for
First Horizon Pharmaceutical® Corporation
Alpharetta, GA 30005
Manufactured by Patheon Inc.
Mississauga, ON L5N 7K9
Made in Canada
For inquiries call 1-800-849-9707

ROBINUL® and ROBINUL® FORTE ℞
(Glycopyrrolate tablets, USP)

DESCRIPTION

Robinul® and Robinul® Forte tablets contain the synthetic anticholinergic, glycopyrrolate. Glycopyrrolate is a quaternary ammonium compound with the following chemical name: 3-[(cyclopentylhydroxyphenylacetyl)oxy]-1, 1-dimethylpyrrolidinium bromide.

Robinul tablets are scored, compressed white tablets engraved HPC 200. Each tablet contains:
Glycopyrrolate, USP .... 1 mg

Robinul Forte tablets are scored, compressed white tablets engraved HORIZON 205. Each tablet contains:
Glycopyrrolate, USP .... 2 mg

Inactive Ingredients: Dibasic Calcium Phosphate, Lactose, Magnesium Stearate, Povidone, Sodium Starch Glycolate.

HOW SUPPLIED

Robinul® (glycopyrrolate, 1 mg) tablets in bottles of 100 (NDC 59630-200-10).

Robinul® Forte (glycopyrrolate, 2 mg) tablets in bottles of 100 (NDC 59630-205-10).

Store at controlled room temperature, 20°C to 25°C (68°F to 77°F).

Dispense in tight container.

Manufactured by:
MIKART, INC.
Atlanta, GA 30318
Manufactured for:
First Horizon Pharmaceutical™ Corporation
Roswell, GA 30076
℞ only
Rev. 01/03 Code 883A00

SULAR® ℞
[su-lar]
(Nisoldipine)
Extended Release Tablets
For Oral Use

DESCRIPTION

SULAR® (nisoldipine) is an extended release tablet dosage form of the dihydropyridine calcium channel blocker nisoldipine. Nisoldipine is 3,5-pyridinedicarboxylic acid, 1,4-dihydro-2,6-dimethyl-4-(2-nitrophenyl)-, methyl 2-methylpropyl ester, $C_{20}H_{24}N_2O_6$, and has the structural formula:

Nisoldipine is a yellow crystalline substance, practically insoluble in water but soluble in ethanol. It has a molecular weight of 388.4. SULAR tablets consist of an external coat and an internal core. Both coat and core contain nisoldipine, the coat as a slow release formulation and the core as a fast release formulation. SULAR tablets contain either 10, 20, 30 or 40 mg of nisoldipine for once-a-day oral administration.

Inert ingredients in the formulation are: hydroxypropylcellulose, lactose, corn starch, crospovidone, microcrystalline cellulose, sodium lauryl sulfate, povidone and magnesium stearate. The inert ingredients in the film coating are: hypromellose, polyethylene glycol, ferric oxide, and titanium dioxide.

CLINICAL PHARMACOLOGY

Mechanism of Action

Nisoldipine is a member of the dihydropyridine class of calcium channel antagonists (calcium ion antagonists or slow channel blockers) that inhibit the transmembrane influx of calcium into vascular smooth muscle and cardiac muscle. It reversibly competes with other dihydropyridines for binding to the calcium channel. Because the contractile process of vascular smooth muscle is dependent upon the movement of extracellular calcium into the muscle through specific ion channels, inhibition of the calcium channel results in dilation of the arterioles. *In vitro* studies show that the effects of nisoldipine on contractile processes are selective, with greater potency on vascular smooth muscle than on cardiac muscle. Although, like other dihydropyridine calcium channel blockers, nisoldipine has negative inotropic effects *in vitro*, studies conducted in intact anesthetized animals have shown that the vasodilating effect occurs at doses lower than those that affect cardiac contractility.

The effect of nisoldipine on blood pressure is principally a consequence of a dose-related decrease of peripheral vascular resistance. While nisoldipine, like other dihydropyridines, exhibits a mild diuretic effect, most of the antihypertensive activity is attributed to its effect on peripheral vascular resistance.

Pharmacokinetics and Metabolism

Nisoldipine pharmacokinetics are independent of the dose in the range of 20 to 60 mg, with plasma concentrations proportional to dose. Nisoldipine accumulation, during multiple dosing, is predictable from a single dose.

Nisoldipine is relatively well absorbed into the systemic circulation with 87% of the radiolabeled drug recovered in urine and feces. The absolute bioavailability of nisoldipine is about 5%. Nisoldipine's low bioavailability is due, in part, to pre-systemic metabolism in the gut wall, and this metabolism decreases from the proximal to the distal parts of the intestine. Food with a high fat content has a pronounced effect on the release of nisoldipine from the coat-core formulation and results in a significant increase in peak concentration (C_{max}) by up to 300%. Total exposure, however, is decreased about 25%, presumably because more of the drug is released proximally. This effect appears to be specific for nisoldipine in the controlled release formulation, as a less pronounced food effect was seen with the immediate release tablet. Concomitant intake of a high fat meal with SULAR should be avoided.

Maximal plasma concentrations of nisoldipine are reached 6 to 12 hours after dosing. The terminal elimination half-life (reflecting post absorption clearance of nisoldipine) ranges from 7 to 12 hours. C_{max} and AUC increase by factors of approximately 1.3 and 1.5, respectively, from first dose to steady state. After oral administration, the concentration of (+) nisoldipine, the active enantiomer, is about 6 times higher than the (−) inactive enantiomer. The plasma protein binding of nisoldipine is very high, with less than 1% unbound over the plasma concentration range of 100 ng/mL to 10 mcg/mL.

Nisoldipine is highly metabolized; 5 major urinary metabolites have been identified. Although 60-80% of an oral dose undergoes urinary excretion, only traces of unchanged nisoldipine are found in urine. The major biotransformation pathway appears to be the hydroxylation of the isobutyl ester. A hydroxylated derivative of the side chain, present in plasma at concentrations approximately equal to the parent compound, appears to be the only active metabolite, and has about 10% of the activity of the parent compound. Cytochrome P_{450} enzymes are believed to play a major role in the metabolism of nisoldipine. The particular isoenzyme system responsible for its metabolism has not been identified, but other dihydropyridines are metabolized by cytochrome P_{450} IIIA4. Nisoldipine should not be administered with grapefruit juice as this has been shown, in a study of 12 subjects, to interfere with nisoldipine metabolism, resulting in a mean increase in C_{max} of about 3-fold (ranging up to about 7-fold) and AUC of almost 2-fold (ranging up to about 5-fold). A similar phenomenon has been seen with several other dihydropyridine calcium channel blockers.

Special Populations

Renal Dysfunction: Because renal elimination is not an important pathway, bioavailability and pharmacokinetics of SULAR were not significantly different in patients with various degrees of renal impairment. Dosing adjustments in patients with mild to moderate renal impairment are not necessary.

Geriatric: Elderly patients have been found to have 2 to 3 fold higher plasma concentrations (C_{max} and AUC) than young subjects. This should be reflected in more cautious dosing (See DOSAGE AND ADMINISTRATION).

Hepatic Insufficiency: In patients with liver cirrhosis given 10 mg SULAR, plasma concentrations of the parent compound were 4 to 5 times higher than those in healthy young subjects. Lower starting and maintenance doses should be used in cirrhotic patients (See DOSAGE AND ADMINISTRATION).

Gender and Race: The effect of gender or race on the pharmacokinetics of nisoldipine has not been investigated.

Disease States: Hypertension does not significantly alter the pharmacokinetics of nisoldipine.

Pharmacodynamics

Hemodynamic Effects

Administration of a single dose of nisoldipine leads to decreased systemic vascular resistance and blood pressure with a transient increase in heart rate. The change in heart rate is greater with immediate release nisoldipine preparations. The effect on blood pressure is directly related to the initial degree of elevation above normal. Chronic administration of nisoldipine results in a sustained decrease in vascular resistance and small increases in stroke index and left ventricular ejection fraction. A study of the immediate release formulation showed no effect of nisoldipine on the renin-angiotensin-aldosterone system or on plasma norepinephrine concentration in normals. Changes in blood pressure in hypertensive patients given SULAR were dose related over the range of 10-60 mg/day.

Nisoldipine does not appear to have significant negative inotropic activity in intact animals or humans, and did not lead to worsening of clinical heart failure in three small studies of patients with asymptomatic and symptomatic left ventricular dysfunction. There is little information, however, in patients with severe congestive heart failure, and all calcium channel blockers should be used with caution in any patient with heart failure.

Electrophysiologic Effects

Nisoldipine has no clinically important chronotropic effects. Except for mild shortening of sinus cycle, SA conduction time and AH intervals, single oral doses up to 20 mg of immediate release nisoldipine did not significantly change other conduction parameters. Similar electrophysiologic effects were seen with single iv doses, which could be blunted in patients pre-treated with beta-blockers. Dose and plasma level related flattening or inversion of T-waves have been observed in a few small studies. Such reports were concentrated in patients receiving rapidly increased high doses in one study; the phenomenon has not been a cause of safety concern in large clinical trials.

Clinical Studies in Hypertension

The antihypertensive efficacy of SULAR was studied in 5 double-blind, placebo-controlled, randomized studies, in which over 600 patients were treated with SULAR as monotherapy and about 300 with placebo; 4 of the five studies compared 2 or 3 fixed doses while the fifth allowed titration from 10-40 mg. Once daily administration of SULAR produced sustained reductions in systolic and diastolic blood pressures over the 24 hour dosing interval in both supine and standing positions. The mean placebo-subtracted reductions in supine systolic and diastolic blood pressure at trough, 24 hours post-dose, in these studies, are shown below. Changes in standing blood pressure were similar:

MEAN SUPINE THROUGH SYSTOLIC AND DIASTOLIC BLOOD PRESSURE CHANGES (mm Hg)

SULAR Dose (mg/day)	10 mg	20 mg	30 mg	40 mg	60 mg	10-40 mg titrated
Systolic	8	11	11	14	15	15
Diastolic	3	5	7	7	10	8

In patients receiving atenolol, supine blood pressure reductions with SULAR at 20, 40 and 60 mg once daily were 12/6, 19/8 and 22/10 mm Hg, respectively. The sustained antihypertensive effect of SULAR was demonstrated by 24 hour blood pressure monitoring and examination of peak and trough effects. The trough/peak ratios ranged from 70 to 100% for diastolic and systolic blood pressure. The mean change in heart rate in these studies was less than one beat per minute. In 4 of the 5 studies, patients received initial doses of 20-30 mg SULAR without incident (excessive effects on blood pressure or heart rate). The fifth study started patients on lower doses of SULAR.

Patient race and gender did not influence the blood pressure lowering effect of SULAR. Despite the higher plasma concentration of nisoldipine in the elderly, there was no consistent difference in their blood pressure response except that the 10 mg dose was somewhat more effective than in non-elderly patients. No postural effect on blood pressure was apparent and there was no evidence of tolerance to the antihypertensive effect of SULAR in patients treated for up to one year.

INDICATIONS AND USAGE

SULAR is indicated for the treatment of hypertension. It may be used alone or in combination with other antihypertensive agents.

CONTRAINDICATIONS

SULAR is contraindicated in patients with known hypersensitivity to dihydropyridine calcium channel blockers.

WARNINGS

Increased angina and/or myocardial infarction in patients with coronary artery disease: Rarely, patients, particularly those with severe obstructive coronary artery disease, have developed increased frequency, duration and/or severity of angina, or acute myocardial infarction on starting calcium channel blocker therapy or at the time of dosage increase. The mechanism of this effect has not been established. In controlled studies of SULAR in patients with angina this was seen about 1.5% of the time in patients given nisoldipine, compared with 0.9% in patients given placebo.

PRECAUTIONS

General

Hypotension: Because nisoldipine, like other vasodilators, decreases peripheral vascular resistance, careful monitoring of blood pressure during the initial administration and titration of SULAR is recommended. Close observation is especially important for patients already taking medications that are known to lower blood pressure. Although in most patients the hypotensive effect of SULAR is modest and well tolerated, occasional patients have had excessive and poorly tolerated hypotension. These responses have usually occurred during initial titration or at the time of subsequent upward dosage adjustment.

Congestive Heart Failure: Although acute hemodynamic studies of nisoldipine in patients with NYHA Class II-IV heart failure have not demonstrated negative inotropic effects, safety of SULAR in patients with heart failure has not been established. Caution therefore should be exercised when using SULAR in patients with heart failure or compromised ventricular function, particularly in combination with a beta-blocker.

Patients with Hepatic Impairment: Because nisoldipine is extensively metabolized by the liver and, in patients with cirrhosis, it reaches blood concentrations about 5 times those in normals, SULAR should be administered cautiously in patients with severe hepatic dysfunction (See DOSAGE AND ADMINISTRATION).

Information for Patients: SULAR is an extended release tablet and should be swallowed whole. Tablets should not be chewed, divided or crushed. SULAR should not be administered with a high fat meal. Grapefruit juice, which has been shown to increase significantly the bioavailability of nisoldipine and other dihydropyridine type calcium channel blockers, should not be taken with SULAR.

Laboratory Tests: SULAR is not known to interfere with the interpretation of laboratory tests.

Drug Interactions: A 30 to 45% increase in AUC and C_{max} of nisoldipine was observed with concomitant administration of cimetidine 400 mg twice daily. Ranitidine 150 mg twice daily did not interact significantly with nisoldipine (AUC was decreased by 15-20%). No pharmacodynamic effects of either histamine H_2 receptor antagonist were observed.

Coadministration of phenytoin with 40 mg SULAR tablets in epileptic patients lowered the nisoldipine plasma concentrations to undetectable levels. Coadministration of SULAR with phenytoin or any known CYP3A4 inducer should be avoided and alternative antihypertensive therapy should be considered. Pharmacokinetic interactions between nisoldipine and beta-blockers (atenolol, propranolol) were variable and not significant. Propranolol attenuated the heart rate increase following administration of immediate release nisoldipine. The blood pressure effect of SULAR tended to be greater in patients on atenolol than in patients on no other antihypertensive therapy. Quinidine at 648 mg bid decreased the bioavailability (AUC) of nisoldipine by 26%, but not the peak concentration. The immediate release, but not the coat-core formulation of nisoldipine increased plasma quinidine concentrations by about 20%. This interaction was not accompanied by ECG changes and its clinical significance is not known. No significant interactions were found between nisoldipine and warfarin or digoxin.

Carcinogenesis, Mutagenesis, Impairment of Fertility: Dietary administration of nisoldipine to male and female rats for up to 24 months (mean doses up to 82 and 111 mg/kg/day, 16 and 19 times the maximum recommended human dose (MRHD) on a mg/m^2 basis, respectively) and female mice for up to 21 months (mean doses of up to 217 mg/kg/day, 20 times the MRHD on a mg/m^2 basis) revealed no evidence of tumorigenic effect of nisoldipine. In male mice receiving a mean dose of 163 mg nisoldipine/kg/day (16 times the MRHD of 60 mg/day on a mg/m^2 basis), an increased frequency of stomach papilloma, but still within the historical range, was observed. No evidence of stomach neoplasia was observed at lower doses (up to 58 mg/kg/day). Nisoldipine was negative when tested in a battery of genotoxicity assays including the Ames test and the CHO/HGRPT assay for mutagenicity and the *in vivo* mouse micronucleus test and *in vitro* CHO cell test for clastogenicity. When administered to male and female rats at doses of up to 30 mg/kg/day (about 5 times the MRHD on a mg/m^2 basis) nisoldipine had no effect on fertility.

Pregnancy Category C: Nisoldipine was neither teratogenic nor fetotoxic at doses that were not maternally toxic. Nisoldipine was fetotoxic but not teratogenic in rats and rabbits at doses resulting in maternal toxicity (reduced maternal body weight gain). In pregnant rats, increased fetal resorption (postimplantation loss) was observed at 100 mg/kg/day and decreased fetal weight was observed at both 30 and 100 mg/kg/day. These doses are, respectively, about 5 and 16 times the MRHD when compared on a mg/m^2 basis. In pregnant rabbits, decreased fetal and placental weights were observed at a dose of 30 mg/kg/day, about 10 times the MRHD when compared on a mg/m^2 basis. In a study in which pregnant monkeys (both treated and control) had high rates of abortion and mortality, the only surviving fetus from a group exposed to a maternal dose of 100 mg nisoldipine/kg/day (about 30 times the MRHD when compared on a mg/m^2 basis) presented with forelimb and vertebral abnormalities not previously seen in control monkeys of the same strain. There are no adequate and well controlled studies in pregnant women. SULAR should be used in pregnancy only if the potential benefit justifies the potential risk to the fetus.

Nursing Mothers: It is not known whether nisoldipine is excreted in human milk. Because many drugs are excreted in human milk, a decision should be made to discontinue nursing, or to discontinue SULAR, taking into account the importance of the drug to the mother.

Pediatric Use: Safety and effectiveness in pediatric patients have not been established.

Geriatric Use: Clinical studies of nisoldipine did not include sufficient numbers of subjects aged 65 and over to determine whether they respond differently from younger subjects. Other reported clinical experience has not identified differences in responses between the elderly and younger patients. Patients over 65 are expected to develop higher plasma concentrations of nisoldipine. In general, dose selection for an elderly patient should be cautious, usually starting at the low end of the dosing range, reflecting the greater frequency of decreased hepatic, renal or cardiac function, and of concomitant disease or other drug therapy.

ADVERSE EXPERIENCES

More than 6000 patients world-wide have received nisoldipine in clinical trials for the treatment of hypertension, either as the immediate release or the SULAR extended release formulation. Of about 1,500 patients who received

SULAR in hypertension studies, about 55% were exposed for at least 2 months and about one third were exposed for over 6 months, the great majority at doses of 20 to 60 mg daily.

SULAR is generally well-tolerated. In the U.S. clinical trials of SULAR in hypertension, 10.9% of the 921 SULAR patients discontinued treatment due to adverse events compared with 2.9% of 280 placebo patients. The frequency of discontinuations due to adverse experiences was related to dose, with a 5.4% discontinuation rate at 10 mg daily and a 10.9% discontinuation rate at 60 mg daily.

The most frequently occurring adverse experiences with SULAR are those related to its vasodilator properties; these are generally mild and only occasionally lead to patient withdrawal from treatment. The table below, from U.S. placebo-controlled parallel dose response trials of SULAR using doses from 10-60 mg once daily in patients with hypertension, lists all of the adverse events, regardless of the causal relationship to SULAR, for which the overall incidence on SULAR was both >1% and greater with SULAR than with placebo.

Adverse Event	Nisoldipine (%) (n=663)	Placebo (%) (n=280)
Peripheral Edema	22	10
Headache	22	15
Dizziness	5	4
Pharyngitis	5	4
Vasodilation	4	2
Sinusitis	3	2
Palpitation	3	1
Chest Pain	2	1
Nausea	2	1
Rash	2	1

Only peripheral edema and possibly dizziness appear to be dose related.

Adverse Event	Placebo	SULAR 10 mg	20 mg	30 mg	40 mg	60 mg
(Rates in %)	N=280	N=30	N=170	N=105	N=139	N=137
Peripheral Edema	10	7	15	20	27	29
Dizziness	4	7	3	3	4	10

The common adverse events occurred at about the same rate in men as in women, and at a similar rate in patients over age 65 as in those under that age, except that headache was much less common in older patients. Except for peripheral edema and vasodilation, which were more common in whites, adverse event rates were similar in blacks and whites.

The following adverse events occurred in ≤1% of all patients treated for hypertension in U.S. and foreign clinical trials, or with unspecified incidence in other studies. Although a causal relationship of SULAR to these events cannot be established, they are listed to alert the physician to a possible relationship with SULAR treatment.

Body As A Whole: cellulitis, chills, facial edema, fever, flu syndrome, malaise

Cardiovascular: atrial fibrillation, cerebrovascular accident, congestive heart failure, first degree AV block, hypertension, hypotension, jugular venous distension, migraine, myocardial infarction, postural hypotension, ventricular extrasystoles, supraventricular tachycardia, syncope, systolic ejection murmur, T wave abnormalities on ECG (flattening, inversion, nonspecific changes), venous insufficiency

Digestive: abnormal liver function tests, anorexia, colitis, diarrhea, dry mouth, dyspepsia, dysphagia, flatulence, gastritis, gastrointestinal hemorrhage, gingival hyperplasia, glossitis, hepatomegaly, increased appetite, melena, mouth ulceration

Endocrine: diabetes mellitus, thyroiditis

Hemic and Lymphatic: anemia, ecchymoses, leukopenia, petechiae

Metabolic and Nutritional: gout, hypokalemia, increased serum creatine kinase, increased nonprotein nitrogen, weight gain, weight loss

Musculoskeletal: arthralgia, arthritis, leg cramps, myalgia, myasthenia, myositis, tenosynovitis

Nervous: abnormal dreams, abnormal thinking and confusion, amnesia, anxiety, ataxia, cerebral ischemia, decreased libido, depression, hypesthesia, hypertonia, insomnia, nervousness, paresthesia, somnolence, tremor, vertigo

Respiratory: asthma, dyspnea, end inspiratory wheeze and fine rales, epistaxis, increased cough, laryngitis, pharyngitis, pleural effusion, rhinitis, sinusitis

Skin and Appendages: acne, alopecia, dry skin, exfoliative dermatitis, fungal dermatitis, herpes simplex, herpes zoster, maculopapular rash, pruritus, pustular rash, skin discoloration, skin ulcer, sweating, urticaria

Special Senses: abnormal vision, amblyopia, blepharitis, conjunctivitis, ear pain, glaucoma, itchy eyes, keratoconjunctivitis, otitis media, retinal detachment, tinnitus, watery eyes, taste disturbance, temporary unilateral loss of vision, vitreous floater

Urogenital: dysuria, hematuria, impotence, nocturia, urinary frequency, increased BUN and serum creatinine, vaginal hemorrhage, vaginitis.

The following postmarketing event has been reported very rarely in patients receiving SULAR: systemic hypersensitivity reaction which may include one or more of the following; angioedema, shortness of breath, tachycardia, chest tightness, hypotension, and rash. A definite causal relationship with SULAR has not been established. An unusual event observed with immediate release nisoldipine but not observed with SULAR was one case of photosensitivity. Gynecomastia has been associated with the use of calcium channel blockers.

OVERDOSAGE

There is no experience with nisoldipine overdosage. Generally, overdosage with other dihydropyridines leading to pronounced hypotension calls for active cardiovascular support including monitoring of cardiovascular and respiratory function, elevation of extremities, judicious use of calcium infusion, pressor agents and fluids. Clearance of nisoldipine would be expected to be slowed in patients with impaired liver function. Since nisoldipine is highly protein bound, dialysis is not likely to be of any benefit; however, plasmapheresis may be beneficial.

DOSAGE AND ADMINISTRATION

The dosage of SULAR must be adjusted to each patient's needs. Therapy usually should be initiated with 20 mg orally once daily, then increased by 10 mg per week or longer intervals, to attain adequate control of blood pressure. Usual maintenance dosage is 20 to 40 mg once daily. Blood pressure response increases over the 10-60 mg daily dose range but adverse event rates also increase. Doses beyond 60 mg once daily are not recommended. SULAR has been used safely with diuretics, ACE inhibitors, and beta-blocking agents. Patients over age 65, or patients with impaired liver function are expected to develop higher plasma concentrations of nisoldipine. Their blood pressure should be monitored closely during any dosage adjustment. A starting dose not exceeding 10 mg daily is recommended in these patient groups. SULAR tablets should be administered orally once daily. Administration with a high fat meal can lead to excessive peak drug concentration and should be avoided. Grapefruit products should be avoided before and after dosing. SULAR is an extended release dosage form and tablets should be swallowed whole, not bitten, divided or crushed.

HOW SUPPLIED

SULAR extended release tablets are supplied as 10 mg, 20 mg, 30 mg, and 40 mg round film coated tablets. The different strengths can be identified as follows:

Strength	Color	Markings
10 mg	Oyster	440 on one side and FH 10 on the other side.
20 mg	Yellow Cream	441 on one side and FH 20 on the other side.
30 mg	Mustard	442 on one side and FH 30 on the other side.
40 mg	Burnt Orange	443 on one side and FH 40 on the other side.

SULAR Tablets are supplied in:

	Strength	NDC Code
Bottles of 100	10 mg	59630-440-10
	20 mg	59630-441-10
	30 mg	59630-442-10
	40 mg	59630-443-10

Protect from light and moisture. Store at 20-25°C (68-77°F); excursions permitted to 15-30°C (59-86°F) [See USP Controlled Room Temperature]. Dispense in tight, light-resistant containers.

℞ **Only**

Continued on next page

Sular—Cont.

SULAR® is a trademark of
First Horizon Pharmaceutical™ Corporation

Manufactured for:
First Horizon Pharmaceutical™ Corporation
Alpharetta, GA 30005
By: Bayer AG, Leverkusen, Germany
Made in Germany SUL-PI-3 Rev 03/04
Code 953A00 Printed in U.S.A.

TANAFED DMX™ SUSPENSION ℞

[tă-nă-fĕd]
℞ Only

DESCRIPTION

Each 5 mL contains:

Dexchlorpheniramine tannate	2.5 mg
Pseudoephedrine tannate	75.0 mg
Dextromethorphan tannate	25.0 mg

in a blue, cotton candy flavored, homogeneous suspension. Inactive ingredients: citric acid, FD&C Blue #1, flavor, glycerin, magnesium aluminum silicate, methylparaben, sodium benzoate, sodium citrate, sodium saccharin, sucrose, purified water, xanthan gum.

HOW SUPPLIED

Tanafed DMX™ Suspension, each teaspoonful (5mL) of which contains dexchlorpheniramine tannate 2.5 mg; dextromethorphan tannate 25.0 mg; and pseudoephedrine tannate 75.0 mg is supplied as a blue colored, cotton candy flavored homogeneous suspension. Tanafed DMX™ Suspension is available in bottles of 16 fl oz (473 mL) NDC 59630-470-16; in bottles of 4 fl oz (118 mL) NDC 59630- 470-04; and in bottles of 20 mL NDC 59630-470-20.

Dispense in a tight, light-resistant container with a child-resistant closure. Shake well before use.

Store at 20–25°C (68–77°F); excursions permitted to 15°–30° C (59°–86° F) [See USP Controlled Room Temperature]. Protect from freezing.

Keep this and all drugs out of the reach of children. In case of accidental overdose, seek professional assistance or contact a Poison Control Center immediately.

Manufactured by:
ELGE, INC.
Rosenberg, TX 77471
Manufactured for:
FIRST HORIZON PHARMACEUTICAL® CORPORATION
Alpharetta, GA 30005
U.S. Patent 5,663,415; 6,509,492; 6,670,370;
Other patents pending

Rev. 2/04

TANAFED DP™ SUSPENSION ℞

[tă-nă-fĕd]
℞ Only

DESCRIPTION

Each 5 mL contains:

Dexchlorpheniramine tannate	2.5 mg
Pseudoephedrine tannate	75.0 mg

in a red, strawberry-banana flavored, homogeneous suspension. Inactive ingredients: citric acid, FD&C Red #40, flavor, glycerin, magnesium aluminum silicate, methyl- paraben, sodium benzoate, sodium citrate, sodium saccharin, sucrose, purified water, xanthan gum.

HOW SUPPLIED

Tanafed DP™ Suspension, each teaspoonful (5mL) of which contains dexchlorpheniramine tannate 2.5 mg and pseudoephedrine tannate 75.0 mg, is supplied as a red colored, strawberry-banana fla- vored homogeneous suspension. Tanafed DP™ Suspension is available in bottles of 16 fl oz (473 mL) NDC 59630-465-16; in bottles of 4 fl oz (118 mL) NDC 59630-465-04; and in bottles of 20 mL NDC 59630-465-20.

Dispense in a tight, light-resistant container with a child-resistant closure. Shake well before use.

Store at 20–25°C (68–77°F); excursions permitted to 15–30°C (59–86°F) [See USP Controlled Room Temperature]. Protect from freezing.

Keep this and all drugs out of the reach of children. In case of accidental overdose, seek profes- sional assistance or contact a Poison Control Center immediately.

Manufactured by:
ELGE, INC.
Rosenberg, TX 77471
Manufactured For:
FIRST HORIZON PHARMACEUTICAL® CORPORATION
Alpharetta, GA 30005
U.S. Patent 5,663,415; 6,509,492;
Other patents pending

Rev. 2/04

C. B. Fleet Co., Inc.

4615 MURRAY PLACE
LYNCHBURG, VA 24502

Direct Inquiries to:
Joseph A. Kanapka, Ph.D.
Director of Product Safety
(434) 528-4000

FLEET® GLYCERIN LAXATIVES: SUPPOSITORIES AND LIQUID GLYCERIN SUPPOSITORIES OTC

(glycerin USP)

COMPOSITION

FLEET® Babylax®—Each rectal applicator delivers 2.3 g of glycerin USP.

FLEET® Liquid Glycerin Suppositories for Adults and Children 6 years of age and over—Each rectal applicator delivers 5.6 g of glycerin USP.

FLEET® Maximum-Strength Glycerin Suppositories for Adults—Each suppository contains 3 g of glycerin USP.

FLEET® Glycerin Suppositories for Adults—Each suppository contains 2 g of glycerin USP.

FLEET® Glycerin Suppositories for Children 2 years to under 6—Each suppository contains 1 g of glycerin USP.

ACTIONS AND USES

Glycerin is a hyperosmotic laxative, which is given rectally, and it usually produces a bowel movement within 15 minutes to 1 hour. The hyperosmotic laxative effect of glycerin attracts water into the stool. These products are used for fast, predictable relief of occasional constipation. However, rectal irritation may occur with its use.

GENERAL LAXATIVE WARNINGS

INFORMATION FOR PATIENT

Do not use a laxative product when nausea, vomiting or abdominal pain is present unless directed by a physician. If you notice a sudden change in bowel habits that persists over a period of 2 weeks, consult a physician before using a laxative. Rectal bleeding or failure to have a bowel movement after use of a laxative may indicate a serious condition. Discontinue use and consult a physician. Laxative products should not be used longer than 1 week unless directed by a physician. This product may cause rectal discomfort or a burning sensation.

Keep this and all drugs out of the reach of children. In case of accidental overdose or ingestion, seek professional assistance or contact a Poison Control Center immediately.

DOSAGE AND ADMINISTRATION

FLEET® Babylax®—Children 2 to under 6 years: 1 unit or as directed by a physician. Children under 2 years: Consult a physician.

Preferred position: Place child on left side with knees bent and arms resting comfortably, or have child kneel, then lower head and chest forward until left side of face is resting on surface with left arm folded comfortably.

CAUTION: REMOVE ORANGE PROTECTIVE SHIELD FROM TIP BEFORE INSERTING. Hold the unit upright, grasping the bulb with fingers. Grasp the orange protective shield with the other hand; pull gently to remove. With steady pressure, gently insert the tip into the rectum with a slight side-to-side movement, with the tip pointing towards navel. **DISCONTINUE USE IF RESISTANCE IS ENCOUNTERED. FORCING THE TIP CAN RESULT IN INJURY.** Insertion may be easier if child receiving suppository bears down as if having a bowel movement. This helps relax the muscles around the anus. Squeeze the bulb until nearly all liquid has been expelled. While continuing to squeeze the bulb, remove the tip from the rectum and discard the unit. It is not necessary to empty the unit completely. The unit contains more than the amount of liquid needed for effective use. A small amount of liquid will remain in the unit after squeezing.

FLEET® Liquid Glycerin Suppositories for Adults and Children 6 years of age and older: One unit or as directed by a physician. Children 2 years to under 6 use Fleet® Babylax®. Children under 2 years, consult a physician.

Preferred position: Lie on left side with right knee bent and arms resting comfortably, or kneel, then lower head and chest forward until left side of face is resting on surface with left arm folded comfortably.

CAUTION: REMOVE ORANGE PROTECTIVE SHIELD BEFORE INSERTING. Hold the unit upright, grasping the bulb with fingers. Grasp the orange protective shield with the other hand; pull gently to remove. With steady pressure, insert the tip into the rectum with a slight side-to-side movement, with the tip pointing toward the navel. **DISCONTINUE USE IF RESISTANCE IS ENCOUNTERED. FORCING THE TIP CAN RESULT IN INJURY.** Insertion may be easier if person receiving suppository bears down as if having a bowel movement. This helps relax the muscles around the anus. Squeeze the bulb until nearly all liquid has been expelled. While continuing to squeeze the bulb, remove the tip from the rectum and discard the unit. It is not necessary to empty the unit completely. The unit contains more than the amount of liquid needed for use. A small amount of liquid will remain in the unit after squeezing.

FLEET® Maximum-Strength Glycerin Suppositories—Adults and Children 6 years of age and older: One suppository.

Remove the foil wrapper and insert one suppository well up into the rectum. The suppository need not melt completely to produce laxative action. Keep away from excessive heat.

FLEET® Glycerin Suppositories—Adults and Children 6 years of age and older: One suppository.

If foil-wrapped, remove the foil wrapper. Insert one suppository well up into the rectum. The suppository need not melt completely to produce laxative action. Store the container tightly closed and keep away from excessive heat.

FLEET® Glycerin Suppositories Child Size—Children 2 to under 6 years: One suppository.

Children under 2 years: Consult a physician.

Insert suppository well up into the rectum. The suppository need not melt completely to produce laxative action. Store the container tightly closed and keep away from excessive heat.

HOW SUPPLIED

FLEET® Babylax® for children 2 to under 6 years—Each box contains 6 child rectal applicators (4 mL each).

FLEET® Liquid Glycerin Suppositories for Adults and Children 6 years of age and over—Each box contains 4 adult rectal applicators (7.5 mL each).

FLEET® Maximum-Strength Glycerin Suppositories—Each box contains 18 individually foil-wrapped adult suppositories.

FLEET® Glycerin Suppositories—Available in jars of 12, 24, and 50 adult suppositories as well as a box containing 12 individually foil-wrapped adult suppositories.

FLEET® Glycerin Suppositories Child Size—Available in jars of 12.

IS THIS PRODUCT OTC?
Yes.

FLEET® BISACODYL LAXATIVES: ENEMA, SUPPOSITORIES, AND TABLETS OTC

(bisacodyl USP)

COMPOSITION

Latex-free FLEET® Bisacodyl Enema - 10 mg bisacodyl USP enema solution in a 37-mL ready-to-use squeeze bottle with a 2 inch, pre-lubricated Comfortip®. It is disposable after a single use.

FLEET® Stimulant Laxative Tablets - Enteric-coated 5 mg bisacodyl USP each tablet.

FLEET® Laxative Suppositories - 10 mg bisacodyl USP each suppository.

ACTION AND USES

Bisacodyl is a stimulant laxative, given either orally or rectally, acting directly on the colonic mucosa-where it stimulates sensory nerve endings to produce parasympathetic reflexes resulting in increased peristaltic contractions of the colon. The contact action of the drug is restricted to the colon, and motility in the small intestine is not appreciably influenced. FLEET® Stimulant Laxative Tablets usually work within 6–12 hours. FLEET® Laxative Suppositories produce a bowel movement within 15 minutes to 1 hour, and the **latex-free** FLEET® Bisacodyl Enema produces a bowel movement within 5–20 minutes. Bisacodyl is useful as a laxative for occasional relief of constipation and in bowel cleansing in preparation for x-ray or endoscopic examination. Bisacodyl may be used as a laxative in postoperative, antepartum, or postpartum care or in preparation for delivery.

Store at temperatures not above 86°F (30°C)

GENERAL LAXATIVE WARNINGS

INFORMATION FOR PATIENT

Do not use a laxative product when nausea, vomiting or abdominal pain is present unless directed by a physician. If you notice a sudden change in bowel habits that persists over a period of 2 weeks, consult a physician before using a laxative. Rectal bleeding or failure to have a bowel movement after use of a laxative may indicate a serious condition. Discontinue use and consult a physician. Laxative products should not be used longer than 1 week unless directed by a physician. As with any drug, if you are pregnant or nursing a baby, seek the advice of a healthcare professional before using this product. This product may cause abdominal discomfort, faintness, and cramps.

Keep this and all drugs out of the reach of children. In case of accidental overdose or ingestion, seek professional assistance or contact a Poison Control Center immediately.

DOSAGE AND ADMINISTRATION

Enema

SHAKE BEFORE USING.

REMOVE ORANGE PROTECTIVE SHIELD FROM TIP BEFORE ADMINISTERING.

Dosage:

Adults and children 12 years of age and over: Use one 1.25 fl. oz. bottle (30-mL delivered dose) in a single daily dose. Children under 12 years of age: DO NOT USE.

Preferred position: Lie on left side with left knee slightly bent and the right leg drawn up, or in knee-chest position. The diaphragm at base of tube prevents reflux and assures controlled flow of the enema solution. Bisacodyl Enema should be used at room temperature.

Tablets
Adults and children 12 years of age and over: Take 2 to 3 tablets (usually 2) in a single dose once daily.
Children 6 to under 12 years of age: Take 1 tablet once daily. Expect results in 6–12 hours if taken at bedtime or within 6 hours if taken before breakfast. Swallow tablets whole. Do not chew or crush tablets. Do not administer tablets within 1 hour after taking an antacid, milk, or milk products.
Children under 6 years of age: Consult your physician.
Suppositories
Adults and children 12 years of age and over: Use 1 suppository once daily. Remove foil wrapper. Lie on your side and, with pointed end first, insert the suppository towards the navel and well up into the rectum. Make sure the suppository touches the bowel wall.
Children 6 to under 12 years of age: One half of one 10 mg suppository once daily.
Children under 6 years of age: Consult your physician.

PROFESSIONAL ADMINISTRATION
See FLEET® Ready-to-Use Enema and FLEET® Prep Kits.

HOW SUPPLIED
Enema
FLEET® Bisacodyl Enema is supplied in a 1.25 fl. oz. (37-mL) ready-to-use squeeze bottle.
IMPORTANT: FLEET® Bisacodyl Enema IS NOT INTENDED FOR ORAL CONSUMPTION in any dosage size.
Tablets
FLEET® Stimulant Laxative Tablets are supplied in cartons of 25 tablets (5 mg each tablet) wrapped in a foil seal.
Suppositories
FLEET® Bisacodyl Suppositories are supplied in cartons of 4 individually foil-wrapped suppositories (10 mg each suppository).
IS THIS PRODUCT OTC?
Yes.

FLEET® ENEMA, A SALINE LAXATIVE OTC
FLEET® ENEMA FOR CHILDREN, A SALINE LAXATIVE

COMPOSITION
FLEET® ENEMA: Each 118-mL delivered dose contains 19 g monobasic sodium phosphate monohydrate and 7 g dibasic sodium phosphate heptahydrate. The **latex-free** FLEET® Enema unit, with a 2 inch, pre-lubricated Comfortip®, contains 4.5 fl. oz. (133 mL) of enema solution in a ready-to-use squeeze bottle. FLEET® ENEMA FOR CHILDREN: Each 59-mL delivered dose contains 9.5 g monobasic sodium phosphate monohydrate and 3.5 g dibasic sodium phosphate heptahydrate. The **latex-free** FLEET® Enema for Children unit, with a 2 inch, pre-lubricated Comfortip®, contains 2.25 fl. oz. (66 mL) of enema solution in a ready-to-use squeeze bottle. Fleet® Enema is designed for quick, convenient administration by nurse or patient according to instructions. It is disposable after a single use.

ELEMENTAL AND ELECTROLYTIC CONTENT	
mEq Phosphate (PO_4) per mL	4.15
mEq Sodium (Na) per mL	1.61
mg Sodium (Na) per mL	37
mmole Phosphorus (P) per mL	1.38

ACTION AND USES
FLEET® Enema is useful as a laxative in the relief of occasional constipation and as part of a bowel cleansing regimen in preparing the colon for surgery, x-ray or endoscopic examination. Used as directed, FLEET® Enema provides thorough yet safe cleansing action and induces complete emptying of the left colon, usually within 1 to 5 minutes, without pain or spasm.

GENERAL LAXATIVE WARNINGS
INFORMATION FOR PATIENT
Using more than one enema in 24 hours can be harmful.
Do not use laxative products when nausea, vomiting or abdominal pain is present unless directed by a physician. If you notice a sudden change in bowel habits that persists over a period of 2 weeks, consult a physician. Rectal bleeding or failure to have a bowel movement after use of a laxative may indicate a serious condition. Discontinue use and consult a physician. Laxative products should not be used longer than 1 week unless directed by a physician. As with any drug, if you are pregnant or nursing a baby, seek the advice of a healthcare professional before using this product.
Keep this and all drugs out of the reach of children. In case of accidental overdose or ingestion, seek professional assistance or contact a Poison Control Center immediately.

PROFESSIONAL USE WARNINGS
Do not use in patients with megacolon, gastrointestinal obstruction, imperforate anus or congestive heart failure.
Use with caution in patients with impaired renal function or pre-existing electrolyte disturbances, or in patients on diuretics or other medications which may affect electrolyte levels or where colostomy exists.
Since FLEET® Enema contains sodium phosphates, there is a risk of elevated serum levels of sodium and phosphate and decreased levels of calcium and potassium, and consequently hypernatremia, hyperphosphatemia, hypocalcemia, hypokalemia and acidosis may occur. This is of particular concern in children with megacolon or any other condition where there is retention of enema solution.
Additional fluids by mouth are recommended with all bowel cleansing dosages.
SINCE FLEET® BRAND ENEMAS ARE AVAILABLE IN ADULT AND CHILDREN'S SIZES, PRESCRIBE CAREFULLY.

PRECAUTIONS
DO NOT ADMINISTER THE 4.5 FL. OZ. ADULT SIZE TO CHILDREN UNDER 12 YEARS OF AGE.
DO NOT ADMINISTER A FULL 2.25 FL. OZ. CHILDREN'S SIZE TO CHILDREN UNDER 5 YEARS OF AGE. FOR CHILDREN 2 TO UNDER 5 YEARS, USE ONE-HALF BOTTLE (SEE **DOSAGE AND ADMINISTRATION**).
DO NOT USE IN CHILDREN UNDER 2 YEARS OF AGE.
IF AFTER THE ENEMA SOLUTION IS ADMINISTERED THERE IS NO RETURN OF LIQUID, CONTACT A PHYSICIAN IMMEDIATELY, AS DEHYDRATION COULD OCCUR.

OVERDOSAGE
Overdosage or retention may lead to severe electrolyte disturbances, including hypernatremia, hyperphosphatemia, hypocalcemia, and hypokalemia, as well as dehydration and hypovolemia, with attendant signs and symptoms of these disturbances (such as metabolic acidosis, renal failure, and tetany). Certain severe electrolyte disturbances may lead to cardiac arrhythmia and death. The patient who has taken an overdose should be monitored carefully. **Treatment of electrolyte imbalance may require immediate medical intervention with appropriate electrolyte and fluid replacement.**

DOSAGE AND ADMINISTRATION
Dosage: FLEET® Enema (Adult size):
Do not use more unless directed by a doctor. See Warnings.

adults and children 12 years and older	one bottle
children 2 to 11 years	use Fleet Enema for Children
children under 2 years	DO NOT USE

REMOVE ORANGE PROTECTIVE SHIELD FROM TIP BEFORE INSERTING.
Preferred position: Lie on left side with knee slightly bent and the right leg drawn up, or in knee-chest position.
The diaphragm at base of tube prevents reflux and assures controlled flow of the enema solution. FLEET® Enema should be used at room temperature.
Dosage: FLEET® Enema for Children:
Do not use more unless directed by a doctor. See Warnings.

children 5 to 11 years	one bottle or as directed by a doctor
children 2 to under 5 years	one-half bottle (see below)
children under 2 years	DO NOT USE

One-half bottle preparation: Unscrew cap and remove 2 Tablespoons of liquid with a measuring spoon. Replace cap and follow DIRECTIONS on back of carton.
REMOVE ORANGE PROTECTIVE SHIELD FROM TIP BEFORE INSERTING.
Preferred position: Lie on left side with knee slightly bent and the right leg drawn up, or in knee-chest position.
The diaphragm at base of tube prevents reflux and assures controlled flow of the enema solution. FLEET® Enema for Children should be used at room temperature.

PROFESSIONAL DOSAGE AND ADMINISTRATION
FLEET® Enema (Adult size) should not be used in children under 12 years of age. In those cases where complications are reported, infants and young children are often involved. FLEET® Enema for Children should be used with caution in children of any age. Careful consideration of the use of enemas in children in general is recommended. See **DOSAGE AND ADMINISTRATION** for dosing detail.
Proper and safe use of FLEET® Enema also requires that the product be administered according to the Directions. Healthcare professionals should remember, when administering the product, to gently insert the enema into the rectum with the tip pointing toward the navel. Insertion may be made easier by having the patient bear down as if having a bowel movement. Care during insertion is necessary due to lack of sensory innervation of the rectum and due to possibility of bowel perforation. Once inserted, squeeze the bottle until nearly all the liquid is expelled. If resistance is encountered on insertion of the nozzle or in administering the solution, the procedure should be discontinued. **Forcing the enema can result in perforation and/or abrasion of the rectum.**
If an enema containing phosphate or sodium is not advised, use FLEET® Bisacodyl Enema.

HOW SUPPLIED
FLEET® Enema is supplied in a 4.5 fl. oz. (133-mL) ready-to-use squeeze bottle. The children's size is 2.25 fl. oz. (66 mL). IMPORTANT: FLEET® Enema (Adult size) and Fleet Enema for Children ARE NOT INTENDED FOR ORAL CONSUMPTION in any dosage size.

IS THIS PRODUCT OTC?
Yes.

FLEET® MINERAL OIL ENEMA OTC
A LUBRICANT LAXATIVE

COMPOSITION
Latex-free FLEET® Mineral Oil Enema unit, with a 2 inch, pre-lubricated Comfortip®, delivers 118 mL of mineral oil USP in a ready-to-use squeeze bottle. FLEET® Mineral Oil Enema is sodium-free. The unit is disposable after a single use.

ACTION AND USES
FLEET® Mineral Oil Enema serves to soften and lubricate hard stools, easing their passage without irritating the mucosa. Results approximate a normal bowel movement in that only the rectum, sigmoid, and part or all of the descending colon are evacuated. FLEET® Mineral Oil Enema is indicated for relief of fecal impaction; is valuable in relief of occasional constipation when straining must be avoided (in hypertension, coronary occlusion, proctologic procedures, or postoperative care); is indicated for removal of barium sulfate residues from the colon after barium administration and is indicated for obtaining the laxative benefits of mineral oil while avoiding possible untoward effects of oral administration such as (1) interference with intestinal absorption of fat-soluble vitamins A, D, E and K and other nutrients, (2) danger of systemic absorption, or (3) possible risk of lipid pneumonia due to aspiration. It is generally effective in 2 to 15 minutes.

GENERAL LAXATIVE WARNINGS
INFORMATION FOR PATIENT
Do not use laxative products when nausea, vomiting or abdominal pain is present unless directed by a physician. If you notice a sudden change in bowel habits that persists over a period of 2 weeks, consult a physician before using a laxative. Rectal bleeding or failure to have a bowel movement after use of a laxative may indicate a serious condition. Discontinue use and consult a physician. Laxative products should not be used longer than 1 week unless directed by a physician. As with any drug, if you are pregnant or nursing a baby, seek the advice of a healthcare professional before using this product.
Keep this and all drugs out of the reach of children. In case of accidental overdose or ingestion, seek professional assistance or contact a Poison Control Center immediately.

PRECAUTIONS
DO NOT ADMINISTER TO CHILDREN UNDER 2 YEARS OF AGE.

DOSAGE AND ADMINISTRATION
Dosage: Adults and children 12 years of age and over—one 4.5 fl. oz. bottle (118-mL delivered dose) in a single daily dose. Children 2 to under 12 years of age—½ bottle (59-mL delivered dose) in a single daily dose.
REMOVE ORANGE PROTECTIVE SHIELD FROM TIP BEFORE INSERTING.
Preferred position: Lie on left side with knee slightly bent and the right leg drawn up, or in knee-chest position.
The diaphragm at base of tube prevents reflux and assures controlled flow of the enema solution. The enema should be used at room temperature. For more thorough cleansing, follow with FLEET® Enema—**according to dosage instructions contained in PDR.**

PROFESSIONAL DOSAGE AND ADMINISTRATION
FLEET® Mineral Oil Enema should not be used in children under 2 years of age and should be used with caution in children of any age. Careful consideration of the use of enemas in children in general is recommended.
Proper and safe use of FLEET® Mineral Oil Enema also requires that the product be administered according to the Directions. Healthcare professionals should remember, when administering the product, to gently insert the enema into the rectum with the tip pointing toward the navel. Insertion may be made easier by having the patient bear down as if having a bowel movement. Care during insertion is necessary due to lack of sensory innervation of the rectum and due to the possibility of bowel perforation. Once inserted, squeeze the bottle until nearly all the liquid is expelled. If resistance is encountered on insertion of the nozzle or in administering the solution, the procedure should be discontinued. **Forcing the enema can result in perforation and/or abrasion of the rectum.**

Continued on next page

Fleet Mineral Oil—Cont.

HOW SUPPLIED

FLEET® Mineral Oil Enema is supplied in 4.5 fl. oz. (133-mL) ready-to-use squeeze bottle.

IS THIS PRODUCT OTC?

Yes.

FLEET® PHOSPHO-SODA® OTC
AN ORAL SALINE LAXATIVE

COMPOSITION

Each 5 mL of Unflavored or Natural Ginger-lemon flavor FLEET® Phospho-soda® contains 2.4 g monobasic sodium phosphate monohydrate and 0.9 g dibasic sodium phosphate heptahydrate in a stable, buffered aqueous solution.

ELEMENTAL AND ELECTROLYTIC CONTENT

mEq Phosphate (PO_4) per mL	12.45
mEq Sodium (Na) per mL	4.82
mg Sodium (Na) per mL	111
mmole Phosphorus (P) per mL	4.15

INDICATIONS

As a laxative, for the relief of occasional constipation. For use as part of a bowel cleansing regimen in preparing the colon for surgery, x-ray or endoscopic examination.

ACTION AND USES

Versatile in action as a gentle laxative or purgative, according to dosage. This product produces a bowel movement in 1/2 to 6 hours, depending on dosage.

PROFESSIONAL USE WARNINGS AND PRECAUTIONS. Do not use in patients with megacolon, gastrointestinal obstruction, ascites, congestive heart failure, kidney disease or in children under 5 years of age. **Use with caution** in patients with impaired renal function, heart disease, acute myocardial infarction, unstable angina, preexisting electrolyte disturbances, increased risk for electrolyte disturbances (e.g., dehydration, gastric retention, bowel perforation, colitis, ileus, inability to take adequate oral fluid, concomitant use of diuretics or other medications that affect electrolytes), with debilitated or elderly patients or with patients who are taking medications known to prolong the QT interval. **In at-risk patients, including elderly patients, consider obtaining baseline and post-treatment sodium, potassium, calcium, chloride, bicarbonate, phosphate, blood urea nitrogen and creatinine values, and consider using the lower end of the dosage range.** There is a risk of elevated serum levels of sodium and phosphate and decreased levels of calcium and potassium; consequently, hypernatremia, hyperphosphatemia, hypocalcemia, hypokalemia, and acidosis may occur. **Additional fluids by mouth are recommended with all bowel cleansing dosages.** Encourage patients to drink large amounts of clear liquids to prevent dehydration. Drinking large amounts of clear liquids also helps ensure that the patient's bowel will be clean for the procedure. No other sodium phosphate preparations should be given concomitantly.

OVERDOSAGE

Overdosage or retention may lead to severe electrolyte disturbances, including hyperphosphatemia, hypernatremia, hypocalcemia, and hypokalemia, as well as dehydration and hypovolemia, with attendant signs and symptoms of these disturbances (such as metabolic acidosis, renal failure, and tetany). Certain severe electrolyte disturbances may lead to cardiac arrhythmia and death. The patient who has taken an overdose should be monitored carefully. **Treatment of electrolyte imbalance may require immediate medical intervention with appropriate electrolyte and fluid replacement.**

WARNINGS

TAKING MORE THAN THE RECOMMENDED DOSE IN 24 HOURS CAN BE HARMFUL. IF THERE IS NO BOWEL MOVEMENT AFTER MAXIMUM DOSAGE, CONTACT A PHYSICIAN, AS DEHYDRATION COULD OCCUR.

SINCE FLEET® PHOSPHO-SODA® IS AVAILABLE IN TWO SIZES, PRESCRIBE BY VOLUME. DO NOT PRESCRIBE "BY THE BOTTLE," AS SERIOUS SIDE EFFECTS FROM OVERDOSAGE MAY OCCUR.

INFORMATION FOR PATIENT

Ask a doctor before using this product if you are on a sodium-restricted diet, have a kidney disease, or are pregnant or nursing a baby. Ask a doctor before using any laxative if you have nausea, vomiting or abdominal pain; have a sudden change in bowel habits lasting more than 2 weeks; or have already used a laxative for more than 1 week. Stop using this product and consult a doctor if you have rectal bleeding or have no bowel movement after use, as dehydration may occur. These symptoms may indicate a serious condition.

Keep this and all drugs out of the reach of children. In case of overdose or accidental ingestion, seek professional assistance or contact a Poison Control Center immediately.

DOSAGE AND ADMINISTRATION

Dilute recommended dose with at least one-half glass (4 fl. oz.) of cold water or other clear liquid. Drink, then follow with at least two additional glasses (8 fl. oz. each) of water or other clear liquid.

DOSAGE: DO NOT EXCEED RECOMMENDED DOSAGE, AS SERIOUS SIDE EFFECTS MAY OCCUR.

SINGLE DAILY DOSAGE: DO NOT TAKE MORE UNLESS DIRECTED BY A DOCTOR. SEE WARNINGS.

adults and children 12 years and older	20 to 45 mL* (4 to 9 teaspoons*)
children 10 and 11 years	10 to 20 mL* (2 to 4 teaspoons*)
children 5 to 9 years	5 to 10 mL* (1 to 2 teaspoons*)
children under 5 years	**DO NOT USE**

* DO NOT TAKE MORE THAN THIS AMOUNT IN A 24-HOUR PERIOD.

HYDRATION AND DIET:

Clear liquid beverages may be consumed throughout the day and should be encouraged.

During bowel preparation you will lose significant amounts of fluid. THIS IS NORMAL. It is very important that you replace this fluid to prevent dehydration. Drink large amounts of clear liquids. Drinking large amounts of clear liquids also helps ensure that your bowel will be clean for the examination. (See "Clear Liquids Diet List" below).

Day before the exam – eat a regular breakfast.

DO NOT DRINK OR EAT ANYTHING COLORED RED OR PURPLE.

Low residue lunch (must be eaten before 2 PM). Lunch may include any of the following items:

- Main entrée – choose one of the following:
  - 3 oz. of skinless chicken, turkey, fish or seafood
  - 1 large or 2 medium eggs
  - 1 can of chicken noodle soup without vegetables
- Vegetable / Fruit – choose one of the following
  - ½ cup applesauce
  - ½ cup of cooked or canned vegetables without seeds. ***No corn.***
- Bread – choose one of the following:
  - 1 white potato roll
  - 2 slices of white bread
  - 1 cup of cooked white rice or 1 cup of cooked pasta
  - 1 small skinless potato
- Condiments – choose one of the following:
  - 2 tsp. of soft tub margarine
  - 1 tsp. mustard or mayonnaise
- Dessert – choose one of the following:
  - 4 vanilla wafers
  - ¼ cup pretzels
  - ½ cup sherbet
- Any items from the "Clear Liquids Diet List" below:

CLEAR LIQUIDS DIET LIST:

BEVERAGES:

- Water, tea or coffee (no milk or non-dairy creamer); sweeteners are okay to use
- Soft drinks (orange, ginger ale, cola, Sprite®, 7-Up®, etc.), Gatorade®, Kool-Aid®
- Strained fruit juices without pulp (apple, white grape, orange, lemonade, etc.)

Dosing:

The timing of the two 1.5 fl. oz. doses of diluted Fleet® Phospho-soda® should be as directed by the physician. See References.

Dilution Alternatives:

1) Mix 1.5 fl. oz. (3 Tablespoons) Fleet® Phospho-soda® with 4 fl. oz. of cold clear liquid. Then follow with at least 16 fl. oz. of clear liquid.

OR

2) Mix 1.5 fl. oz. (3 Tablespoons) Fleet® Phospho-soda® with three 8 fl. oz. glasses cold clear liquid (one Tablespoon of Fleet® Phospho-soda® per glass). Drink all three glasses within 30 minutes.

The taste of Fleet® Phospho-soda® is improved by mixing it with ginger ale, apple juice, or lemon-lime type drinks.

HOW SUPPLIED

Unflavored or Natural Ginger-lemon flavor, in bottles of 1.5 fl. oz. and 3 fl. oz. FLEET® Phospho-soda® should not be confused with FLEET® Enema, a sodium phosphates disposable ready-to-use enema. FLEET® Enema and Fleet® Enema for Children ARE NOT INTENDED FOR ORAL CONSUMPTION in any dosage size.

IS THIS PRODUCT OTC?

Yes.

REFERENCES

1. Balaban, D.H. et al. Low Volume Bowel Preparation for Colonoscopy: Randomized, Endoscopist-Blinded Trial of Liquid Sodium Phosphate versus Tablet Sodium Phosphate. The American Journal of Gastroenterology, 2003; 98(4):827
2. Cohen, S.M. et al. Prospective, Randomized, Endoscopic-Blinded Trial Comparing Precolonoscopy Bowel Cleansing Methods. Diseases of the Colon & Rectum. 1994; 37(7):689.
3. Hookey, L.C. et al. The Safety Profile of Oral Sodium Phosphate for Colonic Cleansing before Colonoscopy in Adults. Gastrointestinal Endoscopy, 2002; 56(6):895
4. Barclay, R.L. et al. Carbohydrate-electrolyte Rehydration Protects against Intravascular Volume Contraction during Colonic Cleansing with Orally Administered Sodium Phosphate. Gastrointestinal Endoscopy, 2002. 56(5):633
5. Allaire, J. et al. A Quality Improvement Project Comparing Two Regimens of Medication for Colonoscopy Preparation. Gastroenterology Nursing, 2003. 27(1):3
6. Oliveira, L. et al. Mechanical Bowel Preparation for Elective Colorectal Surgery. Diseases of the Colon & Rectum. 1997; 40(5):585.
7. Vanner, S. J. et al. A Randomized Prospective Trial Comparing Oral Sodium Phosphate with Standard Polyethylene Glycol-Based Lavage Solution (Golytely) in the Preparation of Patients for Colonoscopy. The American Journal of Gastroenterology. 1990; 85(4):422.

FLEET® PHOSPHO-SODA® ACCU-PREP® OTC

DESCRIPTION

COMPOSITION OF FLEET® PHOSPHO-SODA® ACCU-PREP® BOWEL CLEANSING SYSTEM

Fleet® Phospho-soda® ACCU-PREP® contains:

1. Six 15-mL (1/2 fl. oz.) units of Fleet® Phospho-soda®, net contents 3 fl. oz. (90 mL).
   Active Ingredients: Each Unit (15-mL) contains dibasic sodium phosphate/monobasic sodium phosphate 9.9 g.
2. Four Fleet® Relief Pre-Moistened Anorectal Wipes.
   Active Ingredients: Each pad is moistened with Pramoxine hydrochloride 1% and Glycerin 12%.
3. Patient mixing instructions.

Fleet® Phospho-soda®

COMPOSITION

Each 15-mL of Natural Ginger-lemon flavor Fleet® Phospho-soda® contains 7.2 g monobasic sodium phosphate monohydrate and 2.7 g dibasic sodium phosphate heptahydrate in a stable, aqueous solution.

ELEMENTAL AND ELECTROLYTIC CONTENT:

mEq Phosphate (PO_4) per 15 mL	186.75
mEq Sodium (Na) per 15 mL	72.30
mg Sodium (Na) per 15 mL	1668
mmole Phosphorus (P) per 15 mL	62.25

ACTIONS

Fleet® Phospho-soda® is an oral saline laxative.

INDICATIONS AND USES

For use as part of a bowel cleansing regimen in preparing the colon for surgery, x-ray or endoscopic examination. See DOSAGE AND ADMINISTRATION. This product generally produces a bowel movement in ½ to 6 hours.

PROFESSIONAL USE WARNINGS

Do not use in patients with megacolon, gastrointestinal obstruction, ascites, congestive heart failure, kidney disease or in children under 5 years of age. **Use with caution** in patients with impaired renal function, heart disease, acute myocardial infarction, unstable angina, pre-existing electrolyte disturbances, increased risk for electrolyte disturbances (e.g., dehydration, gastric retention, bowel perforation, colitis, ileus, inability to take adequate oral fluid, concomitant use of diuretics or other medications that affect electrolytes), with debilitated or elderly patients or with patients who are taking medications known to prolong the QT interval. **In at-risk patients, including elderly patients, consider obtaining baseline and post-treatment sodium, potassium, calcium, chloride, bicarbonate, phosphate, blood urea nitrogen and creatinine values, and consider using the lower end of the dosage range.** There is a risk of elevated serum levels of sodium and phosphate and decreased levels of calcium and potassium; consequently, hypernatremia, hyperphosphatemia, hypocalcemia, hypokalemia, and acidosis may occur. **Additional fluids by mouth are recommended with all bowel cleansing dosages.** Encourage patients to drink large amounts of clear liquids to prevent dehydration. Drinking large amounts of clear liquids also helps ensure that the patient's bowel will be clean for the procedure. No other sodium phosphate preparations should be given concomitantly.

OVERDOSAGE

Overdosage or retention may lead to severe electrolyte disturbances, including hypernatremia, hyperphosphatemia, hypocalcemia and hypokalemia, as well as dehydration and hypovolemia, with attendant signs and symptoms of these disturbances (such as metabolic acidosis, renal failure, and tetany). Certain severe electrolyte disturbances may lead to cardiac arrhythmia and death. The patient who has taken an overdose should be monitored carefully. **Treatment of**

electrolyte imbalance may require immediate medical intervention with appropriate electrolyte and fluid replacement.

PRECAUTIONS

GENERAL

Taking more than the recommended dose in 24 hours can be harmful.

The patient should be instructed to open and read directions at least two days in advance of the examination.

Instruct the patient to contact a physician if there is no bowel movement after maximum dosage as dehydration can occur.

INFORMATION FOR PATIENT

Patients should ask a doctor before using this product if they are on a sodium-restricted diet, have a kidney disease, or are pregnant or nursing a baby. Patients should contact a doctor before using any laxative if they have nausea, vomiting or abdominal pain; have a sudden change in bowel habits lasting more than 2 weeks or have already used a laxative for more than 1 week. Patients should stop using the product and call a doctor if they have rectal bleeding, or have no bowel movement with use, as dehydration may occur. These symptoms may indicate a serious condition.

Keep this and all drugs out of the reach of children. In case of overdose or accidental ingestion, seek professional assistance or contact a Poison Control Center immediately.

DOSAGE AND ADMINISTRATION

Each of the two doses consists of 2–3 pre-measured 15-mL (1/2 fl. oz.) units of Phospho-soda. Dilute each pre-measured 15-mL (1/2 fl. oz.) unit in an 8 fl. oz. glass of clear liquid. Repeat for each pre-measured unit (2–3 units) according to the doctor's instructions, at the prescribed times. Drink at least 3 additional 8 fl. oz. glasses of clear liquid after the first dose.

adults and children 12 years & over	2–3 15-mL pre-measured units*
children 5 to 11 years	ask a doctor
children under 5 years	**DO NOT USE**

***DO NOT TAKE MORE THAN 3 PRE-MEASURED UNITS IN EACH DOSE.**

HYDRATION AND DIET

Clear liquid beverages may be consumed throughout the day and should be encouraged. (See "Clear Liquids Diet List" below).

During bowel preparation you will lose significant amounts of fluid. THIS IS NORMAL. It is very important that you replace this fluid to prevent dehydration. Drink large amounts of clear liquids. Drinking large amounts of clear liquids also helps ensure that your bowel will be clean for the examination.

Day before the exam – eat a regular breakfast.

DO NOT DRINK OR EAT ANYTHING COLORED RED OR PURPLE.

Low residue lunch (must be eaten before 2 PM). Lunch may include any of the following items:

- Main entrée – choose one of the following:
  - 3 oz. of skinless chicken, turkey, fish or seafood
  - 1 large or 2 medium eggs
  - 1 can of chicken noodle soup without vegetables
- Vegetable/Fruit – choose one of the following
  - ½ cup applesauce
  - ½ cup of cooked or canned vegetables without seeds. ***No corn.***
- Bread – choose one of the following:
  - 1 white potato roll
  - 2 slices of white bread
  - 1 cup of cooked white rice or 1 cup of cooked pasta
  - 1 small skinless potato
- Condiments – choose one of the following:
  - 2 tsp. of soft tub margarine
  - 1 tsp. mustard or mayonnaise
- Dessert – choose one of the following:
  - 4 vanilla wafers
  - ¼ cup pretzels
  - ½ cup sherbet
- Any items from the "Clear Liquids Diet List" below:

CLEAR LIQUIDS DIET LIST:

BEVERAGES:

- Water, tea or coffee (no milk or non-dairy creamer); sweeteners are okay to use
- Soft drinks (orange, ginger ale, cola, Sprite®, 7-Up®, etc.), Gatorade®, Kool-Aid®
- Strained fruit juices without pulp (apple, white grape, orange, lemonade, etc.)

Fleet® Relief Pre-Moistened Anorectal Wipes

COMPOSITION

Each wipe is moistened with Pramoxine hydrochloride 1%; Glycerin 12%.

ACTIONS

Fleet® Relief Pre-Moistened Anorectal Wipes act as a local anesthetic and protectant for temporary relief of pain, soreness or burning.

INDICATIONS AND USES

For the temporary relief of local itching and discomfort associated with hemorrhoids. Temporarily forms a protective coating over inflamed tissues to help prevent drying of tissues and temporarily provides a coating for relief of anorectal discomfort.

WARNINGS

FOR EXTERNAL USE ONLY

INFORMATION FOR THE PATIENT

Do not exceed the recommended daily dosage. Consult a doctor promptly in case of bleeding. Do not put the product into the rectum by using fingers or any mechanical device or applicator.

Stop use and ask a doctor if the condition worsens or does not improve within 7 days; or if redness, irritation, swelling, pain or other symptoms develop or increase. Certain persons can develop allergic reactions to ingredients in this product.

DIRECTIONS

Adults & children 12 years & over: When practical, cleanse the affected area with mild soap and warm water and rinse thoroughly. Gently dry by patting or blotting with toilet tissue or a soft cloth. Open the sealed pouch and remove one Fleet® Relief Wipe and gently apply to the affected area. Apply after each bowel movement, up to 5 times daily. Discard the wipe after use. There are four Fleet® Relief Wipes. They can be used after a bowel movement or whenever anorectal discomfort is felt.

HOW SUPPLIED

This complete, simple, convenient bowel cleansing kit includes six 15-mL units of Phospho-soda® (Natural ginger-lemon flavor) and four Fleet® Relief Pre-Moistened Anorectal Wipes. Fleet® Phospho-soda® ACCU-PREP® is available in 12 units per case.

Fleet® Phospho-soda® ACCU-PREP® should not be confused with Fleet® Enema, a sodium phosphates disposable ready-to-use enema. Fleet® Enemas, Adult and Children size, ARE NOT INTENDED FOR ORAL CONSUMPTION in any dosage size.

IS THIS PRODUCT OTC?

Yes. Fleet® Phospho-soda® ACCU-PREP® is an OTC product, but it will be stocked behind the pharmacy counter. Patients should be directed to ask their pharmacists for Fleet® Phospho-soda® ACCU-PREP®.

FLEET® PREP KITS OTC

Bowel Evacuant

COMPOSITION

FLEET® Prep Kit 1 contains:

1. FLEET® Phospho-soda®—1.5 fl. oz. (45 mL). Active Ingredients: Each teaspoon (5 mL) contains monobasic sodium phosphate monohydrate 2.4 g and dibasic sodium phosphate heptahydrate 0.9 g. Natural ginger-lemon flavoring.
2. FLEET® Bisacodyl Tablets—4 laxative tablets. Active Ingredient: Each enteric-coated tablet contains 5 mg bisacodyl USP.
3. FLEET® Bisacodyl Suppository—1 laxative suppository. Active Ingredient: Each suppository contains 10 mg bisacodyl USP.
4. 1 Patient Instruction Sheet.

FLEET® Prep Kit 2 contains:

1. FLEET® Phospho-soda®—1.5 fl. oz. (45 mL).
2. FLEET® Bisacodyl Tablets—4 laxative tablets.
3. FLEET® Bagenema—1.
4. 1 Patient Instruction Sheet.

FLEET® Prep Kit 3 contains:

1. FLEET® Phospho-soda® —1.5 fl. oz. (45 mL).
2. FLEET® Bisacodyl Tablets—4 laxative tablets.
3. FLEET® Bisacodyl Enema 1.25 fl. oz. (37 mL)—1 laxative enema. Active Ingredient: Each 30-mL delivered dose contains 10 mg bisacodyl USP.
4. 1 Patient Instruction Sheet.

FLEET PrepKit 3 should not be used in children under 12 years.

Each recommended dose (1.5 fl. oz.) (45 mL) of FLEET® Phospho-soda® contains 5004 mg sodium.

ACTIONS AND USES

Bowel Cleansing System

INDICATIONS

For use as part of a bowel cleansing regimen in preparing the colon for surgery, x-ray or endoscopic examination.

PRECAUTIONS

GENERAL

Bisacodyl products may cause abdominal discomfort, faintness, and cramps. Bisacodyl Tablets should be swallowed whole. Do not prescribe to patients who cannot swallow without chewing unless directed by a physician.

Store at temperatures not above 86°F (30°C)

INFORMATION FOR PATIENT

DO NOT EXCEED RECOMMENDED DOSE UNLESS DIRECTED BY A PHYSICIAN. SERIOUS SIDE EFFECTS MAY OCCUR FROM EXCESS DOSAGE. IF THERE IS NO BOWEL MOVEMENT AFTER MAXIMUM DOSAGE, CONTACT A PHYSICIAN, AS DEHYDRATION COULD OCCUR.

During bowel preparation you will lose significant amounts of fluid. THIS IS NORMAL. It is very important that you replace this fluid to prevent dehydration. Drink large amounts of clear liquids. Drinking large amounts of clear liquids also helps ensure that your bowel will be clean for the examination.

Swallow tablets whole; do not chew tablets unless directed by a physician. Do not take tablets within one hour after taking antacids, milk, or milk products.

Ask a doctor before using this product if you are on a sodium-restricted diet, have a kidney disease, or are pregnant or nursing a baby. Ask a doctor before using any laxative if you have nausea, vomiting or abdominal pain; have a sudden change in bowel habits lasting more than 2 weeks; or have already used a laxative for more than 1 week. Stop using this product and consult a doctor if you have rectal bleeding or have no bowel movement after use, as dehydration may occur. These symptoms may indicate a serious condition.

Keep this and all drugs out of the reach of children. In case of accidental overdose or ingestion, seek professional assistance or contact a Poison Control Center immediately.

PROFESSIONAL USE WARNINGS **Do not use** in patients with megacolon, gastrointestinal obstruction, ascites, congestive heart failure, kidney disease or in children under 5 years of age. **Use with caution** in patients with impaired renal function, heart disease, acute myocardial infarction, unstable angina, pre-existing electrolyte disturbances, increased risk for electrolyte disturbances (e.g., dehydration, gastric retention, bowel perforation, colitis, ileus, inability to take adequate oral fluid, concomitant use of diuretics or other medications that affect electrolytes), with debilitated or elderly patients or with patients who are taking medications known to prolong the QT interval. **In at-risk patients, including elderly patients, consider obtaining baseline and post-treatment sodium, potassium, calcium, chloride, bicarbonate, phosphate, blood urea nitrogen and creatinine values.** There is a risk of elevated serum levels of sodium and phosphate and decreased levels of calcium and potassium; consequently, hypernatremia, hyperphosphatemia, hypocalcemia, hypokalemia, and acidosis may occur. **Additional fluids by mouth are recommended with all bowel cleansing dosages.** Encourage your patients to drink large amounts of clear liquids to prevent dehydration. Drinking large amounts of clear liquids also helps ensure that your patient's bowel will be clean for the procedure. No other sodium phosphate preparations should be given concomitantly.

See individual listings for FLEET® Phospho-soda®, and FLEET® Bisacodyl Laxatives for additional warnings.

PREP KITS SHOULD NOT BE USED IN CHILDREN UNDER 5 YEARS.

OVERDOSAGE

Overdosage or retention may lead to severe electrolyte disturbances, including hypernatremia, hyperphosphatemia, hypocalcemia, and hypokalemia, as well as dehydration and hypovolemia, with attendant signs and symptoms of these disturbances (such as metabolic acidosis, renal failure, and tetany). Certain severe electrolyte disturbances may lead to cardiac arrhythmia and death. The patient who has taken an overdose should be monitored carefully. **Treatment of electrolyte imbalance may require immediate medical intervention with appropriate electrolyte and fluid replacement.**

DOSAGE AND ADMINISTRATION

SEE PATIENT INSTRUCTION SHEET FOR 18-, AND 24-HOUR PREPARATION SCHEDULE IN EACH KIT. The patient should open and read the enclosed directions and labels at least 48 hours in advance of examination.

HOW SUPPLIED

See "Description" for contents of each kit.

Shipping Unit: 48 FLEET® Prep Kits per case.

For full prescribing information on specific products, see individual listings (FLEET® Phospho-soda®, FLEET® Bisacodyl Laxatives).

IS THIS PRODUCT OTC?

Yes.

Fleming & Company

1733 GILSINN LANE
FENTON, MO 63026

Direct Inquiries to:
Fleming & Company
PH: 636-343-8200
FAX: 636-343-5322
email: custserv@flemingcompany.com

EXTENDRYL SR/JR EXTENDED-RELEASE CAPSULES, SYRUP, CHEWABLE TABLETS ℞
Decongestant, antihistamine, anticholinergic

DESCRIPTION
[See table below]

CLINICAL PHARMACOLOGY
Chlorpheniramine maleate is an alkylamine antihistamine which possesses anticholinergic and sedative effects. Phenylephrine HCl is a sympathomimetic which acts predominantly on alpha receptors and has little action on beta receptors, with a mild central stimulant effect. Methscopolamine nitrate is a derivative of scopolamine, which possesses the peripheral actions of the belladonna alkaloids, but does not exhibit the central actions because of its inability to cross the blood-brain barrier.

INDICATIONS AND USAGE
Relief of respiratory congestion, allergic rhinitis, vasomotor rhinitis, and allergic skin reactions of urticaria and angioedema.

CONTRAINDICATIONS
Contraindicated in patients receiving MAO inhibitors, in patients with a known hypersensitivity to any of the ingredients, and in patients with glaucoma, hypertension, cardiac disease, or hyperthyroidism.

PRECAUTIONS
General: Use cautiously, if at all, in the presence of pyloric obstruction. Use with caution in those over 40 years of age, in the presence of diabetes mellitus or urinary retention, and in men with prostatic hypertrophy or a history of bladder difficulty. If disturbances in urination occur, medication should be discontinued for 1 or 2 days and then resumed at a lower dosage. Antihistamines may cause excitability, especially in children. *Information for patients:* Because this product may cause blurring of vision or drowsiness, patients should be cautioned against driving or operating machinery. *Drug interactions:* MAO inhibitors and beta adrenergic blockers increase the effects of sympathomimetics. Sympathomimetics may reduce the antihypertensive effects of methyldopa, guanethidine, mecamylamine, reserpine and veratrum alkaloids. Concomitant use of antihistamines with alcohol or other CNS depressants may have an additive effect. *Pregnancy:* Pregnancy Category C. It is also not known whether the product can cause fetal harm when administered to a pregnant woman or can affect reproduction capacity. The product should be given to a pregnant woman only if clearly needed. *Nursing mothers:* It is not known whether these drugs are excreted in human milk. Because many drugs are excreted in human milk, caution should be exercised when this product is administered to a nursing woman. *Pediatric use:* Safety and effectiveness in children below the age of 6 have not been established.
Geriatric use: Anticholinergic and CNS stimulant effects more likely to occur in older patients; danger of precipitating undiagnosed glaucoma; possible impairment of memory.

ADVERSE REACTIONS
Side effects include xerostomia, blurred vision, bradycardia, mydriasis, flushing, palpitation, dizziness, constipation, urinary retention, drowsiness, increased irritability or excitability, nausea or dysphagia.

OVERDOSAGE
The stomach should be emptied promptly by lavage or by induction of emesis (syrup of ipecac recommended). The installation of activated charcoal into the stomach also should be considered. If respiratory depression is present, treat promptly with oxygen and/or mechanical support of ventilation. If convulsions or marked CNS excitement occurs, only short-acting benzodiazepine-type drugs should be used.

DOSAGE AND ADMINISTRATION
Extended-Release Capsules: Adults and children 12 years of age and older: One SR. capsule every 12 hours. Children 6 to under 12 years of age: One JR. capsule every 12 hours. *Syrup:* Adults and children 12 years of age and older: 1 or 2 teaspoonfuls every 3 or 4 hours. Children 6 to under 12 years of age: $^1/_2$ to 1 teaspoonful depending on age and body weight, may be repeated every 4 hours. *Tablets:* Adults and children 12 years of age and older: 1 or 2 tablets every 4 hours. Children 6 to under 12 years of age: 1 tablet every 4 hours. Do not exceed 4 doses in 24 hours.

HOW SUPPLIED
Capsules and tablets in bottles of 100, syrup in pints.
Supplied as green/red Extendryl Extended-Release Sr/Jr capsules in bottles of 100: "SR," NDC 0256-0111-01; "JR," NDC 0256-0177-01.
Extendryl Syrup as root beer flavored syrup in pints, NDC 0256-0127-01.
Extendryl Chewable Tablets: convex, tan colored, scored on one side in bottles of 100, NDC 0256-0133-01.
Rev. 8/99

Each dose contains:	Phenylephrine HCl	Chlorpheniramine Maleate	Methscopolamine Nitrate
Extendryl SR Capsule	20 mg	8 mg	2.50 mg
Extendryl JR Capsule	10 mg	4 mg	1.25 mg
Extendryl Chewable Tablet (Root beer flavored)	10 mg	2 mg	1.25 mg
Extendryl Syrup (5 mL) (Root beer flavored)	10 mg	2 mg	1.25 mg

MAGONATE® Tablets OTC
MAGONATE® Liquid
Magnesium Gluconate (Dihydrate), USP
(Dietary Supplement)

DESCRIPTION
Each 2 tablets contain magnesium 54 mg (from 1000 mg magnesium gluconate dihydrate) calcium 175 mg and phosphorous 132 mg (from 752 mg dibasic calcium phosphate dihydrate). Each 5 mL of MAGONATE® liquid contains magnesium (elemental) 54 mg. (Each 5 ml contains the same amount of magnesium as contained in 1000 mg of magnesium gluconate dihydrate).

SUGGESTED USES
Magonate® Tablets and Liquid are indicated to maintain magnesium levels when the dietary intake of magnesium is inadequate or when excretion and loss are excessive.

PRECAUTIONS
Excessive dosage may cause loose stools.

CONTRAINDICATIONS
Patients with kidney disease should not take magnesium supplements without the supervision of a physician.

DOSAGES AND ADMINISTRATION
Two Magonate® tablets or 1 teaspoon Magonate® Liquid three times a day (mid-morning, mid-afternoon and bedtime) on an empty stomach with a glass of water.

HOW SUPPLIED
Magonate® Tablets are orange scored, and supplied in bottles of 100 (256-0172-01), and 1000 (256-0172-02) tablets. Magonate® Liquid is supplied in pints, (256-0184-01).
Rev. 11/02

NEPHROCAPS® ℞
Dialysis/Stress Vitamin Supplement

DESCRIPTION
Each black softgel contains:
Vitamin C 100 mg (ascorbic acid); folate 1 mg; niacin 20 mg (niacinamide) thiamine 1.5 mg (thiamine mononitrate); riboflavin 1.7 mg; Vitamin B-6 10 mg (pyridoxine HCl); Vitamin B-12 6 mcg (cyanocobalamin); pantothenic acid 5 mg (calcium pantothenate); and biotin 150 mcg.

INDICATIONS AND USAGE
In the wasting syndrome in chronic renal failure; uremia; impaired metabolic functions of the kidney and to maintain levels when the dietary intake of vitamins is inadequate or excretion and loss are excessive. **Also, highly effective as a stress vitamin.**

PRECAUTIONS
Folic acid may mask the symptoms of pernicious anemia in that hematologic remission may occur while neurologic manifestations remain progressive.

DOSAGE AND ADMINISTRATION
One softgel daily or as directed by a physician. If on dialysis, take after treatment.

HOW SUPPLIED
Plastic bottles of 100 black, oval softgels, NDC 0256-0185-01. Plastic bottles of 30, NDC 0256-0185-04
Contains FD&C yellow # 6. Rev. 11/01

OCEAN® Nasal Spray OTC
(buffered isotonic saline)

USE
For dry nasal membranes squeeze twice in each nostril as needed.
Upright delivers a spray; horizontally a stream; upside down a drop.

HOW SUPPLIED
White plastic 45cc bottle with orange cap (0256-0152-01). Also in pints (NDC 0256-0152-02).
(See PDR For Nonprescription Drugs.)
11/02

RUM–K ℞
(potassium chloride 15% conc, not USP)

DESCRIPTION
Each two teaspoonfuls supply 20 mEq. of potassium and chloride in a butter/rum flavored base that is alcohol and sugar free.

HOW SUPPLIED
Pint bottles NDC 0256-0160-01
℞ only
Rev. 12/99

Forest Pharmaceuticals, Inc.

(Subsidiary of Forest Laboratories, Inc.)
13600 SHORELINE DRIVE
ST. LOUIS, MO 63045

Direct Inquiries to:
Professional Affairs Department
13600 Shoreline Drive
St. Louis, MO 63045
(800) 678-1605

AEROBID® ℞
AEROBID®-M
[aər-ō-bĭd]
(flunisolide)
Inhaler System
For oral inhalation only
℞ only

DESCRIPTION
Flunisolide, the active component of **AEROBID** Inhaler System, is an anti-inflammatory steroid having the chemical name 6α-fluoro-11β, 16α, 17, 21-tetrahydroxypregna-1, 4-diene-3, 20-dione cyclic-16, 17-acetal with acetone.
It has the following structure:

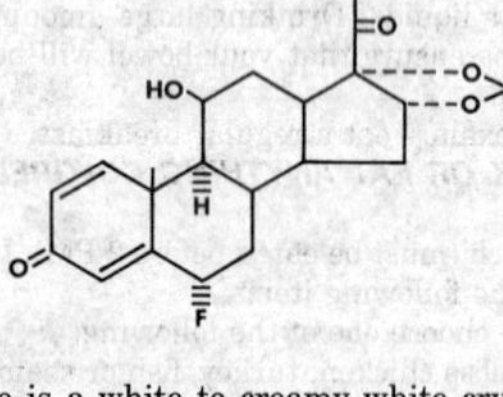

Flunisolide is a white to creamy white crystalline powder with a molecular weight of 434.49. It is soluble in acetone, sparingly soluble in chloroform, slightly soluble in methanol, and practically insoluble in water. It has a melting point of about 245°C.
AEROBID Inhaler is delivered in a metered-dose aerosol system containing a microcrystalline suspension of flunisolide as the hemihydrate in propellants (trichloromonofluoromethane, dichlorodifluoromethane and dichlorotetrafluoroethane) with sorbitan trioleate as a dispersing agent. **AEROBID-M** also contains menthol as a flavoring agent. Each activation delivers approximately 250 mcg of flunisolide to the patient. One **AEROBID** Inhaler System is designed to deliver at least 100 metered inhalations.

CLINICAL PHARMACOLOGY
Flunisolide has demonstrated marked anti-inflammatory and anti-allergic activity in classical test systems. It is a corticosteroid that is several hundred times more potent in animal anti-inflammatory assays than the cortisol standard. The molar dose of each activation of flunisolide in this preparation is approximately 2.5 to 7 times that of comparable inhaled corticosteroid products marketed for the same indication. The dose of flunisolide delivered per activation in this preparation is 10 times that per activation of Nasalide® (flunisolide) nasal solution. Clinical studies have shown therapeutic activity on bronchial mucosa with minimal evidence of systemic activity at recommended doses.
After oral inhalation of 1 mg flunisolide, total systemic availability was 40%. The flunisolide that is swallowed is rapidly and extensively converted to the 6β-OH metabolite and to water-soluble conjugates during the first pass through the liver. This offers a metabolic explanation for the low systemic activity of oral flunisolide itself since the metabolite has the low corticosteroid potency (on the order of the cortisol standard). The inhaled flunisolide absorbed through the bronchial tree is converted to the same metabolites. Repeated inhalation of 2.0 mg of flunisolide per day (the maximum recommended dose) for 14 days did not show accumulation of the drug in plasma. The plasma half-life of flunisolide is approximately 1.8 hours.

The following observations relevant to systemic absorption were made in clinical studies. In one uncontrolled study a statistically significant decrease in responsiveness to metyrapone was noted in 15 adult steroid-independent patients treated with 2.0 mg of flunisolide per day (the maximum recommended dose) for 3 months. A small but statistically significant drop in eosinophils from 11.5% to 7.4% of total circulating leucocytes was noted in another study in children who were not taking oral corticosteroids simultaneously. A 5% incidence of menstrual disturbances was reported during open studies, in which there were no control groups for comparison.
Aerosol administration of flunisolide 2.0 mg twice daily for one week to 6 healthy male subjects revealed neither suppression of adrenal function as measured by early morning cortisol levels nor impairment of HPA axis function as determined by insulin hypoglycemia tests.
Controlled clinical studies have included over 500 patients with asthma, among them 150 children age 6 and over. More than 120 patients have been treated in open trials for two years or more. No significant adrenal suppression attributed to flunisolide was seen in these studies.
Significant decreases of systemic steroid dosages have been possible in flunisolide-treated patients. Recommended doses of flunisolide appear to be the therapeutic equivalent of an average of 10 mg/day of oral prednisone. Asthma patients have had further symptomatic improvement with flunisolide treatment even while reducing concomitant medication.

INDICATIONS AND USAGE

AEROBID (flunisolide) Inhaler is indicated in the maintenance treatment of asthma as prophylactic therapy. **AEROBID** is also indicated for asthma patients who require systemic corticosteroid administration, where adding **AEROBID** may reduce or eliminate the need for the systemic corticosteroids.
AEROBID Inhaler is NOT indicated for the relief of acute bronchospasm.

CONTRAINDICATIONS

AEROBID (flunisolide) Inhaler is contraindicated in the primary treatment of status asthmaticus or other acute episodes of asthma where intensive measures are required.
Hypersensitivity to any of the ingredients of this preparation contraindicates its use.

WARNINGS

Particular care is needed in patients who are transferred from systemically active corticosteroids to **AEROBID** Inhaler because deaths due to adrenal insufficiency have occurred in asthmatic patients during and after transfer from systemic corticosteroids to aerosol corticosteroids. After withdrawal from systemic corticosteroids, a number of months are required for recovery of hypothalamic-pituitary-adrenal (HPA) function. During this period of HPA suppression, patients may exhibit signs and symptoms of adrenal insufficiency when exposed to trauma, surgery or infections, particularly gastroenteritis. Although **AEROBID** Inhaler may provide control of asthmatic symptoms during these episodes, it does NOT provide the systemic steroid that is necessary for coping with these emergencies. During periods of stress or a severe asthmatic attack, patients who have been withdrawn from systemic corticosteroids should be instructed to resume systemic steroids (in large doses) immediately and to contact their physician for further instruction. These patients should also be instructed to carry a warning card indicating that they may need supplementary systemic steroids during periods of stress or a severe asthma attack. To assess the risk of adrenal insufficiency in emergency situations, routine tests of adrenal cortical function, including measurement of early morning resting cortisol levels, should be performed periodically in all patients. An early morning resting cortisol level may be accepted as normal if it falls at or near the normal mean level.
Localized infections with *Candida albicans* or *Aspergillus niger* have occurred in the mouth and pharynx and occasionally in the larynx. Positive cultures for oral *Candida* may be present in up to 34% of patients. Although the frequency of clinically apparent infection is considerably lower, these infections may require treatment with appropriate antifungal therapy or discontinuance of treatment with **AEROBID** Inhaler.
AEROBID Inhaler is not to be regarded as a bronchodilator and is not indicated for relief of bronchospasm.
Patients should be instructed to contact their physician immediately when episodes of asthma that are not responsive to bronchodilators occur during the course of treatment. During such episodes, patients may require therapy with systemic corticosteroids. Theoretically, the use of inhaled corticosteroids with alternate day prednisone systemic treatment should be accompanied by more HPA suppression than a therapeutically equivalent regimen of either alone.
Transfer of patients from systemic steroid therapy to **AEROBID** Inhaler may unmask allergic conditions previously suppressed by the systemic steroid therapy, e.g. rhinitis, conjunctivitis, and eczema.
Persons who are on drugs which suppress the immune system are more susceptible to infections than healthy individuals. Chicken pox and measles, for example, can have a more serious or even fatal course in non-immune children or adults on corticosteroids. In such children or adults who have not had these diseases, particular care should be taken to avoid exposure. How the dose, route and duration of corticosteroid administration affects the risk of developing a disseminated infection is not known. The contribution of the underlying disease and/or prior corticosteroid treatment to the risk is also not known. If exposed to chicken pox, prophylaxis with varicella zoster immune globulin (VZIG) may be indicated. If exposed to measles, prophylaxis with pooled intramuscular immunoglobulin (IG) may be indicated. (See the respective package inserts for complete VZIG and IG prescribing information.) If chicken pox develops, treatment with antiviral agents may be considered.

PRECAUTIONS

General: Because of the relatively high molar dose of flunisolide per activation in this preparation, and because of the evidence suggesting higher levels of systemic absorption with flunisolide than with other comparable inhaled corticosteroids (see CLINICAL PHARMACOLOGY section), patients treated with **AEROBID** (flunisolide) should be observed carefully for any evidence of systemic corticosteroid effect, including suppression of bone growth in children. Particular care should be taken in observing patients postoperatively or during periods of stress for evidence of a decrease in adrenal function. During withdrawal from oral steroids, some patients may experience symptoms of systemically active steroid withdrawal, e.g. joint and/or muscular pain, lassitude and depression, despite maintenance or even improvement of respiratory function. (See DOSAGE AND ADMINISTRATION for details.)
In responsive patients, flunisolide may permit control of asthmatic symptoms without suppression of HPA function. Since flunisolide is absorbed into the circulation and can be systemically active, the beneficial effects of **AEROBID** Inhaler in minimizing or preventing HPA dysfunction may be expected only when recommended dosages are not exceeded.
The long-term local and systemic effects of **AEROBID** (flunisolide) in human subjects are still not fully known. In particular, the effects resulting from chronic use of **AEROBID** on developmental or immunologic processes in the mouth, pharynx, trachea, and lung are unknown.
Inhaled corticosteroids should be used with caution, if at all, in patients with active or quiescent tuberculosis infection of the respiratory tract; untreated systemic fungal, bacterial, parasitic or viral infections; or ocular herpes simplex.
Pulmonary infiltrates with eosinophilia may occur in patients on **AEROBID** Inhaler therapy. Although it is possible that in some patients this state may become manifest because of systemic steroid withdrawal when inhalational steroids are administered, a causative role for the drug and/or its vehicle cannot be ruled out.

Information for Patients:
Since the relief from **AEROBID** Inhaler depends on its regular use and on proper inhalation technique, patients must be instructed to take inhalations at regular intervals. They should also be instructed in the correct method of use. (See Patient Instruction Leaflet.)
Patients whose systemic corticosteroids have been reduced or withdrawn should be instructed to carry a warning card indicating they may need supplemental systemic steroids during periods of stress or a severe asthmatic attack that is not responsive to bronchodilators.
Persons who are on immunosuppressant doses of corticosteroids should be warned to avoid exposure to chicken pox or measles. Patients should also be advised that if they are exposed, medical advice should be sought without delay.
An illustrated leaflet of patient instructions for proper use accompanies each **AEROBID** Inhaler System.
CONTENTS UNDER PRESSURE
Do not puncture. Do not use or store near heat or open flame. Exposure to temperatures above 120°F (49°C) may cause container to explode. Never throw container into fire or incinerator. Keep out of reach of children.
Carcinogenesis: Long-term studies were conducted in mice and rats using oral administration to evaluate the carcinogenic potential of the drug. There was an increase in the incidence of pulmonary adenomas in mice, but not in rats. Female rats receiving the highest oral dose had an increased incidence of mammary adenocarcinoma compared to control rats. An increased incidence of this tumor type has been reported for other corticosteroids.
Impairment of Fertility: Female rats receiving high doses of flunisolide (200 mcg/kg/day) showed some evidence of impaired fertility. Reproductive performance in the low- (8 mcg/kg/day) and mid-dose (40 mcg/kg/day) groups was comparable to controls.
Pregnancy: Pregnancy Category C. As with other corticosteroids, flunisolide has been shown to be teratogenic in rabbits and rats at doses of 40 and 200 mcg/kg/day respectively. It was also fetotoxic in these animal reproductive studies. There are no adequate and well-controlled studies in pregnant women. Flunisolide should be used during pregnancy only if the potential benefit justifies the potential risk to the fetus.
Nursing Mothers: It is not known whether this drug is excreted in human milk. Because other corticosteroids are excreted in human milk, caution should be exercised when flunisolide is administered to nursing women.
Pediatric Use: Safety and effectiveness have not been established in children below the age of 6. Oral corticoids have been shown to cause growth suppression in children and adolescents, particularly with higher doses over extended periods. If a child or adolescent on any corticoid appears to have growth suppression, the possibility that they are particularly sensitive to this effect of steroids should be considered.

ADVERSE REACTIONS

Adverse events reported in controlled clinical trials and long-term open studies in 514 patients treated with **AEROBID** (flunisolide) are described below. Of those patients, 463 were treated for 3 months or longer, 407 for 6 months or longer, 287 for 1 year or longer, and 122 for 2 years or longer.
Musculoskeletal reactions were reported in 35% of steroid-dependent patients in whom the dose of oral steroid was being tapered. This is a well-known effect of steroid withdrawal.

Incidence 10% or greater:
Gastrointestinal: diarrhea (10%), nausea and/or vomiting (25%), upset stomach (10%)
General: flu (10%)
Mouth and Throat: sore throat (20%)
Nervous System: headache (25%)
Respiratory: cold symptoms (15%), nasal congestion (15%), upper respiratory infection (25%)
Special Senses: unpleasant taste (10%)

Incidence 3-9%
Cardiovascular: palpitations
Gastrointestinal: abdominal pain, heartburn
General: chest pain, decreased appetite, edema, fever
Mouth and Throat: *Candida* infection
Nervous System: dizziness, irritability, nervousness, shakiness
Reproductive: menstrual disturbances
Respiratory: chest congestion, cough*, hoarseness, rhinitis, runny nose, sinus congestion, sinus drainage, sinus infection, sinusitis, sneezing, sputum, wheezing*
Skin: eczema, itching (pruritus), rash
Special Senses: ear infection, loss of smell or taste

Incidence 1-3%
General: chills, increased appetite and weight gain, malaise, peripheral edema, sweating, weakness
Cardiovascular: hypertension, tachycardia
Gastrointestinal: constipation, dyspepsia, gas
Hemic/Lymph: capillary fragility, enlarged lymph nodes
Mouth and Throat: dry throat, glossitis, mouth irritation, pharyngitis, phlegm, throat irritation
Nervous System: anxiety, depression, faintness, fatigue, hyperactivity, hypoactivity, insomnia, moodiness, numbness, vertigo
Respiratory: bronchitis, chest tightness*, dyspnea, epistaxis, head stuffiness, laryngitis, nasal irritation, pleurisy, pneumonia, sinus discomfort
Skin: acne, hives or urticaria
Special Senses: blurred vision, earache, eye discomfort, eye infection

Incidence less than 1%, judged by investigators as possibly or probably drug related: abdominal fullness, shortness of breath.

---

*The incidences as shown of cough, wheezing, and chest tightness were judged by investigators to be possibly or probably drug related. In placebo-controlled trials, the *overall* incidences of these adverse events (regardless of investigators' judgement of drug relationship) were similar for drug and placebo-treated groups. They may be related to the vehicle or delivery system.

DOSAGE AND ADMINISTRATION

The **AEROBID** (flunisolide) Inhaler System is for oral inhalation only.
Adults: The recommended starting dose is 2 inhalations twice daily, morning and evening, for a total daily dose of 1 mg. The maximum daily dose should not exceed 4 inhalations twice a day for a total daily dose of 2 mg. When the drug is used chronically at 2 mg/day, patients should be monitored periodically for effects on the hypothalamic-pituitary-adrenal (HPA) axis.
Pediatric Patients: For children and adolescents 6-15 years of age, two inhalations may be administered twice daily for a total daily dose of 1 mg. Higher doses have not been studied. Insufficient information is available to warrant use in children under age 6. With chronic use, pediatric patients should be monitored for growth as well as for effects on the HPA axis.
Rinsing the mouth after inhalation is advised.
Different considerations must be given to the following groups of patients in order to obtain the full therapeutic benefit of **AEROBID** (flunisolide) Inhaler.
Patients Not Receiving Systemic Corticosteroids:
Patients who require maintenance therapy of their asthma may benefit from treatment with **AEROBID** at the doses recommended above. In patients who respond to **AEROBID**, improvement in pulmonary function is usually apparent within one to four weeks after the start of therapy. Once the desired effect is achieved, consideration should be given to tapering to the lowest effective dose.
Patients Maintained on Systemic Corticosteroids:
Clinical studies have shown that **AEROBID** may be effective in the management of asthmatics dependent or maintained on systemic corticosteroids and may permit replacement or significant reduction in the dosage of systemic corticosteroids.
The patient's asthma should be reasonably stable before treatment with **AEROBID** is started. Initially, **AEROBID** should be used concurrently with the patient's usual maintenance dose of systemic corticosteroid. After approximately one week, gradual withdrawal of the systemic corticosteroid

Continued on next page

Aerobid—Cont.

is started by reducing the daily or alternate daily dose. Reductions may be made after an interval of one or two weeks, depending on the response of the patient. A slow rate of withdrawal is strongly recommended. Generally, these decrements should not exceed 2.5 mg of prednisone or its equivalent. During withdrawal, some patients may experience symptoms of systemic corticosteroid withdrawal; e.g. joint and/or muscular pain, lassitude and depression, despite maintenance or even improvement in pulmonary function. Such patients should be encouraged to continue with the inhaler but should be monitored for objective signs of adrenal insufficiency. If evidence of adrenal insufficiency occurs, the systemic corticosteroid doses should be increased temporarily and thereafter withdrawal should continue more slowly. During periods of stress or a severe asthma attack, transfer patients may require supplementary treatment with systemic corticosteroids.

HOW SUPPLIED

AEROBID (flunisolide) Inhaler Systems are available in canisters of 100 metered inhalations.
NDC 0456-0672-99 **AEROBID**
NDC 0456-0670-99 **AEROBID-M**

"Note: The indented statement below is required by the Federal government's Clean Air Act for all products containing or manufactured with chlorofluorocarbons (CFC's)."

> WARNING: Contains trichloromonofluoromethane, dichlorodifluoromethane and dichlorotetrafluoroethane, substances which harm public health and environment by destroying ozone in the upper atmosphere.

"A notice similar to the above WARNING has been placed in the information for the patient of this product pursuant to EPA regulations."

mfd for Revised 3/02
FOREST PHARMACEUTICALS, INC.
St. Louis, MO 63045
mfd by
3M Pharmaceuticals
St. Paul, MN 624200

How to use your
AEROBID®
AEROBID®-M
(flunisolide)
Inhaler System
DIRECTIONS FOR USE:

Before using your new **AEROBID** Inhaler System, it is important that you read over the following simple instructions and familiarize yourself with the inhaler and its metal cartridge.

As your doctor has probably told you, the **AEROBID** Inhaler System must be used for a few days before it begins working, and then should be used regularly to help reduce the frequency and severity of your asthma attacks. It is not a bronchodilator and will not provide relief during an actual asthmatic attack, but it can cut down the number of bad attacks if used regularly every day.

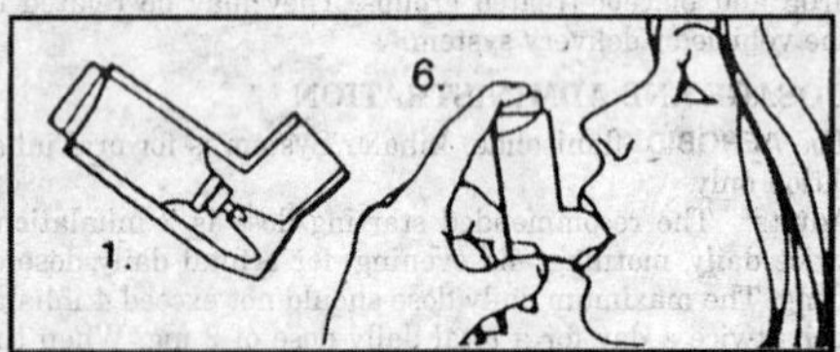

1. Before the first use, place the **AEROBID** metal cartridge inside the plastic container as shown.
2. Shake the inhaler system before each inhalation.
3. Before each use, remove dustcap and inspect mouthpiece for foreign objects.
4. Replace dustcap after each use.
5. Breathe out as completely as possible.
6. Hold the inhaler system upright and put plastic mouthpiece in your mouth as shown, being sure to close your lips tightly around the mouthpiece.
7. Breathe in slowly through your mouth. At the same time firmly press down on the metal cartridge with your index finger.
8. Hold your breath as long as you can.
9. While holding your breath, stop pressing on the cartridge and remove mouthpiece from your mouth.
10. If your doctor has prescribed two or more inhalations at each use, wait a minute to allow pressure to build up again in the metal canister, then repeat steps two through nine (2–9). Be sure to shake the inhaler system *again* before each inhalation.
11. After the prescribed number of inhalations, rinse out your mouth thoroughly with water.
12. Clean the inhaler system every few days. To do so, remove the metal cartridge, then rinse the plastic inhaler and cap with briskly running warm water. Dry thoroughly. Replace the cartridge and cap.

NOTE: If your mouth becomes sore or develops a rash, be sure to mention this to your doctor, but do not stop using your inhaler system unless he tells you.

WARNING: The contents of the metal cartridge are under pressure. Do not puncture. Do not use or store near heat or open flame. Exposure to temperature above 120°F (49°C) may cause cartridge to explode. Never throw cartridge into fire or incinerator. Use by children should always be supervised by an adult.

mfd by
3M Pharmaceuticals, Inc.
St. Paul, MN
For:
FOREST PHARMACEUTICALS, INC.
SUBSIDIARY OF FOREST LABORATORIES, INC.
ST. LOUIS, MISSOURI 63045

Shown in Product Identification Guide, page 312

AEROCHAMBER PLUS™ ℞
AEROCHAMBER PLUS™ with *Mask—Small*
AEROCHAMBER PLUS™ with *Mask*
AEROCHAMBER PLUS™ with *Mask—Large*
Valved Holding Chamber with *FLOWSIGnal®* Whistle/ Valved Holding Chamber with *FLOWSIGnal®* Whistle with *ComfortSeal™* Mask

Directions for Use (Single Patient Use Only)

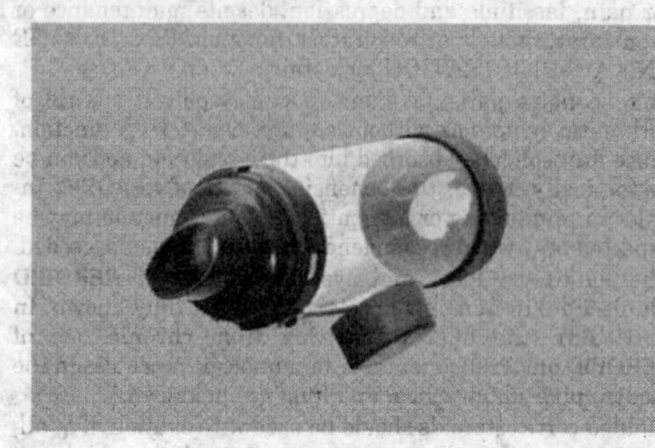

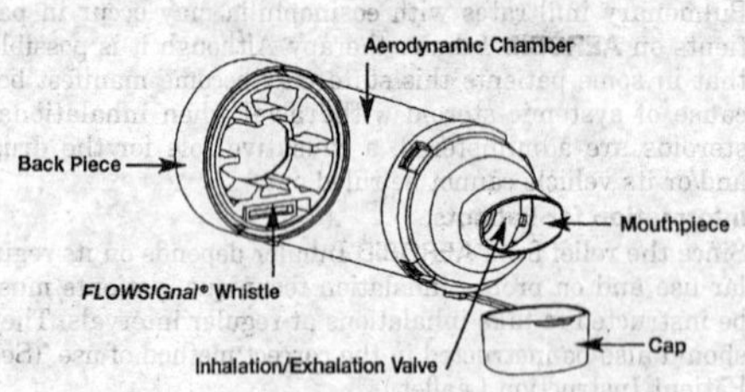

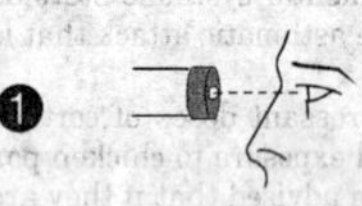

1. Carefully examine the product for damage, missing parts or foreign objects. Any foreign objects should be removed. The product should be replaced IMMEDIATELY if there are any damaged or missing parts. If necessary, use the inhaler (MDI) alone until a replacement is obtained. If your symptoms worsen, please seek immediate medical attention.

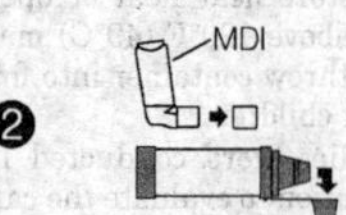

2. Before use, make sure that instructions supplied with inhaler (MDI) have been read. Remove cap(s).

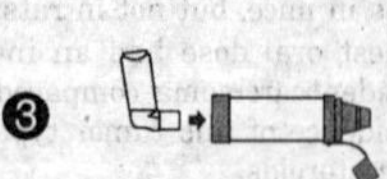

3. Shake the inhaler (MDI) well immediately before each use. Insert the inhaler (MDI) into the back piece of the chamber.

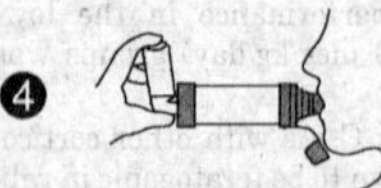

4. Put mouthpiece into mouth.

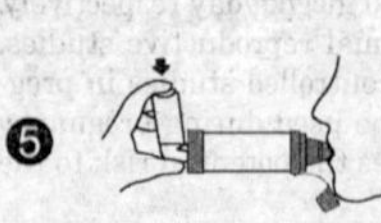

5. Depress inhaler (MDI) at beginning of slow deep inhalation. Hold breath as long as possible, up to 10 seconds before breathing out.
If patient has difficulty with slow deep breaths, an alternative is to keep mouth tight on mouthpiece and breathe slowly 2–3 times after depressing inhaler (MDI).
Administer one (1) puff at a time.

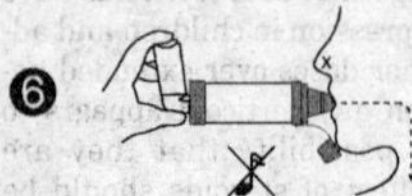

6. Slow down inhalation if you hear the *FLOWSIGnal®* Whistle sound.

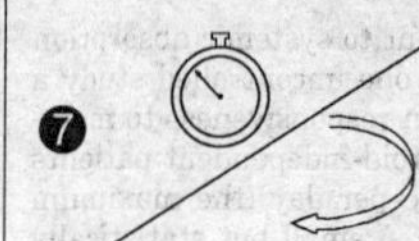

7. Follow instructions supplied with the inhaler (MDI) on amount of time to wait before repeating steps 3–6 as prescribed.

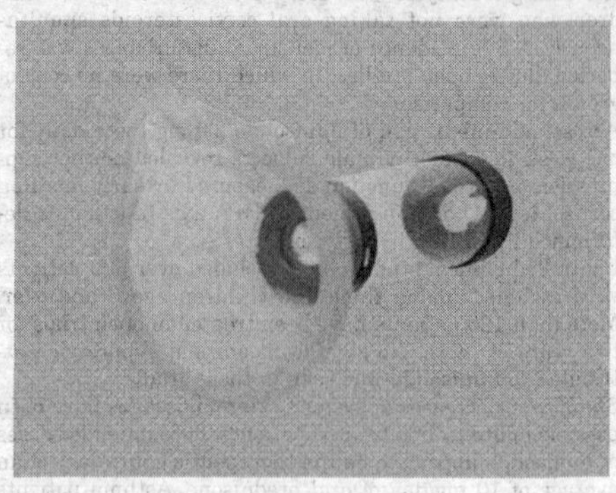

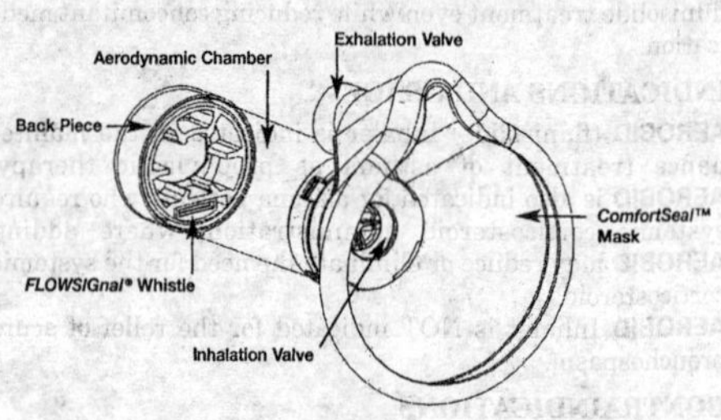

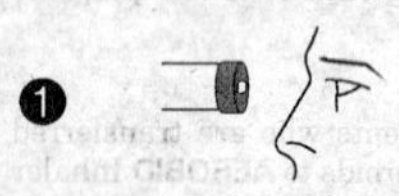

1. Carefully examine the product for damage, missing parts or foreign objects. Any foreign objects should be removed. The product should be replaced IMMEDIATELY if there are any damaged or missing parts. If necessary, use the inhaler (MDI) alone until a replacement is obtained. If your symptoms worsen, please seek immediate medical attention.

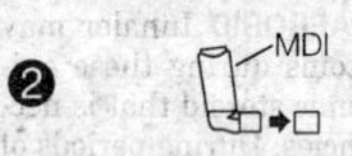

2. Before use, make sure that instructions supplied with inhaler (MDI) have been read. Remove cap.

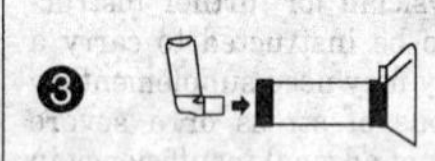

3. Shake the inhaler (MDI) well immediately before each use. Insert the inhaler (MDI) into the back piece of the chamber.

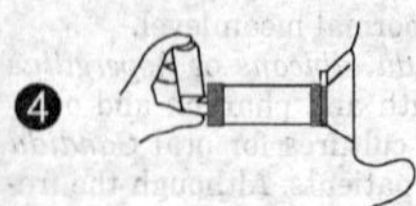

4. Apply mask to face and ensure that there is a good seal.

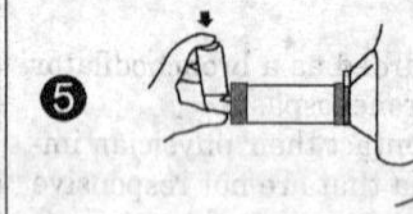

5. Depress inhaler (MDI) at beginning of slow inhalation. Maintain seal with mask for 2–3 breaths after depressing inhaler (MDI).
Administer one (1) puff at a time.

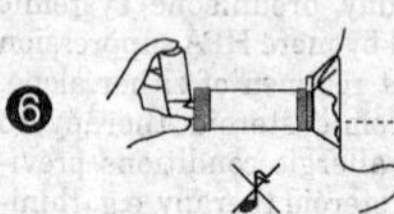

6. Slow down inhalation if you hear the *FLOWSIGnal®* Whistle sound.

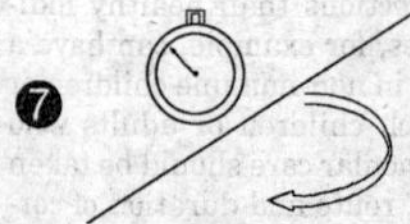

7. Follow instructions supplied with the inhaler (MDI) on amount of time to wait before repeating steps 3–6 as prescribed.

Cleaning Instructions

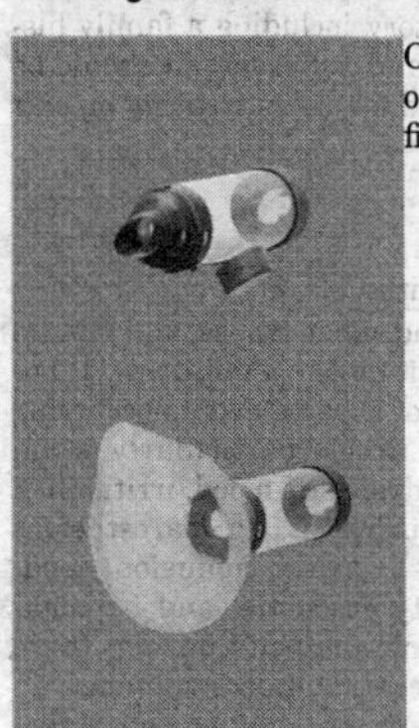

Clean ***AeroChamber Plus™*** VHC only as per instructions before first use, then weekly.

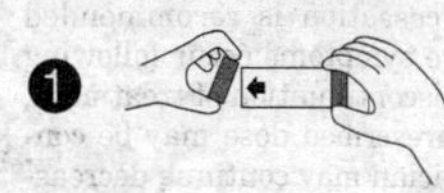

Remove back piece only. (Do not remove mask)

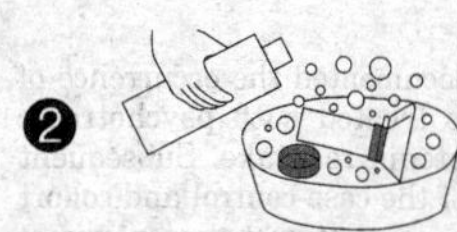

Soak both parts for 15 minutes in lukewarm water with liquid detergent. Agitate gently.

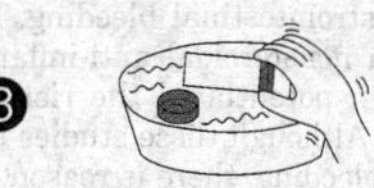

Rinse in clean water.

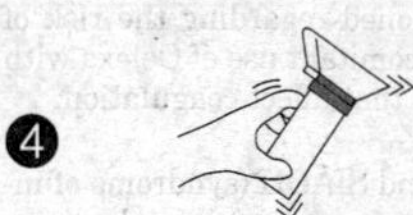

Shake out excess water. **Do not rub dry.**

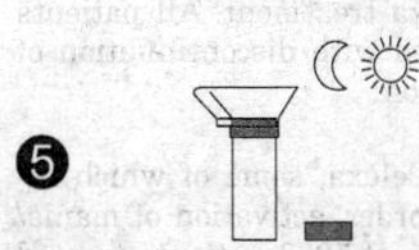

Let air dry in vertical position.

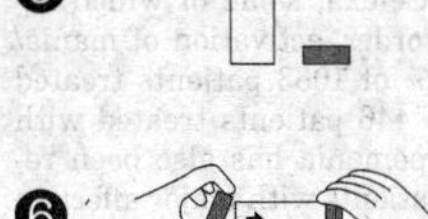

Replace back piece when unit is completely dry and ready for use.

Cautions

— Read all instructions before use.

— Do not leave ***AeroChamber Plus™*** VHC unattended with children. This is a medical device, not a toy.

— Do not disassemble the product beyond what is recommended in the Cleaning Instructions or damage may result.

— If unsure on how to use this product, talk to your physician or pharmacist.

Notes

— VHC = Valved Holding Chamber

— This product contains no latex.

Indications for Use: The ***AeroChamber Plus™*** Valved Holding Chamber ("VHC") is intended to be used by patients who are under the care or treatment of a licensed health care professional or physician. The device is intended to be used by these patients to administer aerosolized medication from most pressurized Metered Dose Inhalers, prescribed by a physician or health care professional. The intended environments for use include the home, hospitals and clinics. **Rx only**

Distributed by:

Forest Pharmaceuticals, Inc.

Subsidiary of Forest Laboratories, Inc. St. Louis, MO 63045

Monaghan Medical Corporation, P.O. Box 2805, Plattsburgh, NY 12901

Covered by one or more of the following Patents 5,042,467; 5,645,049; 5,848,588; 6,345,617; 6,293,279; and patents pending

Printed in USA RMC 5263 and 6209 Revision: 04/02

AeroChamber Plus™ and *ComfortSeal*™ are registered trademarks used under license.

Shown in Product Identification Guide, page 312

ARMOUR® THYROID Tablets ℞

[*thī 'roid*]

(THYROID TABLETS, USP)

DESCRIPTION

Armour® Thyroid (thyroid tablets, USP) for oral use is a natural preparation derived from porcine thyroid glands and has a strong, characteristic odor. (T_3 liothyronine is approximately four times as potent as T_4 levothyroxine on a microgram for microgram basis.) They provide 38 mcg levothyroxine (T_4) and 9 mcg liothyronine (T_3) per grain of thyroid. The inactive ingredients are calcium stearate, dextrose microcrystalline cellulose, sodium starch glycolate and opadry white.

HOW SUPPLIED

Armour Thyroid Tablets (thyroid tablets, USP) are supplied as follows:

Size	Available in	NDC No.
15 mg (1/4 gr)	Bottles of 100	0456-0457-01
30 mg (1/2 gr)	Bottles of 100	0456-0458-01
	Bottles of 1000	0456-0458-00
	Drums of 50,000	0456-0458-69
	Unit dose cartons of 100	0456-0458-63
60 mg (1 gr)	Bottles of 100	0456-0459-01
	Bottles of 1000	0456-0459-00
	Bottles of 5000	0456-0459-51
	Drums of 50,000	0456-0459-69
	Unit dose cartons of 100	0456-0459-63
90 mg (1 1/2 gr)	Bottles of 100	0456-0460-01
120 mg (2 gr)	Bottles of 100	0456-0461-01
	Bottles of 1000	0456-0461-00
	Drums of 50,000	0456-0461-69
	Unit dose cartons of 100	0456-0461-63
180 mg (3 gr)	Bottles of 100	0456-0462-01
	Bottles of 1000	0456-0462-00
240 mg (4 gr)	Bottles of 100	0456-0463-01
300 mg (5 gr)	Bottles of 100	0456-0464-01

The bottles of 100 are special dispensing bottles with child-resistant closures.

Note: (T_3 liothyronine is approximately four times as potent as T_4 levothyroxine on a microgram-for-microgram basis.)

Tablets should be stored at controlled room temperature, 59°–86°F (15°–30°C), in capped bottles or unbroken plastic strip packing.

Forest Pharmaceuticals, Inc.

A Subsidiary of Forest Laboratories, Inc.

St. Louis, MO 63045

REV 11/02 11841102

Shown in Product Identification Guide, page 312

CELEXA® ℞

[*sĕ-lĕk-să*]

(citalopram hydrobromide)

Tablets/Oral Solution

Rx Only

DESCRIPTION

Celexa® (citalopram HBr) is an orally administered selective serotonin reuptake inhibitor (SSRI) with a chemical structure unrelated to that of other SSRIs or of tricyclic, tetracyclic, or other available antidepressant agents. Citalopram HBr is a racemic bicyclic phthalane derivative designated (±)-1-(3-dimethylaminopropyl)-1-(4-fluorophenyl)-1,3-dihydroisobenzofuran-5-carbonitrile, HBr with the following structural formula:

The molecular formula is $C_{20}H_{22}BrFN_2O$ and its molecular weight is 405.35.

Citalopram HBr occurs as a fine, white to off-white powder. Citalopram HBr is sparingly soluble in water and soluble in ethanol.

Celexa (citalopram hydrobromide) is available as tablets or as an oral solution.

Celexa 10 mg tablets are film-coated, oval tablets containing citalopram HBr in strengths equivalent to 10 mg citalopram base. Celexa 20 mg and 40 mg tablets are film-coated, oval, scored tablets containing citalopram HBr in strengths equivalent to 20 mg or 40 mg citalopram base. The tablets also contain the following inactive ingredients: copolyvidone, corn starch, crosscarmellose sodium, glycerin, lactose monohydrate, magnesium stearate, hypromellose, microcrystalline cellulose, polyethylene glycol, and titanium dioxide. Iron oxides are used as coloring agents in the beige (10 mg) and pink (20 mg) tablets.

Celexa oral solution contains citalopram HBr equivalent to 2 mg/mL citalopram base. It also contains the following inactive ingredients: sorbitol, purified water, propylene glycol, methylparaben, natural peppermint flavor, and propylparaben.

CLINICAL PHARMACOLOGY

Pharmacodynamics

The mechanism of action of citalopram HBr as an antidepressant is presumed to be linked to potentiation of serotonergic activity in the central nervous system (CNS) resulting from its inhibition of CNS neuronal reuptake of serotonin (5-HT). *In vitro* and *in vivo* studies in animals suggest that citalopram is a highly selective serotonin reuptake inhibitor (SSRI) with minimal effects on norepinephrine (NE) and dopamine (DA) neuronal reuptake. Tolerance to the inhibition of 5-HT uptake is not induced by long-term (14-day) treatment of rats with citalopram. Citalopram is a racemic mixture (50/50), and the inhibition of 5-HT reuptake by citalopram is primarily due to the (S)-enantiomer. Citalopram has no or very low affinity for 5-HT_{1A}, 5-HT_{2A}, dopamine D_1 and D_2, α_1-, α_2-, and β-adrenergic, histamine H_1, gamma aminobutyric acid (GABA), muscarinic cholinergic, and benzodiazepine receptors. Antagonism of muscarinic, histaminergic, and adrenergic receptors has been hypothesized to be associated with various anticholinergic, sedative, and cardiovascular effects of other psychotropic drugs.

Pharmacokinetics

The single- and multiple-dose pharmacokinetics of citalopram are linear and dose-proportional in a dose range of 10–60 mg/day. Biotransformation of citalopram is mainly hepatic, with a mean terminal half-life of about 35 hours. With once daily dosing, steady state plasma concentrations are achieved within approximately one week. At steady state, the extent of accumulation of citalopram in plasma, based on the half-life, is expected to be 2.5 times the plasma concentrations observed after a single dose. The tablet and oral solution dosage forms of citalopram HBr are bioequivalent.

Absorption and Distribution

Following a single oral dose (40 mg tablet) of citalopram, peak blood levels occur at about 4 hours. The absolute bioavailability of citalopram was about 80% relative to an intravenous dose, and absorption is not affected by food. The volume of distribution of citalopram is about 12 L/kg and the binding of citalopram (CT), demethylcitalopram (DCT) and didemethylcitalopram (DDCT) to human plasma proteins is about 80%.

Metabolism and Elimination

Following intravenous administrations of citalopram, the fraction of drug recovered in the urine as citalopram and DCT was about 10% and 5%, respectively. The systemic clearance of citalopram was 330 mL/min, with approximately 20% of that due to renal clearance.

Citalopram is metabolized to demethylcitalopram (DCT), didemethylcitalopram (DDCT), citalopram-N-oxide, and a deaminated propionic acid derivative. In humans, unchanged citalopram is the predominant compound in plasma. At steady state, the concentrations of citalopram's metabolites, DCT and DDCT, in plasma are approximately one-half and one-tenth, respectively, that of the parent drug. *In vitro* studies show that citalopram is at least 8 times more potent than its metabolites in the inhibition of serotonin reuptake, suggesting that the metabolites evaluated do not likely contribute significantly to the antidepressant actions of citalopram.

In vitro studies using human liver microsomes indicated that CYP3A4 and CYP2C19 are the primary isozymes involved in the N-demethylation of citalopram.

Population Subgroups

Age - Citalopram pharmacokinetics in subjects ≥60 years of age were compared to younger subjects in two normal volunteer studies. In a single-dose study, citalopram AUC and half-life were increased in the elderly subjects by 30% and 50%, respectively, whereas in a multiple-dose study they were increased by 23% and 30%, respectively. 20 mg is the recommended dose for most elderly patients (see **DOSAGE AND ADMINISTRATION**).

Gender - In three pharmacokinetic studies (total N=32), citalopram AUC in women was one and a half to two times that in men. This difference was not observed in five other pharmacokinetic studies (total N=114). In clinical studies, no differences in steady state serum citalopram levels were seen between men (N=237) and women (N=388). There were no gender differences in the pharmacokinetics of DCT and DDCT. No adjustment of dosage on the basis of gender is recommended.

Reduced hepatic function - Citalopram oral clearance was reduced by 37% and half-life was doubled in patients with reduced hepatic function compared to normal subjects. 20 mg is the recommended dose for most hepatically impaired patients (see **DOSAGE AND ADMINISTRATION**).

Reduced renal function - In patients with mild to moderate renal function impairment, oral clearance of citalopram was reduced by 17% compared to normal subjects. No adjustment of dosage for such patients is recommended. No infor-

Continued on next page

Celexa—Cont.

mation is available about the pharmacokinetics of citalopram in patients with severely reduced renal function (creatinine clearance < 20 mL/min).

Drug-Drug Interactions

In vitro enzyme inhibition data did not reveal an inhibitory effect of citalopram on CYP3A4, -2C9, or -2E1, but did suggest that it is a weak inhibitor of CYP1A2, -2D6, and -2C19. Citalopram would be expected to have little inhibitory effect on *in vivo* metabolism mediated by these cytochromes. However, *in vivo* data to address this question are limited.

Since CYP3A4 and 2C19 are the primary enzymes involved in the metabolism of citalopram, it is expected that potent inhibitors of 3A4 (e.g., ketoconazole, itraconazole, and macrolide antibiotics) and potent inhibitors of CYP2C19 (e.g., omeprazole) might decrease the clearance of citalopram. However, coadministration of citalopram and the potent 3A4 inhibitor ketoconazole did not significantly affect the pharmacokinetics of citalopram. Because citalopram is metabolized by multiple enzyme systems, inhibition of a single enzyme may not appreciably decrease citalopram clearance. Citalopram steady state levels were not significantly different in poor metabolizers and extensive 2D6 metabolizers after multiple-dose administration of Celexa, suggesting that coadministration, with Celexa, of a drug that inhibits CYP2D6, is unlikely to have clinically significant effects on citalopram metabolism. See **Drug Interactions** under **PRECAUTIONS** for more detailed information on available drug interaction data.

Clinical Efficacy Trials

The efficacy of Celexa as a treatment for depression was established in two placebo-controlled studies (of 4 to 6 weeks in duration) in adult outpatients (ages 18–66) meeting DSM-III or DSM-III-R criteria for major depression. Study 1, a 6-week trial in which patients received fixed Celexa doses of 10, 20, 40, and 60 mg/day, showed that Celexa at doses of 40 and 60 mg/day was effective as measured by the Hamilton Depression Rating Scale (HAMD) total score, the HAMD depressed mood item (Item 1), the Montgomery Asberg Depression Rating Scale, and the Clinical Global Impression (CGI) Severity scale. This study showed no clear effect of the 10 and 20 mg/day doses, and the 60 mg/day dose was not more effective than the 40 mg/day dose. In study 2, a 4-week, placebo-controlled trial in depressed patients, of whom 85% met criteria for melancholia, the initial dose was 20 mg/day, followed by titration to the maximum tolerated dose or a maximum dose of 80 mg/day. Patients treated with Celexa showed significantly greater improvement than placebo patients on the HAMD total score, HAMD item 1, and the CGI Severity score. In three additional placebo-controlled depression trials, the difference in response to treatment between patients receiving Celexa and patients receiving placebo was not statistically significant, possibly due to high spontaneous response rate, smaller sample size, or, in the case of one study, too low a dose.

In two long-term studies, depressed patients who had responded to Celexa during an initial 6 or 8 weeks of acute treatment (fixed doses of 20 or 40 mg/day in one study and flexible doses of 20–60 mg/day in the second study) were randomized to continuation of Celexa or to placebo. In both studies, patients receiving continued Celexa treatment experienced significantly lower relapse rates over the subsequent 6 months compared to those receiving placebo. In the fixed-dose study, the decreased rate of depression relapse was similar in patients receiving 20 or 40 mg/day of Celexa.

Analyses of the relationship between treatment outcome and age, gender, and race did not suggest any differential responsiveness on the basis of these patient characteristics.

Comparison of Clinical Trial Results

Highly variable results have been seen in the clinical development of all antidepressant drugs. Furthermore, in those circumstances when the drugs have not been studied in the same controlled clinical trial(s), comparisons among the results of studies evaluating the effectiveness of different antidepressant drug products are inherently unreliable. Because conditions of testing (e.g., patient samples, investigators, doses of the treatments administered and compared, outcome measures, etc.) vary among trials, it is virtually impossible to distinguish a difference in drug effect from a difference due to one of the confounding factors just enumerated.

INDICATIONS AND USAGE

Celexa (citalopram HBr) is indicated for the treatment of depression.

The efficacy of Celexa in the treatment of depression was established in 4-6 week, controlled trials of outpatients whose diagnosis corresponded most closely to the DSM-III and DSM-III-R category of major depressive disorder (see **CLINICAL PHARMACOLOGY**).

A major depressive episode (DSM-IV) implies a prominent and relatively persistent (nearly every day for at least 2 weeks) depressed or dysphoric mood that usually interferes with daily functioning, and includes at least five of the following nine symptoms: depressed mood, loss of interest in usual activities, significant change in weight and/or appetite, insomnia or hypersomnia, psychomotor agitation or retardation, increased fatigue, feelings of guilt or worthlessness, slowed thinking or impaired concentration, a suicide attempt or suicidal ideation.

The antidepressant action of Celexa in hospitalized depressed patients has not been adequately studied.

The efficacy of Celexa in maintaining an antidepressant response for up to 24 weeks following 6 to 8 weeks of acute treatment was demonstrated in two placebo-controlled trials (see **CLINICAL PHARMACOLOGY**). Nevertheless, the physician who elects to use Celexa for extended periods should periodically re-evaluate the long-term usefulness of the drug for the individual patient.

CONTRAINDICATIONS

Concomitant use in patients taking monoamine oxidase inhibitors (MAOIs) is contraindicated (see **WARNINGS**).

Celexa is contraindicated in patients with a hypersensitivity to citalopram or any of the inactive ingredients in Celexa.

WARNINGS

Potential for Interaction with Monoamine Oxidase Inhibitors

In patients receiving serotonin reuptake inhibitor drugs in combination with a monoamine oxidase inhibitor (MAOI), there have been reports of serious, sometimes fatal, reactions including hyperthermia, rigidity, myoclonus, autonomic instability with possible rapid fluctuations of vital signs, and mental status changes that include extreme agitation progressing to delirium and coma. These reactions have also been reported in patients who have recently discontinued SSRI treatment and have been started on an MAOI. Some cases presented with features resembling neuroleptic malignant syndrome. Furthermore, limited animal data on the effects of combined use of SSRIs and MAOIs suggest that these drugs may act synergistically to elevate blood pressure and evoke behavioral excitation. Therefore, it is recommended that Celexa should not be used in combination with an MAOI, or within 14 days of discontinuing treatment with an MAOI. Similarly, at least 14 days should be allowed after stopping Celexa before starting an MAOI.

Clinical Worsening and Suicide Risk

Patients with major depressive disorder, both adult and pediatric, may experience worsening of their depression and/or the emergence of suicidal ideation and behavior (suicidality), whether or not they are taking antidepressant medications, and this risk may persist until significant remission occurs. Although there has been a long-standing concern that antidepressants may have a role in inducing worsening of depression and the emergence of suicidality in certain patients, a causal role for antidepressants in inducing such behaviors has not been established. **Nevertheless, patients being treated with antidepressants should be observed closely for clinical worsening and suicidality, especially at the beginning of a course of drug therapy, or at the time of dose changes, either increases or decreases.** Consideration should be given to changing the therapeutic regimen, including possibly discontinuing the medication, in patients whose depression is persistently worse or whose emergent suicidality is severe, abrupt in onset, or was not part of the patient's presenting symptoms.

Because of the possibility of co-morbitity between major depressive disorder and other psychiatric and nonpsychiatric disorders, the same precautions observed when treating patients with major depressive disorder should be observed when treating patients with other psychiatric and nonpsychiatric disorders.

The following symptoms, anxiety, agitation, panic attacks, insomnia, irritability, hostility (aggressiveness), impulsivity, akathisia (psychomotor restlessness), hypomania, and mania, have been reported in adult and pediatric patients being treated with antidepressants for major depressive disorder as well as for other indications, both psychiatric and nonpsychiatric. Although a causal link between the emergence of such symptoms and either the worsening of depression and/or the emergence of suicidal impulses has not been established, consideration should be given to changing the therapeutic regimen, including possibly discontinuing the medication, in patients for whom such symptoms are severe, abrupt in onset, or were not part of the patient's presenting symptoms.

Families and caregivers of patients being treated with antidepressants for major depressive disorder or other indications, both psychiatric and nonpsychiatric, should be alerted about the need to monitor patients for the emergence of agitation, irritability, and the other symptoms described above, as well as the emergence of suicidality, and to report such symptoms immediately to healthcare providers. Prescriptions for Celexa should be written for the smallest quantity of tablets consistent with good patient management, in order to reduce the risk of overdose.

If the decision has been made to discontinue treatment, medication should be tapered, as rapidly as is feasible, but with recognition that abrupt discontinuation can be associated with certain symptoms (see **PRECAUTIONS** and **DOSAGE AND ADMINISTRATION**, **Discontinuation of Treatment with Celexa**, for a description of the risks of discontinuation of Celexa).

It should be noted that Celexa is not approved for use in treating any indications in the pediatric population.

A major depressive episode may be the initial presentation of bipolar disorder. It is generally believed (though not established in controlled trials) that treating such an episode with an antidepressant alone may increase the likelihood of precipitation of a mixed/manic episode in patients at risk for bipolar disorder. Whether any of the symptoms described above represent such a conversion is unknown. However, prior to initiating treatment with an antidepressant, patients should be adequately screened to determine if they are at risk for bipolar disorder; such screening should include a detailed psychiatric history, including a family history of suicide, bipolar disorder, and depression. It should be noted that Celexa is not approved for use in treating bipolar depression.

PRECAUTIONS

General

Discontinuation of Treatment with Celexa

During marketing of Celexa and other SSRIs and SNRIs (serotonin and norepinephrine reuptake inhibitors), there have been spontaneous reports of adverse events occurring upon discontinuation of these drugs, particularly when abrupt, including the following: dysphoric mood, irritability, agitation, dizziness, sensory disturbances (e.g., paresthesias such as electric shock sensations), anxiety, confusion, headache, lethargy, emotional lability, insomnia, and hypomania. While these events are generally self-limiting, there have been reports of serious discontinuation symptoms.

Patients should be monitored for these symptoms when discontinuing treatment with Celexa. A gradual reduction in the dose rather than abrupt cessation is recommended whenever possible. If intolerable symptoms occur following a decrease in the dose or upon discontinuation of treatment, then resuming the previously prescribed dose may be considered. Subsequently, the physician may continue decreasing the dose but at a more gradual rate (see **DOSAGE AND ADMINISTRATION**).

Abnormal Bleeding

Published case reports have documented the occurrence of bleeding episodes in patients treated with psychotropic drugs that interfere with serotonin reuptake. Subsequent epidemiological studies, both of the case-control and cohort design, have demonstrated an association between use of psychotropic drugs that interfere with serotonin reuptake and the occurrence of upper gastrointestinal bleeding. In two studies, concurrent use of a nonsteroidal anti-inflammatory drug (NSAID) or aspirin potentiated the risk of bleeding (see **Drug Interactions**). Although these studies focused on upper gastrointestinal bleeding, there is reason to believe that bleeding at other sites may be similarly potentiated. Patients should be cautioned regarding the risk of bleeding associated with the concomitant use of Celexa with NSAIDs, aspirin, or other drugs that affect coagulation.

Hyponatremia

Several cases of hyponatremia and SIADH (syndrome of inappropriate antidiuretic hormone secretion) have been reported in association with Celexa treatment. All patients with these events have recovered with discontinuation of Celexa and/or medical intervention.

Activation of Mania/Hypomania

In placebo-controlled trials of Celexa, some of which included patients with bipolar disorder, activation of mania/hypomania was reported in 0.2% of 1063 patients treated with Celexa and in none of the 446 patients treated with placebo. Activation of mania/hypomania has also been reported in a small proportion of patients with major affective disorders treated with other marketed antidepressants. As with all antidepressants, Celexa should be used cautiously in patients with a history of mania.

Seizures

Although anticonvulsant effects of citalopram have been observed in animal studies, Celexa has not been systematically evaluated in patients with a seizure disorder. These patients were excluded from clinical studies during the product's premarketing testing. In clinical trials of Celexa, seizures occurred in 0.3% of patients treated with Celexa (a rate of one patient per 98 years of exposure) and 0.5% of patients treated with placebo (a rate of one patient per 50 years of exposure). Like other antidepressants, Celexa should be introduced with care in patients with a history of seizure disorder.

Interference with Cognitive and Motor Performance

In studies in normal volunteers, Celexa in doses of 40 mg/day did not produce impairment of intellectual function or psychomotor performance. Because any psychoactive drug may impair judgment, thinking, or motor skills, however, patients should be cautioned about operating hazardous machinery, including automobiles, until they are reasonably certain that Celexa therapy does not affect their ability to engage in such activities.

Use in Patients with Concomitant Illness

Clinical experience with Celexa in patients with certain concomitant systemic illnesses is limited. Caution is advisable in using Celexa in patients with diseases or conditions that produce altered metabolism or hemodynamic responses.

Celexa has not been systematically evaluated in patients with a recent history of myocardial infarction or unstable heart disease. Patients with these diagnoses were generally excluded from clinical studies during the product's premarketing testing. However, the electrocardiograms of 1116 patients who received Celexa in clinical trials were evaluated and the data indicate that Celexa is not associated with the development of clinically significant ECG abnormalities.

In subjects with hepatic impairment, citalopram clearance was decreased and plasma concentrations were increased. The use of Celexa in hepatically impaired patients should be approached with caution and a lower maximum dosage is recommended (see **DOSAGE AND ADMINISTRATION**).

Because citalopram is extensively metabolized, excretion of unchanged drug in urine is a minor route of elimination. Until adequate numbers of patients with severe renal impairment have been evaluated during chronic treatment with Celexa, however, it should be used with caution in such patients (see **DOSAGE AND ADMINISTRATION**).

Information for Patients

Physicians are advised to discuss the following issues with patients for whom they prescribe Celexa.

Although in controlled studies Celexa has not been shown to impair psychomotor performance, any psychoactive drug may impair judgment, thinking, or motor skills, so patients should be cautioned about operating hazardous machinery, including automobiles, until they are reasonably certain that Celexa therapy does not affect their ability to engage in such activities.

Patients should be told that, although Celexa has not been shown in experiments with normal subjects to increase the mental and motor skill impairments caused by alcohol, the concomitant use of Celexa and alcohol in depressed patients is not advised.

Patients should be advised to inform their physician if they are taking, or plan to take, any prescription or over-the-counter drugs, as there is a potential for interactions.

Patients should be cautioned about the concomitant use of Celexa and NSAIDs, aspirin, or other drugs that affect coagulation since the combined use of psychotropic drugs that interfere with serotonin reuptake and these agents has been associated with an increased risk of bleeding.

Patients should be advised to notify their physician if they become pregnant or intend to become pregnant during therapy.

Patients should be advised to notify their physician if they are breastfeeding an infant.

While patients may notice improvement with Celexa therapy in 1 to 4 weeks, they should be advised to continue therapy as directed.

Patients and their families should be encouraged to be alert to the emergence of anxiety, agitation, panic attacks, insomnia, irritability, hostility, impulsivity, akathisia, hypomania, mania, worsening of depression, and suicidal ideation, especially early during antidepressant treatment. Such symptoms should be reported to the patient's physician, especially if they are severe, abrupt in onset, or were not part of the patient's presenting symptoms.

Laboratory Tests

There are no specific laboratory tests recommended.

Drug Interactions

CNS Drugs - Given the primary CNS effects of citalopram, caution should be used when it is taken in combination with other centrally acting drugs.

Alcohol - Although citalopram did not potentiate the cognitive and motor effects of alcohol in a clinical trial, as with other psychotropic medications, the use of alcohol by depressed patients taking Celexa is not recommended.

Monoamine Oxidase Inhibitors (MAOIs) - See **CONTRAINDICATIONS** and **WARNINGS**.

Drugs That Interfere With Hemostasis (NSAIDs, Aspirin, Warfarin, etc.) - Serotonin release by platelets plays an important role in hemostasis. Epidemiological studies of the case-control and cohort design that have demonstrated an association between use of psychotropic drugs that interfere with serotonin reuptake and the occurrence of upper gastrointestinal bleeding have also shown that concurrent use of an NSAID or aspirin potentiated the risk of bleeding. Thus, patients should be cautioned about the use of such drugs concurrently with Celexa.

Cimetidine - In subjects who had received 21 days of 40 mg/day Celexa, combined administration of 400 mg/day cimetidine for 8 days resulted in an increase in citalopram AUC and C_{max} of 43% and 39%, respectively. The clinical significance of these findings is unknown.

Digoxin - In subjects who had received 21 days of 40 mg/day Celexa, combined administration of Celexa and digoxin (single dose of 1 mg) did not significantly affect the pharmacokinetics of either citalopram or digoxin.

Lithium - Coadministration of Celexa (40 mg/day for 10 days) and lithium (30 mmol/day for 5 days) had no significant effect on the pharmacokinetics of citalopram or lithium. Nevertheless, plasma lithium levels should be monitored with appropriate adjustment to the lithium dose in accordance with standard clinical practice. Because lithium may enhance the serotonergic effects of citalopram, caution should be exercised when Celexa and lithium are coadministered.

Theophylline - Combined administration of Celexa (40 mg/day for 21 days) and the CYP1A2 substrate theophylline (single dose of 300 mg) did not affect the pharmacokinetics of theophylline. The effect of theophylline on the pharmacokinetics of citalopram was not evaluated.

Sumatriptan - There have been rare postmarketing reports describing patients with weakness, hyperreflexia, and incoordination following the use of an SSRI and sumatriptan. If concomitant treatment with sumatriptan and an SSRI (e.g., fluoxetine, fluvoxamine, paroxetine, sertraline, citalopram) is clinically warranted, appropriate observation of the patient is advised.

Warfarin - Administration of 40 mg/day Celexa for 21 days did not affect the pharmacokinetics of warfarin, a CYP3A4 substrate. Prothrombin time was increased by 5%, the clinical significance of which is unknown.

Carbamazepine - Combined administration of Celexa (40 mg/day for 14 days) and carbamazepine (titrated to 400 mg/day for 35 days) did not significantly affect the pharmacokinetics of carbamazepine, a CYP3A4 substrate. Although trough citalopram plasma levels were unaffected, given the enzyme-inducing properties of carbamazepine, the possibility that carbamazepine might increase the clearance of citalopram should be considered if the two drugs are coadministered.

Triazolam - Combined administration of Celexa (titrated to 40 mg/day for 28 days) and the CYP3A4 substrate triazolam (single dose of 0.25 mg) did not significantly affect the pharmacokinetics of either citalopram or triazolam.

Ketoconazole - Combined administration of Celexa (40 mg) and ketoconazole (200 mg) decreased the C_{max} and AUC of ketoconazole by 21% and 10%, respectively, and did not significantly affect the pharmacokinetics of citalopram.

CYP3A4 and 2C19 Inhibitors - *In vitro* studies indicated that CYP3A4 and 2C19 are the primary enzymes involved in the metabolism of citalopram. However, coadministration of citalopram (40 mg) and ketoconazole (200 mg), a potent inhibitor of CYP3A4, did not significantly affect the pharmacokinetics of citalopram. Because citalopram is metabolized by multiple enzyme systems, inhibition of a single enzyme may not appreciably decrease citalopram clearance.

Metoprolol - Administration of 40 mg/day Celexa for 22 days resulted in a two-fold increase in the plasma levels of the beta-adrenergic blocker metoprolol. Increased metoprolol plasma levels have been associated with decreased cardioselectivity. Coadministration of Celexa and metoprolol had no clinically significant effects on blood pressure or heart rate.

Imipramine and Other Tricyclic Antidepressants (TCAs) - *In vitro* studies suggest that citalopram is a relatively weak inhibitor of CYP2D6. Coadministration of Celexa (40 mg/day for 10 days) with the TCA imipramine (single dose of 100 mg), a substrate for CYP2D6, did not significantly affect the plasma concentrations of imipramine or citalopram. However, the concentration of the imipramine metabolite desipramine was increased by approximately 50%. The clinical significance of the desipramine change is unknown. Nevertheless, caution is indicated in the coadministration of TCAs with Celexa.

Electroconvulsive Therapy (ECT) - There are no clinical studies of the combined use of electroconvulsive therapy (ECT) and Celexa.

Carcinogenesis, Mutagenesis, Impairment of Fertility

Carcinogenesis

Citalopram was administered in the diet to NMRI/BOM strain mice and COBS WI strain rats for 18 and 24 months, respectively. There was no evidence for carcinogenicity of citalopram in mice receiving up to 240 mg/kg/day, which is equivalent to 20 times the maximum recommended human daily dose (MRHD) of 60 mg on a surface area (mg/m^2) basis. There was an increased incidence of small intestine carcinoma in rats receiving 8 or 24 mg/kg/day, doses which are approximately 1.3 and 4 times the MRHD, respectively, on a mg/m^2 basis. A no-effect dose for this finding was not established. The relevance of these findings to humans is unknown.

Mutagenesis

Citalopram was mutagenic in the *in vitro* bacterial reverse mutation assay (Ames test) in 2 of 5 bacterial strains (Salmonella TA98 and TA1537) in the absence of metabolic activation. It was clastogenic in the *in vitro* Chinese hamster lung cell assay for chromosomal aberrations in the presence and absence of metabolic activation. Citalopram was not mutagenic in the *in vitro* mammalian forward gene mutation assay (HPRT) in mouse lymphoma cells or in a coupled *in vitro/in vivo* unscheduled DNA synthesis (UDS) assay in rat liver. It was not clastogenic in the *in vitro* chromosomal aberration assay in human lymphocytes or in two *in vivo* mouse micronucleus assays.

Impairment of Fertility

When citalopram was administered orally to 16 male and 24 female rats prior to and throughout mating and gestation at doses of 32, 48, and 72 mg/kg/day, mating was decreased at all doses, and fertility was decreased at doses ≥ 32 mg/kg/day, approximately 5 times the MRHD of 60 mg/day on a body surface area (mg/m^2) basis. Gestation duration was increased at 48 mg/kg/day, approximately 8 times the MRHD.

Pregnancy

Pregnancy Category C

In animal reproduction studies, citalopram has been shown to have adverse effects on embryo/fetal and postnatal development, including teratogenic effects, when administered at doses greater than human therapeutic doses.

In two rat embryo/fetal development studies, oral administration of citalopram (32, 56, or 112 mg/kg/day) to pregnant animals during the period of organogenesis resulted in decreased embryo/fetal growth and survival and an increased incidence of fetal abnormalities (including cardiovascular and skeletal defects) at the high dose, which is approximately 18 times the MRHD of 60 mg/day on a body surface area (mg/m^2) basis. This dose was also associated with maternal toxicity (clinical signs, decreased body weight gain). The developmental, no-effect dose of 56 mg/kg/day is approximately 9 times the MRHD on a mg/m^2 basis. In a rabbit study, no adverse effects on embryo/fetal development were observed at doses of up to 16 mg/kg/day, or approximately 5 times the MRHD on a mg/m^2 basis. Thus, teratogenic effects were observed at a maternally toxic dose in the rat and were not observed in the rabbit.

When female rats were treated with citalopram (4.8, 12.8, or 32 mg/kg/day) from late gestation through weaning, increased offspring mortality during the first 4 days after birth and persistent offspring growth retardation were observed at the highest dose, which is approximately 5 times the MRHD on a mg/m^2 basis. The no-effect dose of 12.8 mg/kg/day is approximately 2 times the MRHD on a mg/m^2 basis. Similar effects on offspring mortality and growth were seen when dams were treated throughout gestation and early lactation at doses ≥ 24 mg/kg/day, approximately 4 times the MRHD on a mg/m^2 basis. A no-effect dose was not determined in that study.

There are no adequate and well-controlled studies in pregnant women; therefore, citalopram should be used during pregnancy only if the potential benefit justifies the potential risk to the fetus.

Pregnancy-Nonteratogenic Effects

Neonates exposed to Celexa and other SSRIs or SNRIs, late in the third trimester, have developed complications requiring prolonged hospitalization, respiratory support, and tube feeding. Such complications can arise immediately upon delivery. Reported clinical findings have included respiratory distress, cyanosis, apnea, seizures, temperature instability, feeding difficulty, vomiting, hypoglycemia, hypotonia, hypertonia, hyperreflexia, tremor, jitteriness, irritability, and constant crying. These features are consistent with either a direct toxic effect of SSRIs and SNRIs or, possibly, a drug discontinuation syndrome. It should be noted that, in some cases, the clinical picture is consistent with serotonin syndrome (see **WARNINGS**).

When treating a pregnant woman with Celexa during the third trimester, the physician should carefully consider the potential risks and benefits of treatment (see **DOSAGE AND ADMINISTRATION**).

Labor and Delivery

The effect of Celexa on labor and delivery in humans is unknown.

Nursing Mothers

As has been found to occur with many other drugs, citalopram is excreted in human breast milk. There have been two reports of infants experiencing excessive somnolence, decreased feeding, and weight loss in association with breastfeeding from a citalopram-treated mother; in one case, the infant was reported to recover completely upon discontinuation of citalopram by its mother and in the second case, no follow-up information was available. The decision whether to continue or discontinue either nursing or Celexa therapy should take into account the risks of citalopram exposure for the infant and the benefits of Celexa treatment for the mother.

Pediatric Use

Safety and effectiveness in pediatric patients have not been established (see **WARNINGS – Clinical Worsening and Suicide Risk**)

Geriatric Use

Of 4422 patients in clinical studies of Celexa, 1357 were 60 and over, 1034 were 65 and over, and 457 were 75 and over. No overall differences in safety or effectiveness were observed between these subjects and younger subjects, and other reported clinical experience has not identified differences in responses between the elderly and younger patients, but greater sensitivity of some older individuals cannot be ruled out. Most elderly patients treated with Celexa in clinical trials received daily doses between 20 and 40 mg (see **DOSAGE AND ADMINISTRATION**).

In two pharmacokinetic studies, citalopram AUC was increased by 23% and 30%, respectively, in elderly subjects as compared to younger subjects, and its half-life was increased by 30% and 50%, respectively (see **CLINICAL PHARMACOLOGY**).

20 mg/day is the recommended dose for most elderly patients (see **DOSAGE AND ADMINISTRATION**).

ADVERSE REACTIONS

The premarketing development program for Celexa included citalopram exposures in patients and/or normal subjects from 3 different groups of studies: 429 normal subjects in clinical pharmacology/pharmacokinetic studies; 4422 exposures from patients in controlled and uncontrolled clinical trials, corresponding to approximately 1370 patient-exposure years. There were, in addition, over 19,000 exposures from mostly open-label, European postmarketing studies. The conditions and duration of treatment with Celexa varied greatly and included (in overlapping categories) open-label and double-blind studies, inpatient and outpatient studies, fixed-dose and dose-titration studies, and short-term and long-term exposure. Adverse reactions were assessed by collecting adverse events, results of physical examinations, vital signs, weights, laboratory analyses, ECGs, and results of ophthalmologic examinations.

Adverse events during exposure were obtained primarily by general inquiry and recorded by clinical investigators using terminology of their own choosing. Consequently, it is not possible to provide a meaningful estimate of the proportion of individuals experiencing adverse events without first grouping similar types of events into a smaller number of standardized event categories. In the tables and tabulations that follow, standard World Health Organization (WHO) terminology has been used to classify reported adverse events.

The stated frequencies of adverse events represent the proportion of individuals who experienced, at least once, a treatment-emergent adverse event of the type listed. An event was considered treatment-emergent if it occurred for the first time or worsened while receiving therapy following baseline evaluation.

Adverse Findings Observed in Short-Term, Placebo-Controlled Trials

Adverse Events Associated with Discontinuation of Treatment

Among 1063 depressed patients who received Celexa at doses ranging from 10 to 80 mg/day in placebo-controlled

Continued on next page

Celexa—Cont.

trials of up to 6 weeks in duration, 16% discontinued treatment due to an adverse event, as compared to 8% of 446 patients receiving placebo. The adverse events associated with discontinuation and considered drug-related (i.e., associated with discontinuation in at least 1% of Celexa-treated patients at a rate at least twice that of placebo) are shown in **TABLE 1**. It should be noted that one patient can report more than one reason for discontinuation and be counted more than once in this table.

TABLE 1
Adverse Events Associated with Discontinuation of Treatment in Short-Term, Placebo-Controlled, Depression Trials

Body System/Adverse Event	Percentage of Patients Discontinuing Due to Adverse Event	
	Citalopram (N=1063)	Placebo (N=446)
General		
Asthenia	1%	<1%
Gastrointestinal Disorders		
Nausea	4%	0%
Dry Mouth	1%	<1%
Vomiting	1%	0%
Central and Peripheral Nervous System Disorders		
Dizziness	2%	<1%
Psychiatric Disorders		
Insomnia	3%	1%
Somnolence	2%	1%
Agitation	1%	<1%

Adverse Events Occurring at an Incidence of 2% or More Among Celexa-Treated Patients

Table 2 enumerates the incidence, rounded to the nearest percent, of treatment-emergent adverse events that occurred among 1063 depressed patients who received Celexa at doses ranging from 10 to 80 mg/day in placebo-controlled trials of up to 6 weeks in duration. Events included are those occurring in 2% or more of patients treated with Celexa and for which the incidence in patients treated with Celexa was greater than the incidence in placebo-treated patients.

The prescriber should be aware that these figures cannot be used to predict the incidence of adverse events in the course of usual medical practice where patient characteristics and other factors differ from those which prevailed in the clinical trials. Similarly, the cited frequencies cannot be compared with figures obtained from other clinical investigations involving different treatments, uses, and investigators. The cited figures, however, do provide the prescribing physician with some basis for estimating the relative contribution of drug and non-drug factors to the adverse event incidence rate in the population studied.

The only commonly observed adverse event that occurred in Celexa patients with an incidence of 5% or greater and at least twice the incidence in placebo patients was ejaculation disorder (primarily ejaculatory delay) in male patients (see **TABLE 2**).

TABLE 2
Treatment-Emergent Adverse Events: Incidence in Placebo-Controlled Clinical Trials*

Body System/Adverse Event	(Percentage of Patients Reporting Event)	
	Celexa (N=1063)	Placebo (N=446)
Autonomic Nervous System Disorders		
Dry Mouth	20%	14%
Sweating Increased	11%	9%
Central & Peripheral Nervous System Disorders		
Tremor	8%	6%
Gastrointestinal Disorders		
Nausea	21%	14%
Diarrhea	8%	5%
Dyspepsia	5%	4%
Vomiting	4%	3%
Abdominal Pain	3%	2%
General		
Fatigue	5%	3%
Fever	2%	<1%
Musculoskeletal System Disorders		
Arthralgia	2%	1%
Myalgia	2%	1%
Psychiatric Disorders		
Somnolence	18%	10%
Insomnia	15%	14%
Anxiety	4%	3%
Anorexia	4%	2%
Agitation	3%	1%
Dysmenorrhea[1]	3%	2%
Libido Decreased	2%	<1%
Yawning	2%	<1%
Respiratory System Disorders		
Upper Respiratory Tract Infection	5%	4%
Rhinitis	5%	3%
Sinusitis	3%	<1%
Urogenital		
Ejaculation Disorder[2,3]	6%	1%
Impotence[3]	3%	<1%

*Events reported by at least 2% of patients treated with Celexa are reported, except for the following events which had an incidence on placebo ≥ Celexa: headache, asthenia, dizziness, constipation, palpitation, vision abnormal, sleep disorder, nervousness, pharyngitis, micturition disorder, back pain.

[1] Denominator used was for females only (N=638 Celexa; N=252 placebo).

[2] Primarily ejaculatory delay.

[3] Denominator used was for males only (N=425 Celexa; N=194 placebo).

Dose Dependency of Adverse Events

The potential relationship between the dose of Celexa administered and the incidence of adverse events was examined in a fixed-dose study in depressed patients receiving placebo or Celexa 10, 20, 40, and 60 mg. Jonckheere's trend test revealed a positive dose response ($p<0.05$) for the following adverse events: fatigue, impotence, insomnia, sweating increased, somnolence, and yawning.

Male and Female Sexual Dysfunction with SSRIs

Although changes in sexual desire, sexual performance, and sexual satisfaction often occur as manifestations of a psychiatric disorder, they may also be a consequence of pharmacologic treatment. In particular, some evidence suggests that SSRIs can cause such untoward sexual experiences.

Reliable estimates of the incidence and severity of untoward experiences involving sexual desire, performance, and satisfaction are difficult to obtain, however, in part because patients and physicians may be reluctant to discuss them. Accordingly, estimates of the incidence of untoward sexual experience and performance cited in product labeling, are likely to underestimate their actual incidence.

The table below displays the incidence of sexual side effects reported by at least 2% of patients taking Celexa in a pool of placebo-controlled clinical trials in patients with depression.

Treatment	Celexa (425 males)	Placebo (194 males)
Abnormal Ejaculation (mostly ejaculatory delay)	6.1% (males only)	1% (males only)
Libido Decreased	3.8% (males only)	<1% (males only)
Impotence	2.8% (males only)	<1% (males only)

In female depressed patients receiving Celexa, the reported incidence of decreased libido and anorgasmia was 1.3% (n=638 females) and 1.1% (n=252 females), respectively.

There are no adequately designed studies examining sexual dysfunction with citalopram treatment.

Priapism has been reported with all SSRIs.

While it is difficult to know the precise risk of sexual dysfunction associated with the use of SSRIs, physicians should routinely inquire about such possible side effects.

Vital Sign Changes

Celexa and placebo groups were compared with respect to (1) mean change from baseline in vital signs (pulse, systolic blood pressure, and diastolic blood pressure) and (2) the incidence of patients meeting criteria for potentially clinically significant changes from baseline in these variables. These analyses did not reveal any clinically important changes in vital signs associated with Celexa treatment. In addition, a comparison of supine and standing vital sign measures for Celexa and placebo treatments indicated that Celexa treatment is not associated with orthostatic changes.

Weight Changes

Patients treated with Celexa in controlled trials experienced a weight loss of about 0.5 kg compared to no change for placebo patients.

Laboratory Changes

Celexa and placebo groups were compared with respect to (1) mean change from baseline in various serum chemistry, hematology, and urinalysis variables, and (2) the incidence of patients meeting criteria for potentially clinically significant changes from baseline in these variables. These analyses revealed no clinically important changes in laboratory test parameters associated with Celexa treatment.

ECG Changes

Electrocardiograms from Celexa (N=802) and placebo (N=241) groups were compared with respect to (1) mean change from baseline in various ECG parameters, and (2) the incidence of patients meeting criteria for potentially clinically significant changes from baseline in these variables. The only statistically significant drug-placebo difference observed was a decrease in heart rate for Celexa of 1.7 bpm compared to no change in heart rate for placebo. There were no observed differences in QT or other ECG intervals.

Other Events Observed During the Premarketing Evaluation of Celexa (citalopram HBr)

Following is a list of WHO terms that reflect treatment-emergent adverse events, as defined in the introduction to the **ADVERSE REACTIONS** section, reported by patients treated with Celexa at multiple doses in a range of 10 to 80 mg/day during any phase of a trial within the premarketing database of 4422 patients. All reported events are included except those already listed in Table 2 or elsewhere in labeling, those events for which a drug cause was remote, those event terms which were so general as to be uninformative, and those occurring in only one patient. It is important to emphasize that, although the events reported occurred during treatment with Celexa, they were not necessarily caused by it.

Events are further categorized by body system and listed in order of decreasing frequency according to the following definitions: frequent adverse events are those occurring on one or more occasions in at least 1/100 patients; infrequent adverse events are those occurring in less than 1/100 patients but at least 1/1000 patients; rare events are those occurring in fewer than 1/1000 patients.

Cardiovascular - *Frequent*: tachycardia, postural hypotension, hypotension. *Infrequent*: hypertension, bradycardia, edema (extremities), angina pectoris, extrasystoles, cardiac failure, flushing, myocardial infarction, cerebrovascular accident, myocardial ischemia. *Rare*: transient ischemic attack, phlebitis, atrial fibrillation, cardiac arrest, bundle branch block.

Central and Peripheral Nervous System Disorders - *Frequent*: paresthesia, migraine. *Infrequent*: hyperkinesia, vertigo, hypertonia, extrapyramidal disorder, leg cramps, involuntary muscle contractions, hypokinesia, neuralgia, dystonia, abnormal gait, hypesthesia, ataxia. *Rare*: abnormal coordination, hyperesthesia, ptosis, stupor.

Endocrine Disorders - *Rare*: hypothyroidism, goiter, gynecomastia.

Gastrointestinal Disorders - *Frequent*: saliva increased, flatulence. *Infrequent*: gastritis, gastroenteritis, stomatitis, eructation, hemorrhoids, dysphagia, teeth grinding, gingivitis, esophagitis. *Rare*: colitis, gastric ulcer, cholecystitis, cholelithiasis, duodenal ulcer, gastroesophageal reflux, glossitis, jaundice, diverticulitis, rectal hemorrhage, hiccups.

General - *Infrequent*: hot flushes, rigors, alcohol intolerance, syncope, influenza-like symptoms. *Rare*: hayfever.

Hemic and Lymphatic Disorders - *Infrequent*: purpura, anemia, epistaxis, leukocytosis, leucopenia, lymphadenopathy. *Rare*: pulmonary embolism, granulocytopenia, lymphocytosis, lymphopenia, hypochromic anemia, coagulation disorder, gingival bleeding.

Metabolic and Nutritional Disorders - *Frequent*: decreased weight, increased weight. *Infrequent*: increased hepatic enzymes, thirst, dry eyes, increased alkaline phosphatase, abnormal glucose tolerance. *Rare*: bilirubinemia, hypokalemia, obesity, hypoglycemia, hepatitis, dehydration.

Musculoskeletal System Disorders - *Infrequent*: arthritis, muscle weakness, skeletal pain. *Rare*: bursitis, osteoporosis.

Psychiatric Disorders - *Frequent*: impaired concentration, amnesia, apathy, depression, increased appetite, aggravated depression, suicide attempt, confusion. *Infrequent*: increased libido, aggressive reaction, paroniria, drug dependence, depersonalization, hallucination, euphoria, psychotic depression, delusion, paranoid reaction, emotional lability, panic reaction, psychosis. *Rare*: catatonic reaction, melancholia.

Reproductive Disorders/Female* - *Frequent*: amenorrhea. *Infrequent*: galactorrhea, breast pain, breast enlargement, vaginal hemorrhage.

*% based on female subjects only: 2955

Respiratory System Disorders - *Frequent*: coughing. *Infrequent*: bronchitis, dyspnea, pneumonia. *Rare*: asthma, laryngitis, bronchospasm, pneumonitis, sputum increased.

Skin and Appendages Disorders - *Frequent*: rash, pruritus. *Infrequent*: photosensitivity reaction, urticaria, acne, skin discoloration, eczema, alopecia, dermatitis, skin dry, psoriasis. *Rare*: hypertrichosis, decreased sweating, melanosis, keratitis, cellulitis, pruritus ani.

Special Senses - *Frequent*: accommodation abnormal, taste perversion. *Infrequent*: tinnitus, conjunctivitis, eye pain. *Rare*: mydriasis, photophobia, diplopia, abnormal lacrimation, cataract, taste loss.

Urinary System Disorders - *Frequent*: polyuria. *Infrequent*: micturition frequency, urinary incontinence, urinary retention, dysuria. *Rare*: facial edema, hematuria, oliguria, pyelonephritis, renal calculus, renal pain.

Other Events Observed During the Postmarketing Evaluation of Celexa (citalopram HBr)

It is estimated that over 30 million patients have been treated with Celexa since market introduction. Although no causal relationship to Celexa treatment has been found, the following adverse events have been reported to be temporally associated with Celexa treatment, and have not been described elsewhere in labeling: acute renal failure, akathisia, allergic reaction, anaphylaxis, angioedema, choreoathetosis, chest pain, delirium, dyskinesia, ecchymosis, epidermal necrolysis, erythema multiforme, gastrointestinal hemorrhage, grand mal convulsions, hemolytic anemia, hepatic necrosis, myoclonus, neuroleptic malignant syndrome, nystagmus, pancreatitis, priapism, prolactinemia, prothrombin decreased, QT prolonged, rhabdomyolysis, serotonin syndrome, spontaneous abortion, thrombocytopenia, thrombosis, ventricular arrhythmia, torsades de pointes, and withdrawal syndrome.

DRUG ABUSE AND DEPENDENCE

Controlled Substance Class

Celexa (citalopram HBr) is not a controlled substance.

Physical and Psychological Dependence

Animal studies suggest that the abuse liability of Celexa is low. Celexa has not been systematically studied in humans for its potential for abuse, tolerance, or physical dependence. The premarketing clinical experience with Celexa did not reveal any drug-seeking behavior. However, these observations were not systematic and it is not possible to predict, on the basis of this limited experience, the extent to which a CNS-active drug will be misused, diverted, and/or abused once marketed. Consequently, physicians should carefully evaluate Celexa patients for history of drug abuse and follow such patients closely, observing them for signs of misuse or abuse (e.g., development of tolerance, incrementations of dose, drug-seeking behavior).

OVERDOSAGE

Human Experience

Although there were no reports of fatal citalopram overdose in clinical trials involving overdoses of up to 2000 mg, postmarketing reports of drug overdoses involving citalopram have included 12 fatalities, 10 in combination with other drugs and/or alcohol and 2 with citalopram alone (3920 mg and 2800 mg), as well as non-fatal overdoses of up to 6000 mg. Symptoms most often accompanying citalopram overdose, alone or in combination with other drugs and/or alcohol, included dizziness, sweating, nausea, vomiting, tremor, somnolence, and sinus tachycardia. In more rare cases, observed symptoms included amnesia, confusion, coma, convulsions, hyperventilation, cyanosis, rhabdomyolysis, and ECG changes (including QTc prolongation, nodal rhythm, ventricular arrhythmia, and one possible case of torsades de pointes).

Management of Overdose

Establish and maintain an airway to ensure adequate ventilation and oxygenation. Gastric evacuation by lavage and use of activated charcoal should be considered. Careful observation and cardiac and vital sign monitoring are recommended, along with general symptomatic and supportive care. Due to the large volume of distribution of citalopram, forced diuresis, dialysis, hemoperfusion, and exchange transfusion are unlikely to be of benefit. There are no specific antidotes for Celexa.

In managing overdosage, consider the possibility of multiple-drug involvement. The physician should consider contacting a poison control center for additional information on the treatment of any overdose.

DOSAGE AND ADMINISTRATION

Initial Treatment

Celexa (citalopram HBr) should be administered at an initial dose of 20 mg once daily, generally with an increase to a dose of 40 mg/day. Dose increases should usually occur in increments of 20 mg at intervals of no less than one week. Although certain patients may require a dose of 60 mg/day, the only study pertinent to dose response for effectiveness did not demonstrate an advantage for the 60 mg/day dose over the 40 mg/day dose; doses above 40 mg are therefore not ordinarily recommended.

Celexa should be administered once daily, in the morning or evening, with or without food.

Special Populations

20 mg/day is the recommended dose for most elderly patients and patients with hepatic impairment, with titration to 40 mg/day only for nonresponding patients.

No dosage adjustment is necessary for patients with mild or moderate renal impairment. Celexa should be used with caution in patients with severe renal impairment.

Treatment of Pregnant Women During the Third Trimester

Neonates exposed to Celexa and other SSRIs or SNRIs, late in the third trimester, have developed complications requiring prolonged hospitalization, respiratory support, and tube feeding (see **PRECAUTIONS**). When treating pregnant women with Celexa during the third trimester, the physician should carefully consider the potential risks and benefits of treatment. The physician may consider tapering Celexa in the third trimester.

Maintenance Treatment

It is generally agreed that acute episodes of depression require several months or longer of sustained pharmacologic therapy. Systematic evaluation of Celexa in two studies has shown that its antidepressant efficacy is maintained for periods of up to 24 weeks following 6 or 8 weeks of initial treatment (32 weeks total). In one study, patients were assigned randomly to placebo or to the same dose of Celexa (20–60 mg/day) during maintenance treatment as they had received during the acute stabilization phase, while in the other study, patients were assigned randomly to continuation of Celexa 20 or 40 mg/day, or placebo, for maintenance treatment. In the latter study, the rates of relapse to depression were similar for the two dose groups (see **Clinical Trials** under **CLINICAL PHARMACOLOGY**). Based on these limited data, it is not known whether the dose of citalopram needed to maintain euthymia is identical to the dose needed to induce remission. If adverse reactions are bothersome, a decrease in dose to 20 mg/day can be considered.

Discontinuation of Treatment with Celexa

Symptoms associated with discontinuation of Celexa and other SSRIs and SNRIs have been reported (see **PRECAUTIONS**). Patients should be monitored for these symptoms when discontinuing treatment. A gradual reduction in the dose rather than abrupt cessation is recommended whenever possible. If intolerable symptoms occur following a decrease in the dose or upon discontinuation of treatment, then resuming the previously prescribed dose may be considered. Subsequently, the physician may continue decreasing the dose but at a more gradual rate.

Switching Patients To or From a Monoamine Oxidase Inhibitor

At least 14 days should elapse between discontinuation of an MAOI and initiation of Celexa therapy. Similarly, at least 14 days should be allowed after stopping Celexa before starting an MAOI (see **CONTRAINDICATIONS** and **WARNINGS**).

HOW SUPPLIED

Tablets:

10 mg	Bottle of 100	NDC # 0456-4010-01

Beige, oval, film-coated.

Imprint on one side with "FP". Imprint on the other side with "10 mg".

20 mg	Bottle of 100	NDC # 0456-4020-01
	10 × 10 Unit Dose	NDC # 0456-4020-63

Pink, oval, scored, film-coated.

Imprint on scored side with "F" on the left side and "P" on the right side.

Imprint on the non-scored side with "20 mg".

40 mg	Bottle of 100	NDC # 0456-4040-01
	10 × 10 Unit Dose	NDC # 0456-4040-63

White, oval, scored, film-coated.

Imprint on scored side with "F" on the left side and "P" on the right side.

Imprint on the non-scored side with "40 mg".

Oral Solution:

10 mg/5 mL, peppermint flavor (240 mL) NDC 0456-4130-08

Store at 25°C (77°F); excursions permitted to 15–30°C (59–86°F).

ANIMAL TOXICOLOGY

Retinal Changes in Rats

Pathologic changes (degeneration/atrophy) were observed in the retinas of albino rats in the 2-year carcinogenicity study with citalopram. There was an increase in both incidence and severity of retinal pathology in both male and female rats receiving 80 mg/kg/day (13 times the maximum recommended daily human dose of 60 mg on a mg/m^2 basis). Similar findings were not present in rats receiving 24 mg/kg/day for two years, in mice treated for 18 months at doses up to 240 mg/kg/day, or in dogs treated for one year at doses up to 20 mg/kg/day (4, 20, and 10 times, respectively, the maximum recommended daily human dose on a mg/m^2 basis).

Additional studies to investigate the mechanism for this pathology have not been performed, and the potential significance of this effect in humans has not been established.

Cardiovascular Changes in Dogs

In a one-year toxicology study, 5 of 10 beagle dogs receiving oral doses of 8 mg/kg/day (4 times the maximum recommended daily human dose of 60 mg on a mg/m^2 basis) died suddenly between weeks 17 and 31 following initiation of treatment. Although appropriate data from that study are not available to directly compare plasma levels of citalopram (CT) and its metabolites, demethylcitalopram (DCT) and didemethylcitalopram (DDCT), to levels that have been achieved in humans, pharmacokinetic data indicate that the relative dog-to-human exposure was greater for the metabolites than for citalopram. Sudden deaths were not observed in rats at doses up to 120 mg/kg/day, which produced plasma levels of CT, DCT, and DDCT similar to those observed in dogs at doses of 8 mg/kg/day. A subsequent intravenous dosing study demonstrated that in beagle dogs, DDCT caused QT prolongation, a known risk factor for the observed outcome in dogs. This effect occurred in dogs at doses producing peak DDCT plasma levels of 810 to 3250 nM (39–155 times the mean steady state DDCT plasma level measured at the maximum recommended human daily dose of 60 mg). In dogs, peak DDCT plasma concentrations are approximately equal to peak CT plasma concentrations, whereas in humans, steady state DDCT plasma concentrations are less than 10% of steady state CT plasma concentrations. Assays of DDCT plasma concentrations in 2020 citalopram-treated individuals demonstrated that DDCT levels rarely exceeded 70 nM; the highest measured level of DDCT in human overdose was 138 nM. While DDCT is ordinarily present in humans at lower levels than in dogs, it is unknown whether there are individuals who may achieve higher DDCT levels. The possibility that DCT, a principal metabolite in humans, may prolong the QT interval in dogs has not been directly examined because DCT is rapidly converted to DDCT in that species.

Forest Pharmaceuticals, Inc.
Subsidiary of Forest Laboratories, Inc.
St. Louis, MO 63045 USA
Licensed from H. Lundbeck A/S
Rev. 06/04

MG #13940(17)

Shown in Product Identification Guide, page 312

CERVIDIL® ℞

Brand of dinoprostone vaginal insert
Rx only

DESCRIPTION

Dinoprostone vaginal insert is a thin, flat, polymeric slab which is rectangular in shape with rounded corners contained within the pouch of a knitted polyester retrieval system, an integral part of which is a long tape. Each slab is buff colored, semitransparent and contains 10 mg of dinoprostone. The hydrogel insert is contained within the pouch of an off-white knitted polyester retrieval system designed to aid retrieval at the end of the dosing interval. The finished product is a controlled release formulation which has been found to release dinoprostone *in vivo* at a rate of approximately 0.3 mg/hr.

The chemical name for dinoprostone (commonly known as prostaglandin E_2 or PGE_2) is 11α, 15S-dihydroxy-9-oxo-prosta-5Z, 13E-dien-1-oic acid and the structural formula is represented below:

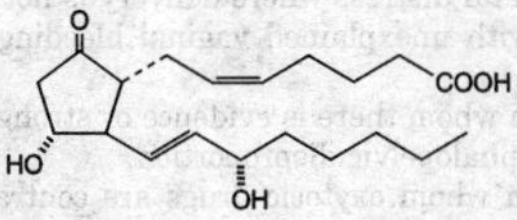

The molecular formula is $C_{20}H_{32}O_5$ and its molecular weight is 352.5. Dinoprostone occurs as a white to off-white crystalline powder. It has a melting point within the range of 65° to 69°C. Dinoprostone is soluble in ethanol and in 25% ethanol in water. Each insert contains 10 mg of dinoprostone in 241 mg of a cross-linked polyethylene oxide/urethane polymer which is a semi-opaque, beige colored, flat rectangular slab measuring 29 mm by 9.5 mm and 0.8 mm in thickness. The insert and its retrieval system, made of polyester yarn, are non-toxic and when placed in a moist environment, absorb water, swell, and release dinoprostone.

CLINICAL PHARMACOLOGY

Dinoprostone (PGE_2) is a naturally-occurring biomolecule. It is found in low concentrations in most tissues of the body and functions as a local hormone (1–3). As with any local hormone, it is very rapidly metabolized in the tissues of synthesis (the half-life estimated to be 2.5–5 minutes). The rate limiting step for inactivation is regulated by the enzyme 15-hydroxyprostaglandin dehydrogenase (PGDH) (1,4). Any PGE_2 that escapes local inactivation is rapidly cleared to the extent of 95% on the first pass through the pulmonary circulation (1,2).

In pregnancy, PGE_2 is secreted continuously by the fetal membranes and placenta and plays an important role in the final events leading to the initiation of labor (1,2). It is known that PGE_2 stimulates the production of $PGF_2\alpha$ which in turn sensitizes the myometrium to endogenous or exogenously administrated oxytocin. Although PGE_2 is capable of initiating uterine contractions and may interact with oxytocin to increase uterine contractility, the available evidence indicates that, in the concentrations found during the early part of labor, PGE_2 plays an important role in cervical ripening without affecting uterine contractions (5–7). This distinction serves as the basis for considering cervical ripening and induction of labor, usually by the use of oxytocin (8–10), as two separate processes.

PGE_2 plays an important role in the complex set of biochemical and structural alterations involved in cervical ripening. Cervical ripening involves a marked relaxation of the cervical smooth muscle fibers of the uterine cervix which must be transformed from a rigid structure to a softened, yielding and dilated configuration to allow passage of the fetus through the birth canal (11–13). This process involves activation of the enzyme collagenase, which is responsible for digestion of some of the structural collagen network of the cervix (1,14). This is associated with a concomitant increase in the amount of hydrophilic glycosaminoglycan, hyaluronic acid, and a decrease in dermatan sulfate (1). Failure of the cervix to undergo these natural physiologic changes, usually assessed by the method described by Bishop (15,16), prior to the onset of effective uterine contractions, results in an unfavorable outcome for successful vaginal delivery and may result in fetal compromise. It is estimated that in approximately 5% of pregnancies the cervix does not ripen normally (17). In an additional 10–11% of pregnancies, labor must be induced for medical or obstetric reasons prior to the time of cervical ripening (17).

The delivery rate of PGE_2 *in vivo* is about 0.3 mg/hour over a period of 12 hours. The controlled release of PGE_2 from the hydrogel insert is an attempt to provide sufficient quantities of PGE_2 to the local receptors to satisfy hormonal requirements. In the majority of patients, these local effects are manifested by changes in the consistency, dilatation and effacement of the cervix as measured by the Bishop score. Although some patients experience uterine hyperstimulation as a result of direct PGE_2- or $PGF_2\alpha$-mediated sensitization of the myometrium to oxytocin, systemic effects of PGE_2 are rarely encountered. The insert is fitted with a biocompatible retrieval system which facilitates removal at the conclusion of therapy or in the event of an adverse reaction.

No correlation could be established between PGE_2 release and plasma concentrations of PGE_m. The relative contributions of endogenously and exogenously released PGE_2 to the plasma levels of the metabolite PGE_m could not be determined. Moreover, it is uncertain as to whether the measured concentrations of PGE_m reflect the natural progression of PGE_m concentrations in blood as birth approaches or to what extent the measured concentrations following PGE_2 administration represent an increase over basal levels that might be measured in control patients.

Continued on next page

Cervidil—Cont.

INDICATIONS AND USAGE

Cervidil Vaginal Insert (dinoprostone, 10 mg) is indicated for the initiation and/or continuation of cervical ripening in patients at or near term in whom there is a medical or obstetrical indication for the induction of labor.

CONTRAINDICATIONS

Cervidil is contraindicated in:
- Patients with known hypersensitivity to prostaglandins.
- Patients in whom there is clinical suspicion or definite evidence of fetal distress where delivery is not imminent.
- Patients with unexplained vaginal bleeding during this pregnancy.
- Patients in whom there is evidence or strong suspicion of marked cephalopelvic disproportion.
- Patients in whom oxytocic drugs are contraindicated or when prolonged contraction of the uterus may be detrimental to fetal safety or uterine integrity, such as previous cesarean section or major uterine surgery (see **PRECAUTIONS** and **ADVERSE REACTIONS**).
- Patients already receiving intravenous oxytocic drugs.
- Multipara with 6 or more previous term pregnancies.

WARNINGS

For hospital use only

Cervidil should be administered only by trained obstetrical personnel in a hospital setting with appropriate obstetrical care facilities.

PRECAUTIONS

1. General Precautions: Since prostaglandins potentiate the effect of oxytocin, Cervidil must be removed before oxytocin administration is initiated and the patient's uterine activity carefully monitored for uterine hyperstimulation. If uterine hyperstimulation is encountered or if labor commences, the vaginal insert should be removed. Cervidil should also be removed prior to amniotomy.

Cervidil is contraindicated when prolonged contraction of the uterus may be detrimental to fetal safety and uterine integrity. Therefore, Cervidil should not be administered to patients with a history of previous cesarean section or uterine surgery given the potential risk for uterine rupture and associated obstetrical complications.

Caution should be exercised in the administration of Cervidil for cervical ripening in patients with ruptured membranes, in cases of non-vertex, or non-singleton presentation, and in patients with a history of previous uterine hypertony, glaucoma, or a history of childhood asthma, even though there have been no asthma attacks in adulthood.

Uterine activity, fetal status and the progression of cervical dilatation and effacement should be carefully monitored whenever the dinoprostone vaginal insert is in place. Any evidence of uterine hyperstimulation, sustained uterine contractions, fetal distress, or other fetal or maternal adverse reactions, should be a cause for consideration of removal of the insert.

2. Drug Interactions: Cervidil may augment the activity of oxytocic agents and their concomitant use is not recommended. A dosing interval of at least 30 minutes is recommended for the sequential use of oxytocin following the removal of the dinoprostone vaginal insert. No other drug interactions have been identified.

3. Carcinogenesis, Mutagenesis, Impairment of Fertility: Long-term carcinogenicity and fertility studies have not been conducted with Cervidil (dinoprostone) Vaginal Insert. No evidence of mutagenicity has been observed with prostaglandin E_2 in the Unscheduled DNA Synthesis Assay, the Micronucleus Test, or Ames Assay.

4. Pregnancy, Teratogenic Effects:
Pregnancy Category C:
Prostaglandin E_2 has produced an increase in skeletal anomalies in rats and rabbits. No effect would be expected clinically, when used as indicated, since Cervidil (dinoprostone) Vaginal Insert is administered after the period of organogenesis. Prostaglandin E_2 has been shown to be embryotoxic in rats and rabbits, and any dose that produces sustained increased uterine tone could put the embryo or fetus at risk.

5. Pediatric Use: The safety and efficacy of Cervidil has been established in women of a reproductive age and women who are pregnant. Although safety and efficacy has not been established in pediatric patients, safety and efficacy are expected to be the same for adolescents.

ADVERSE REACTIONS

Cervidil is well tolerated. In placebo-controlled trials in which 658 women were entered and 320 received active therapy (218 without retrieval system, 102 with retrieval system), the following events were reported.
[See table 1 above]
In Postmarketing Experience Reports, uterine rupture has been reported in association with the use of Cervidil.

Drug related fever, nausea, vomiting, diarrhea, and abdominal pain were noted in less than 1% of patients who received Cervidil.

In study 101–801 (with the retrieval system) cases of hyperstimulation reversed within 2 to 13 minutes of removal of the product. Tocolytics were required in one of the five cases.

Table 1
Total Cervidil-Treated Drug Related Adverse Events

	Controlled Studies[1]		STUDY 101–801[2]	
	Active	Placebo	Active	Placebo
Uterine hyperstimulation with fetal distress	2.8%	0.3%	2.9%	0%
Uterine hyperstimulation without fetal distress	4.7%	0%	2.0%	0%
Fetal Distress without uterine hyperstimulation	3.8%	1.2%	2.9%	1.0%
N	320	338	102	104

[1] Controlled Studies (with and without retrieval system)
[2] Controlled Study (with retrieval system)

Table 2
Efficacy of Cervidil in Double Blind Studies

Parameter	Study #	Primip/Nullip Cervidil	Primip/Nullip Placebo	Multip Cervidil	Multip Placebo	P-Value
Treatment Success*	101–103 (N=81)	65%	28%	87%	29%	<0.001
	101–003 (N=371)	68%	24%	77%	24%	<0.001
	101–801 (N=206)	72%	48%	55%	41%	0.003
Time to Delivery (hours)						
Average	101–103 (N=81)	33.7	48.6	14.0	28.6	
Median		25.7	34.5	12.3	24.6	0.001
Average	101–801 (N=206)	31.1	51.8	52.3	45.9	
Median		25.5	37.2	20.8	27.4	<0.001
Time to Onset of Labor (hours)						
Average	101–103 (N=81)	19.9	39.4	6.8	22.4	
Median		12.0	19.2	6.9	18.3	<0.001

* Treatment success was defined as Bishop score increase at 12 hours of ≥3, vaginal delivery within 12 hours or Bishop score at 12 hours ≥6. These studies were not designed with the power to show differences in cesarean section rates between Cervidil and placebo groups and none were noted.

In cases of fetal distress, when product removal was thought advisable there was a return to normal rhythm and no neonatal sequelae.

Five minute Apgar scores were 7 or above in 98.2% (646/658) of studied neonates whose mothers received Cervidil. In a report of a 3 year pediatric follow-up study in 121 infants, 51 of whose mothers received Cervidil, there were no deleterious effects on physical examination or psychomotor evaluation (18).

DRUG ABUSE AND DEPENDENCE

No drug abuse or dependence has been seen with the use of Cervidil.

OVERDOSAGE

Cervidil is used as a single dosage in a single application. Overdosage is usually manifested by uterine hyperstimulation which may be accompanied by fetal distress and is responsive to removal of the insert. Other treatment must be symptomatic since, to date, clinical experience with prostaglandin antagonists is insufficient.

The use of beta-adrenergic agents should be considered in the event of undesirable increased uterine activity.

DOSAGE AND ADMINISTRATION

The dosage of dinoprostone in the vaginal insert is 10 mg designed to be released at approximately 0.3 mg/hour over a 12 hour period. Cervidil should be removed upon onset of active labor or 12 hours after insertion.

One Cervidil is placed transversely in the posterior fornix of the vagina immediately after removal from its foil package. The insertion of the vaginal insert does not require sterile conditions. The vaginal insert must not be used without its retrieval system. There is no need for previous warming of the product. A minimal amount of K-Y® jelly (or other water-miscible lubricant) may be used to assist in insertion of Cervidil. Care should be taken not to permit excess contact or coating with the lubricant and thus prevent optimal swelling and release of dinoprostone from the vaginal insert. Patients should remain in the recumbent position for 2 hours following insertion, but thereafter may be ambulatory.

HOW SUPPLIED

Cervidil (NDC 0456-4123-63) contains 10 mg dinoprostone. The product is wound and enclosed in an aluminum/polyethylene pack.

Store in a freezer: between −20°C and −10°C (−4°F and 14°F). Cervidil is packed in foil and is stable when stored in a freezer for a period of three years. Vaginal inserts exposed to high humidity will absorb moisture from the air and thereby alter the release characteristics of dinoprostone. Once used, the vaginal insert should be discarded.

CLINICAL STUDIES

[See table 2 above]

REFERENCES

1. Physiology of Labor. In: Williams Obstetrics. Eds. Pritchard, J.A., MacDonald, P.C., and Gant, N.F. Appleton-Century-Crofts, Conn, Pp 295-321, (1985).
2. Rall, T.W. and Schliefer, L.S. Oxytocin, prostaglandin, ergot alkaloids, and other drugs; tocolytics agents, In: The Pharmacological Basis of Therapeutics. Eds. Gilman, A.G., Goodman, L.S., Rall, T.W., and Murad, F. MacMillan Publ. Co., New York, Pp 926-945, (1985).
3. Casey, M.L. and MacDonald, P.C. The initiation of labor in women: Regulation of phospholipid and arachidonic acid metabolism and of prostaglandin production. Semin. Perinat. 10: 270-275, (1986).
4. Casey, M.L., MacDonald, P.C. and Mitchell, M.D. Stimulation of prostaglandin E_2 production in amnion cells in culture by a substance(s) in human fetal urine. Biochem. Biophys. Res. Comm. 114:1056, (1983).
5. Olson, C.M., Lye, S.J., Skinner, K., and Challis, J.R.G. Prostanoid concentrations in maternal/fetal plasma and amniotic fluid and intrauterine tissue prostanoid output in relation to myometrial contractility during the onset of Endocrinology. 116: 389-397, (1985).
6. Ledger, W.L., Ellwood, D.A., and Taylor, M.J. Cervical softening in late pregnant sheep by infusion of prostaglandin E-2 into cervical artery. J. Reprod. Fert. 69, 511-515, (1983).
7. Olson, D.M., Lye, S.J., Skinner, K., and Challis, J.R.G. Early changes in prostaglandin concentrations in ovine maternal and fetal plasma, amniotic fluid and from dispersed cells of intrauterine tissues before the onset of ACTH-induced pre-term labor. J. Reprod. Fert. 71: 45-55, (1984).
8. Caldero-Garcia, R. and Posiero, J. Oxytocin and the contractility of the human uterus, Ann, N.Y. Acad. Sci. 75: 813, (1959).
9. Posiero, J. and Noriega-Guerra, L. Dose-response relationships in uterine effects of oxytocin infusion. Oxytocin. Eds., Caldero-Garcia, R. and Heller, J. Pergamon Press, New York, (1961).
10. Cibils, L. Enhancement of induction of labor. In: Risks in the Practice of Modern Obstetrics. Aldjem, S. Ed. Mosby Publishing, St. Louis, (1972).
11. Bryman, I., Lindblom, B., and Norstrom, A. Extreme sensitivity of cervical musculature to prostaglandin E_2 in early pregnancy. Lancet, 2:1471, (1982).
12. Thiery, M. Induction of labor with prostaglandins. In: Human Parturition. Eds. Keirse, M.J.N.C., Anderson, A.B.M.; and Gravenhorst, J.B. Martinus Nijhoff Publ., Boston, 155-164, (1979).
13. Thiery, M. and Amy, J.J. Induction of labor with prostaglandins. In: Advances in Prostaglandin Research. Prostaglandin and Reproduction. Karim, S.M.M., Ed., MTP, Lancaster, Pp. 149-228, (1975).
14. MacLennan, A.H., Katz, M., and Creasey, R. The morphologic characteristics of cervical ripening induced by the hormones relaxin and prostaglandin F_2 in a rabbit model. Am. J. Obstet. Gynecol, 152: 910696, (1985).
15. Bishop, E. Elective induction of labor. Obstet. & Gynecol. 5: 519-527, (1955).
16. Bishop, E. Pelvic scoring for elective induction. Obstet. & Gynecol. 24: 266-268. (1969).
17. Thiery, M. Preinduction cervical ripening. In: Obstetrics and Gynecology Annual, Vol. 12 Ed. Wynn, R.M. Appleton-Century-Crofts, New York, Pp. 103-146, (1983).
18. MacKenzie, I.; Information on File: Controlled Therapeutics (Scotland).

Mfg by:
Controlled Therapeutics
East Kilbride, Scotland G74 5PB

Made in the U.K.

Distributed by:
FOREST PHARMACEUTICALS, INC.
Subsidiary of Forest Laboratories, Inc.
St. Louis, MO 63045 USA
Rev. 5/01 RMC226

Shown in Product Identification Guide, page 312

ESGIC® Capsules ℞
[*es 'jik*]
(Butalbital, Acetaminophen and Caffeine Capsules, USP)
50 mg/325 mg/40 mg

ESGIC® Tablets ℞
(Butalbital, Acetaminophen and Caffeine Tablets, USP)
50 mg/325 mg/40 mg

ESGIC-PLUS™ Tablets ℞
(Butalbital, Acetaminophen and Caffeine Tablets, USP)
50 mg/500 mg/40 mg

DESCRIPTION

Each Esgic-plus™ Tablet contains:
Butalbital .... 50 mg
Warning: May be habit-forming
Acetaminophen .... 500 mg
Caffeine .... 40 mg

In addition, each tablet contains the following inactive ingredients: colloidal silicon dioxide, croscarmellose sodium, crospovidone, microcrystalline cellulose, povidone, pregelatinized cornstarch, and stearic acid.

HOW SUPPLIED

Esgic-plus™ Tablets, containing butalbital 50 mg **(Warning: May be habit-forming)**, acetaminophen 500 mg and caffeine 40 mg, are white, capsule-shaped, single-scored, and are debossed "FOREST" on one side and "678" on the other side. They are supplied in bottles of 100, NDC 0456-0678-01.

Storage: Store at controlled room temperature, 15° to 30°C (59° to 86°F) (See USP).

Dispense in a tight, light-resistant container with a child-resistant closure.

*Trademark of Medical Economics Company, Inc.

Rx only
Manufactured by:
MIKART, INC.
Atlanta, GA 30318
Distributed by:
FOREST PHARMACEUTICALS, INC.
Subsidiary of
Forest Laboratories, Inc.
St. Louis, Missouri 63045
Rev. 08/02 Code 823A00

Shown in Product Identification Guide, page 312

FLUMADINE® TABLETS ℞
[*flu 'mă-dīne*]
(rimantadine hydrochloride tablets)

FLUMADINE® SYRUP ℞
(rimantadine hydrochloride syrup)

DESCRIPTION

Flumadine® (rimantadine hydrochloride) is a synthetic antiviral drug available as a 100 mg film-coated tablet and as a syrup for oral administration. Each film-coated tablet contains 100 mg of rimantadine hydrochloride plus hydroxypropyl methylcellulose, magnesium stearate, microcrystalline cellulose, sodium starch glycolate, FD&C Yellow No. 6 Lake and FD&C Yellow No. 6. The film coat contains hydroxypropyl methylcellulose and polyethylene glycol. Each teaspoonful (5 mL) of the syrup contains 50 mg of rimantadine hydrochloride in a dye-free, aqueous solution containing citric acid, parabens (methyl and propyl), saccharin sodium, sorbitol and flavors.

Rimantadine hydrochloride is a white to off-white crystalline powder which is freely soluble in water (50 mg/mL at 20°C). Chemically, rimantadine hydrochloride is alpha-methyltricyclo-[3.3.1.1/3.7]decane-1-methanamine hydrochloride, with an empirical formula of $C_{12}H_{21}N{\cdot}HCl$, a molecular weight of 215.77 and the following structural formula:

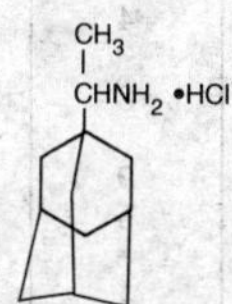

CLINICAL PHARMACOLOGY

MECHANISM OF ACTION: The mechanism of action of rimantadine is not fully understood. Rimantadine appears to exert its inhibitory effect early in the viral replicative cycle, possibly inhibiting the uncoating of the virus. Genetic studies suggest that a virus protein specified by the virion M_2 gene plays an important role in the susceptibility of influenza A virus to inhibition by rimantadine.

MICROBIOLOGY: Rimantadine is inhibitory to the *in vitro* replication of influenza A virus isolates from each of the three antigenic subtypes, *i.e.*, H1N1, H2N2 and H3N2, that have been isolated from man. Rimantadine has little or no activity against influenza B virus (Ref. 1,2). Rimantadine does not appear to interfere with the immunogenicity of inactivated influenza A vaccine.

A quantitative relationship between the *in vitro* susceptibility of influenza A virus to rimantadine and clinical response to therapy has not been established.

Susceptibility test results, expressed as the concentration of the drug required to inhibit virus replication by 50% or more in a cell culture system, vary greatly (from 4 ng/mL to 20 μg/mL) depending upon the assay protocol used, size of the virus inoculum, isolates of the influenza A virus strains tested, and the cell types used (Ref. 2).

Rimantadine-resistant strains of influenza A virus have emerged among freshly isolated epidemic strains in closed settings where rimantadine has been used. Resistant viruses have been shown to be transmissible and to cause typical influenza illness. (Ref. 3).

PHARMACOKINETICS: Although the pharmacokinetic profile of Flumadine has been described, no pharmacodynamic data establishing a correlation between plasma concentration and its antiviral effect are available.

The tablet and syrup formulations of Flumadine are equally absorbed after oral administration. The mean ± SD peak plasma concentration after a single 100 mg dose of Flumadine was 74 ± 22 ng/mL (range: 45 to 138 ng/mL). The time to peak concentration was 6 ± 1 hours in healthy adults (age 20 to 44 years). The single dose elimination half-life in this population was 25.4 ± 6.3 hours (range: 13 to 65 hours). The single dose elimination half-life in a group of healthy 71 to 79 year-old subjects was 32 ± 16 hours (range: 20 to 65 hours).

After the administration of rimantadine 100 mg twice daily to healthy volunteers (age 18 to 70 years) for 10 days, area under the curve (AUC) values were approximately 30% greater than predicted from a single dose. Plasma trough levels at steady state ranged between 118 and 468 ng/mL. In these patients no age-related differences in pharmacokinetics were detected. However, in a comparison of three groups of healthy older subjects (age 50–60, 61–70 and 71–79 years), the 71 to 79 year-old group had average AUC values, peak concentrations and elimination half-life values at steady state that were 20 to 30% higher than the other two groups. Steady-state concentrations in elderly nursing home patients (age 68 to 102 years) were 2- to 4-fold higher than those seen in healthy young and elderly adults.

The pharmacokinetic profile of rimantadine in children has not been established. In a group (n=10) of children 4 to 8 years old who were given a single dose (6.6 mg/kg) of Flumadine syrup, plasma concentrations of rimantadine ranged from 446 to 988 ng/mL at 5 to 6 hours and from 170 to 424 ng/mL at 24 hours. In some children drug was detected in plasma 72 hours after the last dose.

Following oral administration, rimantadine is extensively metabolized in the liver with less than 25% of the dose excreted in the urine as unchanged drug. Three hydroxylated metabolites have been found in plasma. These metabolites, an additional conjugated metabolite and parent drug account for 74 ± 10% (n=4) of a single 200 mg dose of rimantadine excreted in urine over 72 hours.

In a group (n=14) of patients with chronic liver disease, the majority of whom were stabilized cirrhotics, the pharmacokinetics of rimantadine were not appreciably altered following a single 200 mg oral dose compared to 6 healthy subjects who were sex, age and weight matched to 6 of the patients with liver disease. After administration of a single 200 mg dose to patients (n=10) with severe hepatic dysfunction, AUC was approximately 3-fold larger, elimination half-life was approximately 2-fold longer and apparent clearance was about 50% lower when compared to historic data from healthy subjects.

Studies of the effects of renal insufficiency on the pharmacokinetics of rimantadine have given inconsistent results. Following administration of a single 200 mg oral dose of rimantadine to 8 patients with a creatinine clearance (CLcr) of 31–50 mL/min and 6 patients with a CLcr of 11–30 mL/min, the apparent clearance was 37% and 16% lower, respectively, and plasma metabolite concentrations were higher when compared to weight-, age-, and sex-matched healthy subjects (n=9, CLcr > 50 mL/min). After a single 200 mg oral dose of rimantadine was given to 8 hemodialysis patients (CLcr 0–10 mL/min), there was a 1.6-fold increase in the elimination half-life and a 40% decrease in apparent clearance compared to age-matched healthy subjects. Hemodialysis did not contribute to the clearance of rimantadine.

The in vitro human plasma protein binding of rimantadine is about 40% over typical plasma concentrations. Albumin is the major binding protein.

INDICATIONS AND USAGE

Flumadine is indicated for the prophylaxis and treatment of illness caused by various strains of influenza A virus in adults.

Flumadine is indicated for prophylaxis against influenza A virus in children.

PROPHYLAXIS: In controlled studies of children over the age of 1 year, healthy adults and elderly patients, Flumadine has been shown to be safe and effective in preventing signs and symptoms of infection caused by various strains of influenza A virus. Early vaccination on an annual basis as recommended by the Centers of Disease Control's Immunization Practices Advisory Committee is the method of choice in the prophylaxis of influenza unless vaccination is contraindicated, not available or not feasible. Since Flumadine does not completely prevent the host immune response to influenza A infection, individuals who take this drug may still develop immune responses to natural disease or vaccination and may be protected when later exposed to antigenically-related viruses. Following vaccination during an influenza outbreak, Flumadine prophylaxis should be considered for the 2 to 4 week time period required to develop an antibody response. However, the safety and effectiveness of Flumadine prophylaxis have not been demonstrated for longer than 6 weeks.

TREATMENT: Flumadine therapy should be considered for adults who develop an influenza-like illness during known or suspected influenza A infection in the community. When administered within 48 hours after onset of signs and symptoms of infection caused by influenza A virus strains, Flumadine has been shown to reduce the duration of fever and systemic symptoms.

CONTRAINDICATIONS

Flumadine is contraindicated in patients with known hypersensitivity to drugs of the adamantane class, including rimantadine and amantadine.

PRECAUTIONS

GENERAL: An increased incidence of seizures has been reported in patients with a history of epilepsy who received the related drug amantadine. In clinical trials of Flumadine, the occurrence of seizure-like activity was observed in a small number of patients with a history of seizures who were not receiving anticonvulsant medication while taking Flumadine. If seizures develop, Flumadine should be discontinued.

The safety and pharmacokinetics of rimantadine in renal and hepatic insufficiency have only been evaluated after single-dose administration. In a single dose study of patients with anuric renal failure, the apparent clearance of rimantadine was approximately 40% lower and the elimination half-life was 1.6-fold greater than that in healthy age-matched controls. In a study of 14 persons with chronic liver disease (mostly stabilized cirrhotics), no alterations in the pharmacokinetics were observed after the administration of a single dose of rimantadine. However, the apparent clearance of rimantadine following a single dose to 10 patients with severe liver dysfunction was 50% lower than reported for healthy subjects. Because of the potential for accumulation of rimantadine and its metabolites in plasma, caution should be exercised when patients with renal or hepatic insufficiency are treated with rimantadine.

Transmission of rimantadine resistant virus should be considered when treating patients whose contacts are at high risk for influenza A illness. Influenza A virus strains resistant to rimantadine can emerge during treatment and such resistant strains have been shown to be transmissible and to cause typical influenza illness (Ref. 3). Although the frequency, rapidity, and clinical significance of the emergence of drug-resistant virus are not yet established, several small studies have demonstrated that 10% to 30% of patients with initially sensitive-virus, upon treatment with rimantadine, shed rimantadine resistant virus. (Ref. 3, 4, 5, 6)

Clinical response to rimantadine, although slower in those patients who subsequently shed resistant virus, was not significantly different from those who did not shed resistant virus. (Ref. 3) No data are available in humans that address the activity or effectiveness of rimantadine therapy in subjects infected with resistant virus.

DRUG INTERACTIONS: Cimetidine: The effects of chronic cimetidine use on the metabolism of rimantadine are not known. When a single 100 mg dose of Flumadine was administered one hour after the initiation of cimetidine (300 mg four times a day), the apparent total rimantadine clearance of this single dose in mormal healthy adults was reduced by 18% (compared to the apparent total rimantadine clearance in the same subjects in the absence of cimetidine).

Acetaminophen: Flumadine, 100 mg, was given twice daily for 13 days to 12 healthy volunteers. On day 11, acetaminophen (650 mg four times daily) was started and continued for 8 days. The pharmacokinetics of rimantadine were assessed on days 11 and 13. Coadministration with acetaminophen reduced the peak concentration and AUC values for rimantadine by approximately 11%.

Aspirin: Flumadine, 100 mg, was given twice daily for 13 days to 12 healthy volunteers. On day 11, aspirin (650 mg, four times daily) was started and continued for 8 days. The pharmacokinetics of rimantadine were assessed on days 11 and 13. Peak plasma concentrations and AUC of rimantadine were reduced approximately 10% in the presence of aspirin.

CARCINOGENESIS, MUTAGENESIS, AND IMPAIRMENT OF FERTILITY: Carcinogenesis: Carcinogenicity studies in animals have not been performed.

Mutagenesis: No mutagenic effects were seen when rimantadine was evaluated in several standard assays for mutagenicity.

Continued on next page

Flumadine—Cont.

Impairment of Fertility: A reproduction study in male and female rats did not show detectable impairment of fertility at dosages up to 60 mg/kg/day (3 times the maximum human dose based on body surface area comparisons).

PREGNANCY: Teratogenic Effects: Pregnancy Category C. There are no adequate and well-controlled studies in pregnant women. Rimantadine is reported to cross the placenta in mice. Rimantadine has been shown to be embryotoxic in rats when given at a dose of 200 mg/kg/day (11 times the recommended human dose based on body surface area comparisons). At this dose the embryotoxic effect consisted of increased fetal resorption in rats; this dose also produced a variety of maternal effects including ataxia, tremors, convulsions and significantly reduced weight gain. No embryotoxicity was observed when rabbits were given doses up to 50 mg/kg/day (5 times the recommended human dose based on body surface area comparisons). However, there was evidence of a developmental abnormality in the form of a change in the ratio of fetuses with 12 or 13 ribs. This ratio is normally about 50:50 in a litter but was 80:20 after rimantadine treatment.

Nonteratogenic Effects: Rimantadine was administered to pregnant rats in a peri- and postnatal reproduction toxicity study at doses of 30, 60 and 120 mg/kg/day (1.7, 3.4 and 6.8 times the recommended human dose based on body surface area comparisons). Maternal toxicity during gestation was noted at the two higher doses of rimantadine, and at the highest dose, 120 mg/kg/day, there was an increase in pup mortality during the first 2 to 4 days postpartum. Decreased fertility of the F1 generation was also noted for the two higher doses.

For these reasons, Flumadine should be used during pregnancy only if the potential benefit justifies the risk to the fetus.

NURSING MOTHERS: Flumadine should not be administered to nursing mothers because of the adverse effects noted in offspring of rats treated with rimantadine during the nursing period. Rimantadine is concentrated in rat milk in a dose-related manner: 2 to 3 hours following administration of rimantadine, rat breast milk levels were approximately twice those observed in the serum.

PEDIATRIC USE: In children, Flumadine is recommended for the prophylaxis of influenza A. The safety and effectiveness of Flumadine in the treatment of symptomatic influenza infection in children have not been established. Prophylaxis studies with Flumadine have not been performed in children below the age of 1 year.

ADVERSE REACTIONS

In 1,027 patients treated with Flumadine in controlled clinical trials at the recommended dose of 200 mg daily, the most frequently reported adverse events involved the gastrointestinal and nervous systems.

Incidence >1%: Adverse events reported most frequently (1–3%) at the recommended dose in controlled clinical trials are shown in the table below.

	Rimantadine (n=1027)	Control (n=986)
Nervous System		
Insomnia	2.1%	0.9%
Dizziness	1.9%	1.1%
Headache	1.4%	1.3%
Nervousness	1.3%	0.6%
Fatigue	1.0%	0.9%
Gastrointestinal System		
Nausea	2.8%	1.6%
Vomiting	1.7%	0.6%
Anorexia	1.6%	0.8%
Dry mouth	1.5%	0.6%
Abdominal Pain	1.4%	0.8%
Body as a Whole		
Asthenia	1.4%	0.5%

Less frequent adverse events (0.3 to 1%) at the recommended dose in controlled clinical trials were: *Gastrointestinal System:* diarrhea, dyspepsia; *Nervous System:* impairment of concentration, ataxia, somnolence, agitation, depression; *Skin and Appendages:* rash; *Hearing and Vestibular:* tinnitus; *Respiratory:* dyspena.

Additional adverse events (less than 0.3%) reported at recommended doses in controlled clinical trials were: Nervous System: gait abnormality, euphoria, hyperkinesia, tremor, hallucination, confusion, convulsions; *Respiratory:* bronchospasm, cough; *Cardiovascular:* pallor, palpitation, hypertension, cerebrovascular disorder, cardiac failure, pedal edema, heart block, tachycardia, syncope; *Reproduction:* non-puerperal lactation; *Special Senses:* taste loss/change, parosmia.

Rates of adverse events, particularly those involving the gastrointestinal and nervous systems, increased significantly in controlled studies using higher than recommended doses of Flumadine. In most cases, symptoms resolved rapidly with discontinuation of treatment. In addition to the adverse events reported above, the following were also reported at higher than recommended doses: increased lacrimation, increased micturition frequency, fever, rigors, agitation, constipation, diaphoresis, dysphagia, stomatitis, hypesthesia and eye pain.

Adverse Reactions in Trials of Rimantadine and Amantadine: In a six-week prophylaxis study of 436 healthy adults comparing rimantadine with amantadine and placebo, the following adverse reactions were reported with an incidence >1%.

	Rimantadine 200 mg/day (n=145)	Placebo (n=143)	Amantadine 200 mg/day (n=148)
Nervous System			
Insomnia	3.4%	0.7%	7.0%
Nervousness	2.1%	0.7%	2.8%
Impaired Concentration	2.1%	1.4%	2.1%
Dizziness	0.7%	0.0%	2.1%
Depression	0.7%	0.7%	3.5%
Total % of subjects with adverse reactions	6.9%	4.1%	14.7%
Total % of subjects withdrawn due to adverse reactions	6.9%	3.4%	14.0%

GERIATRIC USE:

Approximately 200 patients over the age of 64 were evaluated for safety in controlled clinical trials with Flumadine® (rimantadine hydrochloride). Geriatric subjects who received either 200 mg or 400 mg of rimantadine daily for 1 to 50 days experienced considerably more central nervous system and gastrointestinal adverse events than comparable geriatric subjects receiving placebo. Central nervous system events including dizziness, headache, anxiety, asthenia, and fatigue, occurred up to two times more often in subjects treated with rimantadine than in those treated with placebo. Gastrointestinal symptoms, particularly nausea, vomiting, and abdominal pain occurred at least twice as frequently in subjects receiving rimantadine than in those receiving placebo. The gastrointestinal symptoms appeared to be dose related. In patients over 64, the recommended dose is 100 mg, daily (see Clinical Pharmacology and Dosage and Administration).

OVERDOSAGE

As with any overdose, supportive therapy should be administered as indicated. Overdoses of a related drug, amantadine, have been reported with adverse reactions consisting of agitation, hallucinations, cardiac arrhythmia and death. The administration of intravenous physostigmine (a cholinergic agent) at doses of 1 to 2 mg in adults (Ref. 7) and 0.5 mg in children (Ref. 8) repeated as needed as long as the dose did not exceed 2 mg/hour has been reported anecdotally to be beneficial in patients with central nervous system effects from overdoses of amantadine.

DOSAGE AND ADMINISTRATION

FOR PROPHYLAXIS IN ADULTS AND CHILDREN:

Adults: The recommended adult dose of Flumadine is 100 mg twice a day. In patients with severe hepatic dysfunction, renal failure (CrCl ≤ 10 mL/min.) and elderly nursing home patients, a dose reduction to 100 mg daily is recommended. There are currently no data available regarding the safety of rimantadine during multiple dosing in subjects with renal or hepatic impairment. Because of the potential for accumulation of rimantadine metabolites during multiple dosing, patients with any degree of renal insufficiency should be monitored for adverse effects, with dosage adjustments being made as necessary.

Children: In children less than 10 years of age, Flumadine should be administered once a day, at a dose of 5 mg/kg but not exceeding 150 mg. For children 10 years of age or older, use the adult dose.

FOR TREATMENT IN ADULTS: The recommended adult dose of Flumadine is 100 mg twice a day. In patients with severe hepatic dysfunction, renal failure (CrCl ≤ 10 mL/min) and elderly nursing home patients, a dose reduction to 100 mg daily is recommended. There are currently no data available regarding the safety of rimantadine during multiple dosing in subjects with renal or hepatic impairment. Because of the potential for accumulation of rimantadine metabolites during multiple dosing, patients with any degree of renal insufficiency should be monitored for adverse effects, with dosage adjustments being made as necessary.

Flumadine therapy should be initiated as soon as possible, preferably within 48 hours after onset of signs and symptoms of influenza A infection. Therapy should be continued for approximately seven days from the initial onset of symptoms.

HOW SUPPLIED

Flumadine® tablets (rimantadine hydrochloride tablets) are supplied as 100 mg tablets (orange, oval-shaped, film-coated) in bottles of 100 (NDC 0456-0521-01). Imprint on tablets: (Front) FLUMADINE 100; (Back) FOREST.

Flumadine® syrup (rimantadine hydrochloride syrup) containing 50 mg of rimantadine hydrochloride per teaspoonful (5 mL) (clear, colorless, raspberry-flavored) is supplied in bottles of 8 oz (NDC 0456-0527-08).

Tablets and syrup should be stored at 15°–30°C (59°–86°F).

Rx only

REFERENCES

1. Belshe, R.B., Burk, B., Newman, F., Cerruti, R.L. and Sim, I.S. (1989) J. Infect. Dis. 159, 430–435.
2. Sim, I.S., Cerruti, R.L. and Connell, E.V., (1989) J. Resp. Dis. (Suppl.), S46–S51.
3. Hayden, F.G., Belshe, R.B., Clover, R.D. et al (1989) N.Engl. J. Med. 321 (25), 1696–1702.
4. Hall, C.B., Dolin, R., Gala, C.L., et al (1987) Pediatrics 80, 275–282.
5. Thompson, J., Fleet, W., Lawrence, E. et al (1987) J.Med. Vir. 21, 249–255.
6. Belshe, R.B., Smith, M.H., Hall, C.B., et al (1988) J. Virol. 62, 1508–1512.
7. Casey, D.F. N. Engl. J. Med. 1978:298:516.
8. Berkowitz, C.D. J. Pediatrics. 1979:95:144.

Rev. 5/02

FOREST PHARMACEUTICALS, INC.
Subsidiary of Forest Laboratories, Inc.
St Louis, MO 63045

Shown in Product Identification Guide, page 312

INFASURF® ℞

[ĭn'fă-surf]
(calfactant)
Intratracheal Suspension
Sterile Suspension for Intratracheal Use Only
Rx Only

DESCRIPTION

Infasurf® (calfactant) Intratracheal Suspension is a sterile, non-pyrogenic lung surfactant intended for intratracheal instillation only. It is an extract of natural surfactant from calf lungs which includes phospholipids, neutral lipids, and hydrophobic surfactant-associated proteins B and C (SP-B and SP-C). It contains no preservatives.

Infasurf is an off-white suspension of calfactant in 0.9% aqueous sodium chloride solution. It has a pH of 5.0–6.2 (target pH 5.7). Each milliliter of Infasurf contains 35 mg total phospholipids (including 26 mg phosphatidylcholine of which 16 mg is disaturated phosphatidylcholine) and 0.65 mg proteins including 0.26 mg of SP-B.

CLINICAL PHARMACOLOGY

Endogenous lung surfactant is essential for effective ventilation because it modifies alveolar surface tension thereby stabilizing the alveoli. Lung surfactant deficiency is the cause of Respiratory Distress Syndrome (RDS) in premature infants. Infasurf restores surface activity to the lungs of these infants.

Activity: Infasurf adsorbs rapidly to the surface of the air: liquid interface and modifies surface tension similarly to natural lung surfactant. A minimum surface tension of ≤3 mN/m is produced *in vitro* by Infasurf as measured on a pulsating bubble surfactometer. *Ex vivo,* Infasurf restores the pressure volume mechanics and compliance of surfactant-deficient rat lungs. *In vivo,* Infasurf improves lung compliance, respiratory gas exchange, and survival in preterm lambs with profound surfactant deficiency.

Animal Metabolism: Infasurf is administered directly to the lung lumen surface, its site of action. No human studies of absorption, biotransformation, or excretion of Infasurf have been performed. The administration of Infasurf with radiolabeled phospholipids into the lungs of adult rabbits results in the persistence of 50% of radioactivity in the lung alveolar lining and 25% of radioactivity in the lung tissue 24 hours later. Less than 5% of the radioactivity is found in other organs. In premature lambs with lethal surfactant deficiency, less than 30% of instilled Infasurf is present in the lung lining after 24 hours.

Clinical Studies: The efficacy of Infasurf was demonstrated in two multiple-dose controlled clinical trials involving approximately 2,000 infants treated with Infasurf (approximately 100 mg phospholipid/kg) or Exosurf Neonatal®. In addition, two controlled trials of Infasurf versus Survanta®, and four uncontrolled trials were conducted that involved approximately 15,500 patients treated with Infasurf.

Infasurf versus Exosurf Neonatal®
Treatment Trial

A total of 1,126 infants ≤72 hours of age with RDS who required endotracheal intubation and had an a/A $PO_2 < 0.22$ were enrolled into a multiple-dose, randomized, double-blind treatment trial comparing Infasurf (3mL/kg) and Exosurf Neonatal® (5mL/kg). Patients were given an initial dose and one repeat dose 12 hours later if intubation was still required. The dose was instilled in two aliquots through a side port adapter into the proximal end of the endotracheal tube. Each aliquot was given in small bursts over 20-30 inspiratory cycles. After each aliquot was instilled, the infant was positioned with either the right or the left side dependent. Results for efficacy parameters evaluated at 28 days or to discharge for all treated patients from this treatment trial are shown in Table 1.

Table 1 - Infasurf vs Exosurf Neonatal®
Treatment Trial

Efficacy Parameter	Infasurf (N=570) %	Exosurf Neonatal® (N=556) %	p-Value
Incidence of air leaks[a]	11	22	≤0.001
Death due to RDS	4	4	0.95
Any death to 28 days	8	10	0.21
Any death before discharge	9	12	0.07
BPD[b]	5	6	0.41
Crossover to other surfactant[c]	4	4	1

[a] Pneumothorax and/or pulmonary interstitial emphysema.
[b] BPD is bronchopulmonary dysplasia, diagnosed by positive X-ray and oxygen dependence at 28 days.

[c] Protocol permitted use of comparator surfactant in patients who failed to respond to therapy with the initial randomized surfactant if the infant was < 96 hours of age, had received a full course of the randomized surfactant, and had an a/A PO_2 ratio < 0.10

Prophylaxis Trial

A total of 853 infants <29 weeks gestation were enrolled into a multiple-dose, randomized, double-blind prophylaxis trial comparing Infasurf (3mL/kg) and Exosurf Neonatal® (5mL/kg). The initial dose was administered within 30 minutes of birth. Repeat doses were administered at 12 and 24 hours if the patient remained intubated. Each dose was administered divided in 2 equal aliquots, and given through a side port adapter into the proximal end of the endotracheal tube. Each aliquot was given in small bursts over 20-30 inspiratory cycles. After each aliquot was instilled, the infant was positioned with either the right or the left side dependent. Results for efficacy parameters evaluated to day 28 or to discharge for all treated patients from this prophylaxis trial are shown in Table 2.

Table 2 - Infasurf vs Exosurf Neonatal® Prophylaxis Trial

Efficacy Parameter	Infasurf (N=431) %	Exosurf Neonatal® (N=422) %	p-Value
Incidence of RDS	15	47	≤0.001
Incidence of air leaks[a]	10	15	0.01
Death due to RDS	2	5	≤0.01
Any death to 28 days	12	16	0.10
Any death before discharge	18	19	0.56
BPD[b]	16	17	0.60
Crossover to other surfactant[c]	0.2	3	≤0.001

[a] Pneumothorax and/or pulmonary interstitial emphysema.
[b] BPD is bronchopulmonary dysplasia, diagnosed by positive X-ray and oxygen dependence at 28 days.
[c] Protocol permitted use of comparator surfactant in patients who failed to respond to therapy with the initial randomized surfactant if the infant was < 72 hours of age, had received a full course of the randomized surfactant, and had an a/A PO_2 ratio < 0.10

Infasurf versus Survanta®

Treatment Trial

A total of 662 infants with RDS who required endotracheal intubation and had an a/A PO_2 <0.22 were enrolled into a multiple-dose, randomized, double-blind treatment trial comparing Infasurf (4mL/kg of a formulation that contained 25 mg of phospholipids/mL rather than the 35 mg/mL in the marketed formulation) and Survanta® (4mL/kg). Repeat doses were allowed ≥6 hours following the previous treatment (for up to three doses before 96 hours of age) if the patient required ≥30% oxygen. The surfactant was given through a 5 French feeding catheter inserted into the endotracheal tube. The total dose was instilled in four equal aliquots with the catheter removed between each of the instillations and mechanical ventilation resumed for 0.5 to 2 minutes. Each of the aliquots was administered with the patient in one of four different positions (prone, supine, right, and left lateral) to facilitate even distribution of the surfactant. Results for the major efficacy parameters evaluated at 28 days or to discharge (incidence of air leaks, death due to respiratory causes or to any cause, BPD, or treatment failure) for all treated patients from this treatment trial were not significantly different between Infasurf and Survanta®.

Prophylaxis Trial

A total of 457 infants ≤30 weeks gestation and <1251 grams birth weight were enrolled into a multiple-dose, randomized, double-blind trial comparing Infasurf (4mL/kg of a formulation that contained 25 mg of phospholipids/mL rather than the 35 mg/mL in the marketed formulation) and Survanta® (4mL/kg). The initial dose was administered within 15 minutes of birth and repeat doses were allowed ≥6 hours following the previous treatment (for up to three doses before 96 hours of age) if the patient required ≥30% oxygen. The surfactant was given through a 5 French feeding catheter inserted into the endotracheal tube. The total dose was instilled in four equal aliquots with the catheter removed between each of the instillations and mechanical ventilation resumed for 0.5 to 2 minutes. Each of the aliquots was administered with the patient in one of four different positions (prone, supine, right, and left lateral).

Results for efficacy endpoints evaluated at 28 days or to discharge for all treated patients from this prophylaxis trial showed an increase in mortality from any cause at 28 days (p=0.03) and in death due to respiratory causes (p=0.005) in Infasurf-treated infants. For evaluable patients (patients who met the protocol-defined entry criteria), mortality from any cause and mortality due to respiratory causes were also higher in the Infasurf group (p = 0.07 and 0.03, respectively). However, these observations have not been replicated in other adequate and well-controlled trials and their relevance to the intended population is unknown. All other efficacy outcomes (incidence of RDS, air leaks, BPD, and treatment failure) were not significantly different between Infasurf and Survanta® when analyzed for all treated patients and for evaluable patients.

Table 3 - Common Complications of Prematurity and RDS in Controlled Trials

Complication	Infasurf (N=1001) %	Exosurf Neonatal® (N=978) %	Infasurf (N=553) %	Survanta® (N=566) %
Apnea	61	61	76	76
Patent ductus arteriosus	47	48	45	48
Intracranial hemorrhage	29	31	36	36
Severe intracranial hemorrhage[a]	12	10	9	7
IVH and PVL[b]	7	3	5	5
Sepsis	20	22	28	27
Pulmonary air leaks	12	22	15	15
Pulmonary interstitial emphysema	7	17	10	10
Pulmonary hemorrhage	7	7	7	6
Necrotizing enterocolitis	5	5	17	18

[a] Grade III and IV by the method of Papile.
[b] Patients with both intraventricular hemorrhage and periventricular leukomalacia.

Acute Clinical Effects: As with other surfactants, marked improvements in oxygenation and lung compliance may occur shortly after the administration of Infasurf. All controlled clinical trials with Infasurf demonstrated significant improvements in fraction of inspired oxygen (F_iO_2) and mean airway pressure (MAP) during the first 24 to 48 hours following initiation of Infasurf therapy.

INDICATIONS AND USAGE

Infasurf is indicated for the prevention of Respiratory Distress Syndrome (RDS) in premature infants at high risk for RDS and for the treatment ("rescue") of premature infants who develop RDS. Infasurf decreases the incidence of RDS, mortality due to RDS, and air leaks associated with RDS.

Prophylaxis

Prophylaxis therapy at birth with Infasurf is indicated for premature infants <29 weeks of gestational age at significant risk for RDS. Infasurf prophylaxis should be administered as soon as possible, preferably within 30 minutes after birth.

Treatment

Infasurf therapy is indicated for infants ≤72 hours of age with RDS (confirmed by clinical and radiologic findings) and requiring endotracheal intubation.

WARNINGS

Infasurf is intended for intratracheal use only.

THE ADMINISTRATION OF EXOGENOUS SURFACTANTS, INCLUDING INFASURF, OFTEN RAPIDLY IMPROVES OXYGENATION AND LUNG COMPLIANCE. Following administration of Infasurf, patients should be carefully monitored so that oxygen therapy and ventilatory support can be modified in response to changes in respiratory status.

Infasurf therapy is not a substitute for neonatal intensive care. Optimal care of premature infants at risk for RDS and newborn infants with RDS who need endotracheal intubation requires an acute care unit organized, staffed, equipped, and experienced with intubation, ventilator management, and general care of these patients.

TRANSIENT EPISODES OF REFLUX OF INFASURF INTO THE ENDOTRACHEAL TUBE, CYANOSIS, BRADYCARDIA, OR AIRWAY OBSTRUCTION HAVE OCCURRED DURING THE DOSING PROCEDURES. These events require stopping Infasurf administration and taking appropriate measures to alleviate the condition. After the patient is stable, dosing can proceed with appropriate monitoring.

PRECAUTIONS

When repeat dosing was given at fixed 12-hour intervals in the Infasurf vs. Exosurf Neonatal® trials, transient episodes of cyanosis, bradycardia, reflux of surfactant into the endotracheal tube, and airway obstruction were observed more frequently among infants in the Infasurf-treated group.

An increased proportion of patients with both intraventricular hemorrhage (IVH) and periventricular leukomalacia (PVL) was observed in Infasurf-treated infants in the Infasurf-Exosurf Neonatal® controlled trials. These observations were not associated with increased mortality.

No data are available on the use of Infasurf in conjunction with experimental therapies of RDS, e.g., high-frequency ventilation.

Data from controlled trials on the efficacy of Infasurf are limited to doses of approximately 100 mg phospholipid/kg body weight and up to a total of 4 doses.

Carcinogenesis, Mutagenesis, Impairment of Fertility

Carcinogenesis studies and animal reproduction studies have not been performed with Infasurf. A single mutagenicity study (Ames assay) was negative.

ADVERSE REACTIONS

The most common adverse reactions associated with Infasurf dosing procedures in the controlled trials were cyanosis (65%), airway obstruction (39%), bradycardia (34%), reflux of surfactant into the endotracheal tube (21%), requirement for manual ventilation (16%), and reintubation (3%). These events were generally transient and not associated with serious complications or death.

The incidence of common complications of prematurity and RDS in the four controlled Infasurf trials are presented in Table 3. Prophylaxis and treatment study results for each surfactant are combined.

[See table 3 above]

Follow-up Evaluations

Two-year follow-up data of neurodevelopmental outcomes in 415 infants enrolled in 5 centers that participated in the Infasurf vs. Exosurf Neonatal® controlled trials demonstrated significant developmental delays in equal percentages of Infasurf and Exosurf Neonatal® patients.

OVERDOSAGE

There have been no reports of overdosage with Infasurf. While there are no known adverse effects of excess lung surfactant, overdosage would result in overloading the lungs with an isotonic solution. Ventilation should be supported until clearance of the liquid is accomplished.

DOSAGE AND ADMINISTRATION

FOR INTRATRACHEAL ADMINISTRATION ONLY

Infasurf should be administered under the supervision of clinicians experienced in the acute care of newborn infants with respiratory failure who require intubation.

Rapid and substantial increases in blood oxygenation and improved lung compliance often follow Infasurf instillation. Close clinical monitoring and surveillance following administration may be needed to adjust oxygen therapy and ventilator pressures appropriately.

Dosage

Each dose of Infasurf is 3 mL/kg body weight at birth. Infasurf has been administered every 12 hours for a total of up to 3 doses.

Directions for Use

Infasurf is a suspension which settles during storage. Gentle swirling or agitation of the vial is often necessary for redispersion. DO NOT SHAKE. Visible flecks in the suspension and foaming at the surface are normal for Infasurf.

Infasurf should be stored at refrigerated temperature 2° to 8°C (36° to 46°F). THE 3mL VIAL MUST BE STORED UPRIGHT. Date and time need to be recorded on the carton when Infasurf is removed from the refrigerator. Warming of Infasurf before administration is not necessary.

Unopened, unused vials of Infasurf that have warmed to room temperature can be returned to refrigerated storage within 24 hours for future use. **Infasurf should not be removed from the refrigerator for more than 24 hours. Infasurf should not be returned to the refrigerator more than once.** Repeated warming to room temperature should be avoided. Each single-use vial should be entered only once and the vial with any unused material should be discarded after the initial entry.

INFASURF DOES NOT REQUIRE RECONSTITUTION. DO NOT DILUTE OR SONICATE.

Dosing Procedures

General

Infasurf should only be administered intratracheally through an endotracheal tube. The dose of Infasurf is 3 mL/kg birth weight. The dose is drawn into a syringe from the single-use vial using a 20-gauge or larger needle with care taken to avoid excessive foaming. Administration is made by instillation of the Infasurf suspension into the endotracheal tube.

Administration for Treatment of RDS

Initial Dose

Infasurf should be administered intratracheally through a side-port adapter into the endotracheal tube. Two attendants, one to instill the Infasurf, the other to monitor the patient and assist in positioning, facilitate the dosing. The dose (3 mL/kg) should be administered in two aliquots of 1.5 mL/kg each. After each aliquot is instilled, the infant should be positioned with either the right or the left side dependent. Administration is made while ventilation is continued over 20–30 breaths for each aliquot, with small bursts timed only during the inspiratory cycles. A pause followed by evaluation of the respiratory status and repositioning should separate the two aliquots.

Repeat Doses

Repeat doses of 3 mL/kg of birth weight, up to a total of 3 doses 12 hours apart, have been given in the Infasurf controlled clinical trials if the patient was still intubated.

In the Infasurf vs. Survanta® trials, Infasurf was administered through a 5 French feeding catheter inserted into the endotracheal tube. The total dose was instilled in four equal aliquots with the catheter removed between each of the instillations and mechanical ventilation resumed for 0.5 to 2 minutes. Each of the aliquots was administered with the patient in one of four different positions (prone, supine, right, and left lateral) to facilitate even distribution of the surfactant. Repeat doses were administered as early as 6 hours

Continued on next page

Infasurf—Cont.

after the previous dose for a total of up to 4 doses if the infant was still intubated and required at least 30% inspired oxygen to maintain a $P_aO_2 \leq 80$ torr.

Administration for Prophylaxis of RDS at Birth

The amount of a prophylaxis dose of Infasurf should be based on the infant's birth weight. Administration of Infasurf should be given as soon as possible after birth. Usually the immediate care and stabilization of the premature infant born with hypoxemia and/or bradycardia should precede Infasurf prophylaxis.

The dosing procedures are described under Administration for Treatment of RDS.

Dosing Precautions

During administration of Infasurf liquid suspension into the airway, infants often experience bradycardia, reflux of Infasurf into the endotracheal tube, airway obstruction, cyanosis, dislodgement of the endotracheal tube, or hypoventilation. If any of these events occur, the administration should be interrupted and the infant's condition should be stabilized using appropriate interventions before the administration of Infasurf is resumed. Endotracheal suctioning or reintubation is sometimes needed when there are signs of airway obstruction during the administration of the surfactant.

HOW SUPPLIED

Infasurf (calfactant) Intratracheal Suspension is supplied sterile in single-use, rubber-stoppered glass vials containing 3 mL (NDC 0456-4600-03) and 6 mL (NDC 0456-4600-06) off-white suspension.

Store Infasurf (calfactant) Intratracheal Suspension at refrigerated temperature 2° to 8°C (36° to 46°F) and protect from light. **THE 3mL VIAL MUST BE STORED UPRIGHT.** Vials are for single use only. After opening, discard unused drug.

Rx only

Manufactured for:
FOREST PHARMACEUTICALS, INC.
Subsidiary of Forest Laboratories, Inc.
St. Louis, MO 63045
by:
ONY, Inc.
Amherst, NY 14228
RMC 235 Rev. 06/03

Shown in Product Identification Guide, page 312

LEVOTHROID® ℞

[lĕv'o-throid"]
(levothyroxine sodium tablets, USP)
Rx Only

DESCRIPTION

LEVOTHROID® (levothyroxine sodium tablets, USP) contains synthetic crystalline L-3,3',5,5'-tetraiodothyronine sodium salt [levothyroxine (T_4) sodium]. Synthetic T_4 is identical to that produced in the human thyroid gland. Levothyroxine (T_4) sodium has an empirical formula of $C_{15}H_{10}I_4N\ NaO_4 \times H_2O$, molecular weight of 798.86 g/mol (anhydrous), and structural formula as shown:

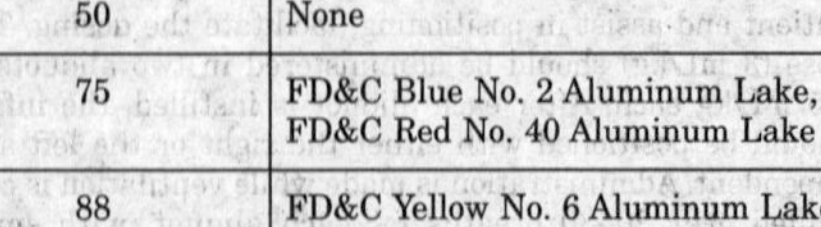

Inactive Ingredients: Microcrystalline cellulose, calcium phosphate dibasic, povidone and magnesium stearate. The following are the coloring additives per tablet strength.

Strength (mcg)	Color Additive(s)
25	FD&C Yellow No. 6 Aluminum Lake
50	None
75	FD&C Blue No. 2 Aluminum Lake, FD&C Red No. 40 Aluminum Lake
88	FD&C Yellow No. 6 Aluminum Lake, FD&C Blue No. 1 Aluminum Lake, D&C Yellow No. 10 Aluminum Lake
100	FD&C Yellow No. 6 Aluminum Lake, D&C Yellow No. 10 Aluminum Lake
112	D&C Red No. 27 Aluminum Lake, D&C Red No. 30 Aluminum Lake
125	FD&C Blue No. 1 Aluminum Lake, FD&C Red No. 40 Aluminum Lake, FD&C Yellow No. 6 Aluminum Lake
150	FD&C Blue No. 2 Aluminum Lake
175	FD&C Blue No. 1 Aluminum Lake, D&C Red No. 30 Aluminum Lake, D&C Red No. 27 Aluminum Lake
200	FD&C Red No. 40 Aluminum Lake
300	FD&C Yellow No. 6 Aluminum Lake, FD&C Blue No.1 Aluminum Lake, D&C Yellow No. 10 Aluminum Lake

CLINICAL PHARMACOLOGY

Thyroid hormone synthesis and secretion is regulated by the hypothalamic-pituitary-thyroid axis. Thyrotropin-releasing hormone (TRH) released from the hypothalamus stimulates secretion of thyrotropin-stimulating hormone, TSH, from the anterior pituitary. TSH, in turn, is the physiologic stimulus for the synthesis and secretion of thyroid hormones, L-thyroxine (T_4) and L-triiodothyronine (T_3), by the thyroid gland. Circulating serum T_3 and T_4 levels exert a feedback effect on both TRH and TSH secretion. When serum T_3 and T_4 levels increase, TRH and TSH secretion decrease. When thyroid hormone levels decrease, TRH and TSH secretion increase. The mechanisms by which thyroid hormones exert their physiologic actions are not completely understood, but it is thought that their principal effects are exerted through control of DNA transcription and protein synthesis. T_3 and T_4 diffuse into the cell nucleus and bind to thyroid receptor proteins attached to DNA. This hormone nuclear receptor complex activates gene transcription and synthesis of messenger RNA and cytoplasmic proteins.

Thyroid hormones regulate multiple metabolic processes and play an essential role in normal growth and development, and normal maturation of the central nervous system and bone. The metabolic actions of thyroid hormones include augmentation of cellular respiration and thermogenesis, as well as metabolism of proteins, carbohydrates and lipids. The protein anabolic effects of thyroid hormones are essential to normal growth and development.

The physiological actions of thyroid hormones are produced predominantly by T_3, the majority of which (approximately 80%) is derived from T_4 by deiodination in peripheral tissues.

Levothyroxine, at doses individualized according to patient response, is effective as replacement or supplemental therapy in hypothyroidism of any etiology, except transient hypothyroidism during the recovery phase of subacute thyroiditis.

Levothyroxine is also effective in the suppression of pituitary TSH secretion in the treatment or prevention of various types of euthyroid goiters, including thyroid nodules, Hashimoto's thyroiditis, multinodular goiter and, as adjunctive therapy in the management of thyrotropin-dependent well-differentiated thyroid cancer (see **INDICATIONS AND USAGE, PRECAUTIONS, DOSAGE AND ADMINISTRATION**).

PHARMACOKINETICS

Absorption - Absorption of orally administered T_4 from the gastrointestinal (GI) tract ranges from 40% to 80%. The majority of the levothyroxine dose is absorbed from the jejunum and upper ileum. The relative bioavailability of LEVOTHROID® tablets, compared to an equal nominal dose of oral levothyroxine sodium solution, is approximately 94%. T_4 absorption is increased by fasting, and decreased in malabsorption syndromes and by certain foods such as soybean infant formula. Dietary fiber decreases bioavailability of T_4. Absorption may also decrease with age. In addition, many drugs and foods affect T_4 absorption (see **PRECAUTIONS, Drug Interactions** and **Drug-Food Interactions**).

Distribution - Circulating thyroid hormones are greater than 99% bound to plasma proteins, including thyroxine-binding globulin (TBG), thyroxine-binding prealbumin (TBPA), and albumin (TBA), whose capacities and affinities vary for each hormone. The higher affinity of both TBG and TBPA for T_4 partially explains the higher serum levels, slower metabolic clearance, and longer half-life of T_4 compared to T_3. Protein-bound thyroid hormones exist in reverse equilibrium with small amounts of free hormone. Only unbound hormone is metabolically active. Many drugs and physiologic conditions affect the binding of thyroid hormones to serum proteins (see **PRECAUTIONS, Drug Interactions** and **Drug-Laboratory Test Interactions**). Thyroid hormones do not readily cross the placental barrier (see **PRECAUTIONS, Pregnancy**).

Metabolism - T_4 is slowly eliminated (see **Table 1**). The major pathway of thyroid hormone metabolism is through sequential deiodination. Approximately eighty-percent of circulating T_3 is derived from peripheral T_4 by monodeiodination. The liver is the major site of degradation for both T_4 and T_3, with T_4 deiodination also occurring at a number of additional sites, including the kidney and other tissues. Approximately 80% of the daily dose of T_4 is deiodinated to yield equal amounts of T_3 and reverse T_3 (rT_3). T_3 and rT_3 are further deiodinated to diiodothyronine. Thyroid hormones are also metabolized via conjugation with glucuronides and sulfates and excreted directly into the bile and gut where they undergo enterohepatic recirculation.

Elimination - Thyroid hormones are primarily eliminated by the kidneys. A portion of the conjugated hormone reaches the colon unchanged and is eliminated in the feces. Approximately 20% of T_4 is eliminated in the stool. Urinary excretion of T_4 decreases with age.

Table 1: Pharmacokinetic Parameters of Thyroid Hormones in Euthyroid Patients

Hormone	Ratio in Thyroglobulin	Biologic Potency	$t_{1/2}$ (days)	Protein Binding (%)[2]
Levothyroxine (T_4)	10-20	1	6-7[1]	99.96
Liothyronine (T_3)	1	4	≤2	99.5

[1] 3 to 4 days in hyperthyroidism, 9 to 10 days in hypothyroidism; [2] Includes TBG, TBPA, and TBA

INDICATIONS AND USAGE

Levothyroxine sodium is used for the following indications:

Hypothyroidism - As replacement or supplemental therapy in congenital or acquired hypothyroidism of any etiology, except transient hypothyroidism during the recovery phase of subacute thyroiditis. Specific indications include: primary (thyroidal), secondary (pituitary), and tertiary (hypothalamic) hypothyroidism and subclinical hypothyroidism. Primary hypothyroidism may result from functional deficiency, primary atrophy, partial or total congenital absence of the thyroid gland, or from the effects of surgery, radiation, or drugs, with or without the presence of goiter.

Pituitary TSH Suppression - In the treatment or prevention of various types of euthyroid goiters (see **WARNINGS** and **PRECAUTIONS**), including thyroid nodules (see **WARNINGS** and **PRECAUTIONS**), subacute or chronic lymphocytic thyroiditis (Hashimoto's thyroiditis), multinodular goiter (see **WARNINGS** and **PRECAUTIONS**) and, as an adjunct to surgery and radioiodine therapy in the management of thyrotropin-dependent well-differentiated thyroid cancer.

CONTRAINDICATIONS

Levothyroxine is contraindicated in patients with untreated subclinical (suppressed serum TSH level with normal T_3 and T_4 levels) or overt thyrotoxicosis of any etiology and in patients with acute myocardial infarction. Levothyroxine is contraindicated in patients with uncorrected adrenal insufficiency since thyroid hormones may precipitate an acute adrenal crisis by increasing the metabolic clearance of glucocorticoids (see **PRECAUTIONS**). LEVOTHROID® is contraindicated in patients with hypersensitivity to any of the inactive ingredients in LEVOTHROID® tablets (see **DESCRIPTION, Inactive Ingredients**).

WARNINGS

WARNING: Thyroid hormones, including LEVOTHROID®, either alone or with other therapeutic agents, should not be used for the treatment of obesity or for weight loss. In euthyroid patients, doses within the range of daily hormonal requirements are ineffective for weight reduction. Larger doses may produce serious or even life threatening manifestations of toxicity, particularly when given in association with sympathomimetic amines such as those used for their anorectic effects.

Levothyroxine sodium should not be used in the treatment of male or female infertility unless this condition is associated with hypothyroidism.

In patients with nontoxic diffuse goiter or nodular thyroid disease, particularly the elderly or those with underlying cardiovascular disease, levothyroxine sodium therapy is contraindicated if the serum TSH level is already suppressed due to the risk of precipitating overt thyrotoxicosis (see **CONTRAINDICATIONS**). If the serum TSH level is not suppressed, LEVOTHROID® should be used with caution in conjunction with careful monitoring of thyroid function for evidence of hyperthyroidism and clinical monitoring for potential associated adverse cardiovascular signs and symptoms of hyperthyroidism.

PRECAUTIONS

General

Levothyroxine has a narrow therapeutic index. Regardless of the indication for use, careful dosage titration is necessary to avoid the consequences of over- or under-treatment. These consequences include, among others, effects on growth and development, cardiovascular function, bone metabolism, reproductive function, cognitive function, emotional state, gastrointestinal function, and on glucose and lipid metabolism. Many drugs interact with levothyroxine sodium, necessitating adjustments in dosing to maintain therapeutic response (see **Drug Interactions**).

Effects on bone mineral density - In women, long-term levothyroxine sodium therapy has been associated with increased bone resorption, thereby decreasing bone mineral density, especially in post-menopausal women on greater than replacement doses or in women who are receiving suppressive doses of levothyroxine sodium. The increased bone resorption may be associated with increased serum levels and urinary excretion of calcium and phosphorous, elevations in bone alkaline phosphatase and suppressed serum parathyroid hormone levels. Therefore, it is recommended that patients receiving levothyroxine sodium be given the minimum dose necessary to achieve the desired clinical and biochemical response.

Patients with underlying cardiovascular disease - Exercise caution when administering levothyroxine to patients with cardiovascular disorders and to the elderly in whom there is an increased risk of occult cardiac disease. In these patients, levothyroxine therapy should be initiated at lower doses than those recommended in younger individuals or in patients without cardiac disease (see **WARNINGS; PRECAUTIONS, Geriatric Use**; and **DOSAGE AND ADMINISTRATION**). If cardiac symptoms develop or worsen, the levothyroxine dose should be reduced or withheld for one week and then cautiously restarted at a lower dose. Overtreatment with levothyroxine sodium may have adverse cardiovascular effects such as an increase in heart rate, cardiac wall thickness, and cardiac contractility and may precipitate angina or arrhythmias. Patients with coronary artery disease who are receiving levothyroxine therapy should be monitored closely during surgical procedures, since the possibility of precipitating cardiac arrhythmias may be greater in those treated with levothyroxine. Concomitant administration of levothyroxine and sympathomimetic agents to patients with coronary artery disease may precipitate coronary insufficiency.

Patients with nontoxic diffuse goiter or nodular thyroid disease - Exercise caution when administering levothyroxine to patients with nontoxic diffuse goiter or nodular thyroid disease in order to prevent precipitation of thyrotoxicosis (see **WARNINGS**). If the serum TSH is already suppressed, levothyroxine sodium should not be administered (see **CONTRAINDICATIONS**).

Associated endocrine disorders

Hypothalamic/pituitary hormone deficiencies - In patients with secondary or tertiary hypothyroidism, additional hypothalamic/pituitary hormone deficiencies should be considered, and, if diagnosed, treated (see **PRECAUTIONS, Autoimmune polyglandular syndrome** for adrenal insufficiency).

Autoimmune polyglandular syndrome - Occasionally, chronic autoimmune thyroiditis may occur in association with other autoimmune disorders such as adrenal insufficiency, pernicious anemia, and insulin-dependent diabetes mellitus. Patients with concomitant adrenal insufficiency should be treated with replacement glucocorticoids prior to initiation of treatment with levothyroxine sodium. Failure to do so may precipitate an acute adrenal crisis when thyroid hormone therapy is initiated, due to increased metabolic clearance of glucocorticoids by thyroid hormone. Patients with diabetes mellitus may require upward adjustments of their antidiabetic therapeutic regimens when treated with levothyroxine (see **PRECAUTIONS, Drug Interactions**).

Other associated medical conditions

Infants with congenital hypothyroidism appear to be at increased risk for other congenital anomalies, with cardiovascular anomalies (pulmonary stenosis, atrial septal defect, and ventricular septal defect) being the most common association.

Information for Patients

Patients should be informed of the following information to aid in the safe and effective use of LEVOTHROID®:

1. Notify your physician if you are allergic to any foods or medicines, are pregnant or intend to become pregnant, are breast-feeding or are taking any other medications, including prescription and over-the-counter preparations.
2. Notify your physician of any other medical conditions you may have, particularly heart disease, diabetes, clotting disorders, and adrenal or pituitary gland problems. Your dose of medications used to control these other conditions may need to be adjusted while you are taking LEVOTHROID®. If you have diabetes, monitor your blood and/or urinary glucose levels as directed by your physician and immediately report any changes to your physician. If you are taking anticoagulants (blood thinners), your clotting status should be checked frequently.
3. Use LEVOTHROID® only as prescribed by your physician. Do not discontinue or change the amount you take or how often you take it, unless directed to do so by your physician.
4. The levothyroxine in LEVOTHROID® is intended to replace a hormone that is normally produced by your thyroid gland. Generally, replacement therapy is to be taken for life, except in cases of transient hypothyroidism, which is usually associated with an inflammation of the thyroid gland (thyroiditis).
5. Take LEVOTHROID® as a single dose, preferably on an empty stomach, one-half to one hour before breakfast. Levothyroxine absorption is increased on an empty stomach.
6. It may take several weeks before you notice an improvement in your symptoms.
7. Notify your physician if you experience any of the following symptoms: rapid or irregular heartbeat, chest pain, shortness of breath, leg cramps, headache, nervousness, irritability, sleeplessness, tremors, change in appetite, weight gain or loss, vomiting, diarrhea, excessive sweating, heat intolerance, fever, changes in menstrual periods, hives or skin rash, or any other unusual medical event.
8. Notify your physician if you become pregnant while taking LEVOTHROID®. It is likely that your dose of LEVOTHROID® will need to be increased while you are pregnant.
9. Notify your physician or dentist that you are taking LEVOTHROID® prior to any surgery.

Table 2: Drug-Thyroidal Axis Interactions

Drugs that may reduce TSH secretion -the reduction is not sustained; therefore, hypothyroidism does not occur

Drug or Drug Class		
Dopamine / Dopamine Agonists	Glucocorticoids	Octreotide

Effect - Use of these agents may result in a transient reduction in TSH secretion when administered at the following doses: Dopamine ($\geq$1 µg/kg/min); Glucocorticoids (hydrocortisone $\geq$100 mg/day or equivalent); Octreotide (>100 µg/day).

Drugs that alter thyroid hormone secretion

Drugs that may decrease thyroid hormone secretion, which may result in hypothyroidism

Drug or Drug Class		
Aminoglutethimide	Iodide	Methimazole
Amiodarone	(including iodine-containing	Propylthiouracil (PTU)
	Radiographic contrast agents)	Sulfonamides
	Lithium	Tolbutamide

Effect - Long-term lithium therapy can result in goiter in up to 50% of patients, and either subclinical or overt hypothyroidism, each in up to 20% of patients. The fetus, neonate, elderly and euthyroid patients with underlying thyroid disease (e.g., Hashimoto's thyroiditis or with Grave's disease previously treated with radioiodine or surgery) are among those individuals who are particularly susceptible to iodine-induced hypothyroidism. Oral cholecystographic agents and amiodarone are slowly excreted, producing more prolonged hypothyroidism than parenterally administered iodinated contrast agents. Long-term aminoglutethimide therapy may minimally decrease T_4 and T_3 levels and increase TSH, although all values remain within normal limits in most patients.

Drugs that may increase thyroid hormone secretion, which may result in hyperthyroidism

Drug or Drug Class

Amiodarone

Iodide (including iodine-containing Radiographic contrast agents)

Effect - Iodide and drugs that contain pharmacological amounts of iodide may cause hyperthyroidism in euthyroid patients with Grave's disease previously treated with antithyroid drugs or in euthyroid patients with thyroid autonomy (e.g., multinodular goiter or hyperfunctioning thyroid adenoma). Hyperthyroidism may develop over several weeks and may persist for several months after therapy discontinuation. Amiodarone may induce hyperthyroidism by causing thyroiditis.

Drugs that may decrease T_4 absorption, which may result in hypothyroidism

Drug or Drug Class		
Antacids	Bile Acid Sequestrants	Cation Exchange Resins
- Aluminum & Magnesium	- Cholestyramine	- Kayexalate
Hydroxides	- Colestipol	Ferrous Sulfate
- Simethicone	Calcium Carbonate	Sucralfate

Effect - Concurrent use may reduce the efficacy of levothyroxine by binding and delaying or preventing absorption, potentially resulting in hypothyroidism. Calcium carbonate may form an insoluble chelate with levothyroxine, and ferrous sulfate likely forms a ferric-thyroxine complex. Administer levothyroxine at least 4 hours apart from these agents.

Drugs that may alter T_4 and T_3 serum transport - but FT_4 concentration remains normal; and, therefore, the patient remains euthyroid

Drugs that may increase serum TBG concentration

Clofibrate	Estrogens (oral)	Mitotane
Estrogen-containing	Heroin/Methadone	Tamoxifen
oral contraceptives	5-Flourouracil	

Drugs that may decrease serum TBG concentration

Androgens / Anabolic Steroids	Glucocorticoids
Asparaginase	Slow-Release Nicotinic Acid

Drugs that may cause protein-binding site displacement

Drug or Drug Class	
Furosemide (> 80 mg IV)	Non Steroidal Anti-Inflammatory Drugs
Heparin	- Fenamates
Hydantoins	- Phenylbutazone
	Salicylates (>2 g/day)

Effect - Administration of these agents with levothyroxine results in an initial transient increase in FT_4. Continued administration results in a decrease in serum T_4 and normal FT_4 and TSH concentrations and, therefore, patients are clinically euthyroid. Salicylates inhibit binding of T_4 and T_3 to TBG and transthyretin. An initial increase in serum FT_4 is followed by return of FT_4 to normal levels with sustained therapeutic serum salicylate concentrations, although total-T_4 levels may decrease by as much as 30%.

Drugs that may alter T_4 and T_3 metabolism

Drugs that may increase hepatic metabolism, which may result in hypothyroidism

Drug or Drug Class			
Carbamazepine	Hydantoins	Phenobarbital	Rifampin

Effect - Stimulation of hepatic microsomal drug-metabolizing enzyme activity may cause increased hepatic degradation of levothyroxine, resulting in increased levothyroxine requirements. Phenytoin and carbamazepine reduce serum protein binding of levothyroxine, and total- and free-T_4 may be reduced by 20% to 40%, but most patients have normal serum TSH levels and are clinically euthyroid.

(Table continued on next page)

10. Partial hair loss may occur rarely during the first few months of LEVOTHROID® therapy, but this is usually temporary.
11. LEVOTHROID® should not be used as a primary or adjunctive therapy in a weight control program.
12. Keep LEVOTHROID® out of the reach of children. Store LEVOTHROID® away from heat, moisture, and light.

Laboratory Tests

General

The diagnosis of hypothyroidism is confirmed by measuring TSH levels using a sensitive assay (second generation assay sensitivity $\leq$0.1 mIU/L or third generation assay sensitivity $\leq$0.01 mIU/L) and measurement of free-T_4.

The adequacy of therapy is determined by periodic assessment of appropriate laboratory tests and clinical evaluation. The choice of laboratory tests depends on various factors including the etiology of the underlying thyroid disease, the presence of concomitant medical conditions, including pregnancy, and the use of concomitant medications (see **PRECAUTIONS, Drug Interactions** and **Drug-Laboratory Test Interactions**). Persistent clinical and laboratory evidence of hypothyroidism despite an apparent adequate replacement dose of LEVOTHROID® may be evidence of inadequate absorption, poor compliance, drug interactions, or decreased T_4 potency of the drug product.

Adults

In adult patients with primary (thyroidal) hypothyroidism, serum TSH levels (using a sensitive assay) alone may be used to monitor therapy. The frequency of TSH monitoring during levothyroxine dose titration depends on the clinical

Continued on next page

Levothroid—Cont.

situation but it is generally recommended at 6-8 week intervals until normalization. For patients who have recently initiated levothyroxine therapy and whose serum TSH has normalized or in patients who have had their dosage or brand of levothyroxine changed, the serum TSH concentration should be measured after 8-12 weeks. When the optimum replacement dose has been attained, clinical (physical examination) and biochemical monitoring may be performed every 6-12 months, depending on the clinical situation, and whenever there is a change in the patient's status. It is recommended that a physical examination and a serum TSH measurement be performed at least annually in patients receiving LEVOTHROID® (see **WARNINGS, PRECAUTIONS,** and **DOSAGE AND ADMINISTRATION**).

Pediatrics

In patients with congenital hypothyroidism, the adequacy of replacement therapy should be assessed by measuring both serum TSH (using a sensitive assay) and total- or free-T_4. During the first three years of life, the serum total- or free-T_4 should be maintained at all times in the upper half of the normal range. While the aim of therapy is to also normalize the serum TSH level, this is not always possible in a small percentage of patients, particularly in the first few months of therapy. TSH may not normalize due to a resetting of the pituitary-thyroid feedback threshold as a result of *in utero* hypothyroidism. Failure of the serum T_4 to increase into the upper half of the normal range within 2 weeks of initiation of LEVOTHROID® therapy and/or of the serum TSH to decrease below 20mU/L within 4 weeks should alert the physician to the possibility that the child is not receiving adequate therapy. Careful inquiry should then be made regarding compliance, dose of medication administered, and method of administration prior to raising the dose of LEVOTHROID®.

The recommended frequency of monitoring of TSH and total- or free-T_4 in children is as follows: at 2 and 4 weeks after the initiation of treatment; every 1-2 months during the first year of life; every 2-3 months between 1 and 3 years of age; and every 3 to 12 months thereafter until growth is completed. More frequent intervals of monitoring may be necessary if poor compliance is suspected or abnormal values are obtained. It is recommended that TSH and T_4 levels, and a physical examination, if indicated, be performed 2 weeks after any change in LEVOTHROID® dosage. Routine clinical examination, including assessment of mental and physical growth and development, and bone maturation, should be performed at regular intervals (see **PRECAUTIONS, Pediatric Use** and **DOSAGE AND ADMINISTRATION**).

Secondary (pituitary) and tertiary (hypothalamic) hypothyroidism

Adequacy of therapy should be assessed by measuring serum free-T_4 levels, which should be maintained in the upper half of the normal range in these patients.

Drug Interactions

Many drugs affect thyroid hormone pharmacokinetics and metabolism (e.g., absorption, synthesis, secretion, catabolism, protein binding, and target tissue response) and may alter the therapeutic response to LEVOTHROID®. In addition, thyroid hormones and thyroid status have varied effects on the pharmacokinetics and actions of other drugs. A listing of drug-thyroidal axis interactions is contained in Table 2.

The list of drug-thyroidal axis interactions in Table 2 may not be comprehensive due to the introduction of new drugs that interact with the thyroidal axis or the discovery of previously unknown interactions. The prescriber should be aware of this fact and should consult appropriate reference sources (e.g., package inserts of newly approved drugs, medical literature) for additional information if a drug-drug interaction with levothyroxine is suspected.

[See table 2 on previous page and above]

Oral anticoagulants - Levothyroxine increases the response to oral anticoagulant therapy. Therefore, a decrease in the dose of anticoagulant may be warranted with correction of the hypothyroid state or when the LEVOTHROID® dose is increased. Prothrombin time should be closely monitored to permit appropriate and timely dosage adjustments (see **Table 2**).

Digitalis glycosides - The therapeutic effects of digitalis glycosides may be reduced by levothyroxine. Serum digitalis glycoside levels may be decreased when a hypothyroid patient becomes euthyroid, necessitating an increase in the dose of digitalis glycosides (see **Table 2**).

Drug-Food Interactions - Consumption of certain foods may affect levothyroxine absorption thereby necessitating adjustments in dosing. Soybean flour (infant formula), cotton seed meal, walnuts, and dietary fiber may bind and decrease the absorption of levothyroxine sodium from the GI tract.

Drug-Laboratory Test Interactions - Changes in TBG concentration must be considered when interpreting T_4 and T_3 values, which necessitates measurement and evaluation of unbound (free) hormone and/or determination of the free-T_4 index (FT_4I). Pregnancy, infectious hepatitis, estrogens, estrogen-containing oral contraceptives, and acute intermittent porphyria increase TBG concentrations. Decreases in TBG concentrations are observed in nephrosis, severe hypoproteinemia, severe liver disease, acromegaly, and after androgen or corticosteroid therapy (see also **Table 2**). Familial hyper- or hypo-thyroxine binding globulinemias have been described, with the incidence of TBG deficiency approximating 1 in 9000.

Table 2 *(cont.)*: Drug-Thyroidal Axis Interactions

Drug or Drug Class	Effect
Drugs that may decrease T_4 5'-deiodinase activity	
Amiodarone; Beta-adrenergic antagonists - (e.g., Propranolol > 160 mg/day); Glucocorticoids - (e.g., Dexamethasone ≥4 mg/day); - Propylthiouracil (PTU)	Administration of these enzyme inhibitors decreases the peripheral conversion of T_4 to T_3, leading to decreased T_3 levels. However, serum T_4 levels are usually normal but may occasionally be slightly increased. In patients treated with large doses of propranolol (> 160 mg/day), T_3 and T_4 levels change slightly, TSH levels remain normal, and patients are clinically euthyroid. It should be noted that actions of particular beta-adrenergic antagonists may be impaired when the hypothyroid patient is converted to the euthyroid state. Short-term administration of large doses of glucocorticoids may decrease serum T_3 concentrations by 30% with minimal change in serum T_4 levels. However, long-term glucocorticoid therapy may result in slightly decreased T_3 and T_4levels due to decreased TBG production (see above).
Miscellaneous	
Anticoagulants (oral) - Coumarin Derivatives - Indandione Derivatives	Thyroid hormones appear to increase the catabolism of vitamin K-dependent clotting factors, thereby increasing the anticoagulant activity of oral anticoagulants. Concomitant use of these agents impairs the compensatory increases in clotting factor synthesis. Prothrombin time should be carefully monitored in patients taking levothyroxine and oral anticoagulants and the dose of anticoagulant therapy adjusted accordingly.
Antidepressants - Tricyclics (e.g., Amitriptyline) - Tetracyclics (e.g., Maprotiline) - Selective Serotonin Reuptake Inhibitors (SSRIs; e.g., Sertraline)	Concurrent use of tri/tetracyclic antidepressants and levothyroxine may increase the therapeutic and toxic effects of both drugs, possibly due to increased receptor sensitivity to catecholamines. Toxic effects may include increased risk of cardiac arrhythmias and CNS stimulation; onset of action of tricyclics may be accelerated. Administration of sertraline in patients stabilized on levothyroxine may result in increased levothyroxine requirements.
Antidiabetic Agents - Biguanides - Meglitinides - Thiazolidinediones - Sulfonylureas - Insulin	Addition of levothyroxine to antidiabetic or insulin therapy may result in increased antidiabetic agent or insulin requirements. Careful monitoring of diabetic control is recommended, especially when thyroid therapy is started, changed, or discontinued.
Cardiac Glycosides	Serum digitalis glycoside levels may be reduced in hyperthyroidism or when the hypothyroid patient is converted to the euthyroid state. Therapeutic effect of digitalis glycosides may be reduced.
Cytokines - Interferon-α - Interleukin-2	Therapy with interferon-α has been associated with the development of antithyroid microsomal antibodies in 20% of patients and some have transient hypothyroidism, hyperthyroidism, or both. Patients who have antithyroid antibodies before treatment are at higher risk for thyroid dysfunction during treatment. Interleukin-2 has been associated with transient painless thyroiditis in 20% of patients. Interferon-β and -γ have not been reported to cause thyroid dysfunction.
Growth Hormones - Somatrem - Somatropin	Excessive use of thyroid hormones with growth hormones may accelerate epiphyseal closure. However, untreated hypothyroidism may interfere with growth response to growth hormone.
Ketamine	Concurrent use may produce marked hypertension and tachycardia; cautious administration to patients receiving thyroid hormone therapy is recommended.
Methylxanthine Bronchodilators - (e.g., Theophylline)	Decreased theophylline clearance may occur in hypothyroid patients; clearance returns to normal when the euthyroid state is achieved.
Radiographic Agents	Thyroid hormones may reduce the uptake of ^{123}I, ^{131}I, and ^{99m}Tc.
Sympathomimetics	Concurrent use may increase the effects of sympathomimetics or thyroid hormone. Thyroid hormones may increase the risk of coronary insufficiency when sympathomimetic agents are administered to patients with coronary artery disease.
Chloral Hydrate; Diazepam; Ethionamide; Lovastatin; Metoclopramide; 6-Mercaptopurine; Nitroprusside; Para-aminosalicylate sodium; Perphenazine; Resorcinol (excessive topical use); Thiazide Diuretics	These agents have been associated with thyroid hormone and / or TSH level alterations by various mechanisms.

Carcinogenesis, Mutagenesis, and Impairment of Fertility - Animal studies have not been performed to evaluate the carcinogenic potential, mutagenic potential or effects on fertility of levothyroxine. The synthetic T_4 in LEVOTHROID® is identical to that produced naturally by the human thyroid gland. Although there has been a reported association between prolonged thyroid hormone therapy and breast cancer, this has not been confirmed. Patients receiving LEVOTHROID® for appropriate clinical indications should be titrated to the lowest effective replacement dose.

Pregnancy - Category A - Studies in women taking levothyroxine sodium during pregnancy have not shown an increased risk of congenital abnormalities. Therefore, the possibility of fetal harm appears remote. LEVOTHROID® should not be discontinued during pregnancy and hypothyroidism diagnosed during pregnancy should be promptly treated.

Hypothyroidism during pregnancy is associated with a higher rate of complications, including spontaneous abortion, pre-eclampsia, stillbirth and premature delivery. Maternal hypothyroidism may have an adverse effect on fetal and childhood growth and development. During pregnancy, serum T_4 levels may decrease and serum TSH levels increase to values outside the normal range. Since elevations in serum TSH may occur as early as 4 weeks gestation, pregnant women taking LEVOTHROID® should have their TSH measured during each trimester. An elevated serum TSH level should be corrected by an increase in the dose of LEVOTHROID®. Since postpartum TSH levels are similar to preconception values, the LEVOTHROID® dosage should return to the pre-pregnancy dose immediately after delivery. A serum TSH level should be obtained 6-8 weeks postpartum.

Thyroid hormones cross the placental barrier to some extent as evidenced by levels in cord blood of athyreotic fetuses being approximately one-third maternal levels. Transfer of thyroid hormone from the mother to the fetus, however, may not be adequate to prevent *in utero* hypothyroidism.

Nursing Mothers - Although thyroid hormones are excreted only minimally in human milk, caution should be exercised when LEVOTHROID® is administered to a nursing woman. However, adequate replacement doses of levothyroxine are generally needed to maintain normal lactation.

Pediatric Use

General

The goal of treatment in pediatric patients with hypothyroidism is to achieve and maintain normal intellectual and physical growth and development.

The initial dose of levothyroxine varies with age and body weight (see **DOSAGE AND ADMINISTRATION, Table 3**). Dosing adjustments are based on an assessment of the individual patient's clinical and laboratory parameters (see **PRECAUTIONS, Laboratory Tests**).

In children in whom a diagnosis of permanent hypothyroidism has not been established, it is recommended that levothyroxine administration be discontinued for a 30-day trial period, but only after the child is at least 3 years of age. Serum T_4 and TSH levels should then be obtained. If the T_4 is low and the TSH high, the diagnosis of permanent hypothyroidism is established, and levothyroxine therapy should be reinstituted. If the T_4 and TSH levels are normal, euthyroidism may be assumed and, therefore, the hypothyroidism can be considered to have been transient. In this instance, however, the physician should carefully monitor the child and repeat the thyroid function tests if any signs or symptoms of hypothyroidism develop. In this setting, the clinician should have a high index of suspicion of relapse. If the results of the levothyroxine withdrawal test are inconclusive, careful follow-up and subsequent testing will be necessary.

Since some more severely affected children may become clinically hypothyroid when treatment is discontinued for 30 days, an alternate approach is to reduce the replacement dose of levothyroxine by half during the 30-day trial period. If, after 30 days, the serum TSH is elevated above 20 mU/L, the diagnosis of permanent hypothyroidism is confirmed, and full replacement therapy should be resumed. However, if the serum TSH has not risen to greater than 20 mU/L, levothyroxine treatment should be discontinued for another 30-day trial period followed by repeat serum T_4 and TSH testing.

The presence of concomitant medical conditions should be considered in certain clinical circumstances and, if present, appropriately treated (see **PRECAUTIONS**).

Congenital Hypothyroidism (see **PRECAUTIONS, Laboratory Tests** and **DOSAGE AND ADMINISTRATION**)

Rapid restoration of normal serum T_4 concentrations is essential for preventing the adverse effects of congenital hypothyroidism on intellectual development as well as on overall physical growth and maturation. Therefore, LEVOTHROID® therapy should be initiated immediately upon diagnosis and is generally continued for life.

During the first 2 weeks of LEVOTHROID® therapy, infants should be closely monitored for cardiac overload, arrhythmias, and aspiration from avid suckling.

The patient should be monitored closely to avoid undertreatment or overtreatment. Undertreatment may have deleterious effects on intellectual development and linear growth. Overtreatment has been associated with craniosynostosis in infants, and may adversely affect the tempo of brain maturation and accelerate the bone age with resultant premature closure of the epiphyses and compromised adult stature.

Acquired Hypothyroidism in Pediatric Patients

The patient should be monitored closely to avoid undertreatment and overtreatment. Undertreatment may result in poor school performance due to impaired concentration and slowed mentation and in reduced adult height. Overtreatment may accelerate the bone age and result in premature epiphyseal closure and compromised adult stature.

Treated children may manifest a period of catch-up growth, which may be adequate in some cases to normalize adult height. In children with severe or prolonged hypothyroidism, catch-up growth may not be adequate to normalize adult height.

Geriatric Use

Because of the increased prevalence of cardiovascular disease among the elderly, levothyroxine therapy should not be initiated at the full replacement dose (see **WARNINGS, PRECAUTIONS,** and **DOSAGE AND ADMINISTRATION**).

ADVERSE REACTIONS

Adverse reactions associated with levothyroxine therapy are primarily those of hyperthyroidism due to therapeutic overdosage (see **PRECAUTIONS** and **OVERDOSAGE**). They include the following:

General: fatigue, increased appetite, weight loss, heat intolerance, fever, excessive sweating;

Central nervous system: headache, hyperactivity, nervousness, anxiety, irritability, emotional lability, insomnia;

Musculoskeletal: tremors, muscle weakness;

Cardiovascular: palpitations, tachycardia, arrhythmias, increased pulse and blood pressure, heart failure, angina, myocardial infarction, cardiac arrest;

Respiratory: dyspnea;

Gastrointestinal: diarrhea, vomiting, abdominal cramps and elevations in liver function tests;

Dermatologic: hair loss, flushing;

Endocrine: decreased bone mineral density;

Reproductive: menstrual irregularities, impaired fertility.

Pseudotumor cerebri and slipped capital femoral epiphysis have been reported in children receiving levothyroxine therapy. Overtreatment may result in craniosynostosis in infants and premature closure of the epiphyses in children with resultant compromised adult height.

Seizures have been reported rarely with the institution of levothyroxine therapy.

Inadequate levothyroxine dosage will produce or fail to ameliorate the signs and symptoms of hypothyroidism.

Hypersensitivity reactions to inactive ingredients have occurred in patients treated with thyroid hormone products. These include urticaria, pruritus, skin rash, flushing, angioedema, various GI symptoms (abdominal pain, nausea, vomiting and diarrhea), fever, arthralgia, serum sickness and wheezing. Hypersensitivity to levothyroxine itself is not known to occur.

OVERDOSAGE

The signs and symptoms of overdosage are those of hyperthyroidism (see **PRECAUTIONS** and **ADVERSE REACTIONS**). In addition, confusion and disorientation may occur. Cerebral embolism, shock, coma, and death have been reported. Seizures have occurred in a child ingesting 18 mg of levothyroxine. Symptoms may not necessarily be evident or may not appear until several days after ingestion of levothyroxine sodium.

Treatment of Overdosage

Levothyroxine sodium should be reduced in dose or temporarily discontinued if signs or symptoms of overdosage occur.

Acute Massive Overdosage - This may be a life-threatening emergency, therefore, symptomatic and supportive therapy should be instituted immediately. If not contraindicated (e.g., by seizures, coma, or loss of the gag reflex), the stomach should be emptied by emesis or gastric lavage to decrease gastrointestinal absorption. Activated charcoal or cholestyramine may also be used to decrease absorption. Central and peripheral increased sympathetic activity may be treated by administering β-receptor antagonists, e.g., propranolol, provided there are no medical contraindications to their use. Provide respiratory support as needed; control congestive heart failure and arrhythmia; control fever, hypoglycemia, and fluid loss as necessary. Large doses of antithyroid drugs (e.g., methimazole or propylthiouracil) followed in one to two hours by large doses of iodine may be given to inhibit synthesis and release of thyroid hormones. Glucocorticoids may be given to inhibit the conversion of T_4 to T_3. Plasmapheresis, charcoal hemoperfusion and exchange transfusion have been reserved for cases in which continued clinical deterioration occurs despite conventional therapy. Because T_4 is highly protein bound, very little drug will be removed by dialysis.

DOSAGE AND ADMINISTRATION

General Principles

The goal of replacement therapy is to achieve and maintain a clinical and biochemical euthyroid state. The goal of suppressive therapy is to inhibit growth and/or function of abnormal thyroid tissue. The dose of LEVOTHROID® that is adequate to achieve these goals depends on a variety of factors including the patient's age, body weight, cardiovascular status, concomitant medical conditions, including pregnancy, concomitant medications, and the specific nature of the condition being treated (see **WARNINGS** and **PRECAUTIONS**). Hence, the following recommendations serve only as dosing guidelines. Dosing must be individualized and adjustments made based on periodic assessment of the patient's clinical response and laboratory parameters (see **PRECAUTIONS, Laboratory Tests**).

LEVOTHROID® is administered as a single daily dose, preferably one-half to one hour before breakfast. LEVOTHROID® should be taken at least 4 hours apart from drugs that are known to interfere with its absorption (see **PRECAUTIONS, Drug Interactions**).

Due to the long half-life of levothyroxine, the peak therapeutic effect at a given dose of levothyroxine sodium may not be attained for 4-6 weeks.

Caution should be exercised when administering LEVOTHROID® to patients with underlying cardiovascular disease, to the elderly, and to those with concomitant adrenal insufficiency (see **PRECAUTIONS**).

Specific Patient Populations

Hypothyroidism in Adults and in Children in Whom Growth and Puberty are Complete (see **WARNINGS** and **PRECAUTIONS, Laboratory Tests**)

Therapy may begin at full replacement doses in otherwise healthy individuals less than 50 years old and in those older than 50 years who have been recently treated for hyperthyroidism or who have been hypothyroid for only a short time (such as a few months). The average full replacement dose of levothyroxine sodium is approximately 1.7 mcg/kg/day (e.g., **100-125 mcg/day** for a 70 kg adult). Older patients may require less than 1 mcg/kg/day. Levothyroxine sodium doses greater than 200 mcg/day are seldom required. An inadequate response to daily doses ≥300 mcg/day is rare and may indicate poor compliance, malabsorption, and/or drug interactions.

For most patients older than 50 years or for patients under 50 years of age with underlying cardiac disease, an initial starting dose of **25-50 mcg/day** of levothyroxine sodium is recommended, with gradual increments in dose at 6-8 week intervals, as needed. The recommended starting dose of levothyroxine sodium in elderly patients with cardiac disease is **12.5-25 mcg/day**, with gradual dose increments at 4-6 week intervals. The levothyroxine sodium dose is generally adjusted in 12.5-25 mcg increments until the patient with primary hypothyroidism is clinically euthyroid and the serum TSH has normalized.

In patients with severe hypothyroidism, the recommended initial levothyroxine sodium dose is **12.5-25 mcg/day** with increases of 25 mcg/day every 2-4 weeks, accompanied by clinical and laboratory assessment, until the TSH level is normalized.

In patients with secondary (pituitary) or tertiary (hypothalamic) hypothyroidism, the levothyroxine sodium dose should be titrated until the patient is clinically euthyroid and the serum free-T_4 level is restored to the upper half of the normal range.

Pediatric Dosage - Congenital or Acquired Hypothyroidism (see **PRECAUTIONS, Laboratory Tests**)

General Principles

In general, levothyroxine therapy should be instituted at full replacement doses as soon as possible. Delays in diagnosis and institution of therapy may have deleterious effects on the child's intellectual and physical growth and development.

Undertreatment and overtreatment should be avoided (see **PRECAUTIONS, Pediatric Use**). LEVOTHROID® may be administered to infants and children who cannot swallow intact tablets by crushing the tablet and suspending the freshly crushed tablet in a small amount (5-10 mL or 1-2 teaspoons) of water. This suspension can be administered by spoon or dropper. **DO NOT STORE THE SUSPENSION.** Foods that decrease absorption of levothyroxine, such as soybean infant formula, should not be used for administering levothyroxine sodium tablets (see **PRECAUTIONS, Drug-Food Interactions**).

Newborns

The recommended starting dose of levothyroxine sodium in newborn infants is **10-15 mcg/kg/day.** A lower starting dose (e.g., 25 mcg/day) should be considered in infants at risk for cardiac failure, and the dose should be increased in 4-6 weeks as needed based on clinical and laboratory response to treatment. In infants with very low (<5 mcg/dL) or undetectable serum T_4 concentrations, the recommended initial starting dose is **50 mcg/day** of levothyroxine sodium.

Infants and Children

Levothyroxine therapy is usually initiated at full replacement doses, with the recommended dose per body weight decreasing with age (see **Table 3**). However, in children with chronic or severe hypothyroidism, an initial dose of **25 mcg/day** of levothyroxine sodium is recommended with increments of 25 mcg every 2-4 weeks until the desired effect is achieved.

Hyperactivity in an older child can be minimized if the starting dose is one-fourth of the recommended full replacement dose, and the dose is then increased on a weekly basis by an amount equal to one-fourth the full-recommended replacement dose until the full recommended replacement dose is reached.

Table 3: Levothyroxine Sodium Dosing Guidelines for Pediatric Hypothyroidism

AGE	Daily Dose Per Kg Body Weight[a]
0-3 months	10-15 mcg/kg/day
3-6 months	8-10 mcg/kg/day
6-12 months	6-8 mcg/kg/day
1-5 years	5-6 mcg/kg/day
6-12 years	4-5 mcg/kg/day
>12 years but growth and puberty incomplete	2-3 mcg/kg/day
Growth and puberty complete	1.7 mcg/kg/day

[a] The dose should be adjusted based on clinical response and laboratory parameters (see **PRECAUTIONS, Laboratory Tests** and **Pediatric Use**).

Pregnancy - Pregnancy may increase levothyroxine requirements (see **Pregnancy**).

Subclinical Hypothyroidism - If this condition is treated, a lower levothyroxine sodium dose (e.g., **1 mcg/kg/day**) than that used for full replacement may be adequate to normalize the serum TSH level. Patients who are not treated should be monitored yearly for changes in clinical status and thyroid laboratory parameters.

TSH Suppression in Well-differentiated Thyroid Cancer and Thyroid Nodules-The target level for TSH suppression in these conditions has not been established with controlled studies. In addition, the efficacy of TSH suppression for benign nodular disease is controversial. Therefore, the dose of LEVOTHROID® used for TSH suppression should be indi-

Continued on next page

Levothroid—Cont.

vidualized based on the specific disease and the patient being treated.
In the treatment of well-differentiated (papillary and follicular) thyroid cancer, levothyroxine is used as an adjunct to surgery and radioiodine therapy. Generally, TSH is suppressed to <0.1 mU/L, and this usually requires a levothyroxine sodium dose of **greater than 2 mcg/kg/day**. However, in patients with high-risk tumors, the target level for TSH suppression may be <0.01 mU/L.
In the treatment of benign nodules and nontoxic multinodular goiter, TSH is generally suppressed to a higher target (e.g., 0.1 to either 0.5 or 1.0 mU/L) than that used for the treatment of thyroid cancer. Levothyroxine sodium is contraindicated if the serum TSH is already suppressed due to the risk of precipitating overt thyrotoxicosis (see **CONTRAINDICATIONS, WARNINGS** and **PRECAUTIONS**).
Myxedema Coma - Myxedema coma is a life-threatening emergency characterized by poor circulation and hypometabolism, and may result in unpredictable absorption of levothyroxine sodium from the gastrointestinal tract. Therefore, oral thyroid hormone drug products are not recommended to treat this condition. Thyroid hormone drug products formulated for intravenous administration should be administered.

HOW SUPPLIED

LEVOTHROID® (levothyroxine sodium tablets, USP) are caplet-shaped, color-coded, potency marked tablets and are supplied as follows:

Strength (mcg)	Color	NDC # for bottles of 100	NDC # for bottles of 1000
25	Orange	NDC 0456-1320-01	NDC 0456-1320-00
50	White	NDC 0456-1321-01	NDC 0456-1321-00
75	Violet	NDC 0456-1322-01	NDC 0456-1322-00
88	Mint Green	NDC 0456-1329-01	NDC 0456-1329-00
100	Yellow	NDC 0456-1323-01	NDC 0456-1323-00
112	Rose	NDC 0456-1330-01	NDC 0456-1330-00
125	Brown	NDC 0456-1324-01	NDC 0456-1324-00
150	Blue	NDC 0456-1325-01	NDC 0456-1325-00
175	Lilac	NDC 0456-1326-01	NDC 0456-1326-00
200	Pink	NDC 0456-1327-01	NDC 0456-1327-00
300	Green	NDC 0456-1328-01	NDC 0456-1328-00

STORAGE CONDITIONS
Store at 25°C (77°F) with excursions permitted to 15-30°C (59°-86°F).
Protect from moisture and light.
Manufactured for:
Forest Pharmaceuticals, Inc.
Subsidiary of Forest Laboratories, Inc.
St. Louis, Missouri, 63045
by:
Lloyd Pharmaceutical
Division of Lloyd, Inc.
Shenandoah, IA 51601

9/03 MG #19006

LEXAPRO® ℞

[*lěks'ă-prō*]
(escitalopram oxalate)
TABLETS/ORAL SOLUTION
Rx Only

DESCRIPTION

LEXAPRO® (escitalopram oxalate) is an orally administered selective serotonin reuptake inhibitor (SSRI). Escitalopram is the pure S-enantiomer (single isomer) of the racemic bicyclic phthalane derivative citalopram. Escitalopram oxalate is designated S-(+)-1-[3-(dimethyl-amino)propyl]-1-(*p*-fluorophenyl)-5-phthalancarbonitrile oxalate with the following structural formula:
[See chemical structure at top of next column]
The molecular formula is $C_{20}H_{21}FN_2O \bullet C_2H_2O_4$ and the molecular weight is 414.40.

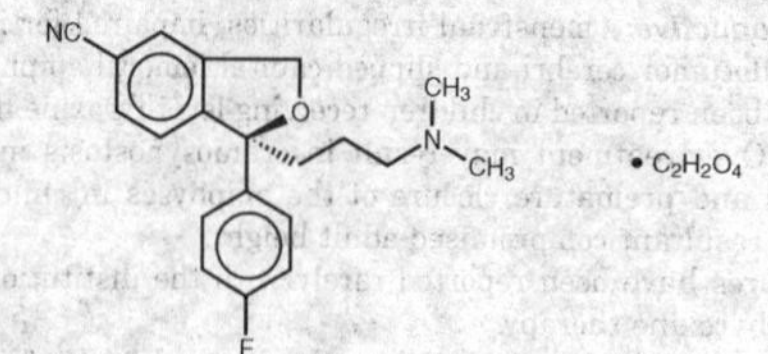

Escitalopram oxalate occurs as a fine, white to slightly-yellow powder and is freely soluble in methanol and dimethyl sulfoxide (DMSO), soluble in isotonic saline solution, sparingly soluble in water and ethanol, slightly soluble in ethyl acetate, and insoluble in heptane.
LEXAPRO (escitalopram oxalate) is available as tablets or as an oral solution. LEXAPRO tablets are film-coated, round tablets containing escitalopram oxalate in strengths equivalent to 5 mg, 10 mg, and 20 mg escitalopram base. The 10 and 20 mg tablets are scored. The tablets also contain the following inactive ingredients: talc, croscarmellose sodium, microcrystalline cellulose/colloidal silicon dioxide, and magnesium stearate. The film coating contains hypromellose, titanium dioxide, and polyethylene glycol.
LEXAPRO oral solution contains escitalopram oxalate equivalent to 1 mg/mL escitalopram base. It also contains the following inactive ingredients: sorbitol, purified water, citric acid, sodium citrate, malic acid, glycerin, propylene glycol, methylparaben, propylparaben, and natural peppermint flavor.

CLINICAL PHARMACOLOGY

Pharmacodynamics
The mechanism of antidepressant action of escitalopram, the S-enantiomer of racemic citalopram, is presumed to be linked to potentiation of serotonergic activity in the central nervous system (CNS) resulting from its inhibition of CNS neuronal reuptake of serotonin (5-HT). *In vitro* and *in vivo* studies in animals suggest that escitalopram is a highly selective serotonin reuptake inhibitor (SSRI) with minimal effects on norepinephrine and dopamine neuronal reuptake. Escitalopram is at least 100-fold more potent than the R-enantiomer with respect to inhibition of 5-HT reuptake and inhibition of 5-HT neuronal firing rate. Tolerance to a model of antidepressant effect in rats was not induced by long-term (up to 5 weeks) treatment with escitalopram. Escitalopram has no or very low affinity for serotonergic ($5\text{-}HT_{1-7}$) or other receptors including alpha- and beta-adrenergic, dopamine (D_{1-5}), histamine (H_{1-3}), muscarinic (M_{1-5}), and benzodiazepine receptors. Escitalopram also does not bind to, or has low affinity for, various ion channels including Na^+, K^+, Cl^-, and Ca^{++} channels. Antagonism of muscarinic, histaminergic, and adrenergic receptors has been hypothesized to be associated with various anticholinergic, sedative, and cardiovascular side effects of other psychotropic drugs.
Pharmacokinetics
The single- and multiple-dose pharmacokinetics of escitalopram are linear and dose-proportional in a dose range of 10 to 30 mg/day. Biotransformation of escitalopram is mainly hepatic, with a mean terminal half-life of about 27-32 hours. With once-daily dosing, steady state plasma concentrations are achieved within approximately one week. At steady state, the extent of accumulation of escitalopram in plasma in young healthy subjects was 2.2-2.5 times the plasma concentrations observed after a single dose. The tablet and the oral solution dosage forms of escitalopram oxalate are bioequivalent.
Absorption and Distribution
Following a single oral dose (20 mg tablet or solution) of escitalopram, peak blood levels occur at about 5 hours. Absorption of escitalopram is not affected by food.
The absolute bioavailability of citalopram is about 80% relative to an intravenous dose, and the volume of distribution of citalopram is about 12 L/kg. Data specific on escitalopram are unavailable.
The binding of escitalopram to human plasma proteins is approximately 56%.
Metabolism and Elimination
Following oral administrations of escitalopram, the fraction of drug recovered in the urine as escitalopram and S-demethylcitalopram (S-DCT) is about 8% and 10%, respectively. The oral clearance of escitalopram is 600 mL/min, with approximately 7% of that due to renal clearance.
Escitalopram is metabolized to S-DCT and S-didemethylcitalopram (S-DDCT). In humans, unchanged escitalopram is the predominant compound in plasma. At steady state, the concentration of the escitalopram metabolite S-DCT in plasma is approximately one-third that of escitalopram. The level of S-DDCT was not detectable in most subjects. *In vitro* studies show that escitalopram is at least 7 and 27 times more potent than S-DCT and S-DDCT, respectively, in the inhibition of serotonin reuptake, suggesting that the metabolites of escitalopram do not contribute significantly to the antidepressant actions of escitalopram. S-DCT and S-DDCT also have no or very low affinity for serotonergic ($5\text{-}HT_{1-7}$) or other receptors including alpha- and beta-adrenergic, dopamine (D_{1-5}), histamine (H_{1-3}), muscarinic (M_{1-5}), and benzodiazepine receptors. S-DCT and S-DDCT also do not bind to various ion channels including Na^+, K^+, Cl^-, and Ca^{++} channels.
In vitro studies using human liver microsomes indicated that CYP3A4 and CYP2C19 are the primary isozymes involved in the N-demethylation of escitalopram.
Population Subgroups
Age—Escitalopram pharmacokinetics in subjects ≥ 65 years of age were compared to younger subjects in a single-dose and a multiple-dose study. Escitalopram AUC and half-life were increased by approximately 50% in elderly subjects, and C_{max} was unchanged. 10 mg is the recommended dose for elderly patients (see **DOSAGE AND ADMINISTRATION**).
Gender—In a multiple-dose study of escitalopram (10 mg/day for 3 weeks) in 18 male (9 elderly and 9 young) and 18 female (9 elderly and 9 young) subjects, there were no differences in AUC, C_{max}, and half-life between the male and female subjects. No adjustment of dosage on the basis of gender is needed.
Reduced hepatic function—Citalopram oral clearance was reduced by 37% and half-life was doubled in patients with reduced hepatic function compared to normal subjects. 10 mg is the recommended dose of escitalopram for most hepatically impaired patients (see **DOSAGE AND ADMINISTRATION**).
Reduced renal function—In patients with mild to moderate renal function impairment, oral clearance of citalopram was reduced by 17% compared to normal subjects. No adjustment of dosage for such patients is recommended. No information is available about the pharmacokinetics of escitalopram in patients with severely reduced renal function (creatinine clearance < 20 mL/min).
Drug-Drug Interactions
In vitro enzyme inhibition data did not reveal an inhibitory effect of escitalopram on CYP3A4, -1A2, -2C9, -2C19, and -2E1. Based on *in vitro* data, escitalopram would be expected to have little inhibitory effect on *in vivo* metabolism mediated by these cytochromes. While *in vivo* data to address this question are limited, results from drug interaction studies suggest that escitalopram, at a dose of 20 mg, has no 3A4 inhibitory effect and a modest 2D6 inhibitory effect. See **Drug Interactions** under **PRECAUTIONS** for more detailed information on available drug interaction data.
Clinical Efficacy Trials
Major Depressive Disorder
The efficacy of LEXAPRO as a treatment for major depressive disorder was established in three, 8-week, placebo-controlled studies conducted in outpatients between 18 and 65 years of age who met DSM-IV criteria for major depressive disorder. The primary outcome in all three studies was change from baseline to endpoint in the Montgomery Asberg Depression Rating Scale (MADRS).
A fixed-dose study compared 10 mg/day LEXAPRO and 20 mg/day LEXAPRO to placebo and 40 mg/day citalopram. The 10 mg/day and 20 mg/day LEXAPRO treatment groups showed significantly greater mean improvement compared to placebo on the MADRS. The 10 mg and 20 mg LEXAPRO groups were similar on this outcome measure.
In a second fixed-dose study of 10 mg/day LEXAPRO and placebo, the 10 mg/day LEXAPRO treatment group showed significantly greater mean improvement compared to placebo on the MADRS.
In a flexible-dose study, comparing LEXAPRO, titrated between 10 and 20 mg/day, to placebo and citalopram, titrated between 20 and 40 mg/day, the LEXAPRO treatment group showed significantly greater mean improvement compared to placebo on the MADRS.
Analyses of the relationship between treatment outcome and age, gender, and race did not suggest any differential responsiveness on the basis of these patient characteristics.
In a longer-term trial, 274 patients meeting (DSM-IV) criteria for major depressive disorder, who had responded during an initial 8-week, open-label treatment phase with LEXAPRO 10 or 20 mg/day, were randomized to continuation of LEXAPRO at their same dose, or to placebo, for up to 36 weeks of observation for relapse. Response during the open-label phase was defined by having a decrease of the MADRS total score to ≤ 12. Relapse during the double-blind phase was defined as an increase of the MADRS total score to ≥ 22, or discontinuation due to insufficient clinical response. Patients receiving continued LEXAPRO experienced a significantly longer time to relapse over the subsequent 36 weeks compared to those receiving placebo.
Generalized Anxiety Disorder
The efficacy of LEXAPRO in the treatment of Generalized Anxiety Disorder (GAD) was demonstrated in three, 8-week, multicenter, flexible-dose, placebo-controlled studies that compared LEXAPRO 10-20 mg/day to placebo in outpatients between 18 and 80 years of age who met DSM-IV criteria for GAD. In all three studies, LEXAPRO showed significantly greater mean improvement compared to placebo on the Hamilton Anxiety Scale (HAM-A).
There were too few patients in differing ethnic and age groups to adequately assess whether or not LEXAPRO has differential effects in these groups. There was no difference in response to LEXAPRO between men and women.

INDICATIONS AND USAGE

Major Depressive Disorder
LEXAPRO (escitalopram) is indicated for the treatment of major depressive disorder.
The efficacy of LEXAPRO in the treatment of major depressive disorder was established in three, 8-week, placebo-controlled trials of outpatients whose diagnoses corresponded most closely to the DSM-IV category of major depressive disorder (see **CLINICAL PHARMACOLOGY**).
A major depressive episode (DSM-IV) implies a prominent and relatively persistent (nearly every day for at least 2

weeks) depressed or dysphoric mood that usually interferes with daily functioning, and includes at least five of the following nine symptoms: depressed mood, loss of interest in usual activities, significant change in weight and/or appetite, insomnia or hypersomnia, psychomotor agitation or retardation, increased fatigue, feelings of guilt or worthlessness, slowed thinking or impaired concentration, a suicide attempt or suicidal ideation.

The efficacy of LEXAPRO in hospitalized patients with major depressive disorders has not been adequately studied.

The efficacy of LEXAPRO in maintaining a response, in patients with major depressive disorder who responded during an 8-week, acute-treatment phase while taking LEXAPRO and were then observed for relapse during a period of up to 36 weeks, was demonstrated in a placebo-controlled trial (see **Clinical Efficacy Trials** under **CLINICAL PHARMACOLOGY**). Nevertheless, the physician who elects to use LEXAPRO for extended periods should periodically re-evaluate the long-term usefulness of the drug for the individual patient (see **DOSAGE AND ADMINISTRATION**).

Generalized Anxiety Disorder

LEXAPRO is indicated for the treatment of Generalized Anxiety Disorder (GAD). The efficacy of LEXAPRO was established in three, 8-week, placebo-controlled trials in patients with GAD (see **CLINICAL PHARMACOLOGY**).

Generalized Anxiety Disorder (DSM-IV) is characterized by excessive anxiety and worry (apprehensive expectation) that is persistent for at least 6 months and which the person finds difficult to control. It must be associated with at least 3 of the following symptoms: restlessness or feeling keyed up or on edge, being easily fatigued, difficulty concentrating or mind going blank, irritability, muscle tension, and sleep disturbance.

The efficacy of LEXAPRO in the long-term treatment of GAD, that is, for more than 8 weeks, has not been systematically evaluated in controlled trials. The physician who elects to use LEXAPRO for extended periods should periodically re-evaluate the long-term usefulness of the drug for the individual patient.

CONTRAINDICATIONS

Concomitant use in patients taking monoamine oxidase inhibitors (MAOIs) is contraindicated (see **WARNINGS**).

LEXAPRO is contraindicated in patients with a hypersensitivity to escitalopram or citalopram or any of the inactive ingredients in LEXAPRO.

WARNINGS

Potential for Interaction with Monoamine Oxidase Inhibitors

In patients receiving serotonin reuptake inhibitor drugs in combination with a monoamine oxidase inhibitor (MAOI), there have been reports of serious, sometimes fatal, reactions including hyperthermia, rigidity, myoclonus, autonomic instability with possible rapid fluctuations of vital signs, and mental status changes that include extreme agitation progressing to delirium and coma. These reactions have also been reported in patients who have recently discontinued SSRI treatment and have been started on an MAOI. Some cases presented with features resembling neuroleptic malignant syndrome. Furthermore, limited animal data on the effects of combined use of SSRIs and MAOIs suggest that these drugs may act synergistically to elevate blood pressure and evoke behavioral excitation. Therefore, it is recommended that LEXAPRO should not be used in combination with an MAOI, or within 14 days of discontinuing treatment with an MAOI. Similarly, at least 14 days should be allowed after stopping LEXAPRO before starting an MAOI.

Serotonin syndrome has been reported in two patients who were concomitantly receiving linezolid, an antibiotic which is a reversible non-selective MAOI.

Clinical Worsening and Suicide Risk

Patients with major depressive disorder, both adult and pediatric, may experience worsening of their depression and/or the emergence of suicidal ideation and behavior (suicidality), whether or not they are taking antidepressant medications, and this risk may persist until significant remission occurs.

Although there has been a long-standing concern that antidepressants may have a role in inducing worsening of depression and the emergence of suicidality in certain patients, a causal role for antidepressants in inducing such behaviors has not been established. **Nevertheless, patients being treated with antidepressants should be observed closely for clinical worsening and suicidality, especially at the beginning of a course of drug therapy, or at the time of dose changes, either increases or decreases.** Consideration should be given to changing the therapeutic regimen, including possibly discontinuing the medication, in patients whose depression is persistently worse or whose emergent suicidality is severe, abrupt in onset, or was not part of the patient's presenting symptoms.

Because of the possibility of co-morbidity between major depressive disorder and other psychiatric and nonpsychiatric disorders, the same precautions observed when treating patients with major depressive disorder should be observed when treating patients with other psychiatric and nonpsychiatric disorders.

The following symptoms, anxiety, agitation, panic attacks, insomnia, irritability, hostility (aggressiveness), impulsivity, akathisia (psychomotor restlessness), hypomania, and mania, have been reported in adult and pediatric patients being treated with antidepressants for major depressive disorder as well as for other indications, both psychiatric and nonpsychiatric. Although a causal link between the emergence of such symptoms and either the worsening of depression and/or the emergence of suicidal impulses has not been established, consideration should be given to changing the therapeutic regimen, including possibly discontinuing the medication, in patients for whom such symptoms are severe, abrupt in onset, or were not part of the patient's presenting symptoms.

Families and caregivers of patients being treated with antidepressants for major depressive disorder or other indications, both psychiatric and nonpsychiatric, should be alerted about the need to monitor patients for the emergence of agitation, irritability, and the other symptoms described above, as well as the emergence of suicidality, and to report such symptoms immediately to healthcare providers. Prescriptions for LEXAPRO should be written for the smallest quantity of tablets consistent with good patient management, in order to reduce the risk of overdose.

If the decision has been made to discontinue treatment, medication should be tapered, as rapidly as is feasible, but with recognition that abrupt discontinuation can be associated with certain symptoms (see **PRECAUTIONS** and **DOSAGE AND ADMINISTRATION, Discontinuation of Treatment with LEXAPRO**, for a description of the risks of discontinuation of LEXAPRO).

It should be noted that LEXAPRO is not approved for use in treating any indications in the pediatric population.

A major depressive episode may be the initial presentation of bipolar disorder. It is generally believed (though not established in controlled trials) that treating such an episode with an antidepressant alone may increase the likelihood of precipitation of a mixed/manic episode in patients at risk for bipolar disorder. Whether any of the symptoms described above represent such a conversion is unknown. However, prior to initiating treatment with an antidepressant, patients should be adequately screened to determine if they are at risk for bipolar disorder; such screening should include a detailed psychiatric history, including a family history of suicide, bipolar disorder, and depression. It should be noted that LEXAPRO is not approved for use in treating bipolar depression.

PRECAUTIONS

General

Discontinuation of Treatment with LEXAPRO

During marketing of Lexapro and other SSRIs and SNRIs (serotonin and norepinephrine reuptake inhibitors), there have been spontaneous reports of adverse events occurring upon discontinuation of these drugs, particularly when abrupt, including the following: dysphoric mood, irritability, agitation, dizziness, sensory disturbances (e.g., paresthesias such as electric shock sensations), anxiety, confusion, headache, lethargy, emotional lability, insomnia, and hypomania. While these events are generally self-limiting, there have been reports of serious discontinuation symptoms.

Patients should be monitored for these symptoms when discontinuing treatment with LEXAPRO. A gradual reduction in the dose rather than abrupt cessation is recommended whenever possible. If intolerable symptoms occur following a decrease in the dose or upon discontinuation of treatment, then resuming the previously prescribed dose may be considered. Subsequently, the physician may continue decreasing the dose but at a more gradual rate (see **DOSAGE AND ADMINISTRATION**).

Abnormal Bleeding

Published case reports have documented the occurrence of bleeding episodes in patients treated with psychotropic drugs that interfere with serotonin reuptake. Subsequent epidemiological studies, both of the case-control and cohort design, have demonstrated an association between use of psychotropic drugs that interfere with serotonin reuptake and the occurrence of upper gastrointestinal bleeding. In two studies, concurrent use of a nonsteroidal anti-inflammatory drug (NSAID) or aspirin potentiated the risk of bleeding (see **Drug Interactions**). Although these studies focused on upper gastrointestinal bleeding, there is reason to believe that bleeding at other sites may be similarly potentiated. Patients should be cautioned regarding the risk of bleeding associated with the concomitant use of LEXAPRO with NSAIDs, aspirin, or other drugs that affect coagulation.

Hyponatremia

One case of hyponatremia has been reported in association with LEXAPRO treatment. Several cases of hyponatremia or SIADH (syndrome of inappropriate antidiuretic hormone secretion) have been reported in association with racemic citalopram. All patients with these events have recovered with discontinuation of escitalopram or citalopram and/or medical intervention. Hyponatremia and SIADH have also been reported in association with other marketed drugs effective in the treatment of major depressive disorder.

Activation of Mania/Hypomania

In placebo-controlled trials of LEXAPRO in major depressive disorder, activation of mania/hypomania was reported in one (0.1%) of 715 patients treated with LEXAPRO and in none of the 592 patients treated with placebo. One additional case of hypomania has been reported in association with LEXAPRO treatment. Activation of mania/hypomania has also been reported in a small proportion of patients with major affective disorders treated with racemic citalopram and other marketed drugs effective in the treatment of major depressive disorder. As with all drugs effective in the treatment of major depressive disorder, LEXAPRO should be used cautiously in patients with a history of mania.

Seizures

Although anticonvulsant effects of racemic citalopram have been observed in animal studies, LEXAPRO has not been systematically evaluated in patients with a seizure disorder. These patients were excluded from clinical studies during the product's premarketing testing. In clinical trials of LEXAPRO, cases of convulsion have been reported in association with LEXAPRO treatment. Like other drugs effective in the treatment of major depressive disorder, LEXAPRO should be introduced with care in patients with a history of seizure disorder.

Interference with Cognitive and Motor Performance

In a study in normal volunteers, LEXAPRO 10 mg/day did not produce impairment of intellectual function or psychomotor performance. Because any psychoactive drug may impair judgment, thinking, or motor skills, however, patients should be cautioned about operating hazardous machinery, including automobiles, until they are reasonably certain that LEXAPRO therapy does not affect their ability to engage in such activities.

Use in Patients with Concomitant Illness

Clinical experience with LEXAPRO in patients with certain concomitant systemic illnesses is limited. Caution is advisable in using LEXAPRO in patients with diseases or conditions that produce altered metabolism or hemodynamic responses.

LEXAPRO has not been systematically evaluated in patients with a recent history of myocardial infarction or unstable heart disease. Patients with these diagnoses were generally excluded from clinical studies during the product's premarketing testing.

In subjects with hepatic impairment, clearance of racemic citalopram was decreased and plasma concentrations were increased. The recommended dose of LEXAPRO in hepatically impaired patients is 10 mg/day (see **DOSAGE AND ADMINISTRATION**).

Because escitalopram is extensively metabolized, excretion of unchanged drug in urine is a minor route of elimination. Until adequate numbers of patients with severe renal impairment have been evaluated during chronic treatment with LEXAPRO, however, it should be used with caution in such patients (see **DOSAGE AND ADMINISTRATION**).

Information for Patients

Physicians are advised to discuss the following issues with patients for whom they prescribe LEXAPRO.

In a study in normal volunteers, LEXAPRO 10 mg/day did not impair psychomotor performance. The effect of LEXAPRO on psychomotor coordination, judgment, or thinking has not been systematically examined in controlled studies. Because psychoactive drugs may impair judgment, thinking, or motor skills, patients should be cautioned about operating hazardous machinery, including automobiles, until they are reasonably certain that LEXAPRO therapy does not affect their ability to engage in such activities.

Patients should be told that, although LEXAPRO has not been shown in experiments with normal subjects to increase the mental and motor skill impairments caused by alcohol, the concomitant use of LEXAPRO and alcohol in depressed patients is not advised.

Patients should be made aware that escitalopram is the active isomer of Celexa (citalopram hydrobromide) and that the two medications should not be taken concomitantly.

Patients should be advised to inform their physician if they are taking, or plan to take, any prescription or over-the-counter drugs, as there is a potential for interactions.

Patients should be cautioned about the concomitant use of LEXAPRO and NSAIDs, aspirin, or other drugs that affect coagulation since the combined use of psychotropic drugs that interfere with serotonin reuptake and these agents has been associated with an increased risk of bleeding.

Patients should be advised to notify their physician if they become pregnant or intend to become pregnant during therapy.

Patients should be advised to notify their physician if they are breastfeeding an infant.

While patients may notice improvement with LEXAPRO therapy in 1 to 4 weeks, they should be advised to continue therapy as directed.

Patients and their families should be encouraged to be alert to the emergence of anxiety, agitation, panic attacks, insomnia, irritability, hostility, impulsivity, akathisia, hypomania, mania, worsening of depression, and suicidal ideation, especially early during antidepressant treatment. Such symptoms should be reported to the patient's physician, especially if they are severe, abrupt in onset, or were not part of the patient's presenting symptoms.

Laboratory Tests

There are no specific laboratory tests recommended.

Concomitant Administration with Racemic Citalopram

Citalopram—Since escitalopram is the active isomer of racemic citalopram (Celexa), the two agents should not be coadministered.

Drug Interactions

CNS Drugs—Given the primary CNS effects of escitalopram, caution should be used when it is taken in combination with other centrally acting drugs.

Alcohol—Although LEXAPRO did not potentiate the cognitive and motor effects of alcohol in a clinical trial, as with other psychotropic medications, the use of alcohol by patients taking LEXAPRO is not recommended.

Continued on next page

Lexapro—Cont.

Monoamine Oxidase Inhibitors (MAOIs)—See **CONTRAINDICATIONS** and **WARNINGS**.

Drugs That Interfere With Hemostasis (NSAIDs, Aspirin, Warfarin, etc.)

Serotonin release by platelets plays an important role in hemostasis. Epidemiological studies of the case-control and cohort design that have demonstrated an association between use of psychotropic drugs that interfere with serotonin reuptake and the occurrence of upper gastrointestinal bleeding have also shown that concurrent use of an NSAID or aspirin potentiated the risk of bleeding. Thus, patients should be cautioned about the use of such drugs concurrently with LEXAPRO.

Cimetidine—In subjects who had received 21 days of 40 mg/day racemic citalopram, combined administration of 400 mg/day cimetidine for 8 days resulted in an increase in citalopram AUC and C_{max} of 43% and 39%, respectively. The clinical significance of these findings is unknown.

Digoxin—In subjects who had received 21 days of 40 mg/day racemic citalopram, combined administration of citalopram and digoxin (single dose of 1 mg) did not significantly affect the pharmacokinetics of either citalopram or digoxin.

Lithium—Coadministration of racemic citalopram (40 mg/day for 10 days) and lithium (30 mmol/day for 5 days) had no significant effect on the pharmacokinetics of citalopram or lithium. Nevertheless, plasma lithium levels should be monitored with appropriate adjustment to the lithium dose in accordance with standard clinical practice. Because lithium may enhance the serotonergic effects of escitalopram, caution should be exercised when LEXAPRO and lithium are coadministered.

Sumatriptan—There have been rare postmarketing reports describing patients with weakness, hyperreflexia, and incoordination following the use of an SSRI and sumatriptan. If concomitant treatment with sumatriptan and an SSRI (e.g., fluoxetine, fluvoxamine, paroxetine, sertraline, citalopram, escitalopram) is clinically warranted, appropriate observation of the patient is advised.

Theophylline—Combined administration of racemic citalopram (40 mg/day for 21 days) and the CYP1A2 substrate theophylline (single dose of 300 mg) did not affect the pharmacokinetics of theophylline. The effect of theophylline on the pharmacokinetics of citalopram was not evaluated.

Warfarin—Administration of 40 mg/day racemic citalopram for 21 days did not affect the pharmacokinetics of warfarin, a CYP3A4 substrate. Prothrombin time was increased by 5%, the clinical significance of which is unknown.

Carbamazepine—Combined administration of racemic citalopram (40 mg/day for 14 days) and carbamazepine (titrated to 400 mg/day for 35 days) did not significantly affect the pharmacokinetics of carbamazepine, a CYP3A4 substrate. Although trough citalopram plasma levels were unaffected, given the enzyme-inducing properties of carbamazepine, the possibility that carbamazepine might increase the clearance of escitalopram should be considered if the two drugs are coadministered.

Triazolam—Combined administration of racemic citalopram (titrated to 40 mg/day for 28 days) and the CYP3A4 substrate triazolam (single dose of 0.25 mg) did not significantly affect the pharmacokinetics of either citalopram or triazolam.

Ketoconazole—Combined administration of racemic citalopram (40 mg) and ketoconazole (200 mg), a potent CYP3A4 inhibitor, decreased the C_{max} and AUC of ketoconazole by 21% and 10%, respectively, and did not significantly affect the pharmacokinetics of citalopram.

Ritonavir—Combined administration of a single dose of ritonavir (600 mg), both a CYP3A4 substrate and a potent inhibitor of CYP3A4, and escitalopram (20 mg) did not affect the pharmacokinetics of either ritonavir or escitalopram.

CYP3A4 and -2C19 Inhibitors—*In vitro* studies indicated that CYP3A4 and -2C19 are the primary enzymes involved in the metabolism of escitalopram. However, coadministration of escitalopram (20 mg) and ritonavir (600 mg), a potent inhibitor of CYP3A4, did not significantly affect the pharmacokinetics of escitalopram. Because escitalopram is metabolized by multiple enzyme systems, inhibition of a single enzyme may not appreciably decrease escitalopram clearance.

Drugs Metabolized by Cytochrome P4502D6—*In vitro* studies did not reveal an inhibitory effect of escitalopram on CYP2D6. In addition, steady state levels of racemic citalopram were not significantly different in poor metabolizers and extensive CYP2D6 metabolizers after multiple-dose administration of citalopram, suggesting that coadministration, with escitalopram, of a drug that inhibits CYP2D6, is unlikely to have clinically significant effects on escitalopram metabolism. However, there are limited *in vivo* data suggesting a modest CYP2D6 inhibitory effect for escitalopram, i.e., coadministration of escitalopram (20 mg/day for 21 days) with the tricyclic antidepressant desipramine (single dose of 50 mg), a substrate for CYP2D6, resulted in a 40% increase in C_{max} and a 100% increase in AUC of desipramine. The clinical significance of this finding is unknown. Nevertheless, caution is indicated in the coadministration of escitalopram and drugs metabolized by CYP2D6.

Metoprolol—Administration of 20 mg/day LEXAPRO for 21 days in healthy volunteers resulted in a 50% increase in C_{max} and 82% increase in AUC of the beta-adrenergic blocker metoprolol (given in a single dose of 100 mg). Increased metoprolol plasma levels have been associated with decreased cardioselectivity. Coadministration of LEXAPRO and metoprolol had no clinically significant effects on blood pressure or heart rate.

Electroconvulsive Therapy (ECT)—There are no clinical studies of the combined use of ECT and escitalopram.

Carcinogenesis, Mutagenesis, Impairment of Fertility

Carcinogenesis

Racemic citalopram was administered in the diet to NMRI/BOM strain mice and COBS WI strain rats for 18 and 24 months, respectively. There was no evidence for carcinogenicity of racemic citalopram in mice receiving up to 240 mg/kg/day. There was an increased incidence of small intestine carcinoma in rats receiving 8 or 24 mg/kg/day racemic citalopram. A no-effect dose for this finding was not established. The relevance of these findings to humans is unknown.

Mutagenesis

Racemic citalopram was mutagenic in the *in vitro* bacterial reverse mutation assay (Ames test) in 2 of 5 bacterial strains (Salmonella TA98 and TA1537) in the absence of metabolic activation. It was clastogenic in the *in vitro* Chinese hamster lung cell assay for chromosomal aberrations in the presence and absence of metabolic activation. Racemic citalopram was not mutagenic in the *in vitro* mammalian forward gene mutation assay (HPRT) in mouse lymphoma cells or in a coupled *in vitro/in vivo* unscheduled DNA synthesis (UDS) assay in rat liver. It was not clastogenic in the *in vitro* chromosomal aberration assay in human lymphocytes or in two *in vivo* mouse micronucleus assays.

Impairment of Fertility

When racemic citalopram was administered orally to 16 male and 24 female rats prior to and throughout mating and gestation at doses of 32, 48, and 72 mg/kg/day, mating was decreased at all doses, and fertility was decreased at doses ≥ 32 mg/kg/day. Gestation duration was increased at 48 mg/kg/day.

Pregnancy

Pregnancy Category C

In a rat embryo/fetal development study, oral administration of escitalopram (56, 112, or 150 mg/kg/day) to pregnant animals during the period of organogenesis resulted in decreased fetal body weight and associated delays in ossification at the two higher doses (approximately ≥ 56 times the maximum recommended human dose [MRHD] of 20 mg/day on a body surface area [mg/m^2] basis). Maternal toxicity (clinical signs and decreased body weight gain and food consumption), mild at 56 mg/kg/day, was present at all dose levels. The developmental no-effect dose of 56 mg/kg/day is approximately 28 times the MRHD on a mg/m^2 basis. No teratogenicity was observed at any of the doses tested (as high as 75 times the MRHD on a mg/m^2 basis).

When female rats were treated with escitalopram (6, 12, 24, or 48 mg/kg/day) during pregnancy and through weaning, slightly increased offspring mortality and growth retardation were noted at 48 mg/kg/day which is approximately 24 times the MRHD on a mg/m^2 basis. Slight maternal toxicity (clinical signs and decreased body weight gain and food consumption) was seen at this dose. Slightly increased offspring mortality was seen at 24 mg/kg/day. The no-effect dose was 12 mg/kg/day which is approximately 6 times the MRHD on a mg/m^2 basis.

In animal reproduction studies, racemic citalopram has been shown to have adverse effects on embryo/fetal and postnatal development, including teratogenic effects, when administered at doses greater than human therapeutic doses.

In two rat embryo/fetal development studies, oral administration of racemic citalopram (32, 56, or 112 mg/kg/day) to pregnant animals during the period of organogenesis resulted in decreased embryo/fetal growth and survival and an increased incidence of fetal abnormalities (including cardiovascular and skeletal defects) at the high dose. This dose was also associated with maternal toxicity (clinical signs, decreased body weight gain). The developmental no-effect dose was 56 mg/kg/day. In a rabbit study, no adverse effects on embryo/fetal development were observed at doses of racemic citalopram of up to 16 mg/kg/day. Thus, teratogenic effects of racemic citalopram were observed at a maternally toxic dose in the rat and were not observed in the rabbit.

When female rats were treated with racemic citalopram (4.8, 12.8, or 32 mg/kg/day) from late gestation through weaning, increased offspring mortality during the first 4 days after birth and persistent offspring growth retardation were observed at the highest dose. The no-effect dose was 12.8 mg/kg/day. Similar effects on offspring mortality and growth were seen when dams were treated throughout gestation and early lactation at doses ≥ 24 mg/kg/day. A no-effect dose was not determined in that study.

There are no adequate and well-controlled studies in pregnant women; therefore, escitalopram should be used during pregnancy only if the potential benefit justifies the potential risk to the fetus.

Pregnancy-Nonteratogenic Effects

Neonates exposed to LEXAPRO and other SSRIs or SNRIs, late in the third trimester, have developed complications requiring prolonged hospitalization, respiratory support, and tube feeding. Such complications can arise immediately upon delivery. Reported clinical findings have included respiratory distress, cyanosis, apnea, seizures, temperature instability, feeding difficulty, vomiting, hypoglycemia, hypotonia, hypertonia, hyperreflexia, tremor, jitteriness, irritability, and constant crying. These features are consistent with either a direct toxic effect of SSRIs and SNRIs or, possibly, a drug discontinuation syndrome. It should be noted that, in some cases, the clinical picture is consistent with serotonin syndrome (see **WARNINGS**).

When treating a pregnant woman with LEXAPRO during the third trimester, the physician should carefully consider the potential risks and benefits of treatment (see **DOSAGE AND ADMINISTRATION**).

Labor and Delivery

The effect of LEXAPRO on labor and delivery in humans is unknown.

Nursing Mothers

Racemic citalopram, like many other drugs, is excreted in human breast milk. There have been two reports of infants experiencing excessive somnolence, decreased feeding, and weight loss in association with breastfeeding from a citalopram-treated mother; in one case, the infant was reported to recover completely upon discontinuation of citalopram by its mother and, in the second case, no follow-up information was available. The decision whether to continue or discontinue either nursing or LEXAPRO therapy should take into account the risks of citalopram exposure for the infant and the benefits of LEXAPRO treatment for the mother.

Pediatric Use

Safety and effectiveness in pediatric patients have not been established (see **WARNINGS—Clinical Worsening and Suicide Risk**).

Geriatric Use

Approximately 6% of the 1144 patients receiving escitalopram in controlled trials of LEXAPRO in major depressive disorder and GAD were 60 years of age or older; elderly patients in these trials received daily doses of LEXAPRO between 10 and 20 mg. The number of elderly patients in these trials was insufficient to adequately assess for possible differential efficacy and safety measures on the basis of age. Nevertheless, greater sensitivity of some elderly individuals to effects of LEXAPRO cannot be ruled out.

In two pharmacokinetic studies, escitalopram half-life was increased by approximately 50% in elderly subjects as compared to young subjects and C_{max} was unchanged (see **CLINICAL PHARMACOLOGY**). 10 mg/day is the recommended dose for elderly patients (see **DOSAGE AND ADMINISTRATION**). Of 4422 patients in clinical studies of racemic citalopram, 1357 were 60 and over, 1034 were 65 and over, and 457 were 75 and over. No overall differences in safety or effectiveness were observed between these subjects and younger subjects, and other reported clinical experience has not identified differences in responses between the elderly and younger patients, but again, greater sensitivity of some elderly individuals cannot be ruled out.

ADVERSE REACTIONS

Adverse event information for LEXAPRO was collected from 715 patients with major depressive disorder who were exposed to escitalopram and from 592 patients who were exposed to placebo in double-blind, placebo-controlled trials. An additional 284 patients with major depressive disorder were newly exposed to escitalopram in open-label trials. The adverse event information for LEXAPRO in patients with GAD was collected from 429 patients exposed to escitalopram and from 427 patients exposed to placebo in double-blind, placebo-controlled trials.

Adverse events during exposure were obtained primarily by general inquiry and recorded by clinical investigators using terminology of their own choosing. Consequently, it is not possible to provide a meaningful estimate of the proportion of individuals experiencing adverse events without first grouping similar types of events into a smaller number of standardized event categories. In the tables and tabulations that follow, standard World Health Organization (WHO) terminology has been used to classify reported adverse events.

The stated frequencies of adverse events represent the proportion of individuals who experienced, at least once, a treatment-emergent adverse event of the type listed. An event was considered treatment-emergent if it occurred for the first time or worsened while receiving therapy following baseline evaluation.

Adverse Events Associated with Discontinuation of Treatment

Major Depressive Disorder

Among the 715 depressed patients who received LEXAPRO in placebo-controlled trials, 6% discontinued treatment due to an adverse event, as compared to 2% of 592 patients receiving placebo. In two fixed-dose studies, the rate of discontinuation for adverse events in patients receiving 10 mg/day LEXAPRO was not significantly different from the rate of discontinuation for adverse events in patients receiving placebo. The rate of discontinuation for adverse events in patients assigned to a fixed dose of 20 mg/day LEXAPRO was 10%, which was significantly different from the rate of discontinuation for adverse events in patients receiving 10 mg/day LEXAPRO (4%) and placebo (3%). Adverse events that were associated with the discontinuation of at least 1% of patients treated with LEXAPRO, and for which the rate was at least twice that of placebo, were nausea (2%) and ejaculation disorder (2% of male patients).

Generalized Anxiety Disorder

Among the 429 GAD patients who received LEXAPRO 10–20 mg/day in placebo-controlled trials, 8% discontinued treatment due to an adverse event, as compared to 4% of 427 patients receiving placebo. Adverse events that were associated with the discontinuation of at least 1% of patients treated with LEXAPRO, and for which the rate was at least twice the placebo rate, were nausea (2%), insomnia (1%), and fatigue (1%).

Incidence of Adverse Events in Placebo-Controlled Clinical Trials

Major Depressive Disorder

Table 1 enumerates the incidence, rounded to the nearest percent, of treatment-emergent adverse events that occurred among 715 depressed patients who received LEXAPRO at doses ranging from 10 to 20 mg/day in placebo-controlled trials. Events included are those occurring in 2% or more of patients treated with LEXAPRO and for which the incidence in patients treated with LEXAPRO was greater than the incidence in placebo-treated patients.

The prescriber should be aware that these figures can not be used to predict the incidence of adverse events in the course of usual medical practice where patient characteristics and other factors differ from those which prevailed in the clinical trials. Similarly, the cited frequencies cannot be compared with figures obtained from other clinical investigations involving different treatments, uses, and investigators. The cited figures, however, do provide the prescribing physician with some basis for estimating the relative contribution of drug and non-drug factors to the adverse event incidence rate in the population studied. The most commonly observed adverse events in LEXAPRO patients (incidence of approximately 5% or greater and approximately twice the incidence in placebo patients) were insomnia, ejaculation disorder (primarily ejaculatory delay), nausea, sweating increased, fatigue, and somnolence (see **TABLE 1**).

TABLE 1
Treatment-Emergent Adverse Events: Incidence in Placebo-Controlled Clinical Trials for Major Depressive Disorder*

Body System/ Adverse Event	(Percentage of Patients Reporting Event) LEXAPRO (N=715)	Placebo (N=592)
Autonomic Nervous System Disorders		
Dry Mouth	6%	5%
Sweating Increased	5%	2%
Central & Peripheral Nervous System Disorders		
Dizziness	5%	3%
Gastrointestinal Disorders		
Nausea	15%	7%
Diarrhea	8%	5%
Constipation	3%	1%
Indigestion	3%	1%
Abdominal Pain	2%	1%
General		
Influenza-like Symptoms	5%	4%
Fatigue	5%	2%
Psychiatric Disorders		
Insomnia	9%	4%
Somnolence	6%	2%
Appetitie Decreased	3%	1%
Libido Decreased	3%	1%
Respiratory System Disorders		
Rhinitis	5%	4%
Sinusitis	3%	2%
Urogenital		
Ejaculation Disorder[1,2]	9%	<1%
Impotence[2]	3%	<1%
Anorgasmia[3]	2%	<1%

*Events reported by at least 2% of patients treated with LEXAPRO are reported, except for the following events which had an incidence on placebo ≥ LEXAPRO: headache, upper respiratory tract infection, back pain, pharyngitis, inflicted injury, anxiety.
[1]Primarily ejaculatory delay.
[2]Denominator used was for males only (N=225 LEXAPRO; N=188 placebo).
[3]Denominator used was for females only (N=490 LEXAPRO; N=404 placebo).

Generalized Anxiety Disorder

Table 2 enumerates the incidence, rounded to the nearest percent of treatment-emergent adverse events that occurred among 429 GAD patients who received LEXAPRO 10 to 20 mg/day in placebo-controlled trials. Events included are those occurring in 2% or more of patients treated with LEXAPRO and for which the incidence in patients treated with LEXAPRO was greater than the incidence in placebo-treated patients.

The most commonly observed adverse events in LEXAPRO patients (incidence of approximately 5% or greater and approximately twice the incidence in placebo patients) were nausea, ejaculation disorder (primarily ejaculatory delay), insomnia, fatigue, decreased libido, and anorgasmia (see **TABLE 2**).

TABLE 2
Treatment-Emergent Adverse Events: Incidence in Placebo-Controlled Clinical Trials for Generalized Anxiety Disorder*

Body System/ Adverse Event	(Percentage of Patients Reporting Event) LEXAPRO (N=429)	Placebo (N=427)
Autonomic Nervous System Disorders		
Dry Mouth	9%	5%
Sweating Increased	4%	1%
Central & Peripheral Nervous System Disorders		
Headache	24%	17%
Paresthesia	2%	1%
Gastrointestinal Disorders		
Nausea	18%	8%
Diarrhea	8%	6%
Constipation	5%	4%
Indigestion	3%	2%
Vomiting	3%	1%
Abdominal Pain	2%	1%
Flatulence	2%	1%
Toothache	2%	0%
General		
Fatigue	8%	2%
Influenza-like Symptoms	5%	4%
Musculoskeletal		
Neck/Shoulder Pain	3%	1%
Psychiatric Disorders		
Somnolence	13%	7%
Insomnia	12%	6%
Libido Decreased	7%	2%
Dreaming Abnormal	3%	2%
Appetitie Decreased	3%	1%
Lethargy	3%	1%
Yawning	2%	1%
Urogenital		
Ejaculation Disorder[1,2]	14%	2%
Anorgasmia[3]	6%	<1%
Menstrual Disorder	2%	1%

*Events reported by at least 2% of patients treated with LEXAPRO are reported, except for the following events which had an incidence on placebo ≥ LEXAPRO: inflicted injury, dizziness, back pain, upper respiratory tract infection, rhinitis, pharyngitis.
[1]Primarily ejaculatory delay.
[2]Denominator used was for males only (N=182 LEXAPRO; N=195 placebo).
[3]Denominator used was for females only (N=247 LEXAPRO; N=232 placebo).

Dose Dependency of Adverse Events

The potential dose dependency of common adverse events (defined as an incidence rate of ≥5% in either the 10 mg or 20 mg LEXAPRO groups) was examined on the basis of the combined incidence of adverse events in two fixed-dose trials. The overall incidence rates of adverse events in 10 mg LEXAPRO-treated patients (66%) was similar to that of the placebo-treated patients (61%), while the incidence rate in 20 mg/day LEXAPRO-treated patients was greater (86%). Table 3 shows common adverse events that occurred in the 20 mg/day LEXAPRO group with an incidence that was approximately twice that of the 10 mg/day LEXAPRO group and approximately twice that of the placebo group.

TABLE 3
Incidence of Common Adverse Events* in Patients With Major Depressive Disorder Receiving Placebo, 10 mg/day LEXAPRO, or 20 mg/day LEXAPRO

Adverse Event	Placebo (N=311)	10 mg/day LEXAPRO (N=310)	20 mg/day LEXAPRO (N=125)
Insomnia	4%	7%	14%
Diarrhea	5%	6%	14%
Dry Mouth	3%	4%	9%
Somnolence	1%	4%	9%
Dizziness	2%	4%	7%
Sweating Increased	<1%	3%	8%
Constipation	1%	3%	6%
Fatigue	2%	2%	6%
Indigestion	1%	2%	6%

*Adverse events with an incidence rate of at least 5% in either of the LEXAPRO groups and with an incidence rate in the 20 mg/day LEXAPRO group that was approximately twice that of the 10 mg/day LEXAPRO group and the placebo group.

Male and Female Sexual Dysfunction with SSRIs

Although changes in sexual desire, sexual performance, and sexual satisfaction often occur as manifestations of a psychiatric disorder, they may also be a consequence of pharmacologic treatment. In particular, some evidence suggests that SSRIs can cause such untoward sexual experiences.

Reliable estimates of the incidence and severity of untoward experiences involving sexual desire, performance, and satisfaction are difficult to obtain, however, in part because patients and physicians may be reluctant to discuss them. Accordingly, estimates of the incidence of untoward sexual experience and performance cited in product labeling are likely to underestimate their actual incidence.

Table 4 shows the incidence rates of sexual side effects in patients with major depressive disorder and GAD in placebo-controlled trials.

TABLE 4
Incidence of Sexual Side Effects in Placebo-Controlled Clinical Trials

Adverse Event	LEXAPRO	Placebo
	In Males Only	
	(N=407)	(N=383)
Ejaculation Disorder (primarily ejaculatory delay)	12%	1%
Libido Decreased	6%	2%
Impotence	2%	<1%
	In Females Only	
	(N=737)	(N=636)
Libido Decreased	3%	1%
Anorgasmia	3%	<1%

There are no adequately designed studies examining sexual dysfunction with escitalopram treatment.

Priapism has been reported with all SSRIs.

While it is difficult to know the precise risk of sexual dysfunction associated with the use of SSRIs, physicians should routinely inquire about such possible side effects.

Vital Sign Changes

LEXAPRO and placebo groups were compared with respect to (1) mean change from baseline in vital signs (pulse, systolic blood pressure, and diastolic blood pressure) and (2) the incidence of patients meeting criteria for potentially clinically significant changes from baseline in these variables. These analyses did not reveal any clinically important changes in vital signs associated with LEXAPRO treatment. In addition, a comparison of supine and standing vital sign measures in subjects receiving LEXAPRO indicated that LEXAPRO treatment is not associated with orthostatic changes.

Weight Changes

Patients treated with LEXAPRO in controlled trials did not differ from placebo-treated patients with regard to clinically important change in body weight.

Laboratory Changes

LEXAPRO and placebo groups were compared with respect to (1) mean change from baseline in various serum chemistry, hematology, and urinalysis variables, and (2) the incidence of patients meeting criteria for potentially clinically significant changes from baseline in these variables. These analyses revealed no clinically important changes in laboratory test parameters associated with LEXAPRO treatment.

ECG Changes

Electrocardiograms from LEXAPRO (N=625), racemic citalopram (N=351), and placebo (N=527) groups were compared with respect to (1) mean change from baseline in various ECG parameters and (2) the incidence of patients meeting criteria for potentially clinically significant changes from baseline in these variables. These analyses revealed (1) a decrease in heart rate of 2.2 bpm for LEXAPRO and 2.7 bpm for racemic citalopram, compared to an increase of 0.3 bpm for placebo and (2) an increase in QTc interval of 3.9 msec for LEXAPRO and 3.7 msec for racemic citalopram, compared to 0.5 msec for placebo. Neither LEXAPRO nor racemic citalopram were associated with the development of clinically significant ECG abnormalities.

Other Events Observed During the Premarketing Evaluation of LEXAPRO

Following is a list of WHO terms that reflect treatment-emergent adverse events, as defined in the introduction to the ADVERSE REACTIONS section, reported by the 1428 patients treated with LEXAPRO for periods of up to one year in double-blind or open-label clinical trials during its premarketing evaluation. All reported events are included except those already listed in Tables 1 & 2, those occurring in only one patient, event terms that are so general as to be uninformative, and those that are unlikely to be drug related. It is important to emphasize that, although the events reported occurred during treatment with LEXAPRO, they were not necessarily caused by it.

Events are further categorized by body system and listed in order of decreasing frequency according to the following definitions: frequent adverse events are those occurring on one or more occasions in at least 1/100 patients; infrequent adverse events are those occurring in less than 1/100 patients but at least 1/1000 patients.

Cardiovascular—*Frequent*: palpitation, hypertension. *Infrequent*: bradycardia, tachycardia, ECG abnormal, flushing, varicose vein.

Central and Peripheral Nervous System Disorders—*Frequent*: light-headed feeling, migraine. *Infrequent*: tremor, vertigo, restless legs, shaking, twitching, dysequilibrium, tics, carpal tunnel syndrome, muscle contractions involuntary, sluggishness, coordination abnormal, faintness, hyperreflexia, muscular tone increased.

Gastrointestinal Disorders—*Frequent*: heartburn, abdominal cramp, gastroenteritis. *Infrequent*: gastroesophageal reflux, bloating, abdominal discomfort, dyspepsia, increased stool frequency, belching, gastritis, hemorrhoids, gagging, polyposis gastric, swallowing difficult.

Continued on next page

Lexapro—Cont.

General—*Frequent*: allergy, pain in limb, fever, hot flushes, chest pain. *Infrequent*: edema of extremities, chills, tightness of chest, leg pain, asthenia, syncope, malaise, anaphylaxis, fall.
Hemic and Lymphatic Disorders—*Infrequent*: bruise, anemia, nosebleed, hematoma, lymphadenopathy cervical.
Metabolic and Nutritional Disorders—*Frequent*: increased weight. *Infrequent*: decreased weight, hyperglycemia, thirst, bilirubin increased, hepatic enzymes increased, gout, hypercholesterolemia.
Musculoskeletal System Disorders—*Frequent*: arthralgia, myalgia. *Infrequent*: jaw stiffness, muscle cramp, muscle stiffness, arthritis, muscle weakness, back discomfort, arthropathy, jaw pain, joint stiffness.
Psychiatric Disorders—*Frequent*: appetite increased, lethargy, irritability, concentration impaired. *Infrequent*: jitteriness, panic reaction, agitation, apathy, forgetfulness, depression aggravated, nervousness, restlessness aggravated, suicide attempt, amnesia, anxiety attack, bruxism, carbohydrate craving, confusion, depersonalization, disorientation, emotional lability, feeling unreal, tremulousness nervous, crying abnormal, depression, excitability, auditory hallucination, suicidal tendency.
Reproductive Disorders/Female*—*Frequent*: menstrual cramps, menstrual disorder. *Infrequent*: menorrhagia, breast neoplasm, pelvic inflammation, premenstrual syndrome, spotting between menses.

*based on female subjects only: N= 905

Respiratory System Disorders—*Frequent*: bronchitis, sinus congestion, coughing, nasal congestion, sinus headache. *Infrequent*: asthma, breath shortness, laryngitis, pneumonia, tracheitis.
Skin and Appendages Disorders—*Frequent*: rash. *Infrequent*: pruritus, acne, alopecia, eczema, dermatitis, dry skin, folliculitis, lipoma, furunculosis, dry lips, skin nodule.
Special Senses—*Frequent*: vision blurred, tinnitus. *Infrequent*: taste alteration, earache, conjunctivitis, vision abnormal, dry eyes, eye irritation, visual disturbance, eye infection, pupils dilated, metallic taste.
Urinary System Disorders—*Frequent*: urinary frequency, urinary tract infection. *Infrequent*: urinary urgency, kidney stone, dysuria, blood in urine.

Events Reported Subsequent to the Marketing of Racemic Citalopram and Escitalopram

Although no causal relationship to racemic citalopram treatment has been found, the following adverse events have been reported to have occurred in patients and to be temporally associated with racemic citalopram treatment and with escitalopram treatment during postmarketing experience and were not observed during the premarketing evaluation of citalopram or escitalopram: acute renal failure, angioedema, toxic epidermal necrolysis, gastrointestinal hemorrhage, grand mal seizures (or convulsions), neuroleptic malignant syndrome, pancreatitis, QT prolongation, rhabdomyolysis, serotonin syndrome, thrombocytopenia, torsades de pointes.

Events Reported Subsequent to the Marketing of Racemic Citalopram (not observed during the postmarketing experience with escitalopram)

Although no causal relationship to racemic citalopram treatment has been found, the following adverse events have been reported to have occurred in patients and to be temporally associated with racemic citalopram treatment and were not observed during the premarketing evaluation of citalopram: akathisia, allergic reaction, anaphylaxis, choreoathetosis, delirium, dyskinesia, ecchymosis, erythema multiforme, hemolytic anemia, hepatic necrosis, myoclonus, nystagmus, priapism, prolactinemia, prothrombin decreased, spontaneous abortion, thrombosis, and ventricular arrhythmia.

Events Reported Subsequent to the Marketing of Escitalopram (not observed during the postmarketing experience with citalopram)

Although no causal relationship to escitalopram treatment has been found, the following adverse events have been reported to have occurred in patients and to be temporally associated with escitalopram treatment and were not observed during the premarketing evaluation of escitalopram: aggression, atrial fibrillation, seizures, diplopia, dystonia, extrapyramidal disorders, abnormal gait, visual hallucinations, hepatitis, hypotension, myocardial infarction, orthostatic hypotension, pulmonary embolism, SIADH, ventricular tachycardia.

DRUG ABUSE AND DEPENDENCE

Controlled Substance Class

LEXAPRO is not a controlled substance.

Physical and Psychological Dependence

Animal studies suggest that the abuse liability of racemic citalopram is low. LEXAPRO has not been systematically studied in humans for its potential for abuse, tolerance, or physical dependence. The premarketing clinical experience with LEXAPRO did not reveal any drug-seeking behavior. However, these observations were not systematic and it is not possible to predict on the basis of this limited experience the extent to which a CNS-active drug will be misused, diverted, and/or abused once marketed. Consequently, physicians should carefully evaluate LEXAPRO patients for history of drug abuse and follow such patients closely, observing them for signs of misuse or abuse (e.g., development of tolerance, incrementations of dose, drug-seeking behavior).

OVERDOSAGE

Human Experience

There have been reports of LEXAPRO overdose involving doses of up to 600 mg. All patients recovered and no symptoms associated with the overdoses were reported. In clinical trials of racemic citalopram, there were no reports of fatal citalopram overdose involving overdoses of up to 2000 mg. During the postmarketing evaluation of citalopram, like other SSRIs, a fatal outcome in a patient who has taken an overdose of citalopram has been rarely reported.
Postmarketing reports of drug overdoses involving citalopram have included 12 fatalities, 10 in combination with other drugs and/or alcohol and 2 with citalopram alone (3920 mg and 2800 mg), as well as non-fatal overdoses of up to 6000 mg. Symptoms most often accompanying citalopram overdose, alone or in combination with other drugs and/or alcohol, included dizziness, sweating, nausea, vomiting, tremor, somnolence, sinus tachycardia, and convulsions. In more rare cases, observed symptoms included amnesia, confusion, coma, hyperventilation, cyanosis, rhabdomyolysis, and ECG changes (including QTc prolongation, nodal rhythm, ventricular arrhythmia, and one possible case of torsades de pointes).

Management of Overdose

Establish and maintain an airway to ensure adequate ventilation and oxygenation. Gastric evacuation by lavage and use of activated charcoal should be considered. Careful observation and cardiac and vital sign monitoring are recommended, along with general symptomatic and supportive care. Due to the large volume of distribution of escitalopram, forced diuresis, dialysis, hemoperfusion, and exchange transfusion are unlikely to be of benefit. There are no specific antidotes for LEXAPRO.
In managing overdosage, consider the possibility of multiple-drug involvement. The physician should consider contacting a poison control center for additional information on the treatment of any overdose.

DOSAGE AND ADMINISTRATION

Major Depressive Disorder

Initial Treatment

The recommended dose of LEXAPRO is 10 mg once daily. A fixed-dose trial of LEXAPRO demonstrated the effectiveness of both 10 mg and 20 mg of LEXAPRO, but failed to demonstrate a greater benefit of 20 mg over 10 mg (see **Clinical Efficacy Trials** under **CLINICAL PHARMACOLOGY**). If the dose is increased to 20 mg, this should occur after a minimum of one week.
LEXAPRO should be administered once daily, in the morning or evening, with or without food.

Special Populations

10 mg/day is the recommended dose for most elderly patients and patients with hepatic impairment.
No dosage adjustment is necessary for patients with mild or moderate renal impairment. LEXAPRO should be used with caution in patients with severe renal impairment.

Treatment of Pregnant Women During the Third Trimester

Neonates exposed to LEXAPRO and other SSRIs or SNRIs, late in the third trimester, have developed complications requiring prolonged hospitalization, respiratory support, and tube feeding (see **PRECAUTIONS**). When treating pregnant women with LEXAPRO during the third trimester, the physician should carefully consider the potential risks and benefits of treatment. The physician may consider tapering LEXAPRO in the third trimester.

Maintenance Treatment

It is generally agreed that acute episodes of major depressive disorder require several months or longer of sustained pharmacological therapy beyond response to the acute episode. Systematic evaluation of continuing LEXAPRO 10 or 20 mg/day for periods of up to 36 weeks in patients with major depressive disorder who responded while taking LEXAPRO during an 8-week, acute-treatment phase demonstrated a benefit of such maintenance treatment (see **Clinical Efficacy Trials** under **CLINICAL PHARMACOLOGY**). Nevertheless, patients should be periodically reassessed to determine the need for maintenance treatment.

Generalized Anxiety Disorder

Initial Treatment

The recommended starting dose of LEXAPRO is 10 mg once daily. If the dose is increased to 20 mg, this should occur after a minimum of one week.
LEXAPRO should be administered once daily, in the morning or evening, with or without food.

Maintenance Treatment

Generalized anxiety disorder is recognized as a chronic condition. The efficacy of LEXAPRO in the treatment of GAD beyond 8 weeks has not been systematically studied. The physician who elects to use LEXAPRO for extended periods should periodically re-evaluate the long-term usefulness of the drug for the individual patient.

Discontinuation of Treatment with LEXAPRO

Symptoms associated with discontinuation of LEXAPRO and other SSRIs and SNRIs have been reported (see **PRECAUTIONS**). Patients should be monitored for these symptoms when discontinuing treatment. A gradual reduction in the dose rather than abrupt cessation is recommended whenever possible. If intolerable symptoms occur following a decrease in the dose or upon discontinuation of treatment, then resuming the previously prescribed dose may be considered. Subsequently, the physician may continue decreasing the dose but at a more gradual rate.

Switching Patients To or From a Monoamine Oxidase Inhibitor

At least 14 days should elapse between discontinuation of an MAOI and initiation of LEXAPRO therapy. Similarly, at least 14 days should be allowed after stopping LEXAPRO before starting an MAOI (see **CONTRAINDICATIONS** and **WARNINGS**).

HOW SUPPLIED

5 mg Tablets:
Bottle of 100 NDC # 0456-2005-01
White to off-white, round, non-scored, film-coated. Imprint "FL" on one side of the tablet and "5" on the other side.
10 mg Tablets:
Bottle of 100 NDC # 0456-2010-01
10 × 10 Unit Dose NDC # 0456-2010-63
White to off-white, round, scored, film-coated. Imprint on scored side with "F" on the left side and "L" on the right side.
Imprint on the non-scored side with "10".
20 mg Tablets:
Bottle of 100 NDC # 0456-2020-01
10 × 10 Unit Dose NDC # 0456-2020-63
White to off-white, round, scored, film-coated. Imprint on scored side with "F" on the left side and "L" on the right side.
Imprint on the non-scored side with "20".
Oral Solution:
5 mg/5 mL, NDC # 0456-2101-08
peppermint flavor (240 mL)
Store at 25°C (77°F); excursions permitted to 15-30°C (59-86°F).

ANIMAL TOXICOLOGY

Retinal Changes in Rats

Pathologic changes (degeneration/atrophy) were observed in the retinas of albino rats in the 2-year carcinogenicity study with racemic citalopram. There was an increase in both incidence and severity of retinal pathology in both male and female rats receiving 80 mg/kg/day. Similar findings were not present in rats receiving 24 mg/kg/day of racemic citalopram for two years, in mice receiving up to 240 mg/kg/day of racemic citalopram for 18 months, or in dogs receiving up to 20 mg/kg/day of racemic citalopram for one year.
Additional studies to investigate the mechanism for this pathology have not been performed, and the potential significance of this effect in humans has not been established.

Cardiovascular Changes in Dogs

In a one-year toxicology study, 5 of 10 beagle dogs receiving oral racemic citalopram doses of 8 mg/kg/day died suddenly between weeks 17 and 31 following initiation of treatment. Sudden deaths were not observed in rats at doses of racemic citalopram up to 120 mg/kg/day, which produced plasma levels of citalopram and its metabolites demethylcitalopram and didemethylcitalopram (DDCT) similar to those observed in dogs at 8 mg/kg/day. A subsequent intravenous dosing study demonstrated that in beagle dogs, racemic DDCT caused QT prolongation, a known risk factor for the observed outcome in dogs.

Forest Pharmaceuticals, Inc.
Subsidiary of Forest Laboratories, Inc.
St. Louis, MO 63045 USA
Licensed from H. Lundbeck A/S
Rev. 06/04

MG #17541(07)
Shown in Product Identification Guide, page 312

LORCET®-HD Ⓒ℞

[*lōr-sét h d*]

HYDROCODONE BITARTRATE and ACETAMINOPHEN CAPSULES 5 mg/500 mg

DESCRIPTION

Each capsule contains:
Hydrocodone Bitartrate 5 mg
Acetaminophen 500 mg

HOW SUPPLIED:

Lorcet-HD Capsules are opaque maroon capsules imprinted with the UAD logo, 1120 and are supplied in bottles of 100 capsules. Each capsule contains Hydrocodone Bitartrate, 5 mg and Acetaminophen (APAP), 500 mg. The NDC number for containers of 100 capsules is 0785-1120-01.
Keep in tight, light-resistant containers.
A Schedule III Narcotic.

Manufactured for
UAD LABORATORIES
Division of Forest Pharmaceuticals, Inc.
St. Louis, MO 63045

LORCET® PLUS Ⓒ℞

[*lōr-sét plus*]

Hydrocodone Bitartrate and Acetaminophen Tablets USP 7.5 mg/650 mg

DESCRIPTION

Each Lorcet® Plus tablet contains:
Hydrocodone Bitartrate .... 7.5 mg

WARNING: May be habit-forming
Acetaminophen .... 650 mg

HOW SUPPLIED

Lorcet® Plus, each tablet of which contains hydrocodone bitartrate 7.5 mg (**WARNING: May be habit-forming**) and acetaminophen 650 mg, are white, capsule-shaped, scored tablets, debossed "U" on one side and "201" on the other side, and are supplied in containers of 100 tablets, NDC #0785-1122-01, containers of 500 tablets, NDC #0785-1122-50, and in unit-dose cartons of 100 tablets (4 cards of 25 tablets per card), NDC #0785-1122-63.

Shown in Product Identification Guide, page 312

LORCET® 10/650 ℞

[*lōr-sét*]

HYDROCODONE BITARTRATE AND ACETAMINOPHEN TABLETS USP
10 mg/650 mg

DESCRIPTION

Each Lorcet® 10/650 tablet contains:
Hydrocodone Bitartrate .... 10 mg
WARNING: May be habit-forming
Acetaminophen .... 650 mg

In addition, each tablet contains the following inactive ingredients: colloidal silicon dioxide, croscarmellose sodium, crospovidone, microcrystalline cellulose, povidone, pregelatinized starch, stearic acid and FD&C Blue #1 Lake.

This product complies with Dissolution Test 1.

HOW SUPPLIED

Lorcet® 10/650, Hydrocodone Bitartrate and Acetaminophen Tablets, each tablet of which contains hydrocodone bitartrate 10 mg (**WARNING: May be habit-forming**) and acetaminophen 650 mg, are light-blue, capsule-shaped, scored tablets, debossed "UAD" on one side and "63 50" on the other side, and are supplied in containers of 100 tablets, NDC 0785-6350-01 and in containers of 500 tablets, NDC 0785-6350-50, and in containers of unit dose (4 × 25's), NDC 0785-6350-63.

Shown in Product Identification Guide, page 312

MONUROL® ℞

[*mon' ur ol*]

(fosfomycin tromethamine)
SACHET
℞ only

DESCRIPTION

MONUROL (fosfomycin tromethamine) sachet contains fosfomycin tromethamine, a synthetic, broad-spectrum, bactericidal antibiotic for oral administration. It is available as a single-dose sachet which contains white granules consisting of 5.631 grams of fosfomycin tromethamine (equivalent to 3 grams of fosfomycin), and the following inactive ingredients: mandarin flavor, orange flavor, saccharin, and sucrose. The contents of the sachet must be dissolved in water. Fosfomycin tromethamine, a phosphonic acid derivative, is available as (1*R*,2*S*)-(1,2-epoxypropyl)phosphonic acid, compound with 2-amino-2-(hydroxymethyl)-1,3-propanediol (1:1). It is a white granular compound with a molecular weight of 259.2. Its empirical formula is $C_3H_7O_4P{\cdot}C_4H_{11}NO_3$, and its chemical structure is as follows:

[chemical structure]

CLINICAL PHARMACOLOGY

Absorption: Fosfomycin tromethamine is rapidly absorbed following oral administration and converted to the free acid, fosfomycin. Absolute oral bioavailability under fasting conditions is 37%. After a single 3-gm dose of MONUROL, the mean (± 1 SD) maximum serum concentration (C_{max}) achieved was 26.1 (± 9.1) μg/mL within 2 hours. The oral bioavailability of fosfomycin is reduced to 30% under fed conditions. Following a single 3-gm oral dose of MONUROL with a high-fat meal, the mean C_{max} achieved was 17.6 (± 4.4) μg/mL within 4 hours.

Cimetidine does not affect the pharmacokinetics of fosfomycin when coadministered with MONUROL. Metoclopramide lowers the serum concentrations and urinary excretion of fosfomycin when coadministered with MONUROL. (See **PRECAUTIONS, Drug Interactions.**)

Distribution: The mean apparent steady-state volume of distribution (V_{SS}) is 136.1 (±44.1) L following oral administration of MONUROL. Fosfomycin is not bound to plasma proteins.

Fosfomycin is distributed to the kidneys, bladder wall, prostate, and seminal vesicles. Following a 50 mg/Kg dose of fosfomycin to patients undergoing urological surgery for bladder carcinoma, the mean concentration of fosfomycin in the bladder, taken at a distance from the neoplastic site, was 18.0 μg per gram of tissue at 3 hours after dosing. Fosfomycin has been shown to cross the placental barrier in animals and man.

Excretion: Fosfomycin is excreted unchanged in both urine and feces. Following oral administration of MONUROL, the mean total body clearance (CL_{TB}) and mean renal clearance (CL_R) of fosfomycin were 16.9 (± 3.5) L/hr and 6.3 (± 1.7) L/hr, respectively. Approximately 38% of a 3-gm dose of MONUROL is recovered from urine, and 18% is recovered from feces. Following intravenous administration, the mean CL_{TB} and mean CL_R of fosfomycin were 6.1 (± 1.0) L/hr and 5.5 (± 1.2) L/hr, respectively.

A mean urine fosfomycin concentration of 706 (± 466) μg/mL was attained within 2–4 hours after a single oral 3-gm dose of MONUROL under fasting conditions. The mean urinary concentration of fosfomycin was 10 μg/mL in samples collected 72–84 hours following a single oral dose of MONUROL.

Following a 3-gm dose of MONUROL administered with a high fat meal, a mean urine fosfomycin concentration of 537 (± 252) μg/mL was attained within 6–8 hours. Although the rate of urinary excretion of fosfomycin was reduced under fed conditions, the cumulative amount of fosfomycin excreted in the urine was the same, 1118 (± 201) mg (fed) vs. 1140 mg (±238) (fasting). Further, urinary concentrations equal to or greater than 100 μg/mL were maintained for the same duration, 26 hours, indicated that MONUROL can be taken without regard to food.

Following oral administration of MONUROL, the mean half-life for elimination ($t_{1/2}$) is 5.7 (± 2.8) hours.

Special Populations:

Geriatric: Based on limited data regarding 24-hour urinary drug concentrations, no differences in urinary excretion of fosfomycin have been observed in elderly subjects. No dosage adjustment is necessary in the elderly.

Gender: There are no gender differences in the pharmacokinetics of fosfomycin.

Renal Insufficiency: In 5 anuric patients undergoing hemodialysis, the $t_{1/2}$ of fosfomycin during hemodialysis was 40 hours. In patients with varying degrees of renal impairment (creatinine clearances varying from 54 mL/min to 7 mL/min), the $t_{1/2}$ of fosfomycin increased from 11 hours to 50 hours. The percent of fosfomycin recovered in urine decreased from 32% to 11% indicating that renal impairment significantly decreases the excretion of fosfomycin.

Microbiology

Fosfomycin (the active component of fosfomycin tromethamine) has *in vitro* activity against a broad range of gram-positive and gram-negative aerobic microorganisms which are associated with uncomplicated urinary tract infections. Fosfomycin is bactericidal in urine at therapeutic doses. The bactericidal action of fosfomycin is due to its inactivation of the enzyme enolpyruvyl transferase, thereby irreversibly blocking the condensation of uridine diphosphate-N-acetylglucosamine with p-enolpyruvate, one of the first steps in bacterial cell wall synthesis. It also reduces adherence of bacteria to uroepithelial cells.

There is generally no cross-resistance between fosfomycin and other classes of antibacterial agents such as beta-lactams and aminoglycosides.

Fosfomycin has been shown to be active against most strains of the following microorganisms, both *in vitro* and in clinical infections as described in the **INDICATIONS AND USAGE** section:

Aerobic gram-positive microorganisms
Enterococcus faecalis

Aerobic gram-negative microorganisms
Escherichia coli

The following *in vitro* data are available, **but their clinical significance is unknown.**

Fosfomycin exhibits *in vitro* minimum inhibitory concentrations (MIC's) of 64 μg/mL or less against most (≥ 90%) strains of the following microorganisms; however, the safety and effectiveness of fosfomycin in treating clinical infections due to these microorganisms has not been established in adequate and well-controlled clinical trials:

Aerobic gram-positive microorganisms
Enterococcus faecium

Aerobic gram-negative microorganisms
Citrobacter diversus
Citrobacter freundii
Enterobacter aerogenes
Klebsiella oxytoca
Klebsiella pneumoniae
Proteus mirabilis
Proteus vulgaris
Serratia marcescens

SUSCEPTIBILITY TESTING

Dilution Techniques:

Quantitative methods are used to determine minimum inhibitory concentrations (MIC's). These MIC's provide estimates of the susceptibility of bacteria to antimicrobial compounds. One such standardized procedure uses a standardized agar dilution method[1] or equivalent with standardized inoculum concentrations and standardized concentrations of fosfomycin tromethamine (in terms of fosfomycin base content) powder supplemented with 25 μg/mL of glucose-6-phosphate. **BROTH DILUTION METHODS SHOULD NOT BE USED TO TEST SUSCEPTIBILITY TO FOSFOMYCIN.** The MIC values obtained should be interpreted according to the following criteria:

MIC (μg/mL)	Interpretation
≤ 64	Susceptible (S)
128	Intermediate (I)
≥ 256	Resistant (R)

A report of "susceptible" indicates that the pathogen is likely to be inhibited by usually achievable concentrations of the antimicrobial compound in the urine. A report of "intermediate" indicates that the result should be considered equivocal, and, if the microorganism is not fully susceptible to alternative, clinically feasible drugs, the test should be repeated. This category provides a buffer zone that prevents small uncontrolled technical factors from causing major discrepancies in interpretation. A report of "resistant" indicates that usually achievable concentrations of the antimicrobial compound in the urine are unlikely to be inhibitory and that other therapy should be selected.

Standardized susceptibility test procedures require the use of laboratory control microorganisms. Standard fosfomycin tromethamine powder should provide the following MIC values for agar dilution testing in media containing 25 μg/mL of glucose-6-phosphate. **[Broth dilution testing should not be performed].**

Microorganism	MIC (μg/mL)
Enterococcus faecalis ATCC 29212	32–128
Escherichia coli ATCC 25922	0.5–2
Pseudomonas aeruginosa ATCC 27853	2–8
Staphylococcus aureus ATCC 29213	0.5–4

Diffusion Techniques:

Quantitative methods that require measurement of zone diameters also provide reproducible estimates of the susceptibility of bacteria to antimicrobial agents. One such standardized procedure[2] requires the use of standardized inoculum concentrations. This procedure uses paper disks impregnated with 200-μg fosfomycin and 50-μg of glucose-6-phosphate to test the susceptibility of microorganisms to fosfomycin.

Reports from the laboratory providing results of the standard single-disk susceptibility test with disks containing 200 μg of fosfomycin and 50 μg of glucose-6-phosphate should be interpreted according to the following criteria:

Zone Diameter (mm)	Interpretation
≥16	Susceptible (S)
13–15	Intermediate (I)
≤12	Resistant (R)

Interpretation should be stated as above for results using dilution techniques. Interpretation involves correlation of the diameter obtained in the disk test with the MIC for fosfomycin.

As with standardized dilution techniques, diffusion methods require use of laboratory control microorganisms that are used to control the technical aspects of the laboratory procedures. For the diffusion technique, the 200-μg fosfomycin disk with the 50-μg of glucose-6-phosphate should provide the following zone diameters in these laboratory quality control strains:

Microorganism	Zone Diameter (mm)
Escherichia coli ATCC 25922	22–30
Staphylococcus aureus ATCC 25923	25–33

INDICATIONS AND USAGE

MONUROL is indicated only for the treatment of uncomplicated urinary tract infections (acute cystitis) in women due to susceptible strains of *Escherichia coli* and *Enterococcus faecalis*. MONUROL is not indicated for the treatment of pyelonephritis or perinephric abscess.

If persistence or reappearance of bacteriuria occurs after treatment with MONUROL, other therapeutic agents should be selected. (See **PRECAUTIONS** and **CLINICAL STUDIES** section.)

CONTRAINDICATIONS

MONUROL is contraindicated in patients with known hypersensitivity to the drug.

PRECAUTIONS

General

Do not use more than one single dose of MONUROL to treat a single episode of acute cystitis. Repeated daily doses of MONUROL did not improve the clinical success or microbiological eradication rates compared to single dose therapy, but did increase the incidence of adverse events.

Urine specimens for culture and susceptibility testing should be obtained before and after completion of therapy.

Information for Patients

Patients should be informed:

- That MONUROL (fosfomycin tromethamine) can be taken with or without food.
- That their symptoms should improve in two to three days after taking MONUROL; if not improved, the patient should contact her health care provider.

Drug Interactions

Metoclopramide: When coadministered with MONUROL, metoclopramide, a drug which increases gastrointestinal motility, lowers the serum concentration and urinary excretion of fosfomycin. Other drugs that increase gastrointestinal motility may produce similar effects.

Cimetidine: Cimetidine does not affect the pharmacokinetics of fosfomycin when coadministered with MONUROL.

Continued on next page

Monurol—Cont.

Carcinogenesis, Mutagenesis, Impairment of Fertility
Long term carcinogenicity studies in rodents have not been conducted because MONUROL is intended for single dose treatment in humans. MONUROL was not mutagenic or genotoxic in the *in vitro* Ames' bacterial reversion test, in cultured human lymphocytes, in Chinese hamster V79 cells, and the *in vivo* mouse micronucleus assay. MONUROL did not affect fertility or reproductive performance in male and female rats.

Pregnancy: Teratogenic Effects
Pregnancy Category B
When administered intramuscularly as the sodium salt at a dose of 1 gm to pregnant women, fosfomycin crosses the placental barrier. MONUROL crosses the placental barrier of rats; it does not produce teratogenic effects in pregnant rats at dosages as high as 1000 mg/kg/day (approximately 9 and 1.4 times the human dose based on body weight and mg/m^2, respectively). When administered to pregnant female rabbits at dosages as high as 1000 mg/kg/day (approximately 9 and 2.7 times the human dose based on body weight and mg/m^2, respectively), fetotoxicities were observed. However, these toxicities were seen at maternally toxic doses and were considered to be due to the sensitivity of the rabbit to changes in the intestinal microflora resulting from the antibiotic administration. There are, however, no adequate and well-controlled studies in pregnant women. Because animal reproduction studies are not always predictive of human response, this drug should be used during pregnancy only if clearly needed.

Nursing Mothers
It is not known whether fosfomycin tromethamine is excreted in human milk. Because many drugs are excreted in human milk and because of the potential for serious adverse reactions in nursing infants from MONUROL, a decision should be made whether to discontinue nursing or to not administer the drug, taking into account the importance of the drug to the mother.

Pediatric Use
Safety and effectiveness in children age 12 years and under have not been established in adequate and well-controlled studies.

Geriatric Use: Clinical studies of Monurol did not include sufficient numbers of subjects aged 65 and over to determine whether they respond differently from younger subjects. Other reported clinical experience has not identified differences in responses between the elderly and younger patients. In general, dose selection for an elderly patient should be cautious, usually starting at the low end of the dosing range, reflecting the greater frequency of decreased hepatic, renal, or cardiac function, and of concomitant disease or other drug therapy.

ADVERSE REACTIONS

Clinical Trials:
In clinical studies, drug related adverse events which were reported in greater than 1% of the fosfomycin-treated study population are listed below:

Drug-Related Adverse Events (%) in Fosfomycin and Comparator Populations

Adverse Events	Fosfomycin N=1233	Nitrofurantoin N=374	Trimethoprim / sulfamethoxazole N=428	Ciprofloxacin N=445
Diarrhea	9.0	6.4	2.3	3.1
Vaginitis	5.5	5.3	4.7	6.3
Nausea	4.1	7.2	8.6	3.4
Headache	3.9	5.9	5.4	3.4
Dizziness	1.3	1.9	2.3	2.2
Asthenia	1.1	0.3	0.5	0.0
Dyspepsia	1.1	2.1	0.7	1.1

In clinical trials, the most frequently reported adverse events occurring in >1% of the study population regardless of drug relationship, were:
diarrhea 10.4%, headache 10.3%, vaginitis 7.6%, nausea 5.2%, rhinitis 4.5%, back pain 3.0%, dysmenorrhea 2.6%, pharyngitis 2.5%, dizziness 2.3%, abdominal pain 2.2%, pain 2.2%, dyspepsia 1.8%, asthenia 1.7%, and rash 1.4%.
The following adverse events occurred in clinical trials at a rate of less than 1%, regardless of drug relationship:
abnormal stools, anorexia, constipation, dry mouth, dysuria, ear disorder, fever, flatulence, flu syndrome, hematuria, infection, insomnia, lymphadenopathy, menstrual disorder, migraine, myalgia, nervousness, paresthesia, pruritus, SGPT increased, skin disorder, somnolence, and vomiting. One patient developed unilateral optic neuritis, an event considered possibly related to MONUROL therapy.

Post-marketing Experience:
Serious adverse events from the marketing experience with MONUROL outside of the United States have been rarely reported and include:
angioedema, aplastic anemia, asthma (exacerbation), cholestatic jaundice, hepatic necrosis, and toxic megacolon.

Laboratory Changes:
Significant laboratory changes reported in U.S. clinical trials of MONUROL without regard to drug relationship include: increased eosinophil count, increased or decreased WBC count, increased bilirubin, increased SGPT, increased SGOT, increased alkaline phosphatase, decreased hematocrit, decreased hemoglobin, increased and decreased platelet count. The changes were generally transient and were not clinically significant.

OVERDOSAGE

In acute toxicology studies, oral administration of high doses of MONUROL up to 5 gm/kg were well-tolerated in mice and rats, produced transient and minor incidences of watery stool in rabbits, and produced diarrhea with anorexia in dogs occurring in 2–3 days after single dose administration. These doses represent 50–125 times the human therapeutic dose.
There have been no reported cases of overdosage. In the event of overdosage, treatment should be symptomatic and supportive.

DOSAGE AND ADMINISTRATION

The recommended dosage for women 18 years of age and older for uncomplicated urinary tract infection (acute cystitis) is one sachet of MONUROL. MONUROL may be taken with or without food.
MONUROL should not be taken in its dry form. Always mix MONUROL with water before ingesting. (See PREPARATION section.)

PREPARATION
MONUROL should be taken orally. Pour the entire contents of a single-dose sachet of MONUROL into 3 to 4 ounces of water (1/2 cup) and stir to dissolve. Do not use hot water. MONUROL should be taken immediately after dissolving in water.

HOW SUPPLIED

MONUROL is available as a single-dose sachet containing the equivalent of 3 grams of fosfomycin.
NDC # 0456-4300-08
Store at controlled room temperature 15° to 30° C (59° to 86°F).
Rx only
Keep this and all drugs out of the reach of children.
Manufactured by:
Inpharzam S.A.
Division of Zambon Group, SpA
Via Industria
6814 Cadempino, Switzerland
Made in Switzerland
Distributed by:
Forest Pharmaceuticals, Inc.
Subsidiary of Forest Laboratories, Inc.
St. Louis, MO 63045

REFERENCES

1. National Committee for Clinical Laboratory Standards, Methods for Dilution. Antimicrobial Susceptibility Tests for Bacteria that Grow Aerobically — Third Edition; Approved Standard NCCLS Document M7-A3, Vol. 13, No. 25 NCCLS, Villanova, PA, December, 1993.
2. National Committee for Clinical Laboratory Standards, Performance Standard for Antimicrobial Disk Susceptibility Tests — Fifth Edition; Approved Standard NCCLS Document M2-A5, Vol. 13, No. 24 NCCLS, Villanova, PA, December, 1993.

CLINICAL STUDIES

In controlled, double-blind studies of acute cystitis performed in the United States, a single-dose of MONUROL was compared to three other oral antibiotics (See table below). The study population consisted of patients with symptoms and signs of acute cystitis of less than 4 days duration, no manifestations of upper tract infection (e.g., flank pain, chills, fever), no history of recurrent urinary tract infections (20% of patients in the clinical studies had a prior episode of acute cystitis within the preceding year), no known structural abnormalities, and no clinical or laboratory evidence of hepatic dysfunction, and no known or suspected CNS disorders, such as epilepsy, or other factors which would predispose to seizures. In these studies, the following clinical success (resolution of symptoms) and microbiologic eradication rates were obtained:
[See table at bottom left]

Treatment Arm	Treatment Duration (days)	Microbiologic Eradication Rate		Clinical Success Rate	Outcome (based on difference in microbiologic eradication rates at 5–11 days post therapy)
		5–11 days post therapy	Study day 12–21		
Fosfomycin	1	630/771 (82%)	591/771 (77%)	542/771 (70%)	
Ciprofloxacin	7	219/222 (98%)	219/222 (98%)	213/222 (96%)	Fosfomycin inferior to ciprofloxacin
Trimethoprim/ sulfamethoxazole	10	194/197 (98%)	194/197 (98%)	186/197 (94%)	Fosfomycin inferior to trimethoprim/ sulfamethoxazole
Nitrofurantoin	7	180/238 (76%)	180/238 (76%)	183/238 (77%)	Fosfomycin equivalent to nitrofurantoin

Pathogen	Fosfomycin 3 gm single dose	Ciprofloxacin 250 mg bid × 7d	Trimethoprim/sulfamethoxazole 160 mg/ 800 mg bid × 10d	Nitrofurantoin 100mg bid × 7d
E. coli	509/644 (79%)	184/187 (98%)	171/174 (98%)	146/187 (78%)
E. faecalis	10/10 (100%)	0/0	4/4 (100%)	1/2 (50%)

Rev. 6/02 RMC 237
Shown in Product Identification Guide, page 312

NAMENDA™ TABLETS ℞

[*nă-měn-dă*]
(memantine hydrochloride)
Rx Only

DESCRIPTION

NAMENDA™ (memantine hydrochloride) is an orally active NMDA receptor antagonist. The chemical name for memantine hydrochloride is 1-amino-3,5-dimethyladamantane hydrochloride with the following structural formula:

$NH_2 \cdot HCl$ … CH_3 … H_3C

The molecular formula is $C_{12}H_{21}N{\bullet}HCl$ and the molecular weight is 215.76.
Memantine HCl occurs as a fine white to off-white powder and is soluble in water. NAMENDA is available for oral administration as capsule-shaped, film-coated tablets containing 5 mg and 10 mg of memantine hydrochloride. The tablets also contain the following inactive ingredients: microcrystalline cellulose, lactose monohydrate, colloidal silicon dioxide, talc and magnesium stearate. In addition the following inactive ingredients are also present as components of the film coat: hypromellose, triacetin, titanium dioxide, FD & C yellow #6 and FD & C blue #2 (5 mg tablets), iron oxide black (10 mg tablets).

CLINICAL PHARMACOLOGY

Mechanism of Action and Pharmacodynamics
Persistent activation of central nervous system N-methyl-D-aspartate (NMDA) receptors by the excitatory amino acid glutamate has been hypothesized to contribute to the symptomatology of Alzheimer's disease. Memantine is postulated to exert its therapeutic effect through its action as a low to moderate affinity uncompetitive (open-channel) NMDA receptor antagonist which binds preferentially to the NMDA receptor-operated cation channels. There is no evidence that memantine prevents or slows neurodegeneration in patients with Alzheimer's disease.
Memantine showed low to negligible affinity for GABA, benzodiazepine, dopamine, adrenergic, histamine and glycine receptors and for voltage-dependent Ca^{2+}, Na^{+} or K^{+} channels. Memantine also showed antagonistic effects at the $5HT_3$ receptor with a potency similar to that for the NMDA receptor and blocked nicotinic acetylcholine receptors with one-sixth to one-tenth the potency.
In vitro studies have shown that memantine does not affect the reversible inhibition of acetylcholinesterase by donepezil, galantamine, or tacrine.

Pharmacokinetics
Memantine is well absorbed after oral administration and has linear pharmacokinetics over the therapeutic dose range. It is excreted predominantly in the urine, unchanged, and has a terminal elimination half-life of about 60-80 hours.

Absorption and Distribution
Following oral administration memantine is highly absorbed with peak concentrations reached in about 3-7 hours. Food has no effect on the absorption of memantine. The mean volume of distribution of memantine is 9-11 L/kg and the plasma protein binding is low (45%).

Metabolism and Elimination
Memantine undergoes little metabolism, with the majority (57-82%) of an administered dose excreted unchanged in urine; the remainder is converted primarily to three polar metabolites: the N-gludantan conjugate, 6-hydroxy memantine, and 1-nitroso-deaminated memantine. These metabolites possess minimal NMDA receptor antagonist activity. The hepatic microsomal CYP450 enzyme system does not play a significant role in the metabolism of memantine. Memantine has a terminal elimination half-life of about 60-80 hours. Renal clearance involves active tubular secretion moderated by pH dependent tubular reabsorption.

Special Populations
Renal Impairment: Adequate information on the effect of renal impairment on the pharmacokinetics of memantine is not available. As the major route of elimination is renal, however, it is very likely that subjects with moderate and severe renal impairment will have significantly higher exposure than normal subjects.
Elderly: The pharmacokinetics of NAMENDA in young and elderly subjects are similar.
Gender: Following multiple dose administration of NAMENDA 20 mg b.i.d., females had about 45% higher exposure than males, but there was no difference in exposure when body weight was taken into account.

Drug-Drug Interactions
Substrates of Microsomal Enzymes: In vitro studies have shown that memantine produces minimal inhibition of CYP450 enzymes CYP1A2, CYP2A6, CYP2C9, CYP2D6, CYP2E1, and CYP3A4. These data indicate that no pharmacokinetic interactions with drugs metabolized by these enzymes are expected.
Inhibitors of Microsomal Enzymes: Since memantine undergoes minimal metabolism, with the majority of the dose excreted unchanged in urine, an interaction between memantine and drugs that are inhibitors of CYP450 enzymes is unlikely. Coadministration of NAMENDA with the AChE inhibitor donepezil HCl does not affect the pharmacokinetics of either compound.
Drugs Eliminated via Renal Mechanisms: Memantine is eliminated in part by tubular secretion. *In vivo* studies have shown that multiple doses of the diuretic hydrochlorothiazide/triamterene (HCTZ/TA) did not affect the AUC of memantine at steady state. Memantine did not affect the bioavailability of TA, and decreased AUC and C_{max} of HCTZ by about 20%.
Drugs that make the urine alkaline: The clearance of memantine was reduced by about 80% under alkaline urine conditions at pH 8. Therefore, alterations of urine pH towards the alkaline state may lead to an accumulation of the drug with a possible increase in adverse effects. Drugs that alkalinize the urine (e.g. carbonic anhydrase inhibitors, sodium bicarbonate) would be expected to reduce renal elimination of memantine.
Drugs highly bound to plasma proteins: Because the plasma protein binding of memantine is low (45%), an interaction with drugs that are highly bound to plasma proteins, such as warfarin and digoxin, is unlikely.

CLINICAL TRIALS

The effectiveness of NAMENDA (memantine hydrochloride) as a treatment for patients with moderate to severe Alzheimer's disease was demonstrated in 2 randomized, double-blind, placebo-controlled clinical studies (Studies 1 and 2) conducted in the United States that assessed both cognitive function and day to day function. The mean age of patients participating in these two trials was 76 with a range of 50-93 years. Approximately 66% of patients were female and 91% of patients were Caucasian.

A third study (Study 3), carried out in Latvia, enrolled patients with severe dementia, but did not assess cognitive function as a planned endpoint.

Study Outcome Measures: In each U.S. study, the effectiveness of NAMENDA was determined using both an instrument designed to evaluate overall function through caregiver-related assessment, and an instrument that measures cognition. Both studies showed that patients on NAMENDA experienced significant improvement on both measures compared to placebo.

Day-to-day function was assessed in both studies using the modified Alzheimer's disease Cooperative Study – Activities of Daily Living inventory (ADCS-ADL). The ADCS-ADL consists of a comprehensive battery of ADL questions used to measure the functional capabilities of patients. Each ADL item is rated from the highest level of independent performance to complete loss. The investigator performs the inventory by interviewing a caregiver familiar with the behavior of the patient. A subset of 19 items, including ratings of the patients' ability to eat, dress, bathe, telephone, travel, shop, and perform other household chores has been validated for the assessment of patients with moderate to severe dementia. This is the modified ADCS-ADL, which has a scoring range of 0 to 54, with the lower scores indicating greater functional impairment.

The ability of NAMENDA to improve cognitive performance was assessed in both studies with the Severe Impairment Battery (SIB), a multi-item instrument that has been validated for the evaluation of cognitive function in patients with moderate to severe dementia. The SIB examines selected aspects of cognitive performance, including elements of attention, orientation, language, memory, visuospatial ability, construction, praxis, and social interaction. The SIB scoring range is from 0 to 100, with lower scores indicating greater cognitive impairment.

Study 1 (Twenty-Eight-Week Study)
In a study of 28 weeks duration, 252 patients with moderate to severe probable Alzheimer's disease (diagnosed by DSM-IV and NINCDS-ADRDA criteria, with Mini-Mental State Examination scores ≥3 and ≤14 and Global Deterioration Scale Stages 5-6) were randomized to NAMENDA or placebo. For patients randomized to NAMENDA, treatment was initiated at 5 mg once daily and increased weekly by 5 mg/day in divided doses to a dose of 20 mg/day (10 mg twice a day).

Effects on the ADCS-ADL:
Figure 1 shows the time course for the change from baseline in the ADCS-ADL score for patients in the two treatment groups completing the 28 weeks of the study. At 28 weeks of treatment, the mean difference in the ADCS-ADL change scores for the NAMENDA-treated patients compared to the patients on placebo was 3.4 units. Using an analysis based on all patients and carrying their last study observation forward (LOCF analysis), NAMENDA treatment was statistically significantly superior to placebo.

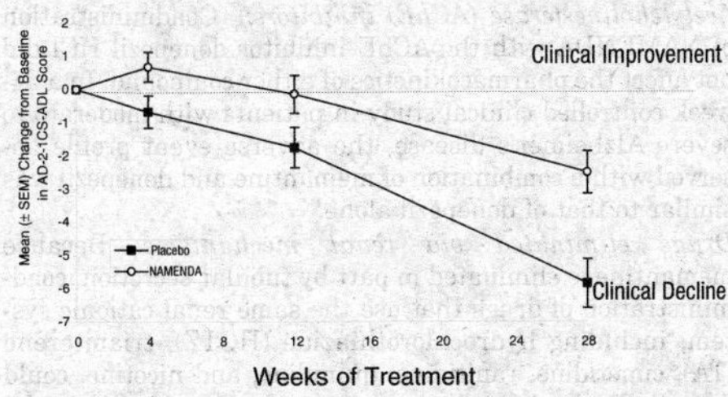

Figure 1: Time course of the change from baseline in ADCS-ADL score for patients completing 28 weeks of treatment.

Figure 2 shows the cumulative percentages of patients from each of the treatment groups who had attained at least the change in the ADCS-ADL shown on the X axis. The curves show that both patients assigned to NAMENDA and placebo have a wide range of responses and generally show deterioration (a negative change in ADCS-ADL compared to baseline), but that the NAMENDA group is more likely to show a smaller decline or an improvement. (In a cumulative distribution display, a curve for an effective treatment would be shifted to the left of the curve for placebo, while an ineffective or deleterious treatment would be superimposed upon or shifted to the right of the curve for placebo.)

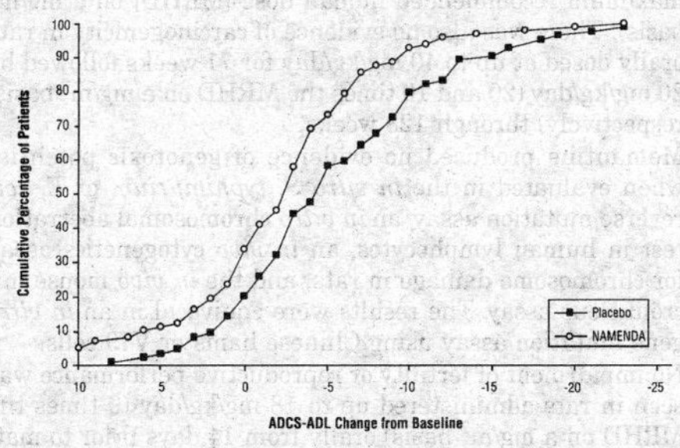

Figure 2: Cumulative percentage of patients completing 28 weeks of double-blind treatment with specified changes from baseline in ADCS-ADL scores.

Effects on the SIB:
Figure 3 shows the time course for the change from baseline in SIB score for the two treatment groups over the 28 weeks of the study. At 28 weeks of treatment, the mean difference in the SIB change scores for the NAMENDA-treated patients compared to the patients on placebo was 5.7 units. Using an LOCF analysis, NAMENDA treatment was statistically significantly superior to placebo.

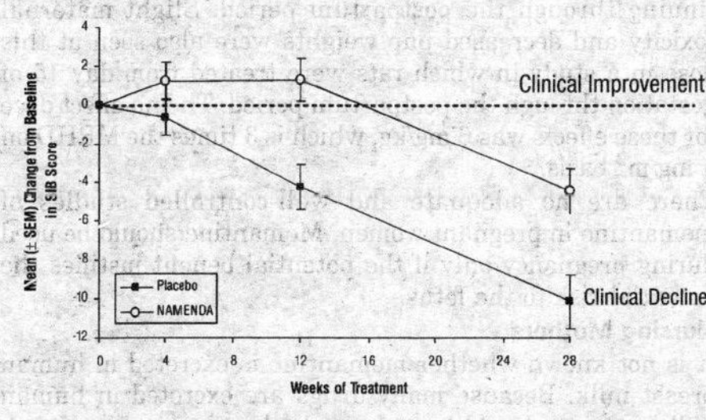

Figure 3: Time course of the change from baseline in SIB score for patients completing 28 weeks of treatment.

Figure 4 shows the cumulative percentages of patients from each treatment group who had attained at least the measure of change in SIB score shown on the X axis.

The curves show that both patients assigned to NAMENDA and placebo have a wide range of responses and generally show deterioration, but that the NAMENDA group is more likely to show a smaller decline or an improvement.

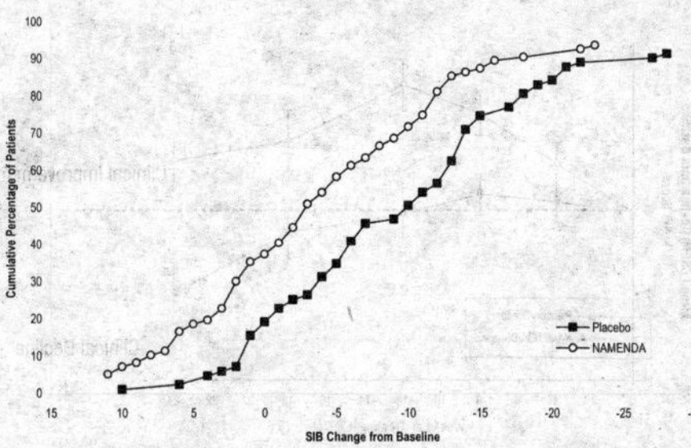

Figure 4: Cumulative percentage of patients completing 28 weeks of double-blind treatment with specified changes from baseline in SIB scores.

Study 2 (Twenty-Four-Week Study)
In a study of 24 weeks duration, 404 patients with moderate to severe probable Alzheimer's disease (diagnosed by NINCDS-ADRDA criteria, with Mini-Mental State Examination scores ≥5 and ≤14) who had been treated with donepezil for at least 6 months and who had been on a stable dose of donepezil for the last 3 months were randomized to NAMENDA or placebo while still receiving donepezil. For patients randomized to NAMENDA, treatment was initiated at 5 mg once daily and increased weekly by 5 mg/day in divided doses to a dose of 20 mg/day (10 mg twice a day).

Effects on the ADCS-ADL:
Figure 5 shows the time course for the change from baseline in the ADCS-ADL score for the two treatment groups over the 24 weeks of the study. At 24 weeks of treatment, the mean difference in the ADCS-ADL change scores for the NAMENDA/donepezil treated patients (combination therapy) compared to the patients on placebo/donepezil (monotherapy) was 1.6 units. Using an LOCF analysis, NAMENDA/donepezil treatment was statistically significantly superior to placebo/donepezil.

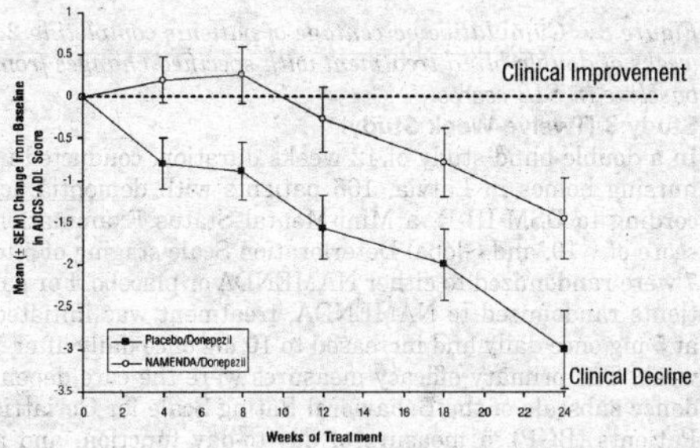

Figure 5: Time course of the change from baseline in ADCS-ADL score for patients completing 24 weeks of treatment.

Figure 6 shows the cumulative percentages of patients from each of the treatment groups who had attained at least the measure of improvement in the ADCS-ADL shown on the X axis.

The curves show that both patients assigned to NAMENDA/donepezil and placebo/donepezil have a wide range of responses and generally show deterioration, but that the NAMENDA/donepezil group is more likely to show a smaller decline or an improvement.

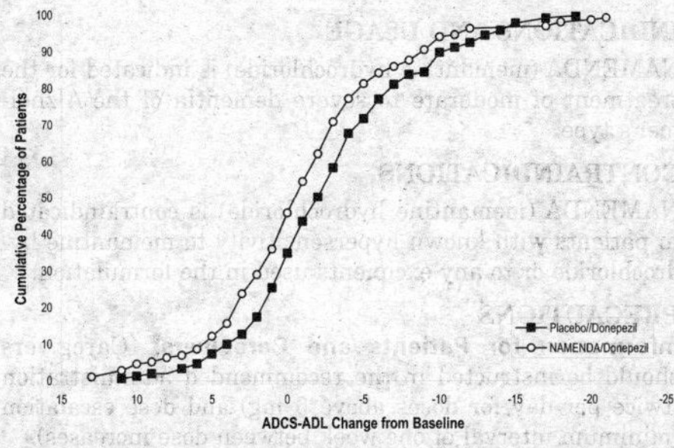

Figure 6: Cumulative percentage of patients completing 24 weeks of double-blind treatment with specified changes from baseline in ADCS-ADL scores.

Effects on the SIB:
Figure 7 shows the time course for the change from baseline in SIB score for the two treatment groups over the 24 weeks of the study. At 24 weeks of treatment, the mean difference in the SIB change scores for the NAMENDA/donepezil-treated patients compared to the patients on placebo/donepezil was 3.3 units. Using an LOCF analysis, NAMENDA/

Continued on next page

Namenda—Cont.

donepezil treatment was statistically significantly superior to placebo/donepezil.

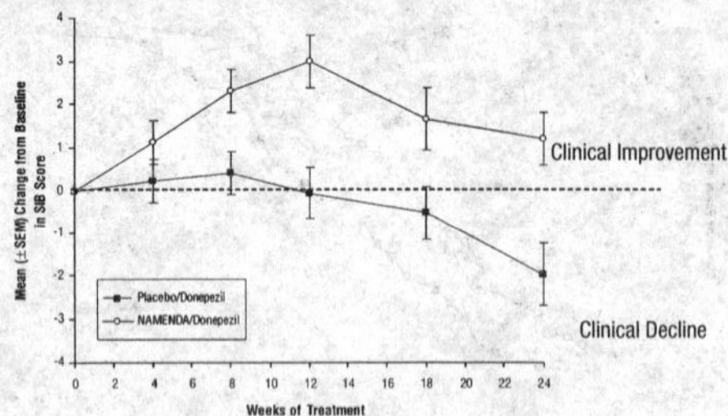

Figure 7: Time course of the change from baseline in SIB score for patients completing 24 weeks of treatment.

Figure 8 shows the cumulative percentages of patients from each treatment group who had attained at least the measure of improvement in SIB score shown on the X axis.

The curves show that both patients assigned to NAMENDA/donepezil and placebo/donepezil have a wide range of responses, but that the NAMENDA/donepezil group is more likely to show an improvement or a smaller decline.

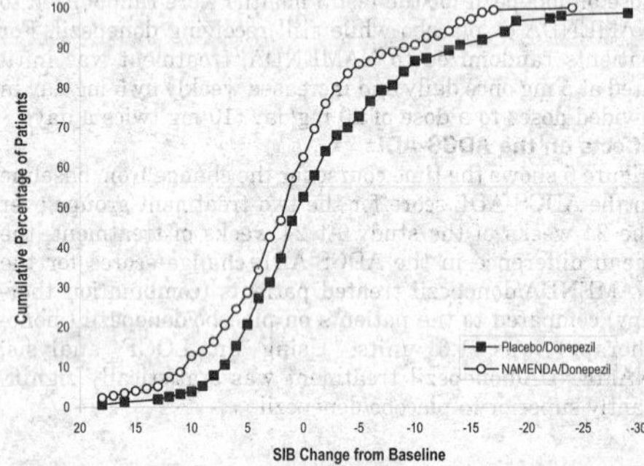

Figure 8: Cumulative percentage of patients completing 24 weeks of double-blind treatment with specified changes from baseline in SIB scores.

Study 3 (Twelve-Week Study)

In a double-blind study of 12 weeks duration, conducted in nursing homes in Latvia, 166 patients with dementia according to DSM-III-R, a Mini-Mental Status Examination score of <10, and Global Deterioration Scale staging of 5 to 7 were randomized to either NAMENDA or placebo. For patients randomized to NAMENDA, treatment was initiated at 5 mg once daily and increased to 10 mg once daily after 1 week. The primary efficacy measures were the care dependency subscale of the Behavioral Rating Scale for Geriatric Patients (BGP), a measure of day-to-day function, and a Clinical Global Impression of Change (CGI-C), a measure of overall clinical effect. No valid measure of cognitive function was used in this study. A statistically significant treatment difference at 12 weeks that favored NAMENDA over placebo was seen on both primary efficacy measures. Because the patients entered were a mixture of Alzheimer's disease and vascular dementia, an attempt was made to distinguish the two groups and all patients were later designated as having either vascular dementia or Alzheimer's disease, based on their scores on the Hachinski Ischemic Scale at study entry. Only about 50% of the patients had computerized tomography of the brain. For the subset designated as having Alzheimer's disease, a statistically significant treatment effect favoring NAMENDA over placebo at 12 weeks was seen on both the BGP and CGI-C.

INDICATIONS AND USAGE

NAMENDA (memantine hydrochloride) is indicated for the treatment of moderate to severe dementia of the Alzheimer's type.

CONTRAINDICATIONS

NAMENDA (memantine hydrochloride) is contraindicated in patients with known hypersensitivity to memantine hydrochloride or to any excipients used in the formulation.

PRECAUTIONS

Information for Patients and Caregivers: Caregivers should be instructed in the recommended administration (twice per day for doses above 5 mg) and dose escalation (minimum interval of one week between dose increases).

Neurological Conditions

Seizures: NAMENDA has not been systematically evaluated in patients with a seizure disorder. In clinical trials of NAMENDA, seizures occurred in 0.2% of patients treated with NAMENDA and 0.5% of patients treated with placebo.

Genitourinary Conditions

Conditions that raise urine pH may decrease the urinary elimination of memantine resulting in increased plasma levels of memantine.

Special Populations

Hepatic Impairment

NAMENDA undergoes partial hepatic metabolism, but the major fraction of a dose (57-82%) is excreted unchanged in urine. The pharmacokinetics of memantine in patients with hepatic impairment have not been investigated, but would be expected to be only modestly affected.

Renal Impairment

There are inadequate data available in patients with mild, moderate, and severe renal impairment but it is likely that patients with moderate renal impairment will have higher exposure than normal subjects. Dose reduction in these patients should be considered. The use of NAMENDA in patients with severe renal impairment is not recommended.

Drug-Drug Interactions

N-methyl-D-aspartate (NMDA) antagonists: The combined use of NAMENDA with other NMDA antagonists (amantadine, ketamine, and dextromethorphan) has not been systematically evaluated and such use should be approached with caution.

Effects of NAMENDA on substrates of microsomal enzymes: In vitro studies conducted with marker substrates of CYP450 enzymes (CYP1A2, -2A6, -2C9, -2D6, -2E1, -3A4) showed minimal inhibition of these enzymes by memantine. No pharmacokinetic interactions with drugs metabolized by these enzymes are expected.

Effects of inhibitors and/or substrates of microsomal enzymes on NAMENDA: Memantine is predominantly renally eliminated, and drugs that are substrates and/or inhibitors of the CYP450 system are not expected to alter the metabolism of memantine.

Acetylcholinesterase (AChE) inhibitors: Coadministration of NAMENDA with the AChE inhibitor donepezil HCl did not affect the pharmacokinetics of either compound. In a 24-week controlled clinical study in patients with moderate to severe Alzheimer's disease, the adverse event profile observed with a combination of memantine and donepezil was similar to that of donepezil alone.

Drugs eliminated via renal mechanisms: Because memantine is eliminated in part by tubular secretion, coadministration of drugs that use the same renal cationic system, including hydrochlorothiazide (HCTZ), triamterene (TA), cimetidine, ranitidine, quinidine, and nicotine, could potentially result in altered plasma levels of both agents. However, coadministration of NAMENDA and HCTZ/TA did not affect the bioavailability of either memantine or TA, and the bioavailability of HCTZ decreased by 20%.

Drugs that make the urine alkaline: The clearance of memantine was reduced by about 80% under alkaline urine conditions at pH 8. Therefore, alterations of urine pH towards the alkaline condition may lead to an accumulation of the drug with a possible increase in adverse effects. Urine pH is altered by diet, drugs (e.g. carbonic anhydrase inhibitors, sodium bicarbonate) and clinical state of the patient (e.g. renal tubular acidosis or severe infections of the urinary tract). Hence, memantine should be used with caution under these conditions.

Carcinogenesis, Mutagenesis and Impairment of Fertility

There was no evidence of carcinogenicity in a 113-week oral study in mice at doses up to 40 mg/kg/day (10 times the maximum recommended human dose [MRHD] on a mg/m^2 basis). There was also no evidence of carcinogenicity in rats orally dosed at up to 40 mg/kg/day for 71 weeks followed by 20 mg/kg/day (20 and 10 times the MRHD on a mg/m^2 basis, respectively) through 128 weeks.

Memantine produced no evidence of genotoxic potential when evaluated in the *in vitro S. typhimurium* or *E. coli* reverse mutation assay, an *in vitro* chromosomal aberration test in human lymphocytes, an *in vivo* cytogenetics assay for chromosome damage in rats, and the *in vivo* mouse micronucleus assay. The results were equivocal in an *in vitro* gene mutation assay using Chinese hamster V79 cells.

No impairment of fertility or reproductive performance was seen in rats administered up to 18 mg/kg/day (9 times the MRHD on a mg/m^2 basis) orally from 14 days prior to mating through gestation and lactation in females, or for 60 days prior to mating in males.

Pregnancy

Pregnancy Category B: Memantine given orally to pregnant rats and pregnant rabbits during the period of organogenesis was not teratogenic up to the highest doses tested (18 mg/kg/day in rats and 30 mg/kg/day in rabbits, which are 9 and 30 times, respectively, the maximum recommended human dose [MRHD] on a mg/m^2 basis).

Slight maternal toxicity, decreased pup weights and an increased incidence of nonossified cervical vertebrae were seen at an oral dose of 18 mg/kg/day in a study in which rats were given oral memantine beginning pre-mating and continuing through the postpartum period. Slight maternal toxicity and decreased pup weights were also seen at this dose in a study in which rats were treated from day 15 of gestation through the postpartum period. The no-effect dose for these effects was 6 mg/kg, which is 3 times the MRHD on a mg/m^2 basis.

There are no adequate and well-controlled studies of memantine in pregnant women. Memantine should be used during pregnancy only if the potential benefit justifies the potential risk to the fetus.

Nursing Mothers

It is not known whether memantine is excreted in human breast milk. Because many drugs are excreted in human milk, caution should be exercised when memantine is administered to a nursing mother.

Pediatric Use

There are no adequate and well-controlled trials documenting the safety and efficacy of memantine in any illness occurring in children.

ADVERSE REACTIONS

The experience described in this section derives from studies in patients with Alzheimer's disease and vascular dementia.

Adverse Events Leading to Discontinuation: In placebo-controlled trials in which dementia patients received doses of NAMENDA up to 20 mg/day, the likelihood of discontinuation because of an adverse event was the same in the NAMENDA group as in the placebo group. No individual adverse event was associated with the discontinuation of treatment in 1% or more of NAMENDA-treated patients and at a rate greater than placebo.

Adverse Events Reported in Controlled Trials: The reported adverse events in NAMENDA (memantine hydrochloride) trials reflect experience gained under closely monitored conditions in a highly selected patient population. In actual practice or in other clinical trials, these frequency estimates may not apply, as the conditions of use, reporting behavior and the types of patients treated may differ. Table 1 lists treatment-emergent signs and symptoms that were reported in at least 2% of patients in placebo-controlled dementia trials and for which the rate of occurrence was greater for patients treated with NAMENDA than for those treated with placebo. No adverse event occurred at a frequency of at least 5% and twice the placebo rate.

Table 1: Adverse Events Reported in Controlled Clinical Trials in at Least 2% of Patients Receiving NAMENDA and at a Higher Frequency than Placebo-treated Patients.

Body System Adverse Event	Placebo (N = 922) %	NAMENDA (N = 940) %
Body as a Whole		
Fatigue	1	2
Pain	1	3
Cardiovascular System		
Hypertension	2	4
Central and Peripheral Nervous System		
Dizziness	5	7
Headache	3	6
Gastrointestinal System		
Constipation	3	5
Vomiting	2	3
Musculoskeletal System		
Back pain	2	3
Psychiatric Disorders		
Confusion	5	6
Somnolence	2	3
Hallucination	2	3
Respiratory System		
Coughing	3	4
Dyspnea	1	2

Other adverse events occurring with an incidence of at least 2% in NAMENDA-treated patients but at a greater or equal rate on placebo were agitation, fall, inflicted injury, urinary incontinence, diarrhea, bronchitis, insomnia, urinary tract infection, influenza-like symptoms, gait abnormal, depression, upper respiratory tract infection, anxiety, peripheral edema, nausea, anorexia, and arthralgia.

The overall profile of adverse events and the incidence rates for individual adverse events in the subpopulation of patients with moderate to severe Alzheimer's disease were not different from the profile and incidence rates described above for the overall dementia population.

Vital Sign Changes: NAMENDA and placebo groups were compared with respect to (1) mean change from baseline in vital signs (pulse, systolic blood pressure, diastolic blood pressure, and weight) and (2) the incidence of patients meeting criteria for potentially clinically significant changes from baseline in these variables. There were no clinically important changes in vital signs in patients treated with NAMENDA. A comparison of supine and standing vital sign measures for NAMENDA and placebo in elderly normal subjects indicated that NAMENDA treatment is not associated with orthostatic changes.

Laboratory Changes: NAMENDA and placebo groups were compared with respect to (1) mean change from baseline in various serum chemistry, hematology, and urinalysis variables and (2) the incidence of patients meeting criteria for potentially clinically significant changes from baseline in these variables. These analyses revealed no clinically important changes in laboratory test parameters associated with NAMENDA treatment.

ECG Changes: NAMENDA and placebo groups were compared with respect to (1) mean change from baseline in various ECG parameters and (2) the incidence of patients meeting criteria for potentially clinically significant changes from baseline in these variables. These analyses revealed no clinically important changes in ECG parameters associated with NAMENDA treatment.

Other Adverse Events Observed During Clinical Trials

NAMENDA has been administered to approximately 1350 patients with dementia, of whom more than 1200 received the maximum recommended dose of 20 mg/day. Patients received NAMENDA treatment for periods of up to 884 days, with 862 patients receiving at least 24 weeks of treatment and 387 patients receiving 48 weeks or more of treatment.

Treatment emergent signs and symptoms that occurred during 8 controlled clinical trials and 4 open-label trials were recorded as adverse events by the clinical investigators using terminology of their own choosing. To provide an overall estimate of the proportion of individuals having similar types of events, the events were grouped into a smaller number of standardized categories using WHO terminology, and event frequencies were calculated across all studies.

All adverse events occurring in at least two patients are included, except for those already listed in Table 1, WHO terms too general to be informative, minor symptoms or events unlikely to be drug-caused, e.g., because they are common in the study population. Events are classified by body system and listed using the following definitions: frequent adverse events – those occurring in at least 1/100 patients; infrequent adverse events – those occurring in 1/100 to 1/1000 patients. These adverse events are not necessarily related to NAMENDA treatment and in most cases were observed at a similar frequency in placebo-treated patients in the controlled studies.

Body as a Whole: *Frequent:* syncope. *Infrequent:* hypothermia, allergic reaction.

Cardiovascular System: *Frequent:* cardiac failure. *Infrequent:* angina pectoris, bradycardia, myocardial infarction, thrombophlebitis, atrial fibrillation, hypotension, cardiac arrest, postural hypotension, pulmonary embolism, pulmonary edema.

Central and Peripheral Nervous System: *Frequent:* transient ischemic attack, cerebrovascular accident, vertigo, ataxia, hypokinesia. *Infrequent:* paresthesia, convulsions, extrapyramidal disorder, hypertonia, tremor, aphasia, hypoesthesia, abnormal coordination, hemiplegia, hyperkinesia, involuntary muscle contractions, stupor, cerebral hemorrhage, neuralgia, ptosis, neuropathy.

Gastrointestinal System: *Infrequent:* gastroenteritis, diverticulitis, gastrointestinal hemorrhage, melena, esophageal ulceration.

Hemic and Lymphatic Disorders: *Frequent:* anemia. *Infrequent:* leukopenia.

Metabolic and Nutritional Disorders: *Frequent:* increased alkaline phosphatase, decreased weight. *Infrequent:* dehydration, hyponatremia, aggravated diabetes mellitus.

Psychiatric Disorders: *Frequent:* aggressive reaction. *Infrequent:* delusion, personality disorder, emotional lability, nervousness, sleep disorder, libido increased, psychosis, amnesia, apathy, paranoid reaction, thinking abnormal, crying abnormal, appetite increased, paroniria, delirium, depersonalization, neurosis, suicide attempt.

Respiratory System: *Frequent:* pneumonia. *Infrequent:* apnea, asthma, hemoptysis.

Skin and Appendages: *Frequent:* rash. *Infrequent:* skin ulceration, pruritus, cellulitis, eczema, dermatitis, erythematous rash, alopecia, urticaria

Special Senses: *Frequent:* cataract, conjunctivitis. *Infrequent:* macula lutea degeneration, decreased visual acuity, decreased hearing, tinnitus, blepharitis, blurred vision, corneal opacity, glaucoma, conjunctival hemorrhage, eye pain, retinal hemorrhage, xerophthalmia, diplopia, abnormal lacrimation, myopia, retinal detachment.

Urinary System: *Frequent:* frequent micturition. *Infrequent:* dysuria, hematuria, urinary retention

ADVERSE EVENTS FROM OTHER SOURCES

Memantine has been commercially available outside the United States since 1982, and has been evaluated in clinical trials including trials in patients with neuropathic pain, Parkinson's disease, organic brain syndrome, and spasticity. The following adverse events of possible importance for which there is inadequate data to determine the causal relationship have been reported to be temporally associated with memantine treatment in more than one patient and are not described elsewhere in labeling: acne, bone fracture, carpal tunnel syndrome, claudication, hyperlipidemia, impotence, otitis media, thrombocytopenia.

ANIMAL TOXICOLOGY

Memantine induced neuronal lesions (vacuolation and necrosis) in the multipolar and pyramidal cells in cortical layers III and IV of the posterior cingulate and retrosplenial neocortices in rats, similar to those which are known to occur in rodents administered other NMDA receptor antagonists. Lesions were seen after a single dose of memantine. In a study in which rats were given daily oral doses of memantine for 14 days, the no-effect dose for neuronal necrosis was 6 times the maximum recommended human dose on a mg/m^2 basis. The potential for induction of central neuronal vacuolation and necrosis by NMDA receptor antagonists in humans is unknown.

DRUG ABUSE AND DEPENDENCE

Controlled Substance Class: Memantine HCl is not a controlled substance.

Physical and Psychological Dependence: Memantine HCl is a low to moderate affinity uncompetitive NMDA antagonist that did not produce any evidence of drug-seeking behavior or withdrawal symptoms upon discontinuation in 2,504 patients who participated in clinical trials at therapeutic doses. Post marketing data, outside the U.S., retrospectively collected, has provided no evidence of drug abuse or dependence.

OVERDOSAGE

Because strategies for the management of overdose are continually evolving, it is advisable to contact a poison control center to determine the latest recommendations for the management of an overdose of any drug.

As in any cases of overdose, general supportive measures should be utilized, and treatment should be symptomatic. Elimination of memantine can be enhanced by acidification of urine. In a documented case of an overdosage with up to 400 mg of memantine, the patient experienced restlessness, psychosis, visual hallucinations, somnolence, stupor and loss of consciousness. The patient recovered without permanent sequelae.

DOSAGE AND ADMINISTRATION

The dosage of NAMENDA (memantine hydrochloride) shown to be effective in controlled clinical trials is 20 mg/day.

The recommended starting dose of NAMENDA is 5 mg once daily. The recommended target dose is 20 mg/day. The dose should be increased in 5 mg increments to 10 mg/day (5 mg twice a day), 15 mg/day (5 mg and 10 mg as separate doses), and 20 mg/day (10 mg twice a day). The minimum recommended interval between dose increases is one week.

NAMENDA can be taken with or without food.

Doses in Special Populations

Dose reduction in patients with moderate renal impairment should be considered. In patients with severe renal impairment the use of NAMENDA has not been systematically evaluated and is not recommended. (See Clinical Pharmacology-Pharmacokinetics)

HOW SUPPLIED

5 mg Tablet:

Bottle of 60 NDC #0456-3205-60
10 × 10 Unit Dose NDC #0456-3205-63

The capsule-shaped, film-coated tablets are tan, with the strength (5) debossed on one side and FL on the other.

10 mg Tablet:

Bottle of 60 NDC #0456-3210-60
10 × 10 Unit Dose NDC #0456-3210-63

The capsule-shaped, film-coated tablets are gray, with the strength (10) debossed on one side and FL on the other.

Titration Pak:

PVC/Aluminum Blister package containing 49 tablets. 28 × 5 mg and 21 × 10 mg tablets. NDC #0456-3200-14

The 5 mg capsule-shaped, film-coated tablets are tan, with the strength (5) debossed on one side and FL on the other. The 10 mg capsule-shaped, film-coated tablets are gray, with the strength (10) debossed on one side and FL on the other.

Store at 25°C (77°F); excursions permitted to 15-30°C (59-86°F)[see USP Controlled Room Temperature]

Forest Pharmaceuticals, Inc.
Subsidiary of Forest Laboratories, Inc.
St. Louis, MO 63045
Licensed from Merz Pharmaceuticals GmbH
10/03

TESSALON® ℞
(benzonatate, USP)
100 mg Perles/
200 mg Capsules
℞ only

DESCRIPTION

TESSALON, a non-narcotic oral antitussive agent, is 2, 5, 8, 11, 14, 17, 20, 23, 26-nonaoxaoctacosan-28-yl p-(butylamino) benzoate; with a molecular weight of 603.7.

$$CH_3(CH_2)_2CH_2NH-C_6H_4-COOCH_2CH_2(OCH_2CH_2)_nOCH_3$$

$$C_{30}H_{53}NO_{11}$$

Each TESSALON Perle contains:
Benzonatate, USP 100 mg
Each TESSALON Capsule contains:
Benzonatate, USP 200 mg

TESSALON Capsules also contain: D&C Yellow 10, gelatin, glycerin, methylparaben and propylparaben.

CLINICAL PHARMACOLOGY

TESSALON acts peripherally by anesthetizing the stretch receptors located in the respiratory passages, lungs, and pleura by dampening their activity and thereby reducing the cough reflex at its source. It begins to act within 15 to 20 minutes and its effect lasts for 3 to 8 hours. TESSALON has no inhibitory effect on the respiratory center in recommended dosage.

INDICATIONS AND USAGE

TESSALON is indicated for the symptomatic relief of cough.

CONTRAINDICATIONS

Hypersensitivity to benzonatate or related compounds.

WARNINGS

Severe hypersensitivity reactions (including bronchospasm, laryngospasm and cardiovascular collapse) have been reported which are possibly related to local anesthesia from sucking or chewing the perle instead of swallowing it. Severe reactions have required intervention with vasopressor agents and supportive measures.

Isolated instances of bizarre behavior, including mental confusion and visual hallucinations, have also been reported in patients taking TESSALON in combination with other prescribed drugs.

PRECAUTIONS

Benzonatate is chemically related to anesthetic agents of the para-amino-benzoic acid class (e.g., procaine; tetracaine) and has been associated with adverse CNS effects possibly related to a prior sensitivity to related agents or interaction with concomitant medication.

Information for Patients: Release of TESSALON from the capsule in the mouth can produce a temporary local anesthesia of the oral mucosa and choking could occur. Therefore, the capsules should be swallowed without chewing.

Usage in Pregnancy: Pregnancy Category C. Animal reproduction studies have not been conducted with TESSALON. It is also not known whether TESSALON can cause fetal harm when administered to a pregnant woman or can affect reproduction capacity. TESSALON should be given to a pregnant woman only if clearly needed.

Nursing Mothers: It is not known whether this drug is excreted in human milk. Because many drugs are excreted in human milk caution should be exercised when TESSALON is administered to a nursing woman.

Carcinogenesis, Mutagenesis, Impairment of Fertility: Carcinogenicity, mutagenicity, and reproduction studies have not been conducted with TESSALON.

Pediatric Use: Safety and effectiveness in children below the age of 10 has not been established.

ADVERSE REACTIONS

Potential Adverse Reactions to TESSALON may include:

Hypersensitivity reactions including bronchospasm, laryngospasm, cardiovascular collapse possibly related to local anesthesia from chewing or sucking the capsule.

CNS: sedation; headache; dizziness; mental confusion; visual hallucinations.

GI: constipation, nausea, GI upset.

Dermatologic: pruritus; skin eruptions.

Other: nasal congestion; sensation of burning in the eyes; vague "chilly" sensation; numbness of the chest; hypersensitivity.

Rare instances of deliberate or accidental overdose have resulted in death.

OVERDOSAGE

Overdose may result in death.

The drug is chemically related to tetracaine and other topical anesthetics and shares various aspects of their pharmacology and toxicology. Drugs of this type are generally well absorbed after ingestion.

Signs and Symptoms:

If capsules are chewed or dissolved in the mouth, oropharyngeal anesthesia will develop rapidly. CNS stimulation may cause restlessness and tremors which may proceed to clonic convulsions followed by profound CNS depression.

Treatment:

Evacuate gastric contents and administer copious amounts of activated charcoal slurry. Even in the conscious patient, cough and gag reflexes may be so depressed as to necessitate special attention to protection against aspiration of gastric contents and orally administered materials. Convulsions should be treated with a short-acting barbiturate given intravenously and carefully titrated for the smallest effective dosage. Intensive support of respiration and cardiovascular-renal function is an essential feature of the treatment of severe intoxication from overdosage.

Do not use CNS stimulants.

DOSAGE AND ADMINISTRATION

Adults and Children over 10: Usual dose is one 100 mg or 200 mg capsule t.i.d. as required. If necessary, up to 600 mg daily may be given.

HOW SUPPLIED

Perles, 100 mg (yellow); bottles of 100
NDC 0456-0688-01 Imprint: T.
Perles, 100 mg (yellow); bottles of 500
NDC 0456-0688-02 Imprint: T.
Capsules, 200 mg (yellow); bottles of 100
NDC 0456-0698-01 Imprint: 0698.
Capsules, 200 mg (yellow); bottles of 500
NDC 0456-0698-02 Imprint: 0698.

Store at 25°C (77°F); excursions permitted to 15–30°C (59–86°F) [see USP Controlled Room Temperature].

Rev. 3/03 (04)

Mfd by
Cardinal Health
St. Petersburg, Florida 33716
for
FOREST PHARMACEUTICALS, INC.
SUBSIDIARY OF FOREST LABORATORIES, INC.
ST. LOUIS, MISSOURI 63045

Shown in Product Identification Guide, page 312

Continued on next page

THYROLAR® Tablets

Name	Composition (T_3/T_4 per tablet)	Color	Armacode®	NDC
Thyrolar—1/4	3.1 mcg/12.5 mcg	Violet/White	YC	0456–0040–01
Thyrolar—1/2	6.25 mcg/25 mcg	Peach/White	YD	0456–0045–01
Thyrolar—1	12.5 mcg/50 mcg	Pink/White	YE	0456–0050–01
Thyrolar—2	25 mcg/100 mcg	Green/White	YF	0456–0055–01
Thyrolar—3	37.5 mcg/150 mcg	Yellow/White	YH	0456–0060–01

THYROLAR® Tablets ℞
[thī-rō-lär]
(Liotrix Tablets, USP)

DESCRIPTION

Thyrolar Tablets (Liotrix Tablets, USP) contain triiodothyronine (T_3 liothyronine) sodium and tetraiodothyronine (T_4 levothyroxine) sodium in the amounts listed in the "How Supplied" section. (T_3 liothyronine sodium is approximately four times as potent as T_4 thyroxine on a microgram for microgram basis.)
The inactive ingredients are calcium phosphate, colloidal silicon dioxide, corn starch, lactose, and magnesium stearate. The tablets also contain the following dyes: Thyrolar 1/4-FD&C Blue #1 and FD&C Red #40; Thyrolar 1/2-FD&C Red #40 and D&C Yellow #10; Thyrolar 1-FD&C Red #40; Thyrolar 2-FD&C Blue #1, FD&C Red #40, and D&C Yellow #10; Thyrolar 3-FD&C Red #40 and D&C Yellow #10.

STRUCTURAL FORMULAS

Liothyronine (T_3) Sodium

Levothyroxine (T_4) Sodium

HOW SUPPLIED

Thyrolar Tablets (Liotrix Tablets, USP) are available in five potencies coded as follows:
[See table above]
Supplied in bottles of 100, two-layered compressed tablets. Tablets should be stored at cold temperature, between 36° and 46°F (2° and 8°C) in a tight, light-resistant container.
Note: (T_3 liothyronine sodium is approximately four times as potent as T_4 thyroxine on a microgram for microgram basis.)
Rev. 11/02 14361102
FOREST PHARMACEUTICALS, INC.
A Subsidiary of Forest Laboratories, Inc.
St. Louis, MO 63045

Shown in Product Identification Guide, page 312

TIAZAC® ℞
(diltiazem hydrochloride)
Extended Release Capsules
USP Drug Release Test 6

DESCRIPTION

Tiazac® (diltiazem hydrochloride) is a calcium ion cellular influx inhibitor (slow channel blocker). Chemically, diltiazem hydrochloride is 1,5-Benzothiazepin-4(5H)-one, 3-(acetyloxy)-5[2-(dimethylamino)ethyl]-2,-3-dihydro-2(4-methoxyphenyl)-, mono-hydrochloride, (+)-cis. The chemical structure is:

Diltiazem hydrochloride is a white to off-white crystalline powder with a bitter taste. It is soluble in water, methanol and chloroform and has a molecular weight of 450.98. Tiazac® capsules contain diltiazem hydrochloride in extended release beads at doses of 120, 180, 240, 300, 360 and 420 mg.
Tiazac® also contains: Microcrystalline Cellulose NF, Sucrose Stearate, Eudragit, Povidone USP, Talc USP, Magnesium Stearate NF, Hypromellose USP, Titanium Dioxide USP, Polysorbate NF, Simethicone USP, Gelatin NF, FD&C Blue #1, FD&C Red #40, D&C Red #28, FD&C Green #3, Black Iron Oxide USP, and other solids.
For oral administration.

CLINICAL PHARMACOLOGY

The therapeutic effects of diltiazem hydrochloride are believed to be related to its ability to inhibit the cellular influx of calcium ions during membrane depolarization of cardiac and vascular smooth muscle.
Mechanisms of Action.
Hypertension: Diltiazem produces its antihypertensive effect primarily by relaxation of vascular smooth muscle and the resultant decrease in peripheral vascular resistance. The magnitude of blood pressure reduction is related to the degree of hypertension: thus hypertensive individuals experience an antihypertensive effect, whereas there is only a modest fall in blood pressure in normotensives.
Angina: Diltiazem HCl has been shown to produce increases in exercise tolerance, probably due to its ability to reduce myocardial oxygen demand. This is accomplished via reductions in heart rate and systemic blood pressure at submaximal and maximal work loads.
Diltiazem has been shown to be a potent dilator of coronary arteries, both epicardial and subendocardial. Spontaneous and ergonovine-induced coronary artery spasm are inhibited by diltiazem.
In animal models, diltiazem interferes with the slow inward (depolarizing) current in excitable tissue. It causes excitation-contraction uncoupling in various myocardial tissues without changes in the configuration of the action potential. Diltiazem produces relaxation of the coronary vascular smooth muscle and dilation of both large and small coronary vascular smooth muscle and dilation of both large and small coronary arteries at drug levels which cause little or no negative inotropic effect. The resultant increases in coronary blood flow (epicardial and subendocardial) occur in ischemic and nonischemic models and are accompanied by dose-dependent decreases in systemic blood pressure and decreases in peripheral resistance.
Hemodynamic and Electrophysiologic Effects. Like other calcium channel antagonists, diltiazem decreases sinoatrial and atrioventricular conduction in isolated tissues and has a negative inotropic effect in isolated preparations. In the intact animal, prolongation of the AH interval can be seen at higher doses.
In man, diltiazem prevents spontaneous and ergonovine-provoked coronary artery spasm. It causes a decrease in peripheral vascular resistance and a modest fall in blood pressure in normotensive individuals and, in exercise tolerance studies in patients with ischemic heart disease, reduces the heart rate-blood pressure product for any given work load. Studies to date, primarily in patients with good ventricular function, have not revealed evidence of a negative inotropic effect; cardiac output, ejection fraction, and left ventricular end diastolic pressure have not been affected. Such data have no predictive value with respect to effects in patients with poor ventricular function, and increased heart failure has been reported in patients with preexisting impairment of ventricular function. There are as yet few data on the interaction of diltiazem and beta-blockers in patients with poor ventricular function. Resting heart rate is usually slightly reduced by diltiazem.
Tiazac® produces antihypertensive effects both in the supine and standing positions. Postural hypotension is infrequently noted upon suddenly assuming an upright position. No reflex tachycardia is associated with the chronic antihypertensive effects.
Diltiazem hydrochloride decreases vascular resistance, increases cardiac output (by increasing stroke volume), and produces a slight decrease or no change in heart rate. During dynamic exercise, increases in diastolic pressure are inhibited while maximum achievable systolic pressure is usually reduced. Chronic therapy with diltiazem hydrochloride produces no change or an increase in plasma catecholamines. No increased activity of the renin-angiotensin-aldosterone axis has been observed. Diltiazem hydrochloride reduces the renal and peripheral effects of angiotensin II. Hypertensive animal models respond to diltiazem with reductions in blood pressure and increased urinary output and natriuresis without a change in urinary sodium/potassium ratio. In man, transient natriuresis and kaliuresis have been reported, but only in high intravenous doses of 0.5 mg/kg of body weight.
Diltiazem-associated prolongation of the AH interval is not more pronounced in patients with first degree heart block. In patients with sick sinus syndrome, diltiazem significantly prolongs sinus cycle length (up to 50% in some cases). Intravenous diltiazem in doses of 20 mg prolongs AH conduction time and AV node functional and effective refractory periods by approximately 20%.
In two short-term, double-blind, placebo-controlled studies in 256 hypertensive patients with doses up to 540 mg/day, Tiazac® showed a clinically unimportant but statistically significant, dose-related increase in PR interval (0.008 seconds). There were no instances of greater than first-degree AV block in any of the clinical trials (see WARNINGS).

Pharmacodynamics.
Hypertension: In short-term, double-blind, placebo-controlled clinical trials Tiazac® demonstrated a dose-related antihypertensive response among patients with mild to moderate hypertension. In one parallel-group study of 198 patients Tiazac® was given for four weeks. The changes in diastolic blood pressure measured at trough (24 hours after the dose) for placebo, 90mg, 180mg, 360mg and 540mg were -5.4, -6.3, -6.2, -8.2, and -11.8mm Hg, respectively. Supine diastolic blood pressure as well as standing diastolic and systolic blood pressures also showed statistically significant linear dose response effects.
In another clinical trial that followed a dose-escalation design, Tiazac® also reduced blood pressure in a linear dose-related manner. Supine diastolic blood pressure measured following two week intervals of treatment was reduced by -3.7mm Hg with 120 mg/day versus -2.0mm Hg with placebo, by -7.6mm Hg after escalation to 240 mg/day versus -2.3mm Hg with placebo, by -8.1mm Hg after escalation to 360 mg/day versus -0.9mm Hg with placebo, and by -10.8mm Hg after escalation to 480/540 mg/day versus -2.2mm Hg with placebo.
Angina: In a double-blind, parallel-group, placebo-controlled trial (approximately 50 patients/group, in patients with chronic stable angina), Tiazac® at doses of 120–540/day increased exercise tolerance time. At trough, 24 hours after dosing, exercise tolerance times using a Bruce exercise protocol, increased by 14, 26, 41, 33 and 32 seconds over baseline for placebo and the 120 mg, 240 mg, 360 mg, and 540 mg/day treated patient groups, respectively. At peak, 8 hours after dosing, exercise tolerance times relative to baseline were statistically significantly increased by 13, 38, 64, 55 and 42 seconds for placebo and 120 mg, 240 mg, 360 mg, and 540 mg/day Tiazac® treated patients, respectively. Compared to baseline, Tiazac® treated patients experienced statistically significant reductions in anginal attacks and decreased nitroglycerin requirements when compared to placebo treated patients.
Pharmacokinetics and Metabolism. Diltiazem is well absorbed from the gastrointestinal tract but undergoes substantial hepatic first-pass effect. The absolute bioavailability of an oral dose of an immediate release formulation (compared to intravenous administration) is approximately 40%. Only 2% to 4% of unchanged diltiazem appears in the urine. The plasma elimination half-life of diltiazem is approximately 3.0–4.5 h. Drugs which induce or inhibit hepatic microsomal enzymes may alter diltiazem disposition. Therapeutic blood levels of diltiazem appear to be in the range of 40–200 ng/mL. There is a departure from linearity when dose strengths are increased; the half-life is slightly increased with dose.
The two primary metabolites of diltiazem are desacetyldiltiazem and desmethyldiltiazem. The desacetyl metabolite is approximately 25% to 50% as potent a coronary vasodilator as diltiazem and is present in plasma at concentrations of 10% to 20% of parent diltiazem. However, recent studies employing sensitive and specific analytical methods have confirmed the existence of several sequential metabolic pathways of diltiazem. As many as nine diltiazem metabolites have been identified in the urine of humans. Total radioactivity measurements following single intravenous dose administration in healthy volunteers suggest the presence of other unidentified metabolites. These metabolites are more slowly excreted, (with a half-life of total radioactivity of approximately 20 hours) and attain concentrations in excess of diltiazem.
In vitro binding studies show diltiazem HCl is 70% to 80% bound to plasma proteins. Competitive *in vitro* ligand binding studies have also shown diltiazem HCl binding is not altered by therapeutic concentrations of digoxin, hydrochlorothiazide, phenylbutazone, propranolol, salicylic acid, or warfarin. A study that compared patients with normal hepatic function to patients with cirrhosis who received immediate release diltiazem found an increase in diltiazem elimination half-life and a 69% increase in bioavailability in the hepatically impaired patients. Patients with severely impaired renal function (creatinine clearance <50 mL/min) who received immediate release diltiazem had modestly increased diltiazem concentrations compared to patients with normal renal function.
Tiazac® Capsules. When compared to a regimen of immediate-release tablets at steady-state, approximately 93% of drug is absorbed from the Tiazac® formulation. When Tiazac® was coadministered with a high fat content breakfast, the extent of diltiazem absorption was not affected; T_{max}, however, occurred slightly earlier. The apparent elimination half-life after single or multiple dosing is 4 to 9.5 hours (mean 6.5 hours).
Tiazac® demonstrates non-linear pharmacokinetics. As the daily dose of Tiazac® capsules is increased from 120 to 540 mg, there was a more than proportional increase in diltiazem plasma concentrations as evidenced by an increase of AUC, C_{max} and C_{min} of 6.8, 6 and 8.6 times, respectively, for a 4.5 times increase in dose.

INDICATIONS AND USAGE

Hypertension:
Tiazac® is indicated for the treatment of hypertension. It may be used alone or in combination with other antihypertensive medications.
Chronic Stable Angina:
Tiazac® is indicated for the treatment of chronic stable angina.

MOST COMMON ADVERSE EVENTS IN DOUBLE-BLIND PLACEBO-CONTROLLED HYPERTENSION TRIALS*

Adverse Events (COSTART Term)	Placebo n = 57 # pts(%)	Tiazac® Up to 360 mg n = 149 # pts(%)	Tiazac® 480–540 mg n = 48 # pts(%)	Adverse Events (COSTART Term)	Placebo n = 57 # pts(%)	Tiazac® Up to 360 mg n = 149 # pts(%)	Tiazac® 480–540 mg n = 48 # pts(%)
edema, peripheral	1 (2)	8 (5)	7 (15)	rash	0 (0)	3 (2)	0 (0)
dizziness	4 (7)	6 (4)	2 (4)	infection	2 (4)	2 (1)	3 (6)
vasodilation	1 (2)	5 (3)	1 (2)	diarrhea	0 (0)	2 (1)	1 (2)
dyspepsia	0 (0)	7 (5)	0 (0)	palpitations	0 (0)	2 (1)	1 (2)
pharyngitis	2 (4)	3 (2)	3 (6)	nervousness	0 (0)	3 (2)	0 (0)

MOST COMMON ADVERSE EVENTS IN DOUBLE-BLIND PLACEBO-CONTROLLED ANGINA TRIALS*

Adverse Events (COSTART Term)	Placebo n = 50 # pts(%)	Tiazac® Up to 360 mg n = 158 # pts(%)	Tiazac® 540 mg n = 49 # pts(%)	Adverse Events (COSTART Term)	Placebo n = 50 # pts(%)	Tiazac® Up to 360 mg n = 158 # pts(%)	Tiazac® 540 mg n = 49 # pts(%)
headache	1 (2)	13 (8)	4 (8)	flu syndrome	0 (0)	0 (0)	1 (2)
edema, peripheral	1 (2)	3 (2)	5 (10)	cough increase	0 (0)	2 (1)	1 (2)
pain	1 (2)	10 (6)	3 (6)	extrasystoles	0 (0)	0 (0)	1 (2)
dizziness	0 (0)	5 (3)	5 (10)	gout	0 (0)	2 (1)	1 (2)
asthenia	0 (0)	1 (1)	2 (4)	myalgia	0 (0)	0 (0)	1 (2)
dyspepsia	0 (0)	2 (1)	3 (6)	impotence	0 (0)	0 (0)	1 (2)
dyspnea	0 (0)	1 (1)	3 (6)	conjunctivitis	0 (0)	0 (0)	1 (2)
bronchitis	0 (0)	1 (1)	2 (4)	rash	0 (0)	2 (1)	1 (2)
AV block	0 (0)	0 (0)	2 (4)	abdominal enlargement	0 (0)	0 (0)	1 (2)
infection	0 (0)	2 (1)	1 (2)				

* Adverse events occurring in treated patients at 2% or more than placebo-treated patients.

CONTRAINDICATIONS

Diltiazem is contraindicated in (1) patients with sick sinus syndrome except in the presence of a functioning ventricular pacemaker, (2) patients with second- or third-degree AV block except in the presence of a functioning ventricular pacemaker, (3) patients with severe hypotension (less than 90 mm Hg systolic), (4) patients who have demonstrated hypersensitivity to the drug, and (5) patients with acute myocardial infarction and pulmonary congestion documented by x-ray on admission.

WARNINGS

1. Cardiac Conduction. Diltiazem hydrochloride prolongs AV node refractory periods without significantly prolonging sinus node recovery time, except in patients with sick sinus syndrome. This effect may rarely result in abnormally slow heart rates (particularly in patients with sick sinus syndrome) or second- or third-degree AV block (13 of 3007 patients or 0.43%). Concomitant use of diltiazem with beta-blockers or digitalis may result in additive effects on cardiac conduction. A patient with Prinzmetal's angina developed periods of asystole (2 to 5 seconds) after a single dose of 60 mg of diltiazem.

2. Congestive Heart Failure. Although diltiazem has a negative inotropic effect in isolated animal tissue preparations, hemodynamic studies in humans with normal ventricular function have not shown a reduction in cardiac index nor consistent negative effects on contractility (dp/dt). An acute study of oral diltiazem in patients with impaired ventricular function (ejection fraction 24% ± 6%) showed improvement in indices of ventricular function without significant decrease in contractile function (dp/dt). Worsening of congestive heart failure has been reported in patients with preexisting impairment of ventricular function. Experience with the use of diltiazem hydrochloride in combination with beta-blockers in patients with impaired ventricular function is limited. Caution should be exercised when using this combination.

3. Hypotension. Decreases in blood pressure associated with diltiazem hydrochloride therapy may occasionally result in symptomatic hypotension.

4. Acute Hepatic Injury. Mild elevations of transaminases with and without concomitant elevation in alkaline phosphatase and bilirubin have been observed in clinical studies. Such elevations were usually transient and frequently resolved even with continued diltiazem treatment. In rare instances, significant elevations in enzymes such as alkaline phosphatase, LDH, SGOT, and SGPT, and other phenomena consistent with acute hepatic injury have been noted. These reactions tended to occur early after therapy initiation (1 to 8 weeks) and have been reversible upon discontinuation of drug therapy. The relationship to diltiazem hydrochloride is uncertain in some cases, but probable in some (see PRECAUTIONS).

PRECAUTIONS

General. Diltiazem hydrochloride is extensively metabolized by the liver and excreted by the kidneys and in bile. As with any drug given over prolonged periods, laboratory parameters of renal and hepatic function should be monitored at regular intervals. The drug should be used with caution in patients with impaired renal or hepatic function. In subacute and chronic dog and rat studies designed to produce toxicity, high doses of diltiazem were associated with hepatic damage. In special subacute hepatic studies, oral doses of 125 mg/kg and higher in rats were associated with histological changes in the liver which were reversible when the drug was discontinued. In dogs, doses of 20 mg/kg were also associated with hepatic changes; however, these changes were reversible with continued dosing.

Dermatological events (see ADVERSE REACTIONS section) may be transient and may disappear despite continued use of diltiazem hydrochloride. However, skin eruptions progressing to erythema multiforme and/or exfoliative dermatitis have also been infrequently reported. Should a dermatologic reaction persist, the drug should be discontinued.

Drug Interactions. Due to the potential for additive effects, caution and careful titration are warranted in patients receiving diltiazem hydrochloride concomitantly with other agents known to affect cardiac contractility and/or conduction (see WARNINGS). Pharmacologic studies indicate that there may be additive effects in prolonging AV conduction when using beta-blockers or digitalis concomitantly with Tiazac® (see WARNINGS). As with all drugs, care should be exercised when treating patients with multiple medications. Diltiazem is both a substrate and an inhibitor of the cytochrome P-450 3A4 enzyme system. Other drugs that are specific substrates, inhibitors, or inducers of the enzyme system may have a significant impact on the efficacy and side effect profile of diltiazem. Patients taking other drugs that are substrates of CYP450 3A4 , especially patients with renal and/or hepatic impairment, may require dosage adjustment when starting or stopping concomitantly administered diltiazem in order to maintain optimum therapeutic blood levels.

Beta Blockers. Controlled and uncontrolled domestic studies suggest that concomitant use of diltiazem hydrochloride and beta-blockers is usually well tolerated, but available data are not sufficient to predict the effects of concomitant treatment in patients with left ventricular dysfunction or cardiac conduction abnormalities. Administration of diltiazem hydrochloride concomitantly with propranolol in five normal volunteers resulted in increased propranolol levels in all subjects and bioavailability of propranolol was increased approximately 50%. *In vitro*, propranolol appears to be displaced from its binding sites by diltiazem. If combination therapy is initiated or withdrawn in conjunction with propranolol, an adjustment in the propranolol dose may be warranted (see WARNINGS).

Cimetidine. A study in six healthy volunteers has shown a significant increase in peak diltiazem plasma levels (58%) and area-under-the-curve (53%) after a 1-week course of cimetidine 1200 mg per day and a single dose of diltiazem 60 mg. Ranitidine produced smaller, nonsignificant increases. The effect may be mediated by cimetidine's known inhibition of hepatic cytochrome P-450, the enzyme system responsible for the first-pass metabolism of diltiazem. Patients currently receiving diltiazem therapy should be carefully monitored for a change in pharmacological effect when initiating and discontinuing therapy with cimetidine. An adjustment in the diltiazem dose may be warranted.

Digitalis. Administration of diltiazem hydrochloride with digoxin in 24 healthy male subjects increased plasma digoxin concentrations approximately 20%. Another investigator found no increase in digoxin levels in 12 patients with coronary artery disease. Since there have been conflicting results regarding the effect of digoxin levels, it is recommended that digoxin levels be monitored when initiating, adjusting, and discontinuing diltiazem hydrochloride therapy to avoid possible over- or under-digitalization (see WARNINGS).

Anesthetics. The depression of cardiac contractility, conductivity, and automaticity as well as the vascular dilation associated with anesthetics may be potentiated by calcium channel blockers. When used concomitantly, anesthetics and calcium blockers should be titrated carefully.

Cyclosporine. A pharmacokinetic interaction between diltiazem and cyclosporine has been observed during studies involving renal and cardiac transplant patients. In renal and cardiac transplant recipients, a reduction of cyclosporine dose ranging from 15% to 48% was necessary to maintain cyclosporine trough concentrations similar to those seen prior to the addition of diltiazem. If these agents are to be administered concurrently, cyclosporine concentrations should be monitored, especially when diltiazem therapy is initiated, adjusted, or discontinued.

The effect of cyclosporine on diltiazem plasma concentrations has not been evaluated.

Carbamazepine. Concomitant administration of diltiazem with carbamazepine has been reported to result in elevated serum levels of carbamazepine (40% to 72% increase), resulting in toxicity in some cases. Patients receiving these drugs concurrently should be monitored for a potential drug interaction.

Benzodiazepines. Studies showed that diltiazem increased the AUC of midazolam and triazolam by 3–4 fold and the C_{max} by 2–fold, compared to placebo. The elimination half life of midazolam and triazolam also increased (1.5–2.5 fold) during coadministration with diltiazem. These pharmacokinetic effects seen during diltiazem coadministration can result in increased clinical effects (e.g., prolonged sodation) of both midazolam and triazolam.

Lovastatin. In a ten-subject study, coadministration of diltiazem (120 mg bid) with lovastatin resulted in a 3–4 times increase in mean lovastatin AUC and C_{max} vs. lovastatin alone; no change in pravastatin AUC and C_{max} was observed during diltiazem coadministration. Diltiazem plasma levels were not significantly affected by lovastatin or pravastatin.

Rifampin. Coadministration of rifampin with diltiazem lowered the diltiazem plasma concentrations to undetectable levels. Coadministration of diltiazem with rifampin or any known CYP3A4 inducer should be avoided when possible, and alternative therapy considered.

Carcinogenesis, Mutagenesis, Impairment of Fertility. A 24-month study in rats at oral dosage levels of up to 100 mg/kg/day and a 21-month study in mice at oral dosage levels of up to 30 mg/kg/day showed no evidence of carcinogenicity. There was also no mutagenic response *in vitro* or *in vivo* in mammalian cell assays or *in vitro* in bacteria. No evidence of impaired fertility was observed in a study performed in male and female rats at oral dosages of up to 100 mg/kg/day.

Pregnancy. Category C. Reproduction studies have been conducted in mice, rats, and rabbits. Administration of doses ranging from 4 to 6 times (depending on species) the upper limit of the optimum dosage range in clinical trials (480 mg q.d. or 8 mg/kg q.d. for a 60 kg patient) resulted in embryo and fetal lethality. These studies revealed, in one species or another, a propensity to cause abnormalities of the skeleton, heart, retina, and tongue. Also observed were reductions in early individual pup weights and pup survival, prolonged delivery and increased incidence of stillbirths. There are no well-controlled studies in pregnant women; therefore, use diltiazem hydrochloride in pregnant women only if the potential benefit justifies the potential risk to the fetus.

Nursing Mothers. Diltiazem is excreted in human milk. One report suggests that concentrations in breast milk may approximate serum levels. If use of Tiazac® is deemed essential, an alternative method of infant feeding should be instituted.

Pediatric Use. Safety and effectiveness in children have not been established.

Geriatric Use. Clinical studies of diltiazem did not include sufficient numbers of subjects aged 65 and over to determine whether they respond differently from younger subjects. Other reported clinical experience has not identified differences in responses between the elderly and younger patients. In general, dose selection for an elderly patient should be cautious, usually starting at the low end of the dosing range, reflecting the greater frequency of decreased hepatic, renal, or cardiac function, and of concomitant disease or other drug therapy.

ADVERSE REACTIONS

Serious adverse reactions have been rare in studies with Tiazac®, as well as with other diltiazem formulations. It should be recognized that patients with impaired ventricular function and cardiac conduction abnormalities have usually been excluded from these studies. A total of 256 hypertensives were treated for between 4 and 8 weeks; a total of 207 patients with chronic stable angina were treated for 3 weeks with doses of Tiazac® ranging from 120–540 mg once daily. Two patients experienced first-degree AV block at 540 mg dose. The following table presents the most common adverse reactions, whether or not drug-related, reported in placebo-controlled trials in patients receiving Tiazac® up to 360 mg and up to 540 mg with rates in placebo patients shown for comparison.

[See first table above]

[See second table above]

In addition, the following events have been reported infrequently (less than 2%) in clinical trials with other diltiazem products:

Cardiovascular. Angina, arrhythmia, AV block (second- or third-degree), bundle branch block, congestive heart failure,

Continued on next page

Tiazac—Cont.

ECG abnormalities, hypotension, palpitations, syncope, tachycardia, ventricular extrasystoles.
Nervous System. Abnormal dreams, amnesia, depression, gait abnormality, hallucinations, insomnia, nervousness, paresthesia, personality change, somnolence, tinnitus, tremor.
Gastrointestinal. Anorexia, constipation, diarrhea, dry mouth, dysgeusia, mild elevations of SGOT, SGPT, LDH, and alkaline phosphatase (see hepatic warnings), nausea, thirst, vomiting, weight increase.
Dermatological. Petechiae, photosensitivity, pruritus.
Other. Albuminuria, allergic reaction, amblyopia, asthenia, CPK increase, crystalluria, dyspnea, edema, epistaxis, eye irritation, headache, hyperglycemia, hyperuricemia, impotence, muscle cramps, nasal congestion, neck rigidity, nocturia, osteoarticular pain, pain, polyuria, rhinitis, sexual difficulties, gynecomastia.
In addition, the following postmarketing events have been reported infrequently in patients receiving diltiazem hydrochloride: alopecia, erythema multiforme, exfoliative dermatitis, Stevens-Johnson syndrome, toxic epidermal necrolysis, extrapyramidal symptoms, gingival hyperplasia, hemolytic anemia, increased bleeding time, leukopenia, purpura, retinopathy, and thrombocytopenia. In addition, events such as myocardial infarction have been observed which are not readily distinguishable from the natural history of the disease in these patients. A number of well-documented cases of generalized rash, characterized as leukocytoclastic vasculitis, have been reported. However, a definitive cause and effect relationship between these events and diltiazem hydrochloride therapy is yet to be established.

OVERDOSAGE

The oral LD50's in mice and rats range from 415 to 740 mg/kg and from 560 to 810 mg/kg, respectively. The intravenous LD50's in these species were 60 and 38 mg/kg, respectively. The oral LD50 in dogs is considered to be in excess of 50 mg/kg, while lethality was seen in monkeys at 360 mg/kg.
The toxic dose in man is not known. Due to extensive metabolism, blood levels after a standard dose of diltiazem can vary over tenfold, limiting the usefulness of blood levels in overdose cases. There have been 29 reports of diltiazem overdose in doses ranging from less than 1 gm to 10.8 gm. Sixteen of these reports involved multiple drug ingestions. Twenty-two reports indicated patients had recovered from diltiazem overdose ranging from less than 1 gm to 10.8 gm. There were seven reports with a fatal outcome; although the amount of diltiazem ingested was unknown, multiple drug ingestions were confirmed in six of the seven reports.
Events observed following diltiazem overdose included bradycardia, hypotension, heart block, and cardiac failure. Most reports of overdose described some supportive medical measure and/or drug treatment. Bradycardia frequently responded favorably to atropine as did heart block, although cardiac pacing was also frequently utilized to treat heart block. Fluids and vasopressors were used to maintain blood pressure, and in cases of cardiac failure, inotropic agents were administered. In addition, some patients received treatment with ventilatory support, activated charcoal, and/or intravenous calcium. Evidence of the effectiveness of intravenous calcium administration to reverse the pharmacological effects of diltiazem overdose was conflicting.
In the event of overdose or exaggerated response, appropriate supportive measures should be employed in addition to gastrointestinal decontamination. Diltiazem does not appear to be removed by peritoneal or hemodialysis. Based on the known pharmacological effects of diltiazem and/or reported clinical experiences, the following measures may be considered:
Bradycardia: Administer atropine (0.60 to 1.0 mg). If there is no response to vagal blockage, administer isoproterenol cautiously.
High-Degree AV Block: Treat as for bradycardia above. Fixed high-degree AV block should be treated with cardiac pacing.
Cardiac Failure: Administer inotropic agents (isoproterenol, dopamine, or dobutamine) and diuretics.
Hypotension: Vasopressors (e.g., dopamine or levarterenol bitartrate). Actual treatment and dosage should depend on the severity of the clinical situation and the judgment and experience of the treating physician.
In a few reported cases, overdose with calcium channel blockers has been associated with hypotension and bradycardia, initially refractory to atropine but becoming more responsive to this treatment when the patients received large doses (close to 1 gram/hour for more than 24 hours) of calcium chloride.
Due to extensive metabolism, plasma concentrations after a standard dose of diltiazem can vary over tenfold, which significantly limits their value in evaluation cases of overdosage.
Charcoal hemoperfusion has been used successfully as an adjunct therapy to hasten drug elimination. Overdoses with as much as 10.8 gm of oral diltiazem have been successfully treated using appropriate supportive care.

DOSAGE AND ADMINISTRATION

Hypertension: Dosage needs to be adjusted by titration to individual patient needs. When used as monotherapy, usual starting doses are 120 to 240 mg once daily. Maximum antihypertensive effect is usually observed by 14 days of chronic therapy; therefore, dosage adjustments should be scheduled accordingly. The usual dosage range studied in clinical trials was 120 to 540 mg once daily. Current clinical experience with 540 mg dose is limited; however, the dose may be increased to 540 mg once daily.
Angina: Dosages for the treatment of angina should be adjusted to each patient's needs, starting with a dose of 120 mg to 180 mg once daily. Individual patients may respond to higher doses of up to 540 mg once daily. When necessary, titration should be carried out over 7 to 14 days.
Concomitant use with Other Cardiovascular Agents.
1. Sublingual Nitroglycerin may be taken as required to abort acute anginal attacks during diltiazem hydrochloride therapy.
2. Prophylactic Nitrate Therapy — Diltiazem hydrochloride may be safely co-administered with short- and long-acting nitrates.
3. Beta-blockers. (See WARNINGS and PRECAUTIONS.)
4. Antihypertensives — Diltiazem hydrochloride has an additive antihypertensive effect when used with other antihypertensive agents. Therefore, the dosage of diltiazem hydrochloride or the concomitant antihypertensives may need to be adjusted when adding one to the other.
Hypertensive or anginal patients who are treated with other formulations of diltiazem can safely be switched to Tiazac capsules at the nearest equivalent total daily dose. Subsequent titration to higher or lower doses may, however, be necessary and should be initiated as clinically indicated.

Strength	Description	Quantity	NDC#
120 mg	#3 lavender/lavender capsule imprinted: Tiazac 120	7's	0456-2612-07
		30's	0456-2612-30
		90's	0456-2612-90
		1000's	0456-2612-00
		HUD's	0456-2612-63
180 mg	#2 white/blue-green capsule imprinted: Tiazac 180	7's	0456-2613-07
		30's	0456-2613-30
		90's	0456-2613-90
		1000's	0456-2613-00
		HUD's	0456-2613-63
240 mg	#1 blue-green/lavender capsule imprinted: Tiazac 240	7's	0456-2614-07
		30's	0456-2614-30
		90's	0456-2614-90
		1000's	0456-2614-00
		HUD's	0456-2614-63
300 mg	#0 white/lavender capsule imprinted: Tiazac 300	7's	0456-2615-07
		30's	0456-2615-30
		90's	0456-2615-90
		1000's	0456-2615-00
		HUD's	0456-2615-63
360 mg	#0 blue-green/blue-green capsule imprinted: Tiazac 360	7's	0456-2616-07
		30's	0456-2616-30
		90's	0456-2616-90
		1000's	0456-2616-00
		HUD's	0456-2616-63
420 mg	#00 white/white capsule imprinted: Tiazac 420	7's	0456-2617-07
		30's	0456-2617-30
		90's	0456-2617-90
		1000's	0456-2617-00

Sprinkling the Capsule Contents on Food
Tiazac® (diltiazem hydrochloride) Extended-release Capsules may also be administered by carefully opening the capsule and sprinkling the capsule contents on a spoonful of applesauce. The applesauce should be swallowed immediately without chewing and followed with a glass of cool water to ensure complete swallowing of the capsule contents. The applesauce should not be hot, and it should be soft enough to be swallowed without chewing. Any capsule contents/applesauce mixture should be used immediately and not stored for future use. Subdividing the contents of a Tiazac® (diltiazem hydrochloride) Extended-release Capsule is not recommended.

HOW SUPPLIED

Tiazac® (diltiazem hydrochloride) Extended-Release Capsules
[See table below]
Storage conditions: Store at controlled room temperature 20°–25°C (68°–77°F). Avoid excessive humidity.
℞ Only.

Manufactured by:
Biovail Corporation
Mississauga, Ontario CANADA L5N 8M5
Manufactured for:
Forest Pharmaceuticals, Inc.
Subsidiary of Forest Laboratories, Inc.
St. Louis, Missouri 63045
Rev: 07/03 LB-0001-08
Shown in Product Identification Guide, page 312

Fujisawa Healthcare, Inc.

THREE PARKWAY NORTH
DEERFIELD, IL 60015-2548

For Medical Information Contact:
Generally:
Medical and Scientific Information
(800) 727-7003
In Emergencies:
Medical and Scientific Information
(800) 727-7003

ADENOCARD® IV ℞

(adenosine injection)
FOR RAPID BOLUS INTRAVENOUS USE

DESCRIPTION

Adenosine is an endogenous nucleoside occurring in all cells of the body. It is chemically 6-amino-9-β-D-ribofuranosyl-9-H-purine and has the following structural formula:

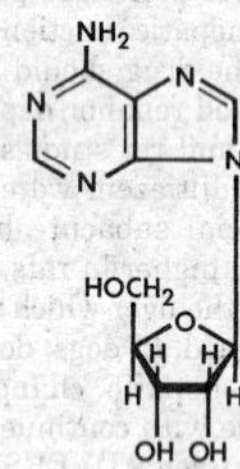

$C_{10}H_{13}N_5O_4$ 267.24

Adenosine is a white crystalline powder. It is soluble in water and practically insoluble in alcohol. Solubility increases by warming and lowering the pH. Adenosine is not chemically related to other antiarrhythmic drugs. Adenocard® (adenosine injection) is a sterile, nonpyrogenic solution for rapid bolus intravenous injection. Each mL contains 3 mg adenosine and 9 mg sodium chloride in Water for Injection. The pH of the solution is between 4.5 and 7.5.
The ***Ansyr®*** plastic syringe is molded from a specially formulated polypropylene. Water permeates from inside the container at an extremely slow rate which will have an insignificant effect on solution concentration over the expected shelf life.
Solutions in contact with the plastic container may leach out certain chemical components from the plastic in very small amounts; however, biological testing was supportive of the safety of the syringe material.

CLINICAL PHARMACOLOGY

Mechanism of Action
Adenocard (adenosine injection) slows conduction time through the A-V node, can interrupt the reentry pathways through the A-V node, and can restore normal sinus rhythm in patients with paroxysmal supraventricular tachycardia (PSVT), including PSVT associated with Wolff-Parkinson-White Syndrome.
Adenocard is antagonized competitively by methylxanthines such as caffeine and theophylline, and potentiated by blockers of nucleoside transport such as dipyridamole. Adenocard is not blocked by atropine.
Hemodynamics
The intravenous bolus dose of 6 or 12 mg Adenocard (adenosine injection) usually has no systemic hemodynamic ef-

fects. When larger doses are given by infusion, adenosine decreases blood pressure by decreasing peripheral resistance.

Pharmacokinetics

Intravenously administered adenosine is rapidly cleared from the circulation via cellular uptake, primarily by erythrocytes and vascular endothelial cells. This process involves a specific transmembrane nucleoside carrier system that is reversible, nonconcentrative, and bidirectionally symmetrical. Intracellular adenosine is rapidly metabolized either via phosphorylation to adenosine monophosphate by adenosine kinase, or via deamination to inosine by adenosine deaminase in the cytosol. Since adenosine kinase has a lower K_m and V_{max} than adenosine deaminase, deamination plays a significant role only when cytosolic adenosine saturates the phosphorylation pathway. Inosine formed by deamination of adenosine can leave the cell intact or can be degraded to hypoxanthine, xanthine, and ultimately uric acid. Adenosine monophosphate formed by phosphorylation of adenosine is incorporated into the high-energy phosphate pool. While extracellular adenosine is primarily cleared by cellular uptake with a half-life of less than 10 seconds in whole blood, excessive amounts may be deaminated by an ecto-form of adenosine deaminase. As Adenocard requires no hepatic or renal function for its activation or inactivation, hepatic and renal failure would not be expected to alter its effectiveness or tolerability.

Clinical Trial Results

In controlled studies in the United States, bolus doses of 3, 6, 9, and 12 mg were studied. A cumulative 60% of patients with paroxysmal supraventricular tachycardia had converted to normal sinus rhythm within one minute after an intravenous bolus dose of 6 mg Adenocard (some converted on 3 mg and failures were given 6 mg), and a cumulative 92% converted after a bolus dose of 12 mg. Seven to sixteen percent of patients converted after 1–4 placebo bolus injections. Similar responses were seen in a variety of patient subsets, including those using or not using digoxin, those with Wolff-Parkinson-White Syndrome, males, females, blacks, Caucasians, and Hispanics.

Adenosine is not effective in converting rhythms other than PSVT, such as atrial flutter, atrial fibrillation, or ventricular tachycardia, to normal sinus rhythm. To date, such patients have not had adverse consequences following administration of adenosine.

INDICATIONS AND USAGE

Intravenous Adenocard (adenosine injection) is indicated for the following.

Conversion to sinus rhythm of paroxysmal supraventricular tachycardia (PSVT), including that associated with accessory bypass tracts (Wolff-Parkinson-White Syndrome). When clinically advisable, appropriate vagal maneuvers (e.g., Valsalva maneuver), should be attempted prior to Adenocard administration.

It is important to be sure the Adenocard solution actually reaches the systemic circulation (see **DOSAGE AND ADMINISTRATION**).

Adenocard does not convert atrial flutter, atrial fibrillation, or ventricular tachycardia to normal sinus rhythm. In the presence of atrial flutter or atrial fibrillation, a transient modest slowing of ventricular response may occur immediately following Adenocard administration.

CONTRAINDICATIONS

Intravenous Adenocard (adenosine injection) is contraindicated in:

1. Second- or third-degree A-V block (except in patients with a functioning artificial pacemaker).
2. Sinus node disease, such as sick sinus syndrome or symptomatic bradycardia (except in patients with a functioning artificial pacemaker).
3. Known hypersensitivity to adenosine.

WARNINGS

Heart Block

Adenocard (adenosine injection) exerts its effect by decreasing conduction through the A-V node and may produce a short lasting first-, second- or third-degree heart block. Appropriate therapy should be instituted as needed. Patients who develop high-level block on one dose of Adenocard should not be given additional doses. Because of the very short half-life of adenosine, these effects are generally self-limiting.

Transient or prolonged episodes of asystole have been reported with fatal outcomes in some cases. Rarely, ventricular fibrillation has been reported following Adenocard administration, including both resuscitated and fatal events. In most instances, these cases were associated with the concomitant use of digoxin and, less frequently with digoxin and verapamil. Although no causal relationship or drug-drug interaction has been established, Adenocard should be used with caution in patients receiving digoxin or digoxin and verapamil in combination. Appropriate resuscitative measures should be available.

Arrhythmias at Time of Conversion

At the time of conversion to normal sinus rhythm, a variety of new rhythms may appear on the electrocardiogram. They generally last only a few seconds without intervention, and may take the form of premature ventricular contractions, atrial premature contractions, sinus bradycardia, sinus tachycardia, skipped beats, and varying degrees of A-V nodal block. Such findings were seen in 55% of patients.

Bronchoconstriction

Adenocard (adenosine injection) is a respiratory stimulant (probably through activation of carotid body chemoreceptors) and intravenous administration in man has been shown to increase minute ventilation (Ve) and reduce arterial PCO_2 causing respiratory alkalosis.

Adenosine administered by inhalation has been reported to cause bronchoconstriction in asthmatic patients, presumably due to mast cell degranulation and histamine release. These effects have not been observed in normal subjects. Adenocard has been administered to a limited number of patients with asthma and mild to moderate exacerbation of their symptoms has been reported. Respiratory compromise has occurred during adenosine infusion in patients with obstructive pulmonary disease. Adenocard should be used with caution in patients with obstructive lung disease not associated with bronchoconstriction (e.g., emphysema, bronchitis, etc.) and should be avoided in patients with bronchoconstriction or bronchospasm (e.g., asthma). Adenocard should be discontinued in any patient who develops severe respiratory difficulties.

PRECAUTIONS

Drug Interactions

Intravenous Adenocard (adenosine injection) has been effectively administered in the presence of other cardioactive drugs, such as quinidine, beta-adrenergic blocking agents, calcium channel blocking agents, and angiotensin converting enzyme inhibitors, without any change in the adverse reaction profile. Digoxin and verapamil use may be rarely associated with ventricular fibrillation when combined with Adenocard (see **WARNINGS**). Because of the potential for additive or synergistic depressant effects on the SA and AV nodes, however, Adenocard should be used with caution in the presence of these agents. The use of Adenocard in patients receiving digitalis may be rarely associated with ventricular fibrillation (see **WARNINGS**).

The effects of adenosine are antagonized by methylxanthines such as caffeine and theophylline. In the presence of these methylxanthines, larger doses of adenosine may be required or adenosine may not be effective. Adenosine effects are potentiated by dipyridamole. Thus, smaller doses of adenosine may be effective in the presence of dipyridamole. Carbamazepine has been reported to increase the degree of heart block produced by other agents. As the primary effect of adenosine is to decrease conduction through the A-V node, higher degrees of heart block may be produced in the presence of carbamazepine.

Carcinogenesis, Mutagenesis, Impairment of Fertility

Studies in animals have not been performed to evaluate the carcinogenic potential of Adenocard (adenosine injection). Adenosine was negative for genotoxic potential in the Salmonella (Ames Test) and Mammalian Microsome Assay.

Adenosine, however, like other nucleosides at millimolar concentrations present for several doubling times of cells in culture, is known to produce a variety of chromosomal alterations. Fertility studies in animals have not been conducted with adenosine.

Pregnancy Category C

Animal reproduction studies have not been conducted with adenosine; nor have studies been performed in pregnant women. As adenosine is a naturally occurring material, widely dispersed throughout the body, no fetal effects would be anticipated. However, since it is not known whether Adenocard can cause fetal harm when administered to pregnant women, Adenocard should be used during pregnancy only if clearly needed.

Pediatric Use

No controlled studies have been conducted in pediatric patients to establish the safety and efficacy of Adenocard for the conversion of paroxysmal supraventricular tachycardia (PSVT). However, intravenous adenosine has been used for the treatment of PSVT in neonates, infants, children and adolescents (see **DOSAGE AND ADMINISTRATION**).[1]

Geriatric Use

Clinical studies of Adenocard did not include sufficient numbers of subjects aged 65 and over to determine whether they respond differently from younger subjects. Other reported clinical experience has not identified differences in responses between elderly and younger patients. In general, Adenocard in geriatric patients should be used with caution since this population may have a diminished cardiac function, nodal dysfunction, concomitant diseases or drug therapy that may alter hemodynamic function and produce severe bradycardia or AV block.

ADVERSE REACTIONS

The following reactions were reported with intravenous Adenocard (adenosine injection) used in controlled U.S. clinical trials. The placebo group had a less than 1% rate of all of these reactions.

Cardiovascular	Facial flushing (18%), headache (2%), sweating, palpitations, chest pain, hypotension (less than 1%).
Respiratory	Shortness of breath/ dyspnea (12%), chest pressure (7%), hyperventilation, head pressure (less than 1%).
Central Nervous System	Lightheadedness (2%), dizziness, tingling in arms, numbness (1%), apprehension, blurred vision, burning sensation, heaviness in arms, neck and back pain (less than 1%).
Gastrointestinal	Nausea (3%), metallic taste, tightness in throat, pressure in groin (less than 1%).

Also, in post-market clinical experience with Adenocard, cases of prolonged asystole, ventricular tachycardia, ventricular fibrillation, transient increase in blood pressure, bradycardia, atrial fibrillation, and bronchospasm, in association with Adenocard use, have been reported (see **WARNINGS**).

OVERDOSAGE

The half-life of Adenocard (adenosine injection) is less than 10 seconds. Thus, adverse effects are generally rapidly self-limiting. Treatment of any prolonged adverse effects should be individualized and be directed toward the specific effect. Methylxanthines, such as caffeine and theophylline, are competitive antagonists of adenosine.

DOSAGE AND ADMINISTRATION

For rapid bolus intravenous use only.

Adenocard (adenosine injection) should be given as a rapid bolus by the peripheral intravenous route. To be certain the solution reaches the systemic circulation, it should be administered either directly into a vein or, if given into an IV line, it should be given as close to the patient as possible and followed by a rapid saline flush.

Adult Patients

The dose recommendation is based on clinical studies with peripheral venous bolus dosing. Central venous (CVP or other) administration of Adenocard has not been systematically studied.

The recommended intravenous doses for adults are as follows:

Initial dose: 6 mg given as a rapid intravenous bolus (administered over a 1–2 second period).

Repeat administration: If the first dose does not result in elimination of the supraventricular tachycardia within 1–2 minutes, 12 mg should be given as a rapid intravenous bolus. This 12 mg dose may be repeated a second time if required.

Pediatric Patients

The dosages used in neonates, infants, children and adolescents were equivalent to those administered to adults on a weight basis.

Pediatric Patients with a Body Weight <50 kg:

Initial dose: Give 0.05 to 0.1 mg/kg as a rapid IV bolus given either centrally or peripherally. A saline flush should follow.

Repeat administration: If conversion of PSVT does not occur within 1–2 minutes, additional bolus injections of adenosine can be administered at incrementally higher doses, increasing the amount given by 0.05 to 0.1 mg/kg. Follow each bolus with a saline flush. This process should continue until sinus rhythm is established or a maximum single dose of 0.3 mg/kg is used.

Pediatric Patients with a Body Weight ≥50 kg:

Administer the adult dose.

Doses greater than 12 mg are not recommended for adult and pediatric patients.

NOTE: Parenteral drug products should be inspected visually for particulate matter and discoloration prior to administration.

HOW SUPPLIED

Adenocard® (adenosine injection) is supplied as a sterile non-pyrogenic solution in normal saline.

NDC 0469-0872-02 Product Code 87102 6 mg/2 mL (3mg/mL) in 2 mL flip-top vials, packaged in 10's.

NDC 0469-8234-12 Product Code 823412 6 mg/2 mL (3 mg/mL) in a 2 mL (fill volume) ***Ansyr®*** plastic disposable syringe, in a package of ten.

NDC 0469-8234-14 Product Code 823414 12 mg/4 mL (3mg/mL) in a 4 mL (fill volume) ***Ansyr®*** plastic disposable syringe, in a package of ten.

Store at controlled room temperature 15°–30°C (59°–86°F). **DO NOT REFRIGERATE** as crystallization may occur. If crystallization has occurred, dissolve crystals by warming to room temperature. The solution must be clear at the time of use.

Contains no preservatives. Discard unused portion.

May require needle or blunt. To prevent needle-stick injuries, needles should not be recapped, purposely bent or broken by hand.

℞ only

REFERENCE

1. Paul T., Pfammatter. J-P. Adenosine: an effective and safe antiarrhythmic drug in pediatrics. Pediatric Cardiology 1997; 18:118–126.

Ansyr® is a registered trademark of Abbott Laboratories

Manufactured for:

Fujisawa Healthcare, Inc., Deerfield IL 60015

Revised: September 2001

Shown in Product Identification Guide, page 312

Continued on next page

ADENOSCAN® ℞

(adenosine injection)
For Intravenous Infusion Only

DESCRIPTION

Adenosine is an endogenous nucleoside occurring in all cells of the body. It is chemically 6-amino-9-beta-D-ribofuranosyl-9-H-purine and has the following structural formula:

$C_{10}H_{13}N_5O_4$ 267.24

Adenosine is a white crystalline powder. It is soluble in water and practically insoluble in alcohol. Solubility increases by warming and lowering the pH of the solution.

Each Adenoscan vial contains a sterile, nonpyrogenic solution of adenosine 3 mg/mL and sodium chloride 9 mg/mL in Water for Injection, q.s. The pH of the solution is between 4.5 and 7.5.

CLINICAL PHARMACOLOGY

Mechanism of Action

Adenosine is a potent vasodilator in most vascular beds, except in renal afferent arterioles and hepatic veins where it produces vasoconstriction. Adenosine is thought to exert its pharmacological effects through activation of purine receptors (cell-surface A_1 and A_2 adenosine receptors). Although the exact mechanism by which adenosine receptor activation relaxes vascular smooth muscle is not known, there is evidence to support both inhibition of the slow inward calcium current reducing calcium uptake, and activation of adenylate cyclase through A_2 receptors in smooth muscle cells. Adenosine may also lessen vascular tone by modulating sympathetic neurotransmission. The intracellular uptake of adenosine is mediated by a specific transmembrane nucleoside transport system. Once inside the cell, adenosine is rapidly phosphorylated by adenosine kinase to adenosine monophosphate, or deaminated by adenosine deaminase to inosine. These intracellular metabolites of adenosine are not vasoactive.

Myocardial uptake of thallium-201 is directly proportional to coronary blood flow. Since Adenoscan significantly increases blood flow in normal coronary arteries with little or no increase in stenotic arteries, Adenoscan causes relatively less thallium-201 uptake in vascular territories supplied by stenotic coronary arteries i.e., a greater difference is seen after Adenoscan between areas served by normal and areas served by stenotic vessels than is seen prior to Adenoscan.

Hemodynamics

Adenosine produces a direct negative chronotropic, dromotropic and inotropic effect on the heart, presumably due to A_1-receptor agonism, and produces peripheral vasodilation, presumably due to A_2-receptor agonism. The net effect of Adenoscan in humans is typically a mild to moderate reduction in systolic, diastolic and mean arterial blood pressure associated with a reflex increase in heart rate. Rarely, significant hypotension and tachycardia have been observed.

Pharmacokinetics

Intravenously administered adenosine is rapidly cleared from the circulation via cellular uptake, primarily by erythrocytes and vascular endothelial cells. This process involves a specific transmembrane nucleoside carrier system that is reversible, nonconcentrative, and bidirectionally symmetrical. Intracellular adenosine is rapidly metabolized either via phosphorylation to adenosine monophosphate by adenosine kinase, or via deamination to inosine by adenosine deaminase in the cytosol. Since adenosine kinase has a lower K_m and V_{max} than adenosine deaminase, deamination plays a significant role only when cytosolic adenosine saturates the phosphorylation pathway. Inosine formed by deamination of adenosine can leave the cell intact or can be degraded to hypoxanthine, xanthine, and ultimately uric acid. Adenosine monophosphate formed by phosphorylation of adenosine is incorporated into the high-energy phosphate pool. While extracellular adenosine is primarily cleared by cellular uptake with a half-life of less than 10 seconds in whole blood, excessive amounts may be deaminated by an ecto-form of adenosine deaminase. As Adenoscan requires no hepatic or renal function for its activation or inactivation, hepatic and renal failure would not be expected to alter its effectiveness or tolerability.

Clinical Trials

In two crossover comparative studies involving 319 subjects who could exercise (including 106 healthy volunteers and 213 patients with known or suspected coronary disease), Adenoscan and exercise thallium images were compared by blinded observers. The images were concordant for the presence of perfusion defects in 85.5% of cases by global analysis (patient by patient) and up to 93% of cases based on vascular territories. In these two studies, 193 patients also had recent coronary arteriography for comparison (healthy volunteers were not catheterized). The sensitivity (true positive Adenoscan divided by the number of patients with positive (abnormal) angiography) for detecting angiographically significant disease (≥50% reduction in the luminal diameter of at least one major vessel) was 64% for Adenoscan and 64% for exercise testing, while the specificity (true negative divided by the number of patients with negative angiograms) was 54% for Adenoscan and 65% for exercise testing. The 95% confidence limits for Adenoscan sensitivity were 56% to 78% and for specificity were 37% to 71%.

Intracoronary Doppler flow catheter studies have demonstrated that a dose of intravenous Adenoscan of 140 mcg/kg/min produces maximum coronary hyperemia (relative to intracoronary papaverine) in approximately 95% of cases within two to three minutes of the onset of the infusion. Coronary blood flow velocity returns to basal levels within one to two minutes of discontinuing the Adenoscan infusion.

INDICATIONS AND USAGE

Intravenous Adenoscan is indicated as an adjunct to thallium-201 myocardial perfusion scintigraphy in patients unable to exercise adequately (See **WARNINGS**).

CONTRAINDICATIONS

Intravenous Adenoscan (adenosine injection) should not be administered to individuals with:

1. Second- or third-degree AV block (except in patients with a functioning artificial pacemaker).
2. Sinus node disease, such as sick sinus syndrome or symptomatic bradycardia (except in patients with a functioning artificial pacemaker).
3. Known or suspected bronchoconstrictive or bronchospastic lung disease (e.g., asthma).
4. Known hypersensitivity to adenosine.

WARNINGS

Fatal Cardiac Arrest, Life Threatening Ventricular Arrhythmias, and Myocardial Infarction.

Fatal cardiac arrest, sustained ventricular tachycardia (requiring resuscitation), and nonfatal myocardial infarction have been reported coincident with Adenoscan infusion. Patients with unstable angina may be at greater risk. Appropriate resuscitative measures should be available.

Sinoatrial and Atrioventricular Nodal Block

Adenoscan (adenosine injection) exerts a direct depressant effect on the SA and AV nodes and has the potential to cause first-, second- or third-degree AV block, or sinus bradycardia. Approximately 6.3% of patients develop AV block with Adenoscan, including first-degree (2.9%), second-degree (2.6%) and third-degree (0.8%) heart block. All episodes of AV block have been asymptomatic, transient, and did not require intervention. Adenoscan can cause sinus bradycardia. Adenoscan should be used with caution in patients with pre-existing first-degree AV block or bundle branch block and should be avoided in patients with high-grade AV block or sinus node dysfunction (except in patients with a functioning artificial pacemaker). Adenoscan should be discontinued in any patient who develops persistent or symptomatic high-grade AV block. Sinus pause has been rarely observed with adenosine infusions.

Hypotension

Adenoscan (adenosine injection) is a potent peripheral vasodilator and can cause significant hypotension. Patients with an intact baroreceptor reflex mechanism are able to maintain blood pressure and tissue perfusion in response to Adenoscan by increasing heart rate and cardiac output. However, Adenoscan should be used with caution in patients with autonomic dysfunction, stenotic valvular heart disease, pericarditis or pericardial effusions, stenotic carotid artery disease with cerebrovascular insufficiency, or uncorrected hypovolemia, due to the risk of hypotensive complications in these patients. Adenoscan should be discontinued in any patient who develops persistent or symptomatic hypotension.

Hypertension

Increases in systolic and diastolic pressure have been observed (as great as 140 mm Hg systolic in one case) concomitant with Adenoscan infusion; most increases resolved spontaneously within several minutes, but in some cases, hypertension lasted for several hours.

Bronchoconstriction

Adenoscan (adenosine injection) is a respiratory stimulant (probably through activation of carotid body chemoreceptors) and intravenous administration in man has been shown to increase minute ventilation (Ve) and reduce arterial PCO_2 causing respiratory alkalosis. Approximately 28% of patients experience breathlessness (dyspnea) or an urge to breathe deeply with Adenoscan. These respiratory complaints are transient and only rarely require intervention. Adenosine administered by inhalation has been reported to cause bronchoconstriction in asthmatic patients, presumably due to mast cell degranulation and histamine release. These effects have not been observed in normal subjects. Adenoscan has been administered to a limited number of patients with asthma and mild to moderate exacerbation of their symptoms has been reported. Respiratory compromise has occurred during adenosine infusion in patients with obstructive pulmonary disease. Adenoscan should be used with caution in patients with obstructive lung disease not associated with bronchoconstriction (e.g., emphysema, bronchitis, etc.) and should be avoided in patients with bronchoconstriction or bronchospasm (e.g., asthma). Adenoscan should be discontinued in any patient who develops severe respiratory difficulties.

PRECAUTIONS

Drug Interactions

Intravenous Adenoscan (adenosine injection) has been given with other cardioactive drugs (such as beta adrenergic blocking agents, cardiac glycosides, and calcium channel blockers) without apparent adverse interactions, but its effectiveness with these agents has not been systematically evaluated. Because of the potential for additive or synergistic depressant effects on the SA and AV nodes, however, Adenoscan should be used with caution in the presence of these agents.

The vasoactive effects of the Adenoscan are inhibited by adenosine receptor antagonists, such as methylxanthines (e.g., caffeine and theophylline). The safety and efficacy of Adenoscan in the presence of these agents has not been systematically evaluated.

The vasoactive effects of Adenoscan are potentiated by nucleoside transport inhibitors, such as dipyridamole. The safety and efficacy of Adenoscan in the presence of dipyridamole has not been systematically evaluated.

Whenever possible, drugs that might inhibit or augment the effects of adenosine should be withheld for at least five half-lives prior to the use of Adenoscan.

Carcinogenesis, Mutagenesis, Impairment of Fertility

Studies in animals have not been performed to evaluate the carcinogenic potential of Adenoscan (adenosine injection). Adenosine was negative for genotoxic potential in the Salmonella (Ames Test) and Mammalian Microsome Assay.

Adenosine, however, like other nucleosides at millimolar concentrations present for several doubling times of cells in culture, is known to produce a variety of chromosomal alterations. Fertility studies in animals have not been conducted with adenosine.

Pregnancy Category C

Animal reproduction studies have not been conducted with adenosine; nor have studies been performed in pregnant women. Because it is not known whether Adenoscan can cause fetal harm when administered to pregnant women, Adenoscan should be used during pregnancy only if clearly needed.

Pediatric Use

The safety and effectiveness of Adenoscan in patients less than 18 years of age have not been established.

Geriatric Use

Clinical studies of Adenoscan did not include sufficient numbers of subjects aged younger than 65 years to determine whether they respond differently. Other reported experience has not revealed clinically relevant differences of the response of elderly in comparison to younger patients. Greater sensitivity of some older individuals, however, cannot be ruled out.

ADVERSE REACTIONS

The following reactions with an incidence of at least 1% were reported with intravenous Adenoscan among 1421 patients enrolled in controlled and uncontrolled U.S. clinical trials. Despite the short half-life of adenosine, 10.6% of the side effects occurred not with the infusion of Adenoscan but several hours after the infusion terminated. Also, 8.4% of the side effects that began coincident with the infusion persisted for up to 24 hours after the infusion was complete. In many cases, it is not possible to know whether these late adverse events are the result of Adenoscan infusion.

Flushing	44%
Chest discomfort	40%
Dyspnea or urge to breathe deeply	28%
Headache	18%
Throat, neck or jaw discomfort	15%
Gastrointestinal discomfort	13%
Lightheadedness/dizziness	12%
Upper extremity discomfort	4%
ST segment depression	3%
First-degree AV block	3%
Second-degree AV block	3%
Paresthesia	2%
Hypotension	2%
Nervousness	2%
Arrhythmias	1%

Adverse experiences of any severity reported in less than 1% of patients include:

Body as a Whole: back discomfort; lower extremity discomfort; weakness.

Cardiovascular System: nonfatal myocardial infarction; life-threatening ventricular arrhythmia; third-degree AV block; bradycardia; palpitation; sinus exit block; sinus pause; sweating; T-wave changes, hypertension (systolic blood pressure >200 mm Hg).

Central Nervous System: drowsiness; emotional instability; tremors.

Genital/Urinary System: vaginal pressure; urgency.

Respiratory System: cough.

Special Senses: blurred vision; dry mouth; ear discomfort; metallic taste; nasal congestion; scotomas; tongue discomfort.

OVERDOSAGE

The half-life of adenosine is less than 10 seconds and side effects of Adenoscan (when they occur) usually resolve quickly when the infusion is discontinued, although delayed or persistent effects have been observed. Methylxanthines, such as caffeine and theophylline, are competitive adenosine receptor antagonists and theophylline has been used to effectively terminate persistent side effects. In controlled U.S. clinical trials, theophylline (50-125 mg slow intravenous injection) was needed to abort Adenoscan side effects in less than 2% of patients.

DOSAGE AND ADMINISTRATION

For intravenous infusion only.

Adenoscan should be given as a continuous peripheral intravenous infusion.

The recommended intravenous dose for adults is 140 mcg/kg/min infused for six minutes (total dose of 0.84 mg/kg).

The required dose of thallium-201 should be injected at the midpoint of the Adenoscan infusion (i.e., after the first three minutes of Adenoscan). Thallium-201 is physically compatible with Adenoscan and may be injected directly into the Adenoscan infusion set.

The injection should be as close to the venous access as possible to prevent an inadvertent increase in the dose of Adenoscan (the contents of the IV tubing) being administered.

There are no data on the safety or efficacy of alternative Adenoscan infusion protocols.

The safety and efficacy of Adenoscan administered by the intracoronary route have not been established.

The following Adenoscan infusion nomogram may be used to determine the appropriate infusion rate corrected for total body weight:

Patient Weight		*Infusion Rate*
kg	*lbs*	*mL/min*
45	99	2.1
50	110	2.3
55	121	2.6
60	132	2.8
65	143	3.0
70	154	3.3
75	165	3.5
80	176	3.8
85	187	4.0
90	198	4.2

This nomogram was derived from the following general formula:

$$\frac{0.140\ (\text{mg/kg/min}) \times \text{total body weight (kg)}}{\text{Adenoscan concentration (3 mg/mL)}} = \text{infusion rate (mL/min)}$$

Note: Parenteral drug products should be inspected visually for particulate matter and discoloration prior to administration.

HOW SUPPLIED

Adenoscan (adenosine injection) is supplied as 20 mL and 30 mL vials of sterile nonpyrogenic solution in normal saline.

Product Code	NDC No.	
87120	0469-0871-20	60 mg/20 mL (3 mg/mL) in a 20 mL single-dose, flip-top glass vial, packaged individually and in packages of ten.
87130	0469-0871-30	90 mg/30 mL (3mg/mL) in a 30 mL single-dose, flip-top glass vial, packaged individually and in packages of ten.

Store at controlled room temperature 15°-30°C (59°-86°F). Do not refrigerate as crystallization may occur. If crystallization has occurred, dissolve crystals by warming to room temperature. The solution must be clear at the time of use. Contains no preservative. Discard unused portion.

℞ only

Manufactured for:
Fujisawa Healthcare, Inc.
Deerfield, IL 60015
Revised: April 2004

Shown in Product Identification Guide, page 312

AMBISOME® ℞

[*ăm-bĭ-sōme*]

(amphotericin B) liposome for injection

DESCRIPTION

AmBisome for Injection is a sterile, non-pyrogenic lyophilized product for intravenous infusion. Each vial contains 50 mg of amphotericin B, USP, intercalated into a liposomal membrane consisting of approximately 213 mg hydrogenated soy phosphatidylcholine; 52 mg cholesterol, NF; 84 mg distearoylphosphatidylglycerol; 0.64 mg alpha tocopherol, USP; together with 900 mg sucrose, NF; and 27 mg disodium succinate hexahydrate as buffer. Following reconstitution with Sterile Water for Injection, USP, the resulting pH of the suspension is between 5–6.

AmBisome is a true single bilayer liposomal drug delivery system. Liposomes are closed, spherical vesicles created by mixing specific proportions of amphophilic substances such as phospholipids and cholesterol so that they arrange themselves into multiple concentric bilayer membranes when hydrated in aqueous solutions. Single bilayer liposomes are then formed by microemulsification of multilamellar vesicles using a homogenizer. AmBisome consists of these unilamellar bilayer liposomes with amphotericin B intercalated within the membrane. Due to the nature and quantity of amphophilic substances used, and the lipophilic moiety in the amphotericin B molecule, the drug is an integral part of the overall structure of the AmBisome liposomes. AmBisome contains true liposomes that are less than 100 nm in diameter. A schematic depiction of the liposome is presented below.

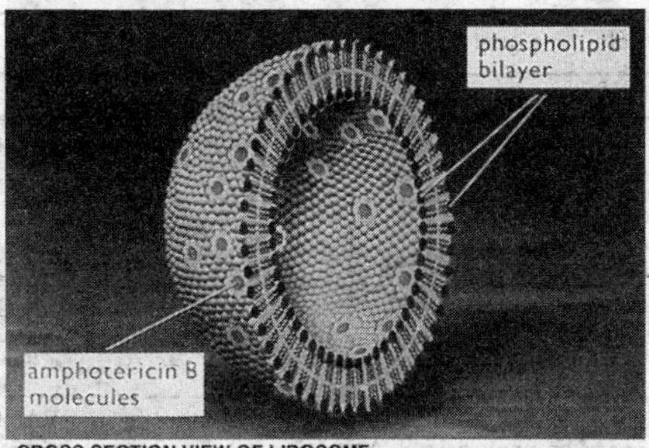

CROSS SECTION VIEW OF LIPOSOME

Note: Liposomal encapsulation or incorporation into a lipid complex can substantially affect a drug's functional properties relative to those of the unencapsulated drug or non-lipid associated drug. In addition, different liposomal or lipid-complex products with a common active ingredient may vary from one another in the chemical composition and physical form of the lipid component. Such differences may affect the functional properties of these drug products.

Amphotericin B is a macrocyclic, polyene, antifungal antibiotic produced from a strain of *Streptomyces nodosus.*

Amphotericin B is designated chemically as: [1R-(1R*,3S*,5R*,6R*,9R*,11R*,15S*,16R*,17R*,18S*,19E,21E,23E,25E,27E,29E,31E,33R*,35S*,36R*,37S*)]-33-[(3-Amino-3,6-dideoxy-β-D-mannopyranosyl)oxy]-1,3,5,6,9,11,17,37-octahydroxy-15,16,18-trimethyl-13-oxo-14,39-dioxabicyclo[33.3.1]nonatriaconta-19,21,23,25,27,29,31-heptaene-36-carboxylic acid (CAS No. 1397-89-3).

Amphotericin B has a molecular formula of $C_{47}H_{73}NO_{17}$ and a molecular weight of 924.09.

The structure of amphotericin B is shown below:

MICROBIOLOGY

Mechanism of Action

Amphotericin B, the active ingredient of AmBisome, acts by binding to the sterol component of a cell membrane leading to alterations in cell permeability and cell death. While amphotericin B has a higher affinity for the ergosterol component of the fungal cell membrane, it can also bind to the cholesterol component of the mammalian cell leading to cytotoxicity. AmBisome, the liposomal preparation of amphotericin B, has been shown to penetrate the cell wall of both extracellular and intracellular forms of susceptible fungi.

Activity *In Vitro* and *In Vivo*

AmBisome has shown *in vitro* activity comparable to amphotericin B against the following organisms: *Aspergillus* species (*A. fumigatus, A. flavus*), *Candida* species (*C. albicans, C. krusei, C. lusitaniae, C. parapsilosis, C. tropicalis*), *Cryptococcus neoformans,* and *Blastomyces dermatitidis.* However, standardized techniques for susceptibility testing of antifungal agents have not been established and results of such studies do not necessarily correlate with clinical outcome.

AmBisome is active in animal models against *Aspergillus fumigatus, Candida albicans, Candida krusei, Candida lusitaniae, Cryptococcus neoformans, Blastomyces dermatitidis, Coccidioides immitis, Histoplasma capsulatum, Paracoccidioides brasiliensis, Leishmania donovani,* and *Leishmania infantum.* The administration of AmBisome in these animal models demonstrated prolonged survival of infected animals, reduction of microorganisms from target organs, or a decrease in lung weight.

Drug Resistance

Mutants with decreased susceptibility to amphotericin B have been isolated from several fungal species after serial passage in culture media containing the drug, and from some patients receiving prolonged therapy. Drug combination studies *in vitro* and *in vivo* suggest that imidazoles may induce resistance to amphotericin B. However, the clinical relevance to drug resistance has not been established.

CLINICAL PHARMACOLOGY

Pharmacokinetics

The assay used to measure amphotericin B in the serum after administration of AmBisome does not distinguish amphotericin B that is complexed with the phospholipids of AmBisome from amphotericin B that is uncomplexed. The pharmacokinetic profile of amphotericin B after administration of AmBisome is based upon total serum concentrations of amphotericin B. The pharmacokinetic profile of amphotericin B was determined in febrile neutropenic cancer and bone marrow transplant patients who received 1–2 hour infusions of 1 to 5 mg/kg/day AmBisome for 3 to 20 days.

The pharmacokinetics of amphotericin B after administration of AmBisome are nonlinear such that there is a greater than proportional increase in serum concentrations with an increase in dose from 1 to 5 mg/kg/day. The pharmacokinetic parameters of total amphotericin B (mean ± SD) after the first dose and at steady state are shown in the table below. [See table above]

Pharmacokinetic Parameters of AmBisome

Dose (mg/kg/day):	1		2.5		5	
Day	1 n = 8	Last n = 7	1 n = 7	Last n = 7	1 n = 12	Last n = 9
Parameters						
C_{max} (mcg/mL)	7.3 ± 3.8	12.2 ± 4.9	17.2 ± 7.1	31.4 ± 17.8	57.6 ± 21	83 ± 35.2
AUC_{0-24} (mcg•hr/mL)	27 ± 14	60 ± 20	65 ± 33	197 ± 183	269 ± 96	555 ± 311
$t_{½}$(hr)	10.7 ± 6.4	7 ± 2.1	8.1 ± 2.3	6.3 ± 2	6.4 ± 2.1	6.8 ± 2.1
V_{ss}(L/kg)	0.44 ± 0.27	0.14 ± 0.05	0.40 ± 0.37	0.16 ± 0.09	0.16 ± 0.10	0.10 ± 0.07
Cl (mL/hr/kg)	39 ± 22	17 ± 6	51 ± 44	22 ± 15	21 ± 14	11 ± 6

Distribution

Based on total amphotericin B concentrations measured within a dosing interval (24 hours) after administration of AmBisome, the mean half-life was 7–10 hours. However, based on total amphotericin B concentration measured up to 49 days after dosing AmBisome, the mean half-life was 100–153 hours. The long terminal elimination half-life is probably a slow redistribution from tissues. Steady state concentrations were generally achieved within 4 days of dosing.

Although variable, mean trough concentrations of amphotericin B remained relatively constant with repeated administration of the same dose over the range of 1 to 5 mg/kg/day, indicating no significant drug accumulation in the serum.

Metabolism

The metabolic pathways of amphotericin B after administration of AmBisome are not known.

Excretion

The mean clearance at steady state was independent of dose. The excretion of amphotericin B after administration of AmBisome has not been studied.

Pharmacokinetics in Special Populations

Renal Impairment

The effect of renal impairment on the disposition of amphotericin B after administration of AmBisome has not been studied. However, AmBisome has been successfully administered to patients with pre-existing renal impairment (see **DESCRIPTION OF CLINICAL STUDIES**).

Hepatic Impairment

The effect of hepatic impairment on the disposition of amphotericin B after administration of AmBisome is not known.

Pediatric and Elderly Patients

The pharmacokinetics of amphotericin B after administration of AmBisome in pediatric and elderly patients have not been studied; however, AmBisome has been used in pediatric and elderly patients (see **DESCRIPTION OF CLINICAL STUDIES**).

Gender and Ethnicity

The effect of gender or ethnicity on the pharmacokinetics of amphotericin B after administration of AmBisome is not known.

INDICATIONS AND USAGE

AmBisome is indicated for the following:

- Empirical therapy for presumed fungal infection in febrile, neutropenic patients.
- Treatment of Cryptococcal Meningitis in HIV infected patients (see **DESCRIPTION OF CLINICAL STUDIES**).

Continued on next page

AmBisome—Cont.

- Treatment of patients with *Aspergillus* species, *Candida* species and/or *Cryptococcus* species infections (see above for the treatment of Cryptococcal Meningitis) refractory to amphotericin B deoxycholate, or in patients where renal impairment or unacceptable toxicity precludes the use of amphotericin B deoxycholate.
- Treatment of visceral leishmaniasis. In immunocompromised patients with visceral leishmaniasis treated with AmBisome, relapse rates were high following initial clearance of parasites (see **DESCRIPTION OF CLINICAL STUDIES**).

See **DOSAGE AND ADMINISTRATION** for recommended doses by indication.

DESCRIPTION OF CLINICAL STUDIES

Eleven clinical studies supporting the efficacy and safety of AmBisome were conducted. This clinical program included both controlled and uncontrolled clinical studies. These studies, which involved 2171 patients, included patients with confirmed systemic mycoses, empirical therapy, and visceral leishmaniasis.

Nineteen hundred and forty-six episodes were evaluable for efficacy, of which 1280 (302 pediatric and 978 adults) were treated with AmBisome.

Three controlled empirical therapy trials compared the efficacy and safety of AmBisome to amphotericin B. One of these studies was conducted in a pediatric population, one in adults, and a third in patients aged 2 years or more. In addition, a controlled empirical therapy trial comparing the safety of AmBisome to Abelcet® (amphotericin B lipid complex) was conducted in patients aged 2 years or more.

One controlled trial compared the efficacy and safety of AmBisome to amphotericin B in HIV patients with cryptococcal meningitis.

One compassionate use study enrolled patients who had failed amphotericin B deoxycholate therapy or who were unable to receive amphotericin B deoxycholate because of renal insufficiency.

Empirical Therapy in Febrile Neutropenic Patients

Study 94-0-002, a randomized, double-blind, comparative multi-center trial, evaluated the efficacy of AmBisome (1.5–6 mg/kg/day) compared with amphotericin B deoxycholate (0.3–1.2 mg/kg/day) in the empirical treatment of 687 adult and pediatric neutropenic patients who were febrile despite having received at least 96 hours of broad spectrum antibacterial therapy. Therapeutic success required (a) resolution of fever during the neutropenic period, (b) absence of an emergent fungal infection, (c) patient survival for at least 7 days post therapy, (d) no discontinuation of therapy due to toxicity or lack of efficacy, and (e) resolution of any study-entry fungal infection.

The overall therapeutic success rates for AmBisome and amphotericin B deoxycholate were equivalent. Results are summarized in the following table. Note: The categories presented below are not mutually exclusive.

[See first table above]

This therapeutic equivalence had no apparent relationship to the use of prestudy antifungal prophylaxis or concomitant granulocytic colony stimulating factors.

The incidence of mycologically confirmed and clinically diagnosed, emergent fungal infections are presented in the following table. AmBisome and amphotericin B were found to be equivalent with respect to the total number of emergent fungal infections.

[See second table at right]

Mycologically confirmed fungal infections at study-entry were cured in 8 of 11 patients in the AmBisome group and 7 of 10 in the amphotericin B group.

Study 97-0-034, a randomized, double-blind, comparative multi-center trial, evaluated the safety of AmBisome (3 and 5 mg/kg/day) compared with amphotericin B lipid complex (5 mg/kg/day) in the empirical treatment of 202 adult and 42 pediatric neutropenic patients. One hundred and sixty-six patients received AmBisome (85 patients received 3 mg/kg/day and 81 received 5 mg/kg/day) and 78 patients received amphotericin B lipid complex. The study patients were febrile despite having received at least 72 hours of broad spectrum antibacterial therapy. The primary endpoint of this study was safety. The study was not designed to draw statistically meaningful conclusions related to comparative efficacy, and in fact, Abelcet is not labeled for this indication.

Two supportive prospective randomized, open label, comparative multi-center studies examined the efficacy of two dosages of AmBisome (1 and 3 mg/kg/day) compared to amphotericin B deoxycholate (1 mg/kg/day) in the treatment of neutropenic patients with presumed fungal infections. These patients were undergoing chemotherapy as part of a bone marrow transplant or had hematological disease. Study 104–10 enrolled adult patients (n=134). Study 104–14 enrolled pediatric patients (n=214). Both studies support the efficacy equivalence of AmBisome and amphotericin B as empirical therapy in febrile neutropenic patients.

Treatment of *Cryptococcal Meningitis in HIV Infected Patients*

Study 94-0-013, a randomized, double-blind, comparative multi-center trial, evaluated the efficacy of AmBisome at doses (3 and 6 mg/kg/day) compared with amphotericin B deoxycholate (0.7 mg/kg/day) for the treatment of cryptococcal meningitis in 266 adult and one pediatric HIV positive patients (the pediatric patient received amphotericin B deoxycholate). Of the 267 treated patients, 86 received AmBisome 3 mg/kg/day, 94 received 6 mg/kg/day and 87 received amphotericin B deoxycholate; cryptococcal meningitis was documented by a positive CSF culture at baseline in 73, 85 and 76 patients, respectively. Patients received study drug once daily for an induction period of 11 to 21 days. Following induction, all patients were switched to oral fluconazole at 400 mg/day for adults and 200 mg/day for patients less than 13 years of age to complete 10 weeks of protocol-directed therapy. For mycologically evaluable patients, defined as all randomized patients who received at least one dose of study drug, had a positive baseline CSF culture, and had at least one follow-up culture, success was evaluated at week 2 (i.e., 14 ± 4 days), and was defined as CSF culture conversion. Success rates at 2 weeks for AmBisome and amphotericin B deoxycholate are summarized in the following table:

[See third table above]

Success at 10 weeks was defined as clinical success at week 10 plus CSF culture conversion at or prior to week 10. Success rates at 10 weeks in patients with positive baseline culture for cryptococcus species are summarized in the following table and show that the efficacy of AmBisome 6 mg/kg/day approximates the efficacy of the amphotericin B deoxycholate regimen. These data do not support the conclusion that AmBisome 3 mg/kg/day is comparable in efficacy to amphotericin B deoxycholate. The table also presents 10-week survival rates for patients treated in this study.

[See fourth table above]

The incidence of infusion-related, cardiovascular and renal adverse events was lower in patients receiving AmBisome compared to amphotericin B deoxycholate (see **ADVERSE REACTIONS** section for details), therefore, the risks and benefits (advantages and disadvantages) of the different amphotericin B formulations should be taken into consideration when selecting a patient treatment regimen.

Empirical Therapy in Febrile Neutropenic Patients: Randomized, Double-Blind Study in 687 Patients

	AmBisome	Amphotericin B
Number of patients receiving at least one dose of study drug	343	344
Overall Success	171 (49.9%)	169 (49.1%)
Fever resolution during neutropenic period	199 (58%)	200 (58.1%)
No treatment emergent fungal infection	300 (87.5%)	301 (87.7%)
Survival through 7 days post study drug	318 (92.7%)	308 (89.5%)
Study drug not prematurely discontinued due to toxicity or lack of efficacy*	294 (85.7%)	280 (81.4%)

* 8 and 10 patients, respectively, were treated as failures due to premature discontinuation alone.

Empirical Therapy in Febrile Neutropenic Patients: Emergent Fungal Infections

	AmBisome	Amphotericin B
Number of patients receiving at least one dose of study drug	343	344
Mycologically confirmed fungal infection	11 (3.2%)	27 (7.8%)
Clinically diagnosed fungal infection	32 (9.3%)	16 (4.7%)
Total emergent fungal infections	43 (12.5%)	43 (12.5%)

Success Rates at 2 weeks (CSF Culture Conversion) Study 94-0-013

	AmBisome 3 mg/kg	AmBisome 6 mg/kg	Amphotericin B 0.7 mg/kg
Success at Week 2	35/60 (58.3%) 97.5% Cl[1]= −9.4%, +31%	36/75 (48%) 97.5% Cl[1]= −18.8%, + 19.8%	29/61 (47.5%)

[1]97.5% Confidence Interval for the difference between AmBisome and amphotericin B success rates. A negative value is in favor of amphotericin B. A positive value is in favor of AmBisome.

Success Rates and Survival Rates at week 10, Study 94-0-013 (see text for definitions)

	AmBisome 3 mg/kg	AmBisome 6 mg/kg	Amphotericin B 0.7 mg/kg
Success in patients with documented cryptococcal meningitis	27/73 (37%) 97.5% Cl[1] = −33.7%, +2.4%	42/85 (49%) 97.5% Cl[1] = −20.9%, + 14.5%	40/76 (53%)
Survival rates	74/86 (86%) 97.5% Cl[1] = −13.8%, +8.9%	85/94 (90%) 97.5% Cl[1] = −8.3%, +12.2%	77/87 (89%)

[1]97.5% Confidence Interval for the difference between AmBisome and amphotericin B success rates. A negative value is in favor of amphotericin B. A positive value is in favor of AmBisome.

Treatment of Patients with *Aspergillus* Species, *Candida* Species and/or *Cryptococcus* Species Infections Refractory to Amphotericin B Deoxycholate, or in Patients Where Renal Impairment or Unacceptable Toxicity Precludes the Use of Amphotericin B Deoxycholate

AmBisome was evaluated in a compassionate use study in hospitalized patients with systemic fungal infections. These patients either had fungal infections refractory to amphotericin B deoxycholate, were intolerant to the use of amphotericin B deoxycholate, or had pre-existing renal insufficiency. Patient recruitment involved 140 infectious episodes in 133 patients, with 53 episodes evaluable for mycological response and 91 episodes evaluable for clinical outcome. Clinical success and mycological eradication occurred in some patients with documented aspergillosis, candidiasis, and cryptococcis.

Treatment of Visceral *Leishmaniasis*

AmBisome was studied in patients with visceral leishmaniasis who were infected in the Mediterranean basin with documented or presumed *Leishmania infantum*. Clinical studies have not provided conclusive data regarding efficacy against *L. donovani* and *L. chagasi*.

AmBisome achieved high rates of acute parasite clearance in immunocompetent patients when total doses of 12–30 mg/kg were administered. Most of these immunocompetent patients remained relapse-free during follow-up periods of 6 months or longer. While acute parasite clearance was achieved in most of the immunocompromised patients who received total doses of 30–40 mg/kg, the majority of these patients were observed to relapse in the 6 months following the completion of therapy. Of the 21 immunocompromised patients studied, 17 were coinfected with HIV; approximately half of the HIV infected patients had AIDS. The following table presents a comparison of efficacy rates among immunocompetent and immunocompromised patients infected in the Mediterranean basin who had no prior treatment or remote prior treatment for visceral leishmaniasis. Efficacy is expressed as both acute parasite clearance

at the end of therapy (EOT) and as overall success (clearance with no relapse) during the follow-up period (F/U) of greater than 6 months for immunocompetent and immunocompromised patients:
[See first table at right]
When followed for 6 months or more after treatment, the overall success rate among immunocompetent patients was 96.5% and the overall success rate among immunocompromised patients was 11.8% due to relapse in the majority of patients. While case reports have suggested there may be a role for long-term therapy to prevent relapses in HIV coinfected patients (Lopez-Dupla, et al. *J. Antimicrob Chemother* 1993;32:657-659), there are no data to date documenting the efficacy or safety of repeat courses of AmBisome or of maintenance therapy with this drug among immunocompromised patients.

CONTRAINDICATIONS

AmBisome is contraindicated in those patients who have demonstrated or have known hypersensitivity to amphotericin B deoxycholate or any other constituents of the product unless, in the opinion of the treating physician, the benefit of therapy outweighs the risk.

WARNINGS

Anaphylaxis has been reported with amphotericin B deoxycholate and other amphotericin B-containing drugs, including AmBisome. If a severe anaphylactic reaction occurs, the infusion should be immediately discontinued and the patient should not receive further infusions of AmBisome.

PRECAUTIONS

General

As with any amphotericin B-containing product the drug should be administered by medically trained personnel. During the initial dosing period, patients should be under close clinical observation. AmBisome has been shown to be significantly less toxic than amphotericin B deoxycholate; however, adverse events may still occur.

Laboratory Tests

Patient management should include laboratory evaluation of renal, hepatic and hematopoietic function, and serum electrolytes (particularly magnesium and potassium).

Drug Interactions

No formal clinical studies of drug interactions have been conducted with AmBisome. However, the following drugs are known to interact with amphotericin B and may interact with AmBisome.

Antineoplastic agents: Concurrent use of antineoplastic agents may enhance the potential for renal toxicity, bronchospasm, and hypotension. Antineoplastic agents should be given concomitantly with caution.

Corticosteroids and corticotropin (ACTH): Concurrent use of corticosteroids and ACTH may potentiate hypokalemia which could predispose the patient to cardiac dysfunction. If used concomitantly, serum electrolytes and cardiac function should be closely monitored.

Digitalis glycosides: Concurrent use may induce hypokalemia and may potentiate digitalis toxicity. When administered concomitantly, serum potassium levels should be closely monitored.

Flucytosine: Concurrent use of flucytosine may increase the toxicity of flucytosine by possibly increasing its cellular uptake and/or impairing its renal excretion.

Azoles (e.g. ketoconazole, miconazole, clotrimazole, fluconazole, etc.): In vitro and *in vivo* animal studies of the combination of amphotericin B and imidazoles suggest that imidazoles may induce fungal resistance to amphotericin B. Combination therapy should be administered with caution, especially in immunocompromised patients.

Leukocyte transfusions: Acute pulmonary toxicity has been reported in patients simultaneously receiving intravenous amphotericin B and leukocyte transfusions.

Other nephrotoxic medications: Concurrent use of amphotericin B and other nephrotoxic medications may enhance the potential for drug-induced renal toxicity. Intensive monitoring of renal function is recommended in patients requiring any combination of nephrotoxic medications.

Skeletal muscle relaxants: Amphotericin B-induced hypokalemia may enhance the curariform effect of skeletal muscle relaxants (e.g. tubocurarine) due to hypokalemia. When administered concomitantly, serum potassium levels should be closely monitored.

Carcinogenesis, Mutagenesis, Impairment of Fertility

No long term studies in animals have been performed to evaluate carcinogenic potential of AmBisome. AmBisome has not been tested to determine its mutagenic potential. A Segment I Reproductive Study in rats found an abnormal estrous cycle (prolonged diestrus) and decreased number of corpora lutea in the high dose groups (10 and 15 mg/kg, doses equivalent to human doses of 1.6 and 2.4 mg/kg based on body surface area considerations). AmBisome did not affect fertility or days to copulation. There were no effects on male reproductive function.

Pregnancy Category B

There have been no adequate and well-controlled studies of AmBisome in pregnant women. Systemic fungal infections have been successfully treated in pregnant women with amphotericin B deoxycholate, but the number of cases reported has been small.

Segment II studies in both rats and rabbits have concluded that AmBisome had no teratogenic potential in these species. In rats, the maternal non-toxic dose of AmBisome was estimated to be 5 mg/kg (equivalent to 0.16 to 0.8 times the recommended human clinical dose range of 1 to 5 mg/kg) and in rabbits, 3 mg/kg (equivalent to 0.2 to 1 times the recommended human clinical dose range), based on body surface area correction. Rabbits receiving the higher doses, (equivalent to 0.5 to 2 times the recommended human dose) of AmBisome experienced a higher rate of spontaneous abortions than did the control groups. AmBisome should only be used during pregnancy if the possible benefits to be derived outweigh the potential risks involved.

AmBisome Efficacy in Visceral Leishmaniasis

Immunocompetent Patients

No. of Patients	Parasite (%) Clearance at EOT	Overall Success (%) at F/U
87	86/87 (98.9)	83/86 (96.5)

Immunocompromised Patients

Regimen	Total Dose	Parasite (%) Clearance at EOT	Overall Success (%) at F/U
100 mg/day X 21 days	29-38.9 mg/kg	10/10 (100)	2/10 (20)
4 mg/kg/day, days 1-5, and 10, 17, 24, 31, 38	40 mg/kg	8/9 (88.9)	0/7 (0)
TOTAL		18/19 (94.7)	2/17 (11.8)

Empirical Therapy Study 94-0-002 Common Adverse Events

Adverse Event by Body System	AmBisome n=343 %	Amphotericin B n=344 %
Body as a Whole		
Abdominal pain	19.8	21.8
Asthenia	13.1	10.8
Back pain	12	7.3
Blood product transfusion react.	18.4	18.6
Chills	47.5	75.9
Infection	11.1	9.3
Pain	14	12.8
Sepsis	14	11.3
Cardiovascular System		
Chest pain	12	11.6
Hypertension	7.9	16.3
Hypotension	14.3	21.5
Tachycardia	13.4	20.9
Digestive System		
Diarrhea	30.3	27.3
Gastrointestinal hemorrhage	9.9	11.3
Nausea	39.7	38.7
Vomiting	31.8	43.9
Metabolic and Nutritional Disorders		
Alkaline phosphatase increased	22.2	19.2
ALT (SGPT) increased	14.6	14
AST (SGOT) increased	12.8	12.8
Bilirubinemia	18.1	19.2
BUN increased	21	31.1
Creatinine increased	22.4	42.2
Edema	14.3	14.8
Hyperglycemia	23	27.9
Hypernatremia	4.1	11
Hypervolemia	12.2	15.4
Hypocalcemia	18.4	20.9
Hypokalemia	42.9	50.6
Hypomagnesemia	20.4	25.6
Peripheral edema	14.6	17.2
Nervous System		
Anxiety	13.7	11
Confusion	11.4	13.4
Headache	19.8	20.9
Insomnia	17.2	14.2
Respiratory System		
Cough increased	17.8	21.8
Dyspnea	23	29.1
Epistaxis	14.9	20.1
Hypoxia	7.6	14.8
Lung disorder	17.8	17.4
Pleural effusion	12.5	9.6
Rhinitis	11.1	11
Skin and Appendages		
Pruritus	10.8	10.2
Rash	24.8	24.4
Sweating	7	10.8
Urogenital System		
Hematuria	14	14

Continued on next page

AmBisome—Cont.

Nursing Mothers
Many drugs are excreted in human milk. However, it is not known whether AmBisome is excreted in human milk. Due to the potential for serious adverse reactions in breast-fed infants, a decision should be made whether to discontinue nursing or whether to discontinue the drug, taking into account the importance of the drug to the mother.

Pediatric Use
Pediatric patients, age 1 month to 16 years, with presumed fungal infection (empirical therapy), confirmed systemic fungal infections or with visceral leishmaniasis have been successfully treated with AmBisome. In studies which included 302 pediatric patients administered AmBisome there was no evidence of any differences in efficacy or safety of AmBisome compared to adults. Since pediatric patients have received AmBisome at doses comparable to those used in adults on a per kilogram body weight basis, no dosage adjustment is required in this population. Safety and effectiveness in pediatric patients below the age of one month has not been established.
(See **DESCRIPTION OF CLINICAL STUDIES—Empirical Therapy in Febrile Neutropenic Patients** and **DOSAGE AND ADMINISTRATION.**)

Elderly Patients
Experience with AmBisome in the elderly (65 years or older) comprised 72 patients. It has not been necessary to alter the dose of AmBisome for this population. As with most other drugs, elderly patients receiving AmBisome should be carefully monitored.

ADVERSE REACTIONS

The following adverse events are based on the experience of 592 adult patients (295 treated with AmBisome and 297 treated with amphotericin B deoxycholate) and 95 pediatric patients (48 treated with AmBisome and 47 treated with amphotericin B deoxycholate) in Study 94-0-002, a randomized double-blind, multi-center study in febrile, neutropenic patients. AmBisome and amphotericin B were infused over two hours.

The incidence of common adverse events (incidence of 10% or greater) occurring with AmBisome compared to amphotericin B deoxycholate, regardless of relationship to study drug, is shown in the following table:
[See second table on previous page]
AmBisome was well tolerated. AmBisome had a lower incidence of chills, hypertension, hypotension, tachycardia, hypoxia, hypokalemia, and various events related to decreased kidney function as compared to amphotericin B deoxycholate.
In pediatric patients (16 years of age or less) in this double-blind study, AmBisome compared to amphotericin B deoxycholate had a lower incidence of hypokalemia (37% versus 55%), chills (29% versus 68%), vomiting (27% versus 55%), and hypertension (10% versus 21%). Similar trends, although with a somewhat lower incidence, were observed in open-label, randomized Study 104-14 involving 205 febrile neutropenic pediatric patients (141 treated with AmBisome and 64 treated with amphotericin B deoxycholate). Pediatric patients appear to have more tolerance than older individuals for the nephrotoxic effects of amphotericin B deoxycholate.
The following adverse events are based on the experience of 244 patients (202 adult and 42 pediatric patients) of whom 85 patients were treated with AmBisome 3 mg/kg, 81 patients were treated with AmBisome 5 mg/kg and 78 patients treated with amphotericin B lipid complex 5 mg/kg in Study 97-0-034, a randomized double-blind, multi-center study in febrile, neutropenic patients. AmBisome and amphotericin B lipid complex were infused over two hours. The incidence of adverse events occurring in more than 10% of subjects in one or more arms regardless of relationship to study drug are summarized in the following table:
[See table below]
The following adverse events are based on the experience of 267 patients (266 adult patients and 1 pediatric patient) of whom 86 patients were treated with AmBisome 3 mg/kg, 94 patients were treated with AmBisome 6 mg/kg and 87 patients treated with amphotericin B deoxycholate 0.7 mg/kg in Study 94-0-013 a randomized, double-blind, comparative multi-center trial, in the treatment of cryptococcal meningitis in HIV positive patients. The incidence of adverse events occurring in more than 10% of subjects in one or more arms regardless of relationship to study drug are summarized in the following table:
[See first table at top of next page]

Infusion Related Reactions
In Study 94-0-002, the large, double-blind study of pediatric and adult febrile neutropenic patients, no premedication to prevent infusion related reaction was administered prior to the first dose of study drug (Day 1). AmBisome-treated patients had a lower incidence of infusion related fever (17% versus 44%), chills/rigors (18% versus 54%), and vomiting (6% versus 8%) on Day 1 as compared to amphotericin B deoxycholate-treated patients.
The incidence of infusion related reactions on Day 1 in pediatric and adult patients is summarized in the following table:
[See second table on next page]
Cardiorespiratory events, except for vasodilatation (flushing), during all study drug infusions were more frequent in amphotericin B-treated patients as summarized in the following table:

Incidence of Infusion Related Cardiorespiratory Events

Event	AmBisome n=343	Amphotericin B n=344
Hypotension	12 (3.5%)	28 (8.1%)
Tachycardia	8 (2.3%)	43 (12.5%)
Hypertension	8 (2.3%)	39 (11.3%)
Vasodilatation	18 (5.2%)	2 (0.6%)
Dyspnea	16 (4.7%)	25 (7.3%)
Hyperventilation	4 (1.2%)	17 (4.9%)
Hypoxia	1 (0.3%)	22 (6.4%)

The percentage of patients who received drugs either for the treatment or prevention of infusion related reactions (e.g., acetaminophen, diphenhydramine, meperidine and hydrocortisone) was lower in AmBisome-treated patients compared with amphotericin B deoxycholate-treated patients.
In the empirical therapy study 97-0-034, on Day 1, where no premedication was administered, the overall incidence of infusion related events of chills/rigors was significantly lower for patients administered AmBisome compared with amphotericin B lipid complex. Fever, chills/rigors and hypoxia were significantly lower for each AmBisome group compared with the amphotericin B lipid complex group. The infusion related event hypoxia was reported for 11.5% of amphotericin B lipid complex-treated patients compared with 0% of patients administered 3 mg/kg per day AmBisome and 1.2% of patients treated with 5 mg/kg per day AmBisome.
[See third table on next page]
Day 1 body temperature increased above the temperature taken within 1 hour prior to infusion (preinfusion temperature) or above the lowest infusion value (no preinfusion temperature recorded).
Patients were not administered premedications to prevent infusion related reactions prior to the Day 1 study drug infusion.
In study 94-0-013, a randomized double-blind multicenter trial comparing AmBisome and amphotericin B deoxycholate as initial therapy for cryptococcal meningitis, premedications to prevent infusion related reactions were permitted. AmBisome treated patients had a lower incidence of fever, chills/rigors and respiratory adverse events as summarized in the following table:
[See first table at top of page 1302]
There have been a few reports of flushing, back pain with or without chest tightness, and chest pain associated with AmBisome administration; on occasion this has been severe. Where these symptoms were noted, the reaction developed within a few minutes after the start of infusion and disappeared rapidly when the infusion was stopped. The symptoms do not occur with every dose and usually do not recur on subsequent administrations when the infusion rate is slowed.

Toxicity and Discontinuation of Dosing
In Study 94-0-002, a significantly lower incidence of grade 3 or 4 toxicity was observed in the AmBisome group compared with the amphotericin B group. In addition, nearly three times as many patients administered amphotericin B required a reduction in dose due to toxicity or discontinuation of study drug due to an infusion related reaction compared with those administered AmBisome.
In empirical therapy study 97-0-034, a greater proportion of patients in the amphotericin B lipid complex group discontinued the study drug due to an adverse event than in the AmBisome groups.

Less Common Adverse Events
The following adverse events also have been reported in 2% to 10% of AmBisome-treated patients receiving chemotherapy or bone marrow transplantation, or had HIV disease in six comparative, clinical trials:
Body as a Whole—abdomen enlarged, allergic reaction, cellulitis, cell mediated immunological reaction, face edema, graft versus host disease, malaise, neck pain, and procedural complication.

Empirical Therapy Study 97-0-034
Common Adverse Events

Adverse Event by Body System	AmBisome 3 mg/kg/day n=85 %	AmBisome 5 mg/kg/day n=81 %	Amphotericin B Lipid Complex 5 mg/kg/day n=78 %
Body as a Whole			
Abdominal pain	12.9	9.9	11.5
Asthenia	8.2	6.2	11.5
Chills/rigors	40	48.1	89.7
Sepsis	12.9	7.4	11.5
Transfusion reaction	10.6	8.6	5.1
Cardiovascular System			
Chest pain	8.2	11.1	6.4
Hypertension	10.6	19.8	23.1
Hypotension	10.6	7.4	19.2
Tachycardia	9.4	18.5	23.1
Digestive System			
Diarrhea	15.3	17.3	14.1
Nausea	25.9	29.6	37.2
Vomiting	22.4	25.9	30.8
Metabolic and Nutritional Disorders			
Alkaline phosphatase increased	7.1	8.6	12.8
Bilirubinemia	16.5	11.1	11.5
BUN increased	20	18.5	28.2
Creatinine increased	20	18.5	48.7
Edema	12.9	12.3	12.8
Hyperglycemia	8.2	8.6	14.1
Hypervolemia	8.2	11.1	14.1
Hypocalcemia	10.6	4.9	5.1
Hypokalemia	37.6	43.2	39.7
Hypomagnesemia	15.3	25.9	15.4
Liver function tests abnormal	10.6	7.4	11.5
Nervous System			
Anxiety	10.6	7.4	9
Confusion	12.9	8.6	3.8
Headache	9.4	17.3	10.3
Respiratory System			
Dyspnea	17.6	22.2	23.1
Epistaxis	10.6	8.6	14.1
Hypoxia	7.1	6.2	20.5
Lung disorder	14.1	13.6	15.4
Skin and Appendages			
Rash	23.5	22.2	14.1

Cryptococcal Meningitis Therapy Study 94-0-013
Common Adverse Events

Adverse Event by Body System	AmBisome 3 mg/kg/day n=86 %	AmBisome 6 mg/kg/day n=94 %	Amphotericin B 0.7 mg/kg/day n=87 %
Body as a Whole			
Abdominal pain	7	7.4	10.3
Infection	12.8	11.7	6.9
Procedural Complication	8.1	9.6	10.3
Cardiovascular System			
Phlebitis	9.3	10.6	25.3
Digestive System			
Anorexia	14	9.6	11.5
Constipation	15.1	14.9	20.7
Diarrhea	10.5	16	10.3
Nausea	16.3	21.3	25.3
Vomiting	10.5	21.3	20.7
Hemic and Lymphatic System			
Anemia	26.7	47.9	43.7
Leukopenia	15.1	17	17.2
Thrombocytopenia	5.8	12.8	6.9
Metabolic and Nutritional Disorders			
Bilirubinemia	0	8.5	12.6
BUN increased	9.3	7.4	10.3
Creatinine increased	18.6	39.4	43.7
Hyperglycemia	9.3	12.8	17.2
Hypocalcemia	12.8	17	13.8
Hypokalemia	31.4	51.1	48.3
Hypomagnesemia	29.1	48.9	40.2
Hyponatremia	11.6	8.5	9.2
Liver Function Tests Abnormal	12.8	4.3	9.2
Nervous System			
Dizziness	7	8.5	10.3
Insomnia	22.1	17	20.7
Respiratory System			
Cough Increased	8.1	2.1	10.3
Skin and Appendages			
Rash	4.7	11.7	4.6

Incidence of Day 1 Infusion Related Reactions (IRR) By Patient Age

	Pediatric Patients (≤ 16 years of age)		Adult Patients (> 16 years of age)	
	AmBisome	Amphotericin B	AmBisome	Amphotericin B
Total number of patients receiving at least one dose of study drug	48	47	295	297
Patients with fever† Increase ≥ 1°C	6 (13%)	22 (47%)	52 (18%)	128 (43%)
Patients with chills/rigors	4 (8%)	22 (47%)	59 (20%)	165 (56%)
Patients with nausea	4 (8%)	4 (9%)	38 (13%)	31 (10%)
Patients with vomiting	2 (4%)	7 (15%)	19 (6%)	21 (7%)
Patients with other reactions	10 (21%)	13 (28%)	47 (16%)	69 (23%)

†Day 1 body temperature increased above the temperature taken within 1 hour prior to infusion (preinfusion temperature) or above the lowest infusion value (no preinfusion temperature recorded).

Incidence of Day 1 Infusion Related Reactions (IRR) Chills/Rigors
Empirical Therapy Study 97-0-034

	AmBisome 3 mg/kg/day	AmBisome 5 mg/kg/day	AmBisome BOTH	Amphotericin B lipid complex 5 mg/kg/day
Total number of patients	85	81	166	78
Patients with Chills/Rigors (Day 1)	16 (18.8%)	19 (23.5%)	35 (21.1%)	62 (79.5%)
Patients with other notable reactions:				
Fever (≥ 1°C increase in temperature)	20 (23.5%)	16 (19.8%)	36 (21.7%)	45 (57.7%)
Nausea	9 (10.6%)	7 (8.6%)	16 (9.6%)	9 (11.5%)
Vomiting	5 (5.9%)	5 (6.2%)	10 (6%)	11 (14.1%)
Hypertension	4 (4.7%)	7 (8.6%)	11 (6.6%)	12 (15.4%)
Tachycardia	2 (2.4%)	8 (9.9%)	10 (6%)	14 (17.9%)
Dyspnea	4 (4.7%)	8 (9.9%)	12 (7.2%)	8 (10.3%)
Hypoxia	0	1 (1.2%)	1 (<1%)	9 (11.5%)

Cardiovascular System—arrhythmia, atrial fibrillation, bradycardia, cardiac arrest, cardiomegaly, hemorrhage, postural hypotension, valvular heart disease, vascular disorder, and vasodilatation (flushing).
Digestive System—anorexia, constipation, dry mouth/nose, dyspepsia, dysphagia, eructation, fecal incontinence, flatulence, hemorrhoids, gum/oral hemorrhage, hematemesis, hepatocellular damage, hepatomegaly, liver function test abnormal, ileus, mucositis, rectal disorder, stomatitis, ulcerative stomatitis, and veno-occlusive liver disease.
Hemic & Lymphatic System—anemia, coagulation disorder, ecchymosis, fluid overload, petechia, prothrombin decreased, prothrombin increased, and thrombocytopenia.
Metabolic & Nutritional Disorders—acidosis, amylase increased, hyperchloremia, hyperkalemia, hypermagnesemia, hyperphosphatemia, hyponatremia, hypophosphatemia, hypoproteinemia, lactate dehydrogenase increased, nonprotein nitrogen (NPN) increased, and respiratory alkalosis.
Musculoskeletal System—arthralgia, bone pain, dystonia, myalgia, and rigors.
Nervous System—agitation, coma, convulsion, cough, depression, dysesthesia, dizziness, hallucinations, nervousness, paresthesia, somnolence, thinking abnormality, and tremor.
Respiratory System—asthma, atelectasis, hemoptysis, hiccup, hyperventilation, influenza-like symptoms, lung edema, pharyngitis, pneumonia, respiratory insufficiency, respiratory failure, and sinusitis.
Skin & Appendages—alopecia, dry skin, herpes simplex, injection site inflammation, maculopapular rash, purpura, skin discoloration, skin disorder, skin ulcer, urticaria, and vesiculobullous rash.
Special Senses—conjunctivitis, dry eyes, and eye hemorrhage.
Urogenital System—abnormal renal function, acute kidney failure, acute renal failure, dysuria, kidney failure, toxic nephropathy, urinary incontinence, and vaginal hemorrhage.

The following infrequent adverse experiences have been reported in post-marketing surveillance, in addition to those mentioned above: angioedema, erythema, urticaria, cyanosis/hypoventilation, pulmonary edema, agranulocytosis, hemorrhagic cystitis.

Clinical Laboratory Values

The effect of AmBisome on renal and hepatic function and on serum electrolytes was assessed from laboratory values measured repeatedly in Study 94-0-002. The frequency and magnitude of hepatic test abnormalities were similar in the AmBisome and amphotericin B groups. Nephrotoxicity was defined as creatinine values increasing 100% or more over pretreatment levels in pediatric patients, and creatinine values increasing 100% or more over pretreatment levels in adult patients provided the peak creatinine concentration was >1.2 mg/dL. Hypokalemia was defined as potassium levels ≤2.5 mmol/L any time during treatment.

Incidence of nephrotoxicity, mean peak serum creatinine concentration, mean change from baseline in serum creatinine, and, incidence of hypokalemia in the double-blind randomized study were lower in the AmBisome group as summarized in the following table:

Study 94-0-002 Laboratory Evidence of Nephrotoxicity

	AmBisome	Amphotericin B
Total number of patients receiving at least one dose of study drug	343	344
Nephrotoxicity	64 (18.7%)	116 (33.7%)
Mean peak creatinine	1.24 mg/dL	1.52 mg/dL
Mean change from baseline in creatinine	0.48 mg/dL	0.77 mg/dL
Hypokalemia	23 (6.7%)	40 (11.6%)

The effect of AmBisome (3 mg/kg/day) vs. amphotericin B (0.6 mg/kg/day) on renal function in adult patients enrolled in this study is illustrated in the following figure:

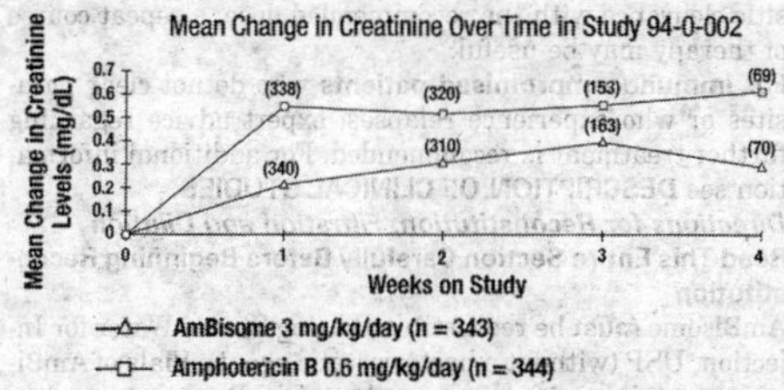

In empirical therapy study 97-0-034, the incidence of nephrotoxicity as measured by increases of serum creatinine from baseline was significantly lower for patients administered AmBisome (individual dose groups and combined) compared with amphotericin B lipid complex.

[See second table on next page]

The following graph shows the average serum creatinine concentrations in the compassionate use study and shows

Continued on next page

AmBisome—Cont.

that there is a drop from pretreatment concentrations for all patients, especially those with elevated (greater than 1.7 mg/dL) pretreatment creatinine concentrations.

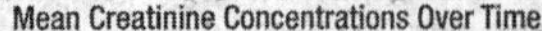

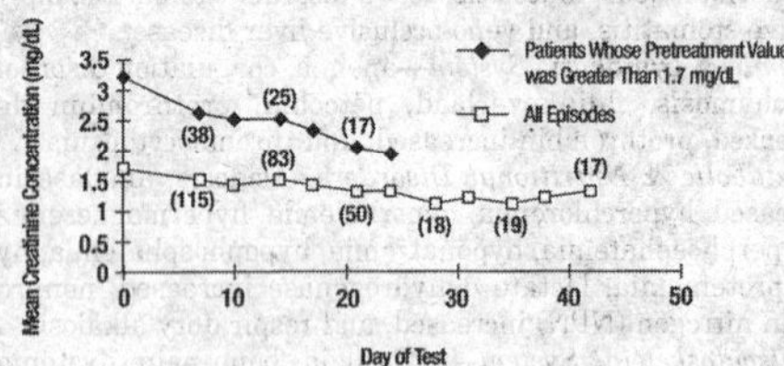

The incidence of nephrotoxicity in Study 94-0-013, comparative trial in cryptococcal meningitis was lower in the AmBisome groups as shown in the following table:
[See third table at right]

Incidence of Infusion-Related Reactions Study 94-0-013

	AmBisome 3 mg/kg	AmBisome 6 mg/kg	Amphotericin B
Total number of patients receiving at least one dose of study drug	86	94	87
Patients with fever increase of >1°C	6 (7%)	8 (9%)	24 (28%)
Patients with chillls/rigors	5 (6%)	8 (9%)	42 (48%)
Patients with nausea	11 (13%)	13 (14%)	18 (20%)
Patients with vomiting	14 (16%)	13 (14%)	16 (18%)
Respiratory adverse events	0	1 (1%)	8 (9%)

Incidence of Nephrotoxicity Empirical Therapy Study 97-0-034

	AmBisome			Amphotericin B lipid complex 5 mg/kg/day
	3 mg/kg/day	5 mg/kg/day	BOTH	
Total number of patients	85	81	166	78
Number with nephrotoxicity				
1.5× baseline serum creatinine value	25 (29.4%)	21 (25.9%)	46 (27.7%)	49 (62.8%)
2× baseline serum creatinine value	12 (14.1%)	12 (14.8%)	24 (14.5%)	33 (42.3%)

Laboratory Evidence of Nephrotoxicity Study 94-0-013

	AmBisome 3 mg/kg	AmBisome 6 mg/kg	Amphotericin B
Total number of patients receiving at least one dose of study drug	86	94	87
Number with Nephrotoxicity (%)			
1.5X baseline serum creatinine	30 (35%)	44 (47%)	52 (60%)
2 X baseline serum creatinine	12 (14%)	20 (21%)	29 (33%)

OVERDOSAGE

The toxicity of AmBisome due to overdose has not been defined. Repeated daily doses up to 10 mg/kg in pediatric patients and 15 mg/kg in adult patients have been administered in clinical trials with no reported dose-related toxicity.
Management—If overdosage should occur, cease administration immediately. Symptomatic supportive measures should be instituted. Particular attention should be given to monitoring renal function.

DOSAGE AND ADMINISTRATION

AmBisome should be administered by intravenous infusion, using a controlled infusion device, over a period of approximately 120 minutes.
An in-line membrane filter may be used for the intravenous infusion of AmBisome; provided **THE MEAN PORE DIAMETER OF THE FILTER IS NOT LESS THAN 1 MICRON.**
NOTE: An existing intravenous line must be flushed with 5% Dextrose Injection prior to infusion of AmBisome. If this is not feasible, AmBisome must be administered through a separate line.
Infusion time may be reduced to approximately 60 minutes in patients in whom the treatment is well-tolerated. If the patient experiences discomfort during infusion, the duration of infusion may be increased.
The recommended initial dose of AmBisome for each indication for adult and pediatric patients is as follows:

Indication	Dose (mg/kg/day)
Empirical therapy	3
Systemic fungal infections: *Aspergillus* *Candida* *Cryptococcus*	3–5
Cryptococcal meningitis in HIV infected patients (see **DESCRIPTION OF CLINICAL STUDIES)**	6

Dosing and rate of infusion should be individualized to the needs of the specific patient to ensure maximum efficacy while minimizing systemic toxicities or adverse events.
Doses recommended for visceral leishmaniasis are presented below:

Visceral Leishmaniasis	Dose (mg/kg/day)
Immunocompetent patients	3 (days 1-5) and 3 on days 14, 21
Immunocompromised patients	4 (days 1-5) and 4 on days 10, 17, 24, 31, 38

For immunocompetent patients who do not achieve parasitic clearance with the recommended dose, a repeat course of therapy may be useful.
For immunocompromised patients who do not clear parasites or who experience relapses, expert advice regarding further treatment is recommended. For additional information see **DESCRIPTION OF CLINICAL STUDIES.**

Directions for Reconstitution, Filtration and Dilution

Read This Entire Section Carefully Before Beginning Reconstitution

AmBisome **must** be reconstituted using Sterile Water for Injection, USP (without a bacteriostatic agent). Vials of AmBisome containing 50 mg of amphotericin B are prepared as follows:

Reconstitution

1. Aseptically add 12 mL of Sterile Water for Injection, USP to each AmBisome vial to yield a preparation containing 4 mg amphotericin B/mL.

CAUTION: DO NOT RECONSTITUTE WITH SALINE OR ADD SALINE TO THE RECONSTITUTED CONCENTRATION, OR MIX WITH OTHER DRUGS. The use of any solution other than those recommended, or the presence of a bacteriostatic agent in the solution, may cause precipitation of AmBisome.

2. **Immediately after the addition of water, SHAKE THE VIAL VIGOROUSLY** for 30 seconds to completely disperse the AmBisome. AmBisome forms a yellow, translucent suspension. Visually inspect the vial for particulate matter and continue shaking until completely dispersed.

Filtration and Dilution

3. Calculate the amount of reconstituted (4 mg/mL) AmBisome to be further diluted.
4. Withdraw this amount of reconstituted AmBisome into a sterile syringe.
5. Attach a 5-micron filter, provided, to the syringe. Inject the syringe contents through the filter, into the appropriate amount of 5% Dextrose Injection. (Use only one filter per vial of AmBisome.)
6. AmBisome must be diluted with 5% Dextrose Injection to a final concentration of 1 to 2 mg/mL prior to administration. Lower concentrations (0.2 to 0.5 mg/mL) may be appropriate for infants and small children to provide sufficient volume for infusion. **DISCARD PARTIALLY USED VIALS.**

STORAGE OF AMBISOME

Unopened vials of lyophilized materials are to be stored at temperatures up to 25° C (77° F).

Storage of Reconstituted Product Concentrate

The reconstituted product concentrate may be stored for up to 24 hours at 2°–8° C (36°–46° F) following reconstitution with Sterile Water for Injection, USP. Do not freeze.

Storage of Diluted Product

Injection of AmBisome should commence within 6 hours of dilution with 5% Dextrose Injection.
As with all parenteral drug products, the reconstituted AmBisome should be inspected visually for particulate matter and discoloration prior to administration, whenever solution and container permit. Do not use material if there is any evidence of precipitation or foreign matter. Aseptic technique must be strictly observed in all handling since no preservative or bacteriostatic agent is present in AmBisome or in the materials specified for reconstitution and dilution.

HOW SUPPLIED

AmBisome for Injection is available as single vial cartons (equivalent to 50 mg amphotericin B) and in packs of ten individual vial cartons (NDC 0469-3051-30).
Each carton contains one pre-packaged, disposable sterile 5 micron filter.
℞ only
Manufactured for:
Fujisawa Healthcare, Inc.
Deerfield, IL 60015-2548
http://www.AmBisome.com
by:
Gilead Sciences, Inc.
San Dimas, CA 91773
AmBisome® is a registered trademark of Gilead Sciences, Inc.
Abelcet® is a registered trademark of the Liposome Company, Inc.
Revised October 2002.
Shown in Product Identification Guide, page 312

PROGRAF® ℞

tacrolimus capsules
tacrolimus injection *(for intravenous infusion only)*

> **WARNING**
> Increased susceptibility to infection and the possible development of lymphoma may result from immunosuppression. Only physicians experienced in immunosuppressive therapy and management of organ transplant patients should prescribe Prograf. Patients receiving the drug should be managed in facilities equipped and staffed with adequate laboratory and supportive medical resources. The physician responsible for maintenance therapy should have complete information requisite for the follow-up of the patient.

DESCRIPTION

Prograf is available for oral administration as capsules (tacrolimus capsules) containing the equivalent of 0.5 mg, 1 mg or 5 mg of anhydrous tacrolimus. Inactive ingredients include lactose, hydroxypropyl methylcellulose, croscarmellose sodium, and magnesium stearate. The 0.5 mg capsule shell contains gelatin, titanium dioxide and ferric oxide, the

1 mg capsule shell contains gelatin and titanium dioxide, and the 5 mg capsule shell contains gelatin, titanium dioxide and ferric oxide.

Prograf is also available as a sterile solution (tacrolimus injection) containing the equivalent of 5 mg anhydrous tacrolimus in 1 mL for administration by intravenous infusion only. Each mL contains polyoxyl 60 hydrogenated castor oil (HCO-60), 200 mg, and dehydrated alcohol, USP, 80.0% v/v. Prograf injection must be diluted with 0.9% Sodium Chloride Injection or 5% Dextrose Injection before use.

Tacrolimus, previously known as FK506, is the active ingredient in Prograf. Tacrolimus is a macrolide immunosuppressant produced by *Streptomyces tsukubaensis*. Chemically, tacrolimus is designated as [3*S*-[3*R**[*E*(1*S**,3*S**,4*S**)], 4*S**,5*R**,8*S**,9*E*,12*R**,14*R**,15*S**,16*R**,18*S**,19*S**,26a*R**]]-5,6,8,11,12,13,14,15,16,17,18,19,24,25,26,26a-hexadecahydro-5,19-dihydroxy-3-[2-(4-hydroxy-3-methoxycyclohexyl)-1-methylethenyl]-14,16-dimethoxy-4,10,12,18-tetramethyl-8-(2-propenyl)-15,19-epoxy-3H-pyrido [2,1-*c*][1,4] oxaazacyclotricosine-1,7,20,21(4H,23H)-tetrone, monohydrate.

The chemical structure of tacrolimus is:

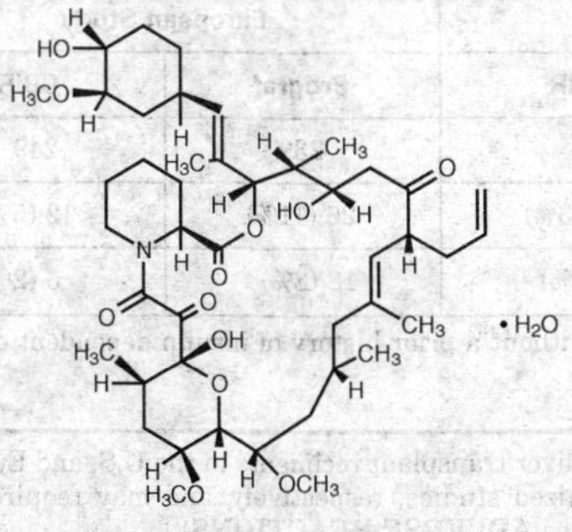

Tacrolimus has an empirical formula of $C_{44}H_{69}NO_{12}\bullet H_2O$ and a formula weight of 822.05. Tacrolimus appears as white crystals or crystalline powder. It is practically insoluble in water, freely soluble in ethanol, and very soluble in methanol and chloroform.

CLINICAL PHARMACOLOGY

Mechanism of Action

Tacrolimus prolongs the survival of the host and transplanted graft in animal transplant models of liver, kidney, heart, bone marrow, small bowel and pancreas, lung and trachea, skin, cornea, and limb.

In animals, tacrolimus has been demonstrated to suppress some humoral immunity and, to a greater extent, cell-mediated reactions such as allograft rejection, delayed type hypersensitivity, collagen-induced arthritis, experimental allergic encephalomyelitis, and graft versus host disease.

Tacrolimus inhibits T-lymphocyte activation, although the exact mechanism of action is not known. Experimental evidence suggests that tacrolimus binds to an intracellular protein, FKBP-12. A complex of tacrolimus-FKBP-12, calcium, calmodulin, and calcineurin is then formed and the phosphatase activity of calcineurin inhibited. This effect may prevent the dephosphorylation and translocation of nuclear factor of activated T-cells (NF-AT), a nuclear component thought to initiate gene transcription for the formation of lymphokines (such as interleukin-2, gamma interferon). The net result is the inhibition of T-lymphocyte activation (i.e., immunosuppression).

Pharmacokinetics

Tacrolimus activity is primarily due to the parent drug. The pharmacokinetic parameters (means ± S.D.) of tacrolimus have been determined following intravenous (IV) and oral (PO) administration in healthy volunteers, kidney transplant and liver transplant patients. (See table below.)

[See first table above]

Population	N	Route (Dose)	Parameters					
			C_{max} (ng/mL)	T_{max} (hr)	AUC (ng•hr/mL)	$t_{1/2}$ (hr)	Cl (L/hr/kg)	V (L/kg)
Healthy Volunteers	8	IV (0.025 mg/kg/4hr)	—	—	598* ± 125	34.2 ± 7.7	0.040 ± 0.009	1.91 ± 0.31
	16	PO (5 mg)	29.7 ± 7.2	1.6 ± 0.7	243** ± 73	34.8 ± 11.4	0.041† ± 0.008	1.94† ± 0.53
Kidney Transplant Pts	26	IV (0.02 mg/kg/12hr)	—	—	294*** ± 262	18.8 ± 16.7	0.083 ± 0.050	1.41 ± 0.66
		PO (0.2 mg/kg/day)	19.2 ± 10.3	3.0	203*** ± 42	#	#	#
		PO (0.3 mg/kg/day)	24.2 ± 15.8	1.5	288*** ± 93	#	#	#
Liver Transplant Pts	17	IV (0.05 mg/kg/12 hr)	—	—	3300*** ± 2130	11.7 ± 3.9	0.053 ± 0.017	0.85 ± 0.30
		PO (0.3 mg/kg/day)	68.5 ± 30.0	2.3 ± 1.5	519*** ± 179	#	#	#

† Corrected for individual bioavailability
* AUC_{0-120}
** AUC_{0-72}
*** AUC_{0-inf}
— not applicable
\# not available

Due to intersubject variability in tacrolimus pharmacokinetics, individualization of dosing regimen is necessary for optimal therapy. (See **DOSAGE AND ADMINISTRATION**). Pharmacokinetic data indicate that whole blood concentrations rather than plasma concentrations serve as the more appropriate sampling compartment to describe tacrolimus pharmacokinetics.

Absorption

Absorption of tacrolimus from the gastrointestinal tract after oral administration is incomplete and variable. The absolute bioavailability of tacrolimus was 17 ± 10% in adult kidney transplant patients (N=26), 22 ± 6% in adult liver transplant patients (N=17), and 18 ± 5% in healthy volunteers (N=16).

A single dose study conducted in 32 healthy volunteers established the bioequivalence of the 1 mg and 5 mg capsules. Another single dose study in 32 healthy volunteers established the bioequivalence of the 0.5 mg and 1 mg capsules. Tacrolimus maximum blood concentrations (C_{max}) and area under the curve (AUC) appeared to increase in a dose-proportional fashion in 18 fasted healthy volunteers receiving a single oral dose of 3, 7 and 10 mg.

In 18 kidney transplant patients, tacrolimus trough concentrations from 3 to 30 ng/mL measured at 10–12 hours post-dose (C_{min}) correlated well with the AUC (correlation coefficient 0.93). In 24 liver transplant patients over a concentration range of 10 to 60 ng/mL, the correlation coefficient was 0.94.

Food Effects: The rate and extent of tacrolimus absorption were greatest under fasted conditions. The presence and composition of food decreased both the rate and extent of tacrolimus absorption when administered to 15 healthy volunteers.

The effect was most pronounced with a high-fat meal (848 kcal, 46% fat): mean AUC and C_{max} were decreased 37% and 77%, respectively; T_{max} was lengthened 5-fold. A high-carbohydrate meal (668 kcal, 85% carbohydrate) decreased mean AUC and mean C_{max} by 28% and 65%, respectively.

In healthy volunteers (N=16), the time of the meal also affected tacrolimus bioavailability. When given immediately following the meal, mean C_{max} was reduced 71%, and mean AUC was reduced 39%, relative to the fasted condition. When administered 1.5 hours following the meal, mean C_{max} was reduced 63%, and mean AUC was reduced 39%, relative to the fasted condition.

In 11 liver transplant patients, Prograf administered 15 minutes after a high fat (400 kcal, 34% fat) breakfast, resulted in decreased AUC (27 ± 18%) and C_{max} (50 ± 19%), as compared to a fasted state.

Population (No. of Patients)	Dose	AUC_{0-t} (ng•hr/mL)	$t_{1/2}$ (hr)	V (L/kg)	Cl (L/hr/kg)
Renal Impairment (n=12)	0.02 mg/kg/4hr IV	393±123 (t=60 hr)	26.3±9.2	1.07 ±0.20	0.038 ±0.014
Mild Hepatic Impairment (n=6)	0.02 mg/kg/4hr IV	367±107 (t=72 hr)	60.6±43.8 Range: 27.8–141	3.1 ±1.6	0.042 ±0.02
	7.7 mg PO	488±320 (t=72 hr)	66.1±44.8 Range: 29.5–138	3.7 ±4.7*	0.034 ±0.019*
Severe Hepatic Impairment (n=6, IV)	0.02 mg/kg/4hr IV (n=2)	762±204 (t=120 hr)	198±158 Range: 81–436	3.9 ±1.0	0.017 ±0.013
	0.01 mg/kg/8hr IV (n=4)	289±117 (t=144 hr)			
(n=5, PO)†	8 mg PO (n=1)	658 (t=120 hr)	119±35 Range: 85–178	3.1 ±3.4*	0.016 ±0.011*
	5 mg PO (n=4)	533±156 (t=144 hr)			
	4 mg PO (n=1)				

*corrected for bioavailability
†1 patient did not receive the PO dose

Distribution

The plasma protein binding of tacrolimus is approximately 99% and is independent of concentration over a range of 5–50 ng/mL. Tacrolimus is bound mainly to albumin and alpha-1-acid glycoprotein, and has a high level of association with erythrocytes. The distribution of tacrolimus between whole blood and plasma depends on several factors, such as hematocrit, temperature at the time of plasma separation, drug concentration, and plasma protein concentration. In a U.S. study, the ratio of whole blood concentration to plasma concentration averaged 35 (range 12 to 67).

Metabolism

Tacrolimus is extensively metabolized by the mixed-function oxidase system, primarily the cytochrome P-450 system (CYP3A). A metabolic pathway leading to the formation of 8 possible metabolites has been proposed. Demethylation and hydroxylation were identified as the primary mechanisms of biotransformation in vitro. The major metabolite identified in incubations with human liver microsomes is 13-demethyl tacrolimus. In in vitro studies, a 31-demethyl metabolite has been reported to have the same activity as tacrolimus.

Excretion

The mean clearance following IV administration of tacrolimus is 0.040, 0.083 and 0.053 L/hr/kg in healthy volunteers, adult kidney transplant patients and adult liver transplant patients, respectively. In man, less than 1% of the dose administered is excreted unchanged in urine.

In a mass balance study of IV administered radiolabeled tacrolimus to 6 healthy volunteers, the mean recovery of radiolabel was 77.8 ± 12.7%. Fecal elimination accounted for 92.4 ± 1.0% and the elimination half-life based on radioactivity was 48.1 ± 15.9 hours whereas it was 43.5 ± 11.6 hours based on tacrolimus concentrations. The mean clearance of radiolabel was 0.029 ± 0.015 L/hr/kg and clearance of tacrolimus was 0.029 ± 0.009 L/hr/kg.

When administered PO, the mean recovery of the radiolabel was 94.9 ± 30.7%. Fecal elimination accounted for 92.6 ± 30.7%, urinary elimination accounted for 2.3 ± 1.1% and the elimination half-life based on radioactivity was 31.9 ± 10.5 hours whereas it was 48.4 ± 12.3 hours based on tacrolimus concentrations. The mean clearance of radiolabel was 0.226 ± 0.116 L/hr/kg and clearance of tacrolimus 0.172 ± 0.088 L/hr/kg.

Special Populations

Pediatric

Pharmacokinetics of tacrolimus have been studied in liver transplantation patients, 0.7 to 13.2 years of age. Following IV administration of a 0.037 mg/kg/day dose to 12 pediatric patients, mean terminal half-life, volume of distribution and clearance were 11.5 ± 3.8 hours, 2.6 ± 2.1 L/kg and 0.138 ± 0.071 L/hr/kg, respectively. Following oral administration to 9 patients, mean AUC and C_{max} were 337 ± 167 ng•hr/mL and 43.4 ± 27.9 ng/mL, respectively. The absolute bioavailability was 31 ± 21%.

Whole blood trough concentrations from 31 patients less than 12 years old showed that pediatric patients needed higher doses than adults to achieve similar tacrolimus trough concentrations. (See **DOSAGE AND ADMINISTRATION**).

Continued on next page

Prograf—Cont.

Renal and Hepatic Insufficiency
The mean pharmacokinetic parameters for tacrolimus following single administrations to patients with renal and hepatic impairment are given in the following table.
[See second table on previous page]
Renal Insufficiency:
Tacrolimus pharmacokinetics following a single IV administration were determined in 12 patients (7 not on dialysis and 5 on dialysis, serum creatinine of 3.9 ± 1.6 and 12.0 ± 2.4 mg/dL, respectively) prior to their kidney transplant. The pharmacokinetic parameters obtained were similar for both groups.
The mean clearance of tacrolimus in patients with renal dysfunction was similar to that in normal volunteers (see previous table).
Hepatic Insufficiency:
Tacrolimus pharmacokinetics have been determined in six patients with mild hepatic dysfunction (mean Pugh score: 6.2) following single IV and oral administrations. The mean clearance of tacrolimus in patients with mild hepatic dysfunction was not substantially different from that in normal volunteers (see previous table). Tracolimus pharmacokinetics were studied in 6 patients with severe hepatic dysfunction (mean Pugh score: >10) The mean clearance was substantially lower in patients with severe hepatic dysfunction, irrespective of the route of administration.
Race
A formal study to evaluate the pharmacokinetic disposition of tacrolimus in Black transplant patients has not been conducted. However, a retrospective comparison of Black and Caucasian kidney transplant patients indicated that Black patients required higher tacrolimus doses to attain similar trough concentrations. (See **DOSAGE AND ADMINISTRATION**).
Gender
A formal study to evaluate the effect of gender on tacrolimus pharmacokinetics has not been conducted, however, there was no difference in dosing by gender in the kidney transplant trial. A retrospective comparison of pharmacokinetics in healthy volunteers, and in kidney and liver transplant patients indicated no gender-based differences.

Clinical Studies

Liver Transplantation

The safety and efficacy of Prograf-based immunosuppression following orthotopic liver transplantation were assessed in two prospective, randomized, non-blinded multicenter studies. The active control groups were treated with a cyclosporine-based immunosuppressive regimen. Both studies used concomitant adrenal corticosteroids as part of the immunosuppressive regimens. These studies were designed to evaluate whether the two regimens were therapeutically equivalent, with patient and graft survival at 12 months following transplantation as the primary endpoints. The Prograf-based immunosuppressive regimen was found to be equivalent to the cyclosporine-based immunosuppressive regimens.
In one trial, 529 patients were enrolled at 12 clinical sites in the United States; prior to surgery, 263 were randomized to the Prograf-based immunosuppressive regimen and 266 to a cyclosporine-based immunosuppressive regimen (CBIR). In 10 of the 12 sites, the same CBIR protocol was used, while 2 sites used different control protocols. This trial excluded patients with renal dysfunction, fulminant hepatic failure with Stage IV encephalopathy, and cancers; pediatric patients (≤ 12 years old) were allowed.
In the second trial, 545 patients were enrolled at 8 clinical sites in Europe; prior to surgery, 270 were randomized to the Prograf-based immunosuppressive regimen and 275 to CBIR. In this study, each center used its local standard CBIR protocol in the active-control arm. This trial excluded pediatric patients, but did allow enrollment of subjects with renal dysfunction, fulminant hepatic failure in Stage IV encephalopathy, and cancers other than primary hepatic with metastases.
One-year patient survival and graft survival in the Prograf-based treatment groups were equivalent to those in the CBIR treatment groups in both studies. The overall one-year patient survival (CBIR and Prograf-based treatment groups combined) was 88% in the U.S. study and 78% in the European study. The overall one-year graft survival (CBIR and Prograf-based treatment groups combined) was 81% in the U.S. study and 73% in the European study. In both studies, the median time to convert from IV to oral Prograf dosing was 2 days.
Because of the nature of the study design, comparisons of differences in secondary endpoints, such as incidence of acute rejection, refractory rejection or use of OKT3 for steroid-resistant rejection, could not be reliably made.

Kidney Transplantation

Prograf-based immunosuppression following kidney transplantation was assessed in a Phase III randomized, multicenter, non-blinded, prospective study. There were 412 kidney transplant patients enrolled at 19 clinical sites in the United States. Study therapy was initiated when renal function was stable as indicated by a serum creatinine ≤ 4 mg/dL (median of 4 days after transplantation, range 1 to 14 days). Patients less than 6 years of age were excluded. There were 205 patients randomized to Prograf-based immunosuppression and 207 patients were randomized to cyclosporine-based immunosuppression. All patients received prophylactic induction therapy consisting of an antilymphocyte antibody preparation, corticosteroids and azathioprine. Overall one year patient and graft survival was 96.1% and 89.6%, respectively and was equivalent between treatment arms.
Because of the nature of the study design, comparisons of differences in secondary endpoints, such as incidence of acute rejection, refractory rejection or use of OKT3 for steroid-resistant rejection, could not be reliably made.

Development of Post Transplant Diabetes Mellitus by Race and by Treatment Group during First Year Post Kidney Transplantation in the Phase III study

Patient Race	Prograf		CBIR	
	No. of Patients at Risk	Patients Who Developed PTDM*	No. of Patients at Risk	Patients Who Developed PTDM*
Black	41	15 (37%)	36	3 (8%)
Hispanic	17	5 (29%)	18	1 (6%)
Caucasian	82	10 (12%)	87	1 (1%)
Other	11	0 (0%)	10	1 (10%)
Total	151	30 (20%)	151	6 (4%)

*use of insulin for 30 or more consecutive days, with < 5 day gap, without a prior history of insulin dependent diabetes mellitus or non insulin dependent diabetes mellitus.

Incidence of Post Transplant Diabetes Mellitus and Insulin Use at One Year in Liver Transplant Recipients

Status of PTDM*	US Study		European Study	
	Prograf	CBIR	Prograf	CBIR
Patients at risk**	239	236	239	249
New Onset PTDM*	42 (18%)	30 (13%)	26 (11%)	12 (5%)
Patients still on insulin at 1 year	23 (10%)	19 (8%)	18 (8%)	6 (2%)

*use of insulin for 30 or more consecutive days, with < 5 day gap, without a prior history of insulin dependent diabetes mellitus or non insulin dependent diabetes mellitus.
**Patients without pretransplant history of diabetes mellitus.

INDICATIONS AND USAGE

Prograf is indicated for the prophylaxis of organ rejection in patients receiving allogeneic liver or kidney transplants. It is recommended that Prograf be used concomitantly with adrenal corticosteroids. Because of the risk of anaphylaxis, Prograf injection should be reserved for patients unable to take Prograf capsules orally.

CONTRAINDICATIONS

Prograf is contraindicated in patients with a hypersensitivity to tacrolimus. Prograf injection is contraindicated in patients with a hypersensitivity to HCO-60 (polyoxyl 60 hydrogenated castor oil).

WARNINGS

(See boxed **WARNING**.)
Insulin-dependent post-transplant diabetes mellitus (PTDM) was reported in 20% of Prograf-treated kidney transplant patients without pretransplant history of diabetes mellitus in the Phase III study (See Tables Below). The median time to onset of PTDM was 68 days. Insulin dependence was reversible in 15% of these PTDM patients at one year and in 50% at two years post transplant. Black and Hispanic kidney transplant patients were at an increased risk of development of PTDM.

Incidence of Post Transplant Diabetes Mellitus and Insulin Use at 2 Years in Kidney Transplant Recipients in the Phase III study

Status of PTDM*	Prograf	CBIR
Patients without pretransplant history of diabetes mellitus	151	151
New onset PTDM*, 1st Year	30/151 (20%)	6/151 (4%)
Still insulin dependent at one year in those without prior history of diabetes.	25/151 (17%)	5/151 (3%)
New onset PTDM* post 1 year	1	0
Patients with PTDM* at 2 years	16/151 (11%)	5/151 (3%)

*use of insulin for 30 or more consecutive days, with < 5 day gap, without a prior history of insulin dependent diabetes mellitus or non insulin dependent diabetes mellitus.

[See first table above]
Insulin-dependent post-transplant diabetes mellitus was reported in 18% and 11% of Prograf-treated liver transplant patients and was reversible in 45% and 31% of these patients at one year post transplant, in the U.S. and European randomized studies, respectively (See Table below). Hyperglycemia was associated with the use of Prograf in 47% and 33% of liver transplant recipients in the U.S. and European randomized studies, respectively, and may require treatment (see **ADVERSE REACTIONS**).
[See second table above]
Prograf can cause neurotoxicity and nephrotoxicity, particularly when used in high doses. Nephrotoxicity was reported in approximately 52% of kidney transplantation patients and in 40% and 36% of liver transplantation patients receiving Prograf in the U.S. and European randomized trials, respectively (see **ADVERSE REACTIONS**). More overt nephrotoxicity is seen early after transplantation, characterized by increasing serum creatinine and a decrease in urine output. Patients with impaired renal function should be monitored closely as the dosage of Prograf may need to be reduced. In patients with persistent elevations of serum creatinine who are unresponsive to dosage adjustments, consideration should be given to changing to another immunosuppressive therapy. Care should be taken in using tacrolimus with other nephrotoxic drugs. **In particular, to avoid excess nephrotoxicity, Prograf should not be used simultaneously with cyclosporine. Prograf or cyclosporine should be discontinued at least 24 hours prior to initiating the other. In the presence of elevated Prograf or cyclosporine concentrations, dosing with the other drug usually should be further delayed.**
Mild to severe hyperkalemia was reported in 31% of kidney transplant recipients and in 45% and 13% of liver transplant recipients treated with Prograf in the U.S. and European randomized trials, respectively, and may require treatment (see **ADVERSE REACTIONS**). **Serum potassium levels should be monitored and potassium-sparing diuretics should not be used during Prograf therapy (see PRECAUTIONS).**
Neurotoxicity, including tremor, headache, and other changes in motor function, mental status, and sensory function were reported in approximately 55% of liver transplant recipients in the two randomized studies. Tremor occurred more often in Prograf-treated kidney transplant patients (54%) compared to cyclosporine-treated patients. The incidence of other neurological events in kidney transplant patients was similar in the two treatment groups (see **ADVERSE REACTIONS**). Tremor and headache have been associated with high whole-blood concentrations of tacrolimus and may respond to dosage adjustment. Seizures have occurred in adult and pediatric patients receiving Prograf (see **ADVERSE REACTIONS**). Coma and delirium also have been associated with high plasma concentrations of tacrolimus.
As in patients receiving other immunosuppressants, patients receiving Prograf are at increased risk of developing lymphomas and other malignancies, particularly of the skin. The risk appears to be related to the intensity and duration of immunosuppression rather than to the use of any specific agent. A lymphoproliferative disorder (LPD) related to Epstein-Barr Virus (EBV) infection has been reported in immunosuppressed organ transplant recipients. The risk of LPD appears greatest in young children who are at risk for primary EBV infection while immunosuppressed or who are switched to Prograf following long-term immunosuppression therapy. Because of the danger of oversuppression of the immune system which can increase susceptibility to infection, combination immunosuppressant therapy should be used with caution.
A few patients receiving Prograf injection have experienced anaphylactic reactions. Although the exact cause of these reactions is not known, other drugs with castor oil derivatives in the formulation have been associated with anaphylaxis in a small percentage of patients. Because of this

potential risk of anaphylaxis, Prograf injection should be reserved for patients who are unable to take Prograf capsules. **Patients receiving Prograf injection should be under continuous observation for at least the first 30 minutes following the start of the infusion and at frequent intervals thereafter. If signs or symptoms of anaphylaxis occur, the infusion should be stopped. An aqueous solution of epinephrine should be available at the bedside as well as a source of oxygen.**

PRECAUTIONS

General

Hypertension is a common adverse effect of Prograf therapy (see **ADVERSE REACTIONS**). Mild or moderate hypertension is more frequently reported than severe hypertension. Antihypertensive therapy may be required; the control of blood pressure can be accomplished with any of the common antihypertensive agents. Since tacrolimus may cause hyperkalemia, potassium-sparing diuretics should be avoided. While calcium-channel blocking agents can be effective in treating Prograf-associated hypertension, care should be taken since interference with tacrolimus metabolism may require a dosage reduction (see ***Drug Interactions***).

Renally and Hepatically Impaired Patients

For patients with renal insufficiency some evidence suggests that lower doses should be used (see **CLINICAL PHARMACOLOGY** and **DOSAGE AND ADMINISTRATION**).

The use of Prograf in liver transplant recipients experiencing post-transplant hepatic impairment may be associated with increased risk of developing renal insufficiency related to high whole-blood levels of tacrolimus. These patients should be monitored closely and dosage adjustments should be considered. Some evidence suggests that lower doses should be used in these patients (see **DOSAGE AND ADMINISTRATION**).

Myocardial Hypertrophy

Myocardial hypertrophy has been reported in association with the administration of Prograf, and is generally manifested by echocardiographically demonstrated concentric increases in left ventricular posterior wall and interventricular septum thickness. Hypertrophy has been observed in infants, children and adults. This condition appears reversible in most cases following dose reduction or discontinuance of therapy. In a group of 20 patients with pre- and post-treatment echocardiograms who showed evidence of myocardial hypertrophy, mean tacrolimus whole blood concentrations during the period prior to diagnosis of myocardial hypertrophy ranged from 11 to 53 ng/mL in infants (N=10, age 0.4 to 2 years), 4 to 46 ng/mL in children (N=7, age 2 to 15 years) and 11 to 24 ng/mL in adults (N=3, age 37 to 53 years).

In patients who develop renal failure or clinical manifestations of ventricular dysfunction while receiving Prograf therapy, echocardiographic evaluation should be considered. If myocardial hypertrophy is diagnosed, dosage reduction or discontinuation of Prograf should be considered.

Information for Patients

Patients should be informed of the need for repeated appropriate laboratory tests while they are receiving Prograf. They should be given complete dosage instructions, advised of the potential risks during pregnancy, and informed of the increased risk of neoplasia. Patients should be informed that changes in dosage should not be undertaken without first consulting their physician.

Patients should be informed that Prograf can cause diabetes mellitus and should be advised of the need to see their physician if they develop frequent urination, increased thirst or hunger.

Laboratory Tests

Serum creatinine, potassium, and fasting glucose should be assessed regularly. Routine monitoring of metabolic and hematologic systems should be performed as clinically warranted.

Drug Interactions

Due to the potential for additive or synergistic impairment of renal function, care should be taken when administering Prograf with drugs that may be associated with renal dysfunction. These include, but are not limited to, aminoglycosides, amphotericin B, and cisplatin. Initial clinical experience with the co-administration of Prograf and cyclosporine resulted in additive/synergistic nephrotoxicity. Patients switched from cyclosporine to Prograf should receive the first Prograf dose no sooner than 24 hours after the last cyclosporine dose. Dosing may be further delayed in the presence of elevated cyclosporine levels.

Drugs That May Alter Tacrolimus Concentrations

Since tacrolimus is metabolized mainly by the CYP3A enzyme systems, substances known to inhibit these enzymes may decrease the metabolism or increase bioavailability of tacrolimus as indicated by increased whole blood or plasma concentrations. Drugs known to induce these enzyme systems may result in an increased metabolism of tacrolimus or decreased bioavailability as indicated by decreased whole blood or plasma concentrations. Monitoring of blood concentrations and appropriate dosage adjustments are essential when such drugs are used concomitantly.

[See first table above]

In a study of 6 normal volunteers, a significant increase in tacrolimus oral bioavailability (14±5% vs. 30±8%) was observed with concomitant ketoconazole administration (200 mg). The apparent oral clearance of tacrolimus during ketoconazole administration was significantly decreased compared to tacrolimus alone (0.430±0.129 L/hr/kg vs. 0.148±0.043 L/hr/kg). Overall, IV clearance of tacrolimus was not significantly changed by ketoconazole co-administration, although it was highly variable between patients.

****Drugs That May Increase Tacrolimus Blood Concentrations:***

Calcium Channel Blockers	Antifungal Agents	Macrolide Antibiotics	Gastrointestinal Prokinetic Agents	Other Drugs
diltiazem	clotrimazole	clarithromycin	cisapride	bromocriptine
nicardipine	fluconazole	erythromycin	metoclopramide	cimetidine
nifedipine	itraconazole	troleandomycin		cyclosporine
verapamil	ketoconazole			danazol
				ethinyl estradiol
				methylprednisolone
				omeprazole
				protease inhibitors
				nefazodone

****Drugs That May Decrease Tacrolimus Blood Concentrations:***

Anticonvulsants	Antibiotics	Herbal Preparations
carbamazepine	rifabutin	St. John's Wort
phenobarbital	rifampin	
phenytoin		

*This table is not all inclusive.

St. John's Wort (*Hypericum perforatum*) induces CYP3A4 and P-glycoprotein. Since tacrolimus is a substrate for CYP3A4, there is the potential that the use of St. John's Wort in patients receiving Prograf could result in reduced tacrolimus levels.

In a study of 6 normal volunteers, a significant decrease in tacrolimus oral bioavailability (14±6% vs. 7±3%) was observed with concomitant rifampin administration (600 mg). In addition, there was a significant increase in tacrolimus clearance (0.036±0.008 L/hr/kg vs. 0.053±0.010 L/hr/kg) with concomitant rifampin administration.

Interaction studies with drugs used in HIV therapy have not been conducted. However, care should be exercised when drugs that are nephrotoxic (e.g., ganciclovir) or that are metabolized by CYP3A (e.g., ritonavir) are administered concomitantly with tacrolimus. Tacrolimus may effect the pharmacokinetics of other drugs (e.g., phenytoin) and increase their concentration. Grapefruit juice affects CYP3A-mediated metabolism and should be avoided (see **DOSAGE AND ADMINISTRATION**).

Other Drug Interactions

Immunosuppressants may affect vaccination. Therefore, during treatment with Prograf, vaccination may be less effective. The use of live vaccines should be avoided; live vaccines may include, but are not limited to measles, mumps, rubella, oral polio, BCG, yellow fever, and TY 21a typhoid.[1]

Carcinogenesis, Mutagenesis and Impairment of Fertility

An increased incidence of malignancy is a recognized complication of immunosuppression in recipients of organ transplants. The most common forms of neoplasms are non-Hodgkin's lymphomas and carcinomas of the skin. As with other immunosuppressive therapies, the risk of malignancies in Prograf recipients may be higher than in the normal, healthy population. Lymphoproliferative disorders associated with Epstein-Barr Virus infection have been seen. It has been reported that reduction or discontinuation of immunosuppression may cause the lesions to regress.

No evidence of genotoxicity was seen in bacterial (*Salmonella* and *E. coli*) or mammalian (Chinese hamster lung-derived cells) in vitro assays of mutagenicity, the in vitro CHO/HGPRT assay of mutagenicity, or in vivo, clastogenicity assays performed in mice; tacrolimus did not cause unscheduled DNA synthesis in rodent hepatocytes.

Carcinogenicity studies were carried out in male and female rats and mice. In the 80-week mouse study and in the 104-week rat study no relationship of tumor incidence to tacrolimus dosage was found. The highest doses used in the mouse and rat studies were 0.8–2.5 times (mice) and 3.5–7.1 times (rats) the recommended clinical dose range of 0.1–0.2 mg/kg/day when corrected for body surface area.

No impairment of fertility was demonstrated in studies of male and female rats. Tacrolimus, given orally at 1.0 mg/kg (0.7–1.4× the recommended clinical dose range of 0.1–0.2 mg/kg/day based on body surface area corrections) to male and female rats, prior to and during mating, as well as to dams during gestation and lactation, was associated with embryolethality and with adverse effects on female reproduction. Effects on female reproductive function (parturition) and embryolethal effects were indicated by a higher rate of pre-implantation loss and increased numbers of undelivered and nonviable pups. When given at 3.2 mg/kg (2.3–4.6× the recommended clinical dose range based on body surface area correction), tacrolimus was associated with maternal and paternal toxicity as well as reproductive toxicity including marked adverse effects on estrus cycles, parturition, pup viability, and pup malformations.

Pregnancy: Category C

In reproduction studies in rats and rabbits, adverse effects on the fetus were observed mainly at dose levels that were toxic to dams. Tacrolimus at oral doses of 0.32 and 1.0 mg/kg during organogenesis in rabbits was associated with maternal toxicity as well as an increase in incidence of abortions; these doses are equivalent to 0.5–1× and 1.6–3.3× the recommended clinical dose range (0.1–0.2 mg/kg) based on body surface area corrections. At the higher dose only, an increased incidence of malformations and developmental variations was also seen. Tacrolimus, at oral doses of 3.2 mg/kg during organogenesis in rats, was associated with maternal toxicity and caused an increase in late resorptions, decreased numbers of live births, and decreased pup weight and viability. Tacrolimus, given orally at 1.0 and 3.2 mg/kg (equivalent to 0.7–1.4× and 2.3–4.6× the recommended clinical dose range based on body surface area corrections) to pregnant rats after organogenesis and during lactation, was associated with reduced pup weights.

No reduction in male or female fertility was evident.

There are no adequate and well-controlled studies in pregnant women. Tacrolimus is transferred across the placenta. The use of tacrolimus during pregnancy has been associated with neonatal hyperkalemia and renal dysfunction. Prograf should be used during pregnancy only if the potential benefit to the mother justifies potential risk to the fetus.

Nursing Mothers

Since tacrolimus is excreted in human milk, nursing should be avoided.

Pediatric Patients

Experience with Prograf in pediatric kidney transplant patients is limited. Successful liver transplants have been performed in pediatric patients (ages up to 16 years) using Prograf. Two randomized active-controlled trials of Prograf in primary liver transplantation included 56 pediatric patients. Thirty-one patients were randomized to Prograf-based and 25 to cyclosporine-based therapies. Additionally, a minimum of 122 pediatric patients were studied in an uncontrolled trial of tacrolimus in living related donor liver transplantation. Pediatric patients generally required higher doses of Prograf to maintain blood trough concentrations of tacrolimus similar to adult patients (see **DOSAGE AND ADMINISTRATION**).

ADVERSE REACTIONS

Liver Transplantation

The principal adverse reactions of Prograf are tremor, headache, diarrhea, hypertension, nausea, and renal dysfunction. These occur with oral and IV administration of Prograf and may respond to a reduction in dosing. Diarrhea was sometimes associated with other gastrointestinal complaints such as nausea and vomiting.

Hyperkalemia and hypomagnesemia have occurred in patients receiving Prograf therapy. Hyperglycemia has been noted in many patients; some may require insulin therapy (see **WARNINGS**).

The incidence of adverse events was determined in two randomized comparative liver transplant trials among 514 patients receiving tacrolimus and steroids and 515 patients receiving a cyclosporine-based regimen (CBIR). The proportion of patients reporting more than one adverse event was 99.8% in the tacrolimus group and 99.6% in the CBIR group. Precautions must be taken when comparing the incidence of adverse events in the U.S. study to that in the European study. The 12-month posttransplant information from the U.S. study and from the European study is presented below. The two studies also included different patient populations and patients were treated with immunosuppressive regimens of differing intensities. Adverse events reported in ≥ 15% in tacrolimus patients (combined study results) are presented below for the two controlled trials in liver transplantation:

[See first table at top of next page]

Less frequently observed adverse reactions in both liver transplantation and kidney transplantation patients are described under the subsection **Less Frequently Reported Adverse Reactions** below.

Kidney Transplantation

The most common adverse reactions reported were infection, tremor, hypertension, decreased renal function, constipation, diarrhea, headache, abdominal pain and insomnia. Adverse events that occurred in ≥ 15% of Prograf-treated kidney transplant patients are presented below:

[See second table on next page]

Less frequently observed adverse reactions in both liver transplantation and kidney transplantation patients are described under the subsection **Less Frequently Reported Adverse Reactions** shown below.

Less Frequently Reported Adverse Reactions

The following adverse events were reported in the range of 3% to less than 15% incidence in either liver or kidney transplant recipients who were treated with tacrolimus in the Phase 3 comparative trials.

NERVOUS SYSTEM: (see **WARNINGS**) abnormal dreams, agitation, amnesia, anxiety, confusion, convulsion, depression, dizziness, emotional lability, encephalopathy, hallucinations, hypertonia, incoordination, myoclonus, nervousness, neuropathy, psychosis, somnolence, thinking abnormal; SPECIAL SENSES: abnormal vision, amblyopia, ear pain, otitis media, tinnitus; GASTROINTESTINAL: an-

Continued on next page

Prograf—Cont.

orexia, cholangitis, cholestatic jaundice, dyspepsia, dysphagia, esophagitis, flatulence, gastritis, gastrointestinal hemorrhage, GGT increase, GI perforation, hepatitis, ileus, increased appetite, jaundice, liver damage, liver function test abnormal, oral moniliasis, rectal disorder, stomatitis; CARDIOVASCULAR: angina pectoris, chest pain, deep thrombophlebitis, abnormal ECG, hemorrhage, hypotension, postural hypotension, peripheral vascular disorder, phlebitis, tachycardia, thrombosis, vasodilatation; UROGENITAL: (see **WARNINGS**) albuminuria, cystitis, dysuria, hematuria, hydronephrosis, kidney failure, kidney tubular necrosis, nocturia, pyuria, toxic nephropathy, oliguria, urinary frequency, urinary incontinence, vaginitis; METABOLIC/NUTRITIONAL: acidosis, alkaline phosphatase increased, alkalosis, ALT (SGPT) increased, AST (SGOT) increased, bicarbonate decreased, bilirubinemia, BUN increased, dehydration, GGT increased, healing abnormal, hypercalcemia, hypercholesterolemia, hyperlipemia, hyperphosphatemia, hyperuricemia, hypervolemia, hypocalcemia, hypoglycemia, hyponatremia, hypophosphatemia, hypoproteinemia, lactic dehydrogenase increase, weight gain; ENDOCRINE: (see **PRECAUTIONS**) Cushing's syndrome, diabetes mellitus; HEMIC/LYMPHATIC: coagulation disorder, ecchymosis, hypochromic anemia, leukocytosis, leukopenia, polycythemia, prothrombin decreased, serum iron decreased, thrombocytopenia; MISCELLANEOUS: abdomen enlarged, abscess, accidental injury, allergic reaction, cellulitis, chills, flu syndrome, generalized edema, hernia, peritonitis, photosensitivity reaction, sepsis; MUSCULOSKELETAL: arthralgia, cramps, generalized spasm, joint disorder, leg cramps, myalgia, myasthenia, osteoporosis; RESPIRATORY: asthma, bronchitis, cough increased, lung disorder, pneumothorax, pulmonary edema, pharyngitis, pneumonia, respiratory disorder, rhinitis, sinusitis, voice alteration; SKIN: acne, alopecia, exfoliative dermatitis, fungal dermatitis, herpes simplex, hirsutism, skin discoloration, skin disorder, skin ulcer, sweating.

There have been rare spontaneous reports of myocardial hypertrophy associated with clinically manifested ventricular dysfunction in patients receiving Prograf therapy (see **PRECAUTIONS**—***Myocardial Hypertrophy***).

Post Marketing

The following have been reported: increased amylase including pancreatitis, hearing loss including deafness, leukoencephalopathy, thrombocytopenic purpura, hemolytic-uremia syndrome, acute renal failure, Stevens-Johnson syndrome, stomach ulcer, glycosuria, cardiac arrhythmia and gastroenteritis.

OVERDOSAGE

Limited overdosage experience is available. Acute overdosages of up to 30 times the intended dose have been reported. Almost all cases have been asymptomatic and all patients recovered with no sequelae. Occasionally, acute overdosage has been followed by adverse reactions consistent with those listed in the **ADVERSE REACTIONS** section except in one case where transient urticaria and lethargy were observed. Based on the poor aqueous solubility and extensive erythrocyte and plasma protein binding, it is anticipated that tacrolimus is not dialyzable to any significant extent; there is no experience with charcoal hemoperfusion. The oral use of activated charcoal has been reported in treating acute overdoses, but experience has not been sufficient to warrant recommending its use. General supportive measures and treatment of specific symptoms should be followed in all cases of overdosage.

In acute oral and IV toxicity studies, mortalities were seen at or above the following doses: in adult rats, 52× the recommended human oral dose; in immature rats, 16× the recommended oral dose; and in adult rats, 16× the recommended human IV dose (all based on body surface area corrections).

DOSAGE AND ADMINISTRATION

Prograf injection (tacrolimus injection)
For IV Infusion Only

NOTE: Anaphylactic reactions have occurred with injectables containing castor oil derivatives. See WARNINGS.

In patients unable to take oral Prograf capsules, therapy may be initiated with Prograf injection. The initial dose of Prograf should be administered no sooner than 6 hours after transplantation. The recommended starting dose of Prograf injection is 0.03–0.05 mg/kg/day as a continuous IV infusion. Adult patients should receive doses at the lower end of the dosing range. Concomitant adrenal corticosteroid therapy is recommended early post-transplantation. Continuous IV infusion of Prograf injection should be continued only until the patient can tolerate oral administration of Prograf capsules.

Preparation for Administration/Stability

Prograf injection must be diluted with 0.9% Sodium Chloride Injection or 5% Dextrose Injection to a concentration between 0.004 mg/mL and 0.02 mg/mL prior to use. Diluted infusion solution should be stored in glass or polyethylene containers and should be discarded after 24 hours. The diluted infusion solution should not be stored in a PVC container due to decreased stability and the potential for extraction of phthalates. In situations where more dilute solutions are utilized (e.g., pediatric dosing, etc.), PVC-free tubing should likewise be used to minimize the potential for significant drug adsorption onto the tubing. Parenteral drug products should be inspected visually for particulate matter and discoloration prior to administration, whenever solution and container permit. Due to the chemical instability of tacrolimus in alkaline media, Prograf injection should not be mixed or co-infused with solutions of pH 9 or greater (e.g., ganciclovir or acyclovir).

Prograf capsules (tacrolimus capsules)

[See third table above]

Liver Transplantation

It is recommended that patients initiate oral therapy with Prograf capsules if possible. If IV therapy is necessary, conversion from IV to oral Prograf is recommended as soon as oral therapy can be tolerated. This usually occurs within 2–3 days. The initial dose of Prograf should be administered no sooner than 6 hours after transplantation. In a patient receiving an IV infusion, the first dose of oral therapy should be given 8–12 hours after discontinuing the IV infusion. The recommended starting oral dose of Prograf capsules is 0.10–0.15 mg/kg/day administered in two divided daily doses every 12 hours. Co-administered grapefruit juice has been reported to increase tacrolimus blood trough concentrations in liver transplant patients. (See ***Drugs That May Alter Tacrolimus Concentrations.***)

LIVER TRANSPLANTATION: ADVERSE EVENTS OCCURRING IN ≥ 15% OF PROGRAF-TREATED PATIENTS

	U.S. STUDY (%) Prograf (N=250)	U.S. STUDY (%) CBIR (N=250)	EUROPEAN STUDY (%) Prograf (N=264)	EUROPEAN STUDY (%) CBIR (N=265)
Nervous System				
Headache (see **WARNINGS**)	64	60	37	26
Tremor (see **WARNINGS**)	56	46	48	32
Insomnia	64	68	32	23
Paresthesia	40	30	17	17
Gastrointestinal				
Diarrhea	72	47	37	27
Nausea	46	37	32	27
Constipation	24	27	23	21
LFT Abnormal	36	30	6	5
Anorexia	34	24	7	5
Vomiting	27	15	14	11
Cardiovascular				
Hypertension (see **PRECAUTIONS**)	47	56	38	43
Urogenital				
Kidney Function Abnormal (see **WARNINGS**)	40	27	36	23
Creatinine Increased (see **WARNINGS**)	39	25	24	19
BUN Increased (see **WARNINGS**)	30	22	12	9
Urinary Tract Infection	16	18	21	19
Oliguria	18	15	19	12
Metabolic and Nutritional				
Hyperkalemia (see **WARNINGS**)	45	26	13	9
Hypokalemia	29	34	13	16
Hyperglycemia (see **WARNINGS**)	47	38	33	22
Hypomagnesemia	48	45	16	9
Hemic and Lymphatic				
Anemia	47	38	5	1
Leukocytosis	32	26	8	8
Thrombocytopenia	24	20	14	19
Miscellaneous				
Abdominal Pain	59	54	29	22
Pain	63	57	24	22
Fever	48	56	19	22
Asthenia	52	48	11	7
Back Pain	30	29	17	17
Ascites	27	22	7	8
Peripheral Edema	26	26	12	14
Respiratory System				
Pleural Effusion	30	32	36	35
Atelectasis	28	30	5	4
Dyspnea	29	23	5	4
Skin and Appendages				
Pruritus	36	20	15	7
Rash	24	19	10	4

KIDNEY TRANSPLANTATION: ADVERSE EVENTS OCCURRING IN ≥ 15% OF PROGRAF-TREATED PATIENTS

	Prograf (N=205)	CBIR (N=207)
Nervous System		
Tremor (See **WARNINGS**)	54	34
Headache (See **WARNINGS**)	44	38
Insomnia	32	30
Paresthesia	23	16
Dizziness	19	16
Gastrointestinal		
Diarrhea	44	41
Nausea	38	36
Constipation	35	43
Vomiting	29	23
Dyspepsia	28	20
Cardiovascular		
Hypertension (See **PRECAUTIONS**)	50	52
Chest Pain	19	13
Urogenital		
Creatinine increased (See **WARNINGS**)	45	42
Urinary Tract Infection	34	35
Metabolic and Nutritional		
Hypophosphatemia	49	53
Hypomagnesemia	34	17
Hyperlipemia	31	38
Hyperkalemia (See **WARNINGS**)	31	32
Diabetes Mellitus (See **WARNINGS**)	24	9
Hypokalemia	22	25
Hyperglycemia (See **WARNINGS**)	22	16
Edema	18	19
Hemic and Lymphatic		
Anemia	30	24
Leukopenia	15	17
Miscellaneous		
Infection	45	49
Peripheral Edema	36	48
Asthenia	34	30
Abdominal Pain	33	31
Pain	32	30
Fever	29	29
Back Pain	24	20
Respiratory System		
Dyspnea	22	18
Cough increased	18	15
Musculoskeletal		
Arthralgia	25	24
Skin		
Rash	17	12
Pruritus	15	7

Summary of Initial Oral Dosage Recommendations and Typical Whole Blood Trough Concentrations

Patient Population	Recommended Initial Oral Dose*	Typical Whole Blood Trough Concentrations
Adult kidney transplant patients	0.2 mg/kg/day	month 1–3 : 7–20 ng/mL month 4–12 : 5–15 ng/mL
Adult liver transplant patients	0.10–0.15 mg/kg/day	month 1–12 : 5–20 ng/mL
Pediatric liver transplant patients	0.15–0.20 mg/kg/day	month 1–12 : 5–20 ng/mL

*Note: two divided doses, q12h

Time After Transplant	Caucasian n = 114 Dose (mg/kg)	Caucasian n = 114 Trough Concentrations (ng/mL)	Black n = 56 Dose (mg/kg)	Black n = 56 Trough Concentrations (ng/mL)
Day 7	0.18	12.0	0.23	10.9
Month 1	0.17	12.8	0.26	12.9
Month 6	0.14	11.8	0.24	11.5
Month 12	0.13	10.1	0.19	11.0

Dosing should be titrated based on clinical assessments of rejection and tolerability. Lower Prograf dosages may be sufficient as maintenance therapy. Adjunct therapy with adrenal corticosteroids is recommended early post transplant.

Dosage and typical tacrolimus whole blood trough concentrations are shown in the table above; blood concentration details are described in **Blood Concentration Monitoring: *Liver Transplantation*** below.

Kidney Transplantation

The recommended starting oral dose of Prograf is 0.2 mg/kg/day administered every 12 hours in two divided doses. The initial dose of Prograf may be administered within 24 hours of transplantation, but should be delayed until renal function has recovered (as indicated for example by a serum creatinine ≤ 4 mg/dL). Black patients may require higher doses to achieve comparable blood concentrations. Dosage and typical tacrolimus whole blood trough concentrations are shown in the table above; blood concentration details are described in **Blood Concentration Monitoring: *Kidney Transplantation*** below.

The data in kidney transplant patients indicate that the Black patients required a higher dose to attain comparable trough concentrations compared to Caucasian patients.

[See fourth table on previous page]

Pediatric Patients

Pediatric liver transplantation patients without pre-existing renal or hepatic dysfunction have required and tolerated higher doses than adults to achieve similar blood concentrations. Therefore, it is recommended that therapy be initiated in pediatric patients at a starting IV dose of 0.03–0.05 mg/kg/day and a starting oral dose of 0.15–0.20 mg/kg/day. Dose adjustments may be required. Experience in pediatric kidney transplantation patients is limited.

Patients with Hepatic or Renal Dysfunction

Due to the reduced clearance and prolonged half-life, patients with severe hepatic impairment (Pugh ≥ 10) may require lower doses of Prograf. Close monitoring of blood concentrations is warranted.

Due to the potential for nephrotoxicity, patients with renal or hepatic impairment should receive doses at the lowest value of the recommended IV and oral dosing ranges. Further reductions in dose below these ranges may be required. Prograf therapy usually should be delayed up to 48 hours or longer in patients with post-operative oliguria.

Conversion from One Immunosuppressive Regimen to Another

Prograf should not be used simultaneously with cyclosporine. Prograf or cyclosporine should be discontinued at least 24 hours before initiating the other. In the presence of elevated Prograf or cyclosporine concentrations, dosing with the other drug usually should be further delayed.

Blood Concentration Monitoring

Monitoring of tacrolimus blood concentrations in conjunction with other laboratory and clinical parameters is considered an essential aid to patient management for the evaluation of rejection, toxicity, dose adjustments and compliance. Factors influencing frequency of monitoring include but are not limited to hepatic or renal dysfunction, the addition or discontinuation of potentially interacting drugs and the posttransplant time. Blood concentration monitoring is not a replacement for renal and liver function monitoring and tissue biopsies.

Two methods have been used for the assay of tacrolimus, a microparticle enzyme immunoassay (MEIA) and an ELISA. Both methods have the same monoclonal antibody for tacrolimus. Comparison of the concentrations in published literature to patient concentrations using the current assays must be made with detailed knowledge of the assay methods and biological matrices employed. Whole blood is the matrix of choice and specimens should be collected into tubes containing ethylene diamine tetraacetic acid (EDTA) anti-coagulant. Heparin anti-coagulation is not recommended because of the tendency to form clots on storage. Samples which are not analyzed immediately should be stored at room temperature or in a refrigerator and assayed within 7 days; if samples are to be kept longer they should be deep frozen at −20°C for up to 12 months.

Liver Transplantation

Although there is a lack of direct correlation between tacrolimus concentrations and drug efficacy, data from Phase II and III studies of liver transplant patients have shown an increasing incidence of adverse events with increasing trough blood concentrations. Most patients are stable when trough whole blood concentrations are maintained between 5 to 20 ng/mL. Long term posttransplant patients often are maintained at the low end of this target range.

Data from the U.S. clinical trial show that tacrolimus whole blood concentrations, as measured by ELISA, were most variable during the first week post-transplantation. After this early period, the median trough blood concentrations, measured at intervals from the second week to one year post-transplantation, ranged from 9.8 ng/mL to 19.4 ng/mL. *Therapeutic Drug Monitoring,* 1995, Volume 17, Number 6 contains a consensus document and several position papers regarding the therapeutic monitoring of tacrolimus from the 1995 International Consensus Conference on Immunosuppressive Drugs. Refer to these manuscripts for further discussions of tacrolimus monitoring.

Kidney Transplantation

Data from the Phase III study indicates that trough concentrations of tacrolimus in whole blood, as measured by IMx®, were most variable during the first week of dosing. During the first three months, 80% of the patients maintained trough concentrations between 7–20 ng/mL, and then between 5–15 ng/mL, through one-year.

The relative risk of toxicity is increased with higher trough concentrations. Therefore, monitoring of whole blood trough concentrations is recommended to assist in the clinical evaluation of toxicity.

HOW SUPPLIED

Prograf capsules (tacrolimus capsules) 0.5 mg

Oblong, light yellow, branded with red "0.5 mg" on the capsule cap and "607" on the capsule body, supplied in 100-count plastic bottles (NDC 0469-0607-73) containing the equivalent of 0.5 mg anhydrous tacrolimus.

Prograf capsules (tacrolimus capsules) 1 mg

Oblong, white, branded with red "1 mg" on the capsule cap and "617" on the capsule body, supplied in 100-count plastic bottles (NDC 0469-0617-73) and 10 blister cards of 10 capsules (NDC 0469-0617-11), containing the equivalent of 1 mg anhydrous tacrolimus.

Prograf capsules (tacrolimus capsules) 5 mg

Oblong, grayish/red, branded with white "5 mg" on the capsule cap and "657" on the capsule body, supplied in 100-count plastic bottles (NDC 0469-0657-73) and 10 blister cards of 10 capsules (NDC 0469-0657-11), containing the equivalent of 5 mg anhydrous tacrolimus.

Made in Japan

Store and Dispense

Store at 25°C (77°F); excursions permitted to 15°C–30°C (59°F–86°F).

Prograf injection (tacrolimus injection) 5 mg (for IV infusion only)

Supplied as a sterile solution in 1 mL ampules containing the equivalent of 5 mg of anhydrous tacrolimus per mL, in boxes of 10 ampules (NDC 0469-3016-01).

Made in Ireland

Store and Dispense

Store between 5°C and 25°C (41°F and 77°F).

℞ only

Manufactured for:
Fujisawa Healthcare, Inc.
Deerfield, IL 60015-2548

REFERENCE

1. CDC: Recommendations of the Advisory Committee on Immunization Practices: Use of vaccines and immune globulins in persons with altered immunocompetence. MMWR 1993;42(RR-4):1–18.

Issued: July 2001

Shown in Product Identification Guide, page 313

PROTOPIC® ℞

(tacrolimus)
Ointment 0.03%
Ointment 0.1%

FOR DERMATOLOGIC USE ONLY
NOT FOR OPHTHALMIC USE

DESCRIPTION

PROTOPIC (tacrolimus) Ointment contains tacrolimus, a macrolide immunosuppressant produced by *Streptomyces tsukubaensis*. It is for topical dermatologic use only. Chemically, tacrolimus is designated as [3S-[3R*[E(1S*,3S*,4S*)],4S*,5R*,8S*,9E,12R*,14R*, 15S*, 16R*,18S*,19S*,26aR*]] - 5,6,8,11,12,13,14,15,16,17,18, 19, 24,25,26,26a-hexadecahydro-5,19-dihydroxy-3-[2-(4-hydroxy-3-methoxycyclohexyl)-1-methylethenyl]-14,16-dimethoxy-4,10,12,18-tetramethyl-8-(2-propenyl)-15, 19-epoxy-3H-pyrido[2,1-*c*][1,4]oxaazacyclotricosine-1,7,20,21(4H,23H)-tetrone, monohydrate. It has the following structural formula:

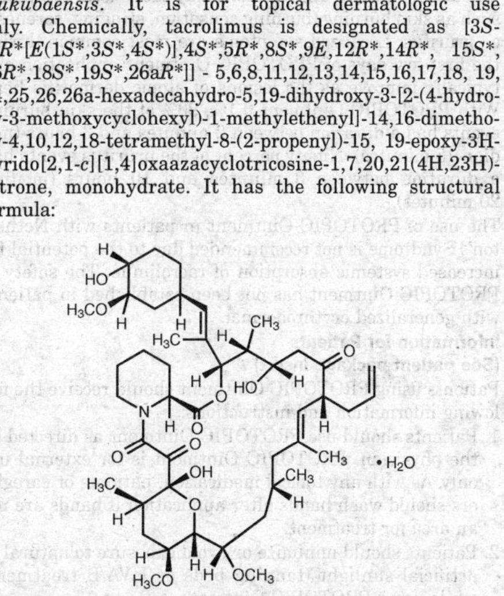

Tacrolimus has an empirical formula of $C_{44}H_{69}NO_{12} \cdot H_2O$ and a formula weight of 822.03. Each gram of PROTOPIC Ointment contains (w/w) either 0.03% or 0.1% of tacrolimus in a base of mineral oil, paraffin, propylene carbonate, white petrolatum and white wax.

CLINICAL PHARMACOLOGY

Mechanism of Action

The mechanism of action of tacrolimus in atopic dermatitis is not known. While the following have been observed, the clinical significance of these observations in atopic dermatitis is not known. It has been demonstrated that tacrolimus inhibits T-lymphocyte activation by first binding to an intracellular protein, FKBP-12. A complex of tacrolimus-FKBP-12, calcium, calmodulin, and calcineurin is then formed and the phosphatase activity of calcineurin is inhibited. This effect has been shown to prevent the dephosphorylation and translocation of nuclear factor of activated T-cells (NF-AT), a nuclear component thought to initiate gene transcription for the formation of lymphokines (such as interleukin-2, gamma interferon). Tacrolimus also inhibits the transcription for genes which encode IL-3, IL-4, IL-5, GM-CSF, and TNF-α, all of which are involved in the early stages of T-cell activation. Additionally, tacrolimus has been shown to inhibit the release of pre-formed mediators from skin mast cells and basophils, and to downregulate the expression of FcεRI on Langerhans cells.

Pharmacokinetics

The pooled results from two pharmacokinetic studies in 49 adult atopic dermatitis patients indicate that tacrolimus is absorbed after the topical application of 0.1% PROTOPIC Ointment. Peak tacrolimus blood concentrations ranged from undetectable to 20 ng/mL after single or multiple doses of 0.1% PROTOPIC Ointment, with 45 of the 49 patients having peak blood concentrations less than 5 ng/mL. The results from a pharmacokinetic study of 0.1% PROTOPIC Ointment in 20 pediatric atopic dermatitis patients (ages 6–13 years), show peak tacrolimus blood concentrations below 1.6 ng/mL in all patients.

There was no evidence based on blood concentrations that tacrolimus accumulates systemically upon intermittent topical application for periods of up to 1 year. The absolute bioavailability of topical tacrolimus is unknown. Using IV historical data for comparison, the bioavailability of tacrolimus from PROTOPIC in atopic dermatitis patients is less than 0.5%. In adults with an average of 53% BSA treated, exposure (i.e., AUC) of tacrolimus from PROTOPIC is approximately 30-fold less than that seen with oral immunosuppressive doses in kidney and liver transplant patients. The lowest tacrolimus blood level at which systemic effects can be observed is not known.

CLINICAL STUDIES

Three randomized, double-blind, vehicle-controlled, multicenter, phase 3 studies were conducted to evaluate PROTOPIC Ointment for the treatment of patients with moderate to severe atopic dermatitis. One (Pediatric) study included 351 patients 2–15 years of age, and the other two (Adult) studies included a total of 632 patients 15–79 years of age. Fifty-five percent (55%) of the patients were women and 27% were black. At baseline, 58% of the patients had severe disease and the mean body surface area (BSA) affected was 46%. Over 80% of patients had atopic dermatitis affecting the face and/or neck region. In these studies, patients applied either PROTOPIC Ointment 0.03%, PROTOPIC Ointment 0.1%, or vehicle ointment twice daily to 10%–100% of their BSA for up to 12 weeks.

In the pediatric study, a significantly greater ($p < 0.001$) percentage of patients achieved at least 90% improvement based on the physician's global evaluation of clinical response (the pre-defined primary efficacy end point) in the PROTOPIC Ointment 0.03% treatment group compared to the vehicle treatment group, but there was insufficient evidence that PROTOPIC Ointment 0.1% provided more efficacy than PROTOPIC Ointment 0.03%.

In both adult studies, a significantly greater ($p < 0.001$) percentage of patients achieved at least 90% improvement based on the physician's global evaluation of clinical response in the PROTOPIC Ointment 0.03% and PROTOPIC Ointment 0.1% treatment groups compared to the vehicle treatment group. There was evidence that PROTOPIC Ointment 0.1% may provide more efficacy than PROTOPIC Ointment 0.03%. The difference in efficacy between PROTOPIC Ointment 0.1% and 0.03% was particularly evident in adult patients with severe disease at baseline, adults with extensive BSA involvement, and black adults. Response rates for each treatment group are shown below by age groups. Because the two adult studies were identically designed, the results from these studies were pooled in this table.

[See table at top of next page]

A statistically significant difference in the percentage of adult patients with ≥ 90% improvement was achieved by week 1 for those treated with PROTOPIC Ointment 0.1%, and by week 3 for those treated with PROTOPIC Ointment 0.03%. A statistically significant difference in the percentage of pediatric patients with ≥ 90% improvement was achieved by week 2 for those treated with PROTOPIC Ointment 0.03%.

In adult patients who had achieved ≥ 90% improvement at the end of treatment, 35% of those treated with PROTOPIC Ointment 0.03% and 41% of those treated with PROTOPIC Ointment 0.1%, regressed from this state of improvement at 2 weeks after end-of-treatment. In pediatric patients who had achieved ≥ 90% improvement, 54% of those treated with PROTOPIC Ointment 0.03% regressed from this state of improvement at 2 weeks after end-of-treatment. Because patients were not followed for longer than 2 weeks after end-of-treatment, it is not known how many additional patients regressed at periods longer than 2 weeks after cessation of therapy.

In both PROTOPIC Ointment treatment groups in adults and in the PROTOPIC Ointment 0.03% treatment group in pediatric patients, a significantly greater improvement compared to vehicle ($p < 0.001$) was observed in the secondary efficacy endpoints of percent body surface area involved, patient evaluation of pruritus, erythema, edema, excoriation,

Continued on next page

Protopic—Cont.

oozing, scaling, and lichenification. The following two graphs depict the time course of improvement in the percent body surface area affected in adult and in pediatric patients as a result of treatment.

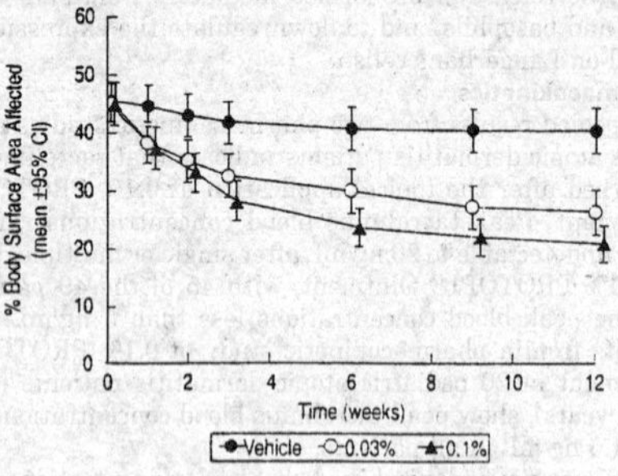

Figure 1 - Adult Patients Body Surface Area Over Time

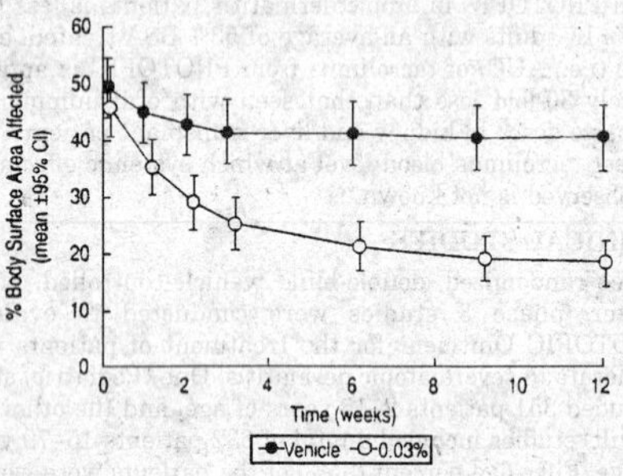

Figure 2 - Pediatric Patients Body Surface Area Over Time

The following two graphs depict the time course of improvement in erythema in adult and in pediatric patients as a result of treatment.

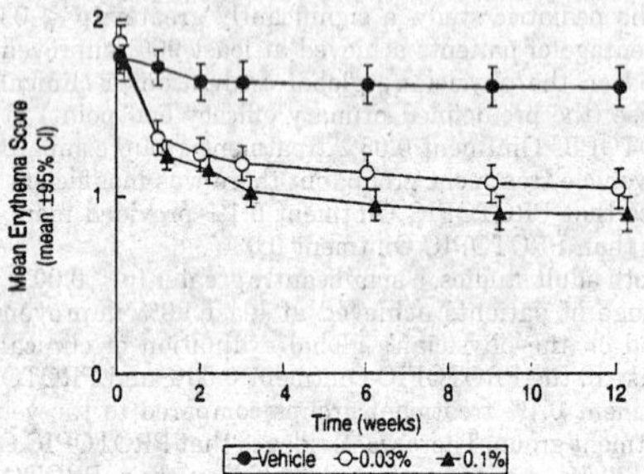

Figure 3 - Adult Patients Mean Erythema Over Time

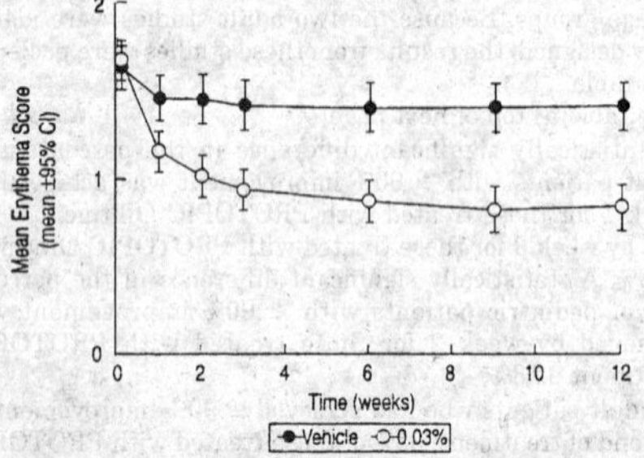

Figure 4 - Pediatric Patients Mean Erythema Over Time

The time course of improvement in the remaining secondary efficacy variables was similar to that of erythema, with improvement in lichenification slightly slower.

A total of 571 patients applied PROTOPIC Ointment 0.1% in long-term adult and pediatric safety studies for up to one year. In the adult study, 246 patients were evaluated for at least 6 months and 68 patients for 12 months. In the pediatric study, 219 patients were evaluated for at least 6 months and 180 patients for 12 months. On average, patients received treatment for 87% of study days.

INDICATIONS AND USAGE

PROTOPIC Ointment, both 0.03% and 0.1% for adults, and only 0.03% for children aged 2 to 15 years, is indicated for short-term and intermittent long-term therapy in the treatment of patients with moderate to severe atopic dermatitis in whom the use of alternative, conventional therapies are

Global Improvement over Baseline at the End-of-Treatment in Three Phase 3 Studies

Physician's Global Evaluation of Clinical Response (% Improvement)	Pediatric Study (2-15 Years of Age)		Adult Studies		
	Vehicle Ointment N = 116	PROTOPIC Ointment 0.03% N = 117	Vehicle Ointment N = 212	PROTOPIC Ointment 0.03% N = 211	PROTOPIC Ointment 0.1% N = 209
100%	4 (3%)	14 (12%)	2 (1%)	21 (10%)	20 (10%)
≥90%	8 (7%)	42 (36%)	14 (7%)	58 (28%)	77 (37%)
≥75%	18 (16%)	65 (56%)	30 (14%)	97 (46%)	117 (56%)
≥50%	31 (27%)	85 (73%)	42 (20%)	130 (62%)	152 (73%)

deemed inadvisable because of potential risks, or in the treatment of patients who are not adequately responsive to or are intolerant of alternative, conventional therapies.

CONTRAINDICATIONS

PROTOPIC Ointment is contraindicated in patients with a history of hypersensitivity to tacrolimus or any other component of the preparation.

PRECAUTIONS

General

Studies have not evaluated the safety and efficacy of PROTOPIC Ointment in the treatment of clinically infected atopic dermatitis. Before commencing treatment with PROTOPIC Ointment, clinical infections at treatment sites should be cleared.

While patients with atopic dermatitis are predisposed to superficial skin infections including eczema herpeticum (Kaposi's varicelliform eruption), treatment with PROTOPIC Ointment may be associated with an increased risk of varicella zoster virus infection (chicken pox or shingles), herpes simplex virus infection, or eczema herpeticum. In the presence of these infections, the balance of risks and benefits associated with PROTOPIC Ointment use should be evaluated.

In clinical studies, 33 cases of lymphadenopathy (0.8%) were reported and were usually related to infections (particularly of the skin) and noted to resolve upon appropriate antibiotic therapy. Of these 33 cases, the majority had either a clear etiology or were known to resolve. Transplant patients receiving immunosuppressive regimens (e.g., systemic tacrolimus) are at increased risk for developing lymphoma; therefore, patients who receive PROTOPIC Ointment and who develop lymphadenopathy should have the etiology of their lymphadenopathy investigated. In the absence of a clear etiology for the lymphadenopathy, or in the presence of acute infectious mononucleosis, discontinuation of PROTOPIC Ointment should be considered. Patients who develop lymphadenopathy should be monitored to ensure that the lymphadenopathy resolves.

The enhancement of ultraviolet carcinogenicity is not necessarily dependent on phototoxic mechanisms. Despite the absence of observed phototoxicity in humans (see **ADVERSE REACTIONS**), PROTOPIC Ointment shortened the time to skin tumor formation in an animal photocarcinogenicity study (see **Carcinogenesis, Mutagenesis, Impairment of Fertility**). Therefore, it is prudent for patients to minimize or avoid natural or artificial sunlight exposure.

The use of PROTOPIC Ointment may cause local symptoms such as skin burning (burning sensation, stinging, soreness) or pruritus. Localized symptoms are most common during the first few days of PROTOPIC Ointment application and typically improve as the lesions of atopic dermatitis heal. With PROTOPIC Ointment 0.1%, 90% of the skin burning events had a duration between 2 minutes and 3 hours (median 15 minutes). Ninety percent of the pruritus events had a duration between 3 minutes and 10 hours (median 20 minutes).

The use of PROTOPIC Ointment in patients with Netherton's Syndrome is not recommended due to the potential for increased systemic absorption of tacrolimus. The safety of PROTOPIC Ointment has not been established in patients with generalized erythroderma.

Information for Patients
(See patient package insert)

Patients using PROTOPIC Ointment should receive the following information and instructions:

1. Patients should use PROTOPIC Ointment as directed by the physician. PROTOPIC Ointment is for external use only. As with any topical medication, patients or caregivers should wash hands after application if hands are not an area for treatment.
2. Patients should minimize or avoid exposure to natural or artificial sunlight (tanning beds or UVA/B treatment) while using PROTOPIC Ointment.
3. Patients should not use this medication for any disorder other than that for which it was prescribed.
4. Patients should report any signs of adverse reactions to their physician.
5. Before applying PROTOPIC Ointment after a bath or shower, be sure your skin is completely dry.

Drug Interactions

Formal topical drug interaction studies with PROTOPIC Ointment have not been conducted. Based on its minimal extent of absorption, interactions of PROTOPIC Ointment with systemically administered drugs are unlikely to occur but cannot be ruled out. The concomitant administration of known CYP3A4 inhibitors in patients with widespread and/or erythrodermic disease should be done with caution. Some examples of such drugs are erythromycin, itraconazole, ketoconazole, fluconazole, calcium channel blockers and cimetidine.

Carcinogenesis, Mutagenesis, Impairment of Fertility

No evidence of genotoxicity was seen in bacterial (*Salmonella* and *E. coli*) or mammalian (Chinese hamster lung-derived cells) *in vitro* assays of mutagenicity, the *in vitro* CHO/HGPRT assay of mutagenicity, or *in vivo* clastogenicity assays performed in mice. Tacrolimus did not cause unscheduled DNA synthesis in rodent hepatocytes.

Oral (feed) carcinogenicity studies have been carried out with systemically administered tacrolimus in male and female rats and mice. In the 80-week mouse study and in the 104-week rat study no relationship of tumor incidence to tacrolimus dosage was found at daily doses up to 3 mg/kg [9X the Maximum Recommended Human Dose (MRHD) based on AUC comparisons] and 5 mg/kg (3X the MRHD based on AUC comparisons), respectively.

A 104-week dermal carcinogenicity study was performed in mice with tacrolimus ointment (0.03%–3%), equivalent to tacrolimus doses of 1.1–118 mg/kg/day or 3.3–354 mg/m^2/day. In the study, the incidence of skin tumors was minimal and the topical application of tacrolimus was not associated with skin tumor formation under ambient room lighting. However, a statistically significant elevation in the incidence of pleomorphic lymphoma in high dose male (25/50) and female animals (27/50) and in the incidence of undifferentiated lymphoma in high dose female animals (13/50) was noted in the mouse dermal carcinogenicity study. Lymphomas were noted in the mouse dermal carcinogenicity study at a daily dose of 3.5 mg/kg (0.1% tacrolimus ointment) (26X MRHD based on AUC comparisons). No drug-related tumors were noted in the mouse dermal carcinogenicity study at a daily dose of 1.1 mg/kg (0.03% tacrolimus ointment) (10X MRHD based on AUC comparisons).

In a 52-week photocarcinogenicity study, the median time to onset of skin tumor formation was decreased in hairless mice following chronic topical dosing with concurrent exposure to UV radiation (40 weeks of treatment followed by 12 weeks of observation) with tacrolimus ointment at ≥0.1% tacrolimus.

Reproductive toxicology studies were not performed with topical tacrolimus. In studies of oral tacrolimus no impairment of fertility was seen in male and female rats. Tacrolimus, given orally at 1.0 mg/kg (0.12X MRHD based on body surface area [BSA]) to male and female rats, prior to and during mating, as well as to dams during gestation and lactation, was associated with embryolethality and with adverse effects on female reproduction. Effects on female reproductive function (parturition) and embryolethal effects were indicated by a higher rate of pre-implantation loss and increased numbers of undelivered and nonviable pups. When given at 3.2 mg/kg (0.43X MRHD based on BSA), tacrolimus was associated with maternal and paternal toxicity as well as reproductive toxicity including marked adverse effects on estrus cycles, parturition, pup viability, and pup malformations.

Pregnancy

Teratogenic Effects: Pregnancy Category C

There are no adequate and well-controlled studies of topically administered tacrolimus in pregnant women. The experience with PROTOPIC Ointment when used by pregnant women is too limited to permit assessment of the safety of its use during pregnancy.

Reproduction studies were carried out with systemically administered tacrolimus in rats and rabbits. Adverse effects on the fetus were observed mainly at oral dose levels that were toxic to dams. Tacrolimus at oral doses of 0.32 and 1.0 mg/kg (0.04X–0.12X MRHD based on BSA) during organogenesis in rabbits was associated with maternal toxicity as well as an increase in incidence of abortions. At the higher dose only, an increased incidence of malformations and developmental variations was also seen. Tacrolimus, at oral doses of 3.2 mg/kg during organogenesis in rats, was associated with maternal toxicity and caused an increase in late resorptions, decreased numbers of live births, and decreased pup weight and viability. Tacrolimus, given orally at 1.0 and 3.2 mg/kg (0.04X–0.12X MRHD based on BSA) to pregnant rats after organogenesis and during lactation, was associated with reduced pup weights.

No reduction in male or female fertility was evident.

There are no adequate and well-controlled studies of systemically administered tacrolimus in pregnant women. Tacrolimus is transferred across the placenta. The use of systemically administered tacrolimus during pregnancy has been associated with neonatal hyperkalemia and renal dysfunction. PROTOPIC Ointment should be used during pregnancy only if the potential benefit to the mother justifies a potential risk to the fetus.

Incidence Of Treatment Emergent Adverse Events

	12-Week Randomized, Double-Blind, Phase 3 Studies 12-Week Adjusted Incidence Rate (%)					Open-Label Studies (up to 1 year) 0.1% Tacrolimus Ointment Incidence(%)	
	Adult			Pediatric		Adult	Pediatric
	Vehicle n=212	0.03% Tacrolimus Ointment n=210	0.1% Tacrolimus Ointment n=209	Vehicle n=116	0.03% Tacrolimus Ointment n=118	n=316	n=255
Skin Burning†	26	46	58	29	43	47	26
Pruritus†	37	46	46	27	41	25	25
Flu-like symptoms†	19	23	31	25	28	22	35
Allergic Reaction	8	12	6	8	4	22	15
Skin Erythema	20	25	28	13	12	12	9
Headache†	11	20	19	8	5	10	18
Skin Infection	11	12	5	14	10	11	11
Fever	4	4	1	13	21	2	18
Infection	1	1	2	9	7	14	8
Cough Increased	2	1	1	14	18	3	15
Asthma	4	6	4	6	6	5	16
Herpes Simplex	4	4	4	2	0	12	5
Eczema Herpeticum	0	1	1	0	2	2	0
Pharyngitis	3	3	4	11	6	5	10
Accidental Injury	4	3	6	3	6	4	12
Pustular Rash	2	3	4	3	2	6	8
Folliculitis†	1	6	4	0	2	11	2
Rhinitis	4	3	2	2	6	5	5
Otitis Media	4	0	1	6	12	1	7
Sinusitis†	1	4	2	8	3	3	7
Diarrhea	3	3	4	2	5	4	6
Urticaria	3	3	6	1	1	5	5
Lack of Drug Effect	1	1	0	1	1	10	2
Bronchitis	0	2	2	3	3	3	6
Vomiting	0	1	1	7	6	1	5
Maculopapular Rash	2	2	2	3	0	4	3
Rash†	1	5	2	4	2	2	5
Abdominal Pain	3	1	1	2	3	1	5
Fungal Dermatitis	0	2	1	3	0	2	6
Gastroenteritis	1	2	2	3	0	4	2
Alcohol Intolerance†	0	3	7	0	0	6	0
Acne†	2	4	7	1	0	2	4
Sunburn	1	2	1	0	0	4	4
Skin Disorder	2	2	1	1	4	1	4
Conjunctivitis	0	2	2	2	1	4	2
Pain	1	2	1	0	1	4	3
Vesiculobullous Rash†	3	3	2	0	4	2	2
Lymphadenopathy	2	2	1	0	3	2	3
Nausea	4	3	2	0	1	1	2
Skin Tingling†	2	3	8	1	2	2	1
Face Edema	2	2	1	2	1	3	1
Dyspepsia†	1	1	4	0	0	1	4
Dry Skin	7	3	3	0	1	0	1
Hyperesthesia†	1	3	7	0	0	3	0
Skin Neoplasm Benign‡‡	1	1	1	0	0	2	3
Back Pain†	0	2	2	1	1	3	1
Peripheral Edema	2	4	3	0	0	2	1
Varicella Zoster/ Herpes Zoster‡	0	1	0	0	5	1	3
Contact Dermatitis	1	3	3	3	4	1	1
Asthenia	1	2	3	0	0	2	1
Pneumonia	0	1	1	2	0	1	2
Eczema	2	2	2	0	0	3	0
Insomnia	3	4	3	1	1	1	0
Exfoliative Dermatitis	3	3	1	0	0	0	2
Dysmenorrhea	2	4	4	0	0	0	2
Periodontal Abscess	1	0	1	0	0	3	0
Myalgia†	0	3	2	0	0	1	0
Cyst†	0	1	3	0	0	0	0

†May be reasonably associated with the use of this drug product.
‡Four cases of chicken pox in the pediatric 12-week study, 1 case of "zoster of the lip" in the adult 12-week study; 7 cases of chicken pox and 1 case of shingles in the open-label pediatric study; 2 cases of herpes zoster in the open-label adult study.
‡‡Generally "warts".

Nursing Mothers

Although systemic absorption of tacrolimus following topical applications of PROTOPIC Ointment is minimal relative to systemic administration, it is known that tacrolimus is excreted in human milk. Because of the potential for serious adverse reactions in nursing infants from tacrolimus, a decision should be made whether to discontinue nursing or to discontinue the drug, taking into account the importance of the drug to the mother.

Pediatric Use

PROTOPIC Ointment 0.03% may be used in pediatric patients 2 years of age and older. Two phase 3 pediatric studies were conducted involving 606 patients 2–15 years of age: one 12-week randomized vehicle-controlled study and one open-label, 1 year, long-term safety study. Three hundred and thirty (330) of these patients were 2 to 6 years of age. The most common adverse events associated with PROTOPIC Ointment application in pediatric patients were skin burning and pruritus (see **ADVERSE REACTIONS**). In addition to skin burning and pruritus, the less common events (<5%) of varicella zoster (mostly children pox), and vesiculobullous rash were more frequent in patients treated with PROTOPIC Ointment 0.03% compared to vehicle. In the long-term 1 year safety study involving 255 pediatric patients using PROTOPIC Ointment, the incidence of adverse events, including infections, did not increase with increased duration of study drug exposure or amount of ointment used. In 491 pediatric patients treated with PROTOPIC Ointment, 3(0.6%) developed eczema herpeticum. Since the safety and efficacy of PROTOPIC Ointment have not been established in pediatric patients below 2 years of age, its use in this age group is not recommended.

Geriatric Use

Twenty-five (25) patients ≥ 65 years old received PROTOPIC Ointment in phase 3 studies. The adverse event profile for these patients was consistent with that for other adult patients.

ADVERSE REACTIONS

No phototoxicity and no photoallergenicity was detected in clinical studies of 12 and 216 normal volunteers, respectively. One out of 198 normal volunteers showed evidence of sensitization in a contact sensitization study.

In three randomized vehicle-controlled studies and two long-term safety studies, 655 and 571 patients respectively, were treated with PROTOPIC Ointment.

The following table depicts the adjusted incidence of adverse events pooled across the 3 identically designed 12 week studies for patients in vehicle, PROTOPIC Ointment 0.03%, and PROTOPIC Ointment 0.1% treatment groups, and the unadjusted incidence of adverse events in two one year long-term safety studies, regardless of relationship to study drug.

[See table above]

Other adverse events which occurred at an incidence greater than or equal to 1% in any clinical study include: alopecia, ALT or AST increased, anaphylactoid reaction, angina pectoris, angioedema, anorexia, anxiety, arrhythmia, arthralgia, arthritis, bilirubinemia, breast pain, cellulitis, cerebrovascular accident, cheilitis, chills, constipation, creatinine increased, dehydration, depression, dizziness, dyspnea, ear pain, ecchymosis, edema, epistaxis, exacerbation of untreated area, eye disorder, eye pain, furunculosis, gastritis, hernia, hyperglycemia, hypertension, hypoglycemia, hypoxia, laryngitis, leukocytosis, leukopenia, liver function tests abnormal, lung disorder, malaise, migraine, neck pain, neuritis, palpitations, paresthesia, peripheral vascular disorder, photosensitivity reaction, procedural complication, routine procedure, skin discoloration, sweating, taste perversion, tooth disorder, unintended pregnancy, vaginal moniliasis, vasodilatation, and vertigo.

OVERDOSAGE

PROTOPIC Ointment is not for oral use. Oral ingestion of PROTOPIC Ointment may lead to adverse effects associated with systemic administration of tacrolimus. If oral ingestion occurs, medical advice should be sought.

DOSAGE AND ADMINISTRATION

ADULT

PROTOPIC Ointment 0.03% and 0.1%

Apply a thin layer of PROTOPIC Ointment 0.03% or 0.1% to the affected skin areas twice daily and rub in gently and completely. Treatment should be continued for one week after clearing of signs and symptoms of atopic dermatitis.

The safety of PROTOPIC Ointment under occlusion which may promote systemic exposure, has not been evaluated. **PROTOPIC Ointment 0.03% and 0.1% should not be used with occlusive dressings.**

PEDIATRIC

PROTOPIC Ointment 0.03%

Apply a thin layer of PROTOPIC Ointment 0.03% to the affected skin areas twice daily and rub in gently and completely. Treatment should be continued for one week after clearing of signs and symptoms of atopic dermatitis. The safety of PROTOPIC Ointment under occlusion, which may promote systemic exposure, has not been evaluated. **PROTOPIC Ointment 0.03% should not be used with occlusive dressings.**

HOW SUPPLIED

PROTOPIC® (tacrolimus) Ointment 0.03%

NDC 0469-5201-30 Product Code 520130
30 gram laminate tube
NDC 0469-5201-60 Product Code 520160
60 gram laminate tube
NDC 0469-5201-11 Product Code 520111
100 gram laminate tube

PROTOPIC® (tacrolimus) Ointment 0.1%

NDC 0469-5202-30 Product Code 520230
30 gram laminate tube
NDC 0469-5202-60 Product Code 520260
60 gram laminate tube
NDC 0469-5202-11 Product Code 520211
100 gram laminate tube

Store at room temperature 25°C (77°F); excursions permitted to 15°–30°C (59°–86°F).

℞ only

Fujisawa Healthcare, Inc.
Issued August 2002/45686
Deerfield, IL 60015–2548 Issued: December 2000

Shown in Product Identification Guide, page 313

IDENTIFICATION PROBLEM?
Turn to the **Product Identification Guide,**
where you'll find more than
1600 products pictured in actual
size and full color.

Galderma Laboratories, L.P.

14501 NORTH FREEWAY
FT. WORTH, TX 76177

Direct Inquiries to:
(800) 582-8225
8:00 am–5:00 pm Central
Monday through Friday
or www.galdermaUSA.com

CAPEX® SHAMPOO ℞

[*kā pĕx*]
(fluocinolone acetonide)
Topical Shampoo, 0.01%
For Dermatological Use Only
Not for Ophthalmic Use
℞ only

DESCRIPTION

Capex® Shampoo 0.01% is supplied as a shampoo formulation with a 12 mg fluocinolone acetonide capsule which is emptied into the shampoo base by the pharmacist at the time of dispensing. After mixing, Capex® Shampoo contains fluocinolone acetonide(6α,9-Difluoro-11β,16α, 17,21-tetrahydroxypregna-1,4-diene-3, 20-dione cyclic 16,17-acetal with acetone), a synthetic fluorinated corticosteroid for topical dermatologic use. The corticosteroids constitute a class of primarily synthetic steroids used topically as an anti-inflammatory and antipruritic agents.
Chemically, Capex® Shampoo mixture is $C_{24}H_{30}F_2O_6$. It has the following structural formula:

Fluocinolone acetonide in Capex® Shampoo has the molecular weight of 452.50. It is a white crystalline powder that is odorless, stable in light and melts at 270°F with decomposition; soluble in alcohol, acetone and methanol; slightly soluble in chloroform; insoluble in water.
Each fluocinolone capsule contains 12 mg of fluocinolone acetonide, 548 mg of dibasic calcium phosphate dihydrate USP, and 240 mg of talc USP. The shampoo base contains aluminum acetate basic, benzalkonium chloride solution, boric acid, citric acid anhydrous, cocamido-ether-sulfate complex, cocoamine oxide, lauramide DEA, magnesium aluminum silicate, methylparaben, oat flour, propylene glycol, propylparaben, purified water, and fragrances, with D&C Yellow #10 and FD&C Blue #1 as coloring.

CLINICAL PHARMACOLOGY

Like other topical corticosteroids, fluocinolone acetonide has anti-inflammatory, antipruritic and vasoconstrictive properties. The mechanism of the anti-inflammatory activity of the topical steroids, in general, is unclear. However corticosteroids are thought to act by the induction of phospholipase A_2 inhibitory proteins, collectively called lipocortins. It is postulated that these proteins control the biosynthesis of potent mediators of inflammation such as prostaglandins and leukotrienes by inhibiting the release of their common precursor arachidonic acid. Arachidonic acid is released from membrane phospholipids by phospholipase A_2.

Pharmacokinetics: The extent of percutaneous absorption of topical corticosteroids is determined by many factors including the vehicle and the integrity of the epidermal barrier. Occlusive dressings with hydrocortisone for up to 24 hours have not been demonstrated to increase penetration; however, occlusion of hydrocortisone for 96 hours markedly enhances penetration. Topical corticosteroids can be absorbed from normal intact skin while inflammation and/or other disease processes in the skin increase percutaneous absorption.
Capex® Shampoo is in the low to medium range of potency as compared with other topical corticosteroids.

CLINICAL STUDIES

In vehicle-controlled studies for the treatment of seborrheic dermatitis of the scalp, after 14 days of treatment, 84% of patients on active treatment and 29% of patients on the drug vehicle had cleared or markedly improved.

INDICATION AND USAGE

Capex® Shampoo is a low to medium potency corticosteroid indicated for the treatment of seborrheic dermatitis of the scalp. This product has not been proven to be effective in other corticosteroid-responsive dermatoses.

CONTRAINDICATIONS

Capex® Shampoo is contraindicated in those patients with a history of hypersensitivity to any of the components of the preparation.

PRECAUTIONS

General: Systemic absorption of topical corticosteroids can produce reversible hypothalamic-pituitary-adrenal (HPA) axis suppression with the potential for glucocorticoid insufficiency after withdrawal of treatment. Manifestations of Cushing's syndrome, hyperglycemia and glucosuria can also be produced in some patients by systemic absorption of topical corticosteroids while on treatment.
Patients applying a topical steroid to a large surface area or to areas under occlusion should be evaluated periodically for evidence of HPA axis suppression. This may be done by using the ACTH stimulation, A.M. plasma cortisol, and urinary free cortisol tests. Patients receiving superpotent corticosteroids should not be treated for more than 2 weeks at a time and only small areas should be treated at any one time due to the increased risk of HPA suppression.
If HPA axis suppression is noted, an attempt should be made to withdraw the drug, to reduce the frequency of application, or to substitute a less potent corticosteroid. Infrequently, signs and symptoms of glucocorticoid insufficiency may occur requiring supplemental systemic corticosteroids. For information on systemic supplementation, see prescribing information for those products.
Pediatric patients may be more susceptible to systemic toxicity from equivalent doses due to their larger skin surface to body mass ratios. (See PRECAUTIONS—Pediatric Use).
If irritation develops, Capex® Shampoo should be discontinued and appropriate therapy instituted. Allergic contact dermatitis with corticosteroids is usually diagnosed by a *failure to heal* rather than noting a clinical exacerbation as with most topical products not containing corticosteroids. Such an observation should be corroborated with appropriate diagnostic patch testing.
If concomitant skin infections are present or develop, an appropriate antifungal or antibacterial agent should be used. If a favorable response does not occur promptly, Capex® Shampoo should be discontinued until the infection has been adequately controlled.
Information for Patients: Patients using topical corticosteroids should receive the following information and instructions:

1. This medication is to be used as directed by the physician. It is for external use only. Avoid contact with the eyes. In case of contact, wash eyes liberally with water.
2. This medication should not be used for any disorder other than that for which it was prescribed.
3. The treated scalp area should not be bandaged or otherwise covered or wrapped so as to be occlusive unless directed by the physician.
4. Patients should report to their physician any signs of local adverse reactions.
5. Discard contents after three (3) months.

Laboratory Tests: The following tests may be helpful in evaluating patients for HPA suppression:
ACTH stimulation test
A.M. plasma cortisol test
Urinary free cortisol test
Carcinogenesis, mutagenesis, and impairment of fertility: Long-term animal studies have not been performed to evaluate the carcinogenic potential or the effect on fertility of Capex® Shampoo.
Pregnancy: Teratogenic effects: Pregnancy category C: Corticosteroids have been shown to be teratogenic in laboratory animals when administered systemically at relatively low dosage levels. Some corticosteroids have been shown to be teratogenic after dermal application in laboratory animals.
There are no adequate and well-controlled studies in pregnant women or teratogenic effects from Capex® Shampoo. Therefore, Capex® Shampoo should be used during pregnancy only if the potential benefit justifies the potential risk to the fetus.
Nursing Mothers: Systemically administered corticosteroids appear in human milk could suppress growth, interfere with endogenous corticosteroid production or cause other untoward effects. It is not known whether topical administration of corticosteroids could result in sufficient systemic absorption to produce detectable quantities in human milk. Because many drugs are secreted in human milk, caution should be exercised when Capex® Shampoo is administered to a nursing woman.
Pediatric Use: Safety and effectiveness in children and infants have not been established. Because of a higher ratio of skin surface area to body mass, pediatric patients are at a greater risk than adults of HPA axis suppression when they are treated with topical corticosteroids. They are therefore also at a greater risk of glucocorticoid insufficiency after withdrawal of treatment and of Cushing's syndrome while on treatment. Adverse effects including striae have been reported with inappropriate use of topical corticosteroids in infants and children.
HPA axis suppression, Cushing's syndrome and intracranial hypertension have be reported in children receiving topical corticosteroids. Manifestations of adrenal suppresion in children include linear growth retardation, delayed weight gain, low plasma cortisol levels and absence of response to ACTH stimulation. Manifestations of intracranial hypertension include bulging fontanelles, headaches and bilateral papilledema.

ADVERSE REACTIONS

The following local adverse reactions have been reported infrequently with topical corticosteroids. They may occur more frequently with the use of occlusive dressings, especially with higher potency corticosteroids. These reactions are listed in an approximate decreasing order of occurrence: dryness, folliculitis, acneform eruptions, perioral dermatitis, allergic contact dermatitis, secondary infection, skin atrophy, striae, miliaria, burning, itching, irritation and hypopigmentation.

OVERDOSAGE

Topically applied Capex® Shampoo can be absorbed in sufficient amount to produce systemic effects (See PRECAUTIONS).

DOSAGE AND ADMINISTRATION

The pharmacist must empty the contents of the enclosed capsule into the shampoo base prior to dispensing to the patient. This product should be shaken well prior to use. No more than approximately one (1) ounce of the medicated shampoo should be applied to the scalp area once daily, worked into a lather and allowed to remain on the scalp for approximately 5 minutes. The hair and scalp should then be rinsed thoroughly with water.

HOW SUPPLIED

Capex® Shampoo is supplied as a two component package: a capsule which contains the active component fluocinolone acetonide 0.01%, and a separate package of liquid shampoo. The pharmacist must mix the content of the capsule into the base at the time of dispensing. Capex® Shampoo is dispensed to the patient in a 6 ounce bottle.
NDC 0299-5500-04
Shake well before using.
Store between 15° and 30°C (59° and 86°F) in tightly closed containers.
Marketed by:
GALDERMA LABORATORIES, L.P.
Fort Worth, Texas 76177 USA
Mfd. by:
Hill Laboratories, Inc. 20002-0700
Sanford, Florida 32773 USA Revised: July 2000
GALDERMA is a registered trademark.

CLINDAGEL® ℞

[*klĭnd-ă-jĕl*]
(clindamycin phosphate gel)
topical gel, 1%
For External Use
℞ Only

DESCRIPTION

Clindagel® (clindamycin phosphate gel) topical gel, 1%, a topical antibiotic, contains clindamycin phosphate, USP, at a concentration equivalent to 10 mg clindamycin per gram in a gel vehicle consisting of carbomer 941, methylparaben, polyethylene glycol 400, propylene glycol, sodium hydroxide, and purified water. Chemically, clindamycin phosphate is a water-soluble ester of the semi-synthetic antibiotic produced by a 7 (S)-chloro-substitution of the 7 (R)-hydroxyl group of the parent antibiotic, lincomycin, and has the structural formula represented below:

The chemical name for clindamycin phosphate is methyl 7-chloro-6,7,8-trideoxy-6-(1-methyl-*trans*-4-propyl-L-2-pyrrolidinecarboxamido)-1-thio-L-*threo*-α-D-*galacto*-octopyranoside 2-(dihydrogen phosphate).

CLINICAL PHARMACOLOGY

Pharmacokinetics: In an open label, parallel group study of 24 patients with acne vulgaris, once-daily topical administration of approximately 3–12 grams/day of **Clindagel®** for five days resulted in peak plasma clindamycin concentrations that were less than 5.5 ng/mL.
Following multiple applications of **Clindagel®** less than 0.04% of the total dose was excreted in the urine.
Microbiology: Although clindamycin phosphate is inactive *in vitro*, rapid *in vitro* hydrolysis converts this compound to clindamycin which has antibacterial activity. Clindamycin inhibits bacteria protein synthesis at the ribosomal level by binding to the 50S ribosomal subunit and affecting the process of peptide chain initiation. *In vitro* studies indicated that clindamycin inhibited all tested *Propionibacterium acnes* cultures at a minimum inhibitory concentration (MIC) of 0.4 µg/mL. Cross-resistance has been demonstrated between clindamycin and erythromycin.

CLINICAL STUDIES

In one 12-week multicenter, randomized, evaluator-blind, vehicle-controlled, parallel comparison clinical trial in which patients used **Clindagel®** (clindamycin phosphate topical gel, 1%) once daily or the vehicle gel once daily, in the treatment of acne vulgaris of mild to moderate severity, **Clindagel®** applied once daily was more effective than the vehicle applied once daily. The mean percent reductions in lesion counts at the end of treatment in this study are shown in the following table:

Lesions	Clindagel® QD N=162	Vehicle Gel QD N=82
Inflammatory	51%	40%*
Noninflammatory	25%	12%*
Total	38%	27%*

*P<0.05

There was a trend in the investigator's global assessment of the results which favored **Clindagel®** QD over the vehicle QD.

In a contact sensitization study, four of the 200 subjects appeared to develop suggestive evidence of allergic contact sensitization to **Clindagel®**. There was no signal for contact sensitization in the clinical trials under normal use conditions.

INDICATIONS AND USAGE

Clindagel® is indicated for topical application in the treatment of acne vulgaris. In view of the potential for diarrhea, bloody diarrhea and pseudomembranous colitis, the physician should consider whether other agents are more appropriate. (See CONTRAINDICATIONS, WARNINGS, and ADVERSE REACTIONS.)

CONTRAINDICATIONS

Clindagel® is contraindicated in individuals with a history of hypersensitivity to preparations containing clindamycin or lincomycin, a history of regional enteritis or ulcerative colitis, or a history of antibiotic-associated colitis.

WARNINGS

Orally and parenterally administered clindamycin has been associated with severe colitis, which may result in patient death. Use of the topical formulation of clindamycin results in absorption of the antibiotic from the skin surface. Diarrhea, bloody diarrhea, and colitis (including pseudomembranous colitis) have been reported with the use of topical and systemic clindamycin.

Studies indicate a toxin(s) produced by *Clostridia* is one primary cause of antibiotic-associated colitis. The colitis is usually characterized by severe persistent diarrhea and severe abdominal cramps and may be associated with the passage of blood and mucus. Endoscopic examination may reveal pseudomembranous colitis. Stool culture for *Clostridium difficile* and stool assay for *C. difficile* toxin may be helpful diagnostically.

When significant diarrhea occurs, the drug should be discontinued. Large bowel endoscopy should be considered to establish a definitive diagnosis in cases of severe diarrhea. Antiperistaltic agents, such as opiates and diphenoxylate with atropine, may prolong and/or worsen the condition.

Diarrhea, colitis, and pseudomembranous colitis have been observed to begin up to several weeks following cessation of oral and parenteral therapy with clindamycin.

PRECAUTIONS

General: **Clindagel®** should be prescribed with caution in atopic individuals.

Drug Interactions: Clindamycin has been shown to have neuromuscular blocking properties that may enhance the action of other neuromuscular blocking agents. Therefore, it should be used with caution in patients receiving such agents.

Carcinogenesis, Mutagenesis, Impairment of Fertility

The carcinogenicity of a 1% clindamycin phosphate gel similar to **Clindagel®** was evaluated by daily application to mice for two years. The daily doses used in this study were approximately 3 and 15 times higher than the human dose of clindamycin phosphate from 5 milliliters of **Clindagel®**, assuming complete absorption and based on a body surface area comparison. No significant increase in tumors was noted in the treated animals.

A 1% clindamycin phosphate gel similar to **Clindagel®** caused a statistically significant shortening of the median time to tumor onset in a study in hairless mice in which tumors were induced by exposure to simulated sunlight.

Genotoxicity tests performed included a rat micronucleus test and an Ames Salmonella reversion test. Both tests were negative. Reproduction studies in rats using oral doses of clindamycin hydrochloride and clindamycin palmitate hydrochloride have revealed no evidence of impaired fertility.

Pregnancy: Teratogenic effects—Pregnancy Category B

Reproduction studies have been performed in rats and mice using subcutaneous and oral doses of clindamycin phosphate, clindamycin hydrochloride and clindamycin palmitate hydrochloride. These studies revealed no evidence of fetal harm. The highest dose used in the rat and mouse teratogenicity studies was equivalent to a clindamycin phosphate dose of 432 mg/kg. For a rat, this dose is 84 fold higher and for a mouse 42 fold higher, than the anticipated human dose of clindamycin phosphate from **Clindagel®** based on a mg/m^2 comparison. There are, however, no adequate and well-controlled studies in pregnant women.

Because animal reproduction studies are not always predictive of human response, this drug should be used during pregnancy only if clearly needed.

Nursing Mothers: It is not known whether clindamycin is excreted in human milk following use of **Clindagel®**. However, orally and parenterally administered clindamycin has been reported to appear in breast milk. Because of the potential for serious adverse reactions in nursing infants, a decision should be made whether to discontinue nursing or to discontinue the drug, taking into account the importance of the drug to the mother.

Pediatric Use: Safety and effectiveness in children under the age of 12 have not been established.

Geriatric Use: The clinical study with **Clindagel®** did not include sufficient numbers of patients aged 65 and over to determine if they respond differently than younger patients.

ADVERSE REACTIONS

In the one well-controlled clinical study comparing **Clindagel®** and its vehicle, the incidence of skin and appendages adverse events occurring in ≥1% of the patients in either group is presented below:

Body System/Adverse Event	Number (%) of Patients Clindagel® QD N=168	Vehicle Gel QD N=84
Skin and appendages disorders		
Dermatitis	0 (0.0)	1 (1.2)
Dermatitis contact	0 (0.0)	1 (1.2)
Dermatitis fungal	0 (0.0)	1 (1.2)
Folliculitis	0 (0.0)	1 (1.2)
Photosensitivity reaction	0 (0.0)	1 (1.2)
Pruritus	1 (0.6)	1 (1.2)
Rash erythematous	0 (0.0)	0 (0.0)
Skin dry	0 (0.0)	0 (0.0)
Peeling	1 (0.6)	0 (0.0)

Orally and parenterally administered clindamycin has been associated with severe colitis, which may end fatally.

Cases of diarrhea, bloody diarrhea, and colitis (including pseudomembranous colitis) have been reported as adverse reactions in patients treated with oral and parenteral formulations of clindamycin and rarely with topical clindamycin (see WARNINGS). Abdominal pain and gastrointestinal disturbances, as well as Gram-negative folliculitis, have also been reported in association with the use of topical formulations of clindamycin.

OVERDOSE

Topically applied **Clindagel®** may be absorbed in sufficient amounts to produce systemic effects (see WARNINGS).

DOSAGE AND ADMINISTRATION

Apply a thin film of **Clindagel®** once daily to the skin where acne lesions appear. Use enough to cover the entire affected area lightly.

Keep container tightly closed.

HOW SUPPLIED

Clindagel® containing clindamycin phosphate equivalent to 10 mg clindamycin per gram, is available in the following sizes:

75 mL bottle - **NDC** 0299-4500-75

40 mL bottle - **NDC** 0299-4500-40

Store under controlled room temperature 20°C–25°C (68°F to 77°F); excursions permitted between 15°C–30°C (59°F to 86°F). Do not store in direct sunlight.

Marketed by:
Galderma Laboratories, L.P.
Fort Worth, Texas 76177 USA
Manufactured by:
DPT Laboratories, Ltd.
San Antonio, Texas 78215 USA
GALDERMA is a registered trademark.
www.clindagel.com
325053-0603 Revised: June 2003

CLOBEX™ ℞

[*klō-bĕks*]

(clobetasol propionate) Lotion, 0.05%

Rx only

For dermatologic use only

Not for ophthalmic, oral or intravaginal use

DESCRIPTION

CLOBEX™ (clobetasol propionate) Lotion, 0.05% contains clobetasol propionate, a synthetic fluorinated corticosteroid, for topical dermatologic use. The corticosteroids constitute a class of primarily synthetic steroids used topically as anti-inflammatory and antipruritic agents.

Clobetasol propionate is 21-chloro-9-fluoro-11β,17-dihydroxy-16β-methylpregna-1,4-diene-3, 20-dione17-propionate, with the empirical formula $C_{25}H_{32}ClFO_5$, a molecular weight of 466.98(CAS Registry Number 25122-46-7).

The following is the chemical structure:

Clobetasol propionate is a white to practically-white crystalline powder insoluble in water. Each gram of CLOBEX™ (clobetasol propionate) Lotion, 0.05% contains 0.5 mg of clobetasol propionate, in a vehicle base composed of hypromellose, propylene glycol, mineral oil, polyoxyethylene glycol 300 isostearate, carbomer 1342, sodium hydroxide and purified water.

CLINICAL PHARMACOLOGY

Like other topical corticosteroids, CLOBEX™ (clobetasol propionate) Lotion, 0.05% has anti-inflammatory, antipruritic, and vasoconstrictive properties. The mechanism of the anti-inflammatory activity of the topical steroids in general is unclear. However, corticosteroids are thought to act by induction of phospholipase A2 inhibitory proteins, collectively called lipocortins. It is postulated that these proteins control the biosynthesis of potent mediators of inflammation such as prostaglandins and leukotrienes by inhibiting the release of their common precursor, arachidonic acid. Arachidonic acid is released from membrane phospholipids by phospholipase A2.

Pharmacokinetics: The extent of percutaneous absorption of topical corticosteroids is determined by many factors, including the vehicle, the integrity of the epidermal barrier and occlusion. For example, occlusive dressing with hydrocortisone for up to 24 hours has not been demonstrated to increase penetration; however, occlusion of hydrocortisone for 96 hours markedly enhances penetration. Topical corticosteroids can be absorbed from normal intact skin. Inflammation and other disease processes in the skin may increase percutaneous absorption.

There are no human data regarding the distribution of corticosteroids to body organs following topical application. Nevertheless, once absorbed through the skin, topical corticosteroids are handled through pharmacokinetic pathways similar to systematically administered corticosteroids. Due to the fact that circulating levels are usually below the level of detection, the use of pharmacodynamic endpoints for assessing the systemic exposure of topical corticosteroids is necessary. They are metabolized, primarily in the liver, and are then excreted by the kidneys. In addition, some corticosteroids and their metabolites are also excreted in the bile.

CLOBEX™ (clobetasol propionate) Lotion, 0.05% is in the super-high range of potency as compared with other topical corticosteroids in vasoconstrictor studies.

In studies evaluating the potential for hypothalamic-pituitary-adrenal (HPA) axis suppression, CLOBEX™ Lotion, 0.05% demonstrated rates of suppression that were numerically higher than those of a clobetasol propionate 0.05% cream (Temovate E® Emollient, 0.05%), (See PRECAUTIONS).

CLINICAL STUDIES

The efficacy of CLOBEX™ (clobetasol propionate) Lotion, 0.05% in psoriasis and atopic dermatitis has been demonstrated in two adequate and well-controlled clinical trials. The first study was conducted in patients with moderate to severe plaque psoriasis. Patients were treated twice daily for 4 weeks with either CLOBEX™ (clobetasol propionate) Lotion, 0.05% or vehicle lotion. Study results demonstrated that the efficacy of CLOBEX™ Lotion, 0.05% in treating moderate to severe plaque psoriasis was superior to that of vehicle. At the end of treatment (4 weeks), 30 of 82 patients (36.6%) treated with CLOBEX™ Lotion, 0.05% compared with 0 of 29 (0%) treated with vehicle achieved success. Success was defined as a score of none or very mild (no or very slight clinical signs or symptoms of erythema, plaque elevation, or scaling) on the Global Severity scale of psoriasis.

The second study was conducted in patients with moderate to severe atopic dermatitis. Patients were treated twice daily for 2 weeks with either CLOBEX™ (clobetasol propionate) Lotion, 0.05% or vehicle lotion. Study results demonstrated that the efficacy of CLOBEX™ Lotion, 0.05% in treating moderate to severe atopic dermatitis was superior to that of vehicle.

At the end of treatment (2 weeks), 41 of 96 patients (42.7%) treated with CLOBEX™ Lotion, 0.05% compared with 4 of 33 (12.1%) treated with vehicle achieved success. Success was defined as a score of none or very mild (no or very slight clinical signs or symptoms of erythema, induration/papulation, oozing/crusting, or pruritus) on the Global Severity scale of atopic dermatitis.

INDICATIONS AND USAGE

CLOBEX™ (clobetasol propionate) Lotion, 0.05% is a super-high potent corticosteroid formulation indicated for the relief of the inflammatory and pruritic manifestations of corticosteroid-responsive dermatoses only in patients 18 years of age or older (see PRECAUTIONS). Treatment should be limited to 2 consecutive weeks. The total dosage should not exceed 50 g (50 mL or 1.75 fl.oz.) per week.

For the treatment of moderate to severe plaque psoriasis, localized lesions (less than 10% body surface area) that have not sufficiently improved after the initial 2-week treatment with CLOBEX™ (clobetasol propionate) Lotion, 0.05% may be treated for up to 2 additional weeks. Any additional benefits of extending treatment should be weighed against the risk of HPA axis suppression before prescribing for more than 2 weeks.

Patients should be instructed to use CLOBEX™ (clobetasol propionate) Lotion, 0.05% for the minimum amount of time necessary to achieve the desired results (see PRECAUTIONS).

Use in patients younger than 18 years of age is not recommended due to numerically high rates of HPA axis suppression (see PRECAUTIONS: Pediatric Use).

CONTRAINDICATIONS

CLOBEX™ (clobetasol propionate) Lotion, 0.05% is contraindicated in patients who are hypersensitive to clobetasol propionate, to other corticosteroids, or to any ingredient in this preparation.

Continued on next page

Clobex Lotion—Cont.

PRECAUTIONS

General: Clobetasol propionate is a highly potent topical corticosteroid that has been shown to suppress the HPA axis at the lowest doses tested.

Systemic absorption of topical corticosteroids has caused reversible adrenal suppression with the potential for glucocorticosteroid insufficiency after withdrawal of treatment. Manifestations of Cushing's syndrome, hyperglycemia, and glucosuria can also be produced in some patients by systemic absorption of topical corticosteroids while on treatment.

Conditions which increase systemic absorption include the application of the more potent steroids, use over large surface areas, prolonged use, and the addition of occlusive dressings. Therefore, patients applying a topical steroid to a large surface area or to areas under occlusion should be evaluated periodically for evidence of adrenal suppression (see laboratory tests below). If adrenal suppression is noted, an attempt should be made to withdraw the drug, to reduce the frequency of application, or to substitute a less potent steroid. Recovery of HPA axis function is generally prompt upon discontinuation of topical corticosteroids. Infrequently, signs and symptoms of glucocorticosteroid insufficiency may occur requiring supplemental systemic corticosteroids. For information on systemic supplementation, see prescribing information for those products.

The effect of CLOBEX™ Lotion, 0.05% on HPA axis function was compared to clobetasol propionate cream 0.05% (Temovate E® Emollient, 0.05%) in adults in two studies, one for psoriasis and one for atopic dermatitis. In total, 8 of 10 evaluable patients with moderate to severe plaque psoriasis experienced adrenal suppression following 4 weeks of CLOBEX™ Lotion, 0.05% therapy (treatment beyond 4 consecutive weeks is not recommended in moderate to severe plaque psoriasis). In follow-up testing, 1 of 2 patients remained suppressed after 8 days. In this comparative study, for clobetasol propionate cream, 0.05% there were 3 of 10 evaluable patients with HPA axis suppression. Furthermore, 5 of 9 evaluable patients with moderate to severe atopic dermatitis experienced adrenal suppression following 2 weeks of CLOBEX™ Lotion, 0.05% therapy (treatment beyond 2 consecutive weeks is not recommended in moderate to severe atopic dermatitis). Of the 3 patients that had follow-up testing, one patient failed to recover adrenal function 7 days post-treatment. For patients treated with clobetasol propionate cream, 0.05%, 4 of 9 evaluable patients experienced adrenal suppression following 2 weeks of treatment. Of the 2 patients that had follow-up testing, both recovered adrenal function 7 days post-treatment. The proportion of subjects suppressed may be underestimated because the adrenal glands were stimulated weekly with cosyntropin in these studies.

The potential increase in systemic exposure does not correlate with any proven benefit, but may lead to an increased potential for hypothalamic-pituitary-adrenal (HPA) axis suppression. Patients with acute illness or injury may have increased morbidity and mortality with intermittent HPA axis suppression. Patients should be instructed to use CLOBEX™ Lotion, 0.05% for the minimum amount of time necessary to achieve the desired results (See INDICATIONS AND USAGE).

If irritation develops, CLOBEX™ Lotion, 0.05% should be discontinued and appropriate therapy instituted. Allergic contact dermatitis with corticosteroids is usually diagnosed by observing a failure to heal rather than noting a clinical exacerbation, as with most topical products not containing corticosteroids.

In the presence of dermatological infections, the use of an appropriate antifungal or antibacterial agent should be instituted. If a favorable response does not occur promptly, use of CLOBEX™ Lotion, 0.05% should be discontinued until the infection has been adequately controlled. CLOBEX™ Lotion, 0.05% should not be used in the treatment of rosacea or perioral dermatitis, and should not be used on the face, groin, or axillae.

Information for Patients: Patients using topical corticosteroids should receive the following information and instructions:

- This medication is to be used as directed by the physician and should not be used longer than the prescribed time period.
- This medication should not be used for any disorder other than that for which it was prescribed.
- The treated skin area should not be bandaged, otherwise covered, or wrapped so as to be occlusive unless directed by the physician.
- Patients should wash their hands after applying the medication.
- Patients should report any signs of local or systemic adverse reactions to the physician.
- Patients should inform their physicians that they are using CLOBEX™ (clobetasol propionate) Lotion, 0.05% if surgery is contemplated.
- This medication is for external use only. It should not be used on the face, underarms, or groin area, and avoid contact with the eyes and lips.
- As with other corticosteroids, therapy should be discontinued when control is achieved. If no improvement is seen within 2 weeks, contact the physician.
- Patients should be informed to not use more than 50 g (50 mL or 1.75 fl.oz.) per week of CLOBEX™ Lotion, 0.05%.

Laboratory Tests: The following tests may be helpful in evaluating patients for HPA axis suppression:

— Cosyntropin stimulation test

— AM plasma cortisol test

Urinary free cortisol test

Carcinogenesis, Mutagenesis, Impairment of Fertility: Long-term animal studies have not been performed to evaluate the carcinogenic potential of clobetasol propionate.

Clobetasol propionate was non-mutagenic in three different test systems: the Ames test, the *Saccharomyces cerevisiae* gene conversion assay, and the *E. coli* B WP2 fluctuation test.

Studies in the rat following subcutaneous administration at dosage levels up to 50 µg/kg per day revealed that the females exhibited an increase in the number of resorbed embryos and a decrease in the number of living fetuses at the highest dose.

Pregnancy: Teratogenic effects: Pregnancy Category C. Corticosteroids have been shown to be teratogenic in laboratory animals when administered systemically at relatively low dosage levels. Some corticosteroids have been shown to be teratogenic after dermal application to laboratory animals.

Clobetasol propionate is absorbed percutaneously, and when administered subcutaneously it was a significant teratogen in both the rabbit and the mouse. Clobetasol propionate has greater teratogenic potential than steroids that are less potent.

Teratogenicity studies in mice using the subcutaneous route resulted in fetotoxicity at the highest dose tested (1 mg/kg) and teratogenicity at all dose levels tested down to 0.03 mg/kg. These doses are approximately 1.4 and 0.04 times, respectively, the human topical dose of CLOBEX™ (clobetasol propionate) Lotion, 0.05%. Abnormalities seen included cleft palate and skeletal abnormalities.

In rabbits, clobetasol propionate was teratogenic at doses of 3 and 10 µg/kg. These doses are approximately 0.02 and 0.05 times, respectively, the human topical dose of CLOBEX™ (clobetasol propionate) Lotion, 0.05%. Abnormalities seen included cleft palate, cranioschisis, and other skeletal abnormalities.

A teratogenicity study in rats using the dermal route resulted in dose related maternal toxicity and fetal effects from 0.05 to 0.5 mg/kg/day of clobetasol propionate. These doses are approximately 0.14 to 1.4 times, respectively, the human topical dose of CLOBEX™ (clobetasol propionate) Lotion, 0.05%. Abnormalities seen included low fetal weights, umbilical herniation, cleft palate, reduced skeletal ossification, and other skeletal abnormalities.

There are no adequate and well-controlled studies of the teratogenic potential of clobetasol propionate in pregnant women. CLOBEX™ (clobetasol propionate) Lotion, 0.05% should be used during pregnancy only if the potential benefit justifies the potential risk to the fetus.

Nursing Mothers: Systemically administered corticosteroids appear in human milk and could suppress growth, interfere with endogenous corticosteroid production, or cause other untoward effects. It is not known whether topical administration of corticosteroids could result in sufficient systemic absorption to produce detectable quanitities in breast milk. Because many drugs are excreted in human milk, caution should be exercised when CLOBEX™ Lotion, 0.05% is administered to a nursing woman.

Pediatric Use: Use of CLOBEX™ Lotion, 0.05% in pediatric patients is not recommended due to the potential for HPA axis suppression (see PRECAUTIONS: General).

The HPA axis suppression potential of CLOBEX™ Lotion, 0.05% has been studied in adolescents (12 to 17 years of age) with moderate to severe atopic dermatitis covering a minimum of 20% of the total body surface area. In total 14 patients were evaluated for HPA axis function. Patients were treated twice daily for 2 weeks with CLOBEX™ Lotion, 0.05%. After 2 weeks of treatment, 9 out of 14 of the patients experienced adrenal suppression. One out of 4 patients treated with CLOBEX™ Lotion, 0.05% who were retested remained suppressed two weeks post-treatment. In comparison, 2 of 10 of the patients treated with clobetasol propionate cream, 0.05% demonstrated HPA axis suppression. One patient who was retested recovered.

None of the patients who developed HPA axis suppression had concomitant clinical signs of adrenal suppression and none of them was discontinued from the study for reasons related to the safety or tolerability of CLOBEX™ Lotion, 0.05%. However patients with acute illness or injury may have increased morbidity and mortality with intermittent HPA axis suppression.

Because of a higher ratio of skin surface area to body mass, pediatric patients are at a greater risk than adults of HPA axis suppression and Cushing's syndrome when they are treated with topical corticosteroids. They are therefore also at greater risk of glucocorticosteroid insufficiency during and/or after withdrawal of treatment. Adverse effects including striae have been reported with inappropriate use of topical corticosteroids in infants and children.

HPA axis suppression, Cushing's syndrome, linear growth retardation, delayed weight gain, and intracranial hypertension have been reported in children receiving topical corticosteroids. Manifestations of adrenal suppression in children include low plasma cortisol levels and absence of response to ACTH stimulation. Manifestations of intracranial hypertension include bulging fontanelles, headaches, and bilateral papilledema.

Geriatric Use: Clinical studies of CLOBEX™ (clobetasol propionate) Lotion, 0.05% did not include sufficient numbers of patients aged 65 and over to determine whether they respond differently than younger patients. In general, dose selection for an elderly patient should be made with caution, usually starting at the low end of the dosing range, reflecting the greater frequency of decreased hepatic, renal or cardiac function, and of concomitant disease or other drug therapy.

ADVERSE REACTIONS

In controlled clinical trials with CLOBEX™ (clobetasol propionate) Lotion, 0.05%, the following adverse reactions have been reported: burning/stinging, skin dryness, irritation, erythema, folliculitis, pruritus, skin atrophy, and telangiectasia.

The pooled incidence of local adverse reactions in trials for psoriasis and atopic dermatitis with CLOBEX™ (clobetasol propionate) Lotion, 0.05% at 1.0% or greater was:

Adverse Reaction	Incidence
Skin Atrophy	4.2%
Telangiectasia	3.2%
Discomfort Skin	1.3%
Skin Dry	1.0%

Other local adverse events occurred at rates less than 1.0%. Similar rates of local adverse reactions were reported in the comparator (clobetasol propionate cream, 0.05%). Most local adverse events were rated as mild to moderate and they are not affected by age, race or gender.

The following additional local adverse reactions have been reported with topical corticosteroids. They may occur more frequently with the use of occlusive dressings and higher potency corticosteroids, including clobetasol propionate. These reactions are listed in an approximate decreasing order of occurrence: irritation, dryness, folliculitis, acneiform eruptions, hypopigmentation, perioral dermatitis, allergic contact dermatitis, secondary infection, striae and miliaria.

OVERDOSAGE

Topically applied CLOBEX™ (clobetasol propionate) Lotion, 0.05% can be absorbed in sufficient amount to produce systemic effects. (See PRECAUTIONS).

DOSAGE AND ADMINISTRATION

CLOBEX™ Lotion, 0.05% should be applied to the affected skin areas twice daily and rubbed in gently and completely. (See INDICATIONS AND USAGE.)

CLOBEX™ Lotion, 0.05% contains a super-high potent topical corticosteroid; therefore treatment should be limited to:

— 2 consecutive weeks for the relief of the inflammatory and pruritic manifestations of corticosteroid-esponsive dermatoses,

— and up to 2 additional weeks in very localized lesions of moderate to severe plaque psoriasis (no more than 10% body surface area) that have not sufficiently improved after the initial 2 weeks of treatment with CLOBEX™ (clobetasol propionate) Lotion 0.05%.

The total dosage should not exceed 50 g (50 mL or 1.75 fl. oz.) per week because of the potential for the drug to suppress the hypothalamic-pituitary-adrenal (HPA) axis.

Therapy should be discontinued when control has been achieved. If no improvement is seen within 2 weeks, reassessment of diagnosis may be necessary.

Use in pediatric patients younger than 18 years is not recommended because of numerically high rates of HPA axis suppression (See PRECAUTIONS: Pediatric Use).

Unless directed by physician, CLOBEX™ Lotion, 0.05% should not be used with occlusive dressings.

HOW SUPPLIED

CLOBEX™ Lotion, 0.05% is supplied in the following sizes:

1 fl. oz./30 mL NDC 0299-3848-01 high density polyethylene bottles.

2 fl. oz./59 mL NDC 0299-3848-02 high density polyethylene bottles.

Store at controlled room temperature 68° to 77°F (20°-25°C). Protect from freezing.

Marketed by:
GALDERMA LABORATORIES, L.P.
Fort Worth, Texas 76177 USA
Manufactured by:
DPT Laboratories, Ltd.
San Antonio, Texas 78215 USA
GALDERMA is a registered trademark.
325054-0703
Revised: July 2003

CLOBEX™
(clobetasol propionate) Lotion, 0.05%

PATIENT INFORMATION

For External Use Only
Not for Ophthalmic (Eye) Use

Read the Patient Information that comes with CLOBEX™ (KLO-bex) Lotion before you start using it and each time you get a refill. There may be new information. This leaflet does not take the place of talking with your doctor about your medical condition or your treatment.

What is CLOBEX™ Lotion?

CLOBEX™ Lotion is a medicine called a topical (skin use only) corticosteroid. It is used for a short time to reduce the inflammation and itching of:

- Moderate to severe skin conditions (atopic dermatitis and other skin problems)
- Moderate to severe plaque psoriasis

CLOBEX™ Lotion is a super-high potent (very strong) topical corticosteroid. It is very important that you use CLOBEX™ Lotion only as directed, in order to avoid serious side effects.

Who should not use CLOBEX™ Lotion?

Do not use CLOBEX™ Lotion if you are allergic to any of its ingredients, or to any other corticosteroid. The active ingredient is clobetasol propionate. See the end of this leaflet for the complete list of other ingredients in CLOBEX™ Lotion. Ask your doctor or pharmacist if you need a list of other corticosteroids.

CLOBEX™ Lotion is not recommended for use on anyone younger than 18 years of age. CLOBEX™ Lotion has not been studied in children under 12 years old. Children have smaller body sizes and have a higher chance of side effects.

What should I tell my doctor before using CLOBEX™ Lotion?

Tell your doctor:

- if you are pregnant, think you are pregnant or plan to be pregnant. Talk with your doctor before using CLOBEX™ Lotion or if you are already using CLOBEX™ Lotion, as it is not known if CLOBEX™ Lotion can harm your unborn child.
- if you are breastfeeding. It is not known if CLOBEX™ Lotion passes into your milk.
- if you think you have a skin infection. You may need another medicine to treat the skin infection before you use CLOBEX™ Lotion.

Tell your doctor about all the other medicines and skin products you use, including prescription and non-prescription medicines, cosmetics, vitamins, and herbal supplements. Some medicines can cause serious side effects if used while you are using CLOBEX™ Lotion.

How should I use CLOBEX™ Lotion?

- Use CLOBEX™ Lotion exactly as directed by your doctor. CLOBEX™ Lotion is for skin use only.
- Apply CLOBEX™ Lotion twice a day, once in the morning and once at night, or as directed by your doctor.

Use only enough to cover the affected areas. Do not apply CLOBEX™ Lotion to your face, neck, groin or armpits. Do not get CLOBEX™ Lotion on your lips or in or near your eyes.

- Make sure your skin is clean and dry before applying CLOBEX™ Lotion.
- Turn the bottle of CLOBEX™ Lotion upside down. Pour a small amount, less than 1 teaspoonful of CLOBEX™ Lotion onto your fingertips, or directly on your affected skin area. Gently, rub the CLOBEX™ Lotion into your affected skin area, until the lotion disappears.
- Wash your hands after using CLOBEX™ Lotion.
- If you forget to apply CLOBEX™ Lotion at the scheduled time, use it as soon as you remember. Then go back to your regular schedule. If it is about time for your next dose, apply just that 1 dose, and continue with your normal application schedule. Do not try to make up for the missed dose. If you miss several doses, tell your doctor.
- Throw away unused CLOBEX™ Lotion.

What should I avoid while using CLOBEX™ Lotion?

Do not do the following while using CLOBEX™ Lotion.

- Do not get CLOBEX™ Lotion on your face, lips, or in or near your eyes because this might cause irritation. If you do, use a lot of water to rinse the CLOBEX™ Lotion off your face, lips, or out of your eyes. If your eyes keep stinging after rinsing them well with water, call your doctor right away.
- Do not apply CLOBEX™ Lotion to your groin or armpits.
- Do not bandage or cover your treated areas unless your doctor tells you to do so.
- Do not wear tight fitting clothes over your treated skin areas.
- Do not use CLOBEX™ Lotion any longer than 2 weeks (14 days) for moderate to severe conditions (atopic dermatitis and other skin problems).
- Do not use CLOBEX™ Lotion any longer than an extra 2 weeks (4 weeks total) for psoriasis on a small area of your body (less than 10 percent of your body surface area) that is not much better after the first 2 weeks of treatment.
- Do not use more than 50 grams (50 mL or 1.75 fluid ounces) of CLOBEX™ Lotion a week. CLOBEX™ Lotion comes in 2 different size bottles, a 1-ounce and a 2-ounce bottle.

What are the possible side effects of CLOBEX™ Lotion?

CLOBEX™ Lotion can pass through your skin. Too much CLOBEX™ Lotion passing through your skin can shut down your adrenal glands. This usually happens if you use too much CLOBEX™ Lotion, or you use it for too long. If this happens, your adrenal glands may not start working immediately once you stop using CLOBEX™ Lotion. Shutting down of the adrenal glands can cause nausea, vomiting, fever, low blood pressure, heart attack, and even death because your body cannot respond to any stress or illness.

Your doctor may do special blood and urine tests to check your adrenal gland function while you are using CLOBEX™ Lotion.

Other possible side effects with CLOBEX™ Lotion include mild burning, stinging, itching, redness, irritation, and dry skin. Also, thinning of the skin, widening of small blood vessels in the skin, and skin discomfort at the site of application may happen. Sometimes your condition will get worse with use of CLOBEX™ Lotion.

If you are ill or injured, or going to have surgery, tell your doctor that you are using CLOBEX™ Lotion.

Tell your doctor if you:

- are going to have surgery
- get sick or don't feel right. Call your doctor right away.
- have irritation of the treated skin area that does not go away.
- have any unusual effects that you do not understand.
- have affected areas that do not seem to be getting better after 2 weeks of using CLOBEX™ Lotion.

These are not all the possible side effects of CLOBEX™ Lotion. For more information, ask your doctor or pharmacist.

General information about the safe and effective use of CLOBEX™ Lotion.

Medicines are sometimes prescribed for conditions that are not mentioned in patient information leaflets. Do not use CLOBEX™ Lotion for a condition for which it was not prescribed. Do not give CLOBEX™ Lotion to other people, even if they have the same symptoms you have. It may harm them. Keep CLOBEX™ Lotion and all medicines out of reach of children.

This leaflet summarizes the most important information about CLOBEX™ Lotion. If you would like more information, talk with your doctor. You can ask your pharmacist or doctor for information about CLOBEX™ Lotion that is written for health professionals.

What are the ingredients of CLOBEX™ Lotion?

Active Ingredient: clobetasol propionate

Inactive Ingredients: hydroxypropyl methylcellulose, propylene glycol, mineral oil, polyoxyethylene glycol 300 isostearate, carbomer 1342, sodium hydroxide and purified water.

Rx only

Marketed by:
GALDERMA LABORATORIES, L.P.
Fort Worth, Texas 76177 USA

Manufactured by:
DPT Laboratories, Ltd.
San Antonio, Texas 78215 USA

GALDERMA is a registered trademark.

325054-0703

Revised: July 2003

CLOBEX™ ℞

[*klō-bĕks*]

(clobetasol propionate)
Shampoo, 0.05%
Rx only
For External Use Only. Not for Ophthalmic Use.

DESCRIPTION

CLOBEX™ (clobetasol propionate) Shampoo, 0.05%, contains clobetasol propionate, a synthetic fluorinated corticosteroid, for topical dermatologic use. The corticosteroids constitute a class of primarily synthetic steroids used topically as anti-inflammatory and antipruritic agents.

The chemical name of clobetasol propionate is 21-chloro-9-fluoro-11β,17-dihydroxy-16β-methylpregna-1, 4-diene-3, 20-dione 17-propionate. It has the following structural formula:

Clobetasol propionate has a molecular weight of 466.97 (CAS Registry Number 25122-46-7). The molecular formula is $C_{25}H_{32}ClFO_5$. Clobetasol propionate is a white to practically white crystalline, odorless powder insoluble in water. Each mL of CLOBEX™ (clobetasol propionate) Shampoo, 0.05%, contains clobetasol propionate, 0.05%, in a shampoo base consisting of alcohol, citric acid, coco-betaine, polyquaternium-10, purified water, sodium citrate, and sodium laureth sulfate.

CLINICAL PHARMACOLOGY

Like other topical corticosteroids, CLOBEX™ (clobetasol propionate) Shampoo, 0.05%, has anti-inflammatory, antipruritic, and vasoconstrictive properties. The mechanism of the anti-inflammatory activity of the topical steroids, in general, is unclear. However, corticosteroids are thought to act by the induction of phospholipase A2 inhibitory proteins, collectively called lipocortins. It is postulated that these proteins control the biosynthesis of potent mediators of inflammation such as prostaglandins and leukotrienes by inhibiting the release of their common precursor, arachidonic acid. Arachidonic acid is released from membrane phospholipids by phospholipase A2.

Pharmacokinetics: The extent of percutaneous absorption of topical corticosteroids is determined by many factors, including the vehicle, the integrity of the epidermal barrier and occlusion. Topical corticosteroids can be absorbed from normal intact skin, while inflammation and/or other disease processes in the skin may increase percutaneous absorption. Due to the fact that circulating levels of corticosteroids are usually below the limit of detection following application, there are no human data regarding the pharmacokinetics of topical corticosteroids. In such cases pharmacodynamic end points, including both hypothalamic-pituitary-adrenal (HPA) axis testing and topical vasoconstriction, are used as surrogates in the assessments of systemic exposure and relative potency, respectively.

In studies evaluating the potential for hypothalamic-pituitary-adrenal (HPA) axis suppression, use of CLOBEX™ (clobetasol propionate) Shampoo, 0.05%, resulted in demonstrable HPA axis suppression in 5 out of 12 (42%) adolescent patients (See PRECAUTIONS).

CLOBEX™ Shampoo is in the super-high range of potency in vasoconstrictor studies.

CLINICAL STUDIES

The safety and efficacy of CLOBEX™ (clobetasol propionate) Shampoo, 0.05%, has been evaluated in two clinical trials involving 290 patients with moderate to severe scalp psoriasis. In both trials, patients were treated with either CLOBEX™ Shampoo or the corresponding vehicle applied once daily for 15 minutes before lathering and rinsing for a period of 4 weeks. Efficacy results are presented in the table below.

[See table below]

Clinical studies of Clobetasol Propionate Shampoo, 0.05%, did not include sufficient numbers of non-Caucasian patients to determine whether they respond differently than Caucasian patients with regards to efficacy and safety.

INDICATIONS AND USAGE

CLOBEX™ (clobetasol propionate) Shampoo, 0.05%, is a super-high potent topical corticosteroid formulation indicated for the treatment of moderate to severe forms of scalp psoriasis in subjects 18 years of age and older (see PRECAUTIONS). Treatment should be limited to 4 consecutive weeks because of the potential for the drug to suppress the hypothalamic-pituitary-adrenal (HPA) axis. The total dosage should not exceed 50 g (50 mL or 1.75 fl. oz.) per week (see DOSAGE and ADMINISTRATION).

Patients should be instructed to use CLOBEX™ Shampoo, 0.05%, for the minimum time period necessary to achieve the desired results (see **PRECAUTIONS**).

Use in patients younger than 18 years of age is not recommended due to numerically high rates of HPA axis suppression (see PRECAUTIONS, Pediatric Use).

Continued on next page

	CLOBEX™ Shampoo n(%)		CLOBEX™ Shampoo Vehicle n(%)	
	Study A	**Study B**	**Study A**	**Study B**
Total Number of Patients	95	99	47	49
Success Rate[1] at Endpoint[2]	40 (42.1%)	28 (28.3%)	1 (2.1%)	5 (10.2%)
Subjects with Scalp Psoriasis Parameter Clear (None) at Endpoint Erythema[3]	17 (17.9%)	12 (12.1%)	3 (6.4%)	1 (2.0%)
Scaling[3]	21 (22.1%)	15 (15.2%)	0 (0%)	2 (4.1%)
Plaque Thickening[3]	35 (36.8%)	34 (34.3%)	5 (10.6%)	5 (10.2%)

[1] Success rate defined as the proportion of patients with a-0 (clear) or 1 (minimal) on a 0 to 5 point physician's Global Severity Scale for scalp psoriasis.
[2] At four (4) weeks or last observation recorded for a subject during the treatment period (baseline if no post-baseline data were available).
[3] Patients with 0 (clear) on a 0 to 3 point scalp psoriasis parameter scale.

Clobex Shampoo—Cont.

There were insufficient numbers of non-Caucasian patients to determine whether they responded differently than Caucasian patients with regards to efficacy and safety.

CONTRAINDICATIONS

Use of CLOBEX™ (clobetasol propionate) Shampoo, 0.05%, is contraindicated in patients who are hypersensitive to clobetasol propionate, to other corticosteroids, or to any ingredient in this preparation.

PRECAUTIONS

General: Clobetasol propionate is a highly potent topical corticosteroid that has been shown to suppress the HPA axis at the lowest doses tested.

Systemic absorption of topical corticosteroids can produce reversible hypothalamic-pituitary-adrenal (HPA) axis suppression with the potential for glucocorticosteroid insufficiency after withdrawal of treatment. Manifestations of Cushing's syndrome, hyperglycemia, and glucosuria can also be produced in some patients by systemic absorption of topical corticosteroids while on treatment.

Conditions which increase systemic absorption include the application of the more potent corticosteroids, use over large surface areas, prolonged use, and the addition of occlusive dressings or use on occluded areas. Therefore, patients applying a topical steroid to a large surface area or to areas under occlusion should be evaluated periodically for evidence of HPA axis suppression. If HPA axis suppression is noted, an attempt should be made to withdraw the drug, to reduce the frequency of application, or to substitute a less potent steroid. Recovery of HPA axis function is generally prompt and complete upon discontinuation of topical corticosteroids. Infrequently, signs and symptoms of glucocorticosteroid insufficiency may occur, requiring supplemental systemic corticosteroids. For information on systemic supplementation, see prescribing information for those products.

The effect of CLOBEX™ (clobetasol propionate) Shampoo, 0.05% on HPA axis suppression was evaluated in one study in adolescents 12 to 17 years of age. In this study, 5 of 12 evaluable subjects developed suppression of their HPA axis following 4 weeks of treatment with CLOBEX™ (clobetasol propionate) Shampoo, 0.05% applied once daily for 15 minutes to a dry scalp before lathering and rinsing.

Pediatric patients may be more susceptible to systemic toxicity from equivalent doses due to their larger skin surface to body mass ratios. (See **PRECAUTIONS - Pediatric Use**).

If irritation develops, CLOBEX™ Shampoo should be discontinued and appropriate therapy instituted. Allergic contact dermatitis with corticosteroids is usually diagnosed by observing a failure to heal rather than noting a clinical exacerbation, as with most topical products not containing corticosteroids. Such an observation should be corroborated with appropriate diagnostic patch testing.

In the presence of dermatological infections, the use of an appropriate antifungal or antibacterial agent should be instituted. If a favorable response does not occur promptly, use of CLOBEX™ Shampoo should be discontinued until the infection has been adequately controlled. Although CLOBEX™ Shampoo is intended for the topical treatment of moderate to severe scalp psoriasis, it should be noted that certain areas of the body, such as the face, groin, and axillae, are more prone to atrophic changes than other areas of the body following treatment with corticosteroids. CLOBEX™ Shampoo should not be used on the face, groin or axillae. Avoid any contact of the drug product with the eyes and lips. In case of contact, rinse thoroughly with water all parts of the body that came in contact with the shampoo.

Information for patients: Patients using topical corticosteroids should receive the following information and instructions:

1. This medication is to be used as directed by the physician and should not be used longer than the prescribed time period. It is for external use only. Avoid contact with the eyes.
2. This medication should not be used for any disorder other than that for which it was prescribed.
3. The scalp area should not be covered while the medication is on the scalp (e.g., shower cap, bathing cap) so as to be occlusive unless directed by the physician.
4. Patients should report any signs of local or systemic adverse reactions to their physician.
5. As with other corticosteroids, therapy should be discontinued when control is achieved. If no improvement is seen within 4 weeks, contact the physician.
6. Patients should wash their hands after applying the medication.
7. Patients should inform their physician(s) that they are using CLOBEX™ Shampoo if surgery is contemplated.
8. Patients should not use more than 50 g (50 mL or 1.75 fl. oz.) per week of CLOBEX™ Shampoo.

Laboratory tests: The cortrosyn stimulation test may be helpful in evaluating patients for HPA axis suppression.

Carcinogenesis, mutagenesis, impairment of fertility: Long-term animal studies have not been performed to evaluate the carcinogenic potential of clobetasol propionate.

Clobetasol propionate did not produce any increase in chromosomal aberrations in Chinese hamster ovary cells *in vitro* in the presence or absence of metabolic activation. Clobetasol propionate was also negative in the micronucleus test in mice after oral administration.

Studies of the effect of CLOBEX™ (clobetasol propionate) Shampoo, 0.05% on fertility have not been conducted.

Pregnancy: Teratogenic Effects: Pregnancy Category C: Corticosteroids have been shown to be teratogenic in laboratory animals when administered systemically at relatively low dosage levels. Some corticosteroids have been shown to be teratogenic after dermal application to laboratory animals.

A teratogenicity study of clobetasol propionate in rats using the dermal route resulted in dose related maternal toxicity and fetal effects from 0.05 to 0.5 mg/kg/day. These doses are approximately 0.1 to 1.0 times, respectively, the maximum human topical dose of clobetasol propionate from CLOBEX™ Shampoo. Abnormalities seen included low fetal weights, umbilical herniation, cleft palate, reduced skeletal ossification other skeletal abnormalities. Clobetasol propionate administered to rats subcutaneously at a dose of 0.1 mg/kg from day 17 of gestation to day 21 postpartum was associated with prolongation of gestation, decreased number of offspring, increased perinatal mortality of offspring, delayed eye opening and delayed hair appearance in surviving offspring. Some increase in offspring perinatal mortality was also observed at a dose of 0.05 mg/kg. Doses of 0.05 and 0.1 mg/kg are approximately 0.1 and 0.2 fold the maximum human topical dose of clobetasol propionate from CLOBEX™ Shampoo.

There are no adequate and well-controlled studies of the teratogenic potential of clobetasol propionate in pregnant women. CLOBEX™ Shampoo should be used during pregnancy only if the potential benefit justifies the potential risk to the fetus.

Nursing Mothers: Systemically administered corticosteroids appear in human milk and could suppress growth, interfere with endogenous corticosteroid production, or cause other untoward effects. It is not known whether topical administration of corticosteroids could result in sufficient systemic absorption to produce detectable quanitities in human milk. Because many drugs are excreted in human milk, caution should be exercised when CLOBEX™ Shampoo, 0.05%, is administered to a nursing woman.

Pediatric use: Use of CLOBEX™ Shampoo, 0.05%, in patients under 18 years old is not recommended due to potential for HPA axis suppression (see PRECAUTIONS: General).

The effect of CLOBEX™ (clobetasol propionate) Shampoo, 0.05%, on HPA axis suppression was evaluated in one study in adolescents 12 to 17 years of age. In this study, 5 of 12 evaluable subjects developed suppression of their HPA axis following 4 weeks of treatment with CLOBEX™ (clobetasol propionate) Shampoo, 0.05%, applied once daily for 15 minutes to a dry scalp before lathering and rinsing. Only one of the five subjects who had suppression was tested for recovery of HPA axis, and this subject recovered after 2 weeks.

No studies have been performed in patients under the age of 12. Because of a higher ratio of skin surface area to body mass, pediatric patients are at a greater risk than adults of HPA axis suppression and Cushing's syndrome when they are treated with topical corticosteroids. They are therefore also at greater risk of adrenal insufficiency during and/or after withdrawal of treatment. Adverse effects including striae have been reported with inappropriate use of topical corticosteroids in infants and children.

Therefore, use is not recommended in patients under the age of 18.

HPA axis suppression, Cushing's syndrome, linear growth retardation, delayed weight gain, and intracranial hypertension have been reported in children receiving topical corticosteroids. Manifestations of adrenal suppression in children include low plasma cortisol levels and an absence of response to ACTH stimulation. Manifestations of intracranial hypertension include bulging fontanelles, headaches, and bilateral papilledema.

Geriatric use: Clinical studies of Clobetasol Propionate Shampoo, 0.05%, did not include sufficient numbers of patients aged 65 and over to determine whether they respond differently than younger patients. In general, dose selection for an elderly patient should be made with caution, usually starting at the low end of the dosing range, reflecting the greater frequency of decreased hepatic, renal or cardiac function, and of concomitant disease or other drug therapy.

ADVERSE REACTIONS

In clinical trials with CLOBEX™ Shampoo, the following adverse reactions have been reported: burning/stinging, pruritus, edema, folliculitis, acne, dry skin, irritant dermatitis, alopecia, urticaria, skin atrophy and telangiectasia.

The table below summarizes selected adverse events that occurred in at least 1% of subjects in the Phase 2 and 3 studies for scalp psoriasis.

Summary of Selected Adverse Events ≥ 1% by Body System

Body System	Clobetasol Propionate Shampoo N=558	Vehicle Shampoo N=127
Skin and Appendages	49 (8.8%)	28 (22.0%)
Discomfort Skin	26 (4.7%)	16 (12.6%)
Pruritus	3 (0.5%)	9 (7.1%)
Body As A Whole	33 (5.9%)	12 (9.4%)
Headache	10 (1.8%)	1 (0.8%)

The following additional local adverse reactions have been reported infrequently with other topical corticosteroids, and they may occur more frequently with the use of occlusive dressings, especially with higher potency corticosteroids. These reactions are listed in an approximately decreasing order of occurrence: hypopigmentation, perioral dermatitis, allergic contact dermatitis, secondary infection, skin atrophy, striae, and miliaria.

Systemic absorption of topical corticosteroids has produced reversible HPA axis suppression, manifestations of Cushing's syndrome, hyperglycemia, and glucosuria in some patients.

OVERDOSAGE

Topically applied, CLOBEX™ Shampoo can be absorbed in sufficient amounts to produce systemic effects. (See **PRECAUTIONS**).

DOSAGE AND ADMINISTRATION

CLOBEX™ Shampoo should be applied onto dry (not wet) scalp once a day in a thin film to the affected areas only, and left in place for 15 minutes before lathering and rinsing.

Move the hair away from the scalp so that one of the affected areas is exposed. Position the bottle over the lesion. Apply a small amount of the shampoo directly onto the lesion, letting the product naturally flow from the bottle (gently squeeze the bottle), avoiding any contact of the product with the facial skin, eyes or lips. In case of contact, rinse thoroughly with water. Spread the product so that the entire lesion is covered with a thin uniform film. Massage gently into the lesion and repeat for additional lesion(s). Wash your hands after applying CLOBEX™ Shampoo. Leave the shampoo in place for 15 minutes, then add water, lather and rinse thoroughly all parts of the scalp and body that came in contact with the shampoo (e.g., hands, face, neck and shoulders). Avoid contact with eyes and lips. Minimize contact to non-affected areas of the body. Although no additional shampoo is necessary to cleanse your hair, you may use a non-medicated shampoo if desired.

Treatment should be limited to 4 consecutive weeks. As with other corticosteroids, therapy should be discontinued when control is achieved. If complete disease control is not achieved after four weeks of treatment with CLOBEX™ Shampoo, 0.05%, treatment with a less potent topical steroid may be substituted. If no improvement is seen within 4 weeks, reassessment of the diagnosis may be necessary.

CLOBEX™ Shampoo should not be used with occlusive dressings unless directed by a physician.

HOW SUPPLIED

CLOBEX™ Shampoo is supplied in 4 fl.oz. (118 mL) bottles.
NDC 0299-3847-04

Storage: Keep tightly closed. Store at controlled room temperature 68°F to 77°F (20°C-25°C).

Marketed by:
GALDERMA LABORATORIES, L.P.
Fort Worth, Texas 76177 USA
Manufactured by:
DPT Laboratories, Ltd.
San Antonio, Texas 78215 USA
GALDERMA is a registered trademark.
www.clobex.com
325060-0104
Revised: January, 2004

PATIENT INFORMATION

For External Use Only
Not for Ophthalmic (Eye) Use
CLOBEX™
(clobetasol propionate) Shampoo, 0.05%

Read the Patient Information that comes with CLOBEX™ Shampoo before you start using it and each time you get a refill. There may be new information. This leaflet does not take the place of talking with your doctor about your medical condition or your treatment.

What is the most important information I should know about CLOBEX™ Shampoo?

What is CLOBEX™ Shampoo?

CLOBEX™ Shampoo is a medicine called a topical (skin use only) corticosteroid. It is used for a short time to treat forms of scalp psoriasis. CLOBEX™ Shampoo is a super-high potent (very strong) topical corticosteroid. It is very important that you use CLOBEX™ Shampoo only as directed in order to avoid serious side effects.

Who should not use CLOBEX™ Shampoo?

Do not use CLOBEX™ Shampoo if you are allergic to any of its ingredients, or to any other corticosteroid. The active ingredient is clobetasol propionate. See the end of this leaflet for a complete list of ingredients in CLOBEX™ Shampoo. Ask your doctor or pharmacist if you need a list of other corticosteroids.

CLOBEX™ Shampoo is not recommended for use by patients under 18 years of age. Children have smaller body sizes and have a higher chance of side effects.

What should I tell my doctor before using CLOBEX™ Shampoo?

Tell your doctor:

- if you are pregnant, think you are pregnant, plan to be pregnant. Talk with your doctor before using

CLOBEX™ Shampoo or if you are already using CLOBEX™ Shampoo. It is not known if CLOBEX™ Shampoo can harm your unborn baby.
- if you are breastfeeding. It is not known if CLOBEX™ Shampoo passes into your milk, and if it can harm your baby.
- if you think you have an infection on your scalp. You may need another medicine to treat the scalp infection before you use CLOBEX™ Shampoo.

Tell your doctor about all the other medicines and skin products you use, including prescription and non-prescription medicines, vitamins, herbal supplements, and cosmetics. Some medicines and products can cause serious side effects if used while you are using CLOBEX™ Shampoo.

How should I use CLOBEX™ Shampoo?
- Use CLOBEX™ Shampoo exactly as prescribed by your doctor. CLOBEX™ Shampoo is for use on your scalp only.
- Apply CLOBEX™ Shampoo on affected areas of the scalp once a day. Use only enough to cover the affected areas of your scalp. Do not use CLOBEX™ Shampoo on your face, groin, armpits, lips, or in your eyes.
- Do not wet your hair before using CLOBEX™ Shampoo. Move the hair away from the scalp so that one of the affected areas is exposed. Apply a small amount of the shampoo directly onto the affected area by gently squeezing the bottle. Gently, rub CLOBEX™ Shampoo into the affected area. Repeat for other affected areas on your scalp.
- **Do not cover your head with a shower cap or bathing cap** while CLOBEX™ Shampoo is on your scalp.
- Leave CLOBEX™ Shampoo in place for 15 minutes before adding water, lathering and rinsing hair and scalp completely. No other shampoos are necessary. However, you can use a non-medicated shampoo on your hair after using CLOBEX™ Shampoo if you want to.
- Wash your hands after applying CLOBEX™ Shampoo. Wash any other part of your body that came into contact with CLOBEX™ Shampoo such as your neck and shoulders.
- If you forget to apply CLOBEX™ Shampoo at the scheduled time, use it as soon as you remember. Then go back to your regular schedule. If it is about time for your next dose, apply just that 1 dose, and continue with your regular schedule. Do not make up the missed dose. If you miss several doses, tell your doctor.
- **Do not use more than 50 grams (50 mL or 1.75 fluid ounces) of CLOBEX™ Shampoo per week.**

What should I avoid while using CLOBEX™ Shampoo?

Do not do the following while using CLOBEX™ Shampoo:
- **Do not get CLOBEX™ Shampoo on your lips or in or near your eyes** because this might cause side effects. If you do, use a lot of water to rinse the CLOBEX™ Shampoo off your face, lips, or out of your eyes. If your eyes keep stinging after rinsing them well with water, contact your doctor right away.
- **Do not apply CLOBEX™ Shampoo to your face, groin or armpits.**
- **Do not get CLOBEX™ Shampoo in your mouth.** If you or a child accidentally swallows CLOBEX™ Shampoo, call your Poison Control center or local emergency room right away.
- **Do not cover your head with a shower or bathing cap** while CLOBEX™ Shampoo is on your scalp.
- **Do not use CLOBEX™ Shampoo any longer than 4 weeks (28 days)** for moderate to severe scalp psoriasis.
- **Do not use more than 50 mL (1.75 fluid ounces) of CLOBEX™ Shampoo per week.**

What should I do if I miss an application of CLOBEX™ Shampoo?

If you forget to apply CLOBEX™ Shampoo at the scheduled time, use it as soon as you remember, and then go back to your regular schedule. If you remember at the time of your next application, apply only one dose and continue with your regular schedule. If you miss several doses, tell your doctor.

What are the possible side effects of CLOBEX™ Shampoo?
CLOBEX™ Shampoo can pass through your skin. Too much CLOBEX™ Shampoo passing through your skin can shut down your adrenal glands. This may happen if you use too much CLOBEX™ Shampoo or if you use it for too long, but it can happen with correct use. If your adrenal glands shut down, they may not start working right away after you stop using CLOBEX™ Shampoo. Shutting down of the adrenal glands can cause nausea, vomiting, fever, low blood pressure, heart attack and even death because your body cannot adequately respond to stress or illness.

Your doctor may do special blood and urine tests to check your adrenal gland function while you are using CLOBEX™ Shampoo.

The most common side effects with CLOBEX™ Shampoo include burning or itching at the site of application. Other possible side effects include thinning of the skin and widening of small blood vessels in the skin.

If you go to another doctor for illness, injury or surgery, tell that doctor that you are using CLOBEX™ Shampoo.

Tell your doctor if you:
- are going to have surgery
- get sick or don't feel right. Call your doctor right away.
- have irritation of the treated skin area that does not go away
- have any unusual effects that you do not understand
- have affected areas that do not seem to be healing after 4 weeks of using CLOBEX™ Shampoo.

These are not all the possible side effects of CLOBEX™ Shampoo. For more information, ask your doctor or pharmacist.

How should I store CLOBEX™ Shampoo?
- Store CLOBEX™ Shampoo at room temperature between 68°F to 77°F (20°C–25°C).
- Keep the bottle tightly closed at all times.
- Do not use CLOBEX™ Shampoo after the expiration date shown on bottle.
- **Keep CLOBEX™ Shampoo and all medicines out of the reach of children.**

General information about CLOBEX™ Shampoo

Medicines are sometimes prescribed for conditions that are not mentioned in patient information leaflets. Do not use CLOBEX™ Shampoo for a condition for which it was not prescribed. Do not give CLOBEX™ Shampoo to other people, even if they have the same symptoms you have. It may harm them. This leaflet summarizes the most important information about CLOBEX™ Shampoo. If you would like more information, talk with your doctor. You can ask your pharmacist or doctor for information about CLOBEX™ Shampoo that is written for health professionals.

What are the ingredients in CLOBEX™ Shampoo?

Active ingredient: clobetasol propionate

Excipients (shampoo base): alcohol, citric acid, coco-betaine, polyquaternium-10, purified water, sodium citrate and sodium laureth sulfate.

Rx only

Marketed by:
GALDERMA LABORATORIES, L.P.
Fort Worth, Texas 76177 USA
Manufactured by:
DPT Laboratories, Ltd.
San Antonio, Texas 78215 USA
GALDERMA is a registered trademark.
www.clobex.com
325060-0104
Revised: January 2004

DIFFERIN® ℞
[dĭf-fūr-ĭn]
(adapalene)
Cream, 0.1%
℞ Only

For topical use only. Not for ophthalmic, oral, or intravaginal use.

DESCRIPTION

DIFFERIN® (adapalene) Cream, 0.1%, contains adapalene 0.1% in an aqueous cream emulsion consisting of carbomer 934P, cyclomethicone, edetate disodium, glycerin, methyl glucose sesquistearate, methylparaben, PEG-20 methyl glucose sesquistearate, phenoxyethanol, propylparaben, purified water, squalane, and trolamine.

The chemical name of adapalene is 6-[3-(1-adamantyl)-4-methoxyphenyl]-2-naphthoic acid. It is a white to off-white powder which is soluble in tetrahydrofuran, sparingly soluble in ethanol, and practically insoluble in water. The molecular formula is $C_{28}H_{28}O_3$ and molecular weight is 412.53. Adapalene is represented by the following structural formula.

OH
O
CH₃O

CLINICAL PHARMACOLOGY

Mechanism of Action: Adapalene acts on retinoid receptors. Biochemical and pharmacological profile studies have demonstrated that adapalene is a modulator of cellular differentiation, keratinization, and inflammatory processes all of which represent important features in the pathology of acne vulgaris.

Mechanistically, adapalene binds to specific retinoic acid nuclear receptors but does not bind to the cytosolic receptor protein. Although the exact mode of action of adapalene is unknown, it is suggested that topical adapalene normalizes the differentiation of follicular epithelial cells resulting in decreased microcomedone formation.

Pharmacokinetics: Absorption of adapalene from DIFFERIN® Cream through human skin is low. In a pharmacokinetic study with six acne patients treated once daily for 5 days with 2 grams of DIFFERIN® Cream applied to 1000 cm^2 of acne involved skin, there were no quantifiable amounts (limit of quantification = 0.35 ng/mL) of adapalene in the plasma samples from any patient. Excretion appears to be primarily by the biliary route.

INDICATIONS AND USAGE

DIFFERIN® Cream is indicated for the topical treatment of acne vulgaris.

CLINICAL STUDIES

Two vehicle-controlled clinical studies were conducted in patients 12 to 30 years of age with mild to moderate acne vulgaris, in which DIFFERIN® Cream was compared with its vehicle. Patients were instructed to apply their treatment medication once daily at bedtime for 12 weeks. In one study patients were provided with a soapless cleanser and were encouraged to refrain from using moisturizers. No other topical medications, other than DIFFERIN® Cream, were to be applied to the face during the studies. DIFFERIN® Cream was significantly more effective than its vehicle in the reduction of acne lesion counts. The mean percent reduction in lesion counts from baseline after treatment for 12 weeks are presented in the following table:
[See table below]

The trend in the Investigator's global assessment of severity supported the efficacy of DIFFERIN® Cream when compared to the cream vehicle.

CONTRAINDICATIONS

DIFFERIN® Cream should not be administered to individuals who are hypersensitive to adapalene or any of the components in the cream vehicle.

PRECAUTIONS

General: Certain cutaneous signs and symptoms of treatment such as erythema, dryness, scaling, burning, or pruritus may be experienced with use of DIFFERIN® Cream. These are most likely to occur during the first two to four weeks of treatment, are mostly mild to moderate in intensity, and usually lessen with continued use of the medication. Depending upon the severity of these side effects, patients should be instructed to reduce the frequency of application or discontinue use.

If a reaction suggesting sensitivity or chemical irritation occurs, use of the medication should be discontinued. Exposure to sunlight, including sunlamps, should be minimized during use of adapalene. Patients who normally experience high levels of sun exposure, and those with inherent sensitivity to sun, should be warned to exercise caution. Use of sunscreen products and protective clothing over treated areas is recommended when exposure cannot be avoided. Weather extremes, such as wind or cold, also may be irritating to patients under treatment with adapalene.

Avoid contact with the eyes, lips, angles of the nose, and mucous membranes. The product should not be applied to cuts, abrasions, eczematous or sunburned skin. As with other retinoids, use of "waxing" as a depilatory method should be avoided on skin treated with adapalene.

Information for Patients: Patients using DIFFERIN® Cream should receive the following information and instructions:
1. This medication is to be used only as directed by the physician.
2. It is for external use only.
3. Avoid contact with the eyes, lips, angles of the nose, and mucous membranes.
4. Cleanse area with a mild or soapless cleanser before applying this medication.
5. Moisturizers may be used if necessary; however, products containing alpha hydroxy or glycolic acids should be avoided.
6. Exposure of the eye to this medication may result in reactions such as swelling, conjunctivitis, and eye irritation.
7. This medication should not be applied to cuts, abrasions, eczematous or sunburned skin.
8. Wax epilation should not be performed on treated skin due to the potential for skin erosions.
9. During the early weeks of therapy, an apparent exacerbation of acne may occur. This is due to the action of this medication on previously unseen lesions and should not be considered a reason to discontinue therapy. Overall clinical benefit may be noticed after two weeks of therapy, but at least eight weeks are required to obtain consistent beneficial effects.

Continued on next page

MEAN PERCENT REDUCTION IN LESION COUNTS FROM BASELINE TO WEEK 12

	Study No. 1		Study No. 2	
Efficacy Variable	Adapalene Cream, 0.1% N=119	Cream Vehicle N=118	Adapalene Cream, 0.1% N=175	Cream Vehicle N=175
Non-inflammatory lesions	34%	18%	35%	15%
Inflammatory lesions	32%	17%	14%	6%
Total lesions	34%	18%	30%	15%

Incidence of Local Cutaneous Irritation with DIFFERIN® Cream from Controlled Clinical Studies (N=285)

	None	Mild	Moderate	Severe
Erythema	52% (148)	38% (108)	10% (28)	<1% (1)
Scaling	58% (166)	35% (100)	6% (18)	<1% (1)
Dryness	48% (136)	42% (121)	9% (26)	<1% (2)
Pruritus (persistent)	74% (211)	21% (61)	4% (12)	<1% (1)
Burning/Stinging (persistent)	71% (202)	24% (69)	4% (12)	<1% (2)

Differin Cream—Cont.

Drug Interactions: As DIFFERIN® Cream has the potential to produce local irritation in some patients, concomitant use of other potentially irritating topical products (medicated or abrasive soaps and cleansers, soaps and cosmetics that have a strong drying effect, and products with high concentrations of alcohol, astringents, spices or lime rind) should be approached with caution. Particular caution should be exercised in using preparations containing sulfur, resorcinol, or salicylic acid in combination with DIFFERIN® Cream. If these preparations have been used, it is advisable not to start therapy with DIFFERIN® Cream until the effects of such preparations in the skin have subsided.

Carcinogenesis, Mutagenesis, Impairment of Fertility: Carcinogenicity studies with adapalene have been conducted in mice at topical doses of 0.4, 1.3, and 4.0 mg/kg/day, and in rats at oral doses of 0.15, 0.5, and 1.5 mg/kg/day. These doses are up to 8 times (mice) and 6 times (rats) in terms of mg/m^2/day the maximum potential exposure at the recommended topical human dose (MRHD), assumed to be 2.5 grams DIFFERIN® Cream, which is approximately 1.5 mg/m^2 adapalene. In the oral study, increased incidence of benign and malignant pheochromocytomas in the adrenal medullas of male rats was observed.

No photocarcinogenicity studies were conducted. Animal studies have shown an increased risk of skin neoplasms with the use of pharmacologically similar drugs (e.g., retinoids) when exposed to UV irradiation in the laboratory or to sunlight. Although the significance of these studies to human use is not clear, patients should be advised to avoid or minimize exposure to either sunlight or artificial UV irradiation sources.

Adapalene did not exhibit mutagenic or genotoxic effects *in vivo* (mouse micronucleus test) and *in vitro* (Ames test, Chinese hamster ovary cell assay, mouse lymphoma TK assay) studies.

Reproductive function and fertility studies were conducted in rats administered oral doses of adapalene in amounts up to 20 mg/kg/day (up to 80 times the MRHD based on mg/m^2 comparisons). No effects of adapalene were found on the reproductive performance or fertility of the F_0 males or females. There were also no detectable effects on the growth, development and subsequent reproductive function of the F_1 generation.

***Pregnancy:* Teratogenic effects. Pregnancy Category C.** No teratogenic effects were seen in rats at oral doses of 0.15 to 5.0 mg/kg/day adapalene (up to 20 times the MRHD based on mg/m^2 comparisons). However, adapalene administered orally at doses of ≥25 mg/kg, (100 times the MRHD for rats or 200 times MRHD for rabbits) has been shown to be teratogenic. Cutaneous teratology studies in rats and rabbits at doses of 0.6, 2.0, and 6.0 mg/kg/day (24 times the MRHD for rats or 48 times the MRHD for rabbits) exhibited no fetotoxicity and only minimal increases in supernumerary ribs in rats. There are no adequate and well-controlled studies in pregnant women. Adapalene should be used during pregnancy only if the potential benefit justifies the potential risk to the fetus.

Nursing Mothers: It is not known whether this drug is excreted in human milk. Because many drugs are excreted in human milk, caution should be exercised when DIFFERIN® Cream is administered to a nursing woman.

Pediatric Use: Safety and effectiveness in pediatric patients below the age of 12 have not been established.

Geriatric Use: Clinical studies of DIFFERIN® Cream were conducted in patients 12 to 30 years of age with acne vulgaris and therefore did not include subjects 65 years and older to determine whether they respond differently than younger subjects. Other reported clinical experience has not identified differences in responses between the elderly and younger patients.

ADVERSE REACTIONS

In controlled clinical trials, local cutaneous irritation was monitored in 285 acne patients who used DIFFERIN® Cream once daily for 12 weeks. The frequency and severity of erythema, scaling, dryness, pruritus and burning were assessed during these studies. The incidence of local cutaneous irritation with DIFFERIN® Cream from the controlled clinical studies is provided in the following table:

[See table above]

Other reported local cutaneous adverse events in patients who used DIFFERIN® Cream once daily included: sunburn (2%), skin discomfort-burning and stinging (1%) and skin irritation (1%). Events occurring in less than 1% of patients treated with DIFFERIN® Cream included: acne flare, dermatitis and contact dermatitis, eyelid edema, conjunctivitis, erythema, pruritus, skin discoloration, rash, and eczema.

OVERDOSAGE

DIFFERIN® Cream is intended for cutaneous use only. If the medication is applied excessively, no more rapid or better results will be obtained and marked redness, scaling, or skin discomfort may occur. The acute oral toxicity of DIFFERIN® Cream in mice and rats is greater than 10 mL/kg. Chronic ingestion of the drug may lead to the same side effects as those associated with excessive oral intake of Vitamin A.

DOSAGE AND ADMINISTRATION

DIFFERIN® Cream should be applied to affected areas of the skin, once daily at nighttime. A thin film of the cream should be applied to the skin areas where acne lesions appear, using enough to cover the entire affected areas lightly. A mild transitory sensation of warmth or slight stinging may occur shortly after the application of DIFFERIN® Cream.

HOW SUPPLIED

DIFFERIN® (adapalene) Cream, 0.1% is supplied in the following sizes.

45 g tube—**NDC** 0299-5915-45

Storage: Store at controlled room temperature 68° to 77°F (20°–25°C). Protect from freezing.

Marketed by:
Galderma Laboratories, L.P.
Fort Worth, Texas 76133 USA
Manufactured by:
DPT Laboratories, Ltd.
San Antonio, Texas 78215 USA
GALDERMA is a registered trademark.
www.differin.com
325035-0702
Revised: July 2002

DIFFERIN® ℞
(adapalene gel)
Gel, 0.1%

DESCRIPTION

Differin® Gel, containing adapalene, is used for the topical treatment of acne vulgaris. Each gram of Differin® Gel contains adapalene 0.1% (1mg) in a vehicle consisting of propylene glycol, carbomer 940, poloxamer 182, edetate disodium, methylparaben, sodium hydroxide, and purified water. May contain hydrochloric acid to adjust pH.

The chemical name of adapalene is 6-[3-(1-adamantyl)-4-methoxyphenyl]-2-naphthoic acid. Adapalene is a white to off-white powder which is soluble in tetrahydrofuran, sparingly soluble in ethanol, and practically insoluble in water. The molecular formula is $C_{28}H_{28}O_3$ and molecular weight is 412.52. Adapalene is represented by the following structural formula:

CLINICAL PHARMACOLOGY

Adapalene is a chemically stable, retinoid-like compound. Biochemical and pharmacological profile studies have demonstrated that adapalene is a modulator of cellular differentiation, keratinization, and inflammatory processes all of which represent important features in the pathology of acne vulgaris.

Mechanistically, adapalene binds to specific retinoic acid nuclear receptors but does not bind to the cytosolic receptor protein. Although the exact mode of action of adapalene is unknown, it is suggested that topical adapalene may normalize the differentiation of follicular epithelial cells resulting in decreased microcomedone formation.

Pharmacokinetics: Absorption of adapalene through human skin is low. Only trace amounts (<0.25 ng/mL) of parent substance have been found in the plasma of acne patients following chronic topical application of adapalene in controlled clinical trials. Excretion appears to be primarily by the biliary route.

INDICATIONS AND USAGE

Differin® Gel is indicated for the topical treatment of acne vulgaris.

CONTRAINDICATIONS

Differin® Gel should not be administered to individuals who are hypersensitive to adapalene or any of the components in the vehicle gel.

WARNINGS

Use of Differin® Gel should be discontinued if hypersensitivity to any of the ingredients is noted. Patients with sunburn should be advised not to use the product until fully recovered.

PRECAUTIONS

General: If a reaction suggesting sensitivity or chemical irritation occurs, use of the medication should be discontinued. Exposure to sunlight, including sunlamps, should be minimized during the use of adapalene. Patients who normally experience high levels of sun exposure, and those with inherent sensitivity to sun, should be warned to exercise caution. Use of sunscreen products and protective clothing over treated areas is recommended when exposure cannot be avoided. Weather extremes, such as wind or cold, also may be irritating to patients under treatment with adapalene.

Avoid contact with the eyes, lips, angles of the nose, and mucous membranes. The product should not be applied to cuts, abrasions, eczematous skin, or sunburned skin.

Certain cutaneous signs and symptoms such as erythema, dryness, scaling, burning, or pruritus may be experienced during treatment. These are most likely to occur during the first two to four weeks and will usually lessen with continued use of the medication. Depending upon the severity of adverse events, patients should be instructed to reduce the frequency of application or discontinue use.

Drug Interactions: As Differin® Gel has the potential to produce local irritation in some patients, concomitant use of other potentially irritating topical products (medicated or abrasive soaps and cleansers, soaps and cosmetics that have a strong drying effect, and products with high concentrations of alcohol, astringents, spices, or lime) should be approached with caution. Particular caution should be exercised in using preparations containing sulfur, resorcinol, or salicylic acid in combination with Differin® Gel. If these preparations have been used, it is advisable not to start therapy with Differin® Gel until the effects of such preparations in the skin have subsided.

Carcinogenesis, Mutagenesis, Impairment of Fertility: Carcinogenicity studies with adapalene have been conducted in mice at topical doses of 0.3, 0.9, and 2.6 mg/kg/day and in rats at oral doses of 0.15, 0.5, and 1.5 mg/kg/day, approximately 4–75 times the maximal daily human topical dose. In the oral study, positive linear trends were observed in the incidence of follicular cell adenomas and carcinomas in the thyroid glands of female rats, and in the incidence of benign and malignant pheochromocytomas in the adrenal medullas of male rats.

No photocarcinogenicity studies were conducted. Animal studies have shown an increased tumorigenic risk with the use of pharmacologically similar drugs (e.g., retinoids) when exposed to UV irradiation in the laboratory or to sunlight. Although the significance of these studies to human use is not clear, patients should be advised to avoid or minimize exposure to either sunlight or artificial UV irradiation sources.

In a series of *in vivo* and *in vitro* studies, adapalene did not exhibit mutagenic or genotoxic activities.

Pregnancy: Teratogenic effects. Pregnancy Category C. No teratogenic effects were seen in rats at oral doses of adapalene 0.15 to 5.0 mg/kg/day, up to 120 times the maximal daily human topical dose. Cutaneous route teratology studies conducted in rats and rabbits at doses of 0.6, 2.0, and 6.0 mg/kg/day, up to 150 times the maximal daily human topical dose exhibited no fetotoxicity and only minimal increases in supernumerary ribs in rats. There are no adequate and well-controlled studies in pregnant women. Adapalene should be used during pregnancy only if the potential benefit justifies the potential risk to the fetus.

Nursing Mothers: It is not known whether this drug is excreted in human milk. Because many drugs are excreted in human milk, caution should be exercised when Differin® Gel is administered to a nursing woman.

Pediatric Use: Safety and effectiveness in pediatric patients below the age of 12 have not been established.

ADVERSE REACTIONS

Some adverse effects such as erythema, scaling, dryness, pruritus, and burning will occur in 10–40% of patients. Pruritus or burning immediately after application also occurs in approximately 20% of patients. The following additional adverse experiences were reported in approximately 1% or less of patients: skin irritation, burning/stinging, erythema, sunburn, and acne flares. These are most commonly seen during the first month of therapy and decrease in frequency and severity thereafter. All adverse effects with use of Differin® Gel during clinical trials were reversible upon discontinuation of therapy.

OVERDOSAGE

Differin® Gel is intended for cutaneous use only. If the medication is applied excessively, no more rapid or better results will be obtained and marked redness, peeling, or discomfort may occur. The acute oral toxicity of Differin® Gel in mice and rats is greater than 10 mL/kg. Chronic ingestion of the drug may lead to the same side effects as those associated with excessive oral intake of Vitamin A.

DOSAGE AND ADMINISTRATION

Differin® Gel should be applied once a day to affected areas after washing in the evening before retiring. A thin film of the gel should be applied, avoiding eyes, lips, and mucous membranes.

During the early weeks of therapy, an apparent exacerbation of acne may occur. This is due to the action of the medication on previously unseen lesions and should not be considered a reason to discontinue therapy. Therapeutic results should be noticed after eight to twelve weeks of treatment.

HOW SUPPLIED

Differin® (adapalene gel) Gel, 0.1% is supplied in the following sizes:

45 g laminate tube-**NDC** 0299-5910-45

Storage: Store at controlled room temperature 20°–25°C (68°–77°F).

CAUTION: Federal law prohibits dispensing without prescription.

Marketed by:
GALDERMA Laboratories, L.P.
Fort Worth, Texas 76177 USA
Mfd. by:
DPT Laboratories, Ltd.
San Antonio, Texas 78215 USA
GALDERMA is a registered trademark.
www.differin.com
325034-0903
Revised: September 2003

DIFFERIN® ℞

(adapalene solution)
Solution, 0.1%

DESCRIPTION

DIFFERIN® Solution, containing adapalene, is used for the topical treatment of acne vulgaris. Each mL of DIFFERIN® Solution contains adapalene 0.1% (1 mg) in a vehicle consisting of polyethylene glycol 400 and SD alcohol 40-B, 30% (w/v).

The chemical name of adapalene is 6-[3-(1-adamantyl)-4-methoxyphenyl]-2-naphthoic acid. Adapalene is a white to off-white powder which is soluble in tetrahydrofuran, sparingly soluble in ethanol, and practically insoluble in water. The molecular formula is $C_{28}H_{28}O_3$ and molecular weight is 412.52. Adapalene is represented by the following structural formula:

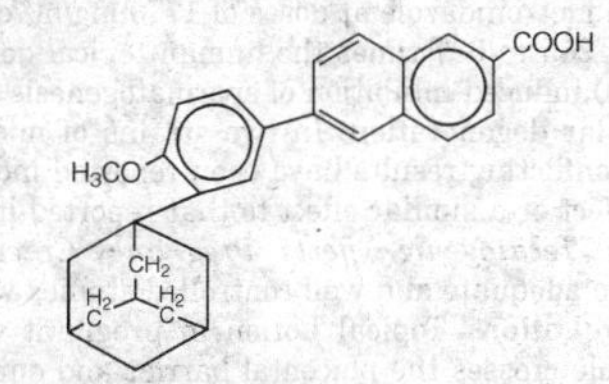

CLINICAL PHARMACOLOGY

Adapalene is a chemically stable, retinoid-like compound. Biochemical and pharmacological profile studies have demonstrated that adapalene is a modulator of cellular differentiation, keratinization, and inflammatory processes all of which represent important features in the pathology of acne vulgaris. Mechanistically, adapalene binds to specific retinoic acid nuclear receptors but does not bind to the cytosolic receptor protein. Although the exact mode of action of adapalene is unknown, it is suggested that topical adapalene may normalize the differentiation of follicular epithelial cells resulting in decreased microcomedone formation.

Pharmacokinetics: Absorption of adapalene through human skin is low. Only trace amounts (< 0.25 ng/mL) of parent substance have been found in the plasma of acne patients following chronic topical application of adapalene in controlled clinical trials. Excretion appears to be primarily by the biliary route.

INDICATIONS AND USAGE

DIFFERIN® Solution is indicated for the topical treatment of acne vulgaris.

CONTRAINDICATIONS

DIFFERIN® Solution should not be administered to individuals who are hypersensitive to adapalene or any of the components in the vehicle solution.

WARNINGS

Use of DIFFERIN® Solution should be discontinued if hypersensitivity to any of the ingredients is noted. Patients with sunburn should be advised not to use the product until fully recovered.

PRECAUTIONS

General: If a reaction suggesting sensitivity or chemical irritation occurs, use of the medication should be discontinued. Exposure to sunlight, including sunlamps, should be minimized during the use of adapalene. Patients who normally experience high levels of sun exposure, and those with inherent sensitivity to sun, should be warned to exercise caution. Use of sunscreen products and protective clothing over treated areas is recommended when exposure cannot be avoided. Weather extremes, such as wind or cold, also may be irritating to patients under treatment with adapalene.

Avoid contact with the eyes, lips, angles of the nose, and mucous membranes. The product should not be applied to cuts, abrasions, eczematous skin, or sunburned skin.

Certain cutaneous signs and symptoms such as erythema, dryness, scaling, burning, or pruritus may be experienced during treatment. These are most likely to occur during the first two to four weeks and will usually lessen with continued use of the medication. Depending upon the severity of adverse events, patients should be instructed to reduce the frequency of application or discontinue use.

Drug Interactions: As DIFFERIN® Solution has the potential to produce local irritation in some patients, concomitant use of other potentially irritating topical products (medicated or abrasive soaps and cleansers, soaps and cosmetics that have a strong drying effect, and products with high concentrations of alcohol, astringents, spices, or lime) should be approached with caution. Particular caution should be exercised in using preparations containing sulfur, resorcinol, or salicylic acid in combination with DIFFERIN® Solution. If these preparations have been used, it is advisable not to start therapy with DIFFERIN® Solution until the effects of such preparations in the skin have subsided.

Carcinogenesis, Mutagenesis, Impairment of Fertility: Carcinogenicity studies with adapalene have been conducted in mice at topical doses of 0.3, 0.9, and 2.6 mg/kg/day and in rats at oral doses of 0.15, 0.5, and 1.5 mg/kg/day, approximately 4–75 times the maximal daily human topical dose. In the oral study, positive linear trends were observed in the incidence of follicular cell adenomas and carcinomas in the thyroid glands of female rats, and in the incidence of benign and malignant pheochromocytomas in the adrenal medullas of male rats.

No photocarcinogenicity studies were conducted. Animal studies have shown an increased tumorigenic risk with the use of pharmacologically similar drugs (e.g., retinoids) when exposed to UV irradiation in the laboratory or to sunlight. Although the significance of these studies to human use is not clear, patients should be advised to avoid or minimize exposure to either sunlight or artificial UV irradiation sources.

In a series of *in vivo* and *in vitro* studies, adapalene did not exhibit mutagenic or genotoxic activities.

Pregnancy: Teratogenic effects. Pregnancy Category C. No teratogenic effects were seen in rats at oral doses of adapalene 0.15 to 5.0 mg/kg/day, up to 120 times the maximal daily human topical dose. Cutaneous route teratology studies conducted in rats and rabbits at doses of 0.6, 2.0, and 6.0 mg/kg/day, up to 150 times the maximal daily human topical dose exhibited no fetotoxicity and only minimal increases in supernumerary ribs in rats. There are no adequate and well-controlled studies in pregnant women. Adapalene should be used during pregnancy only if the potential benefit justifies the potential risk to the fetus.

Nursing Mothers: It is not known whether this drug is excreted in human milk. Because many drugs are excreted in human milk, caution should be exercised when DIFFERIN® Solution is administered to a nursing woman.

Pediatric Use: Safety and effectiveness in pediatric patients below the age of 12 have not been established.

ADVERSE REACTIONS

Some adverse effects such as erythema, scaling, dryness, pruritus, and burning will occur in 30–60% of patients. Pruritus or burning immediately after application also occurs in approximately 30% of patients. The following additional adverse experiences were reported in approximately 1% or less of patients: skin irritation, burning/stinging, erythema, sunburn, and acne flares. These are most commonly seen during the first month of therapy and decrease in frequency and severity thereafter. All adverse effects with use of DIFFERIN® Solution during clinical trials were reversible upon discontinuation of therapy.

OVERDOSAGE

DIFFERIN® Solution is intended for cutaneous use only. If the medication is applied excessively, no more rapid or better results will be obtained and marked redness, peeling, or discomfort may occur. The acute oral toxicity of DIFFERIN® Solution in mice and rats is greater than 10 mL/kg. Chronic ingestion of the drug may lead to the same side effects as those associated with excessive oral intake of Vitamin A.

DOSAGE AND ADMINISTRATION

1. DIFFERIN® Solution should be applied once a day to affected areas.
2. Before retiring in the evening, wash and dry areas to be treated.
3. Apply a thin film of medication to the affected areas. Avoid the eyes, lips, and mucous membranes.

Pledget: Remove pledget from foil just before using. Discard pledget after single use. Do not use if seal is broken.

Glass bottle: Replace cap after each use.

During the early weeks of therapy, an apparent exacerbation of acne may occur. This is due to the action of the medication on previously unseen lesions and should not be considered a reason to discontinue therapy. Therapeutic results should be noticed after eight to twelve weeks of treatment.

HOW SUPPLIED

DIFFERIN® (adapalene solution) Solution, 0.1% is supplied in the following sizes:

30 mL glass bottle with applicator – **NDC** 0299-5905-30
60-count unit-of-use pledget – **NDC** 0299-5905-16

The applicator is designed so that the solution may be applied directly to the involved skin.

Storage: Store at controlled room temperature 20° – 25°C (68° – 77°F). Keep bottle tightly closed and store upright.

Marketed by:
GALDERMA LABORATORIES, L.P.
Fort Worth, Texas 76177 USA
Mfd. by:
DPT Laboratories, Ltd.
San Antonio, Texas 78215 USA
Certain manufacturing operations have been performed by other firms.
www.differin.com
325036-1003
Revised: October 2003

METROGEL® ℞

(metronidazole topical gel)
Topical Gel, 0.75%
FOR TOPICAL USE ONLY
(NOT FOR OPHTHALMIC USE)

DESCRIPTION

MetroGel® Topical Gel contains metronidazole, USP, at a concentration of 7.5 mg per gram (0.75%) in a gel consisting of purified water, methylparaben, propylparaben, propylene glycol, carbomer 940, sodium hydroxide, and edetate disodium. Metronidazole is classified therapeutically as an antiprotozoal and antibacterial agent. Chemically, metronidazole is named 2-methyl-5-nitro-1*H* -imidazole-1-ethanol and has the following structure:

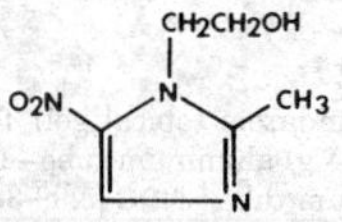

CLINICAL PHARMACOLOGY

Bioavailability studies on the topical administration of 1 gram of **MetroGel®** Topical Gel (7.5 mg of metronidazole) to the face of 10 rosacea patients showed a maximum serum concentration of 66 nanograms per milliliter in one patient. This concentration is approximately 100 times less than concentrations afforded by a single 250 mg oral tablet. The serum metronidazole concentrations were below the detectable limits of the assay at the majority of time points in all patients. Three of the patients had no detectable serum concentrations of metronidazole at any time point. The mean dose of gel applied during clinical studies was 600 mg which represents 4.5 mg of metronidazole per application. Therefore, under normal usage levels, the formulation affords minimal serum concentrations of metronidazole. The mechanisms by which **MetroGel®** (metronidazole topical gel) Topical Gel acts in the treatment of rosacea are unknown, but appear to include an anti-inflammatory effect.

INDICATIONS AND USAGE

MetroGel® Topical Gel is indicated for topical application in the treatment of inflammatory papules and pustules of rosacea.

CONTRAINDICATIONS

MetroGel® Topical Gel is contraindicated in individuals with a history of hypersensitivity to metronidazole, parabens, or other ingredients of the formulation.

PRECAUTIONS

General: MetroGel® Topical Gel has been reported to cause tearing of the eyes. Therefore, contact with the eyes should be avoided. If a reaction suggesting local irritation occurs, patients should be directed to use the medication less frequently or discontinue use. Metronidazole is a nitroimidazole and should be used with care in patients with evidence of, or history of blood dyscrasia.

Information for patients: This medication is to be used as directed by the physician. It is for external use only. Avoid contact with the eyes.

Drug Interactions: Oral metronidazole has been reported to potentiate the anticoagulant effect of coumarin and warfarin resulting in a prolongation of prothrombin time. The effect of topical metronidazole on prothrombin time is not known.

Carcinogenesis, mutagenesis, impairment of fertility: Metronidazole has shown evidence of carcinogenic activity in a number of studies involving chronic, oral administration in mice and rats but not in studies involving hamsters.

Metronidazole has shown evidence of mutagenic activity in several *in vitro* bacterial assay systems. In addition, a dose-response increase in the frequency of micronuclei was ob-

Continued on next page

MetroGel—Cont.

served in mice after intraperitoneal injections and an increase in chromosome aberrations have been reported in patients with Crohn's disease who were treated with 200–1200 mg/day of metronidazole for 1 to 24 months. However, no excess chromosomal aberrations in circulating human lymphocytes have been observed in patients treated for 8 months.

Pregnancy: ***Teratogenic effects: Pregnancy category B:*** There has been no experience to date with the use of **MetroGel®** (metronidazole topical gel) Topical Gel in pregnant patients. Metronidazole crosses the placental barrier and enters the fetal circulation rapidly. No fetotoxicity was observed after oral metronidazole in rats or mice. However, because animal reproduction studies are not always predictive of human response and since oral metronidazole has been shown to be a carcinogen in some rodents, this drug should be used during pregnancy only if clearly needed.

Nursing mothers: After oral administration, metronidazole is secreted in breast milk in concentrations similar to those found in the plasma. Even though **MetroGel®** Topical Gel blood levels are significantly lower than those achieved after oral metronidazole, a decision should be made whether to discontinue nursing or to discontinue the drug, taking into account the importance of the drug to the mother.

Pediatric use: Safety and effectiveness in pediatric patients have not been established.

ADVERSE REACTIONS

The following adverse experiences have been reported with the topical use of metronidazole: burning, skin irritation, dryness, transient redness, metallic taste, tingling or numbness of extremities and nausea.

DOSAGE AND ADMINISTRATION

Apply and rub in a thin film of **MetroGel®** Topical Gel twice daily, morning and evening, to entire affected areas after washing.

Areas to be treated should be cleansed before application of **MetroGel®** (metronidazole topical gel) Topical Gel. Patients may use cosmetics after application of **MetroGel®** Topical Gel.

HOW SUPPLIED

MetroGel® (metronidazole topical gel) Topical Gel is supplied in a 1 oz (28.4 g) aluminum tube—**NDC** 0299-3835-28 and a 45 g aluminum tube—**NDC** 0299-3835-45.

Storage conditions: STORE AT CONTROLLED ROOM TEMPERATURE: 59° to 86°F (15° to 30°C).

Caution: Federal law prohibits dispensing without prescription.

Marketed by:
GALDERMA Laboratories L.P., Fort Worth, Texas 76177 USA
Manufactured by: DPT Laboratories, Ltd.
San Antonio, Texas 78215 USA
GALDERMA is a registered trademark.
225032-0895
www.metrogel.com
Revised: August 1995

METROLOTION® ℞
(metronidazole lotion)
Topical Lotion, 0.75%
Rx only

FOR TOPICAL USE ONLY
(NOT FOR OPHTHALMIC USE)

DESCRIPTION

MetroLotion® (metronidazole lotion) Topical Lotion contains metronidazole, USP, at a concentration of 7.5 mg per gram (0.75% w/w) in a lotion consisting of benzyl alcohol, carbomer 941, cyclomethicone, glycerin, glyceryl stearate, light mineral oil, PEG-100 stearate, polyethylene glycol 400, potassium sorbate, purified water, steareth-21, stearyl alcohol, and sodium hydroxide and/or lactic acid to adjust pH.

Metronidazole is an imidazole and is classified therapeutically as an antiprotozoal and antibacterial agent. Chemically, metronidazole is 2-methyl-5-nitro-1*H*-imidazole-1-ethanol. The molecular formula is $C_6H_9N_3O_3$ and molecular weight is 171.16. Metronidazole is represented by the following structural formula:

CH_2CH_2OH
O_2N — N — CH_3
N

CLINICAL PHARMACOLOGY

The mechanisms by which metronidazole acts in the treatment of rosacea are unknown, but appear to include an anti-inflammatory effect.

Pharmacokinetics: Absorption of metronidazole after topical application of **MetroLotion®** Topical Lotion is less complete and more prolonged than after oral administration. Detectable plasma levels were found in all subjects following the administration of a single 1 gram dose of **MetroLotion®** Topical Lotion (containing 7.5 mg of metronidazole) to the faces of 12 healthy volunteers. The highest concentration (64 ng/mL) seen was approximately 100 times lower than the peak concentrations produced by a single 250 mg tablet of metronidazole. The mean relative bioavailability of metronidazole from **MetroLotion®** Topical Lotion was 47.4%.

Efficacy Outcomes at Week 12

Mean Percent Reduction in Inflammatory Lesion Counts from Baseline

MetroLotion® Topical Lotion N=65	Vehicle Lotion N=60
55%	20%

Investigators' Global Assessment of Improvement (percent change from baseline)

	Worse	No Change	Minimal Improvement	Definite Improvement	Marked Improvement	Clear
MetroLotion® Topical Lotion N=65	5%	12%	11%	32%	32%	8%
Vehicle Lotion N=60	15%	27%	23%	15%	20%	0%

INDICATIONS AND USAGE

MetroLotion® Topical Lotion is indicated for topical application in the treatment of inflammatory papules and pustules of rosacea.

CLINICAL STUDIES

A controlled clinical study was conducted in 144 patients with moderate to severe rosacea, in which **MetroLotion®** Topical Lotion was compared with its vehicle. Applications were made twice daily for 12 weeks during which patients were instructed to avoid spicy foods, thermally hot foods and drinks, alcoholic beverages, and caffeine. Patients were also provided samples of a soapless cleansing lotion and, if requested, a moisturizer. **MetroLotion®** Topical Lotion was significantly more effective than its vehicle in mean percent reduction of inflammatory lesions associated with rosacea and in the investigators' global assessment of improvement. The results of the mean percent reduction in inflammatory lesion counts from baseline after 12 weeks of treatment and the investigators' global assessment of improvement at week 12 are presented in the following table:

[See table above]

The scale is based on the following definitions:

Worse:
Exacerbation of either erythema or quantitative assessment of papules and/or pustules.

No Change:
Condition remains the same.

Minimal Improvement:
Slight improvement in the quantitative assessment of papules and/or pustules, and/or slight improvement in erythema.

Definite Improvement:
More pronounced improvement in the quantitative assessment of papules and/or pustules, and/or more pronounced improvement in erythema.

Marked Improvement:
Obvious improvement in the quantitative assessment of papules and/or pustules, and/or obvious improvement in erythema.

Clear:
No papules or pustules and minimal residual or no erythema.

CONTRAINDICATIONS

MetroLotion® Topical Lotion is contraindicated in individuals with a history of hypersensitivity to metronidazole or to other ingredients of the formulation.

PRECAUTIONS

General: Topical metronidazole formulations have been reported to cause tearing of the eyes. Therefore, contact with the eyes should be avoided. If a reaction suggesting local irritation occurs, patients should be directed to use the medication less frequently or discontinue use. Metronidazole is a nitroimidazole and should be used with care in patients with evidence or history of blood dyscrasia.

Information for Patients: Patients using **MetroLotion®** Topical Lotion should receive the following information and instructions:

1. This medication is to be used only as directed by the physician.
2. It is for external use only.
3. Avoid contact with the eyes.
4. Cleanse affected area(s) before applying this medication.
5. Patients should report any adverse reaction to their physician.

Drug Interactions: Oral metronidazole has been reported to potentiate the anticoagulant effect of warfarin and coumarin anticoagulants, resulting in a prolongation of prothrombin time. The effect of topical metronidazole on prothrombin time is not known.

Carcinogenesis, Mutagenesis, Impairment of Fertility: Metronidazole has shown evidence of carcinogenic activity in a number of studies involving chronic, oral administration in mice and rats but not in studies involving hamsters. Neither carcinogenicity nor photocarcinogenicity studies have been performed by the topical route with **MetroLotion®** Topical Lotion or any marketed metronidazole formulations.

In several long-term studies in mice, oral doses of approximately 198 mg/m²/day or greater (approximately 29 to 71 times the human topical dose on a mg/m² basis) were associated with an increase in lung tumors in male mice and lymphomas in female mice.

Several long-term studies by the oral route in rats have shown statistically significant increases in mammary and hepatic tumors in female rats and testicular tumors and pituitary adenomas in male rats at doses (in feed) of 1593 mg/m²/day or greater (approximately 230 to 573 times the human topical dose on a mg/m² basis). In another oral study (by gavage), mammary tumors in female rats were observed with a dose of 177 mg/m²/day (approximately 26 to 64 times the human topical dose on a mg/m² basis).

In a published study, the ultraviolet radiation-induced carcinogenesis was enhanced in albino hairless mice by intraperitoneal administration of 45 mg/m² metronidazole, as shown by a decreased latency period to the development of skin neoplasms. The concentration of metronidazole in the skin following the intraperitoneal administration was not determined. This study did not distinguish whether metronidazole must be present during the exposure to ultraviolet radiation in order to enhance tumor formation or whether metronidazole could promote tumor formation from preexisting ultraviolet radiation-initiated cells. The significance of these results in the topical use of metronidazole for the treatment of rosacea is unclear.

Metronidazole has shown evidence of mutagenic activity in several *in vitro* bacterial assay systems. In addition, a dose-response increase in the frequency of micronuclei was observed in mice after intraperitoneal injections. An increase in chromosome aberrations in peripheral blood lymphocytes was reported in patients with Crohn's disease who were treated with 200–1200 mg/day of metronidazole for 1 to 24 months. However, in another study, no excess chromosomal aberrations in circulating human lymphocytes were observed in patients treated for 8 months.

In rats, oral metronidazole at doses of 1770 mg/m²/day (approximately 255 to 637 times the human topical dose on a mg/m² basis) induced inhibition of spermatogenesis and severe testicular degeneration. In two strains of mice (ICR and CF1), conflicting results have been reported indicating either no effect or a similar effect to that reported in rats.

Pregnancy: *Teratogenic Effects: Pregnancy Category B:* There are no adequate and well-controlled studies with the use of **MetroLotion®** Topical Lotion in pregnant women. Metronidazole crosses the placental barrier and enters the fetal circulation rapidly. No fetotoxicity was observed after oral administration of metronidazole in rats or mice. However, because animal reproduction studies are not always predictive of human response and since oral metronidazole has been shown to be a carcinogen in some rodents, this drug should be used during pregnancy only if clearly needed.

Nursing Mothers: After oral administration, metronidazole is secreted in breast milk in concentrations similar to those found in the plasma. Even though blood levels are significantly lower with topically applied metronidazole than those achieved after oral administration of metronidazole, a decision should be made whether to discontinue nursing or to discontinue the drug, taking into account the importance of the drug to the mother.

Pediatric Use: Safety and effectiveness in pediatric patients have not been established.

ADVERSE REACTIONS

In a controlled clinical trial, safety data from 141 patients who used **MetroLotion®** Topical Lotion (n=71), or the lotion vehicle (n=70), twice daily and experienced a local cutaneous adverse event which may or may not have been related to the treatments include: local allergic reaction, **MetroLotion®** Topical Lotion 2 (3%), lotion vehicle 0; contact dermatitis, **MetroLotion®** Topical Lotion 2 (3%), lotion vehicle 1 (1%); pruritus, **MetroLotion®** Topical Lotion 1 (1%), lotion vehicle 0; skin discomfort (burning and stinging), **MetroLotion®** Topical Lotion 1 (1%), lotion vehicle 2 (3%); erythema, **MetroLotion®** Topical Lotion 4 (6%), lotion vehicle 0; dry skin, **MetroLotion®** Topical Lotion 0, lotion vehicle 1 (1%); and worsening of rosacea, **MetroLotion®** Topical Lotion 1 (1%), lotion vehicle 7 (10%).

The following additional adverse experiences have been reported with the topical use of metronidazole: skin irritation, transient redness, metallic taste, tingling or numbness of extremities, and nausea.

DOSAGE AND ADMINISTRATION

Apply a thin layer to entire affected areas after washing. Use morning and evening or as directed by physician. Avoid application close to the eyes.
Patients may use cosmetics after waiting for the **MetroLotion**® Topical Lotion to dry (not less than 5 minutes).

HOW SUPPLIED

MetroLotion® (metronidazole lotion) Topical Lotion, 0.75% is supplied in the following size:
2 fl. oz. (59 mL) plastic bottle—**NDC** 0299-3838-02
Storage: Store at controlled room temperature 68° to 77°F (20°–25°C). Protect from freezing.
Marketed by:
GALDERMA LABORATORIES, L.P.
Fort Worth, Texas 76177 USA
Manufactured by:
DPT Laboratories, Ltd.
San Antonio, Texas 78215 USA
GALDERMA is a registered trademark.
325055-0803
www.metrogel.com
Revised: August 2003

ROSANIL® CLEANSER ℞

[*rō'să-nĭl*]
(sodium sulfacetamide 10% and sulfur 5%)
℞ Only

DESCRIPTION

Sodium sulfacetamide is a sulfonamide with antibacterial activity while sulfur acts as a keratolytic agent. Chemically sodium sulfacetamide is N-[(4-aminophenyl)sulfonyl]-acetamide, monosodium salt, monohydrate. The structural formula is:

NH_2—(benzene ring)—$SO_2N(Na)COCH_3 \cdot H_2O$

Each gram of **ROSANIL**® (sodium sulfacetamide 10% and sulfur 5%) Cleanser contains: **Active:** sodium sulfacetamide 10% (100 mg), sulfur 5% (50 mg). **Inactive:** butylated hydroxytoluene, edetate disodium, emulsifying wax, hydrochloric acid, light mineral oil, methylparaben, PPG-2 hydroxyethyl coco/isostearamide, propylparaben, purified water, sodium cocoyl isethionate, sodium lauryl sulfoacetate (and) disodium laureth sulfosuccinate, and sodium thiosulfate.

CLINICAL PHARMACOLOGY

The most widely accepted mechanism of action of sulfon amides is the Woods-Fildes theory which is based on the fact that sulfonamides act as competitive antagonists to para-aminobenzoic acid (PABA), an essential component for bacterial growth. While absorption through intact skin has not been determined, sodium sulfacetamide is readily absorbed from the gastrointestinal tract when taken orally and excreted in the urine, largely unchanged. The biological half-life has variously been reported as 7 to 12.8 hours. The exact mode of action of sulfur in the treatment of acne is unknown, but it has been reported that it inhibits the growth of *Propionibacterium acnes* and the formation of free fatty acids.

INDICATIONS

ROSANIL® Cleanser is indicated in the topical control of acne vulgaris, acne rosacea and seborrheic dermatitis.

CONTRAINDICATIONS

ROSANIL® Cleanser is contraindicated for use by patients having known hypersensitivity to sulfonamides, sulfur or any other component of this preparation, **ROSANIL**® Cleanser is not to be used by patients with kidney disease.

WARNINGS

Although rare, sensitivity to sodium sulfacetamide may occur. Therefore, caution and careful supervision should be observed when prescribing this drug for patients who may be prone to hypersensitivity to topical sulfonamides. Systemic toxic reactions such as agranulocytosis, acute hemolytic anemia, purpura hemorrhagica, drug fever, jaundice, and contact dermatitis indicate hypersensitivity to sulfonamides. Particular caution should be employed if areas of denuded or abraded skin are involved.
FOR EXTERNAL USE ONLY. Keep away from eyes. **Keep out of reach of children.** Keep container tightly closed.

PRECAUTIONS

General: If irritation develops, use of the product should be discontinued and appropriate therapy instituted. Patients should be carefully observed for possible local irritation or sensitization during long-term therapy. The object of this therapy is to achieve desquamation without irritation, but sodium sulfacetamide and sulfur can cause reddening and scaling of the epidermis. These side effects are not unusual in the treatment of acne vulgaris, but patients should be cautioned about the possibility.
Information for Patients: Avoid contact with eyes, eyelids, lips and mucous membranes. If accidental contact occurs, rinse with water. If excessive irritation develops, discontinue use and consult your physician.
Carcinogenesis, Mutagenesis and Impairment of Fertility: Long-term studies in animals have not been performed to evaluate carcinogenic potential.
Pregnancy: Category C. Animal reproduction studies have not been conducted with **ROSANIL**® (sodium sulfacetamide 10% and sulfur 5%) Cleanser. It is also not known whether **ROSANIL**® Cleanser can cause fetal harm when administered to a pregnant woman or can affect reproduction capacity. **ROSANIL**® Cleanser should be given to a pregnant woman only if clearly needed.
Nursing Mothers: It is not known whether sodium sulfacetamide is excreted in the human milk following topical use of **ROSANIL**® Cleanser. However, small amounts of orally administered sulfonamides have been reported to be eliminated in human milk. In view of this and because many drugs are excreted in human milk, caution should be exercised when **ROSANIL**® Cleanser is administered to a nursing woman.
Pediatric Use: Safety and effectiveness in children under the age of 12 have not been established.

ADVERSE REACTIONS

Although rare, sodium sulfacetamide may cause local irritation.

DOSAGE AND ADMINISTRATION

Wash affected areas once or twice daily, or as directed by your physician. Avoid contact with eyes or mucous membranes. Wet skin and liberally apply to areas to be cleansed, massage gently into skin for 10–20 seconds working into a full lather, rinse thoroughly and pat dry. If drying occurs, it may be controlled by rinsing cleanser off sooner or using less often.

HOW SUPPLIED

ROSANIL® (sodium sulfacetamide 10% and sulfur 5%) Cleanser is available in the following sizes:
6 oz tube **NDC** 0299-3839-06
13 oz tube **NDC** 0299-3839-13
Store at controlled room temperature 20°–25°C (68°–77°F).
GALDERMA
Marketed by:
GALDERMA LABORATORIES, L.P.
Fort Worth, Texas 76177 USA
Manufactured by:
DPT Laboratories, Ltd.
San Antonio, Texas 78215 USA
GALDERMA is a registered trademark.
www.rosanil.com
325049-1002 Revised: October 2003

SOLAGÉ® ℞

(mequinol 2%, tretinoin 0.01%)
Rx only
Topical Solution

For Dermatologic use only. Not for ophthalmic, oral or intravaginal use.

DESCRIPTION

Solagé® Topical Solution contains mequinol 2% and tretinoin 0.01%, by weight, in a solution base of ethyl alcohol (77.8% v/v), polyethylene glycol 400, butylated hydroxytoluene, ascorbic acid, citric acid, ascorbyl palmitate, edetate disodium and purified water.
Mequinol is 4- hydroxyanisole, the monomethyl ether of hydroquinone or 1-hydroxy-4-methoxybenzene. It has the chemical formula, $C_7H_8O_2$, a molecular weight of 124.14, and the structural formula:

H_3CO—(benzene ring)—OH

The chemical name for tretinoin, a retinoid, is (all-*E*)-3,7-dimethyl-9-(2,6,6-trimethyl-1-cyclohexen-1-yl)-2,4,6,8-nonatetraenoic acid, also referred to as all-*trans*- retinoic acid. It has the chemical formula, $C_{20}H_{28}O_2$, a molecular weight of 300.44, and the structural formula:

COOH

CLINICAL PHARMACOLOGY

Solar lentigines are localized, pigmented, macular lesions of the skin on the areas of the body which have been chronically exposed to sunlight.
Biopsy specimens of solar lentigines were collected in a clinical study with **Solagé**® Solution at baseline, at the end of a 24 week treatment period and at the end of a subsequent 24 week, no treatment, follow-up period. The end of treatment specimens showed a decrease in melanin pigmentation in both melanocytes and keratinocytes, and an increased lymphocytic infiltration, which may have been the result of irritation or an immunologic reaction. The end of follow-up period specimens showed repigmentation of the melanocytes and keratinocytes to a state similar to the baseline specimens. These results indicate that there is no assurance that any improvement obtained would persist upon discontinuation of drug therapy.
The mechanism of action of mequinol is unknown. Although mequinol is a substrate for the enzyme tyrosinase and acts as a competitive inhibitor of the formation of melanin precursors, the clinical significance of these findings is unknown. The mechanism of action of tretinoin as a depigmenting agent also is unknown.

PHARMACOKINETICS

The percutaneous absorption of tretinoin and the systemic exposure to tretinoin and mequinol were assessed in healthy subjects (n=8) following two weeks of twice daily topical treatment of **Solagé**® Solution. Approximately 0.8 mL of **Solagé**® Solution was applied to a 400 cm^2 area of the back, corresponding to a dose of 37.3 $\mu g/cm^2$ for mequinol and 0.23 $\mu g/cm^2$ for tretinoin. The percutaneous absorption of tretinoin was approximately 4.4%, and systemic concentrations did not increase over endogenous levels. The mean C_{max} for mequinol was 9.92 ng/mL (range 4.22 to 23.62 ng/mL) and the T_{max} was 2 hours (range 1 to 2 hours).

INDICATIONS AND USAGE

(To understand fully the indication for this product, please read the entire **INDICATIONS AND USAGE** section of the labeling).
Solagé® (mequinol 2%, tretinoin 0.01%) Topical Solution is indicated for the treatment of solar lentigines.
Solagé® Solution should only be used under medical supervision as an adjunct to a comprehensive skin care and sun avoidance program where the patient should primarily either avoid the sun or use protective clothing.
Neither the safety nor effectiveness of **Solagé**® Solution for the prevention or treatment of melasma or postinflammatory hyperpigmentation has been established.
The efficacy of using **Solagé**® Solution daily for greater than 24 weeks has not been established.
The local cutaneous safety of using Solagé® Solution in non-Caucasians has not been adequately established (see **Clinical Studies** section).

CONTRAINDICATIONS

The combination of mequinol and tretinoin may cause fetal harm when administered to a pregnant woman. Due to the known effects of these active ingredients, **Solagé**® Topical Solution should not be used in women of childbearing potential. In a dermal teratology study in New Zealand White rabbits, there were no statistically significant differences among treatment groups in fetal malformation data; however, marked hydrocephaly with visible doming of the head was observed in one mid-dose litter (12 and 0.06 mg/kg or 132 and 0.66 mg/m^2 of mequinol and tretinoin, respectively) and two fetuses in one high dose litter (40 and 0.2 mg/kg or 440 and 2.2 mg/m^2 of mequinol and tretinoin, respectively) of **Solagé**® Solution, and two high-dose tretinoin (0.2 mg/kg, 2.2 mg/m^2) treated litters. These malformations were considered to be treatment related and due to the known effects of tretinoin. This was further supported by coincident appearance of other malformations associated with tretinoin, such as cleft palate and appendicular skeletal defects. No effects attributed to treatment were observed in rabbits in that study treated topically with mequinol alone (dose 40 mg/kg, 440 mg/m^2). A no-observed-effect level (NOEL) for teratogenicity in rabbits was established at 4 and 0.02 mg/kg (44 and 0.22 mg/m^2 mequinol and tretinoin, respectively) for **Solagé**® Solution which is approximately the maximum possible human daily dose, based on clinical application to 5% of total body surface area. Plasma tretinoin concentrations were not raised above endogenous levels, even at teratogenic doses. Plasma mequinol concentrations in rabbits at the NOEL at one hour after application were 124 ng/mL or approximately twelve times the mean peak plasma concentrations of that substance seen in human subjects in a clinical pharmacokinetic study.
In a repeated study in pregnant rabbits administered the same dose levels as the study described above, additional precautionary measures were taken to prevent ingestion, although there is no evidence to confirm that ingestion occurred in the initial study. Precautionary measures additionally limited transdermal absorption to a six hour exposure period, or approximately one-fourth of the human clinical daily continuous exposure time. This study did not show any significant teratogenic effects at doses up to approximately 13 times the human dose on a mg/m^2 basis. However, a concurrent tretinoin dose group (0.2 mg/kg/day) did include two litters with limb malformations.
In a published study in albino rats (J. Am. Coll. Toxicology 4(5):31–63, 1985), topical application of 5% of mequinol in a cream vehicle during gestation was embryotoxic and embryolethal. Embryonic loss prior to implantation was noted in that study where animals were treated throughout gestation. Coincidentally, mean preimplantation embryonic loss was increased in the first rabbit study in all mequinol treated groups, relative to control, and in the high dose mequinol/tretinoin and tretinoin only treated groups in the second study. In those studies, dosing began at gestation day 6, when implantation is purported to occur. Increased preimplantation loss was also noted at the high combination dose in a study of early embryonic effects in rats, as was decreased body weight in male pups; these findings are consistent with the published study.
Solagé® Solution was not teratogenic in Sprague-Dawley rats when given in topical doses of 80 and 0.4 mg/kg mequinol and tretinoin, respectively (480 and 2.4 mg/m^2 or

Continued on next page

Solagé—Cont.

11 times the maximum human daily dose). The maximum human dose is defined as the amount of solution applied daily to 5% of the total body surface area.

With widespread use of any drug, a small number of birth defect reports associated temporally with the administration of the drug would be expected by chance alone. Thirty cases of temporally-associated congenital malformations have been reported during two decades of clinical use of another formulation of topical tretinoin. Although no definite pattern of teratogenicity and no casual association has been established from these cases, 6 of the reports describe the rare birth defect category holoprosencephaly (defects associated with incomplete midline development of the forebrain). The significance of these spontaneous reports in terms of risk to the fetus is not known.

No adequate or well-controlled trials have been conducted with **Solagé®** Solution in pregnant women.

Solagé® Topical Solution is contraindicated in individuals with a history of sensitivity reactions to any of its ingredients. It should be discontinued if hypersensitivity to any of its ingredients is noted.

WARNINGS

Solagé® Solution is a dermal irritant and the results of continued irritation of the skin for greater than 52 weeks in chronic, long-term use are not known. Tretinoin has been reported to cause severe irritation on eczematous skin and should be used only with utmost caution in patients with this condition.

Safety and effectiveness of **Solagé®** Solution in individuals with moderately or heavily pigmented skin have not been established.

Solagé® Solution should not be administered if the patient is also taking drugs known to be photosensitizers (e.g., thiazides, tetracyclines, fluoroquinolones, phenothiazines, sulfonamides) because of the possibility of augmented phototoxicity.

Because of heightened burning susceptibility, exposure to sunlight (including sunlamps) to treated areas should be avoided or minimized during the use of **Solagé®** Solution. Patients must be advised to use protective clothing and comply with a comprehensive sun avoidance program when using **Solagé®** Solution. Data are not available to establish how or whether **Solagé®** Solution is degraded (either by sunlight or by normal interior lighting) following application to the skin. Patients with sunburn should be advised not to use **Solagé®** Solution until fully recovered. Patients who may have considerable sun exposure due to their occupation and those patients with inherent sensitivity to sunlight should exercise particular caution when using **Solagé®** Solution and ensure that the precautions outlined in the Patient Medication Guide are observed.

Solagé® Solution should be kept out of the eyes, mouth, paranasal creases, and mucous membranes. **Solagé®** Solution may cause skin irritation, erythema, burning, stinging or tingling, peeling, and pruritis. If the degree of such local irritation warrants, patients should be directed to use less medication, decrease the frequency of application, discontinue use temporarily, or discontinue use altogether. The efficacy at reduced frequencies of application has not been established.

Solagé® Solution should be used with caution by patients with a history, or family history, of vitiligo. One patient in the trials, whose brother had vitiligo, experienced hypopigmentation in areas that had not been treated with study medication. Some of these areas continued to worsen for at least one month post treatment with **Solagé®** Solution. Six weeks later the severity of the hypopigmentation had decreased from moderate to mild and 106 days post treatment, the patient had resolution of some but not all lesions.

Application of larger amounts of medication than recommended will not lead to more rapid or better results, and marked redness, peeling, discomfort, or hypopigmentation of the skin may occur.

PRECAUTIONS

General

For external use only.

Solagé® Solution should only be used as an adjunct to a comprehensive skin care and sun avoidance program. (See **INDICATIONS AND USAGE** section).

If a drug sensitivity, chemical irritation, or a systemic adverse reaction develops, use of **Solagé®** Solution should be discontinued.

Weather extremes, such as wind or cold, may be more irritating to patients using **Solagé®** Solution.

Information for patients

Patients require detailed instruction to obtain maximal benefits and to understand all the precautions necessary to use this product with greatest safety. The Patient Medication Guide is attached to this Package Insert.

Drug Interactions

Concomitant topical products with a strong skin drying effect, products with high concentrations of alcohol, astringents, spices or lime, medicated soaps or shampoos, permanent wave solutions, electrolysis, hair depilatories or waxes, or other preparations that might dry or irritate the skin should be used with caution in patients being treated with **Solagé®** Solution because they may increase irritation when used with **Solagé®** Solution.

Solagé® Solution should not be administered if the patient is also taking drugs known to be photosensitizers (e.g., thiazides, tetracyclines, fluoroquinolones, phenothiazines, sulfonamides) because of the possibility of augmented phototoxicity.

Carcinogenesis, Mutagenesis, Impairment of Fertility

Although a dermal carcinogenicity study in CD-1 mice indicated that **Solagé®** Solution applied topically at daily doses up to 80 and 0.4 mg/kg (240 and 1.2 mg/m^2) of mequinol and tretinoin, respectively, representing approximately 5 times the maximum possible systemic human exposure was not carcinogenic, in a photocarcinogenicity study utilizing Crl:Skh-1(hr/hr BR) hairless albino mice, median time to onset of tumors decreased. Also, the number of tumors increased in all dose groups administered 1.4, 4.3 or 14 µl of **Solagé®** Solution/cm^2 of skin (24 and 0.12, 72 and 0.36, or 240 and 1.2 mg/m^2 of mequinol and tretinoin, respectively; 0.6, 1.9, or 6.5 times the daily human dose on a mg/m^2 basis) following chronic topical dosing with intercurrent exposure to ultraviolet radiation for up to 40 weeks. Similar animal studies have shown an increased tumorigenic risk with the use of retinoids when followed by ultraviolet radiation. Although the significance of these studies to human use is not clear, patients using this product should be advised to avoid or minimize exposure to either sunlight or artificial ultraviolet irradiation sources.

Mequinol was non-mutagenic in the Ames/Salmonella assay using strains TA98, TA100, TA1535, and TA1537, all of which are insensitive to mutagenic effects of structurally-related quinones. **Solagé®** Solution was non-genotoxic in an *in vivo* dermal micronucleus assay in rats, but exposure of bone marrow to drug was not demonstrated.

A dermal reproduction study with **Solagé®** Solution in Sprague-Dawley rats at a daily dose of 80 and 0.4 mg/kg (480 and 2.4 mg/m^2) of mequinol and tretinoin, respectively, approximately 11 times the corresponding maximum possible human exposure, assuming 100% bioavailability following topical application to 5% of the total body surface area, showed no impairment of fertility.

Pregnancy: Teratogenic effects: Pregnancy Category X. Although the magnitude of the potential for teratogenicity may not be well-defined, **Solagé®** Solution is labeled as an "X" because the potential risk of the use of this drug to treat this particular indication (solar lentigines) in a pregnant woman clearly outweighs any possible benefit (see **CONTRAINDICATIONS** section).

Nursing Mothers: It is not known to what extent mequinol and/or tretinoin is excreted in human milk. Because many drugs are excreted in human milk, caution should be exercised when **Solagé®** Solution is administered to a nursing woman.

Pediatric Use: The safety and effectiveness of this product have not been established in pediatric patients. **Solagé®** Solution should not be used on children.

Geriatric Use: Of the total number of patients in clinical studies of **Solagé®** Solution, approximately 43% were 65 and older, while approximately 8% were 75 and over. No overall differences in effectiveness or safety were observed between these patients and younger patients.

ADVERSE REACTIONS

In clinical trials, adverse reactions were primarily mild to moderate in intensity, occurring in 66% and 30% of patients, respectively. The majority of these events were limited to the skin and 64% had an onset of a skin related adverse reaction early in treatment (by week 8). The most frequent adverse reactions in patients treated with **Solagé®** Solution were erythema (49% of patients), burning, stinging, or tingling (26%), desquamation (14%), pruritus (12%), and skin irritation (5%).

Some patients experienced temporary hypopigmentation of treated lesions (5%) or of the skin surrounding treated lesions (7%). Ninety-four of 106 patients (89%) had resolution of hypopigmentation upon discontinuation of treatment to the lesion, and/or re-instruction on proper application to the lesion only. Another 8% (9/106) of patients with hypopigmentation events had resolution within 120 days after the end of treatment. Three of the 106 patients (2.8%) had persistence of hypopigmentation beyond 120 days. Approximately 6% of patients discontinued study participation with **Solagé®** Solution due to adverse reactions. These discontinuations were due primarily to skin redness (erythema) or related cutaneous adverse reactions. **Solagé®** Solution was generally well tolerated.

[See table below]

Adverse Events Occurring in >1% of the Population—All Studies

Body System	Solagé® Solution (mequinol 2%, tretinoin 0.01%)		Tretinoin, 0.01%		Mequinol, 2%		Vehicle	
Skin and Appendages	N	%	N	%	N	%	N	%
Erythema	549	44.6	261	55.3	13	5.1	8	4.6
Burning/Stinging/Tingling	270	21.9	173	36.7	26	10.2	20	11.4
Desquamation	155	12.6	93	19.7	7	2.8	2	1.1
Pruritus	135	11.0	66	14.0	12	4.7	3	1.7
Irritation Skin	90	7.3	25	5.3	1	0.4	1	0.6
Halo Hypopigmentation	76	6.2	16	3.4	2	0.8	2	1.1
Hypopigmentation	50	4.1	8	1.7	2	0.8	0	0.0
Skin Dry	38	3.1	18	3.8	3	1.2	1	0.6
Rash	31	2.5	21	4.4	0	0.0	1	0.6
Crusting	30	2.4	18	3.8	0	0.0	1	0.6
Rash Vesicular Bullae	18	2.1	8	1.7	0	0.0	0	0.0
Dermatitis	25	2.0	0	0.0	0	0.0	0	0.0

OVERDOSAGE

If **Solagé®** Solution is applied excessively, no more rapid or better results will be obtained and marked redness, peeling, discomfort, or hypopigmentation may occur. Oral ingestion of the drug may lead to the same adverse effects as those associated with excessive oral intake of vitamin A (hypervitaminosis A). If oral ingestion occurs, the patient should be monitored, and appropriate supportive measures should be administered as necessary. The maximal no-effect level for oral administration of **Solagé®** Solution in rats was 5.0 mL/kg (30 mg/m^2). Clinical signs observed were attributed to the high alcohol content (77%) of the drug formulation.

DOSAGE AND ADMINISTRATION

Patients require detailed instruction to obtain maximal benefits and to understand all the precautions necessary to use this product with greatest safety. The physician should review the Patient Medication Guide.

Apply **Solagé®** Solution to the solar lentigines using the applicator tip while avoiding application to the surrounding skin. Use twice daily, morning and evening at least 8 hours apart, or as directed by a physician. Patients should not shower or bathe the treatment areas for at least 6 hours after application of **Solagé®** Solution. Special caution should be taken when applying **Solagé®** Solution to avoid the eyes, mouth, paranasal creases, and mucous membranes.

Application of **Solagé®** Solution may cause transitory stinging, burning or irritation.

Improvement continues gradually through the course of therapy and should be apparent by 24 weeks. Patients should avoid exposure to sunlight (including sunlamps) or wear protective clothing while using **Solagé®** Solution. Data are not available to establish how or whether **Solagé®** Solution is degraded (either by sunlight or by normal interior lighting) following application to the skin.

With discontinuation of **Solagé®** Solution therapy, a majority of patients will experience some repigmentation over time of their lesions.

Applications of larger amounts of medication or more frequently than recommended will not lead to more rapid or better results, and marked redness, peeling, irritation, or hypopigmentation (abnormal lightening) of the skin may occur.

Patients treated with **Solagé®** Solution may use cosmetics but should wait 30 minutes before applying.

CLINICAL STUDIES

Two adequate and well-controlled trials evaluated changes in treated hyperpigmented lesions on the face, forearms/back of hands in 421 patients treated with **Solagé®** Topical Solution, 422 patients treated with tretinoin topical solution, 209 patients treated with mequinol topical solution and 107 patients treated with vehicle for up to 24 weeks. In these studies, patients were to avoid sun exposure and use protective clothing, and use of suncreens was prohibited. Patients were allowed to apply Moisturel® Lotion 30 minutes after application of **Solagé®** Solution. Physicians assessed the extent of improvement or worsening of all the treated lesions from the baseline condition on a 7 point scale. The results of these evaluations are shown below.

	Face		Forearms/Back of Hands	
	Solagé Solution	Vehicle	Solagé Solution	Vehicle
Moderate Improvement or greater[1]	57%	15%	54%	14%
Slight Improvement	28%	36%	26%	33%
No Change[2]	15%	49%	20%	53%

[1] Includes the following grades: Moderate Improvement, Marked Improvement, Almost Clear, Completely Clear. Moderate Improvement or greater was considered clinically meaningful.

[2] Includes the following grades: No Change, Worse (less than 1% of patients treated with **Solagé®** Solution were rated as worse).

Improvement (lightening) of the solar lentigines occurred gradually over time during the 24 week treatment period. At 24 weeks of treatment, 57% and 54% of patients experienced moderate improvement or greater, and 3% and 1% of patients were completely clear of all treated lesions for the face and forearms/back of hands, respectively. It should be noted that approximately 9% of patients, from both treatment areas in these studies, with moderate improvement or greater also experienced hypopigmentation of the skin surrounding at least one treated lesion. There are no vehicle-controlled effectiveness data on the course of lesions treated beyond 24 weeks.

After 24 weeks of treatment, for the forearm/back of hands treatment site, the percentage of patients treated with tretinoin topical solution with moderate improvement or greater, slight improvement, or no change, were 38%, 37%, and 26%, respectively, and for mequinol topical solution were 24%, 40%, and 36%, respectively. For the face treatment site, the percentage of patients treated with tretinoin topical solution with moderate improvement or greater, slight improvement, or no change, were 46%, 33%, and 21%, repectively, and for mequinol topical solution were 33%, 30%, and 37% respectively.

The duration of effect was investigated during a period of up to 24 weeks following the discontinuation of treatment. Results from these studies showed that patients may maintain the level of clinical improvement of their treated lesions from the end of treatment through the 24 week follow-up period. However, some degree of repigmentation of treated lesions was observed over time, demonstrating reversibility of the depigmenting action of **Solagé®** Solution.

In the clinical studies, some patients experienced temporary hypopigmentation of treated lesions (5%) or of the skin surrounding treated lesions (7%). Hypopigmentation of the skin surrounding treated lesions occurs even in the setting of proper application of the drug within the lesion border. The majority (94/106—89%) resolved upon discontinuation of treatment to the lesion, and/or re-instruction on proper application to the lesion only. Another 8% (9/106) of patients with hypopigmentation events had resolution within 120 days after the end of treatment.

Three of the 106 patients (2.8%) had persistence of hypopigmentation beyond 120 days. This further demonstrates the reversibility of the depigmenting action of **Solagé®** Solution.

Over 150 patients used **Solagé®** Solution twice daily for 52 weeks in an open label clinical study. The safety profile for **Solagé®** Solution in this long-term study was similar to that seen in the 24 week studies although burning/stinging/tingling, desquamation, pruritis, and irritation of the skin occurred at lower rates and halo hypopigmentation and hypopigmentation occurred at a slightly greater rate.

Over 90 patients used **Solagé®** Solution twice daily and a concomitant sunscreen (PreSun® 29) daily for up to 24 weeks in an open label clinical study. The safety profile for **Solagé®** Solution in this study was similar to that seen in studies which prohibited sunscreen use although desquamation, pruritis, and halo hypopigmentation occurred at slightly lower rates.

The clinical studies of **Solagé®** Solution included 1794 individuals of Skin Type I-V, 94.5% of whom were Caucasian. The trials also included 5% of individuals who were Asian/Pacific Islander–1.2%, African-American–0.8%, and Hispanic/Latino–3.5%. Safety in Asian/Pacific Islander, African-American, and Hispanic/Latino individuals has not been adequately established. Safety and effectiveness of **Solagé®** Solution in individuals with Skin Type VI (never burns from the sun, deeply pigmented skin) or women of childbearing potential have not been established (see CONTRAINDICATIONS).

HOW SUPPLIED

Solagé® (mequinol 2%, tretinoin 0.01%) Topical Solution is available in 30 mL plastic bottles with an applicator. **NDC** 0299-5970-30

STORAGE: The bottle should be protected from light by continuing to store in the carton after opening. Store at controlled room temperature, 20°–25° C (68°–77° F).

Note: FLAMMABLE. Keep away from heat and open flame.

Marketed by:
GALDERMA LABORATORIES, L.P.
Fort Worth, Texas 76177 USA
Manufactured by:
Bristol-Myers Squibb, Buffalo, NY 14213 USA
P50488-0 Revised August 2002

Solagé® Topical Solution

(mequinol 2%, tretinoin 0.01%)
Medication Guide
INFORMATION FOR PATIENTS

Please read this Medication Guide carefully before you start to use your medicine. If you have any questions, or are not sure about any of the information on Solagé® Solution, ask your doctor.

The active ingredients in **Solagé®** Solution (pronounced sola-JAY) are mequinol and tretinoin.

Solagé® Solution also contains ethlyl alcohol (77.8% v/v), polyethylene glycol 400, butylated hydroxytoluene, ascorbic acid, citric acid, ascorbyl palmitate, edetate disodium, and purified water.

What is the Most Important Information about Solagé® Solution?

Solagé® Solution is a prescription medication. It should only be used under supervision of your doctor as part of a sun avoidance program. This program should also include avoiding exposure to artificial sunlight (sunlamps) and avoidance of direct sunlight by wearing protective clothing.

Solagé® Solution does not permanently "cure" solar lentigines, also known as brown "age" or "liver" spots. In clinical trials, most patients experienced some degree of darkening of their spots over time.

Follow the instructions for application of **Solagé®** Solution carefully. Avoid getting the medication on your normal-toned skin, in your eyes, nose, or mouth.

Solagé® Solution can cause the side effect, halo hypopigmentation, which is lightening of the skin surrounding the spot being treated, within the 6 month treatment period.

Warning: Solagé® Solution should not be used if you are pregnant, attempting to become pregnant, or at a high risk of pregnancy. Consult your doctor for adequate birth control measures if you are a female of child-bearing potential. Avoid sunlight and any other medicines that may increase your sensitivity to sunlight (see below).

There is very limited information on the safety of **Solagé®** Solution in people with moderately or darkly pigmented skin.

What Can I Expect From Solagé® Solution?

Solagé® Solution is a prescription medication used for the topical treatment of solar lentigines, also known as brown "age" or "liver" spots.

Studies show that after 24 weeks, for lesions of the face, 57% of patients using **Solagé®** Solution had moderate improvement or greater, with 3% experiencing complete clearing of all treated lesions. Another 28% of patients had slight improvement and 15% had no change or worse (less than 1% of patients had worsening of their lesions). After 24 weeks for lesions of the forearms/back of hands, 54% of patients using **Solagé®** Solution experienced moderate improvement or greater, with 1% experiencing complete clearing of all treated lesions. Another 26% had slight improvement and 20% had no change or worse (less than 1% of patients had worsening of their lesions). Approximately 9% of patients who had success in the treatment of their age spots also experienced the side effect, halo hypopigmentation, which is lightening of skin surrounding the treated spot. Evidence has not been established concerning the effectiveness of **Solagé®** Solution in the treatment of other hyperpigmented conditions of the skin.

Improvement in the color of the treated age spots occurs gradually. Don't be discouraged if you see no immediate improvement. Be patient. If **Solagé®** Solution is going to have a beneficial effect for you, it may take up to six months of treatment before full beneficial effects are seen. After stopping treatment with **Solagé®** Solution, the age spots may darken again over time.

The effectiveness of **Solagé®** Solution in treating solar lentigines, also known as brown "age" or "liver" spots, beyond 6 months has not been established.

Who should not use Solagé® Solution?

Solagé® Solution should not be used if you are pregnant, attempting to become pregnant, or at a high risk of pregnancy. Consult your doctor for adequate birth control measures if you are a female of child-bearing potential.

It is not known if **Solagé®** Solution is passed to infants through breast milk. Do not use **Solagé®** Solution if you intend to breast feed, unless advised otherwise by your doctor.

Solagé® Solutuion should not be used on children.

Do not use **Solagé®** Solution if you are allergic to any ingredients in this medicine. If you are allergic to any of the ingredients, tell your doctor.

If you are sunburned, do not use **Solagé®** Solution until you have fully recovered.

Do not use **Solagé®** Solution if you have a skin condition called eczema or other inflamed or irritated chronic skin conditions.

Do not use **Solagé®** Solution if you are inherently sensitive to sunlight or taking other drugs that increase your sensitivity to sunlight. You should tell your physician if you are also using other medicines that increase sensitivity to sunlight. These medications include but are not limited to: thiazides (used to treat high blood pressure), tetracyclines, fluroquinolones or sulfonamides (used to treat infection), and phenothiazines (used to treat serious emotional problems).

If you are taking any prescription medicines, non-prescription medicines or using any facial or skin creams, check with your physician to make sure they do not interact with **Solagé®** Solution.

There is very limited information on the safety of **Solagé®** Solution in people with moderately or darkly pigmented skin. If you, or a family member, have a history of vitiligo (a skin condition consisting of white patches on various parts of the body), consult your doctor before using **Solagé®** Solution.

How should I use Solagé® Solution?

Solagé® Solution is to be used twice daily, at least eight hours apart, or as directed by your doctor. It is a drug for topical use only and is not a cosmetic preparation. Do not use **Solagé®** Solution around your eyes, lips, creases of the nose or mucous membranes. **Solagé®** Solution may cause severe redness, itching, burning, stinging, and peeling if applied to these areas. If the product gets in your eyes, rinse thoroughly with water and contact your doctor.

Apply **Solagé®** Solution to the age spots using the applicator provided with the medication. Avoid application of **Solagé®** Solution to the surrounding, normally colored skin. Only enough **Solagé®** Solution should be applied to make the lesion appear moist – running or dripping of the medication should be avoided. Applications of larger amounts of **Solagé®** Solution, or more frequent applications than recommended, will not lead to more rapid or better results, and marked redness, peeling, irritation or hypopigmentation may occur. You should not shower or bathe the treatment areas for at least 6 hours after application of **Solagé®** Solution.

Stop treating any age spots that become the same color or lighter than your normally colored skin. If the skin surrounding an age spot becomes lighter than your normally colored skin, stop treating that age spot and contact your doctor regarding continued use of **Solagé®** Solution to that age spot.

If you forget or miss a dose of **Solagé®** Solution, do not try to "make it up." Return to your normal application schedule as soon as you can.

If sensitivity or increased irritation occurs, stop use of **Solagé®** Solution and contact your doctor.

If the age spots become darker with treatment, stop use of **Solagé®** Solution and contact your doctor.

Do not use **Solagé®** Solution for any condition other than for which it was prescribed by your doctor. Do not give it to other persons or allow other persons to use it.

You may use cosmetics after applying **Solagé®** Solution but you should wait 30 minutes before applying.

What should I avoid while using Solagé® Solution?

Solagé® Solution increases your sensitivity to sunlight. Sun exposure (natural or artificial) to areas of the skin treated with **Solagé®** Solution should be avoided. Wear protective clothing if exposure to the sun cannot be avoided. Patients using **Solagé®** Solution should practice a comprehensive sun protection program. Following discontinuation of **Solagé®** Solution, patients should continue to practice a comprehensive sun protection program.

Solagé® Solution should be used with caution if you are also using other topical products with a strong drying effect on the skin, products with high concentrations of alcohol, astringents, spices or lime, medicated soaps, or shampoos, permanent wave solutions, electrolysis, hair removal products or waxes, or other preparations or processes that may dry or irritate your skin. If you are using any of these types of products, tell your doctor before using **Solagé®** Solution.

What are the possible or reasonably likely side effects of Solagé® Solution?

Solagé® Solution may cause redness, stinging, burning or irritation on areas of the skin where it is applied. It may also cause peeling and itching of the areas where applied. Excessive or prolonged application of **Solagé®** Solution may cause the treated age spots or surrounding skin to become temporarily lighter than your normally colored skin. Discontinue application of **Solagé®** Solution to any such affected areas.

How can I get additional information?

This leaflet summarizes the most important information about **Solagé®** Solution. If you would like more information, talk to your doctor.

How should Solagé® Solution be stored?

Solagé® Solution should be protected from light by returning the bottle to the carton after each use. Store at room temperature, 20° C–25° C (68° F–77° F).

Solagé® Solution is FLAMMABLE. Keep away from heat or open flame.

Keep this and all medication out of the reach of children.

Marketed by:
GALDERMA LABORATORIES, L.P.
Fort Worth, Texas 76177 USA
Manufactured by:
Bristol-Myers Squibb
Buffalo, NY 14213 USA
www.solage.com
Revised August 2002
P50488-0

Continued on next page

TRI-LUMA® Cream ℞
[trī-lew-mă]
(fluocinolone acetonide 0.01%, hydroquinone 4%, tretinoin 0.05%)
For External Use Only
Not for Ophthalmic Use
Rx only

DESCRIPTION

TRI-LUMA® Cream (fluocinolone acetonide 0.01%, hydroquinone 4%, tretinoin 0.05%) contains fluocinolone acetonide, USP, hydroquinone, USP, and tretinoin, USP, in a hydrophilic cream base for topical application.
Fluocinolone acetonide is a synthetic fluorinated corticosteroid for topical dermatological use and is classified therapeutically as an anti-inflammatory. It is a white crystalline powder that is odorless and stable in light.
The chemical name for fluocinolone acetonide is: (6α,11β,16α)-6,9-difluoro-11,21-dihydroxy-16,17-[(1-methylethylidene)bis(oxy)]-pregna-1,-4-diene-3,20-dione.
The molecular formula is $C_{24}H_{30}F_2O_6$ and molecular weight is 452.50.
Fluocinolone acetonide has the following structural formula:

Hydroquinone is classified therapeutically as a depigmenting agent. It is prepared from the reduction of p-benzoquinone with sodium bisulfite. It occurs as fine white needles that darken on exposure to air.
The chemical name for hydroquinone is: 1,4-benzenediol.
The molecular formula is $C_6H_6O_2$ and molecular weight is 110.11.
Hydroquinone has the following structural formula:

Tretinoin is all-trans-retinoic acid formed from the oxidation of the aldehyde group of retinene to a carboxyl group. It occurs as yellow to light-orange crystals or crystalline powder with a characteristic odor of ensilage. It is highly reactive to light and moisture. Tretinoin is classified therapeutically as a keratolytic.
The chemical name for tretinoin is: ((all-E)-3,7-dimethyl-9-(2,6,6-trimethyl-1-cyclohexen-1-yl)-2,4,6,8-nonatetraenoic acid.
The molecular formula is $C_{20}H_{28}O_2$ and molecular weight is 300.44.
Tretinoin has the following structural formula:

Each gram of TRI-LUMA® Cream contains Active: fluocinolone acetonide 0.01% (0.1 mg), hydroquinone 4% (40 mg), and tretinoin 0.05% (0.5 mg). **Inactive:** butylated hydroxytoluene, cetyl alcohol, citric acid, glycerin, glyceryl stearate, magnesium aluminum silicate, methyl gluceth-10, methylparaben, PEG-100 stearate, propylparaben, purified water, sodium metabisulfite, stearic acid, and stearyl alcohol.

CLINICAL PHARMACOLOGY

One of the components in TRI-LUMA® Cream, hydroquinone, is a depigmenting agent, and may interrupt one or more steps in the tyrosine-tyrosinase pathway of melanin synthesis. However, the mechanism of action of the active ingredients in TRI-LUMA® Cream in the treatment of melasma is unknown.
Pharmacokinetics: Percutaneous absorption of unchanged tretinoin, hydroquinone and fluocinolone acetonide into the systemic circulation of two groups of healthy volunteers (Total n=59) was found to be minimal following 8 weeks of daily application of 1g (Group I, n=45) or 6g (Group II, n=14) of TRI-LUMA® Cream.
For tretinoin quantifiable plasma concentrations were obtained in 57.78% (26 out of 45) of Group I and 57.14% (8 out of 14) of Group II subjects. The exposure to tretinoin as reflected by the C_{max} values ranged from 2.01 to 5.34 ng/mL (Group I) and 2.0 to 4.99 ng/mL (Group II). Thus, daily application of TRI-LUMA® Cream resulted in a minimal increase of normal endogenous levels of tretinoin. The circulating tretinoin levels represent only a portion of total tretinoin-associated retinoids, which would include metabolites of tretinoin and that sequestered into peripheral tissues.
For hydroquinone quantifiable plasma concentrations were obtained in 18% (8 out of 44) Group I subjects. The exposure to hydroquinone as reflected by the C_{max} values ranged from 25.55 to 86.52 ng/mL. All Group II subjects (6g dose) had post-dose plasma hydroquinone concentrations below the quantitation limit. For fluocinolone acetonide, Groups I and II subjects had all post-dose plasma concentrations below quantitation limit.

PRIMARY EFFICACY ANALYSIS:

Investigators' Assessment of Treatment Success* At the End of 8 Weeks of Treatment

		TRI-LUMA®	HQ+RA	FA+RA	FA+HQ
Study No. 1	Number of Patients	85	83	85	85
	No. of Successes	32	12	0	3
	Proportion of Successes	38%	15%	0	4%
	p-value		<0.001	<0.001	<0.001
Study No. 2	Number of Patients	76	75	76	76
	No. of Successes	10	3	3	1
	Proportion of Successes	13%	4%	4%	1%
	p-value		0.045	0.042	0.005

*Treatment success was defined as melasma severity score of zero (melasma lesions cleared of hyperpigmentation).
p-value is from Cochran-Mantel-Haenszel chi-square statistics controlling for pooled investigator and comparing TRI-LUMA® Cream to the other treatment groups.

Investigators' Assessment of Change in Melasma Severity from Baseline to Day 56 of Treatment (combined results from studies 1 and 2)

			Number (%) of Patients at Day 56[a]				
	Baseline		Cleared[b]	Mild[b]	Moderate[b]	Severe[b]	Missing[b]
	Severity Rating	N	N (%)	N (%)	N (%)	N (%)	N (%)
TRI-LUMA® Cream N=161	Moderate	124	36 (29)	63 (51)	18 (15)	0 (0)	7 (6%)
	Severe	37	6 (16)	19 (51)	9 (24)	2 (5)	1 (3%)

[a]Assessment based on patients with severity scores at Day 56. Percentages are based on the total number in the treatment group population.
[b]Does not include patients who cleared before Day 56 or were missing from the Day 56 assessment.

Clinical Studies: Two adequate and well-controlled efficacy and safety studies were conducted in 641 patients between the ages of 21 to 75 years, having skin phototypes I-IV and moderate to severe melasma of the face. TRI-LUMA® Cream was compared with 3 possible combinations of 2 of the 3 active ingredients [(1) hydroquinone 4% (HQ) + tretinoin 0.05% (RA); (2) fluocinolone acetonide 0.01% (FA) + tretinoin 0.05% (RA); (3) fluocinolone acetonide 0.01% (FA) + hydroquinone 4% (HQ)], contained in the same vehicle as TRI-LUMA® Cream. Patients were instructed to apply their study medication each night, after washing their face with a mild soapless cleanser, for 8 weeks. Instructions were given to apply a thin layer of study medication to the hyperpigmented lesion, making sure to cover the entire lesion including the outside borders extending to the normal pigmented skin. Patients were provided a mild moisturizer for use as needed. A sunscreen with SPF 30 was also provided with instructions for daily use. Protective clothing and avoidance of sunlight exposure to the face was recommended.
Patients were evaluated for melasma severity at Baseline and at Weeks 1, 2, 4, and 8 of treatment. Primary efficacy was based on the proportion of patients who had an investigators' assessment of treatment success, defined as the clearing of melasma at the end of the eight-week treatment period. The majority of patients enrolled in the two studies were white (approximately 66%) and female (approximately 98%). TRI-LUMA® Cream was demonstrated to be significantly more effective than any of the other combinations of the active ingredients.
[See first table above]
In the Investigators' assessment of melasma severity at Day 56 of treatment, the following table shows the clinical improvement profile for all patients treated with TRI-LUMA® Cream based on severity of their melasma at the start of treatment.
[See second table above]
Assessment Scale: Cleared (melasma lesions approximately equivalent to surrounding normal skin or with minimal residual hyperpigmentation); Mild (slightly darker than the surrounding normal skin); Moderate (moderately darker than the surrounding normal skin); Severe (markedly darker than the surrounding normal skin).
Patients experienced improvement of their melasma with the use of TRI-LUMA® Cream as early as 4 weeks. Among the 7 patients that cleared at the end of 4 weeks of treatment with TRI-LUMA® Cream at which time treatment was stopped, 3 patients maintained remission while 4 patients had relapse at the final 8th week evaluation point.
After 8 weeks of treatment with the study drug, patients entered into an open-label long-term safety study in which TRI-LUMA® CREAM was given on an as-needed basis for the treatment of melasma. The objective was to provide evidence of local and systemic safety with cumulative use of TRI-LUMA® Cream for longer than 6 months, up to one year.
Patients were instructed to apply TRI-LUMA® Cream once daily at nighttime after washing their face with a mild soapless cleanser, also provided a mild moisturizer for use as needed and a sunscreen with SPF 30 for daily use, in combination with the use of protective clothing and avoidance of sunlight exposure to the face. Patients were treated daily until melasma is resolved, and then retreated when melasma recurred. The majority of patients used TRI-LUMA® for no more than two courses of treatment and these patients experienced longer remissions. Both the duration of treatment and interval of time between treatment courses decreased with increasing number of treatment courses. Additionally, 24 patients (approximately 8%) cleared of melasma without re-occurrence, for a period of one year.

INDICATIONS AND USAGE

TRI-LUMA® Cream is indicated for the short-term intermittent treatment of moderate to severe melasma of the face, in the presence of measures for sun avoidance, including the use of sunscreens.
The following are important statements relating to the indication and usage of TRI-LUMA® Cream:

- TRI-LUMA® Cream, a combination drug product containing corticosteroid, retinoid, and bleaching agent, was proven safe for the intermittent treatment of melasma, with cumulative treatment time of at least 180 days. Because melasma usually recurs upon discontinuation of TRI-LUMA® Cream, patients can be re-treated with TRI-LUMA® until melasma is resolved. Patients need to avoid sunlight exposure, use sunscreen with appropriate SPF, wear protective clothing, and change to non-hormonal forms of birth control, if hormonal methods are used.
- In clinical trials used to support the use of TRI-LUMA® Cream in the treatment of melasma, patients were instructed to avoid sunlight exposure to the face, wear protective clothing and use a sunscreen with SPF 30 each day. They were to apply the study medication each night, after washing their face with a mild soapless cleanser.
- The safety and efficacy of TRI-LUMA® Cream in patients of skin types V and VI have not been studied. Excessive bleaching resulting in undesirable cosmetic effect in patients with darker skin cannot be excluded.
- The safety and efficacy of TRI-LUMA® Cream in the treatment of hyperpigmentation conditions other than melasma of the face have not been studied.
- Because pregnant and lactating women were excluded from, and women of child-bearing potential had to use birth control measures in the clinical trials, the safety and efficacy of TRI-LUMA® Cream in pregnant women and nursing mothers have not been established (See PRECAUTIONS, Pregnancy).

CONTRAINDICATIONS

TRI-LUMA® Cream is contraindicated in individuals with a history of hypersensitivity, allergy, or intolerance to this product or any of its components.

WARNINGS

TRI-LUMA® Cream contains sodium metabisulfite, a sulfite that may cause allergic-type reactions including anaphylactic symptoms and life-threatening asthmatic episodes in susceptible people.
The overall prevalence of sulfite sensitivity in the general population is unknown and probably low. Sulfite sensitivity is seen more frequently in asthmatic than in non-asthmatic people.

TRI-LUMA® Cream contains hydroquinone, which may produce exogenous ochronosis, a gradual blue-black darkening of the skin, whose occurrence should prompt discontinuation of therapy. The majority of patients developing this condition are Black, but it may also occur in Caucasians and Hispanics.
Cutaneous hypersensitivity to the active ingredients of TRI-LUMA® Cream has been reported in the literature. In a patch test study to determine sensitization potential in 221 healthy volunteers, three volunteers developed sensitivity reactions to TRI-LUMA® Cream or its components.

PRECAUTIONS

General: TRI-LUMA® Cream contains hydroquinone and tretinoin that may cause mild to moderate irritation. Local irritation, such as skin reddening, peeling, mild burning sensation, dryness, and pruritus may be expected at the site of application. Transient skin reddening or mild burning sensation does not preclude treatment. If a reaction suggests hypersensitivity or chemical irritation, the use of the medication should be discontinued.
TRI-LUMA® Cream also contains the corticosteroid fluocinolone acetonide. Systemic absorption of topical corticosteroids can produce reversible hypothalamic-pituitary-adrenal (HPA) axis suppression with the potential for glucocorticosteroid insufficiency after withdrawal of treatment. Manifestations of Cushing's syndrome, hyperglycemia, and glucosuria can also be produced by systemic absorption of topical corticosteroid while on treatment. If HPA axis suppression is noted, the use of TRI-LUMA® Cream should be discontinued. Recovery of HPA axis function generally occurs upon discontinuation of topical corticosteroids.

Information for Patients: Exposure to sunlight, sunlamp, or ultraviolet light should be avoided. Patients who are consistently exposed to sunlight or skin irritants either through their work environment or habits should exercise particular caution. Sunscreen and protective covering (such as the use of a hat) over the treated areas should be used. Sunscreen use is an essential aspect of melasma therapy, as even minimal sunlight sustains melanocytic activity.
Weather extremes, such as heat or cold, may be irritating to patients treated with TRI-LUMA® Cream. Because of the drying effect of this medication, a moisturizer may be applied to the face in the morning after washing.
Application of TRI-LUMA® Cream should be kept away from the eyes, nose, or angles of the mouth, because the mucosa is much more sensitive than the skin to the irritant effect. If local irritation persists or becomes severe, application of the medication should be discontinued, and the health care provider consulted. Allergic contact dermatitis, blistering, crusting, and severe burning or swelling of the skin and irritation of the mucous membranes of the eyes, nose, and mouth require medical attention.
If the medication is applied excessively, marked redness, peeling, or discomfort may occur.
This medication is to be used as directed by the health care provider and should not be used for any disorder other than that for which it is prescribed.

Laboratory Tests: The following tests may be helpful in evaluating patients for HPA axis suppression:

ACTH or cosyntropin stimulation test
A.M. plasma cortisol test
Urinary free cortisol test

Drug Interactions: Patients should avoid medicated or abrasive soaps and cleansers, soaps and cosmetics with drying effects, products with high concentration of alcohol and astringent, and other irritants or keratolytic drugs while on TRI-LUMA® Cream treatment. Patients are cautioned on concomitant use of medications that are known to be photosensitizing.

Carcinogenesis, Mutagenesis, Impairment of Fertility: Long-term animal studies to determine the carcinogenic potential of TRI-LUMA® Cream have not been conducted.
Studies of hydroquinone in animals have demonstrated some evidence of carcinogenicity. The carcinogenic potential of hydroquinone in humans is unknown.
Studies in hairless albino mice suggest that concurrent exposure to tretinoin may enhance the tumorigenic potential of carcinogenic doses of UVB and UVA light from a solar simulator. This effect has been confirmed in a later study in pigmented mice, and dark pigmentation did not overcome the enhancement of photocarcinogenesis by 0.05% tretinoin. Although the significance of these studies to humans is not clear, patients should minimize exposure to sunlight or artificial ultraviolet irradiation sources.
Mutagenicity studies were not conducted with this combination of active ingredients. Published studies have demonstrated that hydroquinone is a mutagen and a clastogen. Treatment with hydroquinone has resulted in positive findings for genetic toxicity in the Ames assay in bacterial strains sensitive to oxidizing mutagens, in *in vitro* studies in mammalian cells, and in the *in vivo* mouse micronucleus assay. Tretinoin has been shown to be negative for mutagenesis in the Ames assay. Additional information regarding the genetic toxicity potential of tretinoin and of fluocinolone acetonide is not available.
A dermal reproductive fertility study was conducted in SD rats using a 10-fold dilution of the clinical formulation. No effect was seen on the traditional parameters used to assess fertility, although prolongation of estrus was observed in some females, and there was a trend towards an increase in pre-and post-implantation loss that was not statistically significant. No adequate study of fertility and early embryonic toxicity of the full-strength drug product has been performed. In a six-month study in minipigs, small testes and severe hypospermia were found when males were treated topically with the full strength drug product.

Summary of Most Common Treatment-Related Adverse Events (TRAE)[a] Study 29

Preferred Term	Number (%) of Patients — Treatment Group — TRI-LUMA® All Patients (N=569)	Patients with at least 180 Cumulative Days of TRI-LUMA® Treatment Days (N=314)
Total number of TRAE[a]	326 (57.29)	202 (64.33)
Application site erythema	166 (29.17)	105 (33.44)
Application site desquamation	145 (25.48)	91 (28.98)
Application site dryness	46 (8.08)	27 (8.60)
Application site burning	38 (6.68)	25 (7.96)
Application site inflammation	31 (5.45)	24 (7.64)
Application site reaction nos	31 (5.45)	17 (5.41)
Application site rash	30 (5.27)	18 (5.73)
Application site pruritus	24 (4.22)	18 (5.73)
Application site pigmentation changes	23 (4.04)	18 (5.73)

[a]Defined as "probably" or "possibly" related to study medication
Data source: Section 14.3, Tables 8.1.1, 8.1.2, and 8.1.3

Pregnancy: Teratogenic Effects: Pregnancy Category C: TRI-LUMA® Cream contains the teratogen, tretinoin, which may cause embryo-fetal death, altered fetal growth, congenital malformations, and potential neurologic deficits. It is difficult to interpret the animal studies on teratogenicity with TRI-LUMA® Cream, because the availability of the dermal applications in these studies cannot be assured, and comparison with clinical dosing is not possible. There are no adequate and well-controlled studies in pregnant women. TRI-LUMA® Cream should be used during pregnancy only if the potential benefit justifies the potential risk to the fetus.

Summary Statement on Teratogenic Risk
TRI-LUMA® Cream contains the teratogen, tretinoin, which may cause embryo-fetal death, altered fetal growth, congenital malformations, and potential neurologic deficits. However, human data have not confirmed an increased risk of these developmental abnormalities when tretinoin is administered by the topical route.

Clinical considerations relevant to actual or potential inadvertent exposure during pregnancy:
In clinical trials involving TRI-LUMA® Cream in the treatment of facial melasma, women of child-bearing potential initiated treatment only after having had a negative pregnancy test and used effective birth control measures during therapy. Thus, safety and efficacy of TRI-LUMA® Cream in pregnancy has not been established. In general, use of drugs should be reduced to a minimum in pregnancy. If a patient has been inadvertently exposed to TRI-LUMA® Cream in pregnancy, she should be counseled on the risk of teratogenesis due to this exposure. The risk of teratogenesis due to topical exposure to TRI-LUMA® Cream may be considered low. However, exposure during the period of organogenesis in the first trimester is theoretically more likely to produce adverse outcome than in later pregnancy.

The prescriber should have the following clinical considerations in making prescribing decisions:

- The potential developmental effects of tretinoin are serious but the risk from topical administration is small.
- Exposure during the period for organogenesis in the first trimester is theoretically more likely to produce adverse outcome than in later pregnancy.
- The risk to the mother for not treating melasma should be determined by the physician with the patient. Mild forms of melasma may not necessarily require drug treatment. TRI-LUMA® Cream is indicated for the treatment of moderate to severe melasma. Melasma may also be managed with other forms of therapy such as topical hydroquinone in the presence of sunlight avoidance, or stopping the use of hormonal birth control methods. If possible, delaying treatment with TRI-LUMA® Cream until after delivery should be considered.
- There are no adequate and well-controlled studies in pregnant women. TRI-LUMA® Cream should be used during pregnancy only if the potential benefit justifies the potential risk to the fetus.

Data Discussion: Tretinoin is considered to be highly teratogenic upon systemic administration. Animal reproductive studies are not available with topical hydroquinone. Corticosteroids have been shown to be teratogenic in laboratory animals when administered systemically at relatively low dosage levels. Some corticosteroids have been shown to be teratogenic after dermal application in laboratory animals.

1. Human Data.

- In clinical trials involving TRI-LUMA® Cream in the treatment of facial melasma, women of child-bearing potential initiated treatment only after having had a negative pregnancy test, and used effective birth control measures during therapy. However, 15 women became pregnant during treatment with TRI-LUMA® Cream. Of these pregnancies, 6 resulted in healthy babies, 6 outcomes still unknown, 2 were reported as miscarriages, and 1 case was lost to follow-up.
- Epidemiologic studies have not confirmed an increase in birth defects associated with the use of topical tretinoin. However, there may be limitations to the sensitivity of epidemiologic studies in the detection of certain forms of fetal injury, such as subtle neurologic or intelligence deficits.

2. Animal Data.

- In a dermal application study using TRI-LUMA® Cream in pregnant rabbits, there was an increase in the number of *in utero* deaths and a decrease in fetal weights in litters from dams treated topically with the drug product.
- In a dermal application study in pregnant rats treated with TRI-LUMA® Cream during organogenesis there was evidence of teratogenicity of the type expected with tretinoin. These morphological alterations included cleft palate, protruding tongue, open eyes, umbilical hernia, and retinal folding or dysplasia.
- In a dermal application study on the gestational and postnatal effects of a 10-fold dilution of TRI-LUMA® Cream in rats, an increase in the number of stillborn pups, lower pup body weights, and delay in preputial separation were observed. An increase in overall activity was seen in some treated litters at postnatal day 22 and in all treated litters at five weeks, a pattern consistent with effects previously noted in animals exposed *in utero* with retinoic acids. No adequate study of the late gestational and postnatal effects of the full-strength TRI-LUMA® Cream has been performed.
- It is difficult to interpret these animal studies on teratogenicity with TRI-LUMA® Cream, because the availability of the dermal applications in these studies could not be assured, and comparison with clinical dosing is not possible.

All pregnancies have a risk of birth defect, loss, or other adverse event regardless of drug exposure. Typically, estimates of increased fetal risk from drug exposure rely heavily on animal data. However, animal studies do not always predict effects in humans. Even if human data are available, such data may not be sufficient to determine whether there is an increased risk to the fetus. Drug effects on behavior, cognitive function, and fertility in the offspring are particularly difficult to assess.

Nursing Mothers: Corticosteroids, when systemically administered, appear in human milk. It is not known whether topical application of TRI-LUMA® Cream could result in sufficient systemic absorption to produce detectable quantities of fluocinolone acetonide, hydroquinone, or tretinoin in human milk. Because many drugs are secreted in human milk, caution should be exercised when TRI-LUMA® Cream is administered to a nursing woman. Care should be taken to avoid contact between the infant being nursed and TRI-LUMA® Cream.

Pediatric Use: Safety and effectiveness of TRI-LUMA® Cream in pediatric patients have not been established.

Geriatric Use: Clinical studies of TRI-LUMA® Cream did not include sufficient number of subjects aged 65 and over to

Continued on next page

Tri-Luma—Cont.

determine whether they respond differently from younger subjects. In general, dose selection for an elderly patient should be cautious, usually starting at the low end of the dosing range, reflecting the greater frequency of decreased hepatic, renal or cardiac function, and of concomitant disease or other drug therapy.

ADVERSE REACTIONS

In the controlled clinical trials, adverse events were monitored in the 161 patients who used TRI-LUMA® Cream once daily during an 8-week treatment period. There were 102 (63%) patients who experienced at least one treatment-related adverse event during these studies. In the long-term clinical study, from a total of 314 patients treated with TRI-LUMA® Cream for at least 180 cumulative days, there were 202 (64%) patients who experienced at least one treatment-related adverse event. No significant increase in severity or incidence of the adverse events was observed from long term use of TRI-LUMA® Cream compared with events reported during the 8-week controlled clinical studies. The most frequently reported adverse events that were observed from the controlled clinical trials and the long term safety were erythema, desquamation, and burning, at the site of application. The number and percentages of these events were markedly lower in the long-term study than in the controlled clinical studies. The great majority of these events were mild to moderate in severity.

Adverse events reported by at least 1% of patients and judged by the investigators to be reasonably related to treatment with TRI-LUMA® Cream from the controlled clinical studies and the long-term study are summarized (in decreasing order of frequency).

Incidence and Frequency of Treatment-related Adverse Events with TRI-LUMA Cream in at least 1% or more of Patients (N=161)

Adverse Event	Number (%) of Patients
Erythema	66 (41%)
Desquamation	61 (38%)
Burning	29 (18%)
Dryness	23 (14%)
Pruritus	18 (11%)
Acne	8 (5%)
Paresthesia	5 (3%)
Telangiectasia	5 (3%)
Hyperesthesia	3 (2%)
Pigmentary changes	3 (2%)
Irritation	3 (2%)
Papules	2 (1%)
Acne-like rash	1 (1%)
Rosacea	1 (1%)
Dry Mouth	1 (1%)
Rash	1 (1%)
Vesicles	1 (1%)

In an open-label long-term safety study, patients who have had cumulative treatment of melasma with TRI-LUMA® Cream for 6 months showed a similar pattern of adverse events as in the 8-week studies.

[See table at top of previous page]

The severity, incidence and type of adverse events experienced from 6 months cumulative use were not significantly different from the events reported for all patients.

The incidence of application site pigmentation changes that occurred in both the controlled and long-term safety studies included 11 occurrences of hypopigmentation and 18 occurrences of hyperpigmentation in 27 patients.

The following local adverse reactions have been reported infrequently with topical corticosteroids. They may occur more frequently with the use of occlusive dressings, especially with higher potency corticosteroids. These reactions are listed in an approximate decreasing order of occurrence: burning, itching, irritation, dryness, folliculitis, acneiform eruptions, hypopigmentation, perioral dermatitis, allergic contact dermatitis, secondary infection, skin atrophy, striae, and miliaria.

TRI-LUMA® Cream contains hydroquinone, which may produce exogenous ochronosis, a gradual blue-black darkening of the skin, whose occurrence should prompt discontinuation of therapy.

Cutaneous hypersensitivity to the active ingredients of TRI-LUMA® Cream has been reported in the literature. In a patch test study to determine sensitization potential in 221 healthy volunteers, three volunteers developed sensitivity reactions to TRI-LUMA® Cream or its components.

DOSAGE AND ADMINISTRATION

TRI-LUMA® Cream should be applied once daily at night. It should be applied at least 30 minutes before bedtime.

Gently wash the face and neck with a mild cleanser. Rinse and pat the skin dry. Apply a thin film of the cream to the hyperpigmented areas of melasma including about 1/2 inch of normal appearing skin surrounding each lesion. Rub lightly and uniformly into the skin. Do not use occlusive dressing.

During the day, use a sunscreen of SPF 30, and wear protective clothing. Avoid sunlight exposure. Patients may use moisturizers and/or cosmetics during the day.

Therapeutic effects may be observed as early as 4 weeks. Use TRI-LUMA® Cream daily for as long as the melasma lesions persist. Treatment should be discontinued when melasma is resolved. When melasma recurs, retreat with TRI-LUMA® Cream until the condition clears.

HOW SUPPLIED

TRI-LUMA® Cream is supplied in 30 g aluminum tubes, **NDC** 0299-5950-30.

Storage: Keep tightly closed. Store at controlled room temperature 68° to 77°F (20°-25°C).

Protect from freezing.

Marketed by:
GALDERMA LABORATORIES, L.P., Fort Worth, TX 76177 USA
GALDERMA is a registered trademark.
www.triluma.com
Manufactured by:
Hill Laboratories, Inc., Sanford, FL 32773 USA
20024-1203 Revised: December 2003

GATE Pharmaceuticals

Div. of TEVA Pharmaceuticals USA
650 CATHILL ROAD
SELLERSVILLE, PA 18960

Direct Inquiries to:
1090 Horsham Road
P. O. Box 1090
North Wales, PA 19454
(800) 292-4283

ADIPEX-P® ℂ ℞
(phentermine HCl 37.5 mg)

DESCRIPTION

Phentermine hydrochloride USP has the chemical name of α,α-Dimethylphenethylamine hydrochloride. The structural formula is as follows:

$$C_6H_5-CH_2C(CH_3)_2-NH_2 \cdot HCl$$

$C_{10}H_{15}N \cdot HCl$ M.W. 185.7

Phentermine hydrochloride is a white, odorless, hygroscopic, crystalline powder which is soluble in water and lower alcohols, slightly soluble in chloroform and insoluble in ether.

ADIPEX-P®, an anorectic agent for oral administration, is available as a capsule or tablet containing 37.5 mg of phentermine hydrochloride (equivalent to 30 mg of phentermine base).

ADIPEX-P® Capsules contain the inactive ingredients Corn Starch, Gelatin, Lactose Monohydrate, Magnesium Stearate, Titanium Dioxide, Black Iron Oxide, FD&C Blue #1, FD&C Red #40 and D&C Red #33.

ADIPEX-P® Tablets contain the inactive ingredients Corn Starch, Lactose (Anhydrous), Magnesium Stearate, Microcrystalline Cellulose, Pregelatinized Starch, Sucrose, and FD&C Blue #1.

CLINICAL PHARMACOLOGY

ADIPEX-P® is a sympathomimetic amine with pharmacologic activity similar to the prototype drugs of this class used in obesity, the amphetamines. Actions include central nervous system stimulation and elevation of blood pressure. Tachyphylaxis and tolerance have been demonstrated with all drugs of this class in which these phenomena have been looked for.

Drugs of this class used in obesity are commonly known as "anorectics" or "anorexigenics." It has not been established that the action of such drugs in treating obesity is primarily one of appetite suppression. Other central nervous system actions, or metabolic effects, may be involved, for example.

Adult obese subjects instructed in dietary management and treated with "anorectic" drugs lose more weight on the average than those treated with placebo and diet, as determined in relatively short-term clinical trials.

The magnitude of increased weight loss of drug-treated patients over placebo-treated patients is only a fraction of a pound a week. The rate of weight loss is greatest in the first weeks of therapy for both drug and placebo subjects and tends to decrease in succeeding weeks. The possible origins of the increased weight loss due to the various drug effects are not established. The amount of weight loss associated with the use of an "anorectic" drug varies from trial to trial, and the increased weight loss appears to be related in part to variables other than the drugs prescribed, such as the physician-investigator, the population treated and the diet prescribed. Studies do not permit conclusions as to the relative importance of the drug and non-drug factors on weight loss.

The natural history of obesity is measured in years, whereas the studies cited are restricted to a few weeks' duration; thus, the total impact of drug-induced weight loss over that of diet alone must be considered clinically limited.

INDICATIONS AND USAGE

ADIPEX-P® (phentermine hydrochloride) is indicated as a short-term (a few weeks) adjunct in a regimen of weight reduction based on exercise, behavioral modification and caloric restriction in the management of exogenous obesity for patients with an initial body mass index ≥ 30 kg/m^2, or ≥ 27 kg/m^2 in the presence of other risk factors (e.g., hypertension, diabetes, hyperlipidemia).

Below is a chart of Body Mass Index (BMI) based on various heights and weights.

BMI is calculated by taking the patient's weight, in kilograms (kg), divided by the patient's height, in meters (m), squared. Metric conversions are as follows: pounds ÷ 2.2 = kg; inches × 0.0254 = meters.

BODY MASS INDEX (BMI), kg/m^2

Weight (pounds)	Height (feet, inches)					
	5'0"	5'3"	5'6"	5'9"	6'0"	6'3"
140	27	25	23	21	19	18
150	29	27	24	22	20	19
160	31	28	26	24	22	20
170	33	30	28	25	23	21
180	35	32	29	27	25	23
190	37	34	31	28	26	24
200	39	36	32	30	27	25
210	41	37	34	31	29	26
220	43	39	36	33	30	28
230	45	41	37	34	31	29
240	47	43	39	36	33	30
250	49	44	40	37	34	31

The limited usefulness of agents of this class (see **CLINICAL PHARMACOLOGY**) should be measured against possible risk factors inherent in their use such as those described below.

CONTRAINDICATIONS

Advanced arteriosclerosis, cardiovascular disease, moderate to severe hypertension, hyperthyroidism, known hypersensitivity or idiosyncrasy to the sympathomimetic amines, glaucoma.

Agitated states.

Patients with a history of drug abuse.

During or within 14 days following the administration of monoamine oxidase inhibitors (hypertensive crises may result).

WARNINGS

ADIPEX-P® is indicated only as short-term monotherapy for the management of exogenous obesity. The safety and efficacy of combination therapy with phentermine and any other drug products for weight loss, including selective serotonin reuptake inhibitors (e.g., fluoxetine, sertraline, fluvoxamine, paroxetine), have not been established. Therefore, coadministration of these drug products for weight loss is not recommended.

Primary Pulmonary Hypertension (PPH)—a rare, frequently fatal disease of the lungs—has been reported to occur in patients receiving a combination of phentermine with fenfluramine or dexfenfluramine. The possibility of an association between PPH and the use of phentermine alone cannot be ruled out; there have been rare cases of PPH in patients who reportedly have taken phentermine alone. The initial symptom of PPH is usually dyspnea. Other initial symptoms include: angina pectoris, syncope or lower extremity edema. Patients should be advised to report immediately any deterioration in exercise tolerance. Treatment should be discontinued in patients who develop new, unexplained symptoms of dyspnea, angina pectoris, syncope or lower extremity edema.

Valvular Heart Disease: Serious regurgitant cardiac valvular disease, primarily affecting the mitral, aortic and/or tricuspid valves, has been reported in otherwise healthy persons who had taken a combination of phentermine with fenfluramine or dexfenfluramine for weight loss. The etiology of these valvulopathies has not been established and their course in individuals after the drugs are stopped is not known. The possibility of an association between valvular heart disease and the use of phentermine alone cannot be ruled out; there have been rare cases of valvular heart disease in patients who reportedly have taken phentermine alone.

Tolerance to the anorectic effect usually develops within a few weeks. When this occurs, the recommended dose should not be exceeded in an attempt to increase the effect; rather, the drug should be discontinued.

ADIPEX-P® may impair the ability of the patient to engage in potentially hazardous activities such as operating machinery or driving a motor vehicle; the patient should therefore be cautioned accordingly.

DRUG ABUSE AND DEPENDENCE

ADIPEX-P® is related chemically and pharmacologically to the amphetamines. Amphetamines and related stimulant drugs have been extensively abused, and the possibility of abuse of ADIPEX-P® should be kept in mind when evaluating the desirability of including a drug as part of a weight reduction program. Abuse of amphetamines and related drugs may be associated with intense psychological dependence and severe social dysfunction. There are reports of patients who have increased the dosage to many times that recommended. Abrupt cessation following prolonged high dosage administration results in extreme fatigue and mental depression; changes are also noted on the sleep EEG. Manifestations of chronic intoxication with anorectic drugs include severe dermatoses, marked insomnia, irritability, hyperactivity and personality changes. The most severe manifestation of chronic intoxications is psychosis, often clinically indistinguishable from schizophrenia.

Usage with Alcohol: Concomitant use of alcohol with ADIPEX-P® may result in an adverse drug interaction.

PRECAUTIONS

General

Caution is to be exercised in prescribing ADIPEX-P® (phentermine hydrochloride) for patients with even mild hypertension.

Insulin requirements in diabetes mellitus may be altered in association with the use of ADIPEX-P® and the concomitant dietary regimen.

ADIPEX-P® may decrease the hypotensive effect of guanethidine.

The least amount feasible should be prescribed or dispensed at one time in order to minimize the possibility of overdosage.

Carcinogenesis, Mutagenesis, Impairment of Fertility: Studies have not been performed with ADIPEX-P® (phentermine hydrochloride) to determine the potential for carcinogenesis, mutagenesis or impairment of fertility.

Pregnancy—Teratogenic Effects: Pregnancy Category C. Animal reproduction studies have not been conducted with ADIPEX-P®. It is also not known whether ADIPEX-P® can cause fetal harm when administered to a pregnant woman or can affect reproductive capacity. ADIPEX-P® should be given to a pregnant woman only if clearly needed.

Nursing Mothers

Because of the potential for serious adverse reactions in nursing infants, a decision should be made whether to discontinue nursing or to discontinue the drug, taking into account the importance of the drug to the mother.

Pediatric Use

Safety and effectiveness in pediatric patients have not been established.

ADVERSE REACTIONS

Cardiovascular: Primary pulmonary hypertension and/or regurgitant cardiac valvular disease (see **WARNINGS**), palpitation, tachycardia, elevation of blood pressure.

Central Nervous System:

Overstimulation, restlessness, dizziness, insomnia, euphoria, dysphoria, tremor, headache; rarely psychotic episodes at recommended doses.

Gastrointestinal: Dryness of the mouth, unpleasant taste, diarrhea, constipation, other gastrointestinal disturbances.

Allergic: Urticaria.

Endocrine: Impotence, changes in libido.

OVERDOSAGE

Manifestations of acute overdosage with phentermine include restlessness, tremor, hyperreflexia, rapid respiration, confusion, assaultiveness, hallucinations, panic states. Fatigue and depression usually follow the central stimulation. Cardiovascular effects include arrhythmia, hypertension or hypotension, and circulatory collapse. Gastrointestinal symptoms include nausea, vomiting, diarrhea and abdominal cramps. Fatal poisoning usually terminates in convulsions and coma.

Management of acute phentermine intoxication is largely symptomatic and includes lavage and sedation with a barbiturate. Experience with hemodialysis or peritoneal dialysis is inadequate to permit recommendations in this regard. Acidification of the urine increases phentermine excretion. Intravenous phentolamine (Regitine®, CIBA) has been suggested for possible acute, severe hypertension, if this complicates phentermine overdosage.

DOSAGE AND ADMINISTRATION

Exogenous Obesity: Dosage should be individualized to obtain an adequate response with the lowest effective dose. The usual adult dose is one capsule or tablet (37.5 mg) daily, administered before breakfast or 1–2 hours after breakfast. For tablets, the dosage may be adjusted to the patient's need. For some patients ½ tablet (18.75 mg) daily may be adequate, while in some cases it may be desirable to give ½ tablet (18.75 mg) two times a day.

Late evening medication should be avoided because of the possibility of resulting insomnia.

Phentermine is not recommended for use in patients sixteen (16) years of age and under.

HOW SUPPLIED

Available in tablets and capsules containing 37.5 mg phentermine hydrochloride (equivalent to 30 mg phentermine base). Each blue and white, oblong, scored tablet is debossed with "ADIPEX-P" and "9"-"9". The #3 capsule has an opaque white body and an opaque bright blue cap. Each capsule is imprinted with "ADIPEX-P" - "37.5" on the cap and two stripes on the body using dark blue ink.

Tablets are packaged in bottles of 30 (NDC 57844-009-56); 100 (NDC 57844-009-01); and 1000 (NDC 57844-009-10).

Capsules are packaged in bottles of 100 (NDC 57844-019-01).

Store at controlled room temperature 15°–30°C (59°–86°F) (see USP).

Dispense in a tight container as defined in the USP, with a child-resistant closure (as required).

Manufactured for:
GATE PHARMACEUTICALS
Div. of Teva Pharmaceuticals USA
Sellersville, PA 18960
Manufactured by:
TEVA PHARMACEUTICALS USA
Sellersville, PA 18960 Rev. R 11/2000
Visit GATE Pharmaceuticals at: www.gatepharma.com

LOFIBRA® ℞

[*lō′fĭ-bră*]
[Fenofibrate capsules (micronized)]
℞ Only

DESCRIPTION

LOFIBRA® [Fenofibrate capsules (micronized)] is a lipid regulating agent available as capsules for oral administration. The chemical name for fenofibrate is 2-[4-(4-chlorobenzoyl) phenoxy]-2-methyl-propanoic acid, 1-methylethyl ester with the following structural formula:

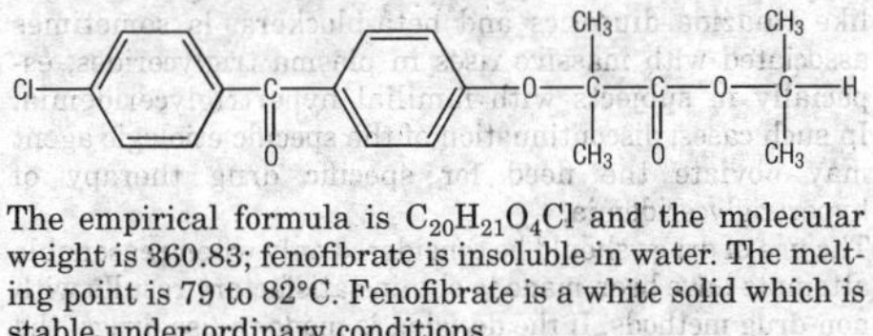

The empirical formula is $C_{20}H_{21}O_4Cl$ and the molecular weight is 360.83; fenofibrate is insoluble in water. The melting point is 79 to 82°C. Fenofibrate is a white solid which is stable under ordinary conditions.

Each 67 mg LOFIBRA® contains the following inactive ingredients: croscarmellose sodium, crospovidone, lactose monohydrate, magnesium stearate, povidone, pregelatinized starch, sodium lauryl sulfate, talc, D&C Red #28, FD&C Blue #1, FD&C Red #40, titanium dioxide and gelatin.

Each 134 mg LOFIBRA® contains the following inactive ingredients: croscarmellose sodium, crospovidone, lactose monohydrate, magnesium stearate, povidone, pregelatinized starch, sodium lauryl sulfate, talc, D&C Red #28, FD&C Blue #1, titanium dioxide and gelatin.

Each 200 mg LOFIBRA® contains the following inactive ingredients: croscarmellose sodium, crospovidone, lactose monohydrate, magnesium stearate, povidone, pregelatinized starch, sodium lauryl sulfate, talc, FD&C Red #40, D&C Red #28, FDA/E172 yellow iron oxide, titanium dioxide and gelatin.

CLINICAL PHARMACOLOGY

A variety of clinical studies have demonstrated that elevated levels of total cholesterol (total-C), low density lipoprotein cholesterol (LDL-C), and apolipoprotein B (apo B), an LDL membrane complex, are associated with human atherosclerosis. Similarly, decreased levels of high density lipoprotein cholesterol (HDL-C) and its transport complex, apolipoprotein A (apo AI and apo AII) are associated with the development of atherosclerosis. Epidemiologic investigations have established that cardiovascular morbidity and mortality vary directly with the level of total-C, LDL-C, and triglycerides, and inversely with the level of HDL-C. The independent effect of raising HDL-C or lowering triglycerides (TG) on the risk of cardiovascular morbidity and mortality has not been determined.

Fenofibric acid, the active metabolite of fenofibrate, produces reductions in total cholesterol, LDL cholesterol, apolipoprotein B, total triglycerides and triglyceride rich lipoprotein (VLDL) in treated patients. In addition, treatment with fenofibrate results in increases in high density lipoprotein (HDL) and apoproteins apo AI and apo AII.

The effects of fenofibric acid seen in clinical practice have been explained *in vivo* in transgenic mice and *in vitro* in human hepatocyte cultures by the activation of peroxisome proliferator activated receptor α (PPARα). Through this mechanism, fenofibrate increases lipolysis and elimination of triglyceride-rich particles from plasma by activating lipoprotein lipase and reducing production of apoproteins C-III (an inhibitor of lipoprotein lipase activity). The resulting fall in triglycerides produces an alteration in the size and composition of LDL from small, dense particles (which are thought to be atherogenic due to their susceptibility to oxidation), to large buoyant particles. These larger particles have a greater affinity for cholesterol receptors and are catabolized rapidly. Activation of PPARa also induces an increase in the synthesis of apoproteins A-I, A-II and HDL-cholesterol.

Fenofibrate also reduces serum uric acid levels in hyperuricemic and normal individuals by increasing the urinary excretion of uric acid.

Pharmacokinetics/Metabolism

Clinical experience has been obtained with two different formulations of fenofibrate: a "micronized" and "non-micronized" formulation, which have been demonstrated to be bioequivalent. Comparisons of blood levels following oral administration of both formulations in healthy volunteers demonstrate that a single capsule containing 67 mg of the "micronized" formulation is bioequivalent to 100 mg of the "non-micronized" formulation. Three capsules containing 67 mg LOFIBRA® are bioequivalent to a single 200 mg LOFIBRA® capsule.

Absorption

The absolute bioavailability of fenofibrate cannot be determined as the compound is virtually insoluble in aqueous media suitable for injection. However, fenofibrate is well absorbed from the gastrointestinal tract. Following oral administration in healthy volunteers, approximately 60% of a single dose of radiolabelled fenofibrate appeared in urine, primarily as fenofibric acid and its glucuronate conjugate, and 25% was excreted in the feces. Peak plasma levels of fenofibric acid occur within 6 to 8 hours after administration.

The absorption of fenofibrate is increased when administered with food. With micronized fenofibrate, the absorption is increased by approximately 35% under fed as compared to fasting conditions.

Distribution

In healthy volunteers, steady-state plasma levels of fenofibric acid were shown to be achieved within 5 days of dosing with single oral doses equivalent to 67 mg fenofibrate and did not demonstrate accumulation across time following multiple dose administration. Serum protein binding was approximately 99% in normal and hyperlipidemic subjects.

Metabolism

Following oral administration, fenofibrate is rapidly hydrolyzed by esterases to the active metabolite, fenofibric acid; no unchanged fenofibrate is detected in plasma.

Fenofibric acid is primarily conjugated with glucuronic acid and then excreted in urine. A small amount of fenofibric acid is reduced at the carbonyl moiety to a benzhydrol metabolite which is, in turn, conjugated with glucuronic acid and excreted in urine.

In vivo metabolism data indicate that neither fenofibrate nor fenofibric acid undergo oxidative metabolism (e.g., cytochrome P450) to a significant extent.

Excretion

After absorption, fenofibrate is mainly excreted in the urine in the form of metabolites, primarily fenofibric acid and fenofibric acid glucuronide. After administration of radiolabelled fenofibrate, approximately 60% of the dose appeared in the urine and 25% was excreted in the feces.

Fenofibric acid is eliminated with a half-life of 20 hours, allowing once daily administration in a clinical setting.

Special populations

Geriatrics

In elderly volunteers 77 to 87 years of age, the oral clearance of fenofibric acid following a single oral dose of fenofibrate was 1.2 L/h, which compares to 1.1 L/h in young adults. This indicates that a similar dosage regimen can be used in the elderly, without increasing accumulation of the drug or metabolites.

Pediatrics

Fenofibrate has not been investigated in adequate and well-controlled trials in pediatric patients.

Gender

No pharmacokinetic difference between males and females has been observed for fenofibrate.

Race

The influence of race on the pharmacokinetics of fenofibrate has not been studied, however fenofibrate is not metabolized by enzymes known for exhibiting inter-ethnic variability. Therefore, inter-ethnic pharmacokinetic differences are very unlikely.

Renal insufficiency

In a study in patients with severe renal impairment (creatinine clearance < 50 mL/min), the rate of clearance of fenofibric acid was greatly reduced, and the compound accumulated during chronic dosage. However, in patients having moderate renal impairment (creatinine clearance of 50 to 90 mL/min), the oral clearance and the oral volume of distribution of fenofibric acid are increased compared to healthy adults (2.1 L/h and 95 L versus 1.1 L/h and 30 L, respectively). Therefore, the dosage of fenofibrate should be minimized in patients who have severe renal impairment, while no modification of dosage is required in patients having moderate renal impairment.

Hepatic insufficiency

No pharmacokinetic studies have been conducted in patients having hepatic insufficiency.

Drug-drug interactions

In vitro studies using human liver microsomes indicate that fenofibrate and fenofibric acid are not inhibitors of cytochrome (CYP) P450 isoforms CYP3A4, CYP2D6, CYP2E1, or CYP1A2. They are weak inhibitors of CYP2C19 and CYP2A6, and mild-to-moderate inhibitors of CYP2C9 at therapeutic concentrations.

Potentiation of coumarin-type anti-coagulants has been observed with prolongation of the prothrombin time/INR.

Bile acid sequestrants have been shown to bind other drugs given concurrently. Therefore, fenofibrate should be taken at least 1 hour before or 4 to 6 hours after a bile acid binding resin to avoid impeding its absorption. (See **WARNINGS** and **PRECAUTIONS**).

Continued on next page

Lofibra—Cont.

Clinical Trials

Hypercholesterolemia (Heterozygous Familial and Nonfamilial) and Mixed Dyslipidemia (Fredrickson Types IIa and IIb)

The effects of fenofibrate at a dose equivalent to 200 mg fenofibrate per day were assessed from four randomized, placebo-controlled, double-blind, parallel-group studies including patients with the following mean baseline lipid values: total-C 306.9 mg/dL; LDL-C 213.8 mg/dL; HDL-C 52.3 mg/dL; and triglycerides 191.0 mg/dL. Fenofibrate therapy lowered LDL-C, total-C, and the LDL-C/HDL-C ratio. Fenofibrate therapy also lowered triglycerides and raised HDL-C (see Table 1).

[See table 1 below]

In a subset of the subjects, measurements of apo B were conducted. Fenofibrate treatment significantly reduced apo B from baseline to endpoint as compared with placebo (-25.1% vs. 2.4%, p<0.0001, n=213 and 143 respectively).

Hypertriglyceridemia (Fredrickson Type IV and V)

The effects of fenofibrate on serum triglycerides were studied in two randomized, double-blind, placebo-controlled clinical trials[1] of 147 hypertriglyceridemia patients (Fredrickson Type IV and V). Patients were treated for eight weeks under protocols that differed only in that one entered patients with baseline triglyceride (TG) levels of 500 to 1500 mg/dL, and the other TG levels of 350 to 500 mg/dL. In patients with hypertriglyceridemia and normal cholesterolemia with or without hyperchylomicronemia (Type IV/V hyperlipidemia), treatment with fenofibrate at dosages equivalent to 200 mg fenofibrate per day decreased primarily very low density lipoprotine (VLDL) triglycerides and VLDL cholesterol. Treatment of patients with type IV hyperlipoproteinemia and elevated triglycerides often results in an increase of low density lipoprotein (LDL) cholesterol (see Table 2).

[See table 2 below]

The effect of fenofibrate on cardiovascular morbidity and mortality has not been determined.

INDICATIONS AND USAGE

Treatment of Hypercholesterolemia

Fenofibrate capsules (micronized) are indicated as adjunctive therapy to diet for the reduction of LDL-C, total-C, Triglycerides and apo B in adult patients with primary hypercholesterolemia or mixed dyslipidemia (Fredrickson Types IIa and IIb. Lipid-altering agents should be used in addition to a diet restricted in saturated fat and cholesterol when response to diet and non-pharmacological interventions alone has been inadequate (see National Cholesterol Education Program [NCEP] Treatment Guidelines, below).

Treatment of Hypertriglyceridemia

Fenofibrate capsules (micronized) are also indicated as adjunctive therapy to diet for treatment of adult patients with hypertriglyceridemia (Fredrickson Types IV and V hyperlipidemia). Improving glycemic control in diabetic patients showing fasting chylomicronemia will usually reduce fasting triglycerides and eliminate chylomicronemia thereby obviating the need for pharmacologic intervention.

Markedly elevated levels of serum triglycerides (e.g. > 2,000 mg/dL) may increase the risk of developing pancreatitis. The effect of fenofibrate therapy on reducing this risk has not been adequately studied.

Drug therapy is not indicated for patients with Type I hyperlipoproteinemia, who have elevations of chylomicrons and plasma triglycerides, but who have normal levels of very low density lipoprotein (VLDL). Inspection of plasma refrigerated for 14 hours is helpful in distinguishing Types I, IV and V hyperlipoproteinemia[2].

The initial treatment for dyslipidemia is dietary therapy specific for the type of lipoprotein abnormality. Excess body weight and excess alcoholic intake may be important factors in hypertriglyceridemia and should be addressed prior to any drug therapy. Physical exercise can be an important ancillary measure. Diseases contributory to hyperlipidemia, such as hypothyroidism or diabetes mellitus should be looked for and adequately treated. Estrogen therapy, like thiazide diuretics and beta-blockers, is sometimes associated with massive rises in plasma triglycerides, especially in subjects with familial hypertriglyceridemia. In such cases, discontinuation of the specific etiologic agent may obviate the need for specific drug therapy of hypertriglyceridemia.

The use of drugs should be considered only when reasonable attempts have been made to obtain satisfactory results with non-drug methods. If the decision is made to use drugs, the patient should be instructed that this does not reduce the importance of adhering to diet (See **WARNINGS** and **PRECAUTIONS**).

Fredrickson Classification of Hyperlipoproteinemias

Type	Lipoprotein Elevated	Lipid Elevation Major	Lipid Elevation Minor
I(rare)	Chylomicrons	TG	↑↔C
IIa	LDL	C	–
IIb	LDL, VLDL	C	TG
III (rare)	IDL	C, TG	–
IV	VLDL	TG	↑↔C
V(rare)	chylomicrons, VLDL	TG	↑↔

C = cholesterol
TG = triglycerides
LDL = low density lipoprotein
VLDL = very low density lipoprotein
IDL = intermediate density lipoprotein

The NCEP Treatment Guidelines

Definite Athero-sclerotic Disease[a]	Two or More Other Risk Factors[b]	LDL-Cholesterol mg/dL (mmol/L) Initiation Level	Goal
No	No	≥190 (≥4.9)	<160 (<4.1)
No	Yes	≥160 (≥4.1)	<130 (<3.4)
Yes	Yes or No	≥130[c] (≥3.4)	<100 (<2.6)

(a) Coronary heart disease or peripheral vascular disease (including symptomatic carotid artery disease).

(b) Other risk factors for coronary heart disease (CHD) include: age (males: ≥45 years; females: ≥55 years or premature menopause without estrogen replacement therapy); family history of premature CHD; current cigarette smoking; hypertension; confirmed HDL-C <35 mg/dL (<0.91 mmol/L); and diabetes mellitus. Subtract 1 risk factor if HDL-C is ≥60 mg/dL (≥1.6 mmol/L).

(c) In CHD patients with LDL-C levels 100 to 129 mg/dL, the physician should exercise clinical judgment in deciding whether to initiate drug treatment.

CONTRAINDICATIONS

LOFIBRA® is contraindicated in patients who exhibit hypersensitivity to fenofibrate.

LOFIBRA® is contraindicated in patients with hepatic or severe renal dysfunction, including primary biliary cirrhosis, and patients with unexplained persistent liver function abnormality.

LOFIBRA® is contraindicated in patients with preexisting gallbladder disease (see **WARNINGS**).

WARNINGS

Liver Function: LOFIBRA® at doses equivalent to 134 mg to 200 mg fenofibrate per day has been associated with increases in serum transaminases [AST (SGOT) or ALT (SGPT)]. In a pooled analysis of 10 placebo-controlled trials, increases to > 3 times the upper limit of normal occurred in 5.3% of patients taking fenofibrate versus 1.1% of patients treated with placebo.

When transaminase determinations were followed either after discontinuation of treatment or during continued treatment, a return to normal limits was usually observed. The incidence of increases in transaminase related to fenofibrate therapy appear to be dose related. In an 8-week dose-ranging study, the incidence of ALT or AST elevations to at least three times the upper limit of normal was 13% in patients receiving dosages equivalent to 134 mg to 200 mg fenofibrate per day and was 0% in those receiving dosages equivalent to 34 mg or 67 mg of fenofibrate per day or placebo. Hepatocellular, chronic active and cholestatic hepatitis associated with fenofibrate therapy have been reported after exposures of weeks to several years. In extremely rare cases, cirrhosis has been reported in association with chronic active hepatitis.

Regular periodic monitoring of liver function, including serum ALT (SGPT) should be performed for the duration of therapy with fenofibrate, and therapy discontinued if enzyme levels persist above three times the normal limit.

Cholelithiasis: Fenofibrate, like clofibrate and gemfibrozil, may increase cholesterol excretion into the bile, leading to cholelithiasis. If cholelithiasis is suspected, gallbladder studies are indicated. Fenofibrate therapy should be discontinued if gallstones are found.

Concomitant Oral Anticoagulants: Caution should be exercised when anticoagulants are given in conjunction with fenofibrate because of the potentiation of coumarin-type anticoagulants in prolonging the prothrombin time/INR. The dosage of the anticoagulant should be reduced to maintain the prothrombin time/INR at the desired level to prevent bleeding complications. Frequent prothrombin time/INR determinations are advisable until it has been definitely determined that the prothrombin time/INR has stabilized.

Concomitant HMG-CoA reductase inhibitors: The combined use of fenofibrate and HMG-CoA reductase inhibitors should be avoided unless the benefit of further alterations in lipid levels is likely to outweigh the increased risk of this drug combination.

In a single-dose drug interaction study in 23 healthy adults the concomitant administration of fenofibrate and pravastatin resulted in no clinically important difference in the pharmacokinetics of fenofibric acid, pravastatin or its active metabolite 3α-hydroxy isopravastatin when compared to either drug given alone.

Table 1

Mean Percent Change in lipid Parameters at End of Treatment†

Treatment Group	Total-C	LDL-C	HDL-C	TG
Pooled Cohort				
Mean baseline lipid values (n=646)	306.9 mg/dL	213.8 mg/dL	52.3 mg/dL	191.0 mg/dL
All FEN (n=361)	-18.7%*	-20.6%*	+11.0%*	-28.9%*
Placebo (n=285)	-0.4%	-2.2%	+0.7%	+7.7%
Baseline LDL-C > 160 mg/dL and TG < 150 mg/dL (Type IIa)				
Mean baseline lipid values (n=334)	307.7 mg/dL	227.7 mg/dL	58.1 mg/dL	101.7 mg/dL
All FEN (n=193)	-22.4%*	-31.4%*	+9.8%	-23.5%*
Placebo (n=141)	+0.2%	-2.2%	+2.6%	+11.7%
Baseline LDL-C > 160 mg/dL and TG < 150 mg/dL (Type IIb)				
Mean baseline lipid values (n=242)	312.8 mg/dL	219.8 mg/dL	46.7 mg/dL	231.9 mg/dL
All FEN (n=126)	-16.8%*	-20.1%*	+14.6%*	-35.9%*
Placebo (n=116)	-3.0%	-6.6%	+2.3%	+0.9%

†Duration of study treatment was 3 to 6 months
*p = <0.05 vs. Placebo

Table 2
Effects of Fenofibrate Capsules (micronized) in Patients With Fredrickson Type IV/V Hyperlipidemia

Study 1	Placebo				Fenofibrate Capsules (micronized)			
Baseline TG Levels 350 to 499 mg/dL	N	Baseline (Mean)	Endpoint (Mean)	% Change (Mean)	N	Baseline (Mean)	Endpoint (Mean)	% Change (Mean)
Triglycerides	28	449	450	-0.5	27	432	223	-46.2*
VLDL Triglycerides	19	367	350	2.7	19	350	178	-44.1*
Total Cholesterol	28	255	261	2.8	27	252	227	-9.1*
HDL Cholesterol	28	35	36	4	27	34	40	19.6*
LDL Cholesterol	28	120	129	12	27	128	137	14.5
VLDL Cholesterol	27	99	99	5.8	27	92	46	-44.7*

Study 2	Placebo				Fenofibrate Capsules (micronized)			
Baseline TG Levels 500 to 1500 mg/dL	N	Baseline (Mean)	Endpoint (Mean)	% Change (Mean)	N	Baseline (Mean)	Endpoint (Mean)	% Change (Mean)
Triglycerides	44	710	750	7.2	48	726	308	-54.5*
VLDL Triglycerides	29	537	571	18.7	33	543	205	-50.6*
Total Cholesterol	44	272	271	0.4	48	261	223	-13.8*
HDL Cholesterol	44	27	28	5.0	48	30	36	22.9*
LDL Cholesterol	42	100	90	-4.2	45	103	131	45.0*
VLDL Cholesterol	42	137	142	11.0	45	126	54	-49.4*

* = p<0.05 vs. Placebo

The combined use of fibric acid derivatives and HMG-CoA reductase inhibitors has been associated, in the absences of a marked pharmacokinetic interaction, in numerous case reports, with rhabdomyolysis, markedly elevated creatine kinase (CK) levels and myoglobinuria, leading in a high proportion of cases to acute renal failure.

The use of fibrates alone, including fenofibrate capsules (micronized) may occasionally be associated with myositis, myopathy, or rhabdomyolysis. Patients receiving fenofibrate and complaining of muscle pain, tenderness, or weakness should have prompt medical evaluation for myopathy, including serum creatine kinase level determination. If myopathy/myositis is suspected or diagnosed, fenofibrate therapy should be stopped.

Mortality: The effect of fenofibrate on coronary heart disease morbidity and mortality and non-cardiovascular mortality has not been established.

Other Considerations: In the Coronary Drug Project, a large study of post myocardial infarction of patients treated for 5 years with clofibrate, there was no difference in mortality seen between the clofibrate group and the placebo group. There was however, a difference in the rate of cholelithiasis and cholecystitis requiring surgery between the two groups (3.0% vs. 1.8%).

Because of chemical, pharmacological, and clinical similarities between fenofibrate, clofibrate, and gemfibrozil, the adverse findings in 4 large randomized, placebo-controlled clinical studies with these other fibrate drugs may also apply to fenofibrate.

In a study conducted by the World Health Organization (WHO), 5000 subjects without known coronary artery disease were treated with placebo or clofibrate for 5 years and followed for an additional one year. There was a statistically significant, higher age-adjusted all-cause mortality in the clofibrate group compared with the placebo group (5.70% vs. 3.96%, p=<0.01). Excess mortality was due to a 33% increase in non-cardiovascular causes, including malignancy, post-cholecystectomy complications, and pancreatitis. This appeared to confirm the higher risk of gallbladder disease seen in clofibrate-treated patients studied in the Coronary Drug Project.

The Helsinki Heart Study was a large (n=4081) study of middle-aged men without a history of coronary artery disease. Subjects received either placebo or gemfibrozil for 5 years, with a 3.5 year open extension afterward. Total mortality was numerically higher in the gemfibrozil randomization group but did not achieve statistical significance (p=0.19, 95% confidence interval for relative risk G:P=.91-1.64). Although cancer deaths trended higher in the gemfibrozil group (p=0.11), cancers (excluding basal cell carcinoma) were diagnosed with equal frequency in both study groups. Due to the limited size of the study, the relative risk of death from any cause was not shown to be different than that seen in the 9 year follow-up data from World Health Organization study (RR=1.29). Similarly, the numerical excess of gallbladder surgeries in the gemfibrozil group did not differ statistically from that observed in the WHO study.

A secondary prevention component of the Helsinki Heart Study enrolled middle-aged men excluded from the primary prevention study because of known or suspected coronary heart disease. Subjects received gemfibrozil or placebo for 5 years. Although cardiac deaths trended higher in the gemfibrozil group, this was not statistically significant (hazard ratio 2.2, 95% confidence interval: 0.94–5.05). The rate of gallbladder surgery was not statistically significant between study groups, but did trend higher in the gemfibrozil group, (1.9% vs. 0.3%, p=0.07). There was a statistically significant difference in the number of appendectomies in the gemfibrozil group (6/311 vs. 0/317, p=0.029).

PRECAUTIONS

Initial therapy: Laboratory studies should be done to ascertain that the lipid levels are consistently abnormal before instituting fenofibrate therapy. Every attempt should be made to control serum lipids with appropriate diet, exercise, weight loss in obese patients, and control of any medical problems such as diabetes mellitus and hypothyroidism that are contributing to the lipid abnormalities. Medications known to exacerbate hypertriglyceridemia (beta-blockers, thiazides, estrogens) should be discontinued or changed if possible prior to consideration of triglyceride-lowering drug therapy.

Continued therapy: Periodic determination of serum lipids should be obtained during initial therapy in order to establish the lowest effective dose of LOFIBRA® [Fenofibrate capsules (micronized)]. Therapy should be withdrawn in patients who do not have an adequate response after two months of treatment with the maximum recommended dose of 200 mg per day.

Pancreatitis: Pancreatitis has been reported in patients taking fenofibrate, gemfibrozil, and clofibrate. This occurrence may represent a failure of efficacy in patients with severe hypertriglyceridemia, a direct drug effect, or a secondary phenomenon mediated through biliary tract stone or sludge formation with obstruction of the common bile duct.

Hypersensitivity Reactions: Acute hypersensitivity reactions including severe skin rashes requiring patient hospitalization and treatment with steroids have occurred very rarely during treatment with fenofibrate, including rare spontaneous reports of Stevens-Johnson syndrome, and toxic epidermal necrolysis. Urticaria was seen in 1.1 vs. 0%, and rash in 1.4 vs. 0.8% of fenofibrate and placebo patients respectively in controlled trials.

Hematologic Changes: Mild to moderate hemoglobin, hematocrit, and white blood cell decreases have been observed in patients following initiation of fenofibrate therapy. However, these levels stabilize during long-term administration. Extremely rare spontaneous reports of thrombocytopenia and agranulocytosis have been received during post-marketing surveillance outside of the U.S. Periodic blood counts are recommended during the first 12 months of fenofibrate administration.

Skeletal muscle: The use of fibrates alone, including fenofibrate, may occasionally be associated with myopathy. Treatment with drugs of the fibrate class has been associated on rare occasions with rhabdomyolysis, usually in patients with impaired renal function. Myopathy should be considered in any patient with diffuse myalgias, muscle tenderness or weakness, and/or marked elevations of creatine phosphokinase levels.

Patients should be advised to report promptly unexplained muscle pain, tenderness or weakness, particularly if accompanied by malaise or fever. CPK levels should be assessed in patients reporting these symptoms, and fenofibrate therapy should be discontinued if markedly elevated CPK levels occur or myopathy is diagnosed.

Drug Interactions

Oral Anticoagulants: CAUTION SHOULD BE EXERCISED WHEN COUMARIN ANTICOAGULANTS ARE GIVEN IN CONJUNCTION WITH LOFIBRA ®. THE DOSAGE OF THE ANTICOAGULANTS SHOULD BE REDUCED TO MAINTAIN THE PROTHROMBIN TIME/INR AT THE DESIRED LEVEL TO PREVENT BLEEDING COMPLICATIONS. FREQUENT PROTHROMBIN TIME/INR DETERMINATIONS ARE ADVISABLE UNTIL IT HAS BEEN DEFINITELY DETERMINED THAT THE PROTHROMBIN TIME/INR HAS STABILIZED.

HMG-CoA reductase inhibitors: The combined use of fenofibrate and HMG-CoA reductase inhibitors should be avoided unless the benefit of further alterations in lipid levels is likely to outweigh the increased risk of this drug combination (see **WARNINGS**).

Resins: Since bile acid sequestrants may bind other drugs given concurrently, patients should take LOFIBRA® at least 1 hour before or 4 to 6 hours after a bile acid binding resin to avoid impeding its absorption.

Cyclosporine: Because cyclosporine can produce nephrotoxicity with decreases in creatinine clearance and rises in serum creatinine, and because renal excretion is the primary elimination route of fibrate drugs including fenofibrate, there is a risk that an interaction will lead to deterioration. The benefits and risks of using fenofibrate with immunosuppressants and other potentially nephrotoxic agents should be carefully considered, and the lowest effective dose employed.

Carcinogenesis, Mutagenesis, Impairment of Fertility: In a 24-month study in rats (10, 45, and 200 mg/kg; 0.3, 1, and 6 times the maximum recommended human dose on the basis of mg/meter^2 of surface area), the incidence of liver carcinoma was significantly increased at 6 times the maximum recommended human dose in males and females. A statistically significant increase in pancreatic carcinomas occurred in males at 1 and 6 times the maximum recommended human dose; there were also increases in pancreatic adenomas and benign testicular interstitial cell tumors at 6 times the maximum recommended human dose in males. In a second 24-month study in a different strain of rats (doses of 10 and 60 mg/kg; 0.3 and 2 times the maximum recommended human dose based on mg/meter^2 surface area), there were significant increases in the incidence of pancreatic acinar adenomas in both sexes and increases in interstitial cell tumors of the testes at 2 times the maximum recommended human dose.

A comparative carcinogenicity study was done in rats comparing three drugs: fenofibrate (10 and 70 mg/kg; 0.3 and 1.6 times the maximum recommended human dose), clofibrate (400 mg/kg; 1.6 times the human dose), and gemfibrozil (250 mg/kg; 1.7 times the human dose) (multiples based on mg/meter^2 surface area). Pancreatic acinar adenomas were increased in males and females on fenofibrate; hepatocellular carcinoma and pancreatic acinar adenomas were increased in males and hepatic neoplastic nodules in females treated with clofibrate; hepatic neoplastic nodules were increased in males and females treated with gemfibrozil while testicular interstitial cell tumors were increased in males on all three drugs.

In a 21-month study in mice at doses of 10, 45, and 200 mg/kg (approximately 0.2, 0.7 and 3 times the maximum recommended human dose on the basis of mg/meter^2 surface area), there were statistically significant increases in liver carcinoma at 3 times the maximum recommended human dose in both males and females. In a second 18-month study at the same doses, there was a significant increase in liver carcinoma in male mice and liver adenoma in female mice at 3 times the maximum recommended human dose.

Electron microscopy studies have demonstrated peroxisomal proliferation following fenofibrate administration to the rat. An adequate study to test for peroxisome proliferation in humans has not been done, but changes in peroxisome morphology and numbers have been observed in humans after treatment with other members of the fibrate class when liver biopsies were compared before and after treatment in the same individual.

Fenofibrate has been demonstrated to be devoid of mutagenic potential in the following tests: Ames, mouse lymphoma, chromosomal aberration and unscheduled DNA synthesis.

Pregnancy Category C: Fenofibrate has been shown to be embryocidal and teratogenic in rats when given in doses 7 to 10 times the maximum recommended human dose and embryocidal in rabbits when given at 9 times the maximum recommended human dose (on the basis of mg/meter^2 surface area). There are no adequate and well-controlled studies in pregnant women. Fenofibrate should be used during pregnancy only if the potential benefit justifies the potential risk to the fetus.

Administration of 9 times the maximum recommended human dose of fenofibrate to female rats before and throughout gestation caused 100% of dams to delay delivery and resulted in a 60% increase in post-implantation loss, a decrease in litter size, a decrease in birth weight, a 40% survival of pups at birth, a 4% survival of pups as neonates, and a 0% survival of pups to weaning, and an increase in spina bifida.

Administration of 10 times the maximum recommended human dose to female rats on days 6 to 15 of gestation caused an increase in gross, visceral and skeletal findings in fetuses (domed head/hunched shoulders/rounded body/abnormal chest, kyphosis, stunted fetuses, elongated sternal ribs, malformed sternebrae, extra foramen in palatine, misshapen vertebrae, supernumerary ribs).

Administration of 7 times the maximum recommended human dose to female rats from day 15 of gestation through weaning caused a delay in delivery, a 40% decrease in live births, a 75% decrease in neonatal survival, and decreases in pup weight, at birth as well as on days 4 and 21 post-partum.

Administration of 9 and 18 times the maximum recommended human dose to female rabbits caused abortions in 10% of dams at 9 times and 25% of dams at 18 times the maximum recommended human dose and death of 7% of fetuses at 18 times the maximum recommended human dose.

Nursing mothers: Fenofibrate should not be used in nursing mothers. Because of the potential for tumorigenicity seen in animal studies, a decision should be made whether to discontinue nursing or to discontinue the drug.

Pediatric Use: Safety and efficacy in pediatric patients have not been established.

Geriatric Use: Fenofibric acid is known to be substantially excreted by the kidney, and the risk of adverse reactions to this drug may be greater in patients with impaired renal function. Because elderly patients are more likely to have decreased renal function, care should be taken in dose selection.

ADVERSE REACTIONS

CLINICAL: Adverse events reported by 2% or more of patients treated with fenofibrate during the double-blind, placebo-controlled trials, regardless of causality, are listed in the table below. Adverse events led to discontinuation of treatment in 5.0% of patients treated with fenofibrate and in 3.0% treated with placebo. Increases in liver function tests were the most frequent events, causing discontinuation of fenofibrate treatment in 1.6% of patients in double-blind trials.

BODY SYSTEM Adverse Event	Fenofibrate* (N=439)	PLACEBO (N=365)
BODY AS A WHOLE		
Abdominal Pain	4.6%	4.4%
Back pain	3.4%	2.5%
Headache	3.2%	2.7%
Asthenia	2.1%	3.0%
Flu Syndrome	2.1%	2.7%
DIGESTIVE		
Liver Function Tests Abnormal	7.5%**	1.4%
Diarrhea	2.3%	4.1%
Nausea	2.3%	1.9%
Constipation	2.1%	1.4%
METABOLIC AND NUTRITIONAL DISORDERS		
SPGT Increased	3.0%	1.6%
Creatine Phosphokinase Increased	3.0%	1.4%
SGOT Increased	3.4%**	0.5%
RESPIRATORY		
Respiratory Disorder	6.2%	5.5%
Rhinitis	2.3%	1.1%

*Dosage equivalent to 200 mg LOFIBRA® [Fenofibrate capsules (micronized)]

**Significantly different from Placebo

Additional adverse events reported by three or more patients in placebo-controlled trials or reported in other controlled or open trials, regardless of causality are listed below.

BODY AS A WHOLE: Chest pain, pain (unspecified), infection, malaise, allergic reaction, cyst, hernia, fever, photosensitivity reaction, and accidental injury.

CARDIOVASCULAR SYSTEM: Angina pectoris, hypertension, vasodilatation, coronary artery disorder, electrocardiogram abnormal, ventricular extrasystoles, myocardial infarct, peripheral vascular disorder, migraine, varicose vein, cardiovascular disorder, hypotension, palpitation, vascular disorder, arrhythmia, phlebitis, tachycardia, extrasystoles, and atrial fibrillation.

DIGESTIVE SYSTEM: Dyspepsia, flatulence, nausea, increased appetite, gastroenteritis, cholelithiasis, rectal disorder, esophagitis, gastritis, colitis, tooth disorder, vomiting, anorexia, gastrointestinal disorder, duodenal ulcer, nausea and vomiting, peptic ulcer, rectal hemorrhage, liver fatty deposit, cholecystitis, eructation, gamma glutamyl transpeptidase, and diarrhea.

ENDOCRINE SYSTEM: Diabetes mellitus

Continued on next page

Lofibra—Cont.

HEMIC AND LYMPHATIC SYSTEM: Anemia, leukopenia, ecchymosis, eosinophilia, lymphadenopathy, and thrombocytopenia.
METABOLIC AND NUTRITIONAL DISORDERS: Creatinine increased, weight gain, hypoglycemia, gout, weight loss, edema, hyperuricemia, and peripheral edema.
MUSCULOSKELETAL SYSTEM: Myositis, myalgia, arthralgia, arthritis, tenosynovitis, joint disorder, arthrosis, leg cramps, bursitis, and myasthenia.
NERVOUS SYSTEM: Dizziness, insomnia, depression, vertigo, libido decreased, anxiety, paresthesia, dry mouth, hypertonia, nervousness, neuralgia, and somnolence.
RESPIRATORY SYSTEM: Pharyngitis, bronchitis, cough increased, dyspnea, asthma, pneumonia, laryngitis, and sinusitis.
SKIN AND APPENDAGES: Rash, pruritus, eczema, herpes zoster, urticaria, acne, sweating, fungal dermatitis, skin disorder, alopecia, contact dermatitis, herpes simplex, maculopapular rash, nail disorder, and skin ulcer.
SPECIAL SENSES: Conjunctivitis, eye disorder, amblyopia, ear pain, otitis media, abnormal vision, cataract specified, and refraction disorder.
UROGENITAL SYSTEM: Urinary frequency, prostatic disorder, dysuria, kidney function abnormal, urolithiasis, gynecomastia, unintended pregnancy, vaginal moniliasis, and cystitis.

OVERDOSAGE

There is no specific treatment for overdose with fenofibrate. General supportive care of the patient is indicated, including monitoring of vital signs and observation of clinical status, should an overdose occur. If indicated, elimination of unabsorbed drug should be achieved by emesis or gastric lavage; usual precautions should be observed to maintain the airway. Because fenofibrate is highly bound to plasma proteins, hemodialysis should not be considered.

DOSAGE AND ADMINISTRATION

Patients should be placed on an appropriate lipid-lowering diet before receiving LOFIBRA® [Fenofibrate capsules (micronized)], and should continue this diet during treatment with LOFIBRA®. LOFIBRA® should be given with meals, thereby optimizing the bioavailability of the medication.
For the treatment of adult patients with primary hypercholesterolemia or mixed hyperlipidemia, the initial dose of LOFIBRA® is 200 mg per day.
For adult patients with hypertriglyceridemia, the initial dose is 67 to 200 mg per day. Dosage should be individualized according to patient response, and should be adjusted if necessary following repeat lipid determinations at 4 to 8 week intervals. The maximum dose is 200 mg per day.
Treatment with LOFIBRA® should be initiated at a dose of 67 mg/day in patients having impaired renal function, and increased only after evaluation of the effects on renal function and lipid levels at this dose. In the elderly, the initial dose should likewise be limited to 67 mg/day.
Lipid levels should be monitored periodically and consideration should be given to reducing the dosage of LOFIBRA® if lipid levels fall significantly below the targeted range.

HOW SUPPLIED

LOFIBRA®, 67 mg are opaque pink cap and body, hard gelatin capsules, printed in black ink **Lofibra** over **67 mg** and **Gate** over **322** on opposing cap and body portions of the capsule. They are supplied as follows:
NDC 57844-322-01 Bottles of 100 capsules
LOFIBRA®, 134 mg are opaque light blue cap and body, hard gelatin capsules, printed in black ink **Lofibra** over **134 mg** and **Gate** over **323** on opposing cap and body portions of the capsule. They are supplied as follows:
NDC 57844-323-01 Bottles of 100 capsules
LOFIBRA®, 200 mg are opaque orange cap and body, hard gelatin capsules, printed in black ink **Lofibra** over **200 mg** and **Gate** over **324** on opposing cap and body portions of the capsule. They are supplied as follows:
NDC 57844-324-01 Bottles of 100 capsules

STORAGE
Store at controlled room temperature, between 20° and 25°C (68° and 77°F) (see USP). Keep out of the reach of children. Protect from moisture.
Manufactured by:
NOVOPHARM LIMITED
Toronto, Canada
M1B 2K9
Manufactured for:
GATE PHARMACEUTICALS
Div. of TEVA PHARMACEUTICALS USA
Sellersville, PA 18960

REFERENCES

1. GOLDBERG AC, *et al.* Fenofibrate for the Treatment of Type IV and V Hyperlipoproteinemias: A Double-Blind, Placebo-Controlled Multicenter US Study. *Clinical Therapeutics*, 11, pp. 69–83, 1989.
2. NIKKILA EA. Familial Lipoprotein Lipase Deficiency and Related Disorders of Chylomicron Metabolism. In Stanbury J.B., *et al.* (eds.): *The Metabolic Basis of Inherited Disease*, 5th edition, McGraw-Hill, 1983, Chap. 30, pp. 622–642.
3. BROWN WV, *et al.* Effects of Fenofibrate on Plasma Lipids: Double-Blind, Multicenter Study In Patients with Type IIA or IIB Hyperlipidemia. *Arteriosclerosis*. 6, pp. 670–678, 1986.

Printed in Canada
72204IN-2600 Rev. 03
Rev. F 7/2003

ORAP® ℞
(pimozide)
Tablets

DESCRIPTION

ORAP® (pimozide) is an orally active antipsychotic agent of the diphenylbutylpiperidine series. The structural formula of pimozide, 1-[1-[4,4-bis(4-fluorophenyl)butyl]-4-piperidinyl]-1, 3-dihydro-2H-benzimidazole-2-one is:

The solubility of pimozide in water is less than 0.01 mg/mL; it is slightly soluble in most organic solvents.
Each white ORAP tablet contains either 1 mg or 2 mg of pimozide and the following inactive ingredients: calcium stearate, microcrystalline cellulose, lactose anhydrous and corn starch.

CLINICAL PHARMACOLOGY

Pharmacodynamic Actions
ORAP (pimozide) is an orally active antipsychotic drug product which shares with other antipsychotics the ability to blockade dopaminergic receptors on neurons in the central nervous system. Although its exact mode of action has not been established, the ability of pimozide to suppress motor and phonic tics in Tourette's Disorder is thought to be a function of its dopaminergic blocking activity. However, receptor blockade is often accompanied by a series of secondary alterations in central dopamine metabolism and function which may contribute to both pimozide's therapeutic and untoward effects. In addition, pimozide, in common with other antipsychotic drugs, has various effects on other central nervous system receptor systems which are not fully characterized.

Metabolism and Pharmacokinetics
More than 50% of a dose of pimozide is absorbed after oral administration. Based on the pharmacokinetic and metabolic profile, pimozide appears to undergo significant first pass metabolism. Peak serum levels occur generally six to eight hours (range 4–12 hours) after dosing.
Pimozide is extensively metabolized, primarily by N-dealkylation in the liver. This metabolism is catalyzed mainly by the cytochrome P450 3A (CYP 3A) enzymatic system and to a lesser extent, by cytochrome P450 1A2 (CYP 1A2). Two major metabolites have been identified, 1-(4-piperidyl)-2-benzimidazolinone and 4,4-bis(4-florophenyl) butyric acid. The antipsychotic activity of these metabolites is undermined. The major route of elimination of pimozide and its metabolites is through the kidney.
The mean serum elimination half-life of pimozide in schizophrenic patients was approximately 55 hours. There was a 13-fold interindividual difference in the area under the serum pimozide level-time curve and an equivalent degree of variation in peak serum levels among patients studied. The significance of this is unclear since there are few correlations between plasma levels and clinical findings.
Effects of food and disease upon the absorption, distribution, metabolism and elimination of pimozide are not known. Effects of concomitant medication on pimozide metabolism are described in the **CONTRAINDICATIONS** section.

INDICATIONS AND USAGE

ORAP (pimozide) is indicated for the suppression of motor and phonic tics in patients with Tourette's Disorder who have failed to respond satisfactorily to standard treatment. ORAP is not intended as a treatment of first choice nor is it intended for the treatment of tics that are merely annoying or cosmetically troublesome. ORAP should be reserved for use in Tourette's Disorder patients whose development and/or daily life function is severely compromised by the presence of motor and phonic tics.
Evidence supporting approval of pimozide for use in Tourette's Disorder was obtained in two controlled clinical investigations which enrolled patients between the ages of 8 and 53 years. Most subjects in the two trials were 12 or older.

CONTAINDICATIONS

1. ORAP (pimozide) is contraindicated in the treatment of simple tics or tics other than those associated with Tourette's Disorder.
2. ORAP should not be used in patients taking drugs that may, themselves, cause motor and phonic tics (e.g., pemoline, methylphenidate and amphetamines) until such patients have been withdrawn from these drugs to determine whether or not the drugs, rather than Tourette's Disorder, are responsible for the tics.
3. Because ORAP prolongs the QT interval of the electrocardiogram it is contraindicated in patients with congenital long QT syndrome, patients with a history of cardiac arrhythmias, or patients taking other drugs which prolong the QT interval of the electrocardiogram (see **PRECAUTIONS—Drug Interactions**).
4. ORAP is contraindicated in patients with severe toxic central nervous system depression or comatose states from any cause.
5. ORAP is contraindicated in patients with hyper-sensitivity to it. As it is not known whether cross-sensitivity exists among the antipsychotics, pimozide should be used with appropriate caution in patients who have demonstrated hypersensitivity to other antipsychotic drugs.
6. Ventricular arrhythmias have been rarely associated with the use of macrolide antibiotics in patients with prolonged QT intervals, as might be produced by ORAP. Specifically, two sudden deaths have been reported when clarithromycin was added to ongoing pimozide therapy. Futhermore, some evidence suggests that pimozide is metabolized partly by the enzyme system cytochrome P450 3A (CYP 3A). Macrolide antibiotics are inhibitors of CYP 3A, and thus could potentially impede pimozide metabolism. For these reasons, ORAP is contraindicated in patients receiving the macrolide antibiotics clarithromycin, erythromycin, azithromycin, dirithromycin, and troleandomycin.
Because azole antifungal agents are also inhibitors of the CYP 3A enzymes and thus may likewise impair pimozide metabolism, ORAP is contraindicated in patients receiving the azole antifungal agents itraconazole and ketoconazole.
Similarly, protease inhibitor drugs are also inhibitors of CYP 3A, and thus ORAP is contraindicated in patients receiving protease inhibitors such as ritonavir, saquinovir, indinavir, and nelfinavir. (See **PRECAUTIONS—Drug Interactions.**)
Nefazone is a potent inhibitor of CYP 3A, and its concomitant use with ORAP is also contraindicated.
Other drugs that are relatively less potent inhibitors of CYP 3A should also be avoided, in view of the risks e.g. zileuton

WARNINGS

The use of ORAP (pimozide) in the treatment of Tourette's Disorder involves different risk/benefit considerations than when antipsychotic drugs are used to treat other conditions. Consequently, a decision to use ORAP should take into consideration the following (see also **PRECAUTIONS—Information for Patients**).

Tardive Dyskinesia
A syndrome consisting of potentially irreversible, involuntary, dyskinetic movements may develop in patients treated with antipsychotic drugs. Although the prevalence of the syndrome appears to be highest among the elderly, especially elderly women, it is impossible to rely upon prevalence estimates to predict, at the inception of antipsychotic treatment, which patients are likely to develop the syndrome. Whether antipsychotic drug products differ in their potential to cause tardive dyskinesia in unknown.
Both the risk of developing tardive dyskinesia and the likelihood that it will become irreversible are believed to increase as the duration of treatment and the total cumulative dose of antipsychotic drugs administered to the patient increase. However, the syndrome can develop, although much less commonly, after relatively brief treatment periods at low doses.
There is no known treatment for established cases of tardive dyskinesia, although the syndrome may remit, partially or completely, if antipsychotic treatment is withdrawn. Antipsychotic treatment itself, however, may suppress (or partially suppress) the signs and symptoms of the syndrome and thereby may possibly mask the underlying process. The effect that symptomatic suppression has upon the long-term course of the syndrome is unknown.
Given these considerations, antipsychotic drugs should be prescribed in a manner that is most likely to minimize the occurrence of tardive dyskinesia. Chronic antipsychotic treatment should generally be reserved for patients who suffer from a chronic illness that, 1) is known to respond to antipsychotic drugs, and 2) for whom alternative, equally effective, but potentially less harmful treatments are not available or appropriate. In patients who do require chronic treatment, the smallest dose and the shortest duration of treatment producing a satisfactory clinical response should be sought. The need for continued treatment should be reassessed periodically.
If signs and symptoms of tardive dyskinesia appear in a patient on antipsychotics, drug discontinuation should be considered. However, some patients may require treatment despite the presence of the syndrome.
(For further information about the description of tardive dyskinesia and its clinical detection, please refer to **ADVERSE REACTIONS** and **PRECAUTIONS—Information for Patients.**)

Neuroleptic Malignant Syndrome (NMS)
A potentially fatal symptom complex sometimes referred to as Neuroleptic Malignant Syndrome (NMS) has been reported in association with antipsychotic drugs. Clinical manifestations of NMS are hyperpyrexia, muscle rigidity, altered mental status (including catatonic signs) and evidence of autonomic instability (irregular pulse or blood pressure, tachycardia, diaphoresis, and cardiac dysrhythmias). Additional signs may include elevated creatine phosphokinase, myoglobinuria (rhabdomyolysis) and acute renal failure.
The diagnostic evaluation of patients with this syndrome is complicated. In arriving at a diagnosis, it is important to identify cases where the clinical presentation includes both serious medical illness (e.g., pneumonia, systemic infection, etc.) and untreated or inadequately treated extrapyramidal signs and symptoms (EPS). Other important considerations

in the differential diagnosis include central anticholinergic toxicity, heat stroke, drug fever and primary central nervous system (CNS) pathology.

The management of NMS should include 1) immediate discontinuation of antipsychotic drugs and other drugs not essential to concurrent therapy, 2) intensive symptomatic treatment and medical monitoring, and 3) treatment of any concomitant serious medical problems for which specific treatments are available. There is no general agreement about specific pharmacological treatment regimens for uncomplicated NMS.

If a patient requires antipsychotic drug treatment after recovery from NMS, the potential reintroduction of drug therapy should be carefully considered. The patient should be carefully monitored, since recurrences of NMS have been reported.

Hyperpyrexia, not associated with the above symptom complex, has been reported with other antipsychotic drugs.

Other

Sudden, unexpected deaths have occurred in experimental studies of conditions other than Tourette's Disorder. These deaths occurred while patients were receiving dosages in the range of 1 mg per kg. One possible mechanism for such deaths is prolongation of the QT interval predisposing patients to ventricular arrhythmia. An electrocardiogram should be performed before ORAP treatment is initiated and periodically thereafter, especially during the period of dose adjustment.

ORAP may have a tumorigenic potential. Based on studies conducted in mice, it is known that pimozide can produce a dose-related increase in pituitary tumors. The full significance of this finding is not known, but should be taken into consideration in the physician's and patient's decisions to use this drug product. This finding should be given special consideration when the patient is young and chronic use of pimozide is anticipated (see **PRECAUTIONS—Carcinogenesis, Mutagenesis, Impairment of Fertility**).

PRECAUTIONS

General

ORAP (pimozide) may impair the mental and/or physical abilities required for the performance of potentially hazardous tasks, such as driving a car or operating machinery, especially during the first few days of therapy.

ORAP produces anticholinergic side effects and should be used with caution in individuals whose conditions may be aggravated by anticholinergic activity.

ORAP should be administered cautiously to patients with impairment of liver or kidney function, because it is metabolized by the liver and excreted by the kidneys.

Antipsychotics should be administered with caution to patients receiving anticonvulsant medication, with a history of seizures, or with EEG abnormalities, because they may lower the convulsive threshold. If indicated, adequate anticonvulsant therapy should be maintained concomitantly.

Information for Patients

Treatment with ORAP exposes the patients to serious risks. A decision to use ORAP chronically in Tourette's Disorder is one that deserves full consideration by the patient (or patient's family) as well as by the treating physician. Because the goal of treatment is symptomatic improvement, the patient's view of the need for treatment and assessment of response are critical in evaluating the impact of therapy and weighing its benefits against the risks. Since the physician is the primary source of information about the use of a drug in any disease, it is recommended that the following information be discussed with patients and/or their families.

ORAP is intended only for use in patients with Tourette's Disorder whose symptoms are severe and who cannot tolerate, or who do not respond to HALDOL* (haloperidol).

Given the likelihood that a proportion of patients exposed chronically to antipsychotics will develop tardive dyskinesia, it is advised that all patients in whom chronic use is contemplated be given, if possible, full information about this risk. The decision to inform patients and/or their guardians must obviously take into account the clinical circumstances and the competency of the patient to understand the information provided.

There is limited information available on the use of ORAP in children under 12 years of age.

The information available on ORAP from foreign marketing experience and from U.S. clinical trials indicates that ORAP has a side effect profile similar to that of other antipsychotic drugs. Patients should be informed that all types of side effects associated with the use of antipsychotics may be associated with the use of ORAP.

In addition, sudden, unexpected deaths have occurred in patients taking high doses of ORAP for conditions other than Tourette's Disorder. These deaths may have been the result of an effect of ORAP upon the heart. Therefore, patients should be instructed not to exceed the prescribed dose of ORAP and they should realize the need for the initial ECG and for follow-up ECGs during treatment.

Also, pimozide, at a dose about 15 times that given humans, caused an increase in the number of benign tumors of the pituitary gland in female mice, it is not possible to say how important this is. Similar tumors were not seen in rats given pimozide, nor at lower doses in mice, which is reassuring. However, any such finding must be considered to suggest a possible risk of long term use of the drug.

Because substances in grapefruit juice may inhibit the metabolism of pimozide by CYP 3A, patients should be advised to avoid grapefruit juice.

Laboratory Tests

An ECG should be done at baseline and periodically thereafter throughout the period of dose adjustment. Any indication of prolongation of QTc interval beyond an absolute limit of 0.47 seconds (children) or 0.52 seconds (adults), or more than 25% above the patient's original baseline should be considered a basis for stopping further dose increase (see **CONTRAINDICATIONS**) and considering a lower dose.

Since hypokalemia has been associated with ventricular arrhythmias, potassium insufficiency, secondary to diuretics, diarrhea, or other cause, should be corrected before ORAP therapy is initiated and normal potassium maintained during therapy.

Drug Interactions

Because ORAP prolongs the QT interval of the electrocardiogram, an additive effect on QT interval would be anticipated if administered with other drugs, such as phenothiazines, tricyclic antidepressants or antiarrhythmic agents, which prolong the QT interval. Also, the use of macrolide antibiotics in patients with prolonged QT intervals has been rarely associated with ventricular arrhythmias. Such concomitant administration should not be undertaken (see **CONTRAINDICATIONS**).

Since ORAP is partly metabolized via CYP 3A, it should not be administered concomitantly with inhibitors of this metabolic system, such as azole antifungal agents and protease inhibitor drugs (see CONTRAINDICATIONS).

As CYP 1A2 may also contribute to the metabolism of ORAP, prescribers should be aware of the theoretical potential of drug interactions with inhibitors of this enzymatic system.

ORAP may be capable of potentiating CNS depressants, including analgesics, sedatives, anxiolytics, and alcohol.

A single case report has suggested possible additive effects of pimozide and fluoxetine leading to bradycardia.

Interaction with Food

Patients should avoid grapefruit juice because it may inhibit the metabolism of pimozide by CYP 3A.

Carcinogenesis, Mutagenesis, Impairment of Fertility

Carcinogenicity studies were conducted in mice and rats. In mice, pimozide causes a dose-related increase in pituitary and mammary tumors.

When mice were treated for up to 18 months with pimozide, pituitary gland changes developed in females only. These changes were characterized as hyperplasia at doses approximating the human dose and adenoma at doses about fifteen times the maximum recommended human dose on a mg per kg basis. The mechanism for the induction of pituitary tumors in mice is not known.

Mammary gland tumors in female mice were also increased, but these tumors are expected in rodents treated with antipsychotic drugs which elevate prolactin levels. Chronic administration of an antipsychotic also causes elevated prolactin levels in humans. Tissue culture experiments indicate that approximately one-third of human breast cancers are prolactin-dependent in *vitro*, a factor of potential importance if the prescription of these drugs is contemplated in a patient with a previously detected breast cancer. Although disturbances such as galactorrhea, amenorrhea, gynecomastia, and impotence have been reported with antipsychotic drugs, the clinical significance of elevated serum prolactin levels is unknown for most patients. Neither clinical studies nor epidemiologic studies conducted to date have shown an association between chronic administration of these drugs and mammary tumorigenesis. The available evidence, however, is considered too limited to be conclusive at this time.

In a 24-month carcinogenicity study in rats, animals received up to 50 times the maximum recommended human dose. No increased incidence of overall tumors or tumors at any site was observed in either sex. Because of the limited number of animals surviving this study, the meaning of these results is unclear.

Pimozide did not have mutagenic activity in the Ames test with four bacterial test strains, in the mouse dominant lethal test or in the micronucleus test is rats.

Reproduction studies in animals were not adequate to assess all aspects of fertility. Nevertheless, female rats administered pimozide had prolonged estrus cycles, an effect also produced by other antipsychotic drugs.

Pregnancy

Category C. Reproduction studies performed in rats and rabbits at oral doses up to 8 times the maximum human dose did not reveal evidence of teratogenicity. In the rat, however, this multiple of the human dose resulted in decreased pregnancies and in the retarded development of fetuses. These effects are thought to be due to an inhibition or delay in implantation which is also observed in rodents administered other antipsychotic drugs. In the rabbit, maternal toxicity, mortality, decreased weight gain, and embryotoxicity including increased resorptions were dose-related. Because animal reproduction studies are not always predictive of human response, pimozide should be given to a pregnant women only if the potential benefits of treatment clearly outweigh the potential risks.

Labor and Delivery

This drug has no recognized use in labor or delivery.

Nursing Mothers

It is not known whether pimozide is excreted in human milk. Because many drugs are excreted in human milk and because of the potential for tumorigenicity and unknown cardiovascular effects in the infant, a decision should be made whether to discontinue nursing or to discontinue the drug, taking into account the importance of the drug to the mother.

Pediatric Use

Although Tourette's Disorder most often has its onset between the ages of 2 and 15 years, information on the use and efficacy of ORAP in patients less than 12 years of age is limited. A 24-week open label study in 36 children between the ages of 2 and 12 demonstrated that pimozide has a similar safety profile in this age group as in older patients and there were no safety findings that would preclude its use in this age group.

Because its use and safety have not been evaluated in other childhood disorders, ORAP is not recommended for use in any condition other than Tourette's Disorder.

ADVERSE REACTIONS

General

Extrapyramidal Reactions: Neuromuscular (extrapyramidal) reactions during the administration of ORAP (pimozide) have been reported frequently, often during the first few days of treatment. In most patients, these reactions involved Parkinson-like symptoms which, then first observed, were usually mild to moderately severe and usually reversible.

Other types of neuromuscular reactions (motor restlessness, dystonia, akathisia, hyperreflexia, opisthotonos, oculgyric crises) have been reported far less frequently. Severe extrapyramidal reactions have been reported to occur at relatively low doses. Generally the occurrence and severity of most extrapyramidal symptoms are dose-related since they occur at relatively high doses and have been shown to disappear or become less severe when the dose is reduced. Administration of antiparkinson drugs such as benztropine mesylate or trihexphenidyl hydrochloride may be required for control of such reactions. It should be noted that persistent extrapyramidal reactions have been reported and that the drug may have to be discontinued in such cases.

Withdrawal Emergent Neurological Signs: Generally, patients receiving short term therapy experience no problems with abrupt discontinuation of antipsychotic drugs. However, some patients on maintenance treatment experience transient dyskinetic signs after abrupt withdrawal. In certain of these cases the dyskinetic movements are indistinguishable from the syndrome described below under "Tardive Dyskinesia" except for duration. It is not known whether gradual withdrawal of antipsychotic drugs with reduce the rate of occurrence of withdrawal emergent neurological signs, but until further evidence becomes available, it seems reasonable to gradually withdraw use of ORAP.

Tardive Dyskinesia: ORAP may be associated with persistent dyskinesias. Tardive dyskinesia, a syndrome consisting of potentially irreversible, involuntary, dyskinetic movements, may appear in some patients on long-term therapy or may occur after drug therapy has been discontinued. The risk appears to be greater in elderly patients on high-dose therapy, especially females. The symptoms are persistent and in some patients appear irreversible. The syndrome is characterized by rhythmical unvoluntary movements of tongue, face, mouth or jaw (e.g., protrusions of tongue, puffing of cheeks, puckering of mouth, chewing movements). Sometimes these may be accompanied by involuntary movements of extremities and the trunk.

There is no known effective treatment for tardive dyskinesia; antiparkinson agents usually do not alleviate the symptoms of this syndrome. It is suggested that all antipsychotic agents be discontinued if these symptoms appear. Should it be necessary to reinstitute treatment, or increase the dosage of the agent, or switch to a different antipsychotic agent, this syndrome may be masked.

It has been reported that fine vermicular movement of the tongue may be an early sign of tardive dyskinesia and if the medication is stopped at that time the syndrome may not develop.

Electrocardiographic Changes: Electrocardiographic changes have been observed in clinical trials of ORAP in Tourette's Disorder and schizophrenia. These have included prolongation of the QT interval, flattening, notching and inversion of the T wave and the appearance of U waves. Sudden, unexpected deaths and grand mal seizure have occurred at doses above 20 mg/day.

Neuroleptic Malignant Syndrome: Neuroleptic malignant syndrome (NMS) has been reported with ORAP. (See **WARNINGS** for further information concerning NMS.)

Hypergyrexia: Hyperpyrexia has been reported with other antipsychotic drugs.

Clinical Trials

The following adverse reaction tabulation was derived from 20 patients in a 6-week long placebo-controlled clinical trial of ORAP in Tourette's Disorder.

Body System/ Adverse Reaction	Pimozide (N = 20)	Placebo (N = 20)
Body as a Whole		
Headache	1	2
Gastrointestinal		
Dry Mouth	5	1
Diarrhea	1	0
Nausea	0	2
Vomiting	0	1
Constipation	4	2

Continued on next page

Orap—Cont.

Eructations	0	1
Thirsty	1	0
Appetite increase	1	0
Endocrine		
Menstrual disorder	0	1
Breast secretions	0	1
Musculoskeletal		
Muscle cramps	0	1
Muscle tightness	3	0
Stooped posture	2	0
CNS		
Drowsiness	7	3
Sedation	14	5
Insomnia	2	2
Dizziness	0	1
Akathisia	8	0
Rigidity	2	0
Speech disorder	2	0
Handwriting change	1	0
Akinesia	8	0
Psychiatric		
Depression	2	3
Excitement	0	1
Nervous	1	0
Adverse behavior effect	5	0
Special Senses		
Visual disturbance	4	0
Taste change	1	0
Sensitivity of eyes to light	1	0
Decrease accommodation	4	1
Spots before eyes	0	1
Urogenital		
Impotence	3	0

The following adverse event tabulation was derived from 36 children (age 2 to 12) in a 24-week open trial of ORAP in Tourette's Disorder.

Body System/ Adverse Reaction	Number of Patients Experiencing Each Event (%)	
	All Events (N=36)	Drug-Related Events (N=36)
Body as a Whole		
Asthenia	9 (25.0)	5 (13.8)
Headache	8 (22.2)	1 (2.7)
Gastrointestinal		
Dysphagia	1 (2.7)	1 (2.7)
Increased Salivation	5 (13.8)	2 (5.5)
Musculoskeletal		
Myalgia	1 (2.7)	1 (2.7)
Central Nervous System		
Dreaming Abnormal	1 (2.7)	1 (2.7)
Hyperkinesia	2 (5.5)	1 (2.7)
Somnolence	10 (27.7)	9 (25.0)
Torticollis	1 (2.7)	1 (2.7)
Tremor, Limbs	1 (2.7)	1 (2.7)
Psychiatric		
Adverse Behavior Effect	10 (27.7)	8 (22.2)
Nervous	3 (8.3)	2 (5.5)
Skin		
Rash	3 (8.3)	1 (2.7)
Special Senses		
Visual disturbance	2 (5.5)	1 (2.7)
Cardiovascular		
ECG Abnormal	1 (2.7)	1 (2.7)

Because clinical investigational experience with ORAP in Tourette's Disorder is limited, uncommon adverse reactions may not have been detected. The physician should consider that other adverse reactions associated with antipsychotics may occur.

Other Adverse Reactions

In addition to the adverse reactions listed above, those listed below have been reported in U.S. clinical trails of ORAP in conditions other than Tourette's Disorder.

Body as a Whole: Asthenia, chest pain, periorbital edema
Cardiovascular/Respiratory: Postural hypotension, hypotension, hypertension, tachycardia, palpitations
Gastrointestinal: Increased salivation, nausea, vomiting, anorexia, GI distress
Endocrine: Loss of libido
Metabolic/Nutritional: Weight gain, weight loss
Central Nervous System: Dizziness, tremor, parkinsonism, fainting, dyskinesia
Psychiatric: Excitement
Skin: Rash, sweating, skin irritation
Special Senses: Blurred vision, cataracts
Urogenital: Nocturia, urinary frequency

Postmarketing Reports

The following experiences were described in spontaneous postmarketing reports. These reports do not provide sufficient information to establish a clear causal relationship will the use of ORAP.
Gastrointestinal: Gingival hyperplasia in one patient
Hematologic: Hemolytic anemia
Metabolic/Nutritional: Hyponatremia
Other: Seizure

OVERDOSAGE

In general, the signs and symptoms of overdosage with ORAP (pimozide) would be an exaggeration of known pharmacologic effects and adverse reactions, the most prominent of which would be: 1) electrocardiographic abnormalities, 2) severe extrapyramidal reactions, 3) hypotension, 4) a comatose state with respiratory depression.
In the event of overdosage, gastric lavage, establishment of a patent airway and, if necessary, mechanically-assisted respiration are advised. Electrocardiographic monitoring should commence immediately and continue until the ECG parameters are within the normal range. Hypotension and circulatory collapse may be counteracted by use of intravenous fluids, plasma, or concentrated albumin, and vasopressor agents such as metaraminol, phenylephrine and norepinephrine. Epinephrine should not be used. In case of severe extrapyramidal reactions, antiparkinson medication should be administered. Because of the long half-life of pimozide, patients who take an overdose should be observed for at least 4 days. As with all drugs, the physician should consider contacting a poison control center for additional information on the treatment of overdose.

DOSAGE AND ADMINISTRATION

General

The suppression of tics by ORAP requires a slow and gradual introduction of the drug. The patient's dose should be carefully adjusted to a point where the suppression of tics and the relief afforded is balanced against the untoward side effects of the drug.
An ECG should be done at baseline and periodically thereafter especially during the period of dose adjustment (see **WARNINGS** and **PRECAUTIONS—Laboratory Tests**).
Periodic attempts should be made to reduce the dosage of ORAP to see whether or not tics persist at the level and extent first identified. In attempts to reduce the dosage of ORAP, consideration should be given to the possibility that increases of tic intensity and frequency may represent a transient, withdrawal-related phenomenon rather than a return of disease symptoms. Specifically, one to two weeks should be allowed to elapse before one concludes that an increase in tic manifestations is a function of the underlying disease syndrome rather than a response to drug withdrawal. A gradual withdrawal is recommended in any case.

Children

Reliable dose response data for the effects of ORAP (pimozide) on tic manifestation in Tourette's Disorder patients below the age of twelve are not available.
Treatment should be initiated at a dose of 0.05 mg/kg preferably taken once at bedtime. The dose may be increased every third day to a maximum of 0.2 mg/kg not to exceed 10 mg/day.

Adults

In general, treatment with ORAP should be initiated with a dose of 1 to 2 mg a day in divided doses. The dose may be increased thereafter every other day. Most patients are maintained at less than 0.2 mg/kg per day, or 10 mg/day, whichever is less. Doses greater than 0.2 mg/kg/day or 10 mg/day are not recommended.

ANIMAL PHARMACOLOGY

A chronic study in dogs indicated that pimozide caused gingival hyperplasia when administered for several months at about 5 times the maximum recommended human dose. This condition was reversible after withdrawal.

HOW SUPPLIED

ORAP® (pimozide) 1 mg tablets are white, oval, scored tablets, debossed "ORAP 1". They are available in bottles of 100 (NDC 57844-151-01).
ORAP® (pimozide) 2 mg tablets are white, oval, scored tablets, debbosed "LEMMON" on one side and "ORAP 2" on the other. They are available in bottles of 100 (NDC 57844-187-01).
Store at controlled room temperature 15°–30°C (59°–86°F).
Dispense in a tight, light-resistant container as defined in the official compendum.
Pharmacist: Dispense in child-resistant container.
Manufactured for:
GATE PHARMACEUTICALS
Div. of TEVA Pharmaceuticals USA
Sellersville, PA 18960

Manufactured by:
TEVA PHARMACEUTICALS USA
Sellersville, PA 18960
Rev. J 8/99

PURINETHOL® ℞

[*pur'in-thawl*]
(mercaptopurine), 50-mg Scored Tablets

CAUTION

PURINETHOL (mercaptopurine) is a potent drug. It should not be used unless a diagnosis of acute lymphatic leukemia has been adequately established and the responsible physician is knowledgeable in assessing response to chemotherapy.

DESCRIPTION

PURINETHOL (mercaptopurine) was synthesized and developed by Hitchings, Elion, and associates at the Wellcome Research Laboratories. It is one of a large series of purine analogues which interfere with nucleic acid biosynthesis and has been found active against human leukemias.
Mercaptopurine, known chemically as 1,7-dihydro-6*H*-purine-6-thione monohydrate, is an analogue of the purine bases adenine and hypoxanthine. Its structural formula is:

PURINETHOL is available in tablet form for oral administration. Each scored tablet contains 50 mg mercaptopurine and the inactive ingredients corn and potato starch, lactose, magnesium stearate, and stearic acid.

CLINICAL PHARMACOLOGY

Clinical studies have shown that the absorption of an oral dose of mercaptopurine in humans is incomplete and variable, averaging approximately 50% of the administered dose. The factors influencing absorption are unknown. Intravenous administration of an investigational preparation of mercaptopurine revealed a plasma half-disappearance time of 21 minutes in pediatric patients and 47 minutes in adults. The volume of distribution usually exceeded that of the total body water.
Following the oral administration of ^{35}S-6-mercaptopurine in one subject, a total of 46% of the dose could be accounted for in the urine (as parent drug and metabolites) in the first 24 hours. Metabolites of mercaptopurine were found in urine within the first 2 hours after administration. Radioactivity (in the form of sulfate) could be found in the urine for weeks afterwards.
There is negligible entry of mercaptopurine into cerebrospinal fluid.
Plasma protein binding averages 19% over the concentration range 10 to 50 mcg/mL (a concentration only achieved by intravenous administration of mercaptopurine at doses exceeding 5 to 10 mg/kg).
Monitoring of plasma levels of mercaptopurine during therapy is of questionable value. There is technical difficulty in determining plasma concentrations which are seldom greater than 1 to 2 mcg/mL after a therapeutic oral dose. More significantly, mercaptopurine enters rapidly into the anabolic and catabolic pathways for purines, and the active intracellular metabolites have appreciably longer half-lives than the parent drug. The biochemical effects of a single dose of mercaptopurine are evident long after the parent drug has disappeared from plasma. Because of this rapid metabolism of mercaptopurine to active intracellular derivatives, hemodialysis would not be expected to appreciably reduce toxicity of the drug. There is no known pharmacologic antagonist to the biochemical actions of mercaptopurine in vivo.
Mercaptopurine competes with hypoxanthine and guanine for the enzyme hypoxanthine-guanine phosphoribosyltransferase (HGPRTase) and is itself converted to thioinosinic acid (TIMP). This intracellular nucleotide inhibits several reactions involving inosinic acid (IMP), including the conversion of IMP to xanthylic acid (XMP) and the conversion of IMP to adenylic acid (AMP) via adenylosuccinate (SAMP). In addition, 6-methylthioinosinate (MTIMP) is formed by the methylation of TIMP. Both TIMP and MTIMP have been reported to inhibit glutamine-5-phosphoribosylpyrophosphate amidotransferase, the first enzyme unique to the de novo pathway for purine ribonucleotide synthesis.
Experiments indicate that radiolabeled mercaptopurine may be recovered from the DNA in the form of deoxythioguanosine. Some mercaptopurine is converted to nucleotide derivatives of 6-thioguanine (6-TG) by the sequential actions of inosinate (IMP) dehydrogenase and xanthylate (XMP) aminase, converting TIMP to thioguanylic acid (TGMP).
Animal tumors that are resistant to mercaptopurine often have lost the ability to convert mercaptopurine to TIMP. However, it is clear that resistance to mercaptopurine may be acquired by other means as well, particularly in human leukemias.
It is not known exactly which of any one or more of the biochemical effects of mercaptopurine and its metabolites are directly or predominantly responsible for cell death.
The catabolism of mercaptopurine and its metabolites is complex. In humans, after oral administration of ^{35}S-6-mercaptopurine, urine contains intact mercaptopurine, thiouric acid (formed by direct oxidation by xanthine oxidase, probably via 6-mercapto-8-hydroxypurine), and a number of 6-methylated thiopurines. The methylthiopurines yield appreciable amounts of inorganic sulfate. The importance of the metabolism by xanthine oxidase relates to the fact that ZYLOPRIM® (allopurinol) inhibits this enzyme and retards the catabolism of mercaptopurine and its active metabolites. A significant reduction in mercaptopurine dosage is mandatory if a potent xanthine oxidase inhibitor and mercaptopurine are used simultaneously in a patient (see PRECAUTIONS).

INDICATIONS AND USAGE

PURINETHOL (mercaptopurine) is indicated for remission induction and maintenance therapy of acute lymphatic leukemia. The response to this agent depends upon the particular subclassification of acute lymphatic leukemia and the age of the patient (pediatric patient or adult).

Acute Lymphatic (Lymphocytic, Lymphoblastic) Leukemia: Given as a single agent for remission induction, PURINETHOL induces complete remission in approximately 25% of pediatric patients and 10% of adults. However, reliance upon PURINETHOL alone is not justified for initial remission induction of acute lymphatic leukemia since combination chemotherapy with vincristine, prednisone, and L-asparaginase results in more frequent complete remission induction than with PURINETHOL alone or in combination. The duration of complete remission induced in acute lymphatic leukemia is so brief without the use of maintenance therapy that some form of drug therapy is considered essential. PURINETHOL, as a single agent, is capable of significantly prolonging complete remission duration; however, combination therapy has produced remission duration longer than that achieved with PURINETHOL alone.

Acute Myelogenous (and Acute Myelomonocytic) Leukemia: As a single agent, PURINETHOL will induce complete remission in approximately 10% of pediatric patients and adults with acute myelogenous leukemia or its subclassifications. These results are inferior to those achieved with combination chemotherapy employing optimum treatment schedules.

Central Nervous System Leukemia: PURINETHOL is not effective for prophylaxis or treatment of central nervous system leukemia.

Other Neoplasms: PURINETHOL is not effective in chronic lymphatic leukemia, the lymphomas (including Hodgkins Disease), or solid tumors.

CONTRAINDICATIONS

PURINETHOL should not be used unless a diagnosis of acute lymphatic leukemia has been adequately established and the responsible physician is knowledgeable in assessing response to chemotherapy.

PURINETHOL should not be used in patients whose disease has demonstrated prior resistance to this drug. In animals and humans, there is usually complete cross-resistance between mercaptopurine and thioguanine.

PURINETHOL should not be used in patients who have a hypersensitivity to mercaptopurine or any component of the formulation.

WARNINGS

SINCE DRUGS USED IN CANCER CHEMOTHERAPY ARE POTENTIALLY HAZARDOUS, IT IS RECOMMENDED THAT ONLY PHYSICIANS EXPERIENCED WITH THE RISKS OF PURINETHOL AND KNOWLEDGEABLE IN THE NATURAL HISTORY OF ACUTE LEUKEMIAS ADMINISTER THIS DRUG.

Bone Marrow Toxicity: The most consistent, dose-related toxicity is bone marrow suppression. This may be manifest by anemia, leukopenia, thrombocytopenia, or any combination of these. Any of these findings may also reflect progression of the underlying disease. Since mercaptopurine may have a delayed effect, it is important to withdraw the medication temporarily at the first sign of an abnormally large fall in any of the formed elements of the blood.

There are individuals with an inherited deficiency of the enzyme thiopurine methyltransferase (TPMT) who may be unusually sensitive to the myelosuppressive effects of mercaptopurine and prone to developing rapid bone marrow suppression following the initiation of treatment. Substantial dosage reductions may be required to avoid the development of life-threatening bone marrow suppression in these patients. This toxicity may be more profound in patients treated with concomitant allopurinol (see PRECAUTIONS: Drug Interactions). This problem could be exacerbated by coadministration with drugs that inhibit TPMT, such as olsalazine, mesalazine, or sulphasalazine.

Hepatotoxicity: Mercaptopurine is hepatotoxic in animals and humans. A small number of deaths have been reported that may have been attributed to hepatic necrosis due to administration of mercaptopurine. Hepatic injury can occur with any dosage, but seems to occur with more frequency when doses of 2.5 mg/kg/day are exceeded. The histologic pattern of mercaptopurine hepatotoxicity includes features of both intrahepatic cholestasis and parenchymal cell necrosis, either of which may predominate. It is not clear how much of the hepatic damage is due to direct toxicity from the drug and how much may be due to a hypersensitivity reaction. In some patients jaundice has cleared following withdrawal of mercaptopurine and reappeared with its reintroduction.

Published reports have cited widely varying incidences of overt hepatotoxicity. In a large series of patients with various neoplastic diseases, mercaptopurine was administered orally in doses ranging from 2.5 mg/kg to 5.0 mg/kg without any evidence of hepatotoxicity. It was noted by the authors that no definite clinical evidence of liver damage could be ascribed to the drug, although an occasional case of serum hepatitis did occur in patients receiving 6-MP who previously had transfusions. In reports of smaller cohorts of adult and pediatric leukemic patients, the incidence of hepatotoxicity ranged from 0% to 6%. In an isolated report by Einhorn and Davidsohn, jaundice was observed more frequently (40%), especially when doses exceeded 2.5 mg/kg. Usually, clinically detectable jaundice appears early in the course of treatment (1 to 2 months). However, jaundice has been reported as early as 1 week and as late as 8 years after the start of treatment with mercaptopurine.

Monitoring of serum transaminase levels, alkaline phosphatase, and bilirubin levels may allow early detection of hepatotoxicity. It is advisable to monitor these liver function tests at weekly intervals when first beginning therapy and at monthly intervals thereafter. Liver function tests may be advisable more frequently in patients who are receiving mercaptopurine with other hepatotoxic drugs or with known pre-existing liver disease.

The concomitant administration of mercaptopurine with other hepatotoxic agents requires especially careful clinical and biochemical monitoring of hepatic function. Combination therapy involving mercaptopurine with other drugs not felt to be hepatotoxic should nevertheless be approached with caution. The combination of mercaptopurine with doxorubicin was reported to be hepatotoxic in 19 of 20 patients undergoing remission-induction therapy for leukemia resistant to previous therapy.

The hepatotoxicity has been associated in some cases with anorexia, diarrhea, jaundice, and ascites. Hepatic encephalopathy has occurred.

The onset of clinical jaundice, hepatomegaly, or anorexia with tenderness in the right hypochondrium are immediate indications for withholding mercaptopurine until the exact etiology can be identified. Likewise, any evidence of deterioration in liver function studies, toxic hepatitis, or biliary stasis should prompt discontinuation of the drug and a search for an etiology of the hepatotoxicity.

Immunosuppression: Mercaptopurine recipients may manifest decreased cellular hypersensitivities and impaired allograft rejection. Induction of immunity to infectious agents or vaccines will be subnormal in these patients; the degree of immunosuppression will depend on antigen dose and temporal relationship to drug. This immunosuppressive effect should be carefully considered with regard to intercurrent infections and risk of subsequent neoplasia.

Pregnancy: Pregnancy Category D. Mercaptopurine can cause fetal harm when administered to a pregnant woman. Women receiving mercaptopurine in the first trimester of pregnancy have an increased incidence of abortion; the risk of malformation in offspring surviving first trimester exposure is not accurately known. In a series of 28 women receiving mercaptopurine after the first trimester of pregnancy, 3 mothers died undelivered, 1 delivered a stillborn child, and 1 aborted; there were no cases of macroscopically abnormal fetuses. Since such experience cannot exclude the possibility of fetal damage, mercaptopurine should be used during pregnancy only if the benefit clearly justifies the possible risk to the fetus, and particular caution should be given to the use of mercaptopurine in the first trimester of pregnancy.

There are no adequate and well-controlled studies in pregnant women. If this drug is used during pregnancy or if the patient becomes pregnant while taking the drug, the patient should be apprised of the potential hazard to the fetus. Women of childbearing potential should be advised to avoid becoming pregnant.

PRECAUTIONS

General: The safe and effective use of PURINETHOL demands a thorough knowledge of the natural history of the condition being treated. After selection of an initial dosage schedule, therapy will frequently need to be modified depending upon the patient's response and manifestations of toxicity.

The most frequent, serious, toxic effect of PURINETHOL is myelosuppression resulting in leukopenia, thrombocytopenia, and anemia. These toxic effects are often unavoidable during the induction phase of adult acute leukemia if remission induction is to be successful. Whether or not these manifestations demand modification or cessation of dosage depends both upon the response of the underlying disease and a careful consideration of supportive facilities (granulocyte and platelet transfusions) which may be available. Life-threatening infections and bleeding have been observed as a consequence of mercaptopurine-induced granulocytopenia and thrombocytopenia. Severe hematologic toxicity may require supportive therapy with platelet transfusions for bleeding, and antibiotics and granulocyte transfusions if sepsis is documented.

If it is not the intent to deliberately induce bone marrow hypoplasia, it is important to discontinue the drug temporarily at the first evidence of an abnormally large fall in white blood cell count, platelet count, or hemoglobin concentration. In many patients with severe depression of the formed elements of the blood due to PURINETHOL, the bone marrow appears hypoplastic on aspiration or biopsy, whereas in other cases it may appear normocellular. The qualitative changes in the erythroid elements toward the megaloblastic series, characteristically seen with the folic acid antagonists and some other antimetabolites, are not seen with this drug.

It is probably advisable to start with smaller dosages in patients with impaired renal function, since the latter might result in slower elimination of the drug and metabolites and a greater cumulative effect.

Information for Patients: Patients should be informed that the major toxicities of PURINETHOL are related to myelosuppression, hepatotoxicity, and gastrointestinal toxicity. Patients should never be allowed to take the drug without medical supervision and should be advised to consult their physician if they experience fever, sore throat, jaundice, nausea, vomiting, signs of local infection, bleeding from any site, or symptoms suggestive of anemia. Women of childbearing potential should be advised to avoid becoming pregnant.

Laboratory Tests: It is recommended that evaluation of the hemoglobin or hematocrit, total white blood cell count and differential count, and quantitative platelet count be obtained weekly while the patient is on therapy with PURINETHOL. In cases where the cause of fluctuations in the formed elements in the peripheral blood is obscure, bone marrow examination may be useful for the evaluation of marrow status. The decision to increase, decrease, continue, or discontinue a given dosage of PURINETHOL must be based not only on the absolute hematologic values, but also upon the rapidity with which changes are occurring. In many instances, particularly during the induction phase of acute leukemia, complete blood counts will need to be done more frequently than once weekly in order to evaluate the effect of the therapy.

Drug Interactions: When allopurinol and mercaptopurine are administered concomitantly, it is imperative that the dose of mercaptopurine be reduced to one third to one quarter of the usual dose. Failure to observe this dosage reduction will result in a delayed catabolism of mercaptopurine and the strong likelihood of inducing severe toxicity.

There is usually complete cross-resistance between mercaptopurine and thioguanine.

The dosage of mercaptopurine may need to be reduced when this agent is combined with other drugs whose primary or secondary toxicity is myelosuppression. Enhanced marrow suppression has been noted in some patients also receiving trimethoprim-sulfamethoxazole.

Inhibition of the anticoagulant effect of warfarin, when given with mercaptopurine, has been reported.

As there is in vitro evidence that aminosalicylate derivatives (e.g., olsalazine, mesalazine, or sulphasalazine) inhibit the TPMT enzyme, they should be administered with caution to patients receiving concurrent mercaptopurine therapy (see WARNINGS).

Carcinogenesis, Mutagenesis, Impairment of Fertility: Mercaptopurine causes chromosomal aberrations in animals and humans and induces dominant-lethal mutations in male mice. In mice, surviving female offspring of mothers who received chronic low doses of mercaptopurine during pregnancy were found sterile, or if they became pregnant, had smaller litters and more dead fetuses as compared to control animals. Carcinogenic potential exists in humans, but the extent of the risk is unknown.

The effect of mercaptopurine on human fertility is unknown for either males or females.

Pregnancy: ***Teratogenic Effects:*** Pregnancy Category D. See WARNINGS section.

Nursing Mothers: It is not known whether this drug is excreted in human milk. Because many drugs are excreted in human milk, and because of the potential for serious adverse reactions in nursing infants from mercaptopurine, a decision should be made whether to discontinue nursing or to discontinue the drug, taking into account the importance of the drug to the mother.

Pediatric Use: See DOSAGE AND ADMINISTRATION section.

ADVERSE REACTIONS

The principal and potentially serious toxic effects of PURINETHOL are bone marrow toxicity and hepatotoxicity (see WARNINGS).

Hematologic: The most frequent adverse reaction to PURINETHOL is myelosuppression. The induction of complete remission of acute lymphatic leukemia frequently is associated with marrow hypoplasia. Maintenance of remission generally involves multiple-drug regimens whose component agents cause myelosuppression. Anemia, leukopenia, and thrombocytopenia are frequently observed. Dosages and schedules are adjusted to prevent life-threatening cytopenias.

Renal: Hyperuricemia and/or hyperuricosuria may occur in patients receiving PURINETHOL as a consequence of rapid cell lysis accompanying the antineoplastic effect. Adverse effects can be minimized by increased hydration, urine alkalinization, and the prophylactic administration of a xanthine oxidase inhibitor such as allopurinol. The dosage of PURINETHOL should be reduced to one third to one quarter of the usual dose if allopurinol is given concurrently.

Gastrointestinal: Intestinal ulceration has been reported. Nausea, vomiting, and anorexia are uncommon during initial administration. Mild diarrhea and sprue-like symptoms have been noted occasionally, but it is difficult at present to attribute these to the medication. Oral lesions are rarely seen, and when they occur they resemble thrush rather than antifolic ulcerations.

An increased risk of pancreatitis may be associated with the investigational use of PURINETHOL in inflammatory bowel disease.

Miscellaneous: While dermatologic reactions can occur as a consequence of disease, the administration of PURINETHOL has been associated with skin rashes and hyperpigmentation. Alopecia has been reported.

Drug fever has been very rarely reported with PURINETHOL. Before attributing fever to PURINETHOL,

Continued on next page

Purinethol—Cont.

every attempt should be made to exclude more common causes of pyrexia, such as sepsis, in patients with acute leukemia.

Oligospermia has been reported.

OVERDOSAGE

Signs and symptoms of overdosage may be immediate such as anorexia, nausea, vomiting, and diarrhea; or delayed such as myelosuppression, liver dysfunction, and gastroenteritis. Dialysis cannot be expected to clear mercaptopurine. Hemodialysis is thought to be of marginal use due to the rapid intracellular incorporation of mercaptopurine into active metabolites with long persistence. The oral LD_{50} of mercaptopurine was determined to be 480 mg/kg in the mouse and 425 mg/kg in the rat.

There is no known pharmacologic antagonist of mercaptopurine. The drug should be discontinued immediately if unintended toxicity occurs during treatment. If a patient is seen immediately following an accidental overdosage of the drug, it may be useful to induce emesis.

DOSAGE AND ADMINISTRATION

Induction Therapy: PURINETHOL is administered orally. The dosage which will be tolerated and be effective varies from patient to patient, and therefore careful titration is necessary to obtain the optimum therapeutic effect without incurring excessive, unintended toxicity. The usual initial dosage for pediatric patients and adults is 2.5 mg/kg of body weight per day (100 to 200 mg in the average adult and 50 mg in an average 5-year-old child). Pediatric patients with acute leukemia have tolerated this dose without difficulty in most cases; it may be continued daily for several weeks or more in some patients. If, after 4 weeks at this dosage, there is no clinical improvement and no definite evidence of leukocyte or platelet depression, the dosage may be increased up to 5 mg/kg daily. A dosage of 2.5 mg/kg/day may result in a rapid fall in leukocyte count within 1 to 2 weeks in some adults with acute lymphatic leukemia and high total leukocyte counts.

The total daily dosage may be given at one time. It is calculated to the nearest multiple of 25 mg. The dosage of PURINETHOL should be reduced to one third to one quarter of the usual dose if allopurinol is given concurrently. Because the drug may have a delayed action, it should be discontinued at the first sign of an abnormally large or rapid fall in the leukocyte or platelet count. If subsequently the leukocyte count or platelet count remains constant for 2 or 3 days, or rises, treatment may be resumed.

Maintenance Therapy: Once a complete hematologic remission is obtained, maintenance therapy is considered essential. Maintenance doses will vary from patient to patient. A usual daily maintenance dose of PURINETHOL is 1.5 to 2.5 mg/kg/day as a single dose. It is to be emphasized that in pediatric patients with acute lymphatic leukemia in remission, superior results have been obtained when PURINETHOL has been combined with other agents (most frequently with methotrexate) for remission maintenance. PURINETHOL should rarely be relied upon as a single agent for the maintenance of remissions induced in acute leukemia.

Procedures for proper handling and disposal of anticancer drugs should be considered. Several guidelines on this subject have been published.[1–8]

There is no general agreement that all of the procedures recommended in the guidelines are necessary or appropriate.

Dosage in Renal Impairment: Consideration should be given to reducing the dosage in patients with impaired renal function.

Dosage in Hepatic Impairment: Consideration should be given to reducing the dosage in patients with impaired hepatic function.

HOW SUPPLIED

Pale yellow to buff, scored tablets containing 50 mg mercaptopurine, imprinted with "PURINETHOL" and "04A"; bottles of 60 (NDC 57844-522-06).

Store at 15° to 25°C (59° to 77°F) in a dry place.

REFERENCES

1. ONS Clinical Practice Committee. Cancer Chemotherapy Guidelines and Recommendations for Practice. Pittsburgh, PA: Oncology Nursing Society;1999:32-41.
2. Recommendations for the safe handling of parenteral antineoplastic drugs. Washington, DC: Division of Safety; Clinical Center Pharmacy Department and Cancer Nursing Services, National Institutes of Health; 1992. US Dept of Health and Human Services. Public Health Service publication NIH 92-2621.
3. AMA Council on Scientific Affairs. Guidelines for handling parenteral antineoplastics. *JAMA.* 1985;253:1590-1591.
4. National Study Commission on Cytotoxic Exposure. Recommendations for handling cytotoxic agents. 1987. Available from Louis P. Jeffrey, Chairman, National Study Commission on Cytotoxic Exposure. Massachusetts College of Pharmacy and Allied Health Sciences, 179 Longwood Avenue, Boston, MA 02115.
5. Clinical Oncological Society of Australia. Guidelines and recommendations for safe handling of antineoplastic agents. *Med J Australia.* 1983;1:426-428.
6. Jones RB, Frank R, Mass T. Safe handling of chemotherapeutic agents: a report from the Mount Sinai Medical Center. *CA-A Cancer J for Clinicians.* 1983;33:258-263.
7. American Society of Hospital Pharmacists. ASHP technical assistance bulletin on handling cytotoxic and hazardous drugs. *Am J Hosp Pharm.* 1990;47:1033-1049.
8. Controlling Occupational Exposure to Hazardous Drugs. (OSHA Work-Practice Guidelines.) *Am J Health-Syst Pharm.* 1996;53:1669-1685.

Manufactured for:
GATE PHARMACEUTICALS
div. of Teva Pharmaceuticals USA
Sellersville, PA 18960
Manufactured by DSM Pharmaceuticals, Inc.
Greenville, NC 27834
Rev. A 10/2003

Genentech, Inc.

1 DNA WAY
SOUTH SAN FRANCISCO, CA 94080-4990

Contact:
Genentech, Inc
1 DNA Way
South San Francisco, CA 94080-4990
(650) 225-1000
www.gene.com
For Medical Information
Contact
1-800-821-8590
medinfo@gene.com
For Customer Service
Contact
1-800-551-2231
For Reimbursement Support
Contact
1-888-249-4918

ACTIVASE® ℞
(Alteplase)

DESCRIPTION

Activase (Alteplase) is a tissue plasminogen activator produced by recombinant DNA technology. It is a sterile, purified glycoprotein of 527 amino acids. It is synthesized using the complementary DNA (cDNA) for natural human tissue-type plasminogen activator obtained from a human melanoma cell line. The manufacturing process involves the secretion of the enzyme alteplase into the culture medium by an established mammalian cell line (Chinese Hamster Ovary cells) into which the cDNA for alteplase has been genetically inserted. Fermentation is carried out in a nutrient medium containing the antibiotic gentamicin, 100 mg/L. However, the presence of the antibiotic is not detectable in the final product.

Phosphoric acid and/or sodium hydroxide may be used prior to lyophilization for pH adjustment.

Activase is a sterile, white to off-white, lyophilized powder for intravenous administration after reconstitution with Sterile Water for Injection, USP.

Quantitative Composition of the Lyophilized Product

	100 mg Vial	50 mg Vial
Alteplase	100 mg (58 million IU)	50 mg (29 million IU)
L-Arginine	3.5 g	1.7 g
Phosphoric Acid	1 g	0.5 g
Polysorbate 80	≤ 11 mg	≤ 4 mg
Vacuum	No	Yes

Biological potency is determined by an in vitro clot lysis assay and is expressed in International Units as tested against the WHO standard. The specific activity of Activase is 580,000 IU/mg.

CLINICAL PHARMACOLOGY

Activase is an enzyme (serine protease) which has the property of fibrin-enhanced conversion of plasminogen to plasmin. It produces limited conversion of plasminogen in the absence of fibrin. When introduced into the systemic circulation at pharmacologic concentration, Activase binds to fibrin in a thrombus and converts the entrapped plasminogen to plasmin. This initiates local fibrinolysis with limited systemic proteolysis. Following administration of 100 mg Activase, there is a decrease (16%–36%) in circulating fibrinogen.[1,2] In a controlled trial, 8 of 73 patients (11%) receiving Activase (1.25 mg/kg body weight over 3 hours) experienced a decrease in fibrinogen to below 100 mg/dL.[2]

The clearance of Alteplase in AMI patients has shown that it is rapidly cleared from the plasma with an initial half-life of less than 5 minutes. There is no difference in the dominant initial plasma half-life between the 3-Hour and accelerated regimens for AMI. The plasma clearance of Alteplase is 380–570 mL/min.[3,4] The clearance is mediated primarily by the liver. The initial volume of distribution approximates plasma volume.

Acute Myocardial Infarction (AMI) Patients

Coronary occlusion due to a thrombus is present in the infarct-related coronary artery in approximately 80% of patients experiencing a transmural myocardial infarction evaluated within 4 hours of onset of symptoms.[5,6]

Two Activase dose regimens have been studied in patients experiencing acute myocardial infarction. (Please see DOSAGE AND ADMINISTRATION.) The comparative efficacy of these two regimens has not been evaluated.

Accelerated Infusion in AMI Patients

Accelerated infusion of Activase was studied in an international, multi-center trial (GUSTO) that randomized 41,021 patients with acute myocardial infarction to four thrombolytic regimens. Entry criteria included onset of chest pain within 6 hours of treatment and ST-segment elevation of ECG. The regimens included accelerated infusion of Activase (≤ 100 mg over 90 minutes, see DOSAGE AND ADMINISTRATION) plus intravenous (IV) heparin (accelerated infusion of Alteplase, n=10,396), or the Kabikinase brand of Streptokinase (1.5 million units over 60 minutes) plus IV heparin (SK [IV], n=10,410), or Streptokinase (as above) plus subcutaneous (SQ) heparin (SK [SQ], n=9841). A fourth regimen combined Alteplase and Streptokinase. Aspirin and heparin use was directed by the GUSTO study protocol as follows: All patients were to receive 160 mg chewable aspirin administered as soon as possible, followed by 160–325 mg daily. IV heparin was directed to be a 5000 U IV bolus initiated as soon as possible, followed by a 1000 U/hour continuous IV infusion for at least 48 hours; subsequent heparin therapy was at the discretion of the attending physician. SQ heparin was directed to be 12,500 U administered 4 hours after initiation of SK therapy, followed by 12,500 U twice daily for 7 days or until discharge, whichever came first. Many of the patients randomized to receive SQ heparin received some IV heparin, usually in response to recurrent chest pain and/or the need for a medical procedure. Some received IV heparin on arrival to the emergency room prior to enrollment and randomization.

Results for the primary endpoint of the study, 30-day mortality, are shown in Table 1. The incidence of 30-day mortality for accelerated infusion of Alteplase was 1.0% lower than for SK (IV) and 1.0% lower than for SK (SQ). The secondary endpoints of combined 30-day mortality or nonfatal stroke, and 24-hour mortality, as well as the safety endpoints of total stroke and intracerebral hemorrhage are also shown in Table 1. The incidence of combined 30-day mortality or nonfatal stroke for the Alteplase accelerated infusion was 1.0% lower than for SK (IV) and 0.8% lower than for SK (SQ).

[See table 1 below]

Subgroup analysis of patients by age, infarct location, time from symptom onset to thrombolytic treatment, and treatment in the U.S. or elsewhere showed consistently lower 30-day mortality for the Alteplase accelerated infusion group. For patients who were over 75 years of age, a predefined subgroup consisting of 12% of patients enrolled, the incidence of stroke was 4.0% for the Alteplase accelerated infusion group, 2.8% for SK (IV), and 3.2% for SK (SQ); the incidence of combined 30-day mortality or nonfatal stroke was 20.6% for accelerated infusion of Alteplase, 21.5% for SK (IV), and 22.0% for SK (SQ).

An angiographic substudy of the GUSTO trial provided data on infarct-related artery patency. Table 2 presents 90-minute, 180-minute, 24-hour, and 5–7 day patency values by TIMI flow grade for the three treatment regimens. Reocclusion rates were similar for all three treatment regimens.

[See table 2 at top of next page]

The exact relationship between coronary artery patency and clinical activity has not been established.

The safety and efficacy of the accelerated infusion of Alteplase have not been evaluated using antithrombotic or antiplatelet regimens other than those used in the GUSTO trial.

3-Hour Infusion in AMI Patients

In patients studied in a controlled trial with coronary angiography at 90 and 120 minutes following infusion of Acti-

Table 1

Event	Accelerated Activase	SK (IV)	p-Value[1]	SK (SQ)	p-Value[1]
30-Day Mortality	6.3%	7.3%	0.003	7.3%	0.007
30-Day Mortality or Nonfatal Stroke	7.2%	8.2%	0.006	8.0%	0.036
24-Hour Mortality	2.4%	2.9%	0.009	2.8%	0.029
Any Stroke	1.6%	1.4%	0.32	1.2%	0.03
Intracerebral Hemorrhage	0.7%	0.6%	0.22	0.5%	0.02

[1] *Two-tailed p-value is for comparison of Accelerated Activase to the respective SK control arm.*

vase, infarct artery patency was observed in 71% and 85% of patients (n=85), respectively.[2] In a second study, where patients received coronary angiography prior to and following infusion of Activase within 6 hours of the onset of symptoms, reperfusion of the obstructed vessel occurred within 90 minutes after the commencement of therapy in 71% of 83 patients.[1]

The exact relationship between coronary artery patency and clinical activity has not been established.

In a double-blind, randomized trial (138 patients) comparing Activase to placebo, patients infused with Activase within 4 hours of onset of symptoms experienced improved left ventricular function at Day 10 compared to the placebo group, when ejection fraction was measured by gated blood pool scan (53.2% vs 46.4%, p=0.018). Relative to baseline (Day 1) values, the net changes in ejection fraction were +3.6% and −4.7% for the treated and placebo groups, respectively (p=0.0001). Also documented was a reduced incidence of clinical congestive heart failure in the treated group (14%) compared to the placebo group (33%) (p=0.009).[7]

In a double-blind, randomized trial (145 patients) comparing Activase to placebo, patients infused with Activase within 2.5 hours of onset of symptoms experienced improved left ventricular function at a mean of 21 days compared to the placebo group, when ejection fraction was measured by gated blood pool scan (52% vs 48%, p=0.08) and by contrast ventriculogram (61% vs 54%, p=0.006). Although the contribution of Activase alone is unclear, the incidence of nonischemic cardiac complications when taken as a group (i.e., congestive heart failure, pericarditis, atrial fibrillation, and conduction disturbance) was reduced when compared to those patients treated with placebo ($p < 0.01$).[8]

In a double-blind, randomized trial (5013 patients) comparing Activase to placebo (ASSET study), patients infused with Activase within 5 hours of the onset of symptoms of acute myocardial infarction experienced improved 30-day survival compared to those treated with placebo. At 1 month, the overall mortality rates were 7.2% for the Activase-treated group and 9.8% for the placebo-treated group (p=0.001).[9,10] This benefit was maintained at 6 months for Activase-treated patients (10.4%) compared to those treated with placebo (13.1%, p=0.008).[10]

In a double-blind, randomized trial (721 patients) comparing Activase to placebo, patients infused with Activase within 5 hours of the onset of symptoms experienced improved ventricular function 10–22 days after treatment compared to the placebo group, when global ejection fraction was measured by contrast ventriculography (50.7% vs 48.5%, p=0.01). Patients treated with Activase had a 19% reduction in infarct size, as measured by cumulative release of HBD (α-hydroxybutyrate dehydrogenase) activity compared to placebo-treated patients (p=0.001). Patients treated with Activase had significantly fewer episodes of cardiogenic shock (p=0.02), ventricular fibrillation ($p < 0.04$) and pericarditis (p=0.01) compared to patients treated with placebo. Mortality at 21 days in Activase-treated patients was reduced to 3.7% compared to 6.3% in placebo-treated patients (1-sided p=0.05).[11] Although these data do not demonstrate unequivocally a significant reduction in mortality for this study, they do indicate a trend that is supported by the results of the ASSET study.

Acute Ischemic Stroke Patients

Two placebo-controlled, double-blind trials (The NINDS t-PA Stroke Trial, Part 1 and Part 2) have been conducted in patients with acute ischemic stroke.[12] Both studies enrolled patients with measurable neurological deficit who could complete screening and begin study treatment within 3 hours from symptom onset. A cranial computerized tomography (CT) scan was performed prior to treatment to rule out the presence of intracranial hemorrhage (ICH). Patients were also excluded for the presence of conditions related to risks of bleeding (see CONTRAINDICATIONS), for minor neurological deficit, for rapidly improving symptoms prior to initiating study treatment, or for blood glucose of < 50 mg/dL or > 400 mg/dL.

Patients were randomized to receive either 0.9 mg/kg Activase (maximum of 90 mg), or placebo. Activase was administered as a 10% initial bolus over 1 minute followed by continuous intravenous infusion of the remainder over 60 minutes (see DOSAGE AND ADMINISTRATION). In patients without recent use of oral anticoagulants or heparin, study treatment was initiated prior to the availability of coagulation study results. However, the infusion was discontinued if either a pretreatment prothrombin time (PT) > 15 seconds or an elevated activated partial thromboplastin time (aPTT) was identified. Although patients with or without prior aspirin use were enrolled, administration of anticoagulants and antiplatelet agents was prohibited for the first 24 hours following symptom onset.

The initial study (NINDS-Part 1, n=291) evaluated neurological improvement at 24 hours after stroke onset. The primary endpoint, the proportion of patients with a 4 or more point improvement in the National Institutes of Health Stroke Scale (NIHSS) score or complete recovery (NIHSS score = 0), was not significantly different between treatment groups. A secondary analysis suggested improved 3-month outcome associated with Activase treatment using the following stroke assessment scales: Barthel Index, Modified Rankin Scale, Glasgow Outcome Scale, and the NIHSS.

A second study (NINDS-Part 2, n=333) assessed clinical outcome at 3 months as the primary outcome. A favorable outcome was defined as minimal or no disability using the four stroke assessment scales: Barthel Index (score ≥ 95), Modified Rankin Scale (score ≤ 1), Glasgow Outcome Scale (score = 1), and NIHSS (score ≤ 1). The results comparing Activase- and placebo-treated patients for the four outcome scales together (Generalized Estimating Equations) and individually are presented in Table 3. In this study, depending upon the scale, the favorable outcome of minimal or no disability occurred in at least 11 per 100 more patients treated with Activase than those receiving placebo. Secondary analyses demonstrated consistent functional and neurological improvement within all four stroke scales as indicated by median scores. These results were highly consistent with the 3-month outcome treatment effects observed in the Part 1 study.

[See table 3 above]

Table 2

Patency (TIMI 2 or 3)	Accelerated Activase	SK (IV)	p-Value	SK (SQ)	p-Value
90-Minute	n=272 81.3%	n=261 59.0%	< 0.0001	n=260 53.5%	< 0.0001
180-Minute	n=80 76.3%	n=76 72.4%	0.58	n=95 71.6%	0.48
24-Hour	n=81 88.9%	n=72 87.5%	0.24	n=67 82.1%	0.79
5–7 Day	n=72 83.3%	n=77 90.9%	0.47	n=75 78.7%	0.17

Table 3
The NINDS t-PA Stroke Trial, Part 2
3-Month Efficacy Outcomes

	Frequency of Favorable Outcome[1]				
Analysis	Placebo (n=165)	Activase (n=168)	Absolute Difference (95% CI)	Relative Frequency[2] (95% CI)	p-Value[3]
Generalized Estimating Equations (Multivariate)	—	—	—	1.34 (1.05, 1.72)	0.02
Barthel Index	37.6%	50.0%	12.4% (3.0, 21.9)	1.33 (1.04, 1.71)	0.02
Modified Rankin Scale	26.1%	38.7%	12.6% (3.7, 21.6)	1.48 (1.08, 2.04)	0.02
Glasgow Outcome Scale	31.5%	44.0%	12.5% (3.3, 21.8)	1.40 (1.05, 1.85)	0.02
NIHSS	20.0%	31.0%	11.0% (2.6, 19.3)	1.55 (1.06, 2.26)	0.02

[1]Favorable Outcome is defined as recovery with minimal or no disability.
[2]Value > 1 indicates frequency of recovery in favor of Activase treatment.
[3]p-Value for Relative Frequency is from Generalized Estimating Equations with log link.

Table 4
The NINDS t-PA Stroke Trial
Safety Outcome

	Part 1 and Part 2 Combined		
	Placebo (n=312)	Activase (n=312)	p-Value[2]
All-Cause 90-day Mortality	64 (20.5%)	54 (17.3%)	0.36
Total ICH[1]	20 (6.4%)	48 (15.4%)	< 0.01
Symptomatic	4 (1.3%)	25 (8.0%)	< 0.01
Asymptomatic	16 (5.1%)	23 (7.4%)	0.32
Symptomatic ICH within 36 hours	2 (0.6%)	20 (6.4%)	< 0.01
New Ischemic Stroke (3-months)	17 (5.4%)	18 (5.8%)	1.00

[1] *Within trial follow-up period. Symptomatic ICH was defined as the occurrence of sudden clinical worsening followed by subsequent verification of ICH on CT scan. Asymptomatic ICH was defined as ICH detected on a routine repeat CT scan without preceding clinical worsening.*
[2]Fisher's Exact Test

The incidences of all-cause 90-day mortality, ICH, and new ischemic stroke following Activase treatment compared to placebo are presented in Table 4 as a combined safety analysis (n=624) for Parts 1 and 2. These data indicated a significant increase in ICH following Activase treatment, particularly symptomatic ICH within 36 hours. In Activase-treated patients, there were no increases compared to placebo in the incidences of 90-day mortality or severe disability.

[See table 4 above]

In a prespecified subgroup analysis in patients receiving aspirin prior to onset of stroke symptoms, there was preserved favorable outcome for Activase-treated patients.

Exploratory, multivariate analyses of both studies combined (n=624) to investigate potential predictors of ICH and treatment effect modifiers were performed. In Activase-treated patients presenting with severe neurological deficit (e.g., NIHSS > 22) or of advanced age (e.g., > 77 years of age), the trends toward increased risk for symptomatic ICH within the first 36 hours were more prominent. Similar trends were also seen for total ICH and for all-cause 90-day mortality in these patients. When risk was assessed by the combination of death and severe disability in these patients, there was no difference between placebo and Activase groups. Analyses for efficacy suggested a reduced but still favorable clinical outcome for Activase-treated patients with severe neurological deficit or advanced age at presentation.

Pulmonary Embolism Patients

In a comparative randomized trial (n=45),[13] 59% of patients (n=22) treated with Activase (100 mg over 2 hours) experienced moderate or marked lysis of pulmonary emboli when assessed by pulmonary angiography 2 hours after treatment initiation. Activase-treated patients also experienced a significant reduction in pulmonary embolism-induced pulmonary hypertension within 2 hours of treatment (p=0.003). Pulmonary perfusion at 24 hours, as assessed by radionuclide scan, was significantly improved (p=0.002).

INDICATIONS AND USAGE

Acute Myocardial Infarction

Activase® (Alteplase) is indicated for use in the management of acute myocardial infarction in adults for the improvement of ventricular function following AMI, the reduction of the incidence of congestive heart failure, and the reduction of mortality associated with AMI. Treatment should be initiated as soon as possible after the onset of AMI symptoms (see CLINICAL PHARMACOLOGY).

Acute Ischemic Stroke

Activase® (Alteplase) is indicated for the management of acute ischemic stroke in adults for improving neurological recovery and reducing the incidence of disability. **Treatment should only be initiated within 3 hours after the onset of stroke symptoms, and after exclusion of intracranial hemorrhage by a cranial computerized tomography (CT) scan or other diagnostic imaging method sensitive for the presence of hemorrhage (see CONTRAINDICATIONS).**

Pulmonary Embolism

Activase® (Alteplase) is indicated in the management of acute massive pulmonary embolism (PE) in adults:

— For the lysis of acute pulmonary emboli, defined as obstruction of blood flow to a lobe or multiple segments of the lungs.

— For the lysis of pulmonary emboli accompanied by unstable hemodynamics, e.g., failure to maintain blood pressure without supportive measures.

The diagnosis should be confirmed by objective means, such as pulmonary angiography or noninvasive procedures such as lung scanning.

Continued on next page

Activase—Cont.

CONTRAINDICATIONS

Acute Myocardial Infarction or Pulmonary Embolism

Activase therapy in patients with acute myocardial infarction or pulmonary embolism is contraindicated in the following situations because of an increased risk of bleeding:

- **Active internal bleeding**
- **History of cerebrovascular accident**
- **Recent intracranial or intraspinal surgery or trauma (see WARNINGS)**
- **Intracranial neoplasm, arteriovenous malformation, or aneurysm**
- **Known bleeding diathesis**
- **Severe uncontrolled hypertension**

Acute Ischemic Stroke

Activase therapy in patients with acute ischemic stroke is contraindicated in the following situations because of an increased risk of bleeding, which could result in significant disability or death:

- **Evidence of intracranial hemorrhage on pretreatment evaluation**
- **Suspicion of subarachnoid hemorrhage on pretreatment evaluation**
- **Recent (within 3 months) intracranial or intraspinal surgery, serious head trauma, or previous stroke**
- **History of intracranial hemorrhage**
- **Uncontrolled hypertension at time of treatment (e.g., > 185 mm Hg systolic or > 110 mm Hg diastolic)**
- **Seizure at the onset of stroke**
- **Active internal bleeding**
- **Intracranial neoplasm, arteriovenous malformation, or aneurysm**
- **Known bleeding diathesis including but not limited to:**
  - **— Current use of oral anticoagulants (e.g., warfarin sodium) or an International Normalized Ratio (INR) >1.7 or a prothrombin time (PT) > 15 seconds**
  - **— Administration of heparin within 48 hours preceding the onset of stroke and have an elevated activated partial thromboplastin time (aPTT) at presentation**
  - **— Platelet count < 100,000/mm^3**

WARNINGS

Bleeding

The most common complication encountered during Activase therapy is bleeding. The type of bleeding associated with thrombolytic therapy can be divided into two broad categories:

- Internal bleeding, involving intracranial and retroperitoneal sites, or the gastrointestinal, genitourinary, or respiratory tracts.
- Superficial or surface bleeding, observed mainly at invaded or disturbed sites (e.g., venous cutdowns, arterial punctures, sites of recent surgical intervention).

The concomitant use of heparin anticoagulation may contribute to bleeding. Some of the hemorrhage episodes occurred 1 or more days after the effects of Activase had dissipated, but while heparin therapy was continuing.

As fibrin is lysed during Activase therapy, bleeding from recent puncture sites may occur. Therefore, thrombolytic therapy requires careful attention to all potential bleeding sites (including catheter insertion sites, arterial and venous puncture sites, cutdown sites, and needle puncture sites).

Intramuscular injections and nonessential handling of the patient should be avoided during treatment with Activase. Venipunctures should be performed carefully and only as required.

Should an arterial puncture be necessary during an infusion of Activase, it is preferable to use an upper extremity vessel that is accessible to manual compression. Pressure should be applied for at least 30 minutes, a pressure dressing applied, and the puncture site checked frequently for evidence of bleeding.

Should serious bleeding (not controllable by local pressure) occur, the infusion of Activase and any concomitant heparin should be terminated immediately.

Each patient being considered for therapy with Activase should be carefully evaluated and anticipated benefits weighed against potential risks associated with therapy.

In the following conditions, the risks of Activase therapy for all approved indications may be increased and should be weighed against the anticipated benefits:

- Recent major surgery, e.g., coronary artery bypass graft, obstetrical delivery, organ biopsy, previous puncture of noncompressible vessels
- Cerebrovascular disease
- Recent gastrointestinal or genitourinary bleeding
- Recent trauma
- Hypertension: systolic BP ≥175 mm Hg and/or diastolic BP ≥110 mm Hg
- High likelihood of left heart thrombus, e.g., mitral stenosis with atrial fibrillation
- Acute pericarditis
- Subacute bacterial endocarditis
- Hemostatic defects including those secondary to severe hepatic or renal disease
- Significant hepatic dysfunction
- Pregnancy
- Diabetic hemorrhagic retinopathy, or other hemorrhagic ophthalmic conditions
- Septic thrombophlebitis or occluded AV cannula at seriously infected site
- Advanced age (e.g., over 75 years old)
- Patients currently receiving oral anticoagulants, e.g., warfarin sodium
- Any other condition in which bleeding constitutes a significant hazard or would be particularly difficult to manage because of its location

Cholesterol Embolization

Cholesterol embolism has been reported rarely in patients treated with all types of thrombolytic agents; the true incidence is unknown. This serious condition, which can be lethal, is also associated with invasive vascular procedures (e.g., cardiac catheterization, angiography, vascular surgery) and/or anticoagulant therapy. Clinical features of cholesterol embolism may include livedo reticularis, "purple toe" syndrome, acute renal failure, gangrenous digits, hypertension, pancreatitis, myocardial infarction, cerebral infarction, spinal cord infarction, retinal artery occlusion, bowel infarction, and rhabdomyolysis.

Use in Acute Myocardial Infarction

In a small subgroup of AMI patients who are at low risk for death from cardiac causes (i.e., no previous myocardial infarction, Killip class I) and who have high blood pressure at the time of presentation, the risk for stroke may offset the survival benefit produced by thrombolytic therapy.[14]

Arrhythmias

Coronary thrombolysis may result in arrhythmias associated with reperfusion. These arrhythmias (such as sinus bradycardia, accelerated idioventricular rhythm, ventricular premature depolarizations, ventricular tachycardia) are not different from those often seen in the ordinary course of acute myocardial infarction and may be managed with standard antiarrhythmic measures. It is recommended that antiarrhythmic therapy for bradycardia and/or ventricular irritability be available when infusions of Activase are administered.

Use in Acute Ischemic Stroke

In addition to the previously listed conditions, the risks of Activase therapy to treat acute ischemic stroke may be increased in the following conditions and should be weighed against the anticipated benefits:

- Patients with severe neurological deficit (e.g., NIHSS > 22) at presentation. There is an increased risk of intracranial hemorrhage in these patients.
- Patients with major early infarct signs on a computerized cranial tomography (CT) scan (e.g., substantial edema, mass effect, or midline shift).

In patients without recent use of oral anticoagulants or heparin, Activase treatment can be initiated prior to the availability of coagulation study results. However, infusion should be discontinued if either a pretreatment International Normalized Ratio (INR) > 1.7 or a prothrombin time (PT) > 15 seconds or an elevated activated partial thromboplastin time (aPTT) is identified.

Treatment should be limited to facilities that can provide appropriate evaluation and management of ICH.

In acute ischemic stroke, neither the incidence of intracranial hemorrhage nor the benefits of therapy are known in patients treated with Activase more than 3 hours after the onset of symptoms. **Therefore, treatment of patients with acute ischemic stroke more than 3 hours after symptom onset is not recommended.**

Due to the increased risk for misdiagnosis of acute ischemic stroke, special diligence is required in making this diagnosis in patients whose blood glucose values are < 50 mg/dL or > 400 mg/dL. The safety and efficacy of treatment with Activase in patients with minor neurological deficit or with rapidly improving symptoms prior to the start of Activase administration has not been evaluated. **Therefore, treatment of patients with minor neurological deficit or with rapidly improving symptoms is not recommended.**

Use in Pulmonary Embolism

It should be recognized that the treatment of pulmonary embolism with Activase has not been shown to constitute adequate clinical treatment of underlying deep vein thrombosis. Furthermore, the possible risk of reembolization due to the lysis of underlying deep venous thrombi should be considered.

PRECAUTIONS

General

Standard management of myocardial infarction or pulmonary embolism should be implemented concomitantly with Activase treatment. Noncompressible arterial puncture must be avoided and internal jugular and subclavian venous punctures should be avoided to minimize bleeding from noncompressible sites. Arterial and venous punctures should be minimized. In the event of serious bleeding, Activase and heparin should be discontinued immediately. Heparin effects can be reversed by protamine.

Orolingual angioedema has been observed in post-market experience in patients treated for acute ischemic stroke and in patients treated for acute myocardial infarction (see PRECAUTIONS: Drug Interactions and ADVERSE REACTIONS: Allergic Reactions). Onset of angioedema occurred during and up to 2 hours after infusion of Activase. In many cases, patients were receiving concomitant Angiotensin-converting enzyme inhibitors. Patients treated with Activase should be monitored during and for several hours after infusion for signs of orolingual angioedema. If angioedema is noted, promptly institute appropriate therapy (e.g. antihistamines, intravenous corticosteroids or epinephrine) and consider discontinuing the Activase infusion. Rare fatal cases of hemorrhage associated with traumatic intubation in patients administered Activase have been reported.

Readministration

There is no experience with readministration of Activase. If an anaphylactoid reaction occurs, the infusion should be discontinued immediately and appropriate therapy initiated.

Although sustained antibody formation in patients receiving one dose of Activase has not been documented, readministration should be undertaken with caution. Detectable levels of antibody (a single point measurement) were reported in one patient, but subsequent antibody test results were negative.

Drug/Laboratory Test Interactions

During Activase therapy, if coagulation tests and/or measures of fibrinolytic activity are performed, the results may be unreliable unless specific precautions are taken to prevent in vitro artifacts. Activase is an enzyme that when present in blood in pharmacologic concentrations remains active under in vitro conditions. This can lead to degradation of fibrinogen in blood samples removed for analysis. Collection of blood samples in the presence of aprotinin (150–200 units/mL) can to some extent mitigate this phenomenon.

Drug Interactions

The interaction of Activase with other cardioactive or cerebroactive drugs has not been studied. In addition to bleeding associated with heparin and vitamin K antagonists, drugs that alter platelet function (such as acetylsalicylic acid, dipyridamole and Abciximab) may increase the risk of bleeding if administered prior to, during, or after Activase therapy.

There have been post-marketing reports of orolingual angioedema associated with the use of Activase. Many patients, primarily acute ischemic stroke patients, were receiving concomitant Angiotensin-converting enzyme inhibitors. (See PRECAUTIONS: General and ADVERSE REACTIONS: Allergic Reactions).

Use of Antithrombotics

Aspirin and heparin have been administered concomitantly with and following infusions of Activase in the management of acute myocardial infarction or pulmonary embolism. Because heparin, aspirin, or Activase may cause bleeding complications, careful monitoring for bleeding is advised, especially at arterial puncture sites.

The concomitant use of heparin or aspirin during the first 24 hours following symptom onset were prohibited in The NINDS t-PA Stroke Trial. The safety of such concomitant use with Activase for the management of acute ischemic stroke is unknown.

Blood Pressure Control

Blood pressure should be monitored frequently and controlled during and following Activase administration in the management of acute ischemic stroke. In The NINDS t-PA Stroke Trial, blood pressure was actively controlled (≤ 185/110 mm Hg) for 24 hours. Blood pressure was monitored during the hospital stay.

Carcinogenesis, Mutagenesis, Impairment of Fertility

Long-term studies in animals have not been performed to evaluate the carcinogenic potential or the effect on fertility. Short-term studies, which evaluated tumorigenicity of Activase and effect on tumor metastases in rodents, were negative.

Studies to determine mutagenicity (Ames test) and chromosomal aberration assays in human lymphocytes were negative at all concentrations tested. Cytotoxicity, as reflected by a decrease in mitotic index, was evidenced only after prolonged exposure and only at the highest concentrations tested.

Pregnancy (Category C)

Activase has been shown to have an embryocidal effect in rabbits when intravenously administered in doses of approximately two times (3 mg/kg) the human dose for AMI. No maternal or fetal toxicity was evident at 0.65 times (1 mg/kg) the human dose in pregnant rats and rabbits dosed during the period of organogenesis. There are no adequate and well-controlled studies in pregnant women. Activase should be used during pregnancy only if the potential benefit justifies the potential risk to the fetus.

Nursing Mothers

It is not known whether Activase is excreted in human milk. Because many drugs are excreted in human milk, caution should be exercised when Activase is administered to a nursing woman.

Pediatric Use

Safety and effectiveness of Activase in pediatric patients have not been established.

ADVERSE REACTIONS

Bleeding

The most frequent adverse reaction associated with Activase in all approved indications is bleeding (see WARNINGS).[15,16]

Should serious bleeding in a critical location (intracranial, gastrointestinal, retroperitoneal, pericardial) occur, Activase therapy should be discontinued immediately, along with any concomitant therapy with heparin. Death and permanent disability are not uncommonly reported in patients that have experienced stroke (including intracranial bleeding) and other serious bleeding episodes.

In the GUSTO trial for the treatment of acute myocardial infarction, using the accelerated infusion regimen the incidence of all strokes for the Activase-treated patients was 1.6%, while the incidence of nonfatal stroke was 0.9%. The incidence of hemorrhagic stroke was 0.7%, not all of which were fatal. The incidence of all strokes, as well as that for hemorrhagic stroke, increased with increasing age (see CLINICAL PHARMACOLOGY: Accelerated Infusion in AMI Patients). Data from previous trials utilizing a 3-hour infusion of ≤ 100 mg indicated that the incidence of total stroke in six randomized, double-blind, placebo-controlled trials[2,7–11,17] was 1.2% (37/3161) in Alteplase-treated patients compared with 0.9% (27/3092) in placebo-treated patients.

For the 3-hour infusion regimen, the incidence of significant internal bleeding (estimated as > 250 cc blood loss) has been reported in studies in over 800 patients. These data do not include patients treated with the Alteplase accelerated infusion.

	Total Dose ≤ 100 mg
gastrointestinal	5%
genitourinary	4%
ecchymosis	1%
retroperitoneal	< 1%
epistaxis	< 1%
gingival	< 1%

The incidence of intracranial hemorrhage (ICH) in acute myocardial infarction patients treated with Activase is as follows:

Dose	Number of Patients	ICH (%)
100 mg, 3-hour	3272	0.4
≤ 100 mg, accelerated	10,396	0.7
150 mg	1779	1.3
1–1.4 mg/kg	237	0.4

These data indicate that a dose of 150 mg of Activase should not be used in the treatment of AMI because it has been associated with an increase in intracranial bleeding.[18]

For acute massive pulmonary embolism, bleeding events were consistent with the general safety profile observed with Activase in acute myocardial infarction patients receiving the 3-hour infusion regimen.

The incidence of ICH, especially symptomatic ICH, in patients with acute ischemic stroke was higher in Activase-treated patients than placebo patients (see CLINICAL PHARMACOLOGY).

A study of another alteplase product, Actilyse, in acute ischemic stroke, suggested that doses greater than 0.9 mg/kg may be associated with an increased incidence of ICH.[19] **Doses greater than 0.9 mg/kg (maximum 90 mg) should not be used in the management of acute ischemic stroke.**

Bleeding events other than ICH were noted in the studies of acute ischemic stroke and were consistent with the general safety profile of Activase. In The NINDS t-PA Stroke Trial (Parts 1 and 2), the frequency of bleeding requiring red blood cell transfusions was 6.4% for Activase-treated patients compared to 3.8% for placebo (p=0.19, using Mantel-Haenszel Chi-Square).

Fibrin which is part of the hemostatic plug formed at needle puncture sites will be lysed during Activase therapy. Therefore, Activase therapy requires careful attention to potential bleeding sites, e.g., catheter insertion sites, and arterial puncture sites.

Allergic Reactions

Allergic-type reactions, e.g., anaphylactoid reaction, laryngeal edema, orolingual angioedema, rash, and urticaria have been reported. A cause and effect relationship to Activase therapy has not been established. When such reactions occur, they usually respond to conventional therapy.

There have been postmarketing reports of orolingual angioedema associated with the use of Activase. Most reports were of patients treated for acute ischemic stroke, some reports were of patients treated for acute myocardial infarctions (see PRECAUTIONS: General). Many of these patients received concomitant angiotensin-converting enzyme inhibitors (see PRECAUTIONS: Drug Interactions). Most cases resolved with prompt treatment; there have been rare fatalities as a result of upper airway hemorrhage from intubation trauma.

Other Adverse Reactions

The following adverse reactions have been reported among patients receiving Activase in clinical trials and in postmarketing experience. These reactions are frequent sequelae of the underlying disease and the effect of Activase on the incidence of these events is unknown.

Use in Acute Myocardial Infarction: Arrhythmias, AV block, cardiogenic shock, heart failure, cardiac arrest, recurrent ischemia, myocardial reinfarction, myocardial rupture, electromechanical dissociation, pericardial effusion, pericarditis, mitral regurgitation, cardiac tamponade, thromboembolism, pulmonary edema. These events may be life threatening and may lead to death. Nausea and/or vomiting, hypotension and fever have also been reported.

Use in Pulmonary Embolism: Pulmonary reembolization, pulmonary edema, pleural effusion, thromboembolism, hypotension. These events may be life threatening and may lead to death. Fever has also been reported.

Use in Acute Ischemic Stroke: Cerebral edema, cerebral herniation, seizure, new ischemic stroke. These events may be life threatening and may lead to death.

DOSAGE AND ADMINISTRATION

Activase is for intravenous administration only. Extravasation of Activase infusion can cause ecchymosis and/or inflammation. Management consists of terminating the infusion at that IV site and application of local therapy.

Acute Myocardial Infarction

Administer Activase as soon as possible after the onset of symptoms. There are two Activase dose regimens for use in the management of acute myocardial infarction; controlled studies to compare clinical outcomes with these regimens have not been conducted.

A DOSE OF 150 mg OF ACTIVASE SHOULD NOT BE USED FOR THE TREATMENT OF ACUTE MYOCARDIAL INFARCTION BECAUSE IT HAS BEEN ASSOCIATED WITH AN INCREASE IN INTRACRANIAL BLEEDING.

Accelerated Infusion

The recommended total dose is based upon patient weight, not to exceed 100 mg. For patients weighing > 67 kg, the recommended dose administered is 100 mg as a 15 mg intravenous bolus, followed by 50 mg infused over the next 30 minutes, and then 35 mg infused over the next 60 minutes. For patients weighing ≤ 67 kg, the recommended dose is administered as a 15 mg intravenous bolus, followed by 0.75 mg/kg infused over the next 30 minutes not to exceed 50 mg, and then 0.50 mg/kg over the next 60 minutes not to exceed 35 mg.

The safety and efficacy of this accelerated infusion of Alteplase regimen has only been investigated with concomitant administration of heparin and aspirin as described in CLINICAL PHARMACOLOGY.

a. The bolus dose may be prepared in one of the following ways:
   1. By removing 15 mL from the vial of reconstituted (1 mg/mL) Activase using a syringe and needle. If this method is used with the 50 mg vials, the syringe should not be primed with air and the needle should be inserted into the Activase vial stopper. If the 100 mg vial is used, the needle should be inserted away from the puncture mark made by the transfer device.
   2. By removing 15 mL from a port (second injection site) on the infusion line after the infusion set is primed.
   3. By programming an infusion pump to deliver a 15 mL (1 mg/mL) bolus at the initiation of the infusion.

b. The remainder of the Activase dose may be administered as follows:

   50 mg vials—administer using either a polyvinyl chloride bag or glass vial and infusion set.

   100 mg vial—insert the spike end of an infusion set through the same puncture site created by the transfer device in the stopper of the vial of reconstituted Activase. Hang the Activase vial from the plastic molded capping attached to the bottom of the vial.

3-Hour Infusion

The recommended dose is 100 mg administered as 60 mg in the first hour (of which 6 to 10 mg is administered as a bolus), 20 mg over the second hour, and 20 mg over the third hour. For smaller patients (< 65 kg), a dose of 1.25 mg/kg administered over 3 hours, as described above, may be used.[15]

Although the value of the use of anticoagulants during and following administration of Activase has not been fully studied, heparin has been administered concomitantly for 24 hours or longer in more than 90% of patients.

Aspirin and/or dipyridamole have been given to patients receiving Alteplase during and/or following heparin treatment.

a. The bolus dose may be prepared in one of the following ways:
   1. By removing 6 to 10 mL from the vial of reconstituted (1 mg/mL) Activase using a syringe and needle. If this method is used with the 50 mg vials, the syringe should not be primed with air and the needle should be inserted into the Activase vial stopper. If the 100 mg vial is used, the needle should be inserted away from the puncture mark made by the transfer device.
   2. By removing 6 to 10 mL from a port (second injection site) on the infusion line after the infusion set is primed.
   3. By programming an infusion pump to deliver a 6 to 10 mL (1 mg/mL) bolus at the initiation of the infusion.

b. The remainder of the Activase dose may be administered as follows:

   50 mg vials—administer using either a polyvinyl chloride bag or glass vial and infusion set.

   100 mg vial—insert the spike end of an infusion set through the same puncture site created by the transfer device in the stopper of the vial of reconstituted Activase. Hang the Activase vial from the plastic molded capping attached to the bottom of the vial.

Acute Ischemic Stroke

THE TOTAL DOSE FOR TREATMENT OF ACUTE ISCHEMIC STROKE SHOULD NOT EXCEED 90 mg.

The recommended dose is 0.9 mg/kg (not to exceed 90 mg total dose) infused over 60 minutes with 10% of the total dose administered as an initial intravenous bolus over 1 minute.

The safety and efficacy of this regimen with concomitant administration of heparin and aspirin during the first 24 hours after symptom onset has not been investigated.

a. The bolus dose may be prepared in one of the following ways:
   1. By removing the appropriate volume from the vial of reconstituted (1 mg/mL) Activase using a syringe and needle. If this method is used with the 50 mg vials, the syringe should not be primed with air and the needle should be inserted into the Activase vial stopper. If the 100 mg vial is used, the needle should be inserted away from the puncture mark made by the transfer device.
   2. By removing the appropriate volume from a port (second injection site) on the infusion line after the infusion set is primed.
   3. By programming an infusion pump to deliver the appropriate volume as a bolus at the initiation of the infusion.

b. The remainder of the Activase dose may be administered as follows:

   50 mg vials—administer using either a polyvinyl chloride bag or glass vial and infusion set.

   100 mg vial—remove from the vial any quantity of drug in excess of that specified for patient treatment. Insert the spike end of an infusion set through the same puncture site created by the transfer device in the stopper of the vial of reconstituted Activase. Hang the Activase vial from the plastic molded capping attached to the bottom of the vial.

Pulmonary Embolism

The recommended dose is 100 mg administered by intravenous infusion over 2 hours. Heparin therapy should be instituted or reinstituted near the end of or immediately following the Activase infusion when the partial thromboplastin time or thrombin time returns to twice normal or less.

The Activase dose may be administered as follows:

50 mg vials—administer using either a polyvinyl chloride bag or glass vial and infusion set.

100 mg vial—insert the spike end of an infusion set through the same puncture site created by the transfer device in the stopper of the vial of reconstituted Activase. Hang the Activase vial from the plastic molded capping attached to the bottom of the vial.

Reconstitution and Dilution

Activase should be reconstituted by aseptically adding the appropriate volume of the accompanying Sterile Water for Injection, USP, to the vial. It is important that Activase be reconstituted only with Sterile Water for Injection, USP, without preservatives. Do not use Bacteriostatic Water for Injection, USP. The reconstituted preparation results in a colorless to pale yellow transparent solution containing Activase 1mg/mL at approximately pH 7.3. The osmolality of this solution is approximately 215 mOsm/kg.

Because Activase contains no antibacterial preservatives, it should be reconstituted immediately before use. The solution may be used for intravenous administration within 8 hours following reconstitution when stored between 2–30°C (36–86°F). Before further dilution or administration, the product should be visually inspected for particulate matter and discoloration prior to administration whenever solution and container permit.

Activase may be administered as reconstituted at 1 mg/mL. As an alternative, the reconstituted solution may be diluted further immediately before administration in an equal volume of 0.9% Sodium Chloride Injection, USP, or 5% Dextrose Injection, USP, to yield a concentration of 0.5 mg/mL. Either polyvinyl chloride bags or glass vials are acceptable. Activase is stable for up to 8 hours in these solutions at room temperature. Exposure to light has no effect on the stability of these solutions. Excessive agitation during dilution should be avoided; mixing should be accomplished with gentle swirling and/or slow inversion. Do not use other infusion solutions, e.g., Sterile Water for Injection, USP, or preservative-containing solutions for further dilution.

50 mg Vials

Reconstitution should be carried out using a large bore needle (e.g., 18 gauge) and a syringe, directing the stream of Sterile Water for Injection, USP, into the lyophilized cake. **DO NOT USE IF VACUUM IS NOT PRESENT.** Slight foaming upon reconstitution is not unusual; standing undisturbed for several minutes is usually sufficient to allow dissipation of any large bubbles.

No other medication should be added to infusion solutions containing Activase. Any unused infusion solution should be discarded.

100 mg Vial

Reconstitution should be carried out using the transfer device provided, adding the contents of the accompanying 100 mL vial of Sterile Water for Injection, USP, to the contents of the 100 mg vial of Activase powder. Slight foaming upon reconstitution is not unusual; standing undisturbed for several minutes is usually sufficient to allow dissipation of any large bubbles. Please refer to the accompanying Instructions for Reconstitution and Administration. **100 mg VIALS DO NOT CONTAIN VACUUM.**

100 mg VIAL RECONSTITUTION

1. Use aseptic technique throughout.
2. Remove the protective flip-caps from one vial of Activase and one vial of Sterile Water for Injection, USP (SWFI).
3. Open the package containing the transfer device by peeling the paper label off the package.
4. Remove the protective cap from one end of the transfer device and keeping the vial of SWFI upright, insert the piercing pin vertically into the center of the stopper of the vial of SWFI.

Continued on next page

Activase—Cont.

5. Remove the protective cap from the other end of the transfer device. **DO NOT INVERT THE VIAL OF SWFI.**
6. Holding the vial of Activase upside-down, position it so that the center of the stopper is directly over the exposed piercing pin of the transfer device.
7. Push the vial of Activase down so that the piercing pin is inserted through the center of the Activase vial stopper.
8. Invert the two vials so that the vial of Activase is on the bottom (upright) and the vial of SWFI is upside-down, allowing the SWFI to flow down through the transfer device. Allow the entire contents of the vial of SWFI to flow into the Activase vial (approximately 0.5 cc of SWFI will remain in the diluent vial). Approximately 2 minutes are required for this procedure.
9. Remove the transfer device and the empty SWFI vial from the Activase vial. Safely discard both the transfer device and the empty diluent vial according to institutional procedures.
10. Swirl gently to dissolve the Activase powder. **DO NOT SHAKE.**

No other medication should be added to infusion solutions containing Activase.

Any unused infusion solution should be discarded.

HOW SUPPLIED

Activase (Alteplase) is supplied as a sterile, lyophilized powder in 50 mg vials containing vacuum and in 100 mg vials without vacuum.

Each 50 mg Activase vial (29 million IU) is packaged with diluent for reconstitution (50 mL Sterile Water for Injection, USP): NDC 50242-044-13.

Each 100 mg Activase vial (58 million IU) is packaged with diluent for reconstitution (100 mL Sterile Water for Injection, USP), and one transfer device: NDC 50242-085-27.

Storage

Store lyophilized Activase at controlled room temperature not to exceed 30°C (86°F), or under refrigeration (2–8°C/36–46°F). Protect the lyophilized material during extended storage from excessive exposure to light.

Do not use beyond the expiration date stamped on the vial.

REFERENCES

1. Mueller H, Rao AK, Forman SA, et al. Thrombolysis in myocardial infarction (TIMI): comparative studies of coronary reperfusion and systemic fibrinogenolysis with two forms of recombinant tissue-type plasminogen activator. *J Am Coll Cardiol.* 1987;10:479–90.
2. Topol EJ, Morriss DC, Smalling RW, et al. A multicenter, randomized, placebo-controlled trial of a new form of intravenous recombinant tissue-type plasminogen activator (Activase®) in acute myocardial infarction. *J Am Coll Cardiol.* 1987;9:1205–13.
3. Seifried E, Tanswell P, Ellbrück D, et al. Pharmacokinetics and haemostatic status during consecutive infusions of recombinant tissue-type plasminogen activator in patients with acute myocardial infarction. *Thromb Haemostas.* 1989;61:497–501.
4. Tanswell P, Tebbe U, Neuhaus K-L, et al. Pharmacokinetics and fibrin specificity of Alteplase during accelerated infusions in acute myocardial infarction. *J Am Coll Cardiol.* 1992;19:1071–5.
5. De Wood MA, Spores J, Notske R, et al. Prevalence of total coronary occlusion during the early hours of transmural myocardial infarction. *New Engl J Med.* 1980;303:897–902.
6. Chesebro JH, Knatterud G, Roberts R, et al. Thrombolysis in myocardial infarction (TIMI) trial, Phase I: a comparison between intravenous tissue plasminogen activator and intravenous streptokinase. *Circulation.* 1987;76(1):142–54.
7. Guerci AD, Gerstenblith G, Brinker JA, et al. A randomized trial of intravenous tissue plasminogen activator for acute myocardial infarction with subsequent randomization to elective coronary angioplasty. *New Engl J Med.* 1987;317:1613-18.
8. O'Rourke M, Baron D, Keogh A, et al. Limitation of myocardial infarction by early infusion of recombinant tissue-plasminogen activator. *Circulation.* 1988;77:1311–15.
9. Wilcox RG, von der Lippe G, Olsson CG, et al. Trial of tissue plasminogen activator for mortality reduction in acute myocardial infarction: ASSET. *Lancet.* 1988;2:525–30.
10. Hampton JR, The University of Nottingham. Personal communication.
11. Van de Werf F, Arnold AER, et al. Effect of intravenous tissue-plasminogen activator on infarct size, left ventricular function and survival in patients with acute myocardial infarction. *Br Med J.* 1988;297:1374–9.
12. The National Institute of Neurological Disorders and Stroke t-PA Stroke Study Group. Tissue plasminogen activator for acute ischemic stroke. *New Engl J Med.* 1995;333:1581–7.
13. Goldhaber SZ, Kessler CM, Heit J, et al. A randomized controlled trial of recombinant tissue plasminogen activator versus urokinase in the treatment of acute pulmonary embolism. *Lancet.* 1988;2:293–8.
14. Aylward P, Wilcox R, Horgan J, White H, Granger C, Califf R, et al. for the GUSTO-I Investigators. Relation of increased arterial blood pressure to mortality and stroke in the context of contemporary thrombolytic therapy for acute myocardial infarction: a randomized trial. *Ann Int Med.* 1996;125:891–900.
15. Califf RM, Topol EJ, George BS, et al. Hemorrhagic complications associated with the use of intravenous tissue plasminogen activator in treatment of acute myocardial infarction. *Am J Med.* 1988;85:353–9.
16. Bovill EG, Terrin ML, Stump DC, et al. Hemorrhagic events during therapy with recombinant tissue-type plasminogen activator, heparin, and aspirin for acute myocardial infarction: results from the thrombolysis in myocardial infarction (TIMI), Phase II trial. *Ann Int Med.* 1991;115(4):256–65.
17. National Heart Foundation of Australia Coronary Thrombolysis Group. Coronary thrombolysis and myocardial infarction salvage by tissue plasminogen activator given up to 4 hours after onset of myocardial infarction. *Lancet.* 1988;1:203–7.
18. Gore JM, Sloan M, Price TR, et al. and the TIMI Investigators. Intracerebral hemorrhage, cerebral infarction, and subdural hematoma after acute myocardial infarction and thrombolytic therapy in the thrombolysis in myocardial infarction study. *Circulation.* 1991;83:448–59.
19. Hacke W, Kaste M, Fieschi C, Toni D, Lesaffre E, von Kummer R, et al. for the ECASS Study Group. Intravenous thrombolysis with recombinant tissue plasminogen activator for acute hemispheric stroke. The European Cooperative Acute Stroke Study (ECASS). *JAMA.* 1995;274:1017–25.

Activase®, (Alteplase) 4800511
Manufactured by Revision Date October 2002
GENENTECH, INC. FDA Approval Date May 2002
1 DNA Way © 2002 Genentech, Inc.
South San Francisco, CA 94080-4990

Shown in Product Identification Guide, page 313

CATHFLO® ACTIVASE® ℞

[*kăth-' flō*]

(ALTEPLASE) 2 mg

Powder for reconstitution for use in central venous access devices

DESCRIPTION

Cathflo® Activase® (Alteplase) is a tissue plasminogen activator (t-PA) produced by recombinant DNA technology. It is a sterile, purified glycoprotein of 527 amino acids. It is synthesized using the complementary DNA (cDNA) for natural human tissue-type plasminogen activator (t-PA) obtained from an established human cell line. The manufacturing process involves secretion of the enzyme Alteplase into the culture medium by an established mammalian cell line (Chinese hamster ovary cells) into which the cDNA for Alteplase has been genetically inserted. Fermentation is carried out in a nutrient medium containing the antibiotic gentamicin sulfate, 100 mg/L. The presence of the antibiotic is not detectable in the final product.

Cathflo Activase is a sterile, white to pale yellow, lyophilized powder for intracatheter instillation for restoration of function to central venous access devices following reconstitution with Sterile Water for Injection, USP.

Each vial of Cathflo Activase contains 2.2 mg of Alteplase (which includes a 10% overfill), 77 mg of L-arginine, 0.2 mg of polysorbate 80, and phosphoric acid for pH adjustment. Each reconstituted vial will deliver 2 mg of Cathflo Activase, at a pH of approximately 7.3.

CLINICAL PHARMACOLOGY

Alteplase is an enzyme (serine protease) that has the property of fibrin-enhanced conversion of plasminogen to plasmin. It produces limited conversion of plasminogen in the absence of fibrin. Alteplase binds to fibrin in a thrombus and converts the entrapped plasminogen to plasmin, thereby initiating local fibrinolysis.[1]

In patients with acute myocardial infarction administered 100 mg of Activase as an accelerated intravenous infusion over 90 minutes, plasma clearance occurred with an initial half-life of less than 5 minutes and a terminal half-life of 72 minutes. Clearance is mediated primarily by the liver.[2]

When Cathflo Activase is administered for restoration of function to central venous access devices according to the instructions in DOSAGE AND ADMINISTRATION, circulating plasma levels of Alteplase are not expected to reach pharmacologic concentrations. If a 2 mg dose of Alteplase were administered by bolus injection directly into the systemic circulation (rather than instilled into the catheter), the concentration of circulating Alteplase would be expected to return to endogenous circulating levels of 5–10 ng/mL within 30 minutes.[1]

CLINICAL STUDIES

Two clinical studies were performed in patients with improperly functioning central venous access devices (CVADs). A placebo-controlled, double-blind, randomized trial (Trial 1) and a larger open-label trial (Trial 2) investigated the use of Alteplase in patients who had an indwelling CVAD for administration of chemotherapy, total parenteral nutrition, or long-term administration of antibiotics or other medications. Both studies enrolled patients whose catheters were not functioning (defined as the inability to withdraw at least 3 cc of blood from the device) but had the ability to instill the necessary volume of study drug. Patients with hemodialysis catheters or a known mechanical occlusion were excluded from both studies. Also excluded were patients considered at high risk for bleeding or embolization (see PRECAUTIONS, Bleeding), as well as patients who were younger than 2 years old or weighed less than 10 kg. Restoration of function was assessed by successful withdrawal of 3 cc of blood and infusion of 5 cc of saline through the catheter.

Trial 1 tested the efficacy of a 2 mg/2 mL Alteplase dose in restoring function to occluded catheters in 150 patients with catheter occlusion up to 24 hours in duration. Patients were randomized to receive either Alteplase or placebo instilled into the lumen of the catheter, and catheter function was assessed at 120 minutes. Restoration of function was assessed by successful withdrawal of 3 cc of blood and infusion of 5 cc of saline through the catheter. All patients whose catheters did not meet these criteria were then administered Alteplase, until function was restored or each patient had received up to two active doses. After the initial dose of study agent, 51 (67%) of 76 patients randomized to Alteplase and 12 (16%) of 74 patients randomized to placebo had catheter function restored. This resulted in a treatment-associated difference of 51% (95% CI is 37% to 64%). A total of 112 (88%) of 127 Alteplase-treated patients had restored function after up to two doses.

Trial 2 was an open-label, single arm trial in 995 patients with catheter dysfunction and included patients with occlusions present for any duration. Patients were treated with Alteplase with up to two doses of 2 mg/2 mL (less for children who weighed less than 30 kg, see DOSAGE AND ADMINISTRATION) instilled into the lumen of the catheter. Assessment for restoration of function was made at 30 minutes after each instillation. If function was not restored, catheter function was re-assessed at 120 minutes. Thirty minutes after instillation of the first dose, 516 (52%) of 995 patients had restored catheter function. One hundred twenty minutes after the instillation of the first dose, 747 (75%) of 995 patients had restored catheter function. If function was not restored after the first dose, a second dose was administered. Two hundred nine patients received a second dose. Thirty minutes after instillation of the second dose, 70 (33%) of 209 patients had restored catheter function. One hundred twenty minutes after the instillation of the second dose, 97 (46%) of 209 patients had restored catheter function. A total of 844 (85%) of 995 patients had function restored after up to 2 doses.

Similar rates of catheter function restoration were seen among all catheter types studied (single-, double-, and triple-lumen, and implanted ports).

There were no gender differences observed in the rate of catheter function restoration. Results were similar across age subgroups, but there was insufficient enrollment of pediatric patients to draw any conclusions regarding relative efficacy in pediatric patients (see PRECAUTIONS, Pediatric Use).

Across both trials, 796 (68%) of 1043 patients with occlusions present for less than 14 days had restored function after one dose, and 902 (88%) had function restored after up to two doses. Of 53 patients with occlusions present for longer than 14 days, 30 (57%) patients had function restored after a single dose, and a total of 38 patients (72%) had restored function after up to two doses.

Three hundred forty-six patients who had successful treatment outcome were evaluated at 30 days after treatment. The incidence of recurrent catheter dysfunction within this period was 26%.

INDICATIONS AND USAGE

Cathflo® Activase® (Alteplase) is indicated for the restoration of function to central venous access devices as assessed by the ability to withdraw blood.

CONTRAINDICATIONS

Cathflo Activase should not be administered to patients with known hypersensitivity to Alteplase or any component of the formulation (see DESCRIPTION).

WARNINGS

None.

PRECAUTIONS

General

Catheter dysfunction may be caused by a variety of conditions other than thrombus formation, such as catheter malposition, mechanical failure, constriction by a suture, and lipid deposits or drug precipitates within the catheter lumen. These types of conditions should be considered before treatment with Cathflo Activase.

Because of the risk of damage to the vascular wall or collapse of soft-walled catheters, vigorous suction should not be applied during attempts to determine catheter occlusion.

Excessive pressure should be avoided when Cathflo Activase is instilled into the catheter. Such force could cause rupture of the catheter or expulsion of the clot into the circulation.

Bleeding

The most frequent adverse reaction associated with all thrombolytics in all approved indications is bleeding.[3,4] Cathflo Activase has not been studied in patients known to be at risk for bleeding events that may be associated with the use of thrombolytics. Caution should be exercised with patients who have active internal bleeding or who have had any of the following within 48 hours: surgery, obstetrical delivery, percutaneous biopsy of viscera or deep tissues, or puncture of non-compressible vessels. In addition, caution should be exercised with patients who have thrombocytopenia, other hemostatic defects (including those secondary to severe hepatic or renal disease), or any condition for which bleeding constitutes a significant hazard or would be particularly difficult to manage because of its location, or who are at high risk for embolic complications (e.g., venous thrombosis in the region of the catheter). Death and permanent disability have been reported in patients who have experienced stroke and other serious bleeding episodes when receiving pharmacologic doses of a thrombolytic.

Should serious bleeding in a critical location (e.g., intracranial, gastrointestinal, retroperitoneal, pericardial) occur, treatment with Cathflo Activase should be stopped and the drug should be withdrawn from the catheter.

Infections

Cathflo Activase should be used with caution in the presence of known or suspected infection in the catheter. Using Cathflo Activase in patients with infected catheters may release a localized infection into the systemic circulation (see ADVERSE REACTIONS). As with all catheterization procedures, care should be used to maintain aseptic technique.

Re-Administration

In clinical trials, patients received up to two 2 mg/2 mL doses (4 mg total) of Alteplase. Additional re-administration of Cathflo Activase has not been studied. Antibody formation in patients receiving one or more doses of Cathflo Activase for restoration of function to CVADs has not been studied.

Drug Interactions

The interaction of Cathflo Activase with other drugs has not been formally studied. Concomitant use of drugs affecting coagulation and/or platelet function has not been studied.

Drug/Laboratory Test Interactions

Potential interactions between Cathflo Activase and laboratory tests have not been studied.

Carcinogenesis, Mutagenesis, Impairment of Fertility

Long-term studies in animals have not been performed to evaluate the carcinogenic potential or the effect on fertility. Short-term studies that evaluated tumorigenicity of Alteplase and effect on tumor metastases were negative in rodents. Studies to determine mutagenicity (Ames test) and chromosomal aberration assays in human lymphocytes were negative at all concentrations tested. Cytotoxicity, as reflected by a decrease in mitotic index, was evidenced only after prolonged exposure at high concentrations exceeding those expected to be achieved with Cathflo® Activase® (Alteplase).

Pregnancy (Category C)

Alteplase has been shown to have an embryocidal effect due to an increased postimplantation loss rate in rabbits when administered intravenously at doses approximately 100 times (3 mg/kg) the human dose for restoration of function to occluded CVADs. No maternal or fetal toxicity was evident at 33 times (1 mg/kg) the human dose for restoration of function to occluded CVADs in pregnant rats and rabbits dosed during the period of organogenesis.

There are no adequate and well-controlled studies in pregnant women. Cathflo Activase should be used during pregnancy only if the potential benefit justifies the potential risk to the fetus.

Nursing Mothers

It is not known whether Cathflo Activase is excreted in human milk. Because many drugs are excreted in human milk, caution should be exercised when Cathflo Activase is administered to a nursing woman.

Pediatric Use

Cathflo Activase has not been studied in patients who are younger than 2 years of age or who weigh less than 10 kg. In Trials 1 and 2, 126 (11%) of 1135 patients treated were from 2 to 16 years of age. No study drug–related adverse events were observed in these patients. A total of 65 patients (6% of all patients treated in the studies) weighed ≥10 kg and <30 kg. These low body weight patients received up to two doses of Alteplase, with each dose equal to 110% of the internal lumen volume of the catheter (to a maximum dose of 2 mg). The rates of catheter function restoration in these subsets of patients were similar to those observed in adult patients. However, there was insufficient enrollment of pediatric patients to draw any conclusions regarding relative efficacy in the pediatric or low weight subgroups, relative efficacy related to catheter types used in these patients, or relative rates of adverse events.

Geriatric Use

In 312 patients enrolled who were age 65 years and over, no incidents of intracranial hemorrhage (ICH), embolic events, or major bleeding events were observed. One hundred three of these patients were age 75 years and over, and 12 were age 85 years and over. The effect of Alteplase on common age-related comorbidities has not been studied. In general, caution should be used in geriatric patients with conditions known to increase the risk of bleeding (see PRECAUTIONS, Bleeding).

ADVERSE REACTIONS

In the clinical trials, the most serious adverse events reported after treatment were sepsis (see PRECAUTIONS, Infections), gastrointestinal bleeding, and venous thrombosis.

Because clinical trials are conducted under widely varying conditions, adverse reaction rates observed in the clinical trials of a drug cannot be directly compared to rates in the clinical trials of another drug and may not reflect the rates observed in practice.

The data described below reflect exposure to Cathflo Activase in 1122 patients, of whom 880 received a single dose and 242 received two sequential doses of Cathflo Activase.

In the Cathflo Activase clinical trials, only limited, focused types of serious adverse events were recorded, including death, major hemorrhage, intracranial hemorrhage, pulmonary or arterial emboli, and other serious adverse events not thought to be attributed to underlying disease or concurrent illness. Major hemorrhage was defined as severe blood loss (>5 mL/kg), blood loss requiring transfusion, or blood loss causing hypotension. Non-serious adverse events and serious events thought to be due to underlying disease or concurrent illness were not recorded. Patients were observed for serious adverse events until catheter function was deemed to be restored or for a maximum of 4 or 6 hours depending on study. For most patients the observation period was 30 minutes to 2 hours. Spontaneously reported deaths and serious adverse events that were not thought to be related to the patient's underlying disease were also recorded during the 30 days following treatment.

Four catheter-related sepsis events occurred from 15 minutes to 1 day after treatment with Alteplase, and a fifth sepsis event occurred on Day 3 after Alteplase treatment. All 5 patients had positive catheter or peripheral blood cultures within 24 hours after symptom onset.

Three patients had a major hemorrhage from a gastrointestinal source from 2 to 3 days after Alteplase treatment. One case of injection site hemorrhage was observed at 4 hours after treatment in a patient with pre-existing thrombocytopenia. These events may have been related to underlying disease and treatments for malignancy, but a contribution to occurrence of the events from Alteplase cannot be ruled out. There were no reports of intracranial hemorrhage.

Three cases of subclavian and upper extremity deep venous thrombosis were reported 3 to 7 days after treatment. These events may have been related to underlying disease or to the long-term presence of an indwelling catheter, but a contribution to occurrence of the events from Alteplase treatment cannot be ruled out. There were no reports of pulmonary emboli.

There were no gender-related differences observed in the rates of adverse reactions. Adverse reactions profiles were similar across age subgroups, but there was insufficient enrollment of pediatric patients to draw any conclusions regarding relative adverse event rates (see PRECAUTIONS, Pediatric Use).

Allergic Reactions

No allergic-type reactions were observed in the trials in patients treated with Alteplase. If an anaphylactic reaction occurs, appropriate therapy should be administered.

DOSAGE AND ADMINISTRATION

Cathflo® Activase® (Alteplase) is for instillation into the dysfunctional catheter at a concentration of 1 mg/mL.

• Patients weighing ≥30 kg:	2 mg in 2 mL
• Patients weighing ≥10 to <30 kg:	110% of the internal lumen volume of the catheter, not to exceed 2 mg in 2 mL

If catheter function is not restored at 120 minutes after 1 dose of Cathflo Activase, a second dose may be instilled (see Instructions for Administration). There is no efficacy or safety information on dosing in excess of 2 mg per dose for this indication. Studies have not been performed with administration of total doses greater than 4 mg (two 2 mg doses).

Instructions for Administration

Preparation of Solution

Reconstitute Cathflo Activase to a final concentration of 1 mg/mL:

1. Aseptically withdraw 2.2 mL of Sterile Water for Injection, USP (diluent is not provided). Do not use Bacteriostatic Water for Injection.
2. Inject the 2.2 mL of Sterile Water for Injection, USP, into the Cathflo Activase vial, directing the diluent stream into the powder. Slight foaming is not unusual; let the vial stand undisturbed to allow large bubbles to dissipate.
3. Mix by gently swirling until the contents are completely dissolved. Complete dissolution should occur within 3 minutes. **DO NOT SHAKE.** The reconstituted preparation results in a colorless to pale yellow transparent solution containing 1 mg/mL Cathflo Activase at a pH of approximately 7.3.
4. Cathflo Activase contains no antibacterial preservatives and should be reconstituted immediately before use. The solution may be used for intracatheter instillation within 8 hours following reconstitution when stored at 2–30°C (36–86°F).

No other medication should be added to solutions containing Cathflo Activase.

Instillation of Solution into the Catheter

1. Inspect the product prior to administration for foreign matter and discoloration.
2. Withdraw 2.0 mL (2.0 mg) of solution from the reconstituted vial.
3. Instill the appropriate dose of Cathflo Activase (see DOSAGE AND ADMINISTRATION) into the occluded catheter.
4. After 30 minutes of dwell time, assess catheter function by attempting to aspirate blood. If the catheter is functional, go to Step 7. If the catheter is not functional, go to Step 5.
5. After 120 minutes of dwell time, assess catheter function by attempting to aspirate blood and catheter contents. If the catheter is functional, go to Step 7. If the catheter is not functional, go to Step 6.
6. If catheter function is not restored after one dose of Cathflo Activase, a second dose may be instilled. Repeat the procedure beginning with Step 1 under Preparation of Solution.
7. If catheter function has been restored, aspirate 4–5 mL of blood to remove Cathflo Activase and residual clot, and gently irrigate the catheter with 0.9% Sodium Chloride, USP.

Any unused solution should be discarded.

Stability and Storage

Store lyophilized Cathflo Activase at refrigerated temperature (2–8°C/36–46°F). Do not use beyond the expiration date on the vial. Protect the lyophilized material during extended storage from excessive exposure to light.

HOW SUPPLIED

Cathflo Activase is supplied as a sterile, lyophilized powder in 2 mg vials.

Each Cathflo® Activase® carton contains one 2 mg vial of Cathflo® Activase® (Alteplase): NDC 50242-041-64.

Each Novaplus™ Cathflo® Activase® carton contains one 2 mg vial of Novaplus™ Cathflo® Activase® (Alteplase): NDC 50242-041-65.

REFERENCES

1. Collen D, Lijnen HR. Fibrinolysis and the control of hemostasis. In: Stamatoyannopoulos G, Nienhui AW, Majerus PW, Varmus H, editors. The molecular basis of blood diseases, 2nd edition. Philadelphia: Saunders, 1994:662–88.
2. Tanswell P, Tebbe U, Neuhaus K-L, Glasle-Schwarz L, Wojick J, Seifried E. Pharmacokinetics and fibrin specificity of alteplase during accelerated infusions in acute myocardial infarction. *J Am Coll Cardiol* 1992;19:1071–5.
3. Califf RM, Topol EJ, George BS, Boswick JM, Abbottsmith C, Sigmon KN, et al., and the Thrombolysis and Angioplasty in Myocardial Infarction Study Group. Hemorrhagic complications associated with the use of intravenous tissue plasminogen activator in the treatment of acute myocardial infarction. *Am J Med* 1988;85:353–9.
4. Bovill EG, Terrin ML, Stump DC, Berke AD, Frederick M, Collen D, et al. Hemorrhagic events during therapy with recombinant tissue-type plasminogen activator, heparin, and aspirin for acute myocardial infarction: results of the thrombolysis in myocardial infarction (TIMI), phase II trial. *Ann Int Med* 1991;115:256–65.

Cathflo® Activase® (Alteplase) 7289101
Manufactured by: LB0551
Genentech, Inc. (4821101)
1 DNA Way Revision Date October 2002
FDA Approval Date September 2001
South San Francisco, CA 94080-4990

Shown in Product Identification Guide, page 313

HERCEPTIN® ℞
[*hər' sĕp-tĭn*]
(Trastuzumab)

WARNINGS:

CARDIOMYOPATHY

HERCEPTIN administration can result in the development of ventricular dysfunction and congestive heart failure. Left ventricular function should be evaluated in all patients prior to and during treatment with HERCEPTIN. Discontinuation of HERCEPTIN treatment should be strongly considered in patients who develop a clinically significant decrease in left ventricular function. The incidence and severity of cardiac dysfunction was particularly high in patients who received HERCEPTIN in combination with anthracyclines and cyclophosphamide. (See WARNINGS.)

HYPERSENSITIVITY REACTIONS INCLUDING ANAPHYLAXIS
INFUSION REACTIONS
PULMONARY EVENTS

HERCEPTIN administration can result in severe hypersensitivity reactions (including anaphylaxis), infusion reactions, and pulmonary events. Rarely, these have been fatal. In most cases, symptoms occurred during or within 24 hours of administration of HERCEPTIN. HERCEPTIN infusion should be interrupted for patients experiencing dyspnea or clinically significant hypotension. Patients should be monitored until signs and symptoms completely resolve. Discontinuation of

Continued on next page

Herceptin—Cont.

HERCEPTIN treatment should be strongly considered for patients who develop anaphylaxis, angioedema, or acute respiratory distress syndrome. (See WARNINGS.)

DESCRIPTION

HERCEPTIN (Trastuzumab) is a recombinant DNA-derived humanized monoclonal antibody that selectively binds with high affinity in a cell-based assay (Kd=5nM) to the extracellular domain of the human epidermal growth factor receptor 2 protein, HER2.[1,2] The antibody is an IgG_1 kappa that contains human framework regions with the complementarity-determining regions of a murine antibody (4D5) that binds to HER2.

The humanized antibody against HER2 is produced by a mammalian cell (Chinese Hamster Ovary [CHO]) suspension culture in a nutrient median containing the antibiotic gentamicin. Gentamicin is not detectable in the final product.

HERCEPTIN is a sterile, white to pale yellow, preservative-free lyophilized powder for intravenous (IV) administration. The nominal content of each HERCEPTIN vial is 440 mg Trastuzumab, 400 mg α, α-trehalose dihydrate, 9.9 mg L-histidine HCl, 6.4 mg L-histidine, and 1.8 mg polysorbate 20, USP. **Reconstitution with 20 mL of the supplied Bacteriostatic Water for Injection (BWFI)**, USP, containing 1.1% benzyl alcohol as a preservative, yields a multi-dose solution containing 21 mg/mL Trastuzumab, at a pH of approximately 6.

CLINICAL PHARMACOLOGY

General

The HER2 (or c-erbB2) proto-oncogene encodes a transmembrane receptor protein of 185 kDa, which is structurally related to the epidermal growth factor receptor.[1] HER2 protein overexpression is observed in 24%–30% of primary breast cancers. HER2 protein overexpression can be determined using immunohistochemistry (IHC) and gene amplification can be determined using fluorescence *in situ* hybridization (FISH) of fixed tumor blocks.[2] In referenced studies where HERCEPTIN use was not studied,[3–5] approximately 96–98% of biopsy specimens that were found to have protein overexpression also had gene amplification and 100% of those with gene amplification also had protein overexpression.[3–5] The precision of the determination of protein overexpression or gene amplification, however, may vary depending on the sensitivity and specificity of the particular assay and assay procedures used (see PRECAUTIONS). When compared to the referenced studies noted above, the correlation between detectable protein overexpression using IHC and detectable gene amplification using FISH was not as high in the studies of HERCEPTIN clinical trial specimens (see CLINICAL STUDIES: HER2 Detection and HER2 Assay Concordance Studies and PRECAUTIONS: HER2 Testing).

Trastuzumab has been shown, in both *in vitro* assays and in animals, to inhibit the proliferation of human tumor cells that overexpress HER2.[6–8]

Trastuzumab is a mediator of antibody-dependent cellular cytotoxicity (ADCC).[9,10] *In vitro*, HERCEPTIN-mediated ADCC has been shown to be preferentially exerted on HER2 overexpressing cancer cells compared with cancer cells that do not overexpress HER2.

Pharmacokinetics

The pharmacokinetics of Trastuzumab were studied in breast cancer patients with metastatic disease. Short duration intravenous infusions of 10 to 500 mg once weekly demonstrated dose-dependent pharmacokinetics. Mean half-life increased and clearance decreased with increasing dose level. The half-life averaged 1.7 and 12 days at the 10 and 500 mg dose levels, respectively. Trastuzumab's volume of distribution was approximately that of serum volume (44 mL/kg). At the highest weekly dose studied (500 mg), mean peak serum concentrations were 377 µg/mL.

In studies using a loading dose of 4 mg/kg followed by a weekly maintenance dose of 2 mg/kg, a mean half-life of 5.8 days (range=1 to 32 days) was observed. Between Weeks 16 and 32, Trastuzumab serum concentrations reached a steady state with mean trough and peak concentrations of approximately 79 µg/mL and 123 µg/mL, respectively.

Detectable concentrations of the circulating extracellular domain of the HER2 receptor (shed antigen) are found in the sera of some patients with HER2 overexpressing tumors. Determination of shed antigen in baseline serum samples revealed that 64% (286/447) of patients had detectable shed antigen, which ranged as high as 1880 ng/mL (median=11 ng/mL) Patients with higher baseline shed antigen levels were more likely to have lower serum trough concentrations. However, with weekly dosing, most patients with elevated shed antigen levels achieved target serum concentrations of Trastuzumab by Week 6.

Data suggest that the disposition of Trastuzumab is not altered based on age or serum creatinine (up to 2.0 mg/dL). No formal interaction studies have been performed.

Mean serum trough concentrations of Trastuzumab when administered in combination with paclitaxel, were consistently elevated approximately 1.5-fold as compared with serum concentrations of Trastuzumab used in combination with anthracycline plus cyclophosphamide. In primate studies, administration of Trastuzumab with paclitaxel resulted in reduction in Trastuzumab clearance. Serum levels of Trastuzumab in combination with cisplatin, doxorubicin or epirubicin plus cyclophosphamide did not suggest any interactions; no formal drug interaction studies were performed.

CLINICAL STUDIES

The safety and efficacy of HERCEPTIN were studied in a randomized, controlled clinical trial in combination with chemotherapy (469 patients) and an open-label single agent clinical trial (222 patients). Both trials studied patients with metastatic breast cancer whose tumors overexpress the HER2 protein. Patients were eligible if they had 2+ or 3+ levels of overexpression (based on a 0 to 3+ scale) by immunohistochemical assessment of tumor tissue performed by a central testing lab.

A multicenter, randomized, controlled clinical trial was conducted in 469 patients with metastatic breast cancer who had not been previously treated with chemotherapy for metastatic disease.[11] Patients were randomized to receive chemotherapy alone or in combination with HERCEPTIN given intravenously as a 4 mg/kg loading dose followed by weekly doses of HERCEPTIN at 2 mg/kg. For those who had received prior anthracycline therapy in the adjuvant setting, chemotherapy consisted of paclitaxel (175 mg/m² over 3 hours every 21 days for at least six cycles); for all other patients, chemotherapy consisted of anthracycline plus cyclophosphamide (AC: doxorubicin 60 mg/m² or epirubicin 75 mg/m² plus 600 mg/m² cyclophosphamide every 21 days for six cycles). Compared with patients in the AC subgroups (n=281), patients in the paclitaxel subgroup (n=188) were more likely to have had the following: poor prognostic factors (premenopausal status, estrogen or progesterone receptor negative tumors, positive lymph nodes), prior therapy (adjuvant chemotherapy, myeloblative chemotherapy, radiotherapy), and a shorter disease-free interval. Sixty-five percent of patients randomized to receive chemotherapy alone in this study received HERCEPTIN at the time of disease progression as part of a separate extension study.

Table 1
Phase III Clinical Efficacy in First-Line Treatment

	Combined Results		Paclitaxel subgroup		AC subgroup	
	HERCEPTIN + All Chemotherapy (n = 235)	All Chemotherapy (n = 234)	HERCEPTIN + Paclitaxel (n = 92)	Paclitaxel (n = 96)	HERCEPTIN + AC[a] (n = 143)	AC (n = 138)
Primary Endpoint						
Time to Progression[b,c]						
Median (months)	7.2	4.5	6.7	2.5	7.6	5.7
95% confidence interval	6.9, 8.2	4.3, 4.9	5.2, 9.9	2.0, 4.3	7.2, 9.1	4.6, 7.1
p-value (log rank)	< 0.0001		< 0.0001		0.002	
Secondary Endpoints						
Overall Response Rate[b]						
Rate (percent)	45	29	38	15	50	38
95% confidence interval	39, 51	23, 35	28, 48	8, 22	42, 58	30, 46
p-value ($_{\chi}2$-test)	< 0.001		< 0.001		0.10	
Duration of Response[b,c]						
Median (months)	8.3	5.8	8.3	4.3	8.4	6.4
25%, 75% quartile	5.5, 14.8	3.9, 8.5	5.1, 11.0	3.7, 7.4	5.8, 14.8	4.5, 8.5
Survival Time[c]						
Median Survival (months)	25.1	20.3	22.1	18.4	26.8	21.4
95% confidence interval	22.2, 29.5	16.8, 24.2	16.9, 28.6	12.7, 24.4	23.3, 32.9	18.3, 26.6
p-value (log rank)	0.05		0.17		0.16	

[a] AC = anthracycline (doxorubicin or epirubicin) and cyclophosphamide.
[b] Assessed by an independent Response Evaluation Committee.
[c] Kaplan-Meier Estimate

Compared with patients randomized to chemotherapy alone, the patients randomized to HERCEPTIN and chemotherapy experienced a significantly longer median time to disease progression, a higher overall response rate (ORR), a longer median duration of response, and a longer median survival (see Table 1). These treatment effects were observed both in patients who received HERCEPTIN plus paclitaxel and in those who received HERCEPTIN plus AC, however the magnitude of the effects was greater in the paclitaxel subgroup (see CLINICAL STUDIES: HER2 Detection).

[See table 1 below]

HERCEPTIN was studied as a single agent in a multicenter, open-label, single-arm clinical trial in patients with HER2 overexpressing metastatic breast cancer who had relapsed following one or two prior chemotherapy regimens for metastatic disease. Of 222 patients enrolled, 66% had received prior adjuvant chemotherapy, 68% had received two prior chemotherapy regimens for metastatic disease, and 25% had received prior myeloablative treatment with hematopoietic rescue. Patients were treated with a loading dose of 4 mg/kg IV followed by weekly doses of HERCEPTIN at 2 mg/kg IV. The ORR (complete response + partial response), as determined by an independent Response Evaluation Committee, was 14%, with a 2% complete response rate and a 12% partial response rate. Complete responses were observed only in patients with disease limited to skin and lymph nodes (see CLINICAL STUDIES: HER2 Detection).

HER2 Detection

(See PRECAUTIONS: HER2 Testing)

Detection of HER2 protein overexpression is necessary for selection of patients appropriate for HERCEPTIN therapy (see INDICATIONS AND USAGE). Overexpression of HER2 by tumors was an entry criterion of the two clinical studies described above. In those studies, a research-use-only IHC assay (referred to as the Clinical Trial Assay, [CTA]) was used.

The commercial assays described below, HercepTest® (IHC assay) and PathVysion® (FISH assay), are appropriate assays to aid in the selection of patients for HERCEPTIN therapy (see HER2 Detection: HER2 Protein Overexpression Detection Methods and HER2 Gene Amplification Detection Methods). The comparability of either assay with regard to the ability to predict clinical benefit from HERCEPTIN therapy has not been prospectively studied. In addition, the utility of either assay in patients whose tumors would score as 0 or 1+ by the Clinical Trial Assay (CTA) has not been established because patients with tumors that scored as 0 or 1+ were excluded from the clinical studies described.

HER2 Protein Overexpression Detection Methods

HER2 protein overexpression can be established by measuring expressed HER2 protein using IHC methodology. In the clinical trial studies described above, specimens were tested with the CTA and scored as 0, 1+, 2+, or 3+ with 3+ indicating the strongest positivity. Only patients with 2+ or 3+ positive tumors were eligible (about 33% of those screened). Data from the randomized trial suggest that the beneficial treatment effects were largely limited to patients with the highest level of HER2 protein overexpression (3+) (see Table 2). In an exploratory analysis, the relative risk (rr) for time to progression was lower in the patients whose tumors tested as CTA 3+ (rr = 0.42 with 95% CI: 0.33, 0.54) than in those tested as CTA 2+ (rr = 0.76 with 95% CI: 0.50, 1.15). The relative risk represents the risk of progression in the HERCEPTIN plus chemotherapy arm versus the chemotherapy arm. Therefore, a lower ratio represents longer time to progression in the HERCEPTIN arm. In the single-arm study of HERCEPTIN as a single agent, the overall response rate in patients whose tumors tested as CTA 3+ was 18% while in those that tested as CTA 2+, it was 6%.

HercepTest®, another IHC assay, was assessed for concordance with the CTA (see HER2 Assay: Concordance Studies), but has not been used to assess tumor specimens from the HERCEPTIN clinical studies described above.

HER2 Gene Amplification Detection Methods

As a surrogate for protein overexpression, measurement of the number of HER2 gene copies using FISH to detect gene amplification may be employed. An exploratory, retrospective assessment of known CTA 2+ or 3+ tumor specimens was performed to detect HER2 gene amplification using PathVysion®, a FISH assay. Data from this retrospective analysis involving 660 of 691 (96%) patients enrolled in the clinical studies (all scoring 2+ or 3+ by the CTA) suggested that the beneficial treatment effects were greater in patients whose tumors tested as FISH (+) than in those that were FISH (−); however, time to progression was prolonged for patients on the HERCEPTIN arm, regardless of the FISH result (see Table 2). In the single arm study of HERCEPTIN as a single agent, the overall response rate in patients whose tumors tested as FISH (+) was 20%, while in those tested as FISH (−), there were no responses.

These data are not sufficient to conclude whether FISH testing can distinguish a subpopulation of CTA 2+ patients who would be unlikely to benefit from HERCEPTIN therapy. In addition, there are no data correlating clinical outcome with FISH test results for patients with tumors that scored as 0 or 1+ by CTA; therefore, conclusions regarding the usefulness of FISH in the general population cannot be made.

[See table 2 at top of next page]

HER2 Assay Concordance Studies
(See PRECAUTIONS: HER2 Testing)
Immunohistochemistry: The DAKO HercepTest®, an IHC test for detecting HER2 protein overexpression, has not been directly studied for its ability to predict HERCEPTIN treatment effect, but has been compared to the CTA on over 500 breast cancer histology specimens obtained from the National Cancer Institute Cooperative Breast Cancer Tissue Resource. Based upon these results, of specimens testing 3+ (strongly positive) on the HercepTest®, 82% were 3+ (i.e., the reading most associated with clinical benefit), 12% were 2+, and 6% were 0 or 1+ on the CTA. The 6% of HercepTest® 3+ specimens that were CTA 0 or 1+ would be expected to represent 2% of the 0 and 1+ population. Of specimens testing 2+ (weakly positive) on the HercepTest®, 14% were 3+, 20% were 2+, and 66% were 0 or 1+ on the CTA. Of specimens testing 0 or 1+ on the HercepTest®, 2% were 3+, 6% were 2+, and 92% were 0 or 1+ on the CTA.
Fluorescence in situ Hybridization: The Vysis PathVysion® HER2 DNA Probe, a FISH test for detecting HER2 gene amplification, was compared with the CTA on over 500 breast cancer histology specimens originally submitted for potential enrollment in the HERCEPTIN trials. A HER2:CEP17 ratio of ≥2 was defined as FISH positive (+). Based on these results, of specimens testing FISH (+) by PathVysion®, 81% were 3+, 10% were 2+, and 9% were 0 or 1+ on the CTA. The 9% of FISH (+) specimens that were CTA 0 or 1+ would be expected to represent 3% of the total CTA 0 or 1+ population. Of specimens testing FISH (−) by PathVysion®, 3% were 3+, 10% were 2+, and 87% were 0 or 1+ on the CTA.

INDICATIONS AND USAGE

HERCEPTIN (Trastuzumab) as a single agent is indicated for the treatment of patients with metastatic breast cancer whose tumors overexpress the HER2 protein and who have received one or more chemotherapy regimens for their metastatic disease. HERCEPTIN in combination with paclitaxel is indicated for treatment of patients with metastatic breast cancer whose tumors overexpress the HER2 protein and who have not received chemotherapy for their metastatic disease. HERCEPTIN should be used in patients whose tumors have been evaluated with an assay validated to predict HER2 protein overexpression (see PRECAUTIONS: HER2 Testing and CLINICAL STUDIES: HER2 Detection).

CONTRAINDICATIONS

None known.

WARNINGS

Cardiotoxicity
Signs and symptoms of cardiac dysfunction, such as dyspnea, increased cough, paroxysmal nocturnal dyspnea, peripheral edema, S_3 gallop, or reduced ejection fraction, have been observed in patients treated with HERCEPTIN. Congested heart failure associated with HERCEPTIN therapy may be severe and has been associated with disabling cardiac failure, death, and mural thrombosis leading to stroke (see BOXED WARNINGS: CARDIOMYOPATHY). The clinical status of patients in the trials who developed congestive heart failure was classified for severity using the New York Heart Association classification system (I-IV, where IV is the most severe level of cardiac failure) (see Table 3).
[See table 3 above]
Candidates for treatment with HERCEPTIN should undergo thorough baseline cardiac assessment including history and physical exam and one or more of the following: EKG, echocardiogram, and MUGA scan. There are no data regarding the most appropriate method of evaluation for the identification of patients at risk for developing cardiotoxicity. Monitoring may not identify all patients who will develop cardiac dysfunction.
Extreme caution should be exercised in treating patients with pre-existing cardiac dysfunction.
Patients receiving HERCEPTIN should undergo frequent monitoring for deteriorating cardiac function.
The probability of cardiac dysfunction was highest in patients who received HERCEPTIN concurrently with anthracyclines. The data suggest that advanced age may increase the probability of cardiac dysfunction.
Pre-existing cardiac disease or prior cardiotoxic therapy (e.g., anthracycline or radiation therapy to the chest) may decrease the ability to tolerate HERCEPTIN therapy; however, the data are not adequate to evaluate the correlation between HERCEPTIN-induced cardiotoxicity and these factors.
Discontinuation of HERCEPTIN therapy should be strongly considered in patients who develop clinically significant congestive heart failure. In the clinical trials, most patients with cardiac dysfunction responded to appropriate medical therapy often including discontinuation of HERCEPTIN. The safety of continuation or resumption of HERCEPTIN in patients who have previously experienced cardiac toxicity has not been studied. There are insufficient data regarding discontinuation of HERCEPTIN therapy in patients with asymptomatic decreases in ejection fraction; such patients should be closely monitored for evidence of clinical deterioration.
Hypersensitivity Reactions Including Anaphylaxis
Severe hypersensitivity reactions have been infrequently reported in patients treated with HERCEPTIN (see BOXED WARNINGS: HYPERSENSITIVITY REACTIONS INCLUDING ANAPHYLAXIS). Signs and symptoms include anaphylaxis, urticaria, bronchospasm, angioedema, and/or hypotension. In some cases, the reactions have been fatal. The onset of symptoms generally occurred during an infusion, but there have also been reports of symptom onset after the completion of an infusion. Reactions were most commonly reported in association with the initial infusion.
HERCEPTIN infusion should be interrupted in all patients with severe hypersensitivity reactions. In the event of a hypersensitivity reaction, appropriate medical therapy should be administered which may include epinephrine, corticosteroids, diphenhydramine, bronchodilators, and oxygen. Patients should be evaluated and carefully monitored until complete resolution of signs and symptoms.
There are no data regarding the most appropriate method of identification of patients who may safely be retreated with HERCEPTIN after experiencing a severe hypersensitivity reaction. HERCEPTIN has been readministered to some patients who fully recovered from a previous severe reaction. Prior to readministration of HERCEPTIN, the majority of these patients were prophylactically treated with pre-medications including antihistamines and/or corticosteroids. While some of these patients tolerated retreatment, others had severe reactions again despite the use of prophylactic pre-medications.
Infusion Reactions
In the postmarketing setting, rare occurrences of severe infusion reactions leading to a fatal outcome have been associated with the use of HERCEPTIN. (See BOXED WARNINGS: INFUSION REACTIONS.)
In clinical trials, infusion reactions consisted of a symptom complex characterized by fever and chills, and on occasion included nausea, vomiting, pain (in some cases at tumor sites), headache, dizziness, dyspnea, hypotension, rash, and asthenia. These reactions were usually mild to moderate in severity. (See ADVERSE REACTIONS.)
However, in postmarketing reports, more severe adverse reactions to HERCEPTIN infusion were observed and included bronchospasm, hypoxia, and severe hypotension. These severe reactions were usually associated with the initial infusion of HERCEPTIN and generally occurred during or immediately following the infusion. However, the onset and clinical course were variable. For some patients, symptoms progressively worsened and led to further pulmonary complications. (See WARNINGS: Pulmonary Events.) In other patients with acute onset of signs and symptoms, initial improvement was followed by clinical deterioration. Delayed post-infusion events with rapid clinical deterioration have also been reported. Rarely, severe infusion reactions culminated in death within hours or up to one week following an infusion.
Some severe reactions have been treated successfully with interruption of the HERCEPTIN infusion and supportive therapy including oxygen, intravenous fluids, beta-agonists, and corticosteroids.
There are no data regarding the most appropriate method of identification of patients who may safely be retreated with HERCEPTIN after experiencing a severe infusion reaction. HERCEPTIN has been readministered to some patients who fully recovered from the previous severe reaction. Prior to readministration of HERCEPTIN, the majority of these patients were prophylactically treated with pre-medications including antihistamines and/or corticosteroids. While some of these patients tolerated retreatment, others had severe reactions again despite the use of prophylactic premedications.
Exacerbation of Chemotherapy-Induced Neutropenia
In randomized, controlled clinical trials designed to assess the impact of the addition of HERCEPTIN on chemotherapy, the per-patient incidences of moderate to severe neutropenia and of febrile neutropenia were higher in patients receiving HERCEPTIN in combination with myelosuppressive chemotherapy as compared to those who received chemotherapy alone. In the postmarketing setting, deaths due to sepsis in patients with severe neutropenia have been reported in patients receiving HERCEPTIN and myelosuppressive chemotherapy, although in controlled clinical trials (pre- and post-marketing), the incidence of septic deaths was not significantly increased. The pathophysiologic basis for exacerbation of neutropenia has not been determined; the effect of HERCEPTIN on the pharmacokinetics of chemotherapeutic agents has not been fully evaluated (see ADVERSE REACTIONS: Anemia and Leukopenia; ADVERSE REACTIONS: Infection).
Pulmonary Events
Severe pulmonary events leading to death have been reported rarely with the use of HERCEPTIN in the postmarketing setting. Signs, symptoms and clinical findings include dyspnea, pulmonary infiltrates, pleural effusions, non-cardiogenic pulmonary edema, pulmonary insufficiency and hypoxia, and acute respiratory distress syndrome. These events may or may not occur as sequelae of infusion reactions. (See WARNINGS: Infusion Reactions.) Patients with symptomatic intrinsic lung disease or with extensive tumor involvement of the lungs, resulting in dyspnea at rest, may be at greater risk of severe reactions.
Other severe events reported rarely in the postmarketing setting include pneumonitis and pulmonary fibrosis.

PRECAUTIONS

General
HERCEPTIN therapy should be used with caution in patients with known hypersensitivity to Trastuzumab, Chinese Hamster Ovary cell proteins, or any component of this product.
HER2 Testing
Assessment for HER2 overexpression should be performed by laboratories with demonstrated proficiency in the specific technology being utilized. Improper assay performance, including use of suboptimally fixed tissue, failure to utilize specified reagents, deviation from specific assay instructions, and failure to include appropriate controls for assay validation, can lead to unreliable results. Refer to the HercepTest® and PathVysion® package inserts for full instructions on assay performance (see CLINICAL STUDIES: HER2 Detection).
Drug Interactions
There have been no formal drug interaction studies performed with HERCEPTIN in humans. Administration of paclitaxel in combination with HERCEPTIN resulted in a two-fold decrease in HERCEPTIN clearance in a non-human primate study and in a 1.5-fold increase in HERCEPTIN serum levels in clinical studies. (see CLINICAL PHARMACOLOGY: Pharmacokinetics.)

Table 2
Treatment Effect versus Level of HER2 Expression
Phase III Randomized Trial (N = 469):
HERCEPTIN Plus Chemotherapy versus Chemotherapy

HER2 Assay Result	Number of Patients (N)	Relative Risk** for Time to Disease Progression (95% CI)	Relative Risk** for Mortality (95% CI)
CTA 2+ or 3+	469	0.49 (0.40, 0.61)	0.80 (0.64, 1.00)
FISH (+)*	325	0.44 (0.34, 0.57)	0.70 (0.53, 0.91)
FISH (−)*	126	0.62 (0.42, 0.94)	1.06 (0.70, 1.63)
CTA 2+	120	0.76 (0.50, 1.15)	1.26 (0.82, 1.94)
FISH (+)	32	0.54 (0.21, 1.35)	1.31 (0.53, 3.27)
FISH (−)	83	0.77 (0.48, 1.25)	1.11 (0.68, 1.82)
CTA 3+	349	0.42 (0.33, 0.54)	0.70 (0.51, 0.90)
FISH (+)	293	0.42 (0.32, 0.55)	0.67 (0.51, 0.89)
FISH (−)	43	0.43 (0.20, 0.94)	0.88 (0.39, 1.98)

* FISH testing results were available for 451 of the 469 patients enrolled on study.
** The relative risk represents the risk of progression or death in the HERCEPTIN plus chemotherapy arm versus the chemotherapy arm.

Table 3
Incidence and Severity of Cardiac Dysfunction

	HERCEPTIN[a] Alone n=213	HERCEPTIN + Paclitaxel[b] n=91	Paclitaxel[b] n=95	HERCEPTIN + Anthracycline+ Cyclophosphamide[b] n=143	Anthracycline + Cyclophosphamide[b] n=135
Any Cardiac Dysfunction	7%	11%	1%	28%	7%
Class III-IV	5%	4%	1%	19%	3%

[a] Open-label, single-agent Phase II study (94% received prior anthracyclines).
[b] Randomized Phase III study comparing chemotherapy plus HERCEPTIN to chemotherapy alone, where chemotherapy is either anthracycline/cyclophosphamide or paclitaxel.

Continued on next page

Herceptin—Cont.

Benzyl Alcohol

For patients with a known hypersensitivity to benzyl alcohol (the preservative in Bacteriostatic Water for Injection) reconstitute HERCEPTIN with Sterile Water for Injection (SWFI), USP. DISCARD THE SWFI-RECONSTITUTED HERCEPTIN VIAL FOLLOWING A SINGLE USE.

Carcinogenesis, Mutagenesis, Impairment of Fertility

Carcinogenesis

HERCEPTIN has not been tested for its carcinogenic potential.

Mutagenesis

No evidence of mutagenic activity was observed in Ames tests using six different test strains of bacteria, with and without metabolic activation, at concentrations of up to 5000 µg/mL Trastuzumab. Human peripheral blood lymphocytes treated *in vitro* at concentrations of up to 5000 µg/plate Trastuzumab, with and without metabolic activation, revealed no evidence of mutagenic potential. In an *in vivo* mutagenic assay (the micronucleus assay), no evidence of chromosomal damage to mouse bone marrow cells was observed following bolus intravenous doses of up to 118 mg/kg Trastuzumab.

Impairment of Fertility

A fertility study has been conducted in female cynomolgus monkeys at doses up to 25 times the weekly human maintenance dose of 2 mg/kg HERCEPTIN and has revealed no evidence of impaired fertility.

Pregnancy Category B

Reproduction studies have been conducted in cynomolgus monkeys at doses up to 25 times the weekly human maintenance dose of 2 mg/kg HERCEPTIN and have revealed no evidence of impaired fertility or harm to the fetus. However, HER2 protein expression is high in many embryonic tissues including cardiac and neural tissues; in mutant mice lacking HER2, embryos died in early gestation.[12] Placental transfer of HERCEPTIN during the early (Days 20–50 of gestation) and late (Days 120–150 of gestation) fetal development period was observed in monkeys. There are, however, no adequate and well-controlled studies in pregnant women. Because animal reproduction studies are not always predictive of human response, this drug should be used during pregnancy only if clearly needed.

Nursing Mothers

A study conducted in lactating cynomolgus monkeys at doses 25 times the weekly human maintenance dose of 2 mg/kg HERCEPTIN demonstrated that Trastuzumab is secreted in the milk. The presence of Trastuzumab in the serum of infant monkeys was not associated with any adverse effects on their growth or development from birth to 3 months of age. It is not known whether HERCEPTIN is secreted in human milk. Because human IgG is secreted in human milk, and the potential for absorption and harm to the infant is unknown, women should be advised to discontinue nursing during HERCEPTIN therapy and for 6 months after the last dose of HERCEPTIN.

Pediatric Use

The safety and effectiveness of HERCEPTIN in pediatric patients have not been established.

Geriatric Use

HERCEPTIN has been administered to 133 patients who were 65 years of age or over. The risk of cardiac dysfunction may be increased in geriatric patients. The reported clinical experience is not adequate to determine whether older patients respond differently from younger patients.

ADVERSE REACTIONS

The most serious adverse reactions caused by HERCEPTIN include cardiomyopathy, hypersensitivity reactions including anaphylaxis, infusion reactions, pulmonary events, and exacerbation of chemotherapy-induced neutropenia. Please refer to the BOXED WARNINGS and/or WARNINGS sections for detailed descriptions of these reactions. The most common adverse reactions associated with HERCEPTIN use are fever, diarrhea, infections, chills, increased cough, headache, rash, and insomnia.

Because clinical trials are conducted under widely varying conditions, adverse reaction rates observed in the clinical trials of a drug cannot be directly compared to rates in the clinical trials of another drug and may not reflect the rates observed in practice. The adverse reaction information from clinical trials does, however, provide a basis for identifying the adverse events that appear to be related to drug use and for approximating rates.

Additional adverse reactions have been identified during post-marketing use of HERCEPTIN. Because these reactions are reported voluntarily from a population of uncertain size, it is not always possible to reliably estimate their frequency or establish a causal relationship to HERCEPTIN exposure. Decisions to include these reactions in labeling are typically based on one or more of the following factors: (1) seriousness of the reaction, (2) frequency of reporting, or (3) strength of causal connection to HERCEPTIN.

Where specific percentages are noted, these data are based on clinical studies of HERCEPTIN alone or in combination with chemotherapy in clinical trials. Data in Table 4 are based on the experience with the recommended dosing regimen for HERCEPTIN in a randomized controlled clinical trial of 234 patients who received HERCEPTIN in combination with chemotherapy and four open-label studies of HERCEPTIN as a single agent in 352 patients at doses of 10–500 mg administered weekly. Data regarding serious adverse events are based on experience in 958 patients enrolled in all clinical trials of HERCEPTIN conducted prior to marketing approval.

Table 4

Adverse Events Occurring in ≥ 5% of Patients or at Increased Incidence in the HERCEPTIN Arm of the Randomized Study (Percent of Patients)

	Single Agent n=352	HERCEPTIN + Paclitaxel n=91	Paclitaxel Alone n=95	HERCEPTIN + AC n=143	AC Alone n=135
Body as a Whole					
Pain	47	61	62	57	42
Asthenia	42	62	57	54	55
Fever	36	49	23	56	34
Chills	32	41	4	35	11
Headache	26	36	28	44	31
Abdominal pain	22	34	22	23	18
Back pain	22	34	30	27	15
Infection	20	47	27	47	31
Flu syndrome	10	12	5	12	6
Accidental injury	6	13	3	9	4
Allergic reaction	3	8	2	4	2
Cardiovascular					
Tachycardia	5	12	4	10	5
Congestive heart failure	7	11	1	28	7
Digestive					
Nausea	33	51	9	76	77
Diarrhea	25	45	29	45	26
Vomiting	23	37	28	53	49
Nausea and vomiting	8	14	11	18	9
Anorexia	14	24	16	31	26
Heme & Lymphatic					
Anemia	4	14	9	36	26
Leukopenia	3	24	17	52	34
Metabolic					
Peripheral edema	10	22	20	20	17
Edema	8	10	8	11	5
Musculoskeletal					
Bone pain	7	24	18	7	7
Arthralgia	6	37	21	8	9
Nervous					
Insomnia	14	25	13	29	15
Dizziness	13	22	24	24	18
Paresthesia	9	48	39	17	11
Depression	6	12	13	20	12
Peripheral neuritis	2	23	16	2	2
Neuropathy	1	13	5	4	4
Respiratory					
Cough increased	26	41	22	43	29
Dyspnea	22	27	26	42	25
Rhinitis	14	22	5	22	16
Pharyngitis	12	22	14	30	18
Sinusitis	9	21	7	13	6
Skin					
Rash	18	38	18	27	17
Herpes simplex	2	12	3	7	9
Acne	2	11	3	3	<1
Urogenital					
Urinary tract infection	5	18	14	13	7

Cardiac Failure/Dysfunction

For a description of cardiac toxicities, see BOXED WARNINGS: CARDIOMYOPATHY and WARNINGS: Cardiotoxicity.

Anemia and Leukopenia

In a randomized, controlled trial (see CLINICAL STUDIES), the per-patient incidences of anemia (30% vs. 21%) and leukopenia (53% vs. 37%) were higher in patients receiving HERCEPTIN in combination with chemotherapy as compared to those receiving chemotherapy alone. The majority of these cytopenic events were mild to moderate in intensity, reversible, and none resulted in discontinuation of therapy with HERCEPTIN.

In a randomized, controlled trial conducted in the post-marketing setting, there were also increased incidences of NCI-CTC Grade 3/4 neutropenia (32% [29/92] vs. 22% [21/94]) and of febrile neutropenia (23% [21/91] vs. 17% [16/94]) in patients randomized to HERCEPTIN in combination with myelosuppressive chemotherapy as compared to chemotherapy alone (see ADVERSE REACTIONS: Infection).

Hematologic toxicity is infrequent following the administration of HERCEPTIN as a single agent, with an incidence of Grade III toxicities for WBC, platelets, hemoglobin all <1%. No Grade IV toxicities were observed.

Diarrhea

Of patients treated with HERCEPTIN as a single agent, 25% experienced diarrhea. An increased incidence of diarrhea, primarily mild to moderate in severity, was observed in patients receiving HERCEPTIN in combination with chemotherapy.

Infection

In a randomized, controlled trial (see CLINICAL STUDIES), the incidence of infections, primarily mild upper respiratory infections of minor clinical significance or catheter infections, was higher (46% vs. 30%) in patients receiving HERCEPTIN in combination with chemotherapy as compared to those receiving chemotherapy alone.

In a randomized, controlled trial conducted in the post-marketing setting, the reported incidence of febrile neutropenia was higher (23% [21/92] vs. 17% [16/94]) in patients receiving HERCEPTIN in combination with myelosuppressive chemotherapy as compared to chemotherapy alone.

In the postmarketing setting, there have also been reports of febrile neutropenia and infection with neutropenia culminating in death associated with the use of HERCEPTIN and myelosuppressive chemotherapy (see WARNINGS: Exacerbation of Chemotherapy-Induced Neutropenia).

Infusion Reactions

During the first infusion with HERCEPTIN, a symptom complex most commonly consisting of chills and/or fever was observed in about 40% of patients in clinical trials. The symptoms were usually mild to moderate in severity and were treated with acetaminophen, diphenhydramine, and meperidine (with or without reduction in the rate of HERCEPTIN infusion). HERCEPTIN discontinuation was infrequent. Other signs and/or symptoms may include nausea, vomiting, pain (in some cases at tumor sites), rigors, headache, dizziness, dyspnea, hypotention, elevated blood pressure, rash and asthenia. The symptoms occurred infrequently with subsequent HERCEPTIN infusions. (See BOXED WARNINGS: INFUSION REACTIONS and WARNINGS: Infusion Reactions.)

Additional adverse reactions have been identified during postmarketing use of HERCEPTIN. Because these reactions are reported voluntarily from a population of uncertain size, it is not always possible to reliably estimate their frequency or establish a causal relationship to HERCEPTIN exposure. Decisions to include these reactions in labeling are typically based on one or more of the following factors: (1) seriousness of the reaction, (2) frequency of reporting, or (3) strength of causal connection to HERCEPTIN.

Hypersensitivity Reactions Including Anaphylaxis Pulmonary Events

In the postmarketing setting, severe hypersensitivity reactions (including anaphylaxis), infusion reactions, and pulmonary adverse events have been reported (see BOXED WARNINGS: HYPERSENSITIVITY REACTIONS INCLUDING ANAPHYLAXIS and WARNINGS: Hypersensitivity Reactions Including Anaphylaxis). These events include anaphylaxis, angioedema, bronchospasm, hypotension, hypoxia, dyspnea, pulmonary infiltrates, pleural effusions, non-cardiogenic pulmonary edema and acute respiratory distress syndrome. For a detailed description, see WARNINGS.

Glomerulopathy
In the postmarketing setting, rare cases of nephrotic syndrome with pathologic evidence of glomerulopathy have been reported. The time to onset ranged from 4 months to approximately 18 months from initiation of HERCEPTIN therapy. Pathologic findings included membranous glomerulonephritis, focal glomerulocleroris and fibrillary glomerulonephritis. Complications included volume overload and congestive heart failure.
[See table 4 at top of previous page]

Other Serious Adverse Events
The following other serious adverse events occurred in at least one of the 958 patients treated with HERCEPTIN in clinical studies:
Body as a Whole: cellulitis, anaphylactoid reaction, ascites, hydrocephalus, radiation injury, deafness, amblyopia
Cardiovascular: vascular thrombosis, pericardial effusion, heart arrest, hypotension, syncope, hemorrhage, shock, arrhythmia
Digestive: hepatic failure, gastroenteritis, hematemesis, ileus, intestinal obstruction, colitis, esophageal ulcer, stomatitis, pancreatitis, hepatitis
Endocrine: hypothyroidism
Hematological: pancytopenia, acute leukemia, coagulation disorder, lymphangitis
Metabolic: hypercalcemia, hypomagnesemia, hyponatremia, hypoglycemia, growth retardation, weight loss
Musculoskeletal: pathological fractures, bone necrosis, myopathy
Nervous: convulsion, ataxia, confusion, manic reaction
Respiratory: apnea, pneumothorax, asthma, hypoxia, laryngitis
Skin: herpes zoster, skin ulceration
Urogenital: hydronephrosis, kidney failure, cervical cancer, hematuria, hemorrhagic cystitis, pyelonephritis

Immunogenicity
Of 903 patients who have been evaluated, human anti-human antibody (HAHA) to Trastuzumab was detected in one patient, who had no allergic manifestations.
The data reflect the percentage of patients whose test results were considered positive for antibodies to HERCEPTIN in the HAHA assay for Trastuzumab, and are highly dependent on the sensitivity and specificity of the assay. Additionally, the observed incidence of antibody positivity in an assay may be influenced by several factors including sample handling, timing of sample collection, concomitant medications, and underlying disease. For these reasons, comparison of the incidence of antibodies to HERCEPTIN with the incidence of antibodies to other products may be misleading.

OVERDOSAGE

There is no experience with overdosage in human clinical trials. Single doses higher than 500 mg have not been tested.

DOSAGE AND ADMINISTRATION

Usual Dose
The recommended initial loading dose is 4 mg/kg Trastuzumab administered as a 90-minute infusion. The recommended weekly maintenance dose is 2 mg/kg Trastuzumab and can be administered as a 30-minute infusion if the initial loading dose was well tolerated. HERCEPTIN may be administered in an outpatient setting. HERCEPTIN is to be diluted in saline for IV infusion. **DO NOT ADMINISTER AS AN IV PUSH OR BOLUS.** (See DOSAGE AND ADMINISTRATION: Administration.)

Preparation for Administration
The diluent provided has been formulated to maintain the stability and sterility of HERCEPTIN for up to 28 days. Other diluents have not been shown to contain effective preservatives for HERCEPTIN. Each vial of HERCEPTIN should be reconstituted with 20 mL of BWFI, USP, 1.1% benzyl alcohol preserved, as supplied, to yield a multi-dose solution containing 21 mg/mL Trastuzumab. Immediately upon reconstitution with BWFI, the vial of HERCEPTIN must be labeled in the area marked "Do not use after:" with the future date that is 28 days from the date of reconstitution.
If the patient has known hypersensitivity to benzyl alcohol, HERCEPTIN must be reconstituted with Sterile Water for Injection. (See PRECAUTIONS.) HERCEPTIN WHICH HAS BEEN RECONSTITUTED WITH SWFI MUST BE USED IMMEDIATELY AND ANY UNUSED PORTION DISCARDED. USE OF OTHER RECONSTITUTION DILUENTS SHOULD BE AVOIDED.
Shaking the reconstituted HERCEPTIN or causing excessive foaming during the addition of diluent may result in problems with dissolution and the amount of HERCEPTIN that can be withdrawn from the vial.
Use appropriate aseptic technique when performing the following reconstitution steps:

a. Using a sterile syringe, slowly inject the 20 mL of diluent into the vial containing the lyophilized cake of Trastuzumab. The stream of diluent should be directed into the lyophilized cake.
b. Swirl the vial gently to aid reconstitution. Trastuzumab may be sensitive to shear-induced stress, e.g., agitation or rapid expulsion from a syringe. **DO NOT SHAKE.**
c. Slight foaming of the product upon reconstitution is not unusual. Allow the vial to stand undisturbed for approximately 5 minutes. The solution should be essentially free of visible particulates, clear to slightly opalescent and colorless to pale yellow.

Determine the number of mg of Trastuzumab needed, based on a loading dose of 4 mg Trastuzumab/kg body weight or a maintenance dose of 2 mg Trastuzumab/kg body weight. Calculate the volume of 21 mg/mL Trastuzumab solution and withdraw this amount from the vial and add it to an infusion bag containing 250 mL of 0.9% Sodium Chloride Injection, USP. **DEXTROSE (5%) SOLUTION SHOULD NOT BE USED.** Gently invert the bag to mix the solution. The reconstituted preparation results in a colorless to pale yellow transparent solution. Parenteral drug products should be inspected visually for particulates and discoloration prior to administration.
No incompatibilities between HERCEPTIN and polyvinylchloride or polyethylene bags have been observed.

Administration
Treatment may be administered in an outpatient setting by administration of a 4 mg/kg Trastuzumab loading dose by intravenous (IV) infusion over 90 minutes. **DO NOT ADMINISTER AS AN IV PUSH OR BOLUS.** Patients should be observed for fever and chills or other infusion-associated symptoms. (See BOXED WARNINGS, WARNINGS, and ADVERSE REACTIONS.) If prior infusions are well tolerated, subsequent weekly doses of 2 mg/kg Trastuzumab may be administered over 30 minutes.
HERCEPTIN should not be mixed or diluted with other drugs. HERCEPTIN infusions should not be administered or mixed with dextrose solutions.

Stability and Storage
Vials of HERCEPTIN are stable at 2–8°C (36–46°F) prior to reconstitution. Do not use beyond the expiration date stamped on the vial. A vial of HERCEPTIN reconstituted with BWFI, as supplied, is stable for 28 days after reconstitution when stored refrigerated at 2–8°C (36–46°F), and the solution is preserved for multiple use. Discard any remaining multi-dose reconstituted solution after 28 days. If unpreserved SWFI (not supplied) is used, the reconstituted HERCEPTIN solution should be used immediately and any unused portion must be discarded. DO NOT FREEZE HERCEPTIN THAT HAS BEEN RECONSTITUTED.
The solution of HERCEPTIN for infusion diluted in polyvinylchloride or polyethylene bags containing 0.9% Sodium Chloride Injection, USP, may be stored at 2–8°C (36–46°F) for up to 24 hours prior to use. Diluted HERCEPTIN has been shown to be stable for up to 24 hours at room temperature (2–25°C). However, because diluted HERCEPTIN contains no effective preservative, the reconstituted and diluted solution should be stored refrigerated (2–8°C).

HOW SUPPLIED

HERCEPTIN (Trastuzumab) is supplied as a lyophilized, sterile powder nominally containing 440 mg Trastuzumab per vial under vacuum.
Each carton contains one vial of 440 mg HERCEPTIN® (Trastuzumab) and one vial containing 20 mL of Bacteriostatic Water for Injection, USP, 1.1% benzyl alcohol. NDC 50242-134-68.

REFERENCES

1. Coussens L. Yang-Feng TL, Liao Y-C, Chen E, Gray A, McGrath J, et al. Tyrosine kinase receptor with extensive homology to EGF receptor shares chromosomal location with neu oncogene. Science 1985;230:1132–9.
2. Press MF, Pike MC, Chazin VR, Hung G, Udove JA, Markowicz M, et al. Her-2/*neu* expression in node-negative breast cancer: direct tissue quantitation by computerized image analysis and association of overexpression with increased risk of recurrent disease. Cancer Res 1993;53:4960–70.
3. Slamon DJ, Godolphin W, Jones LA, Holt JA, Wong SG, Keith DE, et al. Studies of the HER2/*neu* proto-oncogene in human breast and ovarian cancer. Science 1989;244:707–12.
4. Killioniemi OP, Kallioniemi A, Kurisu W, Thor A, Chen L-C, Smith HS, et al. *ERBB2* amplification in breast cancer analyzed by fluorescence in situ hybridization. Proc Natl Acad Sci USA 1992:89:5321–5.
5. Pauletti G, Godolphin W, Press MF, Slamon DJ. Detection and quantitation of HER2/*neu* gene amplification in human breast cancer archival material using fluorescence in situ hybridization. Oncogene 1996;13:63–72.
6. Hudziak RM, Lewis GD, Winget M, Fendly BM, Shepard HM, Ullrich A. p185[HER2] monoclonal antibody has antiproliferative effects *in vitro* and sensitizes human breast tumor cells to tumor necrosis factor. Mol Cell Biol 1989;9:1165–72.
7. Lewis GD, Figari I, Fendly B, Wong WL, Carter P, Gorman C, et al. Differential responses of human tumor cell lines to anti-p185HER2 monoclonal antibodies. Cancer Immunol Immunother 1993;37:255–63.
8. Baselga J, Norton L, Albanell J, Kim Y-M, Mendelsohn J. Recombinant humanized anti-HER2 antibody (Herceptin™) enhances the antitumor activity of paclitaxel and doxorubicin against HER2/*neu* overexpressing human breast cancer xenografts. Cancer Res 1998;58:2825–31.
9. Hotaling TE, Reitz B, Wolfgang-Kimball D, Bauer K. Fox JA. The humanized anti-HER2 antibody rhuMAb HER2 mediates antibody dependent cell-mediated cytotoxicity via FcγR III [abstract]. Proc Am Assoc Cancer Res 1996;37:471. Abstract 3215
10. Pegram MD, Baly D, Wirth C, Gilkerson E, Slamon DJ, Sliwkowski MX, et al. Antibody dependent cell-mediated cytotoxicity in breast cancer patients in Phase III clinical trials of a humanized anti-HER2 antibody [abstract]. Proc Am Assoc Cancer Res 1997;38:602. Abstract 4044
11. Slamon D J., Leyland-Jones B, Shak S., Fuchs H, Paton V, Bajamonde A, et al. Use of chemotherapy plus a monoclonal antibody against HER2 for metastatic breast cancer that overexpresses HER2. N Engl J Med. 2001;344:783–92.
12. Lee, KF, Simon H, Chen H, Bates B, Hung MC, Hauser C. Requirement for neuroregulin receptor, erbB2, in neural and cardiac development. Nature 1995;378:394–8.

HERCEPTIN®
(Trastuzumab)
Manufactured by: 4817405
Genentech, Inc. FDA Approval Date October 2003
1 DNA Way Code revision June 2004
South San Francisco, CA 94080-4990

Shown in Product Identification Guide, page 313

NUTROPIN® ℞

[new-trō-pĭn]
[somatropin (rDNA origin) for injection]

DESCRIPTION

Nutropin is a human growth hormone (hGH) produced by recombinant DNA technology. Nutropin has 191 amino acid residues and a molecular weight of 22,125 daltons. The amino acid sequence of the product is identical to that of pituitary-derived human growth hormone. The protein is synthesized by a specific laboratory strain of *E. coli* as a precursor consisting of the rhGH molecule preceded by the secretion signal from an *E. coli* protein. This precursor is directed to the plasma membrane of the cell. The signal sequence is removed and the native protein is secreted into the periplasm so that the protein is folded appropriately as it is synthesized.
Nutropin is a highly purified preparation. Biological potency is determined using a cell proliferation bioassay.
Nutropin is a sterile, white, lyophilized powder intended for subcutaneous administration after reconstitution with Bacteriostatic Water for Injection, USP (benzyl alcohol preserved). The reconstituted product is nearly isotonic at a concentration of 5 mg/mL growth hormone (GH) and has a pH of approximately 7.4.
Each 5 mg Nutropin vial contains 5 mg (approximately 15 IU) somatropin, lyophilized with 45 mg mannitol, 1.7 mg sodium phosphates (0.4 mg sodium phosphate monobasic and 1.3 mg sodium phosphate dibasic), and 1.7 mg glycine.
Each 10 mg Nutropin vial contains 10 mg (approximately 30 IU) somatropin, lyophilized with 90 mg mannitol, 3.4 mg sodium phosphates (0.8 mg sodium phosphate monobasic and 2.6 mg sodium phosphate dibasic), and 3.4 mg glycine.
Bacteriostatic Water for Injection, USP is sterile water containing 0.9 percent benzyl alcohol per mL as an antimicrobial preservative packaged in a multidose vial. The diluent pH is 4.5–7.0.

CLINICAL PHARMACOLOGY

General
In vitro and in vivo preclinical and clinical testing have demonstrated that Nutropin is therapeutically equivalent to pituitary-derived human GH (hGH). Pediatric patients who lack adequate endogenous GH secretion, patients with chronic renal insufficiency, and patients with Turner syndrome that were treated with Nutropin resulted in an increase in growth rate and an increase in insulin-like growth factor-I (IGF-I) levels similar to that seen with pituitary-derived hGH.
Actions that have been demonstrated for Nutropin, somatrem, and/or pituitary-derived hGH include:

A. Tissue Growth
1) Skeletal Growth: GH stimulates skeletal growth in pediatric patients with growth failure due to a lack of adequate secretion of endogenous GH or secondary to chronic renal insufficiency and in patients with Turner syndrome. Skeletal growth is accomplished at the epiphyseal plates at the ends of a growing bone. Growth and metabolism of epiphyseal plate cells are directly stimulated by GH and one of its mediators, IGF-I. Serum levels of IGF-I are low in children and adolescents who are GH deficient, but increase during treatment with GH. In pediatric patients, new bone is formed at the epiphyses in response to GH and IGF-I. This results in linear growth until these growth plates fuse at the end of puberty. 2) Cell Growth: Treatment with hGH results in an increase in both the number and the size of skeletal muscle cells. 3) Organ Growth: GH influences the size of internal organs, including kidneys, and increases red cell mass. Treatment of hypophysectomized or genetic dwarf rats with GH results in organ growth that is proportional to the overall body growth. In normal rats subjected to nephrectomy-induced uremia, GH promoted skeletal and body growth.

B. Protein Metabolism
Linear growth is facilitated in part by GH-stimulated protein synthesis. This is reflected by nitrogen retention as demonstrated by a decline in urinary nitrogen excretion and blood urea nitrogen during GH therapy.

C. Carbohydrate Metabolism
GH is a modulator of carbohydrate metabolism. For example, patients with inadequate secretion of GH some-

Continued on next page

Nutropin—Cont.

times experience fasting hypoglycemia that is improved by treatment with GH. GH therapy may decrease insulin sensitivity. Untreated patients with chronic renal insufficiency and Turner syndrome have an increased incidence of glucose intolerance. Administration of hGH to adults or children resulted in increases in serum fasting and postprandial insulin levels, more commonly in overweight or obese individuals. In addition, mean fasting and postprandial glucose and hemoglobin A_{1c} levels remained in the normal range.

D. Lipid Metabolism

In GH-deficient patients, administration of GH resulted in lipid mobilization, reduction in body fat stores, increased plasma fatty acids, and decreased plasma cholesterol levels.

E. Mineral Metabolism

The retention of total body potassium in response to GH administration apparently results from cellular growth. Serum levels of inorganic phosphorus may increase slightly in patients with inadequate secretion of endogenous GH, chronic renal insufficiency, or patients with Turner syndrome during GH therapy due to metabolic activity associated with bone growth as well as increased tubular reabsorption of phosphate by the kidney. Serum calcium is not significantly altered in these patients. Sodium retention also occurs. Adults with childhood-onset GH deficiency show low bone mineral density (BMD). GH therapy results in increases in serum alkaline phosphatase. (See PRECAUTIONS: Laboratory Tests.)

F. Connective Tissue Metabolism

GH stimulates the synthesis of chondroitin sulfate and collagen as well as the urinary excretion of hydroxyproline.

Pharmacokinetics

Subcutaneous Absorption—The absolute bioavailability of recombinant human growth hormone (rhGH) after subcutaneous administration in healthy adult males has been determined to be 81±20%. The mean terminal $t_{1/2}$ after subcutaneous administration is significantly longer than that seen after intravenous administration (2.1±0.43 hr vs. 19.5±3.1 min) indicating that the subcutaneous absorption of the compound is slow and rate-limiting.

Distribution—Animal studies with rhGH showed that GH localizes to highly perfused organs, particularly the liver and kidney. The volume of distribution at steady state for rhGH in healthy adult males is about 50 mL/kg body weight, approximating the serum volume.

Metabolism—Both the liver and kidney have been shown to be important metabolizing organs for GH. Animal studies suggest that the kidney is the dominant organ of clearance. GH is filtered at the glomerulus and reabsorbed in the proximal tubules. It is then cleaved within renal cells into its constituent amino acids, which return to the systemic circulation.

Elimination—The mean terminal $t_{1/2}$ after intravenous administration of rhGH in healthy adult males is estimated to be 19.5±3.1 minutes. Clearance of rhGH after intravenous administration in healthy adults and children is reported to be in the range of 116–174 mL/hr/kg.

Bioequivalence of Formulations—Nutropin has been determined to be bioequivalent to Nutropin AQ® [somatropin (rDNA origin) injection] based on the statistical evaluation of AUC and C_{max}.

SPECIAL POPULATIONS

Pediatric—Available literature data suggest that rhGH clearances are similar in adults and children.

Gender—No data are available for exogenously administered rhGH. Available data for methionyl recombinant GH, pituitary-derived GH, and endogenous GH suggest no consistent gender-based differences in GH clearance.

Geriatrics—Limited published data suggest that the plasma clearance and average steady-state plasma concentration of rhGH may not be different between young and elderly patients.

Race—Reported values for half-lives for endogenous GH in normal adult black males are not different from observed values for normal adult white males. No data for other races are available.

Growth Hormone Deficiency (GHD)—Reported values for clearance of rhGH in adults and children with GHD range 138–245 mL/hr/kg and are similar to those observed in healthy adults and children. Mean terminal $t_{1/2}$ values following intravenous and subcutaneous administration in adult and pediatric GHD patients are also similar to those observed in healthy adult males.

Renal Insufficiency—Children and adults with chronic renal failure (CRF) and end-stage renal disease (ESRD) tend to have decreased clearance compared to normals. Endogenous GH production may also increase in some individuals with ESRD. However, no rhGH accumulation has been reported in children with CRF or ESRD dosed with current regimens.

Turner Syndrome—No pharmacokinetic data are available for exogenously administered rhGH. However, reported half-lives, absorption, and elimination rates for endogenous GH in this population are similar to the ranges observed for normal subjects and GHD populations.

Hepatic Insufficiency—A reduction in rhGH clearance has been noted in patients with severe liver dysfunction. The clinical significance of this decrease is unknown.

Summary of Nutropin Pharmacokinetic Parameters in Healthy Adult Males 0.1 mg (approximately 0.3 IU[a])/kg SC

	C_{max} (μg/L)	T_{max} (hr)	$t_{1/2}$ (hr)	$AUC_{0-\infty}$ (μg•hr/L)	CL/F_{SC} (mL/[hr•kg])
MEAN[b]	67.2	6.2	2.1	643	158
CV%	29	37	20	12	12

Abbreviations:
C_{max}=maximum concentration
$t_{1/2}$ =half life
$AUC_{0-\infty}$=area under the curve
CL/F_{SC}=systemic clearance
F_{SC}=subcutaneous bioavailability (not determined)
CV%=coefficient of variation in %; SC=subcutaneous
[a]Based on current International Standard of 3 IU=1 mg
[b]n=36

Single Dose Mean Growth Hormone Concentrations in Healthy Adult Males

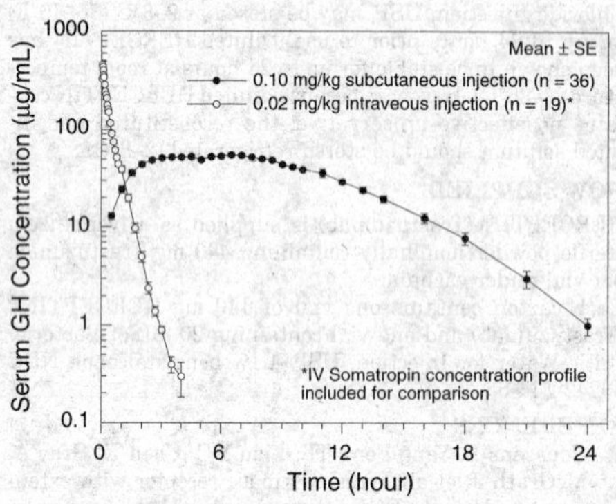

EFFICACY STUDIES

Growth Hormone Deficiency (GHD) in Pubertal Patients

One open-label, multicenter, randomized clinical trial of two dosages of Nutropin was performed in pubertal patients with GHD. Ninety-seven patients (mean age 13.9 years, 83 male, 14 female) currently being treated with approximately 0.3 mg/kg/wk of GH were randomized to 0.3 mg/kg/wk or 0.7 mg/kg/wk Nutropin doses. All patients were already in puberty (Tanner stage ≥2) and had bone ages ≤14 years in males or ≤12 years in females. Mean baseline height standard deviation (SD) score was −1.3.

The mean last measured height in all 97 patients after a mean duration of 2.7±1.2 years, by analysis of covariance (ANCOVA) adjusting for baseline height, is shown below. [See table below]

The mean height SD score at last measured height (n=97) was −0.7±1.0 in the 0.3 mg/kg/wk group and −0.1±1.2 in the 0.7 mg/kg/wk group. For patients completing 3.5 or more years (mean 4.1 years) of Nutropin treatment (15/49 patients in the 0.3 mg/kg/wk group and 16/48 patients in the 0.7 mg/kg/wk group), the mean last measured height was 166.1±8.0 cm in the 0.3 mg/kg/wk group and 171.8±7.1 cm in the 0.7 mg/kg/wk group, adjusting for baseline height and sex.

The mean change in bone age was approximately one year for each year in the study in both dose groups. Patients with baseline height SD scores above −1.0 were able to attain normal adult heights with the 0.3 mg/kg/wk dose of Nutropin (mean height SD score at near-adult height =−0.1, n=15).

Thirty-one patients had bone mineral density (BMD) determined by dual energy x-ray absorptiometry (DEXA) scans at study conclusion. The two dose groups did not differ significantly in mean SD score for total body BMD (−0.9±1.9 in the 0.3 mg/kg/wk group vs. −0.8±1.2 in the 0.7 mg/kg/wk group, n=20) or lumbar spine BMD (−1.0±1.0 in the 0.3 mg/kg/wk group vs. −0.2±1.7 in the 0.7 mg/kg/wk group, n=21).

Over a mean duration of 2.7 years, patients in the 0.7 mg/kg/wk group were more likely to have IGF-I values above the normal range than patients in the 0.3 mg/kg/wk group (27.7% vs. 9.0% of IGF-I measurements for individual patients). The clinical significance of elevated IGF-I values is unknown.

Effects of Nutropin on Growth Failure Due to Chronic Renal Insufficiency (CRI)

Two multicenter, randomized, controlled clinical trials were conducted to determine whether treatment with Nutropin prior to renal transplantation in patients with chronic renal insufficiency could improve their growth rates and height deficits. One study was a double-blind, placebo-controlled trial and the other was an open-label, randomized trial. The dose of Nutropin in both controlled studies was 0.05 mg/kg/day (0.35 mg/kg/week) administered daily by subcutaneous injection. Combining the data from those patients completing two years in the two controlled studies results in 62 patients treated with Nutropin and 28 patients in the control groups (either placebo-treated or untreated). The mean first year growth rate was 10.8 cm/yr for Nutropin-treated patients, compared with a mean growth rate of 6.5 cm/yr for placebo/untreated controls ($p<0.00005$). The mean second year growth rate was 7.8 cm/yr for the Nutropin-treated group, compared with 5.5 cm/yr for controls ($p<0.00005$). There was a significant increase in mean height standard deviation (SD) score in the Nutropin group (–2.9 at baseline to –1.5 at Month 24, n=62) but no significant change in the controls (–2.8 at baseline to –2.9 at Month 24, n=28). The mean third year growth rate of 7.6 cm/yr in the Nutropin-treated patients (n=27) suggests that Nutropin stimulates growth beyond two years. However, there are no control data for the third year because control patients crossed over to Nutropin treatment after two years of participation. The gains in height were accompanied by appropriate advancement of skeletal age. These data demonstrate that Nutropin therapy improves growth rate and corrects the acquired height deficit associated with chronic renal insufficiency. Currently there are insufficient data regarding the benefit of treatment beyond three years. Although predicted final height was improved during Nutropin therapy, the effect of Nutropin on final adult height remains to be determined.

Post-Transplant Growth

The North American Pediatric Renal Transplant Cooperative Study (NAPRTCS) has reported data for growth post-transplant in children who did not receive GH. The average change in height SD score during the initial two years post-transplant was 0.18 (n=300, *J Pediatr*. 1993;122:397–402). Controlled studies of GH treatment for the short stature associated with CRI were not designed to compare the growth of treated or untreated patients after they received renal transplants. However, growth data are available from a small number of patients who have been followed for at least 11 months. Of the 7 control patients, 4 increased their height SD score and 3 had either no significant change or a decrease in height SD score. The 13 patients treated with Nutropin prior to transplant had either no significant change or an increase in height SD score after transplantation, indicating that the individual gains achieved with GH therapy prior to transplant were maintained after transplantation. The differences in the height deficit narrowed between the treated and untreated groups in the post-transplant period.

Turner Syndrome

One long-term, randomized, open-label, multicenter, concurrently controlled study, two long-term, open-label, multicenter, historically controlled studies, and one long-term, randomized, dose-response study were conducted to evaluate the efficacy of GH for the treatment of girls with short stature due to Turner syndrome.

In the randomized study GDCT, comparing GH-treated patients to a concurrent control group who received no GH, the GH-treated patients who received a dose of 0.3 mg/kg/week given 6 times per week from a mean age of 11.7 years for a mean duration of 4.7 years attained a mean near final height of 146.0 cm (n=27) as compared to the control group who attained a near final height of 142.1 cm (n=19). By analysis of covariance, the effect of GH therapy was a mean height increase of 5.4 cm (p=0.001).

In two of the studies (85-023 and 85-044), the effect of long-term GH treatment (0.375 mg/kg/week given either 3 times per week or daily) on adult height was determined by comparing adult heights in the treated patients with those of age-matched historical controls with Turner syndrome who never received any growth-promoting therapy. In Study 85-023, estrogen treatment was delayed until patients were at least age 14. GH therapy resulted in a mean adult height gain of 7.4 cm (mean duration of GH therapy of 7.6 years) vs. matched historical controls by analysis of covariance.

In Study 85-044, patients treated with early GH therapy were randomized to receive estrogen-replacement therapy (conjugated estrogens, 0.3 mg escalating to 0.625 mg daily) at either age 12 or 15 years. Compared with matched his-

Last Measured Height* by Sex and Nutropin Dose

	Age (yr)	Last Measured Height* (cm) 0.3 mg/kg/wk	0.7 mg/kg/wk	Height Difference Between Groups (cm)
	Mean±SD (range)	Mean±SD	Mean±SD	Mean±SE
Male	17.2±1.3 (13.6 to 19.4)	170.9±7.9 (n=42)	174.5±7.9 (n=41)	3.6±1.7
Female	15.8±1.8 (11.9 to 19.3)	154.7±6.3 (n=7)	157.6±6.3 (n=7)	2.9±3.4

*Adjusted for baseline height

torical controls, early GH therapy (mean duration of GH therapy 5.6 years) combined with estrogen replacement at age 12 years resulted in an adult height gain of 5.9 cm (n=26), whereas girls who initiated estrogen at age 15 years (mean duration of GH therapy 6.1 years) had a mean adult height gain of 8.3 cm (n=29). Patients who initiated GH therapy after age 11 (mean age 12.7 years; mean duration of GH therapy 3.8 years) had a mean adult height gain of 5.0 cm (n=51).

Thus, in both studies, 85-023 and 85-044, the greatest improvement in adult height was observed in patients who received early GH treatment and estrogen after age 14 years.

In a randomized, blinded, dose-response study, GDCI, patients were treated from a mean age of 11.1 years for a mean duration of 5.3 years with a weekly dose of either 0.27 mg/kg or 0.36 mg/kg administered 3 or 6 times weekly. The mean near final height of patients receiving growth hormone was 148.7 cm (n=31). This represents a mean gain in adult height of approximately 5 cm compared with previous observations of untreated Turner syndrome girls.

In these studies, Turner syndrome patients (n=181) treated to final adult height achieved statistically significant average estimated adult height gains ranging from 5.0–8.3 cm. [See table above]

Study/Group	Study Design[a]	N at Adult Height	GH Age (yr)	Estrogen Age (yr)	GH Duration (yr)	Adult Height Gain (cm)[b]
GDCT	RCT	27	11.7	13	4.7	5.4
85-023	MHT	17	9.1	15.2	7.6	7.4
85-044: A*	MHT	29	9.4	15.0	6.1	8.3
B*		26	9.6	12.3	5.6	5.9
C*		51	12.7	13.7	3.8	5.0
GDCI	RDT	31	11.1	8–13.5	5.3	~5[c]

[a] RCT: randomized controlled trial; MHT: matched historical controlled trial; RDT: randomized dose-response trial.
[b] Analysis of covariance vs. controls
[c] Compared with historical data
*A= GH age <11 yr, estrogen age 15 yr
B= GH age <11 yr, estrogen age 12 yr
C= GH age >11 yr, estrogen at Month 12

Adult Growth Hormone Deficiency (GHD)

Two multicenter, double-blind, placebo-controlled clinical trials were conducted using Nutropin® [somatropin (rDNA origin) for injection] in GH-deficient adults. One study was conducted in subjects with adult-onset GHD, mean age 48.3 years, n=166, at doses of 0.0125 or 0.00625 mg/kg/day; doses of 0.025 mg/kg/day were not tolerated in these subjects. A second study was conducted in previously treated subjects with childhood-onset GHD, mean age 23.8 years, n=64, at randomly assigned doses of 0.025 or 0.0125 mg/kg/day. The studies were designed to assess the effects of replacement therapy with GH on body composition.

Significant changes from baseline to Month 12 of treatment in body composition (i.e., total body % fat mass, trunk % fat mass, and total body % lean mass by DEXA scan) were seen in all Nutropin groups in both studies ($p<0.0001$ for change from baseline and vs. placebo), whereas no statistically significant changes were seen in either of the placebo groups. In the adult-onset study, the Nutropin group improved mean total body fat from 35.0% to 31.5%, mean trunk fat from 33.9% to 29.5%, and mean lean body mass from 62.2% to 65.7%, whereas the placebo group had mean changes of 0.2% or less (p=not significant). Due to the possible effect of GH-induced fluid retention on DEXA measurements of lean body mass, DEXA scans were repeated approximately 3 weeks after completion of therapy; mean % lean body mass in the Nutropin group was 65.0%, a change of 2.8% from baseline, compared with a change of 0.4% in the placebo group ($p<0.0001$ between groups).

In the childhood-onset study, the high-dose Nutropin group improved mean total body fat from 38.4% to 32.1%, mean trunk fat from 36.7% to 29.0%, and mean lean body mass from 59.1% to 65.5%; the low-dose Nutropin group improved mean total body fat from 37.1% to 31.3%, mean trunk fat from 37.9% to 30.6%, and mean lean body mass from 60.0% to 66.0%; the placebo group had mean changes of 0.6% or less (p=not significant).

[See table below]

In the adult-onset study, significant decreases from baseline to Month 12 in LDL cholesterol and LDL:HDL ratio were seen in the Nutropin group compared to the placebo group, $p<0.02$; there were no statistically significant between-group differences in change from baseline to Month 12 in total cholesterol, HDL cholesterol, or triglycerides. In the childhood-onset study, significant decreases from baseline to Month 12 in total cholesterol, LDL cholesterol, and LDL:HDL ratio were seen in the high-dose Nutropin group only, compared to the placebo group, $p<0.05$. There were no statistically significant between-group differences in HDL cholesterol or triglycerides from baseline to Month 12.

In the childhood-onset study, 55% of the patients had decreased spine bone mineral density (BMD) (z-score <-1) at baseline. The administration of Nutropin (n=16) (0.025 mg/kg/day) for two years resulted in increased spine BMD from baseline when compared to placebo (n=13) (4.6% vs. 1.0%, respectively, $p<0.03$); a transient decrease in spine BMD was seen at six months in the Nutropin-treated patients. Thirty-five percent of subjects treated with this dose had supraphysiological levels of IGF-I at some point during the study, which may carry unknown risks. No significant improvement in total body BMD was found when compared to placebo. A lower GH dose (0.0125 mg/kg/day) did not show significant increments in either of these bone parameters when compared to placebo. No statistically significant effects on BMD were seen in the adult-onset study where patients received GH (0.0125 mg/kg/day) for one year.

Muscle strength, physical endurance, and quality of life measurements were not markedly abnormal at baseline, and no statistically significant effects of Nutropin therapy were observed in the two studies.

INDICATIONS AND USAGE

Pediatric Patients

Nutropin® [somatropin (rDNA origin) for injection] is indicated for the long-term treatment of growth failure due to a lack of adequate endogenous GH secretion.

Nutropin® [somatropin (rDNA origin) for injection] is also indicated for the treatment of growth failure associated with chronic renal insufficiency up to the time of renal transplantation. Nutropin therapy should be used in conjunction with optimal management of chronic renal insufficiency.

Nutropin® [somatropin (rDNA origin) for injection] is also indicated for the long-term treatment of short stature associated with Turner syndrome.

Adult Patients

Nutropin® [somatropin (rDNA origin) for injection] is indicated for the replacement of endogenous GH in patients with adult GH deficiency who meet both of the following two criteria:

1. Biochemical diagnosis of adult GH deficiency by means of a subnormal response to a standard growth hormone stimulation test (peak GH≤5 µg/L), and
2. Adult-onset: Patients who have adult GH deficiency either alone or with multiple hormone deficiencies (hypopituitarism) as a result of pituitary disease, hypothalamic disease, surgery, radiation therapy, or trauma; or

   Childhood-onset: Patients who were GH deficient during childhood, confirmed as an adult before replacement therapy with Nutropin is started.

CONTRAINDICATIONS

Growth hormone should not be initiated to treat patients with acute critical illness due to complications following open heart or abdominal surgery, multiple accidental trauma, or to patients having acute respiratory failure. Two placebo-controlled clinical trials in non-growth hormone-deficient adult patients (n=522) with these conditions revealed a significant increase in mortality (41.9% vs. 19.3%) among somatropin-treated patients (doses 5.3–8 mg/day) compared to those receiving placebo (see WARNINGS).

Nutropin should not be used for growth promotion in pediatric patients with closed epiphyses.

Nutropin should not be used in patients with active neoplasia. GH therapy should be discontinued if evidence of neoplasia develops.

Nutropin, when reconstituted with Bacteriostatic Water for Injection, USP (benzyl alcohol preserved), should not be used in patients with a known sensitivity to benzyl alcohol.

Growth hormone is contraindicated in patients with Prader-Willi syndrome who are severely obese or have severe respiratory impairment (see WARNINGS). Unless patients with Prader-Willi syndrome also have a diagnosis of growth hormone deficiency, Nutropin is not indicated for the long-term treatment of pediatric patients who have growth failure due to genetically confirmed Parader-Willi syndrome.

WARNINGS

See CONTRAINDICATIONS for information on increased mortality in patients with acute critical illnesses in intensive care units due to complications following open heart or abdominal surgery, multiple accidental trauma, or with acute respiratory failure. The safety of continuing growth hormone treatment in patients receiving replacement doses for approved indications who concurrently develop these illnesses has not been established. Therefore, the potential benefit of treatment continuation with growth hormone in patients having acute critical illnesses should be weighed against the potential risk.

Benzyl alcohol as a preservative in Bacteriostatic Water for Injection, USP, has been associated with toxicity in newborns. When administering Nutropin to newborns, reconstitute with Sterile Water for Injection, USP. USE ONLY ONE DOSE PER NUTROPIN VIAL AND DISCARD THE UNUSED PORTION.

There have been reports of fatalities after initiating therapy with growth hormone in pediatric patients with Prader-Willi syndrome who had one or more of the following risk factors: severe obesity, history of upper airway obstruction

Continued on next page

Mean Changes from Baseline to Month 12 in Proportion of Fat and Lean by DEXA for Studies M0431g and M0381g (Adult-onset and Childhood-onset GHD, respectively)

	M0431g			M0381g			
Proportion	Placebo (n=62)	Nutropin (n=63)	Between-Groups t-test p-value	Placebo (n=13)	Nutropin 0.0125 mg/kg/day (n=15)	Nutropin 0.025 mg/kg/day (n=15)	Placebo vs. Pooled Nutropin t-test p-value
Total body percent fat							
Baseline	36.8	35.0	0.38	35.0	37.1	38.4	0.45
Month 12	36.8	31.5		35.2	31.3	32.1	
Baseline to Month 12 change	**−0.1**	**−3.6**	<0.0001	**+0.2**	**−5.8**	**−6.3**	<0.0001
Post-washout	36.4	32.2		N/A	N/A	N/A	
Baseline to post-washout change	**−0.4**	**−2.8**	<0.0001	N/A	N/A	N/A	
Trunk percent fat							
Baseline	35.3	33.9	0.50	32.5	37.9	36.7	0.23
Month 12	35.4	29.5		33.1	30.6	29.0	
Baseline to Month 12 change	**0.0**	**−4.3**	<0.0001	**+0.6**	**−7.3**	**−7.6**	<0.0001
Post-washout	34.9	30.5		N/A	N/A	N/A	
Baseline to post-washout change	**−0.3**	**−3.4**		N/A	N/A	N/A	
Total body percent lean							
Baseline	60.4	62.2	0.37	62.0	60.0	59.1	0.48
Month 12	60.5	65.7		61.8	66.0	65.5	
Baseline to Month 12 change	**+0.2**	**+3.6**	<0.0001	**−0.2**	**+6.0**	**+6.4**	<0.0001
Post-washout	60.9	65.0		N/A	N/A	N/A	
Baseline to post-washout change	**+0.4**	**+2.8**	<0.0001	N/A	N/A	N/A	

Nutropin—Cont.

or sleep apnea, or unidentified respiratory infection. Male patients with one or more of these factors may be at greater risk than females. Patients with Prader-Willi syndrome should be evaluated for signs of upper airway obstruction and sleep apnea before initiation of treatment with growth hormone. If, during treatment with growth hormone, patients show signs of upper airway obstruction (including onset of or increased snoring) and/or new onset sleep apnea, treatment should be interrupted. All patients with Prader-Willi syndrome treated with growth hormone should also have effective weight control and be monitored for signs of respiratory infection, which should be diagnosed as early as possible and treated aggressively (see CONTRAINDICATIONS). Unless patients with Prader-Willi syndrome also have a diagnosis of growth hormone deficiency, Nutropin is not indicated for the long-term treatment of pediatric patients who have growth failure due to genetically confirmed Parader-Willi syndrome.

PRECAUTIONS

General: Nutropin should be prescribed by physicians experienced in the diagnosis and management of patients with GH deficiency, Turner syndrome, or chronic renal insufficiency. No studies have been completed of Nutropin therapy in patients who have received renal transplants. Currently, treatment of patients with functioning renal allografts is not indicated.

Experience with prolonged rhGH treatment in adults is limited.

Geriatric Usage: Clinical studies of Nutropin did not include sufficient numbers of subjects aged 65 and over to determine whether they respond differently from younger subjects. Other reported clinical experience has not identified differences in responses between the elderly and younger patients. In general, dose selection for an elderly patient should be cautious, usually starting at the low end of the dosing range, reflecting the greater frequency of decreased hepatic, renal, or cardiac function, and of concomitant disease or other drug therapy.

Patients with epiphyseal closure who were treated with GH-replacement therapy in childhood should be re-evaluated according to the criteria in the INDICATIONS AND USAGE section before continuation of GH therapy at the reduced dose level recommended for GH-deficient adults.

Because Nutropin may reduce insulin sensitivity, patients should be monitored for evidence of glucose intolerance.

For patients with diabetes mellitus, the insulin dose may require adjustment when GH therapy is instituted. Because GH may reduce insulin sensitivity, particularly in obese individuals, patients should be observed for evidence of glucose intolerance. Patients with diabetes or glucose intolerance should be monitored closely during GH therapy.

Nutropin therapy in adults with GHD of adult onset was associated with an increase of median fasting insulin in the Nutropin 0.0125 mg/kg/day group from 9.0 μU/mL at baseline to 13.0 μU/mL at Month 12 with a return to the baseline median after a 3-week post-washout period off GH therapy. In the placebo group there was no change from 8.0 μU/mL at baseline to Month 12, and after the post-washout the median was 9.0 μU/mL. The between-treatment-groups difference in change from baseline to Month 12 was significant, $p<0.0001$. In childhood-onset subjects, there was a change of median fasting insulin in the Nutropin 0.025 mg/kg/day group from 11.0 μU/mL at baseline to 20.0 μU/mL at Month 12, in the Nutropin 0.0125 mg/kg/day group from 8.5 μU/mL to 11.0 μU/mL, and in the placebo group from 7.0 μU/mL to 8.0 μU/mL. The between-treatment-groups difference for these changes was significant, $p=0.0007$.

In subjects with adult-onset GHD, there was no between-treatment-group difference in changes from baseline to Month 12 in mean HbA_{1c}, $p=0.08$. In childhood-onset, mean HbA_{1c} increased in the Nutropin 0.025 mg/kg/day group from 5.2% at baseline to 5.5% at Month 12, and did not change in the Nutropin 0.0125 mg/kg/day group from 5.1% at baseline or in the placebo group from 5.3% at baseline. The between-treatment-groups difference was significant, $p=0.009$.

Patients with a history of an intracranial lesion should be examined frequently for progression or recurrence of the lesion. In pediatric patients, clinical literature has demonstrated no relationship between GH-replacement therapy and central nervous system (CNS) tumor recurrence or new extracranial tumors. In adults, it is unknown whether there is any relationship between GH-replacement therapy and CNS tumor recurrence.

Patients with growth failure secondary to chronic renal insufficiency should be examined periodically for evidence of progression of renal osteodystrophy. Slipped capital femoral epiphysis or avascular necrosis of the femoral head may be seen in children with advanced renal osteodystrophy, and it is uncertain whether these problems are affected by GH therapy. X-rays of the hip should be obtained prior to initiating GH therapy for CRI patients. Physicians and parents should be alert to the development of a limp or complaints of hip or knee pain in patients treated with Nutropin.

Slipped capital femoral epiphysis may occur more frequently in patients with endocrine disorders or in patients undergoing rapid growth.

Progression of scoliosis can occur in patients who experience rapid growth. Because GH increases growth rate, patients with a history of scoliosis who are treated with GH should be monitored for progression of scoliosis. GH has not been shown to increase the incidence of scoliosis. Skeletal abnormalities including scoliosis are commonly seen in untreated Turner syndrome patients. Physicians should be alert to these abnormalities, which may manifest during GH therapy.

Patients with Turner syndrome should be evaluated carefully for otitis media and other ear disorders since these patients have an increased risk of ear or hearing disorders. In a randomized, controlled trial, there was a statistically significant increase, as compared to untreated controls, in otitis media (43% vs. 26%) and ear disorders (18% vs. 5%) in patients receiving GH. In addition, patients with Turner syndrome should be monitored closely for cardiovascular disorders (e.g., stroke, aortic aneurysm, hypertension) as these patients are also at risk for these conditions.

Intracranial hypertension (IH) with papilledema, visual changes, headache, nausea, and/or vomiting has been reported in a small number of patients treated with GH products. Symptoms usually occurred within the first eight (8) weeks of the initiation of GH therapy. In all reported cases, IH-associated signs and symptoms resolved after termination of therapy or a reduction of the GH dose. Funduscopic examination of patients is recommended at the initiation and periodically during the course of GH therapy. Patients with CRI and Turner syndrome may be at increased risk for development of IH.

See WARNINGS for use of Bacteriostatic Water for Injection, USP, (benzyl alcohol preserved), in newborns.

As with any protein, local or systemic allergic reactions may occur. Parents/Patient should be informed that such reactions are possible and that prompt medical attention should be sought if allergic reactions occur.

Laboratory Tests: Serum levels of inorganic phosphorus, alkaline phosphatase, and parathyroid hormone (PTH) may increase with Nutropin therapy.

Untreated hypothyroidism prevents optimal response to Nutropin. Patients with Turner syndrome have an inherently increased risk of developing autoimmune thyroid disease. Changes in thyroid hormone laboratory measurements may develop during Nutropin treatment. Therefore, patients should have periodic thyroid function tests and should be treated with thyroid hormone when indicated.

Drug Interactions: Excessive glucocorticoid therapy will inhibit the growth-promoting effect of human GH. Patients with ACTH deficiency should have their glucocorticoid-replacement dose carefully adjusted to avoid an inhibitory effect on growth.

The use of Nutropin in patients with chronic renal insufficiency receiving glucocorticoid therapy has not been evaluated. Concomitant glucocorticoid therapy may inhibit the growth-promoting effect of Nutropin. If glucocorticoid replacement is required, the glucocorticoid dose should be carefully adjusted.

There was no evidence in the controlled studies of Nutropin's interaction with drugs commonly used in chronic renal insufficiency patients. Limited published data indicate that GH treatment increases cytochrome P450 (CP450) mediated antipyrine clearance in man. These data suggest that GH administration may alter the clearance of compounds known to be metabolized by CP450 liver enzymes (e.g., corticosteroids, sex steroids, anticonvulsants, cyclosporin). Careful monitoring is advisable when GH is administered in combination with other drugs known to be metabolized by CP450 liver enzymes.

Carcinogenesis, Mutagenesis, Impairment of Fertility: Carcinogenicity, mutagenicity, and reproduction studies have not been conducted with Nutropin.

Pregnancy: Pregnancy (Category C). Animal reproduction studies have not been conducted with Nutropin. It is also not known whether Nutropin can cause fetal harm when administered to a pregnant woman or can affect reproduction capacity. Nutropin should be given to a pregnant woman only if clearly needed.

Nursing Mothers: It is not known whether Nutropin is excreted in human milk. Because many drugs are excreted in human milk, caution should be exercised when Nutropin is administered to a nursing mother.

Information for Patients: Patients being treated with GH and/or their parents should be informed of the potential benefits and risks associated with treatment. If home use is determined to be desirable by the physician, instructions on appropriate use should be given, including a review of the contents of the Patient Information Insert. This information is intended to aid in the safe and effective administration of the medication. It is not a disclosure of all possible adverse or intended effects.

If home use is prescribed, a puncture-resistant container for the disposal of used syringes and needles should be recommended to the patient. Patients and/or parents should be thoroughly instructed in the importance of proper disposal and cautioned against any reuse of needles and syringes (see Patient Information Insert).

ADVERSE REACTIONS

As with all protein pharmaceuticals, a small percentage of patients may develop antibodies to the protein. GH antibody binding capacities below 2 mg/L have not been associated with growth attenuation. In some cases when binding capacity exceeds 2 mg/L, growth attenuation has been observed. In clinical studies of pediatric patients that were treated with Nutropin for the first time, 0/107 growth hormone–deficient (GHD) patients, 0/125 CRI patients, 0/112 Turner syndrome patients, screened for antibody production developed antibodies with binding capacities ≥ 2 mg/L at six months.

Additional short-term immunologic and renal function studies were carried out in a group of patients with chronic renal insufficiency after approximately one year of treatment to detect other potential adverse effects of antibodies to GH. Testing included measurements of C1q, C3, C4, rheumatoid factor, creatinine, creatinine clearance, and BUN. No adverse effects of GH antibodies were noted.

In addition to an evaluation of compliance with the prescribed treatment program and thyroid status, testing for antibodies to GH should be carried out in any patient who fails to respond to therapy.

In studies in patients treated with Nutropin, injection site pain was reported infrequently.

Leukemia has been reported in a small number of GHD patients treated with GH. It is uncertain whether this increased risk is related to the pathology of GH deficiency itself, GH therapy, or other associated treatments such as radiation therapy for intracranial tumors. On the basis of current evidence, experts cannot conclude that GH therapy is responsible for these occurrences. The risk to GHD, CRI, or Turner syndrome patients, if any, remains to be established.

Other adverse drug reactions that have been reported in GH-treated patients include the following: 1) Metabolic: mild, transient peripheral edema. In GHD adults, edema or peripheral edema was reported in 41% of GH-treated patients and 25% of placebo-treated patients; 2) Musculoskeletal: arthralgias; carpal tunnel syndrome. In GHD adults, arthralgias and other joint disorders were reported in 27% of GH-treated patients and 15% of placebo-treated patients; 3) Skin: rare increased growth of pre-existing nevi; patients should be monitored for malignant transformation; and 4) Endocrine: gynecomastia. Rare pancreatitis.

OVERDOSAGE

Acute overdosage could lead to hyperglycemia. Long-term overdosage could result in signs and symptoms of gigantism and/or acromegaly consistent with the known effects of excess GH. (See recommended and maximal dosage instructions given below.)

DOSAGE AND ADMINISTRATION

The Nutropin dosage and administration schedule should be individualized for each patient. Response to growth hormone therapy in pediatric patients tends to decrease with time. However, in pediatric patients failure to increase growth rate, particularly during the first year of therapy, suggests the need for close assessment of compliance and evaluation of other causes of growth failure, such as hypothyroidism, under-nutrition, and advanced bone age.

Dosage

Pediatric Growth Hormone Deficiency (GHD)

A weekly dosage of up to 0.3 mg/kg of body weight divided into daily subcutaneous injection is recommended. In pubertal patients, a weekly dosage of up to 0.7 mg/kg divided daily may be used.

Adult Growth Hormone Deficiency (GHD)

The recommended dosage at the start of therapy is not more than 0.006 mg/kg given as a daily subcutaneous injection. The dose may be increased according to individual patient requirements to a maximum of 0.025 mg/kg daily in patients under 35 years and to a maximum of 0.0125 mg/kg daily in patients over 35 years.

To minimize the occurrence of adverse events in older or overweight patients, lower doses may be necessary. During therapy, dosage should be decreased if required by the occurrence of side effects or excessive IGF-I levels.

Chronic Renal Insufficiency (CRI)

A weekly dosage of up to 0.35 mg/kg of body weight divided into daily subcutaneous injection is recommended.

Nutropin therapy may be continued up to the time of renal transplantation.

In order to optimize therapy for patients who require dialysis, the following guidelines for injection schedule are recommended:

1. Hemodialysis patients should receive their injection at night just prior to going to sleep or at least 3–4 hours after their hemodialysis to prevent hematoma formation due to the heparin.
2. Chronic Cycling Peritoneal Dialysis (CCPD) patients should receive their injection in the morning after they have completed dialysis.
3. Chronic Ambulatory Peritoneal Dialysis (CAPD) patients should receive their injection in the evening at the time of the overnight exchange.

Turner Syndrome

A weekly dosage of up to 0.375 mg/kg of body weight divided into equal doses 3 to 7 times per week by subcutaneous injection is recommended.

Administration

After the dose has been determined, reconstitute as follows: each 5 mg vial should be reconstituted with 1–5 mL of Bacteriostatic Water for Injection, USP (benzyl alcohol preserved); or each 10 mg vial should be reconstituted with 1–10 mL of Bacteriostatic Water for Injection, USP (benzyl alcohol preserved), only. For use in newborns, see WARNINGS. The pH of Nutropin after reconstitution with Bacteriostatic Water for Injection, USP (benzyl alcohol preserved), is approximately 7.4.

To prepare the Nutropin solution, inject the Bacteriostatic Water for Injection, USP (benzyl alcohol preserved) into the Nutropin vial, aiming the stream of liquid against the glass

wall. Then swirl the product vial with a **GENTLE** rotary motion until the contents are completely dissolved. **DO NOT SHAKE**. Because Nutropin is a protein, shaking can result in a cloudy solution. The Nutropin solution should be clear immediately after reconstitution. Occasionally, after refrigeration, you may notice that small colorless particles of protein are present in the Nutropin solution. This is not unusual for solutions containing proteins. If the solution is cloudy immediately after reconstitution or refrigeration, the contents **MUST NOT** be injected.
Before needle insertion, wipe the septum of both the Nutropin and diluent vials with rubbing alcohol or an antiseptic solution to prevent contamination of the contents by microorganisms that may be introduced by repeated needle insertions. It is recommended that Nutropin be administered using sterile, disposable syringes and needles. The syringes should be of small enough volume that the prescribed dose can be drawn from the vial with reasonable accuracy.

STABILITY AND STORAGE
Before Reconstitution—Nutropin and Bacteriostatic Water for Injection, USP (benzyl alcohol preserved), must be stored at 2–8°C/36–46°F (under refrigeration). **Avoid freezing the vials of Nutropin and Bacteriostatic Water for Injection, USP (benzyl alcohol preserved).** Expiration dates are stated on the labels.
After Reconstitution—Vial contents are stable for 14 days when reconstituted with Bacteriostatic Water for Injection, USP (benzyl alcohol preserved), and stored at 2–8°C/36–46°F (under refrigeration). **Avoid freezing the reconstituted vial of Nutropin and the Bacteriostatic Water for Injection, USP (benzyl alcohol preserved).**

HOW SUPPLIED

Nutropin is supplied as 5 mg (approximately 15 IU) or 10 mg (approximately 30 IU) of lyophilized, sterile somatropin per vial.
Each 5 mg carton contains one vial of Nutropin® [somatropin (rDNA origin) for injection] (5 mg per vial) and one 10 mL multiple dose vial of Bacteriostatic Water for Injection, USP (benzyl alcohol preserved). NDC 50242-072-03.
Each 10 mg carton contains one vial of Nutropin® [somatropin (rDNA origin) for injection] (10 mg per vial) and one 10 mL multiple dose vial of Bacteriostatic Water for Injection, USP (benzyl alcohol preserved). NDC 50242-018-21.
Nutropin®
[somatropin (rDNA origin) for injection]
Manufactured by:
Genentech, Inc.
1 DNA Way
South San Francisco, CA 94080–4990
Bacteriostatic Water for Injection, USP
(benzyl alcohol preserved),
Manufactured for:
Genentech, Inc.
(4814405)
FDA Approval Date April 2000
Code Revision Date April 2004

Shown in Product Identification Guide, page 313

NUTROPIN AQ® ℞

[new-trō-pĭn]
[somatropin (rDNA origin) injection]

DESCRIPTION

Nutropin AQ is a human growth hormone (hGH) produced by recombinant DNA technology. Nutropin AQ has 191 amino acid residues and a molecular weight of 22,125 daltons. The amino acid sequence of the product is identical to that of pituitary-derived human growth hormone. The protein is synthesized by a specific laboratory strain of *E. coli* as a precursor consisting of the rhGH molecule preceded by the secretion signal from an *E. coli* protein. This precursor is directed to the plasma membrane of the cell. The signal sequence is removed and the native protein is secreted into the periplasm so that the protein is folded appropriately as it is synthesized.
Nutropin AQ is a highly purified preparation. Biological potency is determined using a cell proliferation bioassay. Nutropin AQ may contain not more than fifteen percent deamidated growth hormone (GH) at expiration. The deamidated form of GH has been extensively characterized and has been shown to be safe and fully active.
Nutropin AQ is a sterile liquid intended for subcutaneous administration. The product is nearly isotonic at a concentration of 5 mg of GH per mL and has a pH of approximately 6.0.
The Nutropin AQ 2 mL vial contains 10 mg (approximately 30 International Units [IU]) somatropin, formulated in 17.4 mg sodium chloride, 5 mg phenol, 4 mg polysorbate 20, and 10 mM sodium citrate.
The Nutropin AQ 2 mL pen cartridge contains 10 mg (approximately 30 International Units) somatropin, formulated in 17.4 mg sodium chloride, 5 mg phenol, 4 mg polysorbate 20, and 10 mM sodium citrate.

CLINICAL PHARMACOLOGY

General
In vitro and in vivo preclinical and clinical testing have demonstrated that Nutropin AQ is therapeutically equivalent to pituitary-derived human GH (hGH). Pediatric patients who lack adequate endogenous GH secretion, patients with chronic renal insufficiency, and patients with Turner syndrome that were treated with Nutropin AQ or Nutropin® [somatropin (rDNA origin) for injection] resulted in an increase in growth rate and an increase in insulin-like growth factor-I (IGF-I) levels similar to that seen with pituitary-derived hGH.
Actions that have been demonstrated for Nutropin AQ, somatropin, somatrem, and/or pituitary-derived hGH include:

A. Tissue Growth
1) Skeletal Growth: GH stimulates skeletal growth in pediatric patients with growth failure due to a lack of adequate secretion of endogenous GH or secondary to chronic renal insufficiency and in patients with Turner syndrome. Skeletal growth is accomplished at the epiphyseal plates at the ends of a growing bone. Growth and metabolism of epiphyseal plate cells are directly stimulated by GH and one of its mediators, IGF-I. Serum levels of IGF-I are low in children and adolescents who are GH deficient, but increase during treatment with GH. In pediatric patients, new bone is formed at the epiphyses in response to GH and IGF-I. This results in linear growth until these growth plates fuse at the end of puberty. 2) Cell Growth: Treatment with hGH results in an increase in both the number and the size of skeletal muscle cells. 3) Organ Growth: GH influences the size of internal organs, including kidneys, and increases red cell mass. Treatment of hypophysectomized or genetic dwarf rats with GH results in organ growth that is proportional to the overall body growth. In normal rats subjected to nephrectomy-induced uremia, GH promoted skeletal and body growth.

B. Protein Metabolism
Linear growth is facilitated in part by GH-stimulated protein synthesis. This is reflected by nitrogen retention as demonstrated by a decline in urinary nitrogen excretion and blood urea nitrogen during GH therapy.

C. Carbohydrate Metabolism
GH is a modulator of carbohydrate metabolism. For example, patients with inadequate secretion of GH sometimes experience fasting hypoglycemia that is improved by treatment with GH. GH therapy may decrease insulin sensitivity. Untreated patients with chronic renal insufficiency and Turner syndrome have an increased incidence of glucose intolerance. Administration of hGH to adults or children resulted in increases in serum fasting and postprandial insulin levels, more commonly in overweight or obese individuals. In addition, mean fasting and postprandial glucose and hemoglobin A_{1c} levels remained in the normal range.

D. Lipid Metabolism
In GH-deficient patients, administration of GH resulted in lipid mobilization, reduction in body fat stores, increased plasma fatty acids, and decreased plasma cholesterol levels.

E. Mineral Metabolism
The retention of total body potassium in response to GH administration apparently results from cellular growth. Serum levels of inorganic phosphorus may increase slightly in patients with inadequate secretion of endogenous GH, chronic renal insufficiency, or patients with Turner syndrome during GH therapy due to metabolic activity associated with bone growth as well as increased tubular reabsorption of phosphate by the kidney. Serum calcium is not significantly altered in these patients. Sodium retention also occurs. Adults with childhood-onset GH deficiency show low bone mineral density (BMD). GH therapy results in increases in serum alkaline phosphatase. (See PRECAUTIONS: Laboratory Tests.)

F. Connective Tissue Metabolism
GH stimulates the synthesis of chondroitin sulfate and collagen as well as the urinary excretion of hydroxyproline.

Pharmacokinetics
Subcutaneous Absorption—The absolute bioavailability of recombinant human growth hormone (rhGH) after subcutaneous administration in healthy adult males has been determined to be 81 ± 20%. The mean terminal $t_{1/2}$ after subcutaneous administration is significantly longer than that seen after intravenous administration (2.1 ± 0.43 hr vs. 19.5 ± 3.1 min) indicating that the subcutaneous absorption of the compound is slow and rate-limiting.
Distribution—Animal studies with rhGH showed that GH localizes to highly perfused organs, particularly the liver and kidney. The volume of distribution at steady state for rhGH in healthy adult males is about 50 mL/kg body weight, approximating the serum volume.
Metabolism—Both the liver and kidney have been shown to be important metabolizing organs for GH. Animal studies suggest that the kidney is the dominant organ of clearance. GH is filtered at the glomerulus and reabsorbed in the proximal tubules. It is then cleaved within renal cells into its constituent amino acids, which return to the systemic circulation.
Elimination—The mean terminal $t_{1/2}$ after intravenous administration of rhGH in healthy adult males is estimated to be 19.5 ± 3.1 minutes. Clearance of rhGH after intravenous administration in healthy adults and children is reported to be in the range of 116–174 mL/hr/kg.
Bioequivalence of Formulations—Nutropin AQ has been determined to be bioequivalent to Nutropin based on the statistical evaluation of AUC and C_{max}.

SPECIAL POPULATIONS
Pediatric—Available literature data suggest that rhGH clearances are similar in adults and children.
Gender—No data are available for exogenously administered rhGH. Available data for methionyl recombinant GH, pituitary-derived GH, and endogenous GH suggest no consistent gender-based differences in GH clearance.
Geriatrics—Limited published data suggest that the plasma clearance and average steady-state plasma concentration of rhGH may not be different between young and elderly patients.
Race—Reported values for half-lives for endogenous GH in normal adult black males are not different from observed values for normal adult white males. No data for other races are available.
Growth Hormone Deficiency (GHD)—Reported values for clearance of rhGH in adults and children with GHD range 138–245 mL/hr/kg and are similar to those observed in healthy adults and children. Mean terminal $t_{1/2}$ values following intravenous and subcutaneous administration in adult and pediatric GHD patients are also similar to those observed in healthy adult males.
Renal Insufficiency—Children and adults with chronic renal failure (CRF) and end-stage renal disease (ESRD) tend to have decreased clearance compared to normal individuals. Endogenous GH production may also increase in some individuals with ESRD. However, no rhGH accumulation has been reported in children with CRF or ESRD dosed with current regimens.
Turner Syndrome—No pharmacokinetic data are available for exogenously administered rhGH. However, reported half-lives, absorption, and elimination rates for endogenous GH in this population are similar to the ranges observed for normal subjects and GHD populations.
Hepatic Insufficiency—A reduction in rhGH clearance has been noted in patients with severe liver dysfunction. The clinical significance of this decrease is unknown.
[See table above]

Summary of Nutropin AQ Pharmacokinetic Parameters in Healthy Adult Males 0.1 mg (approximately 0.3 IU[a])/kg SC

	C_{max} (µg/L)	T_{max} (hr)	$t_{1/2}$ (hr)	$AUC_{0-\infty}$ (µg•hr/L)	CL/F_{sc} (mL/[hr•kg])
MEAN[b]	71.1	3.9	2.3	677	150
CV%	17	56	18	13	13

Abbreviations:
C_{max}=maximum concentration
$t_{1/2}$=half-life
$AUC_{0-\infty}$=area under the curve
CL/F_{sc}=systemic clearance
F_{sc}=subcutaneous bioavailability (not determined)
CV%=coefficient of variation in %; SC=subcutaneous
[a] Based on current International Standard of 3 IU=1 mg
[b] n=36

Single Dose Mean Growth Hormone Concentrations in Healthy Adult Males

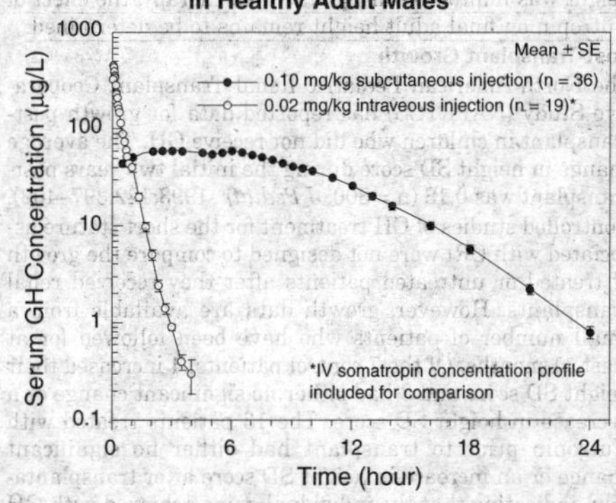

EFFICACY STUDIES

Growth Hormone Deficiency (GHD) in Pubertal Patients
One open label, multicenter, randomized clinical trial of two dosages of Nutropin® [somatropin (rDNA origin) for injection] was performed in pubertal patients with GHD. Ninety-seven patients (mean age 13.9 years, 83 male, 14 female) currently being treated with approximately 0.3 mg/kg/wk of GH were randomized to 0.3 mg/kg/wk or 0.7 mg/kg/wk Nutropin doses. All patients were already in puberty

Continued on next page

Nutropin AQ—Cont.

(Tanner stage ≥ 2) and had bone ages ≤ 14 years in males or ≤12 years in females. Mean baseline height standard deviation (SD) score was −1.3.

The mean last measured height in all 97 patients after a mean duration of 2.7 ± 1.2 years, by analysis of covariance (ANCOVA) adjusting for baseline height, is shown below.

[See first table at right]

The mean height SD score at last measured height (n = 97) was −0.7 ± 1.0 in the 0.3 mg/kg/wk group and −0.1 ± 1.2 in the 0.7 mg/kg/wk group. For patients completing 3.5 or more years (mean 4.1 years) of Nutropin treatment (15/49 patients in the 0.3 mg/kg/wk group and 16/48 patients in the 0.7 mg/kg/wk group), the mean last measured height was 166.1 ± 8.0 cm in the 0.3 mg/kg/wk group and 171.8 ± 7.1 cm in the 0.7 mg/kg/wk group, adjusting for baseline height and sex.

The mean change in bone age was approximately one year for each year in the study in both dose groups. Patients with baseline height SD scores above −1.0 were able to attain normal adult heights with the 0.3 mg/kg/wk dose of Nutropin (mean height SD score at near-adult height = −0.1, n = 15).

Thirty-one patients had bone mineral density (BMD) determined by dual energy x-ray absorptiometry (DEXA) scans at study conclusion. The two dose groups did not differ significantly in mean SD score for total body BMD (−0.9 ± 1.9 in the 0.3 mg/kg/wk group vs. −0.8 ± 1.2 in the 0.7 mg/kg/wk group, n = 20) or lumbar spine BMD (−1.0 ± 1.0 in the 0.3 mg/kg/wk group vs. −0.2 ± 1.7 in the 0.7 mg/kg/wk group, n = 21).

Over a mean duration of 2.7 years, patients in the 0.7 mg/kg/wk group were more likely to have IGF-I values above the normal range than patients in the 0.3 mg/kg/wk group (27.7% vs. 9.0% of IGF-I measurements for individual patients). The clinical significance of elevated IGF-I values is unknown.

Effects of Nutropin on Growth Failure Due to Chronic Renal Insufficiency (CRI)

Two multicenter, randomized, controlled clinical trials were conducted to determine whether treatment with Nutropin prior to renal transplantation in patients with chronic renal insufficiency could improve their growth rates and height deficits. One study was a double-blind, placebo-controlled trial and the other was an open-label, randomized trial. The dose of Nutropin in both controlled studies was 0.05 mg/kg/day (0.35 mg/kg/week) administered daily by subcutaneous injection. Combining the data from those patients completing two years in the two controlled studies results in 62 patients treated with Nutropin and 28 patients in the control groups (either placebo-treated or untreated). The mean first year growth rate was 10.8 cm/yr for Nutropin-treated patients, compared with a mean growth rate of 6.5 cm/yr for placebo/untreated controls ($p < 0.00005$). The mean second year growth rate was 7.8 cm/yr for the Nutropin-treated group, compared with 5.5 cm/yr for controls ($p < 0.00005$). There was a significant increase in mean height standard deviation (SD) score in the Nutropin group (−2.9 at baseline to −1.5 at Month 24, n = 62) but no significant change in the controls (−2.8 at baseline to −2.9 at Month 24, n = 28). The mean third year growth rate of 7.6 cm/yr in the Nutropin-treated patients (n = 27) suggests that Nutropin stimulates growth beyond two years. However, there are no control data for the third year because control patients crossed over to Nutropin treatment after two years of participation. The gains in height were accompanied by appropriate advancement of skeletal age. These data demonstrate that Nutropin therapy improves growth rate and corrects the acquired height deficit associated with chronic renal insufficiency. Currently there are insufficient data regarding the benefit of treatment beyond three years. Although predicted final height was improved during Nutropin therapy, the effect of Nutropin on final adult height remains to be determined.

Post-Transplant Growth

The North American Pediatric Renal Transplant Cooperative Study (NAPRTCS) has reported data for growth post-transplant in children who did not receive GH. The average change in height SD score during the initial two years post-transplant was 0.18 (n = 300, *J Pediatr*. 1993;122:397–402). Controlled studies of GH treatment for the short stature associated with CRI were not designed to compare the growth of treated or untreated patients after they received renal transplants. However, growth data are available from a small number of patients who have been followed for at least 11 months. Of the 7 control patients, 4 increased their height SD score and 3 had either no significant change or a decrease in height SD score. The 13 patients treated with Nutropin prior to transplant had either no significant change or an increase in height SD score after transplantation, indicating that the individual gains achieved with GH therapy prior to transplant were maintained after transplantation. The differences in the height deficit narrowed between the treated and untreated groups in the post-transplant period.

Turner Syndrome

One long-term, randomized, open-label, multicenter, concurrently controlled study, two long-term, open-label, multicenter, historically controlled studies, and one long-term, randomized, dose-response study were conducted to evaluate the efficacy of GH for the treatment of girls with short stature due to Turner syndrome.

Last Measured Height* by Sex and Nutropin Dose

	Age (yr)	Last Measured Height* (cm) 0.3 mg/kg/wk	0.7 mg/kg/wk	Height Difference Between Groups (cm)
	Mean±SD (range)	Mean±SD	Mean±SD	Mean±SE
Male	17.2±1.3 (13.6 to 19.4)	170.9±7.9 (n=42)	174.5±7.9 (n=41)	3.6±1.7
Female	15.8±1.8 (11.9 to 19.3)	154.7±6.3 (n=7)	157.6±6.3 (n=7)	2.9±3.4

*Adjusted for baseline height

Study/ Group	Study Design[a]	N at Adult Height	GH Age (yr)	Estrogen Age (yr)	GH Duration (yr)	Adult Height Gain (cm)[b]
GDCT	RCT	27	11.7	13	4.7	5.4
85-023	MHT	17	9.1	15.2	7.6	7.4
85-044: A*	MHT	29	9.4	15.0	6.1	8.3
B*		26	9.6	12.3	5.6	5.9
C*		51	12.7	13.7	3.8	5.0
GDCI	RDT	31	11.1	8–13.5	5.3	~5[c]

[a] RCT: randomized controlled trial; MHT: matched historical controlled trial; RDT: randomized dose-response trial.
[b] Analysis of covariance vs. controls
[c] Compared with historical data
* A = GH age <11 yr, estrogen age 15 yr
B = GH age <11 yr, estrogen age 12 yr
C = GH age >11 yr, estrogen at Month 12

In the randomized study GDCT, comparing GH-treated patients to a concurrent control group who received no GH, the GH-treated patients who received a dose of 0.3 mg/kg/week given 6 times per week from a mean age of 11.7 years for a mean duration of 4.7 years attained a mean near final height of 146.0 cm (n = 27) as compared to the control group who attained a near final height of 142.1 cm (n = 19). By analysis of covariance, the effect of GH therapy was a mean height increase of 5.4 cm (p = 0.001).

In two of the studies (85-023 and 85-044), the effect of long-term GH treatment (0.375 mg/kg/week given either 3 times per week or daily) on adult height was determined by comparing adult heights in the treated patients with those of age-matched historical controls with Turner syndrome who never received any growth-promoting therapy. In Study 85-023, estrogen treatment was delayed until patients were at least age 14. GH therapy resulted in a mean adult height gain of 7.4 cm (mean duration of GH therapy of 7.6 years) vs. matched historical controls by analysis of covariance.

In Study 85-044, patients treated with early GH therapy were randomized to receive estrogen-replacement therapy (conjugated estrogens, 0.3 mg escalating to 0.625 mg daily) at either age 12 or 15 years. Compared with matched historical controls, early GH therapy (mean duration of GH therapy 5.6 years) combined with estrogen replacement at age 12 years resulted in an adult height gain of 5.9 cm (n = 26), whereas girls who initiated estrogen at age 15 years (mean duration of GH therapy 6.1 years) had a mean adult height gain of 8.3 cm (n = 29). Patients who initiated GH therapy after age 11 (mean age 12.7 years; mean duration of GH therapy 3.8 years) had a mean adult height gain of 5.0 cm (n = 51).

Thus, in both studies, 85-023 and 85-044, the greatest improvement in adult height was observed in patients who received early GH treatment and estrogen after age 14 years.

In a randomized, blinded, dose-response study, GDCI, patients were treated from a mean age of 11.1 years for a mean duration of 5.3 years with a weekly dose of either 0.27 mg/kg or 0.36 mg/kg administered 3 or 6 times weekly. The mean near final height of patients receiving growth hormone was 148.7 cm (n = 31). This represents a mean gain in adult height of approximately 5 cm compared with previous observations of untreated Turner syndrome girls. In these studies, Turner syndrome patients (n = 181) treated to final adult height achieved statistically significant average estimated adult height gains ranging from 5.0–8.3 cm.

[See second table above]

Adult Growth Hormone Deficiency (GHD)

Two multicenter, double-blind, placebo-controlled clinical trials were conducted using Nutropin® [somatropin (rDNA origin) for injection] in GH-deficient adults. One study was conducted in subjects with adult-onset GHD, mean age 48.3 years, n = 166, at doses of 0.0125 or 0.00625 mg/kg/day; doses of 0.025 mg/kg/day were not tolerated in these subjects. A second study was conducted in previously treated subjects with childhood-onset GHD, mean age 23.8 years, n = 64, at randomly assigned doses of 0.025 or 0.0125 mg/kg/day. The studies were designed to assess the effects of replacement therapy with GH on body composition.

Significant changes from baseline to Month 12 of treatment in body composition (i.e., total body % fat mass, trunk % fat mass, and total body % lean mass by DEXA scan) were seen in all Nutropin groups in both studies ($p<0.0001$ for change from baseline and vs. placebo), whereas no statistically significant changes were seen in either of the placebo groups. In the adult-onset study, the Nutropin group improved mean total body fat from 35.0% to 31.5%, mean trunk fat from 33.9% to 29.5%, and mean lean body mass from 62.2% to 65.7%, whereas the placebo group had mean changes of 0.2% or less (p = not significant). Due to the possible effect of GH-induced fluid retention on DEXA measurements of lean body mass, DEXA scans were repeated approximately 3 weeks after completion of therapy; mean % lean body mass in the Nutropin group was 65.0%, a change of 2.8% from baseline, compared with a change of 0.4% in the placebo group ($p<0.0001$ between groups).

In the childhood-onset study, the high-dose Nutropin group improved mean total body fat from 38.4% to 32.1%, mean trunk fat from 36.7% to 29.0%, and mean lean body mass from 59.1% to 65.5%; the low-dose Nutropin group improved mean total body fat from 37.1% to 31.3%, mean trunk fat from 37.9% to 30.6%, and mean lean body mass from 60.0% to 66.0%; the placebo group had mean changes of 0.6% or less (p = not significant).

[See table at top of next page]

In the adult-onset study, significant decreases from baseline to Month 12 in LDL cholesterol and LDL:HDL ratio were seen in the Nutropin group compared to the placebo group, $p<0.02$; there were no statistically significant between-group differences in change from baseline to Month 12 in total cholesterol, HDL cholesterol, or triglycerides. In the childhood-onset study, significant decreases from baseline to Month 12 in total cholesterol, LDL cholesterol, and LDL:HDL ratio were seen in the high-dose Nutropin group only, compared to the placebo group, $p<0.05$. There were no statistically significant between-group differences in HDL cholesterol or triglycerides from baseline to Month 12.

In the childhood-onset study, 55% of the patients had decreased spine bone mineral density (BMD) (z-score < −1) at baseline. The administration of Nutropin (n = 16) (0.025 mg/kg/day) for two years resulted in increased spine BMD from baseline when compared to placebo (n = 13) (4.6% vs. 1.0%, respectively, $p<0.03$); a transient decrease in spine BMD was seen at six months in the Nutropin-treated patients. Thirty-five percent of subjects treated with this dose had supraphysiological levels of IGF-I at some point during the study, which may carry unknown risks. No significant improvement in total body BMD was found when compared to placebo. A lower GH dose (0.0125 mg/kg/day) did not show significant increments in either of these bone parameters when compared to placebo. No statistically significant effects on BMD were seen in the adult-onset study where patients received GH (0.0125 mg/kg/day) for one year.

Muscle strength, physical endurance, and quality of life measurements were not markedly abnormal at baseline, and no statistically significant effects of Nutropin therapy were observed in the two studies.

INDICATIONS AND USAGE

Pediatric Patients

Nutropin AQ® [somatropin (rDNA origin) injection] is indicated for the long-term treatment of growth failure due to a lack of adequate endogenous GH secretion.

Nutropin AQ® [somatropin (rDNA origin) injection] is also indicated for the treatment of growth failure associated with chronic renal insufficiency up to the time of renal transplantation. Nutropin AQ therapy should be used in conjunction with optimal management of chronic renal insufficiency.

Nutropin AQ® [somatropin (rDNA origin) injection] is also indicated for the long-term treatment of short stature associated with Turner syndrome.

Adult Patients

Nutropin AQ® [somatropin (rDNA origin) injection] is indicated for the replacement of endogenous GH in patients with adult GH deficiency who meet both of the following two criteria:

1. Biochemical diagnosis of adult GH deficiency by means of a subnormal response to a standard growth hormone stimulation test (peak GH ≤5 μg/L), and

Mean Changes from Baseline to Month 12 in Proportion of Fat and Lean by DEXA for Studies M0431g and M0381g (Adult-onset and Childhood-onset GHD, respectively)

	M0431g			M0381g			
Proportion	Placebo (n=62)	Nutropin (n=63)	Between-Groups t-test p-value	Placebo (n=13)	Nutropin 0.0125 mg/kg/day (n=15)	Nutropin 0.025 mg/kg/day (n=15)	Placebo vs. Pooled Nutropin t-test p-value
Total body percent fat							
Baseline	36.8	35.0	0.38	35.0	37.1	38.4	0.45
Month 12	36.8	31.5		35.2	31.3	32.1	
Baseline to Month 12 change	**−0.1**	**−3.6**	<0.0001	**+0.2**	**−5.8**	**−6.3**	<0.0001
Post-washout	36.4	32.2		NA	NA	NA	
Baseline to post-washout change	**−0.4**	**−2.8**	<0.0001	NA	NA	NA	
Trunk percent fat							
Baseline	35.3	33.9	0.50	32.5	37.9	36.7	0.23
Month 12	35.4	29.5		33.1	30.6	29.0	
Baseline to Month 12 change	**0.0**	**−4.3**	<0.0001	**+0.6**	**−7.3**	**−7.6**	<0.0001
Post-washout	34.9	30.5		NA	NA	NA	
Baseline to post-washout change	**−0.3**	**−3.4**		NA	NA	NA	
Total body percent lean							
Baseline	60.4	62.2	0.37	62.0	60.0	59.1	0.48
Month 12	60.5	65.7		61.8	66.0	65.5	
Baseline to Month 12 change	**+0.2**	**+3.6**	<0.0001	**−0.2**	**+6.0**	**+6.4**	<0.0001
Post-washout	60.9	65.0		NA	NA	NA	
Baseline to post-washout change	**+0.4**	**+2.8**	<0.0001	NA	NA	NA	

2. Adult-onset: Patients who have adult GH deficiency either alone or with multiple hormone deficiencies (hypopituitarism) as a result of pituitary disease, hypothalamic disease, surgery, radiation therapy, or trauma; or
Childhood-onset: Patients who were GH deficient during childhood, confirmed as an adult before replacement therapy with Nutropin AQ is started.

CONTRAINDICATIONS

Growth hormone should not be initiated to treat patients with acute critical illness due to complications following open heart or abdominal surgery, multiple accidental trauma or to patients having acute respiratory failure. Two placebo-controlled clinical trials in non-growth hormone-deficient adult patients (n = 522) with these conditions revealed a significant increase in mortality (41.9% vs. 19.3%) among somatropin-treated patients (doses 5.3–8 mg/day) compared to those receiving placebo (see WARNINGS).

Nutropin AQ should not be used for growth promotion in pediatric patients with closed epiphyses.

Nutropin AQ should not be used in patients with active neoplasia. GH therapy should be discontinued if evidence of neoplasia develops.

Growth hormone is contraindicated in patients with Prader-Willi syndrome who are severely obese or have severe respiratory impairment (see WARNINGS). Unless patients with Prader-Willi syndrome also have a diagnosis of growth hormone deficiency, Nutropin AQ is not indicated for the long-term treatment of pediatric patients who have growth failure due to genetically confirmed Parader-Willi syndrome.

WARNINGS

See CONTRAINDICATIONS for information on increased mortality in patients with acute critical illnesses in intensive care units due to complications following open heart or abdominal surgery, multiple accidental trauma, or with acute respiratory failure. The safety of continuing growth hormone treatment in patients receiving replacement doses for approved indications who concurrently develop these illnesses has not been established. Therefore, the potential benefit of treatment continuation with growth hormone in patients having acute critical illnesses should be weighed against the potential risk.

There have been reports of fatalities after initiating therapy with growth hormone in pediatric patients with Prader-Willi syndrome who had one or more of the following risk factors: severe obesity, history of upper airway obstruction or sleep apnea, or unidentified respiratory infection. Male patients with one or more of these factors may be at greater risk than females. Patients with Prader-Willi syndrome should be evaluated for signs of upper airway obstruction and sleep apnea before initiation of treatment with growth hormone. If, during treatment with growth hormone, patients show signs of upper airway obstruction (including onset of or increased snoring) and/or new onset sleep apnea, treatment should be interrupted. All patients with Prader-Willi syndrome treated with growth hormone should also have effective weight control and be monitored for signs of respiratory infection, which should be diagnosed as early as possible and treated aggressively (see CONTRAINDICATIONS). Unless patients with Prader-Willi syndrome also have a diagnosis of growth hormone deficiency, Nutropin AQ is not indicated for the long-term treatment of pediatric patients who have growth failure due to genetically confirmed Parader-Willi syndrome.

PRECAUTIONS

General: Nutropin AQ should be prescribed by physicians experienced in the diagnosis and management of patients with GH deficiency, Turner syndrome, or chronic renal insufficiency (CRI). No studies have been completed of Nutropin AQ therapy in patients who have received renal transplants. Currently, treatment of patients with functioning renal allografts is not indicated.

Experience with prolonged rhGH treatment in adults is limited.

Geriatric Usage: Clinical studies of Nutropin AQ did not include sufficient numbers of subjects aged 65 and over to determine whether they respond differently from younger subjects. Other reported clinical experience has not identified differences in responses between the elderly and younger patients. In general, dose selection for an elderly patient should be cautious, usually starting at the low end of the dosing range, reflecting the greater frequency of decreased hepatic, renal, or cardiac function, and of concomitant disease or other drug therapy.

Patients with epiphyseal closure who were treated with GH-replacement therapy in childhood should be re-evaluated according to the criteria in the INDICATIONS AND USAGE section before continuation of GH therapy at the reduced dose level recommended for GH-deficient adults.

Because Nutropin AQ may reduce insulin sensitivity, patients should be monitored for evidence of glucose intolerance.

For patients with diabetes mellitus, the insulin dose may require adjustment when GH therapy is instituted. Because GH may reduce insulin sensitivity, particularly in obese individuals, patients should be observed for evidence of glucose intolerance. Patients with diabetes or glucose intolerance should be monitored closely during GH therapy.

Nutropin therapy in adults with GH deficiency of adult onset was associated with an increase of median fasting insulin in the Nutropin 0.0125 mg/kg/day group from 9.0 μU/mL at baseline to 13.0 μU/mL at Month 12 with a return to the baseline median after a 3-week post-washout period off GH therapy. In the placebo group there was no change from 8.0 μU/mL at baseline to Month 12, and after the post-washout the median was 9.0 μU/mL. The between-treatment-groups difference in change from baseline to Month 12 was significant, $p<0.0001$. In childhood-onset subjects, there was a change of median fasting insulin in the Nutropin 0.025 mg/kg/day group from 11.0 μU/mL at baseline to 20.0 μU/mL at Month 12, in the Nutropin 0.0125 mg/kg/day group from 8.5 μU/mL to 11.0 μU/mL, and in the placebo group from 7.0 μU/mL to 8.0 μU/mL. The between-treatment-groups difference for these changes was significant, $p = 0.0007$.

In subjects with adult-onset GH deficiency, there was no between-treatment-group difference in changes from baseline to Month 12 in mean HbA_{1c}, $p = 0.08$. In childhood-onset mean HbA_{1c} increased in the Nutropin 0.025 mg/kg/day group from 5.2% at baseline to 5.5% at Month 12, and did not change in the Nutropin 0.0125 mg/kg/day group from 5.1% at baseline or in the placebo group from 5.3% at baseline. The between-treatment-groups difference was significant, $p = 0.009$.

Patients with a history of an intracranial lesion should be examined frequently for progression or recurrence of the lesion. In pediatric patients, clinical literature has demonstrated no relationship between GH-replacement therapy and central nervous system (CNS) tumor recurrence or new extracranial tumors. In adults, it is unknown whether there is any relationship between GH-replacement therapy and CNS tumor recurrence.

Patients with growth failure secondary to CRI should be examined periodically for evidence of progression of renal osteodystrophy. Slipped capital femoral epiphysis or avascular necrosis of the femoral head may be seen in children with advanced renal osteodystrophy, and it is uncertain whether these problems are affected by GH therapy. X-rays of the hip should be obtained prior to initiating GH therapy for CRI patients. Physicians and parents should be alert to the development of a limp or complaints of hip or knee pain in patients treated with Nutropin AQ.

Slipped capital femoral epiphysis may occur more frequently in patients with endocrine disorders or in patients undergoing rapid growth.

Progression of scoliosis can occur in patients who experience rapid growth. Because GH increases growth rate, patients with a history of scoliosis who are treated with GH should be monitored for progression of scoliosis. GH has not been shown to increase the incidence of scoliosis. Skeletal abnormalities including scoliosis are commonly seen in untreated Turner syndrome patients. Physicians should be alert to these abnormalities, which may manifest during GH therapy.

Patients with Turner syndrome should be evaluated carefully for otitis media and other ear disorders since these patients have an increased risk of ear or hearing disorders. In a randomized, controlled trial, there was a statistically significant increase, as compared to untreated controls, in otitis media (43% vs. 26%) and ear disorders (18% vs. 5%) in patients receiving GH. In addition, patients with Turner syndrome should be monitored closely for cardiovascular disorders (e.g., stroke, aortic aneurysm, hypertension) as these patients are also at risk for these conditions.

Intracranial hypertension (IH) with papilledema, visual changes, headache, nausea, and/or vomiting has been reported in a small number of patients treated with GH products. Symptoms usually occurred within the first eight (8) weeks of the initiation of GH therapy. In all reported cases, IH-associated signs and symptoms resolved after termination of therapy or a reduction of the GH dose. Funduscopic examination of patients is recommended at the initiation and periodically during the course of GH therapy. Patients with CRI and Turner syndrome may be at increased risk for development of IH.

As with any protein, local or systemic allergic reactions may occur. Parents/Patients should be informed that such reactions are possible and that prompt medical attention should be sought if allergic reactions occur.

Laboratory Tests: Serum levels of inorganic phosphorus, alkaline phosphatase, and parathyroid hormone (PTH) may increase with Nutropin AQ therapy.

Untreated hypothyroidism prevents optimal response to Nutropin AQ. Patients with Turner syndrome have an inherently increased risk of developing autoimmune thyroid disease. Changes in thyroid hormone laboratory measurements may develop during Nutropin AQ treatment. Therefore, patients should have periodic thyroid function tests and should be treated with thyroid hormone when indicated.

Drug Interactions: Excessive glucocorticoid therapy will inhibit the growth-promoting effect of human GH. Patients with ACTH deficiency should have their glucocorticoid-replacement dose carefully adjusted to avoid an inhibitory effect on growth.

The use of Nutropin AQ in patients with CRI receiving glucocorticoid therapy has not been evaluated. Concomitant glucocorticoid therapy may inhibit the growth-promoting effect of Nutropin AQ. If glucocorticoid replacement is required, the glucocorticoid dose should be carefully adjusted.

There was no evidence in the controlled studies of GH's interaction with drugs commonly used in chronic renal insufficiency patients. Limited published data indicate that GH treatment increases cytochrome P450 (CP450) mediated antipyrine clearance in man. These data suggest that GH administration may alter the clearance of compounds known to be metabolized by CP450 liver enzymes (e.g., corticosteroids, sex steroids, anticonvulsants, cyclosporin). Careful monitoring is advisable when GH is administered in combination with other drugs known to be metabolized by CP450 liver enzymes.

Carcinogenesis, Mutagenesis, Impairment of Fertility: Carcinogenicity, mutagenicity, and reproduction studies have not been conducted with Nutropin AQ.

Pregnancy: Pregnancy (Category C). Animal reproduction studies have not been conducted with Nutropin AQ. It is

Continued on next page

Nutropin AQ—Cont.

also not known whether Nutropin AQ can cause fetal harm when administered to a pregnant woman or can affect reproduction capacity. Nutropin AQ should be given to a pregnant woman only if clearly needed.

Nursing Mothers: It is not known whether Nutropin AQ is excreted in human milk. Because many drugs are excreted in human milk, caution should be exercised when Nutropin AQ is administered to a nursing mother.

Information for Patients: Patients being treated with GH and/or their parents should be informed of the potential benefits and risks associated with treatment. If home use is determined to be desirable by the physician, instructions on appropriate use should be given, including a review of the contents of the Patient Information Insert. This information is intended to aid in the safe and effective administration of the medication. It is not a disclosure of all possible adverse or intended effects.

If home use is prescribed, a puncture-resistant container for the disposal of used syringes and needles should be recommended to the patient. Patients and/or parents should be thoroughly instructed in the importance of proper disposal and cautioned against any reuse of needles and syringes (see Patient Information Insert).

ADVERSE REACTIONS

As with all protein pharmaceuticals, a small percentage of patients may develop antibodies to the protein. GH antibody binding capacities below 2 mg/L have not been associated with growth attenuation. In some cases when binding capacity exceeds 2 mg/L, growth attenuation has been observed. In clinical studies of pediatric patients that were treated with Nutropin® [somatropin (rDNA origin) for injection] for the first time, 0/107 growth hormone–deficient (GHD) patients, 0/125 CRI patients, and 0/112 Turner syndrome patients screened for antibody production developed antibodies with binding capacities ≥2 mg/L at six months. In a clinical study of patients that were treated with Nutropin AQ for the first time, 0/38 GHD patients screened for antibody production for up to 15 months developed antibodies with binding capacities ≥2 mg/L.

Additional short-term immunologic and renal function studies were carried out in a group of CRI patients after approximately one year of treatment to detect other potential adverse effects of antibodies to GH. Testing included measurements of C1q, C3, C4, rheumatoid factor, creatinine, creatinine clearance, and BUN. No adverse effects of GH antibodies were noted.

In addition to an evaluation of compliance with the prescribed treatment program and thyroid status, testing for antibodies to GH should be carried out in any patient who fails to respond to therapy.

Injection site discomfort has been reported. This is more commonly observed in children switched from another GH product to Nutropin AQ. Experience with Nutropin AQ in adults is limited.

Leukemia has been reported in a small number of GHD patients treated with GH. It is uncertain whether this increased risk is related to the pathology of GH deficiency itself, GH therapy, or other associated treatments such as radiation therapy for intracranial tumors. On the basis of current evidence, experts cannot conclude that GH therapy is responsible for these occurrences. The risk to GHD, CRI, or Turner syndrome patients, if any, remains to be established.

Other adverse drug reactions that have been reported in GH-treated patients include the following: 1) Metabolic: mild, transient peripheral edema. In GHD adults, edema or peripheral edema was reported in 41% of GH-treated patients and 25% of placebo-treated patients; 2) Musculoskeletal: arthralgias; carpal tunnel syndrome. In GHD adults, arthralgias and other joint disorders were reported in 27% of GH-treated patients and 15% of placebo-treated patients; 3) Skin: rare increased growth of pre-existing nevi; patients should be monitored for malignant transformation; and 4) Endocrine: gynecomastia. Rare pancreatitis.

OVERDOSAGE

Acute overdosage could lead to hyperglycemia. Long-term overdosage could result in signs and symptoms of gigantism and/or acromegaly consistent with the known effects of excess GH. (See recommended and maximal dosage instructions given below.)

DOSAGE AND ADMINISTRATION

The Nutropin AQ dosage and administration schedule should be individualized for each patient. Response to GH therapy in pediatric patients tends to decrease with time. However, in pediatric patients whose failure to increase growth rate, particularly during the first year of therapy, suggests the need for close assessment of compliance and evaluation of other causes of growth failure, such as hypothyroidism, under-nutrition, and advanced bone age.

Dosage

Pediatric Growth Hormone Deficiency (GHD)

A weekly dosage of up to 0.3 mg/kg of body weight divided into daily subcutaneous injection is recommended. In pubertal patients, a weekly dosage of up to 0.7 mg/kg divided daily may be used.

Adult Growth Hormone Deficiency (GHD)

The recommended dosage at the start of therapy is not more than 0.006 mg/kg given as a daily subcutaneous injection. The dose may be increased according to individual patient requirements to a maximum of 0.025 mg/kg daily in patients under 35 years and to a maximum of 0.0125 mg/kg daily in patients over 35 years.

To minimize the occurrence of adverse events in older or overweight patients, lower doses may be necessary. During therapy, dosage should be decreased if required by the occurrence of side effects or excessive IGF-I levels.

Chronic Renal Insufficiency (CRI)

A weekly dosage of up to 0.35 mg/kg of body weight divided into daily subcutaneous injection is recommended.

Nutropin AQ therapy may be continued up to the time of renal transplantation.

In order to optimize therapy for patients who require dialysis, the following guidelines for injection schedule are recommended:

1. Hemodialysis patients should receive their injection at night just prior to going to sleep or at least 3–4 hours after their hemodialysis to prevent hematoma formation due to the heparin.
2. Chronic Cycling Peritoneal Dialysis (CCPD) patients should receive their injection in the morning after they have completed dialysis.
3. Chronic Ambulatory Peritoneal Dialysis (CAPD) patients should receive their injection in the evening at the time of the overnight exchange.

Turner Syndrome

A weekly dosage of up to 0.375 mg/kg of body weight divided into equal doses 3 to 7 times per week by subcutaneous injection is recommended.

Administration

The solution should be clear immediately after removal from the refrigerator. Occasionally, after refrigeration, you may notice that small colorless particles of protein are present in the solution. This is not unusual for solutions containing proteins. Allow the vial or pen cartridge to come to room temperature and gently swirl. If the solution is cloudy, the contents **MUST NOT** be injected.

For Nutropin AQ® Vial

Before needle insertion, wipe the septum of the Nutropin AQ vial with rubbing alcohol or an antiseptic solution to prevent contamination of the contents by microorganisms that may be introduced by repeated needle insertions. It is recommended that Nutropin AQ be administered using sterile, disposable syringes and needles. The syringes should be of small enough volume that the prescribed dose can be drawn from the vial with reasonable accuracy.

For Nutropin AQ Pen® Cartridge

The Nutropin AQ pen cartridge is intended for use only with the Nutropin AQ Pen®. Wipe the septum of the Nutropin AQ pen cartridge with rubbing alcohol or an antiseptic solution to prevent contamination of the contents by microorganisms that may be introduced by repeated needle insertions. It is recommended that Nutropin AQ be administered using sterile, disposable needles. Follow the directions provided in the Nutropin AQ Pen® Instructions for Use.

The Nutropin AQ pen allows for administration of a minimum dose of 0.1 mg to a maximum dose of 4.0 mg, in 0.1 mg increments.

STABILITY AND STORAGE

Vial and cartridge contents are stable for 28 days after initial use when stored at 2–8°C/36–46°F (under refrigeration). **Avoid freezing the vial or the cartridge of Nutropin AQ.** The vials and cartridges of Nutropin AQ are light sensitive and they should be protected from light. Store the vial and cartridge refrigerated in a dark place when they are not in use.

HOW SUPPLIED

Nutropin AQ is supplied as either 10 mg (approximately 30 International Units) of sterile liquid somatropin per vial, or as 10 mg (approximately 30 International Units) of sterile liquid somatropin per pen cartridge.

Each vial carton contains one single vial containing 2 mL of Nutropin AQ® [somatropin (rDNA origin) injection] 10 mg/2 mL (5 mg/mL). NDC 50242-022-20.

Each pen cartridge carton contains one single pen cartridge containing 2 mL of Nutropin AQ® [somatropin (rDNA origin) injection] 10 mg/2 mL (5 mg/mL). NDC 50242-043-14.

Nutropin AQ®
[somatropin (rDNA origin) injection]
Manufactured by:
Genentech, Inc.
1 DNA Way (4814906)
South San Francisco, CA 94080–4990

FDA Approval Date April 2002
Code Revision Date April 2004

Shown in Product Identification Guide, page 313

PULMOZYME® ℞
(dornase alfa)
INHALATION SOLUTION

DESCRIPTION

Pulmozyme® (dornase alfa) Inhalation Solution is a sterile, clear, colorless, highly purified solution of recombinant human deoxyribonuclease I (rhDNase), an enzyme which selectively cleaves DNA. The protein is produced by genetically engineered Chinese Hamster Ovary (CHO) cells containing DNA encoding for the native human protein, deoxyribonuclease I (DNase). Fermentation is carried out in a nutrient medium containing the antibiotic gentamicin, 100-200 mg/L. However, the presence of the antibiotic is not detectable in the final product. The product is purified by tangential flow filtration and column chromatography. The purified glycoprotein contains 260 amino acids with an approximate molecular weight of 37,000 daltons (1). The primary amino acid sequence is identical to that of the native human enzyme.

Pulmozyme is administered by inhalation of an aerosol mist produced by a compressed air driven nebulizer system (see Clinical Experience, DOSAGE AND ADMINISTRATION). Each Pulmozyme single-use ampule will deliver 2.5 mL of the solution to the nebulizer bowl. The aqueous solution contains 1.0 mg/mL dornase alfa, 0.15 mg/mL calcium chloride dihydrate and 8.77 mg/mL sodium chloride. The solution contains no preservative. The nominal pH of the solution is 6.3.

CLINICAL PHARMACOLOGY

General

In cystic fibrosis (CF) patients, retention of viscous purulent secretions in the airways contributes both to reduced pulmonary function and to exacerbations of infection (2,3).

Purulent pulmonary secretions contain very high concentrations of extracellular DNA released by degenerating leukocytes that accumulate in response to infection (4). In vitro, Pulmozyme hydrolyzes the DNA in sputum of CF patients and reduces sputum viscoelasticity (1).

Pharmacokinetics

When 2.5 mg Pulmozyme was administered by inhalation to eighteen CF patients, mean sputum concentrations of 3 µg/mL DNase were measurable within 15 minutes. Mean sputum concentrations declined to an average of 0.6 µg/mL two hours following inhalation. Inhalation of up to 10 mg TID of Pulmozyme by 4 CF patients for six consecutive days, did not result in a significant elevation of serum concentrations of DNase above normal endogenous levels (5,6). After administration of up to 2.5 mg of Pulmozyme twice daily for six months to 321 CF patients, no accumulation of serum DNase was noted.

Pulmozyme, 2.5 mg by inhalation, was administered daily to 98 patients aged 3 months to ≤10 years, and bronchoalveolar lavage (BAL) fluid was obtained within 90 minutes of the first dose. BAL DNase concentrations were detectable in all patients but showed a broad range, from 0.007 to 1.8 µg/mL. Over an average of 14 days of exposure, serum DNase concentrations (mean ± s.d.) increased by 1.3 ± 1.3 ng/mL for the 3 months to <5 year age group and by 0.8 ± 1.2 ng/mL for the 5 to ≤10 year age group. The relationship between BAL or serum DNase concentration and adverse experiences and clinical outcomes is unknown.

Clinical Experience

Pulmozyme has been evaluated in a randomized, placebo-controlled trial of clinically stable cystic fibrosis patients, 5 years of age and older, with baseline forced vital capacity (FVC) greater than or equal to 40% of predicted and receiving standard therapies for cystic fibrosis (7). Patients were treated with placebo (325 patients), 2.5 mg of Pulmozyme once a day (322 patients), or 2.5 mg of Pulmozyme twice a day (321 patients) for six months administered via a Hudson T Up-draft II® nebulizer with a Pulmo-Aide® compressor.

Both doses of Pulmozyme resulted in significant reductions when compared with the placebo group in the number of patients experiencing respiratory tract infections requiring use of parenteral antibiotics. Administration of Pulmozyme reduced the relative risk of developing a respiratory tract infection by 27% and 29% for the 2.5 mg daily dose and the 2.5 mg twice daily dose, respectively (see Table 1). The data suggest that the effects of Pulmozyme on respiratory tract infections in older patients (>21 years) may be smaller than in younger patients, and that twice daily dosing may be required in the older patients. Patients with baseline FVC>85% may also benefit from twice a day dosing (see Table 1). The reduced risk of respiratory infection observed in Pulmozyme treated patients did not directly correlate with improvement in FEV_1 during the initial two weeks of therapy.

Within 8 days of the start of treatment with Pulmozyme, mean FEV_1 increased 7.9% in those treated once a day and 9.0% in those treated twice a day compared to the baseline values. The overall mean FEV_1 during long-term therapy increased 5.8% from baseline at the 2.5 mg daily dose level and 5.6% from baseline at the 2.5 mg twice daily dose level. Placebo recipients did not show significant mean changes in pulmonary function testing (see Figure 1).

For patients 5 years of age or older, with baseline FVC greater than or equal to 40%, administration of Pulmozyme decreased the incidence of occurrence of first respiratory tract infection requiring parenteral antibiotics, and improved mean FEV_1, regardless of age or baseline FVC.

[See table 1 at top of next page]

[See figure 1 at top of next column]

Pulmozyme® (dornase alfa) Inhalation Solution has also been evaluated in a second randomized, placebo-controlled study in clinically stable patients with baseline FVC <40% of predicted (8). Patients were enrolled and treated with placebo (162 patients) or Pulmozyme 2.5 mg QD (158 patients) for twelve weeks. In patients who received Pulmozyme, there was an increase in mean change (as percent of baseline) compared to placebo in FEV_1 (9.4% vs. 2.1%, p< 0.001) and in FVC (12.4% vs. 7.3%, p<0.01). Pulmozyme did not significantly reduce the risk of developing a respiratory tract infection requiring parenteral anti-

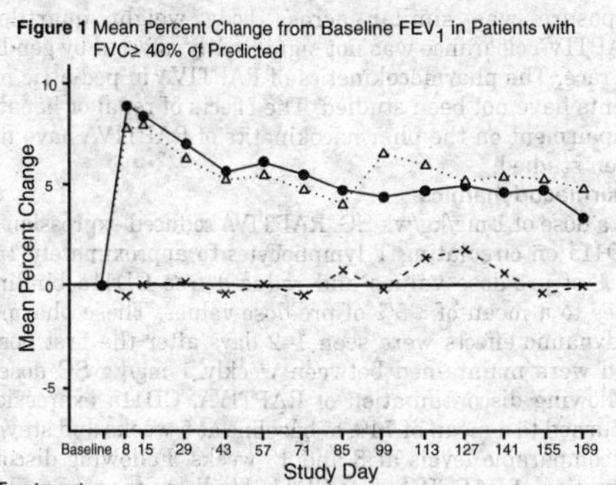

Figure 1 Mean Percent Change from Baseline FEV_1 in Patients with FVC≥ 40% of Predicted

biotics (54% of Pulmozyme patients vs 55% of placebo patients had experienced a respiratory tract infection by 12 weeks, relative risk = .93, p=0.62).

Other Studies

Clinical trials have indicated that Pulmozyme therapy can be continued or initiated during an acute respiratory exacerbation.

Short-term dose ranging studies demonstrated that doses in excess of 2.5 mg BID did not provide further improvement in FEV_1. Patients who have received drug on a cyclical regimen (i.e. administration of Pulmozyme 10 mg BID for 14 days, followed by a 14 day wash out period) showed rapid improvement in FEV_1 with the initiation of each cycle and a return to baseline with each Pulmozyme withdrawal.

INDICATIONS AND USAGE

Daily administration of Pulmozyme® (dornase alfa) Inhalation Solution in conjunction with standard therapies is indicated in the management of cystic fibrosis patients to improve pulmonary function. In patients with an FVC ≥40% of predicted, daily administration of Pulmozyme has also been shown to reduce the risk of respiratory tract infections requiring parenteral antibiotics.

Safety and efficacy of daily administration have not been demonstrated in patients for longer than twelve months.

CONTRAINDICATIONS

Pulmozyme is contraindicated in patients with known hypersensitivity to dornase alfa, Chinese Hamster Ovary cell products, or any component of the product.

WARNINGS

None.

PRECAUTIONS

General

Pulmozyme should be used in conjunction with standard therapies for CF.

Information for Patients

Pulmozyme must be stored in the refrigerator at 2–8°C (36–46°F) and protected from strong light. It should be kept refrigerated during transport and should not be exposed to room temperatures for a total time of 24 hours. The solution should be discarded if it is cloudy or discolored. Pulmozyme contains no preservative and, once opened, the entire contents of the ampule must be used or discarded. Patients should be instructed in the proper use and maintenance of the nebulizer and compressor system used in its delivery.

Pulmozyme should not be diluted or mixed with other drugs in the nebulizer. Mixing of Pulmozyme with other drugs could lead to adverse physicochemical and/or functional changes in Pulmozyme or the admixed compound.

Drug Interactions

Clinical trials have indicated that Pulmozyme can be effectively and safely used in conjunction with standard cystic fibrosis therapies including oral, inhaled and/or parenteral antibiotics, bronchodilators, enzyme supplements, vitamins, oral or inhaled corticosteroids, and analgesics. No formal drug interaction studies have been performed.

Carcinogenesis, Mutagenesis, Impairment of Fertility

Carcinogenesis: Lifetime studies in Sprague Dawley rats showed no carcinogenic effect when Pulmozyme was administered at doses up to 246 µg/kg body weight per day. Pulmozyme was administered to rats as an aerosol for up to 30 minutes per day, daily for two years, with resulting lower respiratory tract doses of up to 246 µg/kg per day, which represents up to a 28.8-fold multiple of the clinical dose. There was no increase in the development of benign or malignant neoplasms and no occurrence of unusual tumor types in rats after lifetime exposure.

Mutagenesis: Ames tests using six different tester strains of bacteria (4 of S. typhimurium and 2 of E. coli) at concentrations up to 5000 µg/plate, a cytogenetic assay using human peripheral blood lymphocytes at concentrations up to 2000 µg/plate, and a mouse lymphoma assay at concentrations up to 1000 µg/plate, with and without metabolic activation, revealed no evidence of mutagenesis potential. Pulmozyme was tested in a micronucleus (in vivo) assay for its potential to produce chromosome damage in bone marrow cells of mice following a bolus intravenous dose of 10 mg/kg on two consecutive days. No evidence of chromosomal damage was noted.

Impairment of Fertility: In studies with rats receiving up to 10 mg/kg/day, a dose representing systemic exposures greater than 600 times that expected following the recommended human dose, fertility and reproductive performance of both males and females was not affected.

Table 1
Incidence of First Respiratory Tract Infection
Requiring Parenteral Antibiotics in Patients with FVC ≥40% of Predicted

	Placebo N=325	2.5 mg QD N=322	2.5 mg BID N=321
Percent of Patients Infected	43%	34%	33%
Relative Risk (vs placebo)		0.73	0.71
p-value (vs placebo)		0.015	0.007
Subgroup by Age and Baseline FVC	**Placebo (N)**	**2.5 mg QD (N)**	**2.5 mg BID (N)**
Age			
5–20 years	42% (201)	25% (199)	28% (184)
21 years and older	44% (124)	48% (123)	39% (137)
Baseline FVC			
40–85% Predicted	54% (194)	41% (201)	44% (203)
>85% Predicted	27% (131)	21% (121)	14% (118)

Table 2
Adverse Events Increased 3% or More in Pulmozyme Treated Patients Over Placebo in CF Clinical Trials

	Trial in Mild to Moderate CF Patients (FVC ≥40% of predicted) treated for 24 weeks			Trial in Advanced CF Patients (FVC <40% of predicted) treated for 12 weeks	
Adverse Event (of any severity or seriousness)	Placebo n=325	Pulmozyme QD n=322	Pulmozyme BID n=321	Placebo n=159	Pulmozyme QD n=161
Voice alteration	7%	12%	16%	6%	18%
Pharyngitis	33%	36%	40%	28%	32%
Rash	7%	10%	12%	1%	3%
Laryngitis	1%	3%	4%	1%	3%
Chest Pain	16%	18%	21%	23%	25%
Conjunctivitis	2%	4%	5%	0%	1%
Rhinitis	Differences were less than 3% for these adverse events in the Trial in mild to moderate CF patients			24%	30%
FVC decrease of ≥10% of predicted°				17%	22%
Fever				28%	32%
Dyspepsia				0%	3%
Dyspnea (when reported as serious)	Difference was less than 3% for this adverse event in the Trial in mild to moderate CF patients			12%†	17%†

°Single measurement only, does not reflect overall FVC changes.
†Total reports of dyspnea (regardless of severity or seriousness) had a difference of less than 3% for the Trial in advanced CF patients.

Pregnancy (Category B)

Reproduction studies have been performed in rats and rabbits with intravenous doses up to 10 mg/kg/day, representing systemic exposures greater than 600 times that expected following the recommended human dose. These studies have revealed no evidence of impaired fertility, harm to the fetus, or effects on development due to Pulmozyme. There are, however, no adequate and well-controlled studies in pregnant women. Because animal reproductive studies are not always predictive of the human response, this drug should be used during pregnancy only if clearly needed.

Nursing Mothers

It is not known whether Pulmozyme® (dornase alfa) Inhalation Solution is excreted in human milk. Small amounts of dornase alfa were detected in maternal milk of cynomolgus monkeys when administered a bolus dose (100 µg/kg) of dornase alfa followed by a six hour intravenous infusion (80 µg/kg/hr). Little or no measurable dornase alfa would be expected in human milk after chronic aerosol administration of recommended doses. Because many drugs are excreted in human milk, caution should still be exercised when Pulmozyme is administered to a nursing woman.

Pediatric Use

Because of the limited experience with the administration of Pulmozyme to patients younger than 5 years of age, its use should be considered only for those patients in whom there is a potential for benefit in pulmonary function or in risk of respiratory tract infection.

Geriatric Use

Cystic fibrosis is primarily a disease of pediatrics and young adults. Clinical studies of Pulmozyme did not include sufficient numbers of subjects aged 65 or older to determine whether they respond differently from younger subjects.

ADVERSE REACTIONS

Patients have been exposed to Pulmozyme for up to 12 months in clinical trials.

In a randomized, placebo-controlled clinical trial in patients with FVC ≥40% of predicted, over 600 patients received Pulmozyme once or twice daily for six months; most adverse events were not more common on Pulmozyme than on placebo and probably reflected the sequelae of the underlying lung disease. In most cases events that were increased were mild, transient in nature, and did not require alterations in dosing. Few patients experienced adverse events resulting in permanent discontinuation from Pulmozyme, and the discontinuation rate was similar for placebo (2%) and Pulmozyme (3%). Events that were more frequent (greater than 3%) in Pulmozyme treated patients than in placebo-treated patients are listed in Table 2.

In a randomized, placebo-controlled trial of patients with advanced disease (FVC <40% of predicted) the safety profile for most adverse events was similar to that reported for the trial in patients with mild to moderate disease. For this study, adverse events that were reported with a higher frequency (greater than 3%) in the Pulmozyme treated patients, are also listed in Table 2.

[See table 2 above]

Events Observed at Similar Rates in Pulmozyme® (dornase alfa) Inhalation Solution and Placebo Treated Patients with FVC ≥40% of Predicted

Body as a Whole	Abdominal pain, Asthenia, Fever, Flu syndrome, Malaise, Sepsis
Digestive System	Intestinal Obstruction, Gall Bladder disease, Liver disease, Pancreatic disease
Metabolic Nutritional System	Diabetes Mellitus, Hypoxia, Weight Loss
Respiratory System	Apnea, Bronchiectasis, Bronchitis, Change in Sputum, Cough Increase, Dyspnea, Hemoptysis, Lung Function Decrease, Nasal Polyps, Pneumonia, Pneumothorax, Rhinitis, Sinusitis, Sputum Increase, Wheeze

Mortality rates observed in controlled trials were similar for the placebo and Pulmozyme treated patients. Causes of death were consistent with progression of cystic fibrosis and included apnea, cardiac arrest, cardiopulmonary arrest, cor pulmonale, heart failure, massive hemoptysis, pneumonia, pneumothorax, and respiratory failure.

Continued on next page

Pulmozyme—Cont.

The safety of Pulmozyme, 2.5 mg by inhalation, was studied with 2 weeks of daily administration in 98 patients with cystic fibrosis (65 aged 3 months to <5 years, 33 aged 5 to ≤10 years). The PARI BABY™ reusable nebulizer (which uses a facemask instead of a mouthpiece) was utilized in patients unable to demonstrate the ability to inhale or exhale orally throughout the entire treatment period (54/65, 83% of the younger and 2/33, 6% of the older patients). The number of patients reporting cough was higher in the younger age group as compared to the older age group (29/65, 45% compared to 10/33, 30%) as was the number reporting moderate to severe cough (24/65, 37% as compared to 6/33, 18%). Other events tended to be of mild to moderate severity. The number of patients reporting rhinitis was higher in the younger age group as compared to the older age group (23/65, 35% compared to 9/33, 27%) as was the number reporting rash (4/65, 6% as compared to 0/33). The nature of adverse events was similar to that seen in the larger trials of Pulmozyme® (dornase alfa) Inhalation Solution.

Allergic Reactions

There have been no reports of anaphylaxis attributed to the administration of Pulmozyme to date. Urticaria, mild to moderate, and mild skin rash have been observed and have been transient. Within all of the studies, a small percentage (average of 2-4%) of patients treated with Pulmozyme developed serum antibodies to Pulmozyme. None of these patients developed anaphylaxis, and the clinical significance of serum antibodies to Pulmozyme is unknown.

OVERDOSAGE

Single-dose inhalation studies in rats and monkeys at doses up to 180-times higher than doses routinely used in clinical studies are well tolerated. Single dose oral administration of Pulmozyme in doses up to 200 mg/kg are also well tolerated by rats.

Cystic fibrosis patients have received up to 20 mg BID for up to 6 days and 10 mg BID intermittently (2 weeks on/2 weeks off drug) for 168 days. These doses were well tolerated.

DOSAGE AND ADMINISTRATION

The recommended dose for use in most cystic fibrosis patients is one 2.5 mg single-use ampule inhaled once daily using a recommended nebulizer. Some patients may benefit from twice daily administraton (see Clinical Experience, Table 1). Clinical trial results and laboratory information are only available to support use of the following nebulizer/compressor systems (see Table 3).

Table 3
Recommended Nebulizer/Compressor Systems

Jet Nebulizer	Compressor
Hudson T Up-draft II® with	Pulmo-Aide®
Marquest Acorn II® with	Pulmo-Aide®
PARI LC Jet⁺ with	PARI PRONEB®
*PARI BABY™ with	PARI PRONEB®
Durable Sidestream® with	MOBILAIRE™
Durable Sidestream® with	Porta-Neb®

*Patients who are unable to inhale or exhale orally throughout the entire nebulization period may use the PARI BABY™ nebulizer.

Patients who use the Sidestream® Nebulizer with the MOBILAIRE™ compressor should turn the compressor control knob fully to the right and then turn on the compressor. At this setting, the needle on the pressure gauge should vibrate between 35 and 45 pounds per square inch (highest pressure output).

No data are currently available that support the administration of Pulmozyme with other nebulizer systems. The patient should follow the manufacturer's instructions on the use and maintenance of the equipment.

Pulmozyme should not be diluted or mixed with other drugs in the nebulizer. Mixing of Pulmozyme with other drugs could lead to adverse physicochemical and/or functional changes in Pulmozyme or the admixed compound. Patients should be advised to squeeze each ampule prior to use in order to check for leaks.

HOW SUPPLIED

Pulmozyme® (dornase alfa) Inhalation Solution is supplied in single-use ampules. Each ampule delivers 2.5 mL of a sterile, clear, colorless, aqueous solution containing 1.0 mg/mL dornase alfa, 0.15 mg/mL calcium chloride dihydrate and 8.77 mg/mL sodium chloride with no preservative. The nominal pH of the solution is 6.3.

Pulmozyme is supplied in:

- 30 unit cartons containing 5 foil pouches of 6 single-use ampules: NDC 50242-100-40.

Storage

Pulmozyme® (dornase alfa) Inhalation Solution should be stored under refrigeration (2–8°C/36–46°F). Ampules should be protected from strong light. Do not use beyond the expiration date stamped on the ampule. Unused ampules should be stored in their protective foil pouch under refrigeration.

REFERENCES

1. Shak S, Capon DJ, Hellmiss R, Marsters SA, Baker CL. Recombinant human DNase I reduces the viscosity of cystic fibrosis sputum. Proc Natl Acad Sci USA 1990;87:9188–92.
2. Boat TF. Cystic Fibrosis. In: Murray JF, Nadel JA, editors. Textbook of respiratory medicine. Philadelphia: Saunders WB, 1988;1:1126-52.
3. Collins FS. Cystic Fibrosis: molecular biology and therapeutic implications. Science 1992;256:774–9.
4. Potter JL, Spector S, Matthews LW, Lemm J. Studies of pulmonary secretions. Am Rev of Respir Dis 1969;99:909–15.
5. Hubbard RC, McElvaney NG, Birrer P, Shak S, Robinson WW, Jolley C, et al. A preliminary study of aerosolized recombinant human deoxyribonuclease I in the treatment of cystic fibrosis. N Eng J Med 1992;326:812–5.
6. Aitken ML, Burke W, McDonald G, Shak S, Montgomery AB, Smith A. Recombinant human DNase inhalation in normal subjects and patients with cystic fibrosis. JAMA 1992;267(14):1947–51.
7. Fuchs HJ, Borowitz DS, Christiansen DH, Morris EM, Nash ML, Ramsey BW, et al. Effect of aerosolized recombinant human DNase on exacerbations of respiratory symptoms and on pulmonary function in patients with cystic fibrosis. N Engl J Med 1994;331:637-42.
8. McCoy K, Hamilton S, Johnson C. Effects of 12-week administration of dornase alfa in patients with advanced cystic fibrosis lung disease. Chest 1996;110:889-95.

Pulmozyme®
(dornase alfa) Revised July 2002
INHALATION SOLUTION

Manufactured by 4806605
GENENTECH, Inc. 4824301
1 DNA Way
South San Francisco, CA 94080-4990
Shown in Product Identification Guide, page 313

RAPTIVA™ ℞

[*răp-tē'vă*]
(efalizumab)
For injection, subcutaneous

DESCRIPTION

RAPTIVA™ (efalizumab) is an immunosuppressive recombinant humanized IgG1 kappa isotype monoclonal antibody that binds to human CD11a (1). Efalizumab has a molecular weight of approximately 150 kilodaltons and is produced in a Chinese hamster ovary mammalian cell expression system in a nutrient medium containing the antibiotic gentamicin. Gentamicin is not detectable in the final product.

RAPTIVA is supplied as a sterile, white to off-white, lyophilized powder in single-use glass vials for subcutaneous (SC) injection. Reconstitution of the single-use vial with 1.3 mL of the supplied sterile water for injection (non-USP) yields approximately 1.5 mL of solution to deliver 125 mg per 1.25 mL (100 mg/mL) of RAPTIVA. The sterile water for injection supplied does not comply with USP requirement for pH. After reconstitution, RAPTIVA is a clear to pale yellow solution with a pH of approximately 6.2. Each single-use vial of RAPTIVA contains 150 mg of efalizumab, 123.2 mg of sucrose, 6.8 mg of L-histidine hydrochloride monohydrate, 4.3 mg of L-histidine and 3 mg of polysorbate 20 and is designed to deliver 125 mg of efalizumab in 1.25 mL.

CLINICAL PHARMACOLOGY

Mechanism of Action

RAPTIVA binds to CD11a, the α subunit of leukocyte function antigen-1 (LFA-1), which is expressed on all leukocytes, and decreases cell surface expression of CD11a. RAPTIVA inhibits the binding of LFA-1 to intercellular adhesion molecule-1 (ICAM-1), thereby inhibiting the adhesion of leukocytes to other cell types. Interaction between LFA-1 and ICAM-1 contributes to the initiation and maintenance of multiple processes, including activation of T lymphocytes, adhesion of T lymphocytes to endothelial cells, and migration of T lymphocytes to sites of inflammation including psoriatic skin. Lymphocyte activation and trafficking to skin play a role in the pathophysiology of chronic plaque psoriasis. In psoriatic skin, ICAM-1 cell surface expression is upregulated on endothelium and keratinocytes. CD11a is also expressed on the surface of B lymphocytes, monocytes, neutrophils, natural killer cells, and other leukocytes. Therefore, the potential exists for RAPTIVA to affect the activation, adhesion, migration, and numbers of cells other than T lymphocytes.

Pharmacokinetics

In patients with moderate to severe plaque psoriasis, following an initial SC RAPTIVA dose of 0.7 mg/kg followed by 11 weekly SC doses of 1 mg/kg/wk, serum concentrations reached a steady-state at 4 weeks with a mean trough concentration of approximately 9 μg/mL (n = 26). After the last dose, the mean peak concentration was approximately 12 μg/mL (n = 25). Mean steady-state clearance was 24 mL/kg/day (range = 5–76 mL/kg/day, n = 25). Mean time to eliminate RAPTIVA after the last steady-state dose was 25 days (range = 13–35 days, n = 17). The mean estimated RAPTIVA SC bioavailability was 50%. In a population pharmacokinetic analysis of 1088 patients, body weight was found to be the most significant covariate affecting RAPTIVA clearance. In patients receiving weekly SC doses of 1 mg/kg, RAPTIVA exposure was similar across body weight quartiles. RAPTIVA clearance was not significantly affected by gender or race. The pharmacokinetics of RAPTIVA in pediatric patients have not been studied. The effects of renal or hepatic impairment on the pharmacokinetics of RAPTIVA have not been studied.

Pharmacodynamics

At a dose of 1 mg/kg/wk SC, RAPTIVA reduced expression of CD11a on circulating T lymphocytes to approximately 15–25% of pre-dose values and reduced free CD11a binding sites to a mean of ≤5% of pre-dose values. These pharmacodynamic effects were seen 1–2 days after the first dose, and were maintained between weekly 1 mg/kg SC doses. Following discontinuation of RAPTIVA, CD11a expression returned to a mean of 74% of baseline at 5 weeks and stayed at comparable levels at 8 and 13 weeks. Following discontinuation of RAPTIVA, free CD11a binding sites returned to a mean of 86% of baseline at 8 weeks and stayed at comparable levels at 13 weeks. No assessments of CD11a expression or free CD11a binding sites were made after 13 weeks.

In clinical trials, RAPTIVA treatment resulted in a mean increase (relative to baseline) in white blood cell (WBC) count of 34%, a doubling of mean lymphocyte counts and an increase in eosinophil counts of 29% due to decreased leukocyte adhesion to blood vessel walls and decreased trafficking from the vascular compartment to tissues. At Day 56 of 1 mg/kg/wk RAPTIVA treatment, 32% (213/676) of patients had a shift in total WBC from low or normal baseline value to above normal, 46% (324/701) had a shift to above normal absolute lymphocyte counts, and 5% (35/675) had a shift to above normal eosinophil counts. Following discontinuation of RAPTIVA treatment, the abnormal elevated lymphocyte counts took approximately 8 weeks to normalize among patients who had above normal lymphocyte counts. Plasma samples collected after first administration of 0.3 mg/kg IV RAPTIVA indicate that at 2 hours TNF-α and IL-6 plasma levels were elevated 9- and 90-fold, respectively, compared with baseline. Plasma samples collected after first administration of 0.7 mg/kg SC RAPTIVA indicate that at 2 days, IL-6 levels were elevated (10 pg/mL as compared with 5 pg/mL at baseline), whereas TNF-α was not detectable. In RAPTIVA-treated patients the mean levels of C reactive protein increased from baseline by 67% and the mean levels of fibrinogen increased by 15%.

CLINICAL STUDIES

RAPTIVA was evaluated in four randomized, double-blind, placebo-controlled studies in adults with chronic (>6 months), stable, plaque psoriasis, who had a minimum body surface area involvement of 10% and who were candidates for, or had previously received systemic therapy or phototherapy. In these studies 54–70% of patients had previously received systemic therapy or phototherapy (PUVA) for psoriasis. Patients with clinically significant flares and patients with guttate, erythrodermic, or pustular psoriasis as the sole form of psoriasis were excluded from the studies.

Patients were randomized to receive doses of 1 mg/kg or 2 mg/kg of RAPTIVA or placebo administered once a week for 12 weeks. Patients randomized to RAPTIVA received 0.7 mg/kg as the first dose prior to receiving the full assigned dose in subsequent weeks. During the studies, patients could receive concomitant low potency topical steroids. No other concomitant psoriasis therapies were allowed during treatment or the follow-up period.

Patients were evaluated using the Psoriasis Area and Severity Index (PASI) during the study. The PASI is a composite score that takes into consideration both the fraction of body surface area affected and the nature and severity of the psoriatic changes within the affected regions (erythema, infiltration/plaque thickness, and desquamation). Both treatment groups in all four studies had baseline median PASI scores of 17. Both treatment groups across all four studies had baseline median body surface area involvement ranging between 22–28%. Compared with placebo, more patients randomized to RAPTIVA had at least a 75% reduction from baseline PASI score (PASI-75) 1 week after the 12-week treatment period (Table 1). RAPTIVA 2 mg/kg was not superior to RAPTIVA 1 mg/kg.

Table 1
Proportion of Patients with ≥75% Improvement in PASI after 12 Weeks of Treatment (PASI-75)

	Placebo	RAPTIVA 1 mg/kg/wk	Difference (95%CI)
Study 1	4% n = 187	27%[a] n = 369	22% (16%, 29%)
Study 2	2% n = 170	39%[a] n = 162	37% (28%, 46%)
Study 3	5% n = 122	22%[a] n = 232	17% (9%, 27%)
Study 4	3% n = 236	24%[a] n = 450	21% (15%, 27%)

[a] p<0.001 for comparison of RAPTIVA group with placebo group using Fisher's exact test within each study.

All three components of the PASI (plaque induration, scaling, and erythema) contributed comparably to the improvement in PASI. Other clinical responses evaluated (Table 2) included the proportion of patients who achieved minimal or clear status by a static Physician Global Assessment (sPGA) and the proportion of patients with a reduction in PASI of at least 50% from baseline (PASI-50) 1 week following the 12-week treatment period. The sPGA is a 6 category scale ranging from "very severe" to "clear" indicating the physician's overall assessment of the psoriasis severity focusing on plaque, scaling and erythema. Treatment success of minimal or clear consisted of none or slight elevation in plaque, none or minimal white color in scaling, and up to moderate definite red coloration in erythema. Across all four studies, the percentage of patients with baseline sPGA classifications of moderate was 48–56%, severe 33–43%, and 3–6% were classified as very severe.

[See table 2 at right]

In Study 1, 12% of RAPTIVA-treated patients achieved a PASI-50 at Week 4 compared with 5% for placebo. The median time to PASI-50 among PASI-75 achievers was approximately 6 weeks. Similar results were observed in Studies 2, 3, and 4.

In Study 3, sustained response to extended RAPTIVA treatment was evaluated. RAPTIVA-treated patients who achieved a PASI-75 response at Week 12 were re-randomized to receive RAPTIVA or placebo for a second contiguous 12-week treatment period. Sixty-one of 79 patients (77%) re-randomized to a second 12-week treatment period with RAPTIVA maintained PASI-75 response compared with 8 of 40 patients (20%) re-randomized to placebo. Sustained responses to RAPTIVA have also been observed in uncontrolled, open-label extension treatment trials when patients received RAPTIVA without interruption for 24 weeks.

In Study 2, response to intermittent RAPTIVA treatment was evaluated among patients who achieved PASI-75 response with 12 weeks of RAPTIVA treatment and were followed off-treatment until relapse of psoriasis (50% loss of treatment response). In patients who resumed RAPTIVA treatment upon relapse of psoriasis, 31% (17/55) re-established a PASI-75 response (compared with the initial baseline). After 12 weeks of treatment, the median duration of a PASI-75 response after RAPTIVA discontinuation was between 1 and 2 months.

The safety and efficacy of RAPTIVA therapy beyond 1 year have not been established.

Table 2
Percentage of Patients Responding after 12 Weeks of Treatment

Outcome Measurement	Study	Placebo	RAPTIVA 1 mg/kg/wk	Difference[a] (95% CI)
sPGA: Minimal or Clear	1	3%	26%	23% (16, 30)
	2	3%	32%	29% (21, 39)
	3	3%	19%	16% (8, 25)
	4	4%	20%	16% (11, 22)
>50% improvement in PASI (PASI-50)	1	14%	59%	45% (37, 53)
	2	15%	61%	46% (37, 56)
	3	16%	52%	36% (26, 47)
	4	14%	52%	38% (31, 45)

The number of patients in each study and treatment group is the same as listed in Table 1.
[a] $p < 0.001$ for comparison of RAPTIVA group to placebo group using Fisher's exact test for all comparisons between groups.

INDICATIONS AND USAGE

RAPTIVA™ (efalizumab) is indicated for the treatment of adult patients (18 years or older) with chronic moderate to severe plaque psoriasis who are candidates for systemic therapy or phototherapy.

CONTRAINDICATIONS

RAPTIVA should not be administered to patients with known hypersensitivity to RAPTIVA or any of its components.

WARNINGS

Serious Infections

RAPTIVA is an immunosuppressive agent and has the potential to increase the risk of infection and reactivate latent, chronic infections. RAPTIVA should not be administered to patients with clinically important infections. Caution should be exercised when considering the use of RAPTIVA in patients with a chronic infection or history of recurrent infections. If a patient develops a serious infection, RAPTIVA should be discontinued. New infections developing during RAPTIVA treatment should be monitored. During the first 12 weeks of controlled trials, serious infections occurred in 7 of 1620 (0.4 %) RAPTIVA-treated patients compared with 1 of 715 (0.1%) placebo-treated patients (see **ADVERSE REACTIONS, Infections**). Serious infections requiring hospitalization included cellulitis, pneumonia, abscess, sepsis, bronchitis, gastroenteritis, aseptic meningitis, Legionnaire's disease, and vertebral osteomyelitis (note some patients had more than one infection).

Malignancies

RAPTIVA is an immunosuppressive agent. Many immunosuppressive agents have the potential to increase the risk of malignancy. The role of RAPTIVA in the development of malignancies is not known. Caution should be exercised when considering the use of RAPTIVA in patients at high risk for malignancy or with a history of malignancy. If a patient develops a malignancy, RAPTIVA should be discontinued (see **ADVERSE REACTIONS, Malignancy**).

Thrombocytopenia

Platelet counts at or below 52,000 cells per µL were observed in 8 (0.3%) RAPTIVA-treated patients during clinical trials compared with none among the placebo-treated patients (see **ADVERSE REACTIONS, Thrombocytopenia**). Five of the 8 patients received a course of systemic steroids for thrombocytopenia. Thrombocytopenia resolved in the 7 patients receiving adequate follow-up (1 patient was lost to follow-up). Physicians should follow patients closely for signs and symptoms of thrombocytopenia. Assessment of platelet counts is recommended during treatment with RAPTIVA (see **PRECAUTIONS, Laboratory Tests**) and RAPTIVA should be discontinued if thrombocytopenia develops.

Psoriasis Worsening and Variants

Worsening of psoriasis can occur during or after discontinuation of RAPTIVA. During clinical studies, 19 of 2589 (0.7%) of RAPTIVA-treated patients had serious worsening of psoriasis during treatment (n = 5) or worsening past baseline after discontinuation of RAPTIVA (n = 14) (see **ADVERSE REACTIONS, Adverse Events of Psoriasis**). In some patients these events took the form of psoriatic erythroderma or pustular psoriasis. Some patients required hospitalization and alternative antipsoriatic therapy to manage the psoriasis worsening. Patients, including those not responding to RAPTIVA treatment, should be closely observed following discontinuation of RAPTIVA, and appropriate psoriasis treatment instituted as necessary.

PRECAUTIONS

Immunosuppression

The safety and efficacy of RAPTIVA in combination with other immunosuppressive agents or phototherapy have not been evaluated. Patients receiving other immunosuppressive agents should not receive concurrent therapy with RAPTIVA because of the possibility of increased risk of infections and malignancies.

Immunizations

The safety and efficacy of vaccines, administered to patients being treated with RAPTIVA have not been studied. In a small clinical study with IV administered RAPTIVA, a single dose of 0.3 mg/kg given before primary immunization with a neoantigen decreased the secondary immune response, and a dose of 1 mg/kg almost completely ablated it. A dose of 0.3 mg/kg IV has comparable pharmacodynamic effects to the recommended dose of 1 mg/kg SC. In chimpanzees exposed to RAPTIVA at ≥10 times the clinical exposure level (based on mean peak plasma levels) antibody responses were decreased following immunization with tetanus toxoid compared with untreated control animals. Acellular, live and live-attenuated vaccines should not be administered during RAPTIVA treatment.

First Dose Reactions

First dose reactions including headache, fever, nausea, and vomiting are associated with RAPTIVA treatment and are dose-level related in incidence and severity (see **ADVERSE REACTIONS**). Therefore, a conditioning dose of 0.7 mg/kg is recommended to reduce the incidence and severity of reactions associated with initial dosing (see **DOSAGE AND ADMINISTRATION**). One case of aseptic meningitis resulting in hospitalization has been observed in association with initial dosing (see **ADVERSE REACTIONS, Inflammatory/Immune-Mediated Reactions**).

Information for Patients

Patients should be informed that their physician may monitor platelet counts during therapy. Patients should be advised to seek immediate medical attention if they develop any of the signs and symptoms associated with severe thrombocytopenia, such as easy bleeding from the gums, bruising, or petechiae. Patients should also be informed that RAPTIVA is an immunosuppressant, and could increase their chances of developing an infection or a malignancy. Patients should be advised to promptly call the prescribing doctor's office if they develop any new signs of, or receive a new diagnosis of infection or malignancy while undergoing treatment with RAPTIVA.

Female patients should also be advised to notify their physicians if they become pregnant while taking RAPTIVA (or within 6 weeks of discontinuing RAPTIVA) and be advised of the existence of and encouraged to enroll in the RAPTIVA Pregnancy Registry.

If a patient or caregiver is to administer RAPTIVA, he/she should be instructed regarding injection techniques and how to measure the correct dose to ensure proper administration of RAPTIVA. Patients should be also referred to the RAPTIVA Patient Package Insert. In addition, patients should have available materials for and be instructed in the proper disposal of needles and syringes to comply with state and local laws. Patients should also be cautioned against reuse of syringes and needles.

Laboratory Tests

Assessment of platelet counts is recommended upon initiating and periodically while receiving RAPTIVA treatment. It is recommended that assessments be more frequent when initiating therapy (e.g., monthly) and may decrease in frequency with continued treatment (e.g., every 3 months). Severe thrombocytopenia has been observed (see **WARNINGS, Thrombocytopenia**).

Drug Interactions

No formal drug interaction studies have been performed with RAPTIVA. RAPTIVA should not be used with other immunosuppressive drugs (see **PRECAUTIONS, Immunosuppression**).

Acellular, live and live-attenuated vaccines should not be administered during RAPTIVA treatment (see **PRECAUTIONS, Immunizations**).

Drug/Laboratory Test Interactions

Increases in lymphocyte counts related to the pharmacologic mechanism of action are frequently observed during RAPTIVA treatment (see **CLINICAL PHARMACOLOGY, Pharmacodynamics**).

Carcinogenesis, Mutagenesis, Impairment of Fertility

Long-term animal studies have not been conducted to evaluate the carcinogenic potential of RAPTIVA.

Subcutaneous injections of male and female mice with an anti-mouse CD11a antibody at up to 30 times the equivalent of the 1 mg/kg clinical dose of RAPTIVA had no adverse effects on mating, fertility, or reproduction parameters. The clinical significance of this observation is uncertain.

Genotoxicity studies were not conducted.

Pregnancy (Category C)

Animal reproduction studies have not been conducted with RAPTIVA. It is also not known whether RAPTIVA can cause fetal harm when administered to a pregnant woman or can affect reproduction capacity. RAPTIVA should be given to a pregnant woman only if clearly needed.

In a developmental toxicity study conducted in mice using an anti-mouse CD11a antibody at up to 30 times the equivalent of the recommended clinical dose of RAPTIVA, no evidence of maternal toxicity, embryotoxicity, or teratogenicity was observed when administered during organogenesis. No adverse effects on behavioral, reproductive, or growth parameters were observed in offspring of female mice subcutaneously treated with an anti-mouse CD11a antibody during gestation and lactation using doses 3- to 30-times the equivalent of the recommended clinical dose of RAPTIVA. At 11 weeks of age, the offspring of these females exhibited a significant reduction in their ability to mount an antibody response, which showed evidence of partial reversibility by 25 weeks of age. Animal studies, however, are not always predictive of human response, and there are no adequate and well-controlled studies in pregnant women.

Since the effects of RAPTIVA on pregnant women and fetal development, including immune system development are not known, healthcare providers are encouraged to enroll patients who become pregnant while taking RAPTIVA (or within 6 weeks of discontinuing RAPTIVA) in the RAPTIVA Pregnancy Registry.

Nursing Mothers

It is not known whether RAPTIVA is excreted in human milk. An anti-mouse CD11a antibody was detected in milk samples of lactating mice exposed to anti-mouse CD11a antibody and the offspring of the exposed females exhibited significant reduction in antibody responses (see **PRECAUTIONS, Pregnancy**). Since maternal immunoglobulins are known to be present in the milk of lactating mothers, and animal data suggest the potential for adverse effects in nursing infants from RAPTIVA, a decision should be made whether to discontinue nursing while taking the drug or to discontinue the use of the drug, taking into account the importance of the drug to the mother.

Pediatric Use

The safety and efficacy of RAPTIVA in pediatric patients have not been studied.

Geriatric Use

Of the 1620 patients who received RAPTIVA in controlled trials, 128 were ≥65 years of age, and 2 were ≥75 years of age. Although no differences in safety or efficacy were observed between older and younger patients, the number of patients aged 65 and over is not sufficient to determine whether they respond differently from younger patients. Because the incidence of infections is higher in the elderly population, in general, caution should be used in treating the elderly.

ADVERSE REACTIONS

The most serious adverse reactions observed during treatment with RAPTIVA were serious infections, malignancies, thrombocytopenia and psoriasis worsening and variants (see **WARNINGS**).

The most common adverse reactions associated with RAPTIVA were a first dose reaction complex that included headache, chills, fever, nausea, and myalgia within two days following the first two injections. These reactions are dose-level related in incidence and severity and were largely mild to moderate in severity when a conditioning dose of 0.7 mg/kg was used as the first dose. In placebo-controlled trials, 29% of patients treated with RAPTIVA 1 mg/kg de-

Continued on next page

Raptiva—Cont.

veloped one or more of these symptoms following the first dose compared with 15% of patients receiving placebo. After the third dose, 4% and 3% of patients receiving RAPTIVA 1 mg/kg and placebo, respectively, experienced these symptoms. Less than 1% of patients discontinued RAPTIVA treatment because of these adverse events.

Other adverse events resulting in discontinuation of RAPTIVA treatment were psoriasis (0.6%), pain (0.4%), arthritis (0.4%), and arthralgia (0.3%).

Because clinical trials are conducted under widely varying conditions, adverse reaction rates observed in the clinical trials of one drug cannot be directly compared to rates in the clinical trials of another drug and may not reflect the rates observed in practice.

The data described below reflect RAPTIVA exposure for 2762 adult psoriasis patients (age range 18 to 75 years), including 2400 patients exposed for three months, 904 for six months, and 218 exposed for one year or more, in all controlled and uncontrolled studies. The median age of patients receiving RAPTIVA was 44 years, with 189 patients above the age of 65; 67% were men, and 89% were Caucasian. These data include patients treated at doses higher than the recommended dose of 1 mg/kg weekly.

Controlled clinical trials provide the most informative basis for estimating the frequency of RAPTIVA-related adverse drug reactions. Table 3 enumerates the adverse events occurring during controlled periods of the clinical trials where the frequency of the adverse events is at least 2% greater in the RAPTIVA-treated group than the placebo group.

Table 3
Adverse Events in Placebo Controlled Study Periods Reported at a ≥2% Higher Rate in the 1 mg/kg/wk RAPTIVA Treatment than Placebo Groups

	Placebo (n = 715)	RAPTIVA 1 mg/kg/wk (n = 1213)
Headache	159 (22%)	391 (32%)
Infection[a]	188 (26%)	350 (29%)
Chills	32 (4%)	154 (13%)
Nausea	51 (7%)	128 (11%)
Pain	38 (5%)	122 (10%)
Myalgia	35 (5%)	102 (8%)
Flu Syndrome	29 (4%)	83 (7%)
Fever	24 (3%)	80 (7%)
Back pain	14 (2%)	50 (4%)
Acne	4 (1%)	45 (4%)

[a] Includes diagnosed infections and other non-specific infections. Most common non-specific infection was upper respiratory infection.

Adverse events occurring at a rate between 1 and 2% greater in the RAPTIVA group compared with placebo were arthralgia, asthenia, peripheral edema, and psoriasis.

The following serious adverse reactions were observed in RAPTIVA-treated patients.

Infections

In the first 12 weeks of placebo-controlled studies, the proportion of patients with serious infection was 0.4% (7/1620) in the RAPTIVA-treated group (5 of these were hospitalized, 0.3%) and 0.1% (1/715) in the placebo group (see **WARNINGS, Serious Infections**). In the complete safety data from both controlled and uncontrolled studies, the overall incidence of hospitalization for infections was 1.6 per 100 patient-years for RAPTIVA-treated patients compared with 1.2 per 100 patient-years for placebo-treated patients. Including both controlled, uncontrolled, and follow-up study treatment periods there were 27 serious infections in 2475 RAPTIVA-treated patients. These infections included cellulitis, pneumonia, abscess, sepsis, sinusitis, bronchitis, gastroenteritis, aseptic meningitis, Legionnaire's disease, septic arthritis, and vertebral osteomyelitis. In controlled trials, the overall rate of infections in RAPTIVA-treated patients was 3% higher than in placebo-treated patients (Table 3).

Malignancies

Among the 2762 psoriasis patients who received RAPTIVA at any dose (median duration 8 months), 31 patients were diagnosed with 37 malignancies (see **WARNINGS, Malignancies**). The overall incidence of malignancies of any kind was 1.8 per 100 patient-years for RAPTIVA-treated patients compared with 1.6 per 100 patient-years for placebo-treated patients. Malignancies observed in the RAPTIVA-treated patients included non-melanoma skin cancer, non-cutaneous solid tumors, Hodgkin's lymphoma and non-Hodgkin's lymphoma, and malignant. The incidence of non-cutaneous solid tumors (8 in 1790 patient-years) and malignant melanoma were within the range expected for the general population.

The majority of the malignancies were non-melanoma skin cancers; 26 cases (13 basal, 13 squamous) in 20 patients (0.7% of 2762 RAPTIVA-treated patients). The incidence was comparable for RAPTIVA-treated and placebo-treated patients. However, the size of the placebo group and duration of follow-up were limited and a difference in rates of non-melanoma skin cancers cannot be excluded.

Thrombocytopenia

In the combined safety database of 2762 RAPTIVA-treated patients, there were eight occurrences (0.3%) of thrombocytopenia of <52,000 cells per µL reported (see **WARNINGS, Thrombocytopenia**). Three of the eight patients were hospitalized for thrombocytopenia, including one patient with heavy uterine bleeding; all cases were consistent with an immune mediated thrombocytopenia. Antiplatelet antibody was evaluated in one patient and was found to be positive. Each case resulted in discontinuation of RAPTIVA. Based on available platelet count measurements, the onset of platelet decline was between 8 and 12 weeks after the first dose of RAPTIVA in 5 of the patients. Onset was more delayed in 3 patients, occurring as late as one year in 1 patient. In these cases, the platelet count nadirs occurred between 12 and 72 weeks after the first dose of RAPTIVA.

Adverse Events of Psoriasis

In the combined safety database from all studies, serious psoriasis adverse events occurred in 19 RAPTIVA-treated patients (0.7%) including hospitalization in 17 patients (see **WARNINGS, Psoriasis Worsening/Variants**). Most of these events (14/19) occurred after discontinuation of study drug and occurred in both patients responding and not responding to RAPTIVA treatment. Serious adverse events of psoriasis included pustular, erythrodermic, and guttate subtypes. During the first 12 weeks of treatment within placebo-controlled studies, the rate of psoriasis adverse events (serious and non-serious) was 3.2% (52/1620) in the RAPTIVA-treated patients and 1.4% (10/715) in the placebo-treated patients.

Hypersensitivity Reactions

Symptoms associated with a hypersensitivity reaction (e.g., dyspnea, asthma, urticaria, angioedema, maculopapular rash) were evaluated by treatment group. In the first 12 weeks of the controlled clinical studies, the proportion of patients reporting at least one hypersensitivity reaction was 8% (95/1213) in the 1 mg/kg/wk group and 7% (49/715) patients in the placebo group. Urticaria was observed in 1% of patients (16/1213) receiving RAPTIVA and 0.4% of patients (3/715) receiving placebo during the initial 12-week treatment period. Other observed adverse events in patients receiving RAPTIVA that may be indicative of hypersensitivity included: laryngospasm, angioedema, erythema multiforme, asthma, and allergic drug eruption. One patient was hospitalized with a serum sickness-like reaction.

Inflammatory/Immune-Mediated Reactions

In the entire RAPTIVA clinical development program of 2762 RAPTIVA-treated patients, inflammatory, potentially immune-mediated adverse events resulting in hospitalization included inflammatory arthritis (12 cases, 0.4% of patients) and interstitial pneumonitis (2 cases). One case each of the following serious adverse reactions was observed: transverse myelitis, bronchiolitis obliterans, aseptic meningitis, idiopathic hepatitis, sialedenitis, and sensorineural hearing loss.

Laboratory Values

In RAPTIVA-treated patients, a mean elevation in alkaline phosphatase (5 Units/L) was observed; 4% of RAPTIVA-treated patients experienced a shift to above normal values compared with 0.6% of placebo-treated patients. The clinical significance of this change is unknown. Higher numbers of RAPTIVA-treated patients experienced elevations above normal in two or more liver function tests than placebo (3.1% vs. 1.5%).

Other laboratory adverse reactions that were observed included thrombocytopenia, (see **WARNINGS**, and **ADVERSE REACTIONS, Thrombocytopenia**), lymphocytosis (40%) (including three cases of transient atypical lymphocytosis), and leukocytosis (26%).

Immunogenicity

In patients evaluated for antibodies to RAPTIVA after RAPTIVA treatment ended, predominantly low-titer antibodies to RAPTIVA or other protein components of the RAPTIVA drug product were detected in 6.3% (67/1063) of patients. The long-term immunogenicity of RAPTIVA is unknown.

The data reflect the percentage of patients whose test results were considered positive for antibodies to RAPTIVA in the ELISA assay, and are highly dependent on the sensitivity and specificity of the assay. Additionally, the observed incidence of antibody positivity in an assay may be influenced by several factors including sample handling, timing of sample collection, concomitant medications, and underlying disease. For these reasons, comparison of the incidence of antibodies to RAPTIVA with the incidence of antibodies to other products may be misleading.

OVERDOSAGE

Doses up to 4 mg/kg/wk SC for 10 weeks following a conditioning (0.7 mg/kg) first dose have been administered without an observed increase in acute toxicity. The maximum administered single dose was 10 mg/kg IV. This was administered to one patient, who subsequently was admitted to the hospital for severe vomiting. In case of overdose, it is recommended that the patient be monitored for 24–48 hours for any acute signs or symptoms of adverse reactions or effects and appropriate treatment instituted.

DOSAGE AND ADMINISTRATION

The recommended dose of RAPTIVA is a single 0.7 mg/kg SC conditioning dose followed by weekly SC doses of 1 mg/kg (maximum single dose not to exceed a total of 200 mg).

RAPTIVA is intended for use under the guidance and supervision of a physician. If it is determined to be appropriate, patients may self-inject RAPTIVA after proper training in the preparation and injection technique and with medical follow-up.

Preparation for Administration

RAPTIVA should be administered using the sterile, disposable syringe and needles provided (see **HOW SUPPLIED** section). Remove the cap from the pre-filled syringe containing sterile water for injection (non-USP) and attach the needle to the syringe. Remove the plastic cap protecting the rubber stopper of the RAPTIVA vial and wipe the top of the rubber stopper with one of the provided alcohol swabs. After cleaning with the alcohol swab, do not touch the top of the vial. To prepare the RAPTIVA solution, using the provided pre-filled diluent syringe slowly inject the 1.3 mL of sterile water for injection (non-USP) into the RAPTIVA vial. Swirl the vial with a GENTLE rotary motion to dissolve the product. DO NOT SHAKE. Shaking will cause foaming of the RAPTIVA solution. Generally, dissolution of RAPTIVA takes less than 5 minutes. RAPTIVA is provided as a single-use vial and contains no antibacterial preservatives. Reconstitute immediately before use and use only once. If the reconstituted RAPTIVA is not used immediately, store the RAPTIVA vial at room temperature and use within 8 hours. The reconstituted solution should be clear to pale yellow and free of particulates.

Administration

Parenteral drug products should be inspected visually for particulate matter and discoloration prior to subcutaneous administration. If particulates or discolorations are noted, the product should not be used. Replace the needle on the syringe with a new needle. Insert the needle into the vial containing the RAPTIVA solution, invert the vial, and keeping the needle below the level of the liquid, withdraw the dose to be given into the syringe.

No other medications should be added to solutions containing RAPTIVA, and RAPTIVA should not be reconstituted with other diluents.

Sites for injection include thigh, abdomen, buttocks, or upper arm. Injection sites should be rotated.

Following administration, discard any unused reconstituted RAPTIVA solution.

Stability and Storage

Do not use a vial beyond the expiration date stamped on the carton or vial label. RAPTIVA (lyophilized powder) must be refrigerated at 2–8°C (36–46°F). Protect the vial from exposure to light. Store in original carton until time of use.

HOW SUPPLIED

RAPTIVA™ (efalizumab) is supplied as a lyophilized, sterile powder to deliver 125 mg of efalizumab per single-use vial. Each RAPTIVA carton contains four trays. Each tray contains one single-use vial designed to deliver 125 mg of efalizumab, one single-use prefilled diluent syringe containing 1.3 mL sterile water for injection (non-USP), two 25 gauge × 5/8 inch needles, two alcohol prep pads, a package insert with an accompanying patient information insert. The NDC number for the four administration dose pack carton is 50242-058-04.

REFERENCES

1. Werther WA, Gonzalez TN, O'Connor SJ, McCabe S, Chan B, Hotaling T, et al. Humanization of an anti-lymphocyte function-associated antigen (LFA)-1 monoclonal antibody and reengineering of the humanized antibody for binding to rhesus LFA-1. J Immunol 1996;157:4986–95.

Patient Information

RAPTIVA (Rap-TEE-vah)
(efalizumab)
for injection, subcutaneous

Read the Patient Information that comes with RAPTIVA™ (efalizumab) before you start using it and each time you get a refill. There may be new information. This information does not take the place of talking with your healthcare provider about your medical condition or treatment. It is important to remain under a healthcare provider's care while using RAPTIVA. **Do not change or stop treatment without first talking with your healthcare provider.** Talk to your healthcare provider or pharmacist if you have any questions about RAPTIVA.

WHAT IS THE MOST IMPORTANT INFORMATION I SHOULD KNOW ABOUT RAPTIVA?

RAPTIVA can decrease the activity of your immune system. Therefore, people using RAPTIVA may have an increased chance of getting:

- **Serious infections.** Some infections could become serious. If you have an infection, tell your healthcare provider before you start using RAPTIVA. If you get an infection that does not go away while taking RAPTIVA, tell your healthcare provider right away.
- **Cancers.** Many drugs that decrease the activity of the immune system can increase the risk of cancer. If you have had cancer you should tell your healthcare provider before you start taking RAPTIVA. The role of RAPTIVA in the development of cancer is not known.
- **Low platelet counts (thrombocytopenia).** Platelets help your blood clot. Low platelets give you a higher chance for bleeding. Call your doctor right away if you have increased bruising or bleeding. Your healthcare provider may do regular blood tests to check your platelets while you are taking RAPTIVA.
- **Worsening of psoriasis.** Some patients have had severe worsening or new forms of psoriasis while taking RAPTIVA or after stopping RAPTIVA. Tell your healthcare provider right away if your psoriasis gets worse or if you see any new rashes during or after treatment with RAPTIVA.

You should not receive vaccines while using RAPTIVA. RAPTIVA may prevent a vaccine from working. Talk to your healthcare provider if you need to receive a vaccine while using RAPTIVA.

WHAT IS RAPTIVA?

RAPTIVA is a medicine used to treat adult patients with moderate to severe plaque psoriasis who can be treated with medicines that affect the whole body (systemic therapy) or with phototherapy.

RAPTIVA is a man-made protein that is like proteins made in the body called antibodies. Antibodies fight disease in the human body. RAPTIVA may decrease the skin changes in the body that are the main problems of moderate to severe plaque psoriasis.

RAPTIVA has not been studied in children under 18 years of age.

WHO SHOULD NOT USE RAPTIVA?

Do not use RAPTIVA if you have ever had an allergic reaction to RAPTIVA.

Before using RAPTIVA, tell your healthcare provider

1. **about the following medical conditions:**
   - **If you are pregnant, planning to become pregnant, or become pregnant while using RAPTIVA.** It is not known if RAPTIVA can harm your unborn baby. If you become pregnant while taking RAPTIVA, notify your healthcare provider immediately. You and your healthcare provider will have to decide if RAPTIVA is right for you during pregnancy. If you use RAPTIVA when you are pregnant, ask your healthcare provider how you can be on the RAPTIVA pregnancy registry.
   - **If you are breast feeding.** It is not known if RAPTIVA passes into your milk. It may harm your baby. You will need to decide whether to use RAPTIVA or breast feed, but you may not do both.
   - **If you have any infections (see WHAT IS THE MOST IMPORTANT INFORMATION I SHOULD KNOW ABOUT RAPTIVA?).**
   - **If you have immune system problems**
2. **about all the medicines you take including prescription and nonprescription medicines, vitamins, and herbal supplements.** It is not known if RAPTIVA and other medicines affect each other. **Especially, tell your healthcare provider if you are using:**
   - **Other medicines or treatments for your psoriasis**
   - **Medicines called immunosuppressives or any medicine that affects your immune system.** Ask your healthcare provider or pharmacist if you are not sure if any of your medicines are immunosuppressives.

HOW SHOULD I USE RAPTIVA?

- RAPTIVA is an injection that you give yourself once a week.
- **See the end of this leaflet for instructions on how to prepare and inject RAPTIVA (HOW DO I PREPARE AND GIVE A RAPTIVA INJECTION?).** Ask your healthcare provider or pharmacist if you have any questions about using RAPTIVA.
- Use RAPTIVA exactly as prescribed by your healthcare provider. Your dose of RAPTIVA is based on your body weight. Tell your healthcare provider if your weight changes. Do not change your dose without talking to your healthcare provider. Do not stop using RAPTIVA without talking to your healthcare provider.
- RAPTIVA is injected under the skin (subcutaneous) of your upper leg (thigh), upper arm, abdomen, or buttocks once a week. Change (rotate) your skin injection site with each injection.
- Use RAPTIVA the same day each week. If you miss your dose of RAPTIVA contact your healthcare provider to find out when to take your next dose of RAPTIVA and what schedule to follow after that.
- If you take more than your regular dose of RAPTIVA, call your healthcare provider right away.
- See your healthcare provider regularly while using RAPTIVA. Do not miss your appointments. Your healthcare provider may do blood tests including platelet counts before and during treatment with RAPTIVA to check its affect on your body.

WHAT SHOULD I AVOID WHILE USING RAPTIVA?

Unless directed by your healthcare provider, do not:

- take other medicines called immunosuppressives.
- take treatments called phototherapy.

You should not receive vaccines while using RAPTIVA. Talk to your healthcare provider if you need to receive a vaccine while taking RAPTIVA (see **WHAT IS THE MOST IMPORTANT INFORMATION I SHOULD KNOW ABOUT RAPTIVA?**).

WHAT ARE THE POSSIBLE SIDE EFFECTS OF RAPTIVA?

RAPTIVA can cause serious side effects including the following (see WHAT IS THE MOST IMPORTANT INFORMATION I SHOULD KNOW ABOUT RAPTIVA?):

RAPTIVA can affect your immune system and might cause:

- **Serious infections**
- **Cancers**
- **Low platelet counts (thrombocytopenia)**
- **Worsening of psoriasis**

The most common side effects of RAPTIVA include headache, chills, fever, nausea, and muscle aches. These reactions usually happen within the first 48 hours following RAPTIVA injection, and often decrease after the first few weeks of use of RAPTIVA. Back pain, joint pain, and swelling of the arms or legs (peripheral edema) can also happen with RAPTIVA. Talk to your healthcare provider about any symptoms that bother you.

If you get any side effect that concerns you or if you get an infection, call your healthcare provider.

These are not all the side effects of RAPTIVA. For more information, ask your healthcare provider or pharmacist.

HOW SHOULD I STORE RAPTIVA?

- Store RAPTIVA vials in the refrigerator at 36° to 46°F (2° to 8°C) until you are ready to prepare your injection. **Do not freeze or store at room temperature.** Once RAPTIVA has been mixed with sterile water, you should use it right away to inject yourself. If you are unable to inject the drug after mixing, the mixture can stay at room temperature for up to 8 hours. Do not use RAPTIVA that was mixed more than 8 hours earlier.

  If you are traveling, be sure to store RAPTIVA at the right temperature. If you have any questions, ask your healthcare provider or pharmacist.
- Protect RAPTIVA vials from light while stored.
- Throw away RAPTIVA vials that are out of date.
- **Keep RAPTIVA and all medicines out of the reach of children.**

GENERAL INFORMATION ABOUT RAPTIVA

Medicines are sometimes prescribed for conditions that are not mentioned in patient information leaflets. Do not use RAPTIVA for a condition for which it was not prescribed. Do not give RAPTIVA to other people, even if they have the same symptoms you have. It may harm them.

This leaflet summarizes the most important information about RAPTIVA. If you would like more information, talk with your healthcare provider. You can ask your healthcare provider or pharmacist for information about RAPTIVA that is written for health professionals. For more information, you can also call 1-877-RAPTIVA (toll free).

HOW DO I PREPARE AND GIVE A RAPTIVA INJECTION?

If your dose amount is more than 1.25 mL, you will need to use 2 RAPTIVA blister trays, and you will give yourself 2 injections of RAPTIVA.

Setting Up the Equipment

1. Take the RAPTIVA blister tray out of the refrigerator, and place it on a flat, well-lit, clean work surface.
2. Wash your hands with soap and warm water before opening the blister tray.
3. Open the tray and lay out the contents. Allow the contents to come to room temperature.

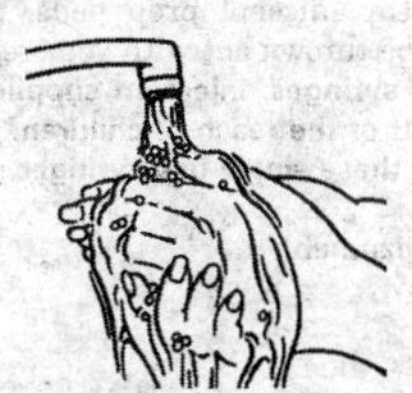

As shown below, the tray contains:

- One RAPTIVA vial
- One 1.3-mL prefilled syringe of sterile water
- Two 25-gauge needles
- Two alcohol prep pads

Contact your healthcare provider or pharmacist if you are missing any of the items listed above.

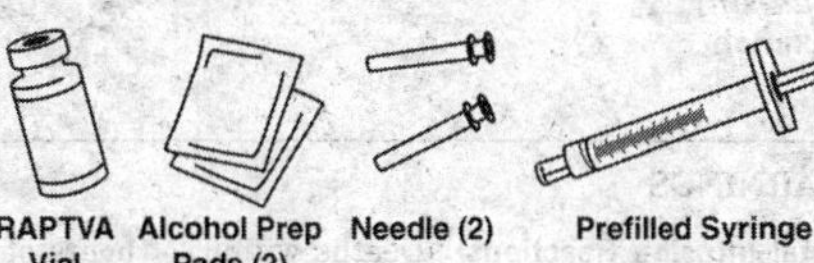

4. Check the expiration (Exp.) date on the RAPTIVA vial label and prefilled syringe label. If the expiration date has passed, do not use the RAPTIVA vial or the prefilled syringe containing the sterile water. Contact your healthcare provider.

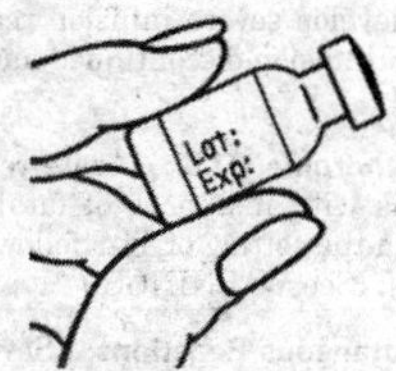

5. Remove the plastic cap protecting the rubber stopper of the RAPTIVA vial. Wipe the rubber stopper with an alcohol prep pad. Do not touch the top of the vial.
6. Remove one of the 25-gauge needles from its package. Remove the cap covering the prefilled syringe tip. Carefully place the capped 25-gauge needle onto the syringe tip. Remove the needle cap. Do not touch the needle.

Mixing RAPTIVA

If your RAPTIVA dose amount is greater than 1.25 mL, repeat Steps 1–3 of this section using a second RAPTIVA blister tray.

1. Keep the RAPTIVA vial upright on a firm surface, and slowly puncture the rubber stopper with the needle. Very slowly push down on the syringe plunger to inject all of the 1.3 mL of sterile water onto the side wall of the vial to cause less foaming. Some foaming may happen; this is normal.

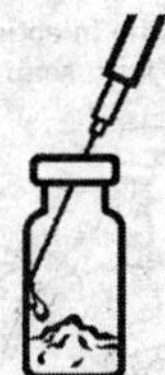

2. With the needle and syringe still in the vial stopper, gently swirl the vial to mix. Wait 5 minutes for the medicine to completely dissolve. To avoid excess foaming, **do not shake the vial.** Very slowly pull out the needle and syringe. Do not use the solution if it is discolored or cloudy or if particles (solid matter) are in the solution. The RAPTIVA solution should be clear to pale yellow.

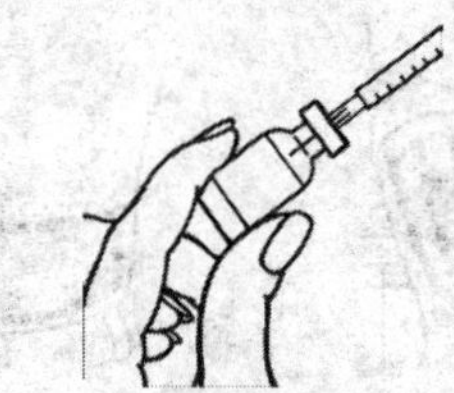

3. Slide the needle into the cap on a flat surface to pick up the cap. To lower the chance of a needlestick injury, do not touch the cap until it covers the needle all the way. Push the cap all the way down over the needle. Twist the capped needle off the syringe and discard it in a puncture-resistant container (see **DISPOSAL OF THE SYRINGE, NEEDLES, AND SUPPLIES). Never reuse a needle.**

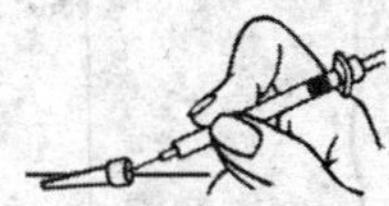

Preparing the RAPTIVA Dose for Injection

If your dose amount is more than 1.25 mL, split the dose evenly and follow Steps 1–8 of this section using the contents of two separate RAPTIVA blister trays.

1. Using an alcohol prep pad, wipe the rubber stopper of the vial containing the mixed RAPTIVA solution.

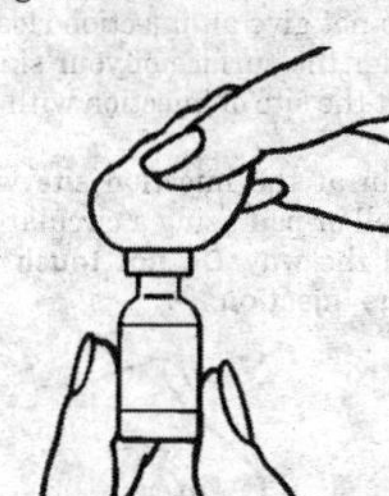

2. Remove the remaining unused needle from its package. Connect this needle to the syringe tip, and carefully remove the needle cap.
3. Keep the RAPTIVA vial in an upright position on a flat surface, and push the needle straight down through the rubber stopper on the vial.
4. Turn the vial upside down, keeping the needle in the vial (The needle will now be pointing upward.). Make sure the tip of the needle is covered all the way by the medicine in the vial. This will make it easier to get the medicine into the syringe.
5. Pull back on the plunger to fill the syringe. Remove the correct dose of medicine by reading the numbers on the syringe.

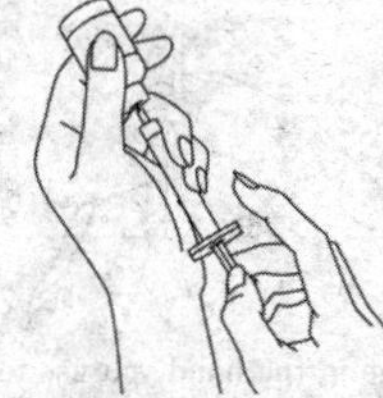

6. Hold the syringe upright and tap the side of the syringe to let air bubbles rise to the top. Gently push in the plunger of the syringe to push the air bubbles out.
7. After removing the bubbles, recheck the dose of medicine in the syringe. Make sure you have the right dose as instructed by your healthcare provider.
8. Slide the needle into the cap on a flat surface to pick up the syringe cap. Do not let the needle touch anything except the inside of the cap. Push the cap all the way down over the needle. Put the syringe down while preparing your skin for injection.

Continued on next page

Raptiva—Cont.

Selecting and Preparing the Injection Site

1. Wash your hands well with soap and water.

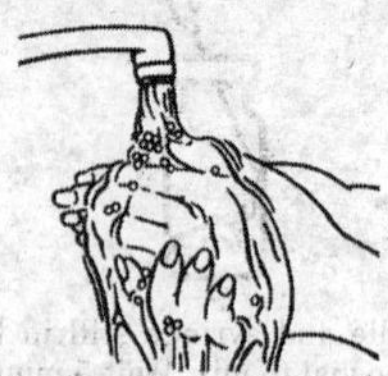

2. Choose an area of the body for the injection. Avoid, if possible, skin involved with psoriasis. Possible injection sites include the following:
   - Outer area of the upper legs (thighs)
   - Stomach area around the belly button

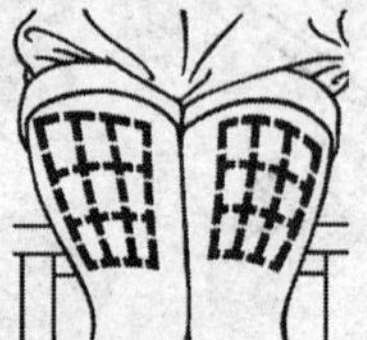

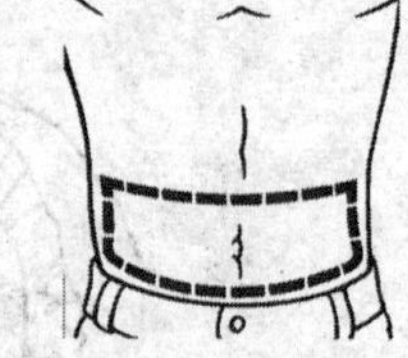

If someone else is giving you an injection, you can also use:
- Back of upper arms
- Buttocks

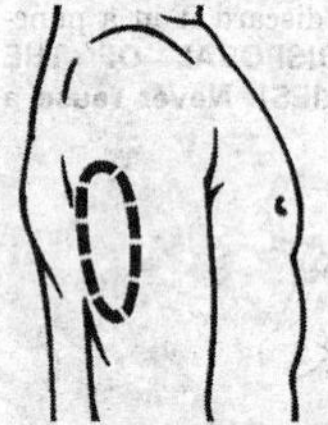

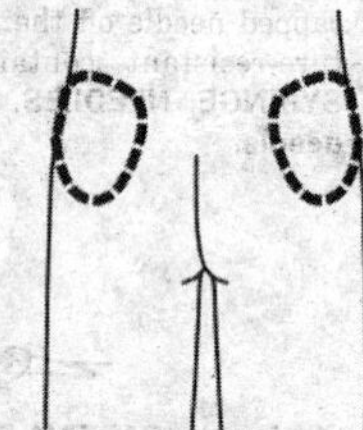

3. It is important to change (rotate) the injection site each time you take RAPTIVA to lower your chances of soreness and redness at the injection site. Changing the injection site will also improve absorption of the medication. Repeat injections given in the same area should be at least 1 inch apart. Do not give an injection close to a vein that you can see under the surface of your skin.
4. Wash the skin at the site of injection with soap and water. Let it air dry.
5. Cleanse the skin at the injection site with an alcohol-soaked cotton ball or pad using a circular motion. Let the area air dry all the way. **Do not touch this area again before giving the injection.**

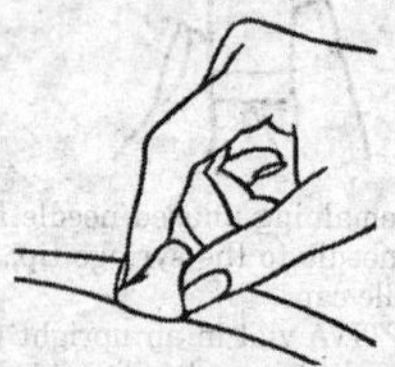

Giving the RAPTIVA Injection under the Skin

Your healthcare provider will teach you how to inject RAPTIVA. Do not inject RAPTIVA unless you have been taught the right way to give the injection.

1. Hold the syringe and remove the needle cover. Twisting the needle cover while pulling will help in the removal. **Do not** touch the needle or allow the needle to touch anything.

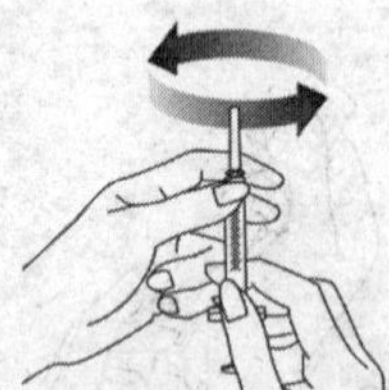

2. Hold the syringe in the hand you use to inject yourself. Use your other hand to pinch a patch of skin at the clean injection site. **Do not** lay the syringe down or allow the needle to touch anything.
3. Hold the syringe firmly between your thumb and fingers so that you have steady control. Insert the needle straight down at a 90-degree angle. This is important to make sure the medicine is injected into fatty tissue. [See first figure at top of next column]
4. After the needle is inserted all the way into the skin, you can gently let go of the pinched skin. Be sure the needle stays in your skin. Slowly and smoothly push the plunger down into the syringe until it stops.
5. When all of the medicine has been injected, remove the needle and do not re-cap it. Press a dry, sterile gauze over

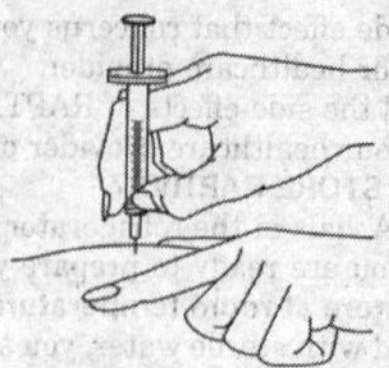

the injection site. Do not use the alcohol prep pad. A small bandage may be put over the injection site.

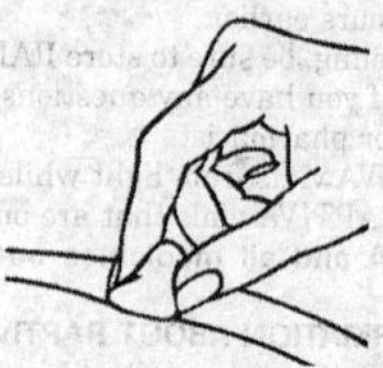

6. If your dose amount is more than 1.25 mL, you will need to give a second injection. Choose the second injection site at least 1 inch from the first injection site.

DISPOSAL OF THE SYRINGE, NEEDLES, AND SUPPLIES

1. Place the used syringe with the attached needle in a puncture-resistant container, like a sharps container. You can buy a sharps container at your local pharmacy.

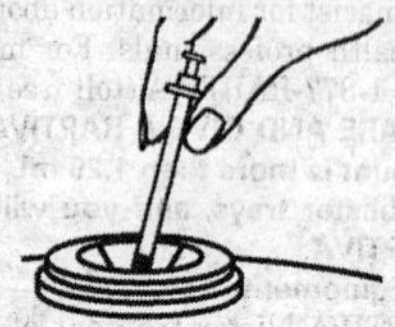

2. Talk to your healthcare provider about how to properly dispose of a filled container of your used syringes and needles. There may be special local and state laws for disposing of used needles and syringes. **Do not throw the filled container in the household trash and do not recycle.**
3. The needle cap, alcohol prep pads, and other used supplies can be thrown out with your regular trash.
4. **Always keep syringes, injection supplies, and disposal containers out of the reach of children.**
5. **Do not reuse these single-use syringes.**

Rx Only

RAPTIVA™ [efalizumab]

Manufactured by:
Genentech, Inc.
1 DNA Way
South San Francisco, CA 94080-4990
4826400
FDA Approval October 2003

Shown in Product Identification Guide, page 313

RITUXAN® ℞

[*rĭ-tŭk-sĭn*]
Rituximab

WARNINGS

Fatal Infusion Reactions: Deaths within 24 hours of RITUXAN infusion have been reported. These fatal reactions followed an infusion reaction complex which included hypoxia, pulmonary infiltrates, acute respiratory distress syndrome, myocardial infarction, ventricular fibrillation or cardiogenic shock. Approximately 80% of fatal infusion reactions occurred in association with the first infusion. (See WARNINGS and ADVERSE REACTIONS.)

Patients who develop severe infusion reactions should have RITUXAN infusion discontinued and receive medical treatment.

Tumor Lysis Syndrome (TLS): Acute renal failure requiring dialysis with instances of fatal outcome has been reported in the setting of TLS following treatment with RITUXAN. (See WARNINGS.)

Severe Mucocutaneous Reactions: Severe mucocutaneous reactions, some with fatal outcome, have been reported in association with RITUXAN treatment. (See WARNINGS and ADVERSE REACTIONS.)

DESCRIPTION

The RITUXAN® (Rituximab) antibody is a genetically engineered chimeric murine/human monoclonal antibody directed against the CD20 antigen found on the surface of normal and malignant B lymphocytes. The antibody is an IgG_1 kappa immunoglobulin containing murine light- and heavy-chain variable region sequences and human constant region sequences. Rituximab is composed of two heavy chains of 451 amino acids and two light chains of 213 amino acids (based on cDNA analysis) and has an approximate molecular weight of 145 kD. Rituximab has a binding affinity for the CD20 antigen of approximately 8.0 nM.

The chimeric anti-CD20 antibody is produced by mammalian cell (Chinese Hamster Ovary) suspension culture in a nutrient medium containing the antibiotic gentamicin. Gentamicin is not detectable in the final product. The anti-CD20 antibody is purified by affinity and ion exchange chromatography. The purification process includes specific viral inactivation and removal procedures. Rituximab drug product is manufactured from either bulk drug substance manufactured by Genentech, Inc. (US License No. 1048) or utilizing formulated bulk Rituximab supplied by IDEC Pharmaceuticals Corporation (US License No. 1235) under a shared manufacturing arrangement.

RITUXAN is a sterile, clear, colorless, preservative-free liquid concentrate for intravenous (IV) administration. RITUXAN is supplied at a concentration of 10 mg/mL in either 100 mg (10 mL) or 500 mg (50 mL) single-use vials. The product is formulated for IV administration in 9.0 mg/mL sodium chloride, 7.35 mg/mL sodium citrate dihydrate, 0.7 mg/mL polysorbate 80, and Sterile Water for Injection. The pH is adjusted to 6.5.

CLINICAL PHARMACOLOGY

General

Rituximab binds specifically to the antigen CD20 (human B-lymphocyte-restricted differentiation antigen, Bp35), a hydrophobic transmembrane protein with a molecular weight of approximately 35 kD located on pre-B and mature B lymphocytes.[1,2] The antigen is also expressed on > 90% of B-cell non-Hodgkin's lymphomas (NHL),[3] but is not found on hematopoietic stem cells, pro-B cells, normal plasma cells or other normal tissues.[4] CD20 regulates an early step(s) in the activation process for cell cycle initiation and differentiation,[4] and possibly functions as a calcium ion channel.[5] CD20 is not shed from the cell surface and does not internalize upon antibody binding.[6] Free CD20 antigen is not found in the circulation.[2]

Preclinical Pharmacology and Toxicology

Mechanism of Action: The Fab domain of Rituximab binds to the CD20 antigen on B lymphocytes, and the Fc domain recruits immune effector functions to mediate B-cell lysis *in vitro*. Possible mechanisms of cell lysis include complement-dependent cytotoxicity (CDC)[7] and antibody-dependent cell mediated cytotoxicity (ADCC). The antibody has been shown to induce apoptosis in the DHL-4 human B-cell lymphoma line.[8]

Normal Tissue Cross-reactivity: Rituximab binding was observed on lymphoid cells in the thymus, the white pulp of the spleen, and a majority of B lymphocytes in peripheral blood and lymph nodes. Little or no binding was observed in the non-lymphoid tissues examined.

Human Pharmacokinetics/Pharmacodynamics

In patients given single doses at 10, 50, 100, 250 or 500 mg/m^2 as an IV infusion, serum levels and the half-life of Rituximab were proportional to dose.[9] In 14 patients given 375 mg/m^2 as an IV infusion for 4 weekly doses, the mean serum half-life was 76.3 hours (range, 31.5 to 152.6 hours) after the first infusion and 205.8 hours (range, 83.9 to 407.0 hours); after the fourth infusion.[10,11,12] The wide range of half-lives may reflect the variable tumor burden among patients and the changes in CD20-positive (normal and malignant) B-cell populations upon repeated administrations.

RITUXAN at a dose of 375 mg/m^2 was administered as an IV infusion at weekly intervals for 4 doses to 203 patients naive to RITUXAN. The mean C_{max} following the fourth infusion was 486 µg/mL (range, 77.5 to 996.6 µg/mL). The peak and trough serum levels of Rituximab were inversely correlated with baseline values for the number of circulating CD20-positive B cells and measures of disease burden. Median steady-state serum levels were higher for responders compared with nonresponders; however, no difference was found in the rate of elimination as measured by serum half-life. Serum levels were higher in patients with International Working Formulation (IWF) subtypes B, C, and D as compared with those with subtype A. Rituximab was detectable in the serum of patients 3 to 6 months after completion of treatment.

RITUXAN at a dose of 375 mg/m^2 was administered as an IV infusion at weekly intervals for 8 doses to 37 patients. The mean C_{max} after 8 infusions was 550 µg/mL (range, 171 to 1177 µg/mL). The mean C_{max} increased with each successive infusion through the eighth infusion (Table 1).

Table 1
Rituximab C_{max} Values

Infusion Number	Mean C_{max} µg/mL	Range µg/mL
1	242.6	16.1–581.9
2	357.5	106.8–948.6
3	381.3	110.5–731.2
4	460.0	138.0–835.8
5	475.3	156.0–929.1
6	515.4	152.7–865.2
7	544.6	187.0–936.8
8	550.0	170.6–1177.0

The pharmacokinetic profile of RITUXAN when administered as 6 infusions of 375 mg/m^2 in combination with 6 cycles of CHOP chemotherapy was similar to that seen with RITUXAN alone.

Administration of RITUXAN resulted in a rapid and sustained depletion of circulating and tissue-based B cells. Lymph node biopsies performed 14 days after therapy showed a decrease in the percentage of B cells in seven of eight patients who had received single doses of Rituximab ≥100 mg/m^2.[9] Among the 166 patients in the pivotal study, circulating B cells (measured as CD19–positive cells) were depleted within the first three doses with sustained depletion for up to 6 to 9 months post-treatment in 83% of patients. Of the responding patients assessed (n = 80), 1% failed to show significant depletion of CD19– positive cells after the third infusion of Rituximab as compared to 19% of the nonresponding patients. B-cell recovery began at approximately 6 months following completion of treatment. Median B-cell levels returned to normal by 12 months following completion of treatment.

There were sustained and statistically significant reductions in both IgM and IgG serum levels observed from 5 through 11 months following Rituximab administration. However, only 14% of patients had reductions in IgM and/or IgG serum levels, resulting in values below the normal range.

CLINICAL STUDIES

Studies with a collective enrollment of 296 patients having relapsed or refractory low-grade or follicular B-cell NHL are described below (Table 2). RITUXAN regimens tested include treatment weekly for 4 doses and treatment weekly for 8 doses. Clinical settings studied were initial treatment, initial treatment of bulky disease, and retreatment.

[See table 2 above]

Table 2
Summary of RITUXAN Efficacy Data by Schedule and Clinical Setting (See ADVERSE REACTIONS for Risk Factors Associated with Increased Rates of Adverse Events.)

	Initial, Weekly × 4 N = 166	Initial, Weekly × 8 N = 37	Initial, Bulky, Weekly × 4 N = 39[1]	Retreatment, Weekly × 4 N = 60
Overall Response Rate	48%	57%	36%	38%
Complete Response Rate	6%	14%	3%	10%
Median Duration Of Response[2,3,4] (Months) [Range]	11.2 [1.9 to 42.1+]	13.4 [2.5 to 36.5+]	6.9 [2.8 to 25.0+]	15.0 [3.0 to 25.1+]

[1]Six of these patients are included in the first column. Thus, data from 296 intent to treat patients are provided in this table.
[2]Kaplan-Meier projected with observed range.
[3]"+" indicates an ongoing response.
[4]Duration of response: interval from the onset of response to disease progression.

Initial Treatment, Weekly for 4 Doses

A multicenter, open-label, single-arm study was conducted in 166 patients with relapsed or refractory low-grade or follicular B-cell NHL who received 375 mg/m^2 of RITUXAN given as an IV infusion weekly for 4 doses.[13] Patients with tumor masses >10 cm or with >5,000 lymphocytes/µL in the peripheral blood were excluded from the study. The overall response rate (ORR) was 48% with 6% complete response (CR) and 42% partial response (PR) rates. The median time to onset of response was 50 days and the median duration of response was 11.2 months (range, 1.9 to 42.1+). Disease-related signs and symptoms (including B-symptoms) were present in 23% (39/166) of patients at study entry and resolved in 64% (25/39) of those patients.

In a multivariate analysis, the ORR was higher in patients with IWF B, C, and D histologic subtypes as compared to IWF subtype A (58% vs. 12%), higher in patients whose largest lesion was <5 cm vs. >7 cm (maximum, 21 cm) in greatest diameter (53% vs. 38%), and higher in patients with chemosensitive relapse as compared with chemoresistant (defined as duration of response <3 months) relapse (53% vs. 36%). ORR in patients previously treated with autologous bone marrow transplant was 78% (18/23). The following adverse prognostic factors were *not* associated with a lower response rate: age ≥60 years, extranodal disease, prior anthracycline therapy, and bone marrow involvement.

Initial Treatment, Weekly for 8 Doses

In a multicenter, single-arm study, 37 patients with relapsed or refractory, low-grade NHL received 375 mg/m^2 of RITUXAN weekly for 8 doses. The ORR was 57% (CR 14%, PR 43%) with a projected median duration of response of 13.4 months (range, 2.5 to 36.5+).[14] (For information on the higher incidence of Grade 3 and 4 adverse events, see ADVERSE REACTIONS, Risk Factors Associated with Increased Rates of Adverse Events.)

Initial Treatment, Bulky Disease, Weekly for 4 Doses

In pooled data from multiple studies of RITUXAN, 39 patients with relapsed or refractory, bulky disease (single lesion >10 cm in diameter), low-grade NHL received 375 mg/m^2 of RITUXAN weekly for 4 doses. The ORR was 36% (CR 3%, PR 33%) with a median duration of response of 6.9 months (range 2.8 to 25.0+). (For information on the higher incidence of Grade 3 and 4 adverse events, see ADVERSE REACTIONS, Risk Factors Associated with Increased Rates of Adverse Events.)

Retreatment, Weekly for 4 Doses

In a multi-center, single-arm study, 60 patients received 375 mg/m^2 of RITUXAN weekly for 4 doses.[15] All patients had relapsed or refractory, low-grade or follicular B-cell NHL and had achieved an objective clinical response to a prior course of RITUXAN. Of these 60 patients, 55 received their second course of RITUXAN, 3 patients received their third course and 2 patients received their second and third courses of RITUXAN in this study. The ORR was 38% (10% CR and 28% PR) with a projected median duration of response of 15 months (range, 3.0 to 25.1+ months).

INDICATIONS AND USAGE

RITUXAN® (Rituximab) is indicated for the treatment of patients with relapsed or refractory, low-grade or follicular, CD20-positive, B-cell non-Hodgkin's lymphoma.

CONTRAINDICATIONS

RITUXAN is contraindicated in patients with known anaphylaxis or IgE-mediated hypersensitivity to murine proteins or to any component of this product. (See WARNINGS.)

WARNINGS (See BOXED WARNINGS)

Severe Infusion Reactions (See BOXED WARNINGS, ADVERSE REACTIONS and Hypersensitivity Reactions): RITUXAN has caused severe infusion reactions. In some cases, these reactions were fatal. These severe reactions typically occurred during the first infusion with time to onset of 30 to 120 minutes. Signs and symptoms of severe infusion reactions may include hypotension, angioedema, hypoxia or bronchospasm, and may require interruption of RITUXAN administration. The most severe manifestations and sequelae include pulmonary infiltrates, acute respiratory distress syndrome, myocardial infarction, ventricular fibrillation, and cardiogenic shock. In the reported cases, the following factors were more frequently associated with fatal outcomes: female gender, pulmonary infiltrates, and chronic lymphocytic leukemia or mantle cell lymphoma.

Management of severe infusion reactions: The RITUXAN infusion should be interrupted for severe reactions and supportive care measures instituted as medically indicated (e.g., intravenous fluids, vasopressors, oxygen, bronchodilators, diphenhydramine, and acetaminophen). In most cases, the infusion can be resumed at a 50% reduction in rate (e.g., from 100 mg/hr to 50 mg/hr) when symptoms have completely resolved. Patients requiring close monitoring during first and all subsequent infusions include those with preexisting cardiac and pulmonary conditions, those with prior clinically significant cardiopulmonary adverse events and those with high numbers of circulating malignant cells (≥ 25,000/mm^3) with or without evidence of high tumor burden.

Tumor Lysis Syndrome (TLS) (See BOXED WARNINGS and ADVERSE REACTIONS): Rapid reduction in tumor volume followed by acute renal failure, hyperkalemia, hypocalcemia, hyperuricemia, or hyperphosphatasemia, have been reported within 12 to 24 hours after the first RITUXAN infusion. Rare instances of fatal outcome have been reported in the setting of TLS following treatment with RITUXAN. The risks of TLS appear to be greater in patients with high numbers of circulating malignant cells (≥ 25,000/mm^3) or high tumor burden. Prophylaxis for TLS should be considered for patients at high risk. Correction of electrolyte abnormalities, monitoring of renal function and fluid balance, and administration of supportive care, including dialysis, should be initiated as indicated. Following complete resolution of the complications of TLS, RITUXAN has been tolerated when re-administered in conjunction with prophylactic therapy for TLS in a limited number of cases.

Hepatitis B Reactivation with Related Fulminant Hepatitis: Hepatitis B virus (HBV) reactivation with fulminant hepatitis, hepatic failure, and death has been reported in some patients with hematologic malignancies treated with RITUXAN. The majority of patients received RITUXAN in combination with chemotherapy. The median time to the diagnosis of hepatitis was approximately 4 months after the initiation of RITUXAN and approximately one month after the last dose.

Persons at high risk of HBV infection should be screened before initiation of RITUXAN. Carriers of hepatitis B should be closely monitored for clinical and laboratory signs of active HBV infection and for signs of hepatitis during and for up to several months following RITUXAN therapy.

In patients who develop viral hepatitis, RITUXAN and any concomitant chemotherapy should be discontinued and appropriate treatment including antiviral therapy initiated. There are insufficient data regarding the safety of resuming RITUXAN therapy in patients who develop hepatitis subsequent to HBV reactivation.

Hypersensitivity Reactions:

RITUXAN has been associated with hypersensitivity reactions (non-IgE-mediated reactions) which may respond to adjustments in the infusion rate and in medical management. Hypotension, bronchospasm, and angioedema have occurred in association with RITUXAN infusion (see Severe Infusion Reactions). RITUXAN infusion should be interrupted for severe hypersensitivity reactions and can be resumed at a 50% reduction in rate (e.g., from 100 mg/hr to 50 mg/hr) when symptoms have completely resolved. Treatment of these symptoms with diphenhydramine and acetaminophen is recommended; additional treatment with bronchodilators or IV saline may be indicated. In most cases, patients who have experienced non-life-threatening hypersensitivity reactions have been able to complete the full course of therapy. (See DOSAGE and ADMINISTRATION.) Medications for the treatment of hypersensitivity reactions, e.g., epinephrine, antihistamines and corticosteroids, should be available for immediate use in the event of a reaction during administration.

Cardiovascular: Infusions should be discontinued in the event of serious or life-threatening cardiac arrhythmias. Patients who develop clinically significant arrhythmias should undergo cardiac monitoring during and after subsequent infusions of RITUXAN. Patients with pre-existing cardiac conditions including arrhythmias and angina have had recurrences of these events during RITUXAN therapy and should be monitored throughout the infusion and immediate post-infusion period.

Renal: RITUXAN administration has been associated with severe renal toxicity including acute renal failure requiring dialysis and in some cases, has led to a fatal outcome. Renal toxicity has occurred in patients with high numbers of circulating malignant cells (>25,000/mm^3) or high tumor burden who experience tumor lysis syndrome (see Tumor Lysis Syndrome) and in patients administered concomitant cisplatin therapy during clinical trials. The combination of cisplatin and RITUXAN is not an approved treatment regimen. If this combination is used in clinical trials *extreme caution* should be exercised; patients should be monitored closely for signs of renal failure. Discontinuation of RITUXAN should be considered for those with rising serum creatinine or oliguria.

Severe Mucocutaneous Reactions (See BOXED WARNINGS and ADVERSE REACTIONS): Mucocutaneous reactions, some with fatal outcome, have been reported in patients treated with RITUXAN. These reports include paraneoplastic pemphigus (an uncommon disorder which is a manifestation of the patient's underlying malignancy),[16] Stevens-Johnson syndrome, lichenoid dermatitis, vesiculobullous dermatitis, and toxic epidermal necrolysis. The onset of the reaction in the reported cases has varied from 1 to 13 weeks following RITUXAN exposure. Patients experiencing a severe mucocutaneous reaction should not receive any further infusions and seek prompt medical evaluation. Skin biopsy may help to distinguish among different mucocutaneous reactions and guide subsequent treatment. The safety of readministration of RITUXAN to patients with any of these mucocutaneous reactions has not been determined.

PRECAUTIONS

Laboratory Monitoring: Because RITUXAN targets all CD20-positive B lymphocytes, malignant and nonmalignant, complete blood counts (CBC) and platelet counts should be obtained at regular intervals during RITUXAN therapy and more frequently in patients who develop cytopenias (see ADVERSE REACTIONS). The duration of cytopenias caused by RITUXAN can extend well beyond the treatment period.

Drug/Laboratory Interactions: There have been no formal drug interaction studies performed with RITUXAN. However, renal toxicity was seen with this drug in combination with cisplatin in clinical trials. (See WARNINGS, Renal.)

HACA Formation: Human antichimeric antibody (HACA) was detected in 4 of 356 patients and 3 had an objective clinical response. The data reflect the percentage of patients whose test results were considered positive for antibodies to RITUXAN using an enzyme-linked immunosorbant assay (limit of detection = 7 ng/mL). The observed incidence of antibody positivity in an assay is highly dependent on the sensitivity and specificity of the assay and may be influenced by several factors including sample handling, concomitant medications, and underlying disease. For these reasons, comparison of the incidence of antibodies to RITUXAN with the incidence of antibodies to other products may be misleading.

Immunization: The safety of immunization with live viral vaccines following RITUXAN therapy has not been studied. The ability to generate a primary or anamnestic humoral response to vaccination is currently being studied.

Carcinogenesis, Mutagenesis, Impairment of Fertility: No long-term animal studies have been performed to establish the carcinogenic or mutagenic potential of RITUXAN, or to determine its effects on fertility in males or females. Individuals of childbearing potential should use effective contraceptive methods during treatment and for up to 12 months following RITUXAN therapy.

Pregnancy Category C: Animal reproduction studies have not been conducted with RITUXAN. It is not known whether RITUXAN can cause fetal harm when administered to a pregnant woman or whether it can affect reproductive capacity. Human IgG is known to pass the placental barrier, and thus may potentially cause fetal B-cell depletion; therefore, RITUXAN should be given to a pregnant woman only if clearly needed.

Nursing Mothers: It is not known whether RITUXAN is excreted in human milk. Because human IgG is excreted in

Continued on next page

Rituxan—Cont.

human milk and the potential for absorption and immunosuppression in the infant is unknown, women should be advised to discontinue nursing until circulating drug levels are no longer detectable. (See CLINICAL PHARMACOLOGY.)

Pediatric Use: The safety and effectiveness of RITUXAN in pediatric patients have not been established.

Geriatric Use: Among the 331 patients enrolled in clinical studies of single agent RITUXAN, 24% were 65 to 75 years old and 5% were 75 years old and older. The overall response rates were higher in older (age ≥ 65 years) vs. younger (age < 65 years) patients (52% vs. 44%, respectively). However, the median duration of response, based on Kaplan-Meier estimates, was shorter in older vs. younger patients: 10.1 months (range, 1.9 to 36.5+) vs. 11.4 months (range, 2.1 to 42.1+), respectively. This shorter duration of response was not statistically significant. Adverse reactions, including incidence, severity and type of adverse reaction were similar between older and younger patients.

ADVERSE REACTIONS

The most serious adverse reactions caused by RITUXAN include infusion reactions, tumor lysis syndrome, mucocutaneous reactions, hypersensitivity reactions, cardiac arrhythmias and angina, and renal failure. Please refer to the BOXED WARNINGS and WARNINGS sections for detailed descriptions of these reactions. Infusion reactions and lymphopenia are the most commonly occurring adverse reactions.

Because clinical trials are conducted under widely varying conditions, adverse reaction rates observed in the clinical trials of a drug cannot be directly compared to rates in the clinical trials of another drug and may not reflect the rates observed in practice. The adverse reaction information from clinical trials does, however, provide a basis for identifying the adverse events that appear to be related to drug use and for approximating rates.

Additional adverse reactions have been identified during postmarketing use of RITUXAN. Because these reactions are reported voluntarily from a population of uncertain size, it is not always possible to reliably estimate their frequency or establish a causal relationship to RITUXAN exposure. Decisions to include these reactions in labeling are typically based on one or more of the following factors: (1) seriousness of the reaction, (2) frequency of reporting, or (3) strength of causal connection to RITUXAN.

Where specific percentages are noted, these data are based on 356 patients treated in nonrandomized, single-arm studies of RITUXAN administered as a single agent. Most patients received RITUXAN 375 mg/m^2 weekly for 4 doses. These include 39 patients with bulky disease (lesions ≥ 10 cm) and 60 patients who received more than 1 course of RITUXAN. Thirty-seven patients received 375 mg/m^2 for 8 doses and 25 patients received doses other than 375 mg/m^2 for 4 doses and up to 500 mg/m^2 single dose in the Phase 1 setting. Adverse events of greater severity are referred to as "Grade 3 and 4 events" defined by the commonly used National Cancer Institute Common Toxicity Criteria.[17]

Table 3
Incidence of Adverse Events ≥ 5% of Patients in Clinical Trials (N = 356) (Adverse Events were followed for a period of 12 months following RITUXAN therapy)

	All Grades (%)	Grade 3 and 4 (%)
Any Adverse Events	**99**	**57**
Body as a Whole	**86**	**10**
Fever	53	1
Chills	33	3
Infection	31	4
Asthenia	26	1
Headache	19	1
Abdominal Pain	14	1
Pain	12	1
Back Pain	10	1
Throat Irritation	9	0
Flushing	5	0
Cardiovascular System	**25**	**3**
Hypotension	10	1
Hypertension	6	1
Digestive System	**37**	**2**
Nausea	23	1
Diarrhea	10	1
Vomiting	10	1
Hemic and Lymphatic System	**67**	**48**
Lymphopenia	48	40
Leukopenia	14	4
Neutropenia	14	6
Thrombocytopenia	12	2
Anemia	8	3
Metabolic and Nutritional Disorders	**38**	**3**
Angioedema	11	1
Hyperglycemia	9	1
Peripheral Edema	8	0
LDH Increase	7	0
Musculoskeletal System	**26**	**3**
Myalgia	10	1
Arthralgia	10	1
Nervous System	**32**	**1**
Dizziness	10	1
Anxiety	5	1
Respiratory System	**38**	**4**
Increased Cough	13	1
Rhinitis	12	1
Bronchospasm	8	1
Dyspnea	7	1
Sinusitis	6	0
Skin and Appendages	**44**	**2**
Night Sweats	15	1
Rash	15	1
Pruritus	14	1
Urticaria	8	1

Risk Factors Associated with Increased Rates of Adverse Events: Administration of RITUXAN weekly for 8 doses resulted in higher rates of Grade 3 and 4 adverse events[17] overall (70%) compared with administration weekly for 4 doses (57%). The incidence of Grade 3 or 4 adverse events was similar in patients retreated with RITUXAN compared with initial treatment (58% and 57%, respectively). The incidence of the following clinically significant adverse events was higher in patients with bulky disease (lesions ≥10 cm) (N = 39) versus patients with lesions < 10 cm (N = 195): abdominal pain, anemia, dyspnea, hypotension, and neutropenia.

Infusion Reactions (See BOXED WARNINGS and WARNINGS): Mild to moderate infusion reactions consisting of fever and chills/rigors occurred in the majority of patients during the first RITUXAN infusion. Other frequent infusion reaction symptoms included nausea, pruritus, angioedema, asthenia, hypotension, headache, bronchospasm, throat irritation, rhinitis, urticaria, rash, vomiting, myalgia, dizziness, and hypertension. These reactions generally occurred within 30 to 120 minutes of beginning the first infusion, and resolved with slowing or interruption of the RITUXAN infusion and with supportive care (diphenhydramine, acetaminophen, IV saline, and vasopressors). In an analysis of data from 356 patients with relapsed or refractory, low-grade NHL who received 4 (N = 319) or 8 (N = 37) weekly infusions of RITUXAN, the incidence of infusion reactions was highest during the first infusion (77%) and decreased with each subsequent infusion (30% with fourth infusion and 14% with eighth infusion).

Infectious Events: RITUXAN induced B-cell depletion in 70% to 80% of patients and was associated with decreased serum immunoglobulins in a minority of patients; the lymphopenia lasted a median of 14 days (range, 1 to 588 days). Infectious events occurred in 31% of patients: 19% of patients had bacterial infections, 10% had viral infections, 1% had fungal infections, and 6% were unknown infections. Incidence is not additive because a single patient may have had more than one type of infection. Serious infectious events (Grade 3 or 4),[17] including sepsis, occurred in 2% of patients.

Hematologic Events: In clinical trials, Grade 3 and 4 cytopenias[17] were reported in 48% of patients treated with RITUXAN; these include: lymphopenia (40%), neutropenia (6%), leukopenia (4%), anemia (3%), and thrombocytopenia (2%). The median duration of lymphopenia was 14 days (range, 1 to 588 days) and of neutropenia was 13 days (range, 2 to 116 days). A single occurrence of transient aplastic anemia (pure red cell aplasia) and two occurrences of hemolytic anemia following RITUXAN therapy were reported.

In addition, there have been a limited number of postmarketing reports of prolonged pancytopenia, marrow hypoplasia, and late onset neutropenia (defined as occurring 40 days after the last dose of RITUXAN) in patients with hematologic malignancies. In reported cases of late onset neutropenia (NCI-CTC Grade 3 and 4), the median duration of neutropenia was 10 days (range 3 to 148 days). Documented resolution of the neutropenia was described in approximately one-half of the reported cases; of those with documented recovery, approximately half received growth factor support. In the remaining cases, information on resolution was not provided. More than half of the reported cases of delayed onset neutropenia occurred in patients who had undergone a prior autologous bone marrow transplantation. In an adequately designed, controlled, clinical trial, the reported incidence of NCI-CTC Grade 3 and 4 neutropenia was higher in patients receiving RITUXAN in combination with fludarabine as compared to those receiving fludarabine alone (76% [39/51] vs.39% [21/53]).[18]

Cardiac Events (See BOXED WARNINGS): Grade 3 or 4 cardiac-related events include hypotension. Rare, fatal cardiac failure with symptomatic onset weeks after RITUXAN has also been reported. Patients who develop clinically significant cardiopulmonary events should have RITUXAN infusion discontinued.

Pulmonary Events (See BOXED WARNINGS): 135 patients (38%) experienced pulmonary events in clinical trials. The most common respiratory system adverse events experienced were increased cough, rhinitis, bronchospasm, dyspnea, and sinusitis. In both clinical studies and postmarketing surveillance, there have been a limited number of reports of bronchiolitis obliterans presenting up to 6 months post-RITUXAN infusion and a limited number of reports of pneumonitis (including interstitial pneumonitis) presenting up to 3 months post-RITUXAN infusion, some of which resulted in fatal outcomes. The safety of resumption or continued administration of RITUXAN in patients with pneumonitis or bronchiolitis obliterans is unknown.

Immune/Autoimmune Events: Immune/autoimmune events have been reported, including uveitis, optic neuritis in a patient with systemic vasculitis, pleuritis in a patient with a lupus-like syndrome, serum sickness with polyarticular arthritis, and vasculitis with rash.

Less Commonly Observed Events: In clinical trials, < 5% and > 1% of the patients experienced the following events regardless of causality assessment: agitation, anorexia, arthritis, conjunctivitis, depression, dyspepsia, edema, hyperkinesia, hypertonia, hypesthesia, hypoglycemia, injection site pain, insomnia, lacrimation disorder, malaise, nervousness, neuritis, neuropathy, paresthesia, somnolence, vertigo, weight decrease.

OVERDOSAGE

There has been no experience with overdosage in human clinical trials. Single doses of up to 500 mg/m^2 have been given in controlled clinical trials.[10]

DOSAGE AND ADMINISTRATION

Initial Therapy:
RITUXAN is given at 375 mg/m^2 IV infusion once weekly for 4 or 8 doses.

Retreatment Therapy: Patients who subsequently develop progressive disease may be safely retreated with RITUXAN 375 mg/m^2 IV infusion once weekly for 4 doses. Currently there are limited data concerning more than 2 courses.

RITUXAN as a Component of Zevalin™ (Ibritumomab Tiuxetan) Therapeutic Regimen: As a required component of the Zevalin therapeutic regimen, RITUXAN 250 mg/m^2 should be infused within 4 hours prior to the administration of Indium-111- (In-111-) Zevalin and within 4 hours prior to the administration of Yttrium-90- (Y-90-) Zevalin. Administration of RITUXAN and In-111-Zevalin should precede RITUXAN and Y-90-Zevalin by 7–9 days. Refer to the Zevalin package insert for full prescribing information regarding the Zevalin therapeutic regimen.

RITUXAN may be administered in an outpatient setting. **DO NOT ADMINISTER AS AN INTRAVENOUS PUSH OR BOLUS. (See Administration.)**

Instructions for Administration

Preparation for Administration: Use appropriate aseptic technique. Withdraw the necessary amount of RITUXAN and dilute to a final concentration of 1 to 4 mg/mL into an infusion bag containing either 0.9% Sodium Chloride, USP, or 5% Dextrose in Water, USP. Gently invert the bag to mix the solution. Discard any unused portion left in the vial. Parenteral drug products should be inspected visually for particulate matter and discoloration prior to administration.

RITUXAN solutions for infusion may be stored at 2–8°C (36–46°F) for 24 hours. RITUXAN solutions for infusion have been shown to be stable for an additional 24 hours at room temperature. However, since RITUXAN solutions do not contain a preservative, diluted solutions should be stored refrigerated (2–8°C). No incompatibilities between RITUXAN and polyvinylchloride or polyethylene bags have been observed.

Administration: DO NOT ADMINISTER AS AN INTRAVENOUS PUSH OR BOLUS.
Infusion and hypersensitivity reactions may occur (see BOXED WARNINGS, WARNINGS, and ADVERSE REACTIONS). Premedication consisting of acetaminophen and diphenhydramine should be considered before each infusion of RITUXAN. Premedication may attenuate infusion reactions. Since transient hypotension may occur during RITUXAN infusion, consideration should be given to withholding antihypertensive medications 12 hours prior to RITUXAN infusion.

First Infusion: The RITUXAN solution for infusion should be administered intravenously at an initial rate of 50 mg/hr. RITUXAN should not be mixed or diluted with other drugs. If hypersensitivity or infusion reactions do not occur, escalate the infusion rate in 50 mg/hr increments every 30 minutes, to a maximum of 400 mg/hr. If a hypersensitivity (non-IgE-mediated) or an infusion reaction develops, the infusion should be temporarily slowed or interrupted (see BOXED WARNINGS and WARNINGS). The infusion can continue at one-half the previous rate upon improvement of patient symptoms.

Subsequent Infusions: If the patient tolerated the first infusion well, subsequent RITUXAN infusions can be administered at an initial rate of 100 mg/hr, and increased by 100 mg/hr increments at 30-minute intervals, to a maximum of 400 mg/hr as tolerated. If the patient did not tolerate the first infusion well, follow the guidelines under First Infusion.

Stability and Storage: RITUXAN vials are stable at 2–8°C (36–46°F). Do not use beyond expiration date stamped on carton. RITUXAN vials should be protected from direct sunlight. Refer to the "Preparation and Administration" section for information on the stability and storage of solutions of RITUXAN diluted for infusion.

HOW SUPPLIED

RITUXAN® (Rituximab) is supplied as 100 mg and 500 mg of sterile, preservative-free, single-use vials.

Single unit 100 mg carton: Contains one 10 mL vial of RITUXAN (10 mg/mL).
NDC 50242-051-21

Single unit 500 mg carton: Contains one 50 mL vial of RITUXAN (10 mg/mL).

NDC 50242-053-06

REFERENCES

1. Valentine MA, Meier KE, Rossie S, et al. Phosphorylation of the CD20 phosphoprotein in resting B lymphocytes. *J Biol Chem* 1989 264(19):11282–11287.
2. Einfeld DA, Brown JP, Valentine MA, et al. Molecular cloning of the human B cell CD20 receptor predicts a hydrophobic protein with multiple transmembrane domains. *EMBO J* 1988 7(3):711–717.
3. Anderson KC, Bates MP, Slaughenhoupt BL, et al. Expression of human B cell-associated antigens on leukemias and lymphomas: A model of human B cell differentiation. *Blood* 1984 63(6):1424–1433.
4. Tedder TF, Boyd AW, Freedman AS, et al. The B cell surface molecule B1 is functionally linked with B cell activation and differentiation. *J Immunol* 1985 135(2):973–979.
5. Tedder TF, Zhou LJ, Bell PD, et al. The CD20 surface molecule of B lymphocytes functions as a calcium channel. *J Cell Biochem* 1990 14D:195.
6. Press OW, Applebaum F, Ledbetter JA, Martin PJ, Zarling J, Kidd P, et al. Monoclonal antibody 1F5 (anti-CD20) serotherapy of human B-cell lymphomas. *Blood* 1987 69(2):584–591.
7. Reff ME, Carner C, Chambers KS, Chinn PC, Leonard JE, Raab R, et al. Depletion of B cells in vivo by a chimeric mouse human monoclonal antibody to CD20. *Blood* 1994 83(2):435–445.
8. Demidem A, Lam T, Alas S, Hariharan K, Hanna N, and Bonavida B. Chimeric anti-CD20 (IDEC-C2B8) monoclonal antibody sensitizes a B cell lymphoma cell line to cell killing by cytotoxic drugs. *Cancer Biotherapy & Radiopharmaceuticals* 1997 12(3):177–186.
9. Maloney DG, Liles TM, Czerwinski C, Waldichuk J, Rosenberg J, Grillo-López A, et al. Phase I clinical trial using escalating single-dose infusion of chimeric anti-CD20 monoclonal antibody (IDEC-C2B8) in patients with recurrent B-cell lymphoma. *Blood* 1994 84(8):2457–2466.
10. Berinstein NL, Grillo-López AJ, White CA, Bence-Bruckler I, Maloney D, Czuczman M, et al. Association of serum Rituximab (IDEC-C2B8) concentration and anti-tumor response in the treatment of recurrent low-grade or follicular non-Hodgkin's lymphoma. *Annals of Oncology* 1998, 9:995–1001.
11. Maloney DG, Grillo-López AJ, Bodkin D, White CA, Liles T-M, Royston I, et al. IDEC-C2B8: Results of a phase I multiple-dose trial in patients with relapsed non-Hodgkin's lymphoma. *J Clin Oncol* 1997 15(10): 3266–3274.
12. Maloney DG, Grillo-López AJ, White CA, Bodkin D, Schilder RJ, Neidhart JA, et al. IDEC-C2B8 (Rituximab) anti-CD20 monoclonal antibody therapy in patients with relapsed low-grade non-Hodgkin's lymphoma. *Blood* 1997 90(6):2188–2195.
13. McLaughlin P, Grillo-López AJ, Link BK, Levy R, Czuczman MS, Williams ME, et al. Rituximab chimeric anti-CD20 monoclonal antibody therapy for relapsed indolent lymphoma: half of patients respond to a four-dose treatment program. *J Clin Oncol* 1998 16(8):2825–2833.
14. Piro LD, White CA, Grillo-López AJ, Janakiraman N, Saven A, Beck TM, et al. Extended Rituximab (anti-CD20 monoclonal antibody) therapy for relapsed or refractory low-grade or follicular non-Hodgkin's lymphoma. *Annals of Oncology* 1999 10:655–661.
15. Davis TA, Grillo-López AJ, White CA, McLaughlin P, Czuczman MS, Link BK, Maloney DG, Weaver RL, Rosenberg J, Levy R. Rituximab anti-CD20 monoclonal antibody therapy in non-hodgkin's lymphoma: safety and efficacy of re-treatment. *J Clin Oncol* 2000 18(17): 3135–3143.
16. Anhalt GJ, Kim SC, Stanley JR, Korman NJ, Jabs DA, Kory M, Izumi H, Ratrie H, Mutasim D, Ariss-Abdo L, Labib RS. Paraneoplastic Pemphigus, an autoimmune mucocutaneous disease associated with neoplasia. *NEJM* 1990 323(25):1729–1735.
17. National Institutes of Health (US), National Cancer Institute. Common Toxicity Criteria. [Bethesda, MD.]: National Institutes of Health, National Cancer Institute; c1998. 73p.
18. Byrd JC, Peterson BL, Morrison VA, Park K, Jacobson R, Hoke E, Vardiman JW, Rai K, Schiffer CA, Larson RA. Randomized phase 2 study of fludarabine with concurrent versus sequential treatment with rituximab in symptomatic, untreated patients with B-cell chronic lymphocytic leukemia: results from Cancer and Leukemia Group B 9712 (CALGB 9712). *Blood* 2003 101(1): 6–14.

Jointly Marketed by:

IDEC Pharmaceuticals Corporation
11011 Torreyana Road
San Diego, CA 92121
Genentech, Inc.
1 DNA Way
South San Francisco, CA 94080-4990
4809705
Revised June 2004

Shown in Product Identification Guide, page 313

TNKase™ ℞
(Tenecteplase)
Full Prescribing Information

DESCRIPTION

Tenecteplase is a tissue plasminogen activator (tPA) produced by recombinant DNA technology using an established mammalian cell line (Chinese Hamster Ovary cells). Tenecteplase is a 527 amino acid glycoprotein developed by introducing the following modifications to the complementary DNA (cDNA) for natural human tPA: a substitution of threonine 103 with asparagine, and a substitution of asparagine 117 with glutamine, both within the kringle 1 domain, and a tetra-alanine substitution at amino acids 296–299 in the protease domain. Cell culture is carried out in nutrient medium containing the antibiotic gentamicin (65 mg/L). However, the presence of the antibiotic is not detectable in the final product (limit of detection is 0.67 µg/vial). TNKase is a sterile, white to off-white, lyophilized powder for single intravenous (IV) bolus administration after reconstitution with Sterile Water for Injection (SWFI), USP. Each vial of TNKase nominally contains 52.5 mg Tenecteplase, 0.55 g L-arginine, 0.17 g phosphoric acid, and 4.3 mg polysorbate 20, which includes a 5% overfill. Each vial will deliver 50 mg of Tenecteplase.

CLINICAL PHARMACOLOGY

General

Tenecteplase is a modified form of human tissue plasminogen activator (tPA) that binds to fibrin and converts plasminogen to plasmin. In the presence of fibrin, *in vitro* studies demonstrate that Tenecteplase conversion of plasminogen to plasmin is increased relative to its conversion in the absence of fibrin. This fibrin specificity decreases systemic activation of plasminogen and the resulting degradation of circulating fibrinogen as compared to a molecule lacking this property. Following administration of 30, 40, or 50 mg of TNKase, there are decreases in circulating fibrinogen (4%–15%) and plasminogen (11%–24%). The clinical significance of fibrin-specificity on safety (e.g., bleeding) or efficacy has not been established. Biological potency is determined by an *in vitro* clot lysis assay and is expressed in Tenecteplase-specific units. The specific activity of Tenecteplase has been defined as 200 units/mg.

Pharmacokinetics

In patients with acute myocardial infarction (AMI), TNKase administered as a single bolus exhibits a biphasic disposition from the plasma. Tenecteplase was cleared from the plasma with an initial half-life of 20 to 24 minutes. The terminal phase half-life of Tenecteplase was 90 to 130 minutes. In 99 of 104 patients treated with Tenecteplase, mean plasma clearance ranged from 99 to 119 mL/min.

The initial volume of distribution is weight related and approximates plasma volume. Liver metabolism is the major clearance mechanism for Tenecteplase.

CLINICAL STUDIES

ASSENT-2 was an international, randomized, double-blind trial that compared 30-day mortality rates in 16,949 patients assigned to receive an IV bolus dose of TNKase or an accelerated infusion of Activase® (Alteplase).[1] Eligibility criteria included onset of chest pain within 6 hours of randomization and ST-segment elevation or left bundle branch block on electrocardiogram (ECG). Patients were to be excluded from the trial if they received GP IIb/IIIa inhibitors within the previous 12 hours. TNKase was dosed using actual or estimated weight in a weight-tiered fashion as described in DOSAGE AND ADMINISTRATION. All patients were to receive 150–325 mg of aspirin administered as soon as possible, followed by 150–325 mg daily. Intravenous heparin was to be administered as soon as possible: for patients weighing ≤ 67 kg, heparin was administered as a 4000 unit IV bolus followed by infusion at 800 U/hr; for patients weighing > 67 kg, heparin was administered as a 5000 unit IV bolus followed by infusion at 1000 U/hr. Heparin was continued for 48 to 72 hours with infusion adjusted to maintain aPTT at 50–75 seconds. The use of GP IIb/IIIa inhibitors was discouraged for the first 24 hours following randomization. The results of the primary endpoint (30-day mortality rates with non-parametric adjustment for the covariates of age, Killip class, heart rate, systolic blood pressure and infarct location) along with selected other 30-day endpoints are shown in Table 1.

[See table 1 above]

Table 1
ASSENT-2
Mortality, Stroke, and Combined Outcome of Death or Stroke Measured at Thirty Days

30-day Events	TNKase (N=8461)	Accelerated Activase (N=8488)	Relative Risk TNKase/Activase (95% CI)
Mortality	6.2%	6.2%	1.00 (0.89, 1.12)
Intracranial Hemorrhage (ICH)	0.9%	0.9%	0.99 (0.73, 1.35)
Any Stroke	1.8%	1.7%	1.07 (0.86, 1.35)
Death or Nonfatal Stroke	7.1%	7.0%	1.01 (0.91, 1.13)

Rates of mortality and the combined endpoint of death or stroke among pre-specified subgroups, including age, gender, time to treatment, infarct location, and history of previous myocardial infarction, demonstrate consistent relative risks across these subgroups. There was insufficient enrollment of non-Caucasian patients to draw any conclusions regarding relative efficacy in racial subsets.

Rates of in-hospital procedures, including percutaneous transluminal coronary angioplasty (PTCA), stent placement, intra-aortic balloon pump (IABP) use, and coronary artery bypass graft (CABG) surgery, were similar between the TNKase and Activase groups.

TIMI 10B was an open-label, controlled, randomized, dose-ranging, angiography study which utilized a blinded core laboratory for review of coronary arteriograms.[2] Patients (n = 837) presenting within 12 hours of symptom onset were treated with fixed doses of 30, 40, or 50 mg of TNKase or the accelerated infusion of Activase and underwent coronary arteriography at 90 minutes. The results showed that the 40 mg and 50 mg doses were similar to accelerated infusion of Activase in restoring patency. TIMI grade 3 flow and TIMI grade 2/3 flow at 90 minutes are shown in Table 2. The exact relationship between coronary artery patency and clinical activity has not been established.

[See table 2 above]

Table 2
TIMI 10B Patency Rates
TIMI Grade Flow at 90 Minutes

	Activase ≤ 100 mg (n=311)	TNKase 30 mg (n=302)	TNKase 40 mg (n=148)	TNKase 50 mg (n=76)
TIMI Grade 3 Flow	63%	54%	63%	66%
TIMI Grade 2/3 Flow	82%	77%	79%	88%
95% CI (TIMI 2/3 Flow)	(77%, 86%)	(72%, 81%)	(72%, 85%)	(79%, 94%)

The angiographic results from TIMI 10B and the safety data from ASSENT-1, an additional uncontrolled safety study of 3,235 TNKase-treated patients, provided the framework to develop a weight-tiered TNKase dose regimen.[3] Exploratory analyses suggested that a weight-adjusted dose of 0.5 mg/kg to 0.6 mg/kg of TNKase resulted in a better patency to bleeding relationship than fixed doses of TNKase across a broad range of patient weights.

INDICATIONS AND USAGE

TNKase is indicated for use in the reduction of mortality associated with acute myocardial infarction (AMI). Treatment should be initiated as soon as possible after the onset of AMI symptoms (see CLINICAL STUDIES).

CONTRAINDICATIONS

TNKase therapy in patients with acute myocardial infarction is contraindicated in the following situations because of an increased risk of bleeding (see WARNINGS):

- **Active internal bleeding**
- **History of cerebrovascular accident**
- **Intracranial or intraspinal surgery or trauma within 2 months**
- **Intracranial neoplasm, arteriovenous malformation, or aneurysm**
- **Known bleeding diathesis**
- **Severe uncontrolled hypertension**

WARNINGS

Bleeding

The most common complication encountered during TNKase therapy is bleeding. The type of bleeding associated with thrombolytic therapy can be divided into two broad categories:

Continued on next page

TNKase—Cont.

- Internal bleeding, involving intracranial and retroperitoneal sites, or the gastrointestinal, genitourinary, or respiratory tracts.
- Superficial or surface bleeding, observed mainly at vascular puncture and access sites (e.g., venous cutdowns, arterial punctures) or sites of recent surgical intervention.

Should serious bleeding (not controlled by local pressure) occur, any concomitant heparin or antiplatelet agents should be discontinued immediately.

In clinical studies of TNKase, patients were treated with both aspirin and heparin. Heparin may contribute to the bleeding risks associated with TNKase. The safety of the use of TNKase with other antiplatelet agents has not been adequately studied (see PRECAUTIONS: Drug Interactions). Intramuscular injections and nonessential handling of the patient should be avoided for the first few hours following treatment with TNKase. Venipunctures should be performed and monitored carefully.

Should an arterial puncture be necessary during the first few hours following TNKase therapy, it is preferable to use an upper extremity vessel that is accessible to manual compression. Pressure should be applied for at least 30 minutes, a pressure dressing applied, and the puncture site checked frequently for evidence of bleeding.

Each patient being considered for therapy with TNKase should be carefully evaluated and anticipated benefits weighed against potential risks associated with therapy. In the following conditions, the risk of TNKase therapy may be increased and should be weighed against the anticipated benefits:

- Recent major surgery, e.g., coronary artery bypass graft, obstetrical delivery, organ biopsy, previous puncture of noncompressible vessels
- Cerebrovascular disease
- Recent gastrointestinal or genitourinary bleeding
- Recent trauma
- Hypertension: systolic BP ≥ 180 mm Hg and/or diastolic BP ≥ 110 mm Hg
- High likelihood of left heart thrombus, e.g., mitral stenosis with atrial fibrillation
- Acute pericarditis
- Subacute bacterial endocarditis
- Hemostatic defects, including those secondary to severe hepatic or renal disease
- Severe hepatic dysfunction
- Pregnancy
- Diabetic hemorrhagic retinopathy or other hemorrhagic ophthalmic conditions
- Septic thrombophlebitis or occluded AV cannula at seriously infected site
- Advanced age (see PRECAUTIONS: Geriatric Use)
- Patients currently receiving oral anticoagulants, e.g., warfarin sodium
- Recent administration of GP IIb/IIIa inhibitors
- Any other condition in which bleeding constitutes a significant hazard or would be particularly difficult to manage because of its location

Cholesterol Embolization

Cholesterol embolism has been reported rarely in patients treated with all types of thrombolytic agents; the true incidence is unknown. This serious condition, which can be lethal, is also associated with invasive vascular procedures (e.g., cardiac catheterization, angiography, vascular surgery) and/or anticoagulant therapy. Clinical features of cholesterol embolism may include livedo reticularis, "purple toe" syndrome, acute renal failure, gangrenous digits, hypertension, pancreatitis, myocardial infarction, cerebral infarction, spinal cord infarction, retinal artery occlusion, bowel infarction, and rhabdomyolysis.

Arrhythmias

Coronary thrombolysis may result in arrhythmias associated with reperfusion. These arrhythmias (such as sinus bradycardia, accelerated idioventricular rhythm, ventricular premature depolarizations, ventricular tachycardia) are not different from those often seen in the ordinary course of acute myocardial infarction and may be managed with standard anti-arrhythmic measures. It is recommended that anti-arrhythmic therapy for bradycardia and/or ventricular irritability be available when TNKase is administered.

PRECAUTIONS

General

Standard management of myocardial infarction should be implemented concomitantly with TNKase treatment. Arterial and venous punctures should be minimized. Noncompressible arterial puncture must be avoided and internal jugular and subclavian venous punctures should be avoided to minimize bleeding from the noncompressible sites. In the event of serious bleeding, heparin and antiplatelet agents should be discontinued immediately. Heparin effects can be reversed by protamine.

Readministration

Readministration of plasminogen activators, including TNKase, to patients who have received prior plasminogen activator therapy has not been systematically studied. Three of 487 patients tested for antibody formation to TNKase had a positive antibody titer at 30 days. The data reflect the percentage of patients whose test results were considered positive for antibodies to TNKase in a radioimmunoprecipitation assay, and are highly dependent on the sensitivity and specificity of the assay. Additionally, the observed incidence of antibody positivity in an assay may be influenced by several factors including sample handling, concomitant medications, and underlying disease. For these reasons, comparison of the incidence of antibodies to TNKase with the incidence of antibodies to other products may be misleading. Although sustained antibody formation in patients receiving one dose of TNKase has not been documented, readministration should be undertaken with caution. If an anaphylactic reaction occurs, appropriate therapy should be administered.

Drug Interactions

Formal interaction studies of TNKase with other drugs have not been performed. Patients studied in clinical trials of TNKase were routinely treated with heparin and aspirin. Anticoagulants (such as heparin and vitamin K antagonists) and drugs that alter platelet function (such as acetylsalicylic acid, dipyridamole, and GP IIb/IIIa inhibitors) may increase the risk of bleeding if administered prior to, during, or after TNKase therapy.

Drug/Laboratory Test Interactions

During TNKase therapy, results of coagulation tests and/or measures of fibrinolytic activity may be unreliable unless specific precautions are taken to prevent *in vitro* artifacts. Tenecteplase is an enzyme that, when present in blood in pharmacologic concentrations, remains active under *in vitro* conditions. This can lead to degradation of fibrinogen in blood samples removed for analysis.

Carcinogenesis, Mutagenesis, Impairment of Fertility

Studies in animals have not been performed to evaluate the carcinogenic potential, mutagenicity, or the effect on fertility.

Pregnancy (Category C)

TNKase has been shown to elicit maternal and embryo toxicity in rabbits given multiple IV administrations. In rabbits administered 0.5, 1.5 and 5.0 mg/kg/day, vaginal hemorrhage resulted in maternal deaths. Subsequent embryonic deaths were secondary to maternal hemorrhage and no fetal anomalies were observed. TNKase does not elicit maternal and embryo toxicity in rabbits following a single IV administration. Thus, in developmental toxicity studies conducted in rabbits, the no observable effect level (NOEL) of a single IV administration of TNKase on maternal or developmental toxicity was 5 mg/kg (approximately 8–10 times the human dose). There are no adequate and well-controlled studies in pregnant women. TNKase should be given to pregnant women only if the potential benefits justify the potential risk to the fetus.

Nursing Mothers

It is not known if TNKase is excreted in human milk. Because many drugs are excreted in human milk, caution should be exercised when TNKase is administered to a nursing woman.

Pediatric Use

The safety and effectiveness of TNKase in pediatric patients have not been established.

Geriatric Use

Of the patients in ASSENT-2 who received TNKase, 4,958 (59%) were under the age of 65; 2,256 (27%) were between the ages of 65 and 74; and 1,244 (15%) were 75 and over. The 30-day mortality rates by age were 2.5% in patients under the age of 65, 8.5% in patients between the ages of 65 and 74, and 16.2% in patients age 75 and over. The ICH rates were 0.4% in patients under the age of 65, 1.6% in patients between the ages of 65 and 74, and 1.7% in patients age 75 and over. The rates of any stroke were 1.0% in patients under the age of 65, 2.9% in patients between the ages of 65 and 74, and 3.0% in patients age 75 and over. Major bleeding rates, defined as bleeding requiring blood transfusion or leading to hemodynamic compromise, were 3.1% in patients under the age of 65, 6.4% in patients between the ages of 65 and 74, and 7.7% in patients age 75 and over. In elderly patients, the benefits of TNKase on mortality should be carefully weighed against the risk of increased adverse events, including bleeding.

ADVERSE REACTIONS

Bleeding

The most frequent adverse reaction associated with TNKase is bleeding (see WARNINGS).

Should serious bleeding occur, concomitant heparin and antiplatelet therapy should be discontinued. Death or permanent disability can occur in patients who experience stroke or serious bleeding episodes.

For TNKase-treated patients in ASSENT-2, the incidence of intracranial hemorrhage was 0.9% and any stroke was 1.8%. The incidence of all strokes, including intracranial bleeding, increases with increasing age (see PRECAUTIONS: Geriatric Use).

In the ASSENT-2 study, the following bleeding events were reported (see Table 3).

[See table 3 below]

Table 3
ASSENT-2
Non-ICH Bleeding Events

	TNKase (N=8461)	Accelerated Activase (N=8488)	Relative Risk TNKase/Activase (95% CI)
Major bleeding[a]	4.7%	5.9%	0.78 (0.69, 0.89)
Minor bleeding	21.8%	23.0%	0.94 (0.89, 1.00)
Units of transfused blood			
Any	4.3%	5.5%	0.77 (0.67, 0.89)
1–2	2.6%	3.2%	
> 2	1.7%	2.2%	

[a]Major bleeding is defined as bleeding requiring blood transfusion or leading to hemodynamic compromise.

Non-intracranial major bleeding and the need for blood transfusions were lower in patients treated with TNKase. Types of major bleeding reported in 1% or more of the patients were hematoma (1.7%) and gastrointestinal tract (1%). Types of major bleeding reported in less than 1% of the patients were urinary tract, puncture site (including cardiac catheterization site), retroperitoneal, respiratory tract, and unspecified. Types of minor bleeding reported in 1% or more of the patients were hematoma (12.3%), urinary tract (3.7%), puncture site (including cardiac catheterization site) (3.6%), pharyngeal (3.1%), gastrointestinal tract (1.9%), epistaxis (1.5%), and unspecified (1.3%).

Allergic Reactions

Allergic-type reactions (e.g., anaphylaxis, angioedema, laryngeal edema, rash, and urticaria) have rarely (< 1%) been reported in patients treated with TNKase. Anaphylaxis was reported in < 0.1% of patients treated with TNKase; however, causality was not established. When such reactions occur, they usually respond to conventional therapy.

Other Adverse Reactions

The following adverse reactions have been reported among patients receiving TNKase in clinical trials. These reactions are frequent sequelae of the underlying disease, and the effect of TNKase on the incidence of these events is unknown. These events include cardiogenic shock, arrhythmias, atrioventricular block, pulmonary edema, heart failure, cardiac arrest, recurrent myocardial ischemia, myocardial reinfarction, myocardial rupture, cardiac tamponade, pericarditis, pericardial effusion, mitral regurgitation, thrombosis, embolism, and electromechanical dissociation. These events can be life-threatening and may lead to death. Nausea and/or vomiting, hypotension, and fever have also been reported.

DOSAGE AND ADMINISTRATION

Dosage

TNKase is for intravenous administration only. The recommended total dose should not exceed 50 mg and is based upon patient weight.

A single bolus dose should be administered over 5 seconds based on patient weight. Treatment should be initiated as soon as possible after the onset of AMI symptoms (see CLINICAL STUDIES).

Dose Information Table

Patient Weight (kg)	TNKase (mg)	Volume TNKase* to be administered (mL)
< 60	30	6
≥ 60 to < 70	35	7
≥ 70 to < 80	40	8
≥ 80 to < 90	45	9
≥ 90	50	10

*From one vial of TNKase reconstituted with 10 mL SWFI.

The safety and efficacy of TNKase has only been investigated with concomitant administration of heparin and aspirin as described in CLINICAL STUDIES.

[See graphic at top of next page]

Reconstitution

NOTE: Read all instructions completely before beginning reconstitution and administration.

1. Remove the shield assembly from the supplied B-D® 10 cc syringe with TwinPak™ Dual Cannula Device (see figure) and aseptically withdraw 10 mL of Sterile Water for Injection (SWFI), USP, from the supplied diluent vial using the red hub cannula syringe filling device. Do not use Bacteriostatic Water for Injection, USP.

The B-D® 10 cc Syringe with TwinPak™ Dual Cannula Device

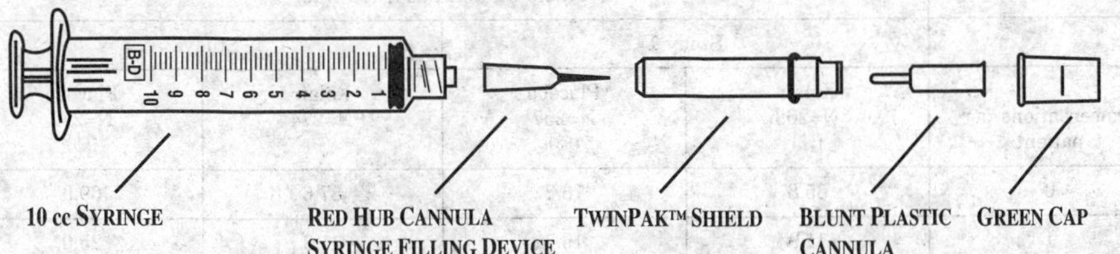

Note: Do not discard the shield assembly.

2. Inject the entire contents of the syringe (10 mL) into the TNKase vial directing the diluent stream into the powder. Slight foaming upon reconstitution is not unusual; any large bubbles will dissipate if the product is allowed to stand undisturbed for several minutes.
3. Gently swirl until contents are completely dissolved. DO NOT SHAKE. The reconstituted preparation results in a colorless to pale yellow transparent solution containing TNKase at 5 mg/mL at a pH of approximately 7.3. The osmolality of this solution is approximately 290 mOsm/kg.
4. Determine the appropriate dose of TNKase (see Dose Information Table) and withdraw this volume (in milliliters) from the reconstituted vial with the syringe. **Any unused solution should be discarded.**
5. Once the appropriate dose of TNKase is drawn into the syringe, stand the shield vertically on a flat surface (with green side down) and passively recap the red hub cannula.
6. Remove the entire shield assembly, including the red hub cannula, by twisting counterclockwise. Note: The shield assembly also contains the clear-ended blunt plastic cannula; retain for split septum IV access.

Administration

1. The product should be visually inspected prior to administration for particulate matter and discoloration. TNKase may be administered as reconstituted at 5 mg/mL.
2. Precipitation may occur when TNKase is administered in an IV line containing dextrose. Dextrose-containing lines should be flushed with a saline-containing solution prior to and following single bolus administration of TNKase.
3. Reconstituted TNKase should be administered as a single IV bolus over 5 seconds.
4. Because TNKase contains no antibacterial preservatives, it should be reconstituted immediately before use. If the reconstituted TNKase is not used immediately, refrigerate the TNKase vial at 2–8°C (36–46°F) and use within 8 hours.
5. Although the supplied syringe is compatible with a conventional needle, this syringe is designed to be used with needleless IV systems. From the information below, follow the instructions applicable to the IV system in use.

Split septum IV system:
- Remove the green cap.
- Attach the clear-ended blunt plastic cannula to the syringe.
- Remove the shield and use the blunt plastic cannula to access the split septum injection port.
- Because the blunt plastic cannula has two side ports, air or fluid expelled through the cannula will exit in two sideways directions; direct away from face or mucous membranes.

Luer-Lok® system: Connect syringe directly to IV port.

Conventional needle (not supplied in this kit): Attach a large bore needle, e.g., 18 gauge, to the syringe's universal Luer-Lok®.

6. Dispose of the syringe, cannula, and shield per established procedures.

HOW SUPPLIED

TNKase is supplied as a sterile, lyophilized powder in a 50 mg vial under partial vacuum. Each 50 mg vial of TNKase is packaged with one 10 mL vial of Sterile Water for Injection, USP, for reconstitution, The B-D® 10 cc syringe with TwinPak™ Dual Cannula Device, and three alcohol prep pads. NDC 50242-038-61.

Stability and Storage

Store lyophilized TNKase at controlled room temperature not to exceed 30°C (86°F) or under refrigeration 2–8°C (36–46°F). Do not use beyond the expiration date stamped on the vial.

REFERENCES

1. ASSENT-2 Investigators. Single-bolus tenecteplase compared with front-loaded alteplase in acute myocardial infarction: the ASSENT-2 double-blind randomised trial. Lancet 1999;354:716-22.
2. Cannon CP, Gibson CM, McCabe CH, Adgey AAJ, Schweiger MJ, Sequeira RF, et al. TNK-tissue plasminogen activator compared with front-loaded alteplase in acute myocardial infarction. Results of the TIMI 10B trial. Circulation 1998;98:2805-14.
3. Van de Werf F, Cannon CP, Luyten A, Houbracken K, McCabe CH, Berioli S, et al. Safety assessment of a single bolus administration of TNK-tissue plasminogen activator in acute myocardial infarction: the ASSENT-1 trial. Am Heart J 1999;137:786-91.

TNKase™
(Tenecteplase)

Manufactured by:
Genentech, Inc. 4819900
1 DNA Way June 2000
South San Francisco, CA 94080-4990

Shown in Product Identification Guide, page 313

XOLAIR® ℞

[*zō′lār*]
Omalizumab
For Subcutaneous Use

DESCRIPTION

Xolair (Omalizumab) is a recombinant DNA-derived humanized IgG1κ monoclonal antibody that selectively binds to human immunoglobulin E (IgE). The antibody has a molecular weight of approximately 149 kilodaltons. Xolair is produced by a Chinese hamster ovary cell suspension culture in a nutrient medium containing the antibiotic gentamicin. Gentamicin is not detectable in the final product.

Xolair is a sterile, white, preservative-free, lyophilized powder contained in a single-use vial that is reconstituted with Sterile Water for Injection (SWFI), USP, and administered as a subcutaneous (SC) injection. A Xolair 75 mg vial contains 129.6 mg of Omalizumab, 93.1 mg sucrose, 1.8 mg L-histidine hydrochloride monohydrate, 1.2 mg L-histidine, and 0.3 mg polysorbate 20, and is designed to deliver 75 mg of Omalizumab in 0.6 mL after reconstitution with 0.9 mL SWFI, USP. A Xolair 150 mg vial contains 202.5 mg of Omalizumab, 145.5 mg sucrose, 2.8 mg L-histidine hydrochloride monohydrate, 1.8 mg L-histidine, and 0.5 mg polysorbate 20, and is designed to deliver 150 mg of Omalizumab in 1.2 mL after reconstitution with 1.4 mL SWFI, USP.

CLINICAL PHARMACOLOGY

Mechanism of Action

Xolair inhibits the binding of IgE to the high-affinity IgE receptor (FcεRI) on the surface of mast cells and basophils. Reduction in surface-bound IgE on FcεRI-bearing cells limits the degree of release of mediators of the allergic response. Treatment with Xolair also reduces the number of FcεRI receptors on basophils in atopic patients.

Pharmacokinetics

After SC administration, Omalizumab is absorbed with an average absolute bioavailability of 62%. Following a single SC dose in adult and adolescent patients with asthma, Omalizumab was absorbed slowly, reaching peak serum concentrations after an average of 7–8 days. The pharmacokinetics of Omalizumab are linear at doses greater than 0.5 mg/kg. Following multiple doses of Omalizumab, areas under the serum concentration-time curve from Day 0 to Day 14 at steady state were up to 6-fold of those after the first dose.

In vitro, Omalizumab forms complexes of limited size with IgE. Precipitating complexes and complexes larger than 1 million daltons in molecular weight are not observed *in vitro* or *in vivo*. Tissue distribution studies in cynomolgus monkeys showed no specific uptake of ^{125}I-Omalizumab by any organ or tissue. The apparent volume of distribution in patients following SC administration was 78±32 mL/kg.

Clearance of Omalizumab involves IgG clearance processes as well as clearance via specific binding and complex formation with its target ligand, IgE. Liver elimination of IgG includes degradation in the liver reticuloendothelial system (RES) and endothelial cells. Intact IgG is also excreted in bile. In studies with mice and monkeys, Omalizumab:IgE complexes were eliminated by interactions with Fcγ receptors within the RES at rates that were generally faster than IgG clearance. In asthma patients Omalizumab serum elimination half-life averaged 26 days, with apparent clearance averaging 2.4±1.1 mL/kg/day. In addition, doubling body weight approximately doubled apparent clearance.

Pharmacodynamics

In clinical studies, serum free IgE levels were reduced in a dose dependent manner within 1 hour following the first dose and maintained between doses. Mean serum free IgE decrease was greater than 96% using recommended doses. Serum total IgE levels (i.e., bound and unbound) increased after the first dose due to the formation of Omalizumab:IgE complexes, which have a slower elimination rate compared with free IgE. At 16 weeks after the first dose, average serum total IgE levels were five-fold higher compared with pre-treatment when using standard assays. After discontinuation of Xolair dosing, the Xolair-induced increase in total IgE and decrease in free IgE were reversible, with no observed rebound in IgE levels after drug washout. Total IgE levels did not return to pre-treatment levels for up to one year after discontinuation of Xolair.

Special Populations

The population pharmacokinetics of Xolair were analyzed to evaluate the effects of demographic characteristics. Analyses of these limited data suggest that no dose adjustments are necessary for age (12–76 years), race, ethnicity, or gender.

CLINICAL STUDIES

The safety and efficacy of Xolair were evaluated in three randomized, double-blind, placebo-controlled, multicenter trials.

The trials enrolled patients 12 to 76 years old, with moderate to severe persistent (NHLBI criteria) asthma for at least one year, and a positive skin test reaction to a perennial aeroallergen. At screening, patients in Studies 1 and 2 had a forced expiratory volume in one second (FEV1) between 40% and 80% predicted, while in Study 3 there was no restriction on screening FEV1. All patients had a FEV1 improvement of at least 12% following beta-agonist administration. All patients were symptomatic and were being treated with inhaled corticosteroids (ICS) and short acting beta-agonists. In Study 3, long-acting beta-agonists were allowed. Study 3 patients were receiving at least 1000 μg/day fluticasone propionate and a subset was also receiving oral corticosteroids. Patients receiving other concomitant controller medications were excluded, and initiation of additional controller medications while on study was prohibited. Patients currently smoking were excluded.

Each study was comprised of a run-in period to achieve a stable conversion to a common ICS (beclomethasone dipropionate, for Studies 1 and 2; fluticasone propionate for Study 3), followed by randomization to Xolair or placebo. In Study 3, patients were stratified by use of ICS-only or ICS with concomitant use of oral steroids. Patients received Xolair for 16 weeks with an unchanged corticosteroid dose unless an acute exacerbation necessitated an increase. Patients then entered an ICS reduction phase of 12 weeks (Studies 1 and 2) or 16 weeks (Study 3) during which ICS (or oral steroid in Study 3 subset) dose reduction was attempted in a step-wise manner.

Xolair dosing was based on body weight and baseline serum total IgE concentration. All patients were required to have a baseline IgE between 30 and 700 IU/mL and body weight not more than 150 kg. Patients were treated according to a dosing table to administer at least 0.016 mg/kg/IU (IgE/mL) of Xolair or a matching volume of placebo over each 4-week period. The maximum Xolair dose per 4 weeks was 750 mg; patients who had a weight-IgE combination that yielded a dose greater than 750 mg were excluded from the studies. Patients who were to receive more than 300 mg within the 4-week period were administered half the total dose every 2 weeks.

The distribution of the number of asthma exacerbations per patient in each group during a study was analyzed separately for the stable steroid and steroid-reduction periods. In all three studies an exacerbation was defined as a worsening of asthma that required treatment with systemic corticosteroids or a doubling of the baseline ICS dose.

In both Studies 1 and 2 the number of exacerbations per patient was reduced in patients treated with Xolair compared with placebo (Table 1). In Study 3 the number of exacerbations in patients treated with Xolair was similar to that in placebo-treated patients (Table 2). The absence of an observed treatment effect in Study 3 may be related to differences in the patient population compared with Studies 1 and 2, study sample size, or other factors. In all three studies most exacerbations were managed in the out-patient setting and the majority were treated with systemic steroids. Hospitalization rates were not significantly different between Xolair and placebo-treated patients; however, the overall hospitalization rate was small. Among those patients who experienced an exacerbation, the distribution of exacerbation severity was similar between treatment groups.

[See table 1 at top of next page]

[See table 2 on next page]

In all three of the studies, a reduction of asthma exacerbations was not observed in the Xolair-treated patients who had FEV1 >80% at the time of randomization. Reductions in exacerbations were not seen in patients who required oral steroids as maintenance therapy.

In Studies 1 and 2 measures of airflow (FEV1) and asthma symptoms were evaluated (Table 3). The clinical relevance of the treatment-associated differences is unknown.

[See table 3 on next page]

Continued on next page

Xolair—Cont.

Results from the stable steroid phase of Study 2 and the steroid reduction phases of both Studies 1 and 2 were similar to those presented in Table 3.

INDICATIONS AND USAGE

Xolair (Omalizumab) is indicated for adults and adolescents (12 years of age and above) with moderate to severe persistent asthma who have a positive skin test or *in vitro* reactivity to a perennial aeroallergen and whose symptoms are inadequately controlled with inhaled corticosteroids. Xolair has been shown to decrease the incidence of asthma exacerbations in these patients. Safety and efficacy have not been established in other allergic conditions.

CONTRAINDICATIONS

Xolair should not be administered to patients who have experienced a severe hypersensitivity reaction to Xolair (see WARNINGS: Anaphylaxis).

WARNINGS

Malignancy

Malignant neoplasms were observed in 20 of 4127 (0.5%) Xolair-treated patients compared with 5 of 2236 (0.2%) control patients in clinical studies of asthma and other allergic disorders. The observed malignancies in Xolair-treated patients were a variety of types, with breast, non-melanoma skin, prostate, melanoma, and parotid occurring more than once, and five other types occurring once each. The majority of patients were observed for less than 1 year. The impact of longer exposure to Xolair or use in patients at higher risk for malignancy (e.g., elderly, current smokers) is not known (see ADVERSE REACTIONS: Malignancy).

Anaphylaxis

Anaphylaxis has occurred within 2 hours of the first or subsequent administration of Xolair in 3 (<0.1%) patients without other identifiable allergic triggers. These events included urticaria and throat and/or tongue edema (see ADVERSE REACTIONS). Patients should be observed after injection of Xolair, and medications for the treatment of severe hypersensitivity reactions including anaphylaxis should be available. If a severe hypersensitivity reaction to Xolair occurs, therapy should be discontinued (see CONTRAINDICATIONS).

PRECAUTIONS

General

Xolair has not been shown to alleviate asthma exacerbations acutely and should not be used for the treatment of acute bronchospasm or status asthmaticus.

Corticosteroid Reduction

Systemic or inhaled corticosteroids should not be abruptly discontinued upon initiation of Xolair therapy. Decreases in corticosteroids should be performed under the direct supervision of a physician and may need to be performed gradually.

Information for Patients

Patients receiving Xolair should be told not to decrease the dose of, or stop taking any other asthma medications unless otherwise instructed by their physician. Patients should be told that they may not see immediate improvement in their asthma after beginning Xolair therapy.

Laboratory Tests

Serum total IgE levels increase following administration of Xolair due to formation of Xolair:IgE complexes (see CLINICAL PHARMACOLOGY, DOSAGE AND ADMINISTRATION). Elevated serum total IgE levels may persist for up to 1 year following discontinuation of Xolair. Serum total IgE levels obtained less than 1 year following discontinuation may not reflect steady state free IgE levels and should not be used to reassess the dosing regimen.

Drug Interactions

No formal drug interaction studies have been performed with Xolair. The concomitant use of Xolair and allergen immunotherapy has not been evaluated.

Carcinogenesis, Mutagenesis, Impairment of Fertility

No long-term studies have been performed in animals to evaluate the carcinogenic potential of Xolair.

No evidence of mutagenic activity was observed in Ames tests using six different strains of bacteria with and without metabolic activation at Omalizumab concentrations up to 5000 μg/mL.

The effects of Omalizumab on male and female fertility have been assessed in cynomolgus monkey studies. Administration of Omalizumab at doses up to and including 75 mg/kg/week did not elicit reproductive toxicity in male cynomolgus monkeys and did not inhibit reproductive capability, including implantation, in female cynomolgus monkeys. These doses provide a 2- to 16-fold safety factor based on total dose and 2- to 5-fold safety factor based on AUC over the range of adult clinical doses.

Pregnancy (Category B)

Reproduction studies in cynomolgus monkeys have been conducted with Omalizumab. Subcutaneous doses up to 75 mg/kg (12-fold the maximum clinical dose) of Omalizumab did not elicit maternal toxicity, embryotoxicity, or teratogenicity when administered throughout organogenesis and did not elicit adverse effects on fetal or neonatal growth when administered throughout late gestation, delivery, and nursing.

IgG molecules are known to cross the placental barrier. There are no adequate and well-controlled studies of Xolair in pregnant women. Because animal reproduction studies are not always predictive of human response, Xolair should be used during pregnancy only if clearly needed.

Table 1
Frequency of Asthma Exacerbations per Patient by Phase in Studies 1 and 2

	Stable Steroid Phase (16 wks)			
	Study 1		Study 2	
Exacerbations per patient	Xolair N=268 (%)	Placebo N=257 (%)	Xolair N=274 (%)	Placebo N=272 (%)
0	85.8	76.7	87.6	69.9
1	11.9	16.7	11.3	25.0
≥2	2.2	6.6	1.1	5.1
p-Value	0.005		<0.001	
Mean number exacerbations/patient	0.2	0.3	0.1	0.4
	Steroid Reduction Phase (12 wks)			
Exacerbations per patient	Xolair N=268 (%)	Placebo N=257 (%)	Xolair N=274 (%)	Placebo N=272 (%)
0	78.7	67.7	83.9	70.2
1	19.0	28.4	14.2	26.1
≥2	2.2	3.9	1.8	3.7
p-Value	0.004		<0.001	
Mean number exacerbations/patient	0.2	0.4	0.2	0.3

Table 2
Percentage of Patients with Asthma Exacerbations by Subgroup and Phase in Study 3

	Stable Steroid Phase (16 wks)			
	Inhaled Only		Oral+Inhaled	
	Xolair N=126	Placebo N=120	Xolair N=50	Placebo N=45
% Patients with ≥1 exacerbations	15.9	15.0	32.0	22.2
Difference (95% CI)	0.9 (−9.7, 13.7)		9.8 (−10.5, 31.4)	
	Steroid Reduction Phase (16 wks)			
	Xolair N=126	Placebo N=120	Xolair N=50	Placebo N=45
% Patients with ≥1 exacerbations	22.2	26.7	42.0	42.2
Difference (95% CI)	−4.4 (−17.6, 7.4)		−0.2 (−22.4, 20.1)	

Table 3
Asthma Symptoms and Pulmonary Function During Stable Steroid Phase of Study 1

	Xolair N=268[a]		Placebo N=257[a]	
Endpoint	Mean Baseline	Median Change (Baseline to Wk 16)	Mean Baseline	Median Change (Baseline to Wk 16)
Total asthma symptom score	4.3	−1.5[b]	4.2	−1.1[b]
Nocturnal asthma score	1.2	−0.4[b]	1.1	−0.2[b]
Daytime asthma score	2.3	−0.9[b]	2.3	−0.6[b]
FEV1 % predicted	68	3[b]	68	0[b]

Asthma symptom scale: total score from 0 (least) to 9 (most); nocturnal and daytime scores from 0 (least) to 4 (most symptoms).

[a] Number of patients available for analysis ranges 255–258 in the Xolair group and 238–239 in the placebo group.

[b] Comparison of Xolair versus placebo ($p<0.05$).

Nursing Mothers

The excretion of Omalizumab in milk was evaluated in female cynomolgus monkeys receiving SC doses of 75 mg/kg/week. Neonatal plasma levels of Omalizumab after *in utero* exposure and 28 days of nursing were between 11% and 94% of the maternal plasma level. Milk levels of Omalizumab were 1.5% of maternal blood concentration. While Xolair presence in human milk has not been studied, IgG is excreted in human milk and therefore it is expected that Xolair will be present in human milk. The potential for Xolair absorption or harm to the infant are unknown; caution should be exercised when administering Xolair to a nursing woman.

Pediatric Use

Safety and effectiveness in pediatric patients below the age of 12 have not been established.

Geriatric Use

In clinical trials 134 patients 65 years of age or older were treated with Xolair. Although there were no apparent age-related differences observed in these studies, the number of patients aged 65 and over is not sufficient to determine whether they respond differently from younger patients.

ADVERSE REACTIONS

The most serious adverse reactions occurring in clinical studies with Xolair are malignancies and anaphylaxis (see WARNINGS). The observed incidence of malignancy among Xolair-treated patients (0.5%) was numerically higher than among patients in control groups (0.2%). Anaphylactic reactions were rare but temporally associated with Xolair administration.

The adverse reactions most commonly observed among patients treated with Xolair included injection site reaction (45%), viral infections (23%), upper respiratory tract infection (20%), sinusitis (16%), headache (15%), and pharyngitis (11%). These events were observed at similar rates in Xolair-treated patients and control patients. These were also the most frequently reported adverse reactions resulting in clinical intervention (e.g., discontinuation of Xolair, or the need for concomitant medication to treat an adverse reaction).

Because clinical trials are conducted under widely varying conditions, adverse reaction rates observed in the clinical trials of one drug cannot be directly compared with rates in the clinical trials of another drug and may not reflect the rates observed in medical practice.

The data described above reflect Xolair exposure for 2076 adult and adolescent patients ages 12 and older, including 1687 patients exposed for six months and 555 exposed for one year or more, in either placebo-controlled or other controlled asthma studies. The mean age of patients receiving Xolair was 42 years, with 134 patients 65 years of age or older; 60% were women, and 85% Caucasian. Patients received Xolair 150 to 375 mg every 2 or 4 weeks or, for patients assigned to control groups, standard therapy with or without a placebo.

Table 4 shows adverse events that occurred ≥ 1% more frequently in patients receiving Xolair than in those receiving placebo in the placebo-controlled asthma studies. Adverse events were classified using preferred terms from the International Medical Nomenclature (IMN) dictionary. Injection site reactions were recorded separately from the reporting of other adverse events and are described following Table 4.

Table 4
Adverse Events ≥1% More Frequent in Xolair-Treated Patients

Adverse event	Xolair n=738 (%)	Placebo n=717 (%)
Body as a whole		
Pain	7	5
Fatigue	3	2
Musculoskeletal system		
Arthralgia	8	6
Fracture	2	1
Leg pain	4	2
Arm pain	2	1
Nervous system		
Dizziness	3	2
Skin and appendages		
Pruritus	2	1
Dermatitis	2	1
Special senses		
Earache	2	1

Age (among patients under age 65), race, and gender did not appear to affect the between group differences in the rates of adverse events.

Injection Site Reactions

Injection site reactions of any severity occurred at a rate of 45% in Xolair-treated patients compared with 43% in placebo-treated patients. The types of injection site reactions included: bruising, redness, warmth, burning, stinging, itching, hive formation, pain, indurations, mass, and inflammation.

Severe injection-site reactions occurred more frequently in Xolair-treated patients compared with patients in the placebo group (12% versus 9%).

The majority of injection site reactions occurred within 1 hour-post injection, lasted less than 8 days, and generally decreased in frequency at subsequent dosing visits.

Immunogenicity

Low titers of antibodies to Xolair were detected in approximately 1 / 1723 (<0.1%) of patients treated with Xolair. The data reflect the percentage of patients whose test results were considered positive for antibodies to Xolair in an ELISA assay and are highly dependent on the sensitivity and specificity of the assay. Additionally, the observed incidence of antibody positivity in the assay may be influenced by several factors including sample handling, timing of sample collection, concomitant medications, and underlying disease. Therefore, comparison of the incidence of antibodies to Xolair with the incidence of antibodies to other products may be misleading.

Table 7
Number of Vials, Number of Injections and Total Injection Volumes for Asthma

Dose (mg)	Number of Vials: 75 mg[a]	150 mg[b]	Number of Injections	Total Volume Injected (mL)
150	0	1	1	1.2
225	1	1	2	1.8
300	0	2	2	2.4
375	1	2	3	3.0

[a] 0.6 mL maximum delivered volume per vial.
[b] 1.2 mL maximum delivered volume per vial.

Allergic symptoms, including urticaria, dermatitis, and pruritus were observed in patients treated with Xolair. There were also 3 cases of anaphylaxis observed within 2 hours of Xolair administration in which there were no other identifiable allergic triggers (see WARNINGS: Anaphylaxis).

OVERDOSAGE

The maximum tolerated dose of Xolair has not been determined. Single intravenous doses of up to 4000 mg have been administered to patients without evidence of dose-limiting toxicities. The highest cumulative dose administered to patients was 44,000 mg over a 20-week period, which was not associated with toxicities.

DOSAGE AND ADMINISTRATION

Xolair (Omalizumab) 150 to 375 mg is administered SC every 2 or 4 weeks. Because the solution is slightly viscous, the injection may take 5-10 seconds to administer. Doses (mg) and dosing frequency are determined by serum total IgE level (IU/mL), measured before the start of treatment, and body weight (kg). See the dose determination charts below (Table 5 and Table 6) for appropriate dose assignment. Doses of more than 150 mg are divided among more than one injection site to limit injections to not more than 150 mg per site.

Table 5
ADMINISTRATION EVERY 4 WEEKS
Xolair Doses (milligrams) Administered by Subcutaneous Injection Every 4 Weeks for Adults and Adolescents (12 Years of Age and Older) with Asthma

Pre-treatment Serum IgE (IU/mL)	Body Weight (kg): 30–60	> 60–70	> 70–90	> 90–150
≥ 30–100	150	150	150	300
> 100–200	300	300	300	
> 200–300	300			
> 300–400	SEE TABLE 6			
> 400–500				
> 500–600				

Table 6
ADMINISTRATION EVERY 2 WEEKS
Xolair Doses (milligrams) Administered by Subcutaneous Injection Every 2 Weeks for Adults and Adolescents (12 Years of Age and Older) with Asthma

Pre-treatment Serum IgE (IU/mL)	Body Weight (kg): 30–60	> 60–70	> 70–90	> 90–150
≥ 30–100	SEE TABLE 5			
> 100–200				225
> 200–300		225	225	300
> 300–400	225	225	300	
> 400–500	300	300	375	
> 500–600	300	375	DO NOT DOSE	
> 600–700	375			

Dosing Adjustments

Total IgE levels are elevated during treatment and remain elevated for up to one year after the discontinuation of treatment. Therefore, re-testing of IgE levels during Xolair treatment cannot be used as a guide for dose determination. Dose determination after treatment interruptions lasting less than 1 year should be based on serum IgE levels obtained at the initial dose determination. Total serum IgE levels may be re-tested for dose determination if treatment with Xolair has been interrupted for one year or more.

Doses should be adjusted for significant changes in body weight. (See Table 5 and Table 6.)

Preparation for Administration

Xolair for SC administration should be prepared using SWFI, USP, ONLY.

Xolair is for single use only and contains no preservatives. The solution should be used for SC administration within 8 hours following reconstitution when stored in the vial at 2–8°C (36–46°F), or within 4 hours of reconstitution when stored at room temperature.

The lyophilized product takes 15–20 minutes to dissolve. The fully reconstituted product will appear clear or slightly opalescent and may have a few small bubbles or foam around the edge of the vial. The reconstituted product is somewhat viscous; in order to obtain the full 0.6 mL (75 mg) or 1.2 mL (150 mg) dose, ALL OF THE PRODUCT MUST BE WITHDRAWN from the vial before expelling any air or excess solution from the syringe.

- **For Xolair 75 mg vial:**

STEP 1: Draw 0.9 mL of SWFI, USP into a 3-cc syringe equipped with a 1-inch, 18-gauge needle.

STEP 2: Place the vial upright on a flat surface and using standard aseptic technique, insert the needle and inject the SWFI, USP directly onto the product.

STEP 3: Keeping the vial upright, gently swirl the upright vial for approximately 1 minute to evenly wet the powder. Do not shake.

STEP 4: After completing STEP 3, gently swirl the vial for 5–10 seconds approximately every 5 minutes in order to dissolve any remaining solids. There should be no visible gel-like particles in the solution. Do not use if foreign particles are present.

Note: Some vials may take longer than 20 minutes to dissolve completely. If this is the case, repeat STEP 4 until there are no visible gel-like particles in the solution. It is acceptable to have small bubbles or foam around the edge of the vial. Do not use if the contents of the vial do not dissolve completely by 40 minutes.

STEP 5: Invert the vial for 15 seconds in order to allow the solution to drain toward the stopper. Using a new 3-cc syringe equipped with a 1-inch, 18-gauge needle, insert the needle into the inverted vial. Position the needle tip at the very bottom of the solution in the vial stopper when drawing the solution into the syringe. Before removing the needle from the vial, pull the plunger all the way back to the end of the syringe barrel in order to remove all of the solution from the inverted vial.

STEP 6: Replace the 18-gauge needle with a 25-gauge needle for subcutaneous injection.

STEP 7: Expel air, large bubbles, and any excess solution in order to obtain the required 0.6 mL dose. A thin layer of small bubbles may remain at the top of the solution in the syringe. Because the solution is slightly viscous, the injection may take 5–10 seconds to administer.

- **For Xolair 150 mg vial:**

STEP 1: Draw 1.4 mL of SWFI, USP into a 3-cc syringe equipped with a 1-inch, 18-gauge needle.

STEP 2: Place the vial upright on a flat surface and using standard aseptic technique, insert the needle and inject the SWFI, USP directly onto the product.

STEP 3: Keeping the vial upright, gently swirl the upright vial for approximately 1 minute to evenly wet the powder. Do not shake.

STEP 4: After completing STEP 3, gently swirl the vial for 5–10 seconds approximately every 5 minutes in order to dissolve any remaining solids. There should be no visible gel-like particles in the solution. Do not use if foreign particles are present.

Note: Some vials may take longer than 20 minutes to dissolve completely. If this is the case, repeat STEP 4 until there are no visible gel-like particles in the solution. It is acceptable to have small bubbles or foam around the edge of the vial. Do not use if the contents of the vial do not dissolve completely by 40 minutes.

STEP 5: Invert the vial for 15 seconds in order to allow the solution to drain toward the stopper. Using a new 3-cc syringe equipped with a 1-inch, 18-gauge needle, insert the needle into the inverted vial. Position the needle tip at the very bottom of the solution in the vial stopper when drawing the solution into the syringe. Before removing the needle from the vial, pull the plunger all the way back to the end of the syringe barrel in order to remove all of the solution from the inverted vial.

STEP 6: Replace the 18-gauge needle with a 25-gauge needle for subcutaneous injection.

STEP 7: Expel air, large bubbles, and any excess solution in order to obtain the required 1.2 mL dose. A thin layer of small bubbles may remain at the top of the solution in the syringe. Because the solution is slightly viscous, the injection may take 5–10 seconds to administer.

A 75 mg vial delivers 0.6 mL (75 mg) of Xolair. A 150 mg vial delivers 1.2 mL (150 mg) of Xolair (see Table 7).

[See table 7 above]

Continued on next page

Xolair—Cont.

Stability and Storage
Xolair should be shipped at controlled ambient temperature (≤30°C [≤86°F]). Xolair should be stored under refrigerated conditions 2–8°C (36–46°F). Do not use beyond the expiration date stamped on carton.
Xolair is for single-use only and contains no preservatives. The solution may be used for SC administration within 8 hours following reconstitution when stored in the vial at 2–8°C (36–46°F), or within 4 hours of reconstitution when stored at room temperature.
Reconstituted Xolair vials should be protected from direct sunlight.

HOW SUPPLIED

Xolair (Omalizumab) is supplied as a lyophilized sterile powder in a single-use 5 cc vial.
The 75 mg vial configuration is designed to deliver 75 mg of Xolair upon reconstitution with 0.9 mL SWFI, USP. Each 75 mg carton contains one single-use vial of Xolair (Omalizumab) NDC 50242-042-01.
The 150 mg vial configuration is designed to deliver 150 mg of Xolair upon reconstitution with 1.4 mL SWFI, USP. Each 150 mg carton contains one single-use vial of Xolair (Omalizumab). NDC 50242-040-62.

XOLAIR®
Omalizumab
For Subcutaneous Use
Manufactured by:
Genentech, Inc.
1 DNA Way
South San Francisco, CA 94080-4990 (4821002)
FDA Approval Date: February 2004
Code Revision Date: September 2004
Jointly marketed by: ©2004 Genentech, Inc.
Genentech, Inc.
1 DNA Way
South San Francisco, CA 94080-4990
Novartis Pharmaceuticals Corporation
One Health Plaza
East Hanover, NJ 07936-1080
Shown in Product Identification Guide, page 313

Genzyme Corporation
500 KENDALL STREET
CAMBRIDGE, MA 02142

Direct Inquiries to:
(800) 745-4447
(617) 768-9000

ALDURAZYME® ℞
[al-dər' ə-zīm]
(laronidase)
Solution for Intravenous Infusion Only

DESCRIPTION

ALDURAZYME® (laronidase) is a polymorphic variant of the human enzyme, α-L-iduronidase that is produced by recombinant DNA technology in a Chinese hamster ovary cell line. α-L-iduronidase (glycosaminoglycan α-L-iduronohydrolase, EC 3.2.1.76) is a lysosomal hydrolase that catalyses the hydrolysis of terminal α-L-iduronic acid residues of dermatan sulfate and heparan sulfate.
Laronidase is a glycoprotein with a molecular weight of approximately 83 kD. The predicted amino acid sequence of the recombinant form, as well as the nucleotide sequence that encodes it, are identical to a polymorphic form of human α-L-iduronidase. The recombinant protein is comprised of 628 amino acids after cleavage of the N-terminus and contains 6 N-linked oligosaccharide modification sites. Two oligosaccharide chains terminate in mannose-6-phosphate sugars. ALDURAZYME has a specific activity of approximately 172 U/mg.
ALDURAZYME, for intravenous infusion, is supplied as a sterile, nonpyrogenic, colorless to pale yellow, clear to slightly opalescent solution that must be diluted prior to administration in 0.9% Sodium Chloride Injection, USP containing 0.1% Albumin (Human). The solution in each vial contains a nominal laronidase concentration of 0.58 mg/mL and a pH of approximately 5.5. The extractable volume of 5.0 mL from each vial provides 2.9 mg laronidase, 43.9 mg sodium chloride, 63.5 mg sodium phosphate monobasic monohydrate, 10.7 mg sodium phosphate dibasic heptahydrate, and 0.05 mg polysorbate 80. ALDURAZYME does not contain preservatives; vials are for single use only.

CLINICAL PHARMACOLOGY

Mechanism of Action
Mucopolysaccharide storage disorders are caused by the deficiency of specific lysosomal enzymes required for the catabolism of glycosaminoglycans (GAG). Mucopolysaccharidosis I (MPS I) is characterized by the deficiency of α-L-iduronidase, a lysosomal hydrolase which catalyses the hydrolysis of terminal α-L-iduronic acid residues of dermatan sulfate and heparan sulfate. Reduced or absent α-L-iduronidase activity results in the accumulation of the GAG substrates, dermatan sulfate and heparan sulfate, throughout the body and leads to widespread cellular, tissue, and organ dysfunction.
The rationale of ALDURAZYME therapy in MPS I is to provide exogenous enzyme for uptake into lysosomes and increase the catabolism of GAG. ALDURAZYME uptake by cells into lysosomes is most likely mediated by the mannose-6-phosphate-terminated oligosaccharide chains of laronidase binding to specific mannose-6-phosphate receptors.
Because many proteins in the blood are restricted from entry into the central nervous system by the blood brain barrier, effects of intravenously administered ALDURAZYME on cells within the central nervous system (CNS) cannot be inferred from activity in sites outside the CNS. The ability of ALDURAZYME to cross the blood brain barrier has not been evaluated in animal models or in clinical trials.

Pharmacokinetics
The pharmacokinetics of laronidase were evaluated in 12 patients with MPS I who received 0.58 mg/kg of ALDURAZYME as a 4 hour infusion. After the 1st, 12th and 26th weekly infusions, the mean maximum plasma concentrations (C_{max}) ranged from 1.2 to 1.7 mcg/mL for the 3 time points. The mean area under the plasma concentration-time curve (AUC_∞) ranged from 4.5 to 6.9 mcg•hour/mL. The mean volume of distribution (V_z) ranged from 0.24 to 0.6 L/kg. Mean plasma clearance (CL) ranged from 1.7 to 2.7 mL/min/kg, and the mean elimination half-life ($t_{1/2}$) ranged from 1.5 to 3.6 hours.

Effects of Antibodies
Most patients who received once-weekly infusions of ALDURAZYME developed antibodies to laronidase by week 12. Between weeks 1 and 12, increases in plasma clearance of laronidase were observed in some patients which appeared to be proportional to the antibody titer. At week 26, plasma clearance of laronidase was comparable to that at week 1, in spite of the continued and, in some cases, increased titers of antibodies.

CLINICAL STUDIES

ALDURAZYME was studied in a randomized, placebo-controlled clinical trial of 45 MPS I patients of whom 1 patient was clinically assessed as having the Hurler form, 37 Hurler-Scheie, and 7 Scheie. All patients had a baseline forced vital capacity (FVC) less than or equal to 77% of predicted. Patients received ALDURAZYME at 0.58 mg/kg or placebo once-weekly for 26 weeks. All patients were treated with antipyretics and antihistamines prior to each infusion. The primary efficacy outcome assessments were FVC and distance walked in 6 minutes (6-minute walk test, 6MWT). After 26 weeks, patients treated with ALDURAZYME showed improvement in FVC and in 6MWT compared to placebo-treated patients (see **Table 1**).
[See table 1 above]

Table 1: Primary Efficacy Outcomes

		ALDURAZYME N = 22	Placebo N = 23
Forced Vital Capacity (percent of predicted normal)			
Baseline	Mean ± s.d.	48 ± 15	54 ± 16
Week 26	Mean ± s.d.	50 ± 17	51 ± 13
Change from baseline to week 26	Mean ± s.d.	1 ± 7	-3 ± 7
	Median	1	-1
Difference between groups	Mean	4	
	Median (95% CI)	2 (0.4, 7) p=0.02*	
6-Minute Walk Distance (meters)			
Baseline	Mean ± s.d.	319 ± 131	367 ± 114
Week 26	Mean ± s.d.	339 ± 127	348 ± 129
Change from baseline to week 26	Mean ± s.d.	20 ± 69	-18 ± 67
	Median	28	-11
Difference between groups	Mean	38	
	Median (95% CI)	39 (-2, 79) p=0.07*	

* By Wilcoxon Rank Sum Test

Evaluations of bioactivity were changes in liver size and urinary GAG levels. Liver size and urinary GAG levels decreased in patients treated with ALDURAZYME compared to patients treated with placebo. No subject in the group receiving ALDURAZYME reached the normal range for urinary GAG levels during this 6-month study.
All 45 patients received open-label ALDURAZYME for 36 weeks following the double-blind period. Maintenance of mean FVC and an additional increase in mean 6MWT distance were observed compared to the start of the open-label period among patients who were initially randomized to and then continued to receive ALDURAZYME. Among patients who had been initially randomized to placebo, improvements from baseline in mean FVC and 6MWT distance were observed compared to the start of the open-label period.

INDICATIONS AND USAGE

ALDURAZYME is indicated for patients with Hurler and Hurler-Scheie forms of Mucopolysaccharidosis I (MPS I) and for patients with the Scheie form who have moderate to severe symptoms. The risks and benefits of treating mildly affected patients with the Scheie form have not been established.
ALDURAZYME has been shown to improve pulmonary function and walking capacity. ALDURAZYME has not been evaluated for effects on the central nervous system manifestations of the disorder.

CONTRAINDICATIONS

There are no known contraindications to the use of ALDURAZYME.

WARNINGS

Hypersensitivity Reactions
Patients treated with ALDURAZYME may develop infusion-related hypersensitivity reactions (see **ADVERSE REACTIONS**). In the clinical studies, one patient developed an anaphylactic reaction approximately three hours after the initiation of the infusion. The reaction consisted of urticaria and airway obstruction. Resuscitation required an emergency tracheostomy. This patient's pre-existing MPS I related upper airway obstruction may have contributed to the severity of this reaction (see **ADVERSE REACTIONS**: **Infusion-Related Reactions** and **Immunogenicity**).
Some infusion-related reactions may be ameliorated by slowing the rate of infusion or treatment with additional antipyretics and/or antihistamines. If severe hypersensitivity or anaphylactic reactions occur, immediately discontinue the infusion of ALDURAZYME and initiate appropriate treatment. Caution should be exercised if epinephrine is being considered for use in patients with MPS I due to the increased prevalence of coronary artery disease in these patients.
The risks and benefits of re-administering ALDURAZYME following a severe hypersensitivity or anaphylactic reaction should be considered. Extreme care should be exercised, with appropriate resuscitation measures available, if the decision is made to re-administer the product.

PRECAUTIONS

General
Patients should receive antipyretics and/or antihistamines prior to infusion (see **WARNINGS** and **ADVERSE REACTIONS**). If an infusion reaction occurs, regardless of pre-treatment, decreasing the infusion rate, temporarily stopping the infusion, and/or administration of additional antipyretics and/or antihistamines may ameliorate the symptoms.

Information for Patients
Patients should be informed that a registry for MPS I patients has been established in order to better understand the variability and progression of MPS I disease, and to continue to monitor and evaluate treatments. Patients should be encouraged to participate and advised that their participation may involve long-term follow-up. Information regarding the registry program may be found at www.MPSIregistry.com or by calling (800) 745-4447.

Drug Interactions
No formal drug interaction studies have been conducted.

Carcinogenesis, Mutagenesis, Impairment of Fertility
Studies to assess the mutagenic and carcinogenic potential of ALDURAZYME have not been conducted.
Reproductive studies in rats have not demonstrated impairment of fertility (see **PRECAUTIONS**: **Pregnancy**).

Pregnancy: Category B
Reproduction studies have been performed in male and female rats at doses up to 6.2 times the human dose and have

revealed no evidence of impaired fertility or harm to the fetus due to ALDURAZYME. However, there are no adequate and well-controlled studies in pregnant women. Because animal reproduction studies are not always predictive of human response, ALDURAZYME should be used during pregnancy only if clearly needed.

Nursing Mothers

It is not known whether the drug is excreted in human milk. Because many drugs are excreted in human milk, caution should be exercised when ALDURAZYME is administered to a nursing woman (See **PRECAUTIONS: Information for Patients** regarding a registry program. Nursing women are encouraged to participate in this program.).

Pediatric Use

Patients younger than 5 were not included in the clinical studies because of inability to comply with efficacy outcome assessments. It is not known if children younger than 5 respond differently from older children.

Geriatric Use

Clinical studies of ALDURAZYME did not include patients aged 65 and over. It is not known whether they respond differently from younger patients.

ADVERSE REACTIONS

The most serious adverse reaction reported with ALDURAZYME was an anaphylactic reaction consisting of urticaria and airway obstruction, which occurred in one patient. Pre-existing upper airway obstruction may have contributed to the severity of the reaction (see **WARNINGS: Hypersensitivity Reactions**).

The most common adverse reactions associated with ALDURAZYME treatment in the clinical studies were upper respiratory tract infection, rash, and injection site reaction.

The most common adverse reactions requiring intervention were infusion-related reactions, particularly flushing. Most infusion-related reactions requiring intervention were ameliorated with slowing of the infusion rate, temporarily stopping the infusion, and/or administering additional antipyretics and/or antihistamines.

The data described below reflect exposure to 0.58 mg/kg of ALDURAZYME for 26 weeks in a placebo-controlled double-blind study in 45 patients with MPS I (N=22 ALDURAZYME, and N=23 placebo). All 45 patients continued into an open-label study of ALDURAZYME treatment for an additional 36 weeks. An additional 10 patients participated in a Phase 1 open-label study with continued infusions for up to 3 years. The population in the placebo-controlled study was evenly distributed for gender (N=23 females and 22 males) and ranged in ages from 6 to 43 years. Of the 45 patients in the placebo-controlled study, 1 was clinically assessed as having Hurler form, 37 Hurler-Scheie, and 7 Scheie. All patients were treated with antipyretics and antihistamines prior to the infusions.

Because clinical trials are conducted under widely varying and controlled conditions, the observed adverse reaction rates may not predict the rates observed in patients in clinical practice.

Table 2 enumerates adverse events and selected laboratory abnormalities that occurred during the placebo-controlled trial in at least 2 patients more in the ALDURAZYME group than was observed in the placebo group. Reported adverse events have been classified using standard WHOART terms. Observed adverse events in the Phase 1 study and the open-label treatment period following the controlled study were not different in nature or severity.

[See table 2 above]

Table 2: Number and (%) of Patients with Adverse Events and Selected Laboratory Abnormalities in the Placebo-Controlled Study

Adverse Event	Placebo (N = 23)	ALDURAZYME (N = 22)
Respiratory System		
Upper respiratory tract infection	4 (17)	7 (32)
Body as a Whole		
Chest pain	0	2 (9)
Nervous System		
Hyperreflexia	0	3 (14)
Paresthesia	1 (4)	3 (14)
Skin and Appendages		
Rash	5 (22)	8 (36)
Resistance Mechanism		
Abscess	0	2 (9)
Liver and Biliary System		
Bilirubinemia	0	2 (9)
Vascular		
Vein disorder	1 (4)	3 (14)
Urinary System		
Facial edema	0	2 (9)
Cardiovascular, General		
Hypotension	0	2 (9)
Dependent edema	0	2 (9)
Vision		
Corneal opacity	0	2 (9)
Application Site		
Injection site pain	0	2 (9)
Injection site reaction	2 (9)	4 (18)
Platelet, Bleeding and Clotting		
Thrombocytopenia	0	2 (9)

Total Volume of ALDURAZYME Infusion = 100 mL	
2 mL/hr × 15 minutes (10 mcg/kg/hr)	Obtain vital signs, if stable then increase the rate to...
4 mL/hr × 15 minutes (20 mcg/kg/hr)	Obtain vital signs, if stable then increase the rate to...
8 mL/hr × 15 minutes (50 mcg/kg/hr)	Obtain vital signs, if stable then increase the rate to...
16 mL/hr × 15 minutes (100 mcg/kg/hr)	Obtain vital signs, if stable then increase the rate to...
32 mL/hr × ~3 hours (200 mcg/kg/hr)	For the remainder of the infusion.

Total Volume of ALDURAZYME Infusion = 250 mL	
5 mL/hr × 15 minutes (10 mcg/kg/hr)	Obtain vital signs, if stable then increase the rate to...
10 mL/hr × 15 minutes (20 mcg/kg/hr)	Obtain vital signs, if stable then increase the rate to...
20 mL/hr × 15 minutes (50 mcg/kg/hr)	Obtain vital signs, if stable then increase the rate to...
40 mL/hr × 15 minutes (100 mcg/kg/hr)	Obtain vital signs, if stable then increase the rate to...
80 mL/hr × ~3 hours (200 mcg/kg/hr)	For the remainder of the infusion.

Infusion-Related Reactions

Infusion-related reactions were reported in 7 of 22 patients treated with ALDURAZYME. Infusion-related reactions were not significantly different between the ALDURAZYME treatment group and the placebo group who received infusions of diluent and all components of ALDURAZYME except the laronidase enzyme. The most common infusion-related reactions included flushing, fever, headache and rash. Flushing occurred in 5 patients (23%) receiving ALDURAZYME; the other reactions were less frequent. All reactions were mild to moderate in severity. The frequency of infusion-related reactions decreased with continued use during the open-label extended use period. There was one case of anaphylaxis during the open-label extension period (see **WARNINGS** and **ADVERSE REACTIONS: Immunogenicity**). Less common infusion-related reactions include cough, bronchospasm, dyspnea, urticaria, angioedema and pruritus.

Immunogenicity

Fifty of 55 patients (91%) treated with ALDURAZYME were positive for antibodies to laronidase. The clinical significance of antibodies to ALDURAZYME is not known, including the potential for product neutralization.

The data reflect the percentage of patients whose test results were considered positive for antibodies to ALDURAZYME using an enzyme-linked immunosorbent assay (ELISA) for laronidase-specific IgG binding antibodies, and are highly dependent on the sensitivity and specificity of the assay. Additionally, the observed incidence of antibodies in an assay may be influenced by several factors including sample handling, timing of sample collection, concomitant medications, and underlying disease. For these reasons, comparison of the incidence of antibodies to ALDURAZYME with the incidence of antibodies to other products may be misleading.

Four patients in the controlled study who experienced severe infusion-related reactions were tested for ALDURAZYME specific IgE antibodies and complement activation. IgE testing was performed by ELISA and complement activation was measured by the Quidel Enzyme Immunoassay. One of the four patients had an anaphylactic reaction consisting of urticaria and airway obstruction and tested positive for both ALDURAZYME specific IgE binding antibodies and complement activation (see **WARNINGS: Hypersensitivity Reactions**).

Other hypersensitivity reactions were also seen in patients receiving ALDURAZYME (see **ADVERSE REACTIONS: Infusion-Related Reactions**).

OVERDOSAGE

There is no experience with overdoses of ALDURAZYME.

DOSAGE AND ADMINISTRATION

The recommended dosage regimen of ALDURAZYME is 0.58 mg/kg of body weight administered once-weekly as an intravenous infusion.

Pretreatment with antipyretics and/or antihistamines is recommended 60 minutes prior to the start of the infusion (see **PRECAUTIONS: General**).

The total volume of the infusion is determined by the patient's body weight and should be delivered over approximately 3 to 4 hours. Patients with a body weight of 20 kg or less should receive a total volume of 100 mL. Patients with a body weight of greater than 20 kg should receive a total volume of 250 mL. The initial infusion rate of 10 mcg/kg/hr may be incrementally increased every 15 minutes during the first hour, as tolerated, until a maximum infusion rate of 200 mcg/kg/hr is reached. The maximum rate is then maintained for the remainder of the infusion (2-3 hours).

For Patients Weighing 20 kg or Less

[See second table above]

For Patients Weighing Greater than 20 kg

[See third table above]

Each vial of ALDURAZYME provides 2.9 mg of laronidase in 5.0 mL of solution and is intended for single use only. Do not use the vial more than one time. The concentrated solution for infusion must be diluted with 0.1% Albumin (Human) in 0.9% Sodium Chloride Injection, USP using aseptic techniques. ALDURAZYME should be prepared using PVC Containers and administered with a PVC infusion set equipped with an in-line, low protein binding 0.2 micrometer (μm) filter. There is no information on the compatibility of diluted ALDURAZYME with glass containers.

Instructions for Use (Aseptic Techniques)

1. Determine the number of vials to be diluted based on the individual patient's weight and the recommended dose of 0.58 mg/kg [Patient's weight (kg) × 1 mL/kg of ALDURAZYME = Total # mL of ALDURAZYME, then Total # of mL of ALDURAZYME ÷ 5 mL per Vial = Total # of Vials]. Round up to the nearest whole vial. Remove the required number of vials from the refrigerator to allow them to reach room temperature. Do not heat or microwave vials.
2. Before withdrawing the ALDURAZYME from the vial, visually inspect each vial for particulate matter and discoloration. The ALDURAZYME solution should be clear to slightly opalescent and colorless to pale yellow. A few translucent particles may be present. Do not use if the solution is discolored or if there is particulate matter in the solution.
3. Determine the total volume of the infusion to be used based on the patient's body weight. The total final volume should be either 100 mL (if weight is less than or equal to 20 kg) or 250 mL (if weight is greater than 20 kg).
4. Using the chart below, prepare an infusion bag of 0.1% Albumin (Human) in 0.9% Sodium Chloride Injection, USP. Remove and discard a volume of 0.9% Sodium Chloride Injection, USP equal to the volume of Albumin (Human) to be added to the infusion bag. Add the appropriate volume of Albumin (Human) to the infusion bag and gently rotate the infusion bag to ensure proper distribution of the Albumin.

Continued on next page

Aldurazyme—Cont.

Total Volume of ALDURAZYME Infusion	Volume of Albumin (Human) 5% to be Added	Volume of Albumin (Human) 25% to be Added
100 mL	2 mL	0.4 mL
250 mL	5 mL	1 mL

5. Withdraw and discard a volume of the 0.1% Albumin (Human) in 0.9% Sodium Chloride Injection, USP from the infusion bag, equal to the volume of ALDURAZYME concentrate to be added.
6. Slowly withdraw the calculated volume of ALDURAZYME from the appropriate number of vials using caution to avoid excessive agitation. Do not use a filter needle, as this may cause agitation. Agitation may denature ALDURAZYME, rendering it biologically inactive.
7. Slowly add the ALDURAZYME solution to the 0.1% Albumin (Human) in 0.9% Sodium Chloride Injection, USP using care to avoid agitation of the solutions. Do not use a filter needle.
8. Gently rotate the infusion bag to ensure proper distribution of ALDURAZYME. Do not shake the solution.

ALDURAZYME does not contain any preservatives, therefore after dilution with saline in the infusion bags, any unused product or waste material should be discarded and disposed of in accordance with local requirements.
ALDURAZYME must not be mixed with other medicinal products in the same infusion.
The compatibility of ALDURAZYME in solution with other products has not been evaluated.

STORAGE
Store ALDURAZYME under refrigeration at 2°C to 8°C (36°F to 46°F). DO NOT FREEZE OR SHAKE. DO NOT USE ALDURAZYME after the expiration date on the vial. This product contains no preservatives.
The diluted solution should be used immediately. If immediate use is not possible, the diluted solution should be stored refrigerated at 2°C to 8°C (36°F to 46°F). The in-use storage should not be longer than 36 hours from the time of preparation to completion of administration. Room temperature storage of diluted solution is not recommended.

HOW SUPPLIED
ALDURAZYME is supplied as a sterile solution in clear Type I glass 5 mL vials (2.9 mg laronidase per 5 mL). The closure consists of a siliconized butyl stopper and an aluminum seal with a plastic flip-off cap.
NDC 58468-0070-1
℞ Only
ALDURAZYME is manufactured by:
BioMarin Pharmaceutical Inc.
371 Bel Marin Keys Blvd.
Suite 210
Novato, CA 94949
US License Number 1649
ALDURAZYME is distributed by:
Genzyme Corporation
One Kendall Square
Cambridge, MA 02139
1-800-745-4447 (phone)
ALDURAZYME is a registered trademark of BioMarin/Genzyme LLC.
5649 (4/03)

CEREZYME® ℞
[se're-zīm]
(imiglucerase for injection)
200 UNITS
400 UNITS

DESCRIPTION
Cerezyme® (imiglucerase for injection) is an analogue of the human enzyme β-glucocerebrosidase, produced by recombinant DNA technology. β-Glucocerebrosidase (β-D-glucosyl-N-acylsphingosine glucohydrolase, E.C. 3.2.1.45) is a lysosomal glycoprotein enzyme which catalyzes the hydrolysis of the glycolipid glucocerebroside to glucose and ceramide.
Cerezyme® is produced by recombinant DNA technology using mammalian cell culture (Chinese hamster ovary). Purified imiglucerase is a monomeric glycoprotein of 497 amino acids, containing 4 N-linked glycosylation sites (Mr = 60,430). Imiglucerase differs from placental glucocerebrosidase by one amino acid at position 495, where histidine is substituted for arginine. The oligosaccharide chains at the glycosylation sites have been modified to terminate in mannose sugars. The modified carbohydrate structures on imiglucerase are somewhat different from those on placental glucocerebrosidase. These mannose-terminated oligosaccharide chains of imiglucerase are specifically recognized by endocytic carbohydrate receptors on macrophages, the cells that accumulate lipid in Gaucher disease.
Cerezyme® is supplied as a sterile, non-pyrogenic, white to off-white lyophilized product. The quantitative composition of the lyophilized drug is provided in the following table:
[See table below]

Ingredient	200 Unit Vial	400 Unit Vial
Imiglucerase (total amount)*	212 units	424 units
Mannitol	170 mg	340 mg
Sodium Citrates (Trisodium Citrate) (Disodium Hydrogen Citrate)	70 mg (52 mg) (18 mg)	140 mg (104 mg) (36 mg)
Polysorbate 80, NF	0.53 mg	1.06 mg

Citric Acid and/or Sodium Hydroxide may have been added at the time of manufacture to adjust pH.

*This provides a respective withdrawal dose of 200 and 400 units of imiglucerase.

An enzyme unit (U) is defined as the amount of enzyme that catalyzes the hydrolysis of 1 micromole of the synthetic substrate para-nitrophenyl-β-D-glucopyranoside (pNP-Glc) per minute at 37°C. The product is stored at 2-8°C (36–46°F). After reconstitution with Sterile Water for Injection, USP, the imiglucerase concentration is 40 U/mL (see **DOSAGE AND ADMINISTRATION** for final concentrations and volumes). Reconstituted solutions have a pH of approximately 6.1.
In addition, Haemaccel® (cross-linked gelatin polypeptides), which is used as a stabilizing agent during the manufacturing process, may also be present in very small amounts in the final product.

CLINICAL PHARMACOLOGY
Mechanism of Action/Pharmacodynamics
Gaucher disease is characterized by a deficiency of β-glucocerebrosidase activity, resulting in accumulation of glucocerebroside in tissue macrophages which become engorged and are typically found in the liver, spleen, and bone marrow and occasionally in lung, kidney, and intestine. Secondary hematologic sequelae include severe anemia and thrombocytopenia in addition to the characteristic progressive hepatosplenomegaly, skeletal complications, including osteonecrosis and osteopenia with secondary pathological fractures. **Cerezyme®** (imiglucerase for injection) catalyzes the hydrolysis of glucocerebroside to glucose and ceramide. In clinical trials, **Cerezyme®** improved anemia and thrombocytopenia, reduced spleen and liver size, and decreased cachexia to a degree similar to that observed with Ceredase® (alglucerase injection).
Pharmacokinetics
During one-hour intravenous infusions of four doses (7.5, 15, 30, 60 U/kg) of **Cerezyme®** (imiglucerase for injection), steady-state enzymatic activity was achieved by 30 minutes. Following infusion, plasma enzymatic activity declined rapidly with a half-life ranging from 3.6 to 10.4 minutes. Plasma clearance ranged from 9.8 to 20.3 mL/min/kg (mean ± S.D., 14.5 ± 4.0 mL/min/kg). The volume of distribution corrected for weight ranged from 0.09 to 0.15 L/kg (0.12 ± 0.02 L/kg). These variables do not appear to be influenced by dose or duration of infusion. However, only one or two patients were studied at each dose level and infusion rate. The pharmacokinetics of **Cerezyme®** do not appear to be different from placental-derived alglucerase (Ceredase®). In patients who developed IgG antibody to **Cerezyme®**, an apparent effect on serum enzyme levels resulted in diminished volume of distribution and clearance and increased elimination half-life compared to patients without antibody (see **WARNINGS**).

INDICATIONS AND USAGE
Cerezyme® (imiglucerase for injection) is indicated for long-term enzyme replacement therapy for pediatric and adult patients with a confirmed diagnosis of Type 1 Gaucher disease that results in one or more of the following conditions:
a. anemia
b. thrombocytopenia
c. bone disease
d. hepatomegaly or splenomegaly

CONTRAINDICATIONS
There are no known contraindications to the use of **Cerezyme®** (imiglucerase for injection). Treatment with **Cerezyme®** should be carefully re-evaluated if there is significant clinical evidence of hypersensitivity to the product.

WARNINGS
Approximately 15% of patients treated and tested to date have developed IgG antibody to **Cerezyme®** (imiglucerase for injection) during the first year of therapy. Patients who developed IgG antibody did so largely within 6 months of treatment and rarely developed antibodies to **Cerezyme®** after 12 months of therapy. Approximately 46% of patients with detectable IgG antibodies experienced symptoms of hypersensitivity.
Patients with antibody to **Cerezyme®** have a higher risk of hypersensitivity reaction. Conversely, not all patients with symptoms of hypersensitivity have detectable IgG antibody. It is suggested that patients be monitored periodically for IgG antibody formation during the first year of treatment. Treatment with **Cerezyme®** should be approached with caution in patients who have exhibited symptoms of hypersensitivity to the product.
Anaphylactoid reaction has been reported in less than 1% of the patient population. Further treatment with imiglucerase should be conducted with caution. Most patients have successfully continued therapy after a reduction in rate of infusion and pretreatment with antihistamines and/or corticosteroids.

PRECAUTIONS
General
In less than 1% of the patient population, pulmonary hypertension and pneumonia have also been observed during treatment with **Cerezyme®** (imiglucerase for injection). Pulmonary hypertension and pneumonia are known complications of Gaucher disease, and have been observed both in patients receiving and not receiving **Cerezyme®**. No causal relationship with **Cerezyme®** has been established. Patients with respiratory symptoms in the absence of fever should be evaluated for the presence of pulmonary hypertension.
Therapy with **Cerezyme®** should be directed by physicians knowledgeable in the management of patients with Gaucher disease.
Caution may be advisable in administration of **Cerezyme®** to patients previously treated with Ceredase® (alglucerase injection) and who have developed antibody to Ceredase® or who have exhibited symptoms of hypersensitivity to Ceredase®.
Carcinogenesis, Mutagenesis, Impairment of Fertility
Studies have not been conducted in either animals or humans to assess the potential effects of **Cerezyme®** (imiglucerase for injection) on carcinogenesis, mutagenesis, or impairment of fertility.
Teratogenic Effects: Pregnancy Category C
Animal reproduction studies have not been conducted with **Cerezyme®** (imiglucerase for injection). It is also not known whether **Cerezyme®** can cause fetal harm when administered to a pregnant woman or can affect reproductive capacity. **Cerezyme®** should not be administered during pregnancy except when the indication and need are clear and the potential benefit is judged by the physician to substantially justify the risk.
Nursing Mothers
It is not known whether this drug is excreted in human milk. Because many drugs are excreted in human milk, caution should be exercised when **Cerezyme®** (imiglucerase for injection) is administered to a nursing woman.
Pediatric Use
The safety and effectiveness of **Cerezyme®** (imiglucerase for injection) have been established in patients between 2 and 16 years of age. Use of **Cerezyme®** in this age group is supported by evidence from adequate and well-controlled studies of **Cerezyme®** and Ceredase® (alglucerase injection) in adults and pediatric patients, with additional data obtained from the medical literature and from long-term post-marketing experience. **Cerezyme®** has been administered to patients younger than 2 years of age, however the safety and effectiveness in patients younger than 2 have not been established.

ADVERSE REACTIONS
Since the approval of **Cerezyme®** (imiglucerase for injection) in May 1994, Genzyme has maintained a worldwide post-marketing database of spontaneously reported adverse events and adverse events discussed in the medical literature. The percentage of events for each reported adverse reaction term has been calculated using the number of patients from these sources as the denominator for total patient exposure to **Cerezyme®** since 1994. Actual patient exposure is difficult to obtain due to the voluntary nature of the database and the continuous accrual and loss of patients over that span of time. The actual number of patients exposed to **Cerezyme®** since 1994 is likely to be greater than estimated from these voluntary sources and, therefore, the percentages calculated for the frequencies of adverse reactions are most likely greater than the actual incidences.
Experience in patients treated with **Cerezyme®** has revealed that approximately 13.8% of patients experienced adverse events which were judged to be related to **Cerezyme®** administration and which occurred with an increase in frequency. Some of the adverse events were related to the route of administration. These include discomfort, pruritus, burning, swelling or sterile abscess at the site of venipuncture. Each of these events was found to occur in < 1% of the total patient population.
Symptoms suggestive of hypersensitivity have been noted in approximately 6.6% of patients. Onset of such symptoms has occurred during or shortly after infusions; these symptoms include pruritus, flushing, urticaria, angioedema,

	200 Unit Vial	400 Unit Vial
Sterile water for reconstitution	5.1 mL	10.2 mL
Final volume of reconstituted product	5.3 mL	10.6 mL
Concentration after reconstitution	40 U/mL	40 U/mL
Withdrawal volume	5.0 mL	10.0 mL
Units of enzyme within final volume	200 units	400 units

chest discomfort, dyspnea, coughing, cyanosis, and hypotension. Anaphylactoid reaction has also been reported (see **WARNINGS**). Each of these events was found to occur in < 1.5% of the total patient population. Pre-treatment with antihistamines and/or corticosteroids and reduced rate of infusion have allowed continued use of **Cerezyme®** in most patients.

Additional adverse reactions that have been reported in approximately 6.5% of patients treated with **Cerezyme®** include: nausea, abdominal pain, vomiting, diarrhea, rash, fatigue, headache, fever, dizziness, chills, backache, and tachycardia. Each of these events was found to occur in < 1.5% of the total patient population.

Incidence rates cannot be calculated from the spontaneously reported adverse events in the post-marketing database. From this database, the most commonly reported adverse events in children (defined as ages 2 – 12 years) included dyspnea, fever, nausea, flushing, vomiting, and coughing, whereas in adolescents (>12 – 16 years) and in adults (>16 years) the most commonly reported events included headache, pruritis, and rash.

In addition to the adverse reactions that have been observed in patients treated with **Cerezyme®**, transient peripheral edema has been reported for this therapeutic class of drug.

OVERDOSE

Experience with doses up to 240 U/kg every 2 weeks have been reported. At that dose there have been no reports of obvious toxicity.

DOSAGE AND ADMINISTRATION

Cerezyme® (imiglucerase for injection) is administered by intravenous infusion over 1–2 hours. Dosage should be individualized to each patient. Initial dosages range from 2.5 U/kg of body weight 3 times a week to 60 U/kg once every 2 weeks. 60 U/kg every 2 weeks is the dosage for which the most data are available. Disease severity may dictate that treatment be initiated at a relatively high dose or relatively frequent administration. Dosage adjustments should be made on an individual basis and may increase or decrease, based on achievement of therapeutic goals as assessed by routine comprehensive evaluations of the patient's clinical manifestations.

Cerezyme® should be stored at 2-8°C (36-46°F). After reconstitution, **Cerezyme®** should be inspected visually before use. Because this is a protein solution, slight flocculation (described as thin translucent fibers) occurs occasionally after dilution. The diluted solution may be filtered through an in-line low protein-binding 0.2 µm filter during administration. Any vials exhibiting opaque particles or discoloration should not be used. DO NOT USE **Cerezyme®** after the expiration date on the vial.

On the day of use, after the correct amount of **Cerezyme®** to be administered to the patient has been determined, the appropriate number of vials are each reconstituted with Sterile Water for Injection, USP. The final concentrations and administration volumes are provided in the following table:

[See table above]

A nominal 5.0 mL for the 200 unit vial (10.0 mL for the 400 unit vial) is withdrawn from each vial. The appropriate amount of **Cerezyme®** for each patient is diluted with 0.9% Sodium Chloride Injection, USP, to a final volume of 100 – 200 mL. **Cerezyme®** is administered by intravenous infusion over 1-2 hours. Aseptic techniques should be used when diluting the dose. Since **Cerezyme®** does not contain any preservative, after reconstitution, vials should be promptly diluted and not stored for subsequent use. **Cerezyme®**, after reconstitution, has been shown to be stable for up to 12 hours when stored at room temperature (25°C) and at 2–8°C. **Cerezyme®**, when diluted, has been shown to be stable for up to 24 hours when stored at 2-8°C.

Relatively low toxicity, combined with the extended time course of response, allows small dosage adjustments to be made occasionally to avoid discarding partially used bottles. Thus, the dosage administered in individual infusions may be slightly increased or decreased to utilize fully each vial as long as the monthly administered dosage remains substantially unaltered.

HOW SUPPLIED

Cerezyme® (imiglucerase for injection) is supplied as a sterile, non-pyrogenic, lyophilized product. It is available as follows:

200 Units per Vial NDC 58468-1983-1
400 Units per Vial NDC 58468-4663-1
Store at 2-8°C (36-46°F).

℞ only

U.S. Patent Numbers: 5,236,838
5,549,892

Cerezyme® (imiglucerase for injection) is manufactured by:
Genzyme Corporation
One Kendall Square
Cambridge, MA 02139 USA

Certain manufacturing operations may have been performed by other firms.
4668 (3/03)

FABRAZYME® ℞

[*fab' rə-zīm*]
agalsidase beta
For intravenous infusion

DESCRIPTION

Fabrazyme® is a recombinant human α-galactosidase A enzyme with the same amino acid sequence as the native enzyme. Purified agalsidase beta is a homodimeric glycoprotein with a molecular weight of approximately 100 KD. The mature protein is comprised of two subunits of 398 amino acids (approximately 51 KD), each of which contains three N-linked glycosylation sites. α-galactosidase A catalyzes the hydrolysis of globotriaosylceramide (GL-3) and other α-galactyl-terminated neutral glycosphingolipids, such as galabiosylceramide and blood group B substances to ceramide dihexoside and galactose. The specific activity of Fabrazyme® is approximately 70 U/mg (one unit is defined as the amount of activity that results in the hydrolysis of 1 µmole of a synthetic substrate, p-nitrophenyl-α-D-galactopyranoside, per minute under the assay conditions).

Fabrazyme® is produced by recombinant DNA technology in a Chinese Hamster Ovary mammalian cell expression system.

Fabrazyme® is intended for intravenous infusion. It is supplied as a sterile, nonpyrogenic, white to off-white, lyophilized cake or powder for reconstitution with Sterile Water for Injection, USP. Each 35 mg vial contains 37 mg of agalsidase beta as well as 222 mg mannitol, 20.4 mg sodium phosphate monobasic monohydrate, and 59.2 mg sodium phosphate dibasic heptahydrate. Following reconstitution as directed, 35 mg of agalsidase beta (7 mL) may be extracted from each 35 mg vial.

Each 5 mg vial contains 5.5 mg of agalsidase beta as well as 33.0 mg mannitol, 3.0 mg sodium phosphate monobasic monohydrate, and 8.8 mg sodium phosphate dibasic heptahydrate. Following reconstitution as directed, 5 mg of agalsidase beta (1 mL) may be extracted from each 5 mg vial.

CLINICAL PHARMACOLOGY

Mechanism of Action

Fabry disease is an X-linked genetic disorder of glycosphingolipid metabolism. Deficiency of the lysosomal enzyme α-galactosidase A leads to progressive accumulation of glycosphingolipids, predominantly GL-3, in many body tissues, occurring over a period of years or decades. Clinical manifestations of Fabry disease include renal failure, cardiomyopathy, and cerebrovascular accidents. Accumulation of GL-3 in renal endothelial cells may play a role in renal failure.

Fabrazyme® is intended to provide an exogenous source of α-galactosidase A in Fabry disease patients. Preclinical and clinical studies evaluating a limited number of cell types indicate that Fabrazyme® will catalyze the hydrolysis of glycosphingolipids including GL-3.

Pharmacokinetics

Plasma profiles of Fabrazyme® were studied at 0.3, 1.0 and 3.0 mg/kg in 15 patients with Fabry disease. The area under the plasma concentration-time curve (AUC_∞) and the clearance did not increase proportionately with increasing doses, demonstrating that the enzyme follows non-linear pharmacokinetics. Terminal half-life was dose independent with a range of 45-102 minutes.

In 11 patients with Fabry disease given 1.0 mg/kg Fabrazyme® every 14 days for a total of 11 infusions, the pharmacokinetic responses following repeated dosing fell into three categories. In some patients, pharmacokinetic responses were maintained with repeated dosing, whereas in other patients, pharmacokinetic values decreased at infusion seven relative to baseline and returned to baseline values by infusion 11. In the remaining patients, AUC declined and failed to return to baseline by infusion 11. In these patients, the average AUC was 25% of its initial level. Some patients with elevated titers of antibody to agalsidase were among those with decreased AUC. The development of antibodies to agalsidase did not influence half-life, but reduced both apparent C_{max} and AUC. The long-term consequence of antibody development to the pharmacokinetics of agalsidase has not been established.

CLINICAL STUDIES

The safety and efficacy of Fabrazyme® were assessed in a randomized, double-blind, placebo-controlled, multinational, multicenter study of 58 Fabry patients (56 males and two females), ages 16 to 61 years, all naive to enzyme replacement therapy. Patients received either 1.0 mg/kg of Fabrazyme® or placebo every two weeks for five months (20 weeks) for a total of 11 infusions. All patients were pretreated with acetaminophen and an antihistamine to decrease or prevent infusion associated reactions. Oral steroids were an additional option to the pretreatment regimen for patients who exhibited severe or recurrent infusion reactions. The primary efficacy endpoint of GL-3 inclusions in renal interstitial capillary endothelial cells, was assessed by light microscopy and was graded on an inclusion severity score ranging from 0 (normal or near normal) to 3 (severe inclusions).

A GL-3 inclusion score of 0 was achieved in 20 of 29 (69%) patients treated with Fabrazyme® compared to 0 of 29 treated with placebo ($p<0.001$). Similar reductions in GL-3 inclusions were observed in the capillary endothelium of the heart and skin (Table 1). No differences between groups in symptoms or renal function were observed during this five month study.

[See table 1 at top of next page]

All 58 patients in the randomized study participated in an open-label extension study of Fabrazyme® at 1.0 mg/kg every two weeks indefinitely. At the end of six months of open-label treatment, most patients achieved a GL-3 inclusion score of 0 in capillary endothelium (Table 1). GL-3 was decreased to normal or near normal levels in mesangial cells, glomerular capillary endothelium, interstitial cells, and non-capillary endothelium. GL-3 deposition was still present in vascular smooth muscle cells, tubular epithelium and podocytes, at variably reduced levels. Plasma GL-3 levels were reduced to levels below the limit of detection and remained so up to 18 months of treatment.

The reduction of GL-3 inclusions suggests that Fabrazyme® may ameliorate disease expression; however, the relationship of GL-3 inclusion reduction to specific clinical manifestations of Fabry disease has not been established.

INDICATIONS AND USAGE

Fabrazyme® (agalsidase beta) is indicated for use in patients with Fabry disease. Fabrazyme® reduces globotriaosylceramide (GL-3) deposition in capillary endothelium of the kidney and certain other cell types (see **CLINICAL STUDIES**).

CONTRAINDICATIONS

No known contraindications.

WARNINGS

Infusion Reactions

Infusion reactions occurred in many patients treated with Fabrazyme® (see **ADVERSE REACTIONS**). Some of the reactions were severe. Infusion reactions included fever, rigors, chest tightness, hypertension, hypotension, pruritus, myalgia, dyspnea, urticaria, abdominal pain, and headache. All patients were pretreated with acetaminophen and an antihistamine. Infusion reactions occurred in some patients after receiving antipyretics, antihistamines, and oral steroids.

Patients should be given antipyretics prior to infusion. If an infusion reaction occurs, regardless of pretreatment, decreasing the infusion rate, temporarily stopping the infusion, and/or administration of additional antipyretics, antihistamines, and/or steroids may ameliorate the symptoms. Because of the potential for severe infusion reactions, appropriate medical support measures should be readily available when Fabrazyme® is administered.

PRECAUTIONS

General

Patients with advanced Fabry disease may have compromised cardiac function, which may predispose them to a higher risk of severe complications from infusion reactions (see **WARNINGS**). Patients with compromised cardiac function should be monitored closely if the decision is made to administer Fabrazyme®.

Most patients develop IgG antibodies to Fabrazyme® (see **ADVERSE REACTIONS: Immunogenicity**). Some patients developed IgE or skin test reactivity specific to Fabrazyme®. Physicians should consider testing for IgE (see **PRECAUTIONS: Laboratory Tests**) in patients who experienced suspected allergic reactions and consider the risks and benefits of continued treatment in patients with anti-Fabrazyme® IgE.

Information for Patients

Patients should be informed that a Registry has been established in order to better understand the variability and progression of Fabry disease in the population as a whole and in women (see **PRECAUTIONS: Responses in Women**), and to monitor and evaluate long-term treatment effects of Fabrazyme®. The Registry will also monitor the effect of Fabrazyme® on pregnant women and their offspring, and determine if Fabrazyme® is excreted in breast milk. Patients should be encouraged to participate and advised that their participation is voluntary and may involve long-term follow-up. For more information visit www.fabryregistry.com or call (800) 745-4447.

Laboratory Tests

There are no marketed tests for antibodies against Fabrazyme®. If testing is warranted, contact your local Genzyme representative or Genzyme Corporation at (800) 745-4447.

Drug Interactions

No drug interaction studies were performed.
No *in vitro* metabolism studies were performed.

Continued on next page

Fabrazyme—Cont.

Carcinogenesis, Mutagenesis, Impairment of Fertility

There are no animal or human studies to assess the carcinogenic or mutagenic potential of Fabrazyme®. There are no studies assessing the potential effect of Fabrazyme® on fertility in humans.

Pregnancy: Category B

Reproduction studies have been performed in rats at doses up to 30 times the human dose and have revealed no evidence of impaired fertility or negative effects on embryo fetal development due to Fabrazyme®. There are, however, no adequate and well-controlled studies in pregnant women. Because animal reproduction studies are not always predictive of human response, this drug should be used during pregnancy only if clearly needed.

Women of childbearing potential should be encouraged to enroll in the Fabry patient registry (see **PRECAUTIONS: Information for Patients**).

Nursing Mothers

It is not known whether Fabrazyme® is excreted in human milk. Because many drugs are excreted in human milk, caution should be exercised when Fabrazyme® is administered to a nursing woman.

Nursing mothers should be encouraged to enroll in the Fabry registry (see **PRECAUTIONS: Information for Patients**).

Responses in Women

Fabry disease is an X-linked genetic disorder. However, some heterozygous women will develop signs and symptoms of Fabry disease due to the variability of the X-chromosome inactivation within cells. Generally, the rates of progression of organ impairment are slower than in male Fabry disease patients and severity of signs and symptoms is variable.

Two women were enrolled in the clinical studies with Fabrazyme®. Therefore, no determination can be made whether symptomatic women respond to Fabrazyme® differently than men. There is also insufficient information to determine whether the relationship between cellular histologic evaluations of biopsies and clinical manifestations differ between women and men.

Pediatric Use

The safety and effectiveness of Fabrazyme® in pediatric patients have not been established.

Geriatric Use

Clinical studies of Fabrazyme® did not include sufficient numbers of subjects aged 65 and over to determine whether they respond differently from younger subjects.

ADVERSE REACTIONS

The most serious and most common adverse reactions reported with Fabrazyme® are infusion reactions. Serious and/or frequently occurring infusion reactions consisted of one or more of the following: tachycardia, hypertension, throat tightness, chest pain/tightness, dyspnea, fever, chills/rigors, abdominal pain, pruritus, urticaria, nausea, vomiting, lip or ear edema, and rash (see **WARNINGS: Infusion Reactions**). Infusion reactions declined in frequency with continued use of Fabrazyme®. However, serious infusion reactions may occur after extended durations of Fabrazyme® treatment.

Other reported serious adverse events included stroke, pain, ataxia, bradycardia, cardiac arrhythmia, cardiac arrest, decreased cardiac output, vertigo, hypoacousia, and nephrotic syndrome. These adverse events also occur as manifestations of Fabry disease; an alteration in frequency or severity cannot be determined from the small numbers of patients studied.

The data described below reflect exposure of 29 patients to 1.0 mg/kg Fabrazyme® every two weeks for 5 months in a placebo-controlled study. All 58 patients continued into an open-label extension study of Fabrazyme® treatment for up to 30 additional months. An additional 28 patients received open-label treatment. All patients were treated with antipyretics and antihistamines prior to the infusions.

Because clinical trials are conducted under widely varying and controlled conditions, the observed adverse reaction rates may not predict the rates observed in patients in clinical practice.

Table 2 enumerates adverse events and selected laboratory abnormalities that occurred during the placebo-controlled trial in at least 2 patients more in the Fabrazyme® group than was observed in the placebo group. Reported adverse events have been classified by organ system. Observed adverse events in the Phase 1/2 study and the open-label treatment period following the controlled study were not different in nature or severity.

Table 2
Incidence (%) of Adverse Events Occurring in the Placebo-Controlled Study

Adverse Event	Placebo (n = 29)	Fabrazyme® (n = 29)
Body as a Whole		
Chest pain	3 (10)	5 (17)
Fever	5 (17)	14 (48)
Pain	3 (10)	6 (21)
Pallor	1 (3)	4 (14)
Rigors	4 (14)	15 (52)
Temperature changed sensation	1 (3)	5 (17)
Cardiovascular		
Cardiomegaly	1 (3)	3 (10)
Hypertension	0	3 (10)
Hypotension	2 (7)	4 (14)
Edema dependent	1 (3)	6 (21)
Central and Peripheral Nervous System		
Dizziness	2 (7)	4 (14)
Headache	11 (38)	13 (45)
Paraesthesia	2 (7)	4 (14)
Gastro-Intestinal System		
Dyspepsia	1 (3)	3 (10)
Nausea	4 (14)	8 (28)
Musculo-Skeletal System		
Arthrosis	0	3 (10)
Skeletal pain	0	6 (21)
Psychiatric		
Anxiety	5 (17)	8 (28)
Depression	1 (3)	3 (10)
Reproductive, Male		
Testicular pain	0	2 (7)
Respiratory System		
Bronchitis	1 (3)	3 (10)
Bronchospasm	0	2 (7)
Laryngitis	0	2 (7)
Pharyngitis	2 (7)	8 (28)
Rhinitis	7 (24)	11 (38)
Sinusitis	0	2 (7)

Table 1
Reduction of GL-3 Inclusions to Normal or Near Normal Levels (0 Score) in the Capillary Endothelium of the Kidney, Heart, and Skin

	5 Months of the Controlled Study		6 Months of the Open-label Extension Study	
	Placebo (n=29)	Fabrazyme® (n=29)	Placebo/Fabrazyme® (n=29)*	Fabrazyme®/Fabrazyme® (n=29)*
Kidney	0/29	20/29	24/24	23/25
Heart	1/29	21/29	13/18	19/22
Skin	1/29	29/29	25/26	26/27

* Results reported where biopsies were available

Immunogenicity

Sixty-three of 71 (89%) patients in the clinical studies treated with Fabrazyme® have developed antibodies to Fabrazyme®. Most patients who develop antibodies do so within the first 3 months of exposure. Antibodies to Fabrazyme® were purified from 15 patients with high antibody titers (≥ 12,800) and studied for inhibition of *in vitro* enzyme activity. Under the conditions of this assay, most of these 15 patients had inhibition of *in vitro* enzyme activity ranging between 14–74% at one or more timepoints during the study. No general pattern was seen in individual patient reactivity over time. The clinical significance of binding and/or inhibitory antibodies to Fabrazyme® is not known. In patients followed in the open-label study, reduction of GL-3 in plasma and GL-3 inclusions in superficial skin capillaries was maintained after antibody formation.

The data reflect the percentage of patients whose test results were considered positive for antibodies to Fabrazyme® using an ELISA and radioimmunoprecipitation (RIP) assay for antibodies. These results are highly dependent on the sensitivity and specificity of the assay. Additionally, the observed incidence of antibodies in an assay may be influenced by several factors including sample handling, timing of sample collection, concomitant medications and underlying disease. For these reasons, comparison of the incidence of antibodies to Fabrazyme® with the incidence of antibodies to other products may be misleading.

OVERDOSAGE

There have been no reports of overdose with Fabrazyme®. In clinical trials, patients received doses up to 3.0 mg/kg body weight.

DOSAGE AND ADMINISTRATION

The recommended dosage of Fabrazyme® is 1.0 mg/kg body weight infused every 2 weeks as an IV infusion.

The initial IV infusion rate should be no more than 0.25 mg/min (15 mg/hr). The infusion rate may be slowed in the event of infusion-associated reactions. After patient tolerance to the infusion is well established, the infusion rate may be increased in increments of 0.05 to 0.08 mg/min (increments of 3 to 5 mg/hr) each subsequent infusion. Thirty-one of 58 (53%) patients have received infusions at rates ≥ 33 mg/hr.

Patients should receive antipyretics prior to infusion (see **WARNINGS**).

Instructions for Use

Fabrazyme® does not contain any preservatives. Vials are for single-use only. Any unused product should be discarded. Shaking or agitation of this product should be avoided. Do not use filter needles during the preparation of the infusion.

Reconstitution and Dilution (using Aseptic Technique)

1. Fabrazyme® vials and diluent should be allowed to reach room temperature prior to reconstitution (approximately 30 minutes). The number of 35 mg and 5 mg vials needed is based on the patient's body weight (kg) and the recommended dose of 1.0 mg/kg.
   Select a combination of 35 mg and 5 mg vials so that the total number of mgs is equal to or greater than the patient's number of kg of body weight.
2. Reconstitute each vial of 35 mg Fabrazyme® by slowly injecting 7.2 mL of Sterile Water for Injection, USP down the inside wall of each vial. Roll and tilt each vial gently. Each vial will yield a 5.0 mg/mL clear, colorless solution (total extractable amount per vial is 35 mg, 7.0 mL).
   Reconstitute each vial of 5 mg Fabrazyme® by slowly injecting 1.1 mL of Sterile Water for Injection, USP down the inside wall of each vial. Roll and tilt each vial gently. Each vial will yield a 5.0 mg/mL clear, colorless solution (total extractable amount per vial is 5 mg, 1.0 mL).
3. Visually inspect the reconstituted vials for particulate matter and discoloration. Do not use the reconstituted solution if there is particulate matter or if it is discolored.
4. The reconstituted solution should be further diluted with 0.9% Sodium Chloride Injection, USP to a final total volume of 500 mL. Prior to adding the volume of reconstituted Fabrazyme® required for the patient dose, remove an equal volume of 0.9% Sodium Chloride for Injection, USP from the 500 mL infusion bag.
   Patient dose (in mg) ÷ 5 mg/mL = Number of mL of reconstituted Fabrazyme® required for patient dose
   Example: Patient dose = 80 mg
   80 mg ÷ 5 mg/mL = 16 mL of Fabrazyme®

   Slowly withdraw the reconstituted solution from each vial up to the total volume required for the patient dose. Inject the reconstituted Fabrazyme® solution directly into the Sodium Chloride solution. Do not inject in the airspace within the infusion bag. Discard any vial with unused reconstituted solution.
5. Gently invert infusion bag to mix the solution, avoiding vigorous shaking and agitation.
6. Fabrazyme® should not be infused in the same intravenous line with other products.
7. The diluted solution may be filtered through an in-line low protein-binding 0.2 µm filter during administration.

Storage

Store Fabrazyme® under refrigeration between 2°–8°C (36°–46°F). DO NOT USE Fabrazyme® after the expiration date on the vial.

Reconstituted and diluted solutions of Fabrazyme® should be used immediately. This product contains no preservatives. If immediate use is not possible, the reconstituted and diluted solution may be stored for up to 24 hours at 2°–8°C (36°–46°F).

HOW SUPPLIED

Fabrazyme® is supplied as a sterile, nonpyrogenic, white to off-white lyophilized cake or powder. Fabrazyme® 35 mg vials are supplied in single-use, clear Type I glass 20 mL (cc) vials. The closure consists of a siliconized butyl stopper and an aluminum seal with a plastic purple flip-off cap.

Fabrazyme® 5 mg vials are supplied in single-use, clear Type I glass 5 mL (cc) vials. The closure consists of a siliconized butyl stopper and an aluminum seal with a plastic gray flip-off cap.

35 mg vial: NDC 58468-0040-1
5 mg vial: NDC 58468-0041-1

Rx Only

U.S. Patent Number: 5,356,804
Fabrazyme® is manufactured and distributed by:
Genzyme Corporation
500 Kendall Street
Cambridge, MA 02142 USA
1-800-745-4447 (phone)
U.S. License Number: 1596
Issued: October 10, 2003
5031 (3/04)

RENAGEL® TABLETS ℞

[*rĕ′na-jəl*]
(sevelamer hydrochloride)
400 and 800 mg
[*se vel′ a mer*]

DESCRIPTION

The active ingredient in Renagel* Tablets is sevelamer hydrochloride, a polymeric phosphate binder intended for oral administration. Sevelamer hydrochloride is poly(allylamine hydrochloride) crosslinked with epichlorohydrin in which forty percent of the amines are protonated. It is known chemically as poly(allylamine-co-N,N′-diallyl-1,3-diamino-2-hydroxypropane) hydrochloride. Sevelamer hydrochloride is hydrophilic, but insoluble in water. The structure is represented below:

Chemical Structure of Sevelamer Hydrochloride

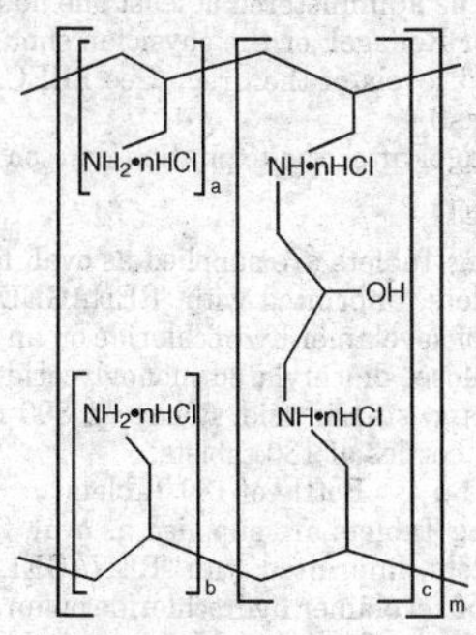

a, b = number of primary amine groups a + b = 9
c = number of crosslinking groups c = 1
n = fraction of protonated amines n = 0.4
m = large number to indicate extended polymer network

The primary amine groups shown in the structure are derived directly from poly(allylamine hydrochloride). The crosslinking groups consist of two secondary amine groups derived from poly(allylamine hydrochloride) and one molecule of epichlorohydrin.

Renagel® Tablets: Each film-coated tablet of Renagel contains either 800 mg or 400 mg of sevelamer hydrochloride on an anhydrous basis. The inactive ingredients are hypromellose, diacetylated monoglyceride, colloidal silicon dioxide, and stearic acid. The tablet imprint contains iron oxide black ink.

*Registered trademark of Genzyme Corporation.

CLINICAL PHARMACOLOGY

Patients with end-stage renal disease (ESRD) retain phosphorus and can develop hyperphosphatemia. High serum phosphorus can precipitate serum calcium resulting in ectopic calcification. When the product of serum calcium and phosphorus concentrations (Ca × P) exceeds 55 mg^2/dL^2, there is an increased risk that ectopic calcification will occur. Hyperphosphatemia plays a role in the development of secondary hyperparathyroidism in renal insufficiency. An increase in parathyroid hormone (PTH) levels is characteristic of patients with chronic renal failure. Increased levels of PTH can lead to osteitis fibrosa, a bone disease. A decrease in serum phosphorus may decrease serum PTH levels.

Treatment of hyperphosphatemia includes reduction in dietary intake of phosphate, inhibition of intestinal phosphate absorption with phosphate binders, and removal of phosphate with dialysis. Renagel taken with meals has been shown to decrease serum phosphorus concentrations in patients with ESRD who are on hemodialysis. *In vitro* studies have shown that the capsule and tablet formulations bind phosphate to a similar extent. Renagel does not contain aluminum or other metals and does not cause aluminum intoxication.

Renagel treatment also results in a lowering of low-density lipoprotein (LDL) and total serum cholesterol levels.

Pharmacokinetics: A mass balance study using ^{14}C-sevelamer hydrochloride in 16 healthy male and female volunteers showed that sevelamer hydrochloride is not systemically absorbed. No absorption studies have been performed in patients with renal disease.

Clinical trials: The ability of Renagel Capsules to lower serum phosphorus in ESRD patients on hemodialysis was demonstrated in six clinical trials: one double-blind placebo controlled 2-week study (renagel N=24); two open-label uncontrolled 8-week studies (renagel N=220) and three active-controlled open-label studies with treatment durations of 8 to 52 weeks (renagel N=256). Two of the active-controlled studies are described here. One trial is a crossover trial with two 8-week periods comparing Renagel to calcium acetate and the other trial is a 52-week parallel design trial comparing Renagel tablets with calcium acetate and calcium carbonate.

Cross-over study of Renagel Capsules and calcium acetate: Eighty-four ESRD patients on hemodialysis who were hyperphosphatemic (serum phosphorus > 6.0 mg/dL) following a two-week phosphate binder washout period were randomized to receive either Renagel Capsules for eight weeks followed by calcium acetate for eight weeks or calcium acetate for eight weeks followed by Renagel Capsules for eight weeks. Treatment periods were separated by a two-week phosphate binder washout period. Patients started on Renagel Capsules or calcium acetate tablets three times per day with meals. Over each eight-week treatment period, at three separate time points the dose of either agent could be titrated up 1 capsule or tablet per meal (3 per day) to control serum phosphorus. Renagel Capsules and calcium acetate both significantly decreased mean serum phosphorus by about 2 mg/dL (Table 1).

Table 1. Mean Serum Phosphorus (mg/dL) at Baseline and Endpoint

	Renagel (N=81)	Calcium (N=83)
Baseline at End of Washout	8.4	8.0
Change from Baseline at Endpoint (95% Confidence Interval)	-2.0* (-2.5, -1.5)	-2.1* (-2.6, -1.7)

*p <0.0001, within treatment group comparison

Figure 1 illustrates that the proportion of patients achieving a given level of serum phosphorus lowering is comparable between the two treatment groups. For example, about half the patients in each group had a decrease of at least 2 mg/dL at endpoint.

Figure 1. Cumulative percent of patients (Y-axis) attaining a phosphorus change from baseline at least as great as the value on the X-axis. A shift to the left of a curve indicates a better response.

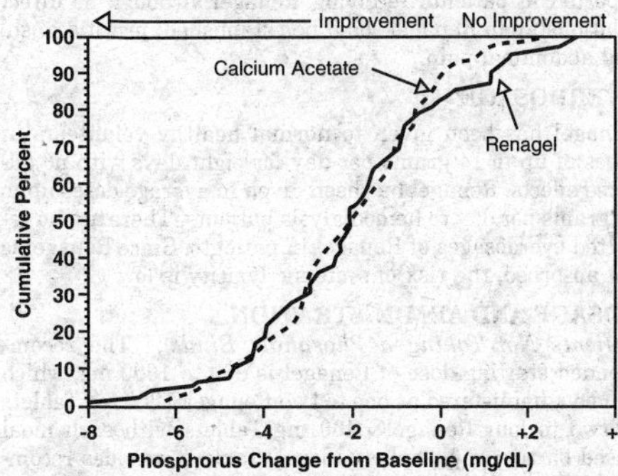

Average daily consumption at the end of treatment was 4.9 g sevelamer hydrochloride (range of 0.0 to 12.6 g) and 5.0 g of calcium acetate (range of 0.0 to 17.8 g). During calcium acetate treatment, 22% of patients developed serum calcium ≥ 11.0 mg/dL on at least one occasion versus 5% for Renagel ($p < 0.05$). Thus the risk of developing hypercalcemia is less with Renagel Capsules compared to calcium acetate.

Mean LDL cholesterol and mean total cholesterol declined significantly on Renagel Capsules treatment (-24% and -15%, respectively). Neither LDL nor total cholesterol changed on calcium acetate treatment. Triglycerides, high-density lipoprotein (HDL) cholesterol, and albumin did not change on either treatment.

Similar reductions in serum phosphorus and LDL cholesterol were observed in an eight-week open-label, uncontrolled study of 172 end stage renal disease patients on hemodialysis.

Parallel study of Renagel and calcium acetate or calcium carbonate: Two hundred ESRD patients on hemodialysis who were hyperphosphatemic (serum phosphorus >5.5 mg/dL) following a two-week phosphate binder washout period were randomized to receive Renagel 800 mg tablets (N=99) or calcium, either calcium acetate (N=54) or calcium carbonate (N=47). Calcium acetate and calcium carbonate produced comparable decreases in serum phosphorus. At week 52, using last-observation-carried-forward, Renagel and Calcium both significantly decreased mean serum phosphorus (Table 2).

Table 2. Mean Serum Phosphorus (mg/dL) and Ion Product at Baseline and End of Treatment

	Renagel (N=94)	Calcium (N=98)
Phosphorus Baseline	7.5	7.3
Change from Baseline at Endpoint	-2.1	-1.8
Ca × Phosphorus Ion Product Baseline	70.5	68.4
Change from Baseline at Endpoint	-19.4	-14.2

Sixty-one percent of Renagel patients and 73% of the calcium patients completed the full 52 weeks of treatment. The major reason for dropout in the Renagel group was gastrointestinal adverse events.

Figure 2, a plot of the phosphorus change from baseline for the completers, illustrates the durability of response for patients who are able to remain on treatment.

Figure 2. Mean Phosphorus Change from Baseline for Patients who Completed 52 Weeks of Treatment

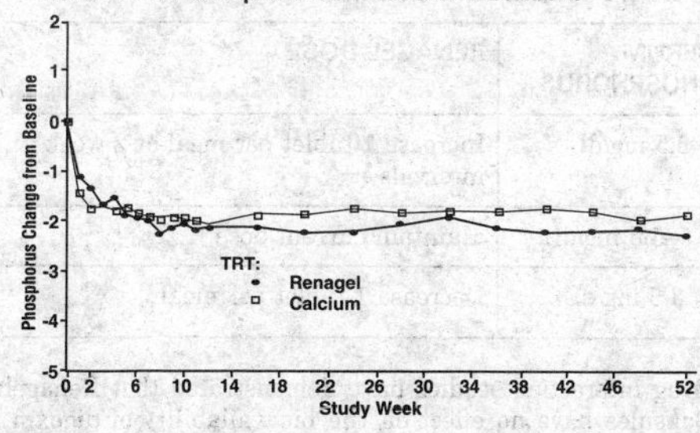

Average daily consumption at the end of treatment was 6.5 g of sevelamer hydrochloride (range of 0.8 to 13 g) or approximately eight 800 mg tablets (range of 1 to 16 tablets), 4.6 g of calcium acetate (range of 0.7 to 9.5 g) and 3.9 g of calcium carbonate (range 1.3 to 9.1 g). During calcium treatment, 34% of patients developed serum calcium corrected for albumin ≥ 11.0 mg/dL on at least one occasion versus 7% for Renagel ($p<0.05$). Thus the risk of developing hypercalcemia is less with Renagel compared to calcium salts.

Mean LDL cholesterol and mean total cholesterol declined significantly ($p<0.05$) on Renagel treatment (-32% and -20%, respectively) compared to calcium (+0.2% and -2%, respectively). Triglycerides, HDL cholesterol, and albumin did not change.

INDICATIONS AND USAGE

Renagel is indicated for the control of serum phosphorus in patients with Chronic Kidney Disease (CKD) on hemodialysis. The safety and efficacy of Renagel in CKD patients who are not on hemodialysis have not been studied. In hemodialysis patients, Renagel decreases the incidence of hypercalcemic episodes relative to patients on calcium treatment.

CONTRAINDICATIONS

Renagel is contraindicated in patients with hypophosphatemia or bowel obstruction. Renagel is contraindicated in patients known to be hypersensitive to sevelamer hydrochloride or any of its constituents.

PRECAUTIONS

General: The safety and efficacy of Renagel in patients with dysphagia, swallowing disorders, severe gastrointestinal (GI) motility disorders, or major GI tract surgery have not been established. Consequently, caution should be exercised when Renagel is used in patients with these GI disorders.

Renagel does not contain calcium or alkali supplementation; serum calcium, bicarbonate, and chloride levels should be monitored.

In preclinical studies in rats and dogs, sevelamer hydrochloride reduced vitamin D, E, K, and folic acid levels at doses of 6–100 times the recommended human dose. In clinical trials, there was no evidence of reduction in serum levels of vitamins with the exception of a one year clinical trial in which Renagel treatment was associated with reduction of 25-hydroxyvitamin D (normal range 10 to 55 mcg/mL) from 39 ± 22 mcg/mL to 34 ± 22 mcg/mL ($p<0.01$). Most (approximately 75%) patients in Renagel clinical trials received vitamin supplements, which is typical of patients on hemodialysis.

Information for the patient: The prescriber should inform patients to take Renagel with meals and adhere to their prescribed diets. Instructions should be given on concomitant medications that should be dosed apart from Renagel. Because the contents of Renagel expand in water, tablets should be swallowed intact and should not be crushed, chewed, broken into pieces, or taken apart prior to administration.

Drug interactions: Renagel Capsules were studied in human drug-drug interaction studies with digoxin, warfarin, enalapril metoprolol and iron.

Digoxin: In 19 healthy subjects receiving 6 Renagel capsules three times a day with meals for 2 days, Renagel did not alter the pharmacokinetics of a single dose of digoxin.

Warfarin: In 14 healthy subjects receiving 6 Renagel capsules three times a day with meals for 2 days, Renagel did not alter the pharmacokinetics of a single dose of warfarin.

Enalapril: In 28 healthy subjects a single dose of 6 Renagel capsules did not alter the pharmacokinetics of a single dose of enalapril.

Metoprolol: In 31 healthy subjects a single dose of 6 Renagel capsules did not alter the pharmacokinetics of a single dose of metoprolol.

Iron: In 23 healthy subjects, a single dose of 7 Renagel capsules did not alter the absorption of a single oral dose of iron as 200 mg exsiccated ferrous sulfate tablet.

However, when administering any other oral medication where a reduction in the bioavailability of that medication would have a clinically significant effect on safety or efficacy, the drug should be administered at least one hour before or three hours after Renagel, or the physician should consider monitoring blood levels of the drug. Patients taking anti-arrhythmic and anti-seizure medications were excluded from the clinical trials. Special precautions should be taken when prescribing Renagel to patients also taking these medications.

Carcinogenesis, mutagenesis, and impairment of fertility: Standard lifetime carcinogenicity bioassays were conducted in mice and rats. Rats were given sevelamer hydrochloride by diet at 0.3, 1, 3 g/kg/day. There was an increased incidence of urinary bladder transitional cell papilloma in male rats (3 g/kg/day) at exposures 2 times the maximum human oral dose of 13 g, based on a comparison of relative body surface area. Mice received mean dietary doses of 0.8, 3, 9 g/kg/day. Increased incidence of tumors was not observed in mice at exposures up to 3 times the maximum human oral dose of 13g, based on a comparison of relative body surface area.

In an *in vitro* mammalian cytogenetic test with metabolic activation, sevelamer hydrochloride caused a statistically significant increase in the number of structural chromosome aberrations. Sevelamer hydrochloride was not mutagenic in the Ames bacterial mutation assay.

Continued on next page

Renagel—Cont.

In a study designed to assess potential impairment of fertility, female rats were given dietary doses of 0.5, 1.5, 4.5 g/kg/day beginning 14 days prior to mating and continuing through gestation. Male rats were given the same doses and treated for 28 days before mating. Sevelamer hydrochloride did not impair fertility in male or female rats at exposures 3 times the maximum human oral dose of 13 g, based on a comparison of relative body surface area.

Pregnancy:

Pregnancy Category C

In pregnant rats given dietary doses of 0.5, 1.5, 4.5 g/kg/day during organogenesis, reduced or irregular ossification of fetal bones, probably due to a reduced absorption of fat-soluble vitamin D occurred in the mid and high dose groups (exposures less than the maximum human dose of 13g, based on a comparison of relative body surface area). In pregnant rabbits given oral doses of 100, 500, 1000 mg/kg/day by gavage during organogenesis an increased incidence of early resorptions occurred at exposures 2 times the maximum human dose of 13 g, based on a comparison of relative body surface area. Requirements for vitamins and other nutrients are increased in pregnancy. The effect of Renagel on the absorption of vitamins and other nutrients has not been studied in pregnant women.

Geriatric use: There is no evidence for special considerations when Renagel is administered to elderly patients.

Pediatric use: The safety and efficacy of Renagel has not been established in pediatric patients.

ADVERSE REACTIONS

In a placebo-controlled study with a treatment duration of two weeks, the adverse events reported for Renagel Capsules (N=24) were similar to those reported for placebo (N=12). In a cross-over study with treatment durations of eight weeks each, the adverse events reported for Renagel Capsules (N=82) were similar to those reported for calcium acetate (N=82) and included headache, infection, pain, hypertension, hypotension, thrombosis, diarrhea, dyspepsia, vomiting, and cough increased. In a parallel design study with treatment duration of 52 weeks, adverse events reported for Renagel Tablets (N=99) were similar to those reported for calcium (calcium acetate and calcium carbonate) (N=101). (Table 3).

Table 3. Treatment-Emergent Adverse Events ≥ 10 % from a Parallel Design Trial of Renagel Tablets versus Calcium for 52 Weeks of Treatment

Adverse Event	Renagel (N=99)	Calcium (N=101)
	Patients %	Patients %
Gastrointestinal Disorders		
Vomiting	22.2	21.8
Nausea	20.2	19.8
Diarrhea	19.2	22.8
Dyspepsia	16.2	6.9
Constipation	8.1	11.9
Infections and Infestations		
Nasopharyngitis	14.1	7.9
Bronchitis	11.1	12.9
Upper Respiratory Tract Infection	5.1	10.9
Musculoskeletal, Connective Tissue and Bone Disorders		
Pain in Limb	13.1	14.9
Arthralgia	12.1	17.8
Back Pain	4.0	17.8
Skin Disorders		
Pruritus	13.1	9.9
Respiratory, Thoracic and Mediastinal Disorders		
Dyspnea	10.1	16.8
Cough	7.1	12.9
Vascular Disorders		
Hypertension	10.1	5.9
Nervous System Disorders		
Headache	9.1	15.8
General Disorders and Site Administration Disorders		
Mechanical Complication of Implant	6.1	10.9
Pyrexia	5.1	10.9

In the parallel design study, the major reason for drop out in the Renagel group was gastrointestinal adverse events. In a long-term, open-label extension trial, adverse events possibly related to Renagel Capsules and which were not dose-related, included nausea (7%), constipation (2%), diarrhea (4%), flatulence (4%), and dyspepsia (5%). During post-marketing experience, the following adverse events have been reported in patients receiving Renagel although no direct relationship to Renagel could be established: pruritis, rash, and abdominal pain.

OVERDOSAGE

Renagel has been given to normal healthy volunteers in doses of up to 14 grams per day for eight days with no adverse effects. Renagel has been given in average doses up to 13 grams per day to hemodialysis patients. There are no reported overdosages of Renagel in patients. Since Renagel is not absorbed, the risk of systemic toxicity is low.

DOSAGE AND ADMINISTRATION

Patients Not Taking a Phosphate Binder. The recommended starting dose of Renagel is 800 to 1600 mg, which can be administered as one to two Renagel® 800 mg Tablets or two to four Renagel® 400 mg Tablets with each meal based on serum phosphorus level. Table 4 provides recommended starting doses of Renagel for patients not taking a phosphate binder.

Table 4. Starting Dose for Patients Not Taking a Phosphate Binder

SERUM PHOSPHORUS	RENAGEL® 800 MG	RENAGEL® 400 MG
> 5.5 and < 7.5 mg/dL	1 tablet three times daily with meals	2 tablets three times daily with meals
≥ 7.5 and < 9.0 mg/dL	2 tablets three times daily with meals	3 tablets three times daily with meals
≥ 9.0 mg/dL	2 tablets three times daily with meals	4 tablets three times daily with meals

Patients Switching From Calcium Acetate. In a study in 84 ESRD patients on hemodialysis, a similar reduction in serum phosphorus was seen with equivalent doses (mg for mg) of Renagel Capsules and calcium acetate. Table 5 gives recommended starting doses of Renagel based on a patient's current calcium acetate dose.

Table 5. Starting Dose for Patients Switching From Calcium Acetate to Renagel

CALCIUM ACETATE 667 MG (TABLETS PER MEAL)	RENAGEL® 800 MG (TABLETS PER MEAL)	RENAGEL® 400 MG (TABLETS PER MEAL)
1 tablet	1 tablet	2 tablets
2 tablets	2 tablets	3 tablets
3 tablets	3 tablets	5 tablets

Dose Titration for All Patients Taking Renagel. Dosage should be adjusted based on the serum phosphorus concentration with a goal of lowering serum phosphorus to 5.5 mg/dL or less. The dose may be increased or decreased by one tablet per meal at two week intervals as necessary. Table 6 gives a dose titration guideline. The average dose in a Phase 3 trial designed to lower serum phosphorus to 5.0 mg/dL or less was approximately three Renagel 800 mg tablets per meal. The maximum average daily Renagel dose studied was 13 grams.

Table 6. Dose Titration Guideline

SERUM PHOSPHORUS	RENAGEL DOSE
> 5.5 mg/dL	Increase 1 tablet per meal at 2 week intervals
3.5–5.5 mg/dL	Maintain current dose
< 3.5 mg/dL	Decrease 1 tablet per meal

Drug interaction studies have demonstrated that Renagel Capsules have no effect on the bioavailability of digoxin, warfarin, enalapril, metoprolol, or iron. When administering any other oral drug for which alteration in blood levels could have a clinically significant effect on safety or efficacy, the drug should be administered at least one hour before or three hours after Renagel, or the physician should consider monitoring blood levels of the drug. (See PRECAUTIONS: Drug interactions.)

Do not use Renagel after the expiration date on the bottle.

HOW SUPPLIED

Renagel® 800 mg Tablets are supplied as oval, film-coated, compressed tablets, imprinted with "RENAGEL 800," containing 800 mg of sevelamer hydrochloride on an anhydrous basis, hypromellose, diacetylated monoglyceride, colloidal silicon dioxide, and stearic acid. Renagel® 800 mg Tablets are packaged in bottles of 180 tablets.

NDC 58468-0021-1 Bottle of 180 Tablets

Renagel® 400 mg Tablets are supplied as oval, film-coated, compressed tablets, imprinted with "RENAGEL 400," containing 400 mg of sevelamer hydrochloride on an anhydrous basis, hypromellose, diacetylated monoglyceride, colloidal silicon dioxide, and stearic acid. Renagel® 400 mg Tablets are packaged in bottles of 360 tablets.

NDC 58468-0020-1 Bottle of 360 Tablets

Storage

Store at 25°C (77°F): excursions permitted to 15–30°C (59–86°F).

[See USP controlled room temperature]

Protect from moisture.

Rx only

Distributed by:

genzyme

Genzyme Corporation
500 Kendall Street
Cambridge, MA 02142
USA
Tel. (800) 847-0069
4777
032204R02
Issued 2/04

Shown in Product Identification Guide, page 313

THYROGEN® ℞

[thī′rō-gen]

(thyrotropin alfa for injection)

DESCRIPTION

Thyrogen® (thyrotropin alfa for injection) contains a highly purified recombinant form of human thyroid stimulating hormone (TSH), a glycoprotein which is produced by recombinant DNA technology. Thyrotropin alfa is synthesized in a genetically modified Chinese hamster ovary cell line.

Thyrotropin alfa is a heterodimeric glycoprotein comprised of two non-covalently linked subunits, an alpha subunit of 92 amino acid residues containing two N-linked glycosylation sites and a beta subunit of 118 residues containing one N-linked glycosylation site. The amino acid sequence of thyrotropin alfa is identical to that of human pituitary thyroid stimulating hormone.

Both thyrotropin alfa and naturally occurring human pituitary thyroid stimulating hormone are synthesized as a mixture of glycosylation variants. Unlike pituitary TSH, which is secreted as a mixture of sialylated and sulfated forms, thyrotropin alfa is sialylated but not sulfated. The biological activity of thyrotropin alfa is determined by a cell-based bioassay. In this assay, cells expressing a functional TSH receptor and a cAMP-responsive element coupled to a heterologous reporter gene, luciferase, enable the measurement of rhTSH activity by measuring the luciferase response. The specific activity of thyrotropin alfa is 4-12 IU/mg using this cell-based bioassay. The specific activity of thyrotropin alfa is determined relative to an internal Genzyme reference material that was calibrated against the World Health Organization (WHO) human pituitary derived TSH reference standard NIBSC 84/703 using an *in vitro* bioassay that measures the amount of cAMP produced by a bovine thyroid microsome preparation in response to rhTSH.

Thyrogen is supplied as a sterile, non-pyrogenic, white to off-white lyophilized product, intended for intramuscular (IM) administration after reconstitution with Sterile Water for Injection, USP. Each vial of Thyrogen contains 1.1 mg thyrotropin alfa (4-12 IU/mg), 36 mg Mannitol, 5.1 mg Sodium Phosphate, and 2.4 mg Sodium Chloride.

After reconstitution with 1.2 mL of Sterile Water for Injection, USP, the thyrotropin alfa concentration is 0.9 mg/mL. The pH of the reconstituted solution is approximately 7.0.

CLINICAL PHARMACOLOGY

Pharmacodynamics

Thyrotropin alfa (recombinant human thyroid stimulating hormone) is a heterodimeric glycoprotein produced by recombinant DNA technology. It has comparable biochemical properties to the human pituitary TSH. Binding of thyrotropin alfa to TSH receptors on normal thyroid epithelial cells or on well-differentiated thyroid cancer tissue stimulates iodine uptake and organification, and synthesis and secretion of thyroglobulin (Tg), triiodothyronine (T_3) and thyroxine (T_4).

In patients with thyroid cancer, a near total or total thyroidectomy is performed and patients are placed on synthetic thyroid hormone supplements to replace endogenous hormone and to suppress serum levels of TSH in order to avoid TSH-stimulated tumor growth. Thereafter, patients are followed up for the presence of remnants or of residual or recurrent cancer by thyroglobulin (Tg) testing while they remain on thyroid hormone suppressive therapy and are euthyroid, or by Tg testing and radioiodine imaging after thyroid hormone withdrawal. Thyrogen is an exogenous source of human TSH that offers an additional diagnostic tool in the follow-up of patients with a history of well-differentiated thyroid cancer.

Pharmacokinetics

The pharmacokinetics of Thyrogen were studied in 16 patients with well-differentiated thyroid cancer given a single 0.9 mg IM dose. Mean peak concentrations of 116 ± 38 mU/L were reached between 3 and 24 hours after injection (median of 10 hours). The mean apparent elimination half-life was 25 ± 10 hours. The organ(s) of TSH clearance in man have not been identified, but studies of pituitary-derived TSH suggest the involvement of the liver and kidneys.

Clinical Trials

Two phase 3 clinical trials were conducted in 358 evaluable patients with well-differentiated thyroid cancer to compare 48-hour radioiodine (^{131}I) whole body scans obtained after Thyrogen to whole body scans after thyroid hormone withdrawal. One of these trials also compared Tg levels obtained after Thyrogen to those on thyroid hormone suppressive therapy, and to those after thyroid hormone withdrawal. All Tg testing was performed in a central laboratory using a radioimmunoassay (RIA) with a functional sensitivity of 2.5 ng/mL. Only successfully ablated patients (defined as patients who have undergone total or near total thyroidectomy with or without radioiodine ablation, and with < 1% uptake in the thyroid bed on a scan after thyroid hormone withdrawal) without detectable anti-thyroglobulin antibodies were included in the Tg data analysis. The maximum Thyrogen Tg value was obtained 72 hours after the final Thyrogen injection, and this value was used in the analysis (see DOSAGE AND ADMINISTRATION).

Radioiodine Whole Body Scan Results

The following table summarizes the scan data in patients with positive scans after withdrawal of thyroid hormone from the phase 3 studies:

[See table above]

Across the two clinical studies, the Thyrogen scan failed to detect remnant and/or cancer localized to the thyroid bed in 16% (20/124) of patients in whom it was detected by a scan after thyroid hormone withdrawal. In addition, the Thyrogen scan failed to detect metastatic disease in 24% (9/38) of patients in whom it was detected by a scan after thyroid hormone withdrawal.

Thyroglobulin (Tg) Results:

Thyrogen Tg Testing Alone and in Combination with Radioiodine Imaging: Comparison with Results after Thyroid Hormone Withdrawal:

In Tg antibody negative patients with a thyroid remnant or cancer as defined by a withdrawal Tg ≥ 2.5 ng/mL or a positive scan (after thyroid hormone withdrawal or after radioiodine therapy), the Thyrogen Tg was ≥ 2.5 ng/mL in 69% (40/58) of patients after 2 doses of Thyrogen, and in 80% (53/66) of patients after 3 doses of Thyrogen. Across both dosage groups, 45% had a Tg ≥ 2.5 ng/mL on thyroid hormone suppressive therapy.

In these same patients, adding the whole body scan increased the detection rate of thyroid remnant or cancer to 84% (49/58) of patients after 2 doses of Thyrogen and 94% (62/66) of patients after 3 doses of Thyrogen.

Thyrogen Tg Testing Alone and in Combination with Radioiodine Imaging in Patients with Confirmed Metastatic Disease:

Metastatic disease was confirmed by a post-treatment scan or by lymph node biopsy in 35 patients. Thyrogen Tg was ≥ 2.5 ng/mL in all 35 patients while Tg on thyroid hormone suppressive therapy was ≥ 2.5 ng/mL in 79% of these patients.

In this same cohort of 35 patients with confirmed metastatic disease, the Thyrogen Tg levels were below 10 ng/mL in 27% (3/11) of patients after 2 doses of Thyrogen and in 13% (3/24) of patients after 3 doses of Thyrogen. The corresponding thyroid hormone withdrawal Tg levels in these 6 patients were 15.6 - 137 ng/mL. The Thyrogen scan detected metastatic disease in 1 of these 6 patients (see INDICATIONS AND USAGE, Considerations in the Use of Thyrogen).

As with thyroid hormone withdrawal, the intra-patient reproducibility of Thyrogen testing with regard to both Tg stimulation and radioiodine imaging has not been studied.

Quality of Life:

Following Thyrogen, no change was observed in any of the 8 domains of the SF-36 Health Survey, a patient-administered quality-of-life measurement instrument. Following thyroid hormone withdrawal, statistically significant negative changes in quality of life parameters were observed in 4 of the 8 SF-36 domains. These 4 domains were: physical functioning, physical role, bodily pain and emotional role. No change was observed in the following scales: general health, vitality, social functioning and mental health.

Hypothyroid Signs and Symptoms:

Thyrogen administration was not associated with the signs and symptoms of hypothyroidism that accompanied thyroid hormone withdrawal as measured by the Billewicz scale. Statistically significant worsening in all signs and symptoms were observed during the hypothyroid phase ($p<0.01$).

[See figure at top of next column]

INDICATIONS AND USAGE

Thyrogen (thyrotropin alfa for injection) is indicated for use as an adjunctive diagnostic tool for serum thyroglobulin

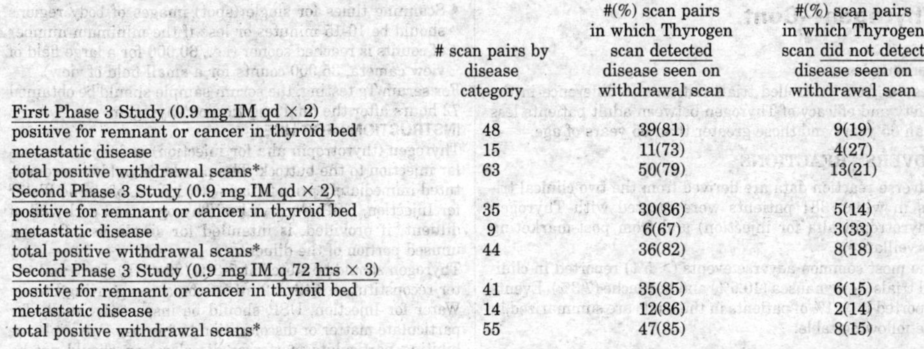

	# scan pairs by disease category	#(%) scan pairs in which Thyrogen scan detected disease seen on withdrawal scan	#(%) scan pairs in which Thyrogen scan did not detect disease seen on withdrawal scan
First Phase 3 Study (0.9 mg IM qd × 2)			
positive for remnant or cancer in thyroid bed	48	39(81)	9(19)
metastatic disease	15	11(73)	4(27)
total positive withdrawal scans*	63	50(79)	13(21)
Second Phase 3 Study (0.9 mg IM qd × 2)			
positive for remnant or cancer in thyroid bed	35	30(86)	5(14)
metastatic disease	9	6(67)	3(33)
total positive withdrawal scans*	44	36(82)	8(18)
Second Phase 3 Study (0.9 mg IM q 72 hrs × 3)			
positive for remnant or cancer in thyroid bed	41	35(85)	6(15)
metastatic disease	14	12(86)	2(14)
total positive withdrawal scans*	55	47(85)	8(15)

* Across all studies, uptake was detected on the Thyrogen scan but not observed on the scan after thyroid hormone withdrawal in 5 patients with remnant or cancer in the thyroid bed.

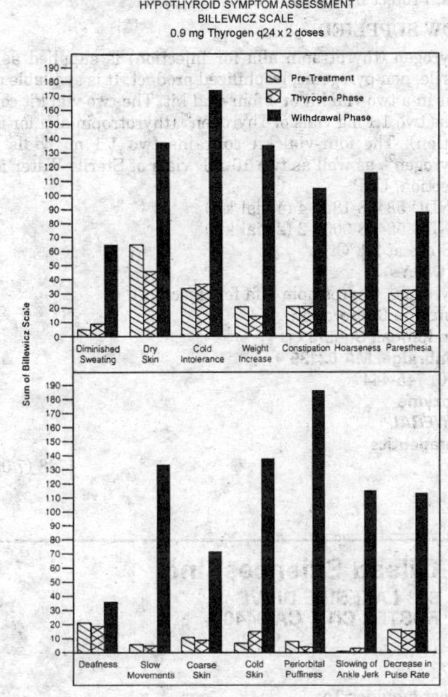

(Tg) testing with or without radioiodine imaging in the follow-up of patients with well-differentiated thyroid cancer.

Potential Clinical Uses:

1) Thyrogen Tg testing may be used in patients with an undetectable Tg on thyroid hormone suppressive therapy to exclude the diagnosis of residual or recurrent thyroid cancer (see CLINICAL PHARMACOLOGY, Clinical Trials, Thyroglobulin (Tg) Results).
2) Thyrogen testing may be used in patients requiring serum Tg testing and radioiodine imaging who are unwilling to undergo thyroid hormone withdrawal testing and whose treating physician believes that use of a less sensitive test is justified.
3) Thyrogen testing may be used in patients who are either unable to mount an adequate endogenous TSH response to thyroid hormone withdrawal or in whom withdrawal is medically contraindicated.

Considerations in the Use of Thyrogen:

1) **Even when Thyrogen-stimulated Tg testing is performed in combination with radioiodine imaging, there remains a meaningful risk of missing a diagnosis of thyroid cancer or of underestimating the extent of disease. Therefore, thyroid hormone withdrawal Tg testing with radioiodine imaging remains the standard diagnostic modality to assess the presence, location and extent of thyroid cancer.**
2) Thyrogen Tg levels are generally lower than, and do not correlate with Tg levels after thyroid hormone withdrawal (see CLINICAL PHARMACOLOGY, Thyroglobulin (Tg) Results).
3) A newly detectable Tg level or a Tg level rising over time after Thyrogen, or a high index of suspicion of metastatic disease, even in the setting of a negative or low-stage Thyrogen radioiodine scan, should prompt further evaluation such as thyroid hormone withdrawal to definitively establish the location and extent of thyroid cancer. On the other hand, none of the 31 patients studied with undetectable Thyrogen Tg levels (< 2.5 ng/mL) had metastatic disease. Therefore, an undetectable Thyrogen Tg level suggests the absence of clinically significant disease (see CLINICAL PHARMACOLOGY, Clinical Trials).
4) The decisions whether to perform a Thyrogen radioiodine scan in conjunction with a Thyrogen serum Tg test and whether and when to withdraw a patient from thyroid hormone are complex. Pertinent factors in these decisions include the sensitivity of the Tg assay used, the Thyrogen Tg level obtained, and the index of suspicion of recurrent or persistent local or metastatic disease. In the clinical trials, combination Tg and scan testing did enhance the diagnostic accuracy of Thyrogen in some cases (see CLINICAL PHARMACOLOGY, Clinical Trials).
5) Thyrogen is not recommended to stimulate radioiodine uptake for the purposes of ablative radiotherapy of thyroid cancer.
6) The signs and symptoms of hypothyroidism which accompany thyroid hormone withdrawal are avoided with Thyrogen (see CLINICAL PHARMACOLOGY, Clinical Trials, Quality of Life, Hypothyroid Signs and Symptoms).

PRECAUTIONS

(see INDICATIONS AND USAGE, Considerations in the Use of Thyrogen)

General

The use of Thyrogen (thyrotropin alfa for injection) should be directed by physicians knowledgeable in the management of patients with thyroid cancer.

Thyroglobulin (Tg) antibodies may confound the Tg assay and render Tg levels uninterpretable. Therefore, in such cases, even with a negative or low-stage Thyrogen radioiodine scan, consideration should be given to evaluating patients further with, for example, a confirmatory thyroid hormone withdrawal scan to determine the location and extent of thyroid cancer.

Thyrogen should be administered intramuscularly only. It should not be administered intravenously.

TSH antibodies have not been reported in patients treated with Thyrogen in the clinical trials, although only 27 patients received Thyrogen on more than one occasion.

Caution should be exercised when Thyrogen is administered to patients who have been previously treated with bovine TSH and, in particular, to those patients who have experienced hypersensitivity reactions to bovine TSH.

Thyrogen is known to cause a transient but significant rise in serum thyroid hormone concentration. Therefore, caution should be exercised in patients with a known history of heart disease and with significant residual thyroid tissue (see ADVERSE REACTIONS).

Drug-Drug Interactions

Formal interaction studies between Thyrogen and other medicinal products have not been performed. In clinical trials, no interactions were observed between Thyrogen and the thyroid hormones triiodothyronine (T_3) and thyroxine (T_4) when administered concurrently.

The use of Thyrogen allows for radioiodine imaging while patients are euthyroid on triiodothyronine (T_3) and/or thyroxine (T_4). Data on radioiodine ^{131}I kinetics indicate that the clearance of radioiodine is approximately 50% greater in euthyroid patients than in hypothyroid patients, who have decreased renal function. Thus radioiodine retention is less in euthyroid patients at the time of imaging and this factor should be considered when selecting the activity of radioiodine for use in radioiodine imaging.

Carcinogenesis, Mutagenesis, Impairment of Fertility

Long-term toxicity studies in animals have not been performed with Thyrogen to evaluate the carcinogenic potential of the drug. Thyrogen was not mutagenic in the bacterial reverse mutation assay. Studies have not been performed with Thyrogen to evaluate the effects on fertility.

Pregnancy Category C

Animal reproduction studies have not been conducted with Thyrogen.

It is also not known whether Thyrogen can cause fetal harm when administered to a pregnant woman or can affect reproductive capacity. Thyrogen should be given to a pregnant woman only if clearly needed.

Nursing Mothers

It is not known whether the drug is excreted in human milk. Because many drugs are excreted in human milk, caution should be exercised when Thyrogen is administered to a nursing woman.

Pediatric Use

Safety and effectiveness in pediatric patients below the age of 16 years have not been established.

Continued on next page

Thyrogen—Cont.

Geriatric Use

Results from controlled trials indicate no difference in the safety and efficacy of Thyrogen between adult patients less than 65 years and those greater than 65 years of age.

ADVERSE REACTIONS

Adverse reaction data are derived from the two clinical trials in which 381 patients were treated with Thyrogen (thyrotropin alfa for injection) and from post-marketing surveillance.

The most common adverse events (> 5%) reported in clinical trials were: nausea (10.5%) and headache (7.3%). Events reported in ≥ 1% of patients in the trials are summarized in the following table:

Summary of Adverse Events During Clinical Studies (≥ 1%)

	% of Patients with Adverse Events (n) (n = 381)
Body as a Whole	
Headache	7.3%(28)
Asthenia	3.4%(13)
Chills	1.0%(4)
Fever	1.0%(4)
Flu Syndrome	1.0%(4)
Digestive System	
Nausea	10.5%(40)
Vomiting	2.1%(8)
Nausea and Vomiting	1.3%(5)
Nervous System	
Dizziness	1.6%(6)
Paresthesia	1.6%(6)

There have been several reports of hypersensitivity reactions including urticaria, rash, pruritus, flushing and respiratory difficulties requiring treatment. However, in clinical trials no patients have developed antibodies to thyrotropin alfa, either after single dose or repeated (27 patients) use of the product.

Four patients out of 55 (7.3%) with CNS metastases who were followed in a special treatment protocol experienced acute hemiplegia, hemiparesis or pain one to three days after Thyrogen administration. The symptoms were attributed to local edema and/or focal hemorrhage at the site of the cerebral or spinal cord metastases. In addition, one case each of acute visual loss and of laryngeal edema with respiratory distress, requiring tracheotomy, with onset of symptoms within 24 hours after Thyrogen administration, have been reported in patients with metastases to the optic nerve and paratracheal areas, respectively. In addition, sudden, rapid and painful enlargement of locally recurring papillary carcinoma has been reported within 12-48 hours of Thyrogen administration. The enlargement was accompanied by dyspnea, stridor or dysphonia. Rapid clinical improvement occurred following glucocorticoid therapy. It is recommended that pretreatment with glucocorticoids be considered for patients in whom local tumor expansion may compromise vital anatomic structures.

A 77 year-old non-thyroidectomized patient with a history of heart disease and spinal metastases who received 4 Thyrogen injections over 6 days in a special treatment protocol experienced a fatal MI 24 hours after he received the last Thyrogen injection. The event was likely related to Thyrogen-induced hyperthyroidism.

OVERDOSAGE

There has been no reported experience of overdose in humans. However, in clinical trials, three patients experienced symptoms after receiving Thyrogen doses higher than those recommended. Two patients had nausea after a 2.7 mg IM dose, and in one of these patients, the event was accompanied by weakness, dizziness and headache. Another patient experienced nausea, vomiting and hot flashes after a 3.6 mg IM dose.

In addition, one patient experienced symptoms after receiving Thyrogen intravenously. This patient received 0.3 mg Thyrogen as a single intravenous bolus and, 15 minutes later experienced severe nausea, vomiting, diaphoresis, hypotension (BP decreased from 115/66 mm Hg to 81/44 mm Hg) and tachycardia (pulse increased from 75 to 117 bpm).

DOSAGE AND ADMINISTRATION

Thyrogen 0.9 mg intramuscularly may be administered every 24 hours for two doses or every 72 hours for three doses. After reconstitution with 1.2 mL Sterile Water for Injection, a 1.0 mL solution (0.9 mg thyrotropin alfa) is administered by intramuscular injection to the buttock.

For radioiodine imaging, radioiodine administration should be given 24 hours following the final Thyrogen injection. Scanning should be performed 48 hours after radioiodine administration (72 hours after the final injection of Thyrogen).

The following parameters utilized in the second Phase 3 study are recommended for radioiodine scanning with Thyrogen:

- A diagnostic activity of 4 mCi (148 MBq) ^{131}I should be used.
- Whole body images should be acquired for a minimum of 30 minutes and/or should contain a minimum of 140,000 counts.
- Scanning times for single (spot) images of body regions should be 10-15 minutes or less if the minimum number of counts is reached sooner (i.e., 60,000 for a large field of view camera, 35,000 counts for a small field of view).

For serum Tg testing, the serum sample should be obtained 72 hours after the final injection of Thyrogen.

INSTRUCTIONS FOR USE

Thyrogen (thyrotropin alfa for injection) is for intramuscular injection to the buttock. The powder should be reconstituted immediately prior to use with 1.2 mL of sterile Water for Injection, USP. Each vial of Thyrogen and each vial of diluent, if provided, is intended for single use. Discard unused portion of the diluent.

Thyrogen should be stored at 2-8°C (36-46°F). Each vial, after reconstitution with 1.2 mL of the accompanying Sterile Water for Injection, USP, should be inspected visually for particulate matter or discoloration before use. Any vials exhibiting particulate matter or discoloration should not be used.

If necessary, the reconstituted solution can be stored for up to 24 hours at a temperature between 2°C and 8°C, while avoiding microbial contamination.

DO NOT USE Thyrogen after the expiration date on the vial. Protect from light.

HOW SUPPLIED

Thyrogen (thyrotropin alfa for injection) is supplied as a sterile, non-pyrogenic, lyophilized product. It is available either in a two-vial kit or a four-vial kit. The two-vial kit contains two 1.1 mg vials of Thyrogen® (thyrotropin alfa for injection). The four-vial kit contains two 1.1 mg vials of Thyrogen®, as well as two 10 mL vials of Sterile Water for Injection, USP.

NDC 58468-1849-4 (4-vial kit)
NDC 58468-0030-2 (2-vial kit)
Store at 2-8°C.

Rx ONLY

Thyrogen® (thyrotropin alfa for injection)

Genzyme Corporation
One Kendall Square
Cambridge, MA 02139
(800) 745-4447
genzyme
GENERAL
therapeutics

4728 (7/03)

Gilead Sciences, Inc.

333 LAKESIDE DRIVE
FOSTER CITY, CA 94404

Direct Inquiries To:
Customer Service
(800) GILEAD5

Medical Emergency Contact:
Medical Information
(800) GILEAD5
FAX: (650) 522-5466

EMTRIVA™ ℞
[*ĕm-trīvă*]
(emtricitabine)
Capsules
℞ Only

WARNING: LACTIC ACIDOSIS AND SEVERE HEPATOMEGALY WITH STEATOSIS, INCLUDING FATAL CASES, HAVE BEEN REPORTED WITH THE USE OF NUCLEOSIDE ANALOGUES ALONE OR IN COMBINATION WITH OTHER ANTIRETROVIRALS (SEE WARNINGS).

DESCRIPTION

EMTRIVA is the brand name of emtricitabine, a synthetic nucleoside analogue with activity against human immunodeficiency virus type 1 (HIV-1) reverse transcriptase.

The chemical name of emtricitabine is 5-fluoro-1-(2*R*,5*S*)-[2-(hydroxymethyl)-1,3-oxathiolan-5-yl]cytosine. Emtricitabine is the (-) enantiomer of a thio analogue of cytidine, which differs from other cytidine analogues in that it has a fluorine in the 5-position.

It has a molecular formula of $C_8H_{10}FN_3O_3S$ and a molecular weight of 247.24. It has the following structural formula:

[structural formula: H_2N, N, O, F, N, O, S, OH]

Emtricitabine is a white to off-white powder with a solubility of approximately 112 mg/mL in water at 25 °C. The log P for emtricitabine is –0.43 and the pKa is 2.65.

EMTRIVA capsules are for oral administration. Each capsule contains 200 mg of emtricitabine and the inactive ingredients, crospovidone, magnesium stearate, microcrystalline cellulose and povidone.

MICROBIOLOGY

Mechanism of Action:

Emtricitabine, a synthetic nucleoside analog of cytosine, is phosphorylated by cellular enzymes to form emtricitabine 5′-triphosphate. Emtricitabine 5′-triphosphate inhibits the activity of the HIV-1 reverse transcriptase by competing with the natural substrate deoxycytidine 5′-triphosphate and by being incorporated into nascent viral DNA which results in chain termination. Emtricitabine 5′-triphosphate is a weak inhibitor of mammalian DNA polymerase α, β, ε and mitochondrial DNA polymerase γ.

Antiviral Activity In Vitro:

The *in vitro* antiviral activity of emtricitabine against laboratory and clinical isolates of HIV was assessed in lymphoblastoid cell lines, the MAGI-CCR5 cell line, and peripheral blood mononuclear cells. The 50% inhibitory concentration (IC_{50}) value for emtricitabine was in the range of 0.0013 to 0.64 μM (0.0003 to 0.158 μg/mL). In drug combination studies of emtricitabine with nucleoside reverse transcriptase inhibitors (abacavir, lamivudine, stavudine, tenofovir, zalcitabine, zidovudine), non-nucleoside reverse transcriptase inhibitors (delavirdine, efavirenz, nevirapine), and protease inhibitors (amprenavir, nelfinavir, ritonavir, saquinavir), additive to synergistic effects were observed. Most of these drug combinations have not been studied in humans. Emtricitabine displayed antiviral activity *in vitro* against HIV-1 clades A, C, D, E, F, and G (IC_{50} values ranged from 0.007 to 0.075 μM) and showed strain specific activity against HIV-2 (IC_{50} values ranged from 0.007 to 1.5 μM).

Drug Resistance:

Emtricitabine-resistant isolates of HIV have been selected *in vitro*. Genotypic analysis of these isolates showed that the reduced susceptibility to emtricitabine was associated with a mutation in the HIV reverse transcriptase gene at codon 184 which resulted in an amino acid substitution of methionine by valine or isoleucine (M184V/I).

Emtricitabine-resistant isolates of HIV have been recovered from some patients treated with emtricitabine alone or in combination with other antiretroviral agents. In a clinical study, viral isolates from 37.5% of treatment-naïve patients with virologic failure showed reduced susceptibility to emtricitabine. Genotypic analysis of these isolates showed that the resistance was due to M184V/I mutations in the HIV reverse transcriptase gene.

Cross Resistance:

Cross-resistance among certain nucleoside analogue reverse transcriptase inhibitors has been recognized. Emtricitabine-resistant isolates (M184V/I) were cross-resistant to lamivudine and zalcitabine but retained sensitivity to abacavir, didanosine, stavudine, tenofovir, zidovudine, and NNRTIs (delavirdine, efavirenz, and nevirapine). HIV-1 isolates containing the K65R mutation, selected *in vivo* by abacavir, didanosine, tenofovir, and zalcitabine, demonstrated reduced susceptibility to inhibition by emtricitabine. Viruses harboring mutations conferring reduced susceptibility to stavudine and zidovudine (M41L, D67N, K70R, L210W, T215Y/F, K219Q/E) or didanosine (L74V) remained sensitive to emtricitabine. HIV-1 containing the K103N mutation associated with resistance to NNRTIs was susceptible to emtricitabine.

CLINICAL PHARMACOLOGY

Pharmacodynamics:

The *in vivo* activity of emtricitabine was evaluated in two clinical trials in which 101 patients were administered 25 to 400 mg a day of EMTRIVA as monotherapy for 10 to 14 days. A dose-related antiviral effect was observed, with a median decrease from baseline in plasma HIV-1 RNA of 1.3 $\log_{10}$ at a dose of 25 mg QD and 1.7 $\log_{10}$ to 1.9 $\log_{10}$ at a dose of 200 mg QD or BID.

Pharmacokinetics:

The pharmacokinetics of emtricitabine were evaluated in healthy volunteers and HIV-infected individuals. Emtricitabine pharmacokinetics are similar between these populations.

Figure 1 shows the mean steady-state plasma emtricitabine concentration-time profile in 20 HIV-infected subjects receiving EMTRIVA.

Figure 1. Mean (± 95% CI) Steady-State Plasma Emtricitabine Concentrations in HIV-Infected Adults (n = 20)

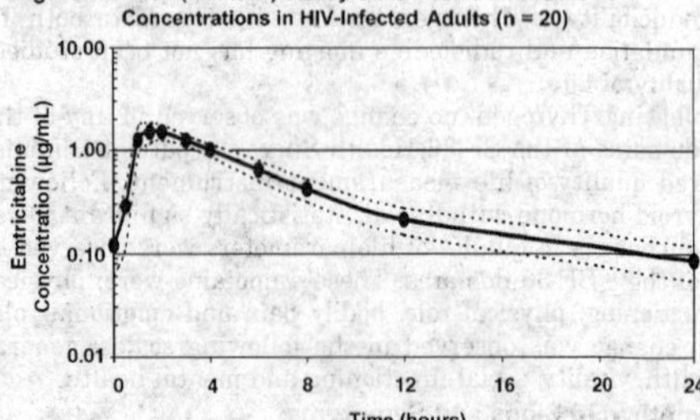

Absorption: Emtricitabine is rapidly and extensively absorbed following oral administration with peak plasma concentrations occurring at 1 to 2 hours post-dose. Following multiple dose oral administration of EMTRIVA to 20 HIV-infected subjects, the (mean ± SD) steady-state plasma emtricitabine peak concentration (C_{max}) was 1.8 ± 0.7 μg/mL and the area-under the plasma concentration-time curve over a 24-hour dosing interval (AUC) was 10.0 ±

3.1 hr*µg/mL. The mean steady state plasma trough concentration at 24 hours post-dose was 0.09 µg/mL. The mean absolute bioavailability of EMTRIVA was 93%.

The multiple dose pharmacokinetics of emtricitabine are dose proportional over a dose range of 25 to 200 mg.

Effects of Food on Oral Absorption: EMTRIVA may be taken with or without food. Emtricitabine systemic exposure (AUC) was unaffected while C_{max} decreased by 29% when EMTRIVA was administered with food (an approximately 1000 kcal high-fat meal).

Distribution: *In vitro* binding of emtricitabine to human plasma proteins was <4% and independent of concentration over the range of 0.02-200 µg/mL. At peak plasma concentration, the mean plasma to blood drug concentration ratio was ~ 1.0 and the mean semen to plasma drug concentration ratio was ~ 4.0.

Metabolism: *In vitro* studies indicate that emtricitabine is not an inhibitor of human CYP450 enzymes. Following administration of ^{14}C-emtricitabine, complete recovery of the dose was achieved in urine (~ 86%) and feces (~ 14%). Thirteen percent (13%) of the dose was recovered in urine as three putative metabolites. The biotransformation of emtricitabine includes oxidation of the thiol moiety to form the 3′-sulfoxide diastereomers (~ 9% of dose) and conjugation with glucuronic acid to form 2′-O-glucuronide (~ 4% of dose). No other metabolites were identifiable.

Elimination: The plasma emtricitabine half-life is approximately 10 hours. The renal clearance of emtricitabine is greater than the estimated creatinine clearance, suggesting elimination by both glomerular filtration and active tubular secretion. There may be competition for elimination with other compounds that are also renally eliminated.

Special Populations:

The pharmacokinetics of emtricitabine were similar in male and female patients and no pharmacokinetic differences due to race have been identified.

The pharmacokinetics of emtricitabine have not been fully evaluated in children or in the elderly.

The pharmacokinetics of emtricitabine have not been studied in patients with hepatic impairment, however, emtricitabine is not metabolized by liver enzymes, so the impact of liver impairment should be limited.

The pharmacokinetics of emtricitabine are altered in patients with renal impairment (See PRECAUTIONS). In patients with creatinine clearance < 50 mL/min or with end-stage renal disease (ESRD) requiring dialysis, C_{max} and AUC of emtricitabine were increased due to a reduction in renal clearance (Table 1). It is recommended that the dosing interval for EMTRIVA be modified in patients with creatinine clearance < 50 mL/min or in patients with ESRD who require dialysis (see DOSAGE AND ADMINISTRATION).

[See table 1 above]

Hemodialysis: Hemodialysis treatment removes approximately 30% of the emtricitabine dose over a 3-hour dialysis period starting within 1.5 hours of emtricitabine dosing (blood flow rate of 400 mL/min and a dialysate flow rate of 600 mL/min). It is not known whether emtricitabine can be removed by peritoneal dialysis.

Drug Interactions

At concentrations up to 14 fold higher than those observed *in vivo*, emtricitabine did not inhibit *in vitro* drug metabolism mediated by any of the following human CYP 450 isoforms: CYP1A2, CYP2A6, CYP2B6, CYP2C9, CYP2C19, CYP2D6 and CYP3A4. Emtricitabine did not inhibit the enzyme responsible for glucuronidation (uridine-5′-disphosphoglucuronyl transferase). Based on the results of these *in vitro* experiments and the known elimination pathways of emtricitabine, the potential for CYP450 mediated interactions involving emtricitabine with other medicinal products is low.

EMTRIVA has been evaluated in healthy volunteers in combination with tenofovir disoproxil fumarate (DF), indinavir, famciclovir, and stavudine. Tables 2 and 3 summarize the pharmacokinetic effects of co-administered drug on emtricitabine pharmacokinetics and effects of emtricitabine on the pharmacokinetics of co-administered drug.

[See table 2 at right]

[See table 3 at right]

Table 1. Mean ± SD Pharmacokinetic Parameters in Patients with Varying Degrees of Renal Function

Creatinine clearance (mL/min)	>80 (n=6)	50-80 (n=6)	30-49 (n=6)	<30 (n=5)	ESRD* <30 (n=5)
Baseline Creatinine clearance (mL/min)	107 ± 21	59.8 ± 6.5	40.9 ± 5.1	22.9 ± 5.3	8.8 ± 1.4
C_{max} (µg/mL)	2.2 ± 0.6	3.8 ± 0.9	3.2 ± 0.6	2.8 ± 0.7	2.8 ± 0.5
AUC (hr•µg/mL)	11.8 ± 2.9	19.9 ± 1.1	25.0 ± 5.7	34.0 ± 2.1	53.2 ± 9.9
CL/F (mL/min)	302 ± 94	168 ± 10	138 ± 28	99 ± 6	64 ± 12
CLr (mL/min)	213.3 ± 89.0	121.4 ± 39.0	68.6 ± 32.1	29.5 ± 11.4	-

*ESRD patients requiring dialysis
"-" = not applicable

Table 2. Drug Interactions: Change in Pharmacokinetic Parameters for Emtricitabine in the Presence of the Co-administered Drug[1]

Co-Administered Drug	Dose of Co-Administered Drug (mg)	Emtricitabine Dose (mg)	N	% Change of Emtricitabine Pharmacokinetic Parameters[2] (90% CI)		
				C_{max}	AUC	C_{min}
Tenofovir DF	300 once daily × 7 days	200 once daily × 7 days	17	↔	↔	↑ 20 (↑ 12 to ↑ 29)
Indinavir	800 × 1	200 × 1	12	↔	↔	-
Famciclovir	500 × 1	200 × 1	12	↔	↔	-
Stavudine	40 × 1	200 × 1	6	↔	↔	-

1. All interaction studies conducted in healthy volunteers
2. ↑ = Increase; ↓ = Decrease; ↔ = no effect; "-" = not applicable

Table 3. Drug Interactions: Change in Pharmacokinetic Parameters for Co-administered Drug in the Presence of the Emtricitabine[1]

Co-Administered Drug	Dose of Co-Administered Drug (mg)	Emtricitabine Dose (mg)	N	% Change of Co-administered Drug Pharmacokinetic Parameters[2] (90% CI)		
				C_{max}	AUC	C_{min}
Tenofovir DF	300 once daily × 7 days	200 once daily × 7 days	17	↔	↔	↔
Indinavir	800 × 1	200 × 1	12	↔	↔	-
Famciclovir	500 × 1	200 × 1	12	↔	↔	-
Stavudine	40 × 1	200 × 1	6	↔	↔	-

1. All interaction studies conducted in healthy volunteers
2. ↑ = Increase; ↓ = Decrease; ↔ = no effect; "-" = not applicable

INDICATION AND USAGE

EMTRIVA is indicated, in combination with other antiretroviral agents, for the treatment of HIV-1 infection in adults. This indication is based on analyses of plasma HIV-1 RNA levels and CD4 cell counts from controlled studies of 48 weeks duration in antiretroviral-naïve patients and antiretroviral-treatment-experienced patients who were virologically suppressed on an HIV treatment regimen.

In antiretroviral-treatment-experienced patients, the use of EMTRIVA may be considered for adults with HIV strains that are expected to be susceptible to EMTRIVA as assessed by genotypic or phenotypic testing. (See MICROBIOLOGY, Drug Resistance and Cross Resistance).

Description of Clinical Studies

Study 301A: EMTRIVA QD + didanosine QD + efavirenz QD compared to stavudine BID + didanosine QD + efavirenz QD

Study 301A was a 48 week double-blind, active-controlled multicenter study comparing EMTRIVA (200 mg QD) administered in combination with didanosine and efavirenz versus stavudine, didanosine and efavirenz in 571 antiretroviral naïve patients. Patients had a mean age of 36 years (range 18 to 69), 85% were male, 52% Caucasian, 16% African-American and 26% Hispanics. Patients had a mean baseline CD4 cell count of 318 cells/mm^3 (range 5–1317) and a median baseline plasma HIV RNA of 4.9 $\log_{10}$ copies/mL (range 2.6–7.0). Thirty-eight percent of patients had baseline viral loads > 100,000 copies/mL and 31% had CD4 cell counts < 200 cells/mL. Treatment outcomes are presented in Table 4 below.

Table 4. Outcomes of Randomized Treatment at Week 48 (Study 301A)

Outcome at Week 48	EMTRIVA+ didanosine+ efavirenz (N=286)	Stavudine+ didanosine+ efavirenz (N=285)
Responder[1]	81% (78%)	68% (59%)
Virologic Failure[2]	3%	11%
Death	0%	<1%
Study Discontinuation Due to Adverse Event	7%	13%
Study Discontinuation For Other Reasons[3]	9%	8%

1. Patients achieved and maintained confirmed HIV RNA < 400 copies/mL (<50 copies/mL) through Week 48.
2. Includes patients who failed to achieve virologic suppression or rebounded after achieving virologic suppression.
3. Includes lost to follow-up, patient withdrawal, noncompliance, protocol violation and other reasons.

The mean increase from baseline in CD4 cell count was 168 cells/mm^3 for the EMTRIVA arm and 134 cells/mm^3 for the stavudine arm.

Through 48 weeks in the EMTRIVA group, 5 patients (1.7%) experienced a new CDC Class C event, compared to 7 patients (2.5%) in the stavudine group.

Study 303: EMTRIVA QD + Stable Background Therapy (SBT) compared to lamivudine BID + SBT

Study 303 was a 48 week, open-label, active-controlled multicenter study comparing EMTRIVA (200 mg QD) to lamivudine, in combination with stavudine or zidovudine and a protease inhibitor or NNRTI in 440 patients who were on a lamivudine-containing triple-antiretroviral drug regimen for at least 12 weeks prior to study entry and had HIV-1 RNA ≤400 copies/mL.

Patients were randomized 1:2 to continue therapy with lamivudine (150 mg BID) or to switch to EMTRIVA (200 mg QD). All patients were maintained on their stable background regimen. Patients had a mean age of 42 years (range 22-80), 86% were male, 64% Caucasian, 21% African-American and 13% Hispanic. Patients had a mean baseline CD4 cell count of 527 cells/mm^3 (range 37-1909), and a median baseline plasma HIV RNA of 1.7 $\log_{10}$ copies/mL (range 1.7–4.0).

The median duration of prior antiretroviral therapy was 27.6 months.

Table 5. Outcomes of Randomized Treatment at Week 48 (Study 303)

Outcome at Week 48	EMTRIVA + ZDV/d4T + NNRTI/PI (N=294)	Lamivudine + ZDV/d4T + NNRTI/PI (N=146)
Responder[1]	77% (67%)	82% (72%)
Virologic Failure[2]	7%	8%
Death	0%	<1%
Study Discontinuation Due to Adverse Event	4%	0%
Study Discontinuation For Other Reasons[3]	12%	10%

1. Patients achieved and maintained confirmed HIV RNA < 400 copies/mL (< 50/mL) through Week 48.
2. Includes patients who failed to achieve virologic suppression or rebounded after achieving virologic suppression.
3. Includes lost to follow-up, patient withdrawal, noncompliance, protocol violation and other reasons.

The mean increase from baseline in CD4 cell count was 29 cells/mm^3 for the EMTRIVA arm and 61 cells/mm^3 for the lamivudine arm.

Continued on next page

Emtriva—Cont.

Through 48 weeks, in the EMTRIVA group 2 patients (0.7%) experienced a new CDC Class C event, compared to 2 patients (1.4%) in the lamivudine group.

CONTRAINDICATIONS

EMTRIVA is contraindicated in patients with previously demonstrated hypersensitivity to any of the components of the products.

WARNINGS

Lactic Acidosis/Severe Hepatomegaly with Steatosis

Lactic acidosis and severe hepatomegaly with steatosis, including fatal cases, have been reported with the use of nucleoside analogues alone or in combination, including emtricitabine and other antiretrovirals. A majority of these cases have been in women. Obesity and prolonged nucleoside exposure may be risk factors. However, cases have also been reported in patients with no known risk factors. Treatment with EMTRIVA should be suspended in any patient who develops clinical or laboratory findings suggestive of lactic acidosis or pronounced hepatotoxicity (which may include hepatomegaly and steatosis even in the absence of marked transaminase elevations).

Post Treatment Exacerbation of Hepatitis

It is recommended that all patients with HIV be tested for the presence of chronic hepatitis B virus (HBV) before initiating antiretroviral therapy. EMTRIVA is not indicated for the treatment of chronic HBV infection and the safety and efficacy of EMTRIVA have not been established in patients co-infected with HBV and HIV. Exacerbations of hepatitis B have been reported in patients after the discontinuation of EMTRIVA. Patients co-infected with HIV and HBV should be closely monitored with both clinical and laboratory follow-up for at least several months after stopping treatment.

PRECAUTIONS

Patients with Impaired Renal Function

Emtricitabine is principally eliminated by the kidney. Reduction of the dosage of EMTRIVA is recommended for patients with impaired renal function (see CLINICAL PHARMACOLOGY and DOSAGE AND ADMINISTRATION).

Drug Interactions

The potential for drug interactions with EMTRIVA has been studied in combination with indinavir, stavudine, famciclovir, and tenofovir disoproxil fumarate. There were no clinically significant drug interactions for any of these drugs (see CLINICAL PHARMACOLOGY, Drug Interactions).

Fat Redistribution

Redistribution/accumulation of body fat including central obesity, dorsocervical fat enlargement (buffalo hump), peripheral wasting, facial wasting, breast enlargement, and "cushingoid appearance" have been observed in patients receiving antiretroviral therapy. The mechanism and long-term consequences of these events are unknown. A causal relationship has not been established.

Information for Patients

EMTRIVA is not a cure for HIV infection and patients may continue to experience illnesses associated with HIV infection, including opportunistic infections. Patients should remain under the care of a physician when using EMTRIVA. Patients should be advised that:

- the use of EMTRIVA has not been shown to reduce the risk of transmission of HIV to others through sexual contact or blood contamination.
- the long term effects of EMTRIVA are unknown.
- EMTRIVA Capsules are for oral ingestion only.
- it is important to take EMTRIVA with combination therapy on a regular dosing schedule to avoid missing doses.
- redistribution or accumulation of body fat may occur in patients receiving antiretroviral therapy and that the cause and long-term health effects of these conditions are not known.

Carcinogenesis, Mutagenesis, Impairment of Fertility

Carcinogenesis: Long-term carcinogenicity studies of emtricitabine in rats and mice are in progress.

Mutagenesis: Emtricitabine was not genotoxic in the reverse mutation bacterial test (Ames test), mouse lymphoma or mouse micronucleus assays.

Impairment of Fertility: Emtricitabine did not affect fertility in male rats at approximately 140-fold or in male and female mice at approximately 60-fold higher exposures (AUC) than in humans given the recommended 200 mg daily dose. Fertility was normal in the offspring of mice exposed daily from before birth (in utero) through sexual maturity at daily exposures (AUC) of approximately 60-fold higher than human exposures at the recommended 200 mg daily dose.

Pregnancy

Pregnancy Category B

The incidence of fetal variations and malformations was not increased in embryofetal toxicity studies performed with emtricitabine in mice at exposures (AUC) approximately 60-fold higher and in rabbits at approximately 120-fold higher than human exposures at the recommended daily dose. There are, however, no adequate and well-controlled studies in pregnant women. Because animal reproduction studies are not always predictive of human response, EMTRIVA should be used during pregnancy only if clearly needed.

Antiretroviral Pregnancy Registry: To monitor fetal outcomes of pregnant women exposed to emtricitabine, an antiretroviral Pregnancy Registry has been established.

Table 6. Selected Treatment-Emergent Adverse Events (All Grades, Regardless of Causality) Reported in ≥ 3% of EMTRIVA-Treated Patients in Either Study 301A or 303 (0-48 weeks)

Adverse event	303		301A	
	EMTRIVA + ZDV/d4T + NNRTI/PI (n=294)	Lamivudine + ZDV/d4T + NNRTI/PI (n=146)	EMTRIVA + didanosine + efavirenz (n=286)	Stavudine + didanosine + efavirenz (n=285)
Body as a Whole				
Abdominal Pain	8%	11%	14%	17%
Asthenia	16%	10%	12%	17%
Headache	13%	6%	22%	25%
Digestive System				
Diarrhea	23%	18%	23%	32%
Dyspepsia	4%	5%	8%	12%
Nausea	18%	12%	13%	23%
Vomiting	9%	7%	9%	12%
Musculoskeletal				
Arthralgia	3%	4%	5%	6%
Myalgia	4%	4%	6%	3%
Nervous System				
Abnormal dreams	2%	<1%	11%	19%
Depressive disorders	6%	10%	9%	13%
Dizziness	4%	5%	25%	26%
Insomnia	7%	3%	16%	21%
Neuritis Neuropathy/Peripheral	4%	3%	4%	13%
Paresthesia	5%	7%	6%	12%
Respiratory				
Increased cough	14%	11%	14%	8%
Rhinitis	18%	12%	12%	10%
Skin				
Rash event[1]	17%	14%	30%	33%

1. Rash event includes rash, pruritus, maculopapular rash, urticaria, vesiculobullous rash, pustular rash, and allergic reaction.

Table 7. Treatment-Emergent Grade 3 / 4 Laboratory Abnormalities Reported in ≥ 1% of EMTRIVA-Treated Patients in Either Study 301A or 303

Number of Patients Treated	303		301A	
	EMTRIVA + ZDV/d4T + NNRTI/PI (n=294)	Lamivudine + ZDV/d4T + NNRTI/PI (n=146)	EMTRIVA + didanosine + efavirenz (n=286)	Stavudine + didanosine + efavirenz (n=285)
Percentage with Grade 3 or Grade 4 laboratory abnormality	31%	28%	34%	38%
ALT (>5.0 × ULN[1])	2%	1%	5%	6%
AST (>5.0 × ULN)	3%	<1%	6%	9%
Bilirubin (>2.5 × ULN)	1%	2%	<1%	<1%
Creatine kinase (>4.0 × ULN)	11%	14%	12%	11%
Neutrophils (<750 mm³)	5%	3%	5%	7%
Pancreatic amylase (>2.0 × ULN)	2%	2%	<1%	1%
Serum amylase (>2.0 × ULN)	2%	2%	5%	10%
Serum glucose (<40 or >250 mg/dL)	3%	3%	2%	3%
Serum lipase (>2.0 × ULN)	<1%	<1%	1%	2%
Triglycerides (>750 mg/dL)	10%	8%	9%	6%

1. ULN=Upper limit of normal

Table 8. Dosing Interval Adjustment in Patients with Renal Impairment

	Creatinine Clearance (mL/min)			
	≥ 50	30-49	15-29	< 15 (including patients requiring hemodialysis)*
Recommended Dose and Dosing Interval	200 mg every 24 hours	200 mg every 48 hours	200 mg every 72 hours	200 mg every 96 hours

*Hemodialysis Patients: If dosing on day of dialysis, give dose after dialysis.

Healthcare providers are encouraged to register patients by calling 1-800-258-4263.

Nursing Mothers: The Centers for Disease Control and Prevention recommend that HIV-infected mothers not breast-feed their infants to avoid risking postnatal transmission of HIV. It is not known whether emtricitabine is secreted into human milk. Because of both the potential for HIV transmission and the potential for serious adverse reactions in nursing infants, **mothers should be instructed not to breast-feed if they are receiving EMTRIVA.**

Pediatric Use:

Safety and effectiveness in pediatric patients have not been established.

Geriatric Use:

Clinical studies of EMTRIVA did not contain sufficient numbers of subjects aged 65 years and over to determine whether they respond differently from younger subjects. In general, dose selection for the elderly patient should be cautious, keeping in mind the greater frequency of decreased hepatic, renal, or cardiac function, and of concomitant disease or other drug therapy (see PRECAUTIONS: Patients with Impaired Renal Function and DOSAGE AND ADMINISTRATION).

ADVERSE REACTIONS

More than 2000 adult patients with HIV infection have been treated with EMTRIVA alone or in combination with

other antiretroviral agents for periods of 10 days to 200 weeks in Phase I-III clinical trials.
Assessment of adverse reactions is based on data from studies 301A and 303 in which 571 treatment naïve (301A) and 440 treatment experienced (303) patients received EMTRIVA 200 mg (n=580) or comparator drug (n=431) for 48 weeks.
The most common adverse events that occurred in patients receiving EMTRIVA with other antiretroviral agents in clinical trials were headache, diarrhea, nausea, and rash, which were generally of mild to moderate severity. Approximately 1% of patients discontinued participation in the clinical studies due to these events. All adverse events were reported with similar frequency in EMTRIVA and control treatment groups with the exception of skin discoloration which was reported with higher frequency in the EMTRIVA treated group.
Skin discoloration, manifested by hyperpigmentation on the palms and/or soles was generally mild and asymptomatic. The mechanism and clinical significance are unknown.
A summary of EMTRIVA treatment emergent clinical adverse events in studies 301A and 303 is provided in Table 6 below.
[See table 6 on previous page]

Laboratory Abnormalities:
Laboratory abnormalities in these studies occurred with similar frequency in the EMTRIVA and comparator groups. A summary of Grade 3 and 4 laboratory abnormalities is provided in Table 7 below.
[See table 7 on previous page]

OVERDOSAGE

There is no known antidote for EMTRIVA. Limited clinical experience is available at doses higher than the therapeutic dose of EMTRIVA. In one clinical pharmacology study single doses of emtricitabine 1200 mg were administered to 11 patients. No severe adverse reactions were reported.
The effects of higher doses are not known. If overdose occurs the patient should be monitored for signs of toxicity, and standard supportive treatment applied as necessary.
Hemodialysis treatment removes approximately 30% of the emtricitabine dose over a 3-hour dialysis period starting within 1.5 hours of emtricitabine dosing (blood flow rate of 400 mL/min and a dialysate flow rate of 600 mL/min). It is not known whether emtricitabine can be removed by peritoneal dialysis.

DOSAGE AND ADMINISTRATION

For adults 18 years of age and older, the dose of EMTRIVA is 200 mg once daily taken orally with or without food.
Dose Adjustment in Patients with Renal Impairment:
Significantly increased drug exposures were seen when EMTRIVA was administered to patients with renal impairment, **(see CLINICAL PHARMACOLOGY: Special Populations)**. Therefore, the dosing interval of EMTRIVA should be adjusted in patients with baseline creatinine clearance < 50 mL/min using the following guidelines (see Table 8). The safety and effectiveness of these dosing interval adjustment guidelines have not been clinically evaluated. Therefore, clinical response to treatment and renal function should be closely monitored in these patients.
[See table 8 on previous page]

HOW SUPPLIED

EMTRIVA is available as capsules. EMTRIVA capsules, 200 mg, are size 1 hard gelatin capsules with a blue cap and white body, printed with "200 mg" in black on the cap and "GILEAD" and the corporate logo in black on the body.
They are packaged in bottles of 30 capsules (NDC 61958-0601-1) with induction sealed child-resistant closures.
Store at 25 °C (77 °F); excursions permitted to 15 °C–30 °C (59 °F–86 °F) [see USP Controlled Room Temperature].
EMTRIVA is manufactured for Gilead Sciences, Inc., Foster City, CA 94404.
July 2003
EMTRIVA™ is a trademark of Gilead Sciences, Inc.

RM-1466
Shown in Product Identification Guide, page 313

HEPSERA™ ℞
[hĕp' sĕră]
adefovir dipivoxil Tablets
℞ Only

WARNINGS

1. SEVERE ACUTE EXACERBATIONS OF HEPATITIS HAVE BEEN REPORTED IN PATIENTS WHO HAVE DISCONTINUED ANTI-HEPATITIS B THERAPY, INCLUDING THERAPY WITH HEPSERA. HEPATIC FUNCTION SHOULD BE MONITORED CLOSELY IN PATIENTS WHO DISCONTINUE ANTI-HEPATITIS B THERAPY. IF APPROPRIATE, RESUMPTION OF ANTI-HEPATITIS B THERAPY MAY BE WARRANTED (SEE WARNINGS).
2. IN PATIENTS AT RISK OF OR HAVING UNDERLYING RENAL DYSFUNCTION, CHRONIC ADMINISTRATION OF HEPSERA MAY RESULT IN NEPHROTOXICITY. THESE PATIENTS SHOULD BE MONITORED CLOSELY FOR RENAL FUNCTION AND MAY REQUIRE DOSE ADJUSTMENT (SEE WARNINGS AND DOSAGE AND ADMINISTRATION).
3. HIV RESISTANCE MAY EMERGE IN CHRONIC HEPATITIS B PATIENTS WITH UNRECOGNIZED OR UNTREATED HUMAN IMMUNODEFICIENCY VIRUS (HIV) INFECTION TREATED WITH ANTI-HEPATITIS B THERAPIES, SUCH AS THERAPY WITH HEPSERA, THAT MAY HAVE ACTIVITY AGAINST HIV (SEE WARNINGS).
4. LACTIC ACIDOSIS AND SEVERE HEPATOMEGALY WITH STEATOSIS, INCLUDING FATAL CASES, HAVE BEEN REPORTED WITH THE USE OF NUCLEOSIDE ANALOGS ALONE OR IN COMBINATION WITH OTHER ANTIRETROVIRALS (SEE WARNINGS).

DESCRIPTION

HEPSERA is the tradename for adefovir dipivoxil, a diester prodrug of adefovir. Adefovir is an acyclic nucleotide analog with activity against human hepatitis B virus (HBV).
The chemical name of adefovir dipivoxil is 9-[2-[bis[(pivaloyloxy)methoxy]phosphinyl]methoxy]ethyl]adenine. It has a molecular formula of $C_{20}H_{32}N_5O_8P$, a molecular weight of 501.48 and the following structural formula:

NH2 N N N N O P O O O O O O O

Adefovir dipivoxil is a white to off-white crystalline powder with an aqueous solubility of 19 mg/mL at pH 2.0 and 0.4 mg/mL at pH 7.2. It has an octanol/aqueous phosphate buffer (pH 7) partition coefficient (log p) of 1.91.
HEPSERA tablets are for oral administration. Each tablet contains 10 mg of adefovir dipivoxil and the following inactive ingredients: croscarmellose sodium, lactose monohydrate, magnesium stearate, pregelatinized starch, and talc.

Microbiology
Mechanism of Action:
Adefovir is an acyclic nucleotide analog of adenosine monophosphate. Adefovir is phosphorylated to the active metabolite, adefovir diphosphate, by cellular kinases. Adefovir diphosphate inhibits HBV DNA polymerase (reverse transcriptase) by competing with the natural substrate deoxyadenosine triphosphate and by causing DNA chain termination after its incorporation into viral DNA. The inhibition constant (K_i) for adefovir diphosphate for HBV DAN polymerase was 0.1 µM. Adefovir diphosphate is a weak inhibitor of human DNA polymerases α and γ with K_i values of 1.18 µM and 0.97 µM, respectively.
Antiviral Activity:
The *in vitro* antiviral activity of adefovir was determined in HBV transfected human hepatoma cell lines. The concentration of adefovir that inhibited 50% of viral DNA synthesis (IC_{50}) varied from 0.2 to 2.5 µM.
Drug Resistance:
Clinical Studies 437 & 438
Genotypic and phenotypic analyses of serum HBV DNA from adefovir dipivoxil (10 mg or 30 mg) treated HBeAg-positive patients (n = 215; study 437) and HBeAg-negative patients (n = 56; study 438) at baseline and week 48 did not identify mutations in the HBV DNA polymerase gene that may confer reduced susceptibility to adefovir. An unconfirmed increase of ≥ 1 log_{10} copies/mL in serum HBV DNA was observed in some patients. The molecular basis and/or the clinical significance for the observed unconfirmed increases are not known.
Cross-resistance:
Recombinant HBV variants containing lamivudine-resistance-associated mutations (L528M, M552I, M552V, L528M + M552V) in the HBV DNA polymerase gene were susceptible to adefovir *in vitro*. Adefovir has also demonstrated anti-HBV activity (median reduction in serum HBV DNA of 4.3 log_{10} copies/mL) against clinical isolates of HBV containing lamivudine-resistance-associated mutations (study 435). HBV variants with DNA polymerase mutations T476N and R or W501Q associated with resistance to hepatitis B immunoglobulin were susceptible to adefovir *in vitro*.

CLINICAL PHARMACOLOGY
Pharmacokinetics
The pharmacokinetics of adefovir have been evaluated in healthy volunteers and patients with chronic hepatitis B. Adefovir pharmacokinetics are similar between these populations.

Table 1. Pharmacokinetic Parameters (Mean ± SD) of Adefovir in Patients with Varying Degrees of Renal Function

Renal Function Group	Unimpaired	Mild	Moderate	Severe
Baseline Creatinine Clearance (mL/min)	> 80 (n = 7)	50 – 80 (n = 8)	30 – 49 (n = 7)	10 – 29 (n = 10)
C_{max} (ng/mL)	17.8 ± 3.22	22.4 ± 4.04	28.5 ± 8.57	51.6 ± 10.3
$AUC_{0-\infty}$ (ng•h/mL)	201 ± 40.8	266 ± 55.7	455 ± 176	1240 ± 629
CL/F (mL/min)	469 ± 99.0	356 ± 85.6	237 ± 118	91.7 ± 51.3
CL_{renal} (mL/min)	231 ± 48.9	148 ± 39.3	83.9 ± 27.5	37.0 ± 18.4

Absorption:
Adefovir dipivoxil is a diester prodrug of the active moiety adefovir. Based on a cross study comparison, the approximate oral bioavailability of adefovir from a 10 mg single dose of HEPSERA is 59%.
Following oral administration of a 10 mg single dose of HEPSERA to chronic hepatitis B patients (n = 14), the peak adefovir plasma concentration (C_{max}) was 18.4 ± 6.26 ng/mL (mean ± SD) and occurred between 0.58 and 4.00 hours (median = 1.75 hours) post dose. The adefovir area under the plasma concentration-time curve ($AUC_{0-\infty}$) was 220 ± 70.0 ng•h/mL. Plasma adefovir concentrations declined in a biexponential manner with a terminal elimination half-life of 7.48 ± 1.65 hours.
The pharmacokinetics of adefovir in subjects with adequate renal function were not affected by once daily dosing of 10 mg HEPSERA over seven days. The impact of long-term once daily administration of 10 mg HEPSERA on adefovir pharmacokinetics has not been evaluated.
Effects of Food on Oral Absorption:
Adefovir exposure was unaffected when a 10 mg single dose of HEPSERA was administered with food (an approximately 1000 kcal high-fat meal). HEPSERA may be taken without regard to food.
Distribution:
In vitro binding of adefovir to human plasma or human serum proteins is ≤ 4% over the adefovir concentration range of 0.1 to 25 µg/mL. The volume of distribution at steady-state following intravenous administration of 1.0 or 3.0 mg/kg/day is 392 ± 75 and 352 ± 9 mL/kg, respectively.
Metabolism and Elimination:
Following oral administration, adefovir dipivoxil is rapidly converted to adefovir. Forty-five percent of the dose is recovered as adefovir in the urine over 24 hours at steady-state following 10 mg oral doses of HEPSERA. Adefovir is renally excreted by a combination of glomerular filtration and active tubular secretion **(See Drug Interactions)**.
Special Populations:
Gender
The pharmacokinetics of adefovir were similar in male and female patients.
Race
Insufficient data are available to determine the effect of race on the pharmacokinetics of adefovir.
Pediatric and Geriatric Patients
Pharmacokinetic studies have not been conducted in children or in the elderly.
Renal Impairment
In subjects with moderately or severely impaired renal function or with end-stage renal disease (ESRD) requiring hemodialysis, C_{max}, AUC, and half-life ($T_{1/2}$) were increased compared to subjects with normal renal function. It is recommended that the dosing interval of HEPSERA be modified in these patients **(See DOSAGE AND ADMINISTRATION)**.
The pharmacokinetics of adefovir in non-chronic hepatitis B patients with varying degrees of renal impairment are described in Table 1. In this study, subjects received a 10 mg single dose of HEPSERA.
[See table 1 above]
A four-hour period of hemodialysis removed approximately 35% of the adefovir dose. The effect of peritoneal dialysis on adefovir removal has not been evaluated.
Hepatic Impairment
The pharmacokinetics of adefovir following a 10 mg single dose of HEPSERA have been studied in non-chronic hepatitis B patients with hepatic impairment. There were no substantial alterations in adefovir pharmacokinetics in patients with moderate and severe hepatic impairment compared to unimpaired patients. No change in HEPSERA dosing is required in patients with hepatic impairment.
Drug Interactions:
Adefovir dipivoxil is rapidly converted to adefovir *in vivo*. At concentrations substantially higher (> 4000 fold) than those observed *in vivo*, adefovir did not inhibit any of the common human CYP450 enzymes, CYP1A2, CYP2C9, CYP2C19, CYP2D6, and CYP3A4. Adefovir is not a substrate for these enzymes. However, the potential for adefovir to induce CYP450 enzymes is unknown. Based on the results of these *in vitro* experiments and the renal elimination pathway of adefovir, the potential for CYP450 mediated interactions involving adefovir as an inhibitor or substrate with other medicinal products is low.
The pharmacokinetics of adefovir have been evaluated following multiple dose administration of HEPSERA (10 mg once daily) in combination with lamivudine (100 mg once daily), trimethoprim/sulfamethoxazole (160/800 mg twice

Continued on next page

Hepsera—Cont.

daily), acetaminophen (1000 mg four times daily) and ibuprofen (800 mg three times daily) in healthy volunteers (n = 18 per study).

Adefovir did not alter the pharmacokinetics of lamivudine, trimethoprim/sulfamethoxazole, acetaminophen and ibuprofen.

The pharmacokinetics of adefovir were unchanged when HEPSERA was co-administered with lamivudine, trimethoprim/sulfamethoxazole and acetaminophen. When HEPSERA was co-administered with ibuprofen (800 mg three times daily) increases in adefovir C_{max} (33%), AUC (23%) and urinary recovery were observed. This increase appears to be due to higher oral bioavailability, not a reduction in renal clearance of adefovir.

INDICATIONS AND USAGE

HEPSERA is indicated for the treatment of chronic hepatitis B in adults with evidence of active viral replication and either evidence of persistent elevations in serum aminotransferases (ALT or AST) or histologically active disease. This indication is based on histological, virological, biochemical, and serological responses in adult patients with HBeAg+ and HBeAg- chronic hepatitis B with compensated liver function, and in adult patients with clinical evidence of lamivudine-resistant hepatitis B virus with either compensated or decompensated liver function.

Description of Clinical Studies

HBeAg-positive Chronic Hepatitis B:

Study 437 was a randomized, double-blind, placebo-controlled, three-arm study in patients with HBeAg-positive chronic hepatitis B that allowed for a comparison between placebo and HEPSERA. The median age of patients was 33 years. Seventy-four percent were male, 59% were Asian, 36% were Caucasian and 24% has prior interferon-α treatment. At baseline, patients had a median total Knodell Histology Activity Index (HAI) score of 10, a median serum HBV DNA level as measured by an experimental polymerase chain reaction assay of 8.36 $\log_{10}$ copies/mL and a median ALT level of 2.3 times the upper limit of normal.

HBeAg-negative (anti-HBe positive/HBV DNA positive) Chronic Hepatitis B:

Study 438 was a randomized, double-blind, placebo-controlled study in patients who were HBeAg-negative at screening, and anti-HBe positive. The median age of patients was 46 years. Eight-three percent were male, 66% were Caucasian, 30% were Asian and 41% had prior interferon-α treatment. At baseline, the median total Knodell HAI score was 10, the median serum HBV DNA level as measured by an experimental polymerase chain reaction assay was 7.08 $\log_{10}$ copies/mL, and the median ALT was 2.3 times the upper limit of normal.

The primary efficacy endpoint in both studies was histological improvement at week 48; results of which are shown in Table 2.

[See table 2 above]

Table 2. Histological Response at Week 48*

	Study 437		Study 438	
	HEPSERA 10 mg	Placebo	HEPSERA 10 mg	Placebo
	(n = 168)	(n = 161)	(n = 121)	(n = 57)
Improvement**	53%	25%	64%	35%
No Improvement	37%	67%	29%	63%
Missing/Unassessable Data	10%	7%	7%	2%

* Intent-to-Treat population (patients with ≥ 1 dose of study drug) with assessable baseline biopsies

** Histological improvement defined as ≥ 2 point decrease in the Knodell necro-inflammatory score with no worsening of the Knodell fibrosis score

Table 3 illustrates the changes in Ishak Fibrosis Score by treatment group.

[See table 3 above]

Table 3. Changes in Ishak Fibrosis Score at Week 48

	Study 437		Study 438	
	HEPSERA 10 mg	Placebo	HEPSERA 10 mg	Placebo
Number of adequate biopsy pairs	(n = 150)	(n = 146)	(n = 112)	(n = 55)
Ishak Fibrosis Score Improved*	34%	19%	34%	14%
Unchanged	55%	60%	62%	50%
Worsened	11%	21%	4%	36%

* Change of 1 point or more in Ishak Fibrosis Score

At week 48, improvement was seen in respect to mean change in serum HBV DNA ($\log_{10}$ copies/mL), normalization of ALT, and HBeAg seroconversion as compared to placebo in patients receiving HEPSERA (Table 4).

[See table 4 at right]

Table 4. Change in Serum HBV DNA, ALT Normalization, and HBeAg Seroconversion at Week 48

	Study 437		Study 438	
	HEPSERA 10 mg	Placebo	HEPSERA 10 mg	Placebo
	(n = 167)	(n = 171)	(n = 123)	(n = 61)
Mean change ± SD in serum HBV DNA from baseline ($\log_{10}$ copies/mL)	−3.57 ± 1.64	−0.98 ± 1.32	−3.65 ± 1.14	−1.32 ± 1.25
ALT Normalization	48%	16%	72%	29%
HBeAg Seroconversion	12%	6%	NA*	NA*

* Patients with HBeAg-negative disease cannot undergo HBeAg seroconversion

In studies 437 and 438, continued treatment with HEPSERA to 72 weeks resulted in continued maintenance of mean reductions in serum HBV DNA observed at week 48. An increase in the proportion of patients with ALT normalization was also observed in study 437. The effect of continued treatment with HEPSERA on seroconversion is unknown.

Pre- and Post-Liver Transplantation Patients:

HEPSERA was also evaluated in an open-label, uncontrolled study of 324 chronic hepatitis B patients pre- (n = 128) and post- (n = 196) liver transplantation with clinical evidence of lamivudine-resistant hepatitis B virus (study 435). The median baseline HBV DNA as measured by an experimental polymerase chain reaction assay was 7.4 and 8.2 $\log_{10}$ copies/mL, and the median baseline ALT was 1.8 and 2.1 times the upper limit of normal in pre- and post-liver transplantation patients, respectively. Results of this study are displayed in Table 5. Treatment with HEPSERA resulted in a similar reduction in serum HBV DNA regardless of the patterns of lamivudine-resistant HBV DNA polymerase mutations at baseline. The clinical significance of these findings as they relate to histological improvement is not known.

Table 5. Efficacy in Pre- and Post-Liver Transplantation Patients at Week 48

Efficacy Parameter	Pre-Liver Transplantation	Post-Liver Transplantation
	(n = 128)	(n = 196)
Mean change ± SD in serum HBV DNA from baseline ($\log_{10}$ copies/mL)	−3.8 ± 1.4	−4.1 ± 1.6
Stable or improved Child-Pugh-Turcotte score	92%*	96%
Normalization of:**		
ALT	76%	49%
Albumin	81%	76%
Bilirubin	50%	75%
Prothrombin time	83%	20%

* 24 week data

** Denominator in patients with abnormal values at baseline

Clinical Evidence of Lamivudine Resistance:

In study 461, an ongoing double-blind, active-controlled study in 59 chronic hepatitis B patients with clinical evidence of lamivudine-resistant hepatitis B virus, patients were randomized to receive either HEPSERA monotherapy or HEPSERA in combination with lamivudine 100 mg or lamivudine 100 mg alone. At week 16, the mean ± SD decrease in serum HBV DNA as measured by an experimental polymerase chain reaction assay was 3.11 ± 0.94 $\log_{10}$ copies/mL for patients treated with HEPSERA and 2.95 ± 0.64 $\log_{10}$ copies/mL for patients treated with HEPSERA in combination with lamivudine. There was a mean decrease in serum HBV DNA of 0.00 ± 0.28 $\log_{10}$ copies/mL in patients receiving lamivudine alone. The clinical significance of these observed changes in serum HBV DNA has not yet been established.

CONTRAINDICATIONS

HEPSERA is contraindicated in patients with previously demonstrated hypersensitivity to any of the components of the product.

WARNINGS

Exacerbations of Hepatitis after Discontinuation of Treatment

Severe acute exacerbation of hepatitis has been reported in patients who have discontinued anti-hepatitis B therapy, including therapy with HEPSERA. Patients who discontinue HEPSERA should be monitored at repeated intervals over a period of time for hepatic function. If appropriate, resumption of anti-hepatitis B therapy may be warranted.

In clinical trials of HEPSERA, exacerbations of hepatitis (ALT elevations 10 times the upper limit of normal or greater) occurred in up to 25% of patients after discontinuation of HEPSERA. Most of these events occurred within 12 weeks of drug discontinuation. These exacerbations generally occurred in the absence of HBeAg seroconversion, and presented as serum ALT elevations in addition to re-emergence of viral replication. In the HBeAg-positive and HBeAg-negative studies in patients with compensated liver function, the exacerbations were not generally accompanied by hepatic decompensation. However, patients with advanced liver disease or cirrhosis may be at higher risk for hepatic decompensation. Although most events appear to have been self-limited or resolved with re-initiation of treatment, severe hepatitis exacerbations, including fatalities, have been reported. Therefore, patients should be closely monitored after stopping treatment.

Nephrotoxicity

Nephrotoxicity characterized by a delayed onset of gradual increases in serum creatinine and decreases in serum phosphorus was historically shown to be the treatment-limiting toxicity of adefovir dipivoxil therapy at substantially higher doses in HIV-infected patients (60 and 120 mg daily) and in chronic hepatitis B patients (30 mg daily). Chronic administration of HEPSERA (10 mg once daily) may result in nephrotoxicity. The overall risk of nephrotoxicity in patients with adequate renal function is low. However, this is of special importance in patients at risk of or having underlying renal dysfunction and patients taking concomitant nephrotoxic agents such as cyclosporine, tacrolimus, aminoglycosides, vancomycin and non-steroidal anti-inflammatory drugs **(See ADVERSE REACTIONS)**.

It is important to monitor renal function for all patients during treatment with HEPSERA, particularly for those with pre-existing or other risks for renal impairment. Patients with renal insufficiency at baseline or during treatment may require dose adjustment **(See DOSAGE AND ADMINISTRATION)**. The risks and benefits of HEPSERA treatment should be carefully evaluated prior to discontinuing HEPSERA in a patient with treatment-emergent nephrotoxicity.

HIV Resistance
Prior to initiating HEPSERA therapy, HIV antibody testing should be offered to all patients. Treatment with anti-hepatitis B therapies, such as HEPSERA, that have activity against HIV in a chronic hepatitis B patient with unrecognized or untreated HIV infection may result in emergence of HIV resistance. HEPSERA has not been shown to suppress HIV RNA in patients; however, there are limited data on the use of HEPSERA to treat patients with chronic hepatitis B co-infected with HIV.

Lactic Acidosis/Severe Hepatomegaly with Steatosis
Lactic acidosis and severe hepatomegaly with steatosis, including fatal cases, have been reported with the use of nucleoside analogs alone or in combination with antiretrovirals.
A majority of these cases have been in women. Obesity and prolonged nucleoside exposure may be risk factors. Particular caution should be exercised when administering nucleoside analogs to any patient with known risk factors for liver disease; however, cases have also been reported in patients with no known risk factors. Treatment with HEPSERA should be suspended in any patient who develops clinical or laboratory findings suggestive of lactic acidosis or pronounced hepatotoxicity (which may include hepatomegaly and steatosis even in the absence of marked transaminase elevations).

PRECAUTIONS

Drug Interactions
Since adefovir is eliminated by the kidney, co-administration of HEPSERA with drugs that reduce renal function or compete for active tubular secretion may increase serum concentrations of either adefovir and/or these co-administered drugs.
Apart from lamivudine, trimethoprim/sulfamethoxazole and acetaminophen, the effects of co-administration of HEPSERA with drugs that are excreted renally, or other drugs known to affect renal function have not been evaluated **(See CLINICAL PHARMACOLOGY)**.
Patients should be monitored closely for adverse events when HEPSERA is co-administered with drugs that are excreted renally or with other drugs known to affect renal function.
Ibuprofen 800 mg three times daily increased adefovir exposure by approximately 23%. The clinical significance of this increase in adefovir exposure is unknown **(See CLINICAL PHARMACOLOGY)**.
While adefovir does not inhibit common CYP450 enzymes, the potential for adefovir to induce CYP450 enzymes is not known.
The effect of adefovir on cyclosporine and tacrolimus concentrations is not known.

Duration of Treatment
The optimal duration of HEPSERA treatment and the relationship between treatment response and long-term outcomes such as hepatocellular carcinoma or decompensated cirrhosis are not known.

Animal Toxicology
Renal tubular nephropathy characterized by histological alterations and/or increases in BUN and serum creatinine was the primary dose-limiting toxicity associated with administration of adefovir dipivoxil in animals. Nephrotoxicity was observed in animals at systemic exposures approximately 3–10 times higher than those in humans at the recommended therapeutic dose of 10 mg/day.

Carcinogenesis, Mutagenesis, Impairment of Fertility
Carcinogenicity studies in mice and rats receiving adefovir have been conducted. In mice, at dose levels of 1, 3, or 10 mg/kg/day, no treatment-related increases in tumor incidence were found at 10 mg/kg/day (systemic exposure was 10 times that achieved in humans at a therapeutic dose of 10 mg/day). In rats dosed at levels of 0.5, 1.5, or 5 mg/kg/day, no drug-related increase in tumor incidence was observed. The exposure at the high dose was four times that at the human therapeutic dose. Adefovir dipivoxil was mutagenic in the *in vitro* mouse lymphoma cell assay (with or without metabolic activation). Adefovir induced chromosomal aberrations in the *in vitro* human peripheral blood lymphocyte assay without metabolic activation. Adefovir was not clastogenic in the *in vivo* mouse micronucleus assay at doses up to 2,000 mg/kg and it was not mutagenic in the Ames bacterial reverse mutation assay using *S. typhimurium* and *E. coli* strains in the presence and absence of metabolic activation. In reproductive toxicology studies, no evidence of impaired fertility was seen in male or female rats at doses up to 30 mg/kg/day (systemic exposure 19 times that achieved in humans at the therapeutic dose).

Pregnancy
Pregnancy Category C:
Reproduction studies conducted with adefovir dipivoxil administered orally have shown no embryotoxicity or teratogenicity in rats at doses up to 35 mg/kg/day (systemic exposure approximately 23 times that achieved in humans at the therapeutic dose of 10 mg/day), or in rabbits at 20 mg/kg/day (systemic exposure 40 times human).
When adefovir was administered intravenously to pregnant rats at doses associated with notable maternal toxicity (20 mg/kg/day, systemic exposure 38 times human), embryotoxicity and an increased incidence of fetal malformations (anasarca, depressed eye bulge, umbilical hernia and kinked tail) were observed. No adverse effects on development were seen with adefovir administered intravenously to pregnant rats at 2.5 mg/kg/day (systemic exposure 12 times human).

Table 8. Dosing Interval Adjustment of HEPSERA in Patients with Renal Impairment

	Creatinine Clearance (mL/min)*			
	≥ 50	20–49	10–19	Hemodialysis Patients
Recommended Dose and Dosing Interval	10 mg every 24 hours	10 mg every 48 hours	10 mg every 72 hours	10 mg every 7 days following dialysis

* Creatinine clearance calculated by Cockcroft-Gault method using lean or ideal body weight

There are no adequate and well-controlled studies in pregnant women. Because animal reproduction studies are not always predictive of human response, HEPSERA should be used during pregnancy only if clearly needed and after careful consideration of the risks and benefits.

Pregnancy Registry
To monitor fetal outcomes of pregnant women exposed to HEPSERA, a pregnancy registry has been established. Healthcare providers are encouraged to register patients by calling 1-800-258-4263.

Labor and Delivery
There are no studies in pregnant women and no data on the effect of HEPSERA on transmission of HBV from mother to infant. Therefore, appropriate infant immunizations should be used to prevent neonatal acquisition of hepatitis B virus.

Lactating Women
It is not known whether adefovir is excreted in human milk. Mothers should be instructed not to breast-feed if they are taking HEPSERA.

Pediatric Use
Safety and effectiveness in pediatric patients have not been established.

Geriatric Use
Clinical studies of HEPSERA did not include sufficient numbers of patients aged 65 and over to determine whether they respond differently from younger patients. In general, caution should be exercised when prescribing to elderly patients since they have greater frequency of decreased renal or cardiac function due to concomitant disease or other drug therapy.

ADVERSE REACTIONS

Assessment of adverse reactions is based on two studies (437 and 438) in which 522 patients with chronic hepatitis B received double-blind treatment with HEPSERA (n = 294) or placebo (n = 228) for 48 weeks. With extended therapy in the second 48 week treatment period, 492 patients were treated for up to 109 weeks, with a median time on treatment of 49 weeks.
In addition to specific adverse events described under the WARNINGS section, all treatment-related clinical adverse events that occurred in 3% or greater of HEPSERA-treated patients compared with placebo are listed in Table 6. A summary of grade 3 and 4 laboratory abnormalities during therapy with HEPSERA compared with placebo is listed in Table 7.

Table 6. Treatment-Related Adverse Events (Grades 1–4) Reported in ≥ 3% of All HEPSERA-Treated Patients in the Pooled 437 – 438 Studies (0–48 Weeks)

	HEPSERA 10 mg	Placebo
	(n = 294)	(n = 228)
Asthenia	13%	14%
Headache	9%	10%
Abdominal pain	9%	11%
Nausea	5%	8%
Flatulence	4%	4%
Diarrhea	3%	4%
Dyspepsia	3%	2%

Laboratory Abnormalities

Table 7. Grade 3–4 Laboratory Abnormalities Reported in ≥ 1% of All HEPSERA-Treated Patients in the Pooled 437 – 438 Studies (0–48 Weeks)

	HEPSERA 10 mg	Placebo
	(n = 294)	(n = 228)
ALT (> 5 × ULN)	20%	41%
Hematuria (≥ 3+)	11%	10%
AST (> 5 × ULN)	8%	23%
Creatine Kinase (> 4 × ULN)	7%	7%
Amylase (> 2 × ULN)	4%	4%
Glycosuria (≥ 3+)	1%	3%

In patients with adequate renal function, increases in serum creatinine ≥ 0.3 mg/dL from baseline were observed in 4% of patients treated with HEPSERA 10 mg daily compared with 2% of patients in the placebo group by week 48. No patients developed a serum creatinine increase ≥ 0.5 mg/dL from baseline by week 48. By week 96, 10% and 2% of HEPSERA-treated patients, by Kaplan-Meier estimate, had increases in serum creatinine ≥ 0.3 mg/dL and ≥ 0.5 mg/dL from baseline, respectively (no placebo-controlled results were available for comparison beyond week 48). Of the 29 of 492 patients with elevations in serum creatinine ≥ 0.3 mg/dL from baseline, 20 out of 29 resolved on continued treatment (≤ 0.2 mg/dL from baseline), 8 of 29 remained unchanged and 1 of 29 resolved on discontinuing treatment **(See Special Risk Patients section below for changes in serum creatinine in patients with underlying renal insufficiency at baseline).**

Special Risk Patients
Pre- (n = 128) and post-liver transplantation patients (n = 196) with chronic hepatitis B and clinical evidence of lamivudine-resistant hepatitis B virus were treated in an open-label study with HEPSERA for up to 129 weeks, with a median time on treatment of 19 and 56 weeks, respectively. The majority of these patients had some degree of underlying renal insufficiency at baseline or other risk factors for renal dysfunction during treatment. Increases in serum creatinine ≥ 0.3 mg/dL from baseline were observed in 26% of these patients by week 48 and 37% by week 96 by Kaplan-Meier estimates. Increases in serum creatinine ≥ 0.5 mg/dL from baseline were observed in 16% of these patients by week 48 and 31% by week 96. Of the 41 of 324 patients with elevations in serum creatinine ≥ 0.5 mg/dL from baseline, 7 of 41 resolved on continued treatment (≤ 0.3 mg/dL from baseline), 18 of 41 remained unchanged and 16 of 41 had not resolved. Additionally, deceases in serum phosphorus were observed in 4% of these patients by week 48, and 6% by week 96 by Kaplan-Meier estimates. One percent (3 of 324) of pre- and post-liver transplantation patients discontinued HEPSERA due to renal events.
Due to the presence of multiple concomitant risk factors for renal dysfunction in these patients, the contributory role of HEPSERA to these changes in serum creatinine and serum phosphorus is difficult to assess.
The most common treatment-related adverse events reported in pre- and post-liver transplantation patients treated with HEPSERA with a 2% frequency or higher include:
Body as a whole: asthenia, abdominal pain, headache, fever
Gastrointestinal: nausea, vomiting, diarrhea, flatulence, hepatic failure
Metabolic and Nutritional: increases in ALT and AST, abnormal liver function
Respiratory: increased cough, pharyngitis, sinusitis
Skin and Appendages: pruritus, rash
Urogenital: increases in creatinine, renal failure, renal insufficiency

OVERDOSAGE

Doses of adefovir dipivoxil 500 mg daily for 2 weeks and 250 mg daily for 12 weeks have been associated with gastrointestinal side effects. If overdose occurs the patient must be monitored for evidence of toxicity, and standard supportive treatment applied as necessary.
Following a 10 mg single dose of HEPSERA, a four-hour hemodialysis session removed approximately 35% of the adefovir dose.

DOSAGE AND ADMINISTRATION

The recommended dose of HEPSERA in chronic hepatitis B patients with adequate renal function is 10 mg, once daily, taken orally, without regard to food. The optimal duration of treatment is unknown.

Dose Adjustment in Renal Impairment
Significantly increased drug exposures were seen when HEPSERA was administered to patients with renal impairment **(See Pharmacokinetics)**. Therefore, the dosing interval of HEPSERA should be adjusted in patients with baseline creatinine clearance < 50 mL/min using the following suggested guidelines (See Table 8). The safety and effectiveness of these dosing interval adjustment guidelines have not been clinically evaluated. Additionally, it is important to note that these guidelines were derived from data in pa-

Continued on next page

Hepsera—Cont.

tients with pre-existing renal impairment at baseline. They may not be appropriate for patients in whom renal insufficiency evolves during treatment with HEPSERA. Therefore, clinical response to treatment and renal function should be closely monitored in these patients.
[See table 8 at top of previous page]
The pharmacokinetics of adefovir have not been evaluated in non-hemodialysis patients with creatinine clearance < 10 mL/min; therefore, no dosing recommendation is available for these patients.

HOW SUPPLIED

HEPSERA is available as tablets. Each tablet contains 10 mg of adefovir dipivoxil. The tablets are white and debossed with "10" and "GILEAD" on one side and the stylized figure of a liver on the other side. They are packaged as follows: Bottles of 30 tablets (NDC 61958-0501-1) containing desiccant (silica gel) and closed with a child-resistant closure.
Store in original container at 25 °C (77 °F), excursions permitted to 15–30 °C (59–86 °F) (See USP Controlled Room Temperature).
Gilead Sciences, Inc.
Foster City, CA 94404
September 2002
HEPSERA™ is a trademark of Gilead Sciences

GILEAD

Shown in Product Identification Guide, page 313

TRUVADA™ ℞

[trew-va-dă]
(emtricitabine and tenofovir disoproxil fumarate)
Tablets
℞ Only

> **WARNING**
> **LACTIC ACIDOSIS AND SEVERE HEPATOMEGALY WITH STEATOSIS, INCLUDING FATAL CASES, HAVE BEEN REPORTED WITH THE USE OF NUCLEOSIDE ANALOGS ALONE OR IN COMBINATION WITH OTHER ANTIRETROVIRALS (SEE WARNINGS).**
> **TRUVADA™ IS NOT INDICATED FOR THE TREATMENT OF CHRONIC HEPATITIS B VIRUS (HBV) INFECTION AND THE SAFETY AND EFFICACY OF TRUVADA HAVE NOT BEEN ESTABLISHED IN PATIENTS CO-INFECTED WITH HBV AND HIV. SEVERE ACUTE EXACERBATIONS OF HEPATITIS B HAVE BEEN REPORTED IN PATIENTS WHO HAVE DISCONTINUED EMTRIVA® or VIREAD®. HEPATIC FUNCTION SHOULD BE MONITORED CLOSELY WITH BOTH CLINICAL AND LABORATORY FOLLOW-UP FOR AT LEAST SEVERAL MONTHS IN PATIENTS WHO DISCONTINUE TRUVADA AND ARE CO-INFECTED WITH HIV AND HBV. IF APPROPRIATE, INITIATION OF ANTI-HEPATITIS B THERAPY MAY BE WARRANTED (SEE WARNINGS).**

DESCRIPTION

TRUVADA Tablets are fixed dose combination tablets containing emtricitabine and tenofovir disoproxil fumarate. EMTRIVA is the brand name for emtricitabine, a synthetic nucleoside analog of cytidine. Tenofovir disoproxil fumarate (VIREAD, also known as tenofovir DF) is converted in vivo to tenofovir, an acyclic nucleoside phosphonate (nucleotide) analog of adenosine 5'-monophosphate. Both emtricitabine and tenofovir exhibit inhibitory activity against HIV-1 reverse transcriptase.
TRUVADA Tablets are for oral administration. Each film-coated tablet contains 200 mg of emtricitabine and 300 mg of tenofovir disoproxil fumarate, (which is equivalent to 245 mg of tenofovir disoproxil), as active ingredients. The tablets also include the following inactive ingredients: croscarmellose sodium, lactose monohydrate, magnesium stearate, microcrystalline cellulose, and pregelatinized starch (gluten free). The tablets are coated with Opadry II Blue Y-30-10701, which contains FD&C Blue #2 aluminum lake, hypromellose, lactose monohydrate, titanium dioxide, and triacetin.

Emtricitabine: The chemical name of emtricitabine is 5-fluoro-1-(2*R*,5*S*)-[2-(hydroxymethyl)-1,3-oxathiolan-5-yl]-cytosine. Emtricitabine is the (-) enantiomer of a thio analog of cytidine, which differs from other cytidine analogs in that it has a fluorine in the 5-position.
It has a molecular formula of $C_8H_{10}FN_3O_3S$ and a molecular weight of 247.24. It has the following structural formula:

Emtricitabine is a white to off-white crystalline powder with a solubility of approximately 112 mg/mL in water at 25°C. The partition coefficient (log p) for emtricitabine is -0.43 and the pKa is 2.65.

Table 1. Single Dose Pharmacokinetic Parameters for Emtricitabine and Tenofovir in Adults[1]

	Emtricitabine	Tenofovir
Fasted Oral Bioavailability[2] (%)	92 (83.1–106.4)	25 (NC–45.0)
Plasma Terminal Elimination Half-Life[2] (hr)	10 (7.4–18.0)	17 (12.0–25.7)
C_{max}[3] (μg/mL)	1.8 ± 0.72[4]	0.30 ± 0.09
AUC[3] (μg·hr/mL)	10.0 ± 3.12[4]	2.29 ± 0.69
CL/F[3] (mL/min)	302 ± 94	1043 ± 115
CL_{renal}[3] (mL/min)	213 ± 89	243 ± 33

1. NC = Not calculated
2. Median (range)
3. Mean (± SD)
4. Data presented as steady state values.

Tenofovir disoproxil fumarate: Tenofovir disoproxil fumarate is a fumaric acid salt of the bis-isopropoxycarbonyloxymethyl ester derivative of tenofovir. The chemical name of tenofovir disoproxil fumarate is 9-[(*R*)-2 [[bis[[(isopropoxycarbonyl)oxy]-methoxy]phosphinyl]methoxy] propyl]adenine fumarate (1:1). It has a molecular formula of $C_{19}H_{30}N_5O_{10}P \cdot C_4H_4O_4$ and a molecular weight of 635.52. It has the following structural formula:

Tenofovir disoproxil fumarate is a white to off-white crystalline powder with a solubility of 13.4 mg/mL in water at 25 °C. The partition coefficient (log p) for tenofovir disoproxil is 1.25 and the pKa is 3.75. All dosages are expressed in terms of tenofovir disoproxil fumarate except where otherwise noted.

MICROBIOLOGY

Mechanism of Action

Emtricitabine: Emtricitabine, a synthetic nucleoside analog of cytidine, is phosphorylated by cellular enzymes to form emtricitabine 5'-triphosphate. Emtricitabine 5'-triphosphate inhibits the activity of the HIV-1 reverse transcriptase (RT) by competing with the natural substrate deoxycytidine 5'-triphosphate and by being incorporated into nascent viral DNA which results in chain termination. Emtricitabine 5'-triphosphate is a weak inhibitor of mammalian DNA polymerase α, β, ε and mitochondrial DNA polymerase γ.

Tenofovir disoproxil fumarate: Tenofovir disoproxil fumarate is an acyclic nucleoside phosphonate diester analog of adenosine monophosphate. Tenofovir disoproxil fumarate requires initial diester hydrolysis for conversion to tenofovir and subsequent phosphorylations by cellular enzymes to form tenofovir diphosphate. Tenofovir diphosphate inhibits the activity of HIV-1 RT by competing with the natural substrate deoxyadenosine 5'-triphosphate and, after incorporation into DNA, by DNA chain termination. Tenofovir diphosphate is a weak inhibitor of mammalian DNA polymerases α, β, and mitochondrial DNA polymerase γ.

Antiviral Activity

Emtricitabine and tenofovir disoproxil fumarate: In combination studies evaluating the in vitro antiviral activity of emtricitabine and tenofovir together, synergistic antiviral effects were observed.

Emtricitabine: The in vitro antiviral activity of emtricitabine against laboratory and clinical isolates of HIV was assessed in lymphoblastoid cell lines, the MAGI-CCR5 cell line, and peripheral blood mononuclear cells. The IC_{50} values for emtricitabine were in the range of 0.0013–0.64 μM (0.0003–0.158 μg/mL). In drug combination studies of emtricitabine with nucleoside reverse transcriptase inhibitors (abacavir, lamivudine, stavudine, zalcitabine, zidovudine), non-nucleoside reverse transcriptase inhibitors (delavirdine, efavirenz, nevirapine), and protease inhibitors (amprenavir, nelfinavir, ritonavir, saquinavir), additive to synergistic effects were observed. Most of these drug combinations have not been studied in humans. Emtricitabine displayed antiviral activity in vitro against HIV-1 clades A, B, C, D, E, F, and G (IC_{50} values ranged from 0.007–0.075 μM) and showed strain specific activity against HIV-2 (IC_{50} values ranged from 0.007–1.5 μM).

Tenofovir disoproxil fumarate: The in vitro antiviral activity of tenofovir against laboratory and clinical isolates of HIV-1 was assessed in lymphoblastoid cell lines, primary monocyte/macrophage cells and peripheral blood lymphocytes. The IC_{50} (50% inhibitory concentration) values for tenofovir were in the range of 0.04–8.5 μM. In drug combination studies of tenofovir with nucleoside reverse transcriptase inhibitors (abacavir, didanosine, lamivudine, stavudine, zalcitabine, zidovudine), non-nucleoside reverse transcriptase inhibitors (delavirdine, efavirenz, nevirapine), and protease inhibitors (amprenavir, indinavir, nelfinavir, ritonavir, saquinavir), additive to synergistic effects were observed. Most of these drug combinations have not been studied in humans. Tenofovir displayed antiviral activity in vitro against HIV-1 clades A, B, C, D, E, F, G and O (IC_{50} values ranged from 0.5–2.2 μM).

Resistance

Emtricitabine and tenofovir disoproxil fumarate: HIV-1 isolates with reduced susceptibility to the combination of emtricitabine and tenofovir have been selected in vitro. Genotypic analysis of these isolates identified the M184I/V and/or K65R amino acid substitutions in the viral RT.

Emtricitabine: Emtricitabine-resistant isolates of HIV have been selected in vitro. Genotypic analysis of these isolates showed that the reduced susceptibility to emtricitabine was associated with a mutation in the HIV RT gene at codon 184 which resulted in an amino acid substitution of methionine by valine or isoleucine (M184V/I).
Emtricitabine-resistant isolates of HIV have been recovered from some patients treated with emtricitabine alone or in combination with other antiretroviral agents. In a clinical study, viral isolates from 6/16 (37.5%) treatment-naïve patients with virologic failure showed >20-fold reduced susceptibility to emtricitabine. Genotypic analysis of these isolates showed that the resistance was due to M184V/I mutations in the HIV RT gene.

Tenofovir disoproxil fumarate: HIV-1 isolates with reduced susceptibility to tenofovir have been selected in vitro. These viruses expressed a K65R mutation in RT and showed a 2–4 fold reduction in susceptibility to tenofovir.
Tenofovir-resistant isolates of HIV-1 have also been recovered from some patients treated with VIREAD in combination with certain antiretroviral agents. In treatment-naïve patients, 7/29 (24%) isolates from patients failing VIREAD + lamivudine + efavirenz at 48 weeks showed >1.4 fold (median 3.4) reduced susceptibility in vitro to tenofovir. In treatment-experienced patients, 14/304 (4.6%, Studies 902 and 907) isolates from patients failing VIREAD at 96 weeks showed >1.4 fold (median 2.7) reduced susceptibility to tenofovir. Genotypic analysis of the resistant isolates showed a mutation in the HIV-1 RT gene resulting in the K65R amino acid substitution.

Cross-resistance

Emtricitabine and tenofovir disoproxil fumarate: Cross-resistance among certain nucleoside reverse transcriptase inhibitors (NRTIs) has been recognized. The M184V/I and/or K65R substitutions selected in vitro by the combination of emtricitabine and tenofovir are also observed in some HIV-1 isolates from subjects failing treatment with tenofovir in combination with either lamivudine or emtricitabine, and either abacavir or didanosine. Therefore, cross-resistance among these drugs may occur in patients whose virus harbors either or both of these amino acid substitutions.

Emtricitabine: Emtricitabine-resistant isolates (M184V/I) were cross-resistant to lamivudine and zalcitabine but retained susceptibility in vitro to didanosine, stavudine, tenofovir, zidovudine, and NNRTIs (delavirdine, efavirenz, and nevirapine). Isolates from heavily treatment-experienced patients containing the M184V/I amino acid substitution in the context of other NRTI resistance-associated substitutions may retain susceptibility to tenofovir. HIV-1 isolates containing the K65R substitution, selected in vivo by abacavir, didanosine, tenofovir, and zalcitabine, demonstrated reduced susceptibility to inhibition by emtricitabine. Viruses harboring mutations conferring reduced susceptibility to stavudine and zidovudine (M41L, D67N, K70R, L210W, T215Y/F, K219Q/E) or didanosine (L74V) remained sensitive to emtricitabine. HIV-1 containing the K103N substitution associated with resistance to NNRTIs was susceptible to emtricitabine.

Tenofovir disoproxil fumarate: HIV-1 isolates from patients (N=20) whose HIV-1 expressed a mean of 3 zidovudine-associated RT amino acid substitutions (M41L, D67N, K70R, L210W, T215Y/F or K219Q/E/N) showed a 3.1-fold decrease in the susceptibility to tenofovir. Multinucleoside resistant HIV-1 with a T69S double insertion mutation in the RT showed reduced susceptibility to tenofovir.

CLINICAL PHARMACOLOGY

Pharmacokinetics in Adults

TRUVADA: One TRUVADA Tablet was bioequivalent to one EMTRIVA Capsule (200 mg) plus one VIREAD Tablet

(300 mg) following single-dose administration to fasting healthy subjects (N=39).

Emtricitabine: The pharmacokinetic properties of emtricitabine are summarized in Table 1. Following oral administration of EMTRIVA, emtricitabine is rapidly absorbed with peak plasma concentrations occurring at 1–2 hours post-dose. In vitro binding of emtricitabine to human plasma proteins is <4% and is independent of concentration over the range of 0.02–200 µg/mL. Following administration of radiolabelled emtricitabine, approximately 86% is recovered in the urine and 13% is recovered as metabolites. The metabolites of emtricitabine include 3′-sulfoxide diastereomers and their glucuronic acid conjugate. Emtricitabine is eliminated by a combination of glomerular filtration and active tubular secretion. Following a single oral dose of EMTRIVA, the plasma emtricitabine half-life is approximately 10 hours.

Tenofovir disoproxil fumarate: The pharmacokinetic properties of tenofovir disoproxil fumarate are summarized in Table 1. Following oral administration of VIREAD, maximum tenofovir serum concentrations are achieved in 1.0 ± 0.4 hour. In vitro binding of tenofovir to human plasma proteins is <0.7% and is independent of concentration over the range of 0.01–25 µg/mL. Approximately 70–80% of the intravenous dose of tenofovir is recovered as unchanged drug in the urine. Tenofovir is eliminated by a combination of glomerular filtration and active tubular secretion. Following a single oral dose of VIREAD, the terminal elimination half-life of tenofovir is approximately 17 hours.

[See table 1 at top of previous page]

Effects of Food on Oral Absorption

TRUVADA may be administered with or without food. Administration of TRUVADA following a high fat meal (784 kcal; 49 grams of fat) or a light meal (373 kcal; 8 grams of fat) delayed the time of tenofovir C_{max} by approximately 0.75 hour. The mean increases in tenofovir AUC and C_{max} were approximately 35% and 15%, respectively, when administered with a high fat or light meal, compared to administration in the fasted state. In previous safety and efficacy studies, VIREAD (tenofovir) was taken under fed conditions. Emtricitabine systemic exposures (AUC and C_{max}) were unaffected when TRUVADA was administered with either a high fat or a light meal.

Special Populations

Race

Emtricitabine: No pharmacokinetic differences due to race have been identified following the administration of EMTRIVA.

Tenofovir disoproxil fumarate: There were insufficient numbers from racial and ethnic groups other than Caucasian to adequately determine potential pharmacokinetic differences among these populations following the administration of VIREAD.

Gender

Emtricitabine and tenofovir disoproxil fumarate: Emtricitabine and tenofovir pharmacokinetics are similar in male and female patients.

Pediatric and Geriatric Patients: Pharmacokinetics of emtricitabine and tenofovir have not been fully evaluated in children (<18 years) or in the elderly (>65 years) (see PRECAUTIONS, Pediatric Use, Geriatric Use).

Patients with Impaired Renal Function: The pharmacokinetics of emtricitabine and tenofovir are altered in patients with renal impairment (see WARNINGS, Renal Impairment). In patients with creatinine clearance <50 mL/min, C_{max}, and $AUC_{0-\infty}$ of emtricitabine and tenofovir were increased. It is recommended that the dosing interval for TRUVADA be modified in patients with creatinine clearance 30–49 mL/min. TRUVADA should not be used in patients with creatinine clearance <30 mL/min and in patients with end-stage renal disease requiring dialysis (see WARNINGS, Renal Impairment).

Patients with Hepatic Impairment: The pharmacokinetics of tenofovir following a 300 mg dose of VIREAD have been studied in non-HIV infected patients with moderate to severe hepatic impairment. There were no substantial alterations in tenofovir pharmacokinetics in patients with hepatic impairment compared with unimpaired patients. The pharmacokinetics of TRUVADA or emtricitabine have not been studied in patients with hepatic impairment; however, emtricitabine is not significantly metabolized by liver enzymes, so the impact of liver impairment should be limited.

Pregnancy: (see PRECAUTIONS, Pregnancy)

Nursing Mothers: (see PRECAUTIONS, Nursing Mothers)

Drug Interactions: (see PRECAUTIONS, Drug Interactions)

TRUVADA: No drug interaction studies have been conducted using TRUVADA Tablets.

Emtricitabine and tenofovir disoproxil fumarate: The steady state pharmacokinetics of emtricitabine and tenofovir were unaffected when emtricitabine and tenofovir disoproxil fumarate were administered together versus each agent dosed alone.

In vitro and clinical pharmacokinetic drug-drug interaction studies have shown the potential for CYP450 mediated interactions involving emtricitabine and tenofovir with other medicinal products is low.

Emtricitabine and tenofovir are primarily excreted by the kidneys by a combination of glomerular filtration and active tubular secretion. No drug-drug interactions due to competition for renal excretion have been observed; however, coadministration of TRUVADA with drugs that are eliminated by active tubular secretion may increase concentrations of emtricitabine, tenofovir, and/or the co-administered drug.

Table 2. Drug Interactions: Changes in Pharmacokinetic Parameters for Emtricitabine in the Presence of the Co-administered Drug[1]

Co-administered Drug	Dose of Co-administered Drug (mg)	Emtricitabine Dose (mg)	N	% Change of Emtricitabine Pharmacokinetic Parameters[2] (90% CI)		
				C_{max}	AUC	C_{min}
Tenofovir DF	300 once daily × 7 days	200 once daily × 7 days	17	⇔	⇔	↑20 (↑12 to ↑29)
Indinavir	800 × 1	200 × 1	12	⇔	⇔	NA
Famciclovir	500 × 1	200 × 1	12	⇔	⇔	NA
Stavudine	40 × 1	200 × 1	6	⇔	⇔	NA

1. All interaction studies conducted in healthy volunteers.
2. ↑ = Increase; ↓ = Decrease; ⇔ = No Effect; NA = Not Applicable

Table 3. Drug Interactions: Changes in Pharmacokinetic Parameters for Co-administered Drug in the Presence of Emtricitabine[1]

Co-administered Drug	Dose of Co-administered Drug (mg)	Emtricitabine Dose (mg)	N	% Change of Co-administered Drug Pharmacokinetic Parameters[2] (90% CI)		
				C_{max}	AUC	C_{min}
Tenofovir DF	300 once daily × 7 days	200 once daily × 7 days	17	⇔	⇔	⇔
Indinavir	800 × 1	200 × 1	12	⇔	⇔	NA
Famciclovir	500 × 1	200 × 1	12	⇔	⇔	NA
Stavudine	40 × 1	200 × 1	6	⇔	⇔	NA

1. All interaction studies conducted in healthy volunteers.
2. ↑ = Increase; ↓ = Decrease; ⇔ = No Effect; NA = Not Applicable

Table 4. Drug Interactions: Changes in Pharmacokinetic Parameters for Tenofovir[1] in the Presence of the Co-administered Drug

Co-administered Drug	Dose of Co-administered Drug (mg)	N	% Change of Tenofovir Pharmacokinetic Parameters[2] (90% CI)		
			C_{max}	AUC	C_{min}
Abacavir	300 once	8	⇔	⇔	NC
Adefovir dipivoxil	10 once	22	⇔	⇔	NC
Atazanavir[3]	400 once daily × 14 days	33	↑14 (↑8 to ↑20)	↑24 (↑21 to ↑28)	↑22 (↑15 to ↑30)
Didanosine (enteric-coated)	400 once	25	⇔	⇔	⇔
Didanosine (buffered)	250 or 400 once daily × 7 days	14	⇔	⇔	⇔
Efavirenz	600 once daily × 14 days	29	⇔	⇔	⇔
Emtricitabine	200 once daily × 7 days	17	⇔	⇔	⇔
Indinavir	800 three times daily × 7 days	13	↑14 (↓3 to ↑33)	⇔	⇔
Lamivudine	150 twice daily × 7 days	15	⇔	⇔	⇔
Lopinavir/ Ritonavir	400/100 twice daily × 14 days	24	⇔	↑32 (↑26 to ↑38)	↑51 (↑32 to ↑66)

1. Patients received VIREAD 300 mg once daily.
2. Increase = ↑; Decrease = ↓; No Effect = ⇔; NC = Not Calculated
3. REYATAZ™ Prescribing Information (Bristol-Myers Squibb)

Drugs that decrease renal function may increase concentrations of emtricitabine and/or tenofovir.

No clinically significant drug interactions have been observed between emtricitabine and famciclovir, indinavir, stavudine, and tenofovir disoproxil fumarate (see Tables 2 and 3). Similarly, no clinically significant drug interactions have been observed between tenofovir disoproxil fumarate and abacavir, adefovir dipivoxil, ribavirin, efavirenz, emtricitabine, indinavir, lamivudine, lopinavir/ritonavir, methadone and oral contraceptives in studies conducted in healthy volunteers (see Tables 4 and 5).

[See table 2 above]
[See table 3 above]
[See table 4 above]
[See table 5 at bottom of next page]

Following multiple dosing to HIV-negative subjects receiving either chronic methadone maintenance therapy or oral contraceptives, or single doses of ribavirin, steady state tenofovir pharmacokinetics were similar to those observed in previous studies, indicating lack of clinically significant drug interactions between these agents and VIREAD.

Co-administration of tenofovir disoproxil fumarate with didanosine results in changes in the pharmacokinetics of didanosine that may be of clinical significance. Table 6 summarizes the effects of tenofovir disoproxil fumarate on the pharmacokinetics of didanosine. Concomitant dosing of tenofovir disoproxil fumarate with didanosine buffered tablets or enteric-coated capsules significantly increases the C_{max} and AUC of didanosine. When didanosine 250 mg enteric-coated capsules were administered with tenofovir disoproxil fumarate, systemic exposures of didanosine were similar to those seen with the 400 mg enteric-coated capsules alone under fasted conditions. The mechanism of this interaction is unknown.

[See table 6 at bottom of next page]

INDICATIONS AND USAGE

TRUVADA is indicated in combination with other antiretroviral agents (such as non-nucleoside reverse transcriptase inhibitors or protease inhibitors) for the treatment of HIV-1 infection in adults. Safety and efficacy studies using TRUVADA Tablets or using EMTRIVA and VIREAD in combination are ongoing.

Both components of TRUVADA have been studied individually, as part of multidrug regimens and have been found to be safe and effective. Since EMTRIVA and lamivudine (3TC) are comparable in their structure, resistance profiles, and efficacy and safety as part of multidrug regimens, existing data from the use of lamivudine and tenofovir in combination have been extrapolated to support use of TRUVADA

Continued on next page

Truvada—Cont.

Tablets for the treatment of HIV-1 infection in adults (see Description of Clinical Studies and Adverse Events). Therefore, in treatment naïve patients, TRUVADA should be considered as an alternative to the combination of VIREAD + EPIVIR® for those patients who might benefit from a once-daily regimen. In treatment experienced patients, the use of TRUVADA should be guided by laboratory testing and treatment history (see Microbiology).

Additional important information regarding the use of TRUVADA for the treatment of HIV-1 infection:

- There are no study results demonstrating the effect of TRUVADA on clinical progression of HIV-1.

Table 5. Drug Interactions: Changes in Pharmacokinetic Parameters for Co-administered Drug in the Presence of Tenofovir

Co-administered Drug	Dose of Co-administered Drug (mg)	N	% Change of Co-administered Drug Pharmacokinetic Parameters[1] (90% CI)		
			C_{max}	AUC	C_{min}
Abacavir	300 once	8	↑12 (↓1 to ↑26)	⇔	NA
Adefovir dipivoxil	10 once	22	⇔	⇔	NA
Atazanavir[2]	400 once daily × 14 days	34	↓21 (↓27 to ↓14)	↓25 (↓30 to ↓19)	↓40 (↓48 to ↓32)
Atazanavir[2]	Atazanavir/ Ritonavir 300/100 once daily × 42 days	10	↓28 (↓50 to ↑5)	↓25[3] (↓42 to ↓3)	↓23[3] (↓46 to ↑10)
Efavirenz	600 once daily × 14 days	30	⇔	⇔	⇔
Emtricitabine	200 once daily × 7 days	17	⇔	⇔	⇔
Indinavir	800 three times daily × 7 days	12	↓11 (↓30 to ↑12)	⇔	⇔
Lamivudine	150 twice daily × 7 days	15	↓24 (↓34 to ↓12)	⇔	⇔
Lopinavir	Lopinavir/Ritonavir 400/100 twice daily × 14 days	24	⇔	⇔	⇔
Methadone[4]	40–110 once daily × 14 days[5]	13	⇔	⇔	⇔
Oral Contraceptives[6]	Ethinyl Estradiol/ Norgestimate (Ortho-Tricyclen®) Once daily × 7 days	20	⇔	⇔	⇔
Ribavirin	600 once	22	⇔	⇔	NA
Ritonavir	Lopinavir/Ritonavir 400/100 twice daily × 14 days	24	⇔	⇔	⇔

1. Increase = ↑; Decrease = ↓; No Effect = ⇔; NA = Not Applicable
2. REYATAZ™ Prescribing Information (Bristol-Myers Squibb)
3. In HIV-infected patients, addition of tenofovir DF to atazanavir 300 mg plus ritonavir 100 mg, resulted in AUC and C_{min} values of atazanavir that were 2.3 and 4-fold higher than the respective values observed for atazanavir 400 mg when given alone.
4. R-(active), S-and total methadone exposures were equivalent when dosed alone or with VIREAD.
5. Individual subjects were maintained on their stable methadone dose. No pharmacodynamic alterations (opiate toxicity or withdrawal signs or symptoms) were reported.
6. Ethinyl estradiol and 17-deacetyl norgestimate (pharmacologically active metabolite) exposures were equivalent when dosed alone or with VIREAD.

Table 6. Drug Interactions: Pharmacokinetic Parameters for Didanosine in the Presence of VIREAD

Didanosine[1] Dose (mg)/ Method of Administration[2]	VIREAD Method of Administration[2]	N	% Difference (90% CI) vs. Didanosine 400 mg Alone, Fasted[3]	
			C_{max}	AUC
Buffered tablets				
400 once daily[4] x 7 days	Fasted 1 hour after didanosine	14	↑28 (↑11 to ↑48)	↑44 (↑31 to ↑59)
Enteric coated capsules				
400 once, fasted	With food, 2 hr after didanosine	26	↑48 (↑25 to ↑76)	↑48 (↑31 to ↑67)
400 once, with food	Simultaneously with didanosine	26	↑64 (↑41 to ↑89)	↑60 (↑44 to ↑79)
250 once, fasted	With food, 2 hr after didanosine	28	↓10 (↓22 to ↑3)	⇔
250 once, fasted	Simultaneously with didanosine	28	⇔	↑14 (0 to ↑31)
250 once, with food	Simultaneously with didanosine	28	↓29 (↓39 to ↓18)	↓11 (↓23 to ↑2)

1. See PRECAUTIONS regarding use of didanosine with VIREAD.
2. Administration with food was with a light meal (~373 kcal, 20% fat).
3. Increase = ↑; Decrease = ↓; No Difference = ⇔
4. Includes 4 subjects weighing <60 kg receiving ddI 250 mg.

- It is not recommended that TRUVADA be used as a component of a triple nucleoside regimen.

Description of Clinical Studies

For safety and efficacy studies using EMTRIVA or VIREAD in combination with other antiretroviral agents, also consult the Prescribing Information for these products.

Safety and efficacy studies using TRUVADA Tablets or using EMTRIVA and VIREAD in combination are ongoing. EMTRIVA and lamivudine (3TC) are both cytosine analogs. They have a similar resistance profile and can each be administered once daily. Multidrug regimens in which EMTRIVA and lamivudine were compared demonstrated similar efficacy and safety (see Studies 303 and 903 below and Adverse Events).

EMTRIVA:

Study 303: EMTRIVA QD + Stable Background Therapy (SBT) Compared to Lamivudine BID + SBT

Study 303 was a 48 week, open-label, active-controlled multicenter study comparing EMTRIVA (200 mg QD) to lamivudine, in combination with stavudine or zidovudine and a protease inhibitor or NNRTI in 440 patients who were on a lamivudine-containing triple-antiretroviral drug regimen for at least 12 weeks prior to study entry and had HIV-1 RNA ≤400 copies/mL.

Patients were randomized 1:2 to continue therapy with lamivudine (150 mg BID) or to switch to EMTRIVA (200 mg QD). All patients were maintained on their stable background regimen. Patients had a mean age of 42 years (range 22–80), 86% were male, 64% Caucasian, 21% African-American and 13% Hispanic. Patients had a mean baseline CD4 cell count of 527 cells/mm^3 (range 37–1909), and a median baseline plasma HIV RNA of 1.7 $\log_{10}$ copies/mL (range 1.7–4.0). The median duration of prior antiretroviral therapy was 27.6 months. Treatment outcomes through 48 weeks are presented in Table 7.

Table 7. Outcomes of Randomized Treatment at Week 48 (Study 303)

Outcome at Week 48	EMTRIVA + ZDV/d4T + NNRTI/PI (N=294)	Lamivudine + ZDV/d4T + NNRTI/PI (N=146)
Responder[1]	77% (67%)	82% (72%)
Virologic Failure[2]	7%	8%
Death	0%	<1%
Study Discontinuation Due to Adverse Event	4%	0%
Study Discontinuation For Other Reasons[3]	12%	10%

1. Patients achieved and maintained confirmed HIV RNA <400 copies/mL (<50 copies/mL) through week 48.
2. Includes patients who failed to achieve virologic suppression or rebounded after achieving virologic suppression.
3. Includes lost to follow-up, patient withdrawal, noncompliance, protocol violation and other reasons.

The mean increase from baseline in CD4 cell count was 29 cells/mm^3 for the EMTRIVA arm and 61 cells/mm^3 for the lamivudine arm. Through 48 weeks, in the EMTRIVA group 2 patients (0.7%) experienced a new CDC Class C event, compared to 2 patients (1.4%) in the lamivudine group.

VIREAD:

Study 903: VIREAD + Lamivudine + Efavirenz Compared with Stavudine + Lamivudine + Efavirenz

Data through 48-weeks are reported for Study 903, a double-blind, active-controlled multicenter study comparing VIREAD (300 mg QD) administered in combination with lamivudine and efavirenz versus stavudine, lamivudine, and efavirenz in 600 antiretroviral-naïve patients. Patients had a mean age of 36 years (range 18–64), 74% were male, 64% were Caucasian and 20% were Black. The mean baseline CD4 cell count was 279 cells/mm^3 (range 3–956) and median baseline plasma HIV-1 RNA was 77,600 copies/mL (range 417–5,130,000). Patients were stratified by baseline HIV-1 RNA and CD4 count. Forty-three percent of patients had baseline viral loads >100,000 copies/mL and 39% had CD4 cell counts <200 cells/mL. Treatment outcomes through 48 weeks are presented in Table 8.

Table 8. Outcomes of Randomized Treatment at Week 48 (Study 903)

Outcome at Week 48	VIREAD + 3TC + EFV (N=299)	Stavudine + 3TC + EFV (N=301)
	%	%
Responder[1]	79% (76%)	82% (79%)
Virologic failure[2]	6%	4%
Rebound	5%	3%

Never Suppressed Through Week 48	0%	1%
Added an Antiretroviral Agent	1%	1%
Death	<1%	1%
Discontinued Due to Adverse Event	6%	6%
Discontinued for Other Reasons[3]	8%	7%

1. Patients achieved and maintained confirmed HIV-1 RNA <400 copies/mL (<50 copies/mL) through week 48.
2. Includes confirmed viral rebound and failure to achieve confirmed <400 copies/mL through week 48.
3. Includes lost to follow-up, patient withdrawal, noncompliance, protocol violation and other reasons.

The mean increase from baseline in CD4 cell count was 169 cells/mm^3 for the VIREAD arm and 167 cells/mm^3 for the stavudine arm. Through 48 weeks, eight patients in the VIREAD group and six patients in the stavudine group experienced a new CDC Class C event.

CONTRAINDICATIONS

TRUVADA is contraindicated in patients with previously demonstrated hypersensitivity to any of the components of the product.

WARNINGS

Lactic Acidosis/Severe Hepatomegaly with Steatosis

Lactic acidosis and severe hepatomegaly with steatosis, including fatal cases, have been reported with the use of nucleoside analogs alone or in combination with other antiretrovirals. A majority of these cases have been in women. Obesity and prolonged nucleoside exposure may be risk factors. Particular caution should be exercised when administering nucleoside analogs to any patient with known risk factors for liver disease; however, cases have also been reported in patients with no known risk factors. Treatment with TRUVADA should be suspended in any patient who develops clinical or laboratory findings suggestive of lactic acidosis or pronounced hepatotoxicity (which may include hepatomegaly and steatosis even in the absence of marked transaminase elevations).

Patients with HIV and Hepatitis B Virus Coinfection

It is recommended that all patients with HIV be tested for the presence of hepatitis B virus (HBV) before initiating antiretroviral therapy. TRUVADA is not indicated for the treatment of chronic HBV infection and the safety and efficacy of TRUVADA have not been established in patients co-infected with HBV and HIV. Severe acute exacerbations of hepatitis B have been reported in patients after the discontinuation of EMTRIVA and VIREAD. Hepatic function should be closely monitored with both clinical and laboratory follow up for at least several months in patients who discontinue TRUVADA and are co-infected with HIV and HBV. If appropriate, initiation of anti-hepatitis B therapy may be warranted.

Renal Impairment

Emtricitabine and tenofovir are principally eliminated by the kidney. Dosing interval adjustment of TRUVADA is recommended in all patients with creatinine clearance 30–49 mL/min, (see **DOSAGE AND ADMINISTRATION**). TRUVADA should not be administered to patients with creatine clearance <30 mL/min or patients requiring hemodialysis.

Renal impairment, including cases of acute renal failure and Fanconi syndrome (renal tubular injury with severe hypophosphatemia), has been reported in association with the use of VIREAD (see ADVERSE REACTIONS-**Post Marketing Experience**). The majority of these cases occurred in patients with underlying systemic or renal disease, or in patients taking nephrotoxic agents, however, some cases occurred in patients without identified risk factors.

TRUVADA should be avoided with concurrent or recent use of a nephrotoxic agent. Patients at risk for, or with a history of, renal dysfunction and patients receiving concomitant nephrotoxic agents should be carefully monitored for changes in serum creatinine and phosphorus.

PRECAUTIONS

Drug Interactions

Tenofovir disoproxil fumarate: When tenofovir disoproxil fumarate was administered with didanosine the C_{max} and AUC of didanosine administered as either the buffered or enteric-coated formulation increased significantly (see Table 6). The mechanism of this interaction is unknown. Higher didanosine concentrations could potentiate didanosine-associated adverse events, including pancreatitis, and neuropathy. In adults weighing >60 kg, the didanosine dose should be reduced to 250 mg when it is co-administered with TRUVADA. Data are not available to recommend a dose adjustment of didanosine for patients weighing <60 kg. When co-administered, TRUVADA and VIDEX EC® may be taken under fasted conditions or with a light meal (<400 kcal, 20% fat). Co-administration of didanosine buffered tablet formulation with TRUVADA should be under fasted conditions. **Co-administration of TRUVADA and didanosine should be undertaken with caution and patients receiving this combination should be monitored closely for didanosine-associated adverse events. Didanosine should be discontinued in patients who develop didanosine-associated adverse events.**

Atazanavir and lopinavir/ritonavir have been shown to increase tenofovir concentrations. The mechanism of this interaction is unknown. **Patients receiving atazanavir and lopinavir/ritonavir and TRUVADA should be monitored for TRUVADA-associated adverse events. TRUVADA should be discontinued in patients who develop TRUVADA-associated adverse events.**

Tenofovir decreases the AUC and C_{min} of atazanavir. When coadministered with TRUVADA, it is recommended that atazanavir 300 mg is given with ritonavir 100 mg. **Atazanavir without ritonavir should not be coadministered with TRUVADA.**

Emtricitabine and tenofovir disoproxil fumarate: Since emtricitabine and tenofovir are primarily eliminated by the kidneys, co-administration of TRUVADA with drugs that reduce renal function or compete for active tubular secretion may increase serum concentrations of emtricitabine, tenofovir, and/or other renally eliminated drugs. Some examples include, but are not limited to adefovir dipivoxil, cidofovir, acyclovir, valacyclovir, ganciclovir and valganciclovir.

TRUVADA is a fixed-dose combination of emtricitabine and tenofovir disoproxil fumarate. TRUVADA should not be co-administered with EMTRIVA or VIREAD. Due to similarities between emtricitabine and lamivudine, TRUVADA should not be co-administered with other drugs containing lamivudine, including COMBIVIR®, EPIVIR, EPIVIR-HBV®, EPZICOM™, or TRIZIVIR®.

Bone Effects

Tenofovir disoproxil fumarate: In study 903 through 48 weeks, decreases from baseline in bone mineral density (BMD) were seen at the lumbar spine and hip in both arms of the study. At 48 weeks, percent decreases in BMD from baseline (mean ± SD) were greater in patients receiving VIREAD + lamivudine + efavirenz (spine, -3.3% ± 3.9; hip, -3.2% ± 3.6) compared with patients receiving stavudine + lamivudine + efavirenz (spine, -2.0% ± 3.5; hip, -1.8% ± 3.3). In addition, there were significant increases in levels of four biochemical markers of bone metabolism (serum bone-specific alkaline phosphatase, serum osteocalcin, serum C-telopeptide and urinary N-telopeptide) in the VIREAD group relative to the stavudine group, suggesting increased bone turnover. Serum parathyroid hormone levels were also higher in the VIREAD group relative to the stavudine group. Except for bone specific alkaline phosphatase, these changes resulted in values that remained within the normal range. There was one bone fracture reported in the VIREAD group compared with four in the stavudine group; no pathologic fractures were identified over 48 weeks of study treatment. The clinical significance of the changes in BMD and biochemical markers is unknown and follow-up is continuing to assess long-term impact.

Bone monitoring should be considered for HIV infected patients who have a history of pathologic bone fracture or are at substantial risk for osteopenia. Although the effect of supplementation with calcium and vitamin D was not studied, such supplementation may be considered for HIV-associated osteopenia or osteoporosis. If bone abnormalities are suspected then appropriate consultation should be obtained.

Fat Redistribution

Redistribution/accumulation of body fat including central obesity, dorsocervical fat enlargement (buffalo hump), peripheral wasting, facial wasting, breast enlargement, and "cushingoid appearance" have been observed in patients receiving antiretroviral therapy. The mechanism and long-term consequences of these events are currently unknown. A causal relationship has not been established.

Information for Patients

TRUVADA is not a cure for HIV infection and patients may continue to experience illnesses associated with HIV infection, including opportunistic infections. Patients should remain under the care of a physician when using TRUVADA.

- Patients should be advised that:
- the use of TRUVADA has not been shown to reduce the risk of transmission of HIV to others through sexual contact or blood contamination,
- the long term effects of TRUVADA are unknown,
- TRUVADA Tablets are for oral ingestion only,
- it is important to take TRUVADA with combination therapy on a regular dosing schedule to avoid missing doses,
- redistribution or accumulation of body fat may occur in patients receiving antiretroviral therapy and that the cause and long-term health effects of these conditions are not known.
- TRUVADA should not be co-administered with EMTRIVA or VIREAD, or drugs containing lamivudine, including COMBIVIR, EPIVIR, EPIVIR-HBV, EPZICOM, or TRIZIVIR.

Animal Toxicology

Tenofovir and tenofovir disoproxil fumarate administered in toxicology studies to rats, dogs and monkeys at exposures (based on AUCs) greater than or equal to 6-fold those observed in humans caused bone toxicity. In monkeys the bone toxicity was diagnosed as osteomalacia. Osteomalacia observed in monkeys appeared to be reversible upon dose reduction or discontinuation of tenofovir. In rats and dogs, the bone toxicity manifested as reduced bone mineral density. The mechanism(s) underlying bone toxicity is unknown.

Evidence of renal toxicity was noted in 4 animal species. Increases in serum creatinine, BUN, glycosuria, proteinuria, phosphaturia and/or calciuria and decreases in serum phosphate were observed to varying degrees in these animals. These toxicities were noted at exposures (based on AUCs) 2–20 times higher than those observed in humans. The relationship of the renal abnormalities, particularly the phosphaturia, to the bone toxicity is not known.

Carcinogenesis, Mutagenesis, Impairment of Fertility

Emtricitabine: Long-term carcinogenicity studies of emtricitabine in rats and mice are in progress.

Emtricitabine was not genotoxic in the reverse mutation bacterial test (Ames test), mouse lymphoma or mouse micronucleus assays.

Emtricitabine did not affect fertility in male rats at approximately 140-fold or in male and female mice at approximately 60-fold higher exposures (AUC) than in humans given the recommended 200 mg daily dose. Fertility was normal in the offspring of mice exposed daily from before birth (in utero) through sexual maturity at daily exposures (AUC) of approximately 60-fold higher than human exposures at the recommended 200 mg daily dose.

Tenofovir disoproxil fumarate: Long-term oral carcinogenicity studies of tenofovir disoproxil fumarate in mice and rats were carried out at exposures up to approximately 16 times (mice) and 5 times (rats) those observed in humans at the therapeutic dose for HIV infection. At the high dose in female mice, liver adenomas were increased at exposures 16 times that in humans. In rats, the study was negative for carcinogenic findings at exposures up to 5 times that observed in humans at the therapeutic dose.

Tenofovir disoproxil fumarate was mutagenic in the in vitro mouse lymphoma assay and negative in an in vitro bacterial mutagenicity test (Ames test). In an in vivo mouse micronucleus assay, tenofovir disoproxil fumarate was negative when administered to male mice.

There were no effects on fertility, mating performance or early embryonic development when tenofovir disoproxil fumarate was administered to male rats at a dose equivalent to 10 times the human dose based on body surface area comparisons for 28 days prior to mating and to female rats for 15 days prior to mating through day seven of gestation. There was, however, an alteration of the estrous cycle in female rats.

Pregnancy

Pregnancy Category B:

Emtricitabine: The incidence of fetal variations and malformations was not increased in embryofetal toxicity studies performed with emtricitabine in mice at exposures (AUC) approximately 60-fold higher and in rabbits at approximately 120-fold higher than human exposures at the recommended daily dose.

Tenofovir disoproxil fumarate: Reproduction studies have been performed in rats and rabbits at doses up to 14 and 19 times the human dose based on body surface area comparisons and revealed no evidence of impaired fertility or harm to the fetus due to tenofovir.

There are, however, no adequate and well-controlled studies in pregnant women. Because animal reproduction studies are not always predictive of human response, TRUVADA should be used during pregnancy only if clearly needed.

Antiretroviral Pregnancy Registry: To monitor fetal outcomes of pregnant women exposed to TRUVADA, an Antiretroviral Pregnancy Registry has been established. Healthcare providers are encouraged to register patients by calling 1-800-258-4263.

Nursing Mothers: The Centers for Disease Control and Prevention recommend that HIV-infected mothers not breast-feed their infants to avoid risking postnatal transmission of HIV. Studies in rats have demonstrated that tenofovir is secreted in milk. It is not known whether tenofovir is excreted in human milk. It is not known whether emtricitabine is excreted in human milk. Because of both the potential for HIV transmission and the potential for serious adverse reactions in nursing infants, **mothers should be instructed not to breast-feed if they are receiving TRUVADA.**

Pediatric Use

Safety and effectiveness in pediatric patients have not been established.

Geriatric Use

Clinical studies of EMTRIVA or VIREAD did not include sufficient numbers of subjects aged 65 and over to determine whether they respond differently from younger subjects. In general, dose selection for the elderly patients should be cautious, keeping in mind the greater frequency of decreased hepatic, renal, or cardiac function, and of concomitant disease or other drug therapy.

ADVERSE REACTIONS

Clinical Trials

TRUVADA: Safety and efficacy studies using TRUVADA tablets or using EMTRIVA and VIREAD in combination are ongoing. Two hundred eighty three HIV-1 infected patients have received combination therapy with EMTRIVA or VIREAD with either a non-nucleoside reverse transcriptase inhibitor or protease inhibitor for 24 to 48 weeks in ongoing clinical studies. Based on these limited data, no new patterns of adverse events were identified and there was no increased frequency of established toxicities.

For additional safety information about EMTRIVA or VIREAD in combination with other antiretroviral agents, also consult the Prescribing Information for these products.

EMTRIVA: Adverse events that occurred in >5% of patients receiving EMTRIVA with other antiretroviral agents in clinical trials include abdominal pain, asthenia, headache, di-

Continued on next page

Truvada—Cont.

arrhea, nausea, vomiting, dizziness, and rash event (including rash, pruritus, maculopapular rash, urticaria, vesiculobullous rash, pustular rash and allergic reaction). Approximately 1% of patients discontinued participation in the clinical studies because of these adverse events.
Other adverse events reported include dyspepsia, arthralgia, myalgia, abnormal dreams, depressive disorder, insomnia, neuropathy, peripheral neuritis, paresthesia, increased cough, and rhinitis.
All adverse events were reported with similar frequency in EMTRIVA and control treatment groups with the exception of skin discoloration which was reported with higher frequency in the EMTRIVA treated group. Skin discoloration, manifested by hyperpigmentation on the palms and/or soles was generally mild and asymptomatic. The mechanism and clinical significance are unknown.
Grade 3/4 elevations of ALT and AST (>5 × ULN), bilirubin (>2.5 × ULN), creatine kinase (>4 × ULN), decreased neutrophils (<750/mm^3), pancreatic amylase (>2.0 × ULN), serum amylase (>2 × ULN), serum glucose (<40 or >250 mg/dL), serum lipase (>2.0 × ULN) and triglycerides (>750 mg/dL) have been reported to occur in 1–12% of patients receiving EMTRIVA.
VIREAD: Adverse events that occurred in >5% of patients receiving VIREAD with other antiretroviral agents in clinical trials included: headache, nausea, diarrhea, vomiting, rash event (including rash, pruritus, maculopapular rash, urticaria, vesiculobullous rash, and pustular rash), and depression. Less than 1% of patients discontinued participation in the clinical studies because of gastrointestinal adverse events.
Other adverse events include asthenia, pain, abdominal pain, back pain, chest pain, fever, flatulence, dizziness, dyspepsia, anorexia, arthralgia, insomnia, abnormal dreams, paresthesia, peripheral neuropathy (including peripheral neuritis and neuropathy), pneumonia, sweating, myalgia and weight loss.
Grade 3/4 elevations of ALT and AST (>5 × ULN), creatine kinase (>4 × ULN), serum amylase (>5 × ULN), urine glucose (≥3+), serum glucose (>250 mg/dL) and serum triglycerides (>750 mg/dL), hematuria (>100 RBC/HPF) and decreased neutrophils (<750/mm^3) have been reported to occur in 2–12% of patients receiving VIREAD.
Post Marketing Experience
EMTRIVA: No additional events have been identified for inclusion in this section.
VIREAD: In addition to adverse events reported from clinical trials, the following events have been identified during post-approval use of VIREAD. Because they are reported voluntarily from a population of unknown size, estimates of frequency cannot be made. These events have been chosen for inclusion because of a combination of their seriousness, frequency of reporting or potential causal connection to VIREAD.
IMMUNE SYSTEM DISORDERS
Allergic reaction
METABOLISM AND NUTRITION DISORDERS
Hypophosphatemia, Lactic acidosis
RESPIRATORY, THORACIC, AND MEDIASTINAL DISORDERS
Dyspnea
GASTROINTESTINAL DISORDERS
Abdominal pain, Pancreatitis
RENAL AND URINARY DISORDERS
Renal insufficiency, Renal failure, Acute renal failure, Fanconi syndrome, Proximal tubulopathy, Proteinuria, Increased creatinine, Acute tubular necrosis

OVERDOSAGE

If overdose occurs the patient must be monitored for evidence of toxicity, and standard supportive treatment applied as necessary.
Emtricitabine: Limited clinical experience is available at doses higher than the therapeutic dose of EMTRIVA. In one clinical pharmacology study single doses of emtricitabine 1200 mg were administered to 11 patients. No severe adverse reactions were reported.
Hemodialysis treatment removes approximately 30% of the emtricitabine dose over a 3-hour dialysis period starting within 1.5 hours of emtricitabine dosing (blood flow rate of 400 mL/min and a dialysate flow rate of 600 mL/min). It is not known whether emtricitabine can be removed by peritoneal dialysis.
Tenofovir disoproxil fumarate: Limited clinical experience at doses higher than the therapeutic dose of VIREAD 300 mg is available. In one study, 600 mg tenofovir disoproxil fumarate was administered to 8 patients orally for 28 days, and no severe adverse reactions were reported. The effects of higher doses are not known.
Tenofovir is efficiently removed by hemodialysis with an extraction coefficient of approximately 54%. Following a single 300 mg dose of VIREAD, a four-hour hemodialysis session removed approximately 10% of the administered tenofovir dose.

DOSAGE AND ADMINISTRATION

The dose of TRUVADA is one tablet (containing 200 mg of emtricitabine and 300 mg of tenofovir disoproxil fumarate) once daily taken orally with or without food.
Dose Adjustment for Renal Impairment:
Significantly increased drug exposures occurred when EMTRIVA or VIREAD were administered to patients with moderate to severe renal impairment (see EMTRIVA or VIREAD Package Insert). Therefore, the dosing interval of TRUVADA should be adjusted in patients with baseline creatinine clearance 30–49 mL/min using the recommendations in Table 9. The safety and effectiveness of these dosing interval adjustment recommendations have not been clinically evaluated, therefore, clinical response to treatment and renal function should be closely monitored in these patients.
[See table 9 below]

Table 9. Dosage Adjustment for Patients with Altered Creatinine Clearance

	Creatinine Clearance (mL/min)[a]		
	≥50	**30–49**	**<30 (Including Patients Requiring Hemodialysis)**
Recommended Dosing Interval	Every 24 hours	Every 48 hours	TRUVADA should not be administered.

[a]Calculated using ideal (lean) body weight.

HOW SUPPLIED

TRUVADA is available as tablets. Each tablet contains 200 mg of emtricitabine and 300 mg of tenofovir disoproxil fumarate (which is equivalent to 245 mg of tenofovir disoproxil). The tablets are blue, capsule-shaped, film-coated, debossed with "GILEAD" on one side and with "701" on the other side. Each bottle contains 30 tablets (NDC 61958-0701-1) and a desiccant (silica gel canister or sachet) and is closed with a child-resistant closure.
Store at 25 °C (77 °F), excursions permitted to 15–30 °C (59–86 °F).
• Keep container tightly closed
• Dispense only in original container
• Do not use if seal over bottle opening is broken or missing.
Gilead Sciences, Inc.
Foster City, CA 94404
August 2004
EMTRIVA, TRUVADA, and VIREAD are trademarks of Gilead Sciences, Inc. REYATAZ and VIDEX are trademarks of Bristol-Myers Squibb. COMBIVIR, EPIVIR, EPIVIR-HBV, EPZICOM, and TRIZIVIR are trademarks of GlaxoSmithKline.

GILEAD

Patient Information

TRUVADA™ (tru-vah-dah) Tablets
Generic name: emtricitabine and tenofovir disoproxil fumarate
(em tri SIT uh bean and te NOÉ fo veer dye soe PROX il FYOU-mar-ate)
Read the Patient Information that comes with TRUVADA before you start taking it and each time you get a refill. There may be new information. This information does not take the place of talking to your healthcare provider about your medical condition or treatment. You should stay under a healthcare provider's care when taking TRUVADA. **Do not change or stop your medicine without first talking with your healthcare provider.** Talk to your healthcare provider or pharmacist if you have any questions about TRUVADA.
What is the most important information I should know about TRUVADA?
- **Some people who have taken medicine like TRUVADA (nucleoside analogs) have developed a serious condition called lactic acidosis** (build up of an acid in the blood). Lactic acidosis can be a medical emergency and may need to be treated in the hospital. **Call your healthcare provider right away if you get the following signs or symptoms of lactic acidosis.**
  • You feel very weak or tired.
  • You have unusual (not normal) muscle pain.
  • You have trouble breathing.
  • You have stomach pain with nausea and vomiting.
  • You feel cold, especially in your arms and legs.
  • You feel dizzy or lightheaded.
  • You have a fast or irregular heartbeat.
- **Some people who have taken medicines like TRUVADA have developed serious liver problems called hepatotoxicity,** with liver enlargement (hepatomegaly) and fat in the liver (steatosis). **Call your healthcare provider right away if you get the following signs or symptoms of liver problems.**
  • Your skin or the white part of your eyes turns yellow (jaundice).
  • Your urine turns dark.
  • Your bowel movements (stools) turn light in color.
  • You don't feel like eating food for several days or longer.
  • You feel sick to your stomach (nausea).
  • You have lower stomach area (abdominal) pain.
- **You may be more likely to get lactic acidosis or liver problems** if you are female, very overweight (obese), or have been taking nucleoside analog medicines, like TRUVADA, for a long time.
- **TRUVADA is not for the treatment of Hepatitis B Virus infection.** Patients infected with both HBV and human immunodeficiency virus (HIV) who take TRUVADA need close medical follow-up for several months after stopping treatment with TRUVADA. Follow-up includes medical exams and blood tests to check for HBV that could be getting worse. **Patients with Hepatitis B Virus infection, who take TRUVADA and then stop it, may get "flare-ups" of their hepatitis. A "flare-up" is when the disease suddenly returns in a worse way than before.**

What is TRUVADA?
TRUVADA is a type of medicine called an HIV (human immunodeficiency virus) nucleoside analog reverse transcriptase inhibitor (NRTI). TRUVADA contains 2 medicines, EMTRIVA® (emtricitabine) and VIREAD® (tenofovir disoproxil fumarate, or tenofovir DF) combined in one pill. TRUVADA is always used with other anti-HIV medicines to treat people with HIV infection. TRUVADA is for adults age 18 and older. TRUVADA has not been studied in children under age 18 or adults over age 65.
HIV infection destroys CD4 (T) cells, which are important to the immune system. The immune system helps fight infection. After a large number of T cells are destroyed, acquired immune deficiency syndrome (AIDS) develops.
TRUVADA helps block HIV reverse transcriptase, a chemical in your body (enzyme) that is needed for HIV to multiply. TRUVADA lowers the amount of HIV in the blood (viral load). TRUVADA may also help to increase the number of T cells (CD4 cells). Lowering the amount of HIV in the blood lowers the chance of death or infections that happen when your immune system is weak (opportunistic infections).
TRUVADA does not cure HIV infection or AIDS. The long-term effects of TRUVADA are not known at this time. People taking TRUVADA may still get opportunistic infections or other conditions that happen with HIV infection. Opportunistic infections are infections that develop because the immune system is weak. Some of these conditions are pneumonia, herpes virus infections, and *Mycobacterium avium complex* (MAC) infection. **It is very important that you see your healthcare provider regularly while taking TRUVADA.**
TRUVADA does not lower your chance of passing HIV to other people through sexual contact, sharing needles, or being exposed to your blood. For your health and the health of others, it is important to always practice safer sex by using a latex or polyurethane condom or other barrier to lower the chance of sexual contact with semen, vaginal secretions, or blood. Never use or share dirty needles.
Who should not take TRUVADA?
Do not take TRUVADA if you are allergic to TRUVADA or any of its ingredients. The active ingredients of TRUVADA are emtricitabine and tenofovir DF. See the end of this leaflet for a complete list of ingredients.
What should I tell my healthcare provider before taking TRUVADA?
Tell your healthcare provider if you:
- **are pregnant or planning to become pregnant.** We do not know if TRUVADA can harm your unborn child. You and your healthcare provider will need to decide if TRUVADA is right for you. If you use TRUVADA while you are pregnant, talk to your healthcare provider about how you can be on the TRUVADA Antiviral Pregnancy Registry.
- **are breast-feeding.** You should not breast feed if you are HIV-positive because of the chance of passing the HIV virus to your baby. Also, it is not known if TRUVADA can pass into your breast milk and if it can harm your baby. If you are a woman who has or will have a baby, talk with your healthcare provider about the best way to feed your baby.
- **have kidney problems or are undergoing kidney dialysis treatment.**
- **have bone problems.**
- **have liver problems including Hepatitis B Virus infection.**

Tell your healthcare provider about all the medicines you take, including prescription and non-prescription medicines, vitamins, and herbal supplements. Especially tell your healthcare provider if you take:
- COMBIVIR®, EMTRIVA, EPIVIR®, EPIVIR-HBV®, EPZICOM™, TRIZIVIR®, or VIREAD. **TRUVADA should not be used with those medicines.**
- Drugs that contain didanosine (VIDEX®, VIDEX EC). Tenofovir DF (a component of TRUVADA) may increase the amount of VIDEX in your blood. **You may need to be followed more carefully if you are taking TRUVADA and VIDEX together.**
- REYATAZ™ (atazanavir sulfate) or KALETRA® (lopinavir/ritonavir). These medicines may increase the amount of tenofovir DF (a component of TRUVADA) in your blood, which could result in more side effects. You may need to be followed more carefully if you are taking TRUVADA and REYATAZ or KALETRA together.

Keep a complete list of all the medicines that you take. Make a new list when medicines are added or stopped. Give copies of this list to all of your healthcare providers and pharmacist every time you visit your healthcare provider or fill a prescription.
How should I take TRUVADA?
- Take TRUVADA exactly as your healthcare provider prescribed it. Follow the directions from your healthcare provider, exactly as written on the label.

- The usual dose of TRUVADA is 1 tablet once a day. TRUVADA is always used with other anti-HIV medicines. If you have kidney problems, you may need to take TRUVADA less often.
- TRUVADA may be taken with or without a meal. Food does not affect how TRUVADA works. Take TRUVADA at the same time each day.
- If you forget to take TRUVADA, take it as soon as you remember that day. **Do not** take more than 1 dose of TRUVADA in a day. **Do not** take 2 doses at the same time. Call your healthcare provider or pharmacist if you are not sure what to do. **It is important that you do not miss any doses of TRUVADA or your anti-HIV medicines.**
- When your TRUVADA supply starts to run low, get more from your healthcare provider or pharmacy. This is very important because the amount of virus in your blood may increase if the medicine is stopped for even a short time. The virus may develop resistance to TRUVADA and become harder to treat.
- Do not change your dose or stop taking TRUVADA without first talking with your healthcare provider. Stay under a healthcare provider's care when taking TRUVADA.
- If you take too much TRUVADA, call your local poison control center or emergency room right away.

What should I avoid while taking TRUVADA?

- **Do not breast-feed.** See "What should I tell my healthcare provider before taking TRUVADA?"
- **Avoid doing things that can spread HIV infection** since TRUVADA does not stop you from passing the HIV infection to others.
  - **Do not share needles or other injection equipment.**
  - **Do not share personal items that can have blood or body fluids on them, like toothbrushes or razor blades.**
  - **Do not have any kind of sex without protection.** Always practice safer sex by using a latex or polyurethane condom or other barrier to reduce the chance of sexual contact with semen, vaginal secretions, or blood.
- COMBIVIR, EMTRIVA, EPIVIR, EPIVIR-HBV, EPZICOM, TRIZIVIR or VIREAD.
  TRUVADA should not be used with these medicines.

What are the possible side effects of TRUVADA?

TRUVADA may cause the following serious side effects (see "What is the most important information I should know about TRUVADA?"):

- **Lactic acidosis** (buildup of an acid in the blood). Lactic acidosis can be a medical emergency and may need to be treated in the hospital. **Call your doctor right away if you get signs of lactic acidosis.** (See "What is the most important information I should know about TRUVADA?")
- **Serious liver problems (hepatotoxicity),** with liver enlargement (hepatomegaly) and fat in the liver (steatosis). Call your healthcare provider right away if you get any signs of liver problems. (See "What is the most important information I should know about TRUVADA?")
- **"Flare-ups" of Hepatitis B Virus infection,** in which the disease suddenly returns in a worse way than before, can occur if you stop taking TRUVADA. Your healthcare provider will monitor your condition for several months after stopping TRUVADA if you have both HIV and HBV infection. TRUVADA is not for the treatment of Hepatitis B Virus infection.
- **Kidney problems** If you have had kidney problems in the past or take other medicines that can cause kidney problems, your healthcare provider should do regular blood tests to check your kidneys.
- **Changes in bone mineral density (thinning bones)** It is not known whether long-term use of TRUVADA will cause damage to your bones. If you have had bone problems in the past, your healthcare provider may need to do tests to check your bone mineral density or may prescribe medicines to help your bone mineral density.

Other side effects with TRUVADA when used with other anti-HIV medicines include:

- Changes in body fat have been seen in some patients taking TRUVADA and other anti-HIV medicines. These changes may include increased amount of fat in the upper back and neck ("buffalo hump"), breast, and around the main part of your body (trunk). Loss of fat from the legs, arms and face may also happen. The cause and long term health effect of these conditions are not known at this time.

The most common side effects of EMTRIVA or VIREAD when used with other anti-HIV medicines are: dizziness, diarrhea, nausea, vomiting, headache, rash, and gas. Skin discoloration (small spots or freckles) may also happen with TRUVADA.

These are not all the side effects of TRUVADA. This list of side effects with TRUVADA is **not complete** at this time because TRUVADA is still being studied. If you have questions about side effects, ask your healthcare provider. Report any new or continuing symptoms to your healthcare provider right away. Your healthcare provider may be able to help you manage these side effects.

How do I store TRUVADA?

- **Keep TRUVADA and all other medicines out of reach of children.**
- Store TRUVADA at room temperature 77 °F (25 °C).
- Keep TRUVADA in its original container and keep the container tightly closed.
- Do not keep medicine that is out of date or that you no longer need. If you throw any medicines away make sure that children will not find them.

General information about TRUVADA:

Medicines are sometimes prescribed for conditions that are not mentioned in patient information leaflets. Do not use TRUVADA for a condition for which it was not prescribed. Do not give TRUVADA to other people, even if they have the same symptoms you have. It may harm them.

This leaflet summarizes the most important information about TRUVADA. If you would like more information, talk with your healthcare provider. You can ask your healthcare provider or pharmacist for information about TRUVADA that is written for health professionals. For more information, you may also call 1-800-GILEAD-5 or access the TRUVADA website at www.TRUVADA.com.

Do not use TRUVADA if seal over bottle opening is broken or missing.

What are the ingredients of TRUVADA?

Active Ingredients: emtricitabine and tenofovir DF

Inactive Ingredients: Croscarmellose sodium, lactose monohydrate, magnesium stearate, microcrystalline cellulose, and pregelatinized starch (gluten free). The tablets are coated with Opadry II Blue Y-30-10701 containing FD&C Blue #2 aluminum lake, hypromellose, lactose monohydrate, titanium dioxide and triacetin.

℞ Only

August 2004

EMTRIVA, TRUVADA, and VIREAD are trademarks of Gilead Sciences, Inc. REYATAZ and VIDEX are trademarks of Bristol-Myers Squibb. KALETRA is a trademark of Abbott Laboratories. COMBIVIR, EPIVIR, EPIVIR-HBV, EPZICOM, and TRIZIVIR are trademarks of GlaxoSmithKline.

Shown in Product Identification Guide, page 313

VIREAD® ℞

[VEER-ee-ad]

(tenofovir disoproxil fumarate) Tablets

Rx Only

WARNING

LACTIC ACIDOSIS AND SEVERE HEPATOMEGALY WITH STEATOSIS, INCLUDING FATAL CASES, HAVE BEEN REPORTED WITH THE USE OF NUCLEOSIDE ANALOGS ALONE OR IN COMBINATION WITH OTHER ANTIRETROVIRALS (SEE WARNINGS).

VIREAD® IS NOT INDICATED FOR THE TREATMENT OF CHRONIC HEPATITIS B VIRUS (HBV) INFECTION AND THE SAFETY AND EFFICACY OF VIREAD HAVE NOT BEEN ESTABLISHED IN PATIENTS CO-INFECTED WITH HBV AND HIV. SEVERE ACUTE EXACERBATIONS OF HEPATITIS B HAVE BEEN REPORTED IN PATIENTS WHO ARE CO-INFECTED WITH HBV AND HIV AND HAVE DISCONTINUED VIREAD. HEPATIC FUNCTION SHOULD BE MONITORED CLOSELY WITH BOTH CLINICAL AND LABORATORY FOLLOW-UP FOR AT LEAST SEVERAL MONTHS IN PATIENTS WHO DISCONTINUE VIREAD AND ARE CO-INFECTED WITH HBV AND HIV. IF APPROPRIATE, INITIATION OF ANTI-HEPATITIS B THERAPY MAY BE WARRANTED (SEE WARNINGS).

DESCRIPTION

VIREAD is the brand name for tenofovir disoproxil fumarate (a prodrug of tenofovir) which is a fumaric acid salt of *bis*-isopropoxycarbonyloxymethyl ester derivative of tenofovir. In vivo tenofovir disoproxil fumarate is converted to tenofovir, an acyclic nucleoside phosphonate (nucleotide) analog of adenosine 5′-monophosphate. Tenofovir exhibits activity against HIV-1 reverse transcriptase.

The chemical name of tenofovir disoproxil fumarate is 9-[(*R*)-2-[[bis[[(isopropoxycarbonyl)oxy]methoxy]phosphinyl]methoxy]propyl]adenine fumarate (1:1). It has a molecular formula of $C_{19}H_{30}N_5O_{10}P \bullet C_4H_4O_4$ and a molecular weight of 635.52. It has the following structural formula:

Tenofovir disoproxil fumarate is a white to off-white crystalline powder with a solubility of 13.4 mg/mL in distilled water at 25 °C. It has an octanol/phosphate buffer (pH 6.5) partition coefficient (log p) of 1.25 at 25 °C.

VIREAD tablets are for oral administration. Each tablet contains 300 mg of tenofovir disoproxil fumarate, which is equivalent to 245 mg of tenofovir disoproxil, and the following inactive ingredients: croscarmellose sodium, lactose monohydrate, magnesium stearate, microcrystalline cellulose, and pregelatinized starch. The tablets are coated with a light blue colored film (Opadry II Y-30-10671-A) that is made of FD&C blue #2 aluminum lake, hydroxypropyl methylcellulose 2910, lactose monohydrate, titanium dioxide, and triacetin.

In this insert, all dosages are expressed in terms of tenofovir disoproxil fumarate except where otherwise noted.

Microbiology

Mechanism of Action: Tenofovir disoproxil fumarate is an acyclic nucleoside phosphonate diester analog of adenosine monophosphate. Tenofovir disoproxil fumarate requires initial diester hydrolysis for conversion to tenofovir and subsequent phosphorylations by cellular enzymes to form tenofovir diphosphate. Tenofovir diphosphate inhibits the activity of HIV-1 reverse transcriptase by competing with the natural substrate deoxyadenosine 5′-triphosphate and, after incorporation into DNA, by DNA chain termination. Tenofovir diphosphate is a weak inhibitor of mammalian DNA polymerases α, β, and mitochondrial DNA polymerase γ.

Antiviral Activity In Vitro: The in vitro antiviral activity of tenofovir against laboratory and clinical isolates of HIV-1 was assessed in lymphoblastoid cell lines, primary monocyte/macrophage cells and peripheral blood lymphocytes. The IC_{50} (50% inhibitory concentration) values for tenofovir were in the range of 0.04 μM to 8.5 μM. In drug combination studies of tenofovir with nucleoside reverse transcriptase inhibitors (abacavir, didanosine, lamivudine, stavudine, zalcitabine, zidovudine), non-nucleoside reverse transcriptase inhibitors (delavirdine, efavirenz, nevirapine), and protease inhibitors (amprenavir, indinavir, nelfinavir, ritonavir, saquinavir), additive to synergistic effects were observed. Most of these drug combinations have not been studied in humans. Tenofovir displayed antiviral activity in vitro against HIV-1 clades A, B, C, D, E, F, G and O (IC_{50} values ranged from 0.5 μM to 2.2 μM).

Drug Resistance: HIV-1 isolates with reduced susceptibility to tenofovir have been selected in vitro. These viruses expressed a K65R mutation in reverse transcriptase and showed a 3–4 fold reduction in susceptibility to tenofovir.

Tenofovir-resistant isolates of HIV-1 have also been recovered from some patients treated with tenofovir in combination with certain antiretroviral agents. In treatment-naïve patients treated with Viread + lamivudine + efavirenz, viral isolates from 7/29 (24%) patients with virologic failure showed reduced susceptibility to tenofovir. In treatment-experienced patients, 14/304 (4.6%) of the VIREAD-treated patients with virologic failure showed reduced susceptibility to tenofovir. Genotypic analysis of the resistant isolates showed a mutation in the HIV-1 reverse transcriptase gene resulting in the K65R amino acid substitution.

Cross-resistance: Cross-resistance among certain reverse transcriptase inhibitors has been recognized. The K65R mutation selected by tenofovir is also selected in some HIV-1 infected subjects treated with abacavir, didanosine, or zalcitabine. HIV isolates with this mutation also show reduced susceptibility to emtricitabine and lamivudine. Therefore, cross-resistance among these drugs may occur in patients whose virus harbors the K65R mutation. HIV-1 isolates from patients (N=20) whose HIV-1 expressed a mean of 3 zidovudine-associated reverse transcriptase mutations (M41L, D67N, K70R, L210W, T215Y/F or K219Q/E/N), showed a 3.1-fold decrease in the susceptibility to tenofovir. Multinucleoside resistant HIV-1 with a T69S double insertion mutation in the reverse transcriptase showed reduced susceptibility to tenofovir.

Pharmacokinetics

The pharmacokinetics of tenofovir disoproxil fumarate have been evaluated in healthy volunteers and HIV-1 infected individuals. Tenofovir pharmacokinetics are similar between these populations.

Absorption: VIREAD is a water soluble diester prodrug of the active ingredient tenofovir. The oral bioavailability of tenofovir from VIREAD in fasted patients is approximately 25%. Following oral administration of a single dose of VIREAD 300 mg to HIV-1 infected patients in the fasted

Continued on next page

Table 1. Pharmacokinetic Parameters (Mean ± SD) of Tenofovir* in Patients with varying Degrees of Renal Function

Baseline Creatinine Clearance (mL/min)	>80 (N=3)	50–80 (N=10)	30–49 (N=8)	12–29 (N=11)
C_{max} (ng/mL)	335.4 ± 31.8	330.4 ± 61.0	372.1 ± 156.1	601.6 ± 185.3
$AUC_{0-\infty}$ (ng•hr/mL)	2184.5 ± 257.4	3063.8 ± 927.0	6008.5 ± 2504.7	15984.7 ± 7223.0
CL/F (mL/min)	1043.7 ± 15.4	807.7 ± 279.2	444.4 ± 209.8	177.0 ± 97.1
CL_{renal} (mL/min)	243.5 ± 33.3	168.6 ± 27.5	100.6 ± 27.5	43.0 ± 31.2

*300 mg, single dose of VIREAD

Viread—Cont.

state, maximum serum concentrations (C_{max}) are achieved in 1.0 ± 0.4 hrs. C_{max} and AUC values are 296 ± 90 ng/mL and 2287 ± 685 ng•h/mL, respectively.

The pharmacokinetics of tenofovir are dose proportional over a VIREAD dose range of 75 to 600 mg and are not affected by repeated dosing.

Effects of Food on Oral Absorption: Administration of VIREAD following a high-fat meal (~700 to 1000 kcal containing 40 to 50% fat) increases the oral bioavailability, with an increase in tenofovir $AUC_{0-\infty}$ of approximately 40% and an increase in C_{max} of approximately 14%. However, administration of VIREAD with a light meal did not have a significant effect on the pharmacokinetics of tenofovir when compared to fasted administration of the drug. Food delays the time to tenofovir C_{max} by approximately 1 hour. C_{max} and AUC of tenofovir are 326 ± 119 ng/mL and 3324 ± 1370 ng•hr/mL following multiple doses of VIREAD 300 mg once daily in the fed state, when meal content was not controlled.

Distribution: In vitro binding of tenofovir to human plasma or serum proteins is less than 0.7 and 7.2%, respectively, over the tenofovir concentration range 0.01 to 25 µg/mL. The volume of distribution at steady-state is 1.3 ± 0.6 L/kg and 1.2 ± 0.4 L/kg, following intravenous administration of tenofovir 1.0 mg/kg and 3.0 mg/kg.

Metabolism and Elimination: In vitro studies indicate that neither tenofovir disoproxil nor tenofovir are substrates of CYP450 enzymes.

Following IV administration of tenofovir, approximately 70-80% of the dose is recovered in the urine as unchanged tenofovir within 72 hours of dosing. Following single dose, oral administration of VIREAD, the terminal elimination half-life of tenofovir is approximately 17 hours. After multiple oral doses of VIREAD 300 mg once daily (under fed conditions), 32 ± 10% of the administered dose is recovered in urine over 24 hours.

Tenofovir is eliminated by a combination of glomerular filtration and active tubular secretion. There may be competition for elimination with other compounds that are also renally eliminated.

Special Populations

There were insufficient numbers from racial and ethnic groups other than Caucasian to adequately determine potential pharmacokinetic differences among these populations.

Tenofovir pharmacokinetics are similar in male and female patients.

Pharmacokinetic studies have not been performed in children (<18 years) or in the elderly (>65 years).

The pharmacokinetics of tenofovir following a 300 mg single dose of VIREAD have been studied in non-HIV infected patients with moderate to severe hepatic impairment. There were no substantial alterations in tenofovir pharmacokinetics in patients with hepatic impairment compared with unimpaired patients. No change in VIREAD dosing is required in patients with hepatic impairment.

The pharmacokinetics of tenofovir are altered in patients with renal impairment (see WARNINGS, Renal Impairment). In patients with creatinine clearance <50 mL/min or with end-stage renal disease (ESRD) requiring dialysis, C_{max}, and $AUC_{0-\infty}$ of tenofovir were increased (Table 1). It is recommended that the dosing interval for VIREAD be modified in patients with creatinine clearance <50 mL/min or in patients with ESRD who require dialysis (see DOSAGE AND ADMINISTRATION).

[See table 1 at bottom of previous page]

Tenofovir is efficiently removed by hemodialysis with an extraction coefficient of approximately 54%. Following a single 300 mg dose of VIREAD, a four-hour hemodialysis session removed approximately 10% of the administered tenofovir dose.

Drug Interactions

At concentrations substantially higher (~300-fold) than those observed in vivo, tenofovir did not inhibit in vitro drug metabolism mediated by any of the following human CYP450 isoforms: CYP3A4, CYP2D6, CYP2C9 or CYP2E1. However, a small (6%) but statistically significant reduction in metabolism of CYP1A substrate was observed. Based on the results of in vitro experiments and the known elimination pathway of tenofovir, the potential for CYP450 mediated interactions involving tenofovir with other medicinal products is low (see Pharmacokinetics).

Tenofovir is primarily excreted by the kidneys by a combination of glomerular filtration and active tubular secretion. Co-administration of VIREAD with drugs that are eliminated by active tubular secretion may increase serum concentrations of either tenofovir or the co-administered drug, due to competition for this elimination pathway. Drugs that decrease renal function may also increase serum concentrations of tenofovir.

VIREAD has been evaluated in healthy volunteers in combination with abacavir, adefovir dipivoxil, atazanavir, didanosine, efavirenz, emtricitabine, indinavir, lamivudine, lopinavir/ritonavir, methadone, oral contraceptives and ribavirin. Tables 2 and 3 summarize pharmacokinetic effects of co-administered drug on tenofovir pharmacokinetics and effects of VIREAD on the pharmacokinetics of co-administered drug.

Table 4 summarizes the drug interaction between VIREAD and didanosine. When administered with multiple doses of VIREAD, the C_{max} and AUC of didanosine 400 mg increased significantly. The mechanism of this interaction is unknown. When didanosine 250 mg enteric-coated capsules were administered with VIREAD, systemic exposures to didanosine were similar to those seen with the 400 mg enteric-coated capsules alone under fasted conditions.

Table 2. Drug Interactions: Changes in Pharmacokinetic Parameters for Tenofovir[1] in the Presence of the Co-administered Drug

Co-administered Drug	Dose of Co-administered Drug (mg)	N	% Change of Tenofovir Pharmacokinetic Parameters[2] (90% CI)		
			C_{max}	AUC	C_{min}
Abacavir	300 once	8	⇔	⇔	NC
Adefovir dipivoxil	10 once	22	⇔	⇔	NC
Atazanavir[3]	400 once daily × 14 days	33	↑ 14 (↑ 8 to ↑ 20)	↑ 24 (↑ 21 to ↑ 28)	↑ 22 (↑ 15 to ↑ 30)
Didanosine (enteric-coated)	400 once	25	⇔	⇔	⇔
Didanosine (buffered)	250 or 400 once daily × 7 days	14	⇔	⇔	⇔
Efavirenz	600 once daily × 14 days	29	⇔	⇔	⇔
Emtricitabine	200 once daily × 7 days	17	⇔	⇔	⇔
Indinavir	800 three times daily × 7 days	13	↑ 14 (↓ 3 to ↑ 33)	⇔	⇔
Lamivudine	150 twice daily × 7 days	15	⇔	⇔	⇔
Lopinavir/ Ritonavir	400/100 twice daily × 14 days	24	⇔	↑ 32 (↑ 26 to ↑ 38)	↑ 51 (↑ 32 to ↑ 66)

1. Patients received VIREAD 300 mg once daily.
2. Increase = ↑; Decrease = ↓; No Effect = ⇔; NC = Not Calculated
3. REYATAZ™ Prescribing Information (Bristol-Myers Squibb)

Table 3. Drug Interactions: Changes in Pharmacokinetic Parameters for Co-administered Drug in the Presence of VIREAD

Co-administered Drug	Dose of Co-administered Drug (mg)	N	% Change of Co-administered Drug Pharmacokinetic Parameters[1] (90% CI)		
			C_{max}	AUC	C_{min}
Abacavir	300 once	8	↑ 12 (↓ 1 to ↑ 26)	⇔	NA
Adefovir dipivoxil	10 once	22	⇔	⇔	NA
Efavirenz	600 once daily × 14 days	30	⇔	⇔	⇔
Emtricitabine	200 once daily × 7 days	17	⇔	⇔	⇔
Indinavir	800 three times daily × 7 days	12	↓ 11 (↓ 30 to ↑ 12)	⇔	⇔
Lamivudine	150 twice daily × 7 days	15	↓ 24 (↓ 34 to ↓ 12)	⇔	⇔
Lopinavir	Lopinavir/Ritonavir 400/100 twice daily × 14 days	24	⇔	⇔	⇔
Methadone[2]	40–110 once daily × 14 days[3]	13	⇔	⇔	⇔
Oral Contraceptives[4]	Ethinyl Estradiol/ Norgestimate (Ortho-Tricyclen®) Once daily × 7 days	20	⇔	⇔	⇔
Ritonavir	Lopinavir/Ritonavir 400/100 twice daily × 14 days	24	⇔	⇔	⇔
Atazanavir[5]	400 once daily × 14 days	34	↓ 21 (↓ 27 to ↓ 14)	↓ 25 (↓ 30 to ↓ 19)	↓ 40 (↓ 48 to ↓ 32)
Atazanavir[5]	Atazanavir/Ritonavir 300/100 once daily × 42 days	10	↓ 28 (↓ 50 to ↑ 5)	↓ 25[6] (↓ 42 to ↓ 3)	↓ 23[6] (↓ 46 to ↑ 10)

1. Increase = ↑; Decrease = ↓; No Effect = ⇔; NA = Not Applicable
2. R-(active), S-and total methadone exposures were equivalent when dosed alone or with VIREAD.
3. Individual subjects were maintained on their stable methadone dose. No pharmacodynamic alterations (opiate toxicity or withdrawal signs or symptoms) were reported.
4. Ethinyl estradiol and 17-deacetyl norgestimate (pharmacologically active metabolite) exposures were equivalent when dosed alone or with VIREAD.
5. REYATAZ™ Prescribing Information (Bristol-Myers Squibb)
6. In HIV-infected patients, addition of tenofovir DF to atazanavir 300 mg plus ritonavir 100 mg, resulted in AUC and C_{min} values of atazanavir that were 2.3 and 4-fold higher than the respective values observed for atazanavir 400 mg when given alone.

[See table 2 at top of previous page]

Following multiple dosing to HIV-negative subjects receiving either chronic methadone maintenance therapy or oral contraceptives, or single doses of ribavirin, steady state tenofovir pharmacokinetics were similar to those observed in previous studies, indicating lack of clinically significant drug interactions between these agents and VIREAD.

[See table 3 on previous page]

[See table 4 above]

INDICATIONS AND USAGE

VIREAD is indicated in combination with other antiretroviral agents for the treatment of HIV-1 infection. This indication is based on analyses of plasma HIV-1 RNA levels and CD4 cell counts in controlled studies of VIREAD in treatment-naïve adults and in treatment-experienced adults.

Additional important information regarding the use of VIREAD for the treatment of HIV-1 infection:

- There are no study results demonstrating the effect of VIREAD on clinical progression of HIV-1.
- The use of VIREAD should be considered for treating adult patients with HIV-1 strains that are expected to be susceptible to tenofovir as assessed by laboratory testing or treatment history (see Description of Clinical Studies).

Description of Clinical Studies

Treatment-Experienced Patients

Study 907: VIREAD + Standard Background Therapy (SBT) Compared to Placebo + SBT

Study 907 was a 24 week, double-blind placebo-controlled multicenter study of VIREAD added to a stable background regimen of antiretroviral agents in 550 treatment-experienced patients. After 24 weeks of blinded study treatment, all patients continuing on study were offered open-label VIREAD for an additional 24 weeks. Patients had a mean baseline CD4 cell count of 427 cells/mm^3 (range 23–1385), median baseline plasma HIV-1 RNA of 2340 (range 50–75,000) copies/mL, and mean duration of prior HIV-1 treatment was 5.4 years. Mean age of the patients was 42 years, 85% were male and 69% were Caucasian, 17% Black and 12% Hispanic.

Changes from baseline in $\log_{10}$ copies/mL plasma HIV-1 RNA levels over time up to week 48 are presented below in Figure 1.

Figure 1
Mean Change from Baseline in Plasma HIV-1 RNA ($\log_{10}$ copies/mL) Through Week 48: Study 907 (All Available Data)[†]

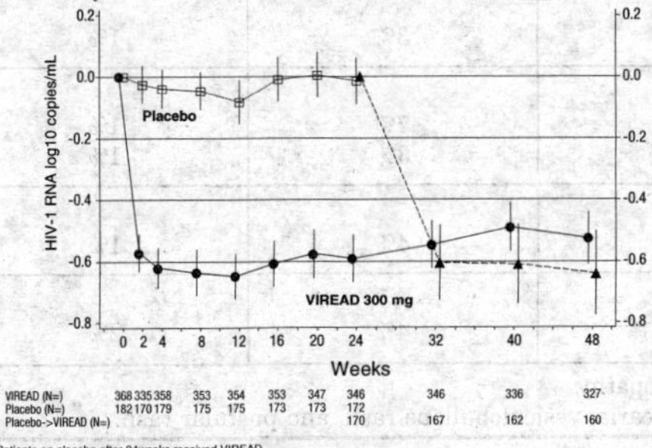

	0	2	4	8	12	16	20	24	32	40	48
● VIREAD (N=)	368	335	358	353	354	353	347	346	346	336	327
□ Placebo (N=)	182	170	179	175	175	173	173	172			
▲ Placebo->VIREAD (N=)								170	167	162	160

[†] Patients on placebo after 24weeks received VIREAD.

The percent of patients with HIV-1 RNA <400 copies/mL and outcomes of patients through 48 weeks are summarized in Table 5.

[See table 5 above]

At 24 weeks of therapy, there was a higher proportion of patients in the VIREAD arm compared to the placebo arm with HIV-1 RNA <50 copies/mL (19% and 1%, respectively). Mean change in absolute CD4 counts by week 24 was +11 cells/mm^3 for the VIREAD group and -5 cells/mm^3 for the placebo group. Mean change in absolute CD4 counts by week 48 was +4 cells/mm^3 for the VIREAD group.

Through week 24, one patient in the VIREAD group and no patients in the placebo arm experienced a new CDC Class C event.

Treatment-Naïve Patients

Study 903: VIREAD + Lamivudine Efavirenz Compared to Stavudine + Lamivudine + Efavirenz

Data through 48-weeks are reported for Study 903, a double-blind, active-controlled multicenter study comparing VIREAD (300 mg QD) administered in combination with lamivudine and efavirenz versus stavudine, lamivudine, and efavirenz in 600 antiretroviral-naïve patients. Patients had a mean age of 36 years (range 18–64), 74% were male, 64% were Caucasian and 20% were Black. The mean baseline CD4 cell count was 279 cells/mm^3 (range 3–956) and median baseline plasma HIV-1 RNA was 77,600 copies/mL (range 417–5,130,000). Patients were stratified by baseline HIV-1 RNA and CD4 count. Forty-three percent of patients had baseline viral loads >100,000 copies/mL and 39% had CD4 cell counts <200 cells/mL. Treatment outcomes through 48 weeks are presented in Table 6 below.

Table 4. Drug Interactions: Pharmacokinetic Parameters for Didanosine in the Presence of VIREAD

Didanosine[1] Dose (mg)/ Method of Administration[2]	VIREAD Method of Administration[2]	N	% Difference (90% CI) vs. Didanosine 400 mg alone, Fasted[3]	
			C_{max}	AUC
Buffered tablets				
400 once daily[4] × 7 days	Fasted 1 hour after didanosine	14	↑ 28 (↑ 11 to ↑ 48)	↑ 44 (↑ 31 to ↑ 59)
Enteric coated capsules				
400 once, fasted	With food, 2 hr after didanosine	26	↑ 48 (↑ 25 to ↑ 76)	↑ 48 (↑ 31 to ↑ 67)
400 once, with food	Simultaneously with didanosine	26	↑ 64 (↑ 41 to ↑ 89)	↑ 60 (↑ 44 to ↑ 79)
250 once, fasted	With food, 2 hr after didanosine	28	↓ 10 (↓ 22 to ↑ 3)	⇔
250 once, fasted	Simultaneously with didanosine	28	⇔	↑ 14 (0 to ↑ 31)
250 once, with food	Simultaneously with didanosine	28	↓ 29 (↓ 39 to ↓ 18)	↓ 11 (↓ 23 to ↑ 2)

1. See PRECAUTIONS regarding use of didanosine with VIREAD.
2. Administration with food was with a light meal (~373 kcal, 20% fat).
3. Increase = ↑; Decrease = ↓; No Difference = ⇔
4. Includes 4 subjects weighing <60 kg receiving ddI 250 mg.

Table 5. Outcomes of Randomized Treatment (Study 907)

Outcomes	0–24 weeks		0–48 weeks	24–48 weeks
	VIREAD (N=368) %	Placebo (N=182) %	VIREAD (N=368) %	Placebo Crossover to VIREAD (N=170) %
HIV-1 RNA <400 copies/mL[1]	40%	11%	28%	30%
Virologic failure[2]	53%	84%	61%	64%
Discontinued due to adverse event	3%	3%	5%	5%
Discontinued for other reasons[3]	3%	3%	5%	1%

1. Patients with HIV-1 RNA <400 copies/mL and no prior study drug discontinuation at week 24 and 48 respectively.
2. Patients with HIV-1 RNA ≥400 copies/mL efficacy failure or missing HIV –1 RNA at week 24 and 48 respectively.
3. Includes lost to follow up, patient withdrawal, noncompliance, protocol violation and other reasons.

Table 6. Outcomes of Randomized Treatment at Week 48 (Study 903)

Outcome at Week 48	VIREAD +3TC+EFV (N=299)	Stavudine +3TC+EFV (N=301)
	%	%
Responder[1]	79%	82%
Virologic failure[2]	6%	4%
Rebound	5%	3%
Never suppressed through week 48	0%	1%
Added an antiretroviral agent	1%	1%
Death	<1%	1%
Discontinued due to adverse event	6%	6%
Discontinued for other reasons[3]	8%	7%

1. Patients achieved and maintained confirmed HIV-1 RNA <400 copies/mL through week 48.
2. Includes confirmed viral rebound and failure to achieve confirmed <400 copies/mL through week 48.
3. Includes lost to follow-up, patient's withdrawal, noncompliance, protocol violation and other reasons.

Achievement of plasma HIV-1 RNA concentrations of less than 400 copies/mL at week 48 was similar between the two treatment groups for the population stratified at baseline on the basis of HIV-1 RNA concentration (< or ≥100,000 copies/mL) and CD4 cell count (< or ≥200 cells/mm^3). Through 48 weeks of therapy, 76% and 79% of patients in the VIREAD and stavudine arms, respectively achieved HIV-1 RNA <50 copies/mL. The mean increase from baseline in CD4 cell count was 169 cells/mm^3 for the VIREAD arm and 167 cells/mm^3 for the stavudine arm.

Through 48 weeks, eight patients in the VIREAD group and six patients in the stavudine group experienced a new CDC Class C event.

Genotypic Analyses of VIREAD in Patients with Previous Antiretroviral Therapy

The virologic response to VIREAD therapy has been evaluated with respect to baseline viral genotype (N=222) in treatment experienced patients participating in two controlled trials.

The use of resistance testing and the clinical interpretation of genotypic mutations is a complex and evolving field. Conclusions regarding the relevance of particular mutations or mutational patterns are subject to change pending additional data.

In two clinical studies, 94% of the participants evaluated had baseline HIV-1 isolates expressing at least one NRTI mutation. These included resistance mutations associated with zidovudine (M41L, D67N, K70R, L210W, T215Y/F or K219Q/E/N), the lamivudine/abacavir-associated mutation (M184V), and others. In addition the majority of participants evaluated had mutations associated with either PI or NNRTI use. Virologic responses for patients in the genotype substudy were similar to the overall study results.

Several exploratory analyses were conducted to evaluate the effect of specific mutations and mutational patterns on virologic outcome. Descriptions of numerical differences in HIV-1 RNA response are displayed in Table 7. Because of the large number of potential comparisons, statistical testing was not conducted.

Varying degrees of cross-resistance of VIREAD to preexisting zidovudine-associated mutations were observed and appeared to depend on the number of specific mutations. VIREAD-treated patients whose HIV-1 expressed 3 or more zidovudine-associated mutations that included either the M41L or L210W reverse transcriptase mutation showed reduced responses to VIREAD therapy; however, these responses were still improved compared with placebo. The presence of the D67N, K70R, T215Y/F or K219Q/E/N mutation did not appear to affect responses to VIREAD therapy. The HIV-1 RNA responses by number and type of baseline zidovudine-associated mutations are shown in Table 7.

[See table 7 at top of next page]

In the protocol defined analyses, virologic response to VIREAD was not reduced in patients with HIV-1 that ex-

Continued on next page

Viread—Cont.

pressed the lamivudine/abacavir-associated M184V mutation. In the absence of zidovudine-associated mutations, patients with the M184V mutation receiving VIREAD showed a −0.84 log10 copies/mL decrease in their HIV-1 RNA relative to placebo. In the presence of zidovudine-associated mutations, the M184V mutation did not affect the mean HIV-1 RNA responses to VIREAD treatment. HIV-1 RNA responses among these patients were durable through week 48.

There were limited data on patients expressing some primary nucleoside reverse transcriptase inhibitor mutations and multi-drug resistant mutations at baseline. However, patients expressing the K65R mutation appeared to have reduced virologic responses to VIREAD.

The presence of at least one HIV-1 protease inhibitor or nonnucleoside reverse transcriptase inhibitor mutation at baseline did not appear to affect the virologic response to VIREAD. Cross-resistance between VIREAD and HIV-1 protease inhibitors is unlikely because of the different enzyme targets involved.

Phenotypic Analyses of VIREAD in Patients with Previous Antiretroviral Therapy

The virologic response to VIREAD therapy has been evaluated with respect to baseline phenotype (N=100) in treatment-experienced patients participating in two controlled trials. Phenotypic analysis of baseline HIV-1 from patients in these studies demonstrated a correlation between baseline susceptibility to VIREAD and response to VIREAD therapy. Table 8 summarizes the HIV-1 RNA response by baseline VIREAD susceptibility.

Table 8. HIV-1 RNA Response at Week 24 by Baseline VIREAD Susceptibility (Intent-To-Treat)[1]

Baseline VIREAD Susceptibility [2]	Change in HIV-1 RNA[3] (N)
≤1	−0.74 (35)
>1 and ≤3	−0.56 (49)
>3 and ≤4	−0.3 (7)
≤4	−0.61 (91)
>4	−0.12 (9)

1. Tenofovir susceptibility was determined by recombinant phenotypic Antivirogram™ assay (Virco).
2. Fold change in susceptibility from wild-type.
3. Average HIV-1 RNA change from baseline through week 24 ($DAVG_{24}$) in log_{10} copies/mL.

CONTRAINDICATIONS

VIREAD is contraindicated in patients with previously demonstrated hypersensitivity to any of the components of the product.

WARNINGS

Lactic Acidosis/Severe Hepatomegaly with Steatosis

Lactic acidosis and severe hepatomegaly with steatosis, including fatal cases, have been reported with the use of nucleoside analogs alone or in combination with other antiretrovirals. A majority of these cases have been in women. Obesity and prolonged nucleoside exposure may be risk factors. Particular caution should be exercised when administering nucleoside analogs to any patient with known risk factors for liver disease; however, cases have also been reported in patients with no known risk factors. Treatment with VIREAD should be suspended in any patient who develops clinical or laboratory findings suggestive of lactic acidosis or pronounced hepatotoxicity (which may include hepatomegaly and steatosis even in the absence of marked transaminase elevations).

Patients Co-infected with HIV and Hepatitis B Virus

It is recommended that all patients with HIV be tested for the presence of chronic hepatitis B virus (HBV) before initiating antiretroviral therapy. VIREAD is not indicated for the treatment of chronic HBV infection and the safety and efficacy of VIREAD have not been established in patients co-infected with HBV and HIV. Severe acute exacerbations of hepatitis B have been reported in patients who are co-infected with HBV and HIV and have discontinued VIREAD. Hepatic function should be monitored closely with both clinical and laboratory follow-up for at least several months in patients who discontinue VIREAD and are co-infected with HIV and HBV. If appropriate, initiation of anti-hepatitis B therapy may be warranted.

Renal Impairment

Tenofovir is principally eliminated by the kidney. Dosing interval adjustment is recommended in all patients with creatinine clearance <50 mL/min (see DOSAGE AND ADMINISTRATION). No safety data are available in patients with renal dysfunction who received VIREAD using these dosing guidelines.

Renal impairment, including cases of acute renal failure and Fanconi syndrome (renal tubular injury with severe hypophosphatemia), has been reported in association with the use of VIREAD (see Adverse Reactions-Post Marketing Experience). The majority of these cases occurred in patients with underlying systemic or renal disease, or in patients taking nephrotoxic agents, however, some cases occurred in patients without identified risk factors.

Table 7. HIV-1 RNA Response At Week 24 by Number of Baseline Zidovudine-Associated Mutations (Intent-To-Treat)[1]

Number of baseline zidovudine-associated mutations[2]	Change in HIV-1 RNA[3] (N)	
	VIREAD 300 mg	Placebo
None	−0.80 (68)	−0.11 (29)
Any	−0.50 (154)	0 (81)
1–2	−0.66 (55)	−0.04 (33)
≥3 including M41L or L210W	−0.21 (57)	+0.01 (29)
≥3 without M41L or L210W	−0.67 (42)	+0.07 (19)

1. Genotypic testing performed by Virco Laboratories and Visible Genetics TruGene™ technology.
2. M41L, D67N, K70R, L210W, T215Y/F or K219Q/E/N in RT.
3. Average HIV-1 RNA change from baseline through week 24 ($DAVG_{24}$) in log_{10} copies/mL.

Table 9. Selected Treatment-Emergent Adverse Events (Grades 2–4) Reported in ≥3% in Any Treatment Group in Study 907 (0–48 weeks)

	VIREAD (N=368) (Week 0–24)	Placebo (N=182) (Week 0–24)	VIREAD (N=368) (Week 0–48)	Placebo Crossover to VIREAD (N=170) (Week 24–48)
Body as a Whole				
Asthenia	7%	6%	11%	1%
Pain	7%	7%	12%	4%
Headache	5%	5%	8%	2%
Abdominal Pain	4%	3%	7%	6%
Back Pain	3%	3%	4%	2%
Chest Pain	3%	1%	3%	2%
Fever	2%	2%	4%	2%
Digestive System				
Diarrhea	11%	10%	16%	11%
Nausea	8%	5%	11%	7%
Vomiting	4%	1%	7%	5%
Anorexia	3%	2%	4%	1%
Dyspepsia	3%	2%	4%	2%
Flatulence	3%	1%	4%	1%
Respiratory				
Pneumonia	2%	0%	3%	2%
Nervous System				
Depression	4%	3%	8%	4%
Insomnia	3%	2%	4%	4%
Peripheral Neuropathy[1]	3%	3%	5%	2%
Dizziness	1%	3%	3%	1%
Skin and Appendage				
Rash Event[2]	5%	4%	7%	1%
Sweating	3%	2%	3%	1%
Musculoskeletal				
Myalgia	3%	3%	4%	1%
Metabolic				
Weight Loss	2%	1%	4%	2%

1. Peripheral neuropathy includes peripheral neuritis and neuropathy.
2. Rash event includes rash, pruritus, maculopapular rash, urticaria, vesiculobullous rash, and pustular rash.

VIREAD should be avoided with concurrent or recent use of a nephrotoxic agent. Patients at risk for, or with a history of, renal dysfunction and patients receiving concomitant nephrotoxic agents should be carefully monitored for changes in serum creatinine and phosphorus.

PRECAUTIONS

Drug Interactions

When administered with VIREAD, C_{max} and AUC of didanosine administered as either the buffered or enteric-coated formulation increased significantly (see Table 4). The mechanism of this interaction is unknown. Higher didanosine concentrations could potentiate didanosine-associated adverse events, including pancreatitis and neuropathy. In adults weighing >60kg, the didanosine dose should be reduced to 250 mg when it is co-administered with VIREAD. Data are not available to recommend a dose adjustment of didanosine for patients weighing <60 kg. When co-administered, VIREAD and didanosine EC may be taken under fasted conditions or with a light meal (<400 kcal, 20% fat). Co-administration of didanosine buffered tablet formulation with VIREAD should be under fasted conditions. **Co-administration of VIREAD and didanosine should be undertaken with caution and patients receiving this combination should be monitored closely for didanosine-associated adverse events. Didanosine should be discontinued in patients who develop didanosine-associated adverse events.**

Since tenofovir is primarily eliminated by the kidneys, co-administration of VIREAD with drugs that reduce renal function or compete for active tubular secretion may increase serum concentrations of tenofovir and/or increase the concentrations of other renally eliminated drugs. Some examples include, but are not limited to adefovir dipivoxil, cidofovir, acyclovir, valacyclovir, ganciclovir and valganciclovir.

Higher tenofovir concentrations could potentiate VIREAD-associated adverse events, including renal disorders.

Atazanavir and lopinavir/ritonavir have been shown to increase tenofovir concentrations. The mechanism of this interaction is unknown. Patients receiving atazanavir and lopinavir/ritonavir and VIREAD should be monitored for VIREAD-associated adverse events. VIREAD should be discontinued in patients who develop VIREAD-associated adverse events.

VIREAD decreases the AUC and C_{min} of atazanavir. When coadministered with VIREAD, it is recommended that atazanavir 300 mg is given with ritonavir 100 mg. Atazanavir without ritonavir should not be coadministered with VIREAD.

Bone Effects

In study 903 through 48 weeks, decreases from baseline in bone mineral density (BMD) were seen at the lumbar spine and hip in both arms of the study. At 48 weeks, percent decreases in BMD from baseline (mean ± SD) were greater in patients receiving VIREAD + lamivudine + efavirenz (spine, −3.3% ± 3.9; hip, −3.2% ± 3.6) compared with patients receiving stavudine + lamivudine + efavirenz (spine, −2.0% ± 3.5; hip. −1.8% ± 3.3). The proportion of patients who met a protocol defined value of BMD loss (5% decrease in spine or 7% decrease in hip) was higher in the VIREAD group than the stavudine group. In addition, there were significant increases in levels of four biochemical markers of bone metabolism (serum bone–specific alkaline phosphatase, serum osteocalcin, serum C-telopeptide and urinary N-telopeptide) in the VIREAD group relative to the stavudine group, suggesting increased bone turnover. Serum parathyroid hormone levels were also higher in the VIREAD group. Except for bone specific alkaline phosphatase, these changes resulted in values that remained within the normal range. There was one bone fracture reported in the VIREAD group compared with four in the stavudine group; no pathologic fractures were identified over 48 weeks of study treatment. The clinical significance of the changes in BMD and biochemical markers is unknown and follow-up is continuing to assess long-term impact.

Bone monitoring should be considered for HIV infected patients who have a history of pathologic bone fracture or are at substantial risk for osteopenia. Although the effect of supplementation with calcium and vitamin D was not studied, such supplementation may be considered for HIV-associated osteopenia or osteoporosis. If bone abnormalities are suspected then appropriate consultation should be obtained.

Fat Redistribution

Redistribution/accumulation of body fat including central obesity, dorsocervical fat enlargement (buffalo hump), peripheral wasting, facial wasting, breast enlargement, and "cushingoid appearance" have been observed in patients receiving antiretroviral therapy. The mechanism and long-term consequences of these events are currently unknown. A causal relationship has not been established.

Animal Toxicology

Tenofovir and tenofovir disoproxil fumarate administered in toxicology studies to rats, dogs and monkeys at exposures (based on AUCs) greater than or equal to 6 fold those observed in humans caused bone toxicity. In monkeys the bone toxicity was diagnosed as osteomalacia. Osteomalacia observed in monkeys appeared to be reversible upon dose reduction or discontinuation of tenofovir. In rats and dogs, the bone toxicity manifested as reduced bone mineral density. The mechanism(s) underlying bone toxicity is unknown.

Evidence of renal toxicity was noted in 4 animal species. Increases in serum creatinine, BUN, glycosuria, proteinuria, phosphaturia and/or calciuria and decreases in serum phosphate were observed to varying degrees in these animals. These toxicities were noted at exposures (based on AUCs) 2–20 times higher than those observed in humans. The relationship of the renal abnormalities, particularly the phosphaturia, to the bone toxicity is not known.

Carcinogenesis, Mutagenesis, Impairment of Fertility

Long-term oral carcinogenicity studies of tenofovir disoproxil fumarate in mice and rats were carried out at exposures up to approximately 16 times (mice) and 5 times (rats) those observed in humans at the therapeutic dose for HIV infection. At the high dose in female mice, liver adenomas were increased at exposures 16 times that in humans. In rats, the study was negative for carcinogenic findings at exposures up to 5 times that observed in humans at the therapeutic dose.

Tenofovir disoproxil fumarate was mutagenic in the in vitro mouse lymphoma assay and negative in an in vitro bacterial mutagenicity test (Ames test). In an in vivo mouse micronucleus assay, tenofovir disoproxil fumarate was negative when administered to male mice.

There were no effects on fertility, mating performance or early embryonic development when tenofovir disoproxil fumarate was administered to male rats at a dose equivalent to 10 times the human dose based on body surface area comparisons for 28 days prior to mating and to female rats for 15 days prior to mating through day seven of gestation. There was, however, an alteration of the estrous cycle in female rats.

Pregnancy

Pregnancy Category B:

Reproduction studies have been performed in rats and rabbits at doses up to 14 and 19 times the human dose based on body surface area comparisons and revealed no evidence of impaired fertility or harm to the fetus due to tenofovir. There are, however, no adequate and well-controlled studies in pregnant women. Because animal reproduction studies are not always predictive of human response, VIREAD should be used during pregnancy only if clearly needed.

Antiretroviral Pregnancy Registry: To monitor fetal outcomes of pregnant women exposed to VIREAD, an Antiretroviral Pregnancy Registry has been established. Healthcare providers are encouraged to register patients by calling 1-800-258-4263.

Nursing Mothers: The Centers for Disease Control and Prevention recommend that HIV-infected mothers not breast-feed their infants to avoid risking postnatal transmission of HIV. Studies in rats have demonstrated that tenofovir is secreted in milk. It is not known whether tenofovir is excreted in human milk. Because of both the potential for HIV transmission and the potential for serious adverse reactions in nursing infants, ***mothers should be instructed not to breast-feed if they are receiving VIREAD.***

Pediatric Use

Safety and effectiveness in pediatric patients have not been established.

Geriatric Use

Clinical studies of VIREAD did not include sufficient numbers of subjects aged 65 and over to determine whether they respond differently from younger subjects. In general, dose selection for the elderly patient should be cautious, keeping in mind the greater frequency of decreased hepatic, renal, or cardiac function, and of concomitant disease or other drug therapy.

ADVERSE REACTIONS

Clinical Trials: More than 12,000 patients have been treated with VIREAD alone or in combination with other antiretroviral medicinal products for periods of 28 days to 215 weeks in Phase I-III clinical trials and expanded access studies. A total of 1,287 patients have received VIREAD 300 mg once daily in Phase I-III clinical trials; over 11,000 patients have received VIREAD in expanded access studies.

Treatment-Experienced Patients

Treatment-Emergent Adverse Events: The most common adverse events that occurred in patients receiving VIREAD with other antiretroviral agents in clinical trials were mild to moderate gastrointestinal events, such as nausea, diarrhea, vomiting and flatulence. Less than 1% of patients discontinued participation in the clinical studies due to gastrointestinal adverse events (Study 907).

A summary of treatment-emergent adverse events that occurred during the first 48 weeks of Study 907 is provided in Table 9 (below).

[See table 9 on previous page]

Laboratory Abnormalities: Laboratory abnormalities observed in this study occurred with similar frequency in the VIREAD and placebo-treated groups. A summary of Grade 3 and 4 laboratory abnormalities is provided in Table 10 below.

[See table 10 above]

Table 10. Grade 3/4 Laboratory Abnormalities Reported in ≥1% of VIREAD-Treated Patients in Study 907 (0–48 weeks)

	VIREAD (N=368) (Week 0–24)	Placebo (N=182) (Week 0–24)	VIREAD (N=368) (Week 0–48)	Placebo Crossover to VIREAD (N=170) (Week 24–48)
	(%)	(%)	(%)	(%)
Any ≥ Grade 3 Laboratory Abnormality	25%	38%	35%	34%
Triglycerides (>750 mg/dL)	8%	13%	11%	9%
Creatine Kinase (M: >990U/L) (F: >845 U/L)	7%	14%	12%	12%
Serum Amylase (>175 U/L)	6%	7%	7%	6%
Urine Glucose(≥3+)	3%	3%	3%	2%
AST (M: >180 U/L) (F: >170 U/L)	3%	3%	4%	5%
ALT (M: >215 U/L) (F: >170 U/L)	2%	2%	4%	5%
Serum Glucose (>250 U/L)	2%	4%	3%	3%
Neutrophils (<750 mg/dL)	1%	1%	2%	1%

Treatment-Naïve Patients

Treatment-Emergent Adverse Events: The adverse reactions seen in a double-blind comparative controlled study in which 600 treatment-naïve patients received VIREAD (N=299) or stavudine (N=301) in combination with lamivudine and efavirenz for 48 weeks (Study 903) were generally consistent, with the addition of dizziness, with those seen in treatment-experienced patients (Table 11).

Mild adverse events (Grade 1) were common with a similar incidence in both arms, and included dizziness, diarrhea and nausea.

Table 11. Selected Treatment-Emergent Adverse Events (Grades 2–4) Reported in ≥3% in Any Treatment Group in Study 903 (0–48 weeks)

	VIREAD +3TC+EFV	d4T+3TC +EFV
	N=299	N=301
Body as a Whole		
Headache	10%	11%
Pain	7%	6%
Fever	5%	6%
Abdominal Pain	4%	8%
Back Pain	4%	3%
Asthenia	3%	5%
Digestive System		
Diarrhea	6%	6%
Nausea	5%	6%
Dyspepsia	3%	2%
Vomiting	3%	6%
Musculoskeletal		
Arthralgia	2%	4%
Nervous System		
Depression	7%	5%
Insomnia	4%	6%
Abnormal Dreams	3%	3%
Dizziness	3%	5%
Paresthesia	2%	3%
Peripheral neuropathy[1]	1%	4%
Respiratory		
Pneumonia	3%	3%
Skin and Appendages		
Rash Event[2]	15%	11%

1. Peripheral neuropathy includes peripheral neuritis and neuropathy
2. Rash event includes rash, pruritus, maculopapular rash, urticaria, vesiculobullous rash, and pustular rash.

Laboratory Abnormalities: With the exception of triglyceride elevations that were more common in the stavudine group (8%) compared with VIREAD (2%), laboratory abnormalities observed in this study occurred with similar frequency in the VIREAD and stavudine treatment arms. A summary of Grade 3 and 4 laboratory abnormalities is provided in Table 12.

Table 12. Grade 3/4 Laboratory Abnormalities Reported in ≥ 1% of VIREAD-Treated Patients in Study 903 (0–48 weeks)

	VIREAD +3TC+EFV	d4T+3TC +EFV
	N=299	N=301
Any ≥ Grade 3 Laboratory Abnormality	28%	31%
Creatine Kinase (M: >990 U/L) (F: >845 U/L)	8%	9%
Serum Amylase (>175 U/L)	7%	6%
AST (M: >180 U/L) (F: >170 U/L)	4%	5%
ALT (M: >215 U/L) (F: >170 U/L)	4%	4%
Hematuria (>100 RBC/ HPF)	4%	4%
Neutrophil (<750/mm^3)	3%	1%
Triglyceride (<750 mg/dL)	2%	8%

Post Marketing Experience: In addition to adverse events reported from clinical trials, the following events have been identified during post-approval use of VIREAD. Because they are reported voluntarily from a population of unknown size, estimates of frequency cannot be made. These events have been chosen for inclusion due to a combination of their seriousness, frequency of reporting or potential causal connection to VIREAD.

IMMUNE SYSTEM DISORDERS
Allergic reaction
METABOLISM AND NUTRITION DISORDERS
Hypophosphatemia, Lactic acidosis
RESPIRATORY, THORACIC, AND MEDIASTINAL DISORDERS
Dyspnea

Continued on next page

Viread—Cont.

GASTROINTESTINAL DISORDERS
Abdominal pain, Pancreatitis
RENAL AND URINARY DISORDERS
Renal insufficiency, Renal failure, Acute renal failure, Fanconi syndrome, Proximal tubulopathy, Proteinuria, Increased creatinine, Acute tubular necrosis

OVERDOSAGE

Limited clinical experience at doses higher than the therapeutic dose of VIREAD 300 mg is available. In Study 901, 600 mg tenofovir disoproxil fumarate was administered to 8 patients orally for 28 days. No severe adverse reactions were reported. The effects of higher doses are not known.
If overdose occurs the patient must be monitored for evidence of toxicity, and standard supportive treatment applied as necessary.
Tenofovir is efficiently removed by hemodialysis with an extraction coefficient of approximately 54%. Following a single 300 mg dose of VIREAD, a four-hour hemodialysis session removed approximately 10% of the administered tenofovir dose.

DOSAGE AND ADMINISTRATION

The dose of VIREAD is 300 mg once daily taken orally, without regard to food.

Dose Adjustment for Renal Impairment

Significantly increased drug exposures occurred when VIREAD was administered to patients with moderate to severe renal impairment (see PHARMACOKINETICS). The dosing interval of VIREAD should be adjusted in patients with baseline creatinine clearance <50 mL/min using the recommendations in Table 13. The safety and effectiveness of these dosing interval adjustment recommendations have not been clinically evaluated, therefore, clinical response to treatment and renal function should be closely monitored in these patients.
[See table 13 above]
The pharmacokinetics of tenofovir have not been evaluated in non-hemodialysis patients with creatinine clearance <10 mL/min; therefore, no dosing recommendation is available for these patients.

Table 13. Dosage Adjustment for Patients with Altered Creatinine Clearance

	Creatinine Clearance (mL/min)[1]			Hemodialysis Patients
	≥50	30–49	10–29	
Recommended 300 mg Dosing Interval	Every 24 hours	Every 48 hours	Twice a week	Every 7 days or after a total of approximately 12 hours of dialysis[2]

1. Calculated using ideal (lean) body weight.
2. Generally once weekly assuming three hemodialysis sessions a week of approximately 4 hours duration. VIREAD should be administered following completion of dialysis.

HOW SUPPLIED

VIREAD is available as tablets. Each tablet contains 300 mg of tenofovir disoproxil fumarate, which is equivalent to 245 mg of tenofovir disoproxil. The tablets are almond-shaped, light blue, film-coated, and debossed with "GILEAD" and "4331" on one side and with "300" on the other side. They are packaged as follows: Bottles of 30 tablets (NDC 61958-0401-1) containing a desiccant (silica gel canister or sachet) and closed with child-resistant closure.
Store at 25 °C (77 °F), excursions permitted to 15–30 °C (59–86 °F) (see USP Controlled Room Temperature).
Do not use if seal over bottle opening is broken or missing.
Gilead Sciences, Inc.
Foster City, CA 94404
June 2004 VIREAD is a registered trademark of Gilead Sciences, Inc

GILEAD

VIREAD®
(tenofovir disoproxil fumarate) Tablets

Patient Information

VIREAD (VEER ee ad)
Generic Name: tenofovir disoproxil fumarate (te NOE' fo veer dye soe PROX il FYOU-mar-ate)
Read this leaflet carefully before you start taking VIREAD. Also, read it each time you get your VIREAD prescription refilled, in case something has changed. This information does not take the place of talking with your healthcare provider when you start this medicine and at check ups. You should stay under a healthcare provider's care when taking VIREAD. Do not change or stop your medicine without first talking with your healthcare provider. Talk to your healthcare provider if you have any questions about VIREAD.

What is VIREAD and how does it work?

VIREAD is a type of medicine called an HIV-1 (human immunodeficiency virus) nucleotide analog reverse transcriptase inhibitor (NRTI). VIREAD is always used in combination with other anti-HIV medicines to treat people with HIV-1 infection. VIREAD is for adults age 18 and older. HIV infection destroys CD4 (T) cells, which are important to the immune system. After a large number of T cells are destroyed, acquired immune deficiency syndrome (AIDS) develops.
VIREAD helps to block HIV-1 reverse transcriptase, a chemical in your body (enzyme) that is needed for HIV-1 to multiply. VIREAD lowers the amount of HIV-1 in the blood (called viral load) and may help to increase the number of T cells (called CD4 cells). Lowering the amount of HIV-1 in the blood lowers the chance of death or infections that happen when your immune system is weak (opportunistic infections).

Does VIREAD cure HIV-1 or AIDS?

VIREAD does not cure HIV-1 infection or AIDS. The long-term effects of VIREAD are not known at this time. People taking VIREAD may still get opportunistic infections or other conditions that happen with HIV-1 infection. Opportunistic infections are infections that develop because the immune system is weak. Some of these conditions are pneumonia, herpes virus infections, and *Mycobacterium avium* complex (MAC) infections.

Does VIREAD reduce the risk of passing HIV-1 to others?

VIREAD does not reduce the risk of passing HIV-1 to others through sexual contact or blood contamination. Continue to practice safe sex and do not use or share dirty needles.

Who should not take VIREAD?

Together with your healthcare provider, you need to decide whether VIREAD is right for you.
Do not take VIREAD if
- you are allergic to VIREAD or any of its ingredients

What should I tell my healthcare provider before taking VIREAD?

Tell your healthcare provider
- *If you are pregnant or planning to become pregnant:* The effects of VIREAD on pregnant women or their unborn babies are not known.
- *If you are breast-feeding:* Do not breast-feed if you are taking VIREAD. Do not breast-feed if you have HIV. If you are a woman who has or will have a baby, talk with your healthcare provider about the best way to feed your baby. If your baby does not already have HIV, there is a chance that the baby can get HIV through breast-feeding.
- **If you have kidney or bone problems**
- **If you have liver problems including Hepatitis B Virus infection**
- **Tell your healthcare provider about all your medical conditions**
- **Tell your healthcare provider about all the medicines you take**, including prescription and non-prescription medicines and dietary supplements. VIREAD may increase the amount of VIDEX® (didanosine) in your blood. You may need to be followed more carefully if you are taking these two drugs together.
  It is a good idea to keep a complete list of all the medicines that you take. Make a new list when medicines are added or stopped. Give copies of this list to all of your healthcare providers **every** time you visit your healthcare provider or fill a prescription.

How should I take VIREAD?

- Stay under a healthcare provider's care when taking VIREAD. Do not change your treatment or stop treatment without first talking with your healthcare provider.
- Take VIREAD every day exactly as your healthcare provider prescribed it. Follow the directions from your healthcare provider, exactly as written on the label. Set up a dosing schedule and follow it carefully.
- The usual dose of VIREAD is 1 tablet once a day, in combination with other anti-HIV medicines. If you have kidney problems, your healthcare provider may recommend that you take VIREAD less frequently.
- VIREAD may be taken with or without a meal.
- When your VIREAD supply starts to run low, get more from your healthcare provider or pharmacy. This is very important because the amount of virus in your blood may increase if the medicine is stopped for even a short time. The virus may develop resistance to VIREAD and become harder to treat.
- Only take medicine that has been prescribed specifically for you. Do not give VIREAD to others or take medicine prescribed for someone else.

What should I do if I miss a dose of VIREAD?

It is important that you do not miss any doses. If you miss a dose of VIREAD, take it as soon as possible and then take your next scheduled dose at its regular time. If it is almost time for your next dose, do not take the missed dose. Wait and take the next dose at the regular time. Do not double the next dose.

What happens if I take too much VIREAD?

If you suspect that you took more than the prescribed dose of VIREAD, contact your local poison control center or emergency room right away.
As with all medicines, VIREAD should be kept out of reach of children.

What should I avoid while taking VIREAD?

- Do not breast-feed. See "What should I tell my healthcare provider before taking VIREAD?"

What are the possible side effects of VIREAD?

- Clinical studies: The most common side effects of VIREAD are: diarrhea, nausea, vomiting, and flatulence (intestinal gas).
- Marketing experience: Other side effects reported since VIREAD has been marketed include: weakness, inflammation of the pancreas, low blood phosphate, dizziness, shortness of breath, and rash.
- Some patients treated with VIREAD have had kidney problems. If you have had kidney problems in the past or need to take another drug that can cause kidney problems, your healthcare provider may need to perform additional blood tests.
- Laboratory tests show changes in the bones of patients treated with VIREAD. It is not known whether long-term use of VIREAD will cause damage to your bones. If you have had bone problems in the past, your healthcare provider may need to perform additional tests or may suggest additional medication.
- Some patients taking antiviral drugs like VIREAD have developed a condition called lactic acidosis (a buildup in the blood of lactic acid, the same substance that causes your muscles to burn during heavy exercise). Symptoms of lactic acidosis include nausea, vomiting, unusual or unexpected stomach discomfort, and weakness. If you notice these symptoms or if your medical condition changes suddenly, call your healthcare provider right away.
- Changes in body fat have been seen in some patients taking anti-HIV medicine. These changes may include increased amount of fat in the upper back and neck ("buffalo hump"), breast, and around the main part of your body (trunk). Loss of fat from the legs, arms and face may also happen. The cause and long term health effects of these conditions are not known at this time.
- If you have hepatitis B virus (HBV) infection, you may have a "flare-up" of hepatitis B, in which the disease suddenly returns in a worse way than before if you stop taking VIREAD. VIREAD is not for the treatment of hepatitis B virus infection.
- There have been other side effects in patients taking VIREAD. However, these side effects may have been due to other medicines that patients were taking or to the illness itself. Some of these side effects can be serious.
- This list of side effects is **not** complete. If you have questions about side effects, ask your healthcare provider. You should report any new or continuing symptoms to your healthcare provider right away. Your healthcare provider may be able to help you manage these side effects.

How do I store VIREAD?

- Keep VIREAD and all other medications out of reach of children.
- Store VIREAD at room temperature 77 °F (25 °C). It should remain stable until the expiration date printed on the label.
- Do not keep your medicine in places that are too hot or cold.
- Do not keep medicine that is out of date or that you no longer need. If you throw any medicines away make sure that children will not find them.

General advice about prescription medicines:

Talk to your healthcare provider if you have any questions about this medicine or your condition. Medicines are sometimes prescribed for purposes other than those listed in a Patient Information Leaflet. If you have any concerns about this medicine, ask your healthcare provider. Your healthcare provider or pharmacist can give you information about this medicine that was written for health care professionals. Do not use this medicine for a condition for which it was not prescribed. Do not share this medicine with other people.
Do not use if seal over bottle opening is broken or missing.
June 2004

GILEAD

Shown in Product Identification Guide, page 313

GlaxoSmithKline

FIVE MOORE DRIVE
RESEARCH TRIANGLE PARK, NC 27709

For Medical Emergencies, Medical Information for Healthcare Professionals, and Consumer Inquiries, Contact:
1-888-825-5249
www.druginfo.gsk.com

ACLOVATE® ℞
[a'klō-vāt]
(alclometasone dipropionate cream)
Cream, 0.05%

ACLOVATE®
(alclometasone dipropionate ointment)
Ointment, 0.05%

For Dermatologic Use Only—
Not for Ophthalmic Use.

DESCRIPTION

ACLOVATE Cream and Ointment contain alclometasone dipropionate (7α-chloro-11β,17,21-trihydroxy-16α-methylpregna-1,4-diene-3,20-dione 17,21-dipropionate), a synthetic corticosteroid for topical dermatologic use. The corticosteroids constitute a class of primarily synthetic steroids

used topically as anti-inflammatory and antipruritic agents. Chemically, alclometasone dipropionate is $C_{28}H_{37}ClO_7$.
Alclometasone dipropionate has the molecular weight of 521. It is a white powder, insoluble in water, slightly soluble in propylene glycol, and moderately soluble in hexylene glycol.
Each gram of ACLOVATE Cream contains 0.5 mg of alclometasone dipropionate in a hydrophilic, emollient cream base of propylene glycol, white petrolatum, cetearyl alcohol, glyceryl stearate, PEG 100 stearate, Ceteth-20, monobasic sodium phosphate, chlorocresol, phosphoric acid, and purified water.
Each gram of ACLOVATE Ointment contains 0.5 mg of alclometasone dipropionate in an ointment base of hexylene glycol, white wax, propylene glycol stearate, and white petrolatum.

CLINICAL PHARMACOLOGY

Like other topical corticosteroids, alclometasone dipropionate has anti-inflammatory, antipruritic, and vasoconstrictive properties. The mechanism of the anti-inflammatory activity of the topical steroids, in general, is unclear. However, corticosteroids are thought to act by the induction of phospholipase A_2 inhibitory proteins, collectively called lipocortins. It is postulated that these proteins control the biosynthesis of potent mediators of inflammation such as prostaglandins and leukotrienes by inhibiting the release of their common precursor, arachidonic acid. Arachidonic acid is released from membrane phospholipids by phospholipase A_2.
Pharmacokinetics: The extent of percutaneous absorption of topical corticosteroids is determined by many factors, including the vehicle and the integrity of the epidermal barrier. Occlusive dressings with hydrocortisone for up to 24 hours have not been demonstrated to increase penetration; however, occlusion of hydrocortisone for 96 hours markedly enhances penetration. Topical corticosteroids can be absorbed from normal intact skin. Inflammation and/or other disease processes in the skin may increase percutaneous absorption. A study utilizing a radiolabeled alclometasone dipropionate ointment formulation was performed to measure systemic absorption and excretion. Results indicated that approximately 3% of the steroid was absorbed during 8 hours of contact with intact skin of normal volunteers.
Studies performed with ACLOVATE Cream and Ointment indicate that these products are in the low to medium range of potency as compared with other topical corticosteroids.

INDICATIONS AND USAGE

ACLOVATE Cream and Ointment are low to medium potency corticosteroids indicated for the relief of the inflammatory and pruritic manifestations of corticosteroid-responsive dermatoses. ACLOVATE Cream and Ointment may be used in pediatric patients 1 year of age or older, although the safety and efficacy of drug use for longer than 3 weeks have not been established (see PRECAUTIONS: Pediatric Use). Since the safety and efficacy of ACLOVATE Cream and Ointment have not been established in pediatric patients below 1 year of age, their use in this age-group is not recommended.

CONTRAINDICATIONS

ACLOVATE Cream and Ointment are contraindicated in those patients with a history of hypersensitivity to any of the components in these preparations.

PRECAUTIONS

General: Systemic absorption of topical corticosteroids can produce reversible hypothalamic-pituitary-adrenal (HPA) axis suppression with the potential for glucocorticosteroid insufficiency after withdrawal of treatment. Manifestations of Cushing syndrome, hyperglycemia, and glucosuria can also be produced in some patients by systemic absorption of topical corticosteroids while on treatment.
Patients applying a topical steroid to a large surface area or to areas under occlusion should be evaluated periodically for evidence of HPA axis suppression. This may be done by using the ACTH stimulation, A.M. plasma cortisol, and urinary free cortisol tests.
The effects of ACLOVATE Cream and Ointment on the HPA axis have been evaluated. In one study, ACLOVATE Cream and Ointment were applied to 30% of the body twice daily for 7 days, and occlusive dressings were used in selected patients either 12 hours or 24 hours daily. In another study, ACLOVATE Cream was applied to 80% of the body surface of normal subjects twice daily for 21 days with daily 12-hour periods of whole body occlusion. Average plasma and urinary free cortisol levels and urinary levels of 17-hydroxysteroids were decreased (about 10%), suggesting suppression of the HPA axis under these conditions. Plasma cortisol levels have also been demonstrated to decrease in pediatric patients treated twice daily for 3 weeks without occlusion.
If HPA axis suppression is noted, an attempt should be made to withdraw the drug, to reduce the frequency of application, or to substitute a less potent corticosteroid. Recovery of HPA axis function is generally prompt upon discontinuation of topical corticosteroids. Infrequently, signs and symptoms of glucocorticosteroid insufficiency may occur, requiring supplemental systemic corticosteroids. For information on systemic supplementation, see prescribing information for those products.
Pediatric patients may be more susceptible to systemic toxicity from equivalent doses due to their larger skin surface area to body mass ratios (see PRECAUTIONS: Pediatric Use).
If irritation develops, ACLOVATE Cream or Ointment should be discontinued and appropriate therapy instituted.
Allergic contact dermatitis with corticosteroids is usually diagnosed by observing *a failure to heal* rather than noting a clinical exacerbation, as with most topical products not containing corticosteroids. Such an observation should be corroborated with appropriate diagnostic patch testing.
If concomitant skin infections are present or develop, an appropriate antifungal or antibacterial agent should be used. If a favorable response does not occur promptly, use of ACLOVATE Cream or Ointment should be discontinued until the infection has been adequately controlled.
Information for Patients: Patients using topical corticosteroids should receive the following information and instructions:

1. This medication is to be used as directed by the physician. It is for external use only. Avoid contact with the eyes.
2. This medication should not be used for any disorder other than that for which it was prescribed.
3. The treated skin area should not be bandaged, otherwise covered or wrapped so as to be occlusive, unless directed by the physician.
4. Patients should report to their physician any signs of local adverse reactions.
5. Parents of pediatric patients should be advised not to use ACLOVATE Cream or Ointment in the treatment of diaper dermatitis. ACLOVATE Cream or Ointment should not be applied in the diaper area as diapers or plastic pants may constitute occlusive dressing (see DOSAGE AND ADMINISTRATION).
6. This medication should not be used on the face, underarms, or groin areas unless directed by the physician.
7. As with other corticosteroids, therapy should be discontinued when control is achieved. If no improvement is seen within 2 weeks, contact the physician.

Laboratory Tests: The following tests may be helpful in evaluating patients for HPA axis suppression:
ACTH stimulation test
A.M. plasma cortisol test
Urinary free cortisol test
Carcinogenesis, Mutagenesis, Impairment of Fertility: Long-term animal studies have not been performed to evaluate the carcinogenic potential or the effect on fertility of topical corticosteroids.
Pregnancy: *Teratogenic Effects:* Pregnancy Category C. Corticosteroids have been shown to be teratogenic in laboratory animals when administered systemically at relatively low dosage levels. Some corticosteroids have been shown to be teratogenic after dermal application in laboratory animals. There are no adequate and well-controlled studies in pregnant women. ACLOVATE Cream or Ointment should be used during pregnancy only if the potential benefit justifies the potential risk to the fetus.
Nursing Mothers: Systemically administered corticosteroids appear in human milk and could suppress growth, interfere with endogenous corticosteroid production, or cause other untoward effects. It is not known whether topical administration of topical corticosteroids could result in sufficient systemic absorption to produce detectable quantities in human milk. Because many drugs are excreted in human milk, caution should be exercised when ACLOVATE Cream or Ointment is administered to a nursing woman.
Pediatric Use: ACLOVATE Cream and Ointment may be used with caution in pediatric patients 1 year of age or older, although the safety and efficacy of drug use for longer than 3 weeks have not been established. Use of ACLOVATE Cream and Ointment is supported by results from adequate and well-controlled studies in pediatric patients with corticosteroid-responsive dermatoses. Since the safety and efficacy of ACLOVATE Cream and Ointment have not been established in pediatric patients below 1 year of age, its use in this age-group is not recommended. Because of a higher ratio of skin surface area to body mass, pediatric patients are at a greater risk than adults of HPA axis suppression and Cushing syndrome when they are treated with topical corticosteroids. They are therefore also at greater risk of adrenal insufficiency during and/or after withdrawal of treatment. Adverse effects, including striae, have been reported with inappropriate use of topical corticosteroids in infants and children. Pediatric patients applying ACLOVATE Cream or Ointment to >20% of the body surface area are at higher risk for HPA axis suppression.
HPA axis suppression, Cushing syndrome, linear growth retardation, delayed weight gain, and intracranial hypertension have been reported in pediatric patients receiving topical corticosteroids. Manifestations of adrenal suppression in pediatric patients include low plasma cortisol levels and absence of response to ACTH stimulation. Manifestations of intracranial hypertension include bulging fontanelles, headaches, and bilateral papilledema.
ACLOVATE Cream or Ointment should not be used in the treatment of diaper dermatitis.
Geriatric Use: A limited number of patients at or above 65 years of age have been treated with ACLOVATE Cream and Ointment in US clinical trials. The number of patients is too small to permit separate analysis of efficacy and safety. No adverse events were reported with ACLOVATE Ointment in geriatric patients, and the single adverse reaction reported with ACLOVATE Cream in this population was similar to those reactions reported by younger patients. Based on available data, no adjustment of dosage of ACLOVATE Cream and Ointment in geriatric patients is warranted.

ADVERSE REACTIONS

The following local adverse reactions have been reported with ACLOVATE Cream in approximately 2% of patients: itching and burning, erythema, dryness, irritation, and papular rashes.
The following local adverse reactions have been reported with ACLOVATE Ointment in approximately 1% of patients: itching, burning, and erythema.
The following additional local adverse reactions have been reported infrequently with topical corticosteroids, but may occur more frequently with the use of occlusive dressings. These reactions are listed in approximate decreasing order of occurrence: folliculitis, acneiform eruptions, hypopigmentation, perioral dermatitis, allergic contact dermatitis, secondary infection, skin atrophy, striae, and miliaria.

OVERDOSAGE

Topically applied ACLOVATE Cream and Ointment can be absorbed in sufficient amounts to produce systemic effects (see PRECAUTIONS).

DOSAGE AND ADMINISTRATION

Apply a thin film of ACLOVATE Cream or Ointment to the affected skin areas 2 or 3 times daily; massage gently until the medication disappears.
ACLOVATE Cream and Ointment may be used in pediatric patients 1 year of age or older. Safety and effectiveness of ACLOVATE Cream or Ointment in pediatric patients for more than 3 weeks of use have not been established. Use in pediatric patients under 1 year of age is not recommended.
As with other corticosteroids, therapy should be discontinued when control is achieved. If no improvement is seen within 2 weeks, reassessment of diagnosis may be necessary.
ACLOVATE Cream or Ointment should not be used with occlusive dressings unless directed by a physician. ACLOVATE Cream or Ointment should not be applied in the diaper area if the child still requires diapers or plastic pants as these garments may constitute occlusive dressing.
Geriatric Use: In studies where geriatric patients (65 years of age or older, see PRECAUTIONS) have been treated with ACLOVATE Cream or Ointment, safety did not differ from that in younger patients; therefore, no dosage adjustment is recommended.

HOW SUPPLIED

ACLOVATE Cream, 0.05% is supplied in:
15-g tubes (NDC 0173-0401-00),
45-g tubes (NDC 0173-0401-01), and
60-g tubes (NDC 0173-0401-06).
ACLOVATE Ointment, 0.05% is supplied in:
15-g tubes (NDC 0173-0402-00),
45-g tubes (NDC 0173-0402-01), and
60-g tubes (NDC 0173-0402-06).
Store between 2° and 30°C (36° and 86°F).
GlaxoSmithKline Consumer Healthcare LP
Pittsburgh, PA 15230

August 2002/RL-1081
Shown in Product Identification Guide, page 313

ADVAIR DISKUS® 100/50 ℞

[*ad'vair disk'us*]
(fluticasone propionate 100 mcg and salmeterol* 50 mcg inhalation powder)

ADVAIR DISKUS® 250/50 ℞

(fluticasone propionate 250 mcg and salmeterol* 50 mcg inhalation powder)

ADVAIR DISKUS® 500/50 ℞

(fluticasone propionate 500 mcg and salmeterol* 50 mcg inhalation powder)

***As salmeterol xinafoate salt 72.5 mcg, equivalent to salmeterol base 50 mcg**
FOR ORAL INHALATION ONLY

WARNING: Data from a large placebo-controlled US study that compared the safety of salmeterol (SEREVENT® Inhalation Aerosol) or placebo added to usual asthma therapy showed a small but significant increase in asthma-related deaths in patients receiving salmeterol (13 deaths out of 13,174 patients treated for 28 weeks) versus those on placebo (4 of 13,179). Subgroup analyses suggest the risk may be greater in African American patients compared to Caucasians (see WARNINGS).

DESCRIPTION

ADVAIR DISKUS 100/50, ADVAIR DISKUS 250/50, and ADVAIR DISKUS 500/50 are combinations of fluticasone propionate and salmeterol xinafoate.
One active component of ADVAIR DISKUS is fluticasone propionate, a corticosteroid having the chemical name *S*-

Continued on next page

Product information on these pages is effective as of August 2004. Further information is available at: GlaxoSmithKline, PO Box 13398, Research Triangle Park, NC 27709. 1-888-825-5249. Corporate Web Site: www.gsk.com

Advair Diskus—Cont.

(fluoromethyl) 6α,9-difluoro-11β,17-dihydroxy-16α-methyl-3-oxoandrosta-1,4-diene-17β-carbothioate, 17-propionate.
Fluticasone propionate is a white to off-white powder with a molecular weight of 500.6, and the empirical formula is $C_{25}H_{31}F_3O_5S$. It is practically insoluble in water, freely soluble in dimethyl sulfoxide and dimethylformamide, and slightly soluble in methanol and 95% ethanol.
The other active component of ADVAIR DISKUS is salmeterol xinafoate, beta$_2$-adrenergic bronchodilator. Salmeterol xinafoate is the racemic form of the 1-hydroxy-2-naphthoic acid salt of salmeterol. The chemical name of salmeterol xinafoate is 4-hydroxy-α^1-[[[6-(4-phenylbutoxy)hexyl]amino]methyl]-1,3-benzenedimethanol, 1-hydroxy-2-naphthalenecarboxylate.
Salmeterol xinafoate is a white to off-white powder with a molecular weight of 603.8, and the empirical formula is $C_{25}H_{37}NO_4 \bullet C_{11}H_8O_3$. It is freely soluble in methanol; slightly soluble in ethanol, chloroform, and isopropanol; and sparingly soluble in water.
ADVAIR DISKUS 100/50, ADVAIR DISKUS 250/50, and ADVAIR DISKUS 500/50 are specially designed plastic devices containing a double-foil blister strip of a powder formulation of fluticasone propionate and salmeterol xinafoate intended for oral inhalation only. Each blister on the double-foil strip within the device contains 100, 250, or 500 mcg of microfine fluticasone propionate and 72.5 mcg of microfine salmeterol xinafoate salt, equivalent to 50 mcg of salmeterol base, in 12.5 mg of formulation containing lactose (which contains milk proteins). Each blister contains 1 complete dose of both medications. After a blister containing medication is opened by activating the device, the medication is dispersed into the airstream created by the patient inhaling through the mouthpiece.
Under standardized in vitro test conditions, ADVAIR DISKUS delivers 93, 233, and 465 mcg of fluticasone propionate and 45 mcg of salmeterol base per blister from ADVAIR DISKUS 100/50, 250/50, and 500/50, respectively, when tested at a flow rate of 60 L/min for 2 seconds. In adult patients with obstructive lung disease and severely compromised lung function (mean forced expiratory volume in 1 second [FEV_1] 20% to 30% of predicted), mean peak inspiratory flow (PIF) through a DISKUS® inhalation device was 82.4 L/min (range, 46.1 to 115.3 L/min).
Inhalation profiles for adolescent (N = 13, aged 12 to 17 years) and adult (N = 17, aged 18 to 50 years) patients with asthma inhaling maximally through the DISKUS device show mean PIF of 122.2 L/min (range, 81.6 to 152.1 L/min).
Inhalation profiles for pediatric patients with asthma inhaling maximally through the DISKUS device show a mean PIF of 75.5 L/min (range, 49.0 to 104.8 L/min) for the 4-year-old patient set (N = 20) and 107.3 L/min (range, 82.8 to 125.6 L/min) for the 8-year-old patient set (N = 20).
The actual amount of drug delivered to the lung will depend on patient factors, such as inspiratory flow profile.

CLINICAL PHARMACOLOGY

Mechanism of Action: ***ADVAIR DISKUS:*** Since ADVAIR DISKUS contains both fluticasone propionate and salmeterol, the mechanisms of action described below for the individual components apply to ADVAIR DISKUS. These drugs represent 2 classes of medications (a synthetic corticosteroid and a selective, long-acting beta-adrenergic receptor agonist) that have different effects on clinical and physiological indices.
Fluticasone Propionate: Fluticasone propionate is a synthetic, trifluorinated corticosteroid with potent anti-inflammatory activity. In vitro assays using human lung cytosol preparations have established fluticasone propionate as a human glucocorticoid receptor agonist with an affinity 18 times greater than dexamethasone, almost twice that of beclomethasone-17-monopropionate (BMP), the active metabolite of beclomethasone dipropionate, and over 3 times that of budesonide. Data from the McKenzie vasoconstrictor assay in man are consistent with these results.
Inflammation is an important component in the pathogenesis of asthma. Corticosteroids have been shown to inhibit multiple cell types (e.g., mast cells, eosinophils, basophils, lymphocytes, macrophages, and neutrophils) and mediator production or secretion (e.g., histamine, eicosanoids, leukotrienes, and cytokines) involved in the asthmatic response. These anti-inflammatory actions of corticosteroids contribute to their efficacy in asthma.
Inflammation is also a component in the pathogenesis of chronic obstructive pulmonary disease (COPD). In contrast to asthma, however, the predominant inflammatory cells in COPD include neutrophils, CD8+ T-lymphocytes, and macrophages. The effects of corticosteroids in the treatment of COPD are not well defined and inhaled corticosteroids and fluticasone propionate when used apart from ADVAIR DISKUS are not indicated for the treatment of COPD.
Salmeterol Xinafoate: Salmeterol is a long-acting beta-adrenergic agonist. In vitro studies and in vivo pharmacologic studies demonstrate that salmeterol is selective for beta$_2$-adrenoceptors compared with isoproterenol, which has approximately equal agonist activity on beta$_1$- and beta$_2$-adrenoceptors. In vitro studies show salmeterol to be at least 50 times more selective for beta$_2$-adrenoceptors than albuterol. Although beta$_2$-adrenoceptors are the predominant adrenergic receptors in bronchial smooth muscle and beta$_1$-adrenoceptors are the predominant receptors in the heart, there are also beta$_2$-adrenoceptors in the human heart comprising 10% to 50% of the total beta-adrenoceptors. The precise function of these receptors has not been established, but they raise the possibility that even highly selective beta$_2$-agonists may have cardiac effects.
The pharmacologic effects of beta$_2$-adrenoceptor agonist drugs, including salmeterol, are at least in part attributable to stimulation of intracellular adenyl cyclase, the enzyme that catalyzes the conversion of adenosine triphosphate (ATP) to cyclic-3',5'-adenosine monophosphate (cyclic AMP). Increased cyclic AMP levels cause relaxation of bronchial smooth muscle and inhibition of release of mediators of immediate hypersensitivity from cells, especially from mast cells.
In vitro tests show that salmeterol is a potent and long-lasting inhibitor of the release of mast cell mediators, such as histamine, leukotrienes, and prostaglandin D_2, from human lung. Salmeterol inhibits histamine-induced plasma protein extravasation and inhibits platelet-activating factor-induced eosinophil accumulation in the lungs of guinea pigs when administered by the inhaled route. In humans, single doses of salmeterol administered via inhalation aerosol attenuate allergen-induced bronchial hyper-responsiveness.
Pharmacokinetics: ***ADVAIR DISKUS: Adult and Adolescent Patients 12 Years of Age and Older:*** Following administration of ADVAIR DISKUS to healthy adult subjects, peak plasma concentrations of fluticasone propionate were achieved in 1 to 2 hours and those of salmeterol were achieved in about 5 minutes.
In a single-dose crossover study, a higher than recommended dose of ADVAIR DISKUS was administered to 14 healthy adult subjects. Two (2) inhalations of the following treatments were administered: ADVAIR DISKUS 500/50, fluticasone propionate powder 500 mcg and salmeterol powder 50 mcg given concurrently, and fluticasone propionate powder 500 mcg alone. Mean peak plasma concentrations of fluticasone propionate averaged 107, 94, and 120 pg/mL, respectively, and of salmeterol averaged 200 and 150 pg/mL, respectively, indicating no significant changes in systemic exposures of fluticasone propionate and salmeterol.
In a repeat-dose study, the highest recommended dose of ADVAIR DISKUS was administered to 45 adolescent and adult patients with asthma. One (1) inhalation twice daily of the following treatments was administered: ADVAIR DISKUS 500/50, fluticasone propionate powder 500 mcg and salmeterol powder 50 mcg given concurrently, or fluticasone propionate powder 500 mcg alone. Mean peak steady-state plasma concentrations of fluticasone propionate averaged 57, 73, and 70 pg/mL, respectively, indicating no significant changes in systemic exposure of fluticasone propionate. No plasma concentrations of salmeterol were measured in this repeat-dose study.
No significant changes in excretion of fluticasone propionate or salmeterol were observed. The terminal half-life of fluticasone propionate averaged 5.33 to 7.65 hours when ADVAIR DISKUS was administered, which is similar to that reported when fluticasone propionate was given concurrently with salmeterol or when fluticasone propionate was given alone (average, 5.30 to 6.91 hours). No terminal half-life of salmeterol was reported upon administration of ADVAIR DISKUS or salmeterol given concurrently with fluticasone propionate.
Pediatric Patients: In a clinical study conducted in patients with asthma aged 4 to 11 years, fluticasone propionate concentrations were obtained in 61 patients at 20 and 40 minutes after dosing with 50 and 100 mcg of fluticasone propionate inhalation powder twice daily using the DISKUS. Plasma concentrations were low and ranged from undetectable (about 80% of the plasma samples) to 88 pg/mL. Mean peak fluticasone propionate plasma concentrations at the 50- and 100-mcg dose levels were 5 and 8 pg/mL, respectively.
Special Populations: Formal pharmacokinetic studies using ADVAIR DISKUS have not been conducted to examine gender differences or in special populations, such as elderly patients or patients with hepatic or renal impairment.
Drug Interactions: In the repeat- and single-dose studies, there was no evidence of significant drug interaction in systemic exposure between fluticasone propionate and salmeterol when given as ADVAIR DISKUS.
Fluticasone Propionate: Absorption: Fluticasone propionate acts locally in the lung; therefore, plasma levels do not predict therapeutic effect. Studies using oral dosing of labeled and unlabeled drug have demonstrated that the oral systemic bioavailability of fluticasone propionate is negligible (<1%), primarily due to incomplete absorption and presystemic metabolism in the gut and liver. In contrast, the majority of the fluticasone propionate delivered to the lung is systemically absorbed. The systemic bioavailability of fluticasone propionate from the DISKUS device in healthy volunteers averages 18%.
Peak steady-state fluticasone propionate plasma concentrations in adult patients with asthma (N = 11) ranged from undetectable to 266 pg/mL after a 500-mcg twice-daily dose of fluticasone propionate inhalation powder using the DISKUS device. The mean fluticasone propionate plasma concentration was 110 pg/mL.
Peak steady-state fluticasone propionate plasma concentrations in subjects with COPD averaged 53 pg/mL (range, 19.3 to 159.3 pg/mL) after treatment with 250 mcg twice daily (N = 30) via the DISKUS device.
Distribution: Following intravenous administration, the initial disposition phase for fluticasone propionate was rapid and consistent with its high lipid solubility and tissue binding. The volume of distribution averaged 4.2 L/kg.
The percentage of fluticasone propionate bound to human plasma proteins averages 91%. Fluticasone propionate is weakly and reversibly bound to erythrocytes and is not significantly bound to human transcortin.
Metabolism: The total clearance of fluticasone propionate is high (average, 1,093 mL/min), with renal clearance accounting for less than 0.02% of the total. The only circulating metabolite detected in man is the 17β-carboxylic acid derivative of fluticasone propionate, which is formed through the cytochrome P450 3A4 pathway. This metabolite had less affinity (approximately 1/2,000) than the parent drug for the glucocorticoid receptor of human lung cytosol in vitro and negligible pharmacological activity in animal studies. Other metabolites detected in vitro using cultured human hepatoma cells have not been detected in man.
Elimination: Following intravenous dosing, fluticasone propionate showed polyexponential kinetics and had a terminal elimination half-life of approximately 7.8 hours. Less than 5% of a radiolabeled oral dose was excreted in the urine as metabolites, with the remainder excreted in the feces as parent drug and metabolites.
Special Populations: Hepatic Impairment: Since fluticasone propionate is predominantly cleared by hepatic metabolism, impairment of liver function may lead to accumulation of fluticasone propionate in plasma. Therefore, patients with hepatic disease should be closely monitored.
Gender: Full pharmacokinetic profiles were obtained from 9 female and 16 male patients with asthma given fluticasone propionate inhalation powder 500 mcg twice daily using the DISKUS device and from 14 female and 43 male patients with COPD given 250 or 500 mcg twice daily. No overall differences in fluticasone propionate pharmacokinetics were observed.
Age: No relationship between fluticasone propionate systemic exposure and age was observed in 57 patients with COPD (aged 40 to 82 years) given 250 or 500 mcg twice daily.
Other: Formal pharmacokinetic studies using fluticasone propionate have not been conducted in other special populations.
Drug Interactions: Fluticasone propionate is a substrate of cytochrome P450 3A4. Coadministration of fluticasone propionate and the highly potent cytochrome P450 3A4 inhibitor ritonavir is not recommended based upon a multiple-dose, crossover drug interaction study in 18 healthy subjects. Fluticasone propionate aqueous nasal spray (200 mcg once daily) was coadministered for 7 days with ritonavir (100 mg twice daily). Plasma fluticasone propionate concentrations following fluticasone propionate aqueous nasal spray alone were undetectable (<10 pg/mL) in most subjects, and when concentrations were detectable peak levels (C_{max} averaged 11.9 pg/mL [range, 10.8 to 14.1 pg/mL] and $AUC_{(0-\tau)}$ averaged 8.43 pg•hr/mL [range, 4.2 to 18.8 pg•hr/mL]). Fluticasone propionate C_{max} and $AUC_{(0-\tau)}$ increased to 318 pg/mL (range, 110 to 648 pg/mL) and 3,102.6 pg•hr/mL (range, 1,207.1 to 5,662.0 pg•hr/mL), respectively, after coadministration of ritonavir with fluticasone propionate aqueous nasal spray. This significant increase in plasma fluticasone propionate exposure resulted in a significant decrease (86%) in plasma cortisol area under the plasma concentration versus time curve (AUC).
Caution should be exercised when other potent cytochrome P450 3A4 inhibitors are coadministered with fluticasone propionate. In a drug interaction study, coadministration of orally inhaled fluticasone propionate (1,000 mcg) and ketoconazole (200 mg once daily) resulted in increased plasma fluticasone propionate exposure and reduced plasma cortisol AUC, but had no effect on urinary excretion of cortisol.
In another multiple-dose drug interaction study, coadministration of orally inhaled fluticasone propionate (500 mcg twice daily) and erythromycin (333 mg 3 times daily) did not affect fluticasone propionate pharmacokinetics.
Salmeterol Xinafoate: Salmeterol xinafoate, an ionic salt, dissociates in solution so that the salmeterol and 1-hydroxy-2-naphthoic acid (xinafoate) moieties are absorbed, distributed, metabolized, and eliminated independently. Salmeterol acts locally in the lung; therefore, plasma levels do not predict therapeutic effect.
Absorption: Because of the small therapeutic dose, systemic levels of salmeterol are low or undetectable after inhalation of recommended doses (50 mcg of salmeterol inhalation powder twice daily). Following chronic administration of an inhaled dose of 50 mcg of salmeterol inhalation powder twice daily, salmeterol was detected in plasma within 5 to 45 minutes in 7 patients with asthma; plasma concentrations were very low, with mean peak concentrations of 167 pg/mL at 20 minutes and no accumulation with repeated doses.
Distribution: The percentage of salmeterol bound to human plasma proteins averages 96% in vitro over the concentration range of 8 to 7,722 ng of salmeterol base per milliliter, much higher concentrations than those achieved following therapeutic doses of salmeterol.
Metabolism: Salmeterol base is extensively metabolized by hydroxylation, with subsequent elimination predominantly in the feces. No significant amount of unchanged salmeterol base was detected in either urine or feces.
Elimination: In 2 healthy adult subjects who received 1 mg of radiolabeled salmeterol (as salmeterol xinafoate) orally, approximately 25% and 60% of the radiolabeled salmeterol was eliminated in urine and feces, respectively, over a pe-

riod of 7 days. The terminal elimination half-life was about 5.5 hours (1 volunteer only).

The xinafoate moiety has no apparent pharmacologic activity. The xinafoate moiety is highly protein bound (>99%) and has a long elimination half-life of 11 days.

Special Populations: Hepatic Impairment: Since salmeterol is predominantly cleared by hepatic metabolism, impairment of liver function may lead to accumulation of salmeterol in plasma. Therefore, patients with hepatic disease should be closely monitored.

Other: Formal pharmacokinetic studies using salmeterol base have not been conducted in other special populations.

Pharmacodynamics: ***ADVAIR DISKUS: Adult and Adolescent Patients:*** Since systemic pharmacodynamic effects of salmeterol are not normally seen at the therapeutic dose, higher doses were used to produce measurable effects. Four (4) studies were conducted in healthy adult subjects: (1) a single-dose crossover study using 2 inhalations of ADVAIR DISKUS 500/50, fluticasone propionate powder 500 mcg and salmeterol powder 50 mcg given concurrently, or fluticasone propionate powder 500 mcg given alone, (2) a cumulative dose study using 50 to 400 mcg of salmeterol powder given alone or as ADVAIR DISKUS 500/50, (3) a repeat-dose study for 11 days using 2 inhalations twice daily of ADVAIR DISKUS 250/50, fluticasone propionate powder 250 mcg, or salmeterol powder 50 mcg, and (4) a single-dose study using 5 inhalations of ADVAIR DISKUS 100/50, fluticasone propionate powder 100 mcg alone, or placebo. In these studies no significant differences were observed in the pharmacodynamic effects of salmeterol (pulse rate, blood pressure, QTc interval, potassium, and glucose) whether the salmeterol was given as ADVAIR DISKUS, concurrently with fluticasone propionate from separate inhalers, or as salmeterol alone. The systemic pharmacodynamic effects of salmeterol were not altered by the presence of fluticasone propionate in ADVAIR DISKUS. The potential effect of salmeterol on the effects of fluticasone propionate on the hypothalamic-pituitary-adrenal (HPA) axis was also evaluated in these studies. No significant differences across treatments were observed in 24-hour urinary cortisol excretion and, where measured, 24-hour plasma cortisol AUC. The systemic pharmacodynamic effects of fluticasone propionate were not altered by the presence of salmeterol in ADVAIR DISKUS in healthy subjects.

Asthma: In clinical studies with ADVAIR DISKUS in adult and adolescent patients 12 years of age and older with asthma, no significant differences were observed in the systemic pharmacodynamic effects of salmeterol (pulse rate, blood pressure, QTc interval, potassium, and glucose) whether the salmeterol was given alone or as ADVAIR DISKUS. In 72 adolescent and adult patients with asthma given either ADVAIR DISKUS 100/50 or ADVAIR DISKUS 250/50, continuous 24-hour electrocardiographic monitoring was performed after the first dose and after 12 weeks of therapy, and no clinically significant dysrhythmias were noted.

In a 28-week study in adolescent and adult patients with asthma, ADVAIR DISKUS 500/50 twice daily was compared with the concurrent use of salmeterol powder 50 mcg plus fluticasone propionate powder 500 mcg from separate inhalers or fluticasone propionate powder 500 mcg alone. No significant differences across treatments were observed in plasma cortisol AUC after 12 weeks of dosing or in 24-hour urinary cortisol excretion after 12 and 28 weeks.

In a 12-week study in adolescent and adult patients with asthma, ADVAIR DISKUS 250/50 twice daily was compared with fluticasone propionate powder 250 mcg alone, salmeterol powder 50 mcg alone, and placebo. For most patients, the ability to increase cortisol production in response to stress, as assessed by 30-minute cosyntropin stimulation, remained intact with ADVAIR DISKUS. One patient (3%) who received ADVAIR DISKUS 250/50 had an abnormal response (peak serum cortisol <18 mcg/dL) after dosing, compared with 2 patients (6%) who received placebo, 2 patients (6%) who received fluticasone propionate 250 mcg, and no patients who received salmeterol.

Chronic Obstructive Pulmonary Disease: In clinical studies with ADVAIR DISKUS in patients with COPD associated with chronic bronchitis, no significant differences were seen in pulse rate, blood pressure, potassium, and glucose between ADVAIR DISKUS, the individual components of ADVAIR DISKUS, and placebo. In a study of ADVAIR DISKUS 250/50, 8 subjects (2 [1.1%] in the group given ADVAIR DISKUS 250/50, 1 [0.5%] in the fluticasone propionate 250 mcg group, 3 [1.7%] in the salmeterol group, and 2 [1.1%] in the placebo group) had QTc intervals >470 msec at least 1 time during the treatment period. Five (5) of these 8 subjects had a prolonged QTc interval at baseline.

In a 24-week study, 130 patients with COPD associated with chronic bronchitis received continuous 24-hour electrocardiographic monitoring prior to the first dose and after 4 weeks of twice-daily treatment with either ADVAIR DISKUS 500/50, fluticasone propionate powder 500 mcg, salmeterol powder 50 mcg, or placebo. No significant differences in ventricular or supraventricular arrhythmias and heart rate were observed among the groups treated with ADVAIR DISKUS 500/50, the individual components, or placebo. One (1) subject in the fluticasone propionate group experienced atrial flutter/atrial fibrillation, and 1 subject in the group given ADVAIR DISKUS 500/50 experienced heart block. There were 3 cases of nonsustained ventricular tachycardia (1 each in the placebo, salmeterol, and fluticasone propionate 500 mcg treatment groups).

Table 1. Percent of Patients Withdrawn Due to Worsening Asthma in Patients Previously Treated With Either Inhaled Corticosteroids or Salmeterol (Study 1)

ADVAIR DISKUS 100/50 (N = 87)	Fluticasone Propionate 100 mcg (N = 85)	Salmeterol 50 mcg (N = 86)	Placebo (N = 77)
3%	11%	35%	49%

Table 2. Peak Expiratory Flow Results for Patients With Asthma Previously Treated With Either Inhaled Corticosteroids or Salmeterol (Study 1)

Efficacy Variable*	ADVAIR DISKUS 100/50 (N = 87)	Fluticasone Propionate 100 mcg (N = 85)	Salmeterol 50 mcg (N = 86)	Placebo (N = 77)
AM PEF (L/min)				
Baseline	393	374	369	382
Change from baseline	53	17	−2	−24
PM PEF (L/min)				
Baseline	418	390	396	398
Change from baseline	35	18	−7	−13

*Change from baseline = change from baseline at Endpoint (last available data).

Short-cosyntropin stimulation testing was performed both at Day 1 and Endpoint in 101 patients with COPD receiving twice-daily ADVAIR DISKUS 250/50, fluticasone propionate powder 250 mcg, salmeterol powder 50 mcg, or placebo. For most patients, the ability to increase cortisol production in response to stress, as assessed by short cosyntropin stimulation, remained intact with ADVAIR DISKUS 250/50. One (1) patient (3%) who received ADVAIR DISKUS 250/50 had an abnormal stimulated cortisol response (peak cortisol <14.5 mcg/dL assessed by high-performance liquid chromatography) after dosing, compared with 2 patients (9%) who received fluticasone propionate 250 mcg, 2 patients (7%) who received salmeterol 50 mcg, and 1 patient (4%) who received placebo following 24 weeks of treatment or early discontinuation from study.

Pediatric Patients: In a 12-week study in patients with asthma aged 4 to 11 years who were receiving inhaled corticosteroids at study entry, ADVAIR DISKUS 100/50 twice daily was compared with fluticasone propionate inhalation powder 100 mcg administered twice daily via the DISKUS. The values for 24-hour urinary cortisol excretion at study entry and after 12 weeks of treatment were similar within each treatment group. After 12 weeks, 24-hour urinary cortisol excretion was also similar between the 2 groups.

Fluticasone Propionate: Asthma: In clinical trials with fluticasone propionate inhalation powder using doses up to and including 250 mcg twice daily, occasional abnormal short cosyntropin tests (peak serum cortisol <18 mcg/dL assessed by radioimmunoassay) were noted both in patients receiving fluticasone propionate and in patients receiving placebo. The incidence of abnormal tests at 500 mcg twice daily was greater than placebo. In a 2-year study carried out with the DISKHALER® inhalation device in 64 patients with mild, persistent asthma (mean FEV_1 91% of predicted) randomized to fluticasone propionate 500 mcg twice daily or placebo, no patient receiving fluticasone propionate had an abnormal response to 6-hour cosyntropin infusion (peak serum cortisol <18 mcg/dL). With a peak cortisol threshold of <35 mcg/dL, 1 patient receiving fluticasone propionate (4%) had an abnormal response at 1 year; repeat testing at 18 months and 2 years was normal. Another patient receiving fluticasone propionate (5%) had an abnormal response at 2 years. No patient on placebo had an abnormal response at 1 or 2 years.

Chronic Obstructive Pulmonary Disease: In a 24-week study, the steady-state fluticasone propionate pharmacokinetics and serum cortisol levels were described in a subset of patients with COPD associated with chronic bronchitis (N = 86) randomized to twice-daily fluticasone propionate inhalation powder via the DISKUS 500 mcg, fluticasone propionate inhalation powder 250 mcg, or placebo. Serial serum cortisol concentrations were measured across a 12-hour dosing interval following at least 4 weeks of dosing. Serum cortisol concentrations following 250 and 500 mcg twice-daily dosing were 10% and 21% lower than placebo, indicating a dose-dependent increase in systemic exposure to fluticasone propionate.

Salmeterol Xinafoate: Inhaled salmeterol, like other beta-adrenergic agonist drugs can produce dose-related cardiovascular effects and effects on blood glucose and/or serum potassium (see PRECAUTIONS: General). The cardiovascular effects (heart rate, blood pressure) associated with salmeterol occur with similar frequency, and are of similar type and severity, as those noted following albuterol administration.

Asthma: The effects of rising doses of salmeterol and standard inhaled doses of albuterol were studied in volunteers and in patients with asthma. Salmeterol doses up to 84 mcg administered as inhalation aerosol resulted in heart rate increases of 3 to 16 beats/min, about the same as albuterol dosed at 180 mcg by inhalation aerosol (4 to 10 beats/min). Adolescent and adult patients receiving 50-mcg doses of salmeterol inhalation powder (N = 60) underwent continuous electrocardiographic monitoring during two 12-hour periods after the first dose and after 1 month of therapy, and no clinically significant dysrhythmias were noted.

Chronic Obstructive Pulmonary Disease: In 24-week clinical studies in patients with COPD associated with chronic bronchitis, the incidence of clinically significant electrocardiogram (ECG) abnormalities (myocardial ischemia, ventricular hypertrophy, clinically significant conduction abnormalities, clinically significant arrhythmias) was lower for patients who received salmeterol (1%, 9 of 688 patients who received either salmeterol 50 mcg or ADVAIR DISKUS) compared with placebo (3%, 10 of 370 subjects).

No significant differences with salmeterol 50 mcg alone or in combination with fluticasone propionate as ADVAIR DISKUS 500/50 was observed on pulse rate and systolic and diastolic blood pressure in a subset of patients with COPD who underwent 12-hour serial vital sign measurements after the first dose (N = 183) and after 12 weeks of therapy (N = 149). Median changes from baseline in pulse rate and systolic and diastolic blood pressure were similar to those seen with placebo (see ADVERSE REACTIONS: Chronic Obstructive Pulmonary Disease Associated With Chronic Bronchitis).

Studies in laboratory animals (minipigs, rodents, and dogs) have demonstrated the occurrence of cardiac arrhythmias and sudden death (with histologic evidence of myocardial necrosis) when beta-agonists and methylxanthines are administered concurrently. The clinical significance of these findings is unknown.

CLINICAL TRIALS

Asthma: ***Adult and Adolescent Patients 12 Years of Age and Older:*** In clinical trials comparing ADVAIR DISKUS with the individual components, improvements in most efficacy endpoints were greater with ADVAIR DISKUS than with the use of either fluticasone propionate or salmeterol alone. In addition, clinical trials showed similar results between ADVAIR DISKUS and the concurrent use of fluticasone propionate plus salmeterol at corresponding doses from separate inhalers.

Studies Comparing ADVAIR DISKUS to Fluticasone Propionate Alone or Salmeterol Alone: Three (3) double-blind, parallel-group clinical trials were conducted with ADVAIR DISKUS in 1,208 adolescent and adult patients (≥ 12 years, baseline FEV_1 63% to 72% of predicted normal) with asthma that was not optimally controlled on their current therapy. All treatments were inhalation powders, given as 1 inhalation from the DISKUS device twice daily, and other maintenance therapies were discontinued.

Study 1: Clinical Trial With ADVAIR DISKUS 100/50: This placebo-controlled, 12-week, US study compared ADVAIR DISKUS 100/50 with its individual components, fluticasone propionate 100 mcg and salmeterol 50 mcg. The study was stratified according to baseline asthma maintenance therapy; patients were using either inhaled corticosteroids (N = 250) (daily doses of beclomethasone dipropionate 252 to 420 mcg; flunisolide 1,000 mcg; fluticasone propionate inhalation aerosol 176 mcg; or triamcinolone acetonide 600 to 1,000 mcg) or salmeterol (N = 106). Baseline FEV_1 measurements were similar across treatments: ADVAIR DISKUS 100/50, 2.17 L; fluticasone propionate 100 mcg, 2.11 L; salmeterol, 2.13 L; and placebo, 2.15 L.

Predefined withdrawal criteria for lack of efficacy, an indicator of worsening asthma, were utilized for this placebo-controlled study. Worsening asthma was defined as a clinically important decrease in FEV_1 or peak expiratory flow (PEF), increase in use of VENTOLIN® (albuterol, USP) Inhalation Aerosol, increase in night awakenings due to asthma, emergency intervention or hospitalization due to asthma, or requirement for asthma medication not allowed by the protocol. As shown in Table 1, statistically signifi-

Continued on next page

Product information on these pages is effective as of August 2004. Further information is available at: GlaxoSmithKline, PO Box 13398, Research Triangle Park, NC 27709. 1-888-825-5249. Corporate Web Site: www.gsk.com

Advair Diskus—Cont.

cantly fewer patients receiving ADVAIR DISKUS 100/50 were withdrawn due to worsening asthma compared with fluticasone propionate, salmeterol, and placebo.

[See table 1 at top of previous page]

The FEV_1 results are displayed in Figure 1. Because this trial used predetermined criteria for worsening asthma, which caused more patients in the placebo group to be withdrawn, FEV_1 results at Endpoint (last available FEV_1 result) are also provided. Patients receiving ADVAIR DISKUS 100/50 had significantly greater improvements in FEV_1 (0.51 L, 25%) compared with fluticasone propionate 100 mcg (0.28 L, 15%), salmeterol (0.11 L, 5%), and placebo (0.01 L, 1%). These improvements in FEV_1 with ADVAIR DISKUS were achieved regardless of baseline asthma maintenance therapy (inhaled corticosteroids or salmeterol).

Figure 1. Mean Percent Change From Baseline in FEV_1 in Patients With Asthma Previously Treated With Either Inhaled Corticosteroids or Salmeterol (Study 1)

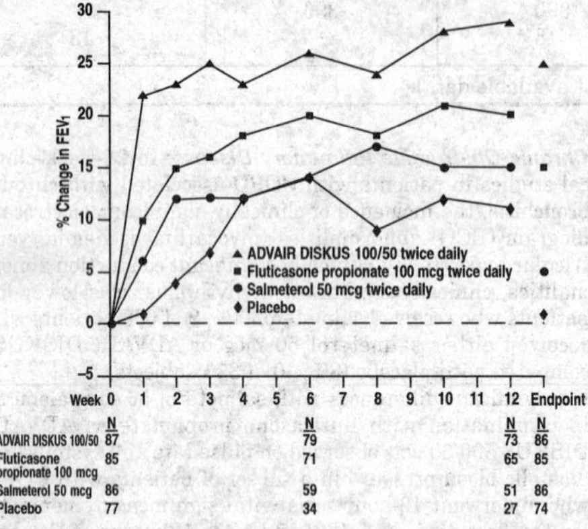

The effect of ADVAIR DISKUS 100/50 on morning and evening PEF endpoints is shown in Table 2.

[See table 2 at top of previous page]

The subjective impact of asthma on patients' perception of health was evaluated through use of an instrument called the Asthma Quality of Life Questionnaire (AQLQ) (based on a 7-point scale where 1 = maximum impairment and 7 = none). Patients receiving ADVAIR DISKUS 100/50 had clinically meaningful improvements in overall asthma-specific quality of life as defined by a difference between groups of ≥0.5 points in change from baseline AQLQ scores (difference in AQLQ score of 1.25 compared to placebo).

Study 2: Clinical Trial With ADVAIR DISKUS 250/50: This placebo-controlled, 12-week, US study compared ADVAIR DISKUS 250/50 with its individual components, fluticasone propionate 250 mcg and salmeterol 50 mcg in 349 patients with asthma using inhaled corticosteroids (daily doses of beclomethasone dipropionate 462 to 672 mcg; flunisolide 1,250 to 2,000 mcg; fluticasone propionate inhalation aerosol 440 mcg; or triamcinolone acetonide 1,100 to 1,600 mcg). Baseline FEV_1 measurements were similar across treatments: ADVAIR DISKUS 250/50, 2.23 L; fluticasone propionate 250 mcg, 2.12 L; salmeterol, 2.20 L; and placebo, 2.19 L.

Efficacy results in this study were similar to those observed in Study 1. Patients receiving ADVAIR DISKUS 250/50 had significantly greater improvements in FEV_1 (0.48 L, 23%) compared with fluticasone propionate 250 mcg (0.25 L, 13%), salmeterol (0.05 L, 4%), and placebo (decrease of 0.11 L, decrease of 5%). Statistically significantly fewer patients receiving ADVAIR DISKUS 250/50 were withdrawn from this study for worsening asthma (4%) compared with fluticasone propionate (22%), salmeterol (38%), and placebo (62%). In addition, ADVAIR DISKUS 250/50 was superior to fluticasone propionate, salmeterol, and placebo for improvements in morning and evening PEF. Patients receiving ADVAIR DISKUS 250/50 also had clinically meaningful improvements in overall asthma-specific quality of life as described in Study 1 (difference in AQLQ score of 1.29 compared to placebo).

Study 3: Clinical Trial With ADVAIR DISKUS 500/50: This 28-week, non-US study compared ADVAIR DISKUS 500/50 with fluticasone propionate 500 mcg alone and concurrent therapy (salmeterol 50 mcg plus fluticasone propionate 500 mcg administered from separate inhalers) twice daily in 503 patients with asthma using inhaled corticosteroids (daily doses of beclomethasone dipropionate 1,260 to 1,680 mcg; budesonide 1,500 to 2,000 mcg; flunisolide 1,500 to 2,000 mcg; or fluticasone propionate inhalation aerosol 660 to 880 mcg [750 to 1,000 mcg inhalation powder]). The primary efficacy parameter, morning PEF, was collected daily for the first 12 weeks of the study. The primary purpose of weeks 13 to 28 was to collect safety data.

Baseline PEF measurements were similar across treatments: ADVAIR DISKUS 500/50, 359 L/min; fluticasone propionate 500 mcg, 351 L/min; and concurrent therapy, 345 L/min. As shown in Figure 2, morning PEF improved significantly with ADVAIR DISKUS 500/50 compared with fluticasone propionate 500 mcg over the 12-week treatment period. Improvements in morning PEF observed with ADVAIR DISKUS 500/50 were similar to improvements observed with concurrent therapy.

Figure 2. Mean Percent Change From Baseline in Morning Peak Expiratory Flow in Patients With Asthma Previously Treated With Inhaled Corticosteroids (Study 3)

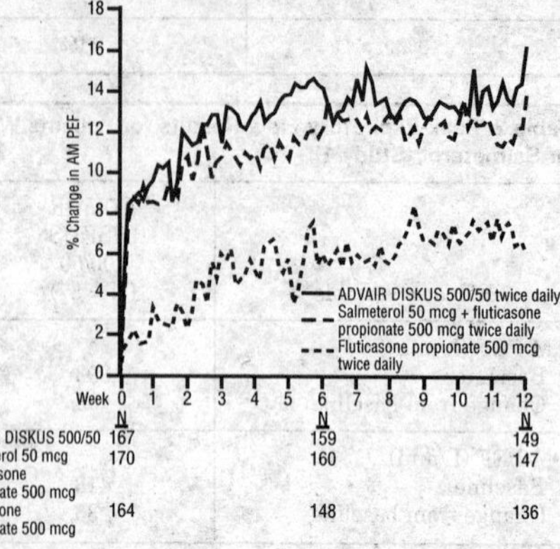

Onset of Action and Progression of Improvement in Asthma Control: The onset of action and progression of improvement in asthma control were evaluated in the 2 placebo-controlled US trials. Following the first dose, the median time to onset of clinically significant bronchodilatation (≥15% improvement in FEV_1) in most patients was seen within 30 to 60 minutes. Maximum improvement in FEV_1 generally occurred within 3 hours, and clinically significant improvement was maintained for 12 hours (see Figure 3).

Following the initial dose, predose FEV_1 relative to Day 1 baseline improved markedly over the first week of treatment and continued to improve over the 12 weeks of treatment in both studies.

No diminution in the 12-hour bronchodilator effect was observed with either ADVAIR DISKUS 100/50 (Figures 3 and 4) or ADVAIR DISKUS 250/50 as assessed by FEV_1 following 12 weeks of therapy.

Figure 3. Percent Change in Serial 12-hour FEV_1 in Patients With Asthma Previously Using Either Inhaled Corticosteroids or Salmeterol (Study 1)

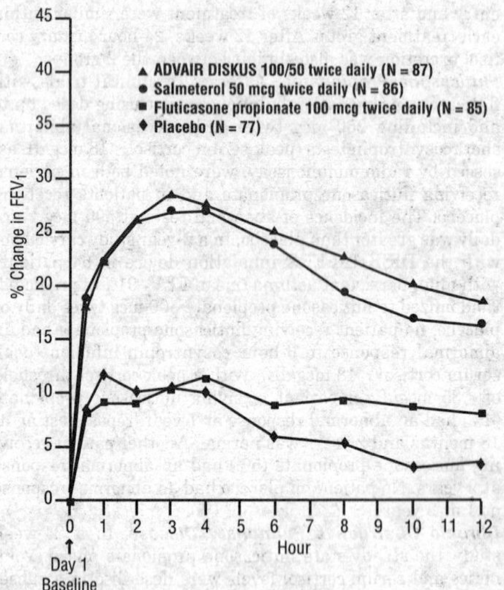

[See figure 4 at top of next column]

Reduction in asthma symptoms, use of rescue VENTOLIN Inhalation Aerosol, and improvement in morning and evening PEF also occurred within the first day of treatment with ADVAIR DISKUS, and continued to improve over the 12 weeks of therapy in both studies.

Pediatric Patients: In a 12-week US study, ADVAIR DISKUS 100/50 twice daily was compared with fluticasone propionate inhalation powder 100 mcg twice daily in 203 children with asthma aged 4 to 11 years. At study entry, the children were symptomatic on low doses of inhaled corticosteroids (beclomethasone dipropionate 252 to 336 mcg/day; budesonide 200 to 400 mcg/day; flunisolide 1,000 mcg/day; triamcinolone acetonide 600 to 1,000 mcg/day; or fluticasone propionate 88 to 250 mcg/day). The primary objective of this study was to determine the safety of ADVAIR DISKUS 100/50 compared with fluticasone propionate inhalation powder 100 mcg in this age-group; however, the study also included secondary efficacy measures of pulmonary function. Morning predose FEV_1 was obtained at baseline and Endpoint (last available FEV_1 result) in children aged 6 to 11 years. In patients receiving ADVAIR DISKUS 100/50, FEV_1 increased from 1.70 L at baseline (N = 79) to 1.88 L at Endpoint (N = 69) compared with an increase from 1.65 L at baseline (N = 83) to 1.77 L at Endpoint (N = 75) in patients receiving fluticasone propionate 100 mcg.

The findings of this study, along with extrapolation of efficacy data from patients 12 years of age and older, support

Figure 4. Percent Change in Serial 12-hour FEV_1 in Patients With Asthma Previously Using Either Inhaled Corticosteroids or Salmeterol (Study 1)

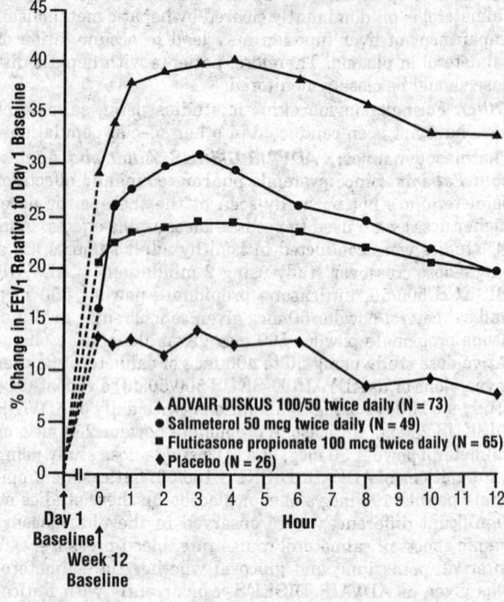

the overall conclusions that ADVAIR DISKUS 100/50 is efficacious in the maintenance treatment of asthma in patients aged 4 to 11 years.

Chronic Obstructive Pulmonary Disease Associated With Chronic Bronchitis: In a clinical trial evaluating twice-daily treatment with ADVAIR DISKUS 250/50 in patients with COPD associated with chronic bronchitis, improvements in lung function (as defined by predose and postdose FEV_1) were significantly greater with ADVAIR DISKUS than with fluticasone propionate 250 mcg, salmeterol 50 mcg, or placebo. The study was a randomized, double-blind, parallel-group, 24-week trial. All patients had a history of cough productive of sputum that was not attributable to another disease process on most days for at least 3 months of the year for at least 2 years. Study treatments were inhalation powders given as 1 inhalation from the DISKUS device twice daily. Maintenance COPD therapies were discontinued, with the exception of theophylline.

Figures 5 and 6 display predose and 2-hour postdose FEV_1 results. To account for patient withdrawals during the study, FEV_1 at Endpoint (last evaluable FEV_1) was evaluated. Patients receiving ADVAIR DISKUS 250/50 had significantly greater improvements in predose FEV_1 at Endpoint (165 mL, 17%) compared with salmeterol 50 mcg (91 mL, 9%) and placebo (1 mL, 1%), demonstrating the contribution of fluticasone propionate to the improvement in lung function with ADVAIR DISKUS (Figure 5). Patients receiving ADVAIR DISKUS 250/50 had significantly greater improvements in postdose FEV_1 at Endpoint (281 mL, 27%) compared with fluticasone propionate 250 mcg (147 mL, 14%) and placebo (58 mL, 6%), demonstrating the contribution of salmeterol to the improvement in lung function with ADVAIR DISKUS (Figure 6).

A similar degree of improvement in lung function was also observed with ADVAIR DISKUS 500/50 twice daily.

Figure 5. Predose FEV_1: Mean Percent Change From Baseline in Patients With COPD Associated With Chronic Bronchitis

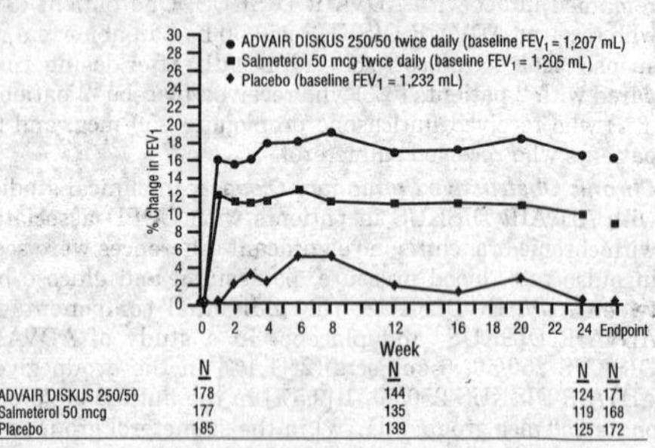

[See figure 6 at top of next column]

Patients treated with ADVAIR DISKUS 250/50 or ADVAIR DISKUS 500/50 did not have a significant reduction in chronic bronchitis symptoms (as measured by the Chronic Bronchitis Symptom Questionnaire) or in COPD exacerbations compared to patients treated with placebo over the 24 weeks of therapy. The improvement in lung function with ADVAIR DISKUS 500/50 was similar to the improvement seen with ADVAIR DISKUS 250/50. Since there is evidence of more systemic exposure to fluticasone propionate from this higher dose and no documented advantage for efficacy, ADVAIR DISKUS 500/50 is not recommended for use in COPD.

The benefit of treatment of patients with COPD associated with chronic bronchitis with ADVAIR DISKUS 250/50 for periods longer than 6 months has not been evaluated.

Figure 6. Two-Hour Postdose FEV_1: Mean Percent Changes From Baseline Over Time in Patients With COPD Associated With Chronic Bronchitis

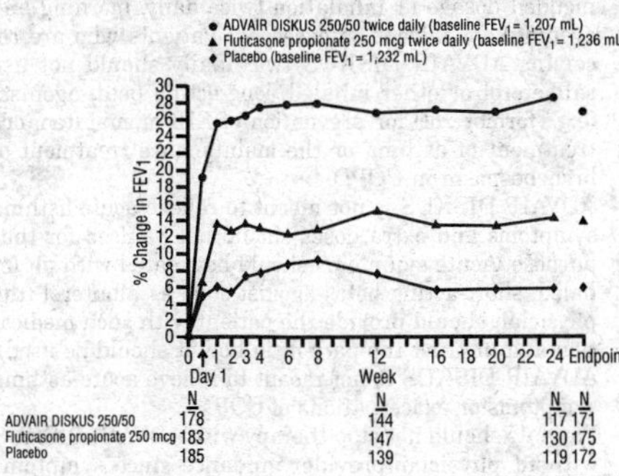

INDICATIONS AND USAGE

Asthma: ADVAIR DISKUS is indicated for the long-term, twice-daily, maintenance treatment of asthma in patients 4 years of age and older.

ADVAIR DISKUS is NOT indicated for the relief of acute bronchospasm.

Chronic Obstructive Pulmonary Disease Associated With Chronic Bronchitis: ADVAIR DISKUS 250/50 is indicated for the twice-daily maintenance treatment of airflow obstruction in patients with COPD associated with chronic bronchitis.

ADVAIR DISKUS 250/50 mcg twice daily is the only approved dosage for the treatment of COPD associated with chronic bronchitis. Higher doses, including ADVAIR DISKUS 500/50, are not recommended (see DOSAGE AND ADMINISTRATION: Chronic Obstructive Pulmonary Disease Associated With Chronic Bronchitis).

The benefit of treating patients with COPD associated with chronic bronchitis with ADVAIR DISKUS 250/50 for periods longer than 6 months has not been evaluated. Patients who are treated with ADVAIR DISKUS 250/50 for COPD associated with chronic bronchitis for periods longer than 6 months should be reevaluated periodically to assess the continuing benefits and potential risks of treatment.

ADVAIR DISKUS is NOT indicated for the relief of acute bronchospasm.

CONTRAINDICATIONS

ADVAIR DISKUS is contraindicated in the primary treatment of status asthmaticus or other acute episodes of asthma or COPD where intensive measures are required.

Hypersensitivity to any of the ingredients of these preparations contraindicates their use (see DESCRIPTION and ADVERSE REACTIONS: Observed During Clinical Practice: *Non-Site Specific*).

WARNINGS

DATA FROM A LARGE PLACEBO-CONTROLLED SAFETY STUDY THAT WAS STOPPED EARLY SUGGEST THAT SALMETEROL, A COMPONENT OF ADVAIR DISKUS, MAY BE ASSOCIATED WITH RARE SERIOUS ASTHMA EPISODES OR ASTHMA-RELATED DEATHS. The Salmeterol Multi-center Asthma Research Trial (SMART) enrolled long-acting $beta_2$-agonist–naive patients with asthma to assess the safety of salmeterol (SEREVENT Inhalation Aerosol) 42 mcg twice daily over 28 weeks compared to placebo, when added to usual asthma therapy. The primary endpoint was the combined number of respiratory-related deaths or respiratory-related life-threatening experiences (intubation and mechanical ventilation). Other endpoints included combined asthma-related deaths or life-threatening experiences and asthma-related deaths.

A planned interim analysis was conducted when approximately half of the intended number of patients had been enrolled (N = 26,353). The anlaysis showed no significant difference for the primary endpoint for the total population. However, a higher number of asthma-related deaths or life-threatening experiences (36 vs. 23) and a higher number of asthma-related deaths (13 vs. 4) occurred in the patients treated with SEREVENT Inhalation Aerosol. Post hoc subgroup analyses revealed no significant increase in respiratory- or asthma-related episodes, including deaths, in Caucasian patients. In African Americans, the study showed a small, though statistically significantly greater, number of primary events (20 vs. 7), asthma-related deaths or life-threatening experiences (19 vs. 4), and asthma-related deaths (8 vs. 1) in patients taking SEREVENT Inhalation Aerosol compared to those taking placebo. Even though SMART did not reach predetermined stopping criteria for the total population, the study was stopped due to the findings in African American patients and difficulties in enrollment. The data from the SMART study are not adequate to determine whether concurrent use of inhaled corticosteroids, such as fluticasone propionate, a component of ADVAIR DISKUS, provides protection from this risk. Therefore, it is not known whether the findings seen with SEREVENT Inhalation Aerosol would apply to ADVAIR DISKUS.

Findings similar to the SMART study findings were reported in a prior 16-week clinical study performed in the United Kingdom, the Salmeterol Nationwide Surveillance (SNS) study. In the SNS study, the incidence of asthma-related death was numerically, though not statistically, greater in patients with asthma treated with salmeterol (42 mcg twice daily) versus albuterol (180 mcg 4 times daily) added to usual asthma therapy.

Given the similar basic mechanisms of action of $beta_2$-agonists, it is possible that the findings seen in the SMART study may be consistent with a class effect.

1. **ADVAIR DISKUS SHOULD NOT BE USED FOR TRANSFERRING PATIENTS FROM SYSTEMIC CORTICOSTEROID THERAPY.** Particular care is needed for patients who have been transferred from systemically active corticosteroids to inhaled corticosteroids because deaths due to adrenal insufficiency have occurred in patients with asthma during and after transfer from systemic corticosteroids to less systemically available inhaled corticosteroids. After withdrawal from systemic corticosteroids, a number of months are required for recovery of HPA function.

Patients who have been previously maintained on 20 mg or more per day of prednisone (or its equivalent) may be most susceptible, particularly when their systemic corticosteroids have been almost completely withdrawn. During this period of HPA suppression, patients may exhibit signs and symptoms of adrenal insufficiency when exposed to trauma, surgery, or infection (particularly gastroenteritis) or other conditions associated with severe electrolyte loss. Although inhaled corticosteroids may provide control of asthma symptoms during these episodes, in recommended doses they supply less than normal physiological amounts of glucocorticoid systemically and do NOT provide the mineralocorticoid activity that is necessary for coping with these emergencies.

During periods of stress or a severe asthma attack, patients who have been withdrawn from systemic corticosteroids should be instructed to resume oral corticosteroids (in large doses) immediately and to contact their physicians for further instruction. These patients should also be instructed to carry a warning card indicating that they may need supplementary systemic corticosteroids during periods of stress or a severe asthma attack.

2. **ADVAIR DISKUS SHOULD NOT BE INITIATED IN PATIENTS DURING RAPIDLY DETERIORATING OR POTENTIALLY LIFE-THREATENING EPISODES OF ASTHMA. Serious acute respiratory events, including fatalities, have been reported both in the United States and worldwide when salmeterol, a component of ADVAIR DISKUS, has been initiated in patients with significantly worsening or acutely deteriorating asthma.** In most cases, these have occurred in patients with severe asthma (e.g., patients with a history of corticosteroid dependence, low pulmonary function, intubation, mechanical ventilation, frequent hospitalizations, or previous life-threatening acute asthma exacerbations) and/or in some patients in whom asthma has been acutely deteriorating (e.g., unresponsive to usual medications; increasing need for inhaled, short-acting $beta_2$-agonists; increasing need for systemic corticosteroids; significant increase in symptoms; recent emergency room visits; sudden or progressive deterioration in pulmonary function). However, they have occurred in a few patients with less severe asthma as well. It was not possible from these reports to determine whether salmeterol contributed to these events or simply failed to relieve the deteriorating asthma.

3. **Drug Interaction With Ritonavir:** A drug interaction study in healthy subjects has shown that ritonavir (a highly potent cytochrome P450 3A4 inhibitor) can significantly increase plasma fluticasone propionate exposure, resulting in significantly reduced serum cortisol concentrations (see CLINICAL PHARMACOLOGY: Pharmacokinetics: *Fluticasone Propionate: Drug Interactions* and PRECAUTIONS: Drug Interactions: *Inhibitors of Cytochrome P450*). During postmarketing use, there have been reports of clinically significant drug interactions in patients receiving fluticasone propionate and ritonavir, resulting in systemic corticosteroid effects including Cushing syndrome and adrenal suppression. Therefore, coadministration of fluticasone propionate and ritonavir is not recommended unless the potential benefit to the patient outweighs the risk of systemic corticosteroid side effects.

4. Do Not Use ADVAIR DISKUS to Treat Acute Symptoms: An inhaled, short-acting $beta_2$-agonist, not ADVAIR DISKUS, should be used to relieve acute symptoms of shortness of breath. When prescribing ADVAIR DISKUS, the physician must also provide the patient with an inhaled, short-acting $beta_2$-agonist (e.g., albuterol) for treatment of shortness of breath that occurs acutely, despite regular twice-daily (morning and evening) use of ADVAIR DISKUS. When beginning treatment with ADVAIR DISKUS, patients who have been taking oral or inhaled, short-acting $beta_2$-agonists on a regular basis (e.g., 4 times a day) should be instructed to discontinue the regular use of these drugs. For patients on ADVAIR DISKUS, inhaled, short-acting $beta_2$-agonists should only be used for symptomatic relief of acute symptoms of shortness of breath (see PRECAUTIONS: Information for Patients).

5. Watch for Increasing Use of Inhaled, Short-Acting $Beta_2$-Agonists, Which Is a Marker of Deteriorating Asthma: Asthma may deteriorate acutely over a period of hours or chronically over several days or longer. If the patient's inhaled, short-acting $beta_2$-agonist becomes less effective, the patient needs more inhalations than usual, or the patient develops a significant decrease in lung function, this may be a marker of destabilization of the disease. In this setting, the patient requires immediate reevaluation with reassessment of the treatment regimen, giving special consideration to the possible need for replacing the current strength of ADVAIR DISKUS with a higher strength, adding additional inhaled corticosteroid, or initiating systemic corticosteroids. Patients should not use more than 1 inhalation twice daily (morning and evening) of ADVAIR DISKUS.

6. Do Not Use an Inhaled, Long-Acting $Beta_2$-Agonist in Conjunction With ADVAIR DISKUS: Patients who are receiving ADVAIR DISKUS twice daily should not use additional salmeterol or other inhaled, long-acting $beta_2$-agonists (e.g., formoterol) for prevention of exercise-induced bronchospasm (EIB) or the maintenance treatment of asthma or the maintenance treatment of bronchospasm associated with COPD. Additional benefit would not be gained from using supplemental salmeterol or formoterol for prevention of EIB since ADVAIR DISKUS already contains an inhaled, long-acting $beta_2$-agonist.

7. Do Not Exceed Recommended Dosage: ADVAIR DISKUS should not be used more often or at higher doses than recommended. Fatalities have been reported in association with excessive use of inhaled sympathomimetic drugs. Large doses of inhaled or oral salmeterol (12 to 20 times the recommended dose) have been associated with clinically significant prolongation of the QTc interval, which has the potential for producing ventricular arrhythmias.

8. Paradoxical Bronchospasm: As with other inhaled asthma and COPD medications, ADVAIR DISKUS can produce paradoxical bronchospasm, which may be life threatening. If paradoxical bronchospasm occurs following dosing with ADVAIR DISKUS, it should be treated immediately with an inhaled, short-acting bronchodilator, ADVAIR DISKUS should be discontinued immediately, and alternative therapy should be instituted.

9. Immediate Hypersensitivity Reactions: Immediate hypersensitivity reactions may occur after administration of ADVAIR DISKUS, as demonstrated by cases of urticaria, angioedema, rash, and bronchospasm.

10. Upper Airway Symptoms: Symptoms of laryngeal spasm, irritation, or swelling, such as stridor and choking, have been reported in patients receiving fluticasone propionate and salmeterol, components of ADVAIR DISKUS.

11. Cardiovascular Disorders: ADVAIR DISKUS, like all products containing sympathomimetic amines, should be used with caution in patients with cardiovascular disorders, especially coronary insufficiency, cardiac arrhythmias, and hypertension. Salmeterol, a component of ADVAIR DISKUS, can produce a clinically significant cardiovascular effect in some patients as measured by pulse rate, blood pressure, and/or symptoms. Although such effects are uncommon after administration of salmeterol at recommended doses, if they occur, the drug may need to be discontinued. In addition, beta-agonists have been reported to produce ECG changes, such as flattening of the T wave, prolongation of the QTc interval, and ST segment depression. The clinical significance of these findings is unknown.

12. Discontinuation of Systemic Corticosteroids: Transfer of patients from systemic corticosteroid therapy to ADVAIR DISKUS may unmask conditions previously suppressed by the systemic corticosteroid therapy, e.g., rhinitis, conjunctivitis, eczema, arthritis, and eosinophilic conditions.

13. Immunosuppression: Persons who are using drugs that suppress the immune system are more susceptible to infections than healthy individuals. Chickenpox and measles, for example, can have a more serious or even fatal course in susceptible children or adults using corticosteroids. In such children or adults who have not had these diseases or been properly immunized, particular care should be taken to avoid exposure. How the dose, route, and duration of corticosteroid administration affect the risk of developing a disseminated infection is not known. The contribution of the underlying disease and/or prior corticosteroid treatment to the risk is also not known. If exposed to chickenpox, prophylaxis with varicella zoster immune globulin (VZIG) may be indicated. If exposed to measles, prophylaxis with pooled intramuscular immunoglobulin (IG) may be indicated. (See the respective package inserts for complete VZIG and IG prescribing information.) If chickenpox develops, treatment with antiviral agents may be considered.

PRECAUTIONS

General: ***Cardiovascular Effects:*** Cardiovascular and central nervous system effects seen with all sympathomimetic drugs (e.g., increased blood pressure, heart rate, excitement) can occur after use of salmeterol, a component of ADVAIR DISKUS, and may require discontinuation of ADVAIR DISKUS. ADVAIR DISKUS, like all medications containing sympathomimetic amines, should be used with caution in patients with cardiovascular disorders, especially coronary insufficiency, cardiac arrhythmias, and hypertension; in patients with convulsive disorders or thyrotoxicosis; and in patients who are unusually responsive to sympathomimetic amines.

As has been described with other beta-adrenergic agonist bronchodilators, clinically significant changes in electrocardiograms (ECGs) have been seen infrequently in individual patients in controlled clinical studies with ADVAIR DISKUS and salmeterol. Clinically significant changes in systolic and/or diastolic blood pressure and pulse rate have

Continued on next page

Product information on these pages is effective as of August 2004. Further information is available at: GlaxoSmithKline, PO Box 13398, Research Triangle Park, NC 27709. 1-888-825-5249. Corporate Web Site: www.gsk.com

Advair Diskus—Cont.

been seen infrequently in individual patients in controlled clinical studies with salmeterol, a component of ADVAIR DISKUS.

Metabolic and Other Effects: Long-term use of orally inhaled corticosteroids may affect normal bone metabolism, resulting in a loss of bone mineral density (BMD). A 2-year study of 160 patients (females 18 to 40 and males 18 to 50 years of age) with asthma receiving chlorofluorocarbon-propelled fluticasone propionate inhalation aerosol 88 or 440 mcg twice daily demonstrated no statistically significant changes in BMD at any time point (24, 52, 76, and 104 weeks of double-blind treatment) as assessed by dual-energy x-ray absorptiometry at lumbar region L1 through L4. Long-term treatment effects of fluticasone propionate on BMD in the COPD population have not been studied.

In patients with major risk factors for decreased bone mineral content, such as tobacco use, advanced age, sedentary lifestyle, poor nutrition, family history of osteoporosis, or chronic use of drugs that can reduce bone mass (e.g., anticonvulsants and corticosteroids), ADVAIR DISKUS may pose an additional risk. Since patients with COPD often have multiple risk factors for reduced BMD, assessment of BMD is recommended, including prior to instituting ADVAIR DISKUS 250/50 and periodically thereafter. If significant reductions in BMD are seen and ADVAIR DISKUS 250/50 is still considered medically important for that patient's COPD therapy, use of medication to treat or prevent osteoporosis should be strongly considered. ADVAIR DISKUS 250/50 mcg twice daily is the only approved dosage for the treatment of COPD associated with chronic bronchitis, and higher doses, including ADVAIR DISKUS 250/50, are not recommended.

Glaucoma, increased intraocular pressure, and cataracts have been reported in patients with asthma and COPD following the long-term administration of inhaled corticosteroids, including fluticasone propionate, a component of ADVAIR DISKUS; therefore, regular eye examinations should be considered.

Lower respiratory tract infections, including pneumonia, have been reported following the inhaled administration of corticosteroids, including fluticasone propionate and ADVAIR DISKUS.

Doses of the related $beta_2$-adrenoceptor agonist albuterol, when administered intravenously, have been reported to aggravate preexisting diabetes mellitus and ketoacidosis. Beta-adrenergic agonist medications may produce significant hypokalemia in some patients, possibly through intracellular shunting, which has the potential to produce adverse cardiovascular effects. The decrease in serum potassium is usually transient, not requiring supplementation.

Clinically significant changes in blood glucose and/or serum potassium were seen infrequently during clinical studies with ADVAIR DISKUS at recommended doses.

During withdrawal from oral corticosteroids, some patients may experience symptoms of systemically active corticosteroid withdrawal, e.g., joint and/or muscular pain, lassitude, and depression, despite maintenance or even improvement of respiratory function.

Fluticasone propionate, a component of ADVAIR DISKUS, will often help control asthma symptoms with less suppression of HPA function than therapeutically equivalent oral doses of prednisone. Since fluticasone propionate is absorbed into the circulation and can be systemically active at higher doses, the beneficial effects of ADVAIR DISKUS in minimizing HPA dysfunction may be expected only when recommended dosages are not exceeded and individual patients are titrated to the lowest effective dose. A relationship between plasma levels of fluticasone propionate and inhibitory effects on stimulated cortisol production has been shown after 4 weeks of treatment with fluticasone propionate inhalation aerosol. Since individual sensitivity to effects on cortisol production exists, physicians should consider this information when prescribing ADVAIR DISKUS.

Because of the possibility of systemic absorption of inhaled corticosteroids, patients treated with ADVAIR DISKUS should be observed carefully for any evidence of systemic corticosteroid effects. Particular care should be taken in observing patients postoperatively or during periods of stress for evidence of inadequate adrenal response.

It is possible that systemic corticosteroid effects such as hypercorticism and adrenal suppression (including adrenal crisis) may appear in a small number of patients, particularly when fluticasone propionate is administered at higher than recommended doses over prolonged periods of time. If such effects occur, the dosage of ADVAIR DISKUS should be reduced slowly, consistent with accepted procedures for reducing systemic corticosteroids and for management of asthma symptoms.

A reduction of growth velocity in children and adolescents may occur as a result of poorly controlled asthma or from the therapeutic use of corticosteroids, including inhaled corticosteroids. The effects of long-term treatment of children and adolescents with inhaled corticosteroids, including fluticasone propionate, on final adult height are not known.

A 52-week, placebo-controlled study to assess the potential growth effects of fluticasone propionate inhalation powder (FLOVENT® ROTADISK®) at 50 and 100 mcg twice daily was conducted in the US in 325 prepubescent children (244 males and 81 females) aged 4 to 11 years. The mean growth velocities at 52 weeks observed in the intent-to-treat population were 6.32 cm/year in the placebo group (N = 76), 6.07 cm/year in the 50-mcg group (N = 98), and 5.66 cm/year in the 100-mcg group (N = 89). An imbalance in the proportion of children entering puberty between groups and a higher dropout rate in the placebo group due to poorly controlled asthma may be confounding factors in interpreting these data. A separate subset analysis of children who remained prepubertal during the study revealed growth rates at 52 weeks of 6.10 cm/year in the placebo group (n = 57), 5.91 cm/year in the 50-mcg group (n = 74), and 5.67 cm/year in the 100-mcg group (n = 79). In children 8.5 years of age, the mean age of children in this study, the range for expected growth velocity is: boys – 3rd percentile = 3.8 cm/year, 50th percentile = 5.4 cm/year, and 97th percentile = 7.0 cm/year; girls – 3rd percentile = 4.2 cm/year, 50th percentile = 5.7 cm/year, and 97th percentile = 7.3 cm/year.

The clinical significance of these growth data is not certain. Physicians should closely follow the growth of children and adolescents taking corticosteroids by any route, and weigh the benefits of corticosteroid therapy against the possibility of growth suppression if growth appears slowed. Patients should be maintained on the lowest dose of inhaled corticosteroid that effectively controls their asthma.

The long-term effects of ADVAIR DISKUS in human subjects are not fully known. In particular, the effects resulting from chronic use of fluticasone propionate on developmental or immunologic processes in the mouth, pharynx, trachea, and lung are unknown. Some patients have received inhaled fluticasone propionate on a continuous basis for periods of 3 years or longer. In clinical studies in patients with asthma treated for 2 years with inhaled fluticasone propionate, no apparent differences in the type or severity of adverse reactions were observed after long- versus short-term treatment.

In clinical studies with ADVAIR DISKUS, the development of localized infections of the pharynx with *Candida albicans* has occurred. When such an infection develops, it should be treated with appropriate local or systemic (i.e., oral antifungal) therapy while remaining on treatment with ADVAIR DISKUS, but at times therapy with ADVAIR DISKUS may need to be interrupted.

Inhaled corticosteroids should be used with caution, if at all, in patients with active or quiescent tuberculosis infections of the respiratory tract; untreated systemic fungal, bacterial, viral, or parasitic infections; or ocular herpes simplex.

Eosinophilic Conditions: In rare cases, patients on inhaled fluticasone propionate, a component of ADVAIR DISKUS, may present with systemic eosinophilic conditions, with some patients presenting with clinical features of vasculitis consistent with Churg-Strauss syndrome, a condition that is often treated with systemic corticosteroid therapy. These events usually, but not always, have been associated with the reduction and/or withdrawal of oral corticosteroid therapy following the introduction of fluticasone propionate. Cases of serious eosinophilic conditions have also been reported with other inhaled corticosteroids in this clinical setting. Physicians should be alert to eosinophilia, vasculitic rash, worsening pulmonary symptoms, cardiac complications, and/or neuropathy presenting in their patients. A causal relationship between fluticasone propionate and these underlying conditions has not been established (see ADVERSE REACTIONS: Observed During Clinical Practice: *Eosinophilic Conditions*).

Chronic Obstructive Pulmonary Disease: ADVAIR DISKUS 250/50 twice daily is the only dosage recommended for the treatment of airflow obstruction in patients with COPD associated with chronic bronchitis. Higher doses, including ADVAIR DISKUS 500/50, are not recommended, as no additional improvement in lung function (defined by predose and postdose FEV_1) was observed in clinical trials and higher doses of corticosteroids increase the risk of systemic effects.

The benefit of treatment of patients with COPD associated with chronic bronchitis with ADVAIR DISKUS 250/50 for periods longer than 6 months has not been evaluated. Patients who are treated with ADVAIR DISKUS 250/50 for COPD associated with chronic bronchitis for periods longer than 6 months should be reevaluated periodically to assess the continuing benefits and potential risks of treatment.

Information for Patients: Patients being treated with ADVAIR DISKUS should receive the following information and instructions. This information is intended to aid them in the safe and effective use of this medication. It is not a disclosure of all possible adverse or intended effects.

It is important that patients understand how to use the DISKUS inhalation device appropriately and how it should be used in relation to other asthma or COPD medications they are taking. Patients should be given the following information:

1. Patients should use ADVAIR DISKUS at regular intervals as directed. Results of clinical trials indicate significant improvement may occur within the first 30 minutes of taking the first dose; however, the full benefit may not be achieved until treatment has been administered for 1 week or longer. The patient should not use more than the prescribed dosage but should contact the physician if symptoms do not improve or if the condition worsens.
2. Most patients are able to taste or feel a dose delivered from ADVAIR DISKUS. However, whether or not patients are able to sense delivery of a dose, you should instruct them not to exceed the recommended dose of 1 inhalation each morning and evening, approximately 12 hours apart. You should instruct them to contact you or the pharmacist if they have questions.
3. The bronchodilation from a single dose of ADVAIR DISKUS may last up to 12 hours or longer. The recommended dosage (1 inhalation twice daily, morning and evening) should not be exceeded. Patients who are receiving ADVAIR DISKUS twice daily should not use salmeterol or other inhaled, long-acting $beta_2$-agonists (e.g., formoterol) for prevention of EIB or maintenance treatment of asthma or the maintenance treatment of bronchospasm in COPD.
4. ADVAIR DISKUS is not meant to relieve acute asthma symptoms and extra doses should not be used for that purpose. Acute symptoms should be treated with an inhaled, short-acting $beta_2$-agonist such as albuterol (the physician should provide the patient with such medication and instruct the patient in how it should be used). ADVAIR DISKUS is not meant to relieve acute asthma symptoms or exacerbations of COPD.
5. Patients should not stop therapy with ADVAIR DISKUS without physician/provider guidance since symptoms may recur after discontinuation.
6. The physician should be notified immediately if any of the following situations occur, which may be a sign of seriously worsening asthma:
   - decreasing effectiveness of inhaled, short-acting $beta_2$-agonists;
   - need for more inhalations than usual of inhaled, short-acting $beta_2$-agonists;
   - significant decrease in lung function as outlined by the physician.
7. Patients should be cautioned regarding common adverse effects associated with $beta_2$-agonists, such as palpitations, chest pain, rapid heart rate, tremor, or nervousness.
8. Patients who are at an increased risk for decreased BMD should be advised that the use of corticosteroids may pose an additional risk and should be told to monitor and, where appropriate, seek treatment for this condition.
9. Long-term use of inhaled corticosteroids, including fluticasone propionate, a component of ADVAIR DISKUS, may increase the risk of some eye problems (cataracts or glaucoma). Regular eye examinations should be considered.
10. When patients are prescribed ADVAIR DISKUS, other medications for asthma and COPD should be used only as directed by their physicians.
11. ADVAIR DISKUS should not be used with a spacer device.
12. Patients who are pregnant or nursing should contact their physicians about the use of ADVAIR DISKUS.
13. Effective and safe use of ADVAIR DISKUS includes an understanding of the way that it should be used:
    - Never exhale into the DISKUS.
    - Never attempt to take the DISKUS apart.
    - Always activate and use the DISKUS in a level, horizontal position.
    - After inhalation, rinse the mouth with water without swallowing.
    - Never wash the mouthpiece or any part of the DISKUS. KEEP IT DRY.
    - Always keep the DISKUS in a dry place.
    - Discard **1 month** after removal from the moisture-protective foil overwrap pouch or after all blisters have been used (when the dose indicator reads "0"), whichever comes first.
14. Patients should be warned to avoid exposure to chickenpox or measles and, if they are exposed, to consult their physicians without delay.
15. For the proper use of ADVAIR DISKUS and to attain maximum improvement, the patient should read and carefully follow the Patient's Instructions for Use accompanying the product.

Drug Interactions: ADVAIR DISKUS has been used concomitantly with other drugs, including short-acting $beta_2$-agonists, methylxanthines, and intranasal corticosteroids, commonly used in patients with asthma or COPD, without adverse drug reactions. No formal drug interaction studies have been performed with ADVAIR DISKUS.

Short-Acting $Beta_2$-Agonists: In clinical trials with patients with asthma, the mean daily need for albuterol by 166 adult and adolescent patients 12 years of age and older using ADVAIR DISKUS was approximately 1.3 inhalations/day, and ranged from 0 to 9 inhalations/day. Five percent (5%) of patients using ADVAIR DISKUS in these trials averaged 6 or more inhalations per day over the course of the 12-week trials. No increase in frequency of cardiovascular adverse reactions was observed among patients who averaged 6 or more inhalations per day.

In a COPD clinical trial, the mean daily need for albuterol for patients using ADVAIR DISKUS 250/50 was 4.1 inhalations/day. Twenty-six percent (26%) of patients using ADVAIR DISKUS 250/50 averaged 6 or more inhalations per day over the course of the 24-week trial. No increase in frequency of cardiovascular adverse reactions was observed among patients who averaged 6 or more inhalations of albuterol per day.

Methylxanthines: The concurrent use of intravenously or orally administered methylxanthines (e.g., aminophylline, theophylline) by adult and adolescent patients 12 years of age and older receiving ADVAIR DISKUS has not been completely evaluated. In clinical trials with patients with asthma, 39 patients receiving ADVAIR DISKUS 100/50, 250/50, or 500/50 twice daily concurrently with a theophylline product had adverse event rates similar to those in 304 patients receiving ADVAIR DISKUS without theophylline. Similar results were observed in patients receiving salmeterol 50 mcg plus fluticasone propionate 500 mcg twice daily concurrently with a theophylline product (N = 39) or without theophylline (N = 132).

In a COPD clinical trial, 17 patients receiving ADVAIR DISKUS 250/50 twice daily concurrently with a theophylline product had adverse event rates similar to those in 161 patients receiving ADVAIR DISKUS without theophylline. Based on the available data, the concomitant administration of methylxanthines with ADVAIR DISKUS did not alter the observed adverse event profile.

Fluticasone Propionate Nasal Spray: In adult and adolescent patients 12 years of age and older taking ADVAIR DISKUS in clinical trials, no difference in the profile of adverse events or HPA axis effects was noted between patients taking FLONASE® (fluticasone propionate) Nasal Spray, 50 mcg concurrently (N = 46) and those who were not (N = 130).

Monoamine Oxidase Inhibitors and Tricyclic Antidepressants: ADVAIR DISKUS should be administered with extreme caution to patients being treated with monoamine oxidase inhibitors or tricyclic antidepressants, or within 2 weeks of discontinuation of such agents, because the action of salmeterol, a component of ADVAIR DISKUS, on the vascular system may be potentiated by these agents.

Beta-Adrenergic Receptor Blocking Agents: Beta-blockers not only block the pulmonary effect of beta-agonists, such as salmeterol, a component of ADVAIR DISKUS, but may produce severe bronchospasm in patients with asthma. Therefore, patients with asthma should not normally be treated with beta-blockers. However, under certain circumstances, there may be no acceptable alternatives to the use of beta-adrenergic blocking agents in patients with asthma. In this setting, cardioselective beta-blockers could be considered, although they should be administered with caution.

Diuretics: The ECG changes and/or hypokalemia that may result from the administration of nonpotassium-sparing diuretics (such as loop or thiazide diuretics) can be acutely worsened by beta-agonists, especially when the recommended dose of the beta-agonist is exceeded. Although the clinical significance of these effects is not known, caution is advised in the coadministration of beta-agonists with nonpotassium-sparing diuretics.

Inhibitors of Cytochrome P450: Fluticasone propionate is a substrate of cytochrome P450 3A4. A drug interaction study with fluticasone propionate aqueous nasal spray in healthy subjects has shown that ritonavir (a highly potent cytochrome P450 3A4 inhibitor) can significantly increase plasma fluticasone propionate exposure, resulting in significantly reduced serum cortisol concentrations (see CLINICAL PHARMACOLOGY: Pharmacokinetics: *Fluticasone Propionate: Drug Interactions*). During postmarketing use, there have been reports of clinically significant drug interactions in patients receiving fluticasone propionate and ritonavir, resulting in systemic corticosteroid effects including Cushing syndrome and adrenal suppression. Therefore, coadministration of fluticasone propionate and ritonavir is not recommended unless the potential benefit to the patient outweighs the risk of systemic corticosteroid side effects.

In a placebo-controlled, crossover study in 8 healthy adult volunteers, coadministration of a single dose of orally inhaled fluticasone propionate (1,000 mcg) with multiple doses of ketoconazole (200 mg) to steady state resulted in increased plasma fluticasone propionate exposure, a reduction in plasma cortisol AUC, and no effect on urinary excretion of cortisol. Caution should be exercised when ADVAIR DISKUS is coadministered with ketoconazole and other known potent cytochrome P450 3A4 inhibitors.

Carcinogenesis, Mutagenesis, Impairment of Fertility: ***Fluticasone Propionate:*** Fluticasone propionate demonstrated no tumorigenic potential in mice at oral doses up to 1,000 mcg/kg (approximately 4 and 10 times, respectively, the maximum recommended daily inhalation dose in adults and children on a mcg/m^2 basis) for 78 weeks or in rats at inhalation doses up to 57 mcg/kg (less than and approximately equivalent to, respectively, the maximum recommended daily inhalation dose in adults and children on a mcg/m^2 basis) for 104 weeks.

Fluticasone propionate did not induce gene mutation in prokaryotic or eukaryotic cells in vitro. No significant clastogenic effect was seen in cultured human peripheral lymphocytes in vitro or in the mouse micronucleus test.

No evidence of impairment of fertility was observed in reproductive studies conducted in male and female rats at subcutaneous doses up to 50 mcg/kg (less than the maximum recommended daily inhalation dose in adults on a mcg/m^2 basis). Prostate weight was significantly reduced at a subcutaneous dose of 50 mcg/kg.

Salmeterol: In an 18-month carcinogenicity study in CD-mice, salmeterol at oral doses of 1.4 mg/kg and above (approximately 20 times the maximum recommended daily inhalation dose in adults and children based on comparison of the plasma area under the curves [AUCs]) caused a dose-related increase in the incidence of smooth muscle hyperplasia, cystic glandular hyperplasia, leiomyomas of the uterus, and cysts in the ovaries. The incidence of leiomyosarcomas was not statistically significant. No tumors were seen at 0.2 mg/kg (approximately 3 times the maximum recommended daily inhalation doses in adults and children based on comparison of the AUCs).

In a 24-month oral and inhalation carcinogenicity study in Sprague Dawley rats, salmeterol caused a dose-related increase in the incidence of mesovarian leiomyomas and ovarian cysts at doses of 0.68 mg/kg and above (approximately 55 and 25 times, respectively, the maximum recommended daily inhalation dose in adults and children on a mg/m^2 basis). No tumors were seen at 0.21 mg/kg (approximately 15 and 8 times, respectively, the maximum recommended daily inhalation dose in adults and children on a mg/m^2 basis). These findings in rodents are similar to those reported previously for other beta-adrenergic agonist drugs. The relevance of these findings to human use is unknown.

Salmeterol produced no detectable or reproducible increases in microbial and mammalian gene mutation in vitro. No clastogenic activity occurred in vitro in human lymphocytes or in vivo in a rat micronucleus test. No effects on fertility were identified in male and female rats treated with salmeterol at oral doses up to 2 mg/kg (approximately 160 times the maximum recommended daily inhalation dose in adults on a mg/m^2 basis).

Pregnancy: ***Teratogenic Effects: ADVAIR DISKUS:*** Pregnancy Category C. From the reproduction toxicity studies in mice and rats, no evidence of enhanced toxicity was seen using combinations of fluticasone propionate and salmeterol compared to toxicity data from the components administered separately. In mice combining 150 mcg/kg subcutaneously of fluticasone propionate (less than the maximum recommended daily inhalation dose in adults on a mcg/m^2 basis) with 10 mg/kg orally of salmeterol (approximately 410 times the maximum recommended daily inhalation dose in adults on a mg/m^2 basis) was teratogenic. Cleft palate, fetal death, increased implantation loss and delayed ossification were seen. These observations are characteristic of glucocorticoids. No developmental toxicity was observed at combination doses up to 40 mcg/kg subcutaneously of fluticasone propionate (less than the maximum recommended daily inhalation dose in adults on a mcg/m^2 basis) and up to 1.4 mg/kg orally of salmeterol (approximately 55 times the maximum recommended daily inhalation dose in adults on a mg/m^2 basis). In rats, no teratogenicity was observed at combination doses up to 30 mcg/kg subcutaneously of fluticasone propionate (less than the maximum recommended daily inhalation dose in adults on a mcg/m^2 basis) and up to 1 mg/kg of salmeterol (approximately 90 times the maximum recommended daily inhalation dose in adults on a mg/m^2 basis). Combining 100 mcg/kg subcutaneously of fluticasone propionate (equivalent to the maximum recommended daily inhalation dose in adults on a mcg/m^2 basis) with 10 mg/kg orally of salmeterol (approximately 810 times the maximum recommended daily inhalation dose in adults on a mg/m^2 basis) produced maternal toxicity, decreased placental weight, decreased fetal weight, umbilical hernia, delayed ossification, and changes in the occipital bone. There are no adequate and well-controlled studies with ADVAIR DISKUS in pregnant women. ADVAIR DISKUS should be used during pregnancy only if the potential benefit justifies the potential risk to the fetus.

Fluticasone Propionate: Pregnancy Category C. Subcutaneous studies in the mouse and rat at 45 and 100 mcg/kg (less than or equivalent to the maximum recommended daily inhalation dose in adults on a mcg/m^2 basis), respectively, revealed fetal toxicity characteristic of potent corticosteroid compounds, including embryonic growth retardation, omphalocele, cleft palate, and retarded cranial ossification.

In the rabbit, fetal weight reduction and cleft palate were observed at a subcutaneous dose of 4 mcg/kg (less than the maximum recommended daily inhalation dose in adults on a mcg/m^2 basis). However, no teratogenic effects were reported at oral doses up to 300 mcg/kg (approximately 5 times the maximum recommended daily inhalation dose in adults on a mcg/m^2 basis) of fluticasone propionate. No fluticasone propionate was detected in the plasma in this study, consistent with the established low bioavailability following oral administration (see CLINICAL PHARMACOLOGY).

Fluticasone propionate crossed the placenta following administration of a subcutaneous dose of 100 mcg/kg to mice (less than the maximum recommended daily inhalation dose in adults on a mcg/m^2 basis), administration of a subcutaneous or an oral dose of 100 mcg/kg to rats (approximately equivalent to the maximum recommended daily inhalation dose in adults on a mcg/m^2 basis), and administration of an oral dose of 300 mcg/kg to rabbits (approximately 5 times the maximum recommended daily inhalation dose in adults on a mcg/m^2 basis).

There are no adequate and well-controlled studies in pregnant women. Fluticasone propionate should be used during pregnancy only if the potential benefit justifies the potential risk to the fetus.

Experience with oral corticosteroids since their introduction in pharmacologic, as opposed to physiologic, doses suggests that rodents are more prone to teratogenic effects from corticosteroids than humans. In addition, because there is a natural increase in corticosteroid production during pregnancy, most women will require a lower exogenous corticosteroid dose and many will not need corticosteroid treatment during pregnancy.

Salmeterol: Pregnancy Category C. No teratogenic effects occurred in rats at oral doses up to 2 mg/kg (approximately 160 times the maximum recommended daily inhalation dose in adults on a mg/m^2 basis). In pregnant Dutch rabbits administered oral doses of 1 mg/kg and above (approximately 50 times the maximum recommended daily inhalation dose in adults based on comparison of the AUCs), salmeterol exhibited fetal toxic effects characteristically resulting from beta-adrenoceptor stimulation. These included precocious eyelid openings, cleft palate, sternebral fusion, limb and paw flexures, and delayed ossification of the frontal cranial bones. No significant effects occurred at an oral dose of 0.6 mg/kg (approximately 20 times the maximum recommended daily inhalation dose in adults based on comparison of the AUCs).

New Zealand White rabbits were less sensitive since only delayed ossification of the frontal bones was seen at an oral dose of 10 mg/kg (approximately 1,600 times the maximum recommended daily inhalation dose in adults on a mg/m^2 basis). Extensive use of other beta-agonists has provided no evidence that these class effects in animals are relevant to their use in humans. There are no adequate and well-controlled studies with salmeterol in pregnant women. Salmeterol should be used during pregnancy only if the potential benefit justifies the potential risk to the fetus.

Salmeterol xinafoate crossed the placenta following oral administration of 10 mg/kg to mice and rats (approximately 410 and 810 times, respectively, the maximum recommended daily inhalation dose in adults on a mg/m^2 basis).

Use in Labor and Delivery: There are no well-controlled human studies that have investigated effects of ADVAIR DISKUS on preterm labor or labor at term. Because of the potential for beta-agonist interference with uterine contractility, use of ADVAIR DISKUS during labor should be restricted to those patients in whom the benefits clearly outweigh the risks.

Nursing Mothers: Plasma levels of salmeterol, a component of ADVAIR DISKUS, after inhaled therapeutic doses are very low. In rats, salmeterol xinafoate is excreted in the milk. There are no data from controlled trials on the use of salmeterol by nursing mothers. It is not known whether fluticasone propionate, a component of ADVAIR DISKUS, is excreted in human breast milk. However, other corticosteroids have been detected in human milk. Subcutaneous administration to lactating rats of 10 mcg/kg tritiated fluticasone propionate (less than the maximum recommended daily inhalation dose in adults on a mcg/m^2 basis) resulted in measurable radioactivity in milk.

Since there are no data from controlled trials on the use of ADVAIR DISKUS by nursing mothers, a decision should be made whether to discontinue nursing or to discontinue ADVAIR DISKUS, taking into account the importance of ADVAIR DISKUS to the mother.

Caution should be exercised when ADVAIR DISKUS is administered to a nursing woman.

Pediatric Use: Use of ADVAIR DISKUS 100/50 in patients 4 to 11 years of age is supported by extrapolation of efficacy data from older patients and by safety and efficacy data from a study of ADVAIR DISKUS 100/50 in children with asthma aged 4 to 11 years (see CLINICAL TRIALS: Asthma: *Pediatric Patients* and ADVERSE REACTIONS: Asthma: *Pediatric Patients*). The safety and effectiveness of ADVAIR DISKUS in children with asthma under 4 years of age have not been established.

Controlled clinical studies have shown that orally inhaled corticosteroids may cause a reduction in growth velocity in pediatric patients. This effect has been observed in the absence of laboratory evidence of HPA axis suppression, suggesting that growth velocity is a more sensitive indicator of systemic corticosteroid exposure in pediatric patients than some commonly used tests of HPA axis function. The long-term effects of this reduction in growth velocity associated with orally inhaled corticosteroids, including the impact on final adult height, are unknown. The potential for "catch-up" growth following discontinuation of treatment with orally inhaled corticosteroids has not been adequately studied.

Inhaled corticosteroids, including fluticasone propionate, a component of ADVAIR DISKUS, may cause a reduction in growth velocity in children and adolescents (see PRECAUTIONS: General: *Metabolic and Other Effects*). The growth of pediatric patients receiving orally inhaled corticosteroids, including ADVAIR DISKUS, should be monitored. If a child or adolescent on any corticosteroid appears to have growth suppression, the possibility that he/she is particularly sensitive to this effect of corticosteroids should be considered. The potential growth effects of prolonged treatment should be weighed against the clinical benefits obtained. To minimize the systemic effects of orally inhaled corticosteroids, including ADVAIR DISKUS, each patient should be titrated to the lowest strength that effectively controls his/her asthma (see DOSAGE AND ADMINISTRATION: Asthma).

Geriatric Use: Of the total number of patients in clinical studies of ADVAIR DISKUS for asthma, 44 were 65 years of age or older and 3 were 75 years of age or older. Of the total number of patients in a clinical study of ADVAIR DISKUS 250/50 for COPD, 85 were 65 years of age or older and 31 were 75 years of age or older. For both diseases, no overall differences in safety were observed between these patients and younger patients, and other reported clinical experience, including studies of the individual components, has not identified differences in responses between the elderly and younger patients, but greater sensitivity of some older individuals cannot be ruled out. As with other products con-

Continued on next page

Product information on these pages is effective as of August 2004. Further information is available at: GlaxoSmithKline, PO Box 13398, Research Triangle Park, NC 27709. 1-888-825-5249. Corporate Web Site: www.gsk.com

Advair Diskus—Cont.

taining $beta_2$-agonists, special caution should be observed when using ADVAIR DISKUS in geriatric patients who have concomitant cardiovascular disease that could be adversely affected by $beta_2$-agonists. Based on available data for ADVAIR DISKUS or its active components, no adjustment of dosage of ADVAIR DISKUS in geriatric patients is warranted.

ADVERSE REACTIONS

Asthma: *Adult and Adolescent Patients 12 Years of Age and Older:* The incidence of common adverse experiences in Table 3 is based upon 2 placebo-controlled, 12-week, US clinical studies (Studies 1 and 2). A total of 705 adolescent and adult patients (349 females and 356 males) previously treated with salmeterol or inhaled corticosteroids were treated twice daily with ADVAIR DISKUS (100/50- or 250/50-mcg doses), fluticasone propionate inhalation powder (100- or 250-mcg doses), salmeterol inhalation powder 50 mcg, or placebo.

[See table 3 below]

Table 3 includes all events (whether considered drug-related or nondrug-related by the investigator) that occurred at a rate of 3% or greater in either of the groups receiving ADVAIR DISKUS and were more common than in the placebo group. In considering these data, differences in average duration of exposure should be taken into account.

Rare cases of immediate and delayed hypersensitivity reactions, including rash and other rare events of angioedema and bronchospasm, have been reported.

These adverse reactions were mostly mild to moderate in severity.

Other adverse events that occurred in the groups receiving ADVAIR DISKUS in these studies with an incidence of 1% to 3% and that occurred at a greater incidence than with placebo were:

Blood and Lymphatic: Lymphatic signs and symptoms.

Cardiovascular: Palpitations.

Drug Interaction, Overdose, and Trauma: Muscle injuries, fractures, wounds and lacerations, contusions and hematomas, burns.

Ear, Nose, and Throat: Rhinorrhea/postnasal drip; ear, nose, and throat infections; ear signs and symptoms; nasal signs and symptoms; nasal sinus disorders; rhinitis; sneezing; nasal irritation; blood in nasal mucosa.

Eye: Keratitis and conjunctivitis, viral eye infections, eye redness.

Gastrointestinal: Dental discomfort and pain, gastrointestinal signs and symptoms, gastrointestinal infections, gastroenteritis, gastrointestinal disorders, oral ulcerations, oral erythema and rashes, constipation, appendicitis, oral discomfort and pain.

Hepatobiliary Tract and Pancreas: Abnormal liver function tests.

Lower Respiratory: Lower respiratory signs and symptoms, pneumonia, lower respiratory infections.

Musculoskeletal: Arthralgia and articular rheumatism; muscle stiffness, tightness, and rigidity; bone and cartilage disorders.

Neurology: Sleep disorders, tremors, hypnagogic effects, compressed nerve syndromes.

Non-Site Specific: Allergies and allergic reactions, congestion, viral infections, pain, chest symptoms, fluid retention, bacterial infections, wheeze and hives, unusual taste.

Skin: Viral skin infections, urticaria, skin flakiness and acquired ichthyosis, disorders of sweat and sebum, sweating.

The incidence of common adverse events reported in Study 3, a 28-week, non-US clinical study of 503 patients previously treated with inhaled corticosteroids who were treated twice daily with ADVAIR DISKUS 500/50, fluticasone propionate inhalation powder 500 mcg and salmeterol inhalation powder 50 mcg used concurrently, or fluticasone propionate inhalation powder 500 mcg was similar to the incidences reported in Table 3.

Pediatric Patients: Pediatric Study: ADVAIR DISKUS 100/50 was well tolerated in clinical trials conducted in children with asthma aged 4 to 11 years. The incidence of common adverse events in Table 4 is based upon a 12-week US study in 203 patients with asthma aged 4 to 11 years (74 females and 129 males) who were receiving inhaled corticosteroids at study entry and were randomized to either ADVAIR DISKUS 100/50 or fluticasone propionate inhalation powder 100 mcg twice daily.

Table 4. Overall Adverse Events With ≥3% Incidence With ADVAIR DISKUS 100/50 in Patients 4 to 11 Years of Age With Asthma

Adverse Event	ADVAIR DISKUS 100/50 (N = 101) %	Fluticasone Propionate 100 mcg (N = 102) %
Ear, nose, & throat		
Upper respiratory tract infection	10	17
Throat irritation	8	7
Ear, nose & throat infections	4	<1
Epistaxis	4	<1
Pharyngitis/throat infection	3	2
Ear signs & symptoms	3	<1
Sinusitis	3	0
Neurology		
Headache	20	20
Gastrointestinal		
Gastrointestinal discomfort & pain	7	5
Nausea & vomiting	5	3
Candidiasis mouth/throat	4	<1
Non-site specific		
Fever	5	13
Chest symptoms	3	<1
Average duration of exposure (days)	74.8	78.8

Table 4 includes all events (whether considered drug-related or nondrug-related by the investigator) that occurred at a rate of 3% or greater in the group receiving ADVAIR DISKUS 100/50.

Chronic Obstructive Pulmonary Disease Associated With Chronic Bronchitis: The incidence of common adverse events in Table 5 is based upon 1 placebo-controlled 24-week, US clinical trial in patients with COPD associated with chronic bronchitis. A total of 723 adult patients (266 females and 457 males) were treated twice daily with ADVAIR DISKUS 250/50, fluticasone propionate inhalation powder 250 mcg, salmeterol inhalation powder 50 mcg, or placebo.

[See table 5 at top of next page]

Table 5 includes all events (whether considered drug-related or nondrug-related by the investigator) that occurred at a rate of 3% or greater in the group receiving ADVAIR DISKUS 250/50 and were more common than in the placebo group.

These adverse reactions were mostly mild to moderate in severity.

Other adverse events that occurred in the groups receiving ADVAIR DISKUS 250/50 with an incidence of 1% to 3% and that occurred at a greater incidence than with placebo were:

Cardiovascular: Syncope.

Drug Interaction, Overdose, and Trauma: Postoperative complications.

Ear, Nose, and Throat: Ear, nose, and throat infections; ear signs and symptoms; laryngitis; nasal congestion/blockage; nasal sinus disorders; pharyngitis/throat infection.

Endocrine and Metabolic: Hypothyroidism.

Eye: Dry eyes, eye infections.

Gastrointestinal: Constipation, gastrointestinal signs and symptoms, oral lesions.

Hepatobiliary Tract and Pancreas: Abnormal liver function tests.

Lower Respiratory: Breathing, disorders, lower respiratory signs and symptoms.

Non-Site Specific: Bacterial infections, candidiasis unspecified site, edema and swelling, nonspecific conditions, viral infections.

Psychiatry: Situational disorders.

Observed During Clinical Practice: In addition to adverse events reported from clinical trials, the following events have been identified during worldwide use of any formulation of ADVAIR, fluticasone propionate, and/or salmeterol regardless of indication. Because they are reported voluntarily from a population of unknown size, estimates of frequency cannot be made. These events have been chosen for inclusion due to either their seriousness, frequency of reporting, or causal connection to ADVAIR DISKUS, fluticasone propionate, and/or salmeterol or a combination of these factors.

In extensive US and worldwide postmarketing experience with salmeterol, a component of ADVAIR DISKUS, serious exacerbations of asthma, including some that have been fatal, have been reported. In most cases, these have occurred in patients with severe asthma and/or in some patients in whom asthma has been acutely deteriorating (see WARNINGS no. 2), but they have also occurred in a few patients with less severe asthma. It was not possible from these reports to determine whether salmeterol contributed to these events or simply failed to relieve the deteriorating asthma.

Cardiovascular: Arrhythmias (including atrial fibrillation, extrasystoles, supraventricular tachycardia), ventricular tachycardia.

Ear, Nose, and Throat: Aphonia, earache, facial and oropharyngeal edema, paranasal sinus pain, throat soreness.

Endocrine and Metabolic: Cushing syndrome, Cushingoid features, growth velocity reduction in children/adolescents, hypercorticism, hyperglycemia, weight gain, osteoporosis.

Eye: Cataracts, glaucoma.

Gastrointestinal: Abdominal pain, dyspepsia, xerostomia.

Musculoskeletal: Back pain, cramps, muscle spasm, myositis.

Table 3. Overall Adverse Effects With ≥3% Incidence in US Controlled Clinical Trials With ADVAIR DISKUS in Patients With Asthma

Adverse Event	ADVAIR DISKUS 100/50 (N = 92) %	ADVAIR DISKUS 250/50 (N = 84) %	Fluticasone Propionate 100 mcg (N = 90) %	Fluticasone Propionate 250 mcg (N = 84) %	Salmeterol 50 mcg (N = 180) %	Placebo (N = 175) %
Ear, nose, & throat						
Upper respiratory tract infection	27	21	29	25	19	14
Pharyngitis	13	10	7	12	8	6
Upper respiratory inflammation	7	6	7	8	8	5
Sinusitis	4	5	6	1	3	4
Hoarseness/dysphonia	5	2	2	4	<1	<1
Oral candidiasis	1	4	2	2	0	0
Lower respiratory						
Viral respiratory infections	4	4	4	10	6	3
Bronchitis	2	8	1	2	2	2
Cough	3	6	0	0	3	2
Neurology						
Headaches	12	13	14	8	10	7
Gastrointestinal						
Nausea & vomiting	4	6	3	4	1	1
Gastrointestinal discomfort & pain	4	1	0	2	1	1
Diarrhea	4	2	2	2	1	1
Viral gastrointestinal infections	3	0	3	1	2	2
Non-site specific						
Candidiasis unspecified site	3	0	1	4	0	1
Musculoskeletal						
Musculoskeletal pain	4	2	1	5	3	3
Average duration of exposure (days)	77.3	78.7	72.4	70.1	60.1	42.3

Neurology: Paresthesia, restlessness.
Non-Site Specific: Immediate and delayed hypersensitivity reaction (including very rare anaphylactic reaction), pallor. Very rare anaphylactic reaction in patients with severe milk protein allergy.
Psychiatry: Agitation, aggression, depression.
Respiratory: Chest congestion; chest tightness; dyspnea; immediate bronchospasm; influenza; paradoxical bronchospasm; tracheitis; wheezing; reports of upper respiratory symptoms of laryngeal spasm, irritation, or swelling such as stridor or choking.
Skin: Contact dermatitis, contusions, ecchymoses, photodermatitis.
Urogenital: Dysmenorrhea, irregular menstrual cycle, pelvic inflammatory disease, vaginal candidiasis, vaginitis, vulvovaginitis.
Eosinophilic Conditions: In rare cases, patients on inhaled fluticasone propionate, a component of ADVAIR DISKUS, may present with systemic eosinophilic conditions, with some patients presenting with clinical features of vasculitis consistent with Churg-Strauss syndrome, a condition that is often treated with systemic corticosteroid therapy. These events usually, but not always, have been associated with the reduction and/or withdrawal of oral corticosteroid therapy following the introduction of fluticasone propionate. Cases of serious eosinophilic conditions have also been reported with other inhaled corticosteroids in this clinical setting. While ADVAIR DISKUS should not be used for transferring patients from systemic corticosteroid therapy, physicians should be alert to eosinophilia, vasculitic rash, worsening pulmonary symptoms, cardiac complications, and/or neuropathy presenting in their patients. A causal relationship between fluticasone propionate and these underlying conditions has not been established (see PRECAUTIONS: General: *Eosinophilic Conditions*).

OVERDOSAGE

ADVAIR DISKUS: No deaths occurred in rats given an inhaled single-dose combination of salmeterol 3.6 mg/kg (approximately 290 and 140 times, respectively, the maximum recommended daily inhalation dose in adults and children on a mg/m^2 basis) and 1.9 mg/kg of fluticasone propionate (approximately 15 and 35 times, respectively, the maximum recommended daily inhalation dose in adults and children on a mg/m^2 basis).
Fluticasone Propionate: Chronic overdosage with fluticasone propionate may result in signs/symptoms of hypercorticism (see PRECAUTIONS: General: *Metabolic and Other Effects*). Inhalation by healthy volunteers of a single dose of 4,000 mcg of fluticasone propionate inhalation powder or single doses of 1,760 or 3,520 mcg of fluticasone propionate inhalation aerosol was well tolerated. Fluticasone propionate given by inhalation aerosol at doses of 1,320 mcg twice daily for 7 to 15 days to healthy human volunteers was also well tolerated. Repeat oral doses up to 80 mg daily for 10 days in healthy volunteers and repeat oral doses up to 20 mg daily for 42 days in patients were well tolerated. Adverse reactions were of mild or moderate severity, and incidences were similar in active and placebo treatment groups. In mice, the oral median lethal dose was >1,000 mg/kg (>4,100 and >9,600 times, respectively, the maximum recommended daily inhalation dose in adults and children on a mg/m^2 basis). In rats the subcutaneous median lethal dose was >1,000 mg/kg (>8,100 and >19,200 times, respectively, the maximum recommended daily inhalation dose in adults and children on a mg/m^2 basis).
Salmeterol: The expected signs and symptoms with overdosage of salmeterol are those of excessive beta-adrenergic stimulation and/or occurrence or exaggeration of any of the signs and symptoms listed under ADVERSE REACTIONS, e.g., seizures, angina, hypertension or hypotension, tachycardia with rates up to 200 beats/min, arrhythmias, nervousness, headache, tremor, muscle cramps, dry mouth, palpitation, nausea, dizziness, fatigue, malaise, and insomnia. Overdosage with salmeterol may be expected to result in exaggeration of the pharmacologic adverse effects associated with beta-adrenoceptor agonists, including tachycardia and/or arrhythmia, tremor, headache, and muscle cramps. Overdosage with salmeterol can lead to clinically significant prolongation of the QTc interval, which can produce ventricular arrhythmias. Other signs of overdosage may include hypokalemia and hyperglycemia.
As with all sympathomimetic medications, cardiac arrest and even death may be associated with abuse of salmeterol. Treatment consists of discontinuation of salmeterol together with appropriate symptomatic therapy. The judicious use of a cardioselective beta-receptor blocker may be considered, bearing in mind that such medication can produce bronchospasm. There is insufficient evidence to determine if dialysis is beneficial for overdosage of salmeterol. Cardiac monitoring is recommended in cases of overdosage.
No deaths were seen in rats given salmeterol at an inhalation dose of 2.9 mg/kg (approximately 240 and 110 times, respectively, the maximum recommended daily inhalation dose in adults and children on a mg/m^2 basis) and in dogs at an inhalation dose of 0.7 mg/kg (approximately 190 and 90 times, respectively, the maximum recommended daily inhalation dose in adults and children on a mg/m^2 basis). By the oral route, no deaths occurred in mice at 150 mg/kg (approximately 6,100 and 2,900 times, respectively, the maximum recommended daily inhalation dose in adults and children on a mg/m^2 basis) and in rats at 1,000 mg/kg (approximately 81,000 and 38,000 times, respectively, the maximum recommended daily inhalation dose in adults and children on a mg/m^2 basis).

Table 5. Overall Adverse Events With ≥3% Incidence With ADVAIR DISKUS 250/50 in Patients With Chronic Obstructive Pulmonary Disease Associated With Chronic Bronchitis

Adverse Event	ADVAIR DISKUS 250/50 (N = 178) %	Fluticasone Propionate 250 mcg (N = 183) %	Salmeterol 50 mcg (N = 177) %	Placebo (N = 185) %
Ear, nose, & throat				
Candidiasis mouth/throat	10	6	3	1
Throat irritation	8	5	4	7
Hoarseness/dysphonia	5	3	<1	0
Sinusitis	3	8	5	3
Lower respiratory				
Viral respiratory infections	6	4	3	3
Neurology				
Headaches	16	11	10	12
Dizziness	4	<1	3	2
Non-site specific				
Fever	4	3	0	3
Malaise & fatigue	3	2	2	3
Musculoskeletal				
Musculoskeletal pain	9	8	12	9
Muscle cramps & spasms	3	3	1	1
Average duration of exposure (days)	141.3	138.5	136.1	131.6

Table 6. Recommended Dosages of ADVAIR DISKUS for Patients With Asthma Aged 12 Years and Older Taking Inhaled Corticosteroids

Current **Daily Dose** of Inhaled Corticosteroid		Recommended Strength and Dosing Schedule of ADVAIR DISKUS
Beclomethasone dipropionate	≤420 mcg 462-840 mcg	100/50 twice daily 250/50 twice daily
Budesonide	≤400 mcg 800-1,200 mcg 1,600 mcg*	100/50 twice daily 250/50 twice daily 500/50 twice daily
Flunisolide	≤1,000 mcg 1,250-2,000 mcg	100/50 twice daily 250/50 twice daily
Fluticasone propionate inhalation aerosol	≤176 mcg 440 mcg 660-880 mcg*	100/50 twice daily 250/50 twice daily 500/50 twice daily
Fluticasone propionate inhalation powder	≤200 mcg 500 mcg 1,000 mcg*	100/50 twice daily 250/50 twice daily 500/50 twice daily
Triamcinolone acetonide	≤1,000 mcg 1,100-1,600 mcg	100/50 twice daily 250/50 twice daily

*ADVAIR DISKUS should not be used for transferring patients from systemic corticosteroid therapy.

DOSAGE AND ADMINISTRATION

ADVAIR DISKUS should be administered by the orally inhaled route only (see Patient's Instructions For Use). After inhalation, the patient should rinse the mouth with water without swallowing. ADVAIR DISKUS should not be used for transferring patients from systemic corticosteroid therapy.
Asthma: ADVAIR DISKUS is available in 3 strengths, ADVAIR DISKUS 100/50, ADVAIR DISKUS 250/50, and ADVAIR DISKUS 500/50, containing 100, 250, and 500 mcg of fluticasone propionate, respectively, and 50 mcg of salmeterol per inhalation.
ADVAIR DISKUS should be administered twice daily every day. More frequent administration (more than twice daily) or a higher number of inhalations (more than 1 inhalation twice daily) of the prescribed strength of ADVAIR DISKUS is not recommended as some patients are more likely to experience adverse effects with higher doses of salmeterol. The safety and efficacy of ADVAIR DISKUS when administered in excess of recommended doses have not been established.
If symptoms arise in the period between doses, an inhaled, short-acting beta$_2$-agonist should be taken for immediate relief.
Patients who are receiving ADVAIR DISKUS twice daily should not use additional salmeterol or other inhaled, long-acting beta$_2$-agonists (e.g., formoterol) for prevention of EIB, or for any other reason.
Adult and Adolescent Patients 12 Years of Age and Older: For patients 12 years of age and older, the dosage is 1 inhalation twice daily (morning and evening, approximately 12 hours apart).
The recommended starting dosages for ADVAIR DISKUS for patients 12 years of age and older are based upon patients' current asthma therapy.

- For patients who are not currently on an inhaled corticosteroid, whose disease severity warrants treatment with 2 maintenance therapies, including patients on non-corticosteroid maintenance therapy, the recommended starting dosage is ADVAIR DISKUS 100/50 twice daily.
- For patients on an inhaled corticosteroid, Table 6 provides the recommended starting dosage. The maximum recommended dosage is ADVAIR DISKUS 500/50 twice daily.

For all patients it is desirable to titrate to the lowest effective strength after adequate asthma stability is achieved.
[See table 6 above]
Improvement in asthma control following inhaled administration of ADVAIR DISKUS can occur within 30 minutes of beginning treatment, although maximum benefit may not be achieved for 1 week or longer after starting treatment. Individual patients will experience a variable time to onset and degree of symptom relief.
For patients who do not respond adequately to the starting dosage after 2 weeks of therapy, replacing the current strength of ADVAIR DISKUS with a higher strength may provide additional improvement in asthma control.
If a previously effective dosage regimen of ADVAIR DISKUS fails to provide adequate improvement in asthma control, the therapeutic regimen should be reevaluated and additional therapeutic options, e.g., replacing the current strength of ADVAIR DISKUS with a higher strength, adding additional inhaled corticosteroid, or initiating oral corticosteroids, should be considered.
Pediatric Patients: For patients aged 4 to 11 years who are symptomatic on an inhaled corticosteroid the dosage is 1 inhalation of ADVAIR DISKUS 100/50 twice daily (morning and evening, approximately 12 hours apart).
Chronic Obstructive Pulmonary Disease Associated With Chronic Bronchitis: The dosage for adults is 1 inhalation (250/50 mcg) twice daily (morning and evening, approximately 12 hours apart).
ADVAIR DISKUS 250/50 mcg twice daily is the only approved dosage for the treatment of COPD associated with

Continued on next page

Product information on these pages is effective as of August 2004. Further information is available at: GlaxoSmithKline, PO Box 13398, Research Triangle Park, NC 27709. 1-888-825-5249. Corporate Web Site: www.gsk.com

Advair Diskus—Cont.

chronic bronchitis. Higher doses, including ADVAIR DISKUS 500/50, are not recommended, as no additional improvement in lung function was observed in clinical trials and higher doses of corticosteroids increase the risk of systemic effects.

If shortness of breath occurs in the period between doses, an inhaled, short-acting beta$_2$-agonist should be taken for immediate relief.

Patients who are receiving ADVAIR DISKUS twice daily should not use additional salmeterol or other inhaled, long-acting beta$_2$-agonist (e.g., formoterol) for the maintenance treatment of COPD or for any other reason.

Geriatric Use: In studies where geriatric patients (65 years of age or older, see PRECAUTIONS: Geriatric Use) have been treated with ADVAIR DISKUS, efficacy and safety did not differ from that in younger patients. Based on available data for ADVAIR DISKUS and its active components, no dosage adjustment is recommended.

Directions for Use: Illustrated Patient's Instructions for Use accompany each package of ADVAIR DISKUS.

HOW SUPPLIED

ADVAIR DISKUS 100/50 is supplied as a disposable, purple device containing 60 blisters. The DISKUS inhalation device is packaged within a purple, plastic-coated, moisture-protective foil pouch (NDC 0173-0695-00). ADVAIR DISKUS 100/50 is also supplied in an institutional pack of 1 purple, disposable DISKUS inhalation device containing 28 blisters. The DISKUS inhalation device is packaged within a purple, plastic-coated, moisture-protective foil pouch (NDC 0173-0695-02).

ADVAIR DISKUS 250/50 is supplied as a disposable, purple device containing 60 blisters. The DISKUS inhalation device is packaged within a purple, plastic-coated, moisture-protective foil pouch (NDC 0173-0696-00). ADVAIR DISKUS 250/50 is also supplied in an institutional pack of 1 purple, disposable DISKUS inhalation device containing 28 blisters. The DISKUS inhalation device is packaged within a purple, plastic-coated, moisture-protective foil pouch (NDC 0173-0696-02).

ADVAIR DISKUS 500/50 is supplied as a disposable, purple device containing 60 blisters. The DISKUS inhalation device is packaged within a purple, plastic-coated, moisture-protective foil pouch (NDC 0173-0697-00). ADVAIR DISKUS 500/50 is also supplied in an institutional pack of 1 purple, disposable DISKUS inhalation device containing 28 blisters. The DISKUS inhalation device is packaged within a purple, plastic-coated, moisture-protective foil pouch (NDC 0173-0697-02).

Store at controlled room temperature (see USP), 20° to 25°C (68° to 77°F), in a dry place away from direct heat or sunlight. Keep out of reach of children. The DISKUS inhalation device is not reusable. The device should be discarded 1 month after removal from the moisture-protective foil overwrap pouch or after all blisters have been used (when the dose indicator reads "0"), whichever comes first. Do not attempt to take the device apart.

GlaxoSmithKline, Research Triangle Park, NC 27709

April 2004/RL-2085

Shown in Product Identification Guide, page 314

AGENERASE® ℞

[a-jin' ə-rās]

(amprenavir)

Capsules

> Because of the potential risk of toxicity from the large amount of the excipient, propylene glycol, contained in **AGENERASE Oral Solution**, that formulation is contraindicated in infants and children below the age of 4 years and certain other patient populations and should be used with caution in others. Consult the complete prescribing information for **AGENERASE Oral Solution** for full information.

DESCRIPTION

AGENERASE (amprenavir) is an inhibitor of the human immunodeficiency virus (HIV) protease. The chemical name of amprenavir is (3*S*)-tetrahydro-3-furyl *N*-[(1*S*,2*R*)-3-(4-amino-*N*-isobutylbenzenesulfonamido)-1-benzyl-2-hydroxypropyl]carbamate. Amprenavir is a single stereoisomer with the (3*S*)(1*S*,2*R*) configuration. It has a molecular formula of $C_{25}H_{35}N_3O_6S$ and a molecular weight of 505.64. Amprenavir is a white to cream-colored solid with a solubility of approximately 0.04 mg/mL in water at 25°C.

AGENERASE Capsules are available for oral administration in strengths of 50 and 150 mg. Each 50-mg capsule contains the inactive ingredients d-alpha tocopheryl polyethylene glycol 1000 succinate (TPGS), polyethylene glycol 400 (PEG 400) 246.7 mg, and propylene glycol 19 mg. Each 150-mg capsule contains the inactive ingredients TPGS, PEG 400 740 mg, and propylene glycol 57 mg. The capsule shell contains the inactive ingredients d-sorbitol and sorbitans solution, gelatin, glycerin, and titanium dioxide. The soft gelatin capsules are printed with edible red ink. Each 150-mg

Table 1. Average (%CV) Pharmacokinetic Parameters After 1,200 mg Twice Daily of Amprenavir Capsules (n = 54)

C_{max} (mcg/mL)	T_{max} (hours)	AUC_{0-12} (mcg•hr/mL)	C_{avg} (mcg/mL)	C_{min} (mcg/mL)	CL/F (mL/min/kg)
7.66 (54%)	1.0 (42%)	17.7 (47%)	1.48 (47%)	0.32 (77%)	19.5 (46%)

Table 2. Average (%CV) Pharmacokinetic Parameters in Children Ages 4 to 12 Years Receiving 20 mg/kg Twice Daily or 15 mg/kg Three Times Daily of AGENERASE Oral Solution

Dose	n	C_{max} (mcg/mL)	T_{max} (hours)	AUC_{ss}* (mcg•hr/mL)	C_{avg} (mcg/mL)	C_{min} (mcg/mL)	CL/F (mL/min/kg)
20 mg/kg b.i.d.	20	6.77 (51%)	1.1 (21%)	15.46 (59%)	1.29 (59%)	0.24 (98%)	29 (58%)
15 mg/kg t.i.d.	17	3.99 (37%)	1.4 (90%)	8.73 (36%)	1.09 (36%)	0.27 (95%)	32 (34%)

*AUC is 0 to 12 hours for b.i.d. and 0 to 8 hours for t.i.d., therefore the C_{avg} is a better comparison of the exposures.

Table 3. Drug Interactions: Pharmacokinetic Parameters for Amprenavir in the Presence of the Coadministered Drug

Coadministered Drug	Dose of Coadministered Drug	Dose of AGENERASE	n	% Change in **Amprenavir** Pharmacokinetic Parameters* (90% CI)		
				C_{max}	AUC	C_{min}
Abacavir	300 mg b.i.d. for 3 weeks	900 mg b.i.d. for 3 weeks	4	↑47 (↓15 to ↑154)	↑29 (↓18 to ↑103)	↑27 (↓46 to ↑197)
Clarithromycin	500 mg b.i.d. for 4 days	1,200 mg b.i.d. for 4 days	12	↑15 (↑1 to ↑31)	↑18 (↑8 to ↑29)	↑39 (↑31 to ↑47)
Delavirdine	600 mg b.i.d. for 10 days	600 mg b.i.d. for 10 days	9	↑40‡	↑130‡	↑125‡
Ethinyl estradiol/ Norethindrone	0.035 mg/1 mg for 1 cycle	1,200 mg b.i.d. for 28 days	10	⇔ (↓20 to ↑3)	↓22 (↓35 to ↓8)	↓20 (↓41 to ↑8)
Indinavir	800 mg t.i.d. for 2 weeks (fasted)	750 or 800 mg t.i.d. for 2 weeks (fasted)	9	↑18 (↓13 to ↑58)	↑33 (↑2 to ↑73)	↑25 (↓27 to ↑116)
Ketoconazole	400 mg single dose	1,200 mg single dose	12	↓16 (↓25 to ↓6)	↑31 (↑20 to ↑42)	NA
Lamivudine	150 mg single dose	600 mg single dose	11	⇔ (↓17 to ↑9)	⇔ (↓15 to ↑14)	NA
Nelfinavir	750 mg t.i.d. for 2 weeks (fed)	750 or 800 mg t.i.d. for 2 weeks (fed)	6	↓14 (↓38 to ↑20)	⇔ (↓19 to ↑47)	↑189 (↑52 to ↑448)
Rifabutin	300 mg q.d. for 10 days	1,200 mg b.i.d. for 10 days	5	⇔ (↓21 to ↑10)	↓15 (↓28 to 0)	↓15 (↓38 to ↑17)
Rifampin	300 mg q.d. for 4 days	1,200 mg b.i.d. for 4 days	11	↓70 (↓76 to ↓62)	↓82 (↓84 to ↓78)	↓92 (↓95 to ↓89)
Ritonavir	100 mg b.i.d. for 2 to 4 weeks	600 mg b.i.d.	18	↓30† (↓44 to ↓14)	↑64† (↑37 to ↑97)	↑508† (↑394 to ↑649)
Ritonavir	200 mg q.d. for 2 to 4 weeks	1,200 mg q.d.	12	⇔† (↓17 to ↑30)	↑62† (↑35 to ↑94)	↑319† (↑190 to ↑508)
Saquinavir	800 mg t.i.d. for 2 weeks (fed)	750 or 800 mg t.i.d. for 2 weeks (fed)	7	↓37 (↓54 to ↓14)	↓32 (↓49 to ↓9)	↓14 (↓52 to ↑54)
Zidovudine	300 mg single dose	600 mg single dose	12	⇔ (↓5 to ↑24)	↑13 (↓2 to ↑31)	NA

*Based on total-drug concentrations.
†Compared to amprenavir 1,200 mg b.i.d. in the same patients.
‡Median percent change; confidence interval not reported.
↑ = Increase; ↓ = Decrease; ⇔ = No change (↑ or ↓ <10%); NA = C_{min} not calculated for single-dose study.

AGENERASE Capsule contains 109 IU vitamin E in the form of TPGS. The total amount of vitamin E in the recommended daily adult dose of AGENERASE is 1744 IU.

MICROBIOLOGY

Mechanism of Action: Amprenavir is an inhibitor of HIV-1 protease. Amprenavir binds to the active site of HIV-1 protease and thereby prevents the processing of viral gag and gag-pol polyprotein precursors, resulting in the formation of immature non-infectious viral particles.

Antiviral Activity in Vitro: The in vitro antiviral activity of amprenavir was evaluated against HIV-1 IIIB in both acutely and chronically infected lymphoblastic cell lines (MT-4, CEM-CCRF, H9) and in peripheral blood lymphocytes. The 50% inhibitory concentration (IC_{50}) of amprenavir ranged from 0.012 to 0.08 µM in acutely infected cells and was 0.41 µM in chronically infected cells (1 µM = 0.50 mcg/mL). Amprenavir exhibited synergistic anti-HIV-1 activity in combination with abacavir, zidovudine, didanosine, or saquinavir, and additive anti-HIV-1 activity in combination with indinavir, nelfinavir, and ritonavir in vitro. These drug combinations have not been adequately studied in humans. The relationship between in vitro anti-HIV-1 activity of amprenavir and the inhibition of HIV-1 replication in humans has not been defined.

Resistance: HIV-1 isolates with a decreased susceptibility to amprenavir have been selected in vitro and obtained from patients treated with amprenavir. Genotypic analysis of isolates from amprenavir-treated patients showed mutations in the HIV-1 protease gene resulting in amino acid substitutions primarily at positions V32I, M46I/L, I47V, I50V, I54L/M, and I84V as well as mutations in the p7/p1 and p1/p6 gag cleavage sites. Phenotypic analysis of HIV-1 isolates from 21 nucleoside reverse transcriptase inhibitor-(NRTI-) experienced, protease inhibitor-naive patients treated with amprenavir in combination with NRTIs for 16 to 48 weeks identified isolates from 15 patients who exhibited a 4- to 17-fold decrease in susceptibility to amprenavir in vitro compared to wild-type virus. Clinical isolates that exhibited a decrease in amprenavir susceptibility harbored one or more amprenavir-associated mutations. The clinical relevance of the genotypic and phenotypic changes associated with amprenavir therapy is under evaluation.

Cross-Resistance: Varying degrees of HIV-1 cross-resistance among protease inhibitors have been observed.

Five of 15 amprenavir-resistant isolates exhibited 4- to 8-fold decrease in susceptibility to ritonavir. However, amprenavir-resistant isolates were susceptible to either indinavir or saquinavir.

CLINICAL PHARMACOLOGY

Pharmacokinetics in Adults: The pharmacokinetic properties of amprenavir have been studied in asymptomatic, HIV-infected adult patients after administration of single oral doses of 150 to 1,200 mg and multiple oral doses of 300 to 1,200 mg twice daily.

Absorption and Bioavailability: Amprenavir was rapidly absorbed after oral administration in HIV-1-infected patients with a time to peak concentration (T_{max}) typically between 1 and 2 hours after a single oral dose. The absolute oral bioavailability of amprenavir in humans has not been established.

Increases in the area under the plasma concentration versus time curve (AUC) after single oral doses between 150 and 1,200 mg were slightly greater than dose proportional. Increases in AUC were dose proportional after 3 weeks of dosing with doses from 300 to 1,200 mg twice daily. The pharmacokinetic parameters after administration of amprenavir 1,200 mg twice daily for 3 weeks to HIV-infected subjects are shown in Table 1.

[See table 1 at top of previous page]

The relative bioavailability of AGENERASE Capsules and Oral Solution was assessed in healthy adults. AGENERASE Oral Solution was 14% less bioavailable compared to the capsules.

Effects of Food on Oral Absorption: The relative bioavailability of AGENERASE Capsules was assessed in the fasting and fed states in healthy volunteers (standardized high-fat meal: 967 kcal, 67 grams fat, 33 grams protein, 58 grams carbohydrate). Administration of a single 1,200-mg dose of amprenavir in the fed state compared to the fasted state was associated with changes in C_{max} (fed: 6.18 ± 2.92 mcg/mL, fasted: 9.72 ± 2.75 mcg/mL), T_{max} (fed: 1.51 ± 0.68, fasted: 1.05 ± 0.63), and $AUC_{0-\infty}$ (fed: 22.06 ± 11.6 mcg•hr/mL, fasted: 28.05 ± 10.1 mcg•hr/mL). AGENERASE may be taken with or without food, but should not be taken with a high-fat meal (see DOSAGE AND ADMINISTRATION).

Distribution: The apparent volume of distribution (V_z/F) is approximately 430 L in healthy adult subjects. In vitro binding is approximately 90% to plasma proteins. The high affinity binding protein for amprenavir is alpha$_1$-acid glycoprotein (AAG). The partitioning of amprenavir into erythrocytes is low, but increases as amprenavir concentrations increase, reflecting the higher amount of unbound drug at higher concentrations.

Metabolism: Amprenavir is metabolized in the liver by the cytochrome P450 3A4 (CYP3A4) enzyme system. The 2 major metabolites result from oxidation of the tetrahydrofuran and aniline moieties. Glucuronide conjugates of oxidized metabolites have been identified as minor metabolites in urine and feces.

Elimination: Excretion of unchanged amprenavir in urine and feces is minimal. Approximately 14% and 75% of an administered single dose of ^{14}C-amprenavir can be accounted for as radiocarbon in urine and feces, respectively. Two metabolites accounted for >90% of the radiocarbon in fecal samples. The plasma elimination half-life of amprenavir ranged from 7.1 to 10.6 hours.

Special Populations: *Hepatic Insufficiency:* AGENERASE has been studied in adult patients with impaired hepatic function using a single 600-mg oral dose. The $AUC_{0-\infty}$ was significantly greater in patients with moderate cirrhosis (25.76 ± 14.68 mcg•hr/mL) compared with healthy volunteers (12.00 ± 4.38 mcg•hr/mL). The $AUC_{0-\infty}$ and C_{max} were significantly greater in patients with severe cirrhosis ($AUC_{0-\infty}$: 38.66 ± 16.08 mcg•hr/mL; C_{max}: 9.43 ± 2.61 mcg/mL) compared with healthy volunteers ($AUC_{0-\infty}$: 12.00 ± 4.38 mcg•hr/mL; C_{max}: 4.90 ± 1.39 mcg/mL). Patients with impaired hepatic function require dosage adjustment (see DOSAGE AND ADMINISTRATION).

Renal Insufficiency: The impact of renal impairment on amprenavir elimination in adult patients has not been studied. The renal elimination of unchanged amprenavir represents <3% of the administered dose.

Pediatric Patients: The pharmacokinetics of amprenavir have been studied after either single or repeat doses of AGENERASE Capsules or Oral Solution in 84 pediatric patients. Twenty HIV-1-infected children ranging in age from 4 to 12 years received single doses from 5 mg/kg to 20 mg/kg using 25-mg or 150-mg capsules. The C_{max} of amprenavir increased less than proportionally with dose. The $AUC_{0-\infty}$ increased proportionally at doses between 5 and 20 mg/kg. Amprenavir is 14% less bioavailable from the liquid formulation than from the capsules; therefore **AGENERASE Capsules and AGENERASE Oral Solution are not interchangeable on a milligram-per-milligram basis.**

AGENERASE Oral Solution is contraindicated in infants and children below the age of 4 years due to the potential risk of toxicity from the large amount of the excipient, propylene glycol. Please see the complete prescribing information for AGENERASE Oral Solution for full information.

[See table 2 at top of previous page]

Geriatric Patients: The pharmacokinetics of amprenavir have not been studied in patients over 65 years of age.

Gender: The pharmacokinetics of amprenavir do not differ between males and females.

Race: The pharmacokinetics of amprenavir do not differ between blacks and non-blacks.

Table 4. Drug Interactions: Pharmacokinetic Parameters for Coadministered Drug in the Presence of Amprenavir

Coadministered Drug	Dose of Coadministered Drug	Dose of AGENERASE	n	% Change in Pharmacokinetic Parameters of **Coadministered Drug** (90% CI) C_{max}	AUC	C_{min}
Clarithromycin	500 mg b.i.d. for 4 days	1,200 mg b.i.d. for 4 days	12	↓10 (↓24 to ↑7)	⇔ (↓17 to ↑11)	⇔ (↓13 to ↑20)
Delavirdine	600 mg b.i.d. for 10 days	600 mg b.i.d. for 10 days	9	↓47*	↓61*	↓88*
Ethinyl estradiol	0.035 mg for 1 cycle	1,200 mg b.i.d. for 28 days	10	⇔ (↓25 to ↑15)	⇔ (↓14 to ↑38)	↑32 (↓3 to ↑79)
Norethindrone	1.0 mg for 1 cycle	1,200 mg b.i.d. for 28 days	10	⇔ (↓20 to ↑18)	↑18 (↑1 to ↑38)	↑45 (↑13 to ↑88)
Ketoconazole	400 mg single dose	1,200 mg single dose	12	↑19 (↑8 to ↑33)	↑44 (↑31 to ↑59)	NA
Lamivudine	150 mg single dose	600 mg single dose	11	⇔ (↓17 to ↑3)	⇔ (↓11 to 0)	NA
Methadone	44 to 100 mg q.d. for >30 days	1,200 mg b.i.d. for 10 days	16	R-Methadone (active)		
				↓25 (↓32 to ↓18)	↓13 (↓21 to ↓5)	↓21 (↓32 to ↓9)
				S-Methadone (inactive)		
				↓48 (↓55 to ↓40)	↓40 (↓46 to ↓32)	↓53 (↓60 to ↓43)
Rifabutin	300 mg q.d. for 10 days	1,200 mg b.i.d. for 10 days	5	↑119 (↑82 to ↑164)	↑193 (↑156 to ↑235)	↑271 (↑171 to ↑409)
Rifampin	300 mg q.d. for 4 days	1,200 mg b.i.d. for 4 days	11	⇔ (↓13 to ↑12)	⇔ (↓10 to ↑13)	ND
Zidovudine	300 mg single dose	600 mg single dose	12	↑40 (↑14 to ↑71)	↑31 (↑19 to ↑45)	NA

*Median percent change; confidence interval not reported.
↑ = Increase; ↓ = Decrease; ⇔ = No change (↑ or ↓ <10%); NA = C_{min} not calculated for single-dose study; ND = Interaction cannot be determined as C_{min} was below the lower limit of quantitation.

Table 5. Outcomes of Randomized Treatment Through Week 48 (PROAB3006)

Outcome	AGENERASE (n = 254)	Indinavir (n = 250)
HIV-1 RNA <400 copies/mL*	30%	49%
HIV-1 RNA ≥400 copies/mL†,‡	38%	26%
Discontinued due to adverse events*,‡	16%	12%
Discontinued due to other reasons‡,§	16%	13%

*Corresponds to rates at Week 48 in Figure 1.
†Virological failures at or before Week 48.
‡Considered to be treatment failure in the analysis.
§Includes discontinuations due to consent withdrawn, loss to follow-up, protocol violations, non-compliance, pregnancy, never treated, and other reasons.

Table 6. Drugs That Are Contraindicated with AGENERASE

Drug Class	Drugs Within Class That Are CONTRAINDICATED with AGENERASE
Ergot derivatives	Dihydroergotamine, ergonovine, ergotamine, methylergonovine
GI motility agent	Cisapride
Neuroleptic	Pimozide
Sedatives/hypnotics	Midazolam, triazolam

Drug Interactions: See also CONTRAINDICATIONS, WARNINGS, and PRECAUTIONS: Drug Interactions.

Amprenavir is metabolized in the liver by the cytochrome P450 enzyme system. Amprenavir inhibits CYP3A4. Caution should be used when coadministering medications that are substrates, inhibitors, or inducers of CYP3A4, or potentially toxic medications that are metabolized by CYP3A4. Amprenavir does not inhibit CYP2D6, CYP1A2, CYP2C9, CYP2C19, CYP2E1, or uridine glucuronosyltransferase (UDPGT).

Drug interaction studies were performed with amprenavir capsules and other drugs likely to be coadministered or drugs commonly used as probes for pharmacokinetic interactions. The effects of coadministration of amprenavir on the AUC, C_{max}, and C_{min} are summarized in Table 3 (effect of other drugs on amprenavir) and Table 4 (effect of amprenavir on other drugs). For information regarding clinical recommendations, see PRECAUTIONS.

[See table 3 on previous page]

[See table 4 above]

Nucleoside Reverse Transcriptase Inhibitors (NRTIs): There was no effect of amprenavir on abacavir in subjects receiving both agents based on historical data.

HIV Protease Inhibitors: The effect of amprenavir on total drug concentrations of other HIV protease inhibitors in subjects receiving both agents was evaluated using comparisons to historical data. Indinavir steady-state C_{max}, AUC, and C_{min} were decreased by 22%, 38%, and 27%, respectively, by concomitant amprenavir. Similar decreases in C_{max} and AUC were seen after the first dose. Saquinavir steady-state C_{max}, AUC, and C_{min} were increased 21%, decreased 19%, and decreased 48%, respectively, by concomitant amprenavir. Nelfinavir steady-state C_{max}, AUC, and C_{min} were increased by 12%, 15%, and 14%, respectively, by concomitant amprenavir.

Methadone: Coadministration of amprenavir and methadone can decrease plasma levels of methadone.

Continued on next page

Product information on these pages is effective as of August 2004. Further information is available at: GlaxoSmithKline, PO Box 13398, Research Triangle Park, NC 27709. 1-888-825-5249. Corporate Web Site: www.gsk.com

Agenerase Capsules—Cont.

Coadministration of amprenavir and methadone as compared to a non-matched historical control group resulted in a 30%, 27%, and 25% decrease in serum amprenavir AUC, C_{max}, and C_{min}, respectively.
For information regarding clinical recommendations, see PRECAUTIONS: Drug Interactions.

INDICATIONS AND USAGE

AGENERASE (amprenavir) is indicated in combination with other antiretroviral agents for the treatment of HIV-1 infection.
The following points should be considered when initiating therapy with AGENERASE:
In a study of NRTI-experienced, protease inhibitor-naive patients, AGENERASE was found to be significantly less effective than indinavir (see Description of Clinical Studies).
Mild to moderate gastrointestinal adverse events led to discontinuation of AGENERASE primarily during the first 12 weeks of therapy (see ADVERSE REACTIONS).
There are no data on response to therapy with AGENERASE in protease inhibitor-experienced patients.
Description of Clinical Studies: ***Therapy-Naive Adults:*** PROAB3001, a randomized, double-blind, placebo-controlled, multicenter study, compared treatment with AGENERASE Capsules (1,200 mg twice daily) plus lamivudine (150 mg twice daily) plus zidovudine (300 mg twice daily) versus lamivudine (150 mg twice daily) plus zidovudine (300 mg twice daily) in 232 patients. Through 24 weeks of therapy, 53% of patients assigned to AGENERASE/zidovudine/lamivudine achieved HIV-1 RNA <400 copies/mL. Through week 48, the antiviral response was 41%. Through 24 weeks of therapy, 11% of patients assigned to zidovudine/lamivudine achieved HIV-1 RNA <400 copies/mL. Antiviral response beyond week 24 is not interpretable because the majority of patients discontinued or changed their antiretroviral therapy.
NRTI-Experienced Adults: PROAB3006, a randomized, open-label multicenter study, compared treatment with AGENERASE Capsules (1,200 mg twice daily) plus NRTIs versus indinavir (800 mg every 8 hours) plus NRTIs in 504 NRTI-experienced, protease inhibitor-naive patients, median age 37 years (range 20 to 71 years), 72% Caucasian, 80% male, with a median CD4 cell count of 404 cells/mm^3 (range 9 to 1,706 cells/mm^3) and a median plasma HIV-1 RNA level of 3.93 $\log_{10}$ copies/mL (range 2.60 to 7.01 $\log_{10}$ copies/mL) at baseline. Through 48 weeks of therapy, the median CD4 cell count increase from baseline in the amprenavir group was significantly lower than in the indinavir group, 97 cells/mm^3 versus 144 cells/mm^3, respectively. There was also a significant difference in the proportions of patients with plasma HIV-1 RNA levels <400 copies/mL through 48 weeks (see Figure 1 and Table 5).

Figure 1. Virologic Response Through Week 48, PROAB3006*,†

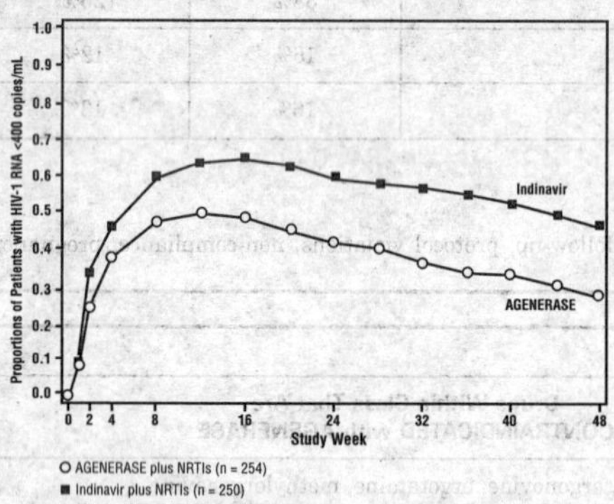

○ AGENERASE plus NRTIs (n = 254)
■ Indinavir plus NRTIs (n = 250)
*Roche AMPLICOR HIV-1 MONITOR assay.
†Discontinuations and missing data were considered as HIV-1 RNA ≥400 copies/mL.

HIV-1 RNA status and reasons for discontinuation of randomized treatment at 48 weeks are summarized (Table 5).
[See table 5 on previous page]

CONTRAINDICATIONS

Coadministration of AGENERASE is contraindicated with drugs that are highly dependent on CYP3A4 for clearance and for which elevated plasma concentrations are associated with serious and/or life-threatening events. These drugs are listed in Table 6.
[See table 6 on previous page]
If AGENERASE is coadministered with ritonavir, the antiarrhythmic agents flecainide and propafenone are also contraindicated.
Because of the potential toxicity from the large amount of the excipient, propylene glycol, contained in **AGENERASE Oral Solution**, that formulation is contraindicated in certain patient populations and should be used with caution in others. Consult the complete prescribing information for **AGENERASE Oral Solution** for full information.
AGENERASE is contraindicated in patients with previously demonstrated clinically significant hypersensitivity to any of the components of this product.

WARNINGS

ALERT: Find out about medicines that should not be taken with AGENERASE.
Serious and/or life-threatening drug interactions could occur between amprenavir and amiodarone, lidocaine (systemic), tricyclic antidepressants, and quinidine. Concentration monitoring of these agents is recommended if these agents are used concomitantly with AGENERASE (see CONTRAINDICATIONS).

Table 7. Drugs That Should Not Be Coadministered with AGENERASE

Drug Class/Drug Name	Clinical Comment
Antimycobacterials: Rifampin*	May lead to loss of virologic response and possible resistance to AGENERASE or to the class of protease inhibitors.
Ergot Derivatives: Dihydroergotamine, ergonovine, ergotamine, methylergonovine	**CONTRAINDICATED** due to potential for serious and/or life-threatening reactions such as acute ergot toxicity characterized by peripheral vasospasm and ischemia of the extremities and other tissues.
GI Motility Agents: Cisapride	**CONTRAINDICATED** due to potential for serious and/or life-threatening reactions such as cardiac arrhythmias.
Herbal Products: St. John's wort (hypericum perforatum)	May lead to loss of virologic response and possible resistance to AGENERASE or to the class of protease inhibitors.
HMG Co-Reductase Inhibitors: Lovastatin, simvastatin	Potential for serious reactions such as risk of myopathy including rhabdomyolysis.
Neuroleptic: Pimozide	**CONTRAINDICATED** due to potential for serious and/or life-threatening reactions such as cardiac arrhythmias.
Non-nucleoside Reverse Transcriptase Inhibitor: Delavirdine*	May lead to loss of virologic response and possible resistance to delavirdine.
Oral Contraceptives: Ethinyl estradiol/norethindrone	May lead to loss of virologic response and possible resistance to AGENERASE. Alternative methods of non-hormonal contraception are recommended.
Sedatives/Hypnotics: Midazolam, triazolam	**CONTRAINDICATED** due to potential for serious and/or life-threatening reactions such as prolonged or increased sedation or respiratory depression.

*See CLINICAL PHARMACOLOGY for magnitude of interaction, Tables 3 and 4.

Table 8. Established and Other Potentially Significant Drug Interactions: Alteration in Dose or Regimen May Be Recommended Based on Drug Interaction Studies or Predicted Interaction

Concomitant Drug Class: Drug Name	Effect on Concentration of Amprenavir or Concomitant Drug	Clinical Comment
	HIV-Antiviral Agents	
Non-nucleoside Reverse Transcriptase Inhibitors: Efavirenz, nevirapine	↓ Amprenavir	Appropriate doses of the combinations with respect to safety and efficacy have not been established.
Nucleoside Reverse Transcriptase Inhibitor: Didanosine (buffered formulation only)	↓ Amprenavir	Take AGENERASE at least 1 hour before or after the buffered formulation of didanosine.
HIV-Protease Inhibitors: Indinavir*, lopinavir/ritonavir, nelfinavir*	↑ Amprenavir Amprenavir's effect on other protease inhibitors is not well established.	Appropriate doses of the combinations with respect to safety and efficacy have not been established.
HIV-Protease Inhibitor: Ritonavir*	↑ Amprenavir	The dose of amprenavir should be reduced when used in combination with ritonavir (see Dosage and Administration). Also, see the full prescribing information for NORVIR for additional drug interaction information.
HIV-Protease Inhibitor: Saquinavir*	↓ Amprenavir Amprenavir's effect on saquinavir is not well established.	Appropriate doses of the combination with respect to safety and efficacy have not been established.

(Table continued on next page)

Rifampin should not be used in combination with amprenavir because it reduces plasma concentrations and AUC of amprenavir by about 90%.
Concomitant use of AGENERASE and St. John's wort (hypericum perforatum) or products containing St. John's wort is not recommended. Coadministration of protease inhibitors, including AGENERASE, with St. John's wort is expected to substantially decrease protease inhibitor concentrations and may result in suboptimal levels of amprenavir and lead to loss of virologic response and possible resistance to AGENERASE or to the class of protease inhibitors.
Concomitant use of AGENERASE with lovastatin or simvastatin is not recommended. Caution should be exercised if HIV protease inhibitors, including AGENERASE, are used concurrently with other HMG-CoA reductase inhibitors that are also metabolized by the CYP3A4 pathway (e.g., atorvastatin). The risk of myopathy, including rhabdomyolysis, may be increased when HIV protease inhibitors, including amprenavir, are used in combination with these drugs.
Particular caution should be used when prescribing sildenafil in patients receiving amprenavir. Coadministration of AGENERASE with sildenafil is expected to substantially increase sildenafil concentrations and may result in an increase in sildenafil-associated adverse events, including hypotension, visual changes, and priapism (see PRECAUTIONS: Drug Interactions and Information for Patients, and the complete prescribing information for sildenafil).
Because of the potential toxicity from the large amount of the excipient, propylene glycol, contained in **AGENERASE Oral Solution**, that formulation is contraindicated in certain patient populations and should be used with caution in others. Consult the complete prescribing information for **AGENERASE Oral Solution** for full information.
Severe and life-threatening skin reactions, including Stevens-Johnson syndrome, have occurred in patients treated with AGENERASE (see ADVERSE REACTIONS).
Acute hemolytic anemia has been reported in a patient treated with AGENERASE.
New onset diabetes mellitus, exacerbation of pre-existing diabetes mellitus, and hyperglycemia have been reported during post-marketing surveillance in HIV-infected patients receiving protease inhibitor therapy. Some patients required either initiation or dose adjustments of insulin or oral hypoglycemic agents for treatment of these events. In some cases, diabetic ketoacidosis has occurred. In those patients who discontinued protease inhibitor therapy, hyperglycemia persisted in some cases. Because these events have been reported voluntarily during clinical practice, estimates of frequency cannot be made and causal relationships between protease inhibitor therapy and these events have not been established.

PRECAUTIONS

General: AGENERASE Capsules and AGENERASE Oral Solution are not interchangeable on a milligram-per-milligram basis (see CLINICAL PHARMACOLOGY: Pediatric Patients).

Amprenavir is a sulfonamide. The potential for cross-sensitivity between drugs in the sulfonamide class and amprenavir is unknown. AGENERASE should be used with caution in patients with a known sulfonamide allergy.

AGENERASE is principally metabolized by the liver. AGENERASE, when used alone and in combination with low-dose ritonavir, has been associated with elevations of SGOT (AST) and SGPT (ALT) in some patients. Caution should be exercised when administering AGENERASE to patients with hepatic impairment (see DOSAGE AND ADMINISTRATION). Appropriate laboratory testing should be conducted prior to initiating therapy with AGENERASE and at periodic intervals during treatment.

Formulations of AGENERASE provide high daily doses of vitamin E (see Information for Patients, DESCRIPTION, and DOSAGE AND ADMINISTRATION). The effects of long-term, high-dose vitamin E administration in humans is not well characterized and has not been specifically studied in HIV-infected individuals. High vitamin E doses may exacerbate the blood coagulation defect of vitamin K deficiency caused by anticoagulant therapy or malabsorption.

Patients with Hemophilia: There have been reports of spontaneous bleeding in patients with hemophilia A and B treated with protease inhibitors. In some patients, additional factor VIII was required. In many of the reported cases, treatment with protease inhibitors was continued or restarted. A causal relationship between protease inhibitor therapy and these episodes has not been established.

Fat Redistribution: Redistribution/accumulation of body fat, including central obesity, dorsocervical fat enlargement (buffalo hump), peripheral wasting, facial wasting, breast enlargement, and "cushingoid appearance," have been observed in patients receiving antiretroviral therapy. The mechanism and long-term consequences of these events are currently unknown. A causal relationship has not been established.

Lipid Elevations: Treatment with AGENERASE alone or in combination with ritonavir has resulted in increases in the concentration of total cholesterol and triglycerides. Triglyceride and cholesterol testing should be performed prior to initiation of therapy with AGENERASE and at periodic intervals during treatment. Lipid disorders should be managed as clinically appropriate. See PRECAUTIONS Table 8: Established and Other Potentially Significant Drug Interactions for additional information on potential drug interactions with AGENERASE and HMG-CoA reductase inhibitors.

Resistance/Cross-Resistance: Because the potential for HIV cross-resistance among protease inhibitors has not been fully explored, it is unknown what effect amprenavir therapy will have on the activity of subsequently administered protease inhibitors. It is also unknown what effect previous treatment with other protease inhibitors will have on the activity of amprenavir (see MICROBIOLOGY).

Information for Patients: A statement to patients and healthcare providers is included on the product's bottle label: **ALERT: Find out about medicines that should NOT be taken with AGENERASE.** A Patient Package Insert (PPI) for AGENERASE Capsules is available for patient information.

Patients treated with AGENERASE Capsules should be cautioned against switching to **AGENERASE Oral Solution** because of the increased risk of adverse events from the large amount of propylene glycol in **AGENERASE Oral Solution**. Please see the complete prescribing information for **AGENERASE Oral Solution** for full information.

Patients should be informed that AGENERASE is not a cure for HIV infection and that they may continue to develop opportunistic infections and other complications associated with HIV disease. The long-term effects of AGENERASE (amprenavir) are unknown at this time. Patients should be told that there are currently no data demonstrating that therapy with AGENERASE can reduce the risk of transmitting HIV to others through sexual contact.

Patients should remain under the care of a physician while using AGENERASE. Patients should be advised to take AGENERASE every day as prescribed. AGENERASE must always be used in combination with other antiretroviral drugs. Patients should not alter the dose or discontinue therapy without consulting their physician. If a dose is missed, patients should take the dose as soon as possible and then return to their normal schedule. However, if a dose is skipped, the patient should not double the next dose.

Patients should inform their doctor if they have a sulfa allergy. The potential for cross-sensitivity between drugs in the sulfonamide class and amprenavir is unknown.

AGENERASE may interact with many drugs; therefore, patients should be advised to report to their doctor the use of any other prescription or nonprescription medication or herbal products, particularly St. John's wort.

Patients taking antacids (or the buffered formulation of didanosine) should take AGENERASE at least 1 hour before or after antacid (or the buffered formulation of didanosine) use.

Patients receiving sildenafil should be advised that they may be at an increased risk of sildenafil-associated adverse events, including hypotension, visual changes, and priapism, and should promptly report any symptoms to their doctor.

Table 8 *(cont.)*. Established and Other Potentially Significant Drug Interactions: Alteration in Dose or Regimen May Be Recommended Based on Drug Interaction Studies or Predicted Interaction

Concomitant Drug Class: Drug Name	Effect on Concentration of Amprenavir or Concomitant Drug	Clinical Comment
	Other Agents	
Antacids	↓ Amprenavir	Take AGENERASE at least 1 hour before or after antacids.
Antiarrhythmics: Amiodarone, lidocaine (systemic), and quinidine	↑ Antiarrhythmics	Caution is warranted and therapeutic concentration monitoring is recommended for antiarrhythmics when coadministered with AGENERASE, if available.
Antiarrhythmic: Bepridil	↑ Bepridil	Use with caution. Increased bepridil exposure may be associated with life-threatening reactions such as cardiac arrhythmias.
Anticoagulant: Warfarin		Concentrations of warfarin may be affected. It is recommended that INR (international normalized ratio) be monitored.
Anticonvulsants: Carbamazepine, phenobarbital, phenytoin	↓ Amprenavir	Use with caution. AGENERASE may be less effective due to decreased amprenavir plasma concentrations in patients taking these agents concomitantly.
Antifungals: Ketoconazole, itraconazole	↑ Ketoconazole ↑ Itraconazole	Increase monitoring for adverse events due to ketoconazole or itraconazole. Dose reduction of ketoconazole or itraconazole may be needed for patients receiving more than 400 mg ketoconazole or itraconazole per day.
Antimycobacterial: Rifabutin*	↑ Rifabutin and rifabutin metabolite	A dosage reduction of rifabutin to at least half the recommended dose is required when AGENERASE and rifabutin are coadministered.*A complete blood count should be performed weekly and as clinically indicated in order to monitor for neutropenia in patients receiving amprenavir and rifabutin.
Benzodiazepines: Alprazolam, clorazepate, diazepam, flurazepam	↑ Benzodiazepines	Clinical significance is unknown; however, a decrease in benzodiazepine dose may be needed.
Calcium Channel Blockers: Diltiazem, felodipine, nifedipine, nicardipine, nimodipine, verapamil, amlodipine, nisoldipine, isradipine	↑ Calcium channel blockers	Caution is warranted and clinical monitoring of patients is recommended.
Corticosteroid: Dexamethasone	↓ Amprenavir	Use with caution. AGENERASE may be less effective due to decreased amprenavir plasma concentrations in patients taking these agents concomitantly.
Erectile Dysfunction Agent: Sildenafil	↑ Sildenafil	Use with caution at reduced doses of 25 mg every 48 hours with increased monitoring for adverse events.
HMG-CoA Reductase Inhibitors: Atorvastatin	↑ Atorvastatin	Use lowest possible dose of atorvastatin with careful monitoring or consider other HMG-CoA reductase inhibitors such as pravastatin or fluvastatin in combination with AGENERASE.
Immunosuppressants: Cyclosporine, tacrolimus, rapamycin	↑ Immunosuppressants	Therapeutic concentration monitoring is recommended for immunosuppressant agents when coadministered with AGENERASE.
Narcotic Analgesics: Methadone*	↓ Amprenavir	AGENERASE may be less effective due to decreased amprenavir plasma concentrations in patients taking these agents concomitantly. Alternative antiretroviral therapy should be considered.
	↓ Methadone	Dosage of methadone may need to be increased when coadministered with AGENERASE.
Tricyclic Antidepressants: Amitriptyline, imipramine	↑ Tricyclics	Therapeutic concentration monitoring is recommended for tricyclic antidepressants when coadministered with AGENERASE.

*See CLINICAL PHARMACOLOGY for magnitude of interaction, Tables 3 and 4.

Patients taking AGENERASE should be instructed **not** to use hormonal contraceptives because some birth control pills (those containing ethinyl estradiol/norethindrone) have been found to decrease the concentration of amprenavir. Therefore, patients receiving hormonal contraceptives should be instructed to use alternate contraceptive measures during therapy with AGENERASE.

High-fat meals may decrease the absorption of AGENERASE and should be avoided. AGENERASE may be taken with meals of normal fat content.

Patients should be informed that redistribution or accumulation of body fat may occur in patients receiving antiretroviral therapy and that the cause and long-term health effects of these conditions are not known at this time.

Adult and pediatric patients should be advised not to take supplemental vitamin E since the vitamin E content of AGENERASE Capsules and Oral Solution exceeds the Reference Daily Intake (adults 30 IU, pediatrics approximately 10 IU).

Laboratory Tests: The combination of AGENERASE and low-dose ritonavir has been associated with elevations of cholesterol and triglycerides, SGOT (AST), and SGPT (ALT) in some patients. Appropriate laboratory testing should be considered prior to initiating combination therapy with AGENERASE and ritonavir and at periodic intervals or if any clinical signs or symptoms of hyperlipidemia or elevated liver function tests occur during therapy. For comprehensive information concerning laboratory test alterations associated with ritonavir, physicians should refer to the complete prescribing information for NORVIR® (ritonavir).

Drug Interactions: See also CONTRAINDICATIONS, WARNINGS, and CLINICAL PHARMACOLOGY: Drug Interactions.

Continued on next page

Product information on these pages is effective as of August 2004. Further information is available at: GlaxoSmithKline, PO Box 13398, Research Triangle Park, NC 27709. 1-888-825-5249. Corporate Web Site: www.gsk.com

Agenerase Capsules—Cont.

AGENERASE is an inhibitor of cytochrome P450 3A4 metabolism and therefore should not be administered concurrently with medications with narrow therapeutic windows that are substrates of CYP3A4. There are other agents that may result in serious and/or life-threatening drug interactions (see CONTRAINDICATIONS and WARNINGS).

[See table 7 at top of page 1398]
[See table 8 on pages 1398 and 1399]

Carcinogenesis and Mutagenesis: Amprenavir was evaluated for carcinogenic potential by oral gavage administration to mice and rats for up to 104 weeks. Daily doses of 50, 275 to 300, and 500 to 600 mg/kg/day were administered to mice and doses of 50, 190, and 750 mg/kg/day were administered to rats. Results showed an increase in the incidence of benign hepatocellular adenomas and an increase in the combined incidence of hepatocellular adenomas plus carcinoma in males of both species at the highest doses tested. Female mice and rats were not affected. These observations were made at systemic exposures equivalent to approximately 2 times (mice) and 4 times (rats) the human exposure (based on $AUC_{0-24\ hr}$ measurement) at the recommended dose of 1,200 mg twice daily. Administration of amprenavir did not cause a statistically significant increase in the incidence of any other benign or malignant neoplasm in mice or rats. It is not known how predictive the results of rodent carcinogenicity studies may be for humans. However, amprenavir was not mutagenic or genotoxic in a battery of in vitro and in vivo assays including bacterial reverse mutation (Ames), mouse lymphoma, rat micronucleus, and chromosome aberrations in human lymphocytes.

Fertility: The effects of amprenavir on fertility and general reproductive performance were investigated in male rats (treated for 28 days before mating at doses producing up to twice the expected clinical exposure based on AUC comparisons) and female rats (treated for 15 days before mating through day 17 of gestation at doses producing up to 2 times the expected clinical exposure). Amprenavir did not impair mating or fertility of male or female rats and did not affect the development and maturation of sperm from treated rats. The reproductive performance of the F1 generation born to female rats given amprenavir was not different from control animals.

Pregnancy and Reproduction: Pregnancy Category C. Embryo/fetal development studies were conducted in rats (dosed from 15 days before pairing to day 17 of gestation) and rabbits (dosed from day 8 to day 20 of gestation). In pregnant rabbits, amprenavir administration was associated with abortions and an increased incidence of 3 minor skeletal variations resulting from deficient ossification of the femur, humerus trochlea, and humerus. Systemic exposure at the highest tested dose was approximately one twentieth of the exposure seen at the recommended human dose. In rat fetuses, thymic elongation and incomplete ossification of bones were attributed to amprenavir. Both findings were seen at systemic exposures that were one half of that associated with the recommended human dose.

Pre- and post-natal developmental studies were performed in rats dosed from day 7 of gestation to day 22 of lactation. Reduced body weights (10% to 20%) were observed in the offspring. The systemic exposure associated with this finding was approximately twice the exposure in humans following administration of the recommended human dose. The subsequent development of these offspring, including fertility and reproductive performance, was not affected by the maternal administration of amprenavir.

There are no adequate and well-controlled studies in pregnant women. AGENERASE should be used during pregnancy only if the potential benefit justifies the potential risk to the fetus.

AGENERASE Oral Solution is contraindicated during pregnancy due to the potential risk of toxicity to the fetus from the high propylene glycol content.

Antiretroviral Pregnancy Registry: To monitor maternal-fetal outcomes of pregnant women exposed to AGENERASE, an Antiretroviral Pregnancy Registry has been established. Physicians are encouraged to register patients by calling 1-800-258-4263.

Nursing Mothers: The Centers for Disease Control and Prevention recommend that HIV-infected mothers not breastfeed their infants to avoid risking postnatal transmission of HIV. Although it is not known if amprenavir is excreted in human milk, amprenavir is secreted into the milk of lactating rats. Because of both the potential for HIV transmission and the potential for serious adverse reactions in nursing infants, **mothers should be instructed not to breastfeed if they are receiving AGENERASE.**

Pediatric Use: Two hundred fifty-one patients aged 4 and above have received amprenavir as single or multiple doses in studies. An adverse event profile similar to that seen in adults was seen in pediatric patients.

AGENERASE Capsules have not been evaluated in pediatric patients below the age of 4 years (see CLINICAL PHARMACOLOGY and DOSAGE AND ADMINISTRATION).

AGENERASE Oral Solution is contraindicated in infants and children below the age of 4 years due to the potential risk of toxicity from the large amount of the excipient, propylene glycol. Please see the complete prescribing information for **AGENERASE Oral Solution** for full information.

Geriatric Use: Clinical studies of AGENERASE did not include sufficient numbers of patients aged 65 and over to determine whether they respond differently from younger adults. In general, dose selection for an elderly patient should be cautious, reflecting the greater frequency of decreased hepatic, renal, or cardiac function, and of concomitant disease or other drug therapy.

Table 9. Selected Clinical Adverse Events of All Grades Reported in >5% of Adult Patients

Adverse Event	PROAB3001 Therapy-Naive Patients: AGENERASE/ Lamivudine/ Zidovudine (n = 113)	PROAB3001 Therapy-Naive Patients: Lamivudine/ Zidovudine (n = 109)	PROAB3006 NRTI-Experienced Patients: AGENERASE/ NRTI (n = 245)	PROAB3006 NRTI-Experienced Patients: Indinavir/NRTI (n = 241)
Digestive				
Nausea	74%	50%	43%	35%
Vomiting	34%	17%	24%	20%
Diarrhea or loose stools	39%	35%	60%	41%
Taste disorders	10%	6%	2%	8%
Skin				
Rash	27%	6%	20%	15%
Nervous				
Paresthesia, oral/perioral	26%	6%	31%	2%
Paresthesia, peripheral	10%	4%	14%	10%
Psychiatric				
Depressive or mood disorders	16%	4%	9%	13%

Table 10. Selected Clinical Adverse Events of All Grades Reported in Adult Patients in Open-Label Clinical Trials of AGENERASE in Combination with Ritonavir

Adverse Event	AGENERASE 1,200 mg plus Ritonavir 200 mg q.d.* (n = 101)	AGENERASE 600 mg plus Ritonavir 100 mg b.i.d.† (n = 239)
Nausea	31%	23%
Diarrhea/loose stools	30%	28%
Headache	16%	12%
Abdominal symptoms	14%	14%
Vomiting	11%	9%
Rash	10%	9%
Paresthesias	9%	11%
Fatigue	7%	14%
Depressive & mood disorders	4%	9%

*Data from 2 open-label studies in treatment-naive patients also receiving abacavir/lamivudine.
† Data from 3 open-label studies in treatment-naive and treatment-experienced patients receiving combination antiretroviral therapy.

Table 11. Grade 3/4 Laboratory Abnormalities Reported in ≥2% of Adult Patients in Open-Label Clinical Trials of AGENERASE in Combination with Ritonavir

Laboratory Abnormality (non-fasting specimens)	AGENERASE 1,200 mg plus Ritonavir 200 mg q.d.* (n = 101)	AGENERASE 600 mg plus Ritonavir 100 mg b.i.d.† (n = 239)
Hypertriglyceridemia (>750 mg/dL)	8%	13%
Hyperglycemia (>251 mg/dL)	2%	3%
AST (>5 × ULN)	3%	5%
AST (>5 × ULN)	4%	4%
Amylase (>2 × ULN)	4%	3%

*Data from 2 open-label studies in treatment-naive patients also receiving abacavir/lamivudine.
† Data from 3 open-label studies in treatment-naive and treatment-experienced patients receiving combination antiretroviral therapy.

ADVERSE REACTIONS

In clinical studies, adverse events leading to amprenavir discontinuation occurred primarily during the first 12 weeks of therapy, and were mostly due to gastrointestinal events (nausea, vomiting, diarrhea, and abdominal pain/discomfort), which were mild to moderate in severity.

Skin rash occurred in 22% of patients treated with amprenavir in studies PROAB3001 and PROAB3006. Rashes were usually maculopapular and of mild or moderate intensity, some with pruritus. Rashes had a median onset of 11 days after amprenavir initiation and a median duration of 10 days. Skin rashes led to amprenavir discontinuation in approximately 3% of patients. In some patients with mild or moderate rash, amprenavir dosing was often continued without interruption; if interrupted, reintroduction of amprenavir generally did not result in rash recurrence.

Severe or life-threatening rash (Grade 3 or 4), including cases of Stevens-Johnson syndrome, occurred in approximately 1% of recipients of AGENERASE (see WARNINGS). Amprenavir therapy should be discontinued for severe or life-threatening rashes and for moderate rashes accompanied by systemic symptoms.

[See table 9 above]

Among amprenavir-treated patients in Phase 3 studies, 2 patients developed de novo diabetes mellitus, 1 patient developed a dorsocervical fat enlargement (buffalo hump), and 9 patients developed fat redistribution.

In studies PROAB3001 and PROAB3006, no increased frequency of Grade 3 or 4 AST, ALT, amylase, or bilirubin elevations was seen compared to controls.

Pediatric Patients: An adverse event profile similar to that seen in adults was seen in pediatric patients.

Concomitant Therapy with Ritonavir: Tables 10 and 11 present adverse clinical events and laboratory abnormalities observed in subjects who received AGENERASE plus ritonavir. Since the trials were small, open-label, of varying duration, and often included different patient populations, direct comparisons to the frequency of events with AGENERASE alone (see Table 9) cannot be made.

[See table 10 above]
[See table 11 above]

OVERDOSAGE

There is no known antidote for AGENERASE. It is not known whether amprenavir can be removed by peritoneal dialysis or hemodialysis. If overdosage occurs, the patient should be monitored for evidence of toxicity and standard supportive treatment applied as necessary.

DOSAGE AND ADMINISTRATION

AGENERASE may be taken with or without food; however, a high-fat meal decreases the absorption of amprenavir and should be avoided (see CLINICAL PHARMACOLOGY: Effects of Food on Oral Absorption). **Adult and pediatric patients should be advised not to take supplemental vitamin E since the vitamin E content of AGENERASE Capsules exceeds the Reference Daily Intake (adults 30 IU, pediatrics approximately 10 IU) (see DESCRIPTION).**

Adults: The recommended oral dose of AGENERASE Capsules for adults is 1,200 mg (eight 150-mg capsules) twice daily in combination with other antiretroviral agents.

Concomitant Therapy: If AGENERASE and ritonavir are used in combination, the recommended dosage regimens are: AGENERASE 1,200 mg with ritonavir 200 mg once daily or AGENERASE 600 mg with ritonavir 100 mg twice daily.

Pediatric Patients: For adolescents (13 to 16 years), the recommended oral dose of AGENERASE Capsules is 1,200 mg (eight 150-mg capsules) twice daily in combination with other antiretroviral agents. For patients between 4 and 12 years of age or for patients 13 to 16 years of age with weight of <50 kg, the recommended oral dose of AGENERASE Capsules is 20 mg/kg twice daily or 15 mg/kg 3 times daily (to a maximum daily dose of 2,400 mg) in combination with other antiretroviral agents. The recommended dose of AGENERASE for use in combination with ritonavir has not been established in pediatric patients.

Before using **AGENERASE Oral Solution**, the complete prescribing information should be consulted.

AGENERASE Capsules and AGENERASE Oral Solution are not interchangeable on a milligram-per-milligram basis (see CLINICAL PHARMACOLOGY).

Patients with Hepatic Impairment: AGENERASE Capsules should be used with caution in patients with moderate or severe hepatic impairment. Patients with a Child-Pugh score ranging from 5 to 8 should receive a reduced dose of AGENERASE Capsules of 450 mg twice daily, and patients with a Child-Pugh score ranging from 9 to 12 should receive a reduced dose of AGENERASE Capsules of 300 mg twice daily (see CLINICAL PHARMACOLOGY: Hepatic Insufficiency).

HOW SUPPLIED

AGENERASE Capsules, 50 mg, are oblong, opaque, off-white to cream-colored soft gelatin capsules printed with "GX CC1" on one side.

Bottles of 480 with child-resistant closures (NDC 0173-0679-00).

AGENERASE Capsules, 150 mg, are oblong, opaque, off-white to cream-colored soft gelatin capsules printed with "GX CC2" on one side.

Bottles of 240 with child-resistant closures (NDC 0173-0672-00).

Store at controlled room temperature of 25°C (77°F) (see USP).

AGENERASE Capsules are manufactured by
R.P. Scherer, Beinheim, France
for GlaxoSmithKline, Research Triangle Park, NC 27709
Licensed from Vertex Pharmaceuticals Incorporated
Cambridge, MA 02139

AGENERASE is a registered trademark of the GlaxoSmithKline group of companies.

February 2004/RL-2070

Shown in Product Identification Guide, page 314

Table 1. Average (%CV) Pharmacokinetic Parameters After 1,200 mg Twice Daily of Amprenavir Capsules (n = 54)

C_{max} (mcg/mL)	T_{max} (hours)	AUC_{0-12} (mcg•hr/mL)	C_{avg} (mcg/mL)	C_{min} (mcg/mL)	CL/F (mL/min/kg)
7.66 (54%)	1.0 (42%)	17.7 (47%)	1.48 (47%)	0.32 (77%)	19.5 (46%)

Table 2. Average (%CV) Pharmacokinetic Parameters in Children Ages 4 to 12 Years Receiving 20 mg/kg Twice Daily or 15 mg/kg Three Times Daily of AGENERASE Oral Solution

Dose	n	C_{max} (mcg/mL)	T_{max} (hours)	AUC_{ss}* (mcg•hr/mL)	C_{avg} (mcg/mL)	C_{min} (mcg/mL)	CL/F (mL/min/kg)
20 mg/kg b.i.d.	20	6.77 (51%)	1.1 (21%)	15.46 (59%)	1.29 (59%)	0.24 (98%)	29 (58%)
15 mg/kg t.i.d.	17	3.99 (37%)	1.4 (90%)	8.73 (36%)	1.09 (36%)	0.27 (95%)	32 (34%)

*AUC is 0 to 12 hours for b.i.d. and 0 to 8 hours for t.i.d., therefore the C_{avg} is a better comparison of the exposures.

Table 3. Drug Interactions: Pharmacokinetic Parameters for Amprenavir in the Presence of the Coadministered Drug

Coadministered Drug	Dose of Coadministered Drug	Dose of AGENERASE	n	% Change in **Amprenavir** Pharmacokinetic Parameters* (90% CI) C_{max}	AUC	C_{min}
Abacavir	300 mg b.i.d. for 3 weeks	900 mg b.i.d. for 3 weeks	4	↑47 (↓15 to ↑154)	↑29 (↓18 to ↑103)	↑27 (↓46 to ↑197)
Clarithromycin	500 mg b.i.d. for 4 days	1,200 mg b.i.d. for 4 days	12	↑15 (↑1 to ↑31)	↑18 (↑8 to ↑29)	↑39 (↑31 to ↑47)
Delavirdine	600 mg b.i.d. for 10 days	600 mg b.i.d. for 10 days	9	↑40‡	↑130‡	↑125‡
Ethinyl estradiol/ Norethindrone	0.035 mg/1 mg for 1 cycle	1,200 mg b.i.d. for 28 days	10	⇔ (↓20 to ↑3)	↓22 (↓35 to ↓8)	↓20 (↓41 to ↑8)
Indinavir	800 mg t.i.d. for 2 weeks (fasted)	750 or 800 mg t.i.d. for 2 weeks (fasted)	9	↑18 (↓13 to ↑58)	↑33 (↑2 to ↑73)	↑25 (↓27 to ↑116)
Ketoconazole	400 mg single dose	1,200 mg single dose	12	↓16 (↓25 to ↓6)	↑31 (↑20 to ↑42)	NA
Lamivudine	150 mg single dose	600 mg single dose	11	⇔ (↓17 to ↑9)	⇔ (↓15 to ↑14)	NA
Nelfinavir	750 mg t.i.d. for 2 weeks (fed)	750 or 800 mg t.i.d. for 2 weeks (fed)	6	↓14 (↓38 to ↑20)	⇔ (↓19 to ↑47)	↑189 (↑52 to ↑448)
Rifabutin	300 mg q.d. for 10 days	1,200 mg b.i.d. for 10 days	5	⇔ (↓21 to ↑10)	↓15 (↓28 to 0)	↓15 (↓38 to ↑17)
Rifampin	300 mg q.d. for 4 days	1,200 mg b.i.d. for 4 days	11	↓70 (↓76 to ↓62)	↓82 (↓84 to ↓78)	↓92 (↓95 to ↓89)
Ritonavir	100 mg b.i.d. for 2 to 4 weeks	600 mg b.i.d.	18	↓30† (↓44 to ↓14)	↑64† (↑37 to ↑97)	↑508† (↑394 to ↑649)
Ritonavir	200 mg q.d. for 2 to 4 weeks	1,200 mg q.d.	12	⇔† (↓17 to ↑30)	↑62† (↑35 to ↑94)	↑319† (↑190 to ↑508)
Saquinavir	800 mg t.i.d. for 2 weeks (fed)	750 or 800 mg t.i.d. for 2 weeks (fed)	7	↓37 (↓54 to ↓14)	↓32 (↓49 to ↓9)	↓14 (↓52 to ↑54)
Zidovudine	300 mg single dose	600 mg single dose	12	⇔ (↓5 to ↑24)	↑13 (↓2 to ↑31)	NA

*Based on total-drug concentrations.
†Compared to amprenavir capsules 1,200 mg b.i.d. in the same patients.
‡Median percent change; confidence interval not reported.
↑ = Increase; ↓ = Decrease; ⇔ = No change (↑ or ↓ <10%); NA = C_{min} not calculated for single-dose study.

AGENERASE® ℞

[əjin'ə-rās]
(amprenavir)
Oral Solution

Because of the potential risk of toxicity from the large amount of the excipient, propylene glycol, AGENERASE Oral Solution is contraindicated in infants and children below the age of 4 years, pregnant women, patients with hepatic or renal failure, and patients treated with disulfiram or metronidazole (see CONTRAINDICATIONS AND WARNINGS).

AGENERASE Oral Solution should be used only when AGENERASE Capsules or other protease inhibitor formulations are not therapeutic options.

DESCRIPTION

AGENERASE (amprenavir) is an inhibitor of the human immunodeficiency virus (HIV) protease. The chemical name of amprenavir is (3*S*)-tetrahydro-3-furyl *N*-[(1*S*,2*R*)-3-(4-amino-*N*-isobutylbenzenesulfonamido)-1-benzyl-2-hydroxypropyl]carbamate. Amprenavir is a single stereoisomer with the (3*S*)(1*S*,2*R*) configuration. It has a molecular formula of $C_{25}H_{35}N_3O_6S$ and a molecular weight of 505.64.

Amprenavir is a white to cream-colored solid with a solubility of approximately 0.04 mg/mL in water at 25°C.

AGENERASE Oral Solution is for oral administration. One milliliter (1 mL) of AGENERASE Oral Solution contains 15 mg of amprenavir in solution and the inactive ingredients acesulfame potassium, artificial grape bubblegum flavor, citric acid (anhydrous), d-alpha tocopheryl polyethylene glycol 1000 succinate (TPGS), menthol, natural peppermint flavor, polyethylene glycol 400 (PEG 400) (170 mg), propylene glycol (550 mg), saccharin sodium, sodium chloride, and sodium citrate (dihydrate). Solutions of sodium hydroxide and/or diluted hydrochloric acid may have been added to adjust pH. Each mL of AGENERASE Oral Solution contains 46 IU vitamin E in the form of TPGS. Propylene glycol is in the formulation to achieve adequate solubility of amprenavir. The recommended daily dose of AGENERASE Oral Solution of 22.5 mg/kg twice daily corresponds to a propylene glycol intake of 1,650 mg/kg/day. Acceptable intake of propylene glycol for pharmaceuticals has not been established.

MICROBIOLOGY

Mechanism of Action: Amprenavir is an inhibitor of HIV-1 protease. Amprenavir binds to the active site of HIV-1 protease and thereby prevents the processing of viral gag and gag-pol polyprotein precursors, resulting in the formation of immature non-infectious viral particles.

Antiviral Activity in Vitro: The in vitro antiviral activity of amprenavir was evaluated against HIV-1 IIIB in both acutely and chronically infected lymphoblastic cell lines (MT-4, CEM-CCRF, H9) and in peripheral blood lymphocytes. The 50% inhibitory concentration (IC_{50}) of amprenavir ranged from 0.012 to 0.08 µM in acutely infected cells and was 0.41 µM in chronically infected cells (1 µM = 0.50 mcg/mL). Amprenavir exhibited synergistic anti-HIV-1 activity in combination with abacavir, zidovudine, didanosine, or saquinavir, and additive anti-HIV-1 activity in combination with indinavir, nelfinavir, and ritonavir in vitro. These drug combinations have not been adequately studied in humans. The relationship between in vitro anti-HIV-1 activity of amprenavir and the inhibition of HIV-1 replication in humans has not been defined.

Resistance: HIV-1 isolates with a decreased susceptibility to amprenavir have been selected in vitro and obtained from patients treated with amprenavir. Genotypic analysis of isolates from amprenavir-treated patients showed mutations in the HIV-1 protease gene resulting in amino acid substitutions primarily at positions V32I, M46I/L, I47V, I50V, I54L/M, and I84V as well as mutations in the p7/p1 and p1/p6 gag cleavage sites. Phenotypic analysis of HIV-1 isolates from 21 nucleoside reverse transcriptase inhibitor-(NRTI-) experienced, protease inhibitor-naive patients treated with amprenavir in combination with NRTIs for 16 to 48 weeks identified isolates from 15 patients who exhibited a 4- to 17-fold decrease in susceptibility to amprenavir in vitro compared to wild-type virus. Clinical isolates that exhibited a decrease in amprenavir susceptibility harbored one or more amprenavir-associated mutations. The clinical

Continued on next page

Product information on these pages is effective as of August 2004. Further information is available at: GlaxoSmithKline, PO Box 13398, Research Triangle Park, NC 27709. 1-888-825-5249. Corporate Web Site: www.gsk.com

Agenerase Oral Solution—Cont.

relevance of the genotypic and phenotypic changes associated with amprenavir therapy is under evaluation.

Cross-Resistance: Varying degrees of HIV-1 cross-resistance among protease inhibitors have been observed. Five of 15 amprenavir-resistant isolates exhibited 4- to 8-fold decrease in susceptibility to ritonavir. However, amprenavir-resistant isolates were susceptible to either indinavir or saquinavir.

CLINICAL PHARMACOLOGY

Pharmacokinetics in Adults: The pharmacokinetic properties of amprenavir have been studied in asymptomatic, HIV-infected adult patients after administration of single oral doses of 150 to 1,200 mg and multiple oral doses of 300 to 1,200 mg twice daily.

Absorption and Bioavailability: Amprenavir was rapidly absorbed after oral administration in HIV-1-infected patients with a time to peak concentration (T_{max}) typically between 1 and 2 hours after a single oral dose. The absolute oral bioavailability of amprenavir in humans has not been established.

Increases in the area under the plasma concentration versus time curve (AUC) after single oral doses between 150 and 1,200 mg were slightly greater than dose proportional. Increases in AUC were dose proportional after 3 weeks of dosing with doses from 300 to 1,200 mg twice daily. The pharmacokinetic parameters after administration of amprenavir 1,200 mg twice daily for 3 weeks to HIV-infected subjects are shown in Table 1.

[See table 1 at top of previous page]

The relative bioavailability of AGENERASE Capsules and Oral Solution was assessed in healthy adults. AGENERASE Oral Solution was 14% less bioavailable compared to the capsules.

Effects of Food on Oral Absorption: The relative bioavailability of AGENERASE Capsules was assessed in the fasting and fed states in healthy volunteers (standardized high-fat meal: 967 kcal, 67 grams fat, 33 grams protein, 58 grams carbohydrate). Administration of a single 1,200-mg dose of amprenavir in the fed state compared to the fasted state was associated with changes in C_{max} (fed: 6.18 ± 2.92 mcg/mL, fasted: 9.72 ± 2.75 mcg/mL), T_{max} (fed: 1.51 ± 0.68, fasted: 1.05 ± 0.63), and $AUC_{0-\infty}$ (fed: 22.06 ± 11.6 mcg•hr/mL, fasted: 28.05 ± 10.1 mcg•hr/mL). AGENERASE may be taken with or without food, but should not be taken with a high-fat meal (see DOSAGE AND ADMINISTRATION).

Distribution: The apparent volume of distribution (V_z/F) is approximately 430 L in healthy adult subjects. In vitro binding is approximately 90% to plasma proteins. The high affinity binding protein for amprenavir is alpha$_1$-acid glycoprotein (AAG). The partitioning of amprenavir into erythrocytes is low, but increases as amprenavir concentrations increase, reflecting the higher amount of unbound drug at higher concentrations.

Metabolism: Amprenavir is metabolized in the liver by the cytochrome P450 3A4 (CYP3A4) enzyme system. The 2 major metabolites result from oxidation of the tetrahydrofuran and aniline moieties. Glucuronide conjugates of oxidized metabolites have been identified as minor metabolites in urine and feces.

AGENERASE Oral Solution contains a large amount of propylene glycol, which is hepatically metabolized by the alcohol and aldehyde dehydrogenase enzyme pathway. Alcohol dehydrogenase (ADH) is present in the human fetal liver at 2 months of gestational age, but at only 3% of adult activity. Although the data are limited, it appears that by 12 to 30 months of postnatal age, ADH activity is equal to or greater than that observed in adults. Additionally, certain patient groups (females, Asians, Eskimos, Native Americans) may be at increased risk of propylene glycol-associated adverse events due to diminished ability to metabolize propylene glycol (see CLINICAL PHARMACOLOGY: Special Populations: Gender and Race).

Elimination: Excretion of unchanged amprenavir in urine and feces is minimal. Approximately 14% and 75% of an administered single dose of ^{14}C-amprenavir can be accounted for as radiocarbon in urine and feces, respectively. Two metabolites accounted for >90% of the radiocarbon in fecal samples. The plasma elimination half-life of amprenavir ranged from 7.1 to 10.6 hours.

Special Populations: ***Hepatic Insufficiency:*** AGENERASE Oral Solution is contraindicated in patients with hepatic failure.

Patients with hepatic impairment are at increased risk of propylene glycol-associated adverse events (see WARNINGS). AGENERASE Oral Solution should be used with caution in patients with hepatic impairment. AGENERASE Capsules have been studied in adult patients with impaired hepatic function using a single 600-mg oral dose. The $AUC_{0-\infty}$ was significantly greater in patients with moderate cirrhosis (25.76 ± 14.68 mcg•hr/mL) compared with healthy volunteers (12.00 ± 4.38 mcg•hr/mL). The $AUC_{0-\infty}$ and C_{max} were significantly greater in patients with severe cirrhosis ($AUC_{0-\infty}$: 38.66 ± 16.08 mcg•hr/mL; C_{max}: 9.43 ± 2.61 mcg/mL) compared with healthy volunteers ($AUC_{0-\infty}$: 12.00 ± 4.38 mcg•hr/mL; C_{max}: 4.90 ± 1.39 mcg/mL). Patients with impaired hepatic function require dosage adjustment (see DOSAGE AND ADMINISTRATION).

Renal Insufficiency: AGENERASE Oral Solution is contraindicated in patients with renal failure.

Table 4. Drug Interactions: Pharmacokinetic Parameters for Coadministered Drug in the Presence of Amprenavir

Coadministered Drug	Dose of Coadministered Drug	Dose of AGENERASE	n	% Change in Pharmacokinetic Parameters of **Coadministered Drug** (90% CI)		
				C_{max}	AUC	C_{min}
Clarithromycin	500 mg b.i.d. for 4 days	1,200 mg b.i.d. for 4 days	12	↓10 (↓24 to ↑7)	⇔ (↓17 to ↑11)	⇔ (↓13 to ↑20)
Delavirdine	600 mg b.i.d. for 10 days	600 mg b.i.d. for 10 days	9	↓47*	↓61*	↓88*
Ethinyl estradiol	0.035 mg for 1 cycle	1,200 mg b.i.d. for 28 days	10	⇔ (↓25 to ↑15)	⇔ (↓14 to ↑38)	↑32 (↓3 to ↑79)
Norethindrone	1.0 mg for 1 cycle	1,200 mg b.i.d. for 28 days	10	⇔ (↓20 to ↑18)	↑18 (↑1 to ↑38)	↑45 (↑13 to ↑88)
Ketoconazole	400 mg single dose	1,200 mg single dose	12	↑19 (↑8 to ↑33)	↑44 (↑31 to ↑59)	NA
Lamivudine	150 mg single dose	600 mg single dose	11	⇔ (↓17 to ↑3)	⇔ (↓11 to 0)	NA
Methadone	44 to 100 mg q.d. for >30 days	1,200 mg b.i.d. for 10 days	16	R-Methadone (active)		
				↓25 (↓32 to ↓18)	↓13 (↓21 to ↓5)	↓21 (↓32 to ↓9)
				S-Methadone (inactive)		
				↓48 (↓55 to ↓40)	↓40 (↓46 to ↓32)	↓53 (↓60 to ↓43)
Rifabutin	300 mg q.d. for 10 days	1,200 mg b.i.d. for 10 days	5	↑119 (↑82 to ↑164)	↑193 (↑156 to ↑235)	↑271 (↑171 to ↑409)
Rifampin	300 mg q.d. for 4 days	1,200 mg b.i.d. for 4 days	11	⇔ (↓13 to ↑12)	⇔ (↓10 to ↑13)	ND
Zidovudine	300 mg single dose	600 mg single dose	12	↑40 (↑14 to ↑71)	↑31 (↑19 to ↑45)	NA

* Median percent change; confidence interval not reported.
↑ = Increase; ↓ = Decrease; ⇔ = No change (↑ or ↓ <10%); NA = C_{min} not calculated for single-dose study; ND = Interaction cannot be determined as C_{min} was below the lower limit of quantitation.

Table 5. Outcomes of Randomized Treatment Through Week 48 (PROAB3006)

Outcome	AGENERASE (n = 254)	Indinavir (n = 250)
HIV-1 RNA <400 copies/mL*	30%	49%
HIV-1 RNA ≥400 copies/mL†,‡	38%	26%
Discontinued due to adverse events*,‡	16%	12%
Discontinued due to other reasons‡,§	16%	13%

*Corresponds to rates at Week 48 in Figure 1.
†Virological failures at or before Week 48.
‡Considered to be treatment failure in the analysis.
§Includes discontinuations due to consent withdrawn, loss to follow-up, protocol violations, non-compliance, pregnancy, never treated, and other reasons.

Patients with renal impairment are at increased risk of propylene glycol-associated adverse events. Additionally, because metabolites of the excipient, propylene glycol, in AGENERASE Oral Solution may alter acid-base balance, patients with renal impairment should be monitored for potential adverse events (see WARNINGS). AGENERASE Oral Solution should be used with caution in patients with renal impairment. The impact of renal impairment on amprenavir elimination has not been studied. The renal elimination of unchanged amprenavir represents <3% of the administered dose.

Pediatric Patients: AGENERASE Oral Solution is contraindicated in infants and children below 4 years of age (see CONTRAINDICATIONS and WARNINGS).

The pharmacokinetics of amprenavir have been studied after either single or repeat doses of AGENERASE Capsules or Oral Solution in 84 pediatric patients. Twenty HIV-1-infected children ranging in age from 4 to 12 years received single doses from 5 mg/kg to 20 mg/kg using 25-mg or 150-mg capsules. The C_{max} of amprenavir increased less than proportionally with dose. The $AUC_{0-\infty}$ increased proportionally at doses between 5 and 20 mg/kg. Amprenavir is 14% less bioavailable from the liquid formulation than from the capsules; therefore **AGENERASE Capsules and AGENERASE Oral Solution are not interchangeable on a milligram-per-milligram basis.**

[See table 2 at top of previous page]

Geriatric Patients: The pharmacokinetics of amprenavir have not been studied in patients over 65 years of age.

Gender: The pharmacokinetics of amprenavir do not differ between males and females. Females may have a lower amount of alcohol dehydrogenase compared with males and may be at increased risk of propylene glycol-associated adverse events; no data are available on propylene glycol metabolism in females.

Race: The pharmacokinetics of amprenavir do not differ between blacks and non-blacks. Certain ethnic populations (Asians, Eskimos, and Native Americans) may be at increased risk of propylene glycol-associated adverse events because of alcohol dehydrogenase polymorphisms; no data are available on propylene glycol metabolism in these groups.

Drug Interactions: See also CONTRAINDICATIONS, WARNINGS, and PRECAUTIONS: Drug Interactions.

Amprenavir is metabolized in the liver by the cytochrome P450 enzyme system. Amprenavir inhibits CYP3A4. Caution should be used when coadministering medications that are substrates, inhibitors, or inducers of CYP3A4, or potentially toxic medications that are metabolized by CYP3A4. Amprenavir does not inhibit CYP2D6, CYP1A2, CYP2C9, CYP2C19, CYP2E1, or uridine glucuronosyltransferase (UDPGT).

Drug interaction studies were performed with amprenavir capsules and other drugs likely to be coadministered or drugs commonly used as probes for pharmacokinetic interactions. The effects of coadministration of amprenavir on the AUC, C_{max}, and C_{min} are summarized in Table 3 (effect of other drugs on amprenavir) and Table 4 (effect of amprenavir on other drugs). For information regarding clinical recommendations, see PRECAUTIONS.

[See table 3 at top of previous page]
[See table 4 above]

Nucleoside Reverse Transcriptase Inhibitors (NRTIs): There was no effect of amprenavir on abacavir in subjects receiving both agents based on historical data.

HIV Protease Inhibitors: Concurrent use of AGENERASE Oral Solution and NORVIR® (ritonavir) Oral Solution is not recommended because the large amount of propylene glycol in AGENERASE Oral Solution and ethanol in NORVIR Oral Solution may compete for the same metabolic pathway for elimination. This combination has not been studied in pediatric patients.

The effect of amprenavir on total drug concentrations of other HIV protease inhibitors in subjects receiving both agents was evaluated using comparisons to historical data. Indinavir steady-state C_{max}, AUC, and C_{min} were decreased by 22%, 38%, and 27%, respectively, by concomitant amprenavir. Similar decreases in C_{max} and AUC were seen after the first dose. Saquinavir steady-state C_{max}, AUC, and C_{min} were increased 21%, decreased 19%, and decreased 48%, respectively, by concomitant amprenavir. Nelfinavir steady-state C_{max}, AUC, and C_{min} were increased by 12%, 15%, and 14%, respectively, by concomitant amprenavir.

Methadone: Coadministration of amprenavir and methadone can decrease plasma levels of methadone.

Coadministration of amprenavir and methadone as compared to a non-matched historical control group resulted in a 30%, 27%, and 25% decrease in serum amprenavir AUC, C_{max}, and C_{min}, respectively.

For information regarding clinical recommendations, see PRECAUTIONS: Drug Interactions.

INDICATIONS AND USAGE

AGENERASE (amprenavir) is indicated in combination with other antiretroviral agents for the treatment of HIV-1 infection.

The following points should be considered when initiating therapy with AGENERASE:

- **In a study of NRTI-experienced, protease inhibitor-naive patients, AGENERASE was found to be significantly less effective than indinavir (see Description of Clinical Studies).**
- **Mild to moderate gastrointestinal adverse events led to discontinuation of AGENERASE primarily during the first 12 weeks of therapy (see ADVERSE REACTIONS).**
- **There are no data on response to therapy with AGENERASE in protease inhibitor-experienced patients.**

AGENERASE Oral Solution should be used only when AGENERASE Capsules or other protease inhibitor formulations are not therapeutic options.

Description of Clinical Studies: *Therapy-Naive Adults:* PROAB3001, a randomized, double-blind, placebo-controlled, multicenter study, compared treatment with AGENERASE Capsules (1,200 mg twice daily) plus lamivudine (150 mg twice daily) plus zidovudine (300 mg twice daily) versus lamivudine (150 mg twice daily) plus zidovudine (300 mg twice daily) in 232 patients. Through 24 weeks of therapy, 53% of patients assigned to AGENERASE/zidovudine/lamivudine achieved HIV-1 RNA <400 copies/mL. Through week 48, the antiviral response was 41%. Through 24 weeks of therapy, 11% of patients assigned to zidovudine/lamivudine achieved HIV-1 RNA <400 copies/mL. Antiviral response beyond week 24 is not interpretable because the majority of patients discontinued or changed their antiretroviral therapy.

NRTI-Experienced Adults: PROAB3006, a randomized, open-label multicenter study, compared treatment with AGENERASE Capsules (1,200 mg twice daily) plus NRTIs versus indinavir (800 mg every 8 hours) plus NRTIs in 504 NRTI-experienced, protease inhibitor-naive patients, median age 37 years (range 20 to 71 years), 72% Caucasian, 80% male, with a median CD4 cell count of 404 cells/mm^3 (range 9 to 1,706 cells/mm^3) and a median plasma HIV-1 RNA level of 3.93 log_{10} copies/mL (range 2.60 to 7.01 log_{10} copies/mL) at baseline. Through 48 weeks of therapy, the median CD4 cell count increase from baseline in the amprenavir group was significantly lower than in the indinavir group, 97 cells/mm^3 versus 144 cells/mm^3, respectively. There was also a significant difference in the proportions of patients with plasma HIV-1 RNA levels <400 copies/mL through 48 weeks (see Figure 1 and Table 5).

Figure 1: Virologic Response Through Week 48, PROAB3006*,†

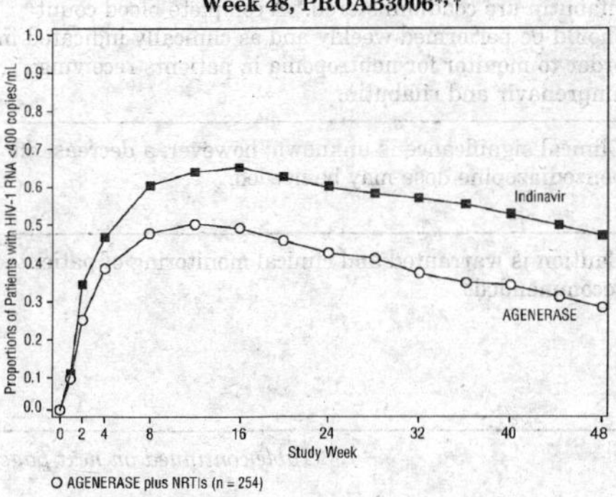

○ AGENERASE plus NRTIs (n = 254)
■ Indinavir plus NRTIs (n = 250)
*Roche AMPLICOR HIV-1 MONITOR assay.
†Discontinuations and missing data were considered as HIV-1 RNA ≥400 copies/mL.

HIV-1 RNA status and reasons for discontinuation of randomized treatment at 48 weeks are summarized (Table 5).

[See table 5 on previous page]

CONTRAINDICATIONS

Because of the potential risk of toxicity from the large amount of the excipient, propylene glycol, AGENERASE Oral Solution is contraindicated in infants and children below the age of 4 years, pregnant women, patients with hepatic or renal failure, and patients treated with disulfiram or metronidazole (see WARNINGS and PRECAUTIONS).

Coadministration of AGENERASE is contraindicated with drugs that are highly dependent on CYP3A4 for clearance and for which elevated plasma concentrations are associated with serious and/or life-threatening events. These drugs are listed in Table 6.

Table 6. Drugs That Are Contraindicated with AGENERASE Oral Solution

Drug Class	Drugs Within Class That Are CONTRAINDICATED with AGENERASE
Alcohol-dependence treatment	Disulfiram
Antibiotic	Metronidazole
Ergot derivatives	Dihydroergotamine, ergonovine, ergotamine, methylergonovine
GI motility agent	Cisapride
Neuroleptic	Pimozide
Sedatives/hypnotics	Midazolam, triazolam

If AGENERASE Capsules are coadministered with ritonavir capsules, the antiarrhythmic agents flecainide and propafenone are also contraindicated.

AGENERASE is contraindicated in patients with previously demonstrated clinically significant hypersensitivity to any of the components of this product.

WARNINGS

ALERT: Find out about medicines that should not be taken with AGENERASE.

Because of the potential risk of toxicity from the large amount of the excipient, propylene glycol, AGENERASE Oral Solution is contraindicated in infants and children below the age of 4 years, pregnant women, patients with hepatic or renal failure, and patients treated with disulfiram or metronidazole (see CLINICAL PHARMACOLOGY, CONTRAINDICATIONS, and PRECAUTIONS).

Because of the possible toxicity associated with the large amount of propylene glycol and the lack of information on chronic exposure to large amounts of propylene glycol, AGENERASE Oral Solution should be used only when AGENERASE Capsules or other protease inhibitor formulations are not therapeutic options. Certain ethnic populations (Asians, Eskimos, Native Americans) and women may be at increased risk of propylene glycol-associated adverse events due to diminished ability to metabolize propylene glycol; no data are available on propylene glycol metabolism in these groups (see CLINICAL PHARMACOLOGY: Special Populations: Gender and Race).

If patients require treatment with AGENERASE Oral Solution, they should be monitored closely for propylene glycol-associated adverse events, including seizures, stupor, tachycardia, hyperosmolality, lactic acidosis, renal toxicity, and hemolysis. Patients should be switched from AGENERASE Oral Solution to AGENERASE Capsules as soon as they are able to take the capsule formulation.

Concurrent use of AGENERASE Oral Solution and NORVIR (ritonavir) Oral Solution is not recommended because the large amount of propylene glycol in AGENERASE Oral Solution and ethanol in NORVIR Oral Solution may compete for the same metabolic pathway for elimination.

Use of alcoholic beverages is not recommended in patients treated with AGENERASE Oral Solution.

Serious and/or life-threatening drug interactions could occur between amprenavir and amiodarone, lidocaine (systemic), tricyclic antidepressants, and quinidine. Concentration monitoring of these agents is recommended if these agents are used concomitantly with AGENERASE (see CONTRAINDICATIONS).

Rifampin should not be used in combination with amprenavir because it reduces plasma concentrations and AUC of amprenavir by about 90%.

Concomitant use of AGENERASE and St. John's wort (hypericum perforatum) or products containing St. John's wort is not recommended. Coadministration of protease inhibitors, including AGENERASE, with St. John's wort is expected to substantially decrease protease inhibitor concentrations and may result in suboptimal levels of amprenavir and lead to loss of virologic response and possible resistance to AGENERASE or to the class of protease inhibitors.

Concomitant use of AGENERASE with lovastatin or simvastatin is not recommended. Caution should be exercised if HIV protease inhibitors, including AGENERASE, are used concurrently with other HMG-CoA reductase inhibitors that are also metabolized by the CYP3A4 pathway (e.g., atorvastatin). The risk of myopathy, including rhabdomyolysis, may be increased when HIV protease inhibitors, including amprenavir, are used in combination with these drugs.

Particular caution should be used when prescribing sildenafil in patients receiving amprenavir. Coadministration of AGENERASE with sildenafil is expected to substantially increase sildenafil concentrations and may result in an increase in sildenafil-associated adverse events, including hypotension, visual changes, and priapism (see PRECAUTIONS: Drug Interactions and Information for Patients, and the complete prescribing information for sildenafil).

Continued on next page

Table 7. Drugs That Should Not Be Coadministered with AGENERASE Oral Solution

Drug Class/Drug Name	Clinical Comment
Alcohol-Dependence Treatment: Disulfiram	**CONTRAINDICATED** due to potential risk of toxicity from the large amount of the excipient, propylene glycol, in AGENERASE Oral Solution.
Antibiotic: Metronidazole	**CONTRAINDICATED** due to potential risk of toxicity from the large amount of the excipient, propylene glycol, in AGENERASE Oral Solution.
Antimycobacterials: Rifampin*	May lead to loss of virologic response and possible resistance to AGENERASE or to the class of protease inhibitors.
Ergot Derivatives: Dihydroergotamine, ergonovine, ergotamine, methylergonovine	**CONTRAINDICATED** due to potential for serious and/or life-threatening reactions such as acute ergot toxicity characterized by peripheral vasospasm and ischemia of the extremities and other tissues.
GI Motility Agents: Cisapride	**CONTRAINDICATED** due to potential for serious and/or life-threatening reactions such as cardiac arrhythmias.
Herbal Products: St. John's wort (hypericum perforatum)	May lead to loss of virologic response and possible resistance to AGENERASE or to the class of protease inhibitors.
HIV-Protease Inhibitor: Ritonavir oral solution	Concurrent use of AGENERASE Oral Solution and NORVIR (ritonavir) Oral Solution is not recommended because the large amount of propylene glycol in AGENERASE Oral Solution and ethanol in NORVIR Oral Solution may compete for the same metabolic pathway for elimination.
HMG Co-Reductase Inhibitors: Lovastatin, simvastatin	Potential for serious reactions such as risk of myopathy including rhabdomyolysis.
Neuroleptic: Pimozide	**CONTRAINDICATED** due to potential for serious and/or life-threatening reactions such as cardiac arrhythmias.
Non-nucleoside Reverse Transcriptase Inhibitor: Delavirdine*	May lead to loss of virologic response and possible resistance to delavirdine.
Oral Contraceptives: Ethinyl estradiol/norethindrone	May lead to loss of virologic response and possible resistance to AGENERASE. Alternative methods of non-hormonal contraception are recommended.
Sedative/Hypnotics: Midazolam, triazolam	**CONTRAINDICATED** due to potential for serious and/or life-threatening reactions such as prolonged or increased sedation or respiratory depression.

*See CLINICAL PHARMACOLOGY for magnitude of interaction, Tables 3 and 4.

Product information on these pages is effective as of August 2004. Further information is available at: GlaxoSmithKline, PO Box 13398, Research Triangle Park, NC 27709. 1-888-825-5249. Corporate Web Site: www.gsk.com

Agenerase Oral Solution—Cont.

Severe and life-threatening skin reactions, including Stevens-Johnson syndrome, have occurred in patients treated with AGENERASE (see ADVERSE REACTIONS). Acute hemolytic anemia has been reported in a patient treated with AGENERASE.

New onset diabetes mellitus, exacerbation of pre-existing diabetes mellitus, and hyperglycemia have been reported during post-marketing surveillance in HIV-infected patients receiving protease inhibitor therapy. Some patients required either initiation or dose adjustments of insulin or oral hypoglycemic agents for treatment of these events. In some cases, diabetic ketoacidosis has occurred. In those patients who discontinued protease inhibitor therapy, hyperglycemia persisted in some cases. Because these events have been reported voluntarily during clinical practice, estimates of frequency cannot be made and causal relationships between protease inhibitor therapy and these events have not been established.

PRECAUTIONS

General: AGENERASE Capsules and AGENERASE Oral Solution are not interchangeable on a milligram-per-milligram basis (see CLINICAL PHARMACOLOGY: Pediatric Patients and CONTRAINDICATIONS).

Amprenavir is a sulfonamide. The potential for cross-sensitivity between drugs in the sulfonamide class and amprenavir is unknown. AGENERASE should be used with caution in patients with a known sulfonamide allergy.

AGENERASE is principally metabolized by the liver. AGENERASE, when used alone and in combination with low-dose ritonavir, has been associated with elevations of SGOT (AST) and SGPT (ALT) in some patients. Caution should be exercised when administering AGENERASE to patients with hepatic impairment (see DOSAGE AND ADMINISTRATION). Appropriate laboratory testing should be conducted prior to initiating therapy with AGENERASE and at periodic intervals during treatment.

Formulations of AGENERASE provide high daily doses of vitamin E (see Information for Patients, DESCRIPTION, and DOSAGE AND ADMINISTRATION). The effects of long-term, high-dose vitamin E administration in humans is not well characterized and has not been specifically studied in HIV-infected individuals. High vitamin E doses may exacerbate the blood coagulation defect of vitamin K deficiency caused by anticoagulant therapy or malabsorption.

Patients with Hemophilia: There have been reports of spontaneous bleeding in patients with hemophilia A and B treated with protease inhibitors. In some patients, additional factor VIII was required. In many of the reported cases, treatment with protease inhibitors was continued or restarted. A causal relationship between protease inhibitor therapy and these episodes has not been established.

Fat Redistribution: Redistribution/accumulation of body fat, including central obesity, dorsocervical fat enlargement (buffalo hump), peripheral wasting, facial wasting, breast enlargement, and "cushingoid appearance," have been observed in patients receiving antiretroviral therapy. The mechanism and long-term consequences of these events are currently unknown. A causal relationship has not been established.

Lipid Elevations: Treatment with AGENERASE alone or in combination with ritonavir capsules has resulted in increases in the concentration of total cholesterol and triglycerides. Triglyceride and cholesterol testing should be performed prior to initiation of therapy with AGENERASE and at periodic intervals during treatment. Lipid disorders should be managed as clinically appropriate. See PRECAUTIONS Table 8: Established and Other Potentially Significant Drug Interactions for additional information on potential drug interactions with AGENERASE and HMG-CoA reductase inhibitors.

Resistance/Cross-Resistance: Because the potential for HIV cross-resistance among protease inhibitors has not been fully explored, it is unknown what effect amprenavir therapy will have on the activity of subsequently administered protease inhibitors. It is also unknown what effect previous treatment with other protease inhibitors will have on the activity of amprenavir (see MICROBIOLOGY).

Information for Patients: A statement to patients and healthcare providers is included on the product's bottle label: **ALERT: Find out about medicines that should NOT be taken with AGENERASE.** A Patient Package Insert (PPI) for AGENERASE Oral Solution is available for patient information.

AGENERASE Oral Solution is contraindicated in infants and children below the age of 4 years, pregnant women, patients with hepatic or renal failure, and patients treated with disulfiram or metronidazole. AGENERASE Oral Solution should be used only when AGENERASE Capsules or other protease inhibitor formulations are not therapeutic options.

Patients treated with AGENERASE Capsules should be cautioned against switching to AGENERASE Oral Solution because of the increased risk of adverse events from the large amount of propylene glycol in AGENERASE Oral Solution.

Women, Asians, Eskimos, or Native Americans, as well as patients who have hepatic or renal insufficiency, should be informed that they may be at increased risk of adverse events from the large amount of propylene glycol in AGENERASE Oral Solution.

Patients should be informed that AGENERASE is not a cure for HIV infection and that they may continue to develop opportunistic infections and other complications associated with HIV disease. The long-term effects of AGENERASE (amprenavir) are unknown at this time. Patients should be told that there are currently no data demonstrating that therapy with AGENERASE can reduce the risk of transmitting HIV to others through sexual contact.

Patients should remain under the care of a physician while using AGENERASE. Patients should be advised to take AGENERASE every day as prescribed. AGENERASE must always be used in combination with other antiretroviral drugs. Patients should not alter the dose or discontinue therapy without consulting their physician. If a dose is missed, patients should take the dose as soon as possible and then return to their normal schedule. However, if a dose is skipped, the patient should not double the next dose.

Patients should inform their doctor if they have a sulfa allergy. The potential for cross-sensitivity between drugs in the sulfonamide class and amprenavir is unknown.

AGENERASE may interact with many drugs; therefore, patients should be advised to report to their doctor the use of any other prescription or nonprescription medication or herbal products, particularly St. John's wort.

Patients taking antacids (or the buffered formulation of didanosine) should take AGENERASE at least 1 hour be-

Table 8. Established and Other Potentially Significant Drug Interactions: Alteration in Dose or Regimen May be Recommended Based on Drug Interaction Studies or Predicted Interaction

Concomitant Drug Class: Drug Name	Effect on Concentration of Amprenavir or Concomitant Drug	Clinical Comment
HIV-Antiviral Agents		
Non-nucleoside Reverse Transcriptase Inhibitor: Efavirenz, nevirapine	↓ Amprenavir	Appropriate doses of the combinations with respect to safety and efficacy have not been established.
Nucleoside Reverse Transcriptase Inhibitor: Didanosine (buffered formulation only)	↓ Amprenavir	Take AGENERASE at least 1 hour before or after the buffered formulation of didanosine.
HIV-Protease Inhibitors: Indinavir*, lopinavir/ritonavir, nelfinavir*	↑ Amprenavir Amprenavir's effect on other protease inhibitors is not well established.	Appropriate doses of the combinations with respect to safety and efficacy have not been established.
HIV-Protease Inhibitor: Ritonavir Capsules*	↑ Amprenavir	The dose of amprenavir should be reduced when used in combination with ritonavir capsules (see Dosage and Administration). Also, see the full prescribing information for NORVIR for additional drug interaction information. Concurrent use of AGENERASE Oral Solution and NORVIR (ritonavir) Oral Solution is not recommended because the large amount of propylene glycol in AGENERASE Oral Solution and ethanol in NORVIR Oral Solution may compete for the same metabolic pathway for elimination.
HIV-Protease Inhibitor: Saquinavir*	↓ Amprenavir Amprenavir's effect on saquinavir is not well established.	Appropriate doses of the combination with respect to safety and efficacy have not been established.
Other Agents		
Antacids	↓ Amprenavir	Take AGENERASE at least 1 hour before or after antacids.
Antiarrhythmics: Amiodarone, lidocaine (systemic), and quinidine	↑ Antiarrhythmics	Caution is warranted and therapeutic concentration monitoring is recommended for antiarrhythmics when coadministered with AGENERASE, if available.
Antiarrhythmic: Bepridil	↑ Bepridil	Use with caution. Increased bepridil exposure may be associated with life-threatening reactions such as cardiac arrhythmias.
Anticoagulant: Warfarin		Concentrations of warfarin may be affected. It is recommended that INR (international normalized ratio) be monitored.
Anticonvulsants: Carbamazepine, phenobarbital, phenytoin	↓ Amprenavir	Use with caution. AGENERASE may be less effective due to decreased amprenavir plasma concentrations in patients taking these agents concomitantly.
Antifungals: Ketoconazole, itraconazole	↑ Ketoconazole ↑ Itraconazole	Increase monitoring for adverse events due to ketoconazole or itraconazole. Dose reduction of ketoconazole or itraconazole may be needed for patients receiving more than 400 mg ketoconazole or itraconazole per day.
Antimycobacterial: Rifabutin*	↑ Rifabutin and rifabutin metabolite	A dosage reduction of rifabutin to at least half the recommended dose is required when AGENERASE and rifabutin are coadministered.* A complete blood count should be performed weekly and as clinically indicated in order to monitor for neutropenia in patients receiving amprenavir and rifabutin.
Benzodiazepines: Alprazolam, clorazepate, diazepam, flurazepam	↑ Benzodiazepines	Clinical significance is unknown; however, a decrease in benzodiazepine dose may be needed.
Calcium Channel Blockers: Diltiazem, felodipine, nifedipine, nicardipine, nimodipine, verapamil, amlodipine, nisoldipine, isradipine	↑ Calcium channel blockers	Caution is warranted and clinical monitoring of patients is recommended.

(Table continued on next page)

Table 8 *(cont.)*. Established and Other Potentially Significant Drug Interactions: Alteration in Dose or Regimen May be Recommended Based on Drug Interaction Studies or Predicted Interaction

Concomitant Drug Class: Drug Name	Effect on Concentration of Amprenavir or Concomitant Drug	Clinical Comment
	Other Agents (cont.)	
Corticosteroid: Dexamethasone	↓ Amprenavir	Use with caution. AGENERASE may be less effective due to decreased amprenavir plasma concentrations in patients taking these agents concomitantly.
Erectile Dysfunction Agent: Sildenafil	↑ Sildenafil	Use with caution at reduced doses of 25 mg every 48 hours with increased monitoring for adverse events.
HMG-CoA Reductase Inhibitors: Atorvastatin	↑ Atorvastatin	Use lowest possible dose of atorvastatin with careful monitoring or consider other HMG-CoA reductase inhibitors such as pravastatin or fluvastatin in combination with AGENERASE.
Immunosuppressants: Cyclosporine, tacrolimus, rapamycin	↑ Immunosuppressants	Therapeutic concentration monitoring is recommended for immunosuppressant agents when coadministered with AGENERASE.
Narcotic Analgesics: Methadone*	↓ Amprenavir ↓ Methadone	AGENERASE may be less effective due to decreased amprenavir plasma concentrations in patients taking these agents concomitantly. Alternative antiretroviral therapy should be considered. Dosage of methadone may need to be increased when coadministered with AGENERASE.
Tricyclic Antidepressants: Amitriptyline, imipramine	↑ Tricyclics	Therapeutic concentration monitoring is recommended for tricyclic antidepressants when coadministered with AGENERASE.

*See CLINICAL PHARMACOLOGY for magnitude of interaction, Tables 3 and 4.

Table 9. Selected Clinical Adverse Events of All Grades Reported in >5% of Adult Patients

	PROAB3001 Therapy-Naive Patients		PROAB3006 NRTI-Experienced Patients	
Adverse Event	AGENERASE*/ Lamivudine/ Zidovudine (n = 113)	Lamivudine/ Zidovudine (n = 109)	AGENERASE*/ NRTI (n = 245)	Indinavir/ NRTI (n = 241)
Digestive				
Nausea	74%	50%	43%	35%
Vomiting	34%	17%	24%	20%
Diarrhea or loose stools	39%	35%	60%	41%
Taste disorders	10%	6%	2%	8%
Skin				
Rash	27%	6%	20%	15%
Nervous				
Paresthesia, oral/perioral	26%	6%	31%	2%
Paresthesia, peripheral	10%	4%	14%	10%
Psychiatric				
Depressive or mood disorders	16%	4%	9%	13%

*AGENERASE Capsules.

Table 10. Selected Clinical Adverse Events of All Grades Reported in Adult Patients in Open-Label Clinical Trials of AGENERASE Capsules in Combination with Ritonavir Capsules

Adverse Event	AGENERASE 1,200 mg plus Ritonavir 200 mg q.d.* (n = 101)	AGENERASE 600 mg plus Ritonavir 100 mg b.i.d.† (n = 239)
Nausea	31%	23%
Diarrhea/loose stools	30%	28%
Headache	16%	12%
Abdominal symptoms	14%	14%
Vomiting	11%	9%
Rash	10%	9%
Paresthesias	9%	11%
Fatigue	7%	14%
Depressive & mood disorders	4%	9%

*Data from 2 open-label studies in treatment-naive patients also receiving abacavir/lamivudine.
† Data from 3 open-label studies in treatment-naive and treatment-experienced patients receiving combination antiretroviral therapy.

fore or after antacid (or the buffered formulation of didanosine) use.
Patients should be advised that drinking alcoholic beverages is not recommended while taking AGENERASE Oral Solution.
Patients receiving sildenafil should be advised that they may be at an increased risk of sildenafil-associated adverse events including hypotension, visual changes, and priapism, and should promptly report any symptoms to their doctor.
Patients taking AGENERASE should be instructed **not** to use hormonal contraceptives because some birth control pills (those containing ethinyl estradiol/norethindrone) have been found to decrease the concentration of amprenavir. Therefore, patients receiving hormonal contraceptives should be instructed to use alternate contraceptive measures during therapy with AGENERASE.
High-fat meals may decrease the absorption of AGENERASE and should be avoided. AGENERASE may be taken with meals of normal fat content.
Patients should be informed that redistribution or accumulation of body fat may occur in patients receiving antiretroviral therapy and that the cause and long-term health effects of these conditions are not known at this time.
Adult and pediatric patients should be advised not to take supplemental vitamin E since the vitamin E content of AGENERASE exceeds the Reference Daily Intake (adults 30 IU, pediatrics approximately 10 IU).
Laboratory Tests: The combination of AGENERASE and low-dose ritonavir has been associated with elevations of cholesterol and triglycerides, SGOT (AST), and SGPT (ALT) in some patients. Appropriate laboratory testing should be considered prior to initiating combination therapy with AGENERASE and ritonavir capsules and at periodic intervals or if any clinical signs or symptoms of hyperlipidemia or elevated liver function tests occur during therapy. For comprehensive information concerning laboratory test alterations associated with ritonavir, physicians should refer to the complete prescribing information for NORVIR (ritonavir).
Drug Interactions: See also CONTRAINDICATIONS, WARNINGS, and CLINICAL PHARMACOLOGY: Drug Interactions.
AGENERASE is an inhibitor of cytochrome P450 3A4 metabolism and therefore should not be administered concurrently with medications with narrow therapeutic windows that are substrates of CYP3A4. There are other agents that may result in serious and/or life-threatening drug interactions (see CONTRAINDICATIONS and WARNINGS).
Use of alcoholic beverages is not recommended in patients treated with AGENERASE Oral Solution.
[See table 7 at top of page 1403]
[See table 8 on previous page and at left]
Carcinogenesis and Mutagenesis: Amprenavir was evaluated for carcinogenic potential by oral gavage administration to mice and rats for up to 104 weeks. Daily doses of 50, 275 to 300, and 500 to 600 mg/kg/day were administered to mice and doses of 50, 190, and 750 mg/kg/day were administered to rats. Results showed an increase in the incidence of benign hepatocellular adenomas and an increase in the combined incidence of hepatocellular adenomas plus carcinoma in males of both species at the highest doses tested. Female mice and rats were not affected. These observations were made at systemic exposures equivalent to approximately 2 times (mice) and 4 times (rats) the human exposure (based on $AUC_{0\text{-}24\ hr}$ measurement) at the recommended dose of 1,200 mg twice daily. Administration of amprenavir did not cause a statistically significant increase in the incidence of any other benign or malignant neoplasm in mice or rats. It is not known how predictive the results of rodent carcinogenicity studies may be for humans. However, amprenavir was not mutagenic or genotoxic in a battery of in vitro and in vivo assays including bacterial reverse mutation (Ames), mouse lymphoma, rat micronucleus, and chromosome aberrations in human lymphocytes.
Fertility: The effects of amprenavir on fertility and general reproductive performance were investigated in male rats (treated for 28 days before mating at doses producing up to twice the expected clinical exposure based on AUC comparisons) and female rats (treated for 15 days before mating through day 17 of gestation at doses producing up to 2 times the expected clinical exposure). Amprenavir did not impair mating or fertility of male or female rats and did not affect the development and maturation of sperm from treated rats. The reproductive performance of the F1 generation born to female rats given amprenavir was not different from control animals.
Pregnancy and Reproduction: AGENERASE Oral Solution is contraindicated during pregnancy due to the potential risk of toxicity to the fetus from the high propylene glycol content. Therefore, if AGENERASE is used in pregnant women, the AGENERASE Capsules formulation should be used (see complete prescribing information for AGENERASE Capsules).
Antiretroviral Pregnancy Registry: To monitor maternal-fetal outcomes of pregnant women exposed to AGENERASE, an Antiretroviral Pregnancy Registry has been established. Physicians are encouraged to register patients by calling 1-800-258-4263.
Nursing Mothers: The Centers for Disease Control and Prevention recommend that HIV-infected mothers not breastfeed their infants to avoid risking postnatal transmission of HIV. Although it is not known if amprenavir is excreted in human milk, amprenavir is secreted into the milk of lactating rats. Because of both the potential for HIV transmission and the potential for serious adverse reactions in nursing infants, **mothers should be instructed not to breastfeed if they are receiving AGENERASE.**
Pediatric Use: AGENERASE Oral Solution is contraindicated in infants and children below the age of 4 years due to the potential risk of toxicity from the excipient, propylene glycol (see CONTRAINDICATIONS and WARNINGS). Alcohol dehydrogenase (ADH), which metabolizes propylene glycol, is present in the human fetal liver at 2 months of gestational age, but at only 3% of adult activity.

Continued on next page

Product information on these pages is effective as of August 2004. Further information is available at: GlaxoSmithKline, PO Box 13398, Research Triangle Park, NC 27709. 1-888-825-5249. Corporate Web Site: www.gsk.com

Table 11. Grade 3/4 Laboratory Abnormalities Reported in ≥2% of Adult Patients in Open-Label Clinical Trials of AGENERASE Capsules in Combination with Ritonavir

Laboratory Abnormality (non-fasting specimens)	AGENERASE 1,200 mg plus Ritonavir 200 mg q.d.* (n = 101)	AGENERASE 600 mg plus Ritonavir 100 mg b.i.d.† (n = 239)
Hypertriglyceridemia (>750 mg/dL)	8%	13%
Hyperglycemia (>251 mg/dL)	2%	3%
AST (>5 × ULN)	3%	5%
ALT (>5 × ULN)	4%	4%
Amylase (>2 × ULN)	4%	3%

*Data from 2 open-label studies in treatment-naive patients also receiving abacavir/lamivudine.
† Data from 3 open-label studies in treatment-naive and treatment-experienced patients receiving combination antiretroviral therapy.

Table 12. Recommended Dosages of AGENERASE Oral Solution

Age/Weight Criteria	Dose b.i.d.	t.i.d.
4-12 years or 13-16 years and <50 kg	22.5 mg/kg (1.5 mL/kg) (maximum dose 2,800 mg per day)	17 mg/kg (1.1 mL/kg) (maximum dose 2,800 mg per day)
13-16 years and ≥50 kg or >16 years	1,400 mg	NA

Agenerase Oral Solution—Cont.

Although the data are limited, it appears that by 12 to 30 months of postnatal age, ADH activity is equal to or greater than that observed in adults.
Two hundred fifty-one patients aged 4 and above have received amprenavir as single or multiple doses in studies. An adverse event profile similar to that seen in adults was seen in pediatric patients.
Concurrent use of AGENERASE Oral Solution and NORVIR (ritonavir) Oral Solution is not recommended because the large amount of propylene glycol in AGENERASE Oral Solution and ethanol in NORVIR Oral Solution may compete for the same metabolic pathway for elimination. This combination has not been studied in pediatric patients.
Geriatric Use: Clinical studies of AGENERASE did not include sufficient numbers of patients aged 65 and over to determine whether they respond differently from younger adults. In general, dose selection for an elderly patient should be cautious, reflecting the greater frequency of decreased hepatic, renal, or cardiac function, and of concomitant disease or other drug therapy.

ADVERSE REACTIONS

In clinical studies, adverse events leading to amprenavir discontinuation occurred primarily during the first 12 weeks of therapy, and were mostly due to gastrointestinal events (nausea, vomiting, diarrhea, and abdominal pain/discomfort), which were mild to moderate in severity.
Skin rash occurred in 22% of patients treated with amprenavir in studies PROAB3001 and PROAB3006. Rashes were usually maculopapular and of mild or moderate intensity, some with pruritus. Rashes had a median onset of 11 days after amprenavir initiation and a median duration of 10 days. Skin rashes led to amprenavir discontinuation in approximately 3% of patients. In some patients with mild or moderate rash, amprenavir dosing was often continued without interruption; if interrupted, reintroduction of amprenavir generally did not result in rash recurrence.
Severe or life-threatening rash (Grade 3 or 4), including cases of Stevens-Johnson syndrome, occurred in approximately 1% of recipients of AGENASE (see WARNINGS). Amprenavir therapy should be discontinued for severe or life-threatening rashes and for moderate rashes accompanied by systemic symptoms.
[See table 9 on previous page]
Among amprenavir-treated patients in Phase 3 studies, 2 patients developed de novo diabetes mellitus, 1 patient developed a dorsocervical fat enlargement (buffalo hump), and 9 patients developed fat redistribution.
In studies PROAB3001 and PROAB3006, no increased frequency of Grade 3 or 4 AST, ALT, amylase, or bilirubin elevations was seen compared to controls.
Pediatric Patients: An adverse event profile similar to that seen in adults was seen in pediatric patients.
Concomitant Therapy with Ritonavir: Tables 10 and 11 present adverse clinical events and laboratory abnormalities observed in subjects who received AGENERASE plus ritonavir. Since the trials were small, open-label, of varying duration, and often included different patient populations, direct comparisons to the frequency of events with AGENERASE Capsules alone (see Table 9) cannot be made.
[See table 10 on previous page]
[See table 11 above]

OVERDOSAGE

There is no known antidote for AGENERASE. It is not known whether amprenavir can be removed by peritoneal dialysis or hemodialysis. If overdosage occurs, the patient should be monitored for evidence of toxicity and standard supportive treatment applied as necessary.
AGENERASE Oral Solution contains large amounts of propylene glycol. In the event of overdosage, monitoring and management of acid-base abnormalities is recommended. Propylene glycol can be removed by hemodialysis.

DOSAGE AND ADMINISTRATION

AGENERASE may be taken with or without food; however, a high-fat meal decreases the absorption of amprenavir and should be avoided (see CLINICAL PHARMACOLOGY: Effects of Food on Oral Absorption). **Adult and pediatric patients should be advised not to take supplemental vitamin E since the vitamin E content of AGENERASE Oral Solution exceeds the Reference Daily Intake (adults 30 IU, pediatrics approximately 10 IU) (see DESCRIPTION).**
The recommended dose of AGENERASE Oral Solution based on body weight and age is shown in Table 12. **Consideration should be given to switching patients from AGENERASE Oral Solution to AGENERASE Capsules as soon as they are able to take the capsule formulation (see WARNINGS).**
[See table 12 above]
Concomitant Therapy: Concurrent use of AGENERASE Oral Solution and NORVIR (ritonavir) Oral Solution is not recommended because the large amount of propylene glycol in AGENERASE Oral Solution and ethanol in NORVIR Oral Solution may compete for the same metabolic pathway for elimination.
Patients with Hepatic Impairment: AGENERASE Oral Solution is contraindicated in patients with hepatic failure (see CONTRAINDICATIONS).
Patients with hepatic impairment are at increased risk of propylene glycol-associated adverse events (see WARNINGS). AGENERASE Oral Solution should be used with caution in patients with hepatic impairment. Based on a study with AGENERASE Capsules, adult patients with a Child-Pugh score ranging from 5 to 8 should receive a reduced dose of AGENERASE Oral Solution of 513 mg (34 mL) twice daily, and adult patients with a Child-Pugh score ranging from 9 to 12 should receive a reduced dose of AGENERASE Oral Solution of 342 mg (23 mL) twice daily (see CLINICAL PHARMACOLOGY: Hepatic Insufficiency). AGENERASE Oral Solution has not been studied in children with hepatic impairment.
Renal Insufficiency: AGENERASE Oral Solution is contraindicated in patients with renal failure (see CONTRAINDICATIONS).
Patients with renal impairment are at increased risk of propylene glycol-associated adverse events. AGENERASE Oral Solution should be used with caution in patients with renal impairment (see WARNINGS).
AGENERASE Capsules and AGENERASE Oral Solution are not interchangeable on a milligram-per-milligram basis (see CLINICAL PHARMACOLOGY).

HOW SUPPLIED

AGENERASE Oral Solution, a clear, pale yellow to yellow, grape-bubblegum-peppermint-flavored liquid, contains 15 mg of amprenavir in each 1 mL.
Bottles of 240 mL with child-resistant closures (NDC 0173-0687-00). This product does not require reconstitution.
Store at controlled room temperature of 25°C (77°F) (see USP).
GlaxoSmithKline, Research Triangle Park, NC 27709
Licensed from Vertex Pharmaceuticals Incorporated
Cambridge, MA 02139

AGENERASE is a registered trademark of the GlaxoSmithKline group of companies.

February 2004/RL-2071
Shown in Product Identification Guide, page 314

ALBENZA® ℞
[al-ben' za]
brand of albendazole
Tablets

DESCRIPTION

Albenza (albendazole) is an orally administered broad-spectrum anthelmintic. Chemically it is Methyl 5-(propylthio)-2-benzimidazolecarbamate. Its molecular formula is $C_{12}H_{15}N_3O_2S$. Its molecular weight is 265.34.
Albendazole is a white to off-white powder. It is soluble in dimethylsulfoxide, strong acids and strong bases. It is slightly soluble in methanol, chloroform, ethyl acetate and acetonitrile. Albendazole is practically insoluble in water. Each white to off-white, film-coated tablet contains 200 mg of albendazole.
Inactive ingredients consist of: carnauba wax, hydroxypropyl methylcellulose, lactose monohydrate, magnesium stearate, microcrystalline cellulose, povidone, sodium lauryl sulfate, sodium saccharin, sodium starch glycolate, and starch.

CLINICAL PHARMACOLOGY

Pharmacokinetics

Absorption and Metabolism

Albendazole is poorly absorbed from the gastrointestinal tract due to its low aqueous solubility. Albendazole concentrations are negligible or undetectable in plasma as it is rapidly converted to the sulfoxide metabolite prior to reaching the systemic circulation. The systemic anthelmintic activity has been attributed to the primary metabolite, albendazole sulfoxide. Oral bioavailability appears to be enhanced when albendazole is coadministered with a fatty meal (estimated fat content 40 g) as evidenced by higher (up to 5-fold on average) plasma concentrations of albendazole sulfoxide as compared to the fasted state.
Maximal plasma concentrations of albendazole sulfoxide are typically achieved 2 to 5 hours after dosing and are on average 1.31 mcg/mL (range 0.46 to 1.58 mcg/mL) following oral doses of albendazole (400 mg) in six hydatid disease patients, when administered with a fatty meal. Plasma concentrations of albendazole sulfoxide increase in a dose-proportional manner over the therapeutic dose range following ingestion of a fatty meal (fat content 43.1 g). The mean apparent terminal elimination half-life of albendazole sulfoxide typically ranges from 8 to 12 hours in twenty-five normal subjects, as well as in fourteen hydatid and eight neurocysticercosis patients.
Following 4 weeks of treatment with albendazole (200 mg three times daily), twelve patients' plasma concentrations of albendazole sulfoxide were approximately 20% lower than those observed during the first half of the treatment period, suggesting that albendazole may induce its own metabolism.

Distribution

Albendazole sulfoxide is 70% bound to plasma protein and is widely distributed throughout the body; it has been detected in urine, bile, liver, cyst wall, cyst fluid, and cerebral spinal fluid (CSF). Concentrations in plasma were 3- to 10-fold and 2- to 4-fold higher than those simultaneously determined in cyst fluid and CSF, respectively. Limited *in vitro* and clinical data suggest that albendazole sulfoxide may be eliminated from cysts at a slower rate than observed in plasma.

Metabolism and Excretion

Albendazole is rapidly converted in the liver to the primary metabolite, albendazole sulfoxide, which is further metabolized to albendazole sulfone and other primary oxidative metabolites that have been identified in human urine. Following oral administration, albendazole has not been detected in human urine. Urinary excretion of albendazole sulfoxide is a minor elimination pathway with less than 1% of the dose recovered in the urine. Biliary elimination presumably accounts for a portion of the elimination as evidenced by biliary concentrations of albendazole sulfoxide similar to those achieved in plasma.

Special Populations

Patients with Impaired Renal Function: The pharmacokinetics of albendazole in patients with impaired renal function have not been studied. However, since renal elimination of albendazole and its primary metabolite, albendazole sulfoxide, is negligible, it is unlikely that clearance of these compounds would be altered in these patients.
Biliary Effects: In patients with evidence of extrahepatic obstruction (n=5), the systemic availability of albendazole sulfoxide was increased, as indicated by a 2-fold increase in maximum serum concentration and a 7-fold increase in area under the curve. The rate of absorption/conversion and elimination of albendazole sulfoxide appeared to be prolonged with mean T_{max} and serum elimination half-life values of 10 hours and 31.7 hours, respectively. Plasma concentrations of parent albendazole were measurable in only one of five patients.
Pediatrics: Following single-dose administration of 200 mg to 300 mg (approximately 10 mg/kg) albendazole to three fasted and two fed pediatric patients with hydatid cyst dis-

ease (age range 6 to 13 years), albendazole sulfoxide pharmacokinetics were similar to those observed in fed adults.

Elderly Patients: Although no studies have investigated the effect of age on albendazole sulfoxide pharmacokinetics, data in twenty-six hydatid cyst patients (up to 79 years) suggest pharmacokinetics similar to those in young healthy subjects.

Microbiology

The principal mode of action for albendazole is by its inhibitory effect on tubulin polymerization which results in the loss of cytoplasmic microtubules.

In the specified treatment indications albendazole appears to be active against the larval forms of the following organisms:

Echinococcus granulosus
Taenia solium

INDICATIONS AND USAGE

Albenza (albendazole) is indicated for the treatment of the following infections:

Neurocysticercosis. *Albenza* is indicated for the treatment of parenchymal neurocysticercosis due to active lesions caused by larval forms of the pork tapeworm, *Taenia solium*.

Lesions considered responsive to albendazole therapy appear as nonenhancing cysts with no surrounding edema on contrast-enhanced computerized tomography. Clinical studies in patients with lesions of this type demonstrate a 74% to 88% reduction in number of cysts; 40% to 70% of albendazole-treated patients showed resolution of all active cysts.

Hydatid disease. *Albenza* is indicated for the treatment of cystic hydatid disease of the liver, lung, and peritoneum, caused by the larval form of the dog tapeworm, *Echinococcus granulosus*.

This indication is based on combined clinical studies which demonstrated non-infectious cyst contents in approximately 80-90% of patients given *Albenza* for 3 cycles of therapy of 28 days each. (See **DOSAGE AND ADMINISTRATION**.)

Clinical cure (disappearance of cysts) was seen in approximately 30% of these patients, and improvement (reduction in cyst diameter of ≥25%) was seen in an additional 40%.

NOTE: When medically feasible, surgery is considered the treatment of choice for hydatid disease. When administering *Albenza* in the pre- or post-surgical setting, optimal killing of cyst contents is achieved when three courses of therapy have been given.

NOTE: The efficacy of albendazole in the therapy of alveolar hydatid disease caused by *Echinococcus multilocularis* has not been clearly demonstrated in clinical studies.

CONTRAINDICATIONS

Albenza (albendazole) is contraindicated in patients with known hypersensitivity to the benzimidazole class of compounds or any components of *Albenza*.

WARNINGS

Rare fatalities associated with the use of *Albenza* have been reported due to granulocytopenia or pancytopenia. (See **PRECAUTIONS**.) Blood counts should be monitored at the beginning of each 28-day cycle of therapy, and every 2 weeks while on therapy with albendazole. Albendazole may be continued if the total white blood cell count and absolute neutrophil count decrease appear modest and do not progress. Albendazole should not be used in pregnant women except in clinical circumstances where no alternative management is appropriate. Patients should not become pregnant for at least 1 month following cessation of albendazole therapy. If a patient becomes pregnant while taking this drug, albendazole should be discontinued immediately. If pregnancy occurs while taking this drug, the patient should be apprised of the potential hazard to the fetus.

PRECAUTIONS

General: Patients being treated for neurocysticercosis should receive appropriate steroid and anticonvulsant therapy as required. Oral or intravenous corticosteroids should be considered to prevent cerebral hypertensive episodes during the first week of anticysticeral therapy.

Cysticercosis may, in rare cases, involve the retina. Before initiating therapy for neurocysticercosis, the patient should be examined for the presence of retinal lesions. If such lesions are visualized, the need for anticysticeral therapy should be weighed against the possibility of retinal damage caused by albendazole-induced changes to the retinal lesion.

Information for Patients

Patients should be advised that:

- Albendazole may cause fetal harm, therefore, women of childbearing age should begin treatment after a negative pregnancy test.
- Women of childbearing age should be cautioned against becoming pregnant while on albendazole or within 1 month of completing treatment.
- During albendazole therapy, because of the possibility of harm to the liver or bone marrow, routine (every 2 weeks) monitoring of blood counts and liver function tests should take place.
- Albendazole should be taken with food.

Laboratory Tests

White Blood Cell Count: Albendazole has been shown to cause occasional (less than 1% of treated patients) reversible reductions in total white blood cell count. Rarely, more significant reductions may be encountered including granulocytopenia, agranulocytosis, or pancytopenia. Blood counts should be performed at the start of each 28-day treatment cycle and every 2 weeks during each 28-day cycle. Albendazole may be continued if the total white blood cell count decrease appears modest and does not progress.

Indication	Patient Weight	Dose	Duration
Hydatid Disease	60 kg or greater	400 mg b.i.d., with meals	28-day cycle followed by a 14-day albendazole-free interval, for a total of 3 cycles
	less than 60 kg	15 mg/kg/day given in divided doses b.i.d. with meals (maximum total daily dose 800 mg)	
	NOTE: When administering *Albenza* in the pre- or post-surgical setting, optimal killing of cyst contents is achieved when three courses of therapy have been given.		
Neurocysticercosis	60 kg or greater	400 mg b.i.d., with meals	8-30 days
	less than 60 kg	15 mg/kg/day given in divided doses b.i.d. with meals (maximum total daily dose 800 mg)	

Liver Function: In clinical trials, treatment with albendazole has been associated with mild to moderate elevations of hepatic enzymes in approximately 16% of patients. These have returned to normal upon discontinuation of therapy.

Liver function tests (transaminases) should be performed before the start of each treatment cycle and at least every 2 weeks during treatment. If enzymes are significantly increased, albendazole therapy should be discontinued. Therapy can be reinstituted when liver enzymes have returned to pretreatment levels, but laboratory tests should be performed frequently during repeat therapy.

Patients with abnormal liver function test results prior to commencing albendazole therapy should be carefully evaluated, since the drug is metabolized by the liver and has been associated with hepatotoxicity in a few patients.

Theophylline: Although single doses of albendazole have been shown not to inhibit theophylline metabolism (see **Drug Interactions**), albendazole does induce cytochrome P450 1A in human hepatoma cells. Therefore, it is recommended that plasma concentrations of theophylline be monitored during and after treatment with Albenza (albendazole).

Drug Interactions

Dexamethasone: Steady-state trough concentrations of albendazole sulfoxide were about 56% higher when 8 mg dexamethasone was coadministered with each dose of albendazole (15 mg/kg/day) in eight neurocysticercosis patients.

Praziquantel: In the fed state, praziquantel (40 mg/kg) increased mean maximum plasma concentration and area under the curve of albendazole sulfoxide by about 50% in healthy subjects (n=10) compared with a separate group of subjects (n=6) given albendazole alone. Mean T_{max} and mean plasma elimination half-life of albendazole sulfoxide were unchanged. The pharmacokinetics of praziquantel were unchanged following coadministration with albendazole (400 mg).

Cimetidine: Albendazole sulfoxide concentrations in bile and cystic fluid were increased (about 2-fold) in hydatid cyst patients treated with cimetidine (10 mg/kg/day) (n=7) compared with albendazole (20 mg/kg/day) alone (n=12). Albendazole sulfoxide plasma concentrations were unchanged 4 hours after dosing.

Theophylline: The pharmacokinetics of theophylline (aminophylline 5.8 mg/kg infused over 20 minutes) were unchanged following a single oral dose of albendazole (400 mg) in 6 healthy subjects.

Carcinogenesis, Mutagenesis, Impairment of Fertility

Long-term carcinogenicity studies were conducted in mice and rats. In the mouse study, albendazole was administered in the diet at doses of 25, 100 and 400 mg/kg/day (0.1, 0.5, and 2 times the recommended human dose based on body surface area in mg/m^2, respectively) for 108 weeks. In the rat study, albendazole was administered in the diet at doses of 3.5, 7, and 20 mg/kg/day (0.04, 0.08, and 0.21 times the recommended human dose based on body surface area in mg/m^2, respectively) for 117 weeks. There was no evidence of increased incidence of tumors in the treated mice and rats when compared to the control group.

In genotoxicity tests, albendazole was found negative in an Ames Salmonella/Microsome Plate mutation assay with and without metabolic activation or with and without preincubation, cell-mediated Chinese Hamster Ovary chromosomal aberration test and *in vivo* mouse micronucleus test. In the *in vitro* BALB/3T3 cells transformation assay, albendazole produced weak activity in the presence of metabolic activation while no activity was found in the absence of metabolic activation.

Albendazole did not adversely affect male or female fertility in the rat at an oral dose of 30 mg/kg/day (0.32 times the recommended human dose based on body surface area in mg/m^2).

Pregnancy

Teratogenic Effects–Pregnancy Category C: Albendazole has been shown to be teratogenic (to cause embryotoxicity and skeletal malformations) in pregnant rats and rabbits. The teratogenic response in the rat was shown at oral doses of 10 and 30 mg/kg/day (0.10 times and 0.32 times the recommended human dose based on body surface area in mg/m^2, respectively) during gestation days 6 to 15 and in pregnant rabbits at oral doses of 30 mg/kg/day (0.60 times the recommended human dose based on body surface area in mg/m^2) administered during gestation days 7 to 19. In the rabbit study, maternal toxicity (33% mortality) was noted at 30 mg/kg/day. In mice, no teratogenic effects were observed at oral doses up to 30 mg/kg/day (0.16 times the recommended human dose based on body surface area in mg/m^2), administered during gestation days 6 to 15.

There are no adequate and well-controlled studies of albendazole administration in pregnant women. Albendazole should be used during pregnancy only if the potential benefit justifies the potential risk to the fetus. (See **WARNINGS**.)

Nursing Mothers: Albendazole is excreted in animal milk. It is not known whether it is excreted in human milk. Because many drugs are excreted in human milk, caution should be exercised when albendazole is administered to a nursing woman.

Pediatric Use: Experience in children under the age of 6 years is limited. In hydatid disease, infection in infants and young children is uncommon, but no problems have been encountered in those who have been treated. In neurocysticercosis, infection is more frequently encountered. In five published studies involving pediatric patients as young as 1 year, no significant problems were encountered, and the efficacy appeared similar to the adult population.

Geriatric Use: Experience in patients 65 years of age or older is limited. The number of patients treated for either hydatid disease or neurocysticercosis is limited, but no problems associated with an older population have been observed.

ADVERSE REACTIONS

The adverse event profile of albendazole differs between hydatid disease and neurocysticercosis. Adverse events occurring with a frequency of ≥1% in either disease are described in the table below.

These symptoms were usually mild and resolved without treatment. Treatment discontinuations were predominantly due to leukopenia (0.7%) or hepatic abnormalities (3.8% in hydatid disease). The following incidence reflects events that were reported by investigators to be at least possibly or probably related to albendazole.

Adverse Event Incidence ≥1% in Hydatid Disease and Neurocysticercosis

Adverse Event	Hydatid Disease	Neurocysticercosis
Abnormal Liver Function Tests	15.6	<1.0
Abdominal Pain	6.0	0
Nausea/Vomiting	3.7	6.2
Headache	1.3	11.0
Dizziness/Vertigo	1.2	<1.0
Raised Intracranial Pressure	0	1.5
Meningeal Signs	0	1.0
Reversible Alopecia	1.6	<1.0
Fever	1.0	0

The following adverse events were observed at an incidence of <1%:

Continued on next page

Product information on these pages is effective as of August 2004. Further information is available at: GlaxoSmithKline, PO Box 13398, Research Triangle Park, NC 27709. 1-888-825-5249. Corporate Web Site: www.gsk.com

Albenza—Cont.

Hematologic: Leukopenia. There have been rare reports of granulocytopenia, pancytopenia, agranulocytosis, or thrombocytopenia. (See **WARNINGS.**)
Dermatologic: Rash, urticaria.
Hypersensitivity: Allergic reactions.
Renal: Acute renal failure related to albendazole therapy has been observed.

OVERDOSAGE

Significant toxicity and mortality were shown in male and female mice at doses exceeding 5,000 mg/kg; in rats, at estimated doses between 1,300 and 2,400 mg/kg; in hamsters, at doses exceeding 10,000 mg/kg; and in rabbits, at estimated doses between 500 and 1,250 mg/kg. In the animals, symptoms were demonstrated in a dose-response relationship and included diarrhea, vomiting, tachycardia, and respiratory distress.
One overdosage has been reported with Albenza (albendazole) in a patient who took at least 16 grams over 12 hours. No untoward effects were reported. In case of overdosage, symptomatic therapy (e.g., gastric lavage and activated charcoal) and general supportive measures are recommended.

DOSAGE AND ADMINISTRATION

Dosing of *Albenza* will vary, depending upon which of the following parasitic infections is being treated.
[See table at top of previous page]
Patients being treated for neurocysticercosis should receive appropriate steroid and anticonvulsant therapy as required. Oral or intravenous corticosteroids should be considered to prevent cerebral hypertensive episodes during the first week of treatment.

HOW SUPPLIED

Albenza (albendazole) is supplied as 200 mg, white to off-white, circular, biconvex, bevel-edged, film-coated Tiltab® tablets in bottles of 112.
NDC 0007-5500-40 .... Bottles of 112
Store between 20° and 25°C (68° and 77°F).
GlaxoSmithKline, Research Triangle Park, NC 27709

September 2001/AL:L3
Shown in Product Identification Guide, page 314

AMERGE® ℞
[ə-merj']
(naratriptan hydrochloride)
Tablets

DESCRIPTION

AMERGE Tablets contain naratriptan as the hydrochloride, which is a selective 5-hydroxytryptamine$_1$ receptor subtype agonist. Naratriptan hydrochloride is chemically designated as N-methyl-3-(1-methyl-4-piperidinyl)-1H-indole-5-ethanesulfonamide monohydrochloride.
The empirical formula is $C_{17}H_{25}N_3O_2S \bullet HCl$, representing a molecular weight of 371.93. Naratriptan hydrochloride is a white to pale yellow powder that is readily soluble in water. Each AMERGE Tablet for oral administration contains 1.11 or 2.78 mg of naratriptan hydrochloride equivalent to 1 or 2.5 mg of naratriptan, respectively. Each tablet also contains the inactive ingredients croscarmellose sodium; hypromellose; lactose; magnesium stearate; microcrystalline cellulose; triacetin; and titanium dioxide, iron oxide yellow, and indigo carmine aluminum lake (FD&C Blue No. 2) for coloring.

CLINICAL PHARMACOLOGY

Mechanism of Action: Naratriptan binds with high affinity to 5-HT_{1D} and 5-HT_{1B} receptors and has no significant affinity or pharmacological activity at 5-HT_{2-4} receptor subtypes or at adrenergic α_1, α_2, or β; dopaminergic D_1 or D_2; muscarinic; or benzodiazepine receptors.
The therapeutic activity of naratriptan in migraine is generally attributed to its agonist activity at 5-$HT_{1D/1B}$ receptors. Two current theories have been proposed to explain the efficacy of 5-$HT_{1D/1B}$ receptor agonists in migraine. One theory suggests that activation of 5-$HT_{1D/1B}$ receptors located on intracranial blood vessels, including those on the arteriovenous anastomoses, leads to vasoconstriction, which is correlated with the relief of migraine headache. The other hypothesis suggests that activation of 5-$HT_{1D/1B}$ receptors on sensory nerve endings in the trigeminal system results in the inhibition of pro-inflammatory neuropeptide release.
In the anesthetized dog, naratriptan has been shown to reduce the carotid arterial blood flow with little or no effect on arterial blood pressure or total peripheral resistance. While the effect on blood flow was selective for the carotid arterial bed, increases in vascular resistance of up to 30% were seen in the coronary arterial bed. Naratriptan has also been shown to inhibit trigeminal nerve activity in rat and cat. In 10 human subjects with suspected coronary artery disease (CAD) undergoing coronary artery catheterization, there was a 1% to 10% reduction in coronary artery diameter following subcutaneous injection of 1.5 mg of naratriptan.
Pharmacokinetics: Naratriptan tablets are well absorbed, with about 70% oral bioavailability. Following administration of a 2.5-mg tablet orally, the peak concentrations are obtained in 2 to 3 hours. After administration of 1- or 2.5-mg tablets, the C_{max} is somewhat (about 50%) higher in women (not corrected for milligram-per-kilogram dose) than in men. During a migraine attack, absorption was slower, with a T_{max} of 3 to 4 hours. Food does not affect the pharmacokinetics of naratriptan. Naratriptan displays linear kinetics over the therapeutic dose range.
The steady-state volume of distribution of naratriptan is 170 L. Plasma protein binding is 28% to 31% over the concentration range of 50 to 1,000 ng/mL.
Naratriptan is predominantly eliminated in urine, with 50% of the dose recovered unchanged and 30% as metabolites in urine. In vitro, naratriptan is metabolized by a wide range of cytochrome P450 isoenzymes into a number of inactive metabolites.
The mean elimination half-life of naratriptan is 6 hours. The systemic clearance of naratriptan is 6.6 mL/min/kg. The renal clearance (220 mL/min) exceeds glomerular filtration rate, indicating active tubular secretion. Repeat administration of naratriptan tablets does not result in drug accumulation.
Special Populations: ***Age:*** A small decrease in clearance (approximately 26%) was observed in healthy elderly subjects (65 to 77 years) compared to younger patients, resulting in slightly higher exposure (see PRECAUTIONS).
Race: The effect of race on the pharmacokinetics of naratriptan has not been examined.
Renal Impairment: Clearance of naratriptan was reduced by 50% in patients with moderate renal impairment (creatinine clearance, 18 to 39 mL/min) compared to the normal group. Decrease in clearances resulted in an increase of mean half-life from 6 hours (healthy) to 11 hours (range, 7 to 20 hours). The mean C_{max} increased by approximately 40%. The effects of severe renal impairment (creatinine clearance, ≤15 mL/min) on the pharmacokinetics of naratriptan has not been assessed (see CONTRAINDICATIONS and DOSAGE AND ADMINISTRATION).
Hepatic Impairment: Clearance of naratriptan was decreased by 30% in patients with moderate hepatic impairment (Child-Pugh grade A or B). This resulted in an approximately 40% increase in the half-life (range, 8 to 16 hours). The effects of severe hepatic impairment (Child-Pugh grade C) on the pharmacokinetics of naratriptan have not been assessed (see CONTRAINDICATIONS and DOSAGE AND ADMINISTRATION).
Drug Interactions: In normal volunteers, coadministration of single doses of naratriptan tablets and alcohol did not result in substantial modification of naratriptan pharmacokinetic parameters.
From population pharmacokinetic analyses, coadministration of naratriptan and fluoxetine, beta-blockers, or tricyclic antidepressants did not affect the clearance of naratriptan.
Naratriptan does not inhibit monoamine oxidase (MAO) enzymes and is a poor inhibitor of P450; metabolic interactions between naratriptan and drugs metabolized by P450 or MAO are therefore unlikely.
Oral Contraceptives: Oral contraceptives reduced clearance by 32% and volume of distribution by 22%, resulting in slightly higher concentrations of naratriptan. Hormone replacement therapy had no effect on pharmacokinetics in older female patients.
Smoking increased the clearance of naratriptan by 30%.

CLINICAL TRIALS

The efficacy of AMERGE Tablets in the acute treatment of migraine headaches was evaluated in 6 randomized, double-blind, placebo-controlled studies of which 4 used the recommended dosing regimen and were conducted as outpatient trials. Three of these studies enrolled adult patients who were predominantly female (86%) and Caucasian (96%) with a mean age of 41 (range, 18 to 65). One study enrolled adolescents with a mean age of 14 (range, 12 to 17). In the adolescent study, 54% of the patients were female and 89% were Caucasian. In all studies, patients were instructed to treat at least 1 moderate to severe headache. Headache response, defined as a reduction in headache severity from moderate or severe pain to mild or no pain, was assessed up to 4 hours after dosing. Associated symptoms such as nausea, vomiting, photophobia, and phonophobia were also assessed. Maintenance of response was assessed for up to 24 hours postdose. A second dose of AMERGE Tablets or other medication was allowed 4 to 24 hours after the initial treatment for recurrent headache. The frequency and time to use of these additional treatments were also determined.
In all 3 trials in adults utilizing the recommended dosage regimen and outpatient use, the percentage of patients achieving headache response 4 hours after treatment, the primary outcome measure, was significantly greater among patients receiving AMERGE compared to those who received placebo. In all studies, response to 2.5 mg was numerically greater than response to 1 mg and in the largest of the 3 studies, there was a statistically significant greater percentage of patients with headache response at 4 hours in the 2.5-mg group compared to the 1-mg group. The results are summarized in Table 1.
[See table 1 below]
In the single study in adolescents, there were no statistically significant differences between any of the treatment groups. The headache response rates at 4 hours (n) were 65% (n = 74), 67% (n = 78), and 64% (n = 70) for placebo, 1-mg, and 2.5-mg groups, respectively.
Comparisons of drug performance based upon results obtained in different clinical trials are never reliable. Because studies are conducted at different times, with different samples of patients, by different investigators, employing different criteria and/or different interpretations of the same criteria, under different conditions (dose, dosing regimen, etc.), quantitative estimates of treatment response and the timing of response may be expected to vary considerably from study to study.
The estimated probability of achieving an initial headache response in adults over the 4 hours following treatment is depicted in Figure 1.

Figure 1. Estimated Probability of Achieving Initial Headache Response Within 4 Hours*

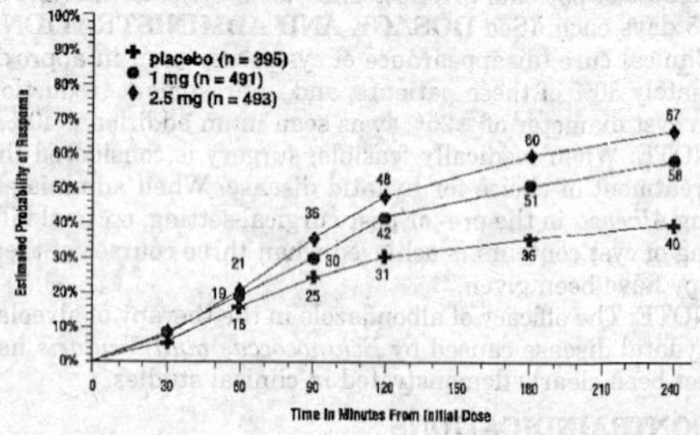

*The figure shows the probability over time of obtaining headache response (no or mild pain) following treatment with AMERGE tablets. The averages displayed are based on pooled data from the 3 controlled clinical trials providing evidence of efficacy (Studies 1, 2, and 3). In this Kaplan-Meier plot, patients not achieving response within 240 minutes were censored at 240 minutes.

For patients with migraine-associated nausea, photophobia, and phonophobia at baseline, there was a lower incidence of these symptoms 4 hours following administration of 1- and 2.5-mg AMERGE Tablets compared to placebo.
Four to 24 hours following the initial dose of study treatment, patients were allowed to use additional treatment for pain relief in the form of a second dose of study treatment or other medication. The estimated probability of patients taking a second dose or other medication for migraine over the 24 hours following the initial dose of study treatment is summarized in Figure 2.

Figure 2. Estimated Prbability of Patients Taking a Second Dose of AMERGE Tablets or Other Medication for Migraine Over the 24 Hours Following the Initial Dose of Study Treatment *

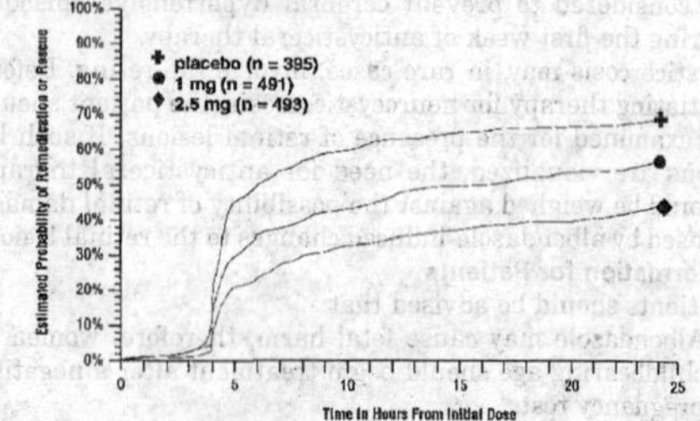

*Kaplan-Meier plot based on data obtained in the 3 controlled clinical trials (Studies 1, 2, and 3) providing evidence of efficacy with patients not using additional treatments censored at 24 hours. The plot also includes patients who had no response to the initial dose. Remedication was discouraged prior to 4 hours postdose.

There is no evidence that doses of 5 mg provide a greater effect than 2.5 mg. There was no evidence to suggest that treatment with AMERGE was associated with an increase in the severity or frequency of migraine attacks. The efficacy of AMERGE Tablets was unaffected by presence of aura; gender, age, or weight of the patient; oral contraceptive use; or concomitant use of common migraine prophylactic drugs

Table 1. Percentage of Adult Patients With Headache Response (Mild or No Headache) 4 Hours Following Treatment

	Placebo	AMERGE 1.0 mg	AMERGE 2.5 mg
Study 1	34% (n = 122)	50%* (n = 117)	60%* (n = 127)
Study 2	27% (n = 104)	52%* (n = 208)	66%*† (n = 199)
Study 3	32% (n = 169)	54%* (n = 166)	65%* (n = 167)

*p<0.05 in comparison with placebo.
†p<0.05 in comparison with 1 mg.

(e.g., beta-blockers, calcium channel blockers, tricyclic antidepressants). There was insufficient data to assess the impact of race on efficacy.

INDICATIONS AND USAGE

AMERGE Tablets are indicated for the acute treatment of migraine attacks with or without aura in adults.

AMERGE Tablets are not intended for the prophylactic therapy of migraine or for use in the management of hemiplegic or basilar migraine (see CONTRAINDICATIONS). Safety and effectiveness of AMERGE Tablets have not been established for cluster headache, which is present in an older, predominantly male population.

CONTRAINDICATIONS

AMERGE Tablets should not be given to patients with history, symptoms, or signs of ischemic cardiac, cerebrovascular, or peripheral vascular syndromes. In addition, patients with other significant underlying cardiovascular diseases should not receive AMERGE Tablets. Ischemic cardiac syndromes include, but are not limited to, angina pectoris of any type (e.g., stable angina of effort and vasospastic forms of angina such as the Prinzmetal variant), all forms of myocardial infarction, and silent myocardial ischemia. Cerebrovascular syndromes include, but are not limited to, strokes of any type as well as transient ischemic attacks. Peripheral vascular disease includes, but is not limited to, ischemic bowel disease (see WARNINGS).

Because AMERGE Tablets may increase blood pressure, they should not be given to patients with uncontrolled hypertension (see WARNINGS).

AMERGE Tablets are contraindicated in patients with severe renal impairment (creatinine clearance, <15 mL/min) (see CLINICAL PHARMACOLOGY and DOSAGE AND ADMINISTRATION).

AMERGE Tablets are contraindicated in patients with severe hepatic impairment (Child-Pugh grade C) (see CLINICAL PHARMACOLOGY and DOSAGE AND ADMINISTRATION).

AMERGE Tablets should not be administered to patients with hemiplegic or basilar migraine.

AMERGE Tablets should not be used within 24 hours of treatment with another 5-HT$_1$ agonist, an ergotamine-containing or ergot-type medication like dihydroergotamine or methysergide.

AMERGE Tablets are contraindicated in patients with hypersensitivity to naratriptan or any of the components.

WARNINGS

AMERGE Tablets should only be used where a clear diagnosis of migraine has been established.

Risk of Myocardial Ischemia and/or Infarction and Other Adverse Cardiac Events: Because of the potential of this class of compounds (5-HT$_{1B/1D}$ agonists) to cause coronary vasospasm, naratriptan should not be given to patients with documented ischemic or vasospastic coronary artery disease (CAD) (see CONTRAINDICATIONS). It is strongly recommended that 5-HT$_1$ agonists (including naratriptan) not be given to patients in whom unrecognized CAD is predicted by the presence of risk factors (e.g., hypertension, hypercholesterolemia, smoker, obesity, diabetes, strong family history of CAD, female with surgical or physiological menopause, or male over 40 years of age) unless a cardiovascular evaluation provides satisfactory clinical evidence that the patient is reasonably free of coronary artery and ischemic myocardial disease or other significant underlying cardiovascular disease. The sensitivity of cardiac diagnostic procedures to detect cardiovascular disease or predisposition to coronary artery vasospasm is modest, at best. If, during the cardiovascular evaluation, the patient's medical history, electrocardiographic, or other investigations reveal findings indicative of, or consistent with, coronary artery vasospasm or myocardial ischemia, naratriptan should not be administered (see CONTRAINDICATIONS).

For patients with risk factors predictive of CAD, who are determined to have a satisfactory cardiovascular evaluation, it is strongly recommended that administration of the first dose of naratriptan take place in the setting of a physician's office or similar medically staffed and equipped facility. Because cardiac ischemia can occur in the absence of clinical symptoms, consideration should be given to obtaining on the first occasion of use an electrocardiogram (ECG) during the interval immediately following administration of AMERGE Tablets, in these patients with risk factors.

It is recommended that patients who are intermittent long-term users of 5-HT$_1$ agonists, including AMERGE Tablets, and who have or acquire risk factors predictive of CAD, as described above, undergo periodic cardiovascular evaluation as they continue to use AMERGE Tablets.

The systematic approach described above is intended to reduce the likelihood that patients with unrecognized cardiovascular disease will be inadvertently exposed to naratriptan.

Cardiac Events and Fatalities Associated With 5-HT$_1$ Agonists: Naratriptan can cause coronary artery vasospasm (see CLINICAL PHARMACOLOGY). Serious adverse cardiac events, including acute myocardial infarction, life-threatening disturbances of cardiac rhythm, and death have been reported within a few hours following the administration of 5-HT$_1$ agonists. Considering the extent of use of 5-HT$_1$ agonists in patients with migraine, the incidence of these events is extremely low.

Premarketing Experience With AMERGE Tablets: Among approximately 3,500 patients with migraine who participated in premarketing clinical trials of naratriptan tablets, 4 patients treated with single oral doses of naratriptan ranging from 1 to 10 mg experienced asymptomatic ischemic ECG changes with at least 1, who took 7.5 mg, likely due to coronary vasospasm.

Cerebrovascular Events and Fatalities With 5-HT$_1$ Agonists: Cerebral hemorrhage, subarachnoid hemorrhage, stroke, and other cerebrovascular events have been reported in patients treated with 5-HT$_1$ agonists, and some have resulted in fatalities. In a number of cases, it appears possible that the cerebrovascular events were primary, the agonist having been administered in the incorrect belief that the symptoms experienced were a consequence of migraine, when they were not. It should be noted that patients with migraine may be at increased risk of certain cerebrovascular events (e.g., stroke, hemorrhage, transient ischemic attack).

Other Vasospasm-Related Events: 5-HT$_1$ agonists may cause vasospastic reactions other than coronary artery spasm. Both peripheral vascular ischemia and colonic ischemia with abdominal pain and bloody diarrhea have been reported with naratriptan.

Increase in Blood Pressure: In healthy volunteers, dose-related increases in systemic blood pressure have been observed after administration of up to 20 mg of oral naratriptan. At the recommended doses, the elevations are generally small, although an increase of systolic pressure of 32 mmHg was seen in 1 patient following a single 2.5-mg dose. The effect may be more pronounced in the elderly and hypertensive patients. A patient who was mildly hypertensive (the baseline blood pressure was 150/98) experienced a significant increase in blood pressure to 204/144 mmHg 225 minutes after administration of a 10-mg oral dose. Significant elevation in blood pressure, including hypertensive crisis, has been reported on rare occasions in patients receiving 5-HT$_1$ agonists with and without a history of hypertension. Naratriptan is contraindicated in patients with uncontrolled hypertension (see CONTRAINDICATIONS).

An 18% increase in mean pulmonary artery pressure and an 8% increase in mean aortic pressure was seen following dosing with 1.5 mg of subcutaneous naratriptan in a study evaluating 10 subjects with suspected CAD undergoing cardiac catheterization.

Hypersensitivity: Hypersensitivity (anaphylaxis/anaphylactoid) reactions may occur in patients receiving naratriptan. Such reactions can be life threatening or fatal. In general, hypersensitivity reactions to drugs are more likely to occur in individuals with a history of sensitivity to multiple allergens (see CONTRAINDICATIONS).

PRECAUTIONS

General: Chest discomfort (including pain, pressure, heaviness, tightness) has been reported after administration of 5-HT$_1$ agonists, including AMERGE Tablets. These events have not been associated with arrhythmias or ischemic ECG changes in clinical trials with AMERGE Tablets. Because naratriptan may cause coronary artery vasospasm, patients who experience signs or symptoms suggestive of angina following naratriptan should be evaluated for the presence of CAD or a predisposition to Prinzmetal variant angina before receiving additional doses of naratriptan, and should be monitored electrocardiographically if dosing is resumed and similar symptoms recur. Similarly, patients who experience other symptoms or signs suggestive of decreased arterial flow, such as ischemic bowel syndrome or Raynaud syndrome following naratriptan administration should be evaluated for atherosclerosis or predisposition to vasospasm (see CONTRAINDICATIONS and WARNINGS).

AMERGE Tablets should also be administered with caution to patients with diseases that may alter the absorption, metabolism, or excretion of drugs, such as impaired renal or hepatic function (see CLINICAL PHARMACOLOGY, CONTRAINDICATIONS, and DOSAGE AND ADMINISTRATION).

Care should be taken to exclude other potentially serious neurological conditions before treating headache in patients not previously diagnosed with migraine or who experience a headache that is atypical for them. There have been rare reports where patients received 5-HT$_1$ agonists for severe headaches that were subsequently shown to have been secondary to an evolving neurologic lesion (see WARNINGS).

For a given attack, if a patient has no response to the first dose of AMERGE, the diagnosis of migraine should be reconsidered before administration of a second dose.

Binding to Melanin-Containing Tissues: In rats treated with a single oral dose (10 mg/kg) of radiolabeled naratriptan, the elimination half-life of radioactivity from the eye was 90 days, suggesting that naratriptan and/or its metabolites may bind to the melanin of the eye. Because there could be accumulation in melanin-rich tissues over time, this raises the possibility that naratriptan could cause toxicity in these tissues after extended use. Although no systematic monitoring of ophthalmologic function was undertaken in clinical trials, and no specific recommendations for ophthalmologic monitoring are offered, prescribers should be aware of the possibility of long-term ophthalmologic effects.

Changes in the Precorneal Tear Film: Dogs receiving oral naratriptan showed transient changes in the precorneal tear film. Corneal stippling was seen at the lowest dose tested, 1 mg/kg/day, and occurred intermittently from day 1 throughout the first 2 to 3 weeks of treatment. Although a no-effect dose was not established, the exposure at the lowest dose tested was approximately 5 times the human exposure after a 5-mg oral dose.

Information for Patients: See PATIENT INFORMATION at the end of this labeling for the text of the separate leaflet provided for patients.

Laboratory Tests: No specific laboratory tests are recommended for monitoring patients prior to and/or after treatment with AMERGE Tablets.

Drug Interactions: Ergot-containing drugs have been reported to cause prolonged vasospastic reactions. Because there is a theoretical basis that these effects may be additive, use of ergotamine-containing or ergot-type medications (like dihydroergotamine or methysergide) and naratriptan within 24 hours is contraindicated (see CONTRAINDICATIONS).

The administration of naratriptan with other 5-HT$_1$ agonists has not been evaluated in migraine patients. Because their vasospastic effects may be additive, coadministration of naratriptan and other 5-HT$_1$ agonists within 24 hours of each other is not recommended (see CONTRAINDICATIONS).

Selective serotonin reuptake inhibitors (SSRIs) (e.g., fluoxetine, fluvoxamine, paroxetine, sertraline) have been reported, rarely, to cause weakness, hyperreflexia, and incoordination when coadministered with 5-HT$_1$ agonists. If concomitant treatment with naratriptan and an SSRI is clinically warranted, appropriate observation of the patient is advised.

Drug/Laboratory Test Interactions: AMERGE Tablets are not known to interfere with commonly employed clinical laboratory tests.

Carcinogenesis, Mutagenesis, Impairment of Fertility: ***Carcinogenesis:*** Lifetime carcinogenicity studies, 104 weeks in duration, were carried out in mice and rats by oral gavage. There was no evidence of an increase in tumors related to naratriptan administration in mice receiving up to 200 mg/kg/day. That dose was associated with a plasma area-under-the-curve (AUC) exposure that was 110 times the exposure in humans receiving the maximum recommended daily dose of 5 mg. Two rat studies were conducted, 1 using a standard diet and the other a nitrite-supplemented diet (naratriptan can be nitrosated in vitro to form a mutagenic product that has been detected in the stomachs of rats fed a high nitrite diet). Doses of 5, 20, and 90 mg/kg were associated with week 13 AUC exposures that in the standard diet study were 7, 40, and 236 times, respectively, and in the nitrite-supplemented diet study were 7, 29, and 180 times, respectively, the exposure attained in humans given the maximum recommended daily dose of 5 mg. In both studies, there was an increase in the incidence of thyroid follicular hyperplasia in high-dose males and females and in thyroid follicular adenomas in high-dose males. In the standard diet study only, there was also an increase in the incidence of benign c-cell adenomas in the thyroid of high-dose males and females. The exposures achieved at the no-effect dose for thyroid tumors were 40 (standard diet) and 29 (nitrite-supplemented diet) times the exposure achieved in humans receiving the maximum recommended daily dose of 5 mg. In the nitrite-supplemented diet study only, the incidence of benign lymphocytic thymoma was increased in all treated groups of females. It was not determined if the nitrosated product is systemically absorbed. However, no changes were seen in the stomachs of rats in that study.

Mutagenesis: Naratriptan was not mutagenic when tested in 2 gene mutation assays, the Ames test and the in vitro thymidine locus mouse lymphoma assay. It was not clastogenic in 2 cytogenetics assays, the in vitro human lymphocyte assay and the in vivo mouse micronucleus assay. Naratriptan can be nitrosated in vitro to form a mutagenic product (WHO nitrosation assay) that has been detected in the stomachs of rats fed a nitrite-supplemented diet.

Impairment of Fertility: In a reproductive toxicity study in which male and female rats were dosed prior to and throughout the mating period with 10, 60, 170, or 340 mg/kg/day (plasma exposures [AUC] approximately 11, 70, 230, and 470 times, respectively, the human exposure at the maximum recommended daily dose [MRDD] of 5 mg), there was a treatment-related decrease in the number of females exhibiting normal estrous cycles at doses of 170 mg/kg/day or greater and an increase in preimplantation loss at 60 mg/kg/day or greater. In high-dose group males, testicular/epididymal atrophy accompanied by spermatozoa depletion reduced mating success and may have contributed to the observed preimplantation loss. The exposures achieved at the no-effect doses for preimplantation loss, anestrus, and testicular effects were approximately 11, 70, and 230 times, respectively, the exposures in humans receiving the MRDD.

In a study in which rats were dosed orally with 10, 60, or 340 mg/kg/day for 6 months, changes in the female reproductive tract including atrophic or cystic ovaries and anestrus were seen at the high dose. The exposure at the no-effect dose of 60 mg/kg was approximately 85 times the exposure in humans receiving the MRDD.

Continued on next page

Product information on these pages is effective as of August 2004. Further information is available at: GlaxoSmithKline, PO Box 13398, Research Triangle Park, NC 27709. 1-888-825-5249. Corporate Web Site: www.gsk.com

Amerge—Cont.

Pregnancy: Pregnancy Category C. There are no adequate and well-controlled studies in pregnant women; therefore, naratriptan should be used during pregnancy only if the potential benefit justifies the potential risk to the fetus.

To monitor fetal outcomes of pregnant women exposed to AMERGE, GlaxoSmithKline maintains a Naratriptan Pregnancy Registry. Healthcare providers are encouraged to register patients by calling (800) 336-2176.

In reproductive toxicity studies in rats and rabbits, oral administration of naratriptan was associated with developmental toxicity (embryolethality, fetal abnormalities, pup mortality, offspring growth retardation) at doses producing maternal plasma drug exposures as low as 11 and 2.5 times, respectively, the exposure in humans receiving the MRDD of 5 mg.

When pregnant rats were administered naratriptan during the period of organogenesis at doses of 10, 60, or 340 mg/kg/day, there was a dose-related increase in embryonic death, with a statistically significant difference at the highest dose, and incidences of fetal structural variations (incomplete/irregular ossification of skull bones, sternebrae, ribs) were increased at all doses. The maternal plasma exposures (AUC) at these doses were approximately 11, 70, and 470 times the exposure in humans at the MRDD. The high dose was maternally toxic, as evidenced by decreased maternal body weight gain during gestation. A no-effect dose for developmental toxicity in rats exposed during organogenesis was not established.

When doses of 1, 5, or 30 mg/kg/day were given to pregnant Dutch rabbits throughout organogenesis, the incidence of a specific fetal skeletal malformation (fused sternebrae) was increased at the high dose, and increased incidences of embryonic death and fetal variations (major blood vessel variations, supernumerary ribs, incomplete skeletal ossification) were observed at all doses (4, 20, and 120 times, respectively, the MRDD on a body surface area basis). Maternal toxicity (decreased body weight gain) was evident at the high dose in this study. In a similar study in New Zealand White rabbits (1, 5, or 30 mg/kg/day throughout organogenesis), decreased fetal weights and increased incidences of fetal skeletal variations were observed at all doses (maternal exposures equivalent to 2.5, 19, and 140 times exposure in humans receiving the MRDD), while maternal body weight gain was reduced at 5 mg/kg or greater. A no-effect dose for developmental toxicity in rabbits exposed during organogenesis was not established.

When female rats were treated with 10, 60, or 340 mg/kg/day during late gestation and lactation, offspring behavioral impairment (tremors) and decreased offspring viability and growth were observed at doses of 60 mg/kg or greater, while maternal toxicity occurred only at the highest dose. Maternal exposures at the no-effect dose for developmental effects in this study were approximately 11 times the exposure in humans receiving the MRDD.

Nursing Mothers: Naratriptan-related material is excreted in the milk of rats. Therefore, caution should be exercised when considering the administration of AMERGE Tablets to a nursing woman.

Pediatric Use: Safety and effectiveness of AMERGE Tablets in pediatric patients (younger than 18 years) have not been established.

One randomized, placebo-controlled clinical trial evaluating oral naratriptan (0.25 to 2.5 mg) in pediatric patients aged 12 to 17 years evaluated a total of 300 adolescent migraineurs. This study did not establish the efficacy of oral naratriptan compared to placebo in the treatment of migraine in adolescents (see CLINICAL TRIALS). Adverse events observed in this clinical trial were similar in nature to those reported in clinical trials in adults.

Geriatric Use: The use of AMERGE Tablets in elderly patients is not recommended.

Naratriptan is known to be substantially excreted by the kidney, and the risk of adverse reactions to this drug may be greater in elderly patients who have reduced renal function. In addition, elderly patients are more likely to have decreased hepatic function; they are at higher risk for CAD; and blood pressure increases may be more pronounced in the elderly. Clinical studies of AMERGE Tablets did not include patients over 65 years of age.

ADVERSE REACTIONS

Serious cardiac events, including some that have been fatal, have occurred following the use of 5-HT$_1$ agonists. These events are extremely rare and most have been reported in patients with risk factors predictive of CAD. Events reported have included coronary artery vasospasm, transient myocardial ischemia, myocardial infarction, ventricular tachycardia, and ventricular fibrillation (see CONTRAINDICATIONS, WARNINGS, and PRECAUTIONS).

Incidence in Controlled Clinical Trials: The most common adverse events were paresthesias, dizziness, drowsiness, malaise/fatigue, and throat/neck symptoms, which occurred at a rate of 2% and at least 2 times placebo rate. Since patients treated only 1 to 3 headaches in the controlled clinical trials, the opportunity for discontinuation of therapy in response to an adverse event was limited. In a long-term, open-label study where patients were allowed to treat multiple migraine attacks for up to 1 year, 15 patients (3.6%) discontinued treatment due to adverse events.

Table 2 lists adverse events that occurred in 5 placebo-controlled clinical trials of approximately 1,752 exposures to placebo and AMERGE Tablets in adult migraine patients. The events cited reflect experience gained under closely monitored conditions of clinical trials in a highly selected patient population. In actual clinical practice or in other clinical trials, these frequency estimates may not apply, as the conditions of use, reporting behavior, and the kinds of patients treated may differ. Only events that occurred at a frequency of 2% or more in the group treated with AMERGE Tablets 2.5 mg and were more frequent in that group than in the placebo group are included in Table 2. From this table, it appears that many of these adverse events are dose related.

[See table 2 below]

One event (vomiting) present in more than 1% of patients receiving AMERGE Tablets occurred more frequently on placebo than on naratriptan 2.5 mg.

AMERGE Tablets are generally well tolerated. Most adverse reactions were mild and transient.

The incidence of adverse events in placebo-controlled clinical trials was not affected by age or weight of the patients, duration of headache prior to treatment, presence of aura, use of prophylactic medications, or tobacco use. There was insufficient data to assess the impact of race on the incidence of adverse events.

Other Events Observed in Association With the Administration of AMERGE Tablets: In the paragraphs that follow, the frequencies of less commonly reported adverse clinical events are presented. Because the reports include events observed in open and uncontrolled studies, the role of AMERGE Tablets in their causation cannot be reliably determined. Furthermore, variability associated with adverse event reporting, the terminology used to describe adverse events, etc. limit the value of the quantitative frequency estimates provided. Event frequencies are calculated as the number of patients reporting an event divided by the total number of patients (n = 3,557) exposed to oral naratriptan doses up to 10 mg. All reported events are included except those already listed in the previous table, those too general to be informative, and those not reasonably associated with the use of the drug. Events are further classified within body system categories and enumerated in order of decreasing frequency using the following definitions: frequent adverse events are those occurring in at least 1/100 patients, infrequent adverse events are those occurring in 1/100 to 1/1,000 patients, and rare adverse events are those occurring in fewer than 1/1,000 patients.

Atypical Sensations: Frequent were warm/cold temperature sensations. Infrequent were feeling strange and burning/stinging sensation.

Cardiovascular: Infrequent were palpitations, increased blood pressure, tachyarrhythmias, and abnormal ECG (PR prolongation, QT$_c$ prolongation, ST/T wave abnormalities, premature ventricular contractions, atrial flutter, or atrial fibrillation), and syncope. Rare were bradycardia, varicosities, hypotension, and heart murmurs.

Ear, Nose, and Throat: Frequent were ear, nose, and throat infections. Infrequent were phonophobia, sinusitis, upper respiratory inflammation, and tinnitus. Rare were allergic rhinitis; labyrinthitis; ear, nose, and throat hemorrhage; and hearing difficulty.

Endocrine and Metabolic: Infrequent were thirst and polydipsia, dehydration, and fluid retention. Rare were hyperlipidemia, hypercholesterolemia, hypothyroidism, hyperglycemia, glycosuria and ketonuria, and parathyroid neoplasm.

Eye: Frequent was photophobia. Infrequent was blurred vision. Rare were eye pain and discomfort, sensation of eye pressure, eye hemorrhage, dry eyes, difficulty focusing, and scotoma.

Gastrointestinal: Frequent were hyposalivation and vomiting. Infrequent were dyspeptic symptoms, diarrhea, gastrointestinal discomfort and pain, gastroenteritis, and constipation. Rare were abnormal liver function tests, abnormal bilirubin levels, hemorrhoids, gastritis, esophagitis, salivary gland inflammation, oral itching and irritation, regurgitation and reflux, and gastric ulcers.

Hematological Disorders: Infrequent was increased white cells. Rare were thrombocytopenia, quantitative red cell or hemoglobin defects, anemia, and purpura.

Lower Respiratory Tract: Infrequent were bronchitis, cough, and pneumonia. Rare were tracheitis, asthma, pleuritis, and airway constriction and obstruction.

Musculoskeletal: Infrequent were muscle pain, arthralgia and articular rheumatism, muscle cramps and spasms, joint and muscle stiffness, tightness, and rigidity. Rare were bone and skeletal pain.

Neurological: Frequent was vertigo. Infrequent were tremors, cognitive function disorders, sleep disorders, and disorders of equilibrium. Rare were compressed nerve syndromes, confusion, sedation, hyperesthesia, coordination disorders, paralysis of cranial nerves, decreased consciousness, dreams, altered sense of taste, neuralgia, neuritis, aphasia, hypoesthesia, motor retardation, muscle twitching and fasciculation, psychomotor restlessness, and convulsions.

Non-Site Specific: Infrequent were chills and/or fever, descriptions of odor or taste, edema and swelling, allergies, and allergic reactions. Rare were spasms and mobility disorders.

Pain and Pressure Sensations: Frequent were pressure/tightness/heaviness sensations.

Psychiatry: Infrequent were anxiety, depressive disorders, and detachment. Rare were aggression and hostility, agitation, hallucinations, panic, and hyperactivity.

Reproduction: Rare were lumps of female reproductive tract, breast inflammation, inflammation of vagina, inflammation of fallopian tube, breast discharge, endometrium disorders, decreased libido, and lumps of breast.

Skin: Infrequent were sweating, skin rashes, pruritus, and urticaria. Rare were skin erythema, dermatitis and dermatosis, hair loss and alopecia, pruritic skin rashes, acne and folliculitis, allergic skin reactions, macular skin/rashes, skin photosensitivity, photodermatitis, skin flakiness, and dry skin.

Urology: Infrequent were bladder inflammation and polyuria and diuresis. Rare were urinary tract hemorrhage, urinary urgency, pyelitis, and urinary incontinence.

Observed During Clinical Practice: The following section enumerates potentially important adverse events that have occurred in clinical practice and that have been reported spontaneously to various surveillance systems. The events enumerated represent reports arising from both domestic and nondomestic use of naratriptan. These events do not include those already listed in the ADVERSE REACTIONS section above. Because the reports cite events reported spontaneously from worldwide postmarketing experience, frequency of events and the role of naratripan in their causation cannot be reliably determined.

Cardiovascular: Angina, myocardial infarction (see WARNINGS).

Gastrointestinal: Colonic ischemia (see WARNINGS).

Lower Respiratory: Dyspnea.

Neurologic: Cerebral vascular accident, including transient ischemic attack, subarachnoid hemorrhage, and cerebral infarction (see WARNINGS).

General: Hypersensitivity, including anaphylaxis/anaphylactoid reactions, in some cases severe (e.g., circulatory collapse) (see WARNINGS).

DRUG ABUSE AND DEPENDENCE

In one clinical study enrolling 12 subjects, all of whom had experience using oral opiates and other psychoactive drugs, AMERGE Tablets produced less intense subjective responses ordinarily associated with many drugs of abuse than did codeine (30 to 90 mg).

OVERDOSAGE

A patient who was mildly hypertensive experienced a significant increase in blood pressure after administration of a 10-mg dose starting at 30 minutes (baseline value of 150/98 to 204/144 mmHg 225 minutes). This event resolved after treatment with antihypertensive therapy. Oral administration of 25 mg of naratriptan in 1 healthy young male subject increased blood pressure from 120/67 mmHg pretreatment up to 191/113 mmHg at approximately 6 hours postdose and resulted in adverse events including lightheadedness, tension in the neck, tiredness, and loss of coordination. Blood pressure returned to near baseline by 8 hours after dosing without any pharmacological intervention.

Another subject experienced asymptomatic ischemic ECG changes likely due to coronary artery vasospasm approximately 2 hours following a 7.5-mg oral dose.

The elimination half-life of naratriptan is about 6 hours (see CLINICAL PHARMACOLOGY), and therefore monitoring of patients after overdose with AMERGE Tablets should continue for at least 24 hours or while symptoms or signs

Table 2. Treatment-Emergent Adverse Events Reported by at Least 2% of Patients in Placebo-Controlled Migraine Trials

Adverse Event Type	Placebo (n = 498)	AMERGE 1 mg (n = 627)	AMERGE 2.5 mg (n = 627)
Atypical sensation	1%	2%	4%
Paresthesias (all types)	<1%	1%	2%
Gastrointestinal	5%	6%	7%
Nausea	4%	4%	5%
Neurologial	3%	4%	7%
Dizziness	1%	1%	2%
Drowsiness	<1%	1%	2%
Malaise/fatigue	1%	2%	2%
Pain and pressure sensation	2%	2%	4%
Throat/neck symptoms	1%	1%	2%

persist. There is no specific antidote to naratriptan. Standard supportive treatment should be applied as required. If the patient presents with chest pain or other symptoms consistent with angina pectoris, ECG monitoring should be performed for evidence of ischemia. It is unknown what effect hemodialysis or peritoneal dialysis has on the serum concentrations of naratriptan.

DOSAGE AND ADMINISTRATION

In controlled clinical trials, single doses of 1 and 2.5 mg of AMERGE Tablets taken with fluid were effective for the acute treatment of migraines in adults. A greater proportion of patients had headache response following a 2.5-mg dose than following a 1-mg dose (see CLINICAL TRIALS). Individuals may vary in response to doses of AMERGE Tablets. The choice of dose should therefore be made on an individual basis, weighing the possible benefit of the 2.5-mg dose with the potential for a greater risk of adverse events. If the headache returns or if the patient has only partial response, the dose may be repeated once after 4 hours, for a maximum dose of 5 mg in a 24-hour period. There is evidence that doses of 5 mg do not provide a greater effect than 2.5 mg. The safety of treating, on average, more than 4 headaches in a 30-day period has not been established.

Renal Impairment: The use of AMERGE is contraindicated in patients with severe renal impairment (creatinine clearance, <15 mL/min) because of decreased clearance of the drug (see CONTRAINDICATIONS and CLINICAL PHARMACOLOGY). In patients with mild to moderate renal impairment, the maximum daily dose should not exceed 2.5 mg over a 24-hour period and a lower starting dose should be considered.

Hepatic Impairment: The use of AMERGE is contraindicated in patients with severe hepatic impairment (Child-Pugh grade C) because of decreased clearance (see CONTRAINDICATIONS and CLINICAL PHARMACOLOGY). In patients with mild or moderate hepatic impairment, the maximum daily dose should not exceed 2.5 mg over a 24-hour period and a lower starting dose should be considered (see CLINICAL PHARMACOLOGY).

HOW SUPPLIED

AMERGE Tablets 1 and 2.5 mg of naratriptan (base) as the hydrochloride. AMERGE Tablets, 1 mg, are white, D-shaped, film-coated tablets debossed with "GX CE3" on one side in blister packs of 9 tablets (NDC 0173-0561-00). AMERGE Tablets, 2.5 mg, are green, D-shaped, film-coated tablets debossed with "GX CE5" on one side in blister packs of 9 tablets (NDC 0173-0562-00).

Store at controlled room temperature, 20° to 25°C (68° to 77°F) (see USP).

PATIENT INFORMATION

The following wording is contained in a separate leaflet provided for patients.

Information for the Patient
AMERGE® (naratriptan hydrochloride) Tablets

Please read this leaflet carefully before you take AMERGE Tablets. This leaflet provides a summary of the information available about your medicine. Please do not throw away this leaflet until you have finished your medicine. You may need to read this leaflet again. This leaflet does not contain all the information on AMERGE Tablets. For further information or advice, ask your doctor or pharmacist.

Information About Your Medicine:
The name of your medicine is AMERGE (naratriptan hydrochloride) Tablets. It can be obtained only by prescription from your doctor. The decision to use AMERGE Tablets is one that you and your doctor should make jointly, taking into account your individual preferences and medical circumstances. If you have risk factors for heart disease (such as high blood pressure, high cholesterol, obesity, diabetes, smoking, strong family history of heart disease, or you are postmenopausal or a male over 40), you should tell your doctor, who should evaluate you for heart disease in order to determine if AMERGE is appropriate for you. The majority of those who have taken AMERGE Tablets have not experienced any significant side effects. Rarely, deaths and/or serious heart problems have been reported with this class of medicines; in all but a few instances, however, these deaths and/or serious heart problems occurred in people with heart disease and it was not clear whether these medicines were a contributing factor.

1. The Purpose of Your Medicine:
AMERGE Tablets are intended to relieve your migraine, but not to prevent or reduce the number of attacks you experience. Use AMERGE Tablets only to treat an actual migraine attack.

2. Important Questions to Consider Before Taking AMERGE Tablets:
If the answer to any of the following questions is **YES** or if you do not know the answer, then please discuss it with your doctor before you use AMERGE Tablets.

- Are you pregnant? Do you think you might be pregnant? Are you trying to become pregnant? Are you not using adequate contraception? Are you breastfeeding?
- Do you have any chest pain, heart disease, shortness of breath, or irregular heartbeats? Have you had a heart attack?
- Do you have risk factors for heart disease (such as high blood pressure, high cholesterol, obesity, diabetes, smoking, strong family history of heart disease, or you are postmenopausal or a male over 40)?
- Have you had a stroke, transient ischemic attacks (TIAs), or Raynaud syndrome?
- Do you have high blood pressure?
- Have you ever had to stop taking this or any other medicine because of an allergy or other problems?
- Are you taking any other migraine medicines, including other 5-HT_1 agonists such as IMITREX® (sumatriptan), or medicines containing ergotamine, dihydroergotamine, or methysergide?
- Are you taking any medicine for depression such as selective serotonin reuptake inhibitors (SSRIs)?
- Have you had, or do you have, any disease of the kidney or liver?
- Is this headache different from your usual migraine attacks?

Remember, if you answered **YES** to any of the above questions, then discuss it with your doctor.

3. The Use of AMERGE Tablets During Pregnancy:
Do not use AMERGE Tablets if you are pregnant, think you might be pregnant, are trying to become pregnant, or are not using adequate contraception, unless you have discussed this with your doctor.

4. How to Use AMERGE Tablets:
For adults, the usual dose is a single tablet taken whole with fluids. It may be given at any time after the headache starts. For an individual attack, if you have no response to the first tablet, do not take a second tablet without first talking to your doctor. If you need more relief due to a partial response or return of your headache after the first tablet, a second tablet may be taken but not sooner than 4 hours following the first tablet. Do not take more than a total of 2 AMERGE Tablets in any 24-hour period. If you have kidney or liver disease, take as directed by your doctor.

5. Side Effects to Watch for:

- Some patients experience pain or tightness in the chest or throat when using AMERGE Tablets. If this happens to you, then discuss it with your doctor before using any more AMERGE Tablets. If the chest pain, tightness, or pressure is severe or does not go away, call your doctor immediately.
- If you have sudden and/or severe abdominal pain following AMERGE Tablets, call your doctor immediately.
- Shortness of breath; wheeziness; heart throbbing, swelling of eyelids, face, or lips; or a skin rash, skin lumps, or hives happens rarely. If it happens to you, then tell your doctor immediately. Do not take any more AMERGE Tablets unless your doctor tells you to do so.
- Some people may have feelings of tingling, heat, flushing (redness of face lasting a short time), heaviness or pressure after treatment with AMERGE Tablets. A few people may feel drowsy, dizzy, tired, or sick. Tell your doctor of these symptoms at your next visit.
- If you feel unwell in any other way or have any symptoms that you do not understand, you should contact your doctor immediately.

6. What to Do if an Overdose Is Taken:
If you have taken more medicine than you have been told, contact either your doctor, hospital emergency department, or nearest poison control center immediately.

7. Storing Your Medicine:
Keep your medicine in a safe place where children cannot reach it. It may be harmful to children. Store your medicine away from heat and light. Do not store at temperatures above 77°F (25°C). If your medicine has expired (the expiration date is printed on the treatment pack), throw it away as instructed. If your doctor decides to stop your treatment, do not keep any leftover medicine unless your doctor tells you to. Throw away your medicine as instructed.

GlaxoSmithKline, Research Triangle Park, NC 27709

May 2003/RL-2007

Shown in Product Identification Guide, page 314

AMOXIL® ℞

[ə-mäx' ĭl]
(amoxicillin capsules, tablets, chewable tablets, and powder for oral suspension)

To reduce the development of drug-resistant bacteria and maintain the effectiveness of AMOXIL (amoxicillin) and other antibacterial drugs, AMOXIL should be used only to treat or prevent infections that are proven or strongly suspected to be caused by bacteria.

DESCRIPTION

Formulations of AMOXIL contain amoxicillin, a semisynthetic antibiotic, an analog of ampicillin, with a broad spectrum of bactericidal activity against many gram-positive and gram-negative microorganisms. Chemically, it is (2*S*,5*R*,6*R*)-6-[(*R*)-(-)-2-amino-2-(*p*-hydroxyphenyl)acetamido]-3,3-dimethyl-7-oxo-4-thia-1-azabicyclo[3.2.0]heptane-2-carboxylic acid trihydrate.

The amoxicillin molecular formula is $C_{16}H_{19}N_3O_5S{\bullet}3H_2O$, and the molecular weight is 419.45.

Capsules, tablets, and powder for oral suspension of AMOXIL are intended for oral administration.

Capsules: Each capsule of AMOXIL, with royal blue opaque cap and pink opaque body, contains 500 mg amoxicillin as the trihydrate. The cap and body of the 500-mg capsule are imprinted with AMOXIL and 500. Inactive ingredients: D&C Red No. 28, FD&C Blue No. 1, FD&C Red No. 40, gelatin, magnesium stearate, and titanium dioxide.

Tablets: Each tablet contains 500 mg or 875 mg amoxicillin as the trihydrate. Each film-coated, capsule-shaped, pink tablet is debossed with AMOXIL centered over 500 or 875, respectively. The 875-mg tablet is scored on the reverse side. Inactive ingredients: Colloidal silicon dioxide, crospovidone, FD&C Red No. 30 aluminum lake, hypromellose, magnesium stearate, microcrystalline cellulose, polyethylene glycol, sodium starch glycolate, and titanium dioxide.

Chewable Tablets: Each cherry-banana-peppermint-flavored tablet contains 200 mg or 400 mg amoxicillin as the trihydrate.

Each 200-mg chewable tablet contains 0.0005 mEq (0.0107 mg) of sodium; the 400-mg chewable tablet contains 0.0009 mEq (0.0215 mg) of sodium. The 200-mg and 400-mg pale pink round tablets are imprinted with the product name AMOXIL and 200 or 400 along the edge of 1 side. Inactive ingredients: Aspartame*, crospovidone NF, FD&C Red No. 40 aluminum lake, flavorings, magnesium stearate, and mannitol.

*See PRECAUTIONS.

Powder for Oral Suspension: Each 5 mL of reconstituted suspension contains 200 mg, 250 mg, or 400 mg amoxicillin as the trihydrate. Each 5 mL of the 250-mg reconstituted suspension contains 0.15 mEq (3.36 mg) of sodium. Each 5 mL of the 200-mg reconstituted suspension contains 0.15 mEq (3.39 mg) of sodium; each 5 mL of the 400-mg reconstituted suspension contains 0.19 mEq (4.33 mg) of sodium.

Pediatric Drops for Oral Suspension: Each mL of reconstituted suspension contains 50 mg amoxicillin as the trihydrate and 0.03 mEq (0.69 mg) of sodium.

Amoxicillin trihydrate for oral suspension 200 mg/5 mL, 250 mg/5 mL (or 50 mg/mL), and 400 mg/5 mL are bubble-gum-flavored pink suspensions. Inactive ingredients: FD&C Red No. 3, flavorings, silica gel, sodium benzoate, sodium citrate, sucrose, and xanthan gum.

CLINICAL PHARMACOLOGY

Amoxicillin is stable in the presence of gastric acid and is rapidly absorbed after oral administration. The effect of food on the absorption of amoxicillin from the tablets and suspension of AMOXIL has been partially investigated. The 400-mg and 875-mg formulations have been studied only when administered at the start of a light meal. However, food effect studies have not been performed with the 200-mg and 500-mg formulations. Amoxicillin diffuses readily into most body tissues and fluids, with the exception of brain and spinal fluid, except when meninges are inflamed. The half-life of amoxicillin is 61.3 minutes. Most of the amoxicillin is excreted unchanged in the urine; its excretion can be delayed by concurrent administration of probenecid. In blood serum, amoxicillin is approximately 20% protein-bound.

Orally administered doses of 250-mg and 500-mg amoxicillin capsules result in average peak blood levels 1 to 2 hours after administration in the range of 3.5 mcg/mL to 5.0 mcg/mL and 5.5 mcg/mL to 7.5 mcg/mL, respectively.

Mean amoxicillin pharmacokinetic parameters from an open, two-part, single-dose crossover bioequivalence study in 27 adults comparing 875 mg of AMOXIL with 875 mg of AUGMENTIN® (amoxicillin/clavulanate potassium) showed that the 875-mg tablet of AMOXIL produces an $AUC_{0-\infty}$ of 35.4 ± 8.1 mcg•hr/mL and a C_{max} of 13.8 ± 4.1 mcg/mL. Dosing was at the start of a light meal following an overnight fast.

Orally administered doses of amoxicillin suspension, 125 mg/5 mL and 250 mg/5 mL, result in average peak blood levels 1 to 2 hours after administration in the range of 1.5 mcg/mL to 3.0 mcg/mL and 3.5 mcg/mL to 5.0 mcg/mL, respectively.

Oral administration of single doses of 400-mg chewable tablets and 400-mg/5 mL suspension of AMOXIL to 24 adult volunteers yielded comparable pharmacokinetic data:

Dose*	$AUC_{0-\infty}$ (mcg•hr/mL)	C_{max} (mcg/mL)†
Amoxicillin	amoxicillin (±S.D.)	amoxicillin (±S.D.)
400 mg (5 mL of suspension)	17.1 (3.1)	5.92 (1.62)
400 mg (1 chewable tablet)	17.9 (2.4)	5.18 (1.64)

* Administered at the start of a light meal.
† Mean values of 24 normal volunteers. Peak concentrations occurred approximately 1 hour after the dose.

Detectable serum levels are observed up to 8 hours after an orally administered dose of amoxicillin. Following a 1-gram dose and utilizing a special skin window technique to determine levels of the antibiotic, it was noted that therapeutic

Continued on next page

Product information on these pages is effective as of August 2004. Further information is available at: GlaxoSmithKline, PO Box 13398, Research Triangle Park, NC 27709. 1-888-825-5249. Corporate Web Site: www.gsk.com

Amoxil—Cont.

levels were found in the interstitial fluid. Approximately 60% of an orally administered dose of amoxicillin is excreted in the urine within 6 to 8 hours.

Microbiology: Amoxicillin is similar to ampicillin in its bactericidal action against susceptible organisms during the stage of active multiplication. It acts through the inhibition of biosynthesis of cell wall mucopeptide. Amoxicillin has been shown to be active against most strains of the following microorganisms, both in vitro and in clinical infections as described in the INDICATIONS AND USAGE section.

Aerobic Gram-Positive Microorganisms:

Enterococcus faecalis
Staphylococcus spp.* (β-lactamase–negative strains only)
Streptococcus pneumoniae
Streptococcus spp. (α- and β-hemolytic strains only)

*Staphylococci which are susceptible to amoxicillin but resistant to methicillin/oxacillin should be considered as resistant to amoxicillin.

Aerobic Gram-Negative Microorganisms:

Escherichia coli (β-lactamase–negative strains only)
Haemophilus influenzae (β-lactamase–negative strains only)
Neisseria gonorrhoeae (β-lactamase–negative strains only)
Proteus mirabilis (β-lactamase–negative strains only)

Helicobacter:

Helicobacter pylori

Susceptibility Tests: *Dilution Techniques:* Quantitative methods are used to determine antimicrobial minimum inhibitory concentrations (MICs). These MICs provide estimates of the susceptibility of bacteria to antimicrobial compounds. The MICs should be determined using a standardized procedure. Standardized procedures are based on a dilution method[1] (broth or agar) or equivalent with standardized inoculum concentrations and standardized concentrations of **ampicillin** powder. Ampicillin is sometimes used to predict susceptibility of *S. pneumoniae* to amoxicillin; however, some intermediate strains have been shown to be susceptible to amoxicillin. Therefore, *S. pneumoniae* susceptibility should be tested using amoxicillin powder. The MIC values should be interpreted according to the following criteria:

For Gram-Positive Aerobes:

Enterococcus

MIC (mcg/mL)	Interpretation
≤8	Susceptible (S)
≥16	Resistant (R)

Staphylococcus[a]

MIC (mcg/mL)	Interpretation
≤0.25	Susceptible (S)
≥0.5	Resistant (R)

Streptococcus (except *S. pneumoniae*)

MIC (mcg/mL)	Interpretation
≤0.25	Susceptible (S)
0.5 to 4	Intermediate (I)
≥8	Resistant (R)

S. pneumoniae[b] from non-meningitis sources.
(**Amoxicillin** powder should be used to determine susceptibility.)

MIC (mcg/mL)	Interpretation
≤2	Susceptible (S)
4	Intermediate (I)
≥8	Resistant (R)

NOTE: These interpretive criteria are based on the recommended doses for respiratory tract infections.

For Gram-Negative Aerobes:

Enterobacteriaceae

MIC (mcg/mL)	Interpretation
≤8	Susceptible (S)
16	Intermediate (I)
≥32	Resistant (R)

H. influenzae[c]

MIC (mcg/mL)	Interpretation
≤1	Susceptible (S)
2	Intermediate (I)
≥4	Resistant (R)

a. Staphylococci which are susceptible to amoxicillin but resistant to methicillin/oxacillin should be considered as resistant to amoxicillin.
b. These interpretive standards are applicable only to broth microdilution susceptibility tests using cation-adjusted Mueller-Hinton broth with 2-5% lysed horse blood.
c. These interpretive standards are applicable only to broth microdilution test with *H. influenzae* using *Haemophilus* Test Medium (HTM).[1]

A report of "Susceptible" indicates that the pathogen is likely to be inhibited if the antimicrobial compound in the blood reaches the concentrations usually achievable. A report of "Intermediate" indicates that the result should be considered equivocal, and, if the microorganism is not fully susceptible to alternative, clinically feasible drugs, the test should be repeated. This category implies possible clinical applicability in body sites where the drug is physiologically concentrated or in situations where high dosage of drug can be used. This category also provides a buffer zone, which prevents small uncontrolled technical factors from causing major discrepancies in interpretation. A report of "Resistant" indicates that the pathogen is not likely to be inhibited if the antimicrobial compound in the blood reaches the concentrations usually achievable; other therapy should be selected.

Standardized susceptibility test procedures require the use of laboratory control microorganisms to control the technical aspects of the laboratory procedures. Standard **ampicillin** powder should provide the following MIC values:

Microorganism		MIC Range (mcg/mL)
E. coli	ATCC 25922	2 to 8
E. faecalis	ATCC 29212	0.5 to 2
H. influenzae	ATCC 49247[d]	2 to 8
S. aureus	ATCC 29213	0.25 to 1

Using **amoxicillin** to determine susceptibility:

Microorganism		MIC Range (mcg/mL)
S. pneumoniae	ATCC 49619[e]	0.03 to 0.12

d. This quality control range is applicable to only *H. influenzae* ATCC 49247 tested by a broth microdilution procedure using HTM.[1]
e. This quality control range is applicable to only *S. pneumoniae* ATCC 49619 tested by the broth microdilution procedure using cation-adjusted Mueller-Hinton broth with 2-5% lysed horse blood.

Diffusion Techniques: Quantitative methods that require measurement of zone diameters also provide reproducible estimates of the susceptibility of bacteria to antimicrobial compounds. One such standardized procedure[2] requires the use of standardized inoculum concentrations. This procedure uses paper disks impregnated with 10 mcg ampicillin to test the susceptibility of microorganisms, except *S. pneumoniae*, to amoxicillin. Interpretation involves correlation of the diameter obtained in the disk test with the MIC for **ampicillin.**

Reports from the laboratory providing results of the standard single-disk susceptibility test with a 10-mcg ampicillin disk should be interpreted according to the following criteria:

For Gram-Positive Aerobes:

Enterococcus

Zone Diameter (mm)	Interpretation
≥17	Susceptible (S)
≤16	Resistant (R)

Staphylococcus[f]

Zone Diameter (mm)	Interpretation
≥29	Susceptible (S)
≤28	Resistant (R)

β-hemolytic streptococci

Zone Diameter (mm)	Interpretation
≥26	Susceptible (S)
19 to 25	Intermediate (I)
≤18	Resistant (R)

NOTE: For streptococci (other than β-hemolytic streptococci and *S. pneumoniae*), an ampicillin MIC should be determined.

S. pneumoniae

S. pneumoniae should be tested using a 1-mcg oxacillin disk. Isolates with oxacillin zone sizes of ≥20 mm are susceptible to amoxicillin. An amoxicillin MIC should be determined on isolates of *S. pneumoniae* with oxacillin zone sizes of ≤19 mm.

For Gram-Negative Aerobes:

Enterobacteriaceae

Zone Diameter (mm)	Interpretation
≥17	Susceptible (S)
14 to 16	Intermediate (I)
≤13	Resistant (R)

H. influenzae[g]

Zone Diameter (mm)	Interpretation
≥22	Susceptible (S)
19 to 21	Intermediate (I)
≤18	Resistant (R)

f. Staphylococci which are susceptible to amoxicillin but resistant to methicillin/oxacillin should be considered as resistant to amoxicillin.
g. These interpretive standards are applicable only to disk diffusion susceptibility tests with *H. influenzae* using *Haemophilus* Test Medium (HTM).[2]

Interpretation should be as stated above for results using dilution techniques.

As with standard dilution techniques, disk diffusion susceptibility test procedures require the use of laboratory control microorganisms. The 10-mcg **ampicillin** disk should provide the following zone diameters in these laboratory test quality control strains:

Microorganism		Zone diameter (mm)
E. coli	ATCC 25922	16 to 22
H. influenzae	ATCC 49247[h]	13 to 21
S. aureus	ATCC 25923	27 to 35

Using 1-mcg **oxacillin** disk:

Microorganism		Zone diameter (mm)
S. pneumoniae	ATCC 49619[i]	8 to 12

h. This quality control range is applicable to only *H. influenzae* ATCC 49247 tested by a disk diffusion procedure using HTM.[2]
i. This quality control range is applicable to only *S. pneumoniae* ATCC 49619 tested by a disk diffusion procedure using Mueller-Hinton agar supplemented with 5% sheep blood and incubated in 5% CO_2.

Susceptibility Testing for *Helicobacter pylori:* In vitro susceptibility testing methods and diagnostic products currently available for determining minimum inhibitory concentrations (MICs) and zone sizes have not been standardized, validated, or approved for testing *H. pylori* microorganisms.

Culture and susceptibility testing should be obtained in patients who fail triple therapy. If clarithromycin resistance is found, a non-clarithromycin-containing regimen should be used.

INDICATIONS AND USAGE

AMOXIL is indicated in the treatment of infections due to susceptible (ONLY β-lactamase–negative) strains of the designated microorganisms in the conditions listed below:

Infections of the ear, nose, and throat—due to *Streptococcus* spp. (α- and β-hemolytic strains only), *S. pneumoniae, Staphylococcus* spp., or *H. influenzae.*

Infections of the genitourinary tract—due to *E. coli, P. mirabilis*, or *E. faecalis.*

Infections of the skin and skin structure—due to *Streptococcus* spp. (α- and β-hemolytic strains only), *Staphylococcus* spp., or *E. coli.*

Infections of the lower respiratory tract—due to *Streptococcus* spp. (α- and β-hemolytic strains only), *S. pneumoniae, Staphylococcus* spp., or *H. influenzae.*

Gonorrhea, acute uncomplicated (ano-genital and urethral infections)—due to *N. gonorrhoeae* (males and females).

H. pylori eradication to reduce the risk of duodenal ulcer recurrence

Triple Therapy: AMOXIL/clarithromycin/lansoprazole

AMOXIL, in combination with clarithromycin plus lansoprazole as triple therapy, is indicated for the treatment of patients with *H. pylori* infection and duodenal ulcer disease (active or 1-year history of a duodenal ulcer) to eradicate *H. pylori*. Eradication of *H. pylori* has been shown to reduce the risk of duodenal ulcer recurrence. (See CLINICAL STUDIES and DOSAGE AND ADMINISTRATION.)

Dual Therapy: AMOXIL/lansoprazole

AMOXIL, in combination with lansoprazole delayed-release capsules as dual therapy, is indicated for the treatment of patients with *H. pylori* infection and duodenal ulcer disease (active or 1-year history of a duodenal ulcer) **who are either allergic or intolerant to clarithromycin or in whom resistance to clarithromycin is known or suspected.** (See the clarithromycin package insert, MICROBIOLOGY.) Eradication of *H. pylori* has been shown to reduce the risk of duodenal ulcer recurrence. (See CLINICAL STUDIES and DOSAGE AND ADMINISTRATION.)

To reduce the development of drug-resistant bacteria and maintain the effectiveness of AMOXIL and other antibacterial drugs, AMOXIL should be used only to treat or prevent infections that are proven or strongly suspected to be caused by susceptible bacteria. When culture and susceptibility information are available, they should be considered in selecting or modifying antibacterial therapy. In the absence of such data, local epidemiology and susceptibility patterns may contribute to the empiric selection of therapy. Indicated surgical procedures should be performed.

CONTRAINDICATIONS

A history of allergic reaction to any of the penicillins is a contraindication.

WARNINGS

SERIOUS AND OCCASIONALLY FATAL HYPERSENSITIVITY (ANAPHYLACTIC) REACTIONS HAVE BEEN REPORTED IN PATIENTS ON PENICILLIN THERAPY. ALTHOUGH ANAPHYLAXIS IS MORE FREQUENT FOLLOWING PARENTERAL THERAPY, IT HAS OCCURRED IN PATIENTS ON ORAL PENICILLINS. THESE REACTIONS ARE MORE LIKELY TO OCCUR IN INDIVIDUALS WITH A HISTORY OF PENICILLIN HYPERSENSITIVITY AND/OR A HISTORY OF SENSITIVITY TO MULTIPLE ALLERGENS. THERE HAVE BEEN REPORTS OF INDIVIDUALS WITH A HISTORY OF PENICILLIN HYPERSENSITIVITY WHO HAVE EXPERIENCED SEVERE REACTIONS WHEN TREATED WITH CEPHALOSPORINS. BEFORE INITIATING THERAPY WITH AMOXIL, CAREFUL INQUIRY SHOULD BE MADE CONCERNING PREVIOUS HYPERSENSITIVITY REACTIONS TO PENICILLINS, CEPHALOSPORINS, OR OTHER ALLERGENS. IF AN ALLERGIC REACTION OCCURS, AMOXIL SHOULD BE DISCONTINUED AND APPROPRIATE THERAPY INSTITUTED. **SERIOUS ANAPHYLACTIC REACTIONS REQUIRE IMMEDIATE EMERGENCY TREATMENT WITH EPINEPHRINE. OXYGEN, INTRAVENOUS STEROIDS, AND AIRWAY MANAGEMENT, INCLUDING INTUBATION, SHOULD ALSO BE ADMINISTERED AS INDICATED.**

Pseudomembranous colitis has been reported with nearly all antibacterial agents, including amoxicillin, and may range in severity from mild to life-threatening. Therefore, it is important to consider this diagnosis in patients who present with diarrhea subsequent to the administration of antibacterial agents.

Treatment with antibacterial agents alters the normal flora of the colon and may permit overgrowth of clostridia. Studies indicate that a toxin produced by *Clostridium difficile* is a primary cause of "antibiotic-associated colitis."

After the diagnosis of pseudomembranous colitis has been established, appropriate therapeutic measures should be initiated. Mild cases of pseudomembranous colitis usually respond to drug discontinuation alone. In moderate-to-severe cases, consideration should be given to management with fluids and electrolytes, protein supplementation, and treatment with an antibacterial drug clinically effective against *C. difficile* colitis.

PRECAUTIONS

General: The possibility of superinfections with mycotic or bacterial pathogens should be kept in mind during therapy. If superinfections occur, amoxicillin should be discontinued and appropriate therapy instituted.

Prescribing AMOXIL in the absence of a proven or strongly suspected bacterial infection or a prophylactic indication is unlikely to provide benefit to the patient and increases the risk of the development of drug-resistant bacteria.

Phenylketonurics: Each 200-mg chewable tablet of AMOXIL contains 1.82 mg phenylalanine; each 400-mg chewable tablet contains 3.64 mg phenylalanine. The suspensions of AMOXIL do not contain phenylalanine and can be used by phenylketonurics.

Laboratory Tests: As with any potent drug, periodic assessment of renal, hepatic, and hematopoietic function should be made during prolonged therapy.

All patients with gonorrhea should have a serologic test for syphilis at the time of diagnosis. Patients treated with amoxicillin should have a follow-up serologic test for syphilis after 3 months.

Drug Interactions: Probenecid decreases the renal tubular secretion of amoxicillin. Concurrent use of amoxicillin and probenecid may result in increased and prolonged blood levels of amoxicillin.

Chloramphenicol, macrolides, sulfonamides, and tetracyclines may interfere with the bactericidal effects of penicillin. This has been demonstrated in vitro; however, the clinical significance of this interaction is not well documented.

Drug/Laboratory Test Interactions: High urine concentrations of ampicillin may result in false-positive reactions when testing for the presence of glucose in urine using CLINITEST®, Benedict's Solution or Fehling's Solution. Since this effect may also occur with amoxicillin, it is recommended that glucose tests based on enzymatic glucose oxidase reactions (such as CLINISTIX®) be used.

Following administration of ampicillin to pregnant women, a transient decrease in plasma concentration of total conjugated estriol, estriol-glucuronide, conjugated estrone, and estradiol has been noted. This effect may also occur with amoxicillin.

Carcinogenesis, Mutagenesis, Impairment of Fertility: Long-term studies in animals have not been performed to evaluate carcinogenic potential. Studies to detect mutagenic potential of amoxicillin alone have not been conducted; however, the following information is available from tests on a 4:1 mixture of amoxicillin and potassium clavulanate (AUGMENTIN). AUGMENTIN was non-mutagenic in the Ames bacterial mutation assay, and the yeast gene conversion assay. AUGMENTIN was weakly positive in the mouse lymphoma assay, but the trend toward increased mutation frequencies in this assay occurred at doses that were also associated with decreased cell survival. AUGMENTIN was negative in the mouse micronucleus test, and in the dominant lethal assay in mice. Potassium clavulanate alone was tested in the Ames bacterial mutation assay and in the mouse micronucleus test, and was negative in each of these assays. In a multi-generation reproduction study in rats, no impairment of fertility or other adverse reproductive effects were seen at doses up to 500 mg/kg (approximately 3 times the human dose in mg/m^2).

Pregnancy: *Teratogenic Effects:* Pregnancy Category B. Reproduction studies have been performed in mice and rats at doses up to 10 times the human dose and have revealed no evidence of impaired fertility or harm to the fetus due to amoxicillin. There are, however, no adequate and well-controlled studies in pregnant women. Because animal reproduction studies are not always predictive of human response, this drug should be used during pregnancy only if clearly needed.

Labor and Delivery: Oral ampicillin-class antibiotics are poorly absorbed during labor. Studies in guinea pigs showed that intravenous administration of ampicillin slightly decreased the uterine tone and frequency of contractions but moderately increased the height and duration of contractions. However, it is not known whether use of amoxicillin in humans during labor or delivery has immediate or delayed adverse effects on the fetus, prolongs the duration of labor, or increases the likelihood that forceps delivery or other obstetrical intervention or resuscitation of the newborn will be necessary.

Nursing Mothers: Penicillins have been shown to be excreted in human milk. Amoxicillin use by nursing mothers may lead to sensitization of infants. Caution should be exercised when amoxicillin is administered to a nursing woman.

Pediatric Use: Because of incompletely developed renal function in neonates and young infants, the elimination of amoxicillin may be delayed. Dosing of AMOXIL should be modified in pediatric patients 12 weeks or younger (≤3 months). (See DOSAGE AND ADMINISTRATION: Neonates and infants.)

Information for Patients: AMOXIL may be taken every 8 hours or every 12 hours, depending on the strength of the product prescribed.

Adults and Pediatric Patients >3 Months:

Infection	Severity*	Usual Adult Dose	Usual Dose for Children >3 Months†‡
Ear/Nose/Throat	Mild/Moderate	500 mg every 12 hours or 250 mg every 8 hours	25 mg/kg/day in divided doses every 12 hours **or** 20 mg/kg/day in divided doses every 8 hours
	Severe	875 mg every 12 hours or 500 mg every 8 hours	45 mg/kg/day in divided doses every 12 hours **or** 40 mg/kg/day in divided doses every 8 hours
Lower Respiratory Tract	Mild/Moderate or Severe	875 mg every 12 hours or 500 mg every 8 hours	45 mg/kg/day in divided doses every 12 hours **or** 40 mg/kg/day in divided doses every 8 hours
Skin/Skin Structure	Mild/Moderate	500 mg every 12 hours or 250 mg every 8 hours	25 mg/kg/day in divided doses every 12 hours **or** 20 mg/kg/day in divided doses every 8 hours
	Severe	875 mg every 12 hours or 500 mg every 8 hours	45 mg/kg/day in divided doses every 12 hours **or** 40 mg/kg/day in divided doses every 8 hours
Genitourinary Tract	Mild/Moderate	500 mg every 12 hours or 250 mg every 8 hours	25 mg/kg/day in divided doses every 12 hours **or** 20 mg/kg/day in divided doses every 8 hours
	Severe	875 mg every 12 hours or 500 mg every 8 hours	45 mg/kg/day in divided doses every 12 hours **or** 40 mg/kg/day in divided doses every 8 hours
Gonorrhea Acute, uncomplicated ano-genital, and urethral infections in males and females		3 grams as single oral dose	Prepubertal children: 50 mg/kg AMOXIL, combined with 25 mg/kg probenecid as a single dose. **NOTE: SINCE PROBENECID IS CONTRAINDICATED IN CHILDREN UNDER 2 YEARS, DO NOT USE THIS REGIMEN IN THESE CASES.**

* Dosing for infections caused by less susceptible organisms should follow the recommendations for severe infections.

† The children's dosage is intended for individuals whose weight is less than 40 kg. Children weighing 40 kg or more should be dosed according to the adult recommendations.

‡ Each strength of the suspension of AMOXIL is available as a chewable tablet for use by older children.

Patients should be counseled that antibacterial drugs, including AMOXIL, should only be used to treat bacterial infections. They do not treat viral infections (e.g., the common cold). When AMOXIL is prescribed to treat a bacterial infection, patients should be told that although it is common to feel better early in the course of therapy, the medication should be taken exactly as directed. Skipping doses or not completing the full course of therapy may: (1) decrease the effectiveness of the immediate treatment, and (2) increase the likelihood that bacteria will develop resistance and will not be treatable by AMOXIL or other antibacterial drugs in the future.

ADVERSE REACTIONS

As with other penicillins, it may be expected that untoward reactions will be essentially limited to sensitivity phenomena. They are more likely to occur in individuals who have previously demonstrated hypersensitivity to penicillins and in those with a history of allergy, asthma, hay fever, or urticaria. The following adverse reactions have been reported as associated with the use of penicillins:

Gastrointestinal: Nausea, vomiting, diarrhea, and hemorrhagic/pseudomembranous colitis.

Onset of pseudomembranous colitis symptoms may occur during or after antibiotic treatment. (See WARNINGS.)

Hypersensitivity Reactions: Serum sickness–like reactions, erythematous maculopapular rashes, erythema multiforme, Stevens-Johnson syndrome, exfoliative dermatitis, toxic epidermal necrolysis, acute generalized exanthematous pustulosis, hypersensitivity vasculitis and urticaria have been reported.

NOTE: These hypersensitivity reactions may be controlled with antihistamines and, if necessary, systemic corticosteroids. Whenever such reactions occur, amoxicillin should be discontinued unless, in the opinion of the physician, the condition being treated is life-threatening and amenable only to amoxicillin therapy.

Liver: A moderate rise in AST (SGOT) and/or ALT (SGPT) has been noted, but the significance of this finding is unknown. Hepatic dysfunction including cholestatic jaundice, hepatic cholestasis and acute cytolytic hepatitis have been reported.

Renal: Crystalluria has also been reported **(see OVERDOSAGE)**.

Hemic and Lymphatic Systems: Anemia, including hemolytic anemia, thrombocytopenia, thrombocytopenic purpura, eosinophilia, leukopenia, and agranulocytosis have been reported during therapy with penicillins. These reactions are usually reversible on discontinuation of therapy and are believed to be hypersensitivity phenomena.

Central Nervous System: Reversible hyperactivity, agitation, anxiety, insomnia, confusion, convulsions, behavioral changes, and/or dizziness have been reported rarely.

Miscellaneous: Tooth discoloration (brown, yellow, or gray staining) has been rarely reported. Most reports occurred in pediatric patients. Discoloration was reduced or eliminated with brushing or dental cleaning in most cases.

Combination Therapy with Clarithromycin and Lansoprazole: In clinical trials using combination therapy with amoxicillin plus clarithromycin and lansoprazole, and amoxicillin plus lansoprazole, no adverse reactions peculiar to these drug combinations were observed. Adverse reactions that have occurred have been limited to those that had been previously reported with amoxicillin, clarithromycin, or lansoprazole.

Triple Therapy: *Amoxicillin/Clarithromycin/Lansoprazole:* The most frequently reported adverse events for patients who received triple therapy were diarrhea (7%), headache (6%), and taste perversion (5%). No treatment-emergent ad-

Continued on next page

Product information on these pages is effective as of August 2004. Further information is available at: GlaxoSmithKline, PO Box 13398, Research Triangle Park, NC 27709. 1-888-825-5249. Corporate Web Site: www.gsk.com

Amoxil—Cont.

verse events were observed at significantly higher rates with triple therapy than with any dual therapy regimen.

Dual Therapy: ***Amoxicillin/Lansoprazole:*** The most frequently reported adverse events for patients who received amoxicillin three times daily plus lansoprazole three times daily dual therapy were diarrhea (8%) and headache (7%). No treatment-emergent adverse events were observed at significantly higher rates with amoxicillin three times daily plus lansoprazole three times daily dual therapy than with lansoprazole alone.

For more information on adverse reactions with clarithromycin or lansoprazole, refer to their package inserts, ADVERSE REACTIONS.

OVERDOSAGE

In case of overdosage, discontinue medication, treat symptomatically, and institute supportive measures as required. If the overdosage is very recent and there is no contraindication, an attempt at emesis or other means of removal of drug from the stomach may be performed. A prospective study of 51 pediatric patients at a poison-control center suggested that overdosages of less than 250 mg/kg of amoxicillin are not associated with significant clinical symptoms and do not require gastric emptying.[3]

Interstitial nephritis resulting in oliguric renal failure has been reported in a small number of patients after overdosage with amoxicillin.

Crystalluria, in some cases leading to renal failure, has also been reported after amoxicillin overdosage in adults and pediatric patients. In case of overdosage, adequate fluid intake and diuresis should be maintained to reduce the risk of amoxicillin crystalluria.

Renal impairment appears to be reversible with cessation of drug administration. High blood levels may occur more readily in patients with impaired renal function because of decreased renal clearance of amoxicillin. Amoxicillin may be removed from circulation by hemodialysis.

DOSAGE AND ADMINISTRATION

Capsules, chewable tablets, and oral suspensions of AMOXIL may be given without regard to meals. The 400-mg suspension, 400-mg chewable tablet, and the 875-mg tablet have been studied only when administered at the start of a light meal. However, food effect studies have not been performed with the 200-mg and 500-mg formulations.

Neonates and Infants Aged ≤12 Weeks (≤3 Months): Due to incompletely developed renal function affecting elimination of amoxicillin in this age group, the recommended upper dose of AMOXIL is 30 mg/kg/day divided q12h.

[See table at top of previous page]

After reconstitution, the required amount of suspension should be placed directly on the child's tongue for swallowing. Alternate means of administration are to add the required amount of suspension to formula, milk, fruit juice, water, ginger ale, or cold drinks. These preparations should then be taken immediately. To be certain the child is receiving full dosage, such preparations should be consumed in entirety.

All patients with gonorrhea should be evaluated for syphilis. (See PRECAUTIONS: Laboratory Tests.)

Larger doses may be required for stubborn or severe infections.

General: It should be recognized that in the treatment of chronic urinary tract infections, frequent bacteriological and clinical appraisals are necessary. Smaller doses than those recommended above should not be used. Even higher doses may be needed at times. In stubborn infections, therapy may be required for several weeks. It may be necessary to continue clinical and/or bacteriological follow-up for several months after cessation of therapy. Except for gonorrhea, treatment should be continued for a minimum of 48 to 72 hours beyond the time that the patient becomes asymptomatic or evidence of bacterial eradication has been obtained. It is recommended that there be at least 10 days' treatment for any infection caused by *Streptococcus pyogenes* to prevent the occurrence of acute rheumatic fever.

H. pylori **Eradication to Reduce the Risk of Duodenal Ulcer Recurrence:** ***Triple Therapy:***
AMOXIL/clarithromycin/lansoprazole

The recommended adult oral dose is 1 gram AMOXIL, 500 mg clarithromycin, and 30 mg lansoprazole, all given twice daily (q12h) for 14 days. (See INDICATIONS AND USAGE.)

Dual Therapy: AMOXIL/lansoprazole

The recommended adult oral dose is 1 gram AMOXIL and 30 mg lansoprazole, each given three times daily (q8h) for 14 days. (See INDICATIONS AND USAGE.)

Please refer to clarithromycin and lansoprazole full prescribing information for CONTRAINDICATIONS and WARNINGS, and for information regarding dosing in elderly and renally impaired patients.

Dosing Recommendations for Adults with Impaired Renal Function: Patients with impaired renal function do not generally require a reduction in dose unless the impairment is severe. Severely impaired patients with a glomerular filtration rate of <30 mL/min. should not receive the 875-mg tablet. Patients with a glomerular filtration rate of 10 to 30 mL/min. should receive 500 mg or 250 mg every 12 hours, depending on the severity of the infection. Patients with a less than 10 mL/min. glomerular filtration rate should receive 500 mg or 250 mg every 24 hours, depending on severity of the infection.

Hemodialysis patients should receive 500 mg or 250 mg every 24 hours, depending on severity of the infection. They should receive an additional dose both during and at the end of dialysis.

There are currently no dosing recommendations for pediatric patients with impaired renal function.

Directions for Mixing Oral Suspension: Prepare suspension at time of dispensing as follows: Tap bottle until all powder flows freely. Add approximately 1/3 of the total amount of water for reconstitution (see table below) and shake vigorously to wet powder. Add remainder of the water and again shake vigorously.

200 mg/5 mL

Bottle Size	Amount of Water Required for Reconstitution
50 mL	39 mL
75 mL	57 mL
100 mL	76 mL

Each teaspoonful (5 mL) will contain 200 mg amoxicillin.

250 mg/5 mL

Bottle Size	Amount of Water Required for Reconstitution
100 mL	74 mL
150 mL	111 mL

Each teaspoonful (5 mL) will contain 250 mg amoxicillin.

400 mg/5 mL

Bottle Size	Amount of Water Required for Reconstitution
50 mL	36 mL
75 mL	54 mL
100 mL	71 mL

Each teaspoonful (5 mL) will contain 400 mg amoxicillin.

Directions for Mixing Pediatric Drops: Prepare pediatric drops at time of dispensing as follows: Add the required amount of water (see table below) to the bottle and shake vigorously. Each mL of suspension will then contain amoxicillin trihydrate equivalent to 50 mg amoxicillin.

Bottle Size	Amount of Water Required for Reconstitution
30 mL	23 mL

NOTE: SHAKE BOTH ORAL SUSPENSION AND PEDIATRIC DROPS WELL BEFORE USING. Keep bottle tightly closed. Any unused portion of the reconstituted suspension must be discarded after 14 days. Refrigeration preferable, but not required.

HOW SUPPLIED

Capsules of AMOXIL: Each capsule contains 500 mg amoxicillin as the trihydrate.

500-mg Capsule

NDC 0029-6007-32 bottles of 500

Tablets of AMOXIL: Each tablet contains 500 mg or 875 mg amoxicillin as the trihydrate.

500-mg Tablet

NDC 0029-6046-20 bottles of 100

875-mg Tablet

NDC 0029-6047-20 bottles of 100

Chewable Tablets of AMOXIL: Each cherry-banana-peppermint-flavored tablet contains 200 mg or 400 mg amoxicillin as the trihydrate.

200-mg Tablet

NDC 0029-6044-12 bottles of 20

400-mg Tablet

NDC 0029-6045-12 bottles of 20
NDC 0029-6045-20 bottles of 100

AMOXIL for Oral Suspension: Each 5 mL of reconstituted bubble-gum-flavored suspension contains 200, 250, or 400 mg amoxicillin as the trihydrate.

200 mg/5 mL

NDC 0029-6048-54 50-mL bottle
NDC 0029-6048-55 75-mL bottle
NDC 0029-6048-59 100-mL bottle

250 mg/5 mL

NDC 0029-6009-23 100-mL bottle
NDC 0029-6009-22 150-mL bottle

400 mg/5 mL

NDC 0029-6049-54 50-mL bottle
NDC 0029-6049-55 75-mL bottle
NDC 0029-6049-59 100-mL bottle

Pediatric Drops of AMOXIL for Oral Suspension: Each mL of bubble-gum-flavored reconstituted suspension contains 50 mg amoxicillin as the trihydrate.

NDC 0029-6038-39 30-mL bottle

Store at or below 20°C (68°F)
- 500-mg capsules
- 250-mg unreconstituted powder

Store at or below 25°C (77°F)
- 200-mg and 400-mg unreconstituted powder
- 200-mg and 400-mg chewable tablets
- 500-mg and 875-mg tablets

Dispense in a tight container.

CLINICAL STUDIES

H. pylori **Eradication to Reduce the Risk of Duodenal Ulcer Recurrence:** Randomized, double-blind clinical studies performed in the United States in patients with *H. pylori* and duodenal ulcer disease (defined as an active ulcer or history of an ulcer within 1 year) evaluated the efficacy of lansoprazole in combination with amoxicillin capsules and clarithromycin tablets as triple 14-day therapy, or in combination with amoxicillin capsules as dual 14-day therapy, for the eradication of *H. pylori*. Based on the results of these studies, the safety and efficacy of 2 different eradication regimens were established:

Triple Therapy: Amoxicillin 1 gram twice daily/clarithromycin 500 mg twice daily/lansoprazole 30 mg twice daily.

Dual Therapy: Amoxicillin 1 gram three times daily/lansoprazole 30 mg three times daily.

All treatments were for 14 days. *H. pylori* eradication was defined as 2 negative tests (culture and histology) at 4 to 6 weeks following the end of treatment.

Triple therapy was shown to be more effective than all possible dual therapy combinations. Dual therapy was shown to be more effective than both monotherapies. Eradication of *H. pylori* has been shown to reduce the risk of duodenal ulcer recurrence.

H. pylori **Eradication Rates—Triple Therapy (amoxicillin/clarithromycin/lansoprazole) Percent of Patients Cured [95% Confidence Interval] (Number of Patients)**

Study	Triple Therapy	Triple Therapy
	Evaluable Analysis*	Intent-to-Treat Analysis†
Study 1	92‡ [80.0-97.7] (n = 48)	86‡ [73.3-93.5] (n = 55)
Study 2	86§ [75.7-93.6] (n = 66)	83§ [72.0-90.8] (n = 70)

* This analysis was based on evaluable patients with confirmed duodenal ulcer (active or within 1 year) and *H. pylori* infection at baseline defined as at least 2 of 3 positive endoscopic tests from CLOtest®, (Delta West Ltd., Bentley, Australia), histology, and/or culture. Patients were included in the analysis if they completed the study. Additionally, if patients dropped out of the study due to an adverse event related to the study drug, they were included in the analysis as failures of therapy.

† Patients were included in the analysis if they had documented *H. pylori* infection at baseline as defined above and had a confirmed duodenal ulcer (active or within 1 year). All dropouts were included as failures of therapy.

‡ ($p<0.05$) versus lansoprazole/amoxicillin and lansoprazole/clarithromycin dual therapy.

§ ($p<0.05$) versus clarithromycin/amoxicillin dual therapy.

H. pylori **Eradication Rates—Dual Therapy (amoxicillin/lansoprazole) Percent of Patients Cured [95% Confidence Interval] (Number of Patients)**

Study	Dual Therapy	Dual Therapy
	Evaluable Analysis*	Intent-to-Treat Analysis†
Study 1	77‡ [62.5-87.2] (n = 51)	70‡ [56.8-81.2] (n = 60)
Study 2	66§ [51.9-77.5] (n = 58)	61§ [48.5-72.9] (n = 67)

* This analysis was based on evaluable patients with confirmed duodenal ulcer (active or within 1 year) and *H. pylori* infection at baseline defined as at least 2 of 3 positive endoscopic tests from CLOtest®, histology and/or culture. Patients were included in the analysis if they completed the study. Additionally, if patients dropped out of the study due to an adverse event related to the study drug, they were included in the analysis as failures of therapy.

† Patients were included in the analysis if they had documented *H. pylori* infection at baseline as defined above and had a confirmed duodenal ulcer (active or within 1 year). All dropouts were included as failures of therapy.

‡ ($p<0.05$) versus lansoprazole alone.

§ ($p<0.05$) versus lansoprazole alone or amoxicillin alone.

REFERENCES

1. National Committee for Clinical Laboratory Standards. Methods for Dilution Antimicrobial Susceptibility Tests for Bacteria that Grow Aerobically–Fourth Edition; Approved Standard NCCLS Document M7-A4, Vol. 17, No. 2. NCCLS, Wayne, PA, January 1997.
2. National Committee for Clinical Laboratory Standards. Performance Standards for Antimicrobial Disk Susceptibility Tests–Sixth Edition; Approved Standard NCCLS Document M2-A6, Vol. 17, No. 1. NCCLS, Wayne, PA, January 1997.
3. Swanson-Bearman B, Dean BS, Lopez G, Krenzelok EP. The effects of penicillin and cephalosporin ingestions in children less than six years of age. *Vet Hum Toxicol.* 1988;30:66-67.

AMOXIL and AUGMENTIN are registered trademarks of GlaxoSmithKline.
CLINITEST is a registered trademark of Miles, Inc.
CLINISTIX is a registered trademark of Bayer Corporation.
CLOtest is a registered trademark of Kimberly-Clark Corporation.
GlaxoSmithKline, Research Triangle Park, NC 27709

June 2004/AM:L27

Shown in Product Identification Guide, page 314

ANCEF® ℞

[*an' sef*]

cefazolin for injection

To reduce the development of drug-resistant bacteria and maintain the effectiveness of ANCEF (cefazolin for injection) and other antibacterial drugs, ANCEF should be used only to treat or prevent infections that are proven or strongly suspected to be caused by bacteria.

DESCRIPTION

ANCEF is a semi-synthetic cephalosporin for parenteral administration. It is the sodium salt of 3-{[(5-methyl-1,3,4-thiadiazol-2-yl)thio]-methyl}-8-oxo-7-[2-(1H-tetrazol-1-yl) acetamido]-5-thia-1-azabicyclo [4.2.0]oct-2-ene-2-carboxylic acid.

Each vial contains 48 mg of sodium/1 gram of cefazolin sodium.

ANCEF in lyophilized form is supplied in vials equivalent to 1 gram of cefazolin; in "Piggyback" Vials for intravenous admixture equivalent to 1 gram of cefazolin; and in Pharmacy Bulk Vials equivalent to 10 grams of cefazolin.

CLINICAL PHARMACOLOGY

After intramuscular administration of ANCEF to normal volunteers, the mean serum concentrations were 37 mcg/mL at 1 hour and 3 mcg/mL at 8 hours following a 500-mg dose, and 64 mcg/mL at 1 hour and 7 mcg/mL at 8 hours following a 1-gram dose.

Studies have shown that following intravenous administration of ANCEF to normal volunteers, mean serum concentrations peaked at approximately 185 mcg/mL and were approximately 4 mcg/mL at 8 hours for a 1-gram dose.

The serum half-life for ANCEF is approximately 1.8 hours following IV administration and approximately 2.0 hours following IM administration.

In a study (using normal volunteers) of constant intravenous infusion with dosages of 3.5 mg/kg for 1 hour (approximately 250 mg) and 1.5 mg/kg the next 2 hours (approximately 100 mg), ANCEF produced a steady serum level at the third hour of approximately 28 mcg/mL.

Studies in patients hospitalized with infections indicate that ANCEF produces mean peak serum levels approximately equivalent to those seen in normal volunteers.

Bile levels in patients without obstructive biliary disease can reach or exceed serum levels by up to 5 times; however, in patients with obstructive biliary disease, bile levels of ANCEF are considerably lower than serum levels (< 1.0 mcg/mL).

In synovial fluid, the level of ANCEF becomes comparable to that reached in serum at about 4 hours after drug administration.

Studies of cord blood show prompt transfer of ANCEF across the placenta. ANCEF is present in very low concentrations in the milk of nursing mothers.

ANCEF is excreted unchanged in the urine. In the first 6 hours approximately 60% of the drug is excreted in the urine and this increases to 70% to 80% within 24 hours. ANCEF achieves peak urine concentrations of approximately 2,400 mcg/mL and 4,000 mcg/mL respectively following 500-mg and 1-gram intramuscular doses.

In patients undergoing peritoneal dialysis (2 L/hr.), ANCEF produced mean serum levels of approximately 10 and 30 mcg/mL after 24 hours' instillation of a dialyzing solution containing 50 mg/L and 150 mg/L, respectively. Mean peak levels were 29 mcg/mL (range 13 to 44 mcg/mL) with 50 mg/L (3 patients), and 72 mcg/mL (range 26 to 142 mcg/mL) with 150 mg/L (6 patients). Intraperitoneal administration of ANCEF is usually well tolerated.

Controlled studies on adult normal volunteers, receiving 1 gram 4 times a day for 10 days, monitoring CBC, SGOT, SGPT, bilirubin, alkaline phosphatase, BUN, creatinine, and urinalysis, indicated no clinically significant changes attributed to ANCEF.

Microbiology: In vitro tests demonstrate that the bactericidal action of cephalosporins results from inhibition of cell wall synthesis. ANCEF is active against the following organisms in vitro and in clinical infections:

Staphylococcus aureus (including penicillinase-producing strains)
Staphylococcus epidermidis
Methicillin-resistant staphylococci are uniformly resistant to cefazolin
Group A beta-hemolytic streptococci and other strains of streptococci (many strains of enterococci are resistant)
Streptococcus pneumoniae
Escherichia coli
Proteus mirabilis
Klebsiella species
Enterobacter aerogenes
Haemophilus influenzae

Most strains of indole positive Proteus (*Proteus vulgaris*), *Enterobacter cloacae, Morganella morganii,* and *Providencia rettgeri* are resistant. *Serratia, Pseudomonas, Mima, Herellea* species are almost uniformly resistant to cefazolin.

Disk Susceptibility Tests: ***Disk Diffusion Technique:*** Quantitative methods that require measurement of zone diameters give the most precise estimates of antibiotic susceptibility. One such procedure[1] has been recommended for use with disks to test susceptibility to cefazolin.

Reports from a laboratory using the standardized single-disk susceptibility test[1] with a 30-mcg cefazolin disk should be interpreted according to the following criteria:

Susceptible organisms produce zones of 18 mm or greater, indicating that the tested organism is likely to respond to therapy.

Organisms of intermediate susceptibility produce zones 15 to 17 mm, indicating that the tested organism would be susceptible if high dosage is used or if the infection is confined to tissues and fluids (e.g., urine), in which high antibiotic levels are attained.

Resistant organisms produce zones of 14 mm or less, indicating that other therapy should be selected.

For gram-positive isolates, a zone of 18 mm is indicative of a cefazolin-susceptible organism when tested with either the cephalosporin-class disk (30 mcg cephalothin) or the cefazolin disk (30 mcg cefazolin).

Gram-negative organisms should be tested with the cefazolin disk (using the above criteria), since cefazolin has been shown by in vitro tests to have activity against certain strains of Enterobacteriaceae found resistant when tested with the cephalothin disk. Gram-negative organisms having zones of less than 18 mm around the cephalothin disk may be susceptible to cefazolin.

Standardized procedures require use of control organisms. The 30-mcg cefazolin disk should give zone diameter between 23 and 29 mm for *E. coli* ATCC 25922 and between 29 and 35 mm for *S. aureus* ATCC 25923.

The cefazolin disk should not be used for testing susceptibility to other cephalosporins.

Dilution Techniques: A bacterial isolate may be considered susceptible if the minimal inhibitory concentration (MIC) for cefazolin is not more than 16 mcg per mL. Organisms are considered resistant if the MIC is equal to or greater than 64 mcg per mL.

The range of MICs for the control strains are as follows:
S. aureus ATCC 25923, 0.25 to 1.0 mcg/mL
E. coli ATCC 25922, 1.0 to 4.0 mcg/mL

INDICATIONS AND USAGE

ANCEF is indicated in the treatment of the following serious infections due to susceptible organisms:

Respiratory Tract Infections: Due to *S. pneumoniae, Klebsiella* species, *H. influenzae, S. aureus* (penicillin-sensitive and penicillin-resistant), and group A beta-hemolytic streptococci.

Injectable benzathine penicillin is considered to be the drug of choice in treatment and prevention of streptococcal infections, including the prophylaxis of rheumatic fever.

ANCEF is effective in the eradication of streptococci from the nasopharynx; however, data establishing the efficacy of ANCEF in the subsequent prevention of rheumatic fever are not available at present.

Urinary Tract Infections: Due to *E. coli, P. mirabilis, Klebsiella* species, and some strains of enterobacter and enterococci.

Skin and Skin Structure Infections: Due to *S. aureus* (penicillin-sensitive and penicillin-resistant), group A beta-hemolytic streptococci, and other strains of streptococci.

Biliary Tract Infections: Due to *E. coli*, various strains of streptococci, *P. mirabilis, Klebsiella* species, and *S. aureus.*

Bone and Joint Infections: Due to *S. aureus.*

Genital Infections: (i.e., prostatitis, epididymitis) due to *E. coli, P. mirabilis, Klebsiella* species, and some strains of enterococci.

Septicemia: Due to *S. pneumoniae, S. aureus* (penicillin-sensitive and penicillin-resistant), *P. mirabilis, E. coli,* and *Klebsiella* species.

Endocarditis: Due to *S. aureus* (penicillin-sensitive and penicillin-resistant) and group A beta-hemolytic streptococci.

Perioperative Prophylaxis: The prophylactic administration of ANCEF preoperatively, intraoperatively, and postoperatively may reduce the incidence of certain postoperative infections in patients undergoing surgical procedures which are classified as contaminated or potentially contaminated (e.g., vaginal hysterectomy, and cholecystectomy in high-risk patients such as those older than 70 years, with acute cholecystitis, obstructive jaundice, or common duct bile stones).

The perioperative use of ANCEF may also be effective in surgical patients in whom infection at the operative site would present a serious risk (e.g., during open-heart surgery and prosthetic arthroplasty).

The prophylactic administration of ANCEF should usually be discontinued within a 24-hour period after the surgical procedure. In surgery where the occurrence of infection may be particularly devastating (e.g., open-heart surgery and prosthetic arthroplasty), the prophylactic administration of ANCEF may be continued for 3 to 5 days following the completion of surgery.

If there are signs of infection, specimens for cultures should be obtained for the identification of the causative organism so that appropriate therapy may be instituted.

(See DOSAGE AND ADMINISTRATION.)

To reduce the development of drug-resistant bacteria and maintain the effectiveness of ANCEF and other antibacterial drugs, ANCEF should be used only to treat or prevent infections that are proven or strongly suspected to be caused by susceptible bacteria. When culture and susceptibility information are available, they should be considered in selecting or modifying antibacterial therapy. In the absence of such data, local epidemiology and susceptibility patterns may contribute to the empiric selection of therapy.

CONTRAINDICATIONS

ANCEF IS CONTRAINDICATED IN PATIENTS WITH KNOWN ALLERGY TO THE CEPHALOSPORIN GROUP OF ANTIBIOTICS.

WARNINGS

BEFORE THERAPY WITH ANCEF IS INSTITUTED, CAREFUL INQUIRY SHOULD BE MADE TO DETERMINE WHETHER THE PATIENT HAS HAD PREVIOUS HYPERSENSITIVITY REACTIONS TO CEFAZOLIN, CEPHALOSPORINS, PENICILLINS, OR OTHER DRUGS. IF THIS PRODUCT IS GIVEN TO PENICILLIN-SENSITIVE PATIENTS, CAUTION SHOULD BE EXERCISED BECAUSE CROSS-HYPERSENSITIVITY AMONG BETA-LACTAM ANTIBIOTICS HAS BEEN CLEARLY DOCUMENTED AND MAY OCCUR IN UP TO 10% OF PATIENTS WITH A HISTORY OF PENICILLIN ALLERGY. IF AN ALLERGIC REACTION TO ANCEF OCCURS, DISCONTINUE TREATMENT WITH THE DRUG. SERIOUS ACUTE HYPERSENSITIVITY REACTIONS MAY REQUIRE TREATMENT WITH EPINEPHRINE AND OTHER EMERGENCY MEASURES, INCLUDING OXYGEN, IV FLUIDS, IV ANTIHISTAMINES, CORTICOSTEROIDS, PRESSOR AMINES, AND AIRWAY MANAGEMENT, AS CLINICALLY INDICATED.

Pseudomembranous colitis has been reported with nearly all antibacterial agents, including cefazolin, and may range in severity from mild to life-threatening. Therefore, it is important to consider this diagnosis in patients who present with diarrhea subsequent to the administration of antibacterial agents.

Treatment with antibacterial agents alters the normal flora of the colon and may permit overgrowth of clostridia. Studies indicate that a toxin produced by *Clostridium difficile* is a primary cause of "antibiotic-associated colitis."

After the diagnosis of pseudomembranous colitis has been established, therapeutic measures should be initiated. Mild cases of pseudomembranous colitis usually respond to drug discontinuation alone. In moderate to severe cases, consideration should be given to management with fluids and electrolytes, protein supplementation, and treatment with an oral antibacterial drug clinically effective against *C. difficile* colitis.

PRECAUTIONS

General: Prolonged use of ANCEF may result in the overgrowth of nonsusceptible organisms. Careful clinical observation of the patient is essential.

When ANCEF is administered to patients with low urinary output because of impaired renal function, lower daily dosage is required (see DOSAGE AND ADMINISTRATION).

As with other β-lactam antibiotics, seizures may occur if inappropriately high doses are administered to patients with impaired renal function (see DOSAGE AND ADMINISTRATION).

ANCEF, as with all cephalosporins, should be prescribed with caution in individuals with a history of gastrointestinal disease, particularly colitis.

Cephalosporins may be associated with a fall in prothrombin activity. Those at risk include patients with renal or hepatic impairment or poor nutritional state, as well as patients receiving a protracted course of antimicrobial therapy, and patients previously stabilized on anticoagulant therapy. Prothrombin time should be monitored in patients at risk and exogenous vitamin K administered as indicated.

Prescribing ANCEF in the absence of a proven or strongly suspected bacterial infection or a prophylactic indication is unlikely to provide benefit to the patient and increases the risk of the development of drug-resistant bacteria.

Drug Interactions: Probenecid may decrease renal tubular secretion of cephalosporins when used concurrently, resulting in increased and more prolonged cephalosporin blood levels.

Drug/Laboratory Test Interactions: A false positive reaction for glucose in the urine may occur with Benedict's solution, Fehling's solution or with CLINITEST® tablets, but not with enzyme-based tests such as CLINISTIX®.

Positive direct and indirect antiglobulin (Coombs) tests have occurred; these may also occur in neonates whose mothers received cephalosporins before delivery.

Information for Patients: Patients should be counseled that antibacterial drugs including ANCEF, should only be used to treat bacterial infections. They do not treat viral infections (e.g., the common cold). When ANCEF is prescribed

Continued on next page

Product information on these pages is effective as of August 2004. Further information is available at: GlaxoSmithKline, PO Box 13398, Research Triangle Park, NC 27709. 1-888-825-5249. Corporate Web Site: www.gsk.com

Ancef—Cont.

to treat a bacterial infection, patients should be told that although it is common to feel better early in the course of therapy, the medication should be taken exactly as directed. Skipping doses or not completing the full course of therapy may: (1) decrease the effectiveness of the immediate treatment, and (2) increase the likelihood that bacteria will develop resistance and will not be treatable by ANCEF or other antibacterial drugs in the future.

Carcinogenesis/Mutagenesis: Mutagenicity studies and long-term studies in animals to determine the carcinogenic potential of ANCEF have not been performed.

Pregnancy: ***Teratogenic Effects:*** Pregnancy Category B. Reproduction studies have been performed in rats, mice, and rabbits at doses up to 25 times the human dose and have revealed no evidence of impaired fertility or harm to the fetus due to ANCEF. There are, however, no adequate and well-controlled studies in pregnant women. Because animal reproduction studies are not always predictive of human response, this drug should be used during pregnancy only if clearly needed.

Labor and Delivery: When cefazolin has been administered prior to caesarean section, drug levels in cord blood have been approximately one quarter to one third of maternal drug levels. The drug appears to have no adverse effect on the fetus.

Nursing Mothers: ANCEF is present in very low concentrations in the milk of nursing mothers. Caution should be exercised when ANCEF is administered to a nursing woman.

Pediatric Use: Safety and effectiveness for use in premature infants and neonates have not been established. See DOSAGE AND ADMINISTRATION for recommended dosage in pediatric patients older than 1 month.

ADVERSE REACTIONS

The following reactions have been reported:

Gastrointestinal: Diarrhea, oral candidiasis (oral thrush), vomiting, nausea, stomach cramps, anorexia, and pseudomembranous colitis. Onset of pseudomembranous colitis symptoms may occur during or after antibiotic treatment (see WARNINGS). Nausea and vomiting have been reported rarely.

Allergic: Anaphylaxis, eosinophilia, itching, drug fever, skin rash, Stevens-Johnson syndrome.

Hematologic: Neutropenia, leukopenia, thrombocytopenia, thrombocythemia.

Hepatic: Transient rise in SGOT, SGPT, and alkaline phosphatase levels has been observed. As with other cephalosporins, reports of hepatitis have been received.

Renal: As with other cephalosporins, reports of increased BUN and creatinine levels, as well as renal failure, have been received.

Local Reactions: Rare instances of phlebitis have been reported at site of injection. Pain at the site of injection after intramuscular administration has occurred infrequently. Some induration has occurred.

Other Reactions: Genital and anal pruritus (including vulvar pruritus, genital moniliasis, and vaginitis).

DOSAGE AND ADMINISTRATION

[See first table above]

Perioperative Prophylactic Use: To prevent postoperative infection in contaminated or potentially contaminated surgery, recommended doses are:

a. 1 gram IV or IM administered 1/2 hour to 1 hour prior to the start of surgery.
b. For lengthy operative procedures (e.g., 2 hours or more), 500 mg to 1 gram IV or IM during surgery (administration modified depending on the duration of the operative procedure).
c. 500 mg to 1 gram IV or IM every 6 to 8 hours for 24 hours postoperatively.

It is important that (1) the preoperative dose be given just (1/2 to 1 hour) prior to the start of surgery so that adequate antibiotic levels are present in the serum and tissues at the time of initial surgical incision; and (2) ANCEF be administered, if necessary, at appropriate intervals during surgery to provide sufficient levels of the antibiotic at the anticipated moments of greatest exposure to infective organisms.

In surgery where the occurrence of infection may be particularly devastating (e.g., open-heart surgery and prosthetic arthroplasty), the prophylactic administration of ANCEF may be continued for 3 to 5 days following the completion of surgery.

Dosage Adjustment for Patients With Reduced Renal Function: ANCEF may be used in patients with reduced renal function with the following dosage adjustments: Patients with a creatinine clearance of 55 mL/min. or greater or a serum creatinine of 1.5 mg % or less can be given full doses. Patients with creatinine clearance rates of 35 to 54 mL/min. or serum creatinine of 1.6 to 3.0 mg % can also be given full doses but dosage should be restricted to at least 8 hour intervals. Patients with creatinine clearance rates of 11 to 34 mL/min. or serum creatinine of 3.1 to 4.5 mg % should be given 1/2 the usual dose every 12 hours. Patients with creatinine clearance rates of 10 mL/min. or less or serum creatinine of 4.6 mg % or greater should be given 1/2 the usual dose every 18 to 24 hours. All reduced dosage recommendations apply after an initial loading dose appropriate to the

Usual Adult Dosage:

Type of Infection	Dose	Frequency
Moderate to severe infections	500 mg to 1 gram	every 6 to 8 hrs.
Mild infections caused by susceptible gram-positive cocci	250 mg to 500 mg	every 8 hours
Acute, uncomplicated urinary tract infections	1 gram	every 12 hours
Pneumococcal pneumonia	500 mg	every 12 hours
Severe, life-threatening infections (e.g., endocarditis, septicemia)*	1 gram to 1.5 grams	every 6 hours

*In rare instances, doses of up to 12 grams of ANCEF per day have been used.

Pediatric Dosage Guide

Weight		25 mg/kg/day Divided into 3 Doses		25 mg/kg/day Divided into 4 Doses	
Lbs	Kg	Approximate Single Dose mg/q8h	Vol. (mL) needed with dilution of 125 mg/mL	Approximate Single Dose mg/q6h	Vol. (mL) needed with dilution of 125 mg/mL
10	4.5	40 mg	0.35 mL	30 mg	0.25 mL
20	9.0	75 mg	0.60 mL	55 mg	0.45 mL
30	13.6	115 mg	0.90 mL	85 mg	0.70 mL
40	18.1	150 mg	1.20 mL	115 mg	0.90 mL
50	22.7	190 mg	1.50 mL	140 mg	1.10 mL

Weight		50 mg/kg/day Divided into 3 Doses		50 mg/kg/day Divided into 4 Doses	
Lbs	Kg	Approximate Single Dose mg/q8h	Vol. (mL) needed with dilution of 225 mg/mL	Approximate Single Dose mg/q6h	Vol. (mL) needed with dilution of 225 mg/mL
10	4.5	75 mg	0.35 mL	55 mg	0.25 mL
20	9.0	150 mg	0.70 mL	110 mg	0.50 mL
30	13.6	225 mg	1.00 mL	170 mg	0.75 mL
40	18.1	300 mg	1.35 mL	225 mg	1.00 mL
50	22.7	375 mg	1.70 mL	285 mg	1.25 mL

severity of the infection. Patients undergoing peritoneal dialysis: See CLINICAL PHARMACOLOGY.

Pediatric Dosage: In pediatric patients, a total daily dosage of 25 to 50 mg per kg (approximately 10 to 20 mg per pound) of body weight, divided into 3 or 4 equal doses, is effective for most mild to moderately severe infections. Total daily dosage may be increased to 100 mg per kg (45 mg per pound) of body weight for severe infections. Since safety for use in premature infants and in neonates has not been established, the use of ANCEF in these patients is not recommended.

[See second table above]

In pediatric patients with mild to moderate renal impairment (creatinine clearance of 70 to 40 mL/min.), 60 percent of the normal daily dose given in equally divided doses every 12 hours should be sufficient. In patients with moderate impairment (creatinine clearance of 40 to 20 mL/min.), 25 percent of the normal daily dose given in equally divided doses every 12 hours should be adequate. Pediatric patients with severe renal impairment (creatinine clearance of 20 to 5 mL/min.) may be given 10 percent of the normal daily dose every 24 hours. All dosage recommendations apply after an initial loading dose.

RECONSTITUTION

Preparation of Parenteral Solution: Parenteral drug products should be SHAKEN WELL when reconstituted, and inspected visually for particulate matter prior to administration. If particulate matter is evident in reconstituted fluids, the drug solutions should be discarded.

When reconstituted or diluted according to the instructions below, ANCEF is stable for 24 hours at room temperature or for 10 days if stored under refrigeration (5°C or 41°F). Reconstituted solutions may range in color from pale yellow to yellow without a change in potency.

Single-Dose Vials: For IM injection, IV direct (bolus) injection or IV infusion, reconstitute with Sterile Water for Injection according to the following table. SHAKE WELL.

Vial Size	Amount of Diluent	Approximate Concentration	Approximate Available Volume
1 gram	2.5 mL	330 mg/mL	3.0 mL

Pharmacy Bulk Vials: Add Sterile Water for Injection, Bacteriostatic Water for Injection, or Sodium Chloride Injection according to the table below. SHAKE WELL. Use promptly. (Discard vial within 4 hours after initial entry.)

Vial Size	Amount of Diluent	Approximate Concentration	Approximate Available Volume
10 grams	45 mL	1 gram/5 mL	51 mL
	96 mL	1 gram/10 mL	102 mL

"Piggyback" Vials: Reconstitute with 50 to 100 mL of Sodium Chloride Injection or other IV solution listed under ADMINISTRATION. When adding diluent to vial, allow air to escape by using a small vent needle or by pumping the syringe. SHAKE WELL. Administer with primary IV fluids, as a single dose.

ADMINISTRATION

Intramuscular Administration: Reconstitute vials with Sterile Water for Injection according to the dilution table above. Shake well until dissolved. ANCEF should be injected into a large muscle mass. Pain on injection is infrequent with ANCEF.

Intravenous Administration: Direct (bolus) injection: Following reconstitution according to the above table, further dilute vials with approximately 5 mL Sterile Water for Injection. Inject the solution slowly over 3 to 5 minutes, directly or through tubing for patients receiving parenteral fluids (see list below).

Intermittent or continuous infusion: Dilute reconstituted ANCEF in 50 to 100 mL of 1 of the following solutions:

- Sodium Chloride Injection, USP
- 5% or 10% Dextrose Injection, USP
- 5% Dextrose in Lactated Ringer's Injection, USP
- 5% Dextrose and 0.9% Sodium Chloride Injection, USP
- 5% Dextrose and 0.45% Sodium Chloride Injection, USP
- 5% Dextrose and 0.2% Sodium Chloride Injection, USP
- Lactated Ringer's Injection, USP
- Invert Sugar 5% or 10% in Sterile Water for Injection
- Ringer's Injection, USP
- 5% Sodium Bicarbonate Injection, USP

HOW SUPPLIED

ANCEF

Each vial contains cefazolin sodium equivalent to 1 gram of cefazolin. NDC 0007-3130-16 (package of 25 vials)

Each vial contains cefazolin sodium equivalent to 1 gram of cefazolin. NDC 0007-3137-05 (package of 10 "piggyback" vials)

As with other cephalosporins, ANCEF tends to darken depending on storage conditions; within the stated recommendations, however, product potency is not adversely affected. Before reconstitution protect from light and store at Controlled Room Temperature 20° to 25°C (68° to 77°F).

REFERENCE

1. Bauer, A.W.; Kirby, W.M.M.; Sherris, J.C., and Turck, M.: Antibiotic Testing by a Standardized Single Disc Method, Am. J. Clin. Path. 45:493, 1966. Standardized Disc Susceptibility Test, Federal Register 39:19182-19184, 1974.

ANCEF is a registered trademark of GlaxoSmithKline.
CLINITEST is a registered trademark of Miles, Inc.
CLINISTIX is a registered trademark of Bayer Corporation.
GlaxoSmithKline, Research Triangle Park, NC 27709

February 2004/AF:L57

Shown in Product Identification Guide, page 314

ARGATROBAN ℞
[är-ga' trō-ban]
Injection

DESCRIPTION

Argatroban is a synthetic direct thrombin inhibitor derived from L-arginine. The chemical name for Argatroban is 1-[5-[(aminoiminomethyl)amino]-1-oxo-2-[[(1,2,3,4-tetrahydro-3-methyl-8-quinolinyl)sulfonyl]amino]pentyl]-4-methyl-2-piperidinecarboxylic acid, monohydrate. Argatroban has 4 asymmetric carbons. One of the asymmetric carbons has an *R* configuration (stereoisomer Type I) and an *S* configuration (stereoisomer Type II). Argatroban consists of a mixture of *R* and *S* stereoisomers at a ratio of approximately 65:35.
The molecular formula of Argatroban is $C_{23}H_{36}N_6O_5S \bullet H_2O$. Its molecular weight is 526.66.
Argatroban is a white, odorless crystalline powder that is freely soluble in glacial acetic acid, slightly soluble in ethanol, and insoluble in acetone, ethyl acetate, and ether. Argatroban Injection is a sterile clear, colorless to pale yellow, slightly viscous solution. Argatroban is available in 250-mg (in 2.5-mL) single-use amber vials, with gray flip-top caps. Each mL of sterile, nonpyrogenic solution contains 100 mg Argatroban. Inert ingredients: 750 mg D-sorbitol, 1,000 mg dehydrated alcohol.

CLINICAL PHARMACOLOGY

Mechanism of Action: Argatroban is a direct thrombin inhibitor that reversibly binds to the thrombin active site. Argatroban does not require the co-factor antithrombin III for antithrombotic activity. Argatroban exerts its anticoagulant effects by inhibiting thrombin-catalyzed or -induced reactions, including fibrin formation; activation of coagulation factors V, VIII, and XIII; activation of protein C; and platelet aggregation.
Argatroban is highly selective for thrombin with an inhibitory constant (K_i) of 0.04 µM. At therapeutic concentrations, Argatroban has little or no effect on related serine proteases (trypsin, factor Xa, plasmin, and kallikrein).
Argatroban is capable of inhibiting the action of both free and clot-associated thrombin.
Argatroban does not interact with heparin-induced antibodies. Evaluation of sera in 12 healthy subjects and 8 patients who received multiple doses of Argatroban did not reveal antibody formation to Argatroban (see CLINICAL STUDIES).
Pharmacokinetics: ***Distribution:*** Argatroban distributes mainly in the extracellular fluid as evidenced by an apparent steady-state volume of distribution of 174 mL/kg (12.18 L in a 70-kg adult). Argatroban is 54% bound to human serum proteins, with binding to albumin and α_1-acid glycoprotein being 20% and 34%, respectively.
Metabolism: The main route of Argatroban metabolism is hydroxylation and aromatization of the 3-methyltetrahydroquinoline ring in the liver. The formation of each of the 4 known metabolites is catalyzed in vitro by the human liver microsomal cytochrome P450 enzymes CYP3A4/5. The primary metabolite (M1) exerts 3- to 5-fold weaker anticoagulant effects than Argatroban. Unchanged Argatroban is the major component in plasma. The plasma concentrations of M1 range between 0% and 20% of that of the parent drug. The other metabolites (M2 to M4) are found only in very low quantities in the urine and have not been detected in plasma or feces. These data, together with the lack of effect of erythromycin (a potent CYP3A4/5 inhibitor) on Argatroban pharmacokinetics, suggest that CYP3A4/5-mediated metabolism is not an important elimination pathway in vivo.
Total body clearance is approximately 5.1 mL/kg/min (0.31 L/kg/hr) for infusion doses up to 40 mcg/kg/min. The terminal elimination half-life of Argatroban ranges between 39 and 51 minutes.
There is no interconversion of the 21–(R):21–(S) diastereoisomers. The plasma ratio of these diastereoisomers is unchanged by metabolism or hepatic impairment, remaining constant at 65:35 (±2%).
Excretion: Argatroban is excreted primarily in the feces, presumably through biliary secretion. In a study in which ^{14}C-Argatroban (5 mcg/kg/min) was infused for 4 hours into healthy subjects, approximately 65% of the radioactivity was recovered in the feces within 6 days of the start of infusion with little or no radioactivity subsequently detected. Approximately 22% of the radioactivity appeared in the urine within 12 hours of the start of infusion. Little or no additional urinary radioactivity was subsequently detected. Average percent recovery of unchanged drug, relative to total dose, was 16% in urine and at least 14% in feces.
Pharmacokinetic/Pharmacodynamic Relationship: When Argatroban is administered by continuous infusion, anticoagulant effects and plasma concentrations of Argatroban follow similar, predictable temporal response profiles, with low intersubject variability. Immediately upon initiation of Argatroban infusion, anticoagulant effects are produced as plasma Argatroban concentrations begin to rise. Steady-state levels of both drug and anticoagulant effect are typically attained within 1 to 3 hours and are maintained until the infusion is discontinued or the dosage adjusted. Steady-state plasma Argatroban concentrations increase proportionally with dose (for infusion doses up to 40 mcg/kg/min in healthy subjects) and are well correlated with steady-state anticoagulant effects. For infusion doses up to 40 mcg/kg/min, Argatroban increases in a dose-dependent fashion, the activated partial thromboplastin time (aPTT), the activated clotting time (ACT), the prothrombin time (PT), the International Normalized Ratio (INR), and the thrombin time (TT) in healthy volunteers and cardiac patients. Representative steady-state plasma Argatroban concentrations and anticoagulant effects are shown below for Argatroban infusion doses up to 10 mcg/kg/min (see Figure 1).

Figure 1. Relationship at Steady State Between Argatroban Dose, Plasma Argatroban Concentration and Anticoagulant Effect

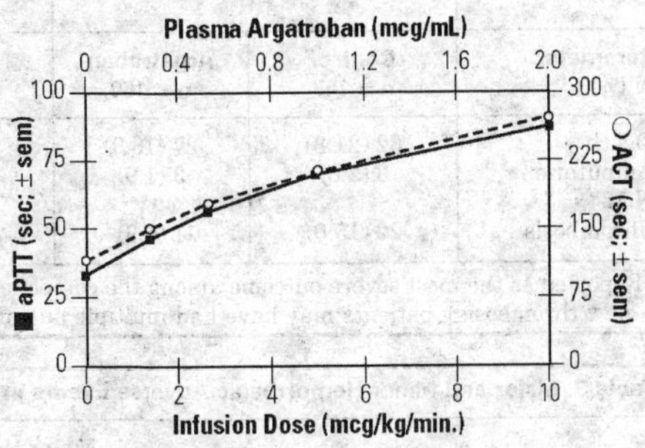

Effect on International Normalized Ratio (INR): Because Argatroban is a direct thrombin inhibitor, co-administration of Argatroban and warfarin produces a combined effect on the laboratory measurement of the INR. However, concurrent therapy, compared to warfarin monotherapy, exerts no additional effect on vitamin K–dependent factor Xa activity. The relationship between INR on co-therapy and warfarin alone is dependent on both the dose of Argatroban and the thromboplastin reagent used. This relationship is influenced by the International Sensitivity Index (ISI) of the thromboplastin. Data for 2 commonly utilized thromboplastins with ISI values of 0.88 (Innovin, Dade) and 1.78 (Thromboplastin C Plus, Dade) are presented in Figure 2 for an Argatroban dose of 2 mcg/kg/min. Thromboplastins with higher ISI values than shown result in higher INRs on combined therapy of warfarin and Argatroban. These data are based on results obtained in normal individuals (see PRECAUTIONS, Drug Interactions and DOSAGE AND ADMINISTRATION, Conversion to Oral Anticoagulant Therapy).

Figure 2. INR Relationship of Argatroban Plus Warfarin Versus Warfarin Alone

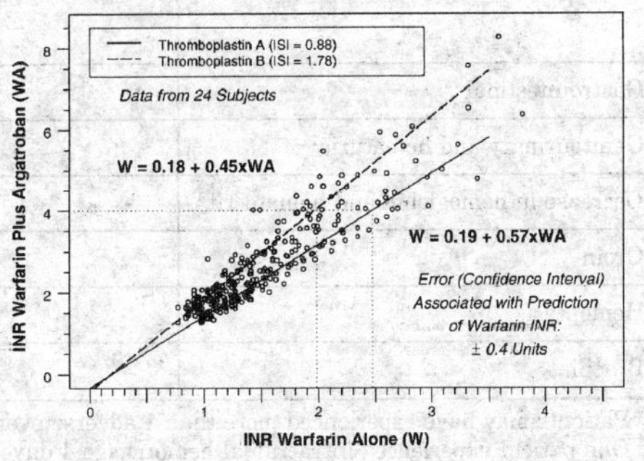

Figure 2 demonstrates the relationship between INR for warfarin alone and INR for warfarin co-administered with Argatroban at a dose of 2 mcg/kg/min. To calculate INR for warfarin alone (INR_W), based on INR for co-therapy of warfarin and Argatroban (INR_{WA}), when the Argatroban dose is 2 mcg/kg/min, use the equation next to the appropriate curve. Example: At a dose of 2 mcg/kg/min and an INR performed with Thromboplastin A, the equation 0.19 + 0.57 (INR_{WA}) = INR_W would allow a prediction of the INR on warfarin alone (INR_W). Thus, using an INR_{WA} value of 4.0 obtained on combined therapy: $INR_W = 0.19 + 0.57\ (4) = 2.47$ as the value for INR on warfarin alone. The error (confidence interval) associated with a prediction is ± 0.4 units. Similar linear relationships and prediction errors exist for Argatroban at a dose of 1 mcg/kg/min. Thus, for Argatroban doses of 1 or 2 mcg/kg/min, INR_W can be predicted from INR_{WA}. For Argatroban doses greater than 2 mcg/kg/min, the error associated with predicting INR_W from INR_{WA} is ±1. Thus, INR_W cannot be reliably predicted from INR_{WA} at doses greater than 2 mcg/kg/min.

SPECIAL POPULATIONS

Renal Impairment: No dosage adjustment is necessary in patients with renal dysfunction. The effect of renal disease on the pharmacokinetics of Argatroban was studied in 6 subjects with normal renal function (mean Clcr = 95 ± 16 mL/min) and in 18 subjects with mild (mean Clcr = 64 ± 10 mL/min), moderate (mean Clcr = 41 ± 5.8 mL/min), and severe (mean Clcr = 5 ± 7 mL/min) renal impairment. The pharmacokinetics and pharmacodynamics of Argatroban at dosages up to 5 mcg/kg/min were not significantly affected by renal dysfunction.
Hepatic Impairment: The dosage of Argatroban should be decreased in patients with hepatic impairment (see PRECAUTIONS and DOSAGE AND ADMINISTRATION). Patients with hepatic impairment were not studied in percutaneous coronary intervention (PCI) trials. At a dose of 2.5 mcg/kg/min, hepatic impairment is associated with decreased clearance and increased elimination half-life of Argatroban (to 1.9 mL/kg/min and 181 minutes, respectively, for patients with a Child-Pugh score >6).
Age, Gender: There are no clinically significant effects of age or gender on the pharmacokinetics or pharmacodynamics (e.g., aPTT) of Argatroban.
Drug-Drug Interactions: ***Digoxin:*** In 12 healthy volunteers, intravenous infusion of Argatroban (2 mcg/kg/min) over 5 days (study days 11 to 15) did not affect the steady-state pharmacokinetics of oral digoxin (0.375 mg daily for 15 days).
Erythromycin: In 10 healthy subjects, orally administered erythromycin (a potent inhibitor of CYP3A4/5) at 500 mg four times daily for 7 days had no effect on the pharmacokinetics of Argatroban at a dose of 1 mcg/kg/min for 5 hours. These data suggest oxidative metabolism by CYP3A4/5 is not an important elimination pathway in vivo for Argatroban.

CLINICAL STUDIES

Heparin-Induced Thrombocytopenia: Heparin-induced thrombocytopenia (HIT) is a potentially serious, immune-mediated complication of heparin therapy that is strongly associated with subsequent venous and arterial thrombosis. Whereas initial treatment of HIT is to discontinue administration of all heparin, patients may require anticoagulation for prevention and treatment of thromboembolic events.
The conclusion that Argatroban is an effective treatment for heparin-induced thrombocytopenia (HIT) and heparin-induced thrombocytopenia and thrombosis syndrome (HITTS) is based upon the data from an historically controlled efficacy and safety study (Study 1) and a follow-on efficacy and safety study (Study 2). These studies were comparable with regard to study design, study objectives, dosing regimens as well as study outline, conduct, and monitoring.
In these studies, 568 adult patients were treated with Argatroban and 193 adult patients made up the historical control group. Patients were required to have a clinical diagnosis of heparin-induced thrombocytopenia, either without thrombosis (HIT) or with thrombosis (HITTS) and be males or non-pregnant females between the age of 18 and 80 years old. HIT/HITTS was defined by a fall in platelet count to less than 100,000/µL or a 50% decrease in platelets after the initiation of heparin therapy with no apparent explanation other than HIT. Patients with HITTS also had presence of an arterial or venous thrombosis documented by appropriate imaging techniques or supported by clinical evidence such as acute myocardial infarction, stroke, pulmonary embolism, or other clinical indications of vascular occlusion. Patients who required anticoagulation with documented histories of positive HIT antibody test were also eligible in the absence of thrombocytopenia or heparin challenge (e.g., patients with latent disease).
Patients with documented unexplained aPTT >200% of control at baseline, documented coagulation disorder or bleeding diathesis unrelated to HITTS, a lumbar puncture within the past 7 days or a history of previous aneurysm, hemorrhagic stroke, or recent thrombotic stroke, within the past 6 months, unrelated to HITTS were excluded from these studies.
The initial dose of Argatroban was 2 mcg/kg/min, not to exceed 10 mcg/kg/min. Two hours after the start of the Argatroban infusion, an aPTT level was obtained and dose adjustments were made to achieve a steady-state aPTT value that was 1.5 to 3.0 times the baseline value, not to exceed 100 seconds. In Study 1, the mean aPTT level for HIT patients was 38 seconds prior to start of Argatroban infusion. At first assessment,* during the Argatroban infusion, mean aPTT level for HIT patients was 64 seconds. Overall the mean aPTT level during the Argatroban infusion for HIT patients was 62.5 seconds. In Study 1, the mean aPTT level for HITTS patients was 34 seconds prior to start of Argatroban infusion. At first assessment,* during the Argatroban infusion, mean aPTT level for HITTS patients was 70 seconds. Overall, the mean aPTT level during the Argatroban infusion for HITTS patients was 64.5 seconds (see DOSAGE AND ADMINISTRATION).

(*First assessment was defined as occurring at least 2 hours post-infusion start time.)

The primary efficacy analysis was based on a comparison of event rates for a composite endpoint that included death (all causes), amputation (all causes) or new thrombosis during the treatment and follow-up period (study days 0 to 37). Secondary analyses included evaluation of the event rates for the components of the composite endpoint as well as time-to-event analyses.

Continued on next page

Product information on these pages is effective as of August 2004. Further information is available at: GlaxoSmithKline, PO Box 13398, Research Triangle Park, NC 27709. 1-888-825-5249. Corporate Web Site: www.gsk.com

Argatroban—Cont.

In Study 1, 304 patients were enrolled having active HIT (129/304, 42%), active HITTS (144/304, 47%), or latent disease (31/304, 10%). Among the 193 historical controls, 139 (72%) had active HIT, 46 (24%) had active HITTS, and 8 (4%) had latent disease. Within each group, those with active HIT and those with latent disease were analyzed together. Positive laboratory confirmation of HIT/HITTS by the heparin-induced platelet aggregation test or serotonin release assay was demonstrated in 174 of 304 (57%) Argatroban-treated patients (i.e., in 80 with HIT or latent disease and 94 with HITTS) and in 149 of 193 (77%) historical controls (i.e., in 119 with HIT or latent disease and 30 with HITTS). The test results for the remainder of the patients and controls were either negative or not determined. A categorical analysis showed a significant improvement in the composite outcome in patients with HIT and HITTS treated with Argatroban versus those in the historical control group (see Table 1). The components of the composite endpoint are shown in Table 2.

[See table 1 at right]
[See table 2 at right]

Time-to-event analyses showed significant improvements in the time-to-first event in patients with HIT or HITTS treated with Argatroban versus those in the historical control group. The between-group differences in the proportion of patients who remained free of death, amputation, or new thrombosis were statistically significant in favor of Argatroban by these analyses (p = 0.007 in patients with HIT and p = 0.018 in patients with HITTS, according to log-rank test).

A time-to-event analysis for the composite endpoint is shown in Figure 3 for patients with HIT and Figure 4 for patients with HITTS.

STUDY 1

Figure 3. Time to First Event for the Composite Efficacy Endpoint: HIT Patients

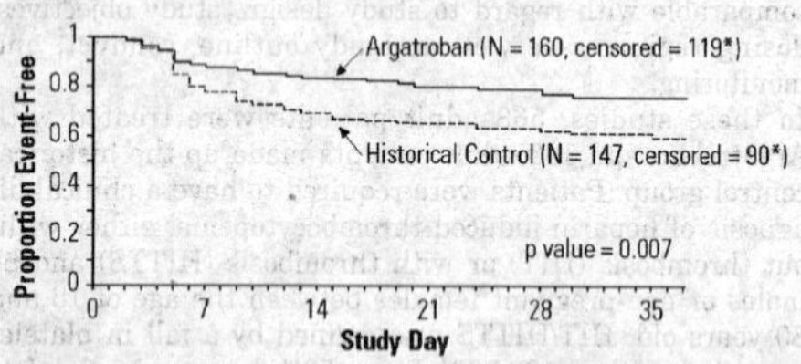

*Censored indicates no clinical endpoint (defined as death, amputation, or new thrombosis) was observed during the follow-up period (maximum period of follow-up was 37 days).

STUDY 1

Figure 4. Time to First Event for the Composite Efficacy Endpoint: HITTS Patients

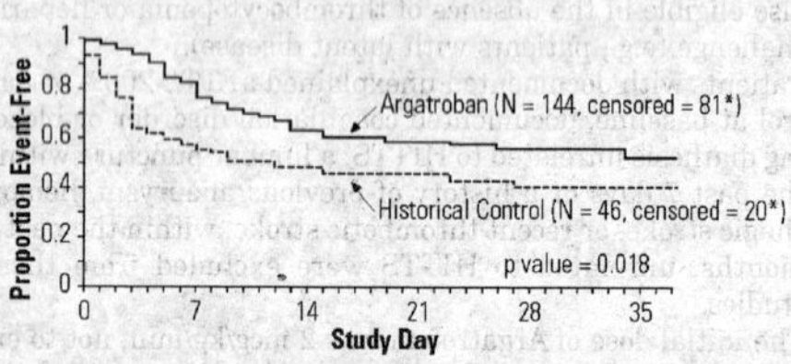

*Censored indicates no clinical endpoint (defined as death, amputation, or new thrombosis) was observed during the follow-up period (maximum period of follow-up was 37 days).

In Study 2, 264 patients were enrolled, having either HIT (125/264, 47.3%) or HITTS (139/264, 52.7%), and then treated with Argatroban. Categorical analysis demonstrated significant improvement in the composite efficacy outcome for Argatroban-treated patients, versus the same historical control group from Study 1, among patients having HIT (25.6% vs. 38.8%), patients having HITTS (41.0% vs. 56.5%), and patients having either HIT or HITTS (33.7% vs. 43.0%). Time-to-event analyses showed significant improvements in the time-to-first event in patients with HIT or HITTS treated with Argatroban versus those in the historical control group. The between-group differences in the proportion of patients who remained free of death, amputation, or new thrombosis were statistically significant in favor of Argatroban.

Anticoagulant Effect: In Study 1, the mean (±SE) dose of Argatroban administered was 2.0 ± 0.1 mcg/kg/min in the HIT arm and 1.9 ± 0.1 mcg/kg/min in the HITTS arm. Seventy-six percent of patients with HIT and 81% of patients with HITTS achieved a target aPTT at least 1.5-fold greater than the baseline aPTT at the first assessment occurring on average at 4.6 hours (HIT) and 3.9 hours (HITTS) following initiation of Argatroban therapy.

No enhancement of aPTT response was observed in subjects receiving repeated administration of Argatroban.

Platelet Count Recovery: In Study 1, the majority of patients, 53% of those with HIT and 58% of those with HITTS, had a recovery of platelet count by day 3. Platelet Count Recovery was defined as an increase in platelet count to >100,000/µL or to at least 1.5-fold greater than the baseline count (platelet count at study initiation) by day 3 of the study.

Table 1. Efficacy Results of Study 1: Composite Endpoint*

	HIT		HITTS		HIT/HITTS	
Parameter, N (%)	**Control n = 147**	**Argatroban n = 160**	**Control n = 46**	**Argatroban n = 144**	**Control n = 193**	**Argatroban n = 304**
Composite Endpoint	57 (38.8)	41 (25.6)	26 (56.5)	63 (43.8)	83 (43.0)	104 (34.2)

*Death (all causes), amputation (all causes), or new thrombosis within 37-day study period.

Table 2. Efficacy Results of Study 1: Components of the Composite Endpoint, Ranked by Severity*

	HIT		HITTS		HIT/HITTS	
Parameter, N (%)	**Control n = 147**	**Argatroban n = 160**	**Control n = 46**	**Argatroban n = 144**	**Control n = 193**	**Argatroban n = 304**
Death	32 (21.8)	27 (16.9)	13 (28.3)	26 (18.1)	45 (23.3)	53 (17.4)
Amputation	3 (2.0)	3 (1.9)	4 (8.7)	16 (11.1)	7 (3.6)	19 (6.2)
New Thrombosis	22 (15.0)	11 (6.9)	9 (19.6)	21 (14.6)	31 (16.1)	32 (10.5)

*Reported as the most severe outcome among the components of composite endpoint (severity ranking: death > amputation > new thrombosis); patients may have had multiple outcomes.

Table 3. Major and Minor Hemorrhagic Adverse Events in HIT/HITTS Patients

Major Hemorrhagic Events*		
	Argatroban-treated Patients (Study 1 and Study 2) (n = 568) %	**Historical Control (n = 193) %**
Overall bleeding	5.3	6.7
Gastrointestinal	2.3	1.6
Genitourinary and hematuria	0.9	0.5
Decrease in hemoglobin and hematocrit	0.7	0
Multisystem hemorrhage and DIC	0.5	1
Limb and BKA stump	0.5	0
Intracranial hemorrhage	0†	0.5
Minor Hemorrhagic Events*		
	Argatroban-treated Patients (Study 1 and Study 2) (n = 568) %	**Historical Control (n = 193) %**
Gastrointestinal	14.4	18.1
Genitourinary and hematuria	11.6	0.8
Decrease in hemoglobin and hematocrit	10.4	0
Groin	5.4	3.1
Hemoptysis	2.9	0.8
Brachial	2.4	0.8

*Patients may have experienced more than 1 adverse event.
† One patient experienced intracranial hemorrhage 4 days after discontinuation of Argatroban and following therapy with urokinase and oral anticoagulation.
DIC = disseminated intravascular coagulation.
BKA = below-the-knee amputation.

Percutaneous Coronary Intervention (PCI) in HIT/HITTS Patients: In 3 similarly designed trials, Argatroban was administered to 91 patients with current or previous clinical diagnosis of HIT/HITTS or heparin-dependent antibodies, who underwent a total of 112 percutaneous coronary interventions (PCIs) including percutaneous transluminal coronary angioplasty (PTCA), coronary stent placement, or atherectomy.

Among the 91 patients undergoing their first PCI with Argatroban, notable ongoing or recent medical history included myocardial infarction (n = 35), unstable angina (n = 23), and chronic angina (n = 34). There were 33 females and 58 males. The average age was 67.6 years (median 70.7, range 44 to 86), and the average weight was 82.5 kg (median 81.0 kg, range 49 to 141).

Due to the history or presence of the heparin-dependent antibody or HIT/HITTS, these patients required alternative anticoagulation. Twenty-one of the 91 patients had a repeat PCI using Argatroban an average of 150 days after their initial PCI. Seven of 91 patients received glycoprotein IIb/IIIa inhibitors. Safety and efficacy were assessed against historical control populations.

Per protocol, all patients received oral aspirin (325 mg) 2 to 24 hours prior to the interventional procedure. After venous or arterial sheaths were in place, anticoagulation was initiated with a bolus of Argatroban of 350 mcg/kg via a large-bore IV line or through the venous sheath over 3 to 5 minutes. Simultaneously, a maintenance infusion of 25 mcg/kg/min was initiated to achieve a therapeutic activated clotting time (ACT) of 300 to 450 seconds. If necessary to achieve this therapeutic range, the maintenance infusion dose was titrated (15 to 40 mcg/kg/min) and/or an additional bolus dose of 150 mcg/kg could be given. Each patient's ACT was checked 5 to 10 minutes following the bolus dose. The ACT was checked as clinically indicated thereafter. Arterial and venous sheaths were removed no sooner than 2 hours after discontinuation of Argatroban and when the ACT was less than 160 seconds.

If a patient required anticoagulation after the procedure, Argatroban could be continued, but at a lower infusion dose between 2.5 and 5 mcg/kg/min. An aPTT was drawn 2 hours after this dose reduction and the dose of Argatroban then adjusted as clinically indicated (not to exceed 10 mcg/kg/min), to reach an aPTT between 1.5 and 3 times baseline value (not to exceed 100 seconds).

Ninety-one patients were treated with Argatroban on their first PCI, and 21 patients were reexposed to Argatroban on subsequent PCIs. In 92 of the 112 interventions (82%), the patient received the initial bolus of 350 mcg/kg and an initial infusion dose of 25 mcg/kg/min. The majority of patients did not require additional bolus dosing during the PCI procedure. The mean value for the initial ACT measurement after the start of dosing for all interventions was 379 sec (median 338 sec; 5th percentile-95th percentile 238 to

675 sec). The mean ACT value per intervention over all measurements taken during the procedure was 416 sec (median 390 sec; 5th percentile-95th percentile 261 to 698 sec). About 65% of patients had ACTs within the recommended range of 300 to 450 seconds throughout the procedure. The investigators did not achieve anticoagulation within the recommended range in about 23% of patients. However, in this small sample, patients with ACTs below 300 seconds did not have more coronary thrombotic events, and patients with ACTs over 450 seconds did not have higher bleeding rates. Acute procedural success was defined as lack of death, emergent coronary artery bypass graft (CABG), or Q-wave myocardial infarction. Acute procedural success was reported in 98.2% of patients who underwent PCIs with Argatroban anticoagulation compared with 94.3% of historical control patients anticoagulated with heparin (p = NS). Among the 112 interventions, 2 patients had emergency CABGs, 3 had repeat PTCAs, 4 had non-Q-wave myocardial infarctions, 3 had myocardial ischemia, 1 had an abrupt closure, and 1 had an impending closure (some patients may have experienced more than 1 event). No patients died. Two patients had protocol-defined major bleeding, 1 of which was retroperitoneal and the other gastrointestinal. Minor bleeding, defined as spontaneous and observed with hemoglobin decreasing >3g/dL or with no bleeding site and hemoglobin decreasing >4g/dL, occurred in 4.5% of interventions.

Additional Information: ***Cardiac Therapy:*** The safety and effectiveness of Argatroban for cardiac indications outside of percutaneous coronary intervention in patients with HIT have not been established.

Reexposure and Lack of Antibody Formation: Plasma from 12 healthy volunteers treated with Argatroban over 6 days showed no evidence of neutralizing antibodies. Repeated administration of Argatroban to more than 40 patients was tolerated with no loss of anticoagulant activity. No change in the dose is required.

INDICATIONS AND USAGE

Argatroban is indicated as an anticoagulant for prophylaxis or treatment of thrombosis in patients with heparin-induced thrombocytopenia.

Argatroban is indicated as an anticoagulant in patients with or at risk for heparin-induced thrombocytopenia undergoing percutaneous coronary intervention (PCI).

CONTRAINDICATIONS

Argatroban is contraindicated in patients with overt major bleeding, or in patients hypersensitive to this product or any of its components (see WARNINGS).

WARNINGS

Argatroban is intended for intravenous administration. All parenteral anticoagulants should be discontinued before administration of Argatroban.

Hemorrhage: Hemorrhage can occur at any site in the body in patients receiving Argatroban. An unexplained fall in hematocrit, a fall in blood pressure, or any other unexplained symptom should lead to consideration of a hemorrhagic event. Argatroban should be used with extreme caution in disease states and other circumstances in which there is an increased danger of hemorrhage. These include severe hypertension; immediately following lumbar puncture; spinal anesthesia; major surgery, especially involving the brain, spinal cord, or eye; hematologic conditions associated with increased bleeding tendencies such as congenital or acquired bleeding disorders and gastrointestinal lesions such as ulcerations.

PRECAUTIONS

Hepatic Impairment: Caution should be exercised when administering Argatroban to patients with hepatic disease, by starting with a lower dose and carefully titrating until the desired level of anticoagulation is achieved. Also, upon cessation of Argatroban infusion in the hepatically impaired patient, full reversal of anticoagulant effects may require longer than 4 hours due to decreased clearance and increased elimination half-life of Argatroban (see DOSAGE AND ADMINISTRATION).

Use of high doses of Argatroban in PCI patients with clinically significant hepatic disease or AST/ALT levels ≥3 times the upper limit of normal should be avoided. Such patients were not studied in PCI trials.

Laboratory Tests: Anticoagulation effects associated with Argatroban infusion at doses up to 40 mcg/kg/min correlate with increases of the activated partial thromboplastin time (aPTT).

Although other global clot-based tests including prothrombin time (PT), the International Normalized Ratio (INR), and thrombin time (TT) are affected by Argatroban, the therapeutic ranges for these tests have not been identified for Argatroban therapy. Plasma Argatroban concentrations also correlate well with anticoagulant effects (see CLINICAL PHARMACOLOGY).

In clinical trials in PCI, the activated clotting time (ACT) was used for monitoring Argatroban anticoagulant activity during the procedure.

The concomitant use of Argatroban and warfarin results in prolongation of the PT and INR beyond that produced by warfarin alone. Alternative approaches for monitoring concurrent Argatroban and warfarin therapy are described in a subsequent section (see DOSAGE AND ADMINISTRATION).

Drug Interactions: ***Heparin:*** Since heparin is contraindicated in patients with heparin-induced thrombocytopenia, the co-administration of Argatroban and heparin is unlikely for this indication. However, if Argatroban is to be initiated after cessation of heparin therapy, allow sufficient time for heparin's effect on the aPTT to decrease prior to initiation of Argatroban therapy.

Aspirin/Acetaminophen: Pharmacokinetic or pharmacodynamic drug-drug interactions have not been demonstrated between Argatroban and concomitantly administered aspirin (162.5 mg orally given 26 and 2 hours prior to initiation of Argatroban 1 mcg/kg/min over 4 hours) or acetaminophen (1,000 mg orally given 12, 6, and 0 hours prior to, and 6 and 12 hours subsequent to, initiation of Argatroban 1.5 mcg/kg/min over 18 hours).

Oral Anticoagulant Agents: Pharmacokinetic drug-drug interactions between Argatroban and warfarin (7.5 mg single oral dose) have not been demonstrated. However, the concomitant use of Argatroban and warfarin (5 to 7.5 mg initial oral dose, followed by 2.5 to 6 mg/day orally for 6 to 10 days) results in prolongation of the prothrombin time (PT) and International Normalized Ratio (INR) (see CLINICAL PHARMACOLOGY and DOSAGE AND ADMINISTRATION).

Thrombolytic Agents: The safety and effectiveness of Argatroban with thrombolytic agents have not been established (see ADVERSE REACTIONS, *Intracranial Bleeding*).

Glycoprotein IIb/IIIa Antagonists: The safety and effectiveness of Argatroban with glycoprotein IIb/IIIa antagonists have not been established.

Co-Administration: Concomitant use of Argatroban with antiplatelet agents, thrombolytics, and other anticoagulants may increase the risk of bleeding (see WARNINGS). Drug-drug interactions have not been observed between Argatroban and digoxin or erythromycin (see CLINICAL PHARMACOLOGY, Drug-Drug Interactions).

Carcinogenesis, Mutagenesis, Impairment of Fertility: No long-term studies in animals have been performed to evaluate the carcinogenic potential of Argatroban.

Argatroban was not genotoxic in the Ames test, the Chinese hamster ovary cell (CHO/HGPRT) forward mutation test, the Chinese hamster lung fibroblast chromosome aberration test, the rat hepatocyte, and WI-38 human fetal lung cell unscheduled DNA synthesis (UDS) tests, or the mouse micronucleus test.

Argatroban at intravenous doses up to 27 mg/kg/day (0.3 times the recommended maximum human dose based on body surface area) was found to have no effect on fertility and reproductive performance of male and female rats.

Pregnancy: Teratogenic Effects: Pregnancy Category B. Teratology studies have been performed in rats with intravenous doses up to 27 mg/kg/day (0.3 times the recommended maximum human dose based on body surface area) and rabbits at intravenous doses up to 10.8 mg/kg/day (0.2 times the recommended maximum human dose based on body surface area) and have revealed no evidence of impaired fertility or harm to the fetus due to Argatroban. There are, however, no adequate and well-controlled studies in pregnant women. Because animal reproduction studies are not always predictive of human response, this drug should be used during pregnancy only if clearly needed.

Nursing Mothers: Experiments in rats show that Argatroban is detected in milk. It is not known whether this drug is excreted in human milk. Because many drugs are excreted in human milk and because of the potential for serious adverse reactions in nursing infants from Argatroban, a decision should be made whether to discontinue nursing or to discontinue the drug, taking into account the importance of the drug to the mother.

Geriatric Use: In the clinical studies of adult patients with HIT or HITTS, the effectiveness of Argatroban was not affected by age.

Pediatric Use: The safety and effectiveness of Argatroban in patients below the age of 18 years have not been established.

ADVERSE REACTIONS

Adverse Events Reported in HIT/HITTS Patients: The following safety information is based on all 568 patients treated with Argatroban in Study 1 and Study 2. The safety profile of the patients from these studies is compared with that of 193 historical controls in which the adverse events were collected retrospectively. The adverse events reported in this section include all events regardless of relationship to treatment. Adverse events are separated into hemorrhagic and non-hemorrhagic events.

Major bleeding was defined as bleeding that was overt and associated with a hemoglobin decrease ≥2 g/dL, that led to a transfusion of ≥2 units, or that was intracranial, retroperitoneal, or into a major prosthetic joint. Minor bleeding was overt bleeding that did not meet the criteria for major bleeding.

Table 3 gives an overview of the most frequently observed hemorrhagic events, presented separately by major and minor bleeding, sorted by decreasing occurrence among Argatroban-treated HIT/HITTS patients.

[See table 3 on previous page]

Table 4 gives an overview of the most frequently observed non-hemorrhagic events sorted by decreasing frequency of occurrence (≥ 2%) among Argatroban-treated HIT/HITTS patients.

[See table 4 above]

Table 4. Non-hemorrhagic Adverse Events in HIT/HITTS Patients*

	Argatroban-treated Patients (Study 1 and Study 2) (n = 568) %	Historical Control (n = 193) %
Dyspnea	8.1	8.8
Hypotension	7.2	2.6
Fever	6.9	2.1
Diarrhea	6.2	1.6
Sepsis	6.0	12.4
Cardiac arrest	5.8	3.1
Nausea	4.8	0.5
Ventricular tachycardia	4.8	3.1
Pain	4.6	3.1
Urinary tract infection	4.6	5.2
Vomiting	4.2	0
Infection	3.7	3.6
Pneumonia	3.3	9.3
Atrial fibrillation	3.0	11.4
Coughing	2.8	1.6
Abnormal renal function	2.8	4.7
Abdominal pain	2.6	1.6
Cerebrovascular disorder	2.3	4.1

*Patients may have experienced more than 1 adverse event.

Adverse Events Reported in HIT/HITTS Patients Undergoing PCI: The following safety information is based on 91 patients initially treated with Argatroban and 21 patients subsequently re-exposed to Argatroban for a total of 112 PCIs with Argatroban anticoagulation. The adverse events reported in this section include all events regardless of relationship to treatment. Adverse events are separated into hemorrhagic (Table 5) and non-hemorrhagic (Table 6) events.

Major bleeding was defined as bleeding that was overt and associated with a hemoglobin decrease ≥5 g/dL, that led to a transfusion of ≥2 units, or that was intracranial, retroperitoneal, or into a major prosthetic joint.

Continued on next page

Product information on these pages is effective as of August 2004. Further information is available at: GlaxoSmithKline, PO Box 13398, Research Triangle Park, NC 27709. 1-888-825-5249. Corporate Web Site: www.gsk.com

Argatroban—Cont.

The rate of major bleeding events and intracranial hemorrhage in the PCI trials was 1.8% and in the placebo arm of the EPILOG trial (placebo plus standard dose, weight-adjusted heparin) was 3.1%.

Table 5. Major and Minor Hemorrhagic Adverse Events in HIT/HITTS Patients Undergoing PCI

Major Hemorrhagic Events*	
	Argatroban-treated Patients (n = 112)† %
Retroperitoneal	0.9
Gastrointestinal	0.9
Intracranial	0
Minor Hemorrhagic Events*	
	Argatroban-treated Patients (n = 112)† %
Groin (bleeding or hematoma)	3.6
Gastrointestinal (includes hematemesis)	2.6
Genitourinary (includes hematuria)	1.8
Decrease in hemoglobin and/or hematocrit	1.8
CABG (coronary arteries)	1.8
Access site	0.9
Hemoptysis	0.9
Other	0.9

* Patients may have experienced more than 1 adverse event.
† 91 patients who underwent 112 interventions.
CABG = coronary artery bypass graft.

Table 6 gives an overview of the most frequently observed non-hemorrhagic events (>2%), sorted by decreasing frequency of occurrence among Argatroban-treated PCI patients.

Table 6. Non-hemorrhagic Adverse Events* in HIT/HITTS Patients Undergoing PCI

	Argatroban Procedures* (n = 112)† %	Controls (n = 2226)‡ %
Chest pain	15.2	9.3
Hypotension	10.7	10.3
Back pain	8.0	13.7
Nausea	7.1	11.5
Vomiting	6.3	6.8
Headache	5.4	5.5
Bradycardia	4.5	3.5
Abdominal pain	3.6	2.2
Fever	3.6	<0.5
Myocardial infarction	3.6	NR§

* Patients may have experienced more than 1 adverse event.
† 91 patients who underwent 112 interventions.
‡ Controls from EPIC (Evaluation of c7E3 Fab in the Prevention of Ischemic Complications), EPILOG (Evaluation in PTCA to Improve Long-Term Outcome with Abciximab GP IIb/IIIa Blockade Study) and CAPTURE (Chimeric 7E3 Antiplatelet Therapy in Unstable angina Refractory to standard treatment) trials. Source: ReoPro® Prescribing Information.
§ NR = not reported.

There were 22 serious adverse events in 17 PCI patients (19.6% in 112 interventions). The types of events, which are listed regardless of relationship to treatment, are shown in Table 7. Table 7 lists the serious adverse events occurring in Argatroban-treated HIT/HITTS patients undergoing PCI.

Table 7. Serious Adverse Events in HIT/HITTS Patients Undergoing PCI*

Coded Term	Argatroban Procedures† (n = 112)
Chest pain	1 (0.9%)
Fever	1 (0.9%)
Retroperitoneal hemorrhage	1 (0.9%)
Angina pectoris	2 (1.8%)
Aortic stenosis	1 (0.9%)
Coronary thrombosis	2 (1.8%)
Arterial thrombosis	1 (0.9%)
Myocardial infarction	4 (3.5%)
Myocardial ischemia	2 (1.8%)
Occlusion coronary	2 (1.8%)
Gastrointestinal hemorrhage	1 (0.9%)
Gastrointestinal disorder (GERD)	1 (0.9%)
Cerebrovascular disorder	1 (0.9%)
Lung edema	1 (0.9%)
Vascular disorder	1 (0.9%)

* Individual events may also have been reported elsewhere (see Table 5 and 6).
† 91 patients underwent 112 procedures. Some patients may have experienced more than 1 event.

Adverse Events Reported in Other Populations: The following safety information is based on a total of 1,127 individuals who were treated with Argatroban in clinical pharmacology studies (n = 211) or for various clinical indications (n = 916).

Intracranial Bleeding: Intracranial bleeding only occurred in patients with acute myocardial infarction who were started on both Argatroban and thrombolytic therapy with streptokinase. The overall frequency of this potentially life-threatening complication among patients receiving both Argatroban and thrombolytic therapy (streptokinase or tissue plasminogen activator) was 1% (8 out of 810 patients). Intracranial bleeding was not observed in 317 subjects or patients who did not receive concomitant thrombolysis (see PRECAUTIONS, Drug Interactions).

Intracranial bleeding was also observed in a prospective, placebo-controlled study of Argatroban in patients who had onset of acute stroke within 12 hours of study entry. Symptomatic intracranial hemorrhage was reported in 5 of 117 patients (4.3%) who received Argatroban and in none of the 54 patients who received placebo. Asymptomatic intracranial hemorrhage occurred in 5 (4.3%) and 2 (3.7%) of the patients, respectively.

Allergic Reactions: 156 allergic reactions or suspected allergic reactions were observed in 1,127 individuals who were treated with Argatroban in clinical pharmacology studies or for various clinical indications. About 95% (148/156) of these reactions occurred in patients who concomitantly received thrombolytic therapy (e.g., streptokinase) for acute myocardial infarction and/or contrast media for coronary angiography.

Allergic reactions or suspected allergic reactions in populations other than HIT/HITTS patients include (in descending order of frequency*):

- Airway reactions (coughing, dyspnea): 10% or more
- Skin reactions (rash, bullous eruption): 1 to <10%
- General reactions (vasodilation): 1 to 10%

* The CIOMS (Council for International Organization of Medical Sciences) III standard categories are used for classification of frequencies.

OVERDOSAGE

Symptoms/Treatment: Excessive anticoagulation, with or without bleeding, may be controlled by discontinuing Argatroban or by decreasing the Argatroban infusion dosage (see WARNINGS). In clinical studies at therapeutic levels, anticoagulation parameters generally return to baseline within 2 to 4 hours after discontinuation of the drug. Reversal of anticoagulant effect may take longer in patients with hepatic impairment.

No specific antidote to Argatroban is available; if life-threatening bleeding occurs and excessive plasma levels of Argatroban are suspected, Argatroban should be discontinued immediately, aPTT and other coagulation tests should be determined. Symptomatic and supportive therapy should be provided to the patient (see WARNINGS).

Single intravenous doses of Argatroban at 200, 124, 150, and 200 mg/kg were lethal to mice, rats, rabbits, and dogs, respectively. The symptoms of acute toxicity were loss of righting reflex, tremors, clonic convulsions, paralysis of hind limbs, and coma.

DOSAGE AND ADMINISTRATION

Each 2.5-mL vial contains 250 mg of Argatroban; and, as supplied, is a concentrated drug (100 mg/mL), which must be diluted 100-fold prior to infusion. Argatroban should not be mixed with other drugs prior to dilution in a suitable intravenous fluid.

Preparation for Intravenous Administration: Argatroban should be diluted in 0.9% Sodium Chloride Injection, 5% Dextrose Injection, or Lactated Ringer's Injection to a final concentration of 1 mg/mL. The contents of each 2.5-mL vial should be diluted 100-fold by mixing with 250 mL of diluent. Use 250 mg (2.5 mL) per 250 mL of diluent or 500 mg (5 mL) per 500 mL of diluent. The constituted solution must be mixed by repeated inversion of the diluent bag for 1 minute. Upon preparation, the solution may show slight but brief haziness due to the formation of microprecipitates that rapidly dissolve upon mixing. The pH of the intravenous solution prepared as recommended is 3.2 to 7.5.

Heparin-Induced Thrombocytopenia (HIT/HITTS): ***Initial Dosage:*** Before administering Argatroban, discontinue heparin therapy and obtain a baseline aPTT. The recommended initial dose of Argatroban for adult patients without hepatic impairment is 2 mcg/kg/min, administered as a continuous infusion (see Table 8).

Table 8. Recommended Doses and Infusion Rates for 2 mcg/kg/min Dose of Argatroban for Patients With HIT/HITTS (Without Hepatic Impairment) (1 mg/mL Final Concentration)

Body Weight (kg)	Dose (mcg/min)	Infusion Rate (mL/hr)
50	100	6
60	120	7
70	140	8
80	160	10
90	180	11
100	200	12
110	220	13
120	240	14
130	260	16
140	280	17

Monitoring Therapy: In general, therapy with Argatroban is monitored using the aPTT. Tests of anticoagulant effects (including the aPTT) typically attain steady-state levels within 1 to 3 hours following initiation of Argatroban. Dose adjustment may be required to attain the target aPTT. Check the aPTT 2 hours after initiation of therapy to confirm that the patient has attained the desired therapeutic range.

Dosage Adjustment: After the initial dose of Argatroban, the dose can be adjusted as clinically indicated (not to exceed 10 mcg/kg/min), until the steady-state aPTT is 1.5 to 3 times the initial baseline value (not to exceed 100 seconds) (see CLINICAL STUDIES for mean values of aPTT obtained after initial doses of Argatroban). Argatroban therapy should be continued until platelet counts have recovered substantially (i.e., $>100 \times 10^9$/L or to pre-HIT/-HITTS baseline value).

Percutaneous Coronary Interventions (PCI) in HIT/HITTS Patients: ***Initial Dosage:*** An infusion of Argatroban should be started at 25 mcg/kg/min and a bolus of 350 mcg/kg administered via a large bore intravenous (IV) line over 3 to 5 minutes (see Table 9). Activated clotting time (ACT) should be checked 5 to 10 minutes after the bolus dose is completed. The procedure may proceed if the ACT is greater than 300 seconds.

Dosage Adjustment: If the ACT is less than 300 seconds, an additional IV bolus dose of 150 mcg/kg should be administered, the infusion dose increased to 30 mcg/kg/min, and the ACT checked 5 to 10 minutes later (see Table 9). If the ACT is greater than 450 seconds, the infusion rate should be decreased to 15 mcg/kg/min, and the ACT checked 5 to 10 minutes later (see Table 9). Once a therapeutic ACT (between 300 and 450 seconds) has been achieved, this infusion dose should be continued for the duration of the procedure.

[See table 9 at top of next page]

In case of dissection, impending abrupt closure, thrombus formation during the procedure, or inability to achieve or maintain an ACT over 300 seconds, additional bolus doses of 150 mcg/kg may be administered and the infusion dose increased to 40 mcg/kg/min. The ACT should be checked after each additional bolus or change in the rate of infusion.

Monitoring therapy: Therapy with Argatroban is monitored using ACT. ACTs should be obtained before dosing, 5 to 10 minutes after bolus dosing and after change in the infusion rate, and at the end of the PCI procedure. Additional ACTs should be drawn about every 20 to 30 minutes during a prolonged procedure.

Continued Anticoagulation after PCI: If a patient requires anticoagulation after the procedure, Argatroban may be continued, but at a lower infusion dose [see DOSAGE AND ADMINISTRATION, Heparin-Induced Thrombocytopenia

Table 9. Recommended Doses and Infusion Rates of Argatroban for Patients Undergoing PCI (Without Hepatic Impairment) (1 mg/mL Final Concentration)

Body Weight (kg)	For ACT 300-450 seconds Initial Dosage* 25 mcg/kg/min			If ACT <300 seconds Dosage Adjustment† 30 mcg/kg/min			If ACT >450 seconds Dosage Adjustment 15 mcg/kg/min	
	Bolus Dose (mcg)	Infusion Dose (mcg/min)	Infusion Rate (mL/hr)	Bolus Dose (mcg)	Infusion Dose (mcg/min)	Infusion Rate (mL/hr)	Infusion Dose (mcg/min)	Infusion Rate (mL/hr)
50	17500	1250	75	7500	1500	90	750	45
60	21000	1500	90	9000	1800	108	900	54
70	24500	1750	105	10500	2100	126	1050	63
80	28000	2000	120	12000	2400	144	1200	72
90	31500	2250	135	13500	2700	162	1350	81
100	35000	2500	150	15000	3000	180	1500	90
110	38500	2750	165	16500	3300	198	1650	99
120	42000	3000	180	18000	3600	216	1800	108
130	45500	3250	195	19500	3900	234	1950	117
140	49000	3500	210	21000	4200	252	2100	126

NOTE: 1 mg = 1000 mcg; 1 kg = 2.2 lbs

* Initial IV bolus dose of 350 mcg/kg should be administered.

† Additional IV bolus dose of 150 mcg/kg should be administered if ACT <300 seconds.

(HIT/HITTS)]. If the patient has HIT or HITTS, Argatroban therapy should be continued until platelet counts have recovered substantially (i.e., >100 × 10^9/L or to pre-HIT/HITTS baseline value).

Dosing in Special Populations: ***Hepatic Impairment:*** For patients with heparin-induced thrombocytopenia with hepatic impairment, the initial dose of Argatroban should be reduced. For patients with moderate hepatic impairment, an initial dose of 0.5 mcg/kg/min is recommended, based on the approximate 4-fold decrease in Argatroban clearance relative to those with normal hepatic function. The aPTT should be monitored closely, and the dosage should be adjusted as clinically indicated (see PRECAUTIONS).

Hepatic Impairment in HIT/HITTS Patients Undergoing PCI: For hepatically impaired HIT/HITTS patients undergoing PCI, refer to PRECAUTIONS, Hepatic Impairment.

Renal Impairment: No dosage adjustment is necessary in patients with renal impairment (see PRECAUTIONS).

CONVERSION TO ORAL ANTICOAGULANT THERAPY

Initiating Oral Anticoagulant Therapy: Once the decision is made to initiate oral anticoagulant therapy, recognize the potential for combined effects on INR with co-administration of Argatroban and warfarin. (See CLINICAL PHARMACOLOGY, Effect on INR.) Continue to monitor Argatroban using aPTT. Oral anticoagulation therapy (warfarin) should be initiated only after substantial recovery of platelet counts (e.g., >100 × 10^9/L or to pre-HIT/-HITTS baseline value). A loading dose of warfarin should not be used. Initiate therapy using the expected daily dose of warfarin. To avoid prothrombotic effects and to ensure continuous anticoagulation when initiating warfarin, it is recommended to overlap Argatroban and warfarin therapy for 4 or 5 days (see warfarin prescribing information).

Co-Administration of Warfarin and Argatroban at Doses Up to 2 mcg/kg/min: Use of Argatroban with warfarin results in prolongation of INR beyond that produced by warfarin alone. To avoid prothrombotic effects and to ensure continuous anticoagulation when initiating warfarin, it is recommended to continue co-administration for at least 4 or 5 days before discontinuing Argatroban. The previously established relationship between INR and bleeding risk is altered. The combination of Argatroban and warfarin does not cause further reduction in the vitamin K–dependent factor Xa activity than that which is seen with warfarin alone. The relationship between INR obtained on combined therapy and INR obtained on warfarin alone is dependent on both the dose of Argatroban and the thromboplastin reagent used. The INR value on warfarin alone (INR_w) can be calculated from the INR value on combination Argatroban and warfarin therapy (see CLINICAL PHARMACOLOGY, Figure 2 explanation and PRECAUTIONS, Drug Interactions). INR should be measured daily while Argatroban and warfarin are co-administered. In general, with doses of Argatroban up to 2 mcg/kg/min, Argatroban can be discontinued when the INR is >4 on combined therapy. After Argatroban is discontinued, repeat the INR measurement in 4 to 6 hours. If the repeat INR is below the desired therapeutic range, resume the infusion of Argatroban and repeat the procedure daily until the desired therapeutic range on warfarin alone is reached.

Co-Administration of Warfarin and Argatroban at Doses Greater than 2 mcg/kg/min: For doses greater than 2 mcg/kg/min, the relationship of INR between warfarin alone to the INR on warfarin plus Argatroban is less predictable. In this case, in order to predict the INR on warfarin alone, temporarily reduce the dose of Argatroban to a dose of 2 mcg/kg/min. Repeat the INR on Argatroban and warfarin 4 to 6 hours after reduction of the Argatroban dose and follow the process outlined above for administering Argatroban at doses up to 2 mcg/kg/min.

STABILITY/COMPATIBILITY

Argatroban is a clear, colorless to pale yellow, slightly viscous solution. If the solution is cloudy, or if an insoluble precipitate is noted, the vial should be discarded.

Solutions prepared as recommended are stable at 25°C (77°F), with excursions permitted to 15° to 30°C (59° to 86°F) in ambient indoor light for 24 hours; therefore, light-resistant measures such as foil protection for intravenous lines are unnecessary. Solutions are physically and chemically stable for up to 48 hours when stored at 2° to 8°C in the dark. Prepared solutions should not be exposed to direct sunlight. No significant potency losses have been noted following simulated delivery of the solution through intravenous tubing.

HOW SUPPLIED

Argatroban Injection is supplied in 2.5-mL solution in single-use vials at the concentration of 100 mg/mL. Each vial contains 250 mg of Argatroban.

NDC 0007-4407-01 (Package of 1)

Storage: Store the vials in original cartons at room temperature [25°C (77°F), with excursions permitted to 15° to 30°C (59° to 86°F)]. Do not freeze. Retain in the original carton to protect from light.

Manufactured by Abbott Laboratories, North Chicago, IL 60064

Distributed by GlaxoSmithKline, Research Triangle Park, NC 27709 for

Encysive Pharmaceuticals Inc., Bellaire, TX 77401

November 2003/AR:L54

Shown in Product Identification Guide, page 314

AUGMENTIN® ℞

[äg-min' tin]

(Amoxicillin/Clavulanate Potassium)
Powder for Oral Suspension
and Chewable Tablets

To reduce the development of drug-resistant bacteria and maintain the effectiveness of AUGMENTIN (amoxicillin/clavulanate potassium) and other antibacterial drugs, AUGMENTIN should be used only to treat or prevent infections that are proven or strongly suspected to be caused by bacteria.

DESCRIPTION

AUGMENTIN is an oral antibacterial combination consisting of the semisynthetic antibiotic amoxicillin and the β-lactamase inhibitor, clavulanate potassium (the potassium salt of clavulanic acid). Amoxicillin is an analog of ampicillin, derived from the basic penicillin nucleus, 6-aminopenicillanic acid. The amoxicillin molecular formula is $C_{16}H_{19}N_3O_5S \cdot 3H_2O$, and the molecular weight is 419.46. Chemically, amoxicillin is (2*S*,5*R*,6*R*)-6-[(*R*)-(-)-2-Amino-2-(*p*-hydroxyphenyl)acetamido]-3,3-dimethyl-7-oxo-4-thia-1-azabicyclo[3.2.0]heptane-2-carboxylic acid trihydrate.

Clavulanic acid is produced by the fermentation of *Streptomyces clavuligerus*. It is a β-lactam structurally related to the penicillins and possesses the ability to inactivate a wide variety of β-lactamases by blocking the active sites of these enzymes. Clavulanic acid is particularly active against the clinically important plasmid-mediated β-lactamases frequently responsible for transferred drug resistance to penicillins and cephalosporins. The clavulanate potassium molecular formula is $C_8H_8KNO_5$, and the molecular weight is 237.25. Chemically, clavulanate potassium is potassium (*Z*)-(2*R*,5*R*)-3-(2-hydroxyethylidene)-7-oxo-4-oxa-1-azabicyclo[3.2.0]-heptane-2-carboxylate.

Inactive Ingredients: Powder for Oral Suspension—Colloidal silicon dioxide, flavorings (see HOW SUPPLIED), xanthan gum, and 1 or more of the following: Aspartame•, hypromellose, mannitol, silica gel, silicon dioxide, and sodium saccharin. Chewable Tablets—Colloidal silicon dioxide, flavorings (see HOW SUPPLIED), magnesium stearate, mannitol, and 1 or more of the following: Aspartame•, D&C Yellow No. 10, FD&C Red No. 40, glycine, sodium saccharin and succinic acid.

•See PRECAUTIONS—Information for the Patient.

Each 125-mg chewable tablet and each 5 mL of reconstituted 125 mg/5 mL oral suspension of AUGMENTIN contains 0.16 mEq potassium. Each 250-mg chewable tablet and each 5 mL of reconstituted 250 mg/5 mL oral suspension of AUGMENTIN contains 0.32 mEq potassium. Each 200-mg chewable tablet and each 5 mL of reconstituted 200 mg/5 mL oral suspension of AUGMENTIN contains 0.14 mEq potassium. Each 400-mg chewable tablet and each 5 mL of reconstituted 400 mg/5 mL oral suspension of AUGMENTIN contains 0.29 mEq of potassium.

CLINICAL PHARMACOLOGY

Amoxicillin and clavulanate potassium are well absorbed from the gastrointestinal tract after oral administration of AUGMENTIN. Dosing in the fasted or fed state has minimal effect on the pharmacokinetics of amoxicillin. While AUGMENTIN can be given without regard to meals, absorption of clavulanate potassium when taken with food is greater relative to the fasted state. In 1 study, the relative bioavailability of clavulanate was reduced when AUGMENTIN was dosed at 30 and 150 minutes after the start of a high-fat breakfast. The safety and efficacy of AUGMENTIN have been established in clinical trials where AUGMENTIN was taken without regard to meals.

Oral administration of single doses of 400-mg chewable tablets of AUGMENTIN and 400 mg/5 mL suspension to 28 adult volunteers yielded comparable pharmacokinetic data:

[See table at top of next page]

Oral administration of 5 mL of 250 mg/5 mL suspension of AUGMENTIN or the equivalent dose of 10 mL 125 mg/5 mL suspension of AUGMENTIN provides average peak serum concentrations approximately 1 hour after dosing of 6.9 mcg/mL for amoxicillin and 1.6 mcg/mL for clavulanic acid. The areas under the serum concentration curves obtained during the first 4 hours after dosing were 12.6 mcg.hr/mL for amoxicillin and 2.9 mcg.hr/mL for clavulanic acid when 5 mL of 250 mg/5 mL suspension of AUGMENTIN or equivalent dose of 10 mL of 125 mg/5 mL suspension of AUGMENTIN was administered to adult volunteers. One 250-mg chewable tablet of AUGMENTIN or two 125-mg chewable tablets of AUGMENTIN are equivalent to 5 mL of 250 mg/5 mL suspension of AUGMENTIN and provide similar serum levels of amoxicillin and clavulanic acid.

Amoxicillin serum concentrations achieved with AUGMENTIN are similar to those produced by the oral administration of equivalent doses of amoxicillin alone. The half-life of amoxicillin after the oral administration of AUGMENTIN is 1.3 hours and that of clavulanic acid is 1.0 hour. Time above the minimum inhibitory concentration of 1.0 mcg/mL for amoxicillin has been shown to be similar after corresponding q12h and q8h dosing regimens of AUGMENTIN in adults and children.

Approximately 50% to 70% of the amoxicillin and approximately 25% to 40% of the clavulanic acid are excreted unchanged in urine during the first 6 hours after administration of 10 mL of 250 mg/5 mL suspension of AUGMENTIN.

Concurrent administration of probenecid delays amoxicillin excretion but does not delay renal excretion of clavulanic acid.

Neither component in AUGMENTIN is highly protein-bound; clavulanic acid has been found to be approximately 25% bound to human serum and amoxicillin approximately 18% bound.

Amoxicillin diffuses readily into most body tissues and fluids with the exception of the brain and spinal fluid. The results of experiments involving the administration of clavulanic acid to animals suggest that this compound, like amoxicillin, is well distributed in body tissues.

Two hours after oral administration of a single 35 mg/kg dose of suspension of AUGMENTIN to fasting children, average concentrations of 3.0 mcg/mL of amoxicillin and 0.5 mcg/mL of clavulanic acid were detected in middle ear effusions.

Microbiology: Amoxicillin is a semisynthetic antibiotic with a broad spectrum of bactericidal activity against many gram-positive and gram-negative microorganisms. Amoxicillin is, however, susceptible to degradation by β-lactamases, and therefore, the spectrum of activity does not include organisms which produce these enzymes. Clavulanic acid is a β-lactam, structurally related to the penicillins, which possesses the ability to inactivate a wide range of β-lactamase enzymes commonly found in microorganisms

Continued on next page

Product information on these pages is effective as of August 2004. Further information is available at: GlaxoSmithKline, PO Box 13398, Research Triangle Park, NC 27709. 1-888-825-5249. Corporate Web Site: www.gsk.com

Augmentin Powder/Chewable—Cont.

resistant to penicillins and cephalosporins. In particular, it has good activity against the clinically important plasmid-mediated β-lactamases frequently responsible for transferred drug resistance.

The formulation of amoxicillin and clavulanic acid in AUGMENTIN protects amoxicillin from degradation by β-lactamase enzymes and effectively extends the antibiotic spectrum of amoxicillin to include many bacteria normally resistant to amoxicillin and other β-lactam antibiotics. Thus, AUGMENTIN possesses the distinctive properties of a broad-spectrum antibiotic and a β-lactamase inhibitor.

Amoxicillin/clavulanic acid has been shown to be active against most strains of the following microorganisms, both in vitro and in clinical infections as described in INDICATIONS AND USAGE.

Gram-Positive Aerobes:

Staphylococcus aureus (β-lactamase and non–β-lactamase–producing)[§]

[§] Staphylococci which are resistant to methicillin/oxacillin must be considered resistant to amoxicillin/clavulanic acid.

Gram-Negative Aerobes:

Enterobacter species (Although most strains of *Enterobacter* species are resistant in vitro, clinical efficacy has been demonstrated with AUGMENTIN in urinary tract infections caused by these organisms.)

Escherichia coli (β-lactamase and non–β-lactamase–producing)

Haemophilus influenzae (β-lactamase and non–β-lactamase–producing)

Klebsiella species (All known strains are β-lactamase–producing.)

Moraxella catarrhalis (β-lactamase and non–β-lactamase–producing)

The following in vitro data are available, **but their clinical significance is unknown**.

Amoxicillin/clavulanic acid exhibits in vitro minimal inhibitory concentrations (MICs) of 2 mcg/mL or less against most (≥90%) strains of *Streptococcus pneumoniae*[||]; MICs of 0.06 mcg/mL or less against most (≥90%) strains of *Neisseria gonorrhoeae*; MICs of 4 mcg/mL or less against most (≥90%) strains of staphylococci and anaerobic bacteria; MICs of 8 mcg/mL or less against most (≥90%) strains of other listed organisms. However, with the exception of organisms shown to respond to amoxicillin alone, the safety and effectiveness of amoxicillin/clavulanic acid in treating clinical infections due to these microorganisms have not been established in adequate and well-controlled clinical trials.

[||] Because amoxicillin has greater in vitro activity against *S. pneumoniae* than does ampicillin or penicillin, the majority of *S. pneumoniae* strains with intermediate susceptibility to ampicillin or penicillin are fully susceptible to amoxicillin.

Gram-Positive Aerobes:

Enterococcus faecalis[¶]

Staphylococcus epidermidis (β-lactamase and non-β-lactamase–producing)

Staphylococcus saprophyticus (β-lactamase and non–β-lactamase–producing)

Streptococcus pneumoniae[¶**]

Streptococcus pyogenes[¶**]

viridans group Streptococcus[¶**]

Gram-Negative Aerobes:

Eikenella corrodens (β-lactamase and non–β-lactamase–producing)

Neisseria gonorrhoeae[¶] (β-lactamase and non–β-lactamase–producing)

Proteus mirabilis[¶] (β-lactamase and non–β-lactamase–producing)

Anaerobic Bacteria

Bacteroides species, including *Bacteroides fragilis* (β-lactamase and non–β-lactamase–producing)

Fusobacterium species (β-lactamase and non–β-lactamase–producing)

Peptostreptococcus species**

[¶] Adequate and well-controlled clinical trials have established the effectiveness of amoxicillin alone in treating certain clinical infections due to these organisms.

**These are non–β-lactamase–producing organisms, and therefore, are susceptible to amoxicillin alone.

Susceptibility Testing: ***Dilution Techniques:*** Quantitative methods are used to determine antimicrobial MICs. These MICs provide estimates of the susceptibility of bacteria to antimicrobial compounds. The MICs should be determined using a standardized procedure. Standardized procedures are based on a dilution method[1] (broth or agar) or equivalent with standardized inoculum concentrations and standardized concentrations of amoxicillin/clavulanate potassium powder.

The recommended dilution pattern utilizes a constant amoxicillin/clavulanate potassium ratio of 2 to 1 in all tubes with varying amounts of amoxicillin. MICs are expressed in terms of the amoxicillin concentration in the presence of clavulanic acid at a constant 2 parts amoxicillin to 1 part clavulanic acid. The MIC values should be interpreted according to the following criteria:

Dose* (amoxicillin/clavulanate potassium)	AUC $_{0-\infty}$ (mcg.hr/mL) amoxicillin (±S.D.)	AUC $_{0-\infty}$ (mcg.hr/mL) clavulanate potassium (±S.D.)	C_{max} (mcg/mL)† amoxicillin (±S.D.)	C_{max} (mcg/mL)† clavulanate potassium (±S.D.)
400/57 mg (5 mL of suspension)	17.29 ±2.28	2.34 ±0.94	6.94 ±1.24	1.10 ±0.42
400/57 mg (1 chewable tablet)	17.24 ±2.64	2.17 ±0.73	6.67 ±1.37	1.03 ±0.33

* Administered at the start of a light meal.

† Mean values of 28 normal volunteers. Peak concentrations occurred approximately 1 hour after the dose.

RECOMMENDED RANGES FOR AMOXICILLIN/CLAVULANIC ACID SUSCEPTIBILITY TESTING

For Gram-Negative Enteric Aerobes:

MIC (mcg/mL)	Interpretation
≤8/4	Susceptible (S)
16/8	Intermediate (I)
≥32/16	Resistant (R)

For *Staphylococcus*[††] and *Haemophilus* species:

MIC (mcg/mL)	Interpretation
≤4/2	Susceptible (S)
≥8/4	Resistant (R)

[††] Staphylococci which are susceptible to amoxicillin/clavulanic acid but resistant to methicillin/oxacillin must be considered as resistant.

For *S. pneumoniae* from non-meningitis sources: Isolates should be tested using amoxicillin/clavulanic acid and the following criteria should be used:

MIC (mcg/mL)	Interpretation
≤2/1	Susceptible (S)
4/2	Intermediate (I)
≥8/4	Resistant (R)

Note: These interpretive criteria are based on the recommended doses for respiratory tract infections.

A report of "Susceptible" indicates that the pathogen is likely to be inhibited if the antimicrobial compound in the blood reaches the concentration usually achievable. A report of "Intermediate" indicates that the result should be considered equivocal, and, if the microorganism is not fully susceptible to alternative, clinically feasible drugs, the test should be repeated. This category implies possible clinical applicability in body sites where the drug is physiologically concentrated or in situations where high dosage of drug can be used. This category also provides a buffer zone that prevents small uncontrolled technical factors from causing major discrepancies in interpretation. A report of "Resistant" indicates that the pathogen is not likely to be inhibited if the antimicrobial compound in the blood reaches the concentrations usually achievable; other therapy should be selected.

Standardized susceptibility test procedures require the use of laboratory control microorganisms to control the technical aspects of the laboratory procedures. Standard amoxicillin/clavulanate potassium powder should provide the following MIC values:

Microorganism	MIC Range (mcg/mL)‡‡
E. coli ATCC 25922	2 to 8
E. coli ATCC 35218	4 to 16
E. faecalis ATCC 29212	0.25 to 1.0
H. influenzae ATCC 49247	2 to 16
S. aureus ATCC 29213	0.12 to 0.5
S. pneumoniae ATCC 49619	0.03 to 0.12

[‡‡] Expressed as concentration of amoxicillin in the presence of clavulanic acid at a constant 2 parts amoxicillin to 1 part clavulanic acid.

Diffusion Techniques: Quantitative methods that require measurement of zone diameters also provide reproducible estimates of the susceptibility of bacteria to antimicrobial compounds. One such standardized procedure[2] requires the use of standardized inoculum concentrations. This procedure uses paper disks impregnated with 30 mcg of amoxicillin/clavulanate potassium (20 mcg amoxicillin plus 10 mcg clavulanate potassium) to test the susceptibility of microorganisms to amoxicillin/clavulanic acid.

Reports from the laboratory providing results of the standard single-disk susceptibility test with a 30-mcg amoxicillin/clavulanate potassium (20 mcg amoxicillin plus 10 mcg clavulanate potassium) disk should be interpreted according to the following criteria:

RECOMMENDED RANGES FOR AMOXICILLIN/CLAVULANIC ACID SUSCEPTIBILITY TESTING

For *Staphylococcus*[§§] species and *H. influenzae*[a]:

Zone Diameter (mm)	Interpretation
≥20	Susceptible (S)
≤19	Resistant (R)

For Other Organisms Except *S. pneumoniae*[b] and *N. gonorrhoeae*[c]:

Zone Diameter (mm)	Interpretation
≥18	Susceptible (S)
14 to 17	Intermediate (I)
≤13	Resistant (R)

[§§] Staphylococci which are resistant to methicillin/oxacillin must be considered as resistant to amoxicillin/clavulanic acid.

[a] A broth microdilution method should be used for testing *H. influenzae*. Beta-lactamase–negative, ampicillin-resistant strains must be considered resistant to amoxicillin/clavulanic acid.

[b] Susceptibility of *S. pneumoniae* should be determined using a 1 mcg oxacillin disk. Isolates with oxacillin zone sizes of ≥20 mm are susceptible to amoxicillin/clavulanic acid. An amoxicillin/clavulanic acid MIC should be determined on isolates of *S. pneumoniae* with oxacillin zone sizes of ≤19 mm.

[c] A broth microdilution method should be used for testing *N. gonorrhoeae* and interpreted according to penicillin breakpoints.

Interpretation should be as stated above for results using dilution techniques. Interpretation involves correlation of the diameter obtained in the disk test with the MIC for amoxicillin/clavulanic acid.

As with standardized dilution techniques, diffusion methods require the use of laboratory control microorganisms that are used to control the technical aspects of the laboratory procedures. For the diffusion technique, the 30-mcg amoxicillin/clavulanate potassium (20 mcg amoxicillin plus 10 mcg clavulanate potassium) disk should provide the following zone diameters in these laboratory quality control strains:

Microorganism	Zone Diameter (mm)
E. coli ATCC 25922	19 to 25 mm
E. coli ATCC 35218	18 to 22 mm
S. aureus ATCC 25923	28 to 36 mm

INDICATIONS AND USAGE

AUGMENTIN is indicated in the treatment of infections caused by susceptible strains of the designated organisms in the conditions listed below:

Lower Respiratory Tract Infections–caused by β-lactamase–producing strains of *H. influenzae* and *M. catarrhalis.*

Otitis Media–caused by β-lactamase–producing strains of *H. influenzae* and *M. catarrhalis.*

Sinusitis–caused by β-lactamase–producing strains of *H. influenzae* and *M. catarrhalis.*

Skin and Skin Structure Infections–caused by β-lactamase–producing strains of *S. aureus, E. coli* and *Klebsiella* spp.

Urinary Tract Infections–caused by β-lactamase–producing strains of *E. coli, Klebsiella* spp. and *Enterobacter* spp.

While AUGMENTIN is indicated only for the conditions listed above, infections caused by ampicillin-susceptible organisms are also amenable to treatment with AUGMENTIN due to its amoxicillin content. Therefore, mixed infections caused by ampicillin-susceptible organisms and β-lactamase–producing organisms susceptible to AUGMENTIN should not require the addition of another antibiotic. Because amoxicillin has greater in vitro activity against *S. pneumoniae* than does ampicillin or penicillin, the majority of *S. pneumoniae* strains with intermediate susceptibility to ampicillin or penicillin are fully susceptible to amoxicillin and AUGMENTIN. (See Microbiology.)

To reduce the development of drug-resistant bacteria and maintain the effectiveness of AUGMENTIN and other antibacterial drugs, AUGMENTIN should be used only to treat or prevent infections that are proven or strongly suspected to be caused by susceptible bacteria. When culture and susceptibility information are available, they should be considered in selecting or modifying antibacterial therapy. In the absence of such data, local epidemiology and susceptibility patterns may contribute to the empiric selection of therapy.

Bacteriological studies, to determine the causative organisms and their susceptibility to AUGMENTIN, should be performed together with any indicated surgical procedures.

CONTRAINDICATIONS

AUGMENTIN is contraindicated in patients with a history of allergic reactions to any penicillin. It is also contraindicated in patients with a previous history of cholestatic jaundice/hepatic dysfunction associated with AUGMENTIN.

WARNINGS

SERIOUS AND OCCASIONALLY FATAL HYPERSENSITIVITY (ANAPHYLACTIC) REACTIONS HAVE BEEN REPORTED IN PATIENTS ON PENICILLIN THERAPY. THESE REACTIONS ARE MORE LIKELY TO OCCUR IN INDIVIDUALS WITH A HISTORY OF PENICILLIN HYPERSENSITIVITY AND/OR A HISTORY OF SENSITIVITY TO MULTIPLE ALLERGENS. THERE HAVE BEEN REPORTS OF INDIVIDUALS WITH A HISTORY OF PENICILLIN HYPERSENSITIVITY WHO HAVE EXPERIENCED SEVERE REACTIONS WHEN TREATED WITH CEPHALOSPORINS. BEFORE INITIATING THERAPY WITH AUGMENTIN, CAREFUL INQUIRY SHOULD BE MADE CONCERNING PREVIOUS HYPERSENSITIVITY REACTIONS TO PENICILLINS, CEPHALOSPORINS, OR OTHER ALLERGENS. IF AN ALLERGIC REACTION OCCURS, AUGMENTIN SHOULD BE DISCONTINUED AND THE APPROPRIATE THERAPY INSTITUTED. **SERIOUS ANAPHYLACTIC REACTIONS REQUIRE IMMEDIATE EMERGENCY TREATMENT WITH EPINEPHRINE. OXYGEN, INTRAVENOUS STEROIDS, AND AIRWAY MANAGEMENT, INCLUDING INTUBATION, SHOULD ALSO BE ADMINISTERED AS INDICATED.**

Pseudomembranous colitis has been reported with nearly all antibacterial agents, including AUGMENTIN, and has ranged in severity from mild to life-threatening. Therefore, it is important to consider this diagnosis in patients who present with diarrhea subsequent to the administration of antibacterial agents.

Treatment with antibacterial agents alters the normal flora of the colon and may permit overgrowth of clostridia. Studies indicate that a toxin produced by *Clostridium difficile* is one primary cause of "antibiotic-associated colitis."

After the diagnosis of pseudomembranous colitis has been established, appropriate therapeutic measures should be initiated. Mild cases of pseudomembranous colitis usually respond to drug discontinuation alone. In moderate to severe cases, consideration should be given to management with fluids and electrolytes, protein supplementation, and treatment with an antibacterial drug clinically effective against *C. difficile* colitis.

AUGMENTIN should be used with caution in patients with evidence of hepatic dysfunction. Hepatic toxicity associated with the use of AUGMENTIN is usually reversible. On rare occasions, deaths have been reported (less than 1 death reported per estimated 4 million prescriptions worldwide). These have generally been cases associated with serious underlying diseases or concomitant medications. (See CONTRAINDICATIONS and ADVERSE REACTIONS–Liver.)

PRECAUTIONS

General: While AUGMENTIN possesses the characteristic low toxicity of the penicillin group of antibiotics, periodic assessment of organ system functions, including renal, hepatic, and hematopoietic function, is advisable during prolonged therapy.

A high percentage of patients with mononucleosis who receive ampicillin develop an erythematous skin rash. Thus, ampicillin-class antibiotics should not be administered to patients with mononucleosis.

The possibility of superinfections with mycotic or bacterial pathogens should be kept in mind during therapy. If superinfections occur (usually involving *Pseudomonas* or *Candida*), the drug should be discontinued and/or appropriate therapy instituted.

Prescribing AUGMENTIN in the absence of a proven or strongly suspected bacterial infection or a prophylactic indication is unlikely to provide benefit to the patient and increases the risk of the development of drug-resistant bacteria.

Information for the Patient: AUGMENTIN may be taken every 8 hours or every 12 hours, depending on the strength of the product prescribed. Each dose should be taken with a meal or snack to reduce the possibility of gastrointestinal upset. Many antibiotics can cause diarrhea. If diarrhea is severe or lasts more than 2 or 3 days, call your doctor.

Keep suspension refrigerated. Shake well before using. When dosing a child with the suspension (liquid) of AUGMENTIN, use a dosing spoon or medicine dropper. Be sure to rinse the spoon or dropper after each use. Bottles of suspension of AUGMENTIN may contain more liquid than required. Follow your doctor's instructions about the amount to use and the days of treatment your child requires. Discard any unused medicine.

Patients should be counseled that antibacterial drugs including AUGMENTIN, should only be used to treat bacterial infections. They do not treat viral infections (e.g., the common cold). When AUGMENTIN is prescribed to treat a bacterial infection, patients should be told that although it is common to feel better early in the course of therapy, the medication should be taken exactly as directed. Skipping doses or not completing the full course of therapy may: (1) decrease the effectiveness of the immediate treatment, and (2) increase the likelihood that bacteria will develop resistance and will not be treatable by AUGMENTIN or other antibacterial drugs in the future.

Phenylketonurics: Each 200-mg chewable tablet of AUGMENTIN contains 2.1 mg phenylalanine; each 400-mg chewable tablet contains 4.2 mg phenylalanine; each 5 mL of either the 200 mg/5 mL or 400 mg/5 mL oral suspension contains 7 mg phenylalanine. The other products of AUGMENTIN do not contain phenylalanine and can be used by phenylketonurics. Contact your physician or pharmacist.

Drug Interactions: Probenecid decreases the renal tubular secretion of amoxicillin. Concurrent use with AUGMENTIN may result in increased and prolonged blood levels of amoxicillin. Co-administration of probenecid cannot be recommended.

The concurrent administration of allopurinol and ampicillin increases substantially the incidence of rashes in patients receiving both drugs as compared to patients receiving ampicillin alone. It is not known whether this potentiation of ampicillin rashes is due to allopurinol or the hyperuricemia present in these patients. There are no data with AUGMENTIN and allopurinol administered concurrently.

In common with other broad-spectrum antibiotics, AUGMENTIN may reduce the efficacy of oral contraceptives.

Drug/Laboratory Test Interactions: Oral administration of AUGMENTIN will result in high urine concentrations of amoxicillin. High urine concentrations of ampicillin may result in false-positive reactions when testing for the presence of glucose in urine using CLINITEST®, Benedict's Solution, or Fehling's Solution. Since this effect may also occur with amoxicillin and therefore AUGMENTIN, it is recommended that glucose tests based on enzymatic glucose oxidase reactions (such as CLINISTIX®) be used.

Following administration of ampicillin to pregnant women, a transient decrease in plasma concentration of total conjugated estriol, estriol-glucuronide, conjugated estrone, and estradiol has been noted. This effect may also occur with amoxicillin and therefore AUGMENTIN.

Carcinogenesis, Mutagenesis, Impairment of Fertility: Long-term studies in animals have not been performed to evaluate carcinogenic potential.

Mutagenesis: The mutagenic potential of AUGMENTIN was investigated in vitro with an Ames test, a human lymphocyte cytogenetic assay, a yeast test and a mouse lymphoma forward mutation assay, and in vivo with mouse micronucleus tests and a dominant lethal test. All were negative apart from the in vitro mouse lymphoma assay where weak activity was found at very high, cytotoxic concentrations.

Impairment of Fertility: AUGMENTIN at oral doses of up to 1,200 mg/kg/day (5.7 times the maximum human dose, 1,480 mg/m^2/day, based on body surface area) was found to have no effect on fertility and reproductive performance in rats, dosed with a 2:1 ratio formulation of amoxicillin: clavulanate.

Teratogenic effects. Pregnancy (Category B): Reproduction studies performed in pregnant rats and mice given AUGMENTIN at oral dosages up to 1,200 mg/kg/day, equivalent to 7,200 and 4,080 mg/m^2/day, respectively (4.9 and 2.8 times the maximum human oral dose based on body surface area), revealed no evidence of harm to the fetus due to AUGMENTIN. There are, however, no adequate and well-controlled studies in pregnant women. Because animal reproduction studies are not always predictive of human response, this drug should be used during pregnancy only if clearly needed.

Labor and Delivery: Oral ampicillin-class antibiotics are generally poorly absorbed during labor. Studies in guinea pigs have shown that intravenous administration of ampicillin decreased the uterine tone, frequency of contractions, height of contractions, and duration of contractions. However, it is not known whether the use of AUGMENTIN in humans during labor or delivery has immediate or delayed adverse effects on the fetus, prolongs the duration of labor, or increases the likelihood that forceps delivery or other obstetrical intervention or resuscitation of the newborn will be necessary. In a single study in women with premature rupture of fetal membranes, it was reported that prophylactic treatment with AUGMENTIN may be associated with an increased risk of necrotizing enterocolitis in neonates.

Nursing Mothers: Ampicillin-class antibiotics are excreted in the milk; therefore, caution should be exercised when AUGMENTIN is administered to a nursing woman.

Pediatric Use: Because of incompletely developed renal function in neonates and young infants, the elimination of amoxicillin may be delayed. Dosing of AUGMENTIN should be modified in pediatric patients younger than 12 weeks (3 months). (See DOSAGE AND ADMINISTRATION—Pediatric.)

ADVERSE REACTIONS

AUGMENTIN is generally well tolerated. The majority of side effects observed in clinical trials were of a mild and transient nature and less than 3% of patients discontinued therapy because of drug-related side effects. From the original premarketing studies, where both pediatric and adult patients were enrolled, the most frequently reported adverse effects were diarrhea/loose stools (9%), nausea (3%), skin rashes and urticaria (3%), vomiting (1%) and vaginitis (1%). The overall incidence of side effects, and in particular diarrhea, increased with the higher recommended dose. Other less frequently reported reactions include: Abdominal discomfort, flatulence, and headache.

In pediatric patients (aged 2 months to 12 years), 1 US/Canadian clinical trial was conducted which compared 45/6.4 mg/kg/day (divided q12h) of AUGMENTIN for 10 days versus 40/10 mg/kg/day (divided q8h) of AUGMENTIN for 10 days in the treatment of acute otitis media. A total of 575 patients were enrolled, and only the suspension formulations were used in this trial. Overall, the adverse event profile seen was comparable to that noted above; however, there were differences in the rates of diarrhea, skin rashes/urticaria, and diaper area rashes. (See CLINICAL STUDIES.)

The following adverse reactions have been reported for ampicillin-class antibiotics:

Gastrointestinal: Diarrhea, nausea, vomiting, indigestion, gastritis, stomatitis, glossitis, black "hairy" tongue, mucocutaneous candidiasis, enterocolitis, and hemorrhagic/pseudomembranous colitis. Onset of pseudomembranous colitis symptoms may occur during or after antibiotic treatment. (See WARNINGS.)

Hypersensitivity Reactions: Skin rashes, pruritus, urticaria, angioedema, serum sickness-like reactions (urticaria or skin rash accompanied by arthritis, arthralgia, myalgia, and frequently fever), erythema multiforme (rarely Stevens-Johnson syndrome), acute generalized exanthematous pustulosis and an occasional case of exfoliative dermatitis (including toxic epidermal necrolysis) have been reported. These reactions may be controlled with antihistamines and, if necessary, systemic corticosteroids. Whenever such reactions occur, the drug should be discontinued, unless the opinion of the physician dictates otherwise. Serious and occasional fatal hypersensitivity (anaphylactic) reactions can occur with oral penicillin. (See WARNINGS.)

Liver: A moderate rise in AST (SGOT) and/or ALT (SGPT) has been noted in patients treated with ampicillin-class antibiotics, but the significance of these findings is unknown. Hepatic dysfunction, including increases in serum transaminases (AST and/or ALT), serum bilirubin and/or alkaline phosphatase, has been infrequently reported with AUGMENTIN. It has been reported more commonly in the elderly, in males, or in patients on prolonged treatment. The histologic findings on liver biopsy have consisted of predominantly cholestatic, hepatocellular, or mixed cholestatic-hepatocellular changes. The onset of signs/symptoms of hepatic dysfunction may occur during or several weeks after therapy has been discontinued. The hepatic dysfunction, which may be severe, is usually reversible. On rare occasions, deaths have been reported (less than 1 death reported per estimated 4 million prescriptions worldwide). These have generally been cases associated with serious underlying diseases or concomitant medications.

Renal: Interstitial nephritis and hematuria have been reported rarely. Crystalluria has also been reported (see **OVERDOSAGE**).

Hemic and Lymphatic Systems: Anemia, including hemolytic anemia, thrombocytopenia, thrombocytopenic purpura, eosinophilia, leukopenia, and agranulocytosis have been reported during therapy with penicillins. These reactions are usually reversible on discontinuation of therapy and are believed to be hypersensitivity phenomena. A slight thrombocytosis was noted in less than 1% of the patients treated with AUGMENTIN. There have been reports of increased prothrombin time in patients receiving AUGMENTIN and anticoagulant therapy concomitantly.

Central Nervous System: Agitation, anxiety, behavioral changes, confusion, convulsions, dizziness, insomnia, and reversible hyperactivity have been reported rarely.

Miscellaneous: Tooth discoloration (brown, yellow, or gray staining) has been rarely reported. Most reports occurred in pediatric patients. Discoloration was reduced or eliminated with brushing or dental cleaning in most cases.

OVERDOSAGE

Following overdosage, patients have experienced primarily gastrointestinal symptoms including stomach and abdominal pain, vomiting, and diarrhea. Rash, hyperactivity, or drowsiness have also been observed in a small number of patients.

In the case of overdosage, discontinue AUGMENTIN, treat symptomatically, and institute supportive measures as required. If the overdosage is very recent and there is no contraindication, an attempt at emesis or other means of removal of drug from the stomach may be performed. A prospective study of 51 pediatric patients at a poison center suggested that overdosages of less than 250 mg/kg of amoxicillin are not associated with significant clinical symptoms and do not require gastric emptying.[3]

Interstitial nephritis resulting in oliguric renal failure has been reported in a small number of patients after overdosage with amoxicillin. Crystalluria, in some cases leading to renal failure, has also been reported after amoxicillin overdosage in adults and pediatric patients. In case of overdosage, adequate fluid intake and diuresis should be maintained to reduce the risk of amoxicillin crystalluria.

Renal impairment appears to be reversible with cessation of drug administration. High blood levels may occur more readily in patients with impaired renal function because of decreased renal clearance of both amoxicillin and clavulanate. Both amoxicillin and clavulanate are removed from the circulation by hemodialysis.

DOSAGE AND ADMINISTRATION

Dosage:

Pediatric Patients: Based on the amoxicillin component, AUGMENTIN should be dosed as follows:

Neonates and infants aged <12 weeks (3 months):

Due to incompletely developed renal function affecting elimination of amoxicillin in this age group, the recommended

Continued on next page

Product information on these pages is effective as of August 2004. Further information is available at: GlaxoSmithKline, PO Box 13398, Research Triangle Park, NC 27709. 1-888-825-5249. Corporate Web Site: www.gsk.com

Augmentin Powder/Chewable—Cont.

dose of AUGMENTIN is 30 mg/kg/day divided q12h, based on the amoxicillin component. Clavulanate elimination is unaltered in this age group. Experience with the 200 mg/5 mL formulation in this age group is limited and, thus, use of the 125 mg/5 mL oral suspension is recommended.

Patients aged 12 weeks (3 months) and older

INFECTIONS	DOSING REGIMEN	
	q12h*	q8h
	200 mg/5 mL or 400 mg/5 mL oral suspension†	125 mg/5 mL or 250 mg/5 mL oral suspension
Otitis media‡, sinusitis, lower respiratory tract infections, and more severe infections	45 mg/kg/day q12h	40 mg/kg/day q8h
Less severe infections	25 mg/kg/day q12h	20 mg/kg/day q8h

* The q12h regimen is recommended as it is associated with significantly less diarrhea. (See CLINICAL STUDIES.) However, the q12h formulations (200 mg and 400 mg) contain aspartame and should not be used by phenylketonurics.

† Each strength of suspension of AUGMENTIN is available as a chewable tablet for use by older children.

‡ Duration of therapy studied and recommended for acute otitis media is 10 days.

Pediatric Patients Weighing 40 kg and More: Should be dosed according to the following adult recommendations: The usual adult dose is one 500-mg tablet of AUGMENTIN every 12 hours or one 250-mg tablet of AUGMENTIN every 8 hours. For more severe infections and infections of the respiratory tract, the dose should be one 875-mg tablet of AUGMENTIN every 12 hours or one 500-mg tablet of AUGMENTIN every 8 hours. Among adults treated with 875 mg every 12 hours, significantly fewer experienced severe diarrhea or withdrawals with diarrhea versus adults treated with 500 mg every 8 hours. For detailed adult dosage recommendations, please see complete prescribing information for tablets of AUGMENTIN.

Hepatically impaired patients should be dosed with caution and hepatic function monitored at regular intervals. (See WARNINGS.)

Adults: Adults who have difficulty swallowing may be given the 125 mg/5 mL or 250 mg/5 mL suspension in place of the 500-mg tablet. The 200 mg/5 mL suspension or the 400 mg/5 mL suspension may be used in place of the 875-mg tablet. See dosage recommendations above for children weighing 40 kg or more.

The 250-mg tablet of AUGMENTIN and the 250-mg chewable tablet do not contain the same amount of clavulanic acid (as the potassium salt). The 250-mg tablet of AUGMENTIN contains 125 mg of clavulanic acid, whereas the 250-mg chewable tablet contains 62.5 mg of clavulanic acid. Therefore, the 250-mg tablet of AUGMENTIN and the 250-mg chewable tablet should *not* be substituted for each other, as they are not interchangeable.

Due to the different amoxicillin to clavulanic acid ratios in the 250-mg tablet of AUGMENTIN (250/125) versus the 250-mg chewable tablet of AUGMENTIN (250/62.5), the 250-mg tablet of AUGMENTIN should not be used until the child weighs at least 40 kg and more.

Directions for Mixing Oral Suspension: Prepare a suspension at time of dispensing as follows: Tap bottle until all the powder flows freely. Add approximately 2/3 of the total amount of water for reconstitution (see table below) and shake vigorously to suspend powder. Add remainder of the water and again shake vigorously.

AUGMENTIN 125 mg/5 mL Suspension

Bottle Size	Amount of Water Required for Reconstitution
75 mL	67 mL
100 mL	90 mL
150 mL	134 mL

Each teaspoonful (5 mL) will contain 125 mg amoxicillin and 31.25 mg of clavulanic acid as the potassium salt.

AUGMENTIN 200 mg/5 mL Suspension

Bottle Size	Amount of Water Required for Reconstitution
50 mL	50 mL
75 mL	75 mL
100 mL	95 mL

Each teaspoonful (5 mL) will contain 200 mg amoxicillin and 28.5 mg of clavulanic acid as the potassium salt.

AUGMENTIN 250 mg/5 mL Suspension

Bottle Size	Amount of Water Required for Reconstitution
75 mL	65 mL
100 mL	87 mL
150 mL	130 mL

Each teaspoonful (5 mL) will contain 250 mg amoxicillin and 62.5 mg of clavulanic acid as the potassium salt.

AUGMENTIN 400 mg/5 mL Suspension

Bottle Size	Amount of Water Required for Reconstitution
50 mL	50 mL
75 mL	70 mL
100 mL	90 mL

Each teaspoonful (5 mL) will contain 400 mg amoxicillin and 57.0 mg of clavulanic acid as the potassium salt.

Note: SHAKE ORAL SUSPENSION WELL BEFORE USING.

Reconstituted suspension must be stored under refrigeration and discarded after 10 days.

Administration: AUGMENTIN may be taken without regard to meals; however, absorption of clavulanate potassium is enhanced when AUGMENTIN is administered at the start of a meal. To minimize the potential for gastrointestinal intolerance, AUGMENTIN should be taken at the start of a meal.

HOW SUPPLIED

AUGMENTIN 125 mg/5 mL for Oral Suspension: Each 5 mL of reconstituted banana-flavored suspension contains 125 mg amoxicillin and 31.25 mg clavulanic acid as the potassium salt.

NDC 0029-6085-39 .... 75 mL bottle
NDC 0029-6085-23 .... 100 mL bottle
NDC 0029-6085-22 .... 150 mL bottle

AUGMENTIN 200 mg/5 mL for Oral Suspension: Each 5 mL of reconstituted orange-flavored suspension contains 200 mg amoxicillin and 28.5 mg clavulanic acid as the potassium salt.

NDC 0029-6087-29 .... 50 mL bottle
NDC 0029-6087-39 .... 75 mL bottle
NDC 0029-6087-51 .... 100 mL bottle

AUGMENTIN 250 mg/5 mL for Oral Suspension: Each 5 mL of reconstituted orange-flavored suspension contains 250 mg amoxicillin and 62.5 mg clavulanic acid as the potassium salt.

NDC 0029-6090-39 .... 75 mL bottle
NDC 0029-6090-23 .... 100 mL bottle
NDC 0029-6090-22 .... 150 mL bottle

AUGMENTIN 400 mg/5 mL for Oral Suspension: Each 5 mL of reconstituted orange-flavored suspension contains 400 mg amoxicillin and 57 mg clavulanic acid as the potassium salt.

NDC 0029-6092-29 .... 50 mL bottle
NDC 0029-6092-39 .... 75 mL bottle
NDC 0029-6092-51 .... 100 mL bottle

AUGMENTIN 125-mg Chewable Tablets: Each mottled yellow, round, lemon-lime-flavored tablet, debossed with BMP 189, contains 125 mg amoxicillin as the trihydrate and 31.25 mg clavulanic acid as the potassium salt.

NDC 0029-6073-47 .... carton of 30 tablets

AUGMENTIN 200-mg Chewable Tablets: Each mottled pink, round, biconvex, cherry-banana-flavored tablet contains 200 mg amoxicillin as the trihydrate and 28.5 mg clavulanic acid as the potassium salt.

NDC 0029-6071-12 .... carton of 20 tablets

AUGMENTIN 250-mg Chewable Tablets: Each mottled yellow, round, lemon-lime-flavored tablet, debossed with BMP 190, contains 250 mg amoxicillin as the trihydrate and 62.5 mg clavulanic acid as the potassium salt.

NDC 0029-6074-47 .... carton of 30 tablets

AUGMENTIN 400-mg Chewable Tablets: Each mottled pink, round, biconvex, cherry-banana-flavored tablet contains 400 mg amoxicillin as the trihydrate and 57.0 mg clavulanic acid as the potassium salt.

NDC 0029-6072-12 .... carton of 20 tablets

AUGMENTIN is Also Supplied as:

AUGMENTIN 250-mg Tablets (250 mg amoxicillin/125 mg clavulanic acid):

NDC 0029-6075-27 bottles of 30 NDC 0029-6075-31 100 Unit Dose tablets

AUGMENTIN 500-mg Tablets (500 mg amoxicillin/125 mg clavulanic acid):

NDC 0029-6080-12 bottles of 20 NDC 0029-6080-31 100 Unit Dose tablets

AUGMENTIN 875-mg Tablets (875 mg amoxicillin/125 mg clavulanic acid):

NDC 0029-6086-12 bottles of 20 NDC 0029-6086-21 100 Unit Dose tablets

Store tablets and dry powder at or below 25°C (77°F). Dispense in original containers. Store reconstituted suspension under refrigeration. Discard unused suspension after 10 days.

CLINICAL STUDIES

In pediatric patients (aged 2 months to 12 years), 1 US/Canadian clinical trial was conducted which compared 45/6.4 mg/kg/day (divided q12h) of AUGMENTIN for 10 days versus 40/10 mg/kg/day (divided q8h) of AUGMENTIN for 10 days in the treatment of acute otitis media. Only the suspension formulations were used in this trial. A total of 575 patients were enrolled, with an even distribution among the 2 treatment groups and a comparable number of patients were evaluable (i.e., ≥84%) per treatment group. Strict otitis media-specific criteria were required for eligibility and a strong correlation was found at the end of therapy and follow-up between these criteria and physician assessment of clinical response. The clinical efficacy rates at the end of therapy visit (defined as 2-4 days after the completion of therapy) and at the follow-up visit (defined as 22-28 days post-completion of therapy) were comparable for the 2 treatment groups, with the following cure rates obtained for the evaluable patients: At end of therapy, 87.2% (n = 265) and 82.3% (n = 260) for 45 mg/kg/day q12h and 40 mg/kg/day q8h, respectively. At follow-up, 67.1% (n = 249) and 68.7% (n = 243) for 45 mg/kg/day q12h and 40 mg/kg/day q8h, respectively.

The incidence of diarrhea††† was significantly lower in patients in the q12h treatment group compared to patients who received the q8h regimen (14.3% and 34.3%, respectively). In addition, the number of patients with either severe diarrhea or who were withdrawn with diarrhea was significantly lower in the q12h treatment group (3.1% and 7.6% for the q12h/10 day and q8h/10 day, respectively). In the q12h treatment group, 3 patients (1.0%) were withdrawn with an allergic reaction, while 1 patient (0.3%) in the q8h group was withdrawn for this reason. The number of patients with a candidal infection of the diaper area was 3.8% and 6.2% for the q12h and q8h groups, respectively.

It is not known if the finding of a statistically significant reduction in diarrhea with the oral suspensions dosed q12h, versus suspensions dosed q8h, can be extrapolated to the chewable tablets. The presence of mannitol in the chewable tablets may contribute to a different diarrhea profile. The q12h oral suspensions are sweetened with aspartame only.

††† Diarrhea was defined as either: (a) 3 or more watery or 4 or more loose/watery stools in 1 day; OR (b) 2 watery stools per day or 3 loose/watery stools per day for 2 consecutive days.

REFERENCES

1. National Committee for Clinical Laboratory Standards. Methods for Dilution Antimicrobial Susceptibility Tests for Bacteria That Grow Aerobically – Third Edition. Approved Standard NCCLS Document M7-A3, Vol. 13, No. 25. NCCLS, Villanova, PA, Dec. 1993.
2. National Committee for Clinical Laboratory Standards. Performance Standard for Antimicrobial Disk Susceptibility Tests – Fifth Edition. Approved Standard NCCLS Document M2-A5, Vol. 13, No. 24. NCCLS, Villanova, PA, Dec. 1993.
3. Swanson-Bearman B, Dean BS, Lopez G, Krenzelok EP. The effects of penicillin and cephalosporin ingestions in children less than six years of age. *Vet Hum Toxicol* 1988;30:66-67.

AUGMENTIN is a registered trademark of GlaxoSmithKline.
CLINITEST is a registered trademark of Miles, Inc.
CLINISTIX is a registered trademark of Bayer Corporation.
GlaxoSmithKline, Research Triangle Park, NC 27709

June 2004/AG:PL15

Shown in Product Identification Guide, page 314

AUGMENTIN® ℞

[*äg-mint'in*]

(amoxicillin/clavulanate potassium)

Tablets

To reduce the development of drug-resistant bacteria and maintain the effectiveness of AUGMENTIN (amoxicillin/clavulanate potassium) and other antibacterial drugs, AUGMENTIN should be used only to treat or prevent infections that are proven or strongly suspected to be caused by bacteria.

DESCRIPTION

AUGMENTIN is an oral antibacterial combination consisting of the semisynthetic antibiotic amoxicillin and the β-lactamase inhibitor, clavulanate potassium (the potassium salt of clavulanic acid). Amoxicillin is an analog of ampicillin, derived from the basic penicillin nucleus, 6-aminopenicillanic acid. The amoxicillin molecular formula is $C_{16}H_{19}N_3O_5S \bullet 3H_2O$, and the molecular weight is 419.46. Chemically, amoxicillin is (2*S*,5*R*,6*R*)-6-[(*R*)-(-)-2-Amino-2-(*p*-hydroxyphenyl)acetamido]-3,3-dimethyl-7-oxo-4-thia-1-azabicyclo[3.2.0]heptane-2-carboxylic acid trihydrate.

Clavulanic acid is produced by the fermentation of *Streptomyces clavuligerus*. It is a β-lactam structurally related to the penicillins and possesses the ability to inactivate a wide variety of β-lactamases by blocking the active sites of these enzymes. Clavulanic acid is particularly active against the clinically important plasmid-mediated β-lactamases frequently responsible for transferred drug resistance to penicillins and cephalosporins. The clavulanate potassium molecular formula is $C_8H_8KNO_5$, and the molecular weight is 237.25. Chemically, clavulanate potassium is potassium (Z)-(2*R*,5*R*)-3-(2-hydroxyethylidene)-7-oxo-4-oxa-1-azabicyclo[3.2.0]-heptane-2-carboxylate.

Inactive Ingredients: Colloidal silicon dioxide, hypromellose, magnesium stearate, microcrystalline cellulose, polyethylene glycol, sodium starch glycolate, and titanium dioxide.

Each tablet of AUGMENTIN contains 0.63 mEq potassium.

CLINICAL PHARMACOLOGY

Amoxicillin and clavulanate potassium are well absorbed from the gastrointestinal tract after oral administration of AUGMENTIN. Dosing in the fasted or fed state has minimal effect on the pharmacokinetics of amoxicillin. While AUGMENTIN can be given without regard to meals, absorption of clavulanate potassium when taken with food is greater relative to the fasted state. In 1 study, the relative bioavailability of clavulanate was reduced when

Dose[†] and regimen	AUC$_{0-24}$ (mcg•hr/mL)		C$_{max}$ (mcg/mL)	
amoxicillin/ clavulanate potassium	amoxicillin (±S.D.)	clavulanate potassium (±S.D.)	amoxicillin (±S.D.)	clavulanate potassium (±S.D.)
250/125 mg q8h	26.7 ± 4.56	12.6 ± 3.25	3.3 ± 1.12	1.5 ± 0.70
500/125 mg q12h	33.4 ± 6.76	8.6 ± 1.95	6.5 ± 1.41	1.8 ± 0.61
500/125 mg q8h	53.4 ± 8.87	15.7 ± 3.86	7.2 ± 2.26	2.4 ± 0.83
875/125 mg q12h	53.5 ± 12.31	10.2 ± 3.04	11.6 ± 2.78	2.2 ± 0.99

*Mean values of 14 normal volunteers (n = 15 for clavulanate potassium in the low-dose regimens). Peak concentrations occurred approximately 1.5 hours after the dose.

[†] Administered at the start of a light meal.

AUGMENTIN was dosed at 30 and 150 minutes after the start of a high-fat breakfast. The safety and efficacy of AUGMENTIN have been established in clinical trials where AUGMENTIN was taken without regard to meals.

Mean* amoxicillin and clavulanate potassium pharmacokinetic parameters are shown in the table below:

[See table above]

Amoxicillin serum concentrations achieved with AUGMENTIN are similar to those produced by the oral administration of equivalent doses of amoxicillin alone. The half-life of amoxicillin after the oral administration of AUGMENTIN is 1.3 hours and that of clavulanic acid is 1.0 hour.

Approximately 50% to 70% of the amoxicillin and approximately 25% to 40% of the clavulanic acid are excreted unchanged in urine during the first 6 hours after administration of a single 250-mg or 500-mg tablet of AUGMENTIN.

Concurrent administration of probenecid delays amoxicillin excretion but does not delay renal excretion of clavulanic acid.

Neither component in AUGMENTIN is highly protein-bound; clavulanic acid has been found to be approximately 25% bound to human serum and amoxicillin approximately 18% bound.

Amoxicillin diffuses readily into most body tissues and fluids with the exception of the brain and spinal fluid. The results of experiments involving the administration of clavulanic acid to animals suggest that this compound, like amoxicillin, is well distributed in body tissues.

Microbiology: Amoxicillin is a semisynthetic antibiotic with a broad spectrum of bactericidal activity against many gram-positive and gram-negative microorganisms. Amoxicillin is, however, susceptible to degradation by β-lactamases, and therefore, the spectrum of activity does not include organisms which produce these enzymes. Clavulanic acid is a β-lactam, structurally related to the penicillins, which possesses the ability to inactivate a wide range of β-lactamase enzymes commonly found in microorganisms resistant to penicillins and cephalosporins. In particular, it has good activity against the clinically important plasmid-mediated β-lactamases frequently responsible for transferred drug resistance.

The formulation of amoxicillin and clavulanic acid in AUGMENTIN protects amoxicillin from degradation by β-lactamase enzymes and effectively extends the antibiotic spectrum of amoxicillin to include many bacteria normally resistant to amoxicillin and other β-lactam antibiotics. Thus, AUGMENTIN possesses the properties of a broad-spectrum antibiotic and a β-lactamase inhibitor.

Amoxicillin/clavulanic acid has been shown to be active against most strains of the following microorganisms, both in vitro and in clinical infections as described in INDICATIONS AND USAGE.

Gram-Positive Aerobes:

Staphylococcus aureus (β-lactamase and non–β-lactamase producing)[‡]

[‡] Staphylococci which are resistant to methicillin/oxacillin must be considered resistant to amoxicillin/clavulanic acid.

Gram-Negative Aerobes:

Enterobacter species (Although most strains of *Enterobacter* species are resistant in vitro, clinical efficacy has been demonstrated with AUGMENTIN in urinary tract infections caused by these organisms.)

Escherichia coli (β-lactamase and non–β-lactamase-producing)

Haemophilus influenzae (β-lactamase and non–β-lactamase–producing)

Klebsiella species (All known strains are β-lactamase-producing.)

Moraxella catarrhalis (β-lactamase and non–β-lactamase-producing)

The following in vitro data are available, **but their clinical significance is unknown.**

Amoxicillin/clavulanic acid exhibits in vitro minimal inhibitory concentrations (MICs) of 2 mcg/mL or less against most (≥90%) strains of *Streptococcus pneumoniae*[§]; MICs of 0.06 mcg/mL or less against most (≥90%) strains of *Neisseria gonorrhoeae*; MICs of 4 mcg/mL or less against most (≥90%) strains of staphylococci and anaerobic bacteria; and MICs of 8 mcg/mL or less against most (≥90%) strains of other listed organisms. However, with the exception of organisms shown to respond to amoxicillin alone, the safety and effectiveness of amoxicillin/clavulanic acid in treating clinical infections due to these microorganisms have not been established in adequate and well-controlled clinical trials.

[§] Because amoxicillin has greater in vitro activity against *S. pneumoniae* than does ampicillin or penicillin, the majority of *S. pneumoniae* strains with intermediate susceptibility to ampicillin or penicillin are fully susceptible to amoxicillin.

Gram-Positive Aerobes:

Enterococcus faecalis[||]

Staphylococcus epidermidis (β-lactamase and non–β-lactamase–producing)

Staphylococcus saprophyticus (β-lactamase and non–β-lactamase–producing)

Streptococcus pneumoniae[||] [¶]

Streptococcus pyogenes[||] [¶]

viridans group *Streptococcus*[||] [¶]

Gram-Negative Aerobes:

Eikenella corrodens (β-lactamase and non–β-lactamase–producing)

Neisseria gonorrhoeae[||] (β-lactamase and non–β-lactamase–producing)

Proteus mirabilis[||] (β-lactamase and non–β-lactamase–producing)

Anaerobic Bacteria:

Bacteroides species, including *Bacteroides fragilis* (β-lactamase and non–β-lactamase–producing)

Fusobacterium species (β-lactamase and non–β-lactamase–producing)

Peptostreptococcus species[¶]

[||] Adequate and well-controlled clinical trials have established the effectiveness of amoxicillin alone in treating certain clinical infections due to these organisms.

[¶] These are non–β-lactamase–producing organisms, and therefore, are susceptible to amoxicillin alone.

Susceptibility Testing: ***Dilution Techniques:*** Quantitative methods are used to determine antimicrobial MICs. These MICs provide estimates of the susceptibility of bacteria to antimicrobial compounds. The MICs should be determined using a standardized procedure. Standardized procedures are based on a dilution method[1] (broth or agar) or equivalent with standardized inoculum concentrations and standardized concentrations of amoxicillin/clavulanate potassium powder.

The recommended dilution pattern utilizes a constant amoxicillin/clavulanate potassium ratio of 2 to 1 in all tubes with varying amounts of amoxicillin. MICs are expressed in terms of the amoxicillin concentration in the presence of clavulanic acid at a constant 2 parts amoxicillin to 1 part clavulanic acid. The MIC values should be interpreted according to the following criteria:

RECOMMENDED RANGES FOR AMOXICILLIN/ CLAVULANIC ACID SUSCEPTIBILITY TESTING

For Gram-Negative Enteric Aerobes:

MIC (mcg/mL)	Interpretation
≤8/4	Susceptible (S)
16/8	Intermediate (I)
≥32/16	Resistant (R)

For *Staphylococcus* and *Haemophilus* species:**

MIC (mcg/mL)	Interpretation
≤4/2	Susceptible (S)
≥8/4	Resistant (R)

**Staphylococci which are susceptible to amoxicillin/clavulanic acid but resistant to methicillin/oxacillin must be considered as resistant.

For *S. pneumoniae* from non-meningitis sources: Isolates should be tested using amoxicillin/clavulanic acid and the following criteria should be used:

MIC (mcg/mL)	Interpretation
≤2.1	Susceptible (S)
4/2	Intermediate (I)
≥8/4	Resistant (R)

Note: These interpretive criteria are based on the recommended doses for respiratory tract infections.

A report of "Susceptible" indicates that the pathogen is likely to be inhibited if the antimicrobial compound in the blood reaches the concentration usually achievable. A report of "Intermediate" indicates that the result should be considered equivocal, and, if the microorganism is not fully susceptible to alternative, clinically feasible drugs, the test should be repeated. This category implies possible clinical applicability in body sites where the drug is physiologically concentrated or in situations where high dosage of drug can be used. This category also provides a buffer zone, which prevents small uncontrolled technical factors from causing major discrepancies in interpretation. A report of "Resistant" indicates that the pathogen is not likely to be inhibited if the antimicrobial compound in the blood reaches the concentrations usually achievable; other therapy should be selected.

Standardized susceptibility test procedures require the use of laboratory control microorganisms to control the technical aspects of the laboratory procedures. Standard amoxicillin/clavulanate potassium powder should provide the following MIC values:

Microorganism	MIC Range (mcg/mL)[††]
Escherichia coli ATCC 25922	2 to 8
Escherichia coli ATCC 35218	4 to 16
Enterococcus faecalis ATCC 29212	0.25 to 1.0
Haemophilus influenzae ATCC 49247	2 to 16
Staphylococcus aureus ATCC 29213	0.12 to 0.5
Streptococcus pneumoniae ATCC 49619	0.03 to 0.12

[††] Expressed as concentration of amoxicillin in the presence of clavulanic acid at a constant 2 parts amoxicillin to 1 part clavulanic acid.

Diffusion Techniques: Quantitative methods that require measurement of zone diameters also provide reproducible estimates of the susceptibility of bacteria to antimicrobial compounds. One such standardized procedure[2] requires the use of standardized inoculum concentrations. This procedure uses paper disks impregnated with 30 mcg of amoxicillin/clavulanate potassium (20 mcg amoxicillin plus 10 mcg clavulanate potassium) to test the susceptibility of microorganisms to amoxicillin/clavulanic acid.

Reports from the laboratory providing results of the standard single-disk susceptibility test with a 30-mcg amoxicillin/clavulanate acid (20 mcg amoxicillin plus 10 mcg clavulanate potassium) disk should be interpreted according to the following criteria:

RECOMMENDED RANGES FOR AMOXICILLIN/ CLAVULANIC ACID SUSCEPTIBILITY TESTING

For *Staphylococcus*[‡‡] species and *H. influenzae*[a]:

Zone Diameter (mm)	Interpretation
≥20	Susceptible (S)
≤19	Resistant (R)

For Other Organisms Except *S. pneumoniae*[b] and *N. gonorrhoeae*[c]:

Zone Diameter (mm)	Interpretation
≥18	Susceptible (S)
14 to 17	Intermediate (I)
≤13	Resistant (R)

[‡‡] Staphylococci which are resistant to methicillin/oxacillin must be considered as resistant to amoxicillin/clavulanic acid.

[a] A broth microdilution method should be used for testing *H. influenzae*. Beta-lactamase–negative, ampicillin-resistant strains must be considered resistant to amoxicillin/ clavulanic acid.

[b] Susceptibility of *S. pneumoniae* should be determined using a 1 mcg oxacillin disk. Isolates with oxacillin zone sizes of ≥20 mm are susceptible to amoxicillin/clavulanic acid. An amoxicillin/clavulanic acid MIC should be determined on isolates of *S. pneumoniae* with oxacillin zone sizes of ≤19 mm.

[c] A broth microdilution method should be used for testing *N. gonorrhoeae* and interpreted according to penicillin breakpoints.

Interpretation should be as stated above for results using dilution techniques. Interpretation involves correlation of the diameter obtained in the disk test with the MIC for amoxicillin/clavulanic acid.

As with standardized dilution techniques, diffusion methods require the use of laboratory control microorganisms that are used to control the technical aspects of the laboratory procedures. For the diffusion technique, the 30-mcg amoxicillin/clavulanate potassium (20-mcg amoxicillin plus 10-mcg clavulanate potassium) disk should provide the following zone diameters in these laboratory quality control strains:

Continued on next page

Product information on these pages is effective as of August 2004. Further information is available at: GlaxoSmithKline, PO Box 13398, Research Triangle Park, NC 27709. 1-888-825-5249. Corporate Web Site: www.gsk.com

Augmentin Tablets—Cont.

Microorganism	Zone Diameter (mm)
Escherichia coli ATCC 25922	19 to 25
Escherichia coli ATCC 35218	18 to 22
Staphylococcus aureus ATCC 25923	28 to 36

INDICATIONS AND USAGE

AUGMENTIN is indicated in the treatment of infections caused by susceptible strains of the designated organisms in the conditions listed below:

Lower Respiratory Tract Infections–caused by β-lactamase–producing strains of *H. influenzae* and *M. catarrhalis.*

Otitis Media–caused by β-lactamase–producing strains of *H. influenzae* and *M. catarrhalis.*

Sinusitis–caused by β-lactamase–producing strains of *H. influenzae* and *M. catarrhalis.*

Skin and Skin Structure Infections–caused by β-lactamase–producing strains of *S. aureus, E. coli,* and *Klebsiella* spp.

Urinary Tract Infections–caused by β-lactamase–producing strains of *E. coli, Klebsiella* spp., and *Enterobacter* spp.

While AUGMENTIN is indicated only for the conditions listed above, infections caused by ampicillin-susceptible organisms are also amenable to treatment with AUGMENTIN due to its amoxicillin content; therefore, mixed infections caused by ampicillin-susceptible organisms and β-lactamase–producing organisms susceptible to AUGMENTIN should not require the addition of another antibiotic. Because amoxicillin has greater in vitro activity against *S. pneumoniae* than does ampicillin or penicillin, the majority of *S. pneumoniae* strains with intermediate susceptibility to ampicillin or penicillin are fully susceptible to amoxicillin and AUGMENTIN. (See Microbiology.)

To reduce the development of drug-resistant bacteria and maintain the effectiveness of AUGMENTIN and other antibacterial drugs, AUGMENTIN should be used only to treat or prevent infections that are proven or strongly suspected to be caused by susceptible bacteria. When culture and susceptibility information are available, they should be considered in selecting or modifying antibacterial therapy. In the absence of such data, local epidemiology and susceptibility patterns may contribute to the empiric selection of therapy.

Bacteriological studies, to determine the causative organisms and their susceptibility to AUGMENTIN, should be performed together with any indicated surgical procedures.

CONTRAINDICATIONS

AUGMENTIN is contraindicated in patients with a history of allergic reactions to any penicillin. It is also contraindicated in patients with a previous history of cholestatic jaundice/hepatic dysfunction associated with AUGMENTIN.

WARNINGS

SERIOUS AND OCCASIONALLY FATAL HYPERSENSITIVITY (ANAPHYLACTIC) REACTIONS HAVE BEEN REPORTED IN PATIENTS ON PENICILLIN THERAPY. THESE REACTIONS ARE MORE LIKELY TO OCCUR IN INDIVIDUALS WITH A HISTORY OF PENICILLIN HYPERSENSITIVITY AND/OR A HISTORY OF SENSITIVITY TO MULTIPLE ALLERGENS. THERE HAVE BEEN REPORTS OF INDIVIDUALS WITH A HISTORY OF PENICILLIN HYPERSENSITIVITY WHO HAVE EXPERIENCED SEVERE REACTIONS WHEN TREATED WITH CEPHALOSPORINS. BEFORE INITIATING THERAPY WITH AUGMENTIN, CAREFUL INQUIRY SHOULD BE MADE CONCERNING PREVIOUS HYPERSENSITIVITY REACTIONS TO PENICILLINS, CEPHALOSPORINS, OR OTHER ALLERGENS. IF AN ALLERGIC REACTION OCCURS, AUGMENTIN SHOULD BE DISCONTINUED AND THE APPROPRIATE THERAPY INSTITUTED. **SERIOUS ANAPHYLACTIC REACTIONS REQUIRE IMMEDIATE EMERGENCY TREATMENT WITH EPINEPHRINE. OXYGEN, INTRAVENOUS STEROIDS, AND AIRWAY MANAGEMENT, INCLUDING INTUBATION, SHOULD ALSO BE ADMINISTERED AS INDICATED.**

Pseudomembranous colitis has been reported with nearly all antibacterial agents, including AUGMENTIN, and has ranged in severity from mild to life-threatening; therefore, it is important to consider this diagnosis in patients who present with diarrhea subsequent to the administration of antibacterial agents.

Treatment with antibacterial agents alters the normal flora of the colon and may permit overgrowth of clostridia. Studies indicate that a toxin produced by *Clostridium difficile* is one primary cause of "antibiotic-associated colitis."

After the diagnosis of pseudomembranous colitis has been established, appropriate therapeutic measures should be initiated. Mild cases of pseudomembranous colitis usually respond to drug discontinuation alone. In moderate to severe cases, consideration should be given to management with fluids and electrolytes, protein supplementation, and treatment with an antibacterial drug clinically effective against *C. difficile* colitis.

AUGMENTIN should be used with caution in patients with evidence of hepatic dysfunction. Hepatic toxicity associated with the use of AUGMENTIN is usually reversible. On rare occasions, deaths have been reported (less than 1 death reported per estimated 4 million prescriptions worldwide). These have generally been cases associated with serious underlying diseases or concomitant medications. (See CONTRAINDICATIONS and ADVERSE REACTIONS–Liver.)

PRECAUTIONS

General: While AUGMENTIN possesses the characteristic low toxicity of the penicillin group of antibiotics, periodic assessment of organ system functions, including renal, hepatic, and hematopoietic function, is advisable during prolonged therapy.

A high percentage of patients with mononucleosis who receive ampicillin develop an erythematous skin rash. Thus, ampicillin-class antibiotics should not be administered to patients with mononucleosis.

The possibility of superinfections with mycotic or bacterial pathogens should be kept in mind during therapy. If superinfections occur (usually involving *Pseudomonas* or *Candida*), the drug should be discontinued and/or appropriate therapy instituted.

Prescribing AUGMENTIN in the absence of a proven or strongly suspected bacterial infection or a prophylactic indication is unlikely to provide benefit to the patient and increases the risk of the development of drug-resistant bacteria.

Drug Interactions: Probenecid decreases the renal tubular secretion of amoxicillin. Concurrent use with AUGMENTIN may result in increased and prolonged blood levels of amoxicillin. Co-administration of probenecid cannot be recommended.

The concurrent administration of allopurinol and ampicillin increases substantially the incidence of rashes in patients receiving both drugs as compared to patients receiving ampicillin alone. It is not known whether this potentiation of ampicillin rashes is due to allopurinol or the hyperuricemia present in these patients. There are no data with AUGMENTIN and allopurinol administered concurrently.

In common with other broad-spectrum antibiotics, AUGMENTIN may reduce the efficacy of oral contraceptives.

Drug/Laboratory Test Interactions: Oral administration of AUGMENTIN will result in high urine concentrations of amoxicillin. High urine concentrations of ampicillin may result in false-positive reactions when testing for the presence of glucose in urine using CLINITEST®, Benedict's Solution, or Fehling's Solution. Since this effect may also occur with amoxicillin and therefore AUGMENTIN, it is recommended that glucose tests based on enzymatic glucose oxidase reactions (such as CLINISTIX®) be used.

Following administration of ampicillin to pregnant women, a transient decrease in plasma concentration of total conjugated estriol, estriol-glucuronide, conjugated estrone and estradiol has been noted. This effect may also occur with amoxicillin and therefore AUGMENTIN.

Information for Patients: Patients should be counseled that antibacterial drugs including AUGMENTIN, should only be used to treat bacterial infections. They do not treat viral infections (e.g., the common cold). When AUGMENTIN is prescribed to treat a bacterial infection, patients should be told that although it is common to feel better early in the course of therapy, the medication should be taken exactly as directed. Skipping doses or not completing the full course of therapy may: (1) decrease the effectiveness of the immediate treatment, and (2) increase the likelihood that bacteria will develop resistance and will not be treatable by AUGMENTIN or other antibacterial drugs in the future.

Carcinogenesis, Mutagenesis, Impairment of Fertility: Long-term studies in animals have not been performed to evaluate carcinogenic potential.

Mutagenesis: The mutagenic potential of AUGMENTIN was investigated in vitro with an Ames test, a human lymphocyte cytogenetic assay, a yeast test and a mouse lymphoma forward mutation assay, and in vivo with mouse micronucleus tests and a dominant lethal test. All were negative apart from the in vitro mouse lymphoma assay where weak activity was found at very high, cytotoxic concentrations.

Impairment of Fertility: AUGMENTIN at oral doses of up to 1,200 mg/kg/day (5.7 times the maximum human dose, 1,480 mg/m^2/day, based on body surface area) was found to have no effect on fertility and reproductive performance in rats, dosed with a 2:1 ratio formulation of amoxicillin: clavulanate.

Teratogenic effects: Pregnancy (Category B). Reproduction studies performed in pregnant rats and mice given AUGMENTIN at oral dosages up to 1,200 mg/kg/day, equivalent to 7,200 and 4,080 mg/m^2/day, respectively (4.9 and 2.8 times the maximum human oral dose based on body surface area), revealed no evidence of harm to the fetus due to AUGMENTIN. There are, however, no adequate and well-controlled studies in pregnant women. Because animal reproduction studies are not always predictive of human response, this drug should be used during pregnancy only if clearly needed.

Labor and Delivery: Oral ampicillin-class antibiotics are generally poorly absorbed during labor. Studies in guinea pigs have shown that intravenous administration of ampicillin decreased the uterine tone, frequency of contractions, height of contractions, and duration of contractions; however, it is not known whether the use of AUGMENTIN in humans during labor or delivery has immediate or delayed adverse effects on the fetus, prolongs the duration of labor, or increases the likelihood that forceps delivery or other obstetrical intervention or resuscitation of the newborn will be necessary. In a single study in women with premature rupture of fetal membranes, it was reported that prophylactic treatment with AUGMENTIN may be associated with an increased risk of necrotizing enterocolitis in neonates.

Nursing Mothers: Ampicillin-class antibiotics are excreted in the milk; therefore, caution should be exercised when AUGMENTIN is administered to a nursing woman.

ADVERSE REACTIONS

AUGMENTIN is generally well tolerated. The majority of side effects observed in clinical trials were of a mild and transient nature and less than 3% of patients discontinued therapy because of drug-related side effects. The most frequently reported adverse effects were diarrhea/loose stools (9%), nausea (3%), skin rashes and urticaria (3%), vomiting (1%) and vaginitis (1%). The overall incidence of side effects, and in particular diarrhea, increased with the higher recommended dose. Other less frequently reported reactions include: Abdominal discomfort, flatulence, and headache.

The following adverse reactions have been reported for ampicillin-class antibiotics:

Gastrointestinal: Diarrhea, nausea, vomiting, indigestion, gastritis, stomatitis, glossitis, black "hairy" tongue, mucocutaneous candidiasis, enterocolitis, and hemorrhagic/pseudomembranous colitis. Onset of pseudomembranous colitis symptoms may occur during or after antibiotic treatment. (See WARNINGS.)

Hypersensitivity Reactions: Skin rashes, pruritus, urticaria, angioedema, serum sickness–like reactions (urticaria or skin rash accompanied by arthritis, arthralgia, myalgia, and frequently fever), erythema multiforme (rarely Stevens-Johnson syndrome), acute generalized exanthematous pustulosis, and an occasional case of exfoliative dermatitis (including toxic epidermal necrolysis) have been reported. These reactions may be controlled with antihistamines and, if necessary, systemic corticosteroids. Whenever such reactions occur, the drug should be discontinued, unless the opinion of the physician dictates otherwise. Serious and occasional fatal hypersensitivity (anaphylactic) reactions can occur with oral penicillin. (See WARNINGS.)

Liver: A moderate rise in AST (SGOT) and/or ALT (SGPT) has been noted in patients treated with ampicillin-class antibiotics but the significance of these findings is unknown. Hepatic dysfunction, including increases in serum transaminases (AST and/or ALT), serum bilirubin, and/or alkaline phosphatase, has been infrequently reported with AUGMENTIN. It has been reported more commonly in the elderly, in males, or in patients on prolonged treatment. The histologic findings on liver biopsy have consisted of predominantly cholestatic, hepatocellular, or mixed cholestatic-hepatocellular changes. The onset of signs/symptoms of hepatic dysfunction may occur during or several weeks after therapy has been discontinued. The hepatic dysfunction, which may be severe, is usually reversible. On rare occasions, deaths have been reported (less than 1 death reported per estimated 4 million prescriptions worldwide). These have generally been cases associated with serious underlying diseases or concomitant medications.

Renal: Interstitial nephritis and hematuria have been reported rarely. Crystalluria has also been reported **(see OVERDOSAGE)**.

Hemic and Lymphatic Systems: Anemia, including hemolytic anemia, thrombocytopenia, thrombocytopenic purpura, eosinophilia, leukopenia, and agranulocytosis have been reported during therapy with penicillins. These reactions are usually reversible on discontinuation of therapy and are believed to be hypersensitivity phenomena. A slight thrombocytosis was noted in less than 1% of the patients treated with AUGMENTIN. There have been reports of increased prothrombin time in patients receiving AUGMENTIN and anticoagulant therapy concomitantly.

Central Nervous System: Agitation, anxiety, behavioral changes, confusion, convulsions, dizziness, insomnia, and reversible hyperactivity have been reported rarely.

Miscellaneous: Tooth discoloration (brown, yellow, or gray staining) has been rarely reported. Most reports occurred in pediatric patients. Discoloration was reduced or eliminated with brushing or dental cleaning in most cases.

OVERDOSAGE

Following overdosage, patients have experienced primarily gastrointestinal symptoms including stomach and abdominal pain, vomiting, and diarrhea. Rash, hyperactivity, or drowsiness have also been observed in a small number of patients.

In the case of overdosage, discontinue AUGMENTIN, treat symptomatically, and institute supportive measures as required. If the overdosage is very recent and there is no contraindication, an attempt at emesis or other means of removal of drug from the stomach may be performed. A prospective study of 51 pediatric patients at a poison center suggested that overdosages of less than 250 mg/kg of amoxicillin are not associated with significant clinical symptoms and do not require gastric emptying.[3]

Interstitial nephritis resulting in oliguric renal failure has been reported in a small number of patients after overdosage with amoxicillin.

Crystalluria, in some cases leading to renal failure, has also been reported after amoxicillin overdosage in adult and pediatric patients. In cases of overdosage, adequate fluid intake and diuresis should be maintained to reduce the risk of amoxicillin crystalluria.

Renal impairment appears to be reversible with cessation of drug administration. High blood levels may occur more readily in patients with impaired renal function because of decreased renal clearance of both amoxicillin and clavulanate. Both amoxicillin and clavulanate are removed from the circulation by hemodialysis. (See DOSAGE AND ADMINISTRATION for recommended dosing for patients with impaired renal function.)

DOSAGE AND ADMINISTRATION

Since both the 250-mg and 500-mg tablets of AUGMENTIN contain the same amount of clavulanic acid (125 mg, as the potassium salt), two 250-mg tablets of AUGMENTIN are not equivalent to one 500-mg tablet of AUGMENTIN; therefore, two 250-mg tablets of AUGMENTIN should not be substituted for one 500-mg tablet of AUGMENTIN.

Dosage

Adults: The usual adult dose is one 500-mg tablet of AUGMENTIN every 12 hours or one 250-mg tablet of AUGMENTIN every 8 hours. For more severe infections and infections of the respiratory tract, the dose should be one 875-mg tablet of AUGMENTIN every 12 hours or one 500-mg tablet of AUGMENTIN every 8 hours.

Patients with impaired renal function do not generally require a reduction in dose unless the impairment is severe. Severely impaired patients with a glomerular filtration rate of <30 mL/min. should not receive the 875-mg tablet. Patients with a glomerular filtration rate of 10 to 30 mL/min. should receive 500 mg or 250 mg every 12 hours, depending on the severity of the infection. Patients with a less than 10 mL/min. glomerular filtration rate should receive 500 mg or 250 mg every 24 hours, depending on severity of the infection.

Hemodialysis patients should receive 500 mg or 250 mg every 24 hours, depending on severity of the infection. They should receive an additional dose both during and at the end of dialysis.

Hepatically impaired patients should be dosed with caution and hepatic function monitored at regular intervals. (See WARNINGS.)

Pediatric Patients: Pediatric patients weighing 40 kg or more should be dosed according to the adult recommendations.

Due to the different amoxicillin to clavulanic acid ratios in the 250-mg tablet of AUGMENTIN (250/125) versus the 250-mg chewable tablet of AUGMENTIN (250/62.5), the 250-mg tablet of AUGMENTIN should not be used until the pediatric patient weighs at least 40 kg or more.

Administration: AUGMENTIN may be taken without regard to meals; however, absorption of clavulanate potassium is enhanced when AUGMENTIN is administered at the start of a meal. To minimize the potential for gastrointestinal intolerance, AUGMENTIN should be taken at the start of a meal.

HOW SUPPLIED

AUGMENTIN 250-mg Tablets: Each white oval filmcoated tablet, debossed with AUGMENTIN on 1 side and 250/125 on the other side, contains 250 mg amoxicillin as the trihydrate and 125 mg clavulanic acid as the potassium salt.

NDC 0029-6075-27 .... bottles of 30
NDC 0029-6075-31 .... Unit Dose (10×10) 100 tablets

AUGMENTIN 500-mg TABLETS: Each white oval filmcoated tablet, debossed with AUGMENTIN on 1 side and 500/125 on the other side, contains 500 mg amoxicillin as the trihydrate and 125 mg clavulanic acid as the potassium salt.

NDC 0029-6080-12 .... bottles of 20
NDC 0029-6080-31 .... Unit Dose (10×10) 100 tablets

AUGMENTIN 875-mg Tablets: Each scored white capsule-shaped tablet, debossed with AUGMENTIN 875 on 1 side and scored on the other side, contains 875 mg amoxicillin as the trihydrate and 125 mg clavulanic acid as the potassium salt.

NDC 0029-6086-12 .... bottles of 20
NDC 0029-6086-21 .... Unit Dose (10×10) 100 tablets

AUGMENTIN is Also Supplied as:

AUGMENTIN 125 mg/5 mL (125 mg amoxicillin/31.25 mg clavulanic acid) For Oral Suspension:

NDC 0029-6085-39 .... 75 mL bottle
NDC 0029-6085-23 .... 100 mL bottle
NDC 0029-6085-22 .... 150 mL bottle

AUGMENTIN 200 mg/5 mL (200 mg amoxicillin/28.5 mg clavulanic acid) For Oral Suspension:

NDC 0029-6087-29 .... 50 mL bottle
NDC 0029-6087-39 .... 75 mL bottle
NDC 0029-6087-51 .... 100 mL bottle

AUGMENTIN 250 mg/5 mL (250 mg amoxicillin/62.5 mg clavulanic acid) For Oral Suspension:

NDC 0029-6090-39 .... 75 mL bottle
NDC 0029-6090-23 .... 100 mL bottle
NDC 0029-6090-22 .... 150 mL bottle

AUGMENTIN 400 mg/5 mL (400 mg amoxicillin/57 mg clavulanic acid) For Oral Suspension:

NDC 0029-6092-29 .... 50 mL bottle
NDC 0029-6092-39 .... 75 mL bottle
NDC 0029-6092-51 .... 100 mL bottle

AUGMENTIN 125 mg (125 mg amoxicillin/31.25 mg clavulanic acid) Chewable Tablets:

NDC 0029-6073-47 carton of 30 (5×6) tablets

AUGMENTIN 200 mg (200 mg amoxicillin/28.5 mg clavulanic acid) Chewable Tablets:

NDC 0029-6071-12 carton of 20 tablets

AUGMENTIN 250 mg (250 mg amoxicillin/62.5 mg clavulanic acid) Chewable Tablets:

NDC 0029-6074-47 carton of 30 (5×6) tablets

AUGMENTIN 400 mg (400 mg amoxicillin/57.0 mg clavulanic acid) Chewable Tablets:

NDC 0029-6072-12 carton of 20 tablets

Store tablets and dry powder at or below 25°C (77°F). Dispense in original container.

CLINICAL STUDIES

Data from 2 pivotal studies in 1,191 patients treated for either lower respiratory tract infections or complicated urinary tract infections compared a regimen of 875-mg tablets of AUGMENTIN q12h to 500-mg tablets of AUGMENTIN dosed q8h (584 and 607 patients, respectively). Comparable efficacy was demonstrated between the q12h and q8h dosing regimens. There was no significant difference in the percentage of adverse events in each group. The most frequently reported adverse event was diarrhea; incidence rates were similar for the 875-mg q12h and 500-mg q8h dosing regimens (14.9% and 14.3%, respectively); however, there was a statistically significant difference ($p<0.05$) in rates of severe diarrhea or withdrawals with diarrhea between the regimens: 1.0% for 875-mg q12h dosing versus 2.5% for the 500-mg q8h dosing.

In 1 of these pivotal studies, 629 patients with either pyelonephritis or a complicated urinary tract infection (i.e., patients with abnormalities of the urinary tract that predispose to relapse of bacteriuria following eradication) were randomized to receive either 875-mg tablets of AUGMENTIN q12h or 500-mg tablets of AUGMENTIN q8h in the following distribution:

	875 mg q12h	500 mg q8h
Pyelonephritis	173 patients	188 patients
Complicated UTI	135 patients	133 patients
Total patients	308	321

The number of bacteriologically evaluable patients was comparable between the 2 dosing regimens. AUGMENTIN produced comparable bacteriological success rates in patients assessed 2 to 4 days immediately following end of therapy. The bacteriologic efficacy rates were comparable at 1 of the follow-up visits (5 to 9 days post-therapy) and at a late post-therapy visit (in the majority of cases, this was 2 to 4 weeks post-therapy), as seen in the table below:

	875 mg q12h	500 mg q8h
2 to 4 days	81%, n = 58	80%, n = 54
5 to 9 days	58.5%, n = 41	51.9%, n = 52
2 to 4 weeks	52.5%, n = 101	54.8%, n = 104

As noted before, though there was no significant difference in the percentage of adverse events in each group, there was a statistically significant difference in rates of severe diarrhea or withdrawals with diarrhea between the regimens.

REFERENCES

1. National Committee for Clinical Laboratory Standards. Methods for Dilution Antimicrobial Susceptibility Tests for Bacteria that Grow Aerobically—Third Edition. Approved Standard NCCLS Document M7-A3, Vol. 13, No. 25. NCCLS, Villanova, PA, December 1993.
2. National Committee for Clinical Laboratory Standards. Performance Standards for Antimicrobial Disk Susceptibility Tests—Fifth Edition. Approved Standard NCCLS Document M2-A5, Vol. 13, No. 24. NCCLS, Villanova, PA, December 1993.
3. Swanson-Biearman B, Dean BS, Lopez G, Krenzelok EP. The effects of penicillin and cephalosporin ingestions in children less than six years of age. *Vet Hum Toxicol* 1988;30:66-67.

June 2004/AG:AL13

Shown in Product Identification Guide, page 314

AUGMENTIN ES-600® ℞

[ăg-min' tin]
(amoxicillin/clavulanate potassium)
Powder for Oral Suspension

To reduce the development of drug-resistant bacteria and maintain the effectiveness of AUGMENTIN ES-600 (amoxicillin/clavulanate potassium) and other antibacterial drugs, AUGMENTIN ES-600 should be used only to treat or prevent infections that are proven or strongly suspected to be caused by bacteria.

DESCRIPTION

AUGMENTIN ES-600 is an oral antibacterial combination consisting of the semisynthetic antibiotic amoxicillin and the β-lactamase inhibitor, clavulanate potassium (the potassium salt of clavulanic acid). Amoxicillin is an analog of ampicillin, derived from the basic penicillin nucleus, 6-aminopenicillanic acid. The amoxicillin molecular formula is $C_{16}H_{19}N_3O_5S \cdot 3H_2O$, and the molecular weight is 419.46. Chemically, amoxicillin is (2*S*,5*R*,6*R*)-6-[(*R*)-(-)-2-Amino-2-(*p*-hydroxyphenyl)acetamido]-3,3-dimethyl-7-oxo-4-thia-1-azabicyclo[3.2.0]heptane-2-carboxylic acid trihydrate.

Clavulanic acid is produced by the fermentation of *Streptomyces clavuligerus*. It is a β-lactam structurally related to the penicillins and possesses the ability to inactivate a wide variety of β-lactamases by blocking the active sites of these enzymes. Clavulanic acid is particularly active against the clinically important plasmid-mediated β-lactamases frequently responsible for transferred drug resistance to penicillins and cephalosporins. The clavulanate potassium molecular formula is $C_8H_8KNO_5$ and the molecular weight is 237.25. Chemically, clavulanate potassium is potassium (*Z*)-(2*R*,5*R*)-3-(2-hyrdoxyethylidene)-7-oxo-4-oxa-1-azabicyclo-[3.2.0]-heptane-2-carboxylate.

Inactive Ingredients: Powder for Oral Suspension—Colloidal silicon dioxide, orange flavorings, xanthan gum, aspartame•, hypromellose, and silicon dioxide.

• See PRECAUTIONS—Information for the Patient/Phenylketonurics.

Each 5 mL of reconstituted 600 mg/5 mL oral suspension of AUGMENTIN ES-600 contains 0.23 mEq potassium.

CLINICAL PHARMACOLOGY

The pharmacokinetics of amoxicillin and clavulanate were determined in a study of 19 pediatric patients, 8 months to 11 years, given AUGMENTIN ES-600 at an amoxicillin dose of 45 mg/kg q12h with a snack or meal. The mean plasma amoxicillin and clavulanate pharmacokinetic parameter values are listed in the following table.

[See table 1 at top of next page]

The effect of food on the oral absorption of AUGMENTIN ES-600 has not been studied.

Approximately 50% to 70% of the amoxicillin and approximately 25% to 40% of the clavulanic acid are excreted unchanged in urine during the first 6 hours after administration of 10 mL of 250 mg/5 mL suspension of AUGMENTIN.

Concurrent administration of probenecid delays amoxicillin excretion but does not delay renal excretion of clavulanic acid.

Neither component in AUGMENTIN ES-600 is highly protein-bound; clavulanic acid has been found to be approximately 25% bound to human serum and amoxicillin approximately 18% bound.

Oral administration of a single dose of AUGMENTIN ES-600 at 45 mg/kg (based on the amoxicillin component) to pediatric patients, 9 months to 8 years, yielded the following pharmacokinetic data for amoxicillin in plasma and middle ear fluid (MEF):

[See table 2 at top of next page]

Dose administered immediately prior to eating.

Amoxicillin diffuses readily into most body tissues and fluids with the exception of the brain and spinal fluid. The results of experiments involving the administration of clavulanic acid to animals suggest that this compound, like amoxicillin, is well distributed in body tissues.

Microbiology: Amoxicillin is a semisynthetic antibiotic with a broad spectrum of bactericidal activity against many gram-positive and gram-negative microorganisms. Amoxicillin is, however, susceptible to degradation by β-lactamases, and therefore, the spectrum of activity does not include organisms which produce these enzymes. Clavulanic acid is a β-lactam, structurally related to the penicillins, which possesses the ability to inactivate a wide range of β-lactamase enzymes commonly found in microorganisms resistant to penicillins and cephalosporins. In particular, it has good activity against the clinically important plasmid-mediated β-lactamases frequently responsible for transferred drug resistance.

The clavulanic acid component in AUGMENTIN ES-600 protects amoxicillin from degradation by β-lactamase enzymes and effectively extends the antibiotic spectrum of amoxicillin to include many bacteria normally resistant to amoxicillin and other β-lactam antibiotics. Thus, AUGMENTIN ES-600 possesses the distinctive properties of a broad-spectrum antibiotic and a β-lactamase inhibitor.

Amoxicillin/clavulanic acid has been shown to be active against most strains of the following microorganisms, both in vitro and in clinical infections as described in INDICATIONS AND USAGE.

Aerobic Gram-Positive Microorganisms:

Streptococcus pneumoniae (including isolates with penicillin MICs ≤2 mcg/mL)

Aerobic Gram-Negative Microorganisms:

Haemophilus influenzae (including β-lactamase-producing strains)

Moraxella catarrhalis (including β-lactamase-producing strains)

The following in vitro data are available, but their clinical significance is unknown.

At least 90% of the following microorganisms exhibit an in vitro minimum inhibitory concentration (MIC) less than or equal to the susceptible breakpoint for amoxicillin/clavulanic acid. However, with the exception of organisms shown to respond to amoxicillin alone, the safety and effectiveness of amoxicillin/clavulanic acid in treating clinical infections due to these microorganisms have not been established in adequate and well-controlled clinical trials.

Aerobic Gram-Positive Microorganisms:

Staphylococcus aureus (including β-lactamase-producing strains)

Streptococcus pyogenes

NOTE: Staphylococci which are resistant to methicillin/oxacillin must be considered resistant to amoxicillin/clavulanic acid.

Continued on next page

Product information on these pages is effective as of August 2004. Further information is available at: GlaxoSmithKline, PO Box 13398, Research Triangle Park, NC 27709. 1-888-825-5249. Corporate Web Site: www.gsk.com

Augmentin ES-600—Cont.

NOTE: *S. pyogenes* do not produce β-lactamase, and, therefore, are susceptible to amoxicillin alone. Adequate and well-controlled clinical trials have established the effectiveness of amoxicillin alone in treating certain clinical infections due to *S. pyogenes*.

Susceptibility Testing: *Dilution Techniques:* Quantitative methods are used to determine antimicrobial minimum inhibitory concentrations (MICs). These MICs provide estimates of the susceptibility of bacteria to antimicrobial compounds. The MICs should be determined using a standardized procedure.[1,2] Standardized procedures are based on a dilution method (broth for *S. pneumoniae* and *H. influenzae*) or equivalent with standardized inoculum concentrations and standardized concentrations of amoxicillin/clavulanate potassium powder.

The recommended dilution pattern utilizes a constant amoxicillin/clavulanate potassium ratio of 2 to 1 in all tubes with varying amounts of amoxicillin. MICs are expressed in terms of the amoxicillin concentration in the presence of clavulanic acid at a constant 2 parts amoxicillin to 1 part clavulanic acid. The MIC values should be interpreted according to the following criteria:

For testing *Streptococcus pneumoniae*[a]:

MIC (mcg/mL)	Interpretation
≤2/1	Susceptible (S)
4/2	Intermediate (I)
≥8/4	Resistant (R)

[a] These interpretive standards are applicable only to broth microdilution susceptibility tests using cation-adjusted Mueller-Hinton broth with 2–5% lysed horse blood.[2]

For testing *Haemophilus influenzae*[b]:

MIC (mcg/mL)	Interpretation
≤4/2	Susceptible (S)
≥8/4	Resistant (R)

[b] These interpretive standards are applicable only to broth microdilution susceptibility tests with *Haemophilus* spp. using *Haemophilus* Test Medium (HTM).[2]

A report of "Susceptible" indicates that the pathogen is likely to be inhibited if the antimicrobial compound in the blood reaches the concentration usually achievable. A report of "Intermediate" indicates that the result should be considered equivocal, and, if the microorganism is not fully susceptible to alternative, clinically feasible drugs, the test should be repeated. This category implies possible clinical applicability in body sites where the drug is physiologically concentrated or in situations where high dosage of drug can be used. This category also provides a buffer zone that prevents small uncontrolled technical factors from causing major discrepancies in interpretation. A report of "Resistant" indicates that the pathogen is not likely to be inhibited if the antimicrobial compound in the blood reaches the concentrations usually achievable; other therapy should be selected.

Standardized susceptibility test procedures require the use of laboratory control microorganisms to control the technical aspects of the laboratory procedures. Standard amoxicillin/clavulanate potassium powder should provide the following MIC values:

Microorganism	MIC Range (mcg/mL)[c]
Escherichia coli ATCC 35218 (*H. influenzae* quality control)	4 to 16
Haemophilus influenzae[d] ATCC 49247	2 to 16
Streptococcus pneumoniae[e] ATCC 49619	0.03 to 0.12

[c] Expressed as concentration of amoxicillin in the presence of clavulanic acid at a constant 2 parts amoxicillin to 1 part clavulanic acid.

[d] This quality control range is applicable to *H. influenzae* ATCC 49247 tested by a broth microdilution procedure using HTM[2]

[e] This quality control range is applicable to *S. pneumoniae* ATCC 49619 tested by a broth microdilution procedure using cation-adjusted Mueller-Hinton broth with 2–5% lysed horse blood.[2]

Diffusion Techniques: Quantitative methods that require measurement of zone diameters also provide reproducible estimates of the susceptibility of bacteria to antimicrobial compounds. One such standardized procedure[3] requires the use of standardized inoculum concentrations. This procedure uses paper disks impregnated with 30 mcg of amoxicillin/clavulanate potassium (20 mcg amoxicillin plus 10 mcg clavulanate potassium) to test the susceptibility of microorganisms to amoxicillin/clavulanic acid.

Reports from the laboratory providing results of the standard single-disk susceptibility test with a 30-mcg amoxicillin/clavulanate potassium (20 mcg amoxicillin plus 10 mcg clavulanate potassium) disk should be interpreted according to the following criteria:

For *H. influenzae*[f]:

Zone Diameter (mm)	Interpretation
≥ 20	Susceptible (S)
≤ 19	Resistant (R)

Table 1. Mean (±SD) Plasma Amoxicillin and Clavulanate Pharmacokinetic Parameter Values Following Administration of 45 mg/kg of AUGMENTIN ES-600 Every 12 Hours to Pediatric Patients

Parameter*	Amoxicillin	Clavulanate
C_{max} (mcg/mL)	15.7 ± 7.7	1.7 ± 0.9
T_{max} (hr)	2.0 (1.0 – 4.0)	1.1 (1.0 – 4.0)
AUC_{0-t} (mcg•hr/mL)	59.8 ± 20.0	4.0 ± 1.9
$T_{½}$ (hr)	1.4 ± 0.3	1.1 ± 0.3
CL/F (L/hr/kg)	0.9 ± 0.4	1.1 ± 1.1

*Arithmetic mean ± standard deviation, except T_{max} values which are medians (ranges).

Table 2. Amoxicillin Concentrations in Plasma and Middle Ear Fluid Following Administration of 45 mg/kg of AUGMENTIN ES-600 to Pediatric Patients

Timepoint		Amoxicillin concentration in plasma (mcg/mL)	Amoxicillin concentration in MEF (mcg/mL)
1 hour	mean	7.7	3.2
	median	9.3	3.5
	range	1.5 – 14.0 (n = 5)	0.2 – 5.5 (n = 4)
2 hour	mean	15.7	3.3
	median	13.0	2.4
	range	11.0 – 25.0 (n = 7)	1.9 – 6 (n = 5)
3 hour	mean	13.0	5.8
	median	12.0	6.5
	range	5.5 – 21.0 (n = 5)	3.9 – 7.4 (n = 5)

[f] These zone diameter standards are applicable only to tests conducted with *Haemophilus* spp. using HTM.[2]

NOTE: Beta-lactamase–negative, ampicillin-resistant *H. influenzae* strains must be considered resistant to amoxicillin/clavulanic acid.

For *Streptococcus pneumoniae*:

Susceptibility of *S. pneumoniae* should be determined using a 1-mcg oxacillin disk. Isolates with oxacillin zone sizes of ≥20 mm are susceptible to amoxicillin/clavulanic acid.[g] An amoxicillin/clavulanic acid MIC should be determined on isolates of *S. pneumoniae* with oxacillin zone sizes of ≤19 mm.

[g] These zone diameter standards for *S. pneumoniae* apply only to tests performed using Mueller-Hinton agar supplemented with 5% sheep blood incubated in 5% CO_2.[3]

Interpretation should be as stated above for results using dilution techniques. Interpretation involves correlation of the diameter obtained in the disk test with the MIC for amoxicillin/clavulanic acid.

As with standardized dilution techniques, diffusion methods require the use of laboratory control microorganisms that are used to control the technical aspects of the laboratory procedures. For the diffusion technique, the 30-mcg amoxicillin/clavulanate potassium (20 mcg amoxicillin plus 10 mcg clavulanate potassium) disk should provide the following zone diameters in these laboratory quality control strains:

Microorganism	Zone Diameter (mm)
Escherichia coli ATCC 35218 (*H. influenzae* quality control)	18 to 22
Haemophilus influenzae[h] ATCC 49247	15 to 23

[h] This quality control limit applies only to tests conducted with *H. influenzae* ATCC 49247 using HTM.

INDICATIONS AND USAGE

AUGMENTIN ES-600 is indicated for the treatment of pediatric patients with recurrent or persistent acute otitis media due to *S. pneumoniae* (penicillin MICs ≤2 mcg/mL), *H. influenzae* (including β-lactamase–producing strains), or *M. catarrhalis* (including β-lactamase–producing strains) characterized by the following risk factors:

- antibiotic exposure for acute otitis media within the preceding 3 months, and either of the following:
  - –age ≤2 years
  - –daycare attendance

[See CLINICAL PHARMACOLOGY, Microbiology.]

Note: Acute otitis media due to *S. pneumoniae* alone can be treated with amoxicillin. AUGMENTIN ES-600 is not indicated for the treatment of acute otitis media due to *S. pneumoniae* with penicillin MIC ≥ 4 mcg/mL.

To reduce the development of drug-resistant bacteria and maintain the effectiveness of AUGMENTIN ES-600 and other antibacterial drugs, AUGMENTIN ES-600 should be used only to treat or prevent infections that are proven or strongly suspected to be caused by susceptible bacteria. When culture and susceptibility information are available, they should be considered in selecting or modifying antibacterial therapy. In the absence of such data, local epidemiology and susceptibility patterns may contribute to the empiric selection of therapy when there is reason to believe the infection may involve both *S. pneumoniae* (penicillin MIC ≤2 mcg/mL) and the β-lactamase–producing organisms listed above. Once the results are known, therapy should be adjusted appropriately.

CONTRAINDICATIONS

AUGMENTIN ES-600 is contraindicated in patients with a history of allergic reactions to any penicillin. It is also contraindicated in patients with a previous history of cholestatic jaundice/hepatic dysfunction associated with AUGMENTIN.

WARNINGS

SERIOUS AND OCCASIONALLY FATAL HYPERSENSITIVITY (ANAPHYLACTIC) REACTIONS HAVE BEEN REPORTED IN PATIENTS ON PENICILLIN THERAPY. THESE REACTIONS ARE MORE LIKELY TO OCCUR IN INDIVIDUALS WITH A HISTORY OF PENICILLIN HYPERSENSITIVITY AND/OR A HISTORY OF SENSITIVITY TO MULTIPLE ALLERGENS. THERE HAVE BEEN REPORTS OF INDIVIDUALS WITH A HISTORY OF PENICILLIN HYPERSENSITIVITY WHO HAVE EXPERIENCED SEVERE REACTIONS WHEN TREATED WITH CEPHALOSPORINS. BEFORE INITIATING THERAPY WITH AUGMENTIN ES-600, CAREFUL INQUIRY SHOULD BE MADE CONCERNING PREVIOUS HYPERSENSITIVITY REACTIONS TO PENICILLINS, CEPHALOSPORINS, OR OTHER ALLERGENS. IF AN ALLERGIC REACTION OCCURS, AUGMENTIN ES-600 SHOULD BE DISCONTINUED AND THE APPROPRIATE THERAPY INSTITUTED. **SERIOUS ANAPHYLACTIC REACTIONS REQUIRE IMMEDIATE EMERGENCY TREATMENT WITH EPINEPHRINE. OXYGEN, INTRAVENOUS STEROIDS, AND AIRWAY MANAGEMENT, INCLUDING INTUBATION, SHOULD ALSO BE ADMINISTERED AS INDICATED.**

Pseudomembranous colitis has been reported with nearly all antibacterial agents, including amoxicillin/clavulanate potassium, and has ranged in severity from mild to life-threatening. Therefore, it is important to consider this diagnosis in patients who present with diarrhea subsequent to the administration of antibacterial agents.

Treatment with antibacterial agents alters the normal flora of the colon and may permit overgrowth of clostridia. Studies indicate that a toxin produced by *Clostridium difficile* is one primary cause of "antibiotic-associated colitis."

After the diagnosis of pseudomembranous colitis has been established, appropriate therapeutic measures should be initiated. Mild cases of pseudomembranous colitis usually respond to drug discontinuation alone. In moderate to severe cases, consideration should be given to management with fluids and electrolytes, protein supplementation, and treatment with an antibacterial drug clinically effective against *C. difficile* colitis.

AUGMENTIN ES-600 should be used with caution in patients with evidence of hepatic dysfunction. Hepatic toxicity associated with the use of amoxicillin/clavulanate potassium is usually reversible. On rare occasions, deaths have been reported (less than 1 death reported per estimated 4 million prescriptions worldwide). These have generally been cases associated with serious underlying diseases or concomitant medications. (See CONTRAINDICATIONS and ADVERSE REACTIONS–Liver.)

PRECAUTIONS

General: While amoxicillin/clavulanate possesses the characteristic low toxicity of the penicillin group of antibiotics, periodic assessment of organ system functions, including renal, hepatic, and hematopoietic function, is advisable if therapy is for longer than the drug is approved for administration.

A high percentage of patients with mononucleosis who receive ampicillin develop an erythematous skin rash. Thus, ampicillin-class antibiotics should not be administered to patients with mononucleosis.

The possibility of superinfections with mycotic or bacterial pathogens should be kept in mind during therapy. If superinfections occur (usually involving *Pseudomonas* or *Candida*), the drug should be discontinued and/or appropriate therapy instituted.

Prescribing AUGMENTIN ES-600 in the absence of a proven or strongly suspected bacterial infection or a prophylactic indication is unlikely to provide benefit to the patient and increases the risk of the development of drug-resistant bacteria.

Information for the Patient: AUGMENTIN ES-600 should be taken every 12 hours with a meal or snack to reduce the possibility of gastrointestinal upset. If diarrhea develops and is severe or lasts more than 2 or 3 days, call your doctor. Keep suspension refrigerated. Shake well before using. When dosing a child with the suspension (liquid) of AUGMENTIN ES-600, use a dosing spoon or medicine dropper. Be sure to rinse the spoon or dropper after each use. Bottles of suspension of AUGMENTIN ES-600 may contain more liquid than required. Follow your doctor's instructions about the amount to use and the days of treatment your child requires. Discard any unused medicine.

Patients should be counseled that antibacterial drugs including AUGMENTIN ES-600, should only be used to treat bacterial infections. They do not treat viral infections (e.g., the common cold). When AUGMENTIN ES-600 is prescribed to treat a bacterial infection, patients should be told that although it is common to feel better early in the course of therapy, the medication should be taken exactly as directed. Skipping doses or not completing the full course of therapy may: (1) decrease the effectiveness of the immediate treatment, and (2) increase the likelihood that bacteria will develop resistance and will not be treatable by AUGMENTIN ES-600 or other antibacterial drugs in the future.

Phenylketonurics: Each 5 mL of the 600 mg/5 mL suspension of AUGMENTIN ES-600 contains 7 mg phenylalanine.

Drug Interactions: Probenecid decreases the renal tubular secretion of amoxicillin. Concurrent use with AUGMENTIN ES-600 may result in increased and prolonged blood levels of amoxicillin. Co-administration of probenecid cannot be recommended.

The concurrent administration of allopurinol and ampicillin increases substantially the incidence of rashes in patients receiving both drugs as compared to patients receiving ampicillin alone. It is not known whether this potentiation of ampicillin rashes is due to allopurinol or the hyperuricemia present in these patients. There are no data with AUGMENTIN ES-600 and allopurinol administered concurrently.

In common with other broad-spectrum antibiotics, amoxicillin/clavulanate may reduce the efficacy of oral contraceptives.

Drug/Laboratory Test Interactions: Oral administration of AUGMENTIN will result in high urine concentrations of amoxicillin. High urine concentrations of ampicillin may result in false-positive reactions when testing for the presence of glucose in urine using CLINITEST®, Benedict's Solution, or Fehling's Solution. Since this effect may also occur with amoxicillin and therefore AUGMENTIN ES-600, it is recommended that glucose tests based on enzymatic glucose oxidase reactions (such as CLINISTIX®) be used.

Following administration of ampicillin to pregnant women, a transient decrease in plasma concentration of total conjugated estriol, estriol-glucuronide, conjugated estrone, and estradiol has been noted. This effect may also occur with amoxicillin and therefore AUGMENTIN ES-600.

Carcinogenesis, Mutagenesis, Impairment of Fertility: Long-term studies in animals have not been performed to evaluate carcinogenic potential. The mutagenic potential of AUGMENTIN was investigated in vitro with an Ames test, a human lymphocyte cytogenetic assay, a yeast test, and a mouse lymphoma forward mutation assay, and in vivo with mouse micronucleus tests and a dominant lethal test. All were negative apart from the in vitro mouse lymphoma assay where weak activity was found at very high, cytotoxic concentrations. AUGMENTIN at oral doses of up to 1,200 mg/kg/day (5.7 times the maximum adult human dose based on body surface area) was found to have no effect on fertility and reproductive performance in rats, dosed with a 2:1 ratio formulation of amoxicillin:clavulanate.

Teratogenic Effects: Pregnancy (Category B). Reproduction studies performed in pregnant rats and mice given AUGMENTIN at oral dosages up to 1,200 mg/kg/day (4.9 and 2.8 times the maximum adult human oral dose based on body surface area, respectively), revealed no evidence of harm to the fetus due to AUGMENTIN. There are, however, no adequate and well-controlled studies in pregnant women. Because animal reproduction studies are not always predictive of human response, this drug should be used during pregnancy only if clearly needed.

Labor and Delivery: Oral ampicillin-class antibiotics are generally poorly absorbed during labor. Studies in guinea pigs have shown that intravenous administration of ampicillin decreased the uterine tone, frequency of contractions, height of contractions, and duration of contractions. However, it is not known whether the use of AUGMENTIN in humans during labor or delivery has immediate or delayed adverse effects on the fetus, prolongs the duration of labor, or increases the likelihood that forceps delivery or other obstetrical intervention or resuscitation of the newborn will be necessary. In a single study in women with premature rupture of fetal membranes, it was reported that prophylactic treatment with AUGMENTIN may be associated with an increased risk of necrotizing enterocolitis in neonates.

Nursing Mothers: Ampicillin-class antibiotics are excreted in human milk; therefore, caution should be exercised when AUGMENTIN is administered to a nursing woman.

Pediatric Use: Safety and efficacy of AUGMENTIN ES-600 in infants younger than 3 months have not been established. Safety and efficacy of AUGMENTIN ES-600 have been demonstrated for treatment of acute otitis media in infants and children 3 months to 12 years (see Description of Clinical Studies).

ADVERSE REACTIONS

AUGMENTIN ES-600 is generally well tolerated. The majority of side effects observed in pediatric clinical trials of acute otitis media were either mild or moderate, and transient in nature; 4.4% of patients discontinued therapy because of drug-related side effects. The most commonly reported side effects with probable or suspected relationship to AUGMENTIN ES-600 were contact dermatitis, i.e., diaper rash (3.5%), diarrhea (2.9%), vomiting (2.2%), moniliasis (1.4%), and rash (1.1%). The most common adverse experiences leading to withdrawal that were of probable or suspected relationship to AUGMENTIN ES-600 were diarrhea (2.5%) and vomiting (1.4%).

The following adverse reactions have been reported for ampicillin-class antibiotics:

Gastrointestinal: Diarrhea, nausea, vomiting, indigestion, gastritis, stomatitis, glossitis, black "hairy" tongue, mucocutaneous candidiasis, enterocolitis, and hemorrhagic/pseudomembranous colitis. Onset of pseudomembranous colitis symptoms may occur during or after antibiotic treatment. (See WARNINGS.)

Hypersensitivity Reactions: Skin rashes, pruritus, urticaria, angioedema, serum sickness-like reactions (urticaria or skin rash accompanied by arthritis, arthralgia, myalgia, and frequently fever), erythema multiforme (rarely Stevens-Johnson syndrome), acute generalized exanthematous pustulosis, and an occasional case of exfoliative dermatitis (including toxic epidermal necrolysis) have been reported. These reactions may be controlled with antihistamines and, if necessary, systemic corticosteroids. Whenever such reactions occur, the drug should be discontinued, unless the opinion of the physician dictates otherwise. Serious and occasional fatal hypersensitivity (anaphylactic) reactions can occur with oral penicillin. (See WARNINGS.)

Liver: A moderate rise in AST (SGOT) and/or ALT (SGPT) has been noted in patients treated with ampicillin-class antibiotics, but the significance of these findings is unknown. Hepatic dysfunction, including increases in serum transaminases (AST and/or ALT), serum bilirubin, and/or alkaline phosphatase, has been infrequently reported with AUGMENTIN. It has been reported more commonly in the elderly, in males, or in patients on prolonged treatment. The histologic findings on liver biopsy have consisted of predominantly cholestatic, hepatocellular, or mixed cholestatic-hepatocellular changes. The onset of signs/symptoms of hepatic dysfunction may occur during or several weeks after therapy has been discontinued. The hepatic dysfunction, which may be severe, is usually reversible. On rare occasions, deaths have been reported (less than 1 death reported per estimated 4 million prescriptions worldwide). These have generally been cases associated with serious underlying diseases or concomitant medications.

Renal: Interstitial nephritis and hematuria have been reported rarely. Crystalluria has also been reported **(see OVERDOSAGE)**.

Hemic and Lymphatic Systems: Anemia, including hemolytic anemia, thrombocytopenia, thrombocytopenic purpura, eosinophilia, leukopenia, and agranulocytosis have been reported during therapy with penicillins. These reactions are usually reversible on discontinuation of therapy and are believed to be hypersensitivity phenomena. A slight thrombocytosis was noted in less than 1% of the patients treated with AUGMENTIN. There have been reports of increased prothrombin time in patients receiving AUGMENTIN and anticoagulant therapy concomitantly.

Central Nervous System: Agitation, anxiety, behavioral changes, confusion, convulsions, dizziness, insomnia, and reversible hyperactivity have been reported rarely.

Miscellaneous: Tooth discoloration (brown, yellow, or gray staining) has been rarely reported. Most reports occurred in pediatric patients. Discoloration was reduced or eliminated with brushing or dental cleaning in most cases.

OVERDOSAGE

Following overdosage, patients have experienced primarily gastrointestinal symptoms including stomach and abdominal pain, vomiting, and diarrhea. Rash, hyperactivity, or drowsiness have also been observed in a small number of patients.

In the case of overdosage, discontinue AUGMENTIN ES-600, treat symptomatically, and institute supportive measures as required. If the overdosage is very recent and there is no contraindication, an attempt at emesis or other means of removal of drug from the stomach may be performed. A prospective study of 51 pediatric patients at a poison control center suggested that overdosages of less than 250 mg/kg of amoxicillin are not associated with significant clinical symptoms and do not require gastric emptying.[4]

Interstitial nephritis resulting in oliguric renal failure has been reported in a small number of patients after overdosage with amoxicillin.

Crystalluria, in some cases leading to renal failure, has also been reported after amoxicillin overdosage in adults and pediatric patients. In cases of overdosage, adequate fluid intake and diuresis should be maintained to reduce the risk of amoxicillin crystalluria. Renal impairment appears to be reversible with cessation of drug administration. High blood levels may occur more readily in patients with impaired renal function because of decreased renal clearance of both amoxicillin and clavulanate. Both amoxicillin and clavulanate are removed from the circulation by hemodialysis.

DOSAGE AND ADMINISTRATION

AUGMENTIN ES-600, 600 mg/5 mL, does not contain the same amount of clavulanic acid (as the potassium salt) as any of the other suspensions of AUGMENTIN. AUGMENTIN ES-600 contains 42.9 mg of clavulanic acid per 5 mL, whereas the 200 mg/5 mL suspension of AUGMENTIN contains 28.5 mg of clavulanic acid per 5 mL and the 400 mg/5 mL suspension contains 57 mg of clavulanic acid per 5 mL. Therefore, the 200 mg/5 mL and 400 mg/5 mL suspensions of AUGMENTIN should *not* be substituted for AUGMENTIN ES-600, as they are not interchangeable.

Dosage: ***Pediatric patients 3 months and older:*** Based on the amoxicillin component (600 mg/5 mL), the recommended dose of AUGMENTIN ES-600 is 90 mg/kg/day divided every 12 hours, administered for 10 days (see chart below).

Body Weight (kg)	Volume of AUGMENTIN ES-600 providing 90 mg/kg/day
8	3.0 mL twice daily
12	4.5 mL twice daily
16	6.0 mL twice daily
20	7.5 mL twice daily
24	9.0 mL twice daily
28	10.5 mL twice daily
32	12.0 mL twice daily
36	13.5 mL twice daily

Pediatric patients weighing 40 kg and more: Experience with AUGMENTIN ES-600 (600 mg/5 mL formulation) in this group is not available.

Adults: Experience with AUGMENTIN ES-600 (600 mg/5 mL formulation) in adults is not available and adults who have difficulty swallowing should not be given AUGMENTIN ES-600 (600 mg/5 mL) in place of the 500-mg or 875-mg tablet of AUGMENTIN.

Hepatically impaired patients should be dosed with caution and hepatic function monitored at regular intervals. (See WARNINGS.)

Directions for Mixing Oral Suspension: Prepare a suspension at time of dispensing as follows: Tap bottle until all the powder flows freely. Add approximately 2/3 of the total amount of water for reconstitution (see table below) and shake vigorously to suspend powder. Add remainder of the water and again shake vigorously.

AUGMENTIN ES-600
(600 mg/5 mL Suspension)

Bottle Size	Amount of Water Required for Reconstitution
75 mL	65 mL
125 mL	110 mL
200 mL	175 mL

Each teaspoonful (5 mL) will contain 600 mg amoxicillin as the trihydrate and 42.9 mg of clavulanic acid as the potassium salt.

Note: SHAKE ORAL SUSPENSION WELL BEFORE USING.

Administration: To minimize the potential for gastrointestinal intolerance, AUGMENTIN ES-600 should be taken at the start of a meal. Absorption of clavulanate potassium may be enhanced when AUGMENTIN ES-600 is administered at the start of a meal.

HOW SUPPLIED

AUGMENTIN ES-600, 600 mg/5 mL, for Oral Suspension: Each 5 mL of reconstituted orange-flavored suspension con-

Continued on next page

Product information on these pages is effective as of August 2004. Further information is available at: GlaxoSmithKline, PO Box 13398, Research Triangle Park, NC 27709. 1-888-825-5249. Corporate Web Site: www.gsk.com

Table 3. Bacteriologic Eradication Rates in the Per Protocol Population

Pathogen	Bacteriologic Eradication on Therapy		
	n/N	%	95% CI*
All *S. pneumoniae*	121/123	98.4	(94.3, 99.8)
S. pneumoniae with penicillin MIC = 2 mcg/mL	19/19	100	(82.4, 100.0)
S. pneumoniae with penicillin MIC = 4 mcg/mL	12/14	85.7	(57.2, 98.2)
H. influenzae	75/81	92.6	(84.6, 97.2)
M. catarrhalis	11/11	100	(71.5, 100.0)

*CI=confidence intervals; 95% CIs are not adjusted for multiple comparisons.

Table 4. Clinical Assessments in the Per Protocol Population (Includes *S. pneumoniae* Patients With Penicillin MICs = 2 or 4 mcg/mL*)

Pathogen	2–4 Days Post-Therapy (Primary Endpoint)		
	n/N	%	95% CI†
All *S. pneumoniae*	122/137	89.1	(82.6, 93.7)
S. pneumoniae with penicillin MIC = 2 mcg/mL	17/20	85.0	(62.1, 96.8)
S. pneumoniae with penicillin MIC = 4 mcg/mL	11/14	78.6	(49.2, 95.3)
H. influenzae	141/162	87.0	(80.9, 91.8)
M. catarrhalis	22/26	84.6	(65.1, 95.6)
	15–18 Days Post-Therapy‡ (Secondary Endpoint)		
	N/N	%	95% CI†
All *S. pneumoniae*	95/136	69.9	(61.4, 77.4)
S. pneumoniae with penicillin MIC = 2 mcg/mL	11/20	55.0	(31.5, 76.9)
S. pneumoniae with penicillin MIC = 4 mcg/mL	5/14	35.7	(12.8, 64.9)
H. influenzae	106/156	67.9	(60.0, 75.2)
M. catarrhalis	14/25	56.0	(34.9, 75.6)

* *S. pneumoniae* strains with penicillin MICs of 2 or 4 mcg/mL are considered resistant to penicillin.
† CI = confidence intervals; 95% CIs are not adjusted for multiple comparisons.
‡ Clinical assessments at 15–18 days post-therapy may have been confounded by viral infections and new episodes of acute otitis media with time elapsed post-treatment.

Augmentin ES-600—Cont.

tains 600 mg amoxicillin and 42.9 mg clavulanic acid as the potassium salt.

NDC 0029-6094-39 .... 75 mL bottle
NDC 0029-6094-45 .... 125 mL bottle
NDC 0029-6094-24 .... 200 mL bottle

STORAGE

Store reconstituted suspension under refrigeration. Discard unused suspension after 10 days. Store dry powder for oral suspension at or below 25°C (77°F). Dispense in original container.

Description of Clinical Studies

Two clinical studies were conducted in pediatric patients with acute otitis media.

A non-comparative, open-label study assessed the bacteriologic and clinical efficacy of AUGMENTIN ES-600 (90/6.4 mg/kg/day, divided every 12 hours) for 10 days in 521 pediatric patients (3 to 50 months) with acute otitis media. The primary objective was to assess bacteriological response in children with acute otitis media due to *S. pneumoniae* with amoxicillin/clavulanic acid MICs of 4 mcg/mL. The study sought the enrollment of patients with the following risk factors: Failure of antibiotic therapy for acute otitis media in the previous 3 months, history of recurrent episodes of acute otitis media, ≤2 years, or daycare attendance. Prior to receiving AUGMENTIN ES-600, all patients had tympanocentesis to obtain middle ear fluid for bacteriological evaluation. Patients from whom *S. pneumoniae* (alone or in combination with other bacteria) was isolated had a second tympanocentesis 4 to 6 days after the start of therapy. Clinical assessments were planned for all patients during treatment (4–6 days after starting therapy), as well as 2–4 days post-treatment and 15–18 days post-treatment. Bacteriological success was defined as the absence of the pretreatment pathogen from the on-therapy tympanocentesis specimen. Clinical success was defined as improvement or resolution of signs and symptoms. Clinical failure was defined as lack of improvement or worsening of signs and/or symptoms at any time following at least 72 hours of AUGMENTIN ES-600; patients who received an additional systemic antibacterial drug for otitis media after 3 days of therapy were considered clinical failures. Bacteriological eradication on therapy (day 4–6 visit) in the per protocol population is summarized in the following table:

[See table 3 above]

Clinical assessments were made in the per protocol population 2–4 days post-therapy and 15–18 days post-therapy. Patients who responded to therapy 2–4 days post-therapy were followed for 15–18 days post-therapy to assess them for acute otitis media. Nonresponders at 2–4 days post-therapy were considered failures at the latter timepoint.

[See table 4 above]

In the intent-to-treat analysis, overall clinical outcomes at 2–4 days and 15–18 days post-treatment in patients with *S. pneumoniae* with penicillin MIC = 2 mcg/mL and 4 mcg/mL were 29/41 (71%) and 17/41 (41.5%), respectively.

In the intent-to-treat population of 521 patients, the most frequently reported adverse events were vomiting (6.9%), fever (6.1%), contact dermatitis (i.e., diaper rash) (6.1%), upper respiratory tract infection (4.0%), and diarrhea (3.8%). Protocol-defined diarrhea (i.e., 3 or more watery stools in one day or 2 watery stools per day for 2 consecutive days as recorded on diary cards) occurred in 12.9% of patients.

A double-blind, randomized, clinical study compared AUGMENTIN ES-600 (90/6.4 mg/kg/day, divided every 12 hours) to AUGMENTIN (45/6.4 mg/kg/day, divided every 12 hours) for 10 days in 450 pediatric patients (3 months to 12 years) with acute otitis media. The primary objective of the study was to compare the safety of AUGMENTIN ES-600 to AUGMENTIN. There was no statistically significant difference between treatments in the proportion of patients with 1 or more adverse events. The most frequently reported adverse events for AUGMENTIN ES-600 and the comparator of AUGMENTIN were coughing (11.9% versus 6.8%), vomiting (6.5% versus 7.7%), contact dermatitis (i.e., diaper rash, 6.0% versus 4.8%), fever (5.5% versus 3.9%), and upper respiratory infection (3.0% versus 9.2%), respectively. The frequencies of protocol-defined diarrhea with AUGMENTIN ES-600 (11.1%) and AUGMENTIN (9.4%) were similar (95% confidence interval on difference: −4.2% to 7.7%). Only 2 patients in the group treated with AUGMENTIN ES-600 and 1 patient in the group treated with AUGMENTIN were withdrawn due to diarrhea.

REFERENCES

1. National Committee for Clinical Microbiology Standards. *Methods for Dilution Antimicrobial Susceptibility Tests for Bacteria That Grow Aerobically* – Sixth Edition. Approved Standard. NCCLS Document M7-A6, Vol.23, No. 2. (ISBN-1-56238-486-4). NCCLS, 940 West Valley Road, Suite 1400, Wayne, PA 19087-1898, January 2003.
2. National Committee for Clinical Microbiology Standards. *Performance Standards for Antimicrobial Susceptibility Testing* – Thirteenth Informational Supplement. NCCLS Document M100-S13 (M7), Vol. 23, No. 2. NCCLS, 940 West Valley Road, Suite 1400, Wayne, PA 19087-1898, January 2003.
3. National Committee for Clinical Microbiology Standards. *Performance Standards for Antimicrobial Disk Susceptibility Tests* – Eighth Edition. Approved Standard. NCCLS Document M2-A8, Vol. 23, No. 1. (ISBN-1-56238-485-6). NCCLS, 940 West Valley Road, Suite 1400, Wayne, PA, 19087-1898, January 2003.
4. Swanson-Biearman B, Dean BS, Lopez G, Krenzelok EP. The effects of penicillin and cephalosporin ingestions in children less than six years of age. *Vet Hum Toxicol* 1988; 30:66–67.

AUGMENTIN ES-600 is a registered trademark of GlaxoSmithKline.
CLINITEST is a registered trademark of Miles, Inc.
CLINISTIX is a registered trademark of Bayer Corporation.
GlaxoSmithKline, Research Triangle Park, NC 27709

June 2004/AE:L9
Shown in Product Identification Guide, page 314

AUGMENTIN XR™ ℞

[äg-mint' in]
(amoxicillin/clavulanate potassium)
Extended Release Tablets

To reduce the development of drug-resistant bacteria and maintain the effectiveness of AUGMENTIN XR (amoxicillin/clavulanate potassium) and other antibacterial drugs, AUGMENTIN XR should be used only to treat or prevent infections that are proven or strongly suspected to be caused by bacteria.

DESCRIPTION

AUGMENTIN XR is an oral antibacterial combination consisting of the semisynthetic antibiotic amoxicillin (present as amoxicillin trihydrate and amoxicillin sodium) and the β-lactamase inhibitor clavulanate potassium (the potassium salt of clavulanic acid). Amoxicillin is an analog of ampicillin, derived from the basic penicillin nucleus 6-aminopenicillanic acid. The amoxicillin trihydrate molecular formula is $C_{16}H_{19}N_3O_5S{\bullet}3H_2O$, and the molecular weight is 419.45. Chemically, amoxicillin trihydrate is (2*S*,5*R*,6*R*)-6-[(*R*)-(-)-2-Amino-2-(*p*-hydroxyphenyl)acetamido]-3,3-dimethyl-7-oxo-4-thia-1-azabicyclo[3.2.0]heptane-2-carboxylic acid trihydrate.

The amoxicillin sodium molecular formula is $C_{16}H_{18}N_3NaO_5S$, and the molecular weight is 387.39. Chemically, amoxicillin sodium is [2*S*-[2α,5α,6β(*S**)]]-6-[[Amino(4-hydroxyphenyl)acetyl]amino]-3,3-dimethyl-7-oxo-4-thia-1-azabicyclo[3.2.0]heptane-2-carboxylic acid monosodium salt.

Clavulanic acid is produced by the fermentation of *Streptomyces clavuligerus*. It is a β-lactam structurally related to the penicillins and possesses the ability to inactivate a wide variety of β-lactamases by blocking the active sites of these enzymes. Clavulanic acid is particularly active against the clinically important plasmid-mediated β-lactamases frequently responsible for transferred drug resistance to penicillins and cephalosporins. The clavulanate potassium molecular formula is $C_8H_8KNO_5$, and the molecular weight is 237.25. Chemically, clavulanate potassium is potassium (*Z*)-(2*R*,5*R*)-3-(2-hydroxyethylidene)-7-oxo-4-oxa-1-azabicyclo-[3.2.0]-heptane-2-carboxylate.

Inactive Ingredients: Citric acid, colloidal silicon dioxide, hypromellose, magnesium stearate, microcrystalline cellulose, polyethylene glycol, sodium starch glycolate, titanium dioxide, and xanthan gum.

Each tablet of AUGMENTIN XR contains 12.6 mg (0.32 mEq) of potassium and 29.3 mg (1.27 mEq) of sodium.

CLINICAL PHARMACOLOGY

Amoxicillin and clavulanate potassium are well absorbed from the gastrointestinal tract after oral administration of AUGMENTIN XR.

AUGMENTIN XR is an extended-release formulation which provides sustained plasma concentrations of amoxicillin. Amoxicillin systemic exposure achieved with AUGMENTIN XR is similar to that produced by the oral administration of equivalent doses of amoxicillin alone. In a study of healthy adult volunteers, the pharmacokinetics of AUGMENTIN XR were compared when administered in a fasted state, at the start of a standardized meal (612 kcal, 89.3 g carb, 24.9 g fat, and 14.0 g protein), or 30 minutes after a high-fat meal. When the systemic exposure to both amoxicillin and clavulanate is taken into consideration, AUGMENTIN XR is optimally administered at the start of a standardized meal. Absorption of amoxicillin is decreased in the fasted state. AUGMENTIN XR is not recommended to be taken with a high-fat meal, because clavulanate absorption is decreased. The pharmacokinetics of the components of AUGMENTIN XR following administration of two AUGMENTIN XR tablets at the start of a standardized meal are presented below.

Table 1. Mean (SD) Pharmacokinetic Parameters for Amoxicillin and Clavulanate Following Oral Administration of Two AUGMENTIN XR Tablets (2,000 mg/125 mg) to Healthy Adult Volunteers (n = 55) Fed a Standardized Meal

Parameter (units)	Amoxicillin	Clavulanate
$AUC_{(0\text{-}inf)}$ (mcg•hr/mL)	71.6 (16.5)	5.29 (1.55)

C_{max} (mcg/mL)	17.0 (4.0)	2.05 (0.80)
T_{max} (hours)*	1.50 (1.00-6.00)	1.03 (0.75-3.00)
$T_{1/2}$ (hours)	1.27 (0.20)	1.03 (0.17)

*Median (range).

The half-life of amoxicillin after the oral administration of AUGMENTIN XR is approximately 1.3 hours, and that of clavulanate is approximately 1.0 hour.
Clearance of amoxicillin is predominantly renal, with approximately 60% to 80% of the dose being excreted unchanged in urine, whereas clearance of clavulanate has both a renal (30% to 50%) and a non-renal component.
Concurrent administration of probenecid delays amoxicillin excretion but does not delay renal excretion of clavulanate.
In a study of adults, the pharmacokinetics of amoxicillin and clavulanate were not affected by administration of an antacid (MAALOX®), either simultaneously with or 2 hours after AUGMENTIN XR.
Neither component in AUGMENTIN XR is highly protein-bound; clavulanate has been found to be approximately 25% bound to human serum and amoxicillin approximately 18% bound.
Amoxicillin diffuses readily into most body tissues and fluids, with the exception of the brain and spinal fluid. The results of experiments involving the administration of clavulanic acid to animals suggest that this compound, like amoxicillin, is well distributed in body tissues.

Microbiology: Amoxicillin is a semisynthetic antibiotic with a broad spectrum of bactericidal activity against many gram-positive and gram-negative microorganisms. Amoxicillin is, however, susceptible to degradation by β-lactamases, and therefore, the spectrum of activity does not include organisms which produce these enzymes. Clavulanic acid is a β-lactam, structurally related to the penicillins, that possesses the ability to inactivate a wide range of β-lactamase enzymes commonly found in microorganisms resistant to penicillins and cephalosporins. In particular, it has good activity against the clinically important plasmid-mediated β-lactamases frequently responsible for transferred drug resistance.
The clavulanic acid component in AUGMENTIN XR protects amoxicillin from degradation by β-lactamase enzymes and effectively extends the antibiotic spectrum of amoxicillin to include many bacteria normally resistant to amoxicillin and other β-lactam antibiotics.
Amoxicillin/clavulanic acid has been shown to be active against most strains of the following microorganisms, both in vitro and in clinical infections as described in INDICATIONS AND USAGE.

Aerobic Gram-Positive Microorganisms:
Streptococcus pneumoniae (including isolates with penicillin MICs ≤2 mcg/mL)
Staphylococcus aureus (including β-lactamase–producing strains)

NOTE: Staphylococci which are resistant to methicillin/oxacillin must be considered resistant to amoxicillin/clavulanic acid.

Aerobic Gram-Negative Microorganisms:
Haemophilus influenzae (including β-lactamase–producing strains)
Moraxella catarrhalis (including β-lactamase–producing strains)
Haemophilus parainfluenzae (including β-lactamase–producing strains)
Klebsiella pneumoniae (all known strains are β-lactamase–producing)

The following in vitro data are available, **but their clinical significance is unknown.**
Amoxicillin/clavulanic acid exhibits in vitro minimal inhibitory concentrations (MICs) of 2.0 mcg/mL or less against most (≥90%) strains of *Streptococcus pyogenes* and MICs of 4.0 mcg/mL or less against most (≥90%) strains of the anaerobic bacteria listed below.

Aerobic Gram-Positive Microorganisms:
Streptococcus pyogenes

Anaerobic Microorganisms:
Bacteroides fragilis (including β-lactamase–producing strains)
Fusobacterium nucleatum (including β-lactamase–producing strains)
Peptostreptococcus magnus
Peptostreptococcus micros

NOTE: *S. pyogenes*, *P. magnus*, and *P. micros* do not produce β-lactamase, and therefore, are susceptible to amoxicillin alone. Adequate and well-controlled clinical trials have established the effectiveness of amoxicillin alone in treating certain clinical infections due to *S. pyogenes*.

Susceptibility Testing: ***Dilution Techniques:*** Quantitative methods are used to determine antimicrobial MICs. These MICs provide estimates of the susceptibility of bacteria to antimicrobial compounds. The MICs should be determined using a standardized procedure.[1,2] Standardized procedures are based on a dilution method (broth or agar; broth for *S. pneumoniae* and *Haemophilus* spp.) or equivalent with standardized inoculum concentrations and standardized concentrations of amoxicillin/clavulanate potassium powder.
The recommended dilution pattern utilizes a constant amoxicillin/clavulanate potassium ratio of 2 to 1 in all tubes with varying amounts of amoxicillin. MICs are expressed in terms of the amoxicillin concentration in the presence of clavulanic acid at a constant 2 parts amoxicillin to 1 part clavulanic acid.
The MIC values should be interpreted according to the following criteria:

For testing *Klebsiella pneumoniae:*

MIC (mcg/mL)	Interpretation
≤8/4	Susceptible (S)
16/8	Intermediate (I)
≥32/16	Resistant (R)

For testing *Streptococcus pneumoniae*[a]:

MIC (mcg/mL)	Interpretation
≤2/1	Susceptible (S)
4/2	Intermediate (I)
≥8/4	Resistant (R)

[a] These interpretive standards are applicable only to broth microdilution susceptibility tests using cation-adjusted Mueller-Hinton broth with 2 to 5% lysed horse blood.[2]

For testing *Staphylococcus* spp. and *Haemophilus* spp.[b]:

MIC (mcg/mL)	Interpretation
≤4/2	Susceptible (S)
≥8/4	Resistant (R)

[b] These interpretive standards are applicable only to broth microdilution susceptibility tests with *Haemophilus* spp. using *Haemophilus* Test Medium (HTM).[2]

NOTE: Staphylococci which are resistant to methicillin/oxacillin must be considered resistant to amoxicillin/clavulanic acid.
A report of "Susceptible" indicates that the pathogen is likely to be inhibited if the antimicrobial compound in the blood reaches the concentration usually achievable. A report of "Intermediate" indicates that the result should be considered equivocal, and if the microorganism is not fully susceptible to alternative, clinically feasible drugs, the test should be repeated. This category implies possible clinical applicability in body sites where the drug is physiologically concentrated or in situations where high dosage of drug can be used. This category also provides a buffer zone which prevents small uncontrolled technical factors from causing major discrepancies in interpretation. A report of "Resistant" indicates that the pathogen is not likely to be inhibited if the antimicrobial compound in the blood reaches the concentrations usually achievable; other therapy should be selected.
Standardized susceptibility test procedures require the use of laboratory control microorganisms to control the technical aspects of the laboratory procedures. Standard amoxicillin/clavulanate potassium powder should provide the following MIC values:

Microorganism		MIC Range (mcg/mL)[c]
Escherichia coli	ATCC 35218	4-16
Escherichia coli	ATCC 25922	2-8
Haemophilus influenzae[d]	ATCC 49247	2-16
Staphylococcus aureus	ATCC 29213	0.12-0.5
Streptococcus pneumoniae[e]	ATCC 49619	0.03-0.12

[c] Expressed as concentration of amoxicillin in the presence of clavulanic acid at a constant 2 parts amoxicillin to 1 part clavulanic acid.
[d] This quality control range is applicable to *H. influenzae* ATCC 49247 tested by a broth microdilution procedure using HTM.[2]
[e] This quality control range is applicable to *S. pneumoniae* ATCC 49619 tested by a broth microdilution procedure using cation-adjusted Mueller-Hinton broth with 2 to 5% lysed horse blood.[2]

Diffusion Techniques: Quantitative methods that require measurement of zone diameters also provide reproducible estimates of the susceptibility of bacteria to antimicrobial compounds. One such standardized procedure requires the use of standardized inoculum concentrations.[3] This procedure uses paper disks impregnated with 30 mcg of amoxicillin/clavulanate potassium (20 mcg amoxicillin plus 10 mcg clavulanate potassium) to test the susceptibility of microorganisms to amoxicillin/clavulanic acid.
Reports from the laboratory providing results of the standard single-disk susceptibility test with a 30-mcg amoxicillin/clavulanate potassium (20 mcg amoxicillin plus 10 mcg clavulanate potassium) disk should be interpreted according to the following criteria:

For testing *Klebsiella pneumoniae:*

Zone Diameter (mm)	Interpretation
≥18	Susceptible (S)
14-17	Intermediate (I)
≤13	Resistant (R)

For testing *Staphylococcus* and *Haemophilus*[f] spp.:

Zone Diameter (mm)	Interpretation
≥20	Susceptible (S)
≤19	Resistant (R)

[f] These zone diameter standards are applicable only to tests conducted with *Haemophilus* spp. using HTM.[2]

NOTE: Staphylococci which are resistant to methicillin/oxacillin must be considered resistant to amoxicillin/clavulanic acid.
NOTE: Beta-lactamase–negative, ampicillin-resistant *H. influenzae* strains must be considered resistant to amoxicillin/clavulanic acid.

For testing *S. pneumoniae:* Susceptibility of *S. pneumoniae* should be determined using a 1-mcg oxacillin disk. Isolates with oxacillin zone sizes of ≥20 mm are susceptible to amoxicillin/clavulanic acid.[g] An amoxicillin/clavulanic acid MIC should be determined on isolates of *S. pneumoniae* with oxacillin zone sizes of ≤19 mm.
[g] These zone diameter standards for *S. pneumoniae* apply only to tests performed using Mueller-Hinton agar supplemented with 5% sheep blood incubated in 5% CO_2.[2]

Interpretation should be as stated above for results using dilution techniques.
Interpretation involves correlation of the diameter obtained in the disk test with the MIC for amoxicillin/clavulanic acid.
As with standardized dilution techniques, diffusion methods require the use of laboratory control microorganisms that are used to control the technical aspects of the laboratory procedures. For the diffusion technique, the 30-mcg amoxicillin/clavulanate potassium (20 mcg amoxicillin plus 10 mcg clavulanate potassium) disk should provide the following zone diameters in these laboratory quality control strains:

Microorganism		Zone Diameter (mm)
Escherichia coli	ATCC 35218	17-22
Escherichia coli	ATCC 25922	18-24
Staphylococcus aureus	ATCC 25923	28-36
Haemophilus influenzae[h]	ATCC 49247	15-23

[h] This quality control limit applies only to tests conducted with *H. influenzae* ATCC 49247 using HTM.[2]

INDICATIONS AND USAGE

AUGMENTIN XR Extended Release Tablets are indicated for the treatment of patients with community-acquired pneumonia or acute bacterial sinusitis due to confirmed, or suspected β-lactamase–producing pathogens (i.e., *H. influenzae, M. catarrhalis, H. parainfluenzae, K. pneumoniae*, or methicillin-susceptible *S. aureus*) and *S. pneumoniae* with reduced susceptibility to penicillin (i.e., penicillin MICs = 2 mcg/mL). AUGMENTIN XR is not indicated for the treatment of infections due to *S. pneumoniae* with penicillin MICs ≥4 mcg/mL. Data are limited with regard to infections due to *S. pneumoniae* with penicillin MICs ≥4 mcg/mL (see CLINICAL STUDIES).
Of the common epidemiological risk factors for patients with resistant pneumococcal infections, only age >65 years was studied. Patients with other common risk factors for resistant pneumococcal infections (e.g., alcoholism, immune-suppressive illness, and presence of multiple co-morbid conditions) were not studied.
In patients with community-acquired pneumonia in whom penicillin-resistant *S. pneumoniae* is suspected, bacteriological studies should be performed to determine the causative organisms and their susceptibility when AUGMENTIN XR is prescribed.
Acute bacterial sinusitis or community-acquired pneumonia due to a penicillin-susceptible strain of *S. pneumoniae* plus a β-lactamase–producing pathogen can be treated with another AUGMENTIN® (amoxicillin/clavulanate potassium) product containing lower daily doses of amoxicillin (i.e., 500 mg q8h or 875 mg q12h). Acute bacterial sinusitis or community-acquired pneumonia due to *S. pneumoniae* alone can be treated with amoxicillin.
To reduce the development of drug-resistant bacteria and maintain the effectiveness of AUGMENTIN XR and other antibacterial drugs, AUGMENTIN XR should be used only to treat or prevent infections that are proven or strongly suspected to be caused by susceptible bacteria. When culture and susceptibility information are available, they should be considered in selecting or modifying antibacterial therapy. In the absence of such data, local epidemiology and susceptibility patterns may contribute to the empiric selection of therapy.

CONTRAINDICATIONS

AUGMENTIN XR is contraindicated in patients with a history of allergic reactions to any penicillin. It is also contraindicated in patients with a previous history of cholestatic jaundice/hepatic dysfunction associated with treatment with amoxicillin/clavulanate potassium.
AUGMENTIN XR is contraindicated in patients with severe renal impairment (creatinine clearance <30 mL/min.) and in hemodialysis patients.

WARNINGS

SERIOUS AND OCCASIONALLY FATAL HYPERSENSITIVITY (ANAPHYLACTIC) REACTIONS HAVE BEEN REPORTED IN PATIENTS ON PENICILLIN THERAPY. THESE REACTIONS ARE MORE LIKELY TO OCCUR IN INDIVIDUALS WITH A HISTORY OF PENICILLIN HYPERSENSITIVITY AND/OR A HISTORY OF SENSITIVITY TO MULTIPLE ALLERGENS. THERE HAVE BEEN REPORTS OF INDIVIDUALS WITH A HISTORY OF PENICILLIN HYPERSENSITIVITY WHO HAVE EXPERI-

Continued on next page

Product information on these pages is effective as of August 2004. Further information is available at: GlaxoSmithKline, PO Box 13398, Research Triangle Park, NC 27709. 1-888-825-5249. Corporate Web Site: www.gsk.com

Augmentin XR—Cont.

ENCED SEVERE REACTIONS WHEN TREATED WITH CEPHALOSPORINS. BEFORE INITIATING THERAPY WITH AUGMENTIN XR, CAREFUL INQUIRY SHOULD BE MADE CONCERNING PREVIOUS HYPERSENSITIVITY REACTIONS TO PENICILLINS, CEPHALOSPORINS, OR OTHER ALLERGENS. IF AN ALLERGIC REACTION OCCURS, AUGMENTIN XR SHOULD BE DISCONTINUED AND THE APPROPRIATE THERAPY INSTITUTED. **SERIOUS ANAPHYLACTIC REACTIONS REQUIRE IMMEDIATE EMERGENCY TREATMENT WITH EPINEPHRINE. OXYGEN, INTRAVENOUS STEROIDS, AND AIRWAY MANAGEMENT, INCLUDING INTUBATION, SHOULD ALSO BE ADMINISTERED AS INDICATED.**

Pseudomembranous colitis has been reported with nearly all antibacterial agents, including amoxicillin/clavulanate potassium, and has ranged in severity from mild to life-threatening. Therefore, it is important to consider this diagnosis in patients who present with diarrhea subsequent to the administration of antibacterial agents.

Treatment with antibacterial agents alters the normal flora of the colon and may permit overgrowth of clostridia. Studies indicate that a toxin produced by *Clostridium difficile* is one primary cause of "antibiotic-associated colitis."

After the diagnosis of pseudomembranous colitis has been established, appropriate therapeutic measures should be initiated. Mild cases of pseudomembranous colitis usually respond to drug discontinuation alone. In moderate to severe cases, consideration should be given to management with fluids and electrolytes, protein supplementation, and treatment with an antibacterial drug clinically effective against *C. difficile* colitis.

AUGMENTIN XR should be used with caution in patients with evidence of hepatic dysfunction. Hepatic toxicity associated with the use of amoxicillin/clavulanate potassium is usually reversible. On rare occasions, deaths have been reported (less than 1 death reported per estimated 4 million prescriptions worldwide). These have generally been cases associated with serious underlying diseases or concomitant medications (see CONTRAINDICATIONS and ADVERSE REACTIONS—Liver).

PRECAUTIONS

General: While amoxicillin/clavulanate potassium possesses the characteristic low toxicity of the penicillin group of antibiotics, periodic assessment of organ system functions, including renal, hepatic, and hematopoietic function, is advisable if therapy is for longer than the drug is approved for administration.

A high percentage of patients with mononucleosis who receive ampicillin develop an erythematous skin rash. Thus, ampicillin-class antibiotics should not be administered to patients with mononucleosis.

The possibility of superinfections with mycotic or bacterial pathogens should be kept in mind during therapy. If superinfections occur (usually involving *Pseudomonas* spp. or *Candida* spp.), the drug should be discontinued and/or appropriate therapy instituted.

Prescribing AUGMENTIN XR in the absence of a proven or strongly suspected bacterial infection or a prophylactic indication is unlikely to provide benefit to the patient and increases the risk of the development of drug-resistant bacteria.

Information for Patients: AUGMENTIN XR should be taken every 12 hours with a meal or snack to reduce the possibility of gastrointestinal upset. If diarrhea develops and is severe or lasts more than 2 or 3 days, call your doctor.

Patients should be counseled that antibacterial drugs, including AUGMENTIN XR, should only be used to treat bacterial infections. They do not treat viral infections (e.g., the common cold). When AUGMENTIN XR is prescribed to treat a bacterial infection, patients should be told that although it is common to feel better early in the course of therapy, the medication should be taken exactly as directed. Skipping doses or not completing the full course of therapy may: (1) decrease the effectiveness of the immediate treatment, and (2) increase the likelihood that bacteria will develop resistance and will not be treatable by AUGMENTIN XR or other antibacterial drugs in the future. Discard any unused medicine.

Drug Interactions: Probenecid decreases the renal tubular secretion of amoxicillin. Concurrent use with AUGMENTIN XR may result in increased and prolonged blood levels of amoxicillin. Co-administration of probenecid cannot be recommended.

The concurrent administration of allopurinol and ampicillin increases substantially the incidence of rashes in patients receiving both drugs as compared to patients receiving ampicillin alone. It is not known whether this potentiation of ampicillin rashes is due to allopurinol or the hyperuricemia present in these patients. In controlled clinical trials of AUGMENTIN XR, 22 patients received concomitant allopurinol and AUGMENTIN XR. No rashes were reported in these patients. However, this sample size is too small to allow for any conclusions to be drawn regarding the risk of rashes with concomitant AUGMENTIN XR and allopurinol use.

In common with other broad-spectrum antibiotics, AUGMENTIN XR may reduce the efficacy of oral contraceptives.

Drug/Laboratory Test Interactions: Oral administration of AUGMENTIN XR will result in high urine concentrations of amoxicillin. High urine concentrations of ampicillin may result in false-positive reactions when testing for the presence of glucose in urine using CLINITEST®, Benedict's Solution, or Fehling's Solution. Since this effect may also occur with amoxicillin and therefore AUGMENTIN XR, it is recommended that glucose tests based on enzymatic glucose oxidase reactions (such as CLINISTIX®) be used.

Following administration of ampicillin to pregnant women, a transient decrease in plasma concentration of total conjugated estriol, estriol-glucuronide, conjugated estrone, and estradiol has been noted. This effect may also occur with amoxicillin, and therefore, AUGMENTIN XR.

Carcinogenesis, Mutagenesis, Impairment of Fertility: Long-term studies in animals have not been performed to evaluate carcinogenic potential. The mutagenic potential of AUGMENTIN was investigated in vitro with an Ames test, a human lymphocyte cytogenetic assay, a yeast test, and a mouse lymphoma forward mutation assay, and in vivo with mouse micronucleus tests and a dominant lethal test. All were negative apart from the in vitro mouse lymphoma assay, where weak activity was found at very high, cytotoxic concentrations. AUGMENTIN at oral doses of up to 1,200 mg/kg/day (1.9 times the maximum human dose of amoxicillin and 15 times the maximum human dose of clavulanate based on body surface area) was found to have no effect on fertility and reproductive performance in rats dosed with a 2:1 ratio formulation of amoxicillin: clavulanate.

Pregnancy: ***Teratogenic Effects:*** Pregnancy Category B: Reproduction studies performed in pregnant rats and mice given AUGMENTIN at oral doses up to 1,200 mg/kg/day revealed no evidence of harm to the fetus due to AUGMENTIN. In terms of body surface area, the doses in rats were 1.6 times the maximum human oral dose of amoxicillin and 13 times the maximum human dose for clavulanate. For mice, these doses were 0.9 and 7.4 times the maximum human oral dose of amoxicillin and clavulanate, respectively. There are, however, no adequate and well-controlled studies in pregnant women. Because animal reproduction studies are not always predictive of human response, this drug should be used during pregnancy only if clearly needed.

Labor and Delivery: Oral ampicillin-class antibiotics are generally poorly absorbed during labor. Studies in guinea pigs have shown that intravenous administration of ampicillin decreased the uterine tone, frequency of contractions, height of contractions, and duration of contractions. However, it is not known whether the use of AUGMENTIN XR in humans during labor or delivery has immediate or delayed adverse effects on the fetus, prolongs the duration of labor, or increases the likelihood that forceps delivery or other obstetrical intervention or resuscitation of the newborn will be necessary. In a single study in women with premature rupture of fetal membranes, it was reported that prophylactic treatment with AUGMENTIN may be associated with an increased risk of necrotizing enterocolitis in neonates.

Nursing Mothers: Ampicillin-class antibiotics are excreted in the milk; therefore, caution should be exercised when AUGMENTIN XR is administered to a nursing woman.

Pediatric Use: Safety and effectiveness in pediatric patients younger than 16 years have not been established.

Geriatric Use: Of the total number of subjects in clinical studies of AUGMENTIN XR, 19.2% were 65 years or older and 7.9% were 75 years or older. No overall differences in safety and effectiveness were observed between these subjects and younger subjects, and other clinical experience has not reported differences in responses between the elderly and younger patients, but a greater sensitivity of some older individuals cannot be ruled out.

This drug is known to be substantially excreted by the kidney, and the risk of dose-dependent toxic reactions to this drug may be greater in patients with impaired renal function. Because elderly patients are more likely to have decreased renal function, it may be useful to monitor renal function.

Each tablet of AUGMENTIN XR contains 29.3 mg (1.27 mEq) of sodium.

ADVERSE REACTIONS

In clinical trials, 4,144 patients have been treated with AUGMENTIN XR. The majority of side effects observed in clinical trials were of a mild and transient nature; 2% of patients discontinued therapy because of drug-related side effects. The most frequently reported adverse effects which were suspected or probably drug-related were diarrhea (15.6%), nausea (2.2%), genital moniliasis (2.1%), and abdominal pain (1.6%). AUGMENTIN XR had a higher rate of diarrhea which required corrective therapy (4.0% versus 2.4% for AUGMENTIN XR and all comparators, respectively).

The following adverse reactions have been reported for ampicillin-class antibiotics:

Gastrointestinal: Diarrhea, nausea, vomiting, indigestion, gastritis, stomatitis, glossitis, black "hairy" tongue, mucocutaneous candidiasis, enterocolitis, and hemorrhagic/pseudomembranous colitis. Onset of pseudomembranous colitis symptoms may occur during or after antibiotic treatment (see WARNINGS).

Hypersensitivity Reactions: Skin rashes, pruritus, urticaria, angioedema, serum sickness-like reactions (urticaria or skin rash accompanied by arthritis, arthralgia, myalgia, and frequently fever), erythema multiforme (rarely Stevens-Johnson syndrome), acute generalized exanthematous pustulosis, and an occasional case of exfoliative dermatitis (including toxic epidermal necrolysis) have been reported. Whenever such reactions occur, the drug should be discontinued, unless the opinion of the physician dictates otherwise. Serious and occasional fatal hypersensitivity (anaphylactic) reactions can occur with oral penicillin (see WARNINGS).

Liver: A moderate rise in AST (SGOT) and/or ALT (SGPT) has been noted in patients treated with ampicillin-class antibiotics, but the significance of these findings is unknown. Hepatic dysfunction, including increases in serum transaminases (AST and/or ALT), serum bilirubin, and/or alkaline phosphatase, has been infrequently reported with AUGMENTIN or AUGMENTIN XR. It has been reported more commonly in the elderly, in males, or in patients on prolonged treatment. The histologic findings on liver biopsy have consisted of predominantly cholestatic, hepatocellular, or mixed cholestatic-hepatocellular changes. The onset of signs/symptoms of hepatic dysfunction may occur during or several weeks after therapy has been discontinued. The hepatic dysfunction, which may be severe, is usually reversible. On rare occasions, deaths have been reported (less than 1 death reported per estimated 4 million prescriptions worldwide). These have generally been cases associated with serious underlying diseases or concomitant medications.

Renal: Interstitial nephritis and hematuria have been reported rarely. Crystalluria has also been reported (see OVERDOSAGE).

Hemic and Lymphatic Systems: Anemia, including hemolytic anemia, thrombocytopenia, thrombocytopenic purpura, eosinophilia, leukopenia, and agranulocytosis have been reported during therapy with penicillins. These reactions are usually reversible on discontinuation of therapy and are believed to be hypersensitivity phenomena. Mild to moderate thrombocytosis was noted in $<1\%$ of patients treated with AUGMENTIN and 3.6% of patients treated with AUGMENTIN XR. There have been reports of increased prothrombin time in patients receiving AUGMENTIN and anticoagulant therapy concomitantly.

Central Nervous System: Agitation, anxiety, behavioral changes, confusion, convulsions, dizziness, headache, insomnia, and reversible hyperactivity have been reported rarely.

Miscellaneous: Tooth discoloration (brown, yellow, or gray staining) has been rarely reported. Most reports occurred in pediatric patients. Discoloration was reduced or eliminated with brushing or dental cleaning in most cases.

OVERDOSAGE

Following overdosage, patients have experienced primarily gastrointestinal symptoms including stomach and abdominal pain, vomiting, and diarrhea. Rash, hyperactivity, or drowsiness have also been observed in a small number of patients.

In the case of overdosage, discontinue AUGMENTIN XR, treat symptomatically, and institute supportive measures as required. If the overdosage is very recent and there is no contraindication, an attempt at emesis or other means of removal of drug from the stomach may be performed. A prospective study of 51 pediatric patients at a poison control center suggested that overdosages of less than 250 mg/kg of amoxicillin are not associated with significant clinical symptoms and do not require gastric emptying.[4]

Interstitial nephritis resulting in oliguric renal failure has been reported in a small number of patients after overdosage with amoxicillin.

Crystalluria, in some cases leading to renal failure, has also been reported after amoxicillin overdosage in adult and pediatric patients. In case of overdosage, adequate fluid intake and diuresis should be maintained to reduce the risk of amoxicillin crystalluria.

Renal impairment appears to be reversible with cessation of drug administration. High blood levels may occur more readily in patients with impaired renal function because of decreased renal clearance of both amoxicillin and clavulanate. Both amoxicillin and clavulanate are removed from the circulation by hemodialysis (see DOSAGE AND ADMINISTRATION).

DOSAGE AND ADMINISTRATION

AUGMENTIN XR should be taken at the start of a meal to enhance the absorption of amoxicillin and to minimize the potential for gastrointestinal intolerance. Absorption of the amoxicillin component is decreased when AUGMENTIN XR is taken on an empty stomach (see CLINICAL PHARMACOLOGY).

The recommended dose of AUGMENTIN XR is 4,000 mg/250 mg daily according to the following table:

Indication	Dose	Duration
Acute bacterial sinusitis	2 tablets q12h	10 days
Community-acquired pneumonia	2 tablets q12h	7-10 days

Tablets of AUGMENTIN (250 mg or 500 mg) CANNOT be used to provide the same dosages as AUGMENTIN XR Extended Release Tablets. This is because AUGMENTIN XR contains 62.5 mg of clavulanic acid, while the AUGMENTIN 250-mg and 500-mg tablets each contain 125 mg of clavulanic acid. In addition, the Extended Release Tablet provides an extended time course of plasma amoxicillin con-

Clinical Outcome for CAP due to *S. pneumoniae*

Penicillin MICs of *S. pneumoniae* Isolates	Intent-To-Treat			Clinically Evaluable		
	n/N*	%	95% CI[†]	n/N*	%	95% CI[†]
All *S. pneumoniae*	184/214	86.0	—	157/172	91.3	—
MIC ≥2.0 mcg/mL[‡]	17/20	85.0	62.1, 96.8	14/15	93.3	68.1, 99.8
MIC = 2.0 mcg/mL	13/14	92.9	66.1, 99.8	10/10	100	69.2, 100
MIC = 4.0 mcg/mL	4/6	66.7	22.3, 95.7	4/5	80.0	28.4, 99.5

* n/N = patients with pathogen eradicated or presumed eradicated/total number of patients.
[†] Confidence limits calculated using exact probabilities.
[‡] *S. pneumoniae* strains with penicillin MICs of ≥2 mcg/mL are considered resistant to penicillin.

Clinical Outcome for ABS

Penicillin MICs of *S. pneumoniae* Isolates	Intent-To-Treat			Clinically Evaluable		
	n/N*	%	95% CI[†]	n/N*	%	95% CI[†]
All *S. pneumoniae*	222/240	92.5	—	210/215	97.7	—
MIC ≥2.0 mcg/mL[‡]	25/26	96.2	80.4, 99.9	22/23	95.7	78.1, 99.9
MIC = 2.0 mcg/mL	16/17	94.1	71.3, 99.9	13/14	92.9	66.1, 99.8
MIC ≥4.0 mcg/mL[§]	9/9	100	66.4, 100	9/9	100	66.4, 100
H. influenzae	177/203	87.2	—	160/170	94.1	—
M. catarrhalis	67/74	90.5	—	61/62	98.4	—

* n/N = patients with pathogen eradicated or presumed eradicated/total number of patients.
[†] Confidence limits calculated using exact probabilities.
[‡] *S. pneumoniae* strains with penicillin MICs of ≥2 mcg/mL are considered resistant to penicillin.
[§] Includes one patient each with *S. pneumoniae* penicillin MICs of 8 and 16 mcg/mL.

centrations compared to immediate-release Tablets. Thus, two AUGMENTIN 500-mg tablets are not equivalent to one AUGMENTIN XR tablet.

Scored AUGMENTIN XR Extended Release Tablets are available for greater convenience for adult patients who have difficulty swallowing. The scored tablet is not intended to reduce the dosage of medication taken; as stated in the table above, the recommended dose of AUGMENTIN XR is two tablets twice a day (q12h).

Renally Impaired Patients: The pharmacokinetics of AUGMENTIN XR have not been studied in patients with renal impairment. AUGMENTIN XR is contraindicated in severely impaired patients with a creatinine clearance of <30 mL/min. and in hemodialysis patients (see CONTRAINDICATIONS).

Hepatically Impaired Patients: Hepatically impaired patients should be dosed with caution and hepatic function monitored at regular intervals (see WARNINGS).

Pediatric Use: Safety and effectiveness in pediatric patients younger than 16 years have not been established.

Geriatric Use: No dosage adjustment is required for the elderly (see PRECAUTIONS).

HOW SUPPLIED

AUGMENTIN XR Extended Release Tablets: Each white, oval film-coated bilayer tablet, debossed with AUGMENTIN XR, contains amoxicillin trihydrate and amoxicillin sodium equivalent to a total of 1,000 mg of amoxicillin and clavulanate potassium equivalent to 62.5 mg of clavulanic acid.

NDC 0029-6096-48 Bottles of 28 (7 day XR pack)
NDC 0029-6096-60 Bottles of 40 (10 day XR pack)

STORAGE

Store tablets at or below 25°C (77°F). Dispense in original container.

CLINICAL STUDIES

Community-Acquired Pneumonia: Three randomized, controlled, double-blind clinical studies and one non-comparative study were conducted in adults with community-acquired pneumonia (CAP). In comparative studies, 582 patients received AUGMENTIN XR at a dose of 2,000 mg/125 mg orally every 12 hours for 7 or 10 days. In the non-comparative study to assess both clinical and bacteriological efficacy, 1,122 patients received AUGMENTIN XR 2,000 mg/125 mg orally every 12 hours for 7 days. In the 3 comparative studies, the combined clinical success rate at test of cure ranged from 86.3% to 94.7% in clinically evaluable patients who received AUGMENTIN XR; in the non-comparative study, the clinical success rate was 85.6%.

Data on the efficacy of AUGMENTIN XR in the treatment of community-acquired pneumonia due to *S. pneumoniae* with reduced susceptibility to penicillin were accrued from the 3 controlled clinical studies and the 1 non-comparative study. The majority of these cases were accrued from the non-comparative study.

[See first table above]

Acute Bacterial Sinusitis: Adults with a diagnosis of acute bacterial sinusitis (ABS) were evaluated in 3 clinical studies. In one study, 363 patients were randomized to receive either AUGMENTIN XR 2,000 mg/125 mg orally every 12 hours or levofloxacin 500 mg orally daily for 10 days in a double-blind, multicenter, prospective trial. These patients were clinically and radiologically evaluated at the test of cure (day 17-28) visit. The combined clinical and radiological responses were 83.7% for AUGMENTIN XR and 84.3% for levofloxacin at the test of cure visit in clinically evaluable patients (95% CI for the treatment difference = -9.4, 8.3). The clinical response rates at the test of cure were 87.0% and 88.6%, respectively.

The other 2 trials were non-comparative, multicenter studies designed to assess the bacteriological and clinical efficacy of AUGMENTIN XR (2,000 mg/125 mg orally q12h for 10 days) in the treatment of 1,554 patients with ABS. Evaluation timepoints were the same as in the prior study. Patients underwent maxillary sinus puncture for culture prior to receiving study medication. At test of cure, the clinical success rates were 87.5% and 87.1% (intention-to-treat) and 92.5% and 94.0% (per protocol populations).

Patients with acute bacterial sinusitis due to *S. pneumoniae* with reduced susceptibility to penicillin were accrued through enrollment in these 2 open-label non-comparative clinical trials. Microbiologic eradication rates for key pathogens in these studies are shown in the following table:

[See second table above]

Safety: In a randomized, double-blind, multicenter study, AUGMENTIN XR (2,000 mg/125 mg orally q12h, n = 255) was compared to AUGMENTIN (875 mg/125 mg orally q12h, n = 259), administered for 7 days for the treatment of community-acquired pneumonia. Adverse events, regardless of relationship to test drug, were reported by 49.4% of patients who received AUGMENTIN XR (versus 51.4% in comparator group). Treatment-related adverse events were reported in 25.1% of patients who received AUGMENTIN XR (versus 24.7% in comparator group); most were mild and transient in nature. Adverse events which led to withdrawal were reported by 2.4% of patients who received AUGMENTIN XR (versus 5.4% in comparator group). In each group, the most frequently reported adverse events were diarrhea (18.0% versus 14.3%, p = 0.28), nausea (4.3% versus 5.4%), and headache (4.3% versus 5.0%). Only one patient (0.4%) who received AUGMENTIN XR and 2 patients (0.8%) in the comparator group withdrew due to diarrhea. Serious adverse events considered suspected or probably related to test drug were reported in 0.8% of patients (versus 0.4% in comparator).

REFERENCES

1. National Committee for Clinical Laboratory Standards. Methods for Dilution Antimicrobial Susceptibility Tests for Bacteria that Grow Aerobically – Fifth Edition. Approved Standard NCCLS Document M7-A5, Vol. 20, No. 2. NCCLS, Wayne, PA, Jan. 2000.
2. National Committee for Clinical Laboratory Standards. Performance Standards for Antimicrobial Susceptibility Testing – Twelfth Informational Standard. M100-S12, Vol. 22, No. 1. NCCLS, Wayne, PA, Jan. 2002.
3. National Committee for Clinical Laboratory Standards. Performance Standards for Antimicrobial Disk Susceptibility Tests – Seventh Edition. Approved Standard NCCLS Document M2-A7, Vol. 20, No. 1. NCCLS, Wayne, PA, Jan. 2000.
4. Swanson-Biearman B, Dean BS, Lopez G, Krenzelok EP. The effects of penicillin and cephalosporin ingestions in children less than six years of age. *Vet Hum Toxicol.* 1988;30:66-67.

June 2004/AX:L6

Shown in Product Identification Guide, page 314

AVANDAMET® ℞

[ə-van' də-met]

(rosiglitazone maleate and metformin hydrochloride) Tablets

DESCRIPTION

AVANDAMET (rosiglitazone maleate and metformin HCl) tablets contain 2 oral antihyperglycemic drugs used in the management of type 2 diabetes: Rosiglitazone maleate and metformin hydrochloride. The combination of rosiglitazone maleate and metformin hydrochloride has been previously approved based on clinical trials in people with type 2 diabetes mellitus inadequately controlled on metformin alone. Additional efficacy and safety information about rosiglitazone and metformin monotherapies may be found in the prescribing information for each individual drug.

Rosiglitazone maleate is an oral antidiabetic agent, which acts primarily by increasing insulin sensitivity. Rosiglitazone improves glycemic control while reducing circulating insulin levels. Pharmacologic studies in animal models indicate that rosiglitazone improves sensitivity to insulin in muscle and adipose tissue and inhibits hepatic gluconeogenesis. Rosiglitazone maleate is not chemically or functionally related to the sulfonylureas, the biguanides, or the α-glucosidase inhibitors.

Chemically, rosiglitazone maleate is (±)-5-[[4-[2-(methyl-2-pyridinylamino)ethoxy]phenyl]methyl]-2,4-thiazolidinedione, (Z)-2-butenedioate (1:1) with a molecular weight of 473.52 (357.44 free base). The molecule has a single chiral center and is present as a racemate. Due to rapid interconversion, the enantiomers are functionally indistinguishable. The molecular formula is $C_{18}H_{19}N_3O_3S \bullet C_4H_4O_4$. Rosiglitazone maleate is a white to off-white solid with a melting point range of 122° to 123°C. The pK_a values of rosiglitazone maleate are 6.8 and 6.1. It is readily soluble in ethanol and a buffered aqueous solution with pH of 2.3; solubility decreases with increasing pH in the physiological range.

Metformin hydrochloride (N,N-dimethylimidodicarbonimidic diamide hydrochloride) is not chemically or pharmacologically related to any other classes of oral antihyperglycemic agents. Metformin hydrochloride is a white to off-white crystalline compound with a molecular formula of $C_4H_{11}N_5 \bullet HCl$ and a molecular weight of 165.63. Metformin hydrochloride is freely soluble in water and is practically insoluble in acetone, ether and chloroform. The pK_a of metformin is 12.4. The pH of a 1% aqueous solution of metformin hydrochloride is 6.68.

AVANDAMET is available for oral administration as tablets containing rosiglitazone maleate and metformin hydrochloride equivalent to: 1 mg rosiglitazone with 500 mg metformin hydrochloride (1 mg/500 mg), 2 mg rosiglitazone with 500 mg metformin hydrochloride (2 mg/500 mg), 4 mg rosiglitazone with 500 mg metformin hydrochloride (4 mg/500 mg), 2 mg rosiglitazone with 1,000 mg metformin hydrochloride (2 mg/1,000 mg), and 4 mg rosiglitazone with 1,000 mg metformin hydrochloride (4 mg/1,000 mg). In addition, each tablet contains the following inactive ingredients: Hypromellose 2910, lactose monohydrate, magnesium stearate, microcrystalline cellulose, polyethylene glycol 400, povidone 29-32, sodium starch glycolate, titanium dioxide, and 1 or more of the following: Red and yellow iron oxides.

CLINICAL PHARMACOLOGY

Mechanism of Action: AVANDAMET combines 2 antidiabetic agents with different mechanisms of action to improve glycemic control in patients with type 2 diabetes: Rosiglitazone maleate, a member of the thiazolidinedione class, and metformin hydrochloride, a member of the biguanide class. Thiazolidinediones are insulin sensitizing agents that act primarily by enhancing peripheral glucose utilization, whereas biguanides act primarily by decreasing endogenous hepatic glucose production.

Rosiglitazone, a member of the thiazolidinedione class of antidiabetic agents, improves glycemic control by improving insulin sensitivity while reducing circulating insulin levels. Rosiglitazone is a highly selective and potent agonist for the peroxisome proliferator–activated receptor-gamma (PPARγ). In humans, PPAR receptors are found in key target tissues for insulin action such as adipose tissue, skeletal muscle, and liver. Activation of PPARγ nuclear receptors regulates the transcription of insulin-responsive genes involved in the control of glucose production, transport, and utilization. In addition, PPARγ-responsive genes also participate in the regulation of fatty acid metabolism.

Insulin resistance is a common feature characterizing the pathogenesis of type 2 diabetes. The antidiabetic activity of rosiglitazone has been demonstrated in animal models of

Continued on next page

Product information on these pages is effective as of August 2004. Further information is available at: GlaxoSmithKline, PO Box 13398, Research Triangle Park, NC 27709. 1-888-825-5249. Corporate Web Site: www.gsk.com

Avandamet—Cont.

type 2 diabetes in which hyperglycemia and/or impaired glucose tolerance is a consequence of insulin resistance in target tissues. Rosiglitazone reduces blood glucose concentrations and reduces hyperinsulinemia in the ob/ob obese mouse, db/db diabetic mouse, and fa/fa fatty Zucker rat.

In animal models, rosiglitazone's antidiabetic activity was shown to be mediated by increased sensitivity to insulin's action in the liver, muscle, and adipose tissue. The expression of the insulin-regulated glucose transporter GLUT-4 was increased in adipose tissue. Rosiglitazone did not induce hypoglycemia in animal models of type 2 diabetes and/or impaired glucose tolerance.

Metformin hydrochloride is an antihyperglycemic agent, which improves glucose tolerance in patients with type 2 diabetes, lowering both basal and postprandial plasma glucose. Its pharmacologic mechanisms of action are different from other classes of oral antihyperglycemic agents. Metformin decreases hepatic glucose production, decreases intestinal absorption of glucose, and increases peripheral glucose uptake and utilization. Unlike sulfonylureas, metformin does not produce hypoglycemia in either patients with type 2 diabetes or normal subjects (except in special circumstances, see PRECAUTIONS) and does not cause hyperinsulinemia. With metformin therapy, insulin secretion remains unchanged while fasting insulin levels and day-long plasma insulin response may actually decrease.

Pharmacokinetics: ***Absorption and Bioavailability: AVANDAMET:*** In a bioequivalence and dose proportionality study of AVANDAMET 4 mg/500 mg, both the rosiglitazone component and the metformin component were bioequivalent to coadministered 4 mg rosiglitazone maleate tablet and 500 mg metformin hydrochloride tablet under fasted conditions (see Table 1). In this study, dose proportionality of rosiglitazone in the combination formulations of 1 mg/500 mg and 4 mg/500 mg was demonstrated.

[See table 1 below]

Administration of AVANDAMET 4 mg/500 mg with food resulted in no change in overall exposure (AUC) for either rosiglitazone or metformin. However, there were decreases in C_{max} of both components (22% for rosiglitazone and 15% for metformin, respectively) and a delay in T_{max} of both components (1.5 hours for rosiglitazone and 0.5 hours for metformin, respectively). These changes are not likely to be clinically significant. The pharmacokinetics of both the rosiglitazone component and the metformin component of AVANDAMET when taken with food were similar to the pharmacokinetics of rosiglitazone and metformin when administered concomitantly as separate tablets with food.

Rosiglitazone maleate: The absolute bioavailability of rosiglitazone is 99%. Peak plasma concentrations are observed about 1 hour after dosing. Maximum plasma concentration (C_{max}) and the area under the curve (AUC) of rosiglitazone increase in a dose-proportional manner over the therapeutic dose range. The elimination half-life is 3 to 4 hours and is independent of dose.

Metformin hydrochloride: The absolute bioavailability of a 500 mg metformin hydrochloride tablet given under fasting conditions is approximately 50% to 60%. Studies using single oral doses of metformin hydrochloride tablets of 500 mg and 1,500 mg, and 850 mg to 2,550 mg, indicate that there is a lack of dose proportionality with increasing doses, which is due to decreased absorption rather than an alteration in elimination.

Distribution: Rosiglitazone maleate: The mean (CV%) oral volume of distribution (V_{ss}/F) of rosiglitazone is approximately 17.6 (30%) liters, based on a population pharmacokinetic analysis. Rosiglitazone is approximately 99.8% bound to plasma proteins, primarily albumin.

Metformin hydrochloride: The apparent volume of distribution (V/F) of metformin following single oral doses of 850 mg metformin hydrochloride averaged 654 ± 358 L. Metformin is negligibly bound to plasma proteins. Metformin partitions into erythrocytes, most likely as a function of time. At usual clinical doses and dosing schedules of metformin, steady-state plasma concentrations of metformin are reached within 24 to 48 hours and are generally <1 mcg/mL. During controlled clinical trials, maximum metformin plasma levels did not exceed 5 mcg/mL, even at maximum doses.

Metabolism and Excretion: Rosiglitazone maleate: Rosiglitazone is extensively metabolized with no unchanged drug excreted in the urine. The major routes of metabolism were N-demethylation and hydroxylation, followed by conjugation with sulfate and glucuronic acid. All the circulating metabolites are considerably less potent than parent and, therefore, are not expected to contribute to the insulin-sensitizing activity of rosiglitazone. In vitro data demonstrate that rosiglitazone is predominantly metabolized by cytochrome P450 (CYP) isoenzyme 2C8, with CYP2C9 contributing as a minor pathway. Following oral or intravenous administration of [^{14}C]rosiglitazone maleate, approximately 64% and 23% of the dose was eliminated in the urine and in the feces, respectively. The plasma half-life of [^{14}C]related material ranged from 103 to 158 hours.

Metformin hydrochloride: Intravenous single-dose studies in normal subjects demonstrate that metformin is excreted unchanged in the urine and does not undergo hepatic metabolism (no metabolites have been identified in humans) nor biliary excretion. Renal clearance is approximately 3.5 times greater than creatinine clearance which indicates that tubular secretion is the major route of metformin elimination. Following oral administration, approximately 90% of the absorbed drug is eliminated via the renal route within the first 24 hours, with a plasma elimination half-life of approximately 6.2 hours. In blood, the elimination half-life is approximately 17.6 hours, suggesting that the erythrocyte mass may be a compartment of distribution.

Special Populations: ***Renal Impairment:*** In subjects with decreased renal function (based on measured creatinine clearance), the plasma and blood half-life of metformin is prolonged and the renal clearance is decreased in proportion to the decrease in creatinine clearance (see WARNINGS, also see GLUCOPHAGE® prescribing information, and CLINICAL PHARMACOLOGY, Pharmacokinetics). Since metformin is contraindicated in patients with renal impairment, administration of AVANDAMET is contraindicated in these patients.

Hepatic Impairment: Unbound oral clearance of rosiglitazone was significantly lower in patients with moderate to severe liver disease (Child-Pugh Class B/C) compared to healthy subjects. As a result, unbound C_{max} and AUC_{0-inf} were increased 2- and 3-fold, respectively. Elimination half-life for rosiglitazone was about 2 hours longer in patients with liver disease, compared to healthy subjects. Therapy with AVANDAMET should not be initiated if the patient exhibits clinical evidence of active liver disease or increased serum transaminase levels (ALT >2.5X upper limit of normal) at baseline (see PRECAUTIONS, Hepatic Effects).

No pharmacokinetic studies of metformin have been conducted in subjects with hepatic insufficiency.

Geriatrics: Results of the population pharmacokinetics analysis (n = 716 <65 years; n = 331 ≥65 years) showed that age does not significantly affect the pharmacokinetics of rosiglitazone. However, limited data from controlled pharmacokinetic studies of metformin hydrochloride in healthy elderly subjects suggest that total plasma clearance of metformin is decreased, the half-life is prolonged, and C_{max} is increased, compared to healthy young subjects. From these data, it appears that the change in metformin pharmacokinetics with aging is primarily accounted for by a change in renal function (see GLUCOPHAGE prescribing information and CLINICAL PHARMACOLOGY, Pharmacokinetics). Metformin treatment and therefore treatment with AVANDAMET should not be initiated in patients ≥80 years of age unless measurement of creatinine clearance demonstrates that renal function is not reduced (see WARNINGS and DOSAGE AND ADMINISTRATION).

Gender: Results of the population pharmacokinetics analysis showed that the mean oral clearance of rosiglitazone in female patients (n = 405) was approximately 6% lower compared to male patients of the same body weight (n = 642). In rosiglitazone and metformin combination studies, efficacy was demonstrated with no gender differences in glycemic response.

Metformin pharmacokinetic parameters did not differ significantly between normal subjects and patients with type 2 diabetes when analyzed according to gender (males = 19, females = 16). Similarly, in controlled clinical studies in patients with type 2 diabetes, the antihyperglycemic effect of metformin hydrochloride tablets was comparable in males and females.

Race: Results of a population pharmacokinetic analysis including subjects of white, black, and other ethnic origins indicate that race has no influence on the pharmacokinetics of rosiglitazone.

No studies of metformin pharmacokinetic parameters according to race have been performed. In controlled clinical studies of metformin hydrochloride in patients with type 2 diabetes, the antihyperglycemic effect was comparable in whites (n = 249), blacks (n = 51), and Hispanics (n = 24).

Pediatrics: No pharmacokinetic data from studies in pediatric subjects are available for either rosiglitazone or metformin.

Table 1. Mean (SD) Pharmacokinetic Parameters for Rosiglitazone and Metformin

		Pharmacokinetic Parameter			
Regimen	**N**	**AUC_{0-inf} (ng.h/mL)**	**C_{max} (ng/mL)**	**T_{max}* (h)**	**$T_{1/2}$ (h)**
Rosiglitazone					
A	25	1,442 (324)	242 (70)	0.95 (0.48-2.47)	4.26 (1.18)
B	25	1,398 (340)	254 (69)	0.57 (0.43-2.58)	3.95 (0.81)
C	24	349 (91)	63.0 (15.0)	0.57 (0.47-1.45)	3.87 (0.88)
Metformin					
A	25	7,116 (2,096)	1,106 (329)	2.97 (1.02-4.02)	3.46 (0.96)
B	25	7,413 (1,838)	1,135 (253)	2.50 (1.03-3.98)	3.36 (0.54)
C	24	6,945 (2,045)	1,080 (327)	2.97 (1.00-5.98)	3.35 (0.59)

*Median and range presented for T_{max}

Regimen Key: Regimen A = 4 mg/500 mg AVANDAMET
Regimen B = 4 mg rosiglitazone maleate tablet + 500 mg metformin hydrochloride tablet
Regimen C = 1 mg/500 mg AVANDAMET

CLINICAL STUDIES

There have been no clinical efficacy trials conducted with AVANDAMET tablets. However, studies utilizing the separate components have established the effective and safe use, and the additive benefit of the combination has been shown in patients with diabetes mellitus inadequately controlled with fasting plasma glucose between 140 and 300 mg/dL despite maximal metformin therapy alone (2,500 mg/day). Bioequivalence of AVANDAMET with coadministered rosiglitazone maleate tablets and metformin hydrochloride tablets was demonstrated (see CLINICAL PHARMACOLOGY, Pharmacokinetics).

The addition of rosiglitazone to metformin resulted in significant improvements in glucose concentrations compared to either of these agents alone. These results are consistent with an additive effect on glycemic control when rosiglitazone is used in combination with metformin. No clinical trials have been conducted with combination rosiglitazone and metformin therapy as initial therapy in patients with type 2 diabetes mellitus. No controlled clinical trials have been conducted in which metformin was added to patients inadequately controlled with rosiglitazone alone. The pattern of LDL and HDL changes following therapy with rosiglitazone in combination with metformin was generally similar to those seen with rosiglitazone in monotherapy.

Clinical Trials of Rosiglitazone Add-on Therapy in Patients Not Adequately Controlled on Metformin Alone: A total of 670 patients with type 2 diabetes participated in two 26-week, randomized, double-blind, placebo/active-controlled studies designed to assess the efficacy of rosiglitazone in combination with metformin. Rosiglitazone maleate, administered in either once-daily or twice-daily dosing regimens, was added to the therapy of patients who were inadequately controlled on 2.5 grams/day of metformin hydrochloride.

In one study, patients inadequately controlled on 2.5 grams/day of metformin hydrochloride (mean baseline FPG 216 mg/dL and mean baseline HbA1c 8.8%) were randomized to receive rosiglitazone 4 mg once daily, rosiglitazone 8 mg once daily, or placebo in addition to metformin. A statistically significant improvement in FPG and HbA1c was observed in patients treated with the combinations of metformin and rosiglitazone 4 mg once daily and rosiglitazone 8 mg once daily, versus patients continued on metformin alone (see Table 2).

[See table 2 at top of next page]

In a second 26-week study, patients with type 2 diabetes inadequately controlled on 2.5 grams/day of metformin hydrochloride who were randomized to receive the combination of rosiglitazone 4 mg twice daily and metformin (N = 105) showed a statistically significant improvement in glycemic control with a mean treatment effect for FPG of −56 mg/dL and a mean treatment effect for HbA1c of −0.8% over metformin alone. The combination of metformin and rosiglitazone resulted in lower levels of FPG and HbA1c than either agent alone.

INDICATIONS AND USAGE

AVANDAMET is indicated as an adjunct to diet and exercise to improve glycemic control in patients with type 2 diabetes mellitus who are already treated with combination rosiglitazone and metformin or who are not adequately controlled on metformin alone.

Management of type 2 diabetes mellitus should include diet control. Caloric restriction, weight loss, and exercise are essential for the proper treatment of the diabetic patient because they help improve insulin sensitivity. This is important not only in the primary treatment of type 2 diabetes but also in maintaining the efficacy of drug therapy. Prior to initiation or escalation of oral antidiabetic therapy in patients with type 2 diabetes mellitus, secondary causes of poor glycemic control, e.g., infection, should be investigated and treated.

The safety and efficacy of AVANDAMET as initial pharmacologic therapy for patients with type 2 diabetes mellitus after a trial of caloric restriction, weight loss, and exercise has not been established.

CONTRAINDICATIONS

AVANDAMET tablets are contraindicated in patients with:

1. Renal disease or renal dysfunction (e.g., as suggested by serum creatinine levels ≥1.5 mg/dL [males], ≥1.4 mg/dL [females], or abnormal creatinine clearance), which may also result from conditions such as cardiovascular collapse (shock), acute myocardial infarction, and septicemia (see WARNINGS and PRECAUTIONS).
2. Congestive heart failure requiring pharmacologic treatment.
3. Known hypersensitivity to rosiglitazone maleate or metformin hydrochloride.
4. Acute or chronic metabolic acidosis, including diabetic ketoacidosis, with or without coma. Diabetic ketoacidosis should be treated with insulin.

AVANDAMET should be temporarily discontinued in patients undergoing radiologic studies involving intravascular administration of iodinated contrast materials, because use of such products may result in acute alteration of renal function (see also PRECAUTIONS).

WARNINGS

Metformin hydrochloride

Lactic Acidosis

Lactic acidosis is a rare, but serious, metabolic complication that can occur due to metformin accumulation during treatment with AVANDAMET; when it occurs, it is fatal in approximately 50% of cases. Lactic acidosis may also occur in association with a number of pathophysiologic conditions, including diabetes mellitus, and whenever there is significant tissue hypoperfusion and hypoxemia. Lactic acidosis is characterized by elevated blood lactate levels (>5 mmol/L), decreased blood pH, electrolyte disturbances with an increased anion gap, and an increased lactate/pyruvate ratio. When metformin is implicated as the cause of lactic acidosis, metformin plasma levels >5 mcg/mL are generally found.

The reported incidence of lactic acidosis in patients receiving metformin hydrochloride is very low (approximately 0.03 cases/1,000 patient years of exposure, with approximately 0.015 fatal cases/1,000 patient years of exposure). Reported cases have occurred primarily in diabetic patients with significant renal insufficiency, including both intrinsic renal disease and renal hypoperfusion, often in the setting of multiple concomitant medical/surgical problems and multiple concomitant medications. Patients with congestive heart failure requiring pharmacologic management, in particular those with unstable or acute congestive heart failure who are at risk of hypoperfusion and hypoxemia, are at increased risk of lactic acidosis. The risk of lactic acidosis increases with the degree of renal dysfunction and the patient's age. The risk of lactic acidosis may, therefore, be significantly decreased by regular monitoring of renal function in patients taking AVANDAMET and by use of the minimum effective dose of AVANDAMET. In particular, treatment of the elderly should be accompanied by careful monitoring of renal function. Treatment with AVANDAMET should not be initiated in patients ≥80 years of age unless measurement of creatinine clearance demonstrates that renal function is not reduced, as these patients are more susceptible to developing lactic acidosis. In addition, AVANDAMET should be promptly withheld in the presence of any condition associated with hypoxemia, dehydration, or sepsis. Because impaired hepatic function may significantly limit the ability to clear lactate, AVANDAMET should generally be avoided in patients with clinical or laboratory evidence of hepatic disease. Patients should be cautioned against excessive alcohol intake, either acute or chronic, when taking AVANDAMET, since alcohol potentiates the effects of metformin hydrochloride on lactate metabolism. In addition, AVANDAMET should be temporarily discontinued prior to any intravascular radiocontrast study and for any surgical procedure (see also PRECAUTIONS).

The onset of lactic acidosis often is subtle, and accompanied only by nonspecific symptoms such as malaise, myalgias, respiratory distress, increasing somnolence, and nonspecific abdominal distress. There may be associated hypothermia, hypotension, and resistant bradyarrhythmias with more marked acidosis. The patient and the patient's physician must be aware of the possible importance of such symptoms and the patient should be instructed to notify the physician immediately if they occur (see also PRECAUTIONS). AVANDAMET should be withdrawn until the situation is clarified. Serum electrolytes, ketones, blood glucose and, if indicated, blood pH, lactate levels, and even blood metformin levels may be useful. Once a patient is stabilized on any dose level of AVANDAMET, gastrointestinal symptoms, which are common during initiation of therapy, are unlikely to be drug related. Later occurrence of gastrointestinal symptoms could be due to lactic acidosis or other serious disease.

Levels of fasting venous plasma lactate above the upper limit of normal but less than 5 mmol/L in patients taking AVANDAMET do not necessarily indicate impending lactic acidosis and may be explainable by other mechanisms, such as poorly controlled diabetes or obesity, vigorous physical activity or technical problems in sample handling (see also PRECAUTIONS).

Lactic acidosis should be suspected in any diabetic patient with metabolic acidosis lacking evidence of ketoacidosis (ketonuria and ketonemia).

Lactic acidosis is a medical emergency that must be treated in a hospital setting. In a patient with lactic acidosis who is taking AVANDAMET, the drug should be discontinued immediately and general supportive measures promptly instituted. Because metformin hydrochloride is dialyzable (with a clearance of up to 170 mL/min under good hemodynamic conditions), prompt hemodialysis is recommended to correct the acidosis and remove the accumulated metformin. Such management often results in prompt reversal of symptoms and recovery (see also CONTRAINDICATIONS and PRECAUTIONS).

Table 2. Glycemic Parameters in a 26-Week Rosiglitazone maleate + Metformin hydrochloride Combination Study

	Metformin	Rosiglitazone 4 mg once daily + metformin	Rosiglitazone 8 mg once daily + metformin
N	113	116	110
FPG (mg/dL)			
Baseline (mean)	214	215	220
Change from baseline (mean)	6	-33	-48
Difference from metformin alone (adjusted mean)		-40*	-53*
Responders (≥30 mg/dL decrease from baseline)	20%	45%	61%
HbA1c (%)			
Baseline (mean)	8.6	8.9	8.9
Change from baseline (mean)	0.5	-0.6	-0.8
Difference from metformin alone (adjusted mean)		-1.0*	-1.2*
Responders (≥0.7% decrease from baseline)	11%	45%	52%

*p<0.0001 compared to metformin.

Rosiglitazone maleate

Cardiac Failure and Other Cardiac Effects: Rosiglitazone, like other thiazolidinediones, alone or in combination with other antidiabetic agents, can cause fluid retention, which may exacerbate or lead to heart failure. Patients should be observed for signs and symptoms of heart failure. AVANDAMET should be discontinued if any deterioration in cardiac status occurs.

Patients with New York Heart Association (NYHA) Class 3 and 4 cardiac status were not studied during the clinical trials with rosiglitazone maleate. In patients requiring pharmacologic treatment for congestive heart failure, AVANDAMET should not be used (see CONTRAINDICATIONS).

In combination with insulin, thiazolidinediones may increase the risk of other cardiovascular adverse events. In three 26-week trials in patients with type 2 diabetes, 216 received 4 mg of rosiglitazone plus insulin, 322 received 8 mg of rosiglitazone plus insulin, and 388 received insulin alone. These trials included patients with long-standing diabetes and a high prevalence of pre-existing medical conditions, including peripheral neuropathy, retinopathy, ischemic heart disease, vascular disease, and congestive heart failure. In these clinical studies, an increased incidence of edema, cardiac failure, and other cardiovascular adverse events was seen in patients on rosiglitazone and insulin combination therapy compared to insulin and placebo. Patients who experienced cardiovoascular events were on average older and had a longer duration of diabetes. These cardiovascular events were noted at both the 4 mg and 8 mg daily doses of rosiglitazone. In this population, however, it was not possible to determine specific risk factors that could be used to identify all patients at risk of heart failure and other cardiovascular events on combination therapy. Three of 10 patients who developed cardiac failure on combination therapy during the double-blind part of the fixed-dose studies had no known prior evidence of congestive heart failure, or pre-existing cardiac condition.

In a double-blind study in type 2 diabetes patients with chronic renal failure (112 received 4 mg or 8 mg of rosiglitazone plus insulin and 108 received insulin alone), there was no difference in cardiovascular adverse events with rosiglitazone in combination with insulin compared to insulin alone.

Patients treated with combination AVANDAMET and insulin should be monitored for cardiovascular adverse events. The combination therapy should be discontinued in patients who do not respond as manifested by a reduction in HbA1c or insulin dose after 4 to 5 months of therapy or who develop any significant adverse events (See ADVERSE REACTIONS.)

There are no studies that have evaluated the safety or effectiveness of AVANDAMET in combination with insulin. The use of AVANDAMET in combination with insulin is not indicated.

PRECAUTIONS

General: ***Metformin hydrochloride:*** **Monitoring of renal function:** Metformin is known to be substantially excreted by the kidney, and the risk of metformin accumulation and lactic acidosis increases with the degree of impairment of renal function. Thus, patients with serum creatinine levels above the upper limit of normal for their age should not receive AVANDAMET. In patients with advanced age, AVANDAMET should be carefully titrated to establish the minimum dose for adequate glycemic effect, because aging is associated with reduced renal function. In elderly patients, particularly those ≥80 years of age, renal function should be monitored regularly and, generally, AVANDAMET should not be titrated to the maximum dose of the metformin component, i.e., 2,000 mg (see WARNINGS and DOSAGE AND ADMINISTRATION).

Before initiation of therapy with AVANDAMET and at least annually thereafter, renal function should be assessed and verified as normal. In patients in whom development of renal dysfunction is anticipated, renal function should be assessed more frequently and AVANDAMET discontinued if evidence of renal impairment is present.

Use of concomitant medications that may affect renal function or metformin disposition: Concomitant medication(s) that may affect renal function or result in significant hemodynamic change or may interfere with the disposition of metformin, such as cationic drugs that are eliminated by renal tubular secretion (see PRECAUTIONS, Drug Interactions), should be used with caution.

Radiologic studies involving the use of intravascular iodinated contrast materials (for example, intravenous urogram, intravenous cholangiography, angiography, and computed tomography (CT) scans with contrast materials): Intravascular contrast studies with iodinated materials can lead to acute alteration of renal function and have been associated with lactic acidosis in patients receiving metformin (see CONTRAINDICATIONS). Therefore, in patients in whom any such study is planned, AVANDAMET should be temporarily discontinued at the time of or prior to the procedure, and withheld for 48 hours subsequent to the procedure and reinstituted only after renal function has been re-evaluated and found to be normal.

Hypoxic states: Cardiovascular collapse (shock) from whatever cause, acute congestive heart failure, acute myocardial infarction, and other conditions characterized by hypoxemia have been associated with lactic acidosis and may also cause prerenal azotemia. When such events occur in patients receiving AVANDAMET, the drug should be promptly discontinued.

Surgical procedures: Use of AVANDAMET should be temporarily suspended for any surgical procedure (except minor procedures not associated with restricted intake of food and fluids) and should not be restarted until the patient's oral intake has resumed and renal function has been evaluated as normal.

Alcohol intake: Alcohol is known to potentiate the effect of metformin on lactate metabolism. Patients, therefore, should be warned against excessive alcohol intake, acute or chronic, while receiving AVANDAMET.

Impaired hepatic function: Since impaired hepatic function has been associated with some cases of lactic acidosis, AVANDAMET should generally be avoided in patients with clinical or laboratory evidence of hepatic disease.

Vitamin B_{12} levels: In controlled clinical trials of metformin hydrochloride of 29 weeks' duration, a decrease to subnormal levels of previously normal serum vitamin B_{12} levels, without clinical manifestations, was observed in approximately 7% of patients. Such a decrease, possibly due to interference with B_{12} absorption from the B_{12}-intrinsic factor complex, is, however, very rarely associated with anemia and appears to be rapidly reversible with discontinuation of metformin or vitamin B_{12} supplementation. Measurement of hematologic parameters on an annual basis is advised in patients on AVANDAMET and any apparent abnormalities

Continued on next page

Product information on these pages is effective as of August 2004. Further information is available at: GlaxoSmithKline, PO Box 13398, Research Triangle Park, NC 27709. 1-888-825-5249. Corporate Web Site: www.gsk.com

Avandamet—Cont.

should be appropriately investigated and managed (see PRECAUTIONS, Laboratory Tests). Certain individuals (those with inadequate vitamin B_{12} or calcium intake or absorption) appear to be predisposed to developing subnormal vitamin B_{12} levels. In these patients, routine serum vitamin B_{12} measurements at 2- to 3-year intervals may be useful.

Change in clinical status of previously controlled diabetic: A patient with type 2 diabetes previously well-controlled on AVANDAMET who develops laboratory abnormalities or clinical illness (especially vague and poorly defined illness) should be evaluated promptly for evidence of ketoacidosis or lactic acidosis. Evaluation should include serum electrolytes and ketones, blood glucose and, if indicated, blood pH, lactate, pyruvate, and metformin levels. If acidosis of either form occurs, AVANDAMET must be stopped immediately and other appropriate corrective measures initiated (see also WARNINGS).

Hypoglycemia: Hypoglycemia does not occur in patients receiving metformin hydrochloride alone under usual circumstances of use but could occur when caloric intake is deficient, when strenuous exercise is not compensated by caloric supplementation, or during concomitant use with hypoglycemic agents (such as sulfonylureas or insulin) or ethanol. Elderly, debilitated or malnourished patients, and those with adrenal or pituitary insufficiency or alcohol intoxication are particularly susceptible to hypoglycemic effects. Hypoglycemia may be difficult to recognize in the elderly and in people who are taking β-adrenergic blocking drugs.

Loss of control of blood glucose: When a patient stabilized on any diabetic regimen is exposed to stress such as fever, trauma, infection, or surgery, a temporary loss of glycemic control may occur. At such times, it may be necessary to withhold AVANDAMET and temporarily administer insulin. AVANDAMET may be reinstituted after the acute episode is resolved.

***Rosiglitazone maleate:* General:** Due to its mechanism of action, rosiglitazone is active only in the presence of endogenous insulin. Therefore, AVANDAMET should not be used in patients with type 1 diabetes.

Edema: AVANDAMET should be used with caution in patients with edema. In a clinical study in healthy volunteers who received rosiglitazone 8 mg once daily for 8 weeks, there was a statistically significant increase in median plasma volume compared to placebo. Since thiazolidinediones, including rosiglitazone, can cause fluid retention, which can exacerbate or lead to congestive heart failure, AVANDAMET should be used with caution in patients at risk for heart failure. Patients should be monitored for signs and symptoms of heart failure (see WARNINGS, Cardiac Failure and Other Cardiac Effects and PRECAUTIONS, Information for Patients).

In controlled clinical trials of patients with type 2 diabetes, mild to moderate edema was reported in patients treated with rosiglitazone maleate, and may be dose related. Patients with ongoing edema are more likely to have adverse events associated with edema if started on combination therapy with insulin and rosiglitazone (see ADVERSE REACTIONS).

Weight gain: Dose-related weight gain was seen with rosiglitazone alone or in combination with other hypoglycemic agents (see Table 3). The mechanism of weight gain is unclear but probably involves a combination of fluid retention and fat accumulation.

In postmarketing experience with rosiglitazone alone or in combination with other hypoglycemic agents, there have been rare reports of unusually rapid increases in weight and increases in excess of that generally observed in clinical trials. Patients who experience such increases should be assessed for fluid accumulation and volume-related events such as excessive edema and congestive heart failure.

[See table 3 below]

Hematologic: Across all controlled clinical studies, decreases in hemoglobin and hematocrit (mean decreases in individual studies ≤1.0 gram/dL and ≤3.3%, respectively) were observed for rosiglitazone maleate alone and in combination with other hypoglycemic agents. The changes occurred primarily during the first 3 months following initiation of rosiglitazone therapy or following an increase in rosiglitazone dose. White blood cell counts also decreased slightly in patients treated with rosiglitazone. The observed changes may be related to the increased plasma volume observed with treatment with rosiglitazone and may be dose related (see ADVERSE REACTIONS, Laboratory Abnormalities).

Ovulation: Therapy with rosiglitazone, like other thiazolidinediones, may result in ovulation in some premenopausal anovulatory women. As a result, these patients may be at an increased risk for pregnancy while taking AVANDAMET (see PRECAUTIONS, Pregnancy, Pregnancy Category C). Thus, adequate contraception in premenopausal women should be recommended. This possible effect has not been specifically investigated in clinical studies so the frequency of this occurrence is not known.

Although hormonal imbalance has been seen in preclinical studies (see PRECAUTIONS, Carcinogenesis, Mutagenesis, Impairment of Fertility), the clinical significance of this finding is not known. If unexpected menstrual dysfunction occurs, the benefits of continued therapy with AVANDAMET should be reviewed.

Hepatic Effects: Another drug of the thiazolidinedione class, troglitazone, was associated with idiosyncratic hepatotoxicity, and very rare cases of liver failure, liver transplants, and death were reported during clinical use. In pre-approval controlled clinical trials in patients with type 2 diabetes, troglitazone was more frequently associated with clinically significant elevations in liver enzymes (ALT >3X upper limit of normal) compared to placebo. Very rare cases of reversible jaundice were also reported.

In pre-approval clinical studies in 4,598 patients treated with rosiglitazone maleate, encompassing approximately 3,600 patient years of exposure, there was no signal of drug-induced hepatotoxicity or elevation of ALT levels. In the pre-approval controlled trials, 0.2% of patients treated with rosiglitazone had elevations in ALT >3X the upper limit of normal compared to 0.2% on placebo and 0.5% on active comparators. The ALT elevations in patients treated with rosiglitazone were reversible and were not clearly causally related to therapy with rosiglitazone.

In postmarketing experience with rosiglitazone maleate, reports of hepatitis and of hepatic enzyme elevations to 3 or more times the upper limit of normal have been received. Very rarely, these reports have involved hepatic failure with and without fatal outcome, although causality has not been established. Rosiglitazone is structurally related to troglitazone, a thiazolidinedione no longer marketed in the United States, which was associated with idiosyncratic hepatotoxicity and rare cases of liver failure, liver transplants, and death during clinical use. Pending the availability of the results of additional large, long-term controlled clinical trials and additional postmarketing safety data, it is recommended that patients treated with AVANDAMET undergo periodic monitoring of liver enzymes.

Liver enzymes should be checked prior to the initiation of therapy with AVANDAMET in all patients and periodically thereafter per the clinical judgement of the healthcare professional. Therapy with AVANDAMET should not be initiated in patients with increased baseline liver enzyme levels (ALT >2.5X upper limit of normal). Patients with mildly elevated liver enzymes (ALT levels ≤2.5X upper limit of normal) at baseline or during therapy with AVANDAMET should be evaluated to determine the cause of the liver enzyme elevation. Initiation of, or continuation of, therapy with AVANDAMET in patients with mild liver enzyme elevations should proceed with caution and include close clinical follow-up, including more frequent liver enzyme monitoring, to determine if the liver enzyme elevations resolve or worsen. If at any time ALT levels increase to >3X the upper limit of normal in patients on therapy with AVANDAMET, liver enzyme levels should be rechecked as soon as possible. If ALT levels remain >3X the upper limit of normal, therapy with AVANDAMET should be discontinued.

If any patient develops symptoms suggesting hepatic dysfunction, which may include unexplained nausea, vomiting, abdominal pain, fatigue, anorexia, and/or dark urine, liver enzymes should be checked. If jaundice is observed, drug therapy should be discontinued.

In addition, if the presence of hepatic disease or hepatic dysfunction of sufficient magnitude to predispose to lactic acidosis is confirmed, therapy with AVANDAMET should be discontinued.

Table 3. Weight Changes (kg) From Baseline During Clinical Trials With Rosiglitazone maleate

		Control Group		Rosiglitazone 4 mg	Rosiglitazone 8 mg
Monotherapy	**Duration**		**Median (25th, 75th percentile)**	**Median (25th, 75th percentile)**	**Median (25th, 75th percentile)**
	26 weeks	placebo	−0.9 (−2.8, 0.9)	1.0 (−0.9, 3.6)	3.1 (1.1, 5.8)
	52 weeks	sulfonylurea	2.0 (0, 4.0)	2.0 (−0.6, 4.0)	2.6 (0, 5.3)
Combination therapy					
sulfonylurea	26 weeks	sulfonylurea	0 (−1.3, 1.2)	1.8 (0, 3.1)	–
metformin	26 weeks	metformin	−1.4 (−3.2, 0.2)	0.8 (−1.0, 2.6)	2.1 (0, 4.3)
insulin	26 weeks	insulin	0.9 (−0.5, 2.7)	4.1 (1.4, 6.3)	5.4 (3.4, 7.3)

There are no data available from clinical trials to evaluate the safety of AVANDAMET in patients who experienced liver abnormalities, hepatic dysfunction, or jaundice while on troglitazone. AVANDAMET should not be used in patients who experienced jaundice while taking troglitazone.

Laboratory Tests: Periodic fasting blood glucose and HbA1c measurements should be performed to monitor therapeutic response.

Liver enzyme monitoring is recommended prior to initiation of therapy with AVANDAMET in all patients and periodically thereafter (see PRECAUTIONS, Hepatic Effects and ADVERSE REACTIONS, Laboratory Abnormalities, *Serum Transaminase Levels*).

Initial and periodic monitoring of hematologic parameters (e.g., hemoglobin/hematocrit and red blood cell indices) and renal function (serum creatinine) should be performed, at least on an annual basis. While megaloblastic anemia has rarely been seen with metformin therapy, if this is suspected, vitamin B_{12} deficiency should be excluded.

Information for Patients: Patients should be informed of the potential risks and advantages of AVANDAMET and of alternative modes of therapy. They should also be informed about the importance of adherence to dietary instructions, weight loss, and a regular exercise program because these methods help improve insulin sensitivity. The importance of regular testing of blood glucose, glycosylated hemoglobin (HbA1c), renal function, and hematologic parameters should be emphasized. Patients should be advised that AVANDAMET can begin to take effect 1 to 2 weeks after initiation, however it can take 2 to 3 months to see the full effect of glycemic improvement.

The risks of lactic acidosis, its symptoms, and conditions that predispose to its development, as noted in the WARNINGS and PRECAUTIONS sections, should be explained to patients. Patients should be advised to discontinue AVANDAMET immediately and to promptly notify their health practitioner if unexplained hyperventilation, myalgia, malaise, unusual somnolence, or other nonspecific symptoms occur. Once a patient is stabilized on any dose level of AVANDAMET, gastrointestinal symptoms, which are common during initiation of metformin therapy, are unlikely to be drug related. Later occurrence of gastrointestinal symptoms could be due to lactic acidosis or other serious disease.

Patients should be counselled against excessive alcohol intake, either acute or chronic, while receiving AVANDAMET.

Patients should be informed that blood will be drawn to check their liver function prior to the start of therapy and periodically thereafter per the clinical judgement of the healthcare professional. Patients with unexplained symptoms of nausea, vomiting, abdominal pain, fatigue, anorexia, or dark urine should immediately report these symptoms to their physician.

Patients who experience an unusually rapid increase in weight or edema or who develop shortness of breath or other symptoms of heart failure while on AVANDAMET should immediately report these symptoms to their physician.

Therapy with AVANDAMET, like other thiazolidinediones, may result in ovulation in some premenopausal anovulatory women. As a result, these patients may be at an increased risk for pregnancy while taking AVANDAMET (see PRECAUTIONS, Pregnancy, Pregnancy Category C). Thus, adequate contraception in premenopausal women should be recommended. This possible effect has not been specifically investigated in clinical studies so the frequency of this occurrence is not known.

Drug Interactions: ***Rosiglitazone maleate:*** Drugs Metabolized by Cytochrome P450: In vitro drug metabolism studies suggest that rosiglitazone does not inhibit any of the major P450 enzymes at clinically relevant concentrations. In vitro data demonstrate that rosiglitazone is predominantly metabolized by CYP2C8, and to a lesser extent, 2C9. An inhibitor of CYP2C8 (such as gemfibrozil) may decrease the metabolism of rosiglitazone and an inducer of CYP2C8 (such as rifampin) may increase the metabolism of rosiglitazone. Therefore, if an inhibitor or an inducer of CYP2C8 is started or stopped during treatment with rosiglitazone, changes in diabetes treatment may be needed based upon clinical response.

Rosiglitazone (4 mg twice daily) was shown to have no clinically relevant effect on the pharmacokinetics of nifedipine and oral contraceptives (ethinyl estradiol and norethindrone), which are predominantly metabolized by CYP3A4.

Concomitant administration of gemfibrozil (600 mg twice daily), an inhibitor of CYP2C8, and rosiglitazone (4 mg once daily) for 7 days increased rosiglitazone AUC by 2 fold, compared to the administration of rosiglitazone (4 mg once daily) alone. Given the potential for dose-related adverse events with rosiglitazone, a decrease in the dose of rosiglitazone may be needed when gemfibrozil is introduced.

Metformin hydrochloride: Furosemide: A single-dose, metformin-furosemide drug interaction study in healthy subjects demonstrated that pharmacokinetic parameters of both compounds were affected by coadministration. Furosemide increased the metformin plasma and blood C_{max} by 22% and blood AUC by 15%, without any significant change in metformin renal clearance. When administered with metformin, the C_{max} and AUC of furosemide were 31% and 12% smaller, respectively, than when administered alone, and the terminal half-life was decreased by 32%, without any significant change in furosemide renal clearance. No information is available about the interaction of metformin and furosemide when coadministered chronically.

Nifedipine: A single-dose, metformin-nifedipine drug interaction study in normal healthy volunteers demonstrated that coadministration of nifedipine increased plasma metformin C_{max} and AUC by 20% and 9%, respectively, and increased the amount excreted in the urine. T_{max} and half-life were unaffected. Nifedipine appears to enhance the absorption of metformin. Metformin had minimal effects on nifedipine.

Cationic Drugs: Cationic drugs (e.g., amiloride, digoxin, morphine, procainamide, quinidine, quinine, ranitidine, triamterene, trimethoprim, and vancomycin) that are eliminated by renal tubular secretion theoretically have the potential for interaction with metformin by competing for common renal tubular transport systems. Such interaction between metformin and oral cimetidine has been observed in normal healthy volunteers in both single- and multiple-dose, metformin-cimetidine drug interaction studies, with a 60% increase in peak metformin plasma and whole blood concentrations and a 40% increase in plasma and whole blood metformin AUC. There was no change in elimination half-life in the single-dose study. Metformin had no effect on cimetidine pharmacokinetics. Although such interactions remain theoretical (except for cimetidine), careful patient monitoring and dose adjustment of AVANDAMET and/or the interfering drug is recommended in patients who are taking cationic medications that are excreted via the proximal renal tubular secretory system.

Other: Certain drugs tend to produce hyperglycemia and may lead to loss of glycemic control. These drugs include thiazides and other diuretics, corticosteroids, phenothiazines, thyroid products, estrogens, oral contraceptives, phenytoin, nicotinic acid, sympathomimetics, calcium channel blocking drugs, and isoniazid. When such drugs are administered to a patient receiving AVANDAMET, the patient should be closely observed to maintain adequate glycemic control.

In healthy volunteers, the pharmacokinetics of metformin and propranolol and metformin and ibuprofen were not affected when coadministered in single-dose interaction studies.

Metformin is negligibly bound to plasma proteins and is therefore, less likely to interact with highly protein-bound drugs such as salicylates, sulfonamides, chloramphenicol, and probenecid.

Carcinogenesis, Mutagenesis, Impairment of Fertility: No animal studies have been conducted with the combined products in AVANDAMET. The following data are based on findings in studies performed with rosiglitazone or metformin individually.

Rosiglitazone maleate: A 2-year carcinogenicity study was conducted in Charles River CD-1 mice at doses of 0.4, 1.5, and 6 mg/kg/day in the diet (highest dose equivalent to approximately 12 times human AUC at the maximum recommended human daily dose of the rosiglitazone component of AVANDAMET). Sprague-Dawley rats were dosed for 2 years by oral gavage at doses of 0.05, 0.3, and 2 mg/kg/day (highest dose equivalent to approximately 10 and 20 times human AUC at the maximum recommended human daily dose of the rosiglitazone component of AVANDAMET for male and female rats, respectively).

Rosiglitazone was not carcinogenic in the mouse. There was an increase in incidence of adipose hyperplasia in the mouse at doses ≥1.5 mg/kg/day (approximately 2 times human AUC at the maximum recommended human daily dose of the rosiglitazone component of AVANDAMET). In rats, there was a significant increase in the incidence of benign adipose tissue tumors (lipomas) at doses ≥0.3 mg/kg/day (approximately 2 times human AUC at the maximum recommended human daily dose of the rosiglitazone component of AVANDAMET). These proliferative changes in both species are considered due to the persistent pharmacological overstimulation of adipose tissue.

Rosiglitazone was not mutagenic or clastogenic in the in vitro bacterial assays for gene mutation, the in vitro chromosome aberration test in human lymphocytes, the in vivo mouse micronucleus test, and the in vivo/in vitro rat UDS assay. There was a small (about 2-fold) increase in mutation in the in vitro mouse lymphoma assay in the presence of metabolic activation.

Rosiglitazone had no effects on mating or fertility of male rats given up to 40 mg/kg/day (approximately 116 times human AUC at the maximum recommended human daily dose of the rosiglitazone component of AVANDAMET). Rosiglitazone altered estrous cyclicity (2 mg/kg/day) and reduced fertility (40 mg/kg/day) of female rats in association with lower plasma levels of progesterone and estradiol (approximately 20 and 200 times human AUC at the maximum recommended human daily dose of the rosiglitazone component of AVANDAMET, respectively). No such effects were noted at 0.2 mg/kg/day (approximately 3 times human AUC at the maximum recommended human daily dose of the rosiglitazone component of AVANDAMET). In monkeys, rosiglitazone (0.6 and 4.6 mg/kg/day; approximately 3 and 15 times human AUC at the maximum recommended human daily dose of the rosiglitazone component of AVANDAMET, respectively) diminished the follicular phase rise in serum estradiol with consequential reduction in the luteinizing hormone surge, lower luteal phase progesterone levels, and amenorrhea. The mechanism for these effects appears to be direct inhibition of ovarian steroidogenesis.

Metformin hydrochloride: Long-term carcinogenicity studies have been performed in rats (dosing duration of 104 weeks) and mice (dosing duration of 91 weeks) at doses up to and including 900 mg/kg/day and 1,500 mg/kg/day, respectively. These doses are both approximately 4 times the maximum recommended human daily dose of 2,000 mg of the metformin component of AVANDAMET based on body surface area comparisons. No evidence of carcinogenicity with metformin was found in either male or female mice. Similarly, there was no tumorigenic potential observed with metformin in male rats. There was, however, an increased incidence of benign stromal uterine polyps in female rats treated with 900 mg/kg/day.

There was no evidence of mutagenic potential of metformin in the following in vitro tests: Ames test (*S. typhimurium*), gene mutation test (mouse lymphoma cells), or chromosomal aberrations test (human lymphocytes). Results in the in vivo mouse micronucleus test were also negative.

Fertility of male or female rats was unaffected by metformin when administrated at doses as high as 600 mg/kg/day, which is approximately 3 times the maximum recommended human daily dose of the metformin component of AVANDAMET based on body surface area comparisons.

Animal Toxicology: Heart weights were increased in mice (3 mg/kg/day), rats (5 mg/kg/day), and dogs (2 mg/kg/day) with rosiglitazone treatments (approximately 5, 22, and 2 times human AUC at the maximum recommended human daily dose of the rosiglitazone component of AVANDAMET, respectively). Morphometric measurement indicated that there was hypertrophy in cardiac ventricular tissues, which may be due to increased heart work as a result of plasma volume expansion.

Pregnancy: Pregnancy Category C: Because current information strongly suggests that abnormal blood glucose levels during pregnancy are associated with a higher incidence of congenital anomalies as well as increased neonatal morbidity and mortality, most experts recommend that insulin monotherapy be used during pregnancy to maintain blood glucose levels as close to normal as possible. AVANDAMET should not be used during pregnancy unless the potential benefit justifies the potential risk to the fetus.

There are no adequate and well-controlled studies in pregnant women with AVANDAMET or its individual components. No animal studies have been conducted with the combined products in AVANDAMET. The following data are based on findings in studies performed with rosiglitazone or metformin individually.

Rosiglitazone maleate: There was no effect on implantation or the embryo with rosiglitazone treatment during early pregnancy in rats, but treatment during mid-late gestation was associated with fetal death and growth retardation in both rats and rabbits. Teratogenicity was not observed at doses up to 3 mg/kg in rats and 100 mg/kg in rabbits (approximately 20 and 75 times human AUC at the maximum recommended human daily dose of the rosiglitazone component of AVANDAMET, respectively). Rosiglitazone caused placental pathology in rats (3 mg/kg/day). Treatment of rats during gestation through lactation reduced litter size, neonatal viability, and postnatal growth, with growth retardation reversible after puberty. For effects on the placenta, embryo/fetus, and offspring, the no-effect dose was 0.2 mg/kg/day in rats and 15 mg/kg/day in rabbits. These no-effect levels are approximately 4 times human AUC at the maximum recommended human daily dose of the rosiglitazone component of AVANDAMET.

Metformin hydrochloride: Metformin was not teratogenic in rats and rabbits at doses up to 600 mg/kg/day. This represents an exposure of about 2 and 6 times the maximum recommended human daily dose of 2,000 mg based on body surface area comparisons for rats and rabbits, respectively. Determination of fetal concentrations demonstrated a partial placental barrier to metformin.

Labor and Delivery: The effect of AVANDAMET or its components on labor and delivery in humans is unknown.

Nursing Mothers: No studies have been conducted with the combined components of AVANDAMET. In studies performed with the individual components, both rosiglitazone-related material and metformin were detectable in milk from lactating rats. It is not known whether rosiglitazone and/or metformin is excreted in human milk. Because many drugs are excreted in human milk, AVANDAMET should not be administered to a nursing woman. If AVANDAMET is discontinued, and if diet alone is inadequate for controlling blood glucose, insulin therapy should be considered.

Pediatric Use: Safety and effectiveness of AVANDAMET in pediatric patients have not been established.

Geriatric Use: Metformin is known to be substantially excreted by the kidney and because the risk of serious adverse reactions to the drug is greater in patients with impaired renal function, AVANDAMET should only be used in patients with normal renal function (see CONTRAINDICATIONS, WARNINGS, and CLINICAL PHARMACOLOGY, Pharmacokinetics). Because aging is associated with reduced renal function, AVANDAMET should be used with caution as age increases. Care should be taken in dose selection and should be based on careful and regular monitoring of renal function. Generally, elderly patients should not be titrated to the maximum dose of AVANDAMET (see also WARNINGS and DOSAGE AND ADMINISTRATION).

ADVERSE REACTIONS

The incidence and types of adverse events reported in controlled, 26-week clinical trials in association with rosiglitazone maleate in combination with doses of metformin hydrochloride of 2,500 mg/day in comparison to adverse reactions reported in association with rosiglitazone and metformin monotherapies are shown in Table 4.

[See table 4 above]

Table 4. Adverse Events (≥5% in Any Treatment Group) Reported by Patients in 26-week Double-blind Clinical Trials

	Rosiglitazone monotherapy N = 2,526	Placebo N = 601	Metformin monotherapy N = 225	Rosiglitazone plus metformin N = 338
Preferred term	**%**	**%**	**%**	**%**
Upper respiratory tract infection	9.9	8.7	8.9	16.0
Injury	7.6	4.3	7.6	8.0
Headache	5.9	5.0	8.9	6.5
Back pain	4.0	3.8	4.0	5.0
Hyperglycemia	3.9	5.7	4.4	2.1
Fatigue	3.6	5.0	4.0	5.9
Sinusitis	3.2	4.5	5.3	6.2
Diarrhea	2.3	3.3	15.6	12.7
Viral infection	3.2	4.0	3.6	5.0
Arthralgia	3.0	4.0	2.2	5.0
Anemia	1.9	0.7	2.2	7.1

Reports of hypoglycemia in patients treated with rosiglitazone and maximum metformin combination therapy were more frequent than in patients treated with rosiglitazone or metformin monotherapies. In double-blind studies, hypoglycemia was reported by 3.0% of patients receiving rosiglitazone in combination with maximum doses of metformin, by 1.3% of patients receiving metformin monotherapy, by 0.6% of patients receiving rosiglitazone as monotherapy, and by 0.2% of patients receiving placebo.

There were a small number of patients treated with rosiglitazone who had adverse events of anemia and edema. Overall, these events were generally mild to moderate in severity and usually did not require discontinuation of treatment with rosiglitazone.

Edema was reported in 4.8% of patients receiving rosiglitazone compared to 1.3% on placebo, and 2.2% on metformin monotherapy and 4.4% on rosiglitazone in combination with maximum doses of metformin. Overall, the types of adverse experiences reported when rosiglitazone was used in combination with metformin were similar to those during monotherapy with rosiglitazone. Reports of anemia (7.1%) were greater in patients treated with a combination of rosiglitazone and metformin compared to monotherapy with rosiglitazone.

Lower pre-treatment hemoglobin/hematocrit levels in patients enrolled in the metformin combination clinical trials may have contributed to the higher reporting rate of anemia in these studies (see ADVERSE REACTIONS, Laboratory Abnormalities, *Hematologic*).

In 26-week double-blind, fixed-dose studies, edema was reported with higher frequency in the rosiglitazone plus insulin combination trials (insulin, 5.4%; and rosiglitazone in combination with insulin, 14.7%). Reports of new-onset or exacerbation of congestive heart failure occurred at rates of 1% for insulin alone, and 2% (4 mg) and 3% (8 mg) for insulin in combination with rosiglitazone (see WARNINGS, Cardiac Failure and Other Cardiac Effects).

In postmarketing experience with rosiglitazone maleate, adverse events potentially related to volume expansion (e.g., congestive heart failure, pulmonary edema, and pleural effusions) have been reported.

In postmarketing experience with rosiglitazone maleate, angioedema and urticaria have been reported rarely.

(See also GLUCOPHAGE prescribing information, ADVERSE REACTIONS).

Laboratory Abnormalities: ***Hematologic:*** Decreases in mean hemoglobin and hematocrit occurred in a dose-related fashion in patients treated with rosiglitazone maleate (mean decreases in individual studies up to 1.0 gram/dL hemoglobin and up to 3.3% hematocrit). The time course and magnitude of decreases were similar in patients treated with a combination of rosiglitazone and other hypoglycemic

Continued on next page

Product information on these pages is effective as of August 2004. Further information is available at: GlaxoSmithKline, PO Box 13398, Research Triangle Park, NC 27709. 1-888-825-5249. Corporate Web Site: www.gsk.com

Avandamet—Cont.

agents or rosiglitazone monotherapy. Pre-treatment levels of hemoglobin and hematocrit were lower in patients in metformin combination studies and may have contributed to the higher reporting rate of anemia. White blood cell counts also decreased slightly in patients treated with rosiglitazone. Decreases in hematologic parameters may be related to increased plasma volume observed with rosiglitazone treatment.

In controlled clinical trials of metformin hydrochloride of 29 weeks' duration, a decrease to subnormal levels of previously normal serum vitamin B_{12} levels, without clinical manifestations, was observed in approximately 7% of patients. Such a decrease, possibly due to interference with B_{12} absorption from the B_{12}-intrinsic factor complex, is, however, very rarely associated with anemia and appears to be rapidly reversible with discontinuation of metformin or vitamin B_{12} supplementation.

Lipids: Changes in serum lipids have been observed following treatment with rosiglitazone maleate (see CLINICAL STUDIES).

Serum Transaminase Levels: In clinical studies in 4,598 patients treated with rosiglitazone maleate encompassing approximately 3,600 patient years of exposure, there was no evidence of drug-induced hepatotoxicity or elevated ALT levels.

In controlled trials, 0.2% of patients treated with rosiglitazone maleate had reversible elevations in ALT >3X the upper limit of normal compared to 0.2% on placebo and 0.5% on active comparators. Hyperbilirubinemia was found in 0.3% of patients treated with rosiglitazone compared with 0.9% treated with placebo and 1% in patients treated with active comparators.

In the clinical program including long-term, open-label experience, the rate per 100 patient years of exposure of ALT increase to >3X the upper limit of normal was 0.35 for patients treated with rosiglitazone maleate, 0.59 for placebo-treated patients, and 0.78 for patients treated with active comparator agents.

In pre-approval clinical trials, there were no cases of idiosyncratic drug reactions leading to hepatic failure. In post-marketing experience with rosiglitazone maleate, reports of hepatic enzyme elevations 3 or more times the upper limit of normal and hepatitis have been received (see PRECAUTIONS, Hepatic Effects).

OVERDOSAGE

Rosiglitazone maleate: Limited data are available with regard to overdosage in humans. In clinical studies in volunteers, rosiglitazone has been administered at single oral doses of up to 20 mg and was well tolerated. In the event of an overdose, appropriate supportive treatment should be initiated as dictated by the patients clinical status.

Metformin hydrochloride: Hypoglycemia has not been seen with ingestion of up to 85 grams of metformin hydrochloride, although lactic acidosis has occurred in such circumstances (see WARNINGS). Metformin is dialyzable with a clearance of up to 170 mL/min under good hemodynamic conditions. Therefore, hemodialysis may be useful for removal of accumulated metformin from patients in whom metformin overdosage is suspected.

DOSAGE AND ADMINISTRATION

General: The selection of the dose of AVANDAMET should be based on the patient's current doses of rosiglitazone and/or metformin.

The safety and efficacy of AVANDAMET as initial therapy for patients with type 2 diabetes mellitus have not been established.

The following recommendations regarding the use of AVANDAMET in patients inadequately controlled on rosiglitazone and metformin monotherapies are based on clinical practice experience with rosiglitazone and metformin combination therapy.

- The dosage of antidiabetic therapy with AVANDAMET should be individualized on the basis of effectiveness and tolerability while not exceeding the maximum recommended daily dose of 8 mg/2,000 mg.
- AVANDAMET should be given in divided doses with meals, with gradual dose escalation. This reduces GI side effects (largely due to metformin) and permits determination of the minimum effective dose for the individual patient.
- Sufficient time should be given to assess adequacy of therapeutic response. Fasting plasma glucose (FPG) should be used to determine the therapeutic response to AVANDAMET. After an increase in metformin dosage, dose titration is recommended if patients are not adequately controlled after 1 to 2 weeks. After an increase in rosiglitazone dosage, dose titration is recommended if patients are not adequately controlled after 8 to 12 weeks.

Dosage Recommendations: For patients inadequately controlled on metformin monotherapy, the usual starting dose of AVANDAMET is 4 mg rosiglitazone (total daily dose) plus the dose of metformin already being taken (see Table 5).

For patients inadequately controlled on rosiglitazone monotherapy, the usual starting dose of AVANDAMET is 1,000 mg metformin (total daily dose) plus the dose of rosiglitazone already being taken (see Table 5).

Table 5. AVANDAMET Starting Dose

PRIOR THERAPY	Usual AVANDAMET Starting Dose	
Total daily dose	**Tablet strength**	**Number of tablets**
Metformin HCl*		
1,000 mg/day	2 mg/500 mg	1 tablet twice a day
2,000 mg/day	2 mg/1,000 mg	1 tablet twice a day
Rosiglitazone		
4 mg/day	2 mg/500 mg	1 tablet twice a day
8 mg/day	4 mg/500 mg	1 tablet twice a day

*For patients on doses of metformin HCl between 1,000 and 2,000 mg/day, initiation of AVANDAMET requires individualization of therapy.

When switching from combination therapy of rosiglitazone plus metformin as separate tablets, the usual starting dose of AVANDAMET is the dose of rosiglitazone and metformin already being taken.

If additional glycemic control is needed, the daily dose of AVANDAMET may be increased by increments of 4 mg rosiglitazone and/or 500 mg metformin, up to the maximum recommended total daily dose of 8 mg/2,000 mg.

No studies have been performed specifically examining the safety and efficacy of AVANDAMET in patients previously treated with other oral hypoglycemic agents and switched to AVANDAMET. Any change in therapy of type 2 diabetes should be undertaken with care and appropriate monitoring as changes in glycemic control can occur.

Specific Patient Populations: AVANDAMET is not recommended for use in pregnancy or for use in pediatric patients. The initial and maintenance dosing of AVANDAMET should be conservative in patients with advanced age, due to the potential for decreased renal function in this population. Any dosage adjustment should be based on a careful assessment of renal function. Generally, elderly, debilitated, and malnourished patients should not be titrated to the maximum dose of AVANDAMET. Monitoring of renal function is necessary to aid in prevention of metformin-associated lactic acidosis, particularly in the elderly (see WARNINGS).

Therapy with AVANDAMET should not be initiated if the patient exhibits clinical evidence of active liver disease or increased serum transaminase levels (ALT >2.5X upper limit of normal at start of therapy) (see PRECAUTIONS, Hepatic Effects and CLINICAL PHARMACOLOGY, Hepatic Impairment). Liver enzyme monitoring is recommended in all patients prior to initiation of therapy with AVANDAMET and periodically thereafter (see PRECAUTIONS, Hepatic Effects).

HOW SUPPLIED

Tablets: Each tablet contains rosiglitazone as the maleate and metformin hydrochloride as follows:

1 mg/500 mg — yellow, film-coated oval tablet, debossed with gsk on one side and 1/500 on the other.

2 mg/500 mg — pale pink, film-coated oval tablet, debossed with gsk on one side and 2/500 on the other.

4 mg/500 mg — orange, film-coated oval tablet, debossed with gsk on one side and 4/500 on the other.

2 mg/1,000 mg — yellow, film-coated oval tablet, debossed with gsk on one side and 2/1000 on the other.

4 mg/1,000 mg — pink, film-coated oval tablet, debossed with gsk on one side and 4/1000 on the other.

1 mg/500 mg bottles of 60: NDC 0007-3166-18
1 mg/500 mg bottles of 100: NDC 0007-3166-20
1 mg/500 mg SUP 100s: NDC 0007-3166-21
2 mg/500 mg bottles of 60: NDC 0007-3167-18
2 mg/500 mg bottles of 100: NDC 0007-3167-20
2 mg/500 mg SUP 100s: NDC 0007-3167-21
4 mg/500 mg bottles of 60: NDC 0007-3168-18
4 mg/500 mg bottles of 100: NDC 0007-3168-20
4 mg/500 mg SUP 100s: NDC 0007-3168-21
2 mg/1,000 mg bottles of 60: NDC 0007-3163-18
2 mg/1,000 mg bottles of 100: NDC 0007-3163-20
4 mg/1,000 mg bottles of 60: NDC 0007-3164-18
4 mg/1,000 mg bottles of 100: NDC 0007-3164-20

STORAGE

Store at 25°C (77°F); excursions permitted to 15° to 30°C (59° to 86°F).

Dispense in a tight, light-resistant container.

GLUCOPHAGE is a registered trademark of Merck Santé S.A.S., an associate of Merck KGaA of Darmstadt, Germany. Licensed to Bristol-Myers Squibb Company.

GlaxoSmithKline, Research Triangle Park, NC 27709

AVANDAMET is a registered trademark of GlaxoSmithKline.

August 2004/AT:L6

Shown in Product Identification Guide, page 314

AVANDIA® ℞

[ə-van'dē-ə]
(rosiglitazone maleate)
Tablets

DESCRIPTION

AVANDIA (rosiglitazone maleate) is an oral antidiabetic agent which acts primarily by increasing insulin sensitivity. AVANDIA is used in the management of type 2 diabetes mellitus (also known as non-insulin-dependent diabetes mellitus [NIDDM] or adult-onset diabetes). AVANDIA improves glycemic control while reducing circulating insulin levels.

Pharmacological studies in animal models indicate that rosiglitazone improves sensitivity to insulin in muscle and adipose tissue and inhibits hepatic gluconeogenesis. Rosiglitazone maleate is not chemically or functionally related to the sulfonylureas, the biguanides, or the alpha-glucosidase inhibitors.

Chemically, rosiglitazone maleate is (±)-5-[[4-[2-(methyl-2-pyridinylamino) ethoxy]phenyl]methyl]-2,4-thiazolidinedione, (*Z*)-2-butenedioate (1:1) with a molecular weight of 473.52 (357.44 free base). The molecule has a single chiral center and is present as a racemate. Due to rapid interconversion, the enantiomers are functionally indistinguishable. The molecular formula is $C_{18}H_{19}N_3O_3S \cdot C_4H_4O_4$. Rosiglitazone maleate is a white to off-white solid with a melting point range of 122° to 123°C. The pKa values of rosiglitazone maleate are 6.8 and 6.1. It is readily soluble in ethanol and a buffered aqueous solution with pH of 2.3; solubility decreases with increasing pH in the physiological range.

Each pentagonal film-coated TILTAB® tablet contains rosiglitazone maleate equivalent to rosiglitazone, 2 mg, 4 mg, or 8 mg, for oral administration. Inactive ingredients are: Hypromellose 2910, lactose monohydrate, magnesium stearate, microcrystalline cellulose, polyethylene glycol 3000, sodium starch glycolate, titanium dioxide, triacetin, and 1 or more of the following: Synthetic red and yellow iron oxides and talc.

CLINICAL PHARMACOLOGY

Mechanism of Action: Rosiglitazone, a member of the thiazolidinedione class of antidiabetic agents, improves glycemic control by improving insulin sensitivity. Rosiglitazone is a highly selective and potent agonist for the peroxisome proliferator-activated receptor-gamma (PPARγ). In humans, PPAR receptors are found in key target tissues for insulin action such as adipose tissue, skeletal muscle, and liver. Activation of PPARγ nuclear receptors regulates the transcription of insulin-responsive genes involved in the control of glucose production, transport, and utilization. In addition, PPARγ-responsive genes also participate in the regulation of fatty acid metabolism.

Insulin resistance is a common feature characterizing the pathogenesis of type 2 diabetes. The antidiabetic activity of rosiglitazone has been demonstrated in animal models of type 2 diabetes in which hyperglycemia and/or impaired glucose tolerance is a consequence of insulin resistance in target tissues. Rosiglitazone reduces blood glucose concentrations and reduces hyperinsulinemia in the ob/ob obese mouse, db/db diabetic mouse, and fa/fa fatty Zucker rat.

In animal models, rosiglitazone's antidiabetic activity was shown to be mediated by increased sensitivity to insulin's action in the liver, muscle, and adipose tissues. The expression of the insulin-regulated glucose transporter GLUT-4 was increased in adipose tissue. Rosiglitazone did not induce hypoglycemia in animal models of type 2 diabetes and/or impaired glucose tolerance.

Pharmacokinetics and Drug Metabolism: Maximum plasma concentration (C_{max}) and the area under the curve (AUC) of rosiglitazone increase in a dose-proportional manner over the therapeutic dose range (see Table 1). The elimination half-life is 3 to 4 hours and is independent of dose.

Table 1. Mean (SD) Pharmacokinetic Parameters for Rosiglitazone Following Single Oral Doses (N = 32)

Parameter	1 mg Fasting	2 mg Fasting	8 mg Fasting	8 mg Fed
$AUC_{0\text{-}inf}$ [ng.hr./mL]	358 (112)	733 (184)	2,971 (730)	2,890 (795)
C_{max} [ng/mL]	76 (13)	156 (42)	598 (117)	432 (92)
Half-life [hr.]	3.16 (0.72)	3.15 (0.39)	3.37 (0.63)	3.59 (0.70)
CL/F* [L/hr.]	3.03 (0.87)	2.89 (0.71)	2.85 (0.69)	2.97 (0.81)

*CL/F = Oral clearance.

Absorption: The absolute bioavailability of rosiglitazone is 99%. Peak plasma concentrations are observed about 1 hour after dosing. Administration of rosiglitazone with food resulted in no change in overall exposure (AUC), but there was an approximately 28% decrease in C_{max} and a delay in T_{max} (1.75 hours). These changes are not likely to be clinically significant; therefore, AVANDIA may be administered with or without food.

Distribution: The mean (CV%) oral volume of distribution (Vss/F) of rosiglitazone is approximately 17.6 (30%) liters, based on a population pharmacokinetic analysis. Rosiglitazone is approximately 99.8% bound to plasma proteins, primarily albumin.

Metabolism: Rosiglitazone is extensively metabolized with no unchanged drug excreted in the urine. The major routes of metabolism were N-demethylation and hydroxylation, followed by conjugation with sulfate and glucuronic acid. All the circulating metabolites are considerably less potent than parent and, therefore, are not expected to contribute to the insulin-sensitizing activity of rosiglitazone.

In vitro data demonstrate that rosiglitazone is predominantly metabolized by Cytochrome P_{450} (CYP) isoenzyme 2C8, with CYP2C9 contributing as a minor pathway.

Excretion: Following oral or intravenous administration of [^{14}C]rosiglitazone maleate, approximately 64% and 23% of the dose was eliminated in the urine and in the feces, respectively. The plasma half-life of [^{14}C]related material ranged from 103 to 158 hours.

Population Pharmacokinetics in Patients with Type 2 Diabetes: Population pharmacokinetic analyses from 3 large clinical trials including 642 men and 405 women with type 2 diabetes (aged 35 to 80 years) showed that the pharmacokinetics of rosiglitazone are not influenced by age, race, smoking, or alcohol consumption. Both oral clearance (CL/F) and oral steady-state volume of distribution (Vss/F) were shown to increase with increases in body weight. Over the weight range observed in these analyses (50 to 150 kg), the range of predicted CL/F and Vss/F values varied by <1.7-fold and <2.3-fold, respectively. Additionally, rosiglitazone CL/F was shown to be influenced by both weight and gender, being lower (about 15%) in female patients.

Special Populations: ***Geriatric:*** Results of the population pharmacokinetic analysis (n = 716 <65 years; n = 331 ≥65 years) showed that age does not significantly affect the pharmacokinetics of rosiglitazone.

Gender: Results of the population pharmacokinetic analysis showed that the mean oral clearance of rosiglitazone in female patients (n = 405) was approximately 6% lower compared to male patients of the same body weight (n = 642).

As monotherapy and in combination with metformin, AVANDIA improved glycemic control in both males and females. In metformin combination studies, efficacy was demonstrated with no gender differences in glycemic response. In monotherapy studies, a greater therapeutic response was observed in females; however, in more obese patients, gender differences were less evident. For a given body mass index (BMI), females tend to have a greater fat mass than males. Since the molecular target PPARγ is expressed in adipose tissues, this differentiating characteristic may account, at least in part, for the greater response to AVANDIA in females. Since therapy should be individualized, no dose adjustments are necessary based on gender alone.

Hepatic Impairment: Unbound oral clearance of rosiglitazone was significantly lower in patients with moderate to severe liver disease (Child-Pugh Class B/C) compared to healthy subjects. As a result, unbound C_{max} and AUC_{0-inf} were increased 2- and 3-fold, respectively. Elimination half-life for rosiglitazone was about 2 hours longer in patients with liver disease, compared to healthy subjects.

Therapy with AVANDIA should not be initiated if the patient exhibits clinical evidence of active liver disease or increased serum transaminase levels (ALT >2.5× upper limit of normal) at baseline (see PRECAUTIONS, General, *Hepatic Effects*).

Renal Impairment: There are no clinically relevant differences in the pharmacokinetics of rosiglitazone in patients with mild to severe renal impairment or in hemodialysis-dependent patients compared to subjects with normal renal function. No dosage adjustment is therefore required in such patients receiving AVANDIA. Since metformin is contraindicated in patients with renal impairment, coadministration of metformin with AVANDIA is contraindicated in these patients.

Race: Results of a population pharmacokinetic analysis including subjects of Caucasian, black, and other ethnic origins indicate that race has no influence on the pharmacokinetics of rosiglitazone.

CLINICAL STUDIES

In clinical studies, treatment with AVANDIA resulted in an improvement in glycemic control, as measured by fasting plasma glucose (FPG) and hemoglobin A1c (HbA1c), with a concurrent reduction in insulin and C-peptide. Postprandial glucose and insulin were also reduced. This is consistent with the mechanism of action of AVANDIA as an insulin sensitizer. The improvement in glycemic control was durable, with maintenance of effect for 52 weeks. The maximum recommended daily dose is 8 mg. Dose-ranging studies suggested that no additional benefit was obtained with a total daily dose of 12 mg.

The addition of AVANDIA to either metformin, a sulfonylurea, or insulin resulted in significant reductions in hyperglycemia compared to any of these agents alone. These results are consistent with an additive effect on glycemic control when AVANDIA is used as combination therapy.

Patients with lipid abnormalities were not excluded from clinical trials of AVANDIA. In all 26-week controlled trials, across the recommended dose range, AVANDIA as monotherapy was associated with increases in total cholesterol, LDL, and HDL and decreases in free fatty acids. These changes were statistically significantly different from placebo or glyburide controls (see Table 2).

Increases in LDL occurred primarily during the first 1 to 2 months of therapy with AVANDIA and LDL levels remained elevated above baseline throughout the trials. In contrast, HDL continued to rise over time. As a result, the LDL/HDL ratio peaked after 2 months of therapy and then appeared to decrease over time. Because of the temporal nature of lipid changes, the 52-week glyburide-controlled study is most pertinent to assess long-term effects on lipids. At baseline, week 26, and week 52, mean LDL/HDL ratios were 3.1, 3.2, and 3.0, respectively, for AVANDIA 4 mg twice daily. The corresponding values for glyburide were 3.2, 3.1, and 2.9. The differences in change from baseline between AVANDIA and glyburide at week 52 were statistically significant.

The pattern of LDL and HDL changes following therapy with AVANDIA in combination with other hypoglycemic agents were generally similar to those seen with AVANDIA in monotherapy.

The changes in triglycerides during therapy with AVANDIA were variable and were generally not statistically different from placebo or glyburide controls.

[See table 2 above]

Table 2. Summary of Mean Lipid Changes in 26-Week Placebo-Controlled and 52-Week Glyburide-Controlled Monotherapy Studies

	Placebo-controlled Studies Week 26			Glyburide-controlled Study Week 26 and Week 52			
	Placebo	AVANDIA		Glyburide Titration		AVANDIA 8 mg	
		4 mg daily*	8 mg daily*	Wk 26	Wk 52	Wk 26	Wk 52
Free Fatty Acids							
N	207	428	436	181	168	166	145
Baseline (mean)	18.1	17.5	17.9	26.4	26.4	26.9	26.6
% Change from baseline (mean)	+0.2%	-7.8%	-14.7%	-2.4%	-4.7%	-20.8%	-21.5%
LDL							
N	190	400	374	175	160	161	133
Baseline (mean)	123.7	126.8	125.3	142.7	141.9	142.1	142.1
% Change from baseline (mean)	+4.8%	+14.1%	+18.6%	-0.9%	-0.5%	+11.9%	+12.1%
HDL							
N	208	429	436	184	170	170	145
Baseline (mean)	44.1	44.4	43.0	47.2	47.7	48.4	48.3
% Change from baseline (mean)	+8.0%	+11.4%	+14.2%	+4.3%	+8.7%	+14.0%	+18.5%

*Once daily and twice daily dosing groups were combined.

Monotherapy: A total of 2,315 patients with type 2 diabetes, previously treated with diet alone or antidiabetic medication(s), were treated with AVANDIA as monotherapy in 6 double-blind studies, which included two 26-week placebo-controlled studies, one 52-week glyburide-controlled study, and 3 placebo-controlled dose-ranging studies of 8 to 12 weeks duration. Previous antidiabetic medication(s) were withdrawn and patients entered a 2 to 4 week placebo run-in period prior to randomization.

Two 26-week, double-blind, placebo-controlled trials, in patients with type 2 diabetes with inadequate glycemic control (mean baseline FPG approximately 228 mg/dL and mean baseline HbA1c 8.9%), were conducted. Treatment with AVANDIA produced statistically significant improvements in FPG and HbA1c compared to baseline and relative to placebo (see Table 3).

[See table 3 above]

Table 3. Glycemic Parameters in Two 26-Week Placebo-Controlled Trials

Study A	Placebo	AVANDIA 2 mg twice daily	AVANDIA 4 mg twice daily
N	158	166	169
FPG (mg/dL)			
Baseline (mean)	229	227	220
Change from baseline (mean)	19	-38	-54
Difference from placebo (adjusted mean)		-58*	-76*
Responders (≥30 mg/dL decrease from baseline)	16%	54%	64%
HbA1c (%)			
Baseline (mean)	9.0	9.0	8.8
Change from baseline (mean)	0.9	-0.3	-0.6
Difference from placebo (adjusted mean)	–	-1.2*	-1.5*
Responders (≥0.7% decrease from baseline)	6%	40%	42%

Study B	Placebo	AVANDIA 4 mg once daily	AVANDIA 2 mg twice daily	AVANDIA 8 mg once daily	AVANDIA 4 mg twice daily
N	173	180	186	181	187
FPG (mg/dL)					
Baseline (mean)	225	229	225	228	228
Change from baseline (mean)	8	-25	-35	-42	-55
Difference from placebo (adjusted mean)	–	-31*	-43*	-49*	-62*
Responders (≥30 mg/dL decrease from baseline)	19%	45%	54%	58%	70%
HbA1c (%)					
Baseline (mean)	8.9	8.9	8.9	8.9	9.0
Change from baseline (mean)	0.8	0.0	-0.1	-0.3	-0.7
Difference from placebo (adjusted mean)	–	-0.8*	-0.9*	-1.1*	-1.5*
Responders (≥0.7% decrease from baseline)	9%	28%	29%	39%	54%

*<0.0001 compared to placebo.

When administered at the same total daily dose, AVANDIA was generally more effective in reducing FPG and HbA1c when administered in divided doses twice daily compared to once daily doses. However, for HbA1c, the difference between the 4 mg once daily and 2 mg twice daily doses was not statistically significant.

Long-term maintenance of effect was evaluated in a 52-week, double-blind, glyburide-controlled trial in patients with type 2 diabetes. Patients were randomized to treatment with AVANDIA 2 mg twice daily (N = 195) or AVANDIA 4 mg twice daily (N = 189) or glyburide (N = 202) for 52 weeks. Patients receiving glyburide were given an in-

Continued on next page

Product information on these pages is effective as of August 2004. Further information is available at: GlaxoSmithKline, PO Box 13398, Research Triangle Park, NC 27709. 1-888-825-5249. Corporate Web Site: www.gsk.com

Avandia—Cont.

itial dosage of either 2.5 mg/day or 5.0 mg/day. The dosage was then titrated in 2.5 mg/day increments over the next 12 weeks, to a maximum dosage of 15.0 mg/day in order to optimize glycemic control. Thereafter the glyburide dose was kept constant.

The median titrated dose of glyburide was 7.5 mg. All treatments resulted in a statistically significant improvement in glycemic control from baseline (see Figure 1 and Figure 2). At the end of week 52, the reduction from baseline in FPG and HbA1c was -40.8 mg/dL and -0.53% with AVANDIA 4 mg twice daily; -25.4 mg/dL and -0.27% with AVANDIA 2 mg twice daily; and -30.0 mg/dL and -0.72% with glyburide. For HbA1c, the difference between AVANDIA 4 mg twice daily and glyburide was not statistically significant at week 52. The initial fall in FPG with glyburide was greater than with AVANDIA; however, this effect was less durable over time. The improvement in glycemic control seen with AVANDIA 4 mg twice daily at week 26 was maintained through week 52 of the study.

Figure 1. Mean FPG Over Time in a 52-Week Glyburide-Controlled Study

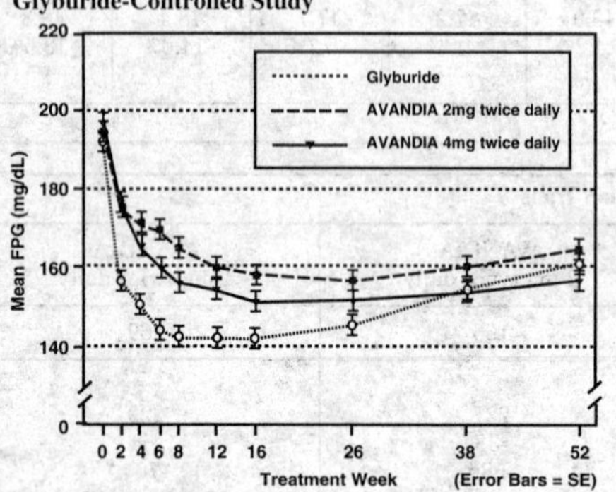

Figure 2. Mean HbA1c Over Time in a 52-Week Glyburide-Controlled Study

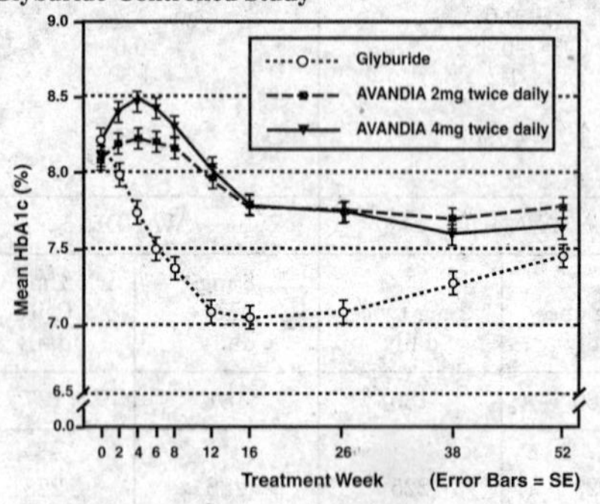

Hypoglycemia was reported in 12.1% of glyburide-treated patients versus 0.5% (2 mg twice daily) and 1.6% (4 mg twice daily) of patients treated with AVANDIA. The improvements in glycemic control were associated with a mean weight gain of 1.75 kg and 2.95 kg for patients treated with 2 mg and 4 mg twice daily of AVANDIA, respectively, versus 1.9 kg in glyburide-treated patients. In patients treated with AVANDIA, C-peptide, insulin, pro-insulin, and pro-insulin split products were significantly reduced in a dose-ordered fashion, compared to an increase in the glyburide-treated patients.

Combination With Metformin: A total of 670 patients with type 2 diabetes participated in two 26-week, randomized, double-blind, placebo/active-controlled studies designed to assess the efficacy of AVANDIA in combination with metformin. AVANDIA, administered in either once daily or twice daily dosing regimens, was added to the therapy of patients who were inadequately controlled on a maximum dose (2.5 grams/day) of metformin.

In one study, patients inadequately controlled on 2.5 grams/day of metformin (mean baseline FPG 216 mg/dL and mean baseline HbA1c 8.8%) were randomized to receive 4 mg of AVANDIA once daily, 8 mg of AVANDIA once daily, or placebo in addition to metformin. A statistically significant improvement in FPG and HbA1c was observed in patients treated with the combinations of metformin and 4 mg of AVANDIA once daily and 8 mg of AVANDIA once daily, versus patients continued on metformin alone (see Table 4).

[See table 4 above]

Table 4. Glycemic Parameters in a 26-Week Combination Study

	Metformin	AVANDIA 4 mg once daily + metformin	AVANDIA 8 mg once daily + metformin
N	113	116	110
FPG (mg/dL)			
Baseline (mean)	214	215	220
Change from baseline (mean)	6	-33	-48
Difference from metformin alone (adjusted mean)	–	-40*	-53*
Responders (≥30 mg/dL decrease from baseline)	20%	45%	61%
HbA1c (%)			
Baseline (mean)	8.6	8.9	8.9
Change from baseline (mean)	0.5	-0.6	-0.8
Difference from metformin alone (adjusted mean)	–	-1.0*	-1.2*
Responders (≥0.7% decrease from baseline)	11%	45%	52%

*<0.0001 compared to metformin.

In a second 26-week study, patients with type 2 diabetes inadequately controlled on 2.5 grams/day of metformin who were randomized to receive the combination of AVANDIA 4 mg twice daily and metformin (N = 105) showed a statistically significant improvement in glycemic control with a mean treatment effect for FPG of -56 mg/dL and a mean treatment effect for HbA1c of -0.8% over metformin alone. The combination of metformin and AVANDIA resulted in lower levels of FPG and HbA1c than either agent alone.

Patients who were inadequately controlled on a maximum dose (2.5 grams/day) of metformin and who were switched to monotherapy with AVANDIA demonstrated loss of glycemic control, as evidenced by increases in FPG and HbA1c. In this group, increases in LDL and VLDL were also seen.

Combination With a Sulfonylurea: A total of 1,216 patients with type 2 diabetes participated in three 26-week randomized, double-blind, placebo/active-controlled studies designed to assess the efficacy and safety of AVANDIA in combination with a sulfonylurea. AVANDIA 2 mg or 4 mg daily, was administered either once daily or in divided doses twice daily, to patients inadequately controlled on a sulfonylurea.

In the two placebo-controlled studies, patients inadequately controlled on sulfonylureas that were randomized to single dose or divided doses of AVANDIA 4 mg daily plus a sulfonylurea showed significantly reduced FPG and HbA1c compared to sulfonylurea plus placebo (see Table 5).

[See table 5 above]

Table 5. Glycemic Parameters in Two 26-Week Combination Studies

Study C (patients on prior sulfonylurea monotherapy)	Sulfonylurea	AVANDIA 2 mg twice daily + sulfonylurea
N	192	183
FPG (mg/dL)		
Baseline (mean)	207	205
Change from baseline (mean)	+6	-38
Difference from sulfonylurea alone (adjusted mean)	–	-44*
Responders (≥30 mg/dL decrease from baseline)	21%	56%
HbA1c (%)		
Baseline (mean)	9.2	9.2
Change from baseline (mean)	+0.2	-0.9
Difference from sulfonylurea alone (adjusted mean)	–	-1.0*
Study D (patients on prior single or multiple therapies)	**Sulfonylurea**	**AVANDIA 4 mg once daily + sulfonylurea**
N	115	116
FPG (mg/dL)		
Baseline (mean)	209	214
Change from baseline (mean)	+23	-25
Difference from sulfonylurea alone (adjusted mean)	–	-47*
Responders (≥30 mg/dL decrease from baseline)	13%	46%
HbA1c (%)		
Baseline (mean)	8.9	9.1
Change from baseline (mean)	+0.6	-0.3
Difference from sulfonylurea alone (adjusted mean)	–	-0.9*

*≤0.0001 compared to sulfonylurea plus placebo.

In the third study, including patients on prior single or multiple therapies, in patients inadequately controlled on the maximal dose of glyburide (20 mg daily), 2 mg of AVANDIA twice daily plus sulfonylurea significantly reduced FPG (n = 98, mean change from baseline of -31 mg/dL) and HbA1c (mean change from baseline of -0.5%) compared to sulfonylurea plus placebo (n = 99, mean change from baseline of FPG of +24 mg/dL and of HbA1c of +0.9%). The combination of sulfonylurea and AVANDIA resulted in lower levels of FPG and HbA1c than either agent alone. Patients who were switched from maximal dose of glyburide to 2 mg of AVANDIA twice daily as monotherapy demonstrated loss of glycemic control, as evidenced by increases in FPG and HbA1c.

Combination With Insulin: In two 26-week randomized, double-blind, fixed-dose studies designed to assess the efficacy and safety of AVANDIA in combination with insulin, patients inadequately controlled on insulin (65 to 76 units/day, mean range at baseline) were randomized to receive AVANDIA 4 mg plus insulin (n = 206) or placebo plus insulin (n = 203). The mean duration of disease in these patients was 12 to 13 years.

Compared to insulin plus placebo, single or divided doses of AVANDIA 4 mg daily plus insulin significantly reduced FPG (mean reduction of 32 to 40 mg/dL) and HbA1c (mean reduction of 0.6% to 0.7%). Approximately 40% of all patients treated with AVANDIA reduced their insulin dose.

INDICATIONS AND USAGE

AVANDIA is indicated as an adjunct to diet and exercise to improve glycemic control in patients with type 2 diabetes mellitus. AVANDIA is indicated as monotherapy. AVANDIA is also indicated for use in combination with a sulfonylurea, metformin, or insulin when diet, exercise, and a single agent do not result in adequate glycemic control. For patients inadequately controlled with a maximum dose of a sulfonylurea or metformin, AVANDIA should be added to, rather than substituted for, a sulfonylurea or metformin.

Management of type 2 diabetes should include diet control. Caloric restriction, weight loss, and exercise are essential for the proper treatment of the diabetic patient because they help improve insulin sensitivity. This is important not only in the primary treatment of type 2 diabetes, but also in maintaining the efficacy of drug therapy. Prior to initiation of therapy with AVANDIA, secondary causes of poor glycemic control, e.g., infection, should be investigated and treated.

CONTRAINDICATIONS

AVANDIA is contraindicated in patients with known hypersensitivity to this product or any of its components.

WARNINGS

Cardiac Failure and Other Cardiac Effects: AVANDIA, like other thiazolidinediones, alone or in combination with other antidiabetic agents, can cause fluid retention, which may exacerbate or lead to heart failure. Patients should be observed for signs and symptoms of heart failure. In combination with insulin, thiazolidinediones may also increase the risk of other cardiovascular adverse events. AVANDIA should be discontinued if any deterioration in cardiac status occurs.

Patients with New York Heart Association (NYHA) Class 3 and 4 cardiac status were not studied during the clinical trials. AVANDIA is not recommended in patients with NYHA Class 3 and 4 cardiac status.

In three 26-week trials in patients with type 2 diabetes, 216 received 4 mg of AVANDIA plus insulin, 322 received 8 mg of AVANDIA plus insulin, and 338 received insulin alone. These trials included patients with long-standing diabetes and a high prevalence of pre-existing medical conditions, including peripheral neuropathy, retinopathy, ischemic heart disease, vascular disease, and congestive heart failure. In these clinical studies an increased incidence of edema, cardiac failure, and other cardiovascular adverse events was seen in patients on AVANDIA and insulin combination therapy compared to insulin and placebo. Patients who experienced cardiovascular events were on average older, and had a longer duration of diabetes. These cardiovascular events were noted at both the 4 mg and 8 mg daily doses of AVANDIA. In this population, however, it was not possible to determine specific risk factors that could be used to identify all patients at risk of heart failure and other cardiovascular events on combination therapy. Three of 10 patients who developed cardiac failure on combination therapy during the double-blind part of the fixed-dose studies had no known prior evidence of congestive heart failure, or pre-existing cardiac condition.

In a double-blind study in type 2 diabetes patients with chronic renal failure (112 received 4 mg or 8 mg of AVANDIA plus insulin and 108 received insulin control), there was no difference in cardiovascular adverse events with AVANDIA in combination with insulin compared to insulin control.

Patients treated with combination AVANDIA and insulin should be monitored for cardiovascular adverse events. This combination therapy should be discontinued in patients who do not respond as manifested by a reduction in HbA1c or insulin dose after 4 to 5 months of therapy or who develop any significant adverse events. (See ADVERSE REACTIONS).

PRECAUTIONS

General: Due to its mechanism of action, AVANDIA is active only in the presence of endogenous insulin. Therefore, AVANDIA should not be used in patients with type 1 diabetes or for the treatment of diabetic ketoacidosis.

Hypoglycemia: Patients receiving AVANDIA in combination with other hypoglycemic agents may be at risk for hypoglycemia, and a reduction in the dose of the concomitant agent may be necessary.

Edema: AVANDIA should be used with caution in patients with edema. In a clinical study in healthy volunteers who received 8 mg of AVANDIA once daily for 8 weeks, there was a statistically significant increase in median plasma volume compared to placebo.

Since thiazolidinediones, including rosiglitazone, can cause fluid retention, which can exacerbate or lead to congestive heart failure, AVANDIA should be used with caution in patients at risk for heart failure. Patients should be monitored for signs and symptoms of heart failure (see WARNINGS, Cardiac Failure and Other Cardiac Effects and PRECAUTIONS, Information for Patients).

In controlled clinical trials of patients with type 2 diabetes, mild to moderate edema was reported in patients treated with AVANDIA, and may be dose related. Patients with ongoing edema are more likely to have adverse events associated with edema if started on combination therapy with insulin and AVANDIA (see ADVERSE REACTIONS).

Weight Gain: Dose-related weight gain was seen with AVANDIA alone and in combination with other hypoglycemic agents (see Table 6). The mechanism of weight gain is unclear but probably involves a combination of fluid retention and fat accumulation.

In postmarketing experience, there have been rare reports of unusually rapid increases in weight and increases in excess of that generally observed in clinical trials. Patients who experience such increases should be assessed for fluid accumulation and volume-related events such as excessive edema and congestive heart failure.

[See table 6 above]

Table 6. Weight Changes (kg) From Baseline During Clinical Trials With AVANDIA

Monotherapy	Duration	Control Group		AVANDIA 4 mg	AVANDIA 8 mg
			Median (25th, 75th percentile)	Median (25th, 75th percentile)	Median (25th, 75th percentile)
	26 weeks	placebo	-0.9 (-2.8, 0.9)	1.0 (-0.9, 3.6)	3.1 (1.1, 5.8)
	52 weeks	sulfonylurea	2.0 (0, 4.0)	2.0 (-0.6, 4.0)	2.6 (0, 5.3)
Combination therapy					
sulfonylurea	26 weeks	sulfonylurea	0 (-1.3, 1.2)	1.8 (0, 3.1)	–
metformin	26 weeks	metformin	-1.4 (-3.2, 0.2)	0.8 (-1.0, 2.6)	2.1 (0, 4.3)
insulin	26 weeks	insulin	0.9 (-0.5, 2.7)	4.1 (1.4, 6.3)	5.4 (3.4, 7.3)

Hematologic: Across all controlled clinical studies, decreases in hemoglobin and hematocrit (mean decreases in individual studies ≤1.0 gram/dL and ≤3.3%, respectively) were observed for AVANDIA alone and in combination with other hypoglycemic agents. The changes occurred primarily during the first 3 months following initiation of therapy with AVANDIA or following a dose increase in AVANDIA. White blood cell counts also decreased slightly in patients treated with AVANDIA. The observed changes may be related to the increased plasma volume observed with treatment with AVANDIA and may be dose related (see ADVERSE REACTIONS, Laboratory Abnormalities, *Hematologic*).

Ovulation: Therapy with AVANDIA, like other thiazolidinediones, may result in ovulation in some premenopausal anovulatory women. As a result, these patients may be at an increased risk for pregnancy while taking AVANDIA (see PRECAUTIONS, Pregnancy, *Pregnancy Category C*). Thus, adequate contraception in premenopausal women should be recommended. This possible effect has not been specifically investigated in clinical studies so the frequency of this occurrence is not known.

Although hormonal imbalance has been seen in preclinical studies (see PRECAUTIONS, Carcinogenesis, Mutagenesis, Impairment of Fertility), the clinical significance of this finding is not known. If unexpected menstrual dysfunction occurs, the benefits of continued therapy with AVANDIA should be reviewed.

Hepatic Effects: Another drug of the thiazolidinedione class, troglitazone, was associated with idiosyncratic hepatotoxicity, and very rare cases of liver failure, liver transplants, and death were reported during clinical use. In pre-approval controlled clinical trials in patients with type 2 diabetes, troglitazone was more frequently associated with clinically significant elevations in liver enzymes (ALT >3× upper limit of normal) compared to placebo. Very rare cases of reversible jaundice were also reported.

In pre-approval clinical studies in 4,598 patients treated with AVANDIA, encompassing approximately 3,600 patient years of exposure, there was no signal of drug-induced hepatotoxicity or elevation of ALT levels. In the pre-approval controlled trials, 0.2% of patients treated with AVANDIA had elevations in ALT >3× the upper limit of normal compared to 0.2% on placebo and 0.5% on active comparators. The ALT elevations in patients treated with AVANDIA were reversible and were not clearly causally related to therapy with AVANDIA.

In postmarketing experience with AVANDIA, reports of hepatitis and of hepatic enzyme elevations to 3 or more times the upper limit of normal have been received. Very rarely, these reports have involved hepatic failure with and without fatal outcome, although causality has not been established. Rosiglitazone is structurally related to troglitazone, a thiazolidinedione no longer marketed in the United States, which was associated with idiosyncratic hepatotoxicity and rare cases of liver failure, liver transplants, and death during clinical use. Pending the availability of the results of additional large, long-term controlled clinical trials and additional postmarketing safety data, it is recommended that patients treated with AVANDIA undergo periodic monitoring of liver enzymes.

Liver enzymes should be checked prior to the initiation of therapy with AVANDIA in all patients and periodically thereafter per the clinical judgement of the healthcare professional. Therapy with AVANDIA should not be initiated in patients with increased baseline liver enzyme levels (ALT >2.5× upper limit of normal). Patients with mildly elevated liver enzymes (ALT levels ≤2.5× upper limit of normal) at baseline or during therapy with AVANDIA should be evaluated to determine the cause of the liver enzyme elevation. Initiation of, or continuation of, therapy with AVANDIA in patients with mild liver enzyme elevations should proceed with caution and include close clinical follow-up, including more frequent liver enzyme monitoring, to determine if the liver enzyme elevations resolve or worsen. If at any time ALT levels increase to >3× the upper limit of normal in patients on therapy with AVANDIA, liver enzyme levels should be rechecked as soon as possible. If ALT levels remain >3× the upper limit of normal, therapy with AVANDIA should be discontinued.

If any patient develops symptoms suggesting hepatic dysfunction, which may include unexplained nausea, vomiting, abdominal pain, fatigue, anorexia and/or dark urine, liver enzymes should be checked. The decision whether to continue the patient on therapy with AVANDIA should be guided by clinical judgment pending laboratory evaluations. If jaundice is observed, drug therapy should be discontinued.

There are no data available from clinical trials to evaluate the safety of AVANDIA in patients who experienced liver abnormalities, hepatic dysfunction, or jaundice while on troglitazone. AVANDIA should not be used in patients who experienced jaundice while taking troglitazone.

Laboratory Tests: Periodic fasting blood glucose and HbA1c measurements should be performed to monitor therapeutic response.

Liver enzyme monitoring is recommended prior to initiation of therapy with AVANDIA in all patients and periodically thereafter (see PRECAUTIONS, General, *Hepatic Effects* and ADVERSE REACTIONS, Laboratory Abnormalities, *Serum Transaminase Levels*).

Information for Patients: Patients should be informed of the following: Management of type 2 diabetes should include diet control. Caloric restriction, weight loss, and exercise are essential for the proper treatment of the diabetic patient because they help improve insulin sensitivity. This is important not only in the primary treatment of type 2 diabetes, but in maintaining the efficacy of drug therapy.

It is important to adhere to dietary instructions and to regularly have blood glucose and glycosylated hemoglobin tested. Patients should be advised that it can take 2 weeks to see a reduction in blood glucose and 2 to 3 months to see full effect. Patients should be informed that blood will be drawn to check their liver function prior to the start of therapy and periodically thereafter per the clinical judgement of the healthcare professional. Patients with unexplained symptoms of nausea, vomiting, abdominal pain, fatigue, anorexia, or dark urine should immediately report these symptoms to their physician. Patients who experience an unusually rapid increase in weight or edema or who develop shortness of breath or other symptoms of heart failure while on AVANDIA should immediately report these symptoms to their physician.

AVANDIA can be taken with or without meals.

When using AVANDIA in combination with other hypoglycemic agents, the risk of hypoglycemia, its symptoms and treatment, and conditions that predispose to its development should be explained to patients and their family members.

Therapy with AVANDIA, like other thiazolidinediones, may result in ovulation in some premenopausal anovulatory women. As a result, these patients may be at an increased risk for pregnancy while taking AVANDIA (see PRECAUTIONS, Pregnancy, *Pregnancy Category C*). Thus, adequate contraception in premenopausal women should be recommended. This possible effect has not been specifically investigated in clinical studies so the frequency of this occurrence is not known.

Drug Interactions: *Drugs Metabolized by Cytochrome P_{450}:* In vitro drug metabolism studies suggest that rosiglitazone does not inhibit any of the major P_{450} enzymes at clinically relevant concentrations. In vitro data demonstrate that rosiglitazone is predominantly metabolized by CYP2C8, and to a lesser extent, 2C9. An inhibitor of CYP2C8 (such as gemfibrozil) may decrease the metabolism of rosiglitazone and an inducer of CYP2C8 (such as rifampin) may increase the metabolism of rosiglitazone. Therefore, if an inhibitor or an inducer of CYP2C8 is started or stopped during treatment with rosiglitazone, changes in diabetes treatment may be based upon clinical response.

AVANDIA (4 mg twice daily) was shown to have no clinically relevant effect on the pharmacokinetics of nifedipine and oral contraceptives (ethinyl estradiol and norethindrone), which are predominantly metabolized by CYP3A4.

Glyburide: AVANDIA (2 mg twice daily) taken concomitantly with glyburide (3.75 to 10 mg/day) for 7 days did not alter the mean steady-state 24-hour plasma glucose concentrations in diabetic patients stabilized on glyburide therapy.

Metformin: Concurrent administration of AVANDIA (2 mg twice daily) and metformin (500 mg twice daily) in healthy volunteers for 4 days had no effect on the steady-state pharmacokinetics of either metformin or rosiglitazone.

Acarbose: Coadministration of acarbose (100 mg three times daily) for 7 days in healthy volunteers had no clinically relevant effect on the pharmacokinetics of a single oral dose of AVANDIA.

Digoxin: Repeat oral dosing of AVANDIA (8 mg once daily) for 14 days did not alter the steady-state pharmacokinetics of digoxin (0.375 mg once daily) in healthy volunteers.

Warfarin: Repeat dosing with AVANDIA had no clinically relevant effect on the steady-state pharmacokinetics of warfarin enantiomers.

Ethanol: A single administration of a moderate amount of alcohol did not increase the risk of acute hypoglycemia in type 2 diabetes mellitus patients treated with AVANDIA.

Ranitidine: Pretreatment with ranitidine (150 mg twice daily for 4 days) did not alter the pharmacokinetics of either single oral or intravenous doses of rosiglitazone in healthy volunteers. These results suggest that the absorption of oral rosiglitazone is not altered in conditions accompanied by increases in gastrointestinal pH.

Continued on next page

Product information on these pages is effective as of August 2004. Further information is available at: GlaxoSmithKline, PO Box 13398, Research Triangle Park, NC 27709. 1-888-825-5249. Corporate Web Site: www.gsk.com

Avandia—Cont.

Gemfibrozil: Concomitant administration of gemfibrozil (600 mg twice daily), an inhibitor of CYP2C8, and rosiglitazone (4 mg once daily) for 7 days increased rosiglitazone AUC by 2 fold, compared to the administration of rosiglitazone (4 mg once daily) alone. Given the potential for dose-related adverse events with rosiglitazone, a decrease in the dose of rosiglitazone may be needed when gemfibrozil is introduced.

Carcinogenesis, Mutagenesis, Impairment of Fertility: ***Carcinogenesis:*** A 2-year carcinogenicity study was conducted in Charles River CD-1 mice at doses of 0.4, 1.5, and 6 mg/kg/day in the diet (highest dose equivalent to approximately 12 times human AUC at the maximum recommended human daily dose). Sprague-Dawley rats were dosed for 2 years by oral gavage at doses of 0.05, 0.3, and 2 mg/kg/day (highest dose equivalent to approximately 10 and 20 times human AUC at the maximum recommended human daily dose for male and female rats, respectively).

Rosiglitazone was not carcinogenic in the mouse. There was an increase in incidence of adipose hyperplasia in the mouse at doses ≥1.5 mg/kg/day (approximately 2 times human AUC at the maximum recommended human daily dose). In rats, there was a significant increase in the incidence of benign adipose tissue tumors (lipomas) at doses ≥0.3 mg/kg/day (approximately 2 times human AUC at the maximum recommended human daily dose). These proliferative changes in both species are considered due to the persistent pharmacological overstimulation of adipose tissue.

Mutagenesis: Rosiglitazone was not mutagenic or clastogenic in the in vitro bacterial assays for gene mutation, the in vitro chromosome aberration test in human lymphocytes, the in vivo mouse micronucleus test, and the in vivo/in vitro rat UDS assay. There was a small (about 2-fold) increase in mutation in the in vitro mouse lymphoma assay in the presence of metabolic activation.

Impairment of Fertility: Rosiglitazone had no effects on mating or fertility of male rats given up to 40 mg/kg/day (approximately 116 times human AUC at the maximum recommended human daily dose). Rosiglitazone altered estrous cyclicity (2 mg/kg/day) and reduced fertility (40 mg/kg/day) of female rats in association with lower plasma levels of progesterone and estradiol (approximately 20 and 200 times human AUC at the maximum recommended human daily dose, respectively). No such effects were noted at 0.2 mg/kg/day (approximately 3 times human AUC at the maximum recommended human daily dose). In monkeys, rosiglitazone (0.6 and 4.6 mg/kg/day; approximately 3 and 15 times human AUC at the maximum recommended human daily dose, respectively) diminished the follicular phase rise in serum estradiol with consequential reduction in the luteinizing hormone surge, lower luteal phase progesterone levels, and amenorrhea. The mechanism for these effects appears to be direct inhibition of ovarian steroidogenesis.

Animal Toxicology: Heart weights were increased in mice (3 mg/kg/day), rats (5 mg/kg/day), and dogs (2 mg/kg/day) with rosiglitazone treatments (approximately 5, 22, and 2 times human AUC at the maximum recommended human daily dose, respectively). Morphometric measurement indicated that there was hypertrophy in cardiac ventricular tissues, which may be due to increased heart work as a result of plasma volume expansion.

Pregnancy: ***Pregnancy Category C:*** There was no effect on implantation or the embryo with rosiglitazone treatment during early pregnancy in rats, but treatment during mid-late gestation was associated with fetal death and growth retardation in both rats and rabbits. Teratogenicity was not observed at doses up to 3 mg/kg in rats and 100 mg/kg in rabbits (approximately 20 and 75 times human AUC at the maximum recommended human daily dose, respectively). Rosiglitazone caused placental pathology in rats (3 mg/kg/day). Treatment of rats during gestation through lactation reduced litter size, neonatal viability, and postnatal growth, with growth retardation reversible after puberty. For effects on the placenta, embryo/fetus, and offspring, the no-effect dose was 0.2 mg/kg/day in rats and 15 mg/kg/day in rabbits. These no-effect levels are approximately 4 times human AUC at the maximum recommended human daily dose.

There are no adequate and well-controlled studies in pregnant women. AVANDIA should not be used during pregnancy unless the potential benefit justifies the potential risk to the fetus.

Because current information strongly suggests that abnormal blood glucose levels during pregnancy are associated with a higher incidence of congenital anomalies as well as increased neonatal morbidity and mortality, most experts recommend that insulin monotherapy be used during pregnancy to maintain blood glucose levels as close to normal as possible.

Labor and Delivery: The effect of rosiglitazone on labor and delivery in humans is not known.

Nursing Mothers: Drug-related material was detected in milk from lactating rats. It is not known whether AVANDIA is excreted in human milk. Because many drugs are excreted in human milk, AVANDIA should not be administered to a nursing woman.

Pediatric Use: The safety and effectiveness of AVANDIA in pediatric patients have not been established.

Geriatric Use: Results of the population pharmacokinetic analysis showed that age does not significantly affect the pharmacokinetics of rosiglitazone (see CLINICAL PHARMACOLOGY, Special Populations). Therefore, no dosage adjustments are required for the elderly. In controlled clinical trials, no overall differences in safety and effectiveness between older (≥65 years) and younger (<65 years) patients were observed.

ADVERSE REACTIONS

In clinical trials, approximately 4,600 patients with type 2 diabetes have been treated with AVANDIA; 3,300 patients were treated for 6 months or longer and 2,000 patients were treated for 12 months or longer.

Trials of AVANDIA as Monotherapy and in Combination With Other Hypoglycemic Agents: The incidence and types of adverse events reported in clinical trials of AVANDIA as monotherapy are shown in Table 7.

[See table 7 below]

There were a small number of patients treated with AVANDIA who had adverse events of anemia and edema. Overall, these events were generally mild to moderate in severity and usually did not require discontinuation of treatment with AVANDIA.

In double-blind studies, anemia was reported in 1.9% of patients receiving AVANDIA compared to 0.7% on placebo, 0.6% on sulfonylureas, and 2.2% on metformin. Edema was reported in 4.8% of patients receiving AVANDIA compared to 1.3% on placebo, 1.0% on sulfonylureas, and 2.2% on metformin. Overall, the types of adverse experiences reported when AVANDIA was used in combination with a sulfonylurea or metformin were similar to those during monotherapy with AVANDIA. Reports of anemia (7.1%) were greater in patients treated with a combination of AVANDIA and metformin compared to monotherapy with AVANDIA or in combination with a sulfonylurea.

Lower pre-treatment hemoglobin/hematocrit levels in patients enrolled in the metformin combination clinical trials may have contributed to the higher reporting rate of anemia in these studies (see ADVERSE REACTIONS, Laboratory Abnormalities, *Hematologic*).

In 26-week double-blind, fixed-dose studies, edema was reported with higher frequency in the AVANDIA plus insulin combination trials (insulin, 5.4%; and AVANDIA in combination with insulin, 14.7%). Reports of new onset or exacerbation of congestive heart failure occurred at rates of 1% for insulin alone, and 2% (4 mg) and 3% (8 mg) for insulin in combination with AVANDIA (see WARNINGS, Cardiac Failure and Other Cardiac Effects).

In postmarketing experience with AVANDIA, adverse events potentially related to volume expansion (e.g., congestive heart failure, pulmonary edema, and pleural effusions) have been reported.

Hypoglycemia was the most frequently reported adverse event in the fixed-dose insulin combination trials, although few patients withdrew for hypoglycemia (4 of 408 for AVANDIA plus insulin and 1 of 203 for insulin alone). Rates of hypoglycemia, confirmed by capillary blood glucose concentration ≤50 mg/dL, were 6% for insulin alone and 12% (4 mg) and 14% (8 mg) for insulin in combination with AVANDIA.

Table 7. Adverse Events (≥5% in Any Treatment Group) Reported by Patients in Double-blind Clinical Trials With AVANDIA as Monotherapy

Preferred Term	AVANDIA Monotherapy N = 2,526	Placebo N = 601	Metformin N = 225	Sulfonylureas* N = 626
	%	%	%	%
Upper respiratory tract infection	9.9	8.7	8.9	7.3
Injury	7.6	4.3	7.6	6.1
Headache	5.9	5.0	8.9	5.4
Back pain	4.0	3.8	4.0	5.0
Hyperglycemia	3.9	5.7	4.4	8.1
Fatigue	3.6	5.0	4.0	1.9
Sinusitis	3.2	4.5	5.3	3.0
Diarrhea	2.3	3.3	15.6	3.0
Hypoglycemia	0.6	0.2	1.3	5.9

*Includes patients receiving glyburide (N = 514), gliclazide (N = 91) or glipizide (N = 21).

In postmarketing experience with AVANDIA, angioedema and urticaria have been reported rarely.

Laboratory Abnormalities: ***Hematologic:*** Decreases in mean hemoglobin and hematocrit occurred in a dose-related fashion in patients treated with AVANDIA (mean decreases in individual studies up to 1.0 gram/dL hemoglobin and up to 3.3% hematocrit). The time course and magnitude of decreases were similar in patients treated with a combination of AVANDIA and other hypoglycemic agents or AVANDIA monotherapy. Pre-treatment levels of hemoglobin and hematocrit were lower in patients in metformin combination studies and may have contributed to the higher reporting rate of anemia. White blood cell counts also decreased slightly in patients treated with AVANDIA. Decreases in hematologic parameters may be related to increased plasma volume observed with treatment with AVANDIA.

Lipids: Changes in serum lipids have been observed following treatment with AVANDIA (see CLINICAL STUDIES).

Serum Transaminase Levels: In clinical studies in 4,598 patients treated with AVANDIA encompassing approximately 3,600 patient years of exposure, there was no evidence of drug-induced hepatotoxicity or elevated ALT levels.

In controlled trials, 0.2% of patients treated with AVANDIA had reversible elevations in ALT >3× the upper limit of normal compared to 0.2% on placebo and 0.5% on active comparators. Hyperbilirubinemia was found in 0.3% of patients treated with AVANDIA compared with 0.9% treated with placebo and 1% in patients treated with active comparators.

In the clinical program including long-term, open-label experience, the rate per 100 patient years exposure of ALT increase to >3× the upper limit of normal was 0.35 for patients treated with AVANDIA, 0.59 for placebo-treated patients, and 0.78 for patients treated with active comparator agents.

In pre-approval clinical trials, there were no cases of idiosyncratic drug reactions leading to hepatic failure. In postmarketing experience with AVANDIA, reports of hepatic enzyme elevations 3 or more times the upper limit of normal and hepatitis have been received (see PRECAUTIONS, General, *Hepatic Effects*).

DOSAGE AND ADMINISTRATION

The management of antidiabetic therapy should be individualized. AVANDIA may be administered either at a starting dose of 4 mg as a single daily dose or divided and administered in the morning and evening. For patients who respond inadequately following 8 to 12 weeks of treatment, as determined by reduction in FPG, the dose may be increased to 8 mg daily as monotherapy or in combination with metformin. Reductions in glycemic parameters by dose and regimen are described under CLINICAL STUDIES. AVANDIA may be taken with or without food.

Monotherapy: The usual starting dose of AVANDIA is 4 mg administered either as a single dose once daily or in divided doses twice daily. In clinical trials, the 4 mg twice daily regimen resulted in the greatest reduction in FPG and HbA1c.

Combination Therapy: When AVANDIA is added to existing therapy, the current dose of a sulfonylurea, metformin, or insulin can be continued upon initiation of AVANDIA therapy.

Sulfonylurea: When used in combination with sulfonylurea, the recommended dose of AVANDIA is 4 mg administered as either a single dose once daily or in divided doses twice daily. If patients report hypoglycemia, the dose of the sulfonylurea should be decreased.

Metformin: The usual starting dose of AVANDIA in combination with metformin is 4 mg administered as either a single dose once daily or in divided doses twice daily. It is unlikely that the dose of metformin will require adjustment due to hypoglycemia during combination therapy with AVANDIA.

Insulin: For patients stabilized on insulin, the insulin dose should be continued upon initiation of therapy with AVANDIA. AVANDIA should be dosed at 4 mg daily. Doses of AVANDIA greater than 4 mg daily in combination with insulin are not currently indicated. It is recommended that the insulin dose be decreased by 10% to 25% if the patient reports hypoglycemia or if FPG concentrations decrease to less than 100 mg/dL. Further adjustments should be individualized based on glucose-lowering response.

Maximum Recommended Dose: The dose of AVANDIA should not exceed 8 mg daily, as a single dose or divided twice daily. The 8 mg daily dose has been shown to be safe and effective in clinical studies as monotherapy and in combination with metformin. Doses of AVANDIA greater than 4 mg daily in combination with a sulfonylurea have not been studied in adequate and well-controlled clinical trials. Doses of AVANDIA greater than 4 mg daily in combination with insulin are not currently indicated.

AVANDIA may be taken with or without food.

No dosage adjustments are required for the elderly.

No dosage adjustment is necessary when AVANDIA is used as monotherapy in patients with renal impairment. Since metformin is contraindicated in such patients, concomitant administration of metformin and AVANDIA is also contraindicated in patients with renal impairment.

Therapy with AVANDIA should not be initiated if the patient exhibits clinical evidence of active liver disease or increased serum transaminase levels (ALT >2.5× upper limit of normal at start of therapy) (see PRECAUTIONS, General, *Hepatic Effects* and CLINICAL PHARMACOLOGY, Special Populations, *Hepatic Impairment*). Liver enzyme

monitoring is recommended in all patients prior to initiation of therapy with AVANDIA and periodically thereafter (see PRECAUTIONS, General, *Hepatic Effects*).
There are no data on the use of AVANDIA in patients younger than 18 years; therefore, use of AVANDIA in pediatric patients is not recommended.

OVERDOSAGE

Limited data are available with regard to overdosage in humans. In clinical studies in volunteers, AVANDIA has been administered at single oral doses of up to 20 mg and was well-tolerated. In the event of an overdose, appropriate supportive treatment should be initiated as dictated by the patient's clinical status.

HOW SUPPLIED

Tablets: Each pentagonal film-coated TILTAB tablet contains rosiglitazone as the maleate as follows: 2 mg–pink, debossed with SB on one side and 2 on the other; 4 mg–orange, debossed with SB on one side and 4 on the other; 8 mg–red-brown, debossed with SB on one side and 8 on the other.
2 mg bottles of 30: NDC 0029-3158-13
2 mg bottles of 60: NDC 0029-3158-18
2 mg bottles of 100: NDC 0029-3158-20
2 mg bottles of 500: NDC 0029-3158-25
2 mg SUP 100s: NDC 0029-3158-21
4 mg bottles of 30: NDC 0029-3159-13
4 mg bottles of 60: NDC 0029-3159-18
4 mg bottles of 100: NDC 0029-3159-20
4 mg bottles of 500: NDC 0029-3159-25
4 mg SUP 100s: NDC 0029-3159-21
8 mg bottles of 30: NDC 0029-3160-13
8 mg bottles of 100: NDC 0029-3160-20
8 mg bottles of 500: NDC 0029-3160-25
8 mg SUP 100s: NDC 0029-3160-21

STORAGE

Store at 25°C (77°F); excursions 15°–30°C (59°–86°F). Dispense in a tight, light-resistant container.
GlaxoSmithKline, Research Triangle Park, NC 27709
AVANDIA and TILTAB are registered trademarks of GlaxoSmithKline.

August 2004/AV:L11
Shown in Product Identification Guide, page 314

AVODART™ ℞

[av' ō dart]
(dutasteride)
Soft Gelatin Capsules

DESCRIPTION

AVODART (dutasteride) is a synthetic 4-azasteroid compound that is a selective inhibitor of both the type 1 and type 2 isoforms of steroid 5α-reductase (5AR), an intracellular enzyme that converts testosterone to 5α-dihydrotestosterone (DHT).
Dutasteride is chemically designated as (5α,17β)-N-{2,5 bis-(trifluoromethyl)phenyl}-3-oxo-4-azaandrost-1-ene-17-carboxamide. The empirical formula of dutasteride is $C_{27}H_{30}F_6N_2O_2$, representing a molecular weight of 528.5.
Dutasteride is a white to pale yellow powder with a melting point of 242° to 250°C. It is soluble in ethanol (44 mg/mL), methanol (64 mg/mL) and polyethylene glycol 400 (3 mg/mL), but it is insoluble in water.
AVODART Soft Gelatin Capsules for oral administration contain 0.5 mg of the active ingredient dutasteride in yellow capsules with red print. Each capsule contains 0.5 mg dutasteride dissolved in a mixture of mono-di-glycerides of caprylic/capric acid and butylated hydroxytoluene. The inactive excipients in the capsule shell are gelatin (from certified BSE-free bovine sources), glycerin, and ferric oxide (yellow). The soft gelatin capsules are printed with edible red ink.

CLINICAL PHARMACOLOGY

Pharmacodynamics: *Mechanism of Action:* Dutasteride inhibits the conversion of testosterone to 5α-dihydrotestosterone (DHT). DHT is the androgen primarily responsible for the initial development and subsequent enlargement of the prostate gland. Testosterone is converted to DHT by the enzyme 5α-reductase, which exists as 2 isoforms, type 1 and type 2. The type 2 isoenzyme is primarily active in the reproductive tissues while the type 1 isoenzyme is also responsible for testosterone conversion in the skin and liver.
Dutasteride is a competitive and specific inhibitor of both type 1 and type 2 5α-reductase isoenzymes, with which it forms a stable enzyme complex. Dissociation from this complex has been evaluated under in vitro and in vivo conditions and is extremely slow. Dutasteride does not bind to the human androgen receptor.
Effect on DHT and Testosterone: The maximum effect of daily doses of dutasteride on the reduction of DHT is dose dependent and is observed within 1 to 2 weeks. After 1 and 2 weeks of daily dosing with dutasteride 0.5 mg, median serum DHT concentrations were reduced by 85% and 90%, respectively. In patients with BPH treated with dutasteride 0.5 mg/day for 2 years, the median decrease in serum DHT was 94% at 1 year and 93% at 2 years. The median increase in serum testosterone was 19% at both 1 and 2 years but remained within the physiologic range.
In BPH patients treated with 5 mg/day of dutasteride or placebo for up to 12 weeks prior to transurethral resection of the prostate, mean DHT concentrations in prostatic tissue were significantly lower in the dutasteride group compared with placebo (784 and 5,793 pg/g, respectively, $p<0.001$). Mean prostatic tissue concentrations of testosterone were significantly higher in the dutasteride group compared with placebo (2,073 and 93 pg/g, respectively, $p<0.001$).
Adult males with genetically inherited type 2 5α-reductase deficiency also have decreased DHT levels. These 5α-reductase deficient males have a small prostate gland throughout life and do not develop BPH. Except for the associated urogenital defects present at birth, no other clinical abnormalities related to 5α-reductase deficiency have been observed in these individuals.
Other Effects: Plasma lipid panel and bone mineral density were evaluated following 52 weeks of dutasteride 0.5 mg once daily in healthy volunteers. There was no change in bone mineral density as measured by dual energy x-ray absorptiometry (DEXA) compared with either placebo or baseline. In addition, the plasma lipid profile (i.e., total cholesterol, low density lipoproteins, high density lipoproteins, and triglycerides) was unaffected by dutasteride. No clinically significant changes in adrenal hormone responses to ACTH stimulation were observed in a subset population (n = 13) of the one-year healthy volunteer study.
Pharmacokinetics: *Absorption:* Following administration of a single 0.5-mg dose of a soft gelatin capsule, time to peak serum concentrations (T_{max}) of dutasteride occurs within 2 to 3 hours. Absolute bioavailability in 5 healthy subjects is approximately 60% (range 40% to 94%). When the drug is administered with food, the maximum serum concentrations were reduced by 10% to 15%. This reduction is of no clinical significance.
Distribution: Pharmacokinetic data following single and repeat oral doses show that dutasteride has a large volume of distribution (300 to 500 L). Dutasteride is highly bound to plasma albumin (99.0%) and alpha-1 acid glycoprotein (96.6%).
In a study of healthy subjects (n = 26) receiving dutasteride 0.5 mg/day for 12 months, semen dutasteride concentrations averaged 3.4 ng/mL (range 0.4 to 14 ng/mL) at 12 months and, similar to serum, achieved steady-state concentrations at 6 months. On average, at 12 months, 11.5% of serum dutasteride concentrations partitioned into semen.
Metabolism and Elimination: Dutasteride is extensively metabolized in humans. While not all metabolic pathways have been identified, in vitro studies showed that dutasteride is metabolized by the CYP3A4 isoenzyme to 2 minor mono-hydroxylated metabolites. Dutasteride is not metabolized in vitro by human cytochrome P450 isoenzymes CYP1A2, CYP2C9, CYP2C19, and CYP2D6 at 2,000 ng/mL (50-fold greater than steady-state serum concentrations). In human serum, following dosing to steady state, unchanged dutasteride, 3 major metabolites (4'-hydroxydutasteride, 1,2-dihydrodutasteride, and 6-hydroxydutasteride), and 2 minor metabolites (6,4'-dihydroxydutasteride and 15-hydroxydutasteride), as assessed by mass spectrometric response, have been detected. The absolute stereochemistry of the hydroxyl additions in the 6 and 15 positions is not known. In vitro, the 4'-hydroxydutasteride and 1,2-dihydrodutasteride metabolites are much less potent than dutasteride against both isoforms of human 5AR. The activity of 6β-hydroxydutasteride is comparable to that of dutasteride.
Dutasteride and its metabolites were excreted mainly in feces. As a percent of dose, there was approximately 5% unchanged dutasteride (~1% to ~15%) and 40% as dutasteride-related metabolites (~2% to ~90%). Only trace amounts of unchanged dutasteride were found in urine (<1%). Therefore, on average, the dose unaccounted for approximated 55% (range 5% to 97%).
The terminal elimination half-life of dutasteride is approximately 5 weeks at steady state. The average steady-state serum dutasteride concentration was 40 ng/mL following 0.5 mg/day for 1 year. Following daily dosing, dutasteride serum concentrations achieve 65% of steady-state concentration after 1 month and approximately 90% after 3 months. Due to the long half-life of dutasteride, serum concentrations remain detectable (greater than 0.1 ng/mL) for up to 4 to 6 months after discontinuation of treatment.
Special Populations: *Pediatric:* Dutasteride pharmacokinetics have not been investigated in subjects less than 18 years of age.
Geriatric: No dose adjustment is necessary in the elderly. The pharmacokinetics and pharmacodynamics of dutasteride were evaluated in 36 healthy male subjects between the ages of 24 and 87 years following administration of a single 5-mg dose of dutasteride. In this single-dose study, dutasteride half-life increased with age (approximately 170 hours in men 20 to 49 years of age, approximately 260 hours in men 50 to 69 years of age, and approximately 300 hours in men over 70 years of age). Of 2,167 men treated with dutasteride in the 3 pivotal studies, 60% were age 65 and over and 15% were age 75 and over. No overall differences in safety or efficacy were observed between these patients and younger patients.
Gender: AVODART is not indicated for use in women (see WARNINGS and PRECAUTIONS). The pharmacokinetics of dutasteride in women have not been studied.
Race: The effect of race on dutasteride pharmacokinetics has not been studied.
Renal Impairment: The effect of renal impairment on dutasteride pharmacokinetics has not been studied. However, less than 0.1% of a steady-state 0.5-mg dose of dutasteride is recovered in human urine, so no adjustment in dosage is anticipated for patients with renal impairment.
Hepatic Impairment: The effect of hepatic impairment on dutasteride pharmacokinetics has not been studied. Because dutasteride is extensively metabolized, exposure could be higher in hepatically impaired patients (see PRECAUTIONS: Use in Hepatic Impairment).
Drug Interactions: In vitro drug metabolism studies reveal that dutasteride is metabolized by human cytochrome P450 isoenzyme CYP3A4. In a human mass balance analysis (n = 8), dutasteride was extensively metabolized. Less than 20% of the dose was excreted unchanged in the feces. No clinical drug interaction studies have been performed to evaluate the impact of CYP3A4 enzyme inhibitors on dutasteride pharmacokinetics. However, based on the in vitro data, blood concentrations of dutasteride may increase in the presence of inhibitors of CYP3A4 such as ritonavir, ketoconazole, verapamil, diltiazem, cimetidine, and ciprofloxacin. Dutasteride is not metabolized in vitro by human cytochrome P450 isoenzymes CYP1A2, CYP2C9, CYP2C19, and CYP2D6 at 2,000 ng/mL (50-fold greater than steady-state serum concentrations).
Clinical drug interaction studies have shown no pharmacokinetic or pharmacodynamic interactions between dutasteride and tamsulosin, terazosin, warfarin, digoxin, and cholestyramine (see PRECAUTIONS: Drug Interactions).
Dutasteride does not inhibit the in vitro metabolism of model substrates for the major human cytochrome P450 isoenzymes (CYP1A2, CYP2C9, CYP2C19, CYP2D6, and CYP3A4) at a concentration of 1,000 ng/mL, 25 times greater than steady-state serum concentrations in humans.

CLINICAL STUDIES

Dutasteride 0.5 mg/day (n = 2,167) or placebo (n = 2,158) was evaluated in male subjects with BPH in three 2-year multicenter, placebo-controlled, double-blind studies, each with 2-year open-label extensions. Data from the first 24 months of the trials are presented. More than 90% of the study population was Caucasian. Subjects were at least 50 years of age with a serum PSA ≥1.5 ng/mL and <10 ng/mL, and BPH diagnosed by medical history and physical examination, including enlarged prostate (≥30 cc) and BPH symptoms that were moderate to severe according to the American Urological Association Symptom Index (AUA-SI). Most of the 4,325 subjects randomly assigned to receive either dutasteride or placebo completed 2 years of treatment (70% and 67%, respectively).
Effect on Symptom Scores: Symptoms were quantified using the AUA-SI, a questionnaire that evaluates urinary symptoms (incomplete emptying, frequency, intermittency, urgency, weak stream, straining, and nocturia) by rating on a 0 to 5 scale for a total possible score of 35. The baseline AUA-SI score across the 3 studies was approximately 17 units in both treatment groups.
Subjects receiving dutasteride achieved statistically significant improvement in symptoms versus placebo by Month 3 in one study, and by Month 12 in the other 2 pivotal studies. At Month 12, the mean decrease from baseline in AUA-SI symptom scores across the 3 studies pooled was −3.3 units for dutasteride and −2.0 units for placebo with a mean difference between the 2 treatment groups of −1.3 (range, −1.1 to −1.5 units in each of the 3 studies, $p<0.001$) and was consistent across the 3 studies. At Month 24, the mean decrease from baseline was −3.8 units for dutasteride and −1.7 units for placebo with a mean difference of −2.1 (range, −1.9 to −2.2 units in each of the 3 studies, $p<0.001$). See Figure 1.
These studies were prospectively designed to evaluate effects on symptoms based on prostate size at baseline. In men with prostate volumes ≥40 cc, the mean decrease was −3.8 units for dutasteride and −1.6 units for placebo with a mean difference between the 2 treatment groups of −2.2 at Month 24. In men with prostate volumes <40 cc, the mean decrease was −3.7 units for dutasteride and −2.2 units for placebo with a mean difference between the 2 treatment groups of −1.5 at Month 24.

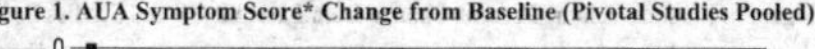
Figure 1. AUA Symptom Score* Change from Baseline (Pivotal Studies Pooled)

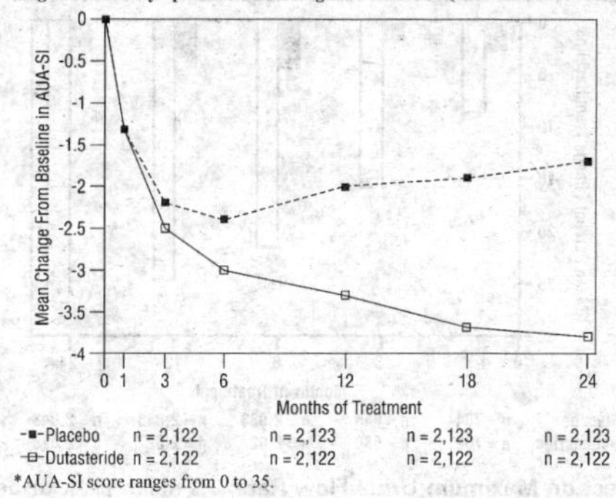

*AUA-SI score ranges from 0 to 35.

Continued on next page

Product information on these pages is effective as of August 2004. Further information is available at: GlaxoSmithKline, PO Box 13398, Research Triangle Park, NC 27709. 1-888-825-5249. Corporate Web Site: www.gsk.com

Avodart—Cont.

Effect on Acute Urinary Retention and the Need for Surgery: Efficacy was also assessed after 2 years of treatment by the incidence of acute urinary retention requiring catheterization and BPH-related urological surgical intervention. Compared with placebo, AVODART was associated with a statistically significantly lower incidence of acute urinary retention (1.8% for AVODART vs. 4.2% for placebo, $p<0.001$; 57% reduction in risk, 95% CI: [38–71%]) and with a statistically significantly lower incidence of surgery (2.2% for AVODART vs. 4.1% for placebo, $p<0.001$; 48% reduction in risk, 95% CI: [26–63%]). See Figures 2 and 3.

Figure 2. Percent of Subjects Developing Acute Urinary Retention Over a 24-Month Period (Pivotal Studies Pooled)

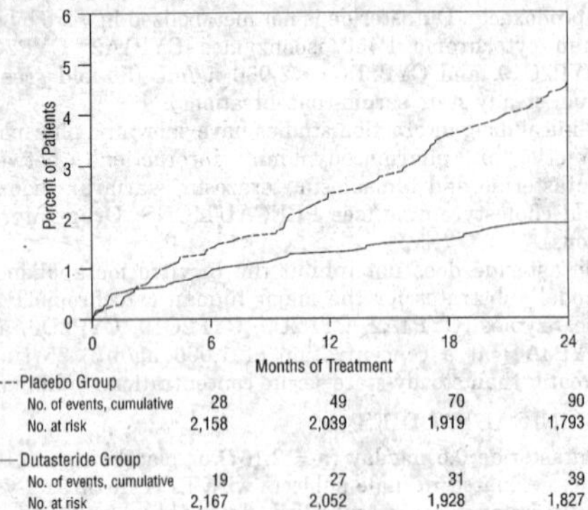

Figure 3. Percent of Subjects Having Surgery for BPH Over a 24-Month Period (Pivotal Studies Pooled)

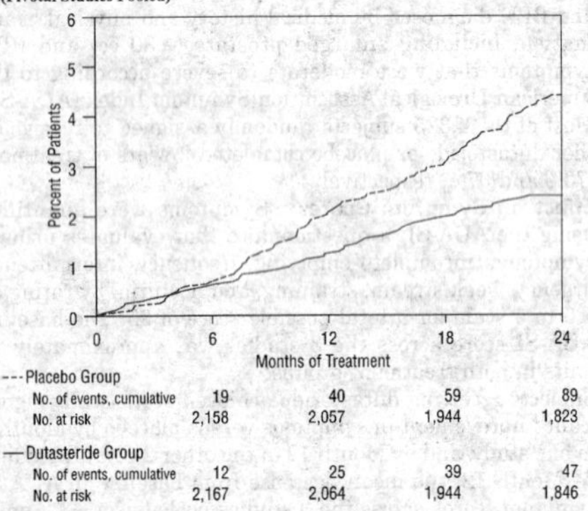

Effect on Prostate Volume: A prostate volume of at least 30 cc measured by transrectal ultrasound was required for study entry. The mean prostate volume at study entry was approximately 54 cc.

Statistically significant differences (dutasteride versus placebo) were noted at the earliest post-treatment prostate volume measurement in each study (Month 1, Month 3, or Month 6) and continued through Month 24. At Month 12, the mean percent change in prostate volume across the 3 studies pooled was −24.7% for dutasteride and −3.4% for placebo; the mean difference (dutasteride minus placebo) was −21.3% (range, −21.0% to −21.6% in each of the 3 studies, $p<0.001$). At Month 24, the mean percent change in prostate volume across the 3 studies pooled was −26.7% for dutasteride and −2.2% for placebo with a mean difference of −24.5% (range −24.0% to −25.1% in each of the 3 studies, $p<0.001$). See Figure 4.

Figure 4. Prostate Volume Percent Change from Baseline (Pivotal Studies Pooled)

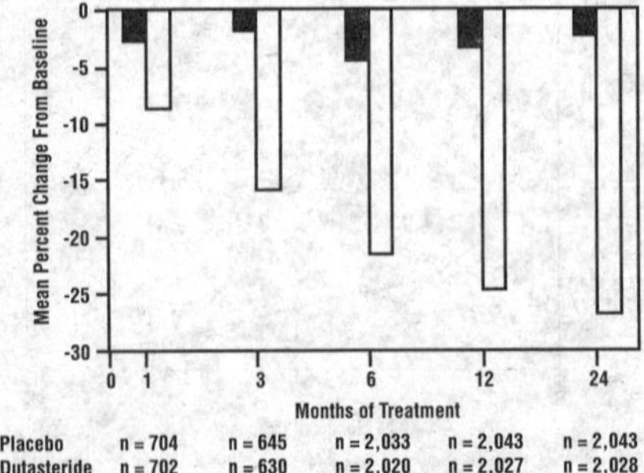

Effect on Maximum Urine Flow Rate: A mean peak urine flow rate (Q_{max}) of ≤15 mL/sec was required for study entry. Q_{max} was approximately 10 mL/sec at baseline across the 3 pivotal studies.

Differences between the 2 groups were statistically significant from baseline at Month 3 in all 3 studies and were maintained through Month 12. At Month 12, the mean increase in Q_{max} across the 3 studies pooled was 1.6 mL/sec for dutasteride and 0.7 mL/sec for placebo; the mean difference (dutasteride minus placebo) was 0.8 mL/sec (range, 0.7 to 1.0 mL/sec in each of the 3 studies, $p<0.001$). At Month 24, the mean increase in Q_{max} was 1.8 mL/sec for dutasteride and 0.7 mL/sec for placebo, with a mean difference of 1.1 mL/sec (range, 1.0 to 1.2 mL/sec in each of the 3 studies, $p<0.001$). See Figure 5.

Figure 5. Q_{max} Change from Baseline (Pivotal Studies Pooled)

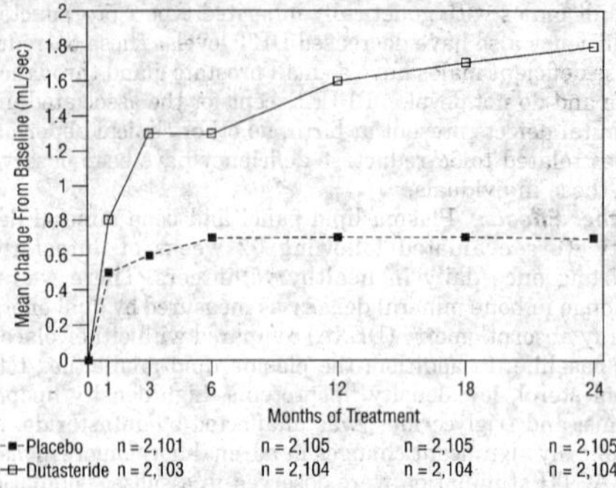

Summary of Clinical Studies: Data from 3 large, well-controlled efficacy studies demonstrate that treatment with AVODART (0.5 mg once daily) reduces the risk of both AUR and BPH-related surgical intervention relative to placebo, improves BPH-related symptoms, decreases prostate volume, and increases maximum urinary flow rates. These data suggest that AVODART arrests the disease process of BPH in men with an enlarged prostate.

INDICATIONS AND USAGE

AVODART is indicated for the treatment of symptomatic benign prostatic hyperplasia (BPH) in men with an enlarged prostate to:

- Improve symptoms
- Reduce the risk of acute urinary retention
- Reduce the risk of the need for BPH-related surgery

CONTRAINDICATIONS

AVODART is contraindicated for use in women and children.

AVODART is contraindicated for patients with known hypersensitivity to dutasteride, other 5α-reductase inhibitors, or any component of the preparation.

WARNINGS

Exposure of Women—Risk to Male Fetus: Dutasteride is absorbed through the skin. Therefore, women who are pregnant or may be pregnant should not handle AVODART Soft Gelatin Capsules because of the possibility of absorption of dutasteride and the potential risk of a fetal anomaly to a male fetus (see CONTRAINDICATIONS). In addition, women should use caution whenever handling AVODART Soft Gelatin Capsules. If contact is made with leaking capsules, the contact area should be washed immediately with soap and water.

PRECAUTIONS

General: Lower urinary tract symptoms of BPH can be indicative of other urological diseases, including prostate cancer. Patients should be assessed to rule out other urological diseases prior to treatment with AVODART. Patients with a large residual urinary volume and/or severely diminished urinary flow may not be good candidates for 5α-reductase inhibitor therapy and should be carefully monitored for obstructive uropathy.

Blood Donation: Men being treated with dutasteride should not donate blood until at least 6 months have passed following their last dose. The purpose of this deferred period is to prevent administration of dutasteride to a pregnant female transfusion recipient.

Use in Hepatic Impairment: The effect of hepatic impairment on dutasteride pharmacokinetics has not been studied. Because dutasteride is extensively metabolized and has a half-life of approximately 5 weeks at steady state, caution should be used in the administration of dutasteride to patients with liver disease.

Use with Potent CYP3A4 Inhibitors: Although dutasteride is extensively metabolized, no metabolically based drug interaction studies have been conducted. The effect of potent CYP3A4 inhibitors has not been studied. Because of the potential for drug-drug interactions, care should be taken when administering dutasteride to patients taking potent, chronic CYP3A4 enzyme inhibitors (e.g., ritonavir).

Effects on PSA and Prostate Cancer Detection: Digital rectal examinations, as well as other evaluations for prostate cancer, should be performed on patients with BPH prior to initiating therapy with AVODART and periodically thereafter.

Dutasteride reduces total serum PSA concentration by approximately 40% following 3 months of treatment and approximately 50% following 6, 12, and 24 months of treatment. This decrease is predictable over the entire range of PSA values, although it may vary in individual patients. Therefore, for interpretation of serial PSAs in a man taking AVODART, a new baseline PSA concentration should be established after 3 to 6 months of treatment, and this new value should be used to assess potentially cancer-related changes in PSA. To interpret an isolated PSA value in a man treated with AVODART for 6 months or more, the PSA value should be doubled for comparison with normal values in untreated men.

Information for Patients: Physicians should instruct their patients to read the Patient Information leaflet before starting therapy with AVODART and to reread it upon prescription renewal for new information regarding the use of AVODART.

AVODART Soft Gelatin Capsules should not be handled by a woman who is pregnant or who may become pregnant because of the potential for absorption of dutasteride and the subsequent potential risk to a developing male fetus (see CONTRAINDICATIONS and WARNINGS: Exposure of Women—Risk to Male Fetus).

Physicians should inform patients that ejaculate volume might be decreased in some patients during treatment with AVODART. This decrease does not appear to interfere with normal sexual function. In clinical trials, impotence and decreased libido, considered by the investigator to be drug-related, occurred in a small number of patients treated with AVODART or placebo (see ADVERSE REACTIONS, Table 1).

Men treated with dutasteride should not donate blood until at least 6 months have passed following their last dose to prevent pregnant women from receiving dutasteride through blood transfusion (see PRECAUTIONS: Blood Donation).

Drug Interactions: Care should be taken when administering dutasteride to patients taking potent, chronic CYP3A4 inhibitors (see PRECAUTIONS: Use with Potent CYP3A4 Inhibitors).

Dutasteride does not inhibit the in vitro metabolism of model substrates for the major human cytochrome P450 isoenzymes (CYP1A2, CYP2C9, CYP2C19, CYP2D6, and CYP3A4) at a concentration of 1,000 ng/mL, 25 times greater than steady-state serum concentrations in humans. In vitro studies demonstrate that dutasteride does not displace warfarin, diazepam, or phenytoin from plasma protein binding sites, nor do these model compounds displace dutasteride.

Digoxin: In a study of 20 healthy volunteers, AVODART did not alter the steady-state pharmacokinetics of digoxin when administered concomitantly at a dose of 0.5 mg/day for 3 weeks.

Warfarin: In a study of 23 healthy volunteers, 3 weeks of treatment with AVODART 0.5 mg/day did not alter the steady-state pharmacokinetics of the S- or R-warfarin isomers or alter the effect of warfarin on prothrombin time when administered with warfarin.

Alpha Adrenergic Blocking Agents: In a single sequence, cross-over study in healthy volunteers, the administration of tamsulosin or terazosin in combination with AVODART had no effect on the steady-state pharmacokinetics of either alpha adrenergic blocker. The percent change in DHT concentrations was similar for AVODART alone compared with the combination treatment.

A clinical trial was conducted in which dutasteride and tamsulosin were administered concomitantly for 24 weeks followed by 12 weeks of treatment with either the dutasteride and tamsulosin combination or dutasteride monotherapy. Results from the second phase of the trial revealed no excess of serious adverse events or discontinuations due to adverse events in the combination group compared to the dutasteride monotherapy group.

Calcium Channel Antagonists: In a population PK analysis, a decrease in clearance of dutasteride was noted when co-administered with the CYP3A4 inhibitors verapamil (−37%, n = 6) and diltiazem (−44%, n = 5). In contrast, no decrease in clearance was seen when amlodipine, another calcium channel antagonist that is not a CYP3A4 inhibitor, was co-administered with dutasteride (+7%, n = 4).

The decrease in clearance and subsequent increase in exposure to dutasteride in the presence of verapamil and diltiazem is not considered to be clinically significant. No dose adjustment is recommended.

Cholestyramine: Administration of a single 5-mg dose of AVODART followed 1 hour later by 12 g cholestyramine did not affect the relative bioavailability of dutasteride in 12 normal volunteers.

Other Concomitant Therapy: Although specific interaction studies were not performed with other compounds, approximately 90% of the subjects in the 3 Phase III pivotal efficacy studies receiving AVODART were taking other medications concomitantly. No clinically significant adverse interactions could be attributed to the combination of AVODART and concurrent therapy when AVODART was co-administered with anti-hyperlipidemics, angiotensin-converting enzyme (ACE) inhibitors, beta-adrenergic blocking agents, calcium channel blockers, corticosteroids, diuretics, nonsteroidal anti-inflammatory drugs (NSAIDs), phosphodiesterase Type V inhibitors, and quinolone antibiotics.

Drug/Laboratory Test Interactions: *Effects on PSA:* PSA levels generally decrease in patients treated with AVODART as the prostate volume decreases. In approximately one-half of the subjects, a 20% decrease in PSA is seen within the first month of therapy. After 6 months of therapy, PSA levels stabilize to a new baseline that is approximately 50% of the pre-treatment value. Results of subjects treated with AVODART for up to 2 years indicate this 50% reduction in PSA is maintained. Therefore, a new baseline PSA concentration should be established after 3 to 6 months of treatment with AVODART (see PRECAUTIONS: Effects on PSA and Prostate Cancer Detection).

Hormone Levels: In healthy volunteers, 52 weeks of treatment with dutasteride 0.5 mg/day (n = 26) resulted in no clinically significant change compared with placebo (n = 23) in sex hormone binding globulin, estradiol, luteinizing hormone, follicle-stimulating hormone, thyroxine (free T4), and dehydroepiandrosterone. Statistically significant, baseline-adjusted mean increases compared with placebo were observed for total testosterone at 8 weeks (97.1 ng/dL, $p<0.003$) and thyroid-stimulating hormone (TSH) at 52 weeks (0.4 mcIU/mL, $p<0.05$). The median percentage changes from baseline within the dutasteride group were 17.9% for testosterone at 8 weeks and 12.4% for TSH at 52 weeks. The mean levels of testosterone and TSH had returned to baseline at the 24-week post-treatment follow-up period in the group of subjects with available data at the visit. In BPH patients treated with dutasteride in a large Phase III trial, there was a median percent increase in luteinizing hormone of 12% at 6 months and 19% at both 12 and 24 months.

Reproductive Function: The effects of dutasteride 0.5 mg/day on reproductive function were evaluated in normal volunteers aged 18 to 52 (n = 26) throughout 52 weeks of treatment. Semen characteristics were evaluated at 3 timepoints and indicated no clinically meaningful changes in sperm concentration, sperm motility, or sperm morphology. A 0.8 mL (25%) mean decrease in ejaculate volume with a concomitant reduction in total sperm per ejaculate was observed at 52 weeks, but remained within the normal range. At the 24-week post-treatment follow-up visit, mean values for both parameters had returned to baseline in the group of subjects with available data at that visit.

CNS Toxicity: In rats and dogs, repeated oral administration of dutasteride resulted in some animals showing signs of non-specific, reversible, centrally mediated toxicity, without associated histopathological changes at exposure 425- and 315-fold the expected clinical exposure (of parent drug), respectively.

Carcinogenesis, Mutagenesis, Impairment of Fertility: ***Carcinogenesis:*** In a 2-year carcinogenicity study in B6C3F1 mice, at doses of 3, 35, 250, and 500 mg/kg/day for males and 3, 35, and 250 mg/kg/day for females. An increased incidence of benign hepatocellular adenomas was noted at 250 mg/kg/day (290-fold the expected clinical exposure to a 0.5 mg daily dose) in females only. Two of the 3 major human metabolites have been detected in mice. The exposure to these metabolites in mice is either lower than in humans or is not known.

In a 2-year carcinogenicity study in Han Wistar rats, at doses of 1.5, 7.5, and 53 mg/kg/day for males and 0.8, 6.3, and 15 mg/kg/day for females there was an increase in Leydig cell adenomas in the testes at 53 mg/kg/day (135-fold the expected clinical exposure). An increased incidence of Leydig cell hyperplasia was present at 7.5 mg/kg/day (52-fold the expected clinical exposure) and 53 mg/kg/day in male rats. A positive correlation between proliferative changes in the Leydig cells and an increase in circulating luteinizing hormone levels has been demonstrated with 5α-reductase inhibitors and is consistent with an effect on the hypothalamic-pituitary-testicular axis following 5α-reductase inhibition. At tumorigenic doses in rats, luteinizing hormone levels in rats were increased by 167%. In this study, the major human metabolites were tested for carcinogenicity at approximately 1 to 3 times the expected clinical exposure.

Mutagenesis: Dutasteride was tested for genotoxicity in a bacterial mutagenesis assay (Ames test), a chromosomal aberration assay in CHO cells, and a micronucleus assay in rats. The results did not indicate any genotoxic potential of the parent drug. Two major human metabolites were also negative in either the Ames test or an abbreviated Ames test.

Impairment of Fertility: Treatment of sexually mature male rats with dutasteride at doses of 0.05, 10, 50, and 500 mg/kg/day (0.1 to 110-fold the expected clinical exposure of parent drug) for up to 31 weeks resulted in dose- and time-dependent decreases in fertility, reduced cauda epididymal (absolute) sperm counts but not sperm concentration (at 50 and 500 mg/kg/day), reduced weights of the epididymis, prostate and seminal vesicles, and microscopic changes in the male reproductive organs. The fertility effects were reversed by recovery week 6 at all doses, and sperm counts were normal at the end of a 14-week recovery period. The 5α-reductase-related changes consisted of cytoplasmic vacuolation of tubular epithelium in the epididymides and decreased cytoplasmic content of epithelium, consistent with decreased secretory activity in the prostate and seminal vesicles. The microscopic changes were no longer present at recovery week 14 in the low-dose group and were partly recovered in the remaining treatment groups. Low levels of dutasteride (0.6 to 17 ng/mL) were detected in the serum of untreated female rats mated to males dosed at 10, 50, or 500 mg/kg/day for 29 to 30 weeks.

In a fertility study in female rats, oral administration of dutasteride at doses of 0.05, 2.5, 12.5, and 30 mg/kg/day resulted in reduced litter size, increased embryo resorption and feminization of male fetuses (decreased anogenital distance) at doses of ≥2.5 mg/kg/day (2- to 10-fold the clinical exposure of parent drug in men). Fetal body weights were also reduced at ≥0.05 mg/kg/day in rats (<0.02-fold the human exposure).

Pregnancy: Pregnancy Category **X** (see CONTRAINDICATIONS). AVODART is contraindicated for use in women. AVODART has not been studied in women because preclinical data suggest that the suppression of circulating levels of dihydrotestosterone may inhibit the development of the external genital organs in a male fetus carried by a woman exposed to dutasteride.

Table 1. Drug-related Adverse Events* Reported in ≥1% Subjects Over a 24-Month Period and More Frequently in the Dutasteride Group than the Placebo Group (Pivotal Studies Pooled)

	Adverse Event Onset			
Adverse Events Dutasteride (n) Placebo (n)	Month 0–6 (n = 2,167) (n = 2,158)	Month 7–12 (n = 1,901) (n = 1,922)	Month 13–18 (n = 1,725) (n = 1,714)	Month 19–24 (n = 1,605) (n = 1,555)
Impotence				
Dutasteride	4.7%	1.4%	1.0%	0.8%
Placebo	1.7%	1.5%	0.5%	0.9%
Decreased libido				
Dutasteride	3.0%	0.7%	0.3%	0.3%
Placebo	1.4%	0.6%	0.2%	0.1%
Ejaculation disorder				
Dutasteride	1.4%	0.5%	0.5%	0.1%
Placebo	0.5%	0.3%	0.1%	0.0%
Gynecomastia†				
Dutasteride	0.5%	0.8%	1.1%	0.6%
Placebo	0.2%	0.3%	0.3%	0.1%

*** A drug-related adverse event is one considered by the investigator to have a reasonable possibility of being caused by the study medication. In assessing causality, investigators were asked to select from one of two options: reasonably related to study medication or unrelated to study medication.**

† Includes breast tenderness and breast enlargement.

In an intravenous embryo-fetal development study in the rhesus monkey (12/group), administration of dutasteride at 400, 780, 1,325, or 2,010 ng/day on gestation days 20 to 100 did not adversely affect development of male external genitalia. Reduction of fetal adrenal weights, reduction in fetal prostate weights, and increases in fetal ovarian and testis weights were observed in monkeys treated with the highest dose. Based on the highest measured semen concentration of dutasteride in treated men (14 ng/mL), these doses represent 0.8 to 16 times based on blood levels of parent drug (32 to 186 times based on a ng/kg daily dose) the potential maximum exposure of a 50-kg human female to 5 mL semen daily from a dutasteride-treated man, assuming 100% absorption. Dutasteride is highly bound to proteins in human semen (>96%), potentially reducing the amount of dutasteride available for vaginal absorption.

In an embryo-fetal development study in female rats, oral administration of dutasteride at doses of 0.05, 2.5, 12.5, and 30 mg/kg/day resulted in feminization of male fetuses (decreased anogenital distance) and male offspring (nipple development, hypospadias, and distended preputial glands) at all doses (0.07- to 111-fold the expected male clinical exposure). An increase in stillborn pups was observed at 30 mg/kg/day, and reduced fetal body weight was observed at doses ≥2.5 mg/kg/day (15- to 111-fold the expected clinical exposure). Increased incidences of skeletal variations considered to be delays in ossification associated with reduced body weight were observed at doses of 12.5 and 30 mg/kg/day (56- to 111-fold the expected clinical exposure).

In an oral pre- and post-natal development study in rats, dutasteride doses of 0.05, 2.5, 12.5, or 30 mg/kg/day were administered. Unequivocal evidence of feminization of the genitalia (i.e., decreased anogenital distance, increased incidence of hypospadias, nipple development) of F1 generation male offspring occurred at doses ≥2.5 mg/kg/day (14- to 90-fold the expected clinical exposure in men). At a daily dose of 0.05 mg/kg/day (0.05-fold the expected clinical exposure), evidence of feminization was limited to a small, but statistically significant, decrease in anogenital distance. Doses of 2.5 to 30 mg/kg/day resulted in prolonged gestation in the parental females and a decrease in time to vaginal patency for female offspring and decrease prostate and seminal vesicle weights in male offspring. Effects on newborn startle response were noted at doses greater than or equal to 12.5 mg/kg/day. Increased stillbirths were noted at 30 mg/kg/day.

Feminization of male fetuses is an expected physiological consequence of inhibition of the conversion of testosterone to DHT by 5α-reductase inhibitors. These results are similar to observations in male infants with genetic 5α-reductase deficiency.

In the rabbit, embryo-fetal study doses of 30, 100, and 200 mg/kg (28- to 93-fold the expected clinical exposure in men) were administered orally on days 7 to 29 of pregnancy to encompass the late period of external genitalia development. Histological evaluation of the genital papilla of fetuses revealed evidence of feminization of the male fetus at all doses. A second embryo-fetal study in rabbits at doses of 0.05, 0.4, 3.0, and 30 mg/kg/day (0.3- to 53-fold the expected clinical exposure) also produced evidence of feminization of the genitalia in male fetuses at all doses. It is not known whether rabbits or rhesus monkeys produce any of the major human metabolites.

Nursing Mothers: AVODART is not indicated for use in women. It is not known whether dutasteride is excreted in human breast milk.

Pediatric Use: AVODART is not indicated for use in the pediatric population. Safety and effectiveness in the pediatric population have not been established.

Geriatric Use: Of 2,167 male subjects treated with AVODART in 3 clinical studies, 60% were 65 and over and 15% were 75 and over. No overall differences in safety or efficacy were observed between these subjects and younger subjects. Other reported clinical experience has not identified differences in responses between the elderly and younger patients.

ADVERSE REACTIONS

Most adverse reactions were mild or moderate and generally resolved while on treatment in both the AVODART and placebo groups. The most common adverse events leading to withdrawal in both treatment groups were associated with the reproductive system.

Over 4,300 male subjects with BPH were randomly assigned to receive placebo or 0.5-mg daily doses of AVODART in 3 identical, placebo-controlled Phase III treatment studies. Of this group, 2,167 male subjects were exposed to AVODART, including 1,772 exposed for 1 year and 1,510 exposed for 2 years. The population was aged 47 to 94 years (mean age 66 years) and greater than 90% Caucasian. Over the 2-year treatment period, 376 subjects (9% of each treatment group) were withdrawn from the studies due to adverse experiences, most commonly associated with the reproductive system. Withdrawals due to adverse events considered by the investigator to have a reasonable possibility of being caused by the study medication occurred in 4% of the subjects receiving AVODART and in 3% of the subjects receiving placebo. Table 1 summarizes clinical adverse reactions that were reported by the investigator as drug-related in at least 1% of subjects receiving AVODART and at a higher incidence than subjects receiving placebo.

[See table 1 above]

Long-Term Treatment: The incidence of most drug-related sexual adverse events (impotence, decreased libido and ejaculation disorder) decreased with duration of treatment. The incidence of drug-related gynecomastia remained constant over the treatment period (see Table 1). The relationship between long-term use of dutasteride and male breast neoplasia is currently unknown.

OVERDOSAGE

In volunteer studies, single doses of dutasteride up to 40 mg (80 times the therapeutic dose) for 7 days have been administered without significant safety concerns. In a clinical study, daily doses of 5 mg (10 times the therapeutic dose) were administered to 60 subjects for 6 months with no additional adverse effects to those seen at therapeutic doses of 0.5 mg.

There is no specific antidote for dutasteride. Therefore, in cases of suspected overdosage symptomatic and supportive treatment should be given as appropriate, taking the long half-life of dutasteride into consideration.

DOSAGE AND ADMINISTRATION

The recommended dose of AVODART is 1 capsule (0.5 mg) taken orally once a day. The capsules should be swallowed whole. AVODART may be administered with or without food.

No dosage adjustment is necessary for subjects with renal impairment or for the elderly (see CLINICAL PHARMACOLOGY: Pharmacokinetics: Geriatric and Renal Impairment). Due to the absence of data in patients with hepatic impairment, no dosage recommendation can be made (see PRECAUTIONS: General).

HOW SUPPLIED

AVODART Soft Gelatin Capsules 0.5 mg are oblong, opaque, dull yellow, gelatin capsules imprinted with "GX CE2" in red ink on one side packaged in bottles of 30 (NDC

Continued on next page

Product information on these pages is effective as of August 2004. Further information is available at: GlaxoSmithKline, PO Box 13398, Research Triangle Park, NC 27709. 1-888-825-5249. Corporate Web Site: www.gsk.com

Avodart—Cont.

0173-0712-15), 100 (NDC 0173-0712-00) with child-resistant closures, and unit dose blister packs of 70 capsules (NDC 0173-0712-01).

Storage and Handling: Store at 25°C (77°F); excursions permitted to 15–30°C (59–86°F) [see USP Controlled Room Temperature].

Dutasteride is absorbed through the skin. AVODART Soft Gelatin capsules should not be handled by women who are pregnant or who may become pregnant because of the potential for absorption of dutasteride and the subsequent potential risk to a developing male fetus (see CLINICAL PHARMACOLOGY: Pharmacokinetics, WARNINGS: Exposure of Women—Risk to Male Fetus, and PRECAUTIONS: Information for Patients and Pregnancy).

Manufactured by: RP Scherer, Beinheim, France for GlaxoSmithKline, Research Triangle Park, NC 27709

July 2003/RL-1180

Shown in Product Identification Guide, page 314

BACTROBAN CREAM® ℞

[bac'trō ban]

brand of mupirocin calcium cream, 2%

For Dermatologic Use

DESCRIPTION

Bactroban Cream (mupirocin calcium cream), 2% contains the dihydrate crystalline calcium hemi-salt of the antibiotic mupirocin. Chemically, it is (α*E*,2*S*,3*R*,4*R*,5*S*)-5-[(2*S*,3*S*,4*S*,5*S*)-2,3-Epoxy-5-hydroxy-4-methylhexyl]tetrahydro-3,4-dihydroxy-β-methyl-2*H*-pyran-2-crotonic acid, ester with 9-hydroxynonanoic acid, calcium salt (2:1), dihydrate.

The molecular formula of mupirocin calcium is $(C_{26}H_{43}O_9)_2Ca \bullet 2H_2O$, and the molecular weight is 1075.3. The molecular weight of mupirocin free acid is 500.6.

Bactroban Cream is a white cream that contains 2.15% w/w mupirocin calcium (equivalent to 2.0% mupirocin free acid) in an oil and water-based emulsion. The inactive ingredients are benzyl alcohol, cetomacrogol 1000, cetyl alcohol, mineral oil, phenoxyethanol, purified water, stearyl alcohol and xanthan gum.

CLINICAL PHARMACOLOGY

Pharmacokinetics

Systemic absorption of mupirocin through intact human skin is minimal. The systemic absorption of mupirocin was studied following application of *Bactroban Cream* three times a day for 5 days to various skin lesions (greater than 10 cm in length or 100 cm² in area) in 16 adults (aged 29 to 60 years) and 10 children (aged 3 to 12 years). Some systemic absorption was observed as evidenced by the detection of the metabolite, monic acid, in urine. Data from this study indicated more frequent occurrence of percutaneous absorption in children (90% of patients) compared to adults (44% of patients). However, the observed urinary concentrations in children (0.07 - 1.3 µg/mL [1 pediatric patient had no detectable level]) are within the observed range (0.08 - 10.03 µg/mL [9 adults had no detectable level]) in the adult population. In general, the degree of percutaneous absorption following multiple dosing appears to be minimal in adults and children. Any mupirocin reaching the systemic circulation is rapidly metabolized, predominantly to inactive monic acid, which is eliminated by renal excretion.

Microbiology

Mupirocin is an antibacterial agent produced by fermentation using the organism *Pseudomonas fluorescens*. It is active against a wide range of gram-positive bacteria including methicillin-resistant *Staphylococcus aureus* (MRSA). It is also active against certain gram-negative bacteria. Mupirocin inhibits bacterial protein synthesis by reversibly and specifically binding to bacterial isoleucyl transfer-RNA synthetase. Due to this unique mode of action, mupirocin demonstrates no *in vitro* cross-resistance with other classes of antimicrobial agents.

Resistance occurs rarely. However, when mupirocin resistance does occur, it appears to result from the production of a modified isoleucyl-tRNA synthetase. High-level plasmid-mediated resistance (MIC >1024 mcg/mL) has been reported in some strains of *S. aureus* and coagulase-negative staphylococci.

Mupirocin is bactericidal at concentrations achieved by topical application. However, the minimum bactericidal concentration (MBC) against relevant pathogens is generally eight-fold to thirty-fold higher than the minimum inhibitory concentration (MIC). In addition, mupirocin is highly protein bound (>97%), and the effect of wound secretions on the MICs of mupirocin has not been determined.

Mupirocin has been shown to be active against most strains of *Staphylococcus aureus* and *Streptococcus pyogenes*, both *in vitro* and in clinical studies. (See **INDICATIONS AND USAGE** section.) The following *in vitro* data are available, BUT THEIR CLINICAL SIGNIFICANCE IS UNKNOWN. Mupirocin is active against most strains of *Staphylococcus epidermidis* and *Staphylococcus saprophyticus.*

INDICATIONS AND USAGE

Bactroban Cream (mupirocin calcium cream), 2% is indicated for the treatment of secondarily infected traumatic skin lesions (up to 10 cm in length or 100 cm² in area) due to susceptible strains of *Staphylococcus aureus* and *Streptococcus pyogenes.*

CONTRAINDICATIONS

Bactroban Cream is contraindicated in patients with known hypersensitivity to any of the constituents of the product.

WARNINGS

Avoid contact with the eyes.

In the event of a sensitization or severe local irritation from *Bactroban Cream*, usage should be discontinued, and appropriate alternative therapy for the infection instituted.

PRECAUTIONS

General

As with other antibacterial products, prolonged use may result in overgrowth of nonsusceptible microorganisms, including fungi. (See **DOSAGE AND ADMINISTRATION**.)

Bactroban Cream is not formulated for use on mucosal surfaces.

Information for Patients

- Use this medication only as directed by your healthcare provider. It is for external use only. Avoid contact with the eyes.
- The treated area may be covered by gauze dressing if desired.
- Report to your healthcare provider any signs of local adverse reactions. The medication should be stopped and your healthcare provider contacted if irritation, severe itching or rash occurs.
- If no improvement is seen in 3 to 5 days, contact your healthcare provider.

Drug Interactions

The effect of the concurrent application of topical mupirocin calcium cream and other topical products has not been studied.

Carcinogenesis, Mutagenesis, Impairment of Fertility

Long-term studies in animals to evaluate carcinogenic potential of mupirocin calcium have not been conducted.

Results of the following studies performed with mupirocin calcium or mupirocin sodium *in vitro* and *in vivo* did not indicate a potential for mutagenicity: rat primary hepatocyte unscheduled DNA synthesis, sediment analysis for DNA strand breaks, *Salmonella* reversion test (Ames), *Escherichia coli* mutation assay, metaphase analysis of human lymphocytes, mouse lymphoma assay, and bone marrow micronuclei assay in mice.

Fertility studies were performed in rats with mupirocin administered subcutaneously at doses up to 49 times a human topical dose of 1 gram/day (approximately 20 mg mupirocin per day) on a mg/m² basis and revealed no evidence of impaired fertility from mupirocin sodium.

Pregnancy

Teratogenic Effects. Pregnancy Category B. Teratology studies have been performed in rats and rabbits with mupirocin administered subcutaneously at doses up to 78 and 154 times, respectively, a human topical dose of 1 gram/day (approximately 20 mg mupirocin per day) on a mg/m² basis and revealed no evidence of harm to the fetus due to mupirocin. There are, however, no adequate and well-controlled studies in pregnant women. Because animal reproduction studies are not always predictive of human response, this drug should be used during pregnancy only if clearly needed.

Nursing Mothers

It is not known whether this drug is excreted in human milk. Because many drugs are excreted in human milk, caution should be exercised when *Bactroban Cream* is administered to a nursing woman.

Pediatric Use

The safety and effectiveness of *Bactroban Cream* have been established in the age groups 3 months to 16 years. Use of *Bactroban Cream* in these age groups is supported by evidence from adequate and well-controlled studies of *Bactroban Cream* in adults with additional data from 93 pediatric patients studied as part of the pivotal trials in adults. (See **CLINICAL STUDIES** section.)

Geriatric Use

In two well-controlled studies, 30 patients over 65 years old were treated with *Bactroban Cream.* No overall difference in the efficacy or safety of *Bactroban Cream* was observed in this patient population when compared to that observed in younger patients.

ADVERSE REACTIONS

In two randomized, double-blind, double-dummy trials, 339 patients were treated with topical *Bactroban Cream* plus oral placebo. Adverse events thought to be possibly or probably drug-related occurred in 28 (8.3%) patients. The incidence of those events that were reported in at least 1% of patients enrolled in these trials were: headache (1.7%), rash and nausea (1.1% each).

Other adverse events thought to be possibly or probably drug-related which occurred in less than 1% of patients were: abdominal pain, burning at application site, cellulitis, dermatitis, dizziness, pruritus, secondary wound infection, and ulcerative stomatitis.

In a supportive study in the treatment of secondarily infected eczema, 82 patients were treated with *Bactroban Cream.* The incidence of adverse events thought to be possibly or probably drug-related was as follows: nausea (4.9%), headache and burning at application site (3.6% each), pruritus (2.4%) and one report each of abdominal pain, bleeding secondary to eczema, pain secondary to eczema, hives, dry skin and rash.

OVERDOSAGE

Intravenous infusions of 252 mg, as well as single oral doses of 500 mg of mupirocin, have been well tolerated in healthy adult subjects. There is no information regarding overdose of *Bactroban Cream.*

DOSAGE AND ADMINISTRATION

A small amount of *Bactroban Cream* should be applied to the affected area three times daily for 10 days. The area treated may be covered with gauze dressing if desired. Patients not showing a clinical response within 3 to 5 days should be re-evaluated.

CLINICAL STUDIES

The efficacy of topical *Bactroban Cream* for the treatment of secondarily infected traumatic skin lesions (e.g., lacerations, sutured wounds and abrasions not more than 10 cm in length or 100 cm² in total area) was compared to that of oral cephalexin in two randomized, double-blind, double-dummy clinical trials. Clinical efficacy rates at follow-up in the per protocol populations (adults and pediatric patients included) were 96.1% for *Bactroban Cream* (n=231) and 93.1% for oral cephalexin (n=219). Pathogen eradication rates at follow-up in the per protocol populations were 100% for both *Bactroban Cream* and oral cephalexin.

Pediatrics

There were 93 pediatric patients aged 2 weeks to 16 years enrolled per protocol in the secondarily infected skin lesion studies, although only 3 were less than 2 years of age in the *Bactroban Cream* treated population. Patients were randomized to either 10 days of topical *Bactroban Cream* t.i.d. or 10 days of oral cephalexin (250 mg q.i.d. for patients >40 kg or 25 mg/kg/day oral suspension in four divided doses for patients ≤40 kg). Clinical efficacy at follow-up (7 to 12 days post-therapy) in the per protocol populations was 97.7% (43/44) for *Bactroban Cream* and 93.9% (46/49) for cephalexin. Only one adverse event (headache) was thought to be possibly or probably related to drug therapy in the *Bactroban Cream* intent-to-treat pediatric population of 70 children (1.4%).

HOW SUPPLIED

Bactroban Cream (mupirocin calcium cream), 2% is supplied in 15 gram and 30 gram tubes.

NDC 0029-1527-22 (15 gram tube)

NDC 0029-1527-25 (30 gram tube)

Store at or below 25°C (77°F). Do not freeze.

GlaxoSmithKline, Research Triangle Park, NC 27709

November 2001/BB:L4

Shown in Product Identification Guide, page 314

BACTROBAN NASAL® ℞

[bac'trō ban]

brand of mupirocin calcium ointment, 2%

for intranasal use only

DESCRIPTION

Bactroban Nasal (mupirocin calcium ointment), 2% contains the dihydrate crystalline calcium hemi-salt of the antibiotic mupirocin. Chemically, it is (α *E*,2*S*,3*R*,4*R*,5*S*)-5-[(2*S*,3*S*,4*S*,5*S*)-2,3-Epoxy-5-hydroxy-4-methylhexyl]tetrahydro-3,4-dihydroxy-β-methyl-2*H*-pyran-2-crotonic acid, ester with 9-hydroxynonanoic acid, calcium salt (2:1), dihydrate.

The molecular formula of mupirocin calcium is $(C_{26}H_{43}O_9)_2Ca \bullet 2H_2O$, and the molecular weight is 1075.3. The molecular weight of mupirocin free acid is 500.6.

Bactroban Nasal is a white to off-white ointment that contains 2.15% w/w mupirocin calcium (equivalent to 2.0% pure mupirocin free acid) in a soft white ointment base. The inactive ingredients are paraffin and a mixture of glycerin esters (Softisan® 649).

CLINICAL PHARMACOLOGY

Pharmacokinetics

Following single or repeated intranasal applications of 0.2 gram of *Bactroban Nasal* t.i.d. for 3 days to five healthy **adult** male subjects, no evidence of systemic absorption of mupirocin was demonstrated. The dosage regimen used in this study was for pharmacokinetic characterization only. (See **DOSAGE AND ADMINISTRATION** for proper clinical dosing information.)

In this study, the concentrations of mupirocin in urine and of monic acid in urine and serum were below the limit of determination of the assay for up to 72 hours after the applications. The lowest levels of determination of the assay used were 50 ng/mL of mupirocin in urine, 75 ng/mL of monic acid in urine, and 10 ng/mL of monic acid in serum. Based on the detectable limit of the urine assay for monic acid, one can extrapolate that a mean of 3.3% (range: 1.2-5.1%) of the applied dose could be systemically absorbed from the nasal mucosa of **adults.**

Data from a report of a pharmacokinetic study in neonates and premature infants indicate that, unlike in adults, significant systemic absorption occurred following intranasal administration of *Bactroban Nasal* in this population. **At this time, the pharmacokinetic properties of mupirocin following intranasal application of *Bactroban Nasal* have not been adequately characterized in neonates or other chil-**

dren less than 12 years of age, and in addition, the safety of the product in children less than 12 years of age has not been established.

The effect of the concurrent application of intranasal mupirocin calcium ointment, 2% with other intranasal products has not been studied. (See **PRECAUTIONS, Drug Interactions.**)

Following intravenous or oral administration, mupirocin is rapidly metabolized. The principal metabolite, monic acid, demonstrates no antibacterial activity. In a study conducted in seven healthy adult male subjects, the elimination half-life after intravenous administration of mupirocin was 20 to 40 minutes for mupirocin and 30 to 80 minutes for monic acid. Monic acid is predominantly eliminated by renal excretion. The pharmacokinetics of mupirocin has not been studied in individuals with renal insufficiency.

Microbiology

Mupirocin is an antibacterial agent produced by fermentation using the organism *Pseudomonas fluorescens.* Mupirocin inhibits bacterial protein synthesis by reversibly and specifically binding to bacterial isoleucyl transfer-RNA synthetase. Due to this mode of action, mupirocin demonstrates no *in vitro* cross-resistance with other classes of antimicrobial agents.

When mupirocin resistance does occur, it appears to result from the production of a modified isoleucyl-tRNA synthetase. High-level plasmid-mediated resistance (MIC >1024 mcg/mL) has been reported in some strains of *S. aureus* and coagulase-negative staphylococci.

Mupirocin is bactericidal at concentrations achieved topically by intranasal administration. However, the minimum bactericidal concentration (MBC) against relevant intranasal pathogens is generally eight-fold to thirty-fold higher than the minimum inhibitory concentration (MIC). In addition, mupirocin is highly protein bound (>97%), and the effect of nasal secretions on the MIC's of intranasally applied mupirocin has not been determined.

Mupirocin has been shown to be active against most strains of methicillin-resistant *S. aureus*, both *in vitro* and in clinical studies of the eradication of nasal colonization. *Bactroban Nasal* only has established clinical utility in nasal eradication as part of a comprehensive program to curtail institutional outbreaks of infections with methicillin-resistant *S. aureus.* (See **INDICATIONS AND USAGE.**)

The following *in vitro* data are available, **but their clinical significance is unknown**. Mupirocin exhibits *in vitro* MIC's of 1 mcg/mL or less against most (>90%) strains of methicillin-susceptible *S. aureus*; however, the safety and effectiveness of mupirocin calcium in eradicating nasal colonization of and preventing subsequent infections due to methicillin-susceptible *S. aureus* have not been established.

INDICATIONS AND USAGE

Bactroban Nasal (mupirocin calcium ointment), 2% is indicated for the eradication of nasal colonization with methicillin-resistant *Staphylococcus aureus* in adult patients and health care workers as part of a comprehensive infection control program to reduce the risk of infection among patients at high risk of methicillin-resistant *S. aureus* infection during institutional outbreaks of infections with this pathogen.

NOTE:

(1) There are insufficient data at this time to establish that this product is safe and effective as part of an intervention program to prevent autoinfection of high-risk patients from their own nasal colonization with *S. aureus*.

(2) There are insufficient data at this time to recommend use of *Bactroban Nasal* for general prophylaxis of any infection in any patient population.

(3) Greater than 90% of subjects/patients in clinical trials had eradication of nasal colonization 2 to 4 days after therapy was completed. Approximately 30% recolonization was reported in one domestic study within 4 weeks after completion of therapy. These eradication rates were clinically and statistically superior to those reported in subjects/patients in the vehicle-treated arms of the adequate and well-controlled studies. Those treated with vehicle had eradication rates of 5% to 30% at 2 to 4 days post-therapy with 85% to 100% recolonization within 4 weeks.

All adequate and well-controlled trials of this product were vehicle-controlled; therefore, no data from direct, head-to-head comparisons with other products are available at this time.

CONTRAINDICATIONS

Bactroban Nasal is contraindicated in patients with known hypersensitivity to any of the constituents of the product.

WARNINGS

AVOID CONTACT WITH THE EYES. Application of *Bactroban Nasal* to the eye under testing conditions has caused severe symptoms such as burning and tearing. These symptoms resolved within days to weeks after discontinuation of the ointment.

In the event of a sensitization or severe local irritation from *Bactroban Nasal*, usage should be discontinued.

PRECAUTIONS

General

As with other antibacterial products, prolonged use may result in overgrowth of nonsusceptible microorganisms, including fungi. (See **DOSAGE AND ADMINISTRATION.**)

Information for Patients

Patients should be given the following instructions:

— Apply approximately one-half of the ointment from the single-use tube directly into one nostril and the other half into the other nostril;
— Avoid contact of the medication with the eyes;
— Discard the tube after using, do not re-use;
— Press the sides of the nose together and gently massage after application to spread the ointment throughout the inside of the nostrils; and
— Discontinue usage of the medication and call your health care practitioner if sensitization or severe local irritation occurs.

Drug Interactions

The effect of the concurrent application of intranasal mupirocin calcium and other intranasal products has not been studied. Until further information is known, mupirocin calcium ointment, 2% should not be applied concurrently with any other intranasal products.

Carcinogenesis, Mutagenesis, Impairment of Fertility

Long-term studies in animals to evaluate carcinogenic potential of mupirocin calcium have not been conducted.

Results of the following studies performed with mupirocin calcium or mupirocin sodium *in vitro* and *in vivo* did not indicate a potential for mutagenicity: rat primary hepatocyte unscheduled DNA synthesis, sediment analysis for DNA strand breaks, *Salmonella* reversion test (Ames), *Escherichia coli* mutation assay, metaphase analysis of human lymphocytes, mouse lymphoma assay, and bone marrow micronuclei assay in mice.

Reproduction studies were performed in rats with mupirocin administered subcutaneously at doses up to **40** times the human intranasal dose (approximately 20 mg mupirocin per day) on a mg/m^2 basis and revealed no evidence of impaired fertility from mupirocin sodium.

Pregnancy

Teratogenic Effects. Pregnancy Category B. Reproduction studies have been performed in rats and rabbits with mupirocin administered subcutaneously at doses up to 65 and 130 times, respectively, the human intranasal dose (approximately 20 mg mupirocin per day) on a mg/m^2 basis and revealed no evidence of harm to the fetus due to mupirocin. There are, however, no adequate and well-controlled studies in pregnant women. Because animal reproduction studies are not always predictive of human response, this drug should be used during pregnancy only if clearly needed.

Nursing Mothers

It is not known whether this drug is excreted in human milk. Because many drugs are excreted in human milk, caution should be exercised when *Bactroban Nasal* is administered to a nursing woman.

Pediatric Use

Safety in children under the age of 12 years has not been established. (See **CLINICAL PHARMACOLOGY.**)

ADVERSE REACTIONS

Clinical Trials

In clinical trials, 210 domestic and 2,130 foreign adult subjects/patients received *Bactroban Nasal* ointment. Less than 1% of domestic or foreign subjects and patients in clinical trials were withdrawn due to adverse events.

The most frequently reported adverse events in foreign clinical trials were as follows: rhinitis (1.0%), taste perversion (0.8%), pharyngitis (0.5%).

In domestic clinical trials, 17% (36/210) of adults treated with *Bactroban Nasal* ointment reported adverse events thought to be at least possibly drug-related. The incidence of adverse events that were reported in at least 1% of adults enrolled in domestic clinical trials were as follows:

ADVERSE EVENTS (≥1% INCIDENCE)-ADULTS IN U.S. TRIALS

	% of Subjects/Patients Experiencing Event *Bactroban Nasal 2%* (n=210)
Headache	9%
Rhinitis	6%
Respiratory disorder, including upper respiratory tract congestion	5%
Pharyngitis	4%
Taste perversion	3%
Burning/Stinging	2%
Cough	2%
Pruritus	1%

The following events thought possibly drug-related were reported in less than 1% of adults enrolled in domestic clinical trials: blepharitis, diarrhea, dry mouth, ear pain, epistaxis, nausea and rash.

All adequate and well-controlled clinical trials have been performed using *Bactroban Nasal* ointment, 2% in one arm and the vehicle ointment in the other arm of the study. No adequate and well-controlled safety data are available from direct, head-to-head comparative studies of this product and other products for this indication.

OVERDOSAGE

Following single or repeated intranasal applications of *Bactroban Nasal* to adults, no evidence for systemic absorption of mupirocin was obtained. Intravenous infusions of 252 mg, as well as single oral doses of 500 mg of mupirocin, have been well tolerated in healthy adult subjects. There is no information regarding local overdose of *Bactroban Nasal* or regarding oral ingestion of the nasal ointment formulation.

DOSAGE AND ADMINISTRATION

(See **INDICATIONS AND USAGE.**)

Adults (12 years of age and older): Approximately one-half of the ointment from the single-use tube should be applied into one nostril and the other half into the other nostril twice daily (morning and evening) for 5 days.

After application, the nostrils should be closed by pressing together and releasing the sides of the nose repetitively for approximately 1 minute. This will spread the ointment throughout the nares.

The single-use 1.0 gram tube will deliver a total of approximately 0.5 grams of the ointment (approximately 0.25 grams/nostril).

The tube should be discarded after usage; it should not be re-used.

The safety and effectiveness of applications of this medication for greater than 5 days have not been established. There are no human clinical or pre-clinical animal data to support the use of this product in a chronic manner or in manners other than those described in this package insert. Until further information is known, *Bactroban Nasal* should not be applied concurrently with any other intranasal products.

HOW SUPPLIED

Bactroban Nasal (mupirocin calcium ointment), 2% is supplied in 1.0 gram tubes packaged in cartons of 10.
NDC 0029-1526-11 (1.0 gram tubes in packages of 10).
Store at or below 25°C (77°F).

REFERENCE

1. National Committee for Clinical Laboratory Standards. Methods for Dilution Antimicrobial Susceptibility Tests for Bacteria That Grow Aerobically—Third Edition; Approved Standard NCCLS Document M7-A3. Vol. 12, No. 25, NCCLS, Villanova, PA, December 1993.

GlaxoSmithKline, Research Triangle Park, NC 27709

August 2001/BN:L4

Shown in Product Identification Guide, page 314

BACTROBAN OINTMENT® ℞

[bac'trō ban]

brand of mupirocin ointment, 2%

For Dermatologic Use

DESCRIPTION

Each gram of Bactroban Ointment (mupirocin ointment), 2% contains 20 mg mupirocin in a bland water miscible ointment base (polyethylene glycol ointment, N.F.) consisting of polyethylene glycol 400 and polyethylene glycol 3350. Mupirocin is a naturally occurring antibiotic. The chemical name is (*E*)-(2*S*,3*R*,4*R*,5*S*)-5-[(2*S*,3*S*,4*S*,5*S*)-2,3-Epoxy-5-hydroxy-4-methylhexyl]tetrahydro-3,4-dihydroxy-β-methyl-2*H*-pyran-2-crotonic acid, ester with 9-hydroxynonanoic acid. The molecular formula of mupirocin is $C_{26}H_{44}O_9$ and the molecular weight is 500.63.

CLINICAL PHARMACOLOGY

Application of ^{14}C-labeled mupirocin ointment to the lower arm of normal male subjects followed by occlusion for 24 hours showed no measurable systemic absorption (<1.1 nanogram mupirocin per milliliter of whole blood). Measurable radioactivity was present in the stratum corneum of these subjects 72 hours after application.

Following intravenous or oral administration, mupirocin is rapidly metabolized. The principal metabolite, monic acid, is eliminated by renal excretion, and demonstrates no antibacterial activity. In a study conducted in seven healthy adult male subjects, the elimination half-life after intravenous administration of mupirocin was 20 to 40 minutes for mupirocin and 30 to 80 minutes for monic acid. The pharmacokinetics of mupirocin has not been studied in individuals with renal insufficiency.

Microbiology: Mupirocin is an antibacterial agent produced by fermentation using the organism *Pseudomonas fluorescens*. It is active against a wide range of gram-positive bacteria including methicillin-resistant *Staphylococcus aureus* (MRSA). It is also active against certain gram-negative bacteria. Mupirocin inhibits bacterial protein synthesis by reversibly and specifically binding to bacterial isoleucyl transfer-RNA synthetase. Due to this unique mode of action, mupirocin demonstrates no *in vitro* cross-resistance with other classes of antimicrobial agents.

Resistance occurs rarely. However, when mupirocin resistance does occur, it appears to result from the production of a modified isoleucyl-tRNA synthetase. High-level plasmid-

Continued on next page

Product information on these pages is effective as of August 2004. Further information is available at: GlaxoSmithKline, PO Box 13398, Research Triangle Park, NC 27709. 1-888-825-5249. Corporate Web Site: www.gsk.com

Bactroban Ointment—Cont.

mediated resistance (MIC >1024 mcg/mL) has been reported in some strains of *S. aureus* and coagulase-negative staphylococci.

Mupirocin is bactericidal at concentrations achieved by topical administration. However, the minimum bactericidal concentration (MBC) against relevant pathogens is generally eight-fold to thirty-fold higher than the minimum inhibitory concentration (MIC). In addition, mupirocin is highly protein bound (>97%), and the effect of wound secretions on the MICs of mupirocin has not been determined.

Mupirocin has been shown to be active against most strains of *Staphylococcus aureus* and *Streptococcus pyogenes*, both *in vitro* and in clinical studies. (See **INDICATIONS AND USAGE.**) The following *in vitro* data are available, BUT THEIR CLINICAL SIGNIFICANCE IS UNKNOWN. Mupirocin is active against most strains of *Staphylococcus epidermidis* and *Staphylococcus saprophyticus.*

INDICATIONS AND USAGE

Bactroban Ointment (mupirocin ointment), 2% is indicated for the topical treatment of impetigo due to: *Staphylococcus aureus* and *Streptococcus pyogenes.*

CONTRAINDICATIONS

This drug is contraindicated in individuals with a history of sensitivity reactions to any of its components.

WARNINGS

Bactroban Ointment is not for ophthalmic use.

PRECAUTIONS

If a reaction suggesting sensitivity or chemical irritation should occur with the use of Bactroban Ointment (mupirocin ointment) 2%, treatment should be discontinued and appropriate alternative therapy for the infection instituted.

As with other antibacterial products, prolonged use may result in overgrowth of nonsusceptible organisms, including fungi.

Bactroban Ointment is not formulated for use on mucosal surfaces. Intranasal use has been associated with isolated reports of stinging and drying. A paraffin-based formulation — Bactroban Nasal® (mupirocin calcium ointment) — is available for intranasal use.

Polyethylene glycol can be absorbed from open wounds and damaged skin and is excreted by the kidneys. In common with other polyethylene glycol-based ointments, *Bactroban Ointment* should not be used in conditions where absorption of large quantities of polyethylene glycol is possible, especially if there is evidence of moderate or severe renal impairment.

Information for Patients: Use this medication only as directed by your healthcare provider. It is for external use only. Avoid contact with the eyes. The medication should be stopped and your healthcare practitioner contacted if irritation, severe itching, or rash occurs.

If impetigo has not improved in 3 to 5 days, contact your healthcare practitioner.

Drug Interactions: The effect of the concurrent application of *Bactroban Ointment* and other drug products has not been studied.

Carcinogenesis, Mutagenesis, Impairment of Fertility: Long-term studies in animals to evaluate carcinogenic potential of mupirocin have not been conducted.

Results of the following studies performed with mupirocin calcium or mupirocin sodium *in vitro* and *in vivo* did not indicate a potential for genotoxicity: rat primary hepatocyte unscheduled DNA synthesis, sediment analysis for DNA strand breaks, *Salmonella* reversion test (Ames), *Escherichia coli* mutation assay, metaphase analysis of human lymphocytes, mouse lymphoma assay, and bone marrow micronuclei assay in mice.

Reproduction studies were performed in male and female rats with mupirocin administered subcutaneously at doses up to 14 times a human topical dose (approximately 60 mg mupirocin per day) on a mg/m^2 basis and revealed no evidence of impaired fertility and reproductive performance from mupirocin.

Pregnancy

Teratogenic Effects.

Pregnancy Category B: Reproduction studies have been performed in rats and rabbits with mupirocin administered subcutaneously at doses up to 22 and 43 times, respectively, the human topical dose (approximately 60 mg mupirocin per day) on a mg/m^2 basis and revealed no evidence of harm to the fetus due to mupirocin. There are, however, no adequate and well-controlled studies in pregnant women. Because animal studies are not always predictive of human response, this drug should be used during pregnancy only if clearly needed.

Nursing Mothers: It is not known whether this drug is excreted in human milk. Because many drugs are excreted in human milk, caution should be exercised when *Bactroban Ointment* is administered to a nursing woman.

Pediatric Use: The safety and effectiveness of *Bactroban Ointment* have been established in the age range of 2 months to 16 years. Use of *Bactroban Ointment* in these age groups is supported by evidence from adequate and well-controlled studies of *Bactroban Ointment* in impetigo in pediatric patients studied as a part of the pivotal clinical trials. (See **CLINICAL STUDIES.**)

ADVERSE REACTIONS

The following local adverse reactions have been reported in connection with the use of *Bactroban Ointment*: burning, stinging, or pain in 1.5% of patients; itching in 1% of patients; rash, nausea, erythema, dry skin, tenderness, swelling, contact dermatitis, and increased exudate in less than 1% of patients. Systemic reactions to *Bactroban Ointment* have occurred rarely.

DOSAGE AND ADMINISTRATION

A small amount of *Bactroban Ointment* should be applied to the affected area three times daily. The area treated may be covered with a gauze dressing if desired. Patients not showing a clinical response within 3 to 5 days should be re-evaluated.

CLINICAL STUDIES

The efficacy of topical *Bactroban Ointment* in impetigo was tested in two studies. In the first, patients with impetigo were randomized to receive either *Bactroban Ointment* or vehicle placebo t.i.d. for 8 to 12 days. Clinical efficacy rates at end of therapy in the evaluable populations (adults and pediatric patients included) were 71% for *Bactroban Ointment* (n=49) and 35% for vehicle placebo (n=51). Pathogen eradication rates in the evaluable populations were 94% for *Bactroban Ointment* and 62% for vehicle placebo. There were no side effects reported in the group receiving *Bactroban Ointment.*

In the second study, patients with impetigo were randomized to receive either *Bactroban Ointment* t.i.d. or 30 to 40 mg/kg oral erythromycin ethylsuccinate per day (this was an unblinded study) for 8 days. There was a follow-up visit 1 week after treatment ended. Clinical efficacy rates at the follow-up visit in the evaluable populations (adults and pediatric patients included) were 93% for *Bactroban Ointment* (n=29) and 78.5% for erythromycin (n=28). Pathogen eradication rates in the evaluable patient populations were 100% for both test groups. There were no side effects reported in the *Bactroban Ointment* group.

Pediatrics

There were 91 pediatric patients aged 2 months to 15 years in the first study described above. Clinical efficacy rates at end of therapy in the evaluable populations were 78% for *Bactroban Ointment* (n=42) and 36% for vehicle placebo (n=49). In the second study described above, all patients were pediatric except two adults in the group receiving *Bactroban Ointment.* The age range of the pediatric patients was 7 months to 13 years. The clinical efficacy rate for *Bactroban Ointment* (n=27) was 96%, and for erythromycin it was unchanged (78.5%).

HOW SUPPLIED

Bactroban Ointment (mupirocin ointment), 2% is supplied in 22 gram tubes.

NDC 0029-1525-44 (22 gram tube)

Store at controlled room temperature 20° to 25°C (68° to 77°F).

GlaxoSmithKline, Research Triangle Park, NC 27709

November 2001/BC:L12C

Shown in Product Identification Guide, page 315

BECONASE AQ® ℞

[be' kō-nāz]

(beclomethasone dipropionate, monohydrate)
Nasal Spray, 42 mcg

For Intranasal Use Only.
SHAKE WELL
BEFORE USE.

DESCRIPTION

Beclomethasone dipropionate, monohydrate, the active component of BECONASE AQ Nasal Spray, is an anti-inflammatory steroid having the chemical name 9-chloro-11β,17,21-trihydroxy-16β-methylpregna-1,4-diene-3,20-dione 17,21-dipropionate, monohydrate.

Beclomethasone 17,21-dipropionate is a diester of beclomethasone, a synthetic halogenated corticosteroid. Beclomethasone dipropionate, monohydrate is a white to creamy-white, odorless powder with a molecular weight of 539.06. It is very slightly soluble in water, very soluble in chloroform, and freely soluble in acetone and in ethanol.

BECONASE AQ Nasal Spray is a metered-dose, manual pump spray unit containing a microcrystalline suspension of beclomethasone dipropionate, monohydrate equivalent to 42 mcg of beclomethasone dipropionate, calculated on the dried basis, in an aqueous medium containing microcrystalline cellulose, carboxymethylcellulose sodium, dextrose, benzalkonium chloride, polysorbate 80, and 0.25% v/w phenylethyl alcohol. The pH through expiry is 5.0 to 6.8.

After initial priming (6 actuations), each actuation of the pump delivers from the nasal adapter 100 mg of suspension containing beclomethasone dipropionate, monohydrate equivalent to 42 mcg of beclomethasone dipropionate. If the pump is not used for 7 days, it should be primed until a fine spray appears. Each 25-g bottle of BECONASE AQ Nasal Spray provides 180 metered sprays.

CLINICAL PHARMACOLOGY

Mechanism of Action: Following topical administration, beclomethasone dipropionate produces anti-inflammatory and vasoconstrictor effects. The mechanisms responsible for the anti-inflammatory action of beclomethasone dipropionate are unknown. Corticosteroids have been shown to have a wide range of effects on multiple cell types (e.g., mast cells, eosinophils, neutrophils, macrophages, and lymphocytes) and mediators (e.g., histamine, eicosanoids, leukotrienes, and cytokines) involved in inflammation. The direct relationship of these findings to the effects of beclomethasone dipropionate on allergic rhinitis symptoms is not known.

Biopsies of nasal mucosa obtained during clinical studies showed no histopathologic changes when beclomethasone dipropionate was administered intranasally.

Beclomethasone dipropionate is a pro-drug with weak glucocorticoid receptor binding affinity. It is hydrolyzed via esterase enzymes to its active metabolite beclomethasone-17-monopropionate (B-17-MP), which has high topical anti-inflammatory activity.

Pharmacokinetics: ***Absorption:*** Beclomethasone dipropionate is sparingly soluble in water. When given by nasal inhalation in the form of an aqueous or aerosolized suspension, the drug is deposited primarily in the nasal passages. The majority of the drug is eventually swallowed. Following intranasal administration of aqueous beclomethasone dipropionate, the systemic absorption was assessed by measuring the plasma concentrations of its active metabolite B-17-MP, for which the absolute bioavailability following intranasal administration is 44% (43% of the administered dose came from the swallowed portion and only 1% of the total dose was bioavailable from the nose). The absorption of unchanged beclomethasone dipropionate following oral and intranasal dosing was undetectable (plasma concentrations <50 pg/mL).

Distribution: The tissue distribution at steady-state for beclomethasone dipropionate is moderate (20 L) but more extensive for B-17-MP (424 L). There is no evidence of tissue storage of beclomethasone dipropionate or its metabolites. Plasma protein binding is moderately high (87%).

Metabolism: Beclomethasone dipropionate is cleared very rapidly from the systemic circulation by metabolism mediated via esterase enzymes that are found in most tissues. The main product of metabolism is the active metabolite (B-17-MP). Minor inactive metabolites, beclomethasone-21-monopropionate (B-21-MP) and beclomethasone (BOH), are also formed, but these contribute little to systemic exposure.

Elimination: The elimination of beclomethasone dipropionate and B-17-MP after intravenous administration are characterized by high plasma clearance (150 and 120 L/hour) with corresponding terminal elimination half-lives of 0.5 and 2.7 hours. Following oral administration of tritiated beclomethasone dipropionate, approximately 60% of the dose was excreted in the feces within 96 hours, mainly as free and conjugated polar metabolites. Approximately 12% of the dose was excreted as free and conjugated polar metabolites in the urine. The renal clearance of beclomethasone dipropionate and its metabolites is negligible.

Pharmacodynamics: The effects of beclomethasone dipropionate on hypothalamic-pituitary-adrenal (HPA) function have been evaluated in adult volunteers by other routes of administration. Studies with beclomethasone dipropionate by the intranasal route may demonstrate that there is more or that there is less absorption by this route of administration. There was no suppression of early morning plasma cortisol concentrations when beclomethasone dipropionate was administered in a dose of 1,000 mcg/day for 1 month as an oral aerosol or for 3 days by intramuscular injection. However, partial suppression of plasma cortisol concentrations was observed when beclomethasone dipropionate was administered in doses of 2,000 mcg/day either by oral aerosol or intramuscular injection. Immediate suppression of plasma cortisol concentrations was observed after single doses of 4,000 mcg of beclomethasone dipropionate. Suppression of HPA function (reduction of early morning plasma cortisol levels) has been reported in adult patients who received 1,600-mcg daily doses of oral beclomethasone dipropionate for 1 month. In clinical studies using beclomethasone dipropionate aerosol intranasally, there was no evidence of adrenal insufficiency. The effect of BECONASE AQ Nasal Spray on HPA function was not evaluated but would not be expected to differ from intranasal beclomethasone dipropionate aerosol.

In 1 study in children with asthma, the administration of inhaled beclomethasone at recommended daily doses for at least 1 year was associated with a reduction in nocturnal cortisol secretion. The clinical significance of this finding is not clear. It reinforces other evidence, however, that topical beclomethasone may be absorbed in amounts that can have systemic effects and that physicians should be alert for evidence of systemic effects, especially in chronically treated patients (see PRECAUTIONS).

INDICATIONS AND USAGE

BECONASE AQ Nasal Spray is indicated for the relief of the symptoms of seasonal or perennial allergic and nonallergic (vasomotor) rhinitis.

Results from 2 clinical trials have shown that significant symptomatic relief was obtained within 3 days. However, symptomatic relief may not occur in some patients for as long as 2 weeks. BECONASE AQ Nasal Spray should not be continued beyond 3 weeks in the absence of significant symptomatic improvement. BECONASE AQ Nasal Spray should not be used in the presence of untreated localized infection involving the nasal mucosa.

BECONASE AQ Nasal Spray is also indicated for the prevention of recurrence of nasal polyps following surgical removal.

Clinical studies have shown that treatment of the symptoms associated with nasal polyps may have to be continued for several weeks or more before a therapeutic result can be fully assessed. Recurrence of symptoms due to polyps can occur after stopping treatment, depending on the severity of the disease.

CONTRAINDICATIONS

Hypersensitivity to any of the ingredients of this preparation contraindicates its use.

WARNINGS

The replacement of a systemic corticosteroid with BECONASE AQ Nasal Spray can be accompanied by signs of adrenal insufficiency.

Careful attention must be given when patients previously treated for prolonged periods with systemic corticosteroids are transferred to BECONASE AQ Nasal Spray. This is particularly important in those patients who have associated asthma or other clinical conditions where too rapid a decrease in systemic corticosteroids may cause a severe exacerbation of their symptoms.

If recommended doses of intranasal beclomethasone are exceeded or if individuals are particularly sensitive or predisposed by virtue of recent systemic steroid therapy, symptoms of hypercorticism may occur, including very rare cases of menstrual irregularities, acneiform lesions, cataracts, and cushingoid features. If such changes occur, BECONASE AQ Nasal Spray should be discontinued slowly consistent with accepted procedures for discontinuing oral steroid therapy.

Persons who are using drugs that suppress the immune system are more susceptible to infections than healthy individuals. Chickenpox and measles, for example, can have a more serious or even fatal course in susceptible children or adults using corticosteroids. In children or adults who have not had these diseases or been properly immunized, particular care should be taken to avoid exposure. How the dose, route, and duration of corticosteroid administration affect the risk of developing a disseminated infection is not known. The contribution of the underlying disease and/or prior corticosteroid treatment to the risk is also not known. If exposed to chickenpox, prophylaxis with varicella zoster immune globulin (VZIG) may be indicated. If exposed to measles, prophylaxis with pooled intramuscular immunoglobulin (IG) may be indicated. (See the respective package inserts for complete VZIG and IG prescribing information.) If chickenpox develops, treatment with antiviral agents may be considered.

Avoid spraying in eyes.

PRECAUTIONS

General: Intranasal corticosteroids may cause a reduction in growth velocity when administered to pediatric patients (see PRECAUTIONS: Pediatric Use).

During withdrawal from oral corticosteroids, some patients may experience symptoms of withdrawal, e.g., joint and/or muscular pain, lassitude, and depression.

Rarely, immediate hypersensitivity reactions may occur after the intranasal administration of beclomethasone (see ADVERSE REACTIONS).

Rare instances of nasal septum perforation have been spontaneously reported.

Rare instances of wheezing, cataracts, glaucoma, and increased intraocular pressure have been reported following the intranasal use of beclomethasone dipropionate.

In clinical studies with beclomethasone dipropionate administered intranasally, the development of localized infections of the nose and pharynx with *Candida albicans* has occurred only rarely. When such an infection develops, it may require treatment with appropriate local therapy and discontinuation of treatment with BECONASE AQ Nasal Spray.

If persistent nasopharyngeal irritation occurs, it may be an indication for stopping BECONASE AQ Nasal Spray.

Beclomethasone dipropionate is absorbed into the circulation. Use of excessive doses of BECONASE AQ Nasal Spray may suppress HPA function.

Intranasal corticosteroids should be used with caution, if at all, in patients with active or quiescent tuberculous infections of the respiratory tract, untreated local or systemic fungal or bacterial infections, systemic viral or parasitic infections, or ocular herpes simplex.

For BECONASE AQ Nasal Spray to be effective in the treatment of nasal polyps, the spray must be able to enter the nose. Therefore, treatment of nasal polyps with BECONASE AQ Nasal Spray should be considered adjunctive therapy to surgical removal and/or the use of other medications that will permit effective penetration of BECONASE AQ Nasal Spray into the nose. Nasal polyps may recur after any form of treatment.

As with any long-term treatment, patients using BECONASE AQ Nasal Spray over several months or longer should be examined periodically for possible changes in the nasal mucosa.

Because of the inhibitory effect of corticosteroids on wound healing, patients who have experienced recent nasal septal ulcers, nasal surgery, or nasal trauma should not use a nasal corticosteroid until healing has occurred.

Although systemic effects have been minimal with recommended doses, this potential increases with excessive doses. Therefore, larger than recommended doses should be avoided.

Information for Patients: Patients being treated with BECONASE AQ Nasal Spray should receive the following information and instructions. This information is intended to aid them in the safe and effective use of this medication. It is not a disclosure of all possible adverse or intended effects.

Patients should use BECONASE AQ Nasal Spray at regular intervals since its effectiveness depends on its regular use. The patient should take the medication as directed. It is not acutely effective, and the prescribed dosage should not be increased. Instead, nasal vasoconstrictors or oral antihistamines may be needed until the effects of BECONASE AQ Nasal Spray are fully manifested. One to 2 weeks may pass before full relief is obtained. The patient should contact the physician if symptoms do not improve, if the condition worsens, or if sneezing or nasal irritation occurs.

For the proper use of BECONASE AQ Nasal Spray and to attain maximum improvement, the patient should read and follow carefully the patient's instructions accompanying the product.

Persons who are using immunosuppressant doses of corticosteroids should be warned to avoid exposure to chickenpox or measles. Patients should also be advised that if they are exposed, medical advice should be sought without delay.

Carcinogenesis, Mutagenesis, Impairment of Fertility: The carcinogenicity of beclomethasone dipropionate was evaluated in rats that were exposed for a total of 95 weeks, 13 weeks at inhalation doses up to 0.4 mg/kg and the remaining 82 weeks at combined oral and inhalation doses up to 2.4 mg/kg. There was no evidence of carcinogenicity in this study at the highest dose, approximately 60 times the maximum recommended daily intranasal dose in adults on a mg/m^2 basis or approximately 35 times the maximum recommended daily intranasal dose in children on a mg/m^2 basis.

Beclomethasone dipropionate did not induce gene mutation in bacterial cells or mammalian Chinese hamster ovary (CHO) cells in vitro. No significant clastogenic effect was seen in cultured CHO cells in vitro or in the mouse micronucleus test in vivo.

In rats, beclomethasone dipropionate caused decreased conception rates at an oral dose of 16 mg/kg (approximately 390 times the maximum recommended daily intranasal dose in adults on a mg/m^2 basis). There was no significant effect of beclomethasone dipropionate on fertility in rats at oral doses of 1.6 mg/kg (approximately 40 times the maximum recommended daily intranasal dose in adults on a mg/m^2 basis). Inhibition of the estrous cycle in dogs was observed following oral dosing at 0.5 mg/kg (approximately 40 times the maximum recommended daily intranasal dose in adults on a mg/m^2 basis). No inhibition of the estrous cycle in dogs was seen following 12 months' exposure at an estimated inhalation dose of 0.33 mg/kg (approximately 25 times the maximum recommended daily intranasal dose in adults on a mg/m^2 basis).

Pregnancy: ***Teratogenic Effects:*** Pregnancy Category C. Like other corticosteroids beclomethasone dipropionate was teratogenic and embryocidal in the mouse and rabbit at a subcutaneous dose of 0.1 mg/kg in mice or 0.025 mg/kg in rabbits (approximately equal to the maximum recommended daily intranasal dose in adults on a mg/m^2 basis). No teratogenicity or embryocidal effects were seen in rats when exposed to an inhalation dose of 0.1 mg/kg plus oral doses of up to 10 mg/kg per day for a combined dose of 10.1 mg/kg (approximately 240 times the maximum recommended daily intranasal dose in adults on a mg/m^2 basis). There are no adequate and well-controlled studies in pregnant women. Beclomethasone dipropionate should be used during pregnancy only if the potential benefit justifies the potential risk to the fetus.

Nonteratogenic Effects: Hypoadrenalism may occur in infants born of mothers receiving corticosteroids during pregnancy. Such infants should be carefully observed.

Nursing Mothers: It is not known whether beclomethasone dipropionate is excreted in human milk. Because other corticosteroids are excreted in human milk, caution should be exercised when BECONASE AQ Nasal Spray is administered to a nursing woman.

Pediatric Use: The safety and effectiveness of BECONASE AQ Nasal Spray have been established in children aged 6 years and above through evidence from extensive clinical use in adult and pediatric patients. The safety and effectiveness of BECONASE AQ Nasal Spray in children below 6 years of age have not been established.

Controlled clinical studies have shown that intranasal corticosteroids may cause a reduction in growth velocity in pediatric patients. This effect has been observed in the absence of laboratory evidence of HPA axis suppression, suggesting that growth velocity is a more sensitive indicator of systemic corticosteroid exposure in pediatric patients than some commonly used tests of HPA axis function. The long-term effects of this reduction in growth velocity associated with intranasal corticosteroids, including the impact on final adult height, are unknown. The potential for "catch-up" growth following discontinuation of treatment with intranasal corticosteroids has not been adequately studied. The growth of pediatric patients receiving intranasal corticosteroids, including BECONASE AQ Nasal Spray, should be monitored routinely (e.g., via stadiometry). The potential growth effects of prolonged treatment should be weighed against the clinical benefits obtained and the risks/benefits of treatment alternatives. To minimize the systemic effects of intranasal corticosteroids, including BECONASE AQ Nasal Spray, each patient should be titrated to the lowest dose that effectively controls his/her symptoms.

In a double-blind, controlled trial, 100 children between the ages of 6 and 9½ years with allergic rhinitis were randomized to receive aqueous intranasal beclomethasone dipropionate 168 mcg twice daily or placebo for 1 year. As measured by stadiometry, children who received beclomethasone dipropionate grew more slowly than those who received placebo. A difference in mean change in height was observed within 1 month of drug initiation. At the end of 12 months, the beclomethasone dipropionate-treated group had a growth velocity on average of 4.75 cm/year compared to 6.20 cm/year in the placebo group ($p<0.01$). While the placebo group had an expected distribution of growth velocity, approximately 50% of the beclomethasone dipropionate-treated children grew below the 10th percentile.

In children 7.3 years of age, the mean age of children in this study, the range for expected growth velocity is: boys – 3rd percentile = 4.1 cm/year, 50th percentile = 5.8 cm/year, and 97th percentile = 7.5 cm/year; girls – 3rd percentile = 4.3 cm/year, 50th percentile = 5.9 cm/year, and 97th percentile = 7.5 cm/year. The potential reversibility of the reduction in growth velocity was not studied. No significant differences were observed between the 2 groups for mean basal plasma cortisol or ACTH-stimulated plasma cortisol levels.

Geriatric Use: Clinical studies of BECONASE AQ Nasal Spray did not include sufficient numbers of subjects aged 65 and over to determine whether they respond differently from younger subjects. Other reported clinical experience has not identified differences in responses between the elderly and younger patients. In general, dose selection for an elderly patient should be cautious, starting at the low end of the dosing range, reflecting the greater frequency of decreased hepatic, renal, or cardiac function, and of concomitant disease or other drug therapy.

ADVERSE REACTIONS

In general, side effects in clinical studies have been primarily associated with irritation of the nasal mucous membranes.

Adverse reactions reported in controlled clinical trials and open studies in patients treated with BECONASE AQ Nasal Spray are described below.

Mild nasopharyngeal irritation following the use of beclomethasone aqueous nasal spray has been reported in up to 24% of patients treated, including occasional sneezing attacks (about 4%) occurring immediately following use of the spray. In patients experiencing these symptoms, none had to discontinue treatment. The incidence of transient irritation and sneezing was approximately the same in the group of patients who received placebo in these studies, implying that these complaints may be related to vehicle components of the formulation.

Fewer than 5 per 100 patients reported headache, nausea, or lightheadedness following the use of BECONASE AQ Nasal Spray. Fewer than 3 per 100 patients reported nasal stuffiness, nosebleeds, rhinorrhea, or tearing eyes.

Rare cases of ulceration of the nasal mucosa and instances of nasal septum perforation have been spontaneously reported (see PRECAUTIONS).

Reports of dryness and irritation of the nose and throat, and unpleasant taste and smell have been received. There are rare reports of loss of taste and smell.

Rare instances of wheezing, cataracts, glaucoma, and increased intraocular pressure have been reported following the use of intranasal beclomethasone dipropionate (see PRECAUTIONS).

Rare cases of immediate and delayed hypersensitivity reactions, including urticaria, angioedema, rash, and bronchospasm, have been reported following the oral and intranasal inhalation of beclomethasone dipropionate.

Cases of growth suppression have been reported for intranasal corticosteroids, including BECONASE AQ (see PRECAUTIONS: Pediatric Use).

OVERDOSAGE

When used at excessive doses, systemic corticosteroid effects such as hypercorticism and adrenal suppression may appear. If such changes occur, BECONASE AQ Nasal Spray should be discontinued slowly consistent with accepted procedures for discontinuing oral steroid therapy. No deaths occurred when beclomethasone dipropionate was given as single oral doses of 3,000 mg/kg to mice (approximately 36,000 times the maximum recommended daily intranasal dose in adults on a mg/m^2 basis, or approximately 21,000 times the maximum recommended daily intranasal dose in children on a mg/m^2 basis) and 2,000 mg/kg to rats (approximately 48,000 times the maximum recommended daily intranasal dose in adults or approximately 29,000 times the maximum recommended daily intranasal dose in children on a mg/m^2 basis). One bottle of BECONASE AQ Nasal Spray contains beclomethasone dipropionate, monohydrate equivalent to 10.5 mg of beclomethasone dipropionate; therefore, acute overdosage is unlikely.

DOSAGE AND ADMINISTRATION

Adults and Children 12 Years of Age and Older: The usual dosage is 1 or 2 nasal inhalations (42 to 84 mcg) in each nostril twice a day (total dose, 168 to 336 mcg/day).

Continued on next page

Product information on these pages is effective as of August 2004. Further information is available at: GlaxoSmithKline, PO Box 13398, Research Triangle Park, NC 27709. 1-888-825-5249. Corporate Web Site: www.gsk.com

Beconase AQ—Cont.

Children 6 to 12 Years of Age: Patients should be started with 1 nasal inhalation in each nostril twice daily; patients not adequately responding to 168 mcg or those with more severe symptoms may use 336 mcg (2 inhalations in each nostril). Once adequate control is achieved, the dosage should be decreased to 84 mcg (1 spray in each nostril) twice daily. BECONASE AQ Nasal Spray is *not* recommended for children below 6 years of age.
The maximum total daily dosage should not exceed 2 sprays in each nostril twice daily (336 mcg/day).
In patients who respond to BECONASE AQ Nasal Spray, an improvement of the symptoms of seasonal or perennial rhinitis usually becomes apparent within a few days after the start of therapy with BECONASE AQ Nasal Spray. However, symptomatic relief may not occur in some patients for as long as 2 weeks. BECONASE AQ Nasal Spray should not be continued beyond 3 weeks in the absence of significant symptomatic improvement.
The therapeutic effects of corticosteroids, unlike those of decongestants, are not immediate. This should be explained to the patient in advance in order to ensure cooperation and continuation of treatment with the prescribed dosage regimen.
In the presence of excessive nasal mucous secretion or edema of the nasal mucosa, the drug may fail to reach the site of intended action. In such cases it is advisable to use a nasal vasoconstrictor during the first 2 to 3 days of therapy with BECONASE AQ Nasal Spray.
Directions for Use: Illustrated Patient's Instructions for Use accompany each package of BECONASE AQ Nasal Spray.

HOW SUPPLIED

BECONASE AQ Nasal Spray, 42 mcg is supplied in an amber glass bottle fitted with a metering atomizing pump and nasal adapter in a box of 1 (NDC 0173-0388-79) with patient's instructions for use. Each bottle contains 25 g of suspension and will provide 180 metered sprays. The correct amount of medication in each spray cannot be assured after 180 sprays even though the bottle is not completely empty. The bottle should be discarded when the labeled number of actuations has been used.
Store between 15° and 30°C (59° and 86°F).
GlaxoSmithKline, Research Triangle Park, NC 27709
December 2002/RL-1175
Shown in Product Identification Guide, page 315

CEFTIN® Tablets ℞
[*sĕf´ tin*]
(cefuroxime axetil tablets)

CEFTIN® for Oral Suspension ℞
(cefuroxime axetil powder for oral suspension)

To reduce the development of drug-resistant bacteria and maintain the effectiveness of CEFTIN and other antibacterial drugs, CEFTIN should be used only to treat or prevent infections that are proven or strongly suspected to be caused by bacteria.

DESCRIPTION

CEFTIN Tablets and CEFTIN for Oral Suspension contain cefuroxime as cefuroxime axetil. CEFTIN is a semisynthetic, broad-spectrum cephalosporin antibiotic for oral administration.
Chemically, cefuroxime axetil, the 1-(acetyloxy) ethyl ester of cefuroxime, is (*RS*)-1-hydroxyethyl (6*R*,7*R*)-7-[2-(2-furyl) glyoxyl-amido]-3-(hydroxymethyl)-8-oxo-5-thia-1-azabicyclo [4.2.0]-oct-2-ene-2-carboxylate, 7^2-(*Z*)-(*O*-methyl-oxime), 1-acetate 3-carbamate. Its molecular formula is $C_{20}H_{22}N_4O_{10}S$, and it has a molecular weight of 510.48.
Cefuroxime axetil is in the amorphous form.
CEFTIN Tablets are film-coated and contain the equivalent of 250 or 500 mg of cefuroxime as cefuroxime axetil. CEFTIN Tablets contain the inactive ingredients colloidal silicon dioxide, croscarmellose sodium, FD&C Blue No. 1, hydrogenated vegetable oil, hypromellose, methylparaben, microcrystalline cellulose, propylene glycol, propylparaben, sodium lauryl sulfate, and titanium dioxide.
CEFTIN for Oral Suspension, when reconstituted with water, provides the equivalent of 125 mg or 250 mg of cefuroxime (as cefuroxime axetil) per 5 mL of suspension. CEFTIN for Oral Suspension contains the inactive ingredients acesulfame potassium, aspartame, povidone K30, stearic acid, sucrose, tutti-frutti flavoring, and xanthan gum.

CLINICAL PHARMACOLOGY

Absorption and Metabolism: After oral administration, cefuroxime axetil is absorbed from the gastrointestinal tract and rapidly hydrolyzed by nonspecific esterases in the intestinal mucosa and blood to cefuroxime. Cefuroxime is subsequently distributed throughout the extracellular fluids. The axetil moiety is metabolized to acetaldehyde and acetic acid.
Pharmacokinetics: Approximately 50% of serum cefuroxime is bound to protein. Serum pharmacokinetic parameters for CEFTIN Tablets and CEFTIN for Oral Suspension are shown in Tables 1 and 2.
[See table 1 above]
[See table 2 above]
Comparative Pharmacokinetic Properties: A 250 mg/5 mL-dose of CEFTIN Suspension is bioequivalent to 2 times 125 mg/5 mL-dose of CEFTIN Suspension when administered with food (see Table 3). **CEFTIN for Oral Suspension was not bioequivalent to CEFTIN Tablets when tested in healthy adults. The tablet and powder for oral suspension formulations are NOT substitutable on a milligram-per-milligram basis.** The area under the curve for the suspension averaged 91% of that for the tablet, and the peak plasma concentration for the suspension averaged 71% of the peak plasma concentration of the tablets. Therefore, the safety and effectiveness of both the tablet and oral suspension formulations had to be established in separate clinical trials.
[See table 3 above]

Table 1. Postprandial Pharmacokinetics of Cefuroxime Administered as CEFTIN Tablets to Adults*

Dose† (Cefuroxime Equivalent)	Peak Plasma Concentration (mcg/mL)	Time of Peak Plasma Concentration (hr)	Mean Elimination Half-Life (hr)	AUC (mcg-hr mL)
125 mg	2.1	2.2	1.2	6.7
250 mg	4.1	2.5	1.2	12.9
500 mg	7.0	3.0	1.2	27.4
1,000 mg	13.6	2.5	1.3	50.0

*Mean values of 12 healthy adult volunteers.
†Drug administered immediately after a meal.

Table 2. Postprandial Pharmacokinetics of Cefuroxime Administered as CEFTIN for Oral Suspension to Pediatric Patients*

Dose† (Cefuroxime Equivalent)	n	Peak Plasma Concentration (mcg/mL)	Time of Peak Plasma Concentration (hr)	Mean Elimination Half-Life (hr)	AUC (mcg-hr mL)
10 mg/kg	8	3.3	3.6	1.4	12.4
15 mg/kg	12	5.1	2.7	1.9	22.5
20 mg/kg	8	7.0	3.1	1.9	32.8

*Mean age = 23 months.
†Drug administered with milk or milk products.

Table 3. Pharmacokinetics of Cefuroxime Administered as 250 mg/5 mL or 2 × 125 mg/5 mL CEFTIN for Oral Suspension to Adults* With Food

Dose (Cefuroxime Equivalent)	Peak Plasma Concentration (mcg/mL)	Time of Peak Plasma Concentration (hr)	Mean Elimination Half-Life (hr)	AUC (mcg-hr mL)
250 mg/5 mL	2.23	3	1.40	8.92
2 × 125 mg/5 mL	2.37	3	1.44	9.75

*Mean values of 18 healthy adult volunteers.

Food Effect on Pharmacokinetics: Absorption of the tablet is greater when taken after food (absolute bioavailability of CEFTIN Tablets increases from 37% to 52%). Despite this difference in absorption, the clinical and bacteriologic responses of patients were independent of food intake at the time of tablet administration in 2 studies where this was assessed.
All pharmacokinetic and clinical effectiveness and safety studies in pediatric patients using the suspension formulation were conducted in the fed state. No data are available on the absorption kinetics of the suspension formulation when administered to fasted pediatric patients.
Renal Excretion: Cefuroxime is excreted unchanged in the urine; in adults, approximately 50% of the administered dose is recovered in the urine within 12 hours. The pharmacokinetics of cefuroxime in the urine of pediatric patients have not been studied at this time. Until further data are available, the renal pharmacokinetic properties of cefuroxime axetil established in adults should not be extrapolated to pediatric patients.
Because cefuroxime is renally excreted, the serum half-life is prolonged in patients with reduced renal function. In a study of 20 elderly patients (mean age = 83.9 years) having a mean creatinine clearance of 34.9 mL/min, the mean serum elimination half-life was 3.5 hours. Despite the lower elimination of cefuroxime in geriatric patients, dosage adjustment based on age is not necessary (see PRECAUTIONS: Geriatric Use).
Microbiology: The in vivo bactericidal activity of cefuroxime axetil is due to cefuroxime's binding to essential target proteins and the resultant inhibition of cell-wall synthesis.
Cefuroxime has bactericidal activity against a wide range of common pathogens, including many beta-lactamase–producing strains. Cefuroxime is stable to many bacterial beta-lactamases, especially plasmid-mediated enzymes that are commonly found in enterobacteriaceae.
Cefuroxime has been demonstrated to be active against most strains of the following microorganisms both in vitro and in clinical infections as described in the INDICATIONS AND USAGE section (see INDICATIONS AND USAGE section).
Aerobic Gram-Positive Microorganisms:
Staphylococcus aureus (including beta-lactamase–producing strains)
Streptococcus pneumoniae
Streptococcus pyogenes
Aerobic Gram-Negative Microorganisms:
Escherichia coli
Haemophilus influenzae (including beta-lactamase–producing strains)
Haemophilus parainfluenzae
Klebsiella pneumoniae
Moraxella catarrhalis (including beta-lactamase–producing strains)
Neisseria gonorrhoeae (including beta-lactamase–producing strains)
Spirochetes:
Borrelia burgdorferi
Cefuroxime has been shown to be active in vitro against most strains of the following microorganisms; however, the clinical significance of these findings is unknown.
Cefuroxime exhibits in vitro minimum inhibitory concentrations (MICs) of 4.0 mcg/mL or less (systemic susceptible breakpoint) against most (≥90%) strains of the following microorganisms; however, the safety and effectiveness of cefuroxime in treating clinical infections due to these microorganisms have not been established in adequate and well-controlled trials.
Aerobic Gram-Positive Microorganisms:
Staphylococcus epidermidis
Staphylococcus saprophyticus
Streptococcus agalactiae
NOTE: Certain strains of enterococci, e.g., *Enterococcus faecalis* (formerly *Streptococcus faecalis*), are resistant to cefuroxime. Methicillin-resistant staphylococci are resistant to cefuroxime.
Aerobic Gram-Negative Microorganisms:
Morganella morganii
Proteus inconstans
Proteus mirabilis
Providencia rettgeri
NOTE: *Pseudomonas* spp., *Campylobacter* spp., *Acinetobacter calcoaceticus*, and most strains of *Serratia* spp. and *Proteus vulgaris* are resistant to most first- and second-generation cephalosporins. Some strains of *Morganella morganii, Enterobacter cloacae,* and *Citrobacter* spp. have been shown by in vitro tests to be resistant to cefuroxime and other cephalosporins.
Anaerobic Microorganisms:
Peptococcus niger
NOTE: Most strains of *Clostridium difficile* and *Bacteroides fragilis* are resistant to cefuroxime.
Susceptibility Tests: *Dilution Techniques:* Quantitative methods that are used to determine MICs provide reproducible estimates of the susceptibility of bacteria to antimicrobial compounds. One such standardized procedure uses a standardized dilution method[1] (broth, agar, or microdilution) or equivalent with cefuroxime powder. The MIC values obtained should be interpreted according to the following criteria:

MIC (mcg/mL)	Interpretation
≤4	(S) Susceptible
8-16	(I) Intermediate
≥32	(R) Resistant

A report of "Susceptible" indicates that the pathogen, if in the blood, is likely to be inhibited by usually achievable concentrations of the antimicrobial compound in blood. A report of "Intermediate" indicates that inhibitory concentrations of the antibiotic may be achieved if high dosage is used or if the infection is confined to tissues or fluids in which high antibiotic concentrations are attained. This category also provides a buffer zone that prevents small, uncontrolled technical factors from causing major discrepancies in interpretation. A report of "Resistant" indicates that usually achievable concentrations of the antimicrobial compound in the blood are unlikely to be inhibitory and that other therapy should be selected.

Standardized susceptibility test procedures require the use of laboratory control microorganisms. Standard cefuroxime powder should give the following MIC values:

Microorganism	MIC (mcg/mL)
Escherichia coli ATCC 25922	2-8
Staphylococcus aureus ATCC 29213	0.5-2

Diffusion Techniques: Quantitative methods that require measurement of zone diameters provide estimates of the susceptibility of bacteria to antimicrobial compounds. One such standardized procedure[2] that has been recommended (for use with disks) to test the susceptibility of microorganisms to cefuroxime uses the 30-mcg cefuroxime disk. Interpretation involves correlation of the diameter obtained in the disk test with the MIC for cefuroxime.

Reports from the laboratory providing results of the standard single-disk susceptibility test with a 30-mcg cefuroxime disk should be interpreted according to the following criteria:

Zone Diameter (mm)	Interpretation
≥23	(S) Susceptible
15-22	(I) Intermediate
≤14	(R) Resistant

Interpretation should be as stated above for results using dilution techniques.

As with standard dilution techniques, diffusion methods require the use of laboratory control microorganisms. The 30-mcg cefuroxime disk provides the following zone diameters in these laboratory test quality control strains:

Microorganism	Zone Diameter (mm)
Escherichia coli ATCC 25922	20-26
Staphylococcus aureus ATCC 25923	27-35

INDICATIONS AND USAGE

NOTE: CEFTIN TABLETS AND CEFTIN FOR ORAL SUSPENSION ARE NOT BIOEQUIVALENT AND ARE NOT SUBSTITUTABLE ON A MILLIGRAM-PER-MILLIGRAM BASIS (SEE CLINICAL PHARMACOLOGY).

CEFTIN Tablets: CEFTIN Tablets are indicated for the treatment of patients with mild to moderate infections caused by susceptible strains of the designated microorganisms in the conditions listed below:

1. **Pharyngitis/Tonsillitis** caused by *Streptococcus pyogenes.*
   NOTE: The usual drug of choice in the treatment and prevention of streptococcal infections, including the prophylaxis of rheumatic fever, is penicillin given by the intramuscular route. CEFTIN Tablets are generally effective in the eradication of streptococci from the nasopharynx; however, substantial data establishing the efficacy of cefuroxime in the subsequent prevention of rheumatic fever are not available. Please also note that in all clinical trials, all isolates had to be sensitive to both penicillin and cefuroxime. There are no data from adequate and well-controlled trials to demonstrate the effectiveness of cefuroxime in the treatment of penicillin-resistant strains of *Streptococcus pyogenes.*
2. **Acute Bacterial Otitis Media** caused by *Streptococcus pneumoniae, Haemophilus influenzae* (including beta-lactamase–producing strains), *Moraxella catarrhalis* (including beta-lactamase–producing strains), or *Streptococcus pyogenes.*
3. **Acute Bacterial Maxillary Sinusitis** caused by *Streptococcus pneumoniae* or *Haemophilus influenzae* (non-beta-lactamase–producing strains only). (See CLINICAL STUDIES section.)
   NOTE: In view of the insufficient numbers of isolates of beta-lactamase–producing strains of *Haemophilus influenzae* and *Moraxella catarrhalis* that were obtained from clinical trials with CEFTIN Tablets for patients with acute bacterial maxillary sinusitis, it was not possible to adequately evaluate the effectiveness of CEFTIN Tablets for sinus infections known, suspected, or considered potentially to be caused by beta-lactamase–producing *Haemophilus influenzae* or *Moraxella catarrhalis.*
4. **Acute Bacterial Exacerbations of Chronic Bronchitis and Secondary Bacterial Infections of Acute Bronchitis** caused by *Streptococcus pneumoniae, Haemophilus influenzae* (beta-lactamase negative strains), or *Haemophilus parainfluenzae* (beta-lactamase negative strains). (See DOSAGE AND ADMINISTRATION section and CLINICAL STUDIES section.)
5. **Uncomplicated Skin and Skin-Structure Infections** caused by *Staphylococcus aureus* (including beta-lactamase–producing strains) or *Streptococcus pyogenes.*
6. **Uncomplicated Urinary Tract Infections** caused by *Escherichia coli* or *Klebsiella pneumoniae.*
7. **Uncomplicated Gonorrhea,** urethral and endocervical, caused by penicillinase-producing and non-penicillinase–producing strains of *Neisseria gonorrhoeae* and uncomplicated gonorrhea, rectal, in females, caused by non-penicillinase–producing strains of *Neisseria gonorrhoeae.*
8. **Early Lyme Disease (erythema migrans)** caused by *Borrelia burgdorferi.*

CEFTIN for Oral Suspension: CEFTIN for Oral Suspension is indicated for the treatment of pediatric patients 3 months to 12 years of age with mild to moderate infections caused by susceptible strains of the designated microorganisms in the conditions listed below. The safety and effectiveness of CEFTIN for Oral Suspension in the treatment of infections other than those specifically listed below have not been established either by adequate and well-controlled trials or by pharmacokinetic data with which to determine an effective and safe dosing regimen.

1. **Pharyngitis/Tonsillitis** caused by *Streptococcus pyogenes.*
   NOTE: The usual drug of choice in the treatment and prevention of streptococcal infections, including the prophylaxis of rheumatic fever, is penicillin given by the intramuscular route. CEFTIN for Oral Suspension is generally effective in the eradication of streptococci from the nasopharynx; however, substantial data establishing the efficacy of cefuroxime in the subsequent prevention of rheumatic fever are not available. Please also note that in all clinical trials, all isolates had to be sensitive to both penicillin and cefuroxime. There are no data from adequate and well-controlled trials to demonstrate the effectiveness of cefuroxime in the treatment of penicillin-resistant strains of *Streptococcus pyogenes.*
2. **Acute Bacterial Otitis Media** caused by *Streptococcus pneumoniae, Haemophilus influenzae* (including beta-lactamase–producing strains), *Moraxella catarrhalis* (including beta-lactamase–producing strains), or *Streptococcus pyogenes.*
3. **Impetigo** caused by *Staphylococcus aureus* (including beta-lactamase–producing strains) or *Streptococcus pyogenes.*

To reduce the development of drug-resistant bacteria and maintain the effectiveness of CEFTIN and other antibacterial drugs, CEFTIN should be used only to treat or prevent infections that are proven or strongly suspected to be caused by susceptible bacteria. When culture and susceptibility information are available, they should be considered in selecting or modifying antibacterial therapy. In the absence of such data, local epidemiology and susceptibility patterns may contribute to the empiric selection of therapy.

CONTRAINDICATIONS

CEFTIN products are contraindicated in patients with known allergy to the cephalosporin group of antibiotics.

WARNINGS

CEFTIN TABLETS AND CEFTIN FOR ORAL SUSPENSION ARE NOT BIOEQUIVALENT AND ARE THEREFORE NOT SUBSTITUTABLE ON A MILLIGRAM-PER-MILLIGRAM BASIS (SEE CLINICAL PHARMACOLOGY).

BEFORE THERAPY WITH CEFTIN PRODUCTS IS INSTITUTED, CAREFUL INQUIRY SHOULD BE MADE TO DETERMINE WHETHER THE PATIENT HAS HAD PREVIOUS HYPERSENSITIVITY REACTIONS TO CEFTIN PRODUCTS, OTHER CEPHALOSPORINS, PENICILLINS, OR OTHER DRUGS. IF THIS PRODUCT IS TO BE GIVEN TO PENICILLIN-SENSITIVE PATIENTS, CAUTION SHOULD BE EXERCISED BECAUSE CROSS-HYPERSENSITIVITY AMONG BETA-LACTAM ANTIBIOTICS HAS BEEN CLEARLY DOCUMENTED AND MAY OCCUR IN UP TO 10% OF PATIENTS WITH A HISTORY OF PENICILLIN ALLERGY. IF A CLINICALLY SIGNIFICANT ALLERGIC REACTION TO CEFTIN PRODUCTS OCCURS, DISCONTINUE THE DRUG AND INSTITUTE APPROPRIATE THERAPY. SERIOUS ACUTE HYPERSENSITIVITY REACTIONS MAY REQUIRE TREATMENT WITH EPINEPHRINE AND OTHER EMERGENCY MEASURES, INCLUDING OXYGEN, INTRAVENOUS FLUIDS, INTRAVENOUS ANTIHISTAMINES, CORTICOSTEROIDS, PRESSOR AMINES, AND AIRWAY MANAGEMENT, AS CLINICALLY INDICATED.

Pseudomembranous colitis has been reported with nearly all antibacterial agents, including cefuroxime, and may range from mild to life threatening. Therefore, it is important to consider this diagnosis in patients who present with diarrhea subsequent to the administration of antibacterial agents.

Treatment with antibacterial agents alters normal flora of the colon and may permit overgrowth of clostridia. Studies indicate that a toxin produced by *Clostridium difficile* is one primary cause of antibiotic-associated colitis.

After the diagnosis of pseudomembranous colitis has been established, appropriate therapeutic measures should be initiated. Mild cases of pseudomembranous colitis usually respond to drug discontinuation alone. In moderate to severe cases, consideration should be given to management with fluids and electrolytes, protein supplementation, and treatment with an antibacterial drug effective against *Clostridium difficile.*

PRECAUTIONS

General: As with other broad-spectrum antibiotics, prolonged administration of cefuroxime axetil may result in overgrowth of nonsusceptible microorganisms. If superinfection occurs during therapy, appropriate measures should be taken.

Cephalosporins, including cefuroxime axetil, should be given with caution to patients receiving concurrent treatment with potent diuretics because these diuretics are suspected of adversely affecting renal function.

Cefuroxime axetil, as with other broad-spectrum antibiotics, should be prescribed with caution in individuals with a history of colitis. The safety and effectiveness of cefuroxime axetil have not been established in patients with gastrointestinal malabsorption. Patients with gastrointestinal malabsorption were excluded from participating in clinical trials of cefuroxime axetil.

Cephalosporins may be associated with a fall in prothrombin activity. Those at risk include patients with renal or hepatic impairment or poor nutritional state, as well as patients receiving a protracted course of antimicrobial therapy, and patients previously stabilized on anticoagulant therapy. Prothrombin time should be monitored in patients at risk and exogenous Vitamin K administered as indicated.

Prescribing CEFTIN in the absence of a proven or strongly suspected bacterial infection or a prophylactic indication is unlikely to provide benefit to the patient and increases the risk of the development of drug-resistant bacteria.

Information for Patients/Caregivers (Pediatric): ***Phenylketonurics:*** CEFTIN for Oral Suspension 125 mg/5 mL contains phenylalanine 11.8 mg per 5 mL (1 teaspoonful) constituted suspension. CEFTIN for Oral Suspension 250 mg/5 mL contains phenylalanine 25.2 mg per 5 mL (1 teaspoonful) constituted suspension.

1. During clinical trials, the tablet was tolerated by pediatric patients old enough to swallow the cefuroxime axetil tablet whole. The crushed tablet has a strong, persistent, bitter taste and should not be administered to pediatric patients in this manner. Pediatric patients who cannot swallow the tablet whole should receive the oral suspension.
2. Discontinuation of therapy due to taste and/or problems of administering this drug occurred in 1.4% of pediatric patients given the oral suspension. Complaints about taste (which may impair compliance) occurred in 5% of pediatric patients.
3. Patients should be counseled that antibacterial drugs, including CEFTIN, should only be used to treat bacterial infections. They do not treat viral infections (e.g., the common cold). When CEFTIN is prescribed to treat a bacterial infection, patients should be told that although it is common to feel better early in the course of therapy, the medication should be taken exactly as directed. Skipping doses or not completing the full course of therapy may: (1) decrease the effectiveness of the immediate treatment, and (2) increase the likelihood that bacteria will develop resistance and will not be treatable by CEFTIN or other antibacterial drugs in the future.

Drug/Laboratory Test Interactions: A false-positive reaction for glucose in the urine may occur with copper reduction tests (Benedict's or Fehling's solution or with CLINITEST® tablets), but not with enzyme-based tests for glycosuria (e.g., CLINISTIX®). As a false-negative result may occur in the ferricyanide test, it is recommended that either the glucose oxidase or hexokinase method be used to determine blood/plasma glucose levels in patients receiving cefuroxime axetil. The presence of cefuroxime does not interfere with the assay of serum and urine creatinine by the alkaline picrate method.

Drug/Drug Interactions: Concomitant administration of probenecid with cefuroxime axetil tablets increases the area under the serum concentration versus time curve by 50%. The peak serum cefuroxime concentration after a 1.5-g single dose is greater when taken with 1 g of probenecid (mean = 14.8 mcg/mL) than without probenecid (mean = 12.2 mcg/mL).

Drugs that reduce gastric acidity may result in a lower bioavailability of CEFTIN compared with that of fasting state and tend to cancel the effect of postprandial absorption.

Carcinogenesis, Mutagenesis, Impairment of Fertility: Although lifetime studies in animals have not been performed to evaluate carcinogenic potential, no mutagenic activity was found for cefuroxime axetil in a battery of bacterial mutation tests. Positive results were obtained in an in vitro chromosome aberration assay; however, negative results were found in an in vivo micronucleus test at doses up to 1.5 g/kg. Reproduction studies in rats at doses up to 1,000 mg/kg/day (9 times the recommended maximum human dose based on mg/m^2) have revealed no impairment of fertility.

Pregnancy: ***Teratogenic Effects:*** Pregnancy Category B. Reproduction studies have been performed in mice at doses up to 3,200 mg/kg/day (14 times the recommended maximum human dose based on mg/m^2) and in rats at doses up to 1,000 mg/kg/day (9 times the recommended maximum human dose based on mg/m^2) and have revealed no evidence of impaired fertility or harm to the fetus due to cefuroxime axetil. There are, however, no adequate and well-controlled studies in pregnant women. Because animal reproduction studies are not always predictive of human response, this drug should be used during pregnancy only if clearly needed.

Continued on next page

Product information on these pages is effective as of August 2004. Further information is available at: GlaxoSmithKline, PO Box 13398, Research Triangle Park, NC 27709. 1-888-825-5249. Corporate Web Site: www.gsk.com

Ceftin—Cont.

Labor and Delivery: Cefuroxime axetil has not been studied for use during labor and delivery.

Nursing Mothers: Because cefuroxime is excreted in human milk, consideration should be given to discontinuing nursing temporarily during treatment with cefuroxime axetil.

Pediatric Use: The safety and effectiveness of CEFTIN have been established for pediatric patients aged 3 months to 12 years for acute bacterial maxillary sinusitis based upon its approval in adults. Use of CEFTIN in pediatric patients is supported by pharmacokinetic and safety data in adults and pediatric patients, and by clinical and microbiological data from adequate and well-controlled studies of the treatment of acute bacterial maxillary sinusitis in adults and of acute otitis media with effusion in pediatric patients. It is also supported by post-marketing adverse events surveillance (see CLINICAL PHARMACOLOGY, INDICATIONS AND USAGE, ADVERSE REACTIONS, DOSAGE AND ADMINISTRATION, and CLINICAL STUDIES).

Geriatric Use: Of the total number of subjects who received cefuroxime axetil in 20 clinical studies of CEFTIN, 375 were 65 and over while 151 were 75 and over. No overall differences in safety or effectiveness were observed between these subjects and younger adult subjects. The geriatric patients reported somewhat fewer gastrointestinal events and less frequent vaginal candidiasis compared with patients aged 12 to 64 years old; however, no clinically significant differences were reported between the elderly and younger adult patients. Other reported clinical experience has not identified differences in responses between the elderly and younger adult patients.

ADVERSE REACTIONS

CEFTIN TABLETS IN CLINICAL TRIALS: Multiple-Dose Dosing Regimens: ***7 to 10 Days Dosing:*** Using multiple doses of cefuroxime axetil tablets, 912 patients were treated with cefuroxime axetil (125 to 500 mg twice daily). There were no deaths or permanent disabilities thought related to drug toxicity. Twenty (2.2%) patients discontinued medication due to adverse events thought by the investigators to be possibly, probably, or almost certainly related to drug toxicity. Seventeen (85%) of the 20 patients who discontinued therapy did so because of gastrointestinal disturbances, including diarrhea, nausea, vomiting, and abdominal pain. The percentage of cefuroxime axetil tablet-treated patients who discontinued study drug because of adverse events was very similar at daily doses of 1,000, 500, and 250 mg (2.3%, 2.1%, and 2.2%, respectively). However, the incidence of gastrointestinal adverse events increased with the higher recommended doses.

The following adverse events were thought by the investigators to be possibly, probably, or almost certainly related to cefuroxime axetil tablets in multiple-dose clinical trials (n = 912 cefuroxime axetil-treated patients).

Table 4. Adverse Reactions—CEFTIN Tablets Multiple-Dose Dosing Regimens—Clinical Trials

Incidence ≥1%	Diarrhea/loose stools	3.7%
	Nausea/vomiting	3.0%
	Transient elevation in AST	2.0%
	Transient elevation in ALT	1.6%
	Eosinophilia	1.1%
	Transient elevation in LDH	1.0%
Incidence <1% but >0.1%	Abdominal pain	
	Abdominal cramps	
	Flatulence	
	Indigestion	
	Headache	
	Vaginitis	
	Vulvar itch	
	Rash	
	Hives	
	Itch	
	Dysuria	
	Chills	
	Chest pain	
	Shortness of breath	
	Mouth ulcers	
	Swollen tongue	
	Sleepiness	
	Thirst	
	Anorexia	
	Positive Coombs test	

5-Day Experience (see CLINICAL STUDIES section): In clinical trials using CEFTIN in a dose of 250 mg twice daily in the treatment of secondary bacterial infections of acute bronchitis, 399 patients were treated for 5 days and 402 patients were treated for 10 days. No difference in the occurrence of adverse events was found between the 2 regimens.

In Clinical Trials for Early Lyme Disease With 20 Days Dosing: Two multicenter trials assessed cefuroxime axetil tablets 500 mg twice a day for 20 days. The most common drug-related adverse experiences were diarrhea (10.6% of patients), Jarisch-Herxheimer reaction (5.6%), and vaginitis (5.4%). Other adverse experiences occurred with frequencies comparable to those reported with 7 to 10 days dosing.

Single-Dose Regimen for Uncomplicated Gonorrhea: In clinical trials using a single dose of cefuroxime axetil tablets, 1,061 patients were treated with the recommended dosage of cefuroxime axetil (1,000 mg) for the treatment of uncomplicated gonorrhea. There were no deaths or permanent disabilities thought related to drug toxicity in these studies.

The following adverse events were thought by the investigators to be possibly, probably, or almost certainly related to cefuroxime axetil in 1,000-mg single-dose clinical trials of cefuroxime axetil tablets in the treatment of uncomplicated gonorrhea conducted in the United States.

Table 5. Adverse Reactions—CEFTIN Tablets 1-g Single-Dose Regimen for Uncomplicated Gonorrhea—Clinical Trials

Incidence ≥1%	Nausea/vomiting	6.8%
	Diarrhea	4.2%
Incidence <1% but >0.1%	Abdominal pain	
	Dyspepsia	
	Erythema	
	Rash	
	Pruritus	
	Vaginal candidiasis	
	Vaginal itch	
	Vaginal discharge	
	Headache	
	Dizziness	
	Somnolence	
	Muscle cramps	
	Muscle stiffness	
	Muscle spasm of neck	
	Tightness/pain in chest	
	Bleeding/pain in urethra	
	Kidney pain	
	Tachycardia	
	Lockjaw-type reaction	

CEFTIN FOR ORAL SUSPENSION IN CLINICAL TRIALS

In clinical trials using multiple doses of cefuroxime axetil powder for oral suspension, pediatric patients (96.7% of whom were younger than 12 years of age) were treated with the recommended dosages of cefuroxime axetil (20 to 30 mg/kg/day divided twice a day up to a maximum dose of 500 or 1,000 mg/day, respectively). There were no deaths or permanent disabilities in any of the patients in these studies. Eleven US patients (1.2%) discontinued medication due to adverse events thought by the investigators to be possibly, probably, or almost certainly related to drug toxicity. The discontinuations were primarily for gastrointestinal disturbances, usually diarrhea or vomiting. During clinical trials, discontinuation of therapy due to the taste and/or problems with administering this drug occurred in 13 (1.4%) pediatric patients enrolled at centers in the United States.

The following adverse events were thought by the investigators to be possibly, probably, or almost certainly related to cefuroxime axetil for oral suspension in multiple-dose clinical trials (n = 931 cefuroxime axetil-treated US patients).

Table 6. Adverse Reactions—CEFTIN for Oral Suspension Multiple-Dose Dosing Regimens—Clinical Trials

Incidence ≥1%	Diarrhea/loose stools	8.6%
	Dislike of taste	5.0%
	Diaper rash	3.4%
	Nausea/vomiting	2.6%
Incidence <1% but >0.1%	Abdominal pain	
	Flatulence	
	Gastrointestinal infection	
	Candidiasis	
	Vaginal irritation	
	Rash	
	Hyperactivity	
	Irritable behavior	
	Eosinophilia	
	Positive direct Coombs test	
	Elevated liver enzymes	
	Viral illness	
	Upper respiratory infection	
	Sinusitis	
	Cough	
	Urinary tract infection	
	Joint swelling	
	Arthralgia	
	Fever	
	Ptyalism	

Table 7. CEFTIN Tablets (May be administered without regard to meals.)

Population/Infection	Dosage	Duration (days)
Adolescents and Adults (13 years and older)		
Pharyngitis/tonsillitis	250 mg b.i.d.	10
Acute bacterial maxillary sinusitis	250 mg b.i.d.	10
Acute bacterial exacerbations of chronic bronchitis	250 or 500 mg b.i.d.	10*
Secondary bacterial infections of acute bronchitis	250 or 500 mg b.i.d.	5–10
Uncomplicated skin and skin-structure infections	250 or 500 mg b.i.d.	10
Uncomplicated urinary tract infections	250 mg b.i.d.	7–10
Uncomplicated gonorrhea	1,000 mg once	single dose
Early Lyme disease	500 mg b.i.d.	20
Pediatric Patients (who can swallow tablets whole)		
Acute otitis media	250 mg b.i.d.	10
Acute bacterial maxillary sinusitis	250 mg b.i.d.	10

*The safety and effectiveness of CEFTIN administered for less than 10 days in patients with acute exacerbations of chronic bronchitis have not been established.

POSTMARKETING EXPERIENCE WITH CEFTIN PRODUCTS

In addition to adverse events reported during clinical trials, the following events have been identified during clinical practice in patients treated with CEFTIN Tablets or with CEFTIN for Oral Suspension and were reported spontaneously. Data are generally insufficient to allow an estimate of incidence or to establish causation.

General: The following hypersensitivity reactions have been reported: anaphylaxis, angioedema, pruritus, rash, serum sickness-like reaction, urticaria.

Gastrointestinal: Pseudomembranous colitis (see WARNINGS).

Hematologic: Hemolytic anemia, leukopenia, pancytopenia, thrombocytopenia, and increased prothrombin time.

Hepatic: Hepatic impairment including hepatitis and cholestasis, jaundice.

Neurologic: Seizure.

Skin: Erythema multiforme, Stevens-Johnson syndrome, toxic epidermal necrolysis.

Urologic: Renal dysfunction.

CEPHALOSPORIN-CLASS ADVERSE REACTIONS

In addition to the adverse reactions listed above that have been observed in patients treated with cefuroxime axetil, the following adverse reactions and altered laboratory tests have been reported for cephalosporin-class antibiotics: toxic nephropathy, aplastic anemia, hemorrhage, increased BUN, increased creatinine, false-positive test for urinary glucose, increased alkaline phosphatase, neutropenia, elevated bilirubin, and agranulocytosis.

Several cephalosporins have been implicated in triggering seizures, particularly in patients with renal impairment when the dosage was not reduced (see DOSAGE AND ADMINISTRATION and OVERDOSAGE). If seizures associated with drug therapy occur, the drug should be discontinued. Anticonvulsant therapy can be given if clinically indicated.

OVERDOSAGE

Overdosage of cephalosporins can cause cerebral irritation leading to convulsions. Serum levels of cefuroxime can be reduced by hemodialysis and peritoneal dialysis.

DOSAGE AND ADMINISTRATION

NOTE: CEFTIN TABLETS AND CEFTIN FOR ORAL SUSPENSION ARE NOT BIOEQUIVALENT AND ARE NOT SUBSTITUTABLE ON A MILLIGRAM-PER-MILLIGRAM BASIS (SEE CLINICAL PHARMACOLOGY).

[See table 7 above]

CEFTIN for Oral Suspension: CEFTIN for Oral Suspension may be administered to pediatric patients ranging in age from 3 months to 12 years, according to dosages in Table 8:

[See table 8 at top of next page]

Patients With Renal Failure: The safety and efficacy of cefuroxime axetil in patients with renal failure have not been established. Since cefuroxime is renally eliminated, its half-life will be prolonged in patients with renal failure.

Directions for Mixing CEFTIN for Oral Suspension: Prepare a suspension at the time of dispensing as follows:

1. Shake the bottle to loosen the powder.
2. Remove the cap.
3. Add the total amount of water for reconstitution (see Table 9) and replace the cap.
4. Invert the bottle and vigorously rock the bottle from side to side so that water rises through the powder.
5. Once the sound of the powder against the bottle disappears, turn the bottle upright and vigorously shake it in a diagonal direction.

[See table 9 at top of next page]

NOTE: SHAKE THE ORAL SUSPENSION WELL BEFORE EACH USE. Replace cap securely after each opening. Store the reconstituted suspension between 2° and 8°C (36° and 16°F) (in a refrigerator). DISCARD AFTER 10 DAYS.

HOW SUPPLIED

CEFTIN Tablets: CEFTIN Tablets, 250 mg of cefuroxime (as cefuroxime axetil), are light blue, capsule-shaped, film-coated tablets engraved with "387" on one side and "Glaxo" on the other side as follows:

20 Tablets/Bottle NDC 0173-0387-00
60 Tablets/Bottle NDC 0173-0387-42
Unit Dose Packs of 100 NDC 0173-0387-01

CEFTIN Tablets, 500 mg of cefuroxime (as cefuroxime axetil), are dark blue, capsule-shaped, film-coated tablets engraved with "394" on one side and "Glaxo" on the other side as follows:

20 Tablets/Bottle NDC 0173-0394-00
60 Tablets/Bottle NDC 0173-0394-42
Unit Dose Packs of 50 NDC 0173-0394-01

Store the tablets between 15° and 30°C (59° and 86°F). Replace cap securely after each opening. Protect unit dose packs from excessive moisture.

CEFTIN for Oral Suspension: CEFTIN for Oral Suspension is provided as dry, white to off-white, tutti-frutti–flavored powder. When reconstituted as directed, CEFTIN for Oral Suspension provides the equivalent of 125 mg or 250 mg of cefuroxime (as cefuroxime axetil) per 5 mL of suspension. It is supplied in amber glass bottles as follows:

125 mg/5 mL: 100-mL Suspension NDC 0173-0740-00
250 mg/5 mL: 50-mL Suspension NDC 0173-0741-10
100-mL Suspension NDC 0173-0741-00

Before reconstitution, store dry powder between 2° and 30°C (36° and 86°F).

After reconstitution, store suspension between 2° and 8°C (36° and 46°F), in a refrigerator. DISCARD AFTER 10 DAYS.

CLINICAL STUDIES

CEFTIN Tablets: ***Acute Bacterial Maxillary Sinusitis:*** One adequate and well-controlled study was performed in patients with acute bacterial maxillary sinusitis. In this study each patient had a maxillary sinus aspirate collected by sinus puncture before treatment was initiated for presumptive acute bacterial sinusitis. All patients had to have radiographic and clinical evidence of acute maxillary sinusitis. As shown in the following summary of the study, the general clinical effectiveness of CEFTIN Tablets was comparable to an oral antimicrobial agent that contained a specific beta-lactamase inhibitor in treating acute maxillary sinusitis. However, sufficient microbiology data were obtained to demonstrate the effectiveness of CEFTIN Tablets in treating acute bacterial maxillary sinusitis due only to *Streptococcus pneumoniae* or non-beta-lactamase–producing *Haemophilus influenzae*. An insufficient number of beta-lactamase–producing *Haemophilus influenzae* and *Moraxella catarrhalis* isolates were obtained in this trial to adequately evaluate the effectiveness of CEFTIN Tablets in the treatment of acute bacterial maxillary sinusitis due to these 2 organisms. This study enrolled 317 adult patients, 132 patients in the United States and 185 patients in South America. Patients were randomized in a 1:1 ratio to cefuroxime axetil 250 mg twice daily or an oral antimicrobial agent that contained a specific beta-lactamase inhibitor. An intent-to-treat analysis of the submitted clinical data yielded the following results:
[See table 10 above]

In this trial and in a supporting maxillary puncture trial, 15 evaluable patients had non-beta-lactamase–producing *Haemophilus influenzae* as the identified pathogen. Ten (10) of these 15 patients (67%) had their pathogen (non-beta-lactamase–producing *Haemophilus influenzae*) eradicated. Eighteen (18) evaluable patients had *Streptococcus pneumoniae* as the identified pathogen. Fifteen (15) of these 18 patients (83%) had their pathogen (*Streptococcus pneumoniae*) eradicated.

Safety: The incidence of drug-related gastrointestinal adverse events was statistically significantly higher in the control arm (an oral antimicrobial agent that contained a specific beta-lactamase inhibitor) versus the cefuroxime axetil arm (12% versus 1%, respectively; $P<.001$), particularly drug-related diarrhea (8% versus 1%, respectively; $P = .001$).

Early Lyme Disease: Two adequate and well-controlled studies were performed in patients with early Lyme disease. In these studies all patients had to present with physician-documented erythema migrans, with or without systemic manifestations of infection. Patients were randomized in a 1:1 ratio to a 20-day course of treatment with cefuroxime axetil 500 mg twice daily or doxycycline 100 mg 3 times daily. Patients were assessed at 1 month posttreatment for success in treating early Lyme disease (Part I) and at 1 year posttreatment for success in preventing the progression to the sequelae of late Lyme disease (Part II).

A total of 355 adult patients (181 treated with cefuroxime axetil and 174 treated with doxycycline) were enrolled in the 2 studies. In order to objectively validate the clinical diagnosis of early Lyme disease in these patients, 2 approaches were used: 1) blinded expert reading of photographs, when available, of the pretreatment erythema migrans skin lesion; and 2) serologic confirmation (using enzyme-linked immunosorbent assay [ELISA] and immunoblot assay ["Western" blot]) of the presence of antibodies specific to *Borrelia burgdorferi*, the etiologic agent of Lyme disease. By these procedures, it was possible to confirm the physician diagnosis of early Lyme disease in 281 (79%) of the 355 study patients. The efficacy data summarized below are specific to this "validated" patient subset, while the safety data summarized below reflect the entire patient population for the 2 studies.

Analysis of the submitted clinical data for evaluable patients in the "validated" patient subset yielded the following results:
[See table 11 above]

CEFTIN and doxycycline were effective in prevention of the development of sequelae of late Lyme disease.

Safety: Drug-related adverse events affecting the skin were reported significantly more frequently by patients treated with doxycycline than by patients treated with cefuroxime axetil (12% versus 3%, respectively; $P = .002$), primarily reflecting the statistically significantly higher incidence of drug-related photosensitivity reactions in the doxycycline arm versus the cefuroxime axetil arm (9% versus 0%, respectively; $P<.001$). While the incidence of drug-related gastrointestinal adverse events was similar in the 2 treatment groups (cefuroxime axetil - 13%; doxycycline - 11%), the incidence of drug-related diarrhea was statistically significantly higher in the cefuroxime axetil arm versus the doxycycline arm (11% versus 3%, respectively; $P = .005$).

Table 8. CEFTIN for Oral Suspension (Must be administered with food. Shake well each time before using.)

Population/Infection	Dosage	Daily Maximum Dose	Duration (days)
Pediatric Patients (3 months to 12 years)			
Pharyngitis/tonsillitis	20 mg/kg/day divided b.i.d.	500 mg	10
Acute otitis media	30 mg/kg/day divided b.i.d.	1,000 mg	10
Acute bacterial maxillary sinusitis	30 mg/kg/day divided b.i.d.	1,000 mg	10
Impetigo	30 mg/kg/day divided b.i.d.	1,000 mg	10

Table 9. Amount of Water Required for Reconstitution of Labeled Volumes of CEFTIN for Oral Suspension

CEFTIN for Oral Suspension	Labeled Volume After Reconstitution	Amount of Water Required for Reconstitution
125 mg/5 mL	100 mL	37 mL
250 mg/5 mL	50 mL	19 mL
	100 mL	35 mL

Table 10. Clinical Effectiveness of CEFTIN Tablets Compared to Beta-Lactamase Inhibitor-Containing Control Drug in the Treatment of Acute Bacterial Maxillary Sinusitis

	US Patients*		South American Patients†	
	CEFTIN (n = 49)	Control (n = 43)	CEFTIN (n = 87)	Control (n = 89)
Clinical success (cure + improvement)	65%	53%	77%	74%
Clinical cure	53%	44%	72%	64%
Clinical improvement	12%	9%	5%	10%

*95% Confidence interval around the success difference [-0.08, +0.32].
† 95% Confidence interval around the success difference [-0.10, +0.16].

Table 11. Clinical Effectiveness of CEFTIN Tablets Compared to Doxycycline in the Treatment of Early Lyme Disease

	Part I (1 Month Posttreatment)*		Part II (1 Year Posttreatment)†	
	CEFTIN (n = 125)	Doxycycline (n = 108)	CEFTIN (n = 105‡)	Doxycycline (n = 83‡)
Satisfactory clinical outcome§	91%	93%	84%	87%
Clinical cure/success	72%	73%	73%	73%
Clinical improvement	19%	19%	10%	13%

*95% confidence interval around the satisfactory difference for Part I (−0.08, +0.05).
† 95% confidence interval around the satisfactory difference for Part II (−0.13, +0.07).
‡ n's include patients assessed as unsatisfactory clinical outcomes (failure + recurrence) in Part I (CEFTIN - 11 [5 failure, 6 recurrence]; doxycycline - 8 [6 failure, 2 recurrence]).
§ Satisfactory clinical outcome includes cure + improvement (Part I) and success + improvement (Part II).

Table 12. Clinical Effectiveness of CEFTIN Tablets 250 mg Twice Daily in Secondary Bacterial Infections of Acute Bronchitis: Comparison of 5 Versus 10 Days' Treatment Duration

	CAE-516 and CAE-517*		CAEA4001 and CAEA4002†	
	5 Day (n = 127)	10 Day (n = 139)	5 Day (n = 173)	10 Day (n = 192)
Clinical success (cure + improvement)	80%	87%	84%	82%
Clinical cure	61%	70%	73%	72%
Clinical improvement	19%	17%	11%	10%

*95% Confidence interval around the success difference [−0.164, +0.029].
† 95% Confidence interval around the success difference [−0.061, +0.103].

Secondary Bacterial Infections of Acute Bronchitis: Four randomized, controlled clinical studies were performed comparing 5 days versus 10 days of CEFTIN for the treatment of patients with secondary bacterial infections of acute bronchitis. These studies enrolled a total of 1,253 patients (CAE-516 n = 360; CAE-517 n = 177; CAEA4001 n = 362; CAEA4002 n = 354). The protocols for CAE-516 and CAE-517 were identical and compared CEFTIN 250 mg twice daily for 5 days, CEFTIN 250 mg twice daily for 10 days, and AUGMENTIN® 500 mg 3 times daily for 10 days. These 2 studies were conducted simultaneously. CAEA4001 and CAEA4002 compared CEFTIN 250 mg twice daily for 5 days, CEFTIN 250 mg twice daily for 10 days, and CECLOR® 250 mg 3 times daily for 10 days. They were otherwise identical to CAE-516 and CAE-517 and were con-

Continued on next page

Product information on these pages is effective as of August 2004. Further information is available at: GlaxoSmithKline, PO Box 13398, Research Triangle Park, NC 27709. 1-888-825-5249. Corporate Web Site: www.gsk.com

Ceftin—Cont.

ducted over the following 2 years. Patients were required to have polymorphonuclear cells present on the Gram stain of their screening sputum specimen, but isolation of a bacterial pathogen from the sputum culture was not required for inclusion. The following table demonstrates the results of the clinical outcome analysis of the pooled studies CAE-516/CAE-517 and CAEA4001/CAEA4002, respectively:

[See table 12 on previous page]

The response rates for patients who were both clinically and bacteriologically evaluable were consistent with those reported for the clinically evaluable patients.

Safety: In these clinical trials, 399 patients were treated with CEFTIN for 5 days and 402 patients with CEFTIN for 10 days. No difference in the occurrence of adverse events was observed between the 2 regimens.

REFERENCES

1. National Committee for Clinical Laboratory Standards. *Methods for Dilution Antimicrobial Susceptibility Tests for Bacteria that Grow Aerobically.* 3rd ed. Approved Standard NCCLS Document M7-A3, Vol. 13, No. 25. Villanova, Pa: NCCLS; 1993.
2. National Committee for Clinical Laboratory Standards. *Performance Standards for Antimicrobial Disk Susceptibility Tests.* 4th ed. Approved Standard NCCLS Document M2-A4, Vol. 10, No. 7. Villanova, Pa: NCCLS; 1990.

GlaxoSmithKline, Research Triangle Park, NC 27709

October 2003/RL-2046

Shown in Product Identification Guide, page 315

COMBIVIR® ℞

[kom' bə-vir]
(lamivudine/zidovudine)
Tablets

> **WARNING**
> **ZIDOVUDINE, ONE OF THE TWO ACTIVE INGREDIENTS IN COMBIVIR, HAS BEEN ASSOCIATED WITH HEMATOLOGIC TOXICITY INCLUDING NEUTROPENIA AND SEVERE ANEMIA, PARTICULARLY IN PATIENTS WITH ADVANCED HIV DISEASE (SEE WARNINGS). PROLONGED USE OF ZIDOVUDINE HAS BEEN ASSOCIATED WITH SYMPTOMATIC MYOPATHY.**
> **LACTIC ACIDOSIS AND SEVERE HEPATOMEGALY WITH STEATOSIS, INCLUDING FATAL CASES, HAVE BEEN REPORTED WITH THE USE OF NUCLEOSIDE ANALOGUES ALONE OR IN COMBINATION, INCLUDING LAMIVUDINE, ZIDOVUDINE, AND OTHER ANTIRETROVIRALS (SEE WARNINGS).**
> **SEVERE ACUTE EXACERBATIONS OF HEPATITIS B HAVE BEEN REPORTED IN PATIENTS WHO ARE CO-INFECTED WITH HEPATITIS B VIRUS (HBV) AND HIV AND HAVE DISCONTINUED LAMIVUDINE, WHICH IS ONE COMPONENT OF COMBIVIR. HEPATIC FUNCTION SHOULD BE MONITORED CLOSELY WITH BOTH CLINICAL AND LABORATORY FOLLOW-UP FOR AT LEAST SEVERAL MONTHS IN PATIENTS WHO DISCONTINUE COMBIVIR AND ARE CO-INFECTED WITH HIV AND HBV. IF APPROPRIATE, INITIATION OF ANTI-HEPATITIS B THERAPY MAY BE WARRANTED (SEE WARNINGS).**

DESCRIPTION

COMBIVIR: COMBIVIR Tablets are combination tablets containing lamivudine and zidovudine. Lamivudine (EPIVIR®, 3TC®) and zidovudine (RETROVIR®, azidothymidine, AZT, or ZDV) are synthetic nucleoside analogues with activity against human immunodeficiency virus (HIV). COMBIVIR Tablets are for oral administration. Each film-coated tablet contains 150 mg of lamivudine, 300 mg of zidovudine, and the inactive ingredients colloidal silicon dioxide, hypromellose, magnesium stearate, microcrystalline cellulose, polyethylene glycol, polysorbate 80, sodium starch glycolate, and titanium dioxide.

Lamivudine: The chemical name of lamivudine is (2R,cis)-4-amino-1-(2-hydroxymethyl-1,3-oxathiolan-5-yl)-(1H)-pyrimidin-2-one. Lamivudine is the (-)enantiomer of a dideoxy analogue of cytidine. Lamivudine has also been referred to as (-)2′,3′-dideoxy, 3′-thiacytidine. It has a molecular formula of $C_8H_{11}N_3O_3S$.

Lamivudine is a white to off-white crystalline solid with a solubility of approximately 70 mg/mL in water at 20°C.

Zidovudine: The chemical name of zidovudine is 3′-azido-3′-deoxythymidine. It has a molecular formula of $C_{10}H_{13}N_5O_4$ and a molecular weight of 267.24.

Zidovudine is a white to beige, odorless, crystalline solid with a solubility of 20.1 mg/mL in water at 25°C.

MICROBIOLOGY

Mechanism of Action: ***Lamivudine:*** Lamivudine is a synthetic nucleoside analogue. Intracellularly, lamivudine is phosphorylated to its active 5′-triphosphate metabolite, lamivudine triphosphate (L-TP). The principal mode of action of L-TP is inhibition of reverse transcriptase (RT) via DNA chain termination after incorporation of the nucleoside analogue. L-TP is a weak inhibitor of mammalian DNA polymerases α and β, and mitochondrial DNA polymerase-γ.

Zidovudine: Zidovudine is a synthetic nucleoside analogue. Intracellularly, zidovudine is phosphorylated to its active 5′-triphosphate metabolite, zidovudine triphosphate (ZDV-TP). The principal mode of action of ZDV-TP is inhibition of RT via DNA chain termination after incorporation of the nucleoside analogue. ZDV-TP is a weak inhibitor of the mammalian DNA polymerase-α and mitochondrial DNA polymerase-γ and has been reported to be incorporated into the DNA of cells in culture.

Antiviral Activity In Vitro: The relationship between in vitro susceptibility of HIV to lamivudine or zidovudine and the inhibition of HIV replication in humans has not been established.

Lamivudine Plus Zidovudine: In HIV-1–infected MT-4 cells, lamivudine in combination with zidovudine had synergistic antiretroviral activity. Synergistic activity of lamivudine and zidovudine was also shown in a variable-ratio study.

Lamivudine: In vitro activity of lamivudine against HIV-1 was assessed in a number of cell lines (including monocytes and fresh human peripheral blood lymphocytes). IC_{50} and IC_{90} values (50% and 90% inhibitory concentrations) for lamivudine were 0.0006 mcg/mL to 0.034 mcg/mL and 0.015 to 0.321 mcg/mL, respectively. Lamivudine had anti–HIV-1 activity in all acute virus-cell infections tested.

Zidovudine: In vitro activity of zidovudine against HIV-1 was assessed in a number of cell lines (including monocytes and fresh human peripheral blood lymphocytes). The IC_{50} and IC_{90} values for zidovudine were 0.003 to 0.013 mcg/mL and 0.03 to 0.13 mcg/mL, respectively. Zidovudine had anti–HIV-1 activity in all acute virus-cell infections tested. However, zidovudine activity was substantially less in chronically infected cell lines. In cell culture drug combination studies with zidovudine, interferon-alpha demonstrated additive activity and zalcitabine, didanosine, saquinavir, indinavir, ritonavir, nelfinavir, nevirapine, and delavirdine demonstrated synergistic activity.

Drug Resistance: Lamivudine Plus Zidovudine Administered As Separate Formulations: In patients receiving lamivudine monotherapy or combination therapy with lamivudine plus zidovudine, HIV-1 isolates from most patients became phenotypically and genotypically resistant to lamivudine within 12 weeks. In some patients harboring zidovudine-resistant virus at baseline, phenotypic sensitivity to zidovudine was restored by 12 weeks of treatment with lamivudine and zidovudine. Combination therapy with lamivudine plus zidovudine delayed the emergence of mutations conferring resistance to zidovudine.

HIV-1 strains resistant to both lamivudine and zidovudine have been isolated from patients after prolonged lamivudine/zidovudine therapy. Dual resistance required the presence of multiple mutations, the most essential of which may be at codon 333 (Gly→Glu). The incidence of dual resistance and the duration of combination therapy required before dual resistance occurs are unknown.

Lamivudine: Lamivudine-resistant isolates of HIV-1 have been selected in vitro and have also been recovered from patients treated with lamivudine or lamivudine plus zidovudine. Genotypic analysis of the resistant isolates showed that the resistance was due to mutations in the HIV-1 reverse transcriptase gene at codon 184 from methionine to either isoleucine or valine.

Zidovudine: HIV isolates with reduced susceptibility to zidovudine have been selected in vitro and were also recovered from patients treated with zidovudine. Genotypic analyses of the isolates showed mutations which result in 5 amino acid substitutions (Met41→Leu, Asp67→Asn, Lys70→Arg, Thr215→Tyr or Phe, and Lys219→Gln) in the HIV-1 reverse transcriptase gene. In general, higher levels of resistance were associated with greater number of mutations.

Cross-Resistance: Cross-resistance among certain reverse transcriptase inhibitors has been recognized.

Lamivudine Plus Zidovudine: Cross-resistance between lamivudine and zidovudine has not been reported. In some patients treated with lamivudine alone or in combination with zidovudine, isolates have emerged with a mutation at codon 184, which confers resistance to lamivudine. In the presence of the 184 mutation, cross-resistance to didanosine and zalcitabine has been seen in some patients; the clinical significance is unknown. In some patients treated with zidovudine plus didanosine or zalcitabine, isolates resistant to multiple drugs, including lamivudine, have emerged (see under Zidovudine below).

Lamivudine: See Lamivudine Plus Zidovudine (above).

Zidovudine: HIV isolates with multidrug resistance to zidovudine, didanosine, zalcitabine, stavudine, and lamivudine were recovered from a small number of patients treated for ≥1 year with zidovudine plus didanosine or zidovudine plus zalcitabine. The pattern of genotypic resistant mutations with such combination therapies was different (Ala62→Val, Val75→Ile, Phe77→Leu, Phe116→Tyr, and Gln151→Met) from the pattern with zidovudine monotherapy, with the 151 mutation being most commonly associated with multidrug resistance. The mutation at codon 151 in combination with the mutations at 62, 75, 77, and 116 results in a virus with reduced susceptibility to zidovudine, didanosine, zalcitabine, stavudine, and lamivudine.

Multiple-drug resistance has been observed in 2 of 39 (5%) patients receiving zidovudine and didanosine combination therapy for 2 years.

CLINICAL PHARMACOLOGY

Pharmacokinetics in Adults: ***COMBIVIR:*** One COMBIVIR Tablet was bioequivalent to one EPIVIR Tablet (150 mg) plus one RETROVIR Tablet (300 mg) following single-dose administration to fasting healthy subjects (n = 24).

Lamivudine: The pharmacokinetic properties of lamivudine in fasting patients are summarized in Table 1. Following oral administration, lamivudine is rapidly absorbed and extensively distributed. Binding to plasma protein is low. Approximately 70% of an intravenous dose of lamivudine is recovered as unchanged drug in the urine. Metabolism of lamivudine is a minor route of elimination. In humans, the only known metabolite is the trans-sulfoxide metabolite (approximately 5% of an oral dose after 12 hours).

Zidovudine: The pharmacokinetic properties of zidovudine in fasting patients are summarized in Table 1. Following oral administration, zidovudine is rapidly absorbed and extensively distributed. Binding to plasma protein is low. Zidovudine is eliminated primarily by hepatic metabolism. The major metabolite of zidovudine is 3′-azido-3′-deoxy-5′-*O*-β-*D*-glucopyranuronosylthymidine (GZDV). GZDV area under the curve (AUC) is about 3-fold greater than the zidovudine AUC. Urinary recovery of zidovudine and GZDV accounts for 14% and 74% of the dose following oral administration, respectively. A second metabolite, 3′-amino-3′-deoxythymidine (AMT), has been identified in plasma. The AMT AUC was one fifth of the zidovudine AUC.

[See table 1 at left]

Effect of Food on Absorption of COMBIVIR: COMBIVIR may be administered with or without food. The extent of lamivudine and zidovudine absorption (AUC) following administration of COMBIVIR with food was similar when compared to fasting healthy subjects (n = 24).

Special Populations: ***Impaired Renal Function: COMBIVIR:*** Because lamivudine and zidovudine require dose adjustment in the presence of renal insufficiency, COMBIVIR is not recommended for patients with impaired renal function (see PRECAUTIONS).

Impaired Hepatic Function: COMBIVIR: A reduction in the daily dose of zidovudine may be necessary in patients with mild to moderate impaired hepatic function or liver cirrhosis. Because COMBIVIR is a fixed-dose combination that cannot be adjusted for this patient population, COMBIVIR is not recommended for patients with impaired hepatic function.

Pregnancy: See PRECAUTIONS: Pregnancy.

COMBIVIR: No data are available.

Zidovudine: Zidovudine pharmacokinetics has been studied in a Phase 1 study of 8 women during the last trimester of pregnancy. As pregnancy progressed, there was no evidence of drug accumulation. The pharmacokinetics of zidovudine was similar to that of nonpregnant adults. Consistent with passive transmission of the drug across the placenta, zidovudine concentrations in neonatal plasma at birth were essentially equal to those in maternal plasma at delivery. Although data are limited, methadone maintenance therapy in 5 pregnant women did not appear to alter zidovudine pharmacokinetics. In a nonpregnant adult population, a potential for interaction has been identified (see CLINICAL PHARMACOLOGY: Drug Interactions).

Nursing Mothers: See PRECAUTIONS: Nursing Mothers.

Lamivudine: Samples of breast milk obtained from 20 mothers receiving lamivudine monotherapy (300 mg twice daily) or combination therapy (150 mg lamivudine twice daily and 300 mg zidovudine twice daily) had measurable concentrations of lamivudine.

COMBIVIR: No data are available.

Table 1. Pharmacokinetic Parameters* for Lamivudine and Zidovudine in Adults

Parameter	Lamivudine		Zidovudine	
Oral bioavailability (%)	86 ± 16	n = 12	64 ± 10	n = 5
Apparent volume of distribution (L/kg)	1.3 ± 0.4	n = 20	1.6 ± 0.6	n = 8
Plasma protein binding (%)	<36		<38	
CSF:plasma ratio†	0.12 [0.04 to 0.47]	n = 38‡	0.60 [0.04 to 2.62]	n = 39§
Systemic clearance (L/hr/kg)	0.33 ± 0.06	n = 20	1.6 ± 0.6	n = 6
Renal clearance (L/hr/kg)	0.22 ± 0.06	n = 20	0.34 ± 0.05	n = 9
Elimination half-life (hr)‖	5 to 7		0.5 to 3	

*Data presented as mean ± standard deviation except where noted.
† Median [range].
‡ Children.
§ Adults.
‖ Approximate range.

Zidovudine: After administration of a single dose of 200 mg zidovudine to 13 HIV-infected women, the mean concentration of zidovudine was similar in human milk and serum.

Pediatric Patients: COMBIVIR: COMBIVIR should not be administered to pediatric patients less than 12 years of age because it is a fixed-dose combination that cannot be adjusted for this patient population.

Gender: COMBIVIR: A pharmacokinetic study in healthy male (n = 12) and female (n = 12) subjects showed no gender differences in zidovudine exposure (AUC∞) or lamivudine AUC∞ normalized for body weight.

Race: Lamivudine: There are no significant racial differences in lamivudine pharmacokinetics.

Drug Interactions: See PRECAUTIONS: Drug Interactions.

COMBIVIR: No drug interaction studies have been conducted using COMBIVIR Tablets.

Lamivudine Plus Zidovudine: No clinically significant alterations in lamivudine or zidovudine pharmacokinetics were observed in 12 asymptomatic HIV-infected adult patients given a single dose of zidovudine (200 mg) in combination with multiple doses of lamivudine (300 mg q 12 hr).
[See table 2 at right]

Table 2. Effect of Coadministered Drugs on Lamivudine and Zidovudine AUC*
Note: ROUTINE DOSE MODIFICATION OF LAMIVUDINE AND ZIDOVUDINE IS NOT WARRANTED WITH COADMINISTRATION OF THE FOLLOWING DRUGS.

Drugs That May Alter Lamivudine Blood Concentrations

Coadministered Drug and Dose	Lamivudine Dose	n	Lamivudine Concentrations		Concentration of Coadministered Drug
			AUC	Variability	
Nelfinavir 750 mg q 8 hr × 7 to 10 days	single 150 mg	11	↑AUC 10%	95% CI: 1% to 20%	↔
Trimethoprim 160 mg/ Sulfamethoxazole 800 mg daily × 5 days	single 300 mg	14	↑AUC 43%	90% CI: 32% to 55%	↔

Drugs That May Alter Zidovudine Blood Concentrations

Coadministered Drug and Dose	Zidovudine Dose	n	Zidovudine Concentrations		Concentration of Coadministered Drug
			AUC	Variability	
Atovaquone 750 mg q 12 hr with food	200 mg q 8 hr	14	↑AUC 31%	Range 23% to 78%†	↔
Fluconazole 400 mg daily	200 mg q 8 hr	12	↑AUC 74%	95% CI: 54% to 98%	Not Reported
Methadone 30 to 90 mg daily	200 mg q 4 hr	9	↑AUC 43%	Range 16% to 64%†	↔
Nelfinavir 750 mg q 8 hr × 7 to 10 days	single 200 mg	11	↓AUC 35%	Range 28% to 41%	↔
Probenecid 500 mg q 6 hr × 2 days	2 mg/kg q 8 hr × 3 days	3	↑AUC 106%	Range 100% to 170%†	Not Assessed
Ritonavir 300 mg q 6 hr × 4 days	200 mg q 8 hr × 4 days	9	↓AUC 25%	95% CI: 15% to 34%	↔
Valproic acid 250 mg or 500 mg q 8 hr × 4 days	100 mg q 8 hr × 4 days	6	↑AUC 80%	Range 64% to 130%†	Not Assessed

↑ = Increase; ↓ = Decrease; ↔ = no significant change; AUC = area under the concentration versus time curve; CI = confidence interval.
* This table is not all inclusive.
† Estimated range of percent difference.

INDICATIONS AND USAGE

COMBIVIR in combination with other antiretroviral agents is indicated for the treatment of HIV infection.

Description of Clinical Studies: ***COMBIVIR:*** There have been no clinical trials conducted with COMBIVIR. See CLINICAL PHARMACOLOGY for information about bioequivalence. One COMBIVIR Tablet given twice daily is an alternative regimen to EPIVIR Tablets 150 mg twice daily plus RETROVIR 600 mg per day in divided doses.

Lamivudine Plus Zidovudine: The NUCB3007 (CAESAR) study was conducted using EPIVIR 150-mg Tablets (150 mg twice daily) and RETROVIR 100-mg Capsules (2 x 100 mg 3 times daily). CAESAR was a multicenter, double-blind, placebo-controlled study comparing continued current therapy [zidovudine alone (62% of patients) or zidovudine with didanosine or zalcitabine (38% of patients)] to the addition of EPIVIR or EPIVIR plus an investigational non-nucleoside reverse transcriptase inhibitor, randomized 1:2:1. A total of 1,816 HIV-infected adults with 25 to 250 (median 122) CD4 cells/mm^3 at baseline were enrolled: median age was 36 years, 87% were male, 84% were nucleoside-experienced, and 16% were therapy-naive. The median duration on study was 12 months. Results are summarized in Table 3.
[See table 3 at right]

Table 3. Number of Patients (%) With At Least 1 HIV Disease-Progression Event or Death

Endpoint	Current Therapy (n = 460)	EPIVIR plus Current Therapy (n = 896)	EPIVIR plus a NNRTI* plus Current Therapy (n = 460)
HIV progression or death	90 (19.6%)	86 (9.6%)	41 (8.9%)
Death	27 (5.9%)	23 (2.6%)	14 (3.0%)

*An investigational non-nucleoside reverse transcriptase inhibitor not approved in the United States.

CONTRAINDICATIONS

COMBIVIR Tablets are contraindicated in patients with previously demonstrated clinically significant hypersensitivity to any of the components of the product.

WARNINGS

COMBIVIR is a fixed-dose combination of lamivudine and zidovudine. Ordinarily, COMBIVIR should not be administered concomitantly with lamivudine, zidovudine, or TRIZIVIR®, a fixed-dose combination of abacavir, lamivudine, and zidovudine.

The complete prescribing information for all agents being considered for use with COMBIVIR should be consulted before combination therapy with COMBIVIR is initiated.

Bone Marrow Suppression: COMBIVIR should be used with caution in patients who have bone marrow compromise evidenced by granulocyte count <1,000 cells/mm^3 or hemoglobin <9.5 g/dL (see ADVERSE REACTIONS).

Frequent blood counts are strongly recommended in patients with advanced HIV disease who are treated with COMBIVIR. For HIV-infected individuals and patients with asymptomatic or early HIV disease, periodic blood counts are recommended.

Lactic Acidosis/Severe Hepatomegaly with Steatosis: Lactic acidosis and severe hepatomegaly with steatosis, including fatal cases, have been reported with the use of nucleoside analogues alone or in combination, including lamivudine, zidovudine, and other antiretrovirals. A majority of these cases have been in women. Obesity and prolonged nucleoside exposure may be risk factors. Particular caution should be exercised when administering COMBIVIR to any patient with known risk factors for liver disease; however, cases have also been reported in patients with no known risk factors. Treatment with COMBIVIR should be suspended in any patient who develops clinical or laboratory findings suggestive of lactic acidosis or pronounced hepatotoxicity (which may include hepatomegaly and steatosis even in the absence of marked transaminase elevations).

Myopathy: Myopathy and myositis, with pathological changes similar to that produced by HIV disease, have been associated with prolonged use of zidovudine, and therefore may occur with therapy with COMBIVIR.

Posttreatment Exacerbations of Hepatitis: In clinical trials in non-HIV-infected patients treated with lamivudine for chronic hepatitis B, clinical and laboratory evidence of exacerbations of hepatitis have occurred after discontinuation of lamivudine. These exacerbations have been detected primarily by serum ALT elevations in addition to re-emergence of hepatitis B viral DNA (HBV DNA). Although most events appear to have been self-limited, fatalities have been reported in some cases. Similar events have been reported from post-marketing experience after changes from lamivudine-containing HIV treatment regimens to non-lamivudine-containing regimens in patients infected with both HIV and HBV. The causal relationship to discontinuation of lamivudine treatment is unknown. Patients should be closely monitored with both clinical and laboratory follow-up for at least several months after stopping treatment. There is insufficient evidence to determine whether re-initiation of lamivudine alters the course of posttreatment exacerbations of hepatitis.

PRECAUTIONS

Patients with HIV and Hepatitis B Virus Coinfection: Safety and efficacy of lamivudine have not been established for treatment of chronic hepatitis B in patients dually infected with HIV and HBV. In non-HIV-infected patients treated with lamivudine for chronic hepatitis B, emergence of lamivudine-resistant HBV has been detected and has been associated with diminished treatment response (see EPIVIR-HBV package insert for additional information). Emergence of hepatitis B virus variants associated with resistance to lamivudine has also been reported in HIV-infected patients who have received lamivudine-containing antiretroviral regimens in the presence of concurrent infection with hepatitis B virus. Posttreatment exacerbations of hepatitis have also been reported (see WARNINGS).

Patients with Impaired Renal Function: Reduction of the dosages of lamivudine and zidovudine is recommended for patients with impaired renal function. Patients with creatinine clearance <50 mL/min should not receive COMBIVIR.

Fat Redistribution: Redistribution/accumulation of body fat including central obesity, dorsocervical fat enlargement (buffalo hump), peripheral wasting, facial wasting, breast enlargement, and "cushingoid appearance" have been observed in patients receiving antiretroviral therapy. The mechanism and long-term consequences of these events are currently unknown. A causal relationship has not been established.

Information for Patients: COMBIVIR is not a cure for HIV infection and patients may continue to experience illnesses associated with HIV infection, including opportunistic infections. Patients should be advised that the use of COMBIVIR has not been shown to reduce the risk of transmission of HIV to others through sexual contact or blood contamination. Patients should be informed that the major toxicities of COMBIVIR are neutropenia and/or anemia. They should be told of the extreme importance of having their blood counts followed closely while on therapy, especially for patients with advanced HIV disease. Patients should be advised of the importance of taking COMBIVIR as it is prescribed.

Patients should be informed that redistribution or accumulation of body fat may occur in patients receiving antiretroviral therapy and that the cause and long-term health effects of these conditions are not known at this time.

Patients co-infected with HIV and HBV should be informed that deterioration of liver disease has occurred in some cases when treatment with lamivudine was discontinued. Patients should be advised to discuss any changes in regimen with their physician.

Drug Interactions: ***Lamivudine:*** Trimethoprim (TMP) 160 mg/sulfamethoxazole (SMX) 800 mg once daily has been shown to increase lamivudine exposure (AUC). The effect of higher doses of TMP/SMX on lamivudine pharmacokinetics has not been investigated (see CLINICAL PHARMACOLOGY). No data are available regarding the potential for in-

Continued on next page

Product information on these pages is effective as of August 2004. Further information is available at: GlaxoSmithKline, PO Box 13398, Research Triangle Park, NC 27709. 1-888-825-5249. Corporate Web Site: www.gsk.com

Combivir—Cont.

teractions with other drugs that have renal clearance mechanisms similar to that of lamivudine.
Lamivudine and zalcitabine may inhibit the intracellular phosphorylation of one another. Therefore, use of COMBIVIR in combination with zalcitabine is not recommended.
Zidovudine: Coadministration of ganciclovir, interferon-alpha, and other bone marrow suppressive or cytotoxic agents may increase the hematologic toxicity of zidovudine. Concomitant use of COMBIVIR with stavudine should be avoided since an antagonistic relationship with zidovudine has been demonstrated in vitro. In addition, concomitant use of zidovudine with doxorubicin or ribavirin should be avoided because an antagonistic relationship has been demonstrated in vitro.
See CLINICAL PHARMACOLOGY for additional drug interactions.
Carcinogenesis, Mutagenesis, and Impairment of Fertility:
Carcinogenicity:
Lamivudine: Long-term carcinogenicity studies with lamivudine in mice and rats showed no evidence of carcinogenic potential at exposures up to 10 times (mice) and 58 times (rats) those observed in humans at the recommended therapeutic dose for HIV infection.
Zidovudine: Zidovudine was administered orally at 3 dosage levels to separate groups of mice and rats (60 females and 60 males in each group). Initial single daily doses were 30, 60, and 120 mg/kg/day in mice and 80, 220, and 600 mg/kg/day in rats. The doses in mice were reduced to 20, 30, and 40 mg/kg/day after day 90 because of treatment-related anemia, whereas in rats only the high dose was reduced to 450 mg/kg/day on day 91 and then to 300 mg/kg/day on day 279.
In mice, 7 late-appearing (after 19 months) vaginal neoplasms (5 nonmetastasizing squamous cell carcinomas, 1 squamous cell papilloma, and 1 squamous polyp) occurred in animals given the highest dose. One late-appearing squamous cell papilloma occurred in the vagina of a middle-dose animal. No vaginal tumors were found at the lowest dose.
In rats, 2 late-appearing (after 20 months), nonmetastasizing vaginal squamous cell carcinomas occurred in animals given the highest dose. No vaginal tumors occurred at the low or middle dose in rats. No other drug-related tumors were observed in either sex of either species.
At doses that produced tumors in mice and rats, the estimated drug exposure (as measured by AUC) was approximately 3 times (mouse) and 24 times (rat) the estimated human exposure at the recommended therapeutic dose of 100 mg every 4 hours.
Two transplacental carcinogenicity studies were conducted in mice. One study administered zidovudine at doses of 20 mg/kg/day or 40 mg/kg/day from gestation day 10 through parturition and lactation with dosing continuing in offspring for 24 months postnatally. The doses of zidovudine employed in this study produced zidovudine exposures approximately 3 times the estimated human exposure at recommended doses. After 24 months at the highest dose, an increase in incidence of vaginal tumors was noted with no increase in tumors in the liver or lung or any other organ in either gender. These findings are consistent with results of the standard oral carcinogenicity study in mice, as described earlier. A second study administered zidovudine at maximum tolerated doses of 12.5 mg/day or 25 mg/day (~1,000 mg/kg nonpregnant body weight or ~450 mg/kg of term body weight) to pregnant mice from days 12 through 18 of gestation. There was an increase in the number of tumors in the lung, liver, and female reproductive tracts in the offspring of mice receiving the higher dose level of zidovudine.
It is not known how predictive the results of rodent carcinogenicity studies may be for humans.
Mutagenicity: Lamivudine: Lamivudine was negative in a microbial mutagenicity screen, in an in vitro cell transformation assay, in a rat micronucleus test, in a rat bone marrow cytogenetic assay, and in an assay for unscheduled DNA synthesis in rat liver. It was mutagenic in an L5178Y/TK$^{+/-}$ mouse lymphoma assay and clastogenic in a cytogenetic assay using cultured human lymphocytes.
Zidovudine: Zidovudine was mutagenic in an L5178Y/TK$^{+/-}$ mouse lymphoma assay, positive in an in vitro cell transformation assay, clastogenic in a cytogenetic assay using cultured human lymphocytes, and positive in mouse and rat micronucleus tests after repeated doses. It was negative in a cytogenetic study in rats given a single dose.
Impairment of Fertility: Lamivudine: In a study of reproductive performance, lamivudine, administered to male and female rats at doses up to 130 times the usual adult dose based on body surface area considerations, revealed no evidence of impaired fertility (judged by conception rates) and no effect on the survival, growth, and development to weaning of the offspring.
Zidovudine: Zidovudine, administered to male and female rats at doses up to 7 times the usual adult dose based on body surface area considerations, had no effect on fertility judged by conception rates.
Pregnancy: Pregnancy Category C.
COMBIVIR: There are no adequate and well-controlled studies of COMBIVIR in pregnant women. Reproduction studies with lamivudine and zidovudine have been performed in animals (see Lamivudine and Zidovudine sections below). COMBIVIR should be used during pregnancy only if the potential benefits outweigh the risks.
Lamivudine: Reproduction studies with orally administered lamivudine have been performed in rats and rabbits at doses up to 4,000 mg/kg/day and 1,000 mg/kg/day, respectively, producing plasma levels up to approximately 35 times that for the adult HIV dose. No evidence of teratogenicity due to lamivudine was observed. Evidence of early embryolethality was seen in the rabbit at exposure levels similar to those observed in humans, but there was no indication of this effect in the rat at exposure levels up to 35 times that in humans. Studies in pregnant rats and rabbits showed that lamivudine is transferred to the fetus through the placenta.
Zidovudine: Reproduction studies with orally administered zidovudine in the rat and in the rabbit at doses up to 500 mg/kg/day revealed no evidence of teratogenicity with zidovudine. Zidovudine treatment resulted in embryo/fetal toxicity as evidenced by an increase in the incidence of fetal resorptions in rats given 150 or 450 mg/kg/day and rabbits given 500 mg/kg/day. The doses used in the teratology studies resulted in peak zidovudine plasma concentrations (after one half of the daily dose) in rats 66 to 226 times, and in rabbits 12 to 87 times, mean steady-state peak human plasma concentrations (after one sixth of the daily dose) achieved with the recommended daily dose (100 mg every 4 hours). In an additional teratology study in rats, a dose of 3,000 mg/kg/day (very near the oral median lethal dose in rats of 3,683 mg/kg) caused marked maternal toxicity and an increase in the incidence of fetal malformations. This dose resulted in peak zidovudine plasma concentrations 350 times peak human plasma concentrations. No evidence of teratogenicity was seen in this experiment at doses of 600 mg/kg/day or less. Two rodent carcinogenicity studies were conducted (see Carcinogenesis, Mutagenesis, Impairment of Fertility).
Antiretroviral Pregnancy Registry: To monitor maternal-fetal outcomes of pregnant women exposed to COMBIVIR and other antiretroviral agents, an Antiretroviral Pregnancy Registry has been established. Physicians are encouraged to register patients by calling 1-800-258-4263.
Nursing Mothers: The Centers for Disease Control and Prevention recommend that HIV-infected mothers not breastfeed their infants to avoid risking postnatal transmission of HIV infection. No specific studies of lamivudine and zidovudine excretion in breast milk after dosing with COMBIVIR have been performed. Zidovudine and lamivudine are excreted in human breast milk (see CLINICAL PHARMACOLOGY: Pharmacokinetics: Nursing Mothers). A study in lactating rats administered 45 mg/kg of lamivudine showed that lamivudine concentrations in milk were slightly greater than those in plasma.
Because of both the potential for HIV transmission and the potential for serious adverse reactions in nursing infants, **mothers should be instructed not to breastfeed if they are receiving COMBIVIR.**
Pediatric Use: COMBIVIR should not be administered to pediatric patients less than 12 years of age because it is a fixed-dose combination that cannot be adjusted for this patient population.
Geriatric Use: Clinical studies of COMBIVIR did not include sufficient numbers of subjects aged 65 and over to determine whether they respond differently from younger subjects. In general, dose selection for an elderly patient should be cautious, reflecting the greater frequency of decreased hepatic, renal, or cardiac function, and of concomitant disease or other drug therapy. COMBIVIR is not recommended for patients with impaired renal function (i.e., creatinine clearance <50 mL/min; see PRECAUTIONS: Patients with Impaired Renal Function and DOSAGE AND ADMINISTRATION).

ADVERSE REACTIONS

Lamivudine Plus Zidovudine Administered As Separate Formulations: In 4 randomized, controlled trials of EPIVIR 300 mg per day plus RETROVIR 600 mg per day, the following selected clinical and laboratory adverse events were observed (see Tables 4 and 5).

Table 4. Selected Clinical Adverse Events (≥5% Frequency) in 4 Controlled Clinical Trials With EPIVIR 300 mg/day and RETROVIR 600 mg/day

Adverse Event	EPIVIR plus RETROVIR (n = 251)
Body as a whole	
Headache	35%
Malaise & fatigue	27%
Fever or chills	10%
Digestive	
Nausea	33%
Diarrhea	18%
Nausea & vomiting	13%
Anorexia and/or decreased appetite	10%
Abdominal pain	9%
Abdominal cramps	6%
Dyspepsia	5%
Nervous system	
Neuropathy	12%
Insomnia & other sleep disorders	11%
Dizziness	10%
Depressive disorders	9%
Respiratory	
Nasal signs & symptoms	20%
Cough	18%
Skin	
Skin rashes	9%
Musculoskeletal	
Musculoskeletal pain	12%
Myalgia	8%
Arthralgia	5%

Pancreatitis was observed in 3 of the 656 adult patients (<0.5%) who received EPIVIR in controlled clinical trials.
Selected laboratory abnormalities observed during therapy are listed in Table 5.
[See table 5 above]

Table 5. Frequencies of Selected Laboratory Abnormalities Among Adults in 4 Controlled Clinical Trials of EPIVIR 300 mg/day plus RETROVIR 600 mg/day*

Test (Abnormal Level)	EPIVIR plus RETROVIR % (n)
Neutropenia (ANC<750/mm^3)	7.2% (237)
Anemia (Hgb<8.0 g/dL)	2.9% (241)
Thrombocytopenia (platelets<50,000/mm^3)	0.4% (240)
ALT (>5.0 × ULN)	3.7% (241)
AST (>5.0 × ULN)	1.7% (241)
Bilirubin (>2.5 × ULN)	0.8% (241)
Amylase (>2.0 × ULN)	4.2% (72)

ULN = Upper limit of normal.
ANC = Absolute neutrophil count.
n = Number of patients assessed.
* Frequencies of these laboratory abnormalities were higher in patients with mild laboratory abnormalities at baseline.

Observed During Clinical Practice: In addition to adverse events reported from clinical trials, the following events have been identified during post-approval use of EPIVIR, RETROVIR, and/or COMBIVIR. Because they are reported voluntarily from a population of unknown size, estimates of frequency cannot be made. These events have been chosen for inclusion due to a combination of their seriousness, frequency of reporting, or potential causal connection to EPIVIR, RETROVIR, and/or COMBIVIR.
Body as a Whole: Redistribution/accumulation of body fat (see PRECAUTIONS: Fat Redistribution).
Cardiovascular: Cardiomyopathy.
Endocrine and Metabolic: Gynecomastia, hyperglycemia.
Gastrointestinal: Oral mucosal pigmentation, stomatitis.
General: Vasculitis, weakness.
Hemic and Lymphatic: Anemia, (including pure red cell aplasia and anemias progressing on therapy), lymphadenopathy, splenomegaly.
Hepatic and Pancreatic: Lactic acidosis and hepatic steatosis, pancreatitis, posttreatment exacerbation of hepatitis B (see WARNINGS).
Hypersensitivity: Sensitization reactions (including anaphylaxis), urticaria.
Musculoskeletal: Muscle weakness, CPK elevation, rhabdomyolysis.
Nervous: Paresthesia, peripheral neuropathy, seizures.
Respiratory: Abnormal breath sounds/wheezing.
Skin: Alopecia, erythema multiforme, Stevens-Johnson syndrome.

OVERDOSAGE

COMBIVIR: There is no known antidote for COMBIVIR.
Lamivudine: One case of an adult ingesting 6 grams of lamivudine was reported; there were no clinical signs or symptoms noted and hematologic tests remained normal. It is not known whether lamivudine can be removed by peritoneal dialysis or hemodialysis.
Zidovudine: Acute overdoses of zidovudine have been reported in pediatric patients and adults. These involved ex-

posures up to 50 grams. The only consistent findings were nausea and vomiting. Other reported occurrences included headache, dizziness, drowsiness, lethargy, confusion, and 1 report of a grand mal seizure. Hematologic changes were transient. All patients recovered. Hemodialysis and peritoneal dialysis appear to have a negligible effect on the removal of zidovudine, while elimination of its primary metabolite, GZDV, is enhanced.

DOSAGE AND ADMINISTRATION

The recommended oral dose of COMBIVIR for adults and adolescents (at least 12 years of age) is 1 tablet (containing 150 mg of lamivudine and 300 mg of zidovudine) twice daily.

Dose Adjustment: Because it is a fixed-dose combination, COMBIVIR should not be prescribed for patients requiring dosage adjustment such as those with reduced renal function (creatinine clearance <50 mL/min) or those experiencing dose-limiting adverse events.

A reduction in the daily dose of zidovudine may be necessary in patients with mild to moderate impaired hepatic function or liver cirrhosis. Because COMBIVIR is a fixed-dose combination that cannot be adjusted for this patient population, COMBIVIR is not recommended for patients with impaired hepatic function.

HOW SUPPLIED

COMBIVIR Tablets, containing 150 mg lamivudine and 300 mg zidovudine, are white, film-coated, modified-capsule-shaped tablets engraved with "GXFC3" on one side. They are available as follows:

60 Tablets/Bottle (NDC 0173-0595-00)
Store between 2° and 30°C (36° and 86°F).
Unit Dose Pack of 120 (NDC 0173-0595-02)
Store between 2° and 30°C (36° and 86°F).

GlaxoSmithKline, Research Triangle Park, NC 27709
Lamivudine is manufactured under agreement from
Shire Pharmaceuticals Group plc, Basingstoke, UK

May 2004/RL-2088

Shown in Product Identification Guide, page 315

COREG® ℞

[kor' eg]
(carvedilol)
Tablets

DESCRIPTION

Carvedilol is a nonselective β-adrenergic blocking agent with α_1-blocking activity. It is (±)-1-(Carbazol-4-yloxy)-3-[[2-(o-methoxyphenoxy)ethyl]amino]-2-propanol. It is a racemic mixture.

Tablets for Oral Administration: COREG (carvedilol) is a white, oval, film-coated tablet containing 3.125 mg, 6.25 mg, 12.5 mg, or 25 mg of carvedilol. The 6.25 mg, 12.5 mg, and 25 mg tablets are TILTAB® tablets. Inactive ingredients consist of colloidal silicon dioxide, crospovidone, hypromellose, lactose, magnesium stearate, polyethylene glycol, polysorbate 80, povidone, sucrose, and titanium dioxide.

Carvedilol is a white to off-white powder with a molecular weight of 406.5 and a molecular formula of $C_{24}H_{26}N_2O_4$. It is freely soluble in dimethylsulfoxide; soluble in methylene chloride and methanol; sparingly soluble in 95% ethanol and isopropanol; slightly soluble in ethyl ether; and practically insoluble in water, gastric fluid (simulated, TS, pH 1.1), and intestinal fluid (simulated, TS without pancreatin, pH 7.5).

CLINICAL PHARMACOLOGY

COREG is a racemic mixture in which nonselective β-adrenoreceptor blocking activity is present in the S(-) enantiomer and α-adrenergic blocking activity is present in both R(+) and S(-) enantiomers at equal potency. COREG has no intrinsic sympathomimetic activity.

Pharmacokinetics: COREG is rapidly and extensively absorbed following oral administration, with absolute bioavailability of approximately 25% to 35% due to a significant degree of first-pass metabolism. Following oral administration, the apparent mean terminal elimination half-life of carvedilol generally ranges from 7 to 10 hours. Plasma concentrations achieved are proportional to the oral dose administered. When administered with food, the rate of absorption is slowed, as evidenced by a delay in the time to reach peak plasma levels, with no significant difference in extent of bioavailability. Taking COREG with food should minimize the risk of orthostatic hypotension.

Carvedilol is extensively metabolized. Following oral administration of radiolabelled carvedilol to healthy volunteers, carvedilol accounted for only about 7% of the total radioactivity in plasma as measured by area under the curve (AUC). Less than 2% of the dose was excreted unchanged in the urine. Carvedilol is metabolized primarily by aromatic ring oxidation and glucuronidation. The oxidative metabolites are further metabolized by conjugation via glucuronidation and sulfation. The metabolites of carvedilol are excreted primarily via the bile into the feces. Demethylation and hydroxylation at the phenol ring produce three active metabolites with β-receptor blocking activity. Based on preclinical studies, the 4'-hydroxyphenyl metabolite is approximately 13 times more potent than carvedilol for β-blockade. Compared to carvedilol, the three active metabolites exhibit weak vasodilating activity. Plasma concentrations of the active metabolites are about one-tenth of those observed for carvedilol and have pharmacokinetics similar to the parent.

Carvedilol undergoes stereoselective first-pass metabolism with plasma levels of R(+)-carvedilol approximately 2 to 3 times higher than S(-)-carvedilol following oral administration in healthy subjects. The mean apparent terminal elimination half-lives for R(+)-carvedilol range from 5 to 9 hours compared with 7 to 11 hours for the S(-)-enantiomer.

The primary P450 enzymes responsible for the metabolism of both R(+) and S(-)-carvedilol in human liver microsomes were CYP2D6 and CYP2C9 and to a lesser extent CYP3A4, 2C19, 1A2, and 2E1. CYP2D6 is thought to be the major enzyme in the 4'- and 5'-hydroxylation of carvedilol, with a potential contribution from 3A4. CYP2C9 is thought to be of primary importance in the O-methylation pathway of S(-)-carvedilol.

Carvedilol is subject to the effects of genetic polymorphism with poor metabolizers of debrisoquin (a marker for cytochrome P450 2D6) exhibiting 2- to 3-fold higher plasma concentrations of R(+)-carvedilol compared to extensive metabolizers. In contrast, plasma levels of S(-)-carvedilol are increased only about 20% to 25% in poor metabolizers, indicating this enantiomer is metabolized to a lesser extent by cytochrome P450 2D6 than R(+)-carvedilol. The pharmacokinetics of carvedilol do not appear to be different in poor metabolizers of S-mephenytoin (patients deficient in cytochrome P450 2C19).

Carvedilol is more than 98% bound to plasma proteins, primarily with albumin. The plasma-protein binding is independent of concentration over the therapeutic range. Carvedilol is a basic, lipophilic compound with a steady-state volume of distribution of approximately 115 L, indicating substantial distribution into extravascular tissues. Plasma clearance ranges from 500 to 700 mL/min.

Congestive Heart Failure: Steady-state plasma concentrations of carvedilol and its enantiomers increased proportionally over the 6.25 to 50 mg dose range in patients with congestive heart failure. Compared to healthy subjects, congestive heart failure patients had increased mean AUC and C_{max} values for carvedilol and its enantiomers, with up to 50% to 100% higher values observed in 6 patients with NYHA class IV heart failure. The mean apparent terminal elimination half-life for carvedilol was similar to that observed in healthy subjects.

Pharmacokinetic Drug-Drug Interactions: Since carvedilol undergoes substantial oxidative metabolism, the metabolism and pharmacokinetics of carvedilol may be affected by induction or inhibition of cytochrome P450 enzymes.

Rifampin: In a pharmacokinetic study conducted in 8 healthy male subjects, rifampin (600 mg daily for 12 days) decreased the AUC and C_{max} of carvedilol by about 70%.

Cimetidine: In a pharmacokinetic study conducted in 10 healthy male subjects, cimetidine (1000 mg/day) increased the steady-state AUC of carvedilol by 30% with no change in C_{max}.

Glyburide: In 12 healthy subjects, combined administration of carvedilol (25 mg once daily) and a single dose of glyburide did not result in a clinically relevant pharmacokinetic interaction for either compound.

Hydrochlorothiazide: A single oral dose of carvedilol 25 mg did not alter the pharmacokinetics of a single oral dose of hydrochlorothiazide 25 mg in 12 patients with hypertension. Likewise, hydrochlorothiazide had no effect on the pharmacokinetics of carvedilol.

Digoxin: Following concomitant administration of carvedilol (25 mg once daily) and digoxin (0.25 mg once daily) for 14 days, steady-state AUC and trough concentrations of digoxin were increased by 14% and 16%, respectively, in 12 hypertensive patients.

Torsemide: In a study of 12 healthy subjects, combined oral administration of carvedilol 25 mg once daily and torsemide 5 mg once daily for 5 days did not result in any significant differences in their pharmacokinetics compared with administration of the drugs alone.

Warfarin: Carvedilol (12.5 mg twice daily) did not have an effect on the steady-state prothrombin time ratios and did not alter the pharmacokinetics of R(+)- and S(-)-warfarin following concomitant administration with warfarin in 9 healthy volunteers.

Special Populations: ***Elderly:*** Plasma levels of carvedilol average about 50% higher in the elderly compared to young subjects.

Hepatic Impairment: Compared to healthy subjects, patients with cirrhotic liver disease exhibit significantly higher concentrations of carvedilol (approximately 4- to 7-fold) following single-dose therapy.

Renal Insufficiency: Although carvedilol is metabolized primarily by the liver, plasma concentrations of carvedilol have been reported to be increased in patients with renal impairment. Based on mean AUC data, approximately 40% to 50% higher plasma concentrations of carvedilol were observed in hypertensive patients with moderate to severe renal impairment compared to a control group of hypertensive patients with normal renal function. However, the ranges of AUC values were similar for both groups. Changes in mean peak plasma levels were less pronounced, approximately 12% to 26% higher in patients with impaired renal function. Consistent with its high degree of plasma protein-binding, carvedilol does not appear to be cleared significantly by hemodialysis.

Pharmacodynamics: ***Congestive Heart Failure:*** The basis for the beneficial effects of COREG in congestive heart failure is not established.

Two placebo-controlled studies compared the acute hemodynamic effects of COREG to baseline measurements in 59 and 49 patients with NYHA class II-IV heart failure receiving diuretics, ACE inhibitors, and digitalis. There were significant reductions in systemic blood pressure, pulmonary artery pressure, pulmonary capillary wedge pressure, and heart rate. Initial effects on cardiac output, stroke volume index, and systemic vascular resistance were small and variable.

These studies measured hemodynamic effects again at 12 to 14 weeks. COREG significantly reduced systemic blood pressure, pulmonary artery pressure, right atrial pressure, systemic vascular resistance, and heart rate, while stroke volume index was increased.

Among 839 patients with NYHA class II-III heart failure treated for 26 to 52 weeks in 4 US placebo-controlled trials, average left ventricular ejection fraction (EF) measured by radionuclide ventriculography increased by 9 EF units (%) in COREG patients and by 2 EF units in placebo patients at a target dose of 25–50 mg twice daily. The effects of carvedilol on ejection fraction were related to dose. Doses of 6.25 mg twice daily, 12.5 mg twice daily, 25 mg twice daily were associated with placebo-corrected increases in EF of 5 EF units, 6 EF units, and 8 EF units, respectively; each of these effects were nominally statistically significant.

Left Ventricular Dysfunction Following Myocardial Infarction: The basis for the beneficial effects of COREG in patients with left ventricular dysfunction following an acute myocardial infarction is not established.

Hypertension: The mechanism by which β-blockade produces an antihypertensive effect has not been established.

β-adrenoreceptor blocking activity has been demonstrated in animal and human studies showing that carvedilol (1) reduces cardiac output in normal subjects; (2) reduces exercise- and/or isoproterenol-induced tachycardia and (3) reduces reflex orthostatic tachycardia. Significant β-adrenoreceptor blocking effect is usually seen within 1 hour of drug administration.

α_1-adrenoreceptor blocking activity has been demonstrated in human and animal studies, showing that carvedilol (1) attenuates the pressor effects of phenylephrine; (2) causes vasodilation and (3) reduces peripheral vascular resistance. These effects contribute to the reduction of blood pressure and usually are seen within 30 minutes of drug administration.

Due to the α_1-receptor blocking activity of carvedilol, blood pressure is lowered more in the standing than in the supine position, and symptoms of postural hypotension (1.8%), including rare instances of syncope, can occur. Following oral administration, when postural hypotension has occurred, it has been transient and is uncommon when COREG is administered with food at the recommended starting dose and titration increments are closely followed (see DOSAGE AND ADMINISTRATION).

In hypertensive patients with normal renal function, therapeutic doses of COREG decreased renal vascular resistance with no change in glomerular filtration rate or renal plasma flow. Changes in excretion of sodium, potassium, uric acid, and phosphorus in hypertensive patients with normal renal function were similar after COREG and placebo.

COREG has little effect on plasma catecholamines, plasma aldosterone, or electrolyte levels, but it does significantly reduce plasma renin activity when given for at least 4 weeks. It also increases levels of atrial natriuretic peptide.

CLINICAL TRIALS

Congestive Heart Failure: A total of 3,946 patients with mild to severe heart failure were evaluated in placebo-controlled studies of carvedilol.

In the largest study (COPERNICUS), 2,289 patients with heart failure at rest or with minimal exertion and left ventricular ejection fraction <25% (mean 20%), despite digitalis (66%), diuretics (99%), and ACE inhibitors (89%) were randomized to placebo or carvedilol. Carvedilol was titrated from a starting dose of 3.125 mg twice daily to the maximum tolerated dose or up to 25 mg twice daily over a minimum of 6 weeks. Most subjects achieved the target dose of 25 mg. The study was conducted in Eastern and Western Europe, the United States, Israel, and Canada. Similar numbers of subjects per group (about 100) withdrew during the titration period.

The primary end point of the trial was all-cause mortality, but cause-specific mortality and the risk of death or hospitalization (total, cardiovascular [CV], or congestive heart failure [CHF]) were also examined. The developing trial data were followed by a data monitoring committee, and mortality analyses were adjusted for these multiple looks. The trial was stopped after a median follow-up of 10 months because of an observed 35% reduction in mortality (from 19.7% per patient year on placebo to 12.8% on carvedilol, hazard ratio 0.65, 95% CI 0.52 – 0.81, p = 0.0014, adjusted) (see Figure 1). The results of COPERNICUS are shown in Table 1.

[See table 1 at top of next page]

[See figure 1 at top of next column]

The effect on mortality was principally the result of a reduction in the rate of sudden death among patients without worsening heart failure.

Continued on next page

Product information on these pages is effective as of August 2004. Further information is available at: GlaxoSmithKline, PO Box 13398, Research Triangle Park, NC 27709. 1-888-825-5249. Corporate Web Site: www.gsk.com

Coreg—Cont.

Figure 1. Survival Analysis for COPERNICUS (intent-to-treat)

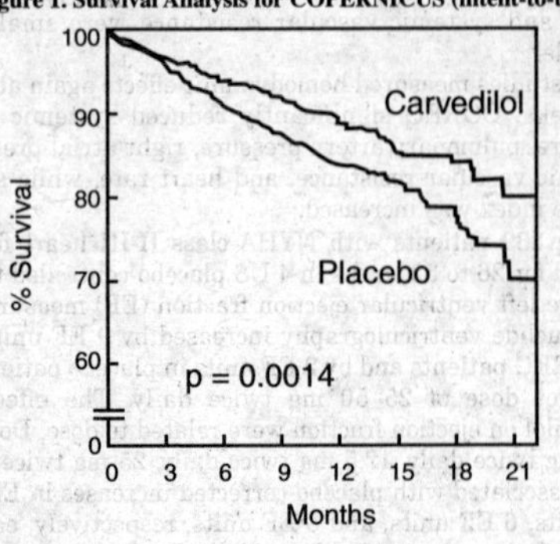

Patients' global assessments, in which carvedilol-treated patients were compared to placebo, were based on pre-specified, periodic patient self-assessments regarding whether clinical status post-treatment showed improvement, worsening or no change compared to baseline. Patients treated with carvedilol showed significant improvement in global assessments compared with those treated with placebo in COPERNICUS.

The protocol also specified that hospitalizations would be assessed. Fewer patients on COREG than on placebo were hospitalized for any reason (198 vs. 268, p = 0.0001), for cardiovascular reasons (246 vs. 314, p = 0.0003), or for worsening heart failure (372 vs. 432, p = 0.0029).

COREG had a consistent and beneficial effect on all-cause mortality as well as the combined end points of all-cause mortality plus hospitalization (total, CV, or for heart failure) in the overall study population and in all subgroups examined, including men and women, elderly and non-elderly, blacks and non-blacks, and diabetics and non-diabetics (see Figure 2).

Figure 2. Effects on Mortality for Subgroups in COPERNICUS

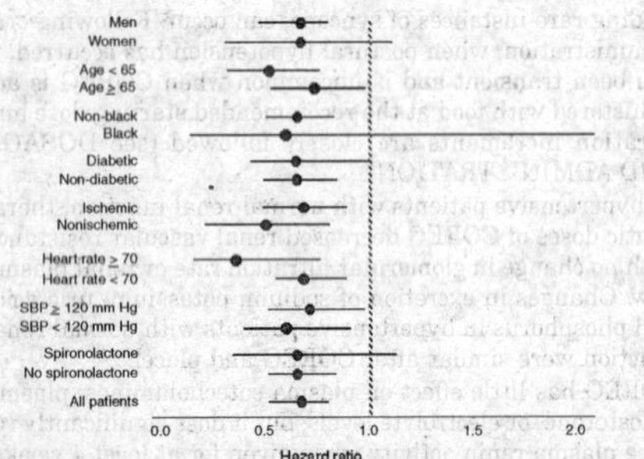

Carvedilol was also studied in five other multicenter, placebo-controlled studies.

Four US multicenter, double-blind, placebo-controlled studies enrolled 1,094 patients (696 randomized to carvedilol) with NYHA class II-III heart failure and ejection fraction <0.35. The vast majority were on digitalis, diuretics, and an ACE inhibitor at study entry. Patients were assigned to the studies based upon exercise ability. An Australia-New Zealand double-blind, placebo-controlled study enrolled 415 patients (half randomized to carvedilol) with less severe heart failure. All protocols excluded patients expected to undergo cardiac transplantation during the 7.5 to 15 months of double-blind follow-up. All randomized patients had tolerated a 2-week course on carvedilol 6.25 mg twice daily.

In each study, there was a primary end point, either progression of heart failure (one US study) or exercise tolerance (two US studies meeting enrollment goals and the Australia-New Zealand study). There were many secondary end points specified in these studies, including NYHA classification, patient and physician global assessments, and cardiovascular hospitalization. Death was not a specified end point in any study, but it was analyzed in all studies. Other analyses not prospectively planned included the sum of deaths and total cardiovascular hospitalizations. In situations where the primary end points of a trial do not show a significant benefit of treatment, assignment of significance values to the other results is complex, and such values need to be interpreted cautiously.

The results of the US and Australia-New Zealand trials were as follows:

Slowing Progression of Heart Failure: One US multicenter study (366 subjects) had as its primary end point the sum of cardiovascular mortality, cardiovascular hospitalization, and sustained increase in heart failure medications. Heart failure progression was reduced, during an average follow-up of 7 months, by 48% (p = 0.008).

In the Australia-New Zealand study, death and total hospitalizations were reduced by about 25% over 18 to 24 months. In the three largest US studies, death and total hospitalizations were reduced by 19%, 39%, and 49%, nominally statistically significant in the last two studies. The Australia-New Zealand results were statistically borderline.

Table 1. Results of COPERNICUS

End point	Placebo N = 1,133	Carvedilol N = 1,156	Hazard ratio (95% CI)	% Reduction	Nominal p value
Mortality	190	130	0.65 (0.52 – 0.81)	35	0.00013
Mortality + all hospitalization	507	425	0.76 (0.67 – 0.87)	24	0.00004
Mortality + CV hospitalization	395	314	0.73 (0.63 – 0.84)	27	0.00002
Mortality + CHF hospitalization	357	271	0.69 (0.59 – 0.81)	31	0.000004

Functional Measures: None of the multicenter studies had NYHA classification as a primary end point, but all such studies had it as a secondary end point. There was at least a trend toward improvement in NYHA class in all studies. Exercise tolerance was the primary end point in 3 studies; in none was a statistically significant effect found.

Subjective Measures: Quality of life, as measured with a standard questionnaire (a primary end point in one study), was unaffected by carvedilol. However, patients' and investigators' global assessments showed significant improvement in most studies.

Mortality: Overall, in these four US trials, mortality was reduced, nominally significantly so in 2 studies.

Left Ventricular Dysfunction Following Myocardial Infarction: CAPRICORN was a double-blind study comparing carvedilol and placebo in 1,959 patients with a recent myocardial infarction (within 21 days) and left ventricular ejection fraction of ≤40%, with (47%) or without symptoms of heart failure. Patients given carvedilol received 6.25 mg twice daily, titrated as tolerated to 25 mg twice daily. Patients had to have a systolic blood pressure >90 mm Hg, a sitting heart rate >60 beats/minute, and no contraindication to β-blocker use. Treatment of the index infarction included aspirin (85%), IV or oral β-blockers (37%), nitrates (73%), heparin (64%), thrombolytics (40%), and acute angioplasty (12%). Background treatment included ACE inhibitors or angiotensin receptor blockers (97%), anticoagulants (20%), lipid-lowering agents (23%), and diuretics (34%). Baseline population characteristics included an average age of 63 years, 74% male, 95% Caucasian, mean blood pressure 121/74 mm Hg, 22% with diabetes, and 54% with a history of hypertension. Mean dosage achieved of carvedilol was 20 mg twice daily; mean duration of follow-up was 15 months.

All-cause mortality was 15% in the placebo group and 12% in the carvedilol group, indicating a 23% risk reduction in patients treated with carvedilol (95% CI 2–40%, p = 0.03), as shown in Figure 3. The effects on mortality in various subgroups are shown in Figure 4. Nearly all deaths were cardiovascular (which were reduced by 25% by carvedilol), and most of these deaths were sudden or related to pump failure (both types of death were reduced by carvedilol). Another study endpoint, total mortality and all-cause hospitalization, did not show a significant improvement.

Figure 3. Survival Analysis for CAPRICORN (intent-to-treat)

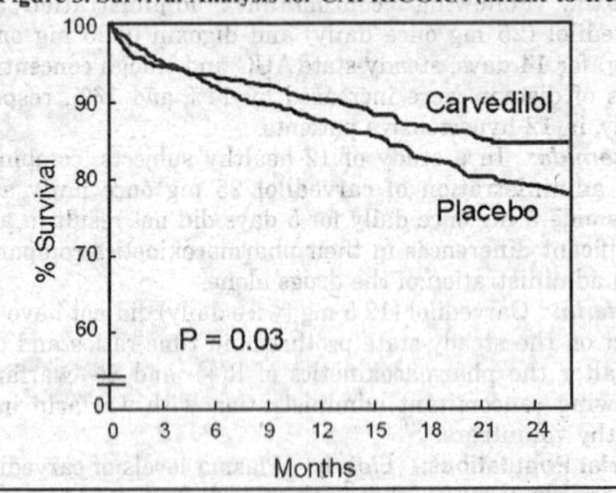

Figure 4. Effects on Mortality for Subgroups in CAPRICORN

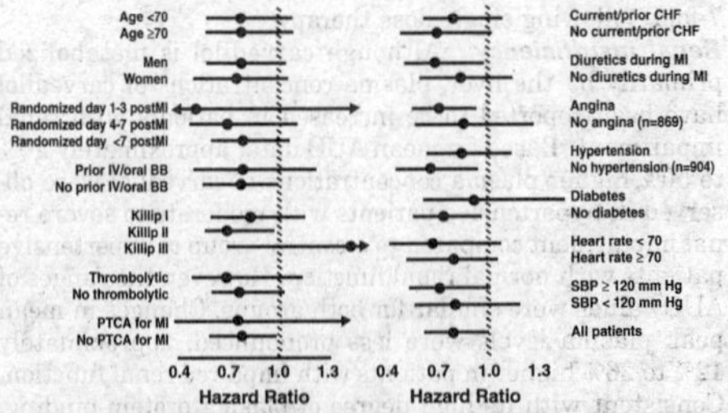

Hypertension: COREG was studied in two placebo-controlled trials that utilized twice-daily dosing, at total daily doses of 12.5 to 50 mg. In these and other studies, the starting dose did not exceed 12.5 mg. At 50 mg/day, COREG reduced sitting trough (12-hour) blood pressure by about 9/5.5 mm Hg; at 25 mg/day the effect was about 7.5/3.5 mm Hg. Comparisons of trough to peak blood pressure showed a trough to peak ratio for blood pressure response of about 65%. Heart rate fell by about 7.5 beats/minute at 50 mg/day. In general, as is true for other β-blockers, responses were smaller in black than non-black patients. There were no age- or gender-related differences in response.

The peak antihypertensive effect occurred 1 to 2 hours after a dose. The dose-related blood pressure response was accompanied by a dose-related increase in adverse effects (see ADVERSE REACTIONS).

INDICATIONS AND USAGE

Congestive Heart Failure: COREG is indicated for the treatment of mild to severe heart failure of ischemic or cardiomyopathic origin, usually in addition to diuretics, ACE inhibitor, and digitalis, to increase survival and, also, to reduce the risk of hospitalization (see CLINICAL TRIALS).

Left Ventricular Dysfunction Following Myocardial Infarction: COREG is indicated to reduce cardiovascular mortality in clinically stable patients who have survived the acute phase of a myocardial infarction and have a left ventricular ejection fraction of ≤40% (with or without symptomatic heart failure) (see CLINICAL TRIALS).

Hypertension: COREG is also indicated for the management of essential hypertension. It can be used alone or in combination with other antihypertensive agents, especially thiazide-type diuretics (see PRECAUTIONS, Drug Interactions).

CONTRAINDICATIONS

COREG is contraindicated in patients with bronchial asthma (two cases of death from status asthmaticus have been reported in patients receiving single doses of COREG) or related bronchospastic conditions, second- or third-degree AV block, sick sinus syndrome or severe bradycardia (unless a permanent pacemaker is in place), or in patients with cardiogenic shock or who have decompensated heart failure requiring the use of intravenous inotropic therapy. Such patients should first be weaned from intravenous therapy before initiating COREG.

Use of COREG in patients with clinically manifest hepatic impairment is not recommended.

COREG is contraindicated in patients with hypersensitivity to any component of the product.

WARNINGS

Cessation of Therapy with COREG: Patients with coronary artery disease, who are being treated with COREG, should be advised against abrupt discontinuation of therapy. Severe exacerbation of angina and the occurrence of myocardial infarction and ventricular arrhythmias have been reported in angina patients following the abrupt discontinuation of therapy with β-blockers. The last two complications may occur with or without preceding exacerbation of the angina pectoris. As with other β-blockers, when discontinuation of COREG is planned, the patients should be carefully observed and advised to limit physical activity to a minimum. COREG should be discontinued over 1 to 2 weeks whenever possible. If the angina worsens or acute coronary insufficiency develops, it is recommended that COREG be promptly reinstituted, at least temporarily. Because coronary artery disease is common and may be unrecognized, it may be prudent not to discontinue COREG therapy abruptly even in patients treated only for hypertension or heart failure (See DOSAGE AND ADMINISTRATION.)

Peripheral Vascular Disease: β-blockers can precipitate or aggravate symptoms of arterial insufficiency in patients with peripheral vascular disease. Caution should be exercised in such individuals.

Anesthesia and Major Surgery: If treatment with COREG is to be continued perioperatively, particular care should be taken when anesthetic agents which depress myocardial function, such as ether, cyclopropane, and trichloroethylene, are used. See OVERDOSAGE for information on treatment of bradycardia and hypertension.

Diabetes and Hypoglycemia: In general, β-blockers may mask some of the manifestations of hypoglycemia, particularly tachycardia. Nonselective β-blockers may potentiate insulin-induced hypoglycemia and delay recovery of serum glucose levels. Patients subject to spontaneous hypoglycemia, or diabetic patients receiving insulin or oral hypoglycemic agents, should be cautioned about these possibilities. In congestive heart failure patients, there is a risk of worsening hyperglycemia (see PRECAUTIONS).

Thyrotoxicosis: β-adrenergic blockade may mask clinical signs of hyperthyroidism, such as tachycardia. Abrupt withdrawal of β-blockade may be followed by an exacerbation of the symptoms of hyperthyroidism or may precipitate thyroid storm.

PRECAUTIONS

General: In clinical trials, COREG caused bradycardia in about 2% of hypertensive patients, 9% of congestive heart failure patients, and 6.5% of myocardial infarction patients with left ventricular dysfunction. If pulse rate drops below 55 beats/minute, the dosage should be reduced.

In clinical trials of primarily mild-to-moderate heart failure, hypotension and postural hypotension occurred in 9.7% and syncope in 3.4% of patients receiving COREG compared to 3.6% and 2.5% of placebo patients, respectively. The risk for these events was highest during the first 30 days of dosing, corresponding to the up-titration period and was a cause for discontinuation of therapy in 0.7% of COREG patients, compared to 0.4% of placebo patients. In a long-term, placebo-controlled trial in severe heart failure (COPERNICUS), hypotension and postural hypotension occurred in 15.1% and syncope in 2.9% of heart failure patients receiving COREG compared to 8.7% and 2.3% of placebo patients, respectively. These events were a cause for discontinuation of therapy in 1.1% of COREG patients, compared to 0.8% of placebo patients.

Postural hypotension occurred in 1.8% and syncope in 0.1% of hypertensive patients, primarily following the initial dose or at the time of dose increase and was a cause for discontinuation of therapy in 1% of patients.

In the CAPRICORN study of survivors of an acute myocardial infarction, hypotension or postural hypotension occurred in 20.2% of patients receiving COREG compared to 12.6% of placebo patients. Syncope was reported in 3.9% and 1.9% of patients, respectively. These events were a cause for discontinuation of therapy in 2.5% of patients receiving COREG, compared to 0.2% of placebo patients.

To decrease the likelihood of syncope or excessive hypotension, treatment should be initiated with 3.125 mg twice daily for congestive heart failure patients and at 6.25 mg twice daily for hypertensive patients and survivors of an acute myocardial infarction with left ventricular dysfunction. Dosage should then be increased slowly, according to recommendations in the DOSAGE AND ADMINISTRATION section, and the drug should be taken with food. During initiation of therapy, the patient should be cautioned to avoid situations such as driving or hazardous tasks, where injury could result should syncope occur.

Rarely, use of carvedilol in patients with congestive heart failure has resulted in deterioration of renal function. Patients at risk appear to be those with low blood pressure (systolic blood pressure <100 mm Hg), ischemic heart disease and diffuse vascular disease, and/or underlying renal insufficiency. Renal function has returned to baseline when carvedilol was stopped. In patients with these risk factors it is recommended that renal function be monitored during up-titration of carvedilol and the drug discontinued or dosage reduced if worsening of renal function occurs.

Worsening heart failure or fluid retention may occur during up-titration of carvedilol. If such symptoms occur, diuretics should be increased and the carvedilol dose should not be advanced until clinical stability resumes (see DOSAGE AND ADMINISTRATION). Occasionally it is necessary to lower the carvedilol dose or temporarily discontinue it. Such episodes do not preclude subsequent successful titration of, or a favorable response to, carvedilol. In a placebo-controlled trial of patients with severe heart failure, worsening heart failure during the first 3 months was reported to a similar degree with carvedilol and with placebo. When treatment was maintained beyond 3 months, worsening heart failure was reported less frequently in patients treated with carvedilol than with placebo. Worsening heart failure observed during long-term therapy is more likely to be related to the patients' underlying disease than to treatment with carvedilol.

In patients with pheochromocytoma, an α-blocking agent should be initiated prior to the use of any β-blocking agent. Although carvedilol has both α- and β-blocking pharmacologic activities, there has been no experience with its use in this condition. Therefore, caution should be taken in the administration of carvedilol to patients suspected of having pheochromocytoma.

Agents with non-selective β-blocking activity may provoke chest pain in patients with Prinzmetal's variant angina. There has been no clinical experience with carvedilol in these patients although the α-blocking activity may prevent such symptoms. However, caution should be taken in the administration of carvedilol to patients suspected of having Prinzmetal's variant angina.

In congestive heart failure patients with diabetes, carvedilol therapy may lead to worsening hyperglycemia, which responds to intensification of hypoglycemic therapy. It is recommended that blood glucose be monitored when carvedilol dosing is initiated, adjusted, or discontinued.

Risk of Anaphylactic Reaction: While taking β-blockers, patients with a history of severe anaphylactic reaction to a variety of allergens may be more reactive to repeated challenge, either accidental, diagnostic, or therapeutic. Such patients may be unresponsive to the usual doses of epinephrine used to treat allergic reaction.

Nonallergic Bronchospasm (e.g., chronic bronchitis and emphysema): Patients with bronchospastic disease should, in general, not receive β-blockers. COREG may be used with caution, however, in patients who do not respond to, or cannot tolerate, other antihypertensive agents. It is prudent, if COREG is used, to use the smallest effective dose, so that inhibition of endogenous or exogenous β-agonists is minimized.

In clinical trials of patients with congestive heart failure, patients with bronchospastic disease were enrolled if they did not require oral or inhaled medication to treat their bronchospastic disease. In such patients, it is recommended that carvedilol be used with caution. The dosing recommendations should be followed closely and the dose should be lowered if any evidence of bronchospasm is observed during up-titration.

Information for Patients: Patients taking COREG should be advised of the following:

- they should not interrupt or discontinue using COREG without a physician's advice.
- congestive heart failure patients should consult their physician if they experience signs or symptoms of worsening heart failure such as weight gain or increasing shortness of breath.
- they may experience a drop in blood pressure when standing, resulting in dizziness and, rarely, fainting. Patients should sit or lie down when these symptoms of lowered blood pressure occur.
- if patients experience dizziness or fatigue, they should avoid driving or hazardous tasks.
- they should consult a physician if they experience dizziness or faintness, in case the dosage should be adjusted.
- they should take COREG with food.
- diabetic patients should report any changes in blood sugar levels to their physician.
- contact lens wearers may experience decreased lacrimation.

Drug Interactions: (Also see CLINICAL PHARMACOLOGY, *Pharmacokinetic Drug-Drug Interactions.*)

Inhibitors of CYP2D6; poor metabolizers of debrisoquin: Interactions of carvedilol with strong inhibitors of CYP2D6 (such as quinidine, fluoxetine, paroxetine, and propafenone) have not been studied, but these drugs would be expected to increase blood levels of the R(+) enantiomer of carvedilol (see CLINICAL PHARMACOLOGY). Retrospective analysis of side effects in clinical trials showed that poor 2D6 metabolizers had a higher rate of dizziness during up-titration, presumably resulting from vasodilating effects of the higher concentrations of the α-blocking R(+) enantiomer.

Catecholamine-depleting agents: Patients taking both agents with β-blocking properties and a drug that can deplete catecholamines (e.g., reserpine and monoamine oxidase inhibitors) should be observed closely for signs of hypotension and/or severe bradycardia.

Clonidine: Concomitant administration of clonidine with agents with β-blocking properties may potentiate blood-pressure- and heart-rate-lowering effects. When concomitant treatment with agents with β-blocking properties and clonidine is to be terminated, the β-blocking agent should be discontinued first. Clonidine therapy can then be discontinued several days later by gradually decreasing the dosage.

Cyclosporin: Modest increases in mean trough cyclosporine concentrations were observed following initiation of carvedilol treatment in 21 renal transplant patients suffering from chronic vascular rejection. In about 30% of patients, the dose of cyclosporine had to be reduced in order to maintain cyclosporine concentrations within the therapeutic range, while in the remainder no adjustment was needed. On the average for the group, the dose of cyclosporine was reduced about 20% in these patients. Due to wide interindividual variability in the dose adjustment required, it is recommended that cyclosporine concentrations be monitored closely after initiation of carvedilol therapy and that the dose of cyclosporine be adjusted as appropriate.

Digoxin: Digoxin concentrations are increased by about 15% when digoxin and carvedilol are administered concomitantly. Both digoxin and COREG slow AV conduction. Therefore, increased monitoring of digoxin is recommended when initiating, adjusting, or discontinuing COREG.

Inducers and inhibitors of hepatic metabolism: Rifampin reduced plasma concentrations of carvedilol by about 70%. Cimetidine increased AUC by about 30% but caused no change in C_{max}.

Calcium channel blockers: Isolated cases of conduction disturbance (rarely with hemodynamic compromise) have been observed when COREG is co-administered with diltiazem. As with other agents with β-blocking properties, if COREG is to be administered orally with calcium channel blockers of the verapamil or diltiazem type, it is recommended that ECG and blood pressure be monitored.

Insulin or oral hypoglycemics: Agents with β-blocking properties may enhance the blood-sugar-reducing effect of insulin and oral hypoglycemics. Therefore, in patients taking insulin or oral hypoglycemics, regular monitoring of blood glucose is recommended.

Carcinogenesis, Mutagenesis, Impairment of Fertility: In 2-year studies conducted in rats given carvedilol at doses up to 75 mg/kg/day (12 times the maximum recommended human dose [MRHD] when compared on a mg/m^2 basis) or in mice given up to 200 mg/kg/day (16 times the MRHD on a mg/m^2 basis), carvedilol had no carcinogenic effect.

Carvedilol was negative when tested in a battery of genotoxicity assays, including the Ames and the CHO/HGPRT assays for mutagenicity and the in vitro hamster micronucleus and in vivo human lymphocyte cell tests for clastogenicity.

At doses ≥200 mg/kg/day (≥32 times the MRHD as mg/m^2) carvedilol was toxic to adult rats (sedation, reduced weight gain) and was associated with a reduced number of successful matings, prolonged mating time, significantly fewer corpora lutea and implants per dam, and complete resorption of 18% of the litters. The no-observed-effect dose level for overt toxicity and impairment of fertility was 60 mg/kg/day (10 times the MRHD as mg/m^2).

Pregnancy: ***Teratogenic Effects.*** Pregnancy Category C. Studies performed in pregnant rats and rabbits given carvedilol revealed increased post-implantation loss in rats at doses of 300 mg/kg/day (50 times the MRHD as mg/m^2) and in rabbits at doses of 75 mg/kg/day (25 times the MRHD as mg/m^2). In the rats, there was also a decrease in fetal body weight at the maternally toxic dose of 300 mg/kg/day (50 times the MRHD as mg/m^2), which was accompanied by an elevation in the frequency of fetuses with delayed skeletal development (missing or stunted 13th rib). In rats the no-observed-effect level for developmental toxicity was 60 mg/kg/day (10 times the MRHD as mg/m^2); in rabbits it was 15 mg/kg/day (5 times the MRHD as mg/m^2). There are no adequate and well-controlled studies in pregnant women. COREG should be used during pregnancy only if the potential benefit justifies the potential risk to the fetus.

Nursing Mothers: It is not known whether this drug is excreted in human milk. Studies in rats have shown that carvedilol and/or its metabolites (as well as other β-blockers) cross the placental barrier and are excreted in breast milk. There was increased mortality at one week post-partum in neonates from rats treated with 60 mg/kg/day (10 times the MRHD as mg/m^2) and above during the last trimester through day 22 of lactation. Because many drugs are excreted in human milk and because of the potential for serious adverse reactions in nursing infants from β-blockers, especially bradycardia, a decision should be made whether to discontinue nursing or to discontinue the drug, taking into account the importance of the drug to the mother. The effects of other α- and β-blocking agents have included perinatal and neonatal distress.

Pediatric Use: Safety and efficacy in patients younger than 18 years of age have not been established.

Geriatric Use: Of the 765 patients with congestive heart failure randomized to COREG in US clinical trials, 31% (235) were 65 years of age or older, and 7.3% (56) were 75 years of age or older. Of the 1,156 patients randomized to COREG in a long-term, placebo-controlled trial in severe heart failure, 47% (547) were 65 years of age or older, and 15% (174) were 75 years of age or older. Of 3,025 patients receiving COREG in congestive heart failure trials worldwide, 42% were 65 years of age or older.

Of the 975 myocardial infarction patients randomized to COREG in the CAPRICORN trial, 48% (468) were 65 years of age or older, and 11% (111) were 75 years of age or older. Of the 2,065 hypertensive patients in US clinical trials of efficacy or safety who were treated with COREG, 21% (436) were 65 years of age or older. Of 3,722 patients receiving COREG in hypertension clinical trials conducted worldwide, 24% were 65 years of age or older.

With the exception of dizziness in hypertensive patients (incidence 8.8% in the elderly vs. 6% in younger patients), no overall differences in the safety or effectiveness (See Figures 2 and 4.) were observed between the older subjects and younger subjects in each of these populations. Similarly, other reported clinical experience has not identified differences in responses between the elderly and younger subjects, but greater sensitivity of some older individuals cannot be ruled out.

ADVERSE REACTIONS

COREG has been evaluated for safety in patients with congestive heart failure (mild, moderate, and severe heart failure), in patients with left ventricular dysfunction following myocardial infarction and in hypertensive patients. The observed adverse event profile was consistent with the pharmacology of the drug and the health status of the patients in the clinical trials. Adverse events reported for each of these patient populations are provided below. Excluded are adverse events considered too general to be informative, and those not reasonably associated with the use of the drug because they were associated with the condition being treated or are very common in the treated population. Rates of adverse events were generally similar across demographic subsets (men and women, elderly and non-elderly, blacks and non-blacks).

Congestive Heart Failure: COREG has been evaluated for safety in congestive heart failure in more than 3,000 patients worldwide of whom more than 2,100 participated in placebo-controlled clinical trials. Approximately 60% of the total treated population received COREG for at least 6 months and 30% received COREG for at least 12 months. Both in US clinical trials in mild-to-moderate heart failure that compared COREG in daily doses up to 100 mg (n = 765) to placebo (n = 437), and in a multinational clinical trial in severe heart failure (COPERNICUS) that compared COREG in daily doses up to 50 mg (n = 1,156) with placebo (n = 1,133), discontinuation rates for adverse experiences were similar in carvedilol and placebo patients. In these databases, the only cause of discontinuation >1%, and occurring more often on carvedilol was dizziness (1.3% on carvedilol, 0.6% on placebo in the COPERNICUS trial).

Continued on next page

Product information on these pages is effective as of August 2004. Further information is available at: GlaxoSmithKline, PO Box 13398, Research Triangle Park, NC 27709. 1-888-825-5249. Corporate Web Site: www.gsk.com

Coreg—Cont.

Table 2 shows adverse events reported in patients with mild-to-moderate heart failure enrolled in US placebo-controlled clinical trials, and with severe heart failure enrolled in the COPERNICUS trial. Shown are adverse events that occurred more frequently in drug-treated patients than placebo-treated patients with an incidence of >3% in patients treated with carvedilol regardless of causality. Median study medication exposure was 6.3 months for both carvedilol and placebo patients in the trials of mild-to-moderate heart failure, and 10.4 months in the trial of severe heart failure patients.

[See table 2 below]

Cardiac failure and dyspnea were also reported in these studies, but the rates were equal or greater in patients who received placebo.

The following adverse events were reported with a frequency of >1% but ≤3% and more frequently with COREG in either the US placebo-controlled trials in patients with mild-to-moderate heart failure, or in patients with severe heart failure in the COPERNICUS trial.

Incidence >1% to ≤3%

Body as a Whole: Allergy, malaise, hypovolemia, fever, leg edema.

Cardiovascular: Fluid overload, postural hypotension, aggravated angina pectoris, AV block, palpitation, hypertension.

Central and Peripheral Nervous System: Hypesthesia, vertigo, paresthesia.

Gastrointestinal: Melena, periodontitis.

Liver and Biliary System: SGPT increased, SGOT increased.

Metabolic and Nutritional: Hyperuricemia, hypoglycemia, hyponatremia, increased alkaline phosphatase, glycosuria, hypervolemia, diabetes mellitus, GGT increased, weight loss, hyperkalemia, creatinine increased.

Musculoskeletal: Muscle cramps.

Platelet, Bleeding and Clotting: Prothrombin decreased, purpura, thrombocytopenia.

Psychiatric: Somnolence.

Reproductive, male: Impotence

Special Senses: Blurred vision.

Urinary System: Renal insufficiency, albuminuria, hematuria.

Left Ventricular Dysfunction Following Myocardial Infarction: COREG has been evaluated for safety in survivors of an acute myocardial infarction with left ventricular dysfunction in the CAPRICORN trial which involved 969 patients who received COREG and 980 who received placebo. Approximately 75% of the patients received COREG for at least 6 months and 53% received COREG for at least 12 months. Patients were treated for an average of 12.9 months and 12.8 months with COREG and placebo, respectively.

The most common adverse events reported with COREG in the CAPRICORN trial were consistent with the profile of the drug in the US heart failure trials and the COPERNICUS trial. The only additional adverse events reported in CAPRICORN in >3% of the patients and more commonly on carvedilol were dyspnea, anemia, and lung edema. The following adverse events were reported with a frequency of >1% but ≤3% and more frequently with COREG: flu syndrome, cerebrovascular accident, peripheral vascular disorder, hypotonia, depression, gastrointestinal pain, arthritis and gout. The overall rates of discontinuations due to adverse events were similar in both groups of patients. In this database, the only cause of discontinuation >1%, and occurring more often on carvedilol was hypotension (1.5% on carvedilol, 0.2% on placebo).

Hypertension: COREG has been evaluated for safety in hypertension in more than 2,193 patients in US clinical trials and in 2,976 patients in international clinical trials. Approximately 36% of the total treated population received COREG for at least 6 months. In general, COREG was well tolerated at doses up to 50 mg daily. Most adverse events reported during COREG therapy were of mild to moderate severity. In US controlled clinical trials directly comparing COREG monotherapy in doses up to 50 mg (n = 1,142) to placebo (n = 462), 4.9% of COREG patients discontinued for adverse events vs. 5.2% of placebo patients. Although there was no overall difference in discontinuation rates, discontinuations were more common in the carvedilol group for postural hypotension (1% vs. 0). The overall incidence of adverse events in US placebo-controlled trials was found to increase with increasing dose of COREG. For individual adverse events this could only be distinguished for dizziness, which increased in frequency from 2% to 5% as total daily dose increased from 6.25 mg to 50 mg.

Table 3 shows adverse events in US placebo-controlled clinical trials for hypertension that occurred with an incidence of >1% regardless of causality, and that were more frequent in drug-treated patients than placebo-treated patients.

Table 3. Adverse Events in US Placebo-Controlled Hypertension Trials Incidence ≥1%, Regardless of Causality

	Adverse Reactions	
	COREG (n = 1,142) % occurrence	Placebo (n = 462) % occurrence
Cardiovascular		
Bradycardia	2	—
Postural hypotension	2	—
Peripheral Edema	1	—
Central Nervous System		
Dizziness	6	5
Insomnia	2	1
Gastrointestinal		
Diarrhea	2	1
Hematologic		
Thrombocytopenia	1	—
Metabolic		
Hypertriglyceridemia	1	—

Dyspnea and fatigue were also reported in these studies, but the rates were equal or greater in patients who received placebo.

The following adverse events not described above were reported as possibly or probably related to COREG in worldwide open or controlled trials with COREG in patients with hypertension or congestive heart failure.

Incidence >0.1% to ≤1%

Cardiovascular: Peripheral ischemia, tachycardia.

Central and Peripheral Nervous System: Hypokinesia.

Gastrointestinal: Bilirubinemia, increased hepatic enzymes (0.2% of hypertension patients and 0.4% of congestive heart failure patients were discontinued from therapy because of increases in hepatic enzymes; see Laboratory Abnormalities.

Psychiatric: Nervousness, sleep disorder, aggravated depression, impaired concentration, abnormal thinking, paroniria, emotional lability.

Respiratory System: Asthma (see CONTRAINDICATIONS).

Reproductive: Male: decreased libido.

Skin and Appendages: Pruritus, rash erythematous, rash maculopapular, rash psoriaform, photosensitivity reaction.

Special Senses: Tinnitus.

Urinary System: Micturition frequency increased.

Autonomic Nervous System: Dry mouth, sweating increased.

Metabolic and Nutritional: Hypokalemia, hypertriglyceridemia.

Hematologic: Anemia, leukopenia.

The following events were reported in ≤0.1% of patients and are potentially important: complete AV block, bundle branch block, myocardial ischemia, cerebrovascular disorder, convulsions, migraine, neuralgia, paresis, anaphylactoid reaction, alopecia, exfoliative dermatitis, amnesia, GI hemorrhage, bronchospasm, pulmonary edema, decreased hearing, respiratory alkalosis, increased BUN, decreased HDL, pancytopenia, and atypical lymphocytes.

Laboratory Abnormalities: Reversible elevations in serum transaminases (ALT or AST) have been observed during treatment with COREG. Rates of transaminase elevations (2- to 3-times the upper limit of normal) observed during controlled clinical trials have generally been similar between patients treated with COREG and those treated with placebo. However, transaminase elevations, confirmed by

Table 2. Adverse Events (% Occurrence) Occurring More Frequently with COREG Than With Placebo in Patients With Mild-to-Moderate Heart Failure Enrolled in US Heart Failure Trials or in Patients With Severe Heart Failure in the COPERNICUS Trial (Incidence >3% in Patients Treated with Carvedilol, Regardless of Causality)

	Mild-to-Moderate HF		Severe Heart Failure	
	COREG	Placebo	COREG	Placebo
	(n = 765)	(n = 437)	(n = 1,156)	(n = 1,133)
Body as a Whole				
Asthenia	7	7	11	9
Fatigue	24	22	—	—
Digoxin level increased	5	4	2	1
Edema generalized	5	3	6	5
Edema dependent	4	2	—	—
Cardiovascular				
Bradycardia	9	1	10	3
Hypotension	9	3	14	8
Syncope	3	3	8	5
Angina Pectoris	2	3	6	4
Central Nervous System				
Dizziness	32	19	24	17
Headache	8	7	5	3
Gastrointestinal				
Diarrhea	12	6	5	3
Nausea	9	5	4	3
Vomiting	6	4	1	2
Metabolic				
Hyperglycemia	12	8	5	3
Weight increase	10	7	12	11
BUN increased	6	5	—	—
NPN increased	6	5	—	—
Hypercholesterolemia	4	3	1	1
Edema peripheral	2	1	7	6
Musculoskeletal				
Arthralgia	6	5	1	1
Respiratory				
Cough Increased	8	9	5	4
Rales	4	4	4	2
Vision				
Vision abnormal	5	2	—	—

rechallenge, have been observed with COREG. In a long-term, placebo-controlled trial in severe heart failure, patients treated with COREG had lower values for hepatic transaminases than patients treated with placebo, possibly because COREG-induced improvements in cardiac function led to less hepatic congestion and/or improved hepatic blood flow.

COREG therapy has not been associated with clinically significant changes in serum potassium, total triglycerides, total cholesterol, HDL cholesterol, uric acid, blood urea nitrogen, or creatinine. No clinically relevant changes were noted in fasting serum glucose in hypertensive patients; fasting serum glucose was not evaluated in the congestive heart failure clinical trials.

Postmarketing Experience: The following adverse reaction has been reported in postmarketing experience: Reports of aplastic anemia have been rare and received only when carvedilol was administered concomitantly with other medications associated with the event.

OVERDOSAGE

The acute oral LD_{50} doses in male and female mice and male and female rats are over 8000 mg/kg. Overdosage may cause severe hypotension, bradycardia, cardiac insufficiency, cardiogenic shock, and cardiac arrest. Respiratory problems, bronchospasms, vomiting, lapses of consciousness, and generalized seizures may also occur.

The patient should be placed in a supine position and, where necessary, kept under observation and treated under intensive-care conditions. Gastric lavage or pharmacologically induced emesis may be used shortly after ingestion.

The following agents may be administered:

for excessive bradycardia: atropine, 2 mg IV.

to support cardiovascular function: glucagon, 5 to 10 mg IV rapidly over 30 seconds, followed by a continuous infusion of 5 mg/hour; sympathomimetics (dobutamine, isoprenaline, adrenaline) at doses according to body weight and effect.

If peripheral vasodilation dominates, it may be necessary to administer adrenaline or noradrenaline with continuous monitoring of circulatory conditions. For therapy-resistant bradycardia, pacemaker therapy should be performed. For bronchospasm, β-sympathomimetics (as aerosol or IV) or aminophylline IV should be given. In the event of seizures, slow IV injection of diazepam or clonazepam is recommended.

NOTE: In the event of severe intoxication where there are symptoms of shock, treatment with antidotes must be continued for a sufficiently long period of time consistent with the 7- to 10-hour half-life of carvedilol.

Cases of overdosage with COREG alone or in combination with other drugs have been reported. Quantities ingested in some cases exceeded 1,000 milligrams. Symptoms experienced included low blood pressure and heart rate. Standard supportive treatment was provided and individuals recovered.

DOSAGE AND ADMINISTRATION

Congestive Heart Failure: DOSAGE MUST BE INDIVIDUALIZED AND CLOSELY MONITORED BY A PHYSICIAN DURING UP-TITRATION. Prior to initiation of COREG, it is recommended that fluid retention be minimized. The recommended starting dose of COREG is 3.125 mg, twice daily for two weeks. Patients who tolerate a dose of 3.125 mg twice daily may have their dose increased to 6.25, 12.5, and 25 mg twice daily over successive intervals of at least two weeks. Patients should be maintained on lower doses if higher doses are not tolerated. A maximum dose of 50 mg twice daily has been administered to patients with mild-to-moderate heart failure weighing over 85 kg (187 lbs).

Patients should be advised that initiation of treatment and (to a lesser extent) dosage increases may be associated with transient symptoms of dizziness or lightheadedness (and rarely syncope) within the first hour after dosing. Thus during these periods they should avoid situations such as driving or hazardous tasks, where symptoms could result in injury. In addition, COREG should be taken with food to slow the rate of absorption. Vasodilatory symptoms often do not require treatment, but it may be useful to separate the time of dosing of COREG from that of the ACE inhibitor or to reduce temporarily the dose of the ACE inhibitor. The dose of COREG should not be increased until symptoms of worsening heart failure or vasodilation have been stabilized.

Fluid retention (with or without transient worsening heart failure symptoms) should be treated by an increase in the dose of diuretics.

The dose of COREG should be reduced if patients experience bradycardia (heart rate <55 beats/minute).

Episodes of dizziness or fluid retention during initiation of COREG can generally be managed without discontinuation of treatment and do not preclude subsequent successful titration of, or a favorable response to, carvedilol.

Left Ventricular Dysfunction Following Myocardial Infarction: DOSAGE MUST BE INDIVIDUALIZED AND MONITORED DURING UP-TITRATION. Treatment with COREG may be started as an inpatient or outpatient and should be started after the patient is hemodynamically stable and fluid retention has been minimized. It is recommended that COREG be started at 6.25 mg twice daily and increased after 3 to 10 days, based on tolerability to 12.5 mg twice daily, then again to the target dose of 25 mg twice daily. A lower starting dose may be used (3.125 mg twice daily) and/or, the rate of up-titration may be slowed if clinically indicated (e.g., due to low blood pressure or heart rate, or fluid retention). Patients should be maintained on lower doses if higher doses are not tolerated. The recommended dosing regimen need not be altered in patients who received treatment with an IV or oral β-blocker during the acute phase of the myocardial infarction.

Hypertension: DOSAGE MUST BE INDIVIDUALIZED. The recommended starting dose of COREG is 6.25 mg twice daily. If this dose is tolerated, using standing systolic pressure measured about 1 hour after dosing as a guide, the dose should be maintained for 7 to 14 days, and then increased to 12.5 mg twice daily if needed, based on trough blood pressure, again using standing systolic pressure one hour after dosing as a guide for tolerance. This dose should also be maintained for 7 to 14 days and can then be adjusted upward to 25 mg twice daily if tolerated and needed. The full antihypertensive effect of COREG is seen within 7 to 14 days. Total daily dose should not exceed 50 mg. COREG should be taken with food to slow the rate of absorption and reduce the incidence of orthostatic effects.

Addition of a diuretic to COREG, or COREG to a diuretic can be expected to produce additive effects and exaggerate the orthostatic component of COREG action.

Use in Patients with Hepatic Impairment: COREG should not be given to patients with severe hepatic impairment (see CONTRAINDICATIONS).

HOW SUPPLIED

Tablets: White, oval, film-coated tablets: 3.125 mg–engraved with 39 and SB, in bottles of 100; 6.25 mg–engraved with 4140 and SB, in bottles of 100; 12.5 mg–engraved with 4141 and SB, in bottles of 100; 25 mg–engraved with 4142 and SB, in bottles of 100. The 6.25 mg, 12.5 mg, and 25 mg tablets are TILTAB tablets.

Store below 30°C (86°F). Protect from moisture. Dispense in a tight, light-resistant container.

3.125 mg 100's: NDC 0007-4139-20
6.25 mg 100's: NDC 0007-4140-20
12.5 mg 100's: NDC 0007-4141-20
25 mg 100's: NDC 0007-4142-20

COREG and TILTAB are registered trademarks of GlaxoSmithKline.

GlaxoSmithKline, Research Triangle Park, NC 27709

October 2003/CO:L8

Shown in Product Identification Guide, page 315

CUTIVATE® ℞
[kyoot'ə-vāt]
(fluticasone propionate cream)
Cream, 0.05%

For Dermatologic Use Only—
Not for Ophthalmic Use.

DESCRIPTION

CUTIVATE (fluticasone propionate cream) Cream, 0.05% contains fluticasone propionate [(6α,11β,16 α,17 α)-6,9,-difluoro-11-hydroxy-16-methyl-3-oxo-17-(1-oxopropoxy)androsta-1,4-diene-17-carbothioic acid, S-fluoromethyl ester], a synthetic fluorinated corticosteroid, for topical dermatologic use. The topical corticosteroids constitute a class of primarily synthetic steroids used as anti-inflammatory and antipruritic agents.

Chemically, fluticasone propionate is $C_{25}H_{31}F_3O_5S$.

Fluticasone propionate has a molecular weight of 500.6. It is a white to off-white powder and is insoluble in water.

Each gram of CUTIVATE Cream contains fluticasone propionate 0.5 mg in a base of propylene glycol, mineral oil, cetostearyl alcohol, Ceteth-20, isopropyl myristate, dibasic sodium phosphate, citric acid, purified water, and imidurea as preservative.

CLINICAL PHARMACOLOGY

Like other topical corticosteroids, fluticasone propionate has anti-inflammatory, antipruritic, and vasoconstrictive properties. The mechanism of the anti-inflammatory activity of the topical steroids, in general, is unclear. However, corticosteroids are thought to act by the induction of phospholipase A_2 inhibitory proteins, collectively called lipocortins. It is postulated that these proteins control the biosynthesis of potent mediators of inflammation such as prostaglandins and leukotrienes by inhibiting the release of their common precursor, arachidonic acid. Arachidonic acid is released from membrane phospholipids by phospholipase A_2.

Fluticasone propionate is lipophilic and has a strong affinity for the glucocorticoid receptor. It has weak affinity for the progesterone receptor, and virtually no affinity for the mineralocorticoid, estrogen, or androgen receptors. The therapeutic potency of glucocorticoids is related to the half-life of the glucocorticoid-receptor complex. The half-life of the fluticasone propionate-glucocorticoid receptor complex is approximately 10 hours.

Studies performed with CUTIVATE Cream indicate that it is in the medium range of potency as compared with other topical corticosteroids.

Pharmacokinetics: ***Absorption:*** The activity of CUTIVATE is due to the parent drug, fluticasone propionate. The extent of percutaneous absorption of topical corticosteroids is determined by many factors, including the vehicle and the integrity of the epidermal barrier. Occlusive dressing enhances penetration. Topical corticosteroids can be absorbed from normal intact skin. Inflammation and/or other disease processes in the skin increase percutaneous absorption.

In a human study of 12 healthy males receiving 12.5 g of 0.05% fluticasone propionate cream twice daily for 3 weeks, plasma levels were generally below the level of quantification (0.05 ng/mL). In another study of 6 healthy males administered 25 g of 0.05% fluticasone propionate cream under occlusion for 5 days, plasma levels of fluticasone ranged from 0.07 to 0.39 ng/mL.

In an animal study using radiolabeled 0.05% fluticasone propionate cream and ointment preparations, rats received a topical dose of 1 g/kg for a 24-hour period. Total recovery of radioactivity was approximately 80% at the end of 7 days. The majority of the dose (73%) was recovered from the surface of the application site. Less than 1% of the dose was recovered in the skin at the application site. Approximately 5% of the dose was absorbed systemically through the skin. Absorption from the skin continued for the duration of the study (7 days), indicating a long retention time at the application site.

Distribution: Following intravenous administration of 1 mg fluticasone propionate in healthy volunteers, the initial disposition phase for fluticasone propionate was rapid and consistent with its high lipid solubility and tissue binding. The apparent volume of distribution averaged 4.2 L/kg (range, 2.3 to 16.7 L/kg). The percentage of fluticasone propionate bound to human plasma proteins averaged 91%. Fluticasone propionate is weakly and reversibly bound to erythrocytes. Fluticasone propionate is not significantly bound to human transcortin.

Metabolism: No metabolites of fluticasone propionate were detected in an in vitro study of radiolabeled fluticasone propionate incubated in a human skin homogenate. The total blood clearance of systemically absorbed fluticasone propionate averages 1,093 mL/min (range, 618 to 1,702 mL/min) after a 1-mg intravenous dose, with renal clearance accounting for less than 0.02% of the total. Fluticasone propionate is metabolized in the liver by cytochrome P450 3A4-mediated hydrolysis of the 5-fluoromethyl carbothioate grouping. This transformation occurs in 1 metabolic step to produce the inactive 17-β-carboxylic acid metabolite, the only known metabolite detected in man. This metabolite has approximately 2,000 times less affinity than the parent drug for the glucocorticoid receptor of human lung cytosol in vitro and negligible pharmacological activity in animal studies. Other metabolites detected in vitro using cultured human hepatoma cells have not been detected in man.

Excretion: Following intravenous dose of 1 mg in healthy volunteers, fluticasone propionate showed polyexponential kinetics and had an average terminal half-life of 7.2 hours (range, 3.2 to 11.2 hours).

INDICATIONS AND USAGE

CUTIVATE Cream is a medium potency corticosteroid indicated for the relief of the inflammatory and pruritic manifestations of corticosteroid-responsive dermatoses. CUTIVATE Cream may be used with caution in pediatric patients 3 months of age or older. The safety and efficacy of drug use for longer than 4 weeks in this population have not been established. The safety and efficacy of CUTIVATE Cream in pediatric patients below 3 months of age have not been established.

CONTRAINDICATIONS

CUTIVATE Cream is contraindicated in those patients with a history of hypersensitivity to any of the components in the preparation.

PRECAUTIONS

General: Systemic absorption of topical corticosteroids can produce reversible hypothalamic-pituitary-adrenal (HPA) axis suppression with the potential for glucocorticosteroid insufficiency after withdrawal from treatment. Manifestations of Cushing's syndrome, hyperglycemia, and glucosuria can also be produced in some patients by systemic absorption of topical corticosteroids while on treatment.

Patients applying a potent topical steroid to a large surface area or to areas under occlusion should be evaluated periodically for evidence of HPA axis suppression. This may be done by using the ACTH stimulation, A.M. plasma cortisol, and urinary free cortisol tests.

If HPA axis suppression is noted, an attempt should be made to withdraw the drug, to reduce the frequency of application, or to substitute a less potent steroid. Recovery of HPA axis function is generally prompt upon discontinuation of topical corticosteroids. Infrequently, signs and symptoms of glucocorticosteroid insufficiency may occur requiring supplemental systemic corticosteroids. For information on systemic supplementation, see prescribing information for those products.

Fluticasone propionate cream, 0.05% caused depression of A.M. plasma cortisol levels in 1 of 6 adult patients when used daily for 7 days in patients with psoriasis or eczema involving at least 30% of the body surface. After 2 days of treatment, this patient developed a 60% decrease from pretreatment values in the A.M. plasma cortisol level.

There was some evidence of corresponding decrease in the 24-hour urinary free cortisol levels. The A.M. plasma cortisol level remained slightly depressed for 48 hours but recovered by day 6 of treatment.

Continued on next page

Product information on these pages is effective as of August 2004. Further information is available at: GlaxoSmithKline, PO Box 13398, Research Triangle Park, NC 27709. 1-888-825-5249. Corporate Web Site: www.gsk.com

Cutivate Cream—Cont.

Fluticasone propionate cream, 0.05%, caused HPA axis suppression in 2 of 43 pediatric patients, ages 2 and 5 years old, who were treated for 4 weeks covering at least 35% of the body surface area. Follow-up testing 12 days after treatment discontinuation, available for 1 of the 2 subjects, demonstrated a normally responsive HPA axis (see PRECAUTIONS: Pediatric Use).

Pediatric patients may be more susceptible to systemic toxicity from equivalent doses due to their larger skin surface to body mass ratios (see PRECAUTIONS: Pediatric Use).

Fluticasone propionate cream, 0.05% may cause local cutaneous adverse reactions (see ADVERSE REACTIONS).

If irritation develops, CUTIVATE Cream should be discontinued and appropriate therapy instituted. Allergic contact dermatitis with corticosteroids is usually diagnosed by observing failure to heal rather than noting a clinical exacerbation as with most topical products not containing corticosteroids. Such an observation should be corroborated with appropriate diagnostic patch testing.

If concomitant skin infections are present or develop, an appropriate antifungal or antibacterial agent should be used. If a favorable response does not occur promptly, use of CUTIVATE Cream should be discontinued until the infection has been adequately controlled.

CUTIVATE Cream should not be used in the presence of preexisting skin atrophy and should not be used where infection is present at the treatment site. CUTIVATE Cream should not be used in the treatment of rosacea and perioral dermatitis.

Information for Patients: Patients using topical corticosteroids should receive the following information and instructions:

1. This medication is to be used as directed by the physician. It is for external use only. Avoid contact with the eyes.
2. This medication should not be used for any disorder other than that for which it was prescribed.
3. The treated skin area should not be bandaged or otherwise covered or wrapped so as to be occlusive unless directed by the physician.
4. Patients should report to their physician any signs of local adverse reactions.
5. Parents of pediatric patients should be advised not to use this medication in the treatment of diaper dermatitis. CUTIVATE Cream should not be applied in the diaper areas as diapers or plastic pants may constitute occlusive dressing (see DOSAGE AND ADMINISTRATION).
6. This medication should not be used on the face, underarms, or groin areas unless directed by a physician.
7. As with other corticosteroids, therapy should be discontinued when control is achieved. If no improvement is seen within 2 weeks, contact the physician.

Laboratory Tests: The following tests may be helpful in evaluating patients for HPA axis suppression:

ACTH stimulation test
A.M. plasma cortisol test
Urinary free cortisol test

Carcinogenesis, Mutagenesis, and Impairment of Fertility: Two 18-month studies were performed in mice to evaluate the carcinogenic potential of fluticasone propionate when given topically (as an 0.05% ointment) and orally. No evidence of carcinogenicity was found in either study.

Fluticasone propionate was not mutagenic in the standard Ames test, *E. coli* fluctuation test, *S. cerevisiae* gene conversion test, or Chinese Hamster ovarian cell assay. It was not clastogenic in mouse micronucleus or cultured human lymphocyte tests.

In a fertility and general reproductive performance study in rats, fluticasone propionate administered subcutaneously to females at up to 50 mcg/kg per day and to males at up to 100 mcg/kg per day (later reduced to 50 mcg/kg per day) had no effect upon mating performance or fertility. These doses are approximately 15 and 30 times, respectively, the human systemic exposure following use of the recommended human topical dose of fluticasone propionate cream, 0.05%, assuming human percutaneous absorption of approximately 3% and the use in a 70-kg person of 15 g/day.

Pregnancy: *Teratogenic Effects:* Pregnancy Category C. Corticosteroids have been shown to be teratogenic in laboratory animals when administered systemically at relatively low dosage levels. Some corticosteroids have been shown to be teratogenic after dermal application in laboratory animals. Teratology studies in the mouse demonstrated fluticasone propionate to be teratogenic (cleft palate) when administered subcutaneously in doses of 45 mcg/kg/day and 150 mcg/kg/day. This dose is approximately 14 and 45 times, respectively, the human topical dose of fluticasone propionate cream, 0.05%. There are no adequate and well-controlled studies in pregnant women. CUTIVATE Cream should be used during pregnancy only if the potential benefit justifies the potential risk to the fetus.

Nursing Mothers: Systemically administered corticosteroids appear in human milk and could suppress growth, interfere with endogenous corticosteroid production, or cause other untoward effects. It is not known whether topical administration of corticosteroids could result in sufficient systemic absorption to produce detectable quantities in human milk. Because many drugs are excreted in human milk, caution should be exercised when CUTIVATE Cream is administered to a nursing woman.

Pediatric Use: CUTIVATE Cream may be used with caution in pediatric patients as young as 3 months of age. The safety and efficacy of drug use for longer than 4 weeks in this population have not been established. The safety and efficacy of CUTIVATE Cream in pediatric patients below 3 months of age have not been established.

Fluticasone propionate cream, 0.05%, caused HPA axis suppression in 2 of 43 pediatric patients, ages 2 and 5 years old, who were treated for 4 weeks covering at least 35% of the body surface area. Follow-up testing 12 days after treatment discontinuation, available for 1 of the 2 subjects, demonstrated a normally responsive HPA axis (see ADVERSE REACTIONS). Adverse effects including striae have been reported with use of topical corticosteroids in pediatric patients.

HPA axis suppression, Cushing syndrome, linear growth retardation, delayed weight gain, and intracranial hypertension have been reported in pediatric patients receiving topical corticosteroids. Manifestations of adrenal suppression in pediatric patients include low plasma cortisol levels to an absence of response to ACTH stimulation. Manifestations of intracranial hypertension include bulging fontanelles, headaches, and bilateral papilledema.

Geriatric Use: A limited number of patients above 65 years of age (n = 126) have been treated with CUTIVATE Cream in US and non-US clinical trials. While the number of patients is too small to permit separate analysis of efficacy and safety, the adverse reactions reported in this population were similar to those reported by younger patients. Based on available data, no adjustment of dosage of CUTIVATE in geriatric patients is warranted.

ADVERSE REACTIONS

In controlled clinical trials of twice-daily administration, the total incidence of adverse reactions associated with the use of CUTIVATE Cream was approximately 4%. These adverse reactions were usually mild; self-limiting; and consisted primarily of pruritus, dryness, numbness of fingers, and burning. These events occurred in 2.9%, 1.2%, 1.0%, and 0.6% of patients, respectively.

Two clinical studies compared once- to twice-daily administration of CUTIVATE Cream for the treatment of moderate to severe eczema. The local drug-related adverse events for the 491 patients enrolled in both studies are shown in Table 1. In the study enrolling both adult and pediatric patients, the incidence of local adverse events in the 119 pediatric patients ages 1 to 12 years was comparable to the 140 patients ages 13 to 62 years.

Fifty-one pediatric patients ages 3 months to 5 years, with moderate to severe eczema, were enrolled in an open-label HPA axis safety study. CUTIVATE Cream was applied twice daily for 3 to 4 weeks over an arithmetic mean body surface area of 64% (range, 35% to 95%). The mean morning cortisol levels with standard deviations before treatment (prestimu-

Table 1. Drug-Related Adverse Events—Skin

Adverse Events	Fluticasone Once Daily (n = 210)	Fluticasone Twice Daily (n = 203)	Vehicle Twice Daily (n = 78)
Skin infection	1 (0.5%)	0	0
Infected eczema	1 (0.5%)	2 (1.0%)	0
Viral warts	0	1 (0.5%)	0
Herpes simplex	0	1 (0.5%)	0
Impetigo	1 (0.5%)	0	0
Atopic dermatitis	1 (0.5%)	0	0
Eczema	1 (0.5%)	0	0
Exacerbation of eczema	4 (1.9%)	1 (0.5%)	1 (1.3%)
Erythema	0	2 (1.0%)	0
Burning	2 (1.0%)	2 (1.0%)	2 (2.6%)
Stinging	0	2 (1.0%)	1 (1.3%)
Skin irritation	6 (2.9%)	2 (1.0%)	0
Pruritus	2 (1.0%)	4 (1.9%)	4 (5.1%)
Exacerbation of pruritus	4 (1.9%)	1 (0.5%)	1 (1.3%)
Folliculitis	1 (0.5%)	1 (0.5%)	0
Blisters	0	1 (0.5%)	0
Dryness of skin	3 (1.4%)	1 (0.5%)	0

Table 2. Adverse Events* From Pediatric Open-Label Trial (n = 51)

Adverse Events	Fluticasone Twice Daily
Burning	1 (2.0%)
Dusky erythema	1 (2.0%)
Erythematous rash	1 (2.0%)
Facial telangiectasia[†]	2 (4.9%)
Non-facial telangiectasia	1 (2.0%)
Urticaria	1 (2.0%)

*See text for additional detail.
[†]n = 41.

Table 3. Physician's Assessment of Clinical Response

	CUTIVATE Cream		Vehicle	
	Study 1 (n = 59)	Study 2 (n = 74)	Study 1 (n = 66)	Study 2 (n = 75)
Cleared	8%	1%	3%	1%
Excellent	29%	28%	11%	17%
Good	27%	34%	20%	28%
Fair	27%	15%	33%	25%
Poor	7%	22%	24%	27%
Worse	2%	0	9%	1%

Table 4. Clinical Signs: Mean Improvements Over Baseline

	CUTIVATE Cream		Vehicle	
	Study 1	Study 2	Study 1	Study 2
Erythema	1.19	1.07	0.55	0.84
Thickening	1.22	1.17	0.81	0.97
Scaling	1.53	1.39	0.95	1.21

Table 5. Physician's Assessment of Clinical Response

	CUTIVATE Cream Once Daily		CUTIVATE Cream Twice Daily	
	Study 1 (n = 64)	Study 2 (n = 106)	Study 1 (n = 65)	Study 2 (n = 100)
Cleared	30%	20%	48%	21%
Excellent	42%	32%	32%	50%
Good	17%	26%	5%	12%
Fair	3%	14%	6%	10%
Poor	5%	3%	8%	4%
Worse	3%	6%	2%	3%

Table 6. Clinical Signs and Symptoms: Mean Improvements Over Baseline

	CUTIVATE Cream Once Daily		CUTIVATE Cream Twice Daily	
	Study 1	Study 2	Study 1	Study 2
Erythema	1.7	1.5	1.8	1.7
Pruritus	2.1	1.6	2.1	1.7
Thickening	1.6	1.3	1.6	1.5
Lichenification	1.2	1.2	1.2	1.3
Vesiculation	0.5	0.4	0.5	0.5
Crusting	0.6	0.7	0.8	0.8

lation mean value = 13.76 ± 6.94 mcg/dL, poststimulation mean value = 30.53 ± 7.23 mcg/dL) and at end treatment (prestimulation mean value = 12.32 ± 6.92 mcg/dL, poststimulation mean value = 28.84 ± 7.16 mcg/dL) showed little change. In 2 of 43 (4.7%) patients with end-treatment results, peak cortisol levels following cosyntropin stimulation testing were ≤18 μg/dL, indicating adrenal suppression. Follow-up testing after treatment discontinuation, available for 1 of the 2 subjects, demonstrated a normally responsive HPA axis. Local drug-related adverse events were transient burning, resolving the same day it was reported; transient urticaria, resolving the same day it was reported; erythematous rash; dusky erythema, resolving within 1 month after cessation of CUTIVATE Cream; and telangiectasia, resolving within 3 months after stopping CUTIVATE Cream.

[See table 1 at top of previous page]

[See table 2 at top of previous page]

The following local adverse reactions have been reported infrequently with topical corticosteroids, and they may occur more frequently with the use of occlusive dressings and higher potency corticosteroids. These reactions are listed in an approximately decreasing order of occurrence: irritation, folliculitis, acneiform eruptions, hypopigmentation, perioral dermatitis, allergic contact dermatitis, secondary infection, skin atrophy, striae, and miliaria. Also, there are reports of the development of pustular psoriasis from chronic plaque psoriasis following reduction or discontinuation of potent topical corticosteroid products.

OVERDOSAGE

Topically applied CUTIVATE Cream can be absorbed in sufficient amounts to produce systemic effects (see PRECAUTIONS).

DOSAGE AND ADMINISTRATION

CUTIVATE Cream may be used in adult and pediatric patients 3 months of age or older. Safety and efficacy of (numbers are realigned in columns below) CUTIVATE Cream in pediatric patients for more than 4 weeks of use have not been established (see PRECAUTIONS: Pediatric Use). The safety and efficacy of CUTIVATE Cream in pediatric patients below 3 months of age have not been established.

Atopic Dermatitis: Apply a thin film of CUTIVATE Cream to the affected skin areas once or twice daily. Rub in gently.

Other Corticosteroid-Responsive Dermatoses: Apply a thin film of CUTIVATE Cream to the affected skin areas twice daily. Rub in gently.

As with other corticosteroids, therapy should be discontinued when control is achieved. If no improvement is seen within 2 weeks, reassessment of diagnosis may be necessary.

CUTIVATE Cream should not be used with occlusive dressings. CUTIVATE Cream should not be applied in the diaper area, as diapers or plastic pants may constitute occlusive dressings.

Geriatric Use: In studies where geriatric patients (65 years of age or older, see PRECAUTIONS) have been treated with CUTIVATE Cream, safety did not differ from that in younger patients; therefore, no dosage adjustment is recommended.

CLINICAL STUDIES

Psoriasis Studies: In 2 vehicle-controlled studies, CUTIVATE Cream applied twice daily was significantly more effective than the vehicle in the treatment of moderate to severe psoriasis. The investigator's global evaluation after 28 days of treatment is shown in Table 3.

[See table 3 on previous page]

The clinical signs of psoriasis were scored on a scale of 0 = absent, 1 = mild, 2 = moderate, and 3 = severe. The mean improvements over baseline in the clinical signs at the end of treatment are shown in Table 4.

[See table 4 on previous page]

Atopic Dermatitis Studies: In 2 controlled 28-day studies, CUTIVATE Cream once daily was equivalent to CUTIVATE Cream twice daily in the treatment of moderate to severe eczema. The investigator's global evaluation after 28 days of treatment is shown in Table 5.

[See table 5 on previous page]

The clinical signs and symptoms of atopic dermatitis were scored on a scale of 0 = absent, 1 = mild, 2 = moderate, and 3 = severe. The mean improvements over baseline at the end of treatment are shown in Table 6.

[See table 6 above]

HOW SUPPLIED

CUTIVATE Cream is supplied in:
15-g tubes (NDC 0173-0430-00),
30-g tubes (NDC 0173-0430-01), and
60-g tubes (NDC 0173-0430-02).
Store between 2° and 30°C (36° and 86°F).

GlaxoSmithKline Consumer Healthcare LP
Pittsburgh, PA 15230

August 2002/RL-1137

Shown in Product Identification Guide, page 315

CUTIVATE® ℞
[kyoot' ə-vāt]
(fluticasone propionate ointment)
Ointment, 0.005%

For Dermatologic Use Only—
Not for Ophthalmic Use.

DESCRIPTION

CUTIVATE (fluticasone propionate ointment) Ointment, 0.005% contains fluticasone propionate [(6α,11β,16α,17α)-6,9,-difluoro-11-hydroxy-16-methyl-3-oxo-17-(1-oxopropoxy)androsta-1,4-diene-17-carbothioic acid, S-fluoromethyl ester], a synthetic fluorinated corticosteroid, for topical dermatologic use. The topical corticosteroids constitute a class of primarily synthetic steroids used as anti-inflammatory and antipruritic agents.

Chemically, fluticasone propionate is $C_{25}H_{31}F_3O_5S$.

Fluticasone propionate has a molecular weight of 500.6. It is a white to off-white powder and is insoluble in water.

Each gram of CUTIVATE Ointment contains fluticasone propionate 0.05 mg in a base of liquid paraffin, microcrystalline wax, propylene glycol, and sorbitan sesquioleate.

CLINICAL PHARMACOLOGY

Like other topical corticosteroids, fluticasone propionate has anti-inflammatory, antipruritic, and vasoconstrictive properties. The mechanism of the anti-inflammatory activity of the topical steroids, in general, is unclear. However, corticosteroids are thought to act by the induction of phospholipase A_2 inhibitory proteins, collectively called lipocortins. It is postulated that these proteins control the biosynthesis of potent mediators of inflammation such as prostaglandins and leukotrienes by inhibiting the release of their common precursor, arachidonic acid. Arachidonic acid is released from membrane phospholipids by phospholipase A_2.

Fluticasone propionate is lipophilic and has a strong affinity for the glucocorticoid receptor. It has weak affinity for the progesterone receptor, and virtually no affinity for the mineralocorticoid, estrogen, or androgen receptors. The therapeutic potency of glucocorticoids is related to the half-life of the glucocorticoid-receptor complex. The half-life of the fluticasone propionate-glucocorticoid receptor complex is approximately 10 hours.

Studies performed with CUTIVATE Ointment indicate that it is in the medium range of potency as compared with other topical corticosteroids.

Pharmacokinetics: ***Absorption:*** The activity of CUTIVATE is due to the parent drug, fluticasone propionate. The extent of percutaneous absorption of topical corticosteroids is determined by many factors, including the vehicle and the integrity of the epidermal barrier. Occlusive dressing enhances penetration. Topical corticosteroids can be absorbed from normal intact skin. Inflammation and/or other disease processes in the skin increase percutaneous absorption.

In a study of 6 healthy volunteers applying 25 g of fluticasone propionate ointment 0.005% twice daily to the trunk and legs for up to 5 days under occlusion, plasma levels of fluticasone ranged from 0.08 to 0.22 ng/mL.

In an animal study using radiolabeled 0.05% fluticasone propionate cream and ointment preparations, rats received a topical dose of 1 g/kg for a 24-hour period. Total recovery of radioactivity was approximately 80% at the end of 7 days. The majority of the dose (73%) was recovered from the surface of the application site. Less than 1% of the dose was recovered in the skin at the application site. Approximately 5% of the dose was absorbed systemically through the skin. Absorption from the skin continued for the duration of the study (7 days), indicating a long retention time at the application site.

Distribution: Following intravenous administration of 1 mg of fluticasone propionate in healthy volunteers, the initial disposition phase for fluticasone propionate was rapid and consistent with its high lipid solubility and tissue binding. The apparent volume of distribution averaged 4.2 L/kg (range, 2.3 to 16.7 L/kg). The percentage of fluticasone propionate bound to human plasma proteins averaged 91%. Fluticasone propionate is weakly and reversibly bound to erythrocytes. Fluticasone propionate is not significantly bound to human transcortin.

Metabolism: No metabolites of fluticasone propionate were detected in an in vitro study of radiolabeled fluticasone propionate incubated in a human skin homogenate. The total blood clearance of systemically absorbed fluticasone propionate averages 1,093 mL/min (range, 618 to 1,702 mL/min) after a 1-mg intravenous dose, with renal clearance accounting for less than 0.02% of the total. Fluticasone propionate is metabolized in the liver by cytochrome P450 3A4-mediated hydrolysis of the 5-fluoromethyl carbothioate grouping. This transformation occurs in 1 metabolic step to produce the inactive 17-β-carboxylic acid metabolite, the only known metabolite detected in man. This metabolite has approximately 2,000 times less affinity than the parent drug for the glucocorticoid receptor of human lung cytosol in vitro and negligible pharmacological activity in animal studies. Other metabolites detected in vitro using cultured human hepatoma cells have not been detected in man.

Excretion: Following an intravenous dose of 1 mg in healthy volunteers, fluticasone propionate showed polyexponential kinetics and had an average terminal half-life of 7.2 hours (range, 3.2 to 11.2 hours).

INDICATIONS AND USAGE

CUTIVATE Ointment is a medium potency corticosteroid indicated for the relief of the inflammatory and pruritic manifestations of corticosteroid-responsive dermatoses in adult patients.

CONTRAINDICATIONS

CUTIVATE Ointment is contraindicated in those patients with a history of hypersensitivity to any of the components in the preparation.

PRECAUTIONS

General: Systemic absorption of topical corticosteroids can produce reversible hypothalamic-pituitary-adrenal (HPA) axis suppression with the potential for glucocorticosteroid insufficiency after withdrawal from treatment. Manifestations of Cushing syndrome, hyperglycemia, and glucosuria can also be produced in some patients by systemic absorption of topical corticosteroids while on treatment.

Patients applying a topical steroid to a large surface area or to areas under occlusion should be evaluated periodically for evidence of HPA axis suppression. This may be done by using the ACTH stimulation, A.M. plasma cortisol, and urinary free cortisol tests.

If HPA axis suppression is noted, an attempt should be made to withdraw the drug, to reduce the frequency of application, or to substitute a less potent corticosteroid. Recovery of HPA axis function is generally prompt upon discontinuation of topical corticosteroids. Infrequently, signs and symptoms of glucocorticosteroid insufficiency may occur, requiring supplemental systemic corticosteroids. For information on systemic supplementation, see prescribing information for those products.

Pediatric patients may be more susceptible to systemic toxicity from equivalent doses due to their larger skin surface to body mass ratios (see PRECAUTIONS: Pediatric Use).

Fluticasone propionate ointment, 0.005% may cause local cutaneous adverse reactions (see ADVERSE REACTIONS).

If irritation develops, CUTIVATE Ointment should be discontinued and appropriate therapy instituted. Allergic contact dermatitis with corticosteroids is usually diagnosed by observing failure to heal rather than noting a clinical exacerbation as with most topical products not containing corticosteroids. Such an observation should be corroborated with appropriate diagnostic patch testing.

If concomitant skin infections are present or develop, an appropriate antifungal or antibacterial agent should be used. If a favorable response does not occur promptly, use of CUTIVATE Ointment should be discontinued until the infection has been adequately controlled.

CUTIVATE Ointment should not be used in the treatment of preexisting skin atrophy and should not be used where infection is present at the treatment site. CUTIVATE Ointment should not be used in the treatment of rosacea and perioral dermatitis.

Information for Patients: Patients using topical corticosteroids should receive the following information and instructions:

1. This medication is to be used as directed by the physician. It is for external use only. Avoid contact with the eyes.
2. This medication should not be used for any disorder other than that for which it was prescribed.
3. The treated skin area should not be bandaged or otherwise covered or wrapped so as to be occlusive unless directed by the physician.
4. Patients should report to their physician any signs of local adverse reactions.
5. This medication should not be used on the face, underarms, or groin areas unless directed by a physician.
6. As with other corticosteroids, therapy should be discontinued when control is achieved. If no improvement is seen within 2 weeks, contact the physician.

Laboratory Tests: The following tests may be helpful in evaluating patients for HPA axis suppression:

ACTH stimulation test
A.M. plasma cortisol test
Urinary free cortisol test

A concentrated fluticasone propionate ointment, 0.05% (10 times that of the marketed fluticasone propionate ointment, 0.005%) suppressed 24-hour urinary free cortisol levels in 2 of 6 patients when used at a dose of 30 g/day for a week in patients with psoriasis or atopic eczema. No suppression of

Continued on next page

Product information on these pages is effective as of August 2004. Further information is available at: GlaxoSmithKline, PO Box 13398, Research Triangle Park, NC 27709. 1-888-825-5249. Corporate Web Site: www.gsk.com

Cutivate Ointment—Cont.

A.M. plasma cortisol was observed. In a second study of the same concentrated formulation of fluticasone propionate ointment, 0.05%, depression of A.M. plasma cortisol levels was noted in 2 of 8 normal volunteers when applied at doses of 50 g/day for 21 days. Morning plasma levels returned to normal levels within 4 days upon discontinuation of fluticasone propionate. In this study there was no corresponding decrease in 24-hour urinary free cortisol levels.
In a study of 35 pediatric patients treated with fluticasone propionate ointment, 0.005% for atopic dermatitis over at least 35% of body surface area, subnormal adrenal function was observed with cosyntropin stimulation testing at the end of 3 to 4 weeks of treatment in 4 patients who had normal testing prior to treatment. It is not known if these patients had recovery of adrenal function because follow-up testing was not performed (see PRECAUTIONS: Pediatric Use and ADVERSE REACTIONS). Adrenal suppression was indicated by either a ≤5 mcg/dL prestimulation cortisol, or a cosyntropin poststimulation cortisol ≤18 mcg/dL, and/or an increase of <7 mcg/dL from the baseline cortisol level.

Carcinogenesis, Mutagenesis, and Impairment of Fertility: Two 18-month studies were performed in mice to evaluate the carcinogenic potential of fluticasone propionate when given topically (as a 0.05% ointment) and orally. No evidence of carcinogenicity was found in either study.
Fluticasone propionate was not mutagenic in the standard Ames test, *E. coli* fluctuation test, *S. cerevisiae* gene conversion test, or Chinese Hamster ovarian cell assay. It was not clastogenic in mouse micronucleus or cultured human lymphocyte tests.
In a fertility and general reproductive performance study in rats, fluticasone propionate administered subcutaneously to females at up to 50 mcg/kg/day and to males at up to 100 mcg/kg/day (later reduced to 50 mcg/kg/day) had no effect upon mating performance or fertility. These doses are approximately 150 and 300 times, respectively, the human systemic exposure following use of the recommended human topical dose of fluticasone propionate ointment, 0.005%, assuming human percutaneous absorption of approximately 3% and the use in a 70-kg person of 15 g/day.

Pregnancy: ***Teratogenic Effects:*** Pregnancy Category C. Corticosteroids have been shown to be teratogenic in laboratory animals when administered systemically at relatively low dosage levels. Some corticosteroids have been shown to be teratogenic after dermal application in laboratory animals. Teratology studies in the mouse demonstrated fluticasone propionate to be teratogenic (cleft palate) when administered subcutaneously in doses of 45 mcg/kg/day and 150 mcg/kg/day. This dose is approximately 140 and 450 times, respectively, the human topical dose of fluticasone propionate ointment, 0.005%. There are no adequate and well-controlled studies in pregnant women. CUTIVATE Ointment should be used during pregnancy only if the potential benefit justifies the potential risk to the fetus.

Nursing Mothers: Systemically administered corticosteroids appear in human milk and could suppress growth, interfere with endogenous corticosteroid production, or cause other untoward effects. It is not known whether topical administration of corticosteroids could result in sufficient systemic absorption to produce detectable quantities in human milk. Because many drugs are excreted in human milk, caution should be exercised when CUTIVATE Ointment is administered to a nursing woman.

Pediatric Use: Use of CUTIVATE Ointment in pediatric patients is not recommended.
In a study of 35 pediatric patients treated with fluticasone propionate ointment, 0.005% for atopic dermatitis over at least 35% of body surface area, subnormal adrenal function was observed with cosyntropin stimulation testing at the end of 3 to 4 weeks of treatment in 4 patients who had normal testing prior to treatment. It is not known if these patients had recovery of adrenal function because follow-up testing was not performed (see PRECAUTIONS: Laboratory Tests and ADVERSE REACTIONS). The decreased responsiveness to cosyntropin testing was not correlated to age of patient, amount of fluticasone propionate ointment used, or serum levels of fluticasone propionate. Plasma fluticasone propionate were not performed in a 6-month-old patient who demonstrated an abnormal response to cosyntropin stimulation testing.
Pediatric patients may demonstrate greater susceptibility to topical corticosteroid-induced HPA axis suppression and Cushing syndrome than mature patients because of a larger skin surface to body weight ratio.
HPA axis suppression, Cushing syndrome, linear growth retardation, delayed weight gain, and intracranial hypertension have been reported in pediatric patients receiving topical corticosteroids. Manifestations of adrenal suppression in pediatric patients include low plasma cortisol levels and an absence of response to ACTH stimulation.
Manifestations of intracranial hypertension include bulging fontanelles, headaches, and bilateral papilledema.

Geriatric Use: A limited number of patients above 65 years of age (n = 203) have been treated with CUTIVATE Ointment in US and non-US clinical trials. While the number of patients is too small to permit separate analysis of efficacy and safety, the adverse reactions reported in this population were similar to those reported by younger patients. Based on available data, no adjustment of dosage of CUTIVATE in geriatric patients is warranted.

ADVERSE REACTIONS

In controlled clinical trials, the total incidence of adverse reactions associated with the use of CUTIVATE Ointment was approximately 4%. These adverse reactions were usually mild, self-limiting, and consisted primarily of pruritus, burning, hypertrichosis, increased erythema, hives, irritation, and lightheadedness. Each of these events occurred individually in less than 1% of patients.
In a study of 35 pediatric patients treated with fluticasone propionate ointment, 0.005% for atopic dermatitis over at least 35% of body surface area, subnormal adrenal function was observed with cosyntropin stimulation testing at the end of 3 to 4 weeks of treatment in 4 patients who had normal testing prior to treatment. It is not known if these patients had recovery of adrenal function because follow-up testing was not performed (see PRECAUTIONS: Laboratory Tests and PRECAUTIONS: Pediatric Use). Telangiectasia on the face was noted in 1 patient on the eighth day of a 4-week treatment period. Facial use was discontinued and the telangiectasia resolved.
The following additional local adverse reactions have been reported infrequently with topical corticosteroids, including fluticasone propionate, and they may occur more frequently with the use of occlusive dressings and higher potency corticosteroids. These reactions are listed in an approximately decreasing order of occurrence: dryness, folliculitis, acneiform eruptions, hypopigmentation, perioral dermatitis, allergic contact dermatitis, secondary infection, skin atrophy, striae, and miliaria. Also, there are reports of the development of pustular psoriasis from chronic plaque psoriasis following reduction or discontinuation of potent topical corticosteroid products.

OVERDOSAGE

Topically applied CUTIVATE Ointment can be absorbed in sufficient amounts to produce systemic effects (see PRECAUTIONS).

DOSAGE AND ADMINISTRATION

Apply a thin film of CUTIVATE Ointment to the affected skin areas twice daily. Rub in gently.
CUTIVATE Ointment should not be used with occlusive dressings.

Geriatric Use: In studies where geriatric patients (65 years of age or older, see PRECAUTIONS) have been treated with CUTIVATE Ointment, safety did not differ from that in younger patients; therefore, no dosage adjustment is recommended.

HOW SUPPLIED

CUTIVATE Ointment, 0.005% is supplied in:
15-g tubes (NDC 59075-431-00)
30-g tubes (NDC 59075-431-01)
60-g tubes (NDC 59075-431-02)
Store between 2° and 30°C (36° and 86°F).
GlaxoSmithKline Consumer Healthcare LP
Pittsburgh, PA 15230

August 2002 RL-1080
Shown in Product Identification Guide, page 315

DARAPRIM® ℞

[*dair' ə-prĭm*]
(pyrimethamine)
25-mg Scored Tablets

DESCRIPTION

DARAPRIM (pyrimethamine) is an antiparasitic compound available in tablet form for oral administration. Each scored tablet contains 25 mg pyrimethamine and the inactive ingredients corn and potato starch, lactose, and magnesium stearate.
Pyrimethamine, known chemically as 5-(4-chlorophenyl)-6-ethyl-2,4-pyrimidinediamine.

CLINICAL PHARMACOLOGY

Pyrimethamine is well absorbed with peak levels occurring between 2 to 6 hours following administration. It is eliminated slowly and has a plasma half-life of approximately 96 hours. Pyrimethamine is 87% bound to human plasma proteins.

Microbiology: Pyrimethamine is a folic acid antagonist and the rationale for its therapeutic action is based on the differential requirement between host and parasite for nucleic acid precursors involved in growth. This activity is highly selective against plasmodia and *Toxoplasma gondii*. Pyrimethamine possesses blood schizonticidal and some tissue schizonticidal activity against malaria parasites of humans. However, the 4-amino-quinoline compounds are more effective against the erythrocytic schizonts. It does not destroy gametocytes, but arrests sporogony in the mosquito.
The action of pyrimethamine against *Toxoplasma gondii* is greatly enhanced when used in conjunction with sulfonamides. This was demonstrated by Eyles and Coleman[1] in the treatment of experimental toxoplasmosis in the mouse. Jacobs et al[2] demonstrated that combination of the 2 drugs effectively prevented the development of severe uveitis in most rabbits following the inoculation of the anterior chamber of the eye with toxoplasma.

INDICATIONS AND USAGE

Treatment of Toxoplasmosis: DARAPRIM is indicated for the treatment of toxoplasmosis when used conjointly with a sulfonamide, since synergism exists with this combination.

Treatment of Acute Malaria: DARAPRIM is also indicated for the treatment of acute malaria. It should not be used alone to treat acute malaria. Fast-acting schizonticides such as chloroquine or quinine are indicated and preferable for the treatment of acute malaria. However, conjoint use of DARAPRIM with a sulfonamide (e.g., sulfadoxine) will initiate transmission control and suppression of susceptible strains of plasmodia.

Chemoprophylaxis of Malaria: DARAPRIM is indicated for the chemoprophylaxis of malaria due to susceptible strains of plasmodia. However, resistance to pyrimethamine is prevalent worldwide. It is not suitable as a prophylactic agent for travelers to most areas.

CONTRAINDICATIONS

Use of DARAPRIM is contraindicated in patients with known hypersensitivity to pyrimethamine or to any component of the formulation. Use of the drug is also contraindicated in patients with documented megaloblastic anemia due to folate deficiency.

WARNINGS

The dosage of pyrimethamine required for the treatment of toxoplasmosis is 10 to 20 times the recommended antimalaria dosage and approaches the toxic level. If signs of folate deficiency develop (see ADVERSE REACTIONS), reduce the dosage or discontinue the drug according to the response of the patient. Folinic acid (leucovorin) should be administered in a dosage of 5 to 15 mg daily (orally, IV, or IM) until normal hematopoiesis is restored.
Data in 2 humans indicate that pyrimethamine may be carcinogenic: a 51-year-old female who developed chronic granulocytic leukemia after taking pyrimethamine for 2 years for toxoplasmosis,[3] and a 56-year-old patient who developed reticulum cell sarcoma after 14 months of pyrimethamine for toxoplasmosis.[4]
Pyrimethamine has been reported to produce a significant increase in the number of lung tumors in mice when given intraperitoneally at doses of 25 mg/kg.[5]
DARAPRIM should be kept out of the reach of infants and children as they are extremely susceptible to adverse effects from an overdose. Deaths in pediatric patients have been reported after accidental ingestion.

PRECAUTIONS

General: The recommended dosage for chemoprophylaxis of malaria should not be exceeded. A small "starting" dose for toxoplasmosis is recommended in patients with convulsive disorders to avoid the potential nervous system toxicity of pyrimethamine. DARAPRIM should be used with caution in patients with impaired renal or hepatic function or in patients with possible folate deficiency, such as individuals with malabsorption syndrome, alcoholism, or pregnancy, and those receiving therapy, such as phenytoin, affecting folate levels (see Pregnancy subsection).

Information for Patients: Patients should be warned that at the first appearance of a skin rash they should stop use of DARAPRIM and seek medical attention immediately. Patients should also be warned that the appearance of sore throat, pallor, purpura, or glossitis may be early indications of serious disorders which require treatment with DARAPRIM to be stopped and medical treatment to be sought.
Women of childbearing potential who are taking DARAPRIM should be warned against becoming pregnant.
Patients should be warned to keep DARAPRIM out of the reach of children. Patients should be advised not to exceed recommended doses. Patients should be warned that if anorexia and vomiting occur, they may be minimized by taking the drug with meals.
Concurrent administration of folinic acid is strongly recommended when used for the treatment of toxoplasmosis in all patients.

Laboratory Tests: In patients receiving high dosage, as for the treatment of toxoplasmosis, semiweekly blood counts, including platelet counts, should be performed.

Drug Interactions: Pyrimethamine may be used with sulfonamides, quinine and other antimalarials, and with other antibiotics. However, the concomitant use of other antifolic drugs, or agents associated with myelosuppression including sulfonamides or trimethoprim-sulfamethoxazole combinations, proguanil, zidovudine, or cytostatic agents (e.g., methotrexate), while the patient is receiving pyrimethamine, may increase the risk of bone marrow suppression. If signs of folate deficiency develop, pyrimethamine should be discontinued. Folinic acid (leucovorin) should be administered until normal hematopoiesis is restored (see WARNINGS). Mild hepatotoxicity has been reported in some patients when lorazepam and pyrimethamine were administered concomitantly.

Carcinogenesis, Mutagenesis, Impairment of Fertility: See WARNINGS section for information on carcinogenesis.

Mutagenesis: Pyrimethamine has been shown to be nonmutagenic in the following in vitro assays: the Ames point mutation assay, the Rec assay, and the *E. coli* WP2 assay. It was positive in the L5178Y/TK +/- mouse lymphoma assay in the absence of exogenous metabolic activation.[6] Human blood lymphocytes cultured in vitro had structural chromosome aberrations induced by pyrimethamine.

In vivo, chromosomes analyzed from the bone marrow of rats dosed with pyrimethamine showed an increased number of structural and numerical aberrations.

Pregnancy: *Teratogenic Effects:* Pregnancy Category C. Pyrimethamine has been shown to be teratogenic in rats when given in oral doses 7 times the human dose for chemoprophylaxis of malaria or 2.5 times the human dose for treatment of toxoplasmosis. At these doses in rats, there was a significant increase in abnormalities such as cleft palate, brachygnathia, oligodactyly, and microphthalmia. Pyrimethamine has also been shown to produce terata such as meningocele in hamsters and cleft palate in miniature pigs when given in oral doses 170 and 5 times the human dose, respectively, for chemoprophylaxis of malaria or for treatment of toxoplasmosis.

There are no adequate and well-controlled studies in pregnant women. DARAPRIM should be used during pregnancy only if the potential benefit justifies the potential risk to the fetus.

Concurrent administration of folinic acid is strongly recommended when used for the treatment of toxoplasmosis during pregnancy.

Nursing Mothers: Pyrimethamine is excreted in human milk. Because of the potential for serious adverse reactions in nursing infants from pyrimethamine and from concurrent use of a sulfonamide with DARAPRIM for treatment of some patients with toxoplasmosis, a decision should be made whether to discontinue nursing or to discontinue the drug, taking into account the importance of the drug to the mother (see WARNINGS and PRECAUTIONS: Pregnancy).

Pediatric Use: See DOSAGE AND ADMINISTRATION section.

Geriatric Use: Clinical studies of DARAPRIM did not include sufficient numbers of subjects aged 65 and over to determine whether they respond differently from younger subjects. Other reported clinical experience has not identified differences in responses between the elderly and younger patients. In general, dose selection for an elderly patient should be cautious, usually starting at the low end of the dosing range, reflecting the greater frequency of decreased hepatic, renal, or cardiac function, and of concomitant disease or other drug therapy.

ADVERSE REACTIONS

Hypersensitivity reactions, occasionally severe (such as Stevens-Johnson syndrome, toxic epidermal necrolysis, erythema multiforme, and anaphylaxis), and hyperphenylalaninemia, can occur particularly when pyrimethamine is administered concomitantly with a sulfonamide. Consult the complete prescribing information for the relevant sulfonamide for sulfonamide-associated adverse events. With doses of pyrimethamine used for the treatment of toxoplasmosis, anorexia and vomiting may occur. Vomiting may be minimized by giving the medication with meals; it usually disappears promptly upon reduction of dosage. Doses used in toxoplasmosis may produce megaloblastic anemia, leukopenia, thrombocytopenia, pancytopenia, atrophic glossitis, hematuria, and disorders of cardiac rhythm. Hematologic effects, however, may also occur at low doses in certain individuals (see PRECAUTIONS: General).

Pulmonary eosinophilia has been reported rarely.

OVERDOSAGE

Following the ingestion of 300 mg or more of pyrimethamine, gastrointestinal and/or central nervous system signs may be present, including convulsions. The initial symptoms are usually gastrointestinal and may include abdominal pain, nausea, severe and repeated vomiting, possibly including hematemesis. Central nervous system toxicity may be manifest by initial excitability, generalized and prolonged convulsions which may be followed by respiratory depression, circulatory collapse, and death within a few hours. Neurological symptoms appear rapidly (30 minutes to 2 hours after drug ingestion), suggesting that in gross overdosage pyrimethamine has a direct toxic effect on the central nervous system.

The fatal dose is variable, with the smallest reported fatal single dose being 375 mg. There are, however, reports of pediatric patients who have recovered after taking 375 to 625 mg.

There is no specific antidote to acute pyrimethamine poisoning. In the event of overdosage, symptomatic and supportive measures should be employed. Gastric lavage is recommended and is effective if carried out very soon after drug ingestion. Parenteral diazepam may be used to control convulsions. Folinic acid should also be administered within 2 hours of drug ingestion to be most effective in counteracting the effects on the hematopoietic system (see WARNINGS). Due to the long half-life of pyrimethamine, daily monitoring of peripheral blood counts is recommended for up to several weeks after the overdose until normal hematologic values are restored.

DOSAGE AND ADMINISTRATION

For Treatment of Toxoplasmosis: The dosage of DARAPRIM for the treatment of toxoplasmosis must be carefully adjusted so as to provide maximum therapeutic effect and a minimum of side effects. At the dosage required, there is a marked variation in the tolerance to the drug. Young patients may tolerate higher doses than older individuals. Concurrent administration of folinic acid is strongly recommended in all patients.

The adult *starting* dose is 50 to 75 mg of the drug daily, together with 1 to 4 g daily of a sulfonamide of the sulfapyrimidine type, e.g., sulfadoxine. This dosage is ordinarily continued for 1 to 3 weeks, depending on the response of the patient and tolerance to therapy. The dosage may then be reduced to about one-half that previously given for each drug and continued for an additional 4 to 5 weeks.

The pediatric dosage of DARAPRIM is 1 mg/kg/day divided into 2 equal daily doses; after 2 to 4 days this dose may be reduced to one half and continued for approximately 1 month. The usual pediatric sulfonamide dosage is used in conjunction with DARAPRIM.

For Treatment of Acute Malaria: DARAPRIM is NOT recommended alone in the treatment of acute malaria. Fast-acting schizonticides, such as chloroquine or quinine, are indicated for treatment of acute malaria. However, DARAPRIM at a dosage of 25 mg daily for 2 days with a sulfonamide will initiate transmission control and suppression of non-falciparum malaria. DARAPRIM is only recommended for patients infected in areas where susceptible plasmodia exist. Should circumstances arise wherein DARAPRIM must be used alone in semi-immune persons, the adult dosage for acute malaria is 50 mg for 2 days; children 4 through 10 years old may be given 25 mg daily for 2 days. In any event, clinical cure should be followed by the once-weekly regimen described below for chemoprophylaxis. Regimens which include suppression should be extended through any characteristic periods of early recrudescence and late relapse, i.e., for at least 10 weeks in each case.

For Chemoprophylaxis of Malaria:

Adults and pediatric patients over 10 years — 25 mg (1 tablet) once weekly

Children 4 through 10 years — 12.5 mg (½ tablet) once weekly

Infants and children under 4 years — 6.25 mg (¼ tablet) once weekly

HOW SUPPLIED

White, scored tablets containing 25 mg pyrimethamine, imprinted with "DARAPRIM" and "A3A" in bottles of 100 (NDC 0173-0201-55).

Store at 15° to 25°C (59° to 77°F) in a dry place and protect from light.

REFERENCES

1. Eyles DE, Coleman N. Synergistic effect of sulfadiazine and Daraprim against experimental toxoplasmosis in the mouse. *Antibiot Chemother.* 1953;3:483-490.
2. Jacobs L, Melton ML, Kaufman HE. Treatment of experimental ocular toxoplasmosis. *Arch Ophthalmol.* 1964;71:111-118.
3. Jim RTS, Elizaga FV. Development of chronic granulocytic leukemia in a patient treated with pyrimethamine. *Hawaii Med J.* 1977;36:173-176.
4. Sadoff L. Antimalarial drugs and Burkitt's lymphoma. *Lancet.* 1973;2:1262-1263.
5. Bahna L. Pyrimethamine. *LARC Monogr Eval Carcinog Risk Chem.* 1977;13:233-242.
6. Clive D, Johnson KO, Spector JKS, et al. Validation and characterization of the L5178Y/TK +/- mouse lymphoma mutagen assay system. *Mut Res.* 1979;59:61-108.

Manufactured by DSM Pharmaceuticals, Inc.
Greenville, NC 27834 for
GlaxoSmithKline, Research Triangle Park, NC 27709

March 2003/RL-1179

Shown in Product Identification Guide, page 315

DEXEDRINE® Ⓒ℞

[*dex ʹə-drēn*]

(dextroamphetamine sulfate)

SPANSULE®

sustained release capsules and Tablets

WARNING

AMPHETAMINES HAVE A HIGH POTENTIAL FOR ABUSE. ADMINISTRATION OF AMPHETAMINES FOR PROLONGED PERIODS OF TIME MAY LEAD TO DRUG DEPENDENCE AND MUST BE AVOIDED. PARTICULAR ATTENTION SHOULD BE PAID TO THE POSSIBILITY OF SUBJECTS OBTAINING AMPHETAMINES FOR NON-THERAPEUTIC USE OR DISTRIBUTION TO OTHERS, AND THE DRUGS SHOULD BE PRESCRIBED OR DISPENSED SPARINGLY.

DESCRIPTION

DEXEDRINE (dextroamphetamine sulfate) is the dextro isomer of the compound *d,l*-amphetamine sulfate, a sympathomimetic amine of the amphetamine group. Chemically, dextroamphetamine is *d*-alpha-methylphenethylamine, and is present in all forms of DEXEDRINE as the neutral sulfate.

SPANSULE capsules: Each SPANSULE sustained-release capsule is so prepared that an initial dose is released promptly and the remaining medication is released gradually over a prolonged period.

Each capsule, with brown cap and clear body, contains dextroamphetamine sulfate. The 5-mg capsule is imprinted 5 mg and 3512 on the brown cap and is imprinted 5 mg and SB on the clear body. The 10-mg capsule is imprinted 10 mg — 3513 — on the brown cap and is imprinted 10 mg — SB — on the clear body. The 15-mg capsule is imprinted 15 mg and 3514 on the brown cap and is imprinted 15 mg and SB on the clear body. A narrow bar appears above and below 15 mg and 3514. Product reformulation in 1996 has caused a minor change in the color of the time-released pellets within each capsule. Inactive ingredients now consist of cetyl alcohol, D&C Yellow No. 10, dibutyl sebacate, ethylcellulose, FD&C Blue No. 1, FD&C Blue No. 1 aluminum lake, FD&C Red No. 40, FD&C Yellow No. 6, gelatin, hypromellose, propylene glycol, povidone, silicon dioxide, sodium lauryl sulfate, sugar spheres, and trace amounts of other inactive ingredients.

Tablets: Each triangular, orange, scored tablet is debossed SKF and E19 and contains dextroamphetamine sulfate, 5 mg. Inactive ingredients consist of calcium sulfate, FD&C Yellow No. 5 (tartrazine), FD&C Yellow No. 6, gelatin, lactose, mineral oil, starch, stearic acid, sucrose, talc, and trace amounts of other inactive ingredients.

CLINICAL PHARMACOLOGY

Amphetamines are noncatecholamine, sympathomimetic amines with CNS stimulant activity. Peripheral actions include elevations of systolic and diastolic blood pressures and weak bronchodilator and respiratory stimulant action.

There is neither specific evidence that clearly establishes the mechanism whereby amphetamines produce mental and behavioral effects in children, nor conclusive evidence regarding how these effects relate to the condition of the central nervous system.

DEXEDRINE SPANSULE capsules are formulated to release the active drug substance in vivo in a more gradual fashion than the standard formulation, as demonstrated by blood levels. The formulation has not been shown superior in effectiveness over the same dosage of the standard, noncontrolled-release formulations given in divided doses.

Pharmacokinetics: The pharmacokinetics of the tablet and sustained-release capsule were compared in 12 healthy subjects. The extent of bioavailability of the sustained-release capsule was similar compared to the immediate-release tablet. Following administration of three 5-mg tablets, average maximal dextroamphetamine plasma concentrations (C_{max}) of 36.6 ng/mL were achieved at approximately 3 hours. Following administration of one 15-mg sustained-release capsule, maximal dextroamphetamine plasma concentrations were obtained approximately 8 hours after dosing. The average C_{max} was 23.5 ng/mL. The average plasma $T_{½}$ was similar for both the tablet and sustained-release capsule and was approximately 12 hours.

In 12 healthy subjects, the rate and extent of dextroamphetamine absorption were similar following administration of the sustained-release capsule formulation in the fed (58 to 75 gm fat) and fasted state.

INDICATIONS AND USAGE

DEXEDRINE is indicated:

1. In Narcolepsy.

2. In Attention Deficit Disorder with Hyperactivity, as an integral part of a total treatment program that typically includes other remedial measures (psychological, educational, social) for a stabilizing effect in pediatric patients (ages 3 years to 16 years) with a behavioral syndrome characterized by the following group of developmentally inappropriate symptoms: Moderate to severe distractibility, short attention span, hyperactivity, emotional lability, and impulsivity. The diagnosis of this syndrome should not be made with finality when these symptoms are only of comparatively recent origin. Nonlocalizing (soft) neurological signs, learning disability, and abnormal EEG may or may not be present, and a diagnosis of central nervous system dysfunction may or may not be warranted.

CONTRAINDICATIONS

Advanced arteriosclerosis, symptomatic cardiovascular disease, moderate to severe hypertension, hyperthyroidism, known hypersensitivity or idiosyncrasy to the sympathomimetic amines, glaucoma.

Agitated states.

Patients with a history of drug abuse.

During or within 14 days following the administration of monoamine oxidase inhibitors (hypertensive crises may result).

PRECAUTIONS

General: Caution is to be exercised in prescribing amphetamines for patients with even mild hypertension.

The least amount feasible should be prescribed or dispensed at 1 time in order to minimize the possibility of overdosage.

The tablets contain FD&C Yellow No. 5 (tartrazine), which may cause allergic-type reactions (including bronchial asthma) in certain susceptible individuals. Although the overall incidence of FD&C Yellow No. 5 (tartrazine) sensitivity in the general population is low, it is frequently seen in patients who also have aspirin hypersensitivity.

Information for Patients: Amphetamines may impair the ability of the patient to engage in potentially hazardous activities such as operating machinery or vehicles; the patient should therefore be cautioned accordingly.

Continued on next page

Product information on these pages is effective as of August 2004. Further information is available at: GlaxoSmithKline, PO Box 13398, Research Triangle Park, NC 27709. 1-888-825-5249. Corporate Web Site: www.gsk.com

Dexedrine —Cont.

Drug Interactions: ***Acidifying agents***—Gastrointestinal acidifying agents (guanethidine, reserpine, glutamic acid HCl, ascorbic acid, fruit juices, etc.) lower absorption of amphetamines. Urinary acidifying agents (ammonium chloride, sodium acid phosphate, etc.) increase the concentration of the ionized species of the amphetamine molecule, thereby increasing urinary excretion. Both groups of agents lower blood levels and efficacy of amphetamines.
Adrenergic blockers—Adrenergic blockers are inhibited by amphetamines.
Alkalinizing agents—Gastrointestinal alkalinizing agents (sodium bicarbonate, etc.) increase absorption of amphetamines. Urinary alkalinizing agents (acetazolamide, some thiazides) increase the concentration of the non-ionized species of the amphetamine molecule, thereby decreasing urinary excretion. Both groups of agents increase blood levels and therefore potentiate the actions of amphetamines.
Antidepressants, tricyclic—Amphetamines may enhance the activity of tricyclic or sympathomimetic agents; d-amphetamine with desipramine or protriptyline and possibly other tricyclics cause striking and sustained increases in the concentration of d-amphetamine in the brain; cardiovascular effects can be potentiated.
MAO inhibitors—MAOI antidepressants, as well as a metabolite of furazolidone, slow amphetamine metabolism. This slowing potentiates amphetamines, increasing their effect on the release of norepinephrine and other monoamines from adrenergic nerve endings; this can cause headaches and other signs of hypertensive crisis. A variety of neurological toxic effects and malignant hyperpyrexia can occur, sometimes with fatal results.
Antihistamines—Amphetamines may counteract the sedative effect of antihistamines.
Antihypertensives—Amphetamines may antagonize the hypotensive effects of antihypertensives.
Chlorpromazine—Chlorpromazine blocks dopamine and norepinephrine reuptake, thus inhibiting the central stimulant effects of amphetamines, and can be used to treat amphetamine poisoning.
Ethosuximide—Amphetamines may delay intestinal absorption of ethosuximide.
Haloperidol—Haloperidol blocks dopamine and norepinephrine reuptake, thus inhibiting the central stimulant effects of amphetamines.
Lithium carbonate—The stimulatory effects of amphetamines may be inhibited by lithium carbonate.
Meperidine—Amphetamines potentiate the analgesic effect of meperidine.
Methenamine therapy—Urinary excretion of amphetamines is increased, and efficacy is reduced, by acidifying agents used in methenamine therapy.
Norepinephrine—Amphetamines enhance the adrenergic effect of norepinephrine.
Phenobarbital—Amphetamines may delay intestinal absorption of phenobarbital; co-administration of phenobarbital may produce a synergistic anticonvulsant action.
Phenytoin—Amphetamines may delay intestinal absorption of phenytoin; co-administration of phenytoin may produce a synergistic anticonvulsant action.
Propoxyphene—In cases of propoxyphene overdosage, amphetamine CNS stimulation is potentiated and fatal convulsions can occur.
Veratrum alkaloids—Amphetamines inhibit the hypotensive effect of veratrum alkaloids.
Drug/Laboratory Test Interactions: Amphetamines can cause a significant elevation in plasma corticosteroid levels. This increase is greatest in the evening.
Amphetamines may interfere with urinary steroid determinations.
Carcinogenesis/Mutagenesis: Mutagenicity studies and long-term studies in animals to determine the carcinogenic potential of DEXEDRINE have not been performed.
Pregnancy—Teratogenic Effects: Pregnancy Category C. DEXEDRINE has been shown to have embryotoxic and teratogenic effects when administered to A/Jax mice and C57BL mice in doses approximately 41 times the maximum human dose. Embryotoxic effects were not seen in New Zealand white rabbits given the drug in doses 7 times the human dose nor in rats given 12.5 times the maximum human dose. While there are no adequate and well-controlled studies in pregnant women, there has been 1 report of severe congenital bony deformity, tracheoesophageal fistula, and anal atresia (VATER association) in a baby born to a woman who took dextroamphetamine sulfate with lovastatin during the first trimester of pregnancy. DEXEDRINE should be used during pregnancy only if the potential benefit justifies the potential risk to the fetus.
Nonteratogenic Effects: Infants born to mothers dependent on amphetamines have an increased risk of premature delivery and low birth weight. Also, these infants may experience symptoms of withdrawal as demonstrated by dysphoria, including agitation, and significant lassitude.
Nursing Mothers: Amphetamines are excreted in human milk. Mothers taking amphetamines should be advised to refrain from nursing.
Pediatric Use: Long-term effects of amphetamines in pediatric patients have not been well established.
Amphetamines are not recommended for use in pediatric patients under 3 years of age with Attention Deficit Disorder with Hyperactivity described under INDICATIONS AND USAGE.
Clinical experience suggests that in psychotic children, administration of amphetamines may exacerbate symptoms of behavior disturbance and thought disorder.
Amphetamines have been reported to exacerbate motor and phonic tics and Tourette's syndrome. Therefore, clinical evaluation for tics and Tourette's syndrome in children and their families should precede use of stimulant medications.
Data are inadequate to determine whether chronic administration of amphetamines may be associated with growth inhibition; therefore, growth should be monitored during treatment.
Drug treatment is not indicated in all cases of Attention Deficit Disorder with Hyperactivity and should be considered only in light of the complete history and evaluation of the child. The decision to prescribe amphetamines should depend on the physician's assessment of the chronicity and severity of the child's symptoms and their appropriateness for his or her age. Prescription should not depend solely on the presence of one or more of the behavioral characteristics.
When these symptoms are associated with acute stress reactions, treatment with amphetamines is usually not indicated.

ADVERSE REACTIONS

Cardiovascular: Palpitations, tachycardia, elevation of blood pressure. There have been isolated reports of cardiomyopathy associated with chronic amphetamine use.
Central Nervous System: Psychotic episodes at recommended doses (rare), overstimulation, restlessness, dizziness, insomnia, euphoria, dyskinesia, dysphoria, tremor, headache, exacerbation of motor and phonic tics, and Tourette's syndrome.
Gastrointestinal: Dryness of the mouth, unpleasant taste, diarrhea, constipation, other gastrointestinal disturbances. Anorexia and weight loss may occur as undesirable effects.
Allergic: Urticaria.
Endocrine: Impotence, changes in libido.

DRUG ABUSE AND DEPENDENCE

Dextroamphetamine sulfate is a Schedule II controlled substance.
Amphetamines have been extensively abused. Tolerance, extreme psychological dependence and severe social disability have occurred. There are reports of patients who have increased the dosage to many times that recommended. Abrupt cessation following prolonged high dosage administration results in extreme fatigue and mental depression; changes are also noted on the sleep EEG.
Manifestations of chronic intoxication with amphetamines include severe dermatoses, marked insomnia, irritability, hyperactivity, and personality changes. The most severe manifestation of chronic intoxication is psychosis, often clinically indistinguishable from schizophrenia. This is rare with oral amphetamines.

OVERDOSAGE

Individual patient response to amphetamines varies widely. While toxic symptoms occasionally occur as an idiosyncrasy at doses as low as 2 mg, they are rare with doses of less than 15 mg; 30 mg can produce severe reactions, yet doses of 400 to 500 mg are not necessarily fatal.
In rats, the oral LD_{50} of dextroamphetamine sulfate is 96.8 mg/kg.
Manifestations of acute overdosage with amphetamines include restlessness, tremor, hyperreflexia, rhabdomyolysis, rapid respiration, hyperpyrexia, confusion, assaultiveness, hallucinations, panic states.
Fatigue and depression usually follow the central stimulation.
Cardiovascular effects include arrhythmias, hypertension or hypotension, and circulatory collapse. Gastrointestinal symptoms include nausea, vomiting, diarrhea, and abdominal cramps. Fatal poisoning is usually preceded by convulsions and coma.

TREATMENT

Consult with a Certified Poison Control Center for up-to-date guidance and advice. Management of acute amphetamine intoxication is largely symptomatic and includes gastric lavage, administration of activated charcoal, administration of a cathartic, and sedation. Experience with hemodialysis or peritoneal dialysis is inadequate to permit recommendation in this regard. Acidification of the urine increases amphetamine excretion, but is believed to increase risk of acute renal failure if myoglobinuria is present. If acute, severe hypertension complicates amphetamine overdosage, administration of intravenous phentolamine (Bedford Laboratories) has been suggested. However, a gradual drop in blood pressure will usually result when sufficient sedation has been achieved.
Chlorpromazine antagonizes the central stimulant effects of amphetamines and can be used to treat amphetamine intoxication.
Since much of the SPANSULE capsule medication is coated for gradual release, therapy directed at reversing the effects of the ingested drug and at supporting the patient should be continued for as long as overdosage symptoms remain. Saline cathartics are useful for hastening the evacuation of pellets that have not already released medication.

DOSAGE AND ADMINISTRATION

Amphetamines should be administered at the lowest effective dosage and dosage should be individually adjusted. Late evening doses—particularly with the SPANSULE capsule form—should be avoided because of the resulting insomnia.
Narcolepsy: Usual dose is 5 to 60 mg per day in divided doses, depending on the individual patient response.
Narcolepsy seldom occurs in children under 12 years of age; however, when it does, DEXEDRINE may be used. The suggested initial dose for patients aged 6 to 12 is 5 mg daily; daily dose may be raised in increments of 5 mg at weekly intervals until an optimal response is obtained. In patients 12 years of age and older, start with 10 mg daily; daily dosage may be raised in increments of 10 mg at weekly intervals until an optimal response is obtained. If bothersome adverse reactions appear (e.g., insomnia or anorexia), dosage should be reduced. SPANSULE capsules may be used for once-a-day dosage wherever appropriate. With tablets, give first dose on awakening; additional doses (1 or 2) at intervals of 4 to 6 hours.
Attention Deficit Disorder with Hyperactivity: Not recommended for pediatric patients under 3 years of age.
In pediatric patients from 3 to 5 years of age, start with 2.5 mg daily, by tablet; daily dosage may be raised in increments of 2.5 mg at weekly intervals until optimal response is obtained.
In pediatric patients 6 years of age and older, start with 5 mg once or twice daily; daily dosage may be raised in increments of 5 mg at weekly intervals until optimal response is obtained. Only in rare cases will it be necessary to exceed a total of 40 mg per day.
SPANSULE capsules may be used for once-a-day dosage wherever appropriate.
With tablets, give first dose on awakening; additional doses (1 or 2) at intervals of 4 to 6 hours.
Where possible, drug administration should be interrupted occasionally to determine if there is a recurrence of behavioral symptoms sufficient to require continued therapy.

HOW SUPPLIED

DEXEDRINE SPANSULE capsules: Each capsule, with brown cap and clear body, contains dextroamphetamine sulfate. The 5-mg capsule is imprinted 5 mg and 3512 on the brown cap and is imprinted 5 mg and SB on the clear body. The 10-mg capsule is imprinted 10 mg — 3513 — on the brown cap and is imprinted 10 mg — SB — on the clear body. The 15-mg capsule is imprinted 15 mg and 3514 on the brown cap and is imprinted 15 mg and SB on the clear body. A narrow bar appears above and below 15 mg and 3514. Available: 5 mg, 10 mg, and 15 mg in bottles of 100.
Store at controlled room temperature between 20° and 25°C (68° and 77°F) [see USP].
Dispense in a tight, light-resistant container.
5 mg 100s: NDC 0007-3512-20
10 mg 100s: NDC 0007-3513-20
15 mg 100s: NDC 0007-3514-20
DEXEDRINE SPANSULE capsules are manufactured by Cardinal Health, Winchester, KY 40391.
DEXEDRINE Tablets: Triangular, orange, scored, debossed SKF and E19. Available: 5 mg in bottles of 100, manufactured by Abbott Laboratories, North Chicago, IL 60064.
Store between 15° and 30°C (59° and 86°F). Dispense in a tight, light-resistant container.
5 mg 100s: NDC 0007-3519-20
GlaxoSmithKline, Research Triangle Park, NC 27709

September 2003/DX:L53
Shown in Product Identification Guide, page 315

DIGIBIND® ℞
[dij ˈə-bīnd]
DIGOXIN IMMUNE FAB (OVINE)

DESCRIPTION

DIGIBIND, Digoxin Immune Fab (Ovine), is a sterile lyophilized powder of antigen binding fragments (Fab) derived from specific antidigoxin antibodies raised in sheep. Production of antibodies specific for digoxin involves conjugation of digoxin as a hapten to human albumin. Sheep are immunized with this material to produce antibodies specific for the antigenic determinants of the digoxin molecule. The antibody is then papain-digested and digoxin-specific Fab fragments of the antibody are isolated and purified by affinity chromatography. These antibody fragments have a molecular weight of approximately 46,200.
Each vial, which will bind approximately 0.5 mg of digoxin (or digitoxin), contains 38 mg of digoxin-specific Fab fragments derived from sheep plus 75 mg of sorbitol as a stabilizer and 28 mg of sodium chloride. The vial contains no preservatives.
DIGIBIND is administered by intravenous injection after reconstitution with Sterile Water for Injection (4 mL per vial).

CLINICAL PHARMACOLOGY

After intravenous injection of Digoxin Immune Fab (Ovine) in the baboon, digoxin-specific Fab fragments are excreted in the urine with a biological half-life of about 9 to 13 hours.[1] In humans with normal renal function, the half-life appears to be 15 to 20 hours.[2] Experimental studies in animals indicate that these antibody fragments have a large volume of distribution in the extracellular space, unlike whole antibody which distributes in a space only about twice the plasma volume.[1] Ordinarily, following administration of DIGIBIND, improvement in signs and symptoms of digitalis intoxication begins within one-half hour or less.[2,3,4,5]

The affinity of DIGIBIND for digoxin is in the range of 10^9 to 10^{11} M^{-1}, which is greater than the affinity of digoxin for (sodium, potassium) ATPase, the presumed receptor for its toxic effects. The affinity of DIGIBIND for digitoxin is about 10^8 to 10^9 M^{-1}.

DIGIBIND binds molecules of digoxin, making them unavailable for binding at their site of action on cells in the body. The Fab fragment-digoxin complex accumulates in the blood, from which it is excreted by the kidney. The net effect is to shift the equilibrium away from binding of digoxin to its receptors in the body, thereby reversing its effects.

INDICATIONS AND USAGE

DIGIBIND, Digoxin Immune Fab (Ovine), is indicated for treatment of potentially life-threatening digoxin intoxication.[3] Although designed specifically to treat life-threatening digoxin overdose, it has also been used successfully to treat life-threatening digitoxin overdose.[3] Since human experience is limited and the consequences of repeated exposures are unknown, DIGIBIND is not indicated for milder cases of digitalis toxicity.

Manifestations of life-threatening toxicity include severe ventricular arrhythmias such as ventricular tachycardia or ventricular fibrillation, or progressive bradyarrhythmias such as severe sinus bradycardia or second or third degree heart block not responsive to atropine.

Ingestion of more than 10 mg of digoxin in previously healthy adults or 4 mg of digoxin in previously healthy children, or ingestion causing steady-state serum concentrations greater than 10 ng/mL, often results in cardiac arrest. Digitalis-induced progressive elevation of the serum potassium concentration also suggests imminent cardiac arrest. If the potassium concentration exceeds 5 mEq/L in the setting of severe digitalis intoxication, therapy with DIGIBIND is indicated.

CONTRAINDICATIONS

There are no known contraindications to the use of DIGIBIND.

WARNINGS

Suicidal ingestion often involves more than one drug; thus, toxicity from other drugs should not be overlooked.

One should consider the possibility of anaphylactic, hypersensitivity, or febrile reactions. If an anaphylactoid reaction occurs, the drug infusion should be discontinued and appropriate therapy initiated using aminophylline, oxygen, volume expansion, diphenhydramine, corticosteroids, and airway management as indicated. The need for epinephrine should be balanced against its potential risk in the setting of digitalis toxicity.

Since the Fab fragment of the antibody lacks the antigenic determinants of the Fc fragment, it should pose less of an immunogenic threat to patients than does an intact immunoglobulin molecule. Patients with known allergies would be particularly at risk, as would individuals who have previously received antibodies or Fab fragments raised in sheep. Papain is used to cleave the whole antibody into Fab and Fc fragments, and traces of papain or inactivated papain residues may be present in DIGIBIND. Patients with allergies to papain, chymopapain, or other papaya extracts also may be particularly at risk.

Skin testing for allergy was performed during the clinical investigation of DIGIBIND. Only one patient developed erythema at the site of skin testing, with no accompanying wheal reaction; this individual had no adverse reaction to systemic treatment with DIGIBIND. Since allergy testing can delay urgently needed therapy, it is not routinely required before treatment of life-threatening digitalis toxicity with DIGIBIND.

Skin testing may be appropriate for high risk individuals, especially patients with known allergies or those previously treated with Digoxin Immune Fab (Ovine). The intradermal skin test can be performed by:

1. Diluting 0.1 mL of reconstituted DIGIBIND (9.5 mg/mL) in 9.9 mL sterile isotonic saline (1:100 dilution, 95 mcg/mL).
2. Injecting 0.1 mL of the 1:100 dilution (9.5 mcg) intradermally and observing for an urticarial wheal surrounded by a zone of erythema. The test should be read at 20 minutes.

The scratch test procedure is performed by placing one drop of a 1:100 dilution of DIGIBIND on the skin and then making a $^1/_4$-inch scratch through the drop with a sterile needle. The scratch site is inspected at 20 minutes for an urticarial wheal surrounded by erythema.

If skin testing causes a systemic reaction, a tourniquet should be applied above the site of testing and measures to treat anaphylaxis should be instituted. Further administration of DIGIBIND should be avoided unless its use is absolutely essential, in which case the patient should be pretreated with corticosteroids and diphenhydramine. The physician should be prepared to treat anaphylaxis.

PRECAUTIONS

General: Standard therapy for digitalis intoxication includes withdrawal of the drug and correction of factors that may contribute to toxicity, such as electrolyte disturbances, hypoxia, acid-base disturbances, and agents such as catecholamines. Also, treatment of arrhythmias may include judicious potassium supplements, lidocaine, phenytoin, procainamide, and/or propranolol; treatment of sinus bradycardia or atrioventricular block may involve atropine or pacemaker insertion. Massive digitalis intoxication can cause hyperkalemia; administration of potassium supplements in the setting of massive intoxication may be hazardous (see Laboratory Tests). After treatment with DIGIBIND, the serum potassium concentration may drop rapidly[2] and must be monitored frequently, especially over the first several hours after DIGIBIND is given (see Laboratory Tests).

The elimination half-life in the setting of renal failure has not been clearly defined. Patients with renal dysfunction have been successfully treated with DIGIBIND.[4] There is no evidence to suggest the time-course of therapeutic effect is any different in these patients than in patients with normal renal function, but excretion of the Fab fragment-digoxin complex from the body is probably delayed. In patients who are functionally anephric, one would anticipate failure to clear the Fab fragment-digoxin complex from the blood by glomerular filtration and renal excretion. Whether failure to eliminate the Fab fragment-digoxin complex in severe renal failure can lead to reintoxication following release of newly unbound digoxin into the blood is uncertain. Such patients should be monitored for a prolonged period for possible recurrence of digitalis toxicity.

Patients with intrinsically poor cardiac function may deteriorate from withdrawal of the inotropic action of digoxin. Studies in animals have shown that the reversal of inotropic effect is relatively gradual, occurring over hours. When needed, additional support can be provided by use of intravenous inotropes, such as dopamine or dobutamine, or vasodilators. One must be careful in using catecholamines not to aggravate digitalis toxic rhythm disturbances. Clearly, other types of digitalis glycosides should not be used in this setting.

Redigitalization should be postponed, if possible, until the Fab fragments have been eliminated from the body, which may require several days. Patients with impaired renal function may require a week or longer.

Laboratory Tests: DIGIBIND will interfere with digitalis immunoassay measurements.[6] Thus, the standard serum digoxin concentration measurement can be clinically misleading until the Fab fragment is eliminated from the body. Serum digoxin or digitoxin concentration should be obtained before administration of DIGIBIND if at all possible. These measurements may be difficult to interpret if drawn soon after the last digitalis dose, since at least 6 to 8 hours are required for equilibration of digoxin between serum and tissue. Patients should be closely monitored, including temperature, blood pressure, electrocardiogram, and potassium concentration, during and after administration of DIGIBIND. The total serum digoxin concentration may rise precipitously following administration of DIGIBIND, but this will be almost entirely bound to the Fab fragment and therefore not able to react with receptors in the body.

Potassium concentrations should be followed carefully. Severe digitalis intoxication can cause life-threatening elevation in serum potassium concentration by shifting potassium from inside to outside the cell. The elevation in serum potassium concentration can lead to increased renal excretion of potassium. Thus, these patients may have hyperkalemia with a total body deficit of potassium. When the effect of digitalis is reversed by DIGIBIND, potassium shifts back inside the cell, with a resulting decline in serum potassium concentration.[4] Hypokalemia may thus develop rapidly. For these reasons, serum potassium concentration should be monitored repeatedly, especially over the first several hours after DIGIBIND is given, and cautiously treated when necessary.

Carcinogenesis, Mutagenesis, Impairment of Fertility: There have been no long-term studies performed in animals to evaluate carcinogenic potential.

Pregnancy: Pregnancy Category C. Animal reproduction studies have not been conducted with DIGIBIND. It is also not known whether DIGIBIND can cause fetal harm when administered to a pregnant woman or can affect reproduction capacity. DIGIBIND should be given to a pregnant woman only if clearly needed.

Nursing Mothers: It is not known whether this drug is excreted in human milk. Because many drugs are excreted in human milk, caution should be exercised when DIGIBIND is administered to a nursing woman.

Pediatric Use: DIGIBIND has been successfully used in infants with no apparent adverse sequelae. As in all other circumstances, use of this drug in infants should be based on careful consideration of the benefits of the drug balanced against the potential risk involved.

Geriatric Use: Of the 150 subjects in an open-label study of DIGIBIND, 42% were 65 and over, while 21% were 75 and over. In a post-marketing surveillance study that enrolled 717 adults, 84% were 60 and over, and 60% were 70 and over. No overall differences in safety or effectiveness were observed between these subjects and younger subjects, and other reported clinical experience has not identified differences in responses between the elderly and younger patients, but greater sensitivity of some older individuals cannot be ruled out.

The kidney excretes the Fab fragment-digoxin complex, and the risk of digoxin release with recurrence of toxicity is potentially increased when excretion of the complex is slowed by renal failure. However, recurrence of toxicity was reported for only 2.8% of patients in the surveillance study and the only factor associated with recurrence of toxicity was inadequacy of initial dose—not renal function. Calculation of dose is the same for patients of all ages and for patients with normal and impaired renal function. Because elderly patients are more likely to have decreased renal function, it may be useful to monitor renal function and to observe for possible recurrence of toxicity.

ADVERSE REACTIONS

Allergic reactions to DIGIBIND have been reported rarely. Patients with a history of allergy, especially to antibiotics, appear to be at particular risk (see WARNINGS). In a few instances, low cardiac output states and congestive heart failure could have been exacerbated by withdrawal of the inotropic effects of digitalis. Hypokalemia may occur from re-activation of (sodium, potassium) ATPase (see Laboratory Tests). Patients with atrial fibrillation may develop a rapid ventricular response from withdrawal of the effects of digitalis on the atrioventricular node.[4]

DOSAGE AND ADMINISTRATION

General Guidelines: The dosage of DIGIBIND varies according to the amount of digoxin (or digitoxin) to be neutralized. The average dose used during clinical testing was 10 vials.

Dosage for Acute Ingestion of Unknown Amount: Twenty (20) vials (760 mg) of DIGIBIND is adequate to treat most life-threatening ingestions in both **adults and children.** However, in children it is important to monitor for volume overload. In general, a large dose of DIGIBIND has a faster onset of effect but may enhance the possibility of a febrile reaction. The physician may consider administering 10 vials, observing the patient's response, and following with an additional 10 vials if clinically indicated.

Dosage for Toxicity During Chronic Therapy: For adults, six vials (228 mg) usually is adequate to reverse most cases of toxicity. This dose can be used in patients who are in acute distress or for whom a serum digoxin or digitoxin concentration is not available. In infants and small children ($\leq$ 20 kg) a single vial usually should suffice.

Methods for calculating the dose of DIGIBIND required to neutralize the known or estimated amount of digoxin or digitoxin in the body are given below (see DOSAGE CALCULATION section).

When determining the dose for DIGIBIND, the following guidelines should be considered:

— Erroneous calculations may result from inaccurate estimates of the amount of digitalis ingested or absorbed or from nonsteady-state serum digitalis concentrations. Inaccurate serum digitalis concentration measurements are a possible source of error. Most serum digoxin assay kits are designed to measure values less than 5 ng/mL. Dilution of samples is required to obtain accurate measures above 5 ng/mL.

— Dosage calculations are based on a steady-state volume of distribution of approximately 5 L/kg for digoxin (0.5 L/kg for digitoxin) to convert serum digitalis concentration to the amount of digitalis in the body. The conversion is based on the principle that body load equals drug steady-state serum concentration multiplied by volume of distribution. These volumes are population averages and vary widely among individuals. Many patients may require higher doses for complete neutralization. Doses should ordinarily be rounded up to the next whole vial.

— If toxicity has not adequately reversed after several hours or appears to recur, readministration of DIGIBIND at a dose guided by clinical judgment may be required.

— Failure to respond to DIGIBIND raises the possibility that the clinical problem is not caused by digitalis intoxication. If there is no response to an adequate dose of DIGIBIND, the diagnosis of digitalis toxicity should be questioned.

DOSAGE CALCULATION

Acute Ingestion of Known Amount: Each vial of DIGIBIND contains 38 mg of purified digoxin-specific Fab fragments which will bind approximately 0.5 mg of digoxin (or digitoxin). Thus one can calculate the total number of vials required by dividing the total digitalis body load in mg by 0.5 mg/vial (see Formula 1).

For toxicity from an acute ingestion, total body load in milligrams will be approximately equal to the amount ingested in milligrams for digoxin capsules and digitoxin, or the amount ingested in milligrams multiplied by 0.80 (to account for incomplete absorption) for digoxin tablets.

Table 1 gives dosage estimates in number of vials for **adults and children** who have ingested a single large dose of digoxin and for whom the approximate number of tablets or capsules is known. The dose of DIGIBIND (in number of vials) represented in Table 1 can be approximated using the following formula:

Formula 1

$$\text{Dose (in \# of vials)} = \frac{\text{Total digitalis body load in mg}}{\text{0.5 mg of digitalis bound/vial}}$$

Continued on next page

Product information on these pages is effective as of August 2004. Further information is available at: GlaxoSmithKline, PO Box 13398, Research Triangle Park, NC 27709. 1-888-825-5249. Corporate Web Site: www.gsk.com

Table 2: Adult Dose Estimate of DIGIBIND (in # of vials) from Steady-State Serum Digoxin Concentration

Patient Weight (kg)	Serum Digoxin Concentration (ng/mL)						
	1	2	4	8	12	16	20
40	0.5 V	1 V	2 V	3 V	5 V	7 V	8 V
60	0.5 V	1 V	3 V	5 V	7 V	10 V	12 V
70	1 V	2 V	3 V	6 V	9 V	11 V	14 V
80	1 V	2 V	3 V	7 V	10 V	13 V	16 V
100	1 V	2 V	4 V	8 V	12 V	16 V	20 V

V = vials

Table 3: Infants and Small Children Dose Estimates of DIGIBIND (in mg) from Steady-State Serum Digoxin Concentration

Patient Weight (kg)	Serum Digoxin Concentration (ng/mL)						
	1	2	4	8	12	16	20
1	0.4* mg	1* mg	1.5* mg	3* mg	5 mg	6 mg	8 mg
3	1* mg	2* mg	5 mg	9 mg	14 mg	18 mg	23 mg
5	2* mg	4 mg	8 mg	15 mg	23 mg	30 mg	38 mg
10	4 mg	8 mg	15 mg	30 mg	46 mg	61 mg	76 mg
20	8 mg	15 mg	30 mg	61 mg	91 mg	122 mg	152 mg

* Dilution of reconstituted vial to 1 mg/mL may be desirable.

Digibind—Cont.

Table 1: Approximate Dose of DIGIBIND for Reversal of a Single Large Digoxin Overdose

Number of Digoxin Tablets or Capsules Ingested*	Dose of DIGIBIND # of Vials
25	10
50	20
75	30
100	40
150	60
200	80

* 0.25 mg tablets with 80% bioavailability or 0.2 mg LANOXICAPS® Capsules with 100% bioavailability.

Calculations Based on Steady-State Serum Digoxin Concentrations: Table 2 gives dosage estimates in number of vials for **adult patients** for whom a steady-state serum digoxin concentration is known. The dose of DIGIBIND (in number of vials) represented in Table 2 can be approximated using the following formula:

Formula 2

$$\text{Dose (in \# of vials)} = \frac{\text{(Serum digoxin concentration in ng/mL) (weight in kg)}}{100}$$

[See table 2 above]

Table 3 gives dosage estimates in milligrams **for infants and small children** based on the steady-state serum digoxin concentration. The dose of DIGIBIND represented in Table 3 can be estimated by multiplying the dose (in number of vials) calculated from Formula 2 by the amount of DIGIBIND contained in a vial (38 mg/vial) (see Formula 3). Since infants and small children can have much smaller dosage requirements, it is recommended that the 38-mg vial be reconstituted as directed and administered with a tuberculin syringe. For very small doses, a reconstituted vial can be diluted with 34 mL of sterile isotonic saline to achieve a concentration of 1 mg/mL.

Formula 3

Dose (in mg) = (Dose [in # of vials]) (38 mg/vial)

[See table 3 above]

Calculation Based on Steady-State Digitoxin Concentration: The dose of DIGIBIND for digitoxin toxicity can be approximated using the following formula:

Formula 4

$$\text{Dose (in \# of vials)} = \frac{\text{(Serum digitoxin concentration in ng/mL) (weight in kg)}}{1000}$$

If the dose based on ingested amount differs substantially from that calculated from the serum digoxin or digitoxin concentration, it may be preferable to use the higher dose.

ADMINISTRATION: The contents in each vial to be used should be dissolved with 4 mL of Sterile Water for Injection, by gentle mixing, to give a clear, colorless, approximately isosmotic solution with a protein concentration of 9.5 mg/mL. Reconstituted product should be used promptly. If it is not used immediately, it may be stored under refrigeration at 2° to 8°C (36° to 46°F) for up to 4 hours. The reconstituted product may be diluted with sterile isotonic saline to a convenient volume. Parenteral drug products should be inspected visually for particulate matter and discoloration prior to administration, whenever solution and container permit.

DIGIBIND, Digoxin Immune Fab (Ovine), is administered by the intravenous route over 30 minutes. It is recommended that it be infused through a 0.22-micron membrane filter to ensure no undissolved particulate matter is administered. If cardiac arrest is imminent, it can be given as a bolus injection.

HOW SUPPLIED

Vials containing 38 mg of purified lyophilized digoxin-specific Fab fragments. Box of 1 (NDC 0173-0230-44).

STORAGE

Refrigerate at 2° to 8°C (36° to 46°F). Unreconstituted vials can be stored at up to 30°C (86°F) for a total of 30 days.

REFERENCES

1. Smith TW, Lloyd BL, Spicer N, Haber E. Immunogenicity and kinetics of distribution and elimination of sheep digoxin-specific IgG and Fab fragments in the rabbit and baboon. *Clin Exp Immunol.* 1979; 36:384-396.
2. Smith TW, Haber E, Yeatman L, Butler VP Jr. Reversal of advanced digoxin intoxication with Fab fragments of digoxin-specific antibodies. *N Engl J Med.* 1976; 294:797-800.
3. Smith TW, Butler VP Jr, Haber E, Fozzard H, Marcus FI, Bremner WF, Schulman IC, Phillips A. Treatment of life-threatening digitalis intoxication with digoxin-specific Fab antibody fragments: Experience in 26 cases. *N Engl J Med.* 1982; 307:1357-1362.
4. Wenger TL, Butler VP Jr, Haber E, Smith TW. Treatment of 63 severely digitalis-toxic patients with digoxin-specific antibody fragments. *J Am Coll Cardiol.* 1985; 5:118A-123A.
5. Spiegel A, Marchlinski FE. Time course for reversal of digoxin toxicity with digoxin-specific antibody fragments. *Am Heart J.* 1985; 109:1397-1399.
6. Gibb I, Adams PC, Parnham AJ, Jennings K. Plasma digoxin: Assay anomalies in Fab-treated patients. *Br J Clin Pharmacol.* 1983; 16:445-447.

THE WELLCOME FOUNDATION LTD., Beckenham, Kent, England BR3 3BS
U.S. License No. 129
Distributed by: GlaxoSmithKline
Research Triangle Park, NC 27709
August 2001/RL-980

Shown in Product Identification Guide, page 315

DYAZIDE® ℞

[dī' ə-zīd]
capsules
diuretic • antihypertensive

DESCRIPTION

Each *Dyazide* capsule for oral use, with opaque red cap and opaque white body, contains hydrochlorothiazide 25 mg and triamterene 37.5 mg, and is imprinted with the product name DYAZIDE and SB. Hydrochlorothiazide is a diuretic/antihypertensive agent and triamterene is an antikaliuretic agent.

Hydrochlorothiazide is slightly soluble in water. It is soluble in dilute ammonia, dilute aqueous sodium hydroxide and dimethylformamide. It is sparingly soluble in methanol.

Hydrochlorothiazide is 6-chloro-3,4-dihydro-2H -1,2,4-benzothiadiazine-7-sulfonamide 1,1-dioxide.

At 50°C, triamterene is practically insoluble in water (less than 0.1%). It is soluble in formic acid, sparingly soluble in methoxyethanol and very slightly soluble in alcohol.

Triamterene is 2,4,7-triamino-6-phenylpteridine.

Inactive ingredients consist of benzyl alcohol, cetylpyridinium chloride, D&C Red No. 33, FD&C Yellow No. 6, gelatin, glycine, lactose, magnesium stearate, microcrystalline cellulose, povidone, polysorbate 80, sodium starch glycolate, titanium dioxide and trace amounts of other inactive ingredients.

Dyazide capsules meet Drug Release Test 3 as published in the USP 23 monograph for Triamterene and Hydrochlorothiazide Capsules.

CLINICAL PHARMACOLOGY

Dyazide is a diuretic/antihypertensive drug product that combines natriuretic and antikaliuretic effects. Each component complements the action of the other. The hydrochlorothiazide component blocks the reabsorption of sodium and chloride ions, and thereby increases the quantity of sodium traversing the distal tubule and the volume of water excreted. A portion of the additional sodium presented to the distal tubule is exchanged there for potassium and hydrogen ions. With continued use of hydrochlorothiazide and depletion of sodium, compensatory mechanisms tend to increase this exchange and may produce excessive loss of potassium, hydrogen and chloride ions. Hydrochlorothiazide also decreases the excretion of calcium and uric acid, may increase the excretion of iodide and may reduce glomerular filtration rate. The exact mechanism of the antihypertensive effect of hydrochlorothiazide is not known.

The triamterene component of *Dyazide* exerts its diuretic effect on the distal renal tubule to inhibit the reabsorption of sodium in exchange for potassium and hydrogen ions. Its natriuretic activity is limited by the amount of sodium reaching its site of action. Although it blocks the increase in this exchange that is stimulated by mineralocorticoids (chiefly aldosterone) it is not a competitive antagonist of aldosterone and its activity can be demonstrated in adrenalectomized rats and patients with Addison's disease. As a result, the dose of triamterene required is not proportionally related to the level of mineralocorticoid activity, but is dictated by the response of the individual patients, and the kaliuretic effect of concomitantly administered drugs. By inhibiting the distal tubular exchange mechanism, triamterene maintains or increases the sodium excretion and reduces the excess loss of potassium, hydrogen and chloride ions induced by hydrochlorothiazide. As with hydrochlorothiazide, triamterene may reduce glomerular filtration and renal plasma flow. Via this mechanism it may reduce uric acid excretion although it has no tubular effect on uric acid reabsorption or secretion. Triamterene does not affect calcium excretion. No predictable antihypertensive effect has been demonstrated for triamterene.

Duration of diuretic activity and effective dosage range of the hydrochlorothiazide and triamterene components of *Dyazide* are similar. Onset of diuresis with *Dyazide* takes place within 1 hour, peaks at 2 to 3 hours and tapers off during the subsequent 7 to 9 hours.

Dyazide capsule is well absorbed.

Upon administration of a single oral dose to fasted normal male volunteers, the following mean pharmacokinetic parameters were determined:

[See table at top of next page]

where AUC(0–48), Cmax, Tmax and Ae represent area under the plasma concentration versus time plot, maximum plasma concentration, time to reach Cmax and amount excreted in urine over 48 hours.

Dyazide capsule is bioequivalent to a single-entity 25 mg hydrochlorothiazide tablet and 37.5 mg triamterene capsule used in the double-blind clinical trial below. (See Clinical Trials.)

In a limited study involving 12 subjects, coadministration of *Dyazide* with a high-fat meal resulted in: (1) an increase in the mean bioavailability of triamterene by about 67% (90% confidence interval = 0.99, 1.90), p-hydroxytriamterene sulfate by about 50% (90% confidence interval = 1.06, 1.77), hydrochlorothiazide by about 17% (90% confidence interval = 0.90, 1.34); (2) increases in the peak concentrations of triamterene and p-hydroxytriamterene; and (3) a delay of up to 2 hours in the absorption of the active constituents.

Clinical Trials

A placebo-controlled, double-blind trial was conducted to evaluate the efficacy of *Dyazide* capsules. This trial demonstrated that *Dyazide* (25 mg hydrochlorothiazide/37.5 mg triamterene) was effective in controlling blood pressure while reducing the incidence of hydrochlorothiazide-induced hypokalemia. This trial involved 636 patients with mild to moderate hypertension controlled by hydrochlorothiazide 25 mg daily and who had hypokalemia (serum potassium <3.5 mEq/L) secondary to the hydrochlorothiazide. Patients were randomly assigned to 4 weeks' treatment with once-daily regimens of 25 mg hydrochlorothiazide plus placebo, or 25 mg hydrochlorothiazide combined with one of the following doses of triamterene: 25 mg, 37.5 mg, 50 mg or 75 mg.

Blood pressure and serum potassium were monitored at baseline and throughout the trial. All five treatment groups had similar mean blood pressure and serum potassium concentrations at baseline (mean systolic blood pressure range: 137±14 mmHg to 140±16 mmHg; mean diastolic blood pressure range: 86±9 mmHg to 88±8 mmHg; mean serum potassium range: 2.3 to 3.4 mEq/L with the majority of patients having values between 3.1 and 3.4 mEq/L).

While all triamterene regimens reversed hypokalemia, at week 4 the 37.5 mg regimen proved optimal compared with the other tested regimens. On this regimen, 81% of the patients had a significant ($p<0.05$) reversal of hypokalemia vs. 59% of patients on the placebo/hydrochlorothiazide regimen. The mean serum potassium concentration on 37.5 mg triamterene went from 3.2±0.2 mEq/L at baseline to 3.7±0.3 mEq/L at week 4, a significantly greater ($p<0.05$) improvement than that achieved with placebo/hydrochlorothiazide (i.e., 3.2±0.2 mEq/L at baseline and 3.5±0.4 mEq/L at week 4). Also, 51% of patients in the 37.5 mg triamterene group had an increase in serum potassium of ≥0.5 mEq/L at week 4 vs. 33% in the placebo group. The 37.5 mg triamterene/25 mg hydrochlorothiazide regimen also maintained control of blood pressure; mean supine systolic blood pressure at week 4 was 138±21 mmHg while mean supine diastolic blood pressure was 87±13 mmHg.

INDICATIONS AND USAGE

This fixed combination drug is not indicated for the initial therapy of edema or hypertension except in individuals in whom the development of hypokalemia cannot be risked.

Dyazide is indicated for the treatment of hypertension or edema in patients who develop hypokalemia on hydrochlorothiazide alone.

Dyazide is also indicated for those patients who require a thiazide diuretic and in whom the development of hypokalemia cannot be risked.

Dyazide may be used alone or as an adjunct to other antihypertensive drugs, such as beta-blockers. Since *Dyazide* may enhance the action of these agents, dosage adjustments may be necessary.

Usage in Pregnancy: The routine use of diuretics in an otherwise healthy woman is inappropriate and exposes mother and fetus to unnecessary hazard. Diuretics do not prevent development of toxemia of pregnancy, and there is no satisfactory evidence that they are useful in the treatment of developed toxemia.

Edema during pregnancy may arise from pathological causes or from the physiologic and mechanical consequences of pregnancy. Diuretics are indicated in pregnancy when edema is due to pathologic causes, just as they are in the absence of pregnancy. Dependent edema in pregnancy resulting from restriction of venous return by the expanded uterus is properly treated through elevation of the lower extremities and use of support hose; use of diuretics to lower intravascular volume in this case is illogical and unnecessary. There is hypervolemia during normal pregnancy which is harmful to neither the fetus nor the mother (in the absence of cardiovascular disease), but which is associated with edema, including generalized edema in the majority of pregnant women. If this edema produces discomfort, increased recumbency will often provide relief. In rare instances this edema may cause extreme discomfort which is not relieved by rest. In these cases a short course of diuretics may provide relief and may be appropriate.

CONTRAINDICATIONS

Antikaliuretic Therapy and Potassium Supplementation

Dyazide should not be given to patients receiving other potassium-sparing agents such as spironolactone, amiloride or other formulations containing triamterene. Concomitant potassium-containing salt substitutes should also not be used. Potassium supplementation should not be used with *Dyazide* except in severe cases of hypokalemia. Such concomitant therapy can be associated with rapid increases in serum potassium levels. If potassium supplementation is used, careful monitoring of the serum potassium level is necessary.

Impaired Renal Function

Dyazide is contraindicated in patients with anuria, acute and chronic renal insufficiency or significant renal impairment.

Hypersensitivity

Hypersensitivity to either drug in the preparation or to other sulfonamide-derived drugs is a contraindication.

Hyperkalemia

Dyazide should not be used in patients with preexisting elevated serum potassium.

WARNINGS

Hyperkalemia

Abnormal elevation of serum potassium levels (greater than or equal to 5.5 mEq/liter) can occur with all potassium-sparing diuretic combinations, including *Dyazide.* Hyperkalemia is more likely to occur in patients with renal impairment and diabetes (even without evidence of renal impairment), and in the elderly or severely ill. Since uncorrected hyperkalemia may be fatal, serum potassium levels must be monitored at frequent intervals especially in patients first receiving *Dyazide,* when dosages are changed or with any illness that may influence renal function.

If hyperkalemia is suspected (warning signs include paresthesias, muscular weakness, fatigue, flaccid paralysis of the extremities, bradycardia and shock), an electrocardiogram (ECG) should be obtained. However, it is important to monitor serum potassium levels because hyperkalemia may not be associated with ECG changes.

If hyperkalemia is present, *Dyazide* should be discontinued immediately and a thiazide alone should be substituted. If the serum potassium exceeds 6.5 mEq/liter more vigorous therapy is required. The clinical situation dictates the procedures to be employed. These include the intravenous administration of calcium chloride solution, sodium bicarbonate solution and/or the oral or parenteral administration of glucose with a rapid-acting insulin preparation. Cationic exchange resins such as sodium polystyrene sulfonate may be orally or rectally administered. Persistent hyperkalemia may require dialysis.

The development of hyperkalemia associated with potassium-sparing diuretics is accentuated in the presence of renal impairment (see CONTRAINDICATIONS section). Patients with mild renal functional impairment should not receive this drug without frequent and continuing monitoring of serum electrolytes. Cumulative drug effects may be observed in patients with impaired renal function. The renal

	AUC (0–48) ng*hrs/mL (±SD)	Cmax ng/mL (±SD)	Median Tmax hrs	Ae Mg (±SD)
triamterene	148.7 (87.9)	46.4 (29.4)	1.1	2.7 (1.4)
hydroxytriamterene sulfate	1865 (471)	720 (364)	1.3	19.7 (6.1)
hydrochlorothiazide	834 (177)	135.1 (35.7)	2.0	14.3 (3.8)

clearances of hydrochlorothiazide and the pharmacologically active metabolite of triamterene, the sulfate ester of hydroxytriamterene, have been shown to be reduced and the plasma levels increased following *Dyazide* administration to elderly patients and patients with impaired renal function.

Hyperkalemia has been reported in diabetic patients with the use of potassium-sparing agents even in the absence of apparent renal impairment. Accordingly, serum electrolytes must be frequently monitored if *Dyazide* is used in diabetic patients.

Metabolic or Respiratory Acidosis

Potassium-sparing therapy should also be avoided in severely ill patients in whom respiratory or metabolic acidosis may occur. Acidosis may be associated with rapid elevations in serum potassium levels. If *Dyazide* is employed, frequent evaluations of acid/base balance and serum electrolytes are necessary.

PRECAUTIONS

Diabetes

Caution should be exercised when administering *Dyazide* to patients with diabetes, since thiazides may cause hyperglycemia, glycosuria and alter insulin requirements in diabetes. Also, diabetes mellitus may become manifest during thiazide administration.

Impaired Hepatic Function

Thiazides should be used with caution in patients with impaired hepatic function. They can precipitate hepatic coma in patients with severe liver disease. Potassium depletion induced by the thiazide may be important in this connection. Administer *Dyazide* cautiously and be alert for such early signs of impending coma as confusion, drowsiness and tremor; if mental confusion increases discontinue *Dyazide* for a few days. Attention must be given to other factors that may precipitate hepatic coma, such as blood in the gastrointestinal tract or preexisting potassium depletion.

Hypokalemia

Hypokalemia is uncommon with *Dyazide*; but, should it develop, corrective measures should be taken such as potassium supplementation or increased intake of potassium-rich foods. Institute such measures cautiously with frequent determinations of serum potassium levels, especially in patients receiving digitalis or with a history of cardiac arrhythmias. If serious hypokalemia (serum potassium less than 3.0 mEq/L) is demonstrated by repeat serum potassium determinations, *Dyazide* should be discontinued and potassium chloride supplementation initiated. Less serious hypokalemia should be evaluated with regard to other coexisting conditions and treated accordingly.

Electrolyte Imbalance

Electrolyte imbalance, often encountered in such conditions as heart failure, renal disease or cirrhosis of the liver, may also be aggravated by diuretics and should be considered during *Dyazide* therapy when using high doses for prolonged periods or in patients on a salt-restricted diet. Serum determinations of electrolytes should be performed, and are particularly important if the patient is vomiting excessively or receiving fluids parenterally. Possible fluid and electrolyte imbalance may be indicated by such warning signs as: dry mouth, thirst, weakness, lethargy, drowsiness, restlessness, muscle pain or cramps, muscular fatigue, hypotension, oliguria, tachycardia and gastrointestinal symptoms.

Hypochloremia

Although any chloride deficit is generally mild and usually does not require specific treatment except under extraordinary circumstances (as in liver disease or renal disease), chloride replacement may be required in the treatment of metabolic alkalosis. Dilutional hyponatremia may occur in edematous patients in hot weather; appropriate therapy is water restriction, rather than administration of salt, except in rare instances when the hyponatremia is life threatening. In actual salt depletion, appropriate replacement is the therapy of choice.

Renal Stones

Triamterene has been found in renal stones in association with the other usual calculus components. *Dyazide* should be used with caution in patients with a history of renal stones.

Laboratory Tests

Serum Potassium: The normal adult range of serum potassium is 3.5 to 5.0 mEq per liter with 4.5 mEq often being used for a reference point. If hypokalemia should develop, corrective measures should be taken such as potassium supplementation or increased dietary intake of potassium-rich foods.

Institute such measures cautiously with frequent determinations of serum potassium levels. Potassium levels persistently above 6 mEq per liter require careful observation and treatment. Serum potassium levels do not necessarily indicate true body potassium concentration. A rise in plasma pH may cause a decrease in plasma potassium concentration and an increase in the intracellular potassium concentration. Discontinue corrective measures for hypokalemia immediately if laboratory determinations reveal an abnormal elevation of serum potassium. Discontinue *Dyazide* and substitute a thiazide diuretic alone until potassium levels return to normal.

Serum Creatinine and BUN: *Dyazide* may produce an elevated blood urea nitrogen level, creatinine level or both. This apparently is secondary to a reversible reduction of glomerular filtration rate or a depletion of intravascular fluid volume (prerenal azotemia) rather than renal toxicity; levels usually return to normal when *Dyazide* is discontinued. If azotemia increases, discontinue *Dyazide*. Periodic BUN or serum creatinine determinations should be made, especially in elderly patients and in patients with suspected or confirmed renal insufficiency.

Serum PBI: Thiazide may decrease serum PBI levels without sign of thyroid disturbance.

Parathyroid Function: Thiazides should be discontinued before carrying out tests for parathyroid function. Calcium excretion is decreased by thiazides. Pathologic changes in the parathyroid glands with hypercalcemia and hypophosphatemia have been observed in a few patients on prolonged thiazide therapy. The common complications of hyperparathyroidism such as bone resorption and peptic ulceration have not been seen.

Drug Interactions

Angiotensin-converting enzyme inhibitors: Potassium-sparing agents should be used with caution in conjunction with angiotensin-converting enzyme (ACE) inhibitors due to an increased risk of hyperkalemia.

Oral hypoglycemic drugs: Concurrent use with chlorpropamide may increase the risk of severe hyponatremia.

Nonsteroidal anti-inflammatory drugs: A possible interaction resulting in acute renal failure has been reported in a few patients on *Dyazide* when treated with indomethacin, a nonsteroidal anti-inflammatory agent. Caution is advised in administering nonsteroidal anti-inflammatory agents with *Dyazide.*

Lithium: Lithium generally should not be given with diuretics because they reduce its renal clearance and increase the risk of lithium toxicity. Read circulars for lithium preparations before use of such concomitant therapy with *Dyazide.*

Surgical considerations: Thiazides have been shown to decrease arterial responsiveness to norepinephrine (an effect attributed to loss of sodium). This diminution is not sufficient to preclude effectiveness of the pressor agent for therapeutic use. Thiazides have also been shown to increase the paralyzing effect of nondepolarizing muscle relaxants such as tubocurarine (an effect attributed to potassium loss); consequently caution should be observed in patients undergoing surgery.

Other Considerations: Concurrent use of hydrochlorothiazide with amphotericin B or corticosteroids or corticotropin (ACTH) may intensify electrolyte imbalance, particularly hypokalemia, although the presence of triamterene minimizes the hypokalemic effect.

Thiazides may add to or potentiate the action of other antihypertensive drugs. See INDICATIONS AND USAGE for concomitant use with other antihypertensive drugs.

The effect of oral anticoagulants may be decreased when used concurrently with hydrochlorothiazide; dosage adjustments may be necessary.

Dyazide may raise the level of blood uric acid; dosage adjustments of antigout medication may be necessary to control hyperuricemia and gout.

The following agents given together with triamterene may promote serum potassium accumulation and possibly result in hyperkalemia because of the potassium-sparing nature of triamterene, especially in patients with renal insufficiency: blood from blood bank (may contain up to 30 mEq of potassium per liter of plasma or up to 65 mEq per liter of whole blood when stored for more than 10 days); low-salt milk (may contain up to 60 mEq of potassium per liter); potassium-containing medications (such as parenteral penicillin G potassium); salt substitutes (most contain substantial amounts of potassium).

Exchange resins, such as sodium polystyrene sulfonate, whether administered orally or rectally, reduce serum potassium levels by sodium replacement of the potassium; fluid retention may occur in some patients because of the increased sodium intake.

Chronic or overuse of laxatives may reduce serum potassium levels by promoting excessive potassium loss from the intestinal tract; laxatives may interfere with the potassium-retaining effects of triamterene.

The effectiveness of methenamine may be decreased when used concurrently with hydrochlorothiazide because of alkalinization of the urine.

Continued on next page

Product information on these pages is effective as of August 2004. Further information is available at: GlaxoSmithKline, PO Box 13398, Research Triangle Park, NC 27709. 1-888-825-5249. Corporate Web Site: www.gsk.com

Dyazide—Cont.

Drug/Laboratory Test Interactions

Triamterene and quinidine have similar fluorescence spectra; thus, *Dyazide* will interfere with the fluorescent measurement of quinidine.

Carcinogenesis, Mutagenesis, Impairment of Fertility

Carcinogenesis

Long-term studies have not been conducted with *Dyazide* (the triamterene/hydrochlorothiazide combination), or with triamterene alone.

Hydrochlorothiazide: Two-year feeding studies in mice and rats, conducted under the auspices of the National Toxicology Program (NTP), treated mice and rats with doses of hydrochlorothiazide up to 600 and 100 mg/kg/day, respectively. On a body-weight basis, these doses are 600 times (in mice) and 100 times (in rats) the Maximum Recommended Human Dose (MRHD) for the hydrochlorothiazide component of *Dyazide* at 50 mg/day (or 1.0 mg/kg/day based on 50 kg individuals). On the basis of body-surface area, these doses are 56 times (in mice) and 21 times (in rats) the MRHD. These studies uncovered no evidence of carcinogenic potential of hydrochlorothiazide in rats or female mice, but there was equivocal evidence of hepatocarcinogenicity in male mice.

Mutagenesis

Studies of the mutagenic potential of *Dyazide* (the triamterene/hydrochlorothiazide combination), or of triamterene alone have not been performed.

Hydrochlorothiazide: Hydrochlorothiazide was not genotoxic in *in vitro* assays using strains TA 98, TA 100, TA 1535, TA 1537 and TA 1538 of *Salmonella typhimurium* (the Ames test); in the Chinese Hamster Ovary (CHO) test for chromosomal aberrations; or in *in vivo* assays using mouse germinal cell chromosomes, Chinese hamster bone marrow chromosomes, and the *Drosophila* sex-linked recessive lethal trait gene. Positive test results were obtained in the *in vitro* CHO Sister Chromatid Exchange (clastogenicity) test, and in the mouse Lymphoma Cell (mutagenicity) assays, using concentrations of hydrochlorothiazide of 43 to 1300 mcg/mL. Positive test results were also obtained in the *Aspergillus nidulans* nondisjunction assay, using an unspecified concentration of hydrochlorothiazide.

Impairment of Fertility

Studies of the effects of *Dyazide* (the triamterene/hydrochlorothiazide combination), or of triamterene alone on animal reproductive function have not been conducted.

Hydrochlorothiazide: Hydrochlorothiazide had no adverse effects on the fertility of mice and rats of either sex in studies wherein these species were exposed, via their diet, to doses of up to 100 and 4 mg/kg/day, respectively, prior to mating and throughout gestation. Corresponding multiples of the MRHD are 100 (mice) and 4 (rats) on the basis of body-weight and 9.4 (mice) and 0.8 (rats) on the basis of body-surface area.

Pregnancy: Category C

Teratogenic Effects

Dyazide: Animal reproduction studies to determine the potential for fetal harm by *Dyazide* have not been conducted. However, a One Generation Study in the rat approximated *Dyazide* composition by using a 1:1 ratio of triamterene to hydrochlorothiazide (30:30 mg/kg/day); there was no evidence of teratogenicity at those doses which were, on a body-weight basis, 15 and 30 times, respectively, the MRHD, and on the basis of body-surface area, 3.1 and 6.2 times, respectively, the MRHD.

The safe use of *Dyazide* in pregnancy has not been established since there are no adequate and well-controlled studies with *Dyazide* in pregnant women. *Dyazide* should be used during pregnancy only if the potential benefit justifies the risk to the fetus.

Triamterene: Reproduction studies have been performed in rats at doses as high as 20 times the MRHD on the basis of body-weight, and 6 times the human dose on the basis of body-surface area without evidence of harm to the fetus due to triamterene.

Because animal reproduction studies are not always predictive of human response, this drug should be used during pregnancy only if clearly needed.

Hydrochlorothiazide: Hydrochlorothiazide was orally administered to pregnant mice and rats during respective periods of major organogenesis at doses up to 3000 and 1000 mg/kg/day, respectively. At these doses, which are multiples of the MRHD equal to 3000 for mice and 1000 for rats, based on body-weight, and equal to 282 for mice and 206 for rats, based on body-surface area, there was no evidence of harm to the fetus.

There are, however, no adequate and well-controlled studies in pregnant women. Because animal reproduction studies are not always predictive of human response, this drug should be used during pregnancy only if clearly needed.

Nonteratogenic Effects —Thiazides and triamterene have been shown to cross the placental barrier and appear in cord blood. The use of thiazides and triamterene in pregnant women requires that the anticipated benefit be weighed against possible hazards to the fetus. These hazards include fetal or neonatal jaundice, pancreatitis, thrombocytopenia and possible other adverse reactions which have occurred in the adult.

Nursing Mothers —Thiazides and triamterene in combination have not been studied in nursing mothers. Triamterene appears in animal milk; this may occur in humans. Thiazides are excreted in human breast milk. If use of the combination drug product is deemed essential, the patient should stop nursing.

Pediatric Use —Safety and effectiveness in pediatric patients have not been established.

ADVERSE REACTIONS

Adverse effects are listed in decreasing order of frequency; however, the most serious adverse effects are listed first regardless of frequency. The serious adverse effects associated with *Dyazide* have commonly occurred in less than 0.1% of patients treated with this product.

Hypersensitivity: anaphylaxis, rash, urticaria, photosensitivity.

Cardiovascular: arrhythmia, postural hypotension.

Metabolic: diabetes mellitus, hyperkalemia, hyperglycemia, glycosuria, hyperuricemia, hypokalemia, hyponatremia, acidosis, hypochloremia.

Gastrointestinal: jaundice and/or liver enzyme abnormalities, pancreatitis, nausea and vomiting, diarrhea, constipation, abdominal pain.

Renal: acute renal failure (one case of irreversible renal failure has been reported), interstitial nephritis, renal stones composed primarily of triamterene, elevated BUN and serum creatinine, abnormal urinary sediment.

Hematologic: leukopenia, thrombocytopenia and purpura, megaloblastic anemia.

Musculoskeletal: muscle cramps.

Central Nervous System: weakness, fatigue, dizziness, headache, dry mouth.

Miscellaneous: impotence, sialadenitis.

Thiazides alone have been shown to cause the following additional adverse reactions:

Central Nervous System: paresthesias, vertigo.

Ophthalmic: xanthopsia, transient blurred vision.

Respiratory: allergic pneumonitis, pulmonary edema, respiratory distress.

Other: necrotizing vasculitis, exacerbation of lupus.

Hematologic: aplastic anemia, agranulocytosis, hemolytic anemia.

Neonate and infancy: thrombocytopenia and pancreatitis—rarely, in newborns whose mothers have received thiazides during pregnancy.

DOSAGE AND ADMINISTRATION

The usual dose of *Dyazide* is one or two capsules given once daily, with appropriate monitoring of serum potassium and of the clinical effect. (See WARNINGS, Hyperkalemia.)

OVERDOSAGE

Electrolyte imbalance is the major concern (see WARNINGS section). Symptoms reported include: polyuria, nausea, vomiting, weakness, lassitude, fever, flushed face and hyperactive deep tendon reflexes. If hypotension occurs, it may be treated with pressor agents such as levarterenol to maintain blood pressure. Carefully evaluate the electrolyte pattern and fluid balance. Induce immediate evacuation of the stomach through emesis or gastric lavage. There is no specific antidote.

Reversible acute renal failure following ingestion of 50 tablets of a product containing a combination of 50 mg triamterene and 25 mg hydrochlorothiazide has been reported.

Although triamterene is largely protein-bound (approximately 67%), there may be some benefit to dialysis in cases of overdosage.

HOW SUPPLIED

Capsules containing 25 mg hydrochlorothiazide and 37.5 mg triamterene, in bottles of 1000 capsules; in Single Unit Packages (unit-dose) of 100 (intended for institutional use only); in Patient-Pak™ unit-of-use bottles of 100.

They are supplied as follows:

NDC 0007-3650-21–Single Unit Packages (unit-dose) of 100 (intended for institutional use only).

NDC 0007-3650-22–in Patient-Pak™ unit-of-use bottles of 100.

NDC 0007-3650-30–bottles of 1000.

Store at controlled room temperature 20° to 25°C (68° to 77°F). Protect from light. Dispense in a tight, light-resistant container.

GlaxoSmithKline, Research Triangle Park, NC 27709

February 1999/DZ:L67

Shown in Product Identification Guide, page 315

ENGERIX-B® ℞

[in'jə-rix]

[Hepatitis B Vaccine (Recombinant)]

DESCRIPTION

ENGERIX-B [Hepatitis B Vaccine (Recombinant)] is a noninfectious recombinant DNA hepatitis B vaccine developed and manufactured by GlaxoSmithKline Biologicals. It contains purified surface antigen of the virus obtained by culturing genetically engineered *Saccharomyces cerevisiae* cells, which carry the surface antigen gene of the hepatitis B virus. The surface antigen expressed in *Saccharomyces cerevisiae* cells is purified by several physicochemical steps and formulated as a suspension of the antigen adsorbed on aluminum hydroxide. The procedures used to manufacture ENGERIX-B result in a product that contains no more than 5% yeast protein. No substances of human origin are used in its manufacture.

ENGERIX-B is supplied as a sterile suspension for intramuscular administration. The vaccine is ready for use without reconstitution; it must be shaken before administration since a fine white deposit with a clear colorless supernatant may form on storage.

Pediatric/Adolescent: Each 0.5-mL dose contains 10 mcg of hepatitis B surface antigen adsorbed on 0.25 mg aluminum as aluminum hydroxide. The pediatric/adolescent vaccine is formulated without preservatives. The pediatric formulation contains a trace amount of thimerosal (<0.5 mcg mercury) from the manufacturing process, sodium chloride (9 mg/mL), and phosphate buffers (disodium phosphate dihydrate, 0.98 mg/mL; sodium dihydrogen phosphate dihydrate, 0.71 mg/mL).

Adult: Each 1-mL adult dose contains 20 mcg of hepatitis B surface antigen adsorbed on 0.5 mg aluminum as aluminum hydroxide. The adult vaccine is formulated without preservatives. The adult formulation contains a trace amount of thimerosal (<1.0 mcg mercury) from the manufacturing process, sodium chloride (9 mg/mL), and phosphate buffers (disodium phosphate dihydrate, 0.98 mg/mL; sodium dihydrogen phosphate dihydrate, 0.71 mg/mL).

CLINICAL PHARMACOLOGY

Several hepatitis viruses are known to cause a systemic infection resulting in major pathologic changes in the liver (e.g., A, B, C, D, E, and G). The estimated lifetime risk of HBV infection in the United States varies from almost 100% for the highest-risk groups to less than 20% for the population as a whole.[1] Hepatitis B infection can have serious consequences including acute massive hepatic necrosis, chronic active hepatitis, and cirrhosis of the liver. Up to 90% of neonates and 6% to 10% of adults who are infected in the United States will become hepatitis B virus carriers.[1] It has been estimated that 200 to 300 million people in the world today are persistently infected with hepatitis B virus.[1] The Centers for Disease Control and Prevention (CDC) estimates that there are approximately 1 to 1.25 million chronic carriers of hepatitis B virus in the United States.[1] Those patients who become chronic carriers can infect others and are at increased risk of developing primary hepatocellular carcinoma. Among other factors, infection with hepatitis B may be the single most important factor for development of this carcinoma.[1,2]

Reduced Risk of Hepatocellular Carcinoma: According to the CDC, the hepatitis B vaccine is recognized as the first anti-cancer vaccine because it can prevent primary liver cancer.[3]

A clear link has been demonstrated between chronic hepatitis B infection and the occurrence of hepatocellular carcinoma. In a Taiwanese study, the institution of universal childhood immunization against hepatitis B virus has been shown to decrease the incidence of hepatocellular carcinoma among children.[4] In a Korean study in adult males, vaccination against hepatitis B virus has been shown to decrease the incidence of, and risk of, developing hepatocellular carcinoma in adults.[5]

Considering the serious consequences of infection, immunization should be considered for all persons at potential risk of exposure to the hepatitis B virus. Mothers infected with hepatitis B virus can infect their infants at, or shortly after, birth if they are carriers of the HBsAg antigen or develop an active infection during the third trimester of pregnancy. Infected infants usually become chronic carriers. Therefore, screening of pregnant women for hepatitis B is recommended.[1] Because a vaccination strategy limited to high-risk individuals has failed to substantially lower the overall incidence of hepatitis B infection, the Advisory Committee on Immunization Practices (ACIP) recommends vaccination of all persons from birth to age 18.[6] The Committee on Infectious Diseases of the American Academy of Pediatrics (AAP) has also endorsed universal infant immunization as part of a comprehensive strategy for the control of hepatitis B infection.[7] The AAP, American Academy of Family Physicians (AAFP), and American Medical Association (AMA) also recommend routine vaccination of adolescents 11 to 12 years of age who have not been vaccinated previously.[8] The AAP further recommends that providers administer hepatitis B vaccine to all previously unvaccinated adolescents.[9] (See INDICATIONS AND USAGE.) There is no specific treatment for acute hepatitis B infection. However, those who develop anti-HBs antibodies after active infection are usually protected against subsequent infection. Antibody titers ≥10 mIU/mL against HBsAg are recognized as conferring protection against hepatitis B.[1] Seroconversion is defined as antibody titers ≥1 mIU/mL.

Protective Efficacy: Protective efficacy with ENGERIX-B has been demonstrated in a clinical trial in neonates at high risk of hepatitis B infection.[10,11] Fifty-eight neonates born of mothers who were both HBsAg and HBeAg positive were given ENGERIX-B (10 mcg at 0, 1, and 2 months) without concomitant hepatitis B immune globulin. Two infants became chronic carriers in the 12-month follow-up period after initial inoculation. Assuming an expected carrier rate of 70%, the protective efficacy rate against the chronic carrier state during the first 12 months of life was 95%.

Immunogenicity in Neonates: Immunization with 10 mcg at 0, 1, and 6 months of age produced seroconversion in 100% of infants by month 7, with a geometric mean antibody titer (GMT) of 713 mIU/mL (N = 52), and the seroprotection rate was 97%.

Clinical trials indicate that administration of hepatitis B immune globulin at birth does not alter the response to ENGERIX-B.

Immunization with 10 mcg at 0, 1, and 2 months of age produced a seroprotection rate of 96% in infants by month 4, with a GMT among seroconverters of 210 mIU/mL (N = 311); an additional dose at month 12 produced a GMT among seroconverters of 2,941 mIU/mL at month 13 (N = 126).

Immunogenicity in Pediatric Patients: In clinical trials with 242 children aged 6 months to, and including, 10 years given 10 mcg at months 0, 1, and 6, the seroprotection rate was 98% 1 to 2 months after the third dose; the GMT of seroconverters was 4,023 mIU/mL.

In a separate clinical trial including both children and adolescents aged 5 to 16 years, 10 mcg of ENGERIX-B was administered at 0, 1, and 6 months (N = 181) or 0, 12, and 24 months (N = 161). Immediately before the third dose of vaccine, seroprotection was achieved in 92.3% of subjects vaccinated on the 0-, 1-, and 6-month schedule and 88.8% of subjects on the 0-, 12-, and 24-month schedule (117.9 mIU/mL versus 162.1 mIU/mL, respectively, p = 0.18). One month following the third dose, seroprotection was achieved in 99.5% of children vaccinated on the 0-, 1-, and 6-month schedule compared to 98.1% of those on the 0-, 12-, and 24-month schedule. GMTs were higher (p = 0.02) for children receiving vaccine on the 0-, 1-, and 6-month schedule compared to those on the 0-, 12-, and 24-month schedule (5,687.4 mIU/mL versus 3,158.7 mIU/mL, respectively). The clinical relevance of this finding is unknown.

Immunogenicity in Adolescents: In clinical trials with healthy adolescent subjects 11 through 19 years of age, immunization with 10 mcg using a 0-, 1-, and 6-month schedule produced a seroprotection rate of 97% at month 8 (N = 119) with a GMT of 1,989 mIU/mL (N = 118, 95% confidence intervals = 1,318-3,020). Immunization with 20 mcg using a 0-, 1-, and 6-month schedule produced a seroprotection rate of 99% at month 8 (N = 122) with a GMT of 7,672 mIU/mL (N = 122, 95% confidence intervals = 5,248-10,965).

Immunogenicity in Healthy Adults and Adolescents: Clinical trials in healthy adult and adolescent subjects have shown that following a course of 3 doses of 20 mcg ENGERIX-B given according to the ACIP-recommended schedule of injections at months 0, 1, and 6, the seroprotection (antibody titers ≥10 mIU/mL) rate for all individuals was 79% at month 6 and 96% at month 7; the GMT for seroconverters at month 7 was 2,204 mIU/mL. On an alternate schedule (injections at months 0, 1, and 2) designed for certain populations (e.g., neonates born of hepatitis B–infected mothers, individuals who have or might have been recently exposed to the virus, and certain travelers to high-risk areas. See INDICATIONS AND USAGE), 99% of all individuals were seroprotected at month 3 and remained protected through month 12. On the alternate schedule, an additional dose at 12 months produced a GMT for seroconverters at month 13 of 9,163 mIU/mL.

Immunogenicity in Older Subjects: Among older subjects given 20 mcg at months 0, 1, and 6, the seroprotection rate 1 month after the third dose was 88%. However, as with other hepatitis B vaccines, in adults over 40 years of age, ENGERIX-B vaccine produced anti-HBs titers that were lower than those in younger adults (GMT among seroconverters 1 month after the third 20-mcg dose with a 0-, 1-, and 6-month schedule: 610 mIU/mL for individuals over 40 years of age, N = 50).

Immunogenicity in Subjects with Chronic Hepatitis C: In a clinical trial of subjects with chronic hepatitis C, 31 subjects received ENGERIX-B on the usual 0-, 1-, and 6-month schedule. All subjects responded with seroprotective titers. The GMT of anti-HBs was 1,260 mIU/mL (95% CI: 709-2,237).

Immunogenicity in Hemodialysis Patients: Hemodialysis patients given hepatitis B vaccines respond with lower titers,[12] which remain at protective levels for shorter durations than in normal subjects. In a study in which patients on chronic hemodialysis (mean time on dialysis was 24 months; N = 562) received 40 mcg of the plasma-derived vaccine at months 0, 1, and 6, approximately 50% of patients achieved antibody titers ≥10 mIU/mL.[12] Since a fourth dose of ENGERIX-B given to healthy adults at month 12 following the 0-, 1-, and 2-month schedule resulted in a substantial increase in the GMT (see above), a 4-dose regimen was studied in hemodialysis patients. In a clinical trial of adults who had been on hemodialysis for a mean of 56 months (N = 43), 67% of patients were seroprotected 2 months after the last dose of 40 mcg of ENGERIX-B (2 × 20 mcg) given on a 0-, 1-, 2-, and 6-month schedule; the GMT among seroconverters was 93 mIU/mL.

Interchangeability With Other Hepatitis B Vaccines: Recombinant DNA vaccines are produced in yeast by expression of a hepatitis B virus gene sequence that codes for the hepatitis B surface antigen. Like plasma-derived vaccine, the yeast-derived vaccines are protein particles visible by electron microscopy and have hepatitis B surface antigen epitopes as determined by monoclonal antibody analyses. Yeast-derived vaccines have been shown by in vitro analyses to induce antibodies (anti-HBs) which are immunologically comparable by epitope specificity and binding affinity to antibodies induced by plasma-derived vaccine.[13] In cross-absorption studies, no differences were detected in the spectra of antibodies induced in man to plasma-derived or to yeast-derived hepatitis B vaccines.[13]

Additionally, patients immunized approximately 3 years previously with plasma-derived vaccine and whose antibody titers were <100 mIU/mL (GMT: 35 mIU/mL; range: 9-94) were given a 20-mcg dose of ENGERIX-B. All patients, including 2 who had not responded to the plasma-derived vaccine, showed a response to ENGERIX-B (GMT: 5,069 mIU/mL; range: 624-15,019). There have been no clinical studies in which a 3-dose vaccine series was initiated with a plasma-derived hepatitis B vaccine and completed with ENGERIX-B, or vice versa. However, because the in vitro and in vivo studies described above indicate the comparability of the antibody produced in response to plasma-derived vaccine and ENGERIX-B, it should be possible to interchange the use of ENGERIX-B and plasma-derived vaccines (but see CONTRAINDICATIONS).

A controlled study (N = 48) demonstrated that completion of a course of immunization with 1 dose of ENGERIX-B (20 mcg, month 6) following 2 doses of RECOMBIVAX HB®* (10 mcg, months 0 and 1) produced a similar GMT (4,077 mIU/mL) to immunization with 3 doses of RECOMBIVAX HB (10 mcg, months 0, 1, and 6; 2,654 mIU/mL). Thus, ENGERIX-B can be used to complete a vaccination course initiated with RECOMBIVAX HB.[14]

Other Clinical Studies: In 1 study, 4 of 244 (1.6%) adults (homosexual men) at high risk of contracting hepatitis B virus became infected during the period prior to completion of 3 doses of ENGERIX-B (20 mcg at 0, 1, and 6 months).[15] No additional patients became infected during the 18-month follow-up period after completion of the immunization course.

INDICATIONS AND USAGE

ENGERIX-B is indicated for immunization against infection caused by all known subtypes of hepatitis B virus. As hepatitis D (caused by the delta virus) does not occur in the absence of hepatitis B infection, it can be expected that hepatitis D will also be prevented by ENGERIX-B vaccination.

ENGERIX-B will not prevent hepatitis caused by other agents, such as hepatitis A, C, and E viruses, or other pathogens known to infect the liver.

Immunization is recommended in persons of all ages, especially those who are, or will be, at increased risk of exposure to hepatitis B virus,[1] for example:

- Infants, Including Those Born of HBsAg-Positive Mothers (*See DOSAGE AND ADMINISTRATION.*)
- Adolescents (*See CLINICAL PHARMACOLOGY.*)
- Healthcare Personnel: *Dentists and oral surgeons. Dental, medical, and nursing students. Physicians, surgeons, and podiatrists. Nurses. Paramedical and ambulance personnel and custodial staff who may be exposed to the virus via blood or other patient specimens. Dental hygienists and dental nurses. Laboratory and blood bank personnel handling blood, blood products, and other patient specimens. Hospital cleaning staff who handle waste.*
- Selected Patients and Patient Contacts: *Patients and staff in hemodialysis units and hematology/oncology units. Patients requiring frequent and/or large volume blood transfusions or clotting factor concentrates (e.g., persons with hemophilia, thalassemia, sickle cell anemia, cirrhosis). Clients (residents) and staff of institutions for the mentally handicapped. Classroom contacts of deinstitutionalized mentally handicapped persons who have persistent hepatitis B surface antigenemia and who show aggressive behavior. Household and other intimate contacts of persons with persistent hepatitis B surface antigenemia.*
- Subpopulations With a Known High Incidence of the Disease, *such as: Alaskan Eskimos. Pacific Islanders. Indochinese immigrants. Haitian immigrants. Refugees from other HBV-endemic areas. All infants of women born in areas where the infection is highly endemic.*
- Individuals With Chronic Hepatitis C: *Risk factors for hepatitis C are similar to those for hepatitis B. Consequently, immunization with hepatitis B vaccine is recommended for individuals with chronic hepatitis C.*
- Persons Who May Be Exposed to the Hepatitis B Virus by Travel to High-Risk Areas (*See ACIP Guidelines, 1990.*)
- Military Personnel Identified as Being at Increased Risk
- Morticians and Embalmers
- Persons at Increased Risk of the Disease Due to Their Sexual Practices,[1,16] *such as: Persons with more than 1 sexual partner in a 6-month period. Persons who have contracted a sexually transmitted disease. Homosexually active males. Female prostitutes.*
- Prisoners
- Users of Illicit Injectable Drugs
- Others: *Police and fire department personnel who render first aid or medical assistance, and any others who, through their work or personal life-style, may be exposed to the hepatitis B virus. Adoptees from countries of high HBV endemicity.*

Use With Other Vaccines: The ACIP states that, in general, simultaneous administration of certain live and inactivated pediatric vaccines has not resulted in impaired antibody responses or increased rates of adverse reactions.[17] Separate sites and syringes should be used for simultaneous administration of injectable vaccines.

CONTRAINDICATIONS

Hypersensitivity to any component of the vaccine, including yeast, is a contraindication (see DESCRIPTION). This vaccine is contraindicated in patients with previous hypersensitivity to any hepatitis B-containing vaccine.

WARNINGS

The vial stopper is latex-free. The tip cap and the rubber plunger of the needleless prefilled syringes contain dry natural latex rubber that may cause allergic reactions in latex sensitive individuals.

Hepatitis B has a long incubation period. Hepatitis B vaccination may not prevent hepatitis B infection in individuals who had an unrecognized hepatitis B infection at the time of vaccine administration. Additionally, it may not prevent infection in individuals who do not achieve protective antibody titers.

PRECAUTIONS

General: As with other vaccines, although a moderate or severe febrile illness is sufficient reason to postpone vaccination, minor illnesses such as mild upper respiratory infections with or without low-grade fever are not contraindications.[17]

Prior to immunization, the patient's medical history should be reviewed. The physician should review the patient's immunization history for possible vaccine sensitivity, previous vaccination-related adverse reactions, and occurrence of any adverse event–related symptoms and/or signs in order to determine the existence of any contraindication to immunization with ENGERIX-B and to allow an assessment of benefits and risks. Epinephrine injection (1:1,000) and other appropriate agents used for the control of immediate allergic reactions must be immediately available should an acute anaphylactic reaction occur.

A separate sterile syringe and needle or a sterile disposable unit should be used for each individual patient to prevent transmission of hepatitis or other infectious agents from one person to another. Needles should be disposed of properly and should not be recapped.

Special care should be taken to prevent injection into a blood vessel.

As with any vaccine administered to immunosuppressed persons or persons receiving immunosuppressive therapy, the expected immune response may not be obtained. For individuals receiving immunosuppressive therapy, deferral of vaccination for at least 3 months after therapy may be considered.[17]

Multiple Sclerosis: Although no causal relationship has been established, rare instances of exacerbation of multiple sclerosis have been reported following administration of hepatitis B vaccines and other vaccines. In persons with multiple sclerosis, the benefit of immunization for prevention of hepatitis B infection and sequelae must be weighed against the risk of exacerbation of the disease.

Information for the Patient:

Patients, parents, or guardians should be informed of the potential benefits and risks of the vaccine, and of the importance of completing the immunization series. As with any vaccine, it is important when a subject returns for the next dose in a series that he or she be questioned concerning occurrence of any symptoms and/or signs of an adverse reaction after a previous dose of the same vaccine. Patients, parents, or guardians should be told to report severe or unusual adverse reactions to their healthcare provider.

The parent or guardian should be given the Vaccine Information Materials, which are required by the National Childhood Vaccine Injury Act of 1986 to be given prior to immunization.

Drug Interactions:

For information regarding simultaneous administration with other vaccines, refer to INDICATIONS AND USAGE.

Carcinogenesis, Mutagenesis, Impairment of Fertility:

ENGERIX-B has not been evaluated for carcinogenic or mutagenic potential, or for impairment of fertility.

Pregnancy: Pregnancy Category C. Animal reproduction studies have not been conducted with ENGERIX-B. It is also not known whether ENGERIX-B can cause fetal harm when administered to a pregnant woman or can affect reproduction capacity. ENGERIX-B should be given to a pregnant woman only if clearly needed.

Nursing Mothers: It is not known whether ENGERIX-B is excreted in human milk. Because many drugs are excreted in human milk, caution should be exercised when ENGERIX-B is administered to a nursing woman.

Pediatric Use: ENGERIX-B has been shown to be well tolerated and highly immunogenic in infants and children of all ages. Newborns also respond well; maternally transferred antibodies do not interfere with the active immune response to the vaccine. (See CLINICAL PHARMACOLOGY for seroconversion rates and titers in neonates and children. See DOSAGE AND ADMINISTRATION for recommended pediatric dosage and for recommended dosage for infants born of HBsAg-positive mothers.)

ADVERSE REACTIONS

ENGERIX-B is generally well tolerated. As with any vaccine, however, it is possible that expanded commercial use of the vaccine could reveal rare adverse reactions.

Ten double-blind studies involving 2,252 subjects showed no significant difference in the frequency or severity of adverse experiences between ENGERIX-B and plasma-derived vaccines. In 36 clinical studies, a total of 13,495 doses of ENGERIX-B were administered to 5,071 healthy adults and children who were initially seronegative for hepatitis B markers, and healthy neonates. All subjects were monitored for 4 days post-administration. Frequency of adverse expe-

Continued on next page

Product information on these pages is effective as of August 2004. Further information is available at: GlaxoSmithKline, PO Box 13398, Research Triangle Park, NC 27709. 1-888-825-5249. Corporate Web Site: www.gsk.com

Engerix-B—Cont.

riences tended to decrease with successive doses of ENGERIX-B. Using a symptom checklist,[†] the most frequently reported adverse reactions were injection site soreness (22%) and fatigue[†] (14%). Other reactions are listed below.

Incidence 1% to 10% of Injections:
Local Reactions at Injection Site: Induration; erythema; swelling.
Body as a Whole: Fever (>37.5°C).
Nervous System: Headache;[†] dizziness.[†]

[†] Parent or guardian completed forms for children and neonates. Neonatal checklist did not include headache, fatigue, or dizziness.

Incidence <1% of Injections:
Local Reactions at Injection Site: Pain; pruritus; ecchymosis.
Body as a Whole: Sweating; malaise; chills; weakness; flushing; tingling.
Cardiovascular System: Hypotension.
Respiratory System: Influenza-like symptoms; upper respiratory tract illnesses.
Gastrointestinal System: Nausea; anorexia; abdominal pain/cramps; vomiting; constipation; diarrhea.
Lymphatic System: Lymphadenopathy.
Musculoskeletal System: Pain/stiffness in arm, shoulder, or neck; arthralgia; myalgia; back pain.
Skin and Appendages: Rash; urticaria; petechiae; pruritus; erythema.
Nervous System: Somnolence; insomnia; irritability; agitation.

Postmarketing Reports: Additional adverse experiences have been reported with the commercial use of ENGERIX-B. Those listed below are to serve as alerting information to physicians.
Hypersensitivity: Anaphylaxis; erythema multiforme including Stevens-Johnson syndrome; angioedema; arthritis. An apparent hypersensitivity syndrome (serum sickness–like) of delayed onset has been reported days to weeks after vaccination, including: arthralgia/arthritis (usually transient), fever, and dermatologic reactions such as urticaria, erythema multiforme, ecchymoses, and erythema nodosum (see CONTRAINDICATIONS).
Cardiovascular System: Tachycardia/palpitations.
Respiratory System: Bronchospasm including asthma-like symptoms.
Gastrointestinal System: Abnormal liver function tests; dyspepsia.
Nervous System: Migraine; syncope; paresis; neuropathy including hypoesthesia, paresthesia, Guillain-Barré syndrome and Bell's palsy, transverse myelitis; optic neuritis; multiple sclerosis; seizures.
Hematologic: Thrombocytopenia.
Skin and Appendages: Eczema; purpura; herpes zoster; erythema nodosum; alopecia.
Special Senses: Conjunctivitis; keratitis; visual disturbances; vertigo; tinnitus; earache.

Reporting Adverse Events: The National Childhood Vaccine Injury Act requires that the manufacturer and lot number of the vaccine administered be recorded by the healthcare provider in the vaccine recipient's permanent medical record, along with the date of administration of the vaccine and the name, address, and title of the person administering the vaccine.[18] The Act further requires the healthcare provider to report to the US Department of Health and Human Services via VAERS the occurrence following immunization of any event set forth in the Vaccine Injury Table including: Anaphylaxis or anaphylactic shock within 4 hours, encephalopathy or encephalitis within 72 hours, or any sequelae thereof (including death).[18,19] In addition, any event considered a contraindication to further doses should be reported. The VAERS toll-free number is 1-800-822-7967.

DOSAGE AND ADMINISTRATION

Injection: ENGERIX-B should be administered by intramuscular injection. *Do not inject intravenously or intradermally.* In adults, the injection should be given in the deltoid region but it may be preferable to inject in the anterolateral thigh in neonates and infants, who have smaller deltoid muscles. ENGERIX-B should not be administered in the gluteal region; such injections may result in suboptimal response. The attending physician should determine final selection of the injection site and needle size, depending upon the patient's age and the size of the target muscle. A 1-inch, 23-gauge needle is sufficient to penetrate the anterolateral thigh in infants younger than 12 months of age. A 5/8-inch, 25-gauge needle may be used to administer the vaccine in the deltoid region of toddlers and children up to, and including, 19 years of age. The 1-inch, 23-gauge needle is appropriate for use in older children and adults.[17]

ENGERIX-B may be administered subcutaneously to persons at risk of hemorrhage (e.g., hemophiliacs). However, hepatitis B vaccines administered subcutaneously are known to result in lower GMTs. Additionally, when other aluminum-adsorbed vaccines have been administered subcutaneously, an increased incidence of local reactions including subcutaneous nodules has been observed. Therefore, subcutaneous administration should be used only in persons who are at risk of hemorrhage with intramuscular injections.

Table 1. Recommended Dosage and Administration Schedules

Group	Dose	Schedules
Infants born of:		
HBsAg-negative mothers	10 mcg/0.5mL	0, 1, 6 months
HBsAg-positive mothers	10 mcg/0.5mL	0, 1, 6 months
Children:		
Birth through 10 years of age	10 mcg/0.5 mL	0, 1, 6 months
Adolescents:		
11 through 19 years of age	10 mcg/0.5 mL	0, 1, 6 months
Adults (>19 years)	20 mcg/1.0 mL	0, 1, 6 months
Adult hemodialysis	40 mcg/2.0 mL*	0, 1, 2, 6 months

*Two × 20 mcg in 1 or 2 injections.

Table 2. Alternate Dosage and Administration Schedules

Group	Dose	Schedules
Infants born of:		
HBsAg-positive mothers	10 mcg/0.5 mL	0, 1, 2, 12 months*
Children:		
Birth through 10 years of age	10 mcg/0.5 mL	0, 1, 2, 12 months*
5 through 10 years of age	10 mcg/0.5 mL	0, 12, 24 months[†]
Adolescents:		
11 through 16 years of age	10 mcg/0.5 mL	0, 12, 24 months[†]
11 through 19 years of age	20 mcg/1.0 mL	0, 1, 6 months
11 through 19 years of age	20 mcg/1.0 mL	0, 1, 2, 12 months[†]
Adults (>19 years)	20 mcg/1.0 mL	0, 1, 2, 12 months[†]

*This schedule is designed for certain populations (e.g., neonates born of hepatitis B–infected mothers, others who have or might have been recently exposed to the virus, certain travelers to high-risk areas. See INDICATIONS AND USAGE). On this alternate schedule, an additional dose at 12 months is recommended for prolonged maintenance of protective titers.
[†] For children and adolescents for whom an extended administration schedule is acceptable based on risk of exposure.

Preparation for Administration: *Shake well before withdrawal and use.* Parenteral drug products should be inspected visually for particulate matter or discoloration prior to administration. With thorough agitation, ENGERIX-B is a slightly turbid white suspension. Discard if it appears otherwise. The vaccine should be used as supplied; no dilution is necessary. The full recommended dose of the vaccine should be used. Any vaccine remaining in a single-dose vial should be discarded.

Dosing Schedules: The usual immunization regimen (see Table 1) consists of 3 doses of vaccine given according to the following schedule: first dose: at elected date; second dose: 1 month later; third dose: 6 months after first dose.
[See table 1 above]
For hemodialysis patients, in whom vaccine-induced protection is less complete and may persist only as long as antibody levels remain above 10 mIU/mL, the need for booster doses should be assessed by annual antibody testing. 40 mcg (2 × 20 mcg) booster doses with ENGERIX-B should be given when antibody levels decline below 10 mIU/mL.[1] Data show individuals given a booster with ENGERIX-B achieve high antibody titers. (See CLINICAL PHARMACOLOGY.)
There are alternate dosing and administration schedules which may be used for specific populations (see Table 2 and accompanying explanations).
[See table 2 above]

Booster Vaccinations: Whenever administration of a booster dose is appropriate, the dose of ENGERIX-B is 10 mcg for children 10 years of age and younger, 20 mcg for adolescents 11 through 19 years of age, and 20 mcg for adults. Studies have demonstrated a substantial increase in antibody titers after ENGERIX-B booster vaccination following an initial course with both plasma- and yeast-derived vaccines. (See CLINICAL PHARMACOLOGY.)
See previous section for discussion on booster vaccination for adult hemodialysis patients.

Known or Presumed Exposure to Hepatitis B Virus: Unprotected individuals with known or presumed exposure to the hepatitis B virus (e.g., neonates born of infected mothers, others experiencing percutaneous or permucosal exposure) should be given hepatitis B immune globulin (HBIG) in addition to ENGERIX-B in accordance with ACIP recommendations[1] and with the package insert for HBIG. ENGERIX-B can be given on either dosing schedule (see above).

STORAGE
Store refrigerated between 2° and 8°C (36° and 46°F). *Do not freeze*; discard if product has been frozen. Do not dilute to administer.

HOW SUPPLIED

ENGERIX-B is supplied as a slightly turbid white suspension in vials and prefilled TIP-LOK® syringes.

Adult Dose
20 mcg/mL in Single-Dose Vials in packages of 1 and 25 vials
NDC 58160-857-01 (package of 1)
NDC 58160-857-16 (package of 25)
20 mcg/mL in Single-Dose Prefilled Disposable TIP-LOK Syringes (packaged without needles)
NDC 58160-857-46 (package of 5)
NDC 58160-857-50 (package of 25)

Pediatric/Adolescent Doses
10 mcg/0.5 mL in Single-Dose Vials in packages of 1 and 10 vials
NDC 58160-856-01 (package of 1)
NDC 58160-856-11 (package of 10)
10 mcg/0.5 mL in Single-Dose Prefilled Disposable TIP-LOK Syringes (packaged without needles)
NDC 58160-856-46 (package of 5)
NDC 58160-856-50 (package of 25)
10 mcg/0.5 mL in Single-Dose Prefilled Disposable TIP-LOK Syringes with 1-inch 25-gauge SAFETYGLIDE™ needles
NDC 58160-856-56 (package of 25)
10 mcg/0.5 mL in Single-Dose Prefilled Disposable TIP-LOK Syringes with 1-inch 23-gauge SAFETYGLIDE needles
NDC 58160-856-58 (package of 25)
10 mcg/0.5 mL in Single-Dose Prefilled Disposable TIP-LOK Syringes with 5/8-inch 25-gauge SAFETYGLIDE needles
NDC 58160-856-57 (package of 25)

REFERENCES

1. Centers for Disease Control and Prevention. Hepatitis B. In: Atkinson W, Wolfe C, Humiston S, Nelson R, eds. *Epidemiology and prevention of vaccine-preventable diseases.* 6th ed. Atlanta, GA: Public Health Foundation; 2000:207-229. **2.** Beasley RP, Hwang L-Y, Stevens CE, et al. Efficacy of hepatitis B immune globulin for prevention of perinatal transmission of hepatitis B virus carrier state: Final report of a randomized double-blind, placebo-controlled trial. *Hepatology* 1983;3(2):135-141. **3.** Centers for Disease Control and Prevention. New vaccine information materials for hepatitis B, haemophilus influenzae type B (Hib), and varicella (chickenpox) vaccines, and revised vaccine information materials for measles, mumps, rubella (MMR) vaccines. *Federal Register* February 23, 1999;64(35):9044-9045. **4.** Chang M-H, Chen C-J, Lai M-S, et al. Universal hepatitis B vaccination in Taiwan and the incidence of hepatocellular carcinoma in children. *N Engl J Med* 1997;336(26):1855-1859. **5.** Lee M-S, Kim D-H, Kim H, et al. Hepatitis B vaccination and reduced risk of primary liver cancer among male adults: A cohort study in Korea. *Int J Epidemiol* 1998;27(2):316-319. **6.** Centers for Disease Control and Prevention. Effectiveness of a Seventh Grade school entry vaccination requirement — Statewide and Orange County, Florida, 1997-1998. *MMWR* 1998;47(34):711-715. **7.** American Academy of Pediatrics. Universal hepatitis B immunization. *Pediatrics* 1992;89(4):795-800. **8.** Centers for Disease Control and Prevention. Immunization of adolescents: Recommendations of the Advisory Committee on Immunization Practices, the American Academy of Pediatrics, the American Academy of Family Physicians, and the American Medical Association. *MMWR* 1996;45(RR-13):1-16. **9.** American Academy of Pediatrics. Immunization of adolescents: Recommendations of the Advisory Committee on Immunization Practices, the American Academy of Pediatrics, the American Academy of Family Physicians, and the American Medical Association. *Pediatrics* 1997;99(3):479-488. **10.** André FE and Safary A. Clinical experience with a yeast-derived hepatitis B vaccine. In: Zuckerman AJ, ed. *Viral hepatitis and liver disease.* New York, NY: Alan R Liss, Inc.; 1988:1025-1030. **11.** Poovorawan Y, Sanpavat S, Pongpunlert W, et al. Protective efficacy of a recombinant DNA hepatitis B vaccine in neonates of HBe antigen-positive mothers. *JAMA* 1989;261(22):3278-3281. **12.** Stevens CE, Alter HJ, Taylor PE, et al. Hepatitis B vaccine in patients receiving hemodialysis. *N Engl J Med*

1984;311(8):496-501. **13.** Hauser P, Voet P, Simoen E, et al. Immunological properties of recombinant HBsAg produced in yeast. *Postgrad Med J* 1987;63(Suppl 2):83-91. **14.** Bush LM, Moonsammy GI, Boscia JA. Evaluation of initiating a hepatitis B vaccination schedule with one vaccine and completing it with another. *Vaccine* 1991;9(11):807-809. **15.** Goilav C, Prinsen H, Safary A, et al. Immunization of homosexual men with a recombinant DNA vaccine against hepatitis B: Immunogenicity and protection. In: Zuckerman AJ, ed. *Viral hepatitis and liver disease.* New York, NY: Alan R Liss, Inc.; 1988:1057-1058. **16.** Centers for Disease Control and Prevention. 1998 Guidelines for treatment of sexually transmitted diseases. *MMWR* 1998;47(RR-1):102. **17.** Centers for Disease Control and Prevention. General Recommendations on Immunization: Recommendations of the Advisory Committee on Immunization Practices (ACIP). *MMWR* 1994;43(RR-1):1-38. **18.** Centers for Disease Control. National Childhood Vaccine Injury Act: Requirements for permanent vaccination records and for reporting of selected events after vaccination. *MMWR* 1988;37 (13):197-200. **19.** Public Health Service. National Vaccine Injury Compensation Program: Revision of the vaccine injury table. *Federal Register* February 8, 1995;60(26):7694.

*Yeast-derived, Hepatitis B Vaccine, MSD.

Manufactured by GlaxoSmithKline Biologicals
Rixensart, Belgium, US License No. 1617
Distributed by GlaxoSmithKline, Research Triangle Park, NC 27709
ENGERIX-B and TIP-LOK are registered trademarks of GlaxoSmithKline
RECOMBIVAX HB is a registered trademark of Merck & Co.
SAFETYGLIDE is a trademark of Becton, Dickinson and Company.

August 2003/EB:L34

Shown in Product Identification Guide, page 315

EPIVIR® Tablets ℞
[*ĕp' ə-vir*]
(lamivudine tablets)

EPIVIR® Oral Solution ℞
(lamivudine oral solution)

WARNING
LACTIC ACIDOSIS AND SEVERE HEPATOMEGALY WITH STEATOSIS, INCLUDING FATAL CASES, HAVE BEEN REPORTED WITH THE USE OF NUCLEOSIDE ANALOGUES ALONE OR IN COMBINATION, INCLUDING LAMIVUDINE AND OTHER ANTIRETROVIRALS (SEE WARNINGS).
EPIVIR TABLETS AND ORAL SOLUTION (USED TO TREAT HIV INFECTION) CONTAIN A HIGHER DOSE OF THE ACTIVE INGREDIENT (LAMIVUDINE) THAN EPIVIR-HBV® TABLETS AND ORAL SOLUTION (USED TO TREAT CHRONIC HEPATITIS B). PATIENTS WITH HIV INFECTION SHOULD RECEIVE ONLY DOSING FORMS APPROPRIATE FOR TREATMENT OF HIV (SEE WARNINGS AND PRECAUTIONS).
SEVERE ACUTE EXACERBATIONS OF HEPATITIS B HAVE BEEN REPORTED IN PATIENTS WHO ARE CO-INFECTED WITH HEPATITIS B VIRUS (HBV) AND HIV AND HAVE DISCONTINUED EPIVIR. HEPATIC FUNCTION SHOULD BE MONITORED CLOSELY WITH BOTH CLINICAL AND LABORATORY FOLLOW-UP FOR AT LEAST SEVERAL MONTHS IN PATIENTS WHO DISCONTINUE EPIVIR AND ARE CO-INFECTED WITH HIV AND HBV. IF APPROPRIATE, INITIATION OF ANTI-HEPATITIS B THERAPY MAY BE WARRANTED (SEE WARNINGS).

DESCRIPTION

EPIVIR (also known as 3TC) is a brand name for lamivudine, a synthetic nucleoside analogue with activity against human immunodeficiency virus-1 (HIV-1) and hepatitis B virus (HBV). The chemical name of lamivudine is (2R,cis)-4-amino-1-(2-hydroxymethyl-1,3-oxathiolan-5-yl)-(1H)-pyrimidin-2-one. Lamivudine is the (-)enantiomer of a dideoxy analogue of cytidine. Lamivudine has also been referred to as (-)2′,3′-dideoxy, 3′-thiacytidine. It has a molecular formula of $C_8H_{11}N_3O_3S$ and a molecular weight of 229.3.

Lamivudine is a white to off-white crystalline solid with a solubility of approximately 70 mg/mL in water at 20°C.

EPIVIR Tablets are for oral administration. Each 150-mg film-coated tablet contains 150 mg of lamivudine and the inactive ingredients hypromellose, magnesium stearate, microcrystalline cellulose, polyethylene glycol, polysorbate 80, sodium starch glycolate, and titanium dioxide.

Each 300-mg film-coated tablet contains 300 mg of lamivudine and the inactive ingredients black iron oxide, hypromellose, magnesium stearate, microcrystalline cellulose, polyethylene glycol, polysorbate 80, sodium starch glycolate, and titanium dioxide.

EPIVIR Oral Solution is for oral administration. One milliliter (1 mL) of EPIVIR Oral Solution contains 10 mg of lamivudine (10 mg/mL) in an aqueous solution and the inactive ingredients artificial strawberry and banana flavors, citric acid (anhydrous), methylparaben, propylene glycol, propylparaben, sodium citrate (dihydrate), and sucrose (200 mg).

MICROBIOLOGY

Mechanism of Action: Lamivudine is a synthetic nucleoside analogue. Intracellularly, lamivudine is phosphorylated to its active 5′-triphosphate metabolite, lamivudine triphosphate (L-TP). The principal mode of action of L-TP is the inhibition of HIV-1 reverse transcriptase (RT) via DNA chain termination after incorporation of the nucleoside analogue into viral DNA. L-TP is a weak inhibitor of mammalian DNA polymerases α and β, and mitochondrial DNA polymerase γ.

Antiviral Activity In Vitro: The in vitro activity of lamivudine against HIV-1 was assessed in a number of cell lines (including monocytes and fresh human peripheral blood lymphocytes) using standard susceptibility assays. IC_{50} values (50% inhibitory concentrations) were in the range of 2 nM to 15 µM. Lamivudine had anti-HIV-1 activity in all acute virus-cell infections tested. In HIV-1–infected MT-4 cells, lamivudine in combination with zidovudine at various ratios exhibited synergistic antiretroviral activity. The relationship between in vitro susceptibility of HIV-1 to lamivudine and the inhibition of HIV-1 replication in humans has not been established. Please see the EPIVIR-HBV package insert for information regarding the inhibitory activity of lamivudine against HBV.

Drug Resistance: Lamivudine-resistant variants of HIV-1 have been selected in vitro. Genotypic analysis showed that the resistance was due to a specific amino acid substitution in the HIV-1 reverse transcriptase at codon 184 changing the methionine residue to either isoleucine or valine.

HIV-1 strains resistant to both lamivudine and zidovudine have been isolated from patients. Susceptibility of clinical isolates to lamivudine and zidovudine was monitored in controlled clinical trials. In patients receiving lamivudine monotherapy or combination therapy with lamivudine plus zidovudine, HIV-1 isolates from most patients became phenotypically and genotypically resistant to lamivudine within 12 weeks. In some patients harboring zidovudine-resistant virus at baseline, phenotypic sensitivity to zidovudine was restored by 12 weeks of treatment with lamivudine and zidovudine. Combination therapy with lamivudine plus zidovudine delayed the emergence of mutations conferring resistance to zidovudine.

Mutations in the HBV polymerase YMDD motif have been associated with reduced susceptibility of HBV to lamivudine in vitro. In studies of non-HIV-infected patients with chronic hepatitis B, HBV isolates with YMDD mutations were detected in some patients who received lamivudine daily for 6 months or more, and were associated with evidence of diminished treatment response; similar HBV mutants have been reported in HIV-infected patients who received lamivudine-containing antiretroviral regimens in the presence of concurrent infection with hepatitis B virus (see PRECAUTIONS and EPIVIR-HBV package insert).

Cross-Resistance: Lamivudine-resistant HIV-1 mutants were cross-resistant to didanosine (ddI) and zalcitabine (ddC). In some patients treated with zidovudine plus didanosine or zalcitabine, isolates resistant to multiple reverse transcriptase inhibitors, including lamivudine, have emerged.

Genotypic and Phenotypic Analysis of On-Therapy HIV-1 Isolates From Patients With Virologic Failure (see INDICATIONS AND USAGE: Description of Clinical Studies): The clinical relevance of genotypic and phenotypic changes associated with lamivudine therapy has not been fully established.

Study EPV20001: Fifty-three of 554 (10%) patients enrolled in EPV20001 were identified as virological failures (plasma HIV-1 RNA level ≥400 copies/mL) by Week 48. Twenty-eight patients were randomized to the lamivudine once-daily treatment group and 25 to the lamivudine twice-daily treatment group. The median baseline plasma HIV-1 RNA levels of patients in the lamivudine once-daily group and lamivudine twice-daily group were 4.9 $\log_{10}$ copies/mL and 4.6 $\log_{10}$ copies/mL, respectively.

Genotypic analysis of on-therapy isolates from 22 patients identified as virologic failures in the lamivudine once-daily group showed that isolates from 0/22 patients contained treatment-emergent mutations associated with zidovudine resistance (M41L, D67N, K70R, L210W, T215Y/F, or K219Q/E), isolates from 10/22 patients contained treatment-emergent mutations associated with efavirenz resistance (L100I, K101E, K103N, V108I, or Y181C), and isolates from 8/22 patients contained a treatment-emergent lamivudine resistance-associated mutation (M184I or M184V).

Genotypic analysis of on-therapy isolates from patients (n = 22) in the lamivudine twice-daily treatment group showed that isolates from 1/22 patients contained treatment-emergent zidovudine resistance mutations, isolates from 7/22 contained treatment-emergent efavirenz resistance mutations, and isolates from 5/22 contained treatment-emergent lamivudine resistance mutations.

Phenotypic analysis of baseline-matched on-therapy HIV-1 isolates from patients (n = 13) receiving lamivudine once daily showed that isolates from 12/13 patients were susceptible to zidovudine; isolates from 8/13 patients exhibited a 25- to 295-fold decrease in susceptibility to efavirenz, and isolates from 7/13 patients showed an 85- to 299-fold decrease in susceptibility to lamivudine.

Phenotypic analysis of baseline-matched on-therapy HIV-1 isolates from patients (n = 13) receiving lamivudine twice daily showed that isolates from all 13 patients were susceptible to zidovudine; isolates from 3/13 patients exhibited a 21- to 342-fold decrease in susceptibility to efavirenz, and isolates from 4/13 patients exhibited a 29- to 159-fold decrease in susceptibility to lamivudine.

Study EPV40001: Fifty patients received zidovudine 300 mg twice daily plus abacavir 300 mg twice daily plus lamivudine 300 mg once daily and 50 patients received zidovudine 300 mg plus abacavir 300 mg plus lamivudine 150 mg all twice daily. The median baseline plasma HIV-1 RNA levels for patients in the 2 groups were 4.79 $\log_{10}$ copies/mL and 4.83 $\log_{10}$ copies/mL, respectively. Fourteen of 50 patients in the lamivudine once-daily treatment group and 9 of 50 patients in the lamivudine twice-daily group were identified as virologic failures.

Genotypic analysis of on-therapy HIV-1 isolates from patients (n = 9) in the lamivudine once-daily treatment group showed that isolates from 6 patients had abacavir and/or lamivudine resistance-associated mutation M184V alone. On-therapy isolates from patients (n = 6) receiving lamivudine twice daily showed that isolates from 2 patients had M184V alone, and isolates from 2 patients harbored the M184V mutation in combination with zidovudine resistance-associated mutations.

Phenotypic analysis of on-therapy isolates from patients (n = 6) receiving lamivudine once daily showed that HIV-1 isolates from 4 patients exhibited a 32- to 53-fold decrease in susceptibility to lamivudine. HIV-1 isolates from these 6 patients were susceptible to zidovudine.

Phenotypic analysis of on-therapy isolates from patients (n = 4) receiving lamivudine twice daily showed that HIV-1 isolates from 1 patient exhibited a 45-fold decrease in susceptibility to lamivudine and a 4.5-fold decrease in susceptibility to zidovudine.

CLINICAL PHARMACOLOGY

Pharmacokinetics in Adults: The steady-state pharmacokinetic properties of the EPIVIR 300-mg tablet once daily for 7 days compared to the EPIVIR 150-mg tablet twice daily for 7 days were assessed in a crossover study in 60 healthy volunteers. EPIVIR 300 mg once daily resulted in lamivudine exposures that were similar to EPIVIR 150 mg twice daily with respect to plasma $AUC_{24,ss}$; however, $C_{max,ss}$ was 66% higher and the trough value was 53% lower compared to the 150-mg twice-daily regimen. Intracellular lamivudine triphosphate exposures in peripheral blood mononuclear cells were also similar with respect to $AUC_{24,ss}$ and $C_{max24,ss}$; however, trough values were lower compared to the 150-mg twice-daily regimen. Inter-subject variability was greater for intracellular lamivudine triphosphate concentrations versus lamivudine plasma trough concentrations. The clinical significance of observed differences for both plasma lamivudine concentrations and intracellular lamivudine triphosphate concentrations is not known.

The pharmacokinetic properties of lamivudine have been studied in asymptomatic, HIV-infected adult patients after administration of single intravenous (IV) doses ranging from 0.25 to 8 mg/kg, as well as single and multiple (twice-daily regimen) oral doses ranging from 0.25 to 10 mg/kg.

The pharmacokinetic properties of lamivudine have also been studied as single and multiple oral doses ranging from 5 mg to 600 mg/day administered to HBV-infected patients.

Absorption and Bioavailability: Lamivudine was rapidly absorbed after oral administration in HIV-infected patients. Absolute bioavailability in 12 adult patients was 86% ± 16% (mean ± SD) for the 150-mg tablet and 87% ± 13% for the oral solution. After oral administration of 2 mg/kg twice a day to 9 adults with HIV, the peak serum lamivudine concentration (C_{max}) was 1.5 ± 0.5 mcg/mL (mean ± SD). The area under the plasma concentration versus time curve (AUC) and C_{max} increased in proportion to oral dose over the range from 0.25 to 10 mg/kg.

An investigational 25-mg dosage form of lamivudine was administered orally to 12 asymptomatic, HIV-infected patients on 2 occasions, once in the fasted state and once with food (1,099 kcal; 75 grams fat, 34 grams protein, 72 grams carbohydrate). Absorption of lamivudine was slower in the fed state (T_{max}: 3.2 ± 1.3 hours) compared with the fasted state (T_{max}: 0.9 ± 0.3 hours); C_{max} in the fed state was 40% ± 23% (mean ± SD) lower than in the fasted state. There was no significant difference in systemic exposure (AUC∞) in the fed and fasted states; therefore, EPIVIR Tablets and Oral Solution may be administered with or without food.

The accumulation ratio of lamivudine in HIV-positive asymptomatic adults with normal renal function was 1.50 following 15 days of oral administration of 2 mg/kg twice daily.

Distribution: The apparent volume of distribution after IV administration of lamivudine to 20 patients was 1.3 ± 0.4 L/kg, suggesting that lamivudine distributes into extravascular spaces. Volume of distribution was independent of dose and did not correlate with body weight.

Binding of lamivudine to human plasma proteins is low (<36%). In vitro studies showed that, over the concentra-

Continued on next page

Product information on these pages is effective as of August 2004. Further information is available at: GlaxoSmithKline, PO Box 13398, Research Triangle Park, NC 27709. 1-888-825-5249. Corporate Web Site: www.gsk.com

Epivir—Cont.

tion range of 0.1 to 100 mcg/mL, the amount of lamivudine associated with erythrocytes ranged from 53% to 57% and was independent of concentration.

Metabolism: Metabolism of lamivudine is a minor route of elimination. In man, the only known metabolite of lamivudine is the trans-sulfoxide metabolite. Within 12 hours after a single oral dose of lamivudine in 6 HIV-infected adults, 5.2% ± 1.4% (mean ± SD) of the dose was excreted as the trans-sulfoxide metabolite in the urine. Serum concentrations of this metabolite have not been determined.

Elimination: The majority of lamivudine is eliminated unchanged in urine by active organic cationic secretion. In 9 healthy subjects given a single 300-mg oral dose of lamivudine, renal clearance was 199.7 ± 56.9 mL/min (mean ± SD). In 20 HIV-infected patients given a single IV dose, renal clearance was 280.4 ± 75.2 mL/min (mean ± SD), representing 71% ± 16% (mean ± SD) of total clearance of lamivudine.

In most single-dose studies in HIV-infected patients, HBV-infected patients, or healthy subjects with serum sampling for 24 hours after dosing, the observed mean elimination half-life ($t_{1/2}$) ranged from 5 to 7 hours. In HIV-infected patients, total clearance was 398.5 ± 69.1 mL/min (mean ± SD). Oral clearance and elimination half-life were independent of dose and body weight over an oral dosing range from 0.25 to 10 mg/kg.

Special Populations: *Adults with Impaired Renal Function:* The pharmacokinetic properties of lamivudine have been determined in a small group of HIV-infected adults with impaired renal function (Table 1).

[See table 1 above]

Table 1. Pharmacokinetic Parameters (Mean ± SD) After a Single 300-mg Oral Dose of Lamivudine in 3 Groups of Adults With Varying Degrees of Renal Function

Parameter	Creatinine Clearance Criterion (Number of Subjects)		
	>60 mL/min (n = 6)	10-30 mL/min (n = 4)	<10 mL/min (n = 6)
Creatinine clearance (mL/min)	111 ± 14	28 ± 8	6 ± 2
C_{max} (mcg/mL)	2.6 ± 0.5	3.6 ± 0.8	5.8 ± 1.2
AUC∞ (mcg•hr/mL)	11.0 ± 1.7	48.0 ± 19	157 ± 74
Cl/F (mL/min)	464 ± 76	114 ± 34	36 ± 11

Exposure (AUC∞), C_{max}, and half-life increased with diminishing renal function (as expressed by creatinine clearance). Apparent total oral clearance (Cl/F) of lamivudine decreased as creatinine clearance decreased. T_{max} was not significantly affected by renal function. Based on these observations, it is recommended that the dosage of lamivudine be modified in patients with renal impairment (see DOSAGE AND ADMINISTRATION).

Based on a study in otherwise healthy subjects with impaired renal function, hemodialysis increased lamivudine clearance from a mean of 64 to 88 mL/min; however, the length of time of hemodialysis (4 hours) was insufficient to significantly alter mean lamivudine exposure after a single-dose administration. Therefore, it is recommended, following correction of dose for creatinine clearance, that no additional dose modification be made after routine hemodialysis. It is not known whether lamivudine can be removed by peritoneal dialysis or continuous (24-hour) hemodialysis.

The effects of renal impairment on lamivudine pharmacokinetics in pediatric patients are not known.

Adults with Impaired Hepatic Function: The pharmacokinetic properties of lamivudine have been determined in adults with impaired hepatic function. Pharmacokinetic parameters were not altered by diminishing hepatic function; therefore, no dose adjustment for lamivudine is required for patients with impaired hepatic function. Safety and efficacy of lamivudine have not been established in the presence of decompensated liver disease.

Pediatric Patients: For pharmacokinetic properties of lamivudine in pediatric patients, see PRECAUTIONS: Pediatric Use.

Gender: There are no significant gender differences in lamivudine pharmacokinetics.

Race: There are no significant racial differences in lamivudine pharmacokinetics.

Drug Interactions: No clinically significant alterations in lamivudine or zidovudine pharmacokinetics were observed in 12 asymptomatic HIV-infected adult patients given a single dose of zidovudine (200 mg) in combination with multiple doses of lamivudine (300 mg q 12 hr).

Lamivudine and trimethoprim/sulfamethoxazole (TMP/SMX) were coadministered to 14 HIV-positive patients in a single-center, open-label, randomized, crossover study. Each patient received treatment with a single 300-mg dose of lamivudine and TMP 160 mg/SMX 800 mg once a day for 5 days with concomitant administration of lamivudine 300 mg with the fifth dose in a crossover design. Coadministration of TMP/SMX with lamivudine resulted in an increase of 44% ± 23% (mean ± SD) in lamivudine AUC∞, a decrease of 29% ± 13% in lamivudine oral clearance, and a decrease of 30% ± 36% in lamivudine renal clearance. The pharmacokinetic properties of TMP and SMX were not altered by coadministration with lamivudine.

Lamivudine and zalcitabine may inhibit the intracellular phosphorylation of one another. Therefore, use of lamivudine in combination with zalcitabine is not recommended.

There was no significant pharmacokinetic interaction between lamivudine and interferon alfa in a study of 19 healthy male subjects.

INDICATIONS AND USAGE

EPIVIR in combination with other antiretroviral agents is indicated for the treatment of HIV infection (see Description of Clinical Studies).

Description of Clinical Studies: The use of EPIVIR is based on the results of clinical studies in HIV-infected patients in combination regimens with other antiretroviral agents. Information from trials with clinical endpoints or a combination of CD4+ cell counts and HIV-1 RNA measurements is included below as documentation of the contribution of lamivudine to a combination regimen in controlled trials.

Clinical Endpoint Study in Adults: B3007 (CAESAR) was a multicenter, double-blind, placebo-controlled study comparing continued current therapy (zidovudine alone [62% of patients] or zidovudine with didanosine or zalcitabine [38% of patients]) to the addition of EPIVIR or EPIVIR plus an investigational non-nucleoside reverse transcriptase inhibitor (NNRTI), randomized 1:2:1. A total of 1,816 HIV-infected adults with 25 to 250 CD4+ cells/mm^3 (median = 122 cells/mm^3) at baseline were enrolled: median age was 36 years, 87% were male, 84% were nucleoside-experienced, and 16% were therapy-naive. The median duration on study was 12 months. Results are summarized in Table 2.

[See table 2 above]

Table 2. Number of Patients (%) With At Least One HIV Disease Progression Event or Death

Endpoint	Current Therapy (n = 460)	EPIVIR plus Current Therapy (n = 896)	EPIVIR plus a NNRTI* plus Current Therapy (n = 460)
HIV progression or death	90 (19.6%)	86 (9.6%)	41 (8.9%)
Death	27 (5.9%)	23 (2.6%)	14 (3.0%)

*An investigational non-nucleoside reverse transcriptase inhibitor not approved in the United States.

Surrogate Endpoint Studies in Adults: Dual Nucleoside Analogue Studies: Principal clinical trials in the initial development of lamivudine compared lamivudine/zidovudine combinations against zidovudine monotherapy or against zidovudine plus zalcitabine. These studies demonstrated the antiviral effect of lamivudine in a 2-drug combination. More recent uses of lamivudine in treatment of HIV infection incorporate it into multiple-drug regimens containing at least 3 antiretroviral drugs for enhanced viral suppression.

Dose Regimen Comparison Surrogate Endpoint Studies in Therapy-Naive Adults: EPV20001 was a multicenter, double-blind, controlled study in which patients were randomized 1:1 to receive EPIVIR 300 mg once daily or EPIVIR 150 mg twice daily, in combination with zidovudine 300 mg twice daily and efavirenz 600 mg once daily. A total of 554 antiretroviral treatment-naive HIV-infected adults enrolled: male (79%), Caucasian (50%), median age of 35 years, baseline CD4+ cell counts of 69 to 1,089 cells/mm^3 (median = 362 cells/mm^3), and median baseline plasma HIV-1 RNA of 4.66 $\log_{10}$ copies/mL. Outcomes of treatment through 48 weeks are summarized in Figure 1 and Table 3.

[See figure 1 at top of next column]

[See table 3 above]

Table 3. Outcomes of Randomized Treatment Through 48 Weeks (Intent-to-Treat)

Outcome	EPIVIR 300 mg Once Daily plus RETROVIR plus Efavirenz (n = 278)	EPIVIR 150 mg Twice Daily plus RETROVIR plus Efavirenz (n = 276)
Responder*	67%	65%
Virologic failure†	8%	8%
Discontinued due to clinical progression	<1%	0%
Discontinued due to adverse events	6%	12%
Discontinued due to other reasons‡	18%	14%

*Achieved confirmed plasma HIV-1 RNA <400 copies/mL and maintained through 48 weeks.

†Achieved suppression but rebounded by Week 48, discontinued due to virologic failure, insufficient viral response according to the investigator, or never suppressed through Week 48.

‡Includes consent withdrawn, lost to followup, protocol violation, data outside the study-defined schedule, and randomized but never initiated treatment.

The proportions of patients with HIV-1 RNA <50 copies/mL (via Roche Ultrasensitive assay) through Week 48 were 61% for patients receiving EPIVIR 300 mg once daily and 63% for patients receiving EPIVIR 150 mg twice daily. Median increases in CD4+ cell counts were 144 cells/mm^3 at Week 48 in patients receiving EPIVIR 300 mg once daily and 146 cells/mm^3 for patients receiving EPIVIR 150 mg twice daily.

A small, randomized, open-label pilot study, EPV40001, was conducted in Thailand. A total of 159 treatment-naive adult patients (male 32%, Asian 100%, median age 30 years, baseline median CD4+ cell count 380 cells/mm^3, median plasma HIV-1 RNA 4.8 $\log_{10}$ copies/mL) were enrolled. Two of the treatment arms in this study provided a comparison between lamivudine 300 mg once daily (n = 54) and lamivudine 150 mg twice daily (n = 52), each in combination with zidovudine 300 mg twice daily and abacavir 300 mg twice daily. In intent-to-treat analyses of 48-week data, the proportions of patients with HIV-1 RNA below 400 copies/mL were 61% (33/54) in the group randomized to once-daily lamivudine and 75% (39/52) in the group randomized to receive all 3 drugs twice daily; the proportions with HIV-1 RNA below 50 copies/mL were 54% (29/54) in the once-daily lamivudine group and 67% (35/52) in the all-twice-daily group; and the median increases in CD4+ cell counts were 166 cells/mm^3 in the once-daily lamivudine group and 216 cells/mm^3 in the all-twice-daily group.

Figure 1: Virologic Response Through Week 48, EPV20001*† (Intent-to-Treat)

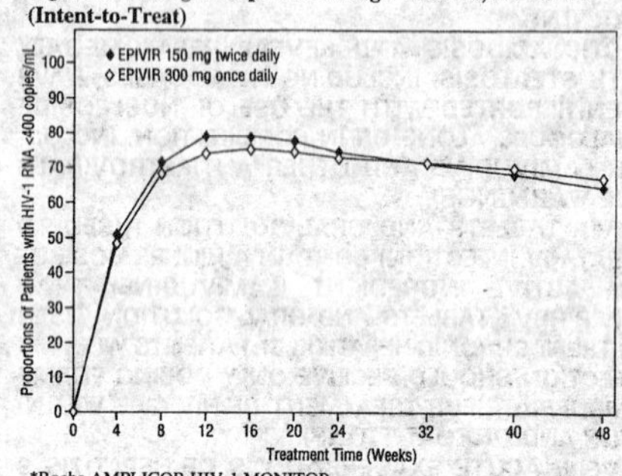

*Roche AMPLICOR HIV-1 MONITOR.

†Responders at each visit are patients who had achieved and maintained HIV-1 RNA <400 copies/mL without discontinuation by that visit.

Clinical Endpoint Study in Pediatric Patients: ACTG300 was a multicenter, randomized, double-blind study that provided for comparison of EPIVIR plus RETROVIR® (zidovudine) to didanosine monotherapy. A total of 471 symptomatic, HIV-infected therapy-naive (≤56 days of antiretroviral therapy) pediatric patients were enrolled in these 2 treatment arms. The median age was 2.7 years (range 6 weeks to 14 years), 58% were female, and 86% were non-Caucasian. The mean baseline CD4+ cell count was 868 cells/mm^3 (mean: 1,060^3 and range: 0 to 4,650 cells/mm^3 for patients ≤5 years of age; mean 419 cells/mm^3 and range: 0 to 1,555 cells/mm^3 for patients >5 years of age) and the mean baseline plasma HIV-1 RNA was 5.0 $\log_{10}$ copies/mL. The median duration on study was 10.1 months for the patients receiving EPIVIR plus RETROVIR and 9.2 months for patients receiving didanosine monotherapy. Results are summarized in Table 4.

[See table 4 at top of next page]

CONTRAINDICATIONS

EPIVIR Tablets and Oral Solution are contraindicated in patients with previously demonstrated clinically significant hypersensitivity to any of the components of the products.

WARNINGS

In pediatric patients with a history of prior antiretroviral nucleoside exposure, a history of pancreatitis, or other significant risk factors for the development of pancreatitis, EPIVIR should be used with caution. Treatment with EPIVIR should be stopped immediately if clinical signs, symptoms, or laboratory abnormalities suggestive of pancreatitis occur (see ADVERSE REACTIONS).

Lactic Acidosis/Severe Hepatomegaly with Steatosis: Lactic acidosis and severe hepatomegaly with steatosis, including fatal cases, have been reported with the use of nucleoside analogues alone or in combination, including lamivudine and other antiretrovirals. A majority of these cases have been in women. Obesity and prolonged nucleoside exposure may be risk factors. Particular caution should be exercised when administering EPIVIR to any patient with known risk factors for liver disease; however, cases have also been reported in patients with no known risk factors. Treatment with EPIVIR should be suspended in any patient who develops clinical or laboratory findings suggestive of lactic acidosis or pronounced hepatotoxicity (which may include hepatomegaly and steatosis even in the absence of marked transaminase elevations).

Important Differences Among Lamivudine-Containing Products: EPIVIR Tablets and Oral Solution contain a higher dose of the same active ingredient (lamivudine) than in EPIVIR-HBV Tablets and Oral Solution. EPIVIR-HBV was developed for patients with chronic hepatitis B. The formulation and dosage of lamivudine in EPIVIR-HBV are not appropriate for patients dually infected with HIV and HBV. Lamivudine has not been adequately studied for treatment of chronic hepatitis B in patients dually infected with HIV and HBV. If treatment with EPIVIR-HBV is prescribed for chronic hepatitis B for a patient with unrecognized or untreated HIV infection, rapid emergence of HIV resistance is likely to result because of the subtherapeutic dose and the inappropriateness of monotherapy HIV treatment. If a decision is made to administer lamivudine to patients dually infected with HIV and HBV, EPIVIR Tablets, EPIVIR Oral Solution, or COMBIVIR® (lamivudine/zidovudine) Tablets should be used as part of an appropriate combination regimen. COMBIVIR (a fixed-dose combination tablet of lamivudine and zidovudine) should not be administered concomitantly with EPIVIR, EPIVIR-HBV, RETROVIR, or TRIZIVIR®.

Posttreatment Exacerbations of Hepatitis: In clinical trials in non-HIV-infected patients treated with lamivudine for chronic hepatitis B, clinical and laboratory evidence of exacerbations of hepatitis have occurred after discontinuation of lamivudine. These exacerbations have been detected primarily by serum ALT elevations in addition to re-emergence of HBV DNA. Although most events appear to have been self-limited, fatalities have been reported in some cases. Similar events have been reported from post-marketing experience after changes from lamivudine-containing HIV treatment regimens to non-lamivudine-containing regimens in patients infected with both HIV and HBV. The causal relationship to discontinuation of lamivudine treatment is unknown. Patients should be closely monitored with both clinical and laboratory followup for at least several months after stopping treatment. There is insufficient evidence to determine whether re-initiation of lamivudine alters the course of posttreatment exacerbations of hepatitis.

PRECAUTIONS

Patients with Impaired Renal Function: Reduction of the dosage of EPIVIR is recommended for patients with impaired renal function (see CLINICAL PHARMACOLOGY and DOSAGE AND ADMINISTRATION).

Patients with HIV and Hepatitis B Virus Coinfection: Safety and efficacy of lamivudine have not been established for treatment of chronic hepatitis B in patients dually infected with HIV and HBV. In non-HIV-infected patients treated with lamivudine for chronic hepatitis B, emergence of lamivudine-resistant HBV has been detected and has been associated with diminished treatment response (see EPIVIR-HBV package insert for additional information). Emergence of hepatitis B virus variants associated with resistance to lamivudine has also been reported in HIV-infected patients who have received lamivudine-containing antiretroviral regimens in the presence of concurrent infection with hepatitis B virus. Posttreatment exacerbations of hepatitis have also been reported (see WARNINGS).

Differences Between Dosing Regimens: Trough levels of lamivudine in plasma and of intracellular lamivudine triphosphate were lower with once-daily dosing than with twice-daily dosing (see CLINICAL PHARMACOLOGY). The clinical significance of this observation is not known.

Fat Redistribution: Redistribution/accumulation of body fat including central obesity, dorsocervical fat enlargement (buffalo hump), peripheral wasting, facial wasting, breast enlargement, and "cushingoid appearance" have been observed in patients receiving antiretroviral therapy. The mechanism and long-term consequences of these events are currently unknown. A causal relationship has not been established.

Information for Patients: EPIVIR is not a cure for HIV infection and patients may continue to experience illnesses associated with HIV infection, including opportunistic infections. Patients should remain under the care of a physician when using EPIVIR. Patients should be advised that the use of EPIVIR has not been shown to reduce the risk of transmission of HIV to others through sexual contact or blood contamination.

Table 4. Number of Patients (%) Reaching a Primary Clinical Endpoint (Disease Progression or Death)

Endpoint	EPIVIR plus RETROVIR (n = 236)	Didanosine (n = 235)
HIV disease progression or death (total)	15 (6.4%)	37 (15.7%)
Physical growth failure	7 (3.0%)	6 (2.6%)
Central nervous system deterioration	4 (1.7%)	12 (5.1%)
CDC Clinical Category C	2 (0.8%)	8 (3.4%)
Death	2 (0.8%)	11 (4.7%)

Patients should be advised that EPIVIR Tablets and Oral Solution contain a higher dose of the same active ingredient (lamivudine) as EPIVIR-HBV Tablets and Oral Solution. If a decision is made to include lamivudine in the HIV treatment regimen of a patient dually infected with HIV and HBV, the formulation and dosage of lamivudine in EPIVIR (not EPIVIR-HBV) should be used.

Patients co-infected with HIV and HBV should be informed that deterioration of liver disease has occurred in some cases when treatment with lamivudine was discontinued. Patients should be advised to discuss any changes in regimen with their physician.

Patients should be advised that the long-term effects of EPIVIR are unknown at this time.

EPIVIR Tablets and Oral Solution are for oral ingestion only.

Patients should be advised of the importance of taking EPIVIR with combination therapy on a regular dosing schedule and to avoid missing doses.

Parents or guardians should be advised to monitor pediatric patients for signs and symptoms of pancreatitis.

Patients should be informed that redistribution or accumulation of body fat may occur in patients receiving antiretroviral therapy and that the cause and long-term health effects of these conditions are not known at this time.

Diabetic patients should be advised that each 15-mL dose of EPIVIR Oral Solution contains 3 grams of sucrose.

Drug Interactions: Lamivudine is predominantly eliminated in the urine by active organic cationic secretion. The possibility of interactions with other drugs administered concurrently should be considered, particularly when their main route of elimination is active renal secretion via the organic cationic transport system (e.g., trimethoprim).

TMP 160 mg/SMX 800 mg once daily has been shown to increase lamivudine exposure (AUC) by 44% (see CLINICAL PHARMACOLOGY). No change in dose of either drug is recommended. There is no information regarding the effect on lamivudine pharmacokinetics of higher doses of TMP/SMX such as those used to treat *Pneumocystis carinii* pneumonia. No data are available regarding interactions with other drugs that have renal clearance mechanisms similar to that of lamivudine.

Lamivudine and zalcitabine may inhibit the intracellular phosphorylation of one another. Therefore, use of lamivudine in combination with zalcitabine is not recommended.

Carcinogenesis, Mutagenesis, and Impairment of Fertility: Long-term carcinogenicity studies with lamivudine in mice and rats showed no evidence of carcinogenic potential at exposures up to 10 times (mice) and 58 times (rats) those observed in humans at the recommended therapeutic dose for HIV infection. Lamivudine was not active in a microbial mutagenicity screen or an in vitro cell transformation assay, but showed weak in vitro mutagenic activity in a cytogenetic assay using cultured human lymphocytes and in the mouse lymphoma assay. However, lamivudine showed no evidence of in vivo genotoxic activity in the rat at oral doses of up to 2,000 mg/kg, producing plasma levels of 35 to 45 times those in humans at the recommended dose for HIV infection. In a study of reproductive performance, lamivudine administered to rats at doses up to 4,000 mg/kg/day, producing plasma levels 47 to 70 times those in humans, revealed no evidence of impaired fertility and no effect on the survival, growth, and development to weaning of the offspring.

Pregnancy: Pregnancy Category C. Reproduction studies have been performed in rats and rabbits at orally administered doses up to 4,000 mg/kg/day and 1,000 mg/kg/day, respectively, producing plasma levels up to approximately 35 times that for the adult HIV dose. No evidence of teratogenicity due to lamivudine was observed. Evidence of early embryolethality was seen in the rabbit at exposure levels similar to those observed in humans, but there was no indication of this effect in the rat at exposure levels up to 35 times that in humans. Studies in pregnant rats and rabbits showed that lamivudine is transferred to the fetus through the placenta.

In 2 clinical studies conducted in South Africa, pharmacokinetic measurements were performed on samples from pregnant women who received lamivudine beginning at week 38 of gestation (10 women who received 150 mg twice daily in combination with zidovudine and 10 who received lamivudine 300 mg twice daily without other antiretrovirals) or beginning at week 36 of gestation (16 women who received lamivudine 150 mg twice daily in combination with zidovudine). These studies were not designed or powered to provide efficacy information. Lamivudine pharmacokinetics in the pregnant women were similar to those obtained following birth and in non-pregnant adults. Lamivudine concentrations were generally similar in maternal, neonatal, and cord serum samples. In a subset of subjects from whom amniotic fluid specimens were obtained following natural rupture of membranes, amniotic fluid concentrations of lamivudine ranged from 1.2 to 2.5 mcg/mL (150 mg twice daily) and 2.1 to 5.2 mcg/mL (300 mg twice daily) and were typically greater than 2 times the maternal serum levels. See the ADVERSE REACTIONS section for the limited late-pregnancy safety information available from these studies. Lamivudine should be used during pregnancy only if the potential benefits outweigh the risks.

Antiretroviral Pregnancy Registry: To monitor maternal-fetal outcomes of pregnant women exposed to lamivudine, a Pregnancy Registry has been established. Physicians are encouraged to register patients by calling 1-800-258-4263.

Nursing Mothers: The Centers for Disease Control and Prevention recommend that HIV-infected mothers not breastfeed their infants to avoid risking postnatal transmission of HIV infection.

A study in lactating rats administered 45 mg/kg of lamivudine showed that lamivudine concentrations in milk were slightly greater than those in plasma. Lamivudine is also excreted in human milk. Samples of breast milk obtained from 20 mothers receiving lamivudine monotherapy (300 mg twice daily) or combination therapy (150 mg lamivudine twice daily and 300 mg zidovudine twice daily) had measurable concentrations of lamivudine.

Because of both the potential for HIV transmission and the potential for serious adverse reactions in nursing infants, **mothers should be instructed not to breastfeed if they are receiving lamivudine.**

Pediatric Use: *HIV:* Limited, uncontrolled pharmacokinetic and safety data are available from administration of lamivudine (and zidovudine) to 36 infants up to 1 week of age in 2 studies in South Africa. In these studies, lamivudine clearance was substantially reduced in 1-week-old neonates relative to pediatric patients (>3 months of age) studied previously. There is insufficient information to establish the time course of changes in clearance between the immediate neonatal period and the age-ranges >3 months old. See the ADVERSE REACTIONS section for the limited safety information available from these studies.

The safety and effectiveness of twice-daily EPIVIR in combination with other antiretroviral agents have been established in pediatric patients 3 months of age and older.

In Study A2002, pharmacokinetic properties of lamivudine were assessed in a subset of 57 HIV-infected pediatric patients (age range: 4.8 months to 16 years, weight range: 5 to 66 kg) after oral and IV administration of 1, 2, 4, 8, 12, and 20 mg/kg/day. In the 9 infants and children (range: 5 months to 12 years of age) receiving oral solution 4 mg/kg twice daily (the usual recommended pediatric dose), absolute bioavailability was 66% ± 26% (mean ± SD), which was less than the 86% ± 16% (mean ± SD) observed in adults. The mechanism for the diminished absolute bioavailability of lamivudine in infants and children is unknown.

Systemic clearance decreased with increasing age in pediatric patients, as shown in Figure 2.

Figure 2: Systemic Clearance (L/hr • kg) of Lamivudine in Relation to Age

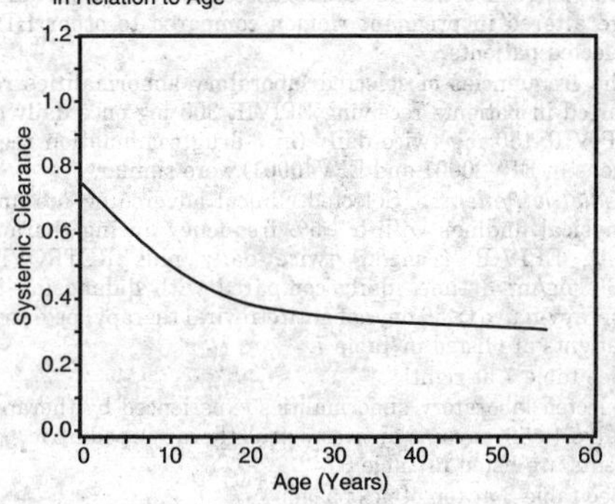

After oral administration of lamivudine 4 mg/kg twice daily to 11 pediatric patients ranging from 4 months to 14 years of age, C_{max} was 1.1 ± 0.6 mcg/mL and half-life was 2.0 ± 0.6 hours. (In adults with similar blood sampling, the half-life was 3.7 ± 1 hours.) Total exposure to lamivudine, as reflected by mean AUC values, was comparable between pediatric patients receiving an 8-mg/kg/day dose and adults receiving a 4-mg/kg/day dose.

Continued on next page

Product information on these pages is effective as of August 2004. Further information is available at: GlaxoSmithKline, PO Box 13398, Research Triangle Park, NC 27709. 1-888-825-5249. Corporate Web Site: www.gsk.com

Epivir—Cont.

Distribution of lamivudine into cerebrospinal fluid (CSF) was assessed in 38 pediatric patients after multiple oral dosing with lamivudine. CSF samples were collected between 2 and 4 hours postdose. At the dose of 8 mg/kg/day, CSF lamivudine concentrations in 8 patients ranged from 5.6% to 30.9% (mean ± SD of 14.2% ± 7.9%) of the concentration in a simultaneous serum sample, with CSF lamivudine concentrations ranging from 0.04 to 0.3 mcg/mL.

The effect of renal impairment on lamivudine pharmacokinetics in pediatric patients is not known.

The safety and pharmacokinetic properties of EPIVIR in combination with antiretroviral agents other than zidovudine have not been established in pediatric patients.

See INDICATIONS AND USAGE: Description of Clinical Studies, CLINICAL PHARMACOLOGY, WARNINGS, ADVERSE REACTIONS, and DOSAGE AND ADMINISTRATION.

HBV: See the complete prescribing information for EPIVIR-HBV Tablets and Oral Solution for additional information on the pharmacokinetics of lamivudine in HBV-infected children.

Geriatric Use: Clinical studies of EPIVIR did not include sufficient numbers of subjects aged 65 and over to determine whether they respond differently from younger subjects. In general, dose selection for an elderly patient should be cautious, reflecting the greater frequency of decreased hepatic, renal, or cardiac function, and of concomitant disease or other drug therapy. In particular, because lamivudine is substantially excreted by the kidney and elderly patients are more likely to have decreased renal function, renal function should be monitored and dosage adjustments should be made accordingly (see PRECAUTIONS: Patients with Impaired Renal Function and DOSAGE AND ADMINISTRATION).

ADVERSE REACTIONS

Clinical Trials in HIV: *Adults:* Selected clinical adverse events with a ≥5% frequency during therapy with EPIVIR 150 mg twice daily plus RETROVIR 200 mg 3 times daily compared with zidovudine are listed in Table 5.

[See table 5 at right]

The types and frequencies of clinical adverse events reported in patients receiving EPIVIR 300 mg once daily or EPIVIR 150 mg twice daily (in 3-drug combination regimens in EPV20001 and EPV40001) were similar. The most common adverse events in both treatment groups were nausea, dizziness, fatigue and/or malaise, headache, dreams, insomnia and other sleep disorders, and skin rash.

Pancreatitis was observed in 9 of the 2,613 adult patients (0.3%) who received EPIVIR in the controlled clinical trials EPV20001, NUCA3001, NUCB3001, NUCA3002, NUCB3002, and B3007.

Selected laboratory abnormalities observed during therapy are summarized in Table 6.

[See table 6 at right]

In small, uncontrolled studies in which pregnant women were given lamivudine alone or in combination with zidovudine beginning in the last few weeks of pregnancy (see PRECAUTIONS: Pregnancy), reported adverse events included anemia, urinary tract infections, and complications of labor and delivery. In postmarketing experience, liver function abnormalities and pancreatitis have been reported in women who received lamivudine in combination with other antiretroviral drugs during pregnancy. It is not known whether risks of adverse events associated with lamivudine are altered in pregnant women compared to other HIV-infected patients.

The frequencies of selected laboratory abnormalities reported in patients receiving EPIVIR 300 mg once daily or EPIVIR 150 mg twice daily (in 3-drug combination regimens in EPV20001 and EPV40001) were similar.

Pediatric Patients: Selected clinical adverse events and physical findings with a ≥5% frequency during therapy with EPIVIR 4 mg/kg twice daily plus RETROVIR 160 mg/m^2 3 times daily compared with didanosine in therapy-naive (≤56 days of antiretroviral therapy) pediatric patients are listed in Table 7.

[See table 7 at right]

Selected laboratory abnormalities experienced by therapy-naive (≤56 days of antiretroviral therapy) pediatric patients are listed in Table 8.

[See table 8 at top of next page]

Pancreatitis, which has been fatal in some cases, has been observed in antiretroviral nucleoside-experienced pediatric patients receiving EPIVIR alone or in combination with other antiretroviral agents. In an open-label dose-escalation study (A2002), 14 patients (14%) developed pancreatitis while receiving monotherapy with EPIVIR. Three of these patients died of complications of pancreatitis. In a second open-label study (A2005), 12 patients (18%) developed pancreatitis. In Study ACTG300, pancreatitis was not observed in 236 patients randomized to EPIVIR plus RETROVIR. Pancreatitis was observed in 1 patient in this study who received open-label EPIVIR in combination with RETROVIR and ritonavir following discontinuation of didanosine monotherapy.

Paresthesias and peripheral neuropathies were reported in 15 patients (15%) in Study A2002, 6 patients (9%) in Study A2005, and 2 patients (<1%) in Study ACTG300.

Table 5. Selected Clinical Adverse Events (≥5% Frequency) in Four Controlled Clinical Trials (A3001, A3002, B3001, B3002)

Adverse Event	EPIVIR 150 mg Twice Daily plus RETROVIR (n = 251)	RETROVIR* (n = 230)
Body as a whole		
Headache	35%	27%
Malaise & fatigue	27%	23%
Fever or chills	10%	12%
Digestive		
Nausea	33%	29%
Diarrhea	18%	22%
Nausea & vomiting	13%	12%
Anorexia and/or decreased appetite	10%	7%
Abdominal pain	9%	11%
Abdominal cramps	6%	3%
Dyspepsia	5%	5%
Nervous system		
Neuropathy	12%	10%
Insomnia & other sleep disorders	11%	7%
Dizziness	10%	4%
Depressive disorders	9%	4%
Respiratory		
Nasal signs & symptoms	20%	11%
Cough	18%	13%
Skin		
Skin rashes	9%	6%
Musculoskeletal		
Musculoskeletal pain	12%	10%
Myalgia	8%	6%
Arthralgia	5%	5%

*Either zidovudine monotherapy or zidovudine in combination with zalcitabine.

Table 6. Frequencies of Selected Laboratory Abnormalities in Adults in Four 24-Week Surrogate Endpoint Studies (A3001, A3002, B3001, B3002) and a Clinical Endpoint Study (B3007)

Test (Threshold Level)	24-Week Surrogate Endpoint Studies*		Clinical Endpoint Study*	
	EPIVIR plus RETROVIR	RETROVIR†	EPIVIR plus Current Therapy	Placebo plus Current Therapy‡
Absolute neutrophil count (<750/mm^3)	7.2%	5.4%	15%	13%
Hemoglobin (<8.0 g/dL)	2.9%	1.8%	2.2%	3.4%
Platelets (<50,000/mm^3)	0.4%	1.3%	2.8%	3.8%
ALT (>5.0 × ULN)	3.7%	3.6%	3.8%	1.9%
AST (>5.0 × ULN)	1.7%	1.8%	4.0%	2.1%
Bilirubin (>2.5 × ULN)	0.8%	0.4%	ND	ND
Amylase (>2.0 × ULN)	4.2%	1.5%	2.2%	1.1%

*The median duration on study was 12 months.
† Either zidovudine monotherapy or zidovudine in combination with zalcitabine.
‡ Current therapy was either zidovudine, zidovudine plus didanosine, or zidovudine plus zalcitabine.
ULN = Upper limit of normal.
ND = Not done.

Table 7. Selected Clinical Adverse Events and Physical Findings (≥5% Frequency) in Pediatric Patients in Study ACTG300

Adverse Event	EPIVIR plus RETROVIR (n = 236)	Didanosine (n = 235)
Body as a whole		
Fever	25%	32%
Digestive		
Hepatomegaly	11%	11%
Nausea & vomiting	8%	7%
Diarrhea	8%	6%
Stomatitis	6%	12%
Splenomegaly	5%	8%
Respiratory		
Cough	15%	18%
Abnormal breath sounds/wheezing	7%	9%
Ear, Nose, and Throat		
Signs or symptoms of ears*	7%	6%
Nasal discharge or congestion	8%	11%
Other		
Skin rashes	12%	14%
Lymphadenopathy	9%	11%

*Includes pain, discharge, erythema, or swelling of an ear.

Limited short-term safety information is available from 2 small, uncontrolled studies in South Africa in neonates receiving lamivudine with or without zidovudine for the first week of life following maternal treatment starting at week 38 or 36 of gestation (see PRECAUTIONS: Pediatric Use). Adverse events reported in these neonates included increased liver function tests, anemia, diarrhea, electrolyte disturbances, hypoglycemia, jaundice and hepatomegaly, rash, respiratory infections, sepsis, and syphilis; 3 neonates died (1 from gastroenteritis with acidosis and convulsions, 1 from traumatic injury, and 1 from unknown causes). Two other nonfatal gastroenteritis or diarrhea cases were reported, including 1 with convulsions; 1 infant had transient renal insufficiency associated with dehydration. The absence of control groups further limits assessments of causality, but it should be assumed that perinatally-exposed infants may be at risk for adverse events comparable to those reported in pediatric and adult HIV-infected patients

Table 8. Frequencies of Selected Laboratory Abnormalities in Pediatric Patients in Study ACTG300

Test (Threshold Level)	EPIVIR plus RETROVIR	Didanosine
Absolute neutrophil count (<400/mm^3)	8%	3%
Hemoglobin (<7.0 g/dL)	4%	2%
Platelets (<50,000/mm^3)	1%	3%
ALT (>10 × ULN)	1%	3%
AST (>10 × ULN)	2%	4%
Lipase (>2.5 × ULN)	3%	3%
Total Amylase (>2.5 × ULN)	3%	3%

ULN = Upper limit of normal.

treated with lamivudine-containing combination regimens. Long-term effects of in utero and infant lamivudine exposure are not known.

Lamivudine in Patients with Chronic Hepatitis B: Clinical trials in chronic hepatitis B used a lower dose of lamivudine (100 mg daily) than the dose used to treat HIV. The most frequent adverse events with lamivudine versus placebo were ear, nose, and throat infections (25% versus 21%); malaise and fatigue (24% versus 28%); and headache (21% versus 21%), respectively. The most frequent laboratory abnormalities reported with lamivudine were elevated ALT, elevated serum lipase, elevated CPK, and posttreatment elevations of liver function tests. Emergence of HBV viral mutants during lamivudine treatment, associated with reduced drug susceptibility and diminished treatment response, was also reported (also see WARNINGS and PRECAUTIONS). Please see the complete prescribing information for EPIVIR-HBV Tablets and Oral Solution for more information.

Observed During Clinical Practice: In addition to adverse events reported from clinical trials, the following events have been identified during post-approval use of lamivudine. Because they are reported voluntarily from a population of unknown size, estimates of frequency cannot be made. These events have been chosen for inclusion due to a combination of their seriousness, frequency of reporting, or potential causal connection to lamivudine.

Body as a Whole: Redistribution/accumulation of body fat (see PRECAUTIONS: Fat Redistribution).

Digestive: Stomatitis.

Endocrine and Metabolic: Hyperglycemia.

General: Weakness.

Hemic and Lymphatic: Anemia (including pure red cell aplasia and severe anemias progressing on therapy), lymphadenopathy, splenomegaly.

Hepatic and Pancreatic: Lactic acidosis and hepatic steatosis, pancreatitis, posttreatment exacerbation of hepatitis B (see WARNINGS and PRECAUTIONS).

Hypersensitivity: Anaphylaxis, urticaria.

Musculoskeletal: Muscle weakness, CPK elevation, rhabdomyolysis.

Nervous: Paresthesia, peripheral neuropathy.

Respiratory: Abnormal breath sounds/wheezing.

Skin: Alopecia, rash, pruritus.

OVERDOSAGE

There is no known antidote for EPIVIR. One case of an adult ingesting 6 g of EPIVIR was reported; there were no clinical signs or symptoms noted and hematologic tests remained normal. Two cases of pediatric overdose were reported in ACTG300. One case was a single dose of 7 mg/kg of EPIVIR; the second case involved use of 5 mg/kg of EPIVIR twice daily for 30 days. There were no clinical signs or symptoms noted in either case. It is not known whether lamivudine can be removed by peritoneal dialysis or hemodialysis. If overdose occurs, the patient should be monitored, and standard supportive treatment applied as required.

DOSAGE AND ADMINISTRATION

Adults: The recommended oral dose of EPIVIR for adults is 300 mg daily, administered as either 150 mg twice daily or 300 mg once daily, in combination with other antiretroviral agents (see DESCRIPTION OF CLINICAL STUDIES, PRECAUTIONS, MICROBIOLOGY, and CLINICAL PHARMACOLOGY). If lamivudine is administered to a patient dually infected with HIV and HBV, the dosage indicated for HIV therapy should be used as part of an appropriate combination regimen (see WARNINGS).

Pediatric Patients: *Infants/Children/Adolescents:* The recommended oral dose of EPIVIR for HIV-infected pediatric patients 3 months up to 16 years of age is 4 mg/kg twice daily (up to a maximum of 150 mg twice a day), administered in combination with other antiretroviral agents.

Dose Adjustment: It is recommended that doses of EPIVIR be adjusted in accordance with renal function (see Table 9) (see CLINICAL PHARMACOLOGY).

Table 9. Adjustment of Dosage of EPIVIR in Adults and Adolescents in Accordance with Creatinine Clearance

Creatinine Clearance (mL/min)	Recommended Dosage of EPIVIR
≥50	150 mg twice daily or 300 mg once daily
30-49	150 mg once daily
15-29	150 mg first dose, then 100 mg once daily
5-14	150 mg first dose, then 50 mg once daily
<5	50 mg first dose, then 25 mg once daily

Insufficient data are available to recommend a dosage of EPIVIR in patients undergoing dialysis. Although there are insufficient data to recommend a specific dose adjustment of EPIVIR in pediatric patients with renal impairment, a reduction in the dose and/or an increase in the dosing interval should be considered.

HOW SUPPLIED

EPIVIR Tablets, 150 mg, are white, modified diamond-shaped, film-coated tablets engraved with "GX CJ7" on one side and plain on the reverse side.

Bottle of 60 tablets (NDC 0173-0470-01) with child-resistant closure.

EPIVIR Tablets, 300 mg, are gray, modified diamond-shaped, film-coated tablets engraved with "GX EJ7" on one side and plain on the reverse side.

Bottle of 30 tablets (NDC 0173-0714-00) with child-resistant closure.

Store at 25°C (77°F); excursions permitted to 15° to 30°C (59° to 86°F) [see USP Controlled Room Temperature].

EPIVIR Oral Solution, a clear, colorless to pale yellow, strawberry-banana flavored liquid, contains 10 mg of lamivudine in each 1 mL in plastic bottles of 240 mL (NDC 0173-0471-00) with child-resistant closures. This product does not require reconstitution.

Store in tightly closed bottles at 25°C (77°F) [see USP Controlled Room Temperature].

GlaxoSmithKline, Research Triangle Park, NC 27709
Manufactured under agreement from
Shire Pharmaceuticals Group plc, Basingstoke, UK

May 2004 RL-2090

Shown in Product Identification Guide, page 315

EPIVIR-HBV® ℞
[ĕp' ə-vir]
(lamivudine)
Tablets

EPIVIR-HBV® ℞
(lamivudine)
Oral Solution

WARNING

LACTIC ACIDOSIS AND SEVERE HEPATOMEGALY WITH STEATOSIS, INCLUDING FATAL CASES, HAVE BEEN REPORTED WITH THE USE OF NUCLEOSIDE ANALOGUES ALONE OR IN COMBINATION, INCLUDING LAMIVUDINE AND OTHER ANTIRETROVIRALS (SEE WARNINGS).

HUMAN IMMUNODEFICIENCY VIRUS (HIV) COUNSELING AND TESTING SHOULD BE OFFERED TO ALL PATIENTS BEFORE BEGINNING EPIVIR-HBV AND PERIODICALLY DURING TREATMENT (SEE WARNINGS), BECAUSE EPIVIR-HBV TABLETS AND ORAL SOLUTION CONTAIN A LOWER DOSE OF THE SAME ACTIVE INGREDIENT (LAMIVUDINE) AS EPIVIR® TABLETS AND ORAL SOLUTION USED TO TREAT HIV INFECTION. IF TREATMENT WITH EPIVIR-HBV IS PRESCRIBED FOR CHRONIC HEPATITIS B FOR A PATIENT WITH UNRECOGNIZED OR UNTREATED HIV INFECTION, RAPID EMERGENCE OF HIV RESISTANCE IS LIKELY BECAUSE OF SUBTHERAPEUTIC DOSE AND INAPPROPRIATE MONOTHERAPY.

SEVERE ACUTE EXACERBATIONS OF HEPATITIS B HAVE BEEN REPORTED IN PATIENTS WHO HAVE DISCONTINUED ANTI-HEPATITIS B THERAPY (INCLUDING EPIVIR-HBV). HEPATIC FUNCTION SHOULD BE MONITORED CLOSELY WITH BOTH CLINICAL AND LABORATORY FOLLOW-UP FOR AT LEAST SEVERAL MONTHS IN PATIENTS WHO DISCONTINUE ANTI-HEPATITIS B THERAPY. IF APPROPRIATE, INITIATION OF ANTI-HEPATITIS B THERAPY MAY BE WARRANTED (SEE WARNINGS).

DESCRIPTION

EPIVIR-HBV is a brand name for lamivudine, a synthetic nucleoside analogue with activity against hepatitis B virus (HBV) and HIV. Lamivudine was initially developed for the treatment of HIV infection as EPIVIR®. Please see the complete prescribing information for EPIVIR Tablets and Oral Solution for additional information. The chemical name of lamivudine is (2R,cis)-4-amino-1-(2-hydroxymethyl-1,3-oxathiolan-5-yl)-(1H)-pyrimidin-2-one. Lamivudine is the (-)enantiomer of a dideoxy analogue of cytidine. Lamivudine has also been referred to as (-)2′,3′-dideoxy, 3′-thiacytidine. It has a molecular formula of $C_8H_{11}N_3O_3S$ and a molecular weight of 229.3.

Lamivudine is a white to off-white crystalline solid with a solubility of approximately 70 mg/mL in water at 20°C.

EPIVIR-HBV Tablets are for oral administration. Each tablet contains 100 mg of lamivudine and the inactive ingredients hypromellose, macrogol 400, magnesium stearate, microcrystalline cellulose, polysorbate 80, red iron oxide, sodium starch glycolate, titanium dioxide, and yellow iron oxide.

EPIVIR-HBV Oral Solution is for oral administration. One milliliter (1 mL) of EPIVIR-HBV Oral Solution contains 5 mg of lamivudine (5 mg/mL) in an aqueous solution and the inactive ingredients artificial strawberry and banana flavors, citric acid (anhydrous), methylparaben, propylene glycol, propylparaben, sodium citrate (dihydrate), and sucrose (200 mg).

MICROBIOLOGY

Mechanism of Action: Lamivudine is a synthetic nucleoside analogue. Lamivudine is phosphorylated intracellularly to lamivudine triphosphate, L-TP. Incorporation of the monophosphate form into viral DNA by HBV polymerase results in DNA chain termination. L-TP also inhibits the RNA- and DNA-dependent DNA polymerase activities of HIV-1 reverse transcriptase (RT). L-TP is a weak inhibitor of mammalian alpha-, beta-, and gamma-DNA polymerases.

Antiviral Activity In Vitro: In vitro activity of lamivudine against HBV was assessed in HBV DNA-transfected 2.2.15 cells, HB611 cells, and infected human primary hepatocytes. IC_{50} values (the concentration of drug needed to reduce the level of extracellular HBV DNA by 50%) varied from 0.01 μM (2.3 ng/mL) to 5.6 μM (1.3 mcg/mL) depending upon the duration of exposure of cells to lamivudine, the cell model system, and the protocol used. See the EPIVIR package insert for information regarding activity of lamivudine against HIV.

Drug Resistance: *HBV:* Genotypic analysis of viral isolates obtained from patients who show renewed evidence of replication of HBV while receiving lamivudine suggests that a reduction in sensitivity of HBV to lamivudine is associated with mutations resulting in a methionine to valine or isoleucine substitution in the YMDD motif of the catalytic domain of HBV polymerase (position 552) and a leucine to methionine substitution at position 528. It is not known whether other HBV mutations may be associated with reduced lamivudine susceptibility in vitro.

In 4 controlled clinical trials in adults, YMDD-mutant HBV were detected in 81 of 335 patients receiving lamivudine 100 mg once daily for 52 weeks. The prevalence of YMDD mutations was less than 10% in each of these trials for patients studied at 24 weeks and increased to an average of 24% (range in 4 studies: 16% to 32%) at 52 weeks. In limited data from a long-term follow-up trial in patients who continued 100 mg/day lamivudine after one of these studies, YMDD mutations further increased from 16% at 1 year to 42% at 2 years. In small numbers of patients receiving lamivudine for longer periods, further increases in the appearance of YMDD mutations were observed.

In a controlled trial in pediatric patients, YMDD-mutant HBV were detected in 31 of 166 (19%) patients receiving lamivudine for 52 weeks. For a subgroup who remained on lamivudine therapy in a follow-up study, YMDD mutations increased from 24% at 12 months to 45% (53 of 118) at 18 months of lamivudine treatment.

Mutant viruses were associated with evidence of diminished treatment response at 52 weeks relative to lamivudine-treated patients without evidence of YMDD mutations in both adult and pediatric studies (see PRECAUTIONS). The long-term clinical significance of YMDD-mutant HBV is not known.

HIV: In studies of HIV-1-infected patients who received lamivudine monotherapy or combination therapy with lamivudine plus zidovudine for at least 12 weeks, HIV-1 isolates with reduced in vitro susceptibility to lamivudine were detected in most patients (see WARNINGS).

CLINICAL PHARMACOLOGY

Pharmacokinetics in Adults: The pharmacokinetic properties of lamivudine have been studied as single and multiple oral doses ranging from 5 to 600 mg per day administered to HBV-infected patients.

The pharmacokinetic properties of lamivudine have also been studied in asymptomatic, HIV-infected adult patients after administration of single intravenous (IV) doses ranging from 0.25 to 8 mg/kg, as well as single and multiple (twice-daily regimen) oral doses ranging from 0.25 to 10 mg/kg.

Absorption and Bioavailability: Lamivudine was rapidly absorbed after oral administration in HBV-infected patients and in healthy subjects. Following single oral doses of 100 mg, the peak serum lamivudine concentration (C_{max}) in HBV-infected patients (steady state) and healthy subjects

Continued on next page

Product information on these pages is effective as of August 2004. Further information is available at: GlaxoSmithKline, PO Box 13398, Research Triangle Park, NC 27709. 1-888-825-5249. Corporate Web Site: www.gsk.com

Epivir-HBV—Cont.

(single dose) was 1.28 ± 0.56 mcg/mL and 1.05 ± 0.32 mcg/mL (mean ± SD), respectively, which occurred between 0.5 and 2 hours after administration. The area under the plasma concentration versus time curve ($AUC_{[0-24\ hr]}$) following 100 mg lamivudine oral single and repeated daily doses to steady state was 4.3 ± 1.4 (mean ± SD) and 4.7 ± 1.7 mcg•hr/mL, respectively. The relative bioavailability of the tablet and solution were then demonstrated in healthy subjects. Although the solution demonstrated a slightly higher peak serum concentration (C_{max}), there was no significant difference in systemic exposure (AUC_∞) between the solution and the tablet. Therefore, the solution and the tablet may be used interchangeably.

After oral administration of lamivudine once daily to HBV-infected adults, the AUC and C_{max} increased in proportion to dose over the range from 5 mg to 600 mg once daily.

The 100-mg tablet was administered orally to 24 healthy subjects on 2 occasions, once in the fasted state and once with food (standard meal: 967 kcal; 67 grams fat, 33 grams protein, 58 grams carbohydrate). There was no significant difference in systemic exposure (AUC_∞) in the fed and fasted states; therefore, EPIVIR-HBV Tablets and Oral Solution may be administered with or without food.

Lamivudine was rapidly absorbed after oral administration in HIV-infected patients. Absolute bioavailability in 12 adult patients was 86% ± 16% (mean ± SD) for the 150-mg tablet and 87% ± 13% for the 10-mg/mL oral solution.

Distribution: The apparent volume of distribution after IV administration of lamivudine to 20 asymptomatic HIV-infected patients was 1.3 ± 0.4 L/kg, suggesting that lamivudine distributes into extravascular spaces. Volume of distribution was independent of dose and did not correlate with body weight.

Binding of lamivudine to human plasma proteins is low (<36%) and independent of dose. In vitro studies showed that over the concentration range of 0.1 to 100 mcg/mL, the amount of lamivudine associated with erythrocytes ranged from 53% to 57% and was independent of concentration.

Metabolism: Metabolism of lamivudine is a minor route of elimination. In man, the only known metabolite of lamivudine is the trans-sulfoxide metabolite. In 9 healthy subjects receiving 300 mg of lamivudine as single oral doses, a total of 4.2% (range 1.5% to 7.5%) of the dose was excreted as the trans-sulfoxide metabolite in the urine, the majority of which was excreted in the first 12 hours.

Serum concentrations of the trans-sulfoxide metabolite have not been determined.

Elimination: The majority of lamivudine is eliminated unchanged in urine by active organic cationic secretion. In 9 healthy subjects given a single 300-mg oral dose of lamivudine, renal clearance was 199.7 ± 56.9 mL/min (mean ± SD). In 20 HIV-infected patients given a single IV dose, renal clearance was 280.4 ± 75.2 mL/min (mean ± SD), representing 71% ± 16% (mean ± SD) of total clearance of lamivudine.

In most single-dose studies in HIV- or HBV-infected patients or healthy subjects with serum sampling for 24 hours after dosing, the observed mean elimination half-life ($t_{½}$) ranged from 5 to 7 hours. In HIV-infected patients, total clearance was 398.5 ± 69.1 mL/min (mean ± SD). Oral clearance and elimination half-life were independent of dose and body weight over an oral dosing range from 0.25 to 10 mg/kg.

Special Populations: Adults With Impaired Renal Function: The pharmacokinetic properties of lamivudine have been determined in healthy subjects and in subjects with impaired renal function, with and without hemodialysis (Table 1):

[See table 1 above]

Table 1. Pharmacokinetic Parameters (Mean ± SD) Dose-Normalized to a Single 100-mg Oral Dose of Lamivudine in Patients With Varying Degrees of Renal Function

Parameter	Creatinine Clearance Criterion (Number of Subjects)		
	≥80 mL/min (n = 9)	20-59 mL/min (n = 8)	<20 mL/min (n = 6)
Creatinine clearance (mL/min)	97 (range 82-117)	39 (range 25-49)	15 (range 13-19)
C_{max} (mcg/mL)	1.31 ± 0.35	1.85 ± 0.40	1.55 ± 0.31
AUC_∞ (mcg•hr/mL)	5.28 ± 1.01	14.67 ± 3.74	27.33 ± 6.56
Cl/F (mL/min)	326.4 ± 63.8	120.1 ± 29.5	64.5 ± 18.3

Exposure (AUC_∞), C_{max}, and half-life increased with diminishing renal function (as expressed by creatinine clearance). Apparent total oral clearance (Cl/F) of lamivudine decreased as creatinine clearance decreased. T_{max} was not significantly affected by renal function. Based on these observations, it is recommended that the dosage of lamivudine be modified in patients with renal impairment (see DOSAGE AND ADMINISTRATION).

Hemodialysis increases lamivudine clearance from a mean of 64 to 88 mL/min; however, the length of time of hemodialysis (4 hours) was insufficient to significantly alter mean lamivudine exposure after a single-dose administration. Therefore, it is recommended, following correction of dose for creatinine clearance, that no additional dose modification is made after routine hemodialysis.

It is not known whether lamivudine can be removed by peritoneal dialysis or continuous (24-hour) hemodialysis.

The effect of renal impairment on lamivudine pharmacokinetics in pediatric patients with chronic hepatitis B is not known.

Adults With Impaired Hepatic Function: The pharmacokinetic properties of lamivudine have been determined in adults with impaired hepatic function (Table 2). Patients were stratified by severity of hepatic functional impairment.

[See table 2 above]

Table 2. Pharmacokinetic Parameters (Mean ± SD) Dose-Normalized to a Single 100-mg Dose of Lamivudine in 3 Groups of Subjects With Normal or Impaired Hepatic Function

Parameter	Normal (n = 8)	Impairment* Moderate (n = 8)	Severe (n = 8)
C_{max} (mcg/mL)	0.92 ± 0.31	1.06 ± 0.58	1.08 ± 0.27
AUC_∞ (mcg•hr/mL)	3.96 ± 0.58	3.97 ± 1.36	4.30 ± 0.63
T_{max} (hr)	1.3 ± 0.8	1.4 ± 0.8	1.4 ± 1.2
Cl/F (mL/min)	424.7 ± 61.9	456.9 ± 129.8	395.2 ± 51.8
Clr (mL/min)	279.2 ± 79.2	323.5 ± 100.9	216.1 ± 58.0

*Hepatic impairment assessed by aminopyrine breath test.

Pharmacokinetic parameters were not altered by diminishing hepatic function. Therefore, no dose adjustment for lamivudine is required for patients with impaired hepatic function. Safety and efficacy of EPIVIR-HBV have not been established in the presence of decompensated liver disease (see PRECAUTIONS).

Post-Hepatic Transplant: Fourteen HBV-infected patients received liver transplant following lamivudine therapy and completed pharmacokinetic assessments at enrollment, 2 weeks after 100-mg once-daily dosing (pre-transplant), and 3 months following transplant; there were no significant differences in pharmacokinetic parameters. The overall exposure of lamivudine is primarily affected by renal dysfunction; consequently, transplant patients with reduced renal function had generally higher exposure than patients with normal renal function. Safety and efficacy of EPIVIR-HBV have not been established in this population (see PRECAUTIONS).

Pediatric Patients: Lamivudine pharmacokinetics were evaluated in a 28-day dose-ranging study in 53 pediatric patients with chronic hepatitis B. Patients aged 2 to 12 years were randomized to receive lamivudine 0.35 mg/kg twice daily, 3 mg/kg once daily, 1.5 mg/kg twice daily, or 4 mg/kg twice daily. Patients aged 13 to 17 years received lamivudine 100 mg once daily. Lamivudine was rapidly absorbed (T_{max} 0.5 to 1 hour). In general, both C_{max} and exposure (AUC) showed dose proportionality in the dosing range studied. Weight-corrected oral clearance was highest at age 2 and declined from 2 to 12 years, where values were then similar to those seen in adults. A dose of 3 mg/kg given once daily produced a steady-state lamivudine AUC (mean 5,953 ng•hr/mL ± 1,562 SD) similar to that associated with a dose of 100 mg/day in adults.

Gender: There are no significant gender differences in lamivudine pharmacokinetics.

Race: There are no significant racial differences in lamivudine pharmacokinetics.

Drug Interactions: Multiple doses of lamivudine and a single dose of interferon were coadministered to 19 healthy male subjects in a pharmacokinetics study. Results indicated a small (10%) reduction in lamivudine AUC, but no change in interferon pharmacokinetic parameters when the 2 drugs were given in combination. All other pharmacokinetic parameters (C_{max}, T_{max}, and $t_{½}$) were unchanged. There was no significant pharmacokinetic interaction between lamivudine and interferon alfa in this study.

Lamivudine and zidovudine were coadministered to 12 asymptomatic HIV-positive adult patients in a single-center, open-label, randomized, crossover study. No significant differences were observed in AUC_∞ or total clearance for lamivudine or zidovudine when the 2 drugs were administered together. Coadministration of lamivudine with zidovudine resulted in an increase of 39% ± 62% (mean ± SD) in C_{max} of zidovudine.

Lamivudine and trimethoprim/sulfamethoxazole (TMP/SMX) were coadministered to 14 HIV-positive patients in a single-center, open-label, randomized, crossover study. Each patient received treatment with a single 300-mg dose of lamivudine and TMP 160 mg/SMX 800 mg once a day for 5 days with concomitant administration of lamivudine 300 mg with the fifth dose in a crossover design. Coadministration of TMP/SMX with lamivudine resulted in an increase of 44% ± 23% (mean ± SD) in lamivudine AUC_∞, a decrease of 29% ± 13% in lamivudine oral clearance, and a decrease of 30% ± 36% in lamivudine renal clearance. The pharmacokinetic properties of TMP and SMX were not altered by coadministration with lamivudine (see PRECAUTIONS: Drug Interactions).

Lamivudine and zalcitabine may inhibit the intracellular phosphorylation of one another. Therefore, use of lamivudine in combination with zalcitabine is not recommended.

INDICATIONS AND USAGE

EPIVIR-HBV is indicated for the treatment of chronic hepatitis B associated with evidence of hepatitis B viral replication and active liver inflammation. This indication is based on 1-year histologic and serologic responses in adult patients with compensated chronic hepatitis B, and more limited information from a study in pediatric patients ages 2 to 17 years (see Description of Clinical Studies below).

Description of Clinical Studies: ***Adults:*** The safety and efficacy of EPIVIR-HBV were evaluated in 4 controlled studies in 967 patients with compensated chronic hepatitis B. All patients were 16 years of age or older and had chronic hepatitis B virus infection (serum HBsAg positive for at least 6 months) accompanied by evidence of HBV replication (serum HBeAg positive and positive for serum HBV DNA, as measured by a research solution-hybridization assay) and persistently elevated ALT levels and/or chronic inflammation on liver biopsy compatible with a diagnosis of chronic viral hepatitis. Three of these studies provided comparisons of EPIVIR-HBV 100 mg once daily versus placebo, and results of these comparisons are summarized below.

- Study 1 was a randomized, double-blind study of EPIVIR-HBV 100 mg once daily versus placebo for 52 weeks followed by a 16-week no-treatment period, in treatment-naive US patients.
- Study 2 was a randomized, double-blind, 3-arm study that compared EPIVIR-HBV 25 mg once daily versus EPIVIR-HBV 100 mg once daily versus placebo for 52 weeks in Asian patients.
- Study 3 was a randomized, partially-blind, 3-arm study conducted primarily in North America and Europe in patients who had ongoing evidence of active chronic hepatitis B despite previous treatment with interferon alfa. The

Table 3. Histologic Response at Week 52 Among Adult Patients Receiving EPIVIR-HBV 100 mg Once Daily or Placebo

Assessment	Study 1		Study 2		Study 3	
	EPIVIR-HBV (n = 62)	Placebo (n = 63)	EPIVIR-HBV (n = 131)	Placebo (n = 68)	EPIVIR-HBV (n = 110)	Placebo (n = 54)
Improvement*	55%	25%	56%	26%	56%	26%
No Improvement	27%	59%	36%	62%	25%	54%
Missing Data	18%	16%	8%	12%	19%	20%

*Improvement was defined as a ≥2-point decrease in the Knodell Histologic Activity Index (HAI)[1] at Week 52 compared with pretreatment HAI. Patients with missing data at baseline were excluded.

study compared EPIVIR-HBV 100 mg once daily for 52 weeks, followed by either EPIVIR-HBV 100 mg or matching placebo once daily for 16 weeks (Arm 1), versus placebo once daily for 68 weeks (Arm 2). (A third arm using a combination of interferon and lamivudine is not presented here because there was not sufficient information to evaluate this regimen.)

Principal endpoint comparisons for the histologic and serologic outcomes in lamivudine (100 mg daily) and placebo recipients in placebo-controlled studies are shown in the following tables.

[See table 3 on previous page]

[See table 4 at right]

Normalization of serum ALT levels was more frequent with lamivudine treatment compared with placebo in Studies 1-3.

The majority of lamivudine-treated patients showed a decrease of HBV DNA to below the assay limit early in the course of therapy. However, reappearance of assay-detectable HBV DNA during lamivudine treatment was observed in approximately one third of patients after this initial response.

Pediatrics: The safety and efficacy of EPIVIR-HBV were evaluated in a double-blind clinical trial in 286 patients ranging from 2 to 17 years of age, who were randomized (2:1) to receive 52 weeks of lamivudine (3 mg/kg once daily to a maximum of 100 mg once daily) or placebo. All patients had compensated chronic hepatitis B accompanied by evidence of hepatitis B virus replication (positive serum HBeAg and positive for serum HBV DNA by a research branched-chain DNA assay) and persistently elevated serum ALT levels. The combination of loss of HBeAg and reduction of HBV DNA to below the assay limit of the research assay, evaluated at Week 52, was observed in 23% of lamivudine subjects and 13% of placebo subjects. Normalization of serum ALT was achieved and maintained to Week 52 more frequently in patients treated with EPIVIR-HBV compared with placebo (55% versus 13%). As in the adult controlled trials, most lamivudine-treated subjects had decreases in HBV DNA below the assay limit early in treatment, but about one third of subjects with this initial response had reappearance of assay-detectable HBV DNA during treatment. Adolescents (ages 13 to 17 years) showed less evidence of treatment effect than younger children.

Table 4. HBeAg Seroconversion* at Week 52 Among Adult Patients Receiving EPIVIR-HBV 100 mg Once Daily or Placebo

	Study 1		Study 2		Study 3	
Seroconversion	EPIVIR-HBV (n = 63)	Placebo (n = 69)	EPIVIR-HBV (n = 140)	Placebo (n = 70)	EPIVIR-HBV (n = 108)	Placebo (n = 53)
Responder	17%	6%	16%	4%	15%	13%
Nonresponder	67%	78%	80%	91%	69%	68%
Missing Data	16%	16%	4%	4%	17%	19%

*Three-component seroconversion was defined as Week 52 values showing loss of HBeAg, gain of HBeAb, and reduction of HBV DNA to below the solution-hybridization assay limit. Subjects with negative baseline HBeAg or HBV DNA assay were excluded from the analysis.

Table 5. Selected Clinical Adverse Events (≥5% Frequency) in 3 Placebo-Controlled Clinical Trials in Adults During Treatment* (Studies 1-3)

Adverse Event	EPIVIR-HBV (n = 332)	Placebo (n = 200)
Non-site specific		
Malaise and fatigue	24%	28%
Fever or chills	7%	9%
Ear, nose, and throat		
Ear, nose, and throat infections	25%	21%
Sore throat	13%	8%
Gastrointestinal		
Nausea and vomiting	15%	17%
Abdominal discomfort and pain	16%	17%
Diarrhea	14%	12%
Musculoskeletal		
Myalgia	14%	17%
Arthralgia	7%	5%
Neurological		
Headache	21%	21%
Skin		
Skin rashes	5%	5%

*Includes patients treated for 52 to 68 weeks.

CONTRAINDICATIONS

EPIVIR-HBV Tablets and EPIVIR-HBV Oral Solution are contraindicated in patients with previously demonstrated clinically significant hypersensitivity to any of the components of the products.

WARNINGS

Lactic Acidosis/Severe Hepatomegaly with Steatosis: Lactic acidosis and severe hepatomegaly with steatosis, including fatal cases, have been reported with the use of nucleoside analogues alone or in combination, including lamivudine and other antiretrovirals. A majority of these cases have been in women. Obesity and prolonged nucleoside exposure may be risk factors. Most of these reports have described patients receiving nucleoside analogues for treatment of HIV infection, but there have been reports of lactic acidosis in patients receiving lamivudine for hepatitis B. Particular caution should be exercised when administering EPIVIR or EPIVIR-HBV to any patient with known risk factors for liver disease; however, cases have also been reported in patients with no known risk factors. Treatment with EPIVIR or EPIVIR-HBV should be suspended in any patient who develops clinical or laboratory findings suggestive of lactic acidosis or pronounced hepatotoxicity (which may include hepatomegaly and steatosis even in the absence of marked transaminase elevations).

Important Differences Between Lamivudine-Containing Products, HIV Testing, and Risk of Emergence of Resistant HIV: EPIVIR-HBV Tablets and Oral Solution contain a lower dose of the same active ingredient (lamivudine) as EPIVIR Tablets and Oral Solution, COMBIVIR® (lamivudine/zidovudine) Tablets, and TRIZIVIR® (abacavir, lamivudine, and zidovudine) Tablets used to treat HIV infection. The formulation and dosage of lamivudine in EPIVIR-HBV are not appropriate for patients dually infected with HBV and HIV. If a decision is made to administer lamivudine to such patients, the higher dosage indicated for HIV therapy should be used as part of an appropriate combination regimen, and the prescribing information for EPIVIR, COMBIVIR, or TRIZIVIR as well as for EPIVIR-HBV should be consulted. HIV counseling and testing should be offered to all patients before beginning EPIVIR-HBV and periodically during treatment because of the risk of rapid emergence of resistant HIV and limitation of treatment options if EPIVIR-HBV is prescribed to treat chronic hepatitis B in a patient who has unrecognized or untreated HIV infection or acquires HIV infection during treatment.

Posttreatment Exacerbations of Hepatitis: Clinical and laboratory evidence of exacerbations of hepatitis have occurred after discontinuation of EPIVIR-HBV (these have been primarily detected by serum ALT elevations, in addition to the re-emergence of HBV DNA commonly observed after stopping treatment; see Table 7 for more information regarding frequency of posttreatment ALT elevations). Although most events appear to have been self-limited, fatalities have been reported in some cases. The causal relationship to discontinuation of lamivudine treatment is unknown. Patients should be closely monitored with both clinical and laboratory follow-up for at least several months after stopping treatment. There is insufficient evidence to determine whether re-initiation of therapy alters the course of posttreatment exacerbations of hepatitis.

Pancreatitis: Pancreatitis has been reported in patients receiving lamivudine, particularly in HIV-infected pediatric patients with prior nucleoside exposure.

PRECAUTIONS

General: Patients should be assessed before beginning treatment with EPIVIR-HBV by a physician experienced in the management of chronic hepatitis B.

Emergence of Resistance-Associated HBV Mutations: In controlled clinical trials, YMDD-mutant HBV were detected in patients with on-lamivudine re-appearance of HBV DNA after an initial decline below the solution-hybridization assay limit (see MICROBIOLOGY: Drug Resistance). These mutations can be detected by a research assay and have been associated with reduced susceptibility to lamivudine in vitro. Lamivudine-treated patients (adult and pediatric) with YMDD-mutant HBV at 52 weeks showed diminished treatment responses in comparison to lamivudine-treated patients without evidence of YMDD mutations, including lower rates of HBeAg seroconversion and HBeAg loss (no greater than placebo recipients), more frequent return of positive HBV DNA by solution-hybridization or branched-chain DNA assay, and more frequent ALT elevations. In the controlled trials, when patients developed YMDD-mutant HBV, they had a rise in HBV DNA and ALT from their own previous on-treatment levels. Progression of hepatitis B, including death, has been reported in some patients with YMDD-mutant HBV, including patients from the liver transplant setting and from other clinical trials. The long-term clinical significance of YMDD-mutant HBV is not known. Increased clinical and laboratory monitoring may aid in treatment decisions if emergence of viral mutants is suspected.

Limitations of Populations Studied: Safety and efficacy of EPIVIR-HBV have not been established in patients with decompensated liver disease or organ transplants; pediatric patients <2 years of age; patients dually infected with HBV and HCV, hepatitis delta, or HIV; or other populations not included in the principal phase III controlled studies. There are no studies in pregnant women and no data regarding effect on vertical transmission, and appropriate infant immunizations should be used to prevent neonatal acquisition of HBV.

Assessing Patients During Treatment: Patients should be monitored regularly during treatment by a physician experienced in the management of chronic hepatitis B. The safety and effectiveness of treatment with EPIVIR-HBV beyond 1 year have not been established. During treatment, combinations of such events such as return of persistently elevated ALT, increasing levels of HBV DNA over time after an initial decline below assay limit, progression of clinical signs or symptoms of hepatic disease, and/or worsening of hepatic necroinflammatory findings may be considered as potentially reflecting loss of therapeutic response. Such observations should be taken into consideration when determining the advisability of continuing therapy with EPIVIR-HBV.

The optimal duration of treatment, the durability of HBeAg seroconversions occurring during treatment, and the relationship between treatment response and long-term outcomes such as hepatocellular carcinoma or decompensated cirrhosis are not known.

Patients with Impaired Renal Function: Reduction of the dosage of EPIVIR-HBV is recommended for patients with impaired renal function (see CLINICAL PHARMACOLOGY and DOSAGE AND ADMINISTRATION).

Information for Patients: A Patient Package Insert (PPI) for EPIVIR-HBV is available for patient information.

Patients should remain under the care of a physician while taking EPIVIR-HBV. They should discuss any new symptoms or concurrent medications with their physician.

Patients should be advised that EPIVIR-HBV is not a cure for hepatitis B, that the long-term treatment benefits of EPIVIR-HBV are unknown at this time, and, in particular, that the relationship of initial treatment response to outcomes such as hepatocellular carcinoma and decompensated cirrhosis is unknown. Patients should be informed that deterioration of liver disease has occurred in some cases when treatment was discontinued. Patients should be advised to discuss any changes in regimen with their physician.

Patients should be informed that emergence of resistant hepatitis B virus and worsening of disease can occur during treatment, and they should promptly report any new symptoms to their physician.

Patients should be counseled on the importance of testing for HIV to avoid inappropriate therapy and development of resistant HIV, and HIV counseling and testing should be offered before starting EPIVIR-HBV and periodically during therapy. Patients should be advised that EPIVIR-HBV Tablets and EPIVIR-HBV Oral Solution contain a lower dose of the same active ingredient (lamivudine) as EPIVIR Tablets, EPIVIR Oral Solution, COMBIVIR Tablets, and TRIZIVIR Tablets. EPIVIR-HBV should not be taken concurrently with EPIVIR, COMBIVIR, or TRIZIVIR (see WARNINGS).

Patients infected with both HBV and HIV who are planning to change their HIV treatment regimen to a regimen that does not include EPIVIR, COMBIVIR, or TRIZIVIR should discuss continued therapy for hepatitis B with their physician.

Patients should be advised that treatment with EPIVIR-HBV has not been shown to reduce the risk of transmission of HBV to others through sexual contact or blood contamination (see Pregnancy section).

Diabetic patients should be advised that each 20-mL dose of EPIVIR-HBV Oral Solution contains 4 grams of sucrose.

Continued on next page

Product information on these pages is effective as of August 2004. Further information is available at: GlaxoSmithKline, PO Box 13398, Research Triangle Park, NC 27709. 1-888-825-5249. Corporate Web Site: www.gsk.com

Epivir-HBV—Cont.

Drug Interactions: Lamivudine is predominantly eliminated in the urine by active organic cationic secretion. The possibility of interactions with other drugs administered concurrently should be considered, particularly when their main route of elimination is active renal secretion via the organic cationic transport system (e.g., trimethoprim).
TMP 160 mg/SMX 800 mg once daily has been shown to increase lamivudine exposure (AUC) by 44% (see CLINICAL PHARMACOLOGY). No change in dose of either drug is recommended. There is no information regarding the effect on lamivudine pharmacokinetics of higher doses of TMP/SMX such as those used to treat *Pneumocystis carinii* pneumonia. No data are available regarding interactions with other drugs that have renal clearance mechanisms similar to that of lamivudine.
Lamivudine and zalcitabine may inhibit the intracellular phosphorylation of one another. Therefore, use of lamivudine in combination with zalcitabine is not recommended.
Carcinogenesis, Mutagenesis, and Impairment of Fertility: Lamivudine long-term carcinogenicity studies in mice and rats showed no evidence of carcinogenic potential at exposures up to 34 times (mice) and 200 times (rats) those observed in humans at the recommended therapeutic dose for chronic hepatitis B. Lamivudine was not active in a microbial mutagenicity screen or an in vitro cell transformation assay, but showed weak in vitro mutagenic activity in a cytogenetic assay using cultured human lymphocytes and in the mouse lymphoma assay. However, lamivudine showed no evidence of in vivo genotoxic activity in the rat at oral doses of up to 2,000 mg/kg producing plasma levels of 60 to 70 times those in humans at the recommended dose for chronic hepatitis B. In a study of reproductive performance, lamivudine administered to rats at doses up to 4,000 mg/kg/day, producing plasma levels 80 to 120 times those in humans, revealed no evidence of impaired fertility and no effect on the survival, growth, and development to weaning of the offspring.
Pregnancy: Pregnancy Category C. Reproduction studies have been performed in rats and rabbits at orally administered doses up to 4,000 mg/kg/day and 1,000 mg/kg/day, respectively, producing plasma levels up to approximately 60 times that for the adult HBV dose. No evidence of teratogenicity due to lamivudine was observed. Evidence of early embryolethality was seen in the rabbit at exposure levels similar to those observed in humans, but there was no indication of this effect in the rat at exposures up to 60 times that in humans. Studies in pregnant rats and rabbits showed that lamivudine is transferred to the fetus through the placenta. There are no adequate and well-controlled studies in pregnant women. Because animal reproductive toxicity studies are not always predictive of human response, lamivudine should be used during pregnancy only if the potential benefits outweigh the risks.
Lamivudine has not been shown to affect the transmission of HBV from mother to infant, and appropriate infant immunizations should be used to prevent neonatal acquisition of HBV.
Pregnancy Registry: To monitor maternal-fetal outcomes of pregnant women exposed to lamivudine, a Pregnancy Registry has been established. Physicians are encouraged to register patients by calling 1-800-258-4263.
Nursing Mothers: A study in lactating rats administered 45 mg/kg of lamivudine showed that lamivudine concentrations in milk were slightly greater than those in plasma. Lamivudine is also excreted in human milk. Samples of breast milk obtained from 20 mothers receiving lamivudine monotherapy (300 mg twice daily) or combination therapy (150 mg lamivudine twice daily and 300 mg zidovudine twice daily) had measurable concentrations of lamivudine. Because of the potential for serious adverse reactions in nursing infants, **mothers should be instructed not to breastfeed if they are receiving lamivudine.**
Pediatric Use: ***HBV:*** Safety and efficacy of lamivudine for treatment of chronic hepatitis B in children have been studied in pediatric patients from 2 to 17 years of age in a controlled clinical trial (see CLINICAL PHARMACOLOGY, INDICATIONS AND USAGE, and DOSAGE AND ADMINISTRATION).
Safety and efficacy in pediatric patients <2 years of age have not been established.
HIV: See the complete prescribing information for EPIVIR Tablets and Oral Solution for additional information on pharmacokinetics of lamivudine in HIV-infected children.
Geriatric Use: Clinical studies of EPIVIR-HBV did not include sufficient numbers of subjects aged 65 and over to determine whether they respond differently from younger subjects. In general, dose selection for an elderly patient should be cautious, reflecting the greater frequency of decreased hepatic, renal, or cardiac function, and of concomitant disease or other drug therapy. In particular, because lamivudine is substantially excreted by the kidney and elderly patients are more likely to have decreased renal function, renal function should be monitored and dosage adjustments should be made accordingly (see PRECAUTIONS: Patients with Impaired Renal Function and DOSAGE AND ADMINISTRATION).

ADVERSE REACTIONS

Several serious adverse events reported with lamivudine (lactic acidosis and severe hepatomegaly with steatosis,

Table 6. Frequencies of Specified Laboratory Abnormalities in 3 Placebo-Controlled Trials in Adults During Treatment* (Studies 1-3)

Test (Abnormal Level)	Patients with Abnormality/Patients with Observations	
	EPIVIR-HBV	Placebo
ALT >3 × baseline†	37/331 (11%)	26/199 (13%)
Albumin <2.5 g/dL	0/331 (0%)	2/199 (1%)
Amylase >3 × baseline	2/259 (<1%)	4/167 (2%)
Serum Lipase ≥2.5 × ULN‡	19/189 (10%)	9/127 (7%)
CPK ≥7 × baseline	31/329 (9%)	9/198 (5%)
Neutrophils <750/mm^3	0/331 (0%)	1/199 (<1%)
Platelets <50,000/mm^3	10/272 (4%)	5/168 (3%)

*Includes patients treated for 52 to 68 weeks.
†See Table 7 for posttreatment ALT values.
‡Includes observations during and after treatment in the 2 placebo-controlled trials that collected this information.
ULN = Upper limit of normal.

Table 7. Posttreatment ALT Elevations in 2 Placebo-Controlled Studies in Adults With No-Active-Treatment Follow-up (Studies 1 and 3)

Abnormal Value	Patients with ALT Elevation/ Patients with Observations*	
	EPIVIR-HBV	Placebo
ALT ≥2 × baseline value	37/137 (27%)	22/116 (19%)
ALT ≥3 × baseline value†	29/137 (21%)	9/116 (8%)
ALT ≥2 × baseline value and absolute ALT >500 IU/L	21/137 (15%)	8/116 (7%)
ALT ≥2 × baseline value; and bilirubin >2 × ULN and ≥2 × baseline value	1/137 (0.7%)	1/116 (0.9%)

*Each patient may be represented in one or more category.
†Comparable to a Grade 3 toxicity in accordance with modified WHO criteria.
ULN = Upper limit of normal.

posttreatment exacerbations of hepatitis B, pancreatitis, and emergence of viral mutants associated with reduced drug susceptibility and diminished treatment response) are also described in WARNINGS and PRECAUTIONS.
Clinical Trials In Chronic Hepatitis B: ***Adults:*** Selected clinical adverse events observed with a ≥5% frequency during therapy with EPIVIR-HBV compared with placebo are listed in Table 5. Frequencies of specified laboratory abnormalities during therapy with EPIVIR-HBV compared with placebo are listed in Table 6.
[See table 5 at top of previous page]
[See table 6 above]
In patients followed for up to 16 weeks after discontinuation of treatment, posttreatment ALT elevations were observed more frequently in patients who had received EPIVIR-HBV than in patients who had received placebo. A comparison of ALT elevations between weeks 52 and 68 in patients who discontinued EPIVIR-HBV at week 52 and patients in the same studies who received placebo throughout the treatment course is shown in Table 7.
[See table 7 above]
Lamivudine in Patients with HIV: In HIV-infected patients, safety information reflects a higher dose of lamivudine (150 mg b.i.d.) than the dose used to treat chronic hepatitis B in HIV-negative patients. In clinical trials using lamivudine as part of a combination regimen for treatment of HIV infection, several clinical adverse events occurred more often in lamivudine-containing treatment arms than in comparator arms. These included nasal signs and symptoms (20% vs. 11%), dizziness (10% vs. 4%), and depressive disorders (9% vs. 4%). Pancreatitis was observed in 9 of the 2,613 adult patients (<0.5%) who received EPIVIR in controlled clinical trials. Laboratory abnormalities reported more often in lamivudine-containing arms included neutropenia and elevations of liver function tests (also more frequent in lamivudine-containing arms for a retrospective analysis of HIV/HBV dually infected patients in one study), and amylase elevations. Please see the complete prescribing information for EPIVIR Tablets and Oral Solution for more information.
Pediatric Patients with Hepatitis B: Most commonly observed adverse events in the pediatric trials were similar to those in adult trials; in addition, respiratory symptoms (cough, bronchitis, and viral respiratory infections) were reported in both lamivudine and placebo recipients. Posttreatment transaminase elevations were observed in some patients followed after cessation of lamivudine.
Pediatric Patients with HIV Infection: In early open-label studies of lamivudine in children with HIV, peripheral neuropathy and neutropenia were reported, and pancreatitis was observed in 14% to 15% of patients.
Observed During Clinical Practice: The following events have been identified during post-approval use of lamivudine in clinical practice. Because they are reported voluntarily from a population of unknown size, estimates of frequency cannot be made. These events have been chosen for inclusion due to either their seriousness, frequency of reporting, potential causal connection to lamivudine, or a combination of these factors. Post-marketing experience with lamivudine at this time is largely limited to use in HIV-infected patients.
Digestive: Stomatitis.
Endocrine and Metabolic: Hyperglycemia.
General: Weakness.
Hemic and Lymphatic: Anemia (including pure red cell aplasia and severe anemias progressing on therapy), lymphadenopathy, splenomegaly.
Hepatic and Pancreatic: Lactic acidosis and steatosis, pancreatitis, posttreatment exacerbation of hepatitis (see WARNINGS and PRECAUTIONS).
Hypersensitivity: Anaphylaxis, urticaria.
Musculoskeletal: Rhabdomyolysis.
Nervous: Paresthesia, peripheral neuropathy.
Respiratory: Abnormal breath sounds/wheezing.
Skin: Alopecia, pruritus, rash.

OVERDOSAGE

There is no known antidote for EPIVIR-HBV. One case of an adult ingesting 6 g of EPIVIR was reported; there were no clinical signs or symptoms noted and hematologic tests remained normal. It is not known whether lamivudine can be removed by peritoneal dialysis or hemodialysis. If overdose occurs, the patient should be monitored, and standard supportive treatment applied as required.

DOSAGE AND ADMINISTRATION

Adults: The recommended oral dose of EPIVIR-HBV for treatment of chronic hepatitis B in adults is 100 mg once daily (see paragraph below and WARNINGS). Safety and effectiveness of treatment beyond 1 year have not been established and the optimum duration of treatment is not known (see PRECAUTIONS).
The formulation and dosage of lamivudine in EPIVIR-HBV are not appropriate for patients dually infected with HBV and HIV. If lamivudine is administered to such patients, the higher dosage indicated for HIV therapy should be used as part of an appropriate combination regimen, and the prescribing information for EPIVIR as well as EPIVIR-HBV should be consulted.
Pediatric Patients: The recommended oral dose of EPIVIR-HBV for pediatric patients 2 to 17 years of age with chronic hepatitis B is 3 mg/kg once daily up to a maximum daily dose of 100 mg. Safety and effectiveness of treatment beyond 1 year have not been established and the optimum duration of treatment is not known (see PRECAUTIONS).
EPIVIR-HBV is available in a 5-mg/mL oral solution when a liquid formulation is needed. (Please see information above regarding distinctions between different lamivudine-containing products.)
Dose Adjustment: It is recommended that doses of EPIVIR-HBV be adjusted in accordance with renal function (Table 8) (see CLINICAL PHARMACOLOGY: Special Populations).

Table 8. Adjustment of Adult Dosage of EPIVIR-HBV in Accordance With Creatinine Clearance

Creatinine Clearance (mL/min)	Recommended Dosage of EPIVIR-HBV
≥50	100 mg once daily
30-49	100 mg first dose, then 50 mg once daily
15-29	100 mg first dose, then 25 mg once daily
5-14	35 mg first dose, then 15 mg once daily
<5	35 mg first dose, then 10 mg once daily

Although there are insufficient data to recommend a specific dose adjustment of EPIVIR-HBV in pediatric patients with renal impairment, a dose reduction should be considered.

No additional dosing of EPIVIR-HBV is required after routine (4-hour) hemodialysis. Insufficient data are available to recommend a dosage of EPIVIR-HBV in patients undergoing peritoneal dialysis (see CLINICAL PHARMACOLOGY: Special Populations).

HOW SUPPLIED

EPIVIR-HBV Tablets, 100 mg, are butterscotch-colored, film-coated, biconvex, capsule-shaped tablets imprinted with "GX CG5" on one side.

Bottles of 60 tablets (NDC 0173-0662-00) with child-resistant closures.

Store at 25°C (77°F), excursions permitted to 15° to 30°C (59° to 86°F) [see USP Controlled Room Temperature].

EPIVIR-HBV Oral Solution, a clear, colorless to pale yellow, strawberry-banana-flavored liquid, contains 5 mg of lamivudine in each 1 mL in plastic bottles of 240 mL.

Bottles of 240 mL (NDC 0173-0663-00) with child-resistant closures. This product does not require reconstitution.

Store at controlled room temperature of 20° to 25°C (68° to 77°F) (see USP) in tightly closed bottles.

REFERENCES

1. Knodell RG, Ishak KG, Black WC, et al. Formulation and application of a numerical scoring system for assessing histological activity in asymptomatic chronic active hepatitis. *Hepatology*. 1982;1:431-435.

GlaxoSmithKline, Research Triangle Park, NC 27709

Manufactured under agreement from

Shire Pharmaceuticals Group plc, Basingstoke, UK

May 2004/RL-2089

Shown in Product Identification Guide, page 315

EPZICOM™ ℞

[*ĕp-zĭ-kŏm*]

(abacavir sulfate and lamivudine)

Tablets

WARNINGS

EPZICOM contains 2 nucleoside analogues (abacavir sulfate and lamivudine) and is intended only for patients whose regimen would otherwise include these 2 components.

Hypersensitivity Reactions: Serious and sometimes fatal hypersensitivity reactions have been associated with abacavir sulfate, a component of EPZICOM. Hypersensitivity to abacavir is a multi-organ clinical syndrome usually characterized by a sign or symptom in 2 or more of the following groups: (1) fever, (2) rash, (3) gastrointestinal (including nausea, vomiting, diarrhea, or abdominal pain), (4) constitutional (including generalized malaise, fatigue, or achiness), and (5) respiratory (including dyspnea, cough, or pharyngitis). Discontinue EPZICOM as soon as a hypersensitivity reaction is suspected. Permanently discontinue EPZICOM if hypersensitivity cannot be ruled out, even when other diagnoses are possible.

Following a hypersensitivity reaction to abacavir, NEVER restart EPZICOM or any other abacavir-containing product because more severe symptoms can occur within hours and may include life-threatening hypotension and death.

Reintroduction of EPZICOM or any other abacavir-containing product, even in patients who have no identified history or unrecognized symptoms of hypersensitivity to abacavir therapy, can result in serious or fatal hypersensitivity reactions. Such reactions can occur within hours (see WARNINGS and PRECAUTIONS: Information for Patients).

Lactic Acidosis and Severe Hepatomegaly: Lactic acidosis and severe hepatomegaly with steatosis, including fatal cases, have been reported with the use of nucleoside analogues alone or in combination, including abacavir, lamivudine, and other antiretrovirals (see WARNINGS).

Exacerbations of Hepatitis B: Severe acute exacerbations of hepatitis B have been reported in patients who are co-infected with hepatitis B virus (HBV) and human immunodeficiency virus (HIV) and have discontinued lamivudine, which is one component of EPZICOM. Hepatic function should be monitored closely with both clinical and laboratory follow-up for at least several months in patients who discontinue EPZICOM and are co-infected with HIV and HBV. If appropriate, initiation of anti-hepatitis B therapy may be warranted (see WARNINGS).

DESCRIPTION

EPZICOM: EPZICOM Tablets contain the following 2 synthetic nucleoside analogues: abacavir sulfate (ZIAGEN®, also a component of TRIZIVIR®) and lamivudine (also known as EPIVIR® or 3TC) with inhibitory activity against HIV.

EPZICOM Tablets are for oral administration. Each orange, film-coated tablet contains the active ingredients 600 mg of abacavir as abacavir sulfate and 300 mg of lamivudine and the inactive ingredients magnesium stearate, microcrystalline cellulose, and sodium starch glycolate. The tablets are coated with a film (Opadry® orange YS-1-13065-A) that is made of FD&C Yellow No. 6, hypromellose, polyethylene glycol 400, polysorbate 80, and titanium dioxide.

Abacavir Sulfate: The chemical name of abacavir sulfate is (1*S*,*cis*)-4-[2-amino-6-(cyclopropylamino)-9*H*-purin-9-yl]-2-cyclopentene-1-methanol sulfate (salt) (2:1). Abacavir sulfate is the enantiomer with *1S, 4R* absolute configuration on the cyclopentene ring. It has a molecular formula of $(C_{14}H_{18}N_6O)_2 \cdot H_2SO_4$ and a molecular weight of 670.76 daltons. It has the following structural formula:

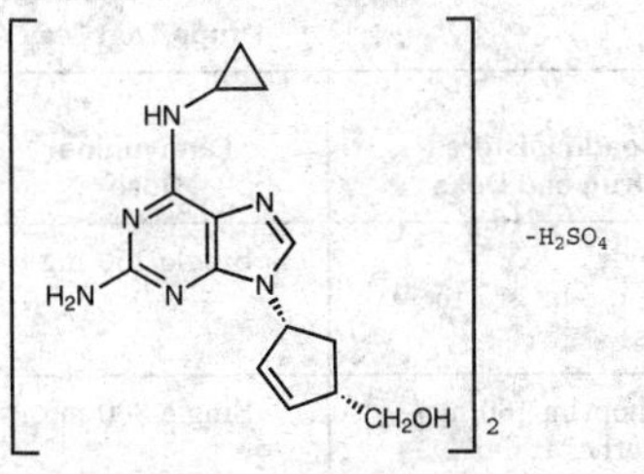

Abacavir sulfate is a white to off-white solid with a solubility of approximately 77 mg/mL in distilled water at 25 °C. In vivo, abacavir sulfate dissociates to its free base, abacavir. All dosages for abacavir sulfate are expressed in terms of abacavir.

Lamivudine: The chemical name of lamivudine is (2R,cis)-4-amino-1-(2-hydroxymethyl-1,3-oxathiolan-5-yl)-(1H)-pyrimidin-2-one. Lamivudine is the (-)enantiomer of a dideoxy analogue of cytidine. Lamivudine has also been referred to as (-)2′,3′-dideoxy, 3′-thiacytidine. It has a molecular formula of $C_8H_{11}N_3O_3S$ and a molecular weight of 229.3 daltons. It has the following structural formula:

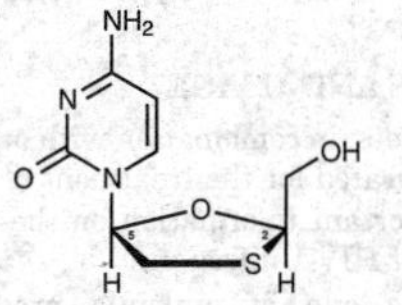

Lamivudine is a white to off-white crystalline solid with a solubility of approximately 70 mg/mL in water at 20 °C.

MICROBIOLOGY

Mechanism of Action: Abacavir is a carbocyclic synthetic nucleoside analogue. Abacavir is converted intracellularly by cellular enzymes to the active metabolite, carbovir triphosphate, an analogue of deoxyguanosine-5′-triphosphate (dGTP). Carbovir triphosphate inhibits the activity of HIV-1 reverse transcriptase (RT) in viral DNA synthesis both by competing with the natural substrate dGTP and by its incorporation into viral DNA resulting in chain termination. Lamivudine is a synthetic nucleoside analogue, which is phosphorylated intracellularly to its active metabolite, lamivudine triphosphate. The principal mode of action of lamivudine triphosphate is inhibition of RT via viral DNA chain termination after incorporation of the nucleoside analogue. Abacavir and lamivudine are weak inhibitors of human DNA polymerases α, β, and γ.

Antiviral Activity: Abacavir had IC_{50} (50% inhibitory concentration) values ranging from 3.7 to 5.8 μM and 0.07 to 1.0 μM against HIV-1_{IIIB} in lymphoblastic cell lines and HIV-1_{BaL} in monocytes/macrophages, respectively, and a mean IC_{50} value of 0.26 μM against 8 clinical isolates in monocytes and peripheral blood mononuclear cells. Lamivudine had IC_{50} values ranging from 0.0026 μM to 15 μM against HIV-1 in monocytes and human peripheral blood lymphocytes. The combination of abacavir and lamivudine has demonstrated antiviral activity in vitro against non-subtype B isolates and HIV-2 isolates with equivalent antiviral activity as for subtype B isolates. Abacavir/lamivudine had additive to synergistic activity in vitro in combination with the nucleoside reverse transcriptase inhibitors (NRTIs: emtricitabine, stavudine, tenofovir, zalcitabine, zidovudine), the non-nucleoside reverse transcriptase inhibitors (NNRTIs: delavirdine, efavirenz, nevirapine), the protease inhibitors (PIs: amprenavir, indinavir, lopinavir, nelfinavir, ritonavir, saquinavir), or the fusion inhibitor, enfuvirtide. Ribavirin, used in combination with interferon for the treatment of HCV infection, decreased the anti-HIV potency of abacavir/lamivudine reproducibly by 2- to 6-fold in vitro.

Resistance: HIV-1 isolates with reduced susceptibility to the combination of abacavir and lamivudine have been selected in vitro and have also been obtained from patients failing abacavir/lamivudine-containing regimens. Genotypic characterization of abacavir/lamivudine-resistant viruses selected in vitro identified amino acid substitutions M184V/I, K65R, L74V, and Y115F in HIV-1 RT.

Genetic analysis of isolates from patients failing an abacavir-containing regimen demonstrated that amino acid substitutions K65R, L74V, Y115F, and M184V in HIV-1 RT contributed to abacavir resistance. Genotypic analysis of isolates recovered from patients failing a lamivudine-containing regimen showed that the resistance was due to the M184V mutation in HIV-1 RT. In a study of therapy-naive adults receiving ZIAGEN 600 mg once daily (n = 384) or 300 mg twice daily (n = 386) in a background regimen of lamivudine 300 mg and efavirenz 600 mg once daily (Study CNA30021), the incidence of virologic failure at 48 weeks was similar between the 2 groups (11% in both arms). Genotypic (n = 38) and phenotypic analyses (n = 35) of virologic failure isolates from this study showed that the RT mutations that emerged during abacavir/lamivudine once-daily and twice-daily therapy were K65R, L74V, Y115F, and M184V/I. The abacavir- and lamivudine-associated resistance mutation M184V/I was the most commonly observed mutation in virologic failure isolates from patients receiving abacavir/lamivudine once daily (56%, 10/18) and twice daily (40%, 8/20).

Thirty-nine percent (7/18) of the isolates from patients who experienced virologic failure in the abacavir once-daily arm had a >2.5-fold decrease in abacavir susceptibility with a median-fold decrease of 1.3 (range 0.5 to 11) compared with 29% (5/17) of the failure isolates in the twice-daily arm with a median-fold decrease of 0.92 (range 0.7 to 13). Fifty-six percent (10/18) of the virologic failure isolates in the once-daily abacavir group compared to 41% (7/17) of the failure isolates in the twice-daily abacavir group had a >2.5-fold decrease in lamivudine susceptibility with median-fold changes of 81 (range 0.79 to >116) and 1.1 (range 0.68 to >116) in the once-daily and twice-daily abacavir arms, respectively.

Cross-Resistance: Cross-resistance has been observed among nucleoside reverse transcriptase inhibitors. Viruses containing abacavir and lamivudine resistance-associated mutations, namely, K65R, L74V, M184V, and Y115F, exhibit cross-resistance to didanosine, emtricitabine, lamivudine, tenofovir, and zalcitabine in vitro and in patients. The K65R mutation can confer resistance to abacavir, didanosine, emtricitabine, lamivudine, stavudine, tenofovir, and zalcitabine; the L74V mutation can confer resistance to abacavir, didanosine, and zalcitabine; and the M184V mutation can confer resistance to abacavir, didanosine, emtricitabine, lamivudine, and zalcitabine.

The combination of abacavir/lamivudine has demonstrated decreased susceptibility to viruses with the mutations K65R with or without the M184V/I mutation, viruses with L74V plus the M184V/I mutation, and viruses with thymidine analog mutations (TAMs: M41L, D67N, K70R, L210W, T215Y/F, K219 E/R/H/Q/N) plus M184V. An increasing number of TAMs is associated with a progressive reduction in abacavir susceptibility.

CLINICAL PHARMACOLOGY

Pharmacokinetics in Adults: *EPZICOM:* In a single-dose, 3-way crossover bioavailability study of 1 EPZICOM tablet versus 2 ZIAGEN Tablets (2 × 300 mg) and 2 EPIVIR Tablets (2 × 150 mg) administered simultaneously in healthy subjects (n = 25), there was no difference in the extent of absorption, as measured by the area under the plasma concentration-time curve (AUC) and maximal peak concentration (C_{max}), of each component.

Abacavir: Following oral administration, abacavir is rapidly absorbed and extensively distributed. After oral administration of a single dose of 600 mg of abacavir in 20 patients, C_{max} was 4.26 ± 1.19 mcg/mL (mean ± SD) and AUC_{∞} was 11.95 ± 2.51 mcg•hr/mL. Binding of abacavir to human plasma proteins is approximately 50% and was independent of concentration. Total blood and plasma drug-related radioactivity concentrations are identical, demonstrating that abacavir readily distributes into erythrocytes. The primary routes of elimination of abacavir are metabolism by alcohol dehydrogenase to form the 5′-carboxylic acid and glucuronyl transferase to form the 5′-glucuronide.

Lamivudine: Following oral administration, lamivudine is rapidly absorbed and extensively distributed. After multiple-dose oral administration of lamivudine 300 mg once daily for 7 days to 60 healthy volunteers, steady-state C_{max} ($C_{max,ss}$) was 2.04 ± 0.54 mcg/mL (mean ± SD) and the 24-hour steady-state AUC ($AUC_{24,ss}$) was 8.87 ± 1.83 mcg•hr/mL. Binding to plasma protein is low. Approximately 70% of an intravenous dose of lamivudine is recovered as unchanged drug in the urine. Metabolism of lamivudine is a

Continued on next page

Product information on these pages is effective as of August 2004. Further information is available at: GlaxoSmithKline, PO Box 13398, Research Triangle Park, NC 27709. 1-888-825-5249. Corporate Web Site: www.gsk.com

Epzicom—Cont.

minor route of elimination. In humans, the only known metabolite is the trans-sulfoxide metabolite (approximately 5% of an oral dose after 12 hours).

The steady-state pharmacokinetic properties of the EPIVIR 300-mg tablet once daily for 7 days compared to the EPIVIR 150-mg tablet twice daily for 7 days were assessed in a crossover study in 60 healthy volunteers. EPIVIR 300 mg once daily resulted in lamivudine exposures that were similar to EPIVIR 150 mg twice daily with respect to plasma $AUC_{24,ss}$; however, $C_{max,ss}$ was 66% higher and the trough value was 53% lower compared to the 150-mg twice-daily regimen. Intracellular lamivudine triphosphate exposures in peripheral blood mononuclear cells were also similar with respect to $AUC_{24,ss}$ and $C_{max24,ss}$; however, trough values were lower compared to the 150-mg twice-daily regimen. Inter-subject variability was greater for intracellular lamivudine triphosphate concentrations versus lamivudine plasma trough concentrations. The clinical significance of observed differences for both plasma lamivudine concentrations and intracellular lamivudine triphosphate concentrations is not known.

In humans, abacavir and lamivudine are not significantly metabolized by cytochrome P450 enzymes.

The pharmacokinetic properties of abacavir and lamivudine in fasting patients are summarized in Table 1.

[See table 1 at right]

Effect of Food on Absorption of EPZICOM: EPZICOM may be administered with or without food. Administration with a high-fat meal in a single-dose bioavailability study resulted in no change in AUC_{last}, AUC_{∞} and C_{max} for lamivudine. Food did not alter the extent of systemic exposure to abacavir (AUC_{∞}), but the rate of absorption (C_{max}) was decreased approximately 24% compared to fasted conditions (n = 25). These results are similar to those from previous studies of the effect of food on abacavir and lamivudine tablets administered separately.

Special Populations: ***Impaired Renal Function:***

EPZICOM: Because lamivudine requires dose adjustment in the presence of renal insufficiency, EPZICOM is not recommended for use in patients with creatinine clearance <50 mL/min (see PRECAUTIONS).

Impaired Hepatic Function: EPZICOM: Abacavir is contraindicated in patients with moderate to severe hepatic impairment and dose reduction is required in patients with mild hepatic impairment. Because EPZICOM is a fixed-dose combination and cannot be dose adjusted, EPZICOM is contraindicated for patients with hepatic impairment.

Pregnancy: See PRECAUTIONS: Pregnancy.

Abacavir and Lamivudine: No data are available on the pharmacokinetics of abacavir or lamivudine during pregnancy.

Nursing Mothers: See PRECAUTIONS: Nursing Mothers.

Abacavir: No data are available on the pharmacokinetics of abacavir in nursing mothers.

Lamivudine: Samples of breast milk obtained from 20 mothers receiving lamivudine monotherapy (300 mg twice daily) or combination therapy (150 mg lamivudine twice daily and 300 mg zidovudine twice daily) had measurable concentrations of lamivudine.

Pediatric Patients: EPZICOM: The pharmacokinetics of EPZICOM in pediatric patients are under investigation. There are insufficient data at this time to recommend a dose (see PRECAUTIONS: Pediatric Use).

Geriatric Patients: The pharmacokinetics of abacavir and lamivudine have not been studied in patients over 65 years of age.

Gender: Abacavir: A population pharmacokinetic analysis in HIV-infected male (n = 304) and female (n = 67) patients showed no gender differences in abacavir AUC normalized for lean body weight.

Lamivudine: A pharmacokinetic study in healthy male (n = 12) and female (n = 12) subjects showed no gender differences in lamivudine AUC∞ normalized for body weight.

Race: Abacavir: There are no significant differences between blacks and Caucasians in abacavir pharmacokinetics.

Lamivudine: There are no significant racial differences in lamivudine pharmacokinetics.

Drug Interactions: See PRECAUTIONS: Drug Interactions. The drug interactions described are based on studies conducted with the individual nucleoside analogues. In humans, abacavir and lamivudine are not significantly metabolized by cytochrome P450 enzymes nor do they inhibit or induce this enzyme system; therefore, it is unlikely that clinically significant drug interactions will occur with drugs metabolized through these pathways.

Abacavir: Fifteen HIV-infected patients were enrolled in a crossover-designed drug interaction study evaluating single doses of abacavir (600 mg), lamivudine (150 mg), and zidovudine (300 mg) alone or in combination. Analysis showed no clinically relevant changes in the pharmacokinetics of abacavir with the addition of lamivudine or zidovudine or the combination of lamivudine and zidovudine. Lamivudine exposure (AUC decreased 15%) and zidovudine exposure (AUC increased 10%) did not show clinically relevant changes with concurrent abacavir.

In a study of 11 HIV-infected patients receiving methadone-maintenance therapy (40 mg and 90 mg daily), with 600 mg of ZIAGEN twice daily (twice the currently recommended dose), oral methadone clearance increased 22% (90% CI 6% to 42%). This alteration will not result in a methadone dose

Table 1. Pharmacokinetic Parameters* for Abacavir and Lamivudine in Adults

Parameter	Abacavir		Lamivudine	
Oral bioavailability (%)	86 ± 25	n = 6	86 ± 16	n = 12
Apparent volume of distribution (L/kg)	0.86 ± 0.15	n = 6	1.3 ± 0.4	n = 20
Systemic clearance (L/hr/kg)	0.80 ± 0.24	n = 6	0.33 ± 0.06	n = 20
Renal clearance (L/hr/kg)	.007 ± .008	n = 6	0.22 ± 0.06	n = 20
Elimination half-life (hr)	1.45 ± 0.32	n = 20	5 to 7†	

*Data presented as mean ± standard deviation except where noted.
† Approximate range.

Table 2. Effect of Coadministered Drugs on Abacavir and Lamivudine AUC*
Note: ROUTINE DOSE MODIFICATION OF ABACAVIR AND LAMIVUDINE IS NOT WARRANTED WITH COADMINISTRATION OF THE FOLLOWING DRUGS.

Drugs That May Alter Abacavir Blood Concentrations

Coadministered Drug and Dose	Abacavir Dose	n	Abacavir Concentrations: AUC	Abacavir Concentrations: Variability	Concentration of Coadministered Drug
Ethanol 0.7 g/kg	Single 600 mg	24	↑41%	90% CI: 35% to 48%	↔

Drugs That May Alter Lamivudine Blood Concentrations

Coadministered Drug and Dose	Lamivudine Dose	n	Lamivudine Concentrations: AUC	Lamivudine Concentrations: Variability	Concentration of Coadministered Drug
Nelfinavir 750 mg q 8 hr × 7 to 10 days	Single 150 mg	11	↑10%	95% CI: 1% to 20%	↔
Trimethoprim 160 mg/ Sulfamethoxazole 800 mg daily× 5 days	Single 300 mg	14	↑43%	90% CI: 32% to 55%	↔

↑ = Increase; ↔ = no significant change; AUC = area under the concentration versus time curve; CI = confidence interval.
*See PRECAUTIONS: Drug Interactions for additional information on drug interactions.

modification in the majority of patients; however, an increased methadone dose may be required in a small number of patients.

Lamivudine: No clinically significant alterations in lamivudine or zidovudine pharmacokinetics were observed in 12 asymptomatic HIV-infected adult patients given a single dose of zidovudine (200 mg) in combination with multiple doses of lamivudine (300 mg q 12 hr). Lamivudine pharmacokinetics are not significantly affected by abacavir.

[See table 2 above]

INDICATIONS AND USAGE

EPZICOM Tablets, in combination with other antiretroviral agents, are indicated for the treatment of HIV-1 infection.

Additional important information on the use of EPZICOM for treatment of HIV-1 infection:

- EPZICOM is one of multiple products containing abacavir. Before starting EPZICOM, review medical history for prior exposure to any abacavir-containing product in order to avoid reintroduction in a patient with a history of hypersensitivity to abacavir.
- In one controlled study (CNA30021), more patients taking ZIAGEN 600 mg once daily had severe hypersensitivity reactions compared to patients taking ZIAGEN 300 mg twice daily.
- As part of a triple-drug regimen, EPZICOM tablets are recommended for use with antiretroviral agents from different pharmacological classes and not with other nucleoside/nucleotide reverse transcriptase inhibitors.

See WARNINGS, ADVERSE REACTIONS, and Description of Clinical Studies.

Description of Clinical Studies: ***EPZICOM:*** There have been no clinical trials conducted with EPZICOM (see CLINICAL PHARMACOLOGY for information about bioequivalence of EPZICOM). One EPZICOM Tablet given once daily is an alternative regimen to EPIVIR Tablets 300 mg once daily plus ZIAGEN Tablets 2 x 300 mg once daily as a component of antiretroviral therapy.

The following study was conducted with the individual components of EPZICOM.

Therapy-Naive Adults: **CNA30021** was an international, multicenter, double-blind, controlled study in which 770 HIV-infected, therapy-naive adults were randomized and received either ZIAGEN 600 mg once daily or ZIAGEN 300 mg twice daily, both in combination with EPIVIR 300 mg once daily and efavirenz 600 mg once daily. The double-blind treatment duration was at least 48 weeks. Study participants had a mean age of 37 years, were: male (81%), Caucasian (54%), black (27%), and American Hispanic (15%). The median baseline CD4+ cell count was 262 cells/mm^3 (range 21 to 918 cells/mm^3) and the median baseline plasma HIV-1 RNA was 4.89 log_{10} copies/mL (range: 2.60 to 6.99 log_{10} copies/mL).

The outcomes of randomized treatment are provided in Table 3.

Table 3. Outcomes of Randomized Treatment Through Week 48 (CNA30021)

Outcome	ZIAGEN 600 mg q.d. plus EPIVIR plus Efavirenz (n = 384)	ZIAGEN 300 mg b.i.d. plus EPIVIR plus Efavirenz (n = 386)
Responder*	64% (71%)	65% (72%)
Virologic failure†	11% (5%)	11% (5%)
Discontinued due to adverse reactions	13%	11%
Discontinued due to other reasons‡	11%	13%

*Patients achieved and maintained confirmed HIV-1 RNA <50 copies/mL (<400 copies/mL) through Week 48 (Roche® AMPLICOR Ultrasensitive HIV-1 MONITOR standard test version 1.0).
† Includes viral rebound, failure to achieve confirmed <50 copies/mL (<400 copies/mL) by Week 48, and insufficient viral load response.
‡ Includes consent withdrawn, lost to follow up, protocol violations, clinical progression, and other.

After 48 weeks of therapy, the median CD4+ cell count increases from baseline were 188 cells/mm^3 in the group receiving ZIAGEN 600 mg once daily and 200 cells/mm^3 in the group receiving ZIAGEN 300 mg twice daily. Through Week 48, 6 subjects (2%) in the group receiving ZIAGEN 600 mg once daily (4 CDC classification C events and 2 deaths) and 10 subjects (3%) in the group receiving ZIAGEN 300 mg twice daily (7 CDC classification C events and 3 deaths) experienced clinical disease progression. None of the deaths were attributed to study medications.

CONTRAINDICATIONS

EPZICOM Tablets are contraindicated in patients with previously demonstrated hypersensitivity to abacavir or to any other component of the product (see WARNINGS). Following a hypersensitivity reaction to abacavir, NEVER restart EPZICOM or any other abacavir-containing product. Fatal rechallenge reactions have been associated with readministration of abacavir to patients with a prior history of a hypersensitivity reaction to abacavir (see WARNINGS and PRECAUTIONS).

EPZICOM Tablets are contraindicated in patients with hepatic impairment (see CLINICAL PHARMACOLOGY).

WARNINGS

Hypersensitivity Reaction: Serious and sometimes fatal hypersensitivity reactions have been associated with EPZICOM and other abacavir-containing products. To min-

imize the risk of a life-threatening hypersensitivity reaction, permanently discontinue EPZICOM if hypersensitivity cannot be ruled out, even when other diagnoses are possible. Important information on signs and symptoms of hypersensitivity, as well as clinical management, is presented below.

Signs and Symptoms of Hypersensitivity: Hypersensitivity to abacavir is a multi-organ clinical syndrome usually characterized by a sign or symptom in 2 or more of the following groups.

Group 1: Fever
Group 2: Rash
Group 3: Gastrointestinal (including nausea, vomiting, diarrhea, or abdominal pain)
Group 4: Constitutional (including generalized malaise, fatigue, or achiness)
Group 5: Respiratory (including dyspnea, cough, or pharyngitis)

Hypersensitivity to abacavir following the presentation of a single sign or symptom has been reported infrequently.

Hypersensitivity to abacavir was reported in approximately 8% of 2,670 patients (n = 206) in 9 clinical trials (range: 2% to 9%) with enrollment from November 1999 to February 2002. Data on time to onset and symptoms of suspected hypersensitivity were collected on a detailed data collection module. The frequencies of symptoms are shown in Figure 1. Symptoms usually appeared within the first 6 weeks of treatment with abacavir, although the reaction may occur at any time during therapy. Median time to onset was 9 days; 89% appeared within the first 6 weeks; 95% of patients reported symptoms from 2 or more of the 5 groups listed above.

Figure 1: Hypersensitivity-Related Symptoms Reported with ≥10% Frequency in Clinical Trials (n = 206 Patients)

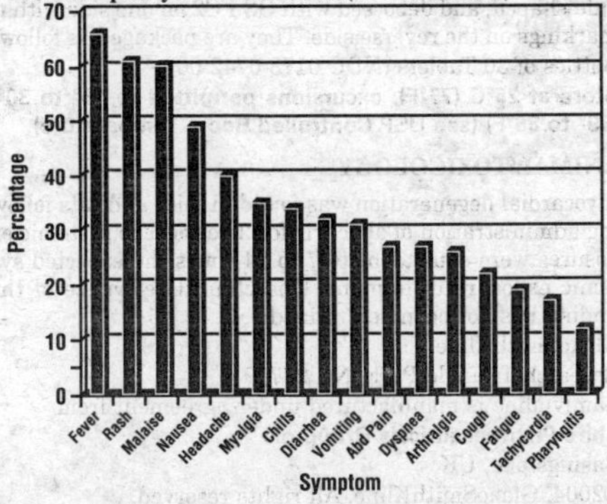

Other less common signs and symptoms of hypersensitivity include lethargy, myolysis, edema, abnormal chest x-ray findings (predominantly infiltrates, which can be localized), and paresthesia. Anaphylaxis, liver failure, renal failure, hypotension, adult respiratory distress syndrome, respiratory failure, and death have occurred in association with hypersensitivity reactions. In one study, 4 patients (11%) receiving ZIAGEN 600 mg once daily experienced hypotension with a hypersensitivity reaction compared with 0 patients receiving ZIAGEN 300 mg twice daily.

Physical findings associated with hypersensitivity to abacavir in some patients include lymphadenopathy, mucous membrane lesions (conjunctivitis and mouth ulcerations), and rash. The rash usually appears maculopapular or urticarial, but may be variable in appearance. There have been reports of erythema multiforme. Hypersensitivity reactions have occurred without rash.

Laboratory abnormalities associated with hypersensitivity to abacavir in some patients include elevated liver function tests, elevated creatine phosphokinase, elevated creatinine, and lymphopenia.

Clinical Management of Hypersensitivity: **Discontinue EPZICOM as soon as a hypersensitivity reaction is suspected. To minimize the risk of a life-threatening hypersensitivity reaction, permanently discontinue EPZICOM if hypersensitivity cannot be ruled out, even when other diagnoses are possible (e.g., acute onset respiratory diseases such as pneumonia, bronchitis, pharyngitis, or influenza; gastroenteritis; or reactions to other medications). Following a hypersensitivity reaction to abacavir, NEVER restart EPZICOM or any other abacavir-containing product because more severe symptoms can occur within hours and may include life-threatening hypotension and death.**

When therapy with EPZICOM has been discontinued for reasons other than symptoms of a hypersensitivity reaction, and if reinitiation of EPZICOM or any other abacavir-containing product is under consideration, carefully evaluate the reason for discontinuation of EPZICOM to ensure that the patient did not have symptoms of a hypersensitivity reaction. If hypersensitivity cannot be ruled out, DO NOT reintroduce EPZICOM or any other abacavir-containing product. If symptoms consistent with hypersensitivity are not identified, reintroduction can be undertaken with continued monitoring for symptoms of a hypersensitivity reaction. Make patients aware that a hypersensitivity reaction can occur with reintroduction of EPZICOM or any other abacavir-containing product and that reintroduction of EPZICOM or introduction of any other abacavir-containing product needs to be undertaken only if medical care can be readily accessed by the patient or others.

Abacavir Hypersensitivity Reaction Registry: To facilitate reporting of hypersensitivity reactions and collection of information on each case, an Abacavir Hypersensitivity Registry has been established. **Physicians should register patients by calling 1-800-270-0425.**

Lactic Acidosis/Severe Hepatomegaly with Steatosis: Lactic acidosis and severe hepatomegaly with steatosis, including fatal cases, have been reported with the use of nucleoside analogues alone or in combination, including abacavir and lamivudine and other antiretrovirals. A majority of these cases have been in women. Obesity and prolonged nucleoside exposure may be risk factors. Particular caution should be exercised when administering EPZICOM to any patient with known risk factors for liver disease; however, cases have also been reported in patients with no known risk factors. Treatment with EPZICOM should be suspended in any patient who develops clinical or laboratory findings suggestive of lactic acidosis or pronounced hepatotoxicity (which may include hepatomegaly and steatosis even in the absence of marked transaminase elevations).

Posttreatment Exacerbations of Hepatitis: In clinical trials in non-HIV-infected patients treated with lamivudine for chronic HBV, clinical and laboratory evidence of exacerbations of hepatitis have occurred after discontinuation of lamivudine. These exacerbations have been detected primarily by serum ALT elevations in addition to re-emergence of HBV DNA. Although most events appear to have been self-limited, fatalities have been reported in some cases. Similar events have been reported from post-marketing experience after changes from lamivudine-containing HIV treatment regimens to non-lamivudine-containing regimens in patients infected with both HIV and HBV. The causal relationship to discontinuation of lamivudine treatment is unknown. Patients should be closely monitored with both clinical and laboratory follow-up for at least several months after stopping treatment. There is insufficient evidence to determine whether re-initiation of lamivudine alters the course of posttreatment exacerbations of hepatitis.

Other: EPZICOM contains fixed doses of 2 nucleoside analogues, abacavir and lamivudine, and should not be administered concomitantly with other abacavir-containing and/or lamivudine-containing products (ZIAGEN, EPIVIR, COMBIVIR®, or TRIZIVIR).

The complete prescribing information for all agents being considered for use with EPZICOM should be consulted before combination therapy with EPZICOM is initiated.

PRECAUTIONS

Therapy-Experienced Patients: *Abacavir:* In clinical trials, patients with prolonged prior NRTI exposure or who had HIV-1 isolates that contained multiple mutations conferring resistance to NRTIs had limited response to abacavir. The potential for cross-resistance between abacavir and other NRTIs should be considered when choosing new therapeutic regimens in therapy-experienced patients (see MICROBIOLOGY: Cross-Resistance).

Patients with HIV and Hepatitis B Virus Coinfection: *Lamivudine:* Safety and efficacy of lamivudine have not been established for treatment of chronic hepatitis B in patients dually infected with HIV and HBV. In non-HIV-infected patients treated with lamivudine for chronic hepatitis B, emergence of lamivudine-resistant HBV has been detected and has been associated with diminished treatment response (see EPIVIR-HBV package insert for additional information). Emergence of hepatitis B virus variants associated with resistance to lamivudine has also been reported in HIV-infected patients who have received lamivudine-containing antiretroviral regimens in the presence of concurrent infection with hepatitis B virus.

Patients with Impaired Renal Function: *EPZICOM:* Since EPZICOM is a fixed-dose tablet and the dosage of the individual components cannot be altered, patients with creatinine clearance <50 mL/min should not receive EPZICOM.

Patients with Impaired Hepatic Function: *EPZICOM:* EPZICOM is contraindicated in patients with hepatic impairment since it is a fixed-dose tablet and the dosage of the individual components cannot be altered.

Fat Redistribution: Redistribution/accumulation of body fat including central obesity, dorsocervical fat enlargement (buffalo hump), peripheral wasting, facial wasting, breast enlargement, and "cushingoid appearance" have been observed in patients receiving antiretroviral therapy. The mechanism and long-term consequences of these events are currently unknown. A causal relationship has not been established.

Information for Patients:

Abacavir: Hypersensitivity Reaction: Inform patients:

- **that a Medication Guide and Warning Card summarizing the symptoms of the abacavir hypersensitivity reaction and other product information will be dispensed by the pharmacist with each new prescription and refill of EPZICOM, and encourage the patient to read the Medication Guide and Warning Card every time to obtain any new information that may be present about EPZICOM. (The complete text of the Medication Guide is reprinted at the end of this document.)**
- **to carry the Warning Card with them.**
- how to identify a hypersensitivity reaction (see WARNINGS and MEDICATION GUIDE).
- that if they develop symptoms consistent with a hypersensitivity reaction to discontinue treatment with EPZICOM and seek medical evaluation immediately.
- that a hypersensitivity reaction can worsen and lead to hospitalization or death if EPZICOM is not immediately discontinued.
- **to not restart EPZICOM or any other abacavir-containing product following a hypersensitivity reaction because more severe symptoms can occur within hours and may include life-threatening hypotension and death.**
- that a hypersensitivity reaction is usually reversible if it is detected promptly and EPZICOM is stopped right away.
- that if they have interrupted EPZICOM for reasons other than symptoms of hypersensitivity (for example, those who have an interruption in drug supply), a serious or fatal hypersensitivity reaction may occur with reintroduction of abacavir.
- that in one study, more severe hypersensitivity reactions were seen when ZIAGEN was dosed 600 mg once daily.
- **to not restart EPZICOM or any other abacavir-containing product without medical consultation and that restarting abacavir needs to be undertaken only if medical care can be readily accessed by the patient or others.**

Lamivudine: Patients co-infected with HIV and HBV should be informed that deterioration of liver disease has occurred in some cases when treatment with lamivudine was discontinued. Patients should be advised to discuss any changes in regimen with their physician.

EPZICOM: Inform patients that some HIV medicines, including EPZICOM, can cause a rare, but serious condition called lactic acidosis with liver enlargement (hepatomegaly).

EPZICOM is not a cure for HIV infection and patients may continue to experience illnesses associated with HIV infection, including opportunistic infections. Patients should remain under the care of a physician when using EPZICOM. Advise patients that the use of EPZICOM has not been shown to reduce the risk of transmission of HIV to others through sexual contact or blood contamination.

Inform patients that redistribution or accumulation of body fat may occur in patients receiving antiretroviral therapy and that the cause and long-term health effects of these conditions are not known at this time.

EPZICOM Tablets are for oral ingestion only.

Patients should be advised of the importance of taking EPZICOM exactly as it is prescribed.

Drug Interactions: *EPZICOM:* No clinically significant changes to pharmacokinetic parameters were observed for abacavir or lamivudine when administered together.

Abacavir: Abacavir has no effect on the pharmacokinetic properties of ethanol. Ethanol decreases the elimination of abacavir causing an increase in overall exposure (see CLINICAL PHARMACOLOGY: Drug Interactions).

The addition of methadone has no clinically significant effect on the pharmacokinetic properties of abacavir. In a study of 11 HIV-infected patients receiving methadone-maintenance therapy (40 mg and 90 mg daily), with 600 mg of ZIAGEN twice daily (twice the currently recommended dose), oral methadone clearance increased 22% (90% CI 6% to 42%). This alteration will not result in a methadone dose modification in the majority of patients; however, an increased methadone dose may be required in a small number of patients.

Lamivudine: Trimethoprim (TMP) 160 mg/sulfamethoxazole (SMX) 800 mg once daily has been shown to increase lamivudine exposure (AUC). No change in dose of either drug is recommended. The effect of higher doses of TMP/SMX on lamivudine pharmacokinetics has not been investigated (see CLINICAL PHARMACOLOGY).

Lamivudine and zalcitabine may inhibit the intracellular phosphorylation of one another. Therefore, use of EPZICOM in combination with zalcitabine is not recommended.

See CLINICAL PHARMACOLOGY for additional drug interactions.

Carcinogenesis, Mutagenesis, Impairment of Fertility: *Carcinogenicity:*

Abacavir: Abacavir was administered orally at 3 dosage levels to separate groups of mice and rats in 2-year carcinogenicity studies. Results showed an increase in the incidence of malignant and non-malignant tumors. Malignant tumors occurred in the preputial gland of males and the clitoral gland of females of both species, and in the liver of female rats. In addition, non-malignant tumors also occurred in the liver and thyroid gland of female rats. These observations were made at systemic exposures in the range of 6 to 32 times the human exposure at the recommended dose.

Lamivudine: Long-term carcinogenicity studies with lamivudine in mice and rats showed no evidence of carcinogenic potential at exposures up to 10 times (mice) and 58 times (rats) those observed in humans at the recommended therapeutic dose for HIV infection.

It is not known how predictive the results of rodent carcinogenicity studies may be for humans.

Mutagenicity: Abacavir: Abacavir induced chromosomal aberrations both in the presence and absence of metabolic

Continued on next page

Product information on these pages is effective as of August 2004. Further information is available at: GlaxoSmithKline, PO Box 13398, Research Triangle Park, NC 27709. 1-888-825-5249. Corporate Web Site: www.gsk.com

Epzicom—Cont.

activation in an in vitro cytogenetic study in human lymphocytes. Abacavir was mutagenic in the absence of metabolic activation, although it was not mutagenic in the presence of metabolic activation in an L5178Y mouse lymphoma assay. Abacavir was clastogenic in males and not clastogenic in females in an in vivo mouse bone marrow micronucleus assay. Abacavir was not mutagenic in bacterial mutagenicity assays in the presence and absence of metabolic activation.

Lamivudine: Lamivudine was mutagenic in an L5178Y mouse lymphoma assay and clastogenic in a cytogenetic assay using cultured human lymphocytes. Lamivudine was not mutagenic in a microbial mutagenicity assay, in an in vitro cell transformation assay, in a rat micronucleus test, in a rat bone marrow cytogenetic assay, and in an assay for unscheduled DNA synthesis in rat liver.

Impairment of Fertility: Abacavir or lamivudine induced no adverse effects on the mating performance or fertility of male and female rats at doses producing systemic exposure levels approximately 8 or 130 times, respectively, higher than those in humans at the recommended dose based on body surface area comparisons.

Pregnancy: Pregnancy Category C. There are no adequate and well-controlled studies of EPZICOM in pregnant women. Reproduction studies with abacavir and lamivudine have been performed in animals (see Abacavir and Lamivudine sections below). EPZICOM should be used during pregnancy only if the potential benefits outweigh the risks.

Abacavir: Studies in pregnant rats showed that abacavir is transferred to the fetus through the placenta. Fetal malformations (increased incidences of fetal anasarca and skeletal malformations) and developmental toxicity (depressed fetal body weight and reduced crown-rump length) were observed in rats at a dose which produced 35 times the human exposure, based on AUC. Embryonic and fetal toxicities (increased resorptions, decreased fetal body weights) and toxicities to the offspring (increased incidence of stillbirth and lower body weights) occurred at half of the above-mentioned dose in separate fertility studies conducted in rats. In the rabbit, no developmental toxicity and no increases in fetal malformations occurred at doses that produced 8.5 times the human exposure at the recommended dose based on AUC.

Lamivudine: Studies in pregnant rats showed that lamivudine is transferred to the fetus through the placenta. Reproduction studies with orally administered lamivudine have been performed in rats and rabbits at doses producing plasma levels up to approximately 35 times that for the recommended adult HIV dose. No evidence of teratogenicity due to lamivudine was observed. Evidence of early embryolethality was seen in the rabbit at exposure levels similar to those observed in humans, but there was no indication of this effect in the rat at exposure levels up to 35 times that in humans.

Antiretroviral Pregnancy Registry: To monitor maternal-fetal outcomes of pregnant women exposed to EPZICOM or other antiretroviral agents, an Antiretroviral Pregnancy Registry has been established. Physicians are encouraged to register patients by calling 1-800-258-4263.

Nursing Mothers: The Centers for Disease Control and Prevention recommend that HIV-infected mothers not breastfeed their infants to avoid risking postnatal transmission of HIV infection.

Abacavir: Abacavir is secreted into the milk of lactating rats.

Lamivudine: Lamivudine is excreted in human breast milk and into the milk of lactating rats.

Because of both the potential for HIV transmission and the potential for serious adverse reactions in nursing infants, **mothers should be instructed not to breastfeed if they are receiving EPZICOM.**

Pediatric Use: Safety and effectiveness of EPZICOM in pediatric patients have not been established.

Geriatric Use: Clinical studies of abacavir and lamivudine did not include sufficient numbers of patients aged 65 and over to determine whether they respond differently from younger patients. In general, dose selection for an elderly patient should be cautious, reflecting the greater frequency of decreased hepatic, renal, or cardiac function, and of concomitant disease or other drug therapy. EPZICOM is not recommended for patients with impaired renal function or impaired hepatic function (see PRECAUTIONS and DOSAGE AND ADMINISTRATION).

ADVERSE REACTIONS

Abacavir: ***Hypersensitivity Reaction:*** **Serious and sometimes fatal hypersensitivity reactions have been associated with abacavir sulfate, a component of EPZICOM.**

In one study, once-daily dosing of ZIAGEN was associated with more severe hypersensitivity reactions (see WARNINGS and PRECAUTIONS: Information for Patients).

Therapy-Naive Adults: Treatment-emergent clinical adverse reactions (rated by the investigator as moderate or severe) with a ≥5% frequency during therapy with ZIAGEN 600 mg once daily or ZIAGEN 300 mg twice daily, both in combination with lamivudine 300 mg once daily and efavirenz 600 mg once daily are listed in Table 4.

Table 4. Treatment-Emergent (All Causality) Adverse Reactions of at Least Moderate Intensity (Grades 2-4, ≥5% Frequency) in Therapy-Naive Adults (CNA30021) Through 48 Weeks of Treatment

Adverse Event	ZIAGEN 600 mg q.d. plus EPIVIR plus Efavirenz (n = 384)	ZIAGEN 300 mg b.i.d. plus EPIVIR plus Efavirenz (n = 386)
Drug hypersensitivity*†	9%	7%
Insomnia	7%	9%
Depression/Depressed mood	7%	7%
Headache/Migraine	7%	6%
Fatigue/Malaise	6%	8%
Dizziness/Vertigo	6%	6%
Nausea	5%	6%
Diarrhea*	5%	6%
Rash	5%	5%
Pyrexia	5%	3%
Abdominal pain/gastritis	4%	5%
Abnormal dreams	4%	5%
Anxiety	3%	5%

* Patients receiving ZIAGEN 600 mg once daily, experienced a significantly higher incidence of severe drug hypersensitivity reactions and severe diarrhea compared to patients who received ZIAGEN 300 mg twice daily. Five percent (5%) of patients receiving ZIAGEN 600 mg once daily had severe drug hypersensitivity reactions compared to 2% of patients receiving ZIAGEN 300 mg twice daily. Two percent (2%) of patients receiving ZIAGEN 600 mg once daily had severe diarrhea while none of the patients receiving ZIAGEN 300 mg twice daily had this event.

† Study **CNA30024** was a multicenter, double-blind, controlled study in which 649 HIV-infected, therapy-naive adults were randomized and received either ZIAGEN (300 mg twice daily), EPIVIR (150 mg twice daily), and efavirenz (600 mg once daily) or zidovudine (300 mg twice daily), EPIVIR (150 mg twice daily), and efavirenz (600 mg once daily). CNA30024 used double-blind ascertainment of suspected hypersensitivity reactions. During the blinded portion of the study, **suspected hypersensitivity to abacavir was reported by investigators in 9% of 324 patients in the abacavir group and 3% of 325 patients in the zidovudine group.**

Laboratory Abnormalities: Laboratory abnormalities observed in clinical studies of ZIAGEN were anemia, neutropenia, liver function test abnormalities, and elevations of CPK, blood glucose, and triglycerides. Additional laboratory abnormalities observed in clinical studies of EPIVIR were thrombocytopenia and elevated levels of bilirubin, amylase, and lipase.

The frequencies of treatment-emergent laboratory abnormalities were comparable between treatment groups in Study CNA30021.

Other Adverse Events: In addition to adverse reactions listed above, other adverse events observed in the expanded access program for abacavir were pancreatitis and increased GGT.

Observed During Clinical Practice: The following reactions have been identified during post-approval use of abacavir and lamivudine. Because they are reported voluntarily from a population of unknown size, estimates of frequency cannot be made. These events have been chosen for inclusion due to a combination of their seriousness, frequency of reporting, or potential causal connection to abacavir and/or lamivudine.

Abacavir: Suspected Stevens-Johnson syndrome (SJS) and toxic epidermal necrolysis (TEN) have been reported in patients receiving abacavir primarily in combination with medications known to be associated with SJS and TEN, respectively. Because of the overlap of clinical signs and symptoms between hypersensitivity to abacavir and SJS and TEN, and the possibility of multiple drug sensitivities in some patients, abacavir should be discontinued and not restarted in such cases.

There have also been reports of erythema multiforme with abacavir use.

Abacavir and Lamivudine:

Body as a Whole: Redistribution/accumulation of body fat (see PRECAUTIONS: Fat Redistribution).

Digestive: Stomatitis.

Endocrine and Metabolic: Hyperglycemia.

General: Weakness.

Hemic and Lymphatic: Aplastic anemia, anemia (including pure red cell aplasia and severe anemias progressing on therapy), lymphadenopathy, splenomegaly.

Hepatic and Pancreatic: Lactic acidosis and hepatic steatosis, pancreatitis, posttreatment exacerbation of hepatitis B (see WARNINGS).

Hypersensitivity: Sensitization reactions (including anaphylaxis), urticaria.

Musculoskeletal: Muscle weakness, CPK elevation, rhabdomyolysis.

Nervous: Paresthesia, peripheral neuropathy, seizures.

Respiratory: Abnormal breath sounds/wheezing.

Skin: Alopecia, erythema multiforme, Stevens-Johnson syndrome.

OVERDOSAGE

Abacavir: There is no known antidote for abacavir. It is not known whether abacavir can be removed by peritoneal dialysis or hemodialysis.

Lamivudine: One case of an adult ingesting 6 grams of lamivudine was reported; there were no clinical signs or symptoms noted and hematologic tests remained normal. It is not known whether lamivudine can be removed by peritoneal dialysis or hemodialysis.

DOSAGE AND ADMINISTRATION

A Medication Guide and Warning Card that provide information about recognition of hypersensitivity reactions should be dispensed with each new prescription and refill. To facilitate reporting of hypersensitivity reactions and collection of information on each case, an Abacavir Hypersensitivity Registry has been established. **Physicians should register patients by calling 1-800-270-0425.**

The recommended oral dose of EPZICOM for adults is one tablet daily, in combination with other antiretroviral agents (see INDICATIONS AND USAGE: Description of Clinical Studies, PRECAUTIONS, MICROBIOLOGY, and CLINICAL PHARMACOLOGY).

EPZICOM can be taken with or without food.

Dose Adjustment: Because it is a fixed-dose tablet, EPZICOM should not be prescribed for patients requiring dosage adjustment such as those with creatinine clearance <50 mL/min, those with hepatic impairment, or those experiencing dose-limiting adverse events. Use of EPIVIR Oral Solution and ZIAGEN Oral Solution may be considered.

HOW SUPPLIED

EPZICOM is available as tablets. Each tablet contains 600 mg of abacavir as abacavir sulfate and 300 mg of lamivudine. The tablets are orange, film-coated, modified capsule-shaped, and debossed with GS FC2 on one side with no markings on the reverse side. They are packaged as follows: Bottles of 30 Tablets (NDC 0173-0742-00).

Store at 25°C (77°F); excursions permitted to 15° to 30°C (59° to 86°F) (see USP Controlled Room Temperature).

ANIMAL TOXICOLOGY

Myocardial degeneration was found in mice and rats following administration of abacavir for 2 years. The systemic exposures were equivalent to 7 to 24 times the expected systemic exposure in humans. The clinical relevance of this finding has not been determined.

GlaxoSmithKline
Research Triangle Park, NC 27709
Lamivudine is manufactured under agreement from
Shire Pharmaceuticals Group plc
Basingstoke, UK

August 2004/RL-2112

MEDICATION GUIDE

EPZICOM™ (ep' zih com) Tablets

Generic name: abacavir sulfate and lamivudine

Read the Medication Guide that comes with Epzicom before you start taking it and each time you get a refill because there may be new information. This information does not take the place of talking to your doctor about your medical condition or your treatment. Be sure to carry your Epzicom Warning Card with you at all times.

What is the most important information I should know about Epzicom?

- **Serious Allergic Reaction to Abacavir. Epzicom contains abacavir (also contained in Ziagen® and Trizivir®).** Patients taking Epzicom may have a serious allergic reaction (hypersensitivity reaction) that can cause death. **If you get a symptom from 2 or more of the following groups while taking Epzicom, stop taking Epzicom and call your doctor right away.**

	Symptom(s)
Group 1	Fever
Group 2	Rash
Group 3	Nausea, vomiting, diarrhea, abdominal (stomach area) pain
Group 4	Generally ill feeling, extreme tiredness, or achiness
Group 5	Shortness of breath, cough, sore throat

A list of these symptoms is on the Warning Card your pharmacist gives you. Carry this Warning Card with you.

If you stop Epzicom because of an allergic reaction, NEVER take Epzicom (abacavir sulfate and lamivudine) or any other abacavir-containing medicine (Ziagen and Trizivir) again. If you take Epzicom or any other abacavir-containing medicine again after you have had an allergic reaction, **WITHIN HOURS** you may get **life-threatening symptoms** that may include **very low blood pressure** or **death.**

If you stop Epzicom for any other reason, even for a few days, and you are not allergic to Epzicom, talk with your doctor before taking it again. Taking Epzicom again can

cause a serious allergic or life-threatening reaction, even if you never had an allergic reaction to it before. If your doctor tells you that you can take Epzicom again, **start taking it when you are around medical help or people who can call a doctor if you need one.**

- **Lactic Acidosis. Some HIV medicines, including Epzicom, can cause a rare but serious condition called lactic acidosis with liver enlargement (hepatomegaly).** Nausea and tiredness that don't get better may be symptoms of lactic acidosis. In some cases this condition can cause death. Women, overweight people, and people who have taken HIV medicines like Epzicom for a long time have a higher chance of getting lactic acidosis and liver enlargement. Lactic acidosis is a medical emergency and must be treated in the hospital.
- **Worsening of hepatitis B virus (HBV) infection.** Patients with HBV infection, who take Epzicom and then stop it, may get "flare-ups" of their hepatitis. "Flare-up" is when the disease suddenly returns in a worse way than before. If you have HBV infection, your doctor should closely monitor your liver function for several months after stopping EPZICOM. You may need to take anti-HBV medicines.

Epzicom can have other serious side effects. Be sure to read the section below entitled "What are the possible side effects of Epzicom?"

What is Epzicom?

Epzicom is a prescription medicine used to treat HIV infection. Epzicom includes 2 medicines: abacavir (Ziagen) and lamivudine or 3TC (Epivir®). See the end of this Medication Guide for a complete list of ingredients in Epzicom. Both of these medicines are called nucleoside analogue reverse transcriptase inhibitors (NRTIs). When used together, they help lower the amount of HIV in your blood. This helps to keep your immune system as healthy as possible so that it can help fight infection.

Different combinations of medicines are used to treat HIV infection. You and your doctor should discuss which combination of medicines is best for you.

- **Epzicom does not cure HIV infection or AIDS.** We do not know if Epzicom will help you live longer or have fewer of the medical problems that people get with HIV or AIDS. It is very important that you see your doctor regularly while you are taking Epzicom.
- **Epzicom does not lower the risk of passing HIV to other people through sexual contact, sharing needles, or being exposed to your blood.** For your health and the health of others, it is important to always practice safe sex by using a latex or polyurethane condom or other barrier method to lower the chance of sexual contact with semen, vaginal secretions, or blood. Never use or share dirty needles.

Who should not take Epzicom?

Do not take Epzicom if you:

- **have ever had a serious allergic reaction (a hypersensitivity reaction) to Epzicom or any other medicine that has abacavir as one of its ingredients (Trizivir and Ziagen).** See the end of this Medication Guide for a complete list of ingredients in Epzicom. If you have had such a reaction, return all of your unused Epzicom to your doctor or pharmacist.
- **have a liver that does not function properly.**
- **are less than 18 years of age.**

Before starting Epzicom tell your doctor about all your medical conditions, including if you:

- **are pregnant or planning to become pregnant.** We do not know if Epzicom will harm your unborn child. You and your doctor will need to decide if Epzicom is right for you. If you use Epzicom while you are pregnant, talk to your doctor about how you can be on the Antiviral Pregnancy Registry for Epzicom.
- **are breastfeeding.** Some of the ingredients in Epzicom can be passed to your baby in your breast milk. It is not known if they could harm your baby. Also, mothers with HIV should not breastfeed because HIV can be passed to the baby in the breast milk.
- **have liver problems including hepatitis B virus infection.**
- **have kidney problems.**

Tell your doctor about all the medicines you take, including prescription and nonprescription medicines, vitamins, and herbal supplements. Especially tell your doctor if you take:

- **methadone**
- **Hivid® (zalcitabine, ddC)**
- **Epivir or Epivir-HBV (lamivudine, 3TC), Ziagen (abacavir sulfate), Combivir® (lamivudine and zidovudine), or Trizivir (abacavir sulfate, lamivudine, and zidovudine).**

How should I take Epzicom?

- **Take Epzicom by mouth exactly as your doctor prescribes it.** The usual dose is 1 tablet once a day. Do not skip doses.
- **You can take Epzicom with or without food.**
- **If you miss a dose of Epzicom, take the missed dose right away. Then, take the next dose at the usual time.**
- **Do not let your Epzicom run out.**
- **Starting Epzicom again can cause a serious allergic or life-threatening reaction, even if you never had an allergic reaction to it before.** If you run out of Epzicom even for a few days, you must ask your doctor if you can start Epzicom again. If your doctor tells you that you can take Epzicom again, start taking it when you are around medical help or people who can call a doctor if you need one.
- If you stop your anti-HIV drugs, even for a short time, the amount of virus in your blood may increase and the virus may become harder to treat.
- **If you take too much Epzicom, call your doctor or poison control center right away.**

What should I avoid while taking Epzicom?

- Do not take Epivir **(lamivudine, 3TC)**, Combivir **(lamivudine and zidovudine)**, Ziagen **(abacavir sulfate)**, or Trizivir **(abacavir sulfate, lamivudine, and zidovudine)** while taking Epzicom. Some of these medicines are already in Epzicom.
- Do not take zalcitabine (Hivid, ddC) while taking Epzicom.

Avoid doing things that can spread HIV infection, as Epzicom does not stop you from passing the HIV infection to others.

- **Do not share needles or other injection equipment.**
- **Do not share personal items that can have blood or body fluids on them, like toothbrushes and razor blades.**
- **Do not have any kind of sex without protection.** Always practice safe sex by using a latex or polyurethane condom or other barrier method to lower the chance of sexual contact with semen, vaginal secretions, or blood.
- **Do not breastfeed.** Epzicom can be passed to babies in breast milk and could harm the baby. Also, mothers with HIV should not breastfeed because HIV can be passed to the baby in the breast milk.

What are the possible side effects of Epzicom?

Epzicom can cause the following serious side effects:

- **Serious allergic reaction that can cause death.** (See "What is the most important information I should know about Epzicom?" at the beginning of this Medication Guide.)
- **Lactic acidosis with liver enlargement (hepatomegaly) that can cause death.** (See "What is the most important information I should know about Epzicom?" at the beginning of this Medication Guide.)
- **Worsening of HBV infection.** (See "What is the most important information I should know about Epzicom?" at the beginning of this Medication Guide.)
- **Changes in body fat.** These changes have happened in patients taking antiretroviral medicines like Epzicom. The changes may include an increased amount of fat in the upper back and neck ("buffalo hump"), breast, and around the back, chest, and stomach area. Loss of fat from the legs, arms, and face may also happen. The cause and long-term health effects of these conditions are not known.

The most common side effects with Epzicom are trouble sleeping, depression, headache, tiredness, dizziness, nausea, diarrhea, rash, fever, stomach pain, abnormal dreams, and anxiety. Most of these side effects did not cause people to stop taking Epzicom.

This list of side effects is not complete. Ask your doctor or pharmacist for more information.

How should I store Epzicom?

- Store Epzicom at room temperature between 59° to 86°F (15° to 30°C).
- Keep Epzicom and all medicines out of the reach of children.

General information for safe and effective use of Epzicom

Medicines are sometimes prescribed for conditions that are not mentioned in Medication Guides. Do not use Epzicom for a condition for which it was not prescribed. Do not give Epzicom to other people, even if they have the same symptoms that you have. It may harm them.

This Medication Guide summarizes the most important information about Epzicom. If you would like more information, talk with your doctor. You can ask your doctor or pharmacist for the information that is written for healthcare professionals or call 1-888-825-5249.

What are the ingredients in Epzicom?

Active ingredients: abacavir sulfate and lamivudine

Inactive ingredients: Each film-coated Epzicom Tablet contains the inactive ingredients magnesium stearate, microcrystalline cellulose, and sodium starch glycolate. The tablets are coated with a film (Opadry® orange YS-1-13065-A) that is made of FD&C Yellow No. 6, hypromellose, polyethylene glycol 400, polysorbate 80, and titanium dioxide.

GlaxoSmithKline
Research Triangle Park, NC 27709

August 2004/MG-027

This Medication Guide has been approved by the US Food and Drug Administration.

ESKALITH® ℞

[es' ka-lith]
(lithium carbonate)
Capsules, 300 mg

ESKALITH CR® ℞

(lithium carbonate)
Controlled-Release Tablets, 450 mg

> **WARNING**
> Lithium toxicity is closely related to serum lithium levels, and can occur at doses close to therapeutic levels. Facilities for prompt and accurate serum lithium determinations should be available before initiating therapy (see DOSAGE AND ADMINISTRATION).

DESCRIPTION

ESKALITH contains lithium carbonate, a white, light alkaline powder with molecular formula Li_2CO_3 and molecular weight 73.89. Lithium is an element of the alkali-metal group with atomic number 3, atomic weight 6.94 and an emission line at 671 nm on the flame photometer.

ESKALITH Capsules: Each capsule, with opaque gray cap and opaque yellow body, is imprinted with the product name ESKALITH and SB and contains lithium carbonate, 300 mg. Inactive ingredients consist of benzyl alcohol, cetylpyridinium chloride, D&C Yellow No. 10, FD&C Green No. 3, FD&C Red No. 40, FD&C Yellow No. 6, gelatin, lactose, magnesium stearate, povidone, sodium lauryl sulfate, titanium dioxide, and trace amounts of other inactive ingredients.

ESKALITH CR Controlled-Release Tablets: Each round, yellow, biconvex tablet, debossed with SKF and J10 on one side and scored on the other side, contains lithium carbonate, 450 mg. Inactive ingredients consist of alginic acid, gelatin, iron oxide, magnesium stearate, and sodium starch glycolate.

ESKALITH CR Tablets 450 mg are designed to release a portion of the dose initially and the remainder gradually; the release pattern of the controlled release tablets reduces the variability in lithium blood levels seen with the immediate release dosage forms.

ACTIONS

Preclinical studies have shown that lithium alters sodium transport in nerve and muscle cells and effects a shift toward intraneuronal metabolism of catecholamines, but the specific biochemical mechanism of lithium action in mania is unknown.

INDICATIONS

ESKALITH (lithium carbonate) is indicated in the treatment of manic episodes of manic-depressive illness. Maintenance therapy prevents or diminishes the intensity of subsequent episodes in those manic-depressive patients with a history of mania.

Typical symptoms of mania include pressure of speech, motor hyperactivity, reduced need for sleep, flight of ideas, grandiosity, elation, poor judgment, aggressiveness and possibly hostility. When given to a patient experiencing a manic episode, ESKALITH may produce a normalization of symptomatology within 1 to 3 weeks.

WARNINGS

Lithium should generally not be given to patients with significant renal or cardiovascular disease, severe debilitation or dehydration, or sodium depletion, since the risk of lithium toxicity is very high in such patients. If the psychiatric indication is life-threatening, and if such a patient fails to respond to other measures, lithium treatment may be undertaken with extreme caution, including daily serum lithium determinations and adjustment to the usually low doses ordinarily tolerated by these individuals. In such instances, hospitalization is a necessity.

Chronic lithium therapy may be associated with diminution of renal concentrating ability, occasionally presenting as nephrogenic diabetes insipidus, with polyuria and polydipsia. Such patients should be carefully managed to avoid dehydration with resulting lithium retention and toxicity. This condition is usually reversible when lithium is discontinued.

Morphologic changes with glomerular and interstitial fibrosis and nephron atrophy have been reported in patients on chronic lithium therapy. Morphologic changes have also been seen in manic-depressive patients never exposed to lithium. The relationship between renal functional and morphologic changes and their association with lithium therapy have not been established.

When kidney function is assessed, for baseline data prior to starting lithium therapy or thereafter, routine urinalysis and other tests may be used to evaluate tubular function (e.g., urine specific gravity or osmolality following a period of water deprivation, or 24-hour urine volume) and glomerular function (e.g., serum creatinine or creatinine clearance). During lithium therapy, progressive or sudden changes in renal function, even within the normal range, indicate the need for reevaluation of treatment.

An encephalopathic syndrome (characterized by weakness, lethargy, fever, tremulousness and confusion, extrapyramidal symptoms, leukocytosis, elevated serum enzymes, BUN and FBS) has occurred in a few patients treated with lithium plus a neuroleptic. In some instances, the syndrome was followed by irreversible brain damage. Because of a possible causal relationship between these events and the concomitant administration of lithium and neuroleptics, patients receiving such combined therapy should be monitored closely for early evidence of neurologic toxicity and treatment discontinued promptly if such signs appear. This en-

Continued on next page

Product information on these pages is effective as of August 2004. Further information is available at: GlaxoSmithKline, PO Box 13398, Research Triangle Park, NC 27709. 1-888-825-5249. Corporate Web Site: www.gsk.com

Eskalith/Eskalith CR—Cont.

cephalopathic syndrome may be similar to or the same as neuroleptic malignant syndrome (NMS).
Lithium toxicity is closely related to serum lithium levels, and can occur at doses close to therapeutic levels (see DOSAGE AND ADMINISTRATION).
Outpatients and their families should be warned that the patient must discontinue lithium carbonate therapy and contact his physician if such clinical signs of lithium toxicity as diarrhea, vomiting, tremor, mild ataxia, drowsiness, or muscular weakness occur.
Lithium carbonate may impair mental and/or physical abilities. Caution patients about activities requiring alertness (e.g., operating vehicles or machinery).
Lithium may prolong the effects of neuromuscular blocking agents. Therefore, neuromuscular blocking agents should be given with caution to patients receiving lithium.
Usage in Pregnancy: Adverse effects on implantation in rats, embryo viability in mice and metabolism *in vitro* of rat testes and human spermatozoa have been attributed to lithium, as have teratogenicity in submammalian species and cleft palates in mice.
In humans, lithium carbonate may cause fetal harm when administered to a pregnant woman. Data from lithium birth registries suggest an increase in cardiac and other anomalies, especially Ebstein's anomaly. If this drug is used in women of childbearing potential, or during pregnancy, or if a patient becomes pregnant while taking this drug, the patient should be apprised of the potential hazard to the fetus.
Usage in Nursing Mothers: Lithium is excreted in human milk. Nursing should not be undertaken during lithium therapy except in rare and unusual circumstances where, in the view of the physician, the potential benefits to the mother outweigh possible hazards to the child.
Usage in Pediatric Patients: Since information regarding the safety and effectiveness of lithium carbonate in children under 12 years of age is not available, its use in such patients is not recommended.
There has been a report of a transient syndrome of acute dystonia and hyperreflexia occurring in a 15 kg child who ingested 300 mg of lithium carbonate.
Usage in the Elderly: Elderly patients often require lower lithium dosages to achieve therapeutic serum levels. They may also exhibit adverse reactions at serum levels ordinarily tolerated by younger patients.

PRECAUTIONS

General: The ability to tolerate lithium is greater during the acute manic phase and decreases when manic symptoms subside (see DOSAGE AND ADMINISTRATION).
The distribution space of lithium approximates that of total body water. Lithium is primarily excreted in urine with insignificant excretion in feces. Renal excretion of lithium is proportional to its plasma concentration. The half-life of elimination of lithium is approximately 24 hours. Lithium decreases sodium reabsorption by the renal tubules which could lead to sodium depletion. Therefore, it is essential for the patient to maintain a normal diet, including salt, and an adequate fluid intake (2,500 to 3,000 mL) at least during the initial stabilization period. Decreased tolerance to lithium has been reported to ensue from protracted sweating or diarrhea and, if such occur, supplemental fluid and salt should be administered under careful medical supervision and lithium intake reduced or suspended until the condition is resolved.
In addition to sweating and diarrhea, concomitant infection with elevated temperatures may also necessitate a temporary reduction or cessation of medication.
Previously existing underlying thyroid disorders do not necessarily constitute a contraindication to lithium treatment; where hypothyroidism exists, careful monitoring of thyroid function during lithium stabilization and maintenance allows for correction of changing thyroid parameters, if any; where hypothyroidism occurs during lithium stabilization and maintenance, supplemental thyroid treatment may be used.
Drug Interactions: Caution should be used when lithium and diuretics are used concomitantly because diuretic-induced sodium loss may reduce the renal clearance of lithium and increase serum lithium levels with risk of lithium toxicity. Patients receiving such combined therapy should have serum lithium levels monitored closely and the lithium dosage adjusted if necessary.
Lithium levels should be closely monitored when patients initiate or discontinue NSAID use. In some cases, lithium toxicity has resulted from interactions between an NSAID and lithium. Indomethacin and piroxicam have been reported to increase significantly steady-state plasma lithium concentrations. There is also evidence that other nonsteroidal anti-inflammatory agents, including the selective cyclooxygenase-2 (COX-2) inhibitors, have the same effect. In a study conducted in healthy subjects, mean steady-state lithium plasma levels increased approximately 17% in subjects receiving lithium 450 mg b.i.d. with celecoxib 200 mg b.i.d. as compared to subjects receiving lithium alone.
Concurrent use of metronidazole with lithium may provoke lithium toxicity due to reduced renal clearance. Patients receiving such combined therapy should be monitored closely.
There is evidence that angiotensin-converting enzyme inhibitors, such as enalapril and captopril, and angiotension II receptor antagonists, such as losartan, may substantially increase steady-state plasma lithium levels, sometimes resulting in lithium toxicity. When such combinations are used, lithium dosage may need to be decreased, and plasma lithium levels should be measured more often.
Concurrent use of calcium channel blocking agents with lithium may increase the risk of neurotoxicity in the form of ataxia, tremors, nausea, vomiting, diarrhea, and/or tinnitus. Caution is recommended.
The concomitant administration of lithium with selective serotonin reuptake inhibitors should be undertaken with caution as this combination has been reported to result in symptoms such as diarrhea, confusion, tremor, dizziness, and agitation.
The following drugs can lower serum lithium concentrations by increasing urinary lithium excretion: acetazolamide, urea, xanthine preparations, and alkalinizing agents such as sodium bicarbonate.
The following have also been shown to interact with lithium: methyldopa, phenytoin, and carbamazepine.

ADVERSE REACTIONS

The occurrence and severity of adverse reactions are generally directly related to serum lithium concentrations as well as to individual patient sensitivity to lithium, and generally occur more frequently and with greater severity at higher concentrations.
Adverse reactions may be encountered at serum lithium levels below 1.5 mEq/L. Mild to moderate adverse reactions may occur at levels from 1.5 to 2.5 mEq/L, and moderate to severe reactions may be seen at levels of 2.0 mEq/L and above.
Fine hand tremor, polyuria, and mild thirst may occur during initial therapy for the acute manic phase, and may persist throughout treatment. Transient and mild nausea and general discomfort may also appear during the first few days of lithium administration.
These side effects usually subside with continued treatment or a temporary reduction or cessation of dosage. If persistent, cessation of lithium therapy may be required.
Diarrhea, vomiting, drowsiness, muscular weakness, and lack of coordination may be early signs of lithium intoxication, and can occur at lithium levels below 2.0 mEq/L. At higher levels, ataxia, giddiness, tinnitus, blurred vision, and a large output of dilute urine may be seen. Serum lithium levels above 3.0 mEq/L may produce a complex clinical picture, involving multiple organs and organ systems. Serum lithium levels should not be permitted to exceed 2.0 mEq/L during the acute treatment phase.
The following reactions have been reported and appear to be related to serum lithium levels, including levels within the therapeutic range:
Neuromuscular/Central Nervous System: Tremor, muscle hyperirritability (fasciculations, twitching, clonic movements of whole limbs), hypertonicity, ataxia, choreoathetotic movements, hyperactive deep tendon reflex, extrapyramidal symptoms including acute dystonia, cogwheel rigidity, blackout spells, epileptiform seizures, slurred speech, dizziness, vertigo, downbeat nystagmus, incontinence of urine or feces, somnolence, psychomotor retardation, restlessness, confusion, stupor, coma, tongue movements, tics, tinnitus, hallucinations, poor memory, slowed intellectual functioning, startled response, worsening of organic brain syndromes, myasthenia gravis (rarely).
Cardiovascular: Cardiac arrhythmia, hypotension, peripheral circulatory collapse, bradycardia, sinus node dysfunction with severe bradycardia (which may result in syncope).
Gastrointestinal: Anorexia, nausea, vomiting, diarrhea, gastritis, salivary gland swelling, abdominal pain, excessive salivation, flatulence, indigestion.
Genitourinary: Glycosuria, decreased creatinine clearance, albuminuria, oliguria, and symptoms of nephrogenic diabetes insipidus including polyuria, thirst and polydipsia.
Dermatologic: Drying and thinning of hair, alopecia, anesthesia of skin, acne, chronic folliculitis, xerosis cutis, psoriasis or its exacerbation, generalized pruritus with or without rash, cutaneous ulcers, angioedema.
Autonomic: Blurred vision, dry mouth, impotence/sexual dysfunction.
Thyroid Abnormalities: Euthyroid goiter and/or hypothyroidism (including myxedema) accompanied by lower T_3 and T_4. I^{131} uptake may be elevated. (See PRECAUTIONS.) Paradoxically, rare cases of hyperthyroidism have been reported.
EEG Changes: Diffuse slowing, widening of the frequency spectrum, potentiation and disorganization of background rhythm.
EKG Changes: Reversible flattening, isoelectricity or inversion of T-waves.
Miscellaneous: Fatigue, lethargy, transient scotomata, exophthalmos, dehydration, weight loss, leukocytosis, headache, transient hyperglycemia, hypercalcemia, hyperparathyroidism, excessive weight gain, edematous swelling of ankles or wrists, metallic taste, dysgeusia/taste distortion, salty taste, thirst, swollen lips, tightness in chest, swollen and/or painful joints, fever, polyarthralgia, dental caries.
Some reports of nephrogenic diabetes insipidus, hyperparathyroidism, and hypothyroidism which persist after lithium discontinuation have been received.
A few reports have been received of the development of painful discoloration of fingers and toes and coldness of the extremities within one day of the starting of treatment with lithium. The mechanism through which these symptoms (resembling Raynaud's syndrome) developed is not known. Recovery followed discontinuance.
Cases of pseudotumor cerebri (increased intracranial pressure and papilledema) have been reported with lithium use. If undetected, this condition may result in enlargement of the blind spot, constriction of visual fields, and eventual blindness due to optic atrophy. Lithium should be discontinued, if clinically possible, if this syndrome occurs.

DOSAGE AND ADMINISTRATION

Immediate-release capsules are usually given t.i.d. or q.i.d. Doses of controlled-release tablets are usually given b.i.d. (approximately 12-hour intervals). When initiating therapy with immediate-release or controlled-release lithium, dosage must be individualized according to serum levels and clinical response.
When switching a patient from immediate-release capsules to ESKALITH CR Controlled-Release Tablets, give the same total daily dose when possible. Most patients on maintenance therapy are stabilized on 900 mg daily, e.g., ESKALITH CR 450 mg b.i.d. When the previous dosage of immediate-release lithium is not a multiple of 450 mg, e.g., 1,500 mg, initiate ESKALITH CR at the multiple of 450 mg nearest to, but *below*, the original daily dose, i.e., 1,350 mg. When the 2 doses are unequal, give the larger dose in the evening. In the above example, with a total daily dose of 1,350 mg, generally 450 mg of ESKALITH CR should be given in the morning and 900 mg of ESKALITH CR in the evening. If desired, the total daily dose of 1,350 mg can be given in 3 equal 450-mg doses of ESKALITH CR. These patients should be monitored at 1- to 2-week intervals, and dosage adjusted if necessary, until stable and satisfactory serum levels and clinical state are achieved.
When patients require closer titration than that available with doses of ESKALITH CR in increments of 450 mg, immediate-release capsules should be used.
Acute Mania: Optimal patient response to ESKALITH can usually be established and maintained with 1,800 mg per day in divided doses. Such doses will normally produce the desired serum lithium level ranging between 1.0 and 1.5 mEq/L.
Dosage must be individualized according to serum levels and clinical response. Regular monitoring of the patient's clinical state and serum lithium levels is necessary. Serum levels should be determined twice per week during the acute phase, and until the serum level and clinical condition of the patient have been stabilized.
Long-Term Control: The desirable serum lithium levels are 0.6 to 1.2 mEq/L. Dosage will vary from one individual to another, but usually 900 mg to 1,200 mg per day in divided doses will maintain this level. Serum lithium levels in uncomplicated cases receiving maintenance therapy during remission should be monitored at least every two months.
Patients unusually sensitive to lithium may exhibit toxic signs at serum levels below 1.0 mEq/L.
N.B.: Blood samples for serum lithium determinations should be drawn immediately prior to the next dose when lithium concentrations are relatively stable (i.e., 8 to 12 hours after the previous dose). Total reliance must not be placed on serum levels alone. Accurate patient evaluation requires both clinical and laboratory analysis.
Elderly patients often respond to reduced dosage, and may exhibit signs of toxicity at serum levels ordinarily tolerated by younger patients.

OVERDOSAGE

The toxic levels for lithium are close to the therapeutic levels. It is therefore important that patients and their families be cautioned to watch for early toxic symptoms and to discontinue the drug and inform the physician should they occur. Toxic symptoms are listed in detail under ADVERSE REACTIONS.
Treatment: No specific antidote for lithium poisoning is known. Early symptoms of lithium toxicity can usually be treated by reduction or cessation of dosage of the drug and resumption of the treatment at a lower dose after 24 to 48 hours. In severe cases of lithium poisoning, the first and foremost goal of treatment consists of elimination of this ion from the patient. Treatment is essentially the same as that used in barbiturate poisoning: 1) gastric lavage, 2) correction of fluid and electrolyte imbalance, and 3) regulation of kidney function. Urea, mannitol and aminophylline all produce significant increases in lithium excretion. Hemodialysis is an effective and rapid means of removing the ion from the severely toxic patient. Infection prophylaxis, regular chest X-rays and preservation of adequate respiration are essential.

HOW SUPPLIED

ESKALITH Capsules 300 mg are gray and yellow capsules imprinted with "ESKALITH" and "SB" on one side of each half of the capsule, in bottles of 100 (NDC 0007-4007-20).
ESKALITH CR Tablets 450 mg are round, yellow, biconvex, controlled-release tablets, debossed with "SKF" and "J10" on one side and scored on the other side, in bottles of 100 (NDC 0007-4010-20).
STORAGE CONDITIONS: Store at 25° C (77° F), excursions permitted to 15-30° C (59-86° F) [see USP Controlled Room Temperature].
Manufactured by Cardinal Health
Winchester, KY 40391
for GlaxoSmithKline, Research Triangle Park, NC 27709

September 2003/EL:L50
Shown in Product Identification Guide, page 315

FLOLAN® ℞

[flō 'lan]

(epoprostenol sodium)

for Injection

DESCRIPTION

FLOLAN (epoprostenol sodium) for Injection is a sterile sodium salt formulated for intravenous (IV) administration. Each vial of FLOLAN contains epoprostenol sodium equivalent to either 0.5 mg (500,000 ng) or 1.5 mg (1,500,000 ng) epoprostenol, 3.76 mg glycine, 2.93 mg sodium chloride, and 50 mg mannitol. Sodium hydroxide may have been added to adjust pH.

Epoprostenol (PGI_2, PGX, prostacyclin), a metabolite of arachidonic acid, is a naturally occurring prostaglandin with potent vasodilatory activity and inhibitory activity of platelet aggregation.

Epoprostenol is (5Z,9α,11α,13*E*,15*S*)-6,9-epoxy-11,15-dihydroxyprosta-5,13-dien-1-oic acid.

Epoprostenol sodium has a molecular weight of 374.45 and a molecular formula of $C_{20}H_{31}NaO_5$.

FLOLAN is a white to off-white powder that must be reconstituted with STERILE DILUENT for FLOLAN. STERILE DILUENT for FLOLAN is supplied in glass vials containing 50 mL of 94 mg glycine, 73.3 mg sodium chloride, sodium hydroxide (added to adjust pH), and Water for Injection, USP.

The reconstituted solution of FLOLAN has a pH of 10.2 to 10.8 and is increasingly unstable at a lower pH.

CLINICAL PHARMACOLOGY

General: Epoprostenol has 2 major pharmacological actions: (1) direct vasodilation of pulmonary and systemic arterial vascular beds, and (2) inhibition of platelet aggregation. In animals, the vasodilatory effects reduce right- and left-ventricular afterload and increase cardiac output and stroke volume. The effect of epoprostenol on heart rate in animals varies with dose. At low doses, there is vagally mediated bradycardia, but at higher doses, epoprostenol causes reflex tachycardia in response to direct vasodilation and hypotension. No major effects on cardiac conduction have been observed. Additional pharmacologic effects of epoprostenol in animals include bronchodilation, inhibition of gastric acid secretion, and decreased gastric emptying.

Pharmacokinetics: Epoprostenol is rapidly hydrolyzed at neutral pH in blood and is also subject to enzymatic degradation. Animal studies using tritium-labeled epoprostenol have indicated a high clearance (93 mL/kg/min), small volume of distribution (357 mL/kg), and a short half-life (2.7 minutes). During infusions in animals, steady-state plasma concentrations of tritium-labeled epoprostenol were reached within 15 minutes and were proportional to infusion rates. No available chemical assay is sufficiently sensitive and specific to assess the in vivo human pharmacokinetics of epoprostenol. The in vitro half-life of epoprostenol in human blood at 37°C and pH 7.4 is approximately 6 minutes; therefore, the in vivo half-life of epoprostenol in humans is expected to be no greater than 6 minutes. The in vitro pharmacologic half-life of epoprostenol in human plasma, based on inhibition of platelet aggregation, was similar for males (n = 954) and females (n = 1,024).

Tritium-labeled epoprostenol has been administered to humans in order to identify the metabolic products of epoprostenol. Epoprostenol is metabolized to 2 primary metabolites: 6-keto-$PGF_{1\alpha}$ (formed by spontaneous degradation) and 6,15-diketo-13,14-dihydro-$PGF_{1\alpha}$ (enzymatically formed), both of which have pharmacological activity orders of magnitude less than epoprostenol in animal test systems. The recovery of radioactivity in urine and feces over a 1-week period was 82% and 4% of the administered dose, respectively. Fourteen additional minor metabolites have been isolated from urine, indicating that epoprostenol is extensively metabolized in humans.

CLINICAL TRIALS IN PULMONARY HYPERTENSION

Acute Hemodynamic Effects: Acute intravenous infusions of FLOLAN for up to 15 minutes in patients with secondary and primary pulmonary hypertension produce dose-related increases in cardiac index (CI) and stroke volume (SV) and dose-related decreases in pulmonary vascular resistance (PVR), total pulmonary resistance (TPR), and mean systemic arterial pressure (SAPm). The effects of FLOLAN on mean pulmonary artery pressure (PAPm) were variable and minor.

Chronic Infusion in Primary Pulmonary Hypertension (PPH): ***Hemodynamic Effects:*** Chronic continuous infusions of FLOLAN in patients with PPH were studied in 2 prospective, open, randomized trials of 8 and 12 weeks' duration comparing FLOLAN plus conventional therapy to conventional therapy alone. Dosage of FLOLAN was determined as described in DOSAGE AND ADMINISTRATION and averaged 9.2 ng/kg/min at study's end. Conventional therapy varied among patients and included some or all of the following: anticoagulants in essentially all patients; oral vasodilators, diuretics, and digoxin in one half to two thirds of patients; and supplemental oxygen in about half the patients. Except for 2 New York Heart Association (NYHA) functional Class II patients, all patients were either functional Class III or Class IV. As results were similar in the 2 studies, the pooled results are described. Chronic hemodynamic effects were generally similar to acute effects. Increases in CI, SV, and arterial oxygen saturation and decreases in PAPm, mean right atrial pressure (RAPm), TPR, and systemic vascular resistance (SVR) were observed in patients who received FLOLAN chronically compared to those who did not. Table 1 illustrates the treatment-related hemodynamic changes in these patients after 8 or 12 weeks of treatment.

[See table 1 above]

Table 1. Hemodynamics During Chronic Administration of FLOLAN in Patients With PPH

Hemodynamic Parameter	Baseline		Mean Change from Baseline at End of Treatment Period*	
	FLOLAN (N = 52)	Standard Therapy (N = 54)	FLOLAN (N = 48)	Standard Therapy (N = 41)
CI (L/min/m²)	2.0	2.0	0.3†	-0.1
PAPm (mm Hg)	60	60	-5†	1
PVR (Wood U)	16	17	-4†	1
SAPm (mm Hg)	89	91	-4	-3
SV (mL/beat)	44	43	6†	-1
TPR (Wood U)	20	21	-5†	1

* At 8 weeks: FLOLAN N = 10, conventional therapy N = 11 (N is the number of patients with hemodynamic data).
At 12 weeks: FLOLAN N = 38, conventional therapy N = 30 (N is the number of patients with hemodynamic data).

† Denotes statistically significant difference between FLOLAN and conventional therapy groups.

CI = cardiac index, PAPm = mean pulmonary arterial pressure, PVR = pulmonary vascular resistance, SAPm = mean systemic arterial pressure, SV = stroke volume, TPR = total pulmonary resistance.

These hemodynamic improvements appeared to persist when FLOLAN was administered for at least 36 months in an open, nonrandomized study.

Clinical Effects: Statistically significant improvement was observed in exercise capacity, as measured by the 6-minute walk test in patients receiving continuous intravenous FLOLAN plus conventional therapy (N = 52) for 8 or 12 weeks compared to those receiving conventional therapy alone (N = 54). Improvements were apparent as early as the first week of therapy. Increases in exercise capacity were accompanied by statistically significant improvement in dyspnea and fatigue, as measured by the Chronic Heart Failure Questionnaire and the Dyspnea Fatigue Index.

Survival was improved in NYHA functional Class III and Class IV PPH patients treated with FLOLAN for 12 weeks in a multicenter, open, randomized, parallel study. At the end of the treatment period, 8 of 40 (20%) patients receiving conventional therapy alone died, whereas none of the 41 patients receiving FLOLAN died (p = 0.003).

Chronic Infusion in Pulmonary Hypertension Associated with the Scleroderma Spectrum of Diseases (PH/SSD): ***Hemodynamic Effects:*** Chronic continuous infusions of FLOLAN in patients with PH/SSD were studied in a prospective, open, randomized trial of 12 weeks' duration comparing FLOLAN plus conventional therapy (N = 56) to conventional therapy alone (N = 55). Except for 5 NYHA functional Class II patients, all patients were either functional Class III or Class IV. Dosage of FLOLAN was determined as described in DOSAGE AND ADMINISTRATION and averaged 11.2 ng/kg/min at study's end. Conventional therapy varied among patients and included some or all of the following: anticoagulants in essentially all patients, supplemental oxygen and diuretics in two thirds of the patients, oral vasodilators in 40% of the patients, and digoxin in a third of the patients. A statistically significant increase in CI, and statistically significant decreases in PAPm, RAPm, PVR, and SAPm after 12 weeks of treatment were observed in patients who received FLOLAN chronically compared to those who did not. Table 2 illustrates the treatment-related hemodynamic changes in these patients after 12 weeks of treatment.

[See table 2 above]

Table 2. Hemodynamics During Chronic Administration of FLOLAN in Patients With PH/SSD

Hemodynamic Parameter	Baseline		Mean Change from Baseline at 12 Weeks	
	FLOLAN (N = 56)	Conventional Therapy (N = 55)	FLOLAN (N = 50)	Conventional Therapy (N = 48)
CI (L/min/m²)	1.9	2.2	0.5*	-0.1
PAPm (mm Hg)	51	49	-5*	1
RAPm (mm Hg)	13	11	-1*	1
PVR (Wood U)	14	11	-5*	1
SAPm (mm Hg)	93	89	-8*	-1

*Denotes statistically significant difference between FLOLAN and conventional therapy groups (N is the number of patients with hemodynamic data).

CI = cardiac index, PAPm = mean pulmonary arterial pressure, RAPm = mean right arterial pressure, PVR = pulmonary vascular resistance, SAPm = mean systemic arterial pressure.

Clinical Effects: Statistically significant improvement was observed in exercise capacity, as measured by the 6-minute walk, in patients receiving continuous intravenous FLOLAN plus conventional therapy for 12 weeks compared to those receiving conventional therapy alone. Improvements were apparent in some patients at the end of the first week of therapy. Increases in exercise capacity were accompanied by statistically significant improvements in dyspnea and fatigue, as measured by the Borg Dyspnea Index and Dyspnea Fatigue Index. At week 12, NYHA functional class improved in 21 of 51 (41%) patients treated with FLOLAN compared to none of the 48 patients treated with conventional therapy alone. However, more patients in both treatment groups (28/51 [55%] with FLOLAN and 35/48 [73%] with conventional therapy alone) showed no change in functional class, and 2/51 (4%) with FLOLAN and 13/48 (27%) with conventional therapy alone worsened. Of the patients randomized, NYHA functional class data at 12 weeks were not available for 5 patients treated with FLOLAN and 7 patients treated with conventional therapy alone.

No statistical difference in survival over 12 weeks was observed in PH/SSD patients treated with FLOLAN as compared to those receiving conventional therapy alone. At the end of the treatment period, 4 of 56 (7%) patients receiving FLOLAN died, whereas 5 of 55 (9%) patients receiving conventional therapy alone died.

No controlled clinical trials with FLOLAN have been performed in patients with pulmonary hypertension associated with other diseases.

Continued on next page

Product information on these pages is effective as of August 2004. Further information is available at: GlaxoSmithKline, PO Box 13398, Research Triangle Park, NC 27709. 1-888-825-5249. Corporate Web Site: www.gsk.com

Flolan—Cont.

INDICATIONS AND USAGE

FLOLAN is indicated for the long-term intravenous treatment of primary pulmonary hypertension and pulmonary hypertension associated with the scleroderma spectrum of disease in NYHA Class III and Class IV patients who do not respond adequately to conventional therapy (see CLINICAL TRIALS IN PULMONARY HYPERTENSION).

CONTRAINDICATIONS

A large study evaluating the effect of FLOLAN on survival in NYHA Class III and IV patients with congestive heart failure due to severe left ventricular systolic dysfunction was terminated after an interim analysis of 471 patients revealed a higher mortality in patients receiving FLOLAN plus conventional therapy than in those receiving conventional therapy alone. The chronic use of FLOLAN in patients with congestive heart failure due to severe left ventricular systolic dysfunction is therefore contraindicated.

Some patients with pulmonary hypertension have developed pulmonary edema during dose initiation, which may be associated with pulmonary veno-occlusive disease. FLOLAN should not be used chronically in patients who develop pulmonary edema during dose initiation.

FLOLAN is also contraindicated in patients with known hypersensitivity to the drug or to structurally related compounds.

WARNINGS

FLOLAN must be reconstituted only as directed using STERILE DILUENT for FLOLAN. FLOLAN must not be reconstituted or mixed with any other parenteral medications or solutions prior to or during administration.

Abrupt Withdrawal: Abrupt withdrawal (including interruptions in drug delivery) or sudden large reductions in dosage of FLOLAN may result in symptoms associated with rebound pulmonary hypertension, including dyspnea, dizziness, and asthenia. In clinical trials, one Class III PPH patient's death was judged attributable to the interruption of FLOLAN. Abrupt withdrawal should be avoided.

Sepsis: See ADVERSE REACTIONS: Adverse Events Attributable to the Drug Delivery System.

PRECAUTIONS

General: FLOLAN should be used only by clinicians experienced in the diagnosis and treatment of pulmonary hypertension. The diagnosis of PPH or PH/SSD should be carefully established.

FLOLAN is a potent pulmonary and systemic vasodilator. Dose initiation with FLOLAN must be performed in a setting with adequate personnel and equipment for physiologic monitoring and emergency care. Dose initiation in controlled PPH clinical trials was performed during right heart catheterization. In uncontrolled PPH and controlled PH/SSD clinical trials, dose initiation was performed without cardiac catheterization. The risk of cardiac catheterization in patients with pulmonary hypertension should be carefully weighed against the potential benefits. During dose initiation, asymptomatic increases in pulmonary artery pressure coincident with increases in cardiac output occurred rarely. In such cases, dose reduction should be considered, but such an increase does not imply that chronic treatment is contraindicated.

During chronic use, FLOLAN is delivered continuously on an ambulatory basis through a permanent indwelling central venous catheter. Unless contraindicated, anticoagulant therapy should be administered to PPH and PH/SSD patients receiving FLOLAN to reduce the risk of pulmonary thromboembolism or systemic embolism through a patent foramen ovale. In order to reduce the risk of infection, aseptic technique must be used in the reconstitution and administration of FLOLAN as well as in routine catheter care. Because FLOLAN is metabolized rapidly, even brief interruptions in the delivery of FLOLAN may result in symptoms associated with rebound pulmonary hypertension including dyspnea, dizziness, and asthenia. The decision to initiate therapy with FLOLAN should be based upon the understanding that there is a high likelihood that intravenous therapy with FLOLAN will be needed for prolonged periods, possibly years, and the patient's ability to accept and care for a permanent intravenous catheter and infusion pump should be carefully considered.

Based on clinical trials, the acute hemodynamic response to FLOLAN did not correlate well with improvement in exercise tolerance or survival during chronic use of FLOLAN. Dosage of FLOLAN during chronic use should be adjusted at the first sign of recurrence or worsening of symptoms attributable to pulmonary hypertension or the occurrence of adverse events associated with FLOLAN (see DOSAGE AND ADMINISTRATION). Following dosage adjustments, standing and supine blood pressure and heart rate should be monitored closely for several hours.

Information for Patients: Patients receiving FLOLAN should receive the following information. **FLOLAN must be reconstituted only with STERILE DILUENT for FLOLAN.** FLOLAN is infused continuously through a permanent indwelling central venous catheter via a small, portable infusion pump. Thus, therapy with FLOLAN requires commitment by the patient to drug reconstitution, drug administration, and care of the permanent central venous catheter. Sterile technique must be adhered to in preparing the drug and in the care of the catheter, and even brief interruptions in the delivery of FLOLAN may result in rapid symptomatic deterioration. A patient's decision to receive FLOLAN should be based upon the understanding that there is a high likelihood that therapy with FLOLAN will be needed for prolonged periods, possibly years. The patient's ability to accept and care for a permanent intravenous catheter and infusion pump should also be carefully considered.

Table 4. Adverse Events Regardless of Attribution Occurring in Patients With PPH With ≥10% Difference Between FLOLAN and Conventional Therapy Alone

Adverse Event	FLOLAN (n = 52)	Conventional Therapy (n = 54)
Occurrence More Common With FLOLAN		
General		
Chills/fever/sepsis/flu-like symptoms	25%	11%
Cardiovascular		
Tachycardia	35%	24%
Flushing	42%	2%
Gastrointestinal		
Diarrhea	37%	6%
Nausea/vomiting	67%	48%
Musculoskeletal		
Jaw pain	54%	0%
Myalgia	44%	31%
Nonspecific musculoskeletal pain	35%	15%
Neurological		
Anxiety/nervousness/tremor	21%	9%
Dizziness	83%	70%
Headache	83%	33%
Hypesthesia, hyperesthesia, paresthesia	12%	2%
Occurrence More Common With Standard Therapy		
Cardiovascular		
Heart failure	31%	52%
Syncope	13%	24%
Shock	0%	13%
Respiratory		
Hypoxia	25%	37%

Drug Interactions: Additional reductions in blood pressure may occur when FLOLAN is administered with diuretics, antihypertensive agents, or other vasodilators. When other antiplatelet agents or anticoagulants are used concomitantly, there is the potential for FLOLAN to increase the risk of bleeding. However, patients receiving infusions of FLOLAN in clinical trials were maintained on anticoagulants without evidence of increased bleeding. In clinical trials, FLOLAN was used with digoxin, diuretics, anticoagulants, oral vasodilators, and supplemental oxygen.

In a pharmacokinetic substudy in patients with congestive heart failure receiving furosemide or digoxin in whom therapy with FLOLAN was initiated, apparent oral clearance values for furosemide (n = 23) and digoxin (n = 30) were decreased by 13% and 15%, respectively, on the second day of therapy and had returned to baseline values by day 87. The change in furosemide clearance value is not likely to be clinically significant. However, patients on digoxin may show elevations of digoxin concentrations after initiation of therapy with FLOLAN, which may be clinically significant in patients prone to digoxin toxicity.

Carcinogenesis, Mutagenesis, Impairment of Fertility: Long-term studies in animals have not been performed to evaluate carcinogenic potential. A micronucleus test in rats revealed no evidence of mutagenicity. The Ames test and DNA elution tests were also negative, although the instability of epoprostenol makes the significance of these tests uncertain. Fertility was not impaired in rats given FLOLAN by subcutaneous injection at doses up to 100 mcg/kg/day (600 mcg/m^2/day, 2.5 times the recommended human dose [4.6 ng/kg/min or 245.1 mcg/m^2/day, IV] based on body surface area).

Pregnancy: Pregnancy Category B. Reproductive studies have been performed in pregnant rats and rabbits at doses up to 100 mcg/kg/day (600 mcg/m^2/day in rats, 2.5 times the recommended human dose, and 1,180 mcg/m^2/day in rabbits, 4.8 times the recommended human dose based on body surface area) and have revealed no evidence of impaired fertility or harm to the fetus due to FLOLAN. There are, however, no adequate and well-controlled studies in pregnant women. Because animal reproduction studies are not always predictive of human response, this drug should be used during pregnancy only if clearly needed.

Labor and Delivery: The use of FLOLAN during labor, vaginal delivery, or cesarean section has not been adequately studied in humans.

Nursing Mothers: It is not known whether this drug is excreted in human milk. Because many drugs are excreted in human milk, caution should be exercised when FLOLAN is administered to a nursing woman.

Pediatric Use: Safety and effectiveness in pediatric patients have not been established.

Geriatric Use: Clinical studies of FLOLAN in pulmonary hypertension did not include sufficient numbers of subjects aged 65 and over to determine whether they respond differently from younger patients. Other reported clinical experience has not identified differences in responses between the elderly and younger patients. In general, dose selection for an elderly patient should be cautious, usually starting at the low end of the dosing range, reflecting the greater frequency of decreased hepatic, renal, or cardiac function and of concomitant disease or other drug therapy.

ADVERSE REACTIONS

During clinical trials, adverse events were classified as follows: (1) adverse events during dose initiation and escalation, (2) adverse events during chronic dosing, and (3) adverse events associated with the drug delivery system.

Adverse Events During Dose Initiation and Escalation: During early clinical trials, FLOLAN was increased in 2-ng/kg/min increments until the patients developed symptomatic intolerance. The most common adverse events and the adverse events that limited further increases in dose were generally related to vasodilation, the major pharmacologic effect of FLOLAN. The most common dose-limiting adverse events (occurring in ≥1% of patients) were nausea, vomiting, headache, hypotension, and flushing, but also include chest pain, anxiety, dizziness, bradycardia, dyspnea, abdominal pain, musculoskeletal pain, and tachycardia. Table 3 lists the adverse events reported during dose initiation and escalation in decreasing order of frequency.

Table 3. Adverse Events During Dose Initiation and Escalation

Adverse Events Occurring in ≥1% of Patients	FLOLAN (n = 391)
Flushing	58%
Headache	49%
Nausea/vomiting	32%
Hypotension	16%
Anxiety, nervousness, agitation	11%
Chest pain	11%
Dizziness	8%
Bradycardia	5%
Abdominal pain	5%
Musculoskeletal pain	3%
Dyspnea	2%
Back pain	2%
Sweating	1%
Dyspepsia	1%
Hypesthesia/paresthesia	1%
Tachycardia	1%

Adverse Events During Chronic Administration: Interpretation of adverse events is complicated by the clinical features of PPH and PH/SSD, which are similar to some of the pharmacologic effects of FLOLAN (e.g., dizziness, syncope). Adverse events probably related to the underlying disease include dyspnea, fatigue, chest pain, edema, hypoxia, right ventricular failure, and pallor. Several adverse events, on the other hand, can clearly be attributed to FLOLAN. These include headache, jaw pain, flushing, diarrhea, nausea and vomiting, flu-like symptoms, and anxiety/nervousness.

Table 5. Adverse Events Regardless of Attribution Occurring in Patients With PPH With <10% Difference Between FLOLAN and Conventional Therapy Alone

Adverse Event	FLOLAN (n = 52)	Conventional Therapy (n = 54)
General		
Asthenia	87%	81%
Cardiovascular		
Angina pectoris	19%	20%
Arrhythmia	27%	20%
Bradycardia	15%	9%
Supraventricular tachycardia	8%	0%
Pallor	21%	30%
Cyanosis	31%	39%
Palpitation	63%	61%
Cerebrovascular accident	4%	0%
Hemorrhage	19%	11%
Hypotension	27%	31%
Myocardial ischemia	2%	6%
Gastrointestinal		
Abdominal pain	27%	31%
Anorexia	25%	30%
Ascites	12%	17%
Constipation	6%	2%
Metabolic		
Edema	60%	63%
Hypokalemia	6%	4%
Weight reduction	27%	24%
Weight gain	6%	4%
Musculoskeletal		
Arthralgia	6%	0%
Bone pain	0%	4%
Chest pain	67%	65%
Neurological		
Confusion	6%	11%
Convulsion	4%	0%
Depression	37%	44%
Insomnia	4%	4%
Respiratory		
Cough increase	38%	46%
Dyspnea	90%	85%
Epistaxis	4%	2%
Pleural effusion	4%	2%
Skin and Appendages		
Pruritus	4%	0%
Rash	10%	13%
Sweating	15%	20%
Special Senses		
Amblyopia	8%	4%
Vision abnormality	4%	0%

Table 6. Adverse Events Regardless of Attribution Occurring in Patients With PH/SSD With ≥10% Difference Between FLOLAN and Conventional Therapy Alone

Adverse Event	FLOLAN (n = 56)	Conventional Therapy (n = 55)
Occurrence More Common With FLOLAN		
Cardiovascular		
Flushing	23%	0%
Hypotension	13%	0%
Gastrointestinal		
Anorexia	66%	47%
Nausea/vomiting	41%	16%
Diarrhea	50%	5%
Musculoskeletal		
Jaw pain	75%	0%
Pain/neck pain/arthralgia	84%	65%
Neurological		
Headache	46%	5%
Skin and Appendages		
Skin ulcer	39%	24%
Eczema/rash/urticaria	25%	4%
Occurrence More Common With Conventional Therapy		
Cardiovascular		
Cyanosis	54%	80%
Pallor	32%	53%
Syncope	7%	20%

(Table continued on next page)

Adverse Events During Chronic Administration for PPH: In an effort to separate the adverse effects of the drug from the adverse effects of the underlying disease, Table 4 lists adverse events that occurred at a rate at least 10% different in the 2 groups in controlled trials for PPH.
[See table 4 at top of previous page]

Thrombocytopenia has been reported during uncontrolled clinical trials in patients receiving FLOLAN.
Table 5 lists additional adverse events reported in PPH patients receiving FLOLAN plus conventional therapy or conventional therapy alone during controlled clinical trials.
[See table 5 above]

Adverse Events During Chronic Administration for PH/SSD: In an effort to separate the adverse effects of the drug from the adverse effects of the underlying disease, Table 6 lists adverse events that occurred at a rate at least 10% different in the 2 groups in the controlled trial for patients with PH/SSD.
[See table 6 below and on next page]
Table 7 lists additional adverse events reported in PH/SSD patients receiving FLOLAN plus conventional therapy or conventional therapy alone during controlled clinical trials.
[See table 7 on pages 1490 and 1491]
Although the relationship to FLOLAN administration has not been established, pulmonary embolism has been reported in several patients taking FLOLAN and there have been reports of hepatic failure.

Adverse Events Attributable to the Drug Delivery System: Chronic infusions of FLOLAN are delivered using a small, portable infusion pump through an indwelling central venous catheter. During controlled PPH trials of up to 12 weeks' duration, up to 21% of patients reported a local infection and up to 13% of patients reported pain at the injection site. During a controlled PH/SSD trial of 12 weeks' duration, 14% of patients reported a local infection and 9% of patients reported pain at the injection site. During long-term follow-up in the clinical trial of PPH, sepsis was reported at least once in 14% of patients and occurred at a rate of 0.32 infections/patient per year in patients treated with FLOLAN. This rate was higher than reported in patients using chronic indwelling central venous catheters to administer parenteral nutrition, but lower than reported in oncology patients using these catheters. Malfunctions in the delivery system resulting in an inadvertent bolus of or a reduction in FLOLAN were associated with symptoms related to excess or insufficient FLOLAN, respectively (see ADVERSE REACTIONS: Adverse Events During Chronic Administration).

Observed During Clinical Practice: In addition to adverse reactions reported from clinical trials, the following events have been identified during post-approval use of FLOLAN. Because they are reported voluntarily from a population of unknown size, estimates of frequency cannot be made. These events have been chosen for inclusion due to a combination of their seriousness, frequency of reporting, or potential causal connection to FLOLAN.

Blood and Lymphatic: Anemia, hypersplenism, pancytopenia, splenomegaly.

Endocrine and Metabolic: Hyperthyroidism.

OVERDOSAGE

Signs and symptoms of excessive doses of FLOLAN during clinical trials are the expected dose-limiting pharmacologic effects of FLOLAN, including flushing, headache, hypotension, tachycardia, nausea, vomiting, and diarrhea. Treatment will ordinarily require dose reduction of FLOLAN.
One patient with secondary pulmonary hypertension accidentally received 50 mL of an unspecified concentration of FLOLAN. The patient vomited and became unconscious with an initially unrecordable blood pressure. FLOLAN was discontinued and the patient regained consciousness within seconds. In clinical practice, fatal occurrences of hypoxemia, hypotension, and respiratory arrest have been reported following overdosage of FLOLAN.
Single intravenous doses of FLOLAN at 10 and 50 mg/kg (2,703 and 27,027 times the recommended acute phase human dose based on body surface area) were lethal to mice and rats, respectively. Symptoms of acute toxicity were hypoactivity, ataxia, loss of righting reflex, deep slow breathing, and hypothermia.

DOSAGE AND ADMINISTRATION

Important Note: FLOLAN must be reconstituted only with STERILE DILUENT for FLOLAN. Reconstituted solutions of FLOLAN must not be diluted or administered with other parenteral solutions or medications (see WARNINGS).

Dosage: Continuous chronic infusion of FLOLAN should be administered through a central venous catheter. Temporary peripheral intravenous infusion may be used until central access is established. Chronic infusion of FLOLAN should be initiated at 2 ng/kg/min and increased in increments of 2 ng/kg/min every 15 minutes or longer until dose-limiting pharmacologic effects are elicited or until a tolerance limit to the drug is established and further increases in the infusion rate are not clinically warranted (see Dosage Adjustments). If dose-limiting pharmacologic effects occur, then the infusion rate should be decreased to an appropriate chronic infusion rate whereby the pharmacologic effects of FLOLAN are tolerated. In clinical trials, the most common dose-limiting adverse events were nausea, vomiting, hypotension, sepsis, headache, abdominal pain, or respiratory disorder (most treatment-limiting adverse events were not serious). If the initial infusion rate of 2 ng/kg/min is not tolerated, a lower dose that is tolerated by the patient should be identified.
In the controlled 12-week trial in PH/SSD, for example, the dose increased from a mean starting dose of 2.2 ng/kg/min. During the first 7 days of treatment, the dose was increased

Continued on next page

Product information on these pages is effective as of August 2004. Further information is available at: GlaxoSmithKline, PO Box 13398, Research Triangle Park, NC 27709. 1-888-825-5249. Corporate Web Site: www.gsk.com

Table 6 *(cont.)*. Adverse Events Regardless of Attribution Occurring in Patients With PH/SSD With ≥10% Difference Between FLOLAN and Conventional Therapy Alone

Adverse Event	FLOLAN (n = 56)	Conventional Therapy (n = 55)
Occurrence More Common With Conventional Therapy (cont.)		
Gastrointestinal		
Ascites	23%	33%
Esophageal reflux/gastritis	61%	73%
Metabolic		
Weight decrease	45%	56%
Neurological		
Dizziness	59%	76%
Respiratory		
Hypoxia	55%	65%

Table 7. Adverse Events Regardless of Attribution Occurring in Patients With PH/SSD With <10% Difference Between FLOLAN and Conventional Therapy Alone

Adverse Event*	FLOLAN (n = 56)	Conventional Therapy (n = 55)
General		
Asthenia	100%	98%
Hemorrhage/hemorrhage injection site/ hemorrhage rectal	11%	2%
Infection/rhinitis	21%	20%
Chills/fever/sepsis/flu-like symptoms	13%	11%
Blood and Lymphatic		
Thrombocytopenia	4%	0%
Cardiovascular		
Heart failure/heart failure right	11%	13%
Myocardial Infarction	4%	0%
Palpitation	63%	71%
Shock	5%	5%
Tachycardia	43%	42%
Vascular disorder peripheral	96%	100%
Vascular disorder	95%	89%
Gastrointestinal		
Abdominal enlargement	4%	0%
Abdominal pain	14%	7%
Constipation	4%	2%
Flatulence	5%	4%
Metabolic		
Edema/edema peripheral/edema genital	79%	87%
Hypercalcemia	48%	51%
Hyperkalemia	4%	0%
Thirst	0%	4%
Musculoskeletal		
Arthritis	52%	45%
Back pain	13%	5%
Chest pain	52%	45%
Cramps leg	5%	7%
Respiratory		
Cough increase	82%	82%
Dyspnea	100%	100%
Epistaxis	9%	7%
Pharyngitis	5%	2%
Pleural effusion	7%	0%
Pneumonia	5%	0%
Pneumothorax	4%	0%
Pulmonary edema	4%	2%
Respiratory disorder	7%	4%
Sinusitis	4%	4%

(Table continued on next page)

Flolan—Cont.

daily to a mean dose of 4.1 ng/kg/min on day 7 of treatment. At the end of week 12, the mean dose was 11.2 ng/kg/min. The mean incremental increase was 2 to 3 ng/kg/min every 3 weeks.

Dosage Adjustments: Changes in the chronic infusion rate should be based on persistence, recurrence, or worsening of the patient's symptoms of pulmonary hypertension and the occurrence of adverse events due to excessive doses of FLOLAN. In general, increases in dose from the initial chronic dose should be expected.

Increments in dose should be considered if symptoms of pulmonary hypertension persist or recur after improving. The infusion should be increased by 1- to 2-ng/kg/min increments at intervals sufficient to allow assessment of clinical response; these intervals should be at least 15 minutes. In clinical trials, incremental increases in dose occurred at intervals of 24 to 48 hours or longer. Following establishment of a new chronic infusion rate, the patient should be observed, and standing and supine blood pressure and heart rate monitored for several hours to ensure that the new dose is tolerated.

During chronic infusion, the occurrence of dose-limiting pharmacological events may necessitate a decrease in infusion rate, but the adverse event may occasionally resolve without dosage adjustment. Dosage decreases should be made gradually in 2-ng/kg/min decrements every 15 minutes or longer until the dose-limiting effects resolve. Abrupt withdrawal of FLOLAN or sudden large reductions in infusion rates should be avoided. Except in life-threatening situations (e.g., unconsciousness, collapse, etc.), infusion rates of FLOLAN should be adjusted only under the direction of a physician.

In patients receiving lung transplants, doses of FLOLAN were tapered after the initiation of cardiopulmonary bypass.

Administration: FLOLAN is administered by continuous intravenous infusion via a central venous catheter using an ambulatory infusion pump. During initiation of treatment, FLOLAN may be administered peripherally.

The ambulatory infusion pump used to administer FLOLAN should: (1) be small and lightweight, (2) be able to adjust infusion rates in 2-ng/kg/min increments, (3) have occlusion, end-of-infusion, and low-battery alarms, (4) be accurate to ±6% of the programmed rate, and (5) be positive pressure-driven (continuous or pulsatile) with intervals between pulses not exceeding 3 minutes at infusion rates used to deliver FLOLAN. The reservoir should be made of polyvinyl chloride, polypropylene, or glass. The infusion pump used in the most recent clinical trials was the CADD-1 HFX 5100 (SIMS Deltec). A 60-inch microbore non-DEHP extension set with proximal antisyphon valve, low priming volume (0.9 mL), and in-line 0.22 micron filter was used during clinical trials.

To avoid potential interruptions in drug delivery, the patient should have access to a backup infusion pump and intravenous infusion sets. A multi-lumen catheter should be considered if other intravenous therapies are routinely administered.

To facilitate extended use at ambient temperatures exceeding 25°C (77°F), a cold pouch with frozen gel packs was used in clinical trials (see DOSAGE AND ADMINISTRATION: Storage and Stability). The cold pouches and gel packs used in clinical trials were obtained from Palco Labs, Palo Alto, California. Any cold pouch used must be capable of maintaining the temperature of reconstituted FLOLAN between 2° and 8°C for 12 hours.

Reconstitution: FLOLAN is stable only when reconstituted with STERILE DILUENT for FLOLAN. FLOLAN must not be reconstituted or mixed with any other parenteral medications or solutions prior to or during administration.

A concentration for the solution of FLOLAN should be selected that is compatible with the infusion pump being used with respect to minimum and maximum flow rates, reservoir capacity, and the infusion pump criteria listed above. FLOLAN, when administered chronically, should be prepared in a drug delivery reservoir appropriate for the infusion pump with a total reservoir volume of at least 100 mL. FLOLAN should be prepared using 2 vials of STERILE DILUENT for FLOLAN for use during a 24-hour period. Table 8 gives directions for preparing several different concentrations of FLOLAN.

[See table 8 at top of next page]

Generally, 3,000 ng/mL and 10,000 ng/mL are satisfactory concentrations to deliver between 2 to 16 ng/kg per minute in adults. Infusion rates may be calculated using the following formula:

Infusion Rate (mL/hr) =

$$\frac{\text{Dose (ng/kg/min)} \times \text{Weight (kg)} \times 60 \text{ min/hr}}{\text{Final Concentration (ng/mL)}}$$

Tables 9 through 12 provide infusion delivery rates for doses up to 16 ng/kg/min based upon patient weight, drug delivery rate, and concentration of the solution of FLOLAN to be used. These tables may be used to select the most appropriate concentration of FLOLAN that will result in an infusion rate between the minimum and maximum flow rates of the infusion pump and that will allow the desired duration of infusion from a given reservoir volume. Higher infusion rates, and therefore, more concentrated solutions may be necessary with long-term administration of FLOLAN.

Table 9. Infusion Rates for FLOLAN at a Concentration of 3,000 ng/mL

Patient Weight (kg)	Dose or Drug Delivery Rate (ng/kg/min) 2	4	6	8	10	12	14	16
	Infusion Delivery Rate (mL/h)							
10	—	—	1.2	1.6	2.0	2.4	2.8	3.2
20	—	1.6	2.4	3.2	4.0	4.8	5.6	6.4
30	1.2	2.4	3.6	4.8	6.0	7.2	8.4	9.6
40	1.6	3.2	4.8	6.4	8.0	9.6	11.2	12.8
50	2.0	4.0	6.0	8.0	10.0	12.0	14.0	16.0
60	2.4	4.8	7.2	9.6	12.0	14.4	16.8	19.2
70	2.8	5.6	8.4	11.2	14.0	16.8	19.6	22.4
80	3.2	6.4	9.6	12.8	16.0	19.2	22.4	25.6
90	3.6	7.2	10.8	14.4	18.0	21.6	25.2	28.8
100	4.0	8.0	12.0	16.0	20.0	24.0	28.0	32.0

Table 10. Infusion Rates for FLOLAN at a Concentration of 5,000 ng/mL

Patient Weight (kg)	Dose or Drug Delivery Rate (ng/kg/min) 2	4	6	8	10	12	14	16
	Infusion Delivery Rate (mL/h)							
10	—	—	—	1.0	1.2	1.4	1.7	1.9
20	—	1.0	1.4	1.9	2.4	2.9	3.4	3.8
30	—	1.4	2.2	2.9	3.6	4.3	5.0	5.8
40	1.0	1.9	2.9	3.8	4.8	5.8	6.7	7.7
50	1.2	2.4	3.6	4.8	6.0	7.2	8.4	9.6
60	1.4	2.9	4.3	5.8	7.2	8.6	10.1	11.5
70	1.7	3.4	5.0	6.7	8.4	10.1	11.8	13.4
80	1.9	3.8	5.8	7.7	9.6	11.5	13.4	15.4
90	2.2	4.3	6.5	8.6	10.8	13.0	15.1	17.3
100	2.4	4.8	7.2	9.6	12.0	14.4	16.8	19.2

Table 7 *(cont.)*. Adverse Events Regardless of Attribution Occurring in Patients With PH/SSD With <10% Difference Between FLOLAN and Conventional Therapy Alone

Adverse Event*	FLOLAN (n = 56)	Conventional Therapy (n = 55)
Neurological		
Anxiety/hyperkinesia/nervousness/tremor	7%	5%
Depression/depression psychotic	13%	4%
Hyperesthesia/hypesthesia/paresthesia	5%	0%
Insomnia	9%	0%
Somnolence	4%	2%
Skin and Appendages		
Collagen disease	82%	84%
Pruritus	4%	2%
Sweat	41%	36%
Urogenital		
Hematuria	5%	0%
Urinary tract infection	7%	0%

*Adverse events that occurred in at least 2 patients in either treatment group.

Table 8. Reconstitution and Dilution Instructions

To make 100 mL of solution with Final Concentration (ng/mL) of:	Directions:
3,000 ng/mL	Dissolve contents of one 0.5-mg vial with 5 mL of STERILE DILUENT for FLOLAN. Withdraw 3 mL and add to sufficient STERILE DILUENT for FLOLAN to make a total of 100 mL.
5,000 ng/mL	Dissolve contents of one 0.5-mg vial with 5 mL of STERILE DILUENT for FLOLAN. Withdraw entire vial contents and add sufficient STERILE DILUENT for FLOLAN to make a total of 100 mL.
10,000 ng/mL	Dissolve contents of two 0.5-mg vials each with 5 mL of STERILE DILUENT for FLOLAN. Withdraw entire vial contents and add sufficient STERILE DILUENT for FLOLAN to make a total of 100 mL.
15,000 ng/mL*	Dissolve contents of one 1.5-mg vial with 5 mL of STERILE DILUENT for FLOLAN. Withdraw entire vial contents and add sufficient STERILE DILUENT for FLOLAN to make a total of 100 mL.

* Higher concentrations may be required for patients who receive FLOLAN long-term.

Table 11. Infusion Rates for FLOLAN at a Concentration of 10,000 ng/mL

Patient Weight (kg)	Dose or Drug Delivery Rate (ng/kg/min) 4	6	8	10	12	14	16
	Infusion Delivery Rate (mL/h)						
20	—	—	1.0	1.2	1.4	1.7	1.9
30	—	1.1	1.4	1.8	2.2	2.5	2.9
40	1.0	1.4	1.9	2.4	2.9	3.4	3.8
50	1.2	1.8	2.4	3.0	3.6	4.2	4.8
60	1.4	2.2	2.9	3.6	4.3	5.0	5.8
70	1.7	2.5	3.4	4.2	5.0	5.9	6.7
80	1.9	2.9	3.8	4.8	5.8	6.7	7.7
90	2.2	3.2	4.3	5.4	6.5	7.6	8.6
100	2.4	3.6	4.8	6.0	7.2	8.4	9.6

Table 12. Infusion Rates for FLOLAN at a Concentration of 15,000 ng/mL

Patient Weight (kg)	Dose or Drug Delivery Rate (ng/kg/min) 4	6	8	10	12	14	16
	Infusion Delivery Rate (mL/h)						
30	—	—	1.0	1.2	1.4	1.7	1.9
40	—	1.0	1.3	1.6	1.9	2.2	2.6
50	—	1.2	1.6	2.0	2.4	2.8	3.2
60	1.0	1.4	1.9	2.4	2.9	3.4	3.8
70	1.1	1.7	2.2	2.8	3.4	3.9	4.5
80	1.3	1.9	2.6	3.2	3.8	4.5	5.1
90	1.4	2.2	2.9	3.6	4.3	5.0	5.8
100	1.6	2.4	3.2	4.0	4.8	5.6	6.4

Storage and Stability: Unopened vials of FLOLAN are stable until the date indicated on the package when stored at 15° to 25°C (59° to 77°F) and protected from light in the carton. Unopened vials of STERILE DILUENT for FLOLAN are stable until the date indicated on the package when stored at 15° to 25°C (59° to 77°F).

Prior to use, reconstituted solutions of FLOLAN must be protected from light and must be refrigerated at 2° to 8°C (36° to 46°F) if not used immediately. **Do not freeze reconstituted solutions of FLOLAN. Discard any reconstituted solution that has been frozen. Discard any reconstituted solution if it has been refrigerated for more than 48 hours.** During use, a single reservoir of reconstituted solution of FLOLAN can be administered at room temperature for a total duration of 8 hours, or it can be used with a cold pouch and administered up to 24 hours with the use of 2 frozen 6-oz gel packs in a cold pouch. When stored or in use, reconstituted FLOLAN must be insulated from temperatures greater than 25°C (77°F) and less than 0°C (32°F), and must not be exposed to direct sunlight.

Use at Room Temperature: Prior to use at room temperature, 15° to 25°C (59° to 77°F), reconstituted solutions of FLOLAN may be stored refrigerated at 2° to 8°C (36° to 46°F) for no longer than 40 hours. When administered at room temperature, reconstituted solutions may be used for no longer than 8 hours. This 48-hour period allows the patient to reconstitute a 2-day supply (200 mL) of FLOLAN. Each 100-mL daily supply may be divided into 3 equal portions. Two of the portions are stored refrigerated at 2° to 8°C (36° to 46°F) until they are used.

Use with a Cold Pouch: Prior to infusion with the use of a cold pouch, solutions may be stored refrigerated at 2° to 8°C (36° to 46°F) for up to 24 hours. When a cold pouch is employed during the infusion, reconstituted solutions of FLOLAN may be used for no longer than 24 hours. The gel packs should be changed every 12 hours. Reconstituted solutions may be kept at 2° to 8°C (36° to 46°F), either in refrigerated storage or in a cold pouch or a combination of the two, for no more than 48 hours.

Parenteral drug products should be inspected visually for particulate matter and discoloration prior to administration whenever solution and container permit. If either occurs, FLOLAN should not be administered.

HOW SUPPLIED

FLOLAN for Injection is supplied as a sterile freeze-dried powder in 17-mL flint glass vials with gray butyl rubber closures, individually packaged in a carton.

17-mL vial containing epoprostenol sodium equivalent to 0.5 mg (500,000 ng), carton of 1 (NDC 0173-0517-00).

17-mL vial containing epoprostenol sodium equivalent to 1.5 mg (1,500,000 ng), carton of 1 (NDC 0173-0519-00).

Store the vials of FLOLAN at 15° to 25°C (59° to 77°F) Protect from light.

The STERILE DILUENT for FLOLAN is supplied in flint glass vials containing 50-mL diluent with fluororesin-faced butyl rubber closures.

50-mL of STERILE DILUENT for FLOLAN, tray of 2 vials (NDC 0173-0518-01).

Store the vials of STERILE DILUENT for FLOLAN at 15° to 25°C (59° to 77°F). DO NOT FREEZE.

GlaxoSmithKline, Research Triangle Park, NC 27709

September 2002/RL-1139

Shown in Product Identification Guide, page 315

FLONASE® ℞

[*flō′ nāz*]

(fluticasone propionate)

Nasal Spray, 50 mcg

For Intranasal Use Only.

SHAKE GENTLY BEFORE USE.

DESCRIPTION

Fluticasone propionate, the active component of FLONASE Nasal Spray, is a synthetic corticosteroid having the chemical name S-(fluoromethyl)6α,9-difluoro-11β-17-dihydroxy-16α-methyl-3-oxoandrosta-1,4-diene-17β-carbothioate, 17-propionate.

Fluticasone propionate is a white to off-white powder with a molecular weight of 500.6, and the empirical formula is $C_{25}H_{31}F_3O_5S$. It is practically insoluble in water, freely soluble in dimethyl sulfoxide and dimethylformamide, and slightly soluble in methanol and 95% ethanol.

FLONASE Nasal Spray, 50 mcg is an aqueous suspension of microfine fluticasone propionate for topical administration to the nasal mucosa by means of a metering, atomizing spray pump. FLONASE Nasal Spray also contains microcrystalline cellulose and carboxymethylcellulose sodium, dextrose, 0.02% w/w benzalkonium chloride, polysorbate 80, and 0.25% w/w phenylethyl alcohol, and has a pH between 5 and 7.

It is necessary to prime the pump before first use or after a period of non-use (1 week or more). After initial priming (6 actuations), each actuation delivers 50 mcg of fluticasone propionate in 100 mg of formulation through the nasal adapter. Each 16-g bottle of FLONASE Nasal Spray provides 120 metered sprays. After 120 metered sprays, the amount of fluticasone propionate delivered per actuation may not be consistent and the unit should be discarded.

CLINICAL PHARMACOLOGY

Mechanism of Action: Fluticasone propionate is a synthetic, trifluorinated corticosteroid with anti-inflammatory activity. In vitro dose response studies on a cloned human glucocorticoid receptor system involving binding and gene expression afforded 50% responses at 1.25 and 0.17 nM concentrations, respectively. Fluticasone propionate was 3-fold to 5-fold more potent than dexamethasone in these assays. Data from the McKenzie vasoconstrictor assay in man also support its potent glucocorticoid activity.

In preclinical studies, fluticasone propionate revealed progesterone-like activity similar to the natural hormone. However, the clinical significance of these findings in relation to the low plasma levels (see Pharmacokinetics) is not known.

The precise mechanism through which fluticasone propionate affects allergic rhinitis symptoms is not known. Corticosteroids have been shown to have a wide range of effects on multiple cell types (e.g., mast cells, eosinophils, neutrophils, macrophages, and lymphocytes) and mediators (e.g., histamine, eicosanoids, leukotrienes, and cytokines) involved in inflammation. In 7 trials in adults, FLONASE Nasal Spray has decreased nasal mucosal eosinophils in 66% (35% for placebo) of patients and basophils in 39% (28% for placebo) of patients. The direct relationship of these findings to long-term symptom relief is not known.

FLONASE Nasal Spray, like other corticosteroids, is an agent that does not have an immediate effect on allergic symptoms. A decrease in nasal symptoms has been noted in some patients 12 hours after initial treatment with FLONASE Nasal Spray. Maximum benefit may not be reached for several days. Similarly, when corticosteroids are discontinued, symptoms may not return for several days.

Pharmacokinetics: *Absorption:* The activity of FLONASE Nasal Spray is due to the parent drug, fluticasone propionate. Indirect calculations indicate that fluticasone propionate delivered by the intranasal route has an absolute bioavailability averaging less than 2%. After intranasal treatment of patients with allergic rhinitis for 3 weeks, fluticasone propionate plasma concentrations were above the level of detection (50 pg/mL) only when recommended doses were exceeded and then only in occasional samples at low plasma levels. Due to the low bioavailability by the intranasal route, the majority of the pharmacokinetic data was obtained via other routes of administration. Studies using oral dosing of radiolabeled drug have demonstrated that fluticasone propionate is highly extracted from plasma and absorption is low. Oral bioavailability is negligible, and the majority of the circulating radioactivity is due to an inactive metabolite.

Distribution: Following intravenous administration, the initial disposition phase for fluticasone propionate was rapid and consistent with its high lipid solubility and tissue binding. The volume of distribution averaged 4.2 L/kg.

The percentage of fluticasone propionate bound to human plasma proteins averaged 91% with no obvious concentration relationship. Fluticasone propionate is weakly and reversibly bound to erythrocytes and freely equilibrates between erythrocytes and plasma. Fluticasone propionate is not significantly bound to human transcortin.

Continued on next page

Product information on these pages is effective as of August 2004. Further information is available at: GlaxoSmithKline, PO Box 13398, Research Triangle Park, NC 27709. 1-888-825-5249. Corporate Web Site: www.gsk.com

Flonase—Cont.

Metabolism: The total blood clearance of fluticasone propionate is high (average, 1,093 mL/min), with renal clearance accounting for less than 0.02% of the total. The only circulating metabolite detected in man is the 17β-carboxylic acid derivative of fluticasone propionate, which is formed through the cytochrome P450 3A4 pathway. This inactive metabolite had less affinity (approximately 1/2,000) than the parent drug for the glucocorticoid receptor of human lung cytosol in vitro and negligible pharmacological activity in animal studies. Other metabolites detected in vitro using cultured human hepatoma cells have not been detected in man.

Elimination: Following intravenous dosing, fluticasone propionate showed polyexponential kinetics and had a terminal elimination half-life of approximately 7.8 hours. Less than 5% of a radiolabeled oral dose was excreted in the urine as metabolites, with the remainder excreted in the feces as parent drug and metabolites.

Special Populations: Fluticasone propionate nasal spray was not studied in any special populations, and no gender-specific pharmacokinetic data have been obtained.

Drug Interactions: Fluticasone propionate is a substrate of cytochrome P450 3A4. Coadministration of fluticasone propionate and the highly potent cytochrome P450 3A4 inhibitor ritonavir is not recommended based upon a multiple-dose, crossover drug interaction study in 18 healthy subjects. Fluticasone propionate aqueous nasal spray (200 mcg once daily) was coadministered for 7 days with ritonavir (100 mg twice daily). Plasma fluticasone propionate concentrations following fluticasone propionate aqueous nasal spray alone were undetectable (<10 pg/mL) in most subjects, and when concentrations were detectable peak levels (C_{max} averaged 11.9 pg/mL [range, 10.8 to 14.1 pg/mL] and $AUC_{(0-\tau)}$ averaged 8.43 pg•hr/mL [range, 4.2 to 18.8 pg•hr/mL]). Fluticasone propionate C_{max} and $AUC_{(0-\tau)}$ increased to 318 pg/mL (range, 110 to 648 pg/mL) and 3,102.6 pg•hr/mL (range, 1,207.1 to 5,662.0 pg•hr/mL), respectively, after coadministration of ritonavir with fluticasone propionate aqueous nasal spray. This significant increase in plasma fluticasone propionate exposure resulted in a significant decrease (86%) in plasma cortisol area under the plasma concentration versus time curve (AUC).

Caution should be exercised when other potent cytochrome P450 3A4 inhibitors are coadministered with fluticasone propionate. In a drug interaction study, coadministration of orally inhaled fluticasone propionate (1,000 mcg) and ketoconazole (200 mg once daily) resulted in increased fluticasone propionate exposure and reduced plasma cortisol AUC, but had no effect on urinary excretion of cortisol.

In another multiple-dose drug interaction study, coadministration of orally inhaled fluticasone propionate (500 mcg twice daily) and erythromycin (333 mg 3 times daily) did not affect fluticasone propionate pharmacokinetics.

Pharmacodynamics: In a trial to evaluate the potential systemic and topical effects of FLONASE Nasal Spray on allergic rhinitis symptoms, the benefits of comparable drug blood levels produced by FLONASE Nasal Spray and oral fluticasone propionate were compared. The doses used were 200 mcg of FLONASE Nasal Spray, the nasal spray vehicle (plus oral placebo), and 5 and 10 mg of oral fluticasone propionate (plus nasal spray vehicle) per day for 14 days. Plasma levels were undetectable in the majority of patients after intranasal dosing, but present at low levels in the majority after oral dosing. FLONASE Nasal Spray was significantly more effective in reducing symptoms of allergic rhinitis than either the oral fluticasone propionate or the nasal vehicle. This trial demonstrated that the therapeutic effect of FLONASE Nasal Spray can be attributed to the topical effects of fluticasone propionate.

In another trial, the potential systemic effects of FLONASE Nasal Spray on the hypothalamic-pituitary-adrenal (HPA) axis were also studied in allergic patients. FLONASE Nasal Spray given as 200 mcg once daily or 400 mcg twice daily was compared with placebo or oral prednisone 7.5 or 15 mg given in the morning. FLONASE Nasal Spray at either dose for 4 weeks did not affect the adrenal response to 6-hour cosyntropin stimulation, while both doses of oral prednisone significantly reduced the response to cosyntropin.

Clinical Trials: A total of 13 randomized, double-blind, parallel-group, multicenter, vehicle placebo-controlled clinical trials were conducted in the United States in adults and pediatric patients (4 years of age and older) to investigate regular use of FLONASE Nasal Spray in patients with seasonal or perennial allergic rhinitis. The trials included 2,633 adults (1,439 men and 1,194 women) with a mean age of 37 (range, 18 to 79 years). A total of 440 adolescents (405 boys and 35 girls), mean age of 14 (range, 12 to 17 years), and 500 children (325 boys and 175 girls), mean age of 9 (range, 4 to 11 years) were also studied. The overall racial distribution was 89% white, 4% black, and 7% other. These trials evaluated the total nasal symptom scores (TNSS) that included rhinorrhea, nasal obstruction, sneezing, and nasal itching in known allergic patients who were treated for 2 to 24 weeks. Subjects treated with FLONASE Nasal Spray exhibited significantly greater decreases in TNSS than vehicle placebo-treated patients. Nasal mucosal basophils and eosinophils were also reduced at the end of treatment in adult studies; however, the clinical significance of this decrease is not known.

There were no significant differences between fluticasone propionate regimens whether administered as a single daily dose of 200 mcg (two 50-mcg sprays in each nostril) or as 100 mcg (one 50-mcg spray in each nostril) twice daily in 6 clinical trials. A clear dose response could not be identified in clinical trials. In 1 trial, 200 mcg/day was slightly more effective than 50 mcg/day during the first few days of treatment; thereafter, no difference was seen.

Two randomized, double-blind, parallel-group, multicenter, vehicle placebo-controlled 28-day trials were conducted in the United States in 732 patients (243 given FLONASE) 12 years of age and older to investigate "as-needed" use of FLONASE Nasal Spray (200 mcg) in patients with seasonal allergic rhinitis. Patients were instructed to take the study medication only on days when they thought they needed the medication for symptom control, not to exceed 2 sprays per nostril on any day, and not more than once daily. "As-needed" use was prospectively defined as average use of study medication no more than 75% of study days. Average use of study medications was 57% to 70% of days for all treatment arms. The studies demonstrated significantly greater reduction in TNSS (sum of nasal congestion, rhinorrhea, sneezing, and nasal itching) with FLONASE Nasal Spray 200 mcg compared to placebo. The relative difference in efficacy with as-needed use as compared to regularly administered doses was not studied.

Three randomized, double-blind, parallel-group, vehicle placebo-controlled trials were conducted in 1,191 patients to investigate regular use of FLONASE Nasal Spray in patients with perennial nonallergic rhinitis. These trials evaluated the patient-rated TNSS (nasal obstruction, postnasal drip, rhinorrhea) in patients treated for 28 days of double-blind therapy and in 1 of the 3 trials for 6 months of open-label treatment. Two of these trials demonstrated that patients treated with FLONASE Nasal Spray at a dose of 100 mcg twice daily exhibited statistically significant decreases in TNSS compared with patients treated with vehicle.

Individualization of Dosage: Patients should use FLONASE Nasal Spray at regular intervals for optimal effect.

Adult patients may be started on a 200-mcg once-daily regimen (two 50-mcg sprays in each nostril once daily). An alternative 200-mcg/day dosage regimen can be given as 100 mcg twice daily (one 50-mcg spray in each nostril twice daily).

Individual patients will experience a variable time to onset and different degree of symptom relief. In 4 randomized, double-blind, vehicle placebo-controlled, parallel-group allergic rhinitis studies and 2 studies of patients in an outdoor "park" setting (park studies), a decrease in nasal symptoms in treated subjects compared to placebo was shown to occur as soon as 12 hours after treatment with a 200-mcg dose of FLONASE Nasal Spray. Maximum effect may take several days. Regular-use patients who have responded may be able to be maintained (after 4 to 7 days) on 100 mcg/day (1 spray in each nostril once daily).

Some patients (12 years of age and older) with seasonal allergic rhinitis may find as-needed use of FLONASE Nasal Spray (not to exceed 200 mcg daily) effective for symptom control (see Clinical Trials). Greater symptom control may be achieved with scheduled regular use. Efficacy of as-needed use of FLONASE Nasal Spray has not been studied in pediatric patients under 12 years of age with seasonal allergic rhinitis, or patients with perennial allergic or nonallergic rhinitis.

Pediatric patients (4 years of age and older) should be started with 100 mcg (1 spray in each nostril once daily). Treatment with 200 mcg (2 sprays in each nostril once daily or 1 spray in each nostril twice daily) should be reserved for pediatric patients not adequately responding to 100 mcg daily. Once adequate control is achieved, the dosage should be decreased to 100 mcg (1 spray in each nostril) daily.

Maximum total daily doses should not exceed 2 sprays in each nostril (total dose, 200 mcg/day). There is no evidence that exceeding the recommended dose is more effective.

INDICATIONS AND USAGE

FLONASE Nasal Spray is indicated for the management of the nasal symptoms of seasonal and perennial allergic and nonallergic rhinitis in adults and pediatric patients 4 years of age and older.

Safety and effectiveness of FLONASE Nasal Spray in children below 4 years of age have not been adequately established.

CONTRAINDICATIONS

FLONASE Nasal Spray is contraindicated in patients with a hypersensitivity to any of its ingredients.

WARNINGS

The replacement of a systemic corticosteroid with a topical corticosteroid can be accompanied by signs of adrenal insufficiency, and in addition some patients may experience symptoms of withdrawal, e.g., joint and/or muscular pain, lassitude, and depression. Patients previously treated for prolonged periods with systemic corticosteroids and transferred to topical corticosteroids should be carefully monitored for acute adrenal insufficiency in response to stress. In those patients who have asthma or other clinical conditions requiring long-term systemic corticosteroid treatment, too rapid a decrease in systemic corticosteroids may cause a severe exacerbation of their symptoms.

The concomitant use of intranasal corticosteroids with other inhaled corticosteroids could increase the risk of signs or symptoms of hypercorticism and/or suppression of the HPA axis.

A drug interaction study in healthy subjects has shown that ritonavir (a highly potent cytochrome P450 3A4 inhibitor) can significantly increase plasma fluticasone propionate exposure, resulting in significantly reduced serum cortisol concentrations (see CLINICAL PHARMACOLOGY: Drug Interactions and PRECAUTIONS: Drug Interactions). During postmarketing use, there have been reports of clinically significant drug interactions in patients receiving fluticasone propionate and ritonavir, resulting in systemic corticosteroid effects including Cushing syndrome and adrenal suppression. Therefore, coadministration of fluticasone propionate and ritonavir is not recommended unless the potential benefit to the patient outweighs the risk of systemic corticosteroid side effects.

Persons who are using drugs that suppress the immune system are more susceptible to infections than healthy individuals. Chickenpox and measles, for example, can have a more serious or even fatal course in susceptible children or adults using corticosteroids. In children or adults who have not had these diseases or been properly immunized, particular care should be taken to avoid exposure. How the dose, route, and duration of corticosteroid administration affect the risk of developing a disseminated infection is not known. The contribution of the underlying disease and/or prior corticosteroid treatment to the risk is also not known. If exposed to chickenpox, prophylaxis with varicella zoster immune globulin (VZIG) may be indicated. If exposed to measles, prophylaxis with pooled intramuscular immunoglobulin (IG) may be indicated. (See the respective package inserts for complete VZIG and IG prescribing information.) If chickenpox develops, treatment with antiviral agents may be considered.

Avoid spraying in eyes.

PRECAUTIONS

General: Intranasal corticosteroids may cause a reduction in growth velocity when administered to pediatric patients (see PRECAUTIONS: Pediatric Use).

Rarely, immediate hypersensitivity reactions or contact dermatitis may occur after the administration of FLONASE Nasal Spray. Rare instances of wheezing, nasal septum perforation, cataracts, glaucoma, and increased intraocular pressure have been reported following the intranasal application of corticosteroids, including fluticasone propionate.

Use of excessive doses of corticosteroids may lead to signs or symptoms of hypercorticism and/or suppression of HPA function.

Although systemic effects have been minimal with recommended doses of FLONASE Nasal Spray, potential risk increases with larger doses. Therefore, larger than recommended doses of FLONASE Nasal Spray should be avoided.

When used at higher than recommended doses or in rare individuals at recommended doses, systemic corticosteroid effects such as hypercorticism and adrenal suppression may appear. If such changes occur, the dosage of FLONASE Nasal Spray should be discontinued slowly consistent with accepted procedures for discontinuing oral corticosteroid therapy.

In clinical studies with fluticasone propionate administered intranasally, the development of localized infections of the nose and pharynx with *Candida albicans* has occurred only rarely. When such an infection develops, it may require treatment with appropriate local therapy and discontinuation of treatment with FLONASE Nasal Spray. Patients using FLONASE Nasal Spray over several months or longer should be examined periodically for evidence of *Candida* infection or other signs of adverse effects on the nasal mucosa.

Intranasal corticosteroids should be used with caution, if at all, in patients with active or quiescent tuberculous infections of the respiratory tract; untreated local or systemic fungal or bacterial infections; systemic viral or parasitic infections; or ocular herpes simplex.

Because of the inhibitory effect of corticosteroids on wound healing, patients who have experienced recent nasal septal ulcers, nasal surgery, or nasal trauma should not use a nasal corticosteroid until healing has occurred.

Information for Patients: Patients being treated with FLONASE Nasal Spray should receive the following information and instructions. This information is intended to aid them in the safe and effective use of this medication. It is not a disclosure of all possible adverse or intended effects. Patients should be warned to avoid exposure to chickenpox or measles and, if exposed, to consult their physician without delay.

Patients should use FLONASE Nasal Spray at regular intervals for optimal effect. Some patients (12 years of age and older) with seasonal allergic rhinitis may find as-needed use of 200 mcg once daily effective for symptom control (see Clinical Trials).

A decrease in nasal symptoms may occur as soon as 12 hours after starting therapy with FLONASE Nasal Spray. Results in several clinical trials indicate statistically significant improvement within the first day or two of treatment; however, the full benefit of FLONASE Nasal Spray may not be achieved until treatment has been administered for several days. The patient should not increase the prescribed dosage but should contact the physician if symptoms do not improve or if the condition worsens.

For the proper use of FLONASE Nasal Spray and to attain maximum improvement, the patient should read and follow carefully the patient's instructions accompanying the product.

Drug Interactions: Fluticasone propionate is a substrate of cytochrome P450 3A4. A drug interaction study with fluticasone propionate aqueous nasal spray in healthy subjects has shown that ritonavir (a highly potent cytochrome P450 3A4 inhibitor) can significantly increase plasma fluticasone propionate exposure, resulting in significantly reduced serum cortisol concentrations (see CLINICAL PHARMACOLOGY: Drug Interactions). During post-marketing use, there have been reports of clinically significant drug interactions in patients receiving fluticasone propionate and ritonavir, resulting in systemic corticosteroid effects including Cushing syndrome and adrenal suppression. Therefore, coadministration of fluticasone propionate and ritonavir is not recommended unless the potential benefit to the patient outweighs the risk of systemic corticosteroid side effects.

In a placebo-controlled, crossover study in 8 healthy volunteers, coadministration of a single dose of orally inhaled fluticasone propionate (1,000 mcg; 5 times the maximum daily intranasal dose) with multiple doses of ketoconazole (200 mg) to steady state resulted in increased plasma fluticasone propionate exposure, a reduction in plasma cortisol AUC, and no effect on urinary excretion of cortisol. Caution should be exercised when FLONASE Nasal Spray is coadministered with ketoconazole and other known potent cytochrome P450 3A4 inhibitors.

Carcinogenesis, Mutagenesis, Impairment of Fertility: Fluticasone propionate demonstrated no tumorigenic potential in mice at oral doses up to 1,000 mcg/kg (approximately 20 times the maximum recommended daily intranasal dose in adults and approximately 10 times the maximum recommended daily intranasal dose in children on a mcg/m^2 basis) for 78 weeks or in rats at inhalation doses up to 57 mcg/kg (approximately 2 times the maximum recommended daily intranasal dose in adults and approximately equivalent to the maximum recommended daily intranasal dose in children on a mcg/m^2 basis) for 104 weeks.

Fluticasone propionate did not induce gene mutation in prokaryotic or eukaryotic cells in vitro. No significant clastogenic effect was seen in cultured human peripheral lymphocytes in vitro or in the mouse micronucleus test.

No evidence of impairment of fertility was observed in reproductive studies conducted in male and female rats at subcutaneous doses up to 50 mcg/kg (approximately 2 times the maximum recommended daily intranasal dose in adults on a mcg/m^2 basis). Prostate weight was significantly reduced at a subcutaneous dose of 50 mcg/kg.

Pregnancy: ***Teratogenic Effects:*** Pregnancy Category C. Subcutaneous studies in the mouse and rat at 45 and 100 mcg/kg, respectively (approximately equivalent to and 4 times the maximum recommended daily intranasal dose in adults on a mcg/m^2 basis, respectively) revealed fetal toxicity characteristic of potent corticosteroid compounds, including embryonic growth retardation, omphalocele, cleft palate, and retarded cranial ossification.

In the rabbit, fetal weight reduction and cleft palate were observed at a subcutaneous dose of 4 mcg/kg (less than the maximum recommended daily intranasal dose in adults on a mcg/m^2 basis). However, no teratogenic effects were reported at oral doses up to 300 mcg/kg (approximately 25 times the maximum recommended daily intranasal dose in adults on a mcg/m^2 basis) of fluticasone propionate to the rabbit. No fluticasone propionate was detected in the plasma in this study, consistent with the established low bioavailability following oral administration (see CLINICAL PHARMACOLOGY).

Fluticasone propionate crossed the placenta following oral administration of 100 mcg/kg to rats or 300 mcg/kg to rabbits (approximately 4 and 25 times, respectively, the maximum recommended daily intranasal dose in adults on a mcg/m^2 basis).

There are no adequate and well-controlled studies in pregnant women. Fluticasone propionate should be used during pregnancy only if the potential benefit justifies the potential risk to the fetus.

Experience with oral corticosteroids since their introduction in pharmacologic, as opposed to physiologic, doses suggests that rodents are more prone to teratogenic effects from corticosteroids than humans. In addition, because there is a natural increase in corticosteroid production during pregnancy, most women will require a lower exogenous corticosteroid dose and many will not need corticosteroid treatment during pregnancy.

Nursing Mothers: It is not known whether fluticasone propionate is excreted in human breast milk. However, other corticosteroids have been detected in human milk. Subcutaneous administration to lactating rats of 10 mcg/kg of tritiated fluticasone propionate (less than the maximum recommended daily intranasal dose in adults on a mcg/m^2 basis) resulted in measurable radioactivity in the milk. Since there are no data from controlled trials on the use of intranasal fluticasone propionate by nursing mothers, caution should be exercised when FLONASE Nasal Spray is administered to a nursing woman.

Pediatric Use: Six hundred fifty (650) patients aged 4 to 11 years and 440 patients aged 12 to 17 years were studied in US clinical trials with fluticasone propionate nasal spray. The safety and effectiveness of FLONASE Nasal Spray in children below 4 years of age have not been established.

Controlled clinical studies have shown that intranasal corticosteroids may cause a reduction in growth velocity in pediatric patients. This effect has been observed in the absence of laboratory evidence of HPA axis suppression, suggesting that growth velocity is a more sensitive indicator of systemic corticosteroid exposure in pediatric patients than some commonly used tests of HPA axis function. The long-term effects of this reduction in growth velocity associated with intranasal corticosteroids, including the impact on final adult height, are unknown. The potential for "catch-up" growth following discontinuation of treatment with intranasal corticosteroids has not been adequately studied.

The growth of pediatric patients receiving intranasal corticosteroids, including FLONASE Nasal Spray, should be monitored routinely (e.g., via stadiometry). The potential growth effects of prolonged treatment should be weighed against the clinical benefits obtained and the risks/benefits of treatment alternatives. To minimize the systemic effects of intranasal corticosteroids, including FLONASE Nasal Spray, each patient should be titrated to the lowest dose that effectively controls his/her symptoms.

A 1-year placebo-controlled clinical growth study was conducted in 150 pediatric patients (ages 3 to 9 years) to assess the effect of FLONASE Nasal Spray (single daily dose of 200 mcg, the maximum approved dose) on growth velocity. From the primary population of 56 patients receiving FLONASE Nasal Spray and 52 receiving placebo, the point estimate for growth velocity with FLONASE Nasal Spray was 0.14 cm/year lower than that noted with placebo (95% confidence interval ranging from 0.54 cm/year lower than placebo to 0.27 cm/year higher than placebo). Thus, no statistically significant effect on growth was noted compared to placebo. No evidence of clinically relevant changes in HPA axis function or bone mineral density was observed as assessed by 12-hour urinary cortisol excretion and dual-energy x-ray absorptiometry, respectively.

The potential for FLONASE Nasal Spray to cause growth suppression in susceptible patients or when given at higher doses cannot be ruled out.

Geriatric Use: A limited number of patients 65 years of age and older (n = 129) or 75 years of age and older (n = 11) have been treated with FLONASE Nasal Spray in US and non-US clinical trials. While the number of patients is too small to permit separate analysis of efficacy and safety, the adverse reactions reported in this population were similar to those reported by younger patients.

ADVERSE REACTIONS

In controlled US studies, more than 3,300 patients with seasonal allergic, perennial allergic, or perennial nonallergic rhinitis received treatment with intranasal fluticasone propionate. In general, adverse reactions in clinical studies have been primarily associated with irritation of the nasal mucous membranes, and the adverse reactions were reported with approximately the same frequency by patients treated with the vehicle itself. The complaints did not usually interfere with treatment. Less than 2% of patients in clinical trials discontinued because of adverse events; this rate was similar for vehicle placebo and active comparators.

Systemic corticosteroid side effects were not reported during controlled clinical studies up to 6 months' duration with FLONASE Nasal Spray. If recommended doses are exceeded, however, or if individuals are particularly sensitive or taking FLONASE Nasal Spray in conjunction with administration of other corticosteroids, symptoms of hypercorticism, e.g., Cushing syndrome, could occur.

The following incidence of common adverse reactions (>3%, where incidence in fluticasone propionate-treated subjects exceeded placebo) is based upon 7 controlled clinical trials in which 536 patients (57 girls and 108 boys aged 4 to 11 years, 137 female and 234 male adolescents and adults) were treated with FLONASE Nasal Spray 200 mcg once daily over 2 to 4 weeks and 2 controlled clinical trials in which 246 patients (119 female and 127 male adolescents and adults) were treated with FLONASE Nasal Spray 200 mcg once daily over 6 months. Also included in the table are adverse events from 2 studies in which 167 children (45 girls and 122 boys aged 4 to 11 years) were treated with FLONASE Nasal Spray 100 mcg once daily for 2 to 4 weeks. [See table above]

Overall Adverse Experiences With >3% Incidence on Fluticasone Propionate in Controlled Clinical Trials With FLONASE Nasal Spray in Patients ≥4 Years With Seasonal or Perennial Allergic Rhinitis

Adverse Experience	Vehicle Placebo (n = 758) %	FLONASE 100 mcg Once Daily (n = 167) %	FLONASE 200 mcg Once Daily (n = 782) %
Headache	14.6	6.6	16.1
Pharyngitis	7.2	6.0	7.8
Epistaxis	5.4	6.0	6.9
Nasal burning/nasal irritation	2.6	2.4	3.2
Nausea/vomiting	2.0	4.8	2.6
Asthma symptoms	2.9	7.2	3.3
Cough	2.8	3.6	3.8

Other adverse events that occurred in ≤3% but ≥1% of patients and that were more common with fluticasone propionate (with uncertain relationship to treatment) included: blood in nasal mucus, runny nose, abdominal pain, diarrhea, fever, flu-like symptoms, aches and pains, dizziness, bronchitis.

Observed During Clinical Practice: In addition to adverse events reported from clinical trials, the following events have been identified during postapproval use of intranasal fluticasone propionate in clinical practice. Because they are reported voluntarily from a population of unknown size, estimates of frequency cannot be made. These events have been chosen for inclusion due to either their seriousness, frequency of reporting, or causal connection to fluticasone propionate or a combination of these factors.

General: Hypersensitivity reactions, including angioedema, skin rash, edema of the face and tongue, pruritus, urticaria, bronchospasm, wheezing, dyspnea, and anaphylaxis/anaphylactoid reactions, which in rare instances were severe.

Ear, Nose, and Throat: Alteration or loss of sense of taste and/or smell and, rarely, nasal septal perforation, nasal ulcer, sore throat, throat irritation and dryness, cough, hoarseness, and voice changes.

Eye: Dryness and irritation, conjunctivitis, blurred vision, glaucoma, increased intraocular pressure, and cataracts.

Cases of growth suppression have been reported for intranasal corticosteroids, including FLONASE (see PRECAUTIONS: Pediatric Use).

OVERDOSAGE

Chronic overdosage may result in signs/symptoms of hypercorticism (see PRECAUTIONS). Intranasal administration of 2 mg (10 times the recommended dose) of fluticasone propionate twice daily for 7 days to healthy human volunteers was well tolerated. Single oral doses up to 16 mg have been studied in human volunteers with no acute toxic effects reported. Repeat oral doses up to 80 mg daily for 10 days in volunteers and repeat oral doses up to 10 mg daily for 14 days in patients were well tolerated. Adverse reactions were of mild or moderate severity, and incidences were similar in active and placebo treatment groups. Acute overdosage with this dosage form is unlikely since 1 bottle of FLONASE Nasal Spray contains approximately 8 mg of fluticasone propionate.

The oral and subcutaneous median lethal doses in mice and rats were >1,000 mg/kg (>20,000 and >41,000 times, respectively, the maximum recommended daily intranasal dose in adults and >10,000 and >20,000 times, respectively, the maximum recommended daily intranasal dose in children on a mg/m^2 basis).

DOSAGE AND ADMINISTRATION

Patients should use FLONASE Nasal Spray at regular intervals for optimal effect.

Adults: The recommended starting dosage in **adults** is 2 sprays (50 mcg of fluticasone propionate each) in each nostril once daily (total daily dose, 200 mcg). The same dosage divided into 100 mcg given twice daily (e.g., 8 a.m. and 8 p.m.) is also effective. After the first few days, patients may be able to reduce their dosage to 100 mcg (1 spray in each nostril) once daily for maintenance therapy. Some patients (12 years of age and older) with seasonal allergic rhinitis may find as-needed use of 200 mcg once daily effective for symptom control (see Clinical Trials). Greater symptom control may be achieved with scheduled regular use.

Adolescents and Children (4 Years of Age and Older): Patients should be started with 100 mcg (1 spray in each nostril once daily). Patients not adequately responding to 100 mcg may use 200 mcg (2 sprays in each nostril). Once adequate control is achieved, the dosage should be decreased to 100 mcg (1 spray in each nostril) daily.

The maximum total daily dosage should not exceed 2 sprays in each nostril (200 mcg/day). (See Individualization of Dosage and Clinical Trials sections.)

FLONASE Nasal Spray is not recommended for children under 4 years of age.

Directions for Use: Illustrated patient's instructions for proper use accompany each package of FLONASE Nasal Spray.

HOW SUPPLIED

FLONASE Nasal Spray 50 mcg is supplied in an amber glass bottle fitted with a white metering atomizing pump, white nasal adapter, and green dust cover in a box of 1 (NDC 0173-0453-01) with patient's instructions for use. Each bottle contains a net fill weight of 16 g and will provide 120 actuations. Each actuation delivers 50 mcg of fluticasone propionate in 100 mg of formulation through the nasal adapter. The correct amount of medication in each spray cannot be assured after 120 sprays even though the bottle is not completely empty. The bottle should be discarded when the labeled number of actuations has been used.

Store between 4° and 30°C (39° and 86°F).

GlaxoSmithKline
Research Triangle Park, NC 27709

March 2004 RL-2066

Shown in Product Identification Guide, page 315

Continued on next page

Product information on these pages is effective as of August 2004. Further information is available at: GlaxoSmithKline, PO Box 13398, Research Triangle Park, NC 27709. 1-888-825-5249. Corporate Web Site: www.gsk.com

FLOVENT® 44 mcg ℞

[flō' vent]

(fluticasone propionate, 44 mcg)
Inhalation Aerosol

FLOVENT® 110 mcg ℞

(fluticasone propionate, 110 mcg)
Inhalation Aerosol

FLOVENT® 220 mcg ℞

(fluticasone propionate, 220 mcg)
Inhalation Aerosol

For Oral Inhalation Only

DESCRIPTION

The active component of FLOVENT 44 mcg Inhalation Aerosol, FLOVENT 110 mcg Inhalation Aerosol, and FLOVENT 220 mcg Inhalation Aerosol is fluticasone propionate, a glucocorticoid having the chemical name S-(fluoromethyl)6α,9-difluoro-11β,17-dihydroxy-16α-methyl-3-oxoandrosta-1,4-diene-17β-carbothioate, 17-propionate.

Fluticasone propionate is a white to off-white powder with a molecular weight of 500.6. It is practically insoluble in water, freely soluble in dimethyl sulfoxide and dimethylformamide, and slightly soluble in methanol and 95% ethanol.

FLOVENT 44 mcg Inhalation Aerosol, FLOVENT 110 mcg Inhalation Aerosol, and FLOVENT 220 mcg Inhalation Aerosol are pressurized, metered-dose aerosol units intended for oral inhalation only. Each unit contains a microcrystalline suspension of fluticasone propionate (micronized) in a mixture of 2 chlorofluorocarbon propellants (trichlorofluoromethane and dichlorodifluoromethane) with soya lecithin. Each actuation of the inhaler delivers 50, 125, or 250 mcg of fluticasone propionate from the valve and 44, 110, or 220 mcg, respectively, of fluticasone propionate from the actuator.

CLINICAL PHARMACOLOGY

Fluticasone propionate is a synthetic, trifluorinated glucocorticoid with potent anti-inflammatory activity. In vitro assays using human lung cytosol preparations have established fluticasone propionate as a human glucocorticoid receptor agonist with an affinity 18 times greater than dexamethasone, almost twice that of beclomethasone-17-monopropionate (BMP), the active metabolite of beclomethasone dipropionate, and over 3 times that of budesonide. Data from the McKenzie vasoconstrictor assay in man are consistent with these results.

The precise mechanisms of glucocorticoid action in asthma are unknown. Inflammation is recognized as an important component in the pathogenesis of asthma. Glucocorticoids have been shown to inhibit multiple cell types (e.g., mast cells, eosinophils, basophils, lymphocytes, macrophages, and neutrophils) and mediator production or secretion (e.g., histamine, eicosanoids, leukotrienes, and cytokines) involved in the asthmatic response. These anti-inflammatory actions of glucocorticoids may contribute to their efficacy in asthma.

Though highly effective for the treatment of asthma, glucocorticoids do not affect asthma symptoms immediately. However, improvement following inhaled administration of fluticasone propionate can occur within 24 hours of beginning treatment, although maximum benefit may not be achieved for 1 to 2 weeks or longer after starting treatment. When glucocorticoids are discontinued, asthma stability may persist for several days or longer.

Pharmacokinetics: ***Absorption:*** The activity of FLOVENT Inhalation Aerosol is due to the parent drug, fluticasone propionate. Studies using oral dosing of labeled and unlabeled drug have demonstrated that the oral systemic bioavailability of fluticasone propionate is negligible (<1%), primarily due to incomplete absorption and presystemic metabolism in the gut and liver. In contrast, the majority of the fluticasone propionate delivered to the lung is systemically absorbed. The systemic bioavailability of fluticasone propionate inhalation aerosol in healthy volunteers averaged about 30% of the dose delivered from the actuator.

Peak plasma concentrations after an 880-mcg inhaled dose ranged from 0.1 to 1.0 ng/mL.

Distribution: Following intravenous administration, the initial disposition phase for fluticasone propionate was rapid and consistent with its high lipid solubility and tissue binding. The volume of distribution averaged 4.2 L/kg. The percentage of fluticasone propionate bound to human plasma proteins averaged 91%. Fluticasone propionate is weakly and reversibly bound to erythrocytes. Fluticasone propionate is not significantly bound to human transcortin.

Metabolism: The total clearance of fluticasone propionate is high (average, 1,093 mL/min), with renal clearance accounting for less than 0.02% of the total. The only circulating metabolite detected in man is the 17β-carboxylic acid derivative of fluticasone propionate, which is formed through the cytochrome P450 3A4 pathway. This metabolite had approximately 2,000 times less affinity than the parent drug for the glucocorticoid receptor of human lung cytosol in vitro and negligible pharmacological activity in animal studies. Other metabolites detected in vitro using cultured human hepatoma cells have not been detected in man.

Excretion: Following intravenous dosing, fluticasone propionate showed polyexponential kinetics and had a terminal elimination half-life of approximately 7.8 hours. Less than 5% of a radiolabeled oral dose was excreted in the urine as metabolites, with the remainder excreted in the feces as parent drug and metabolites.

Special Populations: Formal pharmacokinetic studies using fluticasone propionate were not carried out in any special populations. In a clinical study using fluticasone propionate inhalation powder, trough fluticasone propionate plasma concentrations were collected in 76 males and 74 females after inhaled administration of 100 and 500 mcg twice daily. Full pharmacokinetic profiles were obtained from 7 female patients and 13 male patients at these doses, and no overall differences in pharmacokinetic behavior were found.

Drug Interactions: Fluticasone propionate is a substrate of cytochrome P450 3A4. Coadministration of fluticasone propionate and the highly potent cytochrome P450 3A4 inhibitor ritonavir is not recommended based upon a multiple-dose, crossover drug interaction study in 18 healthy subjects. Fluticasone propionate aqueous nasal spray (200 mcg once daily) was coadministered for 7 days with ritonavir (100 mg twice daily). Plasma fluticasone propionate concentrations following fluticasone propionate aqueous nasal spray alone were undetectable (<10 pg/mL) in most subjects, and when concentrations were detectable peak levels (C_{max} averaged 11.9 pg/mL [range, 10.8 to 14.1 pg/mL] and $AUC_{(0-\tau)}$ averaged 8.43 pg•hr/mL [range, 4.2 to 18.8 pg•hr/mL]). Fluticasone propionate C_{max} and $AUC_{(0-\tau)}$ increased to 318 pg/mL (range, 110 to 648 pg/mL) and 3,102.6 pg•hr/mL (range, 1,207.1 to 5,662.0 pg•hr/mL), respectively, after coadministration of ritonavir with fluticasone propionate aqueous nasal spray. This significant increase in plasma fluticasone propionate exposure resulted in a significant decrease (86%) in plasma cortisol area under the plasma concentration versus time curve (AUC).

Caution should be exercised when other potent cytochrome P450 3A4 inhibitors are coadministered with fluticasone propionate. In a drug interaction study, coadministration of orally inhaled fluticasone propionate (1,000 mcg) and ketoconazole (200 mg once daily) resulted in increased plasma fluticasone propionate exposure and reduced plasma cortisol AUC, but had no effect on urinary excretion of cortisol. In another multiple-dose drug interaction study, coadministration of orally inhaled fluticasone propionate (500 mcg twice daily) and erythromycin (333 mg 3 times daily) did not affect fluticasone propionate pharmacokinetics.

Pharmacodynamics: To confirm that systemic absorption does not play a role in the clinical response to inhaled fluticasone propionate, a double-blind clinical study comparing inhaled and oral fluticasone propionate was conducted. Doses of 100 and 500 mcg twice daily of fluticasone propionate inhalation powder were compared to oral fluticasone propionate, 20,000 mcg given once daily, and placebo for 6 weeks. Plasma levels of fluticasone propionate were detectable in all 3 active groups, but the mean values were highest in the oral group. Both doses of inhaled fluticasone propionate were effective in maintaining asthma stability and improving lung function while oral fluticasone propionate and placebo were ineffective. This demonstrates that the clinical effectiveness of inhaled fluticasone propionate is due to its direct local effect and not to an indirect effect through systemic absorption.

The potential systemic effects of inhaled fluticasone propionate on the hypothalamic-pituitary-adrenal (HPA) axis were also studied in patients with asthma. Fluticasone propionate given by inhalation aerosol at doses of 220, 440, 660, or 880 mcg twice daily was compared with placebo or oral prednisone 10 mg given once daily for 4 weeks. For most patients, the ability to increase cortisol production in response to stress, as assessed by 6-hour cosyntropin stimulation, remained intact with inhaled fluticasone propionate treatment. No patient had an abnormal response (peak less than 18 mcg/dL) after dosing with placebo or 220 mcg twice daily. Ten percent (10%) to 16% of patients treated with fluticasone propionate at doses of 440 mcg or more twice daily had an abnormal response as compared to 29% of patients treated with prednisone.

CLINICAL TRIALS

Double-blind, parallel-group, placebo-controlled, US clinical trials were conducted in 1,818 adolescent and adult patients with asthma to assess the efficacy and/or safety of FLOVENT Inhalation Aerosol in the treatment of asthma. Fixed doses ranging from 22 to 880 mcg twice daily were compared to placebo to provide information about appropriate dosing to cover a range of asthma severity. Patients with asthma included in these studies were those not adequately controlled with beta-agonists alone, those already maintained on daily inhaled corticosteroids, and those requiring oral corticosteroid therapy. In all efficacy trials, at all doses, measures of pulmonary function (forced expiratory volume in 1 second [FEV_1] and morning peak expiratory flow [AM PEF]) were statistically significantly improved as compared with placebo.

In 2 clinical trials of 660 patients with asthma inadequately controlled on bronchodilators alone, FLOVENT Inhalation Aerosol was evaluated at doses of 44 and 88 mcg twice daily. Both doses of FLOVENT Inhalation Aerosol improved asthma control significantly as compared with placebo.

Figure 1 displays results of pulmonary function tests for the recommended starting dosage of FLOVENT Inhalation Aerosol (88 mcg twice daily) and placebo from a 12-week trial in patients with asthma inadequately controlled on bronchodilators alone. Because this trial used predetermined criteria for lack of efficacy, which caused more patients in the placebo group to be withdrawn, pulmonary function results at Endpoint, which is the last evaluable FEV_1 result and includes most patients' lung function data, are also provided. Pulmonary function improved significantly with FLOVENT Inhalation Aerosol compared with placebo by the second week of treatment, and this improvement was maintained over the duration of the trial.

Figure 1. A 12-Week Clinical Trial in Patients Inadequately Controlled on Bronchodilators Alone: Mean Percent Change From Baseline in FEV_1 Prior to AM Dose

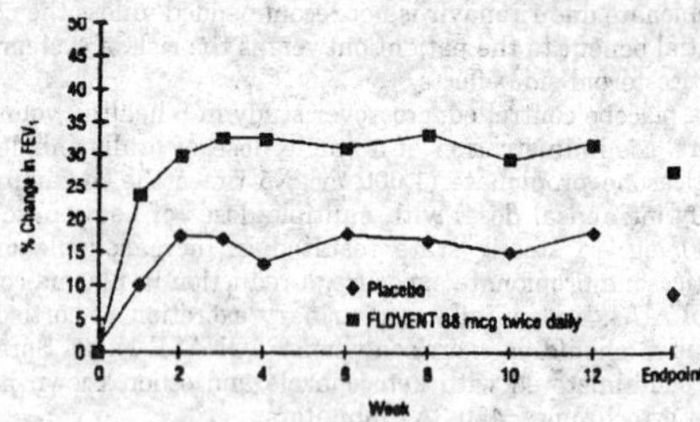

In clinical trials of 924 patients with asthma already receiving daily inhaled corticosteroid therapy (doses of at least 336 mcg/day of beclomethasone dipropionate) in addition to as-needed albuterol and theophylline (46% of all patients), 22- to 440-mcg twice-daily doses of FLOVENT Inhalation Aerosol were also evaluated. All doses of FLOVENT Inhalation Aerosol were efficacious when compared to placebo on major endpoints including lung function and symptom scores. Patients treated with FLOVENT Inhalation Aerosol were also less likely to discontinue study participation due to asthma deterioration (as defined by predetermined criteria for lack of efficacy including lung function and patient-recorded variables such as AM PEF, albuterol use, and nighttime awakenings due to asthma).

Figure 2 displays results of pulmonary function from a 12-week clinical trial in patients with asthma already receiving daily inhaled corticosteroid therapy (beclomethasone dipropionate 336 to 672 mcg/day). The mean percent change from baseline in lung function results for FLOVENT Inhalation Aerosol dosages of 88, 220, and 440 mcg twice daily and placebo are shown over the 12-week trial. Because this trial also used predetermined criteria for lack of efficacy, which caused more patients in the placebo group to be withdrawn, pulmonary function results at Endpoint are included. Pulmonary function improved significantly with FLOVENT Inhalation Aerosol compared with placebo by the first week of treatment, and the improvement was maintained over the duration of the trial. Analysis of the endpoint results that adjusted for differential withdrawal rates indicated that pulmonary function significantly improved with FLOVENT Inhalation Aerosol compared with placebo treatment. Similar improvements in lung function were seen in the other 2 trials in patients treated with inhaled corticosteroids at baseline.

Figure 2. A 12-Week Clinical Trial With Patients Already Receiving Inhaled Corticosteroids: Mean Percent Change From Baseline in FEV_1 Prior to AM Dose

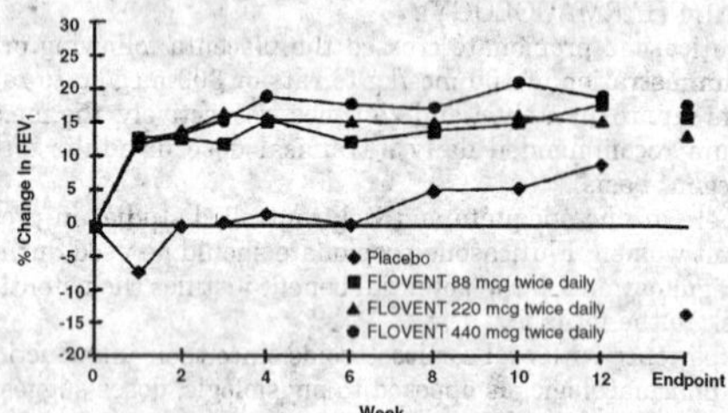

In a clinical trial of 96 patients with severe asthma requiring chronic oral prednisone therapy (average baseline daily prednisone dose was 10 mg), twice-daily doses of 660 and 880 mcg of FLOVENT Inhalation Aerosol were evaluated. Both doses enabled a statistically significantly larger percentage of patients to wean successfully from oral prednisone as compared with placebo (69% of the patients on 660 mcg twice daily and 88% of the patients on 880 mcg twice daily as compared with 3% of patients on placebo). Accompanying the reduction in oral corticosteroid use, patients treated with FLOVENT Inhalation Aerosol had significantly improved lung function and fewer asthma symptoms as compared with the placebo group.

[See figure 3 at top of next column]

INDICATIONS AND USAGE

FLOVENT Inhalation Aerosol is indicated for the maintenance treatment of asthma as prophylactic therapy. It is also indicated for patients requiring oral corticosteroid therapy for asthma. Many of these patients may be able to reduce or eliminate their requirement for oral corticosteroids over time.

FLOVENT Inhalation Aerosol is NOT indicated for the relief of acute bronchospasm.

CONTRAINDICATIONS

FLOVENT Inhalation Aerosol is contraindicated in the primary treatment of status asthmaticus or other acute episodes of asthma where intensive measures are required.

Hypersensitivity to any of the ingredients of these preparations contraindicates their use (see DESCRIPTION).

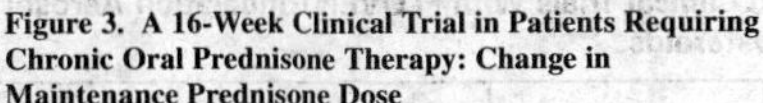

Figure 3. A 16-Week Clinical Trial in Patients Requiring Chronic Oral Prednisone Therapy: Change in Maintenance Prednisone Dose

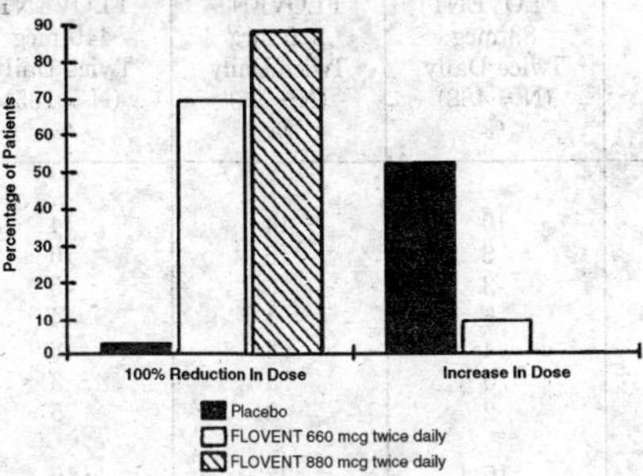

WARNINGS

Particular care is needed for patients who are transferred from systemically active corticosteroids to FLOVENT Inhalation Aerosol because deaths due to adrenal insufficiency have occurred in patients with asthma during and after transfer from systemic corticosteroids to less systemically available inhaled corticosteroids. After withdrawal from systemic corticosteroids, a number of months are required for recovery of HPA function.

Patients who have been previously maintained on 20 mg or more per day of prednisone (or its equivalent) may be most susceptible, particularly when their systemic corticosteroids have been almost completely withdrawn. During this period of HPA suppression, patients may exhibit signs and symptoms of adrenal insufficiency when exposed to trauma, surgery, or infection (particularly gastroenteritis) or other conditions associated with severe electrolyte loss. Although FLOVENT Inhalation Aerosol may provide control of asthma symptoms during these episodes, in recommended doses it supplies less than normal physiological amounts of glucocorticoid systemically and does NOT provide the mineralocorticoid activity that is necessary for coping with these emergencies.

During periods of stress or a severe asthma attack, patients who have been withdrawn from systemic corticosteroids should be instructed to resume oral corticosteroids (in large doses) immediately and to contact their physicians for further instruction. These patients should also be instructed to carry a warning card indicating that they may need supplementary systemic corticosteroids during periods of stress or a severe asthma attack.

A drug interaction study in healthy subjects has shown that ritonavir (a highly potent cytochrome P450 3A4 inhibitor) can significantly increase plasma fluticasone propionate exposure, resulting in significantly reduced serum cortisol concentrations (see CLINICAL PHARMACOLOGY: Drug Interactions and PRECAUTIONS: Drug Interactions). During postmarketing use, there have been reports of clinically significant drug interactions in patients receiving fluticasone propionate and ritonavir, resulting in systemic corticosteroid effects including Cushing syndrome and adrenal suppression. Therefore, coadministration of fluticasone propionate and ritonavir is not recommended unless the potential benefit to the patient outweighs the risk of systemic corticosteroid side effects.

Patients requiring oral corticosteroids should be weaned slowly from systemic corticosteroid use after transferring to FLOVENT Inhalation Aerosol. In a trial of 96 patients, prednisone reduction was successfully accomplished by reducing the daily prednisone dose by 2.5 mg on a weekly basis during transfer to inhaled fluticasone propionate. Successive reduction of prednisone dose was allowed only when lung function, symptoms, and as-needed beta-agonist use were better than or comparable to that seen before initiation of prednisone dose reduction. Lung function (FEV_1 or AM PEF), beta-agonist use, and asthma symptoms should be carefully monitored during withdrawal of oral corticosteroids. In addition to monitoring asthma signs and symptoms, patients should be observed for signs and symptoms of adrenal insufficiency such as fatigue, lassitude, weakness, nausea and vomiting, and hypotension.

Transfer of patients from systemic corticosteroid therapy to FLOVENT Inhalation Aerosol may unmask conditions previously suppressed by the systemic corticosteroid therapy, e.g., rhinitis, conjunctivitis, eczema, and arthritis.

Persons who are on drugs that suppress the immune system are more susceptible to infections than healthy individuals. Chickenpox and measles, for example, can have a more serious or even fatal course in susceptible children or adults on corticosteroids. In such children or adults who have not had these diseases, particular care should be taken to avoid exposure. How the dose, route, and duration of corticosteroid administration affect the risk of developing a disseminated infection is not known. The contribution of the underlying disease and/or prior corticosteroid treatment to the risk is also not known. If exposed to chickenpox, prophylaxis with varicella zoster immune globulin (VZIG) may be indicated. If exposed to measles, prophylaxis with pooled intramuscular immunoglobulin (IG) may be indicated. (See the respective package inserts for complete VZIG and IG prescribing information.) If chickenpox develops, treatment with antiviral agents may be considered.

FLOVENT Inhalation Aerosol is not to be regarded as a bronchodilator and is not indicated for rapid relief of bronchospasm.

As with other inhaled asthma medications, bronchospasm may occur with an immediate increase in wheezing after dosing. If bronchospasm occurs following dosing with FLOVENT Inhalation Aerosol, it should be treated immediately with a fast-acting inhaled bronchodilator. Treatment with FLOVENT Inhalation Aerosol should be discontinued and alternative therapy instituted.

Patients should be instructed to contact their physicians immediately when episodes of asthma that are not responsive to bronchodilators occur during the course of treatment with FLOVENT Inhalation Aerosol. During such episodes, patients may require therapy with oral corticosteroids.

PRECAUTIONS

General: During withdrawal from oral corticosteroids, some patients may experience symptoms of systemically active corticosteroid withdrawal, e.g., joint and/or muscular pain, lassitude, and depression, despite maintenance or even improvement of respiratory function.

Fluticasone propionate will often permit control of asthma symptoms with less suppression of HPA function than therapeutically equivalent oral doses of prednisone. Since fluticasone propionate is absorbed into the circulation and can be systemically active at higher doses, the beneficial effects of FLOVENT Inhalation Aerosol in minimizing HPA dysfunction may be expected only when recommended dosages are not exceeded and individual patients are titrated to the lowest effective dose. A relationship between plasma levels of fluticasone propionate and inhibitory effects on stimulated cortisol production has been shown after 4 weeks of treatment with FLOVENT Inhalation Aerosol. Since individual sensitivity to effects on cortisol production exists, physicians should consider this information when prescribing FLOVENT Inhalation Aerosol.

Because of the possibility of systemic absorption of inhaled corticosteroids, patients treated with these drugs should be observed carefully for any evidence of systemic corticosteroid effects. Particular care should be taken in observing patients postoperatively or during periods of stress for evidence of inadequate adrenal response.

It is possible that systemic corticosteroid effects such as hypercorticism and adrenal suppression (including adrenal crisis) may appear in a small number of patients, particularly when FLOVENT Inhalation Aerosol is administered at higher than recommended doses over prolonged periods of time. If such effects occur, fluticasone propionate inhalation aerosol should be reduced slowly, consistent with accepted procedures for reducing systemic corticosteroids and for management of asthma symptoms.

A reduction of growth velocity in children or teenagers may occur as a result of inadequate control of chronic diseases such as asthma or from use of corticosteroids for treatment. Physicians should closely follow the growth of adolescents taking corticosteroids by any route and weigh the benefits of corticosteroid therapy and asthma control against the possibility of growth suppression if an adolescent's growth appears slowed.

The long-term effects of fluticasone propionate in human subjects are not fully known. In particular, the effects resulting from chronic use of fluticasone propionate on developmental or immunologic processes in the mouth, pharynx, trachea, and lung are unknown. Some patients have received fluticasone propionate inhalation aerosol on a continuous basis for periods of 3 years or longer. In clinical studies with patients treated for nearly 2 years with inhaled fluticasone propionate, no apparent differences in the type or severity of adverse reactions were observed after long- versus short-term treatment.

Rare instances of glaucoma, increased intraocular pressure, and cataracts have been reported following the inhaled administration of corticosteroids, including fluticasone propionate.

In clinical studies with inhaled fluticasone propionate, the development of localized infections of the pharynx with *Candida albicans* has occurred. When such an infection develops, it should be treated with appropriate local or systemic (i.e., oral antifungal) therapy while remaining on treatment with FLOVENT Inhalation Aerosol, but at times therapy with FLOVENT Inhalation Aerosol may need to be interrupted.

Inhaled corticosteroids should be used with caution, if at all, in patients with active or quiescent tuberculosis infection of the respiratory tract; untreated systemic fungal, bacterial, viral or parasitic infections; or ocular herpes simplex.

Eosinophilic Conditions: In rare cases, patients on inhaled fluticasone propionate may present with systemic eosinophilic conditions, with some patients presenting with clinical features of vasculitis consistent with Churg-Strauss syndrome, a condition that is often treated with systemic corticosteroid therapy. These events usually, but not always, have been associated with the reduction and/or withdrawal of oral corticosteroid therapy following the introduction of fluticasone propionate. Cases of serious eosinophilic conditions have also been reported with other inhaled corticosteroids in this clinical setting. Physicians should be alert to eosinophilia, vasculitic rash, worsening pulmonary symptoms, cardiac complications, and/or neuropathy presenting in their patients. A causal relationship between fluticasone propionate and these underlying conditions has not been established (see ADVERSE REACTIONS).

Information for Patients: Patients being treated with FLOVENT Inhalation Aerosol should receive the following information and instructions. This information is intended to aid them in the safe and effective use of this medication. It is not a disclosure of all possible adverse or intended effects.

Patients should use FLOVENT Inhalation Aerosol at regular intervals as directed. Results of clinical trials indicated significant improvement may occur within the first day or two of treatment; however, the full benefit may not be achieved until treatment has been administered for 1 to 2 weeks or longer. The patient should not increase the prescribed dosage but should contact the physician if symptoms do not improve or if the condition worsens.

After inhalation, rinse the mouth with water without swallowing.

Patients should be warned to avoid exposure to chickenpox or measles and, if they are exposed, to consult the physician without delay.

For the proper use of FLOVENT Inhalation Aerosol and to attain maximum improvement, the patient should read and follow carefully the Patient's Instructions for Use accompanying the product.

Drug Interactions: Fluticasone propionate is a substrate of cytochrome P450 3A4. A drug interaction study with fluticasone propionate aqueous nasal spray in healthy subjects has shown that ritonavir (a highly potent cytochrome P450 3A4 inhibitor) can significantly increase plasma fluticasone propionate exposure, resulting in significantly reduced serum cortisol concentrations (see CLINICAL PHARMACOLOGY: Drug Interactions). During postmarketing use, there have been reports of clinically significant drug interactions in patients receiving fluticasone propionate and ritonavir, resulting in systemic corticosteroid effects including Cushing syndrome and adrenal suppression. Therefore, coadministration of fluticasone propionate and ritonavir is not recommended unless the potential benefit to the patient outweighs the risk of systemic corticosteroid side effects.

In a placebo-controlled, crossover study in 8 healthy volunteers, coadministration of a single dose of orally inhaled fluticasone propionate (1,000 mcg) with multiple doses of ketoconazole (200 mg) to steady state resulted in increased mean plasma fluticasone propionate exposure, a reduction in plasma cortisol AUC, and no effect on urinary excretion of cortisol. Caution should be exercised when FLOVENT Inhalation Aerosol is coadministered with ketoconazole and other known potent cytochrome P450 3A4 inhibitors.

Carcinogenesis, Mutagenesis, Impairment of Fertility: Fluticasone propionate demonstrated no tumorigenic potential in studies of oral doses up to 1,000 mcg/kg (approximately 2 times the maximum human daily inhalation dose based on mcg/m^2) for 78 weeks in the mouse or inhalation of up to 57 mcg/kg (approximately 1/4 the maximum human daily inhalation dose based on mcg/m^2) for 104 weeks in the rat.

Fluticasone propionate did not induce gene mutation in prokaryotic or eukaryotic cells in vitro. No significant clastogenic effect was seen in cultured human peripheral lymphocytes in vitro or in the mouse micronucleus test when administered at high doses by the oral or subcutaneous routes. Furthermore, the compound did not delay erythroblast division in bone marrow.

No evidence of impairment of fertility was observed in reproductive studies conducted in rats dosed subcutaneously with doses up to 50 mcg/kg (approximately 1/4 the maximum human daily inhalation dose based on mcg/m^2) in males and females. However, prostate weight was significantly reduced in rats.

Pregnancy: *Teratogenic Effects:* Pregnancy Category C. Subcutaneous studies in the mouse and rat at 45 and 100 mcg/kg, respectively (approximately 1/10 and 1/2 the maximum human daily inhalation dose based on mcg/m^2, respectively), revealed fetal toxicity characteristic of potent glucocorticoid compounds, including embryonic growth retardation, omphalocele, cleft palate, and retarded cranial ossification.

In the rabbit, fetal weight reduction and cleft palate were observed following subcutaneous doses of 4 mcg/kg (approximately 1/25 the maximum human daily inhalation dose based on mcg/m^2). However, following oral administration of up to 300 mcg/kg (approximately 3 times the maximum human daily inhalation dose based on mcg/m^2) of fluticasone propionate to the rabbit, there were no maternal effects nor increased incidence of external, visceral, or skeletal fetal defects. No fluticasone propionate was detected in the plasma in this study, consistent with the established low bioavailability following oral administration (see CLINICAL PHARMACOLOGY).

Less than 0.008% of the administered dose crossed the placenta following oral administration of 100 mcg/kg to rats or 300 mcg/kg to rabbits (approximately 1/2 and 3 times the maximum human daily inhalation dose based on mcg/m^2, respectively).

There are no adequate and well-controlled studies in pregnant women. FLOVENT Inhalation Aerosol should be used during pregnancy only if the potential benefit justifies the potential risk to the fetus.

Experience with oral glucocorticoids since their introduction in pharmacologic, as opposed to physiologic, doses suggests that rodents are more prone to teratogenic effects from glucocorticoids than humans. In addition, because there is a natural increase in glucocorticoid production during pregnancy, most women will require a lower exogenous glucocorticoid dose and many will not need glucocorticoid treatment during pregnancy.

Continued on next page

Product information on these pages is effective as of August 2004. Further information is available at: GlaxoSmithKline, PO Box 13398, Research Triangle Park, NC 27709. 1-888-825-5249. Corporate Web Site: www.gsk.com

Flovent—Cont.

Nursing Mothers: It is not known whether fluticasone propionate is excreted in human breast milk. Subcutaneous administration of 10 mcg/kg tritiated drug to lactating rats (approximately 1/20 the maximum human daily inhalation dose based on mcg/m^2) resulted in measurable radioactivity in both plasma and milk. Because glucocorticoids are excreted in human milk, caution should be exercised when fluticasone propionate inhalation aerosol is administered to a nursing woman.

Pediatric Use: One hundred thirty-seven (137) patients between the ages of 12 and 16 years were treated with FLOVENT Inhalation Aerosol in the US pivotal clinical trials. The safety and effectiveness of FLOVENT Inhalation Aerosol in children below 12 years of age have not been established. Oral corticosteroids have been shown to cause a reduction in growth velocity in children and teenagers with extended use. If a child or teenager on any corticosteroid appears to have growth suppression, the possibility that they are particularly sensitive to this effect of corticosteroids should be considered (see PRECAUTIONS).

Geriatric Use: Five hundred seventy-four (574) patients 65 years of age or older have been treated with FLOVENT Inhalation Aerosol in US and non-US clinical trials. There were no differences in adverse reactions compared to those reported by younger patients.

ADVERSE REACTIONS

The incidence of common adverse events in Table 1 is based upon 7 placebo-controlled US clinical trials in which 1,243 patients (509 female and 734 male adolescents and adults previously treated with as-needed bronchodilators and/or inhaled corticosteroids) were treated with FLOVENT Inhalation Aerosol (doses of 88 to 440 mcg twice daily for up to 12 weeks) or placebo.

[See table 1 above]

Table 1 includes all events (whether considered drug-related or nondrug-related by the investigator) that occurred at a rate of over 3% in groups treated with FLOVENT Inhalation Aerosol and were more common than in the placebo group. In considering these data, differences in average duration of exposure should be taken into account.

These adverse reactions were mostly mild to moderate in severity, with ≤2% of patients discontinuing the studies because of adverse events. Rare cases of immediate and delayed hypersensitivity reactions, including urticaria and rash and other rare events of angioedema and bronchospasm, have been reported.

Systemic glucocorticoid side effects were not reported during controlled clinical trials with FLOVENT Inhalation Aerosol. If recommended doses are exceeded, however, or if individuals are particularly sensitive, symptoms of hypercorticism, e.g., Cushing syndrome, could occur.

Other adverse events that occurred in these clinical trials using FLOVENT Inhalation Aerosol with an incidence of 1% to 3% and that occurred at a greater incidence than with placebo were:

Ear, Nose, and Throat: Pain in nasal sinus(es), rhinitis.
Eye: Irritation of the eye(s).
Gastrointestinal: Nausea and vomiting, diarrhea, dyspepsia and stomach disorder.
Miscellaneous: Fever.
Mouth and Teeth: Dental problem.
Musculoskeletal: Pain in joint, sprain/strain, aches and pains, pain in limb.
Neurological: Dizziness/giddiness.
Respiratory: Bronchitis, chest congestion.
Skin: Dermatitis, rash/skin eruption.
Urogenital: Dysmenorrhea.

In a 16-week study in patients with asthma requiring oral corticosteroids, the effects of FLOVENT Inhalation Aerosol, 660 mcg twice daily (N = 32) and 880 mcg twice daily (N = 32), were compared with placebo. Adverse events (whether considered drug-related or nondrug-related by the investigator) reported by more than 3 patients in either group treated with FLOVENT Inhalation Aerosol and that were more common with FLOVENT than placebo are shown below:

Ear, Nose, and Throat: Pharyngitis (9% and 25%), nasal congestion (19% and 22%), sinusitis (19% and 22%), nasal discharge (16% and 16%), dysphonia (19% and 9%), pain in nasal sinus(es) (13% and 0%), Candida-like oral lesions (16% and 9%), oropharyngeal candidiasis (25% and 19%).
Respiratory: Upper respiratory infection (31% and 19%), influenza (0% and 13%).
Other: Headache (28% and 34%), pain in joint (19% and 13%), nausea and vomiting (22% and 16%), muscular soreness (22% and 13%), malaise/fatigue (22% and 28%), insomnia (3% and 13%).

Observed During Clinical Practice: In addition to adverse events reported from clinical trials, the following events have been identified during postapproval use of fluticasone propionate. Because they are reported voluntarily from a population of unknown size, estimates of frequency cannot be made. These events have been chosen for inclusion due to either their seriousness, frequency of reporting, or causal connection to fluticasone propionate or a combination of these factors.

Ear, Nose, and Throat: Aphonia, facial and oropharyngeal edema, hoarseness, laryngitis, and throat soreness and irritation.

Table 1. Overall Adverse Events With >3% Incidence in US Controlled Clinical Trials With FLOVENT Inhalation Aerosol in Patients Previously Receiving Bronchodilators and/or Inhaled Corticosteroids

Adverse Event	Placebo (N = 475) %	FLOVENT 88 mcg Twice Daily (N = 488) %	FLOVENT 220 mcg Twice Daily (N = 95) %	FLOVENT 440 mcg Twice Daily (N = 185) %
Ear, nose, and throat				
Pharyngitis	7	10	14	14
Nasal congestion	8	8	16	10
Sinusitis	4	3	6	5
Nasal discharge	3	5	4	4
Dysphonia	1	4	3	8
Allergic rhinitis	4	5	3	3
Oral candidiasis	1	2	3	5
Respiratory				
Upper respiratory infection	12	15	22	16
Influenza	2	3	8	5
Neurological				
Headache	14	17	22	17
Average duration of exposure (days)	44	66	64	59

Table 2. Recommended Dosages of FLOVENT Inhalation Aerosol

Previous Therapy	Recommended Starting Dosage	Highest Recommended Dosage
Bronchodilators alone	88 mcg twice daily	440 mcg twice daily
Inhaled corticosteroids	88-220 mcg twice daily*	440 mcg twice daily
Oral corticosteroids†	880 mcg twice daily	880 mcg twice daily

*Starting dosages above 88 mcg twice daily may be considered for patients with poorer asthma control or those who have previously required doses of inhaled corticosteroids that are in the higher range for that specific agent.

NOTE: In all patients, it is desirable to titrate to the lowest effective dosage once asthma stability is achieved.

† **For Patients Currently Receiving Chronic Oral Corticosteroid Therapy:** Prednisone should be reduced no faster than 2.5 mg/day on a weekly basis, beginning after at least 1 week of therapy with FLOVENT Inhalation Aerosol. Patients should be carefully monitored for signs of asthma instability, including serial objective measures of airflow, and for signs of adrenal insufficiency (see WARNINGS). Once prednisone reduction is complete, the dosage of fluticasone propionate should be reduced to the lowest effective dosage.

Endocrine and Metabolic: Cushingoid features, growth velocity reduction in children/adolescents, hyperglycemia, osteoporosis, and weight gain.
Eye: Cataracts.
Non-Site Specific: Very rare anaphylactic reaction.
Psychiatry: Agitation, aggression, depression, and restlessness.
Respiratory: Asthma exacerbation, bronchospasm, chest tightness, cough, dyspnea, immediate bronchospasm, paradoxical bronchospasm, pneumonia, and wheeze.
Skin: Contusions, cutaneous hypersensitivity reactions, ecchymoses, and pruritus.
Eosinophilic Conditions: In rare cases, patients on inhaled fluticasone propionate may present with systemic eosinophilic conditions, with some patients presenting with clinical features of vasculitis consistent with Churg-Strauss syndrome, a condition that is often treated with systemic corticosteroid therapy. These events usually, but not always, have been associated with the reduction and/or withdrawal of oral corticosteroid therapy following the introduction of fluticasone propionate. Cases of serious eosinophilic conditions have also been reported with other inhaled corticosteroids in this clinical setting. Physicians should be alert to eosinophilia, vasculitic rash, worsening pulmonary symptoms, cardiac complications, and/or neuropathy presenting in their patients. A causal relationship between fluticasone propionate and these underlying conditions has not been established (see PRECAUTIONS: Eosinophilic Conditions).

OVERDOSAGE

Chronic overdosage may result in signs/symptoms of hypercorticism (see PRECAUTIONS). Inhalation by healthy volunteers of a single dose of 1,760 or 3,520 mcg of fluticasone propionate inhalation aerosol was well tolerated. Fluticasone propionate given by inhalation aerosol at doses of 1,320 mcg twice daily for 7 to 15 days to healthy human volunteers was also well tolerated. Repeat oral doses up to 80 mg daily for 10 days in healthy volunteers and repeat oral doses up to 20 mg daily for 42 days in patients were well tolerated. Adverse reactions were of mild or moderate severity, and incidences were similar in active and placebo treatment groups. The oral and subcutaneous median lethal doses in rats and mice were >1,000 mg/kg (>2,000 times the maximum human daily inhalation dose based on mg/m^2).

DOSAGE AND ADMINISTRATION

FLOVENT Inhalation Aerosol should be administered by the orally inhaled route in patients 12 years of age and older. Individual patients will experience a variable time to onset and degree of symptom relief. Generally, FLOVENT Inhalation Aerosol has a relatively rapid onset of action for an inhaled glucocorticoid. Improvement in asthma control following inhaled administration of fluticasone propionate can occur within 24 hours of beginning treatment, although maximum benefit may not be achieved for 1 to 2 weeks or longer after starting treatment.

After asthma stability has been achieved (see Table 2), it is always desirable to titrate to the lowest effective dosage to reduce the possibility of side effects. For patients who do not respond adequately to the starting dosage after 2 weeks of therapy, higher dosages may provide additional asthma control. The safety and efficacy of FLOVENT Inhalation Aerosol when administered in excess of recommended dosages have not been established.

The recommended starting dosage and the highest recommended dosage of FLOVENT Inhalation Aerosol, based on prior antiasthma therapy, are listed in Table 2.

[See table 2 above]

Geriatric Use: In studies where geriatric patients (65 years of age or older, see PRECAUTIONS) have been treated with FLOVENT Inhalation Aerosol, efficacy and safety did not differ from that in younger patients. Consequently, no dosage adjustment is recommended.

Directions for Use: Illustrated Patient's Instructions for Use accompany each package of FLOVENT Inhalation Aerosol.

HOW SUPPLIED

FLOVENT 44 mcg Inhalation Aerosol is supplied in 7.9-g canisters containing 60 metered inhalations in institutional pack boxes of 1 (NDC 0173-0497-00) and in 13-g canisters containing 120 metered inhalations in boxes of 1 (NDC 0173-0491-00). Each canister is supplied with a dark orange oral actuator with a peach strapcap and patient's instructions. Each actuation of the inhaler delivers 44 mcg of fluticasone propionate from the actuator.

FLOVENT 110 mcg Inhalation Aerosol is supplied in 7.9-g canisters containing 60 metered inhalations in institutional pack boxes of 1 (NDC 0173-0498-00) and in 13-g canisters containing 120 metered inhalations in boxes of 1 (NDC 0173-0494-00). Each canister is supplied with a dark orange oral actuator with a peach strapcap and patient's instructions. Each actuation of the inhaler delivers 110 mcg of fluticasone propionate from the actuator.

FLOVENT 220 mcg Inhalation Aerosol is supplied in 7.9-g canisters containing 60 metered inhalations in institutional pack boxes of 1 (NDC 0173-0499-00) and in 13-g canisters containing 120 metered inhalations in boxes of 1 (NDC 0173-0495-00). Each canister is supplied with a dark orange oral actuator with a peach strapcap and patient's instructions. Each actuation of the inhaler delivers 220 mcg of fluticasone propionate from the actuator.

FLOVENT canisters are for use with FLOVENT Inhalation Aerosol actuators only. The actuators should not be used with other aerosol medications.

The correct amount of medication in each inhalation cannot be assured after 60 inhalations from the 7.9-g canister or 120 inhalations from the 13-g canister even though the canister is not completely empty. The canister should be discarded when the labeled number of actuations has been used.

Store between 2° and 30°C (36° and 86°F). Store canister with mouthpiece down. Protect from freezing temperatures and direct sunlight.

Avoid spraying in eyes. Contents under pressure. Do not puncture or incinerate. Do not store at temperatures above 120°F. Keep out of reach of children. For best results, the canister should be at room temperature before use. Shake well before using.

GlaxoSmithKline, Research Triangle Park, NC 27709

March 2004/RL-2067

Shown in Product Identification Guide, page 315

FLOVENT® HFA 44 mcg ℞
[flō' vent]
(fluticasone propionate HFA 44 mcg)
Inhalation Aerosol

FLOVENT® HFA 110 mcg
(fluticasone propionate HFA 110 mcg)
Inhalation Aerosol

FLOVENT® HFA 220 mcg
(fluticasone propionate HFA 220 mcg)
Inhalation Aerosol

For Oral Inhalation Only

DESCRIPTION

The active component of FLOVENT HFA 44 mcg Inhalation Aerosol, FLOVENT HFA 110 mcg Inhalation Aerosol, and FLOVENT HFA 220 mcg Inhalation Aerosol is fluticasone propionate, a corticosteroid having the chemical name *S*-(fluoromethyl) 6α,9-difluoro-11β,17-dihydroxy-16α-methyl-3-oxoandrosta-1,4-diene-17β-carbothioate, 17-propionate and the following chemical structure:

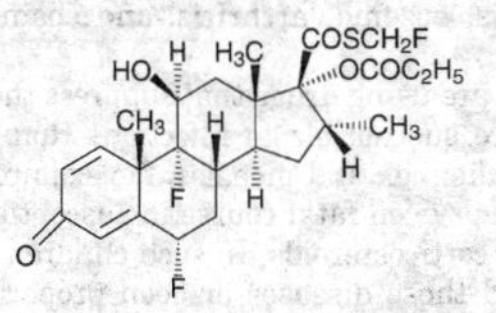

Fluticasone propionate is a white to off-white powder with a molecular weight of 500.6, and the empirical formula is $C_{25}H_{31}F_3O_5S$. It is practically insoluble in water, freely soluble in dimethyl sulfoxide and dimethylformamide, and slightly soluble in methanol and 95% ethanol.

FLOVENT HFA 44 mcg Inhalation Aerosol, FLOVENT HFA 110 mcg Inhalation Aerosol, and FLOVENT HFA 220 mcg Inhalation Aerosol are pressurized, metered-dose aerosol units intended for oral inhalation only. Each unit contains a microcrystalline suspension of fluticasone propionate (micronized) in propellant HFA-134a (1,1,1,2-tetrafluoroethane). It contains no other excipients.

After priming, each actuation of the inhaler delivers 50, 125, or 250 mcg of fluticasone propionate in 60 mg of suspension (for the 44-mcg product) or in 75 mg of suspension (for the 110- and 220-mcg products) from the valve and 44, 110, or 220 mcg, respectively, of fluticasone propionate from the actuator. The actual amount of drug delivered to the lung may depend on patient factors, such as the coordination between the actuation of the device and inspiration through the delivery system.

Each 10.6-g canister (44 mcg) and each 12-g canister (110 and 220 mcg) provides 120 inhalations.

FLOVENT HFA should be primed before using for the first time by releasing 4 test sprays into the air away from the face, shaking well before each spray. In cases where the inhaler has not been used for more than 7 days or when it has been dropped, prime the inhaler again by shaking well and releasing 1 test spray into the air away from the face.

This product does not contain any chlorofluorocarbon (CFC) as the propellant.

CLINICAL PHARMACOLOGY

Mechanism of Action: Fluticasone propionate is a synthetic trifluorinated corticosteroid with potent anti-inflammatory activity. In vitro assays using human lung cytosol preparations have established fluticasone propionate as a human corticosteroid receptor agonist with an affinity 18 times greater than dexamethasone, almost twice that of beclomethasone-17-monopropionate (BMP), the active metabolite of beclomethasone dipropionate, and over 3 times that of budesonide. Data from the McKenzie vasoconstrictor assay in man are consistent with these results. The clinical significance of these findings is unknown.

Inflammation is an important component in the pathogenesis of asthma. Corticosteroids have been shown to inhibit multiple cell types (e.g., mast cells, eosinophils, basophils, lymphocytes, macrophages, and neutrophils) and mediator production or secretion (e.g., histamine, eicosanoids, leukotrienes, and cytokines) involved in the asthmatic response. These anti-inflammatory actions of corticosteroids contribute to their efficacy in asthma.

Though effective for the treatment of asthma, corticosteroids do not affect asthma symptoms immediately. Individual patients will experience a variable time to onset and degree of symptom relief. Maximum benefit may not be achieved for 1 to 2 weeks or longer after starting treatment. When corticosteroids are discontinued, asthma stability may persist for several days or longer.

Studies in patients with asthma have shown a favorable ratio between topical anti-inflammatory activity and systemic corticosteroid effects with recommended doses of orally inhaled fluticasone propionate. This is explained by a combination of a relatively high local anti-inflammatory effect, negligible oral systemic bioavailability (<1%), and the minimal pharmacological activity of the only metabolite detected in man.

Preclinical: Propellant HFA-134a is devoid of pharmacological activity except at very high doses in animals (380 to 1,300 times the maximum human exposure based on comparisons of AUC values), primarily producing ataxia, tremors, dyspnea, or salivation. These are similar to effects produced by the structurally related CFCs, which have been used extensively in metered-dose inhalers.

In animals and humans, propellant HFA-134a was found to be rapidly absorbed and rapidly eliminated, with an elimination half-life of 3 to 27 minutes in animals and 5 to 7 minutes in humans. Time to maximum plasma concentration (T_{max}) and mean residence time are both extremely short, leading to a transient appearance of HFA-134a in the blood with no evidence of accumulation.

Pharmacokinetics: ***Absorption:*** Fluticasone propionate acts locally in the lung; therefore, plasma levels do not predict therapeutic effect. Studies using oral dosing of labeled and unlabeled drug have demonstrated that the oral systemic bioavailability of fluticasone propionate is negligible (<1%), primarily due to incomplete absorption and presystemic metabolism in the gut and liver. In contrast, the majority of the fluticasone propionate delivered to the lung is systemically absorbed. Systemic exposure as measured by AUC in healthy subjects (N = 24) from 8 inhalations, as a single dose, of HFA 134a-propelled fluticasone propionate using the 44-, 110-, and 220-mcg strengths increased proportionally with dose. The geometric means (95% CI) of $AUC_{0\text{-}24\ hr}$ for the 44-, 110-, and 220-mcg strengths were 488 (362 to 657); 1,284 (904 to 1,822); and 2,495 (1,945 to 3,200) pg•hr/mL, respectively, and the geometric means of C_{max} were 126 (108 to 148), 254 (202 to 319), and 421 (338 to 524) pg/mL, respectively. Systemic exposure from the 220-mcg HFA 134a-propelled fluticasone propionate inhaler was 30% lower than that from the CFC 11/12-propelled fluticasone propionate inhaler. Systemic exposure was measured in subjects with asthma from 2 inhalations of HFA 134a-propelled fluticasone propionate using the 44-mcg (N = 20), 110-mcg (N = 15), or 220-mcg (N = 17) strength inhalers twice daily for at least 4 weeks. The geometric means (95% CI) of $AUC_{0\text{-}12\ hr}$ for the 44-, 110-, and 220-mcg strengths were 76 (33 to 175), 298 (191 to 464), and 601 (431 to 838) pg•hr/mL, respectively. C_{max} occurred in about 1 hour, and the geometric means were 25 (18 to 36), 61 (46 to 81), and 103 (73 to 145) pg/mL, respectively.

Distribution: Following intravenous administration, the initial disposition phase for fluticasone propionate was rapid and consistent with its high lipid solubility and tissue binding. The volume of distribution averaged 4.2 L/kg.

The percentage of fluticasone propionate bound to human plasma proteins averages 91%. Fluticasone propionate is weakly and reversibly bound to erythrocytes and is not significantly bound to human transcortin.

Metabolism: The total clearance of fluticasone propionate is high (average, 1,093 mL/min), with renal clearance accounting for less than 0.02% of the total. The only circulating metabolite detected in man is the 17β-carboxylic acid derivative of fluticasone propionate, which is formed through the cytochrome P450 3A4 pathway. This metabolite had less affinity (approximately 1/2,000) than the parent drug for the corticosteroid receptor of human lung cytosol in vitro and negligible pharmacological activity in animal studies. Other metabolites detected in vitro using cultured human hepatoma cells have not been detected in man.

Elimination: Following intravenous dosing, fluticasone propionate showed polyexponential kinetics and had a terminal elimination half-life of approximately 7.8 hours. Less than 5% of a radiolabeled oral dose was excreted in the urine as metabolites, with the remainder excreted in the feces as parent drug and metabolites.

Special Populations: Hepatic Impairment: Since fluticasone propionate is predominantly cleared by hepatic metabolism, impairment of liver function may lead to accumulation of fluticasone propionate in plasma. Therefore, patients with hepatic disease should be closely monitored.

Gender: Systemic exposure for 19 male and 33 female subjects with asthma from 2 inhalations of fluticasone propionate inhalation aerosol using the 44-, 110-, and 220-mcg strengths twice daily was similar.

Other: Formal pharmacokinetic studies using fluticasone propionate have not been conducted in other special populations.

Drug Interactions: Fluticasone propionate is a substrate of cytochrome P450 3A4. Coadministration of fluticasone propionate and the highly potent cytochrome P450 3A4 inhibitor ritonavir is not recommended based upon a multiple-dose, crossover drug interaction study in 18 healthy subjects. Fluticasone propionate aqueous nasal spray (200 mcg once daily) was coadministered for 7 days with ritonavir (100 mg twice daily). Plasma fluticasone propionate concentrations following fluticasone propionate aqueous nasal spray alone were undetectable (<10 pg/mL) in most subjects, and when concentrations were detectable peak levels (C_{max} averaged 11.9 pg/mL [range, 10.8 to 14.1 pg/mL] and $AUC_{(0\text{-}\tau)}$ averaged 8.43 pg•hr/mL [range, 4.2 to 18.8 pg•hr/mL]). Fluticasone propionate C_{max} and $AUC_{(0\text{-}\tau)}$ increased to 318 pg/mL (range, 110 to 648 pg/mL) and 3,102.6 pg•hr/mL (range, 1,207.1 to 5,662.0 pg•hr/mL), respectively, after coadministration of ritonavir with fluticasone propionate aqueous nasal spray. This significant increase in plasma fluticasone propionate exposure resulted in a significant decrease (86%) in plasma cortisol area under the plasma concentration versus time curve (AUC).

Caution should be exercised when other potent cytochrome P450 3A4 inhibitors are coadministered with fluticasone propionate. In a drug interaction study, coadministration of orally inhaled fluticasone propionate (1,000 mcg) and ketoconazole (200 mg once daily) resulted in increased plasma fluticasone propionate exposure and reduced plasma cortisol AUC, but had no effect on urinary excretion of cortisol. In another multiple-dose drug interaction study, coadministration of orally inhaled fluticasone propionate (500 mcg twice daily) and erythromycin (333 mg 3 times daily) did not affect fluticasone propionate pharmacokinetics.

Similar definitive studies with HFA 134a-propelled fluticasone propionate were not performed, but results should be independent of the formulation and drug delivery device.

Pharmacodynamics: Serum cortisol concentrations, urine cortisol excretion, and urine 6-β-hydroxycortisol excretion were collected over 24 hours in 24 healthy subjects following 8 inhalations of HFA 134a-propelled fluticasone propionate (44, 110, and 220 mcg) decreased with increasing dose. However, in subjects with asthma treated with 2 inhalations of HFA 134a-propelled fluticasone propionate (44, 110, and 220 mcg) twice daily for at least 4 weeks, differences in serum cortisol concentrations (N = 65) and urine cortisol excretion (N = 47) compared with placebo were not related to dose and generally not significant. In the study with healthy volunteers, the effect of propellant was also evaluated by comparing results following the 220-mcg strength inhaler containing HFA 134a propellant with the same strength of inhaler containing CFC 11/12 propellant. A lesser effect on the HPA axis with the HFA formulation was observed for serum cortisol, but not urine cortisol and 6-betahydroxy cortisol excretion.

The potential systemic effects of HFA 134a-propelled fluticasone propionate on the hypothalamic-pituitary-adrenal (HPA) axis were also studied in patients with asthma. Fluticasone propionate given by inhalation aerosol at dosages of 440 or 880 mcg twice daily was compared with placebo in oral corticosteroid-dependent subjects with asthma (range of mean dose of prednisone at baseline, 13 to 14 mg/day) in a 16-week study. Consistent with maintenance treatment with oral corticosteroids, abnormal plasma cortisol responses to short cosyntropin stimulation (peak plasma cortisol <18 mcg/dL) were present at baseline in the majority of subjects participating in this study (69% of patients later randomized to placebo and 72% to 78% of patients later randomized to HFA 134a-propelled fluticasone propionate). At week 16, 8 subjects (73%) on placebo compared to 14 (54%) and 13 (68%) subjects receiving HFA 134a-propelled fluticasone propionate (440 and 880 mcg b.i.d., respectively) had post-stimulation cortisol levels of <18 mcg/dL.

To confirm that systemic absorption does not play a role in the clinical response to inhaled fluticasone propionate, a double-blind clinical study comparing inhaled fluticasone propionate powder and oral fluticasone propionate was conducted. Fluticasone propionate inhalation powder in doses of 100 and 500 mcg twice daily was compared to oral fluticasone propionate 20,000 mcg once daily and placebo for 6 weeks. Plasma levels of fluticasone propionate were detectable in all 3 active groups, but the mean values were highest in the oral group. Both dosages of inhaled fluticasone propionate were effective in maintaining asthma stability and improving lung function, while oral fluticasone propionate and placebo were ineffective. This demonstrates that the clinical effectiveness of inhaled fluticasone propionate is due to its direct local effect and not to an indirect effect through systemic absorption.

CLINICAL TRIALS

Three randomized, double-blind, parallel-group, placebo-controlled clinical trials were conducted in the US in 980 adolescent and adult patients (≥12 years of age) with asthma to assess the efficacy and safety of FLOVENT HFA in the treatment of asthma. Fixed dosages of 88, 220, and 440 mcg twice daily (each dose administered as 2 inhalations of the 44-, 110-, and 220-mcg strengths, respectively) and 880 mcg twice daily (administered as 4 inhalations of the 220-mcg strength) were compared with placebo to provide information about appropriate dosing to cover a range of asthma severity. Patients in these studies included those inadequately controlled with bronchodilators alone (Study 1), those already receiving inhaled corticosteroids (Study 2), and those requiring oral corticosteroid therapy (Study 3). In all 3 studies, patients (including placebo-treated patients) were allowed to use VENTOLIN® (albuterol, USP) Inhalation Aerosol as needed for relief of acute asthma symptoms. In Studies 1 and 2, other maintenance asthma therapies were discontinued.

Study 1 enrolled 397 patients with asthma inadequately controlled on bronchodilators alone. FLOVENT HFA was evaluated at dosages of 88, 220, and 440 mcg twice daily for 12 weeks. Baseline FEV_1 values were similar across groups (mean 67% of predicted normal). All 3 dosages of FLOVENT HFA significantly improved asthma control as measured by improvement in AM pre-dose FEV_1 compared with placebo. Pulmonary function (AM pre-dose FEV_1) improved significantly with FLOVENT HFA compared with placebo after the first week of treatment, and this improvement was maintained over the 12-week treatment period.

At Endpoint (last observation), mean change from baseline in AM pre-dose percent predicted FEV_1 was greater in all 3 groups treated with FLOVENT HFA (9.0% to 11.2%) compared with the placebo group (3.4%). The mean differences between the groups treated with FLOVENT HFA 88, 220, and 440 mcg and the placebo group were significant, and the corresponding 95% confidence intervals were (2.2%, 9.2%), (2.8%, 9.9%), and (4.3%, 11.3%), respectively.

Continued on next page

Product information on these pages is effective as of August 2004. Further information is available at: GlaxoSmithKline, PO Box 13398, Research Triangle Park, NC 27709. 1-888-825-5249. Corporate Web Site: www.gsk.com

Flovent HFA—Cont.

Figure 1 displays results of pulmonary function tests (mean percent change from baseline in FEV_1 prior to AM dose) for the recommended starting dosage of FLOVENT HFA (88 mcg twice daily) and placebo from Study 1. This trial used predetermined criteria for lack of efficacy (indicators of worsening asthma), resulting in withdrawal of more patients in the placebo group. Therefore, pulmonary function results at Endpoint (the last evaluable FEV_1 result, including most patients' lung function data) are also displayed.

Figure 1. A 12-Week Clinical Trial in Patients Inadequately Controlled on Bronchodilators Alone: Mean Percent Change From Baseline in FEV_1 Prior to AM Dose (Study 1)

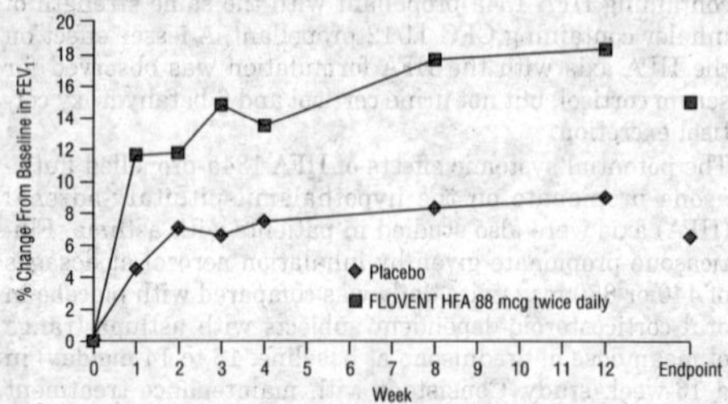

In Study 2, FLOVENT HFA at dosages of 88, 220, and 440 mcg twice daily was evaluated over 12 weeks of treatment in 415 patients with asthma who were already receiving an inhaled corticosteroid at a daily dose within its recommended dose range in addition to as-needed albuterol. Baseline FEV_1 values were similar across groups (mean 65% to 66% of predicted normal). All 3 dosages of FLOVENT HFA significantly improved asthma control (as measured by improvement in FEV1), compared with placebo. Discontinuations from the study for lack of efficacy (defined by a prespecified decrease in FEV_1 or PEF, or an increase in use of VENTOLIN or nighttime awakenings requiring treatment with VENTOLIN) were lower in the groups treated with FLOVENT HFA (6% to 11%) compared to placebo (50%). Pulmonary function (AM pre-dose FEV_1) improved significantly with FLOVENT HFA compared with placebo after the first week of treatment, and the improvement was maintained over the 12-week treatment period.

At Endpoint (last observation), mean change from baseline in AM pre-dose percent predicted FEV_1 was greater in all 3 groups treated with FLOVENT HFA (2.2% to 4.6%) compared with the placebo group (−8.3%). The mean differences between the groups treated with FLOVENT HFA 88, 220, and 440 mcg and the placebo group were significant, and the corresponding 95% confidence intervals were (7.1%, 13.8%), (8.2%, 14.9%), and (9.6%, 16.4%), respectively.

Figure 2 displays the mean percent change from baseline in FEV1 from Week 1 through Week 12. This study used predetermined criteria for lack of efficacy, resulting in withdrawal of more patients in the placebo group; therefore, pulmonary function results at Endpoint are displayed.

Figure 2. A 12-Week Clinical Trial With Patients Already Receiving Daily Inhaled Corticosteroids: Mean Percent Change From Baseline in FEV_1 Prior to AM Dose (Study 2)

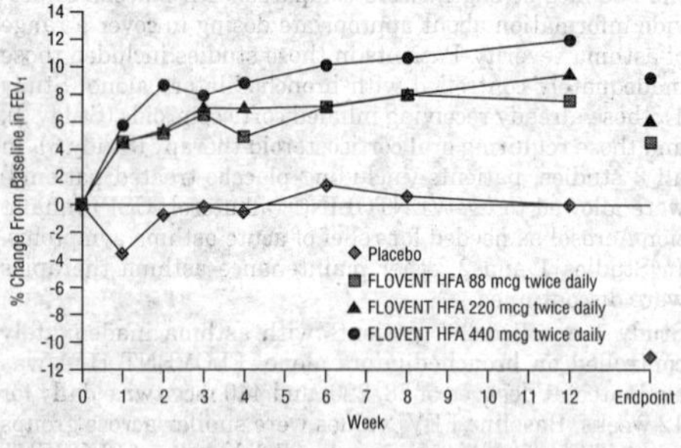

In both studies, use of VENTOLIN, AM and PM PEF, and asthma symptom scores showed numerical improvement with FLOVENT HFA compared to placebo.

Study 3 enrolled 168 patients with asthma requiring oral prednisone therapy (average baseline daily prednisone dose ranged from 13 to 14 mg). FLOVENT HFA at dosages of 440 and 880 mcg twice daily was evaluated over a 16-week treatment period. Baseline FEV_1 values were similar across groups (mean 59% to 62% of predicted normal). Over the course of the study, patients treated with either dosage of FLOVENT HFA required a significantly lower mean daily oral prednisone dose (6 mg) compared with placebo-treated patients (15 mg). Both dosages of FLOVENT HFA enabled a larger percentage of patients (59% and 56% in the groups treated with FLOVENT HFA 440 and 880 mcg, respectively, twice daily) to eliminate oral prednisone as compared with placebo (13%) (see Figure 3). There was no efficacy advantage of FLOVENT HFA 880 mcg twice daily compared to 440 mcg twice daily. Accompanying the reduction in oral corticosteroid use, patients treated with either dosage of FLOVENT HFA had significantly improved lung function, fewer asthma symptoms, and less use of VENTOLIN Inhalation Aerosol compared with the placebo-treatedpatients.

Figure 3. A 16-Week Clinical Trial in Patients Requiring Chronic Oral Prednisone Therapy: Change in Maintenance Prednisone Dose

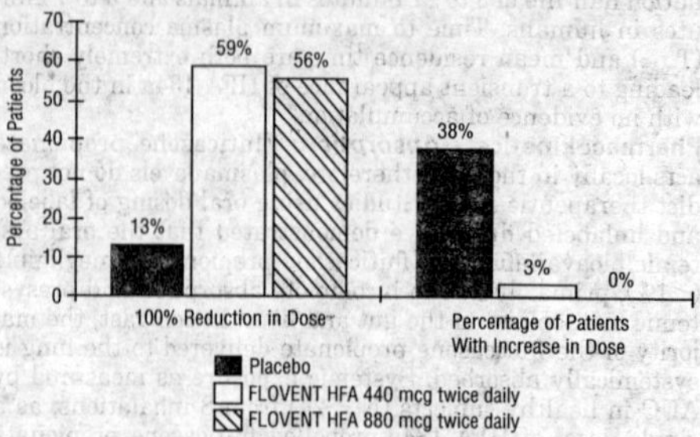

Two long-term safety studies (Study 4 and Study 5) of ≥6 months duration were conducted in 507 adolescent and adult patients with asthma. Study 4 was designed to monitor the safety of 2 doses of FLOVENT HFA, while Study 5 compared HFA 134a-propelled and CFC 11/12-propelled fluticasone propionate. Study 4 enrolled 182 patients who were treated daily with low to high doses of inhaled corticosteroids, beta-agonists (short-acting [as needed or regularly scheduled] or long-acting), theophylline, inhaled cromolyn or nedocromil sodium, leukotriene receptor antagonists, or 5-lipoxygenase inhibitors at baseline. FLOVENT HFA at dosages of 220 and 440 mcg twice daily was evaluated over a 26-week treatment period in 89 and 93 patients, respectively. Study 5 enrolled 325 patients who were treated daily with moderate to high doses of inhaled corticosteroids, with or without concurrent use of salmeterol or albuterol, at baseline. HFA 134a-propelled fluticasone propionate at a dosage of 440 mcg twice daily and CFC 11/12-propelled fluticasone propionate at a dosage of 440 mcg twice daily were evaluated over a 52-week treatment period in 163 and 162 patients, respectively. Baseline FEV_1 values were similar across groups (mean 81% to 84% of predicted normal). Throughout the 52-week treatment period, asthma control was maintained with both formulations of fluticasone propionate compared to baseline. In both studies, none of the patients were withdrawn due to lack of efficacy.

INDICATIONS AND USAGE

FLOVENT HFA Inhalation Aerosol is indicated for the maintenance treatment of asthma as prophylactic therapy in adolescent and adult patients 12 years of age and older. It is also indicated for patients requiring oral corticosteroid therapy for asthma. Many of these patients may be able to reduce or eliminate their requirement for oral corticosteroids over time.

FLOVENT HFA Inhalation Aerosol is NOT indicated for the relief of acute bronchospasm.

CONTRAINDICATIONS

FLOVENT HFA Inhalation Aerosol is contraindicated in the primary treatment of status asthmaticus or other acute episodes of asthma where intensive measures are required.

Hypersensitivity to any of the ingredients (see DESCRIPTION) of these preparations contraindicates their use.

WARNINGS

Particular care is needed for patients who are transferred from systemically active corticosteroids to FLOVENT HFA because deaths due to adrenal insufficiency have occurred in patients with asthma during and after transfer from systemic corticosteroids to less systemically available inhaled corticosteroids. After withdrawal from systemic corticosteroids, a number of months are required for recovery of HPA function.

Patients who have been previously maintained on 20 mg or more per day of prednisone (or its equivalent) may be most susceptible, particularly when their systemic corticosteroids have been almost completely withdrawn. During this period of HPA suppression, patients may exhibit signs and symptoms of adrenal insufficiency when exposed to trauma, surgery, or infection (particularly gastroenteritis) or other conditions associated with severe electrolyte loss. Although FLOVENT HFA may provide control of asthma symptoms during these episodes, in recommended doses it supplies less than normal physiological amounts of glucocorticoid systemically and does NOT provide the mineralocorticoid activity that is necessary for coping with these emergencies.

During periods of stress or a severe asthma attack, patients who have been withdrawn from systemic corticosteroids should be instructed to resume oral corticosteroids (in large doses) immediately and to contact their physicians for further instruction. These patients should also be instructed to carry a warning card indicating that they may need supplementary systemic corticosteroids during periods of stress or a severe asthma attack.

A drug interaction study in healthy subjects has shown that ritonavir (a highly potent cytochrome P450 3A4 inhibitor) can significantly increase plasma fluticasone propionate exposure, resulting in significantly reduced serum cortisol concentrations (see CLINICAL PHARMACOLOGY: Pharmacokinetics: *Drug Interactions* and PRECAUTIONS: Drug Interactions: *Inhibitors of Cytochrome P450*). During postmarketing use, there have been reports of clinically significant drug interactions in patients receiving fluticasone propionate and ritonavir, resulting in systemic corticosteroid effects including Cushing syndrome and adrenal suppression. Therefore, coadministration of fluticasone propionate and ritonavir is not recommended unless the potential benefit to the patient outweighs the risk of systemic corticosteroid side effects.

Patients requiring oral corticosteroids should be weaned slowly from systemic corticosteroid use after transferring to FLOVENT HFA. In a clinical trial of 168 patients, prednisone reduction was successfully accomplished by reducing the daily prednisone dose on a weekly basis following initiation of treatment with FLOVENT HFA. Successive reduction of prednisone dose was allowed only when lung function; symptoms; and as-needed, short-acting beta-agonist use were better than or comparable to that seen before initiation of prednisone dose reduction. Lung function (FEV_1 or AM PEF), beta-agonist use, and asthma symptoms should be carefully monitored during withdrawal of oral corticosteroids. In addition to monitoring asthma signs and symptoms, patients should be observed for signs and symptoms of adrenal insufficiency such as fatigue, lassitude, weakness, nausea and vomiting, and hypotension.

Transfer of patients from systemic corticosteroid therapy to FLOVENT HFA may unmask conditions previously suppressed by the systemic corticosteroid therapy, e.g., rhinitis, conjunctivitis, eczema, arthritis, and eosinophilic conditions.

Persons who are using drugs that suppress the immune system are more susceptible to infections than healthy individuals. Chickenpox and measles, for example, can have a more serious or even fatal course in susceptible children or adults using corticosteroids. In such children or adults who have not had these diseases or been properly immunized, particular care should be taken to avoid exposure. How the dose, route, and duration of corticosteroid administration affect the risk of developing a disseminated infection is not known. The contribution of the underlying disease and/or prior corticosteroid treatment to the risk is also not known. If exposed to chickenpox, prophylaxis with varicella zoster immune globulin (VZIG) may be indicated. If exposed to measles, prophylaxis with pooled intramuscular immunoglobulin (IG) may be indicated. (See the respective package inserts for complete VZIG and IG prescribing information.) If chickenpox develops, treatment with antiviral agents may be considered.

FLOVENT HFA is not to be regarded as a bronchodilator and is not indicated for rapid relief of bronchospasm.

As with other inhaled medications, bronchospasm may occur with an immediate increase in wheezing after dosing. If bronchospasm occurs following dosing with FLOVENT HFA, it should be treated immediately with a fast-acting inhaled bronchodilator. Treatment with FLOVENT HFA should be discontinued and alternative therapy instituted.

Patients should be instructed to contact their physicians immediately when episodes of asthma that are not responsive to bronchodilators occur during the course of treatment with FLOVENT HFA. During such episodes, patients may require therapy with oral corticosteroids.

PRECAUTIONS

General: Orally inhaled corticosteroids may cause a reduction in growth velocity when administered to pediatric patients (see PRECAUTIONS: Pediatric Use).

During withdrawal from systemically active corticosteroids, some patients may experience symptoms of corticosteroid withdrawal, e.g., joint and/or muscular pain, lassitude, and depression, despite maintenance or even improvement of respiratory function.

Fluticasone propionate will often permit control of asthma symptoms with less suppression of HPA function than therapeutically equivalent oral doses of prednisone. Since fluticasone propionate is absorbed into the circulation and can be systemically active at higher doses, the beneficial effects of FLOVENT HFA in minimizing HPA dysfunction may be expected only when recommended dosages are not exceeded and individual patients are titrated to the lowest effective dose. A relationship between plasma levels of fluticasone propionate and inhibitory effects on stimulated cortisol production has been shown after 4 weeks of treatment with fluticasone propionate. Since individual sensitivity to effects on cortisol production exists, physicians should consider this information when prescribing FLOVENT HFA.

Because of the possibility of systemic absorption of inhaled corticosteroids, patients treated with FLOVENT HFA should be observed carefully for any evidence of systemic corticosteroid effects. Particular care should be taken in observing patients postoperatively or during periods of stress for evidence of inadequate adrenal response.

It is possible that systemic corticosteroid effects such as hypercorticism and adrenal suppression (including adrenal crisis) may appear in a small number of patients, particularly when FLOVENT HFA is administered at higher than recommended doses over prolonged periods of time. If such effects occur, the dosage of FLOVENT HFA should be reduced slowly, consistent with accepted procedures for reducing systemic corticosteroids and for management of asthma.

The long-term effects of fluticasone propionate in human subjects are not fully known. In particular, the effects resulting from chronic use of fluticasone propionate on developmental or immunologic processes in the mouth, pharynx, trachea, and lung are unknown. Some patients have received inhaled fluticasone propionate on a continuous basis for periods of 3 years or longer. In clinical studies with patients treated for 2 years with inhaled fluticasone propionate, no apparent differences in the type or severity of adverse reactions were observed after long- versus short-term treatment.

Rare instances of glaucoma, increased intraocular pressure, and cataracts have been reported in patients following the long-term administration of inhaled corticosteroids, including fluticasone propionate.

In clinical studies with inhaled fluticasone propionate, the development of localized infections of the pharynx with *Candida albicans* has occurred. When such an infection develops, it should be treated with appropriate local or systemic (i.e., oral antifungal) therapy while remaining on treatment with FLOVENT HFA, but at times therapy with FLOVENT HFA may need to be interrupted.

Inhaled corticosteroids should be used with caution, if at all, in patients with active or quiescent tuberculosis infection of the respiratory tract; untreated systemic fungal, bacterial, viral or parasitic infections; or ocular herpes simplex.

Eosinophilic Conditions: In rare cases, patients on inhaled fluticasone propionate may present with systemic eosinophilic conditions, with some patients presenting with clinical features of vasculitis consistent with Churg-Strauss syndrome, a condition that is often treated with systemic corticosteroid therapy. These events usually, but not always, have been associated with the reduction and/or withdrawal of oral corticosteroid therapy following the introduction of fluticasone propionate. Cases of serious eosinophilic conditions have also been reported with other inhaled corticosteroids in this clinical setting. Physicians should be alert to eosinophilia, vasculitic rash, worsening pulmonary symptoms, cardiac complications, and/or neuropathy presenting in their patients. A causal relationship between fluticasone propionate and these underlying conditions has not been established (see ADVERSE REACTIONS: Observed During Clinical Practice: *Eosinophilic Conditions*).

Information for Patients: Patients being treated with FLOVENT HFA should receive the following information and instructions. This information is intended to aid them in the safe and effective use of this medication. It is not a disclosure of all possible adverse or intended effects.

It is important that patients understand how to use FLOVENT HFA in relation to other asthma medications they are taking. Patients should be given the following information:

1. Patients should use FLOVENT HFA at regular intervals as directed. Individual patients will experience a variable time to onset and degree of symptom relief and the full benefit may not be achieved until treatment has been administered for 1 to 2 weeks or longer. The patient should not increase the prescribed dosage but should contact the physician if symptoms do not improve or if the condition worsens.
2. Patients who are pregnant or nursing should contact their physicians about the use of FLOVENT HFA.
3. Patients should be warned to avoid exposure to chickenpox or measles and if they are exposed, to consult their physicians without delay.
4. Prime the inhaler before using for the first time by releasing 4 test sprays into the air away from the face, shaking well before each spray. In cases where the inhaler has not been used for more than 7 days or when it has been dropped, prime the inhaler again by shaking well and releasing 1 test spray into the air away from the face.
5. After inhalation, rinse the mouth with water and spit out. Do not swallow.
6. Clean the inhaler at least once a week after the evening dose. Keeping the canister and plastic actuator clean is important to prevent medicine build-up. (See Patient's Instructions for Use leaflet accompanying the product.)
7. Use FLOVENT HFA only with the actuator supplied with the product. Discard the inhaler after the labeled number of inhalations have been used.
8. For the proper use of FLOVENT HFA and to attain maximum improvement, the patient should read and carefully follow the Patient's Instructions for Use leaflet accompanying the product.

Drug Interactions: ***Inhibitors of Cytochrome P450:*** Fluticasone propionate is a substrate of cytochrome P450 3A4. A drug interaction study with fluticasone propionate aqueous nasal spray in healthy subjects has shown that ritonavir (a highly potent cytochrome P450 3A4 inhibitor) can significantly increase plasma fluticasone propionate exposure, resulting in significantly reduced serum cortisol concentrations (see CLINICAL PHARMACOLOGY: Pharmacokinetics: *Drug Interactions*). During postmarketing use, there have been reports of clinically significant drug interactions in patients receiving fluticasone propionate and ritonavir, resulting in systemic corticosteroid effects including Cushing syndrome and adrenal suppression. Therefore, coadministration of fluticasone propionate and ritonavir is not recommended unless the potential benefit to the patient outweighs the risk of systemic corticosteroid side effects.

In a placebo-controlled crossover study in 8 healthy volunteers, coadministration of a single dose of orally inhaled fluticasone propionate (1,000 mcg) with multiple doses of ketoconazole (200 mg) to steady state resulted in increased plasma fluticasone propionate exposure, a reduction in plasma cortisol AUC, and no effect on urinary excretion of cortisol. Caution should be exercised when FLOVENT HFA is coadministered with ketoconazole and other known potent cytochrome P450 3A4 inhibitors.

Carcinogenesis, Mutagenesis, Impairment of Fertility: Fluticasone propionate demonstrated no tumorigenic potential in mice at oral doses up to 1,000 mcg/kg (approximately 2 times the maximum recommended daily inhalation dose on a mcg/m^2 basis) for 78 weeks or in rats at inhalation doses up to 57 mcg/kg (less than the maximum recommended daily inhalation dose on a mcg/m^2 basis) for 104 weeks.

Table 1. Overall Adverse Events With >3% Incidence in US Controlled Clinical Trials With FLOVENT HFA in Patients With Asthma Previously Receiving Bronchodilators and/or Inhaled Corticosteroids

Adverse Event	FLOVENT HFA 44 mcg (N = 203) %	FLOVENT HFA 110 mcg (N = 204) %	FLOVENT HFA 220 mcg (N = 202) %	Placebo (N = 203) %
Ear, nose, and throat				
Upper respiratory tract infection	18	16	16	14
Throat irritation	8	8	10	5
Upper respiratory inflammation	2	5	5	1
Sinusitis/sinus infection	6	7	4	3
Hoarseness/dysphonia	2	3	6	<1
Gastrointestinal				
Candidiasis mouth/throat & non-site specific	4	2	5	<1
Lower respiratory				
Cough	4	6	4	5
Bronchitis	2	2	6	5
Neurological				
Headache	11	7	5	6
Average duration of exposure (days)	73	74	76	60

Fluticasone propionate did not induce gene mutation in prokaryotic or eukaryotic cells in vitro. No significant clastogenic effect was seen in cultured human peripheral lymphocytes in vitro or in the mouse micronucleus test.

No evidence of impairment of fertility was observed in reproductive studies conducted in male and female rats at subcutaneous doses up to 50 mcg/kg (less than the maximum recommended daily inhalation dose in adults on a mcg/m^2 basis). Prostate weight was significantly reduced in rats at a subcutaneous dose of 50 mcg/kg.

Pregnancy: ***Teratogenic Effects:*** Pregnancy Category C. Subcutaneous studies in the mouse and rat at 45 and 100 mcg/kg, respectively (less than the maximum recommended daily inhalation dose in adults on a mcg/m^2 basis), revealed fetal toxicity characteristic of potent corticosteroid compounds, including embryonic growth retardation, omphalocele, cleft palate, and retarded cranial ossification. No teratogenicity was seen in the rat at inhalation doses up to 68.7 mcg/kg (less than the maximum recommended daily inhalation dose in adults on a mcg/m^2 basis).

In the rabbit, fetal weight reduction and cleft palate were observed at a subcutaneous dose of 4 mcg/kg (less than the maximum recommended daily inhalation dose in adults on a mcg/m^2 basis). However, no teratogenic effects were reported at oral doses up to 300 mcg/kg (approximately 3 times the maximum recommended daily inhalation dose in adults on a mcg/m^2 basis) of fluticasone propionate. No fluticasone propionate was detected in the plasma in this study, consistent with the established low bioavailability following oral administration (see CLINICAL PHARMACOLOGY: Pharmacokinetics: *Absorption*).

Fluticasone propionate crossed the placenta following administration of a subcutaneous dose of 100 mcg/kg to mice (less than the maximum recommended daily inhalation dose in adults on a mcg/m^2 basis), a subcutaneous or an oral dose of 100 mcg/kg to rats (less than the maximum recommended daily inhalation dose in adults on a mcg/m^2 basis), and an oral dose of 300 mcg/kg to rabbits (approximately 3 times the maximum recommended daily inhalation dose in adults on a mcg/m^2 basis).

There are no adequate and well-controlled studies in pregnant women. FLOVENT HFA should be used during pregnancy only if the potential benefit justifies the potential risk to the fetus.

Experience with oral corticosteroids since their introduction in pharmacologic, as opposed to physiologic, doses suggests that rodents are more prone to teratogenic effects from corticosteroids than humans. In addition, because there is a natural increase in corticosteroid production during pregnancy, most women will require a lower exogenous corticosteroid dose and many will not need corticosteroid treatment during pregnancy.

Nursing Mothers: It is not known whether fluticasone propionate is excreted in human breast milk. However, other corticosteroids have been detected in human milk. Subcutaneous administration to lactating rats of 10 mcg/kg of tritiated fluticasone propionate (less than the maximum recommended daily inhalation dose in adults on a mcg/m^2 basis) resulted in measurable radioactivity in milk.

Since there are no data from controlled trials on the use of FLOVENT HFA by nursing mothers, a decision should be made whether to discontinue nursing or to discontinue FLOVENT HFA, taking into account the importance of FLOVENT HFA to the mother.

Caution should be exercised when FLOVENT HFA is administered to a nursing woman.

Pediatric Use: Orally inhaled corticosteroids may cause a reduction in growth velocity when administered to pediatric patients. A reduction of growth velocity in children or teenagers may occur as a result of poorly controlled asthma or from use of corticosteroids including inhaled corticosteroids. The effects of long-term treatment of children and adolescents with inhaled corticosteroids, including fluticasone propionate, on final adult height are not known.

Controlled clinical studies have shown that inhaled corticosteroids may cause a reduction in growth in pediatric patients. In these studies, the mean reduction in growth velocity was approximately 1 cm/year (range, 0.3 to 1.8 cm/year) and appears to depend upon dose and duration of exposure. This effect was observed in the absence of laboratory evidence of hypothalamic-pituitary-adrenal (HPA) axis suppression, suggesting that growth velocity is a more sensitive indicator of systemic corticosteroid exposure in pediatric patients than some commonly used tests of HPA axis function. The long-term effects of this reduction in growth velocity associated with orally inhaled corticosteroids, including the impact on final adult height, are unknown. The potential for "catch-up" growth following discontinuation of treatment with orally inhaled corticosteroids has not been adequately studied. The effects on growth velocity of treatment with orally inhaled corticosteroids for over 1 year, including the impact on final adult height, are unknown. The growth of children and adolescents receiving orally inhaled corticosteroids, including FLOVENT HFA, should be monitored routinely (e.g., via stadiometry). The potential growth effects of prolonged treatment should be weighed against the clinical benefits obtained and the risks associated with alternative therapies. To minimize the systemic effects of orally inhaled corticosteroids, including FLOVENT HFA, each patient should be titrated to the lowest dose that effectively controls his/her symptoms.

Since a cross study comparison in adolescent and adult patients (≥12 years of age) indicated that systemic exposure of inhaled fluticasone propionate from FLOVENT HFA would be higher than exposure from FLOVENT® ROTADISK®, results from a study to assess the potential growth effects of FLOVENT® ROTADISK® in pediatric patients (4–11 years of age) are provided.

A 52-week, placebo-controlled study to assess the potential growth effects of fluticasone propionate inhalation powder (FLOVENT® ROTADISK®) at 50 and 100 mcg twice daily was conducted in the US in 325 prepubescent children (244 males and 81 females) aged 4 to 11 years. The mean growth velocities at 52 weeks observed in the intent-to-treat population were 6.32 cm/year in the placebo group (N = 76), 6.07 cm/year in the 50-mcg group (N = 98), and 5.66 cm/year in the 100-mcg group (N = 89). An imbalance in the proportion of children entering puberty between groups and a higher dropout rate in the placebo group due to poorly controlled asthma may be confounding factors in interpreting these data. A separate subset analysis of children who remained prepubertal during the study revealed growth rates at 52 weeks of 6.10 cm/year in the placebo group (n = 57), 5.91 cm/year in the 50-mcg group (n = 74), and 5.67 cm/year in the 100-mcg group (n = 79). In children 8.5 years of age, the mean age of children in this study, the range for expected growth velocity is: boys – 3rd percentile = 3.8 cm/year, 50th percentile = 5.4 cm/year, and 97th percentile = 7.0 cm/year; girls – ± 3rd percentile = 4.2 cm/year, 50th percentile = 5.7 cm/year, and 97th percentile = 7.3 cm/year.

The clinical significance of these growth data is not certain. Physicians should closely follow the growth of children and adolescents taking corticosteroids by any route, and weigh the benefits of corticosteroid therapy against the possibility of growth suppression if growth appears slowed. Patients should be maintained on the lowest dose of inhaled corticosteroid that effectively controls their asthma.

The safety and effectiveness of FLOVENT HFA in children below 12 years of age have not been established.

Continued on next page

Product information on these pages is effective as of August 2004. Further information is available at: GlaxoSmithKline, PO Box 13398, Research Triangle Park, NC 27709. 1-888-825-5249. Corporate Web Site: www.gsk.com

Flovent HFA—Cont.

A total of 73 patients between the ages of 12 to 17 years of age were studied in the US pivotal clinical trials. Improved asthma control (as measured by an improvement in FEV_1) was greater for patients treated with FLOVENT HFA compared to those treated with placebo.

Geriatric Use: Of the total number of patients treated with FLOVENT HFA in US and non-US clinical trials, 173 were 65 years of age or older, 19 of which were 75 years of age or older. No apparent differences in safety or efficacy were observed between these patients and younger patients. No overall differences in safety were observed between these patients and younger patients, and other reported clinical experience has not identified differences in responses between the elderly and younger patients, but greater sensitivity of some older individuals cannot be ruled out. In general, dose selection for an elderly patient should be cautious, reflecting the greater frequency of decreased hepatic function and of concomitant disease or other drug therapy.

ADVERSE REACTIONS

The incidence of common adverse events in Table 1 is based upon 2 placebo-controlled US clinical trials in which 812 adolescent and adult patients (457 females and 355 males) previously treated with as-needed bronchodilators and/or inhaled corticosteroids were treated with FLOVENT HFA (dosages of 88, 220, or 440 mcg twice daily for up to 12 weeks) or placebo.

[See table 1 at top of previous page]

Table 2 includes all events (whether considered drug-related or nondrug-related by the investigator) that occurred at a rate of over 3% in any of the groups treated with FLOVENT HFA and were more common than in the placebo group. In considering these data, differences in average duration of exposure should be taken into account.

These adverse events were mostly mild to moderate in severity. Rare cases of immediate and delayed hypersensitivity reactions, including urticaria and rash, have been reported.

Other adverse events that occurred in the groups receiving FLOVENT HFA in these studies with an incidence of 1% to 3% and that occurred at a greater incidence than with placebo were:

Ear, Nose, and Throat: Sinusitis/sinus infection, rhinitis, pharyngitis/throat infection, rhinorrhea/post-nasal drip, nasal sinus disorders, laryngitis.

Gastrointestinal: Diarrhea, viral gastrointestinal infections, gastrointestinal signs and symptoms, dyspeptic symptoms, gastrointestinal discomfort and pain, hyposalivation.

Musculoskeletal: Musculoskeletal pain, muscle pain, muscle stiffness/tightness/rigidity.

Neurological: Dizziness, migraines.

Non-Site Specific: Fever, viral infections, pain, chest symptoms.

Skin: Viral skin infections.

Trauma: Muscle injuries, soft tissue injuries, injuries.

Urogenital: Urinary infections.

Fluticasone propionate inhalation aerosol (440 or 880 mcg twice daily) was administered for 16 weeks to patients with asthma requiring oral corticosteroids (Study 3). Adverse events not included in Table 2, but reported by >3 patients in either group treated with FLOVENT HFA and more commonly than in the placebo group included rhinitis, nausea and vomiting, arthralgia and articular rheumatism, musculoskeletal pain, muscle pain, malaise and fatigue, and sleep disorders.

In 2 long-term studies (26 and 52 weeks), treatment with FLOVENT HFA at dosages up to 440 mcg twice daily was well tolerated. The pattern of adverse events was similar to that observed in the 12-week studies. There were no new and/or unexpected adverse events with long-term treatment.

Observed During Clinical Practice: In addition to adverse events reported from clinical trials, the following events have been identified during postapproval use of fluticasone propionate. Because they are reported voluntarily from a population of unknown size, estimates of frequency cannot be made. These events have been chosen for inclusion due to either their seriousness, frequency of reporting, or causal connection to fluticasone propionate or a combination of these factors.

Ear, Nose, and Throat: Aphonia, facial and oropharyngeal edema, including angioedema, and throat soreness and irritation.

Endocrine and Metabolic: Cushingoid features, growth velocity reduction in children/adolescents, hyperglycemia, osteoporosis, and weight gain.

Eye: Cataracts.

Non-Site Specific: Very rare anaphylactic reaction.

Psychiatry: Agitation, aggression, depression, and restlessness.

Respiratory: Asthma exacerbation, chest tightness, cough, dyspnea, immediate and delayed bronchospasm, paradoxical bronchospasm, pneumonia, and wheeze.

Skin: Contusions, cutaneous hypersensitivity reactions, ecchymoses, and pruritus.

Eosinophilic Conditions: In rare cases, patients on inhaled fluticasone propionate may present with systemic eosinophilic conditions, with some patients presenting with clinical features of vasculitis consistent with Churg-Strauss syndrome, a condition that is often treated with systemic corticosteroid therapy. These events usually, but not always, have been associated with the reduction and/or withdrawal of oral corticosteroid therapy following the introduction of fluticasone propionate. Cases of serious eosinophilic conditions have also been reported with other inhaled corticosteroids in this clinical setting. Physicians should be alert to eosinophilia, vasculitic rash, worsening pulmonary symptoms, cardiac complications, and/or neuropathy presenting in their patients. A causal relationship between fluticasone propionate and these underlying conditions has not been established (see PRECAUTIONS: Eosinophilic Conditions).

OVERDOSAGE

Chronic overdosage may result in signs/symptoms of hypercorticism (see PRECAUTIONS: General). Inhalation by healthy volunteers of a single dose of 1,760 or 3,520 mcg of CFC 11/12-propelled fluticasone propionate inhalation aerosol was well tolerated. Doses of 1,320 mcg administered to healthy human volunteers twice daily for 7 to 15 days were also well tolerated. Repeat oral doses up to 80 mg daily for 10 days in healthy volunteers and repeat oral doses up to 20 mg daily for 42 days in patients were well tolerated. Adverse reactions were of mild or moderate severity, and incidences were similar in active and placebo treatment groups. The oral and subcutaneous median lethal doses in rats and mice were >1,000 mg/kg (approximately 4,600 and 2,300 times the maximum human daily inhalation dose based on mg/m^2, respectively).

DOSAGE AND ADMINISTRATION

FLOVENT HFA should be administered by the orally inhaled route only in patients 12 years of age and older. Individual patients will experience a variable time to onset and degree of symptom relief. Maximum benefit may not be achieved for 1 to 2 weeks or longer after starting treatment. After asthma stability has been achieved, it is always desirable to titrate to the lowest effective dosage to reduce the possibility of side effects. For patients who do not respond adequately to the starting dosage after 2 weeks of therapy, higher dosages may provide additional asthma control. The safety and efficacy of FLOVENT HFA when administered in excess of recommended dosages have not been established. The recommended starting dosage and the highest recommended dosage of FLOVENT HFA, based on prior asthma therapy, are listed in Table 2.

Table 2. Recommended Dosages of FLOVENT HFA
NOTE: In all patients, it is desirable to titrate to the lowest effective dosage once asthma stability is achieved.

Previous Therapy	Recommended Starting Dosage	Highest Recommended Dosage
Bronchodilators alone	88 mcg twice daily	440 mcg twice daily
Inhaled corticosteroids	88–220 mcg twice daily*	440 mcg twice daily
Oral corticosteroids†	440 mcg twice daily	880 mcg twice daily

*Starting dosages above 88 mcg twice daily may be considered for patients with poorer asthma control or those who have previously required doses of inhaled corticosteroids that are in the higher range for that specific agent.

†**For Patients Currently Receiving Chronic Oral Corticosteroid Therapy:** Prednisone should be reduced no faster than 2.5 to 5 mg/day on a weekly basis, beginning after at least 1 week of therapy with FLOVENT HFA. Patients should be carefully monitored for signs of asthma instability, including serial objective measures of airflow, and for signs of adrenal insufficiency (see WARNINGS). Once prednisone reduction is complete, the dosage of fluticasone propionate HFA should be reduced to the lowest effective dosage.

FLOVENT HFA should be primed before using for the first time by releasing 4 test sprays into the air away from the face, shaking well before each spray. In cases where the inhaler has not been used for more than 7 days or when it has been dropped, prime the inhaler again by shaking well and releasing 1 test spray into the air away from the face.

Geriatric Use: In studies where geriatric patients (65 years of age or older, see PRECAUTIONS: Geriatric Use) have been treated with fluticasone propionate inhalation aerosol, efficacy and safety did not differ from that in younger patients. Based on available data for FLOVENT HFA, no dosage adjustment is recommended.

Directions for Use: Illustrated Patient's Instructions for Use accompany each package of FLOVENT HFA.

HOW SUPPLIED

FLOVENT HFA 44 mcg Inhalation Aerosol is supplied in 10.6-g pressurized aluminum canisters containing 120 metered inhalations in boxes of 1 (NDC 0173-0718-00). Each canister is supplied with a dark orange oral actuator with a peach strapcap packaged within a plastic-coated, moisture-protective foil pouch and patient's instructions. The moisture-protective foil pouch also contains a desiccant that should be discarded when the pouch is opened.

FLOVENT HFA 110 mcg Inhalation Aerosol is supplied in 12-g pressurized aluminum canisters containing 120 metered inhalations in boxes of 1 (NDC 0173-0719-00). Each canister is supplied with a dark orange oral actuator with a peach strapcap packaged within a plastic-coated, moisture-protective foil pouch and patient's instructions. The moisture-protective foil pouch also contains a desiccant that should be discarded when the pouch is opened.

FLOVENT HFA 220 mcg Inhalation Aerosol is supplied in 12-g pressurized aluminum canisters containing 120 metered inhalations in boxes of 1 (NDC 0173-0720-00). Each canister is supplied with a dark orange oral actuator with a peach strapcap packaged within a plastic-coated, moisture-protective foil pouch and patient's instructions. The moisture-protective foil pouch also contains a desiccant that should be discarded when the pouch is opened.

The dark orange actuator supplied with FLOVENT HFA should not be used with any other product canisters, and actuators from other products should not be used with a FLOVENT HFA canister.

The correct amount of medication in each inhalation cannot be assured after 120 inhalations, even though the canister is not completely empty and will continue to operate. The inhaler should be discarded when 120 actuations have been used. Never immerse the canister into water to determine the amount remaining in the canister ("float test").

Keep out of reach of children. Avoid spraying in eyes.

Contents Under Pressure: Do not puncture. Do not use or store near heat or open flame. Exposure to temperatures above 120°F may cause bursting. Never throw into fire or incinerator.

Store at 25°C (77°F); excursions permitted to 15°–30°C (59°–86°F). Store the inhaler with the mouthpiece down. For best results, the inhaler should be at room temperature before use. SHAKE WELL BEFORE USING.

FLOVENT HFA does not contain chlorofluorocarbons (CFCs) as the propellant.

GlaxoSmithKline, Research Triangle Park, NC 27709

May 2004/RL-2098

FLOVENT® ROTADISK® 50 mcg ℞
[flō' vent]
(fluticasone propionate inhalation powder, 50 mcg)

FLOVENT® ROTADISK® 100 mcg ℞
(fluticasone propionate inhalation powder, 100 mcg)

FLOVENT® ROTADISK® 250 mcg ℞
(fluticasone propionate inhalation powder, 250 mcg)

For Oral Inhalation Only
For Use With the DISKHALER® Inhalation Device

DESCRIPTION

The active component of FLOVENT ROTADISK 50 mcg, FLOVENT ROTADISK 100 mcg, and FLOVENT ROTADISK 250 mcg is fluticasone propionate, a corticosteroid having the chemical name S-(fluoromethyl)6α,9-difluoro-11β,17-dihydroxy-16α-methyl-3-oxoandrosta-1,4-diene-17β-carbothioate, 17-propionate.

Fluticasone propionate is a white to off-white powder with a molecular weight of 500.6, and the empirical formula is $C_{25}H_{31}F_3O_5S$. It is practically insoluble in water, freely soluble in dimethyl sulfoxide and dimethylformamide, and slightly soluble in methanol and 95% ethanol.

FLOVENT ROTADISK 50 mcg, FLOVENT ROTADISK 100 mcg, and FLOVENT ROTADISK 250 mcg contain a dry powder presentation of fluticasone propionate intended for oral inhalation only. Each double-foil ROTADISK contains 4 blisters. Each blister contains a mixture of 50, 100, or 250 mcg of microfine fluticasone propionate blended with lactose (which contains milk proteins) to a total weight of 25 mg. The contents of each blister are inhaled using a specially designed plastic device for inhaling powder called the DISKHALER. After a fluticasone propionate ROTADISK is loaded into the DISKHALER, a blister containing medication is pierced and the fluticasone propionate is dispersed into the air stream created when the patient inhales through the mouthpiece.

The amount of drug delivered to the lung will depend on patient factors such as inspiratory flow. Under standardized in vitro testing, FLOVENT ROTADISK delivers 44, 88, or 220 mcg of fluticasone propionate from FLOVENT ROTADISK 50 mcg, FLOVENT ROTADISK 100 mcg, or FLOVENT ROTADISK 250 mcg, respectively, when tested at a flow rate of 60 L/min for 3 seconds. In adult and adolescent patients with asthma, mean peak inspiratory flow (PIF) through the DISKHALER was 123 L/min (range, 88 to 159 L/min), and in pediatric patients 4 to 11 years of age with asthma, mean PIF was 110 L/min (range, 43 to 175 L/min).

CLINICAL PHARMACOLOGY

Fluticasone propionate is a synthetic, trifluorinated corticosteroid with potent anti-inflammatory activity. In vitro assays using human lung cytosol preparations have established fluticasone propionate as a human glucocorticoid receptor agonist with an affinity 18 times greater than dexamethasone, almost twice that of beclomethasone-17-monopropionate (BMP), the active metabolite of beclomethasone dipropionate, and over 3 times that of budesonide. Data from the McKenzie vasoconstrictor assay in man are consistent with these results.

The precise mechanisms of fluticasone propionate action in asthma are unknown. Inflammation is recognized as an important component in the pathogenesis of asthma. Corticosteroids have been shown to inhibit multiple cell types (e.g., mast cells, eosinophils, basophils, lymphocytes, macrophages, and neutrophils) and mediator production or secretion (e.g., histamine, eicosanoids, leukotrienes, and cytokines) involved in the asthmatic response. These anti-inflammatory actions of corticosteroids may contribute to their efficacy in asthma.

Though highly effective for the treatment of asthma, corticosteroids do not affect asthma symptoms immediately. However, improvement following inhaled administration of fluticasone propionate can occur within 24 hours of beginning treatment, although maximum benefit may not be achieved for 1 to 2 weeks or longer after starting treatment. When corticosteroids are discontinued, asthma stability may persist for several days or longer.

Pharmacokinetics: ***Absorption:*** The activity of FLOVENT ROTADISK Inhalation Powder is due to the parent drug, fluticasone propionate. Studies using oral dosing of labeled and unlabeled drug have demonstrated that the oral systemic bioavailability of fluticasone propionate is negligible (<1%), primarily due to incomplete absorption and presystemic metabolism in the gut and liver. In contrast, the majority of the fluticasone propionate delivered to the lung is systemically absorbed. The systemic bioavailability of fluticasone propionate inhalation powder in healthy volunteers averaged about 13.5% of the nominal dose.

Peak plasma concentrations after a 1,000-mcg dose of fluticasone propionate inhalation powder ranged from 0.1 to 1.0 ng/mL.

Distribution: Following intravenous administration, the initial disposition phase for fluticasone propionate was rapid and consistent with its high lipid solubility and tissue binding. The volume of distribution averaged 4.2 L/kg. The percentage of fluticasone propionate bound to human plasma proteins averaged 91%.

Fluticasone propionate is weakly and reversibly bound to erythrocytes. Fluticasone propionate is not significantly bound to human transcortin.

Metabolism: The total clearance of fluticasone propionate is high (average, 1,093 mL/min), with renal clearance accounting for less than 0.02% of the total. The only circulating metabolite detected in man is the 17β-carboxylic acid derivative of fluticasone propionate, which is formed through the cytochrome P450 3A4 pathway. This metabolite had approximately 2,000 times less affinity than the parent drug for the glucocorticoid receptor of human lung cytosol in vitro and negligible pharmacological activity in animal studies. Other metabolites detected in vitro using cultured human hepatoma cells have not been detected in man.

In a multiple-dose drug interaction study, coadministration of fluticasone propionate (500 mcg twice daily) and erythromycin (333 mg 3 times daily) did not affect fluticasone propionate pharmacokinetics.

In a drug interaction study, coadministration of fluticasone propionate (1,000 mcg) and ketoconazole (200 mg once daily) resulted in increased fluticasone propionate concentrations, a reduction in plasma cortisol AUC, and no effect on urinary excretion of cortisol.

Excretion: Following intravenous dosing, fluticasone propionate showed polyexponential kinetics and had a terminal elimination half-life of approximately 7.8 hours. Less than 5% of a radiolabeled oral dose was excreted in the urine as metabolites, with the remainder excreted in the feces as parent drug and metabolites.

Special Populations: Formal pharmacokinetic studies using fluticasone propionate were not carried out in any special populations. In a clinical study using fluticasone propionate inhalation powder, trough fluticasone propionate plasma concentrations were collected in 76 males and 74 females after inhaled administration of 100 and 500 mcg twice daily. Full pharmacokinetic profiles were obtained from 7 female patients and 13 male patients at these doses, and no overall differences in pharmacokinetic behavior were found.

Plasma concentrations of fluticasone propionate were measured 20 and 40 minutes after dosing from 29 children aged 4 to 11 years who were taking either 50 or 100 mcg twice daily of fluticasone propionate inhalation powder. Plasma concentration values ranged from below the limit of quantitation (25 pg/mL) to 117 pg/mL (50-mcg dose) or 154 pg/mL (100-mcg dose). In a study with adults taking the 100-mcg twice-daily dose, the plasma concentrations observed ranged from below the limit of quantitation to 73.1 pg/mL. The median fluticasone propionate plasma concentrations for the 100-mcg dose in children was 58.7 pg/mL; in adults the median plasma concentration was 39.5 pg/mL.

Drug Interactions: Fluticasone propionate is a substrate of cytochrome P450 3A4. Coadministration of fluticasone propionate and the highly potent cytochrome P450 3A4 inhibitor ritonavir is not recommended based upon a multiple-dose, crossover drug interaction study in 18 healthy subjects. Fluticasone propionate aqueous nasal spray (200 mcg once daily) was coadministered for 7 days with ritonavir (100 mg twice daily). Plasma fluticasone propionate concentrations following fluticasone propionate aqueous nasal spray alone were undetectable (<10 pg/mL) in most subjects, and when concentrations were detectable peak levels (C_{max} averaged 11.9 pg/mL [range, 10.8 to 14.1 pg/mL] and $AUC_{(0-\tau)}$ averaged 8.43 pg•hr/mL [range, 4.2 to 18.8 pg•hr/mL]). Fluticasone propionate C_{max} and $AUC_{(0-\tau)}$ increased to 318 pg/mL (range, 110 to 648 pg/mL) and 3,102.6 pg•hr/mL (range, 1,207.1 to 5,662.0 pg•hr/mL), respectively, after coadministration of ritonavir with fluticasone propionate aqueous nasal spray. This significant increase in plasma fluticasone propionate exposure resulted in a significant decrease (86%) in plasma cortisol area under the plasma concentration versus time curve (AUC).

Caution should be exercised when other potent cytochrome P450 3A4 inhibitors are coadministered with fluticasone propionate. In a drug interaction study, coadministration of orally inhaled fluticasone propionate (1,000 mcg) and ketoconazole (200 mg once daily) resulted in increased plasma fluticasone propionate exposure and reduced plasma cortisol AUC, but had no effect on urinary excretion of cortisol. In another multiple-dose drug interaction study, coadministration of orally inhaled fluticasone propionate (500 mcg twice daily) and erythromycin (333 mg 3 times daily) did not affect fluticasone propionate pharmacokinetics.

Pharmacodynamics: To confirm that systemic absorption does not play a role in the clinical response to inhaled fluticasone propionate, a double-blind clinical study comparing inhaled and oral fluticasone propionate was conducted. Doses of 100 and 500 mcg twice daily of fluticasone propionate inhalation powder were compared to oral fluticasone propionate, 20,000 mcg given once daily, and placebo for 6 weeks. Plasma levels of fluticasone propionate were detectable in all 3 active groups, but the mean values were highest in the oral group. Both doses of inhaled fluticasone propionate were effective in maintaining asthma stability and improving lung function while oral fluticasone propionate and placebo were ineffective. This demonstrates that the clinical effectiveness of inhaled fluticasone propionate is due to its direct local effect and not to an indirect effect through systemic absorption.

The potential systemic effects of inhaled fluticasone propionate on the hypothalamic-pituitary-adrenal (HPA) axis were also studied in patients with asthma. Fluticasone propionate given by inhalation aerosol at doses of 220, 440, 660, or 880 mcg twice daily was compared with placebo or oral prednisone 10 mg given once daily for 4 weeks. For most patients, the ability to increase cortisol production in response to stress, as assessed by 6-hour cosyntropin stimulation, remained intact with inhaled fluticasone propionate treatment. No patient had an abnormal response (peak serum cortisol <18 mcg/dL) after dosing with placebo or fluticasone propionate 220 mcg twice daily. For patients treated with 440, 660, and 880 mcg twice daily, 10%, 16%, and 12%, respectively, had an abnormal response as compared to 29% of patients treated with prednisone.

In clinical trials with fluticasone propionate inhalation powder, using doses up to and including 250 mcg twice daily, occasional abnormal short cosyntropin tests (peak serum cortisol <18 mcg/dL) were noted in patients receiving fluticasone propionate or placebo. The incidence of abnormal tests at 500 mcg twice daily was greater than placebo. In a 2-year study carried out in 64 patients randomized to fluticasone propionate 500 mcg twice daily or placebo, 1 patient receiving fluticasone propionate (4%) had an abnormal response to 6-hour cosyntropin infusion at 1 year; repeat testing at 18 months and 2 years was normal. Another patient receiving fluticasone propionate (5%) had an abnormal response at 2 years. No patient on placebo had an abnormal response at 1 or 2 years.

CLINICAL TRIALS

Double-blind, parallel-group, placebo-controlled, US clinical trials were conducted in 1,197 adolescent and adult patients with asthma to assess the efficacy and safety of FLOVENT ROTADISK in the treatment of asthma. Fixed doses of 50, 100, 250, and 500 mcg twice daily were compared to placebo to provide information about appropriate dosing to cover a range of asthma severity. Patients with asthma included in these studies were those not adequately controlled with beta-agonists alone, and those already maintained on daily inhaled corticosteroids. In these efficacy trials, at all doses, measures of pulmonary function (forced expiratory volume in 1 second [FEV_1] and morning peak expiratory flow rate [AM PEF]) were statistically significantly improved as compared with placebo. All doses were delivered by inhalation of the contents of 1 or 2 blisters from the DISKHALER twice daily.

Figure 1 displays results of pulmonary function tests for 2 recommended dosages of FLOVENT ROTADISK (100 and 250 mcg twice daily) and placebo from a 12-week trial in 331 adolescent and adult patients with asthma (baseline FEV_1 = 2.63 L/sec) inadequately controlled on bronchodilators alone. Because this trial used predetermined criteria for lack of efficacy, which caused more patients in the placebo group to be withdrawn, pulmonary function results at Endpoint, which is the last evaluable FEV_1 result and includes most patients' lung function data, are also provided. Pulmonary function at both dosages of FLOVENT ROTADISK improved significantly compared with placebo by the first week of treatment, and this improvement was maintained over the duration of the trial.

[See figure 1 at top of next column]

In a second clinical study of 75 patients, 500 mcg twice daily was evaluated in a similar population. In this trial FLOVENT ROTADISK significantly improved pulmonary function as compared with placebo.

Figure 2 displays results of pulmonary function tests for 2 recommended dosages of FLOVENT ROTADISK (100 and 250 mcg twice daily) and placebo from a 12-week trial in 342 adolescent and adult patients with asthma (baseline FEV_1 = 2.49 L/sec) already receiving daily inhaled corticosteroid therapy (≥336 mcg/day of beclomethasone dipropionate or ≥800 mcg/day of triamcinolone acetonide) in addition to as-

Figure 1. A 12-Week Clinical Trial in Patients Inadequately Controlled on Bronchodilators Alone: Mean Percent Change From Baseline in FEV_1 Prior to AM Dose

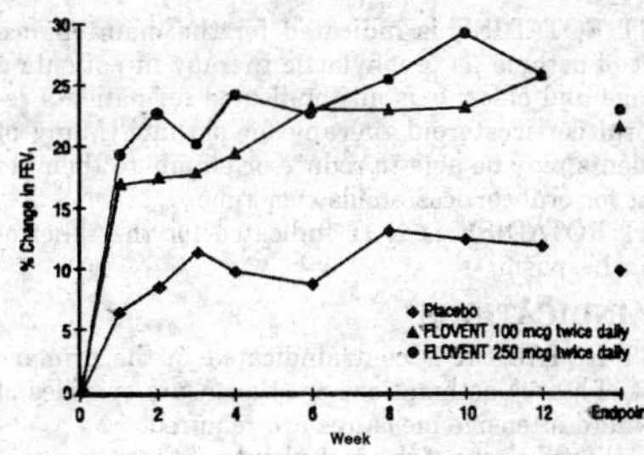

needed albuterol and theophylline (38% of all patients). Because this trial also used predetermined criteria for lack of efficacy, which caused more patients in the placebo group to be withdrawn, pulmonary function results at Endpoint are included. Pulmonary function at both dosages of FLOVENT ROTADISK improved significantly compared with placebo by the first week of treatment and the improvement was maintained over the duration of the trial.

Figure 2. A 12-Week Clinical Trial in Patients Already Receiving Inhaled Corticosteroids: Mean Percent Change From Baseline in FEV_1 Prior to AM Dose

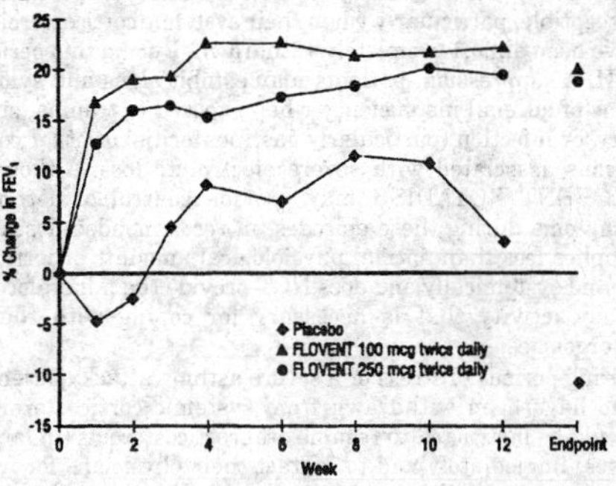

In a second clinical study of 139 patients, treatment with 500 mcg twice daily was evaluated in a similar patient population. In this trial FLOVENT ROTADISK significantly improved pulmonary function as compared with placebo.

In the 4 trials described above, all dosages of FLOVENT ROTADISK were efficacious; however, at higher dosages, patients were less likely to discontinue study participation due to asthma deterioration (as defined by predetermined criteria for lack of efficacy including lung function and patient-recorded variables such as AM PEF, albuterol use, and nighttime awakenings due to asthma).

In a clinical trial of 96 patients with severe asthma requiring chronic oral prednisone therapy (average baseline daily prednisone dose was 10 mg), fluticasone propionate given by inhalation aerosol at doses of 660 and 880 mcg twice daily was evaluated. Both doses enabled a statistically significantly larger percentage of patients to wean successfully from oral prednisone as compared with placebo (69% of the patients on 660 mcg twice daily and 88% of the patients on 880 mcg twice daily as compared with 3% of patients on placebo). Accompanying the reduction in oral corticosteroid use, patients treated with fluticasone propionate had significantly improved lung function and fewer asthma symptoms as compared with the placebo group. These data were obtained from a clinical study using fluticasone propionate inhalation aerosol; no direct assessment of the clinical comparability of equal nominal doses for the FLOVENT ROTADISK and FLOVENT Inhalation Aerosol formulations in this population has been conducted.

Pediatric Experience: In a 12-week, placebo-controlled clinical trial of 263 patients aged 4 to 11 years inadequately controlled on bronchodilators alone (baseline morning peak expiratory flow = 200 L/min), fluticasone propionate inhalation powder doses of 50 and 100 mcg twice daily significantly improved morning peak expiratory flow (28% and 34% change from baseline at Endpoint, respectively) compared to placebo (11% change). In a second placebo-controlled, 52-week trial of 325 patients aged 4 to 11 years, approximately half of whom were receiving inhaled corticosteroids at baseline, doses of fluticasone propionate inhalation powder of 50 and 100 mcg twice daily improved lung function by the first week of treatment, and the improvement continued over 1 year compared to placebo. In both studies, patients on active treatment were significantly less likely to discontinue treatment due to lack of efficacy.

Continued on next page

Product information on these pages is effective as of August 2004. Further information is available at: GlaxoSmithKline, PO Box 13398, Research Triangle Park, NC 27709. 1-888-825-5249. Corporate Web Site: www.gsk.com

Flovent Rotadisk—Cont.

INDICATIONS AND USAGE

FLOVENT ROTADISK is indicated for the maintenance treatment of asthma as prophylactic therapy in patients 4 years of age and older. It is also indicated for patients requiring oral corticosteroid therapy for asthma. Many of these patients may be able to reduce or eliminate their requirement for oral corticosteroids over time.

FLOVENT ROTADISK is NOT indicated for the relief of acute bronchospasm.

CONTRAINDICATIONS

FLOVENT ROTADISK is contraindicated in the primary treatment of status asthmaticus or other acute episodes of asthma where intensive measures are required.

Hypersensitivity to any of the ingredients of these preparations contraindicates their use (see DESCRIPTION and ADVERSE REACTIONS: Observed During Clinical Practice: *Non-Site Specific*).

WARNINGS

Particular care is needed for patients who are transferred from systemically active corticosteroids to FLOVENT ROTADISK because deaths due to adrenal insufficiency have occurred in patients with asthma during and after transfer from systemic corticosteroids to less systemically available inhaled corticosteroids. After withdrawal from systemic corticosteroids, a number of months are required for recovery of HPA function.

Patients who have been previously maintained on 20 mg or more per day of prednisone (or its equivalent) may be most susceptible, particularly when their systemic corticosteroids have been almost completely withdrawn. During this period of HPA suppression, patients may exhibit signs and symptoms of adrenal insufficiency when exposed to trauma, surgery, or infection (particularly gastroenteritis) or other conditions associated with severe electrolyte loss. Although FLOVENT ROTADISK may provide control of asthma symptoms during these episodes, in recommended doses it supplies less than normal physiological amounts of corticosteroid systemically and does NOT provide the mineralocorticoid activity that is necessary for coping with these emergencies.

During periods of stress or a severe asthma attack, patients who have been withdrawn from systemic corticosteroids should be instructed to resume oral corticosteroids (in large doses) immediately and to contact their physicians for further instruction. These patients should also be instructed to carry a warning card indicating that they may need supplementary systemic corticosteroids during periods of stress or a severe asthma attack.

A drug interaction study in healthy subjects has shown that ritonavir (a highly potent cytochrome P450 3A4 inhibitor) can significantly increase plasma fluticasone propionate exposure, resulting in significantly reduced serum cortisol concentrations (see CLINICAL PHARMACOLOGY: Drug Interactions and PRECAUTIONS: Drug Interactions). During postmarketing use, there have been reports of clinically significant drug interactions in patients receiving fluticasone propionate and ritonavir, resulting in systemic corticosteroid effects including Cushing syndrome and adrenal suppression. Therefore, coadministration of fluticasone propionate and ritonavir is not recommended unless the potential benefit to the patient outweighs the risk of systemic corticosteroid side effects.

Patients requiring oral corticosteroids should be weaned slowly from systemic corticosteroid use after transferring to FLOVENT ROTADISK. In a clinical trial of 96 patients, prednisone reduction was successfully accomplished by reducing the daily prednisone dose by 2.5 mg on a weekly basis during transfer to inhaled fluticasone propionate. Successive reduction of prednisone dose was allowed only when lung function, symptoms, and as-needed beta-agonist use were better than or comparable to that seen before initiation of prednisone dose reduction. Lung function (FEV_1 or AM PEF), beta-agonist use, and asthma symptoms should be carefully monitored during withdrawal of oral corticosteroids. In addition to monitoring asthma signs and symptoms, patients should be observed for signs and symptoms of adrenal insufficiency such as fatigue, lassitude, weakness, nausea and vomiting, and hypotension.

Transfer of patients from systemic corticosteroid therapy to FLOVENT ROTADISK may unmask conditions previously suppressed by the systemic corticosteroid therapy, e.g., rhinitis, conjunctivitis, eczema, arthritis.

Persons who are on drugs that suppress the immune system are more susceptible to infections than healthy individuals. Chickenpox and measles, for example, can have a more serious or even fatal course in susceptible children or adults on corticosteroids. In such children or adults who have not had these diseases, particular care should be taken to avoid exposure. How the dose, route, and duration of corticosteroid administration affect the risk of developing a disseminated infection is not known. The contribution of the underlying disease and/or prior corticosteroid treatment to the risk is also not known. If exposed to chickenpox, prophylaxis with varicella zoster immune globulin (VZIG) may be indicated. If exposed to measles, prophylaxis with pooled intramuscular immunoglobulin (IG) may be indicated. (See the respective package inserts for complete VZIG and IG prescribing information.) If chickenpox develops, treatment with antiviral agents may be considered.

FLOVENT ROTADISK is not to be regarded as a bronchodilator and is not indicated for rapid relief of bronchospasm. As with other inhaled asthma medications, bronchospasm may occur with an immediate increase in wheezing after dosing. If bronchospasm occurs following dosing with FLOVENT ROTADISK, it should be treated immediately with a fast-acting inhaled bronchodilator. Treatment with FLOVENT ROTADISK should be discontinued and alternative therapy instituted.

Patients should be instructed to contact their physicians immediately when episodes of asthma that are not responsive to bronchodilators occur during the course of treatment with FLOVENT ROTADISK. During such episodes, patients may require therapy with oral corticosteroids.

PRECAUTIONS

General: During withdrawal from oral corticosteroids, some patients may experience symptoms of systemically active corticosteroid withdrawal, e.g., joint and/or muscular pain, lassitude, and depression, despite maintenance or even improvement of respiratory function.

Fluticasone propionate will often permit control of asthma symptoms with less suppression of HPA function than therapeutically equivalent oral doses of prednisone. Since fluticasone propionate is absorbed into the circulation and can be systemically active at higher doses, the beneficial effects of FLOVENT ROTADISK in minimizing HPA dysfunction may be expected only when recommended dosages are not exceeded and individual patients are titrated to the lowest effective dose. A relationship between plasma levels of fluticasone propionate and inhibitory effects on stimulated cortisol production has been shown after 4 weeks of treatment with FLOVENT Inhalation Aerosol. Since individual sensitivity to effects on cortisol production exists, physicians should consider this information when prescribing FLOVENT ROTADISK.

Because of the possibility of systemic absorption of inhaled corticosteroids, patients treated with these drugs should be observed carefully for any evidence of systemic corticosteroid effects. Particular care should be taken in observing patients postoperatively or during periods of stress for evidence of inadequate adrenal response.

It is possible that systemic corticosteroid effects such as hypercorticism and adrenal suppression (including adrenal crisis) may appear in a small number of patients, particularly when FLOVENT ROTADISK is administered at higher than recommended doses over prolonged periods of time. If such effects occur, FLOVENT ROTADISK should be reduced slowly, consistent with accepted procedures for reducing systemic corticosteroids and for management of asthma symptoms.

A reduction of growth velocity in children or adolescents may occur as a result of poorly controlled asthma or from the therapeutic use of corticosteroids, including inhaled corticosteroids. A 52-week placebo-controlled study to assess the potential growth effects of FLOVENT ROTADISK at 50 and 100 mcg twice daily was conducted in the US in 325 prepubescent children (244 males and 81 females) 4 to 11 years of age. The mean growth velocities at 52 weeks observed in the intent-to-treat population were 6.32 cm/year in the placebo group (n = 76), 6.07 cm/year in the 50-mcg group (n = 98), and 5.66 cm/year in the 100-mcg group (n = 89). An imbalance in the proportion of children entering puberty between groups and a higher dropout rate in the placebo group due to poorly controlled asthma may be confounding factors in interpreting these data. A separate subset analysis of children who remained prepubertal during the study revealed growth rates at 52 weeks of 6.10 cm/year in the placebo group (n = 57), 5.91 cm/year in the 50-mcg group (n = 74), and 5.67 cm/year in the 100-mcg group (n = 79). The clinical significance of these growth data is not certain. In children 8.5 years of age, the mean age of children in this study, the range for expected growth velocity is: boys – 3rd percentile = 3.8 cm/year, 50th percentile = 5.4 cm/year, and 97th percentile = 7.0 cm/year; girls – 3rd percentile = 4.2 cm/year, 50th percentile = 5.7 cm/year, and 97th percentile = 7.3 cm/year. The effects of long-term treatment of children with inhaled corticosteroids, including fluticasone propionate, on final adult height are not known. Physicians should closely follow the growth of children and adolescents taking corticosteroids by any route, and weigh the benefits of corticosteroid therapy against the possibility of growth suppression if growth appears slowed. Patients should be maintained on the lowest dose of inhaled corticosteroid that effectively controls their asthma.

The long-term effects of fluticasone propionate in human subjects are not fully known. In particular, the effects resulting from chronic use of fluticasone propionate on developmental or immunologic processes in the mouth, pharynx, trachea, and lung are unknown. Some patients have received inhaled fluticasone propionate on a continuous basis for periods of 3 years or longer. In clinical studies with patients treated for 2 years with inhaled fluticasone propionate, no apparent differences in the type or severity of adverse reactions were observed after long- versus short-term treatment.

Rare instances of glaucoma, increased intraocular pressure, and cataracts have been reported following the inhaled administration of corticosteroids, including fluticasone propionate.

In clinical studies with inhaled fluticasone propionate, the development of localized infections of the pharynx with *Candida albicans* has occurred. When such an infection develops, it should be treated with appropriate local or systemic (i.e., oral antifungal) therapy while remaining on treatment with FLOVENT ROTADISK, but at times therapy with FLOVENT ROTADISK may need to be interrupted.

Inhaled corticosteroids should be used with caution, if at all, in patients with active or quiescent tuberculous infections of the respiratory tract; untreated systemic fungal, bacterial, viral, or parasitic infections; or ocular herpes simplex.

Eosinophilic Conditions: In rare cases, patients on inhaled fluticasone propionate may present with systemic eosinophilic conditions, with some patients presenting with clinical features of vasculitis consistent with Churg-Strauss syndrome, a condition that is often treated with systemic corticosteroid therapy. These events usually, but not always, have been associated with the reduction and/or withdrawal of oral corticosteroid therapy following the introduction of fluticasone propionate. Cases of serious eosinophilic conditions have also been reported with other inhaled corticosteroids in this clinical setting. Physicians should be alert to eosinophilia, vasculitic rash, worsening pulmonary symptoms, cardiac complications, and/or neuropathy presenting in their patients. A causal relationship between fluticasone propionate and these underlying conditions has not been established (see ADVERSE REACTIONS).

Information for Patients: Patients being treated with FLOVENT ROTADISK should receive the following information and instructions. This information is intended to aid them in the safe and effective use of this medication. It is not a disclosure of all possible adverse or intended effects.

Patients should use FLOVENT ROTADISK at regular intervals as directed. Results of clinical trials indicated significant improvement may occur within the first day or two of treatment; however, the full benefit may not be achieved until treatment has been administered for 1 to 2 weeks or longer. The patient should not increase the prescribed dosage but should contact the physician if symptoms do not improve or if the condition worsens.

Patients should be warned to avoid exposure to chickenpox or measles and, if they are exposed, to consult their physicians without delay.

For the proper use of FLOVENT ROTADISK and to attain maximum improvement, the patient should read and follow carefully the Patient's Instructions for Use accompanying the product.

Drug Interactions: Fluticasone propionate is a substrate of cytochrome P450 3A4. A drug interaction study with fluticasone propionate aqueous nasal spray in healthy subjects has shown that ritonavir (a highly potent cytochrome P450 3A4 inhibitor) can significantly increase plasma fluticasone propionate exposure, resulting in significantly reduced serum cortisol concentrations (see CLINICAL PHARMACOLOGY: Drug Interactions). During postmarketing use, there have been reports of clinically significant drug interactions in patients receiving fluticasone propionate and ritonavir, resulting in systemic corticosteroid effects including Cushing syndrome and adrenal suppression. Therefore, coadministration of fluticasone propionate and ritonavir is not recommended unless the potential benefit to the patient outweighs the risk of systemic corticosteroid side effects.

In a placebo-controlled, crossover study in 8 healthy volunteers, coadministration of a single dose of orally inhaled fluticasone propionate (1,000 mcg) with multiple doses of ketoconazole (200 mg) to steady state resulted in increased plasma fluticasone propionate exposure, a reduction in plasma cortisol AUC, and no effect on urinary excretion of cortisol. Caution should be exercised when FLOVENT ROTADISK is coadministered with ketoconazole and other known potent cytochrome P450 3A4 inhibitors.

Carcinogenesis, Mutagenesis, Impairment of Fertility: Fluticasone propionate demonstrated no tumorigenic potential in mice at oral doses up to 1,000 mcg/kg (approximately 2 times the maximum recommended daily inhalation dose in adults and approximately 10 times the maximum recommended daily inhalation dose in children on a mcg/m^2 basis) for 78 weeks or in rats at inhalation doses up to 57 mcg/kg (approximately 1/4 the maximum recommended daily inhalation dose in adults and comparable to the maximum recommended daily inhalation dose in children on a mcg/m^2 basis) for 104 weeks.

Fluticasone propionate did not induce gene mutation in prokaryotic or eukaryotic cells in vitro. No significant clastogenic effect was seen in cultured human peripheral lymphocytes in vitro or in the mouse micronucleus test when administered at high doses by the oral or subcutaneous routes. Furthermore, the compound did not delay erythroblast division in bone marrow.

No evidence of impairment of fertility was observed in reproductive studies conducted in male and female rats at subcutaneous doses up to 50 mcg/kg (approximately 1/5 the maximum recommended daily inhalation dose in adults on a mcg/m^2 basis). Prostate weight was significantly reduced at a subcutaneous dose of 50 mcg/kg.

Pregnancy: ***Teratogenic Effects:*** Pregnancy Category C. Subcutaneous studies in the mouse and rat at 45 and 100 mcg/kg, respectively (approximately 1/10 and 1/3, respectively, the maximum recommended daily inhalation dose in adults on a mcg/m^2 basis) revealed fetal toxicity characteristic of potent corticosteroid compounds, including embryonic growth retardation, omphalocele, cleft palate, and retarded cranial ossification.

In the rabbit, fetal weight reduction and cleft palate were observed at a subcutaneous dose of 4 mcg/kg (approximately 1/30 the maximum recommended daily inhalation dose in adults on a mcg/m^2 basis). However, no teratogenic effects were reported at oral doses up to 300 mcg/kg (approximately 2 times the maximum recommended daily inhalation dose in adults on a mcg/m^2 basis) of fluticasone propionate. No fluticasone propionate was detected in the plasma in this study, consistent with the established low bioavailability following oral administration (see CLINICAL PHARMACOLOGY).

Fluticasone propionate crossed the placenta following oral administration of 100 mcg/kg to rats or 300 mcg/kg to rabbits (approximately 1/3 and 2 times, respectively, the maximum recommended daily inhalation dose in adults on a mcg/m^2 basis).

There are no adequate and well-controlled studies in pregnant women. FLOVENT ROTADISK should be used during pregnancy only if the potential benefit justifies the potential risk to the fetus.

Experience with oral corticosteroids since their introduction in pharmacologic, as opposed to physiologic, doses suggests that rodents are more prone to teratogenic effects from corticosteroids than humans. In addition, because there is a natural increase in corticosteroid production during pregnancy, most women will require a lower exogenous corticosteroid dose and many will not need corticosteroid treatment during pregnancy.

Nursing Mothers: It is not known whether fluticasone propionate is excreted in human breast milk. Subcutaneous administration to lactating rats of 10 mcg/kg tritiated fluticasone propionate (approximately 1/25 the maximum recommended daily inhalation dose in adults on a mcg/m^2 basis) resulted in measurable radioactivity in milk. Because other corticosteroids are excreted in human milk, caution should be exercised when FLOVENT ROTADISK is administered to a nursing woman.

Pediatric Use: Two hundred fourteen (214) patients 4 to 11 years of age and 142 patients 12 to 16 years of age were treated with FLOVENT ROTADISK in US clinical trials. The safety and effectiveness of FLOVENT ROTADISK Inhalation Powder in children below 4 years of age have not been established.

Inhaled corticosteroids, including fluticasone propionate, may cause a reduction in growth in children and adolescents (see PRECAUTIONS). If a child or adolescent on any corticosteroid appears to have growth suppression, the possibility that they are particularly sensitive to this effect of corticosteroids should be considered. Patients should be maintained on the lowest dose of inhaled corticosteroid that effectively controls their asthma.

Geriatric Use: Safety data have been collected on 280 patients (FLOVENT® DISKUS® N = 83, FLOVENT ROTADISK N = 197) 65 years of age or older and 33 patients (FLOVENT DISKUS N = 14, FLOVENT ROTADISK N = 19) 75 years of age or older who have been treated with fluticasone propionate inhalation powder in US and non-US clinical trials. There were no differences in adverse reactions compared to those reported by younger patients. In addition, there were no apparent differences in efficacy between patients 65 years of age or older and younger patients. Fifteen patients 65 years of age or older and 1 patient 75 years of age or older were included in the efficacy evaluation of US clinical studies.

ADVERSE REACTIONS

The incidence of common adverse events in Table 1 is based upon 6 placebo-controlled clinical trials in which 1,384 patients ≥ 4 years of age (520 females and 864 males) previously treated with as-needed bronchodilators and/or inhaled corticosteroids were treated with FLOVENT ROTADISK (doses of 50 to 500 mcg twice daily for up to 12 weeks) or placebo.

[See table 1 above]

Table 1 includes all events (whether considered drug-related or nondrug-related by the investigator) that occurred at a rate of over 3% in any of the groups treated with FLOVENT ROTADISK and were more common than in the placebo group. In considering these data, differences in average duration of exposure should be taken into account.

These adverse reactions were mostly mild to moderate in severity, with <2% of patients discontinuing the studies because of adverse events. Rare cases of immediate and delayed hypersensitivity reactions, including rash and other rare events of angioedema and bronchospasm, have been reported.

Other adverse events that occurred in these clinical trials using FLOVENT ROTADISK with an incidence of 1% to 3% and that occurred at a greater incidence than with placebo were:

Ear, Nose, and Throat: Otitis media, tonsillitis, nasal discharge, earache, laryngitis, epistaxis, sneezing.

Eye: Conjunctivitis.

Gastrointestinal: Abdominal pain, viral gastroenteritis, gastroenteritis/colitis, abdominal discomfort.

Miscellaneous: Injury.

Mouth and Teeth: Mouth irritation.

Musculoskeletal: Sprain/strain, pain in joint, disorder/symptoms of neck, muscular soreness, aches and pains.

Neurological: Migraine, nervousness.

Respiratory: Chest congestion, acute nasopharyngitis, dyspnea, irritation due to inhalant.

Skin: Dermatitis, urticaria.

Urogenital: Dysmenorrhea, candidiasis of vagina, pelvic inflammatory disease, vaginitis/vulvovaginitis, irregular menstrual cycle.

Table 1. Overall Adverse Events With >3% Incidence in Controlled Clinical Trials With FLOVENT ROTADISK in Patients ≥4 Years Previously Receiving Bronchodilators and/or Inhaled Corticosteroids

Adverse Event	Placebo (N = 438) %	FLOVENT 50 mcg Twice Daily (N = 255) %	FLOVENT 100 mcg Twice Daily (N = 331) %	FLOVENT 250 mcg Twice Daily (N = 176) %	FLOVENT 500 mcg Twice Daily (N = 184) %
Ear, nose, and throat					
Pharyngitis	7	6	8	8	13
Nasal congestion	5	4	4	7	7
Sinusitis	4	5	4	6	4
Rhinitis	4	4	9	2	3
Dysphonia	0	<1	4	6	4
Oral candidiasis	1	3	3	4	11
Respiratory					
Upper respiratory infection	13	16	17	22	16
Influenza	2	3	3	3	4
Bronchitis	2	4	2	1	2
Other					
Headache	11	11	9	14	15
Diarrhea	1	2	2	0	4
Back problems	<1	<1	1	1	4
Fever	3	4	4	2	2
Average duration of exposure (days)	53	77	68	78	60

Table 2. Recommended Dosages of FLOVENT ROTADISK

Previous Therapy	Recommended Starting Dosage	Highest Recommended Dosage
Adults and Adolescents		
Bronchodilators alone	100 mcg twice daily	500 mcg twice daily
Inhaled corticosteroids	100-250 mcg twice daily*	500 mcg twice daily
Oral corticosteroids†	1000 mcg twice daily‡	1000 mcg twice daily‡
Children 4 to 11 Years		
Bronchodilators alone	50 mcg twice daily	100 mcg twice daily
Inhaled corticosteroids	50 mcg twice daily	100 mcg twice daily

* Starting dosages above 100 mcg twice daily for adults and adolescents and 50 mcg twice daily for children 4 to 11 years of age may be considered for patients with poorer asthma control or those who have previously required doses of inhaled corticosteroids that are in the higher range for that specific agent.

NOTE: In all patients, it is desirable to titrate to the lowest effective dosage once asthma stability is achieved.

† **For Patients Currently Receiving Chronic Oral Corticosteroid Therapy:** Prednisone should be reduced no faster than 2.5 mg/day on a weekly basis, beginning after at least 1 week of therapy with FLOVENT ROTADISK. Patients should be carefully monitored for signs of asthma instability, including serial objective measures of airflow, and for signs of adrenal insufficiency (see WARNINGS). Once prednisone reduction is complete, the dosage of fluticasone propionate should be reduced to the lowest effective dosage.

‡ This dosing recommendation is based on clinical data from a study conducted using FLOVENT Inhalation Aerosol. No clinical trials have been conducted in patients on oral corticosteroids using FLOVENT ROTADISK; no direct assessment of the clinical comparability of equal nominal doses for FLOVENT ROTADISK and FLOVENT Inhalation Aerosol in this population has been conducted.

There were no clinically relevant differences in the pattern or severity of adverse events in children compared with those reported in adults.

FLOVENT Inhalation Aerosol (660 or 880 mcg twice daily) was administered for 16 weeks to patients with asthma requiring oral corticosteroids. Adverse events reported more frequently in these patients compared to patients not on oral corticosteroids included sinusitis, nasal discharge, oropharyngeal candidiasis, headache, joint pain, nausea and vomiting, muscular soreness, malaise/fatigue, and insomnia.

Observed During Clinical Practice: In addition to adverse events reported from clinical trials, the following events have been identified during postapproval use of fluticasone propionate in clinical practice. Because they are reported voluntarily from a population of unknown size, estimates of frequency cannot be made. These experiences have been chosen for inclusion due to either their seriousness, frequency of reporting, or causal connection to fluticasone propionate or a combination of these factors.

Ear, Nose, and Throat: Aphonia, facial and oropharyngeal edema, hoarseness, and throat soreness and irritation.

Endocrine and Metabolic: Cushingoid features, growth velocity reduction in children/adolescents, hyperglycemia, osteoporosis, and weight gain.

Eye: Cataracts.

Non-Site Specific: Very rare anaphylactic reaction, very rare anaphylactic reaction in patients with severe milk protein allergy.

Psychiatry: Agitation, aggression, depression, and restlessness.

Respiratory: Asthma exacerbation, bronchospasm, chest tightness, cough, immediate bronchospasm, paradoxical bronchospasm, pneumonia, and wheeze.

Skin: Contusions, ecchymoses, and pruritus.

Eosinophilic Conditions: In rare cases, patients on inhaled fluticasone propionate may present with systemic eosinophilic conditions, with some patients presenting with clinical features of vasculitis consistent with Churg-Strauss syndrome, a condition that is often treated with systemic corticosteroid therapy. These events usually, but not always, have been associated with the reduction and/or withdrawal of oral corticosteroid therapy following the introduction of fluticasone propionate. Cases of serious eosinophilic conditions have also been reported with other inhaled corticosteroids in this clinical setting. Physicians should be alert to eosinophilia, vasculitic rash, worsening pulmonary symptoms, cardiac complications, and/or neuropathy presenting in their patients. A causal relationship between fluticasone propionate and these underlying conditions has not been established (see PRECAUTIONS: Eosinophilic Conditions).

OVERDOSAGE

Chronic overdosage may result in signs/symptoms of hypercorticism (see PRECAUTIONS). Inhalation by healthy volunteers of a single dose of 4,000 mcg of fluticasone propionate inhalation powder or single doses of 1,760 or 3,520 mcg of fluticasone propionate inhalation aerosol was well tolerated. Fluticasone propionate given by inhalation aerosol at doses of 1,320 mcg twice daily for 7 to 15 days to healthy human volunteers was also well tolerated. Repeat oral doses up to 80 mg daily for 10 days in healthy volunteers and repeat oral doses up to 20 mg daily for 42 days in patients were well tolerated. Adverse reactions were of mild or moderate severity, and incidences were similar in active and placebo treatment groups. The oral and subcutaneous median lethal doses in mice and rats were >1,000 mg/kg (>2,000 and >4,100 times, respectively, the maximum recommended daily inhalation dose in adults and >9,600 and >19,000 times, respectively, the maximum recommended daily inhalation dose in children on a mg/m^2 basis).

DOSAGE AND ADMINISTRATION

FLOVENT ROTADISK should be administered by the orally inhaled route in patients 4 years of age and older. Individual patients will experience a variable time to onset and degree of symptom relief. Generally, FLOVENT ROTADISK has a relatively rapid onset of action for an in-

Continued on next page

Product information on these pages is effective as of August 2004. Further information is available at: GlaxoSmithKline, PO Box 13398, Research Triangle Park, NC 27709. 1-888-825-5249. Corporate Web Site: www.gsk.com

Flovent Rotadisk—Cont.

haled corticosteroid. Improvement in asthma control following inhaled administration of fluticasone propionate can occur within 24 hours of beginning treatment, although maximum benefit may not be achieved for 1 to 2 weeks or longer after starting treatment.
After asthma stability has been achieved (see Table 2), it is always desirable to titrate to the lowest effective dosage to reduce the possibility of side effects. Dosages as low as 50 mcg twice daily have been shown to be effective in some patients. For patients who do not respond adequately to the starting dosage after 2 weeks of therapy, higher dosages may provide additional asthma control. The safety and efficacy of FLOVENT ROTADISK when administered in excess of recommended dosages have not been established.
Rinsing the mouth after inhalation is advised.
The recommended starting dosage and the highest recommended dosage of FLOVENT ROTADISK, based on prior anti-asthma therapy, are listed in Table 2.
[See table 2 at top of previous page]
Geriatric Use: In studies where geriatric patients (65 years of age or older, see PRECAUTIONS) have been treated with FLOVENT ROTADISK, efficacy and safety did not differ from that in younger patients. Consequently, no dosage adjustment is recommended.
Directions for Use: Illustrated Patient's Instructions for Use accompany each package of FLOVENT ROTADISK.

HOW SUPPLIED

FLOVENT ROTADISK 50 mcg is a circular double-foil pack containing 4 blisters of the drug. Fifteen (15) ROTADISKS are packaged in a white polypropylene tube, and the tube is packaged in a plastic-coated, moisture-protective foil pouch. A carton contains the foil pouch of 15 ROTADISKS and 1 dark orange and peach DISKHALER inhalation device (NDC 0173-0511-00).
FLOVENT ROTADISK 100 mcg is a circular double-foil pack containing 4 blisters of the drug. Fifteen (15) ROTADISKS are packaged in a white polypropylene tube, and the tube is packaged in a plastic-coated, moisture-protective foil pouch. A carton contains the foil pouch of 15 ROTADISKS and 1 dark orange and peach DISKHALER inhalation device (NDC 0173-0509-00).
FLOVENT ROTADISK 250 mcg is a circular double-foil pack containing 4 blisters of the drug. Fifteen (15) ROTADISKS are packaged in a white polypropylene tube, and the tube is packaged in a plastic-coated, moisture-protective foil pouch. A carton contains the foil pouch of 15 ROTADISKS and 1 dark orange and peach DISKHALER inhalation device (NDC 0173-0504-00).
Store at controlled room temperature (see USP), 20° to 25°C (68° to 77°F) in a dry place. Keep out of reach of children. Do not puncture any fluticasone propionate ROTADISK blister until taking a dose using the DISKHALER. Use the ROTADISK blisters within 2 months after opening of the moisture-protective foil overwrap or before the expiration date, whichever comes first. Place the sticker provided with the product on the tube and enter the date the foil overwrap is opened and the 2-month use date.
GlaxoSmithKline, Research Triangle Park, NC 27709

March 2004/RL-2068
Shown in Product Identification Guide, page 315

FORTAZ® ℞
[for' taz]
(ceftazidime for injection)

FORTAZ® ℞
(ceftazidime injection)

For Intravenous or Intramuscular Use

To reduce the development of drug-resistant bacteria and maintain the effectiveness of FORTAZ and other antibacterial drugs, FORTAZ should be used only to treat or prevent infections that are proven or strongly suspected to be caused by bacteria.

DESCRIPTION

Ceftazidime is a semisynthetic, broad-spectrum, beta-lactam antibiotic for parenteral administration. It is the pentahydrate of pyridinium, 1-[[7-[[(2-amino-4-thiazolyl)[(1-carboxy-1-methylethoxy)imino]acetyl]amino]-2-carboxy-8-oxo-5-thia-1-azabicyclo[4.2.0]oct-2-en-3-yl]methyl]-, hydroxide, inner salt, [6R-[6α,7β(Z)]].
The empirical formula is $C_{22}H_{32}N_6O_{12}S_2$, representing a molecular weight of 636.6.
FORTAZ is a sterile, dry-powdered mixture of ceftazidime pentahydrate and sodium carbonate. The sodium carbonate at a concentration of 118 mg/g of ceftazidime activity has been admixed to facilitate dissolution. The total sodium content of the mixture is approximately 54 mg (2.3 mEq)/g of ceftazidime activity.
FORTAZ in sterile crystalline form is supplied in vials equivalent to 500 mg, 1 g, 2 g, or 6 g of anhydrous ceftazidime and in ADD-Vantage® vials equivalent to 1 or 2 g of anhydrous ceftazidime. Solutions of FORTAZ range in color from light yellow to amber, depending on the diluent and volume used. The pH of freshly constituted solutions usually ranges from 5 to 8.
FORTAZ is available as a frozen, iso-osmotic, sterile, nonpyrogenic solution with 1 or 2 g of ceftazidime as ceftazidime sodium premixed with approximately 2.2 or 1.6 g, respectively, of Dextrose Hydrous, USP. Dextrose has been added to adjust the osmolality. Sodium hydroxide is used to adjust pH and neutralize ceftazidime pentahydrate free acid to the sodium salt. The pH may have been adjusted with hydrochloric acid. Solutions of premixed FORTAZ range in color from light yellow to amber. The solution is intended for intravenous (IV) use after thawing to room temperature. The osmolality of the solution is approximately 300 mOsmol/kg, and the pH of thawed solutions ranges from 5 to 7.5.
The plastic container for the frozen solution is fabricated from a specially designed multilayer plastic, PL 2040. Solutions are in contact with the polyethylene layer of this container and can leach out certain chemical components of the plastic in very small amounts within the expiration period. The suitability of the plastic has been confirmed in tests in animals according to USP biological tests for plastic containers as well as by tissue culture toxicity studies.

CLINICAL PHARMACOLOGY

After IV administration of 500-mg and 1-g doses of ceftazidime over 5 minutes to normal adult male volunteers, mean peak serum concentrations of 45 and 90 mcg/mL, respectively, were achieved. After IV infusion of 500-mg, 1-g, and 2-g doses of ceftazidime over 20 to 30 minutes to normal adult male volunteers, mean peak serum concentrations of 42, 69, and 170 mcg/mL, respectively, were achieved. The average serum concentrations following IV infusion of 500-mg, 1-g, and 2-g doses to these volunteers over an 8-hour interval are given in Table 1.

Table 1. Average Serum Concentrations of Ceftazidime

Ceftazidime IV Dose	Serum Concentrations (mcg/mL)				
	0.5 hr	1 hr	2 hr	4 hr	8 hr
500 mg	42	25	12	6	2
1 g	60	39	23	11	3
2 g	129	75	42	13	5

The absorption and elimination of ceftazidime were directly proportional to the size of the dose. The half-life following IV administration was approximately 1.9 hours. Less than 10% of ceftazidime was protein bound. The degree of protein binding was independent of concentration. There was no evidence of accumulation of ceftazidime in the serum in individuals with normal renal function following multiple IV doses of 1 and 2 g every 8 hours for 10 days.
Following intramuscular (IM) administration of 500-mg and 1-g doses of ceftazidime to normal adult volunteers, the mean peak serum concentrations were 17 and 39 mcg/mL, respectively, at approximately 1 hour. Serum concentrations remained above 4 mcg/mL for 6 and 8 hours after the IM administration of 500-mg and 1-g doses, respectively. The half-life of ceftazidime in these volunteers was approximately 2 hours.
The presence of hepatic dysfunction had no effect on the pharmacokinetics of ceftazidime in individuals administered 2 g intravenously every 8 hours for 5 days. Therefore, a dosage adjustment from the normal recommended dosage is not required for patients with hepatic dysfunction, provided renal function is not impaired.
Approximately 80% to 90% of an IM or IV dose of ceftazidime is excreted unchanged by the kidneys over a 24-hour period. After the IV administration of single 500-mg or 1-g doses, approximately 50% of the dose appeared in the urine in the first 2 hours. An additional 20% was excreted between 2 and 4 hours after dosing, and approximately another 12% of the dose appeared in the urine between 4 and 8 hours later. The elimination of ceftazidime by the kidneys resulted in high therapeutic concentrations in the urine.
The mean renal clearance of ceftazidime was approximately 100 mL/min. The calculated plasma clearance of approximately 115 mL/min indicated nearly complete elimination of ceftazidime by the renal route. Administration of probenecid before dosing had no effect on the elimination kinetics of ceftazidime. This suggested that ceftazidime is eliminated by glomerular filtration and is not actively secreted by renal tubular mechanisms.
Since ceftazidime is eliminated almost solely by the kidneys, its serum half-life is significantly prolonged in patients with impaired renal function. Consequently, dosage adjustments in such patients as described in the DOSAGE AND ADMINISTRATION section are suggested.
Therapeutic concentrations of ceftazidime are achieved in the following body tissues and fluids.
[See table 2 below]

Table 2. Ceftazidime Concentrations in Body Tissues and Fluids

Tissue or Fluid	Dose/Route	No. of Patients	Time of Sample Postdose	Average Tissue or Fluid Level (mcg/mL or mcg/g)
Urine	500 mg IM	6	0-2 hr	2,100.0
	2 g IV	6	0-2 hr	12,000.0
Bile	2 g IV	3	90 min	36.4
Synovial fluid	2 g IV	13	2 hr	25.6
Peritoneal fluid	2 g IV	8	2 hr	48.6
Sputum	1 g IV	8	1 hr	9.0
Cerebrospinal fluid	2 g q8hr IV	5	120 min	9.8
(inflamed meninges)	2 g q8hr IV	6	180 min	9.4
Aqueous humor	2 g IV	13	1-3 hr	11.0
Blister fluid	1 g IV	7	2-3 hr	19.7
Lymphatic fluid	1 g IV	7	2-3 hr	23.4
Bone	2 g IV	8	0.67 hr	31.1
Heart muscle	2 g IV	35	30-280 min	12.7
Skin	2 g IV	22	30-180 min	6.6
Skeletal muscle	2 g IV	35	30-280 min	9.4
Myometrium	2 g IV	31	1-2 hr	18.7

Microbiology: Ceftazidime is bactericidal in action, exerting its effect by inhibition of enzymes responsible for cell-wall synthesis. A wide range of gram-negative organisms is susceptible to ceftazidime in vitro, including strains resistant to gentamicin and other aminoglycosides. In addition, ceftazidime has been shown to be active against gram-positive organisms. It is highly stable to most clinically important beta-lactamases, plasmid or chromosomal, which are produced by both gram-negative and gram-positive organisms and, consequently, is active against many strains resistant to ampicillin and other cephalosporins.
Ceftazidime has been shown to be active against the following organisms both in vitro and in clinical infections (see INDICATIONS AND USAGE).
Aerobes, Gram-negative: *Citrobacter* spp., including *Citrobacter freundii* and *Citrobacter diversus; Enterobacter* spp., including *Enterobacter cloacae* and *Enterobacter aerogenes; Escherichia coli; Haemophilus influenzae,* including ampicillin-resistant strains; *Klebsiella* spp. (including *Klebsiella pneumoniae*); *Neisseria meningitidis; Proteus mirabilis; Proteus vulgaris; Pseudomonas* spp. (including *Pseudomonas aeruginosa*); and *Serratia* spp.
Aerobes, Gram-positive: *Staphylococcus aureus,* including penicillinase- and non–penicillinase-producing strains; *Streptococcus agalactiae* (group B streptococci); *Streptococcus pneumoniae;* and *Streptococcus pyogenes* (group A beta-hemolytic streptococci).
Anaerobes: *Bacteroides* spp. (NOTE: many strains of *Bacteroides fragilis* are resistant).
Ceftazidime has been shown to be active in vitro against most strains of the following organisms; however, the clinical significance of these data is unknown: *Acinetobacter* spp., *Clostridium* spp. (not including *Clostridium difficile*), *Haemophilus parainfluenzae, Morganella morganii* (formerly *Proteus morganii*), *Neisseria gonorrhoeae, Peptococcus* spp., *Peptostreptococcus* spp., *Providencia* spp. (including *Providencia rettgeri,* formerly *Proteus rettgeri*), *Salmonella* spp., *Shigella* spp., *Staphylococcus epidermidis,* and *Yersinia enterocolitica.*
Ceftazidime and the aminoglycosides have been shown to be synergistic in vitro against *Pseudomonas aeruginosa* and the enterobacteriaceae. Ceftazidime and carbenicillin have also been shown to be synergistic in vitro against *Pseudomonas aeruginosa.*
Ceftazidime is not active in vitro against methicillin-resistant staphylococci, *Streptococcus faecalis* and many other enterococci, *Listeria monocytogenes, Campylobacter* spp., or *Clostridium difficile.*
Susceptibility Tests: ***Diffusion Techniques:*** Quantitative methods that require measurement of zone diameters give an estimate of antibiotic susceptibility. One such procedure[1-3] has been recommended for use with disks to test susceptibility to ceftazidime.
Reports from the laboratory giving results of the standard single-disk susceptibility test with a 30-mcg ceftazidime disk should be interpreted according to the following criteria:

Susceptible organisms produce zones of 18 mm or greater, indicating that the test organism is likely to respond to therapy.
Organisms that produce zones of 15 to 17 mm are expected to be susceptible if high dosage is used or if the infection is confined to tissues and fluids (e.g., urine) in which high antibiotic levels are attained.
Resistant organisms produce zones of 14 mm or less, indicating that other therapy should be selected.

Organisms should be tested with the ceftazidime disk since ceftazidime has been shown by in vitro tests to be active against certain strains found resistant when other beta-lactam disks are used.

Standardized procedures require the use of laboratory control organisms. The 30-mcg ceftazidime disk should give zone diameters between 25 and 32 mm for *Escherichia coli* ATCC 25922. For *Pseudomonas aeruginosa* ATCC 27853, the zone diameters should be between 22 and 29 mm. For *Staphylococcus aureus* ATCC 25923, the zone diameters should be between 16 and 20 mm.

Dilution Techniques: In other susceptibility testing procedures, e.g., ICS agar dilution or the equivalent, a bacterial isolate may be considered susceptible if the minimum inhibitory concentration (MIC) value for ceftazidime is not more than 16 mcg/mL. Organisms are considered resistant to ceftazidime if the MIC is ≥64 mcg/mL. Organisms having an MIC value of <64 mcg/mL but >16 mcg/mL are expected to be susceptible if high dosage is used or if the infection is confined to tissues and fluids (e.g., urine) in which high antibiotic levels are attained.

As with standard diffusion methods, dilution procedures require the use of laboratory control organisms. Standard ceftazidime powder should give MIC values in the range of 4 to 16 mcg/mL for *Staphylococcus aureus* ATCC 25923. For *Escherichia coli* ATCC 25922, the MIC range should be between 0.125 and 0.5 mcg/mL. For *Pseudomonas aeruginosa* ATCC 27853, the MIC range should be between 0.5 and 2 mcg/mL.

INDICATIONS AND USAGE

FORTAZ is indicated for the treatment of patients with infections caused by susceptible strains of the designated organisms in the following diseases:

1. **Lower Respiratory Tract Infections,** including pneumonia, caused by *Pseudomonas aeruginosa* and other *Pseudomonas* spp.; *Haemophilus influenzae,* including ampicillin-resistant strains; *Klebsiella* spp.; *Enterobacter* spp.; *Proteus mirabilis; Escherichia coli; Serratia* spp.; *Citrobacter* spp.; *Streptococcus pneumoniae;* and *Staphylococcus aureus* (methicillin-susceptible strains).
2. **Skin and Skin Structure Infections** caused by *Pseudomonas aeruginosa; Klebsiella* spp.; *Escherichia coli; Proteus* spp., including *Proteus mirabilis* and indole-positive *Proteus; Enterobacter* spp.; *Serratia* spp.; *Staphylococcus aureus* (methicillin-susceptible strains); and *Streptococcus pyogenes* (group A beta-hemolytic streptococci).
3. **Urinary Tract Infections,** both complicated and uncomplicated, caused by *Pseudomonas aeruginosa; Enterobacter* spp.; *Proteus* spp., including *Proteus mirabilis* and indole-positive *Proteus; Klebsiella* spp.; and *Escherichia coli.*
4. **Bacterial Septicemia** caused by *Pseudomonas aeruginosa, Klebsiella* spp., *Haemophilus influenzae, Escherichia coli, Serratia* spp., *Streptococcus pneumoniae,* and *Staphylococcus aureus* (methicillin-susceptible strains).
5. **Bone and Joint Infections** caused by *Pseudomonas aeruginosa, Klebsiella* spp., *Enterobacter* spp., and *Staphylococcus aureus* (methicillin-susceptible strains).
6. **Gynecologic Infections,** including endometritis, pelvic cellulitis, and other infections of the female genital tract caused by *Escherichia coli.*
7. **Intra-abdominal Infections,** including peritonitis caused by *Escherichia coli, Klebsiella* spp., and *Staphylococcus aureus* (methicillin-susceptible strains) and polymicrobial infections caused by aerobic and anaerobic organisms and *Bacteroides* spp. (many strains of *Bacteroides fragilis* are resistant).
8. **Central Nervous System Infections,** including meningitis, caused by *Haemophilus influenzae* and *Neisseria meningitidis.* Ceftazidime has also been used successfully in a limited number of cases of meningitis due to *Pseudomonas aeruginosa* and *Streptococcus pneumoniae.*

FORTAZ may be used alone in cases of confirmed or suspected sepsis. Ceftazidime has been used successfully in clinical trials as empiric therapy in cases where various concomitant therapies with other antibiotics have been used.

FORTAZ may also be used concomitantly with other antibiotics, such as aminoglycosides, vancomycin, and clindamycin; in severe and life-threatening infections; and in the immunocompromised patient. When such concomitant treatment is appropriate, prescribing information in the labeling for the other antibiotics should be followed. The dose depends on the severity of the infection and the patient's condition.

To reduce the development of drug-resistant bacteria and maintain the effectiveness of FORTAZ and other antibacterial drugs, FORTAZ should be used only to treat or prevent infections that are proven or strongly suspected to be caused by susceptible bacteria. When culture and susceptibility information are available, they should be considered in selecting or modifying antibacterial therapy. In the absence of such data, local epidemiology and susceptibility patterns may contribute to the empiric selection of therapy.

CONTRAINDICATIONS

FORTAZ is contraindicated in patients who have shown hypersensitivity to ceftazidime or the cephalosporin group of antibiotics.

WARNINGS

BEFORE THERAPY WITH FORTAZ IS INSTITUTED, CAREFUL INQUIRY SHOULD BE MADE TO DETERMINE WHETHER THE PATIENT HAS HAD PREVIOUS HYPERSENSITIVITY REACTIONS TO CEFTAZIDIME, CEPHALOSPORINS, PENICILLINS, OR OTHER DRUGS. IF THIS PRODUCT IS TO BE GIVEN TO PENICILLIN-SENSITIVE PATIENTS, CAUTION SHOULD BE EXERCISED BECAUSE CROSS-HYPERSENSITIVITY AMONG BETA-LACTAM ANTIBIOTICS HAS BEEN CLEARLY DOCUMENTED AND MAY OCCUR IN UP TO 10% OF PATIENTS WITH A HISTORY OF PENICILLIN ALLERGY. IF AN ALLERGIC REACTION TO FORTAZ OCCURS, DISCONTINUE THE DRUG. SERIOUS ACUTE HYPERSENSITIVITY REACTIONS MAY REQUIRE TREATMENT WITH EPINEPHRINE AND OTHER EMERGENCY MEASURES, INCLUDING OXYGEN, IV FLUIDS, IV ANTIHISTAMINES, CORTICOSTEROIDS, PRESSOR AMINES, AND AIRWAY MANAGEMENT, AS CLINICALLY INDICATED.

Pseudomembranous colitis has been reported with nearly all antibacterial agents, including ceftazidime, and may range in severity from mild to life threatening. Therefore, it is important to consider this diagnosis in patients who present with diarrhea subsequent to the administration of antibacterial agents.

Treatment with antibacterial agents alters the normal flora of the colon and may permit overgrowth of clostridia. Studies indicate that a toxin produced by *Clostridium difficile* is one primary cause of "antibiotic-associated colitis."

After the diagnosis of pseudomembranous colitis has been established, appropriate therapeutic measures should be initiated. Mild cases of pseudomembranous colitis usually respond to drug discontinuation alone. In moderate to severe cases, consideration should be given to management with fluids and electrolytes, protein supplementation, and treatment with an antibacterial drug clinically effective against *Clostridium difficile* colitis.

Elevated levels of ceftazidime in patients with renal insufficiency can lead to seizures, encephalopathy, coma, asterixis, neuromuscular excitability, and myoclonia (see PRECAUTIONS).

PRECAUTIONS

General: High and prolonged serum ceftazidime concentrations can occur from usual dosages in patients with transient or persistent reduction of urinary output because of renal insufficiency. The total daily dosage should be reduced when ceftazidime is administered to patients with renal insufficiency (see DOSAGE AND ADMINISTRATION). Elevated levels of ceftazidime in these patients can lead to seizures, encephalopathy, coma, asterixis, neuromuscular excitability, and myoclonia. Continued dosage should be determined by degree of renal impairment, severity of infection, and susceptibility of the causative organisms.

As with other antibiotics, prolonged use of FORTAZ may result in overgrowth of nonsusceptible organisms. Repeated evaluation of the patient's condition is essential. If superinfection occurs during therapy, appropriate measures should be taken.

Inducible type I beta-lactamase resistance has been noted with some organisms (e.g., *Enterobacter* spp., *Pseudomonas* spp., and *Serratia* spp.). As with other extended-spectrum beta-lactam antibiotics, resistance can develop during therapy, leading to clinical failure in some cases. When treating infections caused by these organisms, periodic susceptibility testing should be performed when clinically appropriate. If patients fail to respond to monotherapy, an aminoglycoside or similar agent should be considered.

Cephalosporins may be associated with a fall in prothrombin activity. Those at risk include patients with renal and hepatic impairment, or poor nutritional state, as well as patients receiving a protracted course of antimicrobial therapy. Prothrombin time should be monitored in patients at risk and exogenous vitamin K administered as indicated.

FORTAZ should be prescribed with caution in individuals with a history of gastrointestinal disease, particularly colitis.

Distal necrosis can occur after inadvertent intra-arterial administration of ceftazidime.

Prescribing FORTAZ in the absence of a proven or strongly suspected bacterial infection or a prophylactic indication is unlikely to provide benefit to the patient and increases the risk of the development of drug-resistant bacteria.

Information for Patients: Patients should be counseled that antibacterial drugs, including FORTAZ, should only be used to treat bacterial infections. They do not treat viral infections (e.g., the common cold). When FORTAZ is prescribed to treat a bacterial infection, patients should be told that although it is common to feel better early in the course of therapy, the medication should be taken exactly as directed. Skipping doses or not completing the full course of therapy may: (1) decrease the effectiveness of the immediate treatment, and (2) increase the likelihood that bacteria will develop resistance and will not be treatable by FORTAZ or other antibacterial drugs in the future.

Drug Interactions: Nephrotoxicity has been reported following concomitant administration of cephalosporins with aminoglycoside antibiotics or potent diuretics such as furosemide. Renal function should be carefully monitored, especially if higher dosages of the aminoglycosides are to be administered or if therapy is prolonged, because of the potential nephrotoxicity and ototoxicity of aminoglycosidic antibiotics. Nephrotoxicity and ototoxicity were not noted when ceftazidime was given alone in clinical trials.

Chloramphenicol has been shown to be antagonistic to beta-lactam antibiotics, including ceftazidime, based on in vitro studies and time kill curves with enteric gram-negative bacilli. Due to the possibility of antagonism in vivo, particularly when bactericidal activity is desired, this drug combination should be avoided.

Drug/Laboratory Test Interactions: The administration of ceftazidime may result in a false-positive reaction for glucose in the urine when using CLINITEST® tablets, Benedict's solution, or Fehling's solution. It is recommended that glucose tests based on enzymatic glucose oxidase reactions (such as CLINISTIX®) be used.

Carcinogenesis, Mutagenesis, Impairment of Fertility: Long-term studies in animals have not been performed to evaluate carcinogenic potential. However, a mouse Micronucleus test and an Ames test were both negative for mutagenic effects.

Pregnancy: *Teratogenic Effects:* Pregnancy Category B. Reproduction studies have been performed in mice and rats at doses up to 40 times the human dose and have revealed no evidence of impaired fertility or harm to the fetus due to FORTAZ. There are, however, no adequate and well-controlled studies in pregnant women. Because animal reproduction studies are not always predictive of human response, this drug should be used during pregnancy only if clearly needed.

Nursing Mothers: Ceftazidime is excreted in human milk in low concentrations. Caution should be exercised when FORTAZ is administered to a nursing woman.

Pediatric Use: (see DOSAGE AND ADMINISTRATION).

Geriatric Use: Of the 2,221 subjects who received ceftazidime in 11 clinical studies, 824 (37%) were 65 and over while 391 (18%) were 75 and over. No overall differences in safety or effectiveness were observed between these subjects and younger subjects, and other reported clinical experience has not identified differences in responses between the elderly and younger patients, but greater susceptibility of some older individuals to drug effects cannot be ruled out. This drug is known to be substantially excreted by the kidney, and the risk of toxic reactions to this drug may be greater in patients with impaired renal function. Because elderly patients are more likely to have decreased renal function, care should be taken in dose selection, and it may be useful to monitor renal function (see DOSAGE AND ADMINISTRATION).

ADVERSE REACTIONS

Ceftazidime is generally well tolerated. The incidence of adverse reactions associated with the administration of ceftazidime was low in clinical trials. The most common were local reactions following IV injection and allergic and gastrointestinal reactions. Other adverse reactions were encountered infrequently. No disulfiramlike reactions were reported.

The following adverse effects from clinical trials were considered to be either related to ceftazidime therapy or were of uncertain etiology:

Local Effects, reported in fewer than 2% of patients, were phlebitis and inflammation at the site of injection (1 in 69 patients).

Hypersensitivity Reactions, reported in 2% of patients, were pruritus, rash, and fever. Immediate reactions, generally manifested by rash and/or pruritus, occurred in 1 in 285 patients. Toxic epidermal necrolysis, Stevens-Johnson syndrome, and erythema multiforme have also been reported with cephalosporin antibiotics, including ceftazidime. Angioedema and anaphylaxis (bronchospasm and/or hypotension) have been reported very rarely.

Gastrointestinal Symptoms, reported in fewer than 2% of patients, were diarrhea (1 in 78), nausea (1 in 156), vomiting (1 in 500), and abdominal pain (1 in 416). The onset of pseudomembranous colitis symptoms may occur during or after treatment (see WARNINGS).

Central Nervous System Reactions (fewer than 1%) included headache, dizziness, and paresthesia. Seizures have been reported with several cephalosporins, including ceftazidime. In addition, encephalopathy, coma, asterixis, neuromuscular excitability, and myoclonia have been reported in renally impaired patients treated with unadjusted dosing regimens of ceftazidime (see PRECAUTIONS: General).

Less Frequent Adverse Events (fewer than 1%) were candidiasis (including oral thrush) and vaginitis.

Hematologic: Rare cases of hemolytic anemia have been reported.

Laboratory Test Changes noted during clinical trials with FORTAZ were transient and included: eosinophilia (1 in 13), positive Coombs test without hemolysis (1 in 23), thrombocytosis (1 in 45), and slight elevations in one or more of the hepatic enzymes, aspartate aminotransferase (AST, SGOT) (1 in 16), alanine aminotransferase (ALT, SGPT) (1 in 15), LDH (1 in 18), GGT (1 in 19), and alkaline phosphatase (1 in 23). As with some other cephalosporins, transient elevations of blood urea, blood urea nitrogen, and/or serum creatinine were observed occasionally. Transient leukopenia, neutropenia, agranulocytosis, thrombocytopenia, and lymphocytosis were seen very rarely.

POSTMARKETING EXPERIENCE WITH FORTAZ PRODUCTS

In addition to the adverse events reported during clinical trials, the following events have been observed during clinical practice in patients treated with FORTAZ and were reported spontaneously. For some of these events, data are insufficient to allow an estimate of incidence or to establish causation.

Continued on next page

Product information on these pages is effective as of August 2004. Further information is available at: GlaxoSmithKline, PO Box 13398, Research Triangle Park, NC 27709. 1-888-825-5249. Corporate Web Site: www.gsk.com

Fortaz—Cont.

General: Anaphylaxis; allergic reactions, which, in rare instances, were severe (e.g., cardiopulmonary arrest); urticaria; pain at injection site.
Hepatobiliary Tract: Hyperbilirubinemia, jaundice.
Renal and Genitourinary: Renal impairment.
Cephalosporin-Class Adverse Reactions: In addition to the adverse reactions listed above that have been observed in patients treated with ceftazidime, the following adverse reactions and altered laboratory tests have been reported for cephalosporin-class antibiotics:
Adverse Reactions: Colitis, toxic nephropathy, hepatic dysfunction including cholestasis, aplastic anemia, hemorrhage.
Altered Laboratory Tests: Prolonged prothrombin time, false-positive test for urinary glucose, pancytopenia.

OVERDOSAGE

Ceftazidime overdosage has occurred in patients with renal failure. Reactions have included seizure activity, encephalopathy, asterixis, neuromuscular excitability, and coma. Patients who receive an acute overdosage should be carefully observed and given supportive treatment. In the presence of renal insufficiency, hemodialysis or peritoneal dialysis may aid in the removal of ceftazidime from the body.

DOSAGE AND ADMINISTRATION

Dosage: The usual adult dosage is 1 gram administered intravenously or intramuscularly every 8 to 12 hours. The dosage and route should be determined by the susceptibility of the causative organisms, the severity of infection, and the condition and renal function of the patient.
The guidelines for dosage of FORTAZ are listed in Table 3. The following dosage schedule is recommended.
[See table 3 above]
Impaired Hepatic Function: No adjustment in dosage is required for patients with hepatic dysfunction.
Impaired Renal Function: Ceftazidime is excreted by the kidneys, almost exclusively by glomerular filtration. Therefore, in patients with impaired renal function (glomerular filtration rate [GFR] <50 mL/min), it is recommended that the dosage of ceftazidime be reduced to compensate for its slower excretion. In patients with suspected renal insufficiency, an initial loading dose of 1 gram of FORTAZ may be given. An estimate of GFR should be made to determine the appropriate maintenance dosage. The recommended dosage is presented in Table 4.

Table 4. Recommended Maintenance Dosages of FORTAZ in Renal Insufficiency
NOTE: IF THE DOSE RECOMMENDED IN TABLE 3 ABOVE IS LOWER THAN THAT RECOMMENDED FOR PATIENTS WITH RENAL INSUFFICIENCY AS OUTLINED IN TABLE 4, THE LOWER DOSE SHOULD BE USED.

Creatinine Clearance (mL/min)	Recommended Unit Dose of FORTAZ	Frequency of Dosing
50-31	1 gram	q12hr
30-16	1 gram	q24hr
15-6	500 mg	q24hr
<5	500 mg	q48hr

When only serum creatinine is available, the following formula (Cockcroft's equation)[4] may be used to estimate creatinine clearance. The serum creatinine should represent a steady state of renal function:
[See second table above]
In patients with severe infections who would normally receive 6 grams of FORTAZ daily were it not for renal insufficiency, the unit dose given in the table above may be increased by 50% or the dosing frequency may be increased appropriately. Further dosing should be determined by therapeutic monitoring, severity of the infection, and susceptibility of the causative organism.
In pediatric patients as for adults, the creatinine clearance should be adjusted for body surface area or lean body mass, and the dosing frequency should be reduced in cases of renal insufficiency.
In patients undergoing hemodialysis, a loading dose of 1 gram is recommended, followed by 1 gram after each hemodialysis period.
FORTAZ can also be used in patients undergoing intraperitoneal dialysis and continuous ambulatory peritoneal dialysis. In such patients, a loading dose of 1 gram of FORTAZ may be given, followed by 500 mg every 24 hours. In addition to IV use, FORTAZ can be incorporated in the dialysis fluid at a concentration of 250 mg for 2 L of dialysis fluid.
Note: Generally FORTAZ should be continued for 2 days after the signs and symptoms of infection have disappeared, but in complicated infections longer therapy may be required.
Administration: FORTAZ may be given intravenously or by deep IM injection into a large muscle mass such as the upper outer quadrant of the gluteus maximus or lateral part of the thigh. Intra-arterial administration should be avoided (see PRECAUTIONS).
Intramuscular Administration: For IM administration, FORTAZ should be constituted with one of the following diluents: Sterile Water for Injection, Bacteriostatic Water for Injection, or 0.5% or 1% Lidocaine Hydrochloride Injection. Refer to Table 5.

Table 3. Recommended Dosage Schedule

	Dose	Frequency
Adults		
Usual recommended dosage	**1 gram IV or IM**	**q8-12hr**
Uncomplicated urinary tract infections	250 mg IV or IM	q12hr
Bone and joint infections	2 grams IV	q12hr
Complicated urinary tract infections	500 mg IV or IM	q8-12hr
Uncomplicated pneumonia; mild skin and skin-structure infections	500 mg-1 gram IV or IM	q8hr
Serious gynecologic and intra-abdominal infections	2 grams IV	q8hr
Meningitis	2 grams IV	q8hr
Very severe life-threatening infections, especially in immunocompromised patients	2 grams IV	q8hr
Lung infections caused by *Pseudomonas* spp. in patients with cystic fibrosis with normal renal function*	30-50 mg/kg IV to a maximum of 6 grams per day	q8hr
Neonates (0–4 weeks)	30 mg/kg IV	q12hr
Infants and children (1 month-12 years)	30-50 mg/kg IV to a maximum of 6 grams per day†	q8hr

* Although clinical improvement has been shown, bacteriologic cures cannot be expected in patients with chronic respiratory disease and cystic fibrosis.
† The higher dose should be reserved for immunocompromised pediatric patients or pediatric patients with cystic fibrosis or meningitis.

$$\text{Males: Creatinine clearance (mL/min)} = \frac{\text{Weight (kg)} \times (140 - \text{age})}{72 \times \text{serum creatinine (mg/dL)}}$$

Females: 0.85 × the male value

Table 5. Preparation of Solutions of FORTAZ

Size	Amount of Diluent to be Added (mL)	Approximate Available Volume (mL)	Approximate Ceftazidime Concentration (mg/mL)
Intramuscular			
500-mg vial	1.5	1.8	280
1-gram vial	3.0	3.6	280
Intravenous			
500-mg vial	5.0	5.3	100
1-gram vial	10.0	10.6	100
2-gram vial	10.0	11.5	170
Infusion pack			
1-gram vial	100*	100	10
2-gram vial	100*	100	20
Pharmacy bulk package			
6-gram vial	26	30	200

***Note:** Addition should be in 2 stages (see Instructions for Constitution).

Intravenous Administration: The IV route is preferable for patients with bacterial septicemia, bacterial meningitis, peritonitis, or other severe or life-threatening infections, or for patients who may be poor risks because of lowered resistance resulting from such debilitating conditions as malnutrition, trauma, surgery, diabetes, heart failure, or malignancy, particularly if shock is present or pending.
For direct intermittent IV administration, constitute FORTAZ as directed in Table 5 with Sterile Water for Injection. Slowly inject directly into the vein over a period of 3 to 5 minutes or give through the tubing of an administration set while the patient is also receiving one of the compatible IV fluids (see COMPATIBILITY AND STABILITY).
For IV infusion, constitute the 1- or 2-gram infusion pack with 100 mL of Sterile Water for Injection or one of the compatible IV fluids listed under the COMPATIBILITY AND STABILITY section. Alternatively, constitute the 500-mg, 1-gram, or 2-gram vial and add an appropriate quantity of the resulting solution to an IV container with one of the compatible IV fluids.
Intermittent IV infusion with a Y-type administration set can be accomplished with compatible solutions. However, during infusion of a solution containing ceftazidime, it is desirable to discontinue the other solution.
ADD-Vantage vials are to be constituted only with 50 or 100 mL of 5% Dextrose Injection, 0.9% Sodium Chloride Injection, or 0.45% Sodium Chloride Injection in Abbott ADD-Vantage flexible diluent containers (see Instructions for Constitution). ADD-Vantage vials that have been joined to Abbott ADD-Vantage diluent containers and activated to dissolve the drug are stable for 24 hours at room temperature or for 7 days under refrigeration. Joined vials that have not been activated may be used within a 14-day period; this period corresponds to that for use of Abbott ADD-Vantage containers following removal of the outer packaging (overwrap).
Freezing solutions of FORTAZ in the ADD-Vantage system is not recommended.
[See table 5 above]
All vials of FORTAZ as supplied are under reduced pressure. When FORTAZ is dissolved, carbon dioxide is released and a positive pressure develops. For ease of use please follow the recommended techniques of constitution described on the detachable Instructions for Constitution section of the insert.
Solutions of FORTAZ, like those of most beta-lactam antibiotics, should not be added to solutions of aminoglycoside antibiotics because of potential interaction.
However, if concurrent therapy with FORTAZ and an aminoglycoside is indicated, each of these antibiotics can be administered separately to the same patient.
Directions for Use of FORTAZ Frozen in GALAXY® Plastic Containers: FORTAZ supplied as a frozen, sterile, iso-osmotic, nonpyrogenic solution in plastic containers is to be administered after thawing either as a continuous or intermittent IV infusion. The thawed solution is stable for 24 hours at room temperature or for 7 days if stored under refrigeration. **Do not refreeze.**
Thaw container at room temperature (25°C) or under refrigeration (5°C). Do not force thaw by immersion in water baths or by microwave irradiation. Components of the solution may precipitate in the frozen state and will dissolve upon reaching room temperature with little or no agitation. Potency is not affected. Mix after solution has reached room temperature. Check for minute leaks by squeezing bag firmly. Discard bag if leaks are found as sterility may be impaired. Do not add supplementary medication. Do not use unless solution is clear and seal is intact.
Use sterile equipment.
Caution: Do not use plastic containers in series connections. Such use could result in air embolism due to residual air being drawn from the primary container before administration of the fluid from the secondary container is complete.
Preparation for Administration:
1. Suspend container from eyelet support.
2. Remove protector from outlet port at bottom of container.
3. Attach administration set. Refer to complete directions accompanying set.

COMPATIBILITY AND STABILITY

Intramuscular: FORTAZ, when constituted as directed with Sterile Water for Injection, Bacteriostatic Water for Injection, or 0.5% or 1% Lidocaine Hydrochloride Injection, maintains satisfactory potency for 24 hours at room temperature or for 7 days under refrigeration. Solutions in Sterile Water for Injection that are frozen immediately after constitution in the original container are stable for 3 months when stored at -20°C. Once thawed, solutions should not be refrozen. Thawed solutions may be stored for up to 8 hours at room temperature or for 4 days in a refrigerator.
Intravenous: FORTAZ, when constituted as directed with Sterile Water for Injection, maintains satisfactory potency for 24 hours at room temperature or for 7 days under refrigeration. Solutions in Sterile Water for Injection in the infusion vial or in 0.9% Sodium Chloride Injection in

VIAFLEX® small-volume containers that are frozen immediately after constitution are stable for 6 months when stored at -20°C. Do not force thaw by immersion in water baths or by microwave irradiation. Once thawed, solutions should not be refrozen. Thawed solutions may be stored for up to 24 hours at room temperature or for 7 days in a refrigerator. More concentrated solutions in Sterile Water for Injection in the original container that are frozen immediately after constitution are stable for 3 months when stored at -20°C. Once thawed, solutions should not be refrozen. Thawed solutions may be stored for up to 8 hours at room temperature or for 4 days in a refrigerator.
FORTAZ is compatible with the more commonly used IV infusion fluids. Solutions at concentrations between 1 and 40 mg/mL in 0.9% Sodium Chloride Injection; 1/6 M Sodium Lactate Injection; 5% Dextrose Injection; 5% Dextrose and 0.225% Sodium Chloride Injection; 5% Dextrose and 0.45% Sodium Chloride Injection; 5% Dextrose and 0.9% Sodium Chloride Injection; 10% Dextrose Injection; Ringer's Injection, USP; Lactated Ringer's Injection, USP; 10% Invert Sugar in Water for Injection; and NORMOSOL®-M in 5% Dextrose Injection may be stored for up to 24 hours at room temperature or for 7 days if refrigerated.
The 1- and 2-g FORTAZ ADD-Vantage vials, when diluted in 50 or 100 mL of 5% Dextrose Injection, 0.9% Sodium Chloride Injection, or 0.45% Sodium Chloride Injection, may be stored for up to 24 hours at room temperature or for 7 days under refrigeration.
FORTAZ is less stable in Sodium Bicarbonate Injection than in other IV fluids. It is not recommended as a diluent. Solutions of FORTAZ in 5% Dextrose Injection and 0.9% Sodium Chloride Injection are stable for at least 6 hours at room temperature in plastic tubing, drip chambers, and volume control devices of common IV infusion sets.
Ceftazidime at a concentration of 4 mg/mL has been found compatible for 24 hours at room temperature or for 7 days under refrigeration in 0.9% Sodium Chloride Injection or 5% Dextrose Injection when admixed with: cefuroxime sodium (ZINACEF®) 3 mg/mL; heparin 10 or 50 U/mL; or potassium chloride 10 or 40 mEq/L.
Vancomycin solution exhibits a physical incompatibility when mixed with a number of drugs, including ceftazidime. The likelihood of precipitation with ceftazidime is dependent on the concentrations of vancomycin and ceftazidime present. It is therefore recommended, when both drugs are to be administered by intermittent IV infusion, that they be given separately, flushing the IV lines (with 1 of the compatible IV fluids) between the administration of these 2 agents.
Note: Parenteral drug products should be inspected visually for particulate matter before administration whenever solution and container permit.
As with other cephalosporins, FORTAZ powder as well as solutions tend to darken, depending on storage conditions; within the stated recommendations, however, product potency is not adversely affected.

HOW SUPPLIED

FORTAZ in the dry state should be stored between 15° and 30°C (59° and 86°F) and protected from light. FORTAZ is a dry, white to off-white powder supplied in vials and infusion packs as follows:

NDC 0173-0377-31 500-mg* Vial (Tray of 25)
NDC 0173-0378-35 1-g* Vial (Tray of 25)
NDC 0173-0379-34 2-g* Vial (Tray of 10)
NDC 0173-0380-32 1-g* Infusion Pack (Tray of 10)
NDC 0173-0381-32 2-g* Infusion Pack (Tray of 10)
NDC 0173-0382-37 6-g* Pharmacy Bulk Package (Tray of 6)
NDC 0173-0434-00 1-g ADD-Vantage® Vial (Tray of 25)
NDC 0173-0435-00 2-g ADD-Vantage® Vial (Tray of 10)

(The above ADD-Vantage vials are to be used only with Abbott ADD-Vantage diluent containers.)
FORTAZ frozen as a premixed solution of ceftazidime sodium should not be stored above -20°C. FORTAZ is supplied frozen in 50-mL, single-dose, plastic containers as follows:

NDC 0173-0412-00 1-g* Plastic Container (Carton of 24)
NDC 0173-0413-00 2-g* Plastic Container (Carton of 24)

*Equivalent to anhydrous ceftazidime.

REFERENCES

1. Bauer AW, Kirby WMM, Sherris JC, Turck M. Antibiotic susceptibility testing by a standardized single disk method. *Am J Clin Pathol.* 1966;45:493-496.
2. National Committee for Clinical Laboratory Standards. *Approved Standard: Performance Standards for Antimicrobial Disc Susceptibility Tests.* (M2-A3). December 1984.
3. Certification procedure for antibiotic sensitivity discs (21 CFR 460.1). *Federal Register.* May 30, 1974;39:19182-19184.
4. Cockcroft DW, Gault MH. Prediction of creatinine clearance from serum creatinine. *Nephron.* 1976;16:31-41.

FORTAZ® (ceftazidime for injection):
GlaxoSmithKline, Research Triangle Park, NC 27709
FORTAZ® (ceftazidime injection):
Manufactured for GlaxoSmithKline
Research Triangle Park, NC 27709
by Baxter Healthcare Corporation, Deerfield, IL 60015
FORTAZ and ZINACEF are registered trademarks of GlaxoSmithKline.
ADD-Vantage is a registered trademark of Abbott Laboratories.
CLINITEST and CLINISTIX are registered trademarks of Ames Division, Miles Laboratories, Inc.
GALAXY and VIAFLEX are registered trademarks of Baxter International Inc.
October 2003/RL-2043
Shown in Product Identification Guide, page 316

HAVRIX® ℞

[*hav' rix*]
(Hepatitis A Vaccine, Inactivated)

DESCRIPTION

HAVRIX (Hepatitis A Vaccine, Inactivated) is a noninfectious hepatitis A vaccine developed and manufactured by GlaxoSmithKline Biologicals. The virus (strain HM175) is propagated in MRC_5 human diploid cells. After removal of the cell culture medium, the cells are lysed to form a suspension. This suspension is purified through ultrafiltration and gel permeation chromatography procedures. Treatment of this lysate with formalin ensures viral inactivation. HAVRIX contains a sterile suspension of inactivated virus; viral antigen activity is referenced to a standard using an enzyme linked immunosorbent assay (ELISA), and is therefore expressed in terms of ELISA Units (EL.U.).
HAVRIX is supplied as a sterile suspension for intramuscular administration. The vaccine is ready for use without reconstitution; it must be shaken before administration since a fine white deposit with a clear colorless supernatant may form on storage. After shaking, the vaccine is a slightly turbid white suspension.
Each 1-mL adult dose of vaccine consists of not less than 1440 EL.U. of viral antigen, adsorbed on 0.5 mg of aluminum as aluminum hydroxide.
There are 2 pediatric dose formulations, each with its own dosing schedule (see DOSAGE AND ADMINISTRATION). The formulations are: Not less than 360 EL.U. of viral antigen/0.5 mL; not less than 720 EL.U. of viral antigen/0.5 mL. Each dose is adsorbed onto 0.25 mg of aluminum as aluminum hydroxide.
The vaccine preparations also contain 0.5% (w/v) of 2-phenoxyethanol as a preservative. Other excipients are: Amino acid supplement (0.3% w/v) in a phosphate-buffered saline solution and polysorbate 20 (0.05 mg/mL). Residual MRC_5 cellular proteins (not more than 5 mcg/mL) and traces of formalin (not more than 0.1 mg/mL) are present. Neomycin sulfate, an aminoglycoside antibiotic, is included in the cell growth media; only trace amounts (not more than 40 ng/mL) remain following purification.

CLINICAL PHARMACOLOGY

The hepatitis A virus (HAV) belongs to the picornavirus family. Only one serotype of HAV has been described.[1]
Hepatitis A is highly contagious with the predominant mode of transmission being person-to-person via the fecal-oral route. Infection has been shown to be spread (1) by contaminated water or food; (2) by infected food handlers[2]; (3) after breakdown in usual sanitary conditions or after floods or natural disasters; (4) by ingestion of raw or undercooked shellfish (oysters, clams, mussels) from contaminated waters[3]; (5) during travel to areas of the world with poor hygienic conditions[4,5]; (6) among institutionalized children and adults[6]; (7) in day-care centers where children have not been toilet trained[7]; (8) by parenteral transmission, either blood transfusions or sharing needles with infected people.[1]
The level of economic development influences the prevalence of hepatitis A and the age at which it is most likely to occur. In developing countries with poor hygiene and sanitation, about 90% of children are infected by age 5 years.[1] As conditions improve, the prevalence decreases and the age at which infection occurs increases. Hence it is more likely to occur in adulthood, when disease is generally more severe and more likely to be fatal.[1] In the United States, attack rates for hepatitis A infection are cyclical and vary by population. The rates have increased gradually from 9.2 per 100,000 in 1983 to 14.6 per 100,000 in 1989.[8]
The incubation period for hepatitis A averages 28 days (range: 15 to 50 days).[9] The course of hepatitis A infection is extremely variable, ranging from asymptomatic infection to icteric hepatitis. However, most adults (76% to 97%) become symptomatic.[10] Symptoms range from mild and transient to severe and prolonged and may include fever, nausea, vomiting, and diarrhea in the prodromal phase, followed by jaundice in up to 88% of adults, as well as hepatomegaly and biochemical evidence of hepatocellular damage.[10] Recovery is generally complete and followed by protection against HAV infection. However, illness may be prolonged, and relapse of clinical illness and viral shedding have been described.[11]
Hepatitis A infection is often asymptomatic in children under 2 years of age, who nonetheless excrete the virus in their stool and thereby serve as a source of infection.[10] In older patients and persons with underlying liver disease, it is generally much more severe.[1] This is reflected in mortality rates. While an overall case fatality rate of 0.6% has been reported, a case fatality rate of 2.7% has been reported in patients ≥49 years of age.[1] Indeed, while 67% of cases occur in children, over 70% of deaths occur in those over the age of 49 years.[1]
There is no chronic carrier state. The virus replicates in the liver and is excreted in bile. The highest concentrations of HAV are found in stools of infected persons during the 2-week period immediately before the onset of jaundice and decline after jaundice appears.[12] Children and infants may shed HAV for longer periods than adults, possibly lasting as long as several weeks after the onset of clinical illness.[13] Chronic shedding of HAV in feces has not been demonstrated, but relapses of hepatitis A can occur in as many as 20% of patients,[1,14] and fecal shedding of HAV may recur at this time.[11]
The presence of antibodies to HAV (anti-HAV) confers protection against hepatitis A infection. However, the lowest titer needed to confer protection has not been determined.
In a chimpanzee challenge study, the quality of protection afforded by immune globulin (IG) prepared from initially seronegative human volunteers vaccinated with HAVRIX was comparable to that afforded by commercial IG. In this experiment, chimpanzees immunized with either preparation developed passive-active immunity when challenged with wild-type HAV. No animal in either group developed clinical illness.
In vitro studies in a randomly selected subset of human subjects (n = 80) showed anti-HAV induced by HAVRIX to have functional activity. This was demonstrated by a neutralization assay and a competitive inhibition assay using a panel of monoclonal antibodies known to have neutralizing activity.
Immunogenicity in Adults: In 3 clinical studies involving over 400 healthy adult volunteers given a single 1440 EL.U. dose of HAVRIX, specific humoral antibodies against HAV were elicited in more than 96% of subjects when measured 1 month after vaccination. By day 15, 80% to 98% of vaccinees had already seroconverted (anti-HAV ≥20 mIU/mL [the lower limit of antibody measurement by current assay]). Geometric mean titers (GMTs) of seroconverters ranged from 264 to 339 mIU/mL at day 15 and increased to a range of 335 to 637 mIU/mL by 1 month following vaccination.[15]
The GMTs obtained following a single dose of HAVRIX are at least several times higher than that expected following receipt of IG.
In a clinical study using 2.5 to 5 times the standard dose of IG (standard dose = 0.02 to 0.06 mL/kg), the GMT in recipients was 146 mIU/mL at 5 days post-administration, 77 mIU/mL at month 1, and 63 mIU/mL at month 2.[15]
In 2 clinical trials in which a booster dose of 1440 EL.U. was given 6 months following the initial dose, 100% of vaccinees (n = 269) were seropositive 1 month after the booster dose, with GMTs ranging from 3,318 mIU/mL to 5,925 mIU/mL. The titers obtained from this additional dose approximate those observed several years after natural infection.
In a subset of vaccinees (n = 89), a single dose of HAVRIX 1440 EL.U. elicited specific anti-HAV neutralizing antibodies in more than 94% of vaccinees when measured 1 month after vaccination. These neutralizing antibodies persisted until month 6. One hundred percent of vaccinees had neutralizing antibodies when measured 1 month after a booster dose given at month 6.
Immunogenicity of HAVRIX was studied in subjects with chronic liver disease of various etiologies. 189 healthy adults and 220 adults with either chronic hepatitis B (n = 46), chronic hepatitis C (n = 104), or moderate chronic liver disease of other etiology (n = 70) were vaccinated with HAVRIX 1440 EL.U. on a 0- and 6-month schedule. The last group consisted of alcoholic cirrhosis (n = 17), autoimmune hepatitis (n = 10), chronic hepatitis/cryptogenic cirrhosis (n = 9), hemochromatosis (n = 2), primary biliary cirrhosis (n = 15), primary sclerosing cholangitis (n = 4), and unspecified (n = 13). At each time point, GMTs were lower for subjects with chronic liver disease than for healthy subjects. At month 7, the GMTs ranged from 478 mIU/mL (chronic hepatitis C) to 1,245 mIU/mL (healthy), as determined by a commercial ELISA. The relevance of these data to the duration of protection afforded by HAVRIX is unknown. One month after the first dose, seroconversion rates in adults with chronic liver disease were lower than in healthy adults. However, 1 month after the booster dose at month 6, seroconversion rates were similiar in all groups; rates ranged from 94.7% to 98.1%.
Immunogenicity in Children and Adolescents: In 6 clinical studies involving pediatric vaccinees (n = 762) ranging from 1 to 18 years of age, the GMT following 2 doses of HAVRIX 360 EL.U. given 1 month apart ranged from 197 to 660 mIU/mL. Ninety-nine percent of subjects seroconverted following 2 doses. When a booster (third) dose of HAVRIX 360 EL.U. was administered 6 months following the initial dose, all subjects were seropositive 1 month following the booster dose, with GMTs rising to a range of 3,388 to 4,643 mIU/mL. In 1 study in which children were followed for an additional 6 months, all subjects remained seropositive. Solicited adverse effects were similar in frequency and nature to those seen following administration of ENGERIX-B® [Hepatitis B Vaccine (Recombinant)].

Continued on next page

Product information on these pages is effective as of August 2004. Further information is available at: GlaxoSmithKline, PO Box 13398, Research Triangle Park, NC 27709. 1-888-825-5249. Corporate Web Site: www.gsk.com

Havrix—Cont.

In 4 clinical studies, children and adolescents (n = 314), ranging from 2 to 19 years of age, were immunized with 2 doses of HAVRIX 720 EL.U./0.5 mL given 6 months apart. One month after the first dose, seroconversion ranged from 96.8% to 100%, with GMTs of 194 mIU/mL to 305 mIU/mL. In studies in which sera were obtained 2 weeks following the initial dose, seroconversion ranged from 91.6% to 96.1%. One month following a booster dose at month 6, all subjects were seropositive, with GMTs ranging from 2,495 mIU/mL to 3,644 mIU/mL.[15]

In 1 additional study in which the booster dose was delayed until 1 year following the initial dose, 95.2% of the subjects were seropositive just prior to administration of the booster dose. One month later, all subjects were seropositive, with a GMT of 2,657 mIU/mL.[15]

Also, HAVRIX has been found to be highly efficacious in a clinical study of children at high risk of HAV infection (see below).

At present, the duration of protection afforded by HAVRIX has not been established. Therefore it is unknown if the protection provided to immunized children will last until adulthood.

Protective Efficacy: Protective efficacy with HAVRIX has been demonstrated in a double-blind, randomized controlled study in school children (age 1 to 16 years) in Thailand who were at high risk of HAV infection. A total of 40,119 children were randomized to be vaccinated with either HAVRIX 360 EL.U. or ENGERIX-B at 0, 1, and 12 months. 19,037 children received a primary course (0 and 1 months) of HAVRIX and 19,120 children received a primary course (0 and 1 months) of ENGERIX-B. 38,157 children entered surveillance at day 138 and were observed for an additional 8 months. Using the protocol-defined endpoint (≥2 days absence from school, ALT level >45 U/mL, and a positive result in the HAVAB-M test), 32 cases of clinical hepatitis A occurred in the control group; in the HAVRIX group, 2 cases were identified. These 2 cases were mild both in terms of biochemical and clinical indices of hepatitis A disease. Thus the calculated efficacy rate for prevention of clinical hepatitis A was 94% (95% confidence intervals 74% to 98%).[16]

In outbreak investigations occurring in the trial, 26 clinical cases of hepatitis A (of a total of 34 occurring in the trial) occurred. No cases occurred in HAVRIX vaccinees.

Using additional virological and serological analyses post hoc, the efficacy of HAVRIX was confirmed. Up to 3 additional cases of very mild clinical illness may have occurred in vaccinees. Using available testing, these illnesses could neither be proven nor disproven to have been caused by HAV. By including these as cases, the calculated efficacy rate for prevention of clinical hepatitis A would be 84% (95% confidence intervals 60% to 94%).

In a study designed to interrupt an epidemic of hepatitis A among Native Americans in Alaska, vaccination with a single dose of HAVRIX (1440 EL.U./mL in adults, 720 EL.U./0.5 mL in children and adolescents) appeared to be efficacious.[17]

INDICATIONS AND USAGE

HAVRIX is indicated for active immunization of persons ≥2 years of age against disease caused by hepatitis A virus (HAV).

HAVRIX will not prevent hepatitis caused by other agents such as hepatitis B virus, hepatitis C virus, hepatitis E virus, or other pathogens known to infect the liver.

Immunization with HAVRIX is indicated for those people desiring protection against hepatitis A. Primary immunization should be completed at least 2 weeks prior to expected exposure to HAV. Individuals who are, or will be, at increased risk of infection by HAV include:

- *Travelers:* Persons traveling to areas of higher endemicity for hepatitis A. These areas include, but are not limited to, Africa, Asia (except Japan), the Mediterranean basin, eastern Europe, the Middle East, Central and South America, Mexico, and parts of the Caribbean. Current CDC advisories should be consulted with regard to specific locales.
- *Military Personnel*
- *People Living in, or Relocating to, Areas of High Endemicity*
- *Certain Ethnic and Geographic Populations That Experience Cyclic Hepatitis A Epidemics, such as:* Native peoples of Alaska and the Americas.
- *People With Chronic Liver Disease,* including:
  - — Alcoholic cirrhosis
  - — Chronic hepatitis B
  - — Chronic hepatitis C
  - — Autoimmune hepatitis
  - — Primary biliary cirrhosis
- *Others:*
  - — Persons engaging in high-risk sexual activity (such as men having sex with men)[18]
  - — Residents of a community experiencing an outbreak of hepatitis A
  - — Users of illicit injectable drugs
  - — Persons who have clotting factor disorders (hemophiliacs and other recipients of therapeutic blood products). Hepatitis A transmission has been documented in persons with clotting disorders. Susceptible persons in this category, especially those who receive solvent detergent–treated clotting factor concentrates, should be vaccinated against hepatitis A[19] (see PRECAUTIONS and DOSAGE AND ADMINISTRATION).
  - — Although the epidemiology of hepatitis A does not permit the identification of other specific populations at high risk of disease, outbreaks of hepatitis A or exposure to hepatitis A virus have been described in a variety of populations in which HAVRIX may be useful:
- ■ Certain institutional workers (e.g., caretakers for the developmentally challenged)
- ■ Employees of child day-care centers
- ■ Laboratory workers who handle live hepatitis A virus
- ■ Handlers of primate animals that may be harboring HAV
- ■ *People Exposed to Hepatitis A:*

For those requiring both immediate and long-term protection, HAVRIX may be administered concomitantly with IG.

The Advisory Committee on Immunization Practices (ACIP) has issued the following recommendations regarding food handlers: "Persons who work as food handlers can contract hepatitis A and potentially transmit HAV to others. To decrease the frequency of evaluations of food handlers with hepatitis A and the need for post-exposure prophylaxis of patrons, consideration may be given to vaccination of employees who work in areas where state and local health authorities or private employers determine that such vaccination is cost-effective."[19]

CONTRAINDICATIONS

Hypersensitivity to any component of the vaccine, including neomycin, is a contraindication (see DESCRIPTION). This vaccine is contraindicated in patients with previous hypersensitivity to any hepatitis A-containing vaccine.

WARNINGS

There have been rare reports of anaphylaxis/anaphylactoid reactions following commercial use of the vaccine.

The vial stopper is latex-free. The tip cap and the rubber plunger of the needleless prefilled syringes contain dry natural latex rubber that may cause allergic reactions in latex sensitive individuals.

Hepatitis A has a relatively long incubation period (15 to 50 days). Hepatitis A vaccine may not prevent hepatitis A infection in individuals who have an unrecognized hepatitis A infection at the time of vaccination. Additionally, it may not prevent infection in individuals who do not achieve protective antibody titers (although the lowest titer needed to confer protection has not been determined).

PRECAUTIONS

General: As with any parenteral vaccine, epinephrine should be available for use in case of anaphylaxis or anaphylactoid reaction.

As with any vaccine, administration of HAVRIX should be delayed, if possible, in people with any febrile illness, except when, in the opinion of the physician, withholding vaccine entails the greater risk.

HAVRIX should be administered with caution to people with thrombocytopenia or a bleeding disorder since bleeding may occur following an intramuscular administration to these subjects.

As with any vaccine, if administered to immunosuppressed persons or persons receiving immunosuppressive therapy, the expected immune response may not be obtained.[20]

Care is to be taken by the healthcare provider for the safe and effective use of HAVRIX.

Prior to an injection of any vaccine, all known precautions should be taken to prevent adverse reactions. This includes a review of the patient's history with respect to possible hypersensitivity to the vaccine or similar vaccines.

A separate sterile syringe and needle (for single-dose vial) or a sterile disposable unit (prefilled syringe) must be used for each patient to prevent the transmission of infectious agents from person to person. Needles should not be recapped and should be properly disposed.

Special care should be taken to ensure that HAVRIX is not injected into a blood vessel.

Information for Patients: Patients, parents, or guardians should be fully informed of the benefits and risks of immunization with HAVRIX.

HAVRIX is indicated in a variety of situations (see INDICATIONS AND USAGE). For persons traveling to endemic or epidemic areas, current CDC advisories should be consulted with regard to specific locales.

Travelers should take all necessary precautions to avoid contact with or ingestion of contaminated food or water.

The duration of immunity following a complete schedule of immunization with HAVRIX has not been established.

Drug Interactions: Preliminary results suggest that the concomitant administration of a wide variety of other vaccines is unlikely to interfere with the immune response to HAVRIX.

As with other intramuscular injections, HAVRIX should be given with caution to individuals on anticoagulant therapy. When concomitant administration of other vaccines or IG is required, they should be given with different syringes and at different injection sites.

Carcinogenesis, Mutagenesis, Impairment of Fertility: HAVRIX has not been evaluated for its carcinogenic potential, mutagenic potential, or potential for impairment of fertility.

Pregnancy: Pregnancy Category C. Animal reproduction studies have not been conducted with HAVRIX. It is also not known whether HAVRIX can cause fetal harm when administered to a pregnant woman or can affect reproduction capacity. HAVRIX should be given to a pregnant woman only if clearly needed.

Nursing Mothers: It is not known whether HAVRIX is excreted in human milk. Because many drugs are excreted in human milk, caution should be exercised when HAVRIX is administered to a nursing woman.

Pediatric Use: HAVRIX is well tolerated and highly immunogenic and effective in children ≥2 years of age. (See CLINICAL PHARMACOLOGY for immunogenicity and efficacy data. See DOSAGE AND ADMINISTRATION for recommended dosage.)

ADVERSE REACTIONS

During clinical trials involving more than 31,000 individuals receiving doses ranging from 360 EL.U. to 1440 EL.U. and during extensive postmarketing experience in Europe, HAVRIX has been generally well tolerated. As with all pharmaceuticals, however, it is possible that expanded commercial use of the vaccine could reveal rare adverse events not observed in clinical studies.

The frequency of solicited adverse events tended to decrease with successive doses of HAVRIX. Most events reported were considered by the subjects as mild and did not last for more than 24 hours.

Of solicited adverse events in clinical trials, the most frequently reported by volunteers was injection-site soreness (56% of adults and 21% of children); however, less than 0.5% of soreness was reported as severe. Headache was reported by 14% of adults and less than 9% of children. Other solicited and unsolicited events occurring during clinical trials are listed below:

Incidence 1% to 10% of Injections:

Local Reactions at Injection Site: Induration, redness, swelling.

Body as a Whole: Fatigue, fever (>37.5°C), malaise.

Gastrointestinal: Anorexia, nausea.

Incidence <1% of Injections:

Local Reaction at Injection Site: Hematoma.

Dermatologic: Pruritus, rash, urticaria.

Respiratory: Pharyngitis, other upper respiratory tract infections.

Gastrointestinal: Abdominal pain, diarrhea, dysgeusia, vomiting.

Musculoskeletal: Arthralgia, elevation of creatine phosphokinase, myalgia.

Hematologic: Lymphadenopathy.

Central Nervous System: Hypertonic episode, insomnia, photophobia, vertigo.

Additional Safety Data: Safety data were obtained from 2 additional sources in which large populations were vaccinated. In an outbreak setting in which 4,930 individuals were immunized with a single dose of either 720 EL.U. or 1440 EL.U. of HAVRIX, the vaccine was well tolerated and no serious adverse events due to vaccination were reported. Overall, less than 10% of vaccinees reported solicited general adverse events following the vaccine. The most common solicited local adverse event was pain at the injection site, reported in 22.3% of subjects at 24 hours and decreasing to 2.4% by 72 hours. In a field efficacy trial, 19,037 children received the 360 EL.U. dose of HAVRIX. The most commonly reported adverse events following administration of HAVRIX were injection-site pain (9.5%) and tenderness (8.1%), which were reported following first doses of HAVRIX. Other adverse events were infrequent and comparable to the control vaccine ENGERIX-B. Additionally, no serious adverse events due to the vaccine were reported. The large trial further allowed for analysis of rare adverse events, including hospitalization and death. No significant differences were found between the cohorts.

In subjects with chronic liver disease, HAVRIX was safe and well tolerated. Local injection site reactions were similar among all 4 groups, and no serious adverse reactions attributed to the vaccine were reported in subjects with chronic liver disease.

Postmarketing Reports: Rare voluntary reports of adverse events in people receiving HAVRIX that have been reported since market introduction of the vaccine include the following:

Local: Localized edema.

While no causal relationship has been established, the following rare events have been reported.

Body as a Whole: Anaphylaxis/anaphylactoid reactions, somnolence.

Cardiovascular: Syncope.

Hepatobiliary: Jaundice, hepatitis.

Dermatologic: Erythema multiforme, hyperhydrosis, angioedema.

Respiratory: Dyspnea.

Hematologic: Lymphadenopathy.

Central Nervous System: Convulsions, encephalopathy, dizziness, neuropathy, myelitis, paresthesia, Guillain-Barré syndrome, multiple sclerosis.

Other: Congenital abnormality.

Reporting of Adverse Events: The US Department of Health and Human Services has established the Vaccine Adverse Events Reporting System (VAERS) to accept reports of suspected adverse events after the administration of any vaccine, including, but not limited to, the reporting of events required by the National Childhood Vaccine Injury Act of 1986. The toll-free number for VAERS forms and information is 1-800-822-7967.[21]

DOSAGE AND ADMINISTRATION

HAVRIX should be administered by intramuscular injection. *Do not inject intravenously, intradermally, or subcutaneously.* In adults, the injection should be given in the deltoid region. HAVRIX should not be administered in the gluteal region; such injections may result in suboptimal response.

HAVRIX may be administered concomitantly with IG, although the ultimate antibody titer obtained is likely to be lower than when the vaccine is given alone. HAVRIX has been administered simultaneously with ENGERIX-B without interference with their respective immune responses.

For individuals with clotting factor disorders at risk of hematoma formation following intramuscular injection, the ACIP recommends that when any intramuscular vaccine is indicated for such patients, ". . . the vaccine should be administered intramuscularly if, in the opinion of a physician familiar with the patient's bleeding risk, the vaccine can be administered with reasonable safety by this route. If the patient receives antihemophilia or other similar therapy, intramuscular vaccinations can be scheduled shortly after such therapy is administered. A fine needle (≤23 gauge) should be used for the vaccination and firm pressure applied to the site, without rubbing, for ≥2 minutes. The patient or family should be instructed concerning the risk for hematoma from the injection."[22]

When concomitant administration of other vaccines or IG is required, they should be given with different syringes and at different injection sites.

Preparation for Administration: Shake vial or syringe well before withdrawal and use. Parenteral drug products should be inspected visually for particulate matter or discoloration prior to administration. With thorough agitation, HAVRIX is a slightly turbid white suspension. Discard if it appears otherwise.

The vaccine should be used as supplied; no dilution or reconstitution is necessary. The full recommended dose of the vaccine should be used. After removal of the appropriate volume from a single-dose vial, any vaccine remaining in the vial should be discarded.

Primary immunization for adults consists of a single dose of 1440 EL.U. in 1 mL. Primary immunization for children and adolescents (2 through 18 years of age) may follow either of these 2 schedules:

Group	Dose	Schedule
Children and adolescents (2 through 18 years of age)	Primary course: 360 EL.U./0.5 mL	two doses, given 1 month apart (month 0 and month 1)
	Booster: 360 EL.U./0.5 mL	6 to 12 months after primary course
	OR	
	Primary course: 720 EL.U./0.5 mL	one dose (month 0)
	Booster: 720 EL.U./0.5 mL	6 to 12 months after primary course

Individuals should not be alternated between the 360 EL.U. and 720 EL.U. doses. Those who receive an initial 360 EL.U. dose should continue on the 360 EL.U. dosing schedule. Likewise, those individuals who receive a single 720 EL.U. primary dose should receive a 720 EL.U. booster dose.

For all age groups, a booster dose is recommended anytime between 6 and 12 months after the initiation of the primary dose in order to ensure the highest antibody titers.

In those with an impaired immune system, adequate anti-HAV response may not be obtained after the primary immunization course. Such patients may therefore require administration of additional doses of vaccine.

STORAGE

Store refrigerated between 2° and 8°C (36° and 46°F). Do not freeze; discard if product has been frozen. Do not dilute to administer.

HOW SUPPLIED

HAVRIX is supplied as a slightly turbid white suspension in vials and prefilled TIP-LOK® syringes.

360 EL.U./0.5 mL in Single-Dose Vials

NDC 58160-836-01 Package of 1

720 EL.U./0.5 mL in Single-Dose Vials and Prefilled Syringes

NDC 58160-837-01 Package of 1 Single-Dose Vial

NDC 58160-837-11 Package of 10 Single-Dose Vials

NDC 58160-837-46 Package of 5 Prefilled Disposable TIP-LOK Syringes (packaged without needles)

NDC 58160-837-50 Package of 25 Prefilled Disposable TIP-LOK Syringes (packaged without needles)

NDC 58160-837-56 Package of 25 Prefilled Disposable TIP-LOK Syringes with 1-inch 25-gauge BD SAFETYGLIDE™ Needles

NDC 58160-837-58 Package of 25 Prefilled Disposable TIP-LOK Syringes with 1-inch 23-gauge BD SAFETYGLIDE™ Needles

1440 EL.U./mL in Single-Dose Vials and Prefilled Syringes

NDC 58160-835-01 Package of 1 Single-Dose Vial

NDC 58160-835-41 Package of 1 Prefilled Disposable TIP-LOK Syringe (packaged without needle)

NDC 58160-835-46 Package of 5 Prefilled Disposable TIP-LOK Syringes (packaged without needles)

REFERENCES

1. Hadler SC. Global impact of hepatitis A virus infection changing patterns. In Hollinger FB, Lemon SM, Margolis H, eds. *Viral hepatitis and liver disease.* Baltimore, Williams & Wilkins; 1991:14-20.
2. Dienstag JL, Routenberg JA, Purcell RH, et al. Foodhandler-associated outbreak of hepatitis type A. An immune electron microscopic study. *Ann Intern Med* 1975;83:647-650.
3. Mackowiak PA, Caraway CT, Portnoy BL. Oyster-associated hepatitis: Lessons from the Louisiana experience. *Am J Epidemiol* 1976;103(2):181-191.
4. Woodson RD, Clinton JJ. Hepatitis prophylaxis abroad. Effectiveness of immune serum globulin in protecting Peace Corps volunteers. *JAMA* 1969;209(7):1053-1058.
5. Krugman S, Giles JP. Viral hepatitis. New light on an old disease. *JAMA* 1970;212(6):1019-1029.
6. Mosley JW. Hepatitis types B and non-B. Epidemiologic background. *JAMA* 1975;233(9):967-969.
7. Hadler SC, Erben JJ, Francis DP, et al. Risk factors for hepatitis A in day-care centers. *J Infect Dis* 1982;145(2): 255-261.
8. Shapiro CN, Shaw FE, Mandel EJ, et al. Epidemiology of hepatitis A in the United States. In Hollinger FB, Lemon SM, Margolis H, eds. *Viral hepatitis and liver disease.* Baltimore, Williams & Wilkins; 1991:71-76.
9. Centers for Disease Control. Protection against viral hepatitis: Recommendations of the Immunization Practices Advisory Committee (ACIP). *MMWR* 1990;39 (RR-2):1-26.
10. Lemon SM. Type A viral hepatitis: New developments in an old disease. *N Engl J Med* 1985;313(17):1059-1067.
11. Sjogren MH, Tanno H, Fay O, et al. Hepatitis A virus in stool during clinical relapse. *Ann Intern Med* 1987;106: 221-226.
12. Hollinger FB, Ticehurst J. Hepatitis A virus. In Hollinger FB, Robinson WS, Purcell RH, Gerin JL, Ticehurst J, eds. *Viral hepatitis.* New York, Raven Press, 1990:1-37.
13. Tassopoulos NC, Papaevangelou GJ, Ticehurst JR, et al. Fecal excretion of Greek strains of hepatitis A virus in patients with hepatitis A and in experimentally infected chimpanzees. *J Infect Dis* 1986;154(2):231-237.
14. Chiriaco P, Gaudalupi C, Armigliato M, et al. Polyphasic course of hepatitis type A in children. *J Infect Dis* 1986;153(2):378-379.
15. Data on file, GlaxoSmithKline.
16. Innis BL, Snitbhan R, Kunasol P, et al. Protection against hepatitis A by an inactivated vaccine. *JAMA* 1994;271(17):1328-1334.
17. McMahon BJ, Beller M, Williams J, et al. A program to control an outbreak of hepatitis A in Alaska by using an inactivated hepatitis A vaccine. *Arch Pediatr Adolesc Med* 1996;150:733-739.
18. Centers for Disease Control and Prevention. 1998 Guidelines for treatment of sexually transmitted diseases. *MMWR* 1998;47(RR-1):100.
19. Centers for Disease Control and Prevention. Prevention of hepatitis A through active or passive immunization: Recommendations of the Advisory Committee on Immunization Practices (ACIP). *MMWR* 1999;48(RR-12):26-29.
20. Centers for Disease Control and Prevention. Recommendations of the Advisory Committee on Immunization Practices (ACIP): Use of vaccines and immune globulins in persons with altered immunocompetence. *MMWR* 1993;42 (RR-4):1-18.
21. Centers for Disease Control. Vaccine Adverse Event Reporting System — United States. *MMWR* 1990; 39(41):730-733.
22. Centers for Disease Control and Prevention. General recommendations on immunization: Recommendations of the Advisory Committee on Immunization Practices and the American Academy of Family Physicians. *MMWR* 2002;51(RR-2):23-24.

Manufactured by GlaxoSmithKline Biologicals, Rixensart, Belgium, US License No. 1617

Distributed by GlaxoSmithKline, Research Triangle Park, NC 27709

HAVRIX and TIP-LOK are registered trademarks of GlaxoSmithKline

SAFETYGLIDE is a trademark of Becton, Dickinson and Company.

August 2003/HA:L17

Shown in Product Identification Guide, page 316

HYCAMTIN® ℞

[*hī-kam' tin*]

(topotecan hydrochloride)

For Injection

FOR INTRAVENOUS USE

> **WARNING**
> HYCAMTIN (topotecan hydrochloride) for Injection should be administered under the supervision of a physician experienced in the use of cancer chemotherapeutic agents. Appropriate management of complications is possible only when adequate diagnostic and treatment facilities are readily available.
> Therapy with HYCAMTIN should not be given to patients with baseline neutrophil counts of less than 1,500 cells/mm³. In order to monitor the occurrence of bone marrow suppression, primarily neutropenia, which may be severe and result in infection and death, frequent peripheral blood cell counts should be performed on all patients receiving HYCAMTIN.

DESCRIPTION

HYCAMTIN (topotecan hydrochloride) is a semi-synthetic derivative of camptothecin and is an anti-tumor drug with topoisomerase I-inhibitory activity.

HYCAMTIN for Injection is supplied as a sterile lyophilized, buffered, light yellow to greenish powder available in single-dose vials. Each vial contains topotecan hydrochloride equivalent to 4 mg of topotecan as free base. The reconstituted solution ranges in color from yellow to yellow-green and is intended for administration by intravenous infusion. Inactive ingredients are mannitol, 48 mg, and tartaric acid, 20 mg. Hydrochloric acid and sodium hydroxide may be used to adjust the pH. The solution pH ranges from 2.5 to 3.5.

The chemical name for topotecan hydrochloride is (*S*)-10-[(dimethylamino)methyl]-4-ethyl-4,9-dihydroxy-1*H*-pyrano[3′,4′:6,7] indolizino [1,2-*b*]quinoline-3,14-(4*H*,12*H*)-dione monohydrochloride. It has the molecular formula $C_{23}H_{23}N_3O_5$•HCl and a molecular weight of 457.9.

It is soluble in water and melts with decomposition at 213° to 218°C.

CLINICAL PHARMACOLOGY

Mechanism of Action: Topoisomerase I relieves torsional strain in DNA by inducing reversible single strand breaks. Topotecan binds to the topoisomerase I-DNA complex and prevents religation of these single strand breaks. The cytotoxicity of topotecan is thought to be due to double strand DNA damage produced during DNA synthesis, when replication enzymes interact with the ternary complex formed by topotecan, topoisomerase I, and DNA. Mammalian cells cannot efficiently repair these double strand breaks.

Pharmacokinetics: The pharmacokinetics of topotecan have been evaluated in cancer patients following doses of 0.5 to 1.5 mg/m² administered as a 30-minute infusion. Topotecan exhibits multiexponential pharmacokinetics with a terminal half-life of 2 to 3 hours. Total exposure (AUC) is approximately dose-proportional. Binding of topotecan to plasma proteins is about 35%.

Metabolism and Elimination: Topotecan undergoes a reversible pH dependent hydrolysis of its lactone moiety; it is the lactone form that is pharmacologically active. At pH ≤4, the lactone is exclusively present, whereas the ring-opened hydroxy-acid form predominates at physiologic pH. In vitro studies in human liver microsomes indicate that metabolism of topotecan to an N-demethylated metabolite represents a minor metabolic pathway.

In humans, about 30% of the dose is excreted in the urine and renal clearance is an important determinant of topotecan elimination (see Special Populations).

Special Populations: ***Gender:*** The overall mean topotecan plasma clearance in male patients was approximately 24% higher than that in female patients, largely reflecting difference in body size.

Geriatrics: Topotecan pharmacokinetics have not been specifically studied in an elderly population, but population pharmacokinetic analysis in female patients did not identify age as a significant factor. Decreased renal clearance, which is common in the elderly, is a more important determinant of topotecan clearance (see PRECAUTIONS and DOSAGE AND ADMINISTRATION).

Race: The effect of race on topotecan pharmacokinetics has not been studied.

Renal Impairment: In patients with mild renal impairment (creatinine clearance of 40 to 60 mL/min.), topotecan plasma clearance was decreased to about 67% of the value in patients with normal renal function. In patients with moderate renal impairment (Cl_{cr} of 20 to 39 mL/min.), topotecan plasma clearance was reduced to about 34% of the value in control patients, with an increase in half-life. Mean half-life, estimated in 3 renally impaired patients, was about 5.0 hours. Dosage adjustment is recommended for these patients (see DOSAGE AND ADMINISTRATION).

Continued on next page

Product information on these pages is effective as of August 2004. Further information is available at: GlaxoSmithKline, PO Box 13398, Research Triangle Park, NC 27709. 1-888-825-5249. Corporate Web Site: www.gsk.com

Hycamtin—Cont.

Hepatic Impairment: Plasma clearance in patients with hepatic impairment (serum bilirubin levels between 1.7 and 15.0 mg/dL) was decreased to about 67% of the value in patients without hepatic impairment. Topotecan half-life increased slightly, from 2.0 hours to 2.5 hours, but these hepatically impaired patients tolerated the usual recommended topotecan dosage regimen (see DOSAGE AND ADMINISTRATION).

Drug Interactions: Pharmacokinetic studies of the interaction of topotecan with concomitantly administered medications have not been formally investigated. In vitro inhibition studies using marker substrates known to be metabolized by human P450 CYP1A2, CYP2A6, CYP2C8/9, CYP2C19, CYP2D6, CYP2E, CYP3A, or CYP4A or dihydropyrimidine dehydrogenase indicate that the activities of these enzymes were not altered by topotecan. Enzyme inhibition by topotecan has not been evaluated in vivo.

Pharmacodynamics: The dose-limiting toxicity of topotecan is leukopenia. White blood cell count decreases with increasing topotecan dose or topotecan AUC. When topotecan is administered at a dose of 1.5 mg/m^2/day for 5 days, an 80% to 90% decrease in white blood cell count at nadir is typically observed after the first cycle of therapy.

CLINICAL STUDIES

Ovarian Cancer: HYCAMTIN was studied in 2 clinical trials of 223 patients given topotecan with metastatic ovarian carcinoma. All patients had disease that had recurred on, or was unresponsive to, a platinum-containing regimen. Patients in these 2 studies received an initial dose of 1.5 mg/m^2 given by intravenous infusion over 30 minutes for 5 consecutive days, starting on day 1 of a 21-day course.

One study was a randomized trial of 112 patients treated with HYCAMTIN (1.5 mg/m^2/day × 5 days starting on day 1 of a 21-day course) and 114 patients treated with paclitaxel (175 mg/m^2 over 3 hours on day 1 of a 21-day course). All patients had recurrent ovarian cancer after a platinum-containing regimen or had not responded to at least 1 prior platinum-containing regimen. Patients who did not respond to the study therapy, or who progressed, could be given the alternative treatment.

Response rates, response duration, and time to progression are shown in Table 1.

[See table 1 above]

Table 1. Efficacy of HYCAMTIN Versus Paclitaxel in Ovarian Cancer

Parameter	HYCAMTIN (n = 112)		Paclitaxel (n = 114)
Complete response rate	5%		3%
Partial response rate	16%		11%
Overall response rate	21%		14%
95% Confidence interval	13 to 28%		8 to 20%
(p-value)		(0.20)	
Response duration* (weeks)	n = 23		n = 16
Median	25.9		21.6
95% Confidence interval hazard-ratio	22.1 to 32.9		16.0 to 34.0
(HYCAMTIN:paclitaxel)		0.78	
(p-value)		(0.48)	
Time to progression (weeks)			
Median	18.9		14.7
95% Confidence interval hazard-ratio	12.1 to 23.6		11.9 to 18.3
(HYCAMTIN:paclitaxel)		0.76	
(p-value)		(0.07)	
Survival (weeks)			
Median	63.0		53.0
95% Confidence interval hazard-ratio	46.6 to 71.9		42.3 to 68.7
(HYCAMTIN:paclitaxel)		0.97	
(p-value)		(0.87)	

*The calculation for duration of response was based on the interval between first response and time to progression.

The median time to response was 7.6 weeks (range 3.1 to 21.7) with HYCAMTIN compared to 6.0 weeks (range 2.4 to 18.1) with paclitaxel. Consequently, the efficacy of HYCAMTIN may not be achieved if patients are withdrawn from treatment prematurely.

In the crossover phase, 8 of 61 (13%) patients who received HYCAMTIN after paclitaxel had a partial response and 5 of 49 (10%) patients who received paclitaxel after HYCAMTIN had a response (2 complete responses).

HYCAMTIN was active in ovarian cancer patients who had developed resistance to platinum-containing therapy, defined as tumor progression while on, or tumor relapse within 6 months after completion of, a platinum-containing regimen. One complete and 6 partial responses were seen in 60 patients, for a response rate of 12%. In the same study, there were no complete responders and 4 partial responders on the paclitaxel arm, for a response rate of 7%.

HYCAMTIN was also studied in an open-label, non-comparative trial in 111 patients with recurrent ovarian cancer after treatment with a platinum-containing regimen, or who had not responded to 1 prior platinum-containing regimen. The response rate was 14% (95% CI = 7% to 20%). The median duration of response was 22 weeks (range 4.6 to 41.9 weeks). The time to progression was 11.3 weeks (range 0.7 to 72.1 weeks). The median survival was 67.9 weeks (range 1.4 to 112.9 weeks).

Small Cell Lung Cancer: HYCAMTIN was studied in 426 patients with recurrent or progressive small cell lung cancer in 1 randomized, comparative study and in 3 single-arm studies.

Randomized Comparative Study: In a randomized, comparative, Phase 3 trial, 107 patients were treated with HYCAMTIN (1.5 mg/m^2/day × 5 days starting on day 1 of a 21-day course) and 104 patients were treated with CAV (1,000 mg/m^2 cyclophosphamide, 45 mg/m^2 doxorubicin, 2 mg vincristine administered sequentially on day 1 of a 21-day course). All patients were considered sensitive to first-line chemotherapy (responders who then subsequently progressed ≥60 days after completion of first-line therapy). A total of 77% of patients treated with HYCAMTIN and 79% of patients treated with CAV received platinum/etoposide with or without other agents as first-line chemotherapy.

Response rates, response duration, time to progression, and survival are shown in Table 2.

[See table 2 above]

Table 2. Efficacy of HYCAMTIN Versus CAV (cyclophosphamide-doxorubicin-vincristine) in Small Cell Lung Cancer Patients Sensitive to First-Line Chemotherapy

Parameter	HYCAMTIN (n = 107)		CAV (n = 104)
Complete response rate	0%		1%
Partial response rate	24%		17%
Overall response rate	24%		18%
Difference in overall response rates		6%	
95% Confidence interval of the difference		(−6 to 18%)	
Response duration* (weeks)	n = 26		n = 19
Median	14.4		15.3
95% Confidence interval hazard-ratio	13.1 to 18.0		13.1 to 23.1
(HYCAMTIN:CAV)		1.42 (0.73 to 2.76)	
(p-value)		(0.30)	
Time to progression (weeks)			
Median	13.3		12.3
95% Confidence interval hazard-ratio	11.4 to 16.4		11.0 to 14.1
(HYCAMTIN:CAV)		0.92 (0.69 to 1.22)	
(p-value)		(0.55)	
Survival (weeks)			
Median	25.0		24.7
95% Confidence interval hazard-ratio	20.6 to 29.6		21.7 to 30.3
(HYCAMTIN:CAV)		1.04 (0.78 to 1.39)	
(p-value)		(0.80)	

*The calculation for duration of response was based on the interval between first response and time to progression.

The time to response was similar in both arms: HYCAMTIN median of 6 weeks (range 2.4 to 15.7) versus CAV median 6 weeks (range 5.1 to 18.1).

Changes on a disease-related symptom scale in patients who received HYCAMTIN or who received CAV are presented in Table 3. It should be noted that not all patients had all symptoms, nor did all patients respond to all questions. Each symptom was rated on a 4 category scale with an improvement defined as a change in 1 category from baseline sustained over 2 courses. Limitations in interpretation of the rating scale and responses preclude formal statistical analysis.

[See table 3 above]

Table 3. Percentage of Patients With Symptom Improvement*: HYCAMTIN Versus CAV in Patients With Small Cell Lung Cancer

Symptom	HYCAMTIN (n = 107) n†	(%)	CAV (n = 104) n†	(%)
Shortness of breath	68	(28)	61	(7)
Interference with daily activity	67	(27)	63	(11)
Fatigue	70	(23)	65	(9)
Hoarseness	40	(33)	38	(13)
Cough	69	(25)	61	(15)
Insomnia	57	(33)	53	(19)
Anorexia	56	(32)	57	(16)
Chest pain	44	(25)	41	(17)
Hemoptysis	15	(27)	12	(33)

* Defined as improvement sustained over at least 2 courses compared to baseline.
† Number of patients with baseline and at least 1 post-baseline assessment.

Single Arm Studies: HYCAMTIN was also studied in 3 open-label, non-comparative trials in a total of 319 patients with recurrent or progressive small cell lung cancer after treatment with first-line chemotherapy. In all 3 studies, patients were stratified as either sensitive (responders who then subsequently progressed ≥90 days after completion of first-line therapy) or refractory (no response to first-line chemotherapy or who responded to first-line therapy and then progressed within 90 days of completing first-line therapy). Response rates ranged from 11% to 31% for sensitive patients and 2% to 7% for refractory patients. Median time to progression and median survival were similar in all 3 studies and the comparative study.

INDICATIONS AND USAGE

HYCAMTIN is indicated for the treatment of:

- metastatic carcinoma of the ovary after failure of initial or subsequent chemotherapy.
- small cell lung cancer sensitive disease after failure of first-line chemotherapy. In clinical studies submitted to support approval, sensitive disease was defined as disease responding to chemotherapy but subsequently progressing at least 60 days (in the Phase 3 study) or at least 90 days (in the Phase 2 studies) after chemotherapy (see CLINICAL STUDIES).

CONTRAINDICATIONS

HYCAMTIN is contraindicated in patients who have a history of hypersensitivity reactions to topotecan or to any of its ingredients. HYCAMTIN should not be used in patients who are pregnant or breast-feeding, or those with severe bone marrow depression.

WARNINGS

Bone marrow suppression (primarily neutropenia) is the dose-limiting toxicity of topotecan. Neutropenia is not cumulative over time. The following data on myelosuppression

Table 5. Summary of Non-hematologic Adverse Events in Patients Receiving HYCAMTIN

Non-hematologic Adverse Event	All Grades % Incidence		Grade 3 % Incidence		Grade 4 % Incidence	
	n = 879 Patients	n = 4124 Courses	n = 879 Patients	n = 4124 Courses	n = 879 Patients	n = 4124 Courses
Gastrointestinal						
Nausea	64	42	7	2	1	<1
Vomiting	45	22	4	1	1	<1
Diarrhea	32	14	3	1	1	<1
Constipation	29	15	2	1	1	<1
Abdominal pain	22	10	2	1	2	<1
Stomatitis	18	8	1	<1	<1	<1
Anorexia	19	9	2	1	<1	<1
Body as a Whole						
Fatigue	29	22	5	2	0	0
Fever	28	11	1	<1	<1	<1
Pain*	23	11	2	1	1	<1
Asthenia	25	13	4	1	2	<1
Skin/Appendages						
Alopecia	49	54	NA	NA	NA	NA
Rash†	16	6	1	<1	0	0
Respiratory System						
Dyspnea	22	11	5	2	3	1
Coughing	15	7	1	<1	0	0
CNS/Peripheral Nervous System						
Headache	18	7	1	<1	<1	0

* Pain includes body pain, back pain, and skeletal pain.
† Rash also includes pruritus, rash erythematous, urticaria, dermatitis, bullous eruption, and maculopapular rash.

Table 6. Comparative Toxicity Profiles for Ovarian Cancer Patients Randomized to Receive HYCAMTIN or Paclitaxel

Adverse Event	HYCAMTIN		Paclitaxel	
	Patients n = 112	Courses n = 597	Patients n = 114	Courses n = 589
Hematologic Grade 3/4	%	%	%	%
Grade 4 neutropenia (<500 cells/mL)	80	36	21	9
Grade 3/4 anemia (Hgb < 8 g/dL)	41	16	6	2
Grade 4 thrombocytopenia (<25,000 plts/mL)	27	10	3	<1
Fever/Grade 4 neutropenia	23	6	4	1
Documented sepsis	5	1	2	<1
Death related to sepsis	2	NA	0	NA
Non-hematologic Grade 3/4				
Gastrointestinal				
Abdominal pain	5	1	4	1
Constipation	5	1	0	0
Diarrhea	6	2	1	<1
Intestinal obstruction	5	1	4	1
Nausea	10	3	2	<1
Stomatitis	1	<1	1	<1
Vomiting	10	2	3	<1
Constitutional				
Anorexia	4	1	0	0
Dyspnea	6	2	5	1
Fatigue	7	2	6	2
Malaise	2	<1	2	<1
Neuromuscular				
Arthralgia	1	<1	3	<1
Asthenia	5	2	3	1

(Table continued on next page)

with topotecan is based on the combined experience of 879 patients with metastatic ovarian cancer or small cell lung cancer.

Neutropenia: Grade 4 neutropenia (<500 cells/mm^3) was most common during course 1 of treatment (60% of patients) and occurred in 39% of all courses, with a median duration of 7 days. The nadir neutrophil count occurred at a median of 12 days. Therapy-related sepsis or febrile neutropenia occurred in 23% of patients, and sepsis was fatal in 1%.

Thrombocytopenia: Grade 4 thrombocytopenia (<25,000/mm^3) occurred in 27% of patients and in 9% of courses, with a median duration of 5 days and platelet nadir at a median of 15 days. Platelet transfusions were given to 15% of patients in 4% of courses.

Anemia: Grade 3/4 anemia (<8 g/dL) occurred in 37% of patients and in 14% of courses. Median nadir was at day 15. Transfusions were needed in 52% of patients in 22% of courses.

In ovarian cancer, the overall treatment-related death rate was 1%. In the comparative study in small cell lung cancer, however, the treatment-related death rates were 5% for HYCAMTIN and 4% for CAV.

Monitoring of Bone Marrow Function: HYCAMTIN should be administered only in patients with adequate bone marrow reserves, including baseline neutrophil count of at least 1,500 cells/mm^3 and platelet count at least 100,000/mm^3. Frequent monitoring of peripheral blood cell counts should be instituted during treatment with HYCAMTIN. Patients should not be treated with subsequent courses of HYCAMTIN until neutrophils recover to >1,000 cells/mm^3, platelets recover to >100,000 cells/mm^3, and hemoglobin levels recover to 9.0 g/dL (with transfusion if necessary). Severe myelotoxicity has been reported when HYCAMTIN is used in combination with cisplatin (see Drug Interactions).

Pregnancy: HYCAMTIN may cause fetal harm when administered to a pregnant woman. The effects of topotecan on pregnant women have not been studied. If topotecan is used during a patient's pregnancy, or if a patient becomes pregnant while taking topotecan, she should be warned of the potential hazard to the fetus. Fecund women should be warned to avoid becoming pregnant. In rabbits, a dose of 0.10 mg/kg/day (about equal to the clinical dose on a mg/m^2 basis) given on days 6 through 20 of gestation caused maternal toxicity, embryolethality, and reduced fetal body weight. In the rat, a dose of 0.23 mg/kg/day (about equal to the clinical dose on a mg/m^2 basis) given for 14 days before mating through gestation day 6 caused fetal resorption, microphthalmia, pre-implant loss, and mild maternal toxicity. A dose of 0.10 mg/kg/day (about half the clinical dose on a mg/m^2 basis) given to rats on days 6 through 17 of gestation caused an increase in post-implantation mortality. This dose also caused an increase in total fetal malformations. The most frequent malformations were of the eye (microphthalmia, anophthalmia, rosette formation of the retina, coloboma of the retina, ectopic orbit), brain (dilated lateral and third ventricles), skull, and vertebrae.

PRECAUTIONS

General: Inadvertent extravasation with HYCAMTIN has been associated only with mild local reactions such as erythema and bruising.

Information for Patients: As with other chemotherapeutic agents, HYCAMTIN may cause asthenia or fatigue; if these symptoms occur, caution should be observed when driving or operating machinery.

Hematology: Monitoring of bone marrow function is essential (see WARNINGS and DOSAGE AND ADMINISTRATION).

Carcinogenesis, Mutagenesis, Impairment of Fertility: Carcinogenicity testing of topotecan has not been performed. Topotecan, however, is known to be genotoxic to mammalian cells and is a probable carcinogen. Topotecan was mutagenic to L5178Y mouse lymphoma cells and clastogenic to cultured human lymphocytes with and without metabolic activation. It was also clastogenic to mouse bone marrow. Topotecan did not cause mutations in bacterial cells.

Drug Interactions: Concomitant administration of G-CSF can prolong the duration of neutropenia, so if G-CSF is to be used, it should not be initiated until day 6 of the course of therapy, 24 hours after completion of treatment with HYCAMTIN.

Myelosuppression was more severe when HYCAMTIN was given in combination with cisplatin in Phase 1 studies. In a reported study on concomitant administration of cisplatin 50 mg/m^2 and HYCAMTIN at a dose of 1.25 mg/m^2/day × 5 days, 1 of 3 patients had severe neutropenia for 12 days and a second patient died with neutropenic sepsis. There are no adequate data to define a safe and effective regimen for HYCAMTIN and cisplatin in combination.

Greater myelosuppression is also likely to be seen when HYCAMTIN is used in combination with other cytotoxic agents, thereby necessitating a dose reduction. However, when combining HYCAMTIN with platinum agents (e.g., cisplatin or carboplatin), a distinct sequence-dependent interaction on myelosuppression has been reported. Coadministration of a platinum agent on day 1 of HYCAMTIN dosing required lower doses of each agent compared to coadministration on day 5 of the HYCAMTIN dosing schedule.

Pregnancy: Pregnancy Category D. (See WARNINGS.)

Nursing Mothers: It is not known whether the drug is excreted in human milk. Breast-feeding should be discontinued when women are receiving HYCAMTIN (see CONTRAINDICATIONS).

Pediatric Use: Safety and effectiveness in pediatric patients have not been established.

Geriatric Use: Of the 879 patients with metastatic ovarian cancer or small cell lung cancer in clinical studies of HYCAMTIN, 32% (n = 281) were 65 years of age and older,

Continued on next page

Product information on these pages is effective as of August 2004. Further information is available at: GlaxoSmithKline, PO Box 13398, Research Triangle Park, NC 27709. 1-888-825-5249. Corporate Web Site: www.gsk.com

Hycamtin—Cont.

while 3.8% (n = 33) were 75 years of age and older. No overall differences in effectiveness or safety were observed between these patients and younger adult patients. Other reported clinical experience has not identified differences in responses between the elderly and younger adult patients, but greater sensitivity of some older individuals cannot be ruled out.

There were no apparent differences in the pharmacokinetics of topotecan in elderly patients, once the age-related decrease in renal function was considered (see CLINICAL PHARMACOLOGY).

This drug is known to be substantially excreted by the kidney, and the risk of toxic reactions to this drug may be greater in patients with impaired renal function. Because elderly patients are more likely to have decreased renal function, care should be taken in dose selection, and it may be useful to monitor renal function (see DOSAGE AND ADMINISTRATION).

ADVERSE REACTIONS

Data in the following section are based on the combined experience of 453 patients with metastatic ovarian carcinoma, and 426 patients with small cell lung cancer treated with HYCAMTIN. Table 4 lists the principal hematologic toxicities, and Table 5 lists non-hematologic toxicities occurring in at least 15% of patients.

Table 4. Summary of Hematologic Adverse Events in Patients Receiving HYCAMTIN

Hematologic Adverse Event	Patients n = 879 % Incidence	Courses n = 4124 % Incidence
Neutropenia		
<1,500 cells/mm^3	97	81
<500 cells/mm^3	78	39
Leukopenia		
<3,000 cells/mm^3	97	80
<1,000 cells/mm^3	32	11
Thrombocytopenia		
<75,000 cells/mm^3	69	42
<25,000 cells/mm^3	27	9
Anemia		
<10 g/dL	89	71
<8 g/dL	37	14
Sepsis or fever/infection with grade 4 neutropenia	23	7
Platelet transfusions	15	4
RBC transfusions	52	22

[See table 5 at top of previous page]

Premedications were not routinely used in these clinical studies.

Hematologic: (See WARNINGS.)

Gastrointestinal: The incidence of nausea was 64% (8% grade 3/4), and vomiting occurred in 45% (6% grade 3/4) of patients (see Table 5). The prophylactic use of antiemetics was not routine in patients treated with HYCAMTIN. Thirty-two percent of patients had diarrhea (4% grade 3/4), 29% constipation (2% grade 3/4), and 22% had abdominal pain (4% grade 3/4). Grade 3/4 abdominal pain was 6% in ovarian cancer patients and 2% in small cell lung cancer patients.

Skin/Appendages: Total alopecia (grade 2) occurred in 31% of patients.

Central and Peripheral Nervous System: Headache (18% of patients) was the most frequently reported neurologic toxicity. Paresthesia occurred in 7% of patients but was generally grade 1.

Liver/Biliary: Grade 1 transient elevations in hepatic enzymes occurred in 8% of patients. Greater elevations, grade 3/4, occurred in 4%. Grade 3/4 elevated bilirubin occurred in <2% of patients.

Respiratory: The incidence of grade 3/4 dyspnea was 4% in ovarian cancer patients and 12% in small cell lung cancer patients.

Table 6 shows the grade 3/4 hematologic and major non-hematologic adverse events in the topotecan/paclitaxel comparator trial in ovarian cancer.

[See table 6 on previous page and above]

Premedications were not routinely used in patients randomized to HYCAMTIN, whereas patients receiving paclitaxel received routine pretreatment with corticosteroids, diphenhydramine, and histamine receptor type 2 blockers.

Table 7 shows the grade 3/4 hematologic and major non-hematologic adverse events in the topotecan/CAV comparator trial in small cell lung cancer.

[See table 7 at right]

Premedications were not routinely used in patients randomized to HYCAMTIN, whereas patients receiving CAV received routine pretreatment with corticosteroids, diphenhydramine, and histamine receptor type 2 blockers.

Postmarketing Reports of Adverse Events: Reports of adverse events in patients taking HYCAMTIN received after market introduction, which are not listed above, include the following:

Hematologic: *Rare:* Severe bleeding (in association with thrombocytopenia).

Table 6 *(cont.)*. Comparative Toxicity Profiles for Ovarian Cancer Patients Randomized to Receive HYCAMTIN or Paclitaxel

Adverse Event	HYCAMTIN		Paclitaxel	
	Patients n = 112	Courses n = 597	Patients n = 114	Courses n = 589
Hematologic Grade 3/4	%	%	%	%
Chest pain	2	<1	1	<1
Headache	1	<1	2	1
Myalgia	0	0	3	2
Pain*	5	1	7	2
Skin/Appendages				
Rash†	0	0	1	<1
Liver/Biliary				
Increased hepatic enzymes‡	1	<1	1	<1

*Pain includes body pain, skeletal pain, and back pain.
† Rash also includes pruritus, rash erythematous, urticaria, dermatitis, bullous eruption, and maculopapular rash.
‡ Increased hepatic enzymes includes increased SGOT/AST, increased SGPT/ALT, and increased hepatic enzymes.

Table 7. Comparative Toxicity Profiles for Small Cell Lung Cancer Patients Randomized to Receive HYCAMTIN or CAV

Adverse Event	HYCAMTIN		CAV	
	Patients n = 107	Courses n = 446	Patients n = 104	Courses n = 359
Hematologic Grade 3/4	%	%	%	%
Grade 4 neutropenia (<500 cells/mL)	70	38	72	51
Grade 3/4 anemia (Hgb < 8 g/dL)	42	18	20	7
Grade 4 thrombocytopenia (<25,000 plts/mL)	29	10	5	1
Fever/Grade 4 neutropenia	28	9	26	13
Documented sepsis	5	1	5	1
Death related to sepsis	3	NA	1	NA
Non-hematologic Grade 3/4				
Gastrointestinal				
Abdominal pain	6	1	4	2
Constipation	1	<1	0	0
Diarrhea	1	<1	0	0
Nausea	8	2	6	2
Stomatitis	2	<1	1	<1
Vomiting	3	<1	3	1
Constitutional				
Anorexia	3	1	4	2
Dyspnea	9	5	14	7
Fatigue	6	4	10	3
Neuromuscular				
Asthenia	9	4	7	2
Headache	0	0	2	<1
Pain*	5	2	7	4
Respiratory System				
Coughing	2	1	0	0
Pneumonia	8	2	6	2
Skin/Appendages				
Rash†	1	<1	1	<1
Liver/Biliary				
Increased hepatic enzymes‡	1	<1	0	0

*Pain includes body pain, skeletal pain, and back pain.
† Rash also includes pruritus, rash erythematous, urticaria, dermatitis, bullous eruption, and maculopapular rash.
‡ Increased hepatic enzymes includes increased SGOT/AST, increased SGPT/ALT, and increased hepatic enzymes.

Skin/Appendages: *Rare:* Severe dermatitis, severe pruritus.
Body as a Whole: *Infrequent:* Allergic manifestations; *rare:* Anaphylactoid reactions, angioedema.

OVERDOSAGE

There is no known antidote for overdosage with HYCAMTIN. The primary anticipated complication of overdosage would consist of bone marrow suppression.
One patient on a single-dose regimen of 17.5 mg/m^2 given on day 1 of a 21-day cycle had received a single dose of 35 mg/m^2. This patient experienced severe neutropenia (nadir of 320/mm^3) 14 days later but recovered without incident.
The LD_{10} in mice receiving single intravenous infusions of HYCAMTIN was 75 mg/m^2 (CI 95%: 47 to 97).

DOSAGE AND ADMINISTRATION

Prior to administration of the first course of HYCAMTIN, patients must have a baseline neutrophil count of >1,500 cells/mm^3 and a platelet count of >100,000 cells/mm^3. The recommended dose of HYCAMTIN is 1.5 mg/m^2 by intravenous infusion over 30 minutes daily for 5 consecutive days, starting on day 1 of a 21-day course. In the absence of tumor progression, a minimum of 4 courses is recommended because tumor response may be delayed. The median time to response in 3 ovarian clinical trials was 9 to 12 weeks, and median time to response in 4 small cell lung cancer trials was 5 to 7 weeks. In the event of severe neutropenia during any course, the dose should be reduced by 0.25 mg/m^2 for subsequent courses. Doses should be similarly reduced if the platelet count falls below 25,000 cells/mm^3. Alternatively, in the event of severe neutropenia, G-CSF may be administered following the subsequent course (before resorting to dose reduction) starting from day 6 of the course (24 hours after completion of topotecan administration).
Adjustment of Dose in Special Populations: *Hepatic Impairment:* No dosage adjustment appears to be required for treating patients with impaired hepatic function (plasma bilirubin >1.5 to <10 mg/dL).
Renal Functional Impairment: No dosage adjustment appears to be required for treating patients with mild renal impairment (Cl_{cr} 40 to 60 mL/min.). Dosage adjustment to 0.75 mg/m^2 is recommended for patients with moderate renal impairment (20 to 39 mL/min.). Insufficient data are available in patients with severe renal impairment to provide a dosage recommendation.
Elderly Patients: No dosage adjustment appears to be needed in the elderly other than adjustments related to renal function (see CLINICAL PHARMACOLOGY and PRECAUTIONS).

PREPARATION FOR ADMINISTRATION

Precautions: HYCAMTIN is a cytotoxic anticancer drug. As with other potentially toxic compounds, HYCAMTIN should be prepared under a vertical laminar flow hood while wearing gloves and protective clothing. If HYCAMTIN solution contacts the skin, wash the skin immediately and thoroughly with soap and water. If HYCAMTIN contacts mucous membranes, flush thoroughly with water.
Preparation for Intravenous Administration: Each HYCAMTIN 4-mg vial is reconstituted with 4 mL Sterile Water for Injection. Then the appropriate volume of the reconstituted solution is diluted in either 0.9% Sodium Chloride Intravenous Infusion or 5% Dextrose Intravenous Infusion prior to administration.
Because the lyophilized dosage form contains no antibacterial preservative, the reconstituted product should be used immediately.

STABILITY

Unopened vials of HYCAMTIN are stable until the date indicated on the package when stored between 20° and 25°C (68° and 77°F) [see USP] and protected from light in the original package. Because the vials contain no preservative, contents should be used immediately after reconstitution.
Reconstituted vials of HYCAMTIN diluted for infusion are stable at approximately 20° to 25°C (68° to 77°F) and ambient lighting conditions for 24 hours.

HOW SUPPLIED

HYCAMTIN for Injection is supplied in 4-mg (free base) single-dose vials.
NDC 0007-4201-01 (package of 1)
NDC 0007-4201-05 (package of 5)
Storage: Store the vials protected from light in the original cartons at controlled room temperature between 20° and 25°C (68° and 77°F) [see USP].
Handling and Disposal: Procedures for proper handling and disposal of anticancer drugs should be used. Several guidelines on this subject have been published.[1–8] There is no general agreement that all of the procedures recommended in the guidelines are necessary or appropriate.

REFERENCES

1. Brown KA, Esper P, Kelleher LO, Brace O'Neill JE, Polovich M, White JM, eds. In: *Chemotherapy and Biotherapy Guidelines and Recommendations for Practice.* Pittsburgh, PA: Oncology Nursing Society:2001:55-73.
2. National Institutes of Health Web site. Recommendations for the safe handling of cytotoxic drugs. NIH Publication 92-2621. Available at http://www.nih.gov/od/ors/ds/pubs/cyto/index.htm. Accessed August 21, 2002.
3. AMA Council on Scientific Affairs. Guidelines for handling parenteral antineoplastics. *JAMA.* 1985;253 (11):1590-1591.
4. National Study Commission on Cytotoxic Exposure —Recommendations for handling cytotoxic agents. 1987. Available from Louis P. Jeffrey, Sc.D., Chairman, National Study Commission on Cytotoxic Exposure. Massachusetts College of Pharmacy and Allied Health Sciences, 179 Longwood Avenue, Boston, MA 02115.
5. Clinical Oncological Society of Australia. Guidelines and recommendations for safe handling of antineoplastic agents. *Med J Austr.* 1983;1:426-428.
6. Jones RB, Frank R, Mass T. Safe handling of chemotherapeutic agents: A report from the Mount Sinai Medical Center. *CA-A Cancer for Clin.* 1983;33:258-263.
7. American Society of Hospital Pharmacists. ASHP Technical Assistance Bulletin on Handling Cytotoxic and Hazardous Drugs. *Am J Hosp Pharm.* 1990;47:1033-1049.
8. Controlling Occupational Exposure to Hazardous Drugs. (OSHA Work-Practice Guidelines), *Am J Health-Syst Pharm.* 1996;53:1669-1685.

GlaxoSmithKline, Research Triangle Park, NC 27709

July 2003/HY:L15
Shown in Product Identification Guide, page 316

IMITREX® ℞
[*ĭm'ĭ-trĕx*]
(sumatriptan succinate)
Injection

For Subcutaneous Use Only.

DESCRIPTION

IMITREX (sumatriptan succinate) Injection is a selective 5-hydroxytryptamine$_1$ receptor subtype agonist. Sumatriptan succinate is chemically designated as 3-[2-(dimethylamino)ethyl]-N-methyl-indole-5-methanesulfonamide succinate (1:1).
The empirical formula is $C_{14}H_{21}N_3O_2S \bullet C_4H_6O_4$, representing a molecular weight of 413.5.
Sumatriptan succinate is a white to off-white powder that is readily soluble in water and in saline.
IMITREX Injection is a clear, colorless to pale yellow, sterile, nonpyrogenic solution for subcutaneous injection. Each 0.5 mL of solution contains 6 mg of sumatriptan (base) as the succinate salt and 3.5 mg of sodium chloride, USP in water for injection, USP. The pH range of the solution is approximately 4.2 to 5.3. The osmolality of the injection is 291 mOsmol.

CLINICAL PHARMACOLOGY

Mechanism of Action: Sumatriptan has been demonstrated to be a selective agonist for a vascular 5-hydroxytryptamine$_1$ receptor subtype (probably a member of the $5\text{-}HT_{1D}$ family) with no significant affinity (as measured using standard radioligand binding assays) or pharmacological activity at $5\text{-}HT_2$, $5\text{-}HT_3$ receptor subtypes or at alpha$_1$-, alpha$_2$-, or beta-adrenergic; dopamine$_1$; dopamine$_2$; muscarinic; or benzodiazepine receptors.
The vascular $5\text{-}HT_1$ receptor subtype to which sumatriptan binds selectively, and through which it presumably exerts its antimigrainous effect, has been shown to be present on cranial arteries in both dog and primate, on the human basilar artery, and in the vasculature of the isolated dura mater of humans. In these tissues, sumatriptan activates this receptor to cause vasoconstriction, an action in humans correlating with the relief of migraine and cluster headache. In the anesthetized dog, sumatriptan selectively reduces the carotid arterial blood flow with little or no effect on arterial blood pressure or total peripheral resistance. In the cat, sumatriptan selectively constricts the carotid arteriovenous anastomoses while having little effect on blood flow or resistance in cerebral or extracerebral tissues.
Corneal Opacities: Dogs receiving oral sumatriptan developed corneal opacities and defects in the corneal epithelium. Corneal opacities were seen at the lowest dosage tested, 2 mg/kg/day, and were present after 1 month of treatment. Defects in the corneal epithelium were noted in a 60-week study. Earlier examinations for these toxicities were not conducted and no-effect doses were not established; however, the relative exposure at the lowest dose tested was approximately 5 times the human exposure after a 100-mg oral dose or 3 times the human exposure after a 6-mg subcutaneous dose.
Melanin Binding: In rats with a single subcutaneous dose (0.5 mg/kg) of radiolabeled sumatriptan, the elimination half-life of radioactivity from the eye was 15 days, suggesting that sumatriptan and its metabolites bind to the melanin of the eye. The clinical significance of this binding is unknown.
Pharmacokinetics: Pharmacokinetic parameters following a 6-mg subcutaneous injection into the deltoid area of the arm in 9 males (mean age, 33 years; mean weight, 77 kg) were systemic clearance: 1,194 ± 149 mL/min (mean ± S.D.), distribution half-life: 15 ± 2 minutes, terminal half-life: 115 ± 19 minutes, and volume of distribution central compartment: 50 ± 8 liters. Of this dose, 22% ± 4% was excreted in the urine as unchanged sumatriptan and 38% ± 7% as the indole acetic acid metabolite.
After a single 6-mg subcutaneous manual injection into the deltoid area of the arm in 18 healthy males (age, 24 ± 6 years; weight, 70 kg), the maximum serum concentration (C_{max}) was (mean ± standard deviation) 74 ± 15 ng/mL and the time to peak concentration (T_{max}) was 12 minutes after injection (range, 5 to 20 minutes). In this study, the same dose injected subcutaneously in the thigh gave a C_{max} of 61 ± 15 ng/mL by manual injection versus 52 ± 15 ng/mL by autoinjector techniques. The T_{max} or amount absorbed was not significantly altered by either the site or technique of injection.
The bioavailability of sumatriptan via subcutaneous site injection to 18 healthy male subjects was 97% ± 16% of that obtained following intravenous injection. Protein binding, determined by equilibrium dialysis over the concentration range of 10 to 1,000 ng/mL, is low, approximately 14% to 21%. The effect of sumatriptan on the protein binding of other drugs has not been evaluated.
Special Populations: *Renal Impairment:* The effect of renal impairment on the pharmacokinetics of sumatriptan has not been examined, but little clinical effect would be expected as sumatriptan is largely metabolized to an inactive substance.
Hepatic Impairment: The effect of hepatic disease on the pharmacokinetics of subcutaneously and orally administered sumatriptan has been evaluated. There were no statistically significant differences in the pharmacokinetics of subcutaneously administered sumatriptan in hepatically impaired patients compared to healthy controls. However, the liver plays an important role in the presystemic clearance of orally administered sumatriptan. Accordingly, the bioavailability of sumatriptan following oral administration may be markedly increased in patients with liver disease. In 1 small study of hepatically impaired patients (n = 8) matched for sex, age, and weight with healthy subjects, the hepatically impaired patients had an approximately 70% increase in AUC and C_{max} and a T_{max} 40 minutes earlier compared to the healthy subjects.
Age: The pharmacokinetics of sumatriptan in the elderly (mean age, 72 years, 2 males and 4 females) and in patients with migraine (mean age, 38 years, 25 males and 155 females) were similar to that in healthy male subjects (mean age, 30 years) (see PRECAUTIONS: Geriatric Use).
Race: The systemic clearance and C_{max} of sumatriptan were similar in black (n = 34) and Caucasian (n = 38) healthy male subjects.
Drug Interactions: *Monoamine Oxidase Inhibitors:* In vitro studies with human microsomes suggest that sumatriptan is metabolized by monoamine oxidase (MAO), predominantly the A isoenzyme. In a study of 14 healthy females, pretreatment with MAO-A inhibitor decreased the clearance of sumatriptan. Under the conditions of this experiment, the result was a 2-fold increase in the area under the sumatriptan plasma concentration × time curve (AUC), corresponding to a 40% increase in elimination half-life. No significant effect was seen with an MAO-B inhibitor.
Pharmacodynamics:
Typical Physiologic Responses:
Blood Pressure: (see WARNINGS)
Peripheral (small) Arteries: In healthy volunteers (n = 18), a study evaluating the effects of sumatriptan on peripheral (small vessel) arterial reactivity failed to detect a clinically significant increase in peripheral resistance.
Heart Rate: Transient increases in blood pressure observed in some patients in clinical studies carried out during sumatriptan's development as a treatment for migraine were not accompanied by any clinically significant changes in heart rate.
Respiratory Rate: Experience gained during the clinical development of sumatriptan as a treatment for migraine failed to detect an effect of the drug on respiratory rate.

CLINICAL STUDIES

Migraine: In US controlled clinical trials enrolling more than 1,000 patients during migraine attacks who were experiencing moderate or severe pain and 1 or more of the symptoms enumerated in Table 2 below, onset of relief began as early as 10 minutes following a 6-mg IMITREX Injection. Smaller doses of sumatriptan may also prove effective, although the proportion of patients obtaining adequate relief is decreased and the latency to that relief is greater.
In 1 well-controlled study where placebo (n = 62) was compared to 6 different doses of IMITREX Injection (n = 30 each group) in a single-attack, parallel-group design, the dose response relationship was found to be as shown in Table 1.
[See table 1 at top of next page]
In 2 US well-controlled clinical trials in 1,104 migraine patients with moderate and severe migraine pain, the onset of relief was rapid (less than 10 minutes). Headache relief, as evidenced by a reduction in pain from severe or moderately severe to mild or no headache, was achieved in 70% of the patients within 1 hour of a single 6-mg subcutaneous dose of IMITREX Injection. Headache relief was achieved in approximately 82% of patients within 2 hours, and 65% of all patients were pain free within 2 hours.
Table 2 shows the 1- and 2-hour efficacy results.
[See table 2 at top of next page]
IMITREX Injection also relieved photophobia, phonophobia (sound sensitivity), nausea, and vomiting associated with migraine attacks. Similar efficacy was seen when patients self-administered IMITREX Injection using an autoinjector.

Continued on next page

Product information on these pages is effective as of August 2004. Further information is available at: GlaxoSmithKline, PO Box 13398, Research Triangle Park, NC 27709. 1-888-825-5249. Corporate Web Site: www.gsk.com

Imitrex Injection—Cont.

The efficacy of IMITREX Injection is unaffected by whether or not migraine is associated with aura, duration of attack, gender or age of the patient, or concomitant use of common migraine prophylactic drugs (e.g., beta-blockers).

Cluster Headache: The efficacy of IMITREX Injection in the acute treatment of cluster headache was demonstrated in 2 randomized, double-blind, placebo-controlled, 2-period crossover trials. Patients age 21 to 65 were enrolled and were instructed to treat a moderate to very severe headache within 10 minutes of onset. Headache relief was defined as a reduction in headache severity to mild or no pain. In both trials, the proportion of individuals gaining relief at 10 or 15 minutes was significantly greater among patients receiving 6 mg of IMITREX Injection compared to those who received placebo (see Table 3). One study evaluated a 12-mg dose; there was no statistically significant difference in outcome between patients randomized to the 6- and 12-mg doses.

[See table 3 at right]

The Kaplan-Meier (product limit) Survivorship Plot (Figure 1) provides an estimate of the cumulative probability of a patient with a cluster headache obtaining relief after being treated with either sumatriptan or placebo.

Figure 1. Time to Relief From Time of Injection*

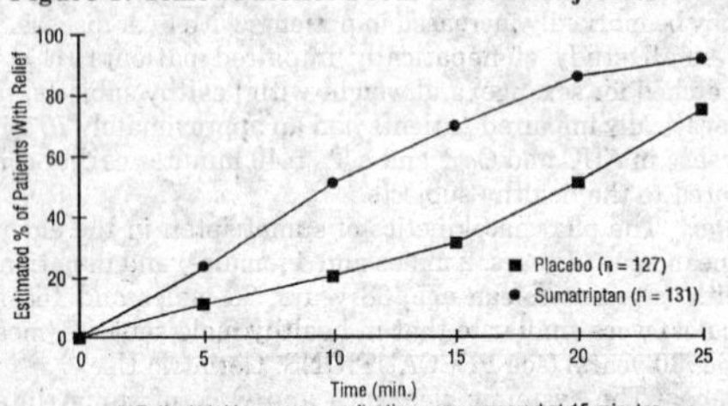

* Patients taking rescue medication were censored at 15 minutes.

The plot was constructed with data from patients who either experienced relief or did not require (request) rescue medication within a period of 2 hours following treatment. As a consequence, the data in the plot are derived from only a subset of the 258 headaches treated (rescue medication was required in 52 of the 127 placebo-treated headaches and 18 of the 131 sumatriptan-treated headaches).

Other data suggest that sumatriptan treatment is not associated with an increase in early recurrence of headache, and that treatment with sumatriptan has little effect on the incidence of later-occurring headaches (i.e., those occurring after 2, but before 18 or 24 hours).

INDICATIONS AND USAGE

IMITREX Injection is indicated for 1) the acute treatment of migraine attacks with or without aura and 2) the acute treatment of cluster headache episodes.

IMITREX Injection is not for use in the management of hemiplegic or basilar migraine (see CONTRAINDICATIONS).

CONTRAINDICATIONS

IMITREX Injection should not be given intravenously because of its potential to cause coronary vasospasm.

IMITREX Injection should not be given to patients with history, symptoms, or signs of ischemic cardiac, cerebrovascular, or peripheral vascular syndromes. In addition, patients with other significant underlying cardiovascular diseases should not receive IMITREX Injection. Ischemic cardiac syndromes include, but are not limited to, angina pectoris of any type (e.g., stable angina of effort and vasospastic forms of angina such as the Prinzmetal variant), all forms of myocardial infarction, and silent myocardial ischemia. Cerebrovascular syndromes include, but are not limited to, strokes of any type as well as transient ischemic attacks. Peripheral vascular disease includes, but is not limited to, ischemic bowel disease (see WARNINGS).

Because IMITREX Injection may increase blood pressure, it should not be given to patients with uncontrolled hypertension.

IMITREX Injection and any ergotamine-containing or ergot-type medication (like dihydroergotamine or methysergide) should not be used within 24 hours of each other, nor should IMITREX Injection and another 5-HT$_1$ agonist.

IMITREX Injection should not be administered to patients with hemiplegic or basilar migraine.

IMITREX Injection is contraindicated in patients with hypersensitivity to sumatriptan or any of its components.

IMITREX Injection is contraindicated in patients with severe hepatic impairment.

WARNINGS

IMITREX Injection should only be used where a clear diagnosis of migraine or cluster headache has been established. The prescriber should be aware that cluster headache patients often possess one or more predictive risk factors for coronary artery disease (CAD).

Risk of Myocardial Ischemia and/or Infarction and Other Adverse Cardiac Events: Sumatriptan should not be given to patients with documented ischemic or vasospastic CAD (see CONTRAINDICATIONS). It is strongly recommended that sumatriptan not be given to patients in whom unrecognized CAD is predicted by the presence of risk factors (e.g., hypertension, hypercholesterolemia, smoker, obesity, diabetes, strong family history of CAD, female with surgical or physiological menopause, or male over 40 years of age) unless a cardiovascular evaluation provides satisfactory clinical evidence that the patient is reasonably free of coronary artery and ischemic myocardial disease or other significant underlying cardiovascular disease. The sensitivity of cardiac diagnostic procedures to detect cardiovascular disease or predisposition to coronary artery vasospasm is modest, at best. If, during the cardiovascular evaluation, the patient's medical history or electrocardiographic investigations reveal findings indicative of or consistent with coronary artery vasospasm or myocardial ischemia, sumatriptan should not be administered (see CONTRAINDICATIONS).

For patients with risk factors predictive of CAD who are determined to have a satisfactory cardiovascular evaluation, it is strongly recommended that administration of the first dose of sumatriptan injection take place in the setting of a physician's office or similar medically staffed and equipped facility. Because cardiac ischemia can occur in the absence of clinical symptoms, consideration should be given to obtaining on the first occasion of use an electrocardiogram (ECG) during the interval immediately following IMITREX Injection, in these patients with risk factors.

It is recommended that patients who are intermittent long-term users of sumatriptan and who have or acquire risk factors predictive of CAD, as described above, undergo periodic interval cardiovascular evaluation as they continue to use sumatriptan. In considering this recommendation for periodic cardiovascular evaluation, it is noted that patients with cluster headache are predominantly male and over 40 years of age, which are risk factors for CAD.

The systematic approach described above is intended to reduce the likelihood that patients with unrecognized cardiovascular disease will be inadvertently exposed to sumatriptan.

Drug-Associated Cardiac Events and Fatalities: Serious adverse cardiac events, including acute myocardial infarction, life-threatening disturbances of cardiac rhythm, and death have been reported within a few hours following the administration of IMITREX Injection or IMITREX® (sumatriptan succinate) Tablets. Considering the extent of use of sumatriptan in patients with migraine, the incidence of these events is extremely low.

The fact that sumatriptan can cause coronary vasospasm, that some of these events have occurred in patients with no prior cardiac disease history and with documented absence of CAD, and the close proximity of the events to sumatriptan use support the conclusion that some of these cases were caused by the drug. In many cases, however, where there has been known underlying CAD, the relationship is uncertain.

Premarketing Experience With Sumatriptan: Among the more than 1,900 patients with migraine who participated in premarketing controlled clinical trials of subcutaneous sumatriptan, there were 8 patients who sustained clinical events during or shortly after receiving sumatriptan that may have reflected coronary artery vasospasm. Six of these 8 patients had ECG changes consistent with transient ischemia, but without accompanying clinical symptoms or signs. Of these 8 patients, 4 had either findings suggestive of CAD or risk factors predictive of CAD prior to study enrollment.

Of 6,348 patients with migraine who participated in premarketing controlled and uncontrolled clinical trials of oral sumatriptan, 2 experienced clinical adverse events shortly after receiving oral sumatriptan that may have reflected coronary vasospasm. Neither of these adverse events was associated with a serious clinical outcome.

Among approximately 4,000 patients with migraine who participated in premarketing controlled and uncontrolled clinical trials of sumatriptan nasal spray, 1 patient experienced an asymptomatic subendocardial infarction possibly subsequent to a coronary vasospastic event.

Postmarketing Experience With Sumatriptan: Serious cardiovascular events, some resulting in death, have been reported in association with the use of IMITREX Injection or IMITREX Tablets. The uncontrolled nature of postmarketing surveillance, however, makes it impossible to determine definitively the proportion of the reported cases that were actually caused by sumatriptan or to reliably assess causation in individual cases. On clinical grounds, the

Table 1. Dose Response Relationship for Efficacy

IMITREX Dose (mg)	% Patients With Relief* at 10 Minutes	% Patients With Relief* at 30 Minutes	% Patients With Relief* at 1 Hour	% Patients With Relief* at 2 Hours	Adverse Events Incidence (%)
placebo	5	15	24	21	55
1	10	40	43	40	63
2	7	23	57	43	63
3	17	47	57	60	77
4	13	37	50	57	80
6	10	63	73	70	83
8	23	57	80	83	93

*Relief is defined as the reduction of moderate or severe pain to no or mild pain after dosing without use of rescue medication.

Table 2. Efficacy Data From US Phase III Trials

	Study 1		Study 2	
1-Hour Data	Placebo (n = 190)	IMITREX 6 mg (n = 384)	Placebo (n = 180)	IMITREX 6 mg (n = 350)
Patients with pain relief (grade 0/1)	18%	70%*	26%	70%*
Patients with no pain	5%	48%*	13%	49%*
Patients without nausea	48%	73%*	50%	73%*
Patients without photophobia	23%	56%*	25%	58%*
Patients with little or no clinical disability§	34%	76%*	34%	76%*
	Study 1		**Study 2**	
2-Hour Data	Placebo†	IMITREX 6 mg‡	Placebo†	IMITREX 6 mg‡
Patients with pain relief (grade 0/1)	31%	81%*	39%	82%*
Patients with no pain	11%	63%*	19%	65%*
Patients without nausea	56%	82%*	63%	81%*
Patients without photophobia	31%	72%*	35%	71%*
Patients with little or no clinical disability§	42%	85%*	49%	84%*

*$P<0.05$ versus placebo.

† Includes patients that may have received an additional placebo injection 1 hour after the initial injection.

‡ Includes patients that may have received an additional 6 mg of IMITREX Injection 1 hour after the initial injection.

§ A successful outcome in terms of clinical disability was defined prospectively as ability to work mildly impaired or ability to work and function normally.

Table 3. Efficacy Data From the Pivotal Cluster Headache Studies

	Study 1		Study 2	
	Placebo (n = 39)	IMITREX 6 mg (n = 39)	Placebo (n = 88)	IMITREX 6 mg (n = 92)
Patients with pain relief (no/mild)				
5 minutes postinjection	8%	21%	7%	23%*
10 minutes postinjection	10%	49%*	25%	49%*
15 minutes postinjection	26%	74%*	35%	75%*

* $p<0.05$.

(n = Number of headaches treated.)

longer the latency between the administration of IMITREX and the onset of the clinical event, the less likely the association is to be causative. Accordingly, interest has focused on events beginning within 1 hour of the administration of IMITREX.

Cardiac events that have been observed to have onset within 1 hour of sumatriptan administration include: coronary artery vasospasm, transient ischemia, myocardial infarction, ventricular tachycardia and ventricular fibrillation, cardiac arrest, and death.

Some of these events occurred in patients who had no findings of CAD and appear to represent consequences of coronary artery vasospasm. However, among domestic reports of serious cardiac events within 1 hour of sumatriptan administration, the majority had risk factors predictive of CAD and the presence of significant underlying CAD was established in most cases (see CONTRAINDICATIONS).

Drug-Associated Cerebrovascular Events and Fatalities: Cerebral hemorrhage, subarachnoid hemorrhage, stroke, and other cerebrovascular events have been reported in patients treated with oral or subcutaneous sumatriptan, and some have resulted in fatalities. The relationship of sumatriptan to these events is uncertain. In a number of cases, it appears possible that the cerebrovascular events were primary, sumatriptan having been administered in the incorrect belief the symptoms experienced were a consequence of migraine when they were not. As with other acute migraine therapies, before treating headaches in patients not previously diagnosed as migraineurs, and in migraineurs who present with atypical symptoms, care should be taken to exclude other potentially serious neurological conditions. It should also be noted that patients with migraine may be at increased risk of certain cerebrovascular events (e.g., cerebrovascular accident, transient ischemic attack).

Other Vasospasm-Related Events: Sumatriptan may cause vasospastic reactions other than coronary artery vasospasm. Both peripheral vascular ischemia and colonic ischemia with abdominal pain and bloody diarrhea have been reported.

Increase in Blood Pressure: Significant elevation in blood pressure, including hypertensive crisis, has been reported on rare occasions in patients with and without a history of hypertension. Sumatriptan is contraindicated in patients with uncontrolled hypertension (see CONTRAINDICATIONS). Sumatriptan should be administered with caution to patients with controlled hypertension as transient increases in blood pressure and peripheral vascular resistance have been observed in a small proportion of patients.

Concomitant Drug Use: In patients taking MAO-A inhibitors, sumatriptan plasma levels attained after treatment with recommended doses are nearly double those obtained under other conditions. Accordingly, the coadministration of sumatriptan and an MAO-A inhibitor is not generally recommended. If such therapy is clinically warranted, however, suitable dose adjustment and appropriate observation of the patient is advised (see CLINICAL PHARMACOLOGY).

Use in Women of Childbearing Potential: (see PRECAUTIONS)

Hypersensitivity: Hypersensitivity (anaphylaxis/anaphylactoid) reactions have occurred on rare occasions in patients receiving sumatriptan. Such reactions can be life threatening or fatal. In general, hypersensitivity reactions to drugs are more likely to occur in individuals with a history of sensitivity to multiple allergens (see CONTRAINDICATIONS).

PRECAUTIONS

General: Chest, jaw, or neck tightness is relatively common after administration of IMITREX Injection. Chest discomfort and jaw or neck tightness have been reported following use of IMITREX Tablets and have also been reported infrequently following the administration of IMITREX® (sumatriptan) Nasal Spray. Only rarely have these symptoms been associated with ischemic ECG changes. However, because sumatriptan may cause coronary artery vasospasm, patients who experience signs or symptoms suggestive of angina following sumatriptan should be evaluated for the presence of CAD or a predisposition to Prinzmetal variant angina before receiving additional doses of sumatriptan and should be monitored electrocardiographically if dosing is resumed and similar symptoms recur. Similarly, patients who experience other symptoms or signs suggestive of decreased arterial flow, such as ischemic bowel syndrome or Raynaud syndrome, following sumatriptan should be evaluated for atherosclerosis or predisposition to vasospasm (see WARNINGS).

IMITREX should also be administered with caution to patients with diseases that may alter the absorption, metabolism, or excretion of drugs, such as impaired hepatic or renal function.

There have been rare reports of seizure following administration of sumatriptan. Sumatriptan should be used with caution in patients with a history of epilepsy or conditions associated with a lowered seizure threshold.

Care should be taken to exclude other potentially serious neurologic conditions before treating headache in patients not previously diagnosed with migraine or cluster headache or who experience a headache that is atypical for them. There have been rare reports where patients received sumatriptan for severe headaches that were subsequently shown to have been secondary to an evolving neurologic lesion (see WARNINGS). For a given attack, if a patient does not respond to the first dose of sumatriptan, the diagnosis of migraine or cluster headache should be reconsidered before administration of a second dose.

Binding to Melanin-Containing Tissues: Because sumatriptan binds to melanin, it could accumulate in melanin-rich tissues (such as the eye) over time. This raises the possibility that sumatriptan could cause toxicity in these tissues after extended use. However, no effects on the retina related to treatment with sumatriptan were noted in any of the toxicity studies. Although no systematic monitoring of ophthalmologic function was undertaken in clinical trials, and no specific recommendations for ophthalmologic function was undertaken in clinical trials, and no specific recommendations for ophthalmologic monitoring are offered, prescribers should be aware of the possibility of long-term ophthalmologic effects (see CLINICAL PHARMACOLOGY).

Corneal Opacities: Sumatriptan causes corneal opacities and defects in the corneal epithelium in dogs; this raises the possibility that these changes may occur in humans. While patients were not systematically evaluated for these changes in clinical trials, and no specific recommendations for monitoring are being offered, prescribers should be aware of the possibility of these changes (see CLINICAL PHARMACOLOGY).

Patients who are advised to self-administer IMITREX Injection in medically unsupervised situations should receive instruction on the proper use of the product from the physician or other suitably qualified health care professional prior to doing so for the first time.

Information for Patients: With the autoinjector, the needle penetrates approximately 1/4 of an inch (5 to 6 mm). Since the injection is intended to be given subcutaneously, intramuscular or intravascular delivery should be avoided. Patients should be directed to use injection sites with an adequate skin and subcutaneous thickness to accommodate the length of the needle. See PATIENT INFORMATION at the end of this labeling for the text of the separate leaflet provided for patients.

Laboratory Tests: No specific laboratory tests are recommended for monitoring patients prior to and/or after treatment with sumatriptan.

Drug Interactions: There is no evidence that concomitant use of migraine prophylactic medications has any effect on the efficacy of sumatriptan. In 2 Phase III trials in the US, a retrospective analysis of 282 patients who had been using prophylactic drugs (verapamil n = 63, amitriptyline n = 57, propranolol n = 94, for 45 other drugs n = 123) were compared to those who had not used prophylaxis (n = 452). There were no differences in relief rates at 60 minutes postdose for IMITREX Injection, whether or not prophylactic medications were used.

Ergot-containing drugs have been reported to cause prolonged vasospastic reactions. Because there is a theoretical basis that these effects may be additive, use of ergotamine-containing or ergot-type medications (like dihydroergotamine or methysergide) and sumatriptan within 24 hours of each other should be avoided (see CONTRAINDICATIONS).

MAO-A inhibitors reduce sumatriptan clearance, significantly increasing systemic exposure. Therefore, the use of sumatriptan in patients receiving MAO-A inhibitors is not ordinarily recommended. If the clinical situation warrants the combined use of sumatriptan and an MAOI, the dose of sumatriptan employed should be reduced (see CLINICAL PHARMACOLOGY and WARNINGS).

Selective serotonin reuptake inhibitors (SSRIs) (e.g., fluoxetine, fluvoxamine, paroxetine, sertraline) have been reported, rarely, to cause weakness, hyperreflexia, and incoordination when coadministered with sumatriptan. If concomitant treatment with sumatriptan and an SSRI is clinically warranted, appropriate observation of the patient is advised.

Drug/Laboratory Test Interactions: IMITREX is not known to interfere with commonly employed clinical laboratory tests.

Carcinogenesis, Mutagenesis, Impairment of Fertility: In carcinogenicity studies, rats and mice were given sumatriptan by oral gavage (rats, 104 weeks) or drinking water (mice, 78 weeks). Average exposures achieved in mice receiving the highest dose were approximately 110 times the exposure attained in humans after the maximum recommended single dose of 6 mg. The highest dose to rats was approximately 260 times the maximum single dose of 6 mg on a mg/m^2 basis. There was no evidence of an increase in tumors in either species related to sumatriptan administration.

Sumatriptan was not mutagenic in the presence or absence of metabolic activation when tested in 2 gene mutation assays (the Ames test and the in vitro mammalian Chinese hamster V79/HGPRT assay). In 2 cytogenetics assays (the in vitro human lymphocyte assay and the in vivo rat micronucleus assay) sumatriptan was not associated with clastogenic activity.

A fertility study (Segment I) by the subcutaneous route, during which male and female rats were dosed daily with sumatriptan prior to and throughout the mating period, has shown no evidence of impaired fertility at doses equivalent to approximately 100 times the maximum recommended single human dose of 6 mg on a mg/m^2 basis. However, following oral administration, a treatment-related decrease in fertility, secondary to a decrease in mating, was seen for rats treated with 50 and 500 mg/kg per day. The no-effect dose for this finding was approximately 8 times the maximum recommended single human dose of 6 mg on a mg/m^2 basis. It is not clear whether the problem is associated with the treatment of males or females or both.

Pregnancy: Pregnancy Category C. Sumatriptan has been shown to be embryolethal in rabbits when given daily at a dose approximately equivalent to the maximum recommended single human subcutaneous dose of 6 mg on a mg/m^2 basis. There is no evidence that establishes that sumatriptan is a human teratogen; however, there are no adequate and well-controlled studies in pregnant women. IMITREX Injection should be used during pregnancy only if the potential benefit justifies the potential risk to the fetus. In assessing this information, the following additional findings should be considered.

Embryolethality: When given intravenously to pregnant rabbits daily throughout the period of organogenesis, sumatriptan caused embryolethality at doses at or close to those producing maternal toxicity. The mechanism of the embryolethality is not known. These doses were approximately equivalent to the maximum single human dose of 6 mg on a mg/m^2 basis.

The intravenous administration of sumatriptan to pregnant rats throughout organogenesis at doses that are approximately 20 times a human dose of 6 mg on a mg/m^2 basis, did not cause embryolethality. Additionally, in a study of pregnant rats given subcutaneous sumatriptan daily prior to and throughout pregnancy, there was no evidence of increased embryo/fetal lethality.

Teratogenicity: Term fetuses from Dutch Stride rabbits treated during organogenesis with oral sumatriptan exhibited an increased incidence of cervicothoracic vascular and skeletal abnormalities. The functional significance of these abnormalities is not known. The highest no-effect dose for these effects was 15 mg/kg/day, approximately 50 times the maximum single dose of 6 mg on a mg/m^2 basis.

In a study in rats dosed daily with subcutaneous sumatriptan prior to and throughout pregnancy, there was no evidence of teratogenicity.

Pregnancy Registry: To monitor fetal outcomes of pregnant women exposed to IMITREX, GlaxoSmithKline maintains a Sumatriptan Pregnancy Registry. Physicians are encouraged to register patients by calling (800) 336-2176.

Nursing Mothers: Sumatriptan is excreted in human breast milk. Therefore, caution should be exercised when considering the administration of IMITREX Injection to a nursing woman.

Pediatric Use: Safety and effectiveness of IMITREX Injection in pediatric patients have not been established.

Completed placebo-controlled clinical trials evaluating oral sumatriptan (25 to 100 mg) in pediatric patients aged 12 to 17 years enrolled a total of 701 adolescent migraineurs. These studies did not establish the efficacy of oral sumatriptan compared to placebo in the treatment of migraine in adolescents. Adverse events observed in these clinical trials were similar in nature to those reported in clinical trials in adults. The frequency of all adverse events in these patients appeared to be both dose- and age-dependent, with younger patients reporting events more commonly than older adolescents. Postmarketing experience includes a limited number of reports that describe pediatric patients who have experienced adverse events, some clinically serious, after use of subcutaneous sumatriptan and/or oral sumatriptan. These reports include events similar in nature to those reported rarely in adults. A myocardial infarct has been reported in a 14-year-old male following the use of oral sumatriptan; clinical signs occurred within 1 day of drug administration. Since clinical data to determine the frequency of serious adverse events in pediatric patients who might receive injectable, oral, or intranasal sumatriptan are not presently available, the use of sumatriptan in patients aged younger than 18 years is not recommended.

Geriatric Use: The use of sumatriptan in elderly patients is not recommended because elderly patients are more likely to have decreased hepatic function, they are at higher risk for CAD, and blood pressure increases may be more pronounced in the elderly (see WARNINGS).

ADVERSE REACTIONS

Serious cardiac events, including some that have been fatal, have occurred following the use of IMITREX Injection or Tablets. These events are extremely rare and most have been reported in patients with risk factors predictive of CAD. Events reported have included coronary artery vasospasm, transient myocardial ischemia, myocardial infarction, ventricular tachycardia, and ventricular fibrillation (see CONTRAINDICATIONS, WARNINGS, and PRECAUTIONS).

Significant hypertensive episodes, including hypertensive crises, have been reported on rare occasions in patients with or without a history of hypertension (see WARNINGS).

Among patients in clinical trials of subcutaneous IMITREX Injection (n = 6,218), up to 3.5% of patients withdrew for reasons related to adverse events.

Incidence in Controlled Clinical Trials of Migraine Headache: Table 4 lists adverse events that occurred in 2 large US, Phase III, placebo-controlled clinical trials in migraine

Continued on next page

Product information on these pages is effective as of August 2004. Further information is available at: GlaxoSmithKline, PO Box 13398, Research Triangle Park, NC 27709. 1-888-825-5249. Corporate Web Site: www.gsk.com

Imitrex Injection—Cont.

patients following either a single dose of IMITREX Injection or placebo. Only events that occurred at a frequency of 1% or more in groups treated with IMITREX Injection and were at least as frequent as in the placebo group are included in Table 4.

[See table 4 at right]

The incidence of adverse events in controlled clinical trials was not affected by gender or age of the patients. There were insufficient data to assess the impact of race on the incidence of adverse events.

Incidence in Controlled Trials of Cluster Headache: In the controlled clinical trials assessing sumatriptan's efficacy as a treatment for cluster headache, no new significant adverse events associated with the use of sumatriptan were detected that had not already been identified in association with the drug's use in migraine.

Overall, the frequency of adverse events reported in the studies of cluster headache were generally lower. Exceptions include reports of paresthesia (5% IMITREX, 0% placebo), nausea and vomiting (4% IMITREX, 0% placebo), and bronchospasm (1% IMITREX, 0% placebo).

Other Events Observed in Association With the Administration of IMITREX Injection: In the paragraphs that follow, the frequencies of less commonly reported adverse clinical events are presented. Because the reports include events observed in open and uncontrolled studies, the role of IMITREX Injection in their causation cannot be reliably determined. Furthermore, variability associated with adverse event reporting, the terminology used to describe adverse events, etc., limit the value of the quantitative frequency estimates provided.

Event frequencies are calculated as the number of patients reporting an event divided by the total number of patients (n = 6,218) exposed to subcutaneous IMITREX Injection. All reported events are included except those already listed in the previous table, those too general to be informative, and those not reasonably associated with the use of the drug. Events are further classified within body system categories and enumerated in order of decreasing frequency using the following definitions: frequent adverse events are defined as those occurring in at least 1/100 patients, infrequent adverse events are those occurring in 1/100 to 1/1,000 patients, and rare adverse events are those occurring in fewer than 1/1,000 patients.

Cardiovascular: Infrequent were hypertension, hypotension, bradycardia, tachycardia, palpitations, pulsating sensations, various transient ECG changes (nonspecific ST or T wave changes, prolongation of PR or QTc intervals, sinus arrhythmia, nonsustained ventricular premature beats, isolated junctional ectopic beats, atrial ectopic beats, delayed activation of the right ventricle), and syncope. Rare were pallor, arrhythmia, abnormal pulse, vasodilatation, and Raynaud syndrome.

Endocrine and Metabolic: Infrequent was thirst. Rare were polydipsia and dehydration.

Eye: Infrequent was irritation of the eye.

Gastrointestinal: Infrequent were gastroesophageal reflux, diarrhea, and disturbances of liver function tests. Rare were peptic ulcer, retching, flatulence/eructation, and gallstones.

Musculoskeletal: Infrequent were various joint disturbances (pain, stiffness, swelling, ache). Rare were muscle stiffness, need to flex calf muscles, backache, muscle tiredness, and swelling of the extremities.

Neurological: Infrequent were mental confusion, euphoria, agitation, relaxation, chills, sensation of lightness, tremor, shivering, disturbances of taste, prickling sensations, paresthesia, stinging sensations, facial pain, photophobia, and lacrimation. Rare were transient hemiplegia, hysteria, globus hystericus, intoxication, depression, myoclonia, monoplegia/diplegia, sleep disturbance, difficulties in concentration, disturbances of smell, hyperesthesia, dysesthesia, simultaneous hot and cold sensations, tickling sensations, dysarthria, yawning, reduced appetite, hunger, and dystonia.

Respiratory: Infrequent was dyspnea. Rare were influenza, diseases of the lower respiratory tract, and hiccoughs.

Skin: Infrequent were erythema, pruritus, and skin rashes and eruptions. Rare was skin tenderness.

Urogenital: Rare were dysuria, frequency, dysmenorrhea, and renal calculus.

Miscellaneous: Infrequent were miscellaneous laboratory abnormalities, including minor disturbances in liver function tests, "serotonin agonist effect," and hypersensitivity to various agents. Rare was fever.

Other Events Observed in the Clinical Development of IMITREX: The following adverse events occurred in clinical trials with IMITREX Tablets and IMITREX Nasal Spray. Because the reports include events observed in open and uncontrolled studies, the role of IMITREX in their causation cannot be reliably determined. All reported events are included except those already listed, those too general to be informative, and those not reasonably associated with the use of the drug.

Breasts: Breast swelling, cysts, disorder of breasts, lumps, masses of breasts, nipple discharge, primary malignant breast neoplasm, and tenderness.

Cardiovascular: Abdominal aortic aneurysm, angina, atherosclerosis, cerebral ischemia, cerebrovascular lesion, heart block, peripheral cyanosis, phlebitis, thrombosis, and transient myocardial ischemia.

Table 4. Treatment-Emergent Adverse Experience Incidence in 2 Large Placebo-Controlled Migraine Clinical Trials: Events Reported by at Least 1% of IMITREX Injection Patients

Adverse Event Type	Percent of Patients Reporting: IMITREX Injection 6 mg Subcutaneous n = 547	Placebo n = 370
Atypical sensations	42.0	9.2
Tingling	13.5	3.0
Warm/hot sensation	10.8	3.5
Burning sensation	7.5	0.3
Feeling of heaviness	7.3	1.1
Pressure sensation	7.1	1.6
Feeling of tightness	5.1	0.3
Numbness	4.6	2.2
Feeling strange	2.2	0.3
Tight feeling in head	2.2	0.3
Cold sensation	1.1	0.5
Cardiovascular		
Flushing	6.6	2.4
Chest discomfort	4.5	1.4
Tightness in chest	2.7	0.5
Pressure in chest	1.8	0.3
Ear, nose, and throat		
Throat discomfort	3.3	0.5
Discomfort: nasal cavity/sinuses	2.2	0.3
Eye		
Vision alterations	1.1	0.0
Gastrointestinal		
Abdominal discomfort	1.3	0.8
Dysphagia	1.1	0.0
Injection site reaction	58.7	23.8
Miscellaneous		
Jaw discomfort	1.8	0.0
Mouth and teeth		
Discomfort of mouth/tongue	4.9	4.6
Musculoskeletal		
Weakness	4.9	0.3
Neck pain/stiffness	4.8	0.5
Myalgia	1.8	0.5
Muscle cramp(s)	1.1	0.0
Neurological		
Dizziness/vertigo	11.9	4.3
Drowsiness/sedation	2.7	2.2
Headache	2.2	0.3
Anxiety	1.1	0.5
Malaise/fatigue	1.1	0.8
Skin		
Sweating	1.6	1.1

The sum of the percentages cited is greater than 100% because patients may experience more than 1 type of adverse event. Only events that occurred at a frequency of 1% or more in groups treated with IMITREX Injection and were at least as frequent in the placebo groups are included.

Ear, Nose, and Throat: Allergic rhinitis; disorder of nasal cavity/sinuses; ear, nose, and throat hemorrhage; ear infection; external otitis; feeling of fullness in the ear(s); hearing disturbances; hearing loss; Meniere disease; nasal inflammation; otalgia; sensitivity to noise; sinusitis; tinnitus; and upper respiratory inflammation.

Endocrine and Metabolic: Elevated thyrotropin stimulating hormone (TSH) levels; endocrine cysts, lumps, and masses; fluid disturbances; galactorrhea; hyperglycemia; hypoglycemia; hypothyroidism; weight gain; and weight loss.

Eye: Accommodation disorders, blindness and low vision, conjunctivitis, disorders of sclera, external ocular muscle disorders, eye edema and swelling, eye hemorrhage, eye itching, eye pain, keratitis, mydriasis, and visual disturbances.

Gastrointestinal: Abdominal distention, colitis, constipation, dental pain, dyspeptic symptoms, feelings of gastrointestinal pressure, gastric symptoms, gastritis, gastroenteritis, gastrointestinal bleeding, gastrointestinal pain, hematemesis, hypersalivation, hyposalivation, intestinal obstruction, melena, nausea and/or vomiting, oral itching and irritation, pancreatitis, salivary gland swelling, and swallowing disorders.

Hematological Disorders: Anemia.

Mouth and Teeth: Disorder of mouth and tongue (e.g., burning of tongue, numbness of tongue, dry mouth).

Musculoskeletal: Acquired musculoskeletal deformity, arthralgia and articular rheumatitis, arthritis, intervertebral disc disorder, muscle atrophy, muscle tightness and rigidity, musculoskeletal inflammation, and tetany.

Neurological: Apathy, aggressiveness, bad/unusual taste, bradylogia, cluster headache, convulsions, depressive disorders, detachment, disturbance of emotions, drug abuse, facial paralysis, hallucinations, heat sensitivity, incoordination, increased alertness, memory disturbance, migraine, motor dysfunction, neoplasm of pituitary, neuralgia, neurotic disorders, paralysis, personality change, phobia, photophobia, psychomotor disorders, radiculopathy, raised intracranial pressure, rigidity, stress, syncope, suicide, and twitching.

Respiratory: Asthma, breathing disorders, bronchitis, cough, and lower respiratory tract infection.

Skin: Dry/scaly skin, eczema, herpes, seborrheic dermatitis, skin nodules, tightness of skin, and wrinkling of skin.

Urogenital: Abnormal menstrual cycle, abortion, bladder inflammation, endometriosis, hematuria, increased urination, inflammation of fallopian tubes, intermenstrual bleeding, menstruation symptoms, micturition disorders, urethritis, and urinary infections.

Miscellaneous: Contusions, difficulty in walking, edema, hematoma, hypersensitivity, fever, fluid retention, lymphadenopathy, overdose, speech disturbance, swelling of extremities, swelling of face, and voice disturbances.

Pain and Other Pressure Sensations: Chest pain and/or heaviness, neck/throat/jaw pain/tightness/pressure, and pain (location specified).

Postmarketing Experience (Reports for Subcutaneous or Oral Sumatriptan): The following section enumerates potentially important adverse events that have occurred in clinical practice and that have been reported spontaneously to various surveillance systems. The events enumerated represent reports arising from both domestic and nondomestic use of oral or subcutaneous dosage forms of sumatriptan. The events enumerated include all except those already listed in the ADVERSE REACTIONS section above or those too general to be informative. Because the reports cite events reported spontaneously from worldwide postmarketing experience, frequency of events and the role of IMITREX Injection in their causation cannot be reliably determined. It is assumed, however, that systemic reactions following sumatriptan use are likely to be similar regardless of route of administration.

Blood: Hemolytic anemia, pancytopenia, thrombocytopenia.

Cardiovascular: Atrial fibrillation, cardiomyopathy, colonic ischemia (see WARNINGS), Prinzmetal variant angina, pulmonary embolism, shock, thrombophlebitis.

Ear, Nose, and Throat: Deafness.
Eye: Ischemic optic neuropathy, retinal artery occlusion, retinal vein thrombosis, loss of vision.
Gastrointestinal: Ischemic colitis with rectal bleeding (see WARNINGS), xerostomia.
Hepatic: Elevated liver function tests.
Neurological: Central nervous system vasculitis, cerebrovascular accident, dysphasia, subarachnoid hemorrhage.
Non-Site Specific: Angioneurotic edema, cyanosis, death (see WARNINGS), temporal arteritis.
Psychiatry: Panic disorder.
Respiratory: Bronchospasm in patients with and without a history of asthma.
Skin: Exacerbation of sunburn, hypersensitivity reactions (allergic vasculitis, erythema, pruritus, rash, shortness of breath, urticaria; in addition, severe anaphylaxis/anaphylactoid reactions have been reported [see WARNINGS]), photosensitivity. Following subcutaneous administration of sumatriptan, pain, redness, stinging, induration, swelling, contusion, subcutaneous bleeding, and, on rare occasions, lipoatrophy (depression in the skin) or lipohypertrophy (enlargement or thickening of tissue) have been reported.
Urogenital: Acute renal failure.

DRUG ABUSE AND DEPENDENCE

The abuse potential of IMITREX Injection cannot be fully delineated in advance of extensive marketing experience. One clinical study enrolling 12 patients with a history of substance abuse failed to induce subjective behavior and/or physiologic response ordinarily associated with drugs that have an established potential for abuse.

OVERDOSAGE

Patients (n = 269) have received single injections of 8 to 12 mg without significant adverse effects. Volunteers (n = 47) have received single subcutaneous doses of up to 16 mg without serious adverse events.
No gross overdoses in clinical practice have been reported. Coronary vasospasm was observed after intravenous administration of IMITREX Injection (see CONTRAINDICATIONS). Overdoses would be expected from animal data (dogs at 0.1 g/kg, rats at 2 g/kg) to possibly cause convulsions, tremor, inactivity, erythema of the extremities, reduced respiratory rate, cyanosis, ataxia, mydriasis, injection site reactions (desquamation, hair loss, and scab formation), and paralysis. The half-life of elimination of sumatriptan is about 2 hours (see CLINICAL PHARMACOLOGY), and therefore monitoring of patients after overdose with IMITREX Injection should continue while symptoms or signs persist, and for at least 10 hours.
It is unknown what effect hemodialysis or peritoneal dialysis has on the serum concentrations of sumatriptan.

DOSAGE AND ADMINISTRATION

The maximum single recommended adult dose of IMITREX Injection is 6 mg injected subcutaneously. Controlled clinical trials have failed to show that clear benefit is associated with the administration of a second 6-mg dose in patients who have failed to respond to a first injection.
The maximum recommended dose that may be given in 24 hours is two 6-mg injections separated by at least 1 hour. Although the recommended dose is 6 mg, if side effects are dose limiting, then lower doses may be used (see CLINICAL PHARMACOLOGY). In patients receiving MAO inhibitors, decreased doses of sumatriptan should be considered (see WARNINGS and CLINICAL PHARMACOLOGY). In patients receiving doses lower than 6 mg, only the single-dose vial dosage form should be used. An autoinjection device is available for use with 6-mg prefilled syringe cartridges to facilitate self-administration in patients in whom this dose is deemed necessary. With this device, the needle penetrates approximately 1/4 inch (5 to 6 mm). Since the injection is intended to be given subcutaneously, intramuscular or intravascular delivery should be avoided. Patients should be directed to use injection sites with an adequate skin and subcutaneous thickness to accommodate the length of the needle.
Parenteral drug products should be inspected visually for particulate matter and discoloration before administration whenever solution and container permit.

HOW SUPPLIED

IMITREX Injection 6 mg (12 mg/mL) containing sumatriptan (base) as the succinate salt is supplied as a clear, colorless to pale yellow, sterile, nonpyrogenic solution as follows: (NDC 0173-0479-00) IMITREX STATdose System® containing 2 prefilled single-dose syringe cartridges, 1 IMITREX STATdose Pen®, and instructions for use.
(NDC 0173-0478-00 IMITREX Injection cartridge pack containing 2 prefilled syringe cartridges for refill of IMITREX STATdose System only.
(NDC 0173-0449-02) 6-mg Single-dose vials (0.5 mL in 2 mL) in cartons of 5 vials.
Store between 2° and 30°C (36° and 86°F). Protect from light.

PATIENT INFORMATION

The following wording is contained in a separate leaflet provided for patients.

Information for the Patient
IMITREX® (sumatriptan succinate) Injection

Please read this leaflet carefully before you take IMITREX Injection. This provides a summary of the information available on your medicine. Please do not throw away this leaflet until you have finished your medicine. You may need to read this leaflet again. This leaflet does not contain all the information on IMITREX Injection. For further information or advice, ask your doctor or pharmacist.

Information About Your Medicine:
The name of your medicine is IMITREX (sumatriptan succinate) Injection. It can be obtained only by prescription from your doctor. The decision to use IMITREX Injection is one that you and your doctor should make jointly, taking into account your individual preferences and medical circumstances. If you have risk factors for heart disease (such as high blood pressure, high cholesterol, obesity, diabetes, smoking, strong family history of heart disease, or you are postmenopausal or a male over 40), you should tell your doctor, who should evaluate you for heart disease in order to determine if IMITREX is appropriate for you. Although the vast majority of those who have taken IMITREX have not experienced any significant side effects, some individuals have experienced serious heart problems and, rarely, considering the extensive use of IMITREX worldwide, deaths have been reported. In all but a few instances, however, serious problems occurred in people with known heart diseases and it was not clear whether IMITREX was a contributory factor in these deaths.

1. The Purpose of Your Medicine:
IMITREX Injection is intended to relieve your migraine or cluster headache, but not to prevent or reduce the number of attacks you experience. Use IMITREX Injection only to treat an actual migraine or cluster headache attack.

2. Important Questions to Consider Before Taking IMITREX Injection:
If the answer to any of the following questions is **YES** or if you do not know the answer, then please discuss with your doctor before you use IMITREX Injection.

- Are you pregnant? Do you think you might be pregnant? Are you trying to become pregnant? Are you using inadequate contraception? Are you breastfeeding?
- Do you have any chest pain, heart disease, shortness of breath, or irregular heartbeats? Have you had a heart attack?
- Do you have risk factors for heart disease (such as high blood pressure, high cholesterol, obesity, diabetes, smoking, strong family history of heart disease, or you are postmenopausal or a male over 40)?
- Have you had a stroke, transient ischemic attacks (TIAs), or Raynaud syndrome?
- Do you have high blood pressure?
- Have you ever had to stop taking this or any other medicine because of an allergy or other problems?
- Are you taking any other migraine medicines, including other 5–HT_1 agonists or any other medicines containing ergotamine, dihydroergotamine, or methysergide?
- Are you taking any medicine for depression (monoamine oxidase inhibitors or selective serotonin reuptake inhibitors [SSRIs])?
- Have you had, or do you have, any disease of the liver or kidney?
- Have you had, or do you have, epilepsy or seizures?
- Is this headache different from your usual migraine attacks?

Remember, if you answered **YES** to any of the above questions, then discuss it with your doctor.

3. The Use of IMITREX Injection During Pregnancy:
Do not use IMITREX Injection if you are pregnant, think you might be pregnant, are trying to become pregnant, or are not using adequate contraception, unless you have discussed this with your doctor.

4. How to Use IMITREX Injection:
Before injecting IMITREX, check with your doctor on acceptable injection sites and see the instructions inside the carton on discarding empty syringes and reloading an autoinjector device.
Never reuse a syringe.
For adults, the usual dose is a single injection given just below the skin. It should be given as soon as the symptoms of your migraine appear, but it may be given at any time during an attack. A second injection may be given if your symptoms of migraine come back. If your symptoms do not improve following the first injection, do not give a second injection for the same attack without first consulting with your doctor. Do not have more than 2 injections in any 24 hours and allow at least 1 hour between each dose.

5. Side Effects to Watch for:

- Some patients experience pain or tightness in the chest or throat when using IMITREX Injection. If this happens to you, then discuss it with your doctor before using any more IMITREX Injection. If the chest pain is severe or does not go away, call your doctor immediately.
- If you have sudden and/or severe abdominal pain following IMITREX Injection, call your doctor immediately.
- Shortness of breath; wheeziness; heart throbbing; swelling of eyelids, face, or lips; or a skin rash, skin lumps, or hives happens rarely. If it happens to you, then tell your doctor immediately. Do not take any more IMITREX Injection unless your doctor tells you to do so.
- Some people may have feelings of tingling, heat, flushing (redness of face lasting a short time), heaviness or pressure after treatment with IMITREX Injection. A few people may feel drowsy, dizzy, tired, or sick. Tell your doctor of these symptoms at your next visit.
- You may experience pain or redness at the site of injection, but this usually lasts less than an hour.
- If you feel unwell in any other way or have any symptoms that you do not understand, you should contact your doctor immediately.

6. What to Do If an Overdose Is Taken:
If you have taken more medicine than you have been told, contact either your doctor, hospital emergency department, or nearest poison control center immediately.

7. Storing Your Medicine:
Keep your medicine in a safe place where children cannot reach it. It may be harmful to children.
Store your medicine away from heat and light. Keep your medicine in the case provided and do not store at temperatures above 86°F (30°C).
If your medicine has expired (the expiration date is printed on the treatment pack), throw it away as instructed. Do not throw away your autoinjector.
If your doctor decides to stop your treatment, do not keep any leftover medicine unless your doctor tells you to. Throw away your medicine as instructed.

GlaxoSmithKline, Research Triangle Park, NC 27709

January 2003/RL-1164
Shown in Product Identification Guide, page 316

IMITREX® ℞
[*ĭm' ĭ-trĕx*]
(sumatriptan)
Nasal Spray

DESCRIPTION

IMITREX (sumatriptan) Nasal Spray contains sumatriptan, a selective 5-hydroxytryptamine$_1$ receptor subtype agonist. Sumatriptan is chemically designated as 3-[2-(dimethylamino)ethyl]-N-methyl-1H-indole-5-methanesulfonamide.
The empirical formula is $C_{14}H_{21}N_3O_2S$, representing a molecular weight of 295.4. Sumatriptan is a white to off-white powder that is readily soluble in water and in saline. Each IMITREX Nasal Spray contains 5 or 20 mg of sumatriptan in a 100-µL unit dose aqueous buffered solution containing monobasic potassium phosphate NF, anhydrous dibasic sodium phosphate USP, sulfuric acid NF, sodium hydroxide NF, and purified water USP. The pH of the solution is approximately 5.5. The osmolality of the solution is 372 or 742 mOsmol for the 5- and 20-mg IMITREX Nasal Spray, respectively.

CLINICAL PHARMACOLOGY

Mechanism of Action: Sumatriptan is an agonist for a vascular 5-hydroxytryptamine$_1$ receptor subtype (probably a member of the 5-HT_{1D} family) having only a weak affinity for 5-HT_{1A}, 5-HT_{5A}, and 5-HT_7 receptors and no significant affinity (as measured using standard radioligand binding assays) or pharmacological activity at 5-HT_2, 5-HT_3, or 5-HT_4 receptor subtypes or at alpha$_1$-, alpha$_2$-, or beta-adrenergic; dopamine$_1$; dopamine$_2$; muscarinic; or benzodiazepine receptors.
The vascular 5-HT_1 receptor subtype that sumatriptan activates is present on cranial arteries in both dog and primate, on the human basilar artery, and in the vasculature of human dura mater and mediates vasoconstriction. This action in humans correlates with the relief of migraine headache. In addition to causing vasoconstriction, experimental data from animal studies show that sumatriptan also activates 5-HT_1 receptors on peripheral terminals of the trigeminal nerve innervating cranial blood vessels. Such an action may contribute to the antimigrainous effect of sumatriptan in humans.
In the anesthetized dog, sumatriptan selectively reduces the carotid arterial blood flow with little or no effect on arterial blood pressure or total peripheral resistance. In the cat, sumatriptan selectively constricts the carotid arteriovenous anastomoses while having little effect on blood flow or resistance in cerebral or extracerebral tissues.
Pharmacokinetics: In a study of 20 female volunteers, the mean maximum concentration following a 5- and 20-mg intranasal dose was 5 and 16 ng/mL, respectively. The mean C_{max} following a 6-mg subcutaneous injection is 71 ng/mL (range, 49 to 110 ng/mL). The mean C_{max} is 18 ng/mL (range, 7 to 47 ng/mL) following oral dosing with 25 mg and 51 ng/mL (range, 28 to 100 ng/mL) following oral dosing with 100 mg of sumatriptan. In a study of 24 male volunteers, the bioavailability relative to subcutaneous injection was low, approximately 17%, primarily due to presystemic metabolism and partly due to incomplete absorption.
Protein binding, determined by equilibrium dialysis over the concentration range of 10 to 1,000 ng/mL, is low, approximately 14% to 21%. The effect of sumatriptan on the protein binding of other drugs has not been evaluated, but would be expected to be minor, given the low rate of protein binding. The mean volume of distribution after subcutaneous dosing is 2.7 L/kg and the total plasma clearance is approximately 1,200 mL/min.
The elimination half-life of sumatriptan administered as a nasal spray is approximately 2 hours, similar to the half-life seen after subcutaneous injection. Only 3% of the dose is

Continued on next page

Product information on these pages is effective as of August 2004. Further information is available at: GlaxoSmithKline, PO Box 13398, Research Triangle Park, NC 27709. 1-888-825-5249. Corporate Web Site: www.gsk.com

Imitrex Nasal Spray—Cont.

excreted in the urine as unchanged sumatriptan; 42% of the dose is excreted as the major metabolite, the indole acetic acid analogue of sumatriptan.
Clinical and pharmacokinetic data indicate that administration of two 5-mg doses, 1 dose in each nostril, is equivalent to administration of a single 10-mg dose in 1 nostril.
Special Populations: ***Renal Impairment:*** The effect of renal impairment on the pharmacokinetics of sumatriptan has not been examined, but little clinical effect would be expected as sumatriptan is largely metabolized to an inactive substance.
Hepatic Impairment: The effect of hepatic disease on the pharmacokinetics of subcutaneously and orally administered sumatriptan has been evaluated, but the intranasal dosage form has not been studied in hepatic impairment. There were no statistically significant differences in the pharmacokinetics of subcutaneously administered sumatriptan in hepatically impaired patients compared to healthy controls. However, the liver plays an important role in the presystemic clearance of orally administered sumatriptan. In 1 small study involving oral sumatriptan in hepatically impaired patients (n = 8) matched for sex, age, and weight with healthy subjects, the hepatically impaired patients had an approximately 70% increase in AUC and C_{max} and a T_{max} 40 minutes earlier compared to the healthy subjects. The bioavailability of nasally absorbed sumatriptan following intranasal administration, which would not undergo first-pass metabolism, should not be altered in hepatically impaired patients. The bioavailability of the swallowed portion of the intranasal sumatriptan dose has not been determined, but would be increased in these patients. The swallowed intranasal dose is small, however, compared to the usual oral dose, so that its impact should be minimal.
Age: The pharmacokinetics of oral sumatriptan in the elderly (mean age; 72 years, 2 males and 4 females) and in patients with migraine (mean age; 38 years, 25 males and 155 females) were similar to that in healthy male subjects (mean age, 30 years). Intranasal sumatriptan has not been evaluated for age differences (see PRECAUTIONS: Geriatric Use).
Race: The systemic clearance and C_{max} of sumatriptan were similar in black (n = 34) and Caucasian (n = 38) healthy male subjects. Intranasal sumatriptan has not been evaluated for race differences.
Drug Interactions: ***Monoamine Oxidase Inhibitors:*** Treatment with monoamine oxidase inhibitors (MAOIs) generally leads to an increase of sumatriptan plasma levels (see CONTRAINDICATIONS and PRECAUTIONS).
MAOI interaction studies have not been performed with intranasal sumatriptan. Due to gut and hepatic metabolic first-pass effects, the increase of systemic exposure after coadministration of an MAO-A inhibitor with oral sumatriptan is greater than after coadministration of the MAOI with subcutaneous sumatriptan. The effects of an MAOI on systemic exposure after intranasal sumatriptan would be expected to be greater than the effect after subcutaneous sumatriptan but smaller than the effect after oral sumatriptan because only swallowed drug would be subject to first-pass effects.
In a study of 14 healthy females, pretreatment with an MAO-A inhibitor decreased the clearance of subcutaneous sumatriptan. Under the conditions of this experiment, the result was a 2-fold increase in the area under the sumatriptan plasma concentration x time curve (AUC), corresponding to a 40% increase in elimination half-life. This interaction was not evident with an MAO-B inhibitor.
A small study evaluating the effect of pretreatment with an MAO-A inhibitor on the bioavailability from a 25-mg oral sumatriptan tablet resulted in an approximately 7-fold increase in systemic exposure.
Xylometazoline: An in vivo drug interaction study indicated that 3 drops of xylometazoline (0.1% w/v), a decongestant, administered 15 minutes prior to a 20-mg nasal dose of sumatriptan did not alter the pharmacokinetics of sumatriptan.

CLINICAL TRIALS

The efficacy of IMITREX Nasal Spray in the acute treatment of migraine headaches was demonstrated in 8, randomized, double-blind, placebo-controlled studies, of which 5 used the recommended dosing regimen and used the marketed formulation. Patients enrolled in these 5 studies were predominately female (86%) and Caucasian (95%), with a mean age of 41 (range of 18 to 65). Patients were instructed to treat a moderate to severe headache. Headache response, defined as a reduction in headache severity from moderate or severe pain to mild or no pain, was assessed up to 2 hours after dosing. Associated symptoms such as nausea, photophobia, and phonophobia were also assessed. Maintenance of response was assessed for up to 24 hours postdose. A second dose of IMITREX Nasal Spray or other medication was allowed 2 to 24 hours after the initial treatment for recurrent headache. The frequency and time to use of these additional treatments were also determined. In all studies, doses of 10 and 20 mg were compared to placebo in the treatment of 1 to 3 migraine attacks. Patients received doses as a single spray into 1 nostril. In 2 studies, a 5-mg dose was also evaluated.
In all 5 trials utilizing the market formulation and recommended dosage regimen, the percentage of patients achieving headache response 2 hours after treatment was significantly greater among patients receiving IMITREX Nasal Spray at all doses (with one exception) compared to those who received placebo. In 4 of the 5 studies, there was a statistically significant greater percentage of patients with headache response at 2 hours in the 20-mg group when compared to the lower dose groups (5 and 10 mg). There were no statistically significant differences between the 5- and 10-mg dose groups in any study. The results from the 5 controlled clinical trials are summarized in Table 1. Note that, in general, comparisons of results obtained in studies conducted under different conditions by different investigators with different samples of patients are ordinarily unreliable for purposes of quantitative comparison.
[See table 1 below]
The estimated probability of achieving an initial headache response over the 2 hours following treatment is depicted in Figure 1.

Figure 1. Estimated Probability of Achieving Initial Headache Response Within 120 Minutes*

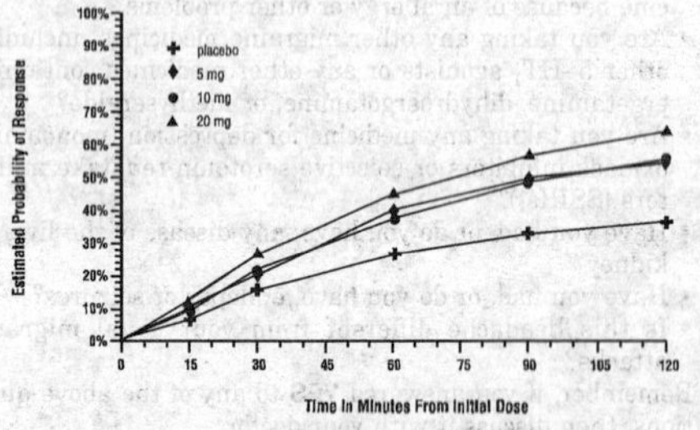

* The figure shows the probability over time of obtaining headache response (no or mild pain) following treatment with intranasal sumatriptan. The averages displayed are based on pooled data from the 5 clinical controlled trials providing evidence of efficacy. Kaplan-Meier plot with patients not achieving response within 120 minutes censored to 120 minutes.

For patients with migraine-associated nausea, photophobia, and phonophobia at baseline, there was a lower incidence of these symptoms at 2 hours following administration of IMITREX Nasal Spray compared to placebo.
Two to 24 hours following the initial dose of study treatment, patients were allowed to use additional treatment for pain relief in the form of a second dose of study treatment or other medication. The estimated probability of patients taking a second dose or other medication for migraine over the 24 hours following the initial dose of study treatment is summarized in Figure 2.

Figure 2. The Estimated Probability of Patients Taking a Second Dose or Other Medication for Migraine Over the 24 Hours Following the Initial Dose of Study Treatment*

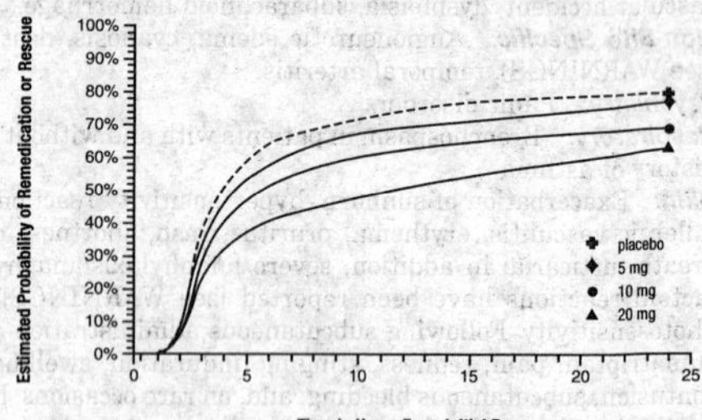

* Kaplan-Meier plot based on data obtained in the 3 clinical controlled trials providing evidence of efficacy with patients not using additional treatments censored to 24 hours. Plot also includes patients who had no response to the initial dose. No remedication was allowed within 2 hours postdose.

There is evidence that doses above 20 mg do not provide a greater effect than 20 mg. There was no evidence to suggest that treatment with sumatriptan was associated with an increase in the severity of recurrent headaches. The efficacy of IMITREX Nasal Spray was unaffected by presence of aura; duration of headache prior to treatment; gender, age, or weight of the patient; or concomitant use of common migraine prophylactic drugs (e.g., beta-blockers, calcium channel blockers, tricyclic antidepressants). There were insufficient data to assess the impact of race on efficacy.

INDICATIONS AND USAGE

IMITREX Nasal Spray is indicated for the acute treatment of migraine attacks with or without aura in adults.
IMITREX Nasal Spray is not intended for the prophylactic therapy of migraine or for use in the management of hemiplegic or basilar migraine (see CONTRAINDICATIONS). Safety and effectiveness of IMITREX Nasal Spray have not been established for cluster headache, which is present in an older, predominantly male population.

CONTRAINDICATIONS

IMITREX Nasal Spray should not be given to patients with history, symptoms, or signs of ischemic cardiac, cerebrovascular, or peripheral vascular syndromes. In addition, patients with other significant underlying cardiovascular diseases should not receive IMITREX Nasal Spray. Ischemic cardiac syndromes include, but are not limited to, angina pectoris of any type (e.g., stable angina of effort and vasospastic forms of angina such as the Prinzmetal variant), all forms of myocardial infarction, and silent myocardial ischemia. Cerebrovascular syndromes include, but are not limited to, strokes of any type as well as transient ischemic attacks. Peripheral vascular disease includes, but is not limited to, ischemic bowel disease (see WARNINGS).
Because IMITREX Nasal Spray may increase blood pressure, it should not be given to patients with uncontrolled hypertension.
Concurrent administration of MAO-A inhibitors or use within 2 weeks of discontinuation of MAO-A inhibitor therapy is contraindicated (see CLINICAL PHARMACOLOGY: Drug Interactions and PRECAUTIONS: Drug Interactions).
IMITREX Nasal Spray and any ergotamine-containing or ergot-type medication (like dihydroergotamine or methysergide) should not be used within 24 hours of each other, nor should IMITREX Nasal Spray and another 5-HT_1 agonist.
IMITREX Nasal Spray should not be administered to patients with hemiplegic or basilar migraine.
IMITREX Nasal Spray is contraindicated in patients with hypersensitivity to sumatriptan or any of its components.
IMITREX Nasal Spray is contraindicated in patients with severe hepatic impairment.

WARNINGS

IMITREX Nasal Spray should only be used where a clear diagnosis of migraine headache has been established.
Risk of Myocardial Ischemia and/or Infarction and Other Adverse Cardiac Events: Sumatriptan should not be given to patients with documented ischemic or vasospastic coronary artery disease (CAD) (see CONTRAINDICATIONS). It is strongly recommended that sumatriptan not be given to patients in whom unrecognized CAD is predicted by the presence of risk factors (e.g., hypertension, hypercholesterolemia, smoker, obesity, diabetes, strong family history of CAD, female with surgical or physiological menopause, or male over 40 years of age) unless a cardiovascular evaluation provides satisfactory clinical evidence that the patient is reasonably free of coronary artery and ischemic myocardial disease or other significant underlying cardiovascular disease. The sensitivity of cardiac diagnostic procedures to detect cardiovascular disease or predisposition to coronary artery vasospasm is modest, at best. If, during the cardiovascular evaluation, the patient's medical history or electrocardiographic investigations reveal findings indicative of, or consistent with, coronary artery vasospasm or myocardial ischemia, sumatriptan should not be administered (see CONTRAINDICATIONS).

Table 1. Percentage of Patients With Headache Response (No or Mild Pain) 2 Hours Following Treatment

	Placebo	IMITREX Nasal Spray 5 mg	IMITREX Nasal Spray 10 mg	IMITREX Nasal Spray 20 mg
Study 1	25% (n = 63)	49%* (n = 121)	46%* (n = 112)	64%*†‡ (n = 118)
Study 2	25% (n = 138)	Not applicable	44%* (n = 273)	55%*† (n = 277)
Study 3	35% (n = 100)	Not applicable	54%* (n = 106)	63%* (n = 202)
Study 4	29% (n = 112)	Not applicable	43% (n = 106)	62%*† (n = 215)
Study 5§	36% (n = 198)	45%* (n = 296)	53%* (n = 291)	60%*‡ (n = 286)

* $p<0.05$ in comparison with placebo.
† $p<0.05$ in comparison with 10 mg.
‡ $p<0.05$ in comparison with 5 mg.
§ Data are for attack 1 only of multiattack study for comparison.

For patients with risk factors predictive of CAD, who are determined to have a satisfactory cardiovascular evaluation, it is strongly recommended that administration of the first dose of sumatriptan nasal spray take place in the setting of a physician's office or similar medically staffed and equipped facility unless the patient has previously received sumatriptan. Because cardiac ischemia can occur in the absence of clinical symptoms, consideration should be given to obtaining on the first occasion of use an electrocardiogram (ECG) during the interval immediately following IMITREX Nasal Spray, in these patients with risk factors.

It is recommended that patients who are intermittent long-term users of sumatriptan and who have or acquire risk factors predictive of CAD, as described above, undergo periodic interval cardiovascular evaluation as they continue to use sumatriptan.

The systematic approach described above is intended to reduce the likelihood that patients with unrecognized cardiovascular disease will be inadvertently exposed to sumatriptan.

Drug-Associated Cardiac Events and Fatalities: Serious adverse cardiac events, including acute myocardial infarction, life-threatening disturbances of cardiac rhythm, and death have been reported within a few hours following the administration of IMITREX® (sumatriptan succinate) Injection or IMITREX® (sumatriptan succinate) Tablets. Considering the extent of use of sumatriptan in patients with migraine, the incidence of these events is extremely low.

The fact that sumatriptan can cause coronary vasospasm, that some of these events have occurred in patients with no prior cardiac disease history and with documented absence of CAD, and the close proximity of the events to sumatriptan use support the conclusion that some of these cases were caused by the drug. In many cases, however, where there has been known underlying coronary artery disease, the relationship is uncertain.

Premarketing Experience With Sumatriptan: Among approximately 4,000 patients with migraine who participated in premarketing controlled and uncontrolled clinical trials of sumatriptan nasal spray, 1 patient experienced an asymptomatic subendocardial infarction possibly subsequent to a coronary vasospastic event.

Of 6,348 patients with migraine who participated in premarketing controlled and uncontrolled clinical trials of oral sumatriptan, 2 experienced clinical adverse events shortly after receiving oral sumatriptan that may have reflected coronary vasospasm. Neither of these adverse events was associated with a serious clinical outcome.

Among the more than 1,900 patients with migraine who participated in premarketing controlled clinical trials of subcutaneous sumatriptan, there were 8 patients who sustained clinical events during or shortly after receiving sumatriptan that may have reflected coronary artery vasospasm. Six of these 8 patients had ECG changes consistent with transient ischemia, but without accompanying clinical symptoms or signs. Of these 8 patients, 4 had either findings suggestive of CAD or risk factors predictive of CAD prior to study enrollment.

Postmarketing Experience With Sumatriptan: Serious cardiovascular events, some resulting in death, have been reported in association with the use of IMITREX Injection or IMITREX Tablets. The uncontrolled nature of postmarketing surveillance, however, makes it impossible to determine definitively the proportion of the reported cases that were actually caused by sumatriptan or to reliably assess causation in individual cases. On clinical grounds, the longer the latency between the administration of IMITREX and the onset of the clinical event, the less likely the association is to be causative. Accordingly, interest has focused on events beginning within 1 hour of the administration of IMITREX.

Cardiac events that have been observed to have onset within 1 hour of sumatriptan administration include: coronary artery vasospasm, transient ischemia, myocardial infarction, ventricular tachycardia and ventricular fibrillation, cardiac arrest, and death.

Some of these events occurred in patients who had no findings of CAD and appear to represent consequences of coronary artery vasospasm. However, among domestic reports of serious cardiac events within 1 hour of sumatriptan administration, almost all of the patients had risk factors predictive of CAD and the presence of significant underlying CAD was established in most cases (see CONTRAINDICATIONS).

Drug-Associated Cerebrovascular Events and Fatalities: Cerebral hemorrhage, subarachnoid hemorrhage, stroke, and other cerebrovascular events have been reported in patients treated with oral or subcutaneous sumatriptan, and some have resulted in fatalities. The relationship of sumatriptan to these events is uncertain. In a number of cases, it appears possible that the cerebrovascular events were primary, sumatriptan having been administered in the incorrect belief that the symptoms experienced were a consequence of migraine when they were not. As with other acute migraine therapies, before treating headaches in patients not previously diagnosed as migraineurs, and in migraineurs who present with atypical symptoms, care should be taken to exclude other potentially serious neurological conditions. It should also be noted that patients with migraine may be at increased risk of certain cerebrovascular events (e.g., cerebrovascular accident, transient ischemic attack).

Other Vasospasm-Related Events: Sumatriptan may cause vasospastic reactions other than coronary artery vasospasm. Both peripheral vascular ischemia and colonic ischemia with abdominal pain and bloody diarrhea have been reported.

Increase in Blood Pressure: Significant elevation in blood pressure, including hypertensive crisis, has been reported on rare occasions in patients with and without a history of hypertension. Sumatriptan is contraindicated in patients with uncontrolled hypertension (see CONTRAINDICATIONS). Sumatriptan should be administered with caution to patients with controlled hypertension as transient increases in blood pressure and peripheral vascular resistance have been observed in a small proportion of patients.

Local Irritation: Of the 3,378 patients using the nasal spray (5-, 10-, or 20-mg doses) on 1 or 2 occasions in controlled clinical studies, approximately 5% noted irritation in the nose and throat. Irritative symptoms such as burning, numbness, paresthesia, discharge, and pain or soreness were noted to be severe in about 1% of patients treated. The symptoms were transient and in approximately 60% of the cases, the symptoms resolved in less than 2 hours. Limited examinations of the nose and throat did not reveal any clinically noticeable injury in these patients. The consequences of extended and repeated use of IMITREX Nasal Spray on the nasal and/or respiratory mucosa have not been systematically evaluated in patients.

No increase in the incidence of local irritation was observed in patients using IMITREX Nasal Spray repeatedly for up to 1 year.

In inhalation studies in rats dosed daily for up to 1 month at exposures as low as one half the maximum daily human exposure (based on dose per surface area of nasal cavity), epithelial hyperplasia (with and without keratinization) and squamous metaplasia were observed in the larynx at all doses tested. These changes were partially reversible after a 2-week drug-free period. When dogs were dosed daily with various formulations by intranasal instillation for up to 13 weeks at exposures of 2 to 4 times the maximum daily human exposure (based on dose per surface area of nasal cavity), respiratory and nasal mucosa exhibited evidence of epithelial hyperplasia, focal squamous metaplasia, granulomata, bronchitis, and fibrosing alveolitis. A no-effect dose was not established. The changes observed in both species are not considered to be signs of either preneoplastic or neoplastic transformation.

Local effects on nasal and respiratory tissues after chronic intranasal dosing in animals have not been studied.

Concomitant Drug Use: In patients taking MAO-A inhibitors, sumatriptan plasma levels attained after treatment with recommended doses are 2-fold (following subcutaneous administration) to 7-fold (following oral administration) higher than those obtained under other conditions. Accordingly, the coadministration of IMITREX Nasal Spray and an MAO-A inhibitor is contraindicated (see CLINICAL PHARMACOLOGY and CONTRAINDICATIONS).

Hypersensitivity: Hypersensitivity (anaphylaxis/anaphylactoid) reactions have occurred on rare occasions in patients receiving sumatriptan. Such reactions can be life threatening or fatal. In general, hypersensitivity reactions to drugs are more likely to occur in individuals with a history of sensitivity to multiple allergens (see CONTRAINDICATIONS).

PRECAUTIONS

General: Chest discomfort and jaw or neck tightness have been reported infrequently following the administration of IMITREX Nasal Spray and have also been reported following use of IMITREX Tablets. Chest, jaw, or neck tightness is relatively common after administration of IMITREX Injection. Only rarely have these symptoms been associated with ischemic ECG changes. However, because sumatriptan may cause coronary artery vasospasm, patients who experience signs or symptoms suggestive of angina following sumatriptan should be evaluated for the presence of CAD or a predisposition to Prinzmetal variant angina before receiving additional doses of sumatriptan, and should be monitored electrocardiographically if dosing is resumed and similar symptoms recur. Similarly, patients who experience other symptoms or signs suggestive of decreased arterial flow, such as ischemic bowel syndrome or Raynaud syndrome following sumatriptan should be evaluated for atherosclerosis or predisposition to vasospasm (see WARNINGS).

IMITREX Nasal Spray should also be administered with caution to patients with diseases that may alter the absorption, metabolism, or excretion of drugs, such as impaired hepatic or renal function.

There have been rare reports of seizure following administration of sumatriptan. Sumatriptan should be used with caution in patients with a history of epilepsy or conditions associated with a lowered seizure threshold.

Care should be taken to exclude other potentially serious neurologic conditions before treating headache in patients not previously diagnosed with migraine headache or who experience a headache that is atypical for them. There have been rare reports where patients received sumatriptan for severe headaches that were subsequently shown to have been secondary to an evolving neurologic lesion (see WARNINGS).

For a given attack, if a patient does not respond to the first dose of sumatriptan, the diagnosis of migraine headache should be reconsidered before administration of a second dose.

Binding to Melanin-Containing Tissues: In rats treated with a single subcutaneous dose (0.5 mg/kg) or oral dose (2 mg/kg) of radiolabeled sumatriptan, the elimination half-life of radioactivity from the eye was 15 and 23 days, respectively, suggesting that sumatriptan and/or its metabolites bind to the melanin of the eye. Comparable studies were not performed by the intranasal route. Because there could be an accumulation in melanin-rich tissues over time, this raises the possibility that sumatriptan could cause toxicity in these tissues after extended use. However, no effects on the retina related to treatment with sumatriptan were noted in any of the oral or subcutaneous toxicity studies. Although no systematic monitoring of ophthalmologic function was undertaken in clinical trials, and no specific recommendations for ophthalmologic monitoring are offered, prescribers should be aware of the possibility of long-term ophthalmologic effects.

Corneal Opacities: Sumatriptan causes corneal opacities and defects in the corneal epithelium in dogs; this raises the possibility that these changes may occur in humans. While patients were not systematically evaluated for these changes in clinical trials, and no specific recommendations for monitoring are being offered, prescribers should be aware of the possibility of these changes (see ANIMAL TOXICOLOGY).

Information for Patients: See PATIENT INFORMATION at the end of this labeling for the text of the separate leaflet provided for patients.

Laboratory Tests: No specific laboratory tests are recommended for monitoring patients prior to and/or after treatment with sumatriptan.

Drug Interactions: Ergot-containing drugs have been reported to cause prolonged vasospastic reactions. Because there is a theoretical basis that these effects may be additive, use of ergotamine-containing or ergot-type medications (like dihydroergotamine or methysergide) and sumatriptan within 24 hours of each other should be avoided (see CONTRAINDICATIONS).

MAO-A inhibitors reduce sumatriptan clearance, significantly increasing systemic exposure. Therefore, the use of IMITREX Nasal Spray in patients receiving MAO-A inhibitors is contraindicated (see CLINICAL PHARMACOLOGY and CONTRAINDICATIONS).

Selective serotonin reuptake inhibitors (SSRIs) (e.g., fluoxetine, fluvoxamine, paroxetine, sertraline) have been reported, rarely, to cause weakness, hyperreflexia, and incoordination when coadministered with sumatriptan. If concomitant treatment with sumatriptan and an SSRI is clinically warranted, appropriate observation of the patient is advised.

Drug/Laboratory Test Interactions: IMITREX Nasal Spray is not known to interfere with commonly employed clinical laboratory tests.

Carcinogenesis, Mutagenesis, Impairment of Fertility: ***Carcinogenesis:*** In carcinogenicity studies, rats and mice were given sumatriptan by oral gavage (rats, 104 weeks) or drinking water (mice, 78 weeks). Average exposures achieved in mice receiving the highest dose (target dose of 160 mg/kg/day) were approximately 184 times the exposure attained in humans after the maximum recommended single intranasal dose of 20 mg. The highest dose administered to rats (160 mg/kg/day, reduced from 360 mg/kg/day during week 21) was approximately 78 times the maximum recommended single intranasal dose of 20 mg on a mg/m^2 basis. There was no evidence of an increase in tumors in either species related to sumatriptan administration. Local effects on nasal and respiratory tissue after chronic intranasal dosing in animals have not been evaluated (see WARNINGS).

Mutagenesis: Sumatriptan was not mutagenic in the presence or absence of metabolic activation when tested in 2 gene mutation assays (the Ames test and the in vitro mammalian Chinese hamster V79/HGPRT assay). In 2 cytogenetics assays (the in vitro human lymphocyte assay and the in vivo rat micronucleus assay) sumatriptan was not associated with clastogenic activity.

Impairment of Fertility: In a study in which male and female rats were dosed daily with oral sumatriptan prior to and throughout the mating period, there was a treatment-related decrease in fertility secondary to a decrease in mating in animals treated with 50 and 500 mg/kg/day. The highest no-effect dose for this finding was 5 mg/kg/day, or approximately twice the maximum recommended single human intranasal dose of 20 mg on a mg/m^2 basis. It is not clear whether the problem is associated with treatment of the males or females or both combined. In a similar study by the subcutaneous route there was no evidence of impaired fertility at 60 mg/kg/day, the maximum dose tested, which is equivalent to approximately 29 times the maximum recommended single human intranasal dose of 20 mg on a mg/m^2 basis. Fertility studies, in which sumatriptan was administered by the intranasal route, were not conducted.

Pregnancy: Pregnancy Category C. In reproductive toxicity studies in rats and rabbits, oral treatment with sumatriptan was associated with embryolethality, fetal abnormalities, and pup mortality. When administered by the intravenous route to rabbits, sumatriptan has been shown to be embryolethal. Reproductive toxicity studies for

Continued on next page

Product information on these pages is effective as of August 2004. Further information is available at: GlaxoSmithKline, PO Box 13398, Research Triangle Park, NC 27709. 1-888-825-5249. Corporate Web Site: www.gsk.com

Imitrex Nasal Spray—Cont.

sumatriptan by the intranasal route have not been conducted.
There are no adequate and well-controlled studies in pregnant women. Therefore, IMITREX Nasal Spray should be used during pregnancy only if the potential benefit justifies the potential risk to the fetus. In assessing this information, the following findings should be considered.
Embryolethality: When given orally or intravenously to pregnant rabbits daily throughout the period of organogenesis, sumatriptan caused embryolethality at doses at or close to those producing maternal toxicity. In the oral studies this dose was 100 mg/kg/day, and in the intravenous studies this dose was 2.0 mg/kg/day. The mechanism of the embryolethality is not known. The highest no-effect dose for embryolethality by the oral route was 50 mg/kg/day, which is approximately 48 times the maximum single recommended human intranasal dose of 20 mg on a mg/m^2 basis. By the intravenous route, the highest no-effect dose was 0.75 mg/kg/day, or approximately 0.7 times the maximum single recommended human intranasal dose of 20 mg on a mg/m^2 basis.
The intravenous administration of sumatriptan to pregnant rats throughout organogenesis at 12.5 mg/kg/day, the maximum dose tested, did not cause embryolethality. This dose is approximately 6 times the maximum single recommended human intranasal dose of 20 mg on a mg/m^2 basis. Additionally, in a study in rats given subcutaneous sumatriptan daily, prior to and throughout pregnancy, at 60 mg/kg/day, the maximum dose tested, there was no evidence of increased embryo/fetal lethality. This dose is equivalent to approximately 29 times the maximum recommended single human intranasal dose of 20 mg on a mg/m^2 basis.
Teratogenicity: Oral treatment of pregnant rats with sumatriptan during the period of organogenesis resulted in an increased incidence of blood vessel abnormalities (cervicothoracic and umbilical) at doses of approximately 250 mg/kg/day or higher. The highest no-effect dose was approximately 60 mg/kg/day, which is approximately 29 times the maximum single recommended human intranasal dose of 20 mg on a mg/m^2 basis. Oral treatment of pregnant rabbits with sumatriptan during the period of organogenesis resulted in an increased incidence of cervicothoracic vascular and skeletal abnormalities. The highest no-effect dose for these effects was 15 mg/kg/day, or approximately 14 times the maximum single recommended human intranasal dose of 20 mg on a mg/m^2 basis.
A study in which rats were dosed daily with oral sumatriptan prior to and throughout gestation demonstrated embryo/fetal toxicity (decreased body weight, decreased ossification, increased incidence of rib variations) and an increased incidence of a syndrome of malformations (short tail/short body and vertebral disorganization) at 500 mg/kg/day. The highest no-effect dose was 50 mg/kg/day, or approximately 24 times the maximum single recommended human intranasal dose of 20 mg on a mg/m^2 basis. In a study in rats dosed daily with subcutaneous sumatriptan prior to and throughout pregnancy, at a dose of 60 mg/kg/day, the maximum dose tested, there was no evidence of teratogenicity. This dose is equivalent to approximately 29 times the maximum recommended single human intranasal dose of 20 mg on a mg/m^2 basis.
Pup Deaths: Oral treatment of pregnant rats with sumatriptan during the period of organogenesis resulted in a decrease in pup survival between birth and postnatal day 4 at doses of approximately 250 mg/kg/day or higher. The highest no-effect dose for this effect was approximately 60 mg/kg/day, or 29 times the maximum single recommended human intranasal dose of 20 mg on a mg/m^2 basis. Oral treatment of pregnant rats with sumatriptan from gestational day 17 through postnatal day 21 demonstrated a decrease in pup survival measured at postnatal days 2, 4, and 20 at the dose of 1,000 mg/kg/day. The highest no-effect dose for this finding was 100 mg/kg/day, approximately 49 times the maximum single recommended human intranasal dose of 20 mg on a mg/m^2 basis. In a similar study in rats by the subcutaneous route there was no increase in pup death at 81 mg/kg/day, the highest dose tested, which is equivalent to 40 times the maximum single recommended human intranasal dose of 20 mg on a mg/m^2 basis.
Pregnancy Registry: To monitor fetal outcomes of pregnant women exposed to IMITREX, GlaxoSmithKline maintains a Sumatriptan Pregnancy Registry. Physicians are encouraged to register patients by calling (800) 336-2176.
Nursing Mothers: Sumatriptan is excreted in human breast milk. Therefore, caution should be exercised when considering the administration of IMITREX Nasal Spray to a nursing woman.
Pediatric Use: Safety and effectiveness of IMITREX Nasal Spray in pediatric patients have not been established.
Completed placebo-controlled clinical trials evaluating oral sumatriptan (25 to 100 mg) in pediatric patients aged 12 to 17 years enrolled a total of 701 adolescent migraineurs. These studies did not establish the efficacy of oral sumatriptan compared to placebo in the treatment of migraine in adolescents. Adverse events observed in these clinical trials were similar in nature to those reported in clinical trials in adults. The frequency of all adverse events in these patients appeared to be both dose- and age-dependent, with younger patients reporting events more commonly than older adolescents. Postmarketing experience includes a limited number of reports that describe pediatric patients who have experienced adverse events, some clinically serious, after use of subcutaneous sumatriptan and/or oral sumatriptan. These reports include events similar in nature to those reported rarely in adults. A myocardial infarct has been reported in a 14-year-old male following the use of oral sumatriptan; clinical signs occurred within 1 day of drug administration. Since clinical data to determine the frequency of serious adverse events in pediatric patients who might receive injectable, oral, or intranasal sumatriptan are not presently available, the use of sumatriptan in patients aged younger than 18 years is not recommended.
Geriatric Use: The use of sumatriptan in elderly patients is not recommended because elderly patients are more likely to have decreased hepatic function, they are at higher risk for CAD, and blood pressure increases may be more pronounced in the elderly (see WARNINGS).

ADVERSE REACTIONS

Serious cardiac events, including some that have been fatal, have occurred following the use of IMITREX Injection or Tablets. These events are extremely rare and most have been reported in patients with risk factors predictive of CAD. Events reported have included coronary artery vasospasm, transient myocardial ischemia, myocardial infarction, ventricular tachycardia, and ventricular fibrillation (see CONTRAINDICATIONS, WARNINGS, and PRECAUTIONS).
Significant hypertensive episodes, including hypertensive crises, have been reported on rare occasions in patients with or without a history of hypertension (see WARNINGS).
Incidence in Controlled Clinical Trials: Among 3,653 patients treated with IMITREX Nasal Spray in active- and placebo-controlled clinical trials, less than 0.4% of patients withdrew for reasons related to adverse events. Table 2 lists adverse events that occurred in worldwide placebo-controlled clinical trials in 3,419 migraineurs. The events cited reflect experience gained under closely monitored conditions of clinical trials in a highly selected patient population. In actual clinical practice or in other clinical trials, these frequency estimates may not apply, as the conditions of use, reporting behavior, and the kinds of patients treated may differ.
Only events that occurred at a frequency of 1% or more in the IMITREX Nasal Spray 20-mg treatment group and were more frequent in that group than in the placebo group are included in Table 2.
[See table 2 below]
Phonophobia also occurred in more than 1% of patients but was more frequent on placebo.
IMITREX Nasal Spray is generally well tolerated. Across all doses, most adverse reactions were mild and transient and did not lead to long-lasting effects. The incidence of adverse events in controlled clinical trials was not affected by gender, weight, or age of the patients; use of prophylactic medications; or presence of aura. There were insufficient data to assess the impact of race on the incidence of adverse events.
Other Events Observed in Association With the Administration of IMITREX Nasal Spray: In the paragraphs that follow, the frequencies of less commonly reported adverse clinical events are presented. Because the reports include events observed in open and uncontrolled studies, the role of IMITREX Nasal Spray in their causation cannot be reliably determined. Furthermore, variability associated with adverse event reporting, the terminology used to describe adverse events, etc., limit the value of the quantitative frequency estimates provided. Event frequencies are calculated as the number of patients who used IMITREX Nasal Spray (5, 10, or 20 mg in controlled and uncontrolled trials) and reported an event divided by the total number of patients (n = 3,711) exposed to IMITREX Nasal Spray. All reported events are included except those already listed in the previous table, those too general to be informative, and those not reasonably associated with the use of the drug. Events are further classified within body system categories and enumerated in order of decreasing frequency using the following definitions: infrequent adverse events are those occurring in 1/100 to 1/1,000 patients and rare adverse events are those occurring in fewer than 1/1,000 patients.
Atypical Sensations: Infrequent were tingling, warm/hot sensation, numbness, pressure sensation, feeling strange, feeling of heaviness, feeling of tightness, paresthesia, cold sensation, and tight feeling in head. Rare were dysesthesia and prickling sensation.
Cardiovascular: Infrequent were flushing and hypertension (see WARNINGS), palpitations, tachycardia, changes in ECG, and arrhythmia (see WARNINGS and PRECAUTIONS). Rare were abdominal aortic aneurysm, hypotension, bradycardia, pallor, and phlebitis.
Chest Symptoms: Infrequent were chest tightness, chest discomfort, and chest pressure/heaviness (see PRECAUTIONS: General).
Ear, Nose, and Throat: Infrequent were disturbance of hearing and ear infection. Rare were otalgia and Meniere disease.
Endocrine and Metabolic: Infrequent was thirst. Rare were galactorrhea, hypothyroidism, and weight loss.
Eye: Infrequent were irritation of eyes and visual disturbance.
Gastrointestinal: Infrequent were abdominal discomfort, diarrhea, dysphagia, and gastroesophageal reflux. Rare were constipation, flatulence/eructation, hematemesis, intestinal obstruction, melena, gastroenteritis, colitis, hemorrhage of gastrointestinal tract, and pancreatitis.
Mouth and Teeth: Infrequent was disorder of mouth and tongue (e.g., burning of tongue, numbness of tongue, dry mouth).
Musculoskeletal: Infrequent were neck pain/stiffness, backache, weakness, joint symptoms, arthritis, and myalgia. Rare were muscle cramps, tetany, intervertebral disc disorder, and muscle stiffness.
Neurological: Infrequent were drowsiness/sedation, anxiety, sleep disturbances, tremors, syncope, shivers, chills, depression, agitation, sensation of lightness, and mental confusion. Rare were difficulty concentrating, hunger, lacrimation, memory disturbances, monoplegia/diplegia, apathy, disturbance of smell, disturbance of emotions, dysarthria, facial pain, intoxication, stress, decreased appetite, difficulty coordinating, euphoria, and neoplasm of pituitary.
Respiratory: Infrequent were dyspnea and lower respiratory tract infection. Rare was asthma.
Skin: Infrequent were rash/skin eruption, pruritus, and erythema. Rare were herpes, swelling of face, sweating, and peeling of skin.
Urogenital: Infrequent were dysuria, disorder of breasts, and dysmenorrhea. Rare were endometriosis and increased urination.
Miscellaneous: Infrequent were cough, edema, and fever. Rare were hypersensitivity, swelling of extremities, voice disturbances, difficulty in walking, and lymphadenopathy.
Other Events Observed in the Clinical Development of IMITREX: The following adverse events occurred in clinical trials with IMITREX Injection and IMITREX Tablets. Because the reports include events observed in open and uncontrolled studies, the role of IMITREX in their causation cannot be reliably determined. All reported events are included except those already listed, those too general to be informative, and those not reasonably associated with the use of the drug.
Breasts: Breast swelling; cysts, lumps, and masses of breasts; nipple discharge; primary malignant breast neoplasm; and tenderness.
Cardiovascular: Abnormal pulse, angina, atherosclerosis, cerebral ischemia, cerebrovascular lesion, heart block, peripheral cyanosis, pulsating sensations, Raynaud syndrome, thrombosis, transient myocardial ischemia, various transient ECG changes (nonspecific ST or T wave changes, prolongation of PR or QTc intervals, sinus arrhythmia, nonsustained ventricular premature beats, isolated junctional ectopic beats, atrial ectopic beats, delayed activation of the right ventricle), and vasodilation.
Ear, Nose, and Throat: Allergic rhinitis; ear, nose, and throat hemorrhage; external otitis; feeling of fullness in the ear(s); hearing disturbances; hearing loss; nasal inflammation; sensitivity to noise; sinusitis; tinnitus; and upper respiratory inflammation.
Endocrine and Metabolic: Dehydration; endocrine cysts, lumps, and masses; elevated thyrotropin stimulating hor-

Table 2. Treatment-Emergent Adverse Events Reported by at Least 1% of Patients in Controlled Migraine Trials

Adverse Event Type	Percent of Patients Reporting			
	Placebo (n = 704)	IMITREX 5 mg (n = 496)	IMITREX 10 mg (n = 1,007)	IMITREX 20 mg (n = 1,212)
Atypical sensations				
Burning sensation	0.1%	0.4%	0.6%	1.4%
Ear, nose, and throat				
Disorder/discomfort of nasal cavity/sinuses	2.4%	2.8%	2.5%	3.8%
Throat discomfort	0.9%	0.8%	1.8%	2.4%
Gastrointestinal				
Nausea and/or vomiting	11.3%	12.2%	11.0%	13.5%
Neurological				
Bad/unusual taste	1.7%	13.5%	19.3%	24.5%
Dizziness/vertigo	0.9%	1.0%	1.7%	1.4%

mone (TSH) levels; fluid disturbances; hyperglycemia; hypoglycemia; polydipsia; and weight gain.
Eye: Accommodation disorders, blindness and low vision, conjunctivitis, disorders of sclera, external ocular muscle disorders, eye edema and swelling, eye itching, eye hemorrhage, eye pain, keratitis, mydriasis, and vision alterations.
Gastrointestinal: Abdominal distention, dental pain, disturbances of liver function tests, dyspeptic symptoms, feelings of gastrointestinal pressure, gallstones, gastric symptoms, gastritis, gastrointestinal pain, hypersalivation, hyposalivation, oral itching and irritation, peptic ulcer, retching, salivary gland swelling, and swallowing disorders.
Hematological Disorders: Anemia.
Injection Site Reaction
Miscellaneous: Contusions, fluid retention, hematoma, hypersensitivity to various agents, jaw discomfort, miscellaneous laboratory abnormalities, overdose, "serotonin agonist effect", and speech disturbance.
Musculoskeletal: Acquired musculoskeletal deformity, arthralgia and articular rheumatitis, muscle atrophy, muscle tiredness, musculoskeletal inflammation, need to flex calf muscles, rigidity, tightness, and various joint disturbances (pain, stiffness, swelling, ache).
Neurological: Aggressiveness, bradylogia, cluster headache, convulsions, detachment, disturbances of taste, drug abuse, dystonia, facial paralysis, globus hystericus, hallucinations, headache, heat sensitivity, hyperesthesia, hysteria, increased alertness, malaise/fatigue, migraine, motor dysfunction, myoclonia, neuralgia, neurotic disorders, paralysis, personality change, phobia, photophobia, psychomotor disorders, radiculopathy, raised intracranial pressure, relaxation, stinging sensations, transient hemiplegia, simultaneous hot and cold sensations, suicide, tickling sensations, twitching, and yawning.
Pain and Other Pressure Sensations: Chest pain, neck tightness/pressure, throat/jaw pain/tightness/pressure, and pain (location specified).
Respiratory: Breathing disorders, bronchitis, diseases of the lower respiratory tract, hiccoughs, and influenza.
Skin: Dry/scaly skin, eczema, seborrheic dermatitis, skin nodules, skin tenderness, tightness of skin, and wrinkling of skin.
Urogenital: Abortion, abnormal menstrual cycle, bladder inflammation, hematuria, inflammation of fallopian tubes, intermenstrual bleeding, menstruation symptoms, micturition disorders, renal calculus, urethritis, urinary frequency, and urinary infections.
Postmarketing Experience (Reports for Subcutaneous or Oral Sumatriptan): The following section enumerates potentially important adverse events that have occurred in clinical practice and that have been reported spontaneously to various surveillance systems. The events enumerated represent reports arising from both domestic and nondomestic use of oral or subcutaneous dosage forms of sumatriptan. The events enumerated include all except those already listed in the ADVERSE REACTIONS section above or those too general to be informative. Because the reports cite events reported spontaneously from worldwide postmarketing experience, frequency of events and the role of sumatriptan in their causation cannot be reliably determined. It is assumed, however, that systemic reactions following sumatriptan use are likely to be similar regardless of route of administration.
Blood: Hemolytic anemia, pancytopenia, thrombocytopenia.
Cardiovascular: Atrial fibrillation, cardiomyopathy, colonic ischemia (see WARNINGS), Prinzmetal variant angina, pulmonary embolism, shock, thrombophlebitis.
Ear, Nose, and Throat: Deafness.
Eye: Ischemic optic neuropathy, retinal artery occlusion, retinal vein thrombosis, loss of vision.
Gastrointestinal: Ischemic colitis with rectal bleeding (see WARNINGS), xerostomia.
Hepatic: Elevated liver function tests.
Neurological: Central nervous system vasculitis, cerebrovascular accident, dysphasia, subarachnoid hemorrhage.
Non-Site Specific: Angioneurotic edema, cyanosis, death (see WARNINGS), temporal arteritis.
Psychiatry: Panic disorder.
Respiratory: Bronchospasm in patients with and without a history of asthma.
Skin: Exacerbation of sunburn, hypersensitivity reactions (allergic vasculitis, erythema, pruritus, rash, shortness of breath, urticaria; in addition, severe anaphylaxis/anaphylactoid reactions have been reported [see WARNINGS]), photosensitivity.
Urogenital: Acute renal failure.

DRUG ABUSE AND DEPENDENCE

One clinical study with IMITREX (sumatriptan succinate) Injection enrolling 12 patients with a history of substance abuse failed to induce subjective behavior and/or physiologic response ordinarily associated with drugs that have an established potential for abuse.

OVERDOSAGE

In clinical trials, the highest single doses of IMITREX Nasal Spray administered without significant adverse effects were 40 mg to 12 volunteers and 40 mg to 85 migraine patients, which is twice the highest single recommended dose. In addition, 12 volunteers were administered a total daily dose of 60 mg (20 mg 3 times daily) for 3.5 days without significant adverse events.
Overdose in animals has been fatal and has been heralded by convulsions, tremor, paralysis, inactivity, ptosis, erythema of the extremities, abnormal respiration, cyanosis, ataxia, mydriasis, salivation, and lacrimation. The elimination half-life of sumatriptan is about 2 hours (see CLINICAL PHARMACOLOGY), and therefore monitoring of patients after overdose with IMITREX Nasal Spray should continue for at least 10 hours or while symptoms or signs persist. It is unknown what effect hemodialysis or peritoneal dialysis has on the serum concentrations of sumatriptan.

DOSAGE AND ADMINISTRATION

In controlled clinical trials, single doses of 5, 10, or 20 mg of IMITREX Nasal Spray administered into 1 nostril were effective for the acute treatment of migraine in adults. A greater proportion of patients had headache response following a 20-mg dose than following a 5- or 10-mg dose (see CLINICAL TRIALS). Individuals may vary in response to doses of IMITREX Nasal Spray. The choice of dose should therefore be made on an individual basis, weighing the possible benefit of the 20-mg dose with the potential for a greater risk of adverse events. A 10-mg dose may be achieved by the administration of a single 5-mg dose in each nostril. There is evidence that doses above 20 mg do not provide a greater effect than 20 mg.
If the headache returns, the dose may be repeated once after 2 hours, not to exceed a total daily dose of 40 mg. The safety of treating an average of more than 4 headaches in a 30-day period has not been established.

HOW SUPPLIED

IMITREX Nasal Spray 5 mg (NDC 0173-0524-00) and 20 mg (NDC 0173-0523-00) are each supplied in boxes of 6 nasal spray devices. Each unit dose spray supplies 5 and 20 mg, respectively, of sumatriptan.
Store between 36° and 86°F (2° and 30°C). Protect from light.

ANIMAL TOXICOLOGY

Corneal Opacities: Dogs receiving oral sumatriptan developed corneal opacities and defects in the corneal epithelium. Corneal opacities were seen at the lowest dosage tested, 2 mg/kg/day, and were present after 1 month of treatment. Defects in the corneal epithelium were noted in a 60-week study. Earlier examinations for these toxicities were not conducted and no-effect doses were not established; however, the relative exposure at the lowest dose tested was approximately 5 times the human exposure after a 100-mg oral dose or 3 times the human exposure after a 6-mg subcutaneous dose or 22 times the human exposure after a single 20-mg intranasal dose. There is evidence of alterations in corneal appearance on the first day of intranasal dosing to dogs. Changes were noted at the lowest dose tested, which was approximately 2 times the maximum single human intranasal dose of 20 mg on a mg/m^2 basis.

PATIENT INFORMATION

The following wording is contained in a separate leaflet provided for patients.

Information for the Patient
IMITREX® (sumatriptan) Nasal Spray

Please read this leaflet carefully before you administer IMITREX Nasal Spray. This leaflet provides a summary of the information available about your medicine. Please do not throw away this leaflet until you have finished your medicine. You may need to read this leaflet again. This leaflet does not contain all the information on IMITREX Nasal Spray. For further information or advice, ask your doctor or pharmacist.
Information About Your Medicine:
The name of your medicine is IMITREX (sumatriptan) Nasal Spray. It can be obtained only by prescription from your doctor. The decision to use IMITREX Nasal Spray is one that you and your doctor should make jointly, taking into account your individual preferences and medical circumstances. If you have risk factors for heart disease (such as high blood pressure, high cholesterol, obesity, diabetes, smoking, strong family history of heart disease, or you are postmenopausal or a male over 40), you should tell your doctor, who should evaluate you for heart disease in order to determine if IMITREX is appropriate for you. Although the vast majority of those who have taken IMITREX have not experienced any significant side effects, some individuals have experienced serious heart problems and, rarely, considering the extensive use of IMITREX worldwide, deaths have been reported. In all but a few instances, however, serious problems occurred in people with known heart disease and it was not clear whether IMITREX was a contributory factor in these deaths.
1. The Purpose of Your Medicine:
IMITREX Nasal Spray is intended to relieve your migraine, but not to prevent or reduce the number of attacks you experience. Use IMITREX Nasal Spray only to treat an actual migraine attack.
2. Important Questions to Consider Before Using IMITREX Nasal Spray:
If the answer to any of the following questions is **YES** or if you do not know the answer, then please discuss it with your doctor before you use IMITREX Nasal Spray.

- Are you pregnant? Do you think you might be pregnant? Are you trying to become pregnant? Are you using inadequate contraception? Are you breastfeeding?
- Do you have any chest pain, heart disease, shortness of breath, or irregular heartbeats? Have you had a heart attack?
- Do you have risk factors for heart disease (such as high blood pressure, high cholesterol, obesity, diabetes, smoking, strong family history of heart disease, or you are postmenopausal or a male over 40)?
- Have you had a stroke, transient ischemic attacks (TIAs), or Raynaud syndrome?
- Do you have high blood pressure?
- Have you ever had to stop taking this or any other medicine because of an allergy or other problems?
- Are you taking any other migraine medicines, including other 5-HT$_1$ agonists or any other medicines containing ergotamine, dihydroergotamine, or methysergide?
- Are you taking any medicines for depression (monoamine oxidase inhibitors or selective serotonin reuptake inhibitors [SSRIs])?
- Have you had, or do you have, any disease of the liver or kidney?
- Have you had, or do you have, epilepsy or seizures?
- Is this headache different from your usual migraine attacks?

Remember, if you answered **YES** to any of the above questions, then discuss it with your doctor.
3. The Use of IMITREX Nasal Spray During Pregnancy:
Do not use IMITREX Nasal Spray if you are pregnant, think you might be pregnant, are trying to become pregnant, or are not using adequate contraception, unless you have discussed this with your doctor.
4. How to Use IMITREX Nasal Spray:
Before using IMITREX Nasal Spray, see the enclosed instruction pamphlet. For adults, the usual dose is a single nasal spray administered into 1 nostril. If your headache comes back, a second nasal spray may be administered anytime after 2 hours of administering the first spray. For any attack where you have no response to the first nasal spray, do not take a second nasal spray without first consulting with your doctor. Do not administer more than a total of 40 mg of IMITREX Nasal Spray in any 24-hour period. The effects of long-term repeated use of IMITREX Nasal Spray on the surfaces of the nose and throat have not been specifically studied. The safety of treating an average of more than 4 headaches in a 30-day period has not been established.
5. Side Effects to Watch for:

- Some patients experience pain or tightness in the chest or throat when using IMITREX Nasal Spray. If this happens to you, then discuss it with your doctor before using any more IMITREX Nasal Spray. If the chest pain is severe or does not go away, call your doctor immediately.
- If you have sudden and/or severe abdominal pain following IMITREX Nasal Spray, call your doctor immediately.
- Shortness of breath; wheeziness; heart throbbing; swelling of eyelids, face, or lips; or a skin rash, skin lumps, or hives happens rarely. If it happens to you, then tell your doctor immediately. Do not take any more IMITREX Nasal Spray unless your doctor tells you to do so.
- Some people may have feelings of tingling, heat, flushing (redness of face lasting a short time), heaviness or pressure after treatment with IMITREX Nasal Spray. A few people may feel drowsy, dizzy, tired, sick, or may experience nasal irritation. Tell your doctor of these symptoms at your next visit.
- If you feel unwell in any other way or have any symptoms that you do not understand, you should contact your doctor immediately.

6. What to Do if an Overdose Is Taken:
If you have taken more medicine than you have been told, contact either your doctor, hospital emergency department, or nearest poison control center immediately.
7. Storing Your Medicine:
Keep your medicine in a safe place where children cannot reach it. It may be harmful to children. Store your medicine away from heat and light. Do not store at temperatures above 86°F (30°C), or below 36°F (2°C). If your medicine has expired (the expiration date is printed on the treatment pack), throw it away as instructed. If your doctor decides to stop your treatment, do not keep any leftover medicine unless your doctor tells you to. Throw away your medicine as instructed.
GlaxoSmithKline, Research Triangle Park, NC 27709

January 2003/RL-1165
Shown in Product Identification Guide, page 316

IMITREX® ℞

[ĭm'ĭ-trĕx]
(sumatriptan succinate)
Tablets

DESCRIPTION

IMITREX Tablets contain sumatriptan (as the succinate), a selective 5-hydroxytryptamine$_1$ receptor subtype agonist. Sumatriptan succinate is chemically designated as 3-[2-(dimethylamino)ethyl]-N-methyl-indole-5-methanesulfonamide succinate (1:1).

Continued on next page

Product information on these pages is effective as of August 2004. Further information is available at: GlaxoSmithKline, PO Box 13398, Research Triangle Park, NC 27709. 1-888-825-5249. Corporate Web Site: www.gsk.com

Imitrex Tablets—Cont.

The empirical formula is $C_{14}H_{21}N_3O_2S•C_4H_6O_4$, representing a molecular weight of 413.5. Sumatriptan succinate is a white to off-white powder that is readily soluble in water and in saline. Each IMITREX Tablet for oral administration contains 35, 70, or 140 mg of sumatriptan succinate equivalent to 25, 50, or 100 mg of sumatriptan, respectively. Each tablet also contains the inactive ingredients croscarmellose sodium, dibasic calcium phosphate, magnesium stearate, microcrystalline cellulose, and sodium bicarbonate. Each 100-mg tablet also contains hypromellose, iron oxide, titanium dioxide, and triacetin.

CLINICAL PHARMACOLOGY

Mechanism of Action: Sumatriptan is an agonist for a vascular 5-hydroxytryptamine$_1$ receptor subtype (probably a member of the 5-HT_{1D} family) having only a weak affinity for 5-HT_{1A}, 5-HT_{5A}, and 5-HT_7 receptors and no significant affinity (as measured using standard radioligand binding assays) or pharmacological activity at 5-HT_2, 5-HT_3, or 5-HT_4 receptor subtypes or at alpha$_1$-, alpha$_2$-, or beta-adrenergic; dopamine$_1$; dopamine$_2$; muscarinic; or benzodiazepine receptors.

The vascular 5-HT_1 receptor subtype that sumatriptan activates is present on cranial arteries in both dog and primate, on the human basilar artery, and in the vasculature of human dura mater and mediates vasoconstriction. This action in humans correlates with the relief of migraine headache. In addition to causing vasoconstriction, experimental data from animal studies show that sumatriptan also activates 5-HT_1 receptors on peripheral terminals of the trigeminal nerve innervating cranial blood vessels. Such an action may also contribute to the antimigrainous effect of sumatriptan in humans.

In the anesthetized dog, sumatriptan selectively reduces the carotid arterial blood flow with little or no effect on arterial blood pressure or total peripheral resistance. In the cat, sumatriptan selectively constricts the carotid arteriovenous anastomoses while having little effect on blood flow or resistance in cerebral or extracerebral tissues.

Pharmacokinetics: The mean maximum concentration following oral dosing with 25 mg is 18 ng/mL (range, 7 to 47 ng/mL) and 51 ng/mL (range, 28 to 100 ng/mL) following oral dosing with 100 mg of sumatriptan. This compares with a C_{max} of 5 and 16 ng/mL following dosing with a 5- and 20-mg intranasal dose, respectively. The mean C_{max} following a 6-mg subcutaneous injection is 71 ng/mL (range, 49 to 110 ng/mL). The bioavailability is approximately 15%, primarily due to presystemic metabolism and partly due to incomplete absorption. The C_{max} is similar during a migraine attack and during a migraine-free period, but the T_{max} is slightly later during the attack, approximately 2.5 hours compared to 2.0 hours. When given as a single dose, sumatriptan displays dose proportionality in its extent of absorption (area under the curve [AUC]) over the dose range of 25 to 200 mg, but the C_{max} after 100 mg is approximately 25% less than expected (based on the 25-mg dose).

A food effect study involving administration of IMITREX Tablets 100 mg to healthy volunteers under fasting conditions and with a high-fat meal indicated that the C_{max} and AUC were increased by 15% and 12%, respectively, when administered in the fed state.

Plasma protein binding is low (14% to 21%). The effect of sumatriptan on the protein binding of other drugs has not been evaluated, but would be expected to be minor, given the low rate of protein binding. The apparent volume of distribution is 2.4 L/kg.

The elimination half-life of sumatriptan is approximately 2.5 hours. Radiolabeled ^{14}C-sumatriptan administered orally is largely renally excreted (about 60%) with about 40% found in the feces. Most of the radiolabeled compound excreted in the urine is the major metabolite, indole acetic acid (IAA), which is inactive, or the IAA glucuronide. Only 3% of the dose can be recovered as unchanged sumatriptan.

In vitro studies with human microsomes suggest that sumatriptan is metabolized by monoamine oxidase (MAO), predominantly the A isoenzyme, and inhibitors of that enzyme may alter sumatriptan pharmacokinetics to increase systemic exposure. No significant effect was seen with an MAO-B inhibitor (see CONTRAINDICATIONS, WARNINGS, and PRECAUTIONS: Drug Interactions).

Special Populations: ***Renal Impairment:*** The effect of renal impairment on the pharmacokinetics of sumatriptan has not been examined, but little clinical effect would be expected as sumatriptan is largely metabolized to an inactive substance.

Hepatic Impairment: The liver plays an important role in the presystemic clearance of orally administered sumatriptan. Accordingly, the bioavailability of sumatriptan following oral administration may be markedly increased in patients with liver disease. In 1 small study of hepatically impaired patients (N = 8) matched for sex, age, and weight with healthy subjects, the hepatically impaired patients had an approximately 70% increase in AUC and C_{max} and a T_{max} 40 minutes earlier compared to the healthy subjects (see DOSAGE AND ADMINISTRATION).

Age: The pharmacokinetics of oral sumatriptan in the elderly (mean age, 72 years; 2 males and 4 females) and in patients with migraine (mean age, 38 years; 25 males and 155 females) were similar to that in healthy male subjects (mean age, 30 years) (see PRECAUTIONS: Geriatric Use).

Gender: In a study comparing females to males, no pharmacokinetic differences were observed between genders for AUC, C_{max}, T_{max}, and half-life.

Race: The systemic clearance and C_{max} of sumatriptan were similar in black (N = 34) and Caucasian (N = 38) healthy male subjects.

Drug Interactions: *Monoamine Oxidase Inhibitors:* Treatment with MAO-A inhibitors generally leads to an increase of sumatriptan plasma levels (see CONTRAINDICATIONS and PRECAUTIONS).

Due to gut and hepatic metabolic first-pass effects, the increase of systemic exposure after coadministration of an MAO-A inhibitor with oral sumatriptan is greater than after coadministration of the monoamine oxidase inhibitors (MAOI) with subcutaneous sumatriptan. In a study of 14 healthy females, pretreatment with an MAO-A inhibitor decreased the clearance of subcutaneous sumatriptan. Under the conditions of this experiment, the result was a 2-fold increase in the area under the sumatriptan plasma concentration x time curve (AUC), corresponding to a 40% increase in elimination half-life. This interaction was not evident with an MAO-B inhibitor.

A small study evaluating the effect of pretreatment with an MAO-A inhibitor on the bioavailability from a 25-mg oral sumatriptan tablet resulted in an approximately 7-fold increase in systemic exposure.

Alcohol: Alcohol consumed 30 minutes prior to sumatriptan ingestion had no effect on the pharmacokinetics of sumatriptan.

CLINICAL STUDIES

The efficacy of IMITREX Tablets in the acute treatment of migraine headaches was demonstrated in 3, randomized, double-blind, placebo-controlled studies. Patients enrolled in these 3 studies were predominately female (87%) and Caucasian (97%), with a mean age of 40 years (range, 18 to 65 years). Patients were instructed to treat a moderate to severe headache. Headache response, defined as a reduction in headache severity from moderate or severe pain to mild or no pain, was assessed up to 4 hours after dosing. Associated symptoms such as nausea, photophobia, and phonophobia were also assessed. Maintenance of response was assessed for up to 24 hours postdose. A second dose of IMITREX Tablets or other medication was allowed 4 to 24 hours after the initial treatment for recurrent headache. Acetaminophen was offered to patients in Studies 2 and 3 beginning at 2 hours after initial treatment if the migraine pain had not improved or worsened. Additional medications were allowed 4 to 24 hours after the initial treatment for recurrent headache or as rescue in all 3 studies. The frequency and time to use of these additional treatments were also determined. In all studies, doses of 25, 50, and 100 mg were compared to placebo in the treatment of migraine attacks. In 1 study, doses of 25, 50, and 100 mg were also compared to each other.

In all 3 trials, the percentage of patients achieving headache response 2 and 4 hours after treatment was significantly greater among patients receiving IMITREX Tablets at all doses compared to those who received placebo. In 1 of the 3 studies, there was a statistically significant greater percentage of patients with headache response at 2 and 4 hours in the 50- or 100-mg group when compared to the 25-mg dose groups. There were no statistically significant differences between the 50- and 100-mg dose groups in any study. The results from the 3 controlled clinical trials are summarized in Table 1.

Comparisons of drug performance based upon results obtained in different clinical trials are never reliable. Because studies are conducted at different times, with different samples of patients, by different investigators, employing different criteria and/or different interpretations of the same criteria, under different conditions (dose, dosing regimen, etc.), quantitative estimates of treatment response and the timing of response may be expected to vary considerably from study to study.

[See table 1 below]

The estimated probability of achieving an initial headache response over the 4 hours following treatment is depicted in Figure 1.

Figure 1. Estimated Probability of Achieving Initial Headache Response Within 240 Minutes*

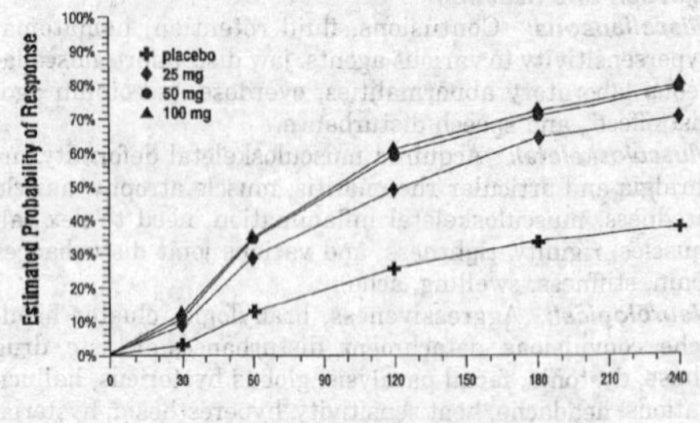

* The figure shows the probability over time of obtaining headache response (no or mild pain) following treatment with sumatriptan. The averages displayed are based on pooled data from the 3 clinical controlled trials providing evidence of efficacy. Kaplan-Meier plot with patients not achieving response and/or taking rescue within 240 minutes censored to 240 minutes.

For patients with migraine-associated nausea, photophobia, and/or phonophobia at baseline, there was a lower incidence of these symptoms at 2 hours (Study 1) and at 4 hours (Studies 1, 2, and 3) following administration of IMITREX Tablets compared to placebo.

As early as 2 hours in Studies 2 and 3 or 4 hours in Study 1, through 24 hours following the initial dose of study treatment, patients were allowed to use additional treatment for pain relief in the form of a second dose of study treatment or other medication. The estimated probability of patients taking a second dose or other medication for migraine over the 24 hours following the initial dose of study treatment is summarized in Figure 2.

Figure 2. The Estimated Probability of Patients Taking a Second Dose or Other Medication for Migraine Over the 24 Hours Following the Initial Dose of Study Treatment*

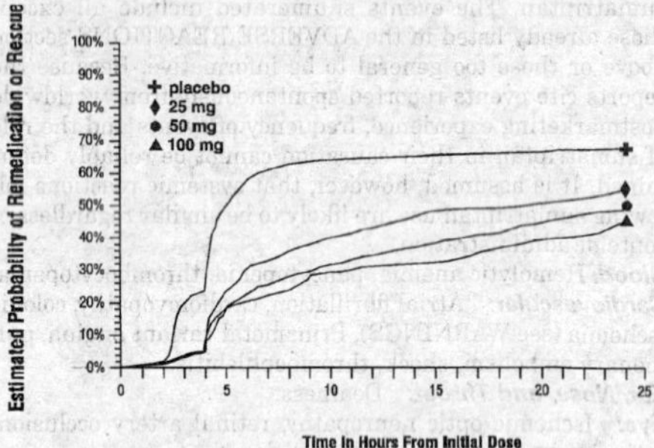

* Kaplan-Meier plot based on data obtained in 3 clinical controlled trials providing evidence of efficacy with patients not using additional treatments censored to 24 hours. Plot also includes patients who had no response to the initial dose. No remedication was allowed within 2 hours postdose.

There is evidence that doses above 50 mg do not provide a greater effect than 50 mg. There was no evidence to suggest that treatment with sumatriptan was associated with an increase in the severity of recurrent headaches. The efficacy of IMITREX Tablets was unaffected by presence of aura; duration of headache prior to treatment; gender, age, or weight of the patient; relationship to menses; or concomitant use of common migraine prophylactic drugs (e.g., beta-blockers, calcium channel blockers, tricyclic antidepressants). There were insufficient data to assess the impact of race on efficacy.

INDICATIONS AND USAGE

IMITREX Tablets are indicated for the acute treatment of migraine attacks with or without aura in adults.

IMITREX Tablets are not intended for the prophylactic therapy of migraine or for use in the management of hemiplegic or basilar migraine (see CONTRAINDICATIONS). Safety and effectiveness of IMITREX Tablets have not been established for cluster headache, which is present in an older, predominantly male population.

CONTRAINDICATIONS

IMITREX Tablets should not be given to patients with history, symptoms, or signs of ischemic cardiac, cerebrovascular, or peripheral vascular syndromes. In addition, patients with other significant underlying cardiovascular diseases should not receive IMITREX Tablets. Ischemic car-

Table 1. Percentage of Patients With Headache Response (No or Mild Pain) 2 and 4 Hours Following Treatment

	Placebo 2 hr	Placebo 4 hr	IMITREX Tablets 25 mg 2 hr	IMITREX Tablets 25 mg 4 hr	IMITREX Tablets 50 mg 2 hr	IMITREX Tablets 50 mg 4 hr	IMITREX Tablets 100 mg 2 hr	IMITREX Tablets 100 mg 4 hr
Study 1	27% (N = 94)	38%	52%* (N = 298)	67%*	61%*† (N = 296)	78%*†	62%*† (N = 296)	79%*†
Study 2	26% (N = 65)	38%	52%* (N = 66)	70%*	50%* (N = 62)	68%*	56%* (N = 66)	71%*
Study 3	17% (N = 47)	19%	52%* (N = 48)	65%*	54%* (N = 46)	72%*	57%* (N = 46)	78%*

* $p<0.05$ in comparison with placebo.
† $p<0.05$ in comparison with 25 mg.

diac syndromes include, but are not limited to, angina pectoris of any type (e.g., stable angina of effort and vasospastic forms of angina such as the Prinzmetal variant), all forms of myocardial infarction, and silent myocardial ischemia. Cerebrovascular syndromes include, but are not limited to, strokes of any type as well as transient ischemic attacks. Peripheral vascular disease includes, but is not limited to, ischemic bowel disease (see WARNINGS).

Because IMITREX Tablets may increase blood pressure, they should not be given to patients with uncontrolled hypertension.

Concurrent administration of MAO-A inhibitors or use within 2 weeks of discontinuation of MAO-A inhibitor therapy is contraindicated (see CLINICAL PHARMACOLOGY: Drug Interactions and PRECAUTIONS: Drug Interactions).

IMITREX Tablets should not be administered to patients with hemiplegic or basilar migraine.

IMITREX Tablets and any ergotamine-containing or ergot-type medication (like dihydroergotamine or methysergide) should not be used within 24 hours of each other, nor should IMITREX and another 5-HT$_1$ agonist.

IMITREX Tablets are contraindicated in patients with hypersensitivity to sumatriptan or any of their components.

IMITREX Tablets are contraindicated in patients with severe hepatic impairment.

WARNINGS

IMITREX Tablets should only be used where a clear diagnosis of migraine headache has been established.

Risk of Myocardial Ischemia and/or Infarction and Other Adverse Cardiac Events: Sumatriptan should not be given to patients with documented ischemic or vasospastic coronary artery disease (CAD) (see CONTRAINDICATIONS). It is strongly recommended that sumatriptan not be given to patients in whom unrecognized CAD is predicted by the presence of risk factors (e.g., hypertension, hypercholesterolemia, smoker, obesity, diabetes, strong family history of CAD, female with surgical or physiological menopause, or male over 40 years of age) unless a cardiovascular evaluation provides satisfactory clinical evidence that the patient is reasonably free of coronary artery and ischemic myocardial disease or other significant underlying cardiovascular disease. The sensitivity of cardiac diagnostic procedures to detect cardiovascular disease or predisposition to coronary artery vasospasm is modest, at best. If, during the cardiovascular evaluation, the patient's medical history or electrocardiographic investigations reveal findings indicative of, or consistent with, coronary artery vasospasm or myocardial ischemia, sumatriptan should not be administered (see CONTRAINDICATIONS).

For patients with risk factors predictive of CAD, who are determined to have a satisfactory cardiovascular evaluation, it is strongly recommended that administration of the first dose of sumatriptan tablets take place in the setting of a physician's office or similar medically staffed and equipped facility unless the patient has previously received sumatriptan. Because cardiac ischemia can occur in the absence of clinical symptoms, consideration should be given to obtaining on the first occasion of use an electrocardiogram (ECG) during the interval immediately following IMITREX Tablets, in these patients with risk factors.

It is recommended that patients who are intermittent long-term users of sumatriptan and who have or acquire risk factors predictive of CAD, as described above, undergo periodic interval cardiovascular evaluation as they continue to use sumatriptan.

The systematic approach described above is intended to reduce the likelihood that patients with unrecognized cardiovascular disease will be inadvertently exposed to sumatriptan.

Drug-Associated Cardiac Events and Fatalities: Serious adverse cardiac events, including acute myocardial infarction, life-threatening disturbances of cardiac rhythm, and death have been reported within a few hours following the administration of IMITREX® (sumatriptan succinate) Injection or IMITREX Tablets. Considering the extent of use of sumatriptan in patients with migraine, the incidence of these events is extremely low.

The fact that sumatriptan can cause coronary vasospasm, that some of these events have occurred in patients with no prior cardiac disease history and with documented absence of CAD, and the close proximity of the events to sumatriptan use support the conclusion that some of these cases were caused by the drug. In many cases, however, where there has been known underlying coronary artery disease, the relationship is uncertain.

Premarketing Experience With Sumatriptan: Of 6,348 patients with migraine who participated in premarketing controlled and uncontrolled clinical trials of oral sumatriptan, 2 experienced clinical adverse events shortly after receiving oral sumatriptan that may have reflected coronary vasospasm. Neither of these adverse events was associated with a serious clinical outcome.

Among the more than 1,900 patients with migraine who participated in premarketing controlled clinical trials of subcutaneous sumatriptan, there were 8 patients who sustained clinical events during or shortly after receiving sumatriptan that may have reflected coronary artery vasospasm. Six of these 8 patients had ECG changes consistent with transient ischemia, but without accompanying clinical symptoms or signs. Of these 8 patients, 4 had either findings suggestive of CAD or risk factors predictive of CAD prior to study enrollment.

Among approximately 4,000 patients with migraine who participated in premarketing controlled and uncontrolled clinical trials of sumatriptan nasal spray, 1 patient experienced an asymptomatic subendocardial infarction possibly subsequent to a coronary vasospastic event.

Postmarketing Experience With Sumatriptan: Serious cardiovascular events, some resulting in death, have been reported in association with the use of IMITREX Injection or IMITREX Tablets. The uncontrolled nature of postmarketing surveillance, however, makes it impossible to determine definitively the proportion of the reported cases that were actually caused by sumatriptan or to reliably assess causation in individual cases. On clinical grounds, the longer the latency between the administration of IMITREX and the onset of the clinical event, the less likely the association is to be causative. Accordingly, interest has focused on events beginning within 1 hour of the administration of IMITREX.

Cardiac events that have been observed to have onset within 1 hour of sumatriptan administration include: coronary artery vasospasm, transient ischemia, myocardial infarction, ventricular tachycardia and ventricular fibrillation, cardiac arrest, and death.

Some of these events occurred in patients who had no findings of CAD and appear to represent consequences of coronary artery vasospasm. However, among domestic reports of serious cardiac events within 1 hour of sumatriptan administration, almost all of the patients had risk factors predictive of CAD and the presence of significant underlying CAD was established in most cases (see CONTRAINDICATIONS).

Drug-Associated Cerebrovascular Events and Fatalities: Cerebral hemorrhage, subarachnoid hemorrhage, stroke, and other cerebrovascular events have been reported in patients treated with oral or subcutaneous sumatriptan, and some have resulted in fatalities. The relationship of sumatriptan to these events is uncertain. In a number of cases, it appears possible that the cerebrovascular events were primary, sumatriptan having been administered in the incorrect belief that the symptoms experienced were a consequence of migraine when they were not. As with other acute migraine therapies, before treating headaches in patients not previously diagnosed as migraineurs, and in migraineurs who present with atypical symptoms, care should be taken to exclude other potentially serious neurological conditions. It should also be noted that patients with migraine may be at increased risk of certain cerebrovascular events (e.g., cerebrovascular accident, transient ischemic attack).

Other Vasospasm-Related Events: Sumatriptan may cause vasospastic reactions other than coronary artery vasospasm. Both peripheral vascular ischemia and colonic ischemia with abdominal pain and bloody diarrhea have been reported.

Increase in Blood Pressure: Significant elevation in blood pressure, including hypertensive crisis, has been reported on rare occasions in patients with and without a history of hypertension. Sumatriptan is contraindicated in patients with uncontrolled hypertension (see CONTRAINDICATIONS). Sumatriptan should be administered with caution to patients with controlled hypertension as transient increases in blood pressure and peripheral vascular resistance have been observed in a small proportion of patients.

Concomitant Drug Use: In patients taking MAO-A inhibitors, sumatriptan plasma levels attained after treatment with recommended doses are 7-fold higher following oral administration than those obtained under other conditions. Accordingly, the coadministration of IMITREX Tablets and an MAO-A inhibitor is contraindicated (see CLINICAL PHARMACOLOGY and CONTRAINDICATIONS).

Hypersensitivity: Hypersensitivity (anaphylaxis/anaphylactoid) reactions have occurred on rare occasions in patients receiving sumatriptan. Such reactions can be life threatening or fatal. In general, hypersensitivity reactions to drugs are more likely to occur in individuals with a history of sensitivity to multiple allergens (see CONTRAINDICATIONS).

PRECAUTIONS

General: Chest discomfort and jaw or neck tightness have been reported following use of IMITREX Tablets and have also been reported infrequently following administration of IMITREX Nasal Spray. Chest, jaw, or neck tightness is relatively common after administration of IMITREX Injection. Only rarely have these symptoms been associated with ischemic ECG changes. However, because sumatriptan may cause coronary artery vasospasm, patients who experience signs or symptoms suggestive of angina following sumatriptan should be evaluated for the presence of CAD or a predisposition to Prinzmetal variant angina before receiving additional doses of sumatriptan, and should be monitored electrocardiographically if dosing is resumed and similar symptoms recur. Similarly, patients who experience other symptoms or signs suggestive of decreased arterial flow, such as ischemic bowel syndrome or Raynaud syndrome following sumatriptan should be evaluated for atherosclerosis or predisposition to vasospasm (see WARNINGS).

IMITREX should also be administered with caution to patients with diseases that may alter the absorption, metabolism, or excretion of drugs, such as impaired hepatic or renal function.

There have been rare reports of seizure following administration of sumatriptan. Sumatriptan should be used with caution in patients with a history of epilepsy or conditions associated with a lowered seizure threshold.

Care should be taken to exclude other potentially serious neurologic conditions before treating headache in patients not previously diagnosed with migraine headache or who experience a headache that is atypical for them. There have been rare reports where patients received sumatriptan for severe headaches that were subsequently shown to have been secondary to an evolving neurologic lesion (see WARNINGS).

For a given attack, if a patient does not respond to the first dose of sumatriptan, the diagnosis of migraine should be reconsidered before administration of a second dose.

Binding to Melanin-Containing Tissues: In rats treated with a single subcutaneous dose (0.5 mg/kg) or oral dose (2 mg/kg) of radiolabeled sumatriptan, the elimination half-life of radioactivity from the eye was 15 and 23 days, respectively, suggesting that sumatriptan and/or its metabolites bind to the melanin of the eye. Because there could be an accumulation in melanin-rich tissues over time, this raises the possibility that sumatriptan could cause toxicity in these tissues after extended use. However, no effects on the retina related to treatment with sumatriptan were noted in any of the oral or subcutaneous toxicity studies. Although no systematic monitoring of ophthalmologic function was undertaken in clinical trials, and no specific recommendations for ophthalmologic monitoring are offered, prescribers should be aware of the possibility of long-term ophthalmologic effects.

Corneal Opacities: Sumatriptan causes corneal opacities and defects in the corneal epithelium in dogs; this raises the possibility that these changes may occur in humans. While patients were not systematically evaluated for these changes in clinical trials, and no specific recommendations for monitoring are being offered, prescribers should be aware of the possibility of these changes (see ANIMAL TOXICOLOGY).

Information for Patients: See PATIENT INFORMATION at the end of this labeling for the text of the separate leaflet provided for patients.

Laboratory Tests: No specific laboratory tests are recommended for monitoring patients prior to and/or after treatment with sumatriptan.

Drug Interactions: Ergot-containing drugs have been reported to cause prolonged vasospastic reactions. Because there is a theoretical basis that these effects may be additive, use of ergotamine-containing or ergot-type medications (like dihydroergotamine or methysergide) and sumatriptan within 24 hours of each other should be avoided (see CONTRAINDICATIONS).

MAO-A inhibitors reduce sumatriptan clearance, significantly increasing systemic exposure. Therefore, the use of IMITREX Tablets in patients receiving MAO-A inhibitors is contraindicated (see CLINICAL PHARMACOLOGY and CONTRAINDICATIONS).

Selective serotonin reuptake inhibitors (SSRIs) (e.g., fluoxetine, fluvoxamine, paroxetine, sertraline) have been reported, rarely, to cause weakness, hyperreflexia, and incoordination when coadministered with sumatriptan. If concomitant treatment with sumatriptan and an SSRI is clinically warranted, appropriate observation of the patient is advised.

Drug/Laboratory Test Interactions: IMITREX Tablets are not known to interfere with commonly employed clinical laboratory tests.

Carcinogenesis, Mutagenesis, Impairment of Fertility: ***Carcinogenesis:*** In carcinogenicity studies, rats and mice were given sumatriptan by oral gavage (rats, 104 weeks) or drinking water (mice, 78 weeks). Average exposures achieved in mice receiving the highest dose (target dose of 160 mg/kg/day) were approximately 40 times the exposure attained in humans after the maximum recommended single oral dose of 100 mg. The highest dose administered to rats (160 mg/kg/day, reduced from 360 mg/kg/day during week 21) was approximately 15 times the maximum recommended single human oral dose of 100 mg on a mg/m^2 basis. There was no evidence of an increase in tumors in either species related to sumatriptan administration.

Mutagenesis: Sumatriptan was not mutagenic in the presence or absence of metabolic activation when tested in 2 gene mutation assays (the Ames test and the in vitro mammalian Chinese hamster V79/HGPRT assay). In 2 cytogenetics assays (the in vitro human lymphocyte assay and the in vivo rat micronucleus assay) sumatriptan was not associated with clastogenic activity.

Impairment of Fertility: In a study in which male and female rats were dosed daily with oral sumatriptan prior to and throughout the mating period, there was a treatment-related decrease in fertility secondary to a decrease in mating in animals treated with 50 and 500 mg/kg/day. The highest no-effect dose for this finding was 5 mg/kg/day, or approximately one half of the maximum recommended single human oral dose of 100 mg on a mg/m^2 basis. It is not clear whether the problem is associated with treatment of the males or females or both combined. In a similar study by the subcutaneous route there was no evidence of impaired fertility at 60 mg/kg/day, the maximum dose tested, which is

Continued on next page

Product information on these pages is effective as of August 2004. Further information is available at: GlaxoSmithKline, PO Box 13398, Research Triangle Park, NC 27709. 1-888-825-5249. Corporate Web Site: www.gsk.com

Imitrex Tablets—Cont.

equivalent to approximately 6 times the maximum recommended single human oral dose of 100 mg on a mg/m^2 basis.

Pregnancy: Pregnancy Category C. In reproductive toxicity studies in rats and rabbits, oral treatment with sumatriptan was associated with embryolethality, fetal abnormalities, and pup mortality. When administered by the intravenous route to rabbits, sumatriptan has been shown to be embryolethal. There are no adequate and well-controlled studies in pregnant women. Therefore, IMITREX should be used during pregnancy only if the potential benefit justifies the potential risk to the fetus. In assessing this information, the following findings should be considered.

Embryolethality: When given orally or intravenously to pregnant rabbits daily throughout the period of organogenesis, sumatriptan caused embryolethality at doses at or close to those producing maternal toxicity. In the oral studies this dose was 100 mg/kg/day, and in the intravenous studies this dose was 2.0 mg/kg/day. The mechanism of the embryolethality is not known. The highest no-effect dose for embryolethality by the oral route was 50 mg/kg/day, which is approximately 9 times the maximum single recommended human oral dose of 100 mg on a mg/m^2 basis. By the intravenous route, the highest no-effect dose was 0.75 mg/kg/day, or approximately one tenth of the maximum single recommended human oral dose of 100 mg on a mg/m^2 basis.

The intravenous administration of sumatriptan to pregnant rats throughout organogenesis at 12.5 mg/kg/day, the maximum dose tested, did not cause embryolethality. This dose is equivalent to the maximum single recommended human oral dose of 100 mg on a mg/m^2 basis. Additionally, in a study in rats given subcutaneous sumatriptan daily prior to and throughout pregnancy at 60 mg/kg/day, the maximum dose tested, there was no evidence of increased embryo/fetal lethality. This dose is equivalent to approximately 6 times the maximum recommended single human oral dose of 100 mg on a mg/m^2 basis.

Teratogenicity: Oral treatment of pregnant rats with sumatriptan during the period of organogenesis resulted in an increased incidence of blood vessel abnormalities (cervicothoracic and umbilical) at doses of approximately 250 mg/kg/day or higher. The highest no-effect dose was approximately 60 mg/kg/day, which is approximately 6 times the maximum single recommended human oral dose of 100 mg on a mg/m^2 basis. Oral treatment of pregnant rabbits with sumatriptan during the period of organogenesis resulted in an increased incidence of cervicothoracic vascular and skeletal abnormalities. The highest no-effect dose for these effects was 15 mg/kg/day, or approximately 3 times the maximum single recommended human oral dose of 100 mg on a mg/m^2 basis.

A study in which rats were dosed daily with oral sumatriptan prior to and throughout gestation demonstrated embryo/fetal toxicity (decreased body weight, decreased ossification, increased incidence of rib variations) and an increased incidence of a syndrome of malformations (short tail/short body and vertebral disorganization) at 500 mg/kg/day. The highest no-effect dose was 50 mg/kg/day, or approximately 5 times the maximum single recommended human oral dose of 100 mg on a mg/m^2 basis. In a study in rats dosed daily with subcutaneous sumatriptan prior to and throughout pregnancy, at a dose of 60 mg/kg/day, the maximum dose tested, there was no evidence of teratogenicity. This dose is equivalent to approximately 6 times the maximum recommended single human oral dose of 100 mg on a mg/m^2 basis.

Pup Deaths: Oral treatment of pregnant rats with sumatriptan during the period of organogenesis resulted in a decrease in pup survival between birth and postnatal day 4 at doses of approximately 250 mg/kg/day or higher. The highest no-effect dose for this effect was approximately 60 mg/kg/day, or 6 times the maximum single recommended human oral dose of 100 mg on a mg/m^2 basis.

Oral treatment of pregnant rats with sumatriptan from gestational day 17 through postnatal day 21 demonstrated a decrease in pup survival measured at postnatal days 2, 4, and 20 at the dose of 1,000 mg/kg/day. The highest no-effect dose for this finding was 100 mg/kg/day, approximately 10 times the maximum single recommended human oral dose of 100 mg on a mg/m^2 basis. In a similar study in rats by the subcutaneous route there was no increase in pup death at 81 mg/kg/day, the highest dose tested, which is equivalent to 8 times the maximum single recommended human oral dose of 100 mg on a mg/m^2 basis.

Pregnancy Registry: To monitor fetal outcomes of pregnant women exposed to IMITREX, GlaxoSmithKline maintains a Sumatriptan Pregnancy Registry. Physicians are encouraged to register patients by calling (800) 336-2176.

Nursing Mothers: Sumatriptan is excreted in human breast milk. Therefore, caution should be exercised when considering the administration of IMITREX Tablets to a nursing woman.

Pediatric Use: Safety and effectiveness of IMITREX Tablets in pediatric patients have not been established.

Completed placebo-controlled clinical trials evaluating oral sumatriptan (25 to 100 mg) in pediatric patients aged 12 to 17 years enrolled a total of 701 adolescent migraineurs. These studies did not establish the efficacy of oral sumatriptan compared to placebo in the treatment of migraine in adolescents. Adverse events observed in these clinical trials were similar in nature to those reported in clinical trials in adults. The frequency of all adverse events in these patients appeared to be both dose- and age-dependent, with younger patients reporting events more commonly than older adolescents. Postmarketing experience includes a limited number of reports that describe pediatric patients who have experienced adverse events, some clinically serious, after use of subcutaneous sumatriptan and/or oral sumatriptan. These reports include events similar in nature to those reported rarely in adults. A myocardial infarct has been reported in a 14-year-old male following the use of oral sumatriptan; clinical signs occurred within 1 day of drug administration. Since clinical data to determine the frequency of serious adverse events in pediatric patients who might receive injectable, oral, or intranasal sumatriptan are not presently available, the use of sumatriptan in patients aged younger than 18 years is not recommended.

Geriatric Use: The use of sumatriptan in elderly patients is not recommended because elderly patients are more likely to have decreased hepatic function, they are at higher risk for CAD, and blood pressure increases may be more pronounced in the elderly (see WARNINGS).

ADVERSE REACTIONS

Serious cardiac events, including some that have been fatal, have occurred following the use of IMITREX Injection or Tablets. These events are extremely rare and most have been reported in patients with risk factors predictive of CAD. Events reported have included coronary artery vasospasm, transient myocardial ischemia, myocardial infarction, ventricular tachycardia, and ventricular fibrillation (see CONTRAINDICATIONS, WARNINGS, and PRECAUTIONS).

Significant hypertensive episodes, including hypertensive crises, have been reported on rare occasions in patients with or without a history of hypertension (see WARNINGS).

Incidence in Controlled Clinical Trials: Table 2 lists adverse events that occurred in placebo-controlled clinical trials in patients who took at least 1 dose of study drug. Only events that occurred at a frequency of 2% or more in any group treated with IMITREX Tablets and were more frequent in that group than in the placebo group are included in Table 2. The events cited reflect experience gained under closely monitored conditions of clinical trials in a highly selected patient population. In actual clinical practice or in other clinical trials, these frequency estimates may not apply, as the conditions of use, reporting behavior, and the kinds of patients treated may differ.

[See table 2 below]

Other events that occurred in more than 1% of patients receiving IMITREX Tablets and at least as often on placebo included nausea and/or vomiting, migraine, headache, hypersalivation, dizziness, and drowsiness/sleepiness.

IMITREX Tablets are generally well tolerated. Across all doses, most adverse reactions were mild and transient and did not lead to long-lasting effects. The incidence of adverse events in controlled clinical trials was not affected by gender or age of the patients. There were insufficient data to assess the impact of race on the incidence of adverse events.

Other Events Observed in Association With the Administration of IMITREX Tablets: In the paragraphs that follow, the frequencies of less commonly reported adverse clinical events are presented. Because the reports include events observed in open and uncontrolled studies, the role of IMITREX Tablets in their causation cannot be reliably determined. Furthermore, variability associated with adverse event reporting, the terminology used to describe adverse events, etc., limit the value of quantitative frequency estimates provided. Event frequencies are calculated as the number of patients who used IMITREX Tablets (25, 50, or 100 mg) and reported an event divided by the total number of patients (N = 6,348) exposed to IMITREX Tablets. All reported events are included except those already listed in the previous table, those too general to be informative, and those not reasonably associated with the use of the drug. Events are further classified within body system categories and enumerated in order of decreasing frequency using the following definitions: frequent adverse events are defined as those occurring in at least 1/100 patients, infrequent adverse events are those occurring in 1/100 to 1/1,000 patients, and rare adverse events are those occurring in fewer than 1/1,000 patients.

Atypical Sensations: Frequent were burning sensation and numbness. Infrequent was tight feeling in head. Rare were dysesthesia.

Cardiovascular: Frequent were palpitations, syncope, decreased blood pressure, and increased blood pressure. Infrequent were arrhythmia, changes in ECG, hypertension, hypotension, pallor, pulsating sensations, and tachycardia. Rare were angina, atherosclerosis, bradycardia, cerebral ischemia, cerebrovascular lesion, heart block, peripheral cyanosis, thrombosis, transient myocardial ischemia, and vasodilation.

Ear, Nose, and Throat: Frequent were sinusitis, tinnitus; allergic rhinitis; upper respiratory inflammation; ear, nose, and throat hemorrhage; external otitis; hearing loss; nasal inflammation; and sensitivity to noise. Infrequent were hearing disturbances and otalgia. Rare was feeling of fullness in the ear(s).

Endocrine and Metabolic: Infrequent was thirst. Rare were elevated thyrotropin stimulating hormone (TSH) levels; galactorrhea; hyperglycemia; hypoglycemia; hypothyroidism; polydipsia; weight gain; weight loss; endocrine cysts, lumps, and masses; and fluid disturbances.

Eye: Rare were disorders of sclera, mydriasis, blindness and low vision, visual disturbances, eye edema and swelling, eye irritation and itching, accommodation disorders, external ocular muscle disorders, eye hemorrhage, eye pain, and keratitis and conjunctivitis.

Gastrointestinal: Frequent were diarrhea and gastric symptoms. Infrequent were constipation, dysphagia, and gastroesophageal reflux. Rare were gastrointestinal bleeding, hematemesis, melena, peptic ulcer, gastrointestinal pain, dyspeptic symptoms, dental pain, feelings of gastrointestinal pressure, gastroesophageal reflux, gastritis, gastroenteritis, hypersalivation, abdominal distention, oral itching and irritation, salivary gland swelling, and swallowing disorders.

Hematological Disorders: Rare was anemia.

Musculoskeletal: Frequent was myalgia. Infrequent was muscle cramps. Rare were tetany; muscle atrophy, weakness, and tiredness; arthralgia and articular rheumatitis; acquired musculoskeletal deformity; muscle stiffness, tightness, and rigidity; and musculoskeletal inflammation.

Neurological: Frequent were phonophobia and photophobia. Infrequent were confusion, depression, difficulty concentrating, disturbance of smell, dysarthria, euphoria, facial pain, heat sensitivity, incoordination, lacrimation, monoplegia, sleep disturbance, shivering, syncope, and tremor. Rare were aggressiveness, apathy, bradylogia, cluster headache, convulsions, decreased appetite, drug abuse, dystonic reaction, facial paralysis, hallucinations, hunger, hyperesthesia, hysteria, increased alertness, memory disturbance, neuralgia, paralysis, personality change, phobia, radiculopathy, rigidity, suicide, twitching, agitation, anxiety, depressive disorders, detachment, motor dysfunction, neurotic disorders, psychomotor disorders, taste disturbances, and raised intracranial pressure.

Respiratory: Frequent was dyspnea. Infrequent was asthma. Rare were hiccoughs, breathing disorders, cough, and bronchitis.

Skin: Frequent was sweating. Infrequent were erythema, pruritus, rash, and skin tenderness. Rare were dry/scaly skin, tightness of skin, wrinkling of skin, eczema, seborrheic dermatitis, and skin nodules.

Breasts: Infrequent was tenderness. Rare were nipple discharge; breast swelling; cysts, lumps, and masses of breasts; and primary malignant breast neoplasm.

Table 2. Treatment-Emergent Adverse Events Reported by at Least 2% of Patients in Controlled Migraine Trials*

	Percent of Patients Reporting			
Adverse Event Type	Placebo (N = 309)	IMITREX 25 mg (N = 417)	IMITREX 50 mg (N = 771)	IMITREX 100 mg (N = 437)
Atypical sensations	4%	5%	6%	6%
Paresthesia (all types)	2%	3%	5%	3%
Sensation warm/cold	2%	3%	2%	3%
Pain and other pressure sensations	4%	6%	6%	8%
Chest - pain/tightness/ pressure and/or heaviness	1%	1%	2%	2%
Neck/throat/jaw - pain/ tightness/pressure	<1%	<1%	2%	3%
Pain - location specified	1%	2%	1%	1%
Other - pressure/tightness/ heaviness	2%	1%	1%	3%
Neurological				
Vertigo	<1%	<1%	<1%	2%
Other				
Malaise/fatigue	<1%	2%	2%	3%

* Events that occurred at a frequency of 2% or more in the group treated with IMITREX Tablets and that occurred more frequently in that group than the placebo group.

Urogenital: Infrequent were dysmenorrhea, increased urination, and intermenstrual bleeding. Rare were abortion and hematuria, urinary frequency, bladder inflammation, micturition disorders, urethritis, urinary infections, menstruation symptoms, abnormal menstrual cycle, inflammation of fallopian tubes, and menstrual cycle symptoms.
Miscellaneous: Frequent was hypersensitivity. Infrequent were fever, fluid retention, and overdose. Rare were edema, hematoma, lymphadenopathy, speech disturbance, voice disturbances, contusions.
Other Events Observed in the Clinical Development of IMITREX: The following adverse events occurred in clinical trials with IMITREX Injection and IMITREX Nasal Spray. Because the reports include events observed in open and uncontrolled studies, the role of IMITREX in their causation cannot be reliably determined. All reported events are included except those already listed, those too general to be informative, and those not reasonably associated with the use of the drug.
Atypical Sensations: Feeling strange, prickling sensation, tingling, and hot sensation.
Cardiovascular: Abdominal aortic aneurysm, abnormal pulse, flushing, phlebitis, Raynaud syndrome, and various transient ECG changes (nonspecific ST or T wave changes, prolongation of PR or QTc intervals, sinus arrhythmia, nonsustained ventricular premature beats, isolated junctional ectopic beats, atrial ectopic beats, delayed activation of the right ventricle).
Chest Symptoms: Chest discomfort.
Endocrine and Metabolic: Dehydration.
Ear, Nose, and Throat: Disorder/discomfort nasal cavity and sinuses, ear infection, Meniere disease, and throat discomfort.
Eye: Vision alterations.
Gastrointestinal: Abdominal discomfort, colitis, disturbance of liver function tests, flatulence/eructation, gallstones, intestinal obstruction, pancreatitis, and retching.
Injection Site Reaction
Miscellaneous: Difficulty in walking, hypersensitivity to various agents, jaw discomfort, miscellaneous laboratory abnormalities, "serotonin agonist effect," swelling of the extremities, and swelling of the face.
Mouth and Teeth: Disorder of mouth and tongue (e.g., burning of tongue, numbness of tongue, dry mouth).
Musculoskeletal: Arthritis, backache, intervertebral disc disorder, neck pain/stiffness, need to flex calf muscles, and various joint disturbances (pain, stiffness, swelling, ache).
Neurological: Bad/unusual taste, chills, diplegia, disturbance of emotions, sedation, globus hystericus, intoxication, myoclonia, neoplasm of pituitary, relaxation, sensation of lightness, simultaneous hot and cold sensations, stinging sensations, stress, tickling sensations, transient hemiplegia, and yawning.
Respiratory: Influenza and diseases of the lower respiratory tract and lower respiratory tract infection.
Skin: Skin eruption, herpes, and peeling of the skin.
Urogenital: Disorder of breasts, endometriosis, and renal calculus.
Postmarketing Experience (Reports for Subcutaneous or Oral Sumatriptan): The following section enumerates potentially important adverse events that have occurred in clinical practice and that have been reported spontaneously to various surveillance systems. The events enumerated represent reports arising from both domestic and nondomestic use of oral or subcutaneous dosage forms of sumatriptan. The events enumerated include all except those already listed in the ADVERSE REACTIONS section above or those too general to be informative. Because the reports cite events reported spontaneously from worldwide postmarketing experience, frequency of events and the role of sumatriptan in their causation cannot be reliably determined. It is assumed, however, that systemic reactions following sumatriptan use are likely to be similar regardless of route of administration.
Blood: Hemolytic anemia, pancytopenia, thrombocytopenia.
Cardiovascular: Atrial fibrillation, cardiomyopathy, colonic ischemia (see WARNINGS), Prinzmetal variant angina, pulmonary embolism, shock, thrombophlebitis.
Ear, Nose, and Throat: Deafness.
Eye: Ischemic optic neuropathy, retinal artery occlusion, retinal vein thrombosis, loss of vision.
Gastrointestinal: Ischemic colitis with rectal bleeding (see WARNINGS), xerostomia.
Hepatic: Elevated liver function tests.
Neurological: Central nervous system vasculitis, cerebrovascular accident, dysphasia, subarachnoid hemorrhage.
Non-Site Specific: Angioneurotic edema, cyanosis, death (see WARNINGS), temporal arteritis.
Psychiatry: Panic disorder.
Respiratory: Bronchospasm in patients with and without a history of asthma.
Skin: Exacerbation of sunburn, hypersensitivity reactions (allergic vasculitis, erythema, pruritus, rash, shortness of breath, urticaria; in addition, severe anaphylaxis/anaphylactoid reactions have been reported [see WARNINGS]), photosensitivity.
Urogenital: Acute renal failure.

DRUG ABUSE AND DEPENDENCE

One clinical study with IMITREX® (sumatriptan succinate) Injection enrolling 12 patients with a history of substance abuse failed to induce subjective behavior and/or physiologic response ordinarily associated with drugs that have an established potential for abuse.

OVERDOSAGE

Patients (N = 670) have received single oral doses of 140 to 300 mg without significant adverse effects. Volunteers (N = 174) have received single oral doses of 140 to 400 mg without serious adverse events.
Overdose in animals has been fatal and has been heralded by convulsions, tremor, paralysis, inactivity, ptosis, erythema of the extremities, abnormal respiration, cyanosis, ataxia, mydriasis, salivation, and lacrimation. The elimination half-life of sumatriptan is approximately 2.5 hours (see CLINICAL PHARMACOLOGY), and therefore monitoring of patients after overdose with IMITREX Tablets should continue for at least 12 hours or while symptoms or signs persist.
It is unknown what effect hemodialysis or peritoneal dialysis has on the serum concentrations of sumatriptan.

DOSAGE AND ADMINISTRATION

In controlled clinical trials, single doses of 25, 50, or 100 mg of IMITREX Tablets were effective for the acute treatment of migraine in adults. There is evidence that doses of 50 and 100 mg may provide a greater effect than 25 mg (see CLINICAL TRIALS). There is also evidence that doses of 100 mg do not provide a greater effect than 50 mg. Individuals may vary in response to doses of IMITREX Tablets. The choice of dose should therefore be made on an individual basis, weighing the possible benefit of a higher dose with the potential for a greater risk of adverse events.
If the headache returns or the patient has a partial response to the initial dose, the dose may be repeated after 2 hours, not to exceed a total daily dose of 200 mg. If a headache returns following an initial treatment with IMITREX Injection, additional single IMITREX Tablets (up to 100 mg/day) may be given with an interval of at least 2 hours between tablet doses. The safety of treating an average of more than 4 headaches in a 30-day period has not been established.
Because of the potential of MAO-A inhibitors to cause unpredictable elevations in the bioavailability of oral sumatriptan, their combined use is contraindicated (see CONTRAINDICATIONS).
Hepatic disease/functional impairment may also cause unpredictable elevations in the bioavailability of orally administered sumatriptan. Consequently, if treatment is deemed advisable in the presence of liver disease, the maximum single dose should in general not exceed 50 mg (see CLINICAL PHARMACOLOGY for the basis of this recommendation).

HOW SUPPLIED

IMITREX Tablets, 25, 50, and 100 mg of sumatriptan (base) as the succinate.
IMITREX Tablets, 25 mg are white, triangular-shaped, film-coated tablets debossed with "I" on one side and "25" on the other in blister packs of 9 tablets (NDC 0173-0735-00).
IMITREX Tablets, 50 mg are white, triangular-shaped, film-coated tablets debossed with "IMITREX 50" on one side and a chevron shape (^) on the other in blister packs of 9 tablets (NDC 0173-0736-01).
IMITREX Tablets, 100 mg, are pink, triangular-shaped, film-coated tablets debossed with "IMITREX 100" on one side and a chevron shape (^) on the other in blister packs of 9 tablets (NDC 0173-0737-01).
Store between 36° and 86°F (2° and 30°C).

ANIMAL TOXICOLOGY

Corneal Opacities: Dogs receiving oral sumatriptan developed corneal opacities and defects in the corneal epithelium. Corneal opacities were seen at the lowest dosage tested, 2 mg/kg/day, and were present after 1 month of treatment. Defects in the corneal epithelium were noted in a 60-week study. Earlier examinations for these toxicities were not conducted and no-effect doses were not established; however, the relative exposure at the lowest dose tested was approximately 5 times the human exposure after a 100-mg oral dose. There is evidence of alterations in corneal appearance on the first day of intranasal dosing to dogs. Changes were noted at the lowest dose tested, which was approximately one half the maximum single human oral dose of 100 mg on a mg/m^2 basis.

PATIENT INFORMATION

The following wording is contained in a separate leaflet provided for patients.

Information for the Patient
IMITREX® (sumatriptan succinate) Tablets

Please read this leaflet carefully before you take IMITREX Tablets. This provides a summary of the information available on your medicine. Please do not throw away this leaflet until you have finished your medicine. You may need to read this leaflet again. This leaflet does not contain all the information on IMITREX Tablets. For further information or advice, ask your doctor or pharmacist.
Information About Your Medicine:
The name of your medicine is IMITREX (sumatriptan succinate) Tablets. It can be obtained only by prescription from your doctor. The decision to use IMITREX Tablets is one that you and your doctor should make jointly, taking into account your individual preferences and medical circumstances. If you have risk factors for heart disease (such as high blood pressure, high cholesterol, obesity, diabetes, smoking, strong family history of heart disease, or you are postmenopausal or a male over 40 years of age), you should tell your doctor, who should evaluate you for heart disease in order to determine if IMITREX is appropriate for you. Although the vast majority of those who have taken IMITREX have not experienced any significant side effects, some individuals have experienced serious heart problems and, rarely, considering the extensiveness of IMITREX use worldwide, deaths have been reported. In all but a few instances, however, serious problems occurred in people with known heart disease and it was not clear whether IMITREX was a contributory factor in these deaths.
1. The Purpose of Your Medicine:
IMITREX Tablets are intended to relieve your migraine, but not to prevent or reduce the number of attacks you experience. Use IMITREX Tablets only to treat an actual migraine attack.
2. Important Questions to Consider Before Taking IMITREX Tablets:
If the answer to any of the following questions is **YES** or if you do not know the answer, then please discuss it with your doctor before you use IMITREX Tablets.

- Are you pregnant? Do you think you might be pregnant? Are you trying to become pregnant? Are you using inadequate contraception? Are you breastfeeding?
- Do you have any chest pain, heart disease, shortness of breath, or irregular heartbeats? Have you had a heart attack?
- Do you have risk factors for heart disease (such as high blood pressure, high cholesterol, obesity, diabetes, smoking, strong family history of heart disease, or you are postmenopausal or a male over 40 years of age)?
- Have you had a stroke, transient ischemic attacks (TIAs), or Raynaud syndrome?
- Do you have high blood pressure?
- Have you ever had to stop taking this or any other medicine because of an allergy or other problems?
- Are you taking any other migraine medicines, including other 5-HT_1 agonists or any other medicines containing ergotamine, dihydroergotamine, or methysergide?
- Are you taking any medicine for depression (monoamine oxidase inhibitors or selective serotonin reuptake inhibitors [SSRIs])?
- Have you had, or do you have, any disease of the liver or kidney?
- Have you had, or do you have, epilepsy or seizures?
- Is this headache different from your usual migraine attacks?

Remember, if you answered **YES** to any of the above questions, then discuss it with your doctor.
3. The Use of IMITREX Tablets During Pregnancy:
Do not use IMITREX Tablets if you are pregnant, think you might be pregnant, are trying to become pregnant, or are not using adequate contraception, unless you have discussed this with your doctor.
4. How to Use IMITREX Tablets:
For adults, the usual dose is a single tablet taken whole with water or other fluids. Do not split tablets.
A second tablet may be taken if your symptoms of migraine come back or if you have a partial response to the initial dose, but not sooner than 2 hours following the first tablet. For a given attack, if you have no response to the first tablet, do not take a second tablet without first consulting with your doctor. Do not take more than a total of 200 mg of IMITREX Tablets in any 24-hour period. The safety of treating an average of more than 4 headaches in a 30-day period has not been established.
5. Side Effects to Watch for:

- Some patients experience pain or tightness in the chest or throat when using IMITREX Tablets. If this happens to you, then discuss it with your doctor before using any more IMITREX Tablets. If the chest pain is severe or does not go away, call your doctor immediately.
- If you have sudden and/or severe abdominal pain following IMITREX Tablets, call your doctor immediately.
- Shortness of breath; wheeziness; heart throbbing; swelling of eyelids, face, or lips; or a skin rash, skin lumps, or hives happens rarely. If it happens to you, then tell your doctor immediately. Do not take any more IMITREX Tablets unless your doctor tells you to do so.
- Some people may have feelings of tingling, heat, flushing (redness of face lasting a short time), heaviness or pressure after treatment with IMITREX Tablets. A few people may feel drowsy, dizzy, tired, or sick. Tell your doctor of these symptoms at your next visit.
- If you feel unwell in any other way or have any symptoms that you do not understand, you should contact your doctor immediately.

6. What to Do if an Overdose is Taken:
If you have taken more medicine than you have been told, contact either your doctor, hospital emergency department, or nearest poison control center immediately.

Continued on next page

Product information on these pages is effective as of August 2004. Further information is available at: GlaxoSmithKline, PO Box 13398, Research Triangle Park, NC 27709. 1-888-825-5249. Corporate Web Site: www.gsk.com

Imitrex Tablets—Cont.

7. Storing Your Medicine:
Keep your medicine in a safe place where children cannot reach it. It may be harmful to children. Do not remove tablets from the packaging until you are ready to use them. Do not store the tablets in any other container.
Store your medicine away from heat and light. Do not store at temperatures above 86°F (30°C), or below 36°F (2°C).
If your medicine has expired (the expiration date is printed on the treatment pack), throw it away as instructed. If your doctor decides to stop your treatment, do not keep any leftover medicine unless your doctor tells you to. Throw away your medicine as instructed.
GlaxoSmithKline, Research Triangle Park, NC 27709

February 2004/RL-2069
Shown in Product Identification Guide, page 316

INFANRIX® ℞

[in' fan-rix]
Diphtheria and Tetanus Toxoids and Acellular Pertussis Vaccine Adsorbed

DESCRIPTION

INFANRIX (Diphtheria and Tetanus Toxoids and Acellular Pertussis Vaccine Adsorbed) is a noninfectious, sterile combination of diphtheria and tetanus toxoids and 3 pertussis antigens [inactivated pertussis toxin (PT), filamentous hemagglutinin (FHA), and pertactin (69 kiloDalton outer membrane protein)] adsorbed onto aluminum hydroxide. INFANRIX is intended for intramuscular injection only.
The diphtheria toxin is produced by growing *Corynebacterium diphtheriae* in Fenton medium containing a bovine extract. Tetanus toxin is produced by growing *Clostridium tetani* in a modified Latham medium derived from bovine casein. The bovine materials used in these extracts are sourced from countries which the United States Department of Agriculture (USDA) has determined neither have nor are at risk of bovine spongiform encephalopathy (BSE). Both toxins are detoxified with formaldehyde, concentrated by ultrafiltration, and purified by precipitation, dialysis, and sterile filtration.
The 3 acellular pertussis antigens (PT, FHA, and pertactin) are isolated from *Bordetella pertussis* culture grown in modified Stainer-Scholte liquid medium. PT and FHA are isolated from the fermentation broth; pertactin is extracted from the cells by heat treatment and flocculation. The antigens are purified in successive chromatographic and precipitation steps. PT is detoxified using glutaraldehyde and formaldehyde. FHA and pertactin are treated with formaldehyde.
Each antigen is individually adsorbed onto aluminum hydroxide. Each 0.5-mL dose is formulated to contain 25 Lf of diphtheria toxoid, 10 Lf of tetanus toxoid, 25 mcg of inactivated PT, 25 mcg of FHA, and 8 mcg of pertactin.
Diphtheria and tetanus toxoid potency is determined by measuring the amount of neutralizing antitoxin in previously immunized guinea pigs. The potency of the acellular pertussis components (PT, FHA, and pertactin) is determined by enzyme-linked immunosorbent assay (ELISA) on sera from previously immunized mice.
Each 0.5-mL dose also contains 2.5 mg of 2-phenoxyethanol as a preservative, 4.5 mg of NaCl, and aluminum adjuvant (not more than 0.625 mg aluminum by assay). Each dose also contains ≤100 mcg of residual formaldehyde and ≤100 mcg of polysorbate 80 (Tween 80). INFANRIX does not contain thimerosal.
The vaccine must be well shaken before administration and is a turbid white suspension after shaking.
Diphtheria and Tetanus Toxoids Adsorbed Bulk Concentrates (For Further Manufacturing) is manufactured by Chiron Behring GmbH & Co, Marburg, Germany. The acellular pertussis antigens are manufactured by GlaxoSmithKline Biologicals, Rixensart, Belgium. Formulation, filling, testing, packaging, and release of the vaccine are performed by GlaxoSmithKline Biologicals Manufacturing (wholly-owned subsidiary of GlaxoSmithKline Biologicals).

CLINICAL PHARMACOLOGY

Simultaneous immunization against diphtheria, tetanus, and pertussis during infancy and childhood has been a routine practice in the United States since the late 1940s. It has played a major role in markedly reducing the incidence of, and deaths from, each of these diseases.
Diphtheria: Diphtheria is an acute toxin-mediated infectious disease caused by toxigenic strains of *C. diphtheriae*. Although the incidence of diphtheria in the United States has decreased from more than 200,000 cases reported in 1921,[1] before the general use of diphtheria toxoid, to only 51 cases of respiratory diphtheria reported from 1980 through 2000,[2] the case-fatality rate has remained constant at about 10%. Of 41 cases reported between 1980 and 1994, 15 (37%) patients had never been immunized, 21 (51%) had been inadequately immunized, and immunization history was unknown for 5 (12%). All 4 (10%) fatalities in this time period occurred in unvaccinated children 9 years and younger.[3] Although diphtheria is rare in the United States, toxigenic *C. diphtheriae* strains continue to circulate in previously endemic areas.[4] Protection against disease is due to the development of neutralizing antibodies to the diphtheria toxin. Following adequate immunization with diphtheria toxoid, it is thought that protection persists for at least 10 years. A serum diphtheria antitoxin level of 0.01 IU/mL is the lowest level giving some degree of protection.[5] Antitoxin levels of at least 0.1 IU/mL are generally regarded as protective.[5] Immunization with diphtheria toxoid does not, however, eliminate carriage of *C. diphtheriae* in the pharynx or nares or on the skin.[1]
Efficacy of diphtheria toxoid used in INFANRIX was determined on the basis of immunogenicity studies. A VERO cell toxin neutralizing test confirmed the ability of infant sera (N = 45), obtained 1 month after a 3-dose primary series, to neutralize diphtheria toxin. Levels of diphtheria antitoxin ≥0.01 IU/mL were achieved in 100% of the sera tested.
Tetanus: Tetanus is a condition manifested primarily by neuromuscular dysfunction caused by a potent exotoxin released by *C. tetani*. Following the introduction of vaccination with tetanus toxoid in the 1940s, the overall incidence of tetanus declined from 0.4 per 100,000 population in 1947 to 0.02 per 100,000 population during the latter half of the 1990s.[6] Adults 60 years of age and older are at greatest risk for tetanus and tetanus-related mortality.[6] Of 124 cases of tetanus reported from 1995 through 1997, 12 (9.7%) occurred among persons younger than 25 years, one of which was a case of neonatal tetanus.[7] Overall, the case-fatality rate was 11%. The disease continues to occur almost exclusively among persons who are unvaccinated, inadequately vaccinated, or whose vaccination histories are unknown or uncertain.[7]
Spores of *C. tetani* are ubiquitous. Naturally acquired immunity to tetanus toxin does not occur. Thus, universal primary immunization and timed booster doses to maintain adequate tetanus antitoxin levels are necessary to protect all age groups.[1] Protection against disease is due to the development of neutralizing antibodies to the tetanus toxin. A serum tetanus antitoxin level of at least 0.01 IU/mL, measured by neutralization assays, is considered the minimum protective level.[8,9] More recently a level ≥0.1 to 0.2 IU/mL has been considered as protective.[10] It is thought that protection persists for at least 10 years.[1]
Efficacy of tetanus toxoid used in INFANRIX was determined on the basis of immunogenicity studies. An in vivo mouse neutralization assay confirmed the ability of infant sera (N = 45), obtained 1 month after a 3-dose primary series, to neutralize tetanus toxin. Levels of tetanus antitoxin ≥0.01 IU/mL were achieved in 100% of the sera tested.
Pertussis: Pertussis (whooping cough) is a disease of the respiratory tract caused by *B. pertussis*. Pertussis is highly communicable (attack rates in unimmunized household contacts of up to 100% have been reported[1,11]) and can cause severe disease, particularly in young infants.[1] Since immunization against pertussis became widespread, the number of reported cases and associated mortality in the United States has declined from an average annual incidence and mortality of 150 cases and 6 deaths per 100,000 population, respectively, in the early 1940s to an annual reported incidence of 2.7 cases per 100,000 population between 1997 and 2000.[12] Of 28,187 cases of pertussis reported among all ages from 1997 to 2000 and for which supplemental clinical information is available, 62 (0.2%) resulted in death.[12] The highest number of pertussis cases (7,867) since 1967 was reported in 2000. From 1997 to 2000, infants younger than 1 year had the highest average annual incidence rate (55.5 cases per 100,000 population). During this period, of the 8,276 pertussis cases reported nationally in infants younger than 1 year, 59% were hospitalized, 11% had pneumonia, 1.3% had seizures, 0.2% had encephalopathy, and 0.7% died. Older children, adolescents, and adults, in whom classic signs are often absent, may go undiagnosed and may serve as reservoirs of disease.[1,13] The incidence of reported pertussis among adolescents and adults increased during the 1980s and 1990s.[12,14]
The role of the different components produced by *B. pertussis* in either the pathogenesis of, or the immunity to, pertussis is not well understood.
Efficacy of a 3-dose primary series of INFANRIX has been assessed in 2 clinical studies.[15,16]
A double-blind, randomized, active Diphtheria and Tetanus Toxoids (DT)-controlled trial conducted in Italy, sponsored by the National Institutes of Health (NIH), assessed the absolute protective efficacy of INFANRIX when administered at 2, 4, and 6 months of age.[15] A total of 15,601 infants were immunized with 1 of 2 acellular DTP (DTaP) vaccines, a US-licensed whole-cell DTP vaccine, or with DT vaccine alone. The mean length of follow-up was 17 months (mean age 24 months), beginning 30 days after the third dose of vaccine. The population used in the primary analysis of the efficacy of INFANRIX included 4,481 infants vaccinated with INFANRIX, and 1,470 DT vaccinees. After 3 doses, the absolute protective efficacy of INFANRIX against WHO-defined typical pertussis (21 days or more of paroxysmal cough with infection confirmed by culture and/or serologic testing) was 84% (95% CI: 76% to 89%). When the definition of pertussis was expanded to include clinically milder disease with respect to type and duration of cough, with infection confirmed by culture and/or serologic testing, the efficacy of INFANRIX was calculated to be 71% (95% CI: 60% to 78%) against >7 days of any cough and 73% (95% CI: 63% to 80%) against ≥14 days of any cough. Vaccine efficacy after 3 doses and with no booster dose in the second year of life was assessed in 2 subsequent follow-up periods. A follow-up period from 24 months to a mean age of 33 months was conducted in a partially unblinded cohort (children who received DT were offered pertussis vaccine and those who declined were retained in the study cohort). During this period, the efficacy of INFANRIX against WHO-defined pertussis was 78% (95% CI: 62% to 87%).[17] During the third follow-up period which was conducted in an unblinded manner among children from 3 to 6 years of age, the efficacy of INFANRIX against WHO-defined pertussis was 86% (95% CI: 79% to 91%). Thus, protection against pertussis in children administered 3 doses of INFANRIX in infancy was sustained to 6 years of age.[18]
A prospective efficacy trial was also conducted in Germany employing a household contact study design.[16] In preparation for this study, 3 doses of INFANRIX were administered at 3, 4, and 5 months of age to more than 22,000 children living in 6 areas of Germany in a safety and immunogenicity study. Infants who did not participate in the safety and immunogenicity study could have received a whole-cell DTP vaccine or DT vaccine. Index cases were identified by spontaneous presentation to a physician. Households with at least one other member (i.e., besides index case) aged 6 through 47 months were enrolled. Household contacts of index cases were monitored for incidence of pertussis by a physician who was blinded to the vaccination status of the household. Calculation of vaccine efficacy was based on attack rates of pertussis in household contacts classified by vaccination status. Of the 173 household contacts who had not received a pertussis vaccine, 96 developed WHO-defined pertussis, as compared to 7 of 112 contacts vaccinated with INFANRIX. The protective efficacy of INFANRIX was calculated to be 89% (95% CI: 77% to 95%), with no indication of waning of protection up until the time of the booster vaccination. The average age of infants vaccinated with INFANRIX at the end of follow-up in this trial was 13 months (range 6 to 25 months). When the definition of pertussis was expanded to include clinically milder disease, with infection confirmed by culture and/or serologic testing, the efficacy of INFANRIX against ≥7 days of any cough was 67% (95% CI: 52% to 78%) and against ≥7 days of paroxysmal cough was 81% (95% CI: 68% to 89%). The corresponding efficacy rates of INFANRIX against ≥14 days of any cough or paroxysmal cough were 73% (95% CI: 59% to 82%) and 84% (95% CI: 71% to 91%), respectively.
Immune Response to INFANRIX Administered as a 3-Dose Primary Series: The immune responses to each of the 3 pertussis antigens contained in INFANRIX were evaluated in sera obtained 1 month after the third dose of vaccine in each of 3 studies (schedule of administration: 2, 4, and 6 months of age in the Italian efficacy study and one US study; 3, 4, and 5 months of age in the German efficacy study). One month after the third dose of INFANRIX, the response rates to each pertussis antigen were similar in all 3 studies. Thus, although a serologic correlate of protection for pertussis has not been established, the antibody responses to these 3 pertussis antigens (PT, FHA, and pertactin) in a US population were similar to those achieved in 2 populations in which efficacy of INFANRIX was demonstrated.
Immune Response to Concomitantly Administered Vaccines: In a clinical trial in the United States, INFANRIX was given concomitantly, at separate sites, with hepatitis B vaccine, *Haemophilus influenzae* type b vaccine (Hib), and poliovirus vaccine live oral (OPV), at 2, 4, and 6 months of age. One month after the third dose of hepatitis B vaccine given simultaneously with INFANRIX, 100% of infants demonstrated anti-HBs antibodies ≥10 mIU/mL (N = 64). Ninety percent of infants who received Hib simultaneously with INFANRIX achieved anti-PRP antibodies ≥1 mcg/mL (N = 72), and 96% to 100% of infants who received OPV simultaneously with INFANRIX showed protective neutralizing antibody to poliovirus Types 1, 2, and 3 (N = 60–61).[19]
In the Italian efficacy trial, 92% of infants received hepatitis B vaccine with the first and second dose of INFANRIX. Ninety-four percent of infants received OPV with the first and second dose of INFANRIX.[15]
No immunogenicity data are available for concurrent administration of INFANRIX with pneumococcal conjugate vaccine, inactivated poliovirus vaccine (IPV), measles, mumps, and rubella vaccine (MMR), or varicella vaccine.

INDICATIONS AND USAGE

INFANRIX is indicated for active immunization against diphtheria, tetanus, and pertussis (whooping cough) as a 5-dose series in infants and children 6 weeks to 7 years of age (prior to seventh birthday). Because of the substantial risks of complications from pertussis disease in infants, completion of the primary series of 3 doses of vaccine early in life is strongly recommended (see DOSAGE AND ADMINISTRATION).[1] INFANRIX should not be administered to any infant before the age of 6 weeks, or to individuals 7 years of age or older.
When passive protection against tetanus or diphtheria is required, Tetanus Immune Globulin or Diphtheria Antitoxin, respectively, should be administered at separate sites.[1]
As with any vaccine, INFANRIX may not protect 100% of individuals receiving the vaccine, and is not recommended for treatment of actual infections.

CONTRAINDICATIONS

Hypersensitivity to any component of the vaccine is a contraindication (see DESCRIPTION).
It is a contraindication to use this vaccine after a serious allergic reaction (e.g., anaphylaxis) temporally associated with a previous dose of this vaccine or with any components

of this vaccine. Because of the uncertainty as to which component of the vaccine might be responsible, no further vaccination with any of these components should be given. Alternatively, such individuals may be referred to an allergist for evaluation if further immunizations are to be considered.[1]

In addition, the following events are contraindications to administration of any pertussis-containing vaccine, including INFANRIX:[10]

- Encephalopathy (e.g., coma, decreased level of consciousness, prolonged seizures) within 7 days of administration of a previous dose of a pertussis-containing vaccine that is not attributable to another identifiable cause;
- Progressive neurologic disorder, including infantile spasms, uncontrolled epilepsy, or progressive encephalopathy. Pertussis vaccine should not be administered to individuals with such conditions until a treatment regimen has been established and the condition has stabilized.

  In instances where the pertussis vaccine component is contraindicated, Diphtheria and Tetanus Toxoids Adsorbed (DT) For Pediatric Use should be administered.[1]

  INFANRIX is not contraindicated for use in individuals with HIV infection.[10,20]

WARNINGS

The vial stopper is latex-free. The tip cap and the rubber plunger of the needleless prefilled syringes contain dry natural latex rubber that may cause allergic reactions in latex sensitive individuals.

If Guillain-Barré syndrome occurs within 6 weeks of receipt of prior vaccine containing tetanus toxoid, the decision to give subsequent doses of INFANRIX or any vaccine containing tetanus toxoid should be based on careful consideration of the potential benefits and possible risks.[10]

If any of the following events occur in temporal relation to receipt of whole-cell DTP or a vaccine containing an acellular pertussis component, the decision to give subsequent doses of INFANRIX or any vaccine containing a pertussis component should be based on careful consideration of the potential benefits and possible risks:[21,22]

- Temperature of ≥40.5°C (105°F) within 48 hours not due to another identifiable cause;
- Collapse or shock-like state (hypotonic-hyporesponsive episode) within 48 hours;
- Persistent, inconsolable crying lasting ≥3 hours, occurring within 48 hours;
- Seizures with or without fever occurring within 3 days.

When a decision is made to withhold pertussis vaccine, Diphtheria and Tetanus Toxoids Adsorbed (DT) For Pediatric Use should be administered.[1]

A committee of the Institute of Medicine (IOM) has concluded that evidence is consistent with a causal relationship between whole-cell DTP vaccine and acute neurologic illness, and under special circumstances, between whole-cell DTP vaccine and chronic neurologic disease in the context of the National Childhood Encephalopathy Study (NCES) report.[23,24] However, the IOM committee concluded that the evidence was insufficient to indicate whether or not whole-cell DTP vaccine increased the overall risk of chronic neurologic disease.[24] Encephalopathy has been reported following INFANRIX (see ADVERSE REACTIONS, Postmarketing Reports), but data are not sufficient to evaluate a causal relationship.

The decision to administer a pertussis-containing vaccine to children with stable CNS disorders must be made by the physician on an individual basis, with consideration of all relevant factors, and assessment of potential risks and benefits for that individual. The Advisory Committee on Immunization Practices (ACIP) and the Committee on Infectious Diseases of the American Academy of Pediatrics (AAP) have issued guidelines for such children.[21,25] The parent or guardian should be advised of the potential increased risk involved (see PRECAUTIONS, Information for Vaccine Recipients and Parents or Guardians).

A family history of seizures or other CNS disorders is not a contraindication to pertussis vaccine.[21]

For children at higher risk for seizures than the general population, an appropriate antipyretic may be administered at the time of vaccination with a vaccine containing an acellular pertussis component (including INFANRIX) and for the ensuing 24 hours according to the respective prescribing information recommended dosage to reduce the possibility of post-vaccination fever.[10,21]

Vaccination should be deferred during the course of a moderate or severe illness with or without fever. Such children should be vaccinated as soon as they have recovered from the acute phase of the illness.[10]

INFANRIX should not be given to infants or children with bleeding disorders such as hemophilia or thrombocytopenia that would contraindicate intramuscular injection, or to children on anticoagulant therapy unless the potential benefit clearly outweighs the risk of administration. If the decision is made to administer INFANRIX in such children, it should be given with caution, with steps taken to avoid the risk of bleeding and hematoma formation following injection.

PRECAUTIONS

Before the injection of any biological, the physician should take all reasonable precautions to prevent allergic or other adverse reactions, including understanding the use of the biological concerned, and the nature of the side effects and adverse reactions that may follow its use.

Table 1.[15] Adverse Events (%) Occurring Within the 3 Days Following Vaccination of Italian Infants With Either INFANRIX or Whole-Cell DTP at 2, 4, and 6 Months of Age

	INFANRIX			Whole-Cell DTP Vaccine		
	Dose 1	Dose 2	Dose 3	Dose 1	Dose 2	Dose 3
No. of infants	4,696	4,560	4,505	4,678	4,474	4,368
Local						
Redness	4.8	8.6	16.0	27.1	24.2	28.0
Redness ≥2.4 cm	1.0	1.3	3.5	12.4	7.3	7.7
Swelling	5.2	8.2	14.5	28.9	23.5	25.8
Swelling ≥2.4 cm	0.7	1.2	2.9	13.1	7.4	8.0
Tenderness	4.7	4.0	5.2	36.0	26.8	25.9
Systemic						
Fever (≥100.4°F)*	7.1	7.9	9.0	46.8	36.1	39.8
Irritability	36.3	34.9	28.8	57.2	50.1	47.2
Drowsiness	34.9	18.8	11.4	54.0	34.1	23.0
Loss of Appetite	16.5	13.9	11.5	31.2	22.8	19.1
Vomiting	5.8†	4.1†	3.3	6.7	4.7	4.8
Crying ≥1 Hour	3.9	3.3	2.2	17.3	11.1	8.2

*Rectal temperatures.

† For the comparison of INFANRIX and whole-cell DTP vaccine, all adverse events reached statistical significance ($p<0.001$) at all doses except vomiting at doses 1 and 2, which was not statistically significant at $p<0.05$.

Table 2.[27] Adverse Events (%) Occurring Within the 3 Days Following Vaccination of US Infants With Either INFANRIX or Whole-Cell DTP at 2, 4, and 6 Months of Age

	INFANRIX			Whole-Cell DTP Vaccine-Lederle			Whole-Cell DTP Vaccine-Connaught		
	Dose 1	Dose 2	Dose 3	Dose 1	Dose 2	Dose 3	Dose 1	Dose 2	Dose 3
No. of infants	407	402	395	74	73	73	76	75	74
Local									
Redness*	10.6	19.4	25.8	28.4	42.5	39.7	35.5	50.7	50.0
Swelling	7.4†¶	12.2†¶	17.5¶	23.0†	26.0†	27.4	30.3¶	37.3¶	31.1¶
Pain*‡	2.7	2.0	1.5	17.6	15.1	9.6	38.2	17.3	14.9
Systemic									
Fever (>101°F)§	0.5†¶	0.7†¶	5.1	12.2†	8.2†	6.8	14.5¶	18.7¶	8.1
Fussiness**	3.9†¶	3.5†¶	4.1	25.7†	13.7†	6.8	21.1¶	16.0¶	8.1
Drowsiness	26.3†¶	16.4†¶	12.9†	51.4†	34.2†	23.3†	52.6¶	28.0¶	18.9
Poor Appetite	8.1†¶	7.7	6.6	31.1†	15.1	9.6	19.7¶	14.7	9.5
Vomiting	6.6	3.7	3.8	8.1	4.1	2.7	7.9	2.7	2.7

‡Moderate or severe = cried or protested to touch or cried when leg moved.

**Moderate or severe = prolonged crying and refusal to play or persistent crying that could not be comforted.

§Rectal temperatures.

*$p<0.05$ for the comparison of INFANRIX and both whole-cell DTP vaccines.

†$p<0.05$ for the comparison of INFANRIX and whole-cell DTP vaccine-Lederle.

¶$p<0.05$ for the comparison of INFANRIX and whole-cell DTP vaccine-Connaught.

Prior to immunization, the patient's current health status and medical history should be reviewed. The physician should review the patient's immunization history for possible vaccine sensitivity, previous vaccination-related adverse reactions, and occurrence of any adverse-event-related symptoms and/or signs, in order to determine the existence of any contraindication to immunization with INFANRIX and to allow an assessment of benefits and risks. Epinephrine injection (1:1,000) and other appropriate agents used for the control of immediate allergic reactions must be immediately available should an acute anaphylactic reaction occur.

A separate sterile syringe and sterile disposable needle or a sterile disposable unit should be used for each individual patient to prevent transmission of hepatitis or other infectious agents from one person to another. Needles should be disposed of properly and should not be recapped.

Special care should be taken to prevent injection into a blood vessel.

As with any vaccine, if administered to immunosuppressed persons, including individuals receiving immunosuppressive therapy, the expected immune response may not be obtained.[20]

Information for Vaccine Recipients and Parents or Guardians: Parents or guardians should be informed by the healthcare provider of the potential benefits and risks of the vaccine, and of the importance of completing the immunization series. When a child returns for the next dose in a series, it is important that the parent or guardian be questioned concerning occurrence of any symptoms and/or signs of an adverse reaction after a previous dose of the same vaccine. The physician should inform the parents or guardians about the potential for adverse reactions that have been temporally associated with administration of INFANRIX or other vaccines containing similar components. The parent or guardian accompanying the recipient should be told to report severe or unusual adverse events to the physician or clinic where the vaccine was administered.

The parent or guardian should be given the Vaccine Information Statements, which are required by the National Childhood Vaccine Injury Act of 1986 to be given prior to immunization. These materials are available free of charge at the CDC website (www.cdc.gov/nip).

The US Department of Health and Human Services has established a Vaccine Adverse Event Reporting System (VAERS) to accept all reports of suspected adverse events after the administration of any vaccine, including but not limited to the reporting of events required by the National

Continued on next page

Product information on these pages is effective as of August 2004. Further information is available at: GlaxoSmithKline, PO Box 13398, Research Triangle Park, NC 27709. 1-888-825-5249. Corporate Web Site: www.gsk.com

Infanrix—Cont.

Childhood Vaccine Injury Act of 1986.[10] The VAERS toll-free number is 1-800-822-7967.

Drug Interactions: For information regarding simultaneous administration with other vaccines, refer to DOSAGE AND ADMINISTRATION and CLINICAL PHARMACOLOGY.

INFANRIX should not be mixed with any other vaccine in the same syringe or vial.

Immunosuppressive therapies, including irradiation, antimetabolites, alkylating agents, cytotoxic drugs, and corticosteroids (used in greater than physiologic doses), may reduce the immune response to vaccines. Although no specific data from studies with INFANRIX under these conditions are available, if immunosuppressive therapy will be discontinued shortly, it would be reasonable to defer immunization until the patient has been off therapy for 3 months; otherwise, the patient should be vaccinated while still on therapy.[1,20] If INFANRIX is administered to a person receiving immunosuppressive therapy, or who received a recent injection of immune globulin, or who has an immunodeficiency disorder, an adequate immunologic response may not be obtained.

Tetanus Immune Globulin or Diphtheria Antitoxin, if needed, should be given at a separate site, with a separate needle and syringe.

Carcinogenesis, Mutagenesis, Impairment of Fertility: INFANRIX has not been evaluated for carcinogenic or mutagenic potential, or for impairment of fertility.

Pregnancy: Pregnancy Category C. INFANRIX is not indicated for women of child-bearing age. Animal reproduction studies have not been conducted with INFANRIX. It is not known whether INFANRIX can cause fetal harm when administered to a pregnant woman or if INFANRIX can affect reproductive capacity.

Geriatric Use: INFANRIX is not indicated for use in adult populations.

Pediatric Use: Safety and effectiveness of INFANRIX in infants younger than 6 weeks of age have not been evaluated (see DOSAGE AND ADMINISTRATION). INFANRIX is not recommended for persons 7 years of age or older. Tetanus and Diphtheria Toxoids Adsorbed For Adult Use (Td) should be used in individuals 7 years of age or older.

ADVERSE REACTIONS

Approximately 92,000 doses of INFANRIX have been administered in clinical studies. In these studies, 28,749 infants have received INFANRIX in primary series studies, 5,830 children have received INFANRIX as a fourth dose following 3 doses of INFANRIX, and 511 children have received INFANRIX as a fifth dose following 4 doses of INFANRIX. In addition, 439 children and 169 children have received INFANRIX as a fourth or fifth dose following 3 or 4 doses of whole-cell DTP vaccine, respectively. In comparative studies, the first 4 doses of INFANRIX have been shown to be followed by fewer of the local and systemic adverse reactions commonly associated with whole-cell DTP vaccination.[26] However, studies have shown that the rate of local injection site reactions (erythema and swelling) and fever increased with successive doses of INFANRIX.

In the double-blind, randomized comparative trial in Italy, safety data in a 3-dose primary series are available for 4,696 infants who received at least one dose of INFANRIX and 4,678 infants who received at least one dose of US-licensed whole-cell DTP vaccine manufactured by Connaught Laboratories, Inc.[15,26] Data were actively collected by parents using standardized diaries for 8 consecutive evenings after each vaccine dose with follow-up telephone calls made by nurses after the eighth day. Table 1 lists adverse events reported during the 3 days after each dose. All common solicited adverse events were less frequent following vaccination with INFANRIX as compared to whole-cell DTP after each 1 of the 3 doses.

[See table 1 at top of previous page]

A similar reduction in adverse events was seen in a randomized, double-blind, comparative trial conducted in the United States when INFANRIX was compared to 2 US-licensed whole-cell DTP vaccines. Adverse events were actively solicited using standardized diaries with follow-up telephone calls made at days 1, 4, and 8 by blinded study personnel. Table 2 summarizes the frequency of adverse events within 3 days of the three primary immunizing doses. The incidence of redness, swelling, pain, fever (rectal temperature >101°F), fussiness, drowsiness, and poor appetite were lower following INFANRIX than following either whole-cell DTP vaccine.

[See table 2 at top of previous page]

The frequencies of adverse events following each dose in children who received INFANRIX at 2, 4, and 6 months of age in a US NIH-sponsored trial are shown in Table 3. Of the 120 infants who received the 3-dose primary series, a subset of 76 received a fourth dose of INFANRIX at 15 to 20 months of age and 22 of the 76 received a fifth dose of INFANRIX at 4 to 6 years of age. Adverse events were actively solicited using standardized diaries with follow-up telephone calls made at day 3 by blinded study personnel.

[See table 3 above]

Of 22,505 children who had previously received 3 doses of INFANRIX at 3, 4, and 5 months of age in the German safety study, 5,361 received a fourth dose at 10 to 36 (mean 20) months of age. Standardized diaries were available on 2,457 children receiving the primary series and 1,809 children receiving the fourth dose. Rates of local and systemic adverse events within 3 days of vaccination for each dose are reported in Table 4. In this study, the rate of erythema, swelling, pain, and fever increased with successive doses of INFANRIX.

[See table 4 above]

INFANRIX administered as a fifth dose in children 4 to 6 years of age previously vaccinated with 4 doses of INFANRIX was evaluated in 2 studies conducted in Germany.[26] Safety data are available for 93 children from Study A, a randomized and single (subject)-blinded trial and for 390 children from Study B, a non-randomized, open trial (see Table 5). Adverse events in both studies were actively solicited using standardized diary cards to record specific adverse events that occurred during the 15 days following vaccination. Note that most children who received a fifth dose of INFANRIX in these studies had received the fourth dose in the German study described earlier. However, the children included in Table 5 may not be the same children who are included in Table 4.

Rates of solicited local and systemic adverse events within 3 days of vaccination are reported in Table 5. Higher rates of local injection site reactions (redness, swelling, and pain) were observed following a fifth dose of INFANRIX compared with the fourth dose (see Table 4 and Table 5). The reported sizes of local redness and swelling tended to be greater following the fifth dose of INFANRIX compared with the fourth dose (see Table 4 and Table 5).

Table 3.[26,28,29,30] Adverse Events (%) Occurring Within the 3 Days Following Vaccination With INFANRIX in US Infants and Children in Which All Doses Were INFANRIX

	Primary (N = 120 infants)			Booster (N = 76 children)	Booster (N = 22 children)
Event	Dose 1 (2 months)	Dose 2 (4 months)	Dose 3 (6 months)	Dose 4 (15 to 20 months)	Dose 5 (4 to 6 years)
Local					
Redness	16.6	15.4	26.3	39.5	59.1
Swelling	12.5	15.4	21.0	32.9	50.0
Pain*	5.0	5.1	0.9	10.5	27.3
Systemic					
Fever (>101.1°F)†	0.0	0.9	3.5	6.6	4.6
Anorexia	7.5	6.0	9.6	11.8	NR
Vomiting	5.8	6.8	3.5	2.6	NR
Drowsiness	37.5	19.7	13.2	6.6	NR
Fussiness‡	3.3	7.7	8.8	9.2	0.0

*Moderate or severe = cried or protested to touch or cried when limb moved.
† Rectal temperatures for primary series and Dose 4; oral temperatures for Dose 5.
‡ Moderate or severe = prolonged crying and refusal to play or persistent crying that could not be comforted. For Dose 5, the solicited adverse event was irritability; however the definition for this term was the same as for fussiness.
NR = not reported in publication.

Table 4.[26] Adverse Events (%) Occurring Within the 3 Days Following Vaccination With INFANRIX in German Infants and Children in Which All Doses Were INFANRIX

	Primary (N = 2,457 infants)			Booster (N = 1,809 children)*
Event	Dose 1 (3 months)	Dose 2 (4 months)	Dose 3 (5 months)	Dose 4 (10 to 36 months)†
Local				
Redness	8.9	23.6	26.6	45.9
Redness >2 cm	0.0	0.5	1.3	13.8
Swelling	3.9	14.1	18.5	35.4
Swelling >2 cm	0.0	0.3	1.3	11.4
Pain	2.0	2.6	3.7	26.3
Systemic				
Fever (≥100.4°F)‡	6.3	8.3	13.3	26.4
Fever (>103.1°F)‡	0.0	0.1	0.1	1.1
Loss of Appetite	8.0	7.4	6.5	11.6
Vomiting	4.3	3.9	3.4	2.9
Restlessness	10.3	9.5	8.6	15.9
Unusual Crying	3.9	4.3	4.1	6.4
Diarrhea	6.0	4.9	4.0	11.0

*May not be same children as in primary series.
† Mean = 20 months.
‡ Rectal temperatures.

Table 5. Adverse Events (%) Occurring Within the 3 Days Following Vaccination* With INFANRIX Administered at 4 to 6 Years of Age in German Children Who Had Previously Received 4 Doses of INFANRIX

	Study A (N = 93)	Study B (N = 390)
Local		
Redness, any	51.6	52.1
Redness, ≥50 mm	23.7	29.2
Redness, ≥110 mm	4.3	6.4
Swelling, any	43.0	49.5
Swelling, ≥50 mm	15.1	20.0
Swelling, ≥110 mm	4.3	5.1
Pain, any	64.5	49.7
Pain, grade 2 or 3	20.4	13.8
Pain, grade 3	1.1	1.5
Systemic		
Fever†, ≥99.5°F	12.9	11.3
Fever†, ≥102.4°F	0.0	0.0
Loss of appetite	14.0	10.3

Vomiting	0.0	2.1
Irritability	18.3	14.1
Diarrhea	4.3	3.8

N = number of infants in a modified intent-to-treat (ITT) cohort (infants who received INFANRIX for their fifth dose of DTaP whose previous 4 doses of DTaP were all with INFANRIX, for whom at least one symptom sheet was completed; 2 subjects from Study B were excluded due to chronic illnesses that could have interefered with safety assessments). Grade 2 pain defined as sufficiently discomforting to interfere with daily activities. Grade 3 pain defined as preventing normal daily activities and needing medical advice.
*Within 3 days of vaccination defined as day of vaccination and the next 2 days.
† Axillary temperatures.

Cases of extensive swelling, of the injected limb, involving an increase in limb circumference, and sometimes involving the entire injected thigh or upper arm, have been reported with INFANRIX.[26,31,32] These reactions have generally begun within 48 hours of vaccination and resolved over an average of 4 days (range 1 to 10 days) without sequelae.[26] In the German study in which 5,361 children received a fourth dose of INFANRIX after 3 doses of the same vaccine, swelling of the injected thigh was reported spontaneously in 62 vaccinees (1.2%).[26] This swelling was associated with pain upon digital pressure in 53% of cases, with rectal temperature ≥100.4°F in 45% of cases, and with injection site redness in 71% of cases (redness of the entire thigh was reported in 17% of such cases). The mean difference in the circumference of the thighs in those subjects in whom this was measured (N = 17) was 2.2 cm (range: 0.5 to 5 cm). In 1,809 children for whom standardized diaries were available, extensive limb swelling was observed in 2.5% of vaccinees. In the two German studies in which subjects received a fifth consecutive dose of INFANRIX, the vaccine was administered in the deltoid muscle in most subjects, and in the thigh in a minority of subjects. In Study A, in which 93 children received a fifth dose of INFANRIX after 4 doses of the same vaccine, extensive swelling of the injected limb was reported spontaneously in 9 vaccinees (9.7%). This swelling was associated with pain and redness in all cases, and with fever in one case. The mean increase in the circumference of the injected limb compared with the opposite limb in those subjects in whom this was measured (N = 8) was 4.4 cm (range: 2 to 7 cm). In 3 cases, the investigators provided additional descriptive information – one case was described as involving the chest, and 2 cases were noted to involve the entire upper arm from the shoulder to the elbow. In Study B, in which 390 children received a fifth dose of INFANRIX after 4 doses of the same vaccine, extensive swelling of the injected limb was reported spontaneously in 25 vaccinees (6.4%). This swelling was associated with redness in all cases, with pain in 88%, and with fever in 12%. The mean increase in the circumference of the injected limb compared with the opposite limb in those subjects in whom this was measured (N = 22) was 3.8 cm (range: 1.2 to 16 cm).[26]

In postmarketing reports, extensive limb swelling also has been reported following administration of each of the first 3 doses of INFANRIX (see ADVERSE REACTIONS, Postmarketing Reports). Extensive limb swelling has also been reported following administration of other acellular DTP vaccines,[32,33] acellular pertussis vaccine alone (without DT),[34] whole-cell DTP vaccine,[35] and other vaccines.[36]

Table 6 lists the frequency of adverse events in US children who received INFANRIX (N = 110) or US-licensed whole-cell DTP vaccine (N = 55) manufactured by Lederle Laboratories at 15 to 20 months of age[37] and in US children who received INFANRIX (N = 115) or US-licensed whole-cell DTP vaccine (N = 57) manufactured by Lederle Laboratories at 4 to 6 years of age.[38] All children had previously received 3 or 4 doses of whole-cell DTP vaccine at approximately 2, 4, 6, and 15-18 months of age. Adverse events were actively solicited using standardized diaries with follow-up telephone calls made at days 1, 4, and 8 by blinded study personnel. Significantly fewer solicited local and general adverse events were reported following INFANRIX than following whole-cell DTP vaccine when administered as the fourth or fifth dose in those previously primed with 3 or 4 doses of whole-cell DTP vaccine.

[See table 6 above]

Severe adverse events reported from the double-blind, randomized comparative Italian study involving 4,696 children administered INFANRIX or 4,678 children administered whole-cell DTP vaccine (manufactured by Connaught Laboratories, Inc.) as a 3-dose primary series are shown in Table 7. The incidence of rectal temperature ≥104°F, hypotonic-hyporesponsive episodes and persistent crying ≥3 hours following administration of INFANRIX was significantly less than that following administration of whole-cell DTP vaccine.[15] Hospitalization rates and death rates within 7 days of vaccination were similar between INFANRIX and DT vaccine recipients.[26]

[See table 7 above]

In the German safety study that enrolled 22,505 infants (66,867 doses of INFANRIX administered as a 3-dose primary series), all subjects were monitored for unsolicited adverse events that occurred within 28 days following vaccination using report cards. In a subset of subjects (N = 2,457), these cards were standardized diaries which solicited specific adverse events that occurred within 8 days of each vaccination in addition to unsolicited adverse events which occurred throughout the course of the entire trial (from study enrollment until approximately 30 days following the third vaccination). Cards from the whole cohort were returned at subsequent visits and were supplemented by spontaneous reporting by parents and a medical history after the first and second doses of vaccine. In the subset of 2,457, adverse events following the third dose of vaccine were reported via standardized diaries and spontaneous reporting at a follow-up visit. Adverse events in the remainder of the cohort were reported via report cards which were returned by mail approximately 28 days after the third dose of vaccine. Adverse events (rates per 1,000 doses) occurring within 7 days following any of the first 3 doses included: unusual crying (0.09), febrile seizure (0.0), afebrile seizure (0.13), and hypotonic-hyporesponsive episodes (0.01).

Table 6.[37,38] Adverse Events (%) Occurring Within the 3 Days Following Vaccination With INFANRIX Administered at 15 to 20 Months and 4 to 6 Years of Age in US Children Who Had Previously Received 3 or 4 Doses of Whole-Cell DTP Vaccine

	15 to 20 months 3 Previous Doses of Whole-Cell DTP Vaccine		4 to 6 years 4 Previous Doses of Whole-Cell DTP Vaccine	
Event	**INFANRIX (N = 110)**	**Whole-Cell DTP Vaccine (N = 55)**	**INFANRIX (N = 115)**	**Whole-Cell DTP Vaccine (N = 57)**
Local				
Redness*	23	45	19	40
Redness†>10 mm	5	31	7	26
Swelling	14	24	15*	33*
Swelling >10 mm	7	15	8	18
Pain†§	5	38	12	40
Systemic				
Fever* (≥99.4°F)‡	25	42	23	47
Fever†(>100.5°F)‡	2	20	1	12
Fussiness	34†	69†	20	30
Drowsiness	9*	24*	11	18
Poor Appetite*	9	20	6	16
Vomiting	2	0	1	4

*p<0.05.
†p<0.0001.
‡Oral temperatures.
§Moderate or severe = cried or protested to touch or cried when arm moved.

Table 7.[15] Severe Adverse Events Occurring Within 48 Hours Following Vaccination With INFANRIX or Whole-Cell DTP in Italian Infants at 2, 4, or 6 Months of Age

	INFANRIX (N = 13,761 Doses)		Whole-Cell DTP Vaccine (N = 13,520 Doses)	
Event	**Number**	**Rate/1,000 Doses**	**Number**	**Rate/1,000 Doses**
Fever (≥104°F)*†	5	0.36	32	2.4
Hypotonic-hyporesponsive episode‡	0	0	9	0.67
Persistent crying ≥3 hours*	6	0.44	54	4.0
Seizures**	1§	0.07	3¶	0.22

*p<0.001.
†Rectal temperatures.
‡p = 0.002.
§Maximum rectal temperature within 72 hours of vaccination = 103.1°F.
¶Maximum rectal temperature within 72 hours of vaccination = 99.5°F, 101.3°F and 102.2°F.
**Not statistically significant at p<0.05.

Rates of serious adverse events that are less common than those reported in this safety study are not known at this time.

In an ongoing US coadministration safety study, INFANRIX was administered concomitantly at separate sites with 7-valent pneumococcal and Hib conjugate vaccines (Lederle Laboratories), Hepatitis B Vaccine (Recombinant) (GlaxoSmithKline Biologicals), and inactivated poliovirus vaccine (IPV) (Aventis Pasteur) at 2, 4, and 6 months of age. Following dose 1 at 2 months of age, fever ≥100.4°F, >101.3°F, >102.2°F, and >103.1°F occurring within 4 days (i.e., day of vaccination and the next 3 days) was reported in 19.8%, 4.5%, 0.3%, and 0.0%, respectively, of infants (N = 333). The frequency of irritability/fussiness, drowsiness, and loss of appetite was 61.5%, 54%, and 27.8%, respectively.

In clinical trials involving more than 29,000 infants and children, 14 deaths in INFANRIX recipients were reported. Causes of deaths included 9 cases of Sudden Infant Death Syndrome (SIDS) and one of each of the following: meal aspiration, hepatoblastoma, neuroblastoma, invasive bacterial infection, and sudden death in a child older than 1 year of age. None of these events was determined to be vaccine-related. The rate of SIDS observed in the German safety study that enrolled 22,505 infants was 0.3/1,000 vaccinated infants. The rate of SIDS in the Italian efficacy trial was 0.4/1,000 infants vaccinated with INFANRIX. The reported rate of SIDS in the United States from 1990 to 1994 was 1.2/1,000 live births.[39] By chance alone, some cases of SIDS can be expected to follow receipt of pertussis-containing vaccines.[22]

As with any vaccine, there is the possibility that broad use of INFANRIX could reveal adverse events not observed in clinical trials.

Additional Adverse Reactions: Rarely, an anaphylactic reaction (i.e., hives, swelling of the mouth, difficulty breathing, hypotension, or shock) has been reported after receiving preparations containing diphtheria, tetanus, and/or pertussis antigens.[22] Arthus-type hypersensitivity reactions, characterized by severe local reactions, may follow receipt of tetanus toxoid. A review by the IOM found evidence for a causal relationship between receipt of tetanus toxoid and both brachial neuritis and Guillain-Barré Syndrome.[40] A few cases of demyelinating diseases of the CNS have been reported following some tetanus toxoid-containing vaccines or tetanus and diphtheria toxoid-containing vaccines, although the IOM concluded that the evidence was inadequate to accept or reject a causal relationship.[40] A few cases of peripheral mononeuropathy and of cranial mononeuropathy have been reported following tetanus toxoid administration, although the IOM concluded that the evidence was inadequate to accept or reject a causal relationship.

Postmarketing Reports: Worldwide voluntary reports of adverse events received for INFANRIX since market introduction are listed below. This list includes adverse events for which 20 or more reports were received with the exception of intussusception, idiopathic thrombocytopenic pur-

Continued on next page

Product information on these pages is effective as of August 2004. Further information is available at: GlaxoSmithKline, PO Box 13398, Research Triangle Park, NC 27709. 1-888-825-5249. Corporate Web Site: www.gsk.com

Infanrix—Cont.

pura, thrombocytopenia, anaphylactic reaction, encephalopathy, and hypotonic-hyporesponsive episode for which fewer than 20 reports were received. These latter events are included either because of the seriousness of the event or the strength of causal connection to components of this or other vaccines or drugs.

Body as a Whole: Fever, Sudden Infant Death Syndrome.
Cardiovascular System: Cyanosis.
Gastrointestinal System: Diarrhea, intussusception, vomiting.
Hematologic/lymphatic: Idiopathic thrombocytopenic purpura, lymphadenopathy, thrombocytopenia.
Hypersensitivity: Anaphylactic reaction, hypersensitivity.
Infections: Cellulitis.
Injection Site Reactions: Injection site reactions.
Musculoskeletal: Limb swelling.
Nervous System: Convulsions, encephalopathy, hypotonia, hypotonic-hyporesponsive episode, somnolence.
Psychiatric: Crying, irritability.
Respiratory System: Respiratory tract infection.
Skin and Appendages: Erythema, pruritus, rash, urticaria.
Special Senses: Ear pain.

These adverse events were reported voluntarily from a population of uncertain size; therefore, it is not always possible to reliably estimate their frequency or establish a causal relationship to vaccination.

Reporting Adverse Events: The National Childhood Vaccine Injury Act requires that the manufacturer and lot number of the vaccine administered be recorded by the healthcare provider in the vaccine recipient's permanent medical record, along with the date of administration of the vaccine and the name, address, and title of the person administering the vaccine.[41] The Act further requires the healthcare provider to report to the US Department of Health and Human Services via VAERS the occurrence following immunization of any event set forth in the Vaccine Injury Table including: Anaphylaxis or anaphylactic shock within 7 days, encephalopathy or encephalitis within 7 days, brachial neuritis within 28 days, or an acute complication or sequelae (including death) of an illness, disability, injury, or condition referred to above, or any events that would contraindicate further doses of vaccine, according to this prescribing information.[41,42] The VAERS toll-free number is 1-800-822-7967.

DOSAGE AND ADMINISTRATION

Preparation for Administration: INFANRIX is an adjuvanted vaccine; therefore shake vigorously to obtain a homogeneous, turbid, white suspension. DO NOT USE IF RESUSPENSION DOES NOT OCCUR WITH VIGOROUS SHAKING. Inspect visually for particulate matter or discoloration prior to administration. After removal of the dose, any vaccine remaining in the vial should be discarded.

INFANRIX should be administered by intramuscular injection. The preferred sites are the anterolateral aspects of the thigh or the deltoid muscle of the upper arm. The vaccine should not be injected in the gluteal area or areas where there may be a major nerve trunk. Before injection, the skin at the injection site should be cleaned and prepared with a suitable germicide. After insertion of the needle, aspirate to ensure that the needle has not entered a blood vessel.

Do not administer this product subcutaneously or intravenously.

Immunization Series: A 0.5 mL dose of INFANRIX is approved for administration in infants and children 6 weeks to 7 years of age (prior to the seventh birthday) as a 5 dose series. The series consists of a primary immunization course of 3 doses administered at 2, 4, and 6 months of age, followed by 2 booster doses, administered at 15 to 20 months of age and at 4 to 6 years of age. The customary age for the first dose is 2 months of age, but it may be given as early as 6 weeks of age. The recommended interval between the first three doses is 8 weeks, with a minimum interval of 4 weeks.[10,21] The recommended interval between the third and fourth dose is 6 to 12 months.[10,21] The fifth dose is recommended before entry into kindergarten or elementary school, and is not needed if the fourth dose was given after the fourth birthday.[21]

Interchanging INFANRIX and DTaP vaccines from different manufacturers for successive doses of the vaccination series is not recommended because data are limited regarding the safety and efficacy of such regimens.

INFANRIX may be used to complete a DTaP immunization series initiated with PEDIARIX™ [Diphtheria and Tetanus Toxoids and Acellular Pertussis Adsorbed, Hepatitis B (Recombinant) and Inactivated Poliovirus Vaccine Combined, manufactured by GlaxoSmithKline Biologicals], because the diphtheria, tetanus, and pertussis components of INFANRIX are the same as those in PEDIARIX. However, the safety and efficacy of INFANRIX in such infants and children have not been evaluated.

INFANRIX may be used to complete the immunization series in infants and children who have received 1 or more doses of whole-cell DTP. However, the safety and efficacy of INFANRIX in such infants and children have not been fully evaluated.

Additional Dosing Information: If any recommended dose of pertussis vaccine cannot be given, DT (For Pediatric Use) should be given as needed to complete the series.

Interruption of the recommended schedule with a delay between doses should not interfere with the final immunity achieved with INFANRIX. There is no need to start the series over again, regardless of the time elapsed between doses.

The use of reduced volume (fractional doses) is not recommended. The effect of such practices on the frequency of serious adverse events and on protection against disease has not been determined.[10]

Preterm infants should be vaccinated according to their chronological age from birth.[10]

Concomitant Vaccine Administration: In clinical trials, INFANRIX was routinely administered, at separate sites, concomitantly with 1 or more of the following vaccines: poliovirus vaccine live oral (OPV), hepatitis B vaccine, and *Haemophilus influenzae* type b vaccine (Hib) (see CLINICAL PHARMACOLOGY). Safety data are available following the first dose of INFANRIX when administered concomitantly at separate sites with Hib and pneumococcal conjugate vaccines, hepatitis B vaccine, and IPV (see ADVERSE EVENTS). No immunogenicity data are available on the simultaneous administration of INFANRIX with pneumococcal conjugate vaccine or IPV.

No immunogenicity or safety data are available on the simultaneous administration of INFANRIX with measles, mumps, and rubella vaccine (MMR) or varicella vaccine.

When concomitant administration of other vaccines is required, they should be given with different syringes and at different injection sites.

STORAGE

Store INFANRIX refrigerated between 2° and 8°C (36° and 46°F). **Do not freeze.** Discard if the vaccine has been frozen. Do not use after expiration date shown on the label.

HOW SUPPLIED

INFANRIX is supplied as a turbid white suspension in single-dose (0.5 mL) vials and disposable prefilled Tip-Lok® syringes.

Single-Dose Vials
NDC 58160-840-01 (package of 1)
NDC 58160-840-11 (package of 10)

Single-Dose Prefilled Disposable Tip-Lok® Syringes (packaged without needles)
NDC 58160-840-46 (package of 5)
NDC 58160-840-50 (package of 25)

Single-Dose Prefilled Disposable Tip-Lok® Syringes with 1-inch 25-gauge BD SafetyGlide™ Needles
NDC 58160-840-56 (package of 25)

Single-Dose Prefilled Disposable Tip-Lok® Syringes with 5/8-inch 25-gauge BD SafetyGlide™ Needles
NDC 58160-840-57 (package of 25)

REFERENCES

1. Centers for Disease Control. Diphtheria, tetanus, and pertussis: Recommendations for vaccine use and other preventive measures — Recommendations of the Immunization Practices Advisory Committee (ACIP). *MMWR* 1991;40(RR-10):1–28. **2.** Centers for Disease Control and Prevention. Diphtheria. In: Atkinson W and Wolfe C, eds. *Epidemiology and prevention of vaccine-preventable diseases.* 7th ed. Atlanta, GA: Public Health Foundation; 2002: 39–48. **3.** Bisgard KM, Hardy I, Popovic T, et al. Respiratory diphtheria in the United States, 1980 through 1995. *Am J Public Health* 1998;88(5):787–791. **4.** Centers for Disease Control and Prevention. Toxigenic *Corynebacterium diphtheriae* — Northern Plains Indian community, August-October 1996. *MMWR* 1997;46(22):506–510. **5.** Mortimer EA and Wharton M. Diphtheria Toxoid. In: Plotkin SA and Orenstein WA, eds. *Vaccines.* 3rd ed. Philadelphia, PA: W.B. Saunders Company; 1999:140–157. **6.** Centers for Disease Control and Prevention. Tetanus — Puerto Rico, 2002. *MMWR* 2002;51(28):613–615. **7.** Centers for Disease Control and Prevention. Tetanus surveillance — United States, 1995–1997. *MMWR* 1998;47(SS-2):1–13. **8.** Wassilak SGF, Orenstein WA, and Sutter RW. Tetanus Toxoid. In: Plotkin SA and Orenstein WA, eds. *Vaccines.* 3rd ed. Philadelphia, PA: W.B. Saunders Company; 1999:441–474. **9.** Department of Health and Human Services, Food and Drug Administration. Biological products; Bacterial vaccines and toxoids; Implementation of efficacy review; Proposed rule. *Federal Register* December 13, 1985;50(240):51002–51117. **10.** Centers for Disease Control and Prevention. General recommendations on immunization: Recommendations of the Advisory Committee on Immunization Practices (ACIP) and the American Academy of Family Physicians (AAFP). *MMWR* 2002;51(RR-2):1–35. **11.** Long SS. Pertussis (*Bordetella pertussis* and *B. parapertussis*). In: Behrman RE, Kliegman RM, Jenson HB, eds. *Nelson Textbook of Pediatrics.* 16th ed. Philadelphia, PA: W.B. Saunders; 2000:838–842. **12.** Centers for Disease Control and Prevention. Pertussis — United States, 1997–2000. *MMWR* 2002;51(4):73–76. **13.** Nennig ME, Shinefield HR, Edwards KM, et al. Prevalence and incidence of adult pertussis in an urban population. *JAMA* 1996;275(21):1672–1674. **14.** Güris D, Strebel PM, Bardenheier B, et al. Changing epidemiology of pertussis in the United States: Increasing reported incidence among adolescents and adults, 1990–1996. *Clin Infect Dis* 1999;28: 1230–1237. **15.** Greco D, Salmaso S, Mastrantonio P, et al. A controlled trial of two acellular vaccines and one whole-cell vaccine against pertussis. *N Engl J Med* 1996;334(6):341–348. **16.** Schmitt H-J, von König CHW, Neiss A, et al. Efficacy of acellular pertussis vaccine in early childhood after household exposure. *JAMA* 1996;275(1):37–41. **17.** Salmaso S, Mastrantonio P, Wassilak SGF, et al. Persistence of protection through 33 months of age provided by immunization in infancy with two three-component acellular pertussis vaccines. *Vaccine* 1998;13(13):1270–1275. **18.** Salmaso S, Mastrantonio P, Tozzi AE, et al. Sustained efficacy during the first 6 years of life of 3-component acellular pertussis vaccines administered in infancy: The Italian experience. *Pediatrics* 2001;108(5):E81. **19.** Blatter M, Reisinger K, Pichichero M, et al. Immunogenicity of diphtheria-tetanus-acellular pertussis (DT-tricomponent Pa), hepatitis B (HB) and *Haemophilus influenzae* type b (Hib) vaccines administered concomitantly at separate sites along with oral poliovirus vaccine (OPV) in infants. In: Abstracts of the 36th Interscience Conference on Antimicrobial Agents and Chemotherapy; September 15–18, 1996; New Orleans, LA. Abstract G102. **20.** Centers for Disease Control and Prevention. Use of vaccines and immune globulins in persons with altered immunocompetence: Recommendations of the Advisory Committee on Immunization Practices (ACIP). *MMWR* 1993;42(RR-4):1–18. **21.** Centers for Disease Control and Prevention. Pertussis vaccination: Use of acellular pertussis vaccines among infants and young children — Recommendations of the Advisory Committee on Immunization Practices (ACIP). *MMWR* 1997;46(RR-7):1–25. **22.** Centers for Disease Control and Prevention. Update: Vaccine side effects, adverse reactions, contraindications, and precautions — Recommendations of the Advisory Committee on Immunization Practices (ACIP). *MMWR* 1996;45(RR-12):1–35. **23.** Institute of Medicine (IOM). Howson CP, Howe CJ, Fineberg HV, eds. *Adverse effects of pertussis and rubella vaccines.* Washington, DC: National Academy Press; 1991. **24.** Institute of Medicine (IOM). Stratton KR, Howe CJ, Johnston RB, eds. *DPT vaccine and chronic nervous system dysfunction: A new analysis.* Washington, DC: National Academy Press; 1994. **25.** American Academy of Pediatrics. Pertussis. In: Pickering LK, ed. *2000 Red Book: Report of the Committee on Infectious Diseases.* 25th ed. Elk Grove Village, IL: American Academy of Pediatrics; 2000:442–448. **26.** Data on File, GlaxoSmithKline. **27.** Bernstein HH, Rothstein EP, Pichichero ME, et al. Reactogenicity and immunogenicity of a three-component acellular pertussis vaccine administered as the primary series to 2, 4 and 6 month-old infants in the United States. *Vaccine* 1995;13(17):1631–1635. **28.** Decker MD, Edwards KM, Steinhoff MC, et al. Comparison of 13 acellular pertussis vaccines: Adverse reactions. *Pediatrics* 1995;96:557–566. **29.** Pichichero ME, Edwards KM, Anderson EL, et al. Safety and immunogenicity of six acellular pertussis vaccines and one whole-cell pertussis vaccine given as a fifth dose in four- to six-year-old children. *Pediatrics* 2000;105(1):e11. **30.** Pichichero ME, Deloria MA, Rennels MB, et al. A safety and immunogenicity comparison of 12 acellular pertussis vaccines and one whole-cell pertussis vaccine given as a fourth dose in 15- to 20-month-old children. *Pediatrics* 1997;100(5):772–788. **31.** Schmitt H-J, Beutel K, Schuind A, et al. Reactogenicity and immunogenicity of a booster dose of a combined diphtheria, tetanus, and tricomponent acellular pertussis vaccine at fourteen to twenty-eight months of age. *J Pediatr* 1997;130:616–623. **32.** Rennels MB, Deloria MA, Pichichero ME, et al. Extensive swelling after booster doses of acellular pertussis-tetanus-diphtheria vaccines. *Pediatrics* 2000;105(1):E12. **33.** Noble GR, Bernier RH, Esber EC, et al. Acellular and whole-cell pertussis vaccines in Japan. Report of a visit by US scientists. *JAMA* 1987;257(10):1351–1356. **34.** Blennow M and Granström M. Adverse reactions and serologic response to a booster dose of acellular pertussis vaccine in children immunized with acellular or whole-cell vaccine as infants. *Pediatrics* 1989;84(1):62–67. **35.** Pim C and Farley J. Local reactions to kindergarten DPT boosters — Cranbrook. *Dis Surveill* 1988;9:230–239. **36.** Gold R, Scheifele D, Barreto L, et al. Safety and immunogenicity of *Haemophilus influenzae* vaccine (tetanus toxoid conjugate) administered concurrently or combined with diphtheria and tetanus toxoids, pertussis vaccine and inactivated poliomyelitis vaccine to healthy infants at two, four and six months of age. *Pediatr Infect Dis J* 1994;13:348–355. **37.** Bernstein HH, Rothstein EP, Reisinger KS, et al. Comparison of a three-component acellular pertussis vaccine with a whole-cell pertussis vaccine in 15- through 20-month-old infants. *Pediatrics* 1994;93(4):656–659. **38.** Annunziato PW, Rothstein EP, Bernstein HH, et al. Comparison of a three-component acellular pertussis vaccine with a whole-cell pertussis vaccine in 4- through 6-year-old children. *Arch Pediatr Adolesc Med* 1994;148:503–507. **39.** Centers for Disease Control and Prevention. Sudden Infant Death Syndrome — United States, 1983-94. *MMWR* 1996;45(40):859–863. **40.** Institute of Medicine (IOM). Stratton KR, Howe CJ, Johnston RB, eds. *Adverse events associated with childhood vaccines. Evidence bearing on causality.* Washington, DC: National Academy Press; 1994. **41.** Centers for Disease Control. National Childhood Vaccine Injury Act: Requirements for permanent vaccination records and for reporting of selected events after vaccination. *MMWR* 1988;37(13):197–200. **42.** National Vaccine Injury Compensation Program: Vaccine injury table. www.hrsa.gov/osp/vicp/table.htm. Accessed April 29, 2002.

Manufactured by GlaxoSmithKline Biologicals
Rixensart, Belgium, US License 1617 and
Chiron Behring GmbH & Co
Marburg, Germany, US License 0097
Distributed by GlaxoSmithKline, Research Triangle Park, NC 27709
INFANRIX and TIP-LOK are registered trademarks of GlaxoSmithKline.
SAFETYGLIDE is a trademark of Becton, Dickinson and Company.

August 2003/IN:L10

Shown in Product Identification Guide, page 316

LAMICTAL® ℞
[la-mik' tal]
(lamotrigine)
Tablets
LAMICTAL® ℞
(lamotrigine)
Chewable Dispersible Tablets

SERIOUS RASHES REQUIRING HOSPITALIZATION AND DISCONTINUATION OF TREATMENT HAVE BEEN REPORTED IN ASSOCIATION WITH THE USE OF LAMICTAL. THE INCIDENCE OF THESE RASHES, WHICH HAVE INCLUDED STEVENS-JOHNSON SYNDROME, IS APPROXIMATELY 0.8% (8 PER 1,000) IN PEDIATRIC PATIENTS (AGE <16 YEARS) RECEIVING LAMICTAL AS ADJUNCTIVE THERAPY FOR EPILEPSY AND 0.3% (3 PER 1,000) IN ADULTS ON ADJUNCTIVE THERAPY FOR EPILEPSY. IN CLINICAL TRIALS OF BIPOLAR AND OTHER MOOD DISORDERS, THE RATE OF SERIOUS RASH WAS 0.08% (0.8 PER 1,000) IN ADULT PATIENTS RECEIVING LAMICTAL AS INITIAL MONOTHERAPY AND 0.13% (1.3 PER 1,000) IN ADULT PATIENTS RECEIVING LAMICTAL AS ADJUNCTIVE THERAPY. IN A PROSPECTIVELY FOLLOWED COHORT OF 1,983 PEDIATRIC PATIENTS WITH EPILEPSY TAKING ADJUNCTIVE LAMICTAL, THERE WAS 1 RASH-RELATED DEATH. IN WORLDWIDE POSTMARKETING EXPERIENCE, RARE CASES OF TOXIC EPIDERMAL NECROLYSIS AND/OR RASH-RELATED DEATH HAVE BEEN REPORTED IN ADULT AND PEDIATRIC PATIENTS, BUT THEIR NUMBERS ARE TOO FEW TO PERMIT A PRECISE ESTIMATE OF THE RATE.
BECAUSE THE RATE OF SERIOUS RASH IS GREATER IN PEDIATRIC PATIENTS THAN IN ADULTS, IT BEARS EMPHASIS THAT LAMICTAL IS APPROVED ONLY FOR USE IN PEDIATRIC PATIENTS BELOW THE AGE OF 16 YEARS WHO HAVE SEIZURES ASSOCIATED WITH THE LENNOX-GASTAUT SYNDROME OR IN PATIENTS WITH PARTIAL SEIZURES (SEE INDICATIONS).
OTHER THAN AGE, THERE ARE AS YET NO FACTORS IDENTIFIED THAT ARE KNOWN TO PREDICT THE RISK OF OCCURRENCE OR THE SEVERITY OF RASH ASSOCIATED WITH LAMICTAL. THERE ARE SUGGESTIONS, YET TO BE PROVEN, THAT THE RISK OF RASH MAY ALSO BE INCREASED BY (1) COADMINISTRATION OF LAMICTAL WITH VALPROATE (INCLUDES VALPROIC ACID AND DIVALPROEX SODIUM), (2) EXCEEDING THE RECOMMENDED INITIAL DOSE OF LAMICTAL, OR (3) EXCEEDING THE RECOMMENDED DOSE ESCALATION FOR LAMICTAL. HOWEVER, CASES HAVE BEEN REPORTED IN THE ABSENCE OF THESE FACTORS.
NEARLY ALL CASES OF LIFE-THREATENING RASHES ASSOCIATED WITH LAMICTAL HAVE OCCURRED WITHIN 2 TO 8 WEEKS OF TREATMENT INITIATION. HOWEVER, ISOLATED CASES HAVE BEEN REPORTED AFTER PROLONGED TREATMENT (E.G., 6 MONTHS). ACCORDINGLY, DURATION OF THERAPY CANNOT BE RELIED UPON AS A MEANS TO PREDICT THE POTENTIAL RISK HERALDED BY THE FIRST APPEARANCE OF A RASH.
ALTHOUGH BENIGN RASHES ALSO OCCUR WITH LAMICTAL, IT IS NOT POSSIBLE TO PREDICT RELIABLY WHICH RASHES WILL PROVE TO BE SERIOUS OR LIFE THREATENING. ACCORDINGLY, LAMICTAL SHOULD ORDINARILY BE DISCONTINUED AT THE FIRST SIGN OF RASH, UNLESS THE RASH IS CLEARLY NOT DRUG RELATED. DISCONTINUATION OF TREATMENT MAY NOT PREVENT A RASH FROM BECOMING LIFE THREATENING OR PERMANENTLY DISABLING OR DISFIGURING.

DESCRIPTION

LAMICTAL (lamotrigine), an antiepileptic drug (AED) of the phenyltriazine class, is chemically unrelated to existing antiepileptic drugs. Its chemical name is 3,5-diamino-6-(2,3-dichlorophenyl)-*as*-triazine, its molecular formula is $C_9H_7N_5Cl_2$, and its molecular weight is 256.09. Lamotrigine is a white to pale cream-colored powder and has a pK_a of 5.7. Lamotrigine is very slightly soluble in water (0.17 mg/mL at 25°C) and slightly soluble in 0.1 M HCl (4.1 mg/mL at 25°C).

LAMICTAL Tablets are supplied for oral administration as 25-mg (white), 100-mg (peach), 150-mg (cream), and 200-mg (blue) tablets. Each tablet contains the labeled amount of lamotrigine and the following inactive ingredients: lactose; magnesium stearate; microcrystalline cellulose; povidone; sodium starch glycolate; FD&C Yellow No. 6 Lake (100-mg tablet only); ferric oxide, yellow (150-mg tablet only); and FD&C Blue No. 2 Lake (200-mg tablet only).

LAMICTAL Chewable Dispersible Tablets are supplied for oral administration. The tablets contain 2 mg (white), 5 mg (white), or 25 mg (white) of lamotrigine and the following inactive ingredients: blackcurrant flavor, calcium carbonate, low-substituted hydroxypropylcellulose, magnesium aluminum silicate, magnesium stearate, povidone, saccharin sodium, and sodium starch glycolate.

CLINICAL PHARMACOLOGY

Mechanism of Action: The precise mechanism(s) by which lamotrigine exerts its anticonvulsant action are unknown. In animal models designed to detect anticonvulsant activity, lamotrigine was effective in preventing seizure spread in the maximum electroshock (MES) and pentylenetetrazol (scMet) tests, and prevented seizures in the visually and electrically evoked after-discharge (EEAD) tests for antiepileptic activity. The relevance of these models to human epilepsy, however, is not known.

One proposed mechanism of action of LAMICTAL, the relevance of which remains to be established in humans, involves an effect on sodium channels. In vitro pharmacological studies suggest that lamotrigine inhibits voltage-sensitive sodium channels, thereby stabilizing neuronal membranes and consequently modulating presynaptic transmitter release of excitatory amino acids (e.g., glutamate and aspartate).

LAMICTAL also displayed inhibitory properties in the kindling model in rats both during kindling development and in the fully kindled state. The relevance of this animal model to specific types of human epilepsy is unclear.

The mechanisms by which lamotrigine exerts its therapeutic action in Bipolar Disorder have not been established.

Pharmacological Properties: Although the relevance for human use is unknown, the following data characterize the performance of LAMICTAL in receptor binding assays. Lamotrigine had a weak inhibitory effect on the serotonin 5-HT_3 receptor (IC_{50} = 18 μM). It does not exhibit high affinity binding (IC_{50}>100 μM) to the following neurotransmitter receptors: adenosine A_1 and A_2; adrenergic α_1, α_2, and β; dopamine D_1 and D_2; γ-aminobutyric acid (GABA) A and B; histamine H_1; kappa opioid; muscarinic acetylcholine; and serotonin 5-HT_2. Studies have failed to detect an effect of lamotrigine on dihydropyridine-sensitive calcium channels. It had weak effects at sigma opioid receptors (IC_{50} = 145 μM). Lamotrigine did not inhibit the uptake of norepinephrine, dopamine, or serotonin, (IC_{50}>200 μM) when tested in rat synaptosomes and/or human platelets in vitro.

Effect of Lamotrigine on N-Methyl d-Aspartate-Receptor Mediated Activity: Lamotrigine did not inhibit N-methyl d-aspartate (NMDA)-induced depolarizations in rat cortical slices or NMDA-induced cyclic GMP formation in immature rat cerebellum, nor did lamotrigine displace compounds that are either competitive or noncompetitive ligands at this glutamate receptor complex (CNQX, CGS, TCHP). The IC_{50} for lamotrigine effects on NMDA-induced currents (in the presence of 3 μM of glycine) in cultured hippocampal neurons exceeded 100 μM.

Folate Metabolism: In vitro, lamotrigine was shown to be an inhibitor of dihydrofolate reductase, the enzyme that catalyzes the reduction of dihydrofolate to tetrahydrofolate. Inhibition of this enzyme may interfere with the biosynthesis of nucleic acids and proteins. When oral daily doses of lamotrigine were given to pregnant rats during organogenesis, fetal, placental, and maternal folate concentrations were reduced. Significantly reduced concentrations of folate are associated with teratogenesis (see PRECAUTIONS: Pregnancy). Folate concentrations were also reduced in male rats given repeated oral doses of lamotrigine. Reduced concentrations were partially returned to normal when supplemented with folinic acid.

Accumulation in Kidneys: Lamotrigine was found to accumulate in the kidney of the male rat, causing chronic progressive nephrosis, necrosis, and mineralization. These findings are attributed to α-2 microglobulin, a species- and sex-specific protein that has not been detected in humans or other animal species.

Melanin Binding: Lamotrigine binds to melanin-containing tissues, e.g., in the eye and pigmented skin. It has been found in the uveal tract up to 52 weeks after a single dose in rodents.

Cardiovascular: In dogs, lamotrigine is extensively metabolized to a 2-N-methyl metabolite. This metabolite causes dose-dependent prolongations of the PR interval, widening of the QRS complex, and, at higher doses, complete AV conduction block. Similar cardiovascular effects are not anticipated in humans because only trace amounts of the 2-N-methyl metabolite (<0.6% of lamotrigine dose) have been found in human urine (see Drug Disposition). However, it is conceivable that plasma concentrations of this metabolite could be increased in patients with a reduced capacity to glucuronidate lamotrigine (e.g., in patients with liver disease).

Pharmacokinetics and Drug Metabolism: The pharmacokinetics of lamotrigine have been studied in patients with epilepsy, healthy young and elderly volunteers, and volunteers with chronic renal failure. Lamotrigine pharmacokinetic parameters for adult and pediatric patients and healthy normal volunteers are summarized in Tables 1 and 2.

[See table 1 above]

Table 1. Mean* Pharmacokinetic Parameters in Healthy Volunteers and Adult Patients With Epilepsy

Adult Study Population	Number of Subjects	T_{max}: Time of Maximum Plasma Concentration (h)	$t_{1/2}$: Elimination Half-life (h)	Cl/F: Apparent Plasma Clearance (mL/min/kg)
Healthy volunteers taking no other medications:				
Single-dose LAMICTAL	179	2.2 (0.25–12.0)	32.8 (14.0–103.0)	0.44 (0.12–1.10)
Multiple-dose LAMICTAL	36	1.7 (0.5–4.0)	25.4 (11.6–61.6)	0.58 (0.24–1.15)
Healthy volunteers taking valproate:				
Single-dose LAMICTAL	6	1.8 (1.0–4.0)	48.3 (31.5–88.6)	0.30 (0.14–0.42)
Multiple-dose LAMICTAL	18	1.9 (0.5–3.5)	70.3 (41.9–113.5)	0.18 (0.12–0.33)
Patients with epilepsy taking valproate only:				
Single-dose LAMICTAL	4	4.8 (1.8–8.4)	58.8 (30.5–88.8)	0.28 (0.16–0.40)
Patients with epilepsy taking carbamazepine, phenytoin, phenobarbital, or primidone† plus valproate:				
Single-dose LAMICTAL	25	3.8 (1.0–10.0)	27.2 (11.2–51.6)	0.53 (0.27–1.04)
Patients with epilepsy taking carbamazepine, phenytoin, phenobarbital, or primidone†:				
Single-dose LAMICTAL	24	2.3 (0.5–5.0)	14.4 (6.4–30.4)	1.10 (0.51–2.22)
Multiple-dose LAMICTAL	17	2.0 (0.75–5.93)	12.6 (7.5–3.1)	1.21 (0.66–1.82)

*The majority of parameter means determined in each study had coefficients of variation between 20% and 40% for half-life and Cl/F and between 30% and 70% for T_{max}. The overall mean values were calculated from individual study means that were weighted based on the number of volunteers/patients in each study. The numbers in parentheses below each parameter mean represent the range of individual volunteer/patient values across studies.

† Carbamazepine, phenobarbital, phenytoin, and primidone have been shown to increase the apparent clearance of lamotrigine. Rifampin has also been shown to increase the apparent clearance of lamotrigine (see CLINICAL PHARMACOLOGY: Drug Interactions and PRECAUTIONS: Drug Interactions).

Absorption: Lamotrigine is rapidly and completely absorbed after oral administration with negligible first-pass metabolism (absolute bioavailability is 98%). The bioavailability is not affected by food. Peak plasma concentrations occur anywhere from 1.4 to 4.8 hours following drug administration. The lamotrigine chewable/dispersible tablets were found to be equivalent, whether they were administered as dispersed in water, chewed and swallowed, or swallowed as whole, to the lamotrigine compressed tablets in terms of rate and extent of absorption.

Distribution: Estimates of the mean apparent volume of distribution (Vd/F) of lamotrigine following oral administration ranged from 0.9 to 1.3 L/kg. Vd/F is independent of dose and is similar following single and multiple doses in both patients with epilepsy and in healthy volunteers.

Continued on next page

Product information on these pages is effective as of August 2004. Further information is available at: GlaxoSmithKline, PO Box 13398, Research Triangle Park, NC 27709. 1-888-825-5249. Corporate Web Site: www.gsk.com

Lamictal—Cont.

Protein Binding: Data from in vitro studies indicate that lamotrigine is approximately 55% bound to human plasma proteins at plasma lamotrigine concentrations from 1 to 10 mcg/mL (10 mcg/mL is 4 to 6 times the trough plasma concentration observed in the controlled efficacy trials). Because lamotrigine is not highly bound to plasma proteins, clinically significant interactions with other drugs through competition for protein binding sites are unlikely. The binding of lamotrigine to plasma proteins did not change in the presence of therapeutic concentrations of phenytoin, phenobarbital, or valproate. Lamotrigine did not displace other AEDs (carbamazepine, phenytoin, phenobarbital) from protein binding sites.

Drug Disposition: Lamotrigine is metabolized predominantly by glucuronic acid conjugation; the major metabolite is an inactive 2-N-glucuronide conjugate. After oral administration of 240 mg of ^{14}C-lamotrigine (15 µCi) to 6 healthy volunteers, 94% was recovered in the urine and 2% was recovered in the feces. The radioactivity in the urine consisted of unchanged lamotrigine (10%), the 2-N-glucuronide (76%), a 5-N-glucuronide (10%), a 2-N-methyl metabolite (0.14%), and other unidentified minor metabolites (4%).

Drug Interactions: **The apparent clearance of lamotrigine is affected by the coadministration of certain medications.** Since lamotrigine is metabolized predominantly by glucuronic acid conjugation, drugs that induce or inhibit glucuronidation may affect the apparent clearance of lamotrigine. Carbamazepine, phenytoin, phenobarbital, and primidone have been shown to increase the apparent clearance of lamotrigine (see DOSAGE AND ADMINISTRATION and PRECAUTIONS: Drug Interactions). Most clinical experience is derived from patients taking these AEDs.

Rifampin also increases the apparent clearance of lamotrigine (see PRECAUTIONS: Drug Interactions).

Valproate decreases the apparent clearance of lamotrigine (i.e., more than doubles the elimination half-life of lamotrigine), whether given with or without carbamazepine, phenytoin, phenobarbital, or primidone. Accordingly, if lamotrigine is to be administered to a patient receiving valproate, lamotrigine must be given at a reduced dosage, of no more than half the dose used in patients not receiving valproate, even in the presence of drugs that increase the apparent clearance of lamotrigine (see DOSAGE AND ADMINISTRATION and PRECAUTIONS: Drug Interactions).

Oxcarbazepine and levetiracetam do not affect the apparent clearance of lamotrigine (see PRECAUTIONS: Drug Interactions).

In vitro inhibition experiments indicated that the formation of the primary metabolite of lamotrigine, the 2-N-glucuronide, was not significantly affected by co-incubation with clozapine, fluoxetine, phenelzine, risperidone, sertraline, or trazodone, and was minimally affected by co-incubation with amitriptyline, bupropion, clonazepam, haloperidol, or lorazepam. In addition, bufuralol metabolism data from human liver microsomes suggested that lamotrigine does not inhibit the metabolism of drugs eliminated predominantly by CYP2D6.

LAMICTAL has no effects on the pharmacokinetics of lithium (see PRECAUTIONS: Drug Interactions).

The pharmacokinetics of LAMICTAL were not changed by co-administration of bupropion (see PRECAUTIONS: Drug Interactions).

Co-administration of olanzapine did not have a clinically relevant effect on LAMICTAL pharmacokinetics (see PRECAUTIONS: Drug Interactions).

Enzyme Induction: The effects of lamotrigine on the induction of specific families of mixed-function oxidase isozymes have not been systematically evaluated.

Following multiple administrations (150 mg twice daily) to normal volunteers taking no other medications, lamotrigine induced its own metabolism, resulting in a 25% decrease in $t_{1/2}$ and a 37% increase in Cl/F at steady state compared to values obtained in the same volunteers following a single dose. Evidence gathered from other sources suggests that self-induction by LAMICTAL may not occur when LAMICTAL is given as adjunctive therapy in patients receiving carbamazepine, phenytoin, phenobarbital, primidone, or rifampin.

Dose Proportionality: In healthy volunteers not receiving any other medications and given single doses, the plasma concentrations of lamotrigine increased in direct proportion to the dose administered over the range of 50 to 400 mg. In 2 small studies (n = 7 and 8) of patients with epilepsy who were maintained on other AEDs, there also was a linear relationship between dose and lamotrigine plasma concentrations at steady state following doses of 50 to 350 mg twice daily.

Elimination: (see Table 1).

Special Populations: Patients With Renal Insufficiency: Twelve volunteers with chronic renal failure (mean creatinine clearance = 13 mL/min; range = 6 to 23) and another 6 individuals undergoing hemodialysis were each given a single 100-mg dose of LAMICTAL. The mean plasma half-lives determined in the study were 42.9 hours (chronic renal failure), 13.0 hours (during hemodialysis), and 57.4 hours (between hemodialysis) compared to 26.2 hours in healthy volunteers. On average, approximately 20% (range = 5.6 to 35.1) of the amount of lamotrigine present in the body was eliminated by hemodialysis during a 4-hour session.

Hepatic Disease: The pharmacokinetics of lamotrigine following a single 100-mg dose of LAMICTAL were evaluated in 24 subjects with moderate to severe hepatic dysfunction and compared with 12 subjects without hepatic impairment. The median apparent clearance of lamotrigine was 0.31, 0.24, or 0.10 mL/kg/min in patients with Grade A, B, or C (Child-Pugh Classification) hepatic impairment, respectively, compared to 0.34 mL/kg/min in the healthy controls. Median half-life of lamotrigine was 36, 60, or 110 hours in patients with Grade A, B, or C hepatic impairment, respectively, versus 32 hours in healthy controls.

Age: Pediatric Patients: The pharmacokinetics of LAMICTAL following a single 2-mg/kg dose were evaluated in 2 studies of pediatric patients (n = 29 for patients aged 10 months to 5.9 years and n = 26 for patients aged 5 to 11 years). Forty-three patients received concomitant therapy with other AEDs and 12 patients received LAMICTAL as monotherapy. Lamotrigine pharmacokinetic parameters for pediatric patients are summarized in Table 2.

Population pharmacokinetic analyses involving patients aged 2 to 18 years demonstrated that lamotrigine clearance was influenced predominantly by total body weight and concurrent AED therapy. The oral clearance of lamotrigine was higher, on a body weight basis, in pediatric patients than in adults. Weight-normalized lamotrigine clearance was higher in those subjects weighing less than 30 kg, compared with those weighing greater than 30 kg. Accordingly, patients weighing less than 30 kg may need an increase of as much as 50% in maintenance doses, based on clinical response, as compared with subjects weighing more than 30 kg being administered the same AEDs (see DOSAGE AND ADMINISTRATION). These analyses also revealed that, after accounting for body weight, lamotrigine clearance was not significantly influenced by age. Thus, the same weight-adjusted doses should be administered to children irrespective of differences in age. Concomitant AEDs which influence lamotrigine clearance in adults were found to have similar effects in children.

[See table 2 below]

Table 2. Mean Pharmacokinetic Parameters in Pediatric Patients With Epilepsy

Pediatric Study Population	Number of Subjects	T_{max} (h)	$t_{1/2}$ (h)	Cl/F (mL/min/kg)
Ages 10 months–5.3 years				
Patients taking carbamazepine, phenytoin, phenobarbital, or primidone*	10	3.0 (1.0–5.9)	7.7 (5.7–11.4)	3.62 (2.44–5.28)
Patients taking antiepileptic drugs (AEDs) with no known effect on the apparent clearance of lamotrigine	7	5.2 (2.9–6.1)	19.0 (12.9–27.1)	1.2 (0.75–2.42)
Patients taking valproate only	8	2.9 (1.0–6.0)	44.9 (29.5–52.5)	0.47 (0.23–0.77)
Ages 5–11 years				
Patients taking carbamazepine, phenytoin, phenobarbital, or primidone*	7	1.6 (1.0–3.0)	7.0 (3.8–9.8)	2.54 (1.35–5.58)
Patients taking carbamazepine, phenytoin, phenobarbital, or primidone* plus valproate	8	3.3 (1.0–6.4)	19.1 (7.0–31.2)	0.89 (0.39–1.93)
Patients taking valproate only†	3	4.5 (3.0–6.0)	65.8 (50.7–73.7)	0.24 (0.21–0.26)
Ages 13–18 years				
Patients taking carbamazepine, phenytoin, phenobarbital, or primidone*	11	†	†	1.3
Patients taking carbamazepine, phenytoin, phenobarbital, or primidone* plus valproate	8	†	†	0.5
Patients taking valproate only	4	†	†	0.3

*Carbamazepine, phenobarbital, phenytoin, and primidone have been shown to increase the apparent clearance of lamotrigine. Rifampin has also been shown to increase the apparent clearance of lamotrigine (see CLINICAL PHARMACOLOGY: Drug Interactions and PRECAUTIONS: Drug Interactions).

† Two subjects were included in the calculation for mean T_{max}.

‡ Parameter not estimated.

Elderly: The pharmacokinetics of lamotrigine following a single 150-mg dose of LAMICTAL were evaluated in 12 elderly volunteers between the ages of 65 and 76 years (mean creatinine clearance = 61 mL/min, range = 33 to 108 mL/min). The mean half-life of lamotrigine in these subjects was 31.2 hours (range, 24.5 to 43.4 hours), and the mean clearance was 0.40 mL/min/kg (range, 0.26 to 0.48 mL/min/kg).

Gender: The clearance of lamotrigine is not affected by gender. However, during dose escalation of LAMICTAL in one clinical trial in patients with epilepsy on a stable dose of valproate (n = 77), mean trough lamotrigine concentrations, unadjusted for weight, were 24% to 45% higher (0.3 to 1.7 mcg/mL) in females than in males.

Race: The apparent oral clearance of lamotrigine was 25% lower in non-Caucasians than Caucasians.

CLINICAL STUDIES

Epilepsy: The results of controlled clinical trials established the efficacy of LAMICTAL as monotherapy in adults with partial onset seizures already receiving treatment with carbamazepine, phenytoin, phenobarbital, or primidone as the single antiepileptic drug (AED), as adjunctive therapy in adults and pediatric patients age 2 to 16 with partial seizures, and as adjunctive therapy in the generalized seizures of Lennox-Gastaut syndrome in pediatric and adult patients.

Monotherapy With LAMICTAL in Adults With Partial Seizures Already Receiving Treatment With Carbamazepine, Phenytoin, Phenobarbital, or Primidone, as the Single AED: The effectiveness of monotherapy with LAMICTAL was established in a multicenter, double-blind clinical trial enrolling 156 adult outpatients with partial seizures. The patients experienced at least 4 simple partial, complex partial, and/or secondarily generalized seizures during each of 2 consecutive 4-week periods while receiving carbamazepine or phenytoin monotherapy during baseline. LAMICTAL (target dose of 500 mg/day) or valproate (1,000 mg/day) was added to either carbamazepine or phenytoin monotherapy over a 4-week period. Patients were then converted to monotherapy with LAMICTAL or valproate during the next 4 weeks, then continued on monotherapy for an additional 12-week period.

Study endpoints were completion of all weeks of study treatment or meeting an escape criterion. Criteria for escape relative to baseline were: (1) doubling of average monthly seizure count, (2) doubling of highest consecutive 2-day seizure frequency, (3) emergence of a new seizure type (defined as a seizure that did not occur during the 8-week baseline) that is more severe than seizure types that occur during study treatment, or (4) clinically significant prolongation of generalized-tonic-clonic (GTC) seizures. The primary efficacy variable was the proportion of patients in each treatment group who met escape criteria.

The percentage of patients who met escape criteria was 42% (32/76) in the LAMICTAL group and 69% (55/80) in the valproate group. The difference in the percentage of patients meeting escape criteria was statistically significant ($p = 0.0012$) in favor of LAMICTAL. No differences in efficacy based on age, sex, or race were detected.

Patients in the control group were intentionally treated with a relatively low dose of valproate; as such, the sole objective of this study was to demonstrate the effectiveness and safety of monotherapy with LAMICTAL, and cannot be interpreted to imply the superiority of LAMICTAL to an adequate dose of valproate.

Adjunctive Therapy With LAMICTAL in Adults With Partial Seizures: The effectiveness of LAMICTAL as adjunctive therapy (added to other AEDs) was established in 3 multicenter, placebo-controlled, double-blind clinical trials in 355 adults with refractory partial seizures. The patients had a history of at least 4 partial seizures per month in spite of receiving one or more AEDs at therapeutic concentrations and, in 2 of the studies, were observed on their established AED regimen during baselines that varied between 8 to 12 weeks. In the third, patients were not observed in a prospective baseline. In patients continuing to have at least 4 seizures per month during the baseline, LAMICTAL or placebo was then added to the existing therapy. In all 3 studies, change from baseline in seizure frequency was the primary measure of effectiveness. The results given below are for all partial seizures in the intent-to-treat population (all patients who received at least one dose of treatment) in each study, unless otherwise indicated. The median seizure frequency at baseline was 3 per week while the mean at baseline was 6.6 per week for all patients enrolled in efficacy studies.

One study (n = 216) was a double-blind, placebo-controlled, parallel trial consisting of a 24-week treatment period. Patients could not be on more than 2 other anticonvulsants and valproate was not allowed. Patients were randomized to receive placebo, a target dose of 300 mg/day of LAMICTAL, or a target dose of 500 mg/day of LAMICTAL. The median reductions in the frequency of all partial seizures relative to baseline were 8% in patients receiving placebo, 20% in patients receiving 300 mg/day of LAMICTAL, and 36% in patients receiving 500 mg/day of LAMICTAL. The seizure frequency reduction was statistically significant in the 500-mg/day group compared to the placebo group, but not in the 300-mg/day group.

A second study (n = 98) was a double-blind, placebo-controlled, randomized, crossover trial consisting of two 14-week treatment periods (the last 2 weeks of which consisted of dose tapering) separated by a 4-week washout period. Patients could not be on more than 2 other anticonvulsants and valproate was not allowed. The target dose of LAMICTAL was 400 mg/day. When the first 12 weeks of the treatment periods were analyzed, the median change in seizure frequency was a 25% reduction on LAMICTAL compared to placebo ($p<0.001$).

The third study (n = 41) was a double-blind, placebo-controlled, crossover trial consisting of two 12-week treatment periods separated by a 4-week washout period. Patients could not be on more than 2 other anticonvulsants. Thirteen patients were on concomitant valproate; these patients received 150 mg/day of LAMICTAL. The 28 other patients had a target dose of 300 mg/day of LAMICTAL. The median change in seizure frequency was a 26% reduction on LAMICTAL compared to placebo ($p<0.01$).

No differences in efficacy based on age, sex, or race, as measured by change in seizure frequency, were detected.

Adjunctive Therapy With LAMICTAL in Pediatric Patients With Partial Seizures: The effectiveness of LAMICTAL as adjunctive therapy in pediatric patients with partial seizures was established in a multicenter, double-blind, placebo-controlled trial in 199 patients aged 2 to 16 years (n = 98 on LAMICTAL, n = 101 on placebo). Following an 8-week baseline phase, patients were randomized to 18 weeks of treatment with LAMICTAL or placebo added to their current AED regimen of up to 2 drugs. Patients were dosed based on body weight and valproate use. Target doses were designed to approximate 5 mg/kg per day for patients taking valproate (maximum dose, 250 mg/day) and 15 mg/kg per day for the patients not taking valproate (maximum dose, 750 mg per day). The primary efficacy endpoint was percentage change from baseline in all partial seizures. For the intent-to-treat population, the median reduction of all partial seizures was 36% in patients treated with LAMICTAL and 7% on placebo, a difference that was statistically significant ($p<0.01$).

Adjunctive Therapy With LAMICTAL in Pediatric and Adult Patients With Lennox-Gastaut Syndrome: The effectiveness of LAMICTAL as adjunctive therapy in patients with Lennox-Gastaut syndrome was established in a multicenter, double-blind, placebo-controlled trial in 169 patients aged 3 to 25 years (n = 79 on LAMICTAL, n = 90 on placebo). Following a 4-week single-blind, placebo phase, patients were randomized to 16 weeks of treatment with LAMICTAL or placebo added to their current AED regimen of up to 3 drugs. Patients were dosed on a fixed-dose regimen based on body weight and valproate use. Target doses were designed to approximate 5 mg/kg per day for patients taking valproate (maximum dose, 200 mg/day) and 15 mg/kg per day for patients not taking valproate (maximum dose, 400 mg/day). The primary efficacy endpoint was percentage change from baseline in major motor seizures (atonic, tonic, major myoclonic, and tonic-clonic seizures). For the intent-to-treat population, the median reduction of major motor seizures was 32% in patients treated with LAMICTAL and 9% on placebo, a difference that was statistically significant ($p<0.05$). Drop attacks were significantly reduced by LAMICTAL (34%) compared to placebo (9%), as were tonic-clonic seizures (36% reduction versus 10% increase for LAMICTAL and placebo, respectively).

Bipolar Disorder: The effectiveness of LAMICTAL in the maintenance treatment of Bipolar I Disorder was established in 2 multicenter, double-blind, placebo-controlled studies in adult patients who met DSM-IV criteria for Bipolar I Disorder. Study 1 enrolled patients with a current or recent (within 60 days) depressive episode as defined by DSM-IV and Study 2 included patients with a current or recent (within 60 days) episode of mania or hypomania as defined by DSM-IV. Both studies included a cohort of patients (30% of 404 patients in Study 1 and 28% of 171 patients in Study 2) with rapid cycling Bipolar Disorder (4 to 6 episodes per year).

In both studies, patients were titrated to a target dose of 200 mg of LAMICTAL, as add-on therapy or as monotherapy, with gradual withdrawal of any psychotropic medications during an 8- to 16-week open-label period. Overall 81% of 1,305 patients participating in the open-label period were receiving 1 or more other psychotropic medications, including benzodiazepines, selective serotonin reuptake inhibitors (SSRIs), atypical antipsychotics (including olanzapine), valproate, or lithium, during titration of LAMICTAL. Patients with a CGI-severity score of 3 or less maintained for at least 4 continuous weeks, including at least the final week on monotherapy with LAMICTAL, were randomized to a placebo-controlled, double-blind treatment period for up to 18 months. The primary endpoint was TIME (time to intervention for a mood episode or one that was emerging, time to discontinuation for either an adverse event that was judged to be related to Bipolar Disorder, or for lack of efficacy). The mood episode could be depression, mania, hypomania, or a mixed episode.

In Study 1, patients received double-blind monotherapy with LAMICTAL, 50 mg/day (n = 50), LAMICTAL 200 mg/day (n = 124), LAMICTAL 400 mg/day (n = 47), or placebo (n = 121). LAMICTAL (200- and 400-mg/day treatment groups combined) was superior to placebo in delaying the time to occurrence of a mood episode. Separate analyses of the 200 and 400 mg/day dose groups revealed no added benefit from the higher dose.

In Study 2, patients received double-blind monotherapy with LAMICTAL (100 to 400 mg/day, n = 59), or placebo (n = 70). LAMICTAL was superior to placebo in delaying time to occurrence of a mood episode. The mean LAMICTAL dose was about 211 mg/day.

Although these studies were not designed to separately evaluate time to the occurrence of depression or mania, a combined analysis for the 2 studies revealed a statistically significant benefit for LAMICTAL over placebo in delaying the time to occurrence of both depression and mania, although the finding was more robust for depression.

INDICATIONS AND USAGE

Epilepsy:

Adjunctive Use: LAMICTAL is indicated as adjunctive therapy for partial seizures in adults and pediatric patients (≥2 years of age).

LAMICTAL is also indicated as adjunctive therapy for the generalized seizures of Lennox-Gastaut syndrome in adult and pediatric patients (≥2 years of age).

Monotherapy Use: LAMICTAL is indicated for conversion to monotherapy in adults with partial seizures who are receiving treatment with carbamazepine, phenytoin, phenobarbital, primidone, or valproate as the single AED.

Safety and effectiveness of LAMICTAL have not been established (1) as initial monotherapy, (2) for conversion to monotherapy from AEDs other than carbamazepine, phenytoin, phenobarbital, primidone, or valproate, or (3) for simultaneous conversion to monotherapy from 2 or more concomitant AEDs (see DOSAGE AND ADMINISTRATION).

Safety and effectiveness in patients below the age of 16 other than those with partial seizures and the generalized seizures of Lennox-Gastaut syndrome have not been established (see BOX WARNING).

Bipolar Disorder: LAMICTAL is indicated for the maintenance treatment of Bipolar I Disorder to delay the time to occurrence of mood episodes (depression, mania, hypomania, mixed episodes) in patients treated for acute mood episodes with standard therapy. The effectiveness of LAMICTAL in the acute treatment of mood episodes has not been established.

The effectiveness of LAMICTAL as maintenance treatment was established in 2 placebo-controlled trials of 18 months' duration in patients with Bipolar I Disorder as defined by DSM-IV (see CLINICAL STUDIES, Bipolar Disorder). The physician who elects to use LAMICTAL for periods extending beyond 18 months should periodically re-evaluate the long-term usefulness of the drug for the individual patient.

CONTRAINDICATIONS

LAMICTAL is contraindicated in patients who have demonstrated hypersensitivity to the drug or its ingredients.

WARNINGS

SEE BOX WARNING REGARDING THE RISK OF SERIOUS RASHES REQUIRING HOSPITALIZATION AND DISCONTINUATION OF LAMICTAL.

ALTHOUGH BENIGN RASHES ALSO OCCUR WITH LAMICTAL, IT IS NOT POSSIBLE TO PREDICT RELIABLY WHICH RASHES WILL PROVE TO BE SERIOUS OR LIFE THREATENING. ACCORDINGLY, LAMICTAL SHOULD ORDINARILY BE DISCONTINUED AT THE FIRST SIGN OF RASH, UNLESS THE RASH IS CLEARLY NOT DRUG RELATED. DISCONTINUATION OF TREATMENT MAY NOT PREVENT A RASH FROM BECOMING LIFE THREATENING OR PERMANENTLY DISABLING OR DISFIGURING.

Serious Rash: ***Pediatric Population:*** The incidence of serious rash associated with hospitalization and discontinuation of LAMICTAL in a prospectively followed cohort of pediatric patients with epilepsy receiving adjunctive therapy was approximately 0.8% (16 of 1,983). When 14 of these cases were reviewed by 3 expert dermatologists, there was considerable disagreement as to their proper classification. To illustrate, one dermatologist considered none of the cases to be Stevens-Johnson syndrome; another assigned 7 of the 14 to this diagnosis. There was 1 rash-related death in this 1,983 patient cohort. Additionally, there have been rare cases of toxic epidermal necrolysis with and without permanent sequelae and/or death in US and foreign postmarketing experience. It bears emphasis, accordingly, that LAMICTAL is only approved for use in those patients below the age of 16 who have partial seizures or generalized seizures associated with the Lennox-Gastaut syndrome (see INDICATIONS).

There is evidence that the inclusion of valproate in a multidrug regimen increases the risk of serious, potentially life-threatening rash in pediatric patients. In pediatric patients who used valproate concomitantly, 1.2% (6 of 482) experienced a serious rash compared to 0.6% (6 of 952) patients not taking valproate.

Adult Population: Serious rash associated with hospitalization and discontinuation of LAMICTAL occurred in 0.3% (11 of 3,348) of adult patients who received LAMICTAL in premarketing clinical trials of epilepsy. In the bipolar and other mood disorders clinical trials, the rate of serious rash was 0.08% (1 of 1,233) of adult patients who received LAMICTAL as initial monotherapy and 0.13% (2 of 1,538) of adult patients who received LAMICTAL as adjunctive therapy. No fatalities occurred among these individuals. However, in worldwide postmarketing experience, rare cases of rash-related death have been reported, but their numbers are too few to permit a precise estimate of the rate.

Among the rashes leading to hospitalization were Stevens-Johnson syndrome, toxic epidermal necrolysis, angioedema, and a rash associated with a variable number of the following systemic manifestations: fever, lymphadenopathy, facial swelling, hematologic, and hepatologic abnormalities.

There is evidence that the inclusion of valproate in a multidrug regimen increases the risk of serious, potentially life-threatening rash in adults. Specifically, of 584 patients administered LAMICTAL with valproate in epilepsy clinical trials, 6 (1%) were hospitalized in association with rash; in contrast, 4 (0.16%) of 2,398 clinical trial patients and volunteers administered LAMICTAL in the absence of valproate were hospitalized.

Other examples of serious and potentially life-threatening rash that did not lead to hospitalization also occurred in premarketing development. Among these, 1 case was reported to be Stevens-Johnson–like.

Hypersensitivity Reactions: Hypersensitivity reactions, some fatal or life threatening, have also occurred. Some of these reactions have included clinical features of multiorgan failure/dysfunction, including hepatic abnormalities and evidence of disseminated intravascular coagulation. It is important to note that early manifestations of hypersensitivity (e.g., fever, lymphadenopathy) may be present even though a rash is not evident. If such signs or symptoms are present, the patient should be evaluated immediately. LAMICTAL should be discontinued if an alternative etiology for the signs or symptoms cannot be established.

Prior to initiation of treatment with LAMICTAL, the patient should be instructed that a rash or other signs or symptoms of hypersensitivity (e.g., fever, lymphadenopathy) may herald a serious medical event and that the patient should report any such occurrence to a physician immediately.

Acute Multiorgan Failure: Multiorgan failure, which in some cases has been fatal or irreversible, has been observed in patients receiving LAMICTAL. Fatalities associated with multiorgan failure and various degrees of hepatic failure have been reported in 2 of 3,796 adult patients and 4 of 2,435 pediatric patients who received LAMICTAL in clinical trials. No such fatalities have been reported in bipolar patients in clinical trials. Rare fatalities from multiorgan failure have also been reported in compassionate plea and postmarketing use. The majority of these deaths occurred in association with other serious medical events, including status epilepticus and overwhelming sepsis, and hantavirus making it difficult to identify the initial cause.

Additionally, 3 patients (a 45-year-old woman, a 3.5-year-old boy, and an 11-year-old girl) developed multiorgan dysfunction and disseminated intravascular coagulation 9 to 14 days after LAMICTAL was added to their AED regimens. Rash and elevated transaminases were also present in all patients and rhabdomyolysis was noted in 2 patients. Both pediatric patients were receiving concomitant therapy with valproate, while the adult patient was being treated with carbamazepine and clonazepam. All patients subsequently recovered with supportive care after treatment with LAMICTAL was discontinued.

Blood Dyscrasias: There have been reports of blood dyscrasias that may or may not be associated with the hypersensitivity syndrome. These have included neutropenia, leukopenia, anemia, thrombocytopenia, pancytopenia, and, rarely, aplastic anemia and pure red cell aplasia.

Withdrawal Seizures: As with other AEDs, LAMICTAL should not be abruptly discontinued. In patients with epilepsy there is a possibility of increasing seizure frequency. In clinical trials in patients with Bipolar Disorder, 2 patients experienced seizures shortly after abrupt withdrawal of LAMICTAL. However, there were confounding factors that may have contributed to the occurrence of seizures in these bipolar patients. Unless safety concerns require a more rapid withdrawal, the dose of LAMICTAL should be tapered over a period of at least 2 weeks (see DOSAGE AND ADMINISTRATION).

PRECAUTIONS

Dermatological Events (see BOX WARNING, WARNINGS): Serious rashes associated with hospitalization and discontinuation of LAMICTAL have been reported. Rare deaths have been reported, but their numbers are too few to permit a precise estimate of the rate. There are suggestions, yet to be proven, that the risk of rash may also be increased by (1) coadministration of LAMICTAL with valproate, (2) exceeding the recommended initial dose of LAMICTAL, or (3) exceeding the recommended dose escalation for LAMICTAL. However, cases have been reported in the absence of these factors.

In epilepsy clinical trials, approximately 10% of all patients exposed to LAMICTAL developed a rash. In the Bipolar Disorder clinical trials, 14% of patients exposed to LAMICTAL developed a rash. Rashes associated with LAMICTAL do not appear to have unique identifying features. Typically, rash occurs in the first 2 to 8 weeks following treatment initia-

Continued on next page

Product information on these pages is effective as of August 2004. Further information is available at: GlaxoSmithKline, PO Box 13398, Research Triangle Park, NC 27709. 1-888-825-5249. Corporate Web Site: www.gsk.com

Lamictal—Cont.

tion. However, isolated cases have been reported after prolonged treatment (e.g., 6 months). Accordingly, duration of therapy cannot be relied upon as a means to predict the potential risk heralded by the first appearance of a rash.

Although most rashes resolved even with continuation of treatment with LAMICTAL, it is not possible to predict reliably which rashes will prove to be serious or life threatening. **ACCORDINGLY, LAMICTAL SHOULD ORDINARILY BE DISCONTINUED AT THE FIRST SIGN OF RASH, UNLESS THE RASH IS CLEARLY NOT DRUG RELATED. DISCONTINUATION OF TREATMENT MAY NOT PREVENT A RASH FROM BECOMING LIFE THREATENING OR PERMANENTLY DISABLING OR DISFIGURING.**

It is recommended that LAMICTAL not be restarted in patients who discontinued due to rash associated with prior treatment with LAMICTAL unless the potential benefits clearly outweigh the risks. If the decision is made to restart a patient who has discontinued LAMICTAL, the need to restart with the initial dosing recommendations should be assessed. The greater the interval of time since the previous dose, the greater consideration should be given to restarting with the initial dosing recommendations. If a patient has discontinued LAMICTAL for a period of more than 5 half-lives, it is recommended that initial dosing recommendations and guidelines be followed. The half-life of LAMICTAL is affected by other concomitant medications (see CLINICAL PHARMACOLOGY Pharmacokinetics and Drug Metabolism, and DOSAGE AND ADMINISTRATION).

Use in Patients With Epilepsy:

Sudden Unexplained Death in Epilepsy (SUDEP): During the premarketing development of LAMICTAL, 20 sudden and unexplained deaths were recorded among a cohort of 4,700 patients with epilepsy (5,747 patient-years of exposure).

Some of these could represent seizure-related deaths in which the seizure was not observed, e.g., at night. This represents an incidence of 0.0035 deaths per patient-year. Although this rate exceeds that expected in a healthy population matched for age and sex, it is within the range of estimates for the incidence of sudden unexplained deaths in patients with epilepsy not receiving LAMICTAL (ranging from 0.0005 for the general population of patients with epilepsy, to 0.004 for a recently studied clinical trial population similar to that in the clinical development program for LAMICTAL, to 0.005 for patients with refractory epilepsy). Consequently, whether these figures are reassuring or suggest concern depends on the comparability of the populations reported upon to the cohort receiving LAMICTAL and the accuracy of the estimates provided. Probably most reassuring is the similarity of estimated SUDEP rates in patients receiving LAMICTAL and those receiving another antiepileptic drug that underwent clinical testing in a similar population at about the same time. Importantly, that drug is chemically unrelated to LAMICTAL. This evidence suggests, although it certainly does not prove, that the high SUDEP rates reflect population rates, not a drug effect.

Status Epilepticus: Valid estimates of the incidence of treatment emergent status epilepticus among patients treated with LAMICTAL are difficult to obtain because reporters participating in clinical trials did not all employ identical rules for identifying cases. At a minimum, 7 of 2,343 adult patients had episodes that could unequivocally be described as status. In addition, a number of reports of variably defined episodes of seizure exacerbation (e.g., seizure clusters, seizure flurries, etc.) were made.

Use in Patients With Bipolar Disorder:

Acute Treatment of Mood Episodes: Safety and effectiveness of LAMICTAL in the acute treatment of mood episodes has not been established.

Suicide: The possibility of a suicide attempt is inherent in Bipolar Disorder, and close supervision of high-risk patients should accompany drug therapy. Prescriptions for LAMICTAL should be written for the smallest quantity of tablets consistent with good patient management, in order to reduce the risk of overdose. Overdoses have been reported for LAMICTAL, some of which have been fatal (see OVERDOSAGE).

Addition of LAMICTAL to a Multidrug Regimen That Includes Valproate (Dosage Reduction): Because valproate reduces the clearance of lamotrigine, the dosage of lamotrigine in the presence of valproate is less than half of that required in its absence (see DOSAGE AND ADMINISTRATION).

Use in Patients With Concomitant Illness: Clinical experience with LAMICTAL in patients with concomitant illness is limited. Caution is advised when using LAMICTAL in patients with diseases or conditions that could affect metabolism or elimination of the drug, such as renal, hepatic, or cardiac functional impairment.

Hepatic metabolism to the glucuronide followed by renal excretion is the principal route of elimination of lamotrigine (see CLINICAL PHARMACOLOGY).

A study in individuals with severe chronic renal failure (mean creatinine clearance = 13 mL/min) not receiving other AEDs indicated that the elimination half-life of unchanged lamotrigine is prolonged relative to individuals with normal renal function. Until adequate numbers of patients with severe renal impairment have been evaluated during chronic treatment with LAMICTAL, it should be used with caution in these patients, generally using a reduced maintenance dose for patients with significant impairment.

Because there is limited experience with the use of LAMICTAL in patients with impaired liver function, the use in such patients may be associated with as yet unrecognized risks (see CLINICAL PHARMACOLOGY and DOSAGE AND ADMINISTRATION

Binding in the Eye and Other Melanin-Containing Tissues: Because lamotrigine binds to melanin, it could accumulate in melanin-rich tissues over time. This raises the possibility that lamotrigine may cause toxicity in these tissues after extended use. Although ophthalmological testing was performed in one controlled clinical trial, the testing was inadequate to exclude subtle effects or injury occurring after long-term exposure. Moreover, the capacity of available tests to detect potentially adverse consequences, if any, of lamotrigine's binding to melanin is unknown.

Accordingly, although there are no specific recommendations for periodic ophthalmological monitoring, prescribers should be aware of the possibility of long-term ophthalmologic effects.

Information for Patients: Prior to initiation of treatment with LAMICTAL, the patient should be instructed that a rash or other signs or symptoms of hypersensitivity (e.g., fever, lymphadenopathy) may herald a serious medical event and that the patient should report any such occurrence to a physician immediately. In addition, the patient should notify his or her physician if worsening of seizure control occurs.

Patients should be advised that LAMICTAL may cause dizziness, somnolence, and other symptoms and signs of central nervous system (CNS) depression. Accordingly, they should be advised neither to drive a car nor to operate other complex machinery until they have gained sufficient experience on LAMICTAL to gauge whether or not it adversely affects their mental and/or motor performance.

Patients should be advised to notify their physicians if they become pregnant or intend to become pregnant during therapy. Patients should be advised to notify their physicians if they intend to breast-feed or are breast-feeding an infant.

Patients should be advised to notify their physician if they stop taking LAMICTAL for any reason and not to resume LAMICTAL without consulting their physician.

Patients should be informed of the availability of a patient information leaflet, and they should be instructed to read the leaflet prior to taking LAMICTAL. See PATIENT INFORMATION at the end of this labeling for the text of the leaflet provided for patients.

Laboratory Tests: The value of monitoring plasma concentrations of LAMICTAL has not been established. Because of the possible pharmacokinetic interactions between LAMICTAL and other AEDs being taken concomitantly (see Table 3), monitoring of the plasma levels of LAMICTAL and concomitant AEDs may be indicated, particularly during dosage adjustments. In general, clinical judgment should be exercised regarding monitoring of plasma levels of LAMICTAL and other anti-seizure drugs and whether or not dosage adjustments are necessary.

Drug Interactions:

Effects of Lamotrigine on the Pharmacokinetics of Other Drugs: (see Table 3).

LAMICTAL Added to Carbamazepine: LAMICTAL has no appreciable effect on steady-state carbamazepine plasma concentration. Limited clinical data suggest there is a higher incidence of dizziness, diplopia, ataxia, and blurred vision in patients receiving carbamazepine with LAMICTAL than in patients receiving other AEDs with LAMICTAL (see ADVERSE REACTIONS). The mechanism of this interaction is unclear. The effect of lamotrigine on plasma concentrations of carbamazepine-epoxide is unclear. In a small subset of patients (n = 7) studied in a placebo-controlled trial, lamotrigine had no effect on carbamazepine-epoxide plasma concentrations, but in a small, uncontrolled study (n = 9), carbamazepine-epoxide levels were seen to increase.

LAMICTAL Added to Oxcarbazepine: The AUC and C_{max} of oxcarbazepine and its active 10-monohydroxy oxcarbazepine metabolite were not significantly different following the addition of oxcarbazepine (600 mg twice daily) to LAMICTAL (200 mg once daily) in healthy male volunteers (n = 13) compared to healthy male volunteers receiving oxcarbazepine alone (n = 13). Limited clinical data suggest a higher incidence of headache, dizziness, nausea, and somnolence with coadministration of LAMICTAL and oxcarbazepine compared to LAMICTAL alone or oxcarbazepine alone.

LAMICTAL Added to Levetiracetam: Potential drug interactions between levetiracetam and lamotrigine were assessed by evaluation serum concentrations of both agents during placebo-controlled clinical trials. These data indicate that lamotrigine does not influence the pharmacokinetics of levetiracetam.

LAMICTAL Added to Valproate: When LAMICTAL was administered to 18 healthy volunteers receiving valproate in a pharmacokinetic study, the trough steady-state valproate concentrations in plasma decreased by an average of 25% over a 3-week period, and then stabilized. However, adding LAMICTAL to the existing therapy did not cause a change in plasma valproate concentrations in either adult or pediatric patients in controlled clinical trials.

LAMICTAL Added to Lithium: The pharmacokinetics of lithium were not altered in healthy subjects (n = 20) by co-administration of 100 mg/day lamotrigine for 6 days.

LAMICTAL Added to Phenytoin: LAMICTAL has no appreciable effect on steady-state phenytoin plasma concentrations in patients with epilepsy.

LAMICTAL Added to Olanzapine: The AUC and C_{max} of olanzapine were similar following the addition of olanzapine (15 mg once daily) to LAMICTAL (200 mg once daily) in healthy male volunteers (n = 16) compared to the AUC and C_{max} in healthy male volunteers receiving olanzapine alone (n = 16).

Results of in vitro experiments suggest that lamotrigine does not reduce the clearance of drugs eliminated predominantly by CYP2D6 (see CLINICAL PHARMACOLOGY).

Effects of Other Drugs on the Pharmacokinetics of Lamotrigine: (see Table 3).

Valproate Added to LAMICTAL: The addition of valproate increases lamotrigine steady-state concentrations in normal volunteers by slightly more than 2-fold. In one study, maximal inhibition of lamotrigine clearance was reached at valproate doses between 250 mg/day and 500 mg/day and did not increase as the valproate dose was further increased.

Carbamazepine, Phenytoin, Phenobarbital, or Primidone) Added to LAMICTAL: The addition of these AEDs decreases lamotrigine steady-state concentrations by approximately 40%.

Oxcarbazepine Added to LAMICTAL: The AUC and C_{max} of lamotrigine were similar following the addition of oxcarbazepine (600 mg twice daily) to LAMICTAL (200 mg once daily) in healthy male volunteers (n = 13) compared to healthy male volunteers receiving LAMICTAL alone (n = 13). Limited clinical data suggest a higher incidence of headache, dizziness, nausea, and somnolence with coadministration of LAMICTAL and oxcarbazepine compared to LAMICTAL alone or oxcarbazepine alone.

Levetiracetam Added to LAMICTAL: Potential drug interactions between levetiracetam and lamotrigine were assessed by evaluating serum concentrations of both agents during placebo-controlled clinical trials. These data indicate that levetiracetam does not influence the pharmacokinetics of lamotrigine.

Bupropion Added to LAMICTAL: The pharmacokinetics of a 100-mg single dose of lamotrigine in 12 healthy volunteers were not changed by co-administration of bupropion at 300 mg/day starting 11 days before the lamotrigine dose.

Olanzapine Added to LAMICTAL: The AUC and C_{max} of lamotrigine was reduced on average by 24% and 20%, respectively, following the addition of olanzapine (15 mg once daily) to LAMICTAL (200 mg once daily) in healthy male volunteers (n = 16) compared to healthy male volunteers receiving LAMICTAL alone (n = 12). This reduction in lamotrigine plasma concentrations is not expected to be clinically relevant.

Other Psychotropic Drugs Added to LAMICTAL: Results of in vitro experiments suggest that clearance of lamotrigine is unlikely to be reduced by concomitant administration of amitriptyline, clonazepam, clozapine, fluoxetine, haloperidol, lorazepam, phenelzine, risperidone, sertraline, or trazodone (see CLINICAL PHARMACOLOGY: Pharmacokinetics and Drug Metabolism).

Rifampin Added to LAMICTAL: In a study in 10 male volunteers, rifampin (600 mg/day for 5 days) significantly increased the apparent clearance of a single 25 mg dose of lamotrigine by approximately 2-fold (AUC decreased by approximately 40%).

Interactions With Folate Inhibitors: Lamotrigine is an inhibitor of dihydrofolate reductase. Prescribers should be aware of this action when prescribing other medications that inhibit folate metabolism.

Interactions With Oral Contraceptives: In women taking lamotrigine, there have been reports of decreased lamotrigine concentrations following introduction of oral contraceptives and reports of increased lamotrigine concentrations following withdrawal of oral contraceptives. Dosage adjustments may be necessary to maintain clinical response when starting or stopping oral contraceptives during lamotrigine therapy.

The net effects of drug interactions with LAMICTAL are summarized in Table 3.

Table 3. Summary of Drug Interactions With LAMICTAL

Drug	Drug Plasma Concentration With Adjunctive LAMICTAL*	Lamotrigine Plasma Concentration With Adjunctive Drugs†
Phenytoin (PHT)	↔	↓
Carbamazepine (CBZ)	↔	↓
CBZ epoxide‡	?	
Valproate	↓	↑
Valproate + PHT and/or CBZ	Not assessed	↔
Oxcarbazepine	↔	↔
10-monohydroxy oxcarbazepine metabolite§	↔	
Levetiracetam	↔	↔
Lithium	↔	Not assessed
Bupropion	Not assessed	↔
Olanzapine	↔	↔‖
Rifampin	Not assessed	↓

*From adjunctive clinical trials and volunteer studies.
† Net effects were estimated by comparing the mean clearance values obtained in adjunctive clinical trials and volunteers studies.

‡ Not administered, but an active metabolite of carbamazepine.
§ Not administered, but an active metabolite of oxcarbazepine
↔ = No significant effect.
? = Conflicting data.
‖ Slight decrease, not expected to be clinically relevant

Drug/Laboratory Test Interactions: None known.

Carcinogenesis, Mutagenesis, Impairment of Fertility: No evidence of carcinogenicity was seen in 1 mouse study or 2 rat studies following oral administration of lamotrigine for up to 2 years at maximum tolerated doses (30 mg/kg per day for mice and 10 to 15 mg/kg per day for rats, doses that are equivalent to 90 mg/m^2 and 60 to 90 mg/m^2 respectively). Steady-state plasma concentrations ranged from 1 to 4 mcg/mL in the mouse study and 1 to 10 mcg/mL in the rat study. Plasma concentrations associated with the recommended human doses of 300 to 500 mg/day are generally in the range of 2 to 5 mcg/mL, but concentrations as high as 19 mcg/mL have been recorded.

Lamotrigine was not mutagenic in the presence or absence of metabolic activation when tested in 2 gene mutation assays (the Ames test and the in vitro mammalian mouse lymphoma assay). In 2 cytogenetic assays (the in vitro human lymphocyte assay and the in vivo rat bone marrow assay), lamotrigine did not increase the incidence of structural or numerical chromosomal abnormalities.

No evidence of impairment of fertility was detected in rats given oral doses of lamotrigine up to 2.4 times the highest usual human maintenance dose of 8.33 mg/kg per day or 0.4 times the human dose on a mg/m^2 basis. The effect of lamotrigine on human fertility is unknown.

Pregnancy: ***Teratogenic Effects:*** Pregnancy Category C. No evidence of teratogenicity was found in mice, rats, or rabbits when lamotrigine was orally administered to pregnant animals during the period of organogenesis at doses up to 1.2, 0.5, and 1.1 times, respectively, on a mg/m^2 basis, the highest usual human maintenance dose (i.e., 500 mg/day). However, maternal toxicity and secondary fetal toxicity producing reduced fetal weight and/or delayed ossification were seen in mice and rats, but not in rabbits at these doses. Teratology studies were also conducted using bolus intravenous administration of the isethionate salt of lamotrigine in rats and rabbits. In rat dams administered an intravenous dose at 0.6 times the highest usual human maintenance dose, the incidence of intrauterine death without signs of teratogenicity was increased.

A behavioral teratology study was conducted in rats dosed during the period of organogenesis. At day 21 postpartum, offspring of dams receiving 5 mg/kg per day or higher displayed a significantly longer latent period for open field exploration and a lower frequency of rearing. In a swimming maze test performed on days 39 to 44 postpartum, time to completion was increased in offspring of dams receiving 25 mg/kg per day. These doses represent 0.1 and 0.5 times the clinical dose on a mg/m basis, respectively.

Lamotrigine did not affect fertility, teratogenesis, or postnatal development when rats were dosed prior to and during mating, and throughout gestation and lactation at doses equivalent to 0.4 times the highest usual human maintenance dose on a mg/m^2 basis.

When pregnant rats were orally dosed at 0.1, 0.14, or 0.3 times the highest human maintenance dose (on a mg/m^2 basis) during the latter part of gestation (days 15 to 20), maternal toxicity and fetal death were seen. In dams, food consumption and weight gain were reduced, and the gestation period was slightly prolonged (22.6 vs. 22.0 days in the control group). Stillborn pups were found in all 3 drug-treated groups with the highest number in the high-dose group. Postnatal death was also seen, but only in the 2 highest doses, and occurred between day 1 and 20. Some of these deaths appear to be drug-related and not secondary to the maternal toxicity. A no-observed-effect level (NOEL) could not be determined for this study.

Although LAMICTAL was not found to be teratogenic in the above studies, lamotrigine decreases fetal folate concentrations in rats, an effect known to be associated with teratogenesis in animals and humans. There are no adequate and well-controlled studies in pregnant women. Because animal reproduction studies are not always predictive of human response, this drug should be used during pregnancy only if the potential benefit justifies the potential risk to the fetus.

Non-Teratogenic Effects: As with other antiepileptic drugs, physiological changes during pregnancy may affect lamotrigine concentrations and/or therapeutic effect. There have been reports of decreased lamotrigine concentrations during pregnancy and restoration of pre-partum concentrations after delivery. Dosage adjustments may be necessary to maintain clinical response.

Pregnancy Exposure Registry: To facilitate monitoring fetal outcomes of pregnant women exposed to lamotrigine, physicians are encouraged to register patients, **before fetal outcome (e.g., ultrasound, results of amniocentesis, birth, etc.) is known,** and can obtain information by calling the Lamotrigine Pregnancy Registry at (800) 336-2176 (toll-free). Patients can enroll themselves in the North American Antiepileptic Drug Pregnancy Registry by calling (888) 233-2334 (toll-free).

Labor and Delivery: The effect of LAMICTAL on labor and delivery in humans is unknown.

Use in Nursing Mothers: Preliminary data indicate that lamotrigine passes into human milk. Because the effects on the infant exposed to LAMICTAL by this route are unknown, breast-feeding while taking LAMICTAL is not recommended.

Pediatric Use: LAMICTAL is indicated as adjunctive therapy for partial seizures in patients above 2 years of age and for the generalized seizures of Lennox-Gastaut syndrome. Safety and effectiveness for other uses in patients with epilepsy below the age of 16 years have not been established (see BOX WARNING).

Safety and effectiveness in patients below the age of 18 years with Bipolar Disorder has not been established.

Geriatric Use: Clinical studies of LAMICTAL for epilepsy and in Bipolar Disorder did not include sufficient numbers of subjects aged 65 and over to determine whether they respond differently from younger subjects. In general, dose selection for an elderly patient should be cautious, usually starting at the low end of the dosing range, reflecting the greater frequency of decreased hepatic, renal, or cardiac function, and of concomitant disease or other drug therapy.

ADVERSE REACTIONS

SERIOUS RASH REQUIRING HOSPITALIZATION AND DISCONTINUATION OF LAMICTAL, INCLUDING STEVENS-JOHNSON SYNDROME AND TOXIC EPIDERMAL NECROLYSIS, HAVE OCCURRED IN ASSOCIATION WITH THERAPY WITH LAMICTAL. RARE DEATHS HAVE BEEN REPORTED, BUT THEIR NUMBERS ARE TOO FEW TO PERMIT A PRECISE ESTIMATE OF THE RATE (see BOX WARNING).

Epilepsy:

Most Common Adverse Events in All Clinical Studies: Adjunctive Therapy in Adults With Epilepsy: The most commonly observed (≥5%) adverse experiences seen in association with LAMICTAL during adjunctive therapy in adults and not seen at an equivalent frequency among placebo-treated patients were: dizziness, ataxia, somnolence, headache, diplopia, blurred vision, nausea, vomiting, and rash. Dizziness, diplopia, ataxia, blurred vision, nausea, and vomiting were dose related. Dizziness, diplopia, ataxia, and blurred vision occurred more commonly in patients receiving carbamazepine with LAMICTAL than in patients receiving other AEDs with LAMICTAL. Clinical data suggest a higher incidence of rash, including serious rash, in patients receiving concomitant valproate than in patients not receiving valproate (see WARNINGS).

Approximately 11% of the 3,378 adult patients who received LAMICTAL as adjunctive therapy in premarketing clinical trials discontinued treatment because of an adverse experience. The adverse events most commonly associated with discontinuation were rash (3.0%), dizziness (2.8%), and headache (2.5%).

In a dose response study in adults, the rate of discontinuation of LAMICTAL for dizziness, ataxia, diplopia, blurred vision, nausea, and vomiting was dose related.

Monotherapy in Adults With Epilepsy: The most commonly observed (≥5%) adverse experiences seen in association with the use of LAMICTAL during the monotherapy phase of the controlled trial in adults not seen at an equivalent rate in the control group were vomiting, coordination abnormality, dyspepsia, nausea, dizziness, rhinitis, anxiety, insomnia, infection, pain, weight decrease, chest pain, and dysmenorrhea. The most commonly observed (≥5%) adverse experiences associated with the use of LAMICTAL during the conversion to monotherapy (add-on) period, not seen at an equivalent frequency among low-dose valproate-treated patients, were dizziness, headache, nausea, asthenia, coordination abnormality, vomiting, rash, somnolence, diplopia, ataxia, accidental injury, tremor, blurred vision, insomnia, nystagmus, diarrhea, lymphadenopathy, pruritus, and sinusitis.

Approximately 10% of the 420 adult patients who received LAMICTAL as monotherapy in premarketing clinical trials discontinued treatment because of an adverse experience. The adverse events most commonly associated with discontinuation were rash (4.5%), headache (3.1%), and asthenia (2.4%).

Adjunctive Therapy in Pediatric Patients With Epilepsy: The most commonly observed (≥5%) adverse experiences seen in association with the use of LAMICTAL as adjunctive treatment in pediatric patients and not seen at an equivalent rate in the control group were infection, vomiting, rash, fever, somnolence, accidental injury, dizziness, diarrhea, abdominal pain, nausea, ataxia, tremor, asthenia, bronchitis, flu syndrome, and diplopia.

In 339 patients age 2 to 16 years, 4.2% of patients on LAMICTAL and 2.9% of patients on placebo discontinued due to adverse experiences. The most commonly reported adverse experiences that led to discontinuation were rash for patients treated with LAMICTAL and deterioration of seizure control for patients treated with placebo.

Approximately 11.5% of the 1,081 pediatric patients who received LAMICTAL as adjunctive therapy in premarketing clinical trials discontinued treatment because of an adverse experience. The adverse events most commonly associated with discontinuation were rash (4.4%), reaction aggravated (1.7%), and ataxia (0.6%).

Incidence in Controlled Clinical Studies of Epilepsy: The prescriber should be aware that the figures in Tables 4, 5, 6, and 7 cannot be used to predict the frequency of adverse experiences in the course of usual medical practice where patient characteristics and other factors may differ from those prevailing during clinical studies. Similarly, the cited frequencies cannot be directly compared with figures obtained from other clinical investigations involving different treatments, uses, or investigators. An inspection of these frequencies, however, does provide the prescriber with one basis to estimate the relative contribution of drug and nondrug factors to the adverse event incidences in the population studied.

Incidence in Controlled Adjunctive Clinical Studies in Adults With Epilepsy: Table 4 lists treatment-emergent signs and symptoms that occurred in at least 2% of adult patients with epilepsy treated with LAMICTAL in placebo-controlled trials and were numerically more common in the patients treated with LAMICTAL. In these studies, either LAMICTAL or placebo was added to the patient's current AED therapy. Adverse events were usually mild to moderate in intensity.

Table 4. Treatment-Emergent Adverse Event Incidence in Placebo-Controlled Adjunctive Trials in Adult Patients With Epilepsy* (Events in at least 2% of patients treated with LAMICTAL and numerically more frequent than in the placebo group.)

Body System/ Adverse Experience†	Percent of Patients Receiving Adjunctive LAMICTAL (n = 711)	Percent of Patients Receiving Adjunctive Placebo (n = 419)
Body as a whole		
Headache	29	19
Flu syndrome	7	6
Fever	6	4
Abdominal pain	5	4
Neck pain	2	1
Reaction aggravated (seizure exacerbation)	2	1
Digestive		
Nausea	19	10
Vomiting	9	4
Diarrhea	6	4
Dyspepsia	5	2
Constipation	4	3
Tooth disorder	3	2
Anorexia	2	1
Musculoskeletal		
Arthralgia	2	0
Nervous		
Dizziness	38	13
Ataxia	22	6
Somnolence	14	7
Incoordination	6	2
Insomnia	6	2
Tremor	4	1
Depression	4	3
Anxiety	4	3
Convulsion	3	1
Irritability	3	2
Speech disorder	3	0
Concentration disturbance	2	1
Respiratory		
Rhinitis	14	9
Pharyngitis	10	9
Cough increased	8	6
Skin and appendages		
Rash	10	5
Pruritus	3	2
Special senses		
Diplopia	28	7
Blurred vision	16	5
Vision abnormality	3	1
Urogenital		
Female patients only	(n = 365)	(n = 207)
Dysmenorrhea	7	6
Vaginitis	4	1
Amenorrhea	2	1

*Patients in these adjunctive studies were receiving 1 to 3 of the following concomitant AEDs (carbamazepine, phenytoin, phenobarbital, or primidone) in addition to LAMICTAL or placebo. Patients may have reported multiple adverse experiences during the study or at discontinuation; thus, patients may be included in more than one category.

†Adverse experiences reported by at least 2% of patients treated with LAMICTAL are included.

In a randomized, parallel study comparing placebo and 300 and 500 mg/day of LAMICTAL, some of the more common drug-related adverse events were dose related (see Table 5).

Continued on next page

Product information on these pages is effective as of August 2004. Further information is available at: GlaxoSmithKline, PO Box 13398, Research Triangle Park, NC 27709. 1-888-825-5249. Corporate Web Site: www.gsk.com

Lamictal—Cont.

Table 5. Dose-Related Adverse Events From a Randomized, Placebo-Controlled Trial in Adults With Epilepsy

Adverse Experience	Percent of Patients Experiencing Adverse Experiences		
	Placebo (n = 73)	LAMICTAL 300 mg (n = 71)	LAMICTAL 500 mg (n = 72)
Ataxia	10	10	28*†
Blurred vision	10	11	25*†
Diplopia	8	24*	49*†
Dizziness	27	31	54*†
Nausea	11	18	25*
Vomiting	4	11	18*

*Significantly greater than placebo group ($p<0.05$).
†Significantly greater than group receiving LAMICTAL 300 mg ($p<0.05$).

Other events that occurred in more than 1% of patients but equally or more frequently in the placebo group included: asthenia, back pain, chest pain, flatulence, menstrual disorder, myalgia, paresthesia, respiratory disorder, and urinary tract infection.

The overall adverse experience profile for LAMICTAL was similar between females and males, and was independent of age. Because the largest non-Caucasian racial subgroup was only 6% of patients exposed to LAMICTAL in placebo-controlled trials, there are insufficient data to support a statement regarding the distribution of adverse experience reports by race. Generally, females receiving either adjunctive LAMICTAL or placebo were more likely to report adverse experiences than males. The only adverse experience for which the reports on LAMICTAL were greater than 10% more frequent in females than males (without a corresponding difference by gender on placebo) was dizziness (difference = 16.5%). There was little difference between females and males in the rates of discontinuation of LAMICTAL for individual adverse experiences.

Incidence in a Controlled Monotherapy Trial in Adults With Partial Seizures: Table 6 lists treatment-emergent signs and symptoms that occurred in at least 5% of patients with epilepsy treated with monotherapy with LAMICTAL in a double-blind trial following discontinuation of either concomitant carbamazepine or phenytoin not seen at an equivalent frequency in the control group.

Table 6. Treatment-Emergent Adverse Event Incidence in Adults With Partial Seizures in a Controlled Monotherapy Trial* (Events in at least 5% of patients treated with LAMICTAL and numerically more frequent than in the valproate group.)

Body System/ Adverse Experience†	Percent of Patients Receiving LAMICTAL Monotherapy‡ (n = 43)	Percent of Patients Receiving Low-Dose Valproate§ Monotherapy (n = 44)
Body as a whole		
Pain	5	0
Infection	5	2
Chest pain	5	2
Digestive		
Vomiting	9	0
Dyspepsia	7	2
Nausea	7	2
Metabolic and nutritional		
Weight decrease	5	2
Nervous		
Coordination abnormality	7	0
Dizziness	7	0
Anxiety	5	0
Insomnia	5	2
Respiratory		
Rhinitis	7	2
Urogenital (female patients only)	(n = 21)	(n = 28)
Dysmenorrhea	5	0

*Patients in these studies were converted to LAMICTAL or valproate monotherapy from adjunctive therapy with carbamazepine or phenytoin. Patients may have reported multiple adverse experiences during the study; thus, patients may be included in more than one category.
†Adverse experiences reported by at least 5% of patients are included.
‡Up to 500 mg/day.
§1,000 mg/day.

Adverse events that occurred with a frequency of less than 5% and greater than 2% of patients receiving LAMICTAL and numerically more frequent than placebo were:
Body as a Whole: Asthenia, fever.
Digestive: Anorexia, dry mouth, rectal hemorrhage, peptic ulcer.
Metabolic and Nutritional: Peripheral edema.
Nervous System: Amnesia, ataxia, depression, hypesthesia, libido increase, decreased reflexes, increased reflexes, nystagmus, irritability, suicidal ideation.
Respiratory: Epistaxis, bronchitis, dyspnea.
Skin and Appendages: Contact dermatitis, dry skin, sweating.
Special Senses: Vision abnormality.
Incidence in Controlled Adjunctive Trials in Pediatric Patients With Epilepsy: Table 7 lists adverse events that occurred in at least 2% of 339 pediatric patients who received LAMICTAL up to 15 mg/kg per day or a maximum of 750 mg per day. Reported adverse events were classified using COSTART terminology.

Table 7. Treatment-Emergent Adverse Event Incidence in Placebo-Controlled Adjunctive Trials in Pediatric Patients With Epilepsy (Events in at least 2% of patients treated with LAMICTAL and numerically more frequent than in the placebo group.)

Body System/ Adverse Experience	Percent of Patients Receiving LAMICTAL (n = 168)	Percent of Patients Receiving Placebo (n = 171)
Body as a whole		
Infection	20	17
Fever	15	14
Accidental injury	14	12
Abdominal pain	10	5
Asthenia	8	4
Flu syndrome	7	6
Pain	5	4
Facial edema	2	1
Photosensitivity	2	0
Cardiovascular		
Hemorrhage	2	1
Digestive		
Vomiting	20	16
Diarrhea	11	9
Nausea	10	2
Constipation	4	2
Dyspepsia	2	1
Tooth disorder	2	1
Hemic and lymphatic		
Lymphadenopathy	2	1
Metabolic and nutritional		
Edema	2	0
Nervous system		
Somnolence	17	15
Dizziness	14	4
Ataxia	11	3
Tremor	10	1
Emotional lability	4	2
Gait abnormality	4	2
Thinking abnormality	3	2
Convulsions	2	1
Nervousness	2	1
Vertigo	2	1
Respiratory		
Pharyngitis	14	11
Bronchitis	7	5
Increased cough	7	6
Sinusitis	2	1
Bronchospasm	2	1
Skin		
Rash	14	12
Eczema	2	1
Pruritus	2	1
Special senses		
Diplopia	5	1
Blurred vision	4	1
Ear disorder	2	1
Visual abnormality	2	0
Urogenital		
Male and female patients		
Urinary tract infection	3	0
Male patients only	n = 93	n = 92
Penis disorder	2	0

Bipolar Disorder: The most commonly observed (≥5%) adverse experiences seen in association with the use of LAMICTAL as monotherapy (100 to 400 mg/day) in Bipolar Disorder in the 2 double-blind, placebo-controlled trials of 18 months' duration, and numerically more frequent than in placebo-treated patients are included in Table 8. Adverse events that occurred in at least 5% of patients and were numerically more common during the dose escalation phase of LAMICTAL in these trials (when patients may have been receiving concomitant medications) compared to the monotherapy phase were: headache (25%), rash (11%), dizziness (10%), diarrhea (8%), dream abnormality (6%), and pruitus (6%).

During the monotherapy phase of the double-blind, placebo-controlled trials of 18 months' duration, 13% of 227 patients who received LAMICTAL (100 to 400 mg/day), 16% of 190 patients who received placebo, and 23% of 166 patients who received lithium discontinued therapy because of an adverse experience. The adverse events which most commonly led to discontinuation of LAMICTAL were rash (3%) and mania/hypomania/mixed mood adverse events (2%). Approximately 16% of 2,401 patients who received LAMICTAL (50 to 500 mg/day) for Bipolar Disorder in premarketing trials discontinued therapy because of an adverse experience; most commonly due to rash (5%) and mania/hypomania/mixed mood adverse events (2%).

Incidence in Controlled Clinical Studies of LAMICTAL for the Maintenance Treatment of Bipolar I Disorder: Table 8 lists treatment-emergent signs and symptoms that occurred in at least 5% of patients with Bipolar Disorder treated with LAMICTAL monotherapy (100 to 400 mg/day), following the discontinuation of other psychotropic drugs, in 2 double-blind, placebo-controlled trials of 18 months' duration and were numerically more frequent than in the placebo group.

Table 8. Treatment-Emergent Adverse Event Incidence in 2 Placebo-Controlled Trials in Adults With Bipolar I Disorder* (Events in at least 5% of patients treated with LAMICTAL monotherapy and numerically more frequent than in the placebo group.)

Body System/ Adverse Experience†	Percent of Patients Receiving LAMICTAL n = 227	Percent of Patients Receiving Placebo n = 190
General		
Back pain	8	6
Fatigue	8	5
Abdominal pain	6	3
Digestive		
Nausea	14	11
Constipation	5	2
Vomiting	5	2
Nervous System		
Insomnia	10	6
Somnolence	9	7
Xerostomia (dry mouth)	6	4
Respiratory		
Rhinitis	7	4
Exacerbation of cough	5	3
Pharyngitis	5	4
Skin		
Rash (non-serious)‡	7	5

*Patients in these studies were converted to LAMICTAL (100 to 400 mg/day) or placebo monotherapy from add-on therapy with other psychotropic medications. Patients may have reported multiple adverse experiences during the study; thus, patients may be included in more than one category.
†Adverse experiences reported by at least 5% of patients are included.
‡In the overall bipolar and other mood disorders clinical trials, the rate of serious rash was 0.08% (1 of 1,233) of adult patients who received LAMICTAL as initial monotherapy and 0.13% (2 of 1,538) of adult patients who received LAMICTAL as adjunctive therapy (see WARNINGS).

These adverse events were usually mild to moderate in intensity.

Other events that occurred in 5% or more patients but equally or more frequently in the placebo group included: dizziness, mania, headache, infection, influenza, pain, accidental injury, diarrhea, and dyspepsia.

Adverse events that occurred with a frequency of less than 5% and greater than 1% of patients receiving LAMICTAL and numerically more frequent than placebo were:
General: Fever, neck pain.
Cardiovascular: Migraine.
Digestive: Flatulence.
Metabolic and Nutritional: Weight gain, edema.
Musculoskeletal: Arthralgia, myalgia.
Nervous System: Amnesia, depression, agitation, emotional lability, dyspraxia, abnormal thoughts, dream abnormality, hypoesthesia.
Respiratory: Sinusitis.
Urogenital: Urinary frequency.
Adverse Events Following Abrupt Discontinuation: In the 2 maintenance trials, there was no increase in the incidence, severity or type of adverse events in Bipolar Disorder patients after abruptly terminating LAMICTAL therapy. In clinical trials in patients with Bipolar Disorder, 2 patients experienced seizures shortly after abrupt withdrawal of LAMICTAL. However, there were confounding factors that may have contributed to the occurrence of seizures in these bipolar patients (see DOSAGE AND ADMINISTRATION).

Mania/Hypomania/Mixed Episodes: During the double-blind, placebo-controlled clinical trials in Bipolar I Disorder in which patients were converted to LAMICTAL monotherapy (100 to 400 mg/day) from other psychotropic medications and followed for durations up to 18 months, the rate of manic or hypomanic or mixed mood episodes reported as adverse experiences was 5% for patients treated with LAMICTAL (n = 227), 4% for patients treated with lithium (n = 166), and 7% for patients treated with placebo (n = 190). In all bipolar controlled trials combined, adverse events of mania (including hypomania and mixed mood episodes) were reported in 5% of patients treated with LAMICTAL (n = 956), 3% of patients treated with lithium (n = 280), and 4% of patients treated with placebo (n = 803). The overall adverse event profile for LAMICTAL was similar between females and males, between elderly and nonelderly patients, and among racial groups.

Other Adverse Events Observed During All Clinical Trials For Pediatric and Adult Patients With Epilepsy or Bipolar Disorder and Other Mood Disorders: LAMICTAL has been administered to 6,694 individuals for whom complete adverse event data was captured during all clinical trials, only some of which were placebo controlled. During these trials, all adverse events were recorded by the clinical investigators using terminology of their own choosing. To provide a meaningful estimate of the proportion of individuals having adverse events, similar types of events were grouped into a smaller number of standardized categories using modified COSTART dictionary terminology. The frequencies presented represent the proportion of the 6,694 individuals exposed to LAMICTAL who experienced an event of the type cited on at least one occasion while receiving LAMICTAL. All reported events are included except those already listed in the previous tables or elsewhere in the labeling, those too general to be informative, and those not reasonably associated with the use of the drug.

Events are further classified within body system categories and enumerated in order of decreasing frequency using the following definitions: *frequent* adverse events are defined as those occurring in at least 1/100 patients; *infrequent* adverse events are those occurring in 1/100 to 1/1,000 patients; *rare* adverse events are those occurring in fewer than 1/1,000 patients.

Body as a Whole: Infrequent: Allergic reaction, chills, halitosis, and malaise. ***Rare:*** Abdomen enlarged, abscess, and suicide/suicide attempt.

Cardiovascular System: Infrequent: Flushing, hot flashes, hypertension, palpitations, postural hypotension, syncope, tachycardia, and vasodilation. ***Rare:*** Angina pectoris, atrial fibrillation, deep thrombophlebitis, ECG abnormality, and myocardial infarction.

Dermatological: Infrequent: Acne, alopecia, hirsutism, maculopapular rash, skin discoloration, and urticaria. ***Rare:*** Angioedema, erythema, exfoliative dermatitis, fungal dermatitis, herpes zoster, leukoderma, multiforme erythema, petechial rash, pustular rash, seborrhea, Stevens-Johnson syndrome, and vesiculobullous rash.

Digestive System: Infrequent: Dysphagia, eructation, gastritis, gingivitis, increased appetite, increased salivation, liver function tests abnormal, and mouth ulceration. ***Rare:*** Gastrointestinal hemorrhage, glossitis, gum hemorrhage, gum hyperplasia, hematemesis, hemorrhagic colitis, hepatitis, melena, stomach ulcer, stomatitis, thirst, and tongue edema.

Endocrine System: Rare: Goiter and hypothyroidism.

Hematologic and Lymphatic System: Infrequent: Ecchymosis and leukopenia. ***Rare:*** Anemia, eosinophilia, fibrin decrease, fibrinogen decrease, iron deficiency anemia, leukocytosis, lymphocytosis, macrocytic anemia, petechia, and thrombocytopenia.

Metabolic and Nutritional Disorders: Infrequent: Aspartate transaminase increased. ***Rare:*** Alcohol intolerance, alkaline phosphatase increase, alanine transaminase increase, bilirubinemia, general edema, gamma glutamyl transpeptidase increase, and hyperglycemia.

Musculoskeletal System: Infrequent: Arthritis, leg cramps, myasthenia, and twitching. ***Rare:*** Bursitis, joint disorder, muscle atrophy, pathological fracture, and tendinous contracture.

Nervous System: Frequent: Confusion and paresthesia. ***Infrequent:*** Akathisia, apathy, aphasia, CNS depression, depersonalization, dysarthria, dyskinesia, euphoria, hallucinations, hostility, hyperkinesia, hypertonia, libido decreased, memory decrease, mind racing, movement disorder, myoclonus, panic attack, paranoid reaction, personality disorder, psychosis, sleep disorder, stupor, and suicidal ideation. ***Rare:*** Cerebellar syndrome, cerebrovascular accident, cerebral sinus thrombosis, choreoathetosis, CNS stimulation, delirium, delusions, dysphoria, dystonia, extrapyramidal syndrome, faintness, grand mal convulsions, hemiplegia, hyperalgesia, hyperesthesia, hypokinesia, hypotonia, manic depression reaction, muscle spasm, neuralgia, neurosis, paralysis, and peripheral neuritis.

Respiratory System: Infrequent: Yawn. ***Rare:*** Hiccup and hyperventilation.

Special Senses: Frequent: Amblyopia. ***Infrequent:*** Abnormality of accommodation, conjunctivitis, dry eyes, ear pain, photophobia, taste perversion, and tinnitus. ***Rare:*** Deafness, lacrimation disorder, oscillopsia, parosmia, ptosis, strabismus, taste loss, uveitis, and visual field defect.

Urogenital System: Infrequent: Abnormal ejaculation, breast pain, hematuria, impotence, menorrhagia, polyuria, urinary incontinence, and urine abnormality. ***Rare:*** Acute kidney failure, anorgasmia, breast abscess, breast neoplasm, creatinine increase, cystitis, dysuria, epididymitis, female lactation, kidney failure, kidney pain, nocturia, urinary retention, urinary urgency, and vaginal moniliasis.

Table 9. LAMICTAL Added to an Antiepileptic Regimen Containing Valproate in Patients 2 to 12 Years of Age

Weeks 1 and 2	0.15 mg/kg/day in 1 or 2 divided doses, rounded down to the nearest whole tablet. Only whole tablets should be used for dosing.
Weeks 3 and 4	0.3 mg/kg/day in 1 or 2 divided doses, rounded down to the nearest whole tablet.

Weight based dosing can be achieved by using the following guide:

If the patient's weight is		Give this daily dose, using the most appropriate combination of LAMICTAL 2-mg and 5-mg tablets	
Greater than	And less than	Weeks 1 and 2	Weeks 3 and 4
6.7 kg	14 kg	2 mg every *other* day	2 mg every day
14.1 kg	27 kg	2 mg every day	4 mg every day
27.1 kg	34 kg	4 mg every day	8 mg every day
34.1 kg	40 kg	5 mg every day	10 mg every day

Usual maintenance dose: 1 to 5 mg/kg/day (maximum 200 mg/day in 1 or 2 divided doses). To achieve the usual maintenance dose, subsequent doses should be increased every 1 to 2 weeks as follows: calculate 0.3 mg/kg/day, round this amount down to the nearest whole tablet, and add this amount to the previously administered daily dose. The usual maintenance dose in patients adding LAMICTAL to valproate alone ranges from 1 to 3 mg/kg/day. Maintenance doses in patients weighing less than 30 kg may need to be increased by as much as 50%, based on clinical response.

Postmarketing and Other Experience: In addition to the adverse experiences reported during clinical testing of LAMICTAL, the following adverse experiences have been reported in patients receiving marketed LAMICTAL and from worldwide noncontrolled investigational use. These adverse experiences have not been listed above, and data are insufficient to support an estimate of their incidence or to establish causation.

Blood and Lymphatic: Agranulocytosis, aplastic anemia, disseminated intravascular coagulation, hemolytic anemia, neutropenia, pancytopenia, red cell aplasia.

Gastrointestinal: Esophagitis.

Hepatobiliary Tract and Pancreas: Pancreatitis.

Immunologic: Lupus-like reaction, vasculitis.

Lower Respiratory: Apnea.

Musculoskeletal: Rhabdomyolysis has been observed in patients experiencing hypersensitivity reactions.

Neurology: Exacerbation of parkinsonian symptoms in patients with pre-existing Parkinson's disease, tics.

Non-site Specific: Hypersensitivity reaction, multiorgan failure, progressive immunosuppression.

DRUG ABUSE AND DEPENDENCE

The abuse and dependence potential of LAMICTAL have not been evaluated in human studies.

OVERDOSAGE

Human Overdose Experience: Overdoses involving quantities up to 15 g have been reported for LAMICTAL, some of which have been fatal. Overdose has resulted in ataxia, nystagmus, increased seizures, decreased level of consciousness, coma, and intraventricular conduction delay.

Management of Overdose: There are no specific antidotes for LAMICTAL. Following a suspected overdose, hospitalization of the patient is advised. General supportive care is indicated, including frequent monitoring of vital signs and close observation of the patient. If indicated, emesis should be induced or gastric lavage should be performed; usual precautions should be taken to protect the airway. It should be kept in mind that lamotrigine is rapidly absorbed (see CLINICAL PHARMACOLOGY). It is uncertain whether hemodialysis is an effective means of removing lamotrigine from the blood. In 6 renal failure patients, about 20% of the amount of lamotrigine in the body was removed by hemodialysis during a 4-hour session. A Poison Control Center should be contacted for information on the management of overdosage of LAMICTAL.

DOSAGE AND ADMINISTRATION

Epilepsy:

Adjunctive Use: LAMICTAL is indicated as adjunctive therapy for partial seizures in adults and pediatric patients (≥2 years of age). LAMICTAL is also indicated as adjunctive therapy for the generalized seizures of Lennox-Gastaut syndrome in adult and pediatric patients (≥2 years of age).

Monotherapy Use: LAMICTAL is indicated for conversion to monotherapy in adults with partial seizures who are receiving treatment with carbamazepine, phenytoin, phenobarbital, primidone, or valproate as the single AED.

Safety and effectiveness of LAMICTAL have not been established (1) as initial monotherapy, (2) for conversion to monotherapy from AEDs other than carbamazepine, phenytoin, phenobarbital, primidone, or valproate, or (3) for simultaneous conversion to monotherapy from 2 or more concomitant AEDs.

Safety and effectiveness in pediatric patients below the age of 16 years other than those with partial seizures and the generalized seizures of Lennox-Gastaut syndrome have not been established (see BOX WARNING).

Bipolar Disorder: LAMICTAL is indicated for the maintenance treatment of Bipolar I Disorder to delay the time to occurrence of mood episodes (depression, mania, hypomania, mixed episodes) in patients treated for acute mood episodes with standard therapy. The effectiveness of LAMICTAL in the acute treatment of mood episodes has not been established.

General Dosing Considerations for Epilepsy and Bipolar Disorder Patients: The risk of nonserious rash is increased when the recommended initial dose and/or the rate of dose escalation of LAMICTAL is exceeded. There are suggestions, yet to be proven, that the risk of severe, potentially life-threatening rash may be increased by (1) coadministration of LAMICTAL with valproate, (2) exceeding the recommended initial dose of LAMICTAL, or (3) exceeding the recommended dose escalation for LAMICTAL. However, cases have been reported in the absence of these factors (see BOX WARNING). Therefore, it is important that the dosing recommendations be followed closely.

It is recommended that LAMICTAL not be restarted in patients who discontinued due to rash associated with prior treatment with LAMICTAL, unless the potential benefits clearly outweigh the risks. If the decision is made to restart a patient who has discontinued LAMICTAL, the need to restart with the initial dosing recommendations should be assessed. The greater the interval of time since the previous dose, the greater consideration should be given to restarting with the initial dosing recommendations. If a patient has discontinued LAMICTAL for a period of more than 5 half-lives, it is recommended that initial dosing recommendations and guidelines be followed. The half-life of LAMICTAL is affected by other concomitant medications (see CLINICAL PHARMACOLOGY: Pharmacokinetics and Drug Metabolism).

Patients With Hepatic Impairment: Experience in patients with hepatic impairment is limited. Based on a clinical pharmacology study in 24 patients with moderate to severe liver dysfunction (see CLINICAL PHARMACOLOGY), the following general recommendations can be made. Initial, escalation, and maintenance doses should generally be reduced by approximately 50% in patients with moderate (Child-Pugh Grade B) and 75% in patients with severe (Child-Pugh Grade C) hepatic impairment. Escalation and maintenance doses should be adjusted according to clinical response.

Patients With Renal Functional Impairment: Initial doses of LAMICTAL should be based on patients' AED regimen (see above); reduced maintenance doses may be effective for patients with significant renal functional impairment (see CLINICAL PHARMACOLOGY). Few patients with severe renal impairment have been evaluated during chronic treatment with LAMICTAL. Because there is inadequate experience in this population, LAMICTAL should be used with caution in these patients.

Epilepsy:

Adjunctive Therapy With LAMICTAL for Epilepsy: This section provides specific dosing recommendations for patients 2 to 12 years of age and patients greater than 12 years of age. Within each of these age-groups, specific dosing recommendations are provided depending upon whether or not the patient is receiving valproate (Tables 9 and 10 for patients 2 to 12 years of age, Tables 11 and 12 for patients greater than 12 years of age). In addition, the section provides a discussion of dosing for those patients receiving concomitant AEDs that have not been systematically evaluated in combination with LAMICTAL.

Patients 2 to 12 Years of Age: LAMICTAL Added to an Antiepileptic Drug Regimen Containing Valproate: Recommended dosing guidelines are summarized in Table 9.

LAMICTAL Added to Carbamazepine, Phenytoin, Phenobarbital, or Primidone: Recommended dosing guidelines are summarized in Table 10.

LAMICTAL Added to Oxcarbazepine or Levetiracetam, or to Antiepileptic Drugs for Which the Interaction With

Continued on next page

Product information on these pages is effective as of August 2004. Further information is available at: GlaxoSmithKline, PO Box 13398, Research Triangle Park, NC 27709. 1-888-825-5249. Corporate Web Site: www.gsk.com

Lamictal—Cont.

Lamotrigine is Not Known: Oxcarbazepine and levetiracetam do not affect the apparent clearance of lamotrigine. Specific dosing guidelines for the addition of LAMICTAL to oxcarbazepine or levetiracetam have not been studied in clinical trials. The effect of AEDs other than those already specified on the metabolism of LAMICTAL is not currently known. Therefore, no specific dosing guidelines can be provided. Conservative starting doses and dose escalations (as with concomitant valproate) would be prudent; maintenance dosing would be expected to fall between the maintenance dose with valproate, which decreases the apparent clearance of lamotrigine, and the maintenance dose without valproate, but with carbamazepine, phenytoin, phenobarbital, or primidone, which increase the apparent clearance of lamotrigine.

Note that the starting doses and dose escalations listed in Tables 9 and 10 are different than those used in clinical trials; however, the maintenance doses are the same as in clinical trials. Smaller starting doses and slower dose escalations than those used in clinical trials are recommended because of the suggestions that the risk of rash may be decreased by smaller starting doses and slower dose escalations. Therefore, maintenance doses will take longer to reach in clinical practice than in clinical trials. It may take several weeks to months to achieve an individualized maintenance dose. Maintenance doses in patients weighing less than 30 kg, regardless of age or concomitant AED, may need to be increased as much as 50%, based on clinical response.

The smallest available strength of LAMICTAL Chewable Dispersible Tablets is 2 mg, and only whole tablets should be administered. If the calculated dose cannot be achieved using whole tablets, the dose should be rounded down to the nearest whole tablet (see HOW SUPPLIED and PATIENT INFORMATION for a description of the available sizes of LAMICTAL Chewable Dispersible Tablets).

[See table 9 at top of previous page]

Table 10. LAMICTAL Added to Carbamazepine, Phenytoin, Phenobarbital, or Primidone* (Without Valproate) in Patients 2 to 12 Years of Age

Weeks 1 and 2	0.6 mg/kg/day in 2 divided doses, rounded down to the nearest whole tablet.
Weeks 3 and 4	1.2 mg/kg/day in 2 divided doses, rounded down to the nearest whole tablet.

Usual maintenance dose: 5 to 15 mg/kg/day (maximum 400 mg/day in 2 divided doses). To achieve the usual maintenance dose, subsequent doses should be increased every 1 to 2 weeks as follows: calculate 1.2 mg/kg/day, round this amount down to the nearest whole tablet, and add this amount to the previously administered daily dose. Maintenance doses in patients weighing less than 30 kg may need to be increased by as much as 50%, based on clinical response.

*Rifampin has also been shown to increase the apparent clearance of lamotrigine (see PRECAUTIONS: Drug Interactions)

Patients Over 12 Years of Age: LAMICTAL Added to an Antiepileptic Drug Regimen Containing Valproate: Recommended dosing guidelines are summarized in Table 11.

LAMICTAL Added to Carbamazepine, Phenytoin, Phenobarbital, or Primidone: Recommended dosing guidelines are summarized in Table 12.

LAMICTAL Added to Oxcarbazepine or Levetiracetam, or to Antiepileptic Drugs for Which the Interaction With Lamotrigine is Not Known: Oxcarbazepine and levetiracetam do not affect the apparent clearance of lamotrigine. Specific dosing guidelines for the addition of LAMICTAL to oxcarbazepine or levetiracetam have not been studied in clinical trials. The effect of AEDs other than those already specified on the metabolism of LAMICTAL is not currently known. Therefore, no specific dosing guidelines can be provided. Conservative starting doses and dose escalations (as with concomitant valproate) would be prudent; maintenance dosing would be expected to fall between the maintenance dose with valproate, which decreases the apparent clearance of lamotrigine, and the maintenance dose without valproate, but with carbamazepine, phenytoin, phenobarbital, or primidone, which increase the apparent clearance of lamotrigine.

Table 11. LAMICTAL Added to an Antiepileptic Drug Regimen Containing Valproate in Patients Over 12 Years of Age

Weeks 1 and 2	25 mg every *other* day
Weeks 3 and 4	25 mg every day

Usual maintenance dose: 100 to 400 mg/day (1 or 2 divided doses). To achieve maintenance, doses may be increased by 25 to 50 mg/day every 1 to 2 weeks. The usual maintenance dose in patients adding LAMICTAL to valproate alone ranges from 100 to 200 mg/day.

Table 12. LAMICTAL Added to Carbamazepine, Phenytoin, Phenobarbital, or Primidone* (Without Valproate) in Patients Over 12 Years of Age

Weeks 1 and 2	50 mg/day
Weeks 3 and 4	100 mg/day in 2 divided doses

Usual maintenance dose: 300 to 500 mg/day (in 2 divided doses). To achieve maintenance, doses may be increased by 100 mg/day every 1 to 2 weeks.

*Rifampin has also been shown to increase the apparent clearance of lamotrigine (see PRECAUTIONS: Drug Interactions)

Conversion From Adjunctive Therapy With Carbamazepine, Phenytoin, Phenobarbital, Primidone, or Valproate as the Single AED to Monotherapy With LAMICTAL in Patients ≥16 Years of Age With Epilepsy: The goal of the transition regimen is to effect the conversion to monotherapy with LAMICTAL under conditions that ensure adequate seizure control while mitigating the risk of serious rash associated with the rapid titration of LAMICTAL.

The recommended maintenance dose of LAMICTAL as monotherapy is 500 mg/day given in 2 divided doses.

To avoid an increased risk of rash, the recommended initial dose and subsequent dose escalations of LAMICTAL should not be exceeded (see BOX WARNING).

Conversion From Adjunctive Therapy With Carbamazepine, Phenytoin, Phenobarbital, or Primidone to Monotherapy With LAMICTAL: After achieving a dose of 500 mg/day of LAMICTAL according to the guidelines in Table 12, the concomitant AED should be withdrawn by 20% decrements each week over a 4-week period. The regimen for the withdrawal of the concomitant AED is based on experience gained in the controlled monotherapy clinical trial.

Conversion From Adjunctive Therapy With Valproate to Monotherapy With LAMICTAL: The conversion regimen involves 4 steps. First, achieve a dose of 200 mg/day of LAMICTAL according to the guidelines in Table 11. Second, while keeping the LAMICTAL dose at 200 mg/day, valproate should be gradually decreased to a dose of 500 mg/day by decrements no greater than 500 mg/day per week. This dosage regimen is then maintained for 1 week. Third, LAMICTAL should then be increased to 300 mg/day while valproate is simultaneously decreased to 250 mg/day. This regimen should be maintained for 1 week. Fourth, valproate should then be discontinued completely and LAMICTAL increased by 100 mg/day every week until the recommended monotherapy dose of 500 mg/day is reached (see Table 13).

Table 13. Conversion From Adjunctive Therapy With Valproate to Monotherapy With LAMICTAL in Patients ≥16 Years of Age.

	LAMICTAL	Valproate
Step 1	Achieve a dose of 200 mg/day according to guidelines in Table 11 (if not already on 200 mg/day).	Maintain previous stable dose.
Step 2	Maintain at 200 mg/day.	Decrease to 500 mg/day by decrements no greater than 500 mg/day per week and then maintain the dose of 500 mg/day for 1 week.
Step 3	Increase to 300 mg/day and maintain for 1 week.	Simultaneously decrease to 250 mg/day and maintain for 1 week.
Step 4	Increase by 100 mg/day every week to achieve maintenance dose of 500 mg/day.	Discontinue.

Conversion From Adjunctive Therapy With Antiepileptic Drugs Other Than Carbamazepine, Phenytoin, Phenobarbital, Primidone, or Valproate to Monotherapy With LAMICTAL: No specific dosing guidelines can be provided for conversion to monotherapy with LAMICTAL with AEDs other than carbamazepine, phenobarbital, phenytoin, primidone, or valproate.

Usual Maintenance Dose for Epilepsy: The usual maintenance doses identified in Tables 9–12 are derived from dosing regimens employed in the placebo-controlled adjunctive studies in which the efficacy of LAMICTAL was established. In patients receiving multidrug regimens employing carbamazepine, phenytoin, phenobarbital, or primidone **without valproate**, maintenance doses of adjunctive LAMICTAL as high as 700 mg/day have been used. In patients receiving **valproate alone,** maintenance doses of adjunctive LAMICTAL as high as 200 mg/day have been used. The advantage of using doses above those recommended in Tables 9-13 has not been established in controlled trials.

Discontinuation Strategy for Patients With Epilepsy: For patients receiving LAMICTAL in combination with other AEDs, a reevaluation of all AEDs in the regimen should be considered if a change in seizure control or an appearance or worsening of adverse experiences is observed.

If a decision is made to discontinue therapy with LAMICTAL, a step-wise reduction of dose over at least 2 weeks (approximately 50% per week) is recommended unless safety concerns require a more rapid withdrawal (see PRECAUTIONS).

Discontinuing carbamazepine, phenytoin, phenobarbital, or primidone should prolong the half-life of lamotrigine; discontinuing valproate should shorten the half-life of lamotrigine.

Target Plasma Levels for Patients With Epilepsy: A therapeutic plasma concentration range has not been established for lamotrigine. Dosing of LAMICTAL should be based on therapeutic response.

Bipolar Disorder: The goal of maintenance treatment with LAMICTAL is to delay the time to occurrence of mood episodes (depression, mania, hypomania, mixed episodes) in patients treated for acute mood episodes with standard therapy. The target dose of LAMICTAL is 200 mg/day (100 mg/day in patients taking valproate, which decreases the apparent clearance of lamotrigine, and 400 mg/day in patients not taking valproate and taking either carbamazepine, phenytoin, phenobarbital, primidone, or rifampin, which increase the apparent clearance of lamotrigine). In the clinical trials, doses up to 400 mg/day as monotherapy were evaluated, however, no additional benefit was seen at 400 mg/day compared to 200 mg/day (see CLINICAL STUDIES: Bipolar Disorder). Accordingly, doses above 200 mg/day are not recommended. Treatment with LAMICTAL is introduced, based on concurrent medications, according to the regimen outlined in Table 14. If other psychotropic medications are withdrawn following stabilization, the dose of LAMICTAL should be adjusted. For patients discontinuing valproate, the dose of LAMICTAL should be doubled over a 2-week period in equal weekly increments (see Table 15). For patients discontinuing carbamazepine, phenytoin, phenobarbital, primidone, or rifampin, the dose of LAMICTAL should remain constant for the first week and then should be decreased by half over a 2-week period in equal weekly decrements (see Table 15). The dose of LAMICTAL may then be further adjusted to the target dose (200 mg) as clinically indicated.

If other drugs are subsequently introduced, the dose of LAMICTAL may need to be adjusted. In particular, the introduction of valproate requires reduction in the dose of LAMICTAL (see CLINICAL PHARMACOLOGY: Drug Interactions).

To avoid an increased risk of rash, the recommended initial dose and subsequent dose escalations of LAMICTAL should not be exceeded (see BOX WARNING).

[See table 14 at top of next page]
[See table 15 on next page]

There is no body of evidence available to answer the question of how long the patient should remain on LAMICTAL therapy. Systematic evaluation of the efficacy of LAMICTAL in patients with either depression or mania who responded to standard therapy during an acute 8 to 16 week treatment phase and were then randomized to LAMICTAL or placebo for up to 76 weeks of observation for affective relapse demonstrated a benefit of such maintenance treatment (see CLINICAL STUDIES: Bipolar Disorder). Nevertheless, patients should be periodically reassessed to determine the need for maintenance treatment.

Discontinuation Strategy in Bipolar Disorder: As with other AEDs, LAMICTAL should not be abruptly discontinued. In the controlled clinical trials, there was no increase in the incidence, type, or severity of adverse experiences following abrupt termination of LAMICTAL. In clinical trials in patients with bipolar disorder, 2 patients experienced seizures shortly after abrupt withdrawal of LAMICTAL. However, there were confounding factors that may have contributed to the occurrence of seizures in these bipolar patients. Discontinuation of LAMICTAL should involve a step-wise reduction of dose over at least 2 weeks (approximately 50% per week) unless safety concerns require a more rapid withdrawal.

Administration of LAMICTAL Chewable Dispersible Tablets: LAMICTAL Chewable Dispersible Tablets may be swallowed whole, chewed, or dispersed in water or diluted fruit juice. If the tablets are chewed, consume a small amount of water or diluted fruit juice to aid in swallowing.

To disperse LAMICTAL Chewable Dispersible Tablets, add the tablets to a small amount of liquid (1 teaspoon, or enough to cover the medication). Approximately 1 minute later, when the tablets are completely dispersed, swirl the solution and consume the entire quantity immediately. *No attempt should be made to administer partial quantities of the dispersed tablets.*

HOW SUPPLIED

LAMICTAL Tablets, 25-mg

White, scored, shield-shaped tablets debossed with "LAMICTAL" and "25", bottles of 100 (NDC 0173-0633-02).

Store at 25°C (77°F); excursions permitted to 15–30°C (59–86°F) [see USP Controlled Room Temperature] in a dry place.

LAMICTAL Tablets, 100-mg

Peach, scored, shield-shaped tablets debossed with "LAMICTAL" and "100", bottles of 100 (NDC 0173-0642-55).

LAMICTAL Tablets, 150-mg

Cream, scored, shield-shaped tablets debossed with "LAMICTAL" and "150", bottles of 60 (NDC 0173-0643-60).

LAMICTAL Tablets, 200-mg

Blue, scored, shield-shaped tablets debossed with "LAMICTAL" and "200", bottles of 60 (NDC 0173-0644-60).

Store at 25°C (77°F); excursions permitted to 15–30°C (59–86°F) [see USP Controlled Room Temperature] in a dry place and protect from light.

LAMICTAL Chewable Dispersible Tablets, 2-mg

White to off-white, round tablets debossed with "LTG" over "2", bottles of 30 (NDC 0173-0699-00). ORDER DIRECTLY FROM GlaxoSmithKline 1-800-334-4153.

LAMICTAL Chewable Dispersible Tablets, 5-mg

White to off-white, caplet-shaped tablets debossed with "GX CL2", bottles of 100 (NDC 0173-0526-00).

LAMICTAL Chewable Dispersible Tablets, 25-mg

White, super elliptical-shaped tablets debossed with "GX CL5", bottles of 100 (NDC 0173-0527-00).

Store at 25°C (77°F); excursions permitted to 15–30°C (59–86°F) [see USP Controlled Room Temperature] in a dry place.

LAMICTAL Starter Kit for Patients Taking Valproate

25-mg, white, scored, shield-shaped tablets debossed with "LAMICTAL" and "25", blisterpack of 35 tablets (NDC 0173-0633-10).

Store at 25°C (77°F); excursions permitted to 15–30°C (59–86°F) [see USP Controlled Room Temperature] in a dry place.

LAMICTAL Starter Kit for Patients Taking Carbamazepine, Phenytoin, Phenobarbital, Primidone, or Rifampin and Not Taking Valproate

25-mg, white, scored, shield-shaped tablets debossed with "LAMICTAL" and "25" and **100-mg,** peach, scored, shield-shaped tablets debossed with "LAMICTAL" and "100", blisterpack of 84, 25-mg tablets and 14, 100-mg tablets (NDC 0173-0594-01)

Store at 25°C (77°F); excursions permitted to 15-30°C (59–86°F) [see USP Controlled Room Temperature] in a dry place and protect from light.

LAMICTAL Starter Kit for Patients Not Taking Carbamazepine, Phenytoin, Phenobarbital, Primidone, Rifampin, or Valproate [FOR USE IN BIPOLAR PATIENTS ONLY]

25-mg, white, scored, shield-shaped tablets debossed with "LAMICTAL" and "25" and **100-mg,** peach, scored, shield-shaped tablets debossed with "LAMICTAL" and "100", blisterpack of 42, 25-mg tablets and 7, 100-mg tablets (NDC 0173-0594-02).

Store at 25°C (77°F); excursions permitted to 15–30°C (59–86°F) [see USP Controlled Room Temperature] in a dry place and protect from light.

PATIENT INFORMATION

The following wording is contained in a separate leaflet provided for patients.

Information for the Patient
LAMICTAL® (lamotrigine) Tablets

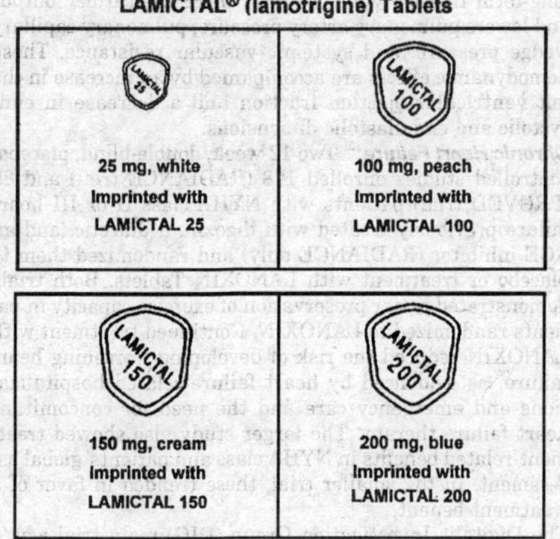

25 mg, white
Imprinted with
LAMICTAL 25
100 mg, peach
Imprinted with
LAMICTAL 100
150 mg, cream
Imprinted with
LAMICTAL 150
200 mg, blue
Imprinted with
LAMICTAL 200

LAMICTAL® (lamotrigine)
Chewable Dispersible Tablets

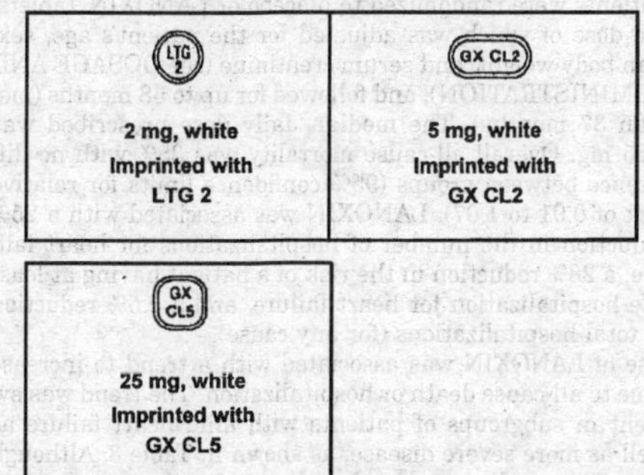

NOTE: The pictures above show actual tablet shape and size and the wording describes the color and printing that is on each strength of LAMICTAL Tablets and Chewable Dispersible Tablets. Before taking your medicine, it is important to compare the tablets you receive from your doctor or pharmacist with these pictures to make sure you have received the correct medicine.

Table 14. Escalation Regimen for LAMICTAL for Patients With Bipolar Disorder*

	For Patients Not Taking Carbamazepine, Phenytoin, Phenobarbital, Primidone, or Rifampin[†] and Not Taking Valproate[‡]	For Patients Taking Valproate	For Patients Taking Carbamazepine, Phenytoin, Phenobarbital, Primidone, or Rifampin[†] and Not Taking Valproate[‡]
Weeks 1 and 2	25 mg daily	25 mg every *other* day	50 mg daily
Weeks 3 and 4	50 mg daily	25 mg daily	100 mg daily, in divided doses
Week 5	100 mg daily	50 mg daily	200 mg daily, in divided doses
Week 6	200 mg daily	100 mg daily	300 mg daily, in divided doses
Week 7	200 mg daily	100 mg daily	up to 400 mg daily, in divided doses

* See CLINICAL PHARMACOLOGY: Drug Interactions and PRECAUTIONS: Drug Interactions for a description of known drug interactions.
[†] Carbamazepine, phenytoin, phenobarbital, primidone, and rifampin have been shown to increase the apparent clearance of lamotrigine.
[‡] Valporate has been shown to decrease the apparent clearance of lamotrigine.

Table 15. Adjustments to LAMICTAL Dosing for Patients With Bipolar Disorder Following Discontinuation of Psychotropic Medications*

	Discontinuation of Psychotropic Drugs (excluding Carbamazepine, Phenytoin, Phenobarbital, Primidone, Rifampin[†], or Valproate[‡])	After Discontinuation of Valproate[‡]	After Discontinuation of Carbamazepine, Phenytoin, Phenobarbital, Primidone, or Rifampin[†]
		Current LAMICTAL dose (mg/day) 100	Current LAMICTAL dose (mg/day) 400
Week 1	Maintain current LAMICTAL dose	150	400
Week 2	Maintain current LAMICTAL dose	200	300
Week 3 onward	Maintain current LAMICTAL dose	200	200

* See CLINICAL PHARMACOLOGY: Drug Interactions and PRECAUTIONS: Drug Interactions for a description of known drug interactions.
[†] Carbamazepine, phenytoin, phenobarbital, primidone, and rifampin have been shown to increase the apparent clearance of lamotrigine.
[‡] Valporate has been shown to decrease the apparent clearance of lamotrigine.

Please read this leaflet carefully before you take LAMICTAL and read the leaflet provided with any refill, in case any information has changed. This leaflet provides a summary of the information about your medicine. Please do not throw away this leaflet until you have finished your medicine. This leaflet does not contain all the information about LAMICTAL and is not meant to take the place of talking with your doctor. If you have any questions about LAMICTAL, ask your doctor or pharmacist.

Information About Your Medicine:

The name of your medicine is LAMICTAL (lamotrigine). The decision to use LAMICTAL is one that you and your doctor should make together. When taking lamotrigine, it is important to follow your doctor's instructions.

1. The Purpose of Your Medicine:

For Patients With Epilepsy: LAMICTAL is intended to be used either alone or in combination with other medicines to treat seizures in people aged 2 years or older.

For Patients With Bipolar Disorder: LAMICTAL is used as maintenance treatment of Bipolar I Disorder to delay the time to occurrence of mood episodes in people aged 18 years or older treated for acute mood episodes with standard therapy.

2. Who Should Not Take LAMICTAL:

You should not take LAMICTAL if you had an allergic reaction to it in the past.

3. Side Effects to Watch for:

- Most people who take LAMICTAL tolerate it well. Common side effects with LAMICTAL include dizziness, headache, blurred or double vision, lack of coordination, sleepiness, nausea, vomiting, insomnia, and rash. LAMICTAL may cause other side effects not listed in this leaflet. If you develop any side effects or symptoms you are concerned about or need more information, call your doctor.
- Although most patients who develop rash while receiving LAMICTAL have mild to moderate symptoms, some individuals may develop a serious skin reaction that requires hospitalization. Rarely, deaths have been reported. These serious skin reactions are most likely to happen within the first 8 weeks of treatment with LAMICTAL. Serious skin reactions occur more often in children than in adults.
- Rashes may be more likely to occur if you: (1) take LAMICTAL in combination with valproate [DEPAKENE® (valproic acid) or DEPAKOTE® (divalproex sodium)], (2) take a higher starting dose of LAMICTAL than your doctor prescribed, or (3) increase your dose of LAMICTAL faster than prescribed.
- It is not possible to predict whether a mild rash will develop into a more serious reaction.
  Therefore, if you experience a skin rash, hives, fever, swollen lymph glands, painful sores in the mouth or around the eyes, or swelling of lips or tongue, tell a doctor immediately, since these symptoms may be the first signs of a serious reaction. A doctor should evaluate your condition and decide if you should continue taking LAMICTAL.

4. The Use of LAMICTAL During Pregnancy and Breast-feeding:

The effects of LAMICTAL during pregnancy are not known at this time. If you are pregnant or are planning to become pregnant, talk to your doctor. Some LAMICTAL passes into breast milk and the effects of this on infants are unknown. Therefore, if you are breast-feeding, you should discuss this with your doctor to determine if you should continue to take LAMICTAL.

5. How to Use LAMICTAL:

- It is important to take LAMICTAL exactly as instructed by your doctor. The dose of LAMICTAL must be increased slowly. It may take several weeks or months before your final dosage can be determined by your doctor, based on your response.
- Do not increase your dose of LAMICTAL or take more frequent doses than those indicated by your doctor. Contact your doctor, if you stop taking LAMICTAL for any reason. Do not restart without consulting your doctor.
- If you miss a dose of LAMICTAL, do not double your next dose.
- Do NOT stop taking LAMICTAL or any of your other medicines unless instructed by your doctor.
- Use caution before driving a car or operating complex, hazardous machinery until you know if LAMICTAL affects your ability to perform these tasks.
- If you have epilepsy, tell your doctor if your seizures get worse or if you have any new types of seizures.
- Always tell your doctor and pharmacist if you are taking or plan to take any other prescription or over-the-counter medicines.

Continued on next page

Product information on these pages is effective as of August 2004. Further information is available at: GlaxoSmithKline, PO Box 13398, Research Triangle Park, NC 27709. 1-888-825-5249. Corporate Web Site: www.gsk.com

Lamictal—Cont.

6. How to Take LAMICTAL:
LAMICTAL Tablets should be swallowed whole. Chewing the tablets may leave a bitter taste.
LAMICTAL Chewable Dispersible Tablets may be swallowed whole, chewed, or mixed in water or diluted fruit juice. If the tablets are chewed, consume a small amount of water or diluted fruit juice to aid in swallowing.
To disperse LAMICTAL Chewable Dispersible Tablets, add the tablets to a small amount of liquid (1 teaspoon, or enough to cover the medication) in a glass or spoon. Approximately 1 minute later, when the tablets are completely dispersed, mix the solution and take the entire amount immediately.
7. Storing Your Medicine:
Store LAMICTAL at room temperature away from heat and light. Always keep your medicines out of the reach of children.
This medicine was prescribed for your use only to treat seizures or to treat Bipolar Disorder. Do not give the drug to others.
If your doctor decides to stop your treatment, do not keep any leftover medicine unless your doctor tells you to. Throw away your medicine as instructed.
Manufactured for GlaxoSmithKline
Research Triangle Park, NC 27709
by DSM Pharmaceuticals, Inc., Greenville, NC 27834 or
GlaxoSmithKline, Research Triangle Park, NC 27709
DEPAKENE and DEPAKOTE are registered trademarks of Abbott Laboratories.

June 2004/RL-2101
Shown in Product Identification Guide, page 316

LANOXICAPS® ℞
[*lă-nŏx' ĭ-kăps*]
(digoxin solution in capsules)
50 mcg (0.05 mg) I.D. Imprint A2C (red)
100 mcg (0.1 mg) I.D. Imprint B2C (yellow)
200 mcg (0.2 mg) I.D. Imprint C2C (green)

DESCRIPTION
LANOXIN (digoxin) is one of the cardiac (or digitalis) glycosides, a closely related group of drugs having in common specific effects on the myocardium. These drugs are found in a number of plants. Digoxin is extracted from the leaves of *Digitalis lanata*. The term "digitalis" is used to designate the whole group of glycosides. The glycosides are composed of two portions: a sugar and a cardenolide (hence "glycosides").
Digoxin is described chemically as (3β,5β,12β)-3-[(*O*-2,6-dideoxy-β-*D*-*ribo*-hexopyranosyl-(1→4)-*O*-2,6-dideoxy-β-*D*-*ribo*-hexopyranosyl-(1→4)-2,6-dideoxy-β-*D*-*ribo*-hexopyranosyl)oxy]-12,14-dihydroxy-card-20(22)-enolide. Its molecular formula is $C_{41}H_{64}O_{14}$, and its molecular weight is 780.95.
Digoxin exists as odorless white crystals that melt with decomposition above 230°C. The drug is practically insoluble in water and in ether; slightly soluble in diluted (50%) alcohol and in chloroform; and freely soluble in pyridine.
LANOXICAPS is a stable solution of digoxin enclosed within a soft gelatin capsule for oral use. Each capsule contains the labeled amount of digoxin USP dissolved in a solvent comprised of polyethylene glycol 400 USP, 8 percent ethyl alcohol, propylene glycol USP, and purified water USP. Inactive ingredients in the capsule shell include FD&C Red No. 40 (0.05-mg Capsule), D&C Yellow No. 10 (0.1-mg and 0.2-mg Capsules), FD&C Blue No. 1 (0.2-mg Capsule), gelatin, glycerin, methylparaben and propylparaben (added as preservatives), purified water, and sorbitol. Capsules are printed with edible ink.

CLINICAL PHARMACOLOGY
Mechanism of Action: Digoxin inhibits sodium-potassium ATPase, an enzyme that regulates the quantity of sodium and potassium inside cells. Inhibition of the enzyme leads to an increase in the intracellular concentration of sodium and thus (by stimulation of sodium-calcium exchange) an increase in the intracellular concentration of calcium. The beneficial effects of digoxin result from direct actions on cardiac muscle, as well as indirect actions on the cardiovascular system mediated by effects on the autonomic nervous system. The autonomic effects include: (1) a vagomimetic action, which is responsible for the effects of digoxin on the sinoatrial and atrioventricular (AV) nodes; and (2) baroreceptor sensitization, which results in increased afferent inhibitory activity and reduced activity of the sympathetic nervous system and renin-angiotensin system for any given increment in mean arterial pressure. The pharmacologic consequences of these direct and indirect effects are: (1) an increase in the force and velocity of myocardial systolic contraction (positive inotropic action); (2) a decrease in the degree of activation of the sympathetic nervous system and renin-angiotensin system (neurohormonal deactivating effect); and (3) slowing of the heart rate and decreased conduction velocity through the AV node (vagomimetic effect). The effects of digoxin in heart failure are mediated by its positive inotropic and neurohormonal deactivating effects, whereas the effects of the drug in atrial arrhythmias are related to its vagomimetic actions. In high doses, digoxin increases sympathetic outflow from the central nervous system (CNS). This increase in sympathetic activity may be an important factor in digitalis toxicity.

Table 1. Comparisons of the Systemic Availability and Equivalent Doses for Preparations of LANOXIN

Product	Absolute Bioavailability	Equivalent Doses (mcg)* Among Dosage Forms			
LANOXIN Tablets	60-80%	62.5	125	250	500
LANOXIN Elixir Pediatric	70-85%	62.5	125	250	500
LANOXICAPS®	90-100%	50	100	200	400
LANOXIN Injection/IV	100%	50	100	200	400

*For example, 125 mcg LANOXIN Tablets equivalent to 125 mcg LANOXIN Elixir Pediatric equivalent to 100 mcg LANOXICAPS equivalent to 100 mcg LANOXIN Injection/IV.

Table 2. Times to Onset of Pharmacologic Effect and to Peak Effect of Preparations of LANOXIN

Product	Time to Onset of Effect*	Time to Peak Effect*
LANOXIN Tablets	0.5-2 hours	2-6 hours
LANOXIN Elixir Pediatric	0.5-2 hours	2-6 hours
LANOXICAPS	0.5-2 hours	2-6 hours
LANOXIN Injection/IV	5-30 minutes†	1-4 hours

*Documented for ventricular response rate in atrial fibrillation, inotropic effects and electrocardiographic changes.
†Depending upon rate of infusion.

Pharmacokinetics: *Absorption:* Absorption of digoxin from LANOXICAPS Capsules has been demonstrated to be 90% to 100% complete compared to an identical intravenous dose of digoxin (absolute bioavailability). In comparison, the absolute bioavailability of conventional digoxin tablets has been demonstrated to be 60% to 80%. The enhanced absorption from LANOXICAPS compared to digoxin tablets and elixir is associated with reduced between-patient and within-patient variability in steady-state serum concentrations. The peak serum concentrations are higher than those observed after tablets. When digoxin tablets or capsules are taken after meals, the rate of absorption is slowed, but the total amount of digoxin absorbed is usually unchanged. When taken with meals high in bran fiber, however, the amount absorbed from an oral dose may be reduced. Comparisons of the systemic availability and equivalent doses for preparations of LANOXIN are shown in Table 1.
[See table 1 above]
In some patients, orally administered digoxin is converted to inactive reduction products (e.g., dihydrodigoxin) by colonic bacteria in the gut. Data suggest that 1 in 10 patients treated with digoxin tablets will degrade 40% or more of the ingested dose. As a result, certain antibiotics may increase the absorption of digoxin in such patients. Although inactivation of these bacteria by antibiotics is rapid, the serum digoxin concentration will rise at a rate consistent with the elimination half-life of digoxin. The magnitude of rise in serum digoxin concentration relates to the extent of bacterial inactivation, and may be as much as 2-fold in some cases. This phenomenon is minimized with LANOXICAPS because they are rapidly absorbed in the upper gastrointestinal tract.
Distribution: Following drug administration, a 6- to 8-hour tissue distribution phase is observed. This is followed by a much more gradual decline in the serum concentration of the drug, which is dependent on the elimination of digoxin from the body. The peak height and slope of the early portion (absorption/distribution phases) of the serum concentration-time curve are dependent upon the route of administration and the absorption characteristics of the formulation. Clinical evidence indicates that the early high serum concentrations (particularly high for digoxin capsules) do not reflect the concentration of digoxin at its site of action, but that with chronic use, the steady-state post-distribution serum levels are in equilibrium with tissue concentrations and correlate with pharmacologic effects. In individual patients, these post-distribution serum concentrations may be useful in evaluating therapeutic and toxic effects (see DOSAGE AND ADMINISTRATION: Serum Digoxin Concentrations).
Digoxin is concentrated in tissues and therefore has a large apparent volume of distribution. Digoxin crosses both the blood-brain barrier and the placenta. At delivery, the serum digoxin concentration in the newborn is similar to the serum concentration in the mother. Approximately 25% of digoxin in the plasma is bound to protein. Serum digoxin concentrations are not significantly altered by large changes in fat tissue weight, so that its distribution space correlates best with lean (i.e., ideal) body weight, not total body weight.
Metabolism: Only a small percentage (16%) of a dose of digoxin is metabolized. The end metabolites, which include 3 β-digoxigenin, 3-keto-digoxigenin, and their glucuronide and sulfate conjugates, are polar in nature and are postulated to be formed via hydrolysis, oxidation, and conjugation. The metabolism of digoxin is not dependent upon the cytochrome P-450 system, and digoxin is not known to induce or inhibit the cytochrome P-450 system.
Excretion: Elimination of digoxin follows first-order kinetics (that is, the quantity of digoxin eliminated at any time is proportional to the total body content). Following intravenous administration to healthy volunteers, 50% to 70% of a digoxin dose is excreted unchanged in the urine. Renal excretion of digoxin is proportional to glomerular filtration rate and is largely independent of urine flow. In healthy volunteers with normal renal function, digoxin has a half-life of 1.5 to 2.0 days. The half-life in anuric patients is prolonged to 3.5 to 5 days. Digoxin is not effectively removed from the body by dialysis, exchange transfusion, or during cardiopulmonary bypass because most of the drug is bound to tissue and does not circulate in the blood.
Special Populations: Race differences in digoxin pharmacokinetics have not been formally studied. Because digoxin is primarily eliminated as unchanged drug via the kidney and because there are no important differences in creatinine clearance among races, pharmacokinetic differences due to race are not expected.
The clearance of digoxin can be primarily correlated with renal function as indicated by creatinine clearance. The Cockcroft and Gault formula for estimation of creatinine clearance includes age, body weight, and gender. A table that provides the usual daily maintenance dose requirements of LANOXICAPS Capsules based on creatinine clearance (per 70 kg) is presented in the DOSAGE AND ADMINISTRATION section.
Plasma digoxin concentration profiles in patients with acute hepatitis generally fell within the range of profiles in a group of healthy subjects.
Pharmacodynamic and Clinical Effects: The times to onset of pharmacologic effect and to peak effect of preparations of LANOXIN are shown in Table 2.
[See table 2 above]
Hemodynamic Effects: Digoxin produces hemodynamic improvement in patients with heart failure. Short- and long-term therapy with the drug increases cardiac output and lowers pulmonary artery pressure, pulmonary capillary wedge pressure, and systemic vascular resistance. These hemodynamic effects are accompanied by an increase in the left ventricular ejection fraction and a decrease in end-systolic and end-diastolic dimensions.
Chronic Heart Failure: Two 12-week, double-blind, placebo-controlled studies enrolled 178 (RADIANCE trial) and 88 (PROVED trial) patients with NYHA class II or III heart failure previously treated with digoxin, a diuretic, and an ACE inhibitor (RADIANCE only) and randomized them to placebo or treatment with LANOXIN Tablets. Both trials demonstrated better preservation of exercise capacity in patients randomized to LANOXIN. Continued treatment with LANOXIN reduced the risk of developing worsening heart failure, as evidenced by heart failure-related hospitalizations and emergency care and the need for concomitant heart failure therapy. The larger study also showed treatment-related benefits in NYHA class and patients' global assessment. In the smaller trial, these trended in favor of a treatment benefit.
The Digitalis Investigation Group (DIG) main trial was a multicenter, randomized, double-blind, placebo-controlled mortality study of 6,801 patients with heart failure and left ventricular ejection fraction ≤0.45. At randomization, 67% were NYHA class I or II, 71% had heart failure of ischemic etiology, 44% had been receiving digoxin, and most were receiving concomitant ACE inhibitor (94%) and diuretic (82%). Patients were randomized to placebo or LANOXIN Tablets, the dose of which was adjusted for the patient's age, sex, lean body weight, and serum creatinine (see DOSAGE AND ADMINISTRATION), and followed for up to 58 months (median 37 months). The median daily dose prescribed was 0.25 mg. Overall all-cause mortality was 35% with no difference between groups (95% confidence limits for relative risk of 0.91 to 1.07). LANOXIN was associated with a 25% reduction in the number of hospitalizations for heart failure, a 28% reduction in the risk of a patient having at least one hospitalization for heart failure, and a 6.5% reduction in total hospitalizations (for any cause).
Use of LANOXIN was associated with a trend to increase time to all-cause death or hospitalization. The trend was evident in subgroups of patients with mild heart failure as well as more severe disease, as shown in Table 3. Although the effect on all-cause death or hospitalization was not statistically significant, much of the apparent benefit derived from effects on mortality and hospitalization attributed to heart failure.
[See table 3 at top of next page]
In situations where there is no statistically significant benefit of treatment evident from a trial's primary endpoint, results pertaining to a secondary endpoint should be interpreted cautiously.

Chronic Atrial Fibrillation: In patients with chronic atrial fibrillation, digoxin slows rapid ventricular response rate in a linear dose-response fashion from 0.25 to 0.75 mg/day. Digoxin should not be used for the treatment of multifocal atrial tachycardia.

INDICATIONS AND USAGE

Heart Failure: LANOXIN is indicated for the treatment of mild to moderate heart failure. LANOXIN increases left ventricular ejection fraction and improves heart failure symptoms as evidenced by exercise capacity and heart failure-related hospitalizations and emergency care, while having no effect on mortality. Where possible, LANOXIN should be used with a diuretic and an angiotensin-converting enzyme inhibitor, but an optimal order for starting these 3 drugs cannot be specified.

Atrial Fibrillation: LANOXIN is indicated for the control of ventricular response rate in patients with chronic atrial fibrillation.

CONTRAINDICATIONS

Digitalis glycosides are contraindicated in patients with ventricular fibrillation or in patients with a known hypersensitivity to digoxin. A hypersensitivity reaction to other digitalis preparations usually constitutes a contraindication to digoxin.

WARNINGS

Sinus Node Disease and AV Block: Because digoxin slows sinoatrial and AV conduction, the drug commonly prolongs the PR interval. The drug may cause severe sinus bradycardia or sinoatrial block in patients with pre-existing sinus node disease and may cause advanced or complete heart block in patients with pre-existing incomplete AV block. In such patients consideration should be given to the insertion of a pacemaker before treatment with digoxin.

Accessory AV Pathway (Wolff-Parkinson-White Syndrome): After intravenous digoxin therapy, some patients with paroxysmal atrial fibrillation or flutter and a coexisting accessory AV pathway have developed increased antegrade conduction across the accessory pathway bypassing the AV node, leading to a very rapid ventricular response or ventricular fibrillation. Unless conduction down the accessory pathway has been blocked (either pharmacologically or by surgery), digoxin should not be used in such patients. The treatment of paroxysmal supraventricular tachycardia in such patients is usually direct-current cardioversion.

Use in Patients with Preserved Left Ventricular Systolic Function: Patients with certain disorders involving heart failure associated with preserved left ventricular ejection fraction may be particularly susceptible to toxicity of the drug. Such disorders include restrictive cardiomyopathy, constrictive pericarditis, amyloid heart disease, and acute cor pulmonale. Patients with idiopathic hypertrophic subaortic stenosis may have worsening of the outflow obstruction due to the inotropic effects of digoxin.

PRECAUTIONS

Use in Patients with Impaired Renal Function: Digoxin is primarily excreted by the kidneys; therefore, patients with impaired renal function require smaller than usual maintenance doses of digoxin (see DOSAGE AND ADMINISTRATION). Because of the prolonged elimination half-life, a longer period of time is required to achieve an initial or new steady-state serum concentration in patients with renal impairment than in patients with normal renal function. If appropriate care is not taken to reduce the dose of digoxin, such patients are at high risk for toxicity, and toxic effects will last longer in such patients than in patients with normal renal function.

Use in Patients with Electrolyte Disorders: In patients with hypokalemia or hypomagnesemia, toxicity may occur despite serum digoxin concentrations below 2.0 ng/mL, because potassium or magnesium depletion sensitizes the myocardium to digoxin. Therefore, it is desirable to maintain normal serum potassium and magnesium concentrations in patients being treated with digoxin. Deficiencies of these electrolytes may result from malnutrition, diarrhea, or prolonged vomiting, as well as the use of the following drugs or procedures: diuretics, amphotericin B, corticosteroids, antacids, dialysis, and mechanical suction of gastrointestinal secretions.

Hypercalcemia from any cause predisposes the patient to digitalis toxicity. Calcium, particularly when administered rapidly by the intravenous route, may produce serious arrhythmias in digitalized patients. On the other hand, hypocalcemia can nullify the effects of digoxin in humans; thus, digoxin may be ineffective until serum calcium is restored to normal. These interactions are related to the fact that digoxin affects contractility and excitability of the heart in a manner similar to that of calcium.

Use in Thyroid Disorders and Hypermetabolic States: Hypothyroidism may reduce the requirements for digoxin. Heart failure and/or atrial arrhythmias resulting from hypermetabolic or hyperdynamic states (e.g., hyperthyroidism, hypoxia, or arteriovenous shunt) are best treated by addressing the underlying condition. Atrial arrhythmias associated with hypermetabolic states are particularly resistant to digoxin treatment. Care must be taken to avoid toxicity if digoxin is used.

Use in Patients with Acute Myocardial Infarction: Digoxin should be used with caution in patients with acute myocardial infarction. The use of inotropic drugs in some patients in this setting may result in undesirable increases in myocardial oxygen demand and ischemia.

Table 3. Subgroup Analyses of Mortality and Hospitalization During the First 2 Years Following Randomization

		Risk of All-Cause Mortality or All-Cause Hospitalization*			Risk of HF-Related Mortality or HF-Related Hospitalization*		
	n	Placebo	LANOXIN	Relative risk†	Placebo	LANOXIN	Relative risk†
All patients (EF ≤0.45)	6,801	604	593	0.94 (0.88–1.00)	294	217	0.69 (0.63–0.76)
NYHA I/II	4,571	549	541	0.96 (0.89–1.04)	242	178	0.70 (0.62–0.80)
EF 0.25–0.45	4,543	568	571	0.99 (0.91–1.07)	244	190	0.74 (0.66–0.84)
CTR ≤0.55	4,455	561	563	0.98 (0.91–1.06)	239	180	0.71 (0.63–0.81)
NYHA III/IV	2,224	719	696	0.88 (0.80–0.97)	402	295	0.65 (0.57–0.75)
EF <0.25	2,258	677	637	0.84 (0.76–0.93)	394	270	0.61 (0.53–0.71)
CTR >0.55	2,346	687	650	0.85 (0.77–0.94)	398	287	0.65 (0.57–0.75)
EF >0.45‡	987	571	585	1.04 (0.88–1.23)	179	136	0.72 (0.53–0.99)

*Number of patients with an event during the first 2 years per 1,000 randomized patients.
†Relative risk (95% confidence interval).
‡DIG Ancillary Study.

Use During Electrical Cardioversion: It may be desirable to reduce the dose of digoxin for 1 to 2 days prior to electrical cardioversion of atrial fibrillation to avoid the induction of ventricular arrhythmias, but physicians must consider the consequences of increasing the ventricular response if digoxin is withdrawn. If digitalis toxicity is suspected, elective cardioversion should be delayed. If it is not prudent to delay cardioversion, the lowest possible energy level should be selected to avoid provoking ventricular arrhythmias.

Laboratory Test Monitoring: Patients receiving digoxin should have their serum electrolytes and renal function (serum creatinine concentrations) assessed periodically; the frequency of assessments will depend on the clinical setting. For discussion of serum digoxin concentrations, see DOSAGE AND ADMINISTRATION.

Drug Interactions: Potassium-depleting *diuretics* are a major contributing factor to digitalis toxicity. *Calcium*, particularly if administered rapidly by the intravenous route, may produce serious arrhythmias in digitalized patients. *Quinidine, verapamil, amiodarone, propafenone, indomethacin, itraconazole, alprazolam,* and *spironolactone* raise the serum digoxin concentration due to a reduction in clearance and/or in volume of distribution of the drug, with the implication that digitalis intoxication may result. *Erythromycin* and *clarithromycin* (and possibly other *macrolide antibiotics*) and *tetracycline* may increase digoxin absorption in patients who inactivate digoxin by bacterial metabolism in the lower intestine, so that digitalis intoxication may result. The risk of this interaction may be reduced if digoxin is given as LANOXICAPS (see CLINICAL PHARMACOLOGY: Absorption). *Propantheline* and *diphenoxylate*, by decreasing gut motility, may increase digoxin absorption. *Antacids, kaolin-pectin, sulfasalazine, neomycin, cholestyramine,* certain *anticancer drugs,* and *metoclopramide* may interfere with intestinal digoxin absorption, resulting in unexpectedly low serum concentrations. *Rifampin* may decrease serum digoxin concentration, especially in patients with renal dysfunction, by increasing the non-renal clearance of digoxin. There have been inconsistent reports regarding the effects of other drugs [e.g., *quinine, penicillamine*] on serum digoxin concentration. *Thyroid* administration to a digitalized, hypothyroid patient may increase the dose requirement of digoxin. Concomitant use of digoxin and *sympathomimetics* increases the risk of cardiac arrhythmias. *Succinylcholine* may cause a sudden extrusion of potassium from muscle cells, and may thereby cause arrhythmias in digitalized patients. Although beta-adrenergic blockers or calcium channel blockers and digoxin may be useful in combination to control atrial fibrillation, their additive effects on AV node conduction can result in advanced or complete heart block.

Due to the considerable variability of these interactions, the dosage of digoxin should be individualized when patients receive these medications concurrently. Furthermore, caution should be exercised when combining digoxin with any drug that may cause a significant deterioration in renal function, since a decline in glomerular filtration or tubular secretion may impair the excretion of digoxin.

Drug/Laboratory Test Interactions: The use of therapeutic doses of digoxin may cause prolongation of the PR interval and depression of the ST segment on the electrocardiogram. Digoxin may produce false positive ST-T changes on the electrocardiogram during exercise testing. These electrophysiologic effects reflect an expected effect of the drug and are not indicative of toxicity.

Carcinogenesis, Mutagenesis, Impairment of Fertility: There have been no long-term studies performed in animals to evaluate carcinogenic potential, nor have studies been conducted to assess the mutagenic potential of digoxin or its potential to affect fertility.

Pregnancy: *Teratogenic Effects:* Pregnancy Category C. Animal reproduction studies have not been conducted with digoxin. It is also not known whether digoxin can cause fetal harm when administered to a pregnant woman or can affect reproduction capacity. Digoxin should be given to a pregnant woman only if clearly needed.

Nursing Mothers: Studies have shown that digoxin concentrations in the mother's serum and milk are similar. However, the estimated exposure of a nursing infant to digoxin via breast feeding will be far below the usual infant maintenance dose. Therefore, this amount should have no pharmacologic effect upon the infant. Nevertheless, caution should be exercised when digoxin is administered to a nursing woman.

Pediatric Use: Newborn infants display considerable variability in their tolerance to digoxin. Premature and immature infants are particularly sensitive to the effects of digoxin, and the dosage of the drug must not only be reduced but must be individualized according to their degree of maturity. Digitalis glycosides can cause poisoning in children due to accidental ingestion.

Geriatric Use: The majority of clinical experience gained with digoxin has been in the elderly population. This experience has not identified differences in response or adverse effects between the elderly and younger patients. However, this drug is known to be substantially excreted by the kidney, and the risk of toxic reactions to this drug may be greater in patients with impaired renal function. Because elderly patients are more likely to have decreased renal function, care should be taken in dose selection, which should be based on renal function, and it may be useful to monitor renal function (see DOSAGE AND ADMINISTRATION).

ADVERSE REACTIONS

In general, the adverse reactions of digoxin are dose-dependent and occur at doses higher than those needed to achieve a therapeutic effect. Hence, adverse reactions are less common when digoxin is used within the recommended dose range or therapeutic serum concentration range and when there is careful attention to concurrent medications and conditions.

Because some patients may be particularly susceptible to side effects with digoxin, the dosage of the drug should always be selected carefully and adjusted as the clinical condition of the patient warrants. In the past, when high doses of digoxin were used and little attention was paid to clinical status or concurrent medications, adverse reactions to digoxin were more frequent and severe. Cardiac adverse reactions accounted for about one half, gastrointestinal disturbances for about one fourth, and CNS and other toxicity for about one fourth of these adverse reactions. However, available evidence suggests that the incidence and severity of digoxin toxicity has decreased substantially in recent years. In recent controlled clinical trials, in patients with predominantly mild to moderate heart failure, the incidence of adverse experiences was comparable in patients taking digoxin and in those taking placebo. In a large mortality trial, the incidence of hospitalization for suspected digoxin toxicity was 2% in patients taking LANOXIN Tablets compared to 0.9% in patients taking placebo. In this trial, the most common manifestations of digoxin toxicity included gastrointestinal and cardiac disturbances; CNS manifestations were less common.

Adults: *Cardiac:* Therapeutic doses of digoxin may cause heart block in patients with pre-existing sinoatrial or AV conduction disorders; heart block can be avoided by adjusting the dose of digoxin. Prophylactic use of a cardiac pacemaker may be considered if the risk of heart block is considered unacceptable. High doses of digoxin may produce a

Continued on next page

Product information on these pages is effective as of August 2004. Further information is available at: GlaxoSmithKline, PO Box 13398, Research Triangle Park, NC 27709. 1-888-825-5249. Corporate Web Site: www.gsk.com

Lanoxicaps—Cont.

variety of rhythm disturbances, such as first-degree, second-degree (Wenckebach), or third-degree heart block (including asystole); atrial tachycardia with block; AV dissociation; accelerated junctional (nodal) rhythm; unifocal or multiform ventricular premature contractions (especially bigeminy or trigeminy); ventricular tachycardia; and ventricular fibrillation. Digoxin produces PR prolongation and ST segment depression which should not by themselves be considered digoxin toxicity. Cardiac toxicity can also occur at therapeutic doses in patients who have conditions which may alter their sensitivity to digoxin (see WARNINGS and PRECAUTIONS).

Gastrointestinal: Digoxin may cause anorexia, nausea, vomiting, and diarrhea. Rarely, the use of digoxin has been associated with abdominal pain, intestinal ischemia, and hemorrhagic necrosis of the intestines.

CNS: Digoxin can produce visual disturbances (blurred or yellow vision), headache, weakness, dizziness, apathy, confusion, and mental disturbances (such as anxiety, depression, delirium, and hallucination).

Other: Gynecomastia has been occasionally observed following the prolonged use of digoxin. Thrombocytopenia and maculopapular rash and other skin reactions have been rarely observed.

The following table summarizes the incidence of those adverse experiences listed above for patients treated with LANOXIN Tablets or placebo from two randomized, double-blind, placebo-controlled withdrawal trials. Patients in these trials were also receiving diuretics with or without angiotensin-converting enzyme inhibitors. These patients had been stable on digoxin, and were randomized to digoxin or placebo. The results shown in Table 4 reflect the experience in patients following dosage titration with the use of serum digoxin concentrations and careful follow-up. These adverse experiences are consistent with results from a large, placebo-controlled mortality trial (DIG trial) wherein over half the patients were not receiving digoxin prior to enrollment. [See table 4 below]

Infants and Children: The side effects of digoxin in infants and children differ from those seen in adults in several respects. Although digoxin may produce anorexia, nausea, vomiting, diarrhea, and CNS disturbances in young patients, these are rarely the initial symptoms of overdosage. Rather, the earliest and most frequent manifestation of excessive dosing with digoxin in infants and children is the appearance of cardiac arrhythmias, including sinus bradycardia. In children, the use of digoxin may produce any arrhythmia. The most common are conduction disturbances or supraventricular tachyarrhythmias, such as atrial tachycardia (with or without block) and junctional (nodal) tachycardia. Ventricular arrhythmias are less common. Sinus bradycardia may be a sign of impending digoxin intoxication, especially in infants, even in the absence of first-degree heart block. Any arrhythmia or alteration in cardiac conduction that develops in a child taking digoxin should be assumed to be caused by digoxin, until further evaluation proves otherwise.

OVERDOSAGE

Treatment of Adverse Reactions Produced by Overdosage: Digoxin should be temporarily discontinued until the adverse reaction resolves. Every effort should also be made to correct factors that may contribute to the adverse reaction (such as electrolyte disturbances or concurrent medications). Once the adverse reaction has resolved, therapy with digoxin may be reinstituted, following a careful reassessment of dose.

Withdrawal of digoxin may be all that is required to treat the adverse reaction. However, when the primary manifestation of digoxin overdosage is a cardiac arrhythmia, additional therapy may be needed.

If the rhythm disturbance is a symptomatic bradyarrhythmia or heart block, consideration should be given to the reversal of toxicity with DIGIBIND® [Digoxin Immune Fab (Ovine)] (see below), the use of atropine, or the insertion of a temporary cardiac pacemaker. However, asymptomatic bradycardia or heart block related to digoxin may require only temporary withdrawal of the drug and cardiac monitoring of the patient.

If the rhythm disturbance is a ventricular arrhythmia, consideration should be given to the correction of electrolyte disorders, particularly if hypokalemia (see below) or hypomagnesemia is present. DIGIBIND is a specific antidote for digoxin and may be used to reverse potentially life-threatening ventricular arrhythmias due to digoxin overdosage.

Administration of Potassium: Every effort should be made to maintain the serum potassium concentration between 4.0 and 5.5 mmol/L. Potassium is usually administered orally, but when correction of the arrhythmia is urgent and the serum potassium concentration is low, potassium may be administered cautiously by the intravenous route. The electrocardiogram should be monitored for any evidence of potassium toxicity (e.g., peaking of T waves) and to observe the effect on the arrhythmia. Potassium salts may be dangerous in patients who manifest bradycardia or heart block due to digoxin (unless primarily related to supraventricular tachycardia) and in the setting of massive digitalis overdosage (see Massive Digitalis Overdosage subsection).

Massive Digitalis Overdosage: Manifestations of life-threatening toxicity include ventricular tachycardia or ventricular fibrillation, or progressive bradyarrhythmias, or heart block. The administration of more than 10 mg of digoxin in a previously healthy adult, or more than 4 mg in a previously healthy child, or a steady-state serum concentration greater than 10 ng/mL, often results in cardiac arrest. DIGIBIND should be used to reverse the toxic effects of ingestion of a massive overdose. The decision to administer DIGIBIND to a patient who has ingested a massive dose of digoxin but who has not yet manifested life-threatening toxicity should depend on the likelihood that life-threatening toxicity will occur (see above).

Patients with massive digitalis ingestion should receive large doses of activated charcoal to prevent absorption and bind digoxin in the gut during enteroenteric recirculation. Emesis or gastric lavage may be indicated especially if ingestion has occurred within 30 minutes of the patient's presentation at the hospital. Emesis should not be induced in patients who are obtunded. If a patient presents more than 2 hours after ingestion or already has toxic manifestations, it may be unsafe to induce vomiting or attempt passage of a gastric tube, because such maneuvers may induce an acute vagal episode that can worsen digitalis-related arrhythmias.

Severe digitalis intoxication can cause a massive shift of potassium from inside to outside the cell, leading to life-threatening hyperkalemia. The administration of potassium supplements in the setting of massive intoxication may be hazardous and should be avoided. Hyperkalemia caused by massive digitalis toxicity is best treated with DIGIBIND; initial treatment with glucose and insulin may also be required if hyperkalemia itself is acutely life-threatening.

Table 4. Adverse Experiences in Two Parallel, Double-Blind, Placebo-Controlled Withdrawal Trials (Number of Patients Reporting)

Adverse Experience	Digoxin Patients (n = 123)	Placebo Patients (n = 125)
Cardiac		
Palpitation	1	4
Ventricular extrasystole	1	1
Tachycardia	2	1
Heart arrest	1	1
Gastrointestinal		
Anorexia	1	4
Nausea	4	2
Vomiting	2	1
Diarrhea	4	1
Abdominal pain	0	6
CNS		
Headache	4	4
Dizziness	6	5
Mental disturbances	5	1
Other		
Rash	2	1
Death	4	3

DOSAGE AND ADMINISTRATION

General: Recommended dosages of digoxin may require considerable modification because of individual sensitivity of the patient to the drug, the presence of associated conditions, or the use of concurrent medications. Due to the more complete absorption of digoxin from soft capsules, recommended oral doses are only 80 percent of those for Tablets and Elixir.

Because the significance of the higher peak serum concentrations associated with once daily capsules is not established, divided daily dosing is presently recommended for:

1. Infants and children under 10 years of age;
2. Patients requiring a daily dose of 300 mcg (0.3 mg) or greater;
3. Patients with a previous history of digitalis toxicity;
4. Patients considered likely to become toxic;
5. Patients in whom compliance is not a problem.

Where compliance is considered a problem, single daily dosing may be appropriate.

In selecting a dose of digoxin, the following factors must be considered:

1. The body weight of the patient. Doses should be calculated based upon lean (i.e., ideal) body weight.
2. The patient's renal function, preferably evaluated on the basis of estimated creatinine clearance.
3. The patient's age. Infants and children require different doses of digoxin than adults. Also, advanced age may be indicative of diminished renal function even in patients with normal serum creatinine concentration (i.e., below 1.5 mg/dL).
4. Concomitant disease states, concurrent medications, or other factors likely to alter the pharmacokinetic or pharmacodynamic profile of digoxin (see PRECAUTIONS).

Serum Digoxin Concentrations: In general, the dose of digoxin used should be determined on clinical grounds. However, measurement of serum digoxin concentrations can be helpful to the clinician in determining the adequacy of digoxin therapy and in assigning certain probabilities to the likelihood of digoxin intoxication. About two thirds of adults considered adequately digitalized (without evidence of toxicity) have serum digoxin concentrations ranging from 0.8 to 2.0 ng/mL. However, digoxin may produce clinical benefits even at serum concentrations below this range. About two thirds of adult patients with clinical toxicity have serum digoxin concentrations greater than 2.0 ng/mL. However, since one third of patients with clinical toxicity have concentrations less than 2.0 ng/mL, values below 2.0 ng/mL do not rule out the possibility that a certain sign or symptom is related to digoxin therapy. Rarely, there are patients who are unable to tolerate digoxin at serum concentrations below 0.8 ng/mL. Consequently, the serum concentration of digoxin should always be interpreted in the overall clinical context, and an isolated measurement should not be used alone as the basis for increasing or decreasing the dose of the drug.

To allow adequate time for equilibration of digoxin between serum and tissue, sampling of serum concentrations should be done just before the next scheduled dose of the drug. If this is not possible, sampling should be done at least 6 to 8 hours after the last dose, regardless of the route of administration or the formulation used. On a once-daily dosing schedule, the concentration of digoxin will be 10% to 25% lower when sampled at 24 versus 8 hours, depending upon the patient's renal function. On a twice-daily dosing schedule, there will be only minor differences in serum digoxin concentrations whether sampling is done at 8 or 12 hours after a dose.

If a discrepancy exists between the reported serum concentration and the observed clinical response, the clinician should consider the following possibilities:

1. Analytical problems in the assay procedure.
2. Inappropriate serum sampling time.
3. Administration of a digitalis glycoside other than digoxin.
4. Conditions (described in WARNINGS and PRECAUTIONS) causing an alteration in the sensitivity of the patient to digoxin.
5. Serum digoxin concentration may decrease acutely during periods of exercise without any associated change in clinical efficacy due to increased binding of digoxin to skeletal muscle.

Heart Failure: ***Adults:*** Digitalization may be accomplished by either of two general approaches that vary in dosage and frequency of administration, but reach the same endpoint in terms of total amount of digoxin accumulated in the body.

1. If rapid digitalization is considered medically appropriate, it may be achieved by administering a loading dose based upon projected peak digoxin body stores. Maintenance dose can be calculated as a percentage of the loading dose.

Table 5. Usual Daily Maintenance Dose Requirements (mcg) of LANOXICAPS Capsules for Estimated Peak Body Stores of 10 mcg/kg

		Lean Body Weight						
Corrected Ccr (mL/min per 70 kg)*	kg	50	60	70	80	90	100	Number of Days Before Steady State Achieved†
	lb	110	132	154	176	198	220	
0		50‡	100	100	100	150	150	22
10		100	100	100	150	150	150	19
20		100	100	150	150	150	200	16
30		100	150	150	150	200	200	14
40		100	150	150	200	200	250	13
50		150	150	200	200	250	250	12
60		150	150	200	200	250	300	11
70		150	200	200	250	250	300	10
80		150	200	200	250	300	300	9
90		150	200	250	250	300	350	8
100		200	200	250	300	300	350	7

*Ccr is creatinine clearance, corrected to 70 kg body weight or 1.73 m^2 body surface area. *For adults,* if only serum creatinine concentrations (Scr) are available, a Ccr (corrected to 70 kg body weight) may be estimated in men as (140 - Age)/Scr. For women, this result should be multiplied by 0.85. *Note: This equation cannot be used for estimating creatinine clearance in infants or children.*

† If no loading dose administered.

‡ 50 mcg = 0.05 mg

Table 6. Usual Digitalizing and Maintenance Dosages for LANOXICAPS in Children With Normal Renal Function Based on Lean Body Weight

Age	Digitalizing* Dose (mcg/kg)	Daily Maintenance Dose† (mcg/kg)
2 to 5 Years	25 to 35	25% to 35% of the oral or I.V. digitalizing dose‡
5 to 10 Years	15 to 30	
Over 10 Years	8 to 12	

*IV digitalizing doses are the same as digitalizing doses of LANOXICAPS.
†Divided daily dosing is recommended for children under 10 years of age.
‡Projected or actual digitalizing dose providing desired clinical response.

2. More gradual digitalization may be obtained by beginning an appropriate maintenance dose, thus allowing digoxin body stores to accumulate slowly. Steady-state serum digoxin concentrations will be achieved in approximately 5 half-lives of the drug for the individual patient. Depending upon the patient's renal function, this will take between 1 and 3 weeks.

Rapid Digitalization with a Loading Dose: Peak digoxin body stores of 8 to 12 mcg/kg should provide therapeutic effect with minimum risk of toxicity in most patients with heart failure and normal sinus rhythm. Because of altered digoxin distribution and elimination, projected peak body stores for patients with renal insufficiency should be conservative (i.e., 6 to 10 mcg/kg) [see PRECAUTIONS].

The loading dose should be administered in several portions, with roughly half the total given as the first dose. Additional fractions of this planned total dose may be given at 6- to 8-hour intervals, **with careful assessment of clinical response before each additional dose.**

If the patient's clinical response necessitates a change from the calculated loading dose of digoxin, then calculation of the maintenance dose should be based upon the amount actually given.

A single initial dose of 400 to 600 mcg (0.4 to 0.6 mg) of LANOXICAPS usually produces a detectable effect in 0.5 to 2 hours that becomes maximal in 2 to 6 hours. Additional doses of 100 to 300 mcg (0.1 to 0.3 mg) may be given cautiously at 6- to 8-hour intervals until clinical evidence of an adequate effect is noted. The usual amount of LANOXICAPS that a 70-kg patient requires to achieve 8 to 12 mcg/kg peak body stores is 600 to 1,000 mcg (0.6 to 1.0 mg).

LANOXIN Injection is frequently used to achieve rapid digitalization, with conversion to LANOXIN Tablets or LANOXICAPS for maintenance therapy. If patients are switched from intravenous to oral digoxin formulations, allowances must be made for differences in bioavailability when calculating maintenance dosages (see Table 1, CLINICAL PHARMACOLOGY).

Maintenance Dosing: The doses of digoxin tablets used in controlled trials in patients with heart failure have ranged from 125 to 500 mcg (0.125 to 0.5 mg) once daily. In these studies, the digoxin dose has been generally titrated according to the patient's age, lean body weight, and renal function. Therapy is generally initiated at a dose of 250 mcg (0.25 mg) once daily in patients under age 70 with good renal function, at a dose of 125 mcg (0.125 mg) once daily in patients over age 70 or with impaired renal function, and at a dose of 62.5 mcg (0.0625 mg) in patients with marked renal impairment. Doses may be increased every 2 weeks according to clinical response.

In a subset of approximately 1,800 patients enrolled in the DIG trial (wherein dosing was based on an algorithm similar to that in Table 5) the mean (±SD) serum digoxin concentrations at 1 month and 12 months were 1.01±0.47 ng/mL and 0.97±0.43 ng/mL, respectively.

The maintenance dose should be based upon the percentage of the peak body stores lost each day through elimination. The following formula has had wide clinical use:

Maintenance Dose = Peak Body Stores (i.e., Loading Dose) x % Daily Loss/100

Where: % Daily Loss = 14 + Ccr/5

(Ccr is creatinine clearance, corrected to 70 kg body weight or 1.73 m^2 body surface area)

Table 5 provides average daily maintenance dose requirements of LANOXICAPS Capsules for patients with heart failure based upon lean body weight and renal function:

[See table 5 above]

Example: Based on the above table, a patient in heart failure with an estimated lean body weight of 70 kg and a Ccr of 60 mL/min, should be given a dose of 200 mcg (0.2 mg) daily of LANOXICAPS, usually taken as a divided dose of one 100-mcg (0.1-mg) capsule after the morning and evening meals. If no loading dose is administered, steady-state serum concentrations in this patient should be anticipated at approximately 11 days.

Infants and Children: In general, divided daily dosing is recommended for infants and young children (under age 10). In these patients, where dosage adjustment is frequent and outside the fixed dosages available, LANOXICAPS may not be the formulation of choice. In the newborn period, renal clearance of digoxin is diminished and suitable dosage adjustments must be observed. This is especially pronounced in the premature infant. Beyond the immediate newborn period, children generally require proportionally larger doses than adults on the basis of body weight or body surface area. Children over 10 years of age require adult dosages in proportion to their body weight. Some researchers have suggested that infants and young children tolerate slightly higher serum concentrations than do adults.

Daily maintenance doses for each age group are given in Table 6 and should provide therapeutic effects with minimum risk of toxicity in most patients with heart failure and normal sinus rhythm. These recommendations assume the presence of normal renal function:

[See table 6 above]

In children with renal disease, digoxin must be carefully titrated based upon clinical response. **It cannot be overemphasized that both the adult and pediatric dosage guidelines provided are based upon average patient response and substantial individual variation can be expected. Accordingly, ultimate dosage selection must be based upon clinical assessment of the patient.**

Atrial Fibrillation: Peak digoxin body stores larger than the 8 to 12 mcg/kg required for most patients with heart failure and normal sinus rhythm have been used for control of ventricular rate in patients with atrial fibrillation. Doses of digoxin used for the treatment of chronic atrial fibrillation should be titrated to the minimum dose that achieves the desired ventricular rate control without causing undesirable side effects. Data are not available to establish the appropriate resting or exercise target rates that should be achieved.

Dosage Adjustment When Changing Preparations: The absolute bioavailability of the capsule formulation is greater than that of the standard tablets and very near that of the intravenous dosage form. As a result, the doses recommended for LANOXICAPS Capsules are the same as those for LANOXIN Injection (see Table 1 in CLINICAL PHARMACOLOGY: Pharmacokinetics). Adjustments in dosage will seldom be necessary when converting a patient from the intravenous formulation to LANOXICAPS. The difference in bioavailability between LANOXIN Injection or LANOXICAPS and LANOXIN Elixir Pediatric or LANOXIN Tablets must be considered when changing patients from one dosage form to another.

Doses of 100 mcg (0.1 mg) and 200 mcg (0.2 mg) of LANOXICAPS are approximately equivalent to 125-mcg (0.125-mg) and 250-mcg (0.25-mg) doses of LANOXIN Tablets and Elixir Pediatric, respectively (see Table 1 in CLINICAL PHARMACOLOGY: Pharmacokinetics).

HOW SUPPLIED

LANOXICAPS (digoxin solution in capsules), 50 mcg (0.05 mg): Bottle of 100 (NDC 0173-0270-55). Imprint A2C (red).

LANOXICAPS (digoxin solution in capsules), 100 mcg (0.1 mg): Bottle of 100 (NDC 0173-0272-55). Imprint B2C (yellow).

LANOXICAPS (digoxin solution in capsules), 200 mcg (0.2 mg): Bottle of 100 (NDC 0173-0274-55). Imprint C2C (green).

Store at 25°C (77°F); excursions permitted to 15 to 30°C (59 to 86°F) [see USP Controlled Room Temperature] in a dry place and protect from light.

Manufactured by Cardinal Health
St. Petersburg, FL 33702
for GlaxoSmithKline, Research Triangle Park, NC 27709

October 2003/RL-2047

Shown in Product Identification Guide, page 316

LANOXIN® ℞

[lă-nŏx'ĭn]
(digoxin)
Elixir Pediatric
50 mcg (0.05 mg) per mL

DESCRIPTION

LANOXIN (digoxin) is one of the cardiac (or digitalis) glycosides, a closely related group of drugs having in common specific effects on the myocardium. These drugs are found in a number of plants. Digoxin is extracted from the leaves of *Digitalis lanata*. The term "digitalis" is used to designate the whole group of glycosides. The glycosides are composed of two portions: a sugar and a cardenolide (hence "glycosides").

Digoxin is described chemically as (3β,5β,12β)-3-[(*O*-2,6-dideoxy-β-*D*-*ribo*-hexopyranosyl-(1→4)-*O*-2,6-dideoxy-β-*D*-*ribo*-hexopyranosyl-(1→4)-2,6-dideoxy-β-*D*-*ribo*-hexopyranosyl)oxy]-12,14-dihydroxy-card-20(22)-enolide. Its molecular formula is $C_{41}H_{64}O_{14}$, its molecular weight is 780.95.

Digoxin exists as odorless white crystals that melt with decomposition above 230°C. The drug is practically insoluble in water and in ether; slightly soluble in diluted (50%) alcohol and in chloroform; and freely soluble in pyridine.

LANOXIN Elixir Pediatric is a stable solution of digoxin specially formulated for oral use in infants and children. Each mL contains 50 mcg (0.05 mg) digoxin, USP. The lime-flavored elixir contains the inactive ingredients alcohol 10%, methylparaben 0.1% (added as a preservative), citric acid, D&C Green No. 5 and Yellow No. 10, flavor, propylene glycol, sodium phosphate, and sucrose. Each package is supplied with a specially calibrated dropper to facilitate the administration of accurate dosage even in premature infants. Starting at 0.2 mL, this 1-mL dropper is marked in divisions of 0.1 mL, each corresponding to 5 mcg (0.005 mg) digoxin.

CLINICAL PHARMACOLOGY

Mechanism of Action: Digoxin inhibits sodium-potassium ATPase, an enzyme that regulates the quantity of sodium and potassium inside cells. Inhibition of the enzyme leads to an increase in the intracellular concentration of sodium and thus (by stimulation of sodium-calcium exchange) an increase in the intracellular concentration of calcium. The beneficial effects of digoxin result from direct actions on cardiac muscle, as well as indirect actions on the cardiovascular system mediated by effects on the autonomic nervous system. The autonomic effects include: (1) a vagomimetic action, which is responsible for the effects of digoxin on the sinoatrial and atrioventricular (AV) nodes; and (2) baroreceptor sensitization, which results in increased afferent inhibitory activity and reduced activity of the sympathetic nervous system and renin-angiotensin system for any given increment in mean arterial pressure. The pharmacologic consequences of these direct and indirect effects are: (1) an increase in the force and velocity of myocardial systolic contraction (positive inotropic action); (2) a decrease in the degree of activation of the sympathetic nervous system and renin-angiotensin system (neurohormonal deactivating ef-

Continued on next page

Product information on these pages is effective as of August 2004. Further information is available at: GlaxoSmithKline, PO Box 13398, Research Triangle Park, NC 27709. 1-888-825-5249. Corporate Web Site: www.gsk.com

Lanoxin Elixir Pediatric—Cont.

fect); and (3) slowing of the heart rate and decreased conduction velocity through the AV node (vagomimetic effect). The effects of digoxin in heart failure are mediated by its positive inotropic and neurohormonal deactivating effects, whereas the effects of the drug in atrial arrhythmias are related to its vagomimetic actions. In high doses, digoxin increases sympathetic outflow from the central nervous system (CNS). This increase in sympathetic activity may be an important factor in digitalis toxicity.

Pharmacokinetics: Note: The following data are from studies performed in adults, unless otherwise stated.

Absorption: Absorption of digoxin from LANOXIN Elixir Pediatric formulation has been demonstrated to be 70% to 85% complete compared to an identical intravenous dose of digoxin (absolute bioavailability). When the elixir is taken after meals, the rate of absorption is slowed, but the total amount of digoxin absorbed is usually unchanged. When taken with meals high in bran fiber, however, the amount absorbed from an oral dose may be reduced. Comparisons of the systemic availability and equivalent doses for preparations of LANOXIN are shown in Table 1:

[See table 1 at right]

Table 1: Comparisons of the Systemic Availability and Equivalent Doses for Preparations of LANOXIN

Product	Absolute Bioavailability	Equivalent Doses (mcg)* Among Dosage Forms			
LANOXIN Tablets	60 – 80%	62.5	125	250	500
LANOXIN Elixir Pediatric	70 – 85%	62.5	125	250	500
LANOXICAPS®	90 – 100%	50	100	200	400
LANOXIN Injection/IV	100%	50	100	200	400

*For example, 125 mcg LANOXIN Tablets equivalent to 125 mcg LANOXIN Elixir Pediatric equivalent to 100 mcg LANOXICAPS equivalent to 100 mcg LANOXIN Injection/IV.

In some patients, orally administered digoxin is converted to inactive reduction products (e.g., dihydrodigoxin) by colonic bacteria in the gut. Data suggest that one in ten patients treated with digoxin tablets will degrade 40% or more of the ingested dose. As a result, certain antibiotics may increase the absorption of digoxin in such patients. Although inactivation of these bacteria by antibiotics is rapid, the serum digoxin concentration will rise at a rate consistent with the elimination half-life of digoxin. The magnitude of rise in serum digoxin concentration relates to the extent of bacterial inactivation, and may be as much as two-fold in some cases.

Distribution: Following drug administration, a 6- to 8-hour tissue distribution phase is observed. This is followed by a much more gradual decline in the serum concentration of the drug, which is dependent on the elimination of digoxin from the body. The peak height and slope of the early portion (absorption/distribution phases) of the serum concentration-time curve are dependent upon the route of administration and the absorption characteristics of the formulation. Clinical evidence indicates that the early high serum concentrations do not reflect the concentration of digoxin at its site of action, but that with chronic use, the steady-state post-distribution serum concentrations are in equilibrium with tissue concentrations and correlate with pharmacologic effects. In individual patients, these post-distribution serum concentrations may be useful in evaluating therapeutic and toxic effects (see DOSAGE AND ADMINISTRATION: Serum Digoxin Concentrations).

Digoxin is concentrated in tissues and therefore has a large apparent volume of distribution. Digoxin crosses both the blood-brain barrier and the placenta. At delivery, the serum digoxin concentration in the newborn is similar to the serum concentration in the mother. Approximately 25% of digoxin in the plasma is bound to protein. Serum digoxin concentrations are not significantly altered by large changes in fat tissue weight, so that its distribution space correlates best with lean (i.e., ideal) body weight, not total body weight.

Metabolism: Only a small percentage (16%) of a dose of digoxin is metabolized. The end metabolites, which include 3β-digoxigenin, 3-keto-digoxigenin, and their glucuronide and sulfate conjugates, are polar in nature and are postulated to be formed via hydrolysis, oxidation, and conjugation. The metabolism of digoxin is not dependent upon the cytochrome P-450 system, and digoxin is not known to induce or inhibit the cytochrome P-450 system.

Excretion: Elimination of digoxin follows first-order kinetics (that is, the quantity of digoxin eliminated at any time is proportional to the total body content). Following intravenous administration to healthy volunteers, 50% to 70% of a digoxin dose is excreted unchanged in the urine. Renal excretion of digoxin is proportional to glomerular filtration rate and is largely independent of urine flow. In healthy volunteers with normal renal function, digoxin has a half-life of 1.5 to 2.0 days. The half-life in anuric patients is prolonged to 3.5 to 5 days. Digoxin is not effectively removed from the body by dialysis, exchange transfusion, or during cardiopulmonary bypass because most of the drug is bound to tissue and does not circulate in the blood.

Special Populations: Race differences in digoxin pharmacokinetics have not been formally studied. Because digoxin is primarily eliminated as unchanged drug via the kidney and because there are no important differences in creatinine clearance among races, pharmacokinetic differences due to race are not expected.

The clearance of digoxin can be primarily correlated with renal function as indicated by creatinine clearance. In children with renal disease, digoxin must be carefully titrated based on clinical response.

Plasma digoxin concentration profiles in patients with acute hepatitis generally fell within the range of profiles in a group of healthy subjects.

Pharmacodynamic and Clinical Effects: The times to onset of pharmacologic effect and to peak effect of preparations of LANOXIN are shown in Table 2:

Table 2: Times to Onset of Pharmacologic Effect and to Peak Effect of Preparations of LANOXIN

Product	Time to Onset of Effect*	Time to Peak Effect*
LANOXIN Tablets	0.5 – 2 hours	2 – 6 hours
LANOXIN Elixir Pediatric	0.5 – 2 hours	2 – 6 hours
LANOXICAPS	0.5 – 2 hours	2 – 6 hours
LANOXIN Injection/IV	5 – 30 minutes†	1 – 4 hours

*Documented for ventricular response rate in atrial fibrillation, inotropic effects and electrocardiographic changes.
†Depending upon rate of infusion.

Hemodynamic Effects: Digoxin produces hemodynamic improvement in patients with heart failure. Short- and long-term therapy with the drug increases cardiac output and lowers pulmonary artery pressure, pulmonary capillary wedge pressure, and systemic vascular resistance. These hemodynamic effects are accompanied by an increase in the left ventricular ejection fraction and a decrease in end-systolic and end-diastolic dimensions.

Chronic Heart Failure: Two 12-week, double-blind, placebo-controlled studies enrolled 178 (RADIANCE trial) and 88 (PROVED trial) adult patients with NYHA class II or III heart failure previously treated with digoxin, a diuretic, and an ACE inhibitor (RADIANCE only) and randomized them to placebo or treatment with LANOXIN. Both trials demonstrated better preservation of exercise capacity in patients randomized to LANOXIN Tablets. Continued treatment with LANOXIN reduced the risk of developing worsening heart failure, as evidenced by heart failure-related hospitalizations and emergency care and the need for concomitant heart failure therapy. The larger study also showed treatment-related benefits in NYHA class and patients' global assessment. In the smaller trial, these trended in favor of a treatment benefit.

The Digitalis Investigation Group (DIG) main trial was a multicenter, randomized, double-blind, placebo-controlled mortality study of 6801 adult patients with heart failure and left ventricular ejection fraction ≤0.45. At randomization, 67% were NYHA class I or II, 71% had heart failure of ischemic etiology, 44% had been receiving digoxin, and most were receiving concomitant ACE inhibitor (94%) and diuretic (82%). Patients were randomized to placebo or LANOXIN Tablets, the dose of which was adjusted for the patient's age, sex, lean body weight, and serum creatinine (see DOSAGE AND ADMINISTRATION), and followed for up to 58 months (median 37 months). The median daily dose prescribed was 0.25 mg. Overall all-cause mortality was 35% with no difference between groups (95% confidence limits for relative risk of 0.91 to 1.07). LANOXIN was associated with a 25% reduction in the number of hospitalizations for heart failure, a 28% reduction in the risk of a patient having at least one hospitalization for heart failure, and a 6.5% reduction in total hospitalizations (for any cause).

Use of LANOXIN was associated with a trend to increase time to all-cause death or hospitalization. The trend was evident in subgroups of patients with mild heart failure as well as more severe disease, as shown in Table 3. Although the effect on all-cause death or hospitalization was not statistically significant, much of the apparent benefit derived from effects on mortality and hospitalization attributed to heart failure.

[See table 3 above]

Table 3: Subgroup Analyses of Mortality and Hospitalization During the First Two Years Following Randomization

	n	Risk of All-Cause Mortality or All-Cause Hospitalization* Placebo	LANOXIN	Relative risk†	Risk of HF-Related Mortality or HF-Related Hospitalization* Placebo	LANOXIN	Relative risk†
All patients (EF ≤0.45)	6801	604	593	0.94 (0.88–1.00)	294	217	0.69 (0.63–0.76)
NYHA I/II	4571	549	541	0.96 (0.89–1.04)	242	178	0.70 (0.62–0.80)
EF 0.25–0.45	4543	568	571	0.99 (0.91–1.07)	244	190	0.74 (0.66–0.84)
CTR ≤0.55	4455	561	563	0.98 (0.91–1.06)	239	180	0.71 (0.63–0.81)
NYHA III/IV	2224	719	696	0.88 (0.80–0.97)	402	295	0.65 (0.57–0.75)
EF <0.25	2258	677	637	0.84 (0.76–0.93)	394	270	0.61 (0.53–0.71)
CTR >0.55	2346	687	650	0.85 (0.77–0.94)	398	287	0.65 (0.57–0.75)
EF >0.45‡	987	571	585	1.04 (0.88–1.23)	179	136	0.72 (0.53–0.99)

*Number of patients with an event during the first 2 years per 1000 randomized patients.
†Relative risk (95% confidence interval).
‡DIG Ancillary Study.

In situations where there is no statistically significant benefit of treatment evident from a trial's primary endpoint, results pertaining to a secondary endpoint should be interpreted cautiously.

Chronic Atrial Fibrillation: In adult patients with chronic atrial fibrillation, digoxin slows rapid ventricular response rate in a linear dose-response fashion from 0.25 to 0.75 mg/day. Digoxin should not be used for the treatment of multifocal atrial tachycardia.

INDICATIONS AND USAGE

Heart Failure: LANOXIN is indicated for the treatment of mild to moderate heart failure. LANOXIN increases left ventricular ejection fraction and improves heart failure symptoms as evidenced by exercise capacity and heart failure-related hospitalizations and emergency care, while having no effect on mortality. Where possible, LANOXIN should be used with a diuretic and an angiotensin-converting enzyme inhibitor, but an optimal order for starting these three drugs cannot be specified.

Atrial Fibrillation: LANOXIN is indicated for the control of ventricular response rate in patients with chronic atrial fibrillation.

CONTRAINDICATIONS

Digitalis glycosides are contraindicated in patients with ventricular fibrillation or in patients with a known hypersensitivity to digoxin. A hypersensitivity reaction to other digitalis preparations usually constitutes a contraindication to digoxin.

WARNINGS

Sinus Node Disease and AV Block: Because digoxin slows sinoatrial and AV conduction, the drug commonly prolongs the PR interval. The drug may cause severe sinus bradycardia or sinoatrial block in patients with pre-existing sinus node disease and may cause advanced or complete heart block in patients with pre-existing incomplete AV block. In such patients consideration should be given to the insertion of a pacemaker before treatment with digoxin.

Accessory AV Pathway (Wolff-Parkinson-White Syndrome): After intravenous digoxin therapy, some patients with paroxysmal atrial fibrillation or flutter and a coexisting accessory AV pathway have developed increased antegrade conduction across the accessory pathway bypassing the AV node, leading to a very rapid ventricular response or ventricular fibrillation. Unless conduction down the accessory pathway has been blocked (either pharmacologically or by surgery), digoxin should not be used in such patients. The treatment of paroxysmal supraventricular tachycardia in such patients is usually direct-current cardioversion.

Use in Patients with Preserved Left Ventricular Systolic Function: Patients with certain disorders involving heart failure associated with preserved left ventricular ejection fraction may be particularly susceptible to toxicity of the drug. Such disorders include restrictive cardiomyopathy, constrictive pericarditis, amyloid heart disease, and acute cor pulmonale. Patients with idiopathic hypertrophic subaortic stenosis may have worsening of the outflow obstruction due to the inotropic effects of digoxin.

PRECAUTIONS

Use in Patients with Impaired Renal Function: Digoxin is primarily excreted by the kidneys; therefore, patients with impaired renal function require smaller than usual maintenance doses of digoxin (see DOSAGE AND ADMINISTRATION). Because of the prolonged elimination half-life, a longer period of time is required to achieve an initial or new steady-state serum concentration in patients with renal impairment than in patients with normal renal function. If appropriate care is not taken to reduce the dose of digoxin, such patients are at high risk for toxicity, and toxic effects will last longer in such patients than in patients with normal renal function.

Use in Patients with Electrolyte Disorders: In patients with hypokalemia or hypomagnesemia, toxicity may occur despite serum digoxin concentrations below 2.0 ng/mL, because potassium or magnesium depletion sensitizes the myocardium to digoxin. Therefore, it is desirable to maintain normal serum potassium and magnesium concentrations in patients being treated with digoxin. Deficiencies of these electrolytes may result from malnutrition, diarrhea, or prolonged vomiting, as well as the use of the following drugs or procedures: diuretics, amphotericin B, corticosteroids, antacids, dialysis, and mechanical suction of gastrointestinal secretions.

Hypercalcemia from any cause predisposes the patient to digitalis toxicity. Calcium, particularly when administered rapidly by the intravenous route, may produce serious arrhythmias in digitalized patients. On the other hand, hypocalcemia can nullify the effects of digoxin in humans; thus, digoxin may be ineffective until serum calcium is restored to normal. These interactions are related to the fact that digoxin affects contractility and excitability of the heart in a manner similar to that of calcium.

Use in Thyroid Disorders and Hypermetabolic States: Hypothyroidism may reduce the requirements for digoxin. Heart failure and/or atrial arrhythmias resulting from hypermetabolic or hyperdynamic states (e.g., hyperthyroidism, hypoxia, or arteriovenous shunt) are best treated by addressing the underlying condition. Atrial arrhythmias associated with hypermetabolic states are particularly resistant to digoxin treatment. Care must be taken to avoid toxicity if digoxin is used.

Use in Patients with Acute Myocardial Infarction: Digoxin should be used with caution in patients with acute myocardial infarction. The use of inotropic drugs in some patients in this setting may result in undesirable increases in myocardial oxygen demand and ischemia.

Use During Electrical Cardioversion: It may be desirable to reduce the dose of digoxin for 1 to 2 days prior to electrical cardioversion of atrial fibrillation to avoid the induction of ventricular arrhythmias, but physicians must consider the consequences of increasing the ventricular response if digoxin is withdrawn. If digitalis toxicity is suspected, elective cardioversion should be delayed. If it is not prudent to delay cardioversion, the lowest possible energy level should be selected to avoid provoking ventricular arrhythmias.

Laboratory Test Monitoring: Patients receiving digoxin should have their serum electrolytes and renal function (serum creatinine concentrations) assessed periodically; the frequency of assessments will depend on the clinical setting. For discussion of serum digoxin concentrations, see DOSAGE AND ADMINISTRATION.

Drug Interactions: Potassium-depleting *diuretics* are a major contributing factor to digitalis toxicity. *Calcium*, particularly if administered rapidly by the intravenous route, may produce serious arrhythmias in digitalized patients. *Quinidine, verapamil, amiodarone, propafenone, indomethacin, itraconazole, alprazolam*, and *spironolactone* raise the serum digoxin concentration due to a reduction in clearance and/or in volume of distribution of the drug, with the implication that digitalis intoxication may result. *Erythromycin* and *clarithromycin* (and possibly other *macrolide antibiotics*) and *tetracycline* may increase digoxin absorption in patients who inactivate digoxin by bacterial metabolism in the lower intestine, so that digitalis intoxication may result (see CLINICAL PHARMACOLOGY: Absorption). *Propantheline* and *diphenoxylate*, by decreasing gut motility, may increase digoxin absorption. *Antacids, kaolin-pectin, sulfasalazine, neomycin, cholestyramine, certain anticancer drugs*, and *metoclopramide* may interfere with intestinal digoxin absorption, resulting in unexpectedly low serum concentrations. *Rifampin* may decrease serum digoxin concentration, especially in patients with renal dysfunction, by increasing the non-renal clearance of digoxin. There have been inconsistent reports regarding the effects of other drugs [e.g., *quinine, penicillamine*] on serum digoxin concentration. *Thyroid* administration to a digitalized, hypothyroid patient may increase the dose requirement of digoxin. Concomitant use of digoxin and *sympathomimetics* increases the risk of cardiac arrhythmias. *Succinylcholine* may cause a sudden extrusion of potassium from muscle cells, and may thereby cause arrhythmias in digitalized patients. Although beta-adrenergic blockers or calcium channel blockers and digoxin may be useful in combination to control atrial fibrillation, their additive effects on AV node conduction can result in advanced or complete heart block.

Due to the considerable variability of these interactions, the dosage of digoxin should be individualized when patients receive these medications concurrently. Furthermore, caution should be exercised when combining digoxin with any drug that may cause a significant deterioration in renal function, since a decline in glomerular filtration or tubular secretion may impair the excretion of digoxin.

Drug/Laboratory Test Interactions: The use of therapeutic doses of digoxin may cause prolongation of the PR interval and depression of the ST segment on the electrocardiogram. Digoxin may produce false positive ST-T changes on the electrocardiogram during exercise testing. These electrophysiologic effects reflect an expected effect of the drug and are not indicative of toxicity.

Carcinogenesis, Mutagenesis, Impairment of Fertility: There have been no long-term studies performed in animals to evaluate carcinogenic potential, nor have studies been conducted to assess the mutagenic potential of digoxin or its potential to affect fertility.

Pregnancy: *Teratogenic Effects:* Pregnancy Category C. Animal reproduction studies have not been conducted with digoxin. It is also not known whether digoxin can cause fetal harm when administered to a pregnant woman or can affect reproduction capacity. Digoxin should be given to a pregnant woman only if clearly needed.

Nursing Mothers: Studies have shown that digoxin concentrations in the mother's serum and milk are similar. However, the estimated exposure of a nursing infant to digoxin via breast feeding will be far below the usual infant maintenance dose. Therefore, this amount should have no pharmacologic effect upon the infant. Nevertheless, caution should be exercised when digoxin is administered to a nursing woman.

Pediatric Use: Newborn infants display considerable variability in their tolerance to digoxin. Premature and immature infants are particularly sensitive to the effects of digoxin, and the dosage of the drug must not only be reduced but must be individualized according to their degree of maturity. Digitalis glycosides can cause poisoning in children due to accidental ingestion.

Geriatric Use: The majority of clinical experience gained with digoxin has been in the elderly population. This experience has not identified differences in response or adverse effects between the elderly and younger patients. However, this drug is known to be substantially excreted by the kidney, and the risk of toxic reactions to this drug may be greater in patients with impaired renal function. Because elderly patients are more likely to have decreased renal function, care should be taken in dose selection, which should be based on renal function, and it may be useful to monitor renal function.

ADVERSE REACTIONS

In general, the adverse reactions of digoxin are dose-dependent and occur at doses higher than those needed to achieve a therapeutic effect. Hence, adverse reactions are less common when digoxin is used within the recommended dose range or therapeutic serum concentration range and when there is careful attention to concurrent medications and conditions.

Because some patients may be particularly susceptible to side effects with digoxin, the dosage of the drug should always be selected carefully and adjusted as the clinical condition of the patient warrants. In the past, when high doses of digoxin were used and little attention was paid to clinical status or concurrent medications, adverse reactions to digoxin were more frequent and severe. Cardiac adverse reactions accounted for about one-half, gastrointestinal disturbances for about one-fourth, and CNS and other toxicity for about one-fourth of these adverse reactions. However, available evidence suggests that the incidence and severity of digoxin toxicity has decreased substantially in recent years. In recent controlled clinical trials, in patients with predominantly mild to moderate heart failure, the incidence of adverse experiences was comparable in patients taking digoxin and in those taking placebo. In a large mortality trial, the incidence of hospitalization for suspected digoxin toxicity was 2% in patients taking LANOXIN Tablets compared to 0.9% in patients taking placebo. In this trial, the most common manifestations of digoxin toxicity included gastrointestinal and cardiac disturbances; CNS manifestations were less common.

Adults: *Cardiac:* Therapeutic doses of digoxin may cause heart block in patients with pre-existing sinoatrial or AV conduction disorders; heart block can be avoided by adjusting the dose of digoxin. Prophylactic use of a cardiac pacemaker may be considered if the risk of heart block is considered unacceptable. High doses of digoxin may produce a variety of rhythm disturbances, such as first-degree, second-degree (Wenckebach), or third-degree heart block (including asystole); atrial tachycardia with block; AV dissociation; accelerated junctional (nodal) rhythm; unifocal or multiform ventricular premature contractions (especially bigeminy or trigeminy); ventricular tachycardia; and ventricular fibrillation. Digoxin produces PR prolongation and ST segment depression which should not by themselves be considered digoxin toxicity. Cardiac toxicity can also occur at therapeutic doses in patients who have conditions which may alter their sensitivity to digoxin (see WARNINGS and PRECAUTIONS).

Gastrointestinal: Digoxin may cause anorexia, nausea, vomiting, and diarrhea. Rarely, the use of digoxin has been associated with abdominal pain, intestinal ischemia, and hemorrhagic necrosis of the intestines.

CNS: Digoxin can produce visual disturbances (blurred or yellow vision), headache, weakness, dizziness, apathy, confusion, and mental disturbances (such as anxiety, depression, delirium, and hallucination).

Other: Gynecomastia has been occasionally observed following the prolonged use of digoxin. Thrombocytopenia and maculopapular rash and other skin reactions have been rarely observed.

Table 4 summarizes the incidence of those adverse experiences listed above for patients treated with LANOXIN Tablets or placebo from two randomized, double-blind, placebo-controlled withdrawal trials. Patients in these trials were also receiving diuretics with or without angiotensin-converting enzyme inhibitors. These patients had been stable on digoxin, and were randomized to digoxin or placebo. The results shown in Table 4 reflect the experience in patients following dosage titration with the use of serum digoxin concentrations and careful follow-up. These adverse experiences are consistent with results from a large, placebo-controlled mortality trial (DIG trial) wherein over half the patients were not receiving digoxin prior to enrollment.

Table 4: Adverse Experiences In Two Parallel, Double-Blind, Placebo-Controlled Withdrawal Trials (Number of Patients Reporting)

Adverse Experience	Digoxin Patients (n = 123)	Placebo Patients (n = 125)
Cardiac		
Palpitation	1	4
Ventricular extrasystole	1	1
Tachycardia	2	1
Heart arrest	1	1
Gastrointestinal		
Anorexia	1	4
Nausea	4	2
Vomiting	2	1
Diarrhea	4	1
Abdominal pain	0	6
CNS		
Headache	4	4
Dizziness	6	5
Mental disturbances	5	1
Other		
Rash	2	1
Death	4	3

Infants and Children: The side effects of digoxin in infants and children differ from those seen in adults in several respects. Although digoxin may produce anorexia, nausea, vomiting, diarrhea, and CNS disturbances in young patients, these are rarely the initial symptoms of overdosage. Rather, the earliest and most frequent manifestation of excessive dosing with digoxin in infants and children is the appearance of cardiac arrhythmias, including sinus bradycardia. In children, the use of digoxin may produce any arrhythmia. The most common are conduction disturbances or supraventricular tachyarrhythmias, such as atrial tachycardia (with or without block) and junctional (nodal) tachycardia. Ventricular arrhythmias are less common. Sinus bradycardia may be a sign of impending digoxin intoxication, especially in infants, even in the absence of first-degree heart block. Any arrhythmia or alteration in cardiac conduction that develops in a child taking digoxin should be assumed to be caused by digoxin, until further evaluation proves otherwise.

OVERDOSAGE

Treatment of Adverse Reactions Produced by Overdosage: Digoxin should be temporarily discontinued until the adverse reaction resolves. Every effort should also be made to correct factors that may contribute to the adverse reaction (such as electrolyte disturbances or concurrent medications). Once the adverse reaction has resolved, therapy with digoxin may be reinstituted, following a careful reassessment of dose.

Withdrawal of digoxin may be all that is required to treat the adverse reaction. However, when the primary manifestation of digoxin overdosage is a cardiac arrhythmia, additional therapy may be needed.

If the rhythm disturbance is a symptomatic bradyarrhythmia or heart block, consideration should be given to the reversal of toxicity with DIGIBIND® [Digoxin Immune Fab (Ovine)] (see below), the use of atropine, or the insertion of a temporary cardiac pacemaker. However, asymptomatic bradycardia or heart block related to digoxin may require only temporary withdrawal of the drug and cardiac monitoring of the patient.

If the rhythm disturbance is a ventricular arrhythmia, consideration should be given to the correction of electrolyte disorders, particularly if hypokalemia (see below) or hypomagnesemia is present. DIGIBIND is a specific antidote for digoxin and may be used to reverse potentially life-threatening ventricular arrhythmias due to digoxin overdosage.

Continued on next page

Product information on these pages is effective as of August 2004. Further information is available at: GlaxoSmithKline, PO Box 13398, Research Triangle Park, NC 27709. 1-888-825-5249. Corporate Web Site: www.gsk.com

Lanoxin Elixir Pediatric—Cont.

Administration of Potassium: Every effort should be made to maintain the serum potassium concentration between 4.0 and 5.5 mmol/L. Potassium is usually administered orally, but when correction of the arrhythmia is urgent and the serum potassium concentration is low, potassium may be administered cautiously by the intravenous route. The electrocardiogram should be monitored for any evidence of potassium toxicity (e.g., peaking of T waves) and to observe the effect on the arrhythmia. Potassium salts may be dangerous in patients who manifest bradycardia or heart block due to digoxin (unless primarily related to supraventricular tachycardia) and in the setting of massive digitalis overdosage (see Massive Digitalis Overdosage subsection).

Massive Digitalis Overdosage: Manifestations of life-threatening toxicity include ventricular tachycardia or ventricular fibrillation, or progressive bradyarrhythmias, or heart block. The administration of more than 10 mg of digoxin in a previously healthy adult or more than 4 mg in a previously healthy child, or a steady-state serum concentration greater than 10 ng/mL often results in cardiac arrest.

DIGIBIND should be used to reverse the toxic effects of ingestion of a massive overdose. The decision to administer DIGIBIND to a patient who has ingested a massive dose of digoxin but who has not yet manifested life-threatening toxicity should depend on the likelihood that life-threatening toxicity will occur (see above).

Patients with massive digitalis ingestion should receive large doses of activated charcoal to prevent absorption and bind digoxin in the gut during enteroenteric recirculation. Emesis or gastric lavage may be indicated especially if ingestion has occurred within 30 minutes of the patient's presentation at the hospital. Emesis should not be induced in patients who are obtunded. If a patient presents more than 2 hours after ingestion or already has toxic manifestations, it may be unsafe to induce vomiting or attempt passage of a gastric tube, because such maneuvers may induce an acute vagal episode that can worsen digitalis-related arrhythmias.

Severe digitalis intoxication can cause a massive shift of potassium from inside to outside the cell, leading to life-threatening hyperkalemia. The administration of potassium supplements in the setting of massive intoxication may be hazardous and should be avoided. Hyperkalemia caused by massive digitalis toxicity is best treated with DIGIBIND; initial treatment with glucose and insulin may also be required if hyperkalemia itself is acutely life-threatening.

DOSAGE AND ADMINISTRATION

General: Recommended dosages of digoxin may require considerable modification because of individual sensitivity of the patient to the drug, the presence of associated conditions, or the use of concurrent medications. In selecting a dose of digoxin, the following factors must be considered:

1. The body weight of the patient. Doses should be calculated based upon lean (i.e., ideal) body weight.
2. The patient's renal function, preferably evaluated on the basis of estimated creatinine clearance.
3. The patient's age. Infants and children require different doses of digoxin than adults. Also, advanced age may be indicative of diminished renal function even in patients with normal serum creatinine concentration (i.e., below 1.5 mg/dL).
4. Concomitant disease states, concurrent medications, or other factors likely to alter the pharmacokinetic or pharmacodynamic profile of digoxin (see PRECAUTIONS).

Serum Digoxin Concentrations: In general, the dose of digoxin used should be determined on clinical grounds. However, measurement of serum digoxin concentrations can be helpful to the clinician in determining the adequacy of digoxin therapy and in assigning certain probabilities to the likelihood of digoxin intoxication. About two-thirds of adults considered adequately digitalized (without evidence of toxicity) have serum digoxin concentrations ranging from 0.8 to 2.0 ng/mL. However, digoxin may produce clinical benefits even at serum concentrations below this range. About two-thirds of adult patients with clinical toxicity have serum digoxin concentrations greater than 2.0 ng/mL. However, since one-third of patients with clinical toxicity have concentrations less than 2.0 ng/mL, values below 2.0 ng/mL do not rule out the possibility that a certain sign or symptom is related to digoxin therapy. Rarely, there are patients who are unable to tolerate digoxin at serum concentrations below 0.8 ng/mL. Consequently, the serum concentration of digoxin should always be interpreted in the overall clinical context, and an isolated measurement should not be used alone as the basis for increasing or decreasing the dose of the drug.

To allow adequate time for equilibration of digoxin between serum and tissue, sampling of serum concentrations should be done just before the next scheduled dose of the drug. If this is not possible, sampling should be done at least 6 to 8 hours after the last dose, regardless of the route of administration or the formulation used. On a once-daily dosing schedule, the concentration of digoxin will be 10% to 25% lower when sampled at 24 versus 8 hours, depending upon the patient's renal function. On a twice-daily dosing schedule, there will be only minor differences in serum digoxin concentrations whether sampling is done at 8 or 12 hours after a dose.

If a discrepancy exists between the reported serum concentration and the observed clinical response, the clinician should consider the following possibilities:

1. Analytical problems in the assay procedure.
2. Inappropriate serum sampling time.
3. Administration of a digitalis glycoside other than digoxin.
4. Conditions (described in WARNINGS and PRECAUTIONS) causing an alteration in the sensitivity of the patient to digoxin.
5. Serum digoxin concentration may decrease acutely during periods of exercise without any associated change in clinical efficacy due to increased binding of digoxin to skeletal muscle.

Heart Failure: Adults: See the LANOXIN Tablets or LANOXICAPS Capsules package insert for specific recommendations.

Infants and Children: In general, divided daily dosing is recommended for infants and young children (under age 10). In the newborn period, renal clearance of digoxin is diminished and suitable dosage adjustments must be observed. This is especially pronounced in the premature infant. Beyond the immediate newborn period, children generally require proportionally larger doses than adults on the basis of body weight or body surface area. Children over 10 years of age require adult dosages in proportion to their body weight. Some researchers have suggested that infants and young children tolerate slightly higher serum concentrations than do adults.

Digitalization may be accomplished by either of two general approaches that vary in dosage and frequency of administration, but reach the same endpoint in terms of total amount of digoxin accumulated in the body.

1. If rapid digitalization is considered medically appropriate, it may be achieved by administering a loading dose based upon projected peak digoxin body stores. Maintenance dose can be calculated as a percentage of the loading dose.
2. More gradual digitalization may be obtained by beginning an appropriate maintenance dose, thus allowing digoxin body stores to accumulate slowly. Steady-state serum digoxin concentrations will be achieved in approximately five half-lives of the drug for the individual patient. Depending upon the patient's renal function, this will take between 1 and 3 weeks.

Rapid Digitalization with a Loading Dose: LANOXIN Injection Pediatric can be used to achieve rapid digitalization, with conversion to an oral formulation of LANOXIN for maintenance therapy. If patients are switched from intravenous to oral digoxin formulations, allowances must be made for differences in bioavailability when calculating maintenance dosages (see Table 1 in CLINICAL PHARMACOLOGY: Pharmacokinetics and dosing Table 5 below).

Peak digoxin body stores of 8 to 12 mcg/kg should provide therapeutic effect with minimum risk of toxicity in most patients with heart failure and normal sinus rhythm. Because of altered digoxin distribution and elimination, projected peak body stores for patients with renal insufficiency should be conservative (i.e., 6 to 10 mcg/kg [see PRECAUTIONS]).

Digitalizing and daily maintenance doses for each age group are given in Table 5 and should provide therapeutic effect with minimum risk of toxicity in most patients with heart failure and normal sinus rhythm. These recommendations assume the presence of normal renal function.

The loading dose should be administered in several portions, with roughly half the total given as the first dose. Additional fractions of this planned total dose may be given at 6- to 8-hour intervals, **with careful assessment of clinical response before each additional dose.** If the patient's clinical response necessitates a change from the calculated loading dose of digoxin, then calculation of the maintenance dose should be based upon the amount actually given.

[See table 5 below]

In children with renal disease, digoxin dosing must be carefully titrated based upon desired clinical response.

Gradual Digitalization With A Maintenance Dose: More gradual digitalization can also be accomplished by beginning an appropriate maintenance dose. The range of percentages provided in Table 5 can be used in calculating this dose for patients with normal renal function.

It cannot be overemphasized that these pediatric dosage guidelines are based upon average patient response and substantial individual variation can be expected. Accordingly, ultimate dosage selection must be based upon clinical assessment of the patient.

Atrial Fibrillation: Peak digoxin body stores larger than the 8 to 12 mcg/kg required for most patients with heart failure and normal sinus rhythm have been used for control of ventricular rate in patients with atrial fibrillation. Doses of digoxin used for the treatment of chronic atrial fibrillation should be titrated to the minimum dose that achieves the desired ventricular rate control without causing undesirable side effects. Data are not available to establish the appropriate resting or exercise target rates that should be achieved.

Dosage Adjustment When Changing Preparations: The difference in bioavailability between LANOXIN Injection or LANOXICAPS and LANOXIN Elixir Pediatric or LANOXIN Tablets must be considered when changing patients from one dosage form to another.

Doses of 100 mcg (0.1 mg) and 200 mcg (0.2 mg) of LANOXICAPS are approximately equivalent to 125-mcg (0.125-mg) and 250-mcg (0.25-mg) doses of LANOXIN Tablets and Elixir Pediatric, respectively (see Table 1 in CLINICAL PHARMACOLOGY: Pharmacokinetics).

HOW SUPPLIED

LANOXIN (digoxin) Elixir Pediatric, 50 mcg (0.05 mg) per mL; Bottle of 60 mL with calibrated dropper (NDC 0173-0264-27).

Store at 25°C (77°F); excursions permitted to 15 to 30°C (59 to 86°F) [see USP Controlled Room Temperature] and protect from light.

GlaxoSmithKline, Research Triangle Park, NC 27709

September 2001/RL-996

Shown in Product Identification Guide, page 316

LANOXIN® ℞

[lă-nŏx'ĭn]

(digoxin)

Injection

500 mcg (0.5 mg) in 2 mL (250 mcg [0.25 mg] per mL)

DESCRIPTION

LANOXIN (digoxin) is one of the cardiac (or digitalis) glycosides, a closely related group of drugs having in common specific effects on the myocardium. These drugs are found in a number of plants. Digoxin is extracted from the leaves of *Digitalis lanata*. The term "digitalis" is used to designate the whole group of glycosides. The glycosides are composed of two portions: a sugar and a cardenolide (hence "glycosides").

Digoxin is described chemically as (3β,5β,12β)-3-[(*O*-2,6-dideoxy-β-*D*-*ribo*-hexopyranosyl-(1→4)-*O*-2,6-dideoxy-β-*D*-*ribo*-hexopyranosyl-(1→4)-2,6-dideoxy-β-*D*-*ribo*-hexopyranosyl)oxy]-12,14-dihydroxy-card-20(22)-enolide. Its molecular formula is $C_{41}H_{64}O_{14}$, its molecular weight is 780.95.

Digoxin exists as odorless white crystals that melt with decomposition above 230°C. The drug is practically insoluble in water and in ether; slightly soluble in diluted (50%) alcohol and in chloroform; and freely soluble in pyridine.

LANOXIN Injection is a sterile solution of digoxin for intravenous or intramuscular injection. The vehicle contains 40% propylene glycol and 10% alcohol. The injection is buffered to a pH of 6.8 to 7.2 with 0.17% dibasic sodium phosphate and 0.08% anhydrous citric acid. Each 2-mL ampul contains 500 mcg (0.5 mg) digoxin (250 mcg [0.25 mg] per mL). Dilution is not required.

CLINICAL PHARMACOLOGY

Mechanism of Action: Digoxin inhibits sodium-potassium ATPase, an enzyme that regulates the quantity of sodium and potassium inside cells. Inhibition of the enzyme leads to an increase in the intracellular concentration of sodium and thus (by stimulation of sodium-calcium exchange) an increase in the intracellular concentration of calcium. The beneficial effects of digoxin result from direct actions on cardiac muscle, as well as indirect actions on the cardiovascular system mediated by effects on the autonomic nervous system. The autonomic effects include: (1) a vagomimetic action, which is responsible for the effects of digoxin on the sinoatrial and atrioventricular (AV) nodes; and (2) baroreceptor sensitization, which results in increased afferent inhibitory activity and reduced activity of the sympathetic nervous system and renin-angiotensin system for any given increment in mean arterial pressure. The pharmacologic consequences of these direct and indirect effects are: (1) an increase in the force and velocity of myocardial systolic con-

Table 5: Usual Digitalizing and Maintenance Dosages for LANOXIN Elixir Pediatric in Children with Normal Renal Function Based on Lean Body Weight

Age	Oral Digitalizing* Dose (mcg/kg)	Daily Maintenance Dose† (mcg/kg)
Premature	20 to 30	20% to 30% of *oral* digitalizing dose‡
Full-Term	25 to 35	
1 to 24 Months	35 to 60	
2 to 5 Years	30 to 40	25% to 35% of *oral* digitalizing dose‡
5 to 10 Years	20 to 35	
Over 10 Years	10 to 15	

*IV digitalizing doses are 80% of oral digitalizing doses.
†Divided daily dosing is recommended for children under 10 years of age.
‡Projected or actual digitalizing dose providing clinical response.

traction (positive inotropic action); (2) a decrease in the degree of activation of the sympathetic nervous system and renin-angiotensin system (neurohormonal deactivating effect); and (3) slowing of the heart rate and decreased conduction velocity through the AV node (vagomimetic effect). The effects of digoxin in heart failure are mediated by its positive inotropic and neurohormonal deactivating effects, whereas the effects of the drug in atrial arrhythmias are related to its vagomimetic actions. In high doses, digoxin increases sympathetic outflow from the central nervous system (CNS). This increase in sympathetic activity may be an important factor in digitalis toxicity.

Pharmacokinetics: Note: the following data are from studies performed in adults, unless otherwise stated.

Absorption: Comparisons of the systemic availability and equivalent doses for preparations of LANOXIN are shown in Table 1.

[See table 1 at right]

Distribution: Following drug administration, a 6- to 8-hour tissue distribution phase is observed. This is followed by a much more gradual decline in the serum concentration of the drug, which is dependent on the elimination of digoxin from the body. The peak height and slope of the early portion (absorption/distribution phases) of the serum concentration-time curve are dependent upon the route of administration and the absorption characteristics of the formulation. Clinical evidence indicates that the early high serum concentrations do not reflect the concentration of digoxin at its site of action, but that with chronic use, the steady-state post-distribution serum concentrations are in equilibrium with tissue concentrations and correlate with pharmacologic effects. In individual patients, these post-distribution serum concentrations may be useful in evaluating therapeutic and toxic effects (see DOSAGE AND ADMINISTRATION: Serum Digoxin Concentrations).

Digoxin is concentrated in tissues and therefore has a large apparent volume of distribution. Digoxin crosses both the blood-brain barrier and the placenta. At delivery, the serum digoxin concentration in the newborn is similar to the serum concentration in the mother. Approximately 25% of digoxin in the plasma is bound to protein. Serum digoxin concentrations are not significantly altered by large changes in fat tissue weight, so that its distribution space correlates best with lean (i.e., ideal) body weight, not total body weight.

Metabolism: Only a small percentage (16%) of a dose of digoxin is metabolized. The end metabolites, which include 3 β-digoxigenin, 3-keto-digoxigenin, and their glucuronide and sulfate conjugates, are polar in nature and are postulated to be formed via hydrolysis, oxidation, and conjugation. The metabolism of digoxin is not dependent upon the cytochrome P-450 system, and digoxin is not known to induce or inhibit the cytochrome P-450 system.

Excretion: Elimination of digoxin follows first-order kinetics (that is, the quantity of digoxin eliminated at any time is proportional to the total body content). Following intravenous administration to healthy volunteers, 50% to 70% of a digoxin dose is excreted unchanged in the urine. Renal excretion of digoxin is proportional to glomerular filtration rate and is largely independent of urine flow. In healthy volunteers with normal renal function, digoxin has a half-life of 1.5 to 2.0 days. The half-life in anuric patients is prolonged to 3.5 to 5 days. Digoxin is not effectively removed from the body by dialysis, exchange transfusion, or during cardiopulmonary bypass because most of the drug is bound to tissue and does not circulate in the blood.

Special Populations: Race differences in digoxin pharmacokinetics have not been formally studied. Because digoxin is primarily eliminated as unchanged drug via the kidney and because there are no important differences in creatinine clearance among races, pharmacokinetic differences due to race are not expected.

The clearance of digoxin can be primarily correlated with renal function as indicated by creatinine clearance. The Cockcroft and Gault formula for estimation of creatinine clearance includes age, body weight, and gender. Table 5 that provides the usual daily maintenance dose requirements of LANOXIN Tablets based on creatinine clearance (per 70 kg) is presented in the DOSAGE AND ADMINISTRATION section.

Plasma digoxin concentration profiles in patients with acute hepatitis generally fell within the range of profiles in a group of healthy subjects.

Pharmacodynamic and Clinical Effects: The times to onset of pharmacologic effect and to peak effect of preparations of LANOXIN are shown in Table 2.

[See table 2 above]

Hemodynamic Effects: Digoxin produces hemodynamic improvement in patients with heart failure. Short- and long-term therapy with the drug increases cardiac output and lowers pulmonary artery pressure, pulmonary capillary wedge pressure, and systemic vascular resistance. These hemodynamic effects are accompanied by an increase in the left ventricular ejection fraction and a decrease in end-systolic and end-diastolic dimensions.

Chronic Heart Failure: Two 12-week, double-blind, placebo-controlled studies enrolled 178 (RADIANCE trial) and 88 (PROVED trial) patients with NYHA class II or III heart failure previously treated with oral digoxin, a diuretic, and an ACE inhibitor (RADIANCE only) and randomized them to placebo or treatment with LANOXIN Tablets. Both trials demonstrated better preservation of exercise capacity in patients randomized to LANOXIN. Continued treatment with LANOXIN reduced the risk of developing worsening heart

Table 1. Comparisons of the Systemic Availability and Equivalent Doses for Preparations of LANOXIN

Product	Absolute Bioavailability	Equivalent Doses (mcg)* Among Dosage Forms			
LANOXIN Tablets	60 - 80%	62.5	125	250	500
LANOXIN Elixir Pediatric	70 - 85%	62.5	125	250	500
LANOXICAPS®	90 - 100%	50	100	200	400
LANOXIN Injection/IV	100%	50	100	200	400

*For example, 125 mcg LANOXIN Tablets equivalent to 125 mcg LANOXIN Elixir Pediatric equivalent to 100 mcg LANOXICAPS equivalent to 100 mcg LANOXIN Injection/IV.

Table 2. Times to Onset of Pharmacologic Effect and to Peak Effect of Preparations of LANOXIN

Product	Time to Onset of Effect*	Time to Peak Effect*
LANOXIN Tablets	0.5 - 2 hours	2 - 6 hours
LANOXIN Elixir Pediatric	0.5 - 2 hours	2 - 6 hours
LANOXICAPS	0.5 - 2 hours	2 - 6 hours
LANOXIN Injection/IV	5 - 30 minutes†	1 - 4 hours

*Documented for ventricular response rate in atrial fibrillation, inotropic effects and electrocardiographic changes.

†Depending upon rate of infusion.

failure, as evidenced by heart failure-related hospitalizations and emergency care and the need for concomitant heart failure therapy. The larger study also showed treatment-related benefits in NYHA class and patients' global assessment. In the smaller trial, these trended in favor of a treatment benefit.

The Digitalis Investigation Group (DIG) main trial was a multicenter, randomized, double-blind, placebo-controlled mortality study of 6,801 patients with heart failure and left ventricular ejection fraction ≤0.45. At randomization, 67% were NYHA class I or II, 71% had heart failure of ischemic etiology, 44% had been receiving digoxin, and most were receiving concomitant ACE inhibitor (94%) and diuretic (82%). Patients were randomized to placebo or LANOXIN Tablets, the dose of which was adjusted for the patient's age, sex, lean body weight, and serum creatinine (see DOSAGE AND ADMINISTRATION), and followed for up to 58 months (median 37 months). The median daily dose prescribed was 0.25 mg. Overall all-cause mortality was 35% with no difference between groups (95% confidence limits for relative risk of 0.91 to 1.07). LANOXIN was associated with a 25% reduction in the number of hospitalizations for heart failure, a 28% reduction in the risk of a patient having at least one hospitalization for heart failure, and a 6.5% reduction in total hospitalizations (for any cause).

Use of LANOXIN was associated with a trend to increase time to all-cause death or hospitalization. The trend was evident in subgroups of patients with mild heart failure as well as more severe disease, as shown in Table 3. Although the effect on all-cause death or hospitalization was not statistically significant, much of the apparent benefit derived from effects on mortality and hospitalization attributed to heart failure.

[See table 3 at bottom of next page]

In situations where there is no statistically significant benefit of treatment evident from a trial's primary endpoint, results pertaining to a secondary endpoint should be interpreted cautiously.

Chronic Atrial Fibrillation: In patients with chronic atrial fibrillation, digoxin slows rapid ventricular response rate in a linear dose-response fashion from 0.25 to 0.75 mg/day. Digoxin should not be used for the treatment of multifocal atrial tachycardia.

INDICATIONS AND USAGE

Heart Failure: LANOXIN is indicated for the treatment of mild to moderate heart failure. LANOXIN increases left ventricular ejection fraction and improves heart failure symptoms as evidenced by exercise capacity and heart failure-related hospitalizations and emergency care, while having no effect on mortality. Where possible, LANOXIN should be used with a diuretic and an angiotensin-converting enzyme inhibitor, but an optimal order for starting these three drugs cannot be specified.

Atrial Fibrillation: LANOXIN is indicated for the control of ventricular response rate in patients with chronic atrial fibrillation.

CONTRAINDICATIONS

Digitalis glycosides are contraindicated in patients with ventricular fibrillation or in patients with a known hypersensitivity to digoxin. A hypersensitivity reaction to other digitalis preparations usually constitutes a contraindication to digoxin.

WARNINGS

Sinus Node Disease and AV Block: Because digoxin slows sinoatrial and AV conduction, the drug commonly prolongs the PR interval. The drug may cause severe sinus bradycardia or sinoatrial block in patients with pre-existing sinus node disease and may cause advanced or complete heart block in patients with pre-existing incomplete AV block. In such patients consideration should be given to the insertion of a pacemaker before treatment with digoxin.

Accessory AV Pathway (Wolff-Parkinson-White Syndrome): After intravenous digoxin therapy, some patients with paroxysmal atrial fibrillation or flutter and a coexisting accessory AV pathway have developed increased antegrade conduction across the accessory pathway bypassing the AV node, leading to a very rapid ventricular response or ventricular fibrillation. Unless conduction down the accessory pathway has been blocked (either pharmacologically or by surgery), digoxin should not be used in such patients. The treatment of paroxysmal supraventricular tachycardia in such patients is usually direct-current cardioversion.

Use in Patients with Preserved Left Ventricular Systolic Function: Patients with certain disorders involving heart failure associated with preserved left ventricular ejection fraction may be particularly susceptible to toxicity of the drug. Such disorders include restrictive cardiomyopathy, constrictive pericarditis, amyloid heart disease, and acute cor pulmonale. Patients with idiopathic hypertrophic subaortic stenosis may have worsening of the outflow obstruction due to the inotropic effects of digoxin.

PRECAUTIONS

Use in Patients with Impaired Renal Function: Digoxin is primarily excreted by the kidneys; therefore, patients with impaired renal function require smaller than usual maintenance doses of digoxin (see DOSAGE AND ADMINISTRATION). Because of the prolonged elimination half-life, a longer period of time is required to achieve an initial or new steady-state serum concentration in patients with renal impairment than in patients with normal renal function. If appropriate care is not taken to reduce the dose of digoxin, such patients are at high risk for toxicity, and toxic effects will last longer in such patients than in patients with normal renal function.

Use in Patients with Electrolyte Disorders: In patients with hypokalemia or hypomagnesemia, toxicity may occur despite serum digoxin concentrations below 2.0 ng/mL, because potassium or magnesium depletion sensitizes the myocardium to digoxin. Therefore, it is desirable to maintain normal serum potassium and magnesium concentrations in patients being treated with digoxin. Deficiencies of these electrolytes may result from malnutrition, diarrhea, or prolonged vomiting, as well as the use of the following drugs or procedures: diuretics, amphotericin B, corticosteroids, antacids, dialysis, and mechanical suction of gastrointestinal secretions.

Hypercalcemia from any cause predisposes the patient to digitalis toxicity. Calcium, particularly when administered rapidly by the intravenous route, may produce serious arrhythmias in digitalized patients. On the other hand, hypocalcemia can nullify the effects of digoxin in humans; thus, digoxin may be ineffective until serum calcium is restored to normal. These interactions are related to the fact that digoxin affects contractility and excitability of the heart in a manner similar to that of calcium.

Use in Thyroid Disorders and Hypermetabolic States: Hypothyroidism may reduce the requirements for digoxin. Heart failure and/or atrial arrhythmias resulting from hypermetabolic or hyperdynamic states (e.g., hyperthyroidism, hypoxia, or arteriovenous shunt) are best treated by addressing the underlying condition. Atrial arrhythmias associated with hypermetabolic states are particularly resistant to digoxin treatment. Care must be taken to avoid toxicity if digoxin is used.

Use in Patients with Acute Myocardial Infarction: Digoxin should be used with caution in patients with acute myocardial infarction. The use of inotropic drugs in some patients in this setting may result in undesirable increases in myocardial oxygen demand and ischemia.

Use During Electrical Cardioversion: It may be desirable to reduce the dose of digoxin for 1 to 2 days prior to electrical cardioversion of atrial fibrillation to avoid the induction of ventricular arrhythmias, but physicians must consider the consequences of increasing the ventricular response if digoxin is withdrawn. If digitalis toxicity is suspected, elective cardioversion should be delayed. If it is not prudent to

Continued on next page

Product information on these pages is effective as of August 2004. Further information is available at: GlaxoSmithKline, PO Box 13398, Research Triangle Park, NC 27709. 1-888-825-5249. Corporate Web Site: www.gsk.com

Lanoxin Injection—Cont.

delay cardioversion, the lowest possible energy level should be selected to avoid provoking ventricular arrhythmias.

Laboratory Test Monitoring: Patients receiving digoxin should have their serum electrolytes and renal function (serum creatinine concentrations) assessed periodically; the frequency of assessments will depend on the clinical setting. For discussion of serum digoxin concentrations, see DOSAGE AND ADMINISTRATION.

Drug Interactions: Potassium-depleting *diuretics* are a major contributing factor to digitalis toxicity. *Calcium*, particularly if administered rapidly by the intravenous route, may produce serious arrhythmias in digitalized patients. *Quinidine, verapamil, amiodarone, propafenone, indomethacin, itraconazole, alprazolam,* and *spironolactone* raise the serum digoxin concentration due to a reduction in clearance and/or in volume of distribution of the drug, with the implication that digitalis intoxication may result. *Erythromycin* and *clarithromycin* (and possibly other *macrolide antibiotics*) and *tetracycline* may increase digoxin absorption in patients who inactivate digoxin by bacterial metabolism in the lower intestine, so that digitalis intoxication may result. *Propantheline* and *diphenoxylate*, by decreasing gut motility, may increase digoxin absorption. *Antacids, kaolin-pectin, sulfasalazine, neomycin, cholestyramine,* certain *anticancer drugs*, and *metoclopramide* may interfere with intestinal digoxin absorption, resulting in unexpectedly low serum concentrations. *Rifampin* may decrease serum digoxin concentration, especially in patients with renal dysfunction, by increasing the non-renal clearance of digoxin. There have been inconsistent reports regarding the effects of other drugs (e.g., *quinine, penicillamine*) on serum digoxin concentration. *Thyroid* administration to a digitalized, hypothyroid patient may increase the dose requirement of digoxin. Concomitant use of digoxin and *sympathomimetics* increases the risk of cardiac arrhythmias. *Succinylcholine* may cause a sudden extrusion of potassium from muscle cells, and may thereby cause arrhythmias in digitalized patients. Although beta-adrenergic blockers or calcium channel blockers and digoxin may be useful in combination to control atrial fibrillation, their additive effects on AV node conduction can result in advanced or complete heart block. Due to the considerable variability of these interactions, the dosage of digoxin should be individualized when patients receive these medications concurrently. Furthermore, caution should be exercised when combining digoxin with any drug that may cause a significant deterioration in renal function, since a decline in glomerular filtration or tubular secretion may impair the excretion of digoxin.

Drug/Laboratory Test Interactions: The use of therapeutic doses of digoxin may cause prolongation of the PR interval and depression of the ST segment on the electrocardiogram. Digoxin may produce false positive ST-T changes on the electrocardiogram during exercise testing. These electrophysiologic effects reflect an expected effect of the drug and are not indicative of toxicity.

Carcinogenesis, Mutagenesis, Impairment of Fertility: There have been no long-term studies performed in animals to evaluate carcinogenic potential, nor have studies been conducted to assess the mutagenic potential of digoxin or its potential to affect fertility.

Pregnancy: ***Teratogenic Effects:*** Pregnancy Category C. Animal reproduction studies have not been conducted with digoxin. It is also not known whether digoxin can cause fetal harm when administered to a pregnant woman or can affect reproduction capacity. Digoxin should be given to a pregnant woman only if clearly needed.

Nursing Mothers: Studies have shown that digoxin concentrations in the mother's serum and milk are similar. However, the estimated exposure of a nursing infant to digoxin via breast feeding will be far below the usual infant maintenance dose. Therefore, this amount should have no pharmacologic effect upon the infant. Nevertheless, caution should be exercised when digoxin is administered to a nursing woman.

Pediatric Use: Newborn infants display considerable variability in their tolerance to digoxin. Premature and immature infants are particularly sensitive to the effects of digoxin, and the dosage of the drug must not only be reduced but must be individualized according to their degree of maturity. Digitalis glycosides can cause poisoning in children due to accidental ingestion.

Geriatric Use: The majority of clinical experience gained with digoxin has been in the elderly population. This experience has not identified differences in response or adverse effects between the elderly and younger patients. However, this drug is known to be substantially excreted by the kidney, and the risk of toxic reactions to this drug may be greater in patients with impaired renal function. Because elderly patients are more likely to have decreased renal function, care should be taken in dose selection, which should be based on renal function, and it may be useful to monitor renal function (see DOSAGE AND ADMINISTRATION).

ADVERSE REACTIONS

In general, the adverse reactions of digoxin are dose-dependent and occur at doses higher than those needed to achieve a therapeutic effect. Hence, adverse reactions are less common when digoxin is used within the recommended dose range or therapeutic serum concentration range and when there is careful attention to concurrent medications and conditions.

Because some patients may be particularly susceptible to side effects with digoxin, the dosage of the drug should always be selected carefully and adjusted as the clinical condition of the patient warrants. In the past, when high doses of digoxin were used and little attention was paid to clinical status or concurrent medications, adverse reactions to digoxin were more frequent and severe. Cardiac adverse reactions accounted for about one-half, gastrointestinal disturbances for about one-fourth, and CNS and other toxicity for about one-fourth of these adverse reactions. However, available evidence suggests that the incidence and severity of digoxin toxicity has decreased substantially in recent years. In recent controlled clinical trials, in patients with predominantly mild to moderate heart failure, the incidence of adverse experiences was comparable in patients taking digoxin and in those taking placebo. In a large mortality trial, the incidence of hospitalization for suspected digoxin toxicity was 2% in patients taking LANOXIN Tablets compared to 0.9% in patients taking placebo. In this trial, the most common manifestations of digoxin toxicity included gastrointestinal and cardiac disturbances; CNS manifestations were less common.

Adults: ***Cardiac:*** Therapeutic doses of digoxin may cause heart block in patients with pre-existing sinoatrial or AV conduction disorders; heart block can be avoided by adjusting the dose of digoxin. Prophylactic use of a cardiac pacemaker may be considered if the risk of heart block is considered unacceptable. High doses of digoxin may produce a variety of rhythm disturbances, such as first-degree, second-degree (Wenckebach), or third-degree heart block (including asystole); atrial tachycardia with block; AV dissociation; accelerated junctional (nodal) rhythm; unifocal or multiform ventricular premature contractions (especially bigeminy or trigeminy); ventricular tachycardia; and ventricular fibrillation. Digoxin produces PR prolongation and ST segment depression which should not by themselves be considered digoxin toxicity. Cardiac toxicity can also occur at therapeutic doses in patients who have conditions which may alter their sensitivity to digoxin (see WARNINGS and PRECAUTIONS).

Gastrointestinal: Digoxin may cause anorexia, nausea, vomiting, and diarrhea. Rarely, the use of digoxin has been associated with abdominal pain, intestinal ischemia, and hemorrhagic necrosis of the intestines.

CNS: Digoxin can produce visual disturbances (blurred or yellow vision), headache, weakness, dizziness, apathy, confusion, and mental disturbances (such as anxiety, depression, delirium, and hallucination).

Other: Gynecomastia has been occasionally observed following the prolonged use of digoxin. Thrombocytopenia and maculopapular rash and other skin reactions have been rarely observed.

The following table summarizes the incidence of those adverse experiences listed above for patients treated with LANOXIN Tablets or placebo from two randomized, double-blind, placebo-controlled withdrawal trials. Patients in these trials were also receiving diuretics with or without angiotensin-converting enzyme inhibitors. These patients had been stable on digoxin, and were randomized to digoxin or placebo. The results shown in Table 4 reflect the experience in patients following dosage titration with the use of serum digoxin concentrations and careful follow-up. These adverse experiences are consistent with results from a large, placebo-controlled mortality trial (DIG trial) wherein over half the patients were not receiving digoxin prior to enrollment.

[See table 4 at top of next page]

Infants and Children: The side effects of digoxin in infants and children differ from those seen in adults in several respects. Although digoxin may produce anorexia, nausea, vomiting, diarrhea, and CNS disturbances in young patients, these are rarely the initial symptoms of overdosage. Rather, the earliest and most frequent manifestation of excessive dosing with digoxin in infants and children is the appearance of cardiac arrhythmias, including sinus bradycardia. In children, the use of digoxin may produce any arrhythmia. The most common are conduction disturbances or supraventricular tachyarrhythmias, such as atrial tachycardia (with or without block) and junctional (nodal) tachycardia. Ventricular arrhythmias are less common. Sinus bradycardia may be a sign of impending digoxin intoxication, especially in infants, even in the absence of first-degree heart block. Any arrhythmia or alteration in cardiac conduction that develops in a child taking digoxin should be assumed to be caused by digoxin, until further evaluation proves otherwise.

OVERDOSAGE

Treatment of Adverse Reactions Produced by Overdosage: Digoxin should be temporarily discontinued until the adverse reaction resolves. Every effort should also be made to correct factors that may contribute to the adverse reaction (such as electrolyte disturbances or concurrent medications). Once the adverse reaction has resolved, therapy with digoxin may be reinstituted, following a careful reassessment of dose.

Withdrawal of digoxin may be all that is required to treat the adverse reaction. However, when the primary manifestation of digoxin overdosage is a cardiac arrhythmia, additional therapy may be needed.

If the rhythm disturbance is a symptomatic bradyarrhythmia or heart block, consideration should be given to the reversal of toxicity with DIGIBIND® [Digoxin Immune Fab (Ovine)] (see below), the use of atropine, or the insertion of a temporary cardiac pacemaker. However, asymptomatic bradycardia or heart block related to digoxin may require only temporary withdrawal of the drug and cardiac monitoring of the patient.

If the rhythm disturbance is a ventricular arrhythmia, consideration should be given to the correction of electrolyte disorders, particularly if hypokalemia (see below) or hypomagnesemia is present. DIGIBIND is a specific antidote for digoxin and may be used to reverse potentially life-threatening ventricular arrhythmias due to digoxin overdosage.

Administration of Potassium: Every effort should be made to maintain the serum potassium concentration between 4.0 and 5.5 mmol/L. Potassium is usually administered orally, but when correction of the arrhythmia is urgent and the

Table 3. Subgroup Analyses of Mortality and Hospitalization During the First Two Years Following Randomization

		Risk of All-Cause Mortality or All-Cause Hospitalization*			Risk of HF-Related Mortality or HF-Related Hospitalization*		
	n	Placebo	LANOXIN	Relative risk†	Placebo	LANOXIN	Relative risk†
All patients (EF ≤0.45)	6,801	604	593	0.94 (0.88-1.00)	294	217	0.69 (0.63-0.76)
NYHA I/II	4,571	549	541	0.96 (0.89-1.04)	242	178	0.70 (0.62-0.80)
EF 0.25-0.45	4,543	568	571	0.99 (0.91-1.07)	244	190	0.74 (0.66-0.84)
CTR ≤0.55	4,455	561	563	0.98 (0.91-1.06)	239	180	0.71 (0.63-0.81)
NYHA III/IV	2,224	719	696	0.88 (0.80-0.97)	402	295	0.65 (0.57-0.75)
EF <0.25	2,258	677	637	0.84 (0.76-0.93)	394	270	0.61 (0.53-0.71)
CTR >0.55	2,346	687	650	0.85 (0.77-0.94)	398	287	0.65 (0.57-0.75)
EF >0.45‡	987	571	585	1.04 (0.88-1.23)	179	136	0.72 (0.53-0.99)

*Number of patients with an event during the first 2 years per 1,000 randomized patients.
†Relative risk (95% confidence interval).
‡DIG Ancillary Study.

serum potassium concentration is low, potassium may be administered cautiously by the intravenous route. The electrocardiogram should be monitored for any evidence of potassium toxicity (e.g., peaking of T waves) and to observe the effect on the arrhythmia. Potassium salts may be dangerous in patients who manifest bradycardia or heart block due to digoxin (unless primarily related to supraventricular tachycardia) and in the setting of massive digitalis overdosage (see Massive Digitalis Overdosage subsection).

Massive Digitalis Overdosage: Manifestations of life-threatening toxicity include ventricular tachycardia or ventricular fibrillation, or progressive bradyarrhythmias, or heart block. The administration of more than 10 mg of digoxin in a previously healthy adult, or more than 4 mg in a previously healthy child, or a steady-state serum concentration greater than 10 ng/mL often results in cardiac arrest.

DIGIBIND should be used to reverse the toxic effects of ingestion of a massive overdose. The decision to administer DIGIBIND to a patient who has ingested a massive dose of digoxin but who has not yet manifested life-threatening toxicity should depend on the likelihood that life-threatening toxicity will occur (see above).

Patients with massive digitalis ingestion should receive large doses of activated charcoal to prevent absorption and bind digoxin in the gut during enteroenteric recirculation. Emesis or gastric lavage may be indicated especially if ingestion has occurred within 30 minutes of the patient's presentation at the hospital. Emesis should not be induced in patients who are obtunded. If a patient presents more than 2 hours after ingestion or already has toxic manifestations, it may be unsafe to induce vomiting or attempt passage of a gastric tube, because such maneuvers may induce an acute vagal episode that can worsen digitalis-related arrhythmias.

Severe digitalis intoxication can cause a massive shift of potassium from inside to outside the cell, leading to life-threatening hyperkalemia. The administration of potassium supplements in the setting of massive intoxication may be hazardous and should be avoided. Hyperkalemia caused by massive digitalis toxicity is best treated with DIGIBIND; initial treatment with glucose and insulin may also be required if hyperkalemia itself is acutely life-threatening.

DOSAGE AND ADMINISTRATION

General: Recommended dosages of digoxin may require considerable modification because of individual sensitivity of the patient to the drug, the presence of associated conditions, or the use of concurrent medications.

Parenteral administration of digoxin should be used only when the need for rapid digitalization is urgent or when the drug cannot be taken orally. Intramuscular injection can lead to severe pain at the injection site, thus intravenous administration is preferred. If the drug must be administered by the intramuscular route, it should be injected deep into the muscle followed by massage. No more than 500 mcg (2 mL) should be injected into a single site.

LANOXIN Injection can be administered undiluted or diluted with a 4-fold or greater volume of Sterile Water for Injection, 0.9% Sodium Chloride Injection, or 5% Dextrose Injection. The use of less than a 4-fold volume of diluent could lead to precipitation of the digoxin. Immediate use of the diluted product is recommended.

If tuberculin syringes are used to measure very small doses, one must be aware of the problem of inadvertent overadministration of digoxin. The syringe should *not* be flushed with the parenteral solution after its contents are expelled into an indwelling vascular catheter.

Slow infusion of LANOXIN Injection is preferable to bolus administration. Rapid infusion of digitalis glycosides has been shown to cause systemic and coronary arteriolar constriction, which may be clinically undesirable. Caution is thus advised and LANOXIN Injection should probably be administered over a period of 5 minutes or longer. Mixing of LANOXIN Injection with other drugs in the same container or simultaneous administration in the same intravenous line is not recommended.

In selecting a dose of digoxin, the following factors must be considered:

1. The body weight of the patient. Doses should be calculated based upon lean (i.e., ideal) body weight.
2. The patient's renal function, preferably evaluated on the basis of estimated creatinine clearance.
3. The patient's age. Infants and children require different doses of digoxin than adults. Also, advanced age may be indicative of diminished renal function even in patients with normal serum creatinine concentration (i.e., below 1.5 mg/dL).
4. Concomitant disease states, concurrent medications, or other factors likely to alter the pharmacokinetic or pharmacodynamic profile of digoxin (see PRECAUTIONS).

Serum Digoxin Concentrations: In general, the dose of digoxin used should be determined on clinical grounds. However, measurement of serum digoxin concentrations can be helpful to the clinician in determining the adequacy of digoxin therapy and in assigning certain probabilities to the likelihood of digoxin intoxication. About two-thirds of adults considered adequately digitalized (without evidence of toxicity) have serum digoxin concentrations ranging from 0.8 to 2.0 ng/mL. However, digoxin may produce clinical benefits even at serum concentrations below this range. About two-thirds of adult patients with clinical toxicity have serum digoxin concentrations greater than 2.0 ng/mL. However,

Table 4. Adverse Experiences In Two Parallel, Double-Blind, Placebo-Controlled Withdrawal Trials (Number of Patients Reporting)

Adverse Experience	Digoxin Patients (n = 123)	Placebo Patients (n = 125)
Cardiac		
Palpitation	1	4
Ventricular extrasystole	1	1
Tachycardia	2	1
Heart arrest	1	1
Gastrointestinal		
Anorexia	1	4
Nausea	4	2
Vomiting	2	1
Diarrhea	4	1
Abdominal pain	0	6
CNS		
Headache	4	4
Dizziness	6	5
Mental disturbances	5	1
Other		
Rash	2	1
Death	4	3

Table 5. Usual Daily Maintenance Dose Requirements (mcg) of LANOXIN Injection for Estimated Peak Body Stores of 10 mcg/kg*

Corrected Ccr (mL/min per 70 kg)[†]	Lean Body Weight kg 50 / lb 110	kg 60 / lb 132	kg 70 / lb 154	kg 80 / lb 176	kg 90 / lb 198	kg 100 / lb 220	Number of Days Before Steady State Achieved[‡]
0	75[§]	75	100	100	125	150	22
10	75	100	100	125	150	150	19
20	100	100	125	150	150	175	16
30	100	125	150	150	175	200	14
40	100	125	150	175	200	225	13
50	125	150	175	200	225	250	12
60	125	150	175	200	225	250	11
70	150	175	200	225	250	275	10
80	150	175	200	250	275	300	9
90	150	200	225	250	300	325	8
100	175	200	250	275	300	350	7

*Daily maintenance doses have been rounded to the nearest 25-mcg increment.
[†] Ccr is creatinine clearance, corrected to 70 kg body weight or 1.73 m^2 body surface area. *For adults,* if only serum creatinine concentrations (Scr) are available, a Ccr (corrected to 70 kg body weight) may be estimated in men as (140 - Age)/Scr. For women, this result should be multiplied by 0.85. *Note: This equation cannot be used for estimating creatinine clearance in infants or children.*
[‡]If no loading dose administered.
[§]75 mcg = 0.075 mg

since one-third of patients with clinical toxicity have concentrations less than 2.0 ng/mL, values below 2.0 ng/mL do not rule out the possibility that a certain sign or symptom is related to digoxin therapy. Rarely, there are patients who are unable to tolerate digoxin at serum concentrations below 0.8 ng/mL. Consequently, the serum concentration of digoxin should always be interpreted in the overall clinical context, and an isolated measurement should not be used alone as the basis for increasing or decreasing the dose of the drug.

To allow adequate time for equilibration of digoxin between serum and tissue, sampling of serum concentrations should be done just before the next scheduled dose of the drug. If this is not possible, sampling should be done at least 6 to 8 hours after the last dose, regardless of the route of administration or the formulation used. On a once-daily dosing schedule, the concentration of digoxin will be 10% to 25% lower when sampled at 24 versus 8 hours, depending upon the patient's renal function. On a twice-daily dosing schedule, there will be only minor differences in serum digoxin concentrations whether sampling is done at 8 or 12 hours after a dose.

If a discrepancy exists between the reported serum concentration and the observed clinical response, the clinician should consider the following possibilities:

1. Analytical problems in the assay procedure.
2. Inappropriate serum sampling time.
3. Administration of a digitalis glycoside other than digoxin.
4. Conditions (described in WARNINGS and PRECAUTIONS) causing an alteration in the sensitivity of the patient to digoxin.
5. Serum digoxin concentration may decrease acutely during periods of exercise without any associated change in clinical efficacy due to increased binding of digoxin to skeletal muscle.

Heart Failure: ***Adults:*** Digitalization may be accomplished by either of two general approaches that vary in dosage and frequency of administration, but reach the same endpoint in terms of total amount of digoxin accumulated in the body.

1. If rapid digitalization is considered medically appropriate, it may be achieved by administering a loading dose based upon projected peak digoxin body stores. Maintenance dose can be calculated as a percentage of the loading dose.
2. More gradual digitalization may be obtained by beginning an appropriate maintenance dose, thus allowing digoxin body stores to accumulate slowly. Steady-state serum digoxin concentrations will be achieved in approximately five half-lives of the drug for the individual patient. Depending upon the patient's renal function, this will take between 1 and 3 weeks.

Rapid Digitalization with a Loading Dose: LANOXIN Injection is frequently used to achieve rapid digitalization, with conversion to LANOXIN Tablets or LANOXICAPS for maintenance therapy. If patients are switched from intravenous to oral digoxin formulations, allowances must be made for differences in bioavailability when calculating maintenance dosages (see Table 1, CLINICAL PHARMACOLOGY: Pharmacokinetics and dosing Table 5).

Intramuscular injection of digoxin is extremely painful and offers no advantages unless other routes of administration are contraindicated.

Peak digoxin body stores of 8 to 12 mcg/kg should provide therapeutic effect with minimum risk of toxicity in most patients with heart failure and normal sinus rhythm. Because of altered digoxin distribution and elimination, projected peak body stores for patients with renal insufficiency should be conservative (i.e., 6 to 10 mcg/kg) [see PRECAUTIONS].

The loading dose should be administered in several portions, with roughly half the total given as the first dose. Additional fractions of this planned total dose may be given at 6- to 8-hour intervals, **with careful assessment of clinical response before each additional dose.** If the patient's clinical response necessitates a change from the calculated loading dose of digoxin, then calculation of the maintenance dose should be based upon the amount actually given.

A single initial intravenous dose of 400 to 600 mcg (0.4 to 0.6 mg) of LANOXIN Injection usually produces a detectable effect in 5 to 30 minutes that becomes maximal in 1 to 4 hours. Additional doses of 100 to 300 mcg (0.1 to 0.3 mg) may be given cautiously at 6- to 8-hour intervals until clin-

Continued on next page

Product information on these pages is effective as of August 2004. Further information is available at: GlaxoSmithKline, PO Box 13398, Research Triangle Park, NC 27709. 1-888-825-5249. Corporate Web Site: www.gsk.com

Lanoxin Injection—Cont.

ical evidence of an adequate effect is noted. The usual amount of LANOXIN Injection that a 70-kg patient requires to achieve 8- to 12-mcg/kg peak body stores is 600 to 1,000 mcg (0.6 to 1.0 mg).

Maintenance Dosing: The doses of oral digoxin used in controlled trials in patients with heart failure have ranged from 125 to 500 mcg (0.125 to 0.5 mg) once daily. In these studies, the digoxin dose has been generally titrated according to the patient's age, lean body weight, and renal function. Therapy is generally initiated at a dose of 250 mcg (0.25 mg) once daily in patients under age 70 with good renal function, at a dose of 125 mcg (0.125 mg) once daily in patients over age 70 or with impaired renal function, and at a dose of 62.5 mcg (0.0625 mg) in patients with marked renal impairment. Doses may be increased every 2 weeks according to clinical response.

In a subset of approximately 1,800 patients enrolled in the DIG trial (wherein dosing was based on an algorithm similar to that in Table 5) the mean (± SD) serum digoxin concentrations at 1 month and 12 months were 1.01 ± 0.47 ng/mL and 0.97 ± 0.43 ng/mL, respectively.

The maintenance dose should be based upon the percentage of the peak body stores lost each day through elimination. The following formula has had wide clinical use:

Maintenance Dose = Peak Body Stores (i.e., Loading Dose) × % Daily Loss/100

Where: % Daily Loss = 14 + Ccr/5

(Ccr is creatinine clearance, corrected to 70 kg body weight or 1.73 m^2 body surface area.)

Table 5 provides average daily maintenance dose requirements of LANOXIN Injection for patients with heart failure based upon lean body weight and renal function:

[See table 5 on previous page]

Example: Based on the above table, a patient in heart failure with an estimated lean body weight of 70 kg and a Ccr of 60 mL/min should be given a dose of 175 mcg (0.175 mg) daily of LANOXIN Injection. If no loading dose is administered, steady-state serum concentrations in this patient should be anticipated at approximately 11 days.

Infants and Children: See the full prescribing information for LANOXIN Injection Pediatric for specific recommendations.

It cannot be overemphasized that dosage guidelines provided are based upon average patient response and substantial individual variation can be expected. Accordingly, ultimate dosage selection must be based upon clinical assessment of the patient.

Atrial Fibrillation: Peak digoxin body stores larger than the 8 to 12 mcg/kg required for most patients with heart failure and normal sinus rhythm have been used for control of ventricular rate in patients with atrial fibrillation. Doses of digoxin used for the treatment of chronic atrial fibrillation should be titrated to the minimum dose that achieves the desired ventricular rate control without causing undesirable side effects. Data are not available to establish the appropriate resting or exercise target rates that should be achieved.

Dosage Adjustment When Changing Preparations: The difference in bioavailability between LANOXIN Injection or LANOXICAPS and LANOXIN Elixir Pediatric or LANOXIN Tablets must be considered when changing patients from one dosage form to another.

Doses of 100 mcg (0.1 mg) and 200 mcg (0.2 mg) of LANOXICAPS are approximately equivalent to 125-mcg (0.125-mg) and 250-mcg (0.25-mg) doses of LANOXIN Tablets and Elixir Pediatric, respectively (see Table 1 in CLINICAL PHARMACOLOGY: Pharmacokinetics).

HOW SUPPLIED

LANOXIN (digoxin) Injection, 500 mcg (0.5 mg) in 2 mL (250 mcg [0.25 mg] per mL); Boxes of 10 (NDC 0173-0260-10) and 50 ampuls (NDC 0173-0260-35).

Store at 25°C (77°F); excursions permitted to 15° to 30°C (59° to 86°F) [see USP Controlled Room Temperature] and protect from light.

Manufactured by Draxis Pharma Inc.
Kirkland, Canada H9H 4J4 for
GlaxoSmithKline, Research Triangle Park, NC 27709

July 2002/RL-1126

Shown in Product Identification Guide, page 316

LANOXIN® ℞
[lă-nŏx'ĭn]
(digoxin)
Injection Pediatric
100 mcg (0.1 mg) in 1 mL

DESCRIPTION

LANOXIN (digoxin) is one of the cardiac (or digitalis) glycosides, a closely related group of drugs having in common specific effects on the myocardium. These drugs are found in a number of plants. Digoxin is extracted from the leaves of *Digitalis lanata.* The term "digitalis" is used to designate the whole group of glycosides. The glycosides are composed of two portions: a sugar and a cardenolide (hence "glycosides").

Digoxin is described chemically as (3β,5β,12β)-3-[(*O*-2,6-dideoxy-β-*D*-*ribo*-hexopyranosyl-(1→4)-*O*-2,6-dideoxy-β-*D*-*ribo*-hexopyranosyl-(1→4)-2,6-dideoxy-β-*D*-*ribo*-hexopyranosyl)oxy]-12,14-dihydroxy-card-20(22)-enolide. Its molecular formula is $C_{41}H_{64}O_{14}$, and its molecular weight is 780.95.

Digoxin exists as odorless white crystals that melt with decomposition above 230°C. The drug is practically insoluble in water and in ether; slightly soluble in diluted (50%) alcohol and in chloroform; and freely soluble in pyridine.

LANOXIN Injection Pediatric is a sterile solution of digoxin for intravenous or intramuscular injection. The vehicle contains 40% propylene glycol and 10% alcohol. The injection is buffered to a pH of 6.8 to 7.2 with 0.17% sodium phosphate and 0.08% anhydrous citric acid. Each 1-mL ampul contains 100 mcg (0.1 mg) digoxin. Dilution is not required.

CLINICAL PHARMACOLOGY

Mechanism of Action: Digoxin inhibits sodium-potassium ATPase, an enzyme that regulates the quantity of sodium and potassium inside cells. Inhibition of the enzyme leads to an increase in the intracellular concentration of sodium and thus (by stimulation of sodium-calcium exchange) an increase in the intracellular concentration of calcium. The beneficial effects of digoxin result from direct actions on cardiac muscle, as well as indirect actions on the cardiovascular system mediated by effects on the autonomic nervous system. The autonomic effects include: (1) a vagomimetic action, which is responsible for the effects of digoxin on the sinoatrial and atrioventricular (AV) nodes; and (2) baroreceptor sensitization, which results in increased afferent inhibitory activity and reduced activity of the sympathetic nervous system and renin-angiotensin system for any given increment in mean arterial pressure. The pharmacologic consequences of these direct and indirect effects are: (1) an increase in the force and velocity of myocardial systolic contraction (positive inotropic action); (2) a decrease in the degree of activation of the sympathetic nervous system and renin-angiotensin system (neurohormonal deactivating effect); and (3) slowing of the heart rate and decreased conduction velocity through the AV node (vagomimetic effect). The effects of digoxin in heart failure are mediated by its positive inotropic and neurohormonal deactivating effects, whereas the effects of the drug in atrial arrhythmias are related to its vagomimetic actions. In high doses, digoxin increases sympathetic outflow from the central nervous system (CNS). This increase in sympathetic activity may be an important factor in digitalis toxicity.

Pharmacokinetics: Note: The following data are from studies performed in adults, unless otherwise stated.

Absorption: Comparisons of the systemic availability and equivalent doses for preparations of digoxin are shown in Table 1.

[See table 1 above]

Table 1. Comparisons of the Systemic Availability and Equivalent Doses for Preparations of LANOXIN

Product	Absolute Bioavailability	Equivalent Doses (mcg)* Among Dosage Forms			
LANOXIN Tablets	60 - 80%	62.5	125	250	500
LANOXIN Elixir Pediatric	70 - 85%	62.5	125	250	500
LANOXICAPS®	90 - 100%	50	100	200	400
LANOXIN Injection/IV	100%	50	100	200	400

*For example, 125 mcg LANOXIN Tablets equivalent to 125 mcg LANOXIN Elixir Pediatric equivalent to 100 mcg LANOXICAPS equivalent to 100 mcg LANOXIN Injection/IV.

Distribution: Following drug administration, a 6- to 8-hour tissue distribution phase is observed. This is followed by a much more gradual decline in the serum concentration of the drug, which is dependent on the elimination of digoxin from the body. The peak height and slope of the early portion (absorption/distribution phases) of the serum concentration-time curve are dependent upon the route of administration and the absorption characteristics of the formulation. Clinical evidence indicates that the early high serum concentrations do not reflect the concentration of digoxin at its site of action, but that with chronic use, the steady-state post-distribution serum concentrations are in equilibrium with tissue concentrations and correlate with pharmacologic effects. In individual patients, these post-distribution serum concentrations may be useful in evaluating therapeutic and toxic effects (see DOSAGE AND ADMINISTRATION: Serum Digoxin Concentrations).

Digoxin is concentrated in tissues and therefore has a large apparent volume of distribution. Digoxin crosses both the blood-brain barrier and the placenta. At delivery, the serum digoxin concentration in the newborn is similar to the serum concentration in the mother. Approximately 25% of digoxin in the plasma is bound to protein. Serum digoxin concentrations are not significantly altered by large changes in fat tissue weight, so that its distribution space correlates best with lean (i.e., ideal) body weight, not total body weight.

Metabolism: Only a small percentage (16%) of a dose of digoxin is metabolized. The end metabolites, which include 3 β-digoxigenin, 3-keto-digoxigenin, and their glucuronide and sulfate conjugates, are polar in nature and are postulated to be formed via hydrolysis, oxidation, and conjugation. The metabolism of digoxin is not dependent upon the cytochrome P-450 system, and digoxin is not known to induce or inhibit the cytochrome P-450 system.

Excretion: Elimination of digoxin follows first-order kinetics (that is, the quantity of digoxin eliminated at any time is proportional to the total body content). Following intravenous administration to healthy volunteers, 50% to 70% of a digoxin dose is excreted unchanged in the urine. Renal excretion of digoxin is proportional to glomerular filtration rate and is largely independent of urine flow. In healthy volunteers with normal renal function, digoxin has a half-life of 1.5 to 2.0 days. The half-life in anuric patients is prolonged to 3.5 to 5 days. Digoxin is not effectively removed from the body by dialysis, exchange transfusion, or during cardiopulmonary bypass because most of the drug is bound to tissue and does not circulate in the blood.

Special Populations: Race differences in digoxin pharmacokinetics have not been formally studied. Because digoxin is primarily eliminated as unchanged drug via the kidney and because there are no important differences in creatinine clearance among races, pharmacokinetic differences due to race are not expected.

The clearance of digoxin can be primarily correlated with renal function as indicated by creatinine clearance. In children with renal disease, digoxin must be carefully titrated based upon clinical response.

Plasma digoxin concentration profiles in patients with acute hepatitis generally fell within the range of profiles in a group of healthy subjects.

Pharmacodynamic and Clinical Effects: The times to onset of pharmacologic effect and to peak effect of preparations of LANOXIN are shown in Table 2.

[See table 2 above]

Table 2. Times to Onset of Pharmacologic Effect and to Peak Effect of Preparations of LANOXIN

Product	Time to Onset of Effect*	Time to Peak Effect*
LANOXIN Tablets	0.5 - 2 hours	2 - 6 hours
LANOXIN Elixir Pediatric	0.5 - 2 hours	2 - 6 hours
LANOXICAPS	0.5 - 2 hours	2 - 6 hours
LANOXIN Injection/IV	5 - 30 minutes†	1 - 4 hours

*Documented for ventricular response rate in atrial fibrillation, inotropic effects and electrocardiographic changes.
†Depending upon rate of infusion.

Hemodynamic Effects: Digoxin produces hemodynamic improvement in patients with heart failure. Short- and long-term therapy with the drug increases cardiac output and lowers pulmonary artery pressure, pulmonary capillary wedge pressure, and systemic vascular resistance. These hemodynamic effects are accompanied by an increase in the left ventricular ejection fraction and a decrease in end-systolic and end-diastolic dimensions.

Chronic Heart Failure: Two 12-week, double-blind, placebo-controlled studies enrolled 178 (RADIANCE trial) and 88 (PROVED trial) adult patients with NYHA class II or III heart failure previously treated with oral digoxin, a diuretic, and an ACE inhibitor (RADIANCE only) and randomized them to placebo or treatment with LANOXIN Tablets. Both trials demonstrated better preservation of exercise capacity in patients randomized to LANOXIN. Continued treatment with LANOXIN reduced the risk of developing worsening heart failure, as evidenced by heart failure-related hospitalizations and emergency care and the need for concomitant heart failure therapy. The larger study also showed treatment-related benefits in NYHA class and patients' global assessment. In the smaller trial, these trended in favor of a treatment benefit.

The Digitalis Investigation Group (DIG) main trial was a multicenter, randomized, double-blind, placebo-controlled mortality study of 6,801 adult patients with heart failure and left ventricular ejection fraction ≤0.45. At randomization, 67% were NYHA class I or II, 71% had heart failure of ischemic etiology, 44% had been receiving digoxin, and most were receiving concomitant ACE inhibitor (94%) and diuretic (82%). Patients were randomized to placebo or LANOXIN Tablets, the dose of which was adjusted for the patient's age, sex, lean body weight, and serum creatinine (see DOSAGE AND ADMINISTRATION), and followed for up to 58 months (median 37 months). The median daily dose prescribed was 0.25 mg. Overall all-cause mortality was 35% with no difference between groups (95% confidence limits for relative risk of 0.91 to 1.07). LANOXIN was associated with a 25% reduction in the number of hospitalizations for heart failure, a 28% reduction in the risk of a patient having at least one hospitalization for heart failure, and a 6.5% reduction in total hospitalizations (for any cause).

Use of LANOXIN was associated with a trend to increase time to all-cause death or hospitalization. The trend was evident in subgroups of patients with mild heart failure as well as more severe disease, as shown in Table 3. Although the effect on all-cause death or hospitalization was not statistically significant, much of the apparent benefit derived from effects on mortality and hospitalization attributed to heart failure.
[See table 3 at right]
In situations where there is no statistically significant benefit of treatment evident from a trial's primary endpoint, results pertaining to a secondary endpoint should be interpreted cautiously.
Chronic Atrial Fibrillation: In adult patients with chronic atrial fibrillation, digoxin slows rapid ventricular response rate in a linear dose-response fashion from 0.25 to 0.75 mg/day. Digoxin should not be used for the treatment of multifocal atrial tachycardia.

INDICATIONS AND USAGE

Heart Failure: LANOXIN is indicated for the treatment of mild to moderate heart failure. LANOXIN increases left ventricular ejection fraction and improves heart failure symptoms as evidenced by exercise capacity and heart failure-related hospitalizations and emergency care, while having no effect on mortality. Where possible, LANOXIN should be used with a diuretic and an angiotensin-converting enzyme inhibitor, but an optimal order for starting these three drugs cannot be specified.
Atrial Fibrillation: LANOXIN is indicated for the control of ventricular response rate in patients with chronic atrial fibrillation.

CONTRAINDICATIONS

Digitalis glycosides are contraindicated in patients with ventricular fibrillation or in patients with a known hypersensitivity to digoxin. A hypersensitivity reaction to other digitalis preparations usually constitutes a contraindication to digoxin.

WARNINGS

Sinus Node Disease and AV Block: Because digoxin slows sinoatrial and AV conduction, the drug commonly prolongs the PR interval. The drug may cause severe sinus bradycardia or sinoatrial block in patients with pre-existing sinus node disease and may cause advanced or complete heart block in patients with pre-existing incomplete AV block. In such patients consideration should be given to the insertion of a pacemaker before treatment with digoxin.
Accessory AV Pathway (Wolff-Parkinson-White Syndrome): After intravenous digoxin therapy, some patients with paroxysmal atrial fibrillation or flutter and a coexisting accessory AV pathway have developed increased antegrade conduction across the accessory pathway bypassing the AV node, leading to a very rapid ventricular response or ventricular fibrillation. Unless conduction down the accessory pathway has been blocked (either pharmacologically or by surgery), digoxin should not be used in such patients. The treatment of paroxysmal supraventricular tachycardia in such patients is usually direct-current cardioversion.
Use in Patients with Preserved Left Ventricular Systolic Function: Patients with certain disorders involving heart failure associated with preserved left ventricular ejection fraction may be particularly susceptible to toxicity of the drug. Such disorders include restrictive cardiomyopathy, constrictive pericarditis, amyloid heart disease, and acute cor pulmonale. Patients with idiopathic hypertrophic subaortic stenosis may have worsening of the outflow obstruction due to the inotropic effects of digoxin.

PRECAUTIONS

Use in Patients with Impaired Renal Function: Digoxin is primarily excreted by the kidneys; therefore, patients with impaired renal function require smaller than usual maintenance doses of digoxin (see DOSAGE AND ADMINISTRATION). Because of the prolonged elimination half-life, a longer period of time is required to achieve an initial or new steady-state serum concentration in patients with renal impairment than in patients with normal renal function. If appropriate care is not taken to reduce the dose of digoxin, such patients are at high risk for toxicity, and toxic effects will last longer in such patients than in patients with normal renal function.
Use in Patients with Electrolyte Disorders: In patients with hypokalemia or hypomagnesemia, toxicity may occur despite serum digoxin concentrations below 2.0 ng/mL, because potassium or magnesium depletion sensitizes the myocardium to digoxin. Therefore, it is desirable to maintain normal serum potassium and magnesium concentrations in patients being treated with digoxin. Deficiencies of these electrolytes may result from malnutrition, diarrhea, or prolonged vomiting, as well as the use of the following drugs or procedures: diuretics, amphotericin B, corticosteroids, antacids, dialysis, and mechanical suction of gastrointestinal secretions.
Hypercalcemia from any cause predisposes the patient to digitalis toxicity. Calcium, particularly when administered rapidly by the intravenous route, may produce serious arrhythmias in digitalized patients. On the other hand, hypocalcemia can nullify the effects of digoxin in humans; thus, digoxin may be ineffective until serum calcium is restored to normal. These interactions are related to the fact that digoxin affects contractility and excitability of the heart in a manner similar to that of calcium.
Use in Thyroid Disorders and Hypermetabolic States: Hypothyroidism may reduce the requirements for digoxin.

Table 3. Subgroup Analyses of Mortality and Hospitalization During the First Two Years Following Randomization

	n	Risk of All-Cause Mortality or All-Cause Hospitalization*			Risk of HF-Related Mortality or HF-Related Hospitalization*		
		Placebo	LANOXIN	Relative risk†	Placebo	LANOXIN	Relative risk†
All patients (EF ≤0.45)	6801	604	593	0.94 (0.88-1.00)	294	217	0.69 (0.63-0.76)
NYHA I/II	4571	549	541	0.96 (0.89-1.04)	242	178	0.70 (0.62-0.80)
EF 0.25-0.45	4543	568	571	0.99 (0.91-1.07)	244	190	0.74 (0.66-0.84)
CTR ≤0.55	4455	561	563	0.98 (0.91-1.06)	239	180	0.71 (0.63-0.81)
NYHA III/IV	2224	719	696	0.88 (0.80-0.97)	402	295	0.65 (0.57-0.75)
EF <0.25	2258	677	637	0.84 (0.76-0.93)	394	270	0.61 (0.53-0.71)
CTR >0.55	2346	687	650	0.85 (0.77-0.94)	398	287	0.65 (0.57-0.75)
EF >0.45‡	987	571	585	1.04 (0.88-1.23)	179	136	0.72 (0.53-0.99)

*Number of patients with an event during the first 2 years per 1000 randomized patients.
†Relative risk (95% confidence interval).
‡DIG Ancillary Study.

Heart failure and/or atrial arrhythmias resulting from hypermetabolic or hyperdynamic states (e.g., hyperthyroidism, hypoxia, or arteriovenous shunt) are best treated by addressing the underlying condition. Atrial arrhythmias associated with hypermetabolic states are particularly resistant to digoxin treatment. Care must be taken to avoid toxicity if digoxin is used.
Use in Patients with Acute Myocardial Infarction: Digoxin should be used with caution in patients with acute myocardial infarction. The use of inotropic drugs in some patients in this setting may result in undesirable increases in myocardial oxygen demand and ischemia.
Use During Electrical Cardioversion: It may be desirable to reduce the dose of digoxin for 1 to 2 days prior to electrical cardioversion of atrial fibrillation to avoid the induction of ventricular arrhythmias, but physicians must consider the consequences of increasing the ventricular response if digoxin is withdrawn. If digitalis toxicity is suspected, elective cardioversion should be delayed. If it is not prudent to delay cardioversion, the lowest possible energy level should be selected to avoid provoking ventricular arrhythmias.
Laboratory Test Monitoring: Patients receiving digoxin should have their serum electrolytes and renal function (serum creatinine concentrations) assessed periodically; the frequency of assessments will depend on the clinical setting. For discussion of serum digoxin concentrations, see DOSAGE AND ADMINISTRATION.
Drug Interactions: Potassium-depleting *diuretics* are a major contributing factor to digitalis toxicity. *Calcium*, particularly if administered rapidly by the intravenous route, may produce serious arrhythmias in digitalized patients. *Quinidine, verapamil, amiodarone, propafenone, indomethacin, itraconazole, alprazolam*, and *spironolactone* raise the serum digoxin concentration due to a reduction in clearance and/or volume of distribution of the drug, with the implication that digitalis intoxication may result. *Erythromycin* and *clarithromycin* (and possibly other *macrolide antibiotics*) and *tetracycline* may increase digoxin absorption in patients who inactivate digoxin by bacterial metabolism in the lower intestine, so that digitalis intoxication may result. *Propantheline* and *diphenoxylate*, by decreasing gut motility, may increase digoxin absorption. *Antacids, kaolin-pectin, sulfasalazine, neomycin, cholestyramine*, certain *anticancer drugs*, and *metoclopramide* may interfere with intestinal digoxin absorption, resulting in unexpectedly low serum concentrations. *Rifampin* may decrease serum digoxin concentration, especially in patients with renal dysfunction, by increasing the non-renal clearance of digoxin. There have been inconsistent reports regarding the effects of other drugs [e.g., *quinine, penicillamine*] on serum digoxin concentration. *Thyroid* administration to a digitalized, hypothyroid patient may increase the dose requirement of digoxin. Concomitant use of digoxin and *sympathomimetics* increases the risk of cardiac arrhythmias. *Succinylcholine* may cause a sudden extrusion of potassium from muscle cells, and may thereby cause arrhythmias in digitalized patients. Although beta-adrenergic blockers or calcium channel blockers and digoxin may be useful in combination to control atrial fibrillation, their additive effects on AV node conduction can result in advanced or complete heart block.
Due to the considerable variability of these interactions, dosage of digoxin should be individualized when patients receive these medications concurrently. Furthermore, caution should be exercised when combining digoxin with any drug that may cause a significant deterioration in renal function, since a decline in glomerular filtration or tubular secretion may impair the excretion of digoxin.
Drug/Laboratory Test Interactions: The use of therapeutic doses of digoxin may cause prolongation of the PR interval and depression of the ST segment on the electrocardiogram. Digoxin may produce false positive ST-T changes on the electrocardiogram during exercise testing. These electrophysiologic effects reflect an expected effect of the drug and are not indicative of toxicity.
Carcinogenesis, Mutagenesis, Impairment of Fertility: There have been no long-term studies performed in animals to evaluate carcinogenic potential, nor have studies been conducted to assess the mutagenic potential of digoxin or its potential to affect fertility.
Pregnancy: ***Teratogenic Effects:*** Pregnancy Category C. Animal reproduction studies have not been conducted with digoxin. It is also not known whether digoxin can cause fetal harm when administered to a pregnant woman or can affect reproductive capacity. Digoxin should be given to a pregnant woman only if clearly needed.
Nursing Mothers: Studies have shown that digoxin concentrations in the mother's serum and milk are similar. However, the estimated exposure of a nursing infant to digoxin via breast feeding will be far below the usual infant maintenance dose. Therefore, this amount should have no pharmacologic effect upon the infant. Nevertheless, caution should be exercised when digoxin is administered to a nursing woman.
Pediatric Use: Newborn infants display considerable variability in their tolerance to digoxin. Premature and immature infants are particularly sensitive to the effects of digoxin, and the dosage of the drug must not only be reduced but must be individualized according to their degree of maturity. Digitalis glycosides can cause poisoning in children due to accidental ingestion.
Geriatric Use: The majority of clinical experience gained with digoxin has been in the elderly population. This experience has not identified differences in response or adverse effects between the elderly and younger patients. However, this drug is known to be substantially excreted by the kidney, and the risk of toxic reactions to this drug may be greater in patients with impaired renal function. Because elderly patients are more likely to have decreased renal function, care should be taken in dose selection, which should be based on renal function, and it may be useful to monitor renal function.

ADVERSE REACTIONS

In general, the adverse reactions of digoxin are dose-dependent and occur at doses higher than those needed to achieve a therapeutic effect. Hence, adverse reactions are less common when digoxin is used within the recommended dose range or therapeutic serum concentration range and when there is careful attention to concurrent medications and conditions.
Because some patients may be particularly susceptible to side effects with digoxin, the dosage of the drug should always be selected carefully and adjusted as the clinical condition of the patient warrants. In the past, when high doses of digoxin were used and little attention was paid to clinical status or concurrent medications, adverse reactions to digoxin were more frequent and severe. Cardiac adverse reactions accounted for about one-half, gastrointestinal disturbances for about one-fourth, and CNS and other toxicity for about one-fourth of these adverse reactions. However, available evidence suggests that the incidence and severity of digoxin toxicity has decreased substantially in recent years. In recent controlled clinical trials, in patients with predominantly mild to moderate heart failure, the incidence of adverse experiences was comparable in patients taking digoxin and in those taking placebo. In a large mortality trial, the incidence of hospitalization for suspected

Continued on next page

Product information on these pages is effective as of August 2004. Further information is available at: GlaxoSmithKline, PO Box 13398, Research Triangle Park, NC 27709. 1-888-825-5249. Corporate Web Site: www.gsk.com

Lanoxin Inj. Pediatric—Cont.

digoxin toxicity was 2% in patients taking LANOXIN Tablets compared to 0.9% in patients taking placebo. In this trial, the most common manifestations of digoxin toxicity included gastrointestinal and cardiac disturbances; CNS manifestations were less common.

Adults: *Cardiac:* Therapeutic doses of digoxin may cause heart block in patients with pre-existing sinoatrial or AV conduction disorders; heart block can be avoided by adjusting the dose of digoxin. Prophylactic use of a cardiac pacemaker may be considered if the risk of heart block is considered unacceptable. High doses of digoxin may produce a variety of rhythm disturbances, such as first-degree, second-degree (Wenckebach), or third-degree heart block (including asystole); atrial tachycardia with block; AV dissociation; accelerated junctional (nodal) rhythm; unifocal or multiform ventricular premature contractions (especially bigeminy or trigeminy); ventricular tachycardia; and ventricular fibrillation. Digoxin produces PR prolongation and ST segment depression which should not by themselves be considered digoxin toxicity. Cardiac toxicity can also occur at therapeutic doses in patients who have conditions which may alter their sensitivity to digoxin (see WARNINGS and PRECAUTIONS).

Gastrointestinal: Digoxin may cause anorexia, nausea, vomiting, and diarrhea. Rarely, the use of digoxin has been associated with abdominal pain, intestinal ischemia, and hemorrhagic necrosis of the intestines.

CNS: Digoxin can produce visual disturbances (blurred or yellow vision), headache, weakness, dizziness, apathy, confusion, and mental disturbances (such as anxiety, depression, delirium, and hallucination).

Other: Gynecomastia has been occasionally observed following the prolonged use of digoxin. Thrombocytopenia and maculopapular rash and other skin reactions have been rarely observed.

The following table summarizes the incidence of those adverse experiences listed above for patients treated with LANOXIN Tablets or placebo from two randomized, double-blind, placebo-controlled withdrawal trials. Patients in these trials were also receiving diuretics with or without angiotensin-converting enzyme inhibitors. These patients had been stable on digoxin, and were randomized to digoxin or placebo. The results shown in Table 4 reflect the experience in patients following dosage titration with the use of serum digoxin concentrations and careful follow-up. These adverse experiences are consistent with results from a large, placebo-controlled mortality trial (DIG trial) wherein over half the patients were not receiving digoxin prior to enrollment. [See table 4 below]

Infants and Children: The side effects of digoxin in infants and children differ from those seen in adults in several respects. Although digoxin may produce anorexia, nausea, vomiting, diarrhea, and CNS disturbances in young patients, these are rarely the initial symptoms of overdosage. Rather, the earliest and most frequent manifestation of excessive dosing with digoxin in infants and children is the appearance of cardiac arrhythmias, including sinus bradycardia. In children, the use of digoxin may produce any arrhythmia. The most common are conduction disturbances or supraventricular tachyarrhythmias, such as atrial tachycardia (with or without block) and junctional (nodal) tachycardia. Ventricular arrhythmias are less common. Sinus bradycardia may be a sign of impending digoxin intoxication, especially in infants, even in the absence of first-degree heart block. Any arrhythmia or alteration in cardiac conduction that develops in a child taking digoxin should be assumed to be caused by digoxin, until further evaluation proves otherwise.

OVERDOSAGE

Treatment of Adverse Reactions Produced by Overdosage: Digoxin should be temporarily discontinued until the adverse reaction resolves. Every effort should also be made to correct factors that may contribute to the adverse reaction (such as electrolyte disturbances or concurrent medications). Once the adverse reaction has resolved, therapy with digoxin may be reinstituted, following a careful reassessment of dose.

Withdrawal of digoxin may be all that is required to treat the adverse reaction. However, when the primary manifestation of digoxin overdosage is a cardiac arrhythmia, additional therapy may be needed.

If the rhythm disturbance is a symptomatic bradyarrhythmia or heart block, consideration should be given to the reversal of toxicity with DIGIBIND® [Digoxin Immune Fab (Ovine)] (see below), the use of atropine, or the insertion of a temporary cardiac pacemaker. However, asymptomatic bradycardia or heart block related to digoxin may require only temporary withdrawal of the drug and cardiac monitoring of the patient.

If the rhythm disturbance is a ventricular arrhythmia, consideration should be given to the correction of electrolyte disorders, particularly if hypokalemia (see below) or hypomagnesemia is present. DIGIBIND is a specific antidote for digoxin and may be used to reverse potentially life-threatening ventricular arrhythmias due to digoxin overdosage.

Administration of Potassium: Every effort should be made to maintain the serum potassium concentration between 4.0 and 5.5 mmol/L. Potassium is usually administered orally, but when correction of the arrhythmia is urgent and the serum potassium concentration is low, potassium may be administered cautiously by the intravenous route. The electrocardiogram should be monitored for any evidence of potassium toxicity (e.g., peaking of T waves) and to observe the effect on the arrhythmia. Potassium salts may be dangerous in patients who manifest bradycardia or heart block due to digoxin (unless primarily related to supraventricular tachycardia) and in the setting of massive digitalis overdosage (see Massive Digitalis Overdosage subsection).

Massive Digitalis Overdosage: Manifestations of life-threatening toxicity include ventricular tachycardia or ventricular fibrillation, or progressive bradyarrhythmias or heart block. The administration of more than 10 mg of digoxin in a previously healthy adult, or more than 4 mg in a previously healthy child, or a steady-state serum concentration greater than 10 ng/mL often results in cardiac arrest.

DIGIBIND should be used to reverse the toxic effects of ingestion of a massive overdose. The decision to administer DIGIBIND to a patient who has ingested a massive dose of digoxin but who has not yet manifested life-threatening toxicity should depend on the likelihood that life-threatening toxicity will occur (see above).

Patients with massive digitalis ingestion should receive large doses of activated charcoal to prevent absorption and bind digoxin in the gut during enteroenteric recirculation. Emesis or gastric lavage may be indicated especially if ingestion has occurred within 30 minutes of the patient's presentation at the hospital. Emesis should not be induced in patients who are obtunded. If a patient presents more than 2 hours after ingestion or already has toxic manifestations, it may be unsafe to induce vomiting or attempt passage of a gastric tube, because such maneuvers may induce an acute vagal episode that can worsen digitalis-related arrhythmias.

Severe digitalis intoxication can cause a massive shift of potassium from inside to outside the cell, leading to life-threatening hyperkalemia. The administration of potassium supplements in the setting of massive intoxication may be hazardous and should be avoided. Hyperkalemia caused by massive digitalis toxicity is best treated with DIGIBIND; initial treatment with glucose and insulin may also be required if hyperkalemia itself is acutely life-threatening.

DOSAGE AND ADMINISTRATION

General: Recommended dosages of digoxin may require considerable modification because of individual sensitivity of the patient to the drug, the presence of associated conditions, or the use of concurrent medications.

Parenteral administration of digoxin should be used only when the need for rapid digitalization is urgent or when the drug cannot be taken orally. Intramuscular injection can lead to severe pain at the injection site, thus intravenous administration is preferred. If the drug must be administered by the intramuscular route, it should be injected deep into the muscle followed by massage. No more than 200 mcg (2 mL) should be injected into a single site.

LANOXIN Injection Pediatric can be administered undiluted or diluted with a 4-fold or greater volume of Sterile Water for Injection, 0.9% Sodium Chloride Injection, or 5% Dextrose Injection. The use of less than a 4-fold volume of diluent could lead to precipitation of the digoxin. Immediate use of the diluted product is recommended.

If tuberculin syringes are used to measure very small doses, one must be aware of the problem of inadvertent overadministration of digoxin. The syringe should *not* be flushed with the parenteral solution after its contents are expelled into an indwelling vascular catheter.

Slow infusion of LANOXIN Injection Pediatric is preferable to bolus administration. Rapid infusion of digitalis glycosides has been shown to cause systemic and coronary arteriolar constriction, which may be clinically undesirable. Caution is thus advised and LANOXIN Injection Pediatric should probably be administered over a period of 5 minutes or longer. Mixing of LANOXIN Injection Pediatric with other drugs in the same container or simultaneous administration in the same intravenous line is not recommended.

In selecting a dose of digoxin, the following factors must be considered:

1. The body weight of the patient. Doses should be calculated based upon lean (i.e., ideal) body weight.
2. The patient's renal function, preferably evaluated on the basis of estimated creatinine clearance.
3. The patient's age. Infants and children require different doses of digoxin than adults. Also, advanced age may be indicative of diminished renal function even in patients with normal serum creatinine concentration (i.e., below 1.5 mg/dL).
4. Concomitant disease states, concurrent medications, or other factors likely to alter the pharmacokinetic or pharmacodynamic profile of digoxin (see PRECAUTIONS).

Serum Digoxin Concentrations: In general, the dose of digoxin used should be determined on clinical grounds. However, measurement of serum digoxin concentrations can be helpful to the clinician in determining the adequacy of digoxin therapy and in assigning certain probabilities to the likelihood of digoxin intoxication. About two-thirds of adults considered adequately digitalized (without evidence of toxicity) have serum digoxin concentrations ranging from 0.8 to 2.0 ng/mL. However, digoxin may produce clinical benefits even at serum concentrations below this range. About two-thirds of adult patients with clinical toxicity have serum digoxin concentrations greater than 2.0 ng/mL. However, since one-third of patients with clinical toxicity have concentrations less than 2.0 ng/mL, values below 2.0 ng/mL do not rule out the possibility that a certain sign or symptom is related to digoxin therapy. Rarely, there are patients who are unable to tolerate digoxin at serum concentrations below 0.8 ng/mL. Consequently, the serum concentration of digoxin should always be interpreted in the overall clinical context, and an isolated measurement should not be used alone as the basis for increasing or decreasing the dose of the drug.

To allow adequate time for equilibration of digoxin between serum and tissue, sampling of serum concentrations should be done just before the next scheduled dose of the drug. If this is not possible, sampling should be done at least 6 to 8 hours after the last dose, regardless of the route of administration or the formulation used. On a once-daily dosing schedule, the concentration of digoxin will be 10% to 25% lower when sampled at 24 versus 8 hours, depending upon the patient's renal function. On a twice-daily dosing schedule, there will be only minor differences in serum digoxin concentrations whether sampling is done at 8 or 12 hours after a dose.

If a discrepancy exists between the reported serum concentration and the observed clinical response, the clinician should consider the following possibilities:

1. Analytical problems in the assay procedure.
2. Inappropriate serum sampling time.
3. Administration of a digitalis glycoside other than digoxin.
4. Conditions (described in WARNINGS and PRECAUTIONS) causing an alteration in the sensitivity of the patient to digoxin.
5. Serum digoxin concentration may decrease acutely during periods of exercise without any associated change in clinical efficacy due to increased binding of digoxin to skeletal muscle.

Heart Failure: *Adults:* See the full prescribing information for LANOXIN Injection for specific recommendations.

Infants and Children: In general, divided daily dosing is recommended for infants and young children (under age 10). In the newborn period, renal clearance of digoxin is diminished and suitable dosage adjustments must be observed. This is especially pronounced in the premature infant. Beyond the immediate newborn period, children generally require proportionally larger doses than adults on the basis of body weight or body surface area. Children over 10 years of age require adult dosages in proportion to their body weight. Some researchers have suggested that infants

Table 4. Adverse Experiences in Two Parallel, Double-Blind, Placebo-Controlled Withdrawal Trials (Number of Patients Reporting)

Adverse Experience	Digoxin Patients (n = 123)	Placebo Patients (n = 125)
Cardiac		
Palpitation	1	4
Ventricular extrasystole	1	1
Tachycardia	2	1
Heart arrest	1	1
Gastrointestinal		
Anorexia	1	4
Nausea	4	2
Vomiting	2	1
Diarrhea	4	1
Abdominal pain	0	6
CNS		
Headache	4	4
Dizziness	6	5
Mental disturbances	5	1
Other		
Rash	2	1
Death	4	3

Table 5. Usual Digitalizing and Maintenance Dosages for LANOXIN® Injection Pediatric in Children with Normal Renal Function Based on Lean Body Weight

Age	IV Digitalizing* Dose (mcg/kg)	Daily IV Maintenance Dose† (mcg/kg)
Premature	15 to 25	20% to 30% of the IV digitalizing dose‡
Full-Term	20 to 30	
1 to 24 Months	30 to 50	
2 to 5 Years	25 to 35	25% to 35% of the IV digitalizing dose‡
5 to 10 Years	15 to 30	
Over 10 Years	8 to 12	

*IV digitalizing doses are 80% of oral digitalizing doses.
†Divided daily dosing is recommended for children under 10 years of age.
‡Projected or actual digitalizing dose providing clinical response.

and young children tolerate slightly higher serum concentrations than do adults.

Digitalization may be accomplished by either of two general approaches that vary in dosage and frequency of administration, but reach the same endpoint in terms of total amount of digoxin accumulated in the body.

1. If rapid digitalization is considered medically appropriate, it may be achieved by administering a loading dose based upon projected peak digoxin body stores. Maintenance dose can be calculated as a percentage of the loading dose.
2. More gradual digitalization may be obtained by beginning an appropriate maintenance dose, thus allowing digoxin body stores to accumulate slowly. Steady-state serum digoxin concentrations will be achieved in approximately five half-lives of the drug for the individual patient. Depending upon the patient's renal function, this will take between 1 and 3 weeks.

Rapid Digitalization with a Loading Dose: LANOXIN Injection Pediatric can be used to achieve rapid digitalization, with conversion to an oral formulation of LANOXIN for maintenance therapy. If patients are switched from intravenous to oral digoxin formulations, allowances must be made for differences in bioavailability when calculating maintenance dosages (see Table 1 in CLINICAL PHARMACOLOGY: Pharmacokinetics and dosing Table 5).

Intramuscular injection of digoxin is extremely painful and offers no advantages unless other routes of administration are contraindicated.

Peak digoxin body stores of 8 to 12 mcg/kg should provide therapeutic effect with minimum risk of toxicity in most patients with heart failure and normal sinus rhythm. Because of altered digoxin distribution and elimination, projected peak body stores for patients with renal insufficiency should be conservative (i.e., 6 to 10 mcg/kg) [see PRECAUTIONS].

Digitalizing and daily maintenance doses for each age group are given in Table 5 and should provide therapeutic effect with minimum risk of toxicity in most patients with heart failure and normal sinus rhythm. These recommendations assume the presence of normal renal function.

The loading dose should be administered in several portions, with roughly half the total given as the first dose. Additional fractions of this planned total dose may be given at 4- to 8-hour intervals, **with careful assessment of clinical response before each additional dose.** If the patient's clinical response necessitates a change from the calculated loading dose of digoxin, then calculation of the maintenance dose should be based upon the amount actually given.

[See table 5 above]

In children with renal disease, digoxin dosing must be carefully titrated based on clinical response.

Gradual Digitalization With A Maintenance Dose: More gradual digitalization can also be accomplished by beginning an appropriate maintenance dose. The range of percentages provided in Table 5 can be used in calculating this dose for patients with normal renal function.

It cannot be overemphasized that these pediatric dosage guidelines are based upon average patient response and substantial individual variation can be expected. Accordingly, ultimate dosage selection must be based upon clinical assessment of the patient.

Atrial Fibrillation: Peak digoxin body stores larger than the 8 to 12 mcg/kg required for most patients with heart failure and normal sinus rhythm have been used for control of ventricular rate in patients with atrial fibrillation. Doses of digoxin used for the treatment of chronic atrial fibrillation should be titrated to the minimum dose that achieves the desired ventricular rate control without causing undesirable side effects. Data are not available to establish the appropriate resting or exercise target rates that should be achieved.

Dosage Adjustment When Changing Preparations: The differences in bioavailability between injectable LANOXIN or LANOXICAPS and LANOXIN Elixir Pediatric or LANOXIN Tablets must be considered when changing patients from one dosage form to another.

Doses of 100 mcg (0.1 mg) and 200 mcg (0.2 mg) of LANOXICAPS are approximately equivalent to 125 mcg (0.125 mg) and 250 mcg (0.25 mg) doses of LANOXIN Tablets and Elixir Pediatric, respectively (see Table 1 in CLINICAL PHARMACOLOGY: Pharmacokinetics).

HOW SUPPLIED

LANOXIN (digoxin) Injection Pediatric, 100 mcg (0.1 mg) in 1 mL; box of 10 ampuls (NDC 0173-0262-10).

Store at 25°C (77°F); excursions permitted to 15 to 30°C (59 to 86°F) [see USP Controlled Room Temperature] and protect from light.

Manufactured by DSM Pharmaceuticals, Inc.
Greenville, NC 27834 for
GlaxoSmithKline, Research Triangle Park, NC 27709

July 2002/RL-1128

Shown in Product Identification Guide, page 316

LANOXIN® ℞

[lă-nŏx ′ in]
(digoxin)
Tablets, USP
125 mcg (0.125 mg) Scored I.D. Imprint Y3B (yellow)
250 mcg (0.25 mg) Scored I.D. Imprint X3A (white)

DESCRIPTION

LANOXIN (digoxin) is one of the cardiac (or digitalis) glycosides, a closely related group of drugs having in common specific effects on the myocardium. These drugs are found in a number of plants. Digoxin is extracted from the leaves of *Digitalis lanata*. The term "digitalis" is used to designate the whole group of glycosides. The glycosides are composed of two portions: a sugar and a cardenolide (hence "glycosides").

Digoxin is described chemically as (3β,5β,12β)-3-[(*O*-2,6-dideoxy-β-*D*-*ribo*-hexopyranosyl-(1→4)-*O*-2,6-dideoxy-β-*D*-*ribo*-hexopyranosyl-(1→4)-2,6-dideoxy-β-*D*-*ribo*-hexopyranosyl)oxy]-12,14-dihydroxy-card-20(22)-enolide. Its molecular formula is $C_{41}H_{64}O_{14}$, its molecular weight is 780.95.

Digoxin exists as odorless white crystals that melt with decomposition above 230°C. The drug is practically insoluble in water and in ether; slightly soluble in diluted (50%) alcohol and in chloroform; and freely soluble in pyridine.

LANOXIN is supplied as 125-mcg (0.125-mg) or 250-mcg (0.25-mg) tablets for oral administration. Each tablet contains the labeled amount of digoxin USP and the following inactive ingredients: corn and potato starches, lactose, and magnesium stearate. In addition, the dyes used in the 125-mcg (0.125-mg) tablets are D&C Yellow No. 10 and FD&C Yellow No. 6.

CLINICAL PHARMACOLOGY

Mechanism of Action: Digoxin inhibits sodium-potassium ATPase, an enzyme that regulates the quantity of sodium and potassium inside cells. Inhibition of the enzyme leads to an increase in the intracellular concentration of sodium and thus (by stimulation of sodium-calcium exchange) an increase in the intracellular concentration of calcium. The beneficial effects of digoxin result from direct actions on cardiac muscle, as well as indirect actions on the cardiovascular system mediated by effects on the autonomic nervous system. The autonomic effects include: (1) a vagomimetic action, which is responsible for the effects of digoxin on the sinoatrial and atrioventricular (AV) nodes; and (2) baroreceptor sensitization, which results in increased afferent inhibitory activity and reduced activity of the sympathetic nervous system and renin-angiotensin system for any given increment in mean arterial pressure. The pharmacologic consequences of these direct and indirect effects are: (1) an increase in the force and velocity of myocardial systolic contraction (positive inotropic action); (2) a decrease in the degree of activation of the sympathetic nervous system and renin-angiotensin system (neurohormonal deactivating effect); and (3) slowing of the heart rate and decreased conduction velocity through the AV node (vagomimetic effect). The effects of digoxin in heart failure are mediated by its positive inotropic and neurohormonal deactivating effects, whereas the effects of the drug in atrial arrhythmias are related to its vagomimetic actions. In high doses, digoxin increases sympathetic outflow from the central nervous system (CNS). This increase in sympathetic activity may be an important factor in digitalis toxicity.

Pharmacokinetics: ***Absorption:*** Following oral administration, peak serum concentrations of digoxin occur at 1 to 3 hours. Absorption of digoxin from LANOXIN Tablets has been demonstrated to be 60% to 80% complete compared to an identical intravenous dose of digoxin (absolute bioavailability) or LANOXICAPS® (relative bioavailability). When LANOXIN Tablets are taken after meals, the rate of absorption is slowed, but the total amount of digoxin absorbed is usually unchanged. When taken with meals high in bran fiber, however, the amount absorbed from an oral dose may be reduced. Comparisons of the systemic availability and equivalent doses for oral preparations of LANOXIN are shown in Table 1.

[See table 1 at top of next page]

In some patients, orally administered digoxin is converted to inactive reduction products (e.g., dihydrodigoxin) by colonic bacteria in the gut. Data suggest that one in ten patients treated with digoxin tablets will degrade 40% or more of the ingested dose. As a result, certain antibiotics may increase the absorption of digoxin in such patients. Although inactivation of these bacteria by antibiotics is rapid, the serum digoxin concentration will rise at a rate consistent with the elimination half-life of digoxin. The magnitude of rise in serum digoxin concentration relates to the extent of bacterial inactivation, and may be as much as two-fold in some cases.

Distribution: Following drug administration, a 6- to 8-hour tissue distribution phase is observed. This is followed by a much more gradual decline in the serum concentration of the drug, which is dependent on the elimination of digoxin from the body. The peak height and slope of the early portion (absorption/distribution phases) of the serum concentration-time curve are dependent upon the route of administration and the absorption characteristics of the formulation. Clinical evidence indicates that the early high serum concentrations do not reflect the concentration of digoxin at its site of action, but that with chronic use, the steady-state post-distribution serum concentrations are in equilibrium with tissue concentrations and correlate with pharmacologic effects. In individual patients, these post-distribution serum concentrations may be useful in evaluating therapeutic and toxic effects (see DOSAGE AND ADMINISTRATION: Serum Digoxin Concentrations).

Digoxin is concentrated in tissues and therefore has a large apparent volume of distribution. Digoxin crosses both the blood-brain barrier and the placenta. At delivery, the serum digoxin concentration in the newborn is similar to the serum concentration in the mother. Approximately 25% of digoxin in the plasma is bound to protein. Serum digoxin concentrations are not significantly altered by large changes in fat tissue weight, so that its distribution space correlates best with lean (i.e., ideal) body weight, not total body weight.

Metabolism: Only a small percentage (16%) of a dose of digoxin is metabolized. The end metabolites, which include 3 β-digoxigenin, 3-keto-digoxigenin, and their glucuronide and sulfate conjugates, are polar in nature and are postulated to be formed via hydrolysis, oxidation, and conjugation. The metabolism of digoxin is not dependent upon the cytochrome P-450 system, and digoxin is not known to induce or inhibit the cytochrome P-450 system.

Excretion: Elimination of digoxin follows first-order kinetics (that is, the quantity of digoxin eliminated at any time is proportional to the total body content). Following intravenous administration to healthy volunteers, 50% to 70% of a digoxin dose is excreted unchanged in the urine. Renal excretion of digoxin is proportional to glomerular filtration rate and is largely independent of urine flow. In healthy volunteers with normal renal function, digoxin has a half-life of 1.5 to 2.0 days. The half-life in anuric patients is prolonged to 3.5 to 5 days. Digoxin is not effectively removed from the body by dialysis, exchange transfusion, or during cardiopulmonary bypass because most of the drug is bound to tissue and does not circulate in the blood.

Special Populations: Race differences in digoxin pharmacokinetics have not been formally studied. Because digoxin is primarily eliminated as unchanged drug via the kidney and because there are no important differences in creatinine clearance among races, pharmacokinetic differences due to race are not expected.

The clearance of digoxin can be primarily correlated with renal function as indicated by creatinine clearance. The Cockcroft and Gault formula for estimation of creatinine clearance includes age, body weight, and gender. Table 5 that provides the usual daily maintenance dose requirements of LANOXIN Tablets based on creatinine clearance (per 70 kg) is presented in the DOSAGE AND ADMINISTRATION section.

Plasma digoxin concentration profiles in patients with acute hepatitis generally fell within the range of profiles in a group of healthy subjects.

Pharmacodynamic and Clinical Effects: The times to onset of pharmacologic effect and to peak effect of preparations of LANOXIN are shown in Table 2.

[See table 2 at top of next page]

Hemodynamic Effects: Digoxin produces hemodynamic improvement in patients with heart failure. Short- and long-term therapy with the drug increases cardiac output and lowers pulmonary artery pressure, pulmonary capillary wedge pressure, and systemic vascular resistance. These hemodynamic effects are accompanied by an increase in the left ventricular ejection fraction and a decrease in end-systolic and end-diastolic dimensions.

Chronic Heart Failure: Two 12-week, double-blind, placebo-controlled studies enrolled 178 (RADIANCE trial) and 88

Continued on next page

Product information on these pages is effective as of August 2004. Further information is available at: GlaxoSmithKline, PO Box 13398, Research Triangle Park, NC 27709. 1-888-825-5249. Corporate Web Site: www.gsk.com

Lanoxin Tablets—Cont.

(PROVED trial) patients with NYHA class II or III heart failure previously treated with digoxin, a diuretic, and an ACE inhibitor (RADIANCE only) and randomized them to placebo or treatment with LANOXIN. Both trials demonstrated better preservation of exercise capacity in patients randomized to LANOXIN. Continued treatment with LANOXIN reduced the risk of developing worsening heart failure, as evidenced by heart failure-related hospitalizations and emergency care and the need for concomitant heart failure therapy. The larger study also showed treatment-related benefits in NYHA class and patients' global assessment. In the smaller trial, these trended in favor of a treatment benefit.

The Digitalis Investigation Group (DIG) main trial was a multicenter, randomized, double-blind, placebo-controlled mortality study of 6801 patients with heart failure and left ventricular ejection fraction ≤0.45. At randomization, 67% were NYHA class I or II, 71% had heart failure of ischemic etiology, 44% had been receiving digoxin, and most were receiving concomitant ACE inhibitor (94%) and diuretic (82%). Patients were randomized to placebo or LANOXIN, the dose of which was adjusted for the patient's age, sex, lean body weight, and serum creatinine (see DOSAGE AND ADMINISTRATION), and followed for up to 58 months (median 37 months). The median daily dose prescribed was 0.25 mg. Overall all-cause mortality was 35% with no difference between groups (95% confidence limits for relative risk of 0.91 to 1.07). LANOXIN was associated with a 25% reduction in the number of hospitalizations for heart failure, a 28% reduction in the risk of a patient having at least one hospitalization for heart failure, and a 6.5% reduction in total hospitalizations (for any cause).

Use of LANOXIN was associated with a trend to increase time to all-cause death or hospitalization. The trend was evident in subgroups of patients with mild heart failure as well as more severe disease, as shown in Table 3. Although the effect on all-cause death or hospitalization was not statistically significant, much of the apparent benefit derived from effects on mortality and hospitalization attributed to heart failure.

[See table 3 at right]

In situations where there is no statistically significant benefit of treatment evident from a trial's primary endpoint, results pertaining to a secondary endpoint should be interpreted cautiously.

Chronic Atrial Fibrillation: In patients with chronic atrial fibrillation, digoxin slows rapid ventricular response rate in a linear dose-response fashion from 0.25 to 0.75 mg/day. Digoxin should not be used for the treatment of multifocal atrial tachycardia.

INDICATIONS AND USAGE

Heart Failure: LANOXIN is indicated for the treatment of mild to moderate heart failure. LANOXIN increases left ventricular ejection fraction and improves heart failure symptoms as evidenced by exercise capacity and heart failure-related hospitalizations and emergency care, while having no effect on mortality. Where possible, LANOXIN should be used with a diuretic and an angiotensin-converting enzyme inhibitor, but an optimal order for starting these three drugs cannot be specified.

Atrial Fibrillation: LANOXIN is indicated for the control of ventricular response rate in patients with chronic atrial fibrillation.

CONTRAINDICATIONS

Digitalis glycosides are contraindicated in patients with ventricular fibrillation or in patients with a known hypersensitivity to digoxin. A hypersensitivity reaction to other digitalis preparations usually constitutes a contraindication to digoxin.

WARNINGS

Sinus Node Disease and AV Block: Because digoxin slows sinoatrial and AV conduction, the drug commonly prolongs the PR interval. The drug may cause severe sinus bradycardia or sinoatrial block in patients with pre-existing sinus node disease and may cause advanced or complete heart block in patients with pre-existing incomplete AV block. In such patients consideration should be given to the insertion of a pacemaker before treatment with digoxin.

Accessory AV Pathway (Wolff-Parkinson-White Syndrome): After intravenous digoxin therapy, some patients with paroxysmal atrial fibrillation or flutter and a coexisting accessory AV pathway have developed increased antegrade conduction across the accessory pathway bypassing the AV node, leading to a very rapid ventricular response or ventricular fibrillation. Unless conduction down the accessory pathway has been blocked (either pharmacologically or by surgery), digoxin should not be used in such patients. The treatment of paroxysmal supraventricular tachycardia in such patients is usually direct-current cardioversion.

Use in Patients with Preserved Left Ventricular Systolic Function: Patients with certain disorders involving heart failure associated with preserved left ventricular ejection fraction may be particularly susceptible to toxicity of the drug. Such disorders include restrictive cardiomyopathy, constrictive pericarditis, amyloid heart disease, and acute cor pulmonale. Patients with idiopathic hypertrophic subaortic stenosis may have worsening of the outflow obstruction due to the inotropic effects of digoxin.

Table 1: Comparisons of the Systemic Availability and Equivalent Doses for Oral Preparations of LANOXIN

Product	Absolute Bioavailability	Equivalent Doses (mcg)* Among Dosage Forms			
LANOXIN Tablets	60–80%	62.5	125	250	500
LANOXIN Elixir Pediatric	70–85%	62.5	125	250	500
LANOXICAPS®	90–100%	50	100	200	400
LANOXIN Injection/IV	100%	50	100	200	400

*For example, 125-mcg LANOXIN Tablets equivalent to 125-mcg LANOXIN Elixir Pediatric equivalent to 100-mcg LANOXICAPS equivalent to 100-mcg LANOXIN Injection/IV.

Table 2: Times to Onset of Pharmacologic Effect and to Peak Effect of Preparations of LANOXIN

Product	Time to Onset of Effect*	Time to Peak Effect*
LANOXIN Tablets	0.5–2 hours	2–6 hours
LANOXIN Elixir Pediatric	0.5–2 hours	2–6 hours
LANOXICAPS	0.5–2 hours	2–6 hours
LANOXIN Injection/IV	5–30 minutes†	1–4 hours

* Documented for ventricular response rate in atrial fibrillation, inotropic effects and electrocardiographic changes.
† Depending upon rate of infusion.

Table 3: Subgroup Analyses of Mortality and Hospitalization During the First Two Years Following Randomization

	n	Risk of All-Cause Mortality or All-Cause Hospitalization*: Placebo	LANOXIN	Relative risk†	Risk of HF-Related Mortality or HF-Related Hospitalization*: Placebo	LANOXIN	Relative risk†
All patients (EF ≤0.45)	6801	604	593	0.94 (0.88–1.00)	294	217	0.69 (0.63–0.76)
NYHA I/II	4571	549	541	0.96 (0.89–1.04)	242	178	0.70 (0.62–0.80)
EF 0.25–0.45	4543	568	571	0.99 (0.91–1.07)	244	190	0.74 (0.66–0.84)
CTR ≤0.55	4455	561	563	0.98 (0.91–1.06)	239	180	0.71 (0.63–0.81)
NYHA III/IV	2224	719	696	0.88 (0.80–0.97)	402	295	0.65 (0.57–0.75)
EF <0.25	2258	677	637	0.84 (0.76–0.93)	394	270	0.61 (0.53–0.71)
CTR >0.55	2346	687	650	0.85 (0.77–0.94)	398	287	0.65 (0.57–0.75)
EF >0.45‡	987	571	585	1.04 (0.88–1.23)	179	136	0.72 (0.53–0.99)

* Number of patients with an event during the first 2 years per 1000 randomized patients.
† Relative risk (95% confidence interval).
‡ DIG Ancillary Study.

PRECAUTIONS

Use in Patients with Impaired Renal Function: Digoxin is primarily excreted by the kidneys; therefore, patients with impaired renal function require smaller than usual maintenance doses of digoxin (see DOSAGE AND ADMINISTRATION). Because of the prolonged elimination half-life, a longer period of time is required to achieve an initial or new steady-state serum concentration in patients with renal impairment than in patients with normal renal function. If appropriate care is not taken to reduce the dose of digoxin, such patients are at high risk for toxicity, and toxic effects will last longer in such patients than in patients with normal renal function.

Use in Patients with Electrolyte Disorders: In patients with hypokalemia or hypomagnesemia, toxicity may occur despite serum digoxin concentrations below 2.0 ng/mL, because potassium or magnesium depletion sensitizes the myocardium to digoxin. Therefore, it is desirable to maintain normal serum potassium and magnesium concentrations in patients being treated with digoxin. Deficiencies of these electrolytes may result from malnutrition, diarrhea, or prolonged vomiting, as well as the use of the following drugs or procedures: diuretics, amphotericin B, corticosteroids, antacids, dialysis, and mechanical suction of gastrointestinal secretions.

Hypercalcemia from any cause predisposes the patient to digitalis toxicity. Calcium, particularly when administered rapidly by the intravenous route, may produce serious arrhythmias in digitalized patients. On the other hand, hypocalcemia can nullify the effects of digoxin in humans; thus, digoxin may be ineffective until serum calcium is restored to normal. These interactions are related to the fact that digoxin affects contractility and excitability of the heart in a manner similar to that of calcium.

Use in Thyroid Disorders and Hypermetabolic States: Hypothyroidism may reduce the requirements for digoxin. Heart failure and/or atrial arrhythmias resulting from hypermetabolic or hyperdynamic states (e.g., hyperthyroidism, hypoxia, or arteriovenous shunt) are best treated by addressing the underlying condition. Atrial arrhythmias associated with hypermetabolic states are particularly resistant to digoxin treatment. Care must be taken to avoid toxicity if digoxin is used.

Use in Patients with Acute Myocardial Infarction: Digoxin should be used with caution in patients with acute myocardial infarction. The use of inotropic drugs in some patients in this setting may result in undesirable increases in myocardial oxygen demand and ischemia.

Use During Electrical Cardioversion: It may be desirable to reduce the dose of digoxin for 1 to 2 days prior to electrical cardioversion of atrial fibrillation to avoid the induction of ventricular arrhythmias, but physicians must consider the consequences of increasing the ventricular response if digoxin is withdrawn. If digitalis toxicity is suspected, elective cardioversion should be delayed. If it is not prudent to delay cardioversion, the lowest possible energy level should be selected to avoid provoking ventricular arrhythmias.

Laboratory Test Monitoring: Patients receiving digoxin should have their serum electrolytes and renal function (serum creatinine concentrations) assessed periodically; the frequency of assessments will depend on the clinical setting. For discussion of serum digoxin concentrations, see DOSAGE AND ADMINISTRATION section.

Drug Interactions: Potassium-depleting *diuretics* are a major contributing factor to digitalis toxicity. *Calcium*, particularly if administered rapidly by the intravenous route, may produce serious arrhythmias in digitalized patients. *Quinidine, verapamil, amiodarone, propafenone, indomethacin, itraconazole, alprazolam,* and *spironolactone* raise the serum digoxin concentration due to a reduction in clearance and/or in volume of distribution of the drug, with the implication that digitalis intoxication may result. *Erythromycin* and *clarithromycin* (and possibly other *macrolide antibiotics*) and *tetracycline* may increase digoxin absorption in patients who inactivate digoxin by bacterial metabolism in the lower intestine, so that digitalis intoxication may result (see CLINICAL PHARMACOLOGY: Absorption). *Propantheline* and *diphenoxylate*, by decreasing gut motility, may increase digoxin absorption. *Antacids, kaolin-pectin, sulfasalazine, neomycin, cholestyramine,* certain *anticancer drugs*, and *metoclopramide* may interfere with intestinal digoxin absorption, resulting in unexpectedly low serum concentrations. *Rifampin* may decrease serum digoxin concentration, especially in patients with renal dysfunction, by increasing the non-renal clearance of digoxin. There have been inconsistent reports regarding the effects of other drugs [e.g., *quinine, penicillamine*] on serum digoxin concentration. *Thyroid* administration to a digitalized, hypothyroid patient may increase the dose requirement of digoxin. Concomitant use of digoxin and *sympathomimetics* increases the risk of cardiac arrhythmias. *Succinylcholine* may cause a sudden extrusion of potassium from muscle cells, and may thereby cause arrhythmias in digitalized patients. Although beta-adrenergic blockers or calcium channel blockers and digoxin may be useful in combination to control atrial fibrillation, their additive effects on AV node conduction can result in advanced or complete heart block.

Due to the considerable variability of these interactions, the dosage of digoxin should be individualized when patients receive these medications concurrently. Furthermore, caution should be exercised when combining digoxin with any drug that may cause a significant deterioration in renal function, since a decline in glomerular filtration or tubular secretion may impair the excretion of digoxin.

Drug/Laboratory Test Interactions: The use of therapeutic doses of digoxin may cause prolongation of the PR interval and depression of the ST segment on the electrocardiogram. Digoxin may produce false positive ST-T changes on the electrocardiogram during exercise testing. These electrophysiologic effects reflect an expected effect of the drug and are not indicative of toxicity.

Carcinogenesis, Mutagenesis, Impairment of Fertility: There have been no long-term studies performed in animals to evaluate carcinogenic potential, nor have studies been conducted to assess the mutagenic potential of digoxin or its potential to affect fertility.

Pregnancy: ***Teratogenic Effects:*** Pregnancy Category C. Animal reproduction studies have not been conducted with digoxin. It is also not known whether digoxin can cause fetal harm when administered to a pregnant woman or can affect reproductive capacity. Digoxin should be given to a pregnant woman only if clearly needed.

Nursing Mothers: Studies have shown that digoxin concentrations in the mother's serum and milk are similar. However, the estimated exposure of a nursing infant to digoxin via breast feeding will be far below the usual infant maintenance dose. Therefore, this amount should have no pharmacologic effect upon the infant. Nevertheless, caution should be exercised when digoxin is administered to a nursing woman.

Pediatric Use: Newborn infants display considerable variability in their tolerance to digoxin. Premature and immature infants are particularly sensitive to the effects of digoxin, and the dosage of the drug must not only be reduced but must be individualized according to their degree of maturity. Digitalis glycosides can cause poisoning in children due to accidental ingestion.

Geriatric Use: The majority of clinical experience gained with digoxin has been in the elderly population. This experience has not identified differences in response or adverse effects between the elderly and younger patients. However, this drug is known to be substantially excreted by the kidney, and the risk of toxic reactions to this drug may be greater in patients with impaired renal function. Because elderly patients are more likely to have decreased renal function, care should be taken in dose selection, which should be based on renal function, and it may be useful to monitor renal function (see DOSAGE AND ADMINISTRATION).

ADVERSE REACTIONS

In general, the adverse reactions of digoxin are dose-dependent and occur at doses higher than those needed to achieve a therapeutic effect. Hence, adverse reactions are less common when digoxin is used within the recommended dose range or therapeutic serum concentration range and when there is careful attention to concurrent medications and conditions.

Because some patients may be particularly susceptible to side effects with digoxin, the dosage of the drug should always be selected carefully and adjusted as the clinical condition of the patient warrants. In the past, when high doses of digoxin were used and little attention was paid to clinical status or concurrent medications, adverse reactions to digoxin were more frequent and severe. Cardiac adverse reactions accounted for about one-half, gastrointestinal disturbances for about one-fourth, and CNS and other toxicity for about one-fourth of these adverse reactions. However, available evidence suggests that the incidence and severity of digoxin toxicity has decreased substantially in recent years. In recent controlled clinical trials, in patients with predominantly mild to moderate heart failure, the incidence of adverse experiences was comparable in patients taking digoxin and in those taking placebo. In a large mortality trial, the incidence of hospitalization for suspected digoxin toxicity was 2% in patients taking LANOXIN compared to 0.9% in patients taking placebo. In this trial, the most common manifestations of digoxin toxicity included gastrointestinal and cardiac disturbances; CNS manifestations were less common.

Adults: ***Cardiac:*** Therapeutic doses of digoxin may cause heart block in patients with pre-existing sinoatrial or AV conduction disorders; heart block can be avoided by adjusting the dose of digoxin. Prophylactic use of a cardiac pacemaker may be considered if the risk of heart block is considered unacceptable. High doses of digoxin may produce a variety of rhythm disturbances, such as first-degree, second-degree (Wenckebach), or third-degree heart block (including asystole); atrial tachycardia with block; AV dissociation; accelerated junctional (nodal) rhythm; unifocal or multiform ventricular premature contractions (especially bigeminy or trigeminy); ventricular tachycardia; and ventricular fibrillation. Digoxin produces PR prolongation and ST segment depression which should not by themselves be considered digoxin toxicity. Cardiac toxicity can also occur at therapeutic doses in patients who have conditions which may alter their sensitivity to digoxin (see WARNINGS and PRECAUTIONS).

Gastrointestinal: Digoxin may cause anorexia, nausea, vomiting, and diarrhea. Rarely, the use of digoxin has been associated with abdominal pain, intestinal ischemia, and hemorrhagic necrosis of the intestines.

CNS: Digoxin can produce visual disturbances (blurred or yellow vision), headache, weakness, dizziness, apathy, confusion, and mental disturbances (such as anxiety, depression, delirium, and hallucination).

Other: Gynecomastia has been occasionally observed following the prolonged use of digoxin. Thrombocytopenia and maculopapular rash and other skin reactions have been rarely observed.

Table 4 summarizes the incidence of those adverse experiences listed above for patients treated with LANOXIN Tablets or placebo from two randomized, double-blind, placebo-controlled withdrawal trials. Patients in these trials were also receiving diuretics with or without angiotensin-converting enzyme inhibitors. These patients had been stable on digoxin, and were randomized to digoxin or placebo. The results shown in Table 4 reflect the experience in patients following dosage titration with the use of serum digoxin concentrations and careful follow-up. These adverse experiences are consistent with results from a large, placebo-controlled mortality trial (DIG trial) wherein over half the patients were not receiving digoxin prior to enrollment.

Table 4: Adverse Experiences In Two Parallel, Double-Blind, Placebo-Controlled Withdrawal Trials (Number of Patients Reporting)

Adverse Experience	Digoxin Patients (n = 123)	Placebo Patients (n = 125)
Cardiac		
Palpitation	1	4
Ventricular extrasystole	1	1
Tachycardia	2	1
Heart arrest	1	1
Gastrointestinal		
Anorexia	1	4
Nausea	4	2
Vomiting	2	1
Diarrhea	4	1
Abdominal pain	0	6
CNS		
Headache	4	4
Dizziness	6	5
Mental disturbances	5	1
Other		
Rash	2	1
Death	4	3

Infants and Children: The side effects of digoxin in infants and children differ from those seen in adults in several respects. Although digoxin may produce anorexia, nausea, vomiting, diarrhea, and CNS disturbances in young patients, these are rarely the initial symptoms of overdosage. Rather, the earliest and most frequent manifestation of excessive dosing with digoxin in infants and children is the appearance of cardiac arrhythmias, including sinus bradycardia. In children, the use of digoxin may produce any arrhythmia. The most common are conduction disturbances or supraventricular tachyarrhythmias, such as atrial tachycardia (with or without block) and junctional (nodal) tachycardia. Ventricular arrhythmias are less common. Sinus bradycardia may be a sign of impending digoxin intoxication, especially in infants, even in the absence of first-degree heart block. Any arrhythmia or alteration in cardiac conduction that develops in a child taking digoxin should be assumed to be caused by digoxin, until further evaluation proves otherwise.

OVERDOSAGE

Treatment of Adverse Reactions Produced by Overdosage: Digoxin should be temporarily discontinued until the adverse reaction resolves. Every effort should also be made to correct factors that may contribute to the adverse reaction (such as electrolyte disturbances or concurrent medications). Once the adverse reaction has resolved, therapy with digoxin may be reinstituted, following a careful reassessment of dose.

Withdrawal of digoxin may be all that is required to treat the adverse reaction. However, when the primary manifestation of digoxin overdosage is a cardiac arrhythmia, additional therapy may be needed.

If the rhythm disturbance is a symptomatic bradyarrhythmia or heart block, consideration should be given to the reversal of toxicity with DIGIBIND® [Digoxin Immune Fab (Ovine)] (see Massive Digitalis Overdosage subsection), the use of atropine, or the insertion of a temporary cardiac pacemaker. However, asymptomatic bradycardia or heart block related to digoxin may require only temporary withdrawal of the drug and cardiac monitoring of the patient.

If the rhythm disturbance is a ventricular arrhythmia, consideration should be given to the correction of electrolyte disorders, particularly if hypokalemia (see Administration of Potassium subsection) or hypomagnesemia is present. DIGIBIND is a specific antidote for digoxin and may be used to reverse potentially life-threatening ventricular arrhythmias due to digoxin overdosage.

Administration of Potassium: Every effort should be made to maintain the serum potassium concentration between 4.0 and 5.5 mmol/L. Potassium is usually administered orally, but when correction of the arrhythmia is urgent and the serum potassium concentration is low, potassium may be administered cautiously by the intravenous route. The electrocardiogram should be monitored for any evidence of potassium toxicity (e.g., peaking of T waves) and to observe the effect on the arrhythmia. Potassium salts may be dangerous in patients who manifest bradycardia or heart block due to digoxin (unless primarily related to supraventricular tachycardia) and in the setting of massive digitalis overdosage (see Massive Digitalis Overdosage subsection).

Massive Digitalis Overdosage: Manifestations of life-threatening toxicity include ventricular tachycardia or ventricular fibrillation, or progressive bradyarrhythmias, or heart block. The administration of more than 10 mg of digoxin in a previously healthy adult, or more than 4 mg in a previously healthy child, or a steady-state serum concentration greater than 10 ng/mL often results in cardiac arrest.

DIGIBIND should be used to reverse the toxic effects of ingestion of a massive overdose. The decision to administer DIGIBIND to a patient who has ingested a massive dose of digoxin but who has not yet manifested life-threatening toxicity should depend on the likelihood that life-threatening toxicity will occur (see above).

Patients with massive digitalis ingestion should receive large doses of activated charcoal to prevent absorption and bind digoxin in the gut during enteroenteric recirculation. Emesis or gastric lavage may be indicated especially if ingestion has occurred within 30 minutes of the patient's presentation at the hospital. Emesis should not be induced in patients who are obtunded. If a patient presents more than 2 hours after ingestion or already has toxic manifestations, it may be unsafe to induce vomiting or attempt passage of a gastric tube, because such maneuvers may induce an acute vagal episode that can worsen digitalis-related arrhythmias.

Severe digitalis intoxication can cause a massive shift of potassium from inside to outside the cell, leading to life-threatening hyperkalemia. The administration of potassium supplements in the setting of massive intoxication may be hazardous and should be avoided. Hyperkalemia caused by massive digitalis toxicity is best treated with DIGIBIND; initial treatment with glucose and insulin may also be required if hyperkalemia itself is acutely life-threatening.

DOSAGE AND ADMINISTRATION

General: Recommended dosages of digoxin may require considerable modification because of individual sensitivity of the patient to the drug, the presence of associated conditions, or the use of concurrent medications. In selecting a dose of digoxin, the following factors must be considered:

1. The body weight of the patient. Doses should be calculated based upon lean (i.e., ideal) body weight.
2. The patient's renal function, preferably evaluated on the basis of estimated creatinine clearance.
3. The patient's age. Infants and children require different doses of digoxin than adults. Also, advanced age may be indicative of diminished renal function even in patients with normal serum creatinine concentration (i.e., below 1.5 mg/dL).
4. Concomitant disease states, concurrent medications, or other factors likely to alter the pharmacokinetic or pharmacodynamic profile of digoxin (see PRECAUTIONS).

Serum Digoxin Concentrations: In general, the dose of digoxin used should be determined on clinical grounds. However, measurement of serum digoxin concentrations can be helpful to the clinician in determining the adequacy of digoxin therapy and in assigning certain probabilities to the likelihood of digoxin intoxication. About two-thirds of adults considered adequately digitalized (without evidence of toxicity) have serum digoxin concentrations ranging from 0.8 to 2.0 ng/mL. However, digoxin may produce clinical benefits even at serum concentrations below this range. About two-thirds of adult patients with clinical toxicity have serum digoxin concentrations greater than 2.0 ng/mL. However, since one-third of patients with clinical toxicity have concentrations less than 2.0 ng/mL, values below 2.0 ng/mL do not rule out the possibility that a certain sign or symptom is related to digoxin therapy. Rarely, there are patients who are unable to tolerate digoxin at serum concentrations below 0.8 ng/mL. Consequently, the serum concentration of digoxin should always be interpreted in the overall clinical context, and an isolated measurement should not be used alone as the basis for increasing or decreasing the dose of the drug.

To allow adequate time for equilibration of digoxin between serum and tissue, sampling of serum concentrations should be done just before the next scheduled dose of the drug. If this is not possible, sampling should be done at least 6 to 8 hours after the last dose, regardless of the route of administration or the formulation used. On a once-daily dosing schedule, the concentration of digoxin will be 10% to 25% lower when sampled at 24 versus 8 hours, depending upon the patient's renal function. On a twice-daily dosing schedule, there will be only minor differences in serum digoxin concentrations whether sampling is done at 8 or 12 hours after a dose.

Continued on next page

Product information on these pages is effective as of August 2004. Further information is available at: GlaxoSmithKline, PO Box 13398, Research Triangle Park, NC 27709. 1-888-825-5249. Corporate Web Site: www.gsk.com

Lanoxin Tablets—Cont.

If a discrepancy exists between the reported serum concentration and the observed clinical response, the clinician should consider the following possibilities:

1. Analytical problems in the assay procedure.
2. Inappropriate serum sampling time.
3. Administration of a digitalis glycoside other than digoxin.
4. Conditions (described in WARNINGS and PRECAUTIONS) causing an alteration in the sensitivity of the patient to digoxin.
5. Serum digoxin concentration may decrease acutely during periods of exercise without any associated change in clinical efficacy due to increased binding of digoxin to skeletal muscle.

Heart Failure: ***Adults:*** Digitalization may be accomplished by either of two general approaches that vary in dosage and frequency of administration, but reach the same endpoint in terms of total amount of digoxin accumulated in the body.

1. If rapid digitalization is considered medically appropriate, it may be achieved by administering a loading dose based upon projected peak digoxin body stores. Maintenance dose can be calculated as a percentage of the loading dose.
2. More gradual digitalization may be obtained by beginning an appropriate maintenance dose, thus allowing digoxin body stores to accumulate slowly. Steady-state serum digoxin concentrations will be achieved in approximately five half-lives of the drug for the individual patient. Depending upon the patient's renal function, this will take between 1 and 3 weeks.

Rapid Digitalization with a Loading Dose: Peak digoxin body stores of 8 to 12 mcg/kg should provide therapeutic effect with minimum risk of toxicity in most patients with heart failure and normal sinus rhythm. Because of altered digoxin distribution and elimination, projected peak body stores for patients with renal insufficiency should be conservative (i.e., 6 to 10 mcg/kg) [see PRECAUTIONS].

The loading dose should be administered in several portions, with roughly half the total given as the first dose. Additional fractions of this planned total dose may be given at 6- to 8-hour intervals, **with careful assessment of clinical response before each additional dose.**

If the patient's clinical response necessitates a change from the calculated loading dose of digoxin, then calculation of the maintenance dose should be based upon the amount actually given.

A single initial dose of 500 to 750 mcg (0.5 to 0.75 mg) of LANOXIN Tablets usually produces a detectable effect in 0.5 to 2 hours that becomes maximal in 2 to 6 hours. Additional doses of 125 to 375 mcg (0.125 to 0.375 mg) may be given cautiously at 6- to 8-hour intervals until clinical evidence of an adequate effect is noted. The usual amount of LANOXIN Tablets that a 70-kg patient requires to achieve 8 to 12 mcg/kg peak body stores is 750 to 1250 mcg (0.75 to 1.25 mg).

LANOXIN Injection is frequently used to achieve rapid digitalization, with conversion to LANOXIN Tablets or LANOXICAPS for maintenance therapy. If patients are switched from intravenous to oral digoxin formulations, allowances must be made for differences in bioavailability when calculating maintenance dosages (see Table 1, CLINICAL PHARMACOLOGY).

Maintenance Dosing: The doses of digoxin used in controlled trials in patients with heart failure have ranged from 125 to 500 mcg (0.125 to 0.5 mg) once daily. In these studies, the digoxin dose has been generally titrated according to the patient's age, lean body weight, and renal function. Therapy is generally initiated at a dose of 250 mcg (0.25 mg) once daily in patients under age 70 with good renal function, at a dose of 125 mcg (0.125 mg) once daily in patients over age 70 or with impaired renal function, and at a dose of 62.5 mcg (0.0625 mg) in patients with marked renal impairment. Doses may be increased every 2 weeks according to clinical response.

In a subset of approximately 1800 patients enrolled in the DIG trial (wherein dosing was based on an algorithm similar to that in Table 5) the mean (± SD) serum digoxin concentrations at 1 month and 12 months were 1.01 ± 0.47 ng/mL and 0.97 ± 0.43 ng/mL, respectively.

The maintenance dose should be based upon the percentage of the peak body stores lost each day through elimination. The following formula has had wide clinical use:

Maintenance Dose = Peak Body Stores
(i.e., Loading Dose) × % Daily Loss/100
Where: % Daily Loss = 14 + Ccr/5

(Ccr is creatinine clearance, corrected to 70 kg body weight or 1.73 m^2 body surface area.)

Table 5 provides average daily maintenance dose requirements of LANOXIN Tablets for patients with heart failure based upon lean body weight and renal function:

[See table 5 below]

Example: Based on Table 5, a patient in heart failure with an estimated lean body weight of 70 kg and a Ccr of 60 mL/min should be given a dose of 250 mcg (0.25 mg) daily of LANOXIN Tablets, usually taken after the morning meal. If no loading dose is administered, steady-state serum concentrations in this patient should be anticipated at approximately 11 days.

Infants and Children: In general, divided daily dosing is recommended for infants and young children (under age 10). In the newborn period, renal clearance of digoxin is diminished and suitable dosage adjustments must be observed. This is especially pronounced in the premature infant. Beyond the immediate newborn period, children generally require proportionally larger doses than adults on the basis of body weight or body surface area. Children over 10 years of age require adult dosages in proportion to their body weight. Some researchers have suggested that infants and young children tolerate slightly higher serum concentrations than do adults.

Daily maintenance doses for each age group are given in Table 6 and should provide therapeutic effects with minimum risk of toxicity in most patients with heart failure and normal sinus rhythm. These recommendations assume the presence of normal renal function:

Table 6: Daily Maintenance Doses in Children with Normal Renal Function

Age	Daily Maintenance Dose (mcg/kg)
2 to 5 Years	10 to 15
5 to 10 Years	7 to 10
Over 10 Years	3 to 5

In children with renal disease, digoxin must be carefully titrated based upon clinical response.

It cannot be overemphasized that both the adult and pediatric dosage guidelines provided are based upon average patient response and substantial individual variation can be expected. Accordingly, ultimate dosage selection must be based upon clinical assessment of the patient.

Atrial Fibrillation: Peak digoxin body stores larger than the 8 to 12 mcg/kg required for most patients with heart failure and normal sinus rhythm have been used for control of ventricular rate in patients with atrial fibrillation. Doses of digoxin used for the treatment of chronic atrial fibrillation should be titrated to the minimum dose that achieves the desired ventricular rate control without causing undesirable side effects. Data are not available to establish the appropriate resting or exercise target rates that should be achieved.

Dosage Adjustment When Changing Preparations: The difference in bioavailability between LANOXIN Injection or LANOXICAPS and LANOXIN Elixir Pediatric or LANOXIN Tablets must be considered when changing patients from one dosage form to another.

Doses of 100 mcg (0.1 mg) and 200 mcg (0.2 mg) of LANOXICAPS are approximately equivalent to 125-mcg (0.125-mg) and 250-mcg (0.25-mg) doses of LANOXIN Tablets and Elixir Pediatric, respectively (see Table 1 in CLINICAL PHARMACOLOGY: Pharmacokinetics).

Table 5: Usual Daily Maintenance Dose Requirements (mcg) of LANOXIN for Estimated Peak Body Stores of 10 mcg/kg

Corrected Ccr	Lean Body Weight						Number of Days Before Steady State Achieved†
	kg 50	60	70	80	90	100	
(mL/min per 70 kg)*	lb 110	132	154	176	198	220	
0	62.5‡	125	125	125	187.5	187.5	22
10	125	125	125	187.5	187.5	187.5	19
20	125	125	187.5	187.5	187.5	250	16
30	125	187.5	187.5	187.5	250	250	14
40	125	187.5	187.5	250	250	250	13
50	187.5	187.5	250	250	250	250	12
60	187.5	187.5	250	250	250	375	11
70	187.5	250	250	250	250	375	10
80	187.5	250	250	250	375	375	9
90	187.5	250	250	250	375	500	8
100	250	250	250	375	375	500	7

* Ccr is creatinine clearance, corrected to 70 kg body weight or 1.73 m^2 body surface area. *For adults*, if only serum creatinine concentrations (Scr) are available, a Ccr (corrected to 70 kg body weight) may be estimated in men as (140 - Age)/Scr. For women, this result should be multiplied by 0.85. *Note*: This equation cannot be used for estimating creatinine clearance in infants or children.
† If no loading dose administered.
‡ 62.5 mcg = 0.0625 mg

HOW SUPPLIED

LANOXIN (digoxin) Tablets, Scored 125 mcg (0.125 mg): Bottles of 100 with child-resistant cap (NDC 0173-0242-55) and 1000 (NDC 0173-0242-75); unit dose pack of 100 (NDC 0173-0242-56). Imprinted with LANOXIN and Y3B (yellow).
Store at 25°C (77°F); excursions permitted to 15 to 30°C (59 to 86°F) [see USP Controlled Room Temperature] in a dry place and protect from light.

LANOXIN (digoxin) Tablets, Scored 250 mcg (0.25 mg): Bottles of 100 with child-resistant cap (NDC 0173-0249-55), 1000 (NDC 0173-0249-75), and 5000 (NDC 0173-0249-80); unit dose pack of 100 (NDC 0173-0249-56). Imprinted with LANOXIN and X3A (white).
Store at 25°C (77°F); excursions permitted to 15 to 30°C (59 to 86°F) [see USP Controlled Room Temperature] in a dry place.

GlaxoSmithKline, Research Triangle Park, NC 27709

August 2001/RL-972

Shown in Product Identification Guide, page 316

LEUKERAN® ℞

[lū 'kŭh-răn]
(chlorambucil)
TABLETS

> **WARNING**
> LEUKERAN (chlorambucil) can severely suppress bone marrow function. Chlorambucil is a carcinogen in humans. Chlorambucil is probably mutagenic and teratogenic in humans. Chlorambucil produces human infertility (see WARNINGS and PRECAUTIONS).

DESCRIPTION

LEUKERAN (chlorambucil) was first synthesized by Everett et al. It is a bifunctional alkylating agent of the nitrogen mustard type that has been found active against selected human neoplastic diseases. Chlorambucil is known chemically as 4-[bis(2-chlorethyl)amino]benzenebutanoic acid.

Chlorambucil hydrolyzes in water and has a pKa of 5.8.

LEUKERAN (chlorambucil) is available in tablet form for oral administration. Each film-coated tablet contains 2 mg chlorambucil and the inactive ingredients colloidal silicon dioxide, hypromellose, lactose (anhydrous), macrogol/PEG 400, microcrystalline cellulose, red iron oxide, stearic acid, titanium dioxide, and yellow iron oxide.

CLINICAL PHARMACOLOGY

Chlorambucil is rapidly and completely absorbed from the gastrointestinal tract. After single oral doses of 0.6 to 1.2 mg/kg, peak plasma chlorambucil levels (C_{max}) are reached within 1 hour and the terminal elimination half-life ($t_{1/2}$) of the parent drug is estimated at 1.5 hours. Chlorambucil undergoes rapid metabolism to phenylacetic acid mustard, the major metabolite, and the combined chlorambucil and phenylacetic acid mustard urinary excretion is extremely low—less than 1% in 24 hours. In a study of 12 patients given single oral doses of 0.2 mg/kg of LEUKERAN, the mean dose (12 mg) adjusted (±SD) plasma chlorambucil C_{max} was 492 ± 160 ng/mL, the AUC was 883 ± 329 ng•h/mL, $t_{1/2}$ was 1.3 ± 0.5 hours, and the t_{max} was 0.83 ± 0.53 hours. For the major metabolite, phenylacetic acid mustard, the mean dose (12 mg) adjusted (±SD) plasma C_{max} was 306 ± 73 ng/mL, the AUC was 1204 ± 285 ng•h/mL, the $t_{1/2}$ was 1.8 ± 0.4 hours, and the t_{max} was 1.9 ± 0.7 hours.

Chlorambucil and its metabolites are extensively bound to plasma and tissue proteins. In vitro, chlorambucil is 99% bound to plasma proteins, specifically albumin. Cerebrospinal fluid levels of chlorambucil have not been determined. Evidence of human teratogenicity suggests that the drug crosses the placenta.

Chlorambucil is extensively metabolized in the liver primarily to phenylacetic acid mustard, which has antineoplastic activity. Chlorambucil and its major metabolite spontaneously degrade in vivo forming monohydroxy and dihydroxy derivatives. After a single dose of radiolabeled chlorambucil (^{14}C), approximately 15% to 60% of the radioactivity appears in the urine after 24 hours. Again, less than 1% of the urinary radioactivity is in the form of chlorambucil or phenylacetic acid mustard. In summary, the pharmacokinetic data suggest that oral chlorambucil undergoes rapid gastrointestinal absorption and plasma clearance and that it is almost completely metabolized, having extremely low urinary excretion.

INDICATIONS AND USAGE

LEUKERAN (chlorambucil) is indicated in the treatment of chronic lymphatic (lymphocytic) leukemia, malignant lymphomas including lymphosarcoma, giant follicular lymphoma, and Hodgkin's disease. It is not curative in any of these disorders but may produce clinically useful palliation.

CONTRAINDICATIONS

Chlorambucil should not be used in patients whose disease has demonstrated a prior resistance to the agent. Patients who have demonstrated hypersensitivity to chlorambucil should not be given the drug. There may be cross-hypersensitivity (skin rash) between chlorambucil and other alkylating agents.

WARNINGS

Because of its carcinogenic properties, chlorambucil should not be given to patients with conditions other than chronic lymphatic leukemia or malignant lymphomas. Convulsions, infertility, leukemia, and secondary malignancies have been observed when chlorambucil was employed in the therapy of malignant and non-malignant diseases.

There are many reports of acute leukemia arising in patients with both malignant and non-malignant diseases following chlorambucil treatment. In many instances, these patients also received other chemotherapeutic agents or some form of radiation therapy. The quantitation of the risk of chlorambucil-induction of leukemia or carcinoma in humans is not possible. Evaluation of published reports of leukemia developing in patients who have received chlorambucil (and other alkylating agents) suggests that the risk of leukemogenesis increases with both chronicity of treatment and large cumulative doses. However, it has proved impossible to define a cumulative dose below which there is no risk of the induction of secondary malignancy. The potential benefits from chlorambucil therapy must be weighed on an individual basis against the possible risk of the induction of a secondary malignancy.

Chlorambucil has been shown to cause chromatid or chromosome damage in humans. Both reversible and permanent sterility have been observed in both sexes receiving chlorambucil.

A high incidence of sterility has been documented when chlorambucil is administered to prepubertal and pubertal males. Prolonged or permanent azoospermia has also been observed in adult males. While most reports of gonadal dysfunction secondary to chlorambucil have related to males, the induction of amenorrhea in females with alkylating agents is well documented and chlorambucil is capable of producing amenorrhea. Autopsy studies of the ovaries from women with malignant lymphoma treated with combination chemotherapy including chlorambucil have shown varying degrees of fibrosis, vasculitis, and depletion of primordial follicles.

Rare instances of skin rash progressing to erythema multiforme, toxic epidermal necrolysis, or Stevens-Johnson syndrome have been reported. Chlorambucil should be discontinued promptly in patients who develop skin reactions.

Pregnancy: Pregnancy Category D. Chlorambucil can cause fetal harm when administered to a pregnant woman. Unilateral renal agenesis has been observed in 2 offspring whose mothers received chlorambucil during the first trimester. Urogenital malformations, including absence of a kidney, were found in fetuses of rats given chlorambucil. There are no adequate and well-controlled studies in pregnant women. If this drug is used during pregnancy, or if the patient becomes pregnant while taking this drug, the patient should be apprised of the potential hazard to the fetus. Women of childbearing potential should be advised to avoid becoming pregnant.

PRECAUTIONS

General: Many patients develop a slowly progressive lymphopenia during treatment. The lymphocyte count usually rapidly returns to normal levels upon completion of drug therapy. Most patients have some neutropenia after the third week of treatment and this may continue for up to 10 days after the last dose. Subsequently, the neutrophil count usually rapidly returns to normal. Severe neutropenia appears to be related to dosage and usually occurs only in patients who have received a total dosage of 6.5 mg/kg or more in one course of therapy with continuous dosing. About one quarter of all patients receiving the continuous-dose schedule, and one third of those receiving this dosage in 8 weeks or less may be expected to develop severe neutropenia.

While it is not necessary to discontinue chlorambucil at the first evidence of a fall in neutrophil count, it must be remembered that the fall may continue for 10 days after the last dose, and that as the total dose approaches 6.5 mg/kg, there is a risk of causing irreversible bone marrow damage. The dose of chlorambucil should be decreased if leukocyte or platelet counts fall below normal values and should be discontinued for more severe depression.

Chlorambucil should **not** be given at full dosages before 4 weeks after a full course of radiation therapy or chemotherapy because of the vulnerability of the bone marrow to damage under these conditions. If the pretherapy leukocyte or platelet counts are depressed from bone marrow disease process prior to institution of therapy, the treatment should be instituted at a reduced dosage.

Persistently low neutrophil and platelet counts or peripheral lymphocytosis suggest bone marrow infiltration. If confirmed by bone marrow examination, the daily dosage of chlorambucil should not exceed 0.1 mg/kg. Chlorambucil appears to be relatively free from gastrointestinal side effects or other evidence of toxicity apart from the bone marrow depressant action. In humans, single oral doses of 20 mg or more may produce nausea and vomiting.

Children with nephrotic syndrome and patients receiving high pulse doses of chlorambucil may have an increased risk of seizures. As with any potentially epileptogenic drug, caution should be exercised when administering chlorambucil to patients with a history of seizure disorder or head trauma, or who are receiving other potentially epileptogenic drugs.

Information for Patients: Patients should be informed that the major toxicities of chlorambucil are related to hypersensitivity, drug fever, myelosuppression, hepatotoxicity, infertility, seizures, gastrointestinal toxicity, and secondary malignancies. Patients should never be allowed to take the drug without medical supervision and should consult their physician if they experience skin rash, bleeding, fever, jaundice, persistent cough, seizures, nausea, vomiting, amenorrhea, or unusual lumps/masses. Women of childbearing potential should be advised to avoid becoming pregnant.

Laboratory Tests: Patients must be followed carefully to avoid life-endangering damage to the bone marrow during treatment. Weekly examination of the blood should be made to determine hemoglobin levels, total and differential leukocyte counts, and quantitative platelet counts. Also, during the first 3 to 6 weeks of therapy, it is recommended that white blood cell counts be made 3 or 4 days after each of the weekly complete blood counts. Galton et al have suggested that in following patients it is helpful to plot the blood counts on a chart at the same time that body weight, temperature, spleen size, etc., are recorded. It is considered dangerous to allow a patient to go more than 2 weeks without hematological and clinical examination during treatment.

Drug Interactions: There are no known drug/drug interactions with chlorambucil.

Carcinogenesis, Mutagenesis, Impairment of Fertility: See WARNINGS section for information on carcinogenesis, mutagenesis, and impairment of fertility.

Pregnancy: ***Teratogenic Effects:*** Pregnancy Category D: See WARNINGS section.

Nursing Mothers: It is not known whether this drug is excreted in human milk. Because many drugs are excreted in human milk and because of the potential for serious adverse reactions in nursing infants from chlorambucil, a decision should be made whether to discontinue nursing or to discontinue the drug, taking into account the importance of the drug to the mother.

Pediatric Use: The safety and effectiveness in pediatric patients have not been established.

Geriatric Use: Clinical studies of chlorambucil did not include sufficient numbers of subjects aged 65 and over to determine whether they respond differently from younger subjects. Other reported clinical experience has not identified differences in responses between the elderly and younger patients. In general, dose selection for an elderly patient should be cautious, usually starting at the low end of the dosing range, reflecting the greater frequency of decreased hepatic, renal, or cardiac function, and of concomitant disease or other drug therapy.

ADVERSE REACTIONS

Hematologic: The most common side effect is bone marrow suppression. Although bone marrow suppression frequently occurs, it is usually reversible if the chlorambucil is withdrawn early enough. However, irreversible bone marrow failure has been reported.

Gastrointestinal: Gastrointestinal disturbances such as nausea and vomiting, diarrhea, and oral ulceration occur infrequently.

CNS: Tremors, muscular twitching, myoclonia, confusion, agitation, ataxia, flaccid paresis, and hallucinations have been reported as rare adverse experiences to chlorambucil which resolve upon discontinuation of drug. Rare, focal and/or generalized seizures have been reported to occur in both children and adults at both therapeutic daily doses and pulse-dosing regimens, and in acute overdose (see PRECAUTIONS: General).

Dermatologic: Allergic reactions such as urticaria and angioneurotic edema have been reported following initial or subsequent dosing. Skin hypersensitivity (including rare reports of skin rash progressing to erythema multiforme, toxic epidermal necrolysis, and Stevens-Johnson syndrome) has been reported (see WARNINGS).

Miscellaneous: Other reported adverse reactions include: pulmonary fibrosis, hepatotoxicity and jaundice, drug fever, peripheral neuropathy, interstitial pneumonia, sterile cystitis, infertility, leukemia, and secondary malignancies (see WARNINGS).

OVERDOSAGE

Reversible pancytopenia was the main finding of inadvertent overdoses of chlorambucil. Neurological toxicity ranging from agitated behavior and ataxia to multiple grand mal seizures has also occurred. As there is no known antidote, the blood picture should be closely monitored and general supportive measures should be instituted, together with appropriate blood transfusions, if necessary. Chlorambucil is not dialyzable.

Oral LD_{50} single doses in mice are 123 mg/kg. In rats, a single intraperitoneal dose of 12.5 mg/kg of chlorambucil produces typical nitrogen-mustard effects; these include atrophy of the intestinal mucous membrane and lymphoid tissues, severe lymphopenia becoming maximal in 4 days, anemia, and thrombocytopenia. After this dose, the animals begin to recover within 3 days and appear normal in about a week, although the bone marrow may not become completely normal for about 3 weeks. An intraperitoneal dose of 18.5 mg/kg kills about 50% of the rats with development of convulsions. As much as 50 mg/kg has been given orally to rats as a single dose, with recovery. Such a dose causes bradycardia, excessive salivation, hematuria, convulsions, and respiratory dysfunction.

DOSAGE AND ADMINISTRATION

The usual oral dosage is 0.1 to 0.2 mg/kg body weight daily for 3 to 6 weeks as required. This usually amounts to 4 to 10 mg per day for the average patient. The entire daily dose may be given at one time. These dosages are for initiation of therapy or for short courses of treatment. The dosage must be carefully adjusted according to the response of the patient and must be reduced as soon as there is an abrupt fall in the white blood cell count. Patients with Hodgkin's disease usually require 0.2 mg/kg daily, whereas patients with other lymphomas or chronic lymphocytic leukemia usually require only 0.1 mg/kg daily. When lymphocytic infiltration of the bone marrow is present, or when the bone marrow is hypoplastic, the daily dose should not exceed 0.1 mg/kg (about 6 mg for the average patient).

Alternate schedules for the treatment of chronic lymphocytic leukemia employing intermittent, biweekly, or once-monthly pulse doses of chlorambucil have been reported. Intermittent schedules of chlorambucil begin with an initial single dose of 0.4 mg/kg. Doses are generally increased by 0.1 mg/kg until control of lymphocytosis or toxicity is observed. Subsequent doses are modified to produce mild hematologic toxicity. It is felt that the response rate of chronic lymphocytic leukemia to the biweekly or once-monthly schedule of chlorambucil administration is similar or better to that previously reported with daily administration and that hematologic toxicity was less than or equal to that encountered in studies using daily chlorambucil.

Radiation and cytotoxic drugs render the bone marrow more vulnerable to damage, and chlorambucil should be used with particular caution within 4 weeks of a full course of radiation therapy or chemotherapy. However, small doses of palliative radiation over isolated foci remote from the bone marrow will not usually depress the neutrophil and platelet count. In these cases chlorambucil may be given in the customary dosage.

It is presently felt that short courses of treatment are safer than continuous maintenance therapy, although both methods have been effective. It must be recognized that continuous therapy may give the appearance of "maintenance" in patients who are actually in remission and have no immediate need for further drug. If maintenance dosage is used, it should not exceed 0.1 mg/kg daily and may well be as low as 0.03 mg/kg daily. A typical maintenance dose is 2 mg to 4 mg daily, or less, depending on the status of the blood counts. It may, therefore, be desirable to withdraw the drug after maximal control has been achieved, since intermittent therapy reinstituted at time of relapse may be as effective as continuous treatment.

Procedures for proper handling and disposal of anticancer drugs should be considered. Several guidelines on this subject have been published.[1–8]

There is no general agreement that all of the procedures recommended in the guidelines are necessary or appropriate.

HOW SUPPLIED

Leukeran is supplied as brown, film-coated, round, biconvex tablets containing 2 mg chlorambucil in amber glass bottles with child-resistant closures. One side is engraved with "GX EG3" and the other side is engraved with an "L."

Bottle of 50 (NDC 0173-0635-35).

Store in a refrigerator, 2° to 8°C (36° to 46°F).

REFERENCES

1. ONS Clinical Practice Committee. Cancer Chemotherapy Guidelines and Recommendations for Practice. Pittsburgh, PA: Oncology Nursing Society; 1999:32-41.
2. Recommendations for the safe handling of parenteral antineoplastic drugs. Washington, DC: Division of Safety, Clinical Center Pharmacy Department and Cancer Nursing Services, National Institutes of Health and Human Services, 1992, US Dept of Health and Human Services, Public Health Service publication NIH 92-2621.
3. AMA Council on Scientific Affairs. Guidelines for handling parenteral antineoplastics. *JAMA*. 1985;253:1590-1591.
4. National Study Commission on Cytotoxic Exposure. Recommendations for handling cytotoxic agents. 1987. Available from Louis P. Jeffrey, Chairman, National Study Commission on Cytotoxic Exposure. Massachusetts College of Pharmacy and Allied Health Sciences, 179 Longwood Avenue, Boston, MA 02115.
5. Clinical Oncological Society of Australia. Guidelines and recommendations for safe handling of antineoplastic agents. *Med J Australia*. 1983;1:426-428.
6. Jones RB, Frank R, Mass T. Safe handling of chemotherapeutic agents: a report from the Mount Sinai Medical Center. *CA-A Cancer J for Clin*. 1983;33:258-263.
7. American Society of Hospital Pharmacists. ASHP technical assistance bulletin on handling cytotoxic and hazardous drugs. *Am J Hosp Pharm*. 1990;47:1033-1049.

Continued on next page

Product information on these pages is effective as of August 2004. Further information is available at: GlaxoSmithKline, PO Box 13398, Research Triangle Park, NC 27709. 1-888-825-5249. Corporate Web Site: www.gsk.com

Leukeran—Cont.

8. Controlling Occupational Exposure to Hazardous Drugs. (OSHA Work-Practice Guidelines.) *Am J Health-Syst Pharm.* 1996;53:1669-1685.

GlaxoSmithKline, Research Triangle Park, NC 27709

November 2003/RL-2054

Shown in Product Identification Guide, page 316

LEXIVA® ℞

[lex-ē' va]

(fosamprenavir calcium)

Tablets

DESCRIPTION

LEXIVA (fosamprenavir calcium) is a prodrug of amprenavir, an inhibitor of human immunodeficiency virus (HIV) protease. The chemical name of fosamprenavir calcium is (3*S*)-tetrahydrofuran-3-yl (1*S*,2*R*)-3-[[(4-aminophenyl) sulfonyl](isobutyl)amino]-1-benzyl-2-(phosphonooxy) propylcarbamate monocalcium salt. Fosamprenavir calcium is a single stereoisomer with the (3*S*)(1*S*,2*R*) configuration. It has a molecular formula of $C_{25}H_{34}CaN_3O_9PS$ and a molecular weight of 623.7. It has the following structural formula:

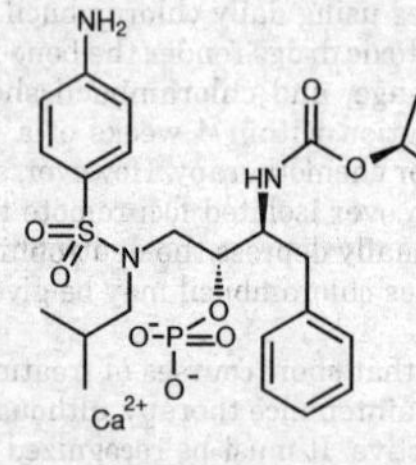

Fosamprenavir calcium is a white to cream-colored solid with a solubility of approximately 0.31 mg/mL in water at 25°C.

LEXIVA Tablets are available for oral administration in a strength of 700 mg of fosamprenavir as fosamprenavir calcium (equivalent to approximately 600 mg of amprenavir). Each 700-mg tablet contains the inactive ingredients colloidal silicon dioxide, croscarmellose sodium, magnesium stearate, microcrystalline cellulose, and povidone K30. The tablet film-coating contains the inactive ingredients hypromellose, iron oxide red, titanium dioxide, and triacetin.

MICROBIOLOGY

Mechanism of Action: Fosamprenavir is rapidly converted to amprenavir by cellular phosphatases in vivo. Amprenavir is an inhibitor of HIV-1 protease. Amprenavir binds to the active site of HIV-1 protease and thereby prevents the processing of viral Gag and Gag-Pol polyprotein precursors, resulting in the formation of immature non-infectious viral particles.

Antiviral Activity in Vitro: Fosamprenavir has little or no antiviral activity in vitro. The in vitro antiviral activity observed with fosamprenavir is not measurable due to trace amounts of amprenavir. The in vitro antiviral activity of amprenavir was evaluated against HIV-1 IIIB in both acutely and chronically infected lymphoblastic cell lines (MT-4, CEM-CCRF, H9) and in peripheral blood lymphocytes. The 50% inhibitory concentration (IC_{50}) of amprenavir ranged from 0.012 to 0.08 μM in acutely infected cells and was 0.41 μM in chronically infected cells (1 μM = 0.50 mcg/mL). Amprenavir exhibited synergistic anti-HIV-1 activity in combination with the nucleoside reverse transcriptase inhibitors (NRTIs) abacavir, didanosine, and zidovudine, and the protease inhibitor (PI) saquinavir, and additive anti-HIV-1 activity in combination with the non-nucleoside reverse transcriptase inhibitor (NNRTI) nevirapine and PIs indinavir, lopinavir, nelfinavir, and ritonavir in vitro. These drug combinations have not been adequately studied in humans. The relationship between in vitro anti-HIV-1 activity of amprenavir and the inhibition of HIV-1 replication in humans has not been defined.

Resistance: HIV-1 isolates with a decreased susceptibility to amprenavir have been selected in vitro and obtained from patients treated with fosamprenavir. Genotypic analysis of isolates from amprenavir-treated patients showed mutations in the HIV-1 protease gene resulting in amino acid substitutions primarily at positions V32I, M46I/L, I47V, I50V, I54L/M, and I84V, as well as mutations in the p7/p1 and p1/p6 Gag and Gag-Pol polyprotein precursor cleavage sites. Some of these amprenavir resistance-associated mutations have also been detected in HIV-1 isolates from antiretroviral-naive patients treated with LEXIVA. Of the 488 antiretroviral-naive patients treated with LEXIVA or LEXIVA/ritonavir, 61 patients (29 receiving LEXIVA and 32 receiving LEXIVA/ritonavir) with virological failure (plasma HIV-1 RNA>1,000 copies/mL on 2 occasions on or after Week 12) were genotyped. Five of the 29 antiretroviral-naive patients (17%) receiving LEXIVA without ritonavir had evidence of genotypic resistance to amprenavir: I54L/M (n = 2), I54L + L33F (n = 1), V32I + I47V (n = 1), and M46I + I47V (n = 1). No amprenavir-associated mutations were detected in antiretroviral-naive patients treated with LEXIVA/ritonavir.

Cross-Resistance: Varying degrees of cross-resistance among HIV-1 protease inhibitors have been observed. An association between virologic response at 48 weeks (HIV-1 RNA level <400 copies/mL) and PI-resistance mutations detected in baseline HIV-1 isolates from PI-experienced patients receiving LEXIVA/ritonavir twice daily (n = 88), or lopinavir/ritonavir twice daily (n = 85) in study APV30003 is shown in Table 1. The majority of subjects had previously received either one (47%) or 2 PIs (36%), most commonly nelfinavir (57%) and indinavir (53%). Out of 102 subjects with baseline phenotypes receiving twice-daily LEXIVA/ritonavir, 54% (55) had resistance to at least one PI, with 98% (54) of those having resistance to nelfinavir. Out of 97 subjects with baseline phenotypes in the lopinavir/ritonavir arm, 60% (58) had resistance to at least one PI, with 97% (56) of those having resistance to nelfinavir.

Table 1. Responders at Study Week 48 by Presence of Baseline PI Resistance-Associated Mutations*

PI-mutations†	LEXIVA/Ritonavir b.i.d. (n = 88)	Lopinavir/ Ritonavir b.i.d. (n = 85)
D30N	21/22 (95%)	17/19 (89%)
N88D/S	20/22 (91%)	12/12 (100%)
L90M	16/31 (52%)	17/29 (59%)
M46I/L	11/22 (50%)	12/24 (50%)
V82A/F/T/S	2/9 (22%)	6/17 (35%)
I54V	2/11 (18%)	6/11 (55%)
I84V	1/6 (17%)	2/5 (40%)

*Results should be interpreted with caution because the subgroups were small.

† Most patients had >1 PI resistance-associated mutation at baseline.

The virologic response based upon baseline phenotype was assessed. Baseline isolates from PI-experienced patients responding to LEXIVA/ritonavir twice daily had a median shift in susceptibility to amprenavir relative to a standard wild-type reference strain of 0.7 (range: 0.1 to 5.4, n = 62), and baseline isolates from individuals failing therapy had a median shift in susceptibility of 1.9 (range: 0.2 to 14, n = 29). Because this was a select patient population, these data do not constitute definitive clinical susceptibility break points. Additional data are needed to determine clinically relevant break points for LEXIVA.

Isolates from 15 of the 20 patients receiving twice-daily LEXIVA/ritonavir and experiencing virologic failure/ongoing replication were subjected to genotypic analysis. The following amprenavir resistance-associated mutations were found either alone or in combination: V32I, M46I/L, I47V, I50V, I54L/M, and I84V.

CLINICAL PHARMACOLOGY

Pharmacokinetics in Adults: Fosamprenavir is a prodrug, which is rapidly hydrolyzed to amprenavir by enzymes in the gut epithelium as it is absorbed.

The pharmacokinetic properties of amprenavir after administration of LEXIVA with or without ritonavir, have been evaluated in both healthy adult volunteers and in HIV-infected patients; no substantial differences in steady-state amprenavir concentrations were observed between the 2 populations.

Absorption and Bioavailability: After administration of a single dose of LEXIVA to HIV-1-infected patients, the time to peak amprenavir concentration (T_{max}) occurred between 1.5 and 4 hours (median 2.5 hours). The absolute oral bioavailability of amprenavir after administration of LEXIVA in humans has not been established.

The pharmacokinetic parameters of amprenavir after administration of LEXIVA (with and without concomitant ritonavir) are shown in Table 2.

[See table 2 below]

The median plasma amprenavir concentrations of the dosing regimens over the dosing intervals are displayed in Figure 1.

Figure 1. Mean (± SD) Steady-State Plasma Amprenavir Concentrations and Mean IC_{50} Values Against HIV from Protease Inhibitor-Naive Patients (in the Absence of Human Serum)

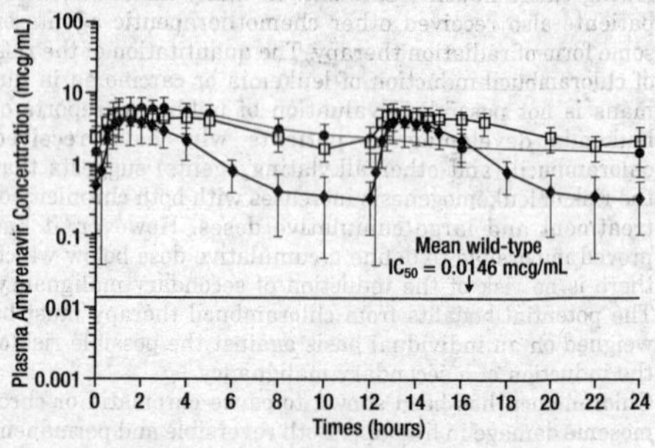

Effects of Food on Oral Absorption: LEXIVA Tablets may be taken with or without food (see DOSAGE AND ADMINISTRATION). Administration of a single 1,400-mg dose of LEXIVA in the fed state (standardized high-fat meal: 967 kcal, 67 grams fat, 33 grams protein, 58 grams carbohydrate) compared to the fasted state was associated with no significant changes in amprenavir C_{max}, T_{max}, or $AUC_{0-\infty}$.

Distribution: In vitro, amprenavir is approximately 90% bound to plasma proteins, primarily to $alpha_1$-acid glycoprotein. In vitro, concentration-dependent binding was observed over the concentration range of 1 to 10 mcg/mL, with decreased binding at higher concentrations. The partitioning of amprenavir into erythrocytes is low, but increases as amprenavir concentrations increase, reflecting the higher amount of unbound drug at higher concentrations.

Metabolism: After oral administration, fosamprenavir is rapidly and almost completely hydrolyzed to amprenavir and inorganic phosphate prior to reaching the systemic circulation. This occurs in the gut epithelium during absorption. Amprenavir is metabolized in the liver by the cytochrome P450 3A4 (CYP3A4) enzyme system. The 2 major metabolites result from oxidation of the tetrahydrofuran and aniline moieties. Glucuronide conjugates of oxidized metabolites have been identified as minor metabolites in urine and feces.

Elimination: Excretion of unchanged amprenavir in urine and feces is minimal. Unchanged amprenavir in urine accounts for approximately 1% of the dose; unchanged amprenavir was not detectable in feces. Approximately 14% and 75% of an administered single dose of ^{14}C-amprenavir can be accounted for as metabolites in urine and feces, respectively. Two metabolites accounted for >90% of the radiocarbon in fecal samples. The plasma elimination half-life of amprenavir is approximately 7.7 hours.

Special Populations: *Hepatic Insufficiency:* The pharmacokinetics of amprenavir after administration of LEXIVA have not been studied in patients with hepatic insufficiency.

The pharmacokinetics of amprenavir have been studied after administration of amprenavir given as AGENERASE® Capsules to adult patients with impaired hepatic function using a single 600-mg oral dose. The $AUC_{0-\infty}$ of amprenavir was significantly greater in patients with moderate cirrhosis (25.76 ± 14.68 mcg•hr/mL) compared with healthy volunteers (12.00 ± 4.38 mcg•hr/mL). The $AUC_{0-\infty}$ and C_{max} were significantly greater in patients with severe cirrhosis ($AUC_{0-\infty}$: 38.66 ± 16.08 mcg•hr/mL; C_{max}: 9.43 ± 2.61 mcg/mL) compared with healthy volunteers ($AUC_{0-\infty}$: 12.00 ± 4.38 mcg•hr/mL; C_{max}: 4.90 ± 1.39 mcg/mL). Based on these data, patients with impaired hepatic function receiving LEXIVA without concurrent ritonavir may require dosage reduction. There are no data on the use of LEXIVA in combination with ritonavir in patients with any degree of hepatic impairment (see PRECAUTIONS and DOSAGE AND ADMINISTRATION).

Renal Insufficiency: The impact of renal impairment on amprenavir elimination in adult patients has not been studied. The renal elimination of unchanged amprenavir represents approximately 1% of the administered dose; therefore, renal impairment is not expected to significantly impact the elimination of amprenavir.

Pediatric Patients: The pharmacokinetics of amprenavir after administration of LEXIVA to pediatric patients are under investigation. There are insufficient data at this time to recommend a dose.

Geriatric Patients: The pharmacokinetics of amprenavir after administration of LEXIVA to patients over 65 years of age have not been studied.

Table 2. Geometric Mean (95% CI) Steady-State Plasma Amprenavir Pharmacokinetic Parameters

Regimen	C_{max} (mcg/mL)	T_{max} (hours)*	AUC_{24} (mcg•hr/mL)	C_{min} (mcg/mL)
LEXIVA 1,400 mg b.i.d.	4.82 (4.06-5.72)	1.3 (0.8-4.0)	33.0 (27.6-39.2)	0.35 (0.27-0.46)
LEXIVA 1,400 mg q.d. plus Ritonavir 200 mg q.d.	7.24 (6.32-8.28)	2.1 (0.8-5.0)	69.4 (59.7-80.8)	1.45 (1.16-1.81)
LEXIVA 700 mg b.i.d. plus Ritonavir 100 mg b.i.d.	6.08 (5.38-6.86)	1.5 (0.75-5.0)	79.2 (69.0-90.6)	2.12 (1.77-2.54)

*Data shown are median (range).

Table 3. Drug Interactions: Pharmacokinetic Parameters for Amprenavir After Administration of LEXIVA in the Presence of the Coadministered Drug(s)

Coadministered Drug(s) and Dose(s)	Dose of **LEXIVA***	n	% Change in **Amprenavir** Pharmacokinetic Parameters (90% CI) C_{max}	AUC	C_{min}
Antacid (MAALOX TC®) 30 mL single dose	1,400 mg single dose	30	↓35 (↓24 to ↓42)	↓18 (↓9 to ↓26)	↑14 (↓7 to ↑39)
Atorvastatin 10 mg q.d. for 4 days	1,400 mg b.i.d. for 2 weeks	16	↓18 (↓34 to ↑1)	↓27 (↓41 to ↓12)	↓12 (↓27 to ↑6)
Atorvastatin 10 mg q.d. for 4 days	700 mg b.i.d. plus ritonavir 100 mg b.i.d. for 2 weeks	16	⇔	⇔	⇔
Efavirenz 600 mg q.d. for 2 weeks	1,400 mg q.d. plus ritonavir 200 mg q.d. for 2 weeks	16	⇔	↓13 (↓30 to ↑7)	↓36 (↓8 to ↓56)
Efavirenz 600 mg q.d. plus additional ritonavir 100 mg q.d for 2 weeks	1,400 mg q.d. plus ritonavir 200 mg q.d. for 2 weeks	16	↑18 (↑1 to ↑38)	↑11 (0 to ↑24)	⇔
Efavirenz 600 mg q.d. for 2 weeks	700 mg b.i.d. plus ritonavir 100 mg b.i.d. for 2 weeks	16	⇔	⇔	↓17 (↓4 to ↓29)
Lopinavir/ritonavir 533 mg/133 mg b.i.d.	1,400 mg b.i.d. for 2 weeks	18	See following section: **HIV Protease Inhibitors**		
Lopinavir/ritonavir 400 mg/100 mg b.i.d. for 2 weeks	700 mg b.i.d. plus ritonavir 100 mg b.i.d. for 2 weeks	18	↓58 (↓42 to ↓70)	↓63 (↓51 to ↓72)	↓65 (↓54 to ↓73)
Ranitidine 300 mg single dose	1,400 mg single dose	30	↓51 (↓43 to ↓58)	↓30 (↓22 to ↓37)	⇔ (↓19 to ↑21)

*Concomitant medication is also shown in this column where appropriate.
↑ = Increase; ↓ = Decrease; ⇔ = No change (↑ or ↓<10%).

Table 4. Drug Interactions: Pharmacokinetic Parameters for Amprenavir After Administration of AGENERASE in the Presence of the Coadministered Drug(s)

Coadministered Drug(s) and Dose(s)	Dose of **AGENERASE***	n	% Change in **Amprenavir** Pharmacokinetic Parameters (90% CI) C_{max}	AUC	C_{min}
Clarithromycin 500 mg b.i.d. for 4 days	1,200 mg b.i.d. for 4 days	12	↑15 (↑1 to ↑31)	↑18 (↑8 to ↑29)	↑39 (↑31 to ↑47)
Delavirdine 600 mg b.i.d. for 10 days	600 mg b.i.d. for 10 days	9	↑40*	↑130*	↑125*
Ethinyl estradiol/ norethindrone 0.035 mg/1 mg for 1 cycle	1,200 mg b.i.d. for 28 days	10	⇔	↓22 (↓35 to ↓8)	↓20 (↓41 to ↑8)
Indinavir 800 mg t.i.d. for 2 weeks (fasted)	750 or 800 mg t.i.d. for 2 weeks (fasted)	9	↑18 (↓13 to ↑58)	↑33 (↑2 to ↑73)	↑25 (↓27 to ↑116)
Ketoconazole 400 mg single dose	1,200 mg single dose	12	↓16 (↓25 to ↓6)	↑31 (↑20 to ↑42)	NA
Lamivudine 150 mg single dose	600 mg single dose	11	⇔	⇔	NA
Nelfinavir 750 mg t.i.d. for 2 weeks (fed)	750 or 800 mg t.i.d. for 2 weeks (fed)	6	↓14 (↓38 to ↑20)	⇔	↑189 (↑52 to ↑448)
Rifabutin 300 mg q.d. for 10 days	1,200 mg b.i.d. for 10 days	5	⇔	↓15 (↓28 to 0)	↓15 (↓38 to ↑17)
Rifampin 300 mg q.d. for 4 days	1,200 mg b.i.d. for 4 days	11	↓70 (↓76 to ↓62)	↓82 (↓84 to ↓78)	↓92 (↓95 to ↓89)
Saquinavir 800 mg t.i.d. for 2 weeks (fed)	750 or 800 mg t.i.d. for 2 weeks (fed)	7	↓37 (↓54 to ↓14)	↓32 (↓49 to ↓9)	↓14 (↓52 to ↑54)
Zidovudine 300 mg single dose	600 single dose	12	⇔	↑13 (↓2 to ↑31)	NA

*Median percent change; confidence interval not reported.
↑ = Increase; ↓ = Decrease; ⇔ = No change (↑ or ↓<10%); NA = C_{min} not calculated for single-dose study.

Gender: The pharmacokinetics of amprenavir after administration of LEXIVA do not differ between males and females.

Race: The pharmacokinetics of amprenavir after administration of LEXIVA do not differ between blacks and non-blacks.

Drug Interactions: See also CONTRAINDICATIONS, WARNINGS, and PRECAUTIONS: Drug Interactions.
Amprenavir, the active metabolite of fosamprenavir, is metabolized in the liver by the cytochrome P450 enzyme system. Amprenavir inhibits CYP3A4. Data also suggest that amprenavir induces CYP3A4. Caution should be used when coadministering medications that are substrates, inhibitors, or inducers of CYP3A4, or potentially toxic medications that are metabolized by CYP3A4. Amprenavir does not inhibit CYP2D6, CYP1A2, CYP2C9, CYP2C19, CYP2E1, or uridine glucuronosyltransferase (UDPGT).

Drug interaction studies were performed with LEXIVA and other drugs likely to be coadministered or drugs commonly used as probes for pharmacokinetic interactions. The effects of coadministration on AUC, C_{max}, and C_{min} values are summarized in Table 3 (effect of other drugs on amprenavir) and Table 5 (effect of LEXIVA on other drugs). In addition, since LEXIVA delivers comparable amprenavir plasma concentrations as AGENERASE, drug interaction data derived from studies with AGENERASE are provided in Tables 4 and 6. For information regarding clinical recommendations, see PRECAUTIONS: Drug Interactions.

[See table 3 at left]
[See table 4 at left]
[See table 5 at top of next page]
[See table 6 on next page]

Nucleoside Reverse Transcriptase Inhibitors: There was no clinically significant effect of amprenavir after administration of AGENERASE on abacavir in subjects receiving both agents based on historical data.

In a Phase III clinical trial (APV30003), plasma amprenavir trough concentrations were similar for subjects receiving tenofovir disoproxil fumarate in combination with LEXIVA and ritonavir as compared to subjects not receiving tenofovir.

HIV Protease Inhibitors: In a 3-arm, randomized, crossover study involving healthy volunteers, amprenavir pharmacokinetics were compared after administration of LEXIVA 1,400 mg twice daily plus lopinavir/ritonavir 533 mg/133 mg twice daily for 2 weeks versus LEXIVA 700 mg twice daily plus ritonavir 100 mg twice daily for 2 weeks. Amprenavir concentrations were lower with the regimen containing lopinavir/ritonavir: C_{max} was 13% lower, AUC was 26% lower, and C_{min} was 42% lower. In the same study, lopinavir pharmacokinetics were compared after administration of LEXIVA 1,400 mg twice daily plus lopinavir/ritonavir 533 mg/133 mg twice daily for 2 weeks versus lopinavir/ritonavir 400 mg/100 mg twice daily for 2 weeks. Lopinavir concentrations were similar (less than 10% change in C_{max}, AUC, and C_{min} values) with these 2 regimens.

The effect of amprenavir after administration of AGENERASE Capsules on concentrations of other HIV protease inhibitors in subjects receiving both agents was evaluated using comparisons to historical data. Indinavir steady-state C_{max}, AUC, and C_{min} were decreased by 22%, 38%, and 27%, respectively, by concomitant amprenavir. Similar decreases in C_{max} and AUC were seen after the first dose. Saquinavir steady-state C_{max}, AUC, and C_{min} were increased 21%, decreased 19%, and decreased 48%, respectively, by concomitant amprenavir. Nelfinavir steady-state C_{max}, AUC, and C_{min} were increased by 12%, 15%, and 14%, respectively, by concomitant amprenavir.

Methadone: Coadministration of amprenavir and methadone can decrease plasma levels of methadone.

Coadministration of amprenavir and methadone as compared to a non-matched historical control group resulted in a 30%, 27%, and 25% decrease in serum amprenavir AUC, C_{max}, and C_{min}, respectively.

INDICATIONS AND USAGE

LEXIVA is indicated in combination with other antiretroviral agents for the treatment of HIV infection in adults.

The following points should be considered when initiating therapy with LEXIVA/ritonavir in protease inhibitor-experienced patients (see Description of Clinical Studies).

- **The protease inhibitor-experienced patient study was not large enough to reach a definitive conclusion that LEXIVA/ritonavir and lopinavir/ritonavir are clinically equivalent.**
- **Once-daily administration of LEXIVA plus ritonavir is not recommended for protease inhibitor-experienced patients.**

Description of Clinical Studies: ***Therapy-Naive Patients: Study APV30001:*** APV30001 was a randomized, open-label study, comparing treatment with LEXIVA Tablets (1,400 mg twice daily) versus nelfinavir (1,250 mg twice daily) in 249 antiretroviral treatment-naive patients. Both groups of patients also received abacavir (300 mg twice daily) and lamivudine (150 mg twice daily).

The mean age of the patients in this study was 37 years (range 17 to 70 years), 69% of the patients were males, 20% were CDC Class C (AIDS), 24% were Caucasian, 32% were black, and 44% were Hispanic. At baseline, the median CD4+ cell count was 212 cells/mm^3 (range: 2 to 1,136 cells/mm^3; 18% of patients had a CD4+ cell count of <50 cells/mm^3 and 30% were in the range of 50 to <200 cells/mm^3). Baseline median HIV-1 RNA was 4.83 $\log_{10}$ copies/mL (range: 1.69 to 7.41 $\log_{10}$ copies/mL; 45% of patients had >100,000 copies/mL).

The outcomes of randomized treatment are provided in Table 7.

Continued on next page

Product information on these pages is effective as of August 2004. Further information is available at: GlaxoSmithKline, PO Box 13398, Research Triangle Park, NC 27709. 1-888-825-5249. Corporate Web Site: www.gsk.com

Lexiva—Cont.

Table 7. Outcomes of Randomized Treatment Through Week 48 (APV30001)

Outcome (Rebound or discontinuation = failure)	LEXIVA 1,400 mg b.i.d. (n = 166)	Nelfinavir 1,250 mg b.i.d. (n = 83)
Responder*	66% (57%)	52% (42%)
Virologic failure	19%	32%
Rebound	16%	19%
Never suppressed through Week 48	3%	13%
Clinical progression	1%	1%
Death	0%	1%
Discontinued due to adverse reactions	4%	2%
Discontinued due to other reasons†	10%	10%

*Patients achieved and maintained confirmed HIV-1 RNA <400 copies/mL (<50 copies/mL) through Week 48 (Roche AMPLICOR HIV-1 MONITOR Assay Version 1.5).

† Includes consent withdrawn, lost to follow up, protocol violations, those with missing data, and other reasons.

Treatment response by viral load strata is shown in Table 8.

Table 8. Proportions of Responders Through Week 48 by Screening Viral Load (APV30001)

Screening Viral Load HIV-1 RNA (copies/mL)	LEXIVA 1,400 mg b.i.d.		Nelfinavir 1,250 mg b.i.d.	
	<400 copies/mL	n	<400 copies/mL	n
≤100,000	65%	93	65%	46
>100,000	67%	73	36%	37

Through 48 weeks of therapy, the median increases from baseline in CD4+ cell counts were 201 cells/mm^3 in the group receiving LEXIVA and 216 cells/mm^3 in the nelfinavir group.

Study APV30002: APV30002 was a randomized, open-label study, comparing treatment with LEXIVA Tablets (1,400 mg once daily) plus ritonavir (200 mg once daily) versus nelfinavir (1,250 mg twice daily) in 649 treatment-naive patients. Both treatment groups also received abacavir (300 mg twice daily) and lamivudine (150 mg twice daily). The mean age of the patients in this study was 37 years (range 18 to 69 years), 73% of the patients were males, 22% were CDC Class C, 53% were Caucasian, 36% were black, and 8% were Hispanic. At baseline, the median CD4+ cell count was 170 cells/mm^3 (range: 1 to 1,055 cells/mm^3; 20% of patients had a CD4+ cell count of <50 cells/mm^3 and 35% were in the range of 50 to <200 cells/mm^3). Baseline median HIV-1 RNA was 4.81 $\log_{10}$ copies/mL (range: 2.65 to 7.29 $\log_{10}$ copies/mL; 43% of patients had >100,000 copies/mL). The outcomes of randomized treatment are provided in Table 9.

Table 9. Outcomes of Randomized Treatment Through Week 48 (APV30002)

Outcome (Rebound or discontinuation = failure)	LEXIVA 1,400 mg q.d./ Ritonavir 200 mg q.d. (n = 322)	Nelfinavir 1,250 mg b.i.d. (n = 327)
Responder*	69% (58%)	68% (55%)
Virologic failure	6%	16%
Rebound	5%	8%
Never suppressed through Week 48	1%	8%
Death	1%	0%
Discontinued due to adverse reactions	9%	6%
Discontinued due to other reasons†	15%	10%

*Patients achieved and maintained confirmed HIV-1 RNA <400 copies/mL (<50 copies/mL) through Week 48 (Roche AMPLICOR HIV-1 MONITOR Assay Version 1.5).

† Includes consent withdrawn, lost to follow up, protocol violations, those with missing data, and other reasons.

Treatment response by viral load strata is shown in Table 10.

Table 5. Drug Interactions: Pharmacokinetic Parameters for Coadministered Drug in the Presence of Amprenavir After Administration of LEXIVA

Coadministered Drug(s) and Dose(s)	Dose of **LEXIVA***	n	% Change in Pharmacokinetic Parameters of **Coadministered Drug** (90% CI) C_{max}	AUC	C_{min}
Atorvastatin 10 mg q.d. for 4 days	1,400 mg b.i.d. for 2 weeks	16	↑304 (↑205 to ↑437)	↑130 (↑100 to ↑164)	↓10 (↓27 to ↑12)
Atorvastatin 10 mg q.d. for 4 days	700 mg b.i.d. plus ritonavir 100 b.i.d. for 2 weeks	16	↑184 (↑126 to ↑257)	↑153 (↑115 to ↑199)	↑73 (↑45 to ↑108)
Lopinavir/ritonavir† 533 mg/133 mg b.i.d. for 2 weeks	1,400 mg b.i.d. for 2 weeks	18	See following section: **HIV Protease Inhibitors**		
Lopinavir/ritonavir† 400 mg/100 mg b.i.d. for 2 weeks	700 mg b.i.d. plus ritonavir 100 mg b.i.d. for 2 weeks	18	↑30 (↓15 to ↑47)	↑37 (↓20 to ↑55)	↑52 (↓28 to ↑82)

*Concomitant medication is also shown in this column where appropriate.
† Data represent lopinavir concentrations.
↑ = Increase; ↓ = Decrease; ⇔ = No change (↑ or ↓<10%).

Table 6. Drug Interactions: Pharmacokinetic Parameters for Coadministered Drug in the Presence of Amprenavir After Administration of AGENERASE

Coadministered Drug(s) and Dose(s)	Dose of **AGENERASE**	n	% Change in Pharmacokinetic Parameters of **Coadministered Drug** (90% CI) C_{max}	AUC	C_{min}
Clarithromycin 500 mg b.i.d. for 4 days	1,200 mg b.i.d. for 4 days	12	↓10 (↓24 to ↑7)	⇔	⇔
Delavirdine 600 mg b.i.d. for 10 days	600 mg b.i.d. for 10 days	9	↓47*	↓61*	↓88*
Ethinyl estradiol 0.035 mg for 1 cycle	1,200 mg b.i.d. for 28 days	10	⇔	⇔	↑32 (↓3 to ↑79)
Ketoconazole 400 mg single dose	1,200 mg single dose	12	↑19 (↑8 to ↑33)	↑44 (↑31 to ↑59)	NA
Lamivudine 150 mg single dose	600 mg single dose	11	⇔	⇔	NA
Methadone 44 to 100 mg q.d. for >30 days	1,200 mg b.i.d. for 10 days	16	R-Methadone (active)		
			↓25 (↓32 to ↓18)	↓13 (↓21 to ↓5)	↓21 (↓32 to ↓9)
			S-Methadone (inactive)		
			↓48 (↓55 to ↓40)	↓40 (↓46 to ↓32)	↓53 (↓60 to ↓43)
Norethindrone 1 mg for 1 cycle	1,200 mg b.i.d. for 28 days	10	⇔	↑18 (↑1 to ↑38)	↑45 (↑13 to ↑88)
Rifabutin 300 mg q.d. for 10 days	1,200 mg b.i.d. for 10 days	5	↑119 (↑82 to ↑164)	↑193 (↑156 to ↑235)	↑271 (↑171 to ↑409)
Rifampin 300 mg q.d. for 4 days	1,200 mg b.i.d. for 4 days	11	⇔	⇔	ND
Zidovudine 300 mg single dose	600 mg single dose	12	↑40 (↑14 to ↑71)	↑31 (↑19 to ↑45)	NA

*Median percent change; confidence interval not reported.
↑ = Increase; ↓ = Decrease; ⇔ = No change (↑ or ↓<10%); NA = C_{min} not calculated for single-dose study; ND = Interaction cannot be determined as C_{min} was below the lower limit of quantitation.

Table 10. Proportions of Responders Through Week 48 by Screening Viral Load (APV30002)

Screening Viral Load HIV-1 RNA (copies/mL)	LEXIVA 1,400 mg q.d./ Ritonavir 200 mg q.d.		Nelfinavir 1,250 mg b.i.d.	
	<400 copies/mL	n	<400 copies/mL	n
≤100,000	72%	197	73%	194
>100,000	66%	125	64%	133

Through 48 weeks of therapy, the median increases from baseline in CD4+ cell counts were 203 cells/mm^3 in the group receiving LEXIVA and 207 cells/mm^3 in the nelfinavir group.

Protease Inhibitor-Experienced Patients: Study APV30003: APV30003 was a randomized, open-label, multicenter study comparing 2 different regimens of LEXIVA plus ritonavir (LEXIVA Tablets 700 mg twice daily plus ritonavir 100 mg twice daily or LEXIVA Tablets 1,400 mg once daily plus ritonavir 200 mg once daily) versus lopinavir/ritonavir (400 mg/100 mg twice daily) in 315 patients who had experienced virologic failure to 1 or 2 prior protease inhibitor-containing regimens.

The mean age of the patients in this study was 42 years (range 24 to 72 years), 85% were male, 33% were CDC Class C, 67% were Caucasian, 24% were black, and 9% were Hispanic. The median CD4+ cell count at baseline was 263 cells/mm^3 (range: 2 to 1,171 cells/mm^3). Baseline median plasma HIV-1 RNA level was 4.14 $\log_{10}$ copies/mL (range: 1.69 to 6.41 $\log_{10}$ copies/mL).

The median durations of prior exposure to NRTIs were 257 weeks for patients receiving LEXIVA/ritonavir twice daily (79% had ≥3 prior NRTIs) and 210 weeks for patients receiving lopinavir/ritonavir (64% had ≥3 prior NRTIs). The median durations of prior exposure to protease inhibitors were 149 weeks for patients receiving LEXIVA/ritonavir twice daily (49% received ≥2 prior PIs) and 130 weeks for patients receiving lopinavir/ritonavir (40% received ≥2 prior PIs).

The time-averaged changes in plasma HIV-1 RNA from baseline (AAUCMB) at 48 weeks (the endpoint on which the study was powered) were -1.4 $\log_{10}$ copies/mL for twice-daily LEXIVA/ritonavir and -1.67 $\log_{10}$ copies/mL for the lopinavir/ritonavir group.

The proportions of patients who achieved and maintained confirmed HIV-1 RNA <400 copies/mL (secondary efficacy endpoint) were 58% with twice-daily LEXIVA/ritonavir and 61% with lopinavir/ritonavir (95% CI for the difference -16.6, 10.1). The proportions of patients with HIV-1 RNA <50 copies/mL with twice-daily LEXIVA/ritonavir and with lopinavir/ritonavir were 46% and 50%, respectively (95% CI for the difference -18.3, 8.9). The proportions of patients who were virologic failures were 29% with twice-daily LEXIVA/ritonavir and 27% with lopinavir/ritonavir.

The frequency of discontinuations due to adverse events and other reasons, and deaths were similar between treatment arms.

Through 48 weeks of therapy, the median increases from baseline in CD4+ cell counts were 81 cells/mm^3 with twice-daily LEXIVA/ritonavir and 91 cells/mm^3 with lopinavir/ritonavir.

This study was not large enough to reach a definitive conclusion that LEXIVA/ritonavir and lopinavir/ritonavir are clinically equivalent.

Once-daily administration of LEXIVA plus ritonavir is **not recommended** for protease inhibitor-experienced patients. Through Week 48, 50% and 37% of patients receiving LEXIVA/ritonavir once daily had plasma HIV-1 RNA <400 copies/mL and <50 copies/mL, respectively.

CONTRAINDICATIONS

LEXIVA is contraindicated in patients with previously demonstrated clinically significant hypersensitivity to any of the components of this product or to amprenavir.

Coadministration of LEXIVA with drugs that are highly dependent on CYP3A4 for clearance and for which elevated plasma concentrations are associated with serious and/or life-threatening events is contraindicated. These drugs are listed in Table 11.

Table 11. Drugs That Are Contraindicated with LEXIVA

Drug Class	Drugs Within Class That Are CONTRAINDICATED with LEXIVA
Ergot derivatives	Dihydroergotamine, ergonovine, ergotamine, methylergonovine
GI motility agent	Cisapride
Neuroleptic	Pimozide
Sedatives/hypnotics	Midazolam, triazolam

If LEXIVA is coadministered with ritonavir, the antiarrhythmic agents flecainide and propafenone are also contraindicated. Also, refer to the full prescribing information for NORVIR® (ritonavir) for other potential drug interactions.

WARNINGS

Serious and/or life-threatening drug interactions could occur between LEXIVA and amiodarone, lidocaine (systemic), tricyclic antidepressants, and quinidine. Concentration monitoring of these agents is recommended if these agents are used concomitantly with LEXIVA (see CONTRAINDICATIONS).

Severe and life-threatening skin reactions, including Stevens-Johnson syndrome, have occurred in patients treated with amprenavir (see ADVERSE REACTIONS).

Acute hemolytic anemia has been reported in a patient treated with amprenavir.

Rifampin should not be used in combination with LEXIVA because it reduces plasma concentrations of amprenavir by about 90%. The effect of rifampin on amprenavir concentrations when rifampin is administered with LEXIVA plus ritonavir is not known.

Concomitant use of LEXIVA and St. John's wort (hypericum perforatum) or products containing St. John's wort is not recommended. Coadministration of protease inhibitors, including LEXIVA, with St. John's wort is expected to substantially decrease protease inhibitor concentrations and may result in suboptimal levels of amprenavir and lead to loss of virologic response and possible resistance to LEXIVA or to the class of protease inhibitors.

Concomitant use of LEXIVA with lovastatin or simvastatin is not recommended. Caution should be exercised if HIV protease inhibitors, including LEXIVA, are used concurrently with other HMG-CoA reductase inhibitors that are also metabolized by the CYP3A4 pathway (e.g., atorvastatin). The risk of myopathy, including rhabdomyolysis, may be increased when HIV protease inhibitors, including LEXIVA, are used in combination with these drugs.

Particular caution should be used when prescribing phosphodiesterase (PDE5) inhibitors for erectile dysfunction (e.g., sildenafil or vardenafil) in patients receiving protease inhibitors, including LEXIVA. Coadministration of a protease inhibitor with a PDE5 inhibitor is expected to substantially increase the PDE5 inhibitor concentration and may result in an increase in PDE5 inhibitor-associated adverse events, including hypotension, visual changes, and priapism (see PRECAUTIONS: Drug Interactions and Information for Patients, and the complete specific PDE5 inhibitor prescribing information).

New onset diabetes mellitus, exacerbation of pre-existing diabetes mellitus, and hyperglycemia have been reported during post-marketing surveillance in HIV-infected patients receiving protease inhibitor therapy. Some patients required either initiation or dose adjustments of insulin or oral hypoglycemic agents for treatment of these events. In some cases, diabetic ketoacidosis has occurred. In those patients who discontinued protease inhibitor therapy, hyperglycemia persisted in some cases. Because these events have been reported voluntarily during clinical practice, estimates of frequency cannot be made and causal relationships between protease inhibitor therapy and these events have not been established.

Table 12. Drugs That Should Not Be Coadministered with LEXIVA

Drug Class/Drug Name	Clinical Comment
Antiarrhythmics: Flecainide, propafenone	**CONTRAINDICATED** if LEXIVA is co-prescribed with **ritonavir** due to potential for serious and/or life-threatening reactions such as cardiac arrhythmias secondary to increases in plasma concentrations of antiarrhythmics.
Antimycobacterials: Rifampin*	May lead to loss of virologic response and possible resistance to LEXIVA or to the class of protease inhibitors.
Ergot derivatives: Dihydroergotamine, ergonovine, ergotamine, methylergonovine	**CONTRAINDICATED** due to potential for serious and/or life-threatening reactions such as acute ergot toxicity characterized by peripheral vasospasm and ischemia of the extremities and other tissues.
GI motility agents: Cisapride	**CONTRAINDICATED**due to potential for serious and/or life-threatening reactions such as cardiac arrhythmias.
Herbal products: St. John's wort (hypericum perforatum)	May lead to loss of virologic response and possible resistance to LEXIVA or to the class of protease inhibitors.
HMG co-reductase inhibitors: Lovastatin, simvastatin	Potential for serious reactions such as risk of myopathy including rhabdomyolysis.
Neuroleptic: Pimozide	**CONTRAINDICATED**due to potential for serious and/or life-threatening reactions such as cardiac arrhythmias.
Non-nucleoside reverse transcriptase inhibitor: Delavirdine*	May lead to loss of virologic response and possible resistance to delavirdine.
Sedative/hypnotics: Midazolam, triazolam	**CONTRAINDICATED** due to potential for serious and/or life-threatening reactions such as prolonged or increased sedation or respiratory depression.

*See CLINICAL PHARMACOLOGY Tables 3, 4, 5, or 6 for magnitude of interaction.

Table 13. Established and Other Potentially Significant Drug Interactions: Alteration in Dose or Regimen May Be Recommended Based on Drug Interaction Studies or Predicted Interaction (Information in the table applies to LEXIVA with or without ritonavir, unless otherwise indicated.)

Concomitant Drug Class: Drug Name	Effect on Concentration of Amprenavir or Concomitant Drug	Clinical Comment
	HIV-Antiviral Agents	
Non-nucleoside reverse transcriptase inhibitors: Efavirenz	**LEXIVA:** ↓ Amprenavir	Appropriate doses of the combinations with respect to safety and efficacy have not been established.
	LEXIVA/ritonavir: ↓ Amprenavir	An additional 100 mg/day (300 mg total) of ritonavir is recommended when efavirenz is administered with LEXIVA/ritonavir once daily. No change in the ritonavir dose is required when efavirenz is administered with LEXIVA plus ritonavir twice daily.
Non-nucleoside reverse transcriptase inhibitor: Nevirapine	↓ Amprenavir	Appropriate doses of the combinations with respect to safety and efficacy have not been established.
HIV protease inhibitors: Indinavir,* nelfinavir*	**LEXIVA:** ↑ Amprenavir Effect on indinavir and nelfinavir is not well established. **LEXIVA/ritonavir:** Interaction has not been evaluated.	Appropriate doses of the combinations with respect to safety and efficacy have not been established.
HIV protease inhibitors: Lopinavir/ritonavir*	↓ Amprenavir ↓ Lopinavir	An increased rate of adverse events has been observed with coadministration of these medications. Appropriate doses of the combinations with respect to safety and efficacy have not been established.
HIV protease inhibitor: Saquinavir*	**LEXIVA:** ↓ Amprenavir Effect on saquinavir is not well established. **LEXIVA/ritonavir:** Interaction has not been evaluated.	Appropriate doses of the combination with respect to safety and efficacy have not been established.

(Table continued on next page)

PRECAUTIONS

Sulfa Allergy: LEXIVA should be used with caution in patients with a known sulfonamide allergy. Fosamprenavir contains a sulfonamide moiety. The potential for cross-sensitivity between drugs in the sulfonamide class and fosamprenavir is unknown. In a clinical study of LEXIVA used as the sole protease inhibitor, rash occurred in 2 of 10 patients (20%) with a history of sulfonamide allergy compared with 42 of 126 patients (33%) with no history of sulfonamide allergy. In 2 clinical studies of LEXIVA plus low-dose ritonavir, rash occurred in 8 of 50 patients (16%) with a history of sulfonamide allergy compared with 50 of 412 patients (12%) with no history of sulfonamide allergy.

Hepatic Impairment and Toxicity: LEXIVA is principally metabolized by the liver; therefore, caution should be exer-

Continued on next page

Product information on these pages is effective as of August 2004. Further information is available at: GlaxoSmithKline, PO Box 13398, Research Triangle Park, NC 27709. 1-888-825-5249. Corporate Web Site: www.gsk.com

Lexiva—Cont.

cised when administering LEXIVA to patients with hepatic impairment because amprenavir concentrations may be increased (see CLINICAL PHARMACOLOGY: Special Populations: Hepatic Insufficiency). Patients with impaired hepatic function receiving LEXIVA without concurrent ritonavir may require dose reduction (see DOSAGE AND ADMINISTRATION). There are no data on the use of LEXIVA in combination with ritonavir in patients with any degree of hepatic impairment.

Patients with underlying hepatitis B or C or marked elevations in transaminases prior to treatment may be at increased risk for developing transaminase elevations. Appropriate laboratory testing should be conducted prior to initiating therapy with LEXIVA and patients should be monitored closely during treatment.

Patients with Hemophilia: There have been reports of spontaneous bleeding in patients with hemophilia A and B treated with protease inhibitors. In some patients, additional factor VIII was required. In many of the reported cases, treatment with protease inhibitors was continued or restarted. A causal relationship between protease inhibitor therapy and these episodes has not been established.

Immune Reconstitution: During the initial phase of treatment, patients responding to antiretroviral therapy may develop an inflammatory response to indolent or residual opportunistic infections (such as MAC, CMV, PCP, and TB), which may necessitate further evaluation and treatment.

Fat Redistribution: Redistribution/accumulation of body fat, including central obesity, dorsocervical fat enlargement (buffalo hump), peripheral wasting, facial wasting, breast enlargement, and "cushingoid appearance," have been observed in patients receiving antiretroviral therapy, including LEXIVA. The mechanism and long-term consequences of these events are currently unknown. A causal relationship has not been established.

Lipid Elevations: Treatment with LEXIVA plus ritonavir has resulted in increases in the concentration of triglycerides (see Tables 16 and 17). Triglyceride and cholesterol testing should be performed prior to initiating therapy with LEXIVA and at periodic intervals during therapy. Lipid disorders should be managed as clinically appropriate. (See PRECAUTIONS: Table 12. Drugs That Should Not Be Coadministered with LEXIVA and Table 13: Established and Other Potentially Significant Drug Interactions for additional information on potential drug interactions with LEXIVA and HMG-CoA reductase inhibitors.)

Resistance/Cross-Resistance: Because the potential for HIV cross-resistance among protease inhibitors has not been fully explored, it is unknown what effect therapy with LEXIVA will have on the activity of subsequently administered protease inhibitors. LEXIVA has been studied in patients who have experienced treatment failure with protease inhibitors (see INDICATIONS AND USAGE: Description of Clinical Studies).

Information for Patients: A statement to patients and healthcare providers is included on the product's bottle label: ALERT: Find out about medicines that should NOT be taken with LEXIVA. **A Patient Information Sheet for LEXIVA Tablets is available for patient information.**

Patients should be informed that LEXIVA is not a cure for HIV infection and that they may continue to develop opportunistic infections and other complications associated with HIV disease. The long-term effects of LEXIVA are unknown at this time. Patients should be told that there are currently no data demonstrating that therapy with LEXIVA can reduce the risk of transmitting HIV to others.

Patients should be told that sustained decreases in plasma HIV-1 RNA have been associated with a reduced risk of progression to AIDS and death. Patients should remain under the care of a physician while using LEXIVA. Patients should be advised to take LEXIVA every day as prescribed. LEXIVA must always be used in combination with other antiretroviral drugs. Patients should not alter the dose or discontinue therapy without consulting their physician. If a dose is missed, patients should take the dose as soon as possible and then return to their normal schedule. However, if a dose is skipped, the patient should not double the next dose.

Patients should inform their healthcare provider if they have a sulfa allergy. The potential for cross-sensitivity between drugs in the sulfonamide class and fosamprenavir is unknown.

LEXIVA may interact with many drugs; therefore, patients should be advised to report to their healthcare provider the use of any other prescription or nonprescription medication or herbal products, particularly St. John's wort.

Patients receiving PDE5 inhibitors should be advised that they may be at an increased risk of PDE5 inhibitor-associated adverse events, including hypotension, visual changes, and priapism, and should promptly report any symptoms to their healthcare provider.

Patients receiving hormonal contraceptives should be instructed to use alternate contraceptive measures during therapy with LEXIVA because hormonal levels may be altered.

Patients should be informed that redistribution or accumulation of body fat may occur in patients receiving antiretroviral therapy, including LEXIVA, and that the cause and long-term health effects of these conditions are not known at this time.

Drug Interactions: See also CONTRAINDICATIONS, WARNINGS, and CLINICAL PHARMACOLOGY: Drug Interactions.

Table 13 ***(cont.).*** **Established and Other Potentially Significant Drug Interactions: Alteration in Dose or Regimen May Be Recommended Based on Drug Interaction Studies or Predicted Interaction (Information in the table applies to LEXIVA with or without ritonavir, unless otherwise indicated.)**

Concomitant Drug Class: Drug Name	Effect on Concentration of Amprenavir or Concomitant Drug	Clinical Comment
Other Agents		
Antiarrhythmics: Amiodarone, lidocaine (systemic), and quinidine	↑ Antiarrhythmics	Caution is warranted and therapeutic concentration monitoring, if available, is recommended for antiarrhythmics when coadministered with LEXIVA.
Antiarrhythmic: Bepridil	↑ Bepridil	Use with caution. Increased bepridil exposure may be associated with life-threatening reactions such as cardiac arrhythmias.
Anticoagulant: Warfarin		Concentrations of warfarin may be affected. It is recommended that INR (international normalized ratio) be monitored.
Anticonvulsants: Carbamazepine, phenobarbital, phenytoin	↓ Amprenavir	Use with caution. LEXIVA may be less effective due to decreased amprenavir plasma concentrations in patients taking these agents concomitantly.
Antifungals: Ketoconazole, itraconazole	↑ Ketoconazole ↑ Itraconazole	Increase monitoring for adverse events due to ketoconazole or itraconazole. **LEXIVA:** Dose reduction of ketoconazole or itraconazole may be needed for patients receiving more than 400 mg ketoconazole or itraconazole per day. **LEXIVA/ritonavir:** High doses of ketoconazole or itraconazole (>200 mg/day) are not recommended.
Antimycobacterial: Rifabutin*	↑ Rifabutin and rifabutin metabolite	A complete blood count should be performed weekly and as clinically indicated in order to monitor for neutropenia in patients receiving LEXIVA and rifabutin. **LEXIVA:** A dosage reduction of rifabutin by at least half the recommended dose is required. **LEXIVA/ritonavir:** Dosage reduction of rifabutin by at least 75% of the usual dose of 300 mg/day is recommended (a maximum dose of 150 mg every other day or 3 times per week).
Benzodiazepines: Alprazolam, clorazepate, diazepam, flurazepam	↑ Benzodiazepines	Clinical significance is unknown; however, a decrease in benzodiazepine dose may be needed.
Calcium channel blockers: Diltiazem, felodipine, nifedipine, nicardipine, nimodipine, verapamil, amlodipine, nisoldipine, isradipine	↑ Calcium channel blockers	Caution is warranted and clinical monitoring of patients is recommended.
Corticosteroid: Dexamethasone	↓ Amprenavir	Use with caution. LEXIVA may be less effective due to decreased amprenavir plasma concentrations in patients taking these agents concomitantly.
Histamine H_2-receptor antagonists and proton-pump inhibitors	**LEXIVA:** ↓ Amprenavir **LEXIVA/ritonavir:** Interaction not evaluated	Use with caution. LEXIVA may be less effective due to decreased amprenavir plasma concentrations in patients taking these agents concomitantly.
HMG-CoA reductase inhibitor: Atorvastatin*	↑ Atorvastatin	Use ≤20 mg/day of atorvastatin with careful monitoring, or consider other HMG-CoA reductase inhibitors such as fluvastatin, pravastatin, or rosuvastatin in combination with LEXIVA.
Immunosuppressants: Cyclosporine, tacrolimus, rapamycin	↑ Immunosuppressants	Therapeutic concentration monitoring is recommended for immunosuppressant agents when coadministered with LEXIVA.
Narcotic analgesic: Methadone	↓ Methadone	Dosage of methadone may need to be increased when coadministered with LEXIVA.
Oral contraceptives: Ethinyl estradiol/ norethindrone	**LEXIVA:** ↑ Ethinyl estradiol/ norethindrone **LEXIVA/ritonavir:** Interaction not evaluated	Because hormonal levels may be altered, alternative methods of non-hormonal contraception are recommended.
PDE5 inhibitors: Sildenafil, vardenafil	↑ Sildenafil ↑ Vardenafil	Use sildenafil with caution at reduced doses of 25 mg every 48 hours with increased monitoring for adverse events. **LEXIVA:** Use vardenafil with caution at reduced doses of no more than 2.5 mg every 24 hours with increased monitoring for adverse events. **LEXIVA/ritonavir:** Use vardenafil with caution at reduced doses of no more than 2.5 mg every 72 hours with increased monitoring for adverse events.
Tricyclic antidepressants: Amitriptyline, imipramine	↑ Tricyclics	Therapeutic concentration monitoring is recommended for tricyclic antidepressants when coadministered with LEXIVA.

*See CLINICAL PHARMACOLOGY Tables 3, 4, 5, or 6 for magnitude of interaction.

Amprenavir, the active metabolite of fosamprenavir, is an inhibitor of cytochrome P450 3A4 metabolism and therefore should not be administered concurrently with medications with narrow therapeutic windows that are substrates of CYP3A4. Data also suggest that amprenavir induces CYP3A4.

Amprenavir is metabolized by CYP3A4. Coadministration of LEXIVA and drugs that induce CYP3A4, such as rifampin, may decrease amprenavir concentrations and reduce its therapeutic effect. Coadministration of LEXIVA and drugs that inhibit CYP3A4 may increase amprenavir concentrations and increase the incidence of adverse effects.

The potential for drug interactions with LEXIVA changes when LEXIVA is coadministered with the potent CYP3A4 inhibitor ritonavir. The magnitude of CYP3A4-mediated drug interactions (effect on amprenavir or effect on coadministered drug) may change when LEXIVA is coadministered with ritonavir. Because ritonavir is a CYP2D6 inhibitor, clinically significant interactions with drugs metabolized by CYP2D6 are possible when coadministered with LEXIVA plus ritonavir.

There are other agents that may result in serious and/or life-threatening drug interactions (see CONTRAINDICATIONS and WARNINGS).

[See table 12 at top of page 1561]
[See table 13 on pages 1561 and 1562]

Carcinogenesis and Mutagenesis: Carcinogenicity studies of fosamprenavir in rats and mice are in progress; however, results are available from carcinogenicity studies with amprenavir. Amprenavir was evaluated for carcinogenic potential by oral gavage administration to mice and rats for up to 104 weeks. Results showed an increase in the incidence of benign hepatocellular adenomas and an increase in the combined incidence of hepatocellular adenomas plus carcinoma in males of both species at the highest doses tested. Female mice and rats were not affected. These observations were made at systemic exposures equivalent to approximately 2 times (mice) and 4 times (rats) the human exposure (based on $AUC_{0\text{-}24/hr}$ measurement) at the recommended dose of 1,200 mg twice daily. Administration of amprenavir did not cause a statistically significant increase in the incidence of any other benign or malignant neoplasm in mice or rats. It is not known how predictive the results of rodent carcinogenicity studies may be for humans.

Fosamprenavir and amprenavir were not mutagenic or genotoxic in a battery of in vitro and in vivo assays. These assays included bacterial reverse mutation (Ames), mouse lymphoma, rat micronucleus, and chromosome aberrations in human lymphocytes.

Impairment of Fertility: The effects of fosamprenavir on fertility and general reproductive performance were investigated in male (treated for 4 weeks before mating) and female rats (treated for 2 weeks before mating through postpartum day 6). Systemic exposures ($AUC_{0\text{-}24/hr}$) to amprenavir in these studies were 3 (males) to 4 (females) times higher than exposures in humans following administration of the maximum recommended human dose (MRHD) of fosamprenavir alone or similar to those seen in humans following administration of fosamprenavir in combination with ritonavir. Fosamprenavir did not impair mating or fertility of male or female rats and did not affect the development and maturation of sperm from treated rats.

Pregnancy and Reproduction: Pregnancy Category C. Embryo/fetal development studies were conducted in rats (dosed from day 6 to day 17 of gestation) and rabbits (dosed from day 7 to day 20 of gestation). Administration of fosamprenavir to pregnant rats and rabbits produced no major effects on embryo-fetal development; however, the incidence of abortion was increased in rabbits that were administered fosamprenavir. Systemic exposures ($AUC_{0\text{-}24/hr}$) to amprenavir at these dosages were 0.8 (rabbits) to 2 (rats) times the exposures in humans following administration of the MRHD of fosamprenavir alone or 0.3 (rabbits) to 0.7 (rats) times the exposures in humans following administration of the MRHD of fosamprenavir in combination with ritonavir. In contrast, administration of amprenavir was associated with abortions and an increased incidence of minor skeletal variations resulting from deficient ossification of the femur, humerus, and trochlea, in pregnant rabbits at the tested dose; approximately one twentieth the exposure seen at the recommended human dose.

The mating and fertility of the F_1 generation born to female rats given fosamprenavir was not different from control animals; however, fosamprenavir did cause a reduction in both pup survival and body weights. Surviving F_1 female rats showed an increased time to successful mating, an increased length of gestation, a reduced number of uterine implantation sites per litter, and reduced gestational body weights compared to control animals. Systemic exposure ($AUC_{0\text{-}24/hr}$) to amprenavir in the F_0 pregnant rats was approximately 2 times higher than exposures in humans following administration of the MRHD of fosamprenavir alone or approximately the same as those seen in humans following administration of the MRHD of fosamprenavir in combination with ritonavir.

There are no adequate and well-controlled studies in pregnant women. LEXIVA should be used during pregnancy only if the potential benefit justifies the potential risk to the fetus.

Antiretroviral Pregnancy Registry: To monitor maternal-fetal outcomes of pregnant women exposed to LEXIVA, an Antiretroviral Pregnancy Registry has been established. Physicians are encouraged to register patients by calling 1-800-258-4263.

Table 14. Selected Clinical Adverse Events Reported in Antiretroviral-Naive Patients

	APV30001*				APV30002*			
	LEXIVA 1,400 mg b.i.d. (n = 166)		Nelfinavir 1,250 mg b.i.d. (n = 83)		LEXIVA 1,400 mg q.d./ Ritonavir 200 mg q.d. (n = 322)		Nelfinavir 1,250 mg b.i.d. (n = 327)	
Adverse Event	Moderate/ Severe Drug-Related	All Grades†	Moderate/ Severe Drug-Related	All Grades†	Moderate/ Severe Drug-Related	All Grades†	Moderate/ Severe Drug-Related	All Grades†
Gastrointestinal								
Diarrhea	5%	34%	18%	63%	10%	52%	18%	72%
Nausea	7%	39%	4%	24%	7%	37%	5%	27%
Vomiting	2%	16%	4%	17%	6%	20%	4%	13%
Abdominal pain	1%	5%	0%	8%	2%	11%	2%	11%
Skin								
Pruritus	0%	7%	0%	11%	<1%	7%	1%	9%
Rash	8%	35%	2%	19%	3%	17%	2%	21%
General disorders								
Fatigue	2%	10%	1%	7%	4%	18%	2%	13%
Nervous system								
Depressive/ mood disorders	1%	8%	0%	8%	<1%	8%	0%	6%
Headache	2%	19%	4%	20%	3%	21%	3%	27%
Paresthesia, oral	0%	2%	0%	0%	<1%	10%	0%	<1%

*All patients also received abacavir and lamivudine twice daily.
† Includes adverse events of all grades regardless of causality reported in >5% of patients.

Table 15. Selected Clinical Adverse Events Reported in Protease Inhibitor-Experienced Patients (Study APV30003)

	LEXIVA 700 mg b.i.d./ Ritonavir 100 mg b.i.d.* (n = 106)		Lopinavir 400 mg b.i.d./ Ritonavir 100 mg b.i.d.* (n = 103)	
Adverse Event	Moderate/Severe Drug-Related	All Grades†	Moderate/Severe Drug-Related	All Grades†
Gastrointestinal				
Diarrhea	13%	38%	11%	47%
Nausea	3%	20%	9%	31%
Vomiting	3%	10%	5%	17%
Abdominal pain	<1%	11%	2%	9%
Skin				
Pruritus	<1%	8%	0%	3%
Rash	3%	9%	0%	22%
General disorders				
Fatigue	<1%	9%	<1%	14%
Nervous system				
Depressive/mood disorders	<1%	11%	<1%	10%
Headache	4%	27%	2%	20%
Paresthesia, oral	0%	<1%	0%	0%

*All patients also received 2 reverse transcriptase inhibitors.
† Includes adverse events of all grades regardless of causality in >5% of patients.

Table 16. Grade 3/4 Laboratory Abnormalities Reported in ≥2% of Antiretroviral-Naive Adult Patients in Studies APV30001 and APV30002

	APV30001*		APV30002*	
Laboratory Abnormality	LEXIVA 1,400 mg b.i.d. (n = 166)	Nelfinavir 1,250 mg b.i.d. (n = 83)	LEXIVA 1,400 mg q.d./ Ritonavir 200 mg q.d. (n = 322)	Nelfinavir 1,250 mg b.i.d. (n = 327)
ALT (>5 × ULN)	6%	5%	8%	8%
AST (>5 × ULN)	6%	6%	6%	7%
Serum lipase (>2 × ULN)	8%	4%	6%	4%
Hypertriglyceridemia† (>750 mg/dL)	0%	1%	6%	2%
Neutropenia (<750 cells/mm^3)	3%	6%	3%	4%

*All patients also received abacavir and lamivudine twice daily.
† Fasting specimens.
ULN = Upper limit of normal.

Nursing Mothers: The Centers for Disease Control and Prevention recommend that HIV-infected mothers not breastfeed their infants to avoid risking postnatal transmission of HIV. Although it is not known if amprenavir is excreted in human milk, amprenavir is secreted into the milk of lactating rats. Because of both the potential for HIV transmission and the potential for serious adverse reactions in nursing infants, **mothers should be instructed not to breastfeed if they are receiving LEXIVA.**

Pediatric Use: The safety and efficacy of LEXIVA Tablets have not been established in pediatric patients.

Geriatric Use: Clinical studies of LEXIVA did not include sufficient numbers of patients aged 65 and over to determine whether they respond differently from younger adults. In general, dose selection for an elderly patient should be cautious, reflecting the greater frequency of decreased hepatic, renal, or cardiac function, and of concomitant disease or other drug therapy.

ADVERSE REACTIONS

LEXIVA was studied in 700 patients in Phase III controlled clinical studies. The most common treatment-emergent adverse events in clinical studies of LEXIVA were diarrhea, nausea, vomiting, headache, and rash and were generally

Continued on next page

Product information on these pages is effective as of August 2004. Further information is available at: GlaxoSmithKline, PO Box 13398, Research Triangle Park, NC 27709. 1-888-825-5249. Corporate Web Site: www.gsk.com

Table 17. Grade 3/4 Laboratory Abnormalities Reported in ≥2% of Protease Inhibitor-Experienced Adult Patients in Study APV30003

Laboratory Abnormality	LEXIVA 700 mg b.i.d./ Ritonavir 100 mg b.i.d.* (n = 104)	Lopinavir 400 mg b.i.d./ Ritonavir 100 mg b.i.d.* (n = 103)
Hypertriglyceridemia† (>750 mg/dL)	11%‡	6%‡
Serum lipase (>2 × ULN)	5%	12%
ALT (>5 × ULN)	4%	4%
AST (>5 × ULN)	4%	2%
Hyperglycemia (>251 mg/dL)	2%‡	2%‡

*All patients also received 2 reverse transcriptase inhibitors.
† Fasting specimens.
‡ n = 100 for LEXIVA/ritonavir, n = 98 for lopinavir/ritonavir.
ULN = Upper limit of normal.

Lexiva—Cont.

mild to moderate in severity. Treatment discontinuation due to adverse events occurred in 6.4% of patients receiving LEXIVA and in 5.9% of patients receiving comparator treatments.

Severe or life-threatening skin reactions, including 1 case of Stevens-Johnson syndrome among 700 patients treated with LEXIVA, were reported in <1% of patients treated with LEXIVA in the clinical studies. Treatment with LEXIVA should be discontinued for severe or life-threatening rashes and for moderate rashes accompanied by systemic symptoms.

Skin rash (without regard to causality) occurred in approximately 19% of patients treated with LEXIVA in the pivotal efficacy studies. Rashes were usually maculopapular and of mild or moderate intensity, some with pruritus. Rash had a median onset of 11 days after initiation of LEXIVA and had a median duration of 13 days. Skin rash led to discontinuation of LEXIVA in <1% of patients. In some patients with mild or moderate rash, dosing with LEXIVA was often continued without interruption; if interrupted, reintroduction of LEXIVA generally did not result in rash recurrence.

Selected adverse events reported during the clinical efficacy studies of LEXIVA are shown in Tables 14 and 15. Each table presents drug-related adverse events of moderate or severe intensity and adverse events of all grades regardless of causality in patients treated with combination therapy for up to 48 weeks.

[See table 14 at top of previous page]
[See table 15 on previous page]

The percentages of patients with Grade 3 or 4 laboratory abnormalities in the clinical efficacy studies of LEXIVA are presented in Tables 16 and 17.

[See table 16 on previous page]

The incidence of Grade 3 or 4 hyperglycemia in antiretroviral-naive patients who received LEXIVA in the pivotal studies was <1%.

[See table 17 above]

OVERDOSAGE

There is no known antidote for LEXIVA. It is not known whether amprenavir can be removed by peritoneal dialysis or hemodialysis. If overdosage occurs, the patient should be monitored for evidence of toxicity and standard supportive treatment applied as necessary.

DOSAGE AND ADMINISTRATION

LEXIVA Tablets may be taken with or without food. The recommended oral dose of LEXIVA, alone or in combination with ritonavir, is as follows:

Therapy-Naive Patients:

- LEXIVA 1,400 mg twice daily (without ritonavir)
- LEXIVA 1,400 mg once daily plus ritonavir 200 mg once daily
- LEXIVA 700 mg twice daily plus ritonavir 100 mg twice daily

The twice-daily plus ritonavir dose is supported by pharmacokinetic and safety data (see CLINICAL PHARMACOLOGY and ADVERSE EVENTS).

Protease Inhibitor-Experienced Patients:

- LEXIVA 700 mg twice daily plus ritonavir 100 mg twice daily

Once-daily administration of LEXIVA plus ritonavir is not recommended in protease inhibitor-experienced patients (see Description of Clinical Studies).

Adjustment of Ritonavir Dose When LEXIVA plus Ritonavir are Administered with Efavirenz: An additional 100 mg/day (300 mg total) of ritonavir is recommended when efavirenz is administered with LEXIVA plus ritonavir once daily (see Table 13. Established and Other Potentially Significant Drug Interactions: Alteration in Dose or Regimen May Be Recommended Based on Drug Interaction Studies or Predicted Interaction).

Prescribers should consult the full prescribing information for NORVIR (ritonavir) when using this agent.

Patients with Hepatic Impairment: LEXIVA Tablets should be used with caution, at a reduced dosage of 700 mg twice daily in patients with mild or moderate hepatic impairment (Child-Pugh score ranging from 5 to 8) receiving LEXIVA without concurrent ritonavir (see CLINICAL PHARMACOLOGY: Hepatic Insufficiency). LEXIVA should not be used in patients with severe hepatic impairment (Child-Pugh score ranging from 9 to 12) because the dose cannot be reduced below 700 mg. There are no data on the use of LEXIVA in combination with ritonavir in patients with any degree of hepatic impairment.

HOW SUPPLIED

LEXIVA Tablets, 700 mg, are pink, film-coated, capsule-shaped, biconvex tablets, with "GX LL7" debossed on one face.

Bottles of 60 with child-resistant closures (NDC 0173-0721-00).

Store at controlled room temperature of 25°C (77°F); excursions permitted to 15° to 30°C (59° to 86°F) (see USP Controlled Room Temperature). Keep container tightly closed.

GlaxoSmithKline, Research Triangle Park, NC 27709
Vertex Pharmaceuticals Incorporated, Cambridge, MA 02139

LEXIVA is a trademark of GlaxoSmithKline.

May 2004/RL-2099

Shown in Product Identification Guide, page 316

LOTRONEX® ℞

[lō' trə-nĕx]
(alosetron hydrochloride)
Tablets

> **WARNING: Serious gastrointestinal adverse events, some fatal, have been reported with the use of LOTRONEX. These events, including ischemic colitis and serious complications of constipation, have resulted in hospitalization, blood transfusion, surgery, and death.**
>
> - **Only physicians who have enrolled in GlaxoSmithKline's Prescribing Program for LOTRONEX, based on their attestation of qualifications and acceptance of responsibilities, should prescribe LOTRONEX (see DOSAGE AND ADMINISTRATION and HOW SUPPLIED).**
> - **LOTRONEX is indicated only for women with severe diarrhea-predominant IBS who have failed to respond to conventional therapy (see INDICATIONS AND USAGE). Less than 5 percent of IBS is considered severe. Before receiving the initial prescription for LOTRONEX, the patient must read and sign the Patient-Physician Agreement (see PRECAUTIONS: Information for Patients).**
> - **LOTRONEX should be discontinued immediately in patients who develop constipation or symptoms of ischemic colitis. Physicians should instruct patients to immediately report constipation or symptoms of ischemic colitis. LOTRONEX should not be resumed in patients who develop ischemic colitis. Physicians should instruct patients who report constipation to immediately contact them if the constipation does not resolve after discontinuation of LOTRONEX. Patients with resolved constipation should resume LOTRONEX only on the advice of their treating physician.**

DESCRIPTION

The active ingredient in LOTRONEX Tablets is alosetron hydrochloride (HCl), a potent and selective antagonist of the serotonin 5-HT3 receptor type. Chemically, alosetron is designated as 2,3,4,5-tetrahydro-5-methyl-2-[(5-methyl-1H-imidazol-4-yl)methyl]-1H-pyrido[4,3-b]indol-1-one, monohydrochloride. Alosetron is achiral and has the empirical formula: $C_{17}H_{18}N_4O \bullet HCl$, representing a molecular weight of 330.8. Alosetron is a white to beige solid that has a solubility of 61 mg/mL in water, 42 mg/mL in 0.1M hydrochloric acid, 0.3 mg/mL in pH 6 phosphate buffer, and <0.1 mg/mL in pH 8 phosphate buffer.

LOTRONEX Tablets are supplied for oral administration as 0.5 mg (white) and 1 mg (blue) tablets. The 0.5 mg tablet contains 0.562 mg alosetron HCl equivalent to 0.5 mg alosetron and the 1 mg tablet contains 1.124 mg alosetron HCl equivalent to 1 mg of alosetron. Each tablet also contains the inactive ingredients: lactose (anhydrous), magnesium stearate, microcrystalline cellulose, and pregelatinized starch. The white film-coat for the 0.5 mg tablet contains hypromellose, titanium dioxide, and triacetin. The blue film-coat for the 1 mg tablet contains hypromellose, titanium dioxide, triacetin, and indigo carmine.

CLINICAL PHARMACOLOGY

Pharmacodynamics: ***Mechanism of Action:*** Alosetron is a potent and selective 5-HT3 receptor antagonist. 5-HT3 receptors are nonselective cation channels that are extensively distributed on enteric neurons in the human gastrointestinal tract, as well as other peripheral and central locations. Activation of these channels and the resulting neuronal depolarization affect the regulation of visceral pain, colonic transit and gastrointestinal secretions, processes that relate to the pathophysiology of irritable bowel syndrome (IBS). 5-HT3 receptor antagonists such as alosetron inhibit activation of non-selective cation channels which results in the modulation of the enteric nervous system.

The cause of IBS is unknown. IBS is characterized by visceral hypersensitivity and hyperactivity of the gastrointestinal tract, which lead to abnormal sensations of pain and motor activity. Following distention of the rectum, IBS patients exhibit pain and discomfort at lower volumes than healthy volunteers. Following such distention, alosetron reduced pain and exaggerated motor responses, possibly due to blockade of 5-HT3 receptors.

In healthy volunteers and IBS patients, alosetron (2 mg orally, twice daily for 8 days) increased colonic transit time without affecting orocecal transit time. In healthy volunteers, alosetron also increased basal jejunal water and sodium absorption after a single 4-mg dose. In IBS patients, multiple oral doses of alosetron (4 mg twice daily for 6.5 days) significantly increased colonic compliance.

Single oral doses of alosetron administered to healthy men produced a dose-dependant reduction in the flare response seen after intradermal injection of serotonin. Urinary 6-β-hydroxycortisol excretion decreased by 52% in elderly subjects after 27.5 days of alosetron 2 mg orally twice daily. This decrease was not statistically significant. In another study utilizing alosetron 1 mg orally twice daily for 4 days, there was a significant decrease in urinary 6-β-hydroxycortisol excretion. However, there was no change in the ratio of 6-β-hydroxycortisol to cortisol, indicating a possible decrease in cortisol production. The clinical significance of these findings is unknown.

Pharmacokinetics: The pharmacokinetics of alosetron have been studied after single oral doses ranging from 0.05 mg to 16 mg in healthy men. The pharmacokinetics of alosetron have also been evaluated in healthy women and men and in patients with IBS after repeated oral doses ranging from 1 mg twice daily to 8 mg twice daily.

Absorption: Alosetron is rapidly absorbed after oral administration with a mean absolute bioavailability of approximately 50% to 60% (approximate range 30% to >90%). After administration of radiolabeled alosetron, only 1% of the dose was recovered in the feces as unchanged drug. Following oral administration of a 1-mg alosetron dose to young men, a peak plasma concentration of approximately 5 ng/mL occurs at 1 hour. In young women, the mean peak plasma concentration is approximately 9 ng/mL, with a similar time to peak.

Food Effects: Alosetron absorption is decreased by approximately 25% by co-administration with food, with a mean delay in time to peak concentration of 15 minutes (see DOSAGE AND ADMINISTRATION).

Distribution: Alosetron demonstrates a volume of distribution of approximately 65 to 95 L. Plasma protein binding is 82% over a concentration range of 20 to 4,000 ng/mL.

Metabolism and Elimination: Plasma concentrations of alosetron increase proportionately with increasing single oral doses up to 8 mg and more than proportionately at a single oral dose of 16 mg. Twice-daily oral dosing of alosetron does not result in accumulation. The terminal elimination half-life of alosetron is approximately 1.5 hours (plasma clearance is approximately 600 mL/min). Population pharmacokinetic analysis in IBS patients confirmed that alosetron clearance is minimally influenced by doses up to 8 mg.

Renal elimination of unchanged alosetron accounts for only 6% of the dose. Renal clearance is approximately 94 mL/min.

Alosetron is extensively metabolized in humans. The biological activity of these metabolites is unknown. A mass balance study was performed utilizing an orally administered dose of unlabeled and ^{14}C-labeled alosetron. This study indicates that on a molar basis, alosetron metabolites reach additive peak plasma concentrations 9-fold greater than alosetron and that the additive metabolite AUCs are 13-fold greater than alosetron's AUC. Plasma radioactivity declined with a half-life 2-fold longer than that of alosetron, indicating the presence of circulating metabolites. Approximately 73% of the radiolabeled dose was recovered in urine with another 24% of the dose recovered in feces. Only 7% of the dose was recovered as unchanged drug. At least 13 metabolites have been detected in urine. The predominant product in urine was a 6-hydroxy metabolite (15% of the dose). This metabolite was secondarily metabolized to a glucuronide that was also present in urine (14% of the dose). Smaller amounts of the 6-hydroxy metabolite and the 6-O-glucuronide also appear to be present in feces. A bis-oxidized dicarbonyl accounted for 14% of the dose and its monocarbonyl precursor accounted for another 4% in urine and 6% in feces. No other urinary metabolite accounted for more than 4% of the dose. Glucuronide or sulfate conjugates of unchanged alosetron were not detected in urine.

In studies of Japanese men, an N-desmethyl metabolite was found circulating in plasma in all subjects and accounted for up to 30% of the dose in one subject when alosetron was administered with food. The clinical significance of this finding is unknown.

Alosetron is metabolized by human microsomal cytochrome P450 (CYP), shown in vitro to involve enzymes 2C9 (30%), 3A4 (18%), and 1A2 (10%). Non-CYP mediated Phase I metabolic conversion also contributes to an extent of about 11% (see PRECAUTIONS: Drug Interactions).

Population Subgroups: ***Age:*** In some studies in healthy men or women, plasma concentrations were elevated by approximately 40% in individuals 65 years and older compared to young adults. However, this effect was not consistently observed in men (see WARNINGS).

Gender: Plasma concentrations are 30% to 50% lower and less variable in men compared to women given the same oral dose. Population pharmacokinetic analysis in IBS patients confirmed that alosetron concentrations were influenced by gender (27% lower in men).

Reduced Hepatic Function: No pharmacokinetic data are available in this patient group (see PRECAUTIONS: Hepatic Insufficiency and DOSAGE AND ADMINISTRATION: Patients with Hepatic Impairment).

Reduced Renal Function: Renal impairment (creatinine clearance 4 to 56 mL/min) has no effect on the renal elimination of alosetron due to the minor contribution of this pathway to elimination. The effect of renal impairment on metabolite kinetics and the effect of end-stage renal disease have not been assessed (see DOSAGE AND ADMINISTRATION: Patients with Renal Impairment).

CLINICAL TRIALS

LOTRONEX 1 mg twice daily was studied in two 12-week U.S. multicenter, randomized, double-blind, placebo-controlled trials of identical design (Studies 1 and 2) in non-constipated women with IBS meeting the Rome Criteria[1] for at least 6 months. Women with severe pain or a history of severe constipation were excluded. A 2-week run-in period established baseline IBS symptoms.

There were a total of 633 women on LOTRONEX and 640 on placebo, about two thirds with diarrhea-predominant IBS. Compared with placebo, 10% to 19% more women with diarrhea-predominant IBS who received LOTRONEX had adequate relief of IBS abdominal pain and discomfort during each month of the study.

Women with Severe Diarrhea-Predominant IBS: LOTRONEX is indicated only for women with severe diarrhea-predominant IBS (see INDICATIONS AND USAGE). The indication has been narrowed to this group of severely affected patients because serious gastrointestinal adverse events, some fatal, have been reported with the use of LOTRONEX. The following prospective and retrospective analyses support efficacy of LOTRONEX in this subset of the population that was studied in clinical trials.

In two 12-week, randomized, double-blind, placebo-controlled trials of women with diarrhea-predominant IBS and bowel urgency on at least 50% of days at entry (Studies 3 and 4), there were a total of 778 women on LOTRONEX and 515 on placebo. Patients on LOTRONEX had significant increases over placebo (13% to 16%) in the median percentage of days with urgency control.

Retrospective Analyses: In analyses of patients from Studies 1 and 2 who had diarrhea-predominant IBS and indicated their baseline run-in IBS symptoms were severe at the start of the trial, LOTRONEX provided greater adequate relief of IBS pain and discomfort than placebo. In further analyses of Studies 1 and 2, 57% of patients had urgency at baseline on 5 or more days per week. In this subset, 32% of patients on LOTRONEX had urgency no more than 1 day in the last week of the trial, compared to 19% of patients on placebo.

In Studies 3 and 4, 66% of patients had urgency at baseline on 5 or more days per week. In this subset, 50% of patients on LOTRONEX had urgency no more than 1 day in the last week of the trial, compared to 29% of patients on placebo. Moreover, in the same subset, 12% on LOTRONEX had urgency no more than 2 days per week in any of the 12 weeks on treatment compared to 1% of placebo patients.

Efficacy in men has not been established.

INDICATIONS AND USAGE

Because of serious gastrointestinal adverse events, some fatal, reported with use of this drug, LOTRONEX is indicated only for women with severe diarrhea-predominant irritable bowel syndrome (IBS) who have:

- chronic IBS symptoms (generally lasting 6 months or longer),
- had anatomic or biochemical abnormalities of the gastrointestinal tract excluded, and
- failed to respond to conventional therapy.

Diarrhea-predominant IBS is severe if it includes diarrhea and one or more of the following:

- frequent and severe abdominal pain/discomfort
- frequent bowel urgency or fecal incontinence
- disability or restriction of daily activities due to IBS

Less than 5 percent of IBS is considered severe.

In men, the safety and effectiveness of LOTRONEX have not been established (see CLINICAL TRIALS).

CONTRAINDICATIONS

LOTRONEX **should not be initiated** in patients with constipation (see WARNINGS).

LOTRONEX is contraindicated in patients:

- With a history of chronic or severe constipation or with a history of sequelae from constipation.
- With a history of intestinal obstruction, stricture, toxic megacolon, gastrointestinal perforation, and/or adhesions.
- With a history of ischemic colitis, impaired intestinal circulation, thrombophlebitis, or hypercoagulable state.
- With current or a history of Crohn's disease or ulcerative colitis.
- With active diverticulitis or a history of diverticulitis.
- Who are unable to understand or comply with the Patient-Physician Agreement.
- With known hypersensitivity to any component of the product.

WARNINGS (See BOXED WARNING and DOSAGE AND ADMINISTRATION.)

Some patients have experienced serious complications of constipation or ischemic colitis without warning.

Constipation: Serious complications of constipation, including obstruction, perforation, impaction, toxic megacolon, secondary colonic ischemia, and death have been reported with use of LOTRONEX. In some cases these complications have required intestinal surgery, including colectomy. **In IBS clinical trials, the incidence of serious complications of constipation in women was approximately 1 per 1,000 patients, but approximately 10% of patients on LOTRONEX withdrew prematurely because of constipation.** Patients who are elderly, debilitated, or taking additional medications that decrease gastrointestinal motility may be at greater risk for complications of constipation.

LOTRONEX should be discontinued immediately in patients who develop constipation (see BOXED WARNING).

Ischemic Colitis: Ischemic colitis has been reported in patients receiving LOTRONEX in clinical trials as well as during marketed use of the drug. **In IBS clinical trials, the cumulative incidence of ischemic colitis in women receiving LOTRONEX was 2 per 1,000 patients (95% confidence interval 1 to 3) over 3 months and was 3 per 1,000 patients (95% confidence interval 1 to 4) over 6 months. Patient experience in controlled clinical trials is insufficient to estimate the incidence of ischemic colitis in patients taking LOTRONEX for longer than 6 months.**

LOTRONEX should be discontinued immediately in patients with signs of ischemic colitis such as rectal bleeding, bloody diarrhea, or new or worsening abdominal pain. Because ischemic colitis can be life-threatening, patients with signs or symptoms of ischemic colitis should be evaluated promptly and have appropriate diagnostic testing performed. Treatment with LOTRONEX should not be resumed in patients who develop ischemic colitis.

PRECAUTIONS

Information for Patients: Patients should be fully counseled on and understand the risks and benefits of LOTRONEX before an initial prescription is written.

PHYSICIANS MUST:

- Be enrolled in GlaxoSmithKline's Prescribing Program for LOTRONEX based on their attestation of qualifications and acceptance of responsibilities. To enroll in the GlaxoSmithKline Prescribing Program for LOTRONEX call 1-888-825-5249 or visit www.LOTRONEX.com.
- Counsel the patient about the risks and benefits of LOTRONEX, in the patients for whom LOTRONEX is indicated, and discuss the impact of IBS symptoms on the patient's life.
- Give the patient a copy of the Medication Guide, which outlines the risks and benefits of LOTRONEX, and instruct the patient to carefully read the Medication Guide. Answer all questions the patient may have about LOTRONEX. The complete text of the Medication Guide is printed at the end of this document.
- Review the Patient-Physician Agreement with the patient, answer all questions, and confirm that the patient has signed the Agreement.
- Sign the Patient-Physician Agreement, give a copy of the signed Agreement to the patient, and put the original in the patient's medical record.
- Provide each patient with appropriate instructions for taking LOTRONEX.

Copies of the Patient-Physician Agreement and additional copies of the Medication Guide are available by contacting GlaxoSmithKline at 1-888-825-5249 or visiting www.LOTRONEX.com.

PATIENTS WHO ARE PRESCRIBED LOTRONEX SHOULD BE INSTRUCTED TO:

- Read the Medication Guide before starting LOTRONEX and each time they refill their prescription.
- Not start taking LOTRONEX if they are constipated.
- Immediately discontinue LOTRONEX and contact their physician if they become constipated, or have symptoms of ischemic colitis such as new or worsening abdominal pain, bloody diarrhea, or blood in the stool. Immediately contact their physician again if their constipation does not resolve after discontinuation of LOTRONEX. Resume LOTRONEX only if their constipation has resolved and after discussion with and the agreement of their treating physician.
- Stop taking LOTRONEX and contact their physician if LOTRONEX does not adequately control IBS symptoms after 4 weeks of taking 1 mg twice a day.

Drug Interactions: In vitro human liver microsome studies and an in vivo metabolic probe study demonstrated that alosetron did not inhibit CYP enzymes 2D6, 3A4, 2C9, or 2C19. In vitro, at total drug concentrations 27-fold higher than peak plasma concentrations observed with the 1-mg dosage, alosetron inhibited CYP enzymes 1A2 (60%) and 2E1 (50%). In an in vivo metabolic probe study, alosetron did not inhibit CYP2E1 but did produce 30% inhibition of both CYP1A2 and N-acetyltransferase. Although not studied with alosetron, inhibition of N-acetyltransferase may have clinically relevant consequences for drugs such as isoniazid, procainamide, and hydralazine. The effect on CYP1A2 was explored further in a clinical interaction study with theophylline and no effect on metabolism was observed. Another study showed that alosetron had no clinically significant effect on plasma concentrations of the oral contraceptive agents ethinyl estradiol and levonorgestrel (CYP3A4 substrates). A clinical interaction study was also conducted with alosetron and the CYP3A4 substrate cisapride. No significant effects on cisapride metabolism or QT interval were noted. The effect of alosetron on monoamine oxidases and on intestinal first pass secondary to high intraluminal concentrations have not been examined. Based on the above data from in vitro and in vivo studies, it is unlikely that alosetron will inhibit the hepatic metabolic clearance of drugs metabolized by the major CYP enzyme 3A4, as well as the CYP enzymes 2D6, 2C9, 2C19, 2E1, or 1A2.

Alosetron does not appear to induce the major cytochrome P450 (CYP) drug metabolizing enzyme 3A. Alosetron also does not appear to induce CYP enzymes 2E1 or 2C19. It is not known whether alosetron might induce other enzymes. Because alosetron is metabolized by a variety of hepatic CYP drug-metabolizing enzymes, inducers or inhibitors of these enzymes may change the clearance of alosetron. The effect of induction or inhibition of these pathways on exposure to alosetron and its metabolites is not known.

Hepatic Insufficiency: Due to the extensive hepatic metabolism of alosetron, increased exposure to alosetron and/or its metabolites is likely to occur in patients with hepatic insufficiency.

Carcinogenesis, Mutagenesis, Impairment of Fertility: In 2-year oral studies, alosetron was not carcinogenic in mice at doses up to 30 mg/kg/day or in rats at doses up to 40 mg/kg/day. These doses are, respectively, about 60 to 160 times the recommended human dose of alosetron of 2 mg/day (1 mg twice daily) based on body surface area. Alosetron was not genotoxic in the Ames tests, the mouse lymphoma cell (L5178Y/TK$^{\pm}$) forward gene mutation test, the human lymphocyte chromosome aberration test, the ex vivo rat hepatocyte unscheduled DNA synthesis (UDS) test, or the in vivo rat micronucleus test for mutagenicity. Alosetron at oral doses up to 40 mg/kg/day (about 160 times the recommended daily human dose based on body surface area) was found to have no effect on fertility and reproductive performance of male or female rats.

Pregnancy: ***Teratogenic Effects:*** Pregnancy Category B. Reproduction studies have been performed in rats at doses up to 40 mg/kg/day (about 160 times the recommended human dose based on body surface area) and rabbits at oral doses up to 30 mg/kg/day (about 240 times the recommended daily human dose based on body surface area). These studies have revealed no evidence of impaired fertility or harm to the fetus due to alosetron. There are, however, no adequate and well-controlled studies in pregnant women. Because animal reproduction studies are not always predictive of human response, LOTRONEX should be used during pregnancy only if clearly needed.

Nursing Mothers: Alosetron and/or metabolites of alosetron are excreted in the breast milk of lactating rats. It is not known whether alosetron is excreted in human milk. Because many drugs are excreted in human milk, caution should be exercised when LOTRONEX is administered to a nursing woman.

Pediatric Use: Safety and effectiveness in pediatric patients have not been established.

Geriatric Use: Postmarketing experience suggests that elderly patients may be at greater risk for complications of constipation (see WARNINGS).

ADVERSE REACTIONS

Table 1 summarizes adverse events from 22 repeat-dose studies in patients with IBS who were treated with 1 mg of LOTRONEX twice daily for 8 to 24 weeks. The adverse events in Table 1 were reported in 1% or more of patients who received LOTRONEX and occurred more frequently on LOTRONEX than on placebo. A statistically significant difference was observed for constipation in patients treated with LOTRONEX compared to placebo ($p<0.0001$).

Table 1. Adverse Events Reported in ≥1% of IBS Patients and More Frequently on LOTRONEX 1 mg B.I.D. than Placebo

Body System Adverse Event	LOTRONEX 1 mg B.I.D. (n = 8,328)	Placebo (n = 2,363)
Gastrointestinal		
Constipation	29%	6%
Abdominal discomfort and pain	7%	4%
Nausea	6%	5%

Continued on next page

Product information on these pages is effective as of August 2004. Further information is available at: GlaxoSmithKline, PO Box 13398, Research Triangle Park, NC 27709. 1-888-825-5249. Corporate Web Site: www.gsk.com

Lotronex—Cont.

Gastrointestinal discomfort and pain	5%	3%
Abdominal distention	2%	1%
Regurgitation and reflux	2%	2%
Hemorrhoids	2%	1%

Gastrointestinal: Constipation is a frequent and dose-related side effect of treatment with LOTRONEX (see WARNINGS). In clinical studies constipation was reported in approximately 29% of IBS patients treated with LOTRONEX 1 mg twice daily (n = 9,316). This effect was statistically significant compared to placebo (p<0.0001). Eleven percent (11%) of patients treated with LOTRONEX 1 mg twice daily withdrew from the studies due to constipation. Although the number of IBS patients treated with LOTRONEX 0.5 mg twice daily is relatively small (n = 243), only 11% of those patients reported constipation and 4% withdrew from clinical studies due to constipation. Among the patients treated with LOTRONEX 1 mg twice daily who reported constipation, 75% reported a single episode and most reports of constipation (70%) occurred during the first month of treatment with the median time to first report of constipation onset of 8 days. Occurrences of constipation in clinical trials were generally mild to moderate in intensity, transient in nature, and resolved either spontaneously with continued treatment or with an interruption of treatment. However, serious complications of constipation have been reported in clinical studies and in postmarketing experience (see BOXED WARNING and WARNINGS). In Studies 1 and 2, 9% of patients treated with LOTRONEX reported constipation and 4 consecutive days with no bowel movement (see CLINICAL TRIALS). Following interruption of treatment, 78% of the affected patients resumed bowel movements within a 2-day period and were able to re-initiate treatment with LOTRONEX.

Hepatic: A similar incidence in elevation of ALT (>2 fold) was seen in patients receiving LOTRONEX or placebo (1.0% vs. 1.2%). A single case of hepatitis (elevated ALT, AST, alkaline phosphatase, and bilirubin) without jaundice was reported in a 12-week study. A causal association with LOTRONEX has not been established.

Long-Term Safety: Patient experience in controlled clinical trials is insufficient to estimate the incidence of ischemic colitis in patients taking LOTRONEX for longer than 6 months.

Other Events Observed During Clinical Evaluation of LOTRONEX: During its assessment in clinical trials, multiple and single doses of LOTRONEX were administered resulting in 11,874 subject-exposures in 86 completed clinical studies. The conditions, dosages, and duration of exposure to LOTRONEX varied between trials, and the studies included healthy male and female volunteers as well as male and female patients with IBS and other indications.

In the listing that follows, reported adverse events were classified using a standardized coding dictionary. Only those events that an investigator believed were possibly related to alosetron, occurred in at least 2 patients, and occurred at a greater frequency during treatment with LOTRONEX than during placebo administration are presented. Serious adverse events occurring in at least 1 patient for which an investigator believed there was reasonable possibility that the event was related to alosetron treatment and which occurred at a greater frequency in LOTRONEX than placebo-treated patients are also presented.

In the following listing, events are categorized by body system. Within each body system, events are presented in descending order of frequency. The following definitions are used: *Infrequent* adverse events are those occurring on one or more occasion in 1/100 to 1/1,000 patients; *Rare* adverse events are those occurring on one or more occasion in fewer than 1/1,000 patients.

Although the events reported occurred during treatment with LOTRONEX, they were not necessarily caused by it.

Blood and Lymphatic: Rare: Quantitative red cell or hemoglobin defects, hemorrhage, and lymphatic signs and symptoms.

Cardiovascular: Infrequent: Tachyarrhythmias. ***Rare:*** Arrhythmias, increased blood pressure, and extrasystoles.

Drug Interaction, Overdose, and Trauma: Rare: Contusions and hematomas.

Ear, Nose, and Throat: Rare: Ear, nose, and throat infections; viral ear, nose, and throat infections; and laryngitis.

Endocrine and Metabolic: Rare: Disorders of calcium and phosphate metabolism, hyperglycemia, hypothalamus/pituitary hypofunction, hypoglycemia, and fluid disturbances.

Eye: Rare: Light sensitivity of eyes.

Gastrointestinal: Infrequent: Hyposalivation, dyspeptic symptoms, gastrointestinal spasms, ischemic colitis (see WARNINGS), and gastrointestinal lesions. ***Rare:*** Abnormal tenderness, colitis, gastrointestinal signs and symptoms, proctitis, diverticulitis, positive fecal occult blood, hyperacidity, decreased gastrointestinal motility and ileus, gastrointestinal obstructions, oral symptoms, gastrointestinal intussusception, gastritis, gastroduodenitis, gastroenteritis, and ulcerative colitis.

Hepatobiliary Tract and Pancreas: Rare: Abnormal bilirubin levels and cholecystitis.

Lower Respiratory: Infrequent: Breathing disorders. ***Rare:*** Viral respiratory infections.

Musculoskeletal: Rare: Muscle pain; muscle stiffness, tightness and rigidity; and bone and skeletal pain.

Neurological: Infrequent: Hypnagogic effects. ***Rare:*** Memory effects, tremors, dreams, cognitive function disorders, disturbances of sense of taste, disorders of equilibrium, confusion, sedation, and hypoesthesia.

Non-site Specific: Infrequent: Malaise and fatigue, cramps, pain, temperature regulation disturbances. ***Rare:*** General signs and symptoms, non-specific conditions, burning sensations, hot and cold sensations, cold sensations, and fungal infections.

Psychiatry: Infrequent: Anxiety. ***Rare:*** Depressive moods.

Reproduction: Rare: Sexual function disorders, female reproductive tract bleeding and hemorrhage, reproductive infections, and fungal reproductive infections.

Skin: Infrequent: Sweating and urticaria. ***Rare:*** Hair loss and alopecia; acne and folliculitis; disorders of sweat and sebum; allergic skin reaction; eczema; skin infections; dermatitis and dermatosis; and nail disorders.

Urology: Infrequent: Urinary frequency. ***Rare:*** Bladder inflammation; polyuria and diuresis; and urinary tract hemorrhage.

Postmarketing Experience: The following events have been identified during use of LOTRONEX in clinical practice. Because they were reported voluntarily from a population of unknown size, estimates of frequency cannot be made. These events have been chosen for inclusion due to a combination of their seriousness, frequency of reporting, or potential causal connection to LOTRONEX.

Gastrointestinal: Constipation, ileus, impaction, obstruction, perforation, ulceration, ischemic colitis, small bowel mesenteric ischemia (see WARNINGS).

Neurological: Headache.

Skin: Rash.

DRUG ABUSE AND DEPENDENCE

LOTRONEX has no known potential for abuse or dependence.

OVERDOSAGE

There is no specific antidote for overdose of LOTRONEX. Patients should be managed with appropriate supportive therapy. Individual oral doses as large as 16 mg have been administered in clinical studies without significant adverse events. This dose is 8 times higher than the recommended total daily dose. Inhibition of the metabolic elimination and reduced first pass of other drugs might occur with overdoses of alosetron (see PRECAUTIONS: Drug Interactions). Single oral doses of LOTRONEX at 15 mg/kg in female mice and 60 mg/kg in female rats (30 and 240 times, respectively, the recommended human dose based on body surface area) were lethal. Symptoms of acute toxicity were labored respiration, subdued behavior, ataxia, tremors, and convulsions.

DOSAGE AND ADMINISTRATION

For safety reasons, LOTRONEX is approved with marketing restrictions. Only physicians who attest to the following qualifications and accept the following responsibilities, and on that basis enroll in the GlaxoSmithKline Prescribing Program for LOTRONEX, should prescribe LOTRONEX.

To enroll, physicians must attest that they are able and willing to:

- diagnose and treat IBS
- diagnose and manage ischemic colitis
- diagnose and manage constipation and complications of constipation
- understand the risks and benefits of treatment with LOTRONEX for severe diarrhea-predominant IBS, including the information in the package insert, Medication Guide, and Patient-Physician Agreement
- educate patients on the risks and benefits of treatment with LOTRONEX and obtain the patient's signature on the Patient-Physician Agreement form, sign it, place the original signed form in the patient's medical record, and give a copy to the patient
- report serious adverse events to GlaxoSmithKline at 1-888-825-5249 or to the Food and Drug Administration's MedWatch Program at 1-800-FDA-1088
- affix program stickers to <u>all</u> prescriptions for LOTRONEX (i.e., the original and all subsequent refill prescriptions). Stickers will be provided as part of the GlaxoSmithKline Prescribing Program for LOTRONEX. No telephone, facsimile, or computerized prescriptions are permitted with this program.

To enroll in the Prescribing Program for LOTRONEX call 1-888-825-5249 or visit www.LOTRONEX.com.

Usual Dose in Adults: For safety reasons, LOTRONEX should be started at a dosage of 1 mg orally once a day for 4 weeks. This dosage may be less constipating than a regimen of 1 mg twice a day (see WARNINGS). If, after 4 weeks, the 1 mg once-a-day dosage is well tolerated but does not adequately control IBS symptoms, then the dosage can be increased to 1 mg twice a day, the dose used in controlled clinical trials (see CLINICAL TRIALS). Although the efficacy of the 1 mg once-a-day dosage in treating diarrhea-predominant IBS has not been evaluated in clinical trials, for safety reasons consideration should be given to continuing this dosage if well tolerated and IBS symptoms in the individual patient are adequately controlled. **LOTRONEX should be discontinued in patients who have not had adequate control of IBS symptoms after 4 weeks of treatment with 1 mg twice a day.**

LOTRONEX should be discontinued immediately in patients who develop constipation or signs of ischemic colitis. LOTRONEX should not be restarted in patients who develop ischemic colitis.

Clinical trial and postmarketing experience suggest that debilitated patients or patients taking additional medications that decrease gastrointestinal motility may be at greater risk of serious complications of constipation. Therefore, appropriate caution and follow-up should be exercised if LOTRONEX is prescribed for these patients (see also Geriatric Patients).

Pediatric Patients: Safety and effectiveness have not been established in pediatric patients (see PRECAUTIONS: Pediatric Use).

Geriatric Patients: Postmarketing experience suggests that elderly patients may be at greater risk for complications of constipation; therefore, appropriate caution and follow-up should be exercised if LOTRONEX is prescribed for these patients (see WARNINGS).

Patients with Renal Impairment: There are insufficient data available on the biological activity of the metabolites of LOTRONEX. It is unknown if dosage adjustment is needed in patients with renal impairment (see CLINICAL PHARMACOLOGY: Reduced Renal Function).

Patients with Hepatic Impairment: No studies have been conducted in patients with hepatic impairment. LOTRONEX is extensively metabolized by the liver and increased exposure to LOTRONEX is likely to occur in patients with hepatic impairment. Increased drug exposure may increase the risk of serious adverse events. LOTRONEX should be used with caution in patients with hepatic impairment (see PRECAUTIONS: Hepatic Insufficiency and CLINICAL PHARMACOLOGY: Population Subgroups: Reduced Hepatic Function).

LOTRONEX can be taken with or without food.

HOW SUPPLIED

The physician must attest to meeting the qualifications and accepting the responsibilities in the DOSAGE AND ADMINISTRATION section of this package insert and submit this attestation to GlaxoSmithKline to be enrolled in the Prescribing Program for LOTRONEX, which utilizes special program stickers that the enrolled physician will affix to <u>all</u> prescriptions for LOTRONEX (i.e., the original and all subsequent refill prescriptions). No telephone, facsimile, or computerized prescriptions are permitted with this program.

LOTRONEX Tablets, 0.5 mg (0.562 mg alosetron HCl equivalent to 0.5 mg alosetron) are white, oval, film-coated tablets debossed with GX EXI on one face. Bottles of 30 (NDC 0173-0738-00) with child-resistant closures.

LOTRONEX Tablets, 1 mg (1.124 mg alosetron HCl equivalent to 1 mg alosetron), are blue, oval, film-coated tablets debossed with GX CT1 on one face. Bottles of 30 (NDC 0173-0690-05) with child-resistant closures.

Store at 25°C (77°F); excursions permitted to 15–30°C (59–86°F) [see USP Controlled Room Temperature]. Protect from light and moisture.

REFERENCE

1. Thompson WG, Creed F, Drossman DA, et al. Functional bowel disease and functional abdominal pain. *Gastroenterol Int.* 1992;5:75-91.

MEDICATION GUIDE

LOTRONEX® (LOW-trah-nex) Tablets
(alosetron hydrochloride)

You MUST do 3 things if you are going to take LOTRONEX:

- **Understand that LOTRONEX has serious risks.**
- **Sign a Patient-Physician Agreement with your doctor.**
- **Follow the directions in this Medication Guide.**

If you can't do ALL of these, you should not take LOTRONEX.

Read this Medication Guide carefully before you sign the Patient-Physician Agreement and before you start to take LOTRONEX. Read the Medication Guide you get with each refill for LOTRONEX. There may be new information. This Medication Guide does not take the place of talking with your doctor.

What is the most important information I should know about LOTRONEX?

Because of serious bowel side effects, including some deaths, seen with use of this drug, LOTRONEX, is only for women who have very bad irritable bowel syndrome and whose main problem is diarrhea (diarrhea-predominant IBS). To decide if you want to use LOTRONEX, you need to know about possible side effects of LOTRONEX and how LOTRONEX may help your IBS. Very few patients have diarrhea-predominant IBS that is bad enough to consider using LOTRONEX.

Do not take LOTRONEX unless all of the things in this list are true about you.

- Your main IBS problem is diarrhea.
- Your IBS has gone on for a long time, 6 months or longer.
- Your doctor has told you that your symptoms are not due to other medical problems.
- You have tried other IBS treatments and none have helped you.

You can tell if your IBS is very bad if you have 1 or more of the following problems:

- You have lots of painful stomach cramps or bloating.
- You often can't control the need to have a bowel movement or have "accidents" where your underwear gets dirty from diarrhea or bowel movements (stools).

- You can't lead a normal home or work life because you need to be near a bathroom.

Unless these things are true about you, you should not consider taking LOTRONEX.

Women whose main IBS problem is constipation should not use LOTRONEX. LOTRONEX has not been shown to help men with IBS.

About 1 woman out of 1,000 women who take LOTRONEX may get serious constipation problems. These constipation problems can lead to being in the hospital, getting blood transfusions, having surgery, or even death.

To lower your chances of getting serious constipation problems

- Do not start taking LOTRONEX if you are constipated.
- If you get constipated while taking LOTRONEX, stop taking it right away and call your doctor.
- If your constipation does not get better after stopping LOTRONEX, call your doctor again.
- Do not start taking LOTRONEX again unless your doctor tells you to do so.

About 1 woman out of 350 women who take LOTRONEX over a 6-month period may get a serious problem where the blood flow to certain parts of the intestines is reduced. This is called ischemic colitis. The risk of ischemic colitis when LOTRONEX is taken for more than 6 months is unknown. If you get ischemic colitis, you may need to go to the hospital, get blood transfusions, or have surgery. It is possible to die from ischemic colitis.

You must stop taking LOTRONEX and call your doctor right away if you have either of these signs of ischemic colitis:

- new or worse pain in your bowels.
- blood in your diarrhea or stool (bowel movements).

Serious problems of constipation or ischemic colitis can happen suddenly. People who are older, who are weak from illness, or who take other constipating medicines may be more likely to have serious constipation problems with LOTRONEX.

Before you take LOTRONEX, be sure you understand the possible risks and benefits of LOTRONEX. Talk with your doctor about how much of a problem IBS is in your life. Talk with your doctor about what else you have tried for IBS and about other things besides LOTRONEX that you may not have tried.

Only doctors who have signed up with the company that makes LOTRONEX should write prescriptions for LOTRONEX. As part of signing up these doctors have said that they know about IBS and the possible side effects of LOTRONEX. They have agreed to use a special sticker on all your prescriptions for LOTRONEX so your pharmacist knows that they have signed up with the company.

Your doctor will ask you to sign a Patient-Physician Agreement after you have read this Medication Guide for the first time. Signing the Agreement means that you understand the risks and benefits of LOTRONEX and that you have read and understand the Medication Guide.

What is LOTRONEX?

LOTRONEX is a medicine that slows the movement of stools (bowel movements) through the bowels. LOTRONEX does not cure IBS and it will not help every person who takes it. For those who are helped, LOTRONEX reduces lower abdominal (stomach area) pain, abdominal discomfort, urgency (sudden need to have a bowel movement), and diarrhea of IBS. If you stop taking LOTRONEX, your IBS symptoms may return within 1 or 2 weeks.

Who should not take LOTRONEX?

LOTRONEX is not right for everyone. Do not ever take LOTRONEX if you:

- are constipated most of the time
- ever had a serious problem from constipation
- ever had serious bowel blockages
- ever had ischemic colitis
- ever had blood flow problems to your bowels
- ever had blood clots
- ever had Crohn's disease, ulcerative colitis, or diverticulitis
- do not understand the Patient-Physician Agreement or are not willing to follow it
- are allergic to LOTRONEX or any of its ingredients. (See the list of ingredients at the end of this Medication Guide.)

If you can take LOTRONEX, do not start taking it if you are constipated.

Before taking LOTRONEX tell your doctor

- about any other illnesses you have or medicines you take or plan to take. This includes prescription and non-prescription medicines, supplements, and herbal remedies. Some illnesses and medicines cause constipation. If you have certain illnesses or take certain medicines, taking LOTRONEX may increase your risk of getting serious side effects from constipation.
- if you are pregnant, planning to get pregnant, or breast feeding.

How should I take LOTRONEX?

- Take LOTRONEX exactly as your doctor prescribes it. You can take LOTRONEX with or without food.
- Begin with no more than 1 mg a day for 4 weeks to see how LOTRONEX affects you. Although the effect of 1 mg once a day on IBS symptoms has not been studied in clinical trials, you and your doctor may decide that you should keep taking this dose if it adequately controls your IBS symptoms and you have not become constipated or had ischemic colitis while taking LOTRONEX.
- If you miss a dose of LOTRONEX, just skip that dose. Do **not** take 2 doses the next time. Wait until the next time you are supposed to take it and then take your normal dose.
- If you try 1 mg once a day for 4 weeks and it does not control your symptoms, does not make you constipated, and does not give you ischemic colitis, tell your doctor. Your doctor may increase your dose up to 1 mg twice a day, the dose that was used in clinical trials.

If 1 mg twice a day does not work after 4 weeks, LOTRONEX is not likely to help you and you should stop using it and call your doctor.

Stop taking LOTRONEX and call your doctor right away if you get constipated or have any signs of low blood flow to parts of your intestines (ischemic colitis) such as new or worse abdominal pain, or blood in your diarrhea or stools.

What are the possible or reasonably likely side effects of LOTRONEX?

LOTRONEX is associated with serious side effects. Read the section "What is the most important information I should know about LOTRONEX?" at the beginning of this Medication Guide for information about the serious side effects associated with LOTRONEX. This tells you what to do if you become constipated or have any signs of ischemic colitis.

This Medication Guide does not tell you about all the possible side effects of LOTRONEX. Your doctor or pharmacist can give you a more complete list.

Medicines are sometimes prescribed for purposes other than those listed in a Medication Guide. If you have any questions or concerns about LOTRONEX, ask your doctor. Do not use LOTRONEX for a condition for which it was not prescribed. Do not share your medicine with other people. Your doctor or pharmacist can give you more information about LOTRONEX that was written for health care professionals.

Active Ingredient: alosetron hydrochloride

Inactive Ingredients: lactose (anhydrous), magnesium stearate, microcrystalline cellulose, and pregelatinized starch. The white film-coat for the 0.5 mg tablet contains hypromellose, titanium dioxide, and triacetin. The blue film-coat for the 1 mg tablet contains hypromellose, titanium dioxide, triacetin, and indigo carmine.

This Medication Guide has been approved by the US Food and Drug Administration.

December 2003 MG-020

PATIENT-PHYSICIAN AGREEMENT FOR LOTRONEX

LOTRONEX® (alosetron hydrochloride) is only for women with very bad irritable bowel syndrome (IBS) whose main problem is diarrhea and who have not been helped by other treatments. Women with constipation as their main IBS problem should **not** use LOTRONEX. LOTRONEX has not been shown to help men with IBS, women with conditions other than IBS, or women under 18.

Some patients taking LOTRONEX develop serious intestinal conditions, including serious constipation and ischemic colitis.

- Serious constipation may happen when the bowels are blocked by stools (bowel movements). **Serious problems resulting from constipation occurred in about 1 in 1,000 women in IBS clinical studies.**
- **Ischemic colitis (which occurred in about 1 in 350 women over a 6-month treatment period in IBS clinical studies) happens when the flow of blood to certain parts of the intestines is reduced.**

Serious problems of constipation or ischemic colitis can happen suddenly. These conditions can lead to hospitalization, blood transfusions, surgery, and even death. Older patients, or patients who have other health problems or who take other medicines that may cause constipation, may be more likely to develop a serious intestinal condition while taking LOTRONEX.

IBS itself does not cause death and generally does not send people to the hospital or lead to surgery. My doctor and I have talked about how bad my IBS problems are and if the benefits of LOTRONEX for me are greater than its risks. Because of serious bowel side effects, including some deaths, seen with use of LOTRONEX, only patients with very bad IBS problems that have not been helped by other treatments should use LOTRONEX. Very few patients have IBS with the main problem being diarrhea that is bad enough to consider using LOTRONEX.

AS A PATIENT:

I know that patients who take LOTRONEX may get serious unwanted bowel side effects. I know that only patients whose IBS is very bad should consider taking LOTRONEX.

I agree that all of the things in this list are true about me:

- My main IBS problem is diarrhea.
- My IBS has gone on for a long time, 6 months or longer.
- My doctor has told me that my symptoms are not due to other medical problems.
- I have tried other IBS treatments and none have helped me.

I can tell that my IBS is very bad because I have 1 or more of the following problems:

- I have lots of painful stomach cramps or bloating.
- I often can't control the need to have a bowel movement or have "accidents" where my underwear gets dirty from diarrhea or bowel movements (stools).
- I can't lead a normal home or work life because I need to be near a bathroom.

Before taking LOTRONEX I will tell my doctor about any illnesses or other medicines, prescription or non-prescription, that I am taking or plan to take. I will also tell my doctor if I

- am constipated now
- am constipated most of the time
- ever had a serious problem from constipation
- ever had serious bowel blockages
- ever had ischemic colitis
- ever had blood flow problems to my bowels
- ever had blood clots
- ever had Crohn's disease, ulcerative colitis, or diverticulitis
- do not understand the Patient-Physician Agreement or am not willing to follow it
- am allergic to LOTRONEX or any of its ingredients. (See the list of ingredients at the end of the Medication Guide.)

- I will stop taking LOTRONEX and call my doctor right away if I get constipated (have no bowel movement, have hard, difficult, or painful bowel movements). If my constipation does not get better, I will call my doctor right away. I will talk to my doctor before I take LOTRONEX again.
- I will stop taking LOTRONEX and call my doctor right away if
  - I have new or worse pain in my bowels.
  - I get blood in my diarrhea or my stool (bowel movements).
- Thirty days after starting LOTRONEX, I will talk to my doctor to recheck my IBS symptoms.
- I will stop taking LOTRONEX and call my doctor if my IBS symptoms have not improved after 4 weeks of taking 1 mg twice a day.

I have read and understand the Medication Guide for LOTRONEX. My doctor answered all my questions about treatment with LOTRONEX. If I see other doctors about my IBS or possible side effects from LOTRONEX, I will tell my doctor who prescribed LOTRONEX. I will take LOTRONEX exactly as my doctor prescribes it. I understand that only doctors who have signed up with the company that makes LOTRONEX should write prescriptions for LOTRONEX. As part of signing up, these doctors have said that they know about IBS and the possible side effects of LOTRONEX. They have agreed to use a special sticker on all my prescriptions for LOTRONEX so my pharmacist knows that they have signed up with the company.

My signature below indicates I have read, understood, and agree with ALL the statements made above. I authorize my doctor to begin treatment with LOTRONEX.

____
Name of Patient (print)

____
Signature Date

SECTION FOR THE PHYSICIAN

I have previously enrolled in the Prescribing Program for LOTRONEX and I reaffirm the attestation of qualifications and acceptance of responsibilities I made at the time of enrollment on the form supplied by GlaxoSmithKline ("PRESCRIBING PROGRAM FOR LOTRONEX: PHYSICIAN ATTESTATION OF QUALIFICATIONS AND ACCEPTANCE OF RESPONSIBILITIES").

I have given the patient named above:

- a copy of the Medication Guide for LOTRONEX, and instructed them to read it carefully before signing this Agreement and to take it home.
- counseling about the risks and benefits of LOTRONEX.
- appropriate instructions for taking LOTRONEX.
- answers to all the patient's questions about treatment with LOTRONEX.
- a prescription for LOTRONEX that has the program sticker affixed on it to alert pharmacists I am enrolled in the Prescribing Program for LOTRONEX.

The patient signed the Patient-Physician Agreement in my presence after I counseled the patient, asked if the patient had any questions about treatment with LOTRONEX, and answered all questions to the best of my ability.

____
Name of Physician (print)

____
Signature Date

After the patient and the physician sign this Patient-Physician Agreement, give a copy to the patient and put the original signed form in the patient's medical record.

PRESCRIBING PROGRAM FOR LOTRONEX™: PHYSICIAN ATTESTATION OF QUALIFICATIONS AND ACCEPTANCE OF RESPONSIBILITIES

I wish to participate in the Prescribing Program for LOTRONEX and by my signature below, attest that I have the qualifications and accept the responsibilities described below.

- I understand that for safety reasons LOTRONEX® (alosetron hydrochloride) is approved with marketing restrictions of which the Prescribing Program for LOTRONEX is a required element.

Continued on next page

Product information on these pages is effective as of August 2004. Further information is available at: GlaxoSmithKline, PO Box 13398, Research Triangle Park, NC 27709. 1-888-825-5249. Corporate Web Site: www.gsk.com

Lotronex—Cont.

- I understand that because of serious gastrointestinal adverse events, some fatal, associated with this drug, LOTRONEX is indicated only for women with severe diarrhea-predominant irritable bowel syndrome (IBS) who have chronic IBS symptoms generally lasting for 6 months or longer, had anatomic or biochemical abnormalities of the gastrointestinal tract excluded, and who have failed to respond to conventional therapy. Diarrhea-predominant IBS is severe if it includes diarrhea and one or more of the following: (1) frequent and severe abdominal pain/discomfort; (2) frequent urgency or fecal incontinence; or (3) disability or restriction of daily activities due to IBS. Less than 5 percent of IBS is considered severe.
- I understand that treatment benefits of LOTRONEX in populations other than adult women with diarrhea-predominant IBS have not been established.
- I have reviewed the complete prescribing information for LOTRONEX and am thoroughly familiar with the important information in the Boxed Warning, Indications and Usage, Contraindications, Warnings, Precautions, Adverse Reactions, Dosage and Administration, and Medication Guide sections. I have also reviewed and am familiar with all the components of the Patient-Physician Agreement for LOTRONEX.
- I can diagnose and treat IBS.
- I can diagnose and manage ischemic colitis.
- I can diagnose and manage constipation and complications of constipation.
- I understand the risks and benefits of treatment with LOTRONEX for severe diarrhea-predominant IBS, including information in the package insert, Medication Guide, and Patient-Physician Agreement.
- I will educate any patient who is considering treatment with LOTRONEX on the risks and benefits of treatment with LOTRONEX and obtain the patient's signature on the Patient-Physician Agreement form, sign it, place the original signed form in the patient's medical record, and give a copy to the patient.
- I will give any patient who is considering treatment with LOTRONEX a copy of the Medication Guide and instruct the patient to read it, and to ask any questions the patient may have, as a preliminary step to completing the Patient-Physician Agreement.
- I will report serious adverse events with LOTRONEX to GlaxoSmithKline at 1-888-825-5249 or to the Food and Drug Administration at 1-800-FDA-1088.
- I will affix program stickers to all prescriptions for LOTRONEX (i.e., the original and all subsequent refill prescriptions). Stickers will be provided as part of the GlaxoSmithKline Prescribing Program for LOTRONEX. I will not prescribe LOTRONEX by telephone, facsimile, or computer.

Name of Physician (print) ____________________

Signature ____________ Date ____________
DEA Number ____________
Office Address: ____________

Office Phone Number: ____________
Office Fax Number: ____________

Upon enrollment, you will receive a prescribing kit for LOTRONEX with the complete prescribing information, Prescription Program stickers, multiple copies of the Medication Guide and Patient-Physician Agreement for LOTRONEX, and instructions for ordering additional supplies of Program materials.

If you have any questions, please call the Prescribing Program for LOTRONEX at 1-888-825-5249 or visit www. LOTRONEX.com.

TO ENROLL, COMPLETE THIS FORM IN ITS ENTIRETY AND MAIL TO THE FOLLOWING ADDRESS:
Prescribing Program for Lotronex
Program Coordinator
12012 Sunset Hills Road
8th Floor
Reston, VA 20190-9870

GlaxoSmithKline, Research Triangle Park, NC 27709

December 2003/RL-1188

Shown in Product Identification Guide, page 316

MALARONE® ℞
[mal' ə-rōn]
(atovaquone and proguanil hydrochloride)
Tablets

MALARONE® ℞
(atovaquone and proguanil hydrochloride)
Pediatric Tablets

DESCRIPTION

MALARONE (atovaquone and proguanil hydrochloride) is a fixed-dose combination of the antimalarial agents atovaquone and proguanil hydrochloride. The chemical name of atovaquone is *trans*-2-[4-(4-chlorophenyl)cyclohexyl]-3-hydroxy-1,4-naphthalenedione. Atovaquone is a yellow crystalline solid that is practically insoluble in water. It has a molecular weight of 366.84 and the molecular formula $C_{22}H_{19}ClO_3$.

The chemical name of proguanil hydrochloride is 1-(4-chlorophenyl)-5-isopropyl-biguanide hydrochloride. Proguanil hydrochloride is a white crystalline solid that is sparingly soluble in water. It has a molecular weight of 290.22 and the molecular formula $C_{11}H_{16}ClN_5 \cdot HCl$.

MALARONE Tablets and MALARONE Pediatric Tablets are for oral administration. Each MALARONE Tablet contains 250 mg of atovaquone and 100 mg of proguanil hydrochloride and each MALARONE Pediatric Tablet contains 62.5 mg of atovaquone and 25 mg of proguanil hydrochloride. The inactive ingredients in both tablets are low-substituted hydroxypropyl cellulose, magnesium stearate, microcrystalline cellulose, poloxamer 188, povidone K30, and sodium starch glycolate. The tablet coating contains hypromellose, polyethylene glycol 400, polyethylene glycol 8000, red iron oxide, and titanium dioxide.

CLINICAL PHARMACOLOGY

Microbiology: ***Mechanism of Action:*** The constituents of MALARONE, atovaquone and proguanil hydrochloride, interfere with 2 different pathways involved in the biosynthesis of pyrimidines required for nucleic acid replication. Atovaquone is a selective inhibitor of parasite mitochondrial electron transport. Proguanil hydrochloride primarily exerts its effect by means of the metabolite cycloguanil, a dihydrofolate reductase inhibitor. Inhibition of dihydrofolate reductase in the malaria parasite disrupts deoxythymidylate synthesis.

Activity In Vitro and In Vivo: Atovaquone and cycloguanil (an active metabolite of proguanil) are active against the erythrocytic and exoerythrocytic stages of *Plasmodium* spp. Enhanced efficacy of the combination compared to either atovaquone or proguanil hydrochloride alone was demonstrated in clinical studies in both immune and nonimmune patients (see CLINICAL STUDIES).

Drug Resistance: Strains of *P. falciparum* with decreased susceptibility to atovaquone or proguanil/cycloguanil alone can be selected in vitro or in vivo. The combination of atovaquone and proguanil hydrochloride may not be effective for treatment of recrudescent malaria that develops after prior therapy with the combination.

Pharmacokinetics: ***Absorption:*** Atovaquone is a highly lipophilic compound with low aqueous solubility. The bioavailability of atovaquone shows considerable inter-individual variability.

Dietary fat taken with atovaquone increases the rate and extent of absorption, increasing AUC 2 to 3 times and C_{max} 5 times over fasting. The absolute bioavailability of the tablet formulation of atovaquone when taken with food is 23%. MALARONE Tablets should be taken with food or a milky drink.

Proguanil hydrochloride is extensively absorbed regardless of food intake.

Distribution: Atovaquone is highly protein bound (>99%) over the concentration range of 1 to 90 mcg/mL. A population pharmacokinetic analysis demonstrated that the apparent volume of distribution of atovaquone (V/F) in adult and pediatric patients after oral administration is approximately 8.8 L/kg.

Proguanil is 75% protein bound. A population pharmacokinetic analysis demonstrated that the apparent V/F of proguanil in adult and pediatric patients >15 years of age with body weights from 31 to 110 kg ranged from 1,617 to 2,502 L. In pediatric patients ≤15 years of age with body weights from 11 to 56 kg, the V/F of proguanil ranged from 462 to 966 L.

In human plasma, the binding of atovaquone and proguanil was unaffected by the presence of the other.

Metabolism: In a study where ^{14}C-labeled atovaquone was administered to healthy volunteers, greater than 94% of the dose was recovered as unchanged atovaquone in the feces over 21 days. There was little or no excretion of atovaquone in the urine (less than 0.6%). There is indirect evidence that atovaquone may undergo limited metabolism; however, a specific metabolite has not been identified. Between 40% to 60% of proguanil is excreted by the kidneys. Proguanil is metabolized to cycloguanil (primarily via CYP2C19) and 4-chlorophenylbiguanide. The main routes of elimination are hepatic biotransformation and renal excretion.

Elimination: The elimination half-life of atovaquone is about 2 to 3 days in adult patients.

The elimination half-life of proguanil is 12 to 21 hours in both adult patients and pediatric patients, but may be longer in individuals who are slow metabolizers.

A population pharmacokinetic analysis in adult and pediatric patients showed that the apparent clearance (CL/F) of both atovaquone and proguanil are related to the body weight. The values CL/F for both atovaquone and proguanil in subjects with body weight ≥11 kg are shown in Table 1. [See table 1 above]

Table 1. Apparent Clearance for Atovaquone and Proguanil in Patients as a Function of Body Weight

Body Weight	Atovaquone N	Atovaquone CL/F (L/hr) Mean ± SD* (range)	Proguanil N	Proguanil CL/F (L/hr) Mean ± SD* (range)
11-20 kg	159	1.34 ± 0.63 (0.52-4.26)	146	29.5 ± 6.5 (10.3-48.3)
21-30 kg	117	1.87 ± 0.81 (0.52-5.38)	113	40.0 ± 7.5 (15.9-62.7)
31-40 kg	95	2.76 ± 2.07 (0.97-12.5)	91	49.5 ± 8.30 (25.8-71.5)
>40 kg	368	6.61 ± 3.92 (1.32-20.3)	282	67.9 ± 19.9 (14.0-145)

*SD = standard deviation

The pharmacokinetics of atovaquone and proguanil in patients with body weight below 11 kg have not been adequately characterized.

Special Populations: ***Pediatrics:*** The pharmacokinetics of proguanil and cycloguanil are similar in adult patients and pediatric patients. However, the elimination half-life of atovaquone is shorter in pediatric patients (1 to 2 days) than in adult patients (2 to 3 days). In clinical trials, plasma trough levels of atovaquone and proguanil in pediatric patients weighing 5 to 40 kg were within the range observed in adults after dosing by body weight.

Geriatrics: In a single-dose study, the pharmacokinetics of atovaquone, proguanil, and cycloguanil were compared in 13 elderly subjects (age 65 to 79 years) to 13 younger subjects (age 30 to 45 years). In the elderly subjects, the extent of systemic exposure (AUC) of cycloguanil was increased (point estimate = 2.36, CI = 1.70, 3.28). T_{max} was longer in elderly subjects (median 8 hours) compared with younger subjects (median 4 hours) and average elimination half-life was longer in elderly subjects (mean 14.9 hours) compared with younger subjects (mean 8.3 hours).

Hepatic Impairment: In a single-dose study, the pharmacokinetics of atovaquone, proguanil, and cycloguanil were compared in 13 subjects with hepatic impairment (9 mild, 4 moderate, as indicated by the Child-Pugh method) to 13 subjects with normal hepatic function. In subjects with mild or moderate hepatic impairment as compared to healthy subjects, there were no marked differences (<50%) in the rate or extent of systemic exposure of atovaquone. However, in subjects with moderate hepatic impairment, the elimination half-life of atovaquone was increased (point estimate = 1.28, 90% CI = 1.00 to 1.63). Proguanil AUC, C_{max}, and its $t_{1/2}$ increased in subjects with mild hepatic impairment when

Table 2. Point Estimates (90% CI) for Proguanil and Cycloguanil Parameters in Subjects with Mild and Moderate Hepatic Impairment Compared to Healthy Volunteers

Parameter	Comparison	Proguanil	Cycloguanil
$AUC_{(0-inf)}$*	mild:healthy	1.96 (1.51, 2.54)	0.32 (0.22, 0.45)
C_{max}*	mild:healthy	1.41 (1.16, 1.71)	0.35 (0.24, 0.50)
$t_{1/2}$†	mild:healthy	1.21 (0.92, 1.60)	0.86 (0.49, 1.48)
$AUC_{(0-inf)}$*	moderate:healthy	1.64 (1.14, 2.34)	ND
C_{max}*	moderate:healthy	0.97 (0.69, 1.36)	ND
$t_{1/2}$†	moderate:healthy	1.46 (1.05, 2.05)	ND

ND = not determined due to lack of quantifiable data.
* Ratio of geometric means.
† Mean difference.

compared to healthy subjects (Table 2). Also, the proguanil AUC and its $t_{½}$ increased in subjects with moderate hepatic impairment when compared to healthy subjects. Consistent with the increase in proguanil AUC, there were marked decreases in the systemic exposure of cycloguanil (C_{max} and AUC) and an increase in its elimination half-life in subjects with mild hepatic impairment when compared to healthy volunteers (Table 2). There were few measurable cycloguanil concentrations in subjects with moderate hepatic impairment (see DOSAGE AND ADMINISTRATION). The pharmacokinetics of atovaquone, proguanil, and cycloguanil after administration of MALARONE have not been studied in patients with severe hepatic impairment.

[See table 2 at top of previous page]

Renal Impairment: In patients with mild to moderate renal impairment, oral clearance and/or AUC data for atovaquone, proguanil, and cycloguanil are within the range of values observed in patients with normal renal function. In patients with severe renal impairment (creatinine clearance <30 mL/min), atovaquone C_{max} and AUC are reduced but the elimination half-lives for proguanil and cycloguanil are prolonged, with corresponding increases in AUC, resulting in the potential of drug accumulation with repeated dosing (see CONTRAINDICATIONS).

Drug Interactions: There are no pharmacokinetic interactions between atovaquone and proguanil at the recommended dose.

Concomitant treatment with **tetracycline** has been associated with approximately a 40% reduction in plasma concentrations of atovaquone.

Concomitant treatment with **metoclopramide** has also been associated with decreased bioavailability of atovaquone.

Concomitant administration of **rifampin** or **rifabutin** is known to reduce atovaquone levels by approximately 50% and 34%, respectively (see PRECAUTIONS: Drug Interactions). The mechanisms of these interactions are unknown.

Atovaquone is highly protein bound (>99%) but does not displace other highly protein-bound drugs in vitro, indicating significant drug interactions arising from displacement are unlikely (see PRECAUTIONS: Drug Interactions). Proguanil is metabolized primarily by CYP2C19. Potential pharmacokinetic interactions with other substrates or inhibitors of this pathway are unknown.

INDICATIONS AND USAGE

Prevention of Malaria: MALARONE is indicated for the prophylaxis of *P. falciparum* malaria, including in areas where chloroquine resistance has been reported (see CLINICAL STUDIES).

Treatment of Malaria: MALARONE is indicated for the treatment of acute, uncomplicated *P. falciparum* malaria. MALARONE has been shown to be effective in regions where the drugs chloroquine, halofantrine, mefloquine, and amodiaquine may have unacceptable failure rates, presumably due to drug resistance.

CONTRAINDICATIONS

MALARONE is contraindicated in individuals with known hypersensitivity to atovaquone or proguanil hydrochloride or any component of the formulation. During clinical trials, 1 case of anaphylaxis following treatment with atovaquone/proguanil was observed.

MALARONE is contraindicated for prophylaxis of *P. falciparum* malaria in patients with severe renal impairment (creatinine clearance <30 mL/min) (see CLINICAL PHARMACOLOGY: Special Populations: Renal Impairment).

PRECAUTIONS

General: MALARONE has not been evaluated for the treatment of cerebral malaria or other severe manifestations of complicated malaria, including hyperparasitemia, pulmonary edema, or renal failure. Patients with severe malaria are not candidates for oral therapy.

Absorption of atovaquone may be reduced in patients with diarrhea or vomiting. If MALARONE is used in patients who are vomiting (see DOSAGE AND ADMINISTRATION), parasitemia should be closely monitored and the use of an antiemetic considered. Vomiting occurred in up to 19% of pediatric patients given treatment doses of MALARONE. In the controlled clinical trials of MALARONE, 15.3% of adults who were treated with atovaquone/proguanil received an antiemetic drug during that part of the trial when they received atovaquone/proguanil. Of these patients, 98.3% were successfully treated. In patients with severe or persistent diarrhea or vomiting, alternative antimalarial therapy may be required.

Parasite relapse occurred commonly when *P. vivax* malaria was treated with MALARONE alone.

In the event of recrudescent *P. falciparum* infections after treatment with MALARONE or failure of chemoprophylaxis with MALARONE, patients should be treated with a different blood schizonticide.

In patients with severe renal impairment (creatinine clearance <30 mL/min) alternatives to MALARONE should be recommended for treatment of acute *P. falciparum* malaria whenever possible (see CONTRAINDICATIONS and CLINICAL PHARMACOLOGY: Special Populations: Renal Impairment). The concomitant administration of MALARONE and any other medication containing proguanil hydrochloride should be avoided.

Information for Patients: Patients should be instructed:

- to take MALARONE tablets at the same time each day with food or a milky drink.
- to take a repeat dose of MALARONE if vomiting occurs within 1 hour after dosing.

Table 3. Adverse Experiences in Placebo-Controlled Clinical Trials of MALARONE for Prophylaxis of Malaria

Adverse Experience	Percent of Subjects With Adverse Experiences (Percent of Subjects With Adverse Experiences Attributable to Therapy)				
	Adults			Children and Adolescents	
	Placebo n = 206	MALARONE* n = 206	MALARONE† n = 381	Placebo n = 140	MALARONE n = 125
Headache	27 (7)	22 (3)	17 (5)	21 (14)	19 (14)
Fever	13 (1)	5 (0)	3 (0)	11 (<1)	6 (0)
Myalgia	11 (0)	12 (0)	7 (0)	0 (0)	0 (0)
Abdominal pain	10 (5)	9 (4)	6 (3)	29 (29)	33 (31)
Cough	8 (<1)	6 (<1)	4 (1)	9 (0)	9 (0)
Diarrhea	8 (3)	6 (2)	4 (1)	3 (1)	2 (0)
Upper respiratory infection	7 (0)	8 (0)	5 (0)	0 (0)	<1 (0)
Dyspepsia	5 (4)	3 (2)	2 (1)	0 (0)	0 (0)
Back pain	4 (0)	8 (0)	4 (0)	0 (0)	0 (0)
Gastritis	3 (2)	3 (3)	2 (2)	0 (0)	0 (0)
Vomiting	2 (<1)	1 (<1)	<1 (<1)	6 (6)	7 (7)
Flu syndrome	1 (0)	2 (0)	4 (0)	6 (0)	9 (0)
Any adverse experience	65 (32)	54 (17)	49 (17)	62 (41)	60 (42)

* Subjects receiving the recommended dose of atovaquone and proguanil hydrochloride in placebo-controlled trials.
† Subjects receiving the recommended dose of atovaquone and proguanil hydrochloride in any trial.

- to take a dose as soon as possible if a dose is missed, then return to their normal dosing schedule. However, if a dose is skipped, the patient should not double the next dose.
- to consult a healthcare professional regarding alternative forms of prophylaxis if prophylaxis with MALARONE is prematurely discontinued for any reason.
- that protective clothing, insect repellents, and bednets are important components of malaria prophylaxis.
- that no chemoprophylactic regimen is 100% effective; therefore, patients should seek medical attention for any febrile illness that occurs during or after return from a malaria-endemic area and inform their healthcare professional that they may have been exposed to malaria.
- that falciparum malaria carries a higher risk of death and serious complications in pregnant women than in the general population. Pregnant women anticipating travel to malarious areas should discuss the risks and benefits of such travel with their physicians (see Pregnancy section).

Drug Interactions: Concomitant treatment with **tetracycline** has been associated with approximately a 40% reduction in plasma concentrations of atovaquone. Parasitemia should be closely monitored in patients receiving tetracycline. While antiemetics may be indicated for patients receiving MALARONE, **metoclopramide** may reduce the bioavailability of atovaquone and should be used only if other antiemetics are not available.

Concomitant administration of **rifampin** or **rifabutin** is known to reduce atovaquone levels by approximately 50% and 34%, respectively. The concomitant administration of MALARONE and rifampin or rifabutin is not recommended.

Atovaquone is highly protein bound (>99%) but does not displace other highly protein-bound drugs in vitro, indicating significant drug interactions arising from displacement are unlikely.

Potential interactions between proguanil or cycloguanil and other drugs that are CYP2C19 substrates or inhibitors are unknown.

Carcinogenesis, Mutagenesis, Impairment of Fertility:
Atovaquone: Carcinogenicity studies in rats were negative; 24-month studies in mice showed treatment-related increases in incidence of hepatocellular adenoma and hepatocellular carcinoma at all doses tested which ranged from approximately 5 to 8 times the average steady-state plasma concentrations in humans during prophylaxis of malaria. Atovaquone alone was negative with or without metabolic activation in the Ames *Salmonella* mutagenicity assay, the Mouse Lymphoma mutagenesis assay, and the Cultured Human Lymphocyte cytogenetic assay. No evidence of genotoxicity was observed in the in vivo Mouse Micronucleus assay.

Proguanil: Carcinogenicity studies with proguanil have not been completed. Proguanil was not genotoxic in in vitro or in vivo studies.

Proguanil alone was negative with or without metabolic activation in the Ames *Salmonella* mutagenicity assay and the Mouse Lymphoma mutagenesis assay. No evidence of genotoxicity was observed in the in vivo Mouse Micronucleus assay.

Genotoxicity studies have not been performed with atovaquone in combination with proguanil. Effects of MALARONE on male and female reproductive performance are unknown.

Pregnancy: Pregnancy Category C. Falciparum malaria carries a higher risk of morbidity and mortality in pregnant women than in the general population. Maternal death and fetal loss are both known complications of falciparum malaria in pregnancy. In pregnant women who must travel to malaria-endemic areas, personal protection against mosquito bites should always be employed (see Information for Patients) in addition to antimalarials.

Atovaquone was not teratogenic and did not cause reproductive toxicity in rats at maternal plasma concentrations up to 5 to 6.5 times the estimated human exposure during treatment of malaria. Following single-dose administration of ^{14}C-labeled atovaquone to pregnant rats, concentrations of radiolabel in rat fetuses were 18% (mid-gestation) and 60% (late gestation) of concurrent maternal plasma concentrations. In rabbits, atovaquone caused maternal toxicity at plasma concentrations that were approximately 0.6 to 1.3 times the estimated human exposure during treatment of malaria. Adverse fetal effects in rabbits, including decreased fetal body lengths and increased early resorptions and post-implantation losses, were observed only in the presence of maternal toxicity. Concentrations of atovaquone in rabbit fetuses averaged 30% of the concurrent maternal plasma concentrations.

The combination of atovaquone and proguanil hydrochloride was not teratogenic in rats at plasma concentrations up to 1.7 and 0.10 times, respectively, the estimated human exposure during treatment of malaria. In rabbits, the combination of atovaquone and proguanil hydrochloride was not teratogenic or embryotoxic to rabbit fetuses at plasma concentrations up to 0.34 and 0.82 times, respectively, the estimated human exposure during treatment of malaria.

While there are no adequate and well-controlled studies of atovaquone and/or proguanil hydrochloride in pregnant women, MALARONE may be used if the potential benefit justifies the potential risk to the fetus. The proguanil component of MALARONE acts by inhibiting the parasitic dihydrofolate reductase (see CLINICAL PHARMACOLOGY: Microbiology: Mechanism of Action). However, there are no clinical data indicating that folate supplementation diminishes drug efficacy, and for women of childbearing age receiving folate supplements to prevent neural tube birth defects, such supplements may be continued while taking MALARONE.

Nursing Mothers: It is not known whether atovaquone is excreted into human milk. In a rat study, atovaquone concentrations in the milk were 30% of the concurrent atovaquone concentrations in the maternal plasma.

Proguanil is excreted into human milk in small quantities. Caution should be exercised when MALARONE is administered to a nursing woman.

Pediatric Use: ***Treatment of Malaria:*** The efficacy and safety of MALARONE for the treatment of malaria have been established in controlled studies involving pediatric patients weighing 5 kg or more (see CLINICAL STUDIES). Safety and effectiveness have not been established in pediatric patients who weigh less than 5 kg.

Prophylaxis of Malaria: The efficacy and safety of MALARONE have been established for the prophylaxis of

Continued on next page

Product information on these pages is effective as of August 2004. Further information is available at: GlaxoSmithKline, PO Box 13398, Research Triangle Park, NC 27709. 1-888-825-5249. Corporate Web Site: www.gsk.com

Malarone—Cont.

malaria in controlled studies involving pediatric patients weighing 11 kg or more (see CLINICAL STUDIES). Safety and effectiveness have not been established in pediatric patients who weigh less than 11 kg.

Geriatric Use: Clinical studies of MALARONE did not include sufficient numbers of subjects aged 65 and over to determine whether they respond differently from younger subjects. In general, dose selection for an elderly patient should be cautious, reflecting the greater frequency of decreased hepatic, renal, or cardiac function, the higher systemic exposure to cycloguanil (see CLINICAL PHARMACOLOGY: Special Populations: Geriatrics), and the greater frequency of concomitant disease or other drug therapy.

ADVERSE REACTIONS

Because MALARONE contains atovaquone and proguanil hydrochloride, the type and severity of adverse reactions associated with each of the compounds may be expected. The higher treatment doses of MALARONE were less well tolerated than the lower prophylactic doses.

Among adults who received MALARONE for treatment of malaria, attributable adverse experiences that occurred in ≥5% of patients were abdominal pain (17%), nausea (12%), vomiting (12%), headache (10%), diarrhea (8%), asthenia (8%), anorexia (5%), and dizziness (5%). Treatment was discontinued prematurely due to an adverse experience in 4 of 436 adults treated with MALARONE.

Among pediatric patients (weighing 11 to 40 kg) who received MALARONE for the treatment of malaria, attributable adverse experiences that occurred in ≥5% of patients were vomiting (10%) and pruritus (6%). Vomiting occurred in 43 of 319 (13%) pediatric patients who did not have symptomatic malaria but were given treatment doses of MALARONE for 3 days in a clinical trial. The design of this clinical trial required that any patient who vomited be withdrawn from the trial. Among pediatric patients with symptomatic malaria treated with MALARONE, treatment was discontinued prematurely due to an adverse experience in 1 of 116 (0.9%).

In a study of 100 pediatric patients (5 to <11 kg body weight) who received MALARONE for the treatment of uncomplicated *P. falciparum* malaria, only diarrhea (6%) occurred in ≥5% of patients as an adverse experience attributable to MALARONE. In 3 patients (3%), treatment was discontinued prematurely due to an adverse experience.

Abnormalities in laboratory tests reported in clinical trials were limited to elevations of transaminases in malaria patients being treated with MALARONE. The frequency of these abnormalities varied substantially across studies of treatment and were not observed in the randomized portions of the prophylaxis trials.

In one phase III trial of malaria treatment in Thai adults, early elevations of ALT and AST were observed to occur more frequently in patients treated with MALARONE compared to patients treated with an active control drug. Rates for patients who had normal baseline levels of these clinical laboratory parameters were: Day 7: ALT 26.7% vs. 15.6%; AST 16.9% vs. 8.6%. By day 14 of this 28-day study, the frequency of transaminase elevations equalized across the 2 groups.

In this and other studies in which transaminase elevations occurred, they were noted to persist for up to 4 weeks following treatment with MALARONE for malaria. None were associated with untoward clinical events.

Among subjects who received MALARONE for prophylaxis of malaria in placebo-controlled trials, adverse experiences occurred in similar proportions of subjects receiving MALARONE or placebo (Table 3). The most commonly reported adverse experiences possibly attributable to MALARONE or placebo were headache and abdominal pain. Prophylaxis with MALARONE was discontinued prematurely due to a treatment-related adverse experience in 3 of 381 adults and 0 of 125 pediatric patients.

[See table 3 at top of previous page]

In an additional placebo-controlled study of malaria prophylaxis with MALARONE involving 330 pediatric patients in a malaria-endemic area (see CLINICAL STUDIES), the safety profile of MALARONE was consistent with that described above. The most common treatment-emergent adverse events with MALARONE were abdominal pain (13%), headache (13%), and cough (10%). Abdominal pain (13% vs. 8%) and vomiting (5% vs. 3%) were reported more often with MALARONE than with placebo, while fever (5% vs. 12%) and diarrhea (1% vs. 5%) were more common with placebo. No patient withdrew from the study due to an adverse experience with MALARONE. No routine laboratory data were obtained during this study.

Among subjects who received MALARONE for prophylaxis of malaria in clinical trials with an active comparator, adverse experiences occurred in a similar or lower proportion of subjects receiving MALARONE than an active comparator (Table 4). The mean durations of dosing and the periods for which the adverse experiences are summarized in Table 4, were 28 days (Study 1) and 26 days (Study 2) for MALARONE, 53 days for mefloquine, and 49 days for chloroquine plus proguanil (reflecting the different recommended dosing regimens). Fewer neuropsychiatric adverse experiences occurred in subjects who received MALARONE than mefloquine. Fewer gastrointestinal adverse experiences occurred in subjects receiving MALARONE than chloroquine/proguanil. Compared with active comparator drugs, subjects receiving MALARONE had fewer adverse experiences overall that were attributed to prophylactic therapy (Table 4). Prophylaxis with MALARONE was discontinued prematurely due to a treatment-related adverse experience in 7 of 1,004 travelers.

[See table 4 below]

In a third active-controlled study, MALARONE (n = 110) was compared with chloroquine/proguanil (n = 111) for the prophylaxis of malaria in 221 non-immune pediatric patients (see CLINICAL STUDIES). The mean duration of exposure was 23 days for MALARONE, 46 days for chloroquine, and 43 days for proguanil, reflecting the different recommended dosage regimens for these products. Fewer patients treated with MALARONE reported abdominal pain (2% vs. 7%) or nausea (<1% vs. 7%) than children who received chloroquine/proguanil. Oral ulceration (2% vs. 2%), vivid dreams (2% vs. <1%), and blurred vision (0% vs. 2%) occurred in similar proportions of patients receiving either MALARONE or chloroquine/proguanil, respectively. Two patients discontinued prophylaxis with chloroquine/proguanil due to adverse events, while none of those receiving MALARONE discontinued due to adverse events.

Post-Marketing Adverse Reactions: In addition to adverse events reported from clinical trials, the following events have been identified during world-wide post-approval use of MALARONE. Because they are reported voluntarily from a population of unknown size, estimates of frequency cannot be made. These events have been chosen for inclusion due to a combination of their seriousness, frequency of reporting, or potential causal connection to MALARONE.

Skin: Cutaneous reactions ranging from rash, photosensitivity, and urticaria to rare cases of erythema multiforme and Stevens-Johnson syndrome.

Central Nervous System: Rare cases of seizures and psychotic events (such as hallucinations); however, a causal relationship has not been established.

OVERDOSAGE

There is limited information regarding overdosage from the administration of MALARONE.

There is no known antidote for atovaquone, and it is currently unknown if atovaquone is dialyzable. The median lethal dose is higher than the maximum oral dose tested in mice and rats (1,825 mg/kg/day). Overdoses up to 31,500 mg of atovaquone have been reported. In one such patient who also took an unspecified dose of dapsone, methemoglobinemia occurred. Rash has also been reported after overdose.

Overdoses of proguanil hydrochloride as large as 1,500 mg have been followed by complete recovery, and doses as high as 700 mg twice daily have been taken for over 2 weeks without serious toxicity. Adverse experiences occasionally associated with proguanil hydrochloride doses of 100 to 200 mg/day, such as epigastric discomfort and vomiting, would be likely to occur with overdose. There are also reports of reversible hair loss and scaling of the skin on the palms and/or soles, reversible aphthous ulceration, and hematologic side effects.

DOSAGE AND ADMINISTRATION

The daily dose should be taken at the same time each day with food or a milky drink. In the event of vomiting within 1 hour after dosing, a repeat dose should be taken.

Prevention of Malaria: Prophylactic treatment with MALARONE should be started 1 or 2 days before entering a malaria-endemic area and continued daily during the stay and for 7 days after return.

Adults: One MALARONE Tablet (adult strength = 250 mg atovaquone/100 mg proguanil hydrochloride) per day.

Pediatric Patients: The dosage for prevention of malaria in pediatric patients is based upon body weight (Table 5).

[See table 5 at top of next page]

Treatment of Acute Malaria: ***Adults:*** Four MALARONE Tablets (adult strength; total daily dose 1 g atovaquone/400 mg proguanil hydrochloride) as a single dose daily for 3 consecutive days.

Pediatric Patients: The dosage for treatment of acute malaria in pediatric patients is based upon body weight (Table 6).

[See table 6 at top of next page]

MALARONE Tablets may be crushed and mixed with condensed milk just prior to administration for children who may have difficulty swallowing tablets.

Patients with Renal Impairment: MALARONE should not be used for malaria prophylaxis in patients with severe renal impairment (creatinine clearance <30 mL/min), and alternatives to MALARONE should be recommended for treatment of acute *P. falciparum* malaria whenever possible (see CONTRAINDICATIONS, PRECAUTIONS: General, and CLINICAL PHARMACOLOGY: Special Populations). No dosage adjustments are needed in patients with mild to moderate renal impairment.

Patients with Hepatic Impairment: No dosage adjustments are needed in patients with mild to moderate hepatic impairment. No studies have been conducted in patients with severe hepatic impairment (see CLINICAL PHARMACOLOGY: Special Populations: Hepatic Impairment).

HOW SUPPLIED

MALARONE Tablets, containing 250 mg atovaquone and 100 mg proguanil hydrochloride, are pink, film-coated, round, biconvex tablets engraved with "GX CM3" on one side.

Bottle of 100 tablets with child-resistant closure (NDC 0173-0675-01).

Unit Dose Pack of 24 (NDC 0173-0675-02).

MALARONE Pediatric Tablets, containing 62.5 mg atovaquone and 25 mg proguanil hydrochloride, are pink, film-coated, round, biconvex tablets engraved with "GX CG7" on one side.

Bottle of 100 tablets with child-resistant closure (NDC 0173-0676-01).

Store at 25°C (77°F); excursions permitted to 15° to 30°C (59° to 86°F) (see USP Controlled Room Temperature).

Table 4. Adverse Experiences in Active-Controlled Clinical Trials of MALARONE for Prophylaxis of Malaria

	Percent of Subjects With Adverse Experiences* (Percent of Subjects With Adverse Experiences Attributable to Therapy)							
	Study 1				Study 2			
Adverse Experience	MALARONE n = 493		Mefloquine n = 483		MALARONE n = 511		Chloroquine plus Proguanil n = 511	
Diarrhea	38	(8)	36	(7)	34	(5)	39	(7)
Nausea	14	(3)	20	(8)	11	(2)	18	(7)
Abdominal pain	17	(5)	16	(5)	14	(3)	22	(6)
Headache	12	(4)	17	(7)	12	(4)	14	(4)
Dreams	7	(7)	16	(14)	6	(4)	7	(3)
Insomnia	5	(3)	16	(13)	4	(2)	5	(2)
Fever	9	(<1)	11	(1)	8	(<1)	8	(<1)
Dizziness	5	(2)	14	(9)	7	(3)	8	(4)
Vomiting	8	(1)	10	(2)	8	(0)	14	(2)
Oral ulcers	9	(6)	6	(4)	5	(4)	7	(5)
Pruritus	4	(2)	5	(2)	3	(1)	2	(<1)
Visual difficulties	2	(2)	5	(3)	3	(2)	3	(2)
Depression	<1	(<1)	5	(4)	<1	(<1)	1	(<1)
Anxiety	1	(<1)	5	(4)	<1	(<1)	1	(<1)
Any adverse experience	64	(30)	69	(42)	58	(22)	66	(28)
Any neuropsychiatric event	20	(14)	37	(29)	16	(10)	20	(10)
Any GI event	49	(16)	50	(19)	43	(12)	54	(20)

*Adverse experiences that started while receiving active study drug.

Table 5. Dosage for Prevention of Malaria in Pediatric Patients

Weight (kg)	Atovaquone/Proguanil HCl Total Daily Dose	Dosage Regimen
11-20	62.5 mg/25 mg	1 MALARONE Pediatric Tablet daily
21-30	125 mg/50 mg	2 MALARONE Pediatric Tablets as a single dose daily
31-40	187.5 mg/75 mg	3 MALARONE Pediatric Tablets as a single dose daily
>40	250 mg/100 mg	1 MALARONE Tablet (adult strength) as a single dose daily

Table 6. Dosage for Treatment of Acute Malaria in Pediatric Patients

Weight (kg)	Atovaquone/ Proguanil HCl Total Daily Dose	Dosage Regimen
5-8	125 mg/50 mg	2 MALARONE Pediatric Tablets daily for 3 consecutive days
9-10	187.5 mg/75 mg	3 MALARONE Pediatric Tablets daily for 3 consecutive days
11-20	250 mg/100 mg	1 MALARONE Tablet (adult strength) daily for 3 consecutive days
21-30	500 mg/200 mg	2 MALARONE Tablets (adult strength) as a single dose daily for 3 consecutive days
31-40	750 mg/300 mg	3 MALARONE Tablets (adult strength) as a single dose daily for 3 consecutive days
>40	1 g/400 mg	4 MALARONE Tablets (adult strength) as a single dose daily for 3 consecutive days

Table 7. Parasitological Response in Clinical Trials of MALARONE for Treatment of *P. falciparum* Malaria

	MALARONE*		Comparator		
Study Site	Evaluable Patients (n)	% Sensitive Response†	Drug(s)	Evaluable Patients (n)	% Sensitive Response†
Brazil	74	98.6%	Quinine and tetracycline	76	100.0%
Thailand	79	100.0%	Mefloquine	79	86.1%
France‡	21	100.0%	Halofantrine	18	100.0%
Kenya‡,§	81	93.8%	Halofantrine	83	90.4%
Zambia	80	100.0%	Pyrimethamine/ sulfadoxine (P/S)	80	98.8%
Gabon†	63	98.4%	Amodiaquine	63	81.0%
Philippines	54	100.0%	Chloroquine (Cq) Cq and P/S	23 32	30.4% 87.5%
Peru	19	100.0%	Chloroquine P/S	13 7	7.7% 100.0%

*MALARONE = 1,000 mg atovaquone and 400 mg proguanil hydrochloride (or equivalent based on body weight for patients weighing ≤40 kg) once daily for 3 days.
† Elimination of parasitemia with no recurrent parasitemia during follow-up for 28 days.
‡ Patients hospitalized only for acute care. Follow-up conducted in outpatients.
§ Study in pediatric patients 3 to 12 years of age.

Table 9. Prevention of Parasitemia in Active-Controlled Clinical Trials of MALARONE for Prophylaxis of *P. falciparum* Malaria in Non-Immune Travelers

	MALARONE	Mefloquine	Chloroquine plus Proguanil
Total number of randomized patients who received study drug	1,004	483	511
Failed to complete study	14	6	4
Developed parasitemia (*P. falciparum*)	0	0	3

ANIMAL TOXICOLOGY

Fibrovascular proliferation in the right atrium, pyelonephritis, bone marrow hypocellularity, lymphoid atrophy, and gastritis/enteritis were observed in dogs treated with proguanil hydrochloride for 6 months at a dose of 12 mg/kg/day (approximately 3.9 times the recommended daily human dose for malaria prophylaxis on a mg/m^2 basis). Bile duct hyperplasia, gall bladder mucosal atrophy, and interstitial pneumonia were observed in dogs treated with proguanil hydrochloride for 6 months at a dose of 4 mg/kg/day (approximately 1.3 times the recommended daily human dose for malaria prophylaxis on a mg/m^2 basis). Mucosal hyperplasia of the cecum and renal tubular basophilia were observed in rats treated with proguanil hydrochloride for 6 months at a dose of 20 mg/kg/day (approximately 1.6 times the recommended daily human dose for malaria prophylaxis on a mg/m^2 basis). Adverse heart, lung, liver, and gall bladder effects observed in dogs and kidney effects observed in rats were not shown to be reversible.

CLINICAL STUDIES

Treatment of Acute Malarial Infections: In 3 phase II clinical trials, atovaquone alone, proguanil hydrochloride alone, and the combination of atovaquone and proguanil hydrochloride were evaluated for the treatment of acute, uncomplicated malaria caused by *P. falciparum*. Among 156 evaluable patients, the parasitological cure rate was 59/89 (66%) with atovaquone alone, 1/17 (6%) with proguanil hydrochloride alone, and 50/50 (100%) with the combination of atovaquone and proguanil hydrochloride.

MALARONE was evaluated for treatment of acute, uncomplicated malaria caused by *P. falciparum* in 8 phase III controlled clinical trials. Among 471 evaluable patients treated with the equivalent of 4 MALARONE Tablets once daily for 3 days, 464 had a sensitive response (elimination of parasitemia with no recurrent parasitemia during follow-up for 28 days) (see Table 7). Seven patients had a response of RI resistance (elimination of parasitemia but with recurrent parasitemia between 7 and 28 days after starting treatment). In these trials, the response to treatment with MALARONE was similar to treatment with the comparator drug in 4 trials, and better than the response to treatment with the comparator drug in the other 4 trials.

The overall efficacy in 521 evaluable patients was 98.7% (see Table 7).

[See table 7 below]

Eighteen of 521 (3.5%) evaluable patients with acute falciparum malaria presented with a pretreatment serum creatinine greater than 2.0 mg/dL (range 2.1 to 4.3 mg/dL). All were successfully treated with MALARONE and 17 of 18 (94.4%) had normal serum creatinine levels by day 7.

Data from a phase II trial of atovaquone conducted in Zambia suggested that approximately 40% of the study population in this country were HIV-infected patients. The enrollment criteria were similar for the phase III trial of MALARONE conducted in Zambia and the results are presented in Table 6. Efficacy rates for MALARONE in this study population were high and comparable to other populations studied.

The efficacy of MALARONE in the treatment of the erythrocytic phase of nonfalciparum malaria was assessed in a small number of patients. Of the 23 patients in Thailand infected with *P. vivax* and treated with atovaquone/proguanil hydrochloride 1,000 mg/400 mg daily for 3 days, parasitemia cleared in 21 (91.3%) at 7 days. Parasite relapse occurred commonly when *P. vivax* malaria was treated with MALARONE alone. Seven patients in Gabon with malaria due to *P. ovale* or *P. malariae* were treated with atovaquone/proguanil hydrochloride 1,000 mg/400 mg daily for 3 days. All 6 evaluable patients (3 with *P. malariae*, 2 with *P. ovale*, and 1 with mixed *P. falciparum* and *P. ovale*) were cured at 28 days. Relapsing malarias including *P. vivax* and *P. ovale* require additional treatment to prevent relapse.

The efficacy of MALARONE in treating acute uncomplicated *P. falciparum* malaria in children weighing ≥5 and <11 kg was examined in an open-label, randomized trial conducted in Gabon. Patients received either MALARONE (2 or 3 MALARONE Pediatric Tablets once daily depending upon body weight) for 3 days (n = 100) or amodiaquine (10 mg/kg/day) for 3 days (n = 100). In this study, the MALARONE Tablets were crushed and mixed with condensed milk just prior to administration. In the per-protocol population, adequate clinical response was obtained in 95% (87/92) of the pediatric patients who received MALARONE and in 53% (41/78) of those who received amodiaquine. A response of RI resistance (elimination of parasitemia but with recurrent parasitemia between 7 and 28 days after starting treatment) was noted in 3% and 40% of the patients, respectively. Two cases of RIII resistance (rising parasite count despite therapy) were reported in the patients receiving MALARONE. There were 4 cases of RIII in the amodiaquine arm.

Prevention of Malaria: MALARONE was evaluated for prophylaxis of malaria in 5 clinical trials in malaria-endemic areas and in 3 active-controlled trials in non-immune travelers to malaria-endemic areas.

Three placebo-controlled studies of 10 to 12 weeks' duration were conducted among residents of malaria-endemic areas in Kenya, Zambia, and Gabon. Of a total of 669 randomized patients (including 264 pediatric patients 5 to 16 years of age), 103 were withdrawn for reasons other than falciparum malaria or drug-related adverse events. (Fifty-five percent of these were lost to follow-up and 45% were withdrawn for protocol violations.) The results are listed in Table 8.

Table 8. Prevention of Parasitemia in Placebo-Controlled Clinical Trials of MALARONE for Prophylaxis of *P. falciparum* Malaria in Residents of Malaria-Endemic Areas

	MALARONE	Placebo
Total number of patients randomized	326	341
Failed to complete study	57	44
Developed parasitemia (*P. falciparum*)	2	92

In another study, 330 Gabonese pediatric patients (weighing 13 to 40 kg, and aged 4 to 14 years) who had received successful open-label radical cure treatment with artesunate, were randomized to receive either MALARONE (dosage based on body weight) or placebo in a double-blind fashion for 12 weeks. Blood smears were obtained weekly and any time malaria was suspected. Nineteen of the 165 children given MALARONE and 18 of 165 patients given placebo withdrew from the study for reasons other than parasitemia (primary reason was lost to follow-up). In the per-protocol population, 1 out of 150 patients (<1%) who received MALARONE developed *P. falciparum* parasitemia while receiving prophylaxis with MALARONE compared with 31 (22%) of the 144 placebo recipients.

Continued on next page

Product information on these pages is effective as of August 2004. Further information is available at: GlaxoSmithKline, PO Box 13398, Research Triangle Park, NC 27709. 1-888-825-5249. Corporate Web Site: www.gsk.com

Malarone—Cont.

In a 10-week study in 175 South African subjects who moved into malaria-endemic areas and were given prophylaxis with 1 MALARONE Tablet daily, parasitemia developed in 1 subject who missed several doses of medication. Since no placebo control was included, the incidence of malaria in this study was not known.

Two active-controlled studies were conducted in non-immune travelers who visited a malaria-endemic area. The mean duration of travel was 18 days (range 2 to 38 days). Of a total of 1,998 randomized patients who received MALARONE or controlled drug, 24 discontinued from the study before follow-up evaluation 60 days after leaving the endemic area. Nine of these were lost to follow-up, 2 withdrew because of an adverse experience, and 13 were discontinued for other reasons. These studies were not large enough to allow for statements of comparative efficacy. In addition, the true exposure rate to *P. falciparum* malaria in both studies is unknown. The results are listed in Table 9.

[See table 9 on previous page]

A third randomized, open-label study was conducted which included 221 otherwise healthy pediatric patients (weighing ≥11 kg and 2 to 17 years of age) who were at risk of contracting malaria by traveling to an endemic area. The mean duration of travel was 15 days (range 1 to 30 days). Prophylaxis with MALARONE (n = 110, dosage based on body weight) began 1 or 2 days before entering the endemic area and lasted until 7 days after leaving the area. A control group (n = 111) received prophylaxis with chloroquine/proguanil dosed according to WHO guidelines. No cases of malaria occurred in either group of children. However, the study was not large enough to allow for statements of comparative efficacy. In addition, the true exposure rate to *P. falciparum* malaria in this study is unknown.

In a malaria challenge study conducted in healthy US volunteers, atovaquone alone prevented malaria in 6 of 6 individuals, whereas 4 of 4 placebo-treated volunteers developed malaria.

Causal Prophylaxis: In separate studies with small numbers of volunteers, atovaquone and proguanil hydrochloride were independently shown to have causal prophylactic activity directed against liver-stage parasites of *P. falciparum*. Six patients given a single dose of atovaquone 250 mg 24 hours prior to malaria challenge were protected from developing malaria, whereas all 4 placebo-treated patients developed malaria.

During the 4 weeks following cessation of prophylaxis in clinical trial participants who remained in malaria-endemic areas and were available for evaluation, malaria developed in 24 of 211 (11.4%) subjects who took placebo and 9 of 328 (2.7%) who took MALARONE. While new infections could not be distinguished from recrudescent infections, all but 1 of the infections in patients treated with MALARONE occurred more than 15 days after stopping therapy, probably representing new infections. The single case occurring on day 8 following cessation of therapy with MALARONE probably represents a failure of prophylaxis with MALARONE.

The possibility that delayed cases of *P. falciparum* malaria may occur some time after stopping prophylaxis with MALARONE cannot be ruled out. Hence, returning travelers developing febrile illnesses should be investigated for malaria.

GlaxoSmithKline, Research Triangle Park, NC 27709

May 2004/RL-2093

Shown in Product Identification Guide, page 316

MEPRON®

℞

[*mĕ'prŏn*]

(atovaquone)

Suspension

DESCRIPTION

MEPRON (atovaquone) is an antiprotozoal agent. The chemical name of atovaquone is *trans*-2-[4-(4-chlorophenyl) cyclohexyl]-3-hydroxy-1,4-naphthalenedione. Atovaquone is a yellow crystalline solid that is practically insoluble in water. It has a molecular weight of 366.84 and the molecular formula $C_{22}H_{19}ClO_3$.

MEPRON Suspension is a formulation of micro-fine particles of atovaquone. The atovaquone particles, reduced in size to facilitate absorption, are significantly smaller than those in the previously marketed tablet formulation. MEPRON Suspension is for oral administration and is bright yellow with a citrus flavor. Each teaspoonful (5 mL) contains 750 mg of atovaquone and the inactive ingredients benzyl alcohol, flavor, poloxamer 188, purified water, saccharin sodium, and xanthan gum.

MICROBIOLOGY

Mechanism of Action: Atovaquone is a hydroxy-1,4-naphthoquinone, an analog of ubiquinone, with antipneumocystis activity. The mechanism of action against *Pneumocystis carinii* has not been fully elucidated. In *Plasmodium* species, the site of action appears to be the cytochrome bc_1 complex (Complex III). Several metabolic enzymes are linked to the mitochondrial electron transport chain via ubiquinone. Inhibition of electron transport by atovaquone will result in indirect inhibition of these enzymes. The ultimate metabolic effects of such blockade may include inhibition of nucleic acid and ATP synthesis.

Table 1. Average Steady-State Plasma Atovaquone Concentrations in Pediatric Patients

Age	Dose of MEPRON Suspension		
	10 mg/kg	30 mg/kg	45 mg/kg
	Average C_{ss} in mcg/mL (mean ± SD)		
1–3 months	5.9 (n = 1)	27.8 ± 5.8 (n = 4)	—
>3–24 months	5.7 ± 5.1 (n = 4)	9.8 ± 3.2 (n = 4)	15.4 ± 6.6 (n = 4)
>2–13 years	16.8 ± 6.4 (n = 4)	37.1 ± 10.9 (n = 3)	—

Table 2. Relationship Between Plasma Atovaquone Concentration and Successful Treatment

Steady-State Plasma Atovaquone Concentrations (mcg/mL)	Successful Treatment* (No. Successes/No. in Group) (%)			
	Observed		Predicted†	
0 to <5	0/6	(0%)	1.5/6	(25%)
5 to <10	18/26	(69%)	14.7/26	(57%)
10 to <15	30/38	(79%)	31.9/38	(84%)
15 to <20	18/19	(95%)	18.1/19	(95%)
20 to <25	18/18	(100%)	17.8/18	(99%)
25+	6/6	(100%)	6/6	(100%)

*Successful treatment was defined as improvement in clinical and respiratory measures persisting at least 4 weeks after cessation of therapy. This was based on data from patients for which both outcome and steady-state plasma atovaquone concentration data are available.

† Based on logistic regression analysis.

Table 3. Confirmed or Presumed/Probable PCP Events (As-Treated Analysis)*

Assessment	Study 115-211: Atovaquone 1,500 mg/day (n = 527)	Study 115-211: Dapsone 100 mg/day (n = 510)	Study 115-213: Atovaquone 750 mg/day (n = 188)	Study 115-213: Atovaquone 1,500 mg/day (n = 172)	Study 115-213: Aerosolized Pentamidine 300 mg/month (n = 169)
%	15%	19%	23%	18%	17%
Relative Risk† (CI)‡	0.77 (0.57, 1.04)		1.47 (0.86, 2.50)	1.14 (0.63, 2.06)	

*Those events occurring during or within 30 days of stopping assigned treatment.

† Relative risk <1 favors atovaquone and values >1 favor comparator. These trials were designed to show superiority of atovaquone to the comparator. This was not shown.

‡ The confidence level of the interval for the dapsone comparative study was 95% and for the pentamidine comparative study was 97.5%.

Activity In Vitro: Several laboratories, using different in vitro methodologies, have shown the IC_{50} (50% inhibitory concentration) of atovaquone against rat *P. carinii* to be in the range of 0.1 to 3.0 mcg/mL.

Drug Resistance: Phenotypic resistance to atovaquone in vitro has not been demonstrated for *P. carinii*. However, in 2 patients who developed *P. carinii* pneumonia (PCP) after prophylaxis with atovaquone, DNA sequence analysis identified mutations in the predicted amino acid sequence of *P. carinii* cytochrome b (a likely target site for atovaquone). The clinical significance of this is unknown.

CLINICAL PHARMACOLOGY

Pharmacokinetics: *Absorption:* Atovaquone is a highly lipophilic compound with low aqueous solubility. The bioavailability of atovaquone is highly dependent on formulation and diet. The suspension formulation provides an approximately 2-fold increase in atovaquone bioavailability in the fasting or fed state compared to the previously marketed tablet formulation. The absolute bioavailability of a 750-mg dose of MEPRON Suspension administered under fed conditions in 9 HIV-infected (CD4 >100 cells/mm^3) volunteers was 47% ± 15%. In the same study, the bioavailability of a 750-mg dose of the previously marketed tablet formulation was 23% ± 11%.

Administering atovaquone with food enhances its absorption by approximately 2 fold. In one study, 16 healthy volunteers received a single dose of 750 mg MEPRON Suspension after an overnight fast and following a standard breakfast (23 g fat: 610 kCal). The mean (±SD) area under the concentration-time curve (AUC) values were 324 ± 115 and 801 ± 320 hr•mcg/mL under fasting and fed conditions, respectively, representing a 2.6 ± 1.0-fold increase. The effect of food (23 g fat: 400 kCal) on plasma atovaquone concentrations was also evaluated in a multiple-dose, randomized, crossover study in 19 HIV-infected volunteers (CD4 <200 cells/mm^3) receiving daily doses of 500 mg MEPRON Suspension. AUC was 280 ± 114 hr•mcg/mL when atovaquone was administered with food as compared to 169 ± 77 hr•mcg/mL under fasting conditions. Maximum plasma atovaquone concentration (C_{max}) was 15.1 ± 6.1 and 8.8 ± 3.7 mcg/mL when atovaquone was administered with food and under fasting conditions, respectively.

Dose Proportionality: Plasma atovaquone concentrations do not increase proportionally with dose. When MEPRON Suspension was administered with food at dosage regimens of 500 mg once daily, 750 mg once daily, and 1,000 mg once daily, average steady-state plasma atovaquone concentrations were 11.7 ± 4.8, 12.5 ± 5.8, and 13.5 ± 5.1 mcg/mL, respectively. The corresponding C_{max} concentrations were 15.1 ± 6.1, 15.3 ± 7.6, and 16.8 ± 6.4 mcg/mL. When MEPRON Suspension was administered to 5 HIV-infected volunteers at a dose of 750 mg twice daily, the average steady-state plasma atovaquone concentration was 21.0 ± 4.9 mcg/mL and C_{max} was 24.0 ± 5.7 mcg/mL. The minimum plasma atovaquone concentration (C_{min}) associated with the 750-mg twice-daily regimen was 16.7 ± 4.6 mcg/mL.

Distribution: Following the intravenous administration of atovaquone, the volume of distribution at steady state (Vd_{ss}) was 0.60 ± 0.17 L/kg (n = 9). Atovaquone is extensively bound to plasma proteins (99.9%) over the concentration range of 1 to 90 mcg/mL. In 3 HIV-infected children who received 750 mg atovaquone as the tablet formulation 4 times daily for 2 weeks, the cerebrospinal fluid concentrations of atovaquone were 0.04, 0.14, and 0.26 mcg/mL, representing less than 1% of the plasma concentration.

Elimination: The plasma clearance of atovaquone following intravenous (IV) administration in 9 HIV-infected volunteers was 10.4 ± 5.5 mL/min (0.15 ± 0.09 mL/min/kg). The half-life of atovaquone was 62.5 ± 35.3 hours after IV administration and ranged from 67.0 ± 33.4 to 77.6 ± 23.1 hours across studies following administration of MEPRON Suspension. The half-life of atovaquone is long due to presumed enterohepatic cycling and eventual fecal elimination. In a study where ^{14}C-labelled atovaquone was administered to healthy volunteers, greater than 94% of the dose was recovered as unchanged atovaquone in the feces over 21 days. There was little or no excretion of atovaquone in the urine (less than 0.6%). There is indirect evidence that atovaquone may undergo limited metabolism; however, a specific metabolite has not been identified.

Special Populations: *Pediatrics:* In a study of MEPRON Suspension in 27 HIV-infected, asymptomatic infants and children between 1 month and 13 years of age, the pharmacokinetics of atovaquone were age dependent. These patients were dosed once daily with food for 12 days. The average steady-state plasma atovaquone concentrations in the 24 patients with available concentration data are shown in Table 1.

[See table 1 above]

Hepatic/Renal Impairment: The pharmacokinetics of atovaquone have not been studied in patients with hepatic or renal impairment.

Drug Interactions: ***Rifampin:*** In a study with 13 HIV-infected volunteers, the oral administration of rifampin 600 mg every 24 hours with MEPRON Suspension 750 mg every 12 hours resulted in a 52% ± 13% decrease in the average steady-state plasma atovaquone concentration and a 37% ± 42% increase in the average steady-state plasma rifampin concentration. The half-life of atovaquone decreased from 82 ± 36 hours when administered without rifampin to 50 ± 16 hours with rifampin.
Rifabutin, another rifamycin, is structurally similar to rifampin and may possibly have some of the same drug interactions as rifampin. No interaction trials have been conducted with MEPRON and rifabutin.
Trimethoprim/Sulfamethoxazole (TMP-SMX): The possible interaction between atovaquone and TMP-SMX was evaluated in 6 HIV-infected adult volunteers as part of a larger multiple-dose, dose-escalation, and chronic dosing study of MEPRON Suspension. In this crossover study, MEPRON Suspension 500 mg once daily, or TMP-SMX tablets (160 mg trimethoprim and 800 mg sulfamethoxazole) twice daily, or the combination were administered with food to achieve steady state. No difference was observed in the average steady-state plasma atovaquone concentration after coadministration with TMP-SMX. Coadministration of MEPRON with TMP-SMX resulted in a 17% and 8% decrease in average steady-state concentrations of trimethoprim and sulfamethoxazole in plasma, respectively. This effect is minor and would not be expected to produce clinically significant events.
Zidovudine: Data from 14 HIV-infected volunteers who were given atovaquone tablets 750 mg every 12 hours with zidovudine 200 mg every 8 hours showed a 24% ± 12% decrease in zidovudine apparent oral clearance, leading to a 35% ± 23% increase in plasma zidovudine AUC. The glucuronide metabolite:parent ratio decreased from a mean of 4.5 when zidovudine was administered alone to 3.1 when zidovudine was administered with atovaquone tablets. This effect is minor and would not be expected to produce clinically significant events. Zidovudine had no effect on atovaquone pharmacokinetics.
Relationship Between Plasma Atovaquone Concentration and Clinical Outcome: In a comparative study of atovaquone tablets with TMP-SMX for oral treatment of mild-to-moderate *Pneumocystis carinii* pneumonia (PCP) (see INDICATIONS AND USAGE), where AIDS patients received 750 mg atovaquone tablets 3 times daily for 21 days, the mean steady-state atovaquone concentration was 13.9 ± 6.9 mcg/mL (n = 133). Analysis of these data established a relationship between plasma atovaquone concentration and successful treatment. This is shown in Table 2.
[See table 2 at top of previous page]
A dosing regimen of MEPRON Suspension for the treatment of mild-to-moderate PCP has been selected to achieve average plasma atovaquone concentrations of approximately 20 mcg/mL, because this plasma concentration was previously shown to be well tolerated and associated with the highest treatment success rates (Table 2). In an open-label PCP treatment study with MEPRON Suspension, dosing regimens of 1,000 mg once daily, 750 mg twice daily, 1,500 mg once daily, and 1,000 mg twice daily were explored. The average steady-state plasma atovaquone concentration achieved at the 750-mg twice-daily dose given with meals was 22.0 ± 10.1 mcg/mL (n = 18).

INDICATIONS AND USAGE

MEPRON Suspension is indicated for the prevention of *Pneumocystis carinii* pneumonia in patients who are intolerant to trimethoprim-sulfamethoxazole (TMP-SMX).
MEPRON Suspension is also indicated for the acute oral treatment of mild-to-moderate PCP in patients who are intolerant to TMP-SMX.
Prevention of PCP: The indication for prevention of PCP is based on the results of 2 clinical trials comparing MEPRON Suspension to dapsone or aerosolized pentamidine in HIV-infected adult and adolescent patients at risk of PCP (CD4 count <200 cells/mm^3 or a prior episode of PCP) and intolerant to TMP-SMX.
Dapsone Comparative Study: This randomized, open-label trial enrolled a total of 1,057 patients at 48 study centers. Patients were randomized to receive 1,500 mg MEPRON Suspension once daily (n = 536) or 100 mg dapsone once daily (n = 521). Median follow-up was 24 months. Patients randomized to the dapsone arm who were seropositive for *Toxoplasma gondii* and had a CD4 count <100 cells/mm^3 also received pyrimethamine and folinic acid. PCP event rates are shown in Table 3. There was no significant difference in mortality rates between the groups.
Aerosolized Pentamidine Comparative Study: This randomized, open-label trial enrolled a total of 549 patients at 35 study centers. Patients were randomized to receive 1,500 mg MEPRON Suspension once daily (n = 175), 750 mg MEPRON Suspension once daily (n = 188), or 300 mg aerosolized pentamidine once monthly (n = 186). Median follow-up was 11.3 months. The results of the PCP event rates appear in Table 3. There were no significant differences in mortality rates among the groups.
[See table 3 on previous page]
An analysis of all PCP events (intent-to-treat analysis) showed results similar to those above.
Treatment of PCP: The indication for treatment of mild-to-moderate PCP is based on the results of comparative pharmacokinetic studies of the suspension and tablet formulations (see CLINICAL PHARMACOLOGY) and clinical efficacy studies of the tablet formulation which established

Table 4. Outcome of Treatment for PCP-Positive Patients Enrolled in the TMP-SMX Comparative Study

	Number of Patients (% of Total)				
Outcome of Therapy*	MEPRON (n = 160)		TMP-SMX (n = 162)		*P* Value
Therapy success	99	(62%)	103	(64%)	0.75
Therapy failure					
–Lack of response	28	(17%)	10	(6%)	<0.01
–Adverse experience	11	(7%)	33	(20%)	<0.01
–Unevaluable	22	(14%)	16	(10%)	0.28
Required alternate PCP therapy during study	55	(34%)	55	(34%)	0.95

*As defined by the protocol and described in study description above.

Table 5. Outcome of Treatment for PCP-Positive Patients Enrolled in the Pentamidine Comparative Study

	Primary Treatment					Salvage Treatment				
Outcome of Therapy	MEPRON (n = 56)		Pentamidine (n = 53)		*P* Value	MEPRON (n = 14)		Pentamidine (n = 11)		*P* Value
Therapy success	32	(57%)	21	(40%)	0.09	13	(93%)	7	(64%)	0.14
Therapy failure										
–Lack of response	16	(29%)	9	(17%)	0.18	0		0		—
–Adverse experience	2	(3.6%)	19	(36%)	<0.01	0		3	(27%)	0.07
–Unevaluable	6	(11%)	4	(8%)	0.75	1	(7%)	1	(9%)	1.00
Required alternate PCP therapy during study	19	(34%)	29	(55%)	0.04	0		4	(36%)	0.03

Table 6. Treatment-Limiting Adverse Experiences in the Dapsone Comparative PCP Prevention Study

	Percentage of Patients with Treatment-Limiting Adverse Experience			
	All Patients		Patients Not Taking Either Drug at Enrollment	
Treatment-Limiting Adverse Experience	MEPRON 1,500 mg/day (n = 536)	Dapsone 100 mg/day (n = 521)	MEPRON 1,500 mg/day (n = 238)	Dapsone 100 mg/day (n = 249)
Any event	24.4%	25.9%	20.2%	43.4%
Rash	6.3%	8.8%	7.6%	16.1%
Nausea	4.1%	0.6%	2.5%	0.8%
Diarrhea	3.2%	0.2%	2.1%	0.4%
Vomiting	2.2%	0.6%	1.3%	0.8%
Allergic reaction	1.1%	2.9%	0.8%	4.8%
Fever	0.6%	2.9%	0%	5.6%
Anemia	0%	1.5%	0%	2.0%

a relationship between plasma atovaquone concentration and successful treatment. The results of a randomized, double-blind trial comparing MEPRON to TMP-SMX in AIDS patients with mild-to-moderate PCP (defined in the study protocol as an alveolar-arterial oxygen diffusion gradient $[(A\text{-}a)DO_2]^1 \leq 45$ mm Hg and $PaO_2 \geq 60$ mm Hg on room air) and a randomized trial comparing MEPRON to IV pentamidine isethionate in patients with mild-to-moderate PCP intolerant to trimethoprim or sulfa-antimicrobials are summarized below:
TMP-SMX Comparative Study: This double-blind, randomized trial initiated in 1990 was designed to compare the safety and efficacy of MEPRON to that of TMP-SMX for the treatment of AIDS patients with histologically confirmed PCP. Only patients with mild-to-moderate PCP were eligible for enrollment.
A total of 408 patients were enrolled into the trial at 37 study centers. Eighty-six patients without histologic confirmation of PCP were excluded from the efficacy analyses. Of the 322 patients with histologically confirmed PCP, 160 were randomized to receive MEPRON and 162 to TMP-SMX.
Study participants randomized to treatment with MEPRON were to receive 750 mg MEPRON (three 250-mg tablets) 3 times daily for 21 days and those randomized to TMP-SMX were to receive 320 mg TMP plus 1,600 mg SMX 3 times daily for 21 days.
Therapy success was defined as improvement in clinical and respiratory measures persisting at least 4 weeks after cessation of therapy. Therapy failures included lack of response, treatment discontinuation due to an adverse experience, and unevaluable.
There was a significant difference (P = 0.03) in mortality rates between the treatment groups. Among the 322 patients with confirmed PCP, 13 of 160 (8%) patients treated with MEPRON and 4 of 162 (2.5%) patients receiving TMP-SMX died during the 21-day treatment course or 8-week follow-up period. In the intent-to-treat analysis for all 408 randomized patients, there were 16 (8%) deaths in the arm treated with MEPRON and 7 (3.4%) deaths in the TMP-SMX arm (P = 0.051). Of the 13 patients treated with MEPRON who died, 4 died of PCP and 5 died with a combination of bacterial infections and PCP; bacterial infections did not appear to be a factor in any of the 4 deaths among TMP-SMX-treated patients.
A correlation between plasma atovaquone concentrations and death was demonstrated; in general, patients with lower plasma concentrations were more likely to die. For those patients for whom day 4 plasma atovaquone concentration data are available, 5 (63%) of the 8 patients with concentrations <5 mcg/mL died during participation in the study. However, only 1 (2.0%) of the 49 patients with day 4 plasma atovaquone concentrations ≥5 mcg/mL died.
Sixty-two percent of patients on MEPRON and 64% of patients on TMP-SMX were classified as protocol-defined therapy successes (Table 4).
[See table 4 above]
The failure rate due to lack of response was significantly larger for patients receiving MEPRON while the failure rate due to adverse experiences was significantly larger for patients receiving TMP-SMX.
There were no significant differences in the effect of either treatment on additional indicators of response (i.e., arterial blood gas measurements, vital signs, serum LDH levels, clinical symptoms, and chest radiographs).
Pentamidine Comparative Study: This unblinded, randomized trial initiated in 1991 was designed to compare the safety and efficacy of MEPRON to that of pentamidine for the treatment of histologically confirmed mild or moderate PCP in AIDS patients. Approximately 80% of the patients either had a history of intolerance to trimethoprim or sulfa-

Continued on next page

Product information on these pages is effective as of August 2004. Further information is available at: GlaxoSmithKline, PO Box 13398, Research Triangle Park, NC 27709. 1-888-825-5249. Corporate Web Site: www.gsk.com

Mepron—Cont.

antimicrobials (the primary therapy group) or were experiencing intolerance to TMP-SMX with treatment of an episode of PCP at the time of enrollment in the study (the salvage treatment group).
Patients randomized to MEPRON were to receive 750 mg atovaquone (three 250-mg tablets) 3 times daily for 21 days and those randomized to pentamidine isethionate were to receive a 3- to 4-mg/kg single IV infusion daily for 21 days. A total of 174 patients were enrolled into the trial at 22 study centers. Thirty-nine patients without histologic confirmation of PCP were excluded from the efficacy analyses. Of the 135 patients with histologically confirmed PCP, 70 were randomized to receive MEPRON and 65 to pentamidine. One hundred and ten (110) of these were in the primary therapy group and 25 were in the salvage therapy group. One patient in the primary therapy group randomized to receive pentamidine did not receive study medication.
There was no difference in mortality rates between the treatment groups. Among the 135 patients with confirmed PCP, 10 of 70 (14%) patients randomized to MEPRON and 9 of 65 (14%) patients randomized to pentamidine died during the 21-day treatment course or 8-week follow-up period. In the intent-to-treat analysis for all randomized patients, there were 11 (12.5%) deaths in the arm treated with MEPRON and 12 (14%) deaths in the pentamidine arm. For those patients for whom day 4 plasma atovaquone concentrations are available, 3 of 5 (60%) patients with concentrations <5 mcg/mL died during participation in the study. However, only 2 of 21 (9%) patients with day 4 plasma concentrations ≥5 mcg/mL died.
The therapeutic outcomes for the 134 patients who received study medication in this trial are presented in Table 5.
[See table 5 at top of previous page]

CONTRAINDICATIONS

MEPRON Suspension is contraindicated for patients who develop or have a history of potentially life-threatening allergic reactions to any of the components of the formulation.

WARNINGS

Clinical experience with MEPRON for the treatment of PCP has been limited to patients with mild-to-moderate PCP [(A-a)DO_2 ≤45 mm Hg]. Treatment of more severe episodes of PCP has not been systematically studied with this agent. Also, the efficacy of MEPRON in patients who are failing therapy with TMP-SMX has not been systematically studied.

PRECAUTIONS

General: Absorption of orally administered MEPRON is limited but can be significantly increased when the drug is taken with food. Plasma atovaquone concentrations have been shown to correlate with the likelihood of successful treatment and survival. Therefore, parenteral therapy with other agents should be considered for patients who have difficulty taking MEPRON with food (see CLINICAL PHARMACOLOGY). Gastrointestinal disorders may limit absorption of orally administered drugs. Patients with these disorders also may not achieve plasma concentrations of atovaquone associated with response to therapy in controlled trials.
Based upon the spectrum of in vitro antimicrobial activity, atovaquone is not effective therapy for concurrent pulmonary conditions such as bacterial, viral, or fungal pneumonia or mycobacterial diseases. Clinical deterioration in patients may be due to infections with other pathogens, as well as progressive PCP. All patients with acute PCP should be carefully evaluated for other possible causes of pulmonary disease and treated with additional agents as appropriate.
If it is necessary to treat patients with severe hepatic impairment, caution is advised and administration should be closely monitored.
Information for Patients: The importance of taking the prescribed dose of MEPRON should be stressed. Patients should be instructed to take their daily doses of MEPRON with meals, as the presence of food will significantly improve the absorption of the drug.
Drug Interactions: Atovaquone is highly bound to plasma protein (>99.9%). Therefore, caution should be used when administering MEPRON concurrently with other highly plasma protein-bound drugs with narrow therapeutic indices, as competition for binding sites may occur. The extent of plasma protein binding of atovaquone in human plasma is not affected by the presence of therapeutic concentrations of phenytoin (15 mcg/mL), nor is the binding of phenytoin affected by the presence of atovaquone.
Rifampin: Coadministration of rifampin and MEPRON Suspension results in a significant decrease in average steady-state plasma atovaquone concentrations (see CLINICAL PHARMACOLOGY: Drug Interactions). Alternatives to rifampin should be considered during the course of PCP treatment with MEPRON.
Rifabutin, another rifamycin, is structurally similar to rifampin and may possibly have some of the same drug interactions as rifampin. No interaction trials have been conducted with MEPRON and rifabutin.
Drug/Laboratory Test Interactions: It is not known if MEPRON interferes with clinical laboratory test or assay results.

Table 7. Treatment-Emergent Adverse Experiences in the Aerosolized Pentamidine Comparative PCP Prevention Study

Treatment-Emergent Adverse Experience	Percentage of Patients with Treatment-Emergent Adverse Experience		
	MEPRON 1,500 mg/day (n = 175)	MEPRON 750 mg/day (n = 188)	Aerosolized Pentamidine (n = 186)
Diarrhea	42%	42%	35%
Rash	39%	46%	28%
Headache	28%	31%	22%
Nausea	26%	32%	23%
Cough increased	25%	25%	31%
Fever	25%	31%	18%
Rhinitis	24%	18%	17%
Asthenia	22%	31%	31%
Infection	22%	18%	19%
Abdominal pain	20%	21%	20%
Dyspnea	15%	21%	16%
Vomiting	15%	22%	11%
Patients discontinuing therapy due to an adverse experience	25%	16%	7%
Patients reporting at least 1 adverse experience	98%	96%	89%

Table 8. Treatment-Emergent Adverse Experiences in the TMP-SMX Comparative PCP Treatment Study

Treatment-Emergent Adverse Experience	Percentage of Patients with Treatment-Emergent Adverse Experience	
	MEPRON (n = 203)	TMP-SMX (n = 205)
Rash (including maculopapular)	23%	34%
Nausea	21%	44%
Diarrhea	19%	7%
Headache	16%	22%
Vomiting	14%	35%
Fever	14%	25%
Insomnia	10%	9%
Asthenia	8%	8%
Pruritus	5%	9%
Monilia, oral	5%	10%
Abdominal pain	4%	7%
Constipation	3%	17%
Dizziness	3%	8%
Patients discontinuing therapy due to an adverse experience	9%	24%
Patients reporting at least 1 adverse experience	63%	65%

Table 9. Treatment-Emergent Laboratory Test Abnormalities in the TMP-SMX Comparative PCP Treatment Study

Laboratory Test Abnormality	Percentage of Patients Developing a Laboratory Test Abnormality	
	MEPRON	TMP-SMX
Anemia (Hgb<8.0 g/dL)	6%	7%
Neutropenia (ANC<750 cells/mm^3)	3%	9%
Elevated ALT (>5 × ULN)	6%	16%
Elevated AST (>5 × ULN)	4%	14%
Elevated alkaline phosphatase (>2.5 × ULN)	8%	6%
Elevated amylase (>1.5 × ULN)	7%	12%
Hyponatremia (<0.96 × LLN)	7%	26%

ULN = upper limit of normal range.
LLN = lower limit of normal range.

Carcinogenesis, Mutagenesis, Impairment of Fertility: Carcinogenicity studies in rats were negative; 24-month studies in mice showed treatment-related increases in incidence of hepatocellular adenoma and hepatocellular carcinoma at all doses tested which ranged from 1.4 to 3.6 times the average steady-state plasma concentrations in humans during acute treatment of *Pneumocystis carinii* pneumonia. Atovaquone was negative with or without metabolic activation in the Ames *Salmonella* mutagenicity assay, the Mouse Lymphoma mutagenesis assay, and the Cultured Human Lymphocyte cytogenetic assay. No evidence of genotoxicity was observed in the in vivo Mouse Micronucleus assay.

Pregnancy: Pregnancy Category C. Atovaquone was not teratogenic and did not cause reproductive toxicity in rats at plasma concentrations up to 2 to 3 times the estimated human exposure. Atovaquone caused maternal toxicity in rabbits at plasma concentrations that were approximately one-half the estimated human exposure. Mean fetal body lengths and weights were decreased and there were higher numbers of early resorption and post-implantation loss per dam. It is not clear whether these effects were caused by atovaquone directly or were secondary to maternal toxicity. Concentrations of atovaquone in rabbit fetuses averaged 30% of the concurrent maternal plasma concentrations. In a separate study in rats given a single ^{14}C-radiolabelled dose, concentrations of radiocarbon in rat fetuses were 18% (middle gestation) and 60% (late gestation) of concurrent maternal plasma concentrations. There are no adequate and well-controlled studies in pregnant women. MEPRON should be used during pregnancy only if the potential benefit justifies the potential risk to the fetus.

Nursing Mothers: It is not known whether atovaquone is excreted into human milk. Because many drugs are excreted into human milk, caution should be exercised when MEPRON is administered to a nursing woman. In a rat study, atovaquone concentrations in the milk were 30% of the concurrent atovaquone concentrations in the maternal plasma.

Pediatric Use: Evidence of safety and effectiveness in pediatric patients has not been established. A relationship between plasma atovaquone concentrations and successful treatment of PCP has been established in adults (see Table 2). In a study of MEPRON Suspension in 27 HIV-infected, asymptomatic infants and children between 1 month and 13 years of age, the pharmacokinetics of atovaquone were age-dependent (see CLINICAL PHARMACOLOGY: Special Populations). No drug-related treatment-limiting adverse events were observed in the pharmacokinetic study.

Geriatric Use: Clinical studies of MEPRON did not include sufficient numbers of subjects aged 65 and over to determine whether they respond differently from younger subjects. Other reported clinical experience has not identified differences in responses between the elderly and younger patients. In general, dose selection for an elderly patient should be cautious, reflecting the greater frequency of decreased hepatic, renal, or cardiac function, and of concomitant disease or other drug therapy.

ADVERSE REACTIONS

Because many patients who participated in clinical trials with MEPRON had complications of advanced HIV disease, it was often difficult to distinguish adverse events caused by MEPRON from those caused by underlying medical conditions. There were no life-threatening or fatal adverse experiences caused by MEPRON.

PCP Prevention Studies: In the dapsone comparative study of MEPRON Suspension, adverse experience data were collected only for treatment-limiting events. Among the entire population (n = 1,057), treatment-limiting events occurred at similar frequencies in patients treated with MEPRON Suspension or dapsone (Table 6). Among patients who were taking neither dapsone nor atovaquone at enrollment (n = 487), treatment-limiting events occurred in 43% of patients treated with dapsone and 20% of patients treated with MEPRON Suspension (P <0.001). In both populations, the type of treatment-limiting events differed between the 2 treatment arms. Hypersensitivity reactions (rash, fever, allergic reaction) and anemia were more common in patients treated with dapsone, while gastrointestinal events (nausea, diarrhea, and vomiting) were more common in patients treated with MEPRON Suspension.

[See table 6 on page 1573]

Table 7 summarizes the clinical adverse experiences reported by ≥20% of patients in any group in the aerosolized pentamidine comparative study of MEPRON Suspension (n = 549), regardless of attribution. The incidence of adverse experiences at the recommended dose was similar to that seen with aerosolized pentamidine. Rash was the only individual adverse experience that occurred significantly more commonly in patients treated with both dosages of MEPRON Suspension (39% to 46%) than in patients treated with aerosolized pentamidine (28%). Among patients treated with MEPRON Suspension, there was no evidence of a dose-related increase in the incidence of adverse experiences. Treatment-limiting adverse experiences occurred less often in patients treated with aerosolized pentamidine (7%) than in patients treated with 1,500 mg MEPRON Suspension once daily (25%, P≤0.001) or 750 mg MEPRON Suspension once daily (16%, P = 0.004). The most common adverse experiences requiring discontinuation of dosing in the group receiving 1,500 mg MEPRON Suspension once daily were rash (6%), diarrhea (4%), and nausea (3%). The most common adverse experience requiring discontinuation of dosing in the group receiving aerosolized pentamidine was bronchospasm (2%).

[See table 7 at top of previous page]

Other events occurring in ≥10% of the patients receiving the recommended dose of MEPRON included sweating, flu syndrome, pain, sinusitis, pruritus, insomnia, depression, and myalgia. Bronchospasm occurred more frequently in patients receiving aerosolized pentamidine (11%) than in patients receiving MEPRON 1,500 mg/day (4%) and MEPRON 750 mg/day (2%).

Neither MEPRON nor aerosolized pentamidine was associated with a substantial change from baseline values in any measured laboratory parameter, nor were there any significant differences in any measured laboratory parameter between MEPRON and aerosolized pentamidine. Some patients had laboratory abnormalities considered serious by the investigator or that contributed to discontinuation of therapy.

PCP Treatment Studies: Table 8 summarizes all the clinical adverse experiences reported by ≥5% of the study population during the TMP-SMX comparative study of MEPRON (n = 408), regardless of attribution. The incidence of adverse experiences with MEPRON Suspension at the recommended dose was similar to that seen with the tablet formulation of atovaquone.

[See table 8 on previous page]

Although an equal percentage of patients receiving MEPRON and TMP-SMX reported at least 1 adverse experience, more patients receiving TMP-SMX required discontinuation of therapy due to an adverse event. Twenty-four percent of patients receiving TMP-SMX were prematurely discontinued from therapy due to an adverse experience versus 9% of patients receiving MEPRON. Four percent of

Continued on next page

Table 10. Treatment-Emergent Adverse Experiences in the Pentamidine Comparative PCP Treatment Study (Primary Therapy Group)

Treatment-Emergent Adverse Experience	Percentage of Patients with Treatment-Emergent Adverse Experience	
	MEPRON (n = 73)	Pentamidine (n = 71)
Fever	40%	25%
Nausea	22%	37%
Rash	22%	13%
Diarrhea	21%	31%
Insomnia	19%	14%
Headache	18%	28%
Vomiting	14%	17%
Cough	14%	1%
Abdominal pain	10%	11%
Pain	10%	10%
Sweat	10%	3%
Monilia, oral	10%	3%
Asthenia	8%	14%
Dizziness	8%	14%
Anxiety	7%	10%
Anorexia	7%	10%
Sinusitis	7%	6%
Dyspepsia	5%	10%
Rhinitis	5%	7%
Taste perversion	3%	13%
Hypoglycemia	1%	15%
Hypotension	1%	10%
Patients discontinuing therapy due to an adverse experience	7%	41%
Patients reporting at least 1 adverse experience	63%	72%

Table 11. Treatment-Emergent Laboratory Test Abnormalities in the Pentamidine Comparative PCP Treatment Study

Laboratory Test Abnormality	Percentage of Patients Developing a Laboratory Test Abnormality	
	MEPRON	Pentamidine
Anemia (Hgb<8.0 g/dL)	4%	9%
Neutropenia (ANC<750 cells/mm^3)	5%	9%
Hyponatremia (<0.96 × LLN)	10%	10%
Hyperkalemia (>1.18 × ULN)	0%	5%
Alkaline phosphatase (>2.5 × ULN)	5%	2%
Hyperglycemia (>1.8 × ULN)	9%	13%
Elevated AST (>5 × ULN)	0%	5%
Elevated amylase (>1.5 × ULN)	8%	4%
Elevated creatinine (>1.5 × ULN)	0%	7%

ULN = upper limit of normal range.
LLN = lower limit of normal range.

Product information on these pages is effective as of August 2004. Further information is available at: GlaxoSmithKline, PO Box 13398, Research Triangle Park, NC 27709. 1-888-825-5249. Corporate Web Site: www.gsk.com

Mepron—Cont.

patients receiving MEPRON had therapy discontinued due to development of rash. The majority of cases of rash among patients receiving MEPRON were mild and did not require the discontinuation of dosing. The only other clinical adverse experience that led to premature discontinuation of dosing of MEPRON by more than 1 patient was vomiting (<1%). The most common adverse experience requiring discontinuation of dosing in the TMP-SMX group was rash (8%).
Laboratory test abnormalities reported for ≥5% of the study population during the treatment period are summarized in Table 9. Two percent of patients treated with MEPRON and 7% of patients treated with TMP-SMX had therapy prematurely discontinued due to elevations in ALT/AST. In general, patients treated with MEPRON developed fewer abnormalities in measures of hepatocellular function (ALT, AST, alkaline phosphatase) or amylase values than patients treated with TMP-SMX.
[See table 9 on page 1574]
Table 10 summarizes the clinical adverse experiences reported by ≥5% of the primary therapy study population (n = 144) during the comparative trial of MEPRON and intravenous pentamidine, regardless of attribution. A slightly lower percentage of patients who received MEPRON reported occurrence of adverse events than did those who received pentamidine (63% vs 72%). However, only 7% of patients discontinued treatment with MEPRON due to adverse events, while 41% of patients who received pentamidine discontinued treatment for this reason (P<0.001). Of the 5 patients who discontinued therapy with MEPRON, 3 reported rash (4%). Rash was not severe in any patient. No other reason for discontinuation of MEPRON was cited more than once. The most frequently cited reasons for discontinuation of pentamidine therapy were hypoglycemia (11%) and vomiting (9%).
[See table 10 at top of previous page]
Laboratory test abnormalities reported in ≥5% of patients in the pentamidine comparative study are presented in Table 11. Laboratory abnormality was reported as the reason for discontinuation of treatment in 2 of 73 patients who received MEPRON. One patient (1%) had elevated creatinine and BUN levels and 1 patient (1%) had elevated amylase levels. Laboratory abnormalities were the sole or contributing factor in 14 patients who prematurely discontinued pentamidine therapy. In the 71 patients who received pentamidine, laboratory parameters most frequently reported as reasons for discontinuation were hypoglycemia (11%), elevated creatinine levels (6%), and leukopenia (4%).
[See table 11 on previous page]
Observed During Clinical Practice: In addition to adverse events reported from clinical trials, the following events have been identified during post-approval use of MEPRON. Because they are reported voluntarily from a population of unknown size, estimates of frequency cannot be made. These events have been chosen for inclusion due to a combination of their seriousness, frequency of reporting, or potential causal connection to MEPRON.
Blood and Lymphatic: Methemoglobinemia, thrombocytopenia.
Eye: Vortex keratopathy.
Hepatobiliary Tract and Pancreas: Pancreatitis.
Skin: Allergic reactions including erythema multiforme.
Urology: Acute renal impairment.

OVERDOSAGE

There is no known antidote for atovaquone, and it is currently unknown if atovaquone is dialyzable. The median lethal dose is higher than the maximum oral dose tested in mice and rats (1,825 mg/kg/day). Overdoses up to 31,500 mg of atovaquone have been reported. In 1 such patient who also took an unspecified dose of dapsone, methemoglobinemia occurred. Rash has also been reported after overdose.

DOSAGE AND ADMINISTRATION

Dosage: ***Prevention of PCP: Adults and Adolescents (13 to 16 Years):*** The recommended oral dose is 1,500 mg (10 mL) once daily administered with a meal.
Treatment of Mild-to-Moderate PCP: Adults and Adolescents (13 to 16 Years): The recommended oral dose is 750 mg (5 mL) administered with meals twice daily for 21 days (total daily dose 1,500 mg).
Note: Failure to administer MEPRON Suspension with meals may result in lower plasma atovaquone concentrations and may limit response to therapy (see CLINICAL PHARMACOLOGY and PRECAUTIONS).
Administration: ***Foil Pouch:*** Open pouch by removing tab at perforation and tear at notch. Take entire contents by mouth. Can be discharged into a dosing spoon or cup or directly into the mouth.
Bottle: SHAKE BOTTLE GENTLY BEFORE USING.

HOW SUPPLIED

MEPRON Suspension (bright yellow, citrus flavored) containing 750 mg atovaquone in each teaspoonful (5 mL).
Bottle of 210 mL with child-resistant cap (NDC 0173-0665-18).
Store at 15° to 25°C (59° to 77°F). DO NOT FREEZE. Dispense in tight container as defined in USP.
5-mL child-resistant foil pouch - unit dose pack of 42 (NDC 0173-0547-00).
Store at 15° to 25°C (59° to 77°F). DO NOT FREEZE.
[1]$(A\text{-}a)DO_2 = [(713 \times FiO_2) - (PaCO_2/0.8)] - PaO_2$ (mm Hg)

GlaxoSmithKline, Research Triangle Park, NC 27709

December 2001/RL-1012
Shown in Product Identification Guide, page 316

MYLERAN® ℞
[*mī 'lə-răn*]
(busulfan)
Tablets

WARNING

MYLERAN is a potent drug. It should not be used unless a diagnosis of chronic myelogenous leukemia has been adequately established and the responsible physician is knowledgeable in assessing response to chemotherapy. MYLERAN can induce severe bone marrow hypoplasia. Reduce or discontinue the dosage immediately at the first sign of any unusual depression of bone marrow function as reflected by an abnormal decrease in any of the formed elements of the blood. A bone marrow examination should be performed if the bone marrow status is uncertain.
SEE WARNINGS FOR INFORMATION REGARDING BUSULFAN-INDUCED LEUKEMOGENESIS IN HUMANS.

DESCRIPTION

MYLERAN (busulfan) is a bifunctional alkylating agent. Busulfan is known chemically as 1,4-butanediol dimethanesulfonate and has the following structural formula:

$$CH_3SO_2O(CH_2)_4OSO_2CH_3$$

Busulfan is *not* a structural analog of the nitrogen mustards. MYLERAN is available in tablet form for oral administration. Each film-coated tablet contains 2 mg busulfan and the inactive ingredients hypromellose, lactose (anhydrous), magnesium stearate, pregelatinized starch, triacetin, and titanium dioxide.
The activity of busulfan in chronic myelogenous leukemia was first reported by D.A.G. Galton in 1953.

CLINICAL PHARMACOLOGY

Busulfan is a small, highly lipophilic molecule that easily crosses the blood brain barrier. Following absorption, 32% and 47% of busulfan are bound to plasma proteins and red blood cells, respectively.
Busulfan absorption from the gastrointestinal tract is essentially complete. This has been demonstrated in radioactive studies after both intravenous and oral administration of ^{35}S-busulfan, ^{14}C-busulfan, and ^{3}H-busulfan. Following intravenous administration of a single therapeutic dose of ^{35}S-busulfan, there was rapid disappearance of radioactivity from the blood and 90% to 95% of the ^{35}S-label disappeared within 3 to 5 minutes after injection. After either oral or intravenous administration of ^{35}S-busulfan, 45% to 60% of the radioactivity was recovered in the urine in the 48 hours after administration; the majority of the total urinary excretion occurring in the first 24 hours. Over 95% of the urinary ^{35}S-label occurs as ^{35}S-methanesulfonic acid. Oral and intravenous administration of 1,4-^{14}C-busulfan showed the same rapid initial disappearance of plasma radioactivity as observed following the administration of ^{35}S-labeled drug. Cumulative radioactivity in the urine after 48 hours was 25% to 30% of the administered dose (contrasting with 45% to 60% for ^{35}S-busulfan), and suggests a slower excretion of the alkylating portion of the molecule and its metabolites than for the sulfonoxymethyl moieties. Regardless of the route of administration, 1,4-^{14}C-busulfan yielded a complex mixture of at least 12 radiolabeled metabolites in urine; the main metabolite being 3-hydroxytetrahydrothiophene-1,1-dioxide. Pharmacokinetic studies employing ^{3}H-busulfan labeled on the tetramethylene chain confirmed a rapid initial clearance of the radioactivity from plasma, irrespective of whether the drug was given orally or intravenously.
A study compared a 2-mg single IV bolus injection to a single oral dose of a 2-mg tablet of nonradioactive busulfan in 8 adult patients 13 to 60 years of age. The study demonstrated that the mean ± SD absolute bioavailability was 80% ± 20% in adults. However, the absolute bioavailability for 8 children 1.5 to 6 years of age was 68% ± 31%.
In another study of 2, 4, and 6 mg of busulfan, given as a single oral dose on consecutive days (starting with the lowest dose) in 5 adult patients, the mean dose-normalized (to 2 mg dose) area under the plasma concentration-time curve (AUC) was about 130 ng•hr/mL, while the mean intra- and inter-patient variability was about 16% and 21%, respectively. Busulfan was eliminated with a plasma terminal elimination half-life ($t_{1/2}$) of about 2.6 hours, and demonstrated linear kinetics within the range of 2 to 6 mg for both the maximum plasma concentration (C_{max}) and AUC. The mean C_{max} for the 2-, 4-, and 6-mg doses (after dose normalization to 2 mg) was about 30 ng/mL. A recent study of 4 to 8 mg as single oral doses in 12 patients showed that the mean ± SD C_{max} (after dose normalization to 4 mg) was 68.2 ± 24.4 ng/mL, occurring at about 0.9 hours and the mean ± SD AUC (after dose normalization to 4 mg) was 269 ± 62 ng•hr/mL. These results are consistent with previous results. In addition, the mean ± SD elimination half-life was 2.69 ± 0.49 hours.
The elimination of busulfan appears to be independent of renal function. This probably reflects the extensive metabolism of the drug in the liver, since less than 2% of the administered dose is excreted in the urine unchanged within 24 hours. The drug is metabolized by enzymatic activity to at least 12 metabolites, among which tetrahydrothiophene, tetrahydrothiophene 12-oxide, sulfolane, and 3-hydroxysulfolane were identified. These metabolites do not have cytotoxic activity.
There is no experience with the use of dialysis in an attempt to modify the clinical toxicity of busulfan. One technical difficulty would derive from the extremely poor water solubility of busulfan. Additionally, all studies of the metabolism of busulfan employing radiolabeled materials indicate rapid chemical reactivity of the parent compound with prolonged retention of some of the metabolites (particularly the metabolites arising from the "alkylating" portion of the molecule). The effectiveness of dialysis at removing significant quantities of unreacted drug would be expected to be minimal in such a situation.
Currently, there are no available data on the effect of food on busulfan bioavailability.
Pharmacokinetics in Hemodialysis Patients: The impact of hemodialysis on the clearance of busulfan was determined in a patient with chronic renal failure undergoing autologous stem cell transplantation. The apparent oral clearance of busulfan during a 4-hour hemodialysis session was increased by 65%, but the 24-hour oral clearance of busulfan was increased by only 11%.
The incidence of veno-occlusive disease was higher (33.3% versus 3.0%) in patients with busulfan $AUC_{0\text{-}6hr}$ >1,500 µM.min (C_{ss} >900 mcg/L) compared to patients with busulfan $AUC_{0\text{-}6hr}$ <1,500 µM.min (C_{ss} <900 mcg/L) (see WARNINGS).
Drug Interactions: Itraconazole reduced busulfan clearance by up to 25% in patients receiving itraconazole compared to patients who did not receive itraconazole. Higher busulfan exposure due to concomitant itraconazole could lead to toxic plasma levels in some patients. Fluconazole had no effect on the clearance of busulfan. Patients treated with concomitant cyclophosphamide and busulfan with phenytoin pretreatment have increased cyclophosphamide and busulfan clearance, which may lead to decreased concentrations of both cyclophosphamide and busulfan. However, busulfan clearance may be reduced in the presence of cyclophosphamide alone, presumably due to competition for glutathione.
Diazepam had no effect on the clearance of busulfan.
No information is available regarding the penetration of busulfan into brain or cerebrospinal fluid.
Biochemical Pharmacology: In aqueous media, busulfan undergoes a wide range of nucleophilic substitution reactions. While this chemical reactivity is relatively non-specific, alkylation of the DNA is felt to be an important biological mechanism for its cytotoxic effect. Coliphage T7 exposed to busulfan was found to have the DNA crosslinked by intrastrand crosslinkages, but no interstrand linkages were found.
The metabolic fate of busulfan has been studied in rats and humans using ^{14}C- and ^{35}S-labeled materials. In humans, as in the rat, almost all of the radioactivity in ^{35}S-labeled busulfan is excreted in the urine in the form of ^{35}S-methanesulfonic acid. Roberts and Warwick demonstrated that the formation of methanesulfonic acid in vivo in the rat is not due to a simple hydrolysis of busulfan to 1,4-butanediol, since only about 4% of 2,3-^{14}C-busulfan was excreted as carbon dioxide, whereas 2,3-^{14}C-1,4-butanediol was converted almost exclusively to carbon dioxide. The predominant reaction of busulfan in the rat is the alkylation of sulfhydryl groups (particularly cysteine and cysteine-containing compounds) to produce a cyclic sulfonium compound which is the precursor of the major urinary metabolite of the 4-carbon portion of the molecule, 3-hydroxytetrahydrothiophene-1,1-dioxide. This has been termed a "sulfur-stripping" action of busulfan and it may modify the function of certain sulfur-containing amino acids, polypeptides, and proteins; whether this action makes an important contribution to the cytotoxicity of busulfan is unknown.
The biochemical basis for acquired resistance to busulfan is largely a matter of speculation. Although altered transport of busulfan into the cell is one possibility, increased intracellular inactivation of the drug before it reaches the DNA is also possible. Experiments with other alkylating agents have shown that resistance to this class of compounds may reflect an acquired ability of the resistant cell to repair alkylation damage more effectively.
Clinical Studies: Although not curative, busulfan reduces the total granulocyte mass, relieves symptoms of the disease, and improves the clinical state of the patient. Approximately 90% of adults with previously untreated chronic myelogenous leukemia will obtain hematologic remission with regression or stabilization of organomegaly following the use of busulfan. It has been shown to be superior to splenic irradiation with respect to survival times and maintenance of hemoglobin levels, and to be equivalent to irradiation at controlling splenomegaly.
It is not clear whether busulfan unequivocally prolongs the survival of responding patients beyond the 31 months experienced by an untreated group of historical controls. Median survival figures of 31 to 42 months have been reported for several groups of patients treated with busulfan, but concurrent control groups of comparable, untreated patients are not available. The median survival figures reported from different studies will be influenced by the percentage of "poor risk" patients initially entered into the particular study. Patients who are alive 2 years following the diagnosis of chronic myelogenous leukemia, and who have been

treated during that period with busulfan, are estimated to have a mean annual mortality rate during the second to fifth year which is approximately two thirds that of patients who received either no treatment, conventional x-ray or ^{32}P-irradiation, or chemotherapy with minimally active drugs.
Busulfan is clearly less effective in patients with chronic myelogenous leukemia who lack the Philadelphia (Ph^1) chromosome. Also, the so-called "juvenile" type of chronic myelogenous leukemia, typically occurring in young children and associated with the absence of a Philadelphia chromosome, responds poorly to busulfan. The drug is of no benefit in patients whose chronic myelogenous leukemia has entered a "blastic" phase.
MYLERAN should not be used in patients whose chronic myelogenous leukemia has demonstrated prior resistance to this drug.
MYLERAN is of no value in chronic lymphocytic leukemia, acute leukemia, or in the "blastic crisis" of chronic myelogenous leukemia.

INDICATIONS AND USAGE

MYLERAN (busulfan) is indicated for the palliative treatment of chronic myelogenous (myeloid, myelocytic, granulocytic) leukemia.

CONTRAINDICATIONS

MYLERAN is contraindicated in patients in whom a definitive diagnosis of chronic myelogenous leukemia has not been firmly established.
MYLERAN is contraindicated in patients who have previously suffered a hypersensitivity reaction to busulfan or any other component of the preparation.

WARNINGS

The most frequent, serious side effect of treatment with busulfan is the induction of bone marrow failure (which may or may not be anatomically hypoplastic) resulting in severe pancytopenia. The pancytopenia caused by busulfan may be more prolonged than that induced with other alkylating agents. It is generally felt that the usual cause of busulfan-induced pancytopenia is the failure to stop administration of the drug soon enough; individual idiosyncrasy to the drug does not seem to be an important factor. *MYLERAN should be used with extreme caution and exceptional vigilance in patients whose bone marrow reserve may have been compromised by prior irradiation or chemotherapy, or whose marrow function is recovering from previous cytotoxic therapy.* Although recovery from busulfan-induced pancytopenia may take from 1 month to 2 years, this complication is potentially reversible, and the patient should be vigorously supported through any period of severe pancytopenia.
A rare, important complication of busulfan therapy is the development of bronchopulmonary dysplasia with pulmonary fibrosis. Symptoms have been reported to occur within 8 months to 10 years after initiation of therapy—the average duration of therapy being 4 years. The histologic findings associated with "busulfan lung" mimic those seen following pulmonary irradiation. Clinically, patients have reported the insidious onset of cough, dyspnea, and low-grade fever. In some cases, however, onset of symptoms may be acute. Pulmonary function studies have revealed diminished diffusion capacity and decreased pulmonary compliance. It is important to exclude more common conditions (such as opportunistic infections or leukemic infiltration of the lungs) with appropriate diagnostic techniques. If measures such as sputum cultures, virologic studies, and exfoliative cytology fail to establish an etiology for the pulmonary infiltrates, lung biopsy may be necessary to establish the diagnosis. Treatment of established busulfan-induced pulmonary fibrosis is unsatisfactory; in most cases the patients have died within 6 months after the diagnosis was established. There is no specific therapy for this complication. MYLERAN should be discontinued if this lung toxicity develops. The administration of corticosteroids has been suggested, but the results have not been impressive or uniformly successful.
Busulfan may cause cellular dysplasia in many organs in addition to the lung. Cytologic abnormalities characterized by giant, hyperchromatic nuclei have been reported in lymph nodes, pancreas, thyroid, adrenal glands, liver, and bone marrow. This cytologic dysplasia may be severe enough to cause difficulty in interpretation of exfoliative cytologic examinations from the lung, bladder, breast, and the uterine cervix.
In addition to the widespread epithelial dysplasia that has been observed during busulfan therapy, chromosome aberrations have been reported in cells from patients receiving busulfan.
Busulfan is mutagenic in mice and, possibly, in humans.
Malignant tumors and acute leukemias have been reported in patients who have received busulfan therapy, and this drug may be a human carcinogen. The World Health Organization has concluded that there is a causal relationship between busulfan exposure and the development of secondary malignancies. Four cases of acute leukemia occurred among 243 patients treated with busulfan as adjuvant chemotherapy following surgical resection of bronchogenic carcinoma. All 4 cases were from a subgroup of 19 of these 243 patients who developed pancytopenia while taking busulfan 5 to 8 years before leukemia became clinically apparent. These findings suggest that busulfan is leukemogenic, although its mode of action is uncertain.
Ovarian suppression and amenorrhea with menopausal symptoms commonly occur during busulfan therapy in premenopausal patients. Busulfan has been associated with ovarian failure including failure to achieve puberty in females. Busulfan interferes with spermatogenesis in experimental animals, and there have been clinical reports of sterility, azoospermia, and testicular atrophy in male patients.
Hepatic veno-occlusive disease, which may be life threatening, has been reported in patients receiving busulfan, usually in combination with cyclophosphamide or other chemotherapeutic agents prior to bone marrow transplantation. Possible risk factors for the development of hepatic veno-occlusive disease include: total busulfan dose exceeding 16 mg/kg based on ideal body weight, and concurrent use of multiple alkylating agents (see CLINICAL PHARMACOLOGY and Drug Interactions).
A clear cause-and-effect relationship with busulfan has not been demonstrated. Periodic measurement of serum transaminases, alkaline phosphatase, and bilirubin is indicated for early detection of hepatotoxicity. A reduced incidence of hepatic veno-occlusive disease and other regimen-related toxicities have been observed in patients treated with high-dose MYLERAN and cyclophosphamide when the first dose of cyclophosphamide has been delayed for >24 hours after the last dose of busulfan (see CLINICAL PHARMACOLOGY and Drug Interactions).
Cardiac tamponade has been reported in a small number of patients with thalassemia (2% in one series) who received busulfan and cyclophosphamide as the preparatory regimen for bone marrow transplantation. In this series, the cardiac tamponade was often fatal. Abdominal pain and vomiting preceded the tamponade in most patients.
Pregnancy: Pregnancy Category D. Busulfan may cause fetal harm when administered to a pregnant woman. Although there have been a number of cases reported where apparently normal children have been born after busulfan treatment during pregnancy, one case has been cited where a malformed baby was delivered by a mother treated with busulfan. During the pregnancy that resulted in the malformed infant, the mother received x-ray therapy early in the first trimester, mercaptopurine until the third month, then busulfan until delivery. In pregnant rats, busulfan produces sterility in both male and female offspring due to the absence of germinal cells in testes and ovaries. Germinal cell aplasia or sterility in offspring of mothers receiving busulfan during pregnancy has not been reported in humans. There are no adequate and well-controlled studies in pregnant women. If this drug is used during pregnancy, or if the patient becomes pregnant while taking this drug, the patient should be apprised of the potential hazard to the fetus. Women of childbearing potential should be advised to avoid becoming pregnant.

PRECAUTIONS

General: The most consistent, dose-related toxicity is bone marrow suppression. This may be manifest by anemia, leukopenia, thrombocytopenia, or any combination of these. It is imperative that patients be instructed to report promptly the development of fever, sore throat, signs of local infection, bleeding from any site, or symptoms suggestive of anemia. Any one of these findings may indicate busulfan toxicity; however, they may also indicate transformation of the disease to an acute "blastic" form. Since busulfan may have a delayed effect, it is important to withdraw the medication temporarily at the first sign of an abnormally large or exceptionally rapid fall in any of the formed elements of the blood. *Patients should never be allowed to take the drug without close medical supervision.*
Seizures have been reported in patients receiving busulfan. As with any potentially epileptogenic drug, caution should be exercised when administering busulfan to patients with a history of seizure disorder, head trauma, or receiving other potentially epileptogenic drugs. Some investigators have used prophylactic anticonvulsant therapy in this setting.
Information for Patients: Patients beginning therapy with busulfan should be informed of the importance of having periodic blood counts and to immediately report any unusual fever or bleeding. Aside from the major toxicity of myelosuppression, patients should be instructed to report any difficulty in breathing, persistent cough, or congestion. They should be told that diffuse pulmonary fibrosis is an infrequent, but serious and potentially life-threatening complication of long-term busulfan therapy. Patients should be alerted to report any signs of abrupt weakness, unusual fatigue, anorexia, weight loss, nausea and vomiting, and melanoderma that could be associated with a syndrome resembling adrenal insufficiency. Patients should never be allowed to take the drug without medical supervision and they should be informed that other encountered toxicities to busulfan include infertility, amenorrhea, skin hyperpigmentation, drug hypersensitivity, dryness of the mucous membranes, and rarely, cataract formation. Women of childbearing potential should be advised to avoid becoming pregnant. The increased risk of a second malignancy should be explained to the patient.
Laboratory Tests: It is recommended that evaluation of the hemoglobin or hematocrit, total white blood cell count and differential count, and quantitative platelet count be obtained weekly while the patient is on busulfan therapy. In cases where the cause of fluctuation in the formed elements of the peripheral blood is obscure, bone marrow examination may be useful for evaluation of marrow status. A decision to increase, decrease, continue, or discontinue a given dose of busulfan must be based not only on the absolute hematologic values, but also on the rapidity with which changes are occurring. The dosage of busulfan may need to be reduced if this agent is combined with other drugs whose primary toxicity is myelosuppression. Occasional patients may be unusually sensitive to busulfan administered at standard dosage and suffer neutropenia or thrombocytopenia after a relatively short exposure to the drug. Busulfan should not be used where facilities for complete blood counts, including quantitative platelet counts, are not available at weekly (or more frequent) intervals.
Drug Interactions: Busulfan may cause additive myelosuppression when used with other myelosuppressive drugs.
In one study, 12 of approximately 330 patients receiving continuous busulfan and thioguanine therapy for treatment of chronic myelogenous leukemia were found to have portal hypertension and esophageal varices associated with abnormal liver function tests. Subsequent liver biopsies were performed in 4 of these patients, all of which showed evidence of nodular regenerative hyperplasia. Duration of combination therapy prior to the appearance of esophageal varices ranged from 6 to 45 months. With the present analysis of the data, no cases of hepatotoxicity have appeared in the busulfan-alone arm of the study. Long-term continuous therapy with thioguanine and busulfan should be used with caution.
Busulfan-induced pulmonary toxicity may be additive to the effects produced by other cytotoxic agents.
The concomitant systemic administration of itraconazole to patients receiving high-dose MYLERAN may result in reduced busulfan clearance (see CLINICAL PHARMACOLOGY). Patients should be monitored for signs of busulfan toxicity when itraconazole is used concomitantly with MYLERAN.
Carcinogenesis, Mutagenesis, Impairment of Fertility: See WARNINGS section. The World Health Organization has concluded that there is a causal relationship between busulfan exposure and the development of secondary malignancies.
Pregnancy: ***Teratogenic Effects:*** Pregnancy Category D. See WARNINGS section.
Nonteratogenic Effects: There have been reports in the literature of small infants being born after the mothers received busulfan during pregnancy, in particular, during the third trimester. One case was reported where an infant had mild anemia and neutropenia at birth after busulfan was administered to the mother from the eighth week of pregnancy to term.
Nursing Mothers: It is not known whether this drug is excreted in human milk. Because of the potential for tumorigenicity shown for busulfan in animal and human studies, a decision should be made whether to discontinue nursing or to discontinue the drug, taking into account the importance of the drug to the mother.
Pediatric Use: See INDICATIONS AND USAGE and DOSAGE AND ADMINISTRATION sections.
Geriatric Use: Clinical studies of busulfan did not include sufficient numbers of subjects aged 65 and over to determine whether they respond differently from younger subjects. Other reported clinical experience has not identified differences in responses between the elderly and younger patients. In general, dose selection for an elderly patient should be cautious, usually starting at the low end of the dosing range, reflecting the greater frequency of decreased hepatic, renal, or cardiac function, and of concomitant disease or other drug therapy.

ADVERSE REACTIONS

Hematological Effects: The most frequent, serious, toxic effect of busulfan is dose-related myelosuppression resulting in leukopenia, thrombocytopenia, and anemia. Myelosuppression is most frequently the result of a failure to discontinue dosage in the face of an undetected decrease in leukocyte or platelet counts.
Aplastic anemia (sometimes irreversible) has been reported rarely, often following long-term conventional doses and also high doses of MYLERAN.
Pulmonary: Interstitial pulmonary fibrosis has been reported rarely, but it is a clinically significant adverse effect when observed and calls for immediate discontinuation of further administration of the drug. The role of corticosteroids in arresting or reversing the fibrosis has been reported to be beneficial in some cases and without effect in others.
Cardiac: Cardiac tamponade has been reported in a small number of patients with thalassemia who received busulfan and cyclophosphamide as the preparatory regimen for bone marrow transplantation (see WARNINGS).
One case of endocardial fibrosis has been reported in a 79-year-old woman who received a total dose of 7,200 mg of busulfan over a period of 9 years for the management of chronic myelogenous leukemia. At autopsy, she was found to have endocardial fibrosis of the left ventricle in addition to interstitial pulmonary fibrosis.
Ocular: Busulfan is capable of inducing cataracts in rats and there have been several reports indicating that this is a rare complication in humans.

Continued on next page

Product information on these pages is effective as of August 2004. Further information is available at: GlaxoSmithKline, PO Box 13398, Research Triangle Park, NC 27709. 1-888-825-5249. Corporate Web Site: www.gsk.com

Myleran—Cont.

Dermatologic: Hyperpigmentation is the most common adverse skin reaction and occurs in 5% to 10% of patients, particularly those with a dark complexion.

Metabolic: In a few cases, a clinical syndrome closely resembling adrenal insufficiency and characterized by weakness, severe fatigue, anorexia, weight loss, nausea and vomiting, and melanoderma has developed after prolonged busulfan therapy. The symptoms have sometimes been reversible when busulfan was withdrawn. Adrenal responsiveness to exogenously administered ACTH has usually been normal. However, pituitary function testing with metyrapone revealed a blunted urinary 17-hydroxycorticosteroid excretion in 2 patients. Following the discontinuation of busulfan (which was associated with clinical improvement), rechallenge with metyrapone revealed normal pituitary-adrenal function.

Hyperuricemia and/or hyperuricosuria are not uncommon in patients with chronic myelogenous leukemia. Additional rapid destruction of granulocytes may accompany the initiation of chemotherapy and increase the urate pool. Adverse effects can be minimized by increased hydration, urine alkalinization, and the prophylactic administration of a xanthine oxidase inhibitor such as allopurinol.

Hepatic Effects: Esophageal varices have been reported in patients receiving continuous busulfan and thioguanine therapy for treatment of chronic myelogenous leukemia (see PRECAUTIONS: Drug Interactions). Hepatic veno-occlusive disease has been observed in patients receiving busulfan (see WARNINGS).

Miscellaneous: Other reported adverse reactions include: urticaria, erythema multiforme, erythema nodosum, alopecia, porphyria cutanea tarda, excessive dryness and fragility of the skin with anhidrosis, dryness of the oral mucous membranes and cheilosis, gynecomastia, cholestatic jaundice, and myasthenia gravis. Most of these are single case reports, and in many, a clear cause-and-effect relationship with busulfan has not been demonstrated.

Seizures (see PRECAUTIONS: General) have been observed in patients receiving higher than recommended doses of busulfan.

Observed During Clinical Practice: The following events have been identified during post-approval use of busulfan. Because they are reported voluntarily from a population of unknown size, estimates of frequency cannot be made. These events have been chosen for inclusion due to a combination of their seriousness, frequency of reporting, or potential causal connection to busulfan.

Blood and Lymphatic: Aplastic anemia.

Eye: Cataracts, corneal thinning, lens changes.

Hepatobiliary Tract and Pancreas: Centrilobular sinusoidal fibrosis, hepatic veno- occlusive disease, hepatocellular atrophy, hepatocellular necrosis, hyperbilirubinemia (see WARNINGS).

Non-site Specific: Infection, mucositis, sepsis.

Respiratory: Pneumonia.

Skin: Rash. An increased local cutaneous reaction has been observed in patients receiving radiotherapy soon after busulfan.

OVERDOSAGE

There is no known antidote to busulfan. The principal toxic effects are bone marrow depression and pancytopenia. The hematologic status should be closely monitored and vigorous supportive measures instituted if necessary. Induction of vomiting or gastric lavage followed by administration of charcoal would be indicated if ingestion were recent. Dialysis may be considered in the management of overdose as there is 1 report of successful dialysis of busulfan (see CLINICAL PHARMACOLOGY).

Gastrointestinal toxicity with mucositis, nausea, vomiting, and diarrhea has been observed when MYLERAN was used in association with bone marrow transplantation.

Oral LD_{50} single doses in mice are 120 mg/kg. Two distinct types of toxic response are seen at median lethal doses given intraperitoneally. Within a matter of hours there are signs of stimulation of the central nervous system with convulsions and death on the first day. Mice are more sensitive to this effect than are rats. With doses at the LD_{50} there is also delayed death due to damage to the bone marrow. At 3 times the LD_{50}, atrophy of the mucosa of the large intestine is found after a week, whereas that of the small intestine is little affected. After doses in the order of 10 times those used therapeutically were added to the diet of rats, irreversible cataracts were produced after several weeks. Small doses had no such effect.

DOSAGE AND ADMINISTRATION

Busulfan is administered orally. The usual adult dose range for *remission induction* is 4 to 8 mg, total dose, daily. Dosing on a weight basis is the same for both pediatric patients and adults, approximately 60 mcg/kg of body weight or 1.8 mg/m^2 of body surface, daily. Since the rate of fall of the leukocyte count is dose related, daily doses exceeding 4 mg per day should be reserved for patients with the most compelling symptoms; the greater the total daily dose, the greater is the possibility of inducing bone marrow aplasia.

A decrease in the leukocyte count is not usually seen during the first 10 to 15 days of treatment; the leukocyte count may actually increase during this period and it should not be interpreted as resistance to the drug, nor should the dose be increased. Since the leukocyte count may continue to fall for more than 1 month after discontinuing the drug, it is important that busulfan be discontinued *prior* to the total leukocyte count falling into the normal range. When the total leukocyte count has declined to approximately 15,000/mcL, the drug should be withheld.

With a constant dose of busulfan, the total leukocyte count declines exponentially; a weekly plot of the leukocyte count on semi-logarithmic graph paper aids in predicting the time when therapy should be discontinued. With the recommended dose of busulfan, a normal leukocyte count is usually achieved in 12 to 20 weeks.

During remission, the patient is examined at monthly intervals and treatment resumed with the induction dosage when the total leukocyte count reaches approximately 50,000/mcL. When remission is shorter than 3 months, maintenance therapy of 1 to 3 mg daily may be advisable in order to keep the hematological status under control and prevent rapid relapse.

Procedures for proper handling and disposal of anticancer drugs should be considered. Several guidelines on this subject have been published.[1–8]

There is no general agreement that all of the procedures recommended in the guidelines are necessary or appropriate.

HOW SUPPLIED

MYLERAN is supplied as white, film-coated, round, biconvex tablets containing 2 mg busulfan in amber glass bottles with child-resistant closures. One side is imprinted with "GX EF3" and the other side is imprinted with an "M."

Bottle of 25 (NDC 0173-0713-25).

Store at 25°C (77°F); excursions permitted to 15° to 30°C (59° to 86°F) (see USP Controlled Room Temperature).

REFERENCES

1. ONS Clinical Practice Committee. Cancer Chemotherapy Guidelines and Recommendations for Practice. Pittsburgh, PA. Oncology Nursing Society; 1999:32-41.
2. Recommendations for the safe handling of parenteral antineoplastic drugs. Washington, DC: Division of Safety, Clinical Center Pharmacy Department and Cancer Nursing Services, National Institutes of Health and Human Services; 1992. US Dept of Health and Human Services, Public Health Service publication NIH 92-2621.
3. AMA Council on Scientific Affairs. Guidelines for handling parenteral antineoplastics. *JAMA.* 1985;253:1590-1591.
4. National Study Commission on Cytotoxic Exposure. Recommendations for handling cytotoxic agents. 1987. Available from Louis P. Jeffrey, Chairman, National Study Commission on Cytotoxic Exposure. Massachusetts College of Pharmacy and Allied Health Sciences, 179 Longwood Avenue, Boston, MA 02115.
5. Clinical Oncological Society of Australia. Guidelines and recommendations for safe handling of antineoplastic agents. *Med J Australia.* 1983;1:426-428.
6. Jones RB, Frank R, Mass T. Safe handling of chemotherapeutic agents: a report from the Mount Sinai Medical Center. *CA-A Cancer J for Clin.* 1983;33:258-263.
7. American Society of Hospital Pharmacists. ASHP technical assistance bulletin on handling cytotoxic and hazardous drugs. *Am J Hosp Pharm.* 1990;47:1033-1049.
8. Controlling Occupational Exposure to Hazardous Drugs. (OSHA Work-Practice Guidelines.) *Am J. Health-Syst Pharm.* 1996:53:1669-1685.

Manufactured by
Heumann Pharma GmbH
90537 Feucht, Germany
for GlaxoSmithKline
Research Triangle Park, NC 27709

January 2004 RL-2065

Shown in Product Identification Guide, page 316

NAVELBINE® ℞

[*na' vəl-bēn*]
(vinorelbine tartrate)
Injection

WARNING

NAVELBINE (vinorelbine tartrate) Injection should be administered under the supervision of a physician experienced in the use of cancer chemotherapeutic agents. This product is for intravenous (IV) use only. Intrathecal administration of other vinca alkaloids has resulted in death. Syringes containing this product should be labeled "WARNING – FOR IV USE ONLY. FATAL if given intrathecally."

Severe granulocytopenia resulting in increased susceptibility to infection may occur. Granulocyte counts should be ≥1,000 cells/mm^3 prior to the administration of NAVELBINE. The dosage should be adjusted according to complete blood counts with differentials obtained on the day of treatment.

Caution - It is extremely important that the intravenous needle or catheter be properly positioned before NAVELBINE is injected. Administration of NAVELBINE may result in extravasation causing local tissue necrosis and/or thrombophlebitis (see DOSAGE AND ADMINISTRATION: Administration Precautions).

DESCRIPTION

NAVELBINE (vinorelbine tartrate) Injection is for intravenous administration. Each vial contains vinorelbine tartrate equivalent to 10 mg (1-mL vial) or 50 mg (5-mL vial) vinorelbine in Water for Injection. No preservatives or other additives are present. The aqueous solution is sterile and nonpyrogenic.

Vinorelbine tartrate is a semi-synthetic vinca alkaloid with antitumor activity. The chemical name is 3′,4′-didehydro-4′-deoxy-*C*′-norvincaleukoblastine [*R*-(*R**,*R**)-2,3- dihydroxybutanedioate (1:2)(salt)].

Vinorelbine tartrate is a white to yellow or light brown amorphous powder with the molecular formula $C_{45}H_{54}N_4O_8{\cdot}2C_4H_6O_6$ and molecular weight of 1079.12. The aqueous solubility is >1,000 mg/mL in distilled water. The pH of NAVELBINE Injection is approximately 3.5.

CLINICAL PHARMACOLOGY

Vinorelbine is a vinca alkaloid that interferes with microtubule assembly. The vinca alkaloids are structurally similar compounds comprised of 2 multiringed units, vindoline and catharanthine. Unlike other vinca alkaloids, the catharanthine unit is the site of structural modification for vinorelbine. The antitumor activity of vinorelbine is thought to be due primarily to inhibition of mitosis at metaphase through its interaction with tubulin. Like other vinca alkaloids, vinorelbine may also interfere with: 1) amino acid, cyclic AMP, and glutathione metabolism, 2) calmodulin-dependent Ca^{++}-transport ATPase activity, 3) cellular respiration, and 4) nucleic acid and lipid biosynthesis. In intact tectal plates from mouse embryos, vinorelbine, vincristine, and vinblastine inhibited mitotic microtubule formation at the same concentration (2 µM), inducing a blockade of cells at metaphase. Vincristine produced depolymerization of axonal microtubules at 5 µM, but vinblastine and vinorelbine did not have this effect until concentrations of 30 µM and 40 µM, respectively. These data suggest relative selectivity of vinorelbine for mitotic microtubules.

Pharmacokinetics: The pharmacokinetics of vinorelbine were studied in 49 patients who received doses of 30 mg/m^2 in 4 clinical trials. Doses were administered by 15- to 20-minute constant-rate infusions. Following intravenous administration, vinorelbine concentration in plasma decays in a triphasic manner. The initial rapid decline primarily represents distribution of drug to peripheral compartments followed by metabolism and excretion of the drug during subsequent phases. The prolonged terminal phase is due to relatively slow efflux of vinorelbine from peripheral compartments. The terminal phase half-life averages 27.7 to 43.6 hours and the mean plasma clearance ranges from 0.97 to 1.26 L/hr/kg. Steady-state volume of distribution (V_{ss}) values range from 25.4 to 40.1 L/kg.

Vinorelbine demonstrated high binding to human platelets and lymphocytes. The free fraction was approximately 0.11 in pooled human plasma over a concentration range of 234 to 1,169 ng/mL. The binding to plasma constituents in cancer patients ranged from 79.6% to 91.2%. Vinorelbine binding was not altered in the presence of cisplatin, 5-fluorouracil, or doxorubicin.

Vinorelbine undergoes substantial hepatic elimination in humans, with large amounts recovered in feces after intravenous administration to humans. Two metabolites of vinorelbine have been identified in human blood, plasma, and urine; vinorelbine N-oxide and deacetylvinorelbine. Deacetylvinorelbine has been demonstrated to be the primary metabolite of vinorelbine in humans, and has been shown to possess antitumor activity similar to vinorelbine. Therapeutic doses of NAVELBINE (30 mg/m^2) yield very small, if any, quantifiable levels of either metabolite in blood or urine. The metabolism of vinca alkaloids has been shown to be mediated by hepatic cytochrome P450 isoenzymes in the CYP3A subfamily. This metabolic pathway may be impaired in patients with hepatic dysfunction or who are taking concomitant potent inhibitors of these isoenzymes (see PRECAUTIONS). The effects of renal or hepatic dysfunction on the disposition of vinorelbine have not been assessed, but based on experience with other anticancer vinca alkaloids, dose adjustments are recommended for patients with impaired hepatic function (see DOSAGE AND ADMINISTRATION).

The disposition of radiolabeled vinorelbine given intravenously was studied in a limited number of patients. Approximately 18% and 46% of the administered dose was recovered in the urine and in the feces, respectively. Incomplete recovery in humans is consistent with results in animals where recovery is incomplete, even after prolonged sampling times. A separate study of the urinary excretion of vinorelbine using specific chromatographic analytical methodology showed that 10.9% ± 0.7% of a 30-mg/m^2 intravenous dose was excreted unchanged in the urine.

The influence of age on the pharmacokinetics of vinorelbine was examined using data from 44 cancer patients (average age, 56.7 ± 7.8 years; range, 41 to 74 years; with 12 patients ≥60 years and 6 patients ≥65 years) in 3 studies. CL (the mean plasma clearance), $t_{1/2}$ (the terminal phase half-life), and V_Z (the volume of distribution during terminal phase) were independent of age. A separate pharmacokinetic study was conducted in 10 elderly patients with metastatic breast cancer (age range, 66 to 81 years; 3 patients >75 years; normal liver function tests) receiving vinorelbine 30 mg/m^2 intravenously. CL, V_{ss}, and $t_{1/2}$ were similar to those reported for younger adult patients in previous studies. No relationship between age, systemic exposure ($AUC_{0-\infty}$), and hematological toxicity was observed.

The pharmacokinetics of vinorelbine are not influenced by the concurrent administration of cisplatin with NAVELBINE (see PRECAUTIONS: Drug Interactions).

Clinical Trials: Data from 1 randomized clinical study (211 evaluable patients) with single-agent NAVELBINE and 2 randomized clinical trials (1,044 patients) using NAVELBINE combined with cisplatin support the use of NAVELBINE in patients with advanced nonsmall cell lung cancer (NSCLC).

Single-Agent NAVELBINE: Single-agent NAVELBINE was studied in a North American, randomized clinical trial in which patients with Stage IV NSCLC, no prior chemotherapy, and Karnofsky Performance Status ≥70 were treated with NAVELBINE (30 mg/m^2) weekly or 5-fluorouracil (5-FU) (425 mg/m^2 IV bolus) plus leucovorin (LV) (20 mg/m^2 IV bolus) daily for 5 days every 4 weeks. A total of 211 patients were randomized at a 2:1 ratio to NAVELBINE (143) or 5-FU/LV (68). NAVELBINE showed improved survival time compared to 5-FU/LV. In an intent-to-treat analysis, the median survival time was 30 weeks versus 22 weeks for patients receiving NAVELBINE versus 5-FU/LV, respectively ($P = 0.06$). The 1-year survival rates were 24% (±4% SE) for NAVELBINE and 16% (±5% SE) for the 5-FU/LV group, using the Kaplan-Meier product-limit estimates. The median survival time with 5-FU/LV was similar to or slightly better than that usually observed in untreated patients with advanced NSCLC, suggesting that the difference was not related to some unknown detrimental effect of 5-FU/LV therapy. The response rates (all partial responses) for NAVELBINE and 5-FU/LV were 12% and 3%, respectively.

NAVELBINE in Combination with Cisplatin: NAVELBINE plus Cisplatin versus Single-Agent Cisplatin: A Phase III open-label, randomized study was conducted which compared NAVELBINE (25 mg/m^2/week) plus cisplatin (100 mg/m^2 every 4 weeks) to single-agent cisplatin (100 mg/m^2 every 4 weeks) in patients with Stage IV or Stage IIIb NSCLC patients with malignant pleural effusion or multiple lesions in more than one lobe who were not previously treated with chemotherapy. Patients included in the study had a performance status of 0 or 1, and 34% had received prior surgery and/or radiotherapy. Characteristics of the 432 randomized patients are provided in Table 1. Two hundred and twelve patients received NAVELBINE plus cisplatin and 210 received single-agent cisplatin. The primary objective of this trial was to compare survival between the 2 treatment groups. Survival (Figure 1) for patients receiving NAVELBINE plus cisplatin was significantly better compared to the patients who received single-agent cisplatin. The results of this trial are summarized in Table 1.

NAVELBINE plus Cisplatin versus Vindesine plus Cisplatin versus Single-Agent NAVELBINE: In a large European clinical trial, 612 patients with Stage III or IV NSCLC, no prior chemotherapy, and WHO Performance Status of 0, 1, or 2 were randomized to treatment with single-agent NAVELBINE (30 mg/m^2/week), NAVELBINE (30 mg/m^2/week) plus cisplatin (120 mg/m^2 days 1 and 29, then every 6 weeks), and vindesine (3 mg/m^2/week for 7 weeks, then every other week) plus cisplatin (120 mg/m^2 days 1 and 29, then every 6 weeks). Patient characteristics are provided in Table 1. Survival was longer in patients treated with NAVELBINE plus cisplatin compared to those treated with vindesine plus cisplatin (Figure 2). Study results are summarized in Table 1.

Dose-Ranging Study: A dose-ranging study of NAVELBINE (20, 25, or 30 mg/m^2/week) plus cisplatin (120 mg/m^2 days 1 and 29, then every 6 weeks) in 32 patients with NSCLC demonstrated a median survival of 10.2 months. There were no responses at the lowest dose level; the response rate was 33% in the 21 patients treated at the 2 highest dose levels.

[See table 1 above]

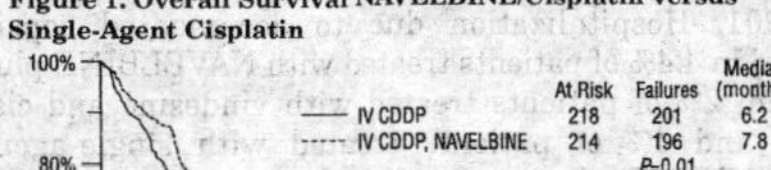

Figure 1. Overall Survival NAVELBINE/Cisplatin versus Single-Agent Cisplatin

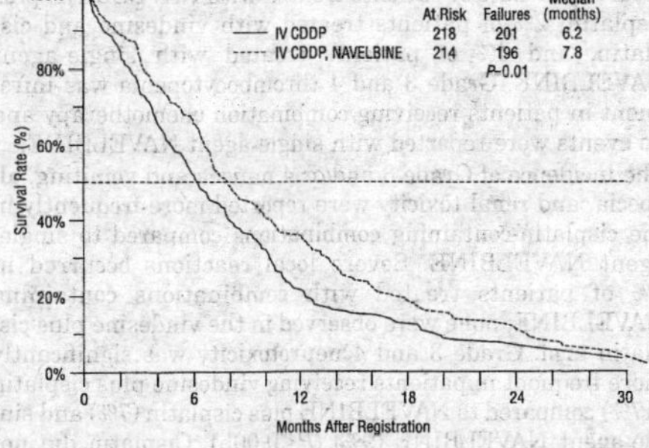

[See figure 2 at top of next column]

INDICATIONS AND USAGE

NAVELBINE is indicated as a single agent or in combination with cisplatin for the first-line treatment of ambulatory patients with unresectable, advanced nonsmall cell lung cancer (NSCLC). In patients with Stage IV NSCLC, NAVELBINE is indicated as a single agent or in combination with cisplatin. In Stage III NSCLC, NAVELBINE is indicated in combination with cisplatin.

Table 1. Randomized Clinical Trials of NAVELBINE in Combination with Cisplatin in NSCLC

	NAVELBINE/Cisplatin vs. Single-Agent Cisplatin		NAVELBINE/Cisplatin vs. Vindesine/Cisplatin vs. Single-Agent NAVELBINE		
	NAVELBINE/ Cisplatin	Cisplatin	NAVELBINE/ Cisplatin	Vindesine/ Cisplatin	NAVELBINE
Demographics					
Number of patients	214	218	206	200	206
Number of males	146	141	182	179	188
Number of females	68	77	24	21	18
Median age (years)	63	64	59	59	60
Range (years)	33-84	37-81	32-75	31-75	30-74
Stage of disease					
Stage IIIA	NA	NA	11%	11%	10%
Stage IIIB	8%	8%	28%	25%	32%
Stage IV	92%	92%	50%	55%	47%
Local recurrence	NA	NA	2%	3%	3%
Metastatic after surgery	NA	NA	9%	8%	9%
Histology					
Adenocarcinoma	54%	52%	32%	40%	28%
Squamous	19%	22%	56%	50%	56%
Large cell	14%	14%	13%	11%	16%
Unspecified	13%	13%	NA	NA	NA
Results					
Median survival (months)	7.8	6.2	9.2*†	7.4	7.2
P value	$P = 0.01$		*$P = 0.09$ vs. vindesine/cisplatin † = 0.05 vs. single-agent NAVELBINE		
12-Month survival rate	38%	22%	35%	27%	30%
Overall response	19%	8%	28%‡§	19%	14%
P value	$P < 0.001$		‡$P = 0.03$ vs. vindesine/cisplatin §$P<0.001$ vs. single-agent NAVELBINE		

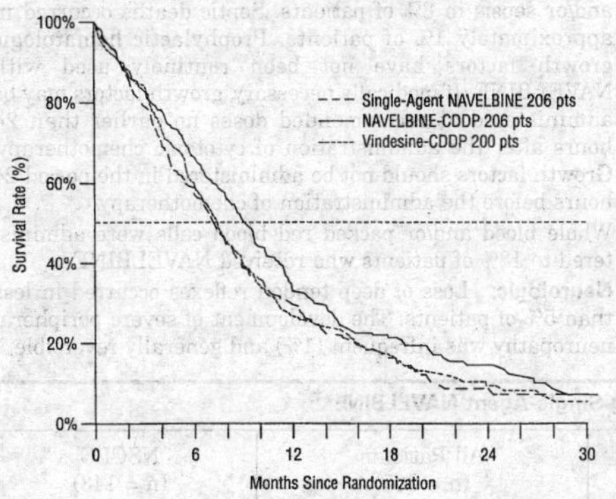

Figure 2. Overall Survival NAVELBINE/Cisplatin versus Vindesine/Cisplatin versus Single-Agent NAVELBINE

CONTRAINDICATIONS

Administration of NAVELBINE is contraindicated in patients with pretreatment granulocyte counts <1,000 cells/mm^3 (see WARNINGS).

WARNINGS

NAVELBINE should be administered in carefully adjusted doses by or under the supervision of a physician experienced in the use of cancer chemotherapeutic agents.

Patients treated with NAVELBINE should be frequently monitored for myelosuppression both during and after therapy. Granulocytopenia is dose-limiting. Granulocyte nadirs occur between 7 and 10 days after dosing with granulocyte count recovery usually within the following 7 to 14 days. Complete blood counts with differentials should be performed and results reviewed prior to administering each dose of NAVELBINE. NAVELBINE should not be administered to patients with granulocyte counts <1,000 cells/mm^3. Patients developing severe granulocytopenia should be monitored carefully for evidence of infection and/or fever. See DOSAGE AND ADMINISTRATION for recommended dose adjustments for granulocytopenia.

Acute shortness of breath and severe bronchospasm have been reported infrequently, following the administration of NAVELBINE and other vinca alkaloids, most commonly when the vinca alkaloid was used in combination with mitomycin. These adverse events may require treatment with supplemental oxygen, bronchodilators, and/or corticosteroids, particularly when there is pre-existing pulmonary dysfunction.

Reported cases of interstitial pulmonary changes and acute respiratory distress syndrome (ARDS), most of which were fatal, occurred in patients treated with single-agent NAVELBINE. The mean time to onset of these symptoms after vinorelbine administration was 1 week (range 3 to 8 days). Patients with alterations in their baseline pulmonary symptoms or with new onset of dyspnea, cough, hypoxia, or other symptoms should be evaluated promptly.

NAVELBINE has been reported to cause severe constipation (e.g., Grade 3-4), paralytic ileus, intestinal obstruction, necrosis, and/or perforation. Some events have been fatal.

Pregnancy: Pregnancy Category D. NAVELBINE may cause fetal harm if administered to a pregnant woman. A single dose of vinorelbine has been shown to be embryo- and/or fetotoxic in mice and rabbits at doses of 9 mg/m^2 and 5.5 mg/m^2, respectively (one third and one sixth the human dose). At nonmaternotoxic doses, fetal weight was reduced and ossification was delayed. There are no studies in pregnant women. If NAVELBINE is used during pregnancy, or if the patient becomes pregnant while receiving this drug, the patient should be apprised of the potential hazard to the fetus. Women of childbearing potential should be advised to avoid becoming pregnant during therapy with NAVELBINE.

PRECAUTIONS

General: Most drug-related adverse events of NAVELBINE are reversible. If severe adverse events occur, NAVELBINE should be reduced in dosage or discontinued and appropriate corrective measures taken. Reinstitution of therapy with NAVELBINE should be carried out with caution and alertness as to possible recurrence of toxicity.

NAVELBINE should be used with extreme caution in patients whose bone marrow reserve may have been compromised by prior irradiation or chemotherapy, or whose marrow function is recovering from the effects of previous chemotherapy (see DOSAGE AND ADMINISTRATION).

Administration of NAVELBINE to patients with prior radiation therapy may result in radiation recall reactions (see ADVERSE REACTIONS and Drug Interactions).

Patients with a prior history or pre-existing neuropathy, regardless of etiology, should be monitored for new or worsening signs and symptoms of neuropathy while receiving NAVELBINE.

Care must be taken to avoid contamination of the eye with concentrations of NAVELBINE used clinically. Severe irritation of the eye has been reported with accidental exposure to another vinca alkaloid. If exposure occurs, the eye should immediately be thoroughly flushed with water.

Information for Patients: Patients should be informed that the major acute toxicities of NAVELBINE are related to bone marrow toxicity, specifically granulocytopenia with increased susceptibility to infection. They should be advised to report fever or chills immediately. Women of childbearing potential should be advised to avoid becoming pregnant during treatment. Patients should be advised to contact their physician if they experience increased shortness of breath, cough, or other new pulmonary symptoms, or if they experience symptoms of abdominal pain or constipation.

Laboratory Tests: Since dose-limiting clinical toxicity is the result of depression of the white blood cell count, it is

Continued on next page

Product information on these pages is effective as of August 2004. Further information is available at: GlaxoSmithKline, PO Box 13398, Research Triangle Park, NC 27709. 1-888-825-5249. Corporate Web Site: www.gsk.com

Navelbine—Cont.

imperative that complete blood counts with differentials be obtained and reviewed on the day of treatment prior to each dose of NAVELBINE (see ADVERSE REACTIONS: Hematologic).

Hepatic: There is no evidence that the toxicity of NAVELBINE is enhanced in patients with elevated liver enzymes. No data are available for patients with severe baseline cholestasis, but the liver plays an important role in the metabolism of NAVELBINE. Because clinical experience in patients with severe liver disease is limited, caution should be exercised when administering NAVELBINE to patients with severe hepatic injury or impairment (see DOSAGE AND ADMINISTRATION).

Drug Interactions: Acute pulmonary reactions have been reported with NAVELBINE and other anticancer vinca alkaloids used in conjunction with mitomycin. Although the pharmacokinetics of vinorelbine are not influenced by the concurrent administration of cisplatin, the incidence of granulocytopenia with NAVELBINE used in combination with cisplatin is significantly higher than with single-agent NAVELBINE. Patients who receive NAVELBINE and paclitaxel, either concomitantly or sequentially, should be monitored for signs and symptoms of neuropathy. Administration of NAVELBINE to patients with prior or concomitant radiation therapy may result in radiosensitizing effects.

Caution should be exercised in patients concurrently taking drugs known to inhibit drug metabolism by hepatic cytochrome P450 isoenzymes in the CYP3A subfamily, or in patients with hepatic dysfunction. Concurrent administration of vinorelbine tartrate with an inhibitor of this metabolic pathway may cause an earlier onset and/or an increased severity of side effects.

Carcinogenesis, Mutagenesis, Impairment of Fertility: The carcinogenic potential of NAVELBINE has not been studied. Vinorelbine has been shown to affect chromosome number and possibly structure in vivo (polyploidy in bone marrow cells from Chinese hamsters and a positive micronucleus test in mice). It was not mutagenic in the Ames test and gave inconclusive results in the mouse lymphoma TK Locus assay. The significance of these or other short-term test results for human risk is unknown. Vinorelbine did not affect fertility to a statistically significant extent when administered to rats on either a once-weekly (9 mg/m^2, approximately one third the human dose) or alternate-day schedule (4.2 mg/m^2, approximately one seventh the human dose) prior to and during mating. However, biweekly administration for 13 or 26 weeks in the rat at 2.1 and 7.2 mg/m^2 (approximately one fifteenth and one fourth the human dose) resulted in decreased spermatogenesis and prostate/seminal vesicle secretion.

Pregnancy: Pregnancy Category D. See WARNINGS section.

Nursing Mothers: It is not known whether the drug is excreted in human milk. Because many drugs are excreted in human milk and because of the potential for serious adverse reactions in nursing infants from NAVELBINE, it is recommended that nursing be discontinued in women who are receiving therapy with NAVELBINE.

Pediatric Use: Safety and effectiveness of NAVELBINE in pediatric patients have not been established. Data from a single-arm study in 46 patients with recurrent solid malignant tumors, including rhabdomyosarcoma/undifferentiated sarcoma, neuroblastoma, and CNS tumors, at doses similar to those used in adults, showed no meaningful clinical activity. Toxicities were similar to those reported in adults.

Geriatric Use: Of the total number of patients in North American clinical studies of IV NAVELBINE, approximately one third were 65 years of age or greater. No overall differences in effectiveness or safety were observed between these patients and younger adult patients. Other reported clinical experience has not identified differences in responses between the elderly and younger adult patients, but greater sensitivity of some older individuals cannot be ruled out.

The pharmacokinetics of vinorelbine in elderly and younger adult patients are similar (see CLINICAL PHARMACOLOGY).

ADVERSE REACTIONS

The pattern of adverse reactions is similar whether NAVELBINE is used as a single agent or in combination. Adverse reactions from studies with single-agent and combination use of NAVELBINE are summarized in Tables 2-4.

Single-Agent NAVELBINE: Data in the following table are based on the experience of 365 patients (143 patients with NSCLC; 222 patients with advanced breast cancer) treated with IV NAVELBINE as a single agent in 3 clinical studies. The dosing schedule in each study was 30 mg/m^2 NAVELBINE on a weekly basis.

[See table 2 below]

Hematologic: Granulocytopenia is the major dose-limiting toxicity with NAVELBINE. Dose adjustments are required for hematologic toxicity and hepatic insufficiency (see DOSAGE AND ADMINISTRATION). Granulocytopenia was generally reversible and not cumulative over time. Granulocyte nadirs occurred 7 to 10 days after the dose, with granulocyte recovery usually within the following 7 to 14 days. Granulocytopenia resulted in hospitalizations for fever and/or sepsis in 8% of patients. Septic deaths occurred in approximately 1% of patients. Prophylactic hematologic growth factors have not been routinely used with NAVELBINE. If medically necessary, growth factors may be administered at recommended doses no earlier than 24 hours after the administration of cytotoxic chemotherapy. Growth factors should not be administered in the period 24 hours before the administration of chemotherapy.

Whole blood and/or packed red blood cells were administered to 18% of patients who received NAVELBINE.

Neurologic: Loss of deep tendon reflexes occurred in less than 5% of patients. The development of severe peripheral neuropathy was infrequent (1%) and generally reversible.

Table 2. Summary of Adverse Events in 365 Patients Receiving Single-Agent NAVELBINE*†

Adverse Event		All Patients (n = 365)	NSCLC (n = 143)
Bone Marrow			
Granulocytopenia	<2,000 cells/mm^3	90%	80%
	<500 cells/mm^3	36%	29%
Leukopenia	<4,000 cells/mm^3	92%	81%
	<1,000 cells/mm^3	15%	12%
Thrombocytopenia	<100,000 cells/mm^3	5%	4%
	<50,000 cells/mm^3	1%	1%
Anemia	<11 g/dL	83%	77%
	<8 g/dL	9%	1%
Hospitalizations due to granulocytopenic complications		9%	8%

Adverse Event	All Grades All Patients	All Grades NSCLC	Grade 3 All Patients	Grade 3 NSCLC	Grade 4 All Patients	Grade 4 NSCLC
Clinical Chemistry Elevations						
Total Bilirubin (n = 351)	13%	9%	4%	3%	3%	2%
SGOT (n = 346)	67%	54%	5%	2%	1%	1%
General						
Asthenia	36%	27%	7%	5%	0%	0%
Injection Site Reactions	28%	38%	2%	5%	0%	0%
Injection Site Pain	16%	13%	2%	1%	0%	0%
Phlebitis	7%	10%	<1%	1%	0%	0%
Digestive						
Nausea	44%	34%	2%	1%	0%	0%
Vomiting	20%	15%	2%	1%	0%	0%
Constipation	35%	29%	3%	2%	0%	0%
Diarrhea	17%	13%	1%	1%	0%	0%
Peripheral Neuropathy‡	25%	20%	1%	1%	<1%	0%
Dyspnea	7%	3%	2%	2%	1%	0%
Alopecia	12%	12%	≤1%	1%	0%	0%

* None of the reported toxicities were influenced by age. Grade based on modified criteria from the National Cancer Institute.

† Patients with NSCLC had not received prior chemotherapy. The majority of the remaining patients had received prior chemotherapy.

‡ Incidence of paresthesia plus hypesthesia.

Skin: Like other anticancer vinca alkaloids, NAVELBINE is a moderate vesicant. Injection site reactions, including erythema, pain at injection site, and vein discoloration, occurred in approximately one third of patients; 5% were severe. Chemical phlebitis along the vein proximal to the site of injection was reported in 10% of patients.

Gastrointestinal: Prophylactic administration of antiemetics was not routine in patients treated with single-agent NAVELBINE. Due to the low incidence of severe nausea and vomiting with single-agent NAVELBINE, the use of serotonin antagonists is generally not required.

Hepatic: Transient elevations of liver enzymes were reported without clinical symptoms.

Cardiovascular: Chest pain was reported in 5% of patients. Most reports of chest pain were in patients who had either a history of cardiovascular disease or tumor within the chest. There have been rare reports of myocardial infarction.

Pulmonary: Shortness of breath was reported in 3% of patients; it was severe in 2% (see WARNINGS). Interstitial pulmonary changes were documented.

Other: Fatigue occurred in 27% of patients. It was usually mild or moderate but tended to increase with cumulative dosing.

Other toxicities that have been reported in less than 5% of patients include jaw pain, myalgia, arthralgia, and rash. Hemorrhagic cystitis and the syndrome of inappropriate ADH secretion were each reported in <1% of patients.

Combination Use: Adverse events for combination use are summarized in Tables 3 and 4.

NAVELBINE in Combination with Cisplatin:

NAVELBINE plus Cisplatin versus Single-Agent Cisplatin (Table 3): Myelosuppression was the predominant toxicity in patients receiving combination therapy, Grade 3 and 4 granulocytopenia of 82% compared to 5% in the single-agent cisplatin arm. Fever and/or sepsis related to granulocytopenia occurred in 11% of patients on NAVELBINE and cisplatin compared to 0% on the cisplatin arm.

Four patients on the combination died of granulocytopenia-related sepsis. During this study, the use of granulocyte colony-stimulating factor ([G-CSF] filgrastim) was permitted, but not mandated, after the first course of treatment for patients who experienced Grade 3 or 4 granulocytopenia (≤1,000 cells/mm^3) or in those who developed neutropenic fever between cycles of chemotherapy. Beginning 24 hours after completion of chemotherapy, G-CSF was started at a dose of 5 mcg/kg/day and continued until the total granulocyte count was >1,000 cells/mm^3 on 2 successive determinations. G-CSF was not administered on the day of treatment.

Grade 3 and 4 anemia occurred more frequently in the combination arm compared to control, 24% vs. 8%, respectively. Thrombocytopenia occurred in 6% of patients treated with NAVELBINE plus cisplatin compared to 2% of patients treated with cisplatin.

The incidence of severe non-hematologic toxicity was similar among the patients in both treatment groups. Patients receiving NAVELBINE plus cisplatin compared to single-agent cisplatin experienced more Grade 3 and/or 4 peripheral numbness (2% vs. <1%), phlebitis/thrombosis/embolism (3% vs. <1%), and infection (6% vs. <1%). Grade 3-4 constipation and/or ileus occurred in 3% of patients treated with combination therapy and in 1% of patients treated with cisplatin.

Seven deaths were reported on the combination arm; 2 were related to cardiac ischemia, 1 massive cerebrovascular accident, 1 multisystem failure due to an overdose of NAVELBINE, and 3 from febrile neutropenia. One death, secondary to respiratory infection unrelated to granulocytopenia, occurred with single-agent cisplatin.

NAVELBINE plus Cisplatin versus Vindesine plus Cisplatin versus Single-Agent NAVELBINE (Table 4): Myelosuppression, specifically Grade 3 and 4 granulocytopenia, was significantly greater with the combination of NAVELBINE plus cisplatin (79%) than with either single-agent NAVELBINE (53%) or vindesine plus cisplatin (48%), $P<0.0001$. Hospitalization due to documented sepsis occurred in 4.4% of patients treated with NAVELBINE plus cisplatin, 2% of patients treated with vindesine and cisplatin, and 4% of patients treated with single-agent NAVELBINE. Grade 3 and 4 thrombocytopenia was infrequent in patients receiving combination chemotherapy and no events were reported with single-agent NAVELBINE.

The incidence of Grade 3 and/or 4 nausea and vomiting, alopecia, and renal toxicity were reported more frequently in the cisplatin-containing combinations compared to single-agent NAVELBINE. Severe local reactions occurred in 2% of patients treated with combinations containing NAVELBINE; none were observed in the vindesine plus cisplatin arm. Grade 3 and 4 neurotoxicity was significantly more frequent in patients receiving vindesine plus cisplatin (17%) compared to NAVELBINE plus cisplatin (7%) and single-agent NAVELBINE (9%) ($P<0.005$). Cisplatin did not appear to increase the incidence of neurotoxicity observed with single-agent NAVELBINE.

[See table 3 on next page]

[See table 4 at bottom of next page]

Observed During Clinical Practice: In addition to the adverse events reported from clinical trials, the following events have been identified during post-approval use of NAVELBINE. Because they are reported voluntarily from a population of unknown size, estimates of frequency cannot be made. These events have been chosen for inclusion due to a combination of their seriousness, frequency of reporting, or potential causal connection to NAVELBINE.

Body as a Whole: Systemic allergic reactions reported as anaphylaxis, pruritus, urticaria, and angioedema; flushing; and radiation recall events such as dermatitis and esophagitis (see PRECAUTIONS) have been reported.

Hematologic: Thromboembolic events, including pulmonary embolus and deep venous thrombosis, have been reported primarily in seriously ill and debilitated patients with known predisposing risk factors for these events.

Neurologic: Peripheral neurotoxicities such as, but not limited to, muscle weakness and disturbance of gait, have been observed in patients with and without prior symptoms. There may be increased potential for neurotoxicity in patients with pre-existing neuropathy, regardless of etiology, who receive NAVELBINE. Vestibular and auditory deficits have been observed with NAVELBINE, usually when used in combination with cisplatin.

Skin: Injection site reactions, including localized rash and urticaria, blister formation, and skin sloughing have been observed in clinical practice. Some of these reactions may be delayed in appearance.

Gastrointestinal: Dysphagia, mucositis, and pancreatitis have been reported.

Cardiovascular: Hypertension, hypotension, vasodilation, tachycardia, and pulmonary edema have been reported.

Pulmonary: Pneumonia has been reported.

Musculoskeletal: Headache has been reported, with and without other musculoskeletal aches and pains.

Other: Pain in tumor-containing tissue, back pain, and abdominal pain have been reported. Electrolyte abnormalities, including hyponatremia with or without the syndrome of inappropriate ADH secretion, have been reported in seriously ill and debilitated patients.

Combination Use: Patients with prior exposure to paclitaxel and who have demonstrated neuropathy should be monitored closely for new or worsening neuropathy. Patients who have experienced neuropathy with previous drug regimens should be monitored for symptoms of neuropathy while receiving NAVELBINE. NAVELBINE may result in radiosensitizing effects with prior or concomitant radiation therapy (see PRECAUTIONS).

OVERDOSAGE

There is no known antidote for overdoses of NAVELBINE. Overdoses involving quantities up to 10 times the recommended dose (30 mg/m^2) have been reported. The toxicities described were consistent with those listed in the ADVERSE REACTIONS section including paralytic ileus, stomatitis, and esophagitis. Bone marrow aplasia, sepsis, and paresis have also been reported. Fatalities have occurred following overdose of NAVELBINE. If overdosage occurs, general supportive measures together with appropriate blood transfusions, growth factors, and antibiotics should be instituted as deemed necessary by the physician.

DOSAGE AND ADMINISTRATION

Single-Agent NAVELBINE: The usual initial dose of single-agent NAVELBINE is 30 mg/m^2 administered weekly. The recommended method of administration is an intravenous injection over 6 to 10 minutes. In controlled trials, single-agent NAVELBINE was given weekly until progression or dose-limiting toxicity.

NAVELBINE in Combination with Cisplatin: NAVELBINE may be administered weekly at a dose of 25 mg/m^2 in combination with cisplatin given every 4 weeks at a dose of 100 mg/m^2.

Blood counts should be checked weekly to determine whether dose reductions of NAVELBINE and/or cisplatin are necessary. In the SWOG study, most patients required a 50% dose reduction of NAVELBINE at day 15 of each cycle and a 50% dose reduction of cisplatin by cycle 3.

NAVELBINE may also be administered weekly at a dose of 30 mg/m^2 in combination with cisplatin, given on days 1 and 29, then every 6 weeks at a dose of 120 mg/m^2.

Dose Modifications for NAVELBINE: The dosage should be adjusted according to hematologic toxicity or hepatic insufficiency, whichever results in the lower dose for the corresponding starting dose of NAVELBINE (see Table 5).

Dose Modifications for Hematologic Toxicity: Granulocyte counts should be ≥1,000 cells/mm^3 prior to the administration of NAVELBINE. Adjustments in the dosage of NAVELBINE should be based on granulocyte counts obtained on the day of treatment according to Table 5.

Table 5. Dose Adjustments Based on Granulocyte Counts

Granulocytes on Day of Treatment (cells/mm^3)	Percentage of Starting Dose of NAVELBINE
≥1,500	100%
1,000 to 1,499	50%
<1,000	Do not administer. Repeat granulocyte count in 1 week. If 3 consecutive weekly doses are held because granulocyte count is <1,000 cells/mm^3, discontinue NAVELBINE.
Note: For patients who, during treatment with NAVELBINE, experienced fever and/or sepsis while granulocytopenic or had 2 consecutive weekly doses held due to granulocytopenia, subsequent doses of NAVELBINE should be:	
≥1,500	75%
1,000 to 1,499	37.5%
<1,000	See above

Dose Modifications for Hepatic Insufficiency: NAVELBINE should be administered with caution to patients with hepatic insufficiency. In patients who develop hyperbilirubinemia during treatment with NAVELBINE, the dose should be adjusted for total bilirubin according to Table 6.

Table 6. Dose Modification Based on Total Bilirubin

Total Bilirubin (mg/dL)	Percentage of Starting Dose of NAVELBINE
≤2.0	100%
2.1 to 3.0	50%
>3.0	25%

Dose Modifications for Concurrent Hematologic Toxicity and Hepatic Insufficiency: In patients with both hematologic toxicity and hepatic insufficiency, the lower of the doses based on the corresponding starting dose of NAVELBINE determined from Table 5 and Table 6 should be administered.

Dose Modifications for Renal Insufficiency: No dose adjustments for NAVELBINE are required for renal insufficiency. Appropriate dose reductions for cisplatin should be made when NAVELBINE is used in combination.

Dose Modifications for Neurotoxicity: If Grade ≥2 neurotoxicity develops, NAVELBINE should be discontinued.

Administration Precautions: Caution - NAVELBINE must be administered intravenously. It is extremely important that the intravenous needle or catheter be properly positioned before any NAVELBINE is injected. Leakage into surrounding tissue during intravenous administration of NAVELBINE may cause considerable irritation, local tissue necrosis, and/or thrombophlebitis. If extravasation occurs, the injection should be discontinued immediately, and any remaining portion of the dose should then be introduced into another vein. Since there are no established guidelines for the treatment of extravasation injuries with

Continued on next page

Table 3. Selected Adverse Events From a Comparative Trial of NAVELBINE plus Cisplatin versus Single-Agent Cisplatin*

	NAVELBINE 25 mg/m^2 plus Cisplatin 100 mg/m^2 (n = 212)			Cisplatin 100 mg/m^2 (n = 210)		
Adverse Event	All Grades	Grade 3	Grade 4	All Grades	Grade 3	Grade 4
Bone Marrow						
Granulocytopenia	89%	22%	60%	26%	4%	1%
Anemia	88%	21%	3%	72%	7%	<1%
Leukopenia	88%	39%	19%	31%	<1%	0%
Thrombocytopenia	29%	4%	1%	21%	1%	<1%
Febrile neutropenia	N/A	N/A	11%	N/A	N/A	0%
Hepatic						
Elevated transaminase	1%	0%	0%	<1%	<1%	0%
Renal						
Elevated creatinine	37%	2%	2%	28%	4%	<1%
Non-Laboratory						
Malaise/fatigue/lethargy	67%	12%	0%	49%	8%	0%
Vomiting	60%	7%	6%	60%	10%	4%
Nausea	58%	14%	0%	57%	12%	0%
Anorexia	46%	0%	0%	37%	0%	0%
Constipation	35%	3%	0%	16%	1%	0%
Alopecia	34%	0%	0%	14%	0%	0%
Weight loss	34%	1%	0%	21%	<1%	0%
Fever without infection	20%	2%	0%	4%	0%	0%
Hearing	18%	4%	0%	18%	3%	<1%
Local (injection site reactions)	17%	<1%	0%	1%	0%	0%
Diarrhea	17%	2%	<1%	11%	1%	<1%
Paresthesias	17%	<1%	0%	10%	<1%	0%
Taste alterations	17%	0%	0%	15%	0%	0%
Peripheral numbness	11%	2%	0%	7%	<1%	0%
Myalgia/arthralgia	12%	<1%	0%	3%	<1%	0%
Phlebitis/thrombosis/embolism	10%	3%	0%	<1%	0%	<1%
Weakness	12%	2%	<1%	7%	2%	0%
Dizziness/vertigo	9%	<1%	0%	3%	<1%	0%
Infection	11%	5%	<1%	<1%	<1%	0%
Respiratory infection	10%	4%	<1%	3%	3%	0%

*Graded according to the standard SWOG criteria.

Table 4. Selected Adverse Events From a Comparative Trial of NAVELBINE Plus Cisplatin versus Vindesine Plus Cisplatin versus Single-Agent NAVELBINE*

	NAVELBINE/Cisplatin[†]			Vindesine/Cisplatin[‡]			NAVELBINE[§]		
Adverse Event	All Grades	Grade 3	Grade 4	All Grades	Grade 3	Grade 4	All Grades	Grade 3	Grade 4
Bone Marrow									
Neutropenia	95%	20%	58%	79%	26%	22%	85%	25%	28%
Leukopenia	94%	40%	17%	82%	24%	3%	83%	26%	6%
Thrombocytopenia	15%	3%	1%	10%	3%	0.5%	3%	0%	0%
Febrile neutropenia	N/A	N/A	4%	N/A	N/A	2%	N/A	N/A	4%
Hepatic									
Elevated bilirubin[‖]	6%	N/A	N/A	5%	N/A	N/A	5%	N/A	N/A
Renal									
Elevated creatinine[‖]	46%	N/A	N/A	37%	N/A	N/A	13%	N/A	N/A
Non-Laboratory									
Nausea/vomiting	74%	27%	3%	72%	24%	1%	31%	1%	1%
Alopecia	51%	7%	0.5%	56%	14%	0%	30%	2%	0%
Ototoxicity	10%	1%	1%	14%	1%	0%	1%	0%	0%
Local reactions	17%	2%	0.5%	7%	0%	0%	22%	2%	0%
Diarrhea	25%	1.5%	0%	24%	1%	0%	12%	0%	0.5%
Neurotoxicity[¶]	44%	7%	0%	58%	16%	1%	44%	8%	0.5%

*Grade based on criteria from the World Health Organization (WHO).

[†] n = 194 to 207; all patients receiving NAVELBINE/cisplatin with laboratory and non-laboratory data.

[‡] n = 173 to 192; all patients receiving vindesine/cisplatin with laboratory and non-laboratory data.

[§] n = 165 to 201; all patients receiving NAVELBINE with laboratory and non-laboratory data.

[‖] Categorical toxicity grade not specified.

[¶] Neurotoxicity includes peripheral neuropathy and constipation.

Product information on these pages is effective as of August 2004. Further information is available at: GlaxoSmithKline, PO Box 13398, Research Triangle Park, NC 27709. 1-888-825-5249. Corporate Web Site: www.gsk.com

Navelbine—Cont.

NAVELBINE, institutional guidelines may be used. The *ONS Chemotherapy Guidelines* provide additional recommendations for the prevention of extravasation injuries.[1]

As with other toxic compounds, caution should be exercised in handling and preparing the solution of NAVELBINE. Skin reactions may occur with accidental exposure. The use of gloves is recommended. If the solution of NAVELBINE contacts the skin or mucosa, immediately wash the skin or mucosa thoroughly with soap and water. Severe irritation of the eye has been reported with accidental contamination of the eye with another vinca alkaloid. If this happens with NAVELBINE, the eye should be flushed with water immediately and thoroughly.

Procedures for proper handling and disposal of anticancer drugs should be used. Several guidelines on this subject have been published.[2–8] There is no general agreement that all of the procedures recommended in the guidelines are necessary or appropriate.

NAVELBINE Injection is a clear, colorless to pale yellow solution. Parenteral drug products should be visually inspected for particulate matter and discoloration prior to administration whenever solution and container permit. If particulate matter is seen, NAVELBINE should not be administered.

Preparation for Administration: NAVELBINE Injection must be diluted in either a syringe or IV bag using one of the recommended solutions. The diluted NAVELBINE should be administered over 6 to 10 minutes into the side port of a free-flowing IV **closest to the IV bag** followed by flushing with at least 75 to 125 mL of one of the solutions. Diluted NAVELBINE may be used for up to 24 hours under normal room light when stored in polypropylene syringes or polyvinyl chloride bags at 5° to 30°C (41° to 86°F).

Syringe: The calculated dose of NAVELBINE should be diluted to a concentration between 1.5 and 3.0 mg/mL. The following solutions may be used for dilution:

5% Dextrose Injection, USP
0.9% Sodium Chloride Injection, USP

IV Bag: The calculated dose of NAVELBINE should be diluted to a concentration between 0.5 and 2 mg/mL. The following solutions may be used for dilution:

5% Dextrose Injection, USP
0.9% Sodium Chloride Injection, USP
0.45% Sodium Chloride Injection, USP
5% Dextrose and 0.45% Sodium Chloride Injection, USP
Ringer's Injection, USP
Lactated Ringer's Injection, USP

Stability: Unopened vials of NAVELBINE are stable until the date indicated on the package when stored under refrigeration at 2° to 8°C (36° to 46°F) and protected from light in the carton. Unopened vials of NAVELBINE are stable at temperatures up to 25°C (77°F) for up to 72 hours. This product should not be frozen.

HOW SUPPLIED

NAVELBINE Injection is a clear, colorless to pale yellow solution in Water for Injection, containing 10 mg vinorelbine per mL. NAVELBINE Injection is available in single-use, clear glass vials with elastomeric stoppers and royal blue caps, individually packaged in a carton in the following vial sizes:

10 mg/1 mL Single-Use Vial, Carton of 1 (NDC 0173-0656-01).
50 mg/5 mL Single-Use Vial, Carton of 1 (NDC 0173-0656-44).

Store the vials under refrigeration at 2° to 8°C (36° to 46°F) in the carton. Protect from light. DO NOT FREEZE.

REFERENCES

1. ONS Clinical Practice Committee. Cancer Chemotherapy Guidelines and Recommendations for Practice. Pittsburgh, Pa: Oncology Nursing Society; 1999:32–41.
2. Recommendations for the safe handling of parenteral antineoplastic drugs. Washington, DC: Division of Safety, National Institutes of Health; 1983. US Dept of Health and Human Services, Public Health Service publication NIH 83–2621.
3. AMA Council on Scientific Affairs. Guidelines for handling parenteral antineoplastics. *JAMA*. 1985;253:1590–1591.
4. National Study Commission on Cytotoxic Exposure. Recommendations for handling cytotoxic agents. 1987. Available from Louis P. Jeffrey, Chairman, National Study Commission on Cytotoxic Exposure. Massachusetts College of Pharmacy and Allied Health Sciences, 179 Longwood Avenue, Boston, MA 02115.
5. Clinical Oncological Society of Australia. Guidelines and recommendations for safe handling of antineoplastic agents. *Med J Australia*. 1983;1:426–428.
6. Jones RB, Frank R, Mass T. Safe handling of chemotherapeutic agents: a report from the Mount Sinai Medical Center. *CA-A Cancer J for Clin*. 1983;33:258–263.
7. American Society of Hospital Pharmacists. ASHP technical assistance bulletin on handling cytotoxic and hazardous drugs. *Am J Hosp Pharm*. 1990;47:1033–1049.
8. Controlling Occupational Exposure to Hazardous Drugs. (OSHA Work-Practice Guidelines.) *Am J Health-Syst Pharm*. 1996;53:1669–1685.

Manufactured by Pierre Fabre Médicament Production
64320 Idron, FRANCE
for GlaxoSmithKline, Research Triangle Park, NC 27709
Under license of Pierre Fabre Médicament –
Centre National de la Recherche Scientifique-France

November 2002/RL-1157

Shown in Product Identification Guide, page 316

OXISTAT® ℞
[*äx 'ē-stát*]
(oxiconazole nitrate cream)
Cream, 1%*

OXISTAT® ℞
(oxiconazole nitrate lotion)
Lotion, 1%*
***Potency expressed as oxiconazole**
FOR TOPICAL DERMATOLOGIC USE ONLY—
NOT FOR OPHTHALMIC OR INTRAVAGINAL USE

DESCRIPTION

OXISTAT Cream and Lotion formulations contain the antifungal active compound oxiconazole nitrate. Both formulations are for topical dermatologic use only.

Chemically, oxiconazole nitrate is 2',4'-dichloro-2-imidazol-1-ylacetophenone (*Z*)-[*0*-(2,4-dichlorobenzyl)oxime], mononitrate. The compound has the empirical formula $C_{18}H_{13}ON_3Cl_4$•HNO_3, a molecular weight of 492.15.

Oxiconazole nitrate is a nearly white crystalline powder, soluble in methanol; sparingly soluble in ethanol, chloroform, and acetone; and very slightly soluble in water.

OXISTAT Cream contains 10 mg of oxiconazole per gram of cream in a white to off-white, opaque cream base of purified water USP, white petrolatum USP, stearyl alcohol NF, propylene glycol USP, polysorbate 60 NF, cetyl alcohol NF, and benzoic acid USP 0.2% as a preservative.

OXISTAT Lotion contains 10 mg of oxiconazole per gram of lotion in a white to off-white, opaque lotion base of purified water USP, white petrolatum USP, stearyl alcohol NF, propylene glycol USP, polysorbate 60 NF, cetyl alcohol NF, and benzoic acid USP 0.2% as a preservative.

CLINICAL PHARMACOLOGY

Pharmacokinetics: The penetration of oxiconazole nitrate into different layers of the skin was assessed using an in vitro permeation technique with human skin. Five hours after application of 2.5 mg/cm² of oxiconazole nitrate cream onto human skin, the concentration of oxiconazole nitrate was demonstrated to be 16.2 µmol in the epidermis, 3.64 µmol in the upper corium, and 1.29 µmol in the deeper corium. Systemic absorption of oxiconazole nitrate is low. Using radiolabeled drug, less than 0.3% of the applied dose of oxiconazole nitrate was recovered in the urine of volunteer subjects up to 5 days after application of the cream formulation.

Neither in vitro nor in vivo studies have been conducted to establish relative activity between the lotion and cream formulations.

Microbiology: Oxiconazole nitrate is an imidazole derivative whose antifungal activity is derived primarily from the inhibition of ergosterol biosynthesis, which is critical for cellular membrane integrity. It has in vitro activity against a wide range of pathogenic fungi.

Oxiconazole has been shown to be active against most strains of the following organisms both in vitro and in clinical infections at indicated body sites (see INDICATIONS AND USAGE):

Epidermophyton floccosum
Trichophyton mentagrophytes
Trichophyton rubrum
Malassezia furfur

The following in vitro data are available; **however, their clinical significance is unknown.** Oxiconazole exhibits satisfactory in vitro minimum inhibitory concentrations (MICs) against most strains of the following organisms; however, the safety and efficacy of oxiconazole in treating clinical infections due to these organisms have not been established in adequate and well-controlled clinical trials:

Candida albicans
Microsporum audouini
Microsporum canis
Microsporum gypseum
Trichophyton tonsurans
Trichophyton violaceum

INDICATIONS AND USAGE

OXISTAT Cream and Lotion are indicated for the topical treatment of the following dermal infections: tinea pedis, tinea cruris, and tinea corporis due to *Trichophyton rubrum, Trichophyton mentagrophytes*, or *Epidermophyton floccosum*. OXISTAT Cream is indicated for the topical treatment of tinea (pityriasis) versicolor due to *Malassezia furfur* (see DOSAGE AND ADMINISTRATION and CLINICAL STUDIES).

OXISTAT Cream may be used in pediatric patients for tinea corporis, tinea cruris, tinea pedis, and tinea (pityriasis) versicolor; however, these indications for which OXISTAT Cream has been shown to be effective rarely occur in children below the age of 12.

CONTRAINDICATIONS

OXISTAT Cream and Lotion are contraindicated in individuals who have shown hypersensitivity to any of their components.

WARNINGS

OXISTAT Cream and Lotion are not for ophthalmic or intravaginal use.

PRECAUTIONS

General: OXISTAT Cream and Lotion are for external dermal use only. Avoid introduction of OXISTAT Cream or Lotion into the eyes or vagina. If a reaction suggesting sensitivity or chemical irritation should occur with the use of OXISTAT Cream or Lotion, treatment should be discontinued and appropriate therapy instituted. If signs of epidermal irritation should occur, the drug should be discontinued.

Information for Patients: The patient should be instructed to:

1. Use OXISTAT as directed by the physician. The hands should be washed after applying the medication to the affected area(s). Avoid contact with the eyes, nose, mouth, and other mucous membranes. OXISTAT is for external use only.
2. Use the medication for the **full** treatment time recommended by the physician, even though symptoms may have improved. Notify the physician if there is no improvement after 2 to 4 weeks, or sooner if the condition worsens (see below).
3. Inform the physician if the area of application shows signs of increased irritation, itching, burning, blistering, swelling, or oozing.
4. Avoid the use of occlusive dressings unless otherwise directed by the physician.
5. Do not use this medication for any disorder other than that for which it was prescribed.

Drug Interactions: Potential drug interactions between OXISTAT and other drugs have not been systematically evaluated.

Carcinogenesis, Mutagenesis, Impairment of Fertility: Although no long-term studies in animals have been performed to evaluate carcinogenic potential, no evidence of mutagenic effect was found in 2 mutation assays (Ames test and Chinese hamster V79 in vitro cell mutation assay) or in 2 cytogenetic assays (human peripheral blood lymphocyte in vitro chromosome aberration assay and in vivo micronucleus assay in mice).

Reproductive studies revealed no impairment of fertility in rats at oral doses of 3 mg/kg/day in females (1 time the human dose based on mg/m²) and 15 mg/kg/day in males (4 times the human dose based on mg/m²). However, at doses above this level, the following effects were observed: a reduction in the fertility parameters of males and females, a reduction in the number of sperm in vaginal smears, extended estrous cycle, and a decrease in mating frequency.

Pregnancy: ***Teratogenic Effects:*** Pregnancy Category B. Reproduction studies have been performed in rabbits, rats, and mice at oral doses up to 100, 150, and 200 mg/kg/day (57, 40, and 27 times the human dose based on mg/m²), respectively, and revealed no evidence of harm to the fetus due to oxiconazole nitrate. There are, however, no adequate and well-controlled studies in pregnant women. Because animal reproduction studies are not always predictive of human response, this drug should be used during pregnancy only if clearly needed.

Nursing Mothers: Because oxiconazole is excreted in human milk, caution should be exercised when the drug is administered to a nursing woman.

Pediatric Use: OXISTAT Cream may be used in pediatric patients for tinea corporis, tinea cruris, tinea pedis, and tinea (pityriasis) versicolor; however, these indications for which OXISTAT Cream has been shown to be effective rarely occur in children below the age of 12.

Geriatric Use: A limited number of patients at or above 65 years of age (n = 508) have been treated with OXISTAT Cream in US and non-US clinical trials, and a limited number (n = 43) have been treated with OXISTAT Lotion in US clinical trials. The number of patients is too small to permit separate analysis of efficacy and safety. No adverse events were reported with OXISTAT Lotion in geriatric patients, and the adverse reactions reported with OXISTAT Cream in this population were similar to those reported by younger patients. Based on available data, no adjustment of dosage of OXISTAT Cream and Lotion in geriatric patients is warranted.

ADVERSE REACTIONS

During clinical trials, of 955 patients treated with oxiconazole nitrate cream, 1%, 41 (4.3%) reported adverse reactions thought to be related to drug therapy. These reactions included pruritus (1.6%); burning (1.4%); irritation and allergic contact dermatitis (0.4% each); folliculitis (0.3%); erythema (0.2%); and papules, fissure, maceration, rash, stinging, and nodules (0.1% each).

In a controlled, multicenter clinical trial of 269 patients treated with oxiconazole nitrate lotion, 1%, 7 (2.6%) reported adverse reactions thought to be related to drug therapy. These reactions included burning and stinging (0.7% each) and pruritus, scaling, tingling, pain, and dyshidrotic eczema (0.4% each).

OVERDOSAGE

When 5% oxiconazole cream (5 times the concentration of the marketed product) was applied at a rate of 1 g/kg to approximately 10% of body surface area of a group of 40 male and female rats for 35 days, 3 deaths and severe dermal inflammation were reported. No overdoses in humans have been reported with use of oxiconazole nitrate cream or lotion.

DOSAGE AND ADMINISTRATION

OXISTAT Cream or Lotion should be applied to affected and immediately surrounding areas once to twice daily in patients with tinea pedis, tinea corporis, or tinea cruris. OXISTAT Cream should be applied once daily in the treatment of tinea (pityriasis) versicolor. Tinea corporis, tinea cruris, and tinea (pityriasis) versicolor should be treated for 2 weeks and tinea pedis for 1 month to reduce the possibility of recurrence. If a patient shows no clinical improvement after the treatment period, the diagnosis should be reviewed.

Note: Tinea (pityriasis) versicolor may give rise to hyperpigmented or hypopigmented patches on the trunk that may extend to the neck, arms, and upper thighs. Treatment of the infection may not immediately result in restoration of pigment to the affected sites. Normalization of pigment following successful therapy is variable and may take months, depending on individual skin type and incidental sun exposure. Although tinea (pityriasis) versicolor is not contagious, it may recur because the organism that causes the disease is part of the normal skin flora.

Geriatric Use: In studies where geriatric patients (65 years of age or older, see PRECAUTIONS) have been treated with OXISTAT Cream or Lotion, safety did not differ from that in younger patients; therefore, no dosage adjustment is recommended.

HOW SUPPLIED

OXISTAT Cream, 1% is supplied in:
15-g tubes (NDC 0173-0423-00),
30-g tubes (NDC 0173-0423-01), and
60-g tubes (NDC 0173-0423-04).
Store between 15° and 30°C (59° and 86°F).

OXISTAT Lotion, 1% is supplied in a 30-mL bottle (NDC 0173-0448-01). **Store between 15° and 30°C (59° and 86°F). Shake well before using.**

CLINICAL STUDIES

The following definitions were applied to the clinical and microbiological outcomes in patients enrolled in the clinical trials that form the basis for the approvals of OXISTAT Lotion and OXISTAT Cream.

Definitions:

1. Mycological Cure: No evidence (culture and KOH preparation) of the baseline (original) pathogen in a specimen from the affected area taken at the 2-week post-treatment visit (for tinea [pityriasis] versicolor, mycological cure was limited to KOH only).
2. Treatment Success: Both a global evaluation of ≥90% clinical improvement and a microbiologic eradication (see above) at the 2-week post-treatment visit.

Tinea Pedis: THERE ARE NO HEAD-TO-HEAD COMPARISON TRIALS OF THE OXISTAT CREAM AND LOTION FORMULATIONS IN THE TREATMENT OF TINEA PEDIS.

Lotion Formulation: The clinical trial for the lotion formulation line extension involved 332 evaluable patients with clinically and microbiologically established tinea pedis. Of these evaluable patients, 64% were diagnosed with hyperkeratotic plantar tinea pedis and 28% with interdigital tinea pedis. Seventy-seven percent (77%) had disease secondary to infection with *Trichophyton rubrum*, 18% had disease secondary to infection with *Trichophyton mentagrophytes*, and 4% had disease secondary to infection with *Epidermophyton floccosum*.

The results of this clinical trial at the 2-week post-treatment follow-up visit are shown in the following table:

Patient Outcome	OXISTAT Lotion		Vehicle
	b.i.d.	q.d.	
Mycological cure	67%	64%	28%
Treatment success	41%	34%	10%

In this study, the improvement and cure rates of the b.i.d.- and q.d.-treated groups did not differ significantly (95% confidence interval) from each other but were statistically (95% confidence interval) superior to the vehicle-treated group.

Cream Formulation: The 2 pivotal trials for the cream formulation involved 281 evaluable patients (total from both trials) with clinically and microbiologically established tinea pedis.

The combined results of these 2 clinical trials at the 2-week post-treatment follow-up visit are shown in the following table:

Patient Outcome	OXISTAT Cream		Vehicle
	b.i.d.	q.d	
Mycological cure	77%	79%	33%
Treatment success	52%	43%	14%

All the improvement and cure rates of the b.i.d.- and q.d.-treated groups did not differ significantly (95% confidence interval) from each other but were statistically (95% confidence interval) superior to the vehicle-treated group.

In addition, pediatric data (95 children ages 10 and under) available with the cream formulation indicate that it is safe and effective for use in children when used as directed. Adverse events were reported in 2 children; 1 child was reported to have reddening of the skin and 1 child was reported to have eczema-like skin alterations.

Tinea (pityriasis) Versicolor: Two pivotal clinical trials of OXISTAT Cream in tinea (pityriasis) versicolor involved 219 evaluable patients in the q day OXISTAT and vehicle arms of the trial with clinical and mycological evidence of tinea (pityriasis) versicolor. Patients were treated for 2 weeks with OXISTAT Cream once daily, or with cream vehicle. The combined results of these clinical trials at the 2-week post-treatment follow-up visit are shown in the following table. These results are based on 207 patients (110 in the OXISTAT group and 97 in the vehicle group) with efficacy evaluations at this visit.

Patient Outcome	OXISTAT Cream q.d.	Vehicle
Mycological cure	88%	67%
Treatment success	83%	62%

Only once a day was shown in both studies to be statistically superior to vehicle for all efficacy parameters at 2 weeks and follow-up.

GlaxoSmithKline Consumer Healthcare LP
Pittsburgh, PA 15230

August 2002/RL-1084
Shown in Product Identification Guide, pages 316 & 317

PARNATE® ℞

[par' nāt]
brand of tranylcypromine sulfate tablets 10 mg

Before prescribing, the physician should be familiar with the entire contents of this prescribing information.

DESCRIPTION

Chemically, tranylcypromine sulfate is (±)-*trans*-2-phenylcyclopropylamine sulfate (2:1).

Each round, rose-red, film-coated tablet is imprinted with the product name PARNATE and SB and contains tranylcypromine sulfate equivalent to 10 mg of tranylcypromine. Inactive ingredients consist of cellulose, citric acid, croscarmellose sodium, D&C Red No. 7, FD&C Blue No. 2, FD&C Red No. 40, FD&C Yellow No. 6, gelatin, iron oxide, lactose, magnesium stearate, talc, titanium dioxide and trace amounts of other inactive ingredients.

ACTION

Tranylcypromine is a non-hydrazine monoamine oxidase inhibitor with a rapid onset of activity. It increases the concentration of epinephrine, norepinephrine and serotonin in storage sites throughout the nervous system and, in theory, this increased concentration of monoamines in the brain stem is the basis for its antidepressant activity. When tranylcypromine is withdrawn, monoamine oxidase activity is recovered in 3 to 5 days, although the drug is excreted in 24 hours.

INDICATIONS

For the treatment of Major Depressive Episode Without Melancholia.

Parnate (tranylcypromine sulfate) should be used in adult patients who can be closely supervised. It should rarely be the first antidepressant drug given. Rather, the drug is suited for patients who have failed to respond to the drugs more commonly administered for depression.

The effectiveness of *Parnate* has been established in adult outpatients, most of whom had a depressive illness which would correspond to a diagnosis of Major Depressive Episode Without Melancholia. As described in the American Psychiatric Association's Diagnostic and Statistical Manual, third edition (DSM III), Major Depressive Episode implies a prominent and relatively persistent (nearly every day for at least 2 weeks) depressed or dysphoric mood that usually interferes with daily functioning and includes at least 4 of the following 8 symptoms: change in appetite, change in sleep, psychomotor agitation or retardation, loss of interest in usual activities or decrease in sexual drive, increased fatigability, feelings of guilt or worthlessness, slowed thinking or impaired concentration and suicidal ideation or attempts.

The effectiveness of *Parnate* in patients who meet the criteria for Major Depressive Episode with Melancholia (endogenous features) has not been established.

SUMMARY OF CONTRAINDICATIONS

Parnate (tranylcypromine sulfate) should not be administered in combination with any of the following: MAO inhibitors or dibenzazepine derivatives; sympathomimetics (including amphetamines); some central nervous system depressants (including narcotics and alcohol); antihypertensive, diuretic, antihistaminic, sedative or anesthetic drugs; bupropion HCl; buspirone HCl; dextromethorphan; cheese or other foods with a high tyramine content; or excessive quantities of caffeine.

Parnate (tranylcypromine sulfate) should not be administered to any patient with a confirmed or suspected cerebrovascular defect or to any patient with cardiovascular disease, hypertension or history of headache.

(For complete discussion of contraindications and warnings, see below.)

CONTRAINDICATIONS

Parnate (tranylcypromine sulfate) is contraindicated:

1. In patients with cerebrovascular defects or cardiovascular disorders

Parnate should not be administered to any patient with a confirmed or suspected cerebrovascular defect or to any patient with cardiovascular disease or hypertension.

2. In the presence of pheochromocytoma

Parnate should not be used in the presence of pheochromocytoma since such tumors secrete pressor substances.

3. In combination with MAO inhibitors or with dibenzazepine-related entities

Parnate (tranylcypromine sulfate) should not be administered together or in rapid succession with other MAO inhibitors or with dibenzazepine-related entities. Hypertensive crises or severe convulsive seizures may occur in patients receiving such combinations.

In patients being transferred to *Parnate* from another MAO inhibitor or from a dibenzazepine-related entity, allow a medication-free interval of at least a week, then initiate *Parnate* using half the normal starting dosage for at least the first week of therapy. Similarly, at least a week should elapse between the discontinuance of *Parnate* and the administration of another MAO inhibitor or a dibenzazepine-related entity, or the readministration of *Parnate*.

The following list includes some other MAO inhibitors, dibenzazepine-related entities and tricyclic antidepressants, and the companies which market them.

Other MAO Inhibitors

Generic Name	Source
Furazolidone	
Isocarboxazid	Marplan® (Oxford Pharm Services)
Pargyline HCl	
Pargyline HCl and methyclothiazide	
Phenelzine sulfate	Nardil® (Parke-Davis)
Procarbazine HCl	Matulane® (Sigma Tau)

Dibenzazepine-Related and Other Tricyclics

Generic Name	Source
Amitriptyline HCl	Elavil® (Zeneca)
Perphenazine and amitriptyline HCl	Etrafon® (Schering) Triavil® (Lotus Biochemical)
Clomipramine hydrochloride	Anafranil® (Geneva)
Desipramine HCl	Norpramin® (Aventis)
Imipramine HCl	Janimine™ (Geneva) Tofranil® (Novartis) (Geneva)
Nortriptyline HCl	Pamelor® (Mallinckrodt)
Protriptyline HCl	Vivactil® (Merck & Co., Inc.)
Doxepin HCl	Sinequan® (Pfizer)
Carbamazepine	Tegretol® (Novartis)
Cyclobenzaprine HCl	Flexeril® (Merck & Co., Inc.)
Amoxapine	(Geneva)
Maprotiline HCl	(Mylan)
Trimipramine maleate	Surmontil® (Wyeth-Ayerst Pharmaceuticals)

4. In combination with bupropion

The concurrent administration of a MAO inhibitor and bupropion hydrochloride (Wellbutrin®, Wellbutrin SR®, Zyban®, GlaxoSmithKline) is contraindicated. At least 14 days should elapse between discontinuation of a MAO inhibitor and initiation of treatment with bupropion hydrochloride.

5. In combination with dexfenfluramine hydrochloride

Because dexfenfluramine hydrochloride is a serotonin releaser and reuptake inhibitor, it should not be used concomitantly with Parnate (tranylcypromine sulfate).

6. In combination with selective serotonin reuptake inhibitors (SSRIs)

As a general rule, *Parnate* should not be administered in combination with any SSRI. There have been reports of serious, sometimes fatal, reactions (including hyperthermia, rigidity, myoclonus, autonomic instability with possible rapid fluctuations of vital signs, and mental status changes that include extreme agitation progressing to delirium and coma) in patients receiving fluoxetine (Prozac®, Eli Lilly and Company) in combination with a monoamine oxidase inhibitor (MAOI), and in patients who have recently discontinued fluoxetine and are then started on a MAOI. Some cases presented with features resembling neuroleptic malignant syndrome. Therefore, fluoxetine and other SSRIs should not be used in combination with a MAOI, or within 14 days of discontinuing therapy with a MAOI. Since fluoxetine and its major metabolite have very long elimination half-lives, at least 5 weeks should be allowed after stopping fluoxetine before starting a MAOI.

Continued on next page

Product information on these pages is effective as of August 2004. Further information is available at: GlaxoSmithKline, PO Box 13398, Research Triangle Park, NC 27709. 1-888-825-5249. Corporate Web Site: www.gsk.com.

Parnate—Cont.

At least 2 weeks should be allowed after stopping sertraline (Zoloft®, Pfizer) or paroxetine (Paxil®, GlaxoSmithKline) before starting a MAOI.

7. In combination with buspirone

Parnate (tranylcypromine sulfate) should not be used in combination with buspirone HCl (BuSpar®, Bristol-Myers Squibb), since several cases of elevated blood pressure have been reported in patients taking MAO inhibitors who were then given buspirone HCl. At least 10 days should elapse between the discontinuation of *Parnate* and the institution of buspirone HCl.

8. In combination with sympathomimetics

Parnate (tranylcypromine sulfate) should not be administered in combination with sympathomimetics, including amphetamines, and over-the-counter drugs such as cold, hay fever or weight-reducing preparations that contain vasoconstrictors.

During *Parnate* therapy, it appears that certain patients are particularly vulnerable to the effects of sympathomimetics when the activity of certain enzymes is inhibited. Use of sympathomimetics and compounds such as guanethidine, methyldopa, reserpine, dopamine, levodopa and tryptophan with *Parnate* may precipitate hypertension, headache and related symptoms. The combination of MAOIs and tryptophan has been reported to cause behavioral and neurologic syndromes including disorientation, confusion, amnesia, delirium, agitation, hypomanic signs, ataxia, myoclonus, hyperreflexia, shivering, ocular oscillations and Babinski's signs.

9. In combination with meperidine

Do not use meperidine concomitantly with MAO inhibitors or within 2 or 3 weeks following MAOI therapy. Serious reactions have been precipitated with concomitant use, including coma, severe hypertension or hypotension, severe respiratory depression, convulsions, malignant hyperpyrexia, excitation, peripheral vascular collapse and death. It is thought that these reactions may be mediated by accumulation of 5-HT (serotonin) consequent to MAO inhibition.

10. In combination with dextromethorphan

The combination of MAO inhibitors and dextromethorphan has been reported to cause brief episodes of psychosis or bizarre behavior.

11. In combination with cheese or other foods with a high tyramine content

Hypertensive crises have sometimes occurred during *Parnate* therapy after ingestion of foods with a high tyramine content. In general, the patient should avoid protein foods in which aging or protein breakdown is used to increase flavor. In particular, patients should be instructed not to take foods such as cheese (particularly strong or aged varieties), sour cream, Chianti wine, sherry, beer (including nonalcoholic beer), liqueurs, pickled herring, anchovies, caviar, liver, canned figs, dried fruits (raisins, prunes, etc.), bananas, raspberries, avocados, overripe fruit, chocolate, soy sauce, sauerkraut, the pods of broad beans (fava beans), yeast extracts, yogurt, meat extracts or meat prepared with tenderizers.

12. In patients undergoing elective surgery

Patients taking *Parnate* should not undergo elective surgery requiring general anesthesia. Also, they should not be given cocaine or local anesthesia containing sympathomimetic vasoconstrictors. The possible combined hypotensive effects of *Parnate* and spinal anesthesia should be kept in mind. *Parnate* should be discontinued at least 10 days prior to elective surgery.

ADDITIONAL CONTRAINDICATIONS

In general, the physician should bear in mind the possibility of a lowered margin of safety when Parnate (tranylcypromine sulfate) is administered in combination with potent drugs.

1. *Parnate* should not be used in combination with some central nervous system depressants such as narcotics and alcohol, or with hypotensive agents. A marked potentiating effect on these classes of drugs has been reported.
2. Anti-parkinsonism drugs should be used with caution in patients receiving *Parnate* since severe reactions have been reported.
3. *Parnate* should not be used in patients with a history of liver disease or in those with abnormal liver function tests.
4. Excessive use of caffeine in any form should be avoided in patients receiving *Parnate*.

WARNING TO PHYSICIANS

Parnate (tranylcypromine sulfate) is a potent agent with the capability of producing serious side effects. *Parnate* is not recommended in those depressive reactions where other antidepressant drugs may be effective. **It should be reserved for patients who can be closely supervised and who have not responded satisfactorily to the drugs more commonly administered for depression.**

Before prescribing, the physician should be completely familiar with the full material on dosage, side effects and contraindications on these pages, with the principles of MAO inhibitor therapy and the side effects of this class of drugs. Also, the physician should be familiar with the symptomatology of mental depressions and alternate methods of treatment to aid in the careful selection of patients for *Parnate* therapy. In depressed patients, the possibility of suicide should always be considered and adequate precautions taken.

Pregnancy Warning: Use of any drug in pregnancy, during lactation or in women of childbearing age requires that the potential benefits of the drug be weighed against its possible hazards to mother and child.

Animal reproductive studies show that *Parnate* passes through the placental barrier into the fetus of the rat, and into the milk of the lactating dog. The absence of a harmful action of *Parnate* on fertility or on postnatal development by either prenatal treatment or from the milk of treated animals has not been demonstrated. Tranylcypromine is excreted in human milk.

WARNING TO THE PATIENT

Patients should be instructed to report promptly the occurrence of headache or other unusual symptoms, i.e., palpitation and/or tachycardia, a sense of constriction in the throat or chest, sweating, dizziness, neck stiffness, nausea or vomiting.

Patients should be warned against eating the foods listed in Section 11 under Contraindications while on Parnate (tranylcypromine sulfate) therapy. Also, they should be told not to drink alcoholic beverages. The patient should also be warned about the possibility of hypotension and faintness, as well as drowsiness sufficient to impair performance of potentially hazardous tasks such as driving a car or operating machinery.

Patients should also be cautioned not to take concomitant medications, whether prescription or over-the-counter drugs such as cold, hay fever or weight-reducing preparations, without the advice of a physician. They should be advised not to consume excessive amounts of caffeine in any form. Likewise, they should inform other physicians, and their dentist, about their use of *Parnate*.

WARNINGS

HYPERTENSIVE CRISES: The most important reaction associated with Parnate (tranylcypromine sulfate) is the occurrence of hypertensive crises which have sometimes been fatal.

These crises are characterized by some or all of the following symptoms: occipital headache which may radiate frontally, palpitation, neck stiffness or soreness, nausea or vomiting, sweating (sometimes with fever and sometimes with cold, clammy skin) and photophobia. Either tachycardia or bradycardia may be present, and associated constricting chest pain and dilated pupils may occur. **Intracranial bleeding, sometimes fatal in outcome, has been reported in association with the paradoxical increase in blood pressure.**

In all patients taking *Parnate* blood pressure should be followed closely to detect evidence of any pressor response. It is emphasized that full reliance should not be placed on blood pressure readings, but that the patient should also be observed frequently.

Therapy should be discontinued immediately upon the occurrence of palpitation or frequent headaches during *Parnate* therapy. These signs may be prodromal of a hypertensive crisis.

Important:
Recommended treatment in hypertensive crises

If a hypertensive crisis occurs, Parnate (tranylcypromine sulfate) should be discontinued and therapy to lower blood pressure should be instituted immediately. Headache tends to abate as blood pressure is lowered. On the basis of present evidence, phentolamine is recommended. (The dosage reported for phentolamine is 5 mg I.V.) Care should be taken to administer this drug slowly in order to avoid producing an excessive hypotensive effect. Fever should be managed by means of external cooling. Other symptomatic and supportive measures may be desirable in particular cases. Do not use parenteral reserpine.

PRECAUTIONS

Hypotension

Hypotension has been observed during Parnate (tranylcypromine sulfate) therapy. Symptoms of postural hypotension are seen most commonly but not exclusively in patients with pre-existent hypertension; blood pressure usually returns rapidly to pretreatment levels upon discontinuation of the drug. At doses above 30 mg daily, postural hypotension is a major side effect and may result in syncope. Dosage increases should be made more gradually in patients showing a tendency toward hypotension at the beginning of therapy. Postural hypotension may be relieved by having the patient lie down until blood pressure returns to normal.

Also, when *Parnate* is combined with those phenothiazine derivatives or other compounds known to cause hypotension, the possibility of additive hypotensive effects should be considered.

OTHER PRECAUTIONS

There have been reports of drug dependency in patients using doses of tranylcypromine significantly in excess of the therapeutic range. Some of these patients had a history of previous substance abuse. The following withdrawal symptoms have been reported: restlessness, anxiety, depression, confusion, hallucinations, headache, weakness and diarrhea.

Drugs which lower the seizure threshold, including MAO inhibitors, should not be used with Amipaque®. As with other MAO inhibitors, Parnate (tranylcypromine sulfate) should be discontinued at least 48 hours before myelography and should not be resumed for at least 24 hours postprocedure.

In depressed patients, the possibility of suicide should always be considered and adequate precautions taken. Exclusive reliance on drug therapy to prevent suicidal attempts is unwarranted, as there may be a delay in the onset of therapeutic effect or an increase in anxiety and agitation. Also, some patients fail to respond to drug therapy or may respond only temporarily.

MAO inhibitors may have the capacity to suppress anginal pain that would otherwise serve as a warning of myocardial ischemia.

The usual precautions should be observed in patients with impaired renal function since there is a possibility of cumulative effects in such patients.

Older patients may suffer more morbidity than younger patients during and following an episode of hypertension or malignant hyperthermia. Older patients have less compensatory reserve to cope with any serious adverse reaction. Therefore, *Parnate* should be used with caution in the elderly population.

Although excretion of *Parnate* is rapid, inhibition of MAO may persist up to 10 days following discontinuation.

Because the influence of *Parnate* on the convulsive threshold is variable in animal experiments, suitable precautions should be taken if epileptic patients are treated.

Some MAO inhibitors have contributed to hypoglycemic episodes in diabetic patients receiving insulin or oral hypoglycemic agents. Therefore, *Parnate* should be used with caution in diabetics using these drugs.

Parnate may aggravate coexisting symptoms in depression, such as anxiety and agitation.

Use Parnate (tranylcypromine sulfate) with caution in hyperthyroid patients because of their increased sensitivity to pressor amines.

Parnate should be administered with caution to patients receiving Antabuse®[†]. In a single study, rats given high intraperitoneal doses of *d* or *l* isomers of tranylcypromine sulfate plus disulfiram experienced severe toxicity including convulsions and death. Additional studies in rats given high oral doses of racemic tranylcypromine sulfate (*Parnate*) and disulfiram produced no adverse interaction.

ADVERSE REACTIONS

Overstimulation which may include increased anxiety, agitation and manic symptoms is usually evidence of excessive therapeutic action. Dosage should be reduced, or a phenothiazine tranquilizer should be administered concomitantly.

Patients may experience restlessness or insomnia; may notice some weakness, drowsiness, episodes of dizziness or dry mouth; or may report nausea, diarrhea, abdominal pain or constipation. Most of these effects can be relieved by lowering the dosage or by giving suitable concomitant medication.

Tachycardia, significant anorexia, edema, palpitation, blurred vision, chills and impotence have each been reported.

Headaches without blood pressure elevation have occurred.

Rare instances of hepatitis, skin rash and alopecia have been reported.

Impaired water excretion compatible with the syndrome of inappropriate secretion of antidiuretic hormone (SIADH) has been reported.

Tinnitus, muscle spasm, tremors, myoclonic jerks, numbness, paresthesia, urinary retention and retarded ejaculation have been reported.

Hematologic disorders including anemia, leukopenia, agranulocytosis and thrombocytopenia have been reported.

Post-Introduction Reports

The following are spontaneously reported adverse events temporally associated with *Parnate* therapy. No clear relationship between *Parnate* and these events has been established. Localized scleroderma, flare-up of cystic acne, ataxia, confusion, disorientation, memory loss, urinary frequency, urinary incontinence, urticaria, fissuring in corner of mouth, akinesia.

DOSAGE AND ADMINISTRATION

Dosage should be adjusted to the requirements of the individual patient. Improvement should be seen within 48 hours to 3 weeks after starting therapy.

The usual effective dosage is 30 mg per day, usually given in divided doses. If there are no signs of improvement after a reasonable period (up to 2 weeks), then the dosage may be increased in 10 mg per day increments at intervals of 1 to 3 weeks; the dosage range may be extended to a maximum of 60 mg per day from the usual 30 mg per day.

OVERDOSAGE

SYMPTOMS: The characteristic symptoms that may be caused by overdosage are usually those described above.

However, an intensification of these symptoms and sometimes severe additional manifestations may be seen, depending on the degree of overdosage and on individual susceptibility. Some patients exhibit insomnia, restlessness and anxiety, progressing in severe cases to agitation, mental confusion and incoherence. Hypotension, dizziness, weakness and drowsiness may occur, progressing in severe cases to extreme dizziness and shock. A few patients have displayed hypertension with severe headache and other symptoms. Rare instances have been reported in which hypertension was accompanied by twitching or myoclonic fibrillation of skeletal muscles with hyperpyrexia, sometimes progressing to generalized rigidity and coma.

TREATMENT: Gastric lavage is helpful if performed early. Treatment should normally consist of general supportive measures, close observation of vital signs and steps to counteract specific symptoms as they occur, since MAO inhibi-

tion may persist. The management of hypertensive crises is described under WARNINGS in the HYPERTENSIVE CRISES section.
External cooling is recommended if hyperpyrexia occurs. Barbiturates have been reported to help relieve myoclonic reactions, but frequency of administration should be controlled carefully because Parnate (tranylcypromine sulfate) may prolong barbiturate activity. When hypotension requires treatment, the standard measures for managing circulatory shock should be initiated. If pressor agents are used, the rate of infusion should be regulated by careful observation of the patient because an exaggerated pressor response sometimes occurs in the presence of MAO inhibition. Remember that the toxic effect of *Parnate* may be delayed or prolonged following the last dose of the drug. Therefore, the patient should be closely observed for at least a week. It is not known if tranylcypromine is dialyzable.

HOW SUPPLIED

Parnate is supplied as round, rose-red, film-coated tablets imprinted with the product name PARNATE and SB and contains tranylcypromine sulfate equivalent to 10 mg of tranylcypromine, in bottles of 100 with a desiccant, manufactured by Abbott Laboratories, North Chicago, IL 60064.
10 mg 100's: NDC 0007-4471-20
Store between 15° and 30°C (59° and 86°F).

*metrizamide, Sanofi-Synthelabo Inc.
†disulfiram, Wyeth-Ayerst Pharmaceuticals.
GlaxoSmithKline, Research Triangle Park, NC 27709

August 2001/PT:L65
Shown in Product Identification Guide, page 317

PAXIL® ℞
[*pax'il*]
(paroxetine hydrochloride)
Tablets and Oral Suspension

DESCRIPTION

PAXIL (paroxetine hydrochloride) is an orally administered psychotropic drug. It is the hydrochloride salt of a phenylpiperidine compound identified chemically as (-)-*trans*-4*R*-(4'-fluorophenyl)-3*S*-[(3',4'-methylenedioxyphenoxy) methyl] piperidine hydrochloride hemihydrate and has the empirical formula of $C_{19}H_{20}FNO_3 \bullet HCl \bullet 1/2H_2O$. The molecular weight is 374.8 (329.4 as free base).
Paroxetine hydrochloride is an odorless, off-white powder, having a melting point range of 120° to 138°C and a solubility of 5.4 mg/mL in water.
Tablets: Each film-coated tablet contains paroxetine hydrochloride equivalent to paroxetine as follows: 10 mg–yellow (scored); 20 mg–pink (scored); 30 mg–blue, 40 mg–green. Inactive ingredients consist of dibasic calcium phosphate dihydrate, hypromellose magnesium stearate, polyethylene glycols, polysorbate 80, sodium starch glycolate, titanium dioxide, and 1 or more of the following: D&C Red No. 30, D&C Yellow No. 10, FD&C Blue No. 2, FD&C Yellow No. 6.
Suspension for Oral Administration: Each 5 mL of orange-colored, orange-flavored liquid contains paroxetine hydrochloride equivalent to paroxetine, 10 mg. Inactive ingredients consist of polacrilin potassium, microcrystalline cellulose, propylene glycol, glycerin, sorbitol, methyl paraben, propyl paraben, sodium citrate dihydrate, citric acid anhydrate, sodium saccharin, flavorings, FD&C Yellow No. 6, and simethicone emulsion, USP.

CLINICAL PHARMACOLOGY

Pharmacodynamics: The efficacy of paroxetine in the treatment of major depressive disorder, social anxiety disorder, obsessive compulsive disorder (OCD), panic disorder (PD), generalized anxiety disorder (GAD), and posttraumatic stress disorder (PTSD) is presumed to be linked to potentiation of serotonergic activity in the central nervous system resulting from inhibition of neuronal reuptake of serotonin (5-hydroxy-tryptamine, 5-HT). Studies at clinically relevant doses in humans have demonstrated that paroxetine blocks the uptake of serotonin into human platelets. In vitro studies in animals also suggest that paroxetine is a potent and highly selective inhibitor of neuronal serotonin reuptake and has only very weak effects on norepinephrine and dopamine neuronal reuptake. *In vitro* radioligand binding studies indicate that paroxetine has little affinity for muscarinic, $alpha_1$-, $alpha_2$-, beta-adrenergic-, dopamine (D_2)-, 5-HT_1-, 5-HT_2-, and histamine (H_1)-receptors; antagonism of muscarinic, histaminergic, and $alpha_1$-adrenergic receptors has been associated with various anticholinergic, sedative, and cardiovascular effects for other psychotropic drugs.
Because the relative potencies of paroxetine's major metabolites are at most 1/50 of the parent compound, they are essentially inactive.
Pharmacokinetics: Paroxetine is equally bioavailable from the oral suspension and tablet.
Paroxetine hydrochloride is completely absorbed after oral dosing of a solution of the hydrochloride salt. In a study in which normal male subjects (n = 15) received 30 mg tablets daily for 30 days, steady-state paroxetine concentrations were achieved by approximately 10 days for most subjects, although it may take substantially longer in an occasional patient. At steady state, mean values of C_{max}, T_{max}, C_{min}, and $T_{1/2}$ were 61.7 ng/mL (CV 45%), 5.2 hr. (CV 10%), 30.7 ng/mL (CV 67%), and 21.0 hr. (CV 32%), respectively. The steady-state C_{max} and C_{min} values were about 6 and 14 times what would be predicted from single-dose studies. Steady-state drug exposure based on AUC_{0-24} was about 8 times greater than would have been predicted from single-dose data in these subjects. The excess accumulation is a consequence of the fact that 1 of the enzymes that metabolizes paroxetine is readily saturable.
In steady-state dose proportionality studies involving elderly and nonelderly patients, at doses of 20 mg to 40 mg daily for the elderly and 20 mg to 50 mg daily for the nonelderly, some nonlinearity was observed in both populations, again reflecting a saturable metabolic pathway. In comparison to C_{min} values after 20 mg daily, values after 40 mg daily were only about 2 to 3 times greater than doubled.
The effects of food on the bioavailability of paroxetine were studied in subjects administered a single dose with and without food. AUC was only slightly increased (6%) when drug was administered with food but the C_{max} was 29% greater, while the time to reach peak plasma concentration decreased from 6.4 hours post-dosing to 4.9 hours.
Paroxetine is extensively metabolized after oral administration. The principal metabolites are polar and conjugated products of oxidation and methylation, which are readily cleared. Conjugates with glucuronic acid and sulfate predominate, and major metabolites have been isolated and identified. Data indicate that the metabolites have no more than 1/50 the potency of the parent compound at inhibiting serotonin uptake. The metabolism of paroxetine is accomplished in part by cytochrome $P_{450}IID_6$. Saturation of this enzyme at clinical doses appears to account for the nonlinearity of paroxetine kinetics with increasing dose and increasing duration of treatment. The role of this enzyme in paroxetine metabolism also suggests potential drug-drug interactions (see PRECAUTIONS).
Approximately 64% of a 30-mg oral solution dose of paroxetine was excreted in the urine with 2% as the parent compound and 62% as metabolites over a 10-day post-dosing period. About 36% was excreted in the feces (probably via the bile), mostly as metabolites and less than 1% as the parent compound over the 10-day post-dosing period.
Distribution: Paroxetine distributes throughout the body, including the CNS, with only 1% remaining in the plasma.
Protein Binding: Approximately 95% and 93% of paroxetine is bound to plasma protein at 100 ng/mL and 400 ng/mL, respectively. Under clinical conditions, paroxetine concentrations would normally be less than 400 ng/mL. Paroxetine does not alter the in vitro protein binding of phenytoin or warfarin.
Renal and Liver Disease: Increased plasma concentrations of paroxetine occur in subjects with renal and hepatic impairment. The mean plasma concentrations in patients with creatinine clearance below 30 mL/min. was approximately 4 times greater than seen in normal volunteers. Patients with creatinine clearance of 30 to 60 mL/min. and patients with hepatic functional impairment had about a 2-fold increase in plasma concentrations (AUC, C_{max}).
The initial dosage should therefore be reduced in patients with severe renal or hepatic impairment, and upward titration, if necessary, should be at increased intervals (see DOSAGE AND ADMINISTRATION).
Elderly Patients: In a multiple-dose study in the elderly at daily paroxetine doses of 20, 30, and 40 mg, C_{min} concentrations were about 70% to 80% greater than the respective C_{min} concentrations in nonelderly subjects. Therefore the initial dosage in the elderly should be reduced (see DOSAGE AND ADMINISTRATION).

Clinical Trials

Major Depressive Disorder: The efficacy of PAXIL as a treatment for major depressive disorder has been established in 6 placebo-controlled studies of patients with major depressive disorder (aged 18 to 73). In these studies, PAXIL was shown to be significantly more effective than placebo in treating major depressive disorder by at least 2 of the following measures: Hamilton Depression Rating Scale (HDRS), the Hamilton depressed mood item, and the Clinical Global Impression (CGI)-Severity of Illness. PAXIL was significantly better than placebo in improvement of the HDRS sub-factor scores, including the depressed mood item, sleep disturbance factor, and anxiety factor.
A study of outpatients with major depressive disorder who had responded to PAXIL (HDRS total score <8) during an initial 8-week open-treatment phase and were then randomized to continuation on PAXIL or placebo for 1 year demonstrated a significantly lower relapse rate for patients taking PAXIL (15%) compared to those on placebo (39%). Effectiveness was similar for male and female patients.
Obsessive Compulsive Disorder: The effectiveness of PAXIL in the treatment of obsessive compulsive disorder (OCD) was demonstrated in two 12-week multicenter placebo-controlled studies of adult outpatients (Studies 1 and 2). Patients in all studies had moderate to severe OCD (DSM-IIIR) with mean baseline ratings on the Yale Brown Obsessive Compulsive Scale (YBOCS) total score ranging from 23 to 26. Study 1, a dose-range finding study where patients were treated with fixed doses of 20, 40, or 60 mg of paroxetine/day demonstrated that daily doses of paroxetine 40 and 60 mg are effective in the treatment of OCD. Patients receiving doses of 40 and 60 mg paroxetine experienced a mean reduction of approximately 6 and 7 points, respectively, on the YBOCS total score which was significantly greater than the approximate 4-point reduction at 20 mg and a 3-point reduction in the placebo-treated patients. Study 2 was a flexible-dose study comparing paroxetine (20 to 60 mg daily) with clomipramine (25 to 250 mg daily). In this study, patients receiving paroxetine experienced a mean reduction of approximately 7 points on the YBOCS total score, which was significantly greater than the mean reduction of approximately 4 points in placebo-treated patients.
The following table provides the outcome classification by treatment group on Global Improvement items of the Clinical Global Impression (CGI) scale for Study 1.
[See table above]

Outcome Classification (%) on CGI-Global Improvement Item for Completers in Study 1

Outcome Classification	Placebo (n = 74)	PAXIL 20 mg (n = 75)	PAXIL 40 mg (n = 66)	PAXIL 60 mg (n = 66)
Worse	14%	7%	7%	3%
No Change	44%	35%	22%	19%
Minimally Improved	24%	33%	29%	34%
Much Improved	11%	18%	22%	24%
Very Much Improved	7%	7%	20%	20%

Subgroup analyses did not indicate that there were any differences in treatment outcomes as a function of age or gender.
The long-term maintenance effects of PAXIL in OCD were demonstrated in a long-term extension to Study 1. Patients who were responders on paroxetine during the 3-month double-blind phase and a 6-month extension on open-label paroxetine (20 to 60 mg/day) were randomized to either paroxetine or placebo in a 6-month double-blind relapse prevention phase. Patients randomized to paroxetine were significantly less likely to relapse than comparably treated patients who were randomized to placebo.
Panic Disorder: The effectiveness of PAXIL in the treatment of panic disorder was demonstrated in three 10- to 12-week multicenter, placebo-controlled studies of adult outpatients (Studies 1-3). Patients in all studies had panic disorder (DSM-IIIR), with or without agoraphobia. In these studies, PAXIL was shown to be significantly more effective than placebo in treating panic disorder by at least 2 out of 3 measures of panic attack frequency and on the Clinical Global Impression Severity of Illness score.
Study 1 was a 10-week dose-range finding study; patients were treated with fixed paroxetine doses of 10, 20, or 40 mg/day or placebo. A significant difference from placebo was observed only for the 40 mg/day group. At endpoint, 76% of patients receiving paroxetine 40 mg/day were free of panic attacks, compared to 44% of placebo-treated patients.
Study 2 was a 12-week flexible-dose study comparing paroxetine (10 to 60 mg daily) and placebo. At endpoint, 51% of paroxetine patients were free of panic attacks compared to 32% of placebo-treated patients.
Study 3 was a 12-week flexible-dose study comparing paroxetine (10 to 60 mg daily) to placebo in patients concurrently receiving standardized cognitive behavioral therapy. At endpoint, 33% of the paroxetine-treated patients showed a reduction to 0 or 1 panic attacks compared to 14% of placebo patients.
In both Studies 2 and 3, the mean paroxetine dose for completers at endpoint was approximately 40 mg/day of paroxetine.
Long-term maintenance effects of PAXIL in panic disorder were demonstrated in an extension to Study 1. Patients who were responders during the 10-week double-blind phase and during a 3-month double-blind extension phase were randomized to either paroxetine (10, 20, or 40 mg/day) or placebo in a 3-month double-blind relapse prevention phase.

Continued on next page

Product information on these pages is effective as of August 2004. Further information is available at: GlaxoSmithKline, PO Box 13398, Research Triangle Park, NC 27709. 1-888-825-5249. Corporate Web Site: www.gsk.com

Paxil—Cont.

Patients randomized to paroxetine were significantly less likely to relapse than comparably treated patients who were randomized to placebo.

Subgroup analyses did not indicate that there were any differences in treatment outcomes as a function of age or gender.

Social Anxiety Disorder: The effectiveness of PAXIL in the treatment of social anxiety disorder was demonstrated in three 12-week, multicenter, placebo-controlled studies (Studies 1, 2, and 3) of adult outpatients with social anxiety disorder (DSM-IV). In these studies, the effectiveness of PAXIL compared to placebo was evaluated on the basis of (1) the proportion of responders, as defined by a Clinical Global Impression (CGI) Improvement score of 1 (very much improved) or 2 (much improved), and (2) change from baseline in the Liebowitz Social Anxiety Scale (LSAS).

Studies 1 and 2 were flexible-dose studies comparing paroxetine (20 to 50 mg daily) and placebo. Paroxetine demonstrated statistically significant superiority over placebo on both the CGI Improvement responder criterion and the Liebowitz Social Anxiety Scale (LSAS). In Study 1, for patients who completed to week 12, 69% of paroxetine-treated patients compared to 29% of placebo-treated patients were CGI Improvement responders. In Study 2, CGI Improvement responders were 77% and 42% for the paroxetine- and placebo-treated patients, respectively.

Study 3 was a 12-week study comparing fixed paroxetine doses of 20, 40, or 60 mg/day with placebo. Paroxetine 20 mg was demonstrated to be significantly superior to placebo on both the LSAS Total Score and the CGI Improvement responder criterion; there were trends for superiority over placebo for the 40 mg and 60 mg/day dose groups. There was no indication in this study of any additional benefit for doses higher than 20 mg/day.

Subgroup analyses generally did not indicate differences in treatment outcomes as a function of age, race, or gender.

Generalized Anxiety Disorder: The effectiveness of PAXIL in the treatment of Generalized Anxiety Disorder (GAD) was demonstrated in two 8-week, multicenter, placebo-controlled studies (Studies 1 and 2) of adult outpatients with Generalized Anxiety Disorder (DSM-IV).

Study 1 was an 8-week study comparing fixed paroxetine doses of 20 mg or 40 mg/day with placebo. Doses of 20 mg or 40 mg of PAXIL were both demonstrated to be significantly superior to placebo on the Hamilton Rating Scale for Anxiety (HAM-A) total score. There was not sufficient evidence in this study to suggest a greater benefit for the 40 mg/day dose compared to the 20 mg/day dose.

Study 2 was a flexible-dose study comparing paroxetine (20 mg to 50 mg daily) and placebo. PAXIL demonstrated statistically significant superiority over placebo on the Hamilton Rating Scale for Anxiety (HAM-A) total score. A third study, also flexible-dose comparing paroxetine (20 mg to 50 mg daily), did not demonstrate statistically significant superiority of PAXIL over placebo on the Hamilton Rating Scale for Anxiety (HAM-A) total score, the primary outcome.

Subgroup analyses did not indicate differences in treatment outcomes as a function of race or gender. There were insufficient elderly patients to conduct subgroup analyses on the basis of age.

In a longer-term trial, 566 patients meeting DSM-IV criteria for Generalized Anxiety Disorder, who had responded during a single-blind, 8-week acute treatment phase with 20 to 50 mg/day of PAXIL, were randomized to continuation of PAXIL at their same dose, or to placebo, for up to 24 weeks of observation for relapse. Response during the single-blind phase was defined by having a decrease of ≥2 points compared to baseline on the CGI-Severity of Illness scale, to a score of ≤3. Relapse during the double-blind phase was defined as an increase of ≥2 points compared to baseline on the CGI-Severity of Illness scale to a score of ≥4, or withdrawal due to lack of efficacy. Patients receiving continued PAXIL experienced a significantly lower relapse rate over the subsequent 24 weeks compared to those receiving placebo.

Posttraumatic Stress Disorder: The effectiveness of PAXIL in the treatment of Posttraumatic Stress Disorder (PTSD) was demonstrated in two 12-week, multicenter, placebo-controlled studies (Studies 1 and 2) of adult outpatients who met DSM-IV criteria for PTSD. The mean duration of PTSD symptoms for the 2 studies combined was 13 years (ranging from .1 year to 57 years). The percentage of patients with secondary major depressive disorder or non-PTSD anxiety disorders in the combined 2 studies was 41% (356 out of 858 patients) and 40% (345 out of 858 patients), respectively. Study outcome was assessed by (i) the Clinician-Administered PTSD Scale Part 2 (CAPS-2) score and (ii) the Clinical Global Impression-Global Improvement Scale (CGI-I). The CAPS-2 is a multi-item instrument that measures 3 aspects of PTSD with the following symptom clusters: Reexperiencing/intrusion, avoidance/numbing and hyperarousal. The 2 primary outcomes for each trial were (i) change from baseline to endpoint on the CAPS-2 total score (17 items), and (ii) proportion of responders on the CGI-I, where responders were defined as patients having a score of 1 (very much improved) or 2 (much improved).

Study 1 was a 12-week study comparing fixed paroxetine doses of 20 mg or 40 mg/day to placebo. Doses of 20 mg and 40 mg of PAXIL were demonstrated to be significantly superior to placebo on change from baseline for the CAPS-2 total score and on proportion of responders on the CGI-I. There was not sufficient evidence in this study to suggest a greater benefit for the 40 mg/day dose compared to the 20 mg/day dose.

Study 2 was a 12-week flexible-dose study comparing paroxetine (20 to 50 mg daily) to placebo. PAXIL was demonstrated to be significantly superior to placebo on change from baseline for the CAPS-2 total score and on proportion of responders on the CGI-I.

A third study, also a flexible-dose study comparing paroxetine (20 to 50 mg daily) to placebo, demonstrated PAXIL to be significantly superior to placebo on change from baseline for CAPS-2 total score, but not on proportion of responders on the CGI-I.

The majority of patients in these trials were women (68% women: 377 out of 551 subjects in Study 1 and 66% women: 202 out of 303 subjects in Study 2). Subgroup analyses did not indicate differences in treatment outcomes as a function of gender. There were an insufficient number of patients who were 65 years and older or were non-Caucasian to conduct subgroup analyses on the basis of age or race, respectively.

INDICATIONS AND USAGE

Major Depressive Disorder: PAXIL is indicated for the treatment of major depressive disorder.

The efficacy of PAXIL in the treatment of a major depressive episode was established in 6-week controlled trials of outpatients whose diagnoses corresponded most closely to the DSM-III category of major depressive disorder (see CLINICAL PHARMACOLOGY—Clinical Trials). A major depressive episode implies a prominent and relatively persistent depressed or dysphoric mood that usually interferes with daily functioning (nearly every day for at least 2 weeks); it should include at least 4 of the following 8 symptoms: Change in appetite, change in sleep, psychomotor agitation or retardation, loss of interest in usual activities or decrease in sexual drive, increased fatigue, feelings of guilt or worthlessness, slowed thinking or impaired concentration, and a suicide attempt or suicidal ideation.

The effects of PAXIL in hospitalized depressed patients have not been adequately studied.

The efficacy of PAXIL in maintaining a response in major depressive disorder for up to 1 year was demonstrated in a placebo-controlled trial (see CLINICAL PHARMACOLOGY—Clinical Trials). Nevertheless, the physician who elects to use PAXIL for extended periods should periodically re-evaluate the long-term usefulness of the drug for the individual patient.

Obsessive Compulsive Disorder: PAXIL is indicated for the treatment of obsessions and compulsions in patients with obsessive compulsive disorder (OCD) as defined in the DSM-IV. The obsessions or compulsions cause marked distress, are time-consuming, or significantly interfere with social or occupational functioning.

The efficacy of PAXIL was established in two 12-week trials with obsessive compulsive outpatients whose diagnoses corresponded most closely to the DSM-IIIR category of obsessive compulsive disorder (see CLINICAL PHARMACOLOGY—Clinical Trials).

Obsessive compulsive disorder is characterized by recurrent and persistent ideas, thoughts, impulses, or images (obsessions) that are ego-dystonic and/or repetitive, purposeful, and intentional behaviors (compulsions) that are recognized by the person as excessive or unreasonable.

Long-term maintenance of efficacy was demonstrated in a 6-month relapse prevention trial. In this trial, patients assigned to paroxetine showed a lower relapse rate compared to patients on placebo (see CLINICAL PHARMACOLOGY—Clinical Trials). Nevertheless, the physician who elects to use PAXIL for extended periods should periodically re-evaluate the long-term usefulness of the drug for the individual patient (see DOSAGE AND ADMINISTRATION).

Panic Disorder: PAXIL is indicated for the treatment of panic disorder, with or without agoraphobia, as defined in DSM-IV. Panic disorder is characterized by the occurrence of unexpected panic attacks and associated concern about having additional attacks, worry about the implications or consequences of the attacks, and/or a significant change in behavior related to the attacks.

The efficacy of PAXIL was established in three 10- to 12-week trials in panic disorder patients whose diagnoses corresponded to the DSM-IIIR category of panic disorder (see CLINICAL PHARMACOLOGY—Clinical Trials).

Panic disorder (DSM-IV) is characterized by recurrent unexpected panic attacks, i.e., a discrete period of intense fear or discomfort in which 4 (or more) of the following symptoms develop abruptly and reach a peak within 10 minutes: (1) palpitations, pounding heart, or accelerated heart rate; (2) sweating; (3) trembling or shaking; (4) sensations of shortness of breath or smothering; (5) feeling of choking; (6) chest pain or discomfort; (7) nausea or abdominal distress; (8) feeling dizzy, unsteady, lightheaded, or faint; (9) derealization (feelings of unreality) or depersonalization (being detached from oneself); (10) fear of losing control; (11) fear of dying; (12) paresthesias (numbness or tingling sensations); (13) chills or hot flushes.

Long-term maintenance of efficacy was demonstrated in a 3-month relapse prevention trial. In this trial, patients with panic disorder assigned to paroxetine demonstrated a lower relapse rate compared to patients on placebo (see CLINICAL PHARMACOLOGY—Clinical Trials). Nevertheless, the physician who prescribes PAXIL for extended periods should periodically re-evaluate the long-term usefulness of the drug for the individual patient.

Social Anxiety Disorder: PAXIL is indicated for the treatment of social anxiety disorder, also known as social phobia, as defined in DSM-IV (300.23). Social anxiety disorder is characterized by a marked and persistent fear of 1 or more social or performance situations in which the person is exposed to unfamiliar people or to possible scrutiny by others. Exposure to the feared situation almost invariably provokes anxiety, which may approach the intensity of a panic attack. The feared situations are avoided or endured with intense anxiety or distress. The avoidance, anxious anticipation, or distress in the feared situation(s) interferes significantly with the person's normal routine, occupational or academic functioning, or social activities or relationships, or there is marked distress about having the phobias. Lesser degrees of performance anxiety or shyness generally do not require psychopharmacological treatment.

The efficacy of PAXIL was established in three 12-week trials in adult patients with social anxiety disorder (DSM-IV). PAXIL has not been studied in children or adolescents with social phobia (see CLINICAL PHARMACOLOGY—Clinical Trials).

The effectiveness of PAXIL in long-term treatment of social anxiety disorder, i.e., for more than 12 weeks, has not been systematically evaluated in adequate and well-controlled trials. Therefore, the physician who elects to prescribe PAXIL for extended periods should periodically re-evaluate the long-term usefulness of the drug for the individual patient (see DOSAGE AND ADMINISTRATION).

Generalized Anxiety Disorder: PAXIL is indicated for the treatment of Generalized Anxiety Disorder (GAD), as defined in DSM-IV. Anxiety or tension associated with the stress of everyday life usually does not require treatment with an anxiolytic.

The efficacy of PAXIL in the treatment of GAD was established in two 8-week placebo-controlled trials in adults with GAD. PAXIL has not been studied in children or adolescents with Generalized Anxiety Disorder (see CLINICAL PHARMACOLOGY—Clinical Trials).

Generalized Anxiety Disorder (DSM-IV) is characterized by excessive anxiety and worry (apprehensive expectation) that is persistent for at least 6 months and which the person finds difficult to control. It must be associated with at least 3 of the following 6 symptoms: Restlessness or feeling keyed up or on edge, being easily fatigued, difficulty concentrating or mind going blank, irritability, muscle tension, sleep disturbance.

The efficacy of PAXIL in maintaining a response in patients with Generalized Anxiety Disorder, who responded during an 8-week acute treatment phase while taking PAXIL and were then observed for relapse during a period of up to 24 weeks, was demonstrated in a placebo-controlled trial (see CLINICAL PHARMACOLOGY—Clinical Trials). Nevertheless, the physician who elects to use PAXIL for extended periods should periodically re-evaluate the long-term usefulness of the drug for the individual patient (see DOSAGE AND ADMINISTRATION).

Posttraumatic Stress Disorder: PAXIL is indicated for the treatment of Posttraumatic Stress Disorder (PTSD).

The efficacy of PAXIL in the treatment of PTSD was established in two 12-week placebo-controlled trials in adults with PTSD (DSM-IV) (see CLINICAL PHARMACOLOGY—Clinical Trials).

PTSD, as defined by DSM-IV, requires exposure to a traumatic event that involved actual or threatened death or serious injury, or threat to the physical integrity of self or others, and a response that involves intense fear, helplessness, or horror. Symptoms that occur as a result of exposure to the traumatic event include reexperiencing of the event in the form of intrusive thoughts, flashbacks, or dreams, and intense psychological distress and physiological reactivity on exposure to cues to the event; avoidance of situations reminiscent of the traumatic event, inability to recall details of the event, and/or numbing of general responsiveness manifested as diminished interest in significant activities, estrangement from others, restricted range of affect, or sense of foreshortened future; and symptoms of autonomic arousal including hypervigilance, exaggerated startle response, sleep disturbance, impaired concentration, and irritability or outbursts of anger. A PTSD diagnosis requires that the symptoms are present for at least a month and that they cause clinically significant distress or impairment in social, occupational, or other important areas of functioning.

The efficacy of PAXIL in longer-term treatment of PTSD, i.e., for more than 12 weeks, has not been systematically evaluated in placebo-controlled trials. Therefore, the physician who elects to prescribe PAXIL for extended periods should periodically re-evaluate the long-term usefulness of the drug for the individual patient (see DOSAGE AND ADMINISTRATION).

CONTRAINDICATIONS

Concomitant use in patients taking either monoamine oxidase inhibitors (MAOIs) or thioridazine is contraindicated (see WARNINGS and PRECAUTIONS).

PAXIL is contraindicated in patients with a hypersensitivity to paroxetine or any of the inactive ingredients in PAXIL.

WARNINGS

Potential for Interaction With Monoamine Oxidase Inhibitors: In patients receiving another serotonin reuptake inhibitor drug in combination with a monoamine oxidase inhibitor (MAOI), there have been reports of serious, sometimes fatal, reactions including hyperthermia, rigidity, myoclonus, autonomic instability with possible rapid fluc-

tuations of vital signs, and mental status changes that include extreme agitation progressing to delirium and coma. These reactions have also been reported in patients who have recently discontinued that drug and have been started on an MAOI. Some cases presented with features resembling neuroleptic malignant syndrome. While there are no human data showing such an interaction with PAXIL, limited animal data on the effects of combined use of paroxetine and MAOIs suggest that these drugs may act synergistically to elevate blood pressure and evoke behavioral excitation. Therefore, it is recommended that PAXIL not be used in combination with an MAOI, or within 14 days of discontinuing treatment with an MAOI. At least 2 weeks should be allowed after stopping PAXIL before starting an MAOI.

Potential Interaction With Thioridazine: Thioridazine administration alone produces prolongation of the QTc interval, which is associated with serious ventricular arrhythmias, such as torsade de pointes-type arrhythmias, and sudden death. This effect appears to be dose related.

An in vivo study suggests that drugs which inhibit $P_{450}IID_6$, such as paroxetine, will elevate plasma levels of thioridazine. Therefore, it is recommended that paroxetine not be used in combination with thioridazine (see CONTRAINDICATIONS and PRECAUTIONS).

Clinical Worsening and Suicide Risk: Patients with major depressive disorder, both adult and pediatric, may experience worsening of their depression and/or the emergence of suicidal ideation and behavior (suicidality), whether or not they are taking antidepressant medications, and this risk may persist until significant remission occurs. Although there has been a long-standing concern that antidepressants may have a role in inducing worsening of depression and the emergence of suicidality in certain patients, a causal role for antidepressants in inducing such behaviors has not been established. **Nevertheless, patients being treated with antidepressants should be observed closely for clinical worsening and suicidality, especially at the beginning of a course of drug therapy, or at the time of dose changes, either increases or decreases.** Consideration should be given to changing the therapeutic regimen, including possibly discontinuing the medication, in patients whose depression is persistently worse or whose emergent suicidality is severe, abrupt in onset, or was not part of the patient's presenting symptoms.

Because of the possibility of co-morbidity between major depressive disorder and other psychiatric and nonpsychiatric disorders, the same precautions observed when treating patients with major depressive disorder should be observed when treating patients with other psychiatric and nonpsychiatric disorders.

The following symptoms, anxiety, agitation, panic attacks, insomnia, irritability, hostility (aggressiveness), impulsivity, akathisia (psychomotor restlessness), hypomania, and mania, have been reported in adult and pediatric patients being treated with antidepressants for major depressive disorder as well as for other indications, both psychiatric and nonpsychiatric. Although a causal link between the emergence of such symptoms and either the worsening of depression and/or the emergence of suicidal impulses has not been established, consideration should be given to changing the therapeutic regimen, including possibly discontinuing the medication, in patients for whom such symptoms are severe, abrupt in onset, or were not part of the patient's presenting symptoms.

Families and caregivers of patients being treated with antidepressants for major depressive disorder or other indications, both psychiatric and nonpsychiatric, should be alerted about the need to monitor patients for the emergence of agitation, irritability, and the other symptoms described above, as well as the emergence of suicidality, and to report such symptoms immediately to health care providers. Prescriptions for PAXIL should be written for the smallest quantity of tablets consistent with good patient management, in order to reduce the risk of overdose.

If the decision has been made to discontinue treatment, medication should be tapered, as rapidly as is feasible, but with recognition that abrupt discontinuation can be associated with certain symptoms (see PRECAUTIONS and DOSAGE AND ADMINISTRATION—Discontinuation of Treatment With PAXIL, for a description of the risks of discontinuation of PAXIL).

It should be noted that PAXIL is not approved for use in treating any indications in the pediatric population.

A major depressive episode may be the initial presentation of bipolar disorder. It is generally believed (though not established in controlled trials) that treating such an episode with an antidepressant alone may increase the likelihood of precipitation of a mixed/manic episode in patients at risk for bipolar disorder. Whether any of the symptoms described above represent such a conversion is unknown. However, prior to initiating treatment with an antidepressant, patients should be adequately screened to determine if they are at risk for bipolar disorder; such screening should include a detailed psychiatric history, including a family history of suicide, bipolar disorder, and depression. It should be noted that PAXIL is not approved for use in treating bipolar depression.

PRECAUTIONS

General: ***Activation of Mania/Hypomania:*** During premarketing testing, hypomania or mania occurred in approximately 1.0% of unipolar patients treated with PAXIL compared to 1.1% of active-control and 0.3% of placebo-treated unipolar patients. In a subset of patients classified as bipolar, the rate of manic episodes was 2.2% for PAXIL and 11.6% for the combined active-control groups. As with all drugs effective in the treatment of major depressive disorder, PAXIL should be used cautiously in patients with a history of mania.

Seizures: During premarketing testing, seizures occurred in 0.1% of patients treated with PAXIL, a rate similar to that associated with other drugs effective in the treatment of major depressive disorder. PAXIL should be used cautiously in patients with a history of seizures. It should be discontinued in any patient who develops seizures.

Discontinuation of Treatment With PAXIL: Recent clinical trials supporting the various approved indications for PAXIL employed a taper-phase regimen, rather than an abrupt discontinuation of treatment. The taper-phase regimen used in GAD and PTSD clinical trials involved an incremental decrease in the daily dose by 10 mg/day at weekly intervals. When a daily dose of 20 mg/day was reached, patients were continued on this dose for 1 week before treatment was stopped.

With this regimen in those studies, the following adverse events were reported at an incidence of 2% or greater for PAXIL and were at least twice that reported for placebo: Abnormal dreams, paresthesia, and dizziness. In the majority of patients, these events were mild to moderate and were self-limiting and did not require medical intervention.

During marketing of PAXIL and other SSRIs and SNRIs (serotonin and norepinephrine reuptake inhibitors), there have been spontaneous reports of adverse events occurring, upon the discontinuation of these drugs (particularly when abrupt), including the following: Dysphoric mood, irritability, agitation, dizziness, sensory disturbances (e.g., paresthesias such as electric shock sensations), anxiety, confusion, headache, lethargy, emotional lability, insomnia, and hypomania. While these events are generally self-limiting, there have been reports of serious discontinuation symptoms.

Patients should be monitored for these symptoms when discontinuing treatment with PAXIL. A gradual reduction in the dose rather than abrupt cessation is recommended whenever possible. If intolerable symptoms occur following a decrease in the dose or upon discontinuation of treatment, then resuming the previously prescribed dose may be considered. Subsequently, the physician may continue decreasing the dose but at a more gradual rate (see DOSAGE AND ADMINISTRATION).

Hyponatremia: Several cases of hyponatremia have been reported. The hyponatremia appeared to be reversible when PAXIL was discontinued. The majority of these occurrences have been in elderly individuals, some in patients taking diuretics or who were otherwise volume depleted.

Abnormal Bleeding: Published case reports have documented the occurrence of bleeding episodes in patients treated with psychotropic agents that interfere with serotonin reuptake. Subsequent epidemiological studies, both of the case-control and cohort design, have demonstrated an association between use of psychotropic drugs that interfere with serotonin reuptake and the occurrence of upper gastrointestinal bleeding. In 2 studies, concurrent use of a nonsteroidal anti-inflammatory drug (NSAID) or aspirin potentiated the risk of bleeding (see Drug Interactions). Although these studies focused on upper gastrointestinal bleeding, there is no reason to believe that bleeding at other sites may be similarly potentiated. Patients should be cautioned regarding the risk of bleeding associated with the concomitant use of paroxetine with NSAIDs, aspirin, or other drugs that affect coagulation.

Use in Patients With Concomitant Illness: Clinical experience with PAXIL in patients with certain concomitant systemic illness is limited. Caution is advisable in using PAXIL in patients with diseases or conditions that could affect metabolism or hemodynamic responses.

As with other SSRIs, mydriasis has been infrequently reported in premarketing studies with PAXIL. A few cases of acute angle closure glaucoma associated with paroxetine therapy have been reported in the literature. As mydriasis can cause acute angle closure in patients with narrow angle glaucoma, caution should be used when PAXIL is prescribed for patients with narrow angle glaucoma.

PAXIL has not been evaluated or used to any appreciable extent in patients with a recent history of myocardial infarction or unstable heart disease. Patients with these diagnoses were excluded from clinical studies during the product's premarket testing. Evaluation of electrocardiograms of 682 patients who received PAXIL in double-blind, placebo-controlled trials, however, did not indicate that PAXIL is associated with the development of significant ECG abnormalities. Similarly, PAXIL does not cause any clinically important changes in heart rate or blood pressure.

Increased plasma concentrations of paroxetine occur in patients with severe renal impairment (creatinine clearance <30 mL/min.) or severe hepatic impairment. A lower starting dose should be used in such patients (see DOSAGE AND ADMINISTRATION).

Information for Patients: Physicians are advised to discuss the following issues with patients for whom they prescribe PAXIL:

Patients and their families should be encouraged to be alert to the emergence of anxiety, agitation, panic attacks, insomnia, irritability, hostility, impulsivity, akathisia, hypomania, mania, worsening of depression, and suicidal ideation, especially early during antidepressant treatment. Such symptoms should be reported to the patient's physician, especially if they are severe, abrupt in onset, or were not part of the patient's presenting symptoms.

Drugs That Interfere With Hemostasis (NSAIDs, Aspirin, Warfarin, etc.): Patients should be cautioned about the concomitant use of paroxetine and NSAIDs, aspirin, or other drugs that affect coagulation since the combined use of psychotropic drugs that interfere with serotonin reuptake and these agents has been associated with an increased risk of bleeding.

Interference With Cognitive and Motor Performance: Any psychoactive drug may impair judgment, thinking, or motor skills. Although in controlled studies PAXIL has not been shown to impair psychomotor performance, patients should be cautioned about operating hazardous machinery, including automobiles, until they are reasonably certain that therapy with PAXIL does not affect their ability to engage in such activities.

Completing Course of Therapy: While patients may notice improvement with treatment with PAXIL in 1 to 4 weeks, they should be advised to continue therapy as directed.

Concomitant Medication: Patients should be advised to inform their physician if they are taking, or plan to take, any prescription or over-the-counter drugs, since there is a potential for interactions.

Alcohol: Although PAXIL has not been shown to increase the impairment of mental and motor skills caused by alcohol, patients should be advised to avoid alcohol while taking PAXIL.

Pregnancy: Patients should be advised to notify their physician if they become pregnant or intend to become pregnant during therapy.

Nursing: Patients should be advised to notify their physician if they are breast-feeding an infant (see PRECAUTIONS—Nursing Mothers).

Laboratory Tests: There are no specific laboratory tests recommended.

Drug Interactions: ***Tryptophan:*** As with other serotonin reuptake inhibitors, an interaction between paroxetine and tryptophan may occur when they are coadministered. Adverse experiences, consisting primarily of headache, nausea, sweating, and dizziness, have been reported when tryptophan was administered to patients taking PAXIL. Consequently, concomitant use of PAXIL with tryptophan is not recommended.

Monoamine Oxidase Inhibitors: See CONTRAINDICATIONS and WARNINGS.

Thioridazine: See CONTRAINDICATIONS and WARNINGS.

Warfarin: Preliminary data suggest that there may be a pharmacodynamic interaction (that causes an increased bleeding diathesis in the face of unaltered prothrombin time) between paroxetine and warfarin. Since there is little clinical experience, the concomitant administration of PAXIL and warfarin should be undertaken with caution (see *Drugs That Interfere With Hemostasis*).

Sumatriptan: There have been rare postmarketing reports describing patients with weakness, hyperreflexia, and incoordination following the use of a selective serotonin reuptake inhibitor (SSRI) and sumatriptan. If concomitant treatment with sumatriptan and an SSRI (e.g., fluoxetine, fluvoxamine, paroxetine, sertraline) is clinically warranted, appropriate observation of the patient is advised.

Drugs Affecting Hepatic Metabolism: The metabolism and pharmacokinetics of paroxetine may be affected by the induction or inhibition of drug-metabolizing enzymes.

Cimetidine: Cimetidine inhibits many cytochrome P_{450} (oxidative) enzymes. In a study where PAXIL (30 mg once daily) was dosed orally for 4 weeks, steady-state plasma concentrations of paroxetine were increased by approximately 50% during coadministration with oral cimetidine (300 mg three times daily) for the final week. Therefore, when these drugs are administered concurrently, dosage adjustment of PAXIL after the 20-mg starting dose should be guided by clinical effect. The effect of paroxetine on cimetidine's pharmacokinetics was not studied.

Phenobarbital: Phenobarbital induces many cytochrome P_{450} (oxidative) enzymes. When a single oral 30-mg dose of PAXIL was administered at phenobarbital steady state (100 mg once daily for 14 days), paroxetine AUC and $T_{1/2}$ were reduced (by an average of 25% and 38%, respectively) compared to paroxetine administered alone. The effect of paroxetine on phenobarbital pharmacokinetics was not studied. Since PAXIL exhibits nonlinear pharmacokinetics, the results of this study may not address the case where the 2 drugs are both being chronically dosed. No initial dosage adjustment of PAXIL is considered necessary when coadministered with phenobarbital; any subsequent adjustment should be guided by clinical effect.

Phenytoin: When a single oral 30-mg dose of PAXIL was administered at phenytoin steady state (300 mg once daily for 14 days), paroxetine AUC and $T_{1/2}$ were reduced (by an average of 50% and 35%, respectively) compared to PAXIL administered alone. In a separate study, when a single oral 300-mg dose of phenytoin was administered at paroxetine

Continued on next page

Product information on these pages is effective as of August 2004. Further information is available at: GlaxoSmithKline, PO Box 13398, Research Triangle Park, NC 27709. 1-888-825-5249. Corporate Web Site: www.gsk.com

Paxil—Cont.

steady state (30 mg once daily for 14 days), phenytoin AUC was slightly reduced (12% on average) compared to phenytoin administered alone. Since both drugs exhibit nonlinear pharmacokinetics, the above studies may not address the case where the 2 drugs are both being chronically dosed. No initial dosage adjustments are considered necessary when these drugs are coadministered; any subsequent adjustments should be guided by clinical effect (see ADVERSE REACTIONS–Postmarketing Reports).

Drugs Metabolized by Cytochrome P_{450} IID_6: Many drugs, including most drugs effective in the treatment of major depressive disorder (paroxetine, other SSRIs and many tricyclics), are metabolized by the cytochrome P_{450} isozyme $P_{450}IID_6$. Like other agents that are metabolized by $P_{450}IID_6$, paroxetine may significantly inhibit the activity of this isozyme. In most patients (>90%), this $P_{450}IID_6$ isozyme is saturated early during dosing with PAXIL. In 1 study, daily dosing of PAXIL (20 mg once daily) under steady-state conditions increased single dose desipramine (100 mg) C_{max}, AUC, and $T_{1/2}$ by an average of approximately 2-, 5-, and 3-fold, respectively. Concomitant use of PAXIL with other drugs metabolized by cytochrome $P_{450}IID_6$ has not been formally studied but may require lower doses than usually prescribed for either PAXIL or the other drug.

Therefore, coadministration of PAXIL with other drugs that are metabolized by this isozyme, including certain drugs effective in the treatment of major depressive disorder (e.g., nortriptyline, amitriptyline, imipramine, desipramine, and fluoxetine), phenothiazines, risperidone, and Type 1C antiarrhythmics (e.g., propafenone, flecainide, and encainide), or that inhibit this enzyme (e.g., quinidine), should be approached with caution.

However, due to the risk of serious ventricular arrhythmias and sudden death potentially associated with elevated plasma levels of thioridazine, paroxetine and thioridazine should not be coadministered (see CONTRAINDICATIONS and WARNINGS).

At steady state, when the $P_{450}IID_6$ pathway is essentially saturated, paroxetine clearance is governed by alternative P_{450} isozymes that, unlike $P_{450}IID_6$, show no evidence of saturation (see PRECAUTIONS—*Tricyclic Antidepressants*).

Drugs Metabolized by Cytochrome P_{450} $IIIA_4$: An in vivo interaction study involving the coadministration under steady-state conditions of paroxetine and terfenadine, a substrate for cytochrome $P_{450}IIIA_4$, revealed no effect of paroxetine on terfenadine pharmacokinetics. In addition, in vitro studies have shown ketoconazole, a potent inhibitor of $P_{450}IIIA_4$ activity, to be at least 100 times more potent than paroxetine as an inhibitor of the metabolism of several substrates for this enzyme, including terfenadine, astemizole, cisapride, triazolam, and cyclosporine. Based on the assumption that the relationship between paroxetine's in vitro K_i and its lack of effect on terfenadine's in vivo clearance predicts its effect on other $IIIA_4$ substrates, paroxetine's extent of inhibition of $IIIA_4$ activity is not likely to be of clinical significance.

Tricyclic Antidepressants (TCAs): Caution is indicated in the coadministration of tricyclic antidepressants (TCAs) with PAXIL, because paroxetine may inhibit TCA metabolism. Plasma TCA concentrations may need to be monitored, and the dose of TCA may need to be reduced, if a TCA is coadministered with PAXIL (see PRECAUTIONS—*Drugs Metabolized by Cytochrome $P_{450}IID_6$*).

Drugs Highly Bound to Plasma Protein: Because paroxetine is highly bound to plasma protein, administration of PAXIL to a patient taking another drug that is highly protein bound may cause increased free concentrations of the other drug, potentially resulting in adverse events. Conversely, adverse effects could result from displacement of paroxetine by other highly bound drugs.

Drugs That Interfere With Hemostasis (NSAIDs, Aspirin, Warfarin, etc.): Serotonin release by platelets plays an important role in hemostasis. Epidemiological studies of the case-control and cohort design that have demonstrated an association between use of psychotropic drugs that interfere with serotonin reuptake and the occurrence of upper gastrointestinal bleeding have also shown that concurrent use of an NSAID or aspirin potentiated the risk of bleeding. Thus, patients should be cautioned about the use of such drugs concurrently with paroxetine.

Alcohol: Although PAXIL does not increase the impairment of mental and motor skills caused by alcohol, patients should be advised to avoid alcohol while taking PAXIL.

Lithium: A multiple-dose study has shown that there is no pharmacokinetic interaction between PAXIL and lithium carbonate. However, since there is little clinical experience, the concurrent administration of paroxetine and lithium should be undertaken with caution.

Digoxin: The steady-state pharmacokinetics of paroxetine was not altered when administered with digoxin at steady state. Mean digoxin AUC at steady state decreased by 15% in the presence of paroxetine. Since there is little clinical experience, the concurrent administration of paroxetine and digoxin should be undertaken with caution.

Diazepam: Under steady-state conditions, diazepam does not appear to affect paroxetine kinetics. The effects of paroxetine on diazepam were not evaluated.

Procyclidine: Daily oral dosing of PAXIL (30 mg once daily) increased steady-state AUC_{0-24}, C_{max}, and C_{min} values of procyclidine (5 mg oral once daily) by 35%, 37%, and 67%, respectively, compared to procyclidine alone at steady state.

	Major Depressive Disorder		OCD		Panic Disorder		Social Anxiety Disorder		Generalized Anxiety Disorder		PTSD	
	PAXIL	Placebo	PAXIL	Placebo	PAXIL	Placebo	PAXIL	Placebo	PAXIL	Placebo	PAXIL	Placebo
CNS												
Somnolence	2.3%	0.7%	—		1.9%	0.3%	3.4%	0.3%	2.0%	0.2%	2.8%	0.6%
Insomnia	—	—	1.7%	0%	1.3%	0.3%	3.1%	0%			—	—
Agitation	1.1%	0.5%	—								—	—
Tremor	1.1%	0.3%	—				1.7%	0%			1.0%	0.2%
Anxiety	—	—	—				1.1%	0%			—	—
Dizziness	—	—	1.5%	0%			1.9%	0%	1.0%	0.2%	—	—
Gastrointestinal												
Constipation	—		1.1%	0%							—	—
Nausea	3.2%	1.1%	1.9%	0%	3.2%	1.2%	4.0%	0.3%	2.0%	0.2%	2.2%	0.6%
Diarrhea	1.0%	0.3%	—									
Dry mouth	1.0%	0.3%	—								—	—
Vomiting	1.0%	0.3%	—				1.0%	0%			—	—
Flatulence							1.0%	0.3%			—	—
Other												
Asthenia	1.6%	0.4%	1.9%	0.4%			2.5%	0.6%	1.8%	0.2%	1.6%	0.2%
Abnormal ejaculation[1]	1.6%	0%	2.1%	0%			4.9%	0.6%	2.5%	0.5%	—	—
Sweating	1.0%	0.3%	—				1.1%	0%	1.1%	0.2%	—	—
Impotence[1]	—		1.5%	0%							—	—
Libido Decreased							1.0%	0%			—	—

Where numbers are not provided the incidence of the adverse events in patients treated with PAXIL was not >1% or was not greater than or equal to 2 times the incidence of placebo.

1. Incidence corrected for gender.

Table 1. Treatment-Emergent Adverse Experience Incidence in Placebo-Controlled Clinical Trials for Major Depressive Disorder[1]

Body System	Preferred Term	PAXIL (n = 421)	Placebo (n = 421)
Body as a Whole	Headache	18%	17%
	Asthenia	15%	6%
Cardiovascular	Palpitation	3%	1%
	Vasodilation	3%	1%
Dermatologic	Sweating	11%	2%
	Rash	2%	1%
Gastrointestinal	Nausea	26%	9%
	Dry Mouth	18%	12%
	Constipation	14%	9%
	Diarrhea	12%	8%
	Decreased Appetite	6%	2%
	Flatulence	4%	2%
	Oropharynx Disorder[2]	2%	0%
	Dyspepsia	2%	1%
Musculoskeletal	Myopathy	2%	1%
	Myalgia	2%	1%
	Myasthenia	1%	0%
Nervous System	Somnolence	23%	9%
	Dizziness	13%	6%
	Insomnia	13%	6%
	Tremor	8%	2%
	Nervousness	5%	3%
	Anxiety	5%	3%
	Paresthesia	4%	2%
	Libido Decreased	3%	0%
	Drugged Feeling	2%	1%
	Confusion	1%	0%
Respiration	Yawn	4%	0%
Special Senses	Blurred Vision	4%	1%
	Taste Perversion	2%	0%
Urogenital System	Ejaculatory Disturbance[3,4]	13%	0%
	Other Male Genital Disorders[3,5]	10%	0%
	Urinary Frequency	3%	1%
	Urination Disorder[6]	3%	0%
	Female Genital Disorders[3,7]	2%	0%

1. Events reported by at least 1% of patients treated with PAXIL are included, except the following events which had an incidence on placebo ≥ PAXIL: Abdominal pain, agitation, back pain, chest pain, CNS stimulation, fever, increased appetite, myoclonus, pharyngitis, postural hypotension, respiratory disorder (includes mostly "cold symptoms" or "URI"), trauma, and vomiting.
2. Includes mostly "lump in throat" and "tightness in throat."
3. Percentage corrected for gender.
4. Mostly "ejaculatory delay."
5. Includes "anorgasmia," "erectile difficulties," "delayed ejaculation/orgasm," and "sexual dysfunction," and "impotence."
6. Includes mostly "difficulty with micturition" and "urinary hesitancy."
7. Includes mostly "anorgasmia" and "difficulty reaching climax/orgasm."

If anticholinergic effects are seen, the dose of procyclidine should be reduced.

Beta-Blockers: In a study where propranolol (80 mg twice daily) was dosed orally for 18 days, the established steady-state plasma concentrations of propranolol were unaltered during coadministration with PAXIL (30 mg once daily) for the final 10 days. The effects of propranolol on paroxetine have not been evaluated (see ADVERSE REACTIONS—Postmarketing Reports).

Theophylline: Reports of elevated theophylline levels associated with treatment with PAXIL have been reported. While this interaction has not been formally studied, it is recommended that theophylline levels be monitored when these drugs are concurrently administered.

Electroconvulsive Therapy (ECT): There are no clinical studies of the combined use of ECT and PAXIL.

Carcinogenesis, Mutagenesis, Impairment of Fertility:

Carcinogenesis: Two-year carcinogenicity studies were conducted in rodents given paroxetine in the diet at 1, 5, and 25 mg/kg/day (mice) and 1, 5, and 20 mg/kg/day (rats). These doses are up to 2.4 (mouse) and 3.9 (rat) times the maximum recommended human dose (MRHD) for major depressive disorder, social anxiety disorder, GAD and PTSD on a mg/m² basis. Because the MRHD for major depressive disorder is slightly less than that for OCD (50 mg versus 60 mg), the doses used in these carcinogenicity studies were only 2.0 (mouse) and 3.2 (rat) times the MRHD for OCD. There was a significantly greater number of male rats in the high-dose group with reticulum cell sarcomas (1/100, 0/50, 0/50, and 4/50 for control, low-, middle-, and high-dose groups, respectively) and a significantly increased linear trend across dose groups for the occurrence of lymphoreticular tumors in male rats. Female rats were not affected. Although there was a dose-related increase in the number of tumors in mice, there was no drug-related increase in the number of mice with tumors. The relevance of these findings to humans is unknown.

Mutagenesis: Paroxetine produced no genotoxic effects in a battery of 5 in vitro and 2 in vivo assays that included the following: Bacterial mutation assay, mouse lymphoma mutation assay, unscheduled DNA synthesis assay, and tests for cytogenetic aberrations in vivo in mouse bone marrow and in vitro in human lymphocytes and in a dominant lethal test in rats.

Impairment of Fertility: A reduced pregnancy rate was found in reproduction studies in rats at a dose of paroxetine of 15 mg/kg/day, which is 2.9 times the MRHD for major depressive disorder, social anxiety disorder, GAD, and PTSD or 2.4 times the MRHD for OCD on a mg/m^2 basis. Irreversible lesions occurred in the reproductive tract of male rats after dosing in toxicity studies for 2 to 52 weeks. These lesions consisted of vacuolation of epididymal tubular epithelium at 50 mg/kg/day and atrophic changes in the seminiferous tubules of the testes with arrested spermatogenesis at 25 mg/kg/day (9.8 and 4.9 times the MRHD for major depressive disorder, social anxiety disorder, and GAD; 8.2 and 4.1 times the MRHD for OCD and PD on a mg/m^2 basis).

Pregnancy: ***Teratogenic Effects:*** Pregnancy Category C. Reproduction studies were performed at doses up to 50 mg/kg/day in rats and 6 mg/kg/day in rabbits administered during organogenesis. These doses are equivalent to 9.7 (rat) and 2.2 (rabbit) times the maximum recommended human dose (MRHD) for major depressive disorder, social anxiety disorder, GAD, and PTSD (50 mg) and 8.1 (rat) and 1.9 (rabbit) times the MRHD for OCD, on an mg/m^2 basis. These studies have revealed no evidence of teratogenic effects. However, in rats, there was an increase in pup deaths during the first 4 days of lactation when dosing occurred during the last trimester of gestation and continued throughout lactation. This effect occurred at a dose of 1 mg/kg/day or 0.19 times (mg/m^2) the MRHD for major depressive disorder, social anxiety disorder, GAD, and PTSD; and at 0.16 times (mg/m^2) the MRHD for OCD. The no-effect dose for rat pup mortality was not determined. The cause of these deaths is not known. There are no adequate and well-controlled studies in pregnant women. Because animal reproduction studies are not always predictive of human response, this drug should be used during pregnancy only if the potential benefit justifies the potential risk to the fetus.

Nonteratogenic Effects: Neonates exposed to PAXIL and other SSRIs or SNRIs, late in the third trimester have developed complications requiring prolonged hospitalization, respiratory support, and tube feeding. Such complications can arise immediately upon delivery. Reported clinical findings have included respiratory distress, cyanosis, apnea, seizures, temperature instability, feeding difficulty, vomiting, hypoglycemia, hypotonia, hypertonia, hyperreflexia, tremor, jitteriness irritability, and constant crying. These features are consistent with either a direct toxic effect of SSRIs and SNRIs or, possibly, a drug discontinuation syndrome. It should be noted, in some cases, the clinical picture is consistent with serotonin syndrome (see WARNINGS—Potential for Interaction With Monoamine Oxidase Inhibitors). When treating a pregnant woman with paroxetine during the third trimester, the physician should carefully consider the potential risks and benefits of treatment (see DOSAGE AND ADMINISTRATION).

Labor and Delivery: The effect of paroxetine on labor and delivery in humans is unknown.

Nursing Mothers: Like many other drugs, paroxetine is secreted in human milk, and caution should be exercised when PAXIL is administered to a nursing woman.

Pediatric Use: Safety and effectiveness in the pediatric population have not been established (see WARNINGS—Clinical Worsening and Suicide Risk).

Geriatric Use: In worldwide premarketing clinical trials with PAXIL, 17% of patients treated with PAXIL (approximately 700) were 65 years of age or older. Pharmacokinetic studies revealed a decreased clearance in the elderly, and a lower starting dose is recommended; there were, however, no overall differences in the adverse event profile between elderly and younger patients, and effectiveness was similar in younger and older patients (see CLINICAL PHARMACOLOGY and DOSAGE AND ADMINISTRATION).

ADVERSE REACTIONS

Associated With Discontinuation of Treatment: Twenty percent (1,199/6,145) of patients treated with PAXIL in worldwide clinical trials in major depressive disorder and 16.1% (84/522), 11.8% (64/542), 9.4% (44/469), 10.7% (79/735), and 11.7% (79/676) of patients treated with PAXIL in worldwide trials in social anxiety disorder, OCD, panic disorder, GAD, and PTSD, respectively, discontinued treatment due to an adverse event. The most common events (≥1%) associated with discontinuation and considered to be drug related (i.e., those events associated with dropout at a rate approximately twice or greater for PAXIL compared to placebo) included the following:

[See first table at top of previous page]

Commonly Observed Adverse Events: ***Major Depressive Disorder:*** The most commonly observed adverse events associated with the use of paroxetine (incidence of 5% or greater and incidence for PAXIL at least twice that for placebo, derived from Table 1) were: Asthenia, sweating, nausea, decreased appetite, somnolence, dizziness, insomnia, tremor, nervousness, ejaculatory disturbance, and other male genital disorders.

Obsessive Compulsive Disorder: The most commonly observed adverse events associated with the use of paroxetine (incidence of 5% or greater and incidence for PAXIL at least twice that of placebo, derived from Table 2) were: Nausea, dry mouth, decreased appetite, constipation, dizziness, somnolence, tremor, sweating, impotence, and abnormal ejaculation.

Table 2. Treatment-Emergent Adverse Experience Incidence in Placebo-Controlled Clinical Trials for Obsessive Compulsive Disorder, Panic Disorder, and Social Anxiety Disorder[1]

		Obsessive Compulsive Disorder		Panic Disorder		Social Anxiety Disorder	
Body System	**Preferred Term**	**PAXIL (n = 542)**	**Placebo (n = 265)**	**PAXIL (n = 469)**	**Placebo (n = 324)**	**PAXIL (n = 425)**	**Placebo (n = 339)**
Body as a Whole	Asthenia	22%	14%	14%	5%	22%	14%
	Abdominal Pain	—	—	4%	3%	—	—
	Chest Pain	3%	2%	—	—	—	—
	Back Pain	—	—	3%	2%	—	—
	Chills	2%	1%	2%	1%	—	—
	Trauma	—	—	—	—	3%	1%
Cardiovascular	Vasodilation	4%	1%	—	—	—	—
	Palpitation	2%	0%	—	—	—	—
Dermatologic	Sweating	9%	3%	14%	6%	9%	2%
	Rash	3%	2%	—	—	—	—
Gastrointestinal	Nausea	23%	10%	23%	17%	25%	7%
	Dry Mouth	18%	9%	18%	11%	9%	3%
	Constipation	16%	6%	8%	5%	5%	2%
	Diarrhea	10%	10%	12%	7%	9%	6%
	Decreased Appetite	9%	3%	7%	3%	8%	2%
	Dyspepsia	—	—	—	—	4%	2%
	Flatulence	—	—	—	—	4%	2%
	Increased Appetite	4%	3%	2%	1%	—	—
	Vomiting	—	—	—	—	2%	1%
Musculoskeletal	Myalgia	—	—	—	—	4%	3%
Nervous System	Insomnia	24%	13%	18%	10%	21%	16%
	Somnolence	24%	7%	19%	11%	22%	5%
	Dizziness	12%	6%	14%	10%	11%	7%
	Tremor	11%	1%	9%	1%	9%	1%
	Nervousness	9%	8%	—	—	8%	7%
	Libido Decreased	7%	4%	9%	1%	12%	1%
	Agitation	—	—	5%	4%	3%	1%
	Anxiety	—	—	5%	4%	5%	4%
	Abnormal Dreams	4%	1%	—	—	—	—
	Concentration Impaired	3%	2%	—	—	4%	1%
	Depersonalization	3%	0%	—	—	—	—
	Myoclonus	3%	0%	3%	2%	2%	1%
	Amnesia	2%	1%	—	—	—	—
Respiratory System	Rhinitis	—	—	3%	0%	—	—
	Pharyngitis	—	—	—	—	4%	2%
	Yawn	—	—	—	—	5%	1%
Special Senses	Abnormal Vision	4%	2%	—	—	4%	1%
	Taste Perversion	2%	0%	—	—	—	—
Urogenital System	Abnormal Ejaculation[2]	23%	1%	21%	1%	28%	1%
	Dysmenorrhea	—	—	—	—	5%	4%
	Female Genital Disorder[2]	3%	0%	9%	1%	9%	1%
	Impotence[2]	8%	1%	5%	0%	5%	1%
	Urinary Frequency	3%	1%	2%	0%	—	—
	Urination Impaired	3%	0%	—	—	—	—
	Urinary Tract Infection	2%	1%	2%	1%	—	—

1. Events reported by at least 2% of OCD, panic disorder, and social anxiety disorder in patients treated with PAXIL are included, except the following events which had an incidence on placebo ≥PAXIL: [OCD]: Abdominal pain, agitation, anxiety, back pain, cough increased, depression, headache, hyperkinesia, infection, paresthesia, pharyngitis, respiratory disorder, rhinitis, and sinusitis. [panic disorder]: Abnormal dreams, abnormal vision, chest pain, cough increased, depersonalization, depression, dysmenorrhea, dyspepsia, flu syndrome, headache, infection, myalgia, nervousness, palpitation, paresthesia, pharyngitis, rash, respiratory disorder, sinusitis, taste perversion, trauma, urination impaired, and vasodilation. [social anxiety disorder]: Abdominal pain, depression, headache, infection, respiratory disorder, and sinusitis.
2. Percentage corrected for gender.

Panic Disorder: The most commonly observed adverse events associated with the use of paroxetine (incidence of 5% or greater and incidence for PAXIL at least twice that for placebo, derived from Table 2) were: Asthenia, sweating, decreased appetite, libido decreased, tremor, abnormal ejaculation, female genital disorders, and impotence.

Social Anxiety Disorder: The most commonly observed adverse events associated with the use of paroxetine (incidence of 5% or greater and incidence for PAXIL at least twice that for placebo, derived from Table 2) were: Sweating, nausea, dry mouth, constipation, decreased appetite, somnolence, tremor, libido decreased, yawn, abnormal ejaculation, female genital disorders, and impotence.

Generalized Anxiety Disorder: The most commonly observed adverse events associated with the use of paroxetine (incidence of 5% or greater and incidence for PAXIL at least twice that for placebo, derived from Table 3) were: Asthenia, infection, constipation, decreased appetite, dry mouth, nausea, libido decreased, somnolence, tremor, sweating, and abnormal ejaculation.

Posttraumatic Stress Disorder: The most commonly observed adverse events associated with the use of paroxetine (incidence of 5% or greater and incidence for PAXIL at least twice that for placebo, derived from Table 3) were: Asthenia, sweating, nausea, dry mouth, diarrhea, decreased appetite, somnolence, libido decreased, abnormal ejaculation, female genital disorders, and impotence.

Incidence in Controlled Clinical Trials: The prescriber should be aware that the figures in the tables following cannot be used to predict the incidence of side effects in the course of usual medical practice where patient characteristics and other factors differ from those that prevailed in the clinical trials. Similarly, the cited frequencies cannot be compared with figures obtained from other clinical investigations involving different treatments, uses, and investigators. The cited figures, however, do provide the prescribing physician with some basis for estimating the relative contribution of drug and nondrug factors to the side effect incidence rate in the populations studied.

Major Depressive Disorder: Table 1 enumerates adverse events that occurred at an incidence of 1% or more among paroxetine-treated patients who participated in short-term (6-week) placebo-controlled trials in which patients were dosed in a range of 20 mg to 50 mg/day. Reported adverse events were classified using a standard COSTART-based Dictionary terminology.

[See table 1 on previous page]

Obsessive Compulsive Disorder, Panic Disorder, and Social Anxiety Disorder: Table 2 enumerates adverse events that occurred at a frequency of 2% or more among OCD patients on PAXIL who participated in placebo-controlled trials of 12-weeks duration in which patients were dosed in a range of 20 mg to 60 mg/day or among patients with panic disorder on PAXIL who participated in placebo-controlled trials of 10- to 12-weeks duration in which patients were dosed in a range of 10 mg to 60 mg/day or among patients with social anxiety disorder on PAXIL who participated in placebo-controlled trials of 12-weeks duration in which patients were dosed in a range of 20 mg to 50 mg/day.

[See table 2 above]

Generalized Anxiety Disorder and Posttraumatic Stress Disorder: Table 3 enumerates adverse events that occurred at a frequency of 2% or more among GAD patients on PAXIL who participated in placebo-controlled trials of

Continued on next page

Product information on these pages is effective as of August 2004. Further information is available at: GlaxoSmithKline, PO Box 13398, Research Triangle Park, NC 27709. 1-888-825-5249. Corporate Web Site: www.gsk.com

Paxil—Cont.

8-weeks duration in which patients were dosed in a range of 10 mg/day to 50 mg/day or among PTSD patients on PAXIL who participated in placebo-controlled trials of 12-weeks duration in which patients were dosed in a range of 20 mg/day to 50 mg/day.
[See table 3 at right]

Dose Dependency of Adverse Events: A comparison of adverse event rates in a fixed-dose study comparing 10, 20, 30, and 40 mg/day of PAXIL with placebo in the treatment of major depressive disorder revealed a clear dose dependency for some of the more common adverse events associated with use of PAXIL, as shown in the following table:
[See table 4 at right]

In a fixed-dose study comparing placebo and 20, 40, and 60 mg of PAXIL in the treatment of OCD, there was no clear relationship between adverse events and the dose of PAXIL to which patients were assigned. No new adverse events were observed in the group treated with 60 mg of PAXIL compared to any of the other treatment groups.

In a fixed-dose study comparing placebo and 10, 20, and 40 mg of PAXIL in the treatment of panic disorder, there was no clear relationship between adverse events and the dose of PAXIL to which patients were assigned, except for asthenia, dry mouth, anxiety, libido decreased, tremor, and abnormal ejaculation. In flexible-dose studies, no new adverse events were observed in patients receiving 60 mg of PAXIL compared to any of the other treatment groups.

In a fixed-dose study comparing placebo and 20, 40, and 60 mg of PAXIL in the treatment of social anxiety disorder, for most of the adverse events, there was no clear relationship between adverse events and the dose of PAXIL to which patients were assigned.

In a fixed-dose study comparing placebo and 20 and 40 mg of PAXIL in the treatment of generalized anxiety disorder, for most of the adverse events, there was no clear relationship between adverse events and the dose of PAXIL to which patients were assigned, except for the following adverse events: Asthenia, constipation, and abnormal ejaculation.

In a fixed-dose study comparing placebo and 20 and 40 mg of PAXIL in the treatment of posttraumatic stress disorder, for most of the adverse events, there was no clear relationship between adverse events and the dose of PAXIL to which patients were assigned, except for impotence and abnormal ejaculation.

Adaptation to Certain Adverse Events: Over a 4- to 6-week period, there was evidence of adaptation to some adverse events with continued therapy (e.g., nausea and dizziness), but less to other effects (e.g., dry mouth, somnolence, and asthenia).

Male and Female Sexual Dysfunction With SSRIs: Although changes in sexual desire, sexual performance, and sexual satisfaction often occur as manifestations of a psychiatric disorder, they may also be a consequence of pharmacologic treatment. In particular, some evidence suggests that selective serotonin reuptake inhibitors (SSRIs) can cause such untoward sexual experiences.

Reliable estimates of the incidence and severity of untoward experiences involving sexual desire, performance, and satisfaction are difficult to obtain, however, in part because patients and physicians may be reluctant to discuss them. Accordingly, estimates of the incidence of untoward sexual experience and performance cited in product labeling, are likely to underestimate their actual incidence.

In placebo-controlled clinical trials involving more than 3,200 patients, the ranges for the reported incidence of sexual side effects in males and females with major depressive disorder, OCD, panic disorder, social anxiety disorder, GAD, and PTSD are displayed in Table 5.
[See table 5 at right]

There are no adequate and well-controlled studies examining sexual dysfunction with paroxetine treatment.

Paroxetine treatment has been associated with several cases of priapism. In those cases with a known outcome, patients recovered without sequelae.

While it is difficult to know the precise risk of sexual dysfunction associated with the use of SSRIs, physicians should routinely inquire about such possible side effects.

Weight and Vital Sign Changes: Significant weight loss may be an undesirable result of treatment with PAXIL for some patients but, on average, patients in controlled trials had minimal (about 1 pound) weight loss versus smaller changes on placebo and active control. No significant changes in vital signs (systolic and diastolic blood pressure, pulse and temperature) were observed in patients treated with PAXIL in controlled clinical trials.

ECG Changes: In an analysis of ECGs obtained in 682 patients treated with PAXIL and 415 patients treated with placebo in controlled clinical trials, no clinically significant changes were seen in the ECGs of either group.

Liver Function Tests: In placebo-controlled clinical trials, patients treated with PAXIL exhibited abnormal values on liver function tests at no greater rate than that seen in placebo-treated patients. In particular, the PAXIL-versus-placebo comparisons for alkaline phosphatase, SGOT, SGPT, and bilirubin revealed no differences in the percentage of patients with marked abnormalities.

Other Events Observed During the Premarketing Evaluation of PAXIL: During its premarketing assessment in major depressive disorder, multiple doses of PAXIL were administered to 6,145 patients in phase 2 and 3 studies. The conditions and duration of exposure to PAXIL varied greatly and included (in overlapping categories) open and double-blind studies, uncontrolled and controlled studies, inpatient and outpatient studies, and fixed-dose, and titration studies. During premarketing clinical trials in OCD, panic disorder, social anxiety disorder, generalized anxiety disorder, and posttraumatic stress disorder, 542, 469, 522, 735, and 676 patients, respectively, received multiple doses of PAXIL. Untoward events associated with this exposure were recorded by clinical investigators using terminology of their own choosing. Consequently, it is not possible to provide a meaningful estimate of the proportion of individuals experiencing adverse events without first grouping similar types of untoward events into a smaller number of standardized event categories.

In the tabulations that follow, reported adverse events were classified using a standard COSTART-based Dictionary terminology. The frequencies presented, therefore, represent the proportion of the 9,089 patients exposed to multiple doses of PAXIL who experienced an event of the type cited on at least 1 occasion while receiving PAXIL. All reported events are included except those already listed in Tables 1 to 3, those reported in terms so general as to be uninformative and those events where a drug cause was remote. It is important to emphasize that although the events reported occurred during treatment with paroxetine, they were not necessarily caused by it.

Events are further categorized by body system and listed in order of decreasing frequency according to the following definitions: Frequent adverse events are those occurring on

Table 3. Treatment-Emergent Adverse Experience Incidence in Placebo-Controlled Clinical Trials for Generalized Anxiety Disorder and Posttraumatic Stress Disorder[1]

		Generalized Anxiety Disorder		Posttraumatic Stress Disorder	
Body System	**Preferred Term**	**PAXIL (n = 735)**	**Placebo (n = 529)**	**PAXIL (n = 676)**	**Placebo (n = 504)**
Body as a Whole	Asthenia	14%	6%	12%	4%
	Headache	17%	14%	—	—
	Infection	6%	3%	5%	4%
	Abdominal Pain			4%	3%
	Trauma			6%	5%
Cardiovascular	Vasodilation	3%	1%	2%	1%
Dermatologic	Sweating	6%	2%	5%	1%
Gastrointestinal	Nausea	20%	5%	19%	8%
	Dry Mouth	11%	5%	10%	5%
	Constipation	10%	2%	5%	3%
	Diarrhea	9%	7%	11%	5%
	Decreased Appetite	5%	1%	6%	3%
	Vomiting	3%	2%	3%	2%
	Dyspepsia	—	—	5%	3%
Nervous System	Insomnia	11%	8%	12%	11%
	Somnolence	15%	5%	16%	5%
	Dizziness	6%	5%	6%	5%
	Tremor	5%	1%	4%	1%
	Nervousness	4%	3%	—	—
	Libido Decreased	9%	2%	5%	2%
	Abnormal Dreams			3%	2%
Respiratory System	Respiratory Disorder	7%	5%	—	—
	Sinusitis	4%	3%	—	—
	Yawn	4%	—	2%	<1%
Special Senses	Abnormal Vision	2%	1%	3%	1%
Urogenital System	Abnormal Ejaculation[2]	25%	2%	13%	2%
	Female Genital Disorder[2]	4%	1%	5%	1%
	Impotence[2]	4%	3%	9%	1%

1. Events reported by at least 2% of GAD and PTSD in patients treated with PAXIL are included, except the following events which had an incidence on placebo ≥PAXIL [GAD]: Abdominal pain, back pain, trauma, dyspepsia, myalgia, and pharyngitis. [PTSD]: Back pain, headache, anxiety, depression, nervousness, respiratory disorder, pharyngitis, and sinusitis.
2. Percentage corrected for gender.

Table 4. Treatment-Emergent Adverse Experience Incidence in a Dose-Comparison Trial in the Treatment of Major Depressive Disorder*

	Placebo	PAXIL			
Body System/ Preferred Term	**n = 51**	**10 mg n = 102**	**20 mg n = 104**	**30 mg n = 101**	**40 mg n = 102**
Body as a Whole					
Asthenia	0.0%	2.9%	10.6%	13.9%	12.7%
Dermatology					
Sweating	2.0%	1.0%	6.7%	8.9%	11.8%
Gastrointestinal					
Constipation	5.9%	4.9%	7.7%	9.9%	12.7%
Decreased Appetite	2.0%	2.0%	5.8%	4.0%	4.9%
Diarrhea	7.8%	9.8%	19.2%	7.9%	14.7%
Dry Mouth	2.0%	10.8%	18.3%	15.8%	20.6%
Nausea	13.7%	14.7%	26.9%	34.7%	36.3%
Nervous System					
Anxiety	0.0%	2.0%	5.8%	5.9%	5.9%
Dizziness	3.9%	6.9%	6.7%	8.9%	12.7%
Nervousness	0.0%	5.9%	5.8%	4.0%	2.9%
Paresthesia	0.0%	2.9%	1.0%	5.0%	5.9%
Somnolence	7.8%	12.7%	18.3%	20.8%	21.6%
Tremor	0.0%	0.0%	7.7%	7.9%	14.7%
Special Senses					
Blurred Vision	2.0%	2.9%	2.9%	2.0%	7.8%
Urogenital System					
Abnormal Ejaculation	0.0%	5.8%	6.5%	10.6%	13.0%
Impotence	0.0%	1.9%	4.3%	6.4%	1.9%
Male Genital Disorders	0.0%	3.8%	8.7%	6.4%	3.7%

*Rule for including adverse events in table: Incidence at least 5% for 1 of paroxetine groups and ≥ twice the placebo incidence for at least 1 paroxetine group.

Table 5. Incidence of Sexual Adverse Events in Controlled Clinical Trials

	PAXIL	Placebo
n (males)	**1446**	**1042**
Decreased Libido	6-15%	0-5%
Ejaculatory Disturbance	13-28%	0-2%
Impotence	2-9%	0-3%
n (females)	**1822**	**1340**
Decreased Libido	0-9%	0-2%
Orgasmic Disturbance	2-9%	0-1%

1 or more occasions in at least 1/100 patients (only those not already listed in the tabulated results from placebo-controlled trials appear in this listing); infrequent adverse events are those occurring in 1/100 to 1/1,000 patients; rare events are those occurring in fewer than 1/1,000 patients. Events of major clinical importance are also described in the PRECAUTIONS section.

Body as a Whole: *Infrequent:* Allergic reaction, chills, face edema, malaise, neck pain; *rare:* Adrenergic syndrome, cellulitis, moniliasis, neck rigidity, pelvic pain, peritonitis, sepsis, ulcer.

Cardiovascular System: *Frequent:* Hypertension, tachycardia; *infrequent:* Bradycardia, hematoma, hypotension, migraine, syncope; *rare:* Angina pectoris, arrhythmia nodal, atrial fibrillation, bundle branch block, cerebral ischemia, cerebrovascular accident, congestive heart failure, heart block, low cardiac output, myocardial infarct, myocardial ischemia, pallor, phlebitis, pulmonary embolus, supraventricular extrasystoles, thrombophlebitis, thrombosis, varicose vein, vascular headache, ventricular extrasystoles.

Digestive System: *Infrequent:* Bruxism, colitis, dysphagia, eructation, gastritis, gastroenteritis, gingivitis, glossitis, increased salivation, liver function tests abnormal, rectal hemorrhage, ulcerative stomatitis; *rare:* Aphthous stomatitis, bloody diarrhea, bulimia, cardiospasm, cholelithiasis, duodenitis, enteritis, esophagitis, fecal impactions, fecal incontinence, gum hemorrhage, hematemesis, hepatitis, ileitis, ileus, intestinal obstruction, jaundice, melena, mouth ulceration, peptic ulcer, salivary gland enlargement, sialadenitis, stomach ulcer, stomatitis, tongue discoloration, tongue edema, tooth caries.

Endocrine System: *Rare:* Diabetes mellitus, goiter, hyperthyroidism, hypothyroidism, thyroiditis.

Hemic and Lymphatic Systems: *Infrequent:* Anemia, leukopenia, lymphadenopathy, purpura; *rare:* Abnormal erythrocytes, basophilia, bleeding time increased, eosinophilia, hypochromic anemia, iron deficiency anemia, leukocytosis, lymphedema, abnormal lymphocytes, lymphocytosis, microcytic anemia, monocytosis, normocytic anemia, thrombocythemia, thrombocytopenia.

Metabolic and Nutritional: *Frequent:* Weight gain; *infrequent:* Edema, peripheral edema, SGOT increased, SGPT increased, thirst, weight loss; *rare:* Alkaline phosphatase increased, bilirubinemia, BUN increased, creatinine phosphokinase increased, dehydration, gamma globulins increased, gout, hypercalcemia, hypercholesteremia, hyperglycemia, hyperkalemia, hyperphosphatemia, hypocalcemia, hypoglycemia, hypokalemia, hyponatremia, ketosis, lactic dehydrogenase increased, non-protein nitrogen (NPN) increased.

Musculoskeletal System: *Frequent:* Arthralgia; *infrequent:* Arthritis, arthrosis; *rare:* Bursitis, myositis, osteoporosis, generalized spasm, tenosynovitis, tetany.

Nervous System: *Frequent:* Emotional lability, vertigo; *infrequent:* Abnormal thinking, alcohol abuse, ataxia, dystonia, dyskinesia, euphoria, hallucinations, hostility, hypertonia, hypesthesia, hypokinesia, incoordination, lack of emotion, libido increased, manic reaction, neurosis, paralysis, paranoid reaction; *rare:* Abnormal gait, akinesia, antisocial reaction, aphasia, choreoathetosis, circumoral paresthesias, convulsion, delirium, delusions, diplopia, drug dependence, dysarthria, extrapyramidal syndrome, fasciculations, grand mal convulsion, hyperalgesia, hysteria, manic-depressive reaction, meningitis, myelitis, neuralgia, neuropathy, nystagmus, peripheral neuritis, psychotic depression, psychosis, reflexes decreased, reflexes increased, stupor, torticollis, trismus, withdrawal syndrome.

Respiratory System: *Infrequent:* Asthma, bronchitis, dyspnea, epistaxis, hyperventilation, pneumonia, respiratory flu; *rare:* Emphysema, hemoptysis, hiccups, lung fibrosis, pulmonary edema, sputum increased, stridor, voice alteration.

Skin and Appendages: *Frequent:* Pruritus; *infrequent:* Acne, alopecia, contact dermatitis, dry skin, ecchymosis, eczema, herpes simplex, photosensitivity, urticaria; *rare:* Angioedema, erythema nodosum, erythema multiforme, exfoliative dermatitis, fungal dermatitis, furunculosis; herpes zoster, hirsutism, maculopapular rash, seborrhea, skin discoloration, skin hypertrophy, skin ulcer, sweating decreased, vesiculobullous rash.

Special Senses: *Frequent:* Tinnitus; *infrequent:* Abnormality of accommodation, conjunctivitis, ear pain, eye pain, keratoconjunctivitis, mydriasis, otitis media; *rare:* Amblyopia, anisocoria, blepharitis, cataract, conjunctival edema, corneal ulcer, deafness, exophthalmos, eye hemorrhage, glaucoma, hyperacusis, night blindness, otitis externa, parosmia, photophobia, ptosis, retinal hemorrhage, taste loss, visual field defect.

Urogenital System: *Infrequent:* Amenorrhea, breast pain, cystitis, dysuria, hematuria, menorrhagia, nocturia, polyuria, pyuria, urinary incontinence, urinary retention, urinary urgency, vaginitis; *rare:* Abortion, breast atrophy, breast enlargement, endometrial disorder, epididymitis, female lactation, fibrocystic breast, kidney calculus, kidney pain, leukorrhea, mastitis, metrorrhagia, nephritis, oliguria, salpingitis, urethritis, urinary casts, uterine spasm, urolith, vaginal hemorrhage, vaginal moniliasis.

Postmarketing Reports: Voluntary reports of adverse events in patients taking PAXIL that have been received since market introduction and not listed above that may have no causal relationship with the drug include acute pancreatitis, elevated liver function tests (the most severe cases were deaths due to liver necrosis, and grossly elevated transaminases associated with severe liver dysfunction), Guillain-Barré syndrome, toxic epidermal necrolysis, priapism, syndrome of inappropriate ADH secretion, symptoms suggestive of prolactinemia and galactorrhea, neuroleptic malignant syndrome-like events; extrapyramidal symptoms which have included akathisia, bradykinesia, cogwheel rigidity, dystonia, hypertonia, oculogyric crisis which has been associated with concomitant use of pimozide; tremor and trismus; serotonin syndrome, associated in some cases with concomitant use of serotonergic drugs and with drugs which may have impaired metabolism of PAXIL (symptoms have included agitation, confusion, diaphoresis, hallucinations, hyperreflexia, myoclonus, shivering, tachycardia, and tremor), status epilepticus, acute renal failure, pulmonary hypertension, allergic alveolitis, anaphylaxis, eclampsia, laryngismus, optic neuritis, porphyria, ventricular fibrillation, ventricular tachycardia (including torsade de pointes), thrombocytopenia, hemolytic anemia, events related to impaired hematopoiesis (including aplastic anemia, pancytopenia, bone marrow aplasia, and agranulocytosis), and vasculitic syndromes (such as Henoch-Schönlein purpura). There has been a case report of an elevated phenytoin level after 4 weeks of PAXIL and phenytoin coadministration. There has been a case report of severe hypotension when PAXIL was added to chronic metoprolol treatment.

DRUG ABUSE AND DEPENDENCE

Controlled Substance Class: PAXIL is not a controlled substance.

Physical and Psychologic Dependence: PAXIL has not been systematically studied in animals or humans for its potential for abuse, tolerance or physical dependence. While the clinical trials did not reveal any tendency for any drug-seeking behavior, these observations were not systematic and it is not possible to predict on the basis of this limited experience the extent to which a CNS-active drug will be misused, diverted, and/or abused once marketed. Consequently, patients should be evaluated carefully for history of drug abuse, and such patients should be observed closely for signs of misuse or abuse of PAXIL (e.g., development of tolerance, incrementations of dose, drug-seeking behavior).

OVERDOSAGE

Human Experience: Since the introduction of PAXIL in the United States, 342 spontaneous cases of deliberate or accidental overdosage during paroxetine treatment have been reported worldwide (circa 1999). These include overdoses with paroxetine alone and in combination with other substances. Of these, 48 cases were fatal and of the fatalities, 17 appeared to involve paroxetine alone. Eight fatal cases that documented the amount of paroxetine ingested were generally confounded by the ingestion of other drugs or alcohol or the presence of significant comorbid conditions. Of 145 non-fatal cases with known outcome, most recovered without sequelae. The largest known ingestion involved 2,000 mg of paroxetine (33 times the maximum recommended daily dose) in a patient who recovered.

Commonly reported adverse events associated with paroxetine overdosage include somnolence, coma, nausea, tremor, tachycardia, confusion, vomiting, and dizziness. Other notable signs and symptoms observed with overdoses involving paroxetine (alone or with other substances) include mydriasis, convulsions (including status epilepticus), ventricular dysrhythmias (including torsade de pointes), hypertension, aggressive reactions, syncope, hypotension, stupor, bradycardia, dystonia, rhabdomyolysis, symptoms of hepatic dysfunction (including hepatic failure, hepatic necrosis, jaundice, hepatitis, and hepatic steatosis), serotonin syndrome, manic reactions, myoclonus, acute renal failure, and urinary retention.

Overdosage Management: Treatment should consist of those general measures employed in the management of overdosage with any drugs effective in the treatment of major depressive disorder.

Ensure an adequate airway, oxygenation, and ventilation. Monitor cardiac rhythm and vital signs. General supportive and symptomatic measures are also recommended. Induction of emesis is not recommended. Gastric lavage with a large-bore orogastric tube with appropriate airway protection, if needed, may be indicated if performed soon after ingestion, or in symptomatic patients.

Activated charcoal should be administered. Due to the large volume of distribution of this drug, forced diuresis, dialysis, hemoperfusion, and exchange transfusion are unlikely to be of benefit. No specific antidotes for paroxetine are known.

A specific caution involves patients who are taking or have recently taken paroxetine who might ingest excessive quantities of a tricyclic antidepressant. In such a case, accumulation of the parent tricyclic and/or an active metabolite may increase the possibility of clinically significant sequelae and extend the time needed for close medical observation (see PRECAUTIONS—*Drugs Metabolized by Cytochrome $P_{450}IID_6$*).

In managing overdosage, consider the possibility of multiple drug involvement. The physician should consider contacting a poison control center for additional information on the treatment of any overdose. Telephone numbers for certified poison control centers are listed in the *Physicians' Desk Reference* (PDR).

DOSAGE AND ADMINISTRATION

Major Depressive Disorder: ***Usual Initial Dosage:*** PAXIL should be administered as a single daily dose with or without food, usually in the morning. The recommended initial dose is 20 mg/day. Patients were dosed in a range of 20 to 50 mg/day in the clinical trials demonstrating the effectiveness of PAXIL in the treatment of major depressive disorder. As with all drugs effective in the treatment of major depressive disorder, the full effect may be delayed. Some patients not responding to a 20-mg dose may benefit from dose increases, in 10-mg/day increments, up to a maximum of 50 mg/day. Dose changes should occur at intervals of at least 1 week.

Maintenance Therapy: There is no body of evidence available to answer the question of how long the patient treated with PAXIL should remain on it. It is generally agreed that acute episodes of major depressive disorder require several months or longer of sustained pharmacologic therapy. Whether the dose needed to induce remission is identical to the dose needed to maintain and/or sustain euthymia is unknown.

Systematic evaluation of the efficacy of PAXIL has shown that efficacy is maintained for periods of up to 1 year with doses that averaged about 30 mg.

Obsessive Compulsive Disorder: ***Usual Initial Dosage:*** PAXIL should be administered as a single daily dose with or without food, usually in the morning. The recommended dose of PAXIL in the treatment of OCD is 40 mg daily. Patients should be started on 20 mg/day and the dose can be increased in 10-mg/day increments. Dose changes should occur at intervals of at least 1 week. Patients were dosed in a range of 20 to 60 mg/day in the clinical trials demonstrating the effectiveness of PAXIL in the treatment of OCD. The maximum dosage should not exceed 60 mg/day.

Maintenance Therapy: Long-term maintenance of efficacy was demonstrated in a 6-month relapse prevention trial. In this trial, patients with OCD assigned to paroxetine demonstrated a lower relapse rate compared to patients on placebo (see CLINICAL PHARMACOLOGY—Clinical Trials). OCD is a chronic condition, and it is reasonable to consider continuation for a responding patient. Dosage adjustments should be made to maintain the patient on the lowest effective dosage, and patients should be periodically reassessed to determine the need for continued treatment.

Panic Disorder: ***Usual Initial Dosage:*** PAXIL should be administered as a single daily dose with or without food, usually in the morning. The target dose of PAXIL in the treatment of panic disorder is 40 mg/day. Patients should be started on 10 mg/day. Dose changes should occur in 10-mg/day increments and at intervals of at least 1 week. Patients were dosed in a range of 10 to 60 mg/day in the clinical trials demonstrating the effectiveness of PAXIL. The maximum dosage should not exceed 60 mg/day.

Maintenance Therapy: Long-term maintenance of efficacy was demonstrated in a 3-month relapse prevention trial. In this trial, patients with panic disorder assigned to paroxetine demonstrated a lower relapse rate compared to patients on placebo (see CLINICAL PHARMACOLOGY—Clinical Trials). Panic disorder is a chronic condition, and it is reasonable to consider continuation for a responding patient. Dosage adjustments should be made to maintain the patient on the lowest effective dosage, and patients should be periodically reassessed to determine the need for continued treatment.

Social Anxiety Disorder: ***Usual Initial Dosage:*** PAXIL should be administered as a single daily dose with or without food, usually in the morning. The recommended and initial dosage is 20 mg/day. In clinical trials the effectiveness of PAXIL was demonstrated in patients dosed in a range of 20 to 60 mg/day. While the safety of PAXIL has been evaluated in patients with social anxiety disorder at doses up to 60 mg/day, available information does not suggest any additional benefit for doses above 20 mg/day. (see CLINICAL PHARMACOLOGY—Clinical Trials).

Maintenance Therapy: There is no body of evidence available to answer the question of how long the patient treated with PAXIL should remain on it. Although the efficacy of PAXIL beyond 12 weeks of dosing has not been demonstrated in controlled clinical trials, social anxiety disorder is recognized as a chronic condition, and it is reasonable to consider continuation of treatment for a responding patient. Dosage adjustments should be made to maintain the patient on the lowest effective dosage, and patients should be periodically reassessed to determine the need for continued treatment.

Generalized Anxiety Disorder: ***Usual Initial Dosage:*** PAXIL should be administered as a single daily dose with or without food, usually in the morning. In clinical trials the effectiveness of PAXIL was demonstrated in patients dosed in a range of 20 to 50 mg/day. The recommended starting dosage and the established effective dosage is 20 mg/day. There is not sufficient evidence to suggest a greater benefit to doses higher than 20 mg/day. Dose changes should occur in 10 mg/day increments and at intervals of at least 1 week.

Maintenance Therapy: Systematic evaluation of continuing PAXIL for periods of up to 24 weeks in patients with Generalized Anxiety Disorder who had responded while taking PAXIL during an 8-week acute treatment phase has demonstrated a benefit of such maintenance (see CLINICAL PHARMACOLOGY—Clinical Trials). Nevertheless, patients should be periodically reassessed to determine the need for maintenance treatment.

Posttraumatic Stress Disorder: ***Usual Initial Dosage:*** PAXIL should be administered as a single daily dose with or

Continued on next page

Product information on these pages is effective as of August 2004. Further information is available at: GlaxoSmithKline, PO Box 13398, Research Triangle Park, NC 27709. 1-888-825-5249. Corporate Web Site: www.gsk.com

Paxil—Cont.

without food, usually in the morning. The recommended starting dosage and the established effective dosage is 20 mg/day. In 1 clinical trial, the effectiveness of PAXIL was demonstrated in patients dosed in a range of 20 to 50 mg/day. However, in a fixed dose study, there was not sufficient evidence to suggest a greater benefit for a dose of 40 mg/day compared to 20 mg/day. Dose changes, if indicated, should occur in 10 mg/day increments and at intervals of at least 1 week.

Maintenance Therapy: There is no body of evidence available to answer the question of how long the patient treated with PAXIL should remain on it. Although the efficacy of PAXIL beyond 12 weeks of dosing has not been demonstrated in controlled clinical trials, PTSD is recognized as a chronic condition, and it is reasonable to consider continuation of treatment for a responding patient. Dosage adjustments should be made to maintain the patient on the lowest effective dosage, and patients should be periodically reassessed to determine the need for continued treatment.

Special Populations: ***Treatment of Pregnant Women During the Third Trimester:*** Neonates exposed to PAXIL and other SSRIs or SNRIs, late in the third trimester have developed complications requiring prolonged hospitalization, respiratory support, and tube feeding (see PRECAUTIONS). When treating pregnant women with paroxetine during the third trimester, the physician should carefully consider the potential risks and benefits of treatment. The physician may consider tapering paroxetine in the third trimester.

Dosage for Elderly or Debilitated Patients, and Patients With Severe Renal or Hepatic Impairment: The recommended initial dose is 10 mg/day for elderly patients, debilitated patients, and/or patients with severe renal or hepatic impairment. Increases may be made if indicated. Dosage should not exceed 40 mg/day.

Switching Patients to or From a Monoamine Oxidase Inhibitor: At least 14 days should elapse between discontinuation of an MAOI and initiation of therapy with PAXIL. Similarly, at least 14 days should be allowed after stopping PAXIL before starting an MAOI.

Discontinuation of Treatment With PAXIL: Symptoms associated with discontinuation of PAXIL have been reported (see PRECAUTIONS). Patients should be monitored for these symptoms when discontinuing treatment, regardless of the indication for which PAXIL is being prescribed. A gradual reduction in the dose rather than abrupt cessation is recommended whenever possible. If intolerable symptoms occur following a decrease in the dose or upon discontinuation of treatment, then resuming the previously prescribed dose may be considered. Subsequently, the physician may continue decreasing the dose but at a more gradual rate.

NOTE: SHAKE SUSPENSION WELL BEFORE USING.

HOW SUPPLIED

Tablets: Film-coated, modified-oval as follows:

10-mg yellow, scored tablets engraved on the front with PAXIL and on the back with 10.
NDC 0029-3210-13 Bottles of 30

20-mg pink, scored tablets engraved on the front with PAXIL and on the back with 20.
NDC 0029-3211-13 Bottles of 30
NDC 0029-3211-20 Bottles of 100
NDC 0029-3211-21 SUP 100's (intended for institutional use only)

30-mg blue tablets engraved on the front with PAXIL and on the back with 30.
NDC 0029-3212-13 Bottles of 30

40-mg green tablets engraved on the front with PAXIL and on the back with 40.
NDC 0029-3213-13 Bottles of 30

Store tablets between 15° and 30°C (59° and 86°F).

Oral Suspension: Orange-colored, orange-flavored, 10 mg/5 mL, in 250 mL white bottles.
NDC 0029-3215-48

Store suspension at or below 25°C (77°F).

PAXIL is a registered trademark of GlaxoSmithKline.
GlaxoSmithKline, Research Triangle Park, NC 27709

April 2004/PX:L31

Shown in Product Identification Guide, page 317

PAXIL CR™ ℞

[pax' il]
(paroxetine hydrochloride)
Controlled-Release Tablets

DESCRIPTION

PAXIL CR (paroxetine hydrochloride) is an orally administered psychotropic drug with a chemical structure unrelated to other selective serotonin reuptake inhibitors or to tricyclic, tetracyclic, or other available antidepressant or antipanic agents. It is the hydrochloride salt of a phenylpiperidine compound identified chemically as (-)-*trans*-4*R*-(4'-fluorophenyl)-3*S*-[(3',4'-methylenedioxyphenoxy) methyl] piperidine hydrochloride hemihydrate and has the empirical formula of $C_{19}H_{20}FNO_3$•HCl•1/2H_2O. The molecular weight is 374.8 (329.4 as free base).

Paroxetine hydrochloride is an odorless, off-white powder, having a melting point range of 120° to 138°C and a solubility of 5.4 mg/mL in water.

Each enteric, film-coated, controlled-release tablet contains paroxetine hydrochloride equivalent to paroxetine as follows: 12.5 mg–yellow, 25 mg–pink, 37.5 mg–blue. One layer of the tablet consists of a degradable barrier layer and the other contains the active material in a hydrophilic matrix. Inactive ingredients consist of hypromellose, polyvinylpyrrolidone, lactose monohydrate, magnesium stearate, colloidal silicon dioxide, glyceryl behenate, methacrylic acid copolymer type C, sodium lauryl sulfate, polysorbate 80, talc, triethyl citrate, and 1 or more of the following colorants: Yellow ferric oxide, red ferric oxide, D&C Red No. 30, D&C Yellow No. 6, D&C Yellow No. 10, FD&C Blue No. 2.

CLINICAL PHARMACOLOGY

Pharmacodynamics: The efficacy of paroxetine in the treatment of major depressive disorder, panic disorder, social anxiety disorder, and premenstrual dysphoric disorder (PMDD) is presumed to be linked to potentiation of serotonergic activity in the central nervous system resulting from inhibition of neuronal reuptake of serotonin (5-hydroxytryptamine, 5-HT). Studies at clinically relevant doses in humans have demonstrated that paroxetine blocks the uptake of serotonin into human platelets. In vitro studies in animals also suggest that paroxetine is a potent and highly selective inhibitor of neuronal serotonin reuptake and has only very weak effects on norepinephrine and dopamine neuronal reuptake. In vitro radioligand binding studies indicate that paroxetine has little affinity for muscarinic, $alpha_1$-, $alpha_2$-, beta-adrenergic-, dopamine (D_2)-, 5-HT_1-, 5-HT_2-, and histamine (H_1)-receptors; antagonism of muscarinic, histaminergic, and $alpha_1$-adrenergic receptors has been associated with various anticholinergic, sedative, and cardiovascular effects for other psychotropic drugs.

Because the relative potencies of paroxetine's major metabolites are at most 1/50 of the parent compound, they are essentially inactive.

Pharmacokinetics: Tablets of PAXIL CR contain a degradable polymeric matrix (GEOMATRIX™) designed to control the dissolution rate of paroxetine over a period of approximately 4 to 5 hours. In addition to controlling the rate of drug release in vivo, an enteric coat delays the start of drug release until tablets of PAXIL CR have left the stomach.

Paroxetine hydrochloride is completely absorbed after oral dosing of a solution of the hydrochloride salt. In a study in which normal male and female subjects (n = 23) received single oral doses of PAXIL CR at 4 dosage strengths (12.5 mg, 25 mg, 37.5 mg, and 50 mg), paroxetine C_{max} and AUC_{0-inf} increased disproportionately with dose (as seen also with immediate-release formulations). Mean C_{max} and AUC_{0-inf} values at these doses were 2.0, 5.5, 9.0, and 12.5 ng/mL, and 121, 261, 338, and 540 ng•hr./mL, respectively. T_{max} was observed typically between 6 and 10 hours post-dose, reflecting a reduction in absorption rate compared with immediate-release formulations. The mean elimination half-life of paroxetine was 15 to 20 hours throughout this range of single doses of PAXIL CR. The bioavailability of 25 mg PAXIL CR is not affected by food.

During repeated administration of PAXIL CR (25 mg once daily), steady state was reached within 2 weeks (i.e., comparable to immediate-release formulations). In a repeat-dose study in which normal male and female subjects (n = 23) received PAXIL CR (25 mg daily), mean steady state C_{max}, C_{min}, and AUC_{0-24} values were 30 ng/mL, 20 ng/mL, and 550 ng•hr./mL, respectively.

Based on studies using immediate-release formulations, steady-state drug exposure based on AUC_{0-24} was several-fold greater than would have been predicted from single-dose data. The excess accumulation is a consequence of the fact that 1 of the enzymes that metabolizes paroxetine is readily saturable.

In steady-state dose proportionality studies involving elderly and nonelderly patients, at doses of the immediate-release formulation of 20 mg to 40 mg daily for the elderly and 20 mg to 50 mg daily for the nonelderly, some nonlinearity was observed in both populations, again reflecting a saturable metabolic pathway. In comparison to C_{min} values after 20 mg daily, values after 40 mg daily were only about 2 to 3 times greater than doubled.

Paroxetine is extensively metabolized after oral administration. The principal metabolites are polar and conjugated products of oxidation and methylation, which are readily cleared. Conjugates with glucuronic acid and sulfate predominate, and major metabolites have been isolated and identified. Data indicate that the metabolites have no more than 1/50 the potency of the parent compound at inhibiting serotonin uptake. The metabolism of paroxetine is accomplished in part by cytochrome $P_{450}IID_6$. Saturation of this enzyme at clinical doses appears to account for the nonlinearity of paroxetine kinetics with increasing dose and increasing duration of treatment. The role of this enzyme in paroxetine metabolism also suggests potential drug-drug interactions (see PRECAUTIONS).

Approximately 64% of a 30-mg oral solution dose of paroxetine was excreted in the urine with 2% as the parent compound and 62% as metabolites over a 10-day post-dosing period. About 36% was excreted in the feces (probably via the bile), mostly as metabolites and less than 1% as the parent compound over the 10-day post-dosing period.

Distribution: Paroxetine distributes throughout the body, including the CNS, with only 1% remaining in the plasma.

Protein Binding: Approximately 95% and 93% of paroxetine is bound to plasma protein at 100 ng/mL and 400 ng/mL, respectively. Under clinical conditions, paroxetine concentrations would normally be less than 400 ng/mL. Paroxetine does not alter the in vitro protein binding of phenytoin or warfarin.

Renal and Liver Disease: Increased plasma concentrations of paroxetine occur in subjects with renal and hepatic impairment. The mean plasma concentrations in patients with creatinine clearance below 30 mL/min. was approximately 4 times greater than seen in normal volunteers. Patients with creatinine clearance of 30 to 60 mL/min. and patients with hepatic functional impairment had about a 2-fold increase in plasma concentrations (AUC, C_{max}).

The initial dosage should therefore be reduced in patients with severe renal or hepatic impairment, and upward titration, if necessary, should be at increased intervals (see DOSAGE AND ADMINISTRATION).

Elderly Patients: In a multiple-dose study in the elderly at daily doses of 20, 30, and 40 mg of the immediate-release formulation, C_{min} concentrations were about 70% to 80% greater than the respective C_{min} concentrations in nonelderly subjects. Therefore the initial dosage in the elderly should be reduced (see DOSAGE AND ADMINISTRATION).

Clinical Trials

Major Depressive Disorder: The efficacy of PAXIL CR controlled-release tablets as a treatment for major depressive disorder has been established in two 12-week, flexible-dose, placebo-controlled studies of patients with DSM-IV Major Depressive Disorder. One study included patients in the age range 18 to 65 years, and a second study included elderly patients, ranging in age from 60 to 88. In both studies, PAXIL CR was shown to be significantly more effective than placebo in treating major depressive disorder as measured by the following: Hamilton Depression Rating Scale (HDRS), the Hamilton depressed mood item, and the Clinical Global Impression (CGI)–Severity of Illness score.

A study of outpatients with major depressive disorder who had responded to immediate-release paroxetine tablets (HDRS total score <8) during an initial 8-week open-treatment phase and were then randomized to continuation on immediate-release paroxetine tablets or placebo for 1 year demonstrated a significantly lower relapse rate for patients taking immediate-release paroxetine tablets (15%) compared to those on placebo (39%). Effectiveness was similar for male and female patients.

Panic Disorder: The effectiveness of PAXIL CR in the treatment of panic disorder was evaluated in three 10-week, multicenter, flexible-dose studies (Studies 1, 2, and 3) comparing paroxetine controlled-release (12.5 to 75 mg daily) to placebo in adult outpatients who had panic disorder (DSM-IV), with or without agoraphobia. These trials were assessed on the basis of their outcomes on 3 variables: (1) the proportions of patients free of full panic attacks at endpoint; (2) change from baseline to endpoint in the median number of full panic attacks; and (3) change from baseline to endpoint in the median Clinical Global Impression Severity score. For Studies 1 and 2, PAXIL CR was consistently superior to placebo on 2 of these 3 variables. Study 3 failed to consistently demonstrate a significant difference between PAXIL CR and placebo on any of these variables.

For all 3 studies, the mean dose of PAXIL CR for completers at endpoint was approximately 50 mg/day. Subgroup analyses did not indicate that there were any differences in treatment outcomes as a function of age or gender.

Long-term maintenance effects of the immediate-release formulation of paroxetine in panic disorder were demonstrated in an extension study. Patients who were responders during a 10-week double-blind phase with immediate-release paroxetine and during a 3-month double-blind extension phase were randomized to either immediate-release paroxetine or placebo in a 3-month double-blind relapse prevention phase. Patients randomized to paroxetine were significantly less likely to relapse than comparably treated patients who were randomized to placebo.

Social Anxiety Disorder: The efficacy of PAXIL CR as a treatment for social anxiety disorder has been established, in part, on the basis of extrapolation from the established effectiveness of the immediate-release formulation of paroxetine. In addition, the effectiveness of PAXIL CR in the treatment of social anxiety disorder was demonstrated in a 12-week, multicenter, double-blind, flexible-dose, placebo-controlled study of adult outpatients with a primary diagnosis of social anxiety disorder (DSM-IV). In the study, the effectiveness of PAXIL CR (12.5 to 37.5 mg daily) compared to placebo was evaluated on the basis of (1) change from baseline in the Liebowitz Social Anxiety Scale (LSAS) total score and (2) the proportion of responders who scored 1 or 2 (very much improved or much improved) on the Clinical Global Impression (CGI) Global Improvement score.

PAXIL CR demonstrated statistically significant superiority over placebo on both the LSAS total score and the CGI Improvement responder criterion. For patients who completed the trial, 64% of patients treated with PAXIL CR compared to 34.7% of patients treated with placebo were CGI Improvement responders.

Subgroup analyses did not indicate that there were any differences in treatment outcomes as a function of gender. Subgroup analyses of studies utilizing the immediate-release formulation of paroxetine generally did not indicate differences in treatment outcomes as a function of age, race, or gender.

Premenstrual Dysphoric Disorder: The effectiveness of PAXIL CR for the treatment of PMDD utilizing a continuous dosing regimen has been established in 2 placebo-controlled trials. Patients in these trials met DSM-IV criteria for PMDD. In a pool of 1,030 patients, treated with daily doses of PAXIL CR 12.5 or 25 mg/day, or placebo the mean duration of the PMDD symptoms was approximately 11 ± 7 years. Patients on systemic hormonal contraceptives were excluded from these trials. Therefore, the efficacy of PAXIL CR in combination with systemic (including oral) hormonal contraceptives for the continuous daily treatment of PMDD is unknown. In both positive studies, patients (N = 672) were treated with 12.5 mg/day or 25 mg/day of PAXIL CR or placebo continuously throughout the menstrual cycle for a period of 3 menstrual cycles. The VAS-Total score is a patient-rated instrument that mirrors the diagnostic criteria of PMDD as identified in the DSM-IV, and includes assessments for mood, physical symptoms, and other symptoms. 12.5 mg/day and 25 mg/day of PAXIL CR were significantly more effective than placebo as measured by change from baseline to the endpoint on the luteal phase VAS-Total score.

In a third study employing intermittent dosing, patients (N = 366) were treated for the 2 weeks prior to the onset of menses (luteal phase dosing, also known as intermittent dosing) with 12.5 mg/day or 25 mg/day of PAXIL CR or placebo for a period of 3 months. 12.5 mg/day and 25 mg/day of PAXIL CR, as luteal phase dosing, was significantly more effective than placebo as measured by change from baseline luteal phase VAS total score.

There is insufficient information to determine the effect of race or age on outcome in these studies.

INDICATIONS AND USAGE

Major Depressive Disorder: PAXIL CR is indicated for the treatment of major depressive disorder.

The efficacy of PAXIL CR in the treatment of a major depressive episode was established in two 12-week controlled trials of outpatients whose diagnoses corresponded to the DSM-IV category of major depressive disorder (see CLINICAL PHARMACOLOGY—Clinical Trials).

A major depressive episode (DSM-IV) implies a prominent and relatively persistent (nearly every day for at least 2 weeks) depressed mood or loss of interest or pleasure in nearly all activities, representing a change from previous functioning, and includes the presence of at least 5 of the following 9 symptoms during the same 2-week period: Depressed mood, markedly diminished interest or pleasure in usual activities, significant change in weight and/or appetite, insomnia or hypersomnia, psychomotor agitation or retardation, increased fatigue, feelings of guilt or worthlessness, slowed thinking or impaired concentration, a suicide attempt, or suicidal ideation.

The antidepressant action of paroxetine in hospitalized depressed patients has not been adequately studied.

PAXIL CR has not been systematically evaluated beyond 12 weeks in controlled clinical trials; however, the effectiveness of immediate-release paroxetine hydrochloride in maintaining a response in major depressive disorder for up to 1 year has been demonstrated in a placebo-controlled trial (see CLINICAL PHARMACOLOGY—Clinical Trials). The physician who elects to use PAXIL CR for extended periods should periodically re-evaluate the long-term usefulness of the drug for the individual patient.

Panic Disorder: PAXIL CR is indicated for the treatment of panic disorder, with or without agoraphobia, as defined in DSM-IV. Panic disorder is characterized by the occurrence of unexpected panic attacks and associated concern about having additional attacks, worry about the implications or consequences of the attacks, and/or a significant change in behavior related to the attacks.

The efficacy of Paxil CR controlled-release tablets was established in two 10-week trials in panic disorder patients whose diagnoses corresponded to the DSM-IV category of panic disorder (see CLINICAL PHARMACOLOGY—Clinical Trials).

Panic disorder (DSM-IV) is characterized by recurrent unexpected panic attacks, i.e., a discrete period of intense fear or discomfort in which 4 (or more) of the following symptoms develop abruptly and reach a peak within 10 minutes: (1) palpitations, pounding heart, or accelerated heart rate; (2) sweating; (3) trembling or shaking; (4) sensations of shortness of breath or smothering; (5) feeling of choking; (6) chest pain or discomfort; (7) nausea or abdominal distress; (8) feeling dizzy, unsteady, lightheaded, or faint; (9) derealization (feelings of unreality) or depersonalization (being detached from oneself); (10) fear of losing control; (11) fear of dying; (12) paresthesias (numbness or tingling sensations); (13) chills or hot flushes.

Long-term maintenance of efficacy with the immediate-release formulation of paroxetine was demonstrated in a 3-month relapse prevention trial. In this trial, patients with panic disorder assigned to immediate-release paroxetine demonstrated a lower relapse rate compared to patients on placebo (see CLINICAL PHARMACOLOGY—Clinical Trials). Nevertheless, the physician who prescribes PAXIL CR for extended periods should periodically re-evaluate the long-term usefulness of the drug for the individual patient.

Social Anxiety Disorder: PAXIL CR is indicated for the treatment of social anxiety disorder, also known as social phobia, as defined in DSM-IV (300.23). Social anxiety disorder is characterized by a marked and persistent fear of 1 or more social or performance situations in which the person is exposed to unfamiliar people or to possible scrutiny by others. Exposure to the feared situation almost invariably provokes anxiety, which may approach the intensity of a panic attack. The feared situations are avoided or endured with intense anxiety or distress. The avoidance, anxious anticipation, or distress in the feared situation(s) interferes significantly with the person's normal routine, occupational or academic functioning, or social activities or relationships, or there is marked distress about having the phobias. Lesser degrees of performance anxiety or shyness generally do not require psychopharmacological treatment.

The efficacy of PAXIL CR as a treatment for social anxiety disorder has been established, in part, on the basis of extrapolation from the established effectiveness of the immediate-release formulation of paroxetine. In addition, the efficacy of PAXIL CR was established in a 12-week trial, in adult outpatients with social anxiety disorder (DSM-IV). PAXIL CR has not been studied in children or adolescents with social phobia (see CLINICAL PHARMACOLOGY—Clinical Trials).

The effectiveness of PAXIL CR in long-term treatment of social anxiety disorder, i.e., for more than 12 weeks, has not been systematically evaluated in adequate and well-controlled trials. Therefore, the physician who elects to prescribe PAXIL CR for extended periods should periodically re-evaluate the long-term usefulness of the drug for the individual patient (see DOSAGE AND ADMINISTRATION).

Premenstrual Dysphoric Disorder: PAXIL CR is indicated for the treatment of PMDD.

The efficacy of PAXIL CR in the treatment of PMDD has been established in 3 placebo-controlled trials (see CLINICAL PHARMACOLOGY—Clinical Trials).

The essential features of PMDD, according to DSM-IV, include markedly depressed mood, anxiety or tension, affective lability, and persistent anger or irritability. Other features include decreased interest in usual activities, difficulty concentrating, lack of energy, change in appetite or sleep, and feeling out of control. Physical symptoms associated with PMDD include breast tenderness, headache, joint and muscle pain, bloating, and weight gain. These symptoms occur regularly during the luteal phase and remit within a few days following the onset of menses; the disturbance markedly interferes with work or school or with usual social activities and relationships with others. In making the diagnosis, care should be taken to rule out other cyclical mood disorders that may be exacerbated by treatment with an antidepressant.

The effectiveness of PAXIL CR in long-term use, that is, for more than 3 menstrual cycles, has not been systematically evaluated in controlled trials. Therefore, the physician who elects to use PAXIL CR for extended periods should periodically re-evaluate the long-term usefulness of the drug for the individual patient.

CONTRAINDICATIONS

Concomitant use in patients taking either monoamine oxidase inhibitors (MAOIs) or thioridazine is contraindicated (see WARNINGS and PRECAUTIONS).

PAXIL CR is contraindicated in patients with a hypersensitivity to paroxetine or to any of the inactive ingredients in PAXIL CR.

WARNINGS

Potential for Interaction With Monoamine Oxidase Inhibitors: In patients receiving another serotonin reuptake inhibitor drug in combination with an MAOI, there have been reports of serious, sometimes fatal, reactions including hyperthermia, rigidity, myoclonus, autonomic instability with possible rapid fluctuations of vital signs, and mental status changes that include extreme agitation progressing to delirium and coma. These reactions have also been reported in patients who have recently discontinued that drug and have been started on an MAOI. Some cases presented with features resembling neuroleptic malignant syndrome. While there are no human data showing such an interaction with paroxetine hydrochloride, limited animal data on the effects of combined use of paroxetine and MAOIs suggest that these drugs may act synergistically to elevate blood pressure and evoke behavioral excitation. Therefore, it is recommended that PAXIL CR not be used in combination with an MAOI, or within 14 days of discontinuing treatment with an MAOI. At least 2 weeks should be allowed after stopping PAXIL CR before starting an MAOI.

Potential Interaction With Thioridazine: Thioridazine administration alone produces prolongation of the QTc interval, which is associated with serious ventricular arrhythmias, such as torsade de pointes-type arrhythmias, and sudden death. This effect appears to be dose related.

An in vivo study suggests that drugs which inhibit $P_{450}IID_6$, such as paroxetine, will elevate plasma levels of thioridazine. Therefore, it is recommended that paroxetine not be used in combination with thioridazine (see CONTRAINDICATIONS and PRECAUTIONS).

Clinical Worsening and Suicide Risk: Patients with major depressive disorder, both adult and pediatric, may experience worsening of their depression and/or the emergence of suicidal ideation and behavior (suicidality), whether or not they are taking antidepressant medications, and this risk may persist until significant remission occurs. Although there has been a long-standing concern that antidepressants may have a role in inducing worsening of depression and the emergence of suicidality in certain patients, a causal role for antidepressants in inducing such behaviors has not been established. **Nevertheless, patients being treated with antidepressants should be observed closely for clinical worsening and suicidality, especially at the beginning of a course of drug therapy, or at the time of dose changes, either increases or decreases.** Consideration should be given to changing the therapeutic regimen, including possibly discontinuing the medication, in patients whose depression is persistently worse or whose emergent suicidality is severe, abrupt in onset, or was not part of the patient's presenting symptoms.

Because of the possibility of co-morbidity between major depressive disorder and other psychiatric and nonpsychiatric disorders, the same precautions observed when treating patients with major depressive disorder should be observed when treating patients with other psychiatric and nonpsychiatric disorders.

The following symptoms, anxiety, agitation, panic attacks, insomnia, irritability, hostility (aggressiveness), impulsivity, akathisia (psychomotor restlessness), hypomania, and mania, have been reported in adult and pediatric patients being treated with antidepressants for major depressive disorder as well as for other indications, both psychiatric and nonpsychiatric. Although a causal link between the emergence of such symptoms and either the worsening of depression and/or the emergence of suicidal impulses has not been established, consideration should be given to changing the therapeutic regimen, including possibly discontinuing the medication, in patients for whom such symptoms are severe, abrupt in onset, or were not part of the patient's presenting symptoms.

Families and caregivers of patients being treated with antidepressants for major depressive disorder or other indications, both psychiatric and nonpsychiatric, should be alerted about the need to monitor patients for the emergence of agitation, irritability, and the other symptoms described above, as well as the emergence of suicidality, and to report such symptoms immediately to health care providers. Prescriptions for PAXIL CR should be written for the smallest quantity of tablets consistent with good patient management, in order to reduce the risk of overdose.

If the decision has been made to discontinue treatment, medication should be tapered, as rapidly as is feasible, but with recognition that abrupt discontinuation can be associated with certain symptoms (see PRECAUTIONS and DOSAGE AND ADMINISTRATION—Discontinuation of Treatment With PAXIL CR, for a description of the risks of discontinuation of PAXIL CR).

It should be noted that PAXIL CR is not approved for use in treating any indications in the pediatric population.

A major depressive episode may be the initial presentation of bipolar disorder. It is generally believed (though not established in controlled trials) that treating such an episode with an antidepressant alone may increase the likelihood of precipitation of a mixed/manic episode in patients at risk for bipolar disorder. Whether any of the symptoms described above represent such a conversion is unknown. However, prior to initiating treatment with an antidepressant, patients should be adequately screened to determine if they are at risk for bipolar disorder; such screening should include a detailed psychiatric history, including a family history of suicide, bipolar disorder, and depression. It should be noted that PAXIL CR is not approved for use in treating bipolar depression.

PRECAUTIONS

General: ***Activation of Mania/Hypomania:*** During premarketing testing of immediate-release paroxetine hydrochloride, hypomania or mania occurred in approximately 1.0% of paroxetine-treated unipolar patients compared to 1.1% of active-control and 0.3% of placebo-treated unipolar patients. In a subset of patients classified as bipolar, the rate of manic episodes was 2.2% for immediate-release paroxetine and 11.6% for the combined active-control groups. Among 1,627 patients with major depressive disorder, panic disorder, social anxiety disorder, or PMDD treated with PAXIL CR in controlled clinical studies, there were no reports of mania or hypomania. As with all drugs effective in the treatment of major depressive disorder, PAXIL CR should be used cautiously in patients with a history of mania.

Seizures: During premarketing testing of immediate-release paroxetine hydrochloride, seizures occurred in 0.1% of paroxetine-treated patients, a rate similar to that associated with other drugs effective in the treatment of major depressive disorder. Among 1,627 patients who received PAXIL CR in controlled clinical trials in major depressive disorder, panic disorder, social anxiety disorder, or PMDD, 1 patient (0.1%) experienced a seizure. PAXIL CR should be used cautiously in patients with a history of seizures. It should be discontinued in any patient who develops seizures.

Discontinuation of Treatment With PAXIL CR: Adverse events while discontinuing therapy with PAXIL CR were not systematically evaluated in most clinical trials; however, in recent placebo-controlled clinical trials utilizing daily doses of PAXIL CR up to 37.5 mg/day, spontaneously reported adverse events while discontinuing therapy with PAXIL CR were evaluated. Patients receiving 37.5 mg/day underwent an incremental decrease in the daily dose by

Continued on next page

Product information on these pages is effective as of August 2004. Further information is available at: GlaxoSmithKline, PO Box 13398, Research Triangle Park, NC 27709. 1-888-825-5249. Corporate Web Site: www.gsk.com

Paxil CR—Cont.

12.5 mg/day to a dose of 25 mg/day for 1 week before treatment was stopped. For patients receiving 25 mg/day or 12.5 mg/day, treatment was stopped without an incremental decrease in dose. With this regimen in those studies, the following adverse events were reported for PAXIL CR, at an incidence of 2% or greater for PAXIL CR and were at least twice that reported for placebo: Dizziness, nausea, nervousness, and additional symptoms described by the investigator as associated with tapering or discontinuing PAXIL CR (e.g., emotional lability, headache, agitation, electric shock sensations, fatigue, and sleep disturbances). These events were reported as serious in 0.3% of patients who discontinued therapy with PAXIL CR.

During marketing of PAXIL CR and other SSRIs (serotonin and norepinephrine reuptake inhibitors), there have been spontaneous reports of adverse events occuring upon discontinuation of these drugs, (particularly when abrupt), including the following: Dysphoric mood, irritability, agitation, dizziness, sensory disturbances (e.g., paresthesias such as electric shock sensations), anxiety, confusion, headache, lethargy, emotional lability, insomnia, and hypomania. While these events are generally self-limiting, there have been reports of serious discontinuation symptoms.

Patients should be monitored for these symptoms when discontinuing treatment with PAXIL CR. A gradual reduction in the dose rather than abrupt cessation is recommended whenever possible. If intolerable symptoms occur following a decrease in the dose or upon discontinuation of treatment, then resuming the previously prescribed dose may be considered. Subsequently, the physician may continue decreasing the dose but at a more gradual rate (see DOSAGE AND ADMINISTRATION).

Hyponatremia: Several cases of hyponatremia have been reported with immediate-release paroxetine hydrochloride. The hyponatremia appeared to be reversible when paroxetine was discontinued. The majority of these occurrences have been in elderly individuals, some in patients taking diuretics or who were otherwise volume depleted.

Abnormal Bleeding: Published case reports have documented the occurrence of bleeding episodes in patients treated with psychotropic drugs that interfere with serotonin reuptake. Subsequent epidemiological studies, both of the case-control and cohort design, have demonstrated an association between use of psychotropic drugs that interfere with serotonin reuptake and the occurrence of upper gastrointestinal bleeding. In 2 studies, concurrent use of a nonsteroidal anti-inflammatory drug (NSAID) or aspirin potentiated the risk of bleeding (see Drug Interactions). Although these studies focused on upper gastrointestinal bleeding, there is reason to believe that bleeding at other sites may be similarly potentiated. Patients should be cautioned regarding the risk of bleeding associated with the concomitant use of paroxetine with NSAIDs, aspirin, or other drugs that affect coagulation.

Use in Patients With Concomitant Illness: Clinical experience with immediate-release paroxetine hydrochloride in patients with certain concomitant systemic illness is limited. Caution is advisable in using PAXIL CR in patients with diseases or conditions that could affect metabolism or hemodynamic responses.

As with other SSRIs, mydriasis has been infrequently reported in premarketing studies with paroxetine hydrochloride. A few cases of acute angle closure glaucoma associated with therapy with immediate-release paroxetine have been reported in the literature. As mydriasis can cause acute angle closure in patients with narrow angle glaucoma, caution should be used when PAXIL CR is prescribed for patients with narrow angle glaucoma.

PAXIL CR or the immediate-release formulation has not been evaluated or used to any appreciable extent in patients with a recent history of myocardial infarction or unstable heart disease. Patients with these diagnoses were excluded from clinical studies during premarket testing. Evaluation of electrocardiograms of 682 patients who received immediate-release paroxetine hydrochloride in double-blind, placebo-controlled trials, however, did not indicate that paroxetine is associated with the development of significant ECG abnormalities. Similarly, paroxetine hydrochloride does not cause any clinically important changes in heart rate or blood pressure.

Increased plasma concentrations of paroxetine occur in patients with severe renal impairment (creatinine clearance <30 mL/min.) or severe hepatic impairment. A lower starting dose should be used in such patients (see DOSAGE AND ADMINISTRATION).

Information For Patients: Physicians are advised to discuss the following issues with patients for whom they prescribe PAXIL CR:

Patients and their families should be encouraged to be alert to the emergence of anxiety, agitation, panic attacks, insomnia, irritability, hostility, impulsivity, akathisia, hypomania, mania, worsening of depression, and suicidal ideation, especially early during antidepressant treatment. Such symptoms should be reported to the patient's physician, especially if they are severe, abrupt in onset, or were not part of the patient's presenting symptoms.

PAXIL CR should not be chewed or crushed, and should be swallowed whole.

Drugs That Interfere With Hemostasis (NSAIDS, Aspirin, Warfarin, etc.): Patients should be cautioned about the concomitant use of paroxetine and NSAIDS, aspirin, or other drugs that affect coagulation since the combined use of psychotropic drugs that interfere with serotonin reuptake and these agents has been associated with an increased risk of bleeding.

Interference With Cognitive and Motor Performance: Any psychoactive drug may impair judgment, thinking, or motor skills. Although in controlled studies immediate-release paroxetine hydrochloride has not been shown to impair psychomotor performance, patients should be cautioned about operating hazardous machinery, including automobiles, until they are reasonably certain that PAXIL CR does not affect their ability to engage in such activities.

Completing Course of Therapy: While patients may notice improvement with use of PAXIL CR in 1 to 4 weeks, they should be advised to continue therapy as directed.

Concomitant Medications: Patients should be advised to inform their physician if they are taking, or plan to take, any prescription or over-the-counter drugs, since there is a potential for interactions.

Alcohol: Although immediate-release paroxetine hydrochloride has not been shown to increase the impairment of mental and motor skills caused by alcohol, patients should be advised to avoid alcohol while taking PAXIL CR.

Pregnancy: Patients should be advised to notify their physician if they become pregnant or intend to become pregnant during therapy.

Nursing: Patients should be advised to notify their physician if they are breast-feeding an infant (see PRECAUTIONS—Nursing Mothers).

Laboratory Tests: There are no specific laboratory tests recommended.

Drug Interactions: ***Tryptophan:*** As with other serotonin reuptake inhibitors, an interaction between paroxetine and tryptophan may occur when they are coadministered. Adverse experiences, consisting primarily of headache, nausea, sweating and dizziness, have been reported when tryptophan was administered to patients taking immediate-release paroxetine. Consequently, concomitant use of PAXIL CR with tryptophan is not recommended.

Monoamine Oxidase Inhibitors: See CONTRAINDICATIONS and WARNINGS.

Thioridazine: See CONTRAINDICATIONS and WARNINGS.

Warfarin: Preliminary data suggest that there may be a pharmacodynamic interaction (that causes an increased bleeding diathesis in the face of unaltered prothrombin time) between paroxetine and warfarin. Since there is little clinical experience, the concomitant administration of PAXIL CR and warfarin should be undertaken with caution (see Drugs That Interfere With Hemostasis).

Sumatriptan: There have been rare postmarketing reports describing patients with weakness, hyperreflexia, and incoordination following the use of an SSRI and sumatriptan. If concomitant treatment with sumatriptan and an SSRI (e.g., fluoxetine, fluvoxamine, paroxetine, sertraline) is clinically warranted, appropriate observation of the patient is advised.

Drugs Affecting Hepatic Metabolism: The metabolism and pharmacokinetics of paroxetine may be affected by the induction or inhibition of drug-metabolizing enzymes.

Cimetidine: Cimetidine inhibits many cytochrome P_{450} (oxidative) enzymes. In a study where immediate-release paroxetine (30 mg once daily) was dosed orally for 4 weeks, steady-state plasma concentrations of paroxetine were increased by approximately 50% during coadministration with oral cimetidine (300 mg three times daily) for the final week. Therefore, when these drugs are administered concurrently, dosage adjustment of PAXIL CR after the starting dose should be guided by clinical effect. The effect of paroxetine on cimetidine's pharmacokinetics was not studied.

Phenobarbital: Phenobarbital induces many cytochrome P_{450} (oxidative) enzymes. When a single oral 30-mg dose of immediate-release paroxetine was administered at phenobarbital steady state (100 mg once daily for 14 days), paroxetine AUC and $T_{1/2}$ were reduced (by an average of 25% and 38%, respectively) compared to paroxetine administered alone. The effect of paroxetine on phenobarbital pharmacokinetics was not studied. Since paroxetine exhibits nonlinear pharmacokinetics, the results of this study may not address the case where the 2 drugs are both being chronically dosed. No initial dosage adjustment with PAXIL CR is considered necessary when coadministered with phenobarbital; any subsequent adjustment should be guided by clinical effect.

Phenytoin: When a single oral 30-mg dose of immediate-release paroxetine was administered at phenytoin steady state (300 mg once daily for 14 days), paroxetine AUC and $T_{1/2}$ were reduced (by an average of 50% and 35%, respectively) compared to immediate-release paroxetine administered alone. In a separate study, when a single oral 300-mg dose of phenytoin was administered at paroxetine steady state (30 mg once daily for 14 days), phenytoin AUC was slightly reduced (12% on average) compared to phenytoin administered alone. Since both drugs exhibit nonlinear pharmacokinetics, the above studies may not address the case where the 2 drugs are both being chronically dosed. No initial dosage adjustments are considered necessary when PAXIL CR is coadministered with phenytoin; any subsequent adjustments should be guided by clinical effect (see ADVERSE REACTIONS–Postmarketing Reports).

Drugs Metabolized by Cytochrome $P_{450}IID_6$: Many drugs, including most drugs effective in the treatment of major depressive disorder (paroxetine, other SSRIs, and many tricyclics), are metabolized by the cytochrome P_{450} isozyme $P_{450}IID_6$. Like other agents that are metabolized by $P_{450}IID_6$, paroxetine may significantly inhibit the activity of this isozyme. In most patients (>90%), this $P_{450}IID_6$ isozyme is saturated early during paroxetine dosing. In 1 study, daily dosing of immediate-release paroxetine (20 mg once daily) under steady-state conditions increased single-dose desipramine (100 mg) C_{max}, AUC, and $T_{½}$ by an average of approximately 2-, 5-, and 3-fold, respectively. Concomitant use of PAXIL CR with other drugs metabolized by cytochrome $P_{450}IID_6$ has not been formally studied but may require lower doses than usually prescribed for either PAXIL CR or the other drug.

Therefore, coadministration of PAXIL CR with other drugs that are metabolized by this isozyme, including certain drugs effective in the treatment of major depressive disorder (e.g., nortriptyline, amitriptyline, imipramine, desipramine, and fluoxetine), phenothiazines, risperidone, and Type 1C antiarrhythmics (e.g., propafenone, flecainide, and encainide), or that inhibit this enzyme (e.g., quinidine), should be approached with caution.

However, due to the risk of serious ventricular arrhythmias and sudden death potentially associated with elevated plasma levels of thioridazine, paroxetine and thioridazine should not be coadministration (see CONTRAINDICATIONS and WARNINGS).

At steady state, when the $P_{450}IID_6$ pathway is essentially saturated, paroxetine clearance is governed by alternative P_{450} isozymes that, unlike $P_{450}IID_6$, show no evidence of saturation (see PRECAUTIONS—Tricyclic Antidepressants).

Drugs Metabolized by Cytochrome $P_{450}IIIA_4$: An in vivo interaction study involving the coadministration under steady-state conditions of paroxetine and terfenadine, a substrate for $P_{450}IIIA_4$, revealed no effect of paroxetine on terfenadine pharmacokinetics. In addition, in vitro studies have shown ketoconazole, a potent inhibitor of $P_{450}IIIA_4$ activity, to be at least 100 times more potent than paroxetine as an inhibitor of the metabolism of several substrates for this enzyme, including terfenadine, astemizole, cisapride, triazolam, and cyclosporine. Based on the assumption that the relationship between paroxetine's in vitro K_i and its lack of effect on terfenadine's in vivo clearance predicts its effect on other $IIIA_4$ substrates, paroxetine's extent of inhibition of $IIIA_4$ activity is not likely to be of clinical significance.

Tricyclic Antidepressants (TCAs): Caution is indicated in the coadministration of TCAs with PAXIL CR, because paroxetine may inhibit TCA metabolism. Plasma TCA concentrations may need to be monitored, and the dose of TCA may need to be reduced, if a TCA is coadministered with PAXIL CR (see PRECAUTIONS—Drugs Metabolized by Cytochrome $P_{450}IID_6$).

Drugs Highly Bound to Plasma Protein: Because paroxetine is highly bound to plasma protein, administration of PAXIL CR to a patient taking another drug that is highly protein bound may cause increased free concentrations of the other drug, potentially resulting in adverse events. Conversely, adverse effects could result from displacement of paroxetine by other highly bound drugs.

Drugs That Interfere With Hemostasis (NSAIDs, Aspirin, Warfarin, etc.): Serotonin release by platelets plays an important role in hemostasis. Epidemiological studies of the case-control and cohort design that have demonstrated an association between use of psychotropic drugs that interfere with serotonin reuptake and the occurrence of upper gastrointestinal bleeding have also shown that concurrent use of an NSAID or aspirin potentiated the risk of bleeding. Thus, patients should be cautioned about the use of such drugs concurrently with paroxetine.

Alcohol: Although paroxetine does not increase the impairment of mental and motor skills caused by alcohol, patients should be advised to avoid alcohol while taking PAXIL CR.

Lithium: A multiple-dose study with immediate-release paroxetine hydrochloride has shown that there is no pharmacokinetic interaction between paroxetine and lithium carbonate. However, since there is little clinical experience, the concurrent administration of PAXIL CR and lithium should be undertaken with caution.

Digoxin: The steady-state pharmacokinetics of paroxetine was not altered when administered with digoxin at steady state. Mean digoxin AUC at steady state decreased by 15% in the presence of paroxetine. Since there is little clinical experience, the concurrent administration of PAXIL CR and digoxin should be undertaken with caution.

Diazepam: Under steady-state conditions, diazepam does not appear to affect paroxetine kinetics. The effects of paroxetine on diazepam were not evaluated.

Procyclidine: Daily oral dosing of immediate-release paroxetine (30 mg once daily) increased steady-state AUC_{0-24}, C_{max}, and C_{min} values of procyclidine (5 mg oral once daily) by 35%, 37% and 67%, respectively, compared to procyclidine alone at steady state. If anticholinergic effects are seen, the dose of procyclidine should be reduced.

Beta-Blockers: In a study where propranolol (80 mg twice daily) was dosed orally for 18 days, the established steady-state plasma concentrations of propranolol were unaltered during coadministration with immediate-release paroxetine (30 mg once daily) for the final 10 days. The effects of propranolol on paroxetine have not been evaluated (see ADVERSE REACTIONS—Postmarketing Reports).

Theophylline: Reports of elevated theophylline levels associated with immediate-release paroxetine treatment have been reported. While this interaction has not been formally studied, it is recommended that theophylline levels be monitored when these drugs are concurrently administered.

Electroconvulsive Therapy (ECT): There are no clinical studies of the combined use of ECT and PAXIL CR.

Carcinogenesis, Mutagenesis, Impairment of Fertility: ***Carcinogenesis:*** Two-year carcinogenicity studies were conducted in rodents given paroxetine in the diet at 1, 5, and 25 mg/kg/day (mice) and 1, 5, and 20 mg/kg/day (rats). These doses are up to approximately 2 (mouse) and 3 (rat) times the maximum recommended human dose (MRHD) on a mg/m^2 basis. There was a significantly greater number of male rats in the high-dose group with reticulum cell sarcomas (1/100, 0/50, 0/50, and 4/50 for control, low-, middle- and high-dose groups, respectively) and a significantly increased linear trend across dose groups for the occurrence of lymphoreticular tumors in male rats. Female rats were not affected. Although there was a dose-related increase in the number of tumors in mice, there was no drug-related increase in the number of mice with tumors. The relevance of these findings to humans is unknown.

Mutagenesis: Paroxetine produced no genotoxic effects in a battery of 5 in vitro and 2 in vivo assays that included the following: Bacterial mutation assay, mouse lymphoma mutation assay, unscheduled DNA synthesis assay, and tests for cytogenetic aberrations in vivo in mouse bone marrow and in vitro in human lymphocytes and in a dominant lethal test in rats.

Impairment of Fertility: A reduced pregnancy rate was found in reproduction studies in rats at a dose of paroxetine of 15 mg/kg/day, which is approximately twice the MRHD on a mg/m^2 basis. Irreversible lesions occurred in the reproductive tract of male rats after dosing in toxicity studies for 2 to 52 weeks. These lesions consisted of vacuolation of epididymal tubular epithelium at 50 mg/kg/day and atrophic changes in the seminiferous tubules of the testes with arrested spermatogenesis at 25 mg/kg/day (approximately 8 and 4 times the MRHD on a mg/m^2 basis).

Pregnancy: Pregnancy Category C. Reproduction studies were performed at doses up to 50 mg/kg/day in rats and 6 mg/kg/day in rabbits administered during organogenesis. These doses are approximately 8 (rat) and 2 (rabbit) times the maximum MRHD on an mg/m^2 basis. These studies have revealed no evidence of teratogenic effects. However, in rats, there was an increase in pup deaths during the first 4 days of lactation when dosing occurred during the last trimester of gestation and continued throughout lactation. This effect occurred at a dose of 1 mg/kg/day or approximately one-sixth of the MRHD on an mg/m^2 basis. The no-effect dose for rat pup mortality was not determined. The cause of these deaths is not known. There are no adequate and well-controlled studies in pregnant women. This drug should be used during pregnancy only if the potential benefit justifies the potential risk to the fetus.

Nonteratogenic Effects: Neonates exposed to PAXIL CR and other SSRIs or SNRIs, late in the third trimester have developed complications requiring prolonged hospitalization, respiratory support, and tube feeding. Such complications can arise immediately upon delivery. Reported clinical findings have included respiratory distress, cyanosis, apnea, seizures, temperature instability, feeding difficulty, vomiting, hypoglycemia, hypotonia, hypertonia, hyperreflexia, tremor, jitteriness, irritability, and constant crying. These features are consistent with either a direct toxic effect of SSRIs and SNRIs or, possibly, a drug discontinuation syndrome. It should be noted that, in some cases, the clinical picture is consistent with serotonin syndrome (see WARNINGS—Potential for Interaction With Monoamine Oxidase Inhibitors). When treating a pregnant woman with paroxetine during the third trimester, the physician should carefully consider the potential risks and benefits of treatment (see DOSAGE AND ADMINISTRATION).

Labor and Delivery: The effect of paroxetine on labor and delivery in humans is unknown.

Nursing Mothers: Like many other drugs, paroxetine is secreted in human milk, and caution should be exercised when PAXIL CR is administered to a nursing woman.

Pediatric Use: Safety and effectiveness in the pediatric population have not been established (see WARNINGS—Clinical Worsening and Suicide Risk).

Geriatric Use: In worldwide premarketing clinical trials with immediate-release paroxetine hydrochloride, 17% of paroxetine-treated patients (approximately 700) were 65 years or older. Pharmacokinetic studies revealed a decreased clearance in the elderly, and a lower starting dose is recommended; there were, however, no overall differences in the adverse event profile between elderly and younger patients, and effectiveness was similar in younger and older patients (see CLINICAL PHARMACOLOGY and DOSAGE AND ADMINISTRATION).

In a controlled study focusing specifically on elderly patients with major depressive disorder, PAXIL CR was demonstrated to be safe and effective in the treatment of elderly patients (>60 years) with major depressive disorder. (See CLINICAL PHARMACOLOGY—Clinical Trials and ADVERSE REACTIONS—Table 2.)

ADVERSE REACTIONS

The information included under the "Adverse Findings Observed in Short-Term, Placebo-Controlled Trials With PAXIL CR" subsection of ADVERSE REACTIONS is based on data from 11 placebo-controlled clinical trials. Three of these studies were conducted in patients with major depressive disorder, 3 studies were done in patients with panic disorder, 1 study was conducted in patients with social anxiety disorder, and 4 studies were done in female patients with PMDD. Two of the studies in major depressive disorder, which enrolled patients in the age range 18 to 65 years, are pooled. Information from a third study of major depressive disorder, which focused on elderly patients (60 to 88 years), is presented separately as is the information from the panic disorder studies and the information from the PMDD studies. Information on additional adverse events associated with PAXIL CR and the immediate-release formulation of paroxetine hydrochloride is included in a separate subsection (see Other Events).

Adverse Findings Observed in Short-Term, Placebo-Controlled Trials with PAXIL CR:

Adverse Events Associated With Discontinuation of Treatment: ***Major Depressive Disorder:*** Ten percent (21/212) of patients treated with PAXIL CR discontinued treatment due to an adverse event in a pool of 2 studies of patients with major depressive disorder. The most common events (≥1%) associated with discontinuation and considered to be drug related (i.e., those events associated with dropout at a rate approximately twice or greater for PAXIL CR compared to placebo) included the following:

	PAXIL CR (n = 212)	Placebo (n = 211)
Nausea	3.7%	0.5%
Asthenia	1.9%	0.5%
Dizziness	1.4%	0.0%
Somnolence	1.4%	0.0%

In a placebo-controlled study of elderly patients with major depressive disorder, 13% (13/104) of patients treated with PAXIL CR discontinued due to an adverse event. Events meeting the above criteria included the following:

	PAXIL CR (n = 104)	Placebo (n = 109)
Nausea	2.9%	0.0%
Headache	1.9%	0.9%
Depression	1.9%	0.0%
LFT's abnormal	1.9%	0.0%

Panic Disorder: Eleven percent (50/444) of patients treated with PAXIL CR in panic disorder studies discontinued treatment due to an adverse event. Events meeting the above criteria included the following:

	PAXIL CR (n = 444)	Placebo (n = 445)
Nausea	2.9%	0.4%
Insomnia	1.8%	0.0%
Headache	1.4%	0.2%
Asthenia	1.1%	0.0%

Social Anxiety Disorder: Three percent (5/186) of patients treated with PAXIL CR in the social anxiety disorder study discontinued treatment due to an adverse event. Events meeting the above criteria included the following:

	PAXIL CR (n = 186)	Placebo (n = 184)
Nausea	2.2%	0.5%
Headache	1.6%	0.5%
Diarrhea	1.1%	0.5%

Premenstrual Dysphoric Disorder: Spontaneously reported adverse events were monitored in studies of both continuous and intermittent dosing of PAXIL CR in the treatment of PMDD. Generally, there were few differences in the adverse event profiles of the 2 dosing regimens. Thirteen percent (88/681) of patients treated with PAXIL CR in PMDD studies of continuous dosing discontinued treatment due to an adverse event.

The most common events (≥1%) associated with discontinuation in either group treated with PAXIL CR with an incidence rate that is at least twice that of placebo in PMDD trials that employed a continuous dosing regimen are shown in the following table. This table also shows those events that were dose dependent (indicated with an asterisk) as defined as events having an incidence rate with 25 mg of PAXIL CR that was at least twice that with 12.5 mg of PAXIL CR (as well as the placebo group).

	PAXIL CR 25 mg (n = 348)	PAXIL CR 12.5 mg (n = 333)	Placebo (n = 349)
TOTAL	15%	9.9%	6.3%
Nausea*	6.0%	2.4%	0.9%
Asthenia	4.9%	3.0%	1.4%
Somnolence*	4.3%	1.8%	0.3%
Insomnia	2.3%	1.5%	0.0%
Concentration Impaired*	2.0%	0.6%	0.3%
Dry mouth*	2.0%	0.6%	0.3%
Dizziness*	1.7%	0.6%	0.6%
Decreased Appetite*	1.4%	0.6%	0.0%
Sweating*	1.4%	0.0%	0.3%
Tremor*	1.4%	0.3%	0.0%
Yawn*	1.1%	0.0%	0.0%
Diarrhea	0.9%	1.2%	0.0%

*Events considered to be dose dependent are defined as events having an incidence rate with 25 mg of PAXIL CR that was at least twice that with 12.5 mg of PAXIL CR (as well as the placebo group).

Commonly Observed Adverse Events: ***Major Depressive Disorder:*** The most commonly observed adverse events associated with the use of PAXIL CR in a pool of 2 trials (incidence of 5.0% or greater and incidence for PAXIL CR at least twice that for placebo, derived from Table 1) were: Abnormal ejaculation, abnormal vision, constipation, decreased libido, diarrhea, dizziness, female genital disorders, nausea, somnolence, sweating, trauma, tremor, and yawning.

Using the same criteria, the adverse events associated with the use of PAXIL CR in a study of elderly patients with major depressive disorder were: Abnormal ejaculation, constipation, decreased appetite, dry mouth, impotence, infection, libido decreased, sweating, and tremor.

Panic Disorder: In the pool of panic disorder studies, the adverse events meeting these criteria were: Abnormal ejaculation, somnolence, impotence, libido decreased, tremor, sweating, and female genital disorders (generally anorgasmia or difficulty achieving orgasm).

Social Anxiety Disorder: In the social anxiety disorder study, the adverse events meeting these criteria were: Nausea, asthenia, abnormal ejaculation, sweating, somnolence, impotence, insomnia, and libido decreased.

Premenstrual Dysphoric Disorder: The most commonly observed adverse events associated with the use of PAXIL CR either during continuous dosing or luteal phase dosing (incidence of 5% or greater and incidence for PAXIL CR at least twice that for placebo, derived from Table 5) were: Nausea, asthenia, libido decreased, somnolence, insomnia, female genital disorders, sweating, dizziness, diarrhea, and constipation.

In the luteal phase dosing PMDD trial, which employed dosing of 12.5 mg/day or 25 mg/day of PAXIL CR limited to the 2 weeks prior to the onset of menses over 3 consecutive menstrual cycles, adverse events were evaluated during the first 14 days of each off-drug phase. When the 3 off-drug phases were combined, the following adverse events were reported at an incidence of 2% or greater for PAXIL CR and were at least twice the rate of that reported for placebo: Infection (5.3% versus 2.5%), depression (2.8% versus 0.8%), insomnia (2.4% versus 0.8%), sinusitis (2.4% versus 0%), and asthenia (2.0% versus 0.8%).

Incidence in Controlled Clinical Trials: Table 1 enumerates adverse events that occurred at an incidence of 1% or more among patients treated with PAXIL CR, aged 18 to 65, who participated in 2 short-term (12-week) placebo-controlled trials in major depressive disorder in which patients were dosed in a range of 25 mg to 62.5 mg/day. Table 2 enumerates adverse events reported at an incidence of 5% or greater among elderly patients (ages 60 to 88) treated with PAXIL CR who participated in a short-term (12-week) placebo-controlled trial in major depressive disorder in which patients were dosed in a range of 12.5 mg to 50 mg/day. Table 3 enumerates adverse events reported at an incidence of 1% or greater among patients (19 to 72 years) treated with PAXIL CR who participated in short-term (10-week) placebo-controlled trials in panic disorder in which patients were dosed in a range of 12.5 mg to 75 mg/day. Table 4 enumerates adverse events reported at an incidence of 1% or greater among adult patients treated with PAXIL CR who participated in a short-term (12-week), double-blind, placebo-controlled trial in social anxiety disorder in which patients were dosed in a range of 12.5 to 37.5 mg/day. Table 5 enumerates adverse events that occurred at an incidence of 1% or more among patients treated with PAXIL CR who participated in three, 12-week, placebo-controlled trials in PMDD in which patients were dosed at 12.5 mg/day or 25 mg/day and in one 12-week placebo-controlled trial in which patients were dosed for 2 weeks prior to the onset of menses (luteal phase dosing) at 12.5 mg/day or 25 mg/day. Reported adverse events were classified using a standard COSTART-based Dictionary terminology.

The prescriber should be aware that these figures cannot be used to predict the incidence of side effects in the course of usual medical practice where patient characteristics and other factors differ from those that prevailed in the clinical trials. Similarly, the cited frequencies cannot be compared with figures obtained from other clinical investigations involving different treatments, uses, and investigators. The cited figures, however, do provide the prescribing physician with some basis for estimating the relative contribution of drug and nondrug factors to the side effect incidence rate in the population studied.

Table 1. Treatment-Emergent Adverse Events Occurring in ≥1% of Patients Treated With PAXIL CR in a Pool of 2 Studies in Major Depressive Disorder[1,2]

	% Reporting Event	
Body System/Adverse Event	**PAXIL CR (n = 212)**	**Placebo (n = 211)**
Body as a Whole		
Headache	27%	20%
Asthenia	14%	9%
Infection[3]	8%	5%
Abdominal Pain	7%	4%
Back Pain	5%	3%

Continued on next page

Product information on these pages is effective as of August 2004. Further information is available at: GlaxoSmithKline, PO Box 13398, Research Triangle Park, NC 27709. 1-888-825-5249. Corporate Web Site: www.gsk.com

Paxil CR—Cont.

Trauma[4]	5%	1%
Pain[5]	3%	1%
Allergic Reaction[6]	2%	1%
Cardiovascular System		
Tachycardia	1%	0%
Vasodilatation[7]	2%	0%
Digestive System		
Nausea	22%	10%
Diarrhea	18%	7%
Dry Mouth	15%	8%
Constipation	10%	4%
Flatulence	6%	4%
Decreased Appetite	4%	2%
Vomiting	2%	1%
Nervous System		
Somnolence	22%	8%
Insomnia	17%	9%
Dizziness	14%	4%
Libido Decreased	7%	3%
Tremor	7%	1%
Hypertonia	3%	1%
Paresthesia	3%	1%
Agitation	2%	1%
Confusion	1%	0%
Respiratory System		
Yawn	5%	0%
Rhinitis	4%	1%
Cough Increased	2%	1%
Bronchitis	1%	0%
Skin and Appendages		
Sweating	6%	2%
Photosensitivity	2%	0%
Special Senses		
Abnormal Vision[8]	5%	1%
Taste Perversion	2%	0%
Urogenital System		
Abnormal Ejaculation[9,10]	26%	1%
Female Genital Disorder[9,11]	10%	<1%
Impotence[9]	5%	3%
Urinary Tract Infection	3%	1%
Menstrual Disorder[9]	2%	<1%
Vaginitis[9]	2%	0%

1. Adverse events for which the PAXIL CR reporting incidence was less than or equal to the placebo incidence are not included. These events are: Abnormal dreams, anxiety, arthralgia, depersonalization, dysmenorrhea, dyspepsia, hyperkinesia, increased appetite, myalgia, nervousness, pharyngitis, purpura, rash, respiratory disorder, sinusitis, urinary frequency, and weight gain.
2. <1% means greater than zero and less than 1%.
3. Mostly flu.
4. A wide variety of injuries with no obvious pattern.
5. Pain in a variety of locations with no obvious pattern.
6. Most frequently seasonal allergic symptoms.
7. Usually flushing.
8. Mostly blurred vision.
9. Based on the number of males or females.
10. Mostly anorgasmia or delayed ejaculation.
11. Mostly anorgasmia or delayed orgasm.

Table 2. Treatment-Emergent Adverse Events Occurring in ≥5% of Patients Treated With PAXIL CR in a Study of Elderly Patients With Major Depressive Disorder[1,2]

	% Reporting Event	
Body System/Adverse Event	**PAXIL CR (n = 104)**	**Placebo (n = 109)**
Body as a Whole		
Headache	17%	13%
Asthenia	15%	14%
Trauma	8%	5%
Infection	6%	2%
Digestive System		
Dry Mouth	18%	7%
Diarrhea	15%	9%
Constipation	13%	5%
Dyspepsia	13%	10%
Decreased Appetite	12%	5%
Flatulence	8%	7%
Nervous System		
Somnolence	21%	12%
Insomnia	10%	8%
Dizziness	9%	5%
Libido Decreased	8%	<1%
Tremor	7%	0%
Skin and Appendages		
Sweating	10%	<1%
Urogenital System		
Abnormal Ejaculation[3,4]	17%	3%
Impotence[3]	9%	3%

1. Adverse events for which the PAXIL CR reporting incidence was less than or equal to the placebo incidence are not included. These events are nausea and respiratory disorder.
2. <1% means greater than zero and less than 1%.
3. Based on the number of males.
4. Mostly anorgasmia or delayed ejaculation.

Table 3. Treatment-Emergent Adverse Events Occurring in ≥1% of Patients Treated With PAXIL CR in a Pool of 3 Panic Disorder Studies[1,2]

	% Reporting Event	
Body System/Adverse Event	**PAXIL CR (n = 444)**	**Placebo (n = 445)**
Body as a Whole		
Asthenia	15%	10%
Abdominal Pain	6%	4%
Trauma[3]	5%	4%
Cardiovascular System		
Vasodilation[4]	3%	2%
Digestive System		
Nausea	23%	17%
Dry Mouth	13%	9%
Diarrhea	12%	9%
Constipation	9%	6%
Decreased Appetite	8%	6%
Metabolic/Nutritional Disorders		
Weight Loss	1%	0%
Musculoskeletal System		
Myalgia	5%	3%
Nervous System		
Insomnia	20%	11%
Somnolence	20%	9%
Libido Decreased	9%	4%
Nervousness	8%	7%
Tremor	8%	2%
Anxiety	5%	4%
Agitation	3%	2%
Hypertonia[5]	2%	<1%
Myoclonus	2%	<1%
Respiratory System		
Sinusitis	8%	5%
Yawn	3%	0%
Skin and Appendages		
Sweating	7%	2%
Special Senses		
Abnormal Vision[6]	3%	<1%
Urogenital System		
Abnormal Ejaculation[7,8]	27%	3%
Impotence[7]	10%	1%
Female Genital Disorders[9,10]	7%	1%
Urinary Frequency	2%	<1%
Urination Impaired	2%	<1%
Vaginitis[9]	1%	<1%

1. Adverse events for which the reporting rate for PAXIL CR was less than or equal to the placebo rate are not included. These events are: Abnormal dreams, allergic reaction, back pain, bronchitis, chest pain, concentration impaired, confusion, cough increased, depression, dizziness, dysmenorrhea, dyspepsia, fever, flatulence, headache, increased appetite, infection, menstrual disorder, migraine, pain, paresthesia, pharyngitis, respiratory disorder, rhinitis, tachycardia, taste perversion, thinking abnormal, urinary tract infection, and vomiting.
2. <1% means greater than zero and less than 1%.
3. Various physical injuries.
4. Mostly flushing.
5. Mostly muscle tightness or stiffness.
6. Mostly blurred vision.
7. Based on the number of male patients.
8. Mostly anorgasmia or delayed ejaculation.
9. Based on the number of female patients.
10. Mostly anorgasmia or difficulty achieving orgasm.

Table 4. Treatment-Emergent Adverse Effects Occurring in ≥1% of Patients Treated With PAXIL CR in a Social Anxiety Disorder Study[1,2]

	% Reporting Event	
Body System/Adverse Event	**PAXIL CR (n = 186)**	**Placebo (n = 184)**
Body as a Whole		
Headache	23%	17%
Asthenia	18%	7%
Abdominal Pain	5%	4%
Back Pain	4%	1%
Trauma[3]	3%	<1%
Allergic Reaction[4]	2%	<1%
Chest Pain	1%	<1%
Cardiovascular System		
Hypertension	2%	0%
Migraine	2%	1%
Tachycardia	2%	1%
Digestive System		
Nausea	22%	6%
Diarrhea	9%	8%
Constipation	5%	2%
Dry Mouth	3%	2%
Dyspepsia	2%	<1%
Decreased Appetite	1%	<1%
Tooth Disorder	1%	0%
Metabolic/Nutritional Disorders		
Weight Gain	3%	1%
Weight Loss	1%	0%
Nervous System		
Insomnia	9%	4%
Somnolence	9%	4%
Libido Decreased	8%	1%
Dizziness	7%	4%
Tremor	4%	2%
Anxiety	2%	1%
Concentration Impaired	2%	0%
Depression	2%	1%
Myoclonus	1%	<1%
Paresthesia	1%	<1%
Respiratory System		
Yawn	2%	0%
Skin and Appendages		
Sweating	14%	3%
Eczema	1%	0%
Special Senses		
Abnormal Vision[5]	2%	0%
Abnormality of Accommodation	2%	0%
Urogenital System		
Abnormal Ejaculation[6,7]	15%	1%
Impotence[6]	9%	0%
Female Genital Disorders[8,9]	3%	0%

1. Adverse events for which the reporting rate for PAXIL CR was less than or equal to the placebo rate are not included. These events are: Dysmenorrhea, flatulence, gastroenteritis, hypertonia, infection, pain, pharyngitis, rash, respiratory disorder, rhinitis, and vomiting.
2. <1% means greater than zero and less than 1%.
3. Various physical injuries.
4. Most frequently seasonal allergic symptoms.
5. Mostly blurred vision.
6. Based on the number of male patients.
7. Mostly anorgasmia or delayed ejaculation.
8. Based on the number of female patients.
9. Mostly anorgasmia or difficulty achieving orgasm.

[See table 5 at top of next page]

Dose Dependency of Adverse Events: The following table shows results in PMDD trials of common adverse events, defined as events with an incidence of ≥1% with 25 mg of PAXIL CR that was at least twice that with 12.5 mg of PAXIL CR and with placebo.

Incidence of Common Adverse Events in Placebo, 12.5 mg and 25 mg of PAXIL CR in a Pool of 3 Fixed-Dose PMDD Trials

Common Adverse Event	**PAXIL CR 25 mg (n = 348)**	**PAXIL CR 12.5 mg (n = 333)**	**Placebo (n = 349)**
Sweating	8.9%	4.2%	0.9%
Tremor	6.0%	1.5%	0.3%
Concentration Impaired	4.3%	1.5%	0.6%
Yawn	3.2%	0.9%	0.3%
Paresthesia	1.4%	0.3%	0.3%
Hyperkinesia	1.1%	0.3%	0.0%
Vaginitis	1.1%	0.3%	0.3%

A comparison of adverse event rates in a fixed-dose study comparing immediate-release paroxetine with placebo in the treatment of major depressive disorder revealed a clear dose dependency for some of the more common adverse events associated with the use of immediate-release paroxetine.

Male and Female Sexual Dysfunction With SSRIs: Although changes in sexual desire, sexual performance, and sexual satisfaction often occur as manifestations of a psychiatric disorder, they may also be a consequence of pharmacologic treatment. In particular, some evidence suggests that SSRIs can cause such untoward sexual experiences.

Reliable estimates of the incidence and severity of untoward experiences involving sexual desire, performance, and satisfaction are difficult to obtain; however, in part because patients and physicians may be reluctant to discuss them. Accordingly, estimates of the incidence of untoward sexual experience and performance cited in product labeling, are likely to underestimate their actual incidence.

The percentage of patients reporting symptoms of sexual dysfunction in the pool of 2 placebo-controlled trials in nonelderly patients with major depressive disorder, in the pool of 3 placebo-controlled trials in patients with panic disorder, in the placebo-controlled trial in patients with social anxiety disorder, and in the intermittent dosing and the pool of 3 placebo-controlled continuous dosing trials in female patients with PMDD are as follows:

[See second table below]

There are no adequate, controlled studies examining sexual dysfunction with paroxetine treatment.

Paroxetine treatment has been associated with several cases of priapism. In those cases with a known outcome, patients recovered without sequelae.

While it is difficult to know the precise risk of sexual dysfunction associated with the use of SSRIs, physicians should routinely inquire about such possible side effects.

Weight and Vital Sign Changes: Significant weight loss may be an undesirable result of treatment with paroxetine for some patients but, on average, patients in controlled trials with PAXIL CR or the immediate-release formulation, had minimal weight loss (about 1 pound). No significant changes in vital signs (systolic and diastolic blood pressure, pulse, and temperature) were observed in patients treated with PAXIL CR, or immediate-release paroxetine hydrochloride, in controlled clinical trials.

ECG Changes: In an analysis of ECGs obtained in 682 patients treated with immediate-release paroxetine and 415 patients treated with placebo in controlled clinical trials, no clinically significant changes were seen in the ECGs of either group.

Liver Function Tests: In a pool of 2 placebo-controlled clinical trials, patients treated with PAXIL CR or placebo exhibited abnormal values on liver function tests at comparable rates. In particular, the controlled-release paroxetine-versus-placebo comparisons for alkaline phosphatase, SGOT, SGPT, and bilirubin revealed no differences in the percentage of patients with marked abnormalities.

In a study of elderly patients with major depressive disorder, 3 of 104 patients treated with PAXIL CR and none of 109 placebo patients experienced liver transaminase elevations of potential clinical concern.

Two of the patients treated with PAXIL CR dropped out of the study due to abnormal liver function tests; the third patient experienced normalization of transaminase levels with continued treatment. Also, in the pool of 3 studies of patients with panic disorder, 4 of 444 patients treated with PAXIL CR and none of 445 placebo patients experienced liver transaminase elevations of potential clinical concern. Elevations in all 4 patients decreased substantially after discontinuation of PAXIL CR. The clinical significance of these findings is unknown.

In placebo-controlled clinical trials with the immediate release formulation of paroxetine, patients exhibited abnormal values on liver function tests at no greater rate than that seen in placebo-treated patients.

Other Events Observed During the Clinical Development of Paroxetine: The following adverse events were reported during the clinical development of PAXIL CR and/or the clinical development of the immediate-release formulation of paroxetine.

Adverse events for which frequencies are provided below occurred in clinical trials with the controlled-release formulation of paroxetine. During its premarketing assessment in major depressive disorder, panic disorder, social anxiety disorder, and PMDD multiple doses of PAXIL CR were administered to 1,627 patients in phase 3 double-blind, controlled, outpatient studies. Untoward events associated with this exposure were recorded by clinical investigators using terminology of their own choosing. Consequently, it is not possible to provide a meaningful estimate of the proportion of individuals experiencing adverse events without first grouping similar types of untoward events into a smaller number of standardized event categories.

In the tabulations that follow, reported adverse events were classified using a COSTART-based dictionary. The frequencies presented, therefore, represent the proportion of the 1,627 patients exposed to PAXIL CR who experienced an event of the type cited on at least 1 occasion while receiving PAXIL CR. All reported events are included except those already listed in Tables 1 through 5 and those events where a drug cause was remote. If the COSTART term for an event was so general as to be uninformative, it was deleted or, when possible, replaced with a more informative term. It is important to emphasize that although the events reported occurred during treatment with paroxetine, they were not necessarily caused by it.

Events are further categorized by body system and listed in order of decreasing frequency according to the following definitions: Frequent adverse events are those occurring on 1 or more occasions in at least 1/100 patients (only those not already listed in the tabulated results from placebo-controlled trials appear in this listing); infrequent adverse events are those occurring in 1/100 to 1/1,000 patients; rare events are those occurring in fewer than 1/1,000 patients.

Adverse events for which frequencies are not provided occurred during the premarketing assessment of immediate-release paroxetine in phase 2 and 3 studies of major depressive disorder, obsessive compulsive disorder, panic disorder, social anxiety disorder, generalized anxiety disorder, and posttraumatic stress disorder. The conditions and duration of exposure to immediate-release paroxetine varied greatly and included (in overlapping categories) open and double-blind studies, uncontrolled and controlled studies, inpatient and outpatient studies, and fixed-dose and titration studies. Only those events not previously listed for controlled-release paroxetine are included. The extent to which these events may be associated with PAXIL CR is unknown.

Events are listed alphabetically within the respective body system. Events of major clinical importance are also described in the PRECAUTIONS section.

Table 5. Treatment-Emergent Adverse Events Occurring in ≥1% of Patients Treated With PAXIL CR in a Pool of 3 Premenstrual Dysphoric Disorder Studies with Continuous Dosing or in 1 Premenstrual Dysphoric Disorder Study with Luteal Phase Dosing[1,2,3]

	% Reporting Event			
	Continuous Dosing		Luteal Phase Dosing	
Body System/Adverse Event	**PAXIL CR (n = 681)**	**Placebo (n = 349)**	**PAXIL CR (n = 246)**	**Placebo (n = 120)**
Body as a Whole				
Asthenia	17%	6%	15%	4%
Headache	15%	12%	-	-
Infection	6%	4%	-	-
Abdominal pain	-	-	3%	0%
Cardiovascular System				
Migraine	1%	<1%	-	-
Digestive System				
Nausea	17%	7%	18%	2%
Diarrhea	6%	2%	6%	0%
Constipation	5%	1%	2%	<1%
Dry Mouth	4%	2%	2%	<1%
Increased Appetite	3%	<1%	-	-
Decreased Appetite	2%	<1%	2%	0%
Dyspepsia	2%	1%	2%	2%
Gingivitis	-	-	1%	0%
Metabolic and Nutritional Disorders				
Generalized Edema	-	-	1%	<1%
Weight Gain	-	-	1%	<1%
Musculoskeletal System				
Arthralgia	2%	1%	-	-
Nervous System				
Libido Decreased	12%	5%	9%	6%
Somnolence	9%	2%	3%	<1%
Insomnia	8%	2%	7%	3%
Dizziness	7%	3%	6%	3%
Tremor	4%	<1%	5%	0%
Concentration Impaired	3%	<1%	1%	0%
Nervousness	2%	<1%	3%	2%
Anxiety	2%	1%	-	-
Lack of Emotion	2%	<1%	-	-
Depression	-	-	2%	<1%
Vertigo	-	-	2%	<1%
Abnormal Dreams	1%	<1%	-	-
Amnesia	-	-	1%	0%
Respiratory System				
Sinusitis	-	-	4%	2%
Yawn	2%	<1%	-	-
Bronchitis	-	-	2%	0%
Cough Increased	1%	<1%	-	-
Skin and Appendages				
Sweating	7%	<1%	6%	<1%
Special Senses				
Abnormal Vision	-	-	1%	0%
Urogenital System				
Female Genital Disorders[4]	8%	1%	2%	0%
Menorrhagia	1%	<1%	-	-
Vaginal Moniliasis	1%	<1%	-	-
Menstrual Disorder	-	-	1%	0%

1. Adverse events for which the reporting rate of PAXIL CR was less than or equal to the placebo rate are not included. These events for continuous dosing are: Abdominal pain, back pain, pain, trauma, weight gain, myalgia, pharyngitis, respiratory disorder, rhinitis, sinusitis, pruritis, dysmenorrhea, menstrual disorder, urinary tract infection, and vomiting. The events for luteal phase dosing are: Allergic reaction, back pain, headache, infection, pain, trauma, myalgia, anxiety, pharyngitis, respiratory disorder, cystitis, and dysmenorrhea.
2. <1% means greater than zero and less than 1%.
3. The luteal phase and continuous dosing PMDD trials were not designed for making direct comparisons between the 2 dosing regimens. Therefore, a comparison between the 2 dosing regimens of the PMDD trials of incidence rates shown in Table 5 should be avoided.
4. Mostly anorgasmia or difficulty achieving orgasm.

	Major Depressive Disorder		**Panic Disorder**		**Social Anxiety Disorder**		**PMDD Continuous Dosing**		**PMDD Luteal Phase Dosing**	
	PAXIL CR	**Placebo**	**PAXIL CR**	**Placebo**	**PAXIL CR**	**Placebo**	**PAXIL CR**	**Placebo**	**PAXIL CR**	**Placebo**
n (males)	**78**	**78**	**162**	**194**	**88**	**97**	**n/a**	**n/a**	**n/a**	**n/a**
Decreased Libido	10%	5%	9%	6%	13%	1%	n/a	n/a	n/a	n/a
Ejaculatory Disturbance	26%	1%	27%	3%	15%	1%	n/a	n/a	n/a	n/a
Impotence	5%	3%	10%	1%	9%	0%	n/a	n/a	n/a	n/a
n (females)	**134**	**133**	**282**	**251**	**98**	**87**	**681**	**349**	**246**	**120**
Decreased Libido	4%	2%	8%	2%	4%	1%	12%	5%	9%	6%
Orgasmic Disturbance	10%	<1%	7%	1%	3%	0%	8%	1%	2%	0%

Continued on next page

Product information on these pages is effective as of August 2004. Further information is available at: GlaxoSmithKline, PO Box 13398, Research Triangle Park, NC 27709. 1-888-825-5249. Corporate Web Site: www.gsk.com

Paxil CR—Cont.

Body as a Whole: Infrequent were chills, face edema, fever, flu syndrome, malaise; rare were abscess, anaphylactoid reaction, anticholinergic syndrome, hypothermia; also observed were adrenergic syndrome, neck rigidity, sepsis.
Cardiovascular System: Infrequent were angina pectoris, bradycardia, hematoma, hypertension, hypotension, palpitation, postural hypotension, supraventricular tachycardia, syncope; rare were bundle branch block; also observed were arrhythmia nodal, atrial fibrillation, cerebrovascular accident, congestive heart failure, low cardiac output, myocardial infarct, myocardial ischemia, pallor, phlebitis, pulmonary embolus, supraventricular extrasystoles, thrombophlebitis, thrombosis, vascular headache, ventricular extrasystoles.
Digestive System: Infrequent were bruxism, dysphagia, eructation, gastritis, gastroenteritis, gastroesophageal reflux, gingivitis, hemorrhoids, liver function test abnormal, melena, pancreatitis, rectal hemorrhage, toothache, ulcerative stomatitis; rare were colitis, glossitis, gum hyperplasia, hepatosplenomegaly, increased salivation, intestinal obstruction, peptic ulcer, stomach ulcer, throat tightness; also observed were aphthous stomatitis, bloody diarrhea, bulimia, cardiospasm, cholelithiasis, duodenitis, enteritis, esophagitis, fecal impactions, fecal incontinence, gum hemorrhage, hematemesis, hepatitis, ileitis, ileus, jaundice, mouth ulceration, salivary gland enlargement, sialadenitis, stomatitis, tongue discoloration, tongue edema.
Endocrine System: Infrequent were ovarian cyst, testes pain; rare were diabetes mellitus, hyperthyroidism; also observed were goiter, hypothyroidism, thyroiditis.
Hemic and Lymphatic System: Infrequent were anemia, eosinophilia, hypochromic anemia, leukocytosis, leukopenia, lymphadenopathy, purpura; rare were thrombocytopenia; also observed were anisocytosis, basophilia, bleeding time increased, lymphedema, lymphocytosis, lymphopenia, microcytic anemia, monocytosis, normocytic anemia, thrombocythemia.
Metabolic and Nutritional Disorders: Infrequent were generalized edema, hyperglycemia, hypokalemia, peripheral edema, SGOT increased, SGPT increased, thirst; rare were bilirubinemia, dehydration, hyperkalemia, obesity; also observed were alkaline phosphatase increased, BUN increased, creatinine phosphokinase increased, gamma globulins increased, gout, hypercalcemia, hypercholesteremia, hyperphosphatemia, hypocalcemia, hypoglycemia, hyponatremia, ketosis, lactic dehydrogenase increased, non-protein nitrogen (NPN) increased.
Musculoskeletal System: Infrequent were arthritis, bursitis, tendonitis; rare were myasthenia, myopathy, myositis; also observed were generalized spasm, osteoporosis, tenosynovitis, tetany.
Nervous System: Frequent were depression; infrequent were amnesia, convulsion, depersonalization, dystonia, emotional lability, hallucinations, hyperkinesia, hypesthesia, hypokinesia, incoordination, libido increased, neuralgia, neuropathy, nystagmus, paralysis, vertigo; rare were ataxia, coma, diplopia, dyskinesia, hostility, paranoid reaction, torticollis, withdrawal syndrome; also observed were abnormal gait, akathisia, akinesia, aphasia, choreoathetosis, circumoral paresthesia, delirium, delusions, dysarthria, euphoria, extrapyramidal syndrome, fasciculations, grand mal convulsion, hyperalgesia, irritability, manic reaction, manic-depressive reaction, meningitis, myelitis, peripheral neuritis, psychosis, psychotic depression, reflexes decreased, reflexes increased, stupor, trismus.
Respiratory System: Frequent were pharyngitis; infrequent were asthma, dyspnea, epistaxis, laryngitis, pneumonia; rare were stridor; also observed were dysphonia, emphysema, hemoptysis, hiccups, hyperventilation, lung fibrosis, pulmonary edema, respiratory flu, sputum increased.
Skin and Appendages: Frequent were rash; infrequent were acne, alopecia, dry skin, eczema, pruritus, urticaria; rare were exfoliative dermatitis, furunculosis, pustular rash, seborrhea; also observed were angioedema, ecchymosis, erythema multiforme, erythema nodosum, hirsutism, maculopapular rash, skin discoloration, skin hypertrophy, skin ulcer, sweating decreased, vesiculobullous rash.
Special Senses: Infrequent were conjunctivitis, earache, keratoconjunctivitis, mydriasis, photophobia, retinal hemorrhage, tinnitus; rare were blepharitis, visual field defect; also observed were amblyopia, anisocoria, blurred vision, cataract, conjunctival edema, corneal ulcer, deafness, exophthalmos, glaucoma, hyperacusis, night blindness, parosmia, ptosis, taste loss.
Urogenital System: Frequent were dysmenorrhea*; infrequent were albuminuria, amenorrhea*, breast pain*, cystitis, dysuria, prostatitis*, urinary retention; rare were breast enlargement*, breast neoplasm*, female lactation, hematuria, kidney calculus, metrorrhagia*, nephritis, nocturia, pregnancy and puerperal disorders*, salpingitis, urinary incontinence, uterine fibroids enlarged*; also observed were breast atrophy, ejaculatory disturbance, endometrial disorder, epididymitis, fibrocystic breast, leukorrhea, mastitis, oliguria, polyuria, pyuria, urethritis, urinary casts, urinary urgency, urolith, uterine spasm, vaginal hemorrhage.

*Based on the number of men and women as appropriate.

Postmarketing Reports: Voluntary reports of adverse events in patients taking immediate-release paroxetine hydrochloride that have been received since market introduction and not listed above that may have no causal relationship with the drug include acute pancreatitis, elevated liver function tests (the most severe cases were deaths due to liver necrosis, and grossly elevated transaminases associated with severe liver dysfunction), Guillain-Barré syndrome, toxic epidermal necrolysis, priapism, syndrome of inappropriate ADH secretion, symptoms suggestive of prolactinemia and galactorrhea, neuroleptic malignant syndrome-like events; extrapyramidal symptoms which have included akathisia, bradykinesia, cogwheel rigidity, dystonia, hypertonia, oculogyric crisis which has been associated with concomitant use of pimozide; tremor and trismus; serotonin syndrome, associated in some cases with concomitant use of serotonergic drugs and with drugs which may have impaired paroxetine metabolism (symptoms have included agitation, confusion, diaphoresis, hallucinations, hyperreflexia, myoclonus, shivering, tachycardia, and tremor); status epilepticus, acute renal failure, pulmonary hypertension, allergic alveolitis, anaphylaxis, eclampsia, laryngismus, optic neuritis, porphyria, ventricular fibrillation, ventricular tachycardia (including torsade de pointes), thrombocytopenia, hemolytic anemia, events related to impaired hematopoiesis (including aplastic anemia, pancytopenia, bone marrow aplasia, and agranulocytosis), and vasculitic syndromes (such as Henoch-Schönlein purpura). There has been a case report of an elevated phenytoin level after 4 weeks of immediate-release paroxetine and phenytoin coadministration. There has been a case report of severe hypotension when immediate-release paroxetine was added to chronic metoprolol treatment.

DRUG ABUSE AND DEPENDENCE

Controlled Substance Class: PAXIL CR is not a controlled substance.
Physical and Psychologic Dependence: PAXIL CR has not been systematically studied in animals or humans for its potential for abuse, tolerance or physical dependence. While the clinical trials did not reveal any tendency for any drug-seeking behavior, these observations were not systematic and it is not possible to predict on the basis of this limited experience the extent to which a CNS-active drug will be misused, diverted, and/or abused once marketed. Consequently, patients should be evaluated carefully for history of drug abuse, and such patients should be observed closely for signs of misuse or abuse of PAXIL CR (e.g., development of tolerance, incrementations of dose, drug-seeking behavior).

OVERDOSAGE

Human Experience: Since the introduction of immediate-release paroxetine hydrochloride in the United States, 342 spontaneous cases of deliberate or accidental overdosage during paroxetine treatment have been reported worldwide (circa 1999). These include overdoses with paroxetine alone and in combination with other substances. Of these, 48 cases were fatal and of the fatalities, 17 appeared to involve paroxetine alone. Eight fatal cases that documented the amount of paroxetine ingested were generally confounded by the ingestion of other drugs or alcohol or the presence of significant comorbid conditions. Of 145 non-fatal cases with known outcome, most recovered without sequelae. The largest known ingestion involved 2,000 mg of paroxetine (33 times the maximum recommended daily dose) in a patient who recovered.
Commonly reported adverse events associated with paroxetine overdosage include somnolence, coma, nausea, tremor, tachycardia, confusion, vomiting, and dizziness. Other notable signs and symptoms observed with overdoses involving paroxetine (alone or with other substances) include mydriasis, convulsions (including status epilepticus), ventricular dysrhythmias (including torsade de pointes), hypertension, aggressive reactions, syncope, hypotension, stupor, bradycardia, dystonia, rhabdomyolysis, symptoms of hepatic dysfunction (including hepatic failure, hepatic necrosis, jaundice, hepatitis, and hepatic steatosis), serotonin syndrome, manic reactions, myoclonus, acute renal failure, and urinary retention.
Overdosage Management: Treatment should consist of those general measures employed in the management of overdosage with any drugs effective in the treatment of major depressive disorder.
Ensure an adequate airway, oxygenation, and ventilation. Monitor cardiac rhythm and vital signs. General supportive and symptomatic measures are also recommended. Induction of emesis is not recommended. Gastric lavage with a large-bore orogastric tube with appropriate airway protection, if needed, may be indicated if performed soon after ingestion, or in symptomatic patients.
Activated charcoal should be administered. Due to the large volume of distribution of this drug, forced diuresis, dialysis, hemoperfusion, and exchange transfusion are unlikely to be of benefit. No specific antidotes for paroxetine are known.
A specific caution involves patients taking or recently having taken paroxetine who might ingest excessive quantities of a tricyclic antidepressant. In such a case, accumulation of the parent tricyclic and an active metabolite may increase the possibility of clinically significant sequelae and extend the time needed for close medical observation (see PRECAUTIONS—Drugs Metabolized by Cytochrome $P_{450}IID_6$).
In managing overdosage, consider the possibility of multiple-drug involvement. The physician should consider contacting a poison control center for additional information on the treatment of any overdose. Telephone numbers for certified poison control centers are listed in the *Physicians' Desk Reference* (PDR).

DOSAGE AND ADMINISTRATION

Major Depressive Disorder: ***Usual Initial Dosage:*** PAXIL CR should be administered as a single daily dose, usually in the morning, with or without food. The recommended initial dose is 25 mg/day. Patients were dosed in a range of 25 mg to 62.5 mg/day in the clinical trials demonstrating the effectiveness of PAXIL CR in the treatment of major depressive disorder. As with all drugs effective in the treatment of major depressive disorder, the full effect may be delayed. Some patients not responding to a 25-mg dose may benefit from dose increases, in 12.5-mg/day increments, up to a maximum of 62.5 mg/day. Dose changes should occur at intervals of at least 1 week.
Patients should be cautioned that PAXIL CR should not be chewed or crushed, and should be swallowed whole.
Maintenance Therapy: There is no body of evidence available to answer the question of how long the patient treated with PAXIL CR should remain on it. It is generally agreed that acute episodes of major depressive disorder require several months or longer of sustained pharmacologic therapy. Whether the dose of an antidepressant needed to induce remission is identical to the dose needed to maintain and/or sustain euthymia is unknown.
Systematic evaluation of the efficacy of immediate-release paroxetine hydrochloride has shown that efficacy is maintained for periods of up to 1 year with doses that averaged about 30 mg, which corresponds to a 37.5-mg dose of PAXIL CR, based on relative bioavailability considerations (see CLINICAL PHARMACOLOGY—Pharmacokinetics).
Panic Disorder: ***Usual Initial Dosage:*** PAXIL CR should be administered as a single daily dose, usually in the morning. Patients should be started on 12.5 mg/day. Dose changes should occur in 12.5-mg/day increments and at intervals of at least 1 week. Patients were dosed in a range of 12.5 to 75 mg/day in the clinical trials demonstrating the effectiveness of PAXIL CR. The maximum dosage should not exceed 75 mg/day.
Patients should be cautioned that PAXIL CR should not be chewed or crushed, and should be swallowed whole.
Maintenance Therapy: Long-term maintenance of efficacy with the immediate-release formulation of paroxetine was demonstrated in a 3-month relapse prevention trial. In this trial, patients with panic disorder assigned to immediate-release paroxetine demonstrated a lower relapse rate compared to patients on placebo. Panic disorder is a chronic condition, and it is reasonable to consider continuation for a responding patient. Dosage adjustments should be made to maintain the patient on the lowest effective dosage, and patients should be periodically reassessed to determine the need for continued treatment.
Social Anxiety Disorder: ***Usual Initial Dosage:*** PAXIL CR should be administered as a single daily dose, usually in the morning, with or without food. The recommended initial dose is 12.5 mg/day. Patients were dosed in a range of 12.5 mg to 37.5 mg/day in the clinical trial demonstrating the effectiveness of PAXIL CR in the treatment of social anxiety disorder. If the dose is increased, this should occur at intervals of at least 1 week, in increments of 12.5 mg/day, up to a maximum of 37.5 mg/day.
Patients should be cautioned that PAXIL CR should not be chewed or crushed, and should be swallowed whole.
Maintenance Therapy: There is no body of evidence available to answer the question of how long the patient treated with PAXIL CR should remain on it. Although the efficacy of PAXIL CR beyond 12 weeks of dosing has not been demonstrated in controlled clinical trials, social anxiety disorder is recognized as a chronic condition, and it is reasonable to consider continuation of treatment for a responding patient. Dosage adjustments should be made to maintain the patient on the lowest effective dosage, and patients should be periodically reassessed to determine the need for continued treatment.
Premenstrual Dysphoric Disorder: ***Usual Initial Dosage:*** PAXIL CR should be administered as a single daily dose, usually in the morning, with or without food. PAXIL CR may be administered either daily throughout the menstrual cycle or limited to the luteal phase of the menstrual cycle, depending on physician assessment. The recommended initial dose is 12.5 mg/day. In clinical trials, both 12.5 mg/day and 25 mg/day were shown to be effective. Dose changes should occur at intervals of at least 1 week.
Patients should be cautioned that PAXIL CR should not be chewed or crushed, and should be swallowed whole.
Maintenance/Continuation Therapy: The effectiveness of PAXIL CR for a period exceeding 3 menstrual cycles has not been systematically evaluated in controlled trials. However, women commonly report that symptoms worsen with age until relieved by the onset of menopause. Therefore, it is reasonable to consider continuation of a responding patient. Patients should be periodically reassessed to determine the need for continued treatment.
Special Populations: ***Treatment of Pregnant Women During the Third Trimester:*** Neonates exposed to PAXIL CR and other SSRIs or SNRIs, late in the third trimester have developed complications requiring prolonged hospitalization, respiratory support, and tube feeding (see PRECAUTIONS). When treating pregnant women with paroxetine during the third trimester, the physician should carefully consider the potential risks and benefits of treatment. The physician may consider tapering paroxetine in the third trimester.
Dosage for Elderly or Debilitated Patients, and Patients With Severe Renal or Hepatic Impairment: The recommended initial dose of PAXIL CR is 12.5 mg/day for elderly

patients, debilitated patients, and/or patients with severe renal or hepatic impairment. Increases may be made if indicated. Dosage should not exceed 50 mg/day.

Switching Patients to or From a Monoamine Oxidase Inhibitor: At least 14 days should elapse between discontinuation of an MAOI and initiation of therapy with PAXIL CR. Similarly, at least 14 days should be allowed after stopping PAXIL CR before starting an MAOI.

Discontinuation of Treatment With PAXIL CR: Symptoms associated with discontinuation of immediate-release paroxetine hydrochloride or PAXIL CR have been reported (see PRECAUTIONS). Patients should be monitored for these symptoms when discontinuing treatment, regardless of the indication for which PAXIL CR is being prescribed. A gradual reduction in the dose rather than abrupt cessation is recommended whenever possible. If intolerable symptoms occur following a decrease in the dose or upon discontinuation of treatment, then resuming the previously prescribed dose may be considered. Subsequently, the physician may continue decreasing the dose but at a more gradual rate.

HOW SUPPLIED

PAXIL CR is supplied as an enteric film-coated, controlled-release, round tablet, as follows:

12.5-mg yellow tablets, engraved with Paxil CR and 12.5
NDC 0029-3206-13 Bottles of 30
NDC 0029-3206-20 Bottles of 100

25-mg pink tablets, engraved with Paxil CR and 25
NDC 0029-3207-13 Bottles of 30
NDC 0029-3207-20 Bottles of 100
NDC 0029-3207-21 SUP 100s (intended for institutional use only)

37.5-mg blue tablets, engraved with Paxil CR and 37.5
NDC 0029-3208-13 Bottles of 30

Store at or below 25°C (77°F) [see USP].

PAXIL CR is a trademark of GlaxoSmithKline.

GEOMATRIX is a trademark of Jago Pharma, Muttenz, Switzerland.

GlaxoSmithKline, Research Triangle Park, NC 27709

April 2004/PC:L10

Shown in Product Identification Guide, page 317

PEDIARIX™ ℞

[*pēd'ē-ə-rix*]

[Diphtheria and Tetanus Toxoids and Acellular Pertussis Adsorbed, Hepatitis B (Recombinant) and Inactivated Poliovirus Vaccine Combined]

DESCRIPTION

PEDIARIX™ [Diphtheria and Tetanus Toxoids and Acellular Pertussis Adsorbed, Hepatitis B (Recombinant) and Inactivated Poliovirus Vaccine Combined] is a noninfectious, sterile, multivalent vaccine for intramuscular administration manufactured by GlaxoSmithKline Biologicals. It contains diphtheria and tetanus toxoids, 3 pertussis antigens (inactivated pertussis toxin [PT], filamentous hemagglutinin [FHA], and pertactin [69 kiloDalton outer membrane protein]), hepatitis B surface antigen, plus poliovirus Type 1 (Mahoney), Type 2 (MEF-1), and Type 3 (Saukett). The diphtheria toxoid, tetanus toxoid, and pertussis antigens are the same as those in INFANRIX® (Diphtheria and Tetanus Toxoids and Acellular Pertussis Vaccine Adsorbed). The hepatitis B surface antigen is the same as that in ENGERIX-B® [Hepatitis B Vaccine (Recombinant)].

The diphtheria toxin is produced by growing *Corynebacterium diphtheriae* in Fenton medium containing a bovine extract. Tetanus toxin is produced by growing *Clostridium tetani* in a modified Latham medium derived from bovine casein. The bovine materials used in these extracts are sourced from countries which the United States Department of Agriculture (USDA) has determined neither have nor are at risk of bovine spongiform encephalopathy (BSE). Both toxins are detoxified with formaldehyde, concentrated by ultrafiltration, and purified by precipitation, dialysis, and sterile filtration.

The 3 acellular pertussis antigens (PT, FHA, and pertactin) are isolated from *Bordetella pertussis* culture grown in modified Stainer-Scholte liquid medium. PT and FHA are isolated from the fermentation broth; pertactin is extracted from the cells by heat treatment and flocculation. The antigens are purified in successive chromatographic and precipitation steps. PT is detoxified using glutaraldehyde and formaldehyde. FHA and pertactin are treated with formaldehyde.

The hepatitis B surface antigen (HBsAg) is obtained by culturing genetically engineered *Saccharomyces cerevisiae* cells, which carry the surface antigen gene of the hepatitis B virus, in synthetic medium. The surface antigen expressed in the *S. cerevisiae* cells is purified by several physiochemical steps, which include precipitation, ion exchange chromatography, and ultrafiltration. The purified HBsAg undergoes dialysis with cysteine to remove residual thimerosal.

The inactivated poliovirus component of PEDIARIX is an enhanced potency component. Each of the 3 strains of poliovirus is individually grown in VERO cells, a continuous line of monkey kidney cells, cultivated on microcarriers. Calf serum and lactalbumin hydrolysate are used during VERO cell culture and/or virus culture. Calf serum is sourced from countries the USDA has determined neither have nor are at risk of BSE. After clarification, each viral suspension is purified by ultrafiltration, diafiltration, and successive chromatographic steps, and inactivated with formaldehyde. The 3 purified viral strains are then pooled to form a trivalent concentrate.

The diphtheria, tetanus, and pertussis antigens are individually adsorbed onto aluminum hydroxide; hepatitis B component is adsorbed onto aluminum phosphate. All antigens are then diluted and combined to produce the final formulated vaccine. Each 0.5-mL dose is formulated to contain 25 Lf of diphtheria toxoid, 10 Lf of tetanus toxoid, 25 mcg of inactivated PT, 25 mcg of FHA, 8 mcg of pertactin, 10 mcg of HBsAg, 40 D-antigen Units (DU) of Type 1 poliovirus, 8 DU of Type 2 poliovirus, and 32 DU of Type 3 poliovirus.

Diphtheria and tetanus toxoid potency is determined by measuring the amount of neutralizing antitoxin in previously immunized guinea pigs. The potency of the acellular pertussis components (PT, FHA, and pertactin) is determined by enzyme-linked immunosorbent assay (ELISA) on sera from previously immunized mice. Potency of the hepatitis B component is established by HBsAg ELISA. The potency of the inactivated poliovirus component is determined by using the D-antigen ELISA and by a poliovirus neutralizing cell culture assay on sera from previously immunized rats.

Each 0.5-mL dose also contains 2.5 mg of 2-phenoxyethanol as a preservative, 4.5 mg of NaCl, and aluminum adjuvant (not more than 0.85 mg aluminum by assay). Each dose also contains ≤100 mcg of residual formaldehyde and ≤100 mcg of polysorbate 80 (Tween 80). Thimerosal is used at the early stages of manufacture and is removed by subsequent purification steps to below the analytical limit of detection (<25 ng of mercury/20 mcg HBsAg) which upon calculation is <12.5 ng mercury per dose. Neomycin sulfate and polymyxin B are used in the polio vaccine manufacturing process and may be present in the final vaccine at ≤0.05 ng neomycin and ≤0.01 ng polymyxin B per dose. The procedures used to manufacture the HBsAg antigen result in a product that contains ≤5% yeast protein.

The vaccine must be well shaken before administration and is a turbid white suspension after shaking.

Diphtheria and Tetanus Toxoids Adsorbed Bulk Concentrate (For Further Manufacturing) is manufactured by Chiron Behring GmbH & Co, Marburg, Germany. The acellular pertussis antigens, the hepatitis B surface antigen, and the inactivated poliovirus antigens are manufactured by GlaxoSmithKline Biologicals, Rixensart, Belgium. Formulation, filling, testing, packaging, and release of the vaccine are performed by GlaxoSmithKline Biologicals Manufacturing (wholly-owned subsidiary of GlaxoSmithKline Biologicals).

CLINICAL PHARMACOLOGY

The efficacy of PEDIARIX is based on the immunogenicity of the individual antigens compared to licensed vaccines. The efficacy of the pertussis component, which does not have a well established correlate of protection, was determined in clinical trials of INFANRIX. The efficacy of the HBsAg was determined in clinical studies of ENGERIX-B. Serological correlates of protection exist for the diphtheria, tetanus, hepatitis B, and poliovirus components.

Diphtheria: Diphtheria is an acute toxin-mediated infectious disease caused by toxigenic strains of *C. diphtheriae*. Although the incidence of diphtheria in the United States has decreased from more than 200,000 cases reported in 1921,[1] before the general use of diphtheria toxoid, to only 51 cases of respiratory diphtheria reported from 1980 through 2000,[2] the case-fatality rate has remained constant at about 10%. Of 41 cases reported between 1980 and 1994, 15 (37%) patients had never been immunized, 21 (51%) had been inadequately immunized, and immunization history was unknown for 5 (12%). All 4 (10%) fatalities in this time period occurred in unvaccinated children 9 years and younger.[3] Although diphtheria is rare in the United States, toxigenic *C. diphtheriae* strains continue to circulate in previously endemic areas.[4] Protection against disease is due to the development of neutralizing antibodies to the diphtheria toxin. Following adequate immunization with diphtheria toxoid, it is thought that protection persists for at least 10 years. A serum diphtheria antitoxin level of 0.01 IU/mL is the lowest level giving some degree of protection.[5] Antitoxin levels of at least 0.1 IU/mL are generally regarded as protective.[5] Immunization with diphtheria toxoid does not, however, eliminate carriage of *C. diphtheriae* in the pharynx or nares or on the skin.[1]

Efficacy of diphtheria toxoid used in INFANRIX was determined on the basis of immunogenicity studies. A VERO cell toxin neutralizing test confirmed the ability of infant sera (N = 45), obtained 1 month after a 3-dose primary series, to neutralize diphtheria toxin. Levels of diphtheria antitoxin ≥0.01 IU/mL were achieved in 100% of the sera tested.

Tetanus: Tetanus is a condition manifested primarily by neuromuscular dysfunction caused by a potent exotoxin released by *C. tetani*. Following the introduction of vaccination with tetanus toxoid in the 1940s, the overall incidence of tetanus declined from 0.4 per 100,000 population in 1947 to 0.02 during the latter half of the 1990s.[6] Adults 60 years of age and older are at greatest risk for tetanus and tetanus-related mortality.[6] Of 124 cases of tetanus reported from 1995 through 1997, 12 (9.7%) occurred among persons younger than 25 years, one of which was a case of neonatal tetanus.[7] Overall, the case-fatality rate was 11%. The disease continues to occur almost exclusively among persons who are unvaccinated, inadequately vaccinated, or whose vaccination histories are unknown or uncertain.[7]

Spores of *C. tetani* are ubiquitous. Naturally acquired immunity to tetanus toxin does not occur. Thus, universal primary immunization and timed booster doses to maintain adequate tetanus antitoxin levels are necessary to protect all age groups.[1] Protection against disease is due to the development of neutralizing antibodies to the tetanus toxin. A serum tetanus antitoxin level of at least 0.01 IU/mL, measured by neutralization assays, is considered the minimum protective level.[8,9] More recently a level ≥0.1 to 0.2 IU/mL has been considered as protective.[10] It is thought that protection persists for at least 10 years.[1]

Efficacy of tetanus toxoid used in INFANRIX was determined on the basis of immunogenicity studies. An in vivo mouse neutralization assay confirmed the ability of infant sera (N = 45), obtained 1 month after a 3-dose primary series, to neutralize tetanus toxin. Levels of tetanus antitoxin ≥0.01 IU/mL were achieved in 100% of the sera tested.

Pertussis: Pertussis (whooping cough) is a disease of the respiratory tract caused by *B. pertussis*. Pertussis is highly communicable (attack rates in unimmunized household contacts of up to 100% have been reported[1,11]) and can cause severe disease, particularly in young infants.[1] Since immunization against pertussis became widespread, the number of reported cases and associated mortality in the United States has declined from an average annual incidence and mortality of 150 cases and 6 deaths per 100,000 population, respectively, in the early 1940s to an annual reported incidence of 2.7 cases per 100,000 population in 2000.[12] Of 28,187 cases of pertussis reported among all ages from 1997 to 2000, 62 (0.2%) resulted in death.[12] The highest number of pertussis cases (7,867) since 1967 was reported in 2000. From 1997 to 2000, infants younger than 1 year had the highest average annual incidence rate (55.5 cases per 100,000 population). During this period, of the 8,276 pertussis cases reported nationally in infants younger than 1 year, 59% were hospitalized, 11% had pneumonia, 1.3% had seizures, 0.2% had encephalopathy, and 0.7% died. Older children, adolescents, and adults, in whom classic signs are often absent, may go undiagnosed and may serve as reservoirs of disease.[1,13] The incidence of reported pertussis among adolescents and adults increased during the 1980s and 1990s.[12,14]

The role of the different components produced by *B. pertussis* in either the pathogenesis of, or the immunity to, pertussis is not well understood.

Efficacy of a 3-dose primary series of INFANRIX has been assessed in 2 clinical studies.[15,16]

A double-blind, randomized, active Diphtheria and Tetanus Toxoids (DT)-controlled trial conducted in Italy, sponsored by the National Institutes of Health (NIH), assessed the absolute protective efficacy of INFANRIX when administered at 2, 4, and 6 months of age.[15] A total of 15,601 infants were immunized with 1 of 2 acellular DTP (DTaP) vaccines, a US-licensed whole-cell DTP vaccine, or with DT vaccine alone. The mean length of follow-up was 17 months (mean age 24 months), beginning 30 days after the third dose of vaccine. The population used in the primary analysis of the efficacy of INFANRIX included 4,481 infants vaccinated with INFANRIX and 1,470 DT vaccinees. After 3 doses, the absolute protective efficacy of INFANRIX against WHO-defined typical pertussis (21 days or more of paroxysmal cough with infection confirmed by culture and/or serologic testing) was 84% (95% CI: 76% to 89%). When the definition of pertussis was expanded to include clinically milder disease with respect to type and duration of cough, with infection confirmed by culture and/or serologic testing, the efficacy of INFANRIX was calculated to be 71% (95% CI: 60% to 78%) against >7 days of any cough and 73% (95% CI: 63% to 80%) against ≥14 days of any cough. A second follow-up period to a mean age of 33 months was conducted in a partially unblinded cohort (children who received DT were offered pertussis vaccine and those who declined were retained in the study cohort). A longer unblinded follow-up period showed that after 3 doses and with no booster dose in the second year of life, the efficacy of INFANRIX against WHO-defined pertussis was 86% (95% CI: 79% to 91%) among children followed to 6 years of age.[17]

A prospective efficacy trial was also conducted in Germany employing a household contact study design.[16] In preparation for this study, 3 doses of INFANRIX were administered at 3, 4, and 5 months of age to more than 22,000 children living in 6 areas of Germany in a safety and immunogenicity study. Infants who did not participate in the safety and immunogenicity study could have received a whole-cell DTP vaccine or DT vaccine. Index cases were identified by spontaneous presentation to a physician. Households with at least one other member (i.e., besides index case) aged 6 through 47 months were enrolled. Household contacts of index cases were monitored for incidence of pertussis by a physician who was blinded to the vaccination status of the household. Calculation of vaccine efficacy was based on attack rates of pertussis in household contacts classified by vaccination status. Of the 173 household contacts who had not received a pertussis vaccine, 96 developed WHO-defined pertussis, as compared to 7 of 112 contacts vaccinated with

Continued on next page

Product information on these pages is effective as of August 2004. Further information is available at: GlaxoSmithKline, PO Box 13398, Research Triangle Park, NC 27709. 1-888-825-5249. Corporate Web Site: www.gsk.com

Pediarix—Cont.

INFANRIX. The protective efficacy of INFANRIX was calculated to be 89% (95% CI: 77% to 95%), with no indication of waning of protection up until the time of the booster vaccination. The average age of infants vaccinated with INFANRIX at the end of follow-up in this trial was 13 months (range 6 to 25 months). When the definition of pertussis was expanded to include clinically milder disease, with infection confirmed by culture and/or serologic testing, the efficacy of INFANRIX against ≥7 days of any cough was 67% (95% CI: 52% to 78%) and against ≥7 days of paroxysmal cough was 81% (95% CI: 68% to 89%). The corresponding efficacy rates of INFANRIX against ≥14 days of any cough or paroxysmal cough were 73% (95% CI: 59% to 82%) and 84% (95% CI: 71% to 91%), respectively.

Hepatitis B: Several hepatitis viruses are known to cause a systemic infection resulting in major pathologic changes in the liver (e.g., A, B, C, D, and E). The estimated lifetime risk of hepatitis B infection in the United States varies from almost 100% for the highest-risk groups to approximately 5% for the population as a whole.[18] The modes of transmission of hepatitis B include sexual contact (contaminated body secretions including semen, vaginal secretions, blood, and saliva); parenteral exposure (e.g., blood transfusions, accidental needlesticks or sharing needles from infected individuals); or maternal-neonatal transmission.[19] Hepatitis B infection can have serious consequences including acute massive hepatic necrosis, chronic active hepatitis, and cirrhosis of the liver. Up to 90% of neonates, 30% to 50% of children aged 1 to 5 years, and 6% to 10% of older children and adults who are infected in the United States will become hepatitis B virus carriers.[19] It has been estimated that 200 to 300 million people in the world are chronically infected with hepatitis B virus,[19] and that there are approximately 1.25 million chronic carriers of hepatitis B virus in the United States.[20] Those patients who become chronic carriers can infect others and are at increased risk of developing primary hepatocellular carcinoma. Among other factors, infection with hepatitis B may be the single most important factor for development of this carcinoma.[20,21]

Mothers infected with hepatitis B virus can infect their infants at, or shortly after, birth if they are carriers of the HBsAg or develop an active infection during the third trimester of pregnancy. Infected infants usually become chronic carriers. Therefore, screening of pregnant women for hepatitis B is recommended.[10] There is no specific treatment for acute hepatitis B infection. Persons who develop anti-HBs antibodies after active infection are usually protected against subsequent infection. Antibody concentrations ≥10 mIU/mL against HBsAg are recognized as conferring protection against hepatitis B.[22]

Protective efficacy with ENGERIX-B has been demonstrated in a clinical trial in neonates at high risk of hepatitis B infection.[23,24] Fifty-eight neonates born of mothers who were both HBsAg- and HBeAg-positive were given ENGERIX-B (10 mcg at 0, 1, and 2 months) without concomitant hepatitis B immune globulin. Two infants became chronic carriers in the 12-month follow-up period after initial inoculation. Assuming an expected carrier rate of 70%, the protective efficacy rate against the chronic carrier state during the first 12 months of life was 95%.

Reduced Risk of Hepatocellular Carcinoma: According to the Centers for Disease Control and Prevention (CDC), hepatitis B vaccine is recognized as the first anti-cancer vaccine because it can prevent primary liver cancer.[25] A clear link has been demonstrated between chronic hepatitis B infection and the occurrence of hepatocellular carcinoma. In a Taiwanese study, the institution of universal childhood immunization against hepatitis B virus has been shown to decrease the incidence of hepatocellular carcinoma among children.[26] In a Korean study in adult males, vaccination against the hepatitis B virus has been shown to decrease the incidence and risk of developing hepatocellular carcinoma in adults.[27]

Poliomyelitis: Poliovirus is an enterovirus that belongs to the picornavirus family.[28] Three serotypes of poliovirus have been identified (Types 1, 2, and 3). Poliovirus is highly contagious with the predominant mode of transmission being person-to-person via the fecal-oral route. The virus may also be spread indirectly through contact with infectious saliva or feces or by contaminated water or sewage.[29]

Replication of poliovirus in the pharynx and intestine is followed by a viremic phase in which involvement of the central nervous system (CNS) can occur. Whereas poliovirus infections are asymptomatic or cause nonspecific symptoms (low-grade fever, malaise, anorexia, and sore throat) in 90% to 95% of individuals, up to 2% of infected persons develop paralytic disease.[28]

As a result of the introduction of poliovirus vaccines in the 1950s and 1960s, and their subsequent widespread use, poliomyelitis control has been achieved in the United States.[30,31] After introduction of conventional (non-enhanced) inactivated poliovirus vaccine (IPV) in 1955, the annual incidence of paralytic disease of 11.4 cases per 100,000 population declined to 0.5 cases per 100,000 population in 1961, when oral poliovirus vaccine (OPV) was introduced. Incidence continued to decline thereafter, with rates of 0.00–0.01 cases per 100,000 population during the years 1990–2000.[32] Evidence suggests that endemic circulation of wild polioviruses ceased in the United States in the 1960s. The last indigenously acquired cases of poliomyelitis caused by wild poliovirus were detected in 1979 and were due to imported viruses. Since then, vaccine-associated paralytic poliomyelitis (VAPP) attributable to live OPV has been the only indigenous form of the disease in the United States.[33] To eliminate the risk for VAPP, since 2000, an all IPV schedule has been recommended for routine childhood polio vaccination in the United States. Although the likelihood of poliovirus importation has decreased substantially since 1997 as a result of decreases in the number of polio cases worldwide, the potential for importation will remain until global eradication is achieved.

IPV induces the production of neutralizing antibodies against each poliovirus serotype; these neutralizing antibodies are recognized as conferring protection against poliomyelitis disease.[34]

Immune Response to PEDIARIX Administered as a 3-Dose Primary Series: In a study conducted in the United States, the immune responses to each of the antigens contained in PEDIARIX were evaluated in sera obtained 1 month after the third dose of vaccine and were compared to those following administration of US-licensed vaccines (INFANRIX and ENGERIX-B concomitantly at separate sites, and OPV [Poliovirus Vaccine Live Oral Trivalent, Lederle Laboratories]).[35] Both groups received a US-licensed *Haemophilus influenzae* type b (Hib) vaccine (Aventis Pasteur) concomitantly at separate sites. The schedule of administration was 2, 4, and 6 months of age. One month after the third dose of PEDIARIX, vaccine response rates for each of the pertussis antigens (with the exception of FHA), geometric mean antibody concentrations for each of the pertussis antigens, and seroprotection rates for diphtheria, tetanus, hepatitis B, and the polioviruses, were shown to be non-inferior to those achieved following separately administered vaccines (see Table 1). The vaccine response to FHA marginally exceeded the 10% limit for non-inferiority.[35]

Table 1. Antibody Responses to Each Antigen Following PEDIARIX as Compared to INFANRIX, ENGERIX-B, and OPV (One Month After Administration of Dose 3) in US Infants Vaccinated at 2, 4, and 6 Months of Age

	PEDIARIX (N = 86-91)	INFANRIX, ENGERIX-B, OPV (N = 73-78)
Anti-Diphtheria		
% ≥0.1 IU/mL*	98.9	100
Anti-Tetanus		
% ≥0.1 IU/mL*	100	100
Anti-PT		
% VR*	98.9	98.7
GMC†	97.1	47.5
Anti-FHA		
% VR	95.6	100
GMC†	119.1	153.2
Anti-Pertactin		
% VR*	95.6	91.0
GMC†	150.4	108.6
Anti-HBsAg		
% ≥10 mIU/mL*	100	100
GMC†	1661.2	804.9
Anti-Polio 1		
% ≥1:8*‡	100	98.6
Anti-Polio 2		
% ≥1:8*‡	98.8	100
Anti-Polio 3		
% ≥1:8*‡	100	100

Both groups received Hib vaccine (Aventis Pasteur) concomitantly at a separate site.
OPV manufactured by Lederle Laboratories.
VR = Vaccine response: In initially seronegative infants, appearance of antibodies (concentration ≥5 EL.U./mL); in initially seropositive infants, at least maintenance of pre-vaccination concentration.
GMC = Geometric mean antibody concentration.
* Seroprotection rate or vaccine response rate to PEDIARIX not inferior to separately administered vaccines (upper limit of 90% CI on the difference for separate administration minus PEDIARIX <10%).
† GMC in the group that received PEDIARIX not inferior to separately administered vaccines (upper limit of 90% CI on the ratio of GMC for separate administration/PEDIARIX <1.5 for anti-PT, anti-FHA, and anti-pertactin, and <2.0 for anti-HBsAg).
‡ Poliovirus neutralizing antibody titer.

Immune Response to Concomitantly Administered Vaccines: In a clinical trial in the United States, PEDIARIX was given concomitantly, at separate sites, with Hib vaccine (Aventis Pasteur) to infants at 2, 4, and 6 months of age.[35] Immunogenicity data are available in 90 infants one month after the third dose of the vaccines; 98.9% (95% CI: 94% to 100%) of infants demonstrated anti-PRP antibodies ≥0.15 mcg/mL and 94.4% (95% CI: 87.5% to 98.2%) demonstrated anti-PRP antibodies ≥1.0 mcg/mL.
Immunogenicity data are not available on the concurrent administration of PEDIARIX with pneumococcal conjugate vaccine.

INDICATIONS AND USAGE

PEDIARIX is indicated for active immunization against diphtheria, tetanus, pertussis (whooping cough), all known subtypes of hepatitis B virus, and poliomyelitis caused by poliovirus Types 1, 2, and 3 as a three-dose primary series in infants born of HBsAg-negative mothers, beginning as early as 6 weeks of age. PEDIARIX should not be administered to any infant before the age of 6 weeks, or to individuals 7 years of age or older.

Infants born of HBsAg-positive mothers should receive Hepatitis B Immune Globulin (Human) (HBIG) and monovalent Hepatitis B Vaccine (Recombinant) within 12 hours of birth and should complete the hepatitis B vaccination series according to a particular schedule.[36] (See manufacturer's prescribing information for Hepatitis B Vaccine [Recombinant]) (see DOSAGE AND ADMINISTRATION).

Infants born of mothers of unknown HBsAg status should receive monovalent Hepatitis B Vaccine (Recombinant) within 12 hours of birth and should complete the hepatitis B vaccination series according to a particular schedule.[36] (See manufacturer's prescribing information for Hepatitis B Vaccine [Recombinant]) (see DOSAGE AND ADMINISTRATION).

PEDIARIX will not prevent hepatitis caused by other agents, such as hepatitis A, C, and E viruses, or other pathogens known to infect the liver. As hepatitis D (caused by the delta virus) does not occur in the absence of hepatitis B infection, hepatitis D will also be prevented by vaccination with PEDIARIX.

Hepatitis B has a long incubation period. Vaccination with PEDIARIX may not prevent hepatitis B infection in individuals who had an unrecognized hepatitis B infection at the time of vaccine administration.

When passive protection against tetanus or diphtheria is required, Tetanus Immune Globulin or Diphtheria Antitoxin, respectively, should be administered at separate sites.[1]

As with any vaccine, PEDIARIX may not protect 100% of individuals receiving the vaccine, and is not recommended for treatment of actual infections.

CONTRAINDICATIONS

Hypersensitivity to any component of the vaccine, including yeast, neomycin, and polymyxin B, is a contraindication (see DESCRIPTION).

It is a contraindication to use this vaccine after a serious allergic reaction (e.g., anaphylaxis) temporally associated with a previous dose of this vaccine or with any components of this vaccine. Because of the uncertainty as to which component of the vaccine might be responsible, no further vaccination with any of these components should be given. Alternatively, such individuals may be referred to an allergist for evaluation if further immunizations are to be considered.[1]

In addition, the following events are contraindications to administration of any pertussis-containing vaccine, including PEDIARIX:[10]

- Encephalopathy (e.g., coma, decreased level of consciousness, prolonged seizures) within 7 days of administration of a previous dose of a pertussis-containing vaccine that is not attributable to another identifiable cause;
- Progressive neurologic disorder, including infantile spasms, uncontrolled epilepsy, or progressive encephalopathy. Pertussis vaccine should not be administered to individuals with such conditions until a treatment regimen has been established and the condition has stabilized.

PEDIARIX is not contraindicated for use in individuals with HIV infection.[10,37]

WARNINGS

Administration of PEDIARIX is associated with higher rates of fever relative to separately administered vaccines. In one study that evaluated medically attended fever after the first dose of PEDIARIX or separately administered vaccines, infants who received PEDIARIX had a higher rate of medical encounters for fever within the first 4 days following vaccination. In some infants, these encounters included the performance of diagnostic studies to evaluate other causes of fever (see ADVERSE REACTIONS).

The vial stopper is latex-free. The tip cap and the rubber plunger of the needleless prefilled syringes contain dry natural latex rubber that may cause allergic reactions in latex sensitive individuals.

If any of the following events occur in temporal relation to receipt of whole-cell DTP or a vaccine containing an acellular pertussis component, the decision to give subsequent doses of PEDIARIX or any vaccine containing a pertussis component should be based on careful consideration of the potential benefits and possible risks:[38,39]

- Temperature of ≥40.5°C (105°F) within 48 hours not due to another identifiable cause;
- Collapse or shock-like state (hypotonic-hyporesponsive episode) within 48 hours;
- Persistent, inconsolable crying lasting ≥3 hours, occurring within 48 hours;
- Seizures with or without fever occurring within 3 days.

When a decision is made to withhold pertussis vaccine, immunization with DT vaccine, hepatitis B vaccine, and IPV should be continued.

If Guillain-Barré syndrome occurs within 6 weeks of receipt of prior vaccine containing tetanus toxoid, the decision to give subsequent doses of PEDIARIX or any vaccine containing tetanus toxoid should be based on careful consideration of the potential benefits and possible risks.[10]

A committee of the Institute of Medicine (IOM) has concluded that evidence is consistent with a causal relationship between whole-cell DTP vaccine and acute neurologic illness, and under special circumstances, between whole-cell DTP vaccine and chronic neurologic disease in the context of the National Childhood Encephalopathy Study (NCES) report.[40,41] However, the IOM committee concluded that the evidence was insufficient to indicate whether or not whole-cell DTP vaccine increased the overall risk of chronic neurologic disease.[41] Acute encephalopathy and permanent neurologic damage have not been reported causally linked or in temporal association with administration of PEDIARIX, but the experience with PEDIARIX is insufficient to rule this out. Encephalopathy has been reported following INFANRIX (see ADVERSE REACTIONS, Postmarketing Reports), but data are not sufficient to evaluate a causal relationship.

The decision to administer a pertussis-containing vaccine to children with stable CNS disorders must be made by the physician on an individual basis, with consideration of all relevant factors, and assessment of potential risks and benefits for that individual. The Advisory Committee on Immunization Practices (ACIP) and the Committee on Infectious Diseases of the American Academy of Pediatrics (AAP) have issued guidelines for such children.[38,42] The parent or guardian should be advised of the potential increased risk involved (see PRECAUTIONS, Information for Vaccine Recipients and Parents or Guardians).

A family history of seizures or other CNS disorders is not a contraindication to pertussis vaccine.[38]

For children at higher risk for seizures than the general population, an appropriate antipyretic may be administered at the time of vaccination with a vaccine containing an acellular pertussis component (including PEDIARIX) and for the ensuing 24 hours according to the respective prescribing information recommended dosage to reduce the possibility of post-vaccination fever.[10,38]

Vaccination should be deferred during the course of a moderate or severe illness with or without fever. Such children should be vaccinated as soon as they have recovered from the acute phase of the illness.[10]

As with other intramuscular injections, PEDIARIX should not be given to children on anticoagulant therapy unless the potential benefit clearly outweighs the risk of administration (see PRECAUTIONS).

PRECAUTIONS

PEDIARIX should be given with caution in children with bleeding disorders such as hemophilia or thrombocytopenia, with steps taken to avoid the risk of hematoma following the injection.

Before the injection of any biological, the physician should take all reasonable precautions to prevent allergic or other adverse reactions, including understanding the use of the biological concerned, and the nature of the side effects and adverse reactions that may follow its use.

Prior to immunization, the patient's current health status and medical history should be reviewed. The physician should review the patient's immunization history for possible vaccine sensitivity, previous vaccination-related adverse reactions and occurrence of any adverse–event-related symptoms and/or signs, in order to determine the existence of any contraindication to immunization with PEDIARIX and to allow an assessment of benefits and risks. Epinephrine injection (1:1000) and other appropriate agents used for the control of immediate allergic reactions must be immediately available should an acute anaphylactic reaction occur.

A separate sterile syringe and sterile disposable needle or a sterile disposable unit should be used for each individual patient to prevent transmission of hepatitis or other infectious agents from one person to another. Needles should be disposed of properly and should not be recapped.

Special care should be taken to prevent injection into a blood vessel.

As with any vaccine, if administered to immunosuppressed persons, including individuals receiving immunosuppressive therapy, the expected immune response may not be obtained.[37]

Information for Vaccine Recipients and Parents or Guardians: Parents or guardians should be informed by the healthcare provider of the potential benefits and risks of the vaccine, and of the importance of completing the immunization series. When a child returns for the next dose in a series, it is important that the parent or guardian be questioned concerning occurrence of any symptoms and/or signs of an adverse reaction after a previous dose of the same vaccine. The physician should inform the parents or guardians about the potential for adverse events that have been temporally associated with administration of PEDIARIX or other vaccines containing similar components. The parent or guardian accompanying the recipient should be told to report severe or unusual adverse events to the physician or clinic where the vaccine was administered.

The parent or guardian should be given the Vaccine Information Statements, which are required by the National Childhood Vaccine Injury Act of 1986 to be given prior to immunization. These materials are available free of charge at the CDC website (www.cdc.gov/nip).

The US Department of Health and Human Services has established a Vaccine Adverse Event Reporting System (VAERS) to accept all reports of suspected adverse events after the administration of any vaccine, including but not limited to the reporting of events required by the National Childhood Vaccine Injury Act of 1986.[10] The VAERS toll-free number is 1-800-822-7967.

Table 2. Percentage of Infants in a German Safety Study With Solicited Local Reactions or Selected Systemic Adverse Events Within 4 Days of Vaccination* at 3, 4, and 5 Months of Age With PEDIARIX Administered Concomitantly With Hib Vaccine or With Separate Concomitant Administration of INFANRIX, Hib Vaccine, and OPV (ITT Cohort)

	PEDIARIX & Hib			INFANRIX, Hib, & OPV		
	Dose 1	**Dose 2**	**Dose 3**	**Dose 1**	**Dose 2**	**Dose 3**
N	**4,666**	**4,619**	**4,574**	**768**	**757**	**750**
Local†						
Pain, any	14.0	10.2	9.9	14.2	9.8	8.1
Pain, grade 2 or 3	2.9	1.2	1.5	3.6	1.7	1.1
Pain, grade 3	0.7	0.3	0.3	1.3	0.4	0.1
Redness, any	18.6	26.6	25.6	16.1	21.4	20.8
Redness, >5 mm	6.7	9.9	9.0	5.9	8.2	7.7
Redness, >20 mm	1.2	1.0	1.1	1.8	0.7	1.1
Swelling, any	12.7	18.5	18.4	9.6	12.9	13.6
Swelling, >5 mm	5.6	7.7	7.8	3.6	5.2	4.8
Swelling, >20 mm	1.2	1.6	1.5	1.3	1.1	1.2
Systemic						
Restlessness, any	41.4	32.0	26.7	46.4	35.0	27.6
Restlessness, grade 2 or 3	14.4	10.0	8.9	20.2	11.5	8.4
Restlessness, grade 3	3.0	1.5	1.6	5.7	3.0	1.7
Fever‡, ≥100.4°F	25.1	19.3	19.7	13.2	13.1	11.2
Fever‡, >101.3°F	5.8	4.1	4.6	2.2	2.8	2.1
Fever‡, >103.1°F	0.3	0.5	0.7	0.3	0.3	0.5
Unusual cry§, any	24.9	16.5	13.1	36.5	19.7	14.3
Unusual cry§, grade 2 or 3	12.7	7.1	5.7	20.8	10.0	5.7
Unusual cry§, grade 3	3.9	1.7	1.4	6.8	2.1	1.1
Loss of appetite, any	17.9	13.3	12.5	19.1	16.2	11.3
Loss of appetite, grade 2 or 3	4.0	2.9	2.7	4.4	2.9	2.3
Loss of appetite, grade 3	0.6	0.5	0.4	0.5	0.7	0.0

N = number of infants in the intent-to-treat (ITT) cohort (infants who received the indicated vaccine and for whom at least one symptom sheet was completed).
Grade 2 defined as sufficiently discomforting to interfere with daily activities.
Grade 3 defined as preventing normal daily activities.
*Within 4 days of vaccination defined as day of vaccination and the next 3 days.
†Local reactions at the injection site for PEDIARIX or INFANRIX.
‡Rectal temperatures.
§Unusual cry lasting >1 hour.

Drug Interactions: For information regarding concomitant administration with other vaccines, refer to DOSAGE AND ADMINISTRATION.

PEDIARIX should not be mixed with any other vaccine in the same syringe or vial.

Immunosuppressive therapies, including irradiation, antimetabolites, alkylating agents, cytotoxic drugs, and corticosteroids (used in greater than physiologic doses), may reduce the immune response to vaccines. Although no specific data from studies with PEDIARIX under these conditions are available, if immunosuppressive therapy will be discontinued shortly, it would be reasonable to defer immunization until the patient has been off therapy for 3 months; otherwise, the patient should be vaccinated while still on therapy.[37] If PEDIARIX is administered to a person receiving immunosuppressive therapy, or who received a recent injection of immune globulin, or who has an immunodeficiency disorder, an adequate immunologic response may not be obtained.

Tetanus Immune Globulin or Diphtheria Antitoxin, if needed, should be given at a separate site, with a separate needle and syringe.

Carcinogenesis, Mutagenesis, Impairment of Fertility: PEDIARIX has not been evaluated for carcinogenic or mutagenic potential, or for impairment of fertility.

Pregnancy: Pregnancy Category C: PEDIARIX is not indicated for women of child-bearing age. Animal reproduction studies have not been conducted with PEDIARIX. It is not known whether PEDIARIX can cause fetal harm when administered to a pregnant woman or if PEDIARIX can affect reproductive capacity.

Geriatric Use: PEDIARIX is not indicated for use in adult populations.

Pediatric Use: Safety and effectiveness of PEDIARIX in infants younger than 6 weeks of age have not been evaluated (see DOSAGE AND ADMINISTRATION). PEDIARIX is not recommended for persons 7 years of age or older. Tetanus and Diphtheria Toxoids Adsorbed (Td) For Adult Use, IPV, and Hepatitis B Vaccine (Recombinant) should be used in individuals 7 years of age or older.

ADVERSE REACTIONS

A total of 20,739 doses of PEDIARIX have been administered to 7,028 infants as a 3-dose primary series. The most common adverse reactions observed in clinical trials were local injection site reactions (pain, redness, or swelling), fever, and fussiness. In comparative studies, administration of PEDIARIX was associated with higher rates of fever relative to separately administered vaccines (see WARNINGS; see ADVERSE REACTIONS Tables 2 and 4). The prevalence of fever was highest on the day of vaccination and the day following vaccination. More than 98% of episodes of fever resolved within the 4-day period following vaccination (i.e., the period including the day of vaccination and the next 3 days). Rates of most other solicited adverse events following PEDIARIX were comparable to rates observed following separately administered US-licensed vaccines (see ADVERSE REACTIONS Table 2).

The adverse event information from clinical trials provides a basis for identifying adverse events that appear to be related to vaccine use and for approximating rates. However, because clinical trials are conducted under widely varying conditions, adverse event rates observed in the clinical trials of a vaccine cannot be directly compared to rates in the clinical trials of another vaccine, and may not reflect the rates observed in practice.

A total of 5,472 infants were enrolled in a German safety study that was originally designed to compare the safety and reactogenicity of PEDIARIX administered concomitantly at separate sites with 1 of 4 Hib vaccines (GlaxoSmithKline Biologicals [not US-licensed]; Lederle Laboratories, Aventis Pasteur, or Merck & Co [all US-licensed]) at 3, 4, and 5 months of age.[43] After enrollment of 1,569 infants, the study was amended to include a control group that received separate US-licensed vaccines (INFANRIX, Hib vaccine [Aventis Pasteur], and OPV [Lederle Laboratories]). Infants in the separate administration group received one less antigen (hepatitis B) than the infants who received PEDIARIX. Safety data were available for 4,666 infants who received PEDIARIX administered concomitantly at separate sites with 1 of 4 Hib vaccines and for 768 infants in the control group that received separate vaccines. Data on adverse events were collected by parents using standardized diary cards for 4 consecutive days following each vaccine dose (i.e., day of vaccination and the next 3 days).

The primary end-point of the study was the percentage of infants with any grade 3 solicited symptom (redness or swelling >20 mm, fever >103.1°F, or crying, pain, vomiting, diarrhea, loss of appetite, or restlessness that prevented normal daily activities) over the 3-dose primary series in infants who received PEDIARIX (4 groups that received PEDIARIX and Hib vaccines pooled) compared to the group that received INFANRIX and Hib vaccine separately with OPV. Analysis for the primary end-point was performed on the according-to-protocol (ATP) cohort that included only those infants who were enrolled after the protocol amendment to include a control group. Of 3,773 infants in the ATP cohort for whom safety data were available, 16.2% (95% CI: 14.9% to 17.5%) of 3,029 infants who received PEDIARIX

Continued on next page

Product information on these pages is effective as of August 2004. Further information is available at: GlaxoSmithKline, PO Box 13398, Research Triangle Park, NC 27709. 1-888-825-5249. Corporate Web Site: www.gsk.com

Pediarix—Cont.

and Hib vaccine compared to 20.3% (95% CI: 17.5% to 23.4%) of 744 infants who received separate vaccines were reported to have had at least one grade 3 solicited symptom within 4 days of vaccination (i.e., day of vaccination and the next 3 days). The difference between groups in the rate of grade 3 symptoms was 4.1% (90% CI: 1.4% to 7.1%).

Data for selected solicited symptoms following each dose in a 3-dose primary series are presented in Table 2 for the intent-to-treat (ITT) cohort (includes all infants enrolled before and after the amendment who received the indicated vaccine and for whom at least one symptom sheet was completed).

[See table 2 at top of previous page]

In this study, infants were also monitored for unsolicited adverse events that occurred within 30 days following vaccination using diaries which were returned at subsequent visits and were supplemented by spontaneous reports and a medical history as reported by parents. Over the entire study period, 6 subjects in the group that received PEDIARIX reported seizures. Two of these subjects had a febrile seizure, 1 of whom also developed afebrile seizures. The remaining 4 subjects had afebrile seizures, including 2 with infantile spasms. Two subjects reported seizures within 7 days following vaccination (1 subject had both febrile and afebrile seizures, and 1 subject had afebrile seizures), corresponding to a rate of 0.22 seizures per 1,000 doses (febrile seizures 0.07 per 1,000 doses, afebrile seizures 0.14 per 1,000 doses). No subject who received concomitant INFANRIX, Hib vaccine, and OPV reported seizures. In a separate German study that evaluated the safety of INFANRIX in 22,505 infants who received 66,867 doses of INFANRIX administered as a 3-dose primary series, the rate of seizures within 7 days of vaccination with INFANRIX was 0.13 per 1,000 doses (febrile seizures 0.0 per 1,000 doses, afebrile seizures 0.13 per 1,000 doses).

No cases of hypotonic-hyporesponsiveness, encephalopathy, or anaphylaxis were reported in the German study that evaluated the safety of PEDIARIX.

Rates of serious adverse events that are less common than those reported in this safety study are not known at this time.

Additional safety data for PEDIARIX are available for 482 infants enrolled in a US study designed to evaluate lot-to-lot consistency and a bridge for a new manufacturing step. Table 3 presents the local reactions and selected adverse events within 4 days of vaccination with PEDIARIX administered concomitantly with a US-licensed Hib vaccine (Aventis Pasteur) at 2, 4, and 6 months of age. Data on adverse events were collected by parents using standardized diaries for 4 consecutive days after each vaccine dose (i.e., day of vaccination and the next 3 days) with follow-up telephone calls made by study personnel between days 1 and 3.

[See table 3 at right]

Post-dose 1 safety data are available from a US study initiated in December 2001, which was designed to assess the safety of PEDIARIX administered concomitantly at separate sites with Hib and pneumococcal conjugate vaccines (Lederle Laboratories), relative to separately administered INFANRIX, ENGERIX-B, IPV (Aventis Pasteur), Hib vaccine (Lederle Laboratories), and pneumococcal conjugate vaccine (Lederle Laboratories) at 2, 4, and 6 months of age. The study was powered to evaluate fever >101.3°F. Enrollment for this study is complete, with 673 infants in the group that received PEDIARIX and 335 infants in the separate vaccines group. Safety data following the second and third doses are expected in 2003. Data for fever within 4 days following dose 1 (i.e., day of vaccination and the next 3 days) are presented in Table 4.

[See table 4 at right]

In this study, medical attention (a visit to or from medical personnel) for fever within 4 days following vaccination was sought for 8 infants who received PEDIARIX (1.2%) and no infants who received separately administered vaccines. Four infants were seen by medical personnel in an office setting; no diagnostic tests were performed in 2 of the infants and a complete blood count (CBC) was done in the other 2 infants. Of 3 infants who were seen in an emergency room, all had a CBC and a blood and urine culture performed; chest X-rays were done in 2 of the infants and a nasopharyngeal specimen was tested for Respiratory Syncytial Virus in one of the infants. One infant was hospitalized for a work-up that included a CBC, blood and urine cultures, a lumbar puncture, and a chest X-ray. All episodes of medically attended fever resolved within 4 days post-vaccination.

In 12 clinical trials, 5 deaths were reported in 7,028 (0.07%) recipients of PEDIARIX and 1 death was reported in 1,764 (0.06%) recipients of comparator vaccines. Causes of death in the group that received PEDIARIX included 2 cases of Sudden Infant Death Syndrome (SIDS) and one case of each of the following: Convulsive disorder, congenital immunodeficiency with sepsis, and neuroblastoma. One case of SIDS was reported in the comparator group. The rate of SIDS among all recipients of PEDIARIX across the 12 trials was 0.3/1,000. The rate of SIDS observed for recipients of PEDIARIX in the German safety study was 0.2/1,000 infants (reported rate of SIDS in Germany in the latter part of the 1990s was 0.7/1,000 newborns).[44] The reported rate of SIDS in the United States from 1990 to 1994 was 1.2/1,000 live births.[45] By chance alone, some cases of SIDS can be expected to follow receipt of pertussis-containing vaccines.[39]

Table 3. Percentage of Infants in a US Lot Consistency Study With Solicited Local Reactions or Selected Systemic Adverse Events Within 4 Days of Vaccination* at 2, 4, and 6 Months of Age With PEDIARIX Administered Concomitantly With Hib Vaccine (ITT Cohort)

	PEDIARIX & Hib		
	Dose 1	**Dose 2**	**Dose 3**
Local†	**N = 482**	**N = 469**	**N = 466**
Pain, any	30.5	25.4	23.0
Pain, grade 2 or 3	6.2	5.5	3.6
Pain, grade 3	1.2	0.6	0.6
Redness, any	25.3	32.6	35.6
Redness, >5 mm	9.3	10.4	8.6
Redness, >20 mm	0.6	1.5	1.3
Swelling, any	15.1	16.6	22.3
Swelling, >5 mm	6.8	6.2	6.4
Swelling, >20 mm	1.0	1.3	1.3
Systemic	**N = 482**	**N = 469**	**N = 467**
Restlessness, any	28.8	30.3	28.5
Restlessness, grade 2 or 3	7.1	9.0	9.4
Restlessness, grade 3	1.0	1.1	0.6
Fever‡, ≥100.4°F	26.6	31.3	25.9
Fever‡, >101.3°F	2.9	6.2	4.7
Fever‡, >103.1°F	0.0	0.2	0.6
Fussiness, any	61.8	63.8	57.0
Fussiness, grade 2 or 3	14.9	21.5	17.1
Fussiness, grade 3	2.7	3.4	1.7
Loss of appetite, any	21.6	19.8	18.8
Loss of appetite, grade 2 or 3	3.1	3.2	2.4
Loss of appetite, grade 3	0.2	0.4	0.0
Sleeping more than usual, any	46.7	31.8	28.1
Sleeping more than usual, grade 2 or 3	10.2	6.0	4.7
Sleeping more than usual, grade 3	1.7	0.4	0.6

N = number of infants in the intent-to-treat (ITT) cohort (infants who received the indicated vaccine and for whom at least one symptom sheet was completed).
Grade 2 defined as sufficiently discomforting to interfere with daily activities.
Grade 3 defined as preventing normal daily activities.
*Within 4 days of vaccination defined as day of vaccination and the next 3 days.
†Local reactions at the injection site for PEDIARIX.
‡Rectal temperatures.

Table 4. Percentage of Infants in a US Coadministration Safety Study With Fever Within 4 Days of Dose 1* at 2 Months of Age With PEDIARIX Administered Concomitantly With Hib Vaccine and Pneumococcal Conjugate Vaccine or With Separate Concomitant Administration of INFANRIX, ENGERIX-B, IPV, Hib Vaccine, and Pneumococcal Conjugate Vaccine

	PEDIARIX, Hib, & Pneumococcal Conjugate (N = 667)	INFANRIX, ENGERIX-B, IPV, Hib, & Pneumococcal Conjugate (N = 333)	Separate Vaccine Group Minus Combination Vaccine Group
Fever†	**%**	**%**	**Difference (95% CI)**
≥100.4°F‡	27.9	19.8	-8.07 (-13.54, -2.60)
>101.3°F	7.0	4.5	-2.54 (-5.50, 0.41)
>102.2°F‡	2.2	0.3	-1.95 (-3.22, -0.68)
>103.1°F	0.4	0.0	-0.45 (-0.96, 0.06)
M.A.‡	1.2	0.0	-1.20 (-2.03, -0.37)

N = number of infants for whom at least one symptom sheet was completed, excluding 3 infants for whom temperature was not measured and 3 infants whose temperature was measured by the tympanic method.
*Within 4 days of dose 1 defined as day of vaccination and the next 3 days.
† Rectal temperatures.
‡ The group that received PEDIARIX compared to separate vaccine group p value <0.05 (2-sided Fisher Exact test) or the 95% confidence interval on the difference between groups does not include 0.
M.A. = Medically attended (a visit to or from medical personnel).

Limited data are available on the safety of administering PEDIARIX after a birth dose of hepatitis B vaccine (see Table 5). In a study conducted in Moldova, 160 infants received a dose of hepatitis B vaccine within 48 hours of birth followed by 3 doses of PEDIARIX at 6, 10, and 14 weeks of age. No information was collected on the HBsAg status of mothers of enrolled infants.

[See table 5 at bottom of next page]

Although there was no comparator group who received PEDIARIX without a birth dose of hepatitis B vaccine, available data suggest that some local adverse events may occur at a higher rate when PEDIARIX is administered after a birth dose of hepatitis B vaccine.

As with any vaccine, there is the possibility that broad use of PEDIARIX could reveal adverse events not observed in clinical trials.

Additional Adverse Events: Rarely, an anaphylactic reaction (i.e., hives, swelling of the mouth, difficulty breathing, hypotension, or shock) has been reported after receiving preparations containing diphtheria, tetanus, and/or pertussis antigens.[39] Arthus-type hypersensitivity reactions, characterized by severe local reactions, may follow receipt of tetanus toxoid. A review by the IOM found evidence for a causal relationship between receipt of tetanus toxoid and both brachial neuritis and Guillain-Barré syndrome.[46] A few cases of demyelinating diseases of the CNS have been reported following some tetanus toxoid-containing vaccines or tetanus and diphtheria toxoid-containing vaccines, although the IOM concluded that the evidence was inadequate to accept or reject a causal relationship.[46] A few cases of peripheral mononeuropathy and of cranial mononeuropathy have been reported following tetanus toxoid administration, although the IOM concluded that the evidence was inadequate to accept or reject a causal relationship.

Postmarketing Reports: Worldwide voluntary reports of adverse events received for INFANRIX and ENGERIX-B in children younger than 7 years of age since market introduction of these US-licensed vaccines are listed below. This list includes adverse events for which 20 or more reports were received with the exception of intussusception, idiopathic thrombocytopenic purpura, thrombocytopenia, anaphylactic reaction, angioedema, encephalopathy, hypotonic-hyporesponsive episode, and alopecia for which fewer than 20 reports were received. These latter events are included either because of the seriousness of the event or the strength of causal connection to components of this or other vaccines or drugs.

Body as a whole: Asthenia[b], fever[a+b], lethargy[b], malaise[b], Sudden Infant Death Syndrome[a+b].
Cardiovascular system: Cyanosis[a+b], edema[b], pallor[b].
Gastrointestinal system: Abdominal pain[b], anorexia[b], diarrhea[a+b], intussusception[a+b], nausea[b], vomiting[a+b].
Hematologic/lymphatic: Idiopathic thrombocytopenic purpura[a+b], lymphadenopathy[a], thrombocytopenia[a+b].
Hepatic: Jaundice[b], liver function tests abnormal[b].
Hypersensitivity: Anaphylactic reaction[a+b], angioedema[b], hypersensitivity[a].
Infections: Cellulitis[a].
Injection site reactions: Injection site reactions[a+b].
Musculoskeletal: Arthralgia[b], limb swelling[a+b].
Nervous system: Convulsions[a+b], encephalopathy[a], headache[b], hypotonia[a+b], hypotonic hyporesponsive episode[a], somnolence[a+b].
Psychiatric: Crying[a+b], irritability[a+b].
Respiratory system: Respiratory tract infection[a].
Skin and appendages: Alopecia[b], erythema[a+b], erythema multiforme[b], petechiae[b], pruritus[a+b], rash[a+b], urticaria[a+b].
Special senses: Ear pain[a].

[a] Following INFANRIX.
[b] Following ENGERIX-B.
[a+b] Following either INFANRIX or ENGERIX-B.

These reactions were reported voluntarily from a population of uncertain size; therefore, it is not always possible to reliably estimate their frequency or establish a causal relationship to vaccination.

Reporting Adverse Events: The National Childhood Vaccine Injury Act requires that the manufacturer and lot number of the vaccine administered be recorded by the healthcare provider in the vaccine recipient's permanent medical record, along with the date of administration of the vaccine and the name, address, and title of the person administering the vaccine.[47] The Act further requires the healthcare provider to report to the US Department of Health and Human Services via VAERS the occurrence following immunization of any event set forth in the Vaccine Injury Table including: Anaphylaxis or anaphylactic shock within 7 days, encephalopathy or encephalitis within 7 days, brachial neuritis within 28 days, or an acute complication or sequelae (including death) of an illness, disability, injury, or condition referred to above, or any events that would contraindicate further doses of vaccine, according to this prescribing information.[47,48] The VAERS toll-free number is 1-800-822-7967.

DOSAGE AND ADMINISTRATION

Preparation for Administration: PEDIARIX contains an adjuvant; therefore shake vigorously to obtain a homogeneous, turbid, white suspension. DO NOT USE IF RESUSPENSION DOES NOT OCCUR WITH VIGOROUS SHAKING. Inspect visually for particulate matter or discoloration prior to administration. After removal of the dose, any vaccine remaining in the vial should be discarded.

PEDIARIX should be administered by intramuscular injection. The preferred sites are the anterolateral aspects of the thigh or the deltoid muscle of the upper arm. The vaccine should not be injected in the gluteal area or areas where there may be a major nerve trunk. Gluteal injections may result in suboptimal hepatitis B immune response. Before injection, the skin at the injection site should be cleaned and prepared with a suitable germicide. After insertion of the needle, aspirate to ensure that the needle has not entered a blood vessel.

Do not administer this product subcutaneously or intravenously.

Recommended Schedule: The primary immunization series for PEDIARIX is 3 doses of 0.5 mL, given intramuscularly, at 6- to 8-week intervals (preferably 8 weeks). The customary age for the first dose is 2 months of age, but it may be given starting at 6 weeks of age.

PEDIARIX should not be administered to any infant before the age of 6 weeks. Only monovalent hepatitis B vaccine can be used for the birth dose.

Infants born of HBsAg-positive mothers should receive HBIG and Hepatitis B Vaccine (Recombinant) within 12 hours of birth at separate sites and should complete the hepatitis B vaccination series according to a particular schedule.[36] (See manufacturer's prescribing information for Hepatitis B Vaccine [Recombinant]).

Infants born of mothers of unknown HBsAg status should receive Hepatitis B Vaccine (Recombinant) within 12 hours of birth and should complete the hepatitis B vaccination series according to a particular schedule.[36] (See manufacturer's prescribing information for Hepatitis B Vaccine [Recombinant]).

The administration of PEDIARIX for completion of the hepatitis B vaccination series in infants who were born of HBsAg-positive mothers and who received monovalent Hepatitis B Vaccine (Recombinant) and HBIG has not been studied.

Modified Schedules: ***Children Previously Vaccinated With One or More Doses of Hepatitis B Vaccine:*** Infants born of HBsAg-negative mothers and who received a dose of hepatitis B vaccine at or shortly after birth may be administered 3 doses of PEDIARIX according to the recommended schedule. However, data are limited regarding the safety of PEDIARIX in such infants (see ADVERSE REACTIONS). There are no data to support the use of a 3-dose series of PEDIARIX in infants who have previously received more than one dose of hepatitis B vaccine. PEDIARIX may be used to complete a hepatitis B vaccination series in infants who have received 1 or more doses of Hepatitis B Vaccine (Recombinant) and who are also scheduled to receive the other vaccine components of PEDIARIX. However, the safety and efficacy of PEDIARIX in such infants have not been studied.

Children Previously Vaccinated With One or More Doses of INFANRIX: PEDIARIX may be used to complete the first 3 doses of the DTaP series in infants who have received 1 or 2 doses of INFANRIX and are also scheduled to receive the other vaccine components of PEDIARIX. However, the safety and efficacy of PEDIARIX in such infants have not been evaluated.

Children Previously Vaccinated With One or More Doses of IPV: PEDIARIX may be used to complete the first 3 doses of the IPV series in infants who have received 1 or 2 doses of IPV and are also scheduled to receive the other vaccine components of PEDIARIX. However, the safety and efficacy of PEDIARIX in such infants have not been studied.

Interchangeability of PEDIARIX and Licensed DTaP, IPV, or Recombinant Hepatitis B Vaccines: It is recommended that PEDIARIX be given for all 3 doses because data are limited regarding the safety and efficacy of using acellular pertussis vaccines from different manufacturers for successive doses of the pertussis vaccination series. PEDIARIX is not recommended for completion of the first 3 doses of the DTaP vaccination series initiated with a DTaP vaccine from a different manufacturer because no data are available regarding the safety or efficacy of using such a regimen.

PEDIARIX may be used to complete a hepatitis B vaccination series initiated with a licensed Hepatitis B Vaccine (Recombinant) vaccine from a different manufacturer.

PEDIARIX may be used to complete the first 3 doses of the IPV vaccination series initiated with IPV from a different manufacturer.

Additional Dosing Information: If any recommended dose of pertussis vaccine cannot be given, DT (For Pediatric Use), Hepatitis B (Recombinant), and inactivated poliovirus vaccines should be given as needed to complete the series.

Interruption of the recommended schedule with a delay between doses should not interfere with the final immunity achieved with PEDIARIX. There is no need to start the series over again, regardless of the time elapsed between doses.

The use of reduced volume (fractional doses) is not recommended. The effect of such practices on the frequency of serious adverse events and on protection against disease has not been determined.[10]

Preterm infants should be vaccinated according to their chronological age from birth.[10]

PEDIARIX is not indicated for use as a booster dose following a 3-dose primary series of PEDIARIX. Children who have received a 3-dose primary series of PEDIARIX should receive a fourth dose of IPV at 4 to 6 years of age and a fourth dose of DTaP vaccine at 15 to 18 months of age. Because the pertussis antigen components of INFANRIX are the same as those components in PEDIARIX, these children should receive INFANRIX as their fourth dose of DTaP. However, data are insufficient to evaluate the safety of INFANRIX following 3 doses of PEDIARIX.

Concomitant Vaccine Administration: In clinical trials, PEDIARIX was routinely administered, at separate sites, concomitantly with Hib vaccine (see CLINICAL PHARMACOLOGY). Safety data are available following the first dose of PEDIARIX administered concomitantly, at separate sites, with Hib and pneumococcal conjugate vaccines (see ADVERSE REACTIONS).

When concomitant administration of other vaccines is required, they should be given with separate syringes and at different injection sites.

STORAGE

Store PEDIARIX refrigerated between 2° and 8°C (36° and 46°F). **Do not freeze.** Discard if the vaccine has been frozen. Do not use after expiration date shown on the label.

HOW SUPPLIED

PEDIARIX is supplied as a turbid white suspension in single-dose (0.5 mL) vials and disposable prefilled Tip-Lok® syringes.

Single-Dose Vials
NDC 58160-841-11 (package of 10)
Single-Dose Prefilled Disposable Tip-Lok® Syringes (packaged without needles)
NDC 58160-841-46 (package of 5)
NDC 58160-841-50 (package of 25)
Single-Dose Prefilled Disposable Tip-Lok® Syringes with 1-inch 25-gauge BD SafetyGlide™ Needles
NDC 58160-841-56 (package of 25)
Single-Dose Prefilled Disposable Tip-Lok® Syringes with 5/8-inch 25-gauge BD SafetyGlide™ Needles
NDC 58160-841-57 (package of 25)

Table 5. Percentage of Infants in a Moldovan Study With Solicited Local Reactions or Selected Systemic Adverse Events Within 4 Days of Vaccination* at 6, 10, and 14 Weeks of Age With PEDIARIX Administered Concomitantly With Hib Vaccine Following a Birth Dose of Hepatitis B Vaccine (ITT Cohort)

	PEDIARIX & Hib		
	Dose 1	Dose 2	Dose 3
N	160	158	157
Local†			
Pain, any	25.6	18.4	14.0
Pain, grade 3	3.1	0.6	1.9
Redness, any	41.9	41.8	47.1
Redness, >20 mm	1.9	2.5	4.5
Swelling, any	20.6	18.4	28.0
Swelling, >20 mm	4.4	2.5	7.0
Systemic			
Restlessness, any	13.1	10.8	8.9
Restlessness, grade 3	1.3	0.6	0.6
Fever‡, ≥100.4°F	14.4	11.4	5.1
Fever‡, >103.1°F	0.0	0.6	0.0
Fussiness, any	25.0	21.5	17.8
Fussiness, grade 3	2.5	0.6	0.6

N = number of infants in the intent-to-treat (ITT) cohort (infants who received the indicated vaccine and for whom at least one symptom sheet was completed).
Grade 3 defined as preventing normal daily activities.
*Within 4 days of vaccination defined as day of vaccination and the next 3 days.
†Local reactions at the injection site for PEDIARIX.
‡Rectal temperatures.

REFERENCES

1. Centers for Disease Control. Diphtheria, tetanus, and pertussis: Recommendations for vaccine use and other preventive measures — Recommendations of the Immunization Practices Advisory Committee (ACIP). *MMWR* 1991;40(RR-10):1-28. **2.** Centers for Disease Control and Prevention. Diphtheria. In: Atkinson W and Wolfe C, eds. *Epidemiology and prevention of vaccine-preventable diseases.* 7th ed. Atlanta, GA: Public Health Foundation; 2002:39-48. **3.** Bisgard KM, Hardy I, Popovic T, et al. Respiratory diphtheria in the United States, 1980 through 1995. *Am J Public Health* 1998;88(5):787-791. **4.** Centers for Disease Control and Prevention. Toxigenic *Corynebacterium diphtheriae* — Northern Plains Indian community, August-October 1996. *MMWR* 1997;46(22):506-510. **5.** Mortimer EA and Wharton M. Diphtheria Toxoid. In: Plotkin SA and Orenstein WA, eds. *Vaccines.* 3rd ed. Philadelphia, PA: W.B. Saunders Company; 1999:140-157. **6.** Centers for Disease Control and Prevention. Tetanus — Puerto Rico, 2002. *MMWR* 2002;51(28):613-615. **7.** Centers for Disease Control and Prevention. Tetanus surveillance — United States, 1995-1997. *MMWR* 1998;47(SS-2):1-13. **8.** Wassilak SGF, Orenstein WA, and Sutter RW. Tetanus Toxoid. In: Plotkin SA and Orenstein WA, eds. *Vaccines.* 3rd ed. Philadelphia, PA: W.B. Saunders Company; 1999:441-474. **9.** Department of Health and Human Services, Food and Drug Administration. Biological products; Bacterial vaccines and toxoids; Implementation of efficacy review; Proposed rule. *Federal Register* December 13, 1985;50(240):51002-51117. **10.** Centers for Disease Control and Prevention. General recommenda-

Continued on next page

Product information on these pages is effective as of August 2004. Further information is available at: GlaxoSmithKline, PO Box 13398, Research Triangle Park, NC 27709. 1-888-825-5249. Corporate Web Site: www.gsk.com

Pediarix—Cont.

tions on immunization: Recommendations of the Advisory Committee on Immunization Practices (ACIP) and the American Academy of Family Physicians (AAFP). *MMWR* 2002;51(RR-2):1-35. **11.** Long SS. Pertussis (*Bordetella pertussis* and *B. parapertussis*). In: Behrman RE, Kliegman RM, Jenson HB, eds. *Nelson Textbook of Pediatrics*. 16th ed. Philadelphia, PA: W.B. Saunders; 2000:838-842. **12.** Centers for Disease Control and Prevention. Pertussis — United States, 1997-2000. *MMWR* 2002;51(4):73-76. **13.** Nennig ME, Shinefield HR, Edwards KM, et al. Prevalence and incidence of adult pertussis in an urban population. *JAMA* 1996;275(21):1672-1674. **14.** Güris D, Strebel PM, Bardenheier B, et al. Changing epidemiology of pertussis in the United States: Increasing reported incidence among adolescents and adults, 1990-1996. *Clin Infect Dis* 1999;28:1230-1237. **15.** Greco D, Salmaso S, Mastrantonio P, et al. A controlled trial of two acellular vaccines and one whole-cell vaccine against pertussis. *N Engl J Med* 1996;334(6):341-348. **16.** Schmitt H-J, von König CHW, Neiss A, et al. Efficacy of acellular pertussis vaccine in early childhood after household exposure. *JAMA* 1996;275(1):37-41. **17.** Salmaso S, Mastrantonio P, Tozzi AE, et al. Sustained efficacy during the first 6 years of life of 3-component acellular pertussis vaccines administered in infancy: The Italian experience. *Pediatrics* 2001;108(5):E81.**18.** Centers for Disease Control. Recommendations for protection against viral hepatitis: Recommendation of the Immunization Practices Advisory Committee (ACIP). *MMWR* 1985;34(22):313-324. **19.** Centers for Disease Control and Prevention. Hepatitis B. In: Atkinson W and Wolfe C, eds. *Epidemiology and prevention of vaccine-preventable diseases*. 7th ed. Atlanta, GA: Public Health Foundation; 2002:169-189. **20.** Lee WM. Hepatitis B virus infection. *N Engl J Med* 1997;337(24):1733-1745. **21.** Centers for Disease Control. Protection against viral hepatitis: Recommendations of the Immunization Practices Advisory Committee (ACIP). *MMWR* 1990;39(RR-2):1-26. **22.** Ambrosch F, Frisch-Niggemeyer W, Kremsner P, et al. Persistence of vaccine-induced antibodies to hepatitis B surface antigen and the need for booster vaccination in adult subjects. *Postgrad Med J* 1987;63(Suppl. 2):129-135. **23.** Andre FE and Safary A. Clinical experience with a yeast-derived hepatitis B vaccine. In: Zuckerman AJ, ed. *Viral hepatitis and liver disease*. New York, NY: Alan R Liss, Inc.; 1988: 1025-1030. **24.** Poovorawan Y, Sanpavat S, Pongpunlert W, et al. Protective efficacy of a recombinant DNA hepatitis B vaccine in neonates of HBe antigen-positive mothers. *JAMA* 1989;261(22):3278-3281. **25.** Centers for Disease Control and Prevention. Proposed vaccine information materials for hepatitis B, Haemophilus influenza type B (Hib), varicella (chickenpox), and measles, mumps, rubella (MMR) vaccines. *Federal Register* September 3, 1998;63(171): 47026-47031. **26.** Chang MH, Chen CJ, Lai MS. Universal hepatitis B vaccination in Taiwan and the incidence of hepatocellular carcinoma in children. *N Engl J Med* 1997;336:1855-1859. **27.** Lee MS, Kim DH, Kim H, et al. Hepatitis B vaccination and reduced risk of primary liver cancer among male adults: A cohort study in Korea. *Int J Epidemiol* 1998;27(2):316-319. **28.** Centers for Disease Control and Prevention. Poliomyelitis. In: Atkinson W and Wolfe C, eds. *Epidemiology and prevention of vaccine-preventable diseases*. 7th ed. Atlanta, GA: Public Health Foundation; 2002:71-82. **29.** Centers for Disease Control and Prevention. Poliomyelitis prevention in the United States: Introduction of a sequential vaccination schedule of inactivated poliovirus vaccine followed by oral poliovirus vaccine — Recommendations of the Advisory Committee on Immunization Practices (ACIP). *MMWR* 1997;46(RR-3):1-25. **30.** Kim-Farley RJ, Bart KJ, Schonberger LP, et al. Poliomyelitis in the USA: Virtual elimination of disease caused by wild virus. *Lancet* 1984;2:1315-1317. **31.** Nathanson N, Martin JR. The epidemiology of poliomyelitis: Enigmas surrounding its appearance, epidemiology, and disappearance. *Am J Epidemiol* 1979;110(6):672-692. **32.** Centers for Disease Control and Prevention. Summary of notifiable diseases, United States, 2000. *MMWR* 2000;49(53):83. **33.** Centers for Disease Control and Prevention. Poliomyelitis prevention in the United States: Updated recommendations of the Advisory Committee on Immunization Practices (ACIP). *MMWR* 2000;49(RR-5):1-22. **34.** Sutter RW, Pallansch MA, Sawyer LA, et al. Defining surrogate serologic tests with respect to predicting protective vaccine efficacy: Poliovirus vaccination. In: Williams JC, Goldenthal KL, Burns DL, Lewis Jr BP, eds. Combined vaccines and simultaneous administration. Current issues and perspectives. New York, NY: The New York Academy of Sciences; 1995:289-299. **35.** Yeh SH, Ward JI, Partridge S, et al. Safety and immunogenicity of a pentavalent diphtheria, tetanus, pertussis, hepatitis B and polio combination vaccine in infants. *Pediatr Infect Dis J* 2001;20:973-980. **36.** Centers for Disease Control and Prevention. Recommended childhood immunization schedule — United States, 2002. *MMWR* 2002;51(2):31-33. **37.** Centers for Disease Control and Prevention. Use of vaccines and immune globulins in persons with altered immunocompetence: Recommendations of the Advisory Committee on Immunization Practices (ACIP). *MMWR* 1993;42(RR-4):1-18. **38.** Centers for Disease Control and Prevention. Pertussis vaccination: Use of acellular pertussis vaccines among infants and young children — Recommendations of the Advisory Committee on Immunization Practices (ACIP). *MMWR* 1997;46(RR-7):1-25. **39.** Centers for Disease Control and Prevention. Update: Vaccine side effects, adverse reactions, contraindications, and precautions — Recommendations of the Advisory Committee on Immunization Practices (ACIP). *MMWR* 1996;45(RR-12):1-35. **40.** Institute of Medicine (IOM). Howson CP, Howe CJ, Fineberg HV, eds. *Adverse effects of pertussis and rubella vaccines*. Washington, DC: National Academy Press; 1991. **41.** Institute of Medicine (IOM). Stratton KR, Howe CJ, Johnston RB, eds. *DPT vaccine and chronic nervous dysfunction: A new analysis*. Washington, DC: National Academy Press; 1994. **42.** American Academy of Pediatrics. Pertussis. In: Pickering LK, ed. *2000 Red Book: Report of the Committee on Infectious Diseases*. 25th ed. Elk Grove Village, IL: American Academy of Pediatrics; 2000:442-448. **43.** Zepp F, Schuind A, Meyer C, et al. Safety and reactogenicity of a novel DTPa-HBV-IPV combined vaccine given along with commercial Hib vaccines in comparison with separate concomitant administration of DTPa, Hib, and OPV vaccines in infants. *Pediatrics* 2002;109(4):E58. **44.** Poets CF. Plötzlicher Säuglingstod. Neue Erkenntnisse. *Pädiat prax* 2001;60:285-292. **45.** Centers for Disease Control and Prevention. Sudden Infant Death Syndrome — United States, 1983-94. *MMWR* 1996;45(40):859-863. **46.** Institute of Medicine (IOM). Stratton KR, Howe CJ, Johnston RB, eds. *Adverse events associated with childhood vaccines. Evidence bearing on causality*. Washington, DC: National Academy Press; 1994. **47.** Centers for Disease Control. National Childhood Vaccine Injury Act: Requirements for permanent vaccination records and for reporting of selected events after vaccination. *MMWR* 1988;37(13):197-200. **48.** National Vaccine Injury Compensation Program: Vaccine injury table. www.hrsa.gov/osp/vicp/table.htm. Accessed April 29, 2002.

Manufactured by GlaxoSmithKline Biologicals
Rixensart, Belgium, US License 1617, and
Chiron Behring GmbH & Co
Marburg, Germany, US License 0097
Distributed by GlaxoSmithKline, Research Triangle Park, NC 27709
PEDIARIX is a trademark and TIP-LOK, INFANRIX, and ENGERIX-B are registered trademarks of GlaxoSmithKline.
SAFETYGLIDE is a trademark of Becton, Dickinson and Company.

August 2003/PE:L2

Shown in Product Identification Guide, page 317

RELAFEN®

℞

[rel 'ə-fen]
brand of nabumetone
tablets

DESCRIPTION

Relafen (nabumetone) is a naphthylalkanone designated chemically as 4-(6-methoxy-2-naphthalenyl)-2-butanone.

Nabumetone is a white to off-white crystalline substance with a molecular weight of 228.3. It is nonacidic and practically insoluble in water, but soluble in alcohol and most organic solvents. It has an n-octanol:phosphate buffer partition coefficient of 2400 at pH 7.4.

Tablets for Oral Administration: Each oval-shaped, film-coated tablet contains 500 mg or 750 mg of nabumetone. Inactive ingredients consist of hydroxypropyl methylcellulose, microcrystalline cellulose, polyethylene glycol, polysorbate 80, sodium lauryl sulfate, sodium starch glycolate and titanium dioxide. The 750 mg tablets also contain iron oxides.

CLINICAL PHARMACOLOGY

Relafen is a nonsteroidal anti-inflammatory drug (NSAID) that exhibits anti-inflammatory, analgesic and antipyretic properties in pharmacologic studies. As with other nonsteroidal anti-inflammatory agents, its mode of action is not known. However, the ability to inhibit prostaglandin synthesis may be involved in the anti-inflammatory effect.

The parent compound is a prodrug, which undergoes hepatic biotransformation to the active component, 6-methoxy-2-naphthylacetic acid (6MNA), that is a potent inhibitor of prostaglandin synthesis.

It is acidic and has an n-octanol:phosphate buffer partition coefficient of 0.5 at pH 7.4.

Pharmacokinetics

After oral administration, approximately 80% of a radiolabelled dose of nabumetone is found in the urine, indicating that nabumetone is well absorbed from the gastrointestinal tract. Nabumetone itself is not detected in the plasma because, after absorption, it undergoes rapid biotransformation to the principal active metabolite, 6-methoxy-2-naphthylacetic acid (6MNA). Approximately 35% of a 1000 mg oral dose of nabumetone is converted to 6MNA and 50% is converted into unidentified metabolites which are subsequently excreted in the urine. Following oral administration of *Relafen,* 6MNA exhibits pharmacokinetic characteristics that generally follow a one-compartment model with first order input and first order elimination.

6MNA is more than 99% bound to plasma proteins. The free fraction is dependent on total concentration of 6MNA and is proportional to dose over the range of 1000 mg to 2000 mg. It is 0.2% to 0.3% at concentrations typically achieved following administration of *Relafen* 1000 mg and is approximately 0.6% to 0.8% of the total concentrations at steady state following daily administration of 2000 mg.

Steady-state plasma concentrations of 6MNA are slightly lower than predicted from single-dose data. This may result from the higher fraction of unbound 6MNA which undergoes greater hepatic clearance.

Coadministration of food increases the rate of absorption and subsequent appearance of 6MNA in the plasma but does not affect the extent of conversion of nabumetone into 6MNA. Peak plasma concentrations of 6MNA are increased by approximately one third.

Coadministration with an aluminum-containing antacid had no significant effect on the bioavailability of 6MNA.

[See table 1 below]

The simulated curves in the graph below illustrate the range of active metabolite plasma concentrations that would be expected from 95% of patients following 1000 mg to 2000 mg doses to steady state. The cross-hatched area represents the expected overlap in plasma concentrations due to intersubject variation following oral administration of 1000 mg to 2000 mg of *Relafen.*

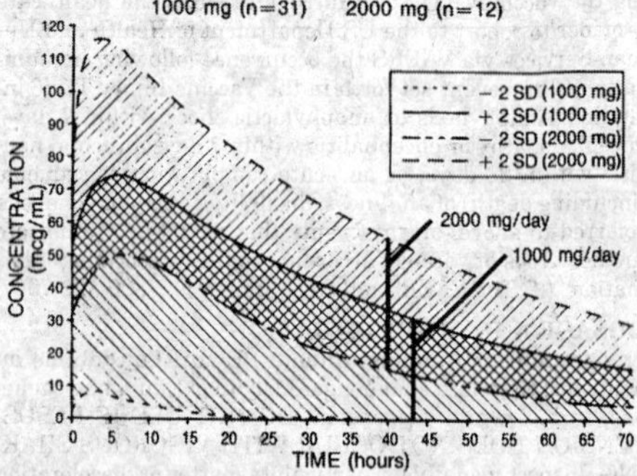

6MNA undergoes biotransformation in the liver, producing inactive metabolites that are eliminated as both free metabolites and conjugates. None of the known metabolites of 6MNA has been detected in plasma. Preliminary *in vivo* and *in vitro* studies suggest that unlike other NSAIDs, there is no evidence of enterohepatic recirculation of the active metabolite. Approximately 75% of a radiolabelled dose was recovered in urine in 48 hours. Approximately 80% was recovered in 168 hours. A further 9% appeared in the feces. In the first 48 hours, metabolites consisted of:

—nabumetone, unchanged	not detectable
—6-methoxy-2-naphthylacetic acid (6MNA), unchanged	<1%
—6MNA, conjugated	11%
—6-hydroxy-2-naphthylacetic acid (6HNA), unchanged	5%
—6HNA, conjugated	7%
—4-(6-hydroxy-2-naphthyl)-butan-2-ol, conjugated	9%
—*O*-desmethyl-nabumetone, conjugated	7%
—unidentified minor metabolites	34%
Total % Dose:	73%

Following oral administration of dosages of 1000 mg to 2000 mg to steady state, the mean plasma clearance of 6MNA is 20 to 30 mL/min. and the elimination half-life is approximately 24 hours.

Elderly Patients: Steady-state plasma concentrations in elderly patients were generally higher than in young healthy subjects. (See Table 1 for summary of pharmacokinetic parameters.)

Renal Insufficiency: In studies of patients with renal insufficiency, the mean terminal half-life of 6MNA was increased in patients with severe renal dysfunction (creatinine clearance <30 mL/min./1.73 m^2). In patients undergoing hemodialysis, steady-state plasma concentra-

Table 1. Mean pharmacokinetic parameters of nabumetone active metabolite (6MNA) at steady state following oral administration of 1000 mg or 2000 mg doses of Relafen (nabumetone)

Abbreviation (units)	Young Adults Mean ± SD 1000 mg n = 31	Young Adults Mean ± SD 2000 mg n = 12	Elderly Mean ± SD 1000 mg n = 27
t_{max} (hours)	3.0 (1.0 to 12.0)	2.5 (1.0 to 8.0)	4.0 (1.0 to 10.0)
$t_{1/2}$ (hours)	22.5 ± 3.7	26.2 ± 3.7	29.8 ± 8.1
CL_{SS}/F (mL/min.)	26.1 ± 17.3	21.0 ± 4.0	18.6 ± 13.4
Vd_{SS}/F (L)	55.4 ± 26.4	53.4 ± 11.3	50.2 ± 25.3

tions of the active metabolite were similar to those observed in healthy subjects. Due to extensive protein-binding, 6MNA is not dialyzable.

Hepatic Impairment: Data in patients with severe hepatic impairment are limited. Biotransformation of nabumetone to 6MNA and the further metabolism of 6MNA to inactive metabolites is dependent on hepatic function and could be reduced in patients with severe hepatic impairment (history of or biopsy-proven cirrhosis).

Special Studies

Gastrointestinal: Relafen (nabumetone) was compared to aspirin in inducing gastrointestinal blood loss. Food intake was not monitored. Studies utilizing ^{51}Cr-tagged red blood cells in healthy males showed no difference in fecal blood loss after 3 or 4 weeks' administration of *Relafen* 1000 mg or 2000 mg daily when compared to either placebo-treated or nontreated subjects. In contrast, aspirin 3600 mg daily produced an increase in fecal blood loss when compared to the *Relafen*-treated, placebo-treated or nontreated subjects. The clinical relevance of the data is unknown.

The following endoscopy trials entered patients who had been previously treated with NSAIDs. These patients had varying baseline scores and different courses of treatment. The trials were not designed to correlate symptoms and endoscopy scores. The clinical relevance of these endoscopy trials, i.e., either G.I. symptoms or serious G.I. events, is not known.

Ten endoscopy studies were conducted in 488 patients who had baseline and post-treatment endoscopy. In 5 clinical trials that compared a total of 194 patients on *Relafen* 1000 mg daily or naproxen 250 mg or 500 mg twice daily for 3 to 12 weeks, *Relafen* treatment resulted in fewer patients with endoscopically detected lesions (>3 mm). In 2 trials a total of 101 patients on *Relafen* 1000 mg or 2000 mg daily or piroxicam 10 mg to 20 mg for 7 to 10 days, there were fewer *Relafen* patients with endoscopically detected lesions. In 3 trials of a total of 47 patients on *Relafen* 1000 mg daily or indomethacin 100 mg to 150 mg daily for 3 to 4 weeks, the endoscopy scores were higher with indomethacin. Another 12-week trial in a total of 171 patients compared the results of treatment with *Relafen* 1000 mg/day to ibuprofen 2400 mg/day and ibuprofen 2400 mg/day plus misoprostol 800 mcg/day. The results showed that patients treated with *Relafen* had a lower number of endoscopically detected lesions (>5 mm) than patients treated with ibuprofen alone but comparable to the combination of ibuprofen plus misoprostol. The results did not correlate with abdominal pain.

Other: In 1-week repeat-dose studies in healthy volunteers, *Relafen* 1000 mg daily had little effect on collagen-induced platelet aggregation and no effect on bleeding time. In comparison, naproxen 500 mg daily suppressed collagen-induced platelet aggregation and significantly increased bleeding time.

CLINICAL TRIALS

Osteoarthritis: The use of *Relafen* in relieving the signs and symptoms of osteoarthritis was assessed in double-blind controlled trials in which 1,047 patients were treated for 6 weeks to 6 months. In these trials, *Relafen* in a dose of 1000 mg/day administered at night was comparable to naproxen 500 mg/day and to aspirin 3600 mg/day.

Rheumatoid Arthritis: The use of *Relafen* in relieving the signs and symptoms of rheumatoid arthritis was assessed in double-blind, randomized, controlled trials in which 770 patients were treated for 3 weeks to 6 months. *Relafen,* in a dose of 1000 mg/day administered at night was comparable to naproxen 500 mg/day and to aspirin 3600 mg/day.

In controlled clinical trials of rheumatoid arthritis patients, *Relafen* has been used in combination with gold, d-penicillamine and corticosteroids.

INDIVIDUALIZATION OF DOSING

There is considerable interpatient variation in response to *Relafen.* Therapy is usually initiated at a *Relafen* dose of 1000 mg daily, then adjusted, if needed, based on clinical response.

In clinical trials with osteoarthritis and rheumatoid arthritis patients, most patients responded to *Relafen* in doses of 1000 mg/day administered nightly; total daily dosages up to 2000 mg were used. In open-labelled studies, 1,490 patients were permitted dosage increases and were followed for approximately 1 year (mode). Twenty percent of patients (n=294) were withdrawn for lack of effectiveness during the first year of these open-labelled studies. The following table provides patient-exposure to doses used in the U.S. clinical trials:

Table 2. Clinical double-blind and open-labelled trials of Relafen (nabumetone) in osteoarthritis and rheumatoid arthritis

	Number of Patients		Mean/Mode Duration of Treatment (yrs.)	
***Relafen* Dose**	**OA**	**RA**	**OA**	**RA**
500 mg	17	6	0.4/–	0.2/–
1000 mg	917	701	1.2/1	1.4/1
1500 mg	645	224	2.3/1	1.7/1
2000 mg	15	100	0.6/1	1.3/1

As with other NSAIDs, the lowest dose should be sought for each patient. Patients weighing under 50 kg may be less likely to require dosages beyond 1000 mg. Therefore, after observing the response to initial therapy, the dose should be adjusted to meet individual patients' requirements.

INDICATIONS AND USAGE

Relafen is indicated for acute and chronic treatment of signs and symptoms of osteoarthritis and rheumatoid arthritis.

CONTRAINDICATIONS

Relafen is contraindicated in patients who have previously exhibited hypersensitivity to it.

Relafen is contraindicated in patients in whom *Relafen,* aspirin or other NSAIDs induce asthma, urticaria or other allergic-type reactions. Fatal asthmatic reactions have been reported in such patients receiving NSAIDs.

WARNINGS

Risk of G.I. Ulceration, Bleeding and Perforation with NSAID Therapy: Serious gastrointestinal toxicity such as bleeding, ulceration and perforation can occur at any time, with or without warning symptoms, in patients treated chronically with NSAID therapy. Although minor upper gastrointestinal problems, such as dyspepsia, are common, usually developing early in therapy, physicians should remain alert for ulceration and bleeding in patients treated chronically with NSAIDs even in the absence of previous G.I. tract symptoms.

In controlled clinical trials involving 1,677 patients treated with *Relafen* (1,140 followed for 1 year and 927 for 2 years), the cumulative incidence of peptic ulcers was 0.3% (95% CI; 0%, 0.6%) at 3 to 6 months, 0.5% (95% CI; 0.1%, 0.9%) at 1 year and 0.8% (95% CI; 0.3%, 1.3%) at 2 years. Physicians should inform patients about the signs and symptoms of serious G.I. toxicity and what steps to take if they occur. In patients with active peptic ulcer, physicians must weigh the benefits of Relafen (nabumetone) therapy against possible hazards, institute an appropriate ulcer treatment regimen and monitor the patients' progress carefully.

Studies to date have not identified any subset of patients not at risk of developing peptic ulceration and bleeding. Except for a prior history of serious G.I. events and other risk factors known to be associated with peptic ulcer disease, such as alcoholism, smoking, etc., no risk factors (e.g., age, sex) have been associated with increased risk. Elderly or debilitated patients seem to tolerate ulceration or bleeding less well than other individuals and most spontaneous reports of fatal G.I. events are in this population.

High doses of any NSAID probably carry a greater risk of these reactions, although controlled clinical trials showing this do not exist in most cases. In considering the use of relatively large doses (within the recommended dosage range), sufficient benefit should be anticipated to offset the potential increased risk of G.I. toxicity.

PRECAUTIONS

General

Renal Effects: As a class, NSAIDs have been associated with renal papillary necrosis and other abnormal renal pathology during long-term administration to animals.

A second form of renal toxicity often associated with NSAIDs is seen in patients with conditions leading to a reduction in renal blood flow or blood volume, where renal prostaglandins have a supportive role in the maintenance of renal perfusion. In these patients, administration of an NSAID results in a dose-dependent decrease in prostaglandin synthesis and, secondarily, in a reduction of renal blood flow, which may precipitate overt renal decompensation. Patients at greatest risk of this reaction are those with impaired renal function, heart failure, liver dysfunction, those taking diuretics, and the elderly. Discontinuation of NSAID therapy is typically followed by recovery to the pretreatment state.

Because nabumetone undergoes extensive hepatic metabolism, no adjustment of *Relafen* dosage is generally necessary in patients with renal insufficiency. However, as with all NSAIDs, patients with impaired renal function should be monitored more closely than patients with normal renal function (see CLINICAL PHARMACOLOGY, Renal Insufficiency). In patients with severe renal impairment (creatinine clearance ≤30 mL/min.), laboratory tests should be performed at baseline and within weeks of starting therapy. Further tests should be carried out as necessary; if the impairment worsens, discontinuation of therapy may be warranted. The oxidized and conjugated metabolites of 6MNA are eliminated primarily by the kidneys. The extent to which these largely inactive metabolites may accumulate in patients with renal failure has not been studied. As with other drugs whose metabolites are excreted by the kidneys, the possibility that adverse reactions (not listed in ADVERSE REACTIONS) may be attributable to these metabolites should be considered.

Hepatic Function: As with other NSAIDs, borderline elevations of one or more liver function tests may occur in up to 15% of patients. These abnormalities may progress, may remain essentially unchanged, or may return to normal with continued therapy. The ALT (SGPT) test is probably the most sensitive indicator of liver dysfunction. Meaningful (3 times the upper limit of normal) elevations of ALT (SGPT) or AST (SGOT) have occurred in controlled clinical trials of Relafen (nabumetone) in less than 1% of patients. A patient with symptoms and/or signs suggesting liver dysfunction, or in whom an abnormal liver test has occurred, should be evaluated for evidence of the development of a more severe hepatic reaction while on *Relafen* therapy. Severe hepatic reactions, including jaundice and fatal hepatitis, have been reported with *Relafen* and other NSAIDs. Although such reactions are rare, if abnormal liver tests persist or worsen, if clinical signs and symptoms consistent with liver disease develop, or if systemic manifestations occur (e.g., eosinophilia, rash, etc.), *Relafen* should be discontinued. Because nabumetone's biotransformation to 6MNA is dependent upon hepatic function, the biotransformation could be decreased in patients with severe hepatic dysfunction. Therefore, *Relafen* should be used with caution in patients with severe hepatic impairment (see Pharmacokinetics, *Hepatic Impairment*).

Fluid Retention and Edema: Fluid retention and edema have been observed in some patients taking *Relafen.* Therefore, as with other NSAIDs, *Relafen* should be used cautiously in patients with a history of congestive heart failure, hypertension or other conditions predisposing to fluid retention.

Photosensitivity: Based on U.V. light photosensitivity testing, *Relafen* may be associated with more reactions to sun exposure than might be expected based on skin tanning types.

Information for Patients: *Relafen,* like other drugs of its class, is not free of side effects. The side effects of these drugs can cause discomfort and, rarely, there are more serious side effects, such as gastrointestinal bleeding, which may result in hospitalization and even fatal outcome.

NSAIDs are often essential agents in the management of arthritis, but they also may be commonly employed for conditions which are less serious. Physicians may wish to discuss with their patients the potential risks (see WARNINGS, PRECAUTIONS and ADVERSE REACTIONS) and likely benefits of NSAID treatment, particularly when the drugs are used for less serious conditions where treatment without NSAIDs may represent an acceptable alternative to both the patient and the physician.

Laboratory Tests: Because severe G.I. tract ulceration and bleeding can occur without warning symptoms, physicians should follow chronically treated patients for signs and symptoms of ulceration and bleeding, and should inform them of the importance of this follow-up (see WARNINGS, Risk of G.I. Ulceration, Bleeding and Perforation with NSAID Therapy).

Drug Interactions: *In vitro* studies have shown that, because of its affinity for protein, 6MNA may displace other protein-bound drugs from their binding site. Caution should be exercised when administering *Relafen* with warfarin since interactions have been seen with other NSAIDs.

Concomitant administration of an aluminum-containing antacid had no significant effect on the bioavailability of 6MNA. When administered with food or milk, there is more rapid absorption; however, the total amount of 6MNA in the plasma is unchanged (see Pharmacokinetics).

Carcinogenesis, Mutagenesis: In two-year studies conducted in mice and rats, nabumetone had no statistically significant tumorigenic effect. Nabumetone did not show mutagenic potential in the Ames test and mouse micronucleus test *in vivo.* However, nabumetone- and 6MNA-treated lymphocytes in culture showed chromosomal aberrations at 80 mcg/mL and higher concentrations (equal to the average human exposure to *Relafen* at the maximum recommended dose).

Impairment of Fertility: Nabumetone did not impair fertility of male or female rats treated orally at doses of 320 mg/kg/day (1888 mg/m^2) before mating.

Pregnancy: Teratogenic Effects. Pregnancy Category C. Nabumetone did not cause any teratogenic effect in rats given up to 400 mg/kg (2360 mg/m^2) and in rabbits up to 300 mg/kg (3540 mg/m^2) orally. However, increased post-implantation loss was observed in rats at 100 mg/kg (590 mg/m^2) orally and at higher doses (equal to the average human exposure to 6MNA at the maximum recommended human dose). There are no adequate, well-controlled studies in pregnant women. This drug should be used during pregnancy only if clearly needed.

Because of the known effect of prostaglandin-synthesis-inhibiting drugs on the human fetal cardiovascular system (closure of ductus arteriosus), use of Relafen (nabumetone) during the third trimester of pregnancy is not recommended.

Labor and Delivery: The effects of *Relafen* on labor and delivery in women are not known. As with other drugs known to inhibit prostaglandin synthesis, an increased incidence of dystocia and delayed parturition occurred in rats treated throughout pregnancy.

Nursing Mothers: *Relafen* is not recommended for use in nursing mothers because of the possible adverse effects of prostaglandin-synthesis-drugs on neonates. It is not known whether nabumetone or its metabolites are excreted in human milk; however, 6MNA is excreted in the milk of lactating rats.

Pediatric Use: Safety and effectiveness in pediatric patients have not been established.

Geriatric Use: Of the 1,677 patients in U.S. clinical studies who were treated with *Relafen,* 411 patients (24%) were 65 years of age or older; 22 patients (1%) were 75 years of age or older. No overall differences in efficacy or safety were ob-

Continued on next page

Product information on these pages is effective as of August 2004. Further information is available at: GlaxoSmithKline, PO Box 13398, Research Triangle Park, NC 27709. 1-888-825-5249. Corporate Web Site: www.gsk.com

Relafen—Cont.

served between these older patients and younger ones. Similar results were observed in a 1-year, non-U.S. postmarketing surveillance study of 10,800 *Relafen* patients, of whom 4,577 patients (42%) were 65 years of age or older.

ADVERSE REACTIONS

Adverse reaction information was derived from blinded-controlled and open-labelled clinical trials and from worldwide marketing experience. In the description below, rates of the more common events (greater than 1%) and many of the less common events (less than 1%) represent results of U.S. clinical studies.

Of the 1,677 patients who received *Relafen* during U.S. clinical trials, 1,524 were treated for at least 1 month, 1,327 for at least 3 months, 929 for at least a year and 750 for at least 2 years. Over 300 patients have been treated for 5 years or longer.

The most frequently reported adverse reactions were related to the gastrointestinal tract. They were diarrhea, dyspepsia and abdominal pain.

Incidence ≥1%—Probably Causally Related

Gastrointestinal: Diarrhea (14%), dyspepsia (13%), abdominal pain (12%), constipation*, flatulence*, nausea*, positive stool guaiac*, dry mouth, gastritis, stomatitis, vomiting.

Central Nervous System: Dizziness*, headache*, fatigue, increased sweating, insomnia, nervousness, somnolence.

Dermatologic: Pruritus*, rash*.

Special Senses: Tinnitus*.

Miscellaneous: Edema*.

*Incidence of reported reaction between 3% and 9%. Reactions occurring in 1% to 3% of the patients are unmarked.

Incidence <1%—Probably Causally Related†

Gastrointestinal: Anorexia, jaundice, duodenal ulcer, dysphagia, gastric ulcer, gastroenteritis, gastrointestinal bleeding, increased appetite, liver function abnormalities, melena, *hepatic failure*

Central Nervous System: Asthenia, agitation, anxiety, confusion, depression, malaise, paresthesia, tremor, vertigo.

Dermatologic: Bullous eruptions, photosensitivity, urticaria, pseudoporphyria cutanea tarda, *toxic epidermal necrolysis, erythema multiforme, Stevens-Johnson Syndrome.*

Cardiovascular: Vasculitis.

Metabolic: Weight gain.

Respiratory: Dyspnea, *eosinophilic pneumonia, hypersensitivity pneumonitis, idiopathic interstitial pneumonitis.*

Genitourinary: Albuminuria, azotemia, *hyperuricemia, interstitial nephritis, nephrotic syndrome, vaginal bleeding, renal failure.*

Special Senses: Abnormal vision.

Hematologic/Lymphatic: *Thrombocytopenia.*

Hypersensitivity: *Anaphylactoid reaction, anaphylaxis,* angioneurotic edema.

†Adverse reactions reported only in worldwide postmarketing experience or in the literature, not seen in clinical trials, are considered rarer and are italicized.

Incidence <1%—Causal Relationship Unknown

Gastrointestinal: Bilirubinuria, duodenitis, eructation, gallstones, gingivitis, glossitis, pancreatitis, rectal bleeding.

Central Nervous System: Nightmares.

Dermatologic: Acne, alopecia.

Cardiovascular: Angina, arrhythmia, hypertension, myocardial infarction, palpitations, syncope, thrombophlebitis.

Respiratory: Asthma, cough.

Genitourinary: Dysuria, hematuria, impotence, renal stones.

Special Senses: Taste disorder.

Body as a Whole: Fever, chills.

Hematologic/Lymphatic: Anemia, leukopenia, granulocytopenia.

Metabolic/Nutritional: Hyperglycemia, hypokalemia, weight loss.

OVERDOSAGE

Symptoms following acute NSAIDs overdoses are usually limited to lethargy, drowsiness, nausea, vomiting, and epigastric pain, which are generally reversible with supportive care. Gastrointestinal bleeding can occur. Hypertension, acute renal failure, respiratory depression and coma may occur, but are rare. Anaphylactoid reactions have been reported with therapeutic ingestion of NSAIDs, and may occur following an overdose.

Patients should be managed by symptomatic and supportive care following a NSAIDs overdose. There are no specific antidotes. Emesis and/or activated charcoal (60 to 100 grams in adults, 1 to 2 grams/kg in children) and/or osmotic cathartic may be indicated in patients seen within 4 hours of ingestion with symptoms or following a large overdose (5 to 10 times the usual dose). Forced diuresis, alkalinization of urine, hemodialysis, or hemoperfusion may not be useful due to high protein binding.

There have been overdoses of up to 25 grams of *Relafen* reported with no long-term sequelae following standard emergency treatment (i.e., activated charcoal, gastric lavage, IV H2-blockers, etc.).

DOSAGE AND ADMINISTRATION

Osteoarthritis and Rheumatoid Arthritis

The recommended starting dose is 1000 mg taken as a single dose with or without food. Some patients may obtain more symptomatic relief from 1500 mg to 2000 mg per day. Relafen (nabumetone) can be given in either a single or twice-daily dose. Dosages over 2000 mg per day have not been studied. The lowest effective dose should be used for chronic treatment.

HOW SUPPLIED

Tablets: Oval-shaped, film-coated: 500 mg–white, imprinted with the product name RELAFEN and 500, in bottles of 100, and in Single Unit Packages of 100 (intended for institutional use only). 750 mg–beige, imprinted with the product name RELAFEN and 750, in bottles of 100, and in Single Unit Packages of 100 (intended for institutional use only).

Store at 25°C (77°F); excursions permitted to 15-30°C (59-86°F) in well-closed container; dispense in light-resistant container.

500 mg 100's: NDC 0029-4851-20
500 mg SUP 100's: NDC 0029-4851-21
750 mg 100's: NDC 0029-4852-20
750 mg SUP 100's: NDC 0029-4852-21

GlaxoSmithKline, Research Triangle Park, NC 27709

October 2001/RL:L12

Shown in Product Identification Guide, page 317

RELENZA® ℞

[*ra-lin' za*]

(zanamivir for inhalation)

For Oral Inhalation Only
For Use with the DISKHALER® Inhalation Device

DESCRIPTION

The active component of RELENZA is zanamivir. The chemical name of zanamivir is 5-(acetylamino)-4-[(aminoiminomethyl)-amino]-2,6-anhydro-3,4,5-trideoxy-D-glycero-D-galacto-non-2-enonic acid. It has a molecular formula of $C_{12}H_{20}N_4O_7$ and a molecular weight of 332.3.

Zanamivir is a white to off-white powder with a solubility of approximately 18 mg/mL in water at 20°C.

RELENZA is for administration to the respiratory tract by oral inhalation only. Each RELENZA ROTADISK® contains 4 regularly spaced double-foil blisters with each blister containing a powder mixture of 5 mg of zanamivir and 20 mg of lactose (which contains milk proteins). The contents of each blister are inhaled using a specially designed breath-activated plastic device for inhaling powder called the DISKHALER. After a RELENZA ROTADISK is loaded into the DISKHALER, a blister that contains medication is pierced and the zanamivir is dispersed into the air stream created when the patient inhales through the mouthpiece. The amount of drug delivered to the respiratory tract will depend on patient factors such as inspiratory flow. Under standardized in vitro testing, RELENZA ROTADISK delivers 4 mg of zanamivir from the DISKHALER device when tested at a pressure drop of 3 kPa (corresponding to a flow rate of about 62 to 65 L/min) for 3 seconds. In a study of 5 adult and 5 adolescent patients with obstructive airway diseases, the combined peak inspiratory flow rates (PIFR) ranged from 66 to 140 L/min. In a separate study of 16 pediatric patients, PIFR results were more variable; 4 did not achieve measurable flow rates, and PIFR for measurable inhalations by 12 children ranged from 30.5 to 122.4 L/min. Only 1 of 4 children under age 8 had a measurable flow rate (see CLINICAL PHARMACOLOGY: Pediatric Patients, INDICATIONS AND USAGE: Description of Clinical Studies, and PRECAUTIONS: Pediatric Use).

MICROBIOLOGY

Mechanism of Action: The proposed mechanism of action of zanamivir is via inhibition of influenza virus neuraminidase with the possibility of alteration of virus particle aggregation and release.

Antiviral Activity In Vitro: The antiviral activity of zanamivir against laboratory and clinical isolates of influenza virus was determined in cell culture assays. The concentrations of zanamivir required for inhibition of influenza virus were highly variable depending on the assay method used and virus isolate tested. The 50% and 90% inhibitory concentrations (IC_{50} and IC_{90}) of zanamivir were in the range of 0.005 to 16.0 µM and 0.05 to >100 µM, respectively (1 µM = 0.33 mcg/mL). The relationship between the in vitro inhibition of influenza virus by zanamivir and the inhibition of influenza virus replication in humans has not been established.

Drug Resistance: Influenza viruses with reduced susceptibility to zanamivir have been recovered in vitro by passage of the virus in the presence of increasing concentrations of the drug. Genetic analysis of these viruses showed that the reduced susceptibility in vitro to zanamivir is associated with mutations that result in amino acid changes in the viral neuraminidase or viral hemagglutinin or both.

In an immunocompromised patient infected with influenza B virus, a variant virus emerged after treatment with an investigational nebulized solution of zanamivir for 2 weeks. Analysis of this variant showed a hemagglutinin mutation (Thr 198 Ile) which resulted in a reduced affinity for human cell receptors, and a mutation in the neuraminidase active site (Arg 152 Lys) which reduced the enzyme's activity to zanamivir by 1000-fold.

Insufficient information is available to characterize the risk of emergence of zanamivir resistance in clinical use.

Cross-Resistance: Cross-resistance has been observed between zanamivir-resistant and oseltamivir-resistant influenza virus mutants generated in vitro. No studies have been performed to assess risk of emergence of cross-resistance during clinical use.

Influenza Vaccine Interaction Study: An interaction study (n = 138) was conducted to evaluate the effects of zanamivir (10 mg once daily) on the serological response to a single dose of trivalent inactivated influenza vaccine, as measured by hemagglutination inhibition titers. There was no clear difference in hemagglutination inhibition antibody titers at 2 weeks and 4 weeks after vaccine administration between zanamivir and placebo recipients.

Influenza Challenge Studies: Antiviral activity of zanamivir was supported for influenza A, and to a more limited extent for influenza B, by Phase 1 studies in volunteers who received intranasal inoculations of challenge strains of influenza virus, and received an intranasal formulation of zanamivir or placebo starting before or shortly after viral inoculation.

CLINICAL PHARMACOLOGY

Pharmacokinetics: ***Absorption and Bioavailability:*** Pharmacokinetic studies of orally inhaled zanamivir indicate that approximately 4% to 17% of the inhaled dose is systemically absorbed. The peak serum concentrations ranged from 17 to 142 ng/mL within 1 to 2 hours following a 10-mg dose. The area under the serum concentration versus time curve (AUC_∞) ranged from 111 to 1,364 ng•hr/mL.

Distribution: Zanamivir has limited plasma protein binding (<10%).

Metabolism: Zanamivir is renally excreted as unchanged drug. No metabolites have been detected in humans.

Elimination: The serum half-life of zanamivir following administration by oral inhalation ranges from 2.5 to 5.1 hours. It is excreted unchanged in the urine with excretion of a single dose completed within 24 hours. Total clearance ranges from 2.5 to 10.9 L/hr. Unabsorbed drug is excreted in the feces.

Special Populations: Impaired Hepatic Function: The pharmacokinetics of zanamivir have not been studied in patients with impaired hepatic function.

Impaired Renal Function: Systemic exposure is limited after inhalation (see Absorption and Bioavailability). After a single intravenous dose of 4 mg or 2 mg of zanamivir in volunteers with mild/moderate or severe renal impairment, respectively, significant decreases in renal clearance (and hence total clearance: normals 5.3 L/hr, mild/moderate 2.7 L/hr, and severe 0.8 L/hr; median values) and significant increases in half-life (normals 3.1 hr, mild/moderate 4.7 hr, and severe 18.5 hr; median values) and systemic exposure were observed. Safety and efficacy have not been documented in the presence of severe renal insufficiency.

Pediatric Patients: The pharmacokinetics of zanamivir were evaluated in pediatric patients with signs and symptoms of respiratory illness. Sixteen patients, 6 to 12 years of age, received a single dose of 10-mg zanamivir dry powder via DISKHALER. Five patients had either undetectable zanamivir serum concentrations or had low drug concentrations (8.32 to 10.38 ng/mL) that were not detectable after 1.5 hours. Eleven patients had C_{max} median values of 43 ng/mL (range 15 to 74) and AUC_∞ median values of 167 ng•hr/mL (range 58 to 279). Low or undetectable serum concentrations were related to lack of measurable PIFR in individual patients (see DESCRIPTION, INDICATIONS AND USAGE: Description of Clinical Studies, and PRECAUTIONS: Pediatric Use).

Geriatric Patients: The pharmacokinetics of zanamivir have not been studied in patients over 65 years of age (see PRECAUTIONS: Geriatric Use).

Gender, Race, and Weight: In a population pharmacokinetic analysis in patient studies, no clinically significant differences in serum concentrations and/or pharmacokinetic parameters (V/F, CL/F, ka, AUC_{0-3}, C_{max}, T_{max}, CL_r, and % excreted in urine) were observed when demographic variables (gender, age, race, and weight) and indices of infection (laboratory evidence of infection, overall symptoms, symptoms of upper respiratory illness, and viral titers) were considered. There were no significant correlations between measures of systemic exposure and safety parameters.

Drug Interactions: No clinically significant pharmacokinetic drug interactions are predicted based on data from in vitro studies.

Zanamivir is not a substrate nor does it affect cytochrome P450 (CYP) isoenzymes (CYP1A1/2, 2A6, 2C9, 2C18, 2D6, 2E1, and 3A4) in human liver microsomes.

INDICATIONS AND USAGE

RELENZA is indicated for treatment of uncomplicated acute illness due to influenza A and B virus in adults and pediatric patients 7 years and older who have been symptomatic for no more than 2 days (see Description of Clinical Studies and PRECAUTIONS).

RELENZA is not recommended for treatment of patients with underlying airways disease (such as asthma or chronic obstructive pulmonary disease) (see WARNINGS and PRECAUTIONS).

Description of Clinical Studies: *Adults and Adolescents:* The efficacy of RELENZA 10 mg inhaled twice daily for 5 days in the treatment of influenza has been evaluated in placebo-controlled studies conducted in North America, the Southern Hemisphere, and Europe during their respective influenza seasons. The magnitude of treatment effect varied between studies, with possible relationships to population-related factors including amount of symptomatic relief medication used.

Populations Studied: The principal Phase 3 studies enrolled 1,588 patients ages 12 years and older (median age 34 years, 49% male, 91% Caucasian), with uncomplicated influenza-like illness within 2 days of symptom onset. Influenza was confirmed by culture, hemagglutination inhibition antibodies, or investigational direct tests. Of 1,164 patients with confirmed influenza, 89% had influenza A and 11% had influenza B. These studies served as the principal basis for efficacy evaluation, with more limited Phase 2 studies providing supporting information where necessary. Following randomization to either zanamivir or placebo (inhaled lactose vehicle), all patients received instruction and supervision by a healthcare professional for the initial dose.

Principal Results: The definition of time to improvement in major symptoms of influenza included no fever and self-assessment of "none" or "mild" for headache, myalgia, cough, and sore throat. A Phase 2 and a Phase 3 study conducted in North America (total of over 600 influenza-positive patients) suggested up to one day of shortening of median time to this defined improvement in symptoms in patients receiving zanamivir compared to placebo, although statistical significance was not reached in either of these studies. In a study conducted in the Southern Hemisphere (321 influenza-positive patients), a 1.5-day difference in median time to symptom improvement was observed. Additional evidence of efficacy was provided by the European study.

Other Findings: There was no consistent difference in treatment effect in patients with influenza A compared to influenza B; however, these trials enrolled smaller numbers of patients with influenza B and thus provided less evidence in support of efficacy in influenza B.

In general, patients with lower temperature (e.g., 38.2°C or less) or investigator-rated as having less severe symptoms at entry derived less benefit from therapy.

No consistent treatment effect was demonstrated in patients with underlying chronic medical conditions, including respiratory or cardiovascular disease (see WARNINGS and PRECAUTIONS).

No consistent differences in rate of development of complications were observed between treatment groups.

Some fluctuation of symptoms was observed after the primary study endpoint in both treatment groups.

Pediatric Patients: The efficacy of RELENZA 10 mg inhaled twice daily for 5 days in the treatment of influenza in pediatric patients has been evaluated in a placebo-controlled study conducted in North America and Europe, enrolling 471 patients, ages 5 to 12 years (55% male, 90% Caucasian), within 36 hours of symptom onset. Of 346 patients with confirmed influenza, 65% had influenza A and 35% had influenza B. The definition of time to improvement included no fever and parental assessment of no or mild cough and absent/minimal muscle and joint aches or pains, sore throat, chills/feverishness, and headache. Median time to symptom improvement was one day shorter in patients receiving zanamivir compared with placebo. No consistent differences in rate of development of complications were observed between treatment groups. Some fluctuation of symptoms was observed after the primary study endpoint in both treatment groups.

Although this study was designed to enroll children ages 5 to 12 years, the product is indicated only for children 7 years of age and older. This evaluation is based on the combination of lower estimates of treatment effect in 5- and 6-year-olds compared with the overall study population, and evidence of inadequate inhalation through the DISKHALER in a pharmacokinetic study (see DESCRIPTION, CLINICAL PHARMACOLOGY: Pediatric Patients, and PRECAUTIONS: Pediatric Use).

CONTRAINDICATIONS

RELENZA is contraindicated in patients with a known hypersensitivity to any component of the formulation (see DESCRIPTION).

WARNINGS

BRONCHOSPASM AND DECLINE IN LUNG FUNCTION HAVE BEEN REPORTED IN SOME PATIENTS RECEIVING RELENZA. MANY BUT NOT ALL OF THESE PATIENTS HAD UNDERLYING AIRWAYS DISEASE SUCH AS ASTHMA OR CHRONIC OBSTRUCTIVE PULMONARY DISEASE. BECAUSE OF THE RISK OF SERIOUS ADVERSE EVENTS AND BECAUSE EFFICACY HAS NOT BEEN DEMONSTRATED IN THIS POPULATION, RELENZA IS NOT GENERALLY RECOMMENDED FOR TREATMENT OF PATIENTS WITH UNDERLYING AIRWAYS DISEASE (SEE PRECAUTIONS). Some patients with serious adverse events during treatment with RELENZA have had fatal outcomes, although causality was difficult to assess.

RELENZA SHOULD BE DISCONTINUED IN ANY PATIENT WHO DEVELOPS BRONCHOSPASM OR DECLINE IN RESPIRATORY FUNCTION; immediate treatment and hospitalization may be required. Some patients without prior pulmonary disease may also have respiratory abnormalities from acute respiratory infection that could resemble adverse drug reactions or increase patient vulnerability to adverse drug reactions.

PRECAUTIONS

General: Patients should be instructed in the use of the delivery system. Instructions should include a demonstration whenever possible. Patients should read and follow carefully the Patient Instructions for Use accompanying the product. Effective and safe use of RELENZA requires proper use of the DISKHALER to inhale the drug.

There is no evidence for efficacy of zanamivir in any illness caused by agents other than influenza virus A and B.

No data are available to support safety or efficacy in patients who begin treatment after 48 hours of symptoms.

Safety and efficacy of repeated treatment courses have not been studied.

Patients with Respiratory Disease: SAFETY AND EFFICACY OF RELENZA HAVE NOT BEEN DEMONSTRATED IN PATIENTS WITH UNDERLYING CHRONIC PULMONARY DISEASE (SEE WARNINGS). IN PARTICULAR, RELENZA HAS NOT BEEN SHOWN TO BE EFFECTIVE IN PATIENTS WITH SEVERE OR DECOMPENSATED CHRONIC OBSTRUCTIVE PULMONARY DISEASE OR ASTHMA, AND SERIOUS ADVERSE EVENTS HAVE BEEN REPORTED IN SUCH PATIENTS. THEREFORE, RELENZA IS NOT GENERALLY RECOMMENDED FOR TREATMENT OF PATIENTS WITH UNDERLYING AIRWAYS DISEASE SUCH AS ASTHMA OR CHRONIC OBSTRUCTIVE PULMONARY DISEASE (SEE WARNINGS).

Bronchospasm was documented following administration of zanamivir in 1 of 13 patients with mild or moderate asthma (but without acute influenza-like illness) in a Phase 1 study. In interim results from an ongoing treatment study in patients with acute influenza-like illness superimposed on underlying asthma or chronic obstructive pulmonary disease, more patients on zanamivir than on placebo experienced greater than 20% decline in FEV_1 or peak expiratory flow rate.

If treatment with RELENZA is considered for a patient with underlying airways disease, the potential risks and benefits should be carefully weighed. If a decision is made to prescribe RELENZA for such a patient, this should be done only under conditions of careful monitoring of respiratory function, close observation, and appropriate supportive care including availability of fast-acting bronchodilators.

Allergic Reactions: Allergic-like reactions, including oropharyngeal edema and serious skin rashes, have been reported in post-marketing experience with RELENZA. RELENZA should be stopped and appropriate treatment instituted if an allergic reaction occurs or is suspected.

Bacterial Infections: Serious bacterial infections may begin with influenza-like symptoms or may coexist with or occur as complications during the course of influenza. RELENZA has not been shown to prevent such complications.

Prevention of Influenza: Use of zanamivir should not affect the evaluation of individuals for annual influenza vaccination in accordance with guidelines of the Centers for Disease Control and Prevention Advisory Committee on Immunization Practices. Safety and efficacy of zanamivir have not been established for prophylactic use of zanamivir to prevent influenza.

Limitations of Populations Studied: Safety and efficacy have not been demonstrated in patients with high-risk underlying medical conditions (see INDICATIONS AND USAGE: Description of Clinical Studies, and WARNINGS). No information is available regarding treatment of influenza in patients with any medical condition sufficiently severe or unstable to be considered at imminent risk of requiring inpatient management.

Information for Patients: Patients should be instructed in use of the delivery system. Instructions should include a demonstration whenever possible.

For the proper use of RELENZA, the patient should read and follow carefully the accompanying Patient Instructions for Use.

Patients should be advised that the use of RELENZA for treatment of influenza has not been shown to reduce the risk of transmission of influenza to others.

Patients should be advised of the risk of bronchospasm, especially in the setting of underlying airways disease, and should stop RELENZA and contact their physician if they experience increased respiratory symptoms during treatment such as worsening wheezing, shortness of breath, or other signs or symptoms of bronchospasm (see WARNINGS). If a decision is made to prescribe RELENZA for a patient with asthma or chronic obstructive pulmonary disease, the patient should be made aware of the risks and should have a fast-acting bronchodilator available. Patients scheduled to take inhaled bronchodilators at the same time as RELENZA should be advised to use their bronchodilators before taking RELENZA.

Drug Interactions: No clinically significant pharmacokinetic drug interactions are predicted based on data from in vitro studies.

Carcinogenesis, Mutagenesis, and Impairment of Fertility:

Carcinogenesis: In 2-year carcinogenicity studies conducted in rats and mice using a powder formulation administered through inhalation, zanamivir induced no statistically significant increases in tumors over controls. The maximum daily exposures in rats and mice were approximately 23 to 25 and 20 to 22 times, respectively, greater than those in humans at the proposed clinical dose based on AUC comparisons.

Mutagenesis: Zanamivir was not mutagenic in in vitro and in vivo genotoxicity assays which included bacterial mutation assays in *S. typhimurium* and *E. coli*, mammalian mutation assays in mouse lymphoma, chromosomal aberration assays in human peripheral blood lymphocytes, and the in vivo mouse bone marrow micronucleus assay.

Impairment of Fertility: The effects of zanamivir on fertility and general reproductive performance were investigated in male (dosed for 10 weeks prior to mating, and throughout mating, gestation/lactation, and shortly after weaning) and female rats (dosed for 3 weeks prior to mating through day 19 of pregnancy, or day 21 post partum) at IV doses 1, 9, and 90 mg/kg/day. Zanamivir did not impair mating or fertility of male or female rats, and did not affect the sperm of treated male rats. The reproductive performance of the F1 generation born to female rats given zanamivir was not affected. Based on a subchronic study in rats at a 90-mg/kg/day IV dose, AUC values ranged between 142 and 199 mcg • hr/mL (>300 times the human exposure at the proposed clinical dose).

Pregnancy: Pregnancy Category C. Embryo/fetal development studies were conducted in rats (dosed from days 6 to 15 of pregnancy) and rabbits (dosed from days 7 to 19 of pregnancy) using the same IV doses. Pre- and post-natal developmental studies were performed in rats (dosed from day 16 of pregnancy until litter day 21 to 23). In all studies, intravenous (1, 9, and 90 mg/kg/day) instead of the inhalational route of drug administration was used. No malformations, maternal toxicity, or embryotoxicity were observed in pregnant rats or rabbits and their fetuses. Because of insufficient blood sampling timepoints in both rat and rabbit reproductive toxicity studies, AUC values were not available. However, in a subchronic study in rats at the 90-mg/kg/day IV dose, the AUC values were greater than 300 times the human exposure at the proposed clinical dose.

An additional embryo/fetal study, in a different strain of rat, was conducted using subcutaneous administration of zanamivir, 3 times daily, at doses of 1, 9, or 80 mg/kg during days 7 to 17 of pregnancy. There was an increase in the incidence rates of a variety of minor skeleton alterations and variants in the exposed offspring in this study. Based on AUC measurements, the high dose in the study produced an exposure greater than 1,000 times the human exposure at the proposed clinical dose. However, the individual incidence rate of each skeletal alteration or variant, in most instances, remained within the background rates of the historical occurrence in the strain studied.

Zanamivir has been shown to cross the placenta in rats and rabbits. In these animals, fetal blood concentrations of zanamivir were significantly lower than zanamivir concentrations in the maternal blood.

There are no adequate and well-controlled studies of zanamivir in pregnant women. Zanamivir should be used during pregnancy only if the potential benefit justifies the potential risk to the fetus.

Nursing Mothers: Studies in rats have demonstrated that zanamivir is excreted in milk. However, nursing mothers should be instructed that it is not known whether zanamivir is excreted in human milk. Because many drugs are excreted in human milk, caution should be exercised when RELENZA is administered to a nursing mother.

Pediatric Use: Safety and effectiveness of RELENZA have not been established in pediatric patients under 7 years of age.

The safety and effectiveness of RELENZA have been studied in a Phase 3 treatment study in pediatric patients, where 471 children 5 to 12 years of age received zanamivir or placebo (see INDICATIONS AND USAGE: Description of Clinical Studies, ADVERSE REACTIONS, and DOSAGE AND ADMINISTRATION). In a Phase 1 study of 16 children ages 6 to 12 years with signs and symptoms of respiratory disease, 4 did not produce a measurable peak inspiratory flow rate (PIFR) through the DISKHALER (3 with no adequate inhalation on request, 1 with missing data), 9 had measurable PIFR on each of 2 inhalations, and 3 achieved measurable PIFR on only 1 of 2 inhalations. Neither of two 6-year-olds and one of two 7-year-olds produced measurable PIFR. Overall, 8 of the 16 children (including all those under 8 years old) either did not produce measurable inspiratory flow through the DISKHALER or produced peak inspiratory flow rates below the 60 L/min considered optimal for the device under standardized in vitro testing; lack of measurable flow rate was related to low or undetectable serum concentrations (see DESCRIPTION, CLINICAL PHARMACOLOGY: Pediatric Patients, and INDICATIONS AND USAGE: Description of Clinical Studies). Prescribers should carefully evaluate the ability of young children to use the delivery system if prescription of RELENZA is considered. When RELENZA is prescribed for children, it should be used only under adult supervision and with attention to proper use of the delivery system.

Adolescents were included in the 3 principal Phase 3 adult treatment studies. In these studies, 67 patients were 12 to 16 years of age. No definite differences in safety and efficacy were observed between these adolescent patients and young adults.

Geriatric Use: Of the total number of patients in 6 clinical treatment studies of RELENZA, 59 were 65 and over, while

Continued on next page

Product information on these pages is effective as of August 2004. Further information is available at: GlaxoSmithKline, PO Box 13398, Research Triangle Park, NC 27709. 1-888-825-5249. Corporate Web Site: www.gsk.com

Relenza—Cont.

24 were 75 and over. No overall differences in safety or effectiveness were observed between these subjects and younger patients, and other reported clinical experience has not identified differences in responses between the elderly and younger patients, but greater sensitivity of some older individuals cannot be ruled out.

ADVERSE REACTIONS

See WARNINGS and PRECAUTIONS for information about risk of serious adverse events such as bronchospasm and allergic-like reactions, and for safety information in patients with underlying respiratory disease.

Clinical Trials in Adults and Adolescents: Adverse events that occurred with an incidence ≥1.5% in treatment studies are listed in Table 1. This table shows adverse events occurring in patients ≥12 years of age receiving RELENZA 10 mg inhaled twice daily, RELENZA in all inhalation regimens, and placebo inhaled twice daily (where placebo consisted of the same lactose vehicle used in RELENZA).

[See table 1 below]

Additional adverse reactions occurring in less than 1.5% of patients receiving RELENZA included malaise, fatigue, fever, abdominal pain, myalgia, arthralgia, and urticaria.

The most frequent laboratory abnormalities in Phase 3 treatment studies included elevations of liver enzymes and CPK, lymphopenia, and neutropenia. These were reported in similar proportions of zanamivir and lactose vehicle placebo recipients with acute influenza-like illness.

Clinical Trials in Pediatric Patients: Adverse events that occurred with an incidence ≥1.5% in children receiving treatment doses of RELENZA in 2 Phase 3 studies are listed in Table 2. This table shows adverse events occurring in pediatric patients 5 to 12 years old receiving RELENZA 10 mg inhaled twice daily, and placebo inhaled twice daily (where placebo consisted of the same lactose vehicle used in RELENZA).

[See table 2 below]

In 1 of the 2 studies described in Table 2, some additional information is available from children (5 to 12 years old) without acute influenza-like illness who received an investigational prophylaxis regimen of RELENZA; 132 children received RELENZA and 145 children received placebo. Among these children, nasal signs and symptoms (zanamivir 20%, placebo 9%), cough (zanamivir 16%, placebo 8%), and throat/tonsil discomfort and pain (zanamivir 11%, placebo 6%) were reported more frequently with RELENZA than placebo. In a subset with chronic respiratory disease, lower respiratory adverse events (described as asthma, cough, or viral respiratory infections which could include influenza-like symptoms) were reported in 7 of 7 zanamivir recipients and 5 of 12 placebo recipients.

Observed During Clinical Practice: In addition to adverse events reported from clinical trials, the following events have been identified during post-marketing use of zanamivir (RELENZA). Because they are reported voluntarily from a population of unknown size, estimates of frequency cannot be made. These events have been chosen for inclusion due to a combination of their seriousness, frequency of reporting, or potential causal connection to zanamivir (RELENZA).

General: Allergic or allergic-like reaction, including oropharyngeal edema (see PRECAUTIONS).

Cardiac: Arrhythmias, syncope.

Neurologic: Seizures.

Respiratory: Bronchospasm, dyspnea (see WARNINGS and PRECAUTIONS).

Skin: Facial edema; rash, including serious cutaneous reactions (see PRECAUTIONS).

OVERDOSAGE

There have been no reports of overdosage from administration of RELENZA. Doses of zanamivir up to 64 mg/day have been administered by nebulizer. Additionally, doses of up to 1,200 mg/day for 5 days have been administered intravenously. Adverse effects were similar to those seen in clinical studies at the recommended dose.

DOSAGE AND ADMINISTRATION

RELENZA is for administration to the respiratory tract by oral inhalation only, using the DISKHALER device provided. **Patients should be instructed in the use of the delivery system. Instructions should include a demonstration whenever possible. If RELENZA is prescribed for children, it should be used only under adult supervision and instruction, and the supervising adult should first be instructed by a healthcare professional (see PRECAUTIONS).**

The recommended dose of RELENZA for treatment of influenza in adults and pediatric patients ages 7 years and older is 2 inhalations (one 5-mg blister per inhalation for a total dose of 10 mg) twice daily (approximately 12 hours apart) for 5 days. Two doses should be taken on the first day of treatment whenever possible provided there is at least 2 hours between doses. On subsequent days, doses should be about 12 hours apart (e.g., morning and evening) at approximately the same time each day. There are no data on the effectiveness of treatment with RELENZA when initiated more than 2 days after the onset of signs or symptoms.

Patients scheduled to use an inhaled bronchodilator at the same time as RELENZA should use their bronchodilator before taking RELENZA. (See WARNINGS and PRECAUTIONS regarding patients with chronic respiratory disease and other medical conditions.)

HOW SUPPLIED

RELENZA is supplied in a circular double-foil pack (a ROTADISK) containing 4 blisters of the drug. Five ROTADISKS are packaged in a white polypropylene tube. The tube is packaged in a carton with 1 blue and gray DISKHALER inhalation device (NDC 0173-0681-01).

Store at 25°C (77°F); excursions permitted to 15° to 30°C (59° to 86°F) (see USP Controlled Room Temperature). Keep out of reach of children. Do not puncture any RELENZA ROTADISK blister until taking a dose using the DISKHALER.

GlaxoSmithKline, Research Triangle Park, NC 27709

April 2003/RL-2000

Shown in Product Identification Guide, page 317

Table 1. Summary of Adverse Events ≥1.5% Incidence During Treatment in Adults and Adolescents

Adverse Event	RELENZA 10 mg b.i.d. **Inhaled** (n = 1,132)	RELENZA All Dosing Regimens* (n = 2,289)	Placebo (Lactose Vehicle†) (n = 1,520)
Body as a whole			
Headaches	2%	2%	3%
Digestive			
Diarrhea	3%	3%	4%
Nausea	3%	3%	3%
Vomiting	1%	1%	2%
Respiratory			
Nasal signs and symptoms	2%	3%	3%
Bronchitis	2%	2%	3%
Cough	2%	2%	3%
Sinusitis	3%	2%	2%
Ear, nose, & throat infections	2%	1%	2%
Nervous system			
Dizziness	2%	1%	<1%

*Includes studies where RELENZA was administered intranasally (6.4 mg 2 to 4 times per day in addition to inhaled preparation) and/or inhaled more frequently (q.i.d.) than the currently recommended dose.
† Because the placebo consisted of inhaled lactose powder, which is also the vehicle for the active drug, some adverse events occurring at similar frequencies in different treatment groups could be related to lactose vehicle inhalation.

Table 2. Summary of Adverse Events ≥1.5% Incidence During Treatment in Pediatric Patients*

Adverse Event	RELENZA 10 mg b.i.d. Inhaled (n = 291)	Placebo (Lactose Vehicle†) (n = 318)
Respiratory		
Ear, nose, & throat infections	5%	5%
Ear, nose, & throat hemorrhage	<1%	2%
Asthma	<1%	2%
Cough	<1%	2%
Digestive		
Vomiting	2%	3%
Diarrhea	2%	2%
Nausea	<1%	2%

*Includes a subset of patients receiving RELENZA for treatment of influenza in a prophylaxis study.
† Because the placebo consisted of inhaled lactose powder, which is also the vehicle for the active drug, some adverse events occurring at similar frequencies in different treatment groups could be related to lactose vehicle inhalation.

REQUIP® ℞

[*rē' kwip*]

brand of ropinirole hydrochloride

Tablets

DESCRIPTION

Requip (ropinirole hydrochloride), an orally administered anti-Parkinsonian drug, is a non-ergoline dopamine agonist. It is the hydrochloride salt of 4-[2-(dipropylamino)-ethyl]-1,3-dihydro-2H-indol-2-one monohydrochloride and has an empirical formula of $C_{16}H_{24}N_2O$•HCl. The molecular weight is 296.84 (260.38 as the free base).

Ropinirole hydrochloride is a white to pale greenish-yellow powder with a melting range of 243° to 250°C and a solubility of 133 mg/mL in water.

Each pentagonal film-coated Tiltab® tablet with beveled edges contains ropinirole hydrochloride equivalent to ropinirole, 0.25 mg, 0.5 mg, 1 mg, 2 mg, 3 mg, 4 mg or 5 mg. Inactive ingredients consist of: croscarmellose sodium, hydrous lactose, magnesium stearate, microcrystalline cellulose, and one or more of the following: carmine, FD&C Blue No. 2 aluminum lake, FD&C Yellow No. 6 aluminum lake, hydroxypropyl methylcellulose, iron oxides, polyethylene glycol, polysorbate 80, titanium dioxide.

CLINICAL PHARMACOLOGY

Mechanism of Action

Requip is a non-ergoline dopamine agonist with high relative *in vitro* specificity and full intrinsic activity at the D_2 and D_3 dopamine receptor subtypes, binding with higher affinity to D_3 than to D_2 or D_4 receptor subtypes. The relevance of D_3 receptor binding in Parkinson's disease is unknown.

Ropinirole has moderate *in vitro* affinity for opioid receptors. Ropinirole and its metabolites have negligible *in vitro* affinity for dopamine D_1, 5-HT_1, 5-HT_2, benzodiazepine, GABA, muscarinic, alpha$_1$-, alpha$_2$-, and beta-adrenoreceptors.

The precise mechanism of action of *Requip* as a treatment for Parkinson's disease is unknown, although it is believed to be due to stimulation of post-synaptic dopamine D_2-type receptors within the caudate-putamen in the brain. This conclusion is supported by studies that show that ropinirole improves motor function in various animal models of Parkinson's disease. In particular, ropinirole attenuates the motor deficits induced by lesioning the ascending nigrostriatal dopaminergic pathway with the neurotoxin 1-methyl-4-phenyl-1,2,3,6-tetrahydropyridine (MPTP) in primates.

Clinical Pharmacology Studies

In healthy normotensive subjects, single oral doses of *Requip* in the range 0.01 to 2.5 mg had little or no effect on supine blood pressure and pulse rates. Upon standing, *Requip* caused decreases in systolic and diastolic blood pressure at doses above 0.25 mg. In some subjects, these changes were associated with the emergence of orthostatic symptoms, bradycardia and, in one case, transient sinus arrest with syncope. The effect of repeat dosing and slow titration of *Requip* was not studied in healthy volunteers.

The mechanism of *Requip*-induced postural hypotension is presumed to be due to a D_2-mediated blunting of the noradrenergic response to standing and subsequent decrease in peripheral vascular resistance. Nausea is a common concomitant of orthostatic signs and symptoms.

At oral doses as low as 0.2 mg, *Requip* suppressed serum prolactin concentrations in healthy male volunteers.

Requip had no dose-related effect on ECG wave form and rhythm in young healthy male volunteers in the range of 0.01 to 2.5 mg.

Pharmacokinetics

Absorption, Distribution, Metabolism and Elimination

Ropinirole is rapidly absorbed after oral administration, reaching peak concentration in approximately 1-2 hours. In clinical studies, over 88% of a radiolabeled dose was recovered in urine and the absolute bioavailability was 55%, indicating a first pass effect. Relative bioavailability from a tablet compared to an oral solution is 85%. Food does not affect the extent of absorption of ropinirole, although its T_{max} is increased by 2.5 hours when the drug is taken with a meal. The clearance of ropinirole after oral administration to patients is 47 L/hr (cv=45%) and its elimination half-life is approximately 6 hours. Ropinirole is extensively metabolized by the liver to inactive metabolites and displays linear kinetics over the therapeutic dosing range of 1 mg to 8 mg t.i.d. Steady-state concentrations are expected to be achieved within 2 days of dosing. Accumulation upon multiple dosing is predictive from single dosing.

Ropinirole is widely distributed throughout the body, with an apparent volume of distribution of 7.5 L/kg (cv=32%). It is up to 40% bound to plasma proteins and has a blood-to-plasma ratio of 1:1.

The major metabolic pathways are N-despropylation and hydroxylation to form the inactive N-despropyl and hydroxy metabolites. *In vitro* studies indicate that the major cytochrome P_{450} isozyme involved in the metabolism of ropinirole is CYP1A2, an enzyme known to be stimulated by smoking and omeprazole, and inhibited by, for example, fluvoxamine, mexiletine, and the older fluoroquinolones, such as ciprofloxacin and norfloxacin. The N-despropyl metabolite is converted to carbamyl glucuronide, carboxylic acid, and N-despropyl hydroxy metabolites. The hydroxy metabolite of ropinirole is rapidly glucuronidated. Less than 10% of the administered dose is excreted as unchanged drug in urine. N-despropyl ropinirole is the predominant metabolite found in urine (40%), followed by the carboxylic acid metabolite (10%), and the glucuronide of the hydroxy metabolite (10%).

P_{450} Interaction: *In vitro* metabolism studies showed that CYP1A2 was the major enzyme responsible for the metabolism of ropinirole. There is thus the potential for inhibitors or substrates of this enzyme to alter its clearance when coadministered with ropinirole. Therefore, if therapy with a drug known to be a potent inhibitor of CYP1A2 is stopped or started during treatment with *Requip*, adjustment of the *Requip* dose may be required.

Population Subgroups

Because therapy with *Requip* is initiated at a subtherapeutic dosage and gradually titrated upward according to clinical tolerability to obtain the optimum therapeutic effect, adjustment of the initial dose based on gender, weight or age is not necessary.

Age: Oral clearance of ropinirole is reduced by 30% in patients above 65 years of age compared to younger patients. Dosage adjustment is not necessary in the elderly (above 65 years) as the dose of ropinirole is to be individually titrated to clinical response.

Gender: Female and male patients showed similar oral clearance.

Race: The influence of race on the pharmacokinetics of ropinirole has not been evaluated.

Cigarette Smoking: The effect of smoking on the oral clearance of ropinirole has not been evaluated. Smoking is expected to increase the clearance of ropinirole since CYP1A2 is known to be induced by smoking.

Renal Impairment: Based on population pharmacokinetic analysis, no difference was observed in the pharmacokinetics of ropinirole in patients with moderate renal impairment (creatinine clearance between 30 to 50 mL/min.) compared to an age-matched population with creatinine clearance above 50 mL/min. Therefore, no dosage adjustment is necessary in moderately renally impaired patients. The use of Requip (ropinirole hydrochloride) in patients with severe renal impairment has not been studied.

The effect of hemodialysis on drug removal is not known, but because of the relatively high apparent volume of distribution of ropinirole (525 L), the removal of the drug by hemodialysis is unlikely.

Hepatic Impairment: The pharmacokinetics of ropinirole have not been studied in hepatically impaired patients. These patients may have higher plasma levels and lower clearance of the drug than patients with normal hepatic function. The drug should be titrated with caution in this population.

Other Diseases: Population pharmacokinetic analysis revealed no change in the oral clearance of ropinirole in patients with concomitant diseases, such as hypertension, depression, osteoporosis/arthritis, and insomnia, compared to patients with Parkinson's disease only.

Clinical Trials

The effectiveness of *Requip* in the treatment of Parkinson's disease was evaluated in a multi-national drug development program consisting of 11 randomized, controlled trials. Four were conducted in patients with early Parkinson's disease and no concomitant L-dopa and 7 were conducted in patients with advanced Parkinson's disease with concomitant L-dopa.

Among these 11 studies, three placebo-controlled studies provide the most persuasive evidence of ropinirole's effectiveness in the management of patients with Parkinson's disease who were and were not receiving concomitant L-dopa. Two of these three trials enrolled patients with early Parkinson's disease (without L-dopa) and one enrolled patients receiving L-dopa.

In these studies a variety of measures were used to assess the effects of treatment (e.g., the Unified Parkinson's Disease Rating Scale [UPDRS], Clinical Global Impression scores, patient diaries recording time "on" and "off," and tolerability of L-dopa dose reductions).

In both studies of early Parkinson's disease (without L-dopa) patients, the motor component (Part III) of the UPDRS was the primary outcome assessment. The UPDRS is a four-part multi-item rating scale intended to evaluate mentation (Part I), activities of daily living (Part II), motor performance (Part III), and complications of therapy (Part IV). Part III of the UPDRS contains 14 items designed to assess the severity of the cardinal motor findings in patients with Parkinson's disease (e.g., tremor, rigidity, bradykinesia, postural instability, etc.) scored for different body regions and has a maximum (worst) score of 108. Responders were defined as patients with at least a 30% reduction in the Part III score.

In the study of advanced Parkinson's disease (with L-dopa) patients, both reduction in percent awake time spent "off" and the ability to reduce the daily use of L-dopa were assessed as a combined endpoint and individually.

Studies in Patients with Early Parkinson's Disease (without L-dopa)

One early therapy study was a 12-week multicenter study in which 63 patients (41 on *Requip*) with idiopathic Parkinson's disease receiving concomitant anti-Parkinson medication (but not L-dopa) were randomized to either *Requip* or placebo. Patients had a mean disease duration of approximately 2 years. Patients were eligible for enrollment if they presented with bradykinesia and at least tremor, rigidity, or postural instability. In addition, they must have been classified as Hoehn & Yahr Stage I-IV. This scale, ranging from I=unilateral involvement with minimal impairment to V=confined to wheelchair or bed, is a standard instrument used for staging patients with Parkinson's disease. The primary outcome measure in this trial was the proportion of patients experiencing a decrease (compared to baseline) of at least 30% in the UPDRS motor score.

Patients were titrated for up to 10 weeks, starting at 0.5 mg b.i.d., with weekly increments of 0.5 mg b.i.d. to a maximum of 5 mg b.i.d. Once patients reached their maximally tolerated dose (or 5 mg b.i.d.), they were maintained on that dose through 12 weeks. The mean dose achieved by patients at study endpoint was 7.4 mg/day. At the end of 12 weeks, 71% of *Requip*-treated patients were responders, compared with 41% of patients in the placebo group (p=0.021).

Statistically significant differences between the percentage of responders on *Requip* compared to placebo were seen after 8 weeks of treatment.

In addition, the mean percentage improvement from baseline in the Total Motor Score was 43% in *Requip*-treated patients compared with 21% in placebo-treated patients (p=0.018).

Statistically significant differences in UPDRS motor score between *Requip* and placebo were seen after 2 weeks of treatment.

The median daily dose at which a 30% reduction in UPDRS motor score was sustained was 4 mg.

The second trial in early Parkinson's disease (without L-dopa) patients was a double-blind, randomized, placebo-controlled 6-month study. Patients were essentially similar to those in the study described above; concomitant use of selegiline was allowed, but patients were not permitted to use anticholinergics or amantadine during the study. Patients had a mean disease duration of 2 years and limited (not more than a 6-week period) or no prior exposure to L-dopa. The starting dose of *Requip* in this trial was 0.25 mg t.i.d. The dose was titrated at weekly intervals by increments of 0.25 mg t.i.d. to a dose of 1.0 mg t.i.d. Further titrations at weekly intervals were at increments of 0.5 mg t.i.d. up to a dose of 3.0 mg t.i.d and then weekly at increments of 1.0 mg t.i.d. Patients were to be titrated to a dose of at least 1.5 mg t.i.d. and then to their maximally tolerated dose, up to a maximum of 8.0 mg t.i.d. The mean dose attained in patients at study endpoint was 15.7 mg/day.

The primary measure of effectiveness was the mean percent reduction (improvement) from baseline in the UPDRS Motor Score. In this study 241 patients were enrolled. At the end of the 6-month study, *Requip*-treated patients had 22% improvement in motor score, compared with a 4% worsening in the placebo group ($p<0.001$).

Statistically significant differences in UPDRS motor score improvement between *Requip* and placebo were seen after 12 weeks of treatment.

Study in Patients with Advanced Parkinson's Disease (with L-dopa)

This double-blind, randomized, placebo-controlled 6-month trial evaluated 148 patients (Hoehn & Yahr II-IV) who were not adequately controlled on L-dopa. Patients in this study had a mean disease duration of approximately 9 years, had been exposed to L-dopa for approximately 7 years, and had experienced "on-off" periods with L-dopa therapy. Patients previously receiving stable doses of selegiline, amantadine and/or anticholinergic agents could continue on these agents during the study. Patients were started at a *Requip* dose of 0.25 mg t.i.d. and titrated upward by weekly intervals until an optimal therapeutic response was achieved. The maximum dose of study medication was 8 mg t.i.d. All patients had to be titrated to at least a dose of 2.5 mg t.i.d. Patients could then be maintained on this dose level or higher for the remainder of the study. Once a dose of 2.5 mg t.i.d. was achieved, patients underwent a mandatory reduction in their L-dopa dose, to be followed by additional mandatory reductions with continued escalation of the *Requip* dose. Reductions in the dosage of L-dopa were also allowed if patients experienced adverse events that the investigator considered related to dopaminergic therapy. The mean dose attained at study endpoint was 16.3 mg/day. The primary outcome was the proportion of responders, defined as patients who were able both to achieve a decrease (compared to baseline) of at least 20% in their L-dopa dose and a decrease of at least 20% in the proportion of the time awake in the "off" condition (a period of time during the day when patients are particularly immobile), as determined by patient diary. In addition, the mean percent change from baseline in daily L-dopa dose was examined.

At the end of 6 months, 28% of *Requip*-treated patients were classified as responders (based on combined endpoint) while 11% of placebo-treated patients were responders (p=0.02). Based on the protocol-mandated reductions in L-dopa dosage with escalating *Requip* doses, *Requip*-treated patients had a 19.4% mean reduction in L-dopa dose while placebo-treated patients had a 3% reduction ($p<0.001$). L-dopa dosage reduction was also allowed during the study if dyskinesias or other dopaminergic effects occurred. Overall, reduction of L-dopa dose was sustained in 87% of *Requip*-treated patients and in 57% of patients on placebo. On average, the L-dopa dose was reduced by 31% in *Requip*-treated patients.

The mean number of "off" hours per day during baseline was 6.4 hours for *Requip*-treated patients and 7.3 hours for patients treated with placebo. At the end of the 6-month study, patients treated with *Requip* had a mean of 4.9 hours per day of "off" time, while placebo-treated patients had a mean of 6.4 hours per day of "off" time.

INDICATIONS AND USAGE

Requip (ropinirole hydrochloride) is indicated for the treatment of the signs and symptoms of idiopathic Parkinson's disease.

The effectiveness of *Requip* was demonstrated in randomized, controlled trials in patients with early Parkinson's disease who were not receiving concomitant L-dopa therapy as well as in patients with advanced disease on concomitant L-dopa (see CLINICAL PHARMACOLOGY, Clinical Trials).

CONTRAINDICATIONS

Requip is contraindicated for patients known to have hypersensitivity to the product.

WARNINGS

Falling Asleep During Activities of Daily Living:

Patients treated with *Requip* have reported falling asleep while engaged in activities of daily living, including the operation of motor vehicles which sometimes resulted in accidents. Although many of these patients reported somnolence while on *Requip*, some perceived that they had no warning signs such as excessive drowsiness, and believed that they were alert immediately prior to the event. Some of these events have been reported as late as one year after initiation of treatment.

Somnolence is a common occurrence in patients receiving *Requip*. Many clinical experts believe that falling asleep while engaged in activities of daily living always occurs in a setting of pre-existing somnolence although patients may not give such a history. For this reason, prescribers should continually reassess patients for drowsiness or sleepiness especially since some of the events occur well after the start of treatment. Prescribers should also be aware that patients may not acknowledge drowsiness or sleepiness until directly questioned about drowsiness or sleepiness during specific activities.

Before initiating treatment with *Requip*, patients should be advised of the potential to develop drowsiness and specifically asked about factors that may increase the risk with *Requip* such as concomitant sedating medications, the presence of sleep disorders, and concomitant medications that increase ropinirole plasma levels (e.g., ciprofloxacin—see PRECAUTIONS, Drug Interactions). If a patient develops significant daytime sleepiness or episodes of falling asleep during activities that require active participation (e.g., conversations, eating, etc.), *Requip* should ordinarily be discontinued. [See DOSAGE AND ADMINISTRATION for guidance in discontinuing *Requip*.] If a decision is made to continue *Requip*, patients should be advised to not drive and to avoid other potentially dangerous activities. There is insufficient information to establish that dose reduction will eliminate episodes of falling asleep while engaged in activities of daily living.

Syncope

Syncope, sometimes associated with bradycardia, was observed in association with ropinirole in both early Parkinson's disease (without L-dopa) patients and advanced Parkinson's disease (with L-dopa) patients. In the two double-blind placebo-controlled studies of *Requip* in patients with Parkinson's disease who were not being treated with L-dopa, 11.5% (18 of 157) of patients on *Requip* had syncope compared to 1.4% (2 of 147) of patients on placebo. Most of these cases occurred more than 4 weeks after initiation of therapy with *Requip*, and were usually associated with a recent increase in dose.

Of 208 patients being treated with both L-dopa and *Requip*, in placebo-controlled advanced Parkinson's disease trials, there were reports of syncope in 6 (2.9%) compared to 2 of 120 (1.7%) of placebo/L-dopa patients.

Because the studies of *Requip* excluded patients with significant cardiovascular disease, it is not known to what extent the estimated incidence figures apply to Parkinson's disease patients as a whole. Therefore, patients with severe cardiovascular disease should be treated with caution.

Two of 47 Parkinson's disease patient volunteers enrolled in phase 1 studies had syncope following a 1 mg dose. In phase 1 studies including 110 healthy volunteers, one patient developed hypotension, bradycardia, and sinus arrest of 26 seconds accompanied by syncope; the patient recovered spontaneously without intervention. One other healthy volunteer reported syncope.

Symptomatic Hypotension

Dopamine agonists, in clinical studies and clinical experience, appear to impair the systemic regulation of blood pressure, with resulting postural hypotension, especially during dose escalation. Parkinson's disease patients, in addition, appear to have an impaired capacity to respond to a postural challenge. For these reasons, Parkinson's patients being treated with dopaminergic agonists ordinarily (1) require careful monitoring for signs and symptoms of postural

Continued on next page

Product information on these pages is effective as of August 2004. Further information is available at: GlaxoSmithKline, PO Box 13398, Research Triangle Park, NC 27709. 1-888-825-5249. Corporate Web Site: www.gsk.com

Requip—Cont.

hypotension, especially during dose escalation, and (2) should be informed of this risk (see PRECAUTIONS, Information for Patients).

Although the clinical trials were not designed to systematically monitor blood pressure, there were individual reported cases of postural hypotension in early Parkinson's disease (without L-dopa) *Requip*-treated patients. Most of these cases occurred more than 4 weeks after initiation of therapy with *Requip*, and were usually associated with a recent increase in dose.

In phase 1 studies of *Requip* that included 110 healthy volunteers, nine subjects had documented symptomatic postural hypotension. These episodes appeared mainly at doses above 0.8 mg and these doses are higher than the starting doses recommended for Parkinson's disease patients. In eight of these nine individuals, the hypotension was accompanied by bradycardia, but did not develop into syncope. (See Syncope above.) None of these events resulted in death or hospitalization.

One of 47 Parkinson's disease patient volunteers enrolled in phase 1 studies had documented hypotension following a 2 mg dose on two occasions.

Hallucinations

In double-blind, placebo-controlled, early therapy studies in patients with Parkinson's disease who were not treated with L-dopa, 5.2% (8 of 157) of patients treated with *Requip* reported hallucinations, compared to 1.4% of patients on placebo (2 of 147). Among those patients receiving both *Requip* and L-dopa, in advanced Parkinson's disease (with L-dopa) studies, 10.1% (21 of 208) were reported to experience hallucinations, compared to 4.2% (5 of 120) of patients treated with placebo and L-dopa.

Hallucinations were of sufficient severity to cause discontinuation of treatment in 1.3% of the early Parkinson's disease (without L-dopa) patients and 1.9% of the advanced Parkinson's disease (with L-dopa) patients compared to 0% and 1.7% of placebo patients, respectively.

PRECAUTIONS

General

Dyskinesia: *Requip* may potentiate the dopaminergic side effects of L-dopa and may cause and/or exacerbate pre-existing dyskinesia. Decreasing the dose of L-dopa may ameliorate this side effect.

Renal and Hepatic: No dosage adjustment is needed in patients with mild to moderate renal impairment (creatinine clearance of 30 to 50 mL/min.). Because the use of *Requip* in patients with severe renal or hepatic impairment has not been studied, administration of *Requip* to such patients should be carried out with caution.

Events Reported with Dopaminergic Therapy:

Withdrawal Emergent Hyperpyrexia and Confusion: Although not reported with *Requip*, a symptom complex resembling the neuroleptic malignant syndrome (characterized by elevated temperature, muscular rigidity, altered consciousness, and autonomic instability), with no other obvious etiology, has been reported in association with rapid dose reduction, withdrawal of, or changes in anti-Parkinsonian therapy.

Fibrotic Complications: Cases of retroperitoneal fibrosis, pulmonary infiltrates, pleural effusion, and pleural thickening have been reported in some patients treated with ergot-derived dopaminergic agents. While these complications may resolve when the drug is discontinued, complete resolution does not always occur.

Although these adverse events are believed to be related to the ergoline structure of these compounds, whether other, nonergot derived dopamine agonists can cause them is unknown.

In the *Requip* development program, a 69-year-old man with obstructive lung disease was treated with *Requip* for 16 months and developed pleural thickening and effusion accompanied by lower extremity edema, cardiomegaly, pleuritic pain, and shortness of breath. Pleural biopsy demonstrated chronic inflammation and sclerosis. The effusion resolved after medical therapy and discontinuation of *Requip*. The patient was lost to follow-up. The relationship of these events to Requip (ropinirole hydrochloride) cannot be established.

Retinal pathology in albino rats: Retinal degeneration was observed in albino rats in the 2-year carcinogenicity study at all doses tested (equivalent to 0.6 to 20 times the maximum recommended human dose on a mg/m^2 basis), but was statistically significant at the highest dose (50 mg/kg/day). Additional studies to further evaluate the specific pathology (e.g., loss of photoreceptor cells) have not been performed. Similar changes were not observed in a 2-year carcinogenicity study in albino mice or in rats or monkeys treated for 1 year.

The potential significance of this effect in humans has not been established, but cannot be disregarded because disruption of a mechanism that is universally present in vertebrates (e.g., disk shedding) may be involved.

Binding to melanin: *Requip* binds to melanin-containing tissues (i.e., eyes, skin) in pigmented rats. After a single dose, long-term retention of drug was demonstrated, with a half-life in the eye of 20 days. It is not known if *Requip* accumulates in these tissues over time.

Information for Patients

Patients should be instructed to take *Requip* only as prescribed.

Requip can be taken with or without food. Since ingestion with food reduces the maximum concentration (C_{max}) of *Requip*, patients should be advised that taking *Requip* with food may reduce the occurrence of nausea. However, this has not been established in controlled clinical trials.

Patients should be informed that hallucinations can occur, and that the elderly are at a higher risk than younger patients with Parkinson's disease.

Patients should be advised that they may develop postural (orthostatic) hypotension with or without symptoms such as dizziness, nausea, syncope, and sometimes sweating. Hypotension and/or orthostatic symptoms may occur more frequently during initial therapy or with an increase in dose at any time (cases have been seen after weeks of treatment). Accordingly, patients should be cautioned against rising rapidly after sitting or lying down, especially if they have been doing so for prolonged periods, and especially at the initiation of treatment with *Requip*.

Patients should be alerted to the potential sedating effects associated with *Requip* including somnolence and the possibility of falling asleep while engaged in activities of daily living. Since somnolence is a frequent adverse event with potentially serious consequences, patients should neither drive a car nor engage in other potentially dangerous activities until they have gained sufficient experience with *Requip* to gauge whether or not it affects their mental and/or motor performance adversely. Patients should be advised that if increased somnolence or episodes of falling asleep during activities of daily living (e.g., watching television, passenger in a car, etc.) are experienced at any time during treatment, they should not drive or participate in potentially dangerous activities until they have contacted their physician. Because of possible additive effects, caution should be advised when patients are taking other sedating medications or alcohol in combination with *Requip* and when taking concomitant medications that increase plasma levels of ropinirole (e.g., ciprofloxacin).

Because of the possible additive sedative effects, caution should also be used when patients are taking alcohol or other CNS depressants (e.g., benzodiazepines, antipsychotics, antidepressants, etc.) in combination with *Requip*.

Because of the possibility that ropinirole may be excreted in breast milk, patients should be advised to notify their physicians if they intend to breast-feed or are breast-feeding an infant.

Because ropinirole has been shown to have adverse effects on embryo-fetal development, including teratogenic effects, in animals, and because experience in humans is limited, patients should be advised to notify their physician if they become pregnant or intend to become pregnant during therapy (see PRECAUTIONS, Pregnancy).

Drug Interactions

P_{450} Interaction: *In vitro* metabolism studies showed that CYP1A2 was the major enzyme responsible for the metabolism of ropinirole. There is thus the potential for substrates or inhibitors of this enzyme when coadministered with ropinirole to alter its clearance. Therefore, if therapy with a drug known to be a potent inhibitor of CYP1A2 is stopped or started during treatment with *Requip*, adjustment of the *Requip* dose may be required.

L-dopa: Co-administration of carbidopa + L-dopa (Sinemet® 10/100 mg b.i.d.) with ropinirole (2.0 mg t.i.d.) had no effect on the steady-state pharmacokinetics of ropinirole (n=28 patients). Oral administration of *Requip* 2.0 mg t.i.d. increased mean steady state C_{max} of L-dopa by 20% but its AUC was unaffected (n=23 patients).

Digoxin: Co-administration of *Requip* (2.0 mg t.i.d.) with digoxin (0.125-0.25 mg q.d.) did not alter the steady-state pharmacokinetics of digoxin in 10 patients.

Theophylline: Administration of theophylline (300 mg b.i.d., a substrate of CYP1A2) did not alter the steady-state pharmacokinetics of ropinirole (2 mg t.i.d.) in 12 patients with Parkinson's disease. Ropinirole (2 mg t.i.d.) did not alter the pharmacokinetics of theophylline (5 mg/kg i.v.) in 12 patients with Parkinson's disease.

Ciprofloxacin: Co-administration of ciprofloxacin (500 mg b.i.d.), an inhibitor of CYP1A2, with ropinirole (2 mg t.i.d.) increased ropinirole AUC by 84% on average, and C_{max} by 60% (n=12 patients).

Estrogens: Population pharmacokinetic analysis revealed that estrogens (mainly ethinylestradiol: intake 0.6-3 mg over 4-month to 23-year period) reduced the oral clearance of ropinirole by 36% in 16 patients. Dosage adjustment may not be needed for *Requip* in patients on estrogen therapy because patients must be carefully titrated with ropinirole to tolerance or adequate effect. However, if estrogen therapy is stopped or started during treatment with *Requip*, then adjustment of the Requip (ropinirole hydrochloride) dose may be required.

Dopamine Antagonists: Since ropinirole is a dopamine agonist, it is possible that dopamine antagonists, such as neuroleptics (phenothiazines, butyrophenones, thioxanthenes) or metoclopramide, may diminish the effectiveness of *Requip*. Patients with major psychotic disorders, treated with neuroleptics, should only be treated with dopamine agonists if the potential benefits outweigh the risks.

Population analysis showed that commonly administered drugs, e.g., selegiline, amantadine, tricyclic antidepressants, benzodiazepines, ibuprofen, thiazides, antihistamines, and anticholinergics did not affect the oral clearance of ropinirole.

Carcinogenesis, Mutagenesis, Impairment of Fertility

Two-year carcinogenicity studies were conducted in Charles River CD-1 mice at doses of 5, 15, and 50 mg/kg/day and in Sprague-Dawley rats at doses of 1.5, 15, and 50 mg/kg/day (top doses equivalent to 10 times and 20 times, respectively, the maximum recommended human dose of 24 mg/day on a mg/m^2 basis). In the male rat, there was a significant increase in testicular Leydig cell adenomas at all doses tested, i.e., ≥1.5 mg/kg (0.6 times the maximum recommended human dose on a mg/m^2 basis). This finding is of questionable significance because the endocrine mechanisms believed to be involved in the production of Leydig cell hyperplasia and adenomas in rats are not relevant to humans. In the female mouse, there was an increase in benign uterine endometrial polyps at a dose of 50 mg/kg/day (10 times the maximum recommended human dose on a mg/m^2 basis).

Ropinirole was not mutagenic or clastogenic in the *in vitro* Ames test, the *in vitro* chromosome aberration test in human lymphocytes, the *in vitro* mouse lymphoma (L1578Y cells) assay, and the *in vivo* mouse micronucleus test.

When administered to female rats prior to and during mating and throughout pregnancy, ropinirole caused disruption of implantation at doses of 20 mg/kg/day (8 times the maximum recommended human dose on a mg/m^2 basis) or greater. This effect is thought to be due to the prolactin-lowering effect of ropinirole. In humans, chorionic gonadotropin, not prolactin, is essential for implantation. In rat studies using low doses (5 mg/kg) during the prolactin-dependent phase of early pregnancy (gestation days 0-8), ropinirole did not affect female fertility at dosages up to 100 mg/kg/day (40 times the maximum recommended human dose on a mg/m^2 basis). No effect on male fertility was observed in rats at dosages up to 125 mg/kg/day (50 times the maximum recommended human dose on a mg/m^2 basis).

Pregnancy

Pregnancy Category C: In animal reproduction studies, ropinirole has been shown to have adverse effects on embryo-fetal development, including teratogenic effects. Ropinirole given to pregnant rats during organogenesis (20 mg/kg on gestation days 6 and 7 followed by 20, 60, 90, 120 or 150 mg/kg on gestation days 8 through 15) resulted in decreased fetal body weight at 60 mg/kg/day, increased fetal death at 90 mg/kg/day, and digital malformations at 150 mg/kg/day (24, 36 and 60 times the maximum recommended clinical dose on a mg/m^2 basis, respectively). The combined administration of ropinirole (10 mg/kg/day; 8 times the maximum recommended human dose on a mg/m^2 basis) and L-dopa (250 mg/kg/day) to pregnant rabbits during organogenesis produced a greater incidence and severity of fetal malformations (primarily digit defects) than were seen in the offspring of rabbits treated with L-dopa alone. No indication of an effect on development of the conceptus was observed in rabbits when a maternally toxic dose of ropinirole was administered alone (20 mg/kg/day: 16 times the maximum recommended human dose on a mg/m^2 basis). In a perinatal-postnatal study in rats, 10 mg/kg/day (4 times the maximum recommended human dose on a mg/m^2 basis) of ropinirole impaired growth and development of nursing offspring and altered neurological development of female offspring.

There are no adequate and well-controlled studies using *Requip* in pregnant women. *Requip* should be used during pregnancy only if the potential benefit outweighs the potential risk to the fetus.

Nursing Mothers

Requip inhibits prolactin secretion in humans and could potentially inhibit lactation.

Studies in rats have shown that *Requip* and/or its metabolite(s) is excreted in breast milk. It is not known whether this drug is excreted in human milk. Because many drugs are excreted in human milk and because of the potential for serious adverse reactions in nursing infants from *Requip*, a decision should be made whether to discontinue nursing or to discontinue the drug, taking into account the importance of the drug to the mother.

Pediatric Use

Safety and effectiveness in the pediatric population have not been established.

ADVERSE REACTIONS

During the pre-marketing development of *Requip*, patients received *Requip* either without L-dopa (early Parkinson's disease studies) or as concomitant therapy with L-dopa (advanced Parkinson's disease studies). Because these 2 populations may have differential risks for various adverse events, this section will, in general, present adverse event data for these 2 populations separately.

Early Parkinson's Disease (without L-dopa)

The most commonly observed adverse events (>5%) in the double-blind, placebo-controlled early Parkinson's disease trials associated with the use of *Requip* (n=157) not seen at an equivalent frequency among the placebo-treated patients (n=147) were, in order of decreasing incidence: nausea, dizziness, somnolence, headache, vomiting, syncope, fatigue, dyspepsia, viral infection, constipation, pain, increased sweating, asthenia, dependent/leg edema, orthostatic symptoms, abdominal pain, pharyngitis, confusion, hallucinations, urinary tract infections, and abnormal vision.

Approximately 24% of 157 *Requip*-treated patients who participated in the double-blind, placebo-controlled early Parkinson's disease (without L-dopa) trials discontinued treatment due to adverse events compared to 13% of 147 patients who received placebo. The adverse events most commonly causing discontinuation of treatment by *Requip*-treated patients were: nausea (6.4%), dizziness (3.8%), aggravated Parkinson's disease (1.3%), hallucinations (1.3%), somnolence (1.3%), vomiting (1.3%) and headache (1.3%). Of these, hallucinations appear to be dose-related. While other adverse events leading to discontinuation may be dose-related, the titration design utilized in these trials precluded an adequate assessment of the dose response. For example, in the larger of the 2 trials described in CLINICAL PHARMACOLOGY, Clinical Trials, the difference in the rate of discontinuations emerged only after 10 weeks of treatment, suggesting, although not proving, that the effect could be related to dose.

Adverse Event Incidence in Controlled Clinical Studies

Table 1 lists treatment-emergent adverse events that occurred in ≥2% of patients with early Parkinson's disease (without L-dopa) treated with *Requip* participating in the double-blind, placebo-controlled studies and were numerically more common in the *Requip* group. In these studies, either Requip (ropinirole hydrochloride) or placebo was used as early therapy (i.e., without L-dopa).

The prescriber should be aware that these figures cannot be used to predict the incidence of adverse events in the course of usual medical practice where patient characteristics and other factors differ from those that prevailed in the clinical studies. Similarly, the cited frequencies cannot be compared with figures obtained from other clinical investigations involving different treatments, uses and investigators. However, the cited figures do provide the prescribing physician with some basis for estimating the relative contribution of drug and non-drug factors to the adverse-events incidence rate in the population studied.

[See table 1 at right]

Other events reported by 1% or more of early Parkinson's disease (without L-dopa) patients treated with *Requip*, but that were equally or more frequent in the placebo group were: headache, upper respiratory infection, insomnia, arthralgia, tremor, back pain, anxiety, dyskinesias, aggravated Parkinsonism, depression, falls, myalgia, leg cramps, paresthesias, nervousness, diarrhea, arthritis, hot flushes, weight loss, rash, cough, hyperglycemia, muscle spasm, arthrosis, abnormal dreams, dystonia, increased salivation, bradycardia, gout, basal cell carcinoma, gingivitis, hematuria, and rigors.

Among the treatment-emergent adverse events in patients treated with *Requip*, hallucinations appear to be dose-related.

The incidence of adverse events was not materially different between women and men.

Advanced Parkinson's Disease (with L-dopa)

The most commonly observed adverse events (>5%), in the double-blind, placebo-controlled advanced Parkinson's disease (with L-dopa) trials associated with the use of *Requip* (n = 208) as an adjunct to L-dopa not seen at an equivalent frequency among the placebo-treated patients (n = 120) were, in order of decreasing incidence: dyskinesias, nausea, dizziness, aggravated Parkinsonism, somnolence, headache, insomnia, injury, hallucinations, falls, abdominal pain, upper respiratory infection, confusion, increased sweating, vomiting, viral infection, increased drug level, arthralgia, tremor, anxiety, urinary tract infection, constipation, dry mouth, pain, hypokinesia, and paresthesia.

Approximately 24% of 208 patients who received Requip (ropinirole hydrochloride) in the double-blind, placebo-controlled advanced Parkinson's disease (with L-dopa) trials discontinued treatment due to adverse events compared to 18% of 120 patients who received placebo. The events most commonly (≥1%) causing discontinuation of treatment by *Requip*-treated patients were: dizziness (2.9%), dyskinesias (2.4%), vomiting (2.4%), confusion (2.4%), nausea (1.9%), hallucinations (1.9%), anxiety (1.9%), and increased sweating (1.4%). Of these, hallucinations and dyskinesias appear to be dose-related.

Adverse Event Incidence in Controlled Clinical Studies

Table 2 lists treatment-emergent adverse events that occurred in ≥2% of patients with advanced Parkinson's disease (with L-dopa) treated with *Requip* who participated in the double-blind, placebo-controlled studies and were numerically more common in the *Requip* group. In these studies, either *Requip* or placebo was used as an adjunct to L-dopa. Adverse events were usually mild or moderate in intensity.

The prescriber should be aware that these figures cannot be used to predict the incidence of adverse events in the course of usual medical practice where patient characteristics and other factors differ from those that prevailed in the clinical studies. Similarly, the cited frequencies cannot be compared with figures obtained from other clinical investigations involving different treatments, uses, and investigators. However, the cited figures do provide the prescribing physician with some basis for estimating the relative contribution of drug and non-drug factors to the adverse-events incidence rate in the population studied.

[See table 2 at bottom of next page]

Other events reported by 1% or more of patients treated with both *Requip* and L-dopa, but equally or more frequent in the placebo/L-dopa group were: myocardial infarction, orthostatic symptoms, virus infections, asthenia, dyspepsia, myalgia, back pain, depression, leg cramps, fatigue, rhinitis, chest pain, hematuria, vertigo, tinnitus, leg edema, hot flushes, abnormal gait, hyperkinesia, and pharyngitis.

Among the treatment-emergent adverse events in patients treated with *Requip*, hallucinations and dyskinesias appear to be dose-related.

Other Adverse Events Observed During All Phase 2/3 Clinical Trials: *Requip* has been administered to 1,599 individuals in clinical trials. During these trials, all adverse events were recorded by the clinical investigators using terminology of their own choosing. To provide a meaningful estimate of the proportion of individuals having adverse events, similar types of events were grouped into a smaller number of standardized categories using modified WHOART dictionary terminology. These categories are used in the listing below. The frequencies presented represent the proportion of the 1,599 individuals exposed to *Requip* who experienced events of the type cited on at least one occasion while receiving *Requip*. All reported events that occurred at least twice (or once for serious or potentially serious events), except those already listed above, trivial events, and terms too vague to be meaningful are included, without regard to determination of a causal relationship to Requip (ropinirole hydrochloride), except that events very unlikely to be drug-related have been deleted.

Events are further classified within body system categories and enumerated in order of decreasing frequency using the following definitions: frequent adverse events are defined as those occurring in at least 1/100 patients and infrequent adverse events are those occurring in 1/100 to 1/1000 patients and rare events are those occurring in fewer than 1/1000 patients.

Body as a Whole: *infrequent* – cellulitis, peripheral edema, fever, influenza-like symptoms, enlarged abdomen, precordial chest pain, and generalized edema; *rare* – ascites.

Cardiovascular: *infrequent* – cardiac failure, bradycardia, tachycardia, supraventricular tachycardia, angina pectoris, bundle branch block, cardiac arrest, cardiomegaly, aneurysm, mitral insufficiency; *rare* – ventricular tachycardia.

Central/Peripheral Nervous System: *frequent* – neuralgia; *infrequent* – involuntary muscle contractions, hypertonia, dysphonia, abnormal coordination, extrapyramidal disorder, migraine, choreoathetosis, coma, stupor, aphasia, convulsions, hypotonia, peripheral neuropathy, paralysis; *rare* – grand mal convulsions, hemiparesis, hemiplegia.

Endocrine: *infrequent* – hypothyroidism, gynecomastia, hyperthyroidism; *rare* – goiter, SIADH.

Gastrointestinal: *infrequent* – increased hepatic enzymes, bilirubinemia, cholecystitis, cholelithiasis colitis, dysphagia, periodontitis, fecal incontinence, gastroesophageal reflux, hemorrhoids, toothache, eructation, gastritis, esophagitis, hiccups, diverticulitis, duodenal ulcer, gastric ulcer, melena, duodenitis, gastrointestinal hemorrhage, glossitis, rectal hemorrhage, pancreatitis, stomatitis and ulcerative stomatitis, tongue edema; *rare* – biliary pain, hemorrhagic gastritis, hematemesis, salivary duct obstruction.

Hematologic: *infrequent* – purpura, thrombocytopenia, hematoma, Vitamin B12 deficiency, hypochromic anemia, eosinophilia, leukocytosis, leukopenia, lymphocytosis, lymphopenia, lymphedema.

Metabolic/Nutritional: *frequent* – increased BUN; *infrequent* – hypoglycemia, increased alkaline phosphatase, increased LDH, weight increase, hyperphosphatemia, hyperuricemia, diabetes mellitus, glycosuria, hypokalemia, hypercholesterolemia, hyperkalemia, acidosis, hyponatre-

Continued on next page

Table 1: Treatment-Emergent Adverse Event[1] Incidence in Double-blind, Placebo-controlled Early Parkinson's Disease (without L-dopa) Trials (Events ≥2% of Patients Treated with *Requip* and Numerically More Frequent than the Placebo Group)

	Requip N = 157 (%)	Placebo N = 147 (%)
Autonomic Nervous System		
Flushing	3	1
Dry Mouth	5	3
Increased Sweating	6	4
Body as a Whole		
Asthenia	6	1
Chest Pain	4	2
Dependent Edema	6	3
Leg Edema	7	1
Fatigue	11	4
Malaise	3	1
Pain	8	4
Cardiovascular General		
Hypertension	5	3
Hypotension	2	0
Orthostatic Symptoms	6	5
Syncope	12	1
Central/Peripheral Nervous System		
Dizziness	40	22
Hyperkinesia	2	1
Hypesthesia	4	2
Vertigo	2	0
Gastrointestinal System		
Abdominal Pain	6	3
Anorexia	4	1
Dyspepsia	10	5
Flatulence	3	1
Nausea	60	22
Vomiting	12	7
Heart Rate/Rhythm		
Extrasystoles	2	1
Atrial Fibrillation	2	0
Palpitation	3	2
Tachycardia	2	0
Metabolic/Nutritional		
Increased Alkaline Phosphatase	3	1
Psychiatric		
Amnesia	3	1
Impaired Concentration	2	0
Confusion	5	1
Hallucination	5	1
Somnolence	40	6
Yawning	3	0
Reproductive Male		
Impotence	3	1
Resistance Mechanism		
Viral Infection	11	3
Respiratory System		
Bronchitis	3	1
Dyspnea	3	0
Pharyngitis	6	4
Rhinitis	4	3
Sinusitis	4	3
Urinary System		
Urinary Tract Infection	5	4
Vascular Extracardiac		
Peripheral Ischemia	3	0
Vision		
Eye Abnormality	3	1
Abnormal Vision	6	3
Xerophthalmia	2	0

1. Patients may have reported multiple adverse experiences during the study or at discontinuation; thus, patients may be included in more than one category.

Product information on these pages is effective as of August 2004. Further information is available at: GlaxoSmithKline, PO Box 13398, Research Triangle Park, NC 27709. 1-888-825-5249. Corporate Web Site: www.gsk.com

Requip—Cont.

mia, thirst, increased CPK, dehydration; *rare* – hypochloremia.
Musculoskeletal: *infrequent* – aggravated arthritis, tendinitis, osteoporosis, bursitis, polymyalgia rheumatica, muscle weakness, skeletal pain, torticollis; *rare* – Dupuytren's contracture requiring surgery.
Neoplasm: *infrequent* – malignant breast neoplasm; *rare* – bladder carcinoma, benign brain neoplasm, esophageal carcinoma, malignant laryngeal neoplasm, lipoma, rectal carcinoma, uterine neoplasm.
Psychiatric: *infrequent* – increased libido, agitation, apathy, impaired concentration, depersonalization, paranoid reaction, personality disorder, euphoria, delirium, dementia, delusion, emotional lability, decreased libido, manic reaction, somnambulism, aggressive reaction, neurosis; *rare* – suicide attempt.
Genito-urinary: *infrequent* – amenorrhea, vaginal hemorrhage, penile disorder, prostatic disorder, balanoposthitis, epididymitis, perineal pain, dysuria, micturition frequency, albuminuria, nocturia, polyuria, renal calculus; *rare* – breast enlargement, mastitis, uterine hemorrhage, ejaculation disorder, Peyronie's Disease, pyelonephritis, acute renal failure, uremia.
Resistance Mechanism: *infrequent* – herpes zoster, otitis media, sepsis, abscess, herpes simplex, fungal infection, genital moniliasis.
Respiratory: *infrequent* – asthma, epistaxis, laryngitis, pleurisy, pulmonary edema.
Skin/Appendage: *infrequent* – pruritis, dermatitis, eczema, skin ulceration, alopecia, skin hypertrophy, skin discoloration, urticaria, fungal dermatitis, furunculosis, hyperkeratosis, photosensitivity reaction, psoriasis, maculopapular rash, psoriaform rash, seborrhea.
Special Senses: *infrequent* – tinnitus, earache, decreased hearing, abnormal lacrimation, conjunctivitis, blepharitis, glaucoma, abnormal accommodation, blepharospasm, eye pain, photophobia; *rare* – scotoma.
Vascular Extracardiac: *infrequent* – varicose veins, phlebitis, peripheral gangrene; *rare* – limb embolism, pulmonary embolism, gangrene, subarachnoid hemorrhage, deep thrombophlebitis, leg thrombophlebitis, thrombosis.
Falling Asleep During Activities of Daily Living: Patients treated with *Requip* have reported falling asleep while engaged in activities of daily living, including operation of a motor vehicle which sometimes resulted in accidents (see bolded WARNING).

DRUG ABUSE AND DEPENDENCE

Controlled Substance Class
Requip is not a controlled substance.
Physical and Psychological Dependence
Animal studies and human clinical trials with Requip (ropinirole hydrochloride) did not reveal any potential for drug-seeking behavior or physical dependence.

OVERDOSAGE

There were no reports of intentional overdose of *Requip* in the premarketing clinical trials. A total of 27 patients accidentally took more than their prescribed dose of *Requip*, with 10 patients ingesting more than 24 mg/day. The largest overdose reported in premarketing clinical trials was 435 mg taken over a 7-day period (62.1 mg/day). Of patients who received a dose greater than 24 mg/day, one experienced mild oro-facial dyskinesia, another patient experienced intermittent nausea. Other symptoms reported with accidental overdoses were: agitation, increased dyskinesia, grogginess, sedation, orthostatic hypotension, chest pain, confusion, vomiting and nausea.
Overdose Management
It is anticipated that the symptoms of *Requip* overdose will be related to its dopaminergic activity. General supportive measures are recommended. Vital signs should be maintained, if necessary. Removal of any unabsorbed material (e.g., by gastric lavage) should be considered.

DOSAGE AND ADMINISTRATION

In all clinical studies, dosage was initiated at a subtherapeutic level and gradually titrated to therapeutic response.

Table 2: Treatment-Emergent Adverse Event[1] Incidence in Double-blind, Placebo-controlled Advanced Parkinson's Disease (with L-dopa) Trials (Events ≥2% of Patients Treated with *Requip* and Numerically More Frequent than the Placebo Group)

	Requip N = 208 (%)	Placebo N = 120 (%)
Autonomic Nervous System		
Dry Mouth	5	1
Increased Sweating	7	2
Body as a Whole		
Increased Drug Level	7	3
Pain	5	3
Cardiovascular General		
Hypotension	2	1
Syncope	3	2
Central/Peripheral Nervous System		
Dizziness	26	16
Dyskinesia	34	13
Falls	10	7
Headache	17	12
Hypokinesia	5	4
Paresis	3	0
Paresthesia	5	3
Tremor	6	3
Gastrointestinal System		
Abdominal Pain	9	8
Constipation	6	3
Diarrhea	5	3
Dysphagia	2	1
Flatulence	2	1
Nausea	30	18
Increased Saliva	2	1
Vomiting	7	4
Metabolic/Nutritional		
Weight Decrease	2	1
Musculoskeletal System		
Arthralgia	7	5
Arthritis	3	1
Psychiatric		
Amnesia	5	1
Anxiety	6	3
Confusion	9	2
Abnormal Dreaming	3	2
Hallucination	10	4
Nervousness	5	3
Somnolence	20	8
Red Blood Cell		
Anemia	2	0
Resistance Mechanism		
Upper Repiratory Tract Infection	9	8
Respiratory System		
Dyspnea	3	2
Urinary System		
Pyuria	2	1
Urinary Incontinence	2	1
Urinary Tract Infection	6	3
Vision		
Diplopia	2	1

1. Patients may have reported multiple adverse experiences during the study or at discontinuation; thus, patients may be included in more than one category.

The dosage should be increased to achieve a maximum therapeutic effect, balanced against the principal side effects of nausea, dizziness, somnolence and dyskinesia.
Requip should be taken three times daily. *Requip* can be taken with or without food. Since ingestion with food reduces the maximum concentration (C_{max}) of *Requip*, patients should be advised that taking *Requip* with food may reduce the occurrence of nausea. However, this has not been established in controlled clinical trials.
The recommended starting dose is 0.25 mg three times daily. Based on individual patient response, dosage should then be titrated with weekly increments as described in the table below. After week 4, if necessary, daily dosage may be increased by 1.5 mg per day on a weekly basis up to a dose of 9 mg per day, and then by up to 3 mg per day weekly to a total dose of 24 mg per day.

Ascending-Dose Schedule of *Requip*

Week	Dosage	Total Daily Dose
1	0.25 mg three times daily	0.75 mg
2	0.5 mg three times daily	1.5 mg
3	0.75 mg three times daily	2.25 mg
4	1.0 mg three times daily	3.0 mg

Doses greater than 24 mg/day have not been tested in clinical trials.
When *Requip* is administered as adjunct therapy to L-dopa, the concurrent dose of L-dopa may be decreased gradually as tolerated. L-dopa dosage reduction was allowed during the advanced Parkinson's disease (with L-dopa) study if dyskinesias or other dopaminergic effects occurred. Overall, reduction of L-dopa dose was sustained in 87% of *Requip*-treated patients and in 57% of patients on placebo. On average the L-dopa dose was reduced by 31% in *Requip*-treated patients.
Requip should be discontinued gradually over a 7-day period. The frequency of administration should be reduced from three times daily to twice daily for 4 days. For the remaining 3 days, the frequency should be reduced to once daily prior to complete withdrawal of Requip (ropinirole hydrochloride).

HOW SUPPLIED

Tablets: Each pentagonal film-coated Tiltab® tablet with beveled edges contains ropinirole hydrochloride as follows: 0.25 mg – white imprinted with SB and 4890; 0.5 mg – yellow imprinted with SB and 4891; 1.0 mg – green imprinted with SB and 4892; 2.0 mg – pale yellowish pink imprinted with SB and 4893; 3.0 mg – pale to moderate reddish-purple imprinted with SB and 4895; 4.0 mg – pale brown imprinted with SB and 4896; 5.0 mg – blue imprinted with SB and 4894.
0.25 mg SUP 30's: NDC 0007-4890-14
0.25 mg bottles of 100: NDC 0007-4890-20
0.5 mg SUP 30's: NDC 0007-4891-14
0.5 mg bottles of 100: NDC 0007-4891-20
1 mg SUP 30's: NDC 0007-4892-14
1 mg bottles of 100: NDC 0007-4892-20
2 mg SUP 30's: NDC 0007-4893-14
2 mg bottles of 100: NDC 0007-4893-20
3 mg bottles of 100: NDC 0007-4895-20
4 mg bottles of 100: NDC 0007-4896-20
5 mg SUP 30's: NDC 0007-4894-14
5 mg bottles of 100: NDC 0007-4894-20
STORAGE
Protect from light and moisture. Close container tightly after each use.
Store at controlled room temperature 20°-25°C (68°-77°F) [see USP].
GlaxoSmithKline, Research Triangle Park, NC 27709

November 2001/RQ:L10
Shown in Product Identification Guide, page 317

RETROVIR® ℞
[re' trō-vir]
(zidovudine)
Tablets

RETROVIR® ℞
(zidovudine)
Capsules

RETROVIR® ℞
(zidovudine)
Syrup

WARNING
RETROVIR (ZIDOVUDINE) HAS BEEN ASSOCIATED WITH HEMATOLOGIC TOXICITY INCLUDING NEUTROPENIA AND SEVERE ANEMIA PARTICULARLY IN PATIENTS WITH ADVANCED HIV DISEASE (SEE WARNINGS). PROLONGED USE OF RETROVIR HAS BEEN ASSOCIATED WITH SYMPTOMATIC MYOPATHY.
LACTIC ACIDOSIS AND SEVERE HEPATOMEGALY WITH STEATOSIS, INCLUDING FATAL CASES, HAVE BEEN REPORTED WITH THE USE OF NUCLEOSIDE ANALOGUES ALONE OR IN COMBINATION, INCLUDING RETROVIR AND OTHER ANTIRETROVIRALS (SEE WARNINGS).

DESCRIPTION

RETROVIR is the brand name for zidovudine (formerly called azidothymidine [AZT]), a pyrimidine nucleoside analogue active against human immunodeficiency virus (HIV).

Tablets: RETROVIR Tablets are for oral administration. Each film-coated tablet contains 300 mg of zidovudine and the inactive ingredients hypromellose, magnesium stearate, microcrystalline cellulose, polyethylene glycol, sodium starch glycolate, and titanium dioxide.

Capsules: RETROVIR Capsules are for oral administration. Each capsule contains 100 mg of zidovudine and the inactive ingredients corn starch, magnesium stearate, microcrystalline cellulose, and sodium starch glycolate. The 100-mg empty hard gelatin capsule, printed with edible black ink, consists of black iron oxide, dimethylpolysiloxane, gelatin, pharmaceutical shellac, soya lecithin, and titanium dioxide. The blue band around the capsule consists of gelatin and FD&C Blue No. 2.

Syrup: RETROVIR Syrup is for oral administration. Each teaspoonful (5 mL) of RETROVIR Syrup contains 50 mg of zidovudine and the inactive ingredients sodium benzoate 0.2% (added as a preservative), citric acid, flavors, glycerin, and liquid sucrose. Sodium hydroxide may be added to adjust pH.

The chemical name of zidovudine is 3′-azido-3′-deoxythymidine.

Zidovudine is a white to beige, odorless, crystalline solid with a molecular weight of 267.24 and a solubility of 20.1 mg/mL in water at 25°C. The molecular formula is $C_{10}H_{13}N_5O_4$.

MICROBIOLOGY

Mechanism of Action: Zidovudine is a synthetic nucleoside analogue of the naturally occurring nucleoside, thymidine, in which the 3′-hydroxy (-OH) group is replaced by an azido ($-N_3$) group. Within cells, zidovudine is converted to the active metabolite, zidovudine 5′-triphosphate (AztTP), by the sequential action of the cellular enzymes. Zidovudine 5′-triphosphate inhibits the activity of the HIV reverse transcriptase both by competing for utilization with the natural substrate, deoxythymidine 5′-triphosphate (dTTP), and by its incorporation into viral DNA. The lack of a 3′-OH group in the incorporated nucleoside analogue prevents the formation of the 5′ to 3′ phosphodiester linkage essential for DNA chain elongation and, therefore, the viral DNA growth is terminated. The active metabolite AztTP is also a weak inhibitor of the cellular DNA polymerase-alpha and mitochondrial polymerase-gamma and has been reported to be incorporated into the DNA of cells in culture.

In Vitro HIV Susceptibility: The in vitro anti-HIV activity of zidovudine was assessed by infecting cell lines of lymphoblastic and monocytic origin and peripheral blood lymphocytes with laboratory and clinical isolates of HIV. The IC_{50} and IC_{90} values (50% and 90% inhibitory concentrations) were 0.003 to 0.013 and 0.03 to 0.13 mcg/mL, respectively (1 nM = 0.27 ng/mL). The IC_{50} and IC_{90} values of HIV isolates recovered from 18 untreated AIDS/ARC patients were in the range of 0.003 to 0.013 mcg/mL and 0.03 to 0.3 mcg/mL, respectively. Zidovudine showed antiviral activity in all acutely infected cell lines; however, activity was substantially less in chronically infected cell lines. In drug combination studies with zalcitabine, didanosine, lamivudine, saquinavir, indinavir, ritonavir, nevirapine, delavirdine, or interferon-alpha, zidovudine showed additive to synergistic activity in cell culture. The relationship between the in vitro susceptibility of HIV to reverse transcriptase inhibitors and the inhibition of HIV replication in humans has not been established.

Drug Resistance: HIV isolates with reduced sensitivity to zidovudine have been selected in vitro and were also recovered from patients treated with RETROVIR. Genetic analysis of the isolates showed mutations that result in 5 amino acid substitutions (Met41→Leu, A67→Asn, Lys70→Arg, Thr215→Tyr or Phe, and Lys219→Gln) in the viral reverse transcriptase. In general, higher levels of resistance were associated with greater number of mutations with 215 mutation being the most significant.

Cross-Resistance: The potential for cross-resistance between HIV reverse transcriptase inhibitors and protease inhibitors is low because of the different enzyme targets involved. Combination therapy with zidovudine plus zalcitabine or didanosine does not appear to prevent the emergence of zidovudine-resistant isolates. Combination therapy with RETROVIR plus EPIVIR® delayed the emergence of mutations conferring resistance to zidovudine. In some patients harboring zidovudine-resistant virus, combination therapy with RETROVIR plus EPIVIR restored phenotypic sensitivity to zidovudine by 12 weeks of treatment. HIV isolates with multidrug resistance to zidovudine, didanosine, zalcitabine, stavudine, and lamivudine were recovered from a small number of patients treated for ≥1 year with the combination of zidovudine and didanosine or zalcitabine. The pattern of resistant mutations in the combination therapy was different (Ala62→Val, Val75→Ile, Phe77→116Tyr, and Gln→151Met) from monotherapy, with mutation 151 being most significant for multidrug resistance. Site-directed mutagenesis studies showed that these mutations could also result in resistance to zalcitabine, lamivudine, and stavudine.

CLINICAL PHARMACOLOGY

Pharmacokinetics: ***Adults:*** The pharmacokinetic properties of zidovudine in fasting patients are summarized in Table 1. Following oral administration, zidovudine is rapidly absorbed and extensively distributed, with peak serum concentrations occurring within 0.5 to 1.5 hours. Binding to plasma protein is low. Zidovudine is primarily eliminated by hepatic metabolism. The major metabolite of zidovudine is 3′-azido-3′-deoxy-5′-*O*-β-*D*-glucopyranuronosylthymidine (GZDV). GZDV area under the curve (AUC) is about 3-fold greater than the zidovudine AUC. Urinary recovery of zidovudine and GZDV accounts for 14% and 74%, respectively, of the dose following oral administration. A second metabolite, 3′-amino-3′-deoxythymidine (AMT), has been identified in the plasma following single-dose intravenous (IV) administration of zidovudine. The AMT AUC was one fifth of the zidovudine AUC. Pharmacokinetics of zidovudine were dose independent at oral dosing regimens ranging from 2 mg/kg every 8 hours to 10 mg/kg every 4 hours.

The extent of absorption (AUC) was equivalent when zidovudine was administered as RETROVIR Tablets or Syrup compared to RETROVIR Capsules.

Table 1. Zidovudine Pharmacokinetic Parameters in Fasting Adult Patients

Parameter	Mean ± SD (except where noted)
Oral bioavailability (%)	64 ± 10 (n = 5)
Apparent volume of distribution (L/kg)	1.6 ± 0.6 (n = 8)
Plasma protein binding (%)	<38
CSF:plasma ratio*	0.6 [0.04 to 2.62] (n =39)
Systemic clearance (L/hr/kg)	1.6 ± 0.6 (n = 6)
Renal clearance (L/hr/kg)	0.34 ± 0.05 (n = 9)
Elimination half-life (hr)†	0.5 to 3 (n = 19)

*Median [range].
†Approximate range.

Adults with Impaired Renal Function: Zidovudine clearance was decreased resulting in increased zidovudine and GZDV half-life and AUC in patients with impaired renal function (n = 14) following a single 200-mg oral dose (Table 2). Plasma concentrations of AMT were not determined. A dose adjustment should not be necessary for patients with creatinine clearance (CrCl) ≥15 mL/min.

[See table 2 above]

Table 2. Zidovudine Pharmacokinetic Parameters in Patients With Severe Renal Impairment*

Parameter	Control Subjects (Normal Renal Function) (n = 6)	Patients With Renal Impairment (n = 14)
CrCl (mL/min)	120 ± 8	18 ± 2
Zidovudine AUC (ng•hr/mL)	1,400 ± 200	3,100 ± 300
Zidovudine half-life (hr)	1.0 ± 0.2	1.4 ± 0.1

*Data are expressed as mean ± standard deviation.

The pharmacokinetics and tolerance of zidovudine were evaluated in a multiple-dose study in patients undergoing hemodialysis (n = 5) or peritoneal dialysis (n = 6) receiving escalating doses up to 200 mg 5 times daily for 8 weeks. Daily doses of 500 mg or less were well tolerated despite significantly elevated GZDV plasma concentrations. Apparent zidovudine oral clearance was approximately 50% of that reported in patients with normal renal function. Hemodialysis and peritoneal dialysis appeared to have a negligible effect on the removal of zidovudine, whereas GZDV elimination was enhanced. A dosage adjustment is recommended for patients undergoing hemodialysis or peritoneal dialysis (see DOSAGE AND ADMINISTRATION: Dose Adjustment).

Adults with Impaired Hepatic Function: Data describing the effect of hepatic impairment on the pharmacokinetics of zidovudine are limited. However, because zidovudine is eliminated primarily by hepatic metabolism, it is expected that zidovudine clearance would be decreased and plasma concentrations would be increased following administration of the recommended adult doses to patients with hepatic impairment (see DOSAGE AND ADMINISTRATION: Dose Adjustment).

Pediatrics: Zidovudine pharmacokinetics have been evaluated in HIV-infected pediatric patients (Table 3).

Patients from 3 Months to 12 Years of Age: Overall, zidovudine pharmacokinetics in pediatric patients greater than 3 months of age are similar to those in adult patients. Proportional increases in plasma zidovudine concentrations were observed following administration of oral solution from 90 to 240 mg/m^2 every 6 hours. Oral bioavailability, terminal half-life, and oral clearance were comparable to adult values. As in adult patients, the major route of elimination was by metabolism to GZDV. After intravenous dosing, about 29% of the dose was excreted in the urine unchanged, and about 45% of the dose was excreted as GZDV (see DOSAGE AND ADMINISTRATION: Pediatrics).

Patients Younger Than 3 Months of Age: Zidovudine pharmacokinetics have been evaluated in pediatric patients from birth to 3 months of life. Zidovudine elimination was determined immediately following birth in 8 neonates who were exposed to zidovudine in utero. The half-life was 13.0 ± 5.8 hours. In neonates ≤14 days old, bioavailability was greater, total body clearance was slower, and half-life was longer than in pediatric patients >14 days old. For dose recommendations for neonates, see DOSAGE AND ADMINISTRATION: Neonatal Dosing.

[See table 3 at top of next page]

Pregnancy: Zidovudine pharmacokinetics have been studied in a Phase 1 study of 8 women during the last trimester of pregnancy. As pregnancy progressed, there was no evidence of drug accumulation. Zidovudine pharmacokinetics were similar to that of nonpregnant adults. Consistent with passive transmission of the drug across the placenta, zidovudine concentrations in neonatal plasma at birth were essentially equal to those in maternal plasma at delivery. Although data are limited, methadone maintenance therapy in 5 pregnant women did not appear to alter zidovudine pharmacokinetics. However, in another patient population, a potential for interaction has been identified (see PRECAUTIONS).

Nursing Mothers: **The Centers for Disease Control and Prevention recommend that HIV-infected mothers not breastfeed their infants to avoid risking postnatal transmission of HIV.** After administration of a single dose of 200 mg zidovudine to 13 HIV-infected women, the mean concentration of zidovudine was similar in human milk and serum (see PRECAUTIONS: Nursing Mothers).

Geriatric Patients: Zidovudine pharmacokinetics have not been studied in patients over 65 years of age.

Gender: A pharmacokinetic study in healthy male (n = 12) and female (n = 12) subjects showed no differences in zidovudine exposure (AUC) when a single dose of zidovudine was administered as the 300-mg RETROVIR Tablet.

Effect of Food on Absorption: RETROVIR may be administered with or without food. The extent of zidovudine absorption (AUC) was similar when a single dose of zidovudine was administered with food.

Drug Interactions: See Table 4 and PRECAUTIONS: Drug Interactions.

Zidovudine Plus Lamivudine: No clinically significant alterations in lamivudine or zidovudine pharmacokinetics were observed in 12 asymptomatic HIV-infected adult patients given a single dose of zidovudine (200 mg) in combination with multiple doses of lamivudine (300 mg every 12 hours).

[See table 4 at top of next page]

INDICATIONS AND USAGE

RETROVIR in combination with other antiretroviral agents is indicated for the treatment of HIV infection.

Maternal-Fetal HIV Transmission: RETROVIR is also indicated for the prevention of maternal-fetal HIV transmission as part of a regimen that includes oral RETROVIR beginning between 14 and 34 weeks of gestation, intravenous RETROVIR during labor, and administration of RETROVIR Syrup to the neonate after birth. The efficacy of this regimen for preventing HIV transmission in women who have received RETROVIR for a prolonged period before pregnancy has not been evaluated. The safety of RETROVIR for the mother or fetus during the first trimester of pregnancy has not been assessed (see Description of Clinical Studies).

Description of Clinical Studies: Therapy with RETROVIR has been shown to prolong survival and decrease the incidence of opportunistic infections in patients with advanced HIV disease and to delay disease progression in asymptomatic HIV-infected patients.

Combination Therapy in Adults: RETROVIR in combination with other antiretroviral agents has been shown to be superior to monotherapy for one or more of the following endpoints: delaying death, delaying development of AIDS, increasing CD4 cell counts, and decreasing plasma HIV RNA. The clinical efficacy of a combination regimen that includes RETROVIR was demonstrated in study ACTG320. This study was a multicenter, randomized, double-blind, placebo-controlled trial that compared RETROVIR 600 mg/day plus EPIVIR 300 mg/day to RETROVIR plus EPIVIR plus indinavir 800 mg t.i.d. The incidence of AIDS-defining events or death was lower in the triple-drug–containing

Continued on next page

Product information on these pages is effective as of August 2004. Further information is available at: GlaxoSmithKline, PO Box 13398, Research Triangle Park, NC 27709. 1-888-825-5249. Corporate Web Site: www.gsk.com

Retrovir Tabs/Capsules/Syrup—Cont.

arm compared to the two-drug–containing arm (6.1% versus 10.9%, respectively).
The complete prescribing information for each drug should be consulted before combination therapy that includes RETROVIR is initiated.

Monotherapy in Adults: In controlled studies of treatment-naive patients conducted between 1986 and 1989, monotherapy with RETROVIR, as compared to placebo, reduced the risk of HIV disease progression, as assessed using endpoints that included the occurrence of HIV-related illnesses, AIDS-defining events, or death. These studies enrolled patients with advanced disease (BW002), and asymptomatic or mildly symptomatic disease in patients with CD4 cell counts between 200 and 500 cells/mm^3 (ACTG016 and ACTG019). A survival benefit for monotherapy with RETROVIR was not demonstrated in the latter 2 studies. Subsequent studies showed that the clinical benefit of monotherapy with RETROVIR was time limited.

Pediatric Patients: ACTG300 was a multicenter, randomized, double-blind study that provided for comparison of EPIVIR plus RETROVIR to didanosine monotherapy. A total of 471 symptomatic, HIV-infected therapy-naive pediatric patients were enrolled in these 2 treatment arms. The median age was 2.7 years (range 6 weeks to 14 years), the mean baseline CD4 cell count was 868 cells/mm^3, and the mean baseline plasma HIV RNA was 5.0 $\log_{10}$ copies/mL. The median duration that patients remained on study was approximately 10 months. Results are summarized in Table 5.

[See table 5 at right]

Pregnant Women and Their Neonates: The utility of RETROVIR for the prevention of maternal-fetal HIV transmission was demonstrated in a randomized, double-blind, placebo-controlled trial (ACTG076) conducted in HIV-infected pregnant women with CD4 cell counts of 200 to 1,818 cells/mm^3 (median in the treated group: 560 cells/mm^3) who had little or no previous exposure to RETROVIR. Oral RETROVIR was initiated between 14 and 34 weeks of gestation (median 11 weeks of therapy) followed by IV administration of RETROVIR during labor and delivery. Following birth, neonates received oral RETROVIR Syrup for 6 weeks. The study showed a statistically significant difference in the incidence of HIV infection in the neonates (based on viral culture from peripheral blood) between the group receiving RETROVIR and the group receiving placebo. Of 363 neonates evaluated in the study, the estimated risk of HIV infection was 7.8% in the group receiving RETROVIR and 24.9% in the placebo group, a relative reduction in transmission risk of 68.7%. RETROVIR was well tolerated by mothers and infants. There was no difference in pregnancy-related adverse events between the treatment groups.

Table 3. Zidovudine Pharmacokinetic Parameters in Pediatric Patients*

Parameter	Birth to 14 Days of Age	14 Days to 3 Months of Age	3 Months to 12 Years of Age
Oral bioavailability (%)	89 ± 19 (n = 15)	61 ± 19 (n = 17)	65 ± 24 (n = 18)
CSF:plasma ratio	no data	no data	0.68 (0.03 to 3.25)[†] (n = 38)
CL (L/hr/kg)	0.65 ± 0.29 (n = 18)	1.14 ± 0.24 (n = 16)	1.85 ± 0.47 (n = 20)
Elimination half-life (hr)	3.1 ± 1.2 (n = 21)	1.9 ± 0.7 (n = 18)	1.5 ± 0.7 (n = 21)

*Data presented as mean ± standard deviation except where noted.
[†]Median [range].

Table 4. Effect of Coadministered Drugs on Zidovudine AUC*
Note: ROUTINE DOSE MODIFICATION OF ZIDOVUDINE IS NOT WARRANTED WITH COADMINISTRATION OF THE FOLLOWING DRUGS.

Coadministered Drug and Dose	Zidovudine Dose	n	Zidovudine Concentrations		Concentration of Coadministered Drug
			AUC	Variability	
Atovaquone 750 mg q 12 hr with food	200 mg q 8 hr	14	↑ AUC 31%	Range 23% to 78%[†]	↔
Fluconazole 400 mg daily	200 mg q 8 hr	12	↑ AUC 74%	95% CI: 54% to 98%	Not Reported
Methadone 30 to 90 mg daily	200 mg q 4 hr	9	↑ AUC 43%	Range 16% to 64%[†]	↔
Nelfinavir 750 mg q 8 hr × 7 to 10 days	single 200 mg	11	↓ AUC 35%	Range 28% to 41%	↔
Probenecid 500 mg q 6 hr × 2 days	2 mg/kg q 8 hr × 3 days	3	↑ AUC 106%	Range 100% to 170%[†]	Not Assessed
Rifampin 600 mg daily × 14 days	200 mg q 8 hr × 14 days	8	↓ AUC 47%	90% CI: 41% to 53%	Not Assessed
Ritonavir 300 mg q 6 hr × 4 days	200 mg q 8 hr × 4 days	9	↓ AUC 25%	95% CI: 15% to 34%	↔
Valproic acid 250 mg or 500 mg q 8 hr × 4 days	100 mg q 8 hr × 4 days	6	↑ AUC 80%	Range 64% to 130%[†]	Not Assessed

↑ = Increase; ↓ = Decrease; ↔ = no significant change; AUC = area under the concentration versus time curve; CI = confidence interval.
*This table is not all inclusive.
[†]Estimated range of percent difference.

Table 5. Number of Patients (%) Reaching a Primary Clinical Endpoint (Disease Progression or Death)

Endpoint	EPIVIR plus RETROVIR (n = 236)	Didanosine (n = 235)
HIV disease progression or death (total)	15 (6.4%)	37 (15.7%)
Physical growth failure	7 (3.0%)	6 (2.6%)
Central nervous system deterioration	4 (1.7%)	12 (5.1%)
CDC Clinical Category C	2 (0.8%)	8 (3.4%)
Death	2 (0.8%)	11 (4.7%)

CONTRAINDICATIONS

RETROVIR Tablets, Capsules, and Syrup are contraindicated for patients who have potentially life-threatening allergic reactions to any of the components of the formulations.

WARNINGS

COMBIVIR and TRIZIVIR are combination product tablets that contain zidovudine as one of their components. RETROVIR should not be administered concomitantly with COMBIVIR or TRIZIVIR.
The incidence of adverse reactions appears to increase with disease progression; patients should be monitored carefully, especially as disease progression occurs.

Bone Marrow Suppression: RETROVIR should be used with caution in patients who have bone marrow compromise evidenced by granulocyte count <1,000 cells/mm^3 or hemoglobin <9.5 g/dL. In patients with advanced symptomatic HIV disease, anemia and neutropenia were the most significant adverse events observed. There have been reports of pancytopenia associated with the use of RETROVIR, which was reversible in most instances after discontinuance of the drug. However, significant anemia, in many cases requiring dose adjustment, discontinuation of RETROVIR, and/or blood transfusions, has occurred during treatment with RETROVIR alone or in combination with other antiretrovirals.
Frequent blood counts are strongly recommended in patients with advanced HIV disease who are treated with RETROVIR. For HIV-infected individuals and patients with asymptomatic or early HIV disease, periodic blood counts are recommended. If anemia or neutropenia develops, dosage adjustments may be necessary (see DOSAGE AND ADMINISTRATION).

Myopathy: Myopathy and myositis with pathological changes, similar to that produced by HIV disease, have been associated with prolonged use of RETROVIR.

Lactic Acidosis/Severe Hepatomegaly with Steatosis: Lactic acidosis and severe hepatomegaly with steatosis, including fatal cases, have been reported with the use of nucleoside analogues alone or in combination, including zidovudine and other antiretrovirals. A majority of these cases have been in women. Obesity and prolonged exposure to antiretroviral nucleoside analogues may be risk factors. Particular caution should be exercised when administering RETROVIR to any patient with known risk factors for liver disease; however, cases have also been reported in patients with no known risk factors. Treatment with RETROVIR should be suspended in any patient who develops clinical or laboratory findings suggestive of lactic acidosis or pronounced hepatotoxicity (which may include hepatomegaly and steatosis even in the absence of marked transaminase elevations).

PRECAUTIONS

General: Zidovudine is eliminated from the body primarily by renal excretion following metabolism in the liver (glucuronidation). In patients with severely impaired renal function (CrCl<15 mL/min), dosage reduction is recommended. Although the data are limited, zidovudine concentrations appear to be increased in patients with severely impaired hepatic function which may increase the risk of hematologic toxicity (see CLINICAL PHARMACOLOGY: Pharmacokinetics and DOSAGE AND ADMINISTRATION).

Fat Redistribution: Redistribution/accumulation of body fat, including central obesity, dorsocervical fat enlargement (buffalo hump), peripheral wasting, facial wasting, breast enlargement, and "cushingoid appearance," have been observed in patients receiving antiretroviral therapy. The mechanism and long-term consequences of these events are currently unknown. A causal relationship has not been established.

Information for Patients: RETROVIR is not a cure for HIV infection, and patients may continue to acquire illnesses associated with HIV infection, including opportunistic infections. Therefore, patients should be advised to seek medical care for any significant change in their health status.
The safety and efficacy of RETROVIR in women, intravenous drug users, and racial minorities is not significantly different than that observed in white males.
Patients should be informed that the major toxicities of RETROVIR are neutropenia and/or anemia. The frequency and severity of these toxicities are greater in patients with more advanced disease and in those who initiate therapy later in the course of their infection. They should be told that if toxicity develops, they may require transfusions or drug discontinuation. They should be told of the extreme importance of having their blood counts followed closely while on therapy, especially for patients with advanced symptomatic HIV disease. They should be cautioned about the use of other medications, including ganciclovir and interferon-alpha, that may exacerbate the toxicity of RETROVIR (see PRECAUTIONS: Drug Interactions). Patients should be informed that other adverse effects of RETROVIR include nausea and vomiting. Patients should also be encouraged to contact their physician if they experience muscle weakness, shortness of breath, symptoms of hepatitis or pancreatitis, or any other unexpected adverse events while being treated with RETROVIR.
RETROVIR Tablets, Capsules, and Syrup are for oral ingestion only. Patients should be told of the importance of taking RETROVIR exactly as prescribed. They should be told not to share medication and not to exceed the recommended dose. Patients should be told that the long-term effects of RETROVIR are unknown at this time.

Pregnant women considering the use of RETROVIR during pregnancy for prevention of HIV-transmission to their infants should be advised that transmission may still occur in some cases despite therapy. The long-term consequences of in utero and infant exposure to RETROVIR are unknown, including the possible risk of cancer.

HIV-infected pregnant women should be advised not to breastfeed to avoid postnatal transmission of HIV to a child who may not yet be infected.

Patients should be advised that therapy with RETROVIR has not been shown to reduce the risk of transmission of HIV to others through sexual contact or blood contamination.

Patients should be informed that redistribution or accumulation of body fat may occur in patients receiving antiretroviral therapy and that the cause and long-term health effects of these conditions are not known at this time.

Drug Interactions: See CLINICAL PHARMACOLOGY section (Table 4) for information on zidovudine concentrations when coadministered with other drugs. For patients experiencing pronounced anemia or other severe zidovudine-associated events while receiving chronic administration of zidovudine and some of the drugs (e.g., fluconazole, valproic acid) listed in Table 4, zidovudine dose reduction may be considered.

Antiretroviral Agents: Concomitant use of zidovudine with stavudine should be avoided since an antagonistic relationship has been demonstrated in vitro.

Some nucleoside analogues affecting DNA replication, such as ribavirin, antagonize the in vitro antiviral activity of RETROVIR against HIV; concomitant use of such drugs should be avoided.

Doxorubicin: Concomitant use of zidovudine with doxorubicin should be avoided since an antagonistic relationship has been demonstrated in vitro (see CLINICAL PHARMACOLOGY for additional drug interactions).

Phenytoin: Phenytoin plasma levels have been reported to be low in some patients receiving RETROVIR, while in one case a high level was documented. However, in a pharmacokinetic interaction study in which 12 HIV-positive volunteers received a single 300-mg phenytoin dose alone and during steady-state zidovudine conditions (200 mg every 4 hours), no change in phenytoin kinetics was observed. Although not designed to optimally assess the effect of phenytoin on zidovudine kinetics, a 30% decrease in oral zidovudine clearance was observed with phenytoin.

Overlapping Toxicities: Coadministration of ganciclovir, interferon-alpha, and other bone marrow suppressive or cytotoxic agents may increase the hematologic toxicity of zidovudine.

Carcinogenesis, Mutagenesis, Impairment of Fertility: Zidovudine was administered orally at 3 dosage levels to separate groups of mice and rats (60 females and 60 males in each group). Initial single daily doses were 30, 60, and 120 mg/kg/day in mice and 80, 220, and 600 mg/kg/day in rats. The doses in mice were reduced to 20, 30, and 40 mg/kg/day after day 90 because of treatment-related anemia, whereas in rats only the high dose was reduced to 450 mg/kg/day on day 91 and then to 300 mg/kg/day on day 279.

In mice, 7 late-appearing (after 19 months) vaginal neoplasms (5 nonmetastasizing squamous cell carcinomas, 1 squamous cell papilloma, and 1 squamous polyp) occurred in animals given the highest dose. One late-appearing squamous cell papilloma occurred in the vagina of a middle-dose animal. No vaginal tumors were found at the lowest dose.

In rats, 2 late-appearing (after 20 months), nonmetastasizing vaginal squamous cell carcinomas occurred in animals given the highest dose. No vaginal tumors occurred at the low or middle dose in rats. No other drug-related tumors were observed in either sex of either species.

At doses that produced tumors in mice and rats, the estimated drug exposure (as measured by AUC) was approximately 3 times (mouse) and 24 times (rat) the estimated human exposure at the recommended therapeutic dose of 100 mg every 4 hours.

Two transplacental carcinogenicity studies were conducted in mice. One study administered zidovudine at doses of 20 mg/kg/day or 40 mg/kg/day from gestation day 10 through parturition and lactation with dosing continuing in offspring for 24 months postnatally. The doses of zidovudine employed in this study produced zidovudine exposures approximately 3 times the estimated human exposure at recommended doses. After 24 months, an increase in incidence of vaginal tumors was noted with no increase in tumors in the liver or lung or any other organ in either gender. These findings are consistent with results of the standard oral carcinogenicity study in mice, as described earlier. A second study administered zidovudine at maximum tolerated doses of 12.5 mg/day or 25 mg/day (~1,000 mg/kg nonpregnant body weight or ~450 mg/kg of term body weight) to pregnant mice from days 12 through 18 of gestation. There was an increase in the number of tumors in the lung, liver, and female reproductive tracts in the offspring of mice receiving the higher dose level of zidovudine.

It is not known how predictive the results of rodent carcinogenicity studies may be for humans.

Zidovudine was mutagenic in a 5178Y/TK$^{+/-}$ mouse lymphoma assay, positive in an in vitro cell transformation assay, clastogenic in a cytogenetic assay using cultured human lymphocytes, and positive in mouse and rat micronucleus tests after repeated doses. It was negative in a cytogenetic study in rats given a single dose.

Table 6. Percentage (%) of Patients with Adverse Events* in Asymptomatic HIV Infection (ACTG019)

Adverse Event	RETROVIR 500 mg/day (n = 453)	Placebo (n = 428)
Body as a whole		
Asthenia	8.6%†	5.8%
Headache	62.5%	52.6%
Malaise	53.2%	44.9%
Gastrointestinal		
Anorexia	20.1%	10.5%
Constipation	6.4%†	3.5%
Nausea	51.4%	29.9%
Vomiting	17.2%	9.8%

*Reported in ≥5% of study population.
†Not statistically significant versus placebo.

Table 7. Frequencies of Selected (Grade 3/4) Laboratory Abnormalities in Patients with Asymptomatic HIV Infection (ACTG019)

Adverse Event	RETROVIR 500 mg/day (n = 453)	Placebo (n = 428)
Anemia (Hgb<8 g/dL)	1.1%	0.2%
Granulocytopenia (<750 cells/mm^3)	1.8%	1.6%
Thrombocytopenia (platelets<50,000/mm^3)	0%	0.5%
ALT (>5 × ULN)	3.1%	2.6%
AST (>5 × ULN)	0.9%	1.6%
Alkaline phosphatase (>5 × ULN)	0%	0%

ULN = Upper limit of normal.

Table 8. Selected Clinical Adverse Events and Physical Findings (≥5% Frequency) in Pediatric Patients in Study ACTG300

Adverse Event	EPIVIR plus RETROVIR (n = 236)	Didanosine (n = 235)
Body as a whole		
Fever	25%	32%
Digestive		
Hepatomegaly	11%	11%
Nausea & vomiting	8%	7%
Diarrhea	8%	6%
Stomatitis	6%	12%
Splenomegaly	5%	8%
Respiratory		
Cough	15%	18%
Abnormal breath sounds/wheezing	7%	9%
Ear, Nose, and Throat		
Signs or symptoms of ears*	7%	6%
Nasal discharge or congestion	8%	11%
Other		
Skin rashes	12%	14%
Lymphadenopathy	9%	11%

*Includes pain, discharge, erythema, or swelling of an ear.

Zidovudine, administered to male and female rats at doses up to 7 times the usual adult dose based on body surface area considerations, had no effect on fertility judged by conception rates.

Pregnancy: Pregnancy Category C. Oral teratology studies in the rat and in the rabbit at doses up to 500 mg/kg/day revealed no evidence of teratogenicity with zidovudine. Zidovudine treatment resulted in embryo/fetal toxicity as evidenced by an increase in the incidence of fetal resorptions in rats given 150 or 450 mg/kg/day and rabbits given 500 mg/kg/day. The doses used in the teratology studies resulted in peak zidovudine plasma concentrations (after one half of the daily dose) in rats 66 to 226 times, and in rabbits 12 to 87 times, mean steady-state peak human plasma concentrations (after one sixth of the daily dose) achieved with the recommended daily dose (100 mg every 4 hours). In an in vitro experiment with fertilized mouse oocytes, zidovudine exposure resulted in a dose-dependent reduction in blastocyst formation. In an additional teratology study in rats, a dose of 3,000 mg/kg/day (very near the oral median lethal dose in rats of 3,683 mg/kg) caused marked maternal toxicity and an increase in the incidence of fetal malformations. This dose resulted in peak zidovudine plasma concentrations 350 times peak human plasma concentrations. (Estimated area-under-the-curve [AUC] in rats at this dose level was 300 times the daily AUC in humans given 600 mg per day.) No evidence of teratogenicity was seen in this experiment at doses of 600 mg/kg/day or less.

Two rodent transplacental carcinogenicity studies were conducted (see Carcinogenesis, Mutagenesis, Impairment of Fertility).

A randomized, double-blind, placebo-controlled trial was conducted in HIV-infected pregnant women to determine the utility of RETROVIR for the prevention of maternal-fetal HIV-transmission (see INDICATIONS AND USAGE: Description of Clinical Studies). Congenital abnormalities occurred with similar frequency between neonates born to mothers who received RETROVIR and neonates born to mothers who received placebo. Abnormalities were either problems in embryogenesis (prior to 14 weeks) or were recognized on ultrasound before or immediately after initiation of study drug.

Antiretroviral Pregnancy Registry: To monitor maternal-fetal outcomes of pregnant women exposed to RETROVIR, an Antiretroviral Pregnancy Registry has been established. Physicians are encouraged to register patients by calling 1-800-258-4263.

Nursing Mothers: The Centers for Disease Control and Prevention recommend that HIV-infected mothers not breastfeed their infants to avoid risking postnatal transmission of HIV. Zidovudine is excreted in human milk (see CLINICAL PHARMACOLOGY: Pharmacokinetics: Nursing Mothers). Because of both the potential for HIV transmission and the potential for serious adverse reactions in nursing infants, **mothers should be instructed not to breastfeed if they are receiving RETROVIR** (see Pediatric Use and INDICATIONS AND USAGE: Maternal-Fetal HIV Transmission).

Pediatric Use: RETROVIR has been studied in HIV-infected pediatric patients over 3 months of age who had HIV-related symptoms or who were asymptomatic with abnormal laboratory values indicating significant HIV-related immunosuppression. RETROVIR has also been studied in neonates perinatally exposed to HIV (see ADVERSE REACTIONS, DOSAGE AND ADMINISTRATION, INDICATIONS AND USAGE: Description of Clinical Studies, and CLINICAL PHARMACOLOGY: Pharmacokinetics).

Geriatric Use: Clinical studies of RETROVIR did not include sufficient numbers of subjects aged 65 and over to de-

Continued on next page

Product information on these pages is effective as of August 2004. Further information is available at: GlaxoSmithKline, PO Box 13398, Research Triangle Park, NC 27709. 1-888-825-5249. Corporate Web Site: www.gsk.com

Retrovir Tabs/Capsules/Syrup—Cont.

termine whether they respond differently from younger subjects. Other reported clinical experience has not identified differences in responses between the elderly and younger patients. In general, dose selection for an elderly patient should be cautious, reflecting the greater frequency of decreased hepatic, renal, or cardiac function, and of concomitant disease or other drug therapy.

ADVERSE REACTIONS

Adults: The frequency and severity of adverse events associated with the use of RETROVIR are greater in patients with more advanced infection at the time of initiation of therapy.

Table 6 summarizes events reported at a statistically significant greater incidence for patients receiving RETROVIR in a monotherapy study:

[See table 6 at top of previous page]

In addition to the adverse events listed in Table 6, other adverse events observed in clinical studies were abdominal cramps, abdominal pain, arthralgia, chills, dyspepsia, fatigue, hyperbilirubinemia, insomnia, musculoskeletal pain, myalgia, and neuropathy.

Selected laboratory abnormalities observed during a clinical study of monotherapy with RETROVIR are shown in Table 7.

[See table 7 at top of previous page]

Pediatric: ***Study ACTG300:*** Selected clinical adverse events and physical findings with a ≥5% frequency during therapy with EPIVIR 4 mg/kg twice daily plus RETROVIR 160 mg/m^2 3 times daily compared with didanosine in therapy-naive (≤56 days of antiretroviral therapy) pediatric patients are listed in Table 8.

[See table 8 on previous page]

Selected laboratory abnormalities experienced by therapy-naive (≤56 days of antiretroviral therapy) pediatric patients are listed in Table 9.

[See table 9 below]

Additional adverse events reported in open-label studies in pediatric patients receiving RETROVIR 180 mg/m^2 every 6 hours were congestive heart failure, decreased reflexes, ECG abnormality, edema, hematuria, left ventricular dilation, macrocytosis, nervousness/irritability, and weight loss. The clinical adverse events reported among adult recipients of RETROVIR may also occur in pediatric patients.

Use for the Prevention of Maternal-Fetal Transmission of HIV: In a randomized, double-blind, placebo-controlled trial in HIV-infected women and their neonates conducted to determine the utility of RETROVIR for the prevention of maternal-fetal HIV transmission, RETROVIR Syrup at 2 mg/kg was administered every 6 hours for 6 weeks to neonates beginning within 12 hours following birth. The most commonly reported adverse experiences were anemia (hemoglobin <9.0 g/dL) and neutropenia (<1,000 cells/mm^3). Anemia occurred in 22% of the neonates who received RETROVIR and in 12% of the neonates who received placebo. The mean difference in hemoglobin values was less than 1.0 g/dL for neonates receiving RETROVIR compared to neonates receiving placebo. No neonates with anemia required transfusion and all hemoglobin values spontaneously returned to normal within 6 weeks after completion of therapy with RETROVIR. Neutropenia was reported with similar frequency in the group that received RETROVIR (21%) and in the group that received placebo (27%). The long-term consequences of in utero and infant exposure to RETROVIR are unknown.

Observed During Clinical Practice: In addition to adverse events reported from clinical trials, the following events have been identified during use of RETROVIR in clinical practice. Because they are reported voluntarily from a population of unknown size, estimates of frequency cannot be made. These events have been chosen for inclusion due to either their seriousness, frequency of reporting, potential causal connection to RETROVIR, or a combination of these factors.

Body as a Whole: Back pain, chest pain, flu-like syndrome, generalized pain, redistribution/accumulation of body fat (see PRECAUTIONS: Fat Redistribution).

Cardiovascular: Cardiomyopathy, syncope.

Endocrine: Gynecomastia.

Eye: Macular edema.

Gastrointestinal: Constipation, dysphagia, flatulence, oral mucosa pigmentation, mouth ulcer.

General: Sensitization reactions including anaphylaxis and angioedema, vasculitis.

Hemic and Lymphatic: Aplastic anemia, hemolytic anemia, leukopenia, lymphadenopathy, pancytopenia with marrow hypoplasia, pure red cell aplasia.

Hepatobiliary Tract and Pancreas: Hepatitis, hepatomegaly with steatosis, jaundice, lactic acidosis, pancreatitis.

Musculoskeletal: Increased CPK, increased LDH, muscle spasm, myopathy and myositis with pathological changes (similar to that produced by HIV disease), rhabdomyolysis, tremor.

Nervous: Anxiety, confusion, depression, dizziness, loss of mental acuity, mania, paresthesia, seizures, somnolence, vertigo.

Respiratory: Cough, dyspnea, rhinitis, sinusitis.

Skin: Changes in skin and nail pigmentation, pruritus, rash, Stevens-Johnson syndrome, toxic epidermal necrolysis, sweat, urticaria.

Special Senses: Amblyopia, hearing loss, photophobia, taste perversion.

Urogenital: Urinary frequency, urinary hesitancy.

OVERDOSAGE

Acute overdoses of zidovudine have been reported in pediatric patients and adults. These involved exposures up to 50 grams. No specific symptoms or signs have been identified following acute overdosage with zidovudine apart from those listed as adverse events such as fatigue, headache, vomiting, and occasional reports of hematological disturbances. All patients recovered without permanent sequelae. Hemodialysis and peritoneal dialysis appear to have a negligible effect on the removal of zidovudine while elimination of its primary metabolite, GZDV, is enhanced.

DOSAGE AND ADMINISTRATION

Adults: The recommended oral dose of RETROVIR is 600 mg per day in divided doses in combination with other antiretroviral agents.

Pediatrics: The recommended dose in pediatric patients 6 weeks to 12 years of age is 160 mg/m^2 every 8 hours (480 mg/m^2/day up to a maximum of 200 mg every 8 hours) in combination with other antiretroviral agents.

Maternal-Fetal HIV Transmission: The recommended dosing regimen for administration to pregnant women (>14 weeks of pregnancy) and their neonates is:

Maternal Dosing: 100 mg orally 5 times per day until the start of labor (see INDICATIONS AND USAGE: Description of Clinical Studies). During labor and delivery, intravenous RETROVIR should be administered at 2 mg/kg (total body weight) over 1 hour followed by a continuous intravenous infusion of 1 mg/kg/hour (total body weight) until clamping of the umbilical cord.

Neonatal Dosing: 2 mg/kg orally every 6 hours starting within 12 hours after birth and continuing through 6 weeks of age. Neonates unable to receive oral dosing may be administered RETROVIR intravenously at 1.5 mg/kg, infused over 30 minutes, every 6 hours. (See PRECAUTIONS if hepatic disease or renal insufficiency is present.)

Monitoring of Patients: Hematologic toxicities appear to be related to pretreatment bone marrow reserve and to dose and duration of therapy. In patients with poor bone marrow reserve, particularly in patients with advanced symptomatic HIV disease, frequent monitoring of hematologic indices is recommended to detect serious anemia or neutropenia (see WARNINGS). In patients who experience hematologic toxicity, reduction in hemoglobin may occur as early as 2 to 4 weeks, and neutropenia usually occurs after 6 to 8 weeks.

Dose Adjustment: ***Anemia:*** Significant anemia (hemoglobin of <7.5 g/dL or reduction of >25% of baseline) and/or significant neutropenia (granulocyte count of <750 cells/mm^3 or reduction of >50% from baseline) may require a dose interruption until evidence of marrow recovery is observed (see WARNINGS). In patients who develop significant anemia, dose interruption does not necessarily eliminate the need for transfusion. If marrow recovery occurs following dose interruption, resumption in dose may be appropriate using adjunctive measures such as epoetin alfa at recommended doses, depending on hematologic indices such as serum erythropoetin level and patient tolerance.

For patients experiencing pronounced anemia while receiving chronic coadministration of zidovudine and some of the drugs (e.g., fluconazole, valproic acid) listed in Table 4, zidovudine dose reduction may be considered.

End-Stage Renal Disease: In patients maintained on hemodialysis or peritoneal dialysis, recommended dosing is 100 mg every 6 to 8 hours (see CLINICAL PHARMACOLOGY: Pharmacokinetics).

Hepatic Impairment: There are insufficient data to recommend dose adjustment of RETROVIR in patients with mild to moderate impaired hepatic function or liver cirrhosis. Since RETROVIR is primarily eliminated by hepatic metabolism, a reduction in the daily dose may be necessary in these patients. Frequent monitoring for hematologic toxicities is advised (see CLINICAL PHARMACOLOGY: Pharmacokinetics and PRECAUTIONS: General).

HOW SUPPLIED

RETROVIR Tablets 300 mg (biconvex, white, round, film-coated) containing 300 mg zidovudine, one side engraved "GX CW3" and "300" on the other side. Bottle of 60 (NDC 0173-0501-00).

Store at 15° to 25°C (59° to 77°F).

RETROVIR Capsules 100 mg (white, opaque cap and body with a dark blue band) containing 100 mg zidovudine and printed with "Wellcome" and unicorn logo on cap and "Y9C" and "100" on body. Bottles of 100 (NDC 0173-0108-55) and Unit Dose Pack of 100 (NDC 0173-0108-56).

Store at 15° to 25°C (59° to 77°F) and protect from moisture.

RETROVIR Syrup (colorless to pale yellow, strawberry-flavored) containing 50 mg zidovudine in each teaspoonful (5 mL). Bottle of 240 mL (NDC 0173-0113-18) with child-resistant cap.

Store at 15° to 25°C (59° to 77°F).

GlaxoSmithKline, Research Triangle Park, NC 27709

April 2003/RL-1194

Shown in Product Identification Guide, page 317

RETROVIR® ℞

[re'trō-vir]

(zidovudine)

IV Infusion

FOR INTRAVENOUS INFUSION ONLY

WARNING

RETROVIR (ZIDOVUDINE) HAS BEEN ASSOCIATED WITH HEMATOLOGIC TOXICITY, INCLUDING NEUTROPENIA AND SEVERE ANEMIA, PARTICULARLY IN PATIENTS WITH ADVANCED HIV DISEASE (SEE WARNINGS). PROLONGED USE OF RETROVIR HAS BEEN ASSOCIATED WITH SYMPTOMATIC MYOPATHY. LACTIC ACIDOSIS AND SEVERE HEPATOMEGALY WITH STEATOSIS, INCLUDING FATAL CASES, HAVE BEEN REPORTED WITH THE USE OF NUCLEOSIDE ANALOGUES ALONE OR IN COMBINATION, INCLUDING RETROVIR AND OTHER ANTIRETROVIRALS (SEE WARNINGS).

DESCRIPTION

RETROVIR is the brand name for zidovudine (formerly called azidothymidine [AZT]), a pyrimidine nucleoside analogue active against human immunodeficiency virus (HIV). RETROVIR IV Infusion is a sterile solution for intravenous infusion only. Each mL contains 10 mg zidovudine in Water for Injection. Hydrochloric acid and/or sodium hydroxide may have been added to adjust the pH to approximately 5.5. RETROVIR IV Infusion contains no preservatives.

The chemical name of zidovudine is 3′-azido-3′-deoxythymidine.

Zidovudine is a white to beige, odorless, crystalline solid with a molecular weight of 267.24 and a solubility of 20.1 mg/mL in water at 25°C. The molecular formula is $C_{10}H_{13}N_5O_4$.

MICROBIOLOGY

Mechanism of Action: Zidovudine is a synthetic nucleoside analogue of the naturally occurring nucleoside, thymidine, in which the 3′-hydroxy (-OH) group is replaced by an azido (-N_3) group.

Within cells, zidovudine is converted to the active metabolite, zidovudine 5′-triphosphate (AztTP), by the sequential action of the cellular enzymes. Zidovudine 5′-triphosphate inhibits the activity of the HIV reverse transcriptase both by competing for utilization with the natural substrate, deoxythymidine 5′-triphosphate (dTTP), and by its incorporation into viral DNA. The lack of a 3′-OH group in the incorporated nucleoside analogue prevents the formation of the 5′ to 3′ phosphodiester linkage essential for DNA chain elongation and, therefore, the viral DNA growth is terminated. The active metabolite AztTP is also a weak inhibitor of the cellular DNA polymerase-alpha and mitochondrial polymerase-gamma and has been reported to be incorporated into the DNA of cells in culture.

In Vitro HIV Susceptibility: The in vitro anti-HIV activity of zidovudine was assessed by infecting cell lines of lymphoblastic and monocytic origin and peripheral blood lymphocytes with laboratory and clinical isolates of HIV. The IC_{50} and IC_{90} values (50% and 90% inhibitory concentrations) were 0.003 to 0.013 and 0.03 to 0.13 mcg/mL, respectively (1 nM = 0.27 ng/mL). The IC_{50} and IC_{90} values of HIV isolates recovered from 18 untreated AIDS/ARC patients were in the range of 0.003 to 0.013 mcg/mL and 0.03 to 0.3 mcg/mL, respectively. Zidovudine showed antiviral activity in all acutely infected cell lines; however, activity was substantially less in chronically infected cell lines. In drug combination studies with zalcitabine, didanosine, lamivudine, saquinavir, indinavir, ritonavir, nevirapine, delavirdine, or interferon-alpha, zidovudine showed additive to synergistic activity in cell culture. The relationship between the in vitro susceptibility of HIV to reverse transcriptase inhibitors and the inhibition of HIV replication in humans has not been established.

Table 9. Frequencies of Selected (Grade 3/4) Laboratory Abnormalities in Pediatric Patients in Study ACTG300

Test (Abnormal Level)	EPIVIR plus RETROVIR	Didanosine
Neutropenia (ANC<400 cells/mm^3)	8%	3%
Anemia (Hgb<7.0 g/dL)	4%	2%
Thrombocytopenia (platelets<50,000/mm^3)	1%	3%
ALT (>10 × ULN)	1%	3%
AST (>10 × ULN)	2%	4%
Lipase (>2.5 × ULN)	3%	3%
Total amylase (>2.5 × ULN)	3%	3%

ULN = Upper limit of normal.
ANC = Absolute neutrophil count.

Drug Resistance: HIV isolates with reduced sensitivity to zidovudine have been selected in vitro and were also recovered from patients treated with RETROVIR. Genetic analysis of the isolates showed mutations that result in 5 amino acid substitutions (Met41→Leu, A67→Asn, Lys70→Arg, Thr215→Tyr or Phe, and Lys219→Gln) in the viral reverse transcriptase. In general, higher levels of resistance were associated with greater number of mutations, with 215 mutation being the most significant.

Cross-Resistance: The potential for cross-resistance between HIV reverse transcriptase inhibitors and protease inhibitors is low because of the different enzyme targets involved. Combination therapy with zidovudine plus zalcitabine or didanosine does not appear to prevent the emergence of zidovudine-resistant isolates. Combination therapy with RETROVIR plus EPIVIR® delayed the emergence of mutations conferring resistance to zidovudine. In some patients harboring zidovudine-resistant virus, combination therapy with RETROVIR plus EPIVIR restored phenotypic sensitivity to zidovudine by 12 weeks of treatment. HIV isolates with multidrug resistance to zidovudine, didanosine, zalcitabine, stavudine, and lamivudine were recovered from a small number of patients treated for ≥1 year with the combination of zidovudine and didanosine or zalcitabine. The pattern of resistant mutations in the combination therapy was different (Ala62→Val, Val75→Ile, Phe77→116Tyr, and Gln→151Met) from monotherapy, with mutation 151 being most significant for multidrug resistance. Site-directed mutagenesis studies showed that these mutations could also result in resistance to zalcitabine, lamivudine, and stavudine.

CLINICAL PHARMACOLOGY

Pharmacokinetics: ***Adults:*** The pharmacokinetics of zidovudine have been evaluated in 22 adult HIV-infected patients in a Phase 1 dose-escalation study. Following intravenous (IV) dosing, dose-independent kinetics was observed over the range of 1 to 5 mg/kg. The major metabolite of zidovudine is 3′-azido-3′-deoxy-5′-*O*-β-*D*-glucopyranuronosylthymidine (GZDV). GZDV area under the curve (AUC) is about 3-fold greater than the zidovudine AUC. Urinary recovery of zidovudine and GZDV accounts for 18% and 60%, respectively, following IV dosing. A second metabolite, 3′-amino-3′-deoxythymidine (AMT), has been identified in the plasma following single-dose IV administration of zidovudine. The AMT AUC was one fifth of the zidovudine AUC.

The mean steady-state peak and trough concentrations of zidovudine at 2.5 mg/kg every 4 hours were 1.06 and 0.12 mcg/mL, respectively.

The zidovudine cerebrospinal fluid (CSF)/plasma concentration ratio was determined in 39 patients receiving chronic therapy with RETROVIR. The median ratio measured in 50 paired samples drawn 1 to 8 hours after the last dose of RETROVIR was 0.6.

Table 1. Zidovudine Pharmacokinetic Parameters Following Intravenous Administration in HIV-Infected Patients

Parameter	Mean ± SD (except where noted)
Apparent volume of distribution (L/kg)	1.6 ± 0.6 (n = 11)
Plasma protein binding (%)	<38
CSF:plasma ratio*	0.6 [0.04 to 2.62] (n = 39)
Systemic clearance (L/hr/kg)	1.6 (0.8 to 2.7) (n = 18)
Renal clearance (L/hr/kg)	0.34 ± 0.05 (n = 16)
Elimination half-life (hr)†	1.1 (0.5 to 2.9) (n = 19)

*Median [range].
†Approximate range.

Adults with Impaired Renal Function: Zidovudine clearance was decreased resulting in increased zidovudine and GZDV half-life and AUC in patients with impaired renal function (n = 14) following a single 200-mg oral dose (Table 2). Plasma concentrations of AMT were not determined. A dose adjustment should not be necessary for patients with creatinine clearance (CrCl) ≥15 mL/min.

[See table 2 above]

The pharmacokinetics and tolerance of oral zidovudine were evaluated in a multiple-dose study in patients undergoing hemodialysis (n = 5) or peritoneal dialysis (n = 6) receiving escalating doses up to 200 mg 5 times daily for 8 weeks. Daily doses of 500 mg or less were well tolerated despite significantly elevated GZDV plasma concentrations. Apparent zidovudine oral clearance was approximately 50% of that reported in patients with normal renal function. Hemodialysis and peritoneal dialysis appeared to have a negligible effect on the removal of zidovudine, whereas GZDV elimination was enhanced. A dosage adjustment is recommended for patients undergoing hemodialysis or peritoneal dialysis (see DOSAGE AND ADMINISTRATION: Dose Adjustment).

Table 2. Zidovudine Pharmacokinetic Parameters in Patients With Severe Renal Impairment*

Parameter	Control Subjects (Normal Renal Function) (n = 6)	Patients With Renal Impairment (n = 14)
CrCl (mL/min)	120 ± 8	18 ± 2
Zidovudine AUC (ng•hr/mL)	1,400 ± 200	3,100 ± 300
Zidovudine half-life (hr)	1.0 ± 0.2	1.4 ± 0.1

*Data are expressed as mean ± standard deviation.

Table 3. Zidovudine Pharmacokinetic Parameters in Pediatric Patients*

Parameter	Birth to 14 Days of Age	14 Days to 3 Months of Age	3 Months to 12 Years of Age
Oral bioavailability (%)	89 ± 19 (n = 15)	61 ± 19 (n = 17)	65 ± 24 (n = 18)
CSF:plasma ratio	no data	no data	0.26 ± 0.17† (n = 28)
CL (L/hr/kg)	0.65 ± 0.29 (n = 18)	1.14 ± 0.24 (n = 16)	1.85 ± 0.47 (n = 20)
Elimination half-life (hr)	3.1 ± 1.2 (n = 21)	1.9 ± 0.7 (n = 18)	1.5 ± 0.7 (n = 21)

*Data presented as mean ± standard deviation except where noted.
†CSF ratio determined at steady-state on constant intravenous infusion.

Adults with Impaired Hepatic Function: Data describing the effect of hepatic impairment on the pharmacokinetics of zidovudine are limited. However, because zidovudine is eliminated primarily by hepatic metabolism, it is expected that zidovudine clearance would be decreased and plasma concentrations would be increased following administration of the recommended adult doses to patients with hepatic impairment (see DOSAGE AND ADMINISTRATION: Dose Adjustment).

Pediatrics: Zidovudine pharmacokinetics have been evaluated in HIV-infected pediatric patients (Table 3).

Patients from 3 Months to 12 Years of Age: Overall, zidovudine pharmacokinetics in pediatric patients >3 months of age are similar to those in adult patients. Proportional increases in plasma zidovudine concentrations were observed following administration of oral solution from 90 to 240 mg/m^2 every 6 hours. Oral bioavailability, terminal half-life, and oral clearance were comparable to adult values. As in adult patients, the major route of elimination was by metabolism to GZDV. After intravenous dosing, about 29% of the dose was excreted in the urine unchanged and about 45% of the dose was excreted as GZDV (see DOSAGE AND ADMINISTRATION: Pediatrics).

Patients Younger Than 3 Months of Age: Zidovudine pharmacokinetics have been evaluated in pediatric patients from birth to 3 months of life. Zidovudine elimination was determined immediately following birth in 8 neonates who were exposed to zidovudine in utero. The half-life was 13.0 ± 5.8 hours. In neonates ≤14 days old, bioavailability was greater, total body clearance was slower, and half-life was longer than in pediatric patients >14 days old. For dose recommendations for neonates, see DOSAGE AND ADMINISTRATION: Neonatal Dosing.

[See table 3 above]

Pregnancy: Zidovudine pharmacokinetics have been studied in a Phase 1 study of 8 women during the last trimester of pregnancy. As pregnancy progressed, there was no evidence of drug accumulation. Zidovudine pharmacokinetics were similar to that of nonpregnant adults. Consistent with passive transmission of the drug across the placenta, zidovudine concentrations in neonatal plasma at birth were essentially equal to those in maternal plasma at delivery. Although data are limited, methadone maintenance therapy in 5 pregnant women did not appear to alter zidovudine pharmacokinetics. However, in another patient population, a potential for interaction has been identified (see PRECAUTIONS).

Nursing Mothers: **The Centers for Disease Control and Prevention recommend that HIV-infected mothers not breastfeed their infants to avoid risking postnatal transmission of HIV.** After administration of a single dose of 200 mg zidovudine to 13 HIV-infected women, the mean concentration of zidovudine was similar in human milk and serum (see PRECAUTIONS: Nursing Mothers).

Geriatric Patients: Zidovudine pharmacokinetics have not been studied in patients over 65 years of age.

Gender: A pharmacokinetic study in healthy male (n = 12) and female (n = 12) subjects showed no differences in zidovudine exposure (AUC) when a single dose of zidovudine was administered as the 300-mg RETROVIR Tablet.

Drug Interactions: See Table 4 and PRECAUTIONS: Drug Interactions.

Zidovudine Plus Lamivudine: No clinically significant alterations in lamivudine or zidovudine pharmacokinetics were observed in 12 asymptomatic HIV-infected adult patients given a single oral dose of zidovudine (200 mg) in combination with multiple oral doses of lamivudine (300 mg every 12 hours).

[See table 4 at top of next page]

INDICATIONS AND USAGE

RETROVIR IV Infusion in combination with other antiretroviral agents is indicated for the treatment of HIV infection.

Maternal-Fetal HIV Transmission: RETROVIR is also indicated for the prevention of maternal-fetal HIV transmission as part of a regimen that includes oral RETROVIR beginning between 14 and 34 weeks of gestation, intravenous RETROVIR during labor, and administration of RETROVIR Syrup to the neonate after birth. The efficacy of this regimen for preventing HIV transmission in women who have received RETROVIR for a prolonged period before pregnancy has not been evaluated. The safety of RETROVIR for the mother or fetus during the first trimester of pregnancy has not been assessed (see Description of Clinical Studies).

Description of Clinical Studies: Therapy with RETROVIR has been shown to prolong survival and decrease the incidence of opportunistic infections in patients with advanced HIV disease at the initiation of therapy and to delay disease progression in asymptomatic HIV-infected patients. RETROVIR in combination with other antiretroviral agents has been shown to be superior to monotherapy in one or more of the following endpoints: delaying death, delaying development of AIDS, increasing CD4 cell counts, and decreasing plasma HIV-1 RNA. The complete prescribing information for each drug should be consulted before combination therapy that includes RETROVIR is initiated.

Pregnant Women and Their Neonates: The utility of RETROVIR for the prevention of maternal-fetal HIV transmission was demonstrated in a randomized, double-blind, placebo-controlled trial (ACTG 076) conducted in HIV-infected pregnant women with CD4 cell counts of 200 to 1,818 cells/mm^3 (median in the treated group: 560 cells/mm^3) who had little or no previous exposure to RETROVIR. Oral RETROVIR was initiated between 14 and 34 weeks of gestation (median 11 weeks of therapy) followed by intravenous administration of RETROVIR during labor and delivery. Following birth, neonates received oral RETROVIR Syrup for 6 weeks. The study showed a statistically significant difference in the incidence of HIV infection in the neonates (based on viral culture from peripheral blood) between the group receiving RETROVIR and the group receiving placebo. Of 363 neonates evaluated in the study, the estimated risk of HIV infection was 7.8% in the group receiving RETROVIR and 24.9% in the placebo group, a relative reduction in transmission risk of 68.7%. RETROVIR was well tolerated by mothers and infants. There was no difference in pregnancy-related adverse events between the treatment groups.

CONTRAINDICATIONS

RETROVIR IV Infusion is contraindicated for patients who have potentially life-threatening allergic reactions to any of the components of the formulation.

WARNINGS

COMBIVIR® and TRIZIVIR® are combination product tablets that contain zidovudine as one of their components. RETROVIR should not be administered concomitantly with COMBIVIR or TRIZIVIR.

The incidence of adverse reactions appears to increase with disease progression; patients should be monitored carefully, especially as disease progression occurs.

Continued on next page

Product information on these pages is effective as of August 2004. Further information is available at: GlaxoSmithKline, PO Box 13398, Research Triangle Park, NC 27709. 1-888-825-5249. Corporate Web Site: www.gsk.com

Retrovir Infusion—Cont.

Bone Marrow Suppression: RETROVIR should be used with caution in patients who have bone marrow compromise evidenced by granulocyte count <1,000 cells/mm^3 or hemoglobin <9.5 g/dL. In patients with advanced symptomatic HIV disease, anemia and neutropenia were the most significant adverse events observed. There have been reports of pancytopenia associated with the use of RETROVIR, which was reversible in most instances, after discontinuance of the drug. However, significant anemia, in many cases requiring dose adjustment, discontinuation of RETROVIR, and/or blood transfusions, has occurred during treatment with RETROVIR alone or in combination with other antiretrovirals.

Frequent blood counts are strongly recommended in patients with advanced HIV disease who are treated with RETROVIR. For HIV-infected individuals and patients with asymptomatic or early HIV disease, periodic blood counts are recommended. If anemia or neutropenia develops, dosage adjustments may be necessary (see DOSAGE AND ADMINISTRATION).

Myopathy: Myopathy and myositis with pathological changes, similar to that produced by HIV disease, have been associated with prolonged use of RETROVIR.

Lactic Acidosis/Severe Hepatomegaly with Steatosis: Lactic acidosis and severe hepatomegaly with steatosis, including fatal cases, have been reported with the use of nucleoside analogues alone or in combination, including zidovudine and other antiretrovirals. A majority of these cases have been in women. Obesity and prolonged exposure to antiretroviral nucleoside analogues may be risk factors. Particular caution should be exercised when administering RETROVIR to any patient with known risk factors for liver disease; however, cases have also been reported in patients with no known risk factors. Treatment with RETROVIR should be suspended in any patient who develops clinical or laboratory findings suggestive of lactic acidosis or pronounced hepatotoxicity (which may include hepatomegaly and steatosis even in the absence of marked transaminase elevations).

PRECAUTIONS

General: Zidovudine is eliminated from the body primarily by renal excretion following metabolism in the liver (glucuronidation). In patients with severely impaired renal function (CrCl<15 mL/min), dosage reduction is recommended. Although the data are limited, zidovudine concentrations appear to be increased in patients with severely impaired hepatic function, which may increase the risk of hematologic toxicity (see CLINICAL PHARMACOLOGY: Pharmacokinetics and DOSAGE AND ADMINISTRATION).

Information for Patients: RETROVIR is not a cure for HIV infection, and patients may continue to acquire illnesses associated with HIV infection, including opportunistic infections. Therefore, patients should be advised to seek medical care for any significant change in their health status.

The safety and efficacy of RETROVIR in treating women, intravenous drug users, and racial minorities is not significantly different than that observed in white males.

Patients should be informed that the major toxicities of RETROVIR are neutropenia and/or anemia. The frequency and severity of these toxicities are greater in patients with more advanced disease and in those who initiate therapy later in the course of their infection. They should be told that if toxicity develops, they may require transfusions or drug discontinuation. They should be told of the extreme importance of having their blood counts followed closely while on therapy, especially for patients with advanced symptomatic HIV disease. They should be cautioned about the use of other medications, including ganciclovir and interferon-alpha, which may exacerbate the toxicity of RETROVIR (see PRECAUTIONS: Drug Interactions). Patients should be informed that other adverse effects of RETROVIR include nausea and vomiting. Patients should also be encouraged to contact their physician if they experience muscle weakness, shortness of breath, symptoms of hepatitis or pancreatitis, or any other unexpected adverse events while being treated with RETROVIR.

Pregnant women considering the use of RETROVIR during pregnancy for prevention of HIV transmission to their infants should be advised that transmission may still occur in some cases despite therapy. The long-term consequences of in utero and neonatal exposure to RETROVIR are unknown, including the possible risk of cancer.

HIV-infected pregnant women should be advised not to breastfeed to avoid postnatal transmission of HIV to a child who may not yet be infected.

Patients should be advised that therapy with RETROVIR has not been shown to reduce the risk of transmission of HIV to others through sexual contact or blood contamination.

Drug Interactions: See CLINICAL PHARMACOLOGY section (Table 4) for information on zidovudine concentrations when coadministered with other drugs. For patients experiencing pronounced anemia or other severe zidovudine-associated events while receiving chronic administration of zidovudine and some of the drugs (e.g., fluconazole, valproic acid) listed in Table 4, zidovudine dose reduction may be considered.

Antiretroviral Agents: Concomitant use of zidovudine with stavudine should be avoided since an antagonistic relationship has been demonstrated in vitro.

Table 4. Effect of Coadministered Drugs on Zidovudine AUC*

Note: ROUTINE DOSE MODIFICATION OF ZIDOVUDINE IS NOT WARRANTED WITH COADMINISTRATION OF THE FOLLOWING DRUGS.

Coadministered Drug and Dose	Zidovudine Oral Dose	n	Zidovudine Concentrations AUC	Zidovudine Concentrations Variability	Concentration of Coadministered Drug
Atovaquone 750 mg q 12 hr with food	200 mg q 8 hr	14	↑AUC 31%	Range 23% to 78%†	↔
Fluconazole 400 mg daily	200 mg q 8 hr	12	↑AUC 74%	95% CI: 54% to 98%	Not Reported
Methadone 30 to 90 mg daily	200 mg q 4 hr	9	↑AUC 43%	Range 16% to 64%†	↔
Nelfinavir 750 mg q 8 hr × 7 to 10 days	single 200 mg	11	↓AUC 35%	Range 28% to 41%	↔
Probenecid 500 mg q 6 hr × 2 days	2 mg/kg q 8 hr × 3 days	3	↑AUC 106%	Range 100% to 170%†	Not Assessed
Rifampin 600 mg daily × 14 days	200 mg q 8 hr × 14 days	8	↓AUC 47%	90% CI: 41% to 53%†	Not Assessed
Ritonavir 300 mg q 6 hr × 4 days	200 mg q 8 hr × 4 days	9	↓AUC 25%	95% CI: 15% to 34%	↔
Valproic acid 250 mg or 500 mg q 8 hr × 4 days	100 mg q 8 hr × 4 days	6	↑AUC 80%	Range 64% to 130%†	Not Assessed

↑ = Increase; ↓ = Decrease; ↔ = no significant change; AUC = area under the concentration versus time curve; CI = confidence interval.
*This table is not all inclusive.
†Estimated range of percent difference.

Some nucleoside analogues affecting DNA replication, such as ribavirin, antagonize the in vitro antiviral activity of RETROVIR against HIV; concomitant use of such drugs should be avoided.

Doxorubicin: Concomitant use of zidovudine with doxorubicin should be avoided since an antagonistic relationship has been demonstrated in vitro (see CLINICAL PHARMACOLOGY for additional drug interactions).

Phenytoin: Phenytoin plasma levels have been reported to be low in some patients receiving RETROVIR, while in 1 case a high level was documented. However, in a pharmacokinetic interaction study in which 12 HIV-positive volunteers received a single 300-mg phenytoin dose alone and during steady-state zidovudine conditions (200 mg every 4 hours), no change in phenytoin kinetics was observed. Although not designed to optimally assess the effect of phenytoin on zidovudine kinetics, a 30% decrease in oral zidovudine clearance was observed with phenytoin.

Overlapping Toxicities: Coadministration of ganciclovir, interferon-alpha, and other bone marrow suppressive or cytotoxic agents may increase the hematologic toxicity of zidovudine.

Carcinogenesis, Mutagenesis, Impairment of Fertility: Zidovudine was administered orally at 3 dosage levels to separate groups of mice and rats (60 females and 60 males in each group). Initial single daily doses were 30, 60, and 120 mg/kg/day in mice and 80, 220, and 600 mg/kg/day in rats. The doses in mice were reduced to 20, 30, and 40 mg/kg/day after day 90 because of treatment-related anemia, whereas in rats only the high dose was reduced to 450 mg/kg/day on day 91, and then to 300 mg/kg/day on day 279.

In mice, 7 late-appearing (after 19 months) vaginal neoplasms (5 nonmetastasizing squamous cell carcinomas, 1 squamous cell papilloma, and 1 squamous polyp) occurred in animals given the highest dose. One late-appearing squamous cell papilloma occurred in the vagina of a middle-dose animal. No vaginal tumors were found at the lowest dose.

In rats, 2 late-appearing (after 20 months), nonmetastasizing vaginal squamous cell carcinomas occurred in animals given the highest dose. No vaginal tumors occurred at the low or middle dose in rats. No other drug-related tumors were observed in either sex of either species.

At doses that produced tumors in mice and rats, the estimated drug exposure (as measured by AUC) was approximately 3 times (mouse) and 24 times (rat) the estimated human exposure at the recommended therapeutic dose of 100 mg every 4 hours.

Two transplacental carcinogenicity studies were conducted in mice. One study administered zidovudine at doses of 20 mg/kg/day or 40 mg/kg/day from gestation day 10 through parturition and lactation with dosing continuing in offspring for 24 months postnatally. The doses of zidovudine employed in this study produced zidovudine exposures approximately 3 times the estimated human exposure at recommended doses. After 24 months, an increase in incidence of vaginal tumors was noted with no increase in tumors in the liver or lung or any other organ in either gender. These findings are consistent with results of the standard oral carcinogenicity study in mice, as described earlier. A second study administered zidovudine at maximum tolerated doses of 12.5 mg/day or 25 mg/day (~1,000 mg/kg nonpregnant body weight or ~450 mg/kg of term body weight) to pregnant mice from days 12 through 18 of gestation. There was an increase in the number of tumors in the lung, liver, and female reproductive tracts in the offspring of mice receiving the higher dose level of zidovudine. It is not known how predictive the results of rodent carcinogenicity studies may be for humans.

Zidovudine was mutagenic in a 5178Y/TK$^{+/-}$ mouse lymphoma assay, positive in an in vitro cell transformation assay, clastogenic in a cytogenetic assay using cultured human lymphocytes, and positive in mouse and rat micronucleus tests after repeated doses. It was negative in a cytogenetic study in rats given a single dose.

Zidovudine, administered to male and female rats at doses up to 7 times the usual adult dose based on body surface area considerations, had no effect on fertility judged by conception rates.

Pregnancy: Pregnancy Category C. Oral teratology studies in the rat and in the rabbit at doses up to 500 mg/kg/day revealed no evidence of teratogenicity with zidovudine. Zidovudine treatment resulted in embryo/fetal toxicity as evidenced by an increase in the incidence of fetal resorptions in rats given 150 or 450 mg/kg/day and rabbits given 500 mg/kg/day. The doses used in the teratology studies resulted in peak zidovudine plasma concentrations (after one half of the daily dose) in rats 66 to 226 times, and in rabbits 12 to 87 times, mean steady-state peak human plasma concentrations (after one sixth of the daily dose) achieved with the recommended daily dose (100 mg every 4 hours). In an in vitro experiment with fertilized mouse oocytes, zidovudine exposure resulted in a dose-dependent reduction in blastocyst formation. In an additional teratology study in rats, a dose of 3,000 mg/kg/day (very near the oral median lethal dose in rats of 3,683 mg/kg) caused marked maternal toxicity and an increase in the incidence of fetal malformations. This dose resulted in peak zidovudine plasma concentrations 350 times peak human plasma concentrations. (Estimated area-under-the-curve [AUC] in rats at this dose level was 300 times the daily AUC in humans given 600 mg per day.) No evidence of teratogenicity was seen in this experiment at doses of 600 mg/kg/day or less.

Two rodent transplacental carcinogenicity studies were conducted (see Carcinogenesis, Mutagenesis, Impairment of Fertility).

A randomized, double-blind, placebo-controlled trial was conducted in HIV-infected pregnant women to determine the utility of RETROVIR for the prevention of maternal-fetal HIV transmission (see INDICATIONS AND USAGE: Description of Clinical Studies). Congenital abnormalities occurred with similar frequency between neonates born to mothers who received RETROVIR and neonates born to mothers who received placebo. Abnormalities were either problems in embryogenesis (prior to 14 weeks) or were recognized on ultrasound before or immediately after initiation of study drug.

Antiretroviral Pregnancy Registry: To monitor maternal-fetal outcomes of pregnant women exposed to RETROVIR, an Antiretroviral Pregnancy Registry has been established. Physicians are encouraged to register patients by calling 1-800-258-4263.

Nursing Mothers: The Centers for Disease Control and Prevention recommend that HIV-infected mothers not breastfeed their infants to avoid risking postnatal transmission of HIV.

Zidovudine is excreted in human milk (see CLINICAL PHARMACOLOGY: Pharmacokinetics: Nursing Mothers). Because of both the potential for HIV transmission and the potential for serious adverse reactions in nursing infants, **mothers should be instructed not to breastfeed if they are receiving RETROVIR** (see Pediatric Use and INDICATIONS AND USAGE: Maternal-Fetal HIV Transmission).

Pediatric Use: RETROVIR has been studied in HIV-infected pediatric patients over 3 months of age who had HIV-related symptoms or who were asymptomatic with abnormal laboratory values indicating significant HIV-related immunosuppression. RETROVIR has also been studied in neonates perinatally exposed to HIV (see ADVERSE REACTIONS, DOSAGE AND ADMINISTRATION, INDICATIONS AND USAGE: Description of Clinical Studies, and CLINICAL PHARMACOLOGY: Pharmacokinetics).

Geriatric Use: Clinical studies of RETROVIR did not include sufficient numbers of subjects aged 65 and over to determine whether they respond differently from younger subjects. Other reported clinical experience has not identified differences in responses between the elderly and younger patients. In general, dose selection for an elderly patient should be cautious, reflecting the greater frequency of decreased hepatic, renal, or cardiac function, and of concomitant disease or other drug therapy.

ADVERSE REACTIONS

The adverse events reported during intravenous administration of RETROVIR IV Infusion are similar to those reported with oral administration; neutropenia and anemia were reported most frequently. Long-term intravenous administration beyond 2 to 4 weeks has not been studied in adults and may enhance hematologic adverse events. Local reaction, pain, and slight irritation during intravenous administration occur infrequently.

Adults: The frequency and severity of adverse events associated with the use of RETROVIR are greater in patients with more advanced infection at the time of initiation of therapy.

Table 5 summarizes events reported at a statistically significantly greater incidence for patients receiving RETROVIR orally in a monotherapy study:

Table 5. Percentage (%) of Patients with Adverse Events* in Asymptomatic HIV Infection (ACTG 019)

Adverse Event	RETROVIR 500 mg/day (n = 453)	Placebo (n = 428)
Body as a Whole		
Asthenia	8.6%	5.8%
Headache	62.5%	52.6%
Malaise	53.2%	44.9%
Gastrointestinal		
Anorexia	20.1%	10.5%
Constipation	6.4%†	3.5%
Nausea	51.4%	29.9%
Vomiting	17.2%	9.8%

*Reported in ≥5% of study population.
†Not statistically significant versus placebo.

In addition to the adverse events listed in Table 5, other adverse events observed in clinical studies were abdominal cramps, abdominal pain, arthralgia, chills, dyspepsia, fatigue, hyperbilirubinemia, insomnia, musculoskeletal pain, myalgia, and neuropathy.

Selected laboratory abnormalities observed during a clinical study of monotherapy with oral RETROVIR are shown in Table 6.

Table 6. Frequencies of Selected (Grade 3/4) Laboratory Abnormalities in Patients with Asymptomatic HIV Infection (ACTG 019)

Adverse Event	RETROVIR 500 mg/day (n = 453)	Placebo (n = 428)
Anemia (Hgb<8 g/dL)	1.1%	0.2%
Granulocytopenia (<750 cells/mm^3)	1.8%	1.6%
Thrombocytopenia (platelets<50,000/mm^3)	0%	0.5%
ALT (>5 × ULN)	3.1%	2.6%
AST (>5 × ULN)	0.9%	1.6%
Alkaline phosphatase (>5 × ULN)	0%	0%

ULN = Upper limit of normal.

Pediatrics: ***Study ACTG300:*** Selected clinical adverse events and physical findings with a ≥5% frequency during therapy with EPIVIR 4 mg/kg twice daily plus RETROVIR 160 mg/m^2 orally 3 times daily compared with didanosine in therapy-naive (≤56 days of antiretroviral therapy) pediatric patients are listed in Table 7.

Table 7. Selected Clinical Adverse Events and Physical Findings (≥5% Frequency) in Pediatric Patients in Study ACTG300

Adverse Event	EPIVIR plus RETROVIR (n = 236)	Didanosine (n = 235)
Body as a Whole		
Fever	25%	32%
Digestive		
Hepatomegaly	11%	11%
Nausea & vomiting	8%	7%
Diarrhea	8%	6%
Stomatitis	6%	12%
Splenomegaly	5%	8%
Respiratory		
Cough	15%	18%
Abnormal breath sounds/ wheezing	7%	9%
Ear, Nose and Throat		
Signs or symptoms of ears*	7%	6%
Nasal discharge or congestion	8%	11%
Other		
Skin rashes	12%	14%
Lymphadenopathy	9%	11%

*Includes pain, discharge, erythema, or swelling of an ear.

Selected laboratory abnormalities experienced by therapy-naive (≤56 days of antiretroviral therapy) pediatric patients are listed in Table 8.

Table 8. Frequencies of Selected (Grade 3/4) Laboratory Abnormalities in Pediatric Patients in Study ACTG300

Test (Abnormal Level)	EPIVIR plus RETROVIR	Didanosine
Neutropenia (ANC<400 cells/mm^3)	8%	3%
Anemia (Hgb<7.0 g/dL)	4%	2%
Thrombocytopenia (platelets<50,000/mm^3)	1%	3%
ALT (>10 × ULN)	1%	3%
AST (>10 × ULN)	2%	4%
Lipase (>2.5 ×ULN)	3%	3%
Total amylase (>2.5 × ULN)	3%	3%

ULN = Upper limit of normal.
ANC = Absolute neutrophil count.

Additional adverse events reported in open-label studies in pediatric patients receiving RETROVIR 180 mg/m^2 every 6 hours were congestive heart failure, decreased reflexes, ECG abnormality, edema, hematuria, left ventricular dilation, macrocytosis, nervousness/irritability, and weight loss. The clinical adverse events reported among adult recipients of RETROVIR may also occur in pediatric patients.

Use for the Prevention of Maternal-Fetal Transmission of HIV: In a randomized, double-blind, placebo-controlled trial in HIV-infected women and their neonates conducted to determine the utility of RETROVIR for the prevention of maternal-fetal HIV transmission, RETROVIR Syrup at 2 mg/kg was administered every 6 hours for 6 weeks to neonates beginning within 12 hours following birth. The most commonly reported adverse experiences were anemia (hemoglobin <9.0 g/dL) and neutropenia (<1,000 cells/mm^3). Anemia occurred in 22% of the neonates who received RETROVIR and in 12% of the neonates who received placebo. The mean difference in hemoglobin values was less than 1.0 g/dL for neonates receiving RETROVIR compared to neonates receiving placebo. No neonates with anemia required transfusion and all hemoglobin values spontaneously returned to normal within 6 weeks after completion of therapy with RETROVIR. Neutropenia was reported with similar frequency in the group that received RETROVIR (21%) and in the group that received placebo (27%). The long-term consequences of in utero and infant exposure to RETROVIR are unknown.

Observed During Clinical Practice: In addition to adverse events reported from clinical trials, the following events have been identified during use of RETROVIR in clinical practice. Because they are reported voluntarily from a population of unknown size, estimates of frequency cannot be made. These events have been chosen for inclusion due to either their seriousness, frequency of reporting, potential causal connection to RETROVIR, or a combination of these factors.

Body as a Whole: Back pain, chest pain, flu-like syndrome, generalized pain.

Cardiovascular: Cardiomyopathy, syncope.

Endocrine: Gynecomastia.

Eye: Macular edema.

Gastrointestinal: Constipation, dysphagia, flatulence, oral mucosal pigmentation, mouth ulcer.

General: Sensitization reactions including anaphylaxis and angioedema, vasculitis.

Hemic and Lymphatic: Aplastic anemia, hemolytic anemia, leukopenia, lymphadenopathy, pancytopenia with marrow hypoplasia, pure red cell aplasia.

Hepatobiliary Tract and Pancreas: Hepatitis, hepatomegaly with steatosis, jaundice, lactic acidosis, pancreatitis.

Musculoskeletal: Increased CPK, increased LDH, muscle spasm, myopathy and myositis with pathological changes (similar to that produced by HIV disease), rhabdomyolysis, tremor.

Nervous: Anxiety, confusion, depression, dizziness, loss of mental acuity, mania, paresthesia, seizures, somnolence, vertigo.

Respiratory: Cough, dyspnea, rhinitis, sinusitis.

Skin: Changes in skin and nail pigmentation, pruritus, rash, Stevens-Johnson syndrome, toxic epidermal necrolysis, sweat, urticaria.

Special Senses: Amblyopia, hearing loss, photophobia, taste perversion.

Urogenital: Urinary frequency, urinary hesitancy.

OVERDOSAGE

Acute overdoses of zidovudine have been reported in pediatric patients and adults. These involved exposures up to 50 grams. No specific symptoms or signs have been identified following acute overdosage with zidovudine apart from those listed as adverse events such as fatigue, headache, vomiting, and occasional reports of hematological disturbances. All patients recovered without permanent sequelae. Hemodialysis and peritoneal dialysis appear to have a negligible effect on the removal of zidovudine, while elimination of its primary metabolite, GZDV, is enhanced.

DOSAGE AND ADMINISTRATION

Adults: The recommended intravenous dose is 1 mg/kg infused over 1 hour. This dose should be administered 5 to 6 times daily (5 to 6 mg/kg daily). The effectiveness of this dose compared to higher dosing regimens in improving the neurologic dysfunction associated with HIV disease is unknown. A small randomized study found a greater effect of higher doses of RETROVIR on improvement of neurological symptoms in patients with pre-existing neurological disease.

Patients should receive RETROVIR IV Infusion only until oral therapy can be administered. The intravenous dosing regimen equivalent to the oral administration of 100 mg every 4 hours is approximately 1 mg/kg intravenously every 4 hours.

Maternal-Fetal HIV Transmission: The recommended dosing regimen for administration to pregnant women (>14 weeks of pregnancy) and their neonates is:

Maternal Dosing: 100 mg orally 5 times per day until the start of labor. During labor and delivery, intravenous RETROVIR should be administered at 2 mg/kg (total body weight) over 1 hour followed by a continuous intravenous infusion of 1 mg/kg/hour (total body weight) until clamping of the umbilical cord.

Neonatal Dosing: 2 mg/kg orally every 6 hours starting within 12 hours after birth and continuing through 6 weeks of age. Neonates unable to receive oral dosing may be administered RETROVIR intravenously at 1.5 mg/kg, infused over 30 minutes, every 6 hours. (See PRECAUTIONS if hepatic disease or renal insufficiency is present.)

Monitoring of Patients: Hematologic toxicities appear to be related to pretreatment bone marrow reserve and to dose and duration of therapy. In patients with poor bone marrow reserve, particularly in patients with advanced symptomatic HIV disease, frequent monitoring of hematologic indices is recommended to detect serious anemia or neutropenia (see WARNINGS). In patients who experience hematologic toxicity, reduction in hemoglobin may occur as early as 2 to 4 weeks, and neutropenia usually occurs after 6 to 8 weeks.

Dose Adjustment: ***Anemia:*** Significant anemia (hemoglobin of <7.5 g/dL or reduction of >25% of baseline) and/or significant neutropenia (granulocyte count of <750 cells/mm^3 or reduction of >50% from baseline) may require a dose interruption until evidence of marrow recovery is observed (see WARNINGS). In patients who develop significant anemia, dose interruption does not necessarily eliminate the need for transfusion. If marrow recovery occurs following dose interruption, resumption in dose may be appropriate using adjunctive measures such as epoetin alfa at recommended doses, depending on hematologic indices such as serum erythropoetin level and patient tolerance.

For patients experiencing pronounced anemia while receiving chronic coadministration of zidovudine and some of the drugs (e.g., fluconazole, valproic acid) listed in Table 4, zidovudine dose reduction may be considered.

End-Stage Renal Disease: In patients maintained on hemodialysis or peritoneal dialysis (CrCl <15 mL/min), recommended dosing is 1 mg/kg every 6 to 8 hours (see CLINICAL PHARMACOLOGY: Pharmacokinetics).

Hepatic Impairment: There are insufficient data to recommend dose adjustment of RETROVIR in patients with mild to moderate impaired hepatic function or liver cirrhosis. Since RETROVIR is primarily eliminated by hepatic metabolism, a reduction in the daily dose may be necessary in these patients. Frequent monitoring of hematologic toxicities is advised (see CLINICAL PHARMACOLOGY: Pharmacokinetics and PRECAUTIONS: General).

Method of Preparation: RETROVIR IV Infusion must be diluted prior to administration. The calculated dose should be removed from the 20-mL vial and added to 5% Dextrose Injection solution to achieve a concentration no greater than 4 mg/mL. Admixture in biologic or colloidal fluids (e.g., blood products, protein solutions, etc.) is not recommended.

After dilution, the solution is physically and chemically stable for 24 hours at room temperature and 48 hours if refrigerated at 2° to 8°C (36° to 46°F). Care should be taken during admixture to prevent inadvertent contamination. As an additional precaution, the diluted solution should be admin-

Continued on next page

Product information on these pages is effective as of August 2004. Further information is available at: GlaxoSmithKline, PO Box 13398, Research Triangle Park, NC 27709. 1-888-825-5249. Corporate Web Site: www.gsk.com

Retrovir Infusion—Cont.

istered within 8 hours if stored at 25°C (77°F) or 24 hours if refrigerated at 2° to 8°C to minimize potential administration of a microbially contaminated solution.

Parenteral drug products should be inspected visually for particulate matter and discoloration prior to administration whenever solution and container permit. Should either be observed, the solution should be discarded and fresh solution prepared.

Administration: RETROVIR IV Infusion is administered intravenously at a constant rate over 1 hour. Rapid infusion or bolus injection should be avoided. RETROVIR IV Infusion should not be given intramuscularly.

HOW SUPPLIED

RETROVIR IV Infusion, 10 mg zidovudine in each mL.
20-mL Single-Use Vial, Tray of 10 (NDC 0173-0107-93).
Store vials at 15° to 25°C (59° to 77°F) and protect from light.
GlaxoSmithKline, Research Triangle Park, NC 27709

August 2003/RL-2029
Shown in Product Identification Guide, page 317

SEREVENT® DISKUS® ℞

[*sĕr' ə-vent dĭsk' us*]
(salmeterol xinafoate inhalation powder)
FOR ORAL INHALATION ONLY

WARNING: Data from a large placebo-controlled US study that compared the safety of salmeterol (SEREVENT® Inhalation Aerosol) or placebo added to usual asthma therapy showed a small but significant increase in asthma-related deaths in patients receiving salmeterol (13 deaths out of 13,174 patients treated for 28 weeks) versus those on placebo (4 of 13,179). Subgroup analyses suggest the risk may be greater in African-American patients compared to Caucasians (see WARNINGS and CLINICAL TRIALS: Asthma: *Salmeterol Multi-center Asthma Research Trial*).

DESCRIPTION

SEREVENT DISKUS (salmeterol xinafoate inhalation powder) contains salmeterol xinafoate as the racemic form of the 1-hydroxy-2-naphthoic acid salt of salmeterol. The active component of the formulation is salmeterol base, a highly selective beta$_2$-adrenergic bronchodilator. The chemical name of salmeterol xinafoate is 4-hydroxy-α^1-[[[6-(4-phenylbutoxy)hexyl]amino]methyl]-1,3-benzenedimethanol, 1-hydroxy-2-naphthalenecarboxylate.

Salmeterol xinafoate is a white to off-white powder with a molecular weight of 603.8, and the empirical formula is $C_{25}H_{37}NO_4 \cdot C_{11}H_8O_3$. It is freely soluble in methanol; slightly soluble in ethanol, chloroform, and isopropanol; and sparingly soluble in water.

SEREVENT DISKUS is a specially designed plastic inhalation delivery system containing a double-foil blister strip of a powder formulation of salmeterol xinafoate intended for oral inhalation only. The DISKUS®, which is the delivery component, is an integral part of the drug product. Each blister on the double-foil strip within the unit contains 50 mcg of salmeterol administered as the salmeterol xinafoate salt in 12.5 mg of formulation containing lactose (which contains milk proteins). After a blister containing medication is opened by activating the DISKUS, the medication is dispersed into the airstream created by the patient inhaling through the mouthpiece.

Under standardized in vitro test conditions, SEREVENT DISKUS delivers 47 mcg when tested at a flow rate of 60 L/min for 2 seconds. In adult patients with obstructive lung disease and severely compromised lung function (mean forced expiratory volume in 1 second [FEV$_1$] 20% to 30% of predicted), mean peak inspiratory flow (PIF) through a DISKUS was 82.4 L/min (range, 46.1 to 115.3 L/min).

The actual amount of drug delivered to the lung will depend on patient factors, such as inspiratory flow profile.

CLINICAL PHARMACOLOGY

Mechanism of Action: Salmeterol is a selective, long-acting beta$_2$-adrenergic agonist. In vitro studies and in vivo pharmacologic studies demonstrate that salmeterol is selective for beta$_2$-adrenoceptors compared with isoproterenol, which has approximately equal agonist activity on beta$_1$- and beta$_2$-adrenoceptors. In vitro studies show salmeterol to be at least 50 times more selective for beta$_2$-adrenoceptors than albuterol. Although beta$_2$-adrenoceptors are the predominant adrenergic receptors in bronchial smooth muscle and beta$_1$-adrenoceptors are the predominant receptors in the heart, there are also beta$_2$-adrenoceptors in the human heart comprising 10% to 50% of the total beta-adrenoceptors. The precise function of these receptors has not been established, but they raise the possibility that even highly selective beta$_2$-agonists may have cardiac effects.

The pharmacologic effects of beta$_2$-adrenoceptor agonist drugs, including salmeterol, are at least in part attributable to stimulation of intracellular adenyl cyclase, the enzyme that catalyzes the conversion of adenosine triphosphate (ATP) to cyclic-3',5'-adenosine monophosphate (cyclic AMP). Increased cyclic AMP levels cause relaxation of bronchial smooth muscle and inhibition of release of mediators of immediate hypersensitivity from cells, especially from mast cells.

In vitro tests show that salmeterol is a potent and long-lasting inhibitor of the release of mast cell mediators, such as histamine, leukotrienes, and prostaglandin D$_2$, from human lung. Salmeterol inhibits histamine-induced plasma protein extravasation and inhibits platelet-activating factor-induced eosinophil accumulation in the lungs of guinea pigs when administered by the inhaled route. In humans, single doses of salmeterol administered via inhalation aerosol attenuate allergen-induced bronchial hyperresponsiveness.

Pharmacokinetics: Salmeterol xinafoate, an ionic salt, dissociates in solution so that the salmeterol and 1-hydroxy-2-naphthoic acid (xinafoate) moieties are absorbed, distributed, metabolized, and excreted independently. Salmeterol acts locally in the lung; therefore, plasma levels do not predict therapeutic effect.

***Absorption*:** Because of the small therapeutic dose, systemic levels of salmeterol are low or undetectable after inhalation of recommended doses (50 mcg of salmeterol inhalation powder twice daily). Following chronic administration of an inhaled dose of 50 mcg of salmeterol inhalation powder twice daily, salmeterol was detected in plasma within 5 to 45 minutes in 7 patients with asthma; plasma concentrations were very low, with mean peak concentrations of 167 pg/mL at 20 minutes and no accumulation with repeated doses.

***Distribution*:** The percentage of salmeterol bound to human plasma proteins averages 96% in vitro over the concentration range of 8 to 7,722 ng of salmeterol base per milliliter, much higher concentrations than those achieved following therapeutic doses of salmeterol.

***Metabolism*:** Salmeterol base is extensively metabolized by hydroxylation, with subsequent elimination predominantly in the feces. No significant amount of unchanged salmeterol base has been detected in either urine or feces.

***Elimination*:** In 2 healthy subjects who received 1 mg of radiolabeled salmeterol (as salmeterol xinafoate) orally, approximately 25% and 60% of the radiolabeled salmeterol was eliminated in urine and feces, respectively, over a period of 7 days. The terminal elimination half-life was about 5.5 hours (1 volunteer only).

The xinafoate moiety has no apparent pharmacologic activity. The xinafoate moiety is highly protein bound (>99%) and has a long elimination half-life of 11 days.

***Special Populations*:** The pharmacokinetics of salmeterol base has not been studied in elderly patients nor in patients with hepatic or renal impairment. Since salmeterol is predominantly cleared by hepatic metabolism, liver function impairment may lead to accumulation of salmeterol in plasma. Therefore, patients with hepatic disease should be closely monitored.

Pharmacodynamics: Inhaled salmeterol, like other beta-adrenergic agonist drugs, can in some patients produce dose-related cardiovascular effects and effects on blood glucose and/or serum potassium (see PRECAUTIONS). The cardiovascular effects (heart rate, blood pressure) associated with salmeterol inhalation aerosol occur with similar frequency, and are of similar type and severity, as those noted following albuterol administration.

The effects of rising doses of salmeterol and standard inhaled doses of albuterol were studied in volunteers and in patients with asthma. Salmeterol doses up to 84 mcg administered as inhalation aerosol resulted in heart rate increases of 3 to 16 beats/min, about the same as albuterol dosed at 180 mcg by inhalation aerosol (4 to 10 beats/min). Adolescent and adult patients receiving 50-mcg doses of salmeterol inhalation powder (N = 60) underwent continuous electrocardiographic monitoring during two 12-hour periods after the first dose and after 1 month of therapy, and no clinically significant dysrhythmias were noted. Also, pediatric patients receiving 50-mcg doses of salmeterol inhalation powder (N = 67) underwent continuous electrocardiographic monitoring during two 12-hour periods after the first dose and after 3 months of therapy, and no clinically significant dysrhythmias were noted.

In 24-week clinical studies in patients with chronic obstructive pulmonary disease (COPD), the incidence of clinically significant abnormalities on the predose electrocardiograms (ECGs) at Weeks 12 and 24 in patients who received salmeterol 50 mcg was not different compared with placebo.

No effect of treatment with salmeterol 50 mcg was observed on pulse rate and systolic and diastolic blood pressure in a subset of patients with COPD who underwent 12-hour serial vital sign measurements after the first dose (N = 91) and after 12 weeks of therapy (N = 74). Median changes from baseline in pulse rate and systolic and diastolic blood pressure were similar for patients receiving either salmeterol or placebo (see ADVERSE REACTIONS).

Studies in laboratory animals (minipigs, rodents, and dogs) have demonstrated the occurrence of cardiac arrhythmias and sudden death (with histologic evidence of myocardial necrosis) when beta-agonists and methylxanthines are administered concurrently. The clinical significance of these findings is unknown.

CLINICAL TRIALS

Asthma: During the initial treatment day in several multiple-dose clinical trials with SEREVENT DISKUS in patients with asthma, the median time to onset of clinically significant bronchodilatation (≥15% improvement in FEV$_1$) ranged from 30 to 48 minutes after a 50-mcg dose.

One hour after a single dose of 50 mcg of SEREVENT DISKUS, the majority of patients had ≥15% improvement in FEV$_1$. Maximum improvement in FEV$_1$ generally occurred within 180 minutes, and clinically significant improvement continued for 12 hours in most patients.

In 2 randomized, double-blind studies, SEREVENT DISKUS was compared with albuterol inhalation aerosol and placebo in adolescent and adult patients with mild-to-moderate asthma (protocol defined as 50% to 80% predicted FEV$_1$, actual mean of 67.7% at baseline), including patients who did and who did not receive concurrent inhaled corticosteroids. The efficacy of SEREVENT DISKUS was demonstrated over the 12-week period with no change in effectiveness over this time period (see Figure 1). There were no gender- or age-related differences in safety or efficacy. No development of tachyphylaxis to the bronchodilator effect was noted in these studies. FEV$_1$ measurements (mean change from baseline) from these two 12-week studies are shown in Figure 1 for both the first and last treatment days.

Figure 1. Serial 12-Hour FEV$_1$ From Two 12-Week Clinical Trials in Patients With Asthma

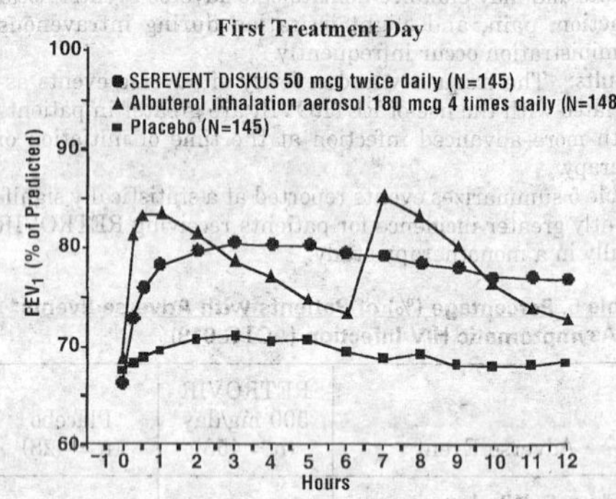

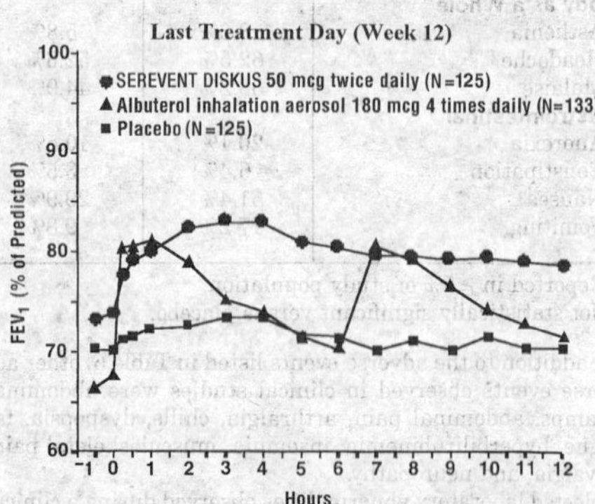

Table 1 shows the treatment effects seen during daily treatment with SEREVENT DISKUS for 12 weeks in adolescent and adult patients with mild-to-moderate asthma.

[See table 1 at top of next page]

Safe usage with maintenance of efficacy for periods up to 1 year has been documented.

SEREVENT DISKUS and SEREVENT® (salmeterol xinafoate) Inhalation Aerosol were compared to placebo in 2 additional randomized, double-blind clinical trials in adolescent and adult patients with mild-to-moderate asthma. SEREVENT DISKUS 50 mcg and SEREVENT Inhalation Aerosol 42 mcg, both administered twice daily, produced significant improvements in pulmonary function compared with placebo over the 12-week period. While no statistically significant differences were observed between the active treatments for any of the efficacy assessments or safety evaluations performed, there were some efficacy measures on which the metered-dose inhaler appeared to provide better results. Similar findings were noted in 2 randomized, single-dose, crossover comparisons of SEREVENT DISKUS and SEREVENT Inhalation Aerosol for the prevention of exercise-induced bronchospasm (EIB). Therefore, while SEREVENT DISKUS was comparable to SEREVENT Inhalation Aerosol in clinical trials in mild-to-moderate patients with asthma, it should not be assumed that they will produce clinically equivalent outcomes in all patients.

In a randomized, double-blind, controlled study (N = 449), 50 mcg of SEREVENT DISKUS was administered twice daily to pediatric patients with asthma who did and who did not receive concurrent inhaled corticosteroids. The efficacy of salmeterol inhalation powder was demonstrated over the 12-week treatment period with respect to periodic serial peak expiratory flow (PEF) (36% to 39% postdose increase from baseline) and FEV$_1$ (32% to 33% postdose increase from baseline). Salmeterol was effective in demographic subgroup analyses (gender and age) and was effective when coadministered with other inhaled asthma medications such as short-acting bronchodilators and inhaled corticosteroids. A second randomized, double-blind, placebo-controlled study (N = 207) with 50 mcg of salmeterol inhalation powder via an alternate device supported the findings of the trial with the DISKUS.

Effects in Patients With Asthma on Concomitant Inhaled Corticosteroids: In 4 clinical trials in adult and adolescent patients with asthma (N = 1,922), the effect of adding salmeterol to inhaled corticosteroid therapy was evaluated. The studies utilized the inhalation aerosol formulation of salmeterol xinafoate for a treatment period of 6 months. They compared the addition of salmeterol therapy to an increase (at least doubling) of the inhaled corticosteroid dose. Two randomized, double-blind, controlled, parallel-group clinical trials (N = 997) enrolled patients (ages 18 to 82 years) with persistent asthma who were previously maintained but not adequately controlled on inhaled corticosteroid therapy. During the 2-week run-in period, all patients were switched to beclomethasone dipropionate 168 mcg twice daily. Patients still not adequately controlled were randomized to either the addition of SEREVENT Inhalational Aerosol 42 mcg twice daily or an increase of beclomethasone dipropionate to 336 mcg twice daily. As compared to the doubled dose of beclomethasone dipropionate, the addition of SEREVENT Inhalation Aerosol resulted in statistically significantly greater improvements in pulmonary function and asthma symptoms, and statistically significantly greater reduction in supplemental albuterol use. The percent of patients who experienced asthma exacerbations overall was not different between groups (i.e., 16.2% in the group receiving SEREVENT Inhalation Aerosol versus 17.9% in the higher dose beclomethasone dipropionate group).

Two randomized, double-blind, parallel-group clinical trials (N = 925) enrolled patients (ages 12 to 78 years) with persistent asthma who were previously maintained but not adequately controlled on prior therapy. During the 2- to 4-week run-in period, all patients were switched to fluticasone propionate 88 mcg twice daily. Patients still not adequately controlled were randomized to either the addition of SEREVENT Inhalation Aerosol 42 mcg twice daily or an increase of fluticasone propionate to 220 mcg twice daily. As compared to the increased (2.5 times) dose of fluticasone propionate, the addition of SEREVENT Inhalation Aerosol resulted in statistically significantly greater improvements in pulmonary function and asthma symptoms, and statistically significantly greater reductions in supplemental albuterol use. Fewer patients receiving SEREVENT Inhalation Aerosol experienced asthma exacerbations than those receiving the higher dose of fluticasone propionate (8.8% versus 13.8%).

Exercise-Induced Bronchospasm: In 2 randomized, single-dose, crossover studies in adolescents and adults with EIB (N = 53), 50 mcg of SEREVENT DISKUS prevented EIB when dosed 30 minutes to exercise. For many patients, this protective effect against prior EIB was still apparent up to 8.5 hours following a single dose.

[See table 2 at right]

In 2 randomized studies in children 4 to 11 years old with asthma and EIB (N = 50), a single 50-mcg dose of SEREVENT DISKUS prevented EIB when dosed 30 minutes prior to exercise, with protection lasting up to 11.5 hours in repeat testing following this single dose in many patients.

Salmeterol Multi-center Asthma Research Trial: The Salmeterol Multi-center Asthma Research Trial (SMART) enrolled long-acting beta$_2$-agonist–naive patients with asthma (average age of 39 years, 71% Caucasian, 18% African-American, 8% Hispanic) to assess the safety of salmeterol (SEREVENT Inhalation Aerosol, 42 mcg twice daily over 28 weeks) compared to placebo when added to usual asthma therapy. The primary endpoint was the combined number of respiratory-related deaths or respiratory-related life-threatening experiences (intubation and mechanical ventilation). Other endpoints included combined asthma-related deaths or life-threatening experiences and asthma-related deaths. A planned interim analysis was conducted when approximately half of the intended number of patients had been enrolled (N = 26,353).

Due to the low rate of primary events in the study, the findings of the planned interim analysis were not conclusive. The analysis showed no significant difference for the primary endpoint for the total population. However, a higher number of asthma-related deaths or life-threatening experiences (36 vs. 23) and a higher number of asthma-related deaths (13 vs. 4) occurred in the patients treated with salmeterol. Post hoc subgroup analyses revealed no significant increase in respiratory- or asthma-related episodes, including deaths, in Caucasian patients. In African-Americans, the study showed a small, though statistically significantly greater, number of primary events (20 vs. 7), asthma-related deaths or life-threatening experiences (19 vs. 4), and asthma-related deaths (8 vs. 1) in patients taking salmeterol compared those taking placebo. The numbers of patients from other ethnic groups were too small to draw any conclusions in these populations. Even though SMART did not reach predetermined stopping criteria for the total population, the study was stopped due to the findings in African-American patients and difficulties in enrollment.

Chronic Obstructive Pulmonary Disease: In 2 clinical trials evaluating twice-daily treatment with SEREVENT DISKUS 50 mcg (N = 336) compared to placebo (N = 366) in patients with chronic bronchitis with airflow limitation, with or without emphysema, improvements in pulmonary function endpoints were greater with salmeterol 50 mcg than with placebo. Treatment with SEREVENT DISKUS did not result in significant improvements in secondary endpoints assessing COPD symptoms in either clinical trial. Both trials were randomized, double-blind, parallel-group

Table 1. Daily Efficacy Measurements in Two 12-Week Clinical Trials (Combined Data)

Parameter	Time	Placebo	SEREVENT DISKUS	Albuterol Inhalation Aerosol
No. of randomized subjects		152	149	148
Mean AM peak expiratory flow (L/min)	baseline 12 weeks	394 396	395 427*	394 394
Mean % days with no asthma symptoms	baseline 12 weeks	14 20	13 33	12 21
Mean % nights with no awakenings	baseline 12 weeks	70 73	63 85*	68 71
Rescue medications (mean no. of inhalations per day)	baseline 12 weeks	4.2 3.3	4.3 1.6†	4.3 2.2
Asthma exacerbations		14%	15%	16%

* Statistically superior to placebo and albuterol ($p<0.001$).
† Statistically superior to placebo ($p<0.001$).

Table 2. Results of 2 Exercise-Induced Bronchospasm Studies in Adolescents and Adults

		Placebo (N = 52)		SEREVENT DISKUS (N = 52)	
		n	% Total	n	% Total
0.5-Hour postdose exercise challenge	% Fall in FEV$_1$				
	<10%	15	29	31	60
	≥10%,<20%	3	6	11	21
	≥20%	34	65	10	19
Mean maximal % fall in FEV$_1$ (SE)		-25% (1.8)		-11% (1.9)	
8.5-Hour postdose exercise challenge	% Fall in FEV$_1$				
	<10%	12	23	26	50
	≥10%,<20%	7	13	12	23
	≥20%	33	63	14	27
Mean maximal % fall in FEV$_1$ (SE)		-27% (1.5)		-16% (2.0)	

studies of 24 weeks' duration and were identical in design, patient entrance criteria, and overall conduct.

Figure 2 displays the integrated 2-hour postdose FEV$_1$ results from the 2 clinical trials. The percent change in FEV$_1$ refers to the change from baseline, defined as the predose value on Treatment Day 1. To account for patient withdrawals during the study, Endpoint (last evaluable FEV$_1$) data are provided. Patients receiving SEREVENT DISKUS 50 mcg had significantly greater improvements in 2-hour postdose FEV$_1$ at Endpoint (216 mL, 20%) compared to placebo (43 mL, 5%). Improvement was apparent on the first day of treatment and maintained throughout the 24 weeks of treatment.

Figure 2. Mean Percent Change From Baseline in Postdose FEV$_1$ Integrated Data From 2 Trials of Patients With Chronic Bronchitis and Airflow Limitation

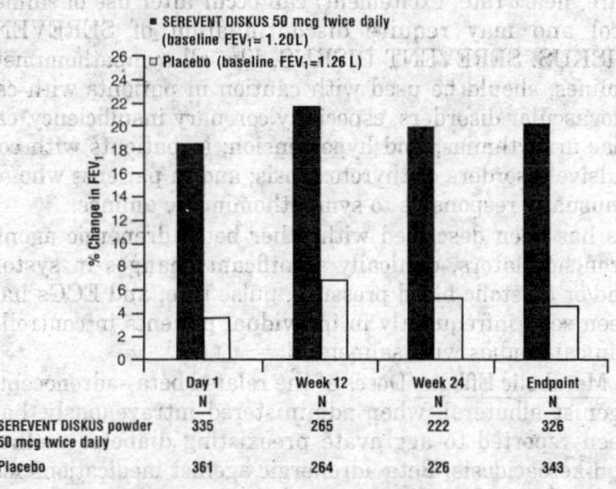

Onset of Action and Duration of Effect: The onset of action and duration of effect of SEREVENT DISKUS were evaluated in a subset of patients (n = 87) from 1 of the 2 clinical trials discussed above. Following the first 50-mcg dose, significant improvement in pulmonary function (mean FEV$_1$ increase of 12% or more and at least 200 mL) occurred at 2 hours. The mean time to peak bronchodilator effect was 4.75 hours. As seen in Figure 3, evidence of bronchodilatation was seen throughout the 12-hour period. Figure 3 also demonstrates that the bronchodilating effect after 12 weeks of treatment was similar to that observed after the first dose. The mean time to peak bronchodilator effect after 12 weeks of treatment was 3.27 hours.

[See figure 3 at top of next column]

INDICATIONS AND USAGE

Asthma: SEREVENT DISKUS is indicated for long-term, twice-daily (morning and evening) administration in the maintenance treatment of asthma and in the prevention of bronchospasm in patients 4 years of age and older with reversible obstructive airway disease, including patients with symptoms of nocturnal asthma, who require regular treatment with inhaled, short-acting beta$_2$-agonists. It is not indicated for patients whose asthma can be managed by occasional use of inhaled, short-acting beta$_2$-agonists.

Figure 3. Serial 12-Hour FEV$_1$ on the First Day and at Week 12 of Treatment

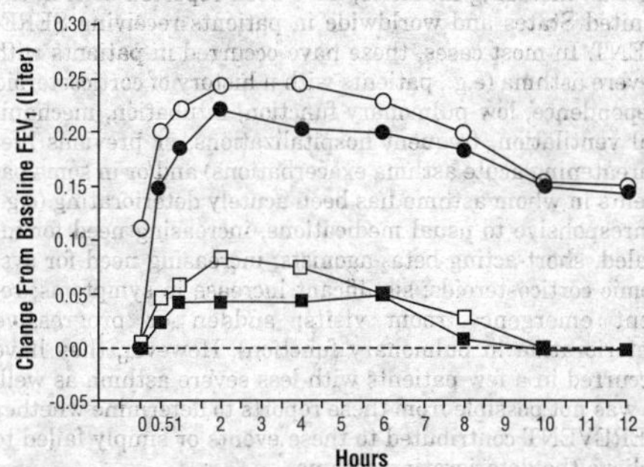

SEREVENT DISKUS is also indicated for prevention of exercise-induced bronchospasm in patients 4 years of age and older.

SEREVENT DISKUS may be used alone or in combination with inhaled or systemic corticosteroid therapy.

Chronic Obstructive Pulmonary Disease: SEREVENT DISKUS is indicated for the long-term, twice-daily (morning and evening) administration in the maintenance treatment of bronchospasm associated with COPD (including emphysema and chronic bronchitis).

CONTRAINDICATIONS

SEREVENT DISKUS is contraindicated in patients with a history of hypersensitivity to salmeterol or any other component of the drug product (see DESCRIPTION and ADVERSE REACTIONS: Observed During Clinical Practice: Non-Site Specific).

WARNINGS

DATA FROM A LARGE PLACEBO-CONTROLLED SAFETY STUDY THAT WAS STOPPED EARLY SUGGEST THAT SALMETEROL MAY BE ASSOCIATED WITH RARE SERIOUS ASTHMA EPISODES OR ASTHMA-

Continued on next page

Product information on these pages is effective as of August 2004. Further information is available at: GlaxoSmithKline, PO Box 13398, Research Triangle Park, NC 27709. 1-888-825-5249. Corporate Web Site: www.gsk.com

Serevent Diskus—Cont.

RELATED DEATHS. Data from this study, called the Salmeterol Multi-center Asthma Research Trial (SMART), further suggest that the risk might be greater in African-American patients, in whom the increased risk was statistically significant at the time of the interim analysis. These results led to stopping the study prematurely (see CLINICAL TRIALS: Asthma: *Salmeterol Multi-center Asthma Research Trial*). The data from the SMART study are not adequate to determine whether concurrent use of inhaled corticosteroids provides protection from this risk. Given the similar basic mechanisms of action of beta$_2$-agonists, it is possible that the findings seen in the SMART study may be consistent with a class effect. Findings similar to the SMART study findings were reported in a prior 16-week clinical study performed in the United Kingdom, the Salmeterol Nationwide Surveillance (SNS) study. In the SNS study, the incidence of asthma-related death was numerically, though not statistically, greater in patients with asthma treated with salmeterol (42 mcg twice daily) versus albuterol (180 mcg 4 times daily) added to usual asthma therapy.

SEREVENT DISKUS SHOULD NOT BE INITIATED IN PATIENTS WITH SIGNIFICANTLY WORSENING OR ACUTELY DETERIORATING ASTHMA, WHICH MAY BE A LIFE-THREATENING CONDITION. Serious acute respiratory events, including fatalities, have been reported both in the United States and worldwide when SEREVENT has been initiated in this situation.

Although it is not possible from these reports to determine whether SEREVENT contributed to these adverse events or simply failed to relieve the deteriorating asthma, the use of SEREVENT DISKUS in this setting is inappropriate.

SEREVENT DISKUS SHOULD NOT BE USED TO TREAT ACUTE SYMPTOMS. It is crucial to inform patients of this and prescribe an inhaled, short-acting beta$_2$-agonist for this purpose as well as warn them that increasing inhaled beta$_2$-agonist use is a signal of deteriorating asthma.

SEREVENT DISKUS IS NOT A SUBSTITUTE FOR INHALED OR ORAL CORTICOSTEROIDS. Corticosteroids should not be stopped or reduced when SEREVENT DISKUS is initiated.

(See PRECAUTIONS: Information for Patients and the Patient's Instructions for Use accompanying the product.)

1. Do Not Introduce SEREVENT DISKUS as a Treatment for Acutely Deteriorating Asthma: SEREVENT DISKUS is intended for the maintenance treatment of asthma (see INDICATIONS AND USAGE) and should not be introduced in acutely deteriorating asthma, which is a potentially life-threatening condition. There are no data demonstrating that SEREVENT DISKUS provides greater efficacy than or additional efficacy to inhaled, short-acting beta$_2$-agonists in patients with worsening asthma. Serious acute respiratory events, including fatalities, have been reported both in the United States and worldwide in patients receiving SEREVENT. In most cases, these have occurred in patients with severe asthma (e.g., patients with a history of corticosteroid dependence, low pulmonary function, intubation, mechanical ventilation, frequent hospitalizations, or previous life-threatening acute asthma exacerbations) and/or in some patients in whom asthma has been acutely deteriorating (e.g., unresponsive to usual medications; increasing need for inhaled, short-acting beta$_2$-agonists; increasing need for systemic corticosteroids; significant increase in symptoms; recent emergency room visits; sudden or progressive deterioration in pulmonary function). However, they have occurred in a few patients with less severe asthma as well. It was not possible from these reports to determine whether SEREVENT contributed to these events or simply failed to relieve the deteriorating asthma.

2. Do Not Use SEREVENT DISKUS to Treat Acute Symptoms: An inhaled, short-acting beta$_2$-agonist, not SEREVENT DISKUS, should be used to relieve acute asthma or COPD symptoms. When prescribing SEREVENT DISKUS, the physician must also provide the patient with an inhaled, short-acting beta$_2$-agonist (e.g., albuterol) for treatment of symptoms that occur acutely, despite regular twice-daily (morning and evening) use of SEREVENT DISKUS.

When beginning treatment with SEREVENT DISKUS, patients who have been taking inhaled, short-acting beta$_2$-agonists on a regular basis (e.g., 4 times a day) should be instructed to discontinue the regular use of these drugs and use them only for symptomatic relief of acute asthma or COPD symptoms (see PRECAUTIONS: Information for Patients).

3. Watch for Increasing Use of Inhaled, Short-Acting Beta$_2$-Agonists, Which Is a Marker of Deteriorating Asthma or COPD: The patient's condition may deteriorate acutely over a period of hours or chronically over several days or longer. If the patient's inhaled, short-acting beta$_2$-agonist becomes less effective, the patient needs more inhalations than usual, or the patient develops a significant decrease in PEF or lung function, these may be markers of destabilization of their disease. In this setting, the patient requires immediate reevaluation with reassessment of the treatment regimen, giving special consideration to the possible need for corticosteroids. If the patient uses 4 or more inhalations per day of an inhaled, short-acting beta$_2$-agonist for 2 or more consecutive days, or if more than 1 canister (200 inhalations per canister) of inhaled, short-acting beta$_2$-agonist is used in an 8-week period in conjunction with SEREVENT DISKUS, then the patient should consult the physician for reevaluation. **Increasing the daily dosage of SEREVENT DISKUS in this situation is not appropriate. SEREVENT DISKUS should not be used more frequently than twice daily (morning and evening) at the recommended dose of 1 inhalation.**

4. Do Not Use SEREVENT DISKUS as a Substitute for Oral or Inhaled Corticosteroids: The use of beta-adrenergic agonist bronchodilators alone may not be adequate to control asthma in many patients. Early consideration should be given to adding anti-inflammatory agents, e.g., corticosteroids. There are no data demonstrating that SEREVENT DISKUS has a clinical anti-inflammatory effect and could be expected to take the place of corticosteroids. Patients who already require oral or inhaled corticosteroids for treatment of asthma should be continued on a suitable dose to maintain clinical stability even if they feel better as a result of initiating SEREVENT DISKUS. Any change in corticosteroid dosage should be made ONLY after clinical evaluation (see PRECAUTIONS: Information for Patients).

5. Do Not Exceed Recommended Dosage: As with other inhaled beta$_2$-adrenergic drugs, SEREVENT DISKUS should not be used more often or at higher doses than recommended. Fatalities have been reported in association with excessive use of inhaled sympathomimetic drugs. Large doses of inhaled or oral salmeterol (12 to 20 times the recommended dose) have been associated with clinically significant prolongation of the QTc interval, which has the potential for producing ventricular arrhythmias.

6. Paradoxical Bronchospasm: As with other inhaled asthma and COPD medications, SEREVENT DISKUS can produce paradoxical bronchospasm, which may be life threatening. If paradoxical bronchospasm occurs following dosing with SEREVENT DISKUS, it should be treated with a short-acting, inhaled bronchodilator; SEREVENT DISKUS should be discontinued immediately; and alternative therapy should be instituted.

7. Immediate Hypersensitivity Reactions: Immediate hypersensitivity reactions may occur after administration of SEREVENT DISKUS, as demonstrated by cases of urticaria, angioedema, rash, and bronchospasm.

8. Upper Airway Symptoms: Symptoms of laryngeal spasm, irritation, or swelling, such as stridor and choking, have been reported in patients receiving SEREVENT DISKUS.

9. Cardiovascular Disorders: SEREVENT DISKUS, like all sympathomimetic amines, should be used with caution in patients with cardiovascular disorders, especially coronary insufficiency, cardiac arrhythmias, and hypertension. SEREVENT DISKUS, like all other beta-adrenergic agonists, can produce a clinically significant cardiovascular effect in some patients as measured by pulse rate, blood pressure, and/or symptoms. Although such effects are uncommon after administration of SEREVENT DISKUS at recommended doses, if they occur, the drug may need to be discontinued. In addition, beta-agonists have been reported to produce ECG changes, such as flattening of the T wave, prolongation of the QTc interval, and ST segment depression. The clinical significance of these findings is unknown.

PRECAUTIONS

General: 1. Cardiovascular and Other Effects: No effect on the cardiovascular system is usually seen after the administration of inhaled salmeterol at recommended doses, but the cardiovascular and central nervous system effects seen with all sympathomimetic drugs (e.g., increased blood pressure, heart rate, excitement) can occur after use of salmeterol and may require discontinuation of SEREVENT DISKUS. SEREVENT DISKUS, like all sympathomimetic amines, should be used with caution in patients with cardiovascular disorders, especially coronary insufficiency, cardiac arrhythmias, and hypertension; in patients with convulsive disorders or thyrotoxicosis; and in patients who are unusually responsive to sympathomimetic amines.

As has been described with other beta-adrenergic agonist bronchodilators, clinically significant changes in systolic and/or diastolic blood pressure, pulse rate, and ECGs have been seen infrequently in individual patients in controlled clinical studies with salmeterol.

2. Metabolic Effects: Doses of the related beta$_2$-adrenoceptor agonist albuterol, when administered intravenously, have been reported to aggravate preexisting diabetes mellitus and ketoacidosis. Beta-adrenergic agonist medications may produce significant hypokalemia in some patients, possibly through intracellular shunting, which has the potential to produce adverse cardiovascular effects. The decrease in serum potassium is usually transient, not requiring supplementation.

Clinically significant changes in blood glucose and/or serum potassium were seen rarely during clinical studies with long-term administration of SEREVENT DISKUS at recommended doses.

Information for Patients: Patients being treated with SEREVENT DISKUS should receive the following information and instructions. This information is intended to aid them in the safe and effective use of this medication. It is not a disclosure of all possible adverse or intended effects. It is important that patients understand how to use the DISKUS appropriately and how to use SEREVENT DISKUS in relation to other asthma or COPD medications they are taking. Patients should be given the following information:

1. The action of SEREVENT DISKUS may last up to 12 hours or longer. The recommended dosage (1 inhalation twice daily, morning and evening) should not be exceeded.
2. Most patients are able to taste or feel a dose delivered from SEREVENT DISKUS. However, whether or not patients are able to sense delivery of a dose, you should instruct them not to exceed the recommended dose of 1 inhalation twice daily, morning and evening. You should instruct them to contact you or the pharmacist if they have questions.
3. SEREVENT DISKUS is not meant to relieve acute asthma or COPD symptoms and extra doses should not be used for that purpose. Acute symptoms should be treated with an inhaled, short-acting bronchodilator (the physician should provide the patient with such medication and instruct the patient in how it should be used).
4. Patients should not stop therapy with SEREVENT DISKUS for asthma or COPD without physician/provider guidance since symptoms may worsen after discontinuation.
5. • When used for the treatment of EIB, 1 inhalation of SEREVENT DISKUS should be taken 30 minutes before exercise.
   • Additional doses of SEREVENT should not be used for 12 hours.
   • Patients who are receiving SEREVENT DISKUS twice daily should not use additional SEREVENT for prevention of EIB.
6. The physician should be notified immediately if any of the following situations occur, which may be a sign of seriously worsening asthma or COPD:
   • Decreasing effectiveness of inhaled, short-acting beta$_2$-agonists
   • Need for more inhalations than usual of inhaled, short-acting beta$_2$-agonists
   • Significant decrease in PEF or lung function as outlined by the physician
   • Use of 4 or more inhalations per day of a short-acting beta$_2$-agonist for 2 or more days consecutively
   • Use of more than 1 canister (200 inhalations per canister) of an inhaled, short-acting beta$_2$-agonist in an 8-week period.
7. SEREVENT DISKUS should not be used as a substitute for oral or inhaled corticosteroids. The dosage of these medications should not be changed and they should not be stopped without consulting the physician, even if the patient feels better after initiating treatment with SEREVENT DISKUS.
8. Patients should be cautioned regarding adverse effects associated with beta$_2$-agonists, such as palpitations, chest pain, rapid heart rate, tremor, or nervousness.
9. When patients are prescribed SEREVENT DISKUS, other medications for asthma and COPD should be used only as directed by the physician.
10. SEREVENT DISKUS should not be used with a spacer device.
11. Patients who are pregnant or nursing should contact the physician about the use of SEREVENT DISKUS.
12. Effective and safe use of SEREVENT DISKUS includes an understanding of the way that it should be used:
    • Never exhale into the DISKUS.
    • Never attempt to take the DISKUS apart.
    • Always activate and use the DISKUS in a level, horizontal position.
    • Never wash the mouthpiece or any part of the DISKUS. KEEP IT DRY.
    • Always keep the DISKUS in a dry place.
    • Discard **6 weeks** after removal from the moisture-protective foil overwrap pouch or after all blisters have been used (when the dose indicator reads "0"), whichever comes first.
13. For the proper use of SEREVENT DISKUS and to attain maximum benefit, the patient should read and follow carefully the Patient's Instructions for Use accompanying the product.

Drug Interactions: ***Short-Acting Beta$_2$-Agonists:*** In two 12-week, repetitive-dose adolescent and adult clinical trials in patients with asthma (N = 149), the mean daily need for additional beta$_2$-agonist in patients using SEREVENT DISKUS was approximately 1½ inhalations/day. Twenty-six percent (26%) of the patients in these trials used between 8 and 24 inhalations of short-acting beta-agonist per day on 1 or more occasions. Nine percent (9%) of the patients in these trials averaged over 4 inhalations/day over the course of the 12-week trials. No increase in frequency of cardiovascular events was observed among the 3 patients who averaged 8 to 11 inhalations/day; however, the safety of concomitant use of more than 8 inhalations/day of short-acting beta$_2$-agonist with SEREVENT DISKUS has not been established. In 29 patients who experienced worsening of asthma while receiving SEREVENT DISKUS during these trials, albuterol therapy administered via either nebulizer or inhalation aerosol (1 dose in most cases) led to improvement in FEV_1 and no increase in occurrence of cardiovascular adverse events.

In 2 clinical trials in patients with COPD, the mean daily need for additional beta$_2$-agonist for patients using SEREVENT DISKUS was approximately 4 inhalations/day. Twenty-four percent (24%) of the patients using SEREVENT DISKUS in these trials averaged 6 or more inhalations of albuterol per day over the course of the 24-week trials. No increase in frequency of cardiovascular events was observed among patients who averaged 6 or more inhalations per day.

Monoamine Oxidase Inhibitors and Tricyclic Antidepressants: Salmeterol should be administered with extreme caution to patients being treated with monoamine oxidase inhibitors or tricyclic antidepressants, or within 2 weeks of discontinuation of such agents, because the action of salmeterol on the vascular system may be potentiated by these agents.

Corticosteroids and Cromoglycate: In clinical trials, inhaled corticosteroids and/or inhaled cromolyn sodium did not alter the safety profile of salmeterol when administered concurrently.

Methylxanthines: The concurrent use of intravenously or orally administered methylxanthines (e.g., aminophylline, theophylline) by patients receiving salmeterol has not been completely evaluated. In 1 clinical asthma trial, 87 patients receiving SEREVENT Inhalation Aerosol 42 mcg twice daily concurrently with a theophylline product had adverse event rates similar to those in 71 patients receiving SEREVENT Inhalation Aerosol without theophylline. Resting heart rates were slightly higher in the patients on theophylline but were little affected by therapy with SEREVENT Inhalation Aerosol.

In 2 clinical trials in patients with COPD, 39 subjects receiving SEREVENT DISKUS concurrently with a theophylline product had adverse event rates similar to those in 302 patients receiving SEREVENT DISKUS without theophylline. Based on the available data, the concomitant administration of methylxanthines with SEREVENT DISKUS did not alter the observed adverse event profile.

Beta-Adrenergic Receptor Blocking Agents: Beta-blockers not only block the pulmonary effect of beta-agonists, such as SEREVENT DISKUS, but may also produce severe bronchospasm in patients with asthma or COPD. Therefore, patients with asthma or COPD should not normally be treated with beta-blockers. However, under certain circumstances, e.g., as prophylaxis after myocardial infarction, there may be no acceptable alternatives to the use of beta-adrenergic blocking agents in patients with asthma or COPD. In this setting, cardioselective beta-blockers could be considered, although they should be administered with caution.

Diuretics: The ECG changes and/or hypokalemia that may result from the administration of nonpotassium-sparing diuretics (such as loop or thiazide diuretics) can be acutely worsened by beta-agonists, especially when the recommended dose of the beta-agonist is exceeded. Although the clinical significance of these effects is not known, caution is advised in the coadministration of beta-agonists with nonpotassium-sparing diuretics.

Carcinogenesis, Mutagenesis, Impairment of Fertility: In an 18-month oral carcinogenicity study in CD-mice, salmeterol xinafoate caused a dose-related increase in the incidence of smooth muscle hyperplasia, cystic glandular hyperplasia, leiomyomas of the uterus, and ovarian cysts at doses of 1.4 mg/kg and above (approximately 20 times the maximum recommended daily inhalation dose in adults and children based on comparison of the area under the plasma concentration versus time curves [AUCs]). The incidence of leiomyosarcomas was not statistically significant. No tumors were seen at 0.2 mg/kg (approximately 3 times the maximum recommended daily inhalation doses in adults and children based on comparison of the AUCs).

In a 24-month oral and inhalation carcinogenicity study in Sprague Dawley rats, salmeterol caused a dose-related increase in the incidence of mesovarian leiomyomas and ovarian cysts at doses of 0.68 mg/kg and above (approximately 55 times the maximum recommended daily inhalation dose in adults and approximately 25 times the maximum recommended daily inhalation dose in children on a mg/m^2 basis). No tumors were seen at 0.21 mg/kg (approximately 15 times the maximum recommended daily inhalation dose in adults and approximately 8 times the maximum recommended daily inhalation dose in children on a mg/m^2 basis). These findings in rodents are similar to those reported previously for other beta-adrenergic agonist drugs. The relevance of these findings to human use is unknown.

Salmeterol produced no detectable or reproducible increases in microbial and mammalian gene mutation in vitro. No clastogenic activity occurred in vitro in human lymphocytes or in vivo in a rat micronucleus test. No effects on fertility were identified in male and female rats treated with salmeterol at oral doses up to 2 mg/kg (approximately 160 times the maximum recommended daily inhalation dose in adults on a mg/m^2 basis).

Pregnancy: ***Teratogenic Effects:*** Pregnancy Category C. No teratogenic effects occurred in rats at oral doses up to 2 mg/kg (approximately 160 times the maximum recommended daily inhalation dose in adults on a mg/m^2 basis). In pregnant Dutch rabbits administered oral doses of 1 mg/kg and above (approximately 50 times the maximum recommended daily inhalation dose in adults based on comparison of the AUCs), salmeterol exhibited fetal toxic effects characteristically resulting from beta-adrenoceptor stimulation. These included precocious eyelid openings, cleft palate, sternebral fusion, limb and paw flexures, and delayed ossification of the frontal cranial bones. No significant effects occurred at an oral dose of 0.6 mg/kg (approximately 20 times the maximum recommended daily inhalation dose in adults based on comparison of the AUCs).

New Zealand White rabbits were less sensitive since only delayed ossification of the frontal bones was seen at an oral dose of 10 mg/kg (approximately 1,600 times the maximum recommended daily inhalation dose in adults on a mg/m^2 basis). Extensive use of other beta-agonists has provided no evidence that these class effects in animals are relevant to their use in humans. There are no adequate and well-controlled studies with SEREVENT DISKUS in pregnant women. SEREVENT DISKUS should be used during pregnancy only if the potential benefit justifies the potential risk to the fetus.

Salmeterol xinafoate crossed the placenta following oral administration of 10 mg/kg to mice and rats (approximately 410 and 810 times, respectively, the maximum recommended daily inhalation dose in adults on a mg/m^2 basis).

Use in Labor and Delivery: There are no well-controlled human studies that have investigated effects of salmeterol on preterm labor or labor at term. Because of the potential for beta-agonist interference with uterine contractility, use of SEREVENT DISKUS during labor should be restricted to those patients in whom the benefits clearly outweigh the risks.

Nursing Mothers: Plasma levels of salmeterol after inhaled therapeutic doses are very low. In rats, salmeterol xinafoate is excreted in the milk. However, since there are no data from controlled trials on the use of salmeterol by nursing mothers, a decision should be made whether to discontinue nursing or to discontinue SEREVENT DISKUS, taking into account the importance of SEREVENT DISKUS to the mother. Caution should be exercised when SEREVENT DISKUS is administered to a nursing woman.

Pediatric Use: The safety and efficacy of SEREVENT DISKUS has been evaluated in over 2,500 patients aged 4 to 11 years with asthma, 346 of whom were administered SEREVENT DISKUS for 1 year. Based on available data, no adjustment of dosage of SEREVENT DISKUS in pediatric patients is warranted for either asthma or EIB (see DOSAGE AND ADMINISTRATION).

In 2 randomized, double-blind, controlled clinical trials of 12 weeks' duration, SEREVENT DISKUS 50-mcg was administered to 211 pediatric patients with asthma who did and who did not receive concurrent inhaled corticosteroids. The efficacy of SEREVENT DISKUS was demonstrated over the 12-week treatment period with respect to PEF and FEV$_1$. SEREVENT DISKUS was effective in demographic subgroups (gender and age) of the population. SEREVENT DISKUS was effective when coadministered with other inhaled asthma medications, such as short-acting bronchodilators and inhaled corticosteroids. SEREVENT DISKUS was well tolerated in the pediatric population, and there were no safety issues identified specific to the administration of SEREVENT DISKUS to pediatric patients.

In 2 randomized studies in children 4 to 11 years old with asthma and EIB, a single 50-mcg dose of SEREVENT DISKUS prevented EIB when dosed 30 minutes prior to exercise, with protection lasting up to 11.5 hours in repeat testing following this single dose in many patients.

Geriatric Use: Of the total number of adolescent and adult patients with asthma who received SEREVENT DISKUS in chronic dosing clinical trials, 209 were 65 years of age and older. Of the total number of patients with COPD who received SEREVENT DISKUS in chronic dosing clinical trials, 167 were 65 years of age or older and 45 were 75 years of age or older. No apparent differences in the safety of SEREVENT DISKUS were observed when geriatric patients were compared with younger patients in clinical trials. As with other beta$_2$-agonists, however, special caution should be observed when using SEREVENT DISKUS in geriatric patients who have concomitant cardiovascular disease that could be adversely affected by this class of drug. Data from the trials in patients with COPD suggested a greater effect on FEV$_1$ of SEREVENT DISKUS in the <65 years age-group, as compared with the ≥65 years age-group. However, based on available data, no adjustment of dosage of SEREVENT DISKUS in geriatric patients is warranted.

ADVERSE REACTIONS

Adverse reactions to salmeterol are similar in nature to reactions to other selective beta$_2$-adrenoceptor agonists, i.e., tachycardia; palpitations; immediate hypersensitivity reactions, including urticaria, angioedema, rash, bronchospasm (see WARNINGS); headache; tremor; nervousness; and paradoxical bronchospasm (see WARNINGS).

Asthma: Two multicenter, 12-week, controlled studies have evaluated twice-daily doses of SEREVENT DISKUS in patients 12 years of age and older with asthma. Table 3 reports the incidence of adverse events in these 2 studies.

Table 3. Adverse Event Incidence in Two 12-Week Adolescent and Adult Clinical Trials in Patients With Asthma

Adverse Event	Percent of Patients: Placebo (N = 152)	SEREVENT DISKUS 50 mcg Twice Daily (N = 149)	Albuterol Inhalation Aerosol 180 mcg 4 Times Daily (N = 150)
Ear, nose, and throat			
Nasal/sinus congestion, pallor	6	9	8
Rhinitis	4	5	4
Neurological			
Headache	9	13	12
Respiratory			
Asthma	1	3	<1
Tracheitis/bronchitis	4	7	3
Influenza	2	5	5

[See table 3 above]

Table 3 includes all events (whether considered drug-related or nondrug-related by the investigator) that occurred at a rate of 3% or greater in the group receiving SEREVENT DISKUS and were more common than in the placebo group.

Pharyngitis, sinusitis, upper respiratory tract infection, and cough occurred at ≥3% but were more common in the placebo group. However, throat irritation has been described at rates exceeding that of placebo in other controlled clinical trials.

Other adverse events that occurred in the group receiving SEREVENT DISKUS in these studies with an incidence of 1% to 3% and that occurred at a greater incidence than with placebo were:

Ear, Nose, and Throat: Sinus headache.

Gastrointestinal: Nausea.

Mouth and Teeth: Oral mucosal abnormality.

Musculoskeletal: Pain in joint.

Neurological: Sleep disturbance, paresthesia.

Skin: Contact dermatitis, eczema.

Miscellaneous: Localized aches and pains, pyrexia of unknown origin.

Two multicenter, 12-week, controlled studies have evaluated twice-daily doses of SEREVENT DISKUS in patients aged 4 to 11 years with asthma. Table 4 includes all events (whether considered drug-related or nondrug-related by the investigator) that occurred at a rate of 3% or greater in the group receiving SEREVENT DISKUS and were more common than in the placebo group.

Table 4. Adverse Event Incidence in Two 12-Week Pediatric Clinical Trials in Patients With Asthma

Adverse Event	Percent of Patients: Placebo (N = 215)	SEREVENT DISKUS 50 mcg Twice Daily (N = 211)	Albuterol Inhalation Powder 200 mcg 4 Times Daily (N = 115)
Ear, nose, and throat			
Ear signs and symptoms	3	4	9
Pharyngitis	3	6	3
Neurological			
Headache	14	17	20
Respiratory			
Asthma	2	4	<1
Skin			
Skin rashes	3	4	2
Urticaria	0	3	2

[See table 4 above]

Continued on next page

Product information on these pages is effective as of August 2004. Further information is available at: GlaxoSmithKline, PO Box 13398, Research Triangle Park, NC 27709. 1-888-825-5249. Corporate Web Site: www.gsk.com

Serevent Diskus—Cont.

The following events were reported at an incidence of 1% to 2% (3 to 4 patients) in the salmeterol group and with a higher incidence than in the albuterol and placebo groups: gastrointestinal signs and symptoms, lower respiratory signs and symptoms, photodermatitis, and arthralgia and articular rheumatism.

In clinical trials evaluating concurrent therapy of salmeterol with inhaled corticosteroids, adverse events were consistent with those previously reported for salmeterol, or might otherwise be expected with the use of inhaled corticosteroids.

Chronic Obstructive Pulmonary Disease: Two multicenter, 24-week, controlled studies have evaluated twice-daily doses of SEREVENT DISKUS in patients with COPD. For presentation (Table 5), the placebo data from a third trial, identical in design, patient entrance criteria, and overall conduct but comparing fluticasone propionate with placebo, were integrated with the placebo data from these 2 studies (total N = 341 for salmeterol and 576 for placebo).

[See table 5 below]

Other events occurring in the group receiving SEREVENT DISKUS that occurred at a frequency of 1% to <3% and were more common than in the placebo group were as follows:

Endocrine and Metabolic: Hyperglycemia.

Eye: Keratitis and conjunctivitis.

Gastrointestinal: Candidiasis mouth/throat, dyspeptic symptoms, hyposalivation, dental discomfort and pain, gastrointestinal infections.

Lower Respiratory: Lower respiratory signs and symptoms.

Musculoskeletal: Arthralgia and articular rheumatism; muscle pain; bone and skeletal pain; musculoskeletal inflammation; muscle stiffness, tightness, and rigidity.

Neurology: Migraines.

Non-Site Specific: Pain, edema and swelling.

Psychiatry: Anxiety.

Skin: Skin rashes.

Observed During Clinical Practice: In addition to adverse events reported from clinical trials, the following events have been identified during postapproval use of salmeterol. Because they are reported voluntarily from a population of unknown size, estimates of frequency cannot be made. These events have been chosen for inclusion due to either their seriousness, frequency of reporting, or causal connection to salmeterol or a combination of these factors.

In extensive US and worldwide postmarketing experience with salmeterol, serious exacerbations of asthma, including some that have been fatal, have been reported. In most cases, these have occurred in patients with severe asthma and/or in some patients in whom asthma has been acutely deteriorating (see WARNINGS no. 1), but they have also occurred in a few patients with less severe asthma. It was not possible from these reports to determine whether salmeterol contributed to these events or simply failed to relieve the deteriorating asthma.

Respiratory: Reports of upper airway symptoms of laryngeal spasm, irritation, or swelling such as stridor or choking; oropharyngeal irritation.

Cardiovascular: Arrhythmias (including atrial fibrillation, supraventricular tachycardia, extrasystoles), and anaphylaxis.

Non-Site Specific: Very rare anaphylactic reaction in patients with severe milk protein allergy.

OVERDOSAGE

The expected signs and symptoms with overdosage of SEREVENT DISKUS are those of excessive beta-adrenergic stimulation and/or occurrence or exaggeration of any of the signs and symptoms listed under ADVERSE REACTIONS, e.g., seizures, angina, hypertension or hypotension, tachycardia with rates up to 200 beats/min, arrhythmias, nervousness, headache, tremor, muscle cramps, dry mouth, palpitation, nausea, dizziness, fatigue, malaise, and insomnia. Overdosage with SEREVENT DISKUS may be expected to result in exaggeration of the pharmacologic adverse effects associated with beta-adrenoceptor agonists, including tachycardia and/or arrhythmia, tremor, headache, and muscle cramps. Overdosage with SEREVENT DISKUS can lead to clinically significant prolongation of the QTc interval, which can produce ventricular arrhythmias. Other signs of overdosage may include hypokalemia and hyperglycemia.

As with all sympathomimetic medications, cardiac arrest and even death may be associated with abuse of SEREVENT DISKUS.

Treatment consists of discontinuation of SEREVENT DISKUS together with appropriate symptomatic therapy. The judicious use of a cardioselective beta-receptor blocker may be considered, bearing in mind that such medication can produce bronchospasm. There is insufficient evidence to determine if dialysis is beneficial for overdosage of SEREVENT DISKUS. Cardiac monitoring is recommended in cases of overdosage.

No deaths were seen in rats at an inhalation dose of 2.9 mg/kg (approximately 240 times the maximum recommended daily inhalation dose in adults and approximately 110 times the maximum recommended daily inhalation dose in children on a mg/m^2 basis) and in dogs at an inhalation dose of 0.7 mg/kg (approximately 190 times the maximum recommended daily inhalation dose in adults and approximately 90 times the maximum recommended daily inhalation dose in children on a mg/m^2 basis). By the oral route, no deaths occurred in mice at 150 mg/kg (approximately 6,100 times the maximum recommended daily inhalation dose in adults and approximately 2,900 times the maximum recommended daily inhalation dose in children on a mg/m^2 basis) and in rats at 1,000 mg/kg (approximately 81,000 times the maximum recommended daily inhalation dose in adults and approximately 38,000 times the maximum recommended daily inhalation dose in children on a mg/m^2 basis).

DOSAGE AND ADMINISTRATION

SEREVENT DISKUS should be administered by the orally inhaled route only (see Patient's Instructions for Use). The patient must not exhale into the DISKUS and the DISKUS should only be activated and used in a level, horizontal position.

Asthma: For maintenance of bronchodilatation and prevention of symptoms of asthma, including the symptoms of nocturnal asthma, the usual dosage for adults and children 4 years of age and older is 1 inhalation (50 mcg) twice daily (morning and evening, approximately 12 hours apart). If a previously effective dosage regimen fails to provide the usual response, medical advice should be sought immediately as this is often a sign of destabilization of asthma. Under these circumstances, the therapeutic regimen should be reevaluated and additional therapeutic options, such as inhaled or systemic corticosteroids, should be considered. If symptoms arise in the period between doses, an inhaled, short-acting beta$_2$-agonist should be taken for immediate relief.

Chronic Obstructive Pulmonary Disease: For maintenance treatment of bronchospasm associated with COPD (including chronic bronchitis and emphysema), the usual dosage for adults is 1 inhalation (50 mcg) twice daily (morning and evening, approximately 12 hours apart).

For both asthma and COPD, adverse effects are more likely to occur with higher doses of salmeterol, and more frequent administration or administration of a larger number of inhalations is not recommended.

To gain full therapeutic benefit, SEREVENT DISKUS should be administered twice daily (morning and evening) in the treatment of reversible airway obstruction.

Geriatric Use: Based on available data for SEREVENT DISKUS, no dosage adjustment is recommended.

Prevention of Exercise-Induced Bronchospasm: One inhalation of SEREVENT DISKUS at least 30 minutes before exercise has been shown to protect patients against EIB. When used intermittently as needed for prevention of EIB, this protection may last up to 9 hours in adolescents and adults and up to 12 hours in patients 4 to 11 years of age. Additional doses of SEREVENT should not be used for 12 hours after the administration of this drug. Patients who are receiving SEREVENT DISKUS twice daily should not use additional SEREVENT for prevention of EIB. If regular, twice-daily dosing is not effective in preventing EIB, other appropriate therapy for EIB should be considered.

HOW SUPPLIED

SEREVENT DISKUS is supplied as a disposable, teal green unit containing 60 blisters. The drug product is packaged within a teal green, plastic-coated, moisture-protective foil pouch (NDC 0173-0521-00).

SEREVENT DISKUS is also supplied in an institutional pack of 1 teal green, disposable unit containing 28 blisters. The drug product is packaged within a teal green, plastic-coated, moisture-protective foil pouch (NDC 0173-0520-00). **Store at controlled room temperature (see USP), 20° to 25°C (68° to 77°F) in a dry place away from direct heat or sunlight. Keep out of reach of children. SEREVENT DISKUS should be discarded 6 weeks after removal from the moisture-protective foil overwrap pouch or after all blisters have been used (when the dose indicator reads "0"), whichever comes first. The DISKUS is not reusable. Do not attempt to take the DISKUS apart.**

GlaxoSmithKline, Research Triangle Park, NC 27709

August 2003/RL-2032

Shown in Product Identification Guide, page 317

Table 5. Adverse Events With ≥3% Incidence in US Controlled Clinical Trials With SEREVENT DISKUS in Patients With Chronic Obstructive Pulmonary Disease*

Adverse Event	Percent of Patients: Placebo (N = 576)	Percent of Patients: SEREVENT DISKUS 50 mcg Twice Daily (N = 341)
Cardiovascular		
Hypertension	2	4
Ear, nose, and throat		
Throat irritation	6	7
Nasal congestion/blockage	3	4
Sinusitis	2	4
Ear signs and symptoms	1	3
Gastrointestinal		
Nausea and vomiting	3	3
Lower respiratory		
Cough	4	5
Rhinitis	2	4
Viral respiratory infection	4	5
Musculoskeletal		
Musculoskeletal pain	10	12
Muscle cramps and spasms	1	3
Neurological		
Headache	11	14
Dizziness	2	4
Average duration of exposure (days)	128.9	138.5

*Table 5 includes all events (whether considered drug-related or nondrug-related by the investigator) that occurred at a rate of 3% or greater in the group receiving SEREVENT DISKUS and were more common in the group receiving SEREVENT DISKUS than in the placebo group.

TABLOID® brand Thioguanine ℞

[*tab' loid*]

40-mg Scored Tablets

CAUTION

TABLOID brand Thioguanine is a potent drug. It should not be used unless a diagnosis of acute nonlymphocytic leukemia has been adequately established and the responsible physician is knowledgeable in assessing response to chemotherapy.

DESCRIPTION

TABLOID brand Thioguanine was synthesized and developed by Hitchings, Elion, and associates at the Wellcome Research Laboratories. It is one of a large series of purine analogues which interfere with nucleic acid biosynthesis, and has been found active against selected human neoplastic diseases.

Thioguanine, known chemically as 2-amino-1,7-dihydro-6*H*-purine-6-thione, is an analogue of the nucleic acid constituent guanine, and is closely related structurally and functionally to PURINETHOL® (mercaptopurine).

TABLOID brand Thioguanine is available in tablets for oral administration. Each scored tablet contains 40 mg thioguanine and the inactive ingredients gum acacia, lactose, magnesium stearate, potato starch, and stearic acid.

CLINICAL PHARMACOLOGY

Clinical studies have shown that the absorption of an oral dose of thioguanine in humans is incomplete and variable, averaging approximately 30% of the administered dose (range: 14% to 46%). Following oral administration of ^{35}S-6-thioguanine, total plasma radioactivity reached a maximum at 8 hours and declined slowly thereafter. Parent drug represented only a very small fraction of the total plasma radioactivity at any time, being virtually undetectable throughout the period of measurements.

The oral administration of radiolabeled thioguanine revealed only trace quantities of parent drug in the urine. However, a methylated metabolite, 2-amino-6-methylthiopurine (MTG), appeared very early, rose to a maximum 6 to 8 hours after drug administration, and was still being excreted after 12 to 22 hours. Radiolabeled sulfate appeared somewhat later than MTG but was the principal metabolite after 8 hours. Thiouric acid and some unidentified products were found in the urine in small amounts. Intravenous administration of ^{35}S-6-thioguanine disclosed a median plasma half-disappearance time of 80 minutes (range: 25 to 240 minutes) when the compound was given in single doses of 65 to 300 mg/m^2. Although initial plasma levels of thioguanine did correlate with the dose level, there was no correlation between the plasma half-disappearance time and the dose.

Thioguanine is incorporated into the DNA and the RNA of human bone marrow cells. Studies with intravenous ^{35}S-6-thioguanine have shown that the amount of thioguanine incorporated into nucleic acids is more than 100 times higher after 5 daily doses than after a single dose. With the 5-dose schedule, from one-half to virtually all of the guanine in the residual DNA was replaced by thioguanine. Tissue distribution studies of ^{35}S-6-thioguanine in mice showed only traces of radioactivity in brain after oral administration. No measurements have been made of thioguanine concentrations in human cerebrospinal fluid (CSF), but observations on tissue distribution in animals, together with the lack of CNS penetration by the closely related compound, mercaptopurine, suggest that thioguanine does not reach therapeutic concentrations in the CSF.

Monitoring of plasma levels of thioguanine during therapy is of questionable value. There is technical difficulty in determining plasma concentrations, which are seldom greater than 1 to 2 mcg/mL after a therapeutic oral dose. More significantly, thioguanine enters rapidly into the anabolic and catabolic pathways for purines, and the active intracellular metabolites have appreciably longer half-lives than the parent drug. The biochemical effects of a single dose of thioguanine are evident long after the parent drug has disappeared from plasma. Because of this rapid metabolism of thioguanine to active intracellular derivatives, hemodialysis would not be expected to appreciably reduce toxicity of the drug.

Thioguanine competes with hypoxanthine and guanine for the enzyme hypoxanthine-guanine phosphoribosyltransferase (HGPRTase) and is itself converted to 6-thioguanylic acid (TGMP). This nucleotide reaches high intracellular concentrations at therapeutic doses. TGMP interferes at several points with the synthesis of guanine nucleotides. It inhibits de novo purine biosynthesis by pseudo-feedback inhibition of glutamine-5-phosphoribosylpyrophosphate amidotransferase—the first enzyme unique to the de novo pathway for purine ribonucleotide synthesis. TGMP also inhibits the conversion of inosinic acid (IMP) to xanthylic acid (XMP) by competition for the enzyme IMP dehydrogenase. At one time TGMP was felt to be a significant inhibitor of ATP:GMP phosphotransferase (guanylate kinase), but recent results have shown this not to be so.

Thioguanylic acid is further converted to the di- and triphosphates, thioguanosine diphosphate (TGDP) and thioguanosine triphosphate (TGTP) (as well as their 2′-deoxyribosyl analogues) by the same enzymes which metabolize guanine nucleotides. Thioguanine nucleotides are incorporated into both the RNA and the DNA by phosphodiester linkages and it has been argued that incorporation of such fraudulent bases contributes to the cytotoxicity of thioguanine.

Thus, thioguanine has multiple metabolic effects and at present it is not possible to designate one major site of action. Its tumor inhibitory properties may be due to one or more of its effects on (a) feedback inhibition of de novo purine synthesis; (b) inhibition of purine nucleotide interconversions; or (c) incorporation into the DNA and the RNA. The net consequence of its actions is a sequential blockade of the synthesis and utilization of the purine nucleotides.

The catabolism of thioguanine and its metabolites is complex and shows significant differences between humans and the mouse. In both humans and mice, after oral administration of ^{35}S-6-thioguanine, urine contains virtually no detectable intact thioguanine. While deamination and subsequent oxidation to thiouric acid occurs only to a small extent in humans, it is the main pathway in mice. The product of deamination by guanase, 6-thioxanthine is inactive, having negligible antitumor activity. This pathway of thioguanine inactivation is not dependent on the action of xanthine oxidase, and an inhibitor of that enzyme (such as allopurinol) will not block the detoxification of thioguanine even though the inactive 6-thioxanthine is normally further oxidized by xanthine oxidase to thiouric acid before it is eliminated. In humans, methylation of thioguanine is much more extensive than in the mouse. The product of methylation, 2-amino-6-methylthiopurine, is also substantially less active and less toxic than thioguanine and its formation is likewise unaffected by the presence of allopurinol. Appreciable amounts of inorganic sulfate are also found in both murine and human urine, presumably arising from further metabolism of the methylated derivatives.

In some animal tumors, resistance to the effect of thioguanine correlates with the loss of HGPRTase activity and the resulting inability to convert thioguanine to thioguanylic acid. However, other resistance mechanisms, such as increased catabolism of TGMP by a nonspecific phosphatase, may be operative. Although not invariable, it is usual to find cross-resistance between thioguanine and its close analogue, PURINETHOL (mercaptopurine).

INDICATIONS AND USAGE

a) Acute Nonlymphocytic Leukemias: TABLOID brand Thioguanine is indicated for remission induction, remission consolidation, and maintenance therapy of acute nonlymphocytic leukemias. The response to this agent depends upon the age of the patient (younger patients faring better than older) and whether thioguanine is used in previously treated or previously untreated patients. Reliance upon thioguanine alone is seldom justified for initial remission induction of acute nonlymphocytic leukemias because combination chemotherapy including thioguanine results in more frequent remission induction and longer duration of remission than thioguanine alone.

b) Other Neoplasms: TABLOID brand Thioguanine is not effective in chronic lymphocytic leukemia, Hodgkin's lymphoma, multiple myeloma, or solid tumors. Although thioguanine is one of several agents with activity in the treatment of the chronic phase of chronic myelogenous leukemia, more objective responses are observed with MYLERAN® (busulfan), and therefore busulfan is usually regarded as the preferred drug.

CONTRAINDICATIONS

Thioguanine should not be used in patients whose disease has demonstrated prior resistance to this drug. In animals and humans, there is usually complete cross-resistance between PURINETHOL (mercaptopurine) and TABLOID brand Thioguanine.

WARNINGS

SINCE DRUGS USED IN CANCER CHEMOTHERAPY ARE POTENTIALLY HAZARDOUS, IT IS RECOMMENDED THAT ONLY PHYSICIANS EXPERIENCED WITH THE RISKS OF THIOGUANINE AND KNOWLEDGEABLE IN THE NATURAL HISTORY OF ACUTE NONLYMPHOCYTIC LEUKEMIAS ADMINISTER THIS DRUG.

The most consistent, dose-related toxicity is bone marrow suppression. This may be manifested by anemia, leukopenia, thrombocytopenia, or any combination of these. Any one of these findings may also reflect progression of the underlying disease. Since thioguanine may have a delayed effect, it is important to withdraw the medication temporarily at the first sign of an abnormally large fall in any of the formed elements of the blood.

There are individuals with an inherited deficiency of the enzyme thiopurine methyltransferase (TPMT) who may be unusually sensitive to the myelosuppressive effects of thioguanine and prone to developing rapid bone marrow suppression following the initiation of treatment. Substantial dosage reductions may be required to avoid the development of life-threatening bone marrow suppression in these patients. Prescribers should be aware that some laboratories offer testing for TPMT deficiency. Since bone marrow suppression may be associated with factors other than TPMT deficiency, TPMT testing may not identify all patients at risk for severe toxicity. Therefore, close monitoring of clinical and hematologic parameters is important. Bone marrow suppression could be exacerbated by coadministration with drugs that inhibit TPMT, such as olsalazine, mesalazine, or sulphasalazine.

It is recommended that evaluation of the hemoglobin concentration or hematocrit, total white blood cell count and differential count, and quantitative platelet count be obtained frequently while the patient is on thioguanine therapy. In cases where the cause of fluctuations in the formed elements in the peripheral blood is obscure, bone marrow examination may be useful for the evaluation of marrow status. The decision to increase, decrease, continue, or discontinue a given dosage of thioguanine must be based not only on the absolute hematologic values, but also upon the rapidity with which changes are occurring. In many instances, particularly during the induction phase of acute leukemia, complete blood counts will need to be done more frequently in order to evaluate the effect of the therapy. The dosage of thioguanine may need to be reduced when this agent is combined with other drugs whose primary toxicity is myelosuppression.

Myelosuppression is often unavoidable during the induction phase of adult acute nonlymphocytic leukemias if remission induction is to be successful. Whether or not this demands modification or cessation of dosage depends both upon the response of the underlying disease and a careful consideration of supportive facilities (granulocyte and platelet transfusions) which may be available. Life-threatening infections and bleeding have been observed as consequences of thioguanine-induced granulocytopenia and thrombocytopenia.

The effect of thioguanine on the immunocompetence of patients is unknown.

Pregnancy: Pregnancy Category D. Drugs such as thioguanine are potential mutagens and teratogens. Thioguanine may cause fetal harm when administered to a pregnant woman. Thioguanine has been shown to be teratogenic in rats when given in doses 5 times the human dose. When given to the rat on the 4th and 5th days of gestation, 13% of surviving placentas did not contain fetuses, and 19% of offspring were malformed or stunted. The malformations noted included generalized edema, cranial defects, and general skeletal hypoplasia, hydrocephalus, ventral hernia, situs inversus, and incomplete development of the limbs. There are no adequate and well-controlled studies in pregnant women. If this drug is used during pregnancy, or if the patient becomes pregnant while taking the drug, the patient should be apprised of the potential hazard to the fetus. Women of childbearing potential should be advised to avoid becoming pregnant.

PRECAUTIONS

General: Although the primary toxicity of thioguanine is myelosuppression, other toxicities have occasionally been observed, particularly when thioguanine is used in combination with other cancer chemotherapeutic agents.

A few cases of jaundice have been reported in patients with leukemia receiving thioguanine. Among these were 2 adult male patients and 4 pediatric patients with acute myelogenous leukemia and an adult male with acute lymphocytic leukemia who developed veno-occlusive hepatic disease while receiving chemotherapy for their leukemia. Six patients had received cytarabine prior to treatment with thioguanine, and some were receiving other chemotherapy in addition to thioguanine when they became symptomatic. While veno-occlusive hepatic disease has not been reported in patients treated with thioguanine alone, it is recommended that thioguanine be withheld if there is evidence of toxic hepatitis or biliary stasis, and that appropriate clinical and laboratory investigations be initiated to establish the etiology of the hepatic dysfunction. Deterioration in liver function studies during thioguanine therapy should prompt discontinuation of treatment and a search for an explanation of the hepatotoxicity.

Information for Patients: Patients should be informed that the major toxicities of thioguanine are related to myelosuppression, hepatotoxicity, and gastrointestinal toxicity. Patients should never be allowed to take the drug without medical supervision and should be advised to consult their physician if they experience fever, sore throat, jaundice, nausea, vomiting, signs of local infection, bleeding from any site, or symptoms suggestive of anemia. Women of childbearing potential should be advised to avoid becoming pregnant.

Laboratory Tests: Prescribers should be aware that some laboratories offer testing for TPMT deficiency (see WARNINGS).

It is advisable to monitor liver function tests (serum transaminases, alkaline phosphatase, bilirubin) at weekly intervals when first beginning therapy and at monthly intervals thereafter. It may be advisable to perform liver function tests more frequently in patients with known pre-existing liver disease or in patients who are receiving thioguanine and other hepatotoxic drugs. Patients should be instructed to discontinue thioguanine immediately if clinical jaundice is detected (see WARNINGS).

Drug Interactions: There is usually complete cross-resistance between PURINETHOL (mercaptopurine) and TABLOID brand Thioguanine.

In one study, 12 of approximately 330 patients receiving continuous busulfan and thioguanine therapy for treatment of chronic myelogenous leukemia were found to have esophageal varices associated with abnormal liver function tests. Subsequent liver biopsies were performed in 4 of these patients, all of which showed evidence of nodular regenerative hyperplasia. Duration of combination therapy prior to the appearance of esophageal varices ranged from 6 to 45 months. With the present analysis of the data, no cases of hepatotoxicity have appeared in the busulfan-alone arm of the study. Long-term continuous therapy with thioguanine and busulfan should be used with caution.

As there is in vitro evidence that aminosalicylate derivatives (e.g., olsalazine, mesalazine, or sulphasalazine) inhibit the TPMT enzyme, they should be administered with caution to patients receiving concurrent thioguanine therapy (see WARNINGS).

Carcinogenesis, Mutagenesis, Impairment of Fertility: In view of its action on cellular DNA, thioguanine is potentially mutagenic and carcinogenic, and consideration should be given to the theoretical risk of carcinogenesis when thioguanine is administered (see WARNINGS).

Pregnancy: ***Teratogenic Effects:*** Pregnancy Category D. See WARNINGS section.

Nursing Mothers: It is not known whether this drug is excreted in human milk. Because of the potential for tumorigenicity shown for thioguanine, a decision should be made whether to discontinue nursing or to discontinue the drug, taking into account the importance of the drug to the mother.

Pediatric Use: See DOSAGE AND ADMINISTRATION section.

Geriatric Use: Clinical studies of thioguanine did not include sufficient numbers of subjects aged 65 and over to determine whether they respond differently from younger subjects. Other reported clinical experience has not identified differences in responses between the elderly and younger patients. In general, dose selection for an elderly patient should be cautious, usually starting at the low end of the dosing range, reflecting the greater frequency of decreased hepatic, renal, or cardiac function, and of concomitant disease or other drug therapy.

ADVERSE REACTIONS

The most frequent adverse reaction to thioguanine is myelosuppression. The induction of complete remission of acute myelogenous leukemia usually requires combination chemotherapy in dosages which produce marrow hypoplasia. Since consolidation and maintenance of remission are also effected by multiple-drug regimens whose component agents cause myelosuppression, pancytopenia is observed in

Continued on next page

Product information on these pages is effective as of August 2004. Further information is available at: GlaxoSmithKline, PO Box 13398, Research Triangle Park, NC 27709. 1-888-825-5249. Corporate Web Site: www.gsk.com

Tabloid—Cont.

nearly all patients. Dosages and schedules must be adjusted to prevent life-threatening cytopenias whenever these adverse reactions are observed.

Hyperuricemia frequently occurs in patients receiving thioguanine as a consequence of rapid cell lysis accompanying the antineoplastic effect. Adverse effects can be minimized by increased hydration, urine alkalinization, and the prophylactic administration of a xanthine oxidase inhibitor such as ZYLOPRIM® (allopurinol). Unlike PURINETHOL (mercaptopurine) and IMURAN® (azathioprine), thioguanine may be continued in the usual dosage when allopurinol is used conjointly to inhibit uric acid formation.

Less frequent adverse reactions include nausea, vomiting, anorexia, and stomatitis. Intestinal necrosis and perforation have been reported in patients who received multiple-drug chemotherapy including thioguanine.

Hepatic Effects: Liver enzyme and other liver function studies are occasionally abnormal. If jaundice, hepatomegaly, or anorexia with tenderness in the right hypochondrium occurs, thioguanine should be withheld until the exact etiology can be determined. There have been reports of veno-occlusive liver disease occurring in patients who received combination chemotherapy including thioguanine. Esophageal varices have been reported in patients receiving continuous busulfan and thioguanine therapy for treatment of chronic myelogenous leukemia (see PRECAUTIONS: Drug Interactions).

OVERDOSAGE

Signs and symptoms of overdosage may be immediate, such as nausea, vomiting, malaise, hypotension, and diaphoresis; or delayed, such as myelosuppression and azotemia. It is not known whether thioguanine is dialyzable. Hemodialysis is thought to be of marginal use due to the rapid intracellular incorporation of thioguanine into active metabolites with long persistence. The oral LD_{50} of thioguanine was determined to be 823 mg/kg ± 50.73 mg/kg and 740 mg/kg ± 45.24 mg/kg for male and female rats, respectively. Symptoms of overdosage may occur after a single dose of as little as 2.0 to 3.0 mg/kg thioguanine. As much as 35 mg/kg has been given in a single oral dose with reversible myelosuppression observed. There is no known pharmacologic antagonist of thioguanine. The drug should be discontinued immediately if unintended toxicity occurs during treatment. Severe hematologic toxicity may require supportive therapy with platelet transfusions for bleeding, and granulocyte transfusions and antibiotics if sepsis is documented. If a patient is seen immediately following an accidental overdosage of the drug, it may be useful to induce emesis.

DOSAGE AND ADMINISTRATION

TABLOID brand Thioguanine is administered orally. The dosage which will be tolerated and effective varies according to the stage and type of neoplastic process being treated. Because the usual therapies for adult and pediatric acute nonlymphocytic leukemias involve the use of thioguanine with other agents in combination, physicians responsible for administering these therapies should be experienced in the use of cancer chemotherapy and in the chosen protocol.

There are individuals with an inherited deficiency of the enzyme thiopurine methyltransferase (TPMT) who may be unusually sensitive to the myelosuppressive effects of thioguanine and prone to developing rapid bone marrow suppression following the initiation of treatment. Substantial dosage reductions may be required to avoid the development of life-threatening bone marrow suppression in these patients (see WARNINGS). Prescribers should be aware that some laboratories offer testing for TPMT deficiency.

Ninety-six (59%) of 163 pediatric patients with previously untreated acute nonlymphocytic leukemia obtained complete remission with a multiple-drug protocol including thioguanine, prednisone, cytarabine, cyclophosphamide, and vincristine. Remission was maintained with daily thioguanine, 4-day pulses of cytarabine and cyclophosphamide, and a single dose of vincristine every 28 days. The median duration of remission was 11.5 months.

Fifty-three percent of previously untreated adults with acute nonlymphocytic leukemias attained remission following use of the combination of thioguanine and cytarabine according to a protocol developed at The Memorial Sloan-Kettering Cancer Center. A median duration of remission of 8.8 months was achieved with the multiple-drug maintenance regimen which included thioguanine.

On those occasions when single-agent chemotherapy with thioguanine may be appropriate, the usual initial dosage for pediatric patients and adults is approximately 2 mg/kg of body weight per day. If, after 4 weeks on this dosage, there is no clinical improvement and no leukocyte or platelet depression, the dosage may be cautiously increased to 3 mg/kg/day. The total daily dose may be given at one time.

The dosage of thioguanine used does not depend on whether or not the patient is receiving ZYLOPRIM (allopurinol); **this is in contradistinction to the dosage reduction which is mandatory when PURINETHOL (mercaptopurine) or IMURAN (azathioprine) is given simultaneously with allopurinol.**

Procedures for proper handling and disposal of anticancer drugs should be considered. Several guidelines on this subject have been published.[1-8]

There is no general agreement that all of the procedures recommended in the guidelines are necessary or appropriate.

HOW SUPPLIED

Greenish-yellow, scored tablets containing 40 mg thioguanine, imprinted with "WELLCOME" and "U3B" on each tablet; in bottles of 25 (NDC 0173-0880-25).

Store at 15° to 25°C (59° to 77°F) in a dry place.

REFERENCES

1. ONS Clinical Practice Committee. Cancer Chemotherapy Guidelines and Recommendations for Practice. Pittsburgh, PA: Oncology Nursing Society; 1999:32-41.
2. Recommendations for the safe handling of parenteral antineoplastic drugs. Washington, DC: Division of Safety, Clinical Center Pharmacy Department and Cancer Nursing Services, National Institutes of Health and Human Services, 1992, US Dept of Health and Human Services, Public Health Service publication NIH 92-2621.
3. AMA Council on Scientific Affairs. Guidelines for handling parenteral antineoplastics. *JAMA.* 1985;253:1590-1591.
4. National Study Commission on Cytotoxic Exposure. Recommendations for handling cytotoxic agents. 1987. Available from Louis P. Jeffrey, Chairman, National Study Commission on Cytotoxic Exposure. Massachusetts College of Pharmacy and Allied Health Sciences, 179 Longwood Avenue, Boston, MA 02115.
5. Clinical Oncological Society of Australia. Guidelines and recommendations for safe handling of antineoplastic agents. *Med J Australia.* 1983;1:426-428.
6. Jones RB, Frank R, Mass T. Safe handling of chemotherapeutic agents: a report from the Mount Sinai Medical Center. *CA-A Cancer J for Clin.* 1983;33:258-263.
7. American Society of Hospital Pharmacists. ASHP technical assistance bulletin on handling cytotoxic and hazardous drugs. *Am J Hosp Pharm.* 1990;47:1033-1049.
8. Controlling Occupational Exposure to Hazardous Drugs. (OSHA Work-Practice Guidelines.) *Am J Health-Syst Pharm.* 1996;53:1669-1685.

Manufactured by DSM Pharmaceuticals, Inc.
Greenville, NC 27834
for GlaxoSmithKline, Research Triangle Park, NC 27709

January 2004/RL-2063

Shown in Product Identification Guide, page 317

TAGAMET® ℞

[tag 'ə-met]
brand of
cimetidine tablets
cimetidine hydrochloride liquid
and cimetidine hydrochloride injection

DESCRIPTION

Tagamet (cimetidine) is a histamine H_2-receptor antagonist. Chemically it is *N''*-cyano- *N* -methyl-*N'*-[2-[[(5-methyl-1*H*-imidazol-4-yl) methyl] thio]-ethyl]-guanidine.

The empirical formula for cimetidine is $C_{10}H_{16}N_6S$ and for cimetidine hydrochloride, $C_{10}H_{16}N_6SHCl$; these represent molecular weights of 252.34 and 288.80, respectively.

Cimetidine contains an imidazole ring, and is chemically related to histamine.

(The liquid and injection dosage forms contain cimetidine as the hydrochloride.)

Cimetidine has a bitter taste and characteristic odor.

Solubility Characteristics: Cimetidine is soluble in alcohol, slightly soluble in water, very slightly soluble in chloroform and insoluble in ether. Cimetidine hydrochloride is freely soluble in water, soluble in alcohol, very slightly soluble in chloroform and practically insoluble in ether.

Tablets for Oral Administration: Each light green, film-coated tablet contains cimetidine as follows: 300 mg–round, debossed with the product name TAGAMET, SB and 300; 400 mg–oval Tiltab®, debossed with the product name TAGAMET, SB and 400; 800 mg–oval Tiltab® tablets, debossed with the product name TAGAMET, SB and 800. Inactive ingredients consist of cellulose, D&C Yellow No. 10, FD&C Blue No. 2, FD&C Red No. 40, FD&C Yellow No. 6, hydroxypropyl methylcellulose, iron oxides, magnesium stearate, povidone, propylene glycol, sodium lauryl sulfate, sodium starch glycolate, starch, titanium dioxide and trace amounts of other inactive ingredients.

Liquid for Oral Administration: Each 5 mL (1 teaspoonful) of clear, light orange, mint-peach flavored liquid contains cimetidine hydrochloride equivalent to cimetidine, 300 mg; alcohol, 2.8%. Inactive ingredients consist of FD&C Yellow No. 6, flavors, methylparaben, polyoxyethylene polyoxypropylene glycol, propylene glycol, propylparaben, saccharin sodium, sodium chloride, sodium phosphate, sorbitol and water.

Injection:

Single-Dose Vials for Intramuscular or Intravenous Administration: Each 2 mL contains, in sterile aqueous solution (pH range 3.8 to 6), cimetidine hydrochloride equivalent to cimetidine, 300 mg; phenol, 10 mg.

Multi-Dose Vials for Intramuscular or Intravenous Administration: 8 mL (300 mg/2 mL): Each 2 mL contains, in sterile aqueous solution (pH range 3.8 to 6), cimetidine hydrochloride equivalent to cimetidine, 300 mg; phenol, 10 mg.

Single-Dose Premixed Plastic Containers for Intravenous Administration: Each 50 mL of sterile aqueous solution (pH range 5 to 7) contains cimetidine hydrochloride equivalent to 300 mg cimetidine and 0.45 grams sodium chloride. No preservative has been added.

The plastic container is fabricated from specially formulated polyvinyl chloride. The amount of water that can permeate from inside the container into the overwrap is insufficient to affect the solution significantly. Solutions in contact with the plastic container can leach out certain of its chemical components in very small amounts within the expiration period, e.g., di 2-ethylhexyl phthalate (DEHP), up to 5 parts per million. However, the safety of the plastic has been confirmed in tests in animals according to the USP biological tests for plastic containers as well as by tissue culture toxicity studies.

ADD-Vantage®* Vials for Intravenous Administration: Each 2 mL contains, in sterile aqueous solution (pH range 3.8 to 6), cimetidine hydrochloride equivalent to cimetidine, 300 mg; phenol, 10 mg.

All of the above injection formulations are pyrogen free, and sodium hydroxide N.F. is used as an ingredient to adjust the pH.

*ADD-Vantage® is a trademark of Abbott Laboratories.

CLINICAL PHARMACOLOGY

Tagamet (cimetidine) competitively inhibits the action of histamine at the histamine H_2 receptors of the parietal cells and thus is a histamine H_2-receptor antagonist.

Tagamet is not an anticholinergic agent. Studies have shown that *Tagamet* inhibits both daytime and nocturnal basal gastric acid secretion. *Tagamet* also inhibits gastric acid secretion stimulated by food, histamine, pentagastrin, caffeine and insulin.

Antisecretory Activity

1) **Acid Secretion:** *Nocturnal: Tagamet* 800 mg orally at bedtime reduces mean hourly H^+ activity by greater than 85% over an 8-hour period in duodenal ulcer patients, with no effect on daytime acid secretion. *Tagamet* 1600 mg orally h.s. produces 100% inhibition of mean hourly H^+ activity over an 8-hour period in duodenal ulcer patients, but also reduces H^+ activity by 35% for an additional 5 hours into the following morning. *Tagamet* 400 mg b.i.d. and 300 mg q.i.d. decrease nocturnal acid secretion in a dose-related manner, i.e., 47% to 83% over a 6- to 8-hour period and 54% over a 9-hour period, respectively.

Food Stimulated: During the first hour after a standard experimental meal, oral *Tagamet* 300 mg inhibited gastric acid secretion in duodenal ulcer patients by at least 50%. During the subsequent 2 hours *Tagamet* inhibited gastric acid secretion by at least 75%.

The effect of a 300 mg breakfast dose of *Tagamet* continued for at least 4 hours and there was partial suppression of the rise in gastric acid secretion following the luncheon meal in duodenal ulcer patients. This suppression of gastric acid output was enhanced and could be maintained by another 300 mg dose of *Tagamet* given with lunch.

In another study, *Tagamet* 300 mg given with the meal increased gastric pH as compared with placebo.

	Mean Gastric pH	
	Tagamet	**Placebo**
1 hour	3.5	2.6
2 hours	3.1	1.6
3 hours	3.8	1.9
4 hours	6.1	2.2

24-Hour Mean H^+ Activity: *Tagamet* 800 mg h.s., 400 mg b.i.d. and 300 mg q.i.d. all provide a similar, moderate (less than 60%) level of 24-hour acid suppression. However, the 800 mg h.s. regimen exerts its entire effect on nocturnal acid, and does not affect daytime gastric physiology.

Chemically Stimulated: Oral Tagamet (cimetidine) significantly inhibited gastric acid secretion stimulated by betazole (an isomer of histamine), pentagastrin, caffeine and insulin as follows:

Stimulant	Stimulant Dose	*Tagamet*	% Inhibition
Betazole	1.5mg/kg (sc)	300mg (po)	85% at 2½ hours
Pentagastrin	6mcg/kg/hr (iv)	100mg/hr (iv)	60% at 1 hour
Caffeine	5mg/kg/hr (iv)	300mg (po)	100% at 1 hour
Insulin	0.03 units/kg/hr (iv)	100mg/hr (iv)	82% at 1 hour

When food and betazole were used to stimulate secretion, inhibition of hydrogen ion concentration usually ranged from 45% to 75% and the inhibition of volume ranged from 30% to 65%.

Parenteral administration also significantly inhibits gastric acid secretion. In a crossover study involving patients with active or healed duodenal or gastric ulcers, either continuous I.V. infusion of *Tagamet* 37.5 mg/hour (900 mg/day) or intermittent injection of *Tagamet* 300 mg q6h (1200 mg/day) maintained gastric pH above 4.0 for more than 50% of the time under steady-state conditions.

2) **Pepsin:** Oral *Tagamet* 300 mg reduced total pepsin output as a result of the decrease in volume of gastric juice.

3) **Intrinsic Factor:** Intrinsic factor secretion was studied with betazole as a stimulant. Oral *Tagamet* 300 mg inhib-

ited the rise in intrinsic factor concentration produced by betazole, but some intrinsic factor was secreted at all times.

Other

Lower Esophageal Sphincter Pressure and Gastric Emptying

Tagamet has no effect on lower esophageal sphincter (LES) pressure or the rate of gastric emptying.

Pharmacokinetics

Tagamet is rapidly absorbed after oral administration and peak levels occur in 45 to 90 minutes. The half-life of *Tagamet* is approximately 2 hours. Both oral and parenteral (I.V. or I.M.) administration provide comparable periods of therapeutically effective blood levels; blood concentrations remain above that required to provide 80% inhibition of basal gastric acid secretion for 4 to 5 hours following a dose of 300 mg.

Steady-state blood concentrations of cimetidine with continuous infusion of *Tagamet* are determined by the infusion rate and clearance of the drug in the individual patient. In a study of peptic ulcer patients with normal renal function, an infusion rate of 37.5 mg/hour produced average steady-state plasma cimetidine concentrations of about 0.9 mcg/mL. Blood levels with other infusion rates will vary in direct proportion to the infusion rate.

The principal route of excretion of *Tagamet* is the urine. Following parenteral administration, most of the drug is excreted as the parent compound; following oral administration, the drug is more extensively metabolized, the sulfoxide being the major metabolite. Following a single oral dose, 48% of the drug is recovered from the urine after 24 hours as the parent compound. Following I.V. or I.M. administration, approximately 75% of the drug is recovered from the urine after 24 hours as the parent compound.

CLINICAL TRIALS

Duodenal Ulcer

Tagamet (cimetidine) has been shown to be effective in the treatment of active duodenal ulcer and, at reduced dosage, in maintenance therapy following healing of active ulcers.

Active Duodenal Ulcer: *Tagamet* accelerates the rate of duodenal ulcer healing. Healing rates reported in U.S. and foreign controlled trials with *Tagamet* are summarized below, beginning with the regimen providing the lowest nocturnal dose.

Duodenal Ulcer Healing Rates with Various *Tagamet* Dosage Regimens*

Regimen	300 mg q.i.d.	400 mg b.i.d.	800 mg h.s.	1600 mg h.s.
week 4	68%	73%	80%	86%
week 6	80%	80%	89%	—
week 8	—	92%	94%	

* Averages from controlled clinical trials.

A U.S., double-blind, placebo-controlled, dose-ranging study demonstrated that all once-daily at bedtime (h.s.) *Tagamet* regimens were superior to placebo in ulcer healing and that *Tagamet* 800 mg h.s. healed 75% of patients at 4 weeks. The healing rate with 800 mg h.s. was significantly superior to 400 mg h.s. (66%) and not significantly different from 1600 mg h.s. (81%).

In the U.S. dose-ranging trial, over 80% of patients receiving *Tagamet* 800 mg h.s. experienced nocturnal pain relief after 1 day. Relief from daytime pain was reported in approximately 70% of patients after 2 days. As with ulcer healing, the 800 mg h.s. dose was superior to 400 mg h.s. and not different from 1600 mg h.s.

In foreign, double-blind studies with *Tagamet* 800 mg h.s., 79% to 85% of patients were healed at 4 weeks.

While short-term treatment with Tagamet (cimetidine) can result in complete healing of the duodenal ulcer, acute therapy will not prevent ulcer recurrence after *Tagamet* has been discontinued. Some follow-up studies have reported that the rate of recurrence once therapy was discontinued was slightly higher for patients healed on *Tagamet* than for patients healed on other forms of therapy; however, the *Tagamet*-treated patients generally had more severe disease.

Maintenance Therapy in Duodenal Ulcer: Treatment with a reduced dose of *Tagamet* has been proven effective as maintenance therapy following healing of active duodenal ulcers.

In numerous placebo-controlled studies conducted worldwide, the percent of patients with observed ulcers at the end of 1 year's therapy with *Tagamet* 400 mg h.s. was significantly lower (10% to 45%) than in patients receiving placebo (44% to 70%). Thus, from 55% to 90% of patients were maintained free of observed ulcers at the end of 1 year with *Tagamet* 400 mg h.s.

Factors such as smoking, duration and severity of disease, gender, and genetic traits may contribute to variations in actual percentages.

Trials of other anti-ulcer therapy, whether placebo-controlled, positive-controlled or open, have demonstrated a range of results similar to that seen with *Tagamet*.

Active Benign Gastric Ulcer

Tagamet has been shown to be effective in the short-term treatment of active benign gastric ulcer.

In a multicenter, double-blind U.S. study, patients with endoscopically confirmed benign gastric ulcer were treated with *Tagamet* 300 mg four times a day or with placebo for 6 weeks. Patients were limited to those with ulcers ranging from 0.5 to 2.5 cm in size. Endoscopically confirmed healing at 6 weeks was seen in significantly* more *Tagamet*-treated patients than in patients receiving placebo, as shown below:

	Tagamet	Placebo
week 2	14/63 (22%)	7/63 (11%)
total at week 6	43/65 (66%)*	30/67 (45%)

*$p<0.05$

In a similar multicenter U.S. study of the 800 mg h.s. oral regimen, the endoscopically confirmed healing rates were:

	Tagamet	Placebo
total at week 6	63/83 (76%)*	44/80 (55%)

*$p = 0.005$

Similarly, in worldwide double-blind clinical studies, endoscopically evaluated benign gastric ulcer healing rates were consistently higher with *Tagamet* than with placebo.

Gastroesophageal Reflux Disease

In two multicenter, double-blind, placebo-controlled studies in patients with gastroesophageal reflux disease (GERD) and endoscopically proven erosions and/or ulcers, *Tagamet* was significantly more effective than placebo in healing lesions. The endoscopically confirmed healing rates were:

Trial		*Tagamet* (800 mg b.i.d.)	*Tagamet* (400 mg q.i.d.)	Placebo	p-Value (800 mg b.i.d. vs. placebo)
1	Week 6	45%	52%	26%	0.02
	Week 12	60%	66%	42%	0.02
2	Week 6	50%		20%	<0.01
	Week 12	67%		36%	<0.01

In these trials *Tagamet* was superior to placebo by most measures in improving symptoms of day- and night-time heartburn, with many of the differences statistically significant. The q.i.d. regimen was generally somewhat better than the b.i.d. regimen where these were compared.

Prevention of Upper Gastrointestinal Bleeding in Critically Ill Patients

A double-blind, placebo-controlled randomized study of continuous infusion cimetidine was performed in 131 critically ill patients (mean APACHE II score = 15.99) to compare the incidence of upper gastrointestinal bleeding, manifested as hematemesis or bright red blood which did not clear after adjustment of the nasogastric tube and a 5 to 10 minute lavage, persistent Gastroccult® positive coffee grounds for 8 consecutive hours which did not clear with 100 cc lavage and/or which were accompanied by a drop in hematocrit of 5 percentage points, or melena, with an endoscopically documented upper gastrointestinal source of bleed. 14% (9/65) of patients treated with cimetidine continuous infusion developed bleeding compared to 33% (22/66) of the placebo group. Coffee grounds was the manifestation of bleeding that accounted for the difference between groups. Another randomized, double-blind placebo-controlled study confirmed these results for an end point of upper gastrointestinal bleeding with a confirmed upper gastrointestinal source noted on endoscopy, and by post hoc analyses of bleeding episodes between groups.

Pathological Hypersecretory Conditions

(such as Zollinger-Ellison Syndrome)

Tagamet significantly inhibited gastric acid secretion and reduced occurrence of diarrhea, anorexia and pain in patients with pathological hypersecretion associated with Zollinger-Ellison Syndrome, systemic mastocytosis and multiple endocrine adenomas. Use of *Tagamet* was also followed by healing of intractable ulcers.

INDICATIONS AND USAGE

Tagamet (cimetidine) is indicated in:

(1) Short-term treatment of active duodenal ulcer. Most patients heal within 4 weeks and there is rarely reason to use *Tagamet* at full dosage for longer than 6 to 8 weeks (see Dosage and Administration–Duodenal Ulcer). Concomitant antacids should be given as needed for relief of pain. However, simultaneous administration of *Tagamet* and antacids is not recommended, since antacids have been reported to interfere with the absorption of *Tagamet*.

(2) Maintenance therapy for duodenal ulcer patients at reduced dosage after healing of active ulcer. Patients have been maintained on continued treatment with *Tagamet* 400 mg h.s. for periods of up to 5 years.

(3) Short-term treatment of active benign gastric ulcer. There is no information concerning usefulness of treatment periods of longer than 8 weeks.

(4) Erosive gastroesophageal reflux disease (GERD). Erosive esophagitis diagnosed by endoscopy. Treatment is indicated for 12 weeks for healing of lesions and control of symptoms. The use of *Tagamet* beyond 12 weeks has not been established (see Dosage and Administration—GERD).

(5) Prevention of upper gastrointestinal bleeding in critically ill patients.

(6) The treatment of pathological hypersecretory conditions (i.e., Zollinger-Ellison Syndrome, systemic mastocytosis, multiple endocrine adenomas).

CONTRAINDICATIONS

Tagamet is contraindicated for patients known to have hypersensitivity to the product.

PRECAUTIONS

General: Rare instances of cardiac arrhythmias and hypotension have been reported following the rapid administration of Tagamet (cimetidine hydrochloride) Injection by intravenous bolus.

Symptomatic response to *Tagamet* therapy does not preclude the presence of a gastric malignancy. There have been rare reports of transient healing of gastric ulcers despite subsequently documented malignancy.

Reversible confusional states (see Adverse Reactions) have been observed on occasion, predominantly, but not exclusively, in severely ill patients. Advancing age (50 or more years) and preexisting liver and/or renal disease appear to be contributing factors. In some patients these confusional states have been mild and have not required discontinuation of *Tagamet* therapy. In cases where discontinuation was judged necessary, the condition usually cleared within 3 to 4 days of drug withdrawal.

Drug Interactions: *Tagamet,* apparently through an effect on certain microsomal enzyme systems, has been reported to reduce the hepatic metabolism of warfarin-type anticoagulants, phenytoin, propranolol, nifedipine, chlordiazepoxide, diazepam, certain tricyclic antidepressants, lidocaine, theophylline and metronidazole, thereby delaying elimination and increasing blood levels of these drugs.

Clinically significant effects have been reported with the warfarin anticoagulants; therefore, close monitoring of prothrombin time is recommended, and adjustment of the anticoagulant dose may be necessary when *Tagamet* is administered concomitantly. Interaction with phenytoin, lidocaine and theophylline has also been reported to produce adverse clinical effects.

However, a crossover study in healthy subjects receiving either *Tagamet* 300 mg q.i.d. or 800 mg h.s. concomitantly with a 300 mg b.i.d. dosage of theophylline (Theo-Dur®, Key Pharmaceuticals, Inc.) demonstrated less alteration in steady-state theophylline peak serum levels with the 800 mg h.s. regimen, particularly in subjects aged 54 years and older. Data beyond 10 days are not available. (Note: All patients receiving theophylline should be monitored appropriately, regardless of concomitant drug therapy.)

Dosage of the drugs mentioned above and other similarly metabolized drugs, particularly those of low therapeutic ratio or in patients with renal and/or hepatic impairment, may require adjustment when starting or stopping concomitantly administered *Tagamet* to maintain optimum therapeutic blood levels.

Alteration of pH may affect absorption of certain drugs (e.g., ketoconazole). If these products are needed, they should be given at least 2 hours before cimetidine administration.

Additional clinical experience may reveal other drugs affected by the concomitant administration of *Tagamet*.

Carcinogenesis, Mutagenesis, Impairment of Fertility: In a 24-month toxicity study conducted in rats, at dose levels of 150, 378 and 950 mg/kg/day (approximately 8 to 48 times the recommended human dose), there was a small increase in the incidence of benign Leydig cell tumors in each dose group; when the combined drug-treated groups and control groups were compared, this increase reached statistical significance. In a subsequent 24-month study, there were no differences between the rats receiving 150 mg/kg/day and the untreated controls. However, a statistically significant increase in benign Leydig cell tumor incidence was seen in the rats that received 378 and 950 mg/kg/day. These tumors were common in control groups as well as treated groups and the difference became apparent only in aged rats.

Tagamet (cimetidine) has demonstrated a weak antiandrogenic effect. In animal studies this was manifested as reduced prostate and seminal vesicle weights. However, there was no impairment of mating performance or fertility, nor any harm to the fetus in these animals at doses 8 to 48 times the full therapeutic dose of *Tagamet,* as compared with controls. The cases of gynecomastia seen in patients treated for 1 month or longer may be related to this effect.

In human studies, *Tagamet* has been shown to have no effect on spermatogenesis, sperm count, motility, morphology or *in vitro* fertilizing capacity.

Pregnancy: Teratogenic Effects. Pregnancy Category B: Reproduction studies have been performed in rats, rabbits and mice at doses up to 40 times the normal human dose and have revealed no evidence of impaired fertility or harm to the fetus due to *Tagamet*. There are, however, no adequate and well-controlled studies in pregnant women. Because animal reproductive studies are not always predictive of human response, this drug should be used during pregnancy only if clearly needed.

Nursing Mothers: Cimetidine is secreted in human milk and, as a general rule, nursing should not be undertaken while a patient is on a drug.

Pediatric Use: Clinical experience in children is limited. Therefore, *Tagamet* therapy cannot be recommended for

Continued on next page

Product information on these pages is effective as of August 2004. Further information is available at: GlaxoSmithKline, PO Box 13398, Research Triangle Park, NC 27709. 1-888-825-5249. Corporate Web Site: www.gsk.com

Tagamet—Cont.

children under 16, unless, in the judgment of the physician, anticipated benefits outweigh the potential risks. In very limited experience, doses of 20 to 40 mg/kg per day have been used.
Immunocompromised Patients: In immunocompromised patients, decreased gastric acidity, including that produced by acid-suppressing agents such as cimetidine, may increase the possibility of a hyperinfection of strongyloidiasis.

ADVERSE REACTIONS

Adverse effects reported in patients taking *Tagamet* are described below by body system. Incidence figures of 1 in 100 and greater are generally derived from controlled clinical studies.
Gastrointestinal: Diarrhea (usually mild) has been reported in approximately 1 in 100 patients.
CNS: Headaches, ranging from mild to severe, have been reported in 3.5% of 924 patients taking 1600 mg/day, 2.1% of 2,225 patients taking 800 mg/day and 2.3% of 1,897 patients taking placebo. Dizziness and somnolence (usually mild) have been reported in approximately 1 in 100 patients on either 1600 mg/day or 800 mg/day.
Reversible confusional states, e.g., mental confusion, agitation, psychosis, depression, anxiety, hallucinations, disorientation, have been reported predominantly, but not exclusively, in severely ill patients. They have usually developed within 2 to 3 days of initiation of *Tagamet* therapy and have cleared within 3 to 4 days of discontinuation of the drug.
Endocrine: Gynecomastia has been reported in patients treated for 1 month or longer. In patients being treated for pathological hypersecretory states, this occurred in about 4% of cases while in all others the incidence was 0.3% to 1% in various studies. No evidence of induced endocrine dysfunction was found, and the condition remained unchanged or returned toward normal with continuing Tagamet (cimetidine) treatment.
Reversible impotence has been reported in patients with pathological hypersecretory disorders, e.g., Zollinger-Ellison Syndrome, receiving *Tagamet*, particularly in high doses, for at least 12 months (range 12 to 79 months, mean 38 months). However, in large-scale surveillance studies at regular dosage, the incidence has not exceeded that commonly reported in the general population.
Hematologic: Decreased white blood cell counts in *Tagamet*-treated patients (approximately 1 per 100,000 patients), including agranulocytosis (approximately 3 per million patients), have been reported, including a few reports of recurrence on rechallenge. Most of these reports were in patients who had serious concomitant illnesses and received drugs and/or treatment known to produce neutropenia. Thrombocytopenia (approximately 3 per million patients) and, very rarely, cases of pancytopenia or aplastic anemia have also been reported. As with some other H_2-receptor antagonists, there have been extremely rare reports of immune hemolytic anemia.
Hepatobiliary: Dose-related increases in serum transaminase have been reported. In most cases they did not progress with continued therapy and returned to normal at the end of therapy. There have been rare reports of cholestatic or mixed cholestatic-hepatocellular effects. These were usually reversible. Because of the predominance of cholestatic features, severe parenchymal injury is considered highly unlikely. However, as in the occasional liver injury with other H_2-receptor antagonists, in exceedingly rare circumstances fatal outcomes have been reported.
There has been reported a single case of biopsy-proven periportal hepatic fibrosis in a patient receiving *Tagamet*.
Rare cases of pancreatitis, which cleared on withdrawal of the drug, have been reported.
Hypersensitivity: Rare cases of fever and allergic reactions including anaphylaxis and hypersensitivity vasculitis, which cleared on withdrawal of the drug, have been reported.
Renal: Small, possibly dose-related increases in plasma creatinine, presumably due to competition for renal tubular secretion, are not uncommon and do not signify deteriorating renal function. Rare cases of interstitial nephritis and urinary retention, which cleared on withdrawal of the drug, have been reported.
Cardiovascular: Rare cases of bradycardia, tachycardia and A-V heart block have been reported with H_2-receptor antagonists.
Musculoskeletal: There have been rare reports of reversible arthralgia and myalgia; exacerbation of joint symptoms in patients with preexisting arthritis has also been reported. Such symptoms have usually been alleviated by a reduction in Tagamet (cimetidine) dosage. Rare cases of polymyositis have been reported, but no causal relationship has been established.
Integumental: Mild rash and, very rarely, cases of severe generalized skin reactions including Stevens-Johnson syndrome, epidermal necrolysis, erythema multiforme, exfoliative dermatitis and generalized exfoliative erythroderma have been reported with H_2-receptor antagonists. Reversible alopecia has been reported very rarely.
Immune Function: There have been extremely rare reports of strongyloidiasis hyperinfection in immunocompromised patients.

OVERDOSAGE

Studies in animals indicate that toxic doses are associated with respiratory failure and tachycardia that may be controlled by assisted respiration and the administration of a beta-blocker.
Reported acute ingestions orally of up to 20 grams have been associated with transient adverse effects similar to those encountered in normal clinical experience. The usual measures to remove unabsorbed material from the gastrointestinal tract, clinical monitoring and supportive therapy should be employed.
There have been reports of severe CNS symptoms, including unresponsiveness, following ingestion of between 20 and 40 grams of cimetidine, and extremely rare reports following concomitant use of multiple CNS-active medications and ingestion of cimetidine at doses less than 20 grams. An elderly, terminally ill dehydrated patient with organic brain syndrome receiving concomitant antipsychotic agents and *Tagamet* 4800 mg intravenously over a 24-hour period experienced mental deterioration with reversal on *Tagamet* discontinuation.
There have been two deaths in adults who were reported to have ingested over 40 grams orally on a single occasion.

DOSAGE AND ADMINISTRATION

Duodenal Ulcer
Active Duodenal Ulcer: Clinical studies have indicated that suppression of nocturnal acid is the most important factor in duodenal ulcer healing (see Clinical Pharmacology–Acid Secretion). This is supported by recent clinical trials (see Clinical Trials–Active Duodenal Ulcer). Therefore, there is no apparent rationale, except for familiarity with use, for treating with anything other than a once-daily at bedtime dosage regimen (h.s.).
In a U.S. dose-ranging study of 400 mg h.s., 800 mg h.s. and 1600 mg h.s., a continuous dose response relationship for ulcer healing was demonstrated.
However, 800 mg h.s. is the dose of choice for most patients, as it provides a high healing rate (the difference between 800 mg h.s. and 1600 mg h.s. being small), maximal pain relief, a decreased potential for drug interactions (see Precautions–Drug Interactions) and maximal patient convenience. Patients unhealed at 4 weeks, or those with persistent symptoms, have been shown to benefit from 2 to 4 weeks of continued therapy.
It has been shown that patients who both have an endoscopically demonstrated ulcer larger than 1.0 cm and are also heavy smokers (i.e., smoke one pack of cigarettes or more per day) are more difficult to heal. There is some evidence which suggests that more rapid healing can be achieved in this subpopulation with *Tagamet* 1600 mg at bedtime. While early pain relief with either 800 mg h.s. or 1600 mg h.s. is equivalent in all patients, 1600 mg h.s. provides an appropriate alternative when it is important to ensure healing within 4 weeks for this subpopulation. Alternatively, approximately 94% of all patients will also heal in 8 weeks with *Tagamet* 800 mg h.s.
Other *Tagamet* regimens in the U.S. which have been shown to be effective are: 300 mg four times daily, with meals and at bedtime, the original regimen with which U.S. physicians have the most experience, and 400 mg twice daily, in the morning and at bedtime (see Clinical Trials–Active Duodenal Ulcer).
Concomitant antacids should be given as needed for relief of pain. However, simultaneous administration of *Tagamet* and antacids is not recommended, since antacids have been reported to interfere with the absorption of Tagamet (cimetidine).
While healing with *Tagamet* often occurs during the first week or two, treatment should be continued for 4 to 6 weeks unless healing has been demonstrated by endoscopic examination.
Maintenance Therapy for Duodenal Ulcer: In those patients requiring maintenance therapy, the recommended adult oral dose is 400 mg at bedtime.
Active Benign Gastric Ulcer
The recommended adult oral dosage for short-term treatment of active benign gastric ulcer is 800 mg h.s., or 300 mg four times a day with meals and at bedtime. Controlled clinical studies were limited to 6 weeks of treatment (see Clinical Trials). 800 mg h.s. is the preferred regimen for most patients based upon convenience and reduced potential for drug interactions. Symptomatic response to *Tagamet* does not preclude the presence of a gastric malignancy. It is important to follow gastric ulcer patients to assure rapid progress to complete healing.
Erosive Gastroesophageal Reflux Disease (GERD)
The recommended adult oral dosage for the treatment of erosive esophagitis that has been diagnosed by endoscopy is 1600 mg daily in divided doses (800 mg b.i.d. or 400 mg q.i.d.) for 12 weeks. The use of *Tagamet* beyond 12 weeks has not been established.
Prevention of Upper Gastrointestinal Bleeding
The recommended adult dosing regimen is continuous I.V. infusion of 50 mg/hour. Patients with creatinine clearance less than 30 cc/min. should receive half the recommended dose. Treatment beyond 7 days has not been studied.
Pathological Hypersecretory Conditions
(such as Zollinger-Ellison Syndrome)
Recommended adult oral dosage: 300 mg four times a day with meals and at bedtime. In some patients it may be necessary to administer higher doses more frequently. Doses should be adjusted to individual patient needs, but should not usually exceed 2400 mg per day and should continue as long as clinically indicated.
Parenteral Administration
In hospitalized patients with pathological hypersecretory conditions or intractable ulcers, or in patients who are unable to take oral medication, *Tagamet* may be administered parenterally.
The doses and regimen for parenteral administration in patients with GERD have not been established.
All parenteral drug products should be inspected visually for particulate matter and discoloration prior to administration.
Recommendations for parenteral administration:
Intramuscular injection: 300 mg q 6 to 8 hours (no dilution necessary). Transient pain at the site of injection has been reported.
Intravenous injection: 300 mg q 6 to 8 hours. In some patients it may be necessary to increase dosage. When this is necessary, the increases should be made by more frequent administration of a 300 mg dose, but should not exceed 2400 mg per day. Dilute Tagamet (cimetidine hydrochloride) Injection, 300 mg, in Sodium Chloride Injection (0.9%) or another compatible I.V. solution (see Stability of *Tagamet* Injection) to a total volume of 20 mL and inject over a period of not less than 5 minutes (see Precautions).
Intermittent intravenous infusion: 300 mg q 6 to 8 hours, infused over 15 to 20 minutes. In some patients it may be necessary to increase dosage. When this is necessary, the increases should be made by more frequent administration of a 300 mg dose, but should not exceed 2400 mg per day.
Vials: Dilute *Tagamet* Injection, 300 mg, in at least 50 mL of 5% Dextrose Injection, or another compatible I.V. solution (see Stability of *Tagamet* Injection). **Plastic containers:** Use premixed *Tagamet* Injection, 300 mg, in 0.9% Sodium Chloride in 50 mL plastic containers. **ADD-Vantage® Vials:** Dilute contents of one vial in an ADD-Vantage® Diluent Container, available in 50 mL and 100 mL sizes of 0.9% Sodium Chloride Injection, and 5% Dextrose Injection.
Continuous intravenous infusion: 37.5 mg/hour (900 mg/day). For patients requiring a more rapid elevation of gastric pH, continuous infusion may be preceded by a 150 mg loading dose administered by I.V. infusion as described above. Dilute 900 mg *Tagamet* Injection in a compatible I.V. fluid (see Stability of *Tagamet* Injection) for constant rate infusion over a 24-hour period. Note: *Tagamet* may be diluted in 100 to 1000 mL; however, a volumetric pump is recommended if the volume for 24-hour infusion is less than 250 mL. In one study in patients with pathological hypersecretory states, the mean infused dose of cimetidine was 160 mg/hour with a range of 40 to 600 mg/hour.
These doses maintained the intragastric acid secretory rate at 10 mEq/hour or less. The infusion rate should be adjusted to individual patient requirements.
DIRECTIONS FOR USE OF TAGAMET (cimetidine hydrochloride) INJECTION IN PLASTIC CONTAINERS
To open: Tear overwrap down side at slit and remove solution containers.
Some opacity of the plastic due to moisture absorption during the sterilization process may be observed. This is normal and does not affect solution quality or safety. The opacity will diminish gradually.
Do not add other drugs to premixed *Tagamet* Injection in plastic containers.
CAUTION: Check for minute leaks by squeezing inner bag firmly. If leaks are found, discard solution as sterility may be impaired. Additives should not be introduced into this solution. Do not use if the solution is cloudy or precipitated or if the seal is not intact.
Do not use plastic containers in series connections. Such use could result in air embolism due to residual air being drawn from the primary container before administration of the fluid from the secondary container is complete.
Use sterile equipment.
Preparation for administration:
1. Suspend container from eyelet support.
2. Remove plastic protector from outlet port at bottom of container.
3. Attach administration set. Refer to complete directions accompanying set.

DIRECTIONS FOR USE OF TAGAMET® INJECTION IN ADD-VANTAGE® VIALS are enclosed in ADD-Vantage® Vial packaging.
Stability of *Tagamet* Injection
When added to or diluted with most commonly used intravenous solutions, e.g., Sodium Chloride Injection (0.9%), Dextrose Injection (5% or 10%), Lactated Ringer's Solution, 5% Sodium Bicarbonate Injection, Tagamet (cimetidine hydrochloride) Injection should not be used after more than 48 hours of storage at room temperature.
Tagamet Injection premixed in plastic containers is stable through the labeled expiration date when stored under the recommended conditions.
Dosage Adjustment for Patients with Impaired Renal Function
Patients with severely impaired renal function have been treated with *Tagamet*. However, such usage has been very limited. On the basis of this experience the recommended dosage is 300 mg q 12 hours orally or by intravenous injection. Should the patient's condition require, the frequency of dosing may be increased to q 8 hours or even further with caution. In severe renal failure, accumulation may occur and the lowest frequency of dosing compatible with an adequate patient response should be used. When liver impairment is also present, further reductions in dosage may be necessary. Hemodialysis reduces the level of circulating *Tagamet*. Ideally, the dosage schedule should be adjusted so that the timing of a scheduled dose coincides with the end of hemodialysis.
Patients with creatinine clearance less than 30 cc/min. who are being treated for prevention of upper gastrointestinal bleeding should receive half the recommended dose.

HOW SUPPLIED

Tablets: Light green, film-coated as follows: 300 mg–round, debossed with the product name TAGAMET, SB and 300–tablets in bottles of 100; 400 mg–oval-shaped Tiltab®, debossed with the product name TAGAMET, SB and 400–tablets in bottles of 60; 800 mg–oval-shaped Tiltab®, debossed with the product name TAGAMET, SB and 800–tablets in bottles of 30.

Store between 15° and 30°C (59° and 86°F); dispense in a tight light-resistant container.

300 mg 100's: NDC 0108-5013-20
400 mg 60's: NDC 0108-5026-18
800 mg 30's: NDC 0108-5027-13

GlaxoSmithKline, Research Triangle Park, NC 27709

June 2002/TG:L93

Shown in Product Identification Guide, page 317

TEMOVATE® ℞
[*tim'ō-vāt*]
(clobetasol propionate cream)
Cream, 0.05%
TEMOVATE® ℞
(clobetasol propionate ointment)
Ointment, 0.05%

FOR TOPICAL DERMATOLOGIC USE ONLY—NOT FOR OPHTHALMIC, ORAL, OR INTRAVAGINAL USE

DESCRIPTION

TEMOVATE (clobetasol propionate cream and ointment) Cream and Ointment contain the active compound clobetasol propionate, a synthetic corticosteroid, for topical dermatologic use. Clobetasol, an analog of prednisolone, has a high degree of glucocorticoid activity and a slight degree of mineralocorticoid activity.

Chemically, clobetasol propionate is (11β,16β)-21-chloro-9-fluoro-11-hydroxy-16-methyl-17-(1-oxopropoxy)-pregna-1,4-diene-3,20-dione.

Clobetasol propionate has the empirical formula $C_{25}H_{32}ClFO_5$ and a molecular weight of 467. It is a white to cream-colored crystalline powder insoluble in water.

TEMOVATE Cream contains clobetasol propionate 0.5 mg/g in a cream base of propylene glycol, glyceryl monostearate, cetostearyl alcohol, glyceryl stearate, PEG 100 stearate, white wax, chlorocresol, sodium citrate, citric acid monohydrate, and purified water.

TEMOVATE Ointment contains clobetasol propionate 0.5 mg/g in a base of propylene glycol, sorbitan sesquioleate, and white petrolatum.

CLINICAL PHARMACOLOGY

Like other topical corticosteroids, clobetasol propionate has anti-inflammatory, antipruritic, and vasoconstrictive properties. The mechanism of the anti-inflammatory activity of the topical steroids, in general, is unclear. However, corticosteroids are thought to act by the induction of phospholipase A_2 inhibitory proteins, collectively called lipocortins. It is postulated that these proteins control the biosynthesis of potent mediators of inflammation such as prostaglandins and leukotrienes by inhibiting the release of their common precursor, arachidonic acid. Arachidonic acid is released from membrane phospholipids by phospholipase A_2.

Pharmacokinetics: The extent of percutaneous absorption of topical corticosteroids is determined by many factors, including the vehicle and the integrity of the epidermal barrier. Occlusive dressing with hydrocortisone for up to 24 hours has not been demonstrated to increase penetration; however, occlusion of hydrocortisone for 96 hours markedly enhances penetration. Topical corticosteroids can be absorbed from normal intact skin. Inflammation and/or other disease processes in the skin may increase percutaneous absorption.

Studies performed with TEMOVATE Cream and Ointment indicate that they are in the super-high range of potency as compared with other topical corticosteroids.

INDICATIONS AND USAGE

TEMOVATE Cream and Ointment are super-high potency corticosteroid formulations indicated for the relief of the inflammatory and pruritic manifestations of corticosteroid-responsive dermatoses. Treatment beyond 2 consecutive weeks is not recommended, and the total dosage should not exceed 50 g/week because of the potential for the drug to suppress the hypothalamic-pituitary-adrenal (HPA) axis. Use in pediatric patients under 12 years of age is not recommended.

As with other highly active corticosteroids, therapy should be discontinued when control has been achieved. If no improvement is seen within 2 weeks, reassessment of the diagnosis may be necessary.

CONTRAINDICATIONS

TEMOVATE Cream and Ointment are contraindicated in those patients with a history of hypersensitivity to any of the components of the preparations.

PRECAUTIONS

General: TEMOVATE Cream and Ointment should not be used in the treatment of rosacea or perioral dermatitis, and should not be used on the face, groin, or axillae.

Systemic absorption of topical corticosteroids can produce reversible HPA axis suppression with the potential for glucocorticosteroid insufficiency after withdrawal from treatment. Manifestations of Cushing syndrome, hyperglycemia, and glucosuria can also be produced in some patients by systemic absorption of topical corticosteroids while on therapy.

Patients applying a topical steroid to a large surface area or to areas under occlusion should be evaluated periodically for evidence of HPA axis suppression. This may be done by using the ACTH stimulation, A.M. plasma cortisol, and urinary free cortisol tests. Patients receiving super-potent corticosteroids should not be treated for more than 2 weeks at a time, and only small areas should be treated at any one time due to the increased risk of HPA suppression.

TEMOVATE Cream and Ointment produced HPA axis suppression when used at doses as low as 2 g/day for 1 week in patients with eczema.

If HPA axis suppression is noted, an attempt should be made to withdraw the drug, to reduce the frequency of application, or to substitute a less potent corticosteroid. Recovery of HPA axis function is generally prompt upon discontinuation of topical corticosteroids. Infrequently, signs and symptoms of glucocorticosteroid insufficiency may occur that require supplemental systemic corticosteroids. For information on systemic supplementation, see prescribing information for those products.

Pediatric patients may be more susceptible to systemic toxicity from equivalent doses due to their larger skin surface to body mass ratios (see PRECAUTIONS: Pediatric Use).

If irritation develops, TEMOVATE Cream and Ointment should be discontinued and appropriate therapy instituted. Allergic contact dermatitis with corticosteroids is usually diagnosed by observing a *failure to heal* rather than noting a clinical exacerbation as with most topical products not containing corticosteroids. Such an observation should be corroborated with appropriate diagnostic patch testing.

If concomitant skin infections are present or develop, an appropriate antifungal or antibacterial agent should be used. If a favorable response does not occur promptly, use of TEMOVATE Cream and Ointment should be discontinued until the infection has been adequately controlled.

Information for Patients: Patients using topical corticosteroids should receive the following information and instructions:

1. This medication is to be used as directed by the physician. It is for external use only. Avoid contact with the eyes.
2. This medication should not be used for any disorder other than that for which it was prescribed.
3. The treated skin area should not be bandaged, otherwise covered, or wrapped so as to be occlusive unless directed by the physician.
4. Patients should report any signs of local adverse reactions to the physician.

Laboratory Tests: The following tests may be helpful in evaluating patients for HPA axis suppression:
ACTH stimulation test
A.M. plasma cortisol test
Urinary free cortisol test

Carcinogenesis, Mutagenesis, Impairment of Fertility: Long-term animal studies have not been performed to evaluate the carcinogenic potential of clobetasol propionate.

Studies in the rat following subcutaneous administration at dosage levels up to 50 mcg/kg/day revealed that the females exhibited an increase in the number of resorbed embryos and a decrease in the number of living fetuses at the highest dose.

Clobetasol propionate was nonmutagenic in 3 different test systems: the Ames test, the *Saccharomyces cerevisiae* gene conversion assay, and the *E. coli* B WP2 fluctuation test.

Pregnancy: ***Teratogenic Effects:*** Pregnancy Category C. Corticosteroids have been shown to be teratogenic in laboratory animals when administered systemically at relatively low dosage levels. Some corticosteroids have been shown to be teratogenic after dermal application to laboratory animals.

Clobetasol propionate has not been tested for teratogenicity when applied topically; however, it is absorbed percutaneously, and when administered subcutaneously it was a significant teratogen in both the rabbit and mouse. Clobetasol propionate has greater teratogenic potential than steroids that are less potent.

Teratogenicity studies in mice using the subcutaneous route resulted in fetotoxicity at the highest dose tested (1 mg/kg) and teratogenicity at all dose levels tested down to 0.03 mg/kg. These doses are approximately 1.4 and 0.04 times, respectively, the human topical dose of TEMOVATE Cream and Ointment. Abnormalities seen included cleft palate and skeletal abnormalities.

In rabbits, clobetasol propionate was teratogenic at doses of 3 and 10 mcg/kg. These doses are approximately 0.02 and 0.05 times, respectively, the human topical dose of TEMOVATE Cream and Ointment. Abnormalities seen included cleft palate, cranioschisis, and other skeletal abnormalities.

There are no adequate and well-controlled studies of the teratogenic potential of clobetasol propionate in pregnant women. TEMOVATE Cream and Ointment should be used during pregnancy only if the potential benefit justifies the potential risk to the fetus.

Nursing Mothers: Systemically administered corticosteroids appear in human milk and could suppress growth, interfere with endogenous corticosteroid production, or cause other untoward effects. It is not known whether topical administration of corticosteroids could result in sufficient systemic absorption to produce detectable quantities in human milk. Because many drugs are excreted in human milk, caution should be exercised when TEMOVATE Cream or Ointment is administered to a nursing woman.

Pediatric Use: Safety and effectiveness of TEMOVATE Cream and Ointment in pediatric patients have not been established. Use in pediatric patients under 12 years of age is not recommended. Because of a higher ratio of skin surface area to body mass, pediatric patients are at a greater risk than adults of HPA axis suppression and Cushing syndrome when they are treated with topical corticosteroids. They are therefore also at greater risk of adrenal insufficiency during or after withdrawal of treatment. Adverse effects including striae have been reported with inappropriate use of topical corticosteroids in infants and children.

HPA axis suppression, Cushing syndrome, linear growth retardation, delayed weight gain, and intracranial hypertension have been reported in children receiving topical corticosteroids. Manifestations of adrenal suppression in children include low plasma cortisol levels and an absence of response to ACTH stimulation. Manifestations of intracranial hypertension include bulging fontanelles, headaches, and bilateral papilledema.

Geriatric Use: A limited number of patients at or above 65 years of age have been treated with TEMOVATE Cream (n = 231) and with TEMOVATE Ointment (n = 101) in US and non-US clinical trials. While the number of patients is too small to permit separate analysis of efficacy and safety, the adverse reactions reported in this population were similar to those reported by younger patients. Based on available data, no adjustment of dosage of TEMOVATE Cream and Ointment in geriatric patients is warranted.

ADVERSE REACTIONS

In controlled clinical trials, the most frequent adverse reactions reported for TEMOVATE Cream were burning and stinging sensation in 1% of treated patients. Less frequent adverse reactions were itching, skin atrophy, and cracking and fissuring of the skin.

In controlled clinical trials, the most frequent adverse events reported for TEMOVATE Ointment were burning sensation, irritation, and itching in 0.5% of treated patients. Less frequent adverse reactions were stinging, cracking, erythema, folliculitis, numbness of fingers, skin atrophy, and telangiectasia.

Cushing syndrome has been reported in infants and adults as a result of prolonged use of topical clobetasol propionate formulations.

The following additional local adverse reactions have been reported with topical corticosteroids, and they may occur more frequently with the use of occlusive dressings and higher potency corticosteroids. These reactions are listed in an approximately decreasing order of occurrence: dryness, acneiform eruptions, hypopigmentation, perioral dermatitis, allergic contact dermatitis, secondary infection, irritation, striae, and miliaria.

OVERDOSAGE

Topically applied TEMOVATE Cream and Ointment can be absorbed in sufficient amounts to produce systemic effects (see PRECAUTIONS).

DOSAGE AND ADMINISTRATION

Apply a thin layer of TEMOVATE Cream or Ointment to the affected skin areas twice daily and rub in gently and completely (see **INDICATIONS AND USAGE**).

TEMOVATE Cream and Ointment are super-high potency topical corticosteroids; therefore, **treatment should be limited to 2 consecutive weeks and amounts greater than 50 g/week should not be used.**

As with other highly active corticosteroids, therapy should be discontinued when control has been achieved. If no improvement is seen within 2 weeks, reassessment of diagnosis may be necessary.

TEMOVATE Cream and Ointment should not be used with occlusive dressings.

Geriatric Use: In studies where geriatric patients (65 years of age or older, see PRECAUTIONS) have been treated with TEMOVATE Cream or Ointment, safety did not differ from that in younger patients; therefore, no dosage adjustment is recommended.

HOW SUPPLIED

TEMOVATE Cream, 0.05% is supplied in:
15-g tubes (NDC 0173-0375-73),
30-g tubes (NDC 0173-0375-72),
45-g tubes (NDC 0173-0375-01), and
60-g tubes (NDC 0173-0375-02).

TEMOVATE Ointment, 0.05% is supplied in:
15-g tubes (NDC 0173-0376-73),
30-g tubes (NDC 0173-0376-72),
45-g tubes (NDC 0173-0376-01), and
60-g tubes (NDC 0173-0376-02).

Store between 15° and 30°C (59° and 86°F). TEMOVATE Cream should not be refrigerated.

GlaxoSmithKline Consumer Healthcare LP,
Pittsburgh, PA 15230

Continued on next page

Product information on these pages is effective as of August 2004. Further information is available at: GlaxoSmithKline, PO Box 13398, Research Triangle Park, NC 27709. 1-888-825-5249. Corporate Web Site: www.gsk.com

Temovate Cream/Ointment—Cont.

August 2002/RL-1085
Shown in Product Identification Guide, page 317

TEMOVATE® ℞

[tim'ō-vāt]
(clobetasol propionate gel)
Gel, 0.05%

FOR TOPICAL DERMATOLOGIC USE ONLY— NOT FOR OPHTHALMIC, ORAL, OR INTRAVAGINAL USE

DESCRIPTION

TEMOVATE (clobetasol propionate gel) Gel contains the active compound clobetasol propionate, a synthetic corticosteroid, for topical dermatologic use. Clobetasol, an analog of prednisolone, has a high degree of glucocorticoid activity and a slight degree of mineralocorticoid activity.
Chemically, clobetasol propionate is (11β,16β)-21-chloro-9-fluoro-11-hydroxy-16-methyl-17-(1-oxopropoxy)-pregna-1,4-diene-3,20-dione.
Clobetasol propionate has the empirical formula $C_{25}H_{32}ClFO_5$ and a molecular weight of 467. It is a white to cream-colored crystalline powder insoluble in water.
TEMOVATE Gel contains clobetasol propionate 0.5 mg/g in a base of propylene glycol, carbomer 934P, sodium hydroxide, and purified water.

CLINICAL PHARMACOLOGY

Like other topical corticosteroids, clobetasol propionate has anti-inflammatory, antipruritic, and vasoconstrictive properties. The mechanism of the anti-inflammatory activity of the topical steroids, in general, is unclear. However, corticosteroids are thought to act by the induction of phospholipase A_2 inhibitory proteins, collectively called lipocortins. It is postulated that these proteins control the biosynthesis of potent mediators of inflammation such as prostaglandins and leukotrienes by inhibiting the release of their common precursor, arachidonic acid. Arachidonic acid is released from membrane phospholipids by phospholipase A_2.
Pharmacokinetics: The extent of percutaneous absorption of topical corticosteroids is determined by many factors, including the vehicle and the integrity of the epidermal barrier. Occlusive dressing with hydrocortisone for up to 24 hours has not been demonstrated to increase penetration; however, occlusion of hydrocortisone for 96 hours markedly enhances penetration. Topical corticosteroids can be absorbed from normal intact skin. Inflammation and/or other disease processes in the skin may increase percutaneous absorption. Greater absorption was observed for the TEMOVATE gel formulation as compared to the cream formulation in in vitro human skin penetration studies.
Studies performed with TEMOVATE Gel indicate that it is in the super-high range of potency as compared with other topical corticosteroids.

INDICATIONS AND USAGE

TEMOVATE Gel is a super-high potency corticosteroid formulation indicated for the relief of the inflammatory and pruritic manifestations of corticosteroid-responsive dermatoses. Treatment beyond 2 consecutive weeks is not recommended, and the total dosage should not exceed 50 g/week because of the potential for the drug to suppress the hypothalamic-pituitary-adrenal (HPA) axis. Use in pediatric patients under 12 years of age is not recommended.

CONTRAINDICATIONS

TEMOVATE Gel is contraindicated in those patients with a history of hypersensitivity to any of the components of the preparation.

PRECAUTIONS

General: Clobetasol propionate is a highly potent topical corticosteroid that has been shown to suppress the HPA axis at doses as low as 2 g/day.
Systemic absorption of topical corticosteroids can produce reversible HPA axis suppression with the potential for glucocorticosteroid insufficiency after withdrawal from treatment. Manifestations of Cushing syndrome, hyperglycemia, and glucosuria can also be produced in some patients by systemic absorption of topical corticosteroids while on therapy.
Patients applying a topical steroid to a large surface area or to areas under occlusion should be evaluated periodically for evidence of HPA axis suppression. This may be done by using the ACTH stimulation, A.M. plasma cortisol, and urinary free cortisol tests. Patients receiving super-potent corticosteroids should not be treated for more than 2 weeks at a time, and only small areas should be treated at any one time due to the increased risk of HPA suppression.
If HPA axis suppression is noted, an attempt should be made to withdraw the drug, to reduce the frequency of application, or to substitute a less potent corticosteroid. Recovery of HPA axis function is generally prompt and complete upon discontinuation of topical corticosteroids. Infrequently, signs and symptoms of glucocorticosteroid insufficiency may occur that require supplemental systemic corticosteroids. For information on systemic supplementation, see prescribing information for those products.
Pediatric patients may be more susceptible to systemic toxicity from equivalent doses due to their larger skin surface to body mass ratios (see PRECAUTIONS: Pediatric Use).
If irritation develops, TEMOVATE Gel should be discontinued and appropriate therapy instituted. Allergic contact dermatitis with corticosteroids is usually diagnosed by observing a *failure to heal* rather than noting a clinical exacerbation as with most topical products not containing corticosteroids. Such an observation should be corroborated with appropriate diagnostic patch testing.
If concomitant skin infections are present or develop, an appropriate antifungal or antibacterial agent should be used. If a favorable response does not occur promptly, use of TEMOVATE Gel should be discontinued until the infection has been adequately controlled.
TEMOVATE Gel should not be used in the treatment of rosacea or perioral dermatitis, and should not be used on the face, groin, or axillae.
Information for Patients: Patients using topical corticosteroids should receive the following information and instructions:

1. This medication is to be used as directed by the physician. It is for external use only. Avoid contact with the eyes.
2. This medication should not be used for any disorder other than that for which it was prescribed.
3. The treated skin area should not be bandaged, otherwise covered, or wrapped so as to be occlusive unless directed by the physician.
4. Patients should report any signs of local adverse reactions to the physician.
5. Patients should inform their physicians that they are using TEMOVATE if surgery is contemplated.

Laboratory Tests: The following tests may be helpful in evaluating patients for HPA axis suppression:
ACTH stimulation test
A.M. plasma cortisol test
Urinary free cortisol test
Carcinogenesis, Mutagenesis, Impairment of Fertility: Long-term animal studies have not been performed to evaluate the carcinogenic potential of clobetasol propionate.
Studies in the rat following subcutaneous administration at dosage levels up to 50 mcg/kg/day revealed that the females exhibited an increase in the number of resorbed embryos and a decrease in the number of living fetuses at the highest dose.
Clobetasol propionate was nonmutagenic in 3 different test systems: the Ames test, the *Saccharomyces cerevisiae* gene conversion assay, and the *E. coli* B WP2 fluctuation test.
Pregnancy: *Teratogenic Effects:* Pregnancy Category C. Corticosteroids have been shown to be teratogenic in laboratory animals when administered systemically at relatively low dosage levels. Some corticosteroids have been shown to be teratogenic after dermal application to laboratory animals.
Clobetasol propionate has not been tested for teratogenicity when applied topically; however, it is absorbed percutaneously, and when administered subcutaneously it was a significant teratogen in both the rabbit and mouse. Clobetasol propionate has greater teratogenic potential than steroids that are less potent.
Teratogenicity studies in mice using the subcutaneous route resulted in fetotoxicity at the highest dose tested (1 mg/kg) and teratogenicity at all dose levels tested down to 0.03 mg/kg. These doses are approximately 1.4 and 0.04 times, respectively, the human topical dose of TEMOVATE Gel. Abnormalities seen included cleft palate and skeletal abnormalities.
In rabbits, clobetasol propionate was teratogenic at doses of 3 and 10 mcg/kg. These doses are approximately 0.02 and 0.05 times, respectively, the human topical dose of TEMOVATE Gel. Abnormalities seen included cleft palate, cranioschisis, and other skeletal abnormalities.
There are no adequate and well-controlled studies of the teratogenic potential of clobetasol propionate in pregnant women. TEMOVATE Gel should be used during pregnancy only if the potential benefit justifies the potential risk to the fetus.
Nursing Mothers: Systemically administered corticosteroids appear in human milk and could suppress growth, interfere with endogenous corticosteroid production, or cause other untoward effects. It is not known whether topical administration of corticosteroids could result in sufficient systemic absorption to produce detectable quantities in human milk. Because many drugs are excreted in human milk, caution should be exercised when TEMOVATE Gel is administered to a nursing woman.
Pediatric Use: Safety and effectiveness of TEMOVATE Gel in children and infants have not been established; therefore, use in children under 12 years of age is not recommended. Because of a higher ratio of skin surface area to body mass, children are at a greater risk than adults of HPA axis suppression when they are treated with topical corticosteroids. They are therefore also at greater risk of adrenal insufficiency after withdrawal of treatment and of Cushing syndrome while on treatment. Adverse effects including striae have been reported with inappropriate use of topical corticosteroids in infants and children (see PRECAUTIONS).
HPA axis suppression, Cushing syndrome, and intracranial hypertension have been reported in children receiving topical corticosteroids. Manifestations of adrenal suppression in children include linear growth retardation, delayed weight gain, low plasma cortisol levels, and absence of response to ACTH stimulation. Manifestations of intracranial hypertension include bulging fontanelles, headaches, and bilateral papilledema.
Geriatric Use: A limited number of patients at or above 65 years of age (n = 37) have been treated with TEMOVATE Gel in US clinical trials. The number of patients is too small to permit separate analysis of efficacy and safety, and no adverse events were reported in geriatric patients. Based on available data, no adjustment of dosage of TEMOVATE Gel in geriatric patients is warranted.

ADVERSE REACTIONS

In a controlled trial with TEMOVATE Gel, the only reported adverse reaction that was considered to be drug related was a report of burning sensation (1.8% of treated patients).
In larger controlled clinical trials with other clobetasol propionate formulations, the most frequently reported adverse reactions have included burning, stinging, irritation, pruritus, erythema, folliculitis, cracking and fissuring of the skin, numbness of fingers, skin atrophy, and telangiectasia (all less than 2%).
Cushing syndrome has been reported in infants and adults as a result of prolonged use of topical clobetasol propionate formulations.
The following additional local adverse reactions are reported infrequently with topical corticosteroids, but may occur more frequently with super-high potency corticosteroids such as TEMOVATE Gel. These reactions are listed in approximate decreasing order of occurrence: dryness, hypertrichosis, acneiform eruptions, hypopigmentation, perioral dermatitis, allergic contact dermatitis, secondary infection, irritation, striae, and miliaria.

OVERDOSAGE

Topically applied TEMOVATE Gel can be absorbed in sufficient amounts to produce systemic effects (see PRECAUTIONS).

DOSAGE AND ADMINISTRATION

Apply a thin layer of TEMOVATE Gel to the affected skin areas twice daily and rub in gently and completely (see INDICATIONS AND USAGE).
TEMOVATE Gel is a super-high potency topical corticosteroid; therefore, **treatment should be limited to 2 consecutive weeks and amounts greater than 50 g/week should not be used.**
As with other highly active corticosteroids, therapy should be discontinued when control has been achieved. If no improvement is seen within 2 weeks, reassessment of diagnosis may be necessary.
TEMOVATE Gel should not be used with occlusive dressings.
Geriatric Use: In studies where geriatric patients (65 years of age or older, see PRECAUTIONS) have been treated with TEMOVATE Gel, safety did not differ from that in younger patients; therefore, no dosage adjustment is recommended.

HOW SUPPLIED

TEMOVATE Gel, 0.05% is supplied in:
15-g tubes (NDC 0173-0455-01),
30-g tubes (NDC 0173-0455-02), and
60-g tubes (NDC 0173-0455-03)
Store between 2° and 30°C (36° and 86°F).
GlaxoSmithKline Consumer Healthcare LP, Pittsburgh, PA 15230

April 2002/RL-1087
Shown in Product Identification Guide, page 317

TEMOVATE® ℞

[tim' ō-vāt]
(clobetasol propionate scalp application)
Scalp Application, 0.05%

FOR TOPICAL DERMATOLOGIC USE ONLY— NOT FOR OPHTHALMIC, ORAL, OR INTRAVAGINAL USE

DESCRIPTION

TEMOVATE (clobetasol propionate scalp application) Scalp Application contains the active compound clobetasol propionate, a synthetic corticosteroid, for topical dermatologic use. Clobetasol, an analog of prednisolone, has a high degree of glucocorticoid activity and a slight degree of mineralocorticoid activity.
Chemically, clobetasol propionate is (11β, 16β)-21-chloro-9-fluoro-11-hydroxy-16-methyl-17-(1-oxopropoxy)pregna-1,4-diene-3,20-dione.
Clobetasol propionate has the empirical formula $C_{25}H_{32}ClFO_5$ and a molecular weight of 467. It is a white to cream-colored crystalline powder insoluble in water.
TEMOVATE Scalp Application contains clobetasol propionate 0.5 mg/g in a base of purified water, isopropyl alcohol (39.3%), carbomer 934P, and sodium hydroxide.

CLINICAL PHARMACOLOGY

The corticosteroids are a class of compounds comprising steroid hormones secreted by the adrenal cortex and their synthetic analogs. In pharmacologic doses, corticosteroids are used primarily for their anti-inflammatory and/or immunosuppressive effects. Topical corticosteroids such as clobetasol propionate are effective in the treatment of corticosteroid-responsive dermatoses primarily because of their anti-inflammatory, antipruritic, and vasoconstrictive actions. However, while the physiologic, pharmacologic, and

clinical effects of the corticosteroids are well known, the exact mechanisms of their actions in each disease are uncertain.
Clobetasol propionate, a corticosteroid, has been shown to have topical (dermatologic) and systemic pharmacologic and metabolic effects characteristic of this class of drugs.
Pharmacokinetics: The extent of percutaneous absorption of topical corticosteroids, including clobetasol propionate, is determined by many factors, including the vehicle, the integrity of the epidermal barrier, and the use of occlusive dressings (see DOSAGE AND ADMINISTRATION).
As with all topical corticosteroids, clobetasol propionate can be absorbed from normal intact skin. Inflammation and/or other disease processes in the skin may increase percutaneous absorption. Occlusive dressings substantially increase the percutaneous absorption of topical corticosteroids (see DOSAGE AND ADMINISTRATION).
Once absorbed through the skin, topical corticosteroids enter pharmacokinetic pathways similarly to systemically administered corticosteroids. Corticosteroids are bound to plasma proteins in varying degrees. Corticosteroids are metabolized primarily in the liver and are then excreted by the kidneys. Some of the topical corticosteroids, including clobetasol propionate and its metabolites, are also excreted into the bile.
Following repeated nonocclusive application in the treatment of scalp psoriasis, there is some evidence that TEMOVATE Scalp Application has the potential to depress plasma cortisol levels in some patients. However, hypothalamic-pituitary-adrenal (HPA) axis effects produced by systemically absorbed clobetasol propionate have been shown to be transient and reversible upon completion of a 2-week course of treatment.

INDICATIONS AND USAGE

TEMOVATE Scalp Application is indicated for short-term topical treatment of inflammatory and pruritic manifestations of moderate to severe corticosteroid-responsive dermatoses of the scalp. Treatment beyond 2 consecutive weeks is not recommended, and the total dosage should not exceed 50 mL/week because of the potential for the drug to suppress the HPA axis.
This product is not recommended for use in pediatric patients under 12 years of age.

CONTRAINDICATIONS

TEMOVATE Scalp Application is contraindicated in patients with primary infections of the scalp, or in patients who are hypersensitive to clobetasol propionate, other corticosteroids, or any ingredient in this preparation.

PRECAUTIONS

General: Clobetasol propionate is a highly potent topical corticosteroid that has been shown to suppress the HPA axis at doses as low as 2 g (of ointment) per day. Systemic absorption of topical corticosteroids has resulted in reversible HPA axis suppression, manifestations of Cushing syndrome, hyperglycemia, and glucosuria in some patients.
Conditions that augment systemic absorption include the application of the more potent corticosteroids, use over large surface areas, prolonged use, and the addition of occlusive dressings. Therefore, patients receiving a large dose of a potent topical steroid applied to a large surface area should be evaluated periodically for evidence of HPA axis suppression by using the urinary free cortisol and ACTH stimulation tests. If HPA axis suppression is noted, an attempt should be made to withdraw the drug, to reduce the frequency of application, or to substitute a less potent steroid.
Recovery of HPA axis function is generally prompt and complete upon discontinuation of the drug. Infrequently, signs and symptoms of steroid withdrawal may occur, requiring supplemental systemic corticosteroids.
Pediatric patients may absorb proportionally larger amounts of topical corticosteroids and thus be more susceptible to systemic toxicity (see PRECAUTIONS: Pediatric Use).
If irritation develops, topical corticosteroids should be discontinued and appropriate therapy instituted. Irritation is possible if TEMOVATE Scalp Application contacts the eye. If that should occur, immediate flushing of the eye with a large volume of water is recommended.
If the inflammatory lesion becomes infected, the use of an appropriate antifungal or antibacterial agent should be instituted. If a favorable response does not occur promptly, the corticosteroid should be discontinued until the infection has been adequately controlled.
Although TEMOVATE Scalp Application is intended for the treatment of inflammatory conditions of the scalp, it should be noted that certain areas of the body, such as the face, groin, and axillae, are more prone to atrophic changes than other areas of the body following treatment with corticosteroids. Frequent observation of the patient is important if these areas are to be treated.
As with other potent topical corticosteroids, TEMOVATE Scalp Application should not be used in the treatment of rosacea and perioral dermatitis. Topical corticosteroids in general should not be used in the treatment of acne or as sole therapy in widespread plaque psoriasis.
Information for Patients: Patients using TEMOVATE Scalp Application should receive the following information and instructions:

1. This medication is to be used as directed by the physician and should not be used longer than the prescribed time period. It is for external use only. Avoid contact with the eyes.
2. This medication should not be used for any disorder other than that for which it was prescribed.
3. The treated skin area should not be bandaged or otherwise covered or wrapped so as to be occlusive.
4. Patients should report any signs of local adverse reactions to the physician.

Laboratory Tests: The following tests may be helpful in evaluating patients for HPA axis suppression:
Urinary free cortisol test
ACTH stimulation test
Carcinogenesis, Mutagenesis, Impairment of Fertility: Long-term animal studies have not been performed to evaluate the carcinogenic potential of clobetasol propionate.
Studies in the rat following subcutaneous administration at dosage levels up to 50 mcg/kg/day revealed that the females exhibited an increase in the number of resorbed embryos and a decrease in the number of living fetuses at the highest dose.
Clobetasol propionate was nonmutagenic in 3 different test systems: the Ames test, the *Saccharomyces cerevisiae* gene conversion assay, and the *E. coli* B WP2 fluctuation test.
Pregnancy: *Teratogenic Effects:* Pregnancy Category C. Corticosteroids have been shown to be teratogenic in laboratory animals when administered systemically at relatively low dosage levels. Some corticosteroids have been shown to be teratogenic after dermal application to laboratory animals.
Clobetasol propionate has not been tested for teratogenicity when applied topically; however, it is absorbed percutaneously, and when administered subcutaneously it was a significant teratogen in both the rabbit and mouse. Clobetasol propionate has greater teratogenic potential than steroids that are less potent.
Teratogenicity studies in mice using the subcutaneous route resulted in fetotoxicity at the highest dose tested (1 mg/kg) and teratogenicity at all dose levels tested down to 0.03 mg/kg. These doses are approximately 1.4 and 0.04 times, respectively, the human topical dose of TEMOVATE Scalp Application. Abnormalities seen included cleft palate and skeletal abnormalities.
In rabbits, clobetasol propionate was teratogenic at doses of 3 and 10 mcg/kg. These doses are approximately 0.02 and 0.05 times, respectively, the human topical dose of TEMOVATE Scalp Application. Abnormalities seen included cleft palate, cranioschisis, and other skeletal abnormalities.
There are no adequate and well-controlled studies of the teratogenic potential of clobetasol propionate in pregnant women. TEMOVATE Scalp Application should be used during pregnancy only if the potential benefit justifies the potential risk to the fetus.
Nursing Mothers: Systemically administered corticosteroids appear in human milk and could suppress growth, interfere with endogenous corticosteroid production, or cause other untoward effects. It is not known whether topical administration of corticosteroids could result in sufficient systemic absorption to produce detectable quantities in human milk. Because many drugs are excreted in human milk, caution should be exercised when TEMOVATE Scalp Application is administered to a nursing woman.
Pediatric Use: Use of TEMOVATE Scalp Application in pediatric patients under 12 years of age is not recommended. **Pediatric patients may demonstrate greater susceptibility to topical corticosteroid-induced HPA axis suppression and Cushing syndrome than mature patients because of a larger skin surface area to body weight ratio.**
HPA axis suppression, Cushing syndrome, linear growth retardation, delayed weight gain, and intracranial hypertension have been reported in children receiving topical corticosteroids. Manifestations of adrenal suppression in children include low plasma cortisol levels and an absence of response to ACTH stimulation. Manifestations of intracranial hypertension include bulging fontanelles, headaches, and bilateral papilledema.
Geriatric Use: A limited number of patients at or above 65 years of age (n = 65) have been treated with TEMOVATE Scalp Application in US and non-US clinical trials. While the number of patients is too small to permit separate analysis of efficacy and safety, the adverse reactions reported in this population were similar to those reported by younger patients. Based on available data, no adjustment of dosage of TEMOVATE Scalp Application in geriatric patients is warranted.

ADVERSE REACTIONS

TEMOVATE Scalp Application is generally well tolerated when used for 2-week treatment periods.
The most frequent adverse events reported for TEMOVATE Scalp Application have been local and have included burning and/or stinging sensation, which occurred in 29 of 294 patients; scalp pustules, which occurred in 3 of 294 patients; and tingling and folliculitis, each of which occurred in 2 of 294 patients. Less frequent adverse events were itching and tightness of the scalp, dermatitis, tenderness, headache, hair loss, and eye irritation, each of which occurred in 1 of 294 patients.
The following local adverse reactions are reported infrequently when topical corticosteroids are used as recommended. These reactions are listed in an approximately decreasing order of occurrence: burning, itching, irritation, dryness, folliculitis, hypertrichosis, acneiform eruptions, hypopigmentation, perioral dermatitis, allergic contact dermatitis, maceration of the skin, secondary infection, skin atrophy, striae, and miliaria. Systemic absorption of topical corticosteroids has produced reversible HPA axis suppression, manifestations of Cushing syndrome, hyperglycemia, and glucosuria in some patients. In rare instances, treatment (or withdrawal of treatment) of psoriasis with corticosteroids is thought to have exacerbated the disease or provoked the pustular form of the disease, so careful patient supervision is recommended.

OVERDOSAGE

Topically applied TEMOVATE Scalp Application can be absorbed in sufficient amounts to produce systemic effects (see PRECAUTIONS).

DOSAGE AND ADMINISTRATION

TEMOVATE Scalp Application should be applied to the affected scalp areas twice daily, once in the morning and once at night.
TEMOVATE Scalp Application is potent; therefore, **treatment must be limited to 2 consecutive weeks and amounts greater than 50 mL/week should not be used.**
TEMOVATE Scalp Application is not to be used with occlusive dressings.
Geriatric Use: In studies where geriatric patients (65 years of age or older, see PRECAUTIONS) have been treated with TEMOVATE Scalp Application, safety did not differ from that in younger patients; therefore, no dosage adjustment is recommended.

HOW SUPPLIED

TEMOVATE Scalp Application, 0.05% is supplied in plastic squeeze bottles, 25 mL (NDC 0173-0432-00) and 50 mL (NDC 0173-0432-01).
Store between 4° and 25°C (39° and 77°F). Do not use near an open flame.
GlaxoSmithKline Consumer Healthcare LP, Pittsburgh, PA 15230

April 2002/RL-1088
Shown in Product Identification Guide, page 317

TEMOVATE E® ℞

[tim'ō-vāt]
(clobetasol propionate emollient cream)
Emollient, 0.05%

FOR TOPICAL DERMATOLOGIC USE ONLY—NOT FOR OPHTHALMIC, ORAL, OR INTRAVAGINAL USE

DESCRIPTION

TEMOVATE E (clobetasol propionate emollient cream) Emollient contains the active compound clobetasol propionate, a synthetic corticosteroid, for topical dermatologic use. Clobetasol, an analog of prednisolone, has a high degree of glucocorticoid activity and a slight degree of mineralocorticoid activity.
Chemically, clobetasol propionate is (11β,16β)-21-chloro-9-fluoro-11-hydroxy-16-methyl-17-(1-oxopropoxy)-pregna-1,4-diene-3,20-dione.
Clobetasol propionate has the empirical formula $C_{25}H_{32}ClFO_5$ and a molecular weight of 467. It is a white to cream-colored crystalline powder insoluble in water.
TEMOVATE E Emollient contains clobetasol propionate 0.5 mg/g in an emollient base of cetostearyl alcohol, isopropyl myristate, propylene glycol, cetomacrogol 1000, dimethicone 360, citric acid, sodium citrate, purified water, and imidurea as a preservative.

CLINICAL PHARMACOLOGY

Like other topical corticosteroids, clobetasol propionate has anti-inflammatory, antipruritic, and vasoconstrictive properties. The mechanism of the anti-inflammatory activity of the topical steroids, in general, is unclear. However, corticosteroids are thought to act by the induction of phospholipase A_2 inhibitory proteins, collectively called lipocortins. It is postulated that these proteins control the biosynthesis of potent mediators of inflammation such as prostaglandins and leukotrienes by inhibiting the release of their common precursor, arachidonic acid. Arachidonic acid is released from membrane phospholipids by phospholipase A_2.
Pharmacokinetics: The extent of percutaneous absorption of topical corticosteroids is determined by many factors, including the vehicle and the integrity of the epidermal barrier. Occlusive dressing with hydrocortisone for up to 24 hours has not been demonstrated to increase penetration; however, occlusion of hydrocortisone for 96 hours markedly enhances penetration. Topical corticosteroids can be absorbed from normal intact skin. Inflammation and/or other disease processes in the skin may increase percutaneous absorption.
Studies performed with TEMOVATE E Emollient indicate that it is in the super-high range of potency as compared with other topical corticosteroids.

Continued on next page

Product information on these pages is effective as of August 2004. Further information is available at: GlaxoSmithKline, PO Box 13398, Research Triangle Park, NC 27709. 1-888-825-5249. Corporate Web Site: www.gsk.com

Temovate E—Cont.

INDICATIONS AND USAGE

TEMOVATE E Emollient is a super-high potency corticosteroid formulation indicated for the relief of the inflammatory and pruritic manifestations of corticosteroid-responsive dermatoses. Treatment beyond 2 consecutive weeks is not recommended, and the total dosage should not exceed 50 g/week because of the potential for the drug to suppress the hypothalamic-pituitary-adrenal (HPA) axis. Use in pediatric patients under 12 years of age is not recommended. In the treatment of moderate to severe plaque-type psoriasis, TEMOVATE E Emollient applied to 5% to 10% of body surface area can be used up to 4 consecutive weeks. The total dosage should not exceed 50 g/week. When dosing for more than 2 weeks, any additional benefits of extending treatment should be weighed against the risk of HPA suppression. Treatment beyond 4 consecutive weeks is not recommended. Patients should be instructed to use TEMOVATE E Emollient for the minimum amount of time necessary to achieve the desired results (see PRECAUTIONS and INDICATIONS AND USAGE). Use in pediatric patients under 16 years of age has not been studied.

CONTRAINDICATIONS

TEMOVATE E Emollient is contraindicated in those patients with a history of hypersensitivity to any of the components of the preparation.

PRECAUTIONS

General: Clobetasol propionate is a highly potent topical corticosteroid that has been shown to suppress the HPA axis at doses as low as 2 g/day.

Systemic absorption of topical corticosteroids can produce reversible HPA axis suppression with the potential for glucocorticosteroid insufficiency after withdrawal from treatment. Manifestations of Cushing syndrome, hyperglycemia, and glucosuria can also be produced in some patients by systemic absorption of topical corticosteroids while on therapy.

Patients applying a topical steroid to a large surface area or to areas under occlusion should be evaluated periodically for evidence of HPA axis suppression. This may be done by using the ACTH stimulation, A.M. plasma cortisol, and urinary free cortisol tests. Patients receiving super-potent corticosteroids should not be treated for more than 2 weeks at a time, and only small areas should be treated at any one time due to the increased risk of HPA suppression.

In a controlled clinical trial involving patients with moderate to severe plaque-type psoriasis, TEMOVATE E Emollient applied to 5% to 10% of body surface area resulted in additional benefits in the treatment of patients for 4 consecutive weeks. In this trial, there were no clobetasol-treated patients with clinically significant decreases in morning cortisol levels after 4 weeks of treatment; however, morning cortisol levels may not identify patients with adrenal dysfunction. Therefore, the additional benefits of extending treatment beyond 2 weeks should be weighed against the potential for HPA suppression. Therapy should be discontinued when control has been achieved. Treatment beyond 4 consecutive weeks is not recommended.

If HPA axis suppression is noted, an attempt should be made to withdraw the drug, to reduce the frequency of application, or to substitute a less potent corticosteroid. Recovery of HPA axis function is generally prompt upon discontinuation of topical corticosteroids. Infrequently, signs and symptoms of glucocorticosteroid insufficiency may occur that require supplemental systemic corticosteroids. For information on systemic supplementation, see prescribing information for those products.

Pediatric patients may be more susceptible to systemic toxicity from equivalent doses due to their larger skin surface to body mass ratios (see PRECAUTIONS: Pediatric Use). The use of TEMOVATE E Emollient, for 4 consecutive weeks has not been studied in pediatric patients under 16 years of age.

If irritation develops, TEMOVATE E Emollient should be discontinued and appropriate therapy instituted. Allergic contact dermatitis with corticosteroids is usually diagnosed by observing a *failure to heal* rather than noting a clinical exacerbation as with most topical products not containing corticosteroids. Such an observation should be corroborated with appropriate diagnostic patch testing.

If concomitant skin infections are present or develop, an appropriate antifungal or antibacterial agent should be used. If a favorable response does not occur promptly, use of TEMOVATE E Emollient should be discontinued until the infection has been adequately controlled.

TEMOVATE E Emollient should not be used in the treatment of rosacea or perioral dermatitis, and should not be used on the face, groin, or axillae.

Information for Patients: Patients using topical corticosteroids should receive the following information and instructions:

1. This medication is to be used as directed by the physician. It is for external use only. Avoid contact with the eyes.
2. This medication should not be used for any disorder other than that for which it was prescribed.
3. The treated skin area should not be bandaged, otherwise covered, or wrapped so as to be occlusive unless directed by the physician.
4. Patients should report any signs of local adverse reactions to the physician.
5. Patients should inform their physicians that they are using TEMOVATE if surgery is contemplated.
6. This medication should not be used on the face, underarms, or groin areas.
7. As with other corticosteroids, therapy should be discontinued when control has been achieved. If no improvement is seen within 2 weeks, contact the physician.

Laboratory Tests: The following tests may be helpful in evaluating patients for HPA axis suppression:

ACTH stimulation test
A.M. plasma cortisol test
Urinary free cortisol test

Carcinogenesis, Mutagenesis, Impairment of Fertility: Long-term animal studies have not been performed to evaluate the carcinogenic potential of clobetasol propionate.

Studies in the rat following subcutaneous administration at dosage levels up to 50 mcg/kg/day revealed that the females exhibited an increase in the number of resorbed embryos and a decrease in the number of living fetuses at the highest dose.

Clobetasol propionate was nonmutagenic in 3 different test systems: the Ames test, the *Saccharomyces cerevisiae* gene conversion assay, and the *E. coli* B WP2 fluctuation test.

Pregnancy: ***Teratogenic Effects:*** Pregnancy Category C. Corticosteroids have been shown to be teratogenic in laboratory animals when administered systemically at relatively low dosage levels. Some corticosteroids have been shown to be teratogenic after dermal application to laboratory animals.

Clobetasol propionate has not been tested for teratogenicity when applied topically; however, it is absorbed percutaneously, and when administered subcutaneously it was a significant teratogen in both the rabbit and mouse. Clobetasol propionate has greater teratogenic potential than steroids that are less potent.

Teratogenicity studies in mice using the subcutaneous route resulted in fetotoxicity at the highest dose tested (1 mg/kg) and teratogenicity at all dose levels tested down to 0.03 mg/kg. These doses are approximately 1.4 and 0.04 times, respectively, the human topical dose of TEMOVATE E Emollient. Abnormalities seen included cleft palate and skeletal abnormalities.

In rabbits, clobetasol propionate was teratogenic at doses of 3 and 10 mcg/kg. These doses are approximately 0.02 and 0.05 times, respectively, the human topical dose of TEMOVATE E Emollient. Abnormalities seen included cleft palate, cranioschisis, and other skeletal abnormalities.

There are no adequate and well-controlled studies of the teratogenic potential of clobetasol propionate in pregnant women. TEMOVATE E Emollient should be used during pregnancy only if the potential benefit justifies the potential risk to the fetus.

Nursing Mothers: Systemically administered corticosteroids appear in human milk and could suppress growth, interfere with endogenous corticosteroid production, or cause other untoward effects. It is not known whether topical administration of corticosteroids could result in sufficient systemic absorption to produce detectable quantities in human milk. Because many drugs are excreted in human milk, caution should be exercised when TEMOVATE E Emollient is administered to a nursing woman.

Pediatric Use: Safety and effectiveness of TEMOVATE E Emollient in pediatric patients have not been established. Use in pediatric patients under 12 years of age is not recommended. For continued use beyond 2 consecutive weeks, the safety of TEMOVATE E Emollient has not been studied. Because of a higher ratio of skin surface area to body mass, pediatric patients are at a greater risk than adults of HPA axis suppression and Cushing syndrome when they are treated with topical corticosteroids. They are therefore also at greater risk of adrenal insufficiency during or after withdrawal of treatment. Adverse effects including striae have been reported with inappropriate use of topical corticosteroids in infants and children.

HPA axis suppression, Cushing syndrome, linear growth retardation, delayed weight gain, and intracranial hypertension have been reported in children receiving topical corticosteroids. Manifestations of adrenal suppression in children include low plasma cortisol levels and absence of response to ACTH stimulation. Manifestations of intracranial hypertension include bulging fontanelles, headaches, and bilateral papilledema.

Geriatric Use: A limited number of patients at or above 65 years of age (n = 34) have been treated with TEMOVATE E Emollient in US clinical trials. While the number of patients is too small to permit separate analysis of efficacy and safety, the single adverse reaction reported in this population was similar to those reactions reported by younger patients. Based on available data, no adjustment of dosage of TEMOVATE E Emollient in geriatric patients is warranted.

ADVERSE REACTIONS

In controlled trials with all clobetasol propionate formulations, the following adverse reactions have been reported: burning/stinging, pruritus, irritation, erythema, folliculitis, cracking and fissuring of the skin, numbness of the fingers, tenderness in the elbow, skin atrophy, and telangiectasia. The incidence of local adverse reactions reported in the trials with TEMOVATE E Emollient was <2% of patients treated with the exception of burning/stinging, which occurred in 5% of treated patients.

Cushing syndrome has been reported in infants and adults as a result of prolonged use of other topical clobetasol propionate formulations.

The following additional local adverse reactions are reported infrequently with topical corticosteroids, but may occur more frequently with super-high potency corticosteroids such as TEMOVATE E Emollient. These reactions are listed in an approximately decreasing order of occurrence: dryness, hypertrichosis, acneiform eruptions, hypopigmentation, perioral dermatitis, allergic contact dermatitis, secondary infection, striae, and miliaria.

OVERDOSAGE

Topically applied TEMOVATE E Emollient can be absorbed in sufficient amounts to produce systemic effects (see PRECAUTIONS).

DOSAGE AND ADMINISTRATION

Apply a thin layer of TEMOVATE E Emollient to the affected skin areas twice daily and rub in gently and completely (see INDICATIONS AND USAGE).

TEMOVATE E Emollient is a super-high potency topical corticosteroid; therefore, **treatment should be limited to 2 consecutive weeks and amounts greater than 50 g/week should not be used.**

In moderate to severe plaque-type psoriasis, TEMOVATE E Emollient applied to 5% to 10% of body surface area can be used up to 4 weeks. The total dosage should not exceed 50 g/week. When dosing for more than 2 weeks, any additional benefits of extending treatment should be weighed against the risk of HPA suppression. As with other highly active corticosteroids, therapy should be discontinued when control has been achieved. If no improvement is seen within 2 weeks, reassessment of diagnosis may be necessary. Treatment beyond 4 consecutive weeks is not recommended. Use in pediatric patients under 16 years of age has not been studied.

TEMOVATE E Emollient should not be used with occlusive dressings.

Geriatric Use: In studies where geriatric patients (65 years of age or older, see PRECAUTIONS) have been treated with TEMOVATE E Emollient, safety did not differ from that in younger patients; therefore, no dosage adjustment is recommended.

HOW SUPPLIED

TEMOVATE E Emollient, 0.05% is supplied in:
15-g tubes (NDC 0173-0454-01),
30-g tubes (NDC 0173-0454-02), and
60-g tubes (NDC 0173-0454-03).

Store between 15° and 30°C (59° and 86°F). TEMOVATE E Emollient should not be refrigerated.

GlaxoSmithKline Consumer Healthcare LP,
Pittsburgh, PA 15230

August 2002/RL-1086

Shown in Product Identification Guide, page 317

TIMENTIN® ℞

[*tī-mĕn' tin*]

(sterile ticarcillin disodium and clavulanate potassium) for Intravenous Administration

To reduce the development of drug-resistant bacteria and maintain the effectiveness of TIMENTIN (ticarcillin disodium and clavulanate potassium) and other antibacterial drugs, TIMENTIN should be used only to treat or prevent infections that are proven or strongly suspected to be caused by bacteria.

DESCRIPTION

TIMENTIN is a sterile injectable antibacterial combination consisting of the semisynthetic antibiotic ticarcillin disodium and the β-lactamase inhibitor clavulanate potassium (the potassium salt of clavulanic acid) for intravenous administration. Ticarcillin is derived from the basic penicillin nucleus, 6-amino-penicillanic acid.

Chemically, ticarcillin disodium is *N*-(2-Carboxy-3,3-dimethyl-7-oxo-4-thia-1-azabicyclo[3.2.0]hept-6-yl)-3-thiophenemalonamic acid disodium salt.

Clavulanic acid is produced by the fermentation of *Streptomyces clavuligerus*. It is a β-lactam structurally related to the penicillins and possesses the ability to inactivate a wide variety of β-lactamases by blocking the active sites of these enzymes. Clavulanic acid is particularly active against the clinically important plasmid-mediated β-lactamases frequently responsible for transferred drug resistance to penicillins and cephalosporins.

Chemically, clavulanate potassium is potassium (*Z*)-(2*R*,5*R*)-3-(2-hydroxyethylidene)-7-oxo-4-oxa-1-azabicyclo[3.2.0]heptane-2-carboxylate.

TIMENTIN is supplied as a white to pale yellow powder for reconstitution. TIMENTIN is very soluble in water, its solubility being greater than 600 mg/mL. The reconstituted solution is clear, colorless or pale yellow, having a pH of 5.5 to 7.5.

For the 3.1-gram dosage of TIMENTIN, the theoretical sodium content is 4.51 mEq (103.6 mg) per gram of TIMENTIN. The theoretical potassium content is 0.15 mEq (6 mg) per gram of TIMENTIN.

CLINICAL PHARMACOLOGY

After an intravenous infusion (30 min.) of 3.1 grams of TIMENTIN, peak serum concentrations of both ticarcillin and clavulanic acid are attained immediately after completion of infusion. Ticarcillin serum levels are similar to those produced by the administration of equivalent amounts of ticarcillin alone with a mean peak serum level of 330 mcg/mL. The corresponding mean peak serum level for clavulanic acid is 8 mcg/mL. (See following table.)

[See table above]

SERUM LEVELS IN ADULTS
AFTER A 30-MINUTE IV INFUSION OF TIMENTIN®

TICARCILLIN SERUM LEVELS (mcg/mL)

Dose	0	15 min.	30 min.	1 hr.	1.5 hr.	3.5 hr.	5.5 hr.
3.1 gram	324 (293 to 388)	223 (184 to 293)	176 (135 to 235)	131 (102 to 195)	90 (65 to 119)	27 (19 to 37)	6 (5 to 7)

CLAVULANIC ACID SERUM LEVELS (mcg/mL)

Dose	0	15 min.	30 min.	1 hr.	1.5 hr.	3.5 hr.	5.5 hr.
3.1 gram	8.0 (5.3 to 10.3)	4.6 (3.0 to 7.6)	2.6 (1.8 to 3.4)	1.8 (1.6 to 2.2)	1.2 (0.8 to 1.6)	0.3 (0.2 to 0.3)	0

The mean area under the serum concentration curve was 485 mcg•hr/mL for ticarcillin and 8.2 mcg•hr/mL for clavulanic acid.

The mean serum half-lives of ticarcillin and clavulanic acid in healthy volunteers are 1.1 hours and 1.1 hours, respectively.

In pediatric patients receiving approximately 50 mg/kg of TIMENTIN (30:1 ratio ticarcillin to clavulanate), mean ticarcillin serum half-lives were 4.4 hours in neonates (n = 18) and 1.0 hour in infants and children (n = 41). The corresponding clavulanate serum half-lives averaged 1.9 hours in neonates (n = 14) and 0.9 hour in infants and children (n = 40). Area under the serum concentration time curves averaged 339 mcg•hr/mL in infants and children (n = 41), whereas the corresponding mean clavulanate area under the serum concentration time curves was approximately 7 mcg•hr/mL in the same population (n = 40).

Approximately 60% to 70% of ticarcillin and approximately 35% to 45% of clavulanic acid are excreted unchanged in urine during the first 6 hours after administration of a single dose of TIMENTIN to normal volunteers with normal renal function. Two hours after an intravenous injection of 3.1 grams of TIMENTIN, concentrations of ticarcillin in urine generally exceed 1,500 mcg/mL. The corresponding concentrations of clavulanic acid in urine generally exceed 40 mcg/mL. By 4 to 6 hours after injection, the urine concentrations of ticarcillin and clavulanic acid usually decline to approximately 190 mcg/mL and 2 mcg/mL, respectively.

Neither component of TIMENTIN is highly protein bound; ticarcillin has been found to be approximately 45% bound to human serum protein and clavulanic acid approximately 25% bound.

Somewhat higher and more prolonged serum levels of ticarcillin can be achieved with the concurrent administration of probenecid; however, probenecid does not enhance the serum levels of clavulanic acid.

Ticarcillin can be detected in tissues and interstitial fluid following parenteral administration.

Penetration of ticarcillin into bile and pleural fluid has been demonstrated. The results of experiments involving the administration of clavulanic acid to animals suggest that this compound, like ticarcillin, is well distributed in body tissues.

An inverse relationship exists between the serum half-life of ticarcillin and creatinine clearance. The dosage of TIMENTIN need only be adjusted in cases of severe renal impairment. (See DOSAGE AND ADMINISTRATION.)

Ticarcillin may be removed from patients undergoing dialysis; the actual amount removed depends on the duration and type of dialysis.

Microbiology: Ticarcillin is a semisynthetic antibiotic with a broad spectrum of bactericidal activity against many gram-positive and gram-negative aerobic and anaerobic bacteria.

Ticarcillin is, however, susceptible to degradation by β-lactamases, and therefore, the spectrum of activity does not normally include organisms which produce these enzymes. Clavulanic acid is a β-lactam, structurally related to the penicillins, which possesses the ability to inactivate a wide range of β-lactamase enzymes commonly found in microorganisms resistant to penicillins and cephalosporins. In particular, it has good activity against the clinically important plasmid-mediated β-lactamases frequently responsible for transferred drug resistance.

The formulation of ticarcillin with clavulanic acid in TIMENTIN protects ticarcillin from degradation by β-lactamase enzymes and effectively extends the antibiotic spectrum of ticarcillin to include many bacteria normally resistant to ticarcillin and other β-lactam antibiotics. Thus, TIMENTIN possesses the distinctive properties of a broad-spectrum antibiotic and a β-lactamase inhibitor. Ticarcillin/clavulanic acid has been shown to be active against most strains of the following microorganisms, both in vitro and in clinical infections as described in the INDICATIONS AND USAGE section.

Gram-Positive Aerobes:

Staphylococcus aureus (β-lactamase and non–β-lactamase–producing)*

Staphylococcus epidermidis (β-lactamase and non–β-lactamase–producing)*

*Staphylococci that are resistant to methicillin/oxacillin must be considered resistant to ticarcillin/clavulanic acid.

Gram-Negative Aerobes:

Citrobacter species (β-lactamase and non–β-lactamase–producing)

Enterobacter species including *E. cloacae* (β-lactamase and non–β-lactamase–producing)

(Although most strains of *Enterobacter* species are resistant in vitro, clinical efficacy has been demonstrated with TIMENTIN in urinary tract infections and gynecologic infections caused by these organisms.)

Escherichia coli (β-lactamase and non–β-lactamase–producing)

Haemophilus influenzae (β-lactamase and non–β-lactamase–producing)†

Klebsiella species including *K. pneumoniae* (β-lactamase and non–β-lactamase–producing)

Pseudomonas species including *P. aeruginosa* (β-lactamase and non–β-lactamase–producing)

Serratia marcescens (β-lactamase and non–β-lactamase–producing)

†β-lactamase–negative, ampicillin-resistant (BLNAR) strains of *H. influenzae* must be considered resistant to ticarcillin/clavulanic acid.

Anaerobic Bacteria:

Bacteroides fragilis group (β-lactamase and non–β-lactamase–producing)

Prevotella (formerly *Bacteroides*) *melaninogenicus* (β-lactamase and non–β-lactamase–producing)

The following in vitro data are available, **but their clinical significance is unknown.**

The following strains exhibit an in vitro minimum inhibitory concentration (MIC) less than or equal to the susceptible breakpoint for ticarcillin/clavulanic acid. However, with the exception of organisms shown to respond to ticarcillin alone, the safety and effectiveness of ticarcillin/clavulanic acid in treating infections due to these microorganisms have not been established in adequate and well-controlled clinical trials.

Gram-Positive Aerobes:

Staphylococcus saprophyticus (β-lactamase and non–β-lactamase–producing)

Streptococcus agalactiae‡ (Group B)

Streptococcus bovis‡

Streptococcus pneumoniae‡ (penicillin-susceptible strains only)

Streptococcus pyogenes‡

Viridans group streptococci‡

Gram-Negative Aerobes:

Acinetobacter baumannii (β-lactamase and non–β-lactamase–producing)

Acinetobacter calcoaceticus (β-lactamase and non–β-lactamase–producing)

Acinetobacter haemolyticus (β-lactamase and non–β-lactamase–producing)

Acinetobacter lwoffi (β-lactamase and non–β-lactamase–producing)

Moraxella catarrhalis (β-lactamase and non–β-lactamase–producing)

Morganella morganii (β-lactamase and non–β-lactamase–producing)

Neisseria gonorrhoeae (β-lactamase and non–β-lactamase–producing)

Pasteurella multocida (β-lactamase and non–β-lactamase–producing)

Proteus mirabilis (β-lactamase and non–β-lactamase–producing)

Proteus penneri (β-lactamase and non–β-lactamase–producing)

Proteus vulgaris (β-lactamase and non–β-lactamase–producing)

Providencia rettgeri (β-lactamase and non–β-lactamase–producing)

Providencia stuartii (β-lactamase and non–β-lactamase–producing)

Stenotrophomonas maltophilia (β-lactamase and non–β-lactamase–producing)

Anaerobic Bacteria:

Clostridium species including *C. perfringens*, *C. difficile*, *C. sporogenes*, *C. ramosum* and *C. bifermentans* (β-lactamase and non–β-lactamase–producing)

Eubacterium species

Fusobacterium species including *F. nucleatum* and *F. necrophorum* (β-lactamase and non–β-lactamase–producing)

Peptostreptococcus species‡

Veillonella species‡

‡These are non–β-lactamase–producing strains, and therefore, are susceptible to ticarcillin.

In vitro synergism between TIMENTIN and gentamicin, tobramycin, or amikacin against multiresistant strains of *Pseudomonas aeruginosa* has been demonstrated.

Susceptibility Testing: *Dilution Techniques:* Quantitative methods are used to determine antimicrobial MICs. These MICs provide estimates of the susceptibility of bacteria to antimicrobial compounds. The MICs should be determined using a standardized procedure. Standardized procedures are based on a dilution method[1,3] (broth or agar) or equivalent with standardized inoculum concentrations and standardized concentrations of ticarcillin/clavulanate potassium powder.

The recommended dilution pattern utilizes a constant level of 2 mcg/mL clavulanic acid in all tubes with varying amounts of ticarcillin. MICs are expressed in terms of the ticarcillin concentration in the presence of clavulanic acid at a constant 2 mcg/mL. The MIC values should be interpreted according to the following criteria:

RECOMMENDED RANGES FOR TICARCILLIN/CLAVULANIC ACID SUSCEPTIBILITY TESTING*

For *Pseudomonas aeruginosa:*

MIC (mcg/mL)	Interpretation	
≤64	Susceptible	(S)
≥128	Resistant	(R)

For Enterobacteriaceae:

MIC (mcg/mL)	Interpretation	
≤16	Susceptible	(S)
32-64	Intermediate	(I)
≥128	Resistant	(R)

For Staphylococci†:

MIC (mcg/mL)	Interpretation	
≤8	Susceptible	(S)
≥16	Resistant	(R)

*Expressed as concentration of ticarcillin in the presence of clavulanic acid at a constant 2 mcg/mL.

†Staphylococci that are susceptible to ticarcillin/clavulanic acid but resistant to methicillin/oxacillin must be considered as resistant.

A report of "Susceptible" indicates that the pathogen is likely to be inhibited if the antimicrobial compound in the blood reaches the concentrations usually achievable. A report of "Intermediate" indicates that the result should be considered equivocal, and, if the microorganism is not fully susceptible to alternative, clinically feasible drugs, the test should be repeated. This category implies possible clinical applicability in body sites where the drug is physiologically concentrated or in situations where high dosage of drug can be used. This category also provides a buffer zone that prevents small uncontrolled technical factors from causing major discrepancies in interpretation. A report of "Resistant" indicates that the pathogen is not likely to be inhibited if the antimicrobial compound in the blood reaches the concentrations usually achievable; other therapy should be selected.

Standardized susceptibility test procedures require the use of laboratory control microorganisms to control the technical aspects of the laboratory procedures. Standard ticarcillin/clavulanate potassium powder should provide the following MIC values:

Microorganism		MIC (mcg/mL)‡
Escherichia coli	ATCC 25922	4-16
Escherichia coli	ATCC 35218	4-16
Pseudomonas aeruginosa	ATCC 27853	8-32
Staphylococcus aureus	ATCC 29213	0.5-2

‡Expressed as concentration of ticarcillin in the presence of clavulanic acid at a constant 2 mcg/mL.

Diffusion Techniques: Quantitative methods that require measurement of zone diameters also provide reproducible estimates of the susceptibility of bacteria to antimicrobial compounds. One such standardized procedure[2,3] requires the use of standardized inoculum concentrations. This procedure uses paper disks impregnated with 85 mcg of ticarcillin/clavulanate potassium (75 mcg ticarcillin plus 10 mcg clavulanate potassium) to test the susceptibility of microorganisms to ticarcillin/clavulanic acid.

Reports from the laboratory providing results of the standard single-disk susceptibility test with an 85 mcg of ticarcillin/clavulanate potassium (75 mcg ticarcillin plus 10 mcg clavulanate potassium) disk should be interpreted according to the following criteria:

RECOMMENDED RANGES FOR TICARCILLIN/CLAVULANIC ACID SUSCEPTIBILITY TESTING

For *Pseudomonas aeruginosa:*

Zone Diameter (mm)	Interpretation	
≥15	Susceptible	(S)
≤14	Resistant	(R)

Continued on next page

Product information on these pages is effective as of August 2004. Further information is available at: GlaxoSmithKline, PO Box 13398, Research Triangle Park, NC 27709. 1-888-825-5249. Corporate Web Site: www.gsk.com

Timentin IV—Cont.

For Enterobacteriaceae:

Zone Diameter (mm)	Interpretation	
≥20	Susceptible	(S)
15-19	Intermediate	(I)
≤14	Resistant	(R)

For Staphylococci§:

Zone Diameter (mm)	Interpretation	
≥23	Susceptible	(S)
≤22	Resistant	(R)

§Staphylococci that are resistant to methicillin/oxacillin must be considered as resistant to ticarcillin/clavulanic acid.

Interpretation should be as stated above for results using dilution techniques. Interpretation involves correlation of the diameter obtained in the disk test with the MIC for ticarcillin/clavulanic acid.

As with standardized dilution techniques, diffusion methods require the use of laboratory control microorganisms that are used to control the technical aspects of the laboratory procedures. For the diffusion technique, the 85 mcg of ticarcillin/clavulanate potassium (75 mcg ticarcillin plus 10 mcg clavulanate potassium) disk should provide the following zone diameters in these laboratory test quality control strains:

Microorganism		Zone Diameter (mm)
Escherichia coli	ATCC 25922	24-30
Escherichia coli	ATCC 35218	21-25
Pseudomonas aeruginosa	ATCC 27853	20-28
Staphylococcus aureus	ATCC 25923	29-37

Anaerobic Techniques: For anaerobic bacteria, the susceptibility to ticarcillin/clavulanic acid can be determined by standardized test methods[3,4]. The MIC values obtained should be interpreted according to the following criteria:

RECOMMENDED RANGES FOR TICARCILLIN/CLAVULANIC ACID SUSCEPTIBILITY TESTING||

MIC (mcg/mL)	Interpretation	
≤32	Susceptible	(S)
64	Intermediate	(I)
≥128	Resistant	(R)

||Expressed as concentration of ticarcillin in the presence of clavulanic acid at a constant 2 mcg/mL.

Interpretation is identical to that stated above for results using dilution techniques.

As with other susceptibility techniques, the use of laboratory control microorganisms is required to control the technical aspects of the laboratory standardized procedures. Standardized ticarcillin/clavulanate potassium powder should provide the following MIC values:

[See table below]

INDICATIONS AND USAGE

TIMENTIN is indicated in the treatment of infections caused by susceptible strains of the designated microorganisms in the conditions listed below:

Septicemia (including bacteremia) caused by β-lactamase–producing strains of *Klebsiella* spp.*, *E. coli**, *S. aureus**, or *P. aeruginosa** (or other *Pseudomonas* species*)

Lower Respiratory Infections caused by β-lactamase–producing strains of *S. aureus*, *H. influenzae**, or *Klebsiella* spp.*

Bone and Joint Infections caused by β-lactamase–producing strains of *S. aureus*

Skin and Skin Structure Infections caused by β-lactamase–producing strains of *S. aureus*, *Klebsiella* spp.*, or *E. coli**

Urinary Tract Infections (complicated and uncomplicated) caused by β-lactamase–producing strains of *E. coli*, *Klebsiella* spp., *P. aeruginosa** (or other *Pseudomonas* spp.*), *Citrobacter* spp.*, *Enterobacter cloacae**, *S. marcescens**, or *S. aureus**

Gynecologic Infections endometritis caused by β-lactamase–producing strains of *P. melaninogenicus**, *Enterobacter* spp. (including *E. cloacae**), *E. coli*, *K. pneumoniae**, *S. aureus*, or *S. epidermidis*

Intra-abdominal Infections peritonitis caused by β-lactamase–producing strains of *E. coli*, *K. pneumoniae*, or *B. fragilis** group

*Efficacy for this organism in this organ system was studied in fewer than 10 infections.

NOTE: For information on use in pediatric patients (≥3 months of age) see PRECAUTIONS—Pediatric Use and CLINICAL STUDIES sections. There are insufficient data to support the use of TIMENTIN in pediatric patients under 3 months of age or for the treatment of septicemia and/or infections in the pediatric population where the suspected or proven pathogen is *H. influenzae* type b.

While TIMENTIN is indicated only for the conditions listed above, infections caused by ticarcillin-susceptible organisms are also amenable to treatment with TIMENTIN due to its ticarcillin content. Therefore, mixed infections caused by ticarcillin-susceptible organisms and β-lactamase–producing organisms susceptible to ticarcillin/clavulanic acid should not require the addition of another antibiotic.

Due to its broad spectrum of bactericidal activity against gram-positive and gram-negative bacteria, TIMENTIN is particularly useful for the treatment of mixed infections and for presumptive therapy prior to the identification of the causative organisms. TIMENTIN has been shown to be effective as single drug therapy in the treatment of some serious infections where normally combination antibiotic therapy might be employed.

Based on the in vitro synergism between ticarcillin/clavulanic acid and aminoglycosides against certain strains of *P. aeruginosa*, combined therapy has been successful, especially in patients with impaired host defenses. Both drugs should be used in full therapeutic doses.

To reduce the development of drug-resistant bacteria and maintain the effectiveness of TIMENTIN and other antibacterial drugs, TIMENTIN should be used only to treat or prevent infections that are proven or strongly suspected to be caused by susceptible bacteria. When culture and susceptibility information are available, they should be considered in selecting or modifying antibacterial therapy. In the absence of such data, local epidemiology and susceptibility patterns may contribute to the empiric selection of therapy.

CONTRAINDICATIONS

TIMENTIN is contraindicated in patients with a history of hypersensitivity reactions to any of the penicillins.

WARNINGS

SERIOUS AND OCCASIONALLY FATAL HYPERSENSITIVITY (ANAPHYLACTIC) REACTIONS HAVE BEEN REPORTED IN PATIENTS ON PENICILLIN THERAPY. THESE REACTIONS ARE MORE LIKELY TO OCCUR IN INDIVIDUALS WITH A HISTORY OF PENICILLIN HYPERSENSITIVITY AND/OR A HISTORY OF SENSITIVITY TO MULTIPLE ALLERGENS. THERE HAVE BEEN REPORTS OF INDIVIDUALS WITH A HISTORY OF PENICILLIN HYPERSENSITIVITY WHO HAVE EXPERIENCED SEVERE REACTIONS WHEN TREATED WITH CEPHALOSPORINS. BEFORE INITIATING THERAPY WITH TIMENTIN, CAREFUL INQUIRY SHOULD BE MADE CONCERNING PREVIOUS HYPERSENSITIVITY REACTIONS TO PENICILLINS, CEPHALOSPORINS, OR OTHER ALLERGENS. IF AN ALLERGIC REACTION OCCURS, TIMENTIN SHOULD BE DISCONTINUED AND THE APPROPRIATE THERAPY INSTITUTED. **SERIOUS ANAPHYLACTIC REACTIONS REQUIRE IMMEDIATE EMERGENCY TREATMENT WITH EPINEPHRINE. OXYGEN, INTRAVENOUS STEROIDS, AND AIRWAY MANAGEMENT, INCLUDING INTUBATION, SHOULD ALSO BE PROVIDED AS INDICATED.**

Pseudomembranous colitis has been reported with nearly all antibacterial agents, including TIMENTIN, and may range in severity from mild to life-threatening. Therefore, it is important to consider this diagnosis in patients who present with diarrhea subsequent to the administration of antibacterial agents.

Treatment with antibacterial agents alters the normal flora of the colon and may permit overgrowth of clostridia. Studies indicate that a toxin produced by *Clostridium difficile* is a primary cause of "antibiotic-associated colitis."

After the diagnosis of pseudomembranous colitis has been established, appropriate therapeutic measures should be initiated. Mild cases of pseudomembranous colitis usually respond to drug discontinuation alone. In moderate to severe cases, consideration should be given to management with fluids and electrolytes, protein supplementation, and treatment with an antibacterial drug clinically effective against *C. difficile* colitis.

When very high doses of TIMENTIN are administered, especially in the presence of impaired renal function, patients may experience convulsions. (See ADVERSE REACTIONS and OVERDOSAGE.)

PRECAUTIONS

General: While TIMENTIN possesses the characteristic low toxicity of the penicillin group of antibiotics, periodic assessment of organ system functions, including renal, hepatic, and hematopoietic function, is advisable during prolonged therapy.

Bleeding manifestations have occurred in some patients receiving β-lactam antibiotics. These reactions have been associated with abnormalities of coagulation tests such as clotting time, platelet aggregation, and prothrombin time and are more likely to occur in patients with renal impairment. If bleeding manifestations appear, treatment with TIMENTIN should be discontinued and appropriate therapy instituted.

TIMENTIN has only rarely been reported to cause hypokalemia; however, the possibility of this occurring should be kept in mind particularly when treating patients with fluid and electrolyte imbalance. Periodic monitoring of serum potassium may be advisable in patients receiving prolonged therapy.

The theoretical sodium content is 4.51 mEq (103.6 mg) per gram of TIMENTIN. This should be considered when treating patients requiring restricted salt intake.

As with any penicillin, an allergic reaction, including anaphylaxis, may occur during administration of TIMENTIN, particularly in a hypersensitive individual.

The possibility of superinfections with mycotic or bacterial pathogens should be kept in mind, particularly during prolonged treatment. If superinfections occur, appropriate measures should be taken.

Prescribing TIMENTIN in the absence of a proven or strongly suspected bacterial infection or a prophylactic indication is unlikely to provide benefit to the patient and increases the risk of the development of drug-resistant bacteria.

Information for Patients: Patients should be counseled that antibacterial drugs, including TIMENTIN, should only be used to treat bacterial infections. They do not treat viral infections (e.g., the common cold). When TIMENTIN is prescribed to treat a bacterial infection, patients should be told that although it is common to feel better early in the course of therapy, the medication should be taken exactly as directed. Skipping doses or not completing the full course of therapy may: (1) decrease the effectiveness of the immediate treatment, and (2) increase the likelihood that bacteria will develop resistance and will not be treatable by TIMENTIN or other antibacterial drugs in the future.

Drug/Laboratory Test Interactions: As with other penicillins, the mixing of TIMENTIN with an aminoglycoside in solutions for parenteral administration can result in substantial inactivation of the aminoglycoside.

Probenecid interferes with the renal tubular secretion of ticarcillin, thereby increasing serum concentrations and prolonging serum half-life of the antibiotic.

High urine concentrations of ticarcillin may produce false-positive protein reactions (pseudoproteinuria) with the following methods: Sulfosalicylic acid and boiling test, acetic acid test, biuret reaction, and nitric acid test. The bromphenol blue (MULTI-STIX®) reagent strip test has been reported to be reliable.

The presence of clavulanic acid in TIMENTIN may cause a nonspecific binding of IgG and albumin by red cell membranes leading to a false-positive Coombs test.

Carcinogenesis, Mutagenesis, Impairment of Fertility: Long-term studies in animals have not been performed to evaluate carcinogenic potential. However, results from assays for gene mutation in vitro using bacteria (Ames tests) and yeast, and for chromosomal effects in vitro in human lymphocytes, and in vivo in mouse bone marrow (micronucleus test) indicate that TIMENTIN is without any mutagenic potential.

Pregnancy (Category B): Reproduction studies have been performed in rats given doses up to 1,050 mg/kg/day and have revealed no evidence of impaired fertility or harm to the fetus due to TIMENTIN. There are, however, no adequate and well-controlled studies in pregnant women. Because animal reproduction studies are not always predictive of human response, this drug should be used during pregnancy only if clearly needed.

Nursing Mothers: It is not known whether this drug is excreted in human milk. Because many drugs are excreted in human milk, caution should be exercised when TIMENTIN is administered to a nursing woman.

Pediatric Use: The safety and effectiveness of TIMENTIN have been established in the age group of 3 months to 16 years. Use of TIMENTIN in these age groups is supported by evidence from adequate and well-controlled studies of TIMENTIN in adults with additional efficacy, safety, and pharmacokinetic data from both comparative and non-comparative studies in pediatric patients. There are insufficient data to support the use of TIMENTIN in pediatric patients under 3 months of age or for the treatment of septicemia and/or infections in the pediatric population where the suspected or proven pathogen is *H. influenzae* type b.

In those patients in whom meningeal seeding from a distant infection site or in whom meningitis is suspected or documented, or in patients who require prophylaxis against central nervous system infection, an alternate agent with demonstrated clinical efficacy in this setting should be used.

ADVERSE REACTIONS

As with other penicillins, the following adverse reactions may occur:

Hypersensitivity Reactions: Skin rash, pruritus, urticaria, arthralgia, myalgia, drug fever, chills, chest discomfort, erythema multiforme, toxic epidermal necrolysis, Stevens-Johnson syndrome, and anaphylactic reactions.

Central Nervous System: Headache, giddiness, neuromuscular hyperirritability, or convulsive seizures.

Gastrointestinal Disturbances: Disturbances of taste and smell, stomatitis, flatulence, nausea, vomiting and diarrhea, epigastric pain, and pseudomembranous colitis have been reported. Onset of pseudomembranous colitis symp-

Microorganism		Agar dilution MIC Range (mcg/mL)||	Broth microdilution MIC Range (mcg/mL)||
Bacteroides thetaiotaomicron	ATCC 29741	0.5-2	0.5-2
Eubacterium lentum	ATCC 43055	16-64	8-32

||Expressed as concentration of ticarcillin in the presence of clavulanic acid at a constant 2 mcg/mL.

toms may occur during or after antibiotic treatment. (See WARNINGS.)

Hemic and Lymphatic Systems: Thrombocytopenia, leukopenia, neutropenia, eosinophilia, reduction of hemoglobin or hematocrit, and prolongation of prothrombin time and bleeding time.

Abnormalities of Hepatic and Renal Function Tests: Elevation of serum aspartate aminotransferase (SGOT), serum alanine aminotransferase (SGPT), serum alkaline phosphatase, serum LDH, serum bilirubin. There have been reports of transient hepatitis and cholestatic jaundice—as with some other penicillins and some cephalosporins. Elevation of serum creatinine and/or BUN, hypernatremia, reduction in serum potassium, and uric acid.

Local Reactions: Pain, burning, swelling, and induration at the injection site and thrombophlebitis with intravenous administration.

Available safety data for pediatric patients treated with TIMENTIN demonstrate a similar adverse event profile to that observed in adult patients.

DRUG ABUSE AND DEPENDENCE

Neither abuse of nor dependence on TIMENTIN has been reported.

OVERDOSAGE

As with other penicillins, neurotoxic reactions may arise when very high doses of TIMENTIN are administered, especially in patients with impaired renal function. (See WARNINGS and ADVERSE REACTIONS—Central Nervous System.)

In case of overdosage, discontinue TIMENTIN, treat symptomatically, and institute supportive measures as required. Ticarcillin may be removed from circulation by hemodialysis. The molecular weight, degree of protein binding, and pharmacokinetic profile of clavulanic acid together with information from a single patient with renal insufficiency all suggest that this compound may also be removed by hemodialysis.

DOSAGE AND ADMINISTRATION

TIMENTIN should be administered by intravenous infusion (30 min.).

Adults: The usual recommended dosage for systemic and urinary tract infections for average (60 kg) adults is 3.1 grams of TIMENTIN (3.1-gram vial containing 3 grams ticarcillin and 100 mg clavulanic acid) given every 4 to 6 hours. For gynecologic infections, TIMENTIN should be administered as follows: Moderate infections, 200 mg/kg/day in divided doses every 6 hours, and for severe infections, 300 mg/kg/day in divided doses every 4 hours. For patients weighing less than 60 kg, the recommended dosage is 200 to 300 mg/kg/day, based on ticarcillin content, given in divided doses every 4 to 6 hours.

Pediatric Patients (≥3 months):

For patients <60 kg: In patients <60 kg, TIMENTIN is dosed at 50 mg/kg/dose based on the ticarcillin component. TIMENTIN should be administered as follows: Mild to moderate infections 200 mg/kg/day in divided doses every 6 hours; for severe infections, 300 mg/kg/day in divided doses every 4 hours.

For patients ≥60 kg: For mild to moderate infections, 3.1 grams of TIMENTIN (3 grams of ticarcillin and 100 mg of clavulanic acid) administered every 6 hours; for severe infections, 3.1 grams every 4 hours.

Renal Impairment: For infections complicated by renal insufficiency[†], an initial loading dose of 3.1 grams should be followed by doses based on creatinine clearance and type of dialysis as indicated below:

[See first table above]

Creatinine clearance mL/min.	Dosage
over 60	3.1 grams every 4 hrs.
30 to 60	2 grams every 4 hrs.
10 to 30	2 grams every 8 hrs.
less than 10	2 grams every 12 hrs.
less than 10 with hepatic dysfunction	2 grams every 24 hrs.
patients on peritoneal dialysis	3.1 grams every 12 hrs.
patients on hemodialysis	2 grams every 12 hrs. supplemented with 3.1 grams after each dialysis

To calculate creatinine clearance[‡] from a serum creatinine value use the following formula.

$$C_{cr} = \frac{(140\text{–Age})\ (\text{wt. in kg})}{72 \times S_{cr}\ (\text{mg}/100\ \text{mL})}$$

This is the calculated creatinine clearance for adult males; for females it is 15% less.

[‡]Cockcroft, D.W., et al: Prediction of Creatinine Clearance from Serum Creatinine. Nephron 16:31-41, 1976.

[†]The half-life of ticarcillin in patients with renal failure is approximately 13 hours.

Dosage for any individual patient must take into consideration the site and severity of infection, the susceptibility of the organisms causing infection, and the status of the patient's host defense mechanisms.

The duration of therapy depends upon the severity of infection. Generally, TIMENTIN should be continued for at least 2 days after the signs and symptoms of infection have disappeared. The usual duration is 10 to 14 days; however, in difficult and complicated infections, more prolonged therapy may be required.

Frequent bacteriologic and clinical appraisals are necessary during therapy of chronic urinary tract infection and may be required for several months after therapy has been completed. Persistent infections may require treatment for several weeks, and doses smaller than those indicated above should not be used.

In certain infections, involving abscess formation, appropriate surgical drainage should be performed in conjunction with antimicrobial therapy.

INTRAVENOUS ADMINISTRATION DIRECTIONS FOR USE

3.1-gram Vials

The 3.1-gram vial should be reconstituted by adding approximately 13 mL of Sterile Water for Injection, USP, or Sodium Chloride Injection, USP, and shaking well. When dissolved, the concentration of ticarcillin will be approximately 200 mg/mL with a corresponding concentration of 6.7 mg/mL for clavulanic acid. Conversely, each 5.0 mL of the 3.1-gram dose reconstituted with approximately 13 mL of diluent will contain approximately 1 gram of ticarcillin and 33 mg of clavulanic acid.

Intravenous Infusion: The dissolved drug should be further diluted to desired volume using the recommended solution listed in the COMPATIBILITY AND STABILITY Section (STABILITY PERIOD) to a concentration between 10 mg/mL to 100 mg/mL. The solution of reconstituted drug may then be administered over a period of 30 minutes by direct infusion or through a Y-type intravenous infusion set. If this method of administration is used, it is advisable to discontinue temporarily the administration of any other solutions during the infusion of TIMENTIN.

Stability: For I.V. solutions, see STABILITY PERIOD below.

When TIMENTIN is given in combination with another antimicrobial, such as an aminoglycoside, each drug should be given separately in accordance with the recommended dosage and routes of administration for each drug.

After reconstitution and prior to administration, TIMENTIN, as with other parenteral drugs, should be inspected visually for particulate matter. If this condition is evident, the solution should be discarded.

The color of reconstituted solutions of TIMENTIN normally ranges from light to dark yellow, depending on concentration, duration, and temperature of storage while maintaining label claim characteristics.

COMPATIBILITY AND STABILITY

3.1-gram Vials

(Dilutions derived from a stock solution of 200 mg/mL)

The concentrated stock solution at 200 mg/mL is stable for up to 6 hours at room temperature 21° to 24°C (70° to 75°F) or up to 72 hours under refrigeration 4°C (40°F).

If the concentrated stock solution (200 mg/mL) is held for up to 6 hours at room temperature 21° to 24°C (70° to 75°F) or up to 72 hours under refrigeration 4°C (40°F) and further diluted to a concentration between 10 mg/mL and 100 mg/mL with any of the diluents listed below, then the following stability periods apply.

STABILITY PERIOD

(3.1-gram Vials)

[See second table above]

Intravenous Solution (ticarcillin concentrations of 10 mg/mL to 100 mg/mL)	Room Temperature 21° to 24°C (70° to 75°F)	Refrigerated 4°C (40°F)
Dextrose Injection 5%, USP	24 hours	3 days
Sodium Chloride Injection, USP	24 hours	7 days
Lactated Ringer's Injection, USP	24 hours	7 days

If the concentrated stock solution (200 mg/mL) is stored for up to 6 hours at room temperature and then further diluted to a concentration between 10 mg/mL and 100 mg/mL, solutions of Sodium Chloride Injection, USP, and Lactated Ringer's Injection, USP, may be stored frozen -18°C (0°F) for up to 30 days. Solutions prepared with Dextrose Injection 5%, USP, may be stored frozen -18°C (0°F) for up to 7 days. All thawed solutions should be used within 8 hours or discarded. Once thawed, solutions should not be refrozen.

NOTE: TIMENTIN is incompatible with Sodium Bicarbonate.

Unused solutions must be discarded after the time periods listed above.

HOW SUPPLIED

Each 3.1-gram vial of TIMENTIN contains sterile ticarcillin disodium equivalent to 3 grams ticarcillin and sterile clavulanate potassium equivalent to 0.1 gram clavulanic acid.

NDC 0029-6571-26 3.1-gram Vial

TIMENTIN is also supplied as:

NDC 0029-6571-40 3.1-gram ADD-Vantage®[§] Antibiotic Vial

Each 31 gram Pharmacy Bulk Package contains sterile ticarcillin disodium equivalent to 30 grams ticarcillin and sterile clavulanate potassium equivalent to 1 gram clavulanic acid.

NDC 0029-6579-21 31 gram Pharmacy Bulk Package

Vials of TIMENTIN should be stored at or below 24°C (75°F).

NDC 0029-6571-31 TIMENTIN as an iso-osmotic, sterile, nonpyrogenic, frozen solution in GALAXY®[||] (PL 2040) Plastic Containers—supplied in 100 mL single-dose containers equivalent to 3 grams ticarcillin and clavulanate potassium equivalent to 0.1 gram clavulanic acid.

CLINICAL STUDIES

TIMENTIN has been studied in a total of 296 pediatric patients (excluding neonates and infants less than 3 months) in 6 controlled clinical trials. The majority of patients studied had intra-abdominal infections, and the primary comparator was clindamycin and gentamicin with or without ampicillin. At the end-of-therapy visit, comparable efficacy was reported in the trial arms using TIMENTIN and an appropriate comparator.

TIMENTIN was also evaluated in an additional 408 pediatric patients (excluding neonates and infants less than 3 months) in 3 uncontrolled US clinical trials. Patients were treated across a broad range of presenting diagnoses including: Infections in bone and joint, skin and skin structure, lower respiratory tract, urinary tract, as well as intra-abdominal and gynecologic infections. Patients received TIMENTIN either 300 mg/kg/day (based on the ticarcillin component) divided q4h for severe infection or 200 mg/kg/day (based on the ticarcillin component) divided q6h for mild to moderate infections. The efficacy rates were comparable to those obtained in the controlled trials.

The adverse event profile in these 704 pediatric patients treated with TIMENTIN was comparable to that seen in adult patients.

REFERENCES

1. National Committee for Clinical Microbiology Standards. *Methods for Dilution Antimicrobial Susceptibility Tests for Bacteria that Grow Aerobically* - Sixth Edition. Approved Standard. NCCLS Document M7-A6, Vol. 23, No. 2 (ISBN-1-56238-486-4). NCCLS, 940 West Valley Road, Suite 1400, Wayne, PA 19087-1898, January, 2003.
2. National Committee for Clinical Microbiology Standards. *Performance Standards for Antimicrobial Disk Susceptibility Tests* - Eighth Edition. Approved Standard. NCCLS Document M2-A8, Vol. 23, No. 1 (ISBN-1-56238-485-6). NCCLS, 940 West Valley Road, Suite 1400, Wayne, PA 19087-1898, January, 2003.
3. National Committee for Clinical Microbiology Standards. *Performance Standards for Antimicrobial Susceptibility Testing* - Thirteenth Informational Supplement. NCCLS Document M100-S13 (M7), Vol. 23, No. 2. NCCLS, 940 West Valley Road, Suite 1400, Wayne, PA 19087-1898, January, 2003.
4. National Committee for Clinical Laboratory Standards. *Methods for Antimicrobial Susceptibility Testing of Anaerobic Bacteria* - Fifth Edition. Approved Standard NCCLS Document M11-A5, Vol. 21, No. 2 (ISBN 1-56238-429-5). NCCLS, 940 West Valley Road, Suite 1400, Wayne, PA 19087-1898, January, 2001.

[§]ADD-VANTAGE is a registered trademark of Abbott Laboratories.

[||]GALAXY is a registered trademark of Baxter International Inc.

MULTI-STIX is a registered trademark of Bayer Corporation.

TIMENTIN is a registered trademark of GlaxoSmithKline.

GlaxoSmithKline, Research Triangle Park, NC 27709

October 2003/TI:L13IV

Shown in Product Identification Guide, page 317

TIMENTIN® ℞

[*tī-mĕn′ tin*]

(sterile ticarcillin disodium and clavulanate potassium) for Intravenous Administration ADD-VANTAGE® ANTIBIOTIC VIAL

To reduce the development of drug-resistant bacteria and maintain the effectiveness of TIMENTIN (ticarcillin disodium and clavulanate potassium) and other antibacterial drugs, TIMENTIN should be used only to treat or prevent infections that are proven or strongly suspected to be caused by bacteria.

Continued on next page

Product information on these pages is effective as of August 2004. Further information is available at: GlaxoSmithKline, PO Box 13398, Research Triangle Park, NC 27709. 1-888-825-5249. Corporate Web Site: www.gsk.com

Timentin ADD-Vantage—Cont.

DESCRIPTION

TIMENTIN is a sterile injectable antibacterial combination consisting of the semisynthetic antibiotic ticarcillin disodium, and the β-lactamase inhibitor clavulanate potassium (the potassium salt of clavulanic acid) for intravenous administration. Ticarcillin is derived from the basic penicillin nucleus, 6-amino-penicillanic acid.

Chemically, ticarcillin disodium is *N*-(2-Carboxy-3,3-dimethyl-7-oxo-4-thia-1- azabicyclo[3.2.0]hept-6-yl)-3-thiophenemalonamic acid disodium salt.

Clavulanic acid is produced by the fermentation of *Streptomyces clavuligerus*. It is a β-lactam structurally related to the penicillins and possesses the ability to inactivate a wide variety of β-lactamases by blocking the active sites of these enzymes. Clavulanic acid is particularly active against the clinically important plasmid-mediated β-lactamases frequently responsible for transferred drug resistance to penicillins and cephalosporins.

Chemically, clavulanate potassium is potassium (*Z*)-(2*R*,5*R*)-3-(2-hydroxyethylidene)-7-oxo-4-oxa-1-azabicyclo [3.2.0]heptane-2-carboxylate.

TIMENTIN is supplied as a white to pale yellow powder for reconstitution. TIMENTIN is very soluble in water, its solubility being greater than 600 mg/mL. The reconstituted solution is clear, colorless or pale yellow, having a pH of 5.5 to 7.5.

For the 3.1-gram dosage of TIMENTIN, the theoretical sodium content is 4.51 mEq (103.6 mg) per gram of TIMENTIN. The theoretical potassium content is 0.15 mEq (6 mg) per gram of TIMENTIN.

CLINICAL PHARMACOLOGY

After an intravenous infusion (30 min.) of 3.1 grams of TIMENTIN, peak serum concentrations of both ticarcillin and clavulanic acid are attained immediately after completion of infusion. Ticarcillin serum levels are similar to those produced by the administration of equivalent amounts of ticarcillin alone with a mean peak serum level of 330 mcg/mL. The corresponding mean peak serum level for clavulanic acid was 8 mcg/mL. (See following table.)

[See table below]

The mean area under the serum concentration curve was 485 mcg•hr/mL for ticarcillin and 8.2 mcg•hr/mL for clavulanic acid.

The mean serum half-lives of ticarcillin and clavulanic acid in healthy volunteers are 1.1 hours and 1.1 hours, respectively.

In pediatric patients receiving approximately 50 mg/kg of TIMENTIN (30:1 ratio ticarcillin to clavulanate), mean ticarcillin serum half-lives were 4.4 hours in neonates (n = 18) and 1.0 hour in infants and children (n = 41). The corresponding clavulanate serum half-lives averaged 1.9 hours in neonates (n = 14) and 0.9 hour in infants and children (n = 40). Area under the serum concentration time curves averaged 339 mcg•hr/mL in infants and children (n = 41), whereas the corresponding mean clavulanate area under the serum concentration time curves was approximately 7 mcg•hr/mL in the same population (n = 40).

Approximately 60% to 70% of ticarcillin and approximately 35% to 45% of clavulanic acid are excreted unchanged in urine during the first 6 hours after administration of a single dose of TIMENTIN to normal volunteers with normal renal function. Two hours after an intravenous injection of 3.1 grams of TIMENTIN, concentrations of ticarcillin in urine generally exceed 1,500 mcg/mL. The corresponding concentrations of clavulanic acid in urine generally exceed 40 mcg/mL. By 4 to 6 hours after injection, the urine concentrations of ticarcillin and clavulanic acid usually decline to approximately 190 mcg/mL and 2 mcg/mL, respectively. Neither component of TIMENTIN is highly protein bound; ticarcillin has been found to be approximately 45% bound to human serum protein and clavulanic acid approximately 25% bound.

Somewhat higher and more prolonged serum levels of ticarcillin can be achieved with the concurrent administration of probenecid; however, probenecid does not enhance the serum levels of clavulanic acid.

Ticarcillin can be detected in tissues and interstitial fluid following parenteral administration.

Penetration of ticarcillin into bile and pleural fluid has been demonstrated. The results of experiments involving the administration of clavulanic acid to animals suggest that this compound, like ticarcillin, is well distributed in body tissues.

An inverse relationship exists between the serum half-life of ticarcillin and creatinine clearance. The dosage of TIMENTIN need only be adjusted in cases of severe renal impairment. (See DOSAGE AND ADMINISTRATION.)

Ticarcillin may be removed from patients undergoing dialysis; the actual amount removed depends on the duration and type of dialysis.

Microbiology: Ticarcillin is a semisynthetic antibiotic with a broad spectrum of bactericidal activity against many gram-positive and gram-negative aerobic and anaerobic bacteria.

Ticarcillin is, however, susceptible to degradation by β-lactamases, and therefore, the spectrum of activity does not normally include organisms which produce these enzymes.

Clavulanic acid is a β-lactam, structurally related to the penicillins, which possesses the ability to inactivate a wide range of β-lactamase enzymes commonly found in microorganisms resistant to penicillins and cephalosporins. In particular, it has good activity against the clinically important plasmid-mediated β-lactamases frequently responsible for transferred drug resistance.

The formulation of ticarcillin with clavulanic acid in TIMENTIN protects ticarcillin from degradation by β-lactamase enzymes and effectively extends the antibiotic spectrum of ticarcillin to include many bacteria normally resistant to ticarcillin and other β-lactam antibiotics. Thus TIMENTIN possesses the distinctive properties of a broad-spectrum antibiotic and a β-lactamase inhibitor. Ticarcillin/clavulanic acid has been shown to be active against most strains of the following microorganisms, both in vitro and in clinical infections as described in the INDICATIONS AND USAGE section.

Gram-Positive Aerobes:

Staphylococcus aureus (β-lactamase and non–β-lactamase–producing)*

Staphylococcus epidermidis (β-lactamase and non–β-lactamase–producing)*

*Staphylococci that are resistant to methicillin/oxacillin must be considered resistant to ticarcillin/clavulanic acid.

Gram-Negative Aerobes:

Citrobacter species (β-lactamase and non–β-lactamase–producing)

Enterobacter species including *E. cloacae* (β-lactamase and non–β-lactamase–producing)

(Although most strains of *Enterobacter* species are resistant in vitro, clinical efficacy has been demonstrated with TIMENTIN in urinary tract infections and gynecologic infections caused by these organisms.)

Escherichia coli (β-lactamase and non–β-lactamase–producing)

Haemophilus influenzae (β-lactamase and non–β-lactamase–producing)†

Klebsiella species including *K. pneumoniae* (β-lactamase and non–β-lactamase–producing)

Pseudomonas species including *P. aeruginosa* (β-lactamase and non–β-lactamase–producing)

Serratia marcescens (β-lactamase and non–β-lactamase–producing)

†β-lactamase–negative, ampicillin-resistant (BLNAR) strains of *Haemophilus influenzae* must be considered resistant to ticarcillin/clavulanic acid.

Anaerobic Bacteria:

Bacteroides fragilis group (β-lactamase and non–β-lactamase–producing)

Prevotella (formerly *Bacteroides*) *melaninogenicus* (β-lactamase and non–β-lactamase–producing)

The following in vitro data are available, **but their clinical significance is unknown.**

The following strains exhibit an in vitro minimum inhibitory concentration (MIC) less than or equal to the susceptible breakpoint for ticarcillin/clavulanic acid. However, with the exception of organisms shown to respond to ticarcillin alone, the safety and effectiveness of ticarcillin/clavulanic acid in treating infections due to these microorganisms have not been established in adequate and well-controlled clinical trials.

Gram-Positive Aerobes:

Staphylococcus saprophyticus (β-lactamase and non–β-lactamase–producing)

Streptococcus agalactiae‡ (Group B)

Streptococcus bovis‡

Streptococcus pneumoniae‡ (penicillin-susceptible strains only)

Streptococcus pyogenes‡

Viridans group streptococci‡

Gram-Negative Aerobes:

Acinetobacter baumannii (β-lactamase and non–β-lactamase–producing)

Acinetobacter calcoaceticus (β-lactamase and non–β-lactamase–producing)

Acinetobacter haemolyticus (β-lactamase and non–β-lactamase–producing)

Acinetobacter lwoffi (β-lactamase and non–β-lactamase–producing)

Moraxella catarrhalis (β-lactamase and non–β-lactamase–producing)

Morganella morganii (β-lactamase and non–β-lactamase–producing)

Neisseria gonorrhoeae (β-lactamase and non–β-lactamase–producing)

Pasteurella multocida (β-lactamase and non–β-lactamase–producing)

Proteus mirabilis (β-lactamase and non–β-lactamase–producing)

Proteus penneri (β-lactamase and non–β-lactamase–producing)

Proteus vulgaris (β-lactamase and non–β-lactamase–producing)

Providencia rettgeri (β-lactamase and non–β-lactamase–producing)

Providencia stuartii (β-lactamase and non–β-lactamase–producing)

Stenotrophomonas maltophilia (β-lactamase and non–β-lactamase–producing)

Anaerobic Bacteria:

Clostridium species including *C. perfringens, C. difficile, C. sporogenes, C. ramosum,* and *C. bifermentans* (β-lactamase and non–β-lactamase–producing)

Eubacterium species

Fusobacterium species including *F. nucleatum* and *F. necrophorum* (β-lactamase and non–β-lactamase–producing)

Peptostreptococcus species‡

Veillonella species‡

‡These are non–β-lactamase–producing strains, and therefore, are susceptible to ticarcillin.

In vitro synergism between TIMENTIN and gentamicin, tobramycin, or amikacin against multiresistant strains of *Pseudomonas aeruginosa* has been demonstrated.

Susceptibility Testing: ***Dilution Techniques:*** Quantitative methods are used to determine antimicrobial MICs. These MICs provide estimates of the susceptibility of bacteria to antimicrobial compounds. The MICs should be determined using a standardized procedure. Standardized procedures are based on a dilution method[1,3] (broth or agar) or equivalent with standardized inoculum concentrations and standardized concentrations of ticarcillin/clavulanate potassium powder.

The recommended dilution pattern utilizes a constant level of 2 mcg/mL clavulanic acid in all tubes with varying amounts of ticarcillin. MICs are expressed in terms of the ticarcillin concentration in the presence of clavulanic acid at a constant 2 mcg/mL. The MIC values should be interpreted according to the following criteria:

RECOMMENDED RANGES FOR TICARCILLIN/CLAVULANIC ACID SUSCEPTIBILITY TESTING*

For *Pseudomonas aeruginosa:*

MIC (mcg/mL)	Interpretation
≤64	Susceptible (S)
≥128	Resistant (R)

For Enterobacteriaceae:

MIC (mcg/mL)	Interpretation
≤16	Susceptible (S)
32–64	Intermediate (I)
≥128	Resistant (R)

For Staphylococci†:

MIC (mcg/mL)	Interpretation
≤8	Susceptible (S)
≥16	Resistant (R)

*Expressed as concentration of ticarcillin in the presence of clavulanic acid at a constant 2 mcg/mL.

†Staphylococci that are susceptible to ticarcillin/clavulanic acid but resistant to methicillin/oxacillin must be considered as resistant.

A report of "Susceptible" indicates that the pathogen is likely to be inhibited if the antimicrobial compound in the blood reaches the concentrations usually achievable. A report of "Intermediate" indicates that the result should be considered equivocal, and if the microorganism is not fully susceptible to alternative, clinically feasible drugs, the test should be repeated. This category implies possible clinical applicability in body sites where the drug is physiologically concentrated or in situations where high dosage of drug can be used. This category also provides a buffer zone that prevents small uncontrolled technical factors from causing major discrepancies in interpretation. A report of "Resistant" indicates that the pathogen is not likely to be inhibited if the antimicrobial compound in the blood reaches the concentrations usually achievable; other therapy should be selected.

Standardized susceptibility test procedures require the use of laboratory control microorganisms to control the techni-

SERUM LEVELS IN ADULTS
AFTER A 30-MINUTE I.V. INFUSION OF TIMENTIN®

TICARCILLIN SERUM LEVELS (mcg/mL)

Dose	0	15 min.	30 min.	1 hr.	1.5 hr.	3.5 hr.	5.5 hr.
3.1 gram	324 (293 to 388)	223 (184 to 293)	176 (135 to 235)	131 (102 to 195)	90 (65 to 119)	27 (19 to 37)	6 (5 to 7)

CLAVULANIC ACID SERUM LEVELS (mcg/mL)

Dose	0	15 min.	30 min.	1 hr.	1.5 hr.	3.5 hr.	5.5 hr.
3.1 gram	8.0 (5.3 to 10.3)	4.6 (3.0 to 7.6)	2.6 (1.8 to 3.4)	1.8 (1.6 to 2.2)	1.2 (0.8 to 1.6)	0.3 (0.2 to 0.3)	0

cal aspects of the laboratory procedures. Standard ticarcillin/clavulanate potassium powder should provide the following MIC values:

Microorganism		MIC (mcg/mL)‡
Escherichia coli	ATCC 25922	4-16
Escherichia coli	ATCC 35218	4-16
Pseudomonas aeruginosa	ATCC 27853	8-32
Staphylococcus aureus	ATCC 29213	0.5-2

‡Expressed as concentration of ticarcillin in the presence of clavulanic acid at a constant 2 mcg/mL.

Diffusion Techniques: Quantitative methods that require measurement of zone diameters also provide reproducible estimates of the susceptibility of bacteria to antimicrobial compounds. One such standardized procedure[2,3] requires the use of standardized inoculum concentrations. This procedure uses paper disks impregnated with 85 mcg of ticarcillin/clavulanate potassium (75 mcg ticarcillin plus 10 mcg clavulanate potassium) to test the susceptibility of microorganisms to ticarcillin/clavulanic acid.

Reports from the laboratory providing results of the standard single-disk susceptibility test with an 85 mcg of ticarcillin/clavulanate potassium (75 mcg ticarcillin plus 10 mcg clavulanate potassium) disk should be interpreted according to the following criteria:

RECOMMENDED RANGES FOR TICARCILLIN/CLAVULANIC ACID SUSCEPTIBILITY TESTING

For *Pseudomonas aeruginosa*:

Zone Diameter (mm)	Interpretation
≥15	Susceptible (S)
≤14	Resistant (R)

For Enterobacteriaceae:

Zone Diameter (mm)	Interpretation
≥20	Susceptible (S)
15-19	Intermediate (I)
≤14	Resistant (R)

For Staphylococci§:

Zone Diameter (mm)	Interpretation
≥23	Susceptible (S)
≤22	Resistant (R)

§Staphylococci that are resistant to methicillin/oxacillin must be considered as resistant to ticarcillin/clavulanic acid.

Interpretation should be as stated above for results using dilution techniques. Interpretation involves correlation of the diameter obtained in the disk test with the MIC for ticarcillin/clavulanic acid.

As with standardized dilution techniques, diffusion methods require the use of laboratory control microorganisms that are used to control the technical aspects of the laboratory procedures. For the diffusion technique, the 85 mcg of ticarcillin/clavulanate potassium (75 mcg ticarcillin plus 10 mcg clavulanate potassium) disk should provide the following zone diameters in these laboratory test quality control strains:

Microorganism		Zone Diameter (mm)
Escherichia coli	ATCC 25922	24-30
Escherichia coli	ATCC 35218	21-25
Pseudomonas aeruginosa	ATCC 27853	20-28
Staphylococcus aureus	ATCC 25923	29-37

Anaerobic Techniques: For anaerobic bacteria, the susceptibility to ticarcillin/clavulanic acid can be determined by standardized test methods[3,4]. The MIC values obtained should be interpreted according to the following criteria:

RECOMMENDED RANGES FOR TICARCILLIN/CLAVULANIC ACID SUSCEPTIBILITY TESTING||

MIC (mcg/mL)	Interpretation
≤32	Susceptible (S)
64	Intermediate (I)
≥128	Resistant (R)

||Expressed as concentration of ticarcillin in the presence of clavulanic acid at a constant 2 mcg/mL.

Interpretation is identical to that stated above for results using dilution techniques.

As with other susceptibility techniques, the use of laboratory control microorganisms is required to control the technical aspects of the laboratory standardized procedures. Standardized ticarcillin/clavulanate potassium powder should provide the following MIC values:

[See table above]

Microorganism		Agar dilution MIC Range (mcg/mL)||	Broth microdilution MIC Range (mcg/mL)||
Bacteroides thetaiotaomicron	ATCC 29741	0.5-2	0.5-2
Eubacterium lentum	ATCC 43055	16-64	8-32

||Expressed as concentration of ticarcillin in the presence of clavulanic acid at a constant 2 mcg/mL.

INDICATIONS AND USAGE

TIMENTIN is indicated in the treatment of infections caused by susceptible strains of the designated microorganisms in the conditions listed below:

Septicemia (including bacteremia) caused by β-lactamase–producing strains of *Klebsiella* spp.*, *E. coli**, *S. aureus* *, or *P. aeruginosa* * (or other *Pseudomonas* species*)

Lower Respiratory Infections caused by β-lactamase–producing strains of *S. aureus, H. influenzae**, or *Klebsiella* spp.*

Bone and Joint Infections caused by β-lactamase–producing strains of *S. aureus*

Skin and Skin Structure Infections caused by β-lactamase–producing strains of *S. aureus, Klebsiella* spp.*, or *E. coli**

Urinary Tract Infections (complicated and uncomplicated) caused by β-lactamase–producing strains of *E. coli, Klebsiella spp., P. aeruginosa** (or other *Pseudomonas* spp.*), *Citrobacter* spp.*, *Enterobacter cloacae**, *S. marcescens**, or *S. aureus**

Gynecologic Infections endometritis caused by β-lactamase–producing strains of *P. melaninogenicus**, *Enterobacter* spp. (including *E. cloacae**), *E. coli, K. pneumoniae**, *S. aureus*, or *S. epidermidis*

Intra-abdominal Infections peritonitis caused by β-lactamase–producing strains of *E. coli, K. pneumoniae*, or *B. fragilis** group

*Efficacy for this organism in this organ system was studied in fewer than 10 infections.

NOTE: For information on use in pediatric patients (≥3 months of age) see PRECAUTIONS-Pediatric Use and CLINICAL STUDIES sections. There are insufficient data to support the use of TIMENTIN in pediatric patients under 3 months of age or for the treatment of septicemia and/or infections in the pediatric population where the suspected or proven pathogen is *H. influenzae* type b.

While TIMENTIN is indicated only for the conditions listed above, infections caused by ticarcillin-susceptible organisms are also amenable to treatment with TIMENTIN due to its ticarcillin content. Therefore, mixed infections caused by ticarcillin-susceptible organisms and β-lactamase–producing organisms susceptible to ticarcillin/clavulanic acid should not require the addition of another antibiotic.

Due to its broad spectrum of bactericidal activity against gram-positive and gram-negative bacteria, TIMENTIN is particularly useful for the treatment of mixed infections and for presumptive therapy prior to the identification of the causative organisms. TIMENTIN has been shown to be effective as single drug therapy in the treatment of some serious infections where normally combination antibiotic therapy might be employed.

Based on the in vitro synergism between ticarcillin/clavulanic acid and aminoglycosides against certain strains of *P. aeruginosa*, combined therapy has been successful, especially in patients with impaired host defenses. Both drugs should be used in full therapeutic doses.

To reduce the development of drug-resistant bacteria and maintain the effectiveness of TIMENTIN and other antibacterial drugs, TIMENTIN should be used only to treat or prevent infections that are proven or strongly suspected to be caused by susceptible bacteria. When culture and susceptibility information are available, they should be considered in selecting or modifying antibacterial therapy. In the absence of such data, local epidemiology and susceptibility patterns may contribute to the empiric selection of therapy.

CONTRAINDICATIONS

TIMENTIN is contraindicated in patients with a history of hypersensitivity reactions to any of the penicillins.

WARNINGS

SERIOUS AND OCCASIONALLY FATAL HYPERSENSITIVITY (ANAPHYLACTIC) REACTIONS HAVE BEEN REPORTED IN PATIENTS ON PENICILLIN THERAPY. THESE REACTIONS ARE MORE LIKELY TO OCCUR IN INDIVIDUALS WITH A HISTORY OF PENICILLIN HYPERSENSITIVITY AND/OR A HISTORY OF SENSITIVITY TO MULTIPLE ALLERGENS. THERE HAVE BEEN REPORTS OF INDIVIDUALS WITH A HISTORY OF PENICILLIN HYPERSENSITIVITY WHO HAVE EXPERIENCED SEVERE REACTIONS WHEN TREATED WITH CEPHALOSPORINS. BEFORE INITIATING THERAPY WITH TIMENTIN CAREFUL INQUIRY SHOULD BE MADE CONCERNING PREVIOUS HYPERSENSITIVITY REACTIONS TO PENICILLINS, CEPHALOSPORINS, OR OTHER ALLERGENS. IF AN ALLERGIC REACTION OCCURS, TIMENTIN SHOULD BE DISCONTINUED AND THE APPROPRIATE THERAPY INSTITUTED. **SERIOUS ANAPHYLACTIC REACTIONS REQUIRE IMMEDIATE EMERGENCY TREATMENT WITH EPINEPHRINE. OXYGEN, INTRAVENOUS STEROIDS, AND AIRWAY MANAGEMENT, INCLUDING INTUBATION, SHOULD ALSO BE PROVIDED AS INDICATED.**

Pseudomembranous colitis has been reported with nearly all antibacterial agents, including TIMENTIN, and may range in severity from mild to life-threatening. Therefore, it is important to consider this diagnosis in patients who present with diarrhea subsequent to the administration of antibacterial agents.

Treatment with antibacterial agents alters the normal flora of the colon and may permit overgrowth of clostridia. Studies indicate that a toxin produced by *Clostridium difficile* is a primary cause of "antibiotic-associated colitis."

After the diagnosis of pseudomembranous colitis has been established, appropriate therapeutic measures should be initiated. Mild cases of pseudomembranous colitis usually respond to drug discontinuation alone. In moderate to severe cases, consideration should be given to management with fluids and electrolytes, protein supplementation, and treatment with an antibacterial drug clinically effective against *C. difficile* colitis.

When very high doses of TIMENTIN are administered, especially in the presence of impaired renal function, patients may experience convulsions. (See ADVERSE REACTIONS and OVERDOSAGE.)

PRECAUTIONS

General: While TIMENTIN possesses the characteristic low toxicity of the penicillin group of antibiotics, periodic assessment of organ system functions, including renal, hepatic, and hematopoietic function, is advisable during prolonged therapy.

Bleeding manifestations have occurred in some patients receiving β-lactam antibiotics. These reactions have been associated with abnormalities of coagulation tests such as clotting time, platelet aggregation, and prothrombin time and are more likely to occur in patients with renal impairment. If bleeding manifestations appear, treatment with TIMENTIN should be discontinued and appropriate therapy instituted.

TIMENTIN has only rarely been reported to cause hypokalemia; however, the possibility of this occurring should be kept in mind particularly when treating patients with fluid and electrolyte imbalance. Periodic monitoring of serum potassium may be advisable in patients receiving prolonged therapy.

The theoretical sodium content is 4.51 mEq (103.6 mg) per gram of TIMENTIN. This should be considered when treating patients requiring restricted salt intake.

As with any penicillin, an allergic reaction, including anaphylaxis, may occur during administration of TIMENTIN, particularly in a hypersensitive individual.

The possibility of superinfections with mycotic or bacterial pathogens should be kept in mind, particularly during prolonged treatment. If superinfections occur, appropriate measures should be taken.

Prescribing TIMENTIN in the absence of a proven or strongly suspected bacterial infection or a prophylactic indication is unlikely to provide benefit to the patient and increases the risk of the development of drug-resistant bacteria.

Information for Patients: Patients should be counseled that antibacterial drugs, including TIMENTIN, should only be used to treat bacterial infections. They do not treat viral infections (e.g., the common cold). When TIMENTIN is prescribed to treat a bacterial infection, patients should be told that although it is common to feel better early in the course of therapy, the medication should be taken exactly as directed. Skipping doses or not completing the full course of therapy may: (1) decrease the effectiveness of the immediate treatment, and (2) increase the likelihood that bacteria will develop resistance and will not be treatable by TIMENTIN or other antibacterial drugs in the future.

Drug/Laboratory Test Interactions: As with other penicillins, the mixing of TIMENTIN with an aminoglycoside in solutions for parenteral administration can result in substantial inactivation of the aminoglycoside.

Probenecid interferes with the renal tubular secretion of ticarcillin, thereby increasing serum concentrations and prolonging serum half-life of the antibiotic.

High urine concentrations of ticarcillin may produce false-positive protein reactions (pseudoproteinuria) with the following methods: Sulfosalicylic acid and boiling test, acetic acid test, biuret reaction and nitric acid test. The bromphenol blue (MULTI-STIX®) reagent strip test has been reported to be reliable.

The presence of clavulanic acid in TIMENTIN may cause a nonspecific binding of IgG and albumin by red cell membranes leading to a false-positive Coombs test.

Carcinogenesis, Mutagenesis, Impairment of Fertility: Long-term studies in animals have not been performed to evaluate carcinogenic potential. However, results from assays for gene mutation in vitro using bacteria (Ames tests) and yeast, and for chromosomal effects in vitro in human lymphocytes, and in vivo in mouse bone marrow (micronu-

Continued on next page

Product information on these pages is effective as of August 2004. Further information is available at: GlaxoSmithKline, PO Box 13398, Research Triangle Park, NC 27709. 1-888-825-5249. Corporate Web Site: www.gsk.com

Timentin ADD-Vantage—Cont.

cleus test) indicate that TIMENTIN is without any mutagenic potential.

Pregnancy (Category B): Reproduction studies have been performed in rats given doses up to 1,050 mg/kg/day and have revealed no evidence of impaired fertility or harm to the fetus due to TIMENTIN. There are, however, no adequate and well-controlled studies in pregnant women. Because animal reproduction studies are not always predictive of human response, this drug should be used during pregnancy only if clearly needed.

Nursing Mothers: It is not known whether this drug is excreted in human milk. Because many drugs are excreted in human milk, caution should be exercised when TIMENTIN is administered to a nursing woman.

Pediatric Use: The safety and effectiveness of TIMENTIN have been established in the age group of 3 months to 16 years. Use of TIMENTIN in these age groups is supported by evidence from adequate and well-controlled studies of TIMENTIN in adults with additional efficacy, safety, and pharmacokinetic data from both comparative and non-comparative studies in pediatric patients. There are insufficient data to support the use of TIMENTIN in pediatric patients under 3 months of age or for the treatment of septicemia and/or infections in the pediatric population where the suspected or proven pathogen is *H. influenzae* type b.

In those patients in whom meningeal seeding from a distant infection site or in whom meningitis is suspected or documented, or in patients who require prophylaxis against central nervous system infection, an alternate agent with demonstrated clinical efficacy in this setting should be used.

ADVERSE REACTIONS

As with other penicillins, the following adverse reactions may occur:

Hypersensitivity Reactions: Skin rash, pruritus, urticaria, arthralgia, myalgia, drug fever, chills, chest discomfort, erythema multiforme, toxic epidermal necrolysis, Stevens-Johnson Syndrome, and anaphylactic reactions.

Central Nervous System: Headache, giddiness, neuromuscular hyperirritability, or convulsive seizures.

Gastrointestinal Disturbances: Disturbances of taste and smell, stomatitis, flatulence, nausea, vomiting and diarrhea, epigastric pain, and pseudomembranous colitis have been reported. Onset of pseudomembranous colitis symptoms may occur during or after antibiotic treatment. (See WARNINGS.)

Hemic and Lymphatic Systems: Thrombocytopenia, leukopenia, neutropenia, eosinophilia, reduction of hemoglobin or hematocrit, and prolongation of prothrombin time and bleeding time.

Abnormalities of Hepatic and Renal Function Tests: Elevation of serum aspartate aminotransferase (SGOT), serum alanine aminotransferase (SGPT), serum alkaline phosphatase, serum LDH, serum bilirubin. There have been reports of transient hepatitis and cholestatic jaundice—as with some other penicillins and some cephalosporins. Elevation of serum creatinine and/or BUN, hypernatremia, reduction in serum potassium and uric acid.

Local reactions: Pain, burning, swelling, and induration at the injection site and thrombophlebitis with intravenous administration.

Available safety data for pediatric patients treated with TIMENTIN demonstrate a similar adverse event profile to that observed in adult patients.

DRUG ABUSE AND DEPENDENCE

Neither abuse of nor dependence on TIMENTIN has been reported.

OVERDOSAGE

As with other penicillins, neurotoxic reactions may arise when very high doses of TIMENTIN are administered, especially in patients with impaired renal function. (See WARNINGS and ADVERSE REACTIONS-Central Nervous System.)

In case of overdosage, discontinue TIMENTIN, treat symptomatically, and institute supportive measures as required. Ticarcillin may be removed from circulation by hemodialysis. The molecular weight, degree of protein binding, and pharmacokinetic profile of clavulanic acid together with information from a single patient with renal insufficiency all suggest that this compound may also be removed by hemodialysis.

DOSAGE AND ADMINISTRATION

TIMENTIN should be administered by intravenous infusion (30 min.).

Adults: The usual recommended dosage for systemic and urinary tract infections for average (60 kg) adults is 3.1 grams of TIMENTIN (3.1-gram vial containing 3 grams ticarcillin and 100 mg clavulanic acid) given every 4 to 6 hours. For gynecologic infections, TIMENTIN should be administered as follows: Moderate infections 200 mg/kg/day in divided doses every 6 hours and for severe infections 300 mg/kg/day in divided doses every 4 hours. For patients weighing less than 60 kg, the recommended dosage is 200 to 300 mg/kg/day, based on ticarcillin content, given in divided doses every 4 to 6 hours.

Pediatric Patients (≥3 months): ***For patients <60 kg:*** In patients <60 kg, TIMENTIN is dosed at 50 mg/kg/dose based on the ticarcillin component. TIMENTIN should be administered as follows: Mild to moderate infections, 200 mg/kg/day in divided doses every 6 hours; for severe infections, 300 mg/kg/day in divided doses every 4 hours.

For patients ≥60 kg: For mild to moderate infections, 3.1 grams of TIMENTIN (3 grams of ticarcillin and 100 mg of clavulanic acid) administered every 6 hours; for severe infections, 3.1 grams every 4 hours.

Renal Impairment: For infections complicated by renal insufficiency[†], an initial loading dose of 3.1 grams should be followed by doses based on creatinine clearance and type of dialysis as indicated below:

[See table above]

Creatinine clearance mL/min.	Dosage
over 60	3.1 grams every 4 hrs.
30 to 60	2 grams every 4 hrs.
10 to 30	2 grams every 8 hrs.
less than 10	2 grams every 12 hrs.
less than 10 with hepatic dysfunction	2 grams every 24 hrs.
patients on peritoneal dialysis	3.1 grams every 12 hrs.
patients on hemodialysis	2 grams every 12 hrs. supplemented with 3.1 grams after each dialysis

To calculate creatinine clearance[‡] from a serum creatinine value use the following formula.

$$C_{cr} = \frac{(140\text{–Age})\ (\text{wt. in kg})}{72 \times S_{cr}\ (\text{mg/100 mL})}$$

This is the calculated creatinine clearance for adult males; for females it is 15% less.

[‡]Cockcroft, D.W., et al: Prediction of Creatinine Clearance from Serum Creatinine. Nephron 16:31-41, 1976.

NOTE: TIMENTIN in the ADD-VANTAGE® system should only be administered for 3.1-gram dosing.

[†]The half-life of ticarcillin in patients with renal failure is approximately 13 hours.

Dosage for any individual patient must take into consideration the site and severity of infection, the susceptibility of the organisms causing infection, and the status of the patient's host defense mechanisms.

The duration of therapy depends upon the severity of infection. Generally, TIMENTIN should be continued for at least 2 days after the signs and symptoms of infection have disappeared. The usual duration is 10 to 14 days; however, in difficult and complicated infections, more prolonged therapy may be required.

Frequent bacteriologic and clinical appraisals are necessary during therapy of chronic urinary tract infection and may be required for several months after therapy has been completed. Persistent infections may require treatment for several weeks, and doses smaller than those indicated above should not be used.

In certain infections, involving abscess formation, appropriate surgical drainage should be performed in conjunction with antimicrobial therapy.

INSTRUCTIONS FOR USE

To Open Diluent Container:

Peel overwrap at corner and remove solution container. Some opacity of the plastic due to moisture absorption during the sterilization process may be observed.

This is normal and does not affect the solution quality or safety. The opacity will diminish gradually.

To Assemble Vial and Flexible Diluent Container:

(Use Aseptic Technique):

1. Remove the protective covers from the top of the vial and the vial port on the diluent container as follows:
   a. To remove the breakaway vial cap, swing the pull ring over the top of the vial and pull down far enough to start the opening (see Figure 1), then pull straight up to remove the cap (see Figure 2).
   NOTE: Do not access vial with syringe.

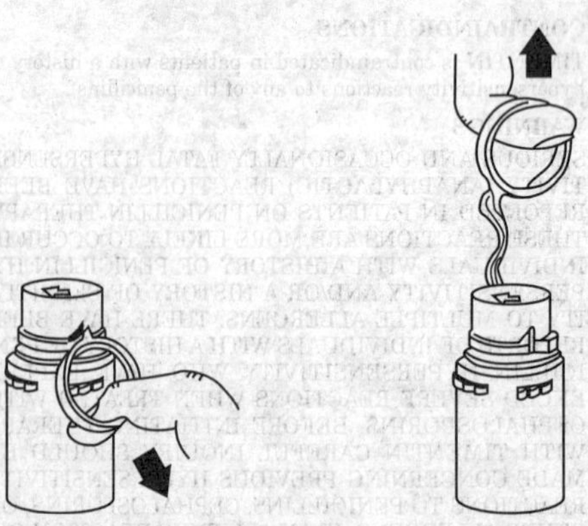

Figure 1 Figure 2

   b. To remove the vial port cover, grasp the tab on the pull ring, pull up to break the 3 tie strings, then pull back to remove the cover (see Figure 3).
2. Screw the vial into the vial port until it will go no further. THE VIAL MUST BE SCREWED IN TIGHTLY TO ASSURE A SEAL. This occurs approximately ½ turn (180°) after the first audible click (see Figure 4). The clicking sound does not assure a seal; the vial must be turned as far as it will go.
   NOTE: Once vial is sealed, do not attempt to remove (see Figure 4).
3. Recheck the vial to assure that it is tight by trying to turn it further in the direction of assembly.
4. Label appropriately.

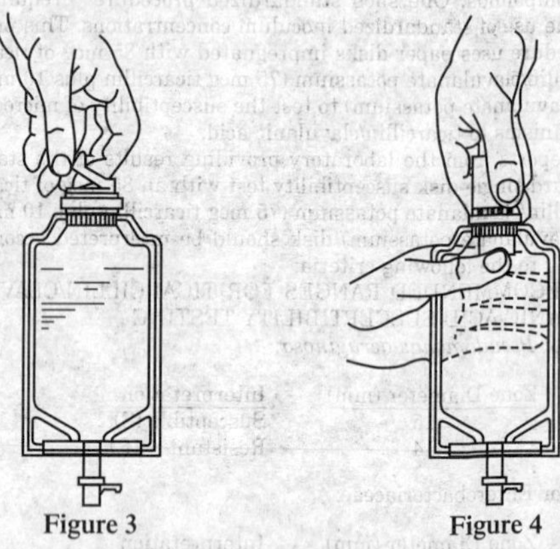

Figure 3 Figure 4

To Reconstitute the Drug:

1. Squeeze the bottom of the diluent container gently to inflate the portion of the container surrounding the end of the drug vial.
2. With the other hand, push the drug vial down into the container telescoping the walls of the container. Grasp the inner cap of the vial through the walls of the container (see Figure 5).
3. Pull the inner cap from the drug vial (see Figure 6). Verify that the rubber stopper has been pulled out, allowing the drug and diluent to mix.
4. Mix container contents thoroughly and use within the specified time.

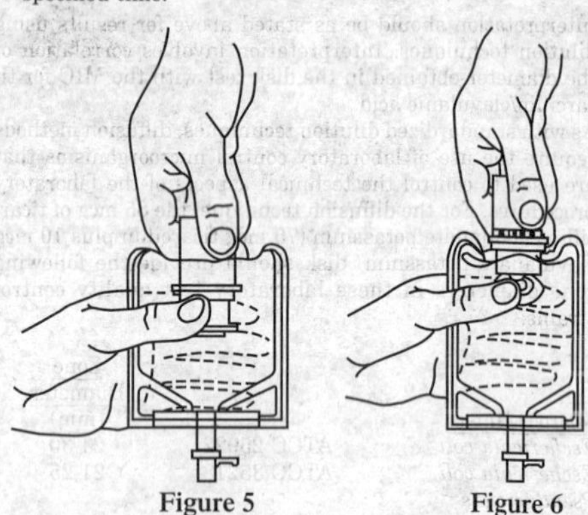

Figure 5 Figure 6

Preparation for Administration:

(Use Aseptic Technique):

1. Confirm the activation and admixture of vial contents.
2. Check for leaks by squeezing container firmly. If leaks are found discard unit as sterility may be impaired.
3. Close flow control clamp of administration set.
4. Remove cover from outlet port at bottom of container.
5. Insert piercing pin of administration set into port with a twisting motion until the pin is firmly seated. **NOTE:** See full directions on administration set carton.
6. Lift the free end of the hanger loop on the bottom of the vial, breaking the 2 tie strings. Bend the loop outward to lock it in the upright position, then suspend container from hanger.
7. Squeeze and release drip chamber to establish proper fluid level in chamber.
8. Open flow control clamp and clear air from set. Close clamp.
9. Attach set to venipuncture device. If device is not indwelling, prime and make venipuncture.
10. Regulate rate of administration with flow control clamp.

WARNING: Do not use flexible container in series connections.

RECONSTITUTION DIRECTIONS

Intravenous Infusion: Use a 50-mL or 100-mL ADD-VANTAGE® DILUENT CONTAINER containing either Sodium Chloride Injection, USP, or 5% Dextrose in Water (refer to INSTRUCTIONS FOR USE section). The resulting concentration of the 3.1-gram dose reconstituted in 50 mL of diluent is approximately 60 mg/mL of ticarcillin

INTRAVENOUS SOLUTION (ticarcillin concentration of ∼30 mg/mL or ∼60 mg/mL)	STABILITY PERIOD ROOM TEMPERATURE 21° to 24°C (70° to 75°F)
Sodium Chloride Injection, USP	24 hours
5% Dextrose in Water	12 hours

and approximately 2 mg/mL of clavulanic acid. The resulting concentration of the 3.1-gram dose reconstituted in 100 mL of diluent is approximately 30 mg/mL of ticarcillin and approximately 1 mg/mL of clavulanic acid.

The solution of reconstituted drug may then be administered over a period of 30 minutes by direct infusion or through a Y-type intravenous infusion set, which may already be in place. If this method or the "piggyback" method of administration is used, it is advisable to discontinue temporarily the administration of any other solutions during the infusion of TIMENTIN. When TIMENTIN is given in combination with another antimicrobial, such as an aminoglycoside, each drug should be given separately in accordance with the recommended dosage and routes of administration for each drug. After reconstitution and prior to administration, TIMENTIN, as with other parenteral drugs, should be inspected visually for particulate matter. If this condition is evident, the solution should be discarded.

The color of reconstituted solutions of TIMENTIN normally ranges from light to dark yellow, depending on concentration, duration, and temperature of storage while maintaining label claim characteristics.

[See table above]

NOTE: TIMENTIN is incompatible with Sodium Bicarbonate.

Unused portions of solutions should be discarded after the time periods listed above.

Avoid excessive heat.

Protect from freezing.

HOW SUPPLIED

Each 3.1-gram vial of TIMENTIN contains sterile ticarcillin disodium equivalent to 3 grams ticarcillin and sterile clavulanate potassium equivalent to 0.1 gram clavulanic acid.

NDC 0029-6571-40 3.1-gram ADD-VANTAGE®§ Antibiotic Vial

TIMENTIN is also supplied as:

NDC 0029-6571-26 3.1-gram Vial

Each 31-gram Pharmacy Bulk Package contains sterile ticarcillin disodium equivalent to 30 grams ticarcillin and sterile clavulanate potassium equivalent to 1 gram clavulanic acid.

NDC 0029-6579-21 31 gram Pharmacy Bulk Package

TIMENTIN should be stored at or below 24°C (75°F).

NDC 0029-6571-31 TIMENTIN as an iso-osmotic, sterile, nonpyrogenic, frozen solution in GALAXY®|| (PL 2040) Plastic Containers—supplied in 100-mL single-dose containers equivalent to 3 grams ticarcillin and clavulanate potassium equivalent to 0.1 gram clavulanic acid.

CLINICAL STUDIES

TIMENTIN has been studied in a total of 296 pediatric patients (excluding neonates and infants less than 3 months) in 6 controlled clinical trials. The majority of patients studied had intra-abdominal infections, and the primary comparator was clindamycin and gentamicin with or without ampicillin. At the end-of-therapy visit, comparable efficacy was reported in the trial arms using TIMENTIN and an appropriate comparator.

TIMENTIN was also evaluated in an additional 408 pediatric patients (excluding neonates and infants less than 3 months) in 3 uncontrolled U.S. clinical trials. Patients were treated across a broad range of presenting diagnoses including: Infections in bone and joint, skin and skin structure, lower respiratory tract, urinary tract, as well as intra-abdominal and gynecologic infections. Patients received TIMENTIN either 300 mg/kg/day (based on the ticarcillin component) divided q4h for severe infection or 200 mg/kg/day (based on the ticarcillin component) divided q6h for mild to moderate infections. The efficacy rates were comparable to those obtained in the controlled trials.

The adverse event profile in these 704 pediatric patients treated with TIMENTIN was comparable to that seen in adult patients.

REFERENCES

1. National Committee for Clinical Laboratory Standards. *Methods for Dilution Antimicrobial Susceptibility Tests for Bacteria that Grow Aerobically* - Sixth Edition. Approved Standard. NCCLS Document M7-A6, Vol. 23, No. 2 (ISBN-1-56238-486-4). NCCLS, 940 West Valley Road, Suite 1400, Wayne, PA 19087-1898, January, 2003.
2. National Committee for Clinical Laboratory Standards. *Performance Standards for Antimicrobial Disk Susceptibility Tests* - Eighth Edition. Approved Standard. NCCLS Document M2-A8, Vol. 23, No. 1 (ISBN-1-56238-485-6). NCCLS, 940 West Valley Road, Suite 1400, Wayne, PA 19087-1898, January, 2003.
3. National Committee for Clinical Laboratory Standards. *Performance Standards for Antimicrobial Susceptibility Testing* - Thirteenth Informational Supplement. NCCLS Document M100-S13 (M7), Vol. 23, No. 2. NCCLS, 940 West Valley Road, Suite 1400, Wayne, PA 19087-1898, January, 2003.
4. National Committee for Clinical Laboratory Standards. *Methods for Antimicrobial Susceptibility Testing of Anaerobic Bacteria* – Fifth Edition. Approved Standard NCCLS Document M11-A5, Vol. 21, No. 2 (ISBN-1-56238-429-5). NCCLS, 940 West Valley Road, Suite 1400, Wayne, PA 19087-1898, January, 2001.

§ADD-VANTAGE is a registered trademark of Abbott Laboratories.

||GALAXY is a registered trademark of Baxter International Inc.

MULTI-STIX is a registered trademark of Bayer Corporation.

TIMENTIN is a registered trademark of GlaxoSmithKline.

GlaxoSmithKline, Research Triangle Park, NC 27709

October 2003/TI:L12AV

Shown in Product Identification Guide, page 317

TIMENTIN® ℞

[*tī-mĕn'tin*]

(sterile ticarcillin disodium and clavulanate potassium) for Intravenous Administration

PHARMACY BULK PACKAGE NOT FOR DIRECT INFUSION

RECONSTITUTED STOCK SOLUTION MUST BE TRANSFERRED AND FURTHER DILUTED FOR IV INFUSION.

To reduce the development of drug-resistant bacteria and maintain the effectiveness of TIMENTIN (ticarcillin disodium and clavulanate potassium) and other antibacterial drugs, TIMENTIN should be used only to treat or prevent infections that are proven or strongly suspected to be caused by bacteria.

PACKAGE DESCRIPTION

TIMENTIN is available in a 31-gram Pharmacy Bulk Package. This sterile dosage form contains multiple-single doses for use in a pharmacy admixture program for the preparation of parenteral fluids.

To reduce the development of drug-resistant bacteria and maintain the effectiveness of TIMENTIN (ticarcillin disodium and clavulanate potassium) and other antibacterial drugs, TIMENTIN should be used only to treat or prevent infections that are proven or strongly suspected to be caused by bacteria.

PRODUCT DESCRIPTION

TIMENTIN is a sterile injectable antibacterial combination consisting of the semisynthetic antibiotic ticarcillin disodium and the β-lactamase inhibitor clavulanate potassium (the potassium salt of clavulanic acid) for intravenous administration. Ticarcillin is derived from the basic penicillin nucleus, 6-amino-penicillanic acid.

Clavulanic acid is produced by the fermentation of *Streptomyces clavuligerus*. It is a β-lactam structurally related to the penicillins and possesses the ability to inactivate a wide variety of β-lactamases by blocking the active sites of these enzymes. Clavulanic acid is particularly active against the clinically important plasmid-mediated β-lactamases frequently responsible for transferred drug resistance to penicillins and cephalosporins.

Chemically, clavulanate potassium is potassium (*Z*)-(2*R*, 5*R*)-3-(2-hydroxyethylidene)-7-oxo-4-oxa-1-azabicyclo[3.2.0]heptane-2-carboxylate.

TIMENTIN is supplied as a white to pale yellow powder for reconstitution. TIMENTIN is very soluble in water, its solubility being greater than 600 mg/mL. The reconstituted solution is clear, colorless or pale yellow, having a pH of 5.5 to 7.5.

For the 3.1-gram dosage of TIMENTIN, the theoretical sodium content is 4.51 mEq (103.6 mg) per gram of TIMENTIN. The theoretical potassium content is 0.15 mEq (6 mg) per gram of TIMENTIN.

CLINICAL PHARMACOLOGY

After an intravenous infusion (30 min.) of 3.1 grams of TIMENTIN, peak serum concentrations of both ticarcillin and clavulanic acid are attained immediately after completion of infusion. Ticarcillin serum levels are similar to those produced by the administration of equivalent amounts of ticarcillin alone with a mean peak serum level of 330 mcg/mL. The corresponding mean peak serum level for clavulanic acid was 8 mcg/mL. (See following table.)

[See first table at top of next page]

The mean area under the serum concentration curve was 485 mcg•hr/mL for ticarcillin and 8.2 mcg•hr/mL for clavulanic acid.

The mean serum half-lives of ticarcillin and clavulanic acid in healthy volunteers are 1.1 hours and 1.1 hours, respectively.

In pediatric patients receiving approximately 50 mg/kg of TIMENTIN (30:1 ratio ticarcillin to clavulanate), mean ticarcillin serum half-lives were 4.4 hours in neonates (n = 18) and 1.0 hour in infants and children (n = 41). The corresponding clavulanate serum half-lives averaged 1.9 hours in neonates (n = 14) and 0.9 hour in infants and children (n = 40). Area under the serum concentration time curves averaged 339 mcg•hr/mL in infants and children (n = 41), whereas the corresponding mean clavulanate area under the serum concentration time curves was approximately 7 mcg•hr/mL in the same population (n = 40).

Approximately 60% to 70% of ticarcillin and approximately 35% to 45% of clavulanic acid are excreted unchanged in urine during the first 6 hours after administration of a single dose of TIMENTIN to normal volunteers with normal renal function. Two hours after an intravenous injection of 3.1 grams of TIMENTIN, concentrations of ticarcillin in urine generally exceed 1,500 mcg/mL. The corresponding concentrations of clavulanic acid in urine generally exceed 40 mcg/mL. By 4 to 6 hours after injection, the urine concentrations of ticarcillin and clavulanic acid usually decline to approximately 190 mcg/mL. Neither component of TIMENTIN is highly protein bound; ticarcillin has been found to be approximately 45% bound to human serum protein and clavulanic acid approximately 25% bound.

Somewhat higher and more prolonged serum levels of ticarcillin can be achieved with the concurrent administration of probenecid; however, probenecid does not enhance the serum levels of clavulanic acid.

Ticarcillin can be detected in tissues and interstitial fluid following parenteral administration.

Penetration of ticarcillin into bile and pleural fluid has been demonstrated. The results of experiments involving the administration of clavulanic acid to animals suggest that this compound, like ticarcillin, is well distributed in body tissues.

An inverse relationship exists between the serum half-life of ticarcillin and creatinine clearance. The dosage of TIMENTIN need only be adjusted in cases of severe renal impairment. (See DOSAGE AND ADMINISTRATION.)

Ticarcillin may be removed from patients undergoing dialysis; the actual amount removed depends on the duration and type of dialysis.

Microbiology: Ticarcillin is a semisynthetic antibiotic with a broad spectrum of bactericidal activity against many gram-positive and gram-negative aerobic and anaerobic bacteria.

Ticarcillin is, however, susceptible to degradation by β-lactamases, and, therefore, the spectrum of activity does not normally include organisms which produce these enzymes.

Clavulanic acid is a β-lactam, structurally related to the penicillins, which possesses the ability to inactivate a wide range of β-lactamase enzymes commonly found in microorganisms resistant to penicillins and cephalosporins. In particular, it has good activity against the clinically important plasmid-mediated β-lactamases frequently responsible for transferred drug resistance.

The formulation of ticarcillin with clavulanic acid in TIMENTIN protects ticarcillin from degradation by β-lactamase enzymes and effectively extends the antibiotic spectrum of ticarcillin to include many bacteria normally resistant to ticarcillin and other β-lactam antibiotics. Thus, TIMENTIN possesses the distinctive properties of a broad-spectrum antibiotic and a β-lactamase inhibitor. Ticarcillin/clavulanic acid has been shown to be active against most strains of the following microorganisms, both in vitro and in clinical infections as described in the INDICATIONS AND USAGE section.

Gram-Positive Aerobes:

Staphylococcus aureus (β-lactamase and non–β-lactamase–producing)*

Staphylococcus epidermidis (β-lactamase and non–β-lactamase–producing)*

*Staphylococci that are resistant to methicillin/oxacillin must be considered resistant to ticarcillin/clavulanic acid.

Gram-Negative Aerobes:

Citrobacter species (β-lactamase and non–β-lactamase–producing)

Enterobacter species including *E. cloacae* (β-lactamase and non–β-lactamase–producing) (Although most strains of *Enterobacter* species are resistant in vitro, clinical efficacy has been demonstrated with TIMENTIN in urinary tract infections and gynecologic infections caused by these organisms.)

Escherichia coli (β-lactamase and non–β-lactamase–producing)

Haemophilus influenzae (β-lactamase and non–β-lactamase–producing)†

Klebsiella species including *K. pneumoniae* (β-lactamase and non–β-lactamase–producing)

Pseudomonas species including *P. aeruginosa* (β-lactamase and non–β-lactamase–producing)

Serratia marcescens (β-lactamase and non–β-lactamase–producing)

†β-lactamase–negative, ampicillin-resistant (BLNAR) strains of *H. influenzae* must be considered resistant to ticarcillin/clavulanic acid.

Continued on next page

Product information on these pages is effective as of August 2004. Further information is available at: GlaxoSmithKline, PO Box 13398, Research Triangle Park, NC 27709. 1-888-825-5249. Corporate Web Site: www.gsk.com

Timentin Pharmacy Bulk—Cont.

Anaerobic Bacteria:
Bacteroides fragilis group (β-lactamase and non–β-lactamase–producing)
Prevotella (formerly *Bacteroides*) *melaninogenicus* (β-lactamase and non–β-lactamase–producing)
The following in vitro data are available, **but their clinical significance is unknown.**
The following strains exhibit an in vitro minimum inhibitory concentration (MIC) less than or equal to the susceptible breakpoint for ticarcillin/clavulanic acid. However, with the exception of organisms shown to respond to ticarcillin alone, the safety and effectiveness of ticarcillin/clavulanic acid in treating infections due to these microorganisms have not been established in adequate and well-controlled clinical trials.
Gram-Positive Aerobes:
Staphylococcus saprophyticus (β-lactamase and non–β-lactamase–producing)
Streptococcus agalactiae‡ (Group B)
Streptococcus bovis‡
Streptococcus pneumoniae‡ (penicillin-susceptible strains only)
Streptococcus pyogenes‡
Viridans group streptococci‡
Gram-Negative Aerobes:
Acinetobacter baumannii (β-lactamase and non–β-lactamase–producing)
Acinetobacter calcoaceticus (β-lactamase and non–β-lactamase–producing)
Acinetobacter haemolyticus (β-lactamase and non–β-lactamase–producing)
Acinetobacter lwoffi (β-lactamase and non–β-lactamase–producing)
Moraxella catarrhalis (β-lactamase and non–β-lactamase–producing)
Morganella morganii (β-lactamase and non–β-lactamase–producing)
Neisseria gonorrhoeae (β-lactamase and non–β-lactamase–producing)
Pasteurella multocida (β-lactamase and non–β-lactamase–producing)
Proteus mirabilis (β-lactamase and non–β-lactamase–producing)
Proteus penneri (β-lactamase and non–β-lactamase–producing)
Proteus vulgaris (β-lactamase and non–β-lactamase–producing)
Providencia rettgeri (β-lactamase and non–β-lactamase–producing)
Providencia stuartii (β-lactamase and non–β-lactamase–producing)
Stenotrophomonas maltophilia (β-lactamase and non–β-lactamase–producing)
Anaerobic Bacteria:
Clostridium species including *C. perfringens, C. difficile, C. sporogenes, C. ramosum,* and *C. bifermentans* (β-lactamase and non–β-lactamase–producing)
Eubacterium species
Fusobacterium species including *F. nucleatum* and *F. necrophorum* (β-lactamase and non–β-lactamase–producing)
Peptostreptococcus species‡
Veillonella species‡

‡These are non–β-lactamase–producing strains, and therefore, are susceptible to ticarcillin.

In vitro synergism between TIMENTIN and gentamicin, tobramycin, or amikacin against multiresistant strains of *Pseudomonas aeruginosa* has been demonstrated.

Susceptibility Testing: *Dilution Techniques:* Quantitative methods are used to determine antimicrobial MICs. These MICs provide estimates of the susceptibility of bacteria to antimicrobial compounds. The MICs should be determined using a standardized procedure. Standardized procedures are based on a dilution method[1,3] (broth or agar) or equivalent with standardized inoculum concentrations and standardized concentrations of ticarcillin/clavulanate potassium powder.
The recommended dilution pattern utilizes a constant level of 2 mcg/mL clavulanic acid in all tubes with varying amounts of ticarcillin. MICs are expressed in terms of the ticarcillin concentration in the presence of clavulanic acid at a constant 2 mcg/mL. The MIC values should be interpreted according to the following criteria:

RECOMMENDED RANGES FOR TICARCILLIN/CLAVULANIC ACID SUSCEPTIBILITY TESTING*

For *Pseudomonas aeruginosa*:

MIC (mcg/mL)	Interpretation	
≤64	Susceptible	(S)
≥128	Resistant	(R)

For Enterobacteriaceae:

MIC (mcg/mL)	Interpretation	
≤16	Susceptible	(S)
32-64	Intermediate	(I)
≥128	Resistant	(R)

For Staphylococci†:

MIC (mcg/mL)	Interpretation	
≤8	Susceptible	(S)
≥16	Resistant	(R)

SERUM LEVELS IN ADULTS
AFTER A 30-MINUTE IV INFUSION OF TIMENTIN®
TICARCILLIN SERUM LEVELS (mcg/mL)

Dose	0	15 min.	30 min.	1 hr.	1.5 hr.	3.5 hr.	5.5 hr.
3.1 gram	324	223	176	131	90	27	6
	(293 to 388)	(184 to 293)	(135 to 235)	(102 to 195)	(65 to 119)	(19 to 37)	(5 to 7)

CLAVULANIC ACID SERUM LEVELS (mcg/mL)

Dose	0	15 min.	30 min.	1 hr.	1.5 hr.	3.5 hr.	5.5 hr.
3.1 gram	8.0	4.6	2.6	1.8	1.2	0.3	0
	(5.3 to 10.3)	(3.0 to 7.6)	(1.8 to 3.4)	(1.6 to 2.2)	(0.8 to 1.6)	(0.2 to 0.3)	

Microorganism		Agar dilution MIC Range (mcg/mL)‖	Broth microdilution MIC Range (mcg/mL)‖
Bacteroides thetaiotaomicron	ATCC 29741	0.5-2	0.5-2
Eubacterium lentum	ATCC 43055	16-64	8-32

‖Expressed as concentration of ticarcillin in the presence of clavulanic acid at a constant 2 mcg/mL.

*Expressed as concentration of ticarcillin in the presence of clavulanic acid at a constant 2 mcg/mL.
†Staphylococci that are susceptible to ticarcillin/clavulanic acid but resistant to methicillin/oxacillin must be considered as resistant.

A report of "Susceptible" indicates that the pathogen is likely to be inhibited if the antimicrobial compound in the blood reaches the concentrations usually achievable. A report of "Intermediate" indicates that the result should be considered equivocal, and, if the microorganism is not fully susceptible to alternative, clinically feasible drugs, the test should be repeated. This category implies possible clinical applicability in body sites where the drug is physiologically concentrated or in situations where high dosage of drug can be used. This category also provides a buffer zone that prevents small uncontrolled technical factors from causing major discrepancies in interpretation. A report of "Resistant" indicates that the pathogen is not likely to be inhibited if the antimicrobial compound in the blood reaches the concentrations usually achievable; other therapy should be selected.
Standardized susceptibility test procedures require the use of laboratory control microorganisms to control the technical aspects of the laboratory procedures. Standard ticarcillin/clavulanate potassium powder should provide the following MIC values:

Microorganism		MIC (mcg/mL)‡
Escherichia coli	ATCC 25922	4-16
Escherichia coli	ATCC 35218	4-16
Pseudomonas aeruginosa	ATCC 27853	8-32
Staphylococcus aureus	ATCC 29213	0.5-2

‡ Expressed as concentration of ticarcillin in the presence of clavulanic acid at a constant 2 mcg/mL.

Diffusion Techniques: Quantitative methods that require measurement of zone diameters also provide reproducible estimates of the susceptibility of bacteria to antimicrobial compounds. One such standardized procedure[2,3] requires the use of standardized inoculum concentrations. This procedure uses paper disks impregnated with 85 mcg of ticarcillin/clavulanate potassium (75 mcg ticarcillin plus 10 mcg clavulanate potassium) to test the susceptibility of microorganisms to ticarcillin/clavulanic acid.
Reports from the laboratory providing results of the standard single-disk susceptibility test with an 85 mcg of ticarcillin/clavulanate potassium (75 mcg ticarcillin plus 10 mcg clavulanate potassium) disk should be interpreted according to the following criteria:

RECOMMENDED RANGES FOR TICARCILLIN/CLAVULANIC ACID SUSCEPTIBILITY TESTING

For *Pseudomonas aeruginosa*:

Zone Diameter (mm)	Interpretation	
≥15	Susceptible	(S)
≤14	Resistant	(R)

For Enterobacteriaceae:

Zone Diameter (mm)	Interpretation	
≥20	Susceptible	(S)
15-19	Intermediate	(I)
≤14	Resistant	(R)

For Staphylococci§:

Zone Diameter (mm)	Interpretation	
≥23	Susceptible	(S)
≤22	Resistant	(R)

§Staphylococci that are resistant to methicillin/oxacillin must be considered as resistant to ticarcillin/clavulanic acid.

Interpretation should be as stated above for results using dilution techniques. Interpretation involves correlation of the diameter obtained in the disk test with the MIC for ticarcillin/clavulanic acid.
As with standardized dilution techniques, diffusion methods require the use of laboratory control microorganisms that are used to control the technical aspects of the laboratory procedures. For the diffusion technique, the 85 mcg of ticarcillin/clavulanate potassium (75 mcg ticarcillin plus 10 mcg clavulanate potassium) disk should provide the following zone diameters in these laboratory test quality control strains:

Microorganism		Zone Diameter (mm)
Escherichia coli	ATCC 25922	24-30
Escherichia coli	ATCC 35218	21-25
Pseudomonas aeruginosa	ATCC 27853	20-28
Staphylococcus aureus	ATCC 25923	29-37

Anaerobic Techniques: For anaerobic bacteria, the susceptibility to ticarcillin/clavulanic acid can be determined by standardized test methods[3,4]. The MIC values obtained should be interpreted according to the following criteria:

RECOMMENDED RANGES FOR TICARCILLIN/CLAVULANIC ACID SUSCEPTIBILITY TESTING‖

MIC (mcg/mL)	Interpretation	
≤32	Susceptible	(S)
64	Intermediate	(I)
≥128	Resistant	(R)

‖Expressed as concentration of ticarcillin in the presence of clavulanic acid at a constant 2 mcg/mL.

Interpretation is identical to that stated above for results using dilution techniques.
As with other susceptibility techniques, the use of laboratory control microorganisms is required to control the technical aspects of the laboratory standardized procedures. Standardized ticarcillin/clavulanate potassium powder should provide the following MIC values:
[See second table above]

INDICATIONS AND USAGE

TIMENTIN is indicated in the treatment of infections caused by susceptible strains of the designated microorganisms in the conditions listed below:
Septicemia (including bacteremia) caused by β-lactamase–producing strains of *Klebsiella* spp.*, *E. coli**, *S. aureus**, or *P. aeruginosa** (or other *Pseudomonas* species*)
Lower Respiratory Infections caused by β-lactamase–producing strains of *S. aureus, H. influenzae**, or *Klebsiella* spp.*
Bone and Joint Infections caused by β-lactamase–producing strains of *S. aureus*
Skin and Skin Structure Infections caused by β-lactamase–producing strains of *S. aureus, Klebsiella spp.**, or *E. coli**
Urinary Tract Infections (complicated and uncomplicated) caused by β-lactamase–producing strains of *E. coli, Klebsiella* spp., *P. aeruginosa** (or other *Pseudomonas* spp.*), *Citrobacter* spp.*, *Enterobacter cloacae**, *S. marcescens**, or *S. aureus**
Gynecologic Infections endometritis caused by β-lactamase–producing strains of *P. melaninogenicus**, *Enterobacter* spp. (including *E. cloacae**), *E. coli, K. pneumoniae**, *S. aureus*, or *S. epidermidis*
Intra-abdominal Infections peritonitis caused by β-lactamase–producing strains of *E. coli, K. pneumoniae,* or *B. fragilis** group

*Efficacy for this organism in this organ system was studied in fewer than 10 infections.

NOTE: For information on use in pediatric patients (≥3 months of age) see PRECAUTIONS-Pediatric Use and CLINICAL STUDIES sections. There are insufficient data to support the use of TIMENTIN in pediatric patients under 3 months of age or for the treatment of septicemia and/or infections in the pediatric population where the suspected or proven pathogen is *H. influenzae* type b.
While TIMENTIN is indicated only for the conditions listed above, infections caused by ticarcillin-susceptible organisms are also amenable to treatment with TIMENTIN due to its ticarcillin content. Therefore, mixed infections caused by ti-

carcillin-susceptible organisms and β-lactamase–producing organisms susceptible to ticarcillin/clavulanic acid should not require the addition of another antibiotic.
Due to its broad spectrum of bactericidal activity against gram-positive and gram-negative bacteria, TIMENTIN is particularly useful for the treatment of mixed infections and for presumptive therapy prior to the identification of the causative organisms. TIMENTIN has been shown to be effective as single drug therapy in the treatment of some serious infections where normally combination antibiotic therapy might be employed.
Based on the in vitro synergism between ticarcillin/clavulanic acid and aminoglycosides against certain strains of *P. aeruginosa*, combined therapy has been successful, especially in patients with impaired host defenses. Both drugs should be used in full therapeutic doses.
To reduce the development of drug-resistant bacteria and maintain the effectiveness of TIMENTIN and other antibacterial drugs, TIMENTIN should be used only to treat or prevent infections that are proven or strongly suspected to be caused by susceptible bacteria. When culture and susceptibility information are available, they should be considered in selecting or modifying antibacterial therapy. In the absence of such data, local epidemiology and susceptibility patterns may contribute to the empiric selection of therapy.

CONTRAINDICATIONS

TIMENTIN is contraindicated in patients with a history of hypersensitivity reactions to any of the penicillins.

WARNINGS

SERIOUS AND OCCASIONALLY FATAL HYPERSENSITIVITY (ANAPHYLACTIC) REACTIONS HAVE BEEN REPORTED IN PATIENTS ON PENICILLIN THERAPY. THESE REACTIONS ARE MORE LIKELY TO OCCUR IN INDIVIDUALS WITH A HISTORY OF PENICILLIN HYPERSENSITIVITY AND/OR A HISTORY OF SENSITIVITY TO MULTIPLE ALLERGENS. THERE HAVE BEEN REPORTS OF INDIVIDUALS WITH A HISTORY OF PENICILLIN HYPERSENSITIVITY WHO HAVE EXPERIENCED SEVERE REACTIONS WHEN TREATED WITH CEPHALOSPORINS. BEFORE INITIATING THERAPY WITH TIMENTIN, CAREFUL INQUIRY SHOULD BE MADE CONCERNING PREVIOUS HYPERSENSITIVITY REACTIONS TO PENICILLINS, CEPHALOSPORINS, OR OTHER ALLERGENS. IF AN ALLERGIC REACTION OCCURS, TIMENTIN SHOULD BE DISCONTINUED AND THE APPROPRIATE THERAPY INSTITUTED. **SERIOUS ANAPHYLACTIC REACTIONS REQUIRE IMMEDIATE EMERGENCY TREATMENT WITH EPINEPHRINE. OXYGEN, INTRAVENOUS STEROIDS, AND AIRWAY MANAGEMENT, INCLUDING INTUBATION, SHOULD ALSO BE PROVIDED AS INDICATED.**
Pseudomembranous colitis has been reported with nearly all antibacterial agents, including TIMENTIN, and may range in severity from mild to life-threatening. Therefore, it is important to consider this diagnosis in patients who present with diarrhea subsequent to the administration of antibacterial agents.
Treatment with antibacterial agents alters the normal flora of the colon and may permit overgrowth of clostridia. Studies indicate that a toxin produced by *Clostridium difficile* is a primary cause of "antibiotic-associated colitis."
After the diagnosis of pseudomembranous colitis has been established, appropriate therapeutic measures should be initiated. Mild cases of pseudomembranous colitis usually respond to drug discontinuation alone. In moderate to severe cases, consideration should be given to management with fluids and electrolytes, protein supplementation and treatment with an antibacterial drug clinically effective against *C. difficile* colitis.
When very high doses of TIMENTIN are administered, especially in the presence of impaired renal function, patients may experience convulsions. (See ADVERSE REACTIONS and OVERDOSAGE.)

PRECAUTIONS

General: While TIMENTIN possesses the characteristic low toxicity of the penicillin group of antibiotics, periodic assessment of organ system functions, including renal, hepatic, and hematopoietic function, is advisable during prolonged therapy.
Bleeding manifestations have occurred in some patients receiving β-lactam antibiotics. These reactions have been associated with abnormalities of coagulation tests such as clotting time, platelet aggregation, and prothrombin time and are more likely to occur in patients with renal impairment. If bleeding manifestations appear, treatment with TIMENTIN should be discontinued and appropriate therapy instituted.
TIMENTIN has only rarely been reported to cause hypokalemia; however, the possibility of this occurring should be kept in mind particularly when treating patients with fluid and electrolyte imbalance. Periodic monitoring of serum potassium may be advisable in patients receiving prolonged therapy.
The theoretical sodium content is 4.51 mEq (103.6 mg) per gram of TIMENTIN. This should be considered when treating patients requiring restricted salt intake.
As with any penicillin, an allergic reaction, including anaphylaxis, may occur during *TIMENTIN* administration, particularly in a hypersensitive individual.
The possibility of superinfections with mycotic or bacterial pathogens should be kept in mind, particularly during prolonged treatment. If superinfections occur, appropriate measures should be taken.

Creatinine clearance mL/min.	Dosage
over 60	3.1 grams every 4 hrs.
30 to 60	2 grams every 4 hrs.
10 to 30	2 grams every 8 hrs.
less than 10	2 grams every 12 hrs.
less than 10 with hepatic dysfunction	2 grams every 24 hrs.
patients on peritoneal dialysis	3.1 grams every 12 hrs.
patients on hemodialysis	2 grams every 12 hrs. supplemented with 3.1 grams after each dialysis

To calculate creatinine clearance[‡] from a serum creatinine value use the following formula.

$$C_{cr} = \frac{(140\text{–Age})\ (\text{wt. in kg})}{72 \times S_{cr}\ (\text{mg/100 mL})}$$

This is the calculated creatinine clearance for adult males; for females it is 15% less.

[‡]Cockcroft, D.W., et al: Prediction of Creatinine Clearance from Serum Creatinine. Nephron 16:31-41, 1976.

Prescribing TIMENTIN in the absence of a proven or strongly suspected bacterial infection or a prophylactic indication is unlikely to provide benefit to the patient and increases the risk of the development of drug-resistant bacteria.
Information for Patients: Patients should be counseled that antibacterial drugs, including TIMENTIN, should only be used to treat bacterial infections. They do not treat viral infections (e.g., the common cold). When TIMENTIN is prescribed to treat a bacterial infection, patients should be told that although it is common to feel better early in the course of therapy, the medication should be taken exactly as directed. Skipping doses or not completing the full course of therapy may: (1) decrease the effectiveness of the immediate treatment, and (2) increase the likelihood that bacteria will develop resistance and will not be treatable by TIMENTIN or other antibacterial drugs in the future.
Drug/Laboratory Test Interactions: As with other penicillins, the mixing of TIMENTIN with an aminoglycoside in solutions for parenteral administration can result in substantial inactivation of the aminoglycoside.
Probenecid interferes with the renal tubular secretion of ticarcillin, thereby increasing serum concentrations and prolonging serum half-life of the antibiotic.
High urine concentrations of ticarcillin may produce false-positive protein reactions (pseudoproteinuria) with the following methods: Sulfosalicylic acid and boiling test, acetic acid test, biuret reaction, and nitric acid test. The bromphenol blue (MULTI-STIX®) reagent strip test has been reported to be reliable.
The presence of clavulanic acid in TIMENTIN may cause a nonspecific binding of IgG and albumin by red cell membranes leading to a false-positive Coombs test.
Carcinogenesis, Mutagenesis, Impairment of Fertility: Long-term studies in animals have not been performed to evaluate carcinogenic potential. However, results from assays for gene mutation in vitro using bacteria (Ames tests) and yeast, and for chromosomal effects in vitro in human lymphocytes, and in vivo in mouse bone marrow (micronucleus test) indicate that TIMENTIN is without any mutagenic potential.
Pregnancy (Category B): Reproduction studies have been performed in rats given doses up to 1,050 mg/kg/day and have revealed no evidence of impaired fertility or harm to the fetus due to TIMENTIN. There are, however, no adequate and well-controlled studies in pregnant women. Because animal reproduction studies are not always predictive of human response, this drug should be used during pregnancy only if clearly needed.
Nursing Mothers: It is not known whether this drug is excreted in human milk. Because many drugs are excreted in human milk, caution should be exercised when TIMENTIN is administered to a nursing woman.
Pediatric Use: The safety and effectiveness of TIMENTIN have been established in the age group of 3 months to 16 years. Use of TIMENTIN in these age groups is supported by evidence from adequate and well-controlled studies of TIMENTIN in adults with additional efficacy, safety, and pharmacokinetic data from both comparative and non-comparative studies in pediatric patients. There are insufficient data to support the use of TIMENTIN in pediatric patients under 3 months of age or for the treatment of septicemia and/or infections in the pediatric population where the suspected or proven pathogen is *H. influenzae* type b.
In those patients in whom meningeal seeding from a distant infection site or in whom meningitis is suspected or documented, or in patients who require prophylaxis against central nervous system infection, an alternate agent with demonstrated clinical efficacy in this setting should be used.

ADVERSE REACTIONS

As with other penicillins, the following adverse reactions may occur:
Hypersensitivity Reactions: Skin rash, pruritus, urticaria, arthralgia, myalgia, drug fever, chills, chest discomfort, erythema multiforme, toxic epidermal necrolysis, Stevens-Johnson syndrome, and anaphylactic reactions.
Central Nervous System: Headache, giddiness, neuromuscular hyperirritability, or convulsive seizures.
Gastrointestinal Disturbances: Disturbances of taste and smell, stomatitis, flatulence, nausea, vomiting and diarrhea, epigastric pain, and pseudomembranous colitis have been reported. Onset of pseudomembranous colitis symptoms may occur during or after antibiotic treatment. (See WARNINGS.)
Hemic and Lymphatic Systems: Thrombocytopenia, leukopenia, neutropenia, eosinophilia, reduction of hemoglobin or hematocrit, and prolongation of prothrombin time and bleeding time.
Abnormalities of Hepatic and Renal Function Tests: Elevation of serum aspartate aminotransferase (SGOT), serum alanine aminotransferase (SGPT), serum alkaline phosphatase, serum LDH, serum bilirubin. There have been reports of transient hepatitis and cholestatic jaundice—as with some other penicillins and some cephalosporins. Elevation of serum creatinine and/or BUN, hypernatremia, reduction in serum potassium and uric acid.
Local Reactions: Pain, burning, swelling, and induration at the injection site and thrombophlebitis with intravenous administration.
Available safety data for pediatric patients treated with TIMENTIN demonstrate a similar adverse event profile to that observed in adult patients.

DRUG ABUSE AND DEPENDENCE

Neither abuse of nor dependence on TIMENTIN has been reported.

OVERDOSAGE

As with other penicillins, neurotoxic reactions may arise when very high doses of TIMENTIN are administered, especially in patients with impaired renal function. (See WARNINGS and ADVERSE REACTIONS-Central Nervous System.)
In case of overdosage, discontinue TIMENTIN, treat symptomatically, and institute supportive measures as required. Ticarcillin may be removed from circulation by hemodialysis. The molecular weight, degree of protein binding, and pharmacokinetic profile of clavulanic acid together with information from a single patient with renal insufficiency all suggest that this compound may also be removed by hemodialysis.

DOSAGE AND ADMINISTRATION

TIMENTIN should be administered by intravenous infusion (30 min.).
Adults: The usual recommended dosage for systemic and urinary tract infections for average (60 kg) adults is 3.1 grams of TIMENTIN (3.1-gram vial containing 3 grams ticarcillin and 100 mg clavulanic acid) given every 4 to 6 hours. For gynecologic infections, TIMENTIN should be administered as follows: Moderate infections 200 mg/kg/day in divided doses every 6 hours, and for severe infections 300 mg/kg/day in divided doses every 4 hours. For patients weighing less than 60 kg, the recommended dosage is 200 to 300 mg/kg/day, based on ticarcillin content, given in divided doses every 4 to 6 hours.
Pediatric Patients (≥3 months): ***For patients <60 kg:*** In patients <60 kg, TIMENTIN is dosed at 50 mg/kg/dose based on the ticarcillin component. TIMENTIN should be administered as follows: Mild to moderate infections 200 mg/kg/day in divided doses every 6 hours; for severe infections, 300 mg/kg/day in divided doses every 4 hours.
For patients ≥60 kg: For mild to moderate infections, 3.1 grams of TIMENTIN (3 grams of ticarcillin and 100 mg of clavulanic acid) administered every 6 hours; for severe infections, 3.1 grams every 4 hours.
Renal Impairment: For infections complicated by renal insufficiency[†], an initial loading dose of 3.1 grams should be followed by doses based on creatinine clearance and type of dialysis as indicated below:
[See table above]

[†]The half-life of ticarcillin in patients with renal failure is approximately 13 hours.

Dosage for any individual patient must take into consideration the site and severity of infection, the susceptibility of the organisms causing infection, and the status of the patient's host defense mechanisms.
The duration of therapy depends upon the severity of infection. Generally, TIMENTIN should be continued for at least 2 days after the signs and symptoms of infection have disappeared. The usual duration is 10 to 14 days; however, in difficult and complicated infections, more prolonged therapy may be required.
Frequent bacteriologic and clinical appraisals are necessary during therapy of chronic urinary tract infection and may

Continued on next page

Product information on these pages is effective as of August 2004. Further information is available at: GlaxoSmithKline, PO Box 13398, Research Triangle Park, NC 27709. 1-888-825-5249. Corporate Web Site: www.gsk.com

Intravenous Solution (ticarcillin concentrations of 10 mg/mL to 100 mg/mL)	STABILITY PERIOD (31-gram Pharmacy Bulk Package) Room Temperature 21° to 24°C (70° to 75°F)	Refrigerated 4°C (40°F)
Dextrose Injection 5%, USP	24 hours	3 days
Sodium Chloride Injection 0.9%, USP	24 hours	4 days
Lactated Ringer's Injection, USP	24 hours	4 days
Sterile Water for Injection, USP	24 hours	4 days

Timentin Pharmacy Bulk—Cont.

be required for several months after therapy has been completed. Persistent infections may require treatment for several weeks, and doses smaller than those indicated above should not be used.

In certain infections, involving abscess formation, appropriate surgical drainage should be performed in conjunction with antimicrobial therapy.

INTRAVENOUS ADMINISTRATION DIRECTIONS FOR PROPER USE OF PHARMACY BULK PACKAGE RECONSTITUTED STOCK SOLUTION MUST BE TRANSFERRED AND FURTHER DILUTED FOR I.V. INFUSION.

The container closure may be penetrated only one time utilizing a suitable sterile transfer device or dispensing set that allows measured distribution of the contents. A sterile substance that must be reconstituted prior to use may require a separate closure entry.

Restrict use of Pharmacy Bulk Packages to an aseptic area such as a laminar flow hood.

Reconstituted contents of the vial should be withdrawn immediately. However, if this is not possible, aliquoting operations must be completed within 4 hours of reconstitution.

Discard the reconstituted stock solution 4 hours after initial entry.

Add 76 mL of Sterile Water for Injection, USP, or Sodium Chloride Injection, USP, to the 31-gram Pharmacy Bulk Package and shake well. For ease of reconstitution, the diluent may be added in 2 portions. Each 1.0 mL of the resulting concentrated stock solution contains approximately 300 mg of ticarcillin and 10 mg of clavulanic acid.

Intravenous Infusion: The desired dosage should be withdrawn from the stock solution and further diluted to desired volume using the recommended solution listed in the COMPATIBILITY AND STABILITY section (STABILITY PERIOD) to a concentration between 10 mg/mL to 100 mg/mL. The solution of reconstituted drug may then be administered over a period of 30 minutes by direct infusion, or through a Y-type intravenous infusion set. If this method, or the "piggyback" method of administration is used, it is advisable to discontinue temporarily the administration of any other solution during the infusion of TIMENTIN.

Stability: For I.V. solutions, see STABILITY PERIOD below.

When TIMENTIN is given in combination with another antimicrobial, such as an aminoglycoside, each drug should be given separately in accordance with the recommended dosage and routes of administration for each drug.

After reconstitution and prior to administration, TIMENTIN, as with other parenteral drugs, should be inspected visually for particulate matter. If this condition is evident, the solution should be discarded.

The color of reconstituted solutions of TIMENTIN normally ranges from light to dark yellow, depending on concentration, duration, and temperature of storage while maintaining label claim characteristics.

COMPATIBILITY AND STABILITY

31-gram Pharmacy Bulk Package

(Dilutions derived from a stock solution of 300 mg/mL)

Aliquots of the reconstituted stock solution at 300 mg/mL are stable for up to 6 hours between 21° and 24°C (70° and 75°F) or up to 72 hours under refrigeration 4°C (40°F). The reconstituted stock solution should be held under refrigeration 4°C (40°F).

If the aliquots of the reconstituted stock solution (300 mg/mL) are held up to 6 hours between 21° and 24°C (70° and 75°F) or up to 72 hours under refrigeration 4°C (40°F) and further diluted to a concentration between 10 mg/mL and 100 mg/mL with any of the diluents listed below, then the following stability periods apply.

[See table above]

If an aliquot of concentrated stock solution (300 mg/mL) is stored for up to 6 hours between 21° and 24°C (70° and 75°F) and then further diluted to a concentration between 10 mg/mL and 100 mg/mL, solutions of Sodium Chloride Injection, USP, Lactated Ringer's Injection, USP, and Sterile Water for Injection, USP, may be stored frozen –18°C (0°F) for up to 30 days. Solutions prepared with Dextrose Injection 5%, USP, may be stored frozen –18°C (0°F) for up to 7 days. All thawed solutions should be used within 8 hours or discarded. Once thawed, solutions should not be refrozen.

NOTE: TIMENTIN is incompatible with Sodium Bicarbonate.

Unused solutions must be discarded after the time periods listed above.

HOW SUPPLIED

TIMENTIN

Each 31-gram vial contains sterile ticarcillin disodium equivalent to 30 grams ticarcillin and sterile clavulanate potassium equivalent to 1 gram clavulanic acid.

NDC 0029-6579-21 31-gram Pharmacy Bulk Package

TIMENTIN is also supplied as:

NDC 0029-6571-26 3.1-gram Vial

NDC 0029-6571-40 3.1-gram ADD-VANTAGE®§ Antibiotic Vial

Vials of TIMENTIN should be stored at or below 24°C (75°F).

NDC 0029-6571-31 TIMENTIN as an iso-osmotic, sterile, nonpyrogenic, frozen solution in GALAXY®|| (PL 2040) Plastic Containers—supplied in 100 mL single-dose containers equivalent to 3 grams ticarcillin and clavulanate potassium equivalent to 0.1 gram clavulanic acid.

CLINICAL STUDIES

TIMENTIN has been studied in a total of 296 pediatric patients (excluding neonates and infants less than 3 months) in 6 controlled clinical trials. The majority of patients studied had intra-abdominal infections, and the primary comparator was clindamycin and gentamicin with or without ampicillin. At the end-of-therapy visit, comparable efficacy was reported in the trial arms using TIMENTIN and an appropriate comparator.

TIMENTIN was also evaluated in an additional 408 pediatric patients (excluding neonates and infants less than 3 months) in 3 uncontrolled U.S. clinical trials. Patients were treated across a broad range of presenting diagnoses including: Infections in bone and joint, skin and skin structure, lower respiratory tract, urinary tract, as well as intra-abdominal and gynecologic infections. Patients received TIMENTIN either 300 mg/kg/day (based on the ticarcillin component) divided q4h for severe infection or 200 mg/kg/day (based on the ticarcillin component) divided q6h for mild to moderate infections. The efficacy rates were comparable to those obtained in the controlled trials.

The adverse event profile in these 704 pediatric patients treated with TIMENTIN was comparable to that seen in adult patients.

REFERENCES

1. National Committee for Clinical Microbiology Standards. *Methods for Dilution Antimicrobial Susceptibility Tests for Bacteria that Grow Aerobically* - Sixth Edition. Approved Standard NCCLS Document M7-A6, Vol. 23, No. 2 (ISBN-1-56238-486-4). NCCLS, 940 West Valley Road, Suite 1400, Wayne, PA 19087-1898, January, 2003.
2. National Committee for Clinical Microbiology Standards. *Performance Standards for Antimicrobial Disk Susceptibility Tests* - Eighth Edition. Approved Standard NCCLS Document M2-A8, Vol. 23, No. 1 (ISBN-1-56238-485-6). NCCLS, 940 West Valley Road, Suite 1400, Wayne, PA 19087-1898, January, 2003.
3. National Committee for Clinical Microbiology Standards. *Performance Standards for Antimicrobial Susceptibility Testing* - Thirteenth Informational Supplement. NCCLS Document M100-S13 (M7), Vol. 23, No. 2 NCCLS, 940 West Valley Road, Suite 1400, Wayne, PA 19087-1898, January, 2003.
4. National Committee for Clinical Laboratory Standards. *Methods for Antimicrobial Susceptibility Testing of Anaerobic Bacteria* – Fifth Edition. Approved Standard NCCLS Document M11-A5, Vol. 21, No. 2 (ISBN-1-56238-429-5). NCCLS, 940 West Valley Road, Suite 1400, Wayne, PA 19087-1898, January, 2001.

§ADD-VANTAGE® is a registered trademark of Abbott Laboratories.

||GALAXY® is a registered trademark of Baxter International Inc.

MULTI-STIX is a registered trademark of Bayer Corporation.

TIMENTIN is a registered trademark of GlaxoSmithKline.

GlaxoSmithKline, Research Triangle Park, NC 27709

October 2003/TI:L13PB

Shown in Product Identification Guide, page 317

TRIZIVIR® ℞

[trī′ zə-vir]

(abacavir sulfate, lamivudine, and zidovudine) Tablets

WARNING

TRIZIVIR contains 3 nucleoside analogs (abacavir sulfate, lamivudine, and zidovudine) and is intended only for patients whose regimen would otherwise include these 3 components.

TRIZIVIR contains abacavir sulfate (ZIAGEN®), which has been associated with fatal hypersensitivity reactions (see WARNINGS). Patients developing signs or symptoms of hypersensitivity (which include fever; skin rash; fatigue; gastrointestinal symptoms such as nausea, vomiting, diarrhea, or abdominal pain; and respiratory symptoms such as pharyngitis, dyspnea, or cough) should discontinue TRIZIVIR as soon as a hypersensitivity reaction is suspected. To avoid a delay in diagnosis and minimize the risk of a life-threatening hypersensitivity reaction, TRIZIVIR should be permanently discontinued if hypersensitivity cannot be ruled out, even when other diagnoses are possible (e.g., acute onset respiratory diseases, gastroenteritis, or reactions to other medications).

Abacavir (as TRIZIVIR OR ZIAGEN) SHOULD NOT be restarted following a hypersensitivity reaction to abacavir because more severe symptoms will recur within hours and may include life-threatening hypotension and death.

Severe or fatal hypersensitivity reactions can occur within hours after reintroduction of abacavir (as TRIZIVIR OR ZIAGEN) in patients who have no identified history or unrecognized symptoms of hypersensitivity to abacavir therapy (see WARNINGS, PRECAUTIONS: Information for Patients, and ADVERSE REACTIONS).

Zidovudine has been associated with hematologic toxicity including neutropenia and severe anemia, particularly in patients with advanced HIV disease (see WARNINGS). Prolonged use of zidovudine has been associated with symptomatic myopathy.

Lactic acidosis and severe hepatomegaly with steatosis, including fatal cases, have been reported with the use of nucleoside analogues alone or in combination, including abacavir, lamivudine, zidovudine, and other antiretrovirals (see WARNINGS).

There are limited data on the use of this triple-combination regimen in patients with higher viral load levels (>100,000 copies/mL) at baseline.

DESCRIPTION

TRIZIVIR: TRIZIVIR Tablets contain the following 3 synthetic nucleoside analogues: abacavir sulfate (ZIAGEN), lamivudine (also known as EPIVIR® or 3TC), and zidovudine (also known as RETROVIR®, azidothymidine, or ZDV) with inhibitory activity against human immunodeficiency virus (HIV).

TRIZIVIR Tablets are for oral administration. Each film-coated tablet contains the active ingredients 300 mg of abacavir as abacavir sulfate, 150 mg of lamivudine, and 300 mg of zidovudine, and the inactive ingredients magnesium stearate, microcrystalline cellulose, and sodium starch glycolate. The tablets are coated with a film (Opadry® green 03B11434) that is made of FD&C Blue No. 2, hypromellose, polyethylene glycol, titanium dioxide, and yellow iron oxide.

Abacavir Sulfate: The chemical name of abacavir sulfate is *(1S,cis)*-4-[2-amino-6-(cyclopropylamino)-*9H*-purin-9-yl]-2-cyclopentene-1-methanol sulfate (salt) (2:1). Abacavir sulfate is the enantiomer with *1S, 4R* absolute configuration on the cyclopentene ring. It has a molecular formula of $(C_{14}H_{18}N_6O)_2 \bullet H_2SO_4$ and a molecular weight of 670.76 daltons.

Abacavir sulfate is a white to off-white solid with a solubility of approximately 77 mg/mL in distilled water at 25°C. In vivo, abacavir sulfate dissociates to its free base, abacavir. In this insert, all dosages for ZIAGEN (abacavir sulfate) are expressed in terms of abacavir.

Lamivudine: The chemical name of lamivudine is (2R,cis)-4-amino-1-(2-hydroxymethyl-1,3-oxathiolan-5-yl)-(1H)-pyrimidin-2-one. Lamivudine is the (-)enantiomer of a dideoxy analogue of cytidine. Lamivudine has also been referred to as (-)2′,3′-dideoxy, 3′-thiacytidine. It has a molecular formula of $C_8H_{11}N_3O_3S$ and a molecular weight of 229.3 daltons.

Lamivudine is a white to off-white crystalline solid with a solubility of approximately 70 mg/mL in water at 20°C.

Zidovudine: The chemical name of zidovudine is 3′-azido-3′-deoxythymidine. It has a molecular formula of $C_{10}H_{13}N_5O_4$ and a molecular weight of 267.24 daltons.

Zidovudine is a white to beige, crystalline solid with a solubility of 20.1 mg/mL in water at 25°C.

MICROBIOLOGY

Mechanism of Action:

Abacavir: Abacavir is a carbocyclic synthetic nucleoside analogue. Intracellularly, abacavir is converted by cellular enzymes to the active metabolite, carbovir triphosphate. Carbovir triphosphate is an analogue of deoxyguanosine-5′-triphosphate (dGTP). Carbovir triphosphate inhibits the activity of HIV-1 reverse transcriptase (RT) both by competing with the natural substrate dGTP and by its incorporation into viral DNA. The lack of a 3′-OH group in the incorporated nucleoside analogue prevents the formation of the 5′ to 3′ phosphodiester linkage essential for DNA chain elongation, and therefore, the viral DNA growth is terminated.

Lamivudine: Lamivudine is a synthetic nucleoside analogue. Intracellularly, lamivudine is phosphorylated to its active 5′-triphosphate metabolite, lamivudine triphosphate (L-TP). The principal mode of action of L-TP is inhibition of RT via DNA chain termination after incorporation of the nucleoside analogue. L-TP is a weak inhibitor of mammalian DNA polymerases-α and -β and mitochondrial DNA polymerase-γ.

Zidovudine: Zidovudine is a synthetic nucleoside analogue. Intracellularly, zidovudine is phosphorylated to its active 5′-triphosphate metabolite, zidovudine triphosphate (ZDV-TP). The principal mode of action of ZDV-TP is inhibition of RT via DNA chain termination after incorporation of the nucleoside analogue. ZDV-TP is a weak inhibitor of the mammalian DNA polymerase-α and mitochondrial DNA polymerase-γ and has been reported to be incorporated into the DNA of cells in culture.

Antiviral Activity In Vitro:
The relationship between in vitro susceptibility of HIV to abacavir, lamivudine, or zidovudine and the inhibition of HIV replication in humans has not been established.

Abacavir: The in vitro anti–HIV-1 activity of abacavir was evaluated against a T-cell tropic laboratory strain HIV-1 IIIB in lymphoblastic cell lines, a monocyte/macrophage tropic laboratory strain HIV-1 BaL in primary monocytes/macrophages, and clinical isolates in peripheral blood mononuclear cells. The concentration of drug necessary to inhibit viral replication by 50 percent (IC_{50}) ranged from 3.7 to 5.8 μM against HIV-1 IIIB, and was 0.26 ± 0.18 μM (1 μM = 0.28 mcg/mL) against 8 clinical isolates. The IC_{50} of abacavir against HIV-1 BaL varied from 0.07 to 1.0 μM. Abacavir had synergistic activity in combination with amprenavir, nevirapine, and zidovudine, and additive activity in combination with didanosine, lamivudine, stavudine, and zalcitabine in vitro. Most of these drug combinations have not been adequately studied in humans.

Lamivudine: In vitro activity of lamivudine against HIV-1 was assessed in a number of cell lines (including monocytes and fresh human peripheral blood lymphocytes). IC_{50} and IC_{90} values (50% and 90% inhibitory concentrations) for lamivudine were 0.0006 mcg/mL to 0.034 mcg/mL and 0.015 to 0.321 mcg/mL, respectively. Lamivudine had anti–HIV-1 activity in all acute virus-cell infections tested.

In HIV-1–infected MT-4 cells, lamivudine in combination with zidovudine had synergistic antiretroviral activity.

Zidovudine: In vitro activity of zidovudine against HIV-1 was assessed in a number of cell lines (including monocytes and fresh human peripheral blood lymphocytes). The IC_{50} and IC_{90} values for zidovudine were 0.003 to 0.013 mcg/mL and 0.03 to 0.13 mcg/mL, respectively. Zidovudine had anti–HIV-1 activity in all acute virus-cell infections tested. However, zidovudine activity was substantially less in chronically infected cell lines. In cell culture drug combination studies, zidovudine demonstrates synergistic activity with delavirdine, didanosine, indinavir, nelfinavir, nevirapine, ritonavir, saquinavir, and zalcitabine, and additive activity with interferon-alpha.

Drug Resistance:
HIV-1 isolates with reduced sensitivity to abacavir, lamivudine, or zidovudine have been selected in vitro and were also obtained from patients treated with abacavir, lamivudine, zidovudine, or lamivudine plus zidovudine. The clinical relevance of genotypic and phenotypic changes associated with abacavir, lamivudine, or zidovudine therapy is currently under evaluation.

Abacavir: Genetic analysis of isolates from abacavir-treated patients showed point mutations in the reverse transcriptase gene that resulted in amino acid substitutions at positions K65R, L74V, Y115F, and M184V. Phenotypic analysis of HIV-1 isolates that harbored abacavir-associated mutations from 17 patients after 12 weeks of abacavir monotherapy exhibited a 3-fold decrease in susceptibility to abacavir in vitro.

Genetic analysis of HIV-1 isolates from 21 previously antiretroviral therapy-naive patients with confirmed virologic failure (plasma HIV-1 RNA ≥400 copies/mL) after 16 to 48 weeks of abacavir/lamivudine/zidovudine therapy showed that 16/21 isolates had abacavir/lamivudine-associated mutation M184V, either alone (11/21), or in combination with Y115F (1/21) or zidovudine-associated (4/21) mutations at the last time point. Phenotypic data available on isolates from 10 patients showed that 7 of the 10 isolates had 25- to 86-fold decreases in susceptibility to lamivudine in vitro. Likewise, isolates from 2 of these 7 patients had 7- to 10-fold decreases in susceptibility to abacavir in vitro.

Lamivudine: Genotypic analysis of isolates selected in vitro and recovered from lamivudine-treated patients showed that the resistance was due to mutations in the HIV-1 reverse transcriptase gene at codon 184 from methionine to either isoleucine or valine.

Zidovudine: Genotypic analyses of the isolates selected in vitro and recovered from zidovudine-treated patients showed mutations, which result in 5 amino acid substitutions (M41L, D67N, K70R, K219Q, T215Y or F) in the HIV-1 reverse transcriptase gene. In general, higher levels of resistance were associated with greater number of mutations. In some patients harboring zidovudine-resistant virus at baseline, phenotypic sensitivity to zidovudine was restored by 12 weeks of treatment with lamivudine and zidovudine. Combination therapy with lamivudine plus zidovudine delayed the emergence of mutations conferring resistance to zidovudine.

Cross-Resistance:
Cross-resistance among certain reverse transcriptase inhibitors has been recognized.

Abacavir: Recombinant laboratory strains of HIV-1 (HXB2) containing multiple reverse transcriptase mutations conferring abacavir resistance exhibited cross-resistance to lamivudine, didanosine, and zalcitabine in vitro. For clinical information in treatment-experienced patients, see INDICATIONS AND USAGE: Description of Clinical Studies and PRECAUTIONS.

Lamivudine: Cross-resistance between lamivudine and zidovudine has not been reported. Cross-resistance to didanosine and zalcitabine has been observed in some patients harboring lamivudine-resistant HIV-1 isolates. In some patients treated with zidovudine plus didanosine or zalcitabine, isolates resistant to multiple drugs, including lamivudine, have emerged (see under Zidovudine below).

Table 1. Pharmacokinetic Parameters* for Abacavir, Lamivudine, and Zidovudine in Adults

Parameter	Abacavir		Lamivudine		Zidovudine	
Oral bioavailability (%)	86 ± 25	n = 6	86 ± 16	n = 12	64 ± 10	n = 5
Apparent volume of distribution (L/kg)	0.86 ± 0.15	n = 6	1.3 ± 0.4	n = 20	1.6 ± 0.6	n = 8
Systemic clearance (L/hr/kg)	0.80 ± 0.24	n = 6	0.33 ± 0.06	n = 20	1.6 ± 0.6	n = 6
Renal clearance (L/hr/kg)	.007 ± .008	n = 6	0.22 ± 0.06	n = 20	0.34 ± 0.05	n = 9
Elimination half-life (hr)†	1.45 ± 0.32	n = 20	5 to 7		0.5 to 3	

*Data presented as mean ± standard deviation except where noted.
†Approximate range.

Zidovudine: HIV isolates with multidrug resistance to didanosine, lamivudine, stavudine, zalcitabine, and zidovudine were recovered from a small number of patients treated for ≥1 year with zidovudine plus didanosine or zidovudine plus zalcitabine. The pattern of genotypic resistant mutations with such combination therapies was different (A62V, V75I, F77L, F116Y, Q151M) from the pattern with zidovudine monotherapy, with the 151 mutation being most commonly associated with multidrug resistance. The mutation at codon 151 in combination with the mutations at 62, 75, 77, and 116 results in a virus with reduced susceptibility to didanosine, lamivudine, stavudine, zalcitabine, and zidovudine.

CLINICAL PHARMACOLOGY

Pharmacokinetics in Adults:

TRIZIVIR: In a single-dose, 3-way crossover bioavailability study of 1 TRIZIVIR tablet versus 1 ZIAGEN tablet (300 mg), 1 EPIVIR tablet (150 mg), plus 1 RETROVIR tablet (300 mg) administered simultaneously in healthy subjects (n = 24), there was no difference in the extent of absorption, as measured by the area under the plasma concentration-time curve (AUC) and maximal peak concentration (C_{max}), of all 3 components. One TRIZIVIR tablet was bioequivalent to 1 ZIAGEN tablet (300 mg), 1 EPIVIR tablet (150 mg), plus 1 RETROVIR tablet (300 mg) following single-dose administration to fasting healthy subjects (n = 24).

Abacavir: Following oral administration, abacavir is rapidly absorbed and extensively distributed. Binding of abacavir to human plasma proteins is approximately 50%. Binding of abacavir to plasma proteins was independent of concentration. Total blood and plasma drug-related radioactivity concentrations are identical, demonstrating that abacavir readily distributes into erythrocytes. The primary routes of elimination of abacavir are metabolism by alcohol dehydrogenase to form the 5′-carboxylic acid and glucuronyl transferase to form the 5′-glucuronide.

Lamivudine: Following oral administration, lamivudine is rapidly absorbed and extensively distributed. Binding to plasma protein is low. Approximately 70% of an intravenous dose of lamivudine is recovered as unchanged drug in the urine. Metabolism of lamivudine is a minor route of elimination. In humans, the only known metabolite is the trans-sulfoxide metabolite (approximately 5% of an oral dose after 12 hours).

Zidovudine: Following oral administration, zidovudine is rapidly absorbed and extensively distributed. Binding to plasma protein is low. Zidovudine is eliminated primarily by hepatic metabolism. The major metabolite of zidovudine is 3′-azido-3′-deoxy-5′-*O*-β-*D*-glucopyranuronosylthymidine (GZDV). GZDV area under the curve (AUC) is about 3-fold greater than the zidovudine AUC. Urinary recovery of zidovudine and GZDV accounts for 14% and 74% of the dose following oral administration, respectively. A second metabolite, 3′-amino-3′-deoxythymidine (AMT), has been identified in plasma. The AMT AUC was one fifth of the zidovudine AUC.

In humans, abacavir, lamivudine, and zidovudine are not significantly metabolized by cytochrome P450 enzymes.

The pharmacokinetic properties of abacavir, lamivudine, and zidovudine in fasting patients are summarized in Table 1.

[See table 1 above]

Effect of Food on Absorption of TRIZIVIR:
TRIZIVIR may be administered with or without food. Administration with food in a single-dose bioavailability study resulted in lower C_{max}, similar to results observed previously for the reference formulations. The average [90% CI] decrease in abacavir, lamivudine, and zidovudine C_{max} was 32% [24% to 38%], 18% [10% to 25%], and 28% [13% to 40%], respectively, when administered with a high-fat meal, compared to administration under fasted conditions. Administration of TRIZIVIR with food did not alter the extent of abacavir, lamivudine, and zidovudine absorption (AUC), as compared to administration under fasted conditions (n = 24).

Special Populations:

Impaired Renal Function:

TRIZIVIR: Because lamivudine and zidovudine require dose adjustment in the presence of renal insufficiency, TRIZIVIR is not recommended for use in patients with creatinine clearance <50 mL/min (see PRECAUTIONS).

Impaired Hepatic Function:

TRIZIVIR: A reduction in the daily dose of zidovudine may be necessary in patients with mild to moderate impaired hepatic function or liver cirrhosis. Because TRIZIVIR is a fixed-dose combination that cannot be adjusted for this patient population, TRIZIVIR is not recommended for patients with impaired hepatic function.

Pregnancy: See PRECAUTIONS: Pregnancy.

Zidovudine: Zidovudine pharmacokinetics have been studied in a Phase 1 study of 8 women during the last trimester of pregnancy. As pregnancy progressed, there was no evidence of drug accumulation. The pharmacokinetics of zidovudine were similar to that of nonpregnant adults. Consistent with passive transmission of the drug across the placenta, zidovudine concentrations in neonatal plasma at birth were essentially equal to those in maternal plasma at delivery. Although data are limited, methadone maintenance therapy in 5 pregnant women did not appear to alter zidovudine pharmacokinetics. In a nonpregnant adult population, a potential for interaction has been identified (see CLINICAL PHARMACOLOGY: Drug Interactions).

Abacavir and Lamivudine: No data are available on the pharmacokinetics of abacavir or lamivudine during pregnancy.

Nursing Mothers: See PRECAUTIONS: Nursing Mothers.

Zidovudine: After administration of a single dose of 200 mg zidovudine to 13 HIV-infected women, the mean concentration of zidovudine was similar in human milk and serum.

Abacavir and Lamivudine: No data are available on the pharmacokinetics of abacavir or lamivudine in nursing mothers.

Pediatric Patients:

TRIZIVIR: TRIZIVIR is not intended for use in pediatric patients. TRIZIVIR should not be administered to adolescents who weigh less than 40 kg because it is a fixed-dose tablet that cannot be dose adjusted for this patient population (see PRECAUTIONS: Pediatric Use).

Geriatric Patients: The pharmacokinetics of abacavir, lamivudine, and zidovudine have not been studied in patients over 65 years of age.

Gender:

Lamivudine and Zidovudine: A pharmacokinetic study in healthy male (n = 12) and female (n = 12) subjects showed no gender differences in zidovudine exposure ($AUC\infty$) or lamivudine $AUC\infty$ normalized for body weight.

Abacavir: The pharmacokinetics of abacavir with respect to gender have not been determined.

Race:

Lamivudine: There are no significant racial differences in lamivudine pharmacokinetics.

Abacavir and Zidovudine: The pharmacokinetics of abacavir and zidovudine with respect to race have not been determined.

Drug Interactions: See PRECAUTIONS: Drug Interactions. The drug interactions described are based on studies conducted with the individual nucleoside analogues. In humans, abacavir, lamivudine, and zidovudine are not significantly metabolized by cytochrome P450 enzymes; therefore, it is unlikely that clinically significant drug interactions will occur with drugs metabolized through these pathways.

Abacavir: Due to their common metabolic pathways via glucuronyl transferase with zidovudine, 15 HIV-infected patients were enrolled in a crossover study evaluating single doses of abacavir (600 mg), lamivudine (150 mg), and zidovudine (300 mg) alone or in combination. Analysis showed no clinically relevant changes in the pharmacokinetics of abacavir with the addition of lamivudine or zidovudine or the combination of lamivudine and zidovudine. Lamivudine exposure (AUC decreased 15%) and zidovudine exposure (AUC increased 10%) did not show clinically relevant changes with concurrent abacavir.

In a study of 11 HIV-infected subjects receiving methadone-maintenance therapy (40 mg and 90 mg daily), with 600 mg of ZIAGEN twice daily (twice the currently recommended dose), oral methadone clearance increased 22% (90% CI 6% to 42%). This alteration will not result in a methadone dose modification in the majority of patients; however, an increased methadone dose may be required in a small number of patients.

Continued on next page

Product information on these pages is effective as of August 2004. Further information is available at: GlaxoSmithKline, PO Box 13398, Research Triangle Park, NC 27709. 1-888-825-5249. Corporate Web Site: www.gsk.com

Trizivir—Cont.

Lamivudine and Zidovudine: No clinically significant alterations in lamivudine or zidovudine pharmacokinetics were observed in 12 asymptomatic HIV-infected adult patients given a single dose of zidovudine (200 mg) in combination with multiple doses of lamivudine (300 mg q 12 hr). [See table 2 below]

INDICATIONS AND USAGE

TRIZIVIR is indicated alone or in combination with other antiretroviral agents for the treatment of HIV-1 infection. The indication for TRIZIVIR is based on 2 controlled trials with abacavir of 16 and 48 weeks in duration that evaluated suppression of HIV RNA and changes in CD4 cell count. At present, there are no results from controlled trials evaluating the effect of abacavir on clinical progression of HIV. There are limited data on the use of this triple-combination regimen in patients with higher viral load levels (>100,000 copies/mL) at baseline (see Description of Clinical Studies for ZIAGEN).

Description of Clinical Studies:

TRIZIVIR: There have been no clinical trials conducted with TRIZIVIR (see CLINICAL PHARMACOLOGY for information about bioequivalence of TRIZIVIR).

The following studies were conducted with the individual components of TRIZIVIR.

ZIAGEN:

Therapy-Naive Adults: CNAAB3003 was a multicenter, double-blind, placebo-controlled study in which 173 HIV-infected, therapy-naive adults were randomized to receive either ZIAGEN (300 mg twice daily), lamivudine (150 mg twice daily), and zidovudine (300 mg twice daily) or lamivudine (150 mg twice daily) and zidovudine (300 mg twice daily). The duration of double-blind treatment was 16 weeks. Study participants were: male (76%), Caucasian (54%), African-American (28%), and Hispanic (16%). The median age was 34 years, the median pretreatment CD4 cell count was 450 cells/mm^3, and median plasma HIV-1 RNA was 4.5 $\log_{10}$ copies/mL. Proportions of patients with plasma HIV-1 RNA <400 copies/mL (using Roche Amplicor HIV-1 MONITOR® Test) through 16 weeks of treatment are summarized in Figure 1.

Figure 1. Proportions of Patients with HIV-1 RNA <400 copies/mL in Study CNAAB3003[1]

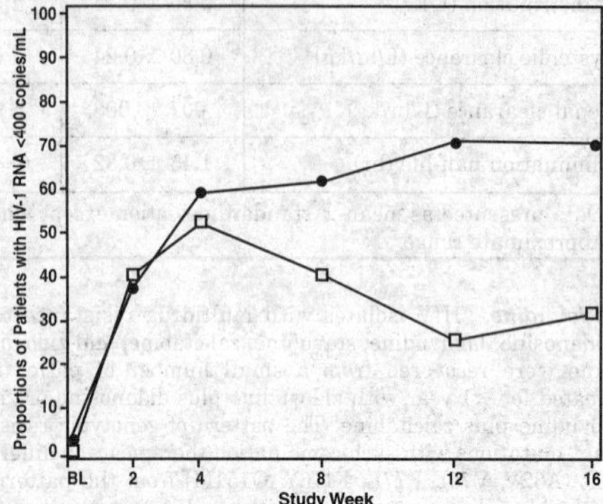

● ZIAGEN/Lamivudine/Zidovudine (n = 87)
□ Lamivudine/Zidovudine (n = 86)
[1]Missing data were considered as HIV-1 RNA ≥ 400 copies/mL.

After 16 weeks of therapy, the median CD4 increases from baseline were 47 cells/mm^3 in the group receiving ZIAGEN and 112 cells/mm^3 in the placebo group.

CNAAB3005 was a multicenter, double-blind, controlled study in which 562 HIV-infected, therapy-naive adults with a pre-entry plasma HIV-1 RNA >10,000 copies/mL were randomized to receive either ZIAGEN (300 mg twice daily) plus COMBIVIR (lamivudine 150 mg/zidovudine 300 mg twice daily), or indinavir (800 mg 3 times a day) plus COMBIVIR twice daily. Study participants were male (87%), Caucasian (73%), African-American (15%), and Hispanic (9%). At baseline the median age was 36 years, the median pretreatment CD4 cell count was 360 cells/mm^3, and median plasma HIV-1 RNA was 4.8 $\log_{10}$ copies/mL. Proportions of patients with plasma HIV-1 RNA <400 copies/mL (using Roche Amplicor HIV-1 MONITOR Test) through 48 weeks of treatment are summarized in Figure 2.

Figure 2. Proportions of Patients with HIV-1 RNA <400 copies/mL in Study CNAAB3005[1]

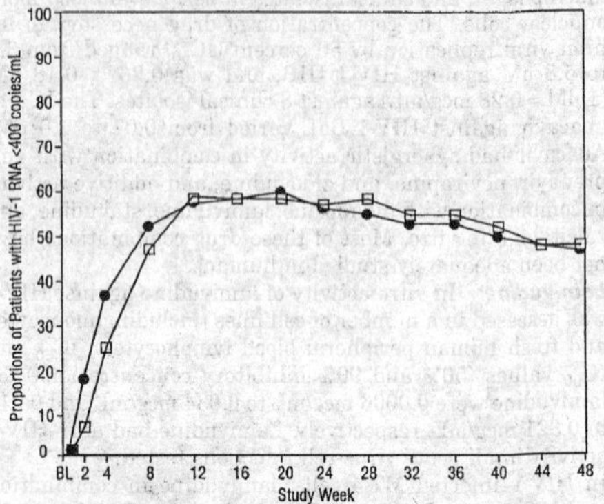

● ZIAGEN/Lamivudine/Zidovudine (n = 282)
□ Indinavir/Lamivudine/Zidovudine (n = 280)
[1]Discontinuations of randomized therapy or missing data were considered as HIV-1 RNA ≥ 400 copies/mL.

Through week 48, an overall mean increase in CD4 cells of about 150 cells/mm^3 was observed in both treatment arms. [See table 3 at top of next page]

Therapy-Experienced Pediatric Patients: A randomized, double-blind study, CNAA3006, compared ZIAGEN plus lamivudine and zidovudine versus lamivudine and zidovudine in pediatric patients, most of whom were extensively pretreated with nucleoside analogue antiretroviral agents. Patients in this study had a limited response to abacavir.

CONTRAINDICATIONS

Abacavir sulfate, one of the components of TRIZIVIR, has been associated with fatal hypersensitivity reactions. ABACAVIR (as TRIZIVIR or ZIAGEN) SHOULD NOT BE RESTARTED FOLLOWING A HYPERSENSITIVITY REACTION TO ABACAVIR (see WARNINGS, PRECAUTIONS, and ADVERSE REACTIONS).

TRIZIVIR Tablets are contraindicated in patients with previously demonstrated hypersensitivity to any of the components of the product (see WARNINGS).

WARNINGS

Hypersensitivity Reaction: TRIZIVIR contains abacavir sulfate (ZIAGEN), which has been associated with fatal hypersensitivity reactions. Patients developing signs or symptoms of hypersensitivity (which include fever; skin rash; fatigue; gastrointestinal symptoms such as nausea, vomiting, diarrhea, or abdominal pain; and respiratory symptoms such as pharyngitis, dyspnea, or cough) should discontinue TRIZIVIR as soon as a hypersensitivity reaction is first suspected, and should seek medical evaluation immediately. To avoid a delay in diagnosis and minimize the risk of a life-threatening hypersensitivity reaction, TRIZIVIR should be permanently discontinued if hypersensitivity cannot be ruled out, even when other diagnoses are possible (e.g., acute onset respiratory diseases, gastroenteritis, or reactions to other medications). Abacavir (as TRIZIVIR or ZIAGEN) SHOULD NOT be restarted following a hypersensitivity reaction to abacavir because more severe symptoms will recur within hours and may include life-threatening hypotension and death.

Severe or fatal hypersensitivity reactions can occur within hours after reintroduction of abacavir (as TRIZIVIR or ZIAGEN) in patients who have no identified history or unrecognized symptoms of hypersensitivity to abacavir therapy.

When therapy with abacavir (as TRIZIVIR or ZIAGEN) has been discontinued for reasons other than symptoms of a hypersensitivity reaction, and if reinitiation of therapy is under consideration, the reason for discontinuation should be evaluated to ensure that the patient did not have symptoms of a hypersensitivity reaction. If hypersensitivity cannot be ruled out, abacavir (as TRIZIVIR or ZIAGEN) should **NOT** be reintroduced. If symptoms consistent with hypersensitivity are not identified, reintroduction can be undertaken with continued monitoring for symptoms of a hypersensitivity reaction. Patients should be made aware that a hypersensitivity reaction can occur with reintroduction of abacavir (as TRIZIVIR or ZIAGEN), and that reintroduction of abacavir (as TRIZIVIR or ZIAGEN) should be undertaken only if medical care can be readily accessed by the patient or others (see ADVERSE REACTIONS).

In clinical trials, hypersensitivity reactions have been reported in approximately 5% of adult and pediatric patients receiving abacavir. Symptoms usually appear within the first 6 weeks of treatment with abacavir although these reactions may occur at any time during therapy (see PRECAUTIONS: Information for Patients and ADVERSE REACTIONS).

Table 2. Effect of Coadministered Drugs on Abacavir, Lamivudine, and Zidovudine AUC*

Note: ROUTINE DOSE MODIFICATION OF ABACAVIR, LAMIVUDINE, AND ZIDOVUDINE IS NOT WARRANTED WITH COADMINISTRATION OF THE FOLLOWING DRUGS.

Drugs That May Alter Lamivudine Blood Concentrations

Coadministered Drug and Dose	Lamivudine Dose	n	Lamivudine Concentrations		Concentration of Coadministered Drug
			AUC	Variability	
Nelfinavir 750 mg q 8 hr × 7 to 10 days	single 150 mg	11	↑ 10%	95% CI: 1% to 20%	↔
Trimethoprim 160 mg/ Sulfamethoxazole 800 mg daily × 5 days	single 300 mg	14	↑ 43%	90% CI: 32% to 55%	↔

Drugs That May Alter Zidovudine Blood Concentrations

Coadministered Drug and Dose	Zidovudine Dose	n	Zidovudine Concentrations		Concentration of Coadministered Drug
			AUC	Variability	
Atovaquone 750 mg q 12 hr with food	200 mg q 8 hr	14	↑ 31%	Range 23% to 78%[†]	↔
Fluconazole 400 mg daily	200 mg q 8 hr	12	↑ 74%	95% CI: 54% to 98%	Not Reported
Methadone 30 to 90 mg daily	200 mg q 4 hr	9	↑ 43%	Range 16% to 64%[†]	↔
Nelfinavir 750 mg q 8 hr × 7 to 10 days	single 200 mg	11	↓ 35%	Range 28% to 41%	↔
Probenecid 500 mg q 6 hr × 2 days	2 mg/kg q 8 hr × 3 days	3	↑ 106%	Range 100% to 170%[†]	Not Assessed
Ritonavir 300 mg q 6 hr × 4 days	200 mg q 8 hr × 4 days	9	↓ 25%	95% CI: 15% to 34%	↔
Valproic acid 250 mg or 500 mg q 8 hr × 4 days	100 mg q 8 hr × 4 days	6	↑ 80%	Range 64% to 130%[†]	Not Assessed

Drugs That May Alter Abacavir Blood Concentrations

Coadministered Drug and Dose	Abacavir Dose	n	Abacavir Concentrations		Concentration of Coadministered Drug
			AUC	Variability	
Ethanol 0.7 g/kg	single 600 mg	24	↑ 41%	90% CI: 35% to 48%	↔

↑ = Increase; ↓ = Decrease; ↔ = no significant change; AUC = area under the concentration versus time curve; CI = confidence interval.
*See PRECAUTIONS: Drug Interactions for additional information on drug interactions.
[†]Estimated range of percent difference.

Abacavir Hypersensitivity Reaction Registry: To facilitate reporting of hypersensitivity reactions and collection of information on each case, an Abacavir Hypersensitivity Registry has been established. Physicians should register patients by calling 1-800-270-0425.

Lactic Acidosis/Severe Hepatomegaly with Steatosis: Lactic acidosis and severe hepatomegaly with steatosis, including fatal cases, have been reported with the use of nucleoside analogues alone or in combination, including abacavir, lamivudine, zidovudine, and other antiretrovirals. A majority of these cases have been in women. Obesity and prolonged nucleoside exposure may be risk factors. Particular caution should be exercised when administering TRIZIVIR to any patient with known risk factors for liver disease; however, cases have also been reported in patients with no known risk factors. Treatment with TRIZIVIR should be suspended in any patient who develops clinical or laboratory findings suggestive of lactic acidosis or pronounced hepatotoxicity (which may include hepatomegaly and steatosis even in the absence of marked transaminase elevations).

Bone Marrow Suppression: Since TRIZIVIR contains zidovudine, TRIZIVIR should be used with caution in patients who have bone marrow compromise evidenced by granulocyte count <1,000 cells/mm^3 or hemoglobin <9.5 g/dL. Frequent blood counts are strongly recommended in patients with advanced HIV disease who are treated with TRIZIVIR. For HIV-infected individuals and patients with asymptomatic or early HIV disease, periodic blood counts are recommended.

Myopathy: Myopathy and myositis, with pathological changes similar to that produced by HIV disease, have been associated with prolonged use of zidovudine, and therefore may occur with therapy with TRIZIVIR.

Posttreatment Exacerbations of Hepatitis: In clinical trials in non-HIV-infected patients treated with lamivudine for chronic hepatitis B (HBV), clinical and laboratory evidence of exacerbations of hepatitis have occurred after discontinuation of lamivudine. These exacerbations have been detected primarily by serum ALT elevations in addition to re-emergence of HBV DNA. Although most events appear to have been self-limited, fatalities have been reported in some cases. Similar events have been reported from post-marketing experience after changes from lamivudine-containing HIV treatment regimens to non-lamivudine-containing regimens in patients infected with both HIV and HBV. The causal relationship to discontinuation of lamivudine treatment is unknown. Patients should be closely monitored with both clinical and laboratory followup for at least several months after stopping treatment. There is insufficient evidence to determine whether re-initiation of lamivudine alters the course of posttreatment exacerbations of hepatitis.

Other: TRIZIVIR contains fixed doses of 3 nucleoside analogues: abacavir, lamivudine, and zidovudine and should not be administered concomitantly with abacavir, lamivudine, or zidovudine.

Because TRIZIVIR is a fixed-dose tablet, it should not be prescribed for adults or adolescents who weigh less than 40 kg or other patients requiring dosage adjustment.

The complete prescribing information for all agents being considered for use with TRIZIVIR should be consulted before combination therapy with TRIZIVIR is initiated.

PRECAUTIONS

Therapy-Experienced Patients:

Abacavir: In clinical trials, patients with prolonged prior nucleoside reverse transcriptase inhibitor (NRTI) exposure or who had HIV-1 isolates that contained multiple mutations conferring resistance to NRTIs had limited response to abacavir. The potential for cross-resistance between abacavir and other NRTIs should be considered when choosing new therapeutic regimens in therapy-experienced patients (see MICROBIOLOGY: Cross-Resistance).

Patients with HIV and Hepatitis B Virus Coinfection:

Lamivudine: Safety and efficacy of lamivudine have not been established for treatment of chronic hepatitis B in patients dually infected with HIV and HBV. In non-HIV-infected patients treated with lamivudine for chronic hepatitis B, emergence of lamivudine-resistant HBV has been detected and has been associated with diminished treatment response (see EPIVIR-HBV package insert for additional information). Emergence of hepatitis B virus variants associated with resistance to lamivudine has also been reported in HIV-infected patients who have received lamivudine-containing antiretroviral regimens in the presence of concurrent infection with hepatitis B virus.

Patients with Impaired Renal Function:

TRIZIVIR: Since TRIZIVIR is a fixed-dose tablet and the dosage of the individual components cannot be altered, patients with creatinine clearance <50 mL/min should not receive TRIZIVIR.

Fat Redistribution: Redistribution/accumulation of body fat including central obesity, dorsocervical fat enlargement (buffalo hump), peripheral wasting, facial wasting, breast enlargement, and "cushingoid appearance" have been observed in patients receiving antiretroviral therapy. The mechanism and long-term consequences of these events are currently unknown. A causal relationship has not been established.

Information for Patients:

Abacavir: **Patients should be advised that a Medication Guide and Warning Card summarizing the symptoms of abacavir hypersensitivity reactions should be dispensed by the pharmacist with each new prescription and refill of TRIZIVIR. The complete text of the Medication Guide is reprinted at the end of this document. Patients should be instructed to carry the Warning Card with them.**

Patients should be advised of the possibility of a hypersensitivity reaction to abacavir (as TRIZIVIR or ZIAGEN) that may result in death. Patients developing signs or symptoms of hypersensitivity (which include fever; skin rash; fatigue; gastrointestinal symptoms such as nausea, vomiting, diarrhea, or abdominal pain; and respiratory symptoms such as sore throat, shortness of breath, or cough) should discontinue treatment with TRIZIVIR and seek medical evaluation immediately. **Abacavir (as TRIZIVIR OR ZIAGEN) SHOULD NOT be restarted following a hypersensitivity reaction to abacavir because more severe symptoms will recur within hours and may include life-threatening hypotension and death.** Patients who have interrupted abacavir (as TRIZIVIR or ZIAGEN) for reasons other than symptoms of hypersensitivity (for example, those who have an interruption in drug supply) should be made aware that a severe or fatal hypersensitivity reaction can occur with reintroduction of abacavir. Patients should be instructed not to reintroduce abacavir (as TRIZIVIR or ZIAGEN) without medical consultation and that reintroduction of abacavir (as TRIZIVIR or ZIAGEN) should be undertaken only if medical care can be readily accessed by the patient or others (see ADVERSE REACTIONS and WARNINGS).

TRIZIVIR: Patients should be informed that TRIZIVIR is not a cure for HIV infection and patients may continue to experience illnesses associated with HIV infection, including opportunistic infections. Patients should be advised that the use of TRIZIVIR has not been shown to reduce the risk of transmission of HIV to others through sexual contact or blood contamination.

Patients should be informed that redistribution or accumulation of body fat may occur in patients receiving antiretroviral therapy and that the cause and long-term health effects of these conditions are not known at this time.

Patients should be advised of the importance of taking TRIZIVIR as it is prescribed.

Zidovudine: Patients should be informed that the important toxicities associated with zidovudine are neutropenia and/or anemia. They should be told of the extreme importance of having their blood counts followed closely while on therapy, especially for patients with advanced HIV disease.

Drug Interactions:

TRIZIVIR: No clinically significant changes to pharmacokinetic parameters were observed for abacavir, lamivudine, or zidovudine when administered together.

Abacavir: Abacavir has no effect on the pharmacokinetic properties of ethanol. Ethanol decreases the elimination of abacavir causing an increase in overall exposure (see CLINICAL PHARMACOLOGY: Drug Interactions).

The addition of methadone has no clinically significant effect on the pharmacokinetic properties of abacavir. In a study of 11 HIV-infected subjects receiving methadone-maintenance therapy (40 mg and 90 mg daily), with 600 mg of ZIAGEN twice daily (twice the currently recommended dose), oral methadone clearance increased 22% (90% CI 6% to 42%). This alteration will not result in a methadone dose modification in the majority of patients; however, an increased methadone dose may be required in a small number of patients.

Lamivudine: Trimethoprim (TMP) 160 mg/sulfamethoxazole (SMX) 800 mg once daily has been shown to increase lamivudine exposure (AUC). The effect of higher doses of TMP/SMX on lamivudine pharmacokinetics has not been investigated (see CLINICAL PHARMACOLOGY).

Lamivudine and zalcitabine may inhibit the intracellular phosphorylation of one another. Therefore, use of TRIZIVIR in combination with zalcitabine is not recommended.

Zidovudine: Coadministration of ganciclovir, interferon-alpha, and other bone marrow suppressive or cytotoxic agents may increase the hematologic toxicity of zidovudine. Concomitant use of zidovudine with stavudine should be avoided since an antagonistic relationship has been demonstrated in vitro. In addition, concomitant use of zidovudine with doxorubicin or ribavirin should be avoided because an antagonistic relationship has also been demonstrated in vitro.

See CLINICAL PHARMACOLOGY for additional drug interactions.

Carcinogenesis, Mutagenesis, and Impairment of Fertility:

Carcinogenicity:

Abacavir: Abacavir was administered orally at 3 dosage levels to separate groups of mice (60 females and 60 males per group) and rats (56 females and 56 males in each group) in carcinogenicity studies. Single doses were 55, 110, and 330 mg/kg/day in mice and 30, 120, and 600 mg/kg/day in rats. Results showed an increase in the incidence of malignant and non-malignant tumors. Malignant tumors occurred in the preputial gland of males and the clitoral gland of females of both species, and in the liver of female rats. In addition, non-malignant tumors also occurred in the liver and thyroid gland of female rats.

Lamivudine: Long-term carcinogenicity studies with lamivudine in mice and rats showed no evidence of carcinogenic potential at exposures up to 10 times (mice) and 58 times (rats) those observed in humans at the recommended therapeutic dose for HIV infection.

Zidovudine: Zidovudine was administered orally at 3 dosage levels to separate groups of mice and rats (60 females and 60 males in each group). Initial single daily doses were 30, 60, and 120 mg/kg/day in mice and 80, 220, and 600 mg/kg/day in rats. The doses in mice were reduced to 20, 30, and 40 mg/kg/day after day 90 because of treatment-related anemia, whereas in rats only the high dose was reduced to 450 mg/kg per day on day 91 and then to 300 mg/kg/day on day 279.

In mice, 7 late-appearing (after 19 months) vaginal neoplasms (5 nonmetastasizing squamous cell carcinomas, 1 squamous cell papilloma, and 1 squamous polyp) occurred in animals given the highest dose. One late-appearing squamous cell papilloma occurred in the vagina of a middle-dose animal. No vaginal tumors were found at the lowest dose.

In rats, 2 late-appearing (after 20 months), nonmetastasizing vaginal squamous cell carcinomas occurred in animals given the highest dose. No vaginal tumors occurred at the low or middle dose in rats. No other drug-related tumors were observed in either sex of either species.

At doses that produced tumors in mice and rats, the estimated drug exposure (as measured by AUC) was approximately 3 times (mouse) and 24 times (rat) the estimated human exposure at the recommended therapeutic dose of 100 mg every 4 hours.

Two transplacental carcinogenicity studies were conducted in mice. One study administered zidovudine at doses of 20 mg/kg/day or 40 mg/kg/day from gestation day 10 through parturition and lactation with dosing continuing in offspring for 24 months postnatally. At these doses, exposures were approximately 3 times the estimated human exposure at the recommended doses. After 24 months at the 40-mg/kg/day dose, an increase in incidence of vaginal tumors was noted with no increase in tumors in the liver or lung or any other organ in either gender. These findings are consistent with results of the standard oral carcinogenicity study in mice, as described earlier. A second study administered zidovudine at maximum tolerated doses of 12.5 mg/day or 25 mg/day (~1,000 mg/kg nonpregnant body weight or ~450 mg/kg of term body weight) to pregnant mice from days 12 through 18 of gestation. There was an increase in the number of tumors in the lung, liver, and female reproductive tracts in the offspring of mice receiving the higher dose level of zidovudine.

It is not known how predictive the results of rodent carcinogenicity studies may be for humans.

Mutagenicity:

Abacavir: Abacavir induced chromosomal aberrations both in the presence and absence of metabolic activation in an in vitro cytogenetic study in human lymphocytes. Abacavir was mutagenic in the absence of metabolic activation, although it was not mutagenic in the presence of metabolic activation in an L5178Y/TK$^{+/-}$ mouse lymphoma assay. At systemic exposures approximately 9 times higher than that in humans at the therapeutic dose, abacavir was clastogenic in males and not clastogenic in females in an in vivo mouse bone marrow micronucleus assay. Abacavir was not mutagenic in bacterial mutagenicity assays in the presence and absence of metabolic activation.

Lamivudine: Lamivudine was mutagenic in an L5178Y/TK$^{+/-}$ mouse lymphoma assay and clastogenic in a cytogenetic assay using cultured human lymphocytes. Lamivudine was negative in a microbial mutagenicity assay, in an in vitro cell transformation assay, in a rat micronucleus test, in a rat bone marrow cytogenetic assay, and in an assay for unscheduled DNA synthesis in rat liver.

Zidovudine: Zidovudine was mutagenic in an L5178Y/TK$^{+/-}$ mouse lymphoma assay, positive in an in vitro cell transformation assay, clastogenic in a cytogenetic assay us-

Continued on next page

Table 3. Outcomes of Randomized Treatment Through Week 48 (CNAAB3005)

Outcome	ZIAGEN/Lamivudine/Zidovudine (n = 282)	Indinavir/Lamivudine/Zidovudine (n = 280)
HIV-1 RNA <400 copies/mL	46%	47%
HIV-1 RNA ≥400 copies/mL*	29%	28%
CDC Class C event	2%	<1%
Discontinued due to adverse reactions	9%	11%
Discontinued due to other reasons†	6%	6%
Randomized but never initiated treatment	7%	5%

*Includes viral rebound and failure to achieve confirmed <400 copies/mL by Week 48.

†Includes consent withdrawn, lost to follow up, protocol violations, those with missing data, and other.

Product information on these pages is effective as of August 2004. Further information is available at: GlaxoSmithKline, PO Box 13398, Research Triangle Park, NC 27709. 1-888-825-5249. Corporate Web Site: www.gsk.com

Trizivir—Cont.

ing cultured human lymphocytes, and positive in mouse and rat micronucleus tests after repeated doses. It was negative in a cytogenetic study in rats given a single dose.

Impairment of Fertility:

Abacavir: Abacavir administered to male and female rats had no adverse effects on fertility judged by conception rates at doses up to approximately 8-fold higher than that in humans at the therapeutic dose based on body surface area comparisons.

Lamivudine: In a study of reproductive performance, lamivudine, administered to male and female rats at doses up to 130 times the usual adult dose based on body surface area considerations, revealed no evidence of impaired fertility judged by conception rates and no effect on the survival, growth, and development to weaning of the offspring.

Zidovudine: Zidovudine, administered to male and female rats at doses up to 7 times the usual adult dose based on body surface area considerations, had no effect on fertility judged by conception rates.

Pregnancy: Pregnancy Category C. There are no adequate and well-controlled studies of TRIZIVIR in pregnant women. Reproduction studies with abacavir, lamivudine, and zidovudine have been performed in animals (see Abacavir, Lamivudine, and Zidovudine sections below). TRIZIVIR should be used during pregnancy only if the potential benefits outweigh the risks.

Abacavir: Studies in pregnant rats showed that abacavir is transferred to the fetus through the placenta. Developmental toxicity (depressed fetal body weight and reduced crown-rump length) and increased incidences of fetal anasarca and skeletal malformations were observed when rats were treated with abacavir at a dose 35 times higher than the human exposure, based on AUC (1,000 mg/kg/day). In a fertility study, evidence of toxicity to the developing embryo and fetuses (increased resorptions, decreased fetal body weights) occurred only at 500 mg/kg/day. The offspring of female rats treated with abacavir at 500 mg/kg/day (beginning at embryo implantation and ending at weaning) showed increased incidence of stillbirth and lower body weights throughout life. In the rabbit, there was no evidence of drug-related developmental toxicity and no increases in fetal malformations at doses up to 8.5 times the human exposure, based on AUC.

Lamivudine: Studies in pregnant rats and rabbits showed that lamivudine is transferred to the fetus through the placenta. Reproduction studies with orally administered lamivudine have been performed in rats and rabbits at doses up to 4,000 mg/kg/day and 1,000 mg/kg/day, respectively, producing plasma levels up to approximately 35 times that for the adult HIV dose. No evidence of teratogenicity due to lamivudine was observed. Evidence of early embryolethality was seen in the rabbit at exposure levels similar to those observed in humans, but there was no indication of this effect in the rat at exposure levels up to 35 times that in humans.

Zidovudine: Reproduction studies with orally administered zidovudine in the rat and in the rabbit at doses up to 500 mg/kg/day revealed no evidence of teratogenicity with zidovudine. Zidovudine treatment resulted in embryo/fetal toxicity as evidenced by an increase in the incidence of fetal resorptions in rats given 150 or 450 mg/kg/day and rabbits given 500 mg/kg/day. The doses used in the teratology studies resulted in peak zidovudine plasma concentrations (after one half of the daily dose) in rats 66 to 226 times, and in rabbits 12 to 87 times, mean steady-state peak human plasma concentrations (after one sixth of the daily dose) achieved with the recommended daily dose (100 mg every 4 hours). In an additional teratology study in rats, a dose of 3,000 mg/kg/day (very near the oral median lethal dose in rats of approximately 3,700 mg/kg) caused marked maternal toxicity and an increase in the incidence of fetal malformations. This dose resulted in peak zidovudine plasma concentrations 350 times peak human plasma concentrations. No evidence of teratogenicity was seen in this experiment at doses of 600 mg/kg/day or less. Two rodent carcinogenicity studies were conducted (see Carcinogenesis, Mutagenesis, and Impairment of Fertility).

Antiretroviral Pregnancy Registry: To monitor maternal-fetal outcomes of pregnant women exposed to TRIZIVIR or other antiretroviral agents, an Antiretroviral Pregnancy Registry has been established. Physicians are encouraged to register patients by calling 1-800-258-4263.

Nursing Mothers: The Centers for Disease Control and Prevention recommend that HIV-infected mothers not breastfeed their infants to avoid risking postnatal transmission of HIV infection.

Abacavir, Lamivudine, and Zidovudine: Zidovudine is excreted in breast milk; abacavir and lamivudine are secreted into the milk of lactating rats.

Because of both the potential for HIV transmission and the potential for serious adverse reactions in nursing infants, **mothers should be instructed not to breastfeed if they are receiving TRIZIVIR.**

Pediatric Use: TRIZIVIR is not intended for use in pediatric patients. TRIZIVIR should not be administered to adolescents who weigh less than 40 kg because it is a fixed-dose tablet that cannot be adjusted for this patient population.

Geriatric Use: Clinical studies of abacavir, lamivudine, and zidovudine did not include sufficient numbers of patients aged 65 and over to determine whether they respond differently from younger patients. In general, dose selection for an elderly patient should be cautious, reflecting the greater frequency of decreased hepatic, renal, or cardiac function, and of concomitant disease or other drug therapy. TRIZIVIR is not recommended for patients with impaired renal function (i.e., creatinine clearance <50 mL/min; see PRECAUTIONS: Patients with Impaired Renal Function and DOSAGE AND ADMINISTRATION).

Table 4. Selected Clinical Adverse Events Grades 1–4 (≥5% Frequency) in Therapy-Naive Adults (CNAAB3003) Through 16 Weeks of Treatment

Adverse Event	ZIAGEN/Lamivudine/Zidovudine (n = 83)	Lamivudine/Zidovudine (n = 81)
Nausea	47%	41%
Nausea and vomiting	16%	11%
Diarrhea	12%	11%
Loss of appetite/anorexia	11%	10%
Insomnia and other sleep disorders	7%	5%

Table 5. Selected Clinical Adverse Events Grades 1–4 (≥5% Frequency) in Therapy-Naive Adults (CNAAB3005) Through 48 Weeks of Treatment

Adverse Event	ZIAGEN/Lamivudine/Zidovudine (n = 262)	Indinavir/Lamivudine/Zidovudine (n = 264)
Nausea	60%	61%
Nausea and vomiting	30%	27%
Diarrhea	26%	27%
Loss of appetite/anorexia	15%	11%
Insomnia and other sleep disorders	13%	12%
Fever and/or chills	20%	13%
Headache	28%	25%
Malaise and/or fatigue	44%	41%

ADVERSE REACTIONS

Abacavir: *Hypersensitivity Reaction:* TRIZIVIR contains abacavir sulfate (ZIAGEN), which has been associated with fatal hypersensitivity reactions. Therapy with abacavir (as TRIZIVIR OR ZIAGEN) SHOULD NOT be restarted following a hypersensitivity reaction because more severe symptoms will recur within hours and may include life-threatening hypotension and death. Patients developing signs or symptoms of hypersensitivity should discontinue treatment as soon as a hypersensitivity reaction is first suspected, and should seek medical evaluation immediately. To avoid a delay in diagnosis and minimize the risk of a life-threatening hypersensitivity reaction, TRIZIVIR should be permanently discontinued if hypersensitivity cannot be ruled out, even when other diagnoses are possible (e.g., acute onset respiratory diseases, gastroenteritis, or reactions to other medications).

Severe or fatal hypersensitivity reactions can occur within hours after reintroduction of abacavir (as TRIZIVIR or ZIAGEN) in patients who have no identified history or unrecognized symptoms of hypersensitivity to abacavir therapy (see WARNINGS and PRECAUTIONS: Information for Patients).

When therapy with abacavir (as TRIZIVIR or ZIAGEN) has been discontinued for reasons other than symptoms of a hypersensitivity reaction, and if reinitiation of therapy is under consideration, the reason for discontinuation should be evaluated to ensure that the patient did not have symptoms of a hypersensitivity reaction. If hypersensitivity cannot be ruled out, abacavir (as TRIZIVIR or ZIAGEN) should **NOT** be reintroduced. If symptoms consistent with hypersensitivity are not identified, reintroduction can be undertaken with continued monitoring for symptoms of hypersensitivity reaction. Patients should be made aware that a hypersensitivity reaction can occur with reintroduction of abacavir (as TRIZIVIR or ZIAGEN), and that reintroduction of abacavir (as TRIZIVIR or ZIAGEN) should be undertaken only if medical care can be readily accessed by the patient or others (see WARNINGS).

In clinical studies, approximately 5% of adult and pediatric patients receiving abacavir developed a hypersensitivity reaction. This reaction is characterized by the appearance of symptoms indicating multi-organ/body system involvement. Symptoms usually appear within the first 6 weeks of treatment with abacavir, although these reactions may occur at any time during therapy. Frequently observed signs and symptoms include fever, skin rash, fatigue, and gastrointestinal symptoms such as nausea, vomiting, diarrhea, or abdominal pain. Other signs and symptoms include malaise, lethargy, myalgia, myolysis, arthralgia, edema, cough, abnormal chest x-ray findings (predominantly infiltrates, which can be localized), dyspnea, headache, and paresthesia. Some patients who experienced a hypersensitivity reaction were initially thought to have acute onset or worsening respiratory disease. The diagnosis of hypersensitivity reaction should be carefully considered for patients presenting with symptoms of acute onset respiratory diseases, even if alternative respiratory diagnoses (pneumonia, bronchitis, flu-like illness) are possible.

Physical findings include lymphadenopathy, mucous membrane lesions (conjunctivitis and mouth ulcerations), and rash. The rash usually appears maculopapular or urticarial but may be variable in appearance. There have been reports of erythema multiforme. Hypersensitivity reactions have occurred without rash.

Laboratory abnormalities include elevated liver function tests, increased creatine phosphokinase or creatinine, and lymphopenia. Anaphylaxis, liver failure, renal failure, hypotension, adult respiratory distress syndrome, respiratory failure, and death have occurred in association with hypersensitivity reactions. Symptoms worsen with continued therapy but often resolve upon discontinuation of abacavir. Risk factors that may predict the occurrence or severity of hypersensitivity to abacavir have not been identified.

Selected clinical adverse events with a ≥5% frequency during therapy with ZIAGEN 300 mg twice daily, EPIVIR 150 mg twice daily, and RETROVIR 300 mg twice daily compared with EPIVIR 150 mg twice daily and RETROVIR 300 mg twice daily from CNAAB3003 are listed in Table 4.

[See table 4 above]

Selected clinical adverse events with a ≥5% frequency during therapy with ZIAGEN 300 mg twice daily, lamivudine 150 mg twice daily, and zidovudine 300 mg twice daily compared with indinavir 800 mg 3 times daily, lamivudine 150 mg twice daily, and zidovudine 300 mg twice daily from CNAAB3005 are listed in Table 5.

[See table 5 above]

Five subjects in the abacavir arm of study CNAAB3005 experienced worsening of pre-existing depression compared to none in the indinavir arm. The background rates of pre-existing depression were similar in the 2 treatment arms.

Laboratory Abnormalities: Laboratory abnormalities (anemia, neutropenia, liver function test abnormalities, and CPK elevations) were observed with similar frequencies in the 2 treatment groups in studies CNAAB3003 and CNAAB3006. Mild elevations of blood glucose were more frequent in subjects receiving abacavir. In study CNAAB3003, triglyceride elevations (all grades) were more common on the abacavir arm (25%) than on the placebo arm (11%). In study CNAAB3005, hyperglycemia and disorders of lipid metabolism occurred with similar frequency in the abacavir and indinavir treatment arms.

Other Adverse Events: In addition to adverse events in Tables 4 and 5, other adverse events observed in the expanded access program for abacavir were pancreatitis and increased GGT.

Lamivudine Plus Zidovudine: In 4 randomized, controlled trials of lamivudine 300 mg per day plus zidovudine 600 mg per day, the following selected clinical and laboratory adverse events were observed (see Tables 6 and 7).

Table 6. Selected Clinical Adverse Events (≥5% Frequency) in 4 Controlled Clinical Trials With Lamivudine 300 mg/day and Zidovudine 600 mg/day

Adverse Event	Lamivudine plus Zidovudine (n = 251)
Body as a whole	
Headache	35%
Malaise & fatigue	27%
Fever or chills	10%
Digestive	
Nausea	33%
Diarrhea	18%
Nausea & vomiting	13%
Anorexia and/or decreased appetite	10%
Abdominal pain	9%
Abdominal cramps	6%
Dyspepsia	5%
Nervous system	
Neuropathy	12%
Insomnia & other sleep disorders	11%
Dizziness	10%
Depressive disorders	9%
Respiratory	
Nasal signs & symptoms	20%
Cough	18%

Skin	
Skin rashes	9%
Musculoskeletal	
Musculoskeletal pain	12%
Myalgia	8%
Arthralgia	5%

Pancreatitis was observed in 3 of the 656 adult patients (<0.5%) who received lamivudine in controlled clinical trials.

Selected laboratory abnormalities observed during therapy are listed in Table 7.

Table 7. Frequencies of Selected Laboratory Abnormalities Among Adults in 4 Controlled Clinical Trials of Lamivudine 300 mg/day plus Zidovudine 600 mg/day*

Test (Abnormal Level)	Lamivudine plus Zidovudine % (n)
Neutropenia (ANC<750/mm^3)	7.2% (237)
Anemia (Hgb <8.0 g/dL)	2.9% (241)
Thrombocytopenia (platelets <50,000/mm^3)	0.4% (240)
ALT (>5.0 × ULN)	3.7% (241)
AST (>5.0 × ULN)	1.7% (241)
Bilirubin (>2.5 × ULN)	0.8% (241)
Amylase (>2.0 × ULN)	4.2% (72)

ULN = Upper limit of normal.
ANC = Absolute neutrophil count.
n = Number of patients assessed.
*Frequencies of these laboratory abnormalities were higher in patients with mild laboratory abnormalities at baseline.

Observed During Clinical Practice: The following events have been identified during post-approval use of abacavir, lamivudine, and/or zidovudine. Because they are reported voluntarily from a population of unknown size, estimates of frequency cannot be made. These events have been chosen for inclusion due to a combination of their seriousness, frequency of reporting, or potential causal connection to lamivudine and/or zidovudine.

Abacavir: Suspected Stevens-Johnson syndrome (SJS) and toxic epidermal necrolysis (TEN) have been reported in patients receiving abacavir primarily in combination with medications known to be associated with SJS and TEN, respectively. Because of the overlap of clinical signs and symptoms between hypersensitivity to abacavir and SJS and TEN, and the possibility of multiple drug sensitivities in some patients, abacavir should be discontinued and not restarted in such cases.

There have also been reports of erythema multiforme with abacavir use.

Abacavir, Lamivudine, and Zidovudine:

Body as a Whole: Redistribution/accumulation of body fat (see PRECAUTIONS: Fat Redistribution).

Cardiovascular: Cardiomyopathy.

Digestive: Stomatitis.

Endocrine and Metabolic: Gynecomastia, hyperglycemia.

Gastrointestinal: Oral mucosal pigmentation.

General: Vasculitis, weakness.

Hemic and Lymphatic: Aplastic anemia, anemia, lymphadenopathy, pure red cell aplasia, splenomegaly.

Hepatic and Pancreatic: Lactic acidosis and hepatic steatosis, pancreatitis, posttreatment exacerbation of hepatitis B (see WARNINGS).

Hypersensitivity: Sensitization reactions (including anaphylaxis), urticaria.

Musculoskeletal: Muscle weakness, CPK elevation, rhabdomyolysis.

Nervous: Paresthesia, peripheral neuropathy, seizures.

Respiratory: Abnormal breath sounds/wheezing.

Skin: Alopecia, erythema multiforme, Stevens-Johnson syndrome.

OVERDOSAGE

Abacavir: There is no known antidote for abacavir. It is not known whether abacavir can be removed by peritoneal dialysis or hemodialysis.

Lamivudine: One case of an adult ingesting 6 grams of lamivudine was reported; there were no clinical signs or symptoms noted and hematologic tests remained normal. It is not known whether lamivudine can be removed by peritoneal dialysis or hemodialysis.

Zidovudine: Acute overdoses of zidovudine have been reported in pediatric patients and adults. These involved exposures up to 50 grams. The only consistent findings were nausea and vomiting. Other reported occurrences included headache, dizziness, drowsiness, lethargy, and confusion. Hematologic changes were transient. All patients recovered. Hemodialysis and peritoneal dialysis appear to have a negligible effect on the removal of zidovudine, while elimination of its primary metabolite, GZDV, is enhanced.

DOSAGE AND ADMINISTRATION

A Medication Guide and Warning Card that provide information about recognition of hypersensitivity reactions should be dispensed with each new prescription and refill. To facilitate reporting of hypersensitivity reactions and collection of information on each case, an Abacavir Hypersensitivity Registry has been established. Physicians should register patients by calling 1-800-270-0425.

The recommended oral dose of TRIZIVIR for adults and adolescents is 1 tablet twice daily. TRIZIVIR is not recommended in adults or adolescents who weigh less than 40 kg because it is a fixed-dose tablet.

Dose Adjustment: Because it is a fixed-dose tablet, TRIZIVIR should not be prescribed for patients requiring dosage adjustment such as those with creatinine clearance <50 mL/min or those experiencing dose-limiting adverse events.

HOW SUPPLIED

TRIZIVIR is available as tablets. Each tablet contains 300 mg of abacavir as abacavir sulfate, 150 mg of lamivudine, and 300 mg of zidovudine. The tablets are blue-green capsule-shaped, film-coated, and imprinted with GX LL1 on one side with no markings on the reverse side. They are packaged as follows:

Bottles of 60 Tablets (NDC 0173-0691-00).

Convenience Pack containing 60 Tablets on one blister roll (NDC 0173-0691-20).

Store at 25°C (77°F); excursions permitted to 15° to 30°C (59° to 86°F) (see USP Controlled Room Temperature).

ANIMAL TOXICOLOGY

Myocardial degeneration was found in mice and rats following administration of abacavir for 2 years. The systemic exposures were equivalent to 7 to 24 times the expected systemic exposure in humans. The clinical relevance of this finding has not been determined.

GlaxoSmithKline, Research Triangle Park, NC 27709
Lamivudine is manufactured under agreement from
Shire Pharmaceuticals Group plc, Basingstoke, UK

November 2003/RL-2056

MEDICATION GUIDE
TRIZIVIR® (TRY-zih-veer) Tablets

Generic name: abacavir sulfate, lamivudine, and zidovudine

Read the Medication Guide you get each time you fill your prescription for Trizivir. There may be new information since you filled your last prescription.

What is the most important information I should know about Trizivir?

Trizivir contains abacavir, which is also called Ziagen®. About 1 in 20 patients (5%) who take abacavir (as Trizivir or Ziagen) will have a **serious allergic reaction** (hypersensitivity reaction) that **may cause death if the drug is not stopped right away.**

You may be having this reaction if:

(1) you get a skin rash, or

(2) you get 1 or more symptoms from at least 2 of the following groups:

- **Fever**
- **Nausea, vomiting, diarrhea, abdominal (stomach area) pain**
- **Extreme tiredness, achiness, generally ill feeling**
- **Sore throat, shortness of breath, cough**

If you think you may be having a reaction, **STOP taking Trizivir and call your doctor right away.**

If you stop treatment with Trizivir because of this serious reaction, **NEVER take abacavir (as Trizivir or Ziagen) again.** If you take any of these medicines again after you have had this serious reaction, **you could die within hours.**

Some patients who have stopped taking abacavir (as Trizivir or Ziagen) and who have then started taking abacavir again have had serious or life-threatening allergic (hypersensitivity) reactions. If you must stop treatment with Trizivir for reasons other than symptoms of hypersensitivity, do not begin taking it again without talking to your health care provider. If your health care provider decides that you may begin taking abacavir (as Trizivir or Ziagen) again, you should do so only in a setting with other people to get access to a doctor if needed.

A written list of these symptoms is on the Warning Card your pharmacist gives you. Carry this Warning Card with you.

Trizivir can have other serious side effects. Be sure to read the section below entitled "What are the possible side effects of Trizivir?"

What is Trizivir?

Trizivir is a medicine used to treat HIV infection. Trizivir includes 3 medicines: Ziagen (abacavir), Epivir® (lamivudine or 3TC), and Retrovir® (zidovudine, AZT, or ZDV).

All 3 of these medicines are called nucleoside analogue reverse transcriptase inhibitors (NRTIs). When used together, they help lower the amount of HIV in your blood. This helps to keep your immune system as healthy as possible so it can fight infection.

Different combinations of medicines are used to treat HIV infection. You and your doctor should discuss which combination of medicines is best for you.

Trizivir does not cure HIV infection or AIDS. Trizivir has not been studied long enough to know if it will help you live longer or have fewer of the medical problems that are associated with HIV infection or AIDS. Therefore, you must see your health care provider regularly.

Who should not take Trizivir?

Do not take Trizivir if you have ever had a serious allergic reaction (a hypersensitivity reaction) to any of the medicines that make up Trizivir, especially Ziagen (abacavir). If you have had such a reaction, return all of your unused Trizivir to your doctor or pharmacist.

Do not take Trizivir if you weigh less than 90 pounds.

How should I take Trizivir?

To help make sure that your anti-HIV therapy is as effective as possible, take your Trizivir exactly as your doctor prescribes it. Do not skip any doses.

The usual dosage is 1 tablet twice a day. You can take Trizivir with food or on an empty stomach.

If you miss a dose of Trizivir, take the missed dose right away. Then, take the next dose at the usual scheduled time. Do not let your Trizivir run out. The amount of virus in your blood may increase if your anti-HIV drugs are stopped, even for a short time. Also, the virus in your body may become harder to treat.

What should I avoid while taking Trizivir?

Do not take Epivir, Retrovir, Combivir®, or Ziagen while taking Trizivir. These medicines are already in Trizivir.

You should avoid taking stavudine (Zerit®) while taking Trizivir. If your doctor prescribes doxorubicin or ribavirin, tell your doctor that you are taking Trizivir.

Practice safe sex while using Trizivir. Do not use or share dirty needles. Trizivir does not reduce the risk of passing HIV to others through sexual contact or blood contamination.

Talk to your doctor if you are pregnant or if you become pregnant while taking Trizivir. Trizivir has not been studied in pregnant women. It is not known whether Trizivir will harm the unborn child.

Mothers with HIV should not breastfeed their babies because HIV is passed to the baby in breast milk. Also, Trizivir can be passed to babies in breast milk and could cause the child to have side effects.

What are the possible side effects of Trizivir?

Life-threatening allergic reaction. Trizivir contains abacavir, which is also called Ziagen. Abacavir has caused some people to have a life-threatening allergic reaction (hypersensitivity reaction) that can cause death. How to recognize a possible reaction and what to do are discussed in "What is the most important information I should know about Trizivir?" at the beginning of this Medication Guide.

Lactic acidosis and severe liver problems. The medicines in Trizivir can cause a serious condition called lactic acidosis and, in some cases, this condition can cause death. Nausea and tiredness that don't get better may be symptoms of lactic acidosis. Women are more likely than men to get this serious side effect.

Blood problems. Retrovir, one of the medicines in Trizivir, can cause serious blood cell problems. These include reduced numbers of white blood cells (neutropenia) and extremely reduced numbers of red blood cells (anemia). These blood cell problems are especially likely to happen in patients with advanced HIV disease or AIDS.

Your doctor should be checking your blood cell counts regularly while you are taking Trizivir. This is especially important if you have advanced HIV or AIDS. This is to make sure that any blood cell problems are found quickly.

Muscle weakness. Retrovir, one of the medicines in Trizivir, can cause muscle weakness. This can be a serious problem.

Other side effects. Trizivir can cause other side effects. The most common side effects of taking the medicines in Trizivir together are nausea, vomiting, diarrhea, loss of appetite, weakness or tiredness, headache, dizziness, pain or tingling of the hands or feet, and muscle and joint pain.

Changes in body fat have been seen in some patients taking antiretroviral therapy. These changes may include increased amount of fat in the upper back and neck ("buffalo hump"), breast, and around the trunk. Loss of fat from the legs, arms, and face may also happen. The cause and long-term health effects of these conditions are not known at this time.

This listing of side effects is not complete. Your doctor or pharmacist can discuss with you a more complete list of side effects with Trizivir.

Ask a health care professional about any concerns about Trizivir. If you want more information, ask your doctor or pharmacist for the labeling for Trizivir that was written for health care professionals.

Do not use Trizivir for a condition for which it was not prescribed. Do not give Trizivir to other persons.

GlaxoSmithKline, Research Triangle Park, NC 27709

July 2002/MG-018

This Medication Guide has been approved by the US Food and Drug Administration.

Shown in Product Identification Guide, page 317

Continued on next page

Product information on these pages is effective as of August 2004. Further information is available at: GlaxoSmithKline, PO Box 13398, Research Triangle Park, NC 27709. 1-888-825-5249. Corporate Web Site: www.gsk.com

TWINRIX® ℞
[*twin'rix*]
[Hepatitis A Inactivated & Hepatitis B (Recombinant) Vaccine]

DESCRIPTION

TWINRIX® [Hepatitis A Inactivated & Hepatitis B (Recombinant) Vaccine] is a sterile bivalent vaccine containing the antigenic components used in producing HAVRIX® (Hepatitis A Vaccine, Inactivated) and ENGERIX-B® [Hepatitis B Vaccine (Recombinant)]. TWINRIX is a sterile suspension of inactivated hepatitis A virus (strain HM175) propagated in MRC_5 cells, and combined with purified surface antigen of the hepatitis B virus. The purified hepatitis B surface antigen (HBsAg) is obtained by culturing genetically engineered *Saccharomyces cerevisiae* cells, which carry the surface antigen gene of the hepatitis B virus, in synthetic media containing inorganic salts, amino acids, dextrose, and vitamins. Bulk preparations of each antigen are adsorbed separately onto aluminum salts and then pooled during formulation.

A 1.0-mL dose of vaccine contains not less than 720 ELISA Units of inactivated hepatitis A virus and 20 mcg of recombinant HBsAg protein. One dose of vaccine also contains 0.45 mg of aluminum in the form of aluminum phosphate and aluminum hydroxide as adjuvants, amino acids, 5.0 mg 2-phenoxyethanol as a preservative, sodium chloride, phosphate buffer, polysorbate 20, Water for Injection, traces of formalin (not more than 0.1 mg), a trace amount of thimerosal (<1 mcg mercury) from the manufacturing process, and residual MRC_5 cellular proteins (not more than 2.5 mcg). Neomycin sulfate, an aminoglycoside antibiotic, is included in the cell growth media; only trace amounts (not more than 20 ng) remain following purification. The manufacturing procedures used to manufacture TWINRIX result in a product that contains no more than 5% yeast protein.

TWINRIX is supplied as a sterile suspension for intramuscular administration. The vaccine is ready for use without reconstitution; it must be shaken before administration since a fine white deposit with a clear colorless supernatant may form on storage. After shaking, the vaccine is a slightly turbid white suspension.

CLINICAL PHARMACOLOGY

Several hepatitis viruses (A, B, C, D, and E) are known to cause a systemic infection resulting in major pathologic changes in the liver. Features of hepatitis A and hepatitis B are described below.

Hepatitis A: The hepatitis A virus (HAV) belongs to the picornavirus family. Only one serotype of HAV has been described.[1]

Hepatitis A is a highly contagious disease with the predominant mode of transmission being person-to-person via the fecal-oral route. Infection has been shown to be spread (1) by contaminated water or food; (2) by infected food handlers[2]; (3) after breakdown in usual sanitary conditions or after floods or natural disasters; (4) by ingestion of raw or undercooked shellfish (oysters, clams, mussels) from contaminated waters[3]; (5) during travel to areas of the world with poor hygienic conditions[4]; (6) among institutionalized children and adults[5]; (7) in day-care centers[6]; and (8) by parenteral transmission, either blood transfusions or sharing needles with infected people.[7]

In the United States, attack rates for hepatitis A disease are cyclical and vary by population. The rates have increased gradually from 10.4 per 100,000 in 1987 to 11.7 per 100,000 in 1996.[8]

The incubation period for hepatitis A averages 28 days (range: 15 to 50 days).[9] The course of hepatitis A infection is extremely variable, ranging from asymptomatic infection to icteric hepatitis. However, most adults (76% to 97%) become symptomatic.[10] Symptoms range from mild and transient to severe and prolonged, and may include fever, nausea, vomiting, and diarrhea in the prodromal phase, followed by jaundice in up to 88% of adults, as well as hepatomegaly and biochemical evidence of hepatocellular damage.[10] Recovery is generally complete and followed by protection against HAV infection. However, illness may be prolonged, and relapse of clinical illness and viral shedding have been described.[11] Up to 22% of adults who contract hepatitis A are hospitalized and approximately 100 patients die annually in the United States from complications of hepatitis A.[12]

Chronic shedding of HAV in feces has not been demonstrated, but relapses of hepatitis A can occur in as many as 20% of patients[11,13] and fecal shedding of HAV may recur at this time.[11] Approximately 70% of pediatric patients less than 6 years of age infected with hepatitis A are asymptomatic, and serve as a reservoir for infection among adults.[12]

The presence of antibodies to HAV, as detected in a standardized assay (HAVAB), is an indication of the presence of protective antibodies against hepatitis A disease. Natural infection provides lifelong immunity even when antibodies to hepatitis A are undetectable. At present, studies show the duration of protection afforded by TWINRIX against hepatitis A lasts at least 4 years.[14]

Hepatitis B: The hepatitis B virus (HBV) belongs to a family of genetically related DNA-containing animal viruses, which are hepatotropic. The incubation period of hepatitis B ranges between 30 and 180 days. The mode of transmission of hepatitis B may be: By contact (contaminated body secretions including semen, vaginal secretions, blood, saliva); percutaneously (usually through accidental needlesticks or by sharing needles with infected people); or by maternal-neonatal transmission.[15]

HBV infection occurs throughout the world with highly variable prevalences. A human reservoir of persistently infected persons is present in nearly all communities of the world. In the United States, parenteral drug abuse, unprotected sexual activity, occupationally acquired infection, or travelers returning from high prevalence countries may be the principal mechanisms of HBV transmission.

Clinical infection with hepatitis B may occur in 2 major forms: Asymptomatic or symptomatic hepatitis. Asymptomatic HBV infection can be subclinical or inapparent. In subclinical infection, patients have abnormal liver enzymes without jaundice, while inapparent asymptomatic infection is identified only by serological testing. One in 4 adults who has symptomatic disease has jaundice (anicteric/icteric hepatitis).

HBV infection can have serious consequences including acute massive hepatic necrosis, chronic active hepatitis, and cirrhosis of the liver. As many as 90% of infants and 6% to 10% of adults who are infected in the United States will become HBV carriers.[12] An estimated 200 to 300 million people are chronic carriers of HBV worldwide.[12] The Centers for Disease Control and Prevention (CDC) estimates that there are approximately 1 million to 1.25 million chronic carriers of HBV in the United States.[12] About 50,000 cases of hepatitis are reported per year, about half of which are hepatitis B. Unreported cases may be 10 times greater. Close contact (sexual contact or household contact) or exposure to blood from infected individuals is associated with increased risk of infection. Those patients who become chronic carriers can infect others and are at increased risk of developing primary hepatocellular carcinoma. Among other factors, infection with HBV may be the single most important factor for development of this carcinoma.[12,16]

Reduced Risk of Hepatocellular Carcinoma: A clear link has been demonstrated between chronic HBV infection and the occurrence of hepatocellular carcinoma. In a Taiwanese study, the institution of universal childhood immunization against HBV has been shown to decrease the incidence of hepatocellular carcinoma among children.[17] In a Korean study in adult males, vaccination against HBV has been shown to decrease the incidence of, and risk of, developing hepatocellular carcinoma in adults.[18]

There is no definitive treatment for acute HBV infection. However, those who develop antibodies to HBsAg after active infection are protected against subsequent infection. Antibody titers ≥10 mIU/mL against HBsAg are recognized as conferring protection against HBV.[19] Seroconversion is defined as an antibody titer ≥1 mIU/mL.

Clinical Trials: ***Immunogenicity in Adults:*** Sera from 1,551 healthy adult volunteers ages 17 to 70, including 555 male subjects and 996 female subjects, in 11 clinical trials were analyzed following administration of 3 doses of TWINRIX on a 0-, 1-, and 6-month schedule. Seroconversion for antibodies against HAV was elicited in 99.9% of vaccinees, and protective antibodies against HBV were detected in 98.5%, 1 month after completion of the 3-dose series.

Table 1. Immunogenicity in TWINRIX Worldwide Clinical Trials

TWINRIX Dose	N	% Seroconversion for Hepatitis A*	% Seroprotection for Hepatitis B†
1	1587	93.8	30.8
2	1571	98.8	78.2
3	1551	99.9	98.5

*Anti-HAV titer ≥assay cut-off: 20 mIU/mL (HAVAB Test) or 33 mIU/mL (ENZYMUN-TEST®).
†Anti-HBsAg titer ≥10 mIU/mL (AUSAB®).

One of the 11 trials was a comparative trial conducted in a US population given either TWINRIX (on a 0-, 1-, and 6-month schedule) or HAVRIX (0- and 6-month schedule) and ENGERIX-B (0-, 1-, and 6-month schedule). The monovalent vaccines were given concurrently in opposite arms. Of a total of 773 adults (ages 18 to 70 years) enrolled in this trial, an immunogenicity analysis was performed in 533 subjects who completed the study according to protocol. Of these, 264 subjects received TWINRIX and 269 subjects received HAVRIX and ENGERIX-B. Seroconversion against HAV and seroprotection against HBV are shown in Table 2.
[See table 2 below]

Since the immune responses to hepatitis A and hepatitis B induced by TWINRIX were non-inferior to the monovalent vaccines, efficacy is expected to be similar to the efficacy for each of the monovalent vaccines (Table 3).
[See table 3 below]

It was noted that the antibody titers achieved 1 month after the final dose of TWINRIX were higher than titers achieved 1 month after the final dose of HAVRIX in these clinical trials. This may have been due to a difference in the recommended dosage regimens for these 2 vaccines, whereby TWINRIX vaccinees received 3 doses of 720 EL.U. of hepatitis A antigen at 0, 1, and 6 months, whereas HAVRIX vaccinees received 2 doses of 1440 EL.U. of the same antigen (at 0 and 6 months). However, these differences in peak titer have not been shown to be clinically significant.

Two clinical trials involving a total of 129 subjects demonstrated that antibodies to both HAV and HBV persisted for at least 4 years after the first vaccine dose in a 3-dose series of TWINRIX, given on a 0-, 1-, and 6-month schedule. For comparison, after the recommended immunization regimens for HAVRIX and ENGERIX-B, respectively, similar studies involving a total of 114 subjects have shown that seropositivity to HAV and HBV also persists for at least 4 years.

The effect of age on immune response to TWINRIX was studied in 2 trials comparing subjects over 40 years of age (n = 183, mean age = 48 in one trial and n = 72, mean age = 50 in the other) with those ≤40 (n = 191; mean age 32.5). The response to the hepatitis A component of TWINRIX declined slightly with age, but >99% of subjects achieved protective antibody levels in both age groups, and antibody titers were comparable to 2 doses of hepatitis A vaccine alone in age matched controls.

The response to hepatitis B immunization is known to decline in vaccinees over 40 years of age. TWINRIX elicited a seroprotective response to hepatitis B in 97% of younger subjects and 93% to 94% of the older subjects, as compared to 92% of older subjects given hepatitis B vaccine alone. Geometric mean titers elicited by TWINRIX were 2,285 in the younger subjects and 1,890 or 1,038 for the older subjects in the 2 trials. Hepatitis B vaccine alone gave titers of 2,896 in younger subjects and 1,157 in those over 40 years of age.

It has been shown in open randomized clinical trials that combining the hepatitis A antigen with the hepatitis B surface antigen in TWINRIX resulted in comparable anti-HAV or anti-HBsAg titers, relative to vaccination with the individual monovalent vaccines or the concomitant administration of each vaccine in opposite arms.

Immune Response to Simultaneously Administered Vaccines: There have been no studies of concomitant administration of TWINRIX with other vaccines.

INDICATIONS AND USAGE

TWINRIX is indicated for active immunization of persons 18 years of age or older against disease caused by hepatitis A virus and infection by all known subtypes of hepatitis B virus. As with any vaccine, vaccination with TWINRIX may not protect 100% of recipients. As hepatitis D (caused by the

Table 2. Percentage of Seroconversion or Seroprotection Rates in the TWINRIX US Clinical Trial

Vaccine	N	Timepoint	% Seroconversion for Hepatitis A* (95% CI)	% Seroprotection for Hepatitis B† (95% CI)
TWINRIX	264	Month 1	91.6	17.9
		Month 2	97.7	61.2
		Month 7	99.6 (97.9-100.0)	95.1 (91.7-97.4)
HAVRIX and ENGERIX-B	269	Month 1	98.1	7.5
		Month 2	98.9	50.4
		Month 7	99.3 (97.3-99.9)	92.2 (88.3-95.1)

*Anti-HAV titer ≥assay cut-off: 33 mIU/mL (ENZYMUN-TEST®).
†Anti-HBsAg titer ≥10 mIU/mL (AUSAB®).

Table 3. Geometric Mean Titers in the TWINRIX US Clinical Trial

Vaccine	N	Timepoint	GMT to Hepatitis A (95% CI)	GMT to Hepatitis B (95% CI)
TWINRIX	263	Month 1	335	8
	259	Month 2	636	23
	264	Month 7	4756 (4152-5448)	2099 (1663-2649)
HAVRIX and ENGERIX-B	268	Month 1	444	6
	269	Month 2	257	18
	269	Month 7	2948 (2638-3294)	1871 (1428-2450)

delta virus) does not occur in the absence of HBV infection, it can be expected that hepatitis D will also be prevented by vaccination with TWINRIX.

TWINRIX will not prevent hepatitis caused by other agents such as hepatitis C virus, hepatitis E virus, or other pathogens known to infect the liver.

Immunization is recommended for all susceptible persons 18 years of age or older who are, or will be, at risk of exposure to both hepatitis A and hepatitis B viruses, including but not limited to:

- *Travelers*: Persons traveling to areas of high/intermediate endemicity for *both* HAV and HBV (see Table 4) *who are at increased risk of HBV infection due to behavioral or occupational factors.* (See CLINICAL PHARMACOLOGY.)

Table 4. Hepatitis A and Hepatitis B Endemicity by Region

Geographic Region	HAV	HBV
Africa	High	High (most)
Caribbean	High	Intermediate
Central America	High	Intermediate
South America (temperate)	High	Intermediate
South America (tropical)	High	High
South and Southeast Asia*	High	High
Middle East†	High	High
Eastern Europe	Intermediate	Intermediate
Southern Europe	Intermediate	Intermediate
Former Soviet Union	Intermediate	Intermediate

*Japan: Low HAV and intermediate HBV endemicity.
†Israel: Intermediate HBV endemicity.

- *Patients With Chronic Liver Disease*, including:
  - — alcoholic cirrhosis
  - — chronic hepatitis C
  - — autoimmune hepatitis
  - — primary biliary cirrhosis
- *Persons at Risk Through Their Work*:
  - — Laboratory workers who handle live hepatitis A and hepatitis B virus
  - — Police and other personnel who render first-aid or medical assistance
  - — Workers who come in contact with feces or sewage
- *Others:*
  - — Healthcare personnel who render first-aid or emergency medical assistance.
  - — Personnel employed in day-care centers and correctional facilities. Residents of drug and alcohol treatment centers. Staff of hemodialysis units.
  - — People living in, or relocating to, areas of high/intermediate endemicity of HAV and who have risk factors for HBV.
  - — Men who have sex with men.
  - — Persons at increased risk of disease due to their sexual practices.[20,21]
  - — Patients frequently receiving blood products including persons who have clotting factor disorders (hemophiliacs and other recipients of therapeutic blood products).
  - — Military recruits and other military personnel at increased risk for HBV.
  - — Users of injectable illicit drugs.
  - — Individuals who are at increased risk for HBV infection and who are close household contacts of patients with acute or relapsing hepatitis A and individuals who are at increased risk for HAV infection and who are close household contacts of individuals with acute or chronic hepatitis B infection.

CONTRAINDICATIONS

Hypersensitivity to any component of the vaccine, including yeast and neomycin, is a contraindication (see DESCRIPTION). This vaccine is contraindicated in patients with previous hypersensitivity to TWINRIX or monovalent hepatitis A or hepatitis B vaccines.

WARNINGS

There have been rare reports of anaphylaxis/anaphylactoid reactions following routine clinical use of TWINRIX. (See CONTRAINDICATIONS.)

The vial stopper is latex-free. The tip cap and the rubber plunger of the needleless prefilled syringes contain dry natural latex rubber that may cause allergic reactions in latex sensitive individuals.

Hepatitis A and hepatitis B have relatively long incubation periods. The vaccine may not prevent hepatitis A or hepatitis B infection in individuals who have an unrecognized hepatitis A or hepatitis B infection at the time of vaccination. Additionally, it may not prevent infection in individuals who do not achieve protective antibody titers.

PRECAUTIONS

General: As with other vaccines, although a moderate or severe acute illness is sufficient reason to postpone vaccination, minor illnesses such as mild upper respiratory infections with or without low-grade fever are not contraindications.[22]

Multiple Sclerosis: Results from 2 clinical studies indicate that there is no association between hepatitis B vaccination and the development of multiple sclerosis,[23] and that vaccination with hepatitis B vaccine does not appear to increase the short-term risk of relapse in multiple sclerosis.[24]

TWINRIX should be administered with caution to people on anticoagulants, and those with thrombocytopenia or a bleeding disorder since bleeding may occur following intramuscular administration to these subjects.

As with any vaccine, if administered to immunosuppressed persons or persons receiving immunosuppressive therapy, the expected immune response may not be obtained.[25]

Before the injection of any vaccine, the physician should take all reasonable precautions to prevent allergic or other adverse reactions, including understanding the use of the vaccine concerned, and the nature of the side effects and adverse reactions that may follow its use.

Prior to immunization with any vaccine, the patient's history should be reviewed. The physician should review the patient's immunization history for possible vaccine sensitivity, previous vaccination-related adverse reactions, and occurrence of any adverse event–related symptoms and/or signs in order to determine the existence of any contraindication to immunization with TWINRIX and to allow an assessment of benefits and risks. As with any parenteral vaccine, epinephrine injection (1:1,000) and other appropriate agents used for the control of immediate allergic reactions must be immediately available should an acute anaphylactic reaction occur.

A separate sterile syringe and needle or a sterile disposable unit must be used for each patient to prevent the transmission of infectious agents from person to person. Needles should be disposed of properly and should not be recapped.

Information for Patients: Patients should be informed of the benefits and risks of immunization with TWINRIX, and of the importance of completing the immunization series. As with any vaccine, it is important when a subject returns for the next dose in a series that he or she be questioned concerning the occurrence of any symptoms and/or signs after a previous dose of the same vaccine and that adverse events be reported. The US Department of Health and Human Services has established the Vaccine Adverse Events Reporting System (VAERS) to accept reports of suspected adverse events after the administration of any vaccine including, but not limited to, the reporting of events required by the National Childhood Vaccine Injury Act of 1986. The toll-free number for VAERS forms and information is 1-800-822-7967.[26]

Carcinogenesis, Mutagenesis, Impairment of Fertility: TWINRIX has not been evaluated for its carcinogenic potential, mutagenic potential, or potential for impairment of fertility.

Pregnancy: Pregnancy Category C. Animal reproduction studies have not been conducted with TWINRIX. It is also not known whether TWINRIX can cause fetal harm when administered to a pregnant woman or can affect reproduction capacity. TWINRIX should be given to a pregnant woman only if clearly indicated (see INDICATIONS AND USAGE).

Pregnancy Exposure Registry: Health care providers are encouraged to register pregnant women who receive TWINRIX in the GlaxoSmithKline vaccination pregnancy registry by calling 1-888-825-5249.

Nursing Mothers It is not known whether TWINRIX is excreted in human milk. Because many drugs are excreted in human milk, caution should be exercised when TWINRIX is administered to a nursing woman.

Pediatric Use: Safety and effectiveness in pediatric patients below the age of 18 years has not been established.

Geriatric Use: Clinical studies of TWINRIX did not include sufficient numbers of subjects aged 65 and over to determine whether they respond differently from younger subjects.

ADVERSE REACTIONS

In clinical trials involving the administration of 6,543 doses to 2,299 individuals and during routine clinical use of the vaccine outside the United States, TWINRIX has been generally well tolerated.

Of 773 volunteers who participated in the comparative trial conducted in the United States, 389 subjects received at least 1 dose of TWINRIX and 384 received at least 1 dose each of ENGERIX-B and HAVRIX as separate but simultaneous injections. Solicited adverse events reported following the administration of TWINRIX are shown in Table 5, compared with adverse events reported after administration of ENGERIX-B and HAVRIX.

[See table 5 above]

[See second table above]

Table 5. Rate of Adverse Events Reported After Administration of TWINRIX or ENGERIX-B and HAVRIX

Adverse Event	TWINRIX			ENGERIX-B			HAVRIX	
	Dose 1	Dose 2	Dose 3	Dose 1	Dose 2	Dose 3	Dose 1	Dose 2
Local	(N = 385) %	(N = 382) %	(N = 374) %	(N = 382) %	(N = 376) %	(N = 369) %	(N = 382) %	(N = 369) %
Soreness	37	35	41	41	25	30	53	47
Redness	8	9	11	6	7	9	7	9
Swelling	4	4	6	3	5	5	5	5

Adverse Event	TWINRIX			ENGERIX-B and HAVRIX		
	Dose 1	Dose 2	Dose 3	Dose 1	Dose 2	Dose 3
General	(N = 385) %	(N = 382) %	(N = 374) %	(N = 382) %	(N = 376) %	(N = 369) %
Headache	22	15	13	19	12	14
Fatigue	14	13	11	14	9	10
Diarrhea	5	4	6	5	3	3
Nausea	4	3	2	7	3	5
Fever	4	3	2	4	2	4
Vomiting	1	1	0	1	1	1

Adverse reactions seen with TWINRIX were similar to those observed after vaccination with the monovalent components. The frequency of solicited adverse events did not increase with successive doses of TWINRIX. Most events reported were considered by the subjects as mild and self-limiting and did not last more than 48 hours.

Among 2,299 subjects in 14 clinical trials, the following adverse experiences were reported to occur within 30 days following vaccination with the frequency shown below.

Incidence 1% to 10% of Injections, Seen in Clinical Trials With TWINRIX:

Local Reactions at Injection Site: Induration.

Respiratory System: Upper respiratory tract infections.

Incidence <1% of Injections, Seen in Clinical Trials With TWINRIX:

Local Reactions at Injection Site: Pruritus, ecchymoses.

Body as a Whole: Sweating, weakness, flushing, influenza-like symptoms.

Cardiovascular System: Syncope.

Gastrointestinal System: Abdominal pain, anorexia, vomiting.

Musculoskeletal System: Arthralgia, myalgia, back pain.

Nervous System: Migraine, paresthesia, vertigo, somnolence, insomnia, irritability, agitation, dizziness.

Respiratory System: Respiratory tract illnesses.

Skin and Appendages: Rash, urticaria, petechiae, erythema.

As with any vaccine, it is possible that expanded routine clinical use of the vaccine could reveal rare adverse events.

Incidence <1% of Injections, Seen in Clinical Trials With HAVRIX[a] and/or ENERGIX-B[b]:

Body as a Whole: Tingling.[b]

Cardiovascular System: Hypotension.[b]

Gastrointestinal: Constipation,[b] dysgeusia.[a]

Hematologic/lymphatic: Lymphadenopathy.[a+b]

Musculoskeletal System: Elevation of creatine phosphokinase.[a]

Nervous System: Hypertonic episode,[a] photophobia.[a]

Post-marketing Reports With HAVRIX and/or ENERGIX-B: Since market introduction, more than 61 million doses of HAVRIX and more than 600 million doses of ENGERIX-B have been distributed worldwide (circa 2000).[27] Voluntary reports of adverse events in people receiving either ENGERIX-B or HAVRIX that have been reported since market introduction of the vaccines include the following:

Body as a Whole: Anaphylaxis/anaphylactoid reactions and allergic reactions.[a]

Hypersensitivity: Erythema multiforme including Stevens-Johnson syndrome,[b] angioedema,[b] arthritis,[b] serum sickness–like syndrome days to weeks after vaccination in-

Continued on next page

Product information on these pages is effective as of August 2004. Further information is available at: GlaxoSmithKline, PO Box 13398, Research Triangle Park, NC 27709. 1-888-825-5249. Corporate Web Site: www.gsk.com

Twinrix—Cont.

cluding arthralgia/arthritis (usually transient), fever, urticaria, erythema multiforme, ecchymoses and erythema nodosum.[b]

Cardiovascular System: Tachycardia/palpitations.[b]

Skin and Appendages: Erythema multiforme,[a] hyperhydrosis,[a] angioedema,[a] eczema,[b] herpes zoster,[b] erythema nodosum,[b] alopecia.[b]

Gastrointestinal System: Jaundice,[a] hepatitis,[a] abnormal liver function tests,[b] dyspepsia.[b]

Hematologic/lymphatic: Thrombocytopenia.[b]

Nervous System: Convulsions,[a] paresis,[b] encephalopathy,[a] neuropathy,[a+b] myelitis,[a] Guillain-Barré syndrome,[a+b] multiple sclerosis,[a+b] Bell's palsy,[b] transverse myelitis,[b] optic neuritis.[b]

Respiratory System: Dyspnea,[a] bronchospasm including asthma-like symptoms.[b]

Special Senses: Conjunctivitis,[b] keratitis,[b] visual disturbances,[b] tinnitus,[b] earache.[b]

Other: Congenital abnormality.[a]

[a] Following HAVRIX.
[b] Following ENGERIX-B.
[a+b] Following either HAVRIX or ENGERIX-B.

DOSAGE AND ADMINISTRATION

TWINRIX should be administered by intramuscular injection. *Do not inject intravenously or intradermally.* In adults, the injection should be given in the deltoid region. TWINRIX should not be administered in the gluteal region; such injections may result in a suboptimal response.

For individuals with clotting factor disorders who are at risk of hemorrhage following intramuscular injection, the ACIP recommends that when any intramuscular vaccine is indicated for such patients, ". . . it should be administered intramuscularly if, in the opinion of a physician familiar with the patient's bleeding risk, the vaccine can be administered with reasonable safety by this route. If the patient receives antihemophilia or other similar therapy, intramuscular vaccination can be scheduled shortly after such therapy is administered. A fine needle (23 gauge or smaller) can be used for the vaccination and firm pressure applied to the site (without rubbing) for at least 2 minutes. The patient should be instructed concerning the risk of hematoma from the injection."[28]

When concomitant administration of other vaccines or immunoglobulin (IG) is required, they should be given with different syringes and at different injection sites.

Preparation for Administration: Shake vial or syringe well before withdrawal and use. Parenteral drug products should be inspected visually for particulate matter or discoloration prior to administration. With thorough agitation, TWINRIX is a slightly turbid white suspension. Discard if it appears otherwise.

The vaccine should be used as supplied; no dilution or reconstitution is necessary. The full recommended dose of the vaccine should be used. After removal of the appropriate volume from a single-dose vial, any vaccine remaining in the vial should be discarded.

Primary immunization for adults consists of 3 doses, given on a 0-, 1-, and 6-month schedule. Each 1-mL dose contains 720 EL.U. of inactivated hepatitis A virus and 20 mcg of hepatitis B surface antigen.

STORAGE

Store refrigerated between 2° and 8° C (36° and 46° F). **DO NOT FREEZE**; discard if product has been frozen. Do not dilute to administer.

HOW SUPPLIED

TWINRIX is supplied as a slightly turbid white suspension in vials and prefilled TIP-LOK® syringes containing a 1.0-mL single dose.

Single-Dose Vials
NDC 58160-850-01 (package of 1)
NDC 58160-850-11 (package of 10)
Single-Dose Prefilled Disposable TIP-LOK® Syringes (packaged without needles)
NDC 58160-850-46 (package of 5)

REFERENCES

1. Day SP, Lemon SM. Hepatitis A virus. In: Gorbach SL, Bartlett JG, Blacklow NR, eds. *Infectious diseases.* Philadelphia, PA: WB Saunders Company; 1992:1787-1791. **2.** Dienstag JL, Routenberg JA, Purcell RH, et al. Foodhandler-associated outbreak of hepatitis type A. An immune electron microscopic study. *Ann Intern Med* 1975;83:647-650. **3.** Mackowiak PA, Caraway CT, Portnoy BL. Oyster-associated hepatitis: Lessons from the Louisiana experience. *Am J Epidemiol* 1976;103(2):181-191. **4.** Woodson RD, Clinton JJ. Hepatitis prophylaxis abroad. Effectiveness of immune serum globulin in protecting Peace Corps volunteers. *JAMA* 1969;209(7):1053-1058. **5.** Krugman S, Giles JP. Viral hepatitis. New light on an old disease. *JAMA* 1970;212(6):1019-1029. **6.** Hadler SC, Erben JJ, Francis DP, et al. Risk factors for hepatitis A in day-care centers. *J Infect Dis* 1982;145(2):255-261. **7.** Hadler SC. Global impact of hepatitis A virus infection changing patterns. In: Hollinger FB, Lemon SM, Margolis H, eds. *Viral hepatitis and liver disease.* Baltimore, MD: Williams & Wilkins; 1991:14-20. **8.** Centers for Disease Control and Prevention. Summary of Notifiable Diseases, United States. 1996. *MMWR* 1997;45(53):73. **9.** Centers for Disease Control and Prevention. Prevention of hepatitis A through active or passive immunization: Recommendations of the Advisory Committee on Immunization Practices (ACIP). *MMWR* 1999;48 (No. RR-12):1-31. **10.** Lemon SM. Type A viral hepatitis. New developments in an old disease. *N Engl J Med* 1985;313(17):1059-1067. **11.** Sjogren MH, Tanno H, Fay O, et al. Hepatitis A virus in stool during clinical relapse. *Ann Intern Med* 1987;106:221-226. **12.** Centers for Disease Control and Prevention. Atkinson W, Wolf C, Humiston S, Nelson R (eds). Epidemiology and prevention of vaccine-preventable diseases. 6th ed. Atlanta, GA: Public Health Foundation: 2000:191-229. **13.** Chiriaco P, Guadalupi C, Armigliato M, et al. Polyphasic course of hepatitis type A in children. *J Infect Dis* 1986; 153(2):378-379. **14.** Data on file (TWR101), GlaxoSmithKline. **15.** Koff RS. Hepatitis B and hepatitis D. In: Gorbach SL, Bartlett JG, Blacklow NR, eds. *Infectious diseases.* Philadelphia, PA: WB Saunders Company; 1992: 709-716. **16.** Beasley RP, Hwang LY, Stevens CE, et al. Efficacy of hepatitis B immune globulin for prevention of perinatal transmission of the hepatitis B virus carrier state: Final report of a randomized double-blind, placebo-controlled trial. *Hepatology* 1983;3(2):135-141. **17.** Chang MH, Chen CJ, Lai MS. Universal hepatitis B vaccination in Taiwan and the incidence of hepatocellular carcinoma in children. *N Engl J Med* 1997;336(26):1855-1859. **18.** Lee MS, Kim DH, Kim H, et al. Hepatitis B vaccination and reduced risk of primary liver cancer among male adults: A cohort study in Korea. *Int J Epidemiol* 1998;27:316-319. **19.** Frisch-Niggemeyer W, Ambrosch F, Hofmann H. The assessment of immunity against hepatitis B after vaccination. *J Bio Stand* 1986;14(3):255-258. **20.** Centers for Disease Control and Prevention. 1998 Guidelines for treatment of sexually transmitted diseases. *MMWR* 1999;47 (RR-1):99-104. **21.** Centers for Disease Control and Prevention. Hepatitis surveillance report No. 57. Atlanta, GA:DHHS; 2000:12. **22.** Centers for Disease Control and Prevention. Health information for international travel, 1999-2000. Atlanta, GA: DHHS. **23.** Ascherio A, Zhang SM, Hernán MA, et al. Hepatitis B vaccination and the risk of multiple sclerosis. *N Engl J Med* 2001;344(5):327-332. **24.** Confavreux C, Suissa S, Saddier P, et al. Vaccination and the risk of relapse in multiple sclerosis. *N Engl J Med* 2001;344(5):319-326. **25.** Centers for Disease Control and Prevention. Recommendations of the Advisory Committee on Immunization Practices (ACIP): Use of vaccines and immune globulins for persons with altered immunocompetence. *MMWR* 1993;42 (RR-4):1-18. **26.** Centers for Disease Control and Prevention. Vaccine adverse event reporting system—United States. *MMWR* 1990;39(41):730-733. **27.** Data on file (TWR201), GlaxoSmithKline. **28.** Centers for Disease Control and Prevention. General recommendations on immunization. Recommendations of the Advisory Committee on Immunization Practices (ACIP). *MMWR* 1994;43(RR-1):23.

Manufactured by GlaxoSmithKline,
Rixensart, Belgium, US License No. 1617
Distributed by GlaxoSmithKline, Research Triangle Park, NC 27709

TWINRIX, HAVRIX, ENGERIX-B, and TIP-LOK are registered trademarks of GlaxoSmithKline. ENZYMUN-TEST is a registered trademark of Boehringer Mannheim Immunodiagnostics. AUSAB is a registered trademark of Abbott Laboratories.

August 2003/TW:L5

Shown in Product Identification Guide, page 317

VALTREX® ℞

[val'trĕx]
(valacyclovir hydrochloride)
Caplets

DESCRIPTION

VALTREX (valacyclovir hydrochloride) is the hydrochloride salt of *L*-valyl ester of the antiviral drug acyclovir (ZOVIRAX® Brand, GlaxoSmithKline).

VALTREX Caplets are for oral administration. Each caplet contains valacyclovir hydrochloride equivalent to 500 mg or 1 gram valacyclovir and the inactive ingredients carnauba wax, colloidal silicon dioxide, crospovidone, FD&C Blue No. 2 Lake, hypromellose, magnesium stearate, microcrystalline cellulose, polyethylene glycol, polysorbate 80, povidone, and titanium dioxide. The blue, film-coated caplets are printed with edible white ink.

The chemical name of valacyclovir hydrochloride is *L*-valine, 2-[(2-amino-1,6-dihydro-6-oxo-9*H*-purin-9-yl)methoxy] ethyl ester, monohydrochloride.

Valacyclovir hydrochloride is a white to off-white powder with the molecular formula $C_{13}H_{20}N_6O_4 \bullet HCl$ and a molecular weight of 360.80. The maximum solubility in water at 25°C is 174 mg/mL. The pk_a's for valacyclovir hydrochloride are 1.90, 7.47, and 9.43.

MICROBIOLOGY

Mechanism of Antiviral Action: Valacyclovir hydrochloride is rapidly converted to acyclovir which has demonstrated antiviral activity against herpes simplex virus types 1 (HSV-1) and 2 (HSV-2) and varicella-zoster virus (VZV) both in vitro and in vivo.

The inhibitory activity of acyclovir is highly selective due to its affinity for the enzyme thymidine kinase (TK) encoded by HSV and VZV. This viral enzyme converts acyclovir into acyclovir monophosphate, a nucleotide analogue. The monophosphate is further converted into diphosphate by cellular guanylate kinase and into triphosphate by a number of cellular enzymes. In vitro, acyclovir triphosphate stops replication of herpes viral DNA. This is accomplished in 3 ways: 1) competitive inhibition of viral DNA polymerase, 2) incorporation and termination of the growing viral DNA chain, and 3) inactivation of the viral DNA polymerase. The greater antiviral activity of acyclovir against HSV compared to VZV is due to its more efficient phosphorylation by the viral TK.

Antiviral Activities: The quantitative relationship between the in vitro susceptibility of herpesviruses to antivirals and the clinical response to therapy has not been established in humans, and virus sensitivity testing has not been standardized. Sensitivity testing results, expressed as the concentration of drug required to inhibit by 50% the growth of virus in cell culture (IC_{50}), vary greatly depending upon a number of factors. Using plaque-reduction assays, the IC_{50} against herpes simplex virus isolates ranges from 0.02 to 13.5 mcg/mL for HSV-1 and from 0.01 to 9.9 mcg/mL for HSV-2. The IC_{50} for acyclovir against most laboratory strains and clinical isolates of VZV ranges from 0.12 to 10.8 mcg/mL. Acyclovir also demonstrates activity against the Oka vaccine strain of VZV with a mean IC_{50} of 1.35 mcg/mL.

Drug Resistance: Resistance of HSV and VZV to acyclovir can result from qualitative and quantitative changes in the viral TK and/or DNA polymerase. Clinical isolates of VZV with reduced susceptibility to acyclovir have been recovered from patients with AIDS. In these cases, TK-deficient mutants of VZV have been recovered.

Resistance of HSV and VZV to acyclovir occurs by the same mechanisms. While most of the acyclovir-resistant mutants isolated thus far from immunocompromised patients have been found to be TK-deficient mutants, other mutants involving the viral TK gene (TK partial and TK altered) and DNA polymerase have also been isolated. TK-negative mutants may cause severe disease in immunocompromised patients. The possibility of viral resistance to valacyclovir (and therefore, to acyclovir) should be considered in patients who show poor clinical response during therapy.

CLINICAL PHARMACOLOGY

After oral administration, valacyclovir hydrochloride is rapidly absorbed from the gastrointestinal tract and nearly completely converted to acyclovir and *L*-valine by first-pass intestinal and/or hepatic metabolism.

Pharmacokinetics: The pharmacokinetics of valacyclovir and acyclovir after oral administration of VALTREX have been investigated in 14 volunteer studies involving 283 adults.

Absorption and Bioavailability: The absolute bioavailability of acyclovir after administration of VALTREX is 54.5% ± 9.1% as determined following a 1-gram oral dose of VALTREX and a 350-mg intravenous acyclovir dose to 12 healthy volunteers. Acyclovir bioavailability from the administration of VALTREX is not altered by administration with food (30 minutes after an 873 Kcal breakfast, which included 51 grams of fat).

There was a lack of dose proportionality in acyclovir maximum concentration (C_{max}) and area under the acyclovir concentration-time curve (AUC) after single-dose administration of 100 mg, 250 mg, 500 mg, 750 mg, and 1 gram of VALTREX to 8 healthy volunteers. The mean C_{max} (± SD) was 0.83 (± 0.14), 2.15 (± 0.50), 3.28 (± 0.83), 4.17 (± 1.14), and 5.65 (± 2.37) mcg/mL, respectively; and the mean AUC (± SD) was 2.28 (± 0.40), 5.76 (± 0.60), 11.59 (± 1.79), 14.11 (± 3.54), and 19.52 (± 6.04) hr•mcg/mL, respectively.

There was also a lack of dose proportionality in acyclovir C_{max} and AUC after the multiple-dose administration of 250 mg, 500 mg, and 1 gram of VALTREX administered 4 times daily for 11 days in parallel groups of 8 healthy volunteers. The mean C_{max} (± SD) was 2.11 (± 0.33), 3.69 (± 0.87), and 4.96 (± 0.64) mcg/mL, respectively, and the mean AUC (± SD) was 5.66 (± 1.09), 9.88 (± 2.01), and 15.70 (± 2.27) hr•mcg/mL, respectively.

There is no accumulation of acyclovir after the administration of valacyclovir at the recommended dosage regimens in healthy volunteers with normal renal function.

Distribution: The binding of valacyclovir to human plasma proteins ranged from 13.5% to 17.9%.

Metabolism: After oral administration, valacyclovir hydrochloride is rapidly absorbed from the gastrointestinal tract. Valacyclovir is converted to acyclovir and *L*-valine by first-pass intestinal and/or hepatic metabolism. Acyclovir is converted to a small extent to inactive metabolites by aldehyde oxidase and by alcohol and aldehyde dehydrogenase. Neither valacyclovir nor acyclovir is metabolized by cytochrome P450 enzymes. Plasma concentrations of unconverted valacyclovir are low and transient, generally becoming non-quantifiable by 3 hours after administration. Peak plasma valacyclovir concentrations are generally less than 0.5 mcg/mL at all doses. After single-dose administration of 1 gram of VALTREX, average plasma valacyclovir concentrations observed were 0.5, 0.4, and 0.8 mcg/mL in patients with hepatic dysfunction, renal insufficiency, and in healthy volunteers who received concomitant cimetidine and probenecid, respectively.

Elimination: The pharmacokinetic disposition of acyclovir delivered by valacyclovir is consistent with previous experience from intravenous and oral acyclovir. Following the oral administration of a single 1-gram dose of radiolabeled valacyclovir to 4 healthy subjects, 45.60% and 47.12% of administered radioactivity was recovered in urine and feces over 96 hours, respectively. Acyclovir accounted for 88.60%

of the radioactivity excreted in the urine. Renal clearance of acyclovir following the administration of a single 1-gram dose of VALTREX to 12 healthy volunteers was approximately 255 ± 86 mL/min which represents 41.9% of total acyclovir apparent plasma clearance.
The plasma elimination half-life of acyclovir typically averaged 2.5 to 3.3 hours in all studies of VALTREX in volunteers with normal renal function.
End-Stage Renal Disease (ESRD): Following administration of VALTREX to volunteers with ESRD, the average acyclovir half-life is approximately 14 hours. During hemodialysis, the acyclovir half-life is approximately 4 hours. Approximately one third of acyclovir in the body is removed by dialysis during a 4-hour hemodialysis session. Apparent plasma clearance of acyclovir in dialysis patients was 86.3 ± 21.3 mL/min/1.73 m^2, compared to 679.16 ± 162.76 mL/min/1.73 m^2 in healthy volunteers.
Reduction in dosage is recommended in patients with renal impairment (see DOSAGE AND ADMINISTRATION).
Geriatrics: After single-dose administration of 1 gram of VALTREX in healthy geriatric volunteers, the half-life of acyclovir was 3.11 ± 0.51 hours, compared to 2.91 ± 0.63 hours in healthy volunteers. The pharmacokinetics of acyclovir following single- and multiple-dose oral administration of VALTREX in geriatric volunteers varied with renal function. Dose reduction may be required in geriatric patients, depending on the underlying renal status of the patient (see PRECAUTIONS and DOSAGE AND ADMINISTRATION).
Pediatrics: Valacyclovir pharmacokinetics have not been evaluated in pediatric patients.
Liver Disease: Administration of VALTREX to patients with moderate (biopsy-proven cirrhosis) or severe (with and without ascites and biopsy-proven cirrhosis) liver disease indicated that the rate but not the extent of conversion of valacyclovir to acyclovir is reduced, and the acyclovir half-life is not affected. Dosage modification is not recommended for patients with cirrhosis.
HIV Disease: In 9 patients with HIV disease and (CD4 cell counts <150 cells/mm^3) who received VALTREX at a dosage of 1 gram 4 times daily for 30 days, the pharmacokinetics of valacyclovir and acyclovir were not different from that observed in healthy volunteers (see WARNINGS).
Drug Interactions: The pharmacokinetics of digoxin was not affected by coadministration of VALTREX 1 gram 3 times daily, and the pharmacokinetics of acyclovir after a single dose of VALTREX (1 gram) was unchanged by coadministration of digoxin (2 doses of 0.75 mg), single doses of antacids (Al^{3+} or Mg^{++}), or multiple doses of thiazide diuretics. Acyclovir C_{max} and AUC following a single dose of VALTREX (1 gram) increased by 8% and 32%, respectively, after a single dose of cimetidine (800 mg), or by 22% and 49%, respectively, after probenecid (1 gram), or by 30% and 78%, respectively, after a combination of cimetidine and probenecid, primarily due to a reduction in renal clearance of acyclovir. These effects are not considered to be of clinical significance in subjects with normal renal function. Therefore, no dosage adjustment is recommended when VALTREX is coadministered with digoxin, antacids, thiazide diuretics, cimetidine, or probenecid in subjects with normal renal function.

CLINICAL TRIALS

Herpes Zoster: Two randomized double-blind clinical trials in immunocompetent adults with localized herpes zoster were conducted. VALTREX was compared to placebo in patients less than 50 years of age, and to ZOVIRAX in patients greater than 50 years of age. All patients were treated within 72 hours of appearance of zoster rash. In patients less than 50 years of age, the median time to cessation of new lesion formation was 2 days for those treated with VALTREX compared to 3 days for those treated with placebo. In patients greater than 50 years of age, the median time to cessation of new lesions was 3 days in patients treated with either VALTREX or ZOVIRAX. In patients less than 50 years of age, no difference was found with respect to the duration of pain after healing (post-herpetic neuralgia) between the recipients of VALTREX and placebo. In patients greater than 50 years of age, among the 83% who reported pain after healing (post-herpetic neuralgia), the median duration of pain after healing [95% confidence interval] in days was: 40 [31, 51], 43 [36, 55], and 59 [41, 77] for 7-day VALTREX, 14-day VALTREX, and 7-day ZOVIRAX, respectively.
Genital Herpes Infections: *Initial Episode:* Six hundred and forty-three immunocompetent adults with first episode genital herpes who presented within 72 hours of symptom onset were randomized in a double-blind trial to receive 10 days of VALTREX 1 gram twice daily (n = 323) or ZOVIRAX 200 mg 5 times a day (n = 320). For both treatment groups: the median time to lesion healing was 9 days, the median time to cessation of pain was 5 days, the median time to cessation of viral shedding was 3 days.
Recurrent Episodes: Three double-blind trials (2 of them placebo-controlled) in immunocompetent adults with recurrent genital herpes were conducted. Patients self-initiated therapy within 24 hours of the first sign or symptom of a recurrent genital herpes episode.
In 1 study, patients were randomized to receive 5 days of treatment with either VALTREX 500 mg twice daily (n = 360) or placebo (n = 259). The median time to lesion healing was 4 days in the group receiving VALTREX 500 mg versus 6 days in the placebo group, and the median time to cessation of viral shedding in patients with at least 1 positive culture (42% of the overall study population) was 2 days in the group receiving VALTREX 500 mg versus 4 days in the placebo group. The median time to cessation of pain was 3 days in the group receiving VALTREX 500 mg versus 4 days in the placebo group. Results supporting efficacy were replicated in a second trial.
In a third study, patients were randomized to receive VALTREX 500 mg twice daily for 5 days (n = 398) or VALTREX 500 mg twice daily for 3 days (and matching placebo twice daily for 2 additional days) (n = 402). The median time to lesion healing was about 4½ days in both treatment groups. The median time to cessation of pain was about 3 days in both treatment groups.
Suppressive Therapy: Two clinical studies were conducted, one in immunocompetent adults and one in HIV-infected adults. A double-blind, 12-month, placebo- and active-controlled study enrolled immunocompetent adults with a history of 6 or more recurrences per year. Outcomes for the overall study population are shown in Table 1.
[See table 1 above]

Table 1. Recurrence Rates in Immunocompetent Adults at 6 and 12 Months

	6 Months			12 Months		
Treatment Arm	VALTREX 1 gram q.d. (n = 269)	ZOVIRAX 400 mg b.i.d. (n = 267)	Placebo (n = 134)	VALTREX 1 gram q.d. (n = 269)	ZOVIRAX 400 mg b.i.d. (n = 267)	Placebo (n = 134)
Recurrence free	55%	54%	7%	34%	34%	4%
Recurrences	35%	36%	83%	46%	46%	85%
Unknowns*	10%	10%	10%	19%	19%	10%

*Includes lost to follow-up, discontinuations due to adverse events, and consent withdrawn.

Subjects with 9 or fewer recurrences per year showed comparable results with VALTREX 500 mg once daily.
In a second study, 293 HIV-infected adults on stable antiretroviral therapy with a history of 4 or more recurrences of ano-genital herpes per year were randomized to receive either VALTREX 500 mg twice daily (n = 194) or matching placebo (n = 99) for 6 months. The median duration of recurrent genital herpes in enrolled subjects was 8 years, and the median number of recurrences in the year prior to enrollment was 5. Overall, the median prestudy HIV-1 RNA was 2.6 $\log_{10}$ copies/mL. Among patients who received VALTREX, the prestudy median CD4 cell count was 336 cells/mm^3; 11% had <100 cells/mm^3, 16% had 100 to 199 cells/mm^3, 42% had 200 to 499 cells/mm^3, and 31% had ≥500 cells/mm^3. Outcomes for the overall study population are shown in Table 2.

Table 2. Recurrence Rates in HIV-Infected Adults at 6 Months

Treatment Arm	VALTREX 500 mg b.i.d. (n = 194)	Placebo (n = 99)
Recurrence free	65%	26%
Recurrences	17%	57%
Unknowns*	18%	17%

*Includes lost to follow-up, discontinuations due to adverse events, and consent withdrawn.

Cold Sores (Herpes Labialis): Two double-blind, placebo-controlled clinical trials were conducted in 1,856 healthy adults and adolescents (≥12 years old) with a history of recurrent cold sores. Patients self-initiated therapy at the earliest symptoms and prior to any signs of a cold sore. The majority of patients initiated treatment within 2 hours of onset of symptoms. Patients were randomized to VALTREX 2 grams twice daily on Day 1 followed by placebo on Day 2, VALTREX 2 grams twice daily on Day 1 followed by 1 gram twice daily on Day 2, or placebo on Days 1 and 2.
The mean duration of cold sore episodes was about 1 day shorter in treated subjects as compared to placebo. The 2-day regimen did not offer additional benefit over the 1-day regimen.
No significant difference was observed between subjects receiving VALTREX or placebo in the prevention of progression of cold sore lesions beyond the papular stage.

INDICATIONS AND USAGE

Herpes Zoster: VALTREX is indicated for the treatment of herpes zoster (shingles).
Genital Herpes: VALTREX is indicated for the treatment or suppression of genital herpes in immunocompetent individuals and for the suppression of recurrent genital herpes in HIV-infected individuals.
Cold Sores (Herpes Labialis): VALTREX is indicated for the treatment of cold sores (herpes labialis).

CONTRAINDICATIONS

VALTREX is contraindicated in patients with a known hypersensitivity or intolerance to valacyclovir, acyclovir, or any component of the formulation.

WARNINGS

Thrombotic thrombocytopenic purpura/hemolytic uremic syndrome (TTP/HUS), in some cases resulting in death, has occurred in patients with advanced HIV disease and also in allogeneic bone marrow transplant and renal transplant recipients participating in clinical trials of VALTREX at doses of 8 grams per day.

PRECAUTIONS

Dosage reduction is recommended when administering VALTREX to patients with renal impairment (see DOSAGE AND ADMINISTRATION). Acute renal failure and central nervous system symptoms have been reported in patients with underlying renal disease who have received inappropriately high doses of VALTREX for their level of renal function. Similar caution should be exercised when administering VALTREX to geriatric patients (see Geriatric Use) and patients receiving potentially nephrotoxic agents.
Given the dosage recommendations for treatment of cold sores, special attention should be paid when prescribing VALTREX for cold sores in patients who are elderly or who have impaired renal function (see DOSAGE AND ADMINISTRATION and Geriatric Use). Treatment should not exceed 1 day (2 doses of 2 grams in 24 hours). Therapy beyond 1 day does not provide additional clinical benefit.
Precipitation of acyclovir in renal tubules may occur when the solubility (2.5 mg/mL) is exceeded in the intratubular fluid. In the event of acute renal failure and anuria, the patient may benefit from hemodialysis until renal function is restored (see DOSAGE AND ADMINISTRATION).
The safety and efficacy of VALTREX have not been established in immunocompromised patients other than for the suppression of genital herpes in HIV-infected patients. The safety and efficacy of VALTREX for suppression of recurrent genital herpes in patients with advanced HIV disease (CD4 cell count <100 cells/mm^3) have not been established. The efficacy of VALTREX for the treatment of genital herpes in HIV-infected patients has not been established. The safety and efficacy of VALTREX have not been established for the treatment of disseminated herpes zoster.
Information for Patients: *Herpes Zoster:* There are no data on treatment initiated more than 72 hours after onset of the zoster rash. Patients should be advised to initiate treatment as soon as possible after a diagnosis of herpes zoster.
Genital Herpes: Patients should be informed that VALTREX is not a cure for genital herpes. There are no data evaluating whether VALTREX will prevent transmission of infection to others. Because genital herpes is a sexually transmitted disease, patients should avoid contact with lesions or intercourse when lesions and/or symptoms are present to avoid infecting partners. Genital herpes can also be transmitted in the absence of symptoms through asymptomatic viral shedding. If medical management of a genital herpes recurrence is indicated, patients should be advised to initiate therapy at the first sign or symptom of an episode.
There are no data on the effectiveness of treatment initiated more than 72 hours after the onset of signs and symptoms of a first episode of genital herpes or more than 24 hours of the onset of signs and symptoms of a recurrent episode.
There are no data on the safety or effectiveness of chronic suppressive therapy of more than 1 year's duration in otherwise healthy patients. There are no data on the safety or effectiveness of chronic suppressive therapy of more than 6 months' duration in HIV-infected patients.
Cold Sores (Herpes Labialis): Patients should be advised to initiate treatment at the earliest symptom of a cold sore (e.g., tingling, itching, or burning). There are no data on the effectiveness of treatment initiated after the development of clinical signs of a cold sore (e.g., papule, vesicle, or ulcer). Patients should be instructed that treatment for cold sores should not exceed 1 day (2 doses) and that their doses should be taken about 12 hours apart. Patients should be informed that VALTREX is not a cure for cold sores (herpes labialis).
Drug Interactions: See CLINICAL PHARMACOLOGY: Pharmacokinetics.
Carcinogenesis, Mutagenesis, Impairment of Fertility: The data presented below include references to the steady-state acyclovir AUC observed in humans treated with 1 gram VALTREX given orally 3 times a day to treat herpes zoster. Plasma drug concentrations in animal studies are expressed as multiples of human exposure to acyclovir (see CLINICAL PHARMACOLOGY: Pharmacokinetics).
Valacyclovir was noncarcinogenic in lifetime carcinogenicity bioassays at single daily doses (gavage) of up to 120 mg/kg/day for mice and 100 mg/kg/day for rats. There was no significant difference in the incidence of tumors between treated and control animals, nor did valacyclovir shorten

Continued on next page

Product information on these pages is effective as of August 2004. Further information is available at: GlaxoSmithKline, PO Box 13398, Research Triangle Park, NC 27709. 1-888-825-5249. Corporate Web Site: www.gsk.com

Valtrex—Cont.

the latency of tumors. Plasma concentrations of acyclovir were equivalent to human levels in the mouse bioassay and 1.4 to 2.3 times human levels in the rat bioassay.

Valacyclovir was tested in 5 genetic toxicity assays. An Ames assay was negative in the absence or presence of metabolic activation. Also negative were an in vitro cytogenetic study with human lymphocytes and a rat cytogenetic study at a single oral dose of 3,000 mg/kg (8 to 9 times human plasma levels).

In the mouse lymphoma assay, valacyclovir was not mutagenic in the absence of metabolic activation. In the presence of metabolic activation (76% to 88% conversion to acyclovir), valacyclovir was mutagenic.

Valacyclovir was not mutagenic in a mouse micronucleus assay at 250 mg/kg but positive at 500 mg/kg (acyclovir concentrations 26 to 51 times human plasma levels).

Valacyclovir did not impair fertility or reproduction in rats at 200 mg/kg/day (6 times human plasma levels).

Pregnancy: ***Teratogenic Effects:*** Pregnancy Category B. Valacyclovir was not teratogenic in rats or rabbits given 400 mg/kg (which results in exposures of 10 and 7 times human plasma levels, respectively) during the period of major organogenesis.

There are no adequate and well-controlled studies of VALTREX or ZOVIRAX in pregnant women. A prospective epidemiologic registry of acyclovir use during pregnancy was established in 1984 and completed in April 1999. There were 749 pregnancies followed in women exposed to systemic acyclovir during the first trimester of pregnancy resulting in 756 outcomes. The occurrence rate of birth defects approximates that found in the general population. However, the small size of the registry is insufficient to evaluate the risk for less common defects or to permit reliable or definitive conclusions regarding the safety of acyclovir in pregnant women and their developing fetuses. VALTREX should be used during pregnancy only if the potential benefit justifies the potential risk to the fetus.

Nursing Mothers: There is no experience with VALTREX. However, acyclovir concentrations have been documented in breast milk in 2 women following oral administration of ZOVIRAX and ranged from 0.6 to 4.1 times corresponding plasma levels. These concentrations would potentially expose the nursing infant to a dose of acyclovir as high as 0.3 mg/kg/day. VALTREX should be administered to a nursing mother with caution and only when indicated.

Pediatric Use: Safety and effectiveness of VALTREX in pre-pubertal pediatric patients have not been established.

Geriatric Use: Of the total number of subjects in clinical studies of VALTREX, 889 were 65 and over, and 350 were 75 and over. In a clinical study of herpes zoster, the duration of pain after healing (post-herpetic neuralgia) was longer in patients 65 and older compared with younger adults. Elderly patients are more likely to have reduced renal function and require dose reduction. Elderly patients are also more likely to have renal or CNS adverse events. With respect to CNS adverse events observed during clinical practice, agitation, hallucinations, confusion, delirium, and encephalopathy were reported more frequently in elderly patients (see CLINICAL PHARMACOLOGY, ADVERSE REACTIONS: Observed During Clinical Practice, and DOSAGE AND ADMINISTRATION).

ADVERSE REACTIONS

Frequently reported adverse events in clinical trials of VALTREX in healthy patients are listed in Tables 3 and 4.

Table 3. Incidence (%) of Adverse Events in Herpes Zoster Study Populations

Adverse Event	VALTREX 1 gram t.i.d. (n = 967)	Placebo (n = 195)
Nausea	15%	8%
Headache	14%	12%
Vomiting	6%	3%
Dizziness	3%	2%
Abdominal pain	3%	2%

[See table 4 above]

Laboratory abnormalities reported in clinical trials of VALTREX in otherwise healthy patients are listed in Table 5.

[See table 5 above]

Suppression of Genital Herpes in HIV-Infected Patients: In HIV-infected patients, frequently reported adverse events for VALTREX (500 mg twice daily; n = 194, median days on therapy = 172) and placebo (n = 99, median days on therapy = 59), respectively, included headache (13% vs. 8%), fatigue (8% vs. 5%), and rash (8% vs. 1%). Post-randomization laboratory abnormalities that were reported more frequently in valacyclovir subjects versus placebo included elevated alkaline phosphatase (4% vs. 2%), elevated ALT (14% vs. 10%), elevated AST (16% vs. 11%), decreased neutrophil counts (18% vs. 10%), and decreased platelet counts (3% vs. 0%).

Cold Sores (Herpes Labialis): In clinical studies for the treatment of cold sores, the adverse events reported by patients receiving VALTREX (n = 609) or placebo (n = 609) included headache (VALTREX 14%, placebo 10%) and dizziness (VALTREX 2%, placebo 1%). The frequencies of abnormal ALT (>2 x ULN) were 1.8% for patients receiving

Table 4. Incidence (%) of Adverse Events in Genital Herpes Study Populations

	Genital Herpes Treatment			Genital Herpes Suppression		
Adverse Event	VALTREX 1 gram b.i.d. (n = 1,194)	VALTREX 500 mg b.i.d. (n = 1,159)	Placebo (n = 439)	VALTREX 1 gram q.d. (n = 269)	VALTREX 500 mg q.d. (n = 266)	Placebo (n = 134)
Nausea	6%	5%	8%	11%	11%	8%
Headache	16%	15%	14%	35%	38%	34%
Vomiting	1%	<1%	<1%	3%	3%	2%
Dizziness	3%	2%	3%	4%	2%	1%
Abdominal pain	2%	1%	3%	11%	9%	6%
Dysmenorrhea	<1%	<1%	1%	8%	5%	4%
Arthralgia	<1%	<1%	<1%	6%	5%	4%
Depression	1%	0%	<1%	7%	5%	5%

Table 5. Incidence (%) of Laboratory Abnormalities in Herpes Zoster and Genital Herpes Study Populations

	Herpes Zoster		Genital Herpes Treatment			Genital Herpes Suppression		
Laboratory Abnormality	VALTREX 1 gram t.i.d.	Placebo	VALTREX 1 gram b.i.d.	VALTREX 500 mg b.i.d.	Placebo	VALTREX 1 gram q.d.	VALTREX 500 mg q.d.	Placebo
Hemoglobin (<0.8 × LLN)	0.8%	0%	0.3%	0.2%	0%	0%	0.8%	0.8%
White blood cells (<0.75 × LLN)	1.3%	0.6%	0.7%	0.6%	0.2%	0.7%	0.8%	1.5%
Platelet count (<100,000/mm³)	1.0%	1.2%	0.3%	0.1%	0.7%	0.4%	1.1%	1.5%
AST (SGOT) (>2 × ULN)	1.0%	0%	1.0%	*	0.5%	4.1%	3.8%	3.0%
Serum Creatinine (>1.5 × ULN)	0.2%	0%	0.7%	0%	0%	0%	0%	0%

*Data were not collected prospectively.
LLN = Lower limit of normal.
ULN = Upper limit of normal.

Table 6. Dosages for Patients with Renal Impairment

Indications	Normal Dosage Regimen (Creatinine Clearance ≥50)	Creatinine Clearance (mL/min) 30-49	10-29	<10
Herpes zoster	1 gram every 8 hours	1 gram every 12 hours	1 gram every 24 hours	500 mg every 24 hours
Genital herpes Initial treatment	1 gram every 12 hours	no reduction	1 gram every 24 hours	500 mg every 24 hours
Genital herpes Recurrent episodes	500 mg every 12 hours	no reduction	500 mg every 24 hours	500 mg every 24 hours
Genital herpes Suppressive therapy	1 gram every 24 hours	no reduction	500 mg every 24 hours	500 mg every 24 hours
	500 mg every 24 hours	no reduction	500 mg every 48 hours	500 mg every 48 hours
Genital herpes Suppressive therapy in HIV-infected patients	500 mg every 12 hours	no reduction	500 mg every 24 hours	500 mg every 24 hours
Herpes labialis (cold sores) **Do not exceed 1 day of treatment.**	Two 2-gram doses taken about 12 hours apart	Two 1-gram doses taken about 12 hours apart	Two 500-mg doses taken about 12 hours apart	500-mg single dose

VALTREX compared with 0.8% for placebo. Other laboratory abnormalities (hemoglobin, white blood cells, alkaline phosphatase, and serum creatinine) occurred with similar frequencies in the 2 groups.

Observed During Clinical Practice: The following events have been identified during post-approval use of VALTREX in clinical practice. Because they are reported voluntarily from a population of unknown size, estimates of frequency cannot be made. These events have been chosen for inclusion due to either their seriousness, frequency of reporting, causal connection to VALTREX, or a combination of these factors.

General: Facial edema, hypertension, tachycardia.

Allergic: Acute hypersensitivity reactions including anaphylaxis, angioedema, dyspnea, pruritus, rash, and urticaria.

CNS Symptoms: Aggressive behavior; agitation; ataxia; coma; confusion; decreased consciousness; dysarthria; encephalopathy; mania: psychosis, including auditory and visual hallucinations; seizures, tremors (see PRECAUTIONS).

Eye: Visual abnormalities.

Gastrointestinal: Diarrhea.

Hepatobiliary Tract and Pancreas: Liver enzyme abnormalities, hepatitis.

Renal: Elevated creatinine, renal failure.

Hematologic: Thrombocytopenia, aplastic anemia, leukocytoclastic vasculitis, TTP/HUS.

Skin: Erythema multiforme, rashes including photosensitivity, alopecia.

Renal Impairment: Renal failure and CNS symptoms have been reported in patients with renal impairment who received VALTREX or acyclovir at greater than the recommended dose. **Dose reduction is recommended in this patient population (see DOSAGE AND ADMINISTRATION).**

OVERDOSAGE

Caution should be exercised to prevent inadvertent overdose (see PRECAUTIONS). Precipitation of acyclovir in renal tubules may occur when the solubility (2.5 mg/mL) is exceeded in the intratubular fluid. In the event of acute renal failure and anuria, the patient may benefit from hemodialysis until renal function is restored (see DOSAGE AND ADMINISTRATION).

DOSAGE AND ADMINISTRATION

VALTREX Caplets may be given without regard to meals.

Herpes Zoster: The recommended dosage of VALTREX for the treatment of herpes zoster is 1 gram orally 3 times daily for 7 days. Therapy should be initiated at the earliest sign or symptom of herpes zoster and is most effective when started within 48 hours of the onset of zoster rash. No data are available on efficacy of treatment started greater than 72 hours after rash onset.

Genital Herpes: ***Initial Episodes:*** The recommended dosage of VALTREX for treatment of initial genital herpes is 1 gram twice daily for 10 days.

There are no data on the effectiveness of treatment with VALTREX when initiated more than 72 hours after the onset of signs and symptoms. Therapy was most effective when administered within 48 hours of the onset of signs and symptoms.

Recurrent Episodes: The recommended dosage of VALTREX for the treatment of recurrent genital herpes is 500 mg twice daily for 3 days.

If medical management of a genital herpes recurrence is indicated, patients should be advised to initiate therapy at the first sign or symptom of an episode. There are no data on the effectiveness of treatment with VALTREX when initiated more than 24 hours after the onset of signs or symptoms.

Suppressive Therapy: The recommended dosage of VALTREX for chronic suppressive therapy of recurrent genital herpes is 1 gram once daily in patients with normal immune function. In patients with a history of 9 or fewer recurrences per year, an alternative dose is 500 mg once daily. The safety and efficacy of therapy with VALTREX beyond 1 year have not been established.

In HIV-infected patients with CD4 cell count ≥100 cells/mm^3, the recommended dosage of VALTREX for chronic suppressive therapy of recurrent genital herpes is 500 mg twice daily. The safety and efficacy of therapy with VALTREX beyond 6 months in patients with HIV infection have not been established.

Cold Sores (Herpes Labialis): The recommended dosage of VALTREX for the treatment of cold sores is 2 grams twice daily for 1 day taken about 12 hours apart. Therapy should be initiated at the earliest symptom of a cold sore (e.g., tingling, itching, or burning). There are no data on the effectiveness of treatment initiated after the development of clinical signs of a cold sore (e.g., papule, vesicle, or ulcer).

Patients with Acute or Chronic Renal Impairment: In patients with reduced renal function, reduction in dosage is recommended (see Table 6).

[See table 6 on previous page]

Hemodialysis: During hemodialysis, the half-life of acyclovir after administration of VALTREX is approximately 4 hours. About one third of acyclovir in the body is removed by dialysis during a 4-hour hemodialysis session. Patients requiring hemodialysis should receive the recommended dose of VALTREX after hemodialysis.

Peritoneal Dialysis: There is no information specific to administration of VALTREX in patients receiving peritoneal dialysis. The effect of chronic ambulatory peritoneal dialysis (CAPD) and continuous arteriovenous hemofiltration/dialysis (CAVHD) on acyclovir pharmacokinetics has been studied. The removal of acyclovir after CAPD and CAVHD is less pronounced than with hemodialysis, and the pharmacokinetic parameters closely resemble those observed in patients with ESRD not receiving hemodialysis. Therefore, supplemental doses of VALTREX should not be required following CAPD or CAVHD.

HOW SUPPLIED

VALTREX Caplets (blue, film-coated, capsule-shaped tablets) containing valacyclovir hydrochloride equivalent to 500 mg valacyclovir and printed with "VALTREX 500 mg". Bottle of 30 (NDC 0173-0933-08) and unit dose pack of 100 (NDC 0173-0933-56).

VALTREX Caplets (blue, film-coated, capsule-shaped tablets) containing valacyclovir hydrochloride equivalent to 1 gram valacyclovir and printed with "VALTREX 1 gram". Bottle of 21 (NDC 0173-0565-02).

Store at 15° to 25°C (59° to 77°F).

GlaxoSmithKline, Research Triangle Park, NC 27709

May 2003/RL-1198

Shown in Product Identification Guide, page 317

VENTOLIN® HFA ℞

[vent'ō-lin]

(albuterol sulfate HFA inhalation aerosol)

Bronchodilator Aerosol
For Oral Inhalation Only

DESCRIPTION

The active component of VENTOLIN HFA (albuterol sulfate HFA inhalation aerosol) is albuterol sulfate, USP, the racemic form of albuterol and a relatively selective beta$_2$-adrenergic bronchodilator. Albuterol sulfate has the chemical name α^1-[(*tert*-butylamino)methyl]-4-hydroxy-*m*-xylene-α, α'-diol sulfate (2:1)(salt).

Albuterol sulfate has a molecular weight of 576.7, and the empirical formula is $(C_{13}H_{21}NO_3)_2 \bullet H_2SO_4$. Albuterol sulfate is a white crystalline powder, soluble in water and slightly soluble in ethanol.

The World Health Organization recommended name for albuterol base is salbutamol.

VENTOLIN HFA is a pressurized metered-dose aerosol unit for oral inhalation. It contains a microcrystalline suspension of albuterol sulfate in propellant HFA-134a (1,1,1,2-tetrafluoroethane). It contains no other excipients.

It is recommended to prime the inhaler before using for the first time and in cases where the inhaler has not been used for more than 2 weeks by releasing 4 test sprays into the air, away from the face. After priming with 4 actuations, each actuation delivers 120 mcg of albuterol sulfate, USP in 75 mg of suspension from the valve and 108 mcg of albuterol sulfate, USP from the mouthpiece (equivalent to 90 mcg of albuterol base from the mouthpiece). Each 18-g canister provides 200 inhalations.

This product does not contain chlorofluorocarbons (CFCs) as the propellant.

CLINICAL PHARMACOLOGY

Mechanism of Action: In vitro studies and in vivo pharmacologic studies have demonstrated that albuterol has a preferential effect on beta$_2$-adrenergic receptors compared with isoproterenol. While it is recognized that beta$_2$-adrenergic receptors are the predominant receptors in bronchial smooth muscle, data indicate that there is a population of beta$_2$-receptors in the human heart existing in a concentration between 10% and 50% of cardiac beta-adrenergic receptors. The precise function of these receptors has not been established (see WARNINGS: Cardiovascular Effects).

Activation of beta$_2$-adrenergic receptors on airway smooth muscle leads to the activation of adenylcyclase and to an increase in the intracellular concentration of cyclic-3′,5′-adenosine monophosphate (cyclic AMP). This increase of cyclic AMP leads to the activation of protein kinase A, which inhibits the phosphorylation of myosin and lowers intracellular ionic calcium concentrations, resulting in relaxation. Albuterol relaxes the smooth muscles of all airways, from the trachea to the terminal bronchioles. Albuterol acts as a functional antagonist to relax the airway irrespective of the spasmogen involved, thus protecting against all bronchoconstrictor challenges. Increased cyclic AMP concentrations are also associated with the inhibition of release of mediators from mast cells in the airway.

Albuterol has been shown in most controlled clinical trials to have more effect on the respiratory tract, in the form of bronchial smooth muscle relaxation, than isoproterenol at comparable doses while producing fewer cardiovascular effects. Controlled clinical studies and other clinical experience have shown that inhaled albuterol, like other beta-adrenergic agonist drugs, can produce a significant cardiovascular effect in some patients, as measured by pulse rate, blood pressure, symptoms, and/or electrocardiographic changes.

Preclinical: Intravenous studies in rats with albuterol sulfate have demonstrated that albuterol crosses the blood-brain barrier and reaches brain concentrations amounting to approximately 5.0% of the plasma concentrations. In structures outside the blood-brain barrier (pineal and pituitary glands), albuterol concentrations were found to be 100 times those in the whole brain.

Studies in laboratory animals (minipigs, rodents, and dogs) have demonstrated the occurrence of cardiac arrhythmias and sudden death (with histologic evidence of myocardial necrosis) when beta-agonists and methylxanthines are administered concurrently. The clinical significance of these findings is unknown.

Propellant HFA-134a is devoid of pharmacological activity except at very high doses in animals (380 to 1,300 times the maximum human exposure based on comparisons of AUC values), primarily producing ataxia, tremors, dyspnea, or salivation. These are similar to effects produced by the structurally related chlorofluorocarbons (CFCs), which have been used extensively in metered-dose inhalers.

In animals and humans, propellant HFA-134a was found to be rapidly absorbed and rapidly eliminated, with an elimination half-life of 3 to 27 minutes in animals and 5 to 7 minutes in humans. Time to maximum plasma concentration (t_{max}) and mean residence time are both extremely short, leading to a transient appearance of HFA-134a in the blood with no evidence of accumulation.

Pharmacokinetics: The systemic levels of albuterol are low after inhalation of recommended doses. A study conducted in 12 healthy male and female subjects using a higher dose (1,080 mcg of albuterol base) showed that mean peak plasma concentrations of approximately 3 ng/mL occurred after dosing when albuterol was delivered using propellant HFA-134a. The mean time to peak concentrations (t_{max}) was delayed after administration of VENTOLIN HFA (t_{max} = 0.42 hours) as compared to CFC-propelled albuterol inhaler (t_{max} = 0.17 hours). Apparent terminal plasma half-life of albuterol is approximately 4.6 hours. No further pharmacokinetic studies for VENTOLIN HFA were conducted in neonates, children, or elderly subjects.

Clinical Trials: In a 12-week, randomized, double-blind study, VENTOLIN HFA (101 patients) was compared to CFC 11/12-propelled albuterol (99 patients) and an HFA-134a placebo inhaler (97 patients) in adolescent and adult patients 12 to 76 years of age with mild to moderate asthma. Serial forced expiratory volume in 1 second (FEV_1) measurements [shown below as percent change from test-day baseline at Day 1 (n = 297) and at Week 12 (n = 249)] demonstrated that 2 inhalations of VENTOLIN HFA produced significantly greater improvement in FEV_1 over the pretreatment value than placebo. Patients taking the HFA-134a placebo inhaler also took VENTOLIN HFA for asthma symptom relief on an as-needed basis.

[See first figure at top of next column]

[See second figure at top of next column]

In the responder population (≥15% increase in FEV_1 within 30 minutes postdose) treated with VENTOLIN HFA, the mean time to onset of a 15% increase in FEV_1 over the pretreatment value was 5.4 minutes, and the mean time to peak effect was 56 minutes. The mean duration of effect as measured by a 15% increase in FEV_1 over the pretreatment value was approximately 4 hours. In some patients, duration of effect was as long as 6 hours.

A second 12-week randomized, double-blind study was conducted to evaluate the efficacy and safety of switching patients from CFC 11/12-propelled albuterol to VENTOLIN HFA. During the 3-week run-in phase of the study, all patients received CFC 11/12-propelled albuterol. During the double-blind treatment phase, VENTOLIN HFA (91 patients) was compared to CFC 11/12-propelled albuterol (100 patients) and an HFA-134a placebo inhaler (95 patients) in adolescent and adult patients with mild to moderate asthma. Serial FEV_1 measurements demonstrated that 2 inhalations of VENTOLIN HFA produced significantly greater improvement in pulmonary function than placebo.

FEV_1 as Percent Change From Predose in a Large, 12-Week Clinical Trial

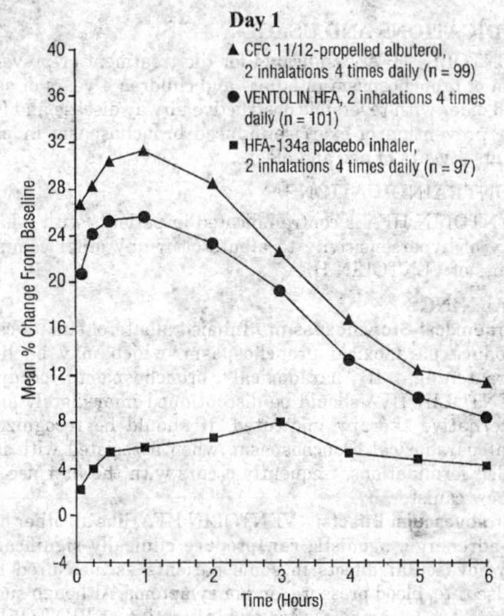

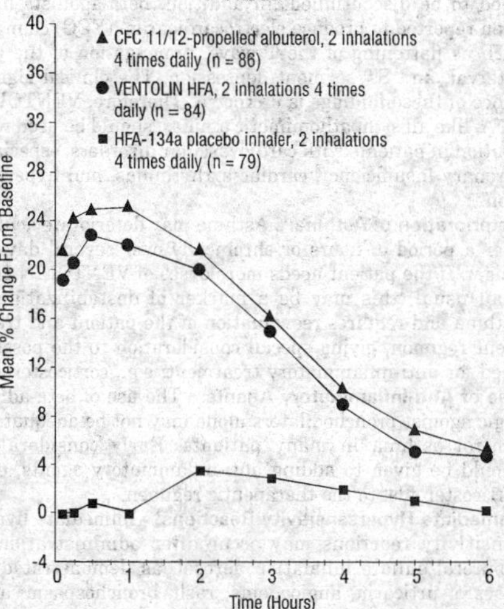

The switching from CFC 11/12-propelled albuterol inhaler to VENTOLIN HFA did not reveal any clinically significant changes in the efficacy profile.

In the 2 adult studies, the efficacy results from VENTOLIN HFA were significantly greater than placebo and were clinically comparable to those achieved with albuterol CFC 11/12-propelled albuterol, although small numerical differences in mean FEV_1 response and other measures were observed. Physicians should recognize that individual responses to beta-adrenergic agonists administered via different propellants may vary and that equivalent responses in individual patients should not be assumed.

In a 2-week, randomized, double-blind study, VENTOLIN HFA was compared to CFC 11/12-propelled albuterol and an HFA-134a placebo inhaler in 135 pediatric patients (4 to 11 years old) with mild to moderate asthma. Serial pulmonary function measurements demonstrated that two inhalations of VENTOLIN HFA produced significantly greater improvement in pulmonary function than placebo and that there were no significant differences between the groups treated with VENTOLIN HFA and CFC 11/12-propelled albuterol. In the responder population treated with VENTOLIN HFA, the mean time to onset of a 15% increase in peak expiratory flow rate (PEFR) over the pretreatment value was 7.8 minutes, and the mean time to peak effect was approximately 90 minutes. The mean duration of effect as measured by a 15% increase in PEFR over the pretreatment value was greater than 3 hours. In some patients, duration of effect was as long as 6 hours.

One controlled clinical study in adult patients with asthma (n = 24) demonstrated that 2 inhalations of VENTOLIN HFA taken approximately 30 minutes prior to exercise significantly prevented exercise-induced bronchospasm (as measured by maximum percentage fall in FEV_1 following exercise) compared to an HFA-134a placebo inhaler. In addition, VENTOLIN HFA was shown to be clinically comparable to a CFC 11/12-propelled albuterol inhaler for this indication.

Some patients who participated in these clinical trials were using concomitant steroid therapy.

Continued on next page

Product information on these pages is effective as of August 2004. Further information is available at: GlaxoSmithKline, PO Box 13398, Research Triangle Park, NC 27709. 1-888-825-5249. Corporate Web Site: www.gsk.com

Ventolin HFA—Cont.

INDICATIONS AND USAGE

VENTOLIN HFA is indicated for the treatment or prevention of bronchospasm in adults and children 4 years of age and older with reversible obstructive airway disease and for the prevention of exercise-induced bronchospasm in patients 4 years of age and older.

CONTRAINDICATIONS

VENTOLIN HFA is contraindicated in patients with a history of hypersensitivity to albuterol or any other components of VENTOLIN HFA.

WARNINGS

Paradoxical Bronchospasm: Inhaled albuterol sulfate can produce paradoxical bronchospasm, which may be life threatening. If paradoxical bronchospasm occurs, VENTOLIN HFA should be discontinued immediately and alternative therapy instituted. It should be recognized that paradoxical bronchospasm, when associated with inhaled formulations, frequently occurs with the first use of a new canister.

Cardiovascular Effects: VENTOLIN HFA, like all other beta-adrenergic agonists, can produce clinically significant cardiovascular effects in some patients as measured by pulse rate, blood pressure, and/or symptoms. Although such effects are uncommon after administration of VENTOLIN HFA at recommended doses, if they occur, the drug may need to be discontinued. In addition, beta-agonists have been reported to produce electrocardiogram (ECG) changes, such as flattening of the T wave, prolongation of the QT_c interval, and ST segment depression. The clinical significance of these findings is unknown. Therefore, VENTOLIN HFA, like all sympathomimetic amines, should be used with caution in patients with cardiovascular disorders, especially coronary insufficiency, cardiac arrhythmias, and hypertension.

Deterioration of Asthma: Asthma may deteriorate acutely over a period of hours or chronically over several days or longer. If the patient needs more doses of VENTOLIN HFA than usual, this may be a marker of destabilization of asthma and requires reevaluation of the patient and treatment regimen, giving special consideration to the possible need for anti-inflammatory treatment, e.g., corticosteroids.

Use of Anti-Inflammatory Agents: The use of beta-adrenergic agonist bronchodilators alone may not be adequate to control asthma in many patients. Early consideration should be given to adding anti-inflammatory agents, e.g., corticosteroids, to the therapeutic regimen.

Immediate Hypersensitivity Reactions: Immediate hypersensitivity reactions may occur after administration of albuterol sulfate inhalation aerosol, as demonstrated by cases of urticaria, angioedema, rash, bronchospasm, anaphylaxis, and oropharyngeal edema.

Do Not Exceed Recommended Dose: Fatalities have been reported in association with excessive use of inhaled sympathomimetic drugs in patients with asthma. The exact cause of death is unknown, but cardiac arrest following an unexpected development of a severe acute asthmatic crisis and subsequent hypoxia is suspected.

PRECAUTIONS

General: Albuterol sulfate, as with all sympathomimetic amines, should be used with caution in patients with cardiovascular disorders, especially coronary insufficiency, hypertension, and cardiac arrhythmia; in patients with convulsive disorders, hyperthyroidism, or diabetes mellitus; and in patients who are unusually responsive to sympathomimetic amines. Clinically significant changes in systolic and diastolic blood pressure have been seen in individual patients and could be expected to occur in some patients after use of any beta-adrenergic bronchodilator.

Large doses of intravenous albuterol have been reported to aggravate preexisting diabetes mellitus and ketoacidosis. As with other beta-agonists, albuterol may produce significant hypokalemia in some patients, possibly through intracellular shunting, which has the potential to produce adverse cardiovascular effects. The decrease is usually transient, not requiring supplementation.

Information for Patients: See illustrated Patient's Instructions for Use accompanying the product. SHAKE WELL BEFORE USING. Patients should be given the following information:

It is recommended to prime the inhaler before using for the first time and in cases where the inhaler has not been used for more than 2 weeks by releasing 4 test sprays into the air, away from the face.

KEEPING THE PLASTIC ACTUATOR CLEAN IS VERY IMPORTANT TO PREVENT MEDICATION BUILD-UP AND BLOCKAGE. THE ACTUATOR SHOULD BE WASHED, SHAKEN TO REMOVE EXCESS WATER, AND AIR-DRIED THOROUGHLY AT LEAST ONCE A WEEK. THE INHALER MAY CEASE TO DELIVER MEDICATION IF NOT PROPERLY CLEANED.

The actuator should be cleaned (with the canister removed) by running warm water through the top and bottom for 30 seconds at least once a week. Do not attempt to clean the metal canister or allow the metal canister to become wet. Never immerse the metal canister in water. The actuator must be shaken to remove excess water, then air-dried thoroughly (such as overnight). Blockage from medication build-up or improper medication delivery may result from failure to clean and thoroughly air-dry the actuator.

If the actuator should become blocked (little or no medication coming out of the mouthpiece), the blockage may be removed by washing the actuator as described above.

If it is necessary to use the inhaler before it is completely dry, shake excess water off the plastic actuator, replace canister, shake well, test spray twice away from face, and take the prescribed dose. After such use, the actuator should be rewashed and allowed to air-dry thoroughly.

The action of VENTOLIN HFA should last up to 4 to 6 hours. VENTOLIN HFA should not be used more frequently than recommended. Do not increase the dose or frequency of doses of VENTOLIN HFA without consulting your physician. If you find that treatment with VENTOLIN HFA becomes less effective for symptomatic relief, your symptoms become worse, and/or you need to use the product more frequently than usual, you should seek medical attention immediately. While you are using VENTOLIN HFA, other inhaled drugs and asthma medications should be taken only as directed by your physician.

Common adverse effects of treatment with inhaled albuterol include palpitations, chest pain, rapid heart rate, tremor, and nervousness. If you are pregnant or nursing, contact your physician about use of VENTOLIN HFA. Effective and safe use of VENTOLIN HFA includes an understanding of the way that it should be administered.

Use VENTOLIN HFA only with the actuator supplied with the product. Discard the canister after 200 sprays have been used or 3 months after removal from the moisture-protective foil pouch, whichever comes first. Never immerse the canister into water to determine how full the canister is ("float test").

In general, the technique for administering VENTOLIN HFA to children is similar to that for adults. Children should use VENTOLIN HFA under adult supervision, as instructed by the patient's physician. (See Patient's Instructions for Use accompanying the product.)

Drug Interactions: Other short-acting sympathomimetic aerosol bronchodilators should not be used concomitantly with albuterol. If additional adrenergic drugs are to be administered by any route, they should be used with caution to avoid deleterious cardiovascular effects.

Monoamine Oxidase Inhibitors or Tricyclic Antidepressants: VENTOLIN HFA should be administered with extreme caution to patients being treated with monoamine oxidase inhibitors or tricyclic antidepressants, or within 2 weeks of discontinuation of such agents, because the action of albuterol on the vascular system may be potentiated.

Beta-Blockers: Beta-adrenergic receptor blocking agents not only block the pulmonary effect of beta-agonists, such as VENTOLIN HFA, but may produce severe bronchospasm in patients with asthma. Therefore, patients with asthma should not normally be treated with beta-blockers. However, under certain circumstances, e.g., as prophylaxis after myocardial infarction, there may be no acceptable alternatives to the use of beta-adrenergic blocking agents in patients with asthma. In this setting, cardioselective beta-blockers should be considered, although they should be administered with caution.

Diuretics: The ECG changes and/or hypokalemia that may result from the administration of nonpotassium-sparing diuretics (such as loop or thiazide diuretics) can be acutely worsened by beta-agonists, especially when the recommended dose of the beta-agonist is exceeded. Although the clinical significance of these effects is not known, caution is advised in the coadministration of beta-agonists with nonpotassium-sparing diuretics.

Digoxin: Mean decreases of 16% to 22% in serum digoxin levels were demonstrated after single-dose intravenous and oral administration of albuterol, respectively, to normal volunteers who had received digoxin for 10 days. The clinical significance of these findings for patients with obstructive airway disease who are receiving albuterol and digoxin on a chronic basis is unclear. Nevertheless, it would be prudent to carefully evaluate the serum digoxin levels in patients who are currently receiving digoxin and albuterol.

Carcinogenesis, Mutagenesis, Impairment of Fertility: In a 2-year study in Sprague-Dawley rats, albuterol sulfate caused a dose-related increase in the incidence of benign leiomyomas of the mesovarium at and above dietary doses of 2.0 mg/kg (approximately 14 times the maximum recommended daily inhalation dose for adults on a mg/m^2 basis and approximately 6 times the maximum recommended daily inhalation dose for children on a mg/m^2 basis). In another study this effect was blocked by the coadministration of propranolol, a non-selective beta-adrenergic antagonist. In an 18-month study in CD-1 mice, albuterol sulfate showed no evidence of tumorigenicity at dietary doses of up to 500 mg/kg (approximately 1,700 times the maximum recommended daily inhalation dose for adults on a mg/m^2 basis and approximately 800 times the maximum recommended daily inhalation dose for children on a mg/m^2 basis). In a 22-month study in Golden hamsters, albuterol sulfate showed no evidence of tumorigenicity at dietary doses of up to 50 mg/kg (approximately 225 times the maximum recommended daily inhalation dose for adults on a mg/m^2 basis and approximately 110 times the maximum recommended daily inhalation dose for children on a mg/m^2 basis).

Albuterol sulfate was not mutagenic in the Ames test or a mutation test in yeast. Albuterol sulfate was not clastogenic in a human peripheral lymphocyte assay or in an AH1 strain mouse micronucleus assay.

Reproduction studies in rats demonstrated no evidence of impaired fertility at oral doses of albuterol sulfate up to 50 mg/kg (approximately 340 times the maximum recommended daily inhalation dose for adults on a mg/m^2 basis).

Pregnancy: *Teratogenic Effects:* Pregnancy Category C. Albuterol sulfate has been shown to be teratogenic in mice. A study in CD-1 mice given albuterol sulfate subcutaneously showed cleft palate formation in 5 of 111 (4.5%) fetuses at 0.25 mg/kg (less than the maximum recommended daily inhalation dose for adults on a mg/m^2 basis) and in 10 of 108 (9.3%) fetuses at 2.5 mg/kg (approximately 8 times the maximum recommended daily inhalation dose for adults on a mg/m^2 basis). The drug did not induce cleft palate formation at a dose of 0.025 mg/kg (less than the maximum recommended daily inhalation dose for adults on a mg/m^2 basis). Cleft palate also occurred in 22 of 72 (30.5%) fetuses from females treated subcutaneously with 2.5 mg/kg of isoproterenol (positive control).

A reproduction study in Stride Dutch rabbits revealed cranioschisis in 7 of 19 fetuses (37%) when albuterol sulfate was administered orally at a 50 mg/kg dose (approximately 680 times the maximum recommended daily inhalation dose for adults on a mg/m^2 basis).

In an inhalation reproduction study in New Zealand white rabbits, albuterol sulfate/HFA-134a formulation exhibited enlargement of the frontal portion of the fetal fontanelles at and above inhalation doses of 0.0193 mg/kg (less than the maximum recommended daily inhalation dose for adults on a mg/m^2 basis).

A study in which pregnant rats were dosed with radiolabeled albuterol sulfate demonstrated that drug-related material is transferred from the maternal circulation to the fetus.

There are no adequate and well-controlled studies of VENTOLIN HFA or albuterol sulfate in pregnant women. VENTOLIN HFA should be used during pregnancy only if the potential benefit justifies the potential risk to the fetus.

During worldwide marketing experience, various congenital anomalies, including cleft palate and limb defects, have been reported in the offspring of patients being treated with albuterol. Some of the mothers were taking multiple medications during their pregnancies. No consistent pattern of defects can be discerned, and a relationship between albuterol use and congenital anomalies has not been established.

Use in Labor and Delivery: Because of the potential for beta-agonist interference with uterine contractility, use of VENTOLIN HFA for relief of bronchospasm during labor should be restricted to those patients in whom the benefits clearly outweigh the risk.

Tocolysis: Albuterol has not been approved for the management of preterm labor. The benefit:risk ratio when albuterol is administered for tocolysis has not been established. Serious adverse reactions, including maternal pulmonary edema, have been reported during or following treatment of premature labor with beta$_2$-agonists, including albuterol.

Nursing Mothers: Plasma levels of albuterol sulfate and HFA-134a after inhaled therapeutic doses are very low in humans, but it is not known whether the components of VENTOLIN HFA are excreted in human milk. Because of the potential for tumorigenicity shown for albuterol in animal studies and lack of experience with the use of VENTOLIN HFA by nursing mothers, a decision should be made whether to discontinue nursing or to discontinue the drug, taking into account the importance of the drug to the mother. Caution should be exercised when albuterol sulfate is administered to a nursing woman.

Pediatric Use: Results from a 2-week, randomized study in pediatric patients 4–11 years old with mild to moderate asthma have shown that VENTOLIN HFA is safe and effective in this population. Safety and effectiveness in children below 4 years of age have not been established.

Geriatrics: Clinical studies of VENTOLIN HFA did not include sufficient numbers of subjects aged 65 and over to determine whether they respond differently from younger subjects. Other reported clinical experience has not identified differences in responses between the elderly and younger patients. In general, dose selection for an elderly patient should be cautious, usually starting at the low end of the dosing range, reflecting the greater frequency of decreased hepatic, renal, or cardiac function, and of concomitant disease or other drug therapy.

ADVERSE REACTIONS

Adverse reaction information concerning VENTOLIN HFA is derived from two 12-week, randomized, double-blind studies in 610 adolescent and adult patients with asthma that compared VENTOLIN HFA, a CFC 11/12-propelled albuterol inhaler, and an HFA-134a placebo inhaler. The following table lists the incidence of all adverse events (whether considered by the investigator to be related or unrelated to drug) from these studies that occurred at a rate of 3% or greater in the group treated with VENTOLIN HFA and more frequently in the group treated with VENTOLIN HFA than in the HFA-134a placebo inhaler group. Overall, the incidence and nature of the adverse events reported for VENTOLIN HFA and a CFC 11/12-propelled albuterol inhaler were comparable. Results in a 2-week pediatric clinical study (n = 135) showed that the adverse event profile was generally similar to that of the adult.

[See table at top of next page]

Adverse events reported by less than 3% of the adolescent and adult patients receiving VENTOLIN HFA and by a greater proportion of patients receiving VENTOLIN HFA than receiving HFA-134a placebo inhaler and that have the

Adverse Experience Incidence (% of Patients) in 2 Large 12-Week Adolescent and Adult Clinical Trials*

Adverse Event Type	Percent of Patients VENTOLIN HFA (n = 202)	CFC 11/12-Propelled Albuterol Inhaler (n = 207)	Placebo HFA-134a (n = 201)
Ear, nose, and throat			
Throat irritation	10	6	7
Upper respiratory inflammation	5	5	2
Lower respiratory			
Viral respiratory infections	7	4	4
Cough	5	2	2
Musculoskeletal			
Musculoskeletal pain	5	5	4

*This table includes all adverse events (whether considered by the investigator to be drug-related or unrelated to drug) that occurred at an incidence rate of at least 3.0% in the group treated with VENTOLIN HFA and more frequently in the group treated with VENTOLIN HFA than in the HFA-134a placebo inhaler group.

potential to be related to VENTOLIN HFA include diarrhea, laryngitis, oropharyngeal edema, cough, lung disorders, tachycardia, and extrasystoles. Palpitation and dizziness have also been observed with VENTOLIN HFA.

Cases of urticaria, angioedema, rash, bronchospasm, hoarseness, and arrhythmias (including atrial fibrillation, supraventricular tachycardia, extrasystoles) have been reported after the use of albuterol, USP.

In addition, albuterol, like other sympathomimetic agents, can cause adverse reactions such as hypertension, angina, vertigo, central nervous system stimulation, sleeplessness, headache, and drying or irritation of the oropharynx.

OVERDOSAGE

The expected symptoms with overdosage are those of excessive beta-adrenergic stimulation and/or occurrence or exaggeration of any of the symptoms listed under ADVERSE REACTIONS, e.g., seizures, angina, hypertension or hypotension, tachycardia with rates up to 200 beats/min, arrhythmias, nervousness, headache, tremor, dry mouth, palpitation, nausea, dizziness, fatigue, malaise, and sleeplessness. Hypokalemia may also occur.

As with all sympathomimetic aerosol medications, cardiac arrest and even death may be associated with abuse of VENTOLIN HFA. Treatment consists of discontinuation of VENTOLIN HFA together with appropriate symptomatic therapy. The judicious use of a cardioselective beta-receptor blocker may be considered, bearing in mind that such medication can produce bronchospasm. There is insufficient evidence to determine if dialysis is beneficial for overdosage of VENTOLIN HFA.

The oral median lethal dose of albuterol sulfate in mice is greater than 2,000 mg/kg (approximately 6,800 times the maximum recommended daily inhalation dose for adults on a mg/m^2 basis and approximately 3,200 times the maximum recommended daily inhalation dose for children on a mg/m^2 basis). In mature rats, the subcutaneous median lethal dose of albuterol sulfate is approximately 450 mg/kg (approximately 3,000 times the maximum recommended daily inhalation dose for adults on a mg/m^2 basis and approximately 1,400 times the maximum recommended daily inhalation dose for children on a mg/m^2 basis). In young rats, the subcutaneous median lethal dose is approximately 2,000 mg/kg (approximately 14,000 times the maximum recommended daily inhalation dose for adults on a mg/m^2 basis and approximately 6,400 times the maximum recommended daily inhalation dose for children on a mg/m^2 basis). The inhalation median lethal dose has not been determined in animals.

DOSAGE AND ADMINISTRATION

Adult and Pediatric Asthma: For treatment of acute episodes of bronchospasm or prevention of asthmatic symptoms, the usual dosage for adults and children 4 years of age and older is 2 inhalations repeated every 4 to 6 hours; in some patients, 1 inhalation every 4 hours may be sufficient. More frequent administration or a larger number of inhalations is not recommended. It is recommended to prime the inhaler before using for the first time and in cases where the inhaler has not been used for more than 2 weeks by releasing 4 test sprays into the air, away from the face.

VENTOLIN HFA can also be used to relieve acute symptoms of asthma. The use of VENTOLIN HFA can be continued as medically indicated to control recurring bouts of bronchospasm. If a previously effective dosage regimen fails to provide the usual response, this may be a marker of destabilization of asthma and requires reevaluation of the patient and the treatment regimen, giving special consideration to the possible need for anti-inflammatory treatment, e.g., corticosteroids.

Safe usage of albuterol for periods extending over several years has been documented.

Exercise-Induced Bronchospasm Prevention: The usual dosage for adults and children 4 years and older is 2 inhalations 15 to 30 minutes before exercise. For treatment, see above.

Cleaning: To maintain proper use of this product, it is important that the actuator be washed and dried thoroughly at least once a week. The inhaler may cease to deliver medication if not properly cleaned and dried thoroughly. **See Information for Patients.** Keeping the plastic actuator clean is very important to prevent medication build-up and blockage. If the actuator becomes blocked with drug, washing the actuator will remove the blockage.

HOW SUPPLIED

VENTOLIN HFA (albuterol sulfate HFA inhalation aerosol) is supplied as a pressurized aluminum canister with a blue plastic actuator and a blue strapcap packaged within a moisture-protective foil pouch, each in boxes of 1 with patient's instructions (NDC 0173-0682-00). The moisture-protective foil pouch also contains a desiccant that should be discarded when the pouch is opened.

It is recommended to prime the inhaler before using for the first time and in cases where the inhaler has not been used for more than 2 weeks by releasing 4 test sprays into the air, away from the face. After priming with 4 actuations, each actuation delivers 120 mcg of albuterol sulfate, USP in 75 mg of suspension from the valve and 108 mcg of albuterol sulfate, USP from the mouthpiece (equivalent to 90 mcg of albuterol base from the mouthpiece). The canister is labeled with a net weight of 18 g and contains 200 metered inhalations.

The blue actuator supplied with VENTOLIN HFA should not be used with any other product canisters, and actuators from other products should not be used with a VENTOLIN HFA canister. The correct amount of medication in each canister cannot be assured after 200 actuations, even though the canister is not completely empty. The canister should be discarded when 200 actuations have been used or 3 months after removal from the moisture-protective foil pouch, whichever comes first. Never immerse the canister into water to determine how full the canister is ("float test").

Contents Under Pressure: Do not puncture. Do not use or store near heat or open flame. Exposure to temperatures above 120°F may cause bursting. Never throw container into fire or incinerator. Keep out of reach of children. Avoid spraying in eyes.

Store between 15° and 25°C (59° and 77°F). Store canister with mouthpiece down. For best results, the canister should be at room temperature before use. SHAKE WELL BEFORE USING.

VENTOLIN HFA does not contain chlorofluorocarbons (CFCs) as the propellant.

GlaxoSmithKline, Research Triangle Park, NC 27709

June 2002/RL-970

Shown in Product Identification Guide, page 317

WELLBUTRIN® ℞

[wel'byū-trin]

(bupropion hydrochloride)

Tablets

DESCRIPTION

WELLBUTRIN (bupropion hydrochloride), an antidepressant of the aminoketone class, is chemically unrelated to tricyclic, tetracyclic, selective serotonin re-uptake inhibitor, or other known antidepressant agents. Its structure closely resembles that of diethylpropion; it is related to phenylethylamines. It is designated as (±)-1-(3-chlorophenyl)-2-[(1,1-dimethylethyl)amino]-1-propanone hydrochloride. The molecular weight is 276.2. The empirical formula is $C_{13}H_{18}ClNO \bullet HCl$. Bupropion hydrochloride powder is white, crystalline, and highly soluble in water. It has a bitter taste and produces the sensation of local anesthesia on the oral mucosa.

WELLBUTRIN is supplied for oral administration as 75-mg (yellow-gold) and 100-mg (red) film-coated tablets. Each tablet contains the labeled amount of bupropion hydrochloride and the inactive ingredients: 75-mg tablet — D&C Yellow No. 10 Lake, FD&C Yellow No. 6 Lake, hydroxypropyl cellulose, hydroxypropyl methylcellulose, microcrystalline cellulose, polyethylene glycol, talc, and titanium dioxide; 100-mg tablet FD&C Red No. 40 Lake, FD&C Yellow No. 6 Lake, hydroxypropyl cellulose, hydroxypropyl methylcellulose, microcrystalline cellulose, polyethylene glycol, talc, and titanium dioxide.

CLINICAL PHARMACOLOGY

Pharmacodynamics: The neurochemical mechanism of the antidepressant effect of bupropion is not known. Bupropion is a relatively weak inhibitor of the neuronal uptake of norepinephrine, serotonin, and dopamine, and does not inhibit monoamine oxidase.

Bupropion produces dose-related central nervous system (CNS) stimulant effects in animals, as evidenced by increased locomotor activity, increased rates of responding in various schedule-controlled operant behavior tasks, and, at high doses, induction of mild stereotyped behavior.

Bupropion causes convulsions in rodents and dogs at doses approximately tenfold the dose recommended as the human antidepressant dose.

Pharmacokinetics: Bupropion is a racemic mixture. The pharmacological activity and pharmacokinetics of the individual enantiomers have not been studied. In humans, following oral administration of WELLBUTRIN, peak plasma bupropion concentrations are usually achieved within 2 hours, followed by a biphasic decline. The terminal phase has a mean half-life of 14 hours, with a range of 8 to 24 hours. The distribution phase has a mean half-life of 3 to 4 hours. The mean elimination half-life (±SD) of bupropion after chronic dosing is 21 (±9) hours, and steady-state plasma concentrations of bupropion are reached within 8 days. Plasma bupropion concentrations are dose-proportional following single doses of 100 to 250 mg; however, it is not known if the proportionality between dose and plasma level is maintained in chronic use.

Absorption: The absolute bioavailability of WELLBUTRIN Tablets in humans has not been determined because an intravenous formulation for human use is not available. However, it appears likely that only a small proportion of any orally administered dose reaches the systemic circulation intact.

Distribution: In vitro tests show that bupropion is 84% bound to human plasma protein at concentrations up to 200 mcg/mL. The extent of protein binding of the hydroxybupropion metabolite is similar to that for bupropion, whereas the extent of protein binding of the threohydrobupropion metabolite is about half that seen with bupropion.

Metabolism: Bupropion is extensively metabolized in humans. Three metabolites have been shown to be active: hydroxybupropion, which is formed via hydroxylation of the *tert*-butyl group of bupropion, and the amino-alcohol isomers threohydrobupropion and erythrohydrobupropion, which are formed via reduction of the carbonyl group. In vitro findings suggest that cytochrome P450IIB6 (CYP2B6) is the principal isoenzyme involved in the formation of hydroxybupropion, while cytochrome P450 isoenzymes are not involved in the formation of threohydrobupropion. Oxidation of the bupropion side chain results in the formation of a glycine conjugate of meta-chlorobenzoic acid, which is then excreted as the major urinary metabolite. The potency and toxicity of the metabolites relative to bupropion have not been fully characterized. However, it has been demonstrated in an antidepressant screening test in mice that hydroxybupropion is one half as potent as bupropion, while threohydrobupropion and erythrohydrobupropion are 5-fold less potent than bupropion. This may be of clinical importance because their plasma concentrations are as high or higher than those of bupropion.

Because bupropion is extensively metabolized, there is the potential for drug-drug interactions, particularly with those agents that are metabolized by the cytochrome P450IIB6 (CYP2B6) isoenzyme. Although bupropion is not metabolized by cytochrome P450IID6 (CYP2D6), there is the potential for drug-drug interactions when bupropion is co-administered with drugs metabolized by this isoenzyme (see PRECAUTIONS: Drug Interactions).

Following a single dose in humans, peak plasma concentrations of hydroxybupropion occur approximately 3 hours after administration of WELLBUTRIN Tablets. Peak plasma concentrations of hydroxybupropion are approximately 10 times the peak level of the parent drug at steady state. The elimination half-life of hydroxybupropion is approximately 20 (±5) hours, and its AUC at steady state is about 17 times that of bupropion. The times to peak concentrations for the erythrohydrobupropion and threohydrobupropion metabolites are similar to that of the hydroxybupropion metabolite. However, their elimination half-lives are longer, 33 (±10) and 37 (±13) hours, respectively, and steady-state AUCs are 1.5 and 7 times that of bupropion, respectively.

Bupropion and its metabolites exhibit linear kinetics following chronic administration of 300 to 450 mg/day.

Elimination: Following oral administration of 200 mg of ^{14}C-bupropion in humans, 87% and 10% of the radioactive dose were recovered in the urine and feces, respectively. However, the fraction of the oral dose of WELLBUTRIN excreted unchanged was only 0.5%, a finding consistent with the extensive metabolism of bupropion.

Populations Subgroups: Factors or conditions altering metabolic capacity (e.g., liver disease, congestive heart failure [CHF], age, concomitant medications, etc.) or elimination may be expected to influence the degree and extent of accumulation of the active metabolites of bupropion. The elimination of the major metabolites of bupropion may be affected by reduced renal or hepatic function because they are moderately polar compounds and are likely to undergo further metabolism or conjugation in the liver prior to urinary excretion.

Hepatic: The effect of hepatic impairment on the pharmacokinetics of bupropion was characterized in 2 single-dose

Continued on next page

Product information on these pages is effective as of August 2004. Further information is available at: GlaxoSmithKline, PO Box 13398, Research Triangle Park, NC 27709. 1-888-825-5249. Corporate Web Site: www.gsk.com

Wellbutrin—Cont.

studies, one in patients with alcoholic liver disease and one in patients with mild to severe cirrhosis. The first study showed that the half-life of hydroxybupropion was significantly longer in 8 patients with alcoholic liver disease than in 8 healthy volunteers (32±14 hours versus 21±5 hours, respectively). Although not statistically significant, the AUCs for bupropion and hydroxybupropion were more variable and tended to be greater (by 53% to 57%) in volunteers with alcoholic liver disease. The differences in half-life for bupropion and the other metabolites in the 2 patient groups were minimal.

The second study showed that there were no statistically significant differences in the pharmacokinetics of bupropion and its active metabolites in 9 patients with mild to moderate hepatic cirrhosis compared to 8 healthy volunteers. However, more variability was observed in some of the pharmacokinetic parameters for bupropion (AUC, C_{max}, and T_{max}) and its active metabolites ($t_{½}$) in patients with mild to moderate hepatic cirrhosis. In addition, in patients with severe hepatic cirrhosis, the bupropion C_{max} and AUC were substantially increased (mean difference: by approximately 70% and 3-fold, respectively) and more variable when compared to values in healthy volunteers; the mean bupropion half-life was also longer (29 hours in patients with severe hepatic cirrhosis vs. 19 hours in healthy subjects). For the metabolite hydroxybupropion, the mean C_{max} was approximately 69% lower. For the combined amino-alcohol isomers threohydrobupropion and erythrohydrobupropion, the mean C_{max} was approximately 31% lower. The mean AUC increased by about 1½-fold for hydroxybupropion and about 2½-fold for threo/erythrohydrobupropion. The median T_{max} was observed 19 hours later for hydroxybupropion and 31 hours later for threo/erythrohydrobupropion. The mean half-lives for hydroxybupropion and threo/erythrohydrobupropion were increased 5- and 2-fold, respectively, in patients with severe hepatic cirrhosis compared to healthy volunteers (see WARNINGS, PRECAUTIONS, and DOSAGE AND ADMINISTRATION).

Renal: The effect of renal disease on the pharmacokinetics of bupropion has not been studied. The elimination of the major metabolites of bupropion may be affected by reduced renal function.

Left Ventricular Dysfunction: During a chronic dosing study in 14 depressed patients with left ventricular dysfunction (history of CHF or an enlarged heart on x-ray), no apparent effect on the pharmacokinetics of bupropion or its metabolites was revealed, compared to healthy volunteers.

Age: The effects of age on the pharmacokinetics of bupropion and its metabolites have not been fully characterized, but an exploration of steady-state bupropion concentrations from several depression efficacy studies involving patients dosed in a range of 300 to 750 mg/day, on a 3 times daily schedule, revealed no relationship between age (18 to 83 years) and plasma concentration of bupropion. A single-dose pharmacokinetic study demonstrated that the disposition of bupropion and its metabolites in elderly subjects was similar to that of younger subjects. These data suggest there is no prominent effect of age on bupropion concentration; however, another pharmacokinetic study, single and multiple dose, has suggested that the elderly are at increased risk for accumulation of bupropion and its metabolites (see PRECAUTIONS: Geriatric Use).

Gender: A single-dose study involving 12 healthy male and 12 healthy female volunteers revealed no sex-related differences in the pharmacokinetic parameters of bupropion.

Smokers: The effects of cigarette smoking on the pharmacokinetics of bupropion were studied in 34 healthy male and female volunteers; 17 were chronic cigarette smokers and 17 were nonsmokers. Following oral administration of a single 150-mg dose of bupropion, there were no statistically significant differences in C_{max}, half-life, T_{max}, AUC or clearance of bupropion or its active metabolites between smokers and nonsmokers.

INDICATIONS AND USAGE

WELLBUTRIN is indicated for the treatment of depression.

A physician considering WELLBUTRIN for the management of a patient's first episode of depression should be aware that the drug may cause generalized seizures in a dose-dependent manner with an approximate incidence of 0.4% (4/1,000). This incidence of seizures may exceed that of other marketed antidepressants by as much as 4-fold. This relative risk is only an approximate estimate because no direct comparative studies have been conducted (see WARNINGS).

The efficacy of WELLBUTRIN has been established in 3 placebo-controlled trials, including 2 of approximately 3 weeks' duration in depressed inpatients and one of approximately 6 weeks' duration in depressed outpatients. The depressive disorder of the patients studied corresponds most closely to the Major Depression category of the APA Diagnostic and Statistical Manual III.

Major Depression implies a prominent and relatively persistent depressed or dysphoric mood that usually interferes with daily functioning (nearly every day for at least 2 weeks); it should include at least 4 of the following 8 symptoms: change in appetite, change in sleep, psychomotor agitation or retardation, loss of interest in usual activities or decrease in sexual drive, increased fatigability, feelings of guilt or worthlessness, slowed thinking or impaired concentration, and suicidal ideation or attempts.

Effectiveness of WELLBUTRIN in long-term use, that is, for more than 6 weeks, has not been systematically evaluated in controlled trials. Therefore, the physician who elects to use WELLBUTRIN for extended periods should periodically reevaluate the long-term usefulness of the drug for the individual patient.

CONTRAINDICATIONS

WELLBUTRIN is contraindicated in patients with a seizure disorder.

WELLBUTRIN is contraindicated in patients treated with ZYBAN® (bupropion hydrochloride) Sustained-Release Tablets, or any other medications that contain bupropion because the incidence of seizure is dose dependent.

WELLBUTRIN is also contraindicated in patients with a current or prior diagnosis of bulimia or anorexia nervosa because of a higher incidence of seizures noted in such patients treated with WELLBUTRIN.

WELLBUTRIN is contraindicated in patients undergoing abrupt discontinuation of alcohol or sedatives (including benzodiazepines).

The concurrent administration of WELLBUTRIN and a monoamine oxidase (MAO) inhibitor is contraindicated. At least 14 days should elapse between discontinuation of an MAO inhibitor and initiation of treatment with WELLBUTRIN.

WELLBUTRIN is contraindicated in patients who have shown an allergic response to bupropion or the other ingredients that make up WELLBUTRIN Tablets.

WARNINGS

Patients should be made aware that WELLBUTRIN contains the same active ingredient found in ZYBAN, used as an aid to smoking cessation treatment, and that WELLBUTRIN should not be used in combination with ZYBAN, or any other medications that contain bupropion.

Seizures: Bupropion is associated with seizures in approximately 0.4% (4/1,000) of patients treated at doses up to 450 mg/day. This incidence of seizures may exceed that of other marketed antidepressants by as much as 4-fold. This relative risk is only an approximate estimate because no direct comparative studies have been conducted. The estimated seizure incidence for WELLBUTRIN increases almost tenfold between 450 and 600 mg/day, which is twice the usually required daily dose (300 mg) and one and one-third the maximum recommended daily dose (450 mg). Given the wide variability among individuals and their capacity to metabolize and eliminate drugs this disproportionate increase in seizure incidence with dose incrementation calls for caution in dosing.

During the initial development, 25 among approximately 2,400 patients treated with WELLBUTRIN experienced seizures. At the time of seizure, 7 patients were receiving daily doses of 450 mg or below for an incidence of 0.33% (3/1,000) within the recommended dose range. Twelve patients experienced seizures at 600 mg/day (2.3% incidence); 6 additional patients had seizures at daily doses between 600 and 900 mg (2.8% incidence).

A separate, prospective study was conducted to determine the incidence of seizure during an 8-week treatment exposure in approximately 3,200 additional patients who received daily doses of up to 450 mg. Patients were permitted to continue treatment beyond 8 weeks if clinically indicated. Eight seizures occurred during the initial 8-week treatment period and 5 seizures were reported in patients continuing treatment beyond 8 weeks, resulting in a total seizure incidence of 0.4%.

The risk of seizure appears to be strongly associated with dose. Sudden and large increments in dose may contribute to increased risk. While many seizures occurred early in the course of treatment, some seizures did occur after several weeks at fixed dose. WELLBUTRIN should be discontinued and not restarted in patients who experience a seizure while on treatment.

The risk of seizure is also related to patient factors, clinical situations, and concomitant medications, which must be considered in selection of patients for therapy with WELLBUTRIN.

- **Patient factors: Predisposing factors that may increase the risk of seizure with bupropion use include history of head trauma or prior seizure, CNS tumor, the presence of severe hepatic cirrhosis, and concomitant medications that lower seizure threshold.**
- **Clinical situations: Circumstances associated with an increased seizure risk include, among others, excessive use of alcohol or sedatives (including benzodiazepines); addiction to opiates, cocaine, or stimulants; use of over-the-counter stimulants and anorectics; and diabetes treated with oral hypoglycemics or insulin.**
- **Concomitant medications: Many medications (e.g., antipsychotics, antidepressants, theophylline, systemic steroids) are known to lower seizure threshold.**

***Recommendations for Reducing the Risk of Seizure:* Retrospective analysis of clinical experience gained during the development of WELLBUTRIN suggests that the risk of seizure may be minimized if**

- **the total daily dose of WELLBUTRIN does *not* exceed 450 mg,**
- **the daily dose is administered 3 times daily, with each single dose *not* to exceed 150 mg to avoid high peak concentrations of bupropion and/or its metabolites, and**
- **the rate of incrementation of dose is very gradual.**

Extreme caution should be used when WELLBUTRIN is administered to patients with a history of seizure, cranial trauma, or other predisposition(s) toward seizure, or prescribed with other agents (e.g., antipsychotics, other antidepressants, theophylline, systemic steroids, etc.) that lower seizure threshold.

Hepatic Impairment: WELLBUTRIN should be used with extreme caution in patients with severe hepatic cirrhosis. In these patients a reduced dose and/or frequency is required, as peak bupropion, as well as AUC, levels are substantially increased and accumulation is likely to occur in such patients to a greater extent than usual. The dose should not exceed 75 mg once a day in these patients (see CLINICAL PHARMACOLOGY, PRECAUTIONS, and DOSAGE AND ADMINISTRATION).

Potential for Hepatotoxicity: In rats receiving large doses of bupropion chronically, there was an increase in incidence of hepatic hyperplastic nodules and hepatocellular hypertrophy. In dogs receiving large doses of bupropion chronically, various histologic changes were seen in the liver, and laboratory tests suggesting mild hepatocellular injury were noted.

Clinical Worsening and Suicide Risk: Patients with major depressive disorder, both adult and pediatric, may experience worsening of their depression and/or the emergence of suicidal ideation and behavior (suicidality), whether or not they are taking antidepressant medications, and this risk may persist until significant remission occurs. Although there has been a long-standing concern that antidepressants may have a role in inducing worsening of depression and the emergence of suicidality in certain patients, a causal role for antidepressants in inducing such behaviors has not been established. **Nevertheless, patients being treated with antidepressants should be observed closely for clinical worsening and suicidality, especially at the beginning of a course of drug therapy, or at the time of dose changes, either increases or decreases.** Consideration should be given to changing the therapeutic regimen, including possibly discontinuing the medication in patients whose depression is persistently worse or whose emergent suicidality is severe, abrupt in onset, or was not part of the patient's presenting symptoms.

Because of the possibility of co-morbidity between major depressive disorder and other psychiatric and nonpsychiatric disorders, the same precautions observed when treating patients with major depressive disorder should be observed when treating patients with other psychiatric and nonpsychiatric disorders.

The following symptoms, anxiety, agitation, panic attacks, insomnia, irritability, hostility (aggressiveness), impulsivity, akathisia (psychomotor restlessness), hypomania, and mania, have been reported in adult and pediatric patients being treated with antidepressants for major depressive disorder as well as for other indications, both psychiatric and nonpsychiatric. Although a causal link between the emergence of such symptoms and either the worsening of depression and/or the emergence of suicidal impulses has not been established, consideration should be given to changing the therapeutic regimen, including possibly discontinuing the medication in patients for whom such symptoms are severe, abrupt in onset, or were not part of the patient's presenting symptoms.

Families and caregivers of patients being treated with antidepressants for major depressive disorder or other indications, both psychiatric and nonpsychiatric, should be alerted about the need to monitor patients for the emergence of agitation, irritability, and the other symptoms described above, as well as the emergence of suicidality, and to report such symptoms immediately to health care providers. Prescriptions for WELLBUTRIN should be written for the smallest quantity of tablets consistent with good patient management, in order to reduce the risk of overdose.

It should be noted that WELLBUTRIN is not approved for use in treating any indications in the pediatric population.

A major depressive episode may be the initial presentation of bipolar disorder. It is generally believed (although not established in controlled trials) that treating such an episode with an antidepressant alone may increase the likelihood of precipitation of a mixed/manic episode in patients at risk for bipolar disorder. Whether any of the symptoms described above represent such a conversion is unknown. However, prior to initiating treatment with an antidepressant, patients should be adequately screened to determine if they are at risk for bipolar disorder; such screening should include a detailed psychiatric history, including a family history of suicide, bipolar disorder, and depression. It should be noted that WELLBUTRIN is not approved for use in treating bipolar depression.

PRECAUTIONS

General: ***Agitation and Insomnia:*** A substantial proportion of patients treated with WELLBUTRIN experience some degree of increased restlessness, agitation, anxiety, and insomnia, especially shortly after initiation of treatment. In clinical studies, these symptoms were sometimes of sufficient magnitude to require treatment with sedative/hypnotic drugs. In approximately 2% of patients, symptoms were sufficiently severe to require discontinuation of treatment with WELLBUTRIN.

Psychosis, Confusion, and Other Neuropsychiatric Phenomena: Patients treated with WELLBUTRIN have been reported to show a variety of neuropsychiatric signs and symptoms including delusions, hallucinations, psychotic episodes, confusion, and paranoia. Because of the uncontrolled nature of many studies, it is impossible to provide a precise estimate of the extent of risk imposed by treatment with WELLBUTRIN. In several cases, neuropsychiatric phenomena abated upon dose reduction and/or withdrawal of treatment.

Activation of Psychosis and/or Mania: Antidepressants can precipitate manic episodes in Bipolar Manic Depressive patients during the depressed phase of their illness and may activate latent psychosis in other susceptible patients. WELLBUTRIN is expected to pose similar risks.

Altered Appetite and Weight: A weight loss of greater than 5 lbs occurred in 28% of patients receiving WELLBUTRIN. This incidence is approximately double that seen in comparable patients treated with tricyclics or placebo. Furthermore, while 34.5% of patients receiving tricyclic antidepressants gained weight, only 9.4% of patients treated with WELLBUTRIN did. Consequently, if weight loss is a major presenting sign of a patient's depressive illness, the anorectic and/or weight reducing potential of WELLBUTRIN should be considered.

Allergic Reactions: Anaphylactoid/anaphylactic reactions characterized by symptoms such as pruritus, urticaria, angioedema, and dyspnea requiring medical treatment have been reported in clinical trials with bupropion. In addition, there have been rare spontaneous postmarketing reports of erythema multiforme, Stevens-Johnson syndrome, and anaphylactic shock associated with bupropion. A patient should stop taking WELLBUTRIN and consult a doctor if experiencing allergic or anaphylactoid/anaphylactic reactions (e.g., skin rash, pruritus, hives, chest pain, edema, and shortness of breath) during treatment.

Arthralgia, myalgia, and fever with rash and other symptoms suggestive of delayed hypersensitivity have been reported in association with bupropion. These symptoms may resemble serum sickness.

Cardiovascular Effects: In clinical practice, hypertension, in some cases severe, requiring acute treatment, has been reported in patients receiving bupropion alone and in combination with nicotine replacement therapy. These events have been observed in both patients with and without evidence of preexisting hypertension.

Data from a comparative study of the sustained-release formulation of bupropion (ZYBAN® Sustained-Release Tablets), nicotine transdermal system (NTS), the combination of sustained-release bupropion plus NTS, and placebo as an aid to smoking cessation suggest a higher incidence of treatment-emergent hypertension in patients treated with the combination of sustained-release bupropion and NTS. In this study, 6.1% of patients treated with the combination of sustained-release bupropion and NTS had treatment-emergent hypertension compared to 2.5%, 1.6%, and 3.1% of patients treated with sustained-release bupropion, NTS, and placebo, respectively. The majority of these patients had evidence of preexisting hypertension. Three patients (1.2%) treated with the combination of ZYBAN and NTS and one patient (0.4%) treated with NTS had study medication discontinued due to hypertension compared to none of the patients treated with ZYBAN or placebo. Monitoring of blood pressure is recommended in patients who receive the combination of bupropion and nicotine replacement.

There is no clinical experience establishing the safety of WELLBUTRIN in patients with a recent history of myocardial infarction or unstable heart disease. Therefore, care should be exercised if it is used in these groups. Bupropion was well tolerated in depressed patients who had previously developed orthostatic hypotension while receiving tricyclic antidepressants and was also generally well tolerated in a group of 36 depressed inpatients with stable congestive heart failure (CHF). However, bupropion was associated with a rise in supine blood pressure in the study of patients with CHF, resulting in discontinuation of treatment in 2 patients for exacerbation of baseline hypertension.

Hepatic Impairment: WELLBUTRIN should be used with extreme caution in patients with severe hepatic cirrhosis. In these patients, a reduced dose and frequency is required. WELLBUTRIN should be used with caution in patients with hepatic impairment (including mild to moderate hepatic cirrhosis) and a reduced frequency and/or dose should be considered in patients with mild to moderate hepatic cirrhosis.

All patients with hepatic impairment should be closely monitored for possible adverse effects that could indicate high drug and metabolite levels (see CLINICAL PHARMACOLOGY, WARNINGS, and DOSAGE AND ADMINISTRATION).

Renal Impairment: No studies have been conducted in patients with renal impairment. Bupropion is extensively metabolized in the liver to active metabolites, which are further metabolized and subsequently excreted by the kidneys. WELLBUTRIN should be used with caution in patients with renal impairment and a reduced frequency and/or dose should be considered as bupropion and its metabolites may accumulate in such patients to a greater extent than usual. The patient should be closely monitored for possible adverse effects that could indicate high drug or metabolite levels.

Information for Patients: See the tear-off leaflet at the end of the labeling accompanying the product for Patient Information.

Patients should be made aware that WELLBUTRIN contains the same active ingredient found in ZYBAN, used as an aid to smoking cessation, and that WELLBUTRIN should not be used in combination with ZYBAN or any other medications that contain bupropion hydrochloride.

Physicians are advised to discuss the following issues with patients:

Patients should be instructed to take WELLBUTRIN in equally divided doses 3 or 4 times a day to minimize the risk of seizure.

Patients should be told that WELLBUTRIN should be discontinued and not restarted if they experience a seizure while on treatment.

Patients should be told that any CNS-active drug like WELLBUTRIN may impair their ability to perform tasks requiring judgment or motor and cognitive skills. Consequently, until they are reasonably certain that WELLBUTRIN does not adversely affect their performance, they should refrain from driving an automobile or operating complex, hazardous machinery.

Patients should be told that the excessive use or abrupt discontinuation of alcohol or sedatives (including benzodiazepines) may alter the seizure threshold. Some patients have reported lower alcohol tolerance during treatment with WELLBUTRIN. Patients should be advised that the consumption of alcohol should be minimized or avoided.

Patients and their families should be encouraged to be alert to the emergence of anxiety, agitation, panic attacks, insomnia, irritability, hostility, impulsivity, akathisia, hypomania, mania, worsening of depression, and suicidal ideation, especially early during antidepressant treatment. Such symptoms should be reported to the patient's physician, especially if they are severe, abrupt in onset, or were not part of the patient's presenting symptoms.

Patients should be advised to inform their physicians if they are taking or plan to take any prescription or over-the-counter drugs. Concern is warranted because WELLBUTRIN and other drugs may affect each other's metabolism.

Patients should be advised to notify their physicians if they become pregnant or intend to become pregnant during therapy.

Laboratory Tests: There are no specific laboratory tests recommended.

Drug Interactions: Few systemic data have been collected on the metabolism of WELLBUTRIN following concomitant administration with other drugs or, alternatively, the effect of concomitant administration of WELLBUTRIN on the metabolism of other drugs.

Because bupropion is extensively metabolized, the coadministration of other drugs may affect its clinical activity. In vitro studies indicate that bupropion is primarily metabolized to hydroxybupropion by the CYP2B6 isoenzyme. Therefore, the potential exists for a drug interaction between WELLBUTRIN and drugs that affect the CYP2B6 isoenzyme (e.g., orphenadrine and cyclophosphamide). The threohydrobupropion metabolite of bupropion does not appear to be produced by the cytochrome P450 isoenzymes. The effects of concomitant administration of cimetidine on the pharmacokinetics of bupropion and its active metabolites were studied in 24 healthy young male volunteers. Following oral administration of two 150-mg sustained-release tablets with and without 800 mg of cimetidine, the pharmacokinetics of bupropion and hydroxybupropion were unaffected. However, there were 16% and 32% increases in the AUC and C_{max}, respectively, of the combined moieties of threohydrobupropion and erythrohydrobupropion.

While not systematically studied, certain drugs may induce the metabolism of bupropion (e.g., carbamazepine, phenobarbital, phenytoin).

Animal data indicated that bupropion may be an inducer of drug-metabolizing enzymes in humans. In one study, following chronic administration of bupropion, 100 mg 3 times daily to 8 healthy male volunteers for 14 days, there was no evidence of induction of its own metabolism. Nevertheless, there may be the potential for clinically important alterations of blood levels of coadministered drugs.

Drugs Metabolized by Cytochrome P450IID6 (CYP2D6): Many drugs, including most antidepressants (SSRIs, many tricyclics), beta-blockers, antiarrhythmics, and antipsychotics are metabolized by the CYP2D6 isoenzyme. Although bupropion is not metabolized by this isoenzyme, bupropion and hydroxybupropion are inhibitors of the CYP2D6 isoenzyme in vitro. In a study of 15 male subjects (ages 19 to 35 years) who were extensive metabolizers of the CYP2D6 isoenzyme, daily doses of bupropion given as 150 mg twice daily followed by a single dose of 50 mg desipramine increased the C_{max}, AUC, and $t_{½}$ of desipramine by an average of approximately 2-, 5- and 2-fold, respectively. The effect was present for at least 7 days after the last dose of bupropion. Concomitant use of bupropion with other drugs metabolized by CYP2D6 has not been formally studied.

Therefore, co-administration of bupropion with drugs that are metabolized by CYP2D6 isoenzyme including certain antidepressants (e.g., nortriptyline, imipramine, desipramine, paroxetine, fluoxetine, sertraline), antipsychotics (e.g., haloperidol, risperidone, thioridazine), beta-blockers (e.g., metoprolol), and Type 1C antiarrhythmics (e.g., propafenone, flecainide), should be approached with caution and should be initiated at the lower end of the dose range of the concomitant medication. If bupropion is added to the treatment regimen of a patient already receiving a drug metabolized by CYP2D6, the need to decrease the dose of the original medication should be considered, particularly for those concomitant medications with a narrow therapeutic index.

MAO Inhibitors: Studies in animals demonstrate that the acute toxicity of bupropion is enhanced by the MAO inhibitor phenelzine (see CONTRAINDICATIONS).

Levodopa and Amantadine: Limited clinical data suggest a higher incidence of adverse experiences in patients receiving bupropion concurrently with either levodopa or amantadine. Administration of WELLBUTRIN Tablets to patients receiving either levodopa or amantadine concurrently should be undertaken with caution, using small initial doses and small gradual dose increases.

Drugs that Lower Seizure Threshold: Concurrent administration of WELLBUTRIN and agents (e.g., antipsychotics, other antidepressants, theophylline, systemic steroids, etc.) that lower seizure threshold should be undertaken only with extreme caution (see WARNINGS). Low initial dosing and small gradual dose increases should be employed.

Nicotine Transdermal System: (see PRECAUTIONS: Cardiovascular Effects).

Alcohol: In post-marketing experience, there have been rare reports of adverse neuropsychiatric events or reduced alcohol tolerance in patients who were drinking alcohol during treatment with WELLBUTRIN. The consumption of alcohol during treatment with WELLBUTRIN should be minimized or avoided (also see CONTRAINDICATIONS).

Carcinogenesis, Mutagenesis, Impairment of Fertility: Lifetime carcinogenicity studies were performed in rats and mice at doses up to 300 and 150 mg/kg/day, respectively. In the rat study there was an increase in nodular proliferative lesions of the liver at doses of 100 to 300 mg/kg/day; lower doses were not tested. The question of whether or not such lesions may be precursors of neoplasms of the liver is currently unresolved. Similar liver lesions were not seen in the mouse study, and no increase in malignant tumors of the liver and other organs was seen in either study.

Bupropion produced a borderline positive response (2 to 3 times control mutation rate) in some strains in the Ames bacterial mutagenicity test, and a high oral dose (300 mg/kg, but not 100 or 200 mg/kg) produced a low incidence of chromosomal aberrations in rats. The relevance of these results in estimating the risk of human exposure to therapeutic doses is unknown.

A fertility study was performed in rats; no evidence of impairment of fertility was encountered at oral doses up to 300 mg/kg/day.

Pregnancy: ***Teratogenic Effects:*** Pregnancy Category B. Reproduction studies have been performed in rabbits and rats at doses up to 15 to 45 times the human daily dose and have revealed no definitive evidence of impaired fertility or harm to the fetus due to bupropion. (In rabbits, a slightly increased incidence of fetal abnormalities was seen in 2 studies, but there was no increase in any specific abnormality). There are no adequate and well-controlled studies in pregnant women. Because animal reproduction studies are not always predictive of human response, this drug should be used during pregnancy only if clearly needed.

To monitor fetal outcomes of pregnant women exposed to WELLBUTRIN, GlaxoSmithKline maintains a Bupropion Pregnancy Registry. Health care providers are encouraged to register patients by calling (800) 336-2176.

Labor and Delivery: The effect of WELLBUTRIN on labor and delivery in humans is unknown.

Nursing Mothers: Like many other drugs, bupropion and its metabolites are secreted in human milk. Because of the potential for serious adverse reactions in nursing infants from WELLBUTRIN, a decision should be made whether to discontinue nursing or to discontinue the drug, taking into account the importance of the drug to the mother.

Pediatric Use: The safety and effectiveness of WELLBUTRIN in pediatric patients under 18 years old have not been established. The immediate-release formulation of bupropion was studied in 104 pediatric patients (age range, 6 to 16) in clinical trials of the drug for other indications. Although generally well tolerated, the limited exposure is insufficient to assess the safety of bupropion in pediatric patients **(see WARNINGS—Clinical Worsening and Suicide Risk).**

Geriatric Use: Of the approximately 6,000 patients who participated in clinical trials with bupropion sustained-release tablets (depression and smoking cessation studies), 275 were 65 and over and 47 were 75 and over. In addition, several hundred patients 65 and over participated in clinical trials using the immediate-release formulation of bupropion (depression studies). No overall differences in safety or effectiveness were observed between these subjects and younger subjects, and other reported clinical experience has not identified differences in responses between the elderly and younger patients, but greater sensitivity of some older individuals cannot be ruled out.

A single-dose pharmacokinetic study demonstrated that the disposition of bupropion and its metabolites in elderly subjects was similar to that of younger subjects; however, another pharmacokinetic study, single and multiple dose, has suggested that the elderly are at increased risk for accumulation of bupropion and its metabolites (see CLINICAL PHARMACOLOGY).

Bupropion is extensively metabolized in the liver to active metabolites, which are further metabolized and excreted by the kidneys. The risk of toxic reaction to this drug may

Continued on next page

Product information on these pages is effective as of August 2004. Further information is available at: GlaxoSmithKline, PO Box 13398, Research Triangle Park, NC 27709. 1-888-825-5249. Corporate Web Site: www.gsk.com

Wellbutrin—Cont.

be greater in patients with impaired renal function. Because elderly patients are more likely to have decreased renal function, care should be taken in dose selection, and it may be useful to monitor renal function (see PRECAUTIONS: Renal Impairment and DOSAGE AND ADMINISTRATION).

ADVERSE REACTIONS (see also WARNINGS and PRECAUTIONS)

Adverse events commonly encountered in patients treated with WELLBUTRIN are agitation, dry mouth, insomnia, headache/migraine, nausea/vomiting, constipation, and tremor.

Adverse events were sufficiently troublesome to cause discontinuation of treatment with WELLBUTRIN in approximately 10% of the 2,400 patients and volunteers who participated in clinical trials during the product's initial development. The more common events causing discontinuation include neuropsychiatric disturbances (3.0%), primarily agitation and abnormalities in mental status; gastrointestinal disturbances (2.1%), primarily nausea and vomiting; neurological disturbances (1.7%), primarily seizures, headaches, and sleep disturbances; and dermatologic problems (1.4%), primarily rashes. It is important to note, however, that many of these events occurred at doses that exceed the recommended daily dose.

Accurate estimates of the incidence of adverse events associated with the use of any drug are difficult to obtain. Estimates are influenced by drug dose, detection technique, setting, physician judgments, etc. Consequently, the table below is presented solely to indicate the relative frequency of adverse events reported in representative controlled clinical studies conducted to evaluate the safety and efficacy of WELLBUTRIN under relatively similar conditions of daily dosage (300 to 600 mg), setting, and duration (3 to 4 weeks). The figures cited cannot be used to predict precisely the incidence of untoward events in the course of usual medical practice where patient characteristics and other factors must differ from those which prevailed in the clinical trials. These incidence figures also cannot be compared with those obtained from other clinical studies involving related drug products as each group of drug trials is conducted under a different set of conditions.

Finally, it is important to emphasize that the tabulation does not reflect the relative severity and/or clinical importance of the events. A better perspective on the serious adverse events associated with the use of WELLBUTRIN is provided in WARNINGS and PRECAUTIONS.

Table 1. Treatment-Emergent Adverse Experience Incidence in Placebo-Controlled Clinical Trials* (Percent of Patients Reporting)

Adverse Experience	WELLBUTRIN Patients (n = 323)	Placebo Patients (n = 185)
Cardiovascular		
Cardiac arrhythmias	5.3	4.3
Dizziness	22.3	16.2
Hypertension	4.3	1.6
Hypotension	2.5	2.2
Palpitations	3.7	2.2
Syncope	1.2	0.5
Tachycardia	10.8	8.6
Dermatologic		
Pruritus	2.2	0.0
Rash	8.0	6.5
Gastrointestinal		
Anorexia	18.3	18.4
Appetite increase	3.7	2.2
Constipation	26.0	17.3
Diarrhea	6.8	8.6
Dyspepsia	3.1	2.2
Nausea/vomiting	22.9	18.9
Weight gain	13.6	22.7
Weight loss	23.2	23.2
Genitourinary		
Impotence	3.4	3.1
Menstrual complaints	4.7	1.1
Urinary frequency	2.5	2.2
Urinary retention	1.9	2.2
Musculoskeletal		
Arthritis	3.1	2.7
Neurological		
Akathisia	1.5	1.1
Akinesia/bradykinesia	8.0	8.6
Cutaneous temperature disturbance	1.9	1.6
Dry mouth	27.6	18.4
Excessive sweating	22.3	14.6
Headache/migraine	25.7	22.2
Impaired sleep quality	4.0	1.6
Increased salivary flow	3.4	3.8
Insomnia	18.6	15.7
Muscle spasms	1.9	3.2
Pseudoparkinsonism	1.5	1.6
Sedation	19.8	19.5
Sensory disturbance	4.0	3.2
Tremor	21.1	7.6
Neuropsychiatric		
Agitation	31.9	22.2
Anxiety	3.1	1.1
Confusion	8.4	4.9
Decreased libido	3.1	1.6
Delusions	1.2	1.1
Disturbed concentration	3.1	3.8
Euphoria	1.2	0.5
Hostility	5.6	3.8
Nonspecific		
Fatigue	5.0	8.6
Fever/chills	1.2	0.5
Respiratory		
Upper respiratory complaints	5.0	11.4
Special Senses		
Auditory disturbance	5.3	3.2
Blurred vision	14.6	10.3
Gustatory disturbance	3.1	1.1

*Events reported by at least 1% of patients receiving WELLBUTRIN are included.

Table 2. Dosing Regimen

Treatment Day	Total Daily Dose	Tablet Strength	Number of Tablets: Morning	Midday	Evening
1	200 mg	100 mg	1	0	1
4	300 mg	100 mg	1	1	1

Other Events Observed During the Development of WELLBUTRIN: The conditions and duration of exposure to WELLBUTRIN varied greatly, and a substantial proportion of the experience was gained in open and uncontrolled clinical settings. During this experience, numerous adverse events were reported; however, without appropriate controls, it is impossible to determine with certainty which events were or were not caused by WELLBUTRIN. The following enumeration is organized by organ system and describes events in terms of their relative frequency of reporting in the data base. Events of major clinical importance are also described in WARNINGS and PRECAUTIONS.

The following definitions of frequency are used: Frequent adverse events are defined as those occurring in at least 1/100 patients. Infrequent adverse events are those occurring in 1/100 to 1/1,000 patients, while rare events are those occurring in less than 1/1,000 patients.

Cardiovascular: Frequent was edema; infrequent were chest pain, electrocardiogram (ECG) abnormalities (premature beats and nonspecific ST-T changes), and shortness of breath/dyspnea; rare were flushing, pallor, phlebitis, and myocardial infarction.

Dermatologic: Frequent were nonspecific rashes; infrequent were alopecia and dry skin; rare were change in hair color, hirsutism, and acne.

Endocrine: Infrequent was gynecomastia; rare were glycosuria and hormone level change.

Gastrointestinal: Infrequent were dysphagia, thirst disturbance, and liver damage/jaundice; rare were rectal complaints, colitis, gastrointestinal bleeding, intestinal perforation, and stomach ulcer.

Genitourinary: Frequent was nocturia; infrequent were vaginal irritation, testicular swelling, urinary tract infection, painful erection, and retarded ejaculation; rare were dysuria, enuresis, urinary incontinence, menopause, ovarian disorder, pelvic infection, cystitis, dyspareunia, and painful ejaculation.

Hematologic/Oncologic: Rare were lymphadenopathy, anemia, and pancytopenia.

Musculoskeletal: Rare was musculoskeletal chest pain.

Neurological: (see WARNINGS) Frequent were ataxia/incoordination, seizure, myoclonus, dyskinesia, and dystonia; infrequent were mydriasis, vertigo, and dysarthria; rare were electroencephalogram (EEG) abnormality, abnormal neurological exam, impaired attention, sciatica, and aphasia.

Neuropsychiatric: (see PRECAUTIONS) Frequent were mania/hypomania, increased libido, hallucinations, decrease in sexual function, and depression; infrequent were memory impairment, depersonalization, psychosis, dysphoria, mood instability, paranoia, formal thought disorder, and frigidity; rare was suicidal ideation.

Oral Complaints: Frequent was stomatitis; infrequent were toothache, bruxism, gum irritation, and oral edema; rare was glossitis.

Respiratory: Infrequent were bronchitis and shortness of breath/dyspnea; rare were epistaxis, rate or rhythm disorder, pneumonia, and pulmonary embolism.

Special Senses: Infrequent was visual disturbance; rare was diplopia.

Nonspecific: Frequent were flu-like symptoms; infrequent was nonspecific pain; rare were body odor, surgically related pain, infection, medication reaction, and overdose.

Postintroduction Reports: Voluntary reports of adverse events temporally associated with bupropion that have been received since market introduction and which may have no causal relationship with the drug include the following:

Body (General): arthralgia, myalgia, and fever with rash and other symptoms suggestive of delayed hypersensitivity. These symptoms may resemble serum sickness (see PRECAUTIONS).

Cardiovascular: hypertension (in some cases severe, see PRECAUTIONS), orthostatic hypotension, third degree heart block

Endocrine: syndrome of inappropriate antidiuretic hormone secretion, hyperglycemia, hypoglycemia

Gastrointestinal: esophagitis, hepatitis, liver damage

Hemic and Lymphatic: ecchymosis, leukocytosis, leukopenia, thrombocytopenia. Altered PT and/or INR, infrequently associated with hemorrhagic or thrombotic complications, were observed when bupropion was coadministered with warfarin.

Musculoskeletal: arthralgia, myalgia, muscle rigidity/fever/rhabdomyolysis, muscle weakness

Nervous: coma, delirium, dream abnormalities, paresthesia, unmasking of tardive dyskinesia

Skin and Appendages: Stevens-Johnson syndrome, angioedema, exfoliative dermatitis, urticaria

Special Senses: tinnitus

DRUG ABUSE AND DEPENDENCE

Humans: Controlled clinical studies conducted in normal volunteers, in subjects with a history of multiple drug abuse, and in depressed patients showed some increase in motor activity and agitation/excitement.

In a population of individuals experienced with drugs of abuse, a single dose of 400 mg of WELLBUTRIN produced mild amphetamine-like activity as compared to placebo on the Morphine-Benzedrine Subscale of the Addiction Research Center Inventories (ARCI) and a score intermediate between placebo and amphetamine on the Liking Scale of the ARCI. These scales measure general feelings of euphoria and drug desirability.

Findings in clinical trials, however, are not known to predict the abuse potential of drugs reliably. Nonetheless, evidence from single-dose studies does suggest that the recommended daily dosage of bupropion when administered in divided doses is not likely to be especially reinforcing to amphetamine or stimulant abusers. However, higher doses, which could not be tested because of the risk of seizure, might be modestly attractive to those who abuse stimulant drugs.

Animals: Studies in rodents have shown that bupropion exhibits some pharmacologic actions common to psychostimulants, including increases in locomotor activity and the production of a mild stereotyped behavior and increases in rates of responding in several schedule-controlled behavior paradigms. Drug discrimination studies in rats showed stimulus generalization between bupropion and amphetamine and other psychostimulants. Rhesus monkeys have been shown to self-administer bupropion intravenously.

OVERDOSAGE

Human Overdose Experience: There has been extensive clinical experience with overdosage of WELLBUTRIN Tablets. Thirteen overdoses occurred during clinical trials. Twelve patients ingested 850 to 4,200 mg and recovered without significant sequelae. Another patient who ingested 9,000 mg of WELLBUTRIN and 300 mg of tranylcypromine experienced a grand mal seizure and recovered without further sequelae.

Since introduction, overdoses of WELLBUTRIN Tablets up to 17,500 mg have been reported. Seizure was reported in approximately one third of all cases. Other serious reactions reported with overdoses of WELLBUTRIN Tablets alone included hallucinations, loss of consciousness, and sinus tachycardia. Fever, muscle rigidity, rhabdomyolysis, hypotension, stupor, coma, and respiratory failure have been reported when WELLBUTRIN Tablets was part of multiple drug overdoses.

Although most patients recovered without sequelae, deaths associated with overdoses of WELLBUTRIN Tablets alone have been reported rarely in patients ingesting massive doses of WELLBUTRIN Tablets. Multiple uncontrolled seizures, bradycardia, cardiac failure, and cardiac arrest prior to death were reported in these patients.

Overdosage Management: Ensure an adequate airway, oxygenation, and ventilation. Monitor cardiac rhythm and vital signs. EEG monitoring is also recommended for the first 48 hours post-ingestion. General supportive and symptomatic measures are also recommended. Induction of emesis is not recommended. Gastric lavage with a large-bore orogastric tube with appropriate airway protection, if needed, may be indicated if performed soon after ingestion or in symptomatic patients.

Activated charcoal should be administered. There is no experience with the use of forced diuresis, dialysis, hemoperfusion, or exchange transfusion in the management of bupropion overdoses. No specific antidotes for bupropion are known.

Due to the dose-related risk of seizures with WELLBUTRIN, hospitalization following suspected overdose should be considered. Based on studies in animals, it is recommended that seizures be treated with intravenous benzodiazepine administration and other supportive measures, as appropriate.

In managing overdosage, consider the possibility of multiple drug involvement. The physician should consider contacting a poison control center for additional information on the treatment of any overdose. Telephone numbers for certified poison control centers are listed in the *Physicians' Desk Reference* (PDR).

DOSAGE AND ADMINISTRATION

General Dosing Considerations: It is particularly important to administer WELLBUTRIN in a manner most likely to minimize the risk of seizure (see WARNINGS). Increases in dose should not exceed 100 mg/day in a 3-day period. Gradual escalation in dosage is also important if agitation, motor restlessness, and insomnia, often seen during the initial days of treatment, are to be minimized. If necessary, these effects may be managed by temporary reduction of dose or the short-term administration of an intermediate to long-acting sedative hypnotic. A sedative hypnotic usually is not required beyond the first week of treatment. Insomnia may also be minimized by avoiding bedtime doses. If distressing, untoward effects supervene, dose escalation should be stopped.

No single dose of WELLBUTRIN should exceed 150 mg. WELLBUTRIN should be administered 3 times daily, preferably with at least 6 hours between successive doses.

Usual Dosage for Adults: The usual adult dose is 300 mg/day, given 3 times daily. Dosing should begin at 200 mg/day, given as 100 mg twice daily. Based on clinical response, this dose may be increased to 300 mg/day, given as 100 mg 3 times daily, no sooner than 3 days after beginning therapy (see table below).

[See table 2 at top of previous page]

Increasing the Dosage Above 300 mg/Day: As with other antidepressants, the full antidepressant effect of WELLBUTRIN may not be evident until 4 weeks of treatment or longer. An increase in dosage, up to a maximum of 450 mg/day, given in divided doses of not more than 150 mg each, may be considered for patients in whom no clinical improvement is noted after several weeks of treatment at 300 mg/day. Dosing above 300 mg/day may be accomplished using the 75- or 100-mg tablets. The 100-mg tablet must be administered 4 times daily with at least 4 hours between successive doses, in order not to exceed the limit of 150 mg in a single dose. WELLBUTRIN should be discontinued in patients who do not demonstrate an adequate response after an appropriate period of treatment at 450 mg/day.

Maintenance: The lowest dose that maintains remission is recommended. Although it is not known how long the patient should remain on WELLBUTRIN, it is generally recognized that acute episodes of depression require several months or longer of antidepressant drug treatment.

Dosage Adjustment for Patients with Impaired Hepatic Function: WELLBUTRIN should be used with extreme caution in patients with severe hepatic cirrhosis. The dose should not exceed 75 mg once a day in these patients. WELLBUTRIN should be used with caution in patients with hepatic impairment (including mild to moderate hepatic cirrhosis) and a reduced frequency and/or dose should be considered in patients with mild to moderate hepatic cirrhosis (see CLINICAL PHARMACOLOGY and PRECAUTIONS).

Dosage Adjustment for Patients with Impaired Renal Function: WELLBUTRIN should be used with caution in patients with renal impairment and a reduced frequency and/or dose should be considered (see CLINICAL PHARMACOLOGY and PRECAUTIONS).

HOW SUPPLIED

WELLBUTRIN Tablets, 75 mg of bupropion hydrochloride, are yellow-gold, round, biconvex tablets printed with "WELLBUTRIN 75" in bottles of 100 (NDC 0173-0177-55).

WELLBUTRIN Tablets, 100 mg of bupropion hydrochloride, are red, round, biconvex tablets printed with "WELLBUTRIN 100" in bottles of 100 (NDC 0173-0178-55).

Store at 15° to 25°C (59° to 77°F). Protect from light and moisture.

Manufactured by DSM Pharmaceuticals, Inc.
Greenville, NC 27834 for
GlaxoSmithKline, Research Triangle Park, NC 27709

April 2004/RL-2076

Shown in Product Identification Guide, page 317

WELLBUTRIN SR® ℞

[wel'byū-trin]
(bupropion hydrochloride)
Sustained-Release Tablets

DESCRIPTION

WELLBUTRIN SR (bupropion hydrochloride), an antidepressant of the aminoketone class, is chemically unrelated to tricyclic, tetracyclic, selective serotonin re-uptake inhibitor, or other known antidepressant agents. Its structure closely resembles that of diethylpropion; it is related to phenylethylamines. It is designated as (±)-1-(3-chlorophenyl)-2-[(1,1-dimethylethyl)amino]-1-propanone hydrochloride. The molecular weight is 276.2. The molecular formula is $C_{13}H_{18}ClNO \bullet HCl$. Bupropion hydrochloride powder is white, crystalline, and highly soluble in water. It has a bitter taste and produces the sensation of local anesthesia on the oral mucosa.

WELLBUTRIN SR Tablets are supplied for oral administration as 100-mg (blue), 150-mg (purple), and 200-mg (light pink), film-coated, sustained-release tablets. Each tablet contains the labeled amount of bupropion hydrochloride and the inactive ingredients: carnauba wax, cysteine hydrochloride, hydroxypropyl methylcellulose, magnesium stearate, microcrystalline cellulose, polyethylene glycol, polysorbate 80, and titanium dioxide and is printed with edible black ink. In addition, the 100-mg tablet contains FD&C Blue No. 1 Lake, the 150-mg tablet contains FD&C Blue No. 2 Lake and FD&C Red No. 40 Lake, and the 200-mg tablet contains FD&C Red No. 40 Lake.

CLINICAL PHARMACOLOGY

Pharmacodynamics: Bupropion is a relatively weak inhibitor of the neuronal uptake of norepinephrine, serotonin, and dopamine, and does not inhibit monoamine oxidase. While the mechanism of action of bupropion, as with other antidepressants, is unknown, it is presumed that this action is mediated by noradrenergic and/or dopaminergic mechanisms.

Pharmacokinetics: Bupropion is a racemic mixture. The pharmacologic activity and pharmacokinetics of the individual enantiomers have not been studied. The mean elimination half-life (±SD) of bupropion after chronic dosing is 21 (±9) hours, and steady-state plasma concentrations of bupropion are reached within 8 days. In a study comparing chronic dosing with WELLBUTRIN SR Tablets 150 mg twice daily to the immediate-release formulation of bupropion at 100 mg 3 times daily, peak plasma concentrations of bupropion at steady state for WELLBUTRIN SR Tablets were approximately 85% of those achieved with the immediate-release formulation. There was equivalence for bupropion AUCs, as well as equivalence for both peak plasma concentration and AUCs for all 3 of the detectable bupropion metabolites. Thus, at steady state, WELLBUTRIN SR Tablets, given twice daily, and the immediate-release formulation of bupropion, given 3 times daily, are essentially bioequivalent for both bupropion and the 3 quantitatively important metabolites.

Absorption: Following oral administration of WELLBUTRIN SR Tablets to healthy volunteers, peak plasma concentrations of bupropion are achieved within 3 hours. Food increased C_{max} and AUC of bupropion by 11% and 17%, respectively, indicating that there is no clinically significant food effect.

Distribution: In vitro tests show that bupropion is 84% bound to human plasma proteins at concentrations up to 200 mcg/mL. The extent of protein binding of the hydroxybupropion metabolite is similar to that for bupropion, whereas the extent of protein binding of the threohydrobupropion metabolite is about half that seen with bupropion.

Metabolism: Bupropion is extensively metabolized in humans. Three metabolites have been shown to be active: hydroxybupropion, which is formed via hydroxylation of the *tert*-butyl group of bupropion, and the amino-alcohol isomers threohydrobupropion and erythrohydrobupropion, which are formed via reduction of the carbonyl group. In vitro findings suggest that cytochrome P450IIB6 (CYP2B6) is the principal isoenzyme involved in the formation of hydroxybupropion, while cytochrome P450 isoenzymes are not involved in the formation of threohydrobupropion. Oxidation of the bupropion side chain results in the formation of a glycine conjugate of meta-chlorobenzoic acid, which is then excreted as the major urinary metabolite. The potency and toxicity of the metabolites relative to bupropion have not been fully characterized. However, it has been demonstrated in an antidepressant screening test in mice that hydroxybupropion is one half as potent as bupropion, while threohydrobupropion and erythrohydrobupropion are 5-fold less potent than bupropion. This may be of clinical importance because the plasma concentrations of the metabolites are as high or higher than those of bupropion.

Because bupropion is extensively metabolized, there is the potential for drug-drug interactions, particularly with those agents that are metabolized by the cytochrome P450IIB6 (CYP2B6) isoenzyme. Although bupropion is not metabolized by cytochrome P450IID6 (CYP2D6), there is the potential for drug-drug interactions when bupropion is co-administered with drugs metabolized by this isoenzyme (see PRECAUTIONS: Drug Interactions).

Following a single dose in humans, peak plasma concentrations of hydroxybupropion occur approximately 6 hours after administration of WELLBUTRIN SR Tablets. Peak plasma concentrations of hydroxybupropion are approximately 10 times the peak level of the parent drug at steady state. The elimination half-life of hydroxybupropion is approximately 20 (±5) hours, and its AUC at steady state is about 17 times that of bupropion. The times to peak concentrations for the erythrohydrobupropion and threohydrobupropion metabolites are similar to that of the hydroxybupropion metabolite. However, their elimination half-lives are longer, 33 (±10) and 37 (±13) hours, respectively, and steady-state AUCs are 1.5 and 7 times that of bupropion, respectively.

Bupropion and its metabolites exhibit linear kinetics following chronic administration of 300 to 450 mg/day.

Elimination: Following oral administration of 200 mg of ^{14}C-bupropion in humans, 87% and 10% of the radioactive dose were recovered in the urine and feces, respectively. However, the fraction of the oral dose of bupropion excreted unchanged was only 0.5%, a finding consistent with the extensive metabolism of bupropion.

Population Subgroups: Factors or conditions altering metabolic capacity (e.g., liver disease, congestive heart failure [CHF], age, concomitant medications, etc.) or elimination may be expected to influence the degree and extent of accumulation of the active metabolites of bupropion. The elimination of the major metabolites of bupropion may be affected by reduced renal or hepatic function because they are moderately polar compounds and are likely to undergo further metabolism or conjugation in the liver prior to urinary excretion.

Hepatic: The effect of hepatic impairment on the pharmacokinetics of bupropion was characterized in 2 single-dose studies, one in patients with alcoholic liver disease and one in patients with mild to severe cirrhosis. The first study showed that the half-life of hydroxybupropion was significantly longer in 8 patients with alcoholic liver disease than in 8 healthy volunteers (32±14 hours versus 21±5 hours, respectively). Although not statistically significant, the AUCs for bupropion and hydroxybupropion were more variable and tended to be greater (by 53% to 57%) in patients with alcoholic liver disease. The differences in half-life for bupropion and the other metabolites in the 2 patient groups were minimal.

The second study showed no statistically significant differences in the pharmacokinetics of bupropion and its active metabolites in 9 patients with mild to moderate hepatic cirrhosis compared to 8 healthy volunteers. However, more variability was observed in some of the pharmacokinetic parameters for bupropion (AUC, C_{max}, and T_{max}) and its active metabolites ($t_{1/2}$) in patients with mild to moderate hepatic cirrhosis. In addition, in patients with severe hepatic cirrhosis, the bupropion C_{max} and AUC were substantially increased (mean difference: by approximately 70% and 3-fold, respectively) and more variable when compared to values in healthy volunteers; the mean bupropion half-life was also longer (29 hours in patients with severe hepatic cirrhosis vs.19 hours in healthy subjects). For the metabolite hydroxybupropion, the mean C_{max} was approximately 69% lower. For the combined amino-alcohol isomers threohydrobupropion and erythrohydrobupropion, the mean C_{max} was approximately 31% lower. The mean AUC increased by about 1½-fold for hydroxybupropion and about 2½-fold for threo/erythrohydrobupropion. The median T_{max} was observed 19 hours later for hydroxybupropion and 31 hours later for threo/erythrohydrobupropion. The mean half-lives for hydroxybupropion and threo/erythrohydrobupropion were increased 5- and 2-fold, respectively, in patients with severe hepatic cirrhosis compared to healthy volunteers (see WARNINGS, PRECAUTIONS, and DOSAGE AND ADMINISTRATION).

Renal: The effect of renal disease on the pharmacokinetics of bupropion has not been studied. The elimination of the major metabolites of bupropion may be affected by reduced renal function.

Left Ventricular Dysfunction: During a chronic dosing study with bupropion in 14 depressed patients with left ventricular dysfunction (history of CHF or an enlarged heart on x-ray), no apparent effect on the pharmacokinetics of bupropion or its metabolites was revealed, compared to healthy volunteers.

Age: The effects of age on the pharmacokinetics of bupropion and its metabolites have not been fully characterized, but an exploration of steady-state bupropion concentrations from several depression efficacy studies involving patients dosed in a range of 300 to 750 mg/day, on a 3 times daily schedule, revealed no relationship between age (18 to 83 years) and plasma concentration of bupropion. A single-dose pharmacokinetic study demonstrated that the disposition of bupropion and its metabolites in elderly subjects was similar to that of younger subjects. These data suggest there is no prominent effect of age on bupropion concentration; however, another pharmacokinetic study, single and multiple dose, has suggested that the elderly are at increased risk for accumulation of bupropion and its metabolites (see PRECAUTIONS: Geriatric Use).

Gender: A single-dose study involving 12 healthy male and 12 healthy female volunteers revealed no sex-related differences in the pharmacokinetic parameters of bupropion.

Smokers: The effects of cigarette smoking on the pharmacokinetics of bupropion were studied in 34 healthy male and female volunteers; 17 were chronic cigarette smokers and 17 were nonsmokers. Following oral administration of a single 150-mg dose of bupropion, there was no statistically significant difference in C_{max}, half-life, T_{max}, AUC, or clearance of bupropion or its active metabolites between smokers and nonsmokers.

CLINICAL TRIALS

The efficacy of the immediate-release formulation of bupropion as a treatment for depression was established in two

Continued on next page

Product information on these pages is effective as of August 2004. Further information is available at: GlaxoSmithKline, PO Box 13398, Research Triangle Park, NC 27709. 1-888-825-5249. Corporate Web Site: www.gsk.com

Wellbutrin SR—Cont.

4-week, placebo-controlled trials in adult inpatients with depression and in one 6-week, placebo-controlled trial in adult outpatients with depression. In the first study, patients were titrated in a bupropion dose range of 300 to 600 mg/day on a 3 times daily schedule; 78% of patients received maximum doses of 450 mg/day or less. This trial demonstrated the effectiveness of the immediate-release formulation of bupropion on the Hamilton Depression Rating Scale (HDRS) total score, the depressed mood item (item 1) from that scale, and the Clinical Global Impressions (CGI) severity score. A second study included 2 fixed doses of the immediate-release formulation of bupropion (300 and 450 mg/day) and placebo. This trial demonstrated the effectiveness of the immediate-release formulation of bupropion, but only at the 450-mg/day dose; the results were positive for the HDRS total score and the CGI severity score, but not for HDRS item 1. In the third study, outpatients received 300 mg/day of the immediate-release formulation of bupropion. This study demonstrated the effectiveness of the immediate-release formulation of bupropion on the HDRS total score, HDRS item 1, the Montgomery-Asberg Depression Rating Scale, the CGI severity score, and the CGI improvement score.

Although there are not as yet independent trials demonstrating the antidepressant effectiveness of the sustained-release formulation of bupropion, studies have demonstrated the bioequivalence of the immediate-release and sustained-release forms of bupropion under steady-state conditions, i.e., bupropion sustained-release 150 mg twice daily was shown to be bioequivalent to 100 mg 3 times daily of the immediate-release formulation of bupropion, with regard to both rate and extent of absorption, for parent drug and metabolites.

In a longer-term study, outpatients meeting DSM-IV criteria for major depressive disorder, recurrent type, who had responded during an 8-week open trial on WELLBUTRIN SR (150 mg twice daily) were randomized to continuation of their same WELLBUTRIN SR dose or placebo, for up to 44 weeks of observation for relapse. Response during the open phase was defined as CGI Improvement score of 1 (very much improved) or 2 (much improved) for each of the final 3 weeks. Relapse during the double-blind phase was defined as the investigator's judgment that drug treatment was needed for worsening depressive symptoms. Patients receiving continued WELLBUTRIN SR treatment experienced significantly lower relapse rates over the subsequent 44 weeks compared to those receiving placebo.

INDICATIONS AND USAGE

WELLBUTRIN SR is indicated for the treatment of depression.

The efficacy of bupropion in the treatment of depression was established in two 4-week controlled trials of depressed inpatients and in one 6-week controlled trial of depressed outpatients whose diagnoses corresponded most closely to the Major Depression category of the APA Diagnostic and Statistical Manual (DSM) (see CLINICAL PHARMACOLOGY).

A major depressive episode (DSM-IV) implies the presence of 1) depressed mood or 2) loss of interest or pleasure; in addition, at least five of the following symptoms have been present during the same 2-week period and represent a change from previous functioning: depressed mood, markedly diminished interest or pleasure in usual activities, significant change in weight and/or appetite, insomnia or hypersomnia, psychomotor agitation or retardation, increased fatigue, feelings of guilt or worthlessness, slowed thinking or impaired concentration, a suicide attempt or suicidal ideation.

The efficacy of WELLBUTRIN SR in maintaining an antidepressant response for up to 44 weeks following 8 weeks of acute treatment was demonstrated in a placebo-controlled trial (see CLINICAL PHARMACOLOGY). Nevertheless, the physician who elects to use WELLBUTRIN SR for extended periods should periodically reevaluate the long-term usefulness of the drug for the individual patient.

CONTRAINDICATIONS

WELLBUTRIN SR is contraindicated in patients with a seizure disorder.

WELLBUTRIN SR is contraindicated in patients treated with ZYBAN® (bupropion hydrochloride) Sustained-Release Tablets, or any other medications that contain bupropion because the incidence of seizure is dose dependent.

WELLBUTRIN SR is contraindicated in patients with a current or prior diagnosis of bulimia or anorexia nervosa because of a higher incidence of seizures noted in patients treated for bulimia with the immediate-release formulation of bupropion.

WELLBUTRIN SR is contraindicated in patients undergoing abrupt discontinuation of alcohol or sedatives (including benzodiazepines).

The concurrent administration of WELLBUTRIN SR Tablets and a monoamine oxidase (MAO) inhibitor is contraindicated. At least 14 days should elapse between discontinuation of an MAO inhibitor and initiation of treatment with WELLBUTRIN SR Tablets.

WELLBUTRIN SR is contraindicated in patients who have shown an allergic response to bupropion or the other ingredients that make up WELLBUTRIN SR Tablets.

WARNINGS

Patients should be made aware that WELLBUTRIN SR contains the same active ingredient found in ZYBAN, used as an aid to smoking cessation treatment, and that WELLBUTRIN SR should not be used in combination with ZYBAN, or any other medications that contain bupropion.

Seizures: Bupropion is associated with a dose-related risk of seizures. The risk of seizures is also related to patient factors, clinical situations, and concomitant medications, which must be considered in selection of patients for therapy with WELLBUTRIN SR.

WELLBUTRIN SR should be discontinued and not restarted in patients who experience a seizure while on treatment.

- **Dose: At doses of WELLBUTRIN SR up to a dose of 300 mg/day, the incidence of seizure is approximately 0.1% (1/1,000) and increases to approximately 0.4% (4/1,000) at the maximum recommended dose of 400 mg/day.**

  Data for the immediate-release formulation of bupropion revealed a seizure incidence of approximately 0.4% (i.e., 13 of 3,200 patients followed prospectively) in patients treated at doses in a range of 300 to 450 mg/day. The 450-mg/day upper limit of this dose range is close to the currently recommended maximum dose of 400 mg/day for WELLBUTRIN SR Tablets. This seizure incidence (0.4%) may exceed that of other marketed antidepressants and WELLBUTRIN SR Tablets up to 300 mg/day by as much as 4-fold. This relative risk is only an approximate estimate because no direct comparative studies have been conducted.

  Additional data accumulated for the immediate-release formulation of bupropion suggested that the estimated seizure incidence increases almost tenfold between 450 and 600 mg/day, which is twice the usual adult dose and one and one-half the maximum recommended daily dose (400 mg) of WELLBUTRIN SR Tablets. This disproportionate increase in seizure incidence with dose incrementation calls for caution in dosing.

  Data for WELLBUTRIN SR Tablets revealed a seizure incidence of approximately 0.1% (i.e., 3 of 3,100 patients followed prospectively) in patients treated at doses in a range of 100 to 300 mg/day. It is not possible to know if the lower seizure incidence observed in this study involving the sustained-release formulation of bupropion resulted from the different formulation or the lower dose used. However, as noted above, the immediate-release and sustained-release formulations are bioequivalent with regard to both rate and extent of absorption during steady state (the most pertinent condition to estimating seizure incidence), since most observed seizures occur under steady-state conditions.
- **Patient factors: Predisposing factors that may increase the risk of seizure with bupropion use include history of head trauma or prior seizure, central nervous system (CNS) tumor, the presence of severe hepatic cirrhosis, and concomitant medications that lower seizure threshold.**
- **Clinical situations: Circumstances associated with an increased seizure risk include, among others, excessive use of alcohol or sedatives (including benzodiazepines); addiction to opiates, cocaine, or stimulants; use of over-the-counter stimulants and anorectics; and diabetes treated with oral hypoglycemics or insulin.**
- **Concomitant medications: Many medications (e.g., antipsychotics, antidepressants, theophylline, systemic steroids) are known to lower seizure threshold.**

***Recommendations for Reducing the Risk of Seizure:* Retrospective analysis of clinical experience gained during the development of bupropion suggests that the risk of seizure may be minimized if**

- **the total daily dose of WELLBUTRIN SR Tablets does *not* exceed 400 mg,**
- **the daily dose is administered twice daily, and**
- **the rate of incrementation of dose is gradual.**
- **No single dose should exceed 200 mg to avoid high peak concentrations of bupropion and/or its metabolites.**

WELLBUTRIN SR should be administered with extreme caution to patients with a history of seizure, cranial trauma, or other predisposition(s) toward seizure, or patients treated with other agents (e.g., antipsychotics, other antidepressants, theophylline, systemic steroids, etc.) that lower seizure threshold.

Hepatic Impairment: WELLBUTRIN SR should be used with extreme caution in patients with severe hepatic cirrhosis. In these patients a reduced frequency and/or dose is required, as peak bupropion, as well as AUC, levels are substantially increased and accumulation is likely to occur in such patients to a greater extent than usual. The dose should not exceed 100 mg every day or 150 mg every other day in these patients (see CLINICAL PHARMACOLOGY, PRECAUTIONS, and DOSAGE AND ADMINISTRATION).

Potential for Hepatotoxicity: In rats receiving large doses of bupropion chronically, there was an increase in incidence of hepatic hyperplastic nodules and hepatocellular hypertrophy. In dogs receiving large doses of bupropion chronically, various histologic changes were seen in the liver, and laboratory tests suggesting mild hepatocellular injury were noted.

Clinical Worsening and Suicide Risk: Patients with major depressive disorder, both adult and pediatric, may experience worsening of their depression and/or the emergence of suicidal ideation and behavior (suicidality), whether or not they are taking antidepressant medications, and this risk may persist until significant remission occurs. Although there has been a long-standing concern that antidepressants may have a role in inducing worsening of depression and the emergence of suicidality in certain patients, a causal role for antidepressants in inducing such behaviors has not been established. **Nevertheless, patients being treated with antidepressants should be observed closely for clinical worsening and suicidality, especially at the beginning of a course of drug therapy, or at the time of dose changes, either increases or decreases.** Consideration should be given to changing the therapeutic regimen, including possibly discontinuing the medication in patients whose depression is persistently worse or whose emergent suicidality is severe, abrupt in onset, or was not part of the patient's presenting symptoms.

Because of the possibility of co-morbidity between major depressive disorder and other psychiatric and nonpsychiatric disorders, the same precautions observed when treating patients with major depressive disorder should be observed when treating patients with other psychiatric and nonpsychiatric disorders.

The following symptoms, anxiety, agitation, panic attacks, insomnia, irritability, hostility (aggressiveness), impulsivity, akathisia (psychomotor restlessness), hypomania, and mania, have been reported in adult and pediatric patients being treated with antidepressants for major depressive disorder as well as for other indications, both psychiatric and nonpsychiatric. Although a causal link between the emergence of such symptoms and either the worsening of depression and/or the emergence of suicidal impulses has not been established, consideration should be given to changing the therapeutic regimen, including possibly discontinuing the medication in patients for whom such symptoms are severe, abrupt in onset, or were not part of the patient's presenting symptoms.

Families and caregivers of patients being treated with antidepressants for major depressive disorder or other indications, both psychiatric and nonpsychiatric, should be alerted about the need to monitor patients for the emergence of agitation, irritability, and the other symptoms described above, as well as the emergence of suicidality, and to report such symptoms immediately to health care providers. Prescriptions for WELLBUTRIN SR should be written for the smallest quantity of tablets consistent with good patient management, in order to reduce the risk of overdose. It should be noted that WELLBUTRIN SR is not approved for use in treating any indications in the pediatric population.

A major depression episode may be the initial presentation of bipolar disorder. It is generally believed (although not established in controlled trials) that treating such an episode with an antidepressant alone may increase the likelihood of precipitation of a mixed/manic episode in patients at risk for bipolar disorder. Whether any of the symptoms described above represent such a conversion is unknown. However, prior to initiating treatment with an antidepressant, patients should be adequately screened to determine if they are at risk for bipolar disorder; such screening should include a detailed psychiatric history, including a family history of suicide, bipolar disorder, and depression. It should be noted that WELLBUTRIN SR is not approved for use in treating bipolar depression.

PRECAUTIONS

General: ***Agitation and Insomnia:*** Patients in placebo-controlled trials with WELLBUTRIN SR Tablets experienced agitation, anxiety, and insomnia as shown in Table 1.

Table 1. Incidence of Agitation, Anxiety, and Insomnia in Placebo-Controlled Trials

Adverse Event Term	WELLBUTRIN SR 300 mg/day (n = 376)	WELLBUTRIN SR 400 mg/day (n = 114)	Placebo (n = 385)
Agitation	3%	9%	2%
Anxiety	5%	6%	3%
Insomnia	11%	16%	6%

In clinical studies, these symptoms were sometimes of sufficient magnitude to require treatment with sedative/hypnotic drugs.

Symptoms were sufficiently severe to require discontinuation of treatment in 1% and 2.6% of patients treated with 300 and 400 mg/day, respectively, of WELLBUTRIN SR Tablets and 0.8% of patients treated with placebo.

Psychosis, Confusion, and Other Neuropsychiatric Phenomena: Depressed patients treated with an immediate-release formulation of bupropion or with WELLBUTRIN SR Tablets have been reported to show a variety of neuropsychiatric signs and symptoms, including delusions, hallucinations, psychosis, concentration disturbance, paranoia, and confusion. In some cases, these symptoms abated upon dose reduction and/or withdrawal of treatment.

Activation of Psychosis and/or Mania: Antidepressants can precipitate manic episodes in bipolar disorder patients during the depressed phase of their illness and may activate latent psychosis in other susceptible patients. WELLBUTRIN SR is expected to pose similar risks.

Altered Appetite and Weight: In placebo-controlled studies, patients experienced weight gain or weight loss as shown in Table 2.

Table 2. Incidence of Weight Gain and Weight Loss in Placebo-Controlled Trials

Weight Change	WELLBUTRIN SR 300 mg/day (n = 339)	WELLBUTRIN SR 400 mg/day (n = 112)	Placebo (n = 347)
Gained >5 lbs	3%	2%	4%
Lost >5 lbs	14%	19%	6%

In studies conducted with the immediate-release formulation of bupropion, 35% of patients receiving tricyclic antidepressants gained weight, compared to 9% of patients treated with the immediate-release formulation of bupropion. If weight loss is a major presenting sign of a patient's depressive illness, the anorectic and/or weight-reducing potential of WELLBUTRIN SR Tablets should be considered.

Allergic Reactions: Anaphylactoid/anaphylactic reactions characterized by symptoms such as pruritus, urticaria, angioedema, and dyspnea requiring medical treatment have been reported in clinical trials with bupropion. In addition, there have been rare spontaneous postmarketing reports of erythema multiforme, Stevens-Johnson syndrome, and anaphylactic shock associated with bupropion. A patient should stop taking WELLBUTRIN SR and consult a doctor if experiencing allergic or anaphylactoid/anaphylactic reactions (e.g., skin rash, pruritus, hives, chest pain, edema, and shortness of breath) during treatment.

Arthralgia, myalgia, and fever with rash and other symptoms suggestive of delayed hypersensitivity have been reported in association with bupropion. These symptoms may resemble serum sickness.

Cardiovascular Effects: In clinical practice, hypertension, in some cases severe, requiring acute treatment, has been reported in patients receiving bupropion alone and in combination with nicotine replacement therapy. These events have been observed in both patients with and without evidence of preexisting hypertension.

Data from a comparative study of the sustained-release formulation of bupropion (ZYBAN® Sustained-Release Tablets), nicotine transdermal system (NTS), the combination of sustained-release bupropion plus NTS, and placebo as an aid to smoking cessation suggest a higher incidence of treatment-emergent hypertension in patients treated with the combination of sustained-release bupropion and NTS. In this study, 6.1% of patients treated with the combination of sustained-release bupropion and NTS had treatment-emergent hypertension compared to 2.5%, 1.6%, and 3.1% of patients treated with sustained-release bupropion, NTS, and placebo, respectively. The majority of these patients had evidence of preexisting hypertension. Three patients (1.2%) treated with the combination of ZYBAN and NTS and one patient (0.4%) treated with NTS had study medication discontinued due to hypertension compared to none of the patients treated with ZYBAN or placebo. Monitoring of blood pressure is recommended in patients who receive the combination of bupropion and nicotine replacement.

There is no clinical experience establishing the safety of WELLBUTRIN SR Tablets in patients with a recent history of myocardial infarction or unstable heart disease. Therefore, care should be exercised if it is used in these groups. Bupropion was well tolerated in depressed patients who had previously developed orthostatic hypotension while receiving tricyclic antidepressants, and was also generally well tolerated in a group of 36 depressed inpatients with stable congestive heart failure (CHF). However, bupropion was associated with a rise in supine blood pressure in the study of patients with CHF, resulting in discontinuation of treatment in 2 patients for exacerbation of baseline hypertension.

Hepatic Impairment: WELLBUTRIN SR should be used with extreme caution in patients with severe hepatic cirrhosis. In these patients, a reduced frequency and/or dose is required. WELLBUTRIN SR should be used with caution in patients with hepatic impairment (including mild to moderate hepatic cirrhosis) and reduced frequency and/or dose should be considered in patients with mild to moderate hepatic cirrhosis.

All patients with hepatic impairment should be closely monitored for possible adverse effects that could indicate high drug and metabolite levels (see CLINICAL PHARMACOLOGY, WARNINGS, and DOSAGE AND ADMINISTRATION).

Renal Impairment: No studies have been conducted in patients with renal impairment. Bupropion is extensively metabolized in the liver to active metabolites, which are further metabolized and subsequently excreted by the kidneys. WELLBUTRIN SR should be used with caution in patients with renal impairment and a reduced frequency and/or dose should be considered as bupropion and its metabolites may accumulate in such patients to a greater extent than usual. The patient should be closely monitored for possible adverse effects that could indicate high drug or metabolite levels.

Information for Patients: See the tear-off leaflet at the end of the labeling accompanying the product for Patient Information.

Patients should be made aware that WELLBUTRIN SR contains the same active ingredient found in ZYBAN, used as an aid to smoking cessation treatment, and that WELLBUTRIN SR should not be used in combination with ZYBAN or any other medications that contain bupropion hydrochloride.

Physicians are advised to discuss the following issues with patients:

As dose is increased during initial titration to doses above 150 mg/day, patients should be instructed to take WELLBUTRIN SR Tablets in 2 divided doses, preferably with at least 8 hours between successive doses, to minimize the risk of seizures.

Patients should be told that WELLBUTRIN SR should be discontinued and not restarted if they experience a seizure while on treatment.

Patients should be told that any CNS-active drug like WELLBUTRIN SR Tablets may impair their ability to perform tasks requiring judgment or motor and cognitive skills. Consequently, until they are reasonably certain that WELLBUTRIN SR Tablets do not adversely affect their performance, they should refrain from driving an automobile or operating complex, hazardous machinery.

Patients should be told that the excessive use or abrupt discontinuation of alcohol or sedatives (including benzodiazepines) may alter the seizure threshold. Some patients have reported lower alcohol tolerance during treatment with WELLBUTRIN SR. Patients should be advised that the consumption of alcohol should be minimized or avoided.

Patients and their families should be encouraged to be alert to the emergence of anxiety, agitation, panic attacks, insomnia, irritability, hostility, impulsivity, akathisia, hypomania, mania, worsening of depression, and suicidal ideation, especially early during antidepressant treatment. Such symptoms should be reported to the patient's physician, especially if they are severe, abrupt in onset, or were not part of the patient's presenting symptoms.

Patients should be advised to inform their physicians if they are taking or plan to take any prescription or over-the-counter drugs. Concern is warranted because WELLBUTRIN SR Tablets and other drugs may affect each other's metabolism.

Patients should be advised to notify their physicians if they become pregnant or intend to become pregnant during therapy.

Patients should be advised to swallow WELLBUTRIN SR Tablets whole so that the release rate is not altered. Do not chew, divide, or crush tablets.

Laboratory Tests: There are no specific laboratory tests recommended.

Drug Interactions: Few systemic data have been collected on the metabolism of WELLBUTRIN SR following concomitant administration with other drugs or, alternatively, the effect of concomitant administration of WELLBUTRIN SR on the metabolism of other drugs.

Because bupropion is extensively metabolized, the coadministration of other drugs may affect its clinical activity. In vitro studies indicate that bupropion is primarily metabolized to hydroxybupropion by the CYP2B6 isoenzyme. Therefore, the potential exists for a drug interaction between WELLBUTRIN SR and drugs that affect the CYP2B6 isoenzyme (e.g., orphenadrine and cyclophosphamide). The threohydrobupropion metabolite of bupropion does not appear to be produced by the cytochrome P450 isoenzymes. The effects of concomitant administration of cimetidine on the pharmacokinetics of bupropion and its active metabolites were studied in 24 healthy young male volunteers. Following oral administration of two 150-mg WELLBUTRIN SR Tablets with and without 800 mg of cimetidine, the pharmacokinetics of bupropion and hydroxybupropion were unaffected. However, there were 16% and 32% increases in the AUC and C_{max}, respectively, of the combined moieties of threohydrobupropion and erythrohydrobupropion.

While not systematically studied, certain drugs may induce the metabolism of bupropion (e.g., carbamazepine, phenobarbital, phenytoin).

Animal data indicated that bupropion may be an inducer of drug-metabolizing enzymes in humans. In one study, following chronic administration of bupropion, 100 mg 3 times daily to 8 healthy male volunteers for 14 days, there was no evidence of induction of its own metabolism. Nevertheless, there may be the potential for clinically important alterations of blood levels of coadministered drugs.

Drugs Metabolized By Cytochrome P450IID6 (CYP2D6): Many drugs, including most antidepressants (SSRIs, many tricyclics), beta-blockers, antiarrhythmics, and antipsychotics are metabolized by the CYP2D6 isoenzyme. Although bupropion is not metabolized by this isoenzyme, bupropion and hydroxybupropion are inhibitors of CYP2D6 isoenzyme in vitro. In a study of 15 male subjects (ages 19 to 35 years) who were extensive metabolizers of the CYP2D6 isoenzyme, daily doses of bupropion given as 150 mg twice daily followed by a single dose of 50 mg desipramine increased the C_{max}, AUC, and $t_{1/2}$ of desipramine by an average of approximately 2-, 5-, and 2-fold, respectively. The effect was present for at least 7 days after the last dose of bupropion. Concomitant use of bupropion with other drugs metabolized by CYP2D6 has not been formally studied.

Therefore, co-administration of bupropion with drugs that are metabolized by CYP2D6 isoenzyme including certain antidepressants (e.g., nortriptyline, imipramine, desipramine, paroxetine, fluoxetine, sertraline), antipsychotics (e.g., haloperidol, risperidone, thioridazine), beta-blockers (e.g., metoprolol), and Type 1C antiarrhythmics (e.g., propafenone, flecainide), should be approached with caution and should be initiated at the lower end of the dose range of the concomitant medication. If bupropion is added to the treatment regimen of a patient already receiving a drug metabolized by CYP2D6, the need to decrease the dose of the original medication should be considered, particularly for those concomitant medications with a narrow therapeutic index.

MAO Inhibitors: Studies in animals demonstrate that the acute toxicity of bupropion is enhanced by the MAO inhibitor phenelzine (see CONTRAINDICATIONS).

Levodopa and Amantadine: Limited clinical data suggest a higher incidence of adverse experiences in patients receiving bupropion concurrently with either levodopa or amantadine. Administration of WELLBUTRIN SR Tablets to patients receiving either levodopa or amantadine concurrently should be undertaken with caution, using small initial doses and gradual dose increases.

Drugs That Lower Seizure Threshold: Concurrent administration of WELLBUTRIN SR Tablets and agents (e.g., antipsychotics, other antidepressants, theophylline, systemic steroids, etc.) that lower seizure threshold should be undertaken only with extreme caution (see WARNINGS). Low initial dosing and gradual dose increases should be employed.

Nicotine Transdermal System: (see PRECAUTIONS: Cardiovascular Effects).

Alcohol: In post-marketing experience, there have been rare reports of adverse neuropsychiatric events or reduced alcohol tolerance in patients who were drinking alcohol during treatment with WELLBUTRIN SR. The consumption of alcohol during treatment with WELLBUTRIN SR should be minimized or avoided (also see CONTRAINDICATIONS).

Carcinogenesis, Mutagenesis, Impairment of Fertility: Lifetime carcinogenicity studies were performed in rats and mice at doses up to 300 and 150 mg/kg/day, respectively. These doses are approximately 7 and 2 times the maximum recommended human dose (MRHD), respectively, on a mg/m^2 basis. In the rat study there was an increase in nodular proliferative lesions of the liver at doses of 100 to 300 mg/kg/day (approximately 2 to 7 times the MRHD on a mg/m^2 basis); lower doses were not tested. The question of whether or not such lesions may be precursors of neoplasms of the liver is currently unresolved. Similar liver lesions were not seen in the mouse study, and no increase in malignant tumors of the liver and other organs was seen in either study.

Bupropion produced a positive response (2 to 3 times control mutation rate) in 2 of 5 strains in the Ames bacterial mutagenicity test and an increase in chromosomal aberrations in 1 of 3 in vivo rat bone marrow cytogenetic studies.

A fertility study in rats at doses up to 300 mg/kg/day revealed no evidence of impaired fertility.

Pregnancy: ***Teratogenic Effects:*** Pregnancy Category B. Teratology studies have been performed at doses up to 450 mg/kg in rats, and at doses up to 150 mg/kg in rabbits (approximately 7 to 11 and 7 times the MRHD, respectively, on a mg/m^2 basis), and have revealed no evidence of harm to the fetus due to bupropion. There are no adequate and well-controlled studies in pregnant women. Because animal reproduction studies are not always predictive of human response, this drug should be used during pregnancy only if clearly needed.

To monitor fetal outcomes of pregnant women exposed to WELLBUTRIN SR, GlaxoSmithKline maintains a Bupropion Pregnancy Registry. Health care providers are encouraged to register patients by calling (800) 336-2176.

Labor and Delivery: The effect of WELLBUTRIN SR Tablets on labor and delivery in humans is unknown.

Nursing Mothers: Like many other drugs, bupropion and its metabolites are secreted in human milk. Because of the potential for serious adverse reactions in nursing infants from WELLBUTRIN SR Tablets, a decision should be made whether to discontinue nursing or to discontinue the drug, taking into account the importance of the drug to the mother.

Pediatric Use: The safety and effectiveness of WELLBUTRIN SR Tablets in pediatric patients below 18 years old have not been established. The immediate-release formulation of bupropion was studied in 104 pediatric patients (age range, 6 to 16) in clinical trials of the drug for other indications. Although generally well tolerated, the limited exposure is insufficient to assess the safety of bupropion in pediatric patients **(see WARNINGS—Clinical Worsening and Suicide Risk)**.

Geriatric Use: Of the approximately 6,000 patients who participated in clinical trials with bupropion sustained-release tablets (depression and smoking cessation studies), 275 were 65 and over and 47 were 75 and over. In addition, several hundred patients 65 and over participated in clinical trials using the immediate-release formulation of bupropion (depression studies). No overall differences in safety or effectiveness were observed between these subjects and younger subjects, and other reported clinical experience has not identified differences in responses between the elderly and younger patients, but greater sensitivity of some older individuals cannot be ruled out.

A single-dose pharmacokinetic study demonstrated that the disposition of bupropion and its metabolites in elderly subjects was similar to that of younger subjects; however, another pharmacokinetic study, single and multiple dose, has

Continued on next page

Product information on these pages is effective as of August 2004. Further information is available at: GlaxoSmithKline, PO Box 13398, Research Triangle Park, NC 27709. 1-888-825-5249. Corporate Web Site: www.gsk.com

Wellbutrin SR—Cont.

suggested that the elderly are at increased risk for accumulation of bupropion and its metabolites (see CLINICAL PHARMACOLOGY).

Bupropion is extensively metabolized in the liver to active metabolites, which are further metabolized and excreted by the kidneys. The risk of toxic reaction to this drug may be greater in patients with impaired renal function. Because elderly patients are more likely to have decreased renal function, care should be taken in dose selection, and it may be useful to monitor renal function (see PRECAUTIONS: Renal Impairment and DOSAGE AND ADMINISTRATION).

ADVERSE REACTIONS (See also WARNINGS and PRECAUTIONS.)

The information included under the Incidence in Controlled Trials subsection of ADVERSE REACTIONS is based primarily on data from controlled clinical trials with WELLBUTRIN SR Tablets. Information on additional adverse events associated with the sustained-release formulation of bupropion in smoking cessation trials, as well as the immediate-release formulation of bupropion, is included in a separate section (see Other Events Observed During the Clinical Development and Postmarketing Experience of Bupropion).

Incidence in Controlled Trials With WELLBUTRIN SR: ***Adverse Events Associated With Discontinuation of Treatment Among Patients Treated With WELLBUTRIN SR Tablets:*** In placebo-controlled clinical trials, 9% and 11% of patients treated with 300 and 400 mg/day, respectively, of WELLBUTRIN SR Tablets and 4% of patients treated with placebo discontinued treatment due to adverse events. The specific adverse events in these trials that led to discontinuation in at least 1% of patients treated with either 300 or 400 mg/day of WELLBUTRIN SR Tablets and at a rate at least twice the placebo rate are listed in Table 3.

Table 3. Treatment Discontinuations Due to Adverse Events in Placebo-Controlled Trials

Adverse Event Term	WELLBUTRIN SR 300 mg/day (n = 376)	WELLBUTRIN SR 400 mg/day (n = 114)	Placebo (n = 385)
Rash	2.4%	0.9%	0.0%
Nausea	0.8%	1.8%	0.3%
Agitation	0.3%	1.8%	0.3%
Migraine	0.0%	1.8%	0.3%

Adverse Events Occurring at an Incidence of 1% or More Among Patients Treated With WELLBUTRIN SR Tablets: Table 4 enumerates treatment-emergent adverse events that occurred among patients treated with 300 and 400 mg/day of WELLBUTRIN SR Tablets and with placebo in placebo-controlled trials. Events that occurred in either the 300- or 400-mg/day group at an incidence of 1% or more and were more frequent than in the placebo group are included. Reported adverse events were classified using a COSTART-based Dictionary.

Accurate estimates of the incidence of adverse events associated with the use of any drug are difficult to obtain. Estimates are influenced by drug dose, detection technique, setting, physician judgments, etc. The figures cited cannot be used to predict precisely the incidence of untoward events in the course of usual medical practice where patient characteristics and other factors differ from those that prevailed in the clinical trials. These incidence figures also cannot be compared with those obtained from other clinical studies involving related drug products as each group of drug trials is conducted under a different set of conditions.

Finally, it is important to emphasize that the tabulation does not reflect the relative severity and/or clinical importance of the events. A better perspective on the serious adverse events associated with the use of WELLBUTRIN SR Tablets is provided in the WARNINGS and PRECAUTIONS sections.

[See table 4 above]

Table 4. Treatment-Emergent Adverse Events in Placebo-Controlled Trials*

Body System/Adverse Event	WELLBUTRIN SR 300 mg/day (n = 376)	WELLBUTRIN SR 400 mg/day (n = 114)	Placebo (n = 385)
Body (General)			
Headache	26%	25%	23%
Infection	8%	9%	6%
Abdominal pain	3%	9%	2%
Asthenia	2%	4%	2%
Chest pain	3%	4%	1%
Pain	2%	3%	2%
Fever	1%	2%	—
Cardiovascular			
Palpitation	2%	6%	2%
Flushing	1%	4%	—
Migraine	1%	4%	1%
Hot flashes	1%	3%	1%
Digestive			
Dry mouth	17%	24%	7%
Nausea	13%	18%	8%
Constipation	10%	5%	7%
Diarrhea	5%	7%	6%
Anorexia	5%	3%	2%
Vomiting	4%	2%	2%
Dysphagia	0%	2%	0%
Musculoskeletal			
Myalgia	2%	6%	3%
Arthralgia	1%	4%	1%
Arthritis	0%	2%	0%
Twitch	1%	2%	—
Nervous system			
Insomnia	11%	16%	6%
Dizziness	7%	11%	5%
Agitation	3%	9%	2%
Anxiety	5%	6%	3%
Tremor	6%	3%	1%
Nervousness	5%	3%	3%
Somnolence	2%	3%	2%
Irritability	3%	2%	2%
Memory decreased	—	3%	1%
Paresthesia	1%	2%	1%
Central nervous system stimulation	2%	1%	1%
Respiratory			
Pharyngitis	3%	11%	2%
Sinusitis	3%	1%	2%
Increased cough	1%	2%	1%
Skin			
Sweating	6%	5%	2%
Rash	5%	4%	1%
Pruritus	2%	4%	2%
Urticaria	2%	1%	0%
Special senses			
Tinnitus	6%	6%	2%
Taste perversion	2%	4%	—
Amblyopia	3%	2%	2%
Urogenital			
Urinary frequency	2%	5%	2%
Urinary urgency	—	2%	0%
Vaginal hemorrhage†	0%	2%	—
Urinary tract infection	1%	0%	—

* Adverse events that occurred in at least 1% of patients treated with either 300 or 400 mg/day of WELLBUTRIN SR Tablets, but equally or more frequently in the placebo group, were: abnormal dreams, accidental injury, acne, appetite increased, back pain, bronchitis, dysmenorrhea, dyspepsia, flatulence, flu syndrome, hypertension, neck pain, respiratory disorder, rhinitis, and tooth disorder.

† Incidence based on the number of female patients.

—Hyphen denotes adverse events occurring in greater than 0 but less than 0.5% of patients.

Incidence of Commonly Observed Adverse Events in Controlled Clinical Trials: Adverse events from Table 4 occurring in at least 5% of patients treated with WELLBUTRIN SR Tablets and at a rate at least twice the placebo rate are listed below for the 300- and 400-mg/day dose groups.

WELLBUTRIN SR 300 mg/day: Anorexia, dry mouth, rash, sweating, tinnitus, and tremor.

WELLBUTRIN SR 400 mg/day: Abdominal pain, agitation, anxiety, dizziness, dry mouth, insomnia, myalgia, nausea, palpitation, pharyngitis, sweating, tinnitus, and urinary frequency.

Other Events Observed During the Clinical Development and Postmarketing Experience of Bupropion: In addition to the adverse events noted above, the following events have been reported in clinical trials and postmarketing experience with the sustained-release formulation of bupropion in depressed patients and in nondepressed smokers, as well as in clinical trials and postmarketing clinical experience with the immediate-release formulation of bupropion.

Adverse events for which frequencies are provided below occurred in clinical trials with the sustained-release formulation of bupropion. The frequencies represent the proportion of patients who experienced a treatment-emergent adverse event on at least one occasion in placebo-controlled studies for depression (n = 987) or smoking cessation (n = 1,013), or patients who experienced an adverse event requiring discontinuation of treatment in an open-label surveillance study with WELLBUTRIN SR Tablets (n = 3,100). All treatment-emergent adverse events are included except those listed in Tables 1 through 4, those events listed in other safety-related sections, those adverse events subsumed under COSTART terms that are either overly general or excessively specific so as to be uninformative, those events not reasonably associated with the use of the drug, and those events that were not serious and occurred in fewer than 2 patients. Events of major clinical importance are described in the WARNINGS and PRECAUTIONS sections of the labeling.

Events are further categorized by body system and listed in order of decreasing frequency according to the following definitions of frequency: Frequent adverse events are defined as those occurring in at least 1/100 patients. Infrequent adverse events are those occurring in 1/100 to 1/1,000 patients, while rare events are those occurring in less than 1/1,000 patients.

Adverse events for which frequencies are not provided occurred in clinical trials or postmarketing experience with bupropion. Only those adverse events not previously listed for sustained-release bupropion are included. The extent to which these events may be associated with WELLBUTRIN SR is unknown.

Body (General): Infrequent were chills, facial edema, musculoskeletal chest pain, and photosensitivity. Rare was malaise. Also observed were arthralgia, myalgia, and fever with rash and other symptoms suggestive of delayed hypersensitivity. These symptoms may resemble serum sickness (see PRECAUTIONS).

Cardiovascular: Infrequent were postural hypotension, stroke, tachycardia, and vasodilation. Rare was syncope. Also observed were complete atrioventricular block, extrasystoles, hypotension, hypertension (in some cases severe, see PRECAUTIONS), myocardial infarction, phlebitis, and pulmonary embolism.

Digestive: Infrequent were abnormal liver function, bruxism, gastric reflux, gingivitis, glossitis, increased salivation, jaundice, mouth ulcers, stomatitis, and thirst. Rare was edema of tongue. Also observed were colitis, esophagitis, gastrointestinal hemorrhage, gum hemorrhage, hepatitis, intestinal perforation, liver damage, pancreatitis, and stomach ulcer.

Endocrine: Also observed were hyperglycemia, hypoglycemia, and syndrome of inappropriate antidiuretic hormone.

Hemic and Lymphatic: Infrequent was ecchymosis. Also observed were anemia, leukocytosis, leukopenia, lymph-

adenopathy, pancytopenia, and thrombocytopenia. Altered PT and/or INR, infrequently associated with hemorrhagic or thrombotic complications, were observed when bupropion was coadministered with warfarin.
Metabolic and Nutritional: Infrequent were edema and peripheral edema. Also observed was glycosuria.
Musculoskeletal: Infrequent were leg cramps. Also observed were muscle rigidity/fever/rhabdomyolysis and muscle weakness.
Nervous System: Infrequent were abnormal coordination, decreased libido, depersonalization, dysphoria, emotional lability, hostility, hyperkinesia, hypertonia, hypesthesia, suicidal ideation, and vertigo. Rare were amnesia, ataxia, derealization, and hypomania. Also observed were abnormal electroencephalogram (EEG), akinesia, aphasia, coma, delirium, dysarthria, dyskinesia, dystonia, euphoria, extrapyramidal syndrome, hallucinations, hypokinesia, increased libido, manic reaction, neuralgia, neuropathy, paranoid reaction, and unmasking tardive dyskinesia.
Respiratory: Rare was bronchospasm. Also observed was pneumonia.
Skin: Rare was maculopapular rash. Also observed were alopecia, angioedema, exfoliative dermatitis, and hirsutism.
Special Senses: Infrequent were accommodation abnormality and dry eye. Also observed were deafness, diplopia, and mydriasis.
Urogenital: Infrequent were impotence, polyuria, and prostate disorder. Also observed were abnormal ejaculation, cystitis, dyspareunia, dysuria, gynecomastia, menopause, painful erection, salpingitis, urinary incontinence, urinary retention, and vaginitis.

DRUG ABUSE AND DEPENDENCE

Controlled Substance Class: Bupropion is not a controlled substance.
Humans: Controlled clinical studies of bupropion conducted in normal volunteers, in subjects with a history of multiple drug abuse, and in depressed patients showed some increase in motor activity and agitation/excitement.
In a population of individuals experienced with drugs of abuse, a single dose of 400 mg of bupropion produced mild amphetamine-like activity as compared to placebo on the Morphine-Benzedrine Subscale of the Addiction Research Center Inventories (ARCI), and a score intermediate between placebo and amphetamine on the Liking Scale of the ARCI. These scales measure general feelings of euphoria and drug desirability.
Findings in clinical trials, however, are not known to reliably predict the abuse potential of drugs. Nonetheless, evidence from single-dose studies does suggest that the recommended daily dosage of bupropion when administered in divided doses is not likely to be especially reinforcing to amphetamine or stimulant abusers. However, higher doses that could not be tested because of the risk of seizure might be modestly attractive to those who abuse stimulant drugs.
Animals: Studies in rodents and primates have shown that bupropion exhibits some pharmacologic actions common to psychostimulants. In rodents, it has been shown to increase locomotor activity, elicit a mild stereotyped behavioral response, and increase rates of responding in several schedule-controlled behavior paradigms. In primate models to assess the positive reinforcing effects of psychoactive drugs, bupropion was self-administered intravenously. In rats, bupropion produced amphetamine-like and cocaine-like discriminative stimulus effects in drug discrimination paradigms used to characterize the subjective effects of psychoactive drugs.

OVERDOSAGE

Human Overdose Experience: There has been very limited experience with overdosage of WELLBUTRIN SR Tablets; 3 cases were reported during clinical trials. One patient ingested 3,000 mg of WELLBUTRIN SR Tablets and vomited quickly after the overdose; the patient experienced blurred vision and lightheadedness. A second patient ingested a "handful" of WELLBUTRIN SR Tablets and experienced confusion, lethargy, nausea, jitteriness, and seizure. A third patient ingested 3,600 mg of WELLBUTRIN SR Tablets and a bottle of wine; the patient experienced nausea, visual hallucinations, and "grogginess." None of the patients experienced further sequelae.
There has been extensive experience with overdosage of the immediate-release formulation of bupropion. Thirteen overdoses occurred during clinical trials. Twelve patients ingested 850 to 4,200 mg and recovered without significant sequelae. Another patient who ingested 9,000 mg of the immediate-release formulation of bupropion and 300 mg of tranylcypromine experienced a grand mal seizure and recovered without further sequelae.
Since introduction, overdoses of up to 17,500 mg of the immediate-release formulation of bupropion have been reported. Seizure was reported in approximately one third of all cases. Other serious reactions reported with overdoses of the immediate-release formulation of bupropion alone included hallucinations, loss of consciousness, and sinus tachycardia. Fever, muscle rigidity, rhabdomyolysis, hypotension, stupor, coma, and respiratory failure have been reported when the immediate-release formulation of bupropion was part of multiple drug overdoses.
Although most patients recovered without sequelae, deaths associated with overdoses of the immediate-release formulation of bupropion alone have been reported rarely in patients ingesting massive doses of the drug. Multiple uncontrolled seizures, bradycardia, cardiac failure, and cardiac arrest prior to death were reported in these patients.
Overdosage Management: Ensure an adequate airway, oxygenation, and ventilation. Monitor cardiac rhythm and vital signs. EEG monitoring is also recommended for the first 48 hours post-ingestion. General supportive and symptomatic measures are also recommended. Induction of emesis is not recommended. Gastric lavage with a large-bore orogastric tube with appropriate airway protection, if needed, may be indicated if performed soon after ingestion or in symptomatic patients.
Activated charcoal should be administered. There is no experience with the use of forced diuresis, dialysis, hemoperfusion, or exchange transfusion in the management of bupropion overdoses. No specific antidotes for bupropion are known.
Due to the dose-related risk of seizures with WELLBUTRIN SR, hospitalization following suspected overdose should be considered. Based on studies in animals, it is recommended that seizures be treated with intravenous benzodiazepine administration and other supportive measures, as appropriate.
In managing overdosage, consider the possibility of multiple drug involvement. The physician should consider contacting a poison control center for additional information on the treatment of any overdose. Telephone numbers for certified poison control centers are listed in the *Physicians' Desk Reference* (PDR).

DOSAGE AND ADMINISTRATION

General Dosing Considerations: It is particularly important to administer WELLBUTRIN SR Tablets in a manner most likely to minimize the risk of seizure (see WARNINGS). Gradual escalation in dosage is also important if agitation, motor restlessness, and insomnia, often seen during the initial days of treatment, are to be minimized. If necessary, these effects may be managed by temporary reduction of dose or the short-term administration of an intermediate to long-acting sedative hypnotic. A sedative hypnotic usually is not required beyond the first week of treatment. Insomnia may also be minimized by avoiding bedtime doses. If distressing, untoward effects supervene, dose escalation should be stopped. WELLBUTRIN SR should be swallowed whole and not crushed, divided, or chewed.
Initial Treatment: The usual adult target dose for WELLBUTRIN SR Tablets is 300 mg/day, given as 150 mg twice daily. Dosing with WELLBUTRIN SR Tablets should begin at 150 mg/day given as a single daily dose in the morning. If the 150-mg initial dose is adequately tolerated, an increase to the 300-mg/day target dose, given as 150 mg twice daily, may be made as early as day 4 of dosing. There should be an interval of at least 8 hours between successive doses.
Increasing the Dosage Above 300 mg/day: As with other antidepressants, the full antidepressant effect of WELLBUTRIN SR Tablets may not be evident until 4 weeks of treatment or longer. An increase in dosage to the maximum of 400 mg/day, given as 200 mg twice daily, may be considered for patients in whom no clinical improvement is noted after several weeks of treatment at 300 mg/day.
Maintenance Treatment: It is generally agreed that acute episodes of depression require several months or longer of sustained pharmacological therapy beyond response to the acute episode. In a study in which patients with major depressive disorder, recurrent type, who had responded during 8 weeks of acute treatment with WELLBUTRIN SR were assigned randomly to placebo or to the same dose of WELLBUTRIN SR (150 mg twice daily) during 44 weeks of maintenance treatment as they had received during the acute stabilization phase, longer-term efficacy was demonstrated (see CLINICAL TRIALS under CLINICAL PHARMACOLOGY). Based on these limited data, it is unknown whether or not the dose of WELLBUTRIN SR needed for maintenance treatment is identical to the dose needed to achieve an initial response. Patients should be periodically reassessed to determine the need for maintenance treatment and the appropriate dose for such treatment.
Dosage Adjustment for Patients with Impaired Hepatic Function: WELLBUTRIN SR should be used with extreme caution in patients with severe hepatic cirrhosis. The dose should not exceed 100 mg every day or 150 mg every other day in these patients. WELLBUTRIN SR should be used with caution in patients with hepatic impairment (including mild to moderate hepatic cirrhosis) and a reduced frequency and/or dose should be considered in patients with mild to moderate hepatic cirrhosis (see CLINICAL PHARMACOLOGY, WARNINGS, and PRECAUTIONS).
Dosage Adjustment for Patients with Impaired Renal Function: WELLBUTRIN SR should be used with caution in patients with renal impairment and a reduced frequency and/or dose should be considered (see CLINICAL PHARMACOLOGY and PRECAUTIONS).

HOW SUPPLIED

WELLBUTRIN SR Sustained-Release Tablets, 100 mg of bupropion hydrochloride, are blue, round, biconvex, film-coated tablets printed with "WELLBUTRIN SR 100" in bottles of 60 (NDC 0173-0947-55) tablets.
WELLBUTRIN SR Sustained-Release Tablets, 150 mg of bupropion hydrochloride, are purple, round, biconvex, film-coated tablets printed with "WELLBUTRIN SR 150" in bottles of 60 (NDC 0173-0135-55) tablets.
WELLBUTRIN SR Sustained-Release Tablets, 200 mg of bupropion hydrochloride, are light pink, round, biconvex, film-coated tablets printed with "WELLBUTRIN SR 200" in bottles of 60 (NDC 0173-0722-00) tablets.
Store at controlled room temperature, 20° to 25°C (68° to 77°F) [see USP]. Dispense in a tight, light-resistant container as defined in the USP.
Distributed by:
GlaxoSmithKline, Research Triangle Park, NC 27709
Manufactured by:
GlaxoSmithKline, Research Triangle Park, NC 27709
or DSM Pharmaceuticals, Inc., Greenville, NC 27834

April 2004/RL-2075
Shown in Product Identification Guide, page 317

WELLBUTRIN XL™ ℞

[wel'byū-trin]
(bupropion hydrochloride extended-release tablets)

DESCRIPTION

WELLBUTRIN XL (bupropion hydrochloride), an antidepressant of the aminoketone class, is chemically unrelated to tricyclic, tetracyclic, selective serotonin re-uptake inhibitor, or other known antidepressant agents. Its structure closely resembles that of diethylpropion; it is related to phenylethylamines. It is designated as (±)-1-(3-chlorophenyl)-2-[(1,1-dimethylethyl)amino]-1-propanone hydrochloride. The molecular weight is 276.2. The molecular formula is $C_{13}H_{18}ClNO \bullet HCl$. Bupropion hydrochloride powder is white, crystalline, and highly soluble in water. It has a bitter taste and produces the sensation of local anesthesia on the oral mucosa. The structural formula is:

NHC(CH$_3$)$_3$
COCHCH$_3$
• HCl
Cl

WELLBUTRIN XL Tablets are supplied for oral administration as 150-mg and 300-mg, creamy-white to pale yellow extended-release tablets. Each tablet contains the labeled amount of bupropion hydrochloride and the inactive ingredients: ethylcellulose aqueous dispersion (NF), glyceryl behenate, methacrylic acid copolymer dispersion (NF), polyvinyl alcohol, polyethylene glycol, povidone, silicon dioxide, and triethyl citrate. The tablets are printed with edible black ink.
The insoluble shell of the extended-release tablet may remain intact during gastrointestinal transit and is eliminated in the feces.

CLINICAL PHARMACOLOGY

Pharmacodynamics: Bupropion is a relatively weak inhibitor of the neuronal uptake of norepinephrine, serotonin, and dopamine, and does not inhibit monoamine oxidase. While the mechanism of action of bupropion, as with other antidepressants, is unknown, it is presumed that this action is mediated by noradrenergic and/or dopaminergic mechanisms.
Pharmacokinetics: Bupropion is a racemic mixture. The pharmacologic activity and pharmacokinetics of the individual enantiomers have not been studied. The mean elimination half-life (±SD) of bupropion after chronic dosing is 21 (±9) hours, and steady-state plasma concentrations of bupropion are reached within 8 days.
In a study comparing 14-day dosing with WELLBUTRIN XL Tablets 300 mg once daily to the immediate-release formulation of bupropion at 100 mg 3 times daily, equivalence was demonstrated for peak plasma concentration and area under the curve for bupropion and the 3 metabolites (hydroxybupropion, threohydrobupropion, and erythrohydrobupropion).
Absorption: Following oral administration of WELLBUTRIN XL Tablets to healthy volunteers, time to peak plasma concentrations for bupropion was approximately 5 hours and food did not affect the C_{max} or AUC of bupropion.
Distribution: In vitro tests show that bupropion is 84% bound to human plasma proteins at concentrations up to 200 mcg/mL. The extent of protein binding of the hydroxybupropion metabolite is similar to that for bupropion, whereas the extent of protein binding of the threohydrobupropion metabolite is about half that seen with bupropion.
Metabolism: Bupropion is extensively metabolized in humans. Three metabolites have been shown to be active: hydroxybupropion, which is formed via hydroxylation of the *tert*-butyl group of bupropion, and the amino-alcohol isomers threohydrobupropion and erythrohydrobupropion, which are formed via reduction of the carbonyl group. In vitro findings suggest that cytochrome P450IIB6 (CYP2B6) is the principal isoenzyme involved in the formation of hydroxybupropion, while cytochrome P450 isoenzymes are not involved in the formation of threohydrobupropion. Oxidation of the bupropion side chain results in the formation of a

Continued on next page

Product information on these pages is effective as of August 2004. Further information is available at: GlaxoSmithKline, PO Box 13398, Research Triangle Park, NC 27709. 1-888-825-5249. Corporate Web Site: www.gsk.com

Wellbutrin XL—Cont.

glycine conjugate of meta-chlorobenzoic acid, which is then excreted as the major urinary metabolite. The potency and toxicity of the metabolites relative to bupropion have not been fully characterized. However, it has been demonstrated in an antidepressant screening test in mice that hydroxybupropion is one half as potent as bupropion, while threohydrobupropion and erythrohydrobupropion are 5-fold less potent than bupropion. This may be of clinical importance because the plasma concentrations of the metabolites are as high or higher than those of bupropion.

Because bupropion is extensively metabolized, there is the potential for drug-drug interactions, particularly with those agents that are metabolized by the cytochrome P450IIB6 (CYP2B6) isoenzyme. Although bupropion is not metabolized by cytochrome P450IID6 (CYP2D6), there is the potential for drug-drug interactions when bupropion is co-administered with drugs metabolized by this isoenzyme (see PRECAUTIONS: Drug Interactions).

In humans, peak plasma concentrations of hydroxybupropion occur approximately 7 hours after administration of WELLBUTRIN XL. Following administration of WELLBUTRIN XL, peak plasma concentrations of hydroxybupropion are approximately 7 times the peak level of the parent drug at steady state. The elimination half-life of hydroxybupropion is approximately 20 (±5) hours, and its AUC at steady state is about 13 times that of bupropion. The times to peak concentrations for the erythrohydrobupropion and threohydrobupropion metabolites are similar to that of the hydroxybupropion metabolite. However, their elimination half-lives are longer, approximately 33 (±10) and 37 (±13) hours, respectively, and steady-state AUCs are 1.4 and 7 times that of bupropion, respectively.

Bupropion and its metabolites exhibit linear kinetics following chronic administration of 300 to 450 mg/day.

Elimination: Following oral administration of 200 mg of ^{14}C-bupropion in humans, 87% and 10% of the radioactive dose were recovered in the urine and feces, respectively. However, the fraction of the oral dose of bupropion excreted unchanged was only 0.5%, a finding consistent with the extensive metabolism of bupropion.

Population Subgroups: Factors or conditions altering metabolic capacity (e.g., liver disease, congestive heart failure [CHF], age, concomitant medications, etc.) or elimination may be expected to influence the degree and extent of accumulation of the active metabolites of bupropion. The elimination of the major metabolites of bupropion may be affected by reduced renal or hepatic function because they are moderately polar compounds and are likely to undergo further metabolism or conjugation in the liver prior to urinary excretion.

Hepatic: The effect of hepatic impairment on the pharmacokinetics of bupropion was characterized in 2 single-dose studies, one in patients with alcoholic liver disease and one in patients with mild to severe cirrhosis. The first study showed that the half-life of hydroxybupropion was significantly longer in 8 patients with alcoholic liver disease than in 8 healthy volunteers (32±14 hours versus 21±5 hours, respectively). Although not statistically significant, the AUCs for bupropion and hydroxybupropion were more variable and tended to be greater (by 53% to 57%) in patients with alcoholic liver disease. The differences in half-life for bupropion and the other metabolites in the 2 patient groups were minimal.

The second study showed no statistically significant differences in the pharmacokinetics of bupropion and its active metabolites in 9 patients with mild to moderate hepatic cirrhosis compared to 8 healthy volunteers. However, more variability was observed in some of the pharmacokinetic parameters for bupropion (AUC, C_{max}, and T_{max}) and its active metabolites ($t_{½}$) in patients with mild to moderate hepatic cirrhosis. In addition, in patients with severe hepatic cirrhosis, the bupropion C_{max} and AUC were substantially increased (mean difference: by approximately 70% and 3-fold, respectively) and more variable when compared to values in healthy volunteers; the mean bupropion half-life was also longer (29 hours in patients with severe hepatic cirrhosis vs 19 hours in healthy subjects). For the metabolite hydroxybupropion, the mean C_{max} was approximately 69% lower. For the combined amino-alcohol isomers threohydrobupropion and erythrohydrobupropion, the mean C_{max} was approximately 31% lower. The mean AUC increased by about 1½-fold for hydroxybupropion and about 2½-fold for threo/erythrohydrobupropion. The median T_{max} was observed 19 hours later for hydroxybupropion and 31 hours later for threo/erythrohydrobupropion. The mean half-lives for hydroxybupropion and threo/erythrohydrobupropion were increased 5- and 2-fold, respectively, in patients with severe hepatic cirrhosis compared to healthy volunteers (see WARNINGS, PRECAUTIONS, and DOSAGE AND ADMINISTRATION).

Renal: The effect of renal disease on the pharmacokinetics of bupropion has not been studied. The elimination of the major metabolites of bupropion may be affected by reduced renal function.

Left Ventricular Dysfunction: During a chronic dosing study with bupropion in 14 depressed patients with left ventricular dysfunction (history of CHF or an enlarged heart on x-ray), no apparent effect on the pharmacokinetics of bupropion or its metabolites was revealed, compared to healthy volunteers.

Age: The effects of age on the pharmacokinetics of bupropion and its metabolites have not been fully characterized, but an exploration of steady-state bupropion concentrations from several depression efficacy studies involving patients dosed in a range of 300 to 750 mg/day, on a 3 times daily schedule, revealed no relationship between age (18 to 83 years) and plasma concentration of bupropion. A single-dose pharmacokinetic study demonstrated that the disposition of bupropion and its metabolites in elderly subjects was similar to that of younger subjects. These data suggest there is no prominent effect of age on bupropion concentration; however, another pharmacokinetic study, single and multiple dose, has suggested that the elderly are at increased risk for accumulation of bupropion and its metabolites (see PRECAUTIONS: Geriatric Use).

Gender: A single-dose study involving 12 healthy male and 12 healthy female volunteers revealed no sex-related differences in the pharmacokinetic parameters of bupropion.

Smokers: The effects of cigarette smoking on the pharmacokinetics of bupropion were studied in 34 healthy male and female volunteers; 17 were chronic cigarette smokers and 17 were nonsmokers. Following oral administration of a single 150-mg dose of bupropion, there was no statistically significant difference in C_{max}, half-life, T_{max}, AUC, or clearance of bupropion or its active metabolites between smokers and nonsmokers.

CLINICAL TRIALS

The efficacy of bupropion as a treatment for major depressive disorder was established with the immediate-release formulation of bupropion in two 4-week, placebo-controlled trials in adult inpatients and in one 6-week, placebo-controlled trial in adult outpatients. In the first study, patients were titrated in a bupropion dose range of 300 to 600 mg/day of the immediate-release formulation on a 3 times daily schedule; 78% of patients received maximum doses of 450 mg/day or less. This trial demonstrated the effectiveness of bupropion on the Hamilton Depression Rating Scale (HDRS) total score, the depressed mood item (item 1) from that scale, and the Clinical Global Impressions (CGI) severity score. A second study included 2 fixed doses of the immediate-release formulation of bupropion (300 and 450 mg/day) and placebo. This trial demonstrated the effectiveness of bupropion, but only at the 450-mg/day dose of the immediate-release formulation; the results were positive for the HDRS total score and the CGI severity score, but not for HDRS item 1. In the third study, outpatients received 300 mg/day of the immediate-release formulation of bupropion. This study demonstrated the effectiveness of bupropion on the HDRS total score, HDRS item 1, the Montgomery-Asberg Depression Rating Scale, the CGI severity score, and the CGI improvement score.

Although there are no independent trials demonstrating the antidepressant effectiveness of WELLBUTRIN XL, studies have demonstrated similar bioavailability of the immediate-release and the extended-release formulations of bupropion under steady-state conditions, i.e., WELLBUTRIN XL 300 mg once daily was shown to have bioavailability that was similar to that of 100 mg 3 times daily of the immediate-release formulation of bupropion, with regard to both rate and extent of absorption, for parent drug and metabolites.

In a longer-term study, outpatients meeting DSM-IV criteria for major depressive disorder, recurrent type, who had responded during an 8-week open trial on bupropion (150 mg twice daily of the sustained-release formulation) were randomized to continuation of their same dose of bupropion or placebo, for up to 44 weeks of observation for relapse. Response during the open phase was defined as CGI Improvement score of 1 (very much improved) or 2 (much improved) for each of the final 3 weeks. Relapse during the double-blind phase was defined as the investigator's judgment that drug treatment was needed for worsening depressive symptoms. Patients receiving continued bupropion treatment experienced significantly lower relapse rates over the subsequent 44 weeks compared to those receiving placebo.

INDICATIONS AND USAGE

WELLBUTRIN XL is indicated for the treatment of major depressive disorder.

The efficacy of bupropion in the treatment of a major depressive episode was established in two 4-week controlled trials of inpatients and in one 6-week controlled trial of outpatients whose diagnoses corresponded most closely to the Major Depression category of the APA Diagnostic and Statistical Manual (DSM) (see CLINICAL PHARMACOLOGY).

A major depressive episode (DSM-IV) implies the presence of 1) depressed mood or 2) loss of interest or pleasure; in addition, at least 5 of the following symptoms have been present during the same 2-week period and represent a change from previous functioning: depressed mood, markedly diminished interest or pleasure in usual activities, significant change in weight and/or appetite, insomnia or hypersomnia, psychomotor agitation or retardation, increased fatigue, feelings of guilt or worthlessness, slowed thinking or impaired concentration, a suicide attempt, or suicidal ideation.

The efficacy of bupropion in maintaining an antidepressant response for up to 44 weeks following 8 weeks of acute treatment was demonstrated in a placebo-controlled trial with the sustained-release formulation of bupropion (see CLINICAL PHARMACOLOGY). Nevertheless, the physician who elects to use WELLBUTRIN XL for extended periods should periodically reevaluate the long-term usefulness of the drug for the individual patient.

CONTRAINDICATIONS

WELLBUTRIN XL is contraindicated in patients with a seizure disorder.

WELLBUTRIN XL is contraindicated in patients treated with ZYBAN® (bupropion hydrochloride) Sustained-Release Tablets, WELLBUTRIN (bupropion hydrochloride) the immediate-release formulation, WELLBUTRIN SR (bupropion hydrochloride) the sustained-release formulation, or any other medications that contain bupropion because the incidence of seizure is dose dependent.

WELLBUTRIN XL is contraindicated in patients with a current or prior diagnosis of bulimia or anorexia nervosa because of a higher incidence of seizures noted in patients treated for bulimia with the immediate-release formulation of bupropion.

WELLBUTRIN XL is contraindicated in patients undergoing abrupt discontinuation of alcohol or sedatives (including benzodiazepines).

The concurrent administration of WELLBUTRIN XL Tablets and a monoamine oxidase (MAO) inhibitor is contraindicated. At least 14 days should elapse between discontinuation of an MAO inhibitor and initiation of treatment with WELLBUTRIN XL Tablets.

WELLBUTRIN XL is contraindicated in patients who have shown an allergic response to bupropion or the other ingredients that make up WELLBUTRIN XL Tablets.

WARNINGS

Patients should be made aware that WELLBUTRIN XL contains the same active ingredient found in ZYBAN, used as an aid to smoking cessation treatment, and that WELLBUTRIN XL should not be used in combination with ZYBAN, or any other medications that contain bupropion, such as WELLBUTRIN SR (bupropion hydrochloride), the sustained-release formulation or WELLBUTRIN (bupropion hydrochloride), the immediate-release formulation.

Seizures: Bupropion is associated with a dose-related risk of seizures. The risk of seizures is also related to patient factors, clinical situations, and concomitant medications, which must be considered in selection of patients for therapy with WELLBUTRIN XL. WELLBUTRIN XL should be discontinued and not restarted in patients who experience a seizure while on treatment.

As both WELLBUTRIN XL and the sustained-release formulation of bupropion (WELLBUTRIN SR) are bioequivalent to the immediate-release formulation of bupropion, the seizure incidence with WELLBUTRIN XL, while not formally evaluated in clinical trials, may be similar to that presented below for the immediate-release and sustained-release formulations of bupropion.

- **Dose: At doses up to 300 mg/day of the sustained-release formulation of bupropion (WELLBUTRIN SR), the incidence of seizure is approximately 0.1% (1/1,000).**
  Data for the immediate-release formulation of bupropion revealed a seizure incidence of approximately 0.4% (i.e., 13 of 3,200 patients followed prospectively) in patients treated at doses in a range of 300 to 450 mg/day. This seizure incidence (0.4%) may exceed that of some other marketed antidepressants.
  Additional data accumulated for the immediate-release formulation of bupropion suggested that the estimated seizure incidence increases almost tenfold between 450 and 600 mg/day. The 600 mg dose is twice the usual adult dose and one and one-third the maximum recommended daily dose (450 mg) of WELLBUTRIN XL Tablets. This disproportionate increase in seizure incidence with dose incrementation calls for caution in dosing.
- **Patient factors: Predisposing factors that may increase the risk of seizure with bupropion use include history of head trauma or prior seizure, central nervous system (CNS) tumor, the presence of severe hepatic cirrhosis, and concomitant medications that lower seizure threshold.**
- **Clinical situations: Circumstances associated with an increased seizure risk include, among others, excessive use of alcohol or sedatives (including benzodiazepines); addiction to opiates, cocaine, or stimulants; use of over-the-counter stimulants and anorectics; and diabetes treated with oral hypoglycemics or insulin.**
- **Concomitant medications: Many medications (e.g., antipsychotics, antidepressants, theophylline, systemic steroids) are known to lower seizure threshold.**

Recommendations for Reducing the Risk of Seizure: **Retrospective analysis of clinical experience gained during the development of bupropion suggests that the risk of seizure may be minimized if**

- **the total daily dose of WELLBUTRIN XL Tablets does *not* exceed 450 mg,**
- **the rate of incrementation of dose is gradual.**

WELLBUTRIN XL should be administered with extreme caution to patients with a history of seizure, cranial trauma, or other predisposition(s) toward seizure, or patients treated with other agents (e.g., antipsychotics, other antidepressants, theophylline, systemic steroids, etc.) that lower seizure threshold.

Hepatic Impairment: WELLBUTRIN XL should be used with extreme caution in patients with severe hepatic cirrhosis. In these patients a reduced frequency and/or dose is required, as peak bupropion, as well as AUC, levels are substantially increased and accumulation is likely to occur in such patients to a greater extent than usual. The dose

should not exceed 150 mg every other day in these patients (see CLINICAL PHARMACOLOGY, PRECAUTIONS, and DOSAGE AND ADMINISTRATION).

Potential for Hepatotoxicity: In rats receiving large doses of bupropion chronically, there was an increase in incidence of hepatic hyperplastic nodules and hepatocellular hypertrophy. In dogs receiving large doses of bupropion chronically, various histologic changes were seen in the liver, and laboratory tests suggesting mild hepatocellular injury were noted.

Clinical Worsening and Suicide Risk: Patients with major depressive disorder, both adult and pediatric, may experience worsening of their depression and/or the emergence of suicidal ideation and behavior (suicidality), whether or not they are taking antidepressant medications, and this risk may persist until significant remission occurs. Although there has been a long-standing concern that antidepressants may have a role in inducing worsening of depression and the emergence of suicidality in certain patients, a causal role for antidepressants in inducing such behaviors has not been established. **Nevertheless, patients being treated with antidepressants should be observed closely for clinical worsening and suicidality, especially at the beginning of a course of drug therapy, or at the time of dose changes, either increases or decreases.** Consideration should be given to changing the therapeutic regimen, including possibly discontinuing the medication in patients whose depression is persistently worse or whose emergent suicidality is severe, abrupt in onset, or was not part of the patient's presenting symptoms.

Because of the possibility of co-morbidity between major depressive disorder and other psychiatric and nonpsychiatric disorders, the same precautions observed when treating patients with major depressive disorder should be observed when treating patients with other psychiatric and nonpsychiatric disorders.

The following symptoms, anxiety, agitation, panic attacks, insomnia, irritability, hostility (aggressiveness), impulsivity, akathisia (psychomotor restlessness), hypomania, and mania, have been reported in adult and pediatric patients being treated with antidepressants for major depressive disorder as well as for other indications, both psychiatric and nonpsychiatric. Although a causal link between the emergence of such symptoms and either the worsening of depression and/or the emergence of suicidal impulses has not been established, consideration should be given to changing the therapeutic regimen, including possibly discontinuing the medication in patients for whom such symptoms are severe, abrupt in onset, or were not part of the patient's presenting symptoms.

Families and caregivers of patients being treated with antidepressants for major depressive disorder or other indications, both psychiatric and nonpsychiatric, should be alerted about the need to monitor patients for the emergence of agitation, irritability, and the other symptoms described above, as well as the emergence of suicidality, and to report such symptoms immediately to health care providers. Prescriptions for WELLBUTRIN XL should be written for the smallest quantity of tablets consistent with good patient management, in order to reduce the risk of overdose.

It should be noted that WELLBUTRIN XL is not approved for use in treating any indications in the pediatric population.

A major depressive episode may be the initial presentation of bipolar disorder. It is generally believed (although not established in controlled trials) that treating such an episode with an antidepressant alone may increase the likelihood of precipitation of a mixed/manic episode in patients at risk for bipolar disorder. Whether any of the symptoms described above represent such a conversion is unknown. However, prior to initiating treatment with an antidepressant, patients should be adequately screened to determine if they are at risk for bipolar disorder; such screening should include a detailed psychiatric history, including a family history of suicide, bipolar disorder, and depression. It should be noted that WELLBUTRIN XL is not approved for use in treating bipolar depression.

PRECAUTIONS

General: ***Agitation and Insomnia:*** Increased restlessness, agitation, anxiety, and insomnia, especially shortly after initiation of treatment, have been associated with treatment with bupropion. Patients in placebo-controlled trials with WELLBUTRIN SR, the sustained-release formulation of bupropion, experienced agitation, anxiety, and insomnia as shown in Table 1.

[See table 1 above]

In clinical studies, these symptoms were sometimes of sufficient magnitude to require treatment with sedative/hypnotic drugs.

Symptoms were sufficiently severe to require discontinuation of treatment in 1% and 2.6% of patients treated with 300 and 400 mg/day, respectively, of bupropion sustained-release tablets and 0.8% of patients treated with placebo.

Psychosis, Confusion, and Other Neuropsychiatric Phenomena: Depressed patients treated with bupropion have been reported to show a variety of neuropsychiatric signs and symptoms, including delusions, hallucinations, psychosis, concentration disturbance, paranoia, and confusion. In some cases, these symptoms abated upon dose reduction and/or withdrawal of treatment.

Activation of Psychosis and/or Mania: Antidepressants can precipitate manic episodes in bipolar disorder patients during the depressed phase of their illness and may activate latent psychosis in other susceptible patients. WELLBUTRIN XL is expected to pose similar risks.

Table 1. Incidence of Agitation, Anxiety, and Insomnia in Placebo-Controlled Trials

Adverse Event Term	WELLBUTRIN SR 300 mg/day (n = 376)	WELLBUTRIN SR 400 mg/day (n = 114)	Placebo (n = 385)
Agitation	3%	9%	2%
Anxiety	5%	6%	3%
Insomnia	11%	16%	6%

Table 2. Incidence of Weight Gain and Weight Loss in Placebo-Controlled Trials

Weight Change	WELLBUTRIN SR 300 mg/day (n = 339)	WELLBUTRIN SR 400 mg/day (n = 112)	Placebo (n = 347)
Gained >5 lbs	3%	2%	4%
Lost >5 lbs	14%	19%	6%

Altered Appetite and Weight: In placebo-controlled studies using WELLBUTRIN SR, the sustained-release formulation of bupropion, patients experienced weight gain or weight loss as shown in Table 2.

[See table 2 above]

In studies conducted with the immediate-release formulation of bupropion, 35% of patients receiving tricyclic antidepressants gained weight, compared to 9% of patients treated with the immediate-release formulation of bupropion. If weight loss is a major presenting sign of a patient's depressive illness, the anorectic and/or weight-reducing potential of WELLBUTRIN XL Tablets should be considered.

Allergic Reactions: Anaphylactoid/anaphylactic reactions characterized by symptoms such as pruritus, urticaria, angioedema, and dyspnea requiring medical treatment have been reported in clinical trials with bupropion. In addition, there have been rare spontaneous postmarketing reports of erythema multiforme, Stevens-Johnson syndrome, and anaphylactic shock associated with bupropion. A patient should stop taking WELLBUTRIN XL and consult a doctor if experiencing allergic or anaphylactoid/anaphylactic reactions (e.g., skin rash, pruritus, hives, chest pain, edema, and shortness of breath) during treatment.

Arthralgia, myalgia, and fever with rash and other symptoms suggestive of delayed hypersensitivity have been reported in association with bupropion. These symptoms may resemble serum sickness.

Cardiovascular Effects: In clinical practice, hypertension, in some cases severe, requiring acute treatment, has been reported in patients receiving bupropion alone and in combination with nicotine replacement therapy. These events have been observed in both patients with and without evidence of pre-existing hypertension.

Data from a comparative study of the sustained-release formulation of bupropion (ZYBAN® Sustained-Release Tablets), nicotine transdermal system (NTS), the combination of sustained-release bupropion plus NTS, and placebo as an aid to smoking cessation suggest a higher incidence of treatment-emergent hypertension in patients treated with the combination of sustained-release bupropion and NTS. In this study, 6.1% of patients treated with the combination of sustained-release bupropion and NTS had treatment-emergent hypertension compared to 2.5%, 1.6%, and 3.1% of patients treated with sustained-release bupropion, NTS, and placebo, respectively. The majority of these patients had evidence of pre-existing hypertension. Three patients (1.2%) treated with the combination of ZYBAN and NTS and 1 patient (0.4%) treated with NTS had study medication discontinued due to hypertension compared to none of the patients treated with ZYBAN or placebo. Monitoring of blood pressure is recommended in patients who receive the combination of bupropion and nicotine replacement.

There is no clinical experience establishing the safety of WELLBUTRIN XL Tablets in patients with a recent history of myocardial infarction or unstable heart disease. Therefore, care should be exercised if it is used in these groups. Bupropion was well tolerated in depressed patients who had previously developed orthostatic hypotension while receiving tricyclic antidepressants, and was also generally well tolerated in a group of 36 depressed inpatients with stable congestive heart failure (CHF). However, bupropion was associated with a rise in supine blood pressure in the study of patients with CHF, resulting in discontinuation of treatment in 2 patients for exacerbation of baseline hypertension.

Hepatic Impairment: WELLBUTRIN XL should be used with extreme caution in patients with severe hepatic cirrhosis. In these patients, a reduced frequency and/or dose is required. WELLBUTRIN XL should be used with caution in patients with hepatic impairment (including mild to moderate hepatic cirrhosis) and reduced frequency and/or dose should be considered in patients with mild to moderate hepatic cirrhosis.

All patients with hepatic impairment should be closely monitored for possible adverse effects that could indicate high drug and metabolite levels (see CLINICAL PHARMACOLOGY, WARNINGS, and DOSAGE AND ADMINISTRATION).

Renal Impairment: No studies have been conducted in patients with renal impairment. Bupropion is extensively metabolized in the liver to active metabolites, which are further metabolized and subsequently excreted by the kidneys. WELLBUTRIN XL should be used with caution in patients with renal impairment and a reduced frequency and/or dose should be considered as bupropion and its metabolites may accumulate in such patients to a greater extent than usual. The patient should be closely monitored for possible adverse effects that could indicate high drug or metabolite levels.

Information for Patients: See the tear-off leaflet accompanying the product for Patient Information.

Patients should be made aware that WELLBUTRIN XL contains the same active ingredient found in ZYBAN, used as an aid to smoking cessation treatment, and that WELLBUTRIN XL should not be used in combination with ZYBAN or any other medications that contain bupropion hydrochloride (such as WELLBUTRIN SR, the sustained-release formulation, and WELLBUTRIN, the immediate-release formulation).

Physicians are advised to discuss the following issues with patients:

Patients should be told that WELLBUTRIN XL should be discontinued and not restarted if they experience a seizure while on treatment.

Patients should be told that any CNS-active drug like WELLBUTRIN XL Tablets may impair their ability to perform tasks requiring judgment or motor and cognitive skills. Consequently, until they are reasonably certain that WELLBUTRIN XL Tablets do not adversely affect their performance, they should refrain from driving an automobile or operating complex, hazardous machinery.

Patients should be told that the excessive use or abrupt discontinuation of alcohol or sedatives (including benzodiazepines) may alter the seizure threshold. Some patients have reported lower alcohol tolerance during treatment with WELLBUTRIN XL. Patients should be advised that the consumption of alcohol should be minimized or avoided.

Patients and their families should be encouraged to be alert to the emergence of anxiety, agitation, panic attacks, insomnia, irritability, hostility, impulsivity, akathisia, hypomania, mania, worsening of depression, and suicidal ideation, especially early during antidepressant treatment. Such symptoms should be reported to the patient's physician, especially if they are severe, abrupt in onset, or were not part of the patient's presenting symptoms.

Patients should be advised to inform their physicians if they are taking or plan to take any prescription or over-the-counter drugs. Concern is warranted because WELLBUTRIN XL Tablets and other drugs may affect each other's metabolism.

Patients should be advised to notify their physicians if they become pregnant or intend to become pregnant during therapy.

Patients should be advised to swallow WELLBUTRIN XL Tablets whole so that the release rate is not altered. Do not chew, divide, or crush tablets.

Patients should be advised that they may notice in their stool something that looks like a tablet. This is normal. The medication in WELLBUTRIN XL is contained in a nonabsorbable shell that has been specially designed to slowly release drug in the body. When this process is completed, the empty shell is eliminated from the body.

Laboratory Tests: There are no specific laboratory tests recommended.

Drug Interactions: Few systemic data have been collected on the metabolism of bupropion following concomitant administration with other drugs or, alternatively, the effect of concomitant administration of bupropion on the metabolism of other drugs.

Because bupropion is extensively metabolized, the coadministration of other drugs may affect its clinical activity. In vitro studies indicate that bupropion is primarily metabolized to hydroxybupropion by the CYP2B6 isoenzyme. Therefore, the potential exists for a drug interaction between WELLBUTRIN XL and drugs that are substrates or inhibitors of the CYP2B6 isoenzyme (e.g., orphenadrine, thiotepa, and cyclophosphamide). In addition, in vitro studies suggest that paroxetine, sertraline, norfluoxetine, and fluvoxamine

Continued on next page

Product information on these pages is effective as of August 2004. Further information is available at: GlaxoSmithKline, PO Box 13398, Research Triangle Park, NC 27709. 1-888-825-5249. Corporate Web Site: www.gsk.com

Wellbutrin XL—Cont.

as well as nelfinavir, ritonavir, and efavirenz inhibit the hydroxylation of bupropion. No clinical studies have been performed to evaluate this finding. The threohydrobupropion metabolite of bupropion does not appear to be produced by the cytochrome P450 isoenzymes. The effects of concomitant administration of cimetidine on the pharmacokinetics of bupropion and its active metabolites were studied in 24 healthy young male volunteers. Following oral administration of two 150-mg tablets of the sustained-release formulation of bupropion with and without 800 mg of cimetidine, the pharmacokinetics of bupropion and hydroxybupropion were unaffected. However, there were 16% and 32% increases in the AUC and C_{max}, respectively, of the combined moieties of threohydrobupropion and erythrohydrobupropion.

While not systematically studied, certain drugs may induce the metabolism of bupropion (e.g., carbamazepine, phenobarbital, phenytoin).

Animal data indicated that bupropion may be an inducer of drug-metabolizing enzymes in humans. In one study, following chronic administration of bupropion, 100 mg 3 times daily to 8 healthy male volunteers for 14 days, there was no evidence of induction of its own metabolism. Nevertheless, there may be the potential for clinically important alterations of blood levels of coadministered drugs.

Drugs Metabolized By Cytochrome P450IID6 (CYP2D6): Many drugs, including most antidepressants (SSRIs, many tricyclics), beta-blockers, antiarrhythmics, and antipsychotics are metabolized by the CYP2D6 isoenzyme. Although bupropion is not metabolized by this isoenzyme, bupropion and hydroxybupropion are inhibitors of CYP2D6 isoenzyme in vitro. In a study of 15 male subjects (ages 19 to 35 years) who were extensive metabolizers of the CYP2D6 isoenzyme, daily doses of bupropion given as 150 mg twice daily followed by a single dose of 50 mg desipramine increased the C_{max}, AUC, and $t_{½}$ of desipramine by an average of approximately 2-, 5-, and 2-fold, respectively. The effect was present for at least 7 days after the last dose of bupropion. Concomitant use of bupropion with other drugs metabolized by CYP2D6 has not been formally studied.

Therefore, co-administration of bupropion with drugs that are metabolized by CYP2D6 isoenzyme including certain antidepressants (e.g., nortriptyline, imipramine, desipramine, paroxetine, fluoxetine, sertraline), antipsychotics (e.g., haloperidol, risperidone, thioridazine), beta-blockers (e.g., metoprolol), and Type 1C antiarrhythmics (e.g., propafenone, flecainide), should be approached with caution and should be initiated at the lower end of the dose range of the concomitant medication. If bupropion is added to the treatment regimen of a patient already receiving a drug metabolized by CYP2D6, the need to decrease the dose of the original medication should be considered, particularly for those concomitant medications with a narrow therapeutic index.

MAO Inhibitors: Studies in animals demonstrate that the acute toxicity of bupropion is enhanced by the MAO inhibitor phenelzine (see CONTRAINDICATIONS).

Levodopa and Amantadine: Limited clinical data suggest a higher incidence of adverse experiences in patients receiving bupropion concurrently with either levodopa or amantadine. Administration of WELLBUTRIN XL Tablets to patients receiving either levodopa or amantadine concurrently should be undertaken with caution, using small initial doses and gradual dose increases.

Drugs That Lower Seizure Threshold: Concurrent administration of WELLBUTRIN XL Tablets and agents (e.g., antipsychotics, other antidepressants, theophylline, systemic steroids, etc.) that lower seizure threshold should be undertaken only with extreme caution (see WARNINGS). Low initial dosing and gradual dose increases should be employed.

Nicotine Transdermal System: (see PRECAUTIONS: Cardiovascular Effects).

Alcohol: In postmarketing experience, there have been rare reports of adverse neuropsychiatric events or reduced alcohol tolerance in patients who were drinking alcohol during treatment with bupropion. The consumption of alcohol during treatment with WELLBUTRIN XL should be minimized or avoided (also see CONTRAINDICATIONS).

Carcinogenesis, Mutagenesis, Impairment of Fertility: Lifetime carcinogenicity studies were performed in rats and mice at doses up to 300 and 150 mg/kg/day, respectively. These doses are approximately 7 and 2 times the maximum recommended human dose (MRHD), respectively, on a mg/m² basis. In the rat study there was an increase in nodular proliferative lesions of the liver at doses of 100 to 300 mg/kg/day (approximately 2 to 7 times the MRHD on a mg/m² basis); lower doses were not tested. The question of whether or not such lesions may be precursors of neoplasms of the liver is currently unresolved. Similar liver lesions were not seen in the mouse study, and no increase in malignant tumors of the liver and other organs was seen in either study.

Bupropion produced a positive response (2 to 3 times control mutation rate) in 2 of 5 strains in the Ames bacterial mutagenicity test and an increase in chromosomal aberrations in 1 of 3 in vivo rat bone marrow cytogenetic studies.

A fertility study in rats at doses up to 300 mg/kg/day revealed no evidence of impaired fertility.

Pregnancy: ***Teratogenic Effects:*** Pregnancy Category B. Teratology studies have been performed with bupropion immediate-release formulation at dosages up to 450 mg/kg in rats, and at doses up to 150 mg/kg in rabbits (approximately 7 to 11 and 7 times the MRHD, respectively, on a mg/m² basis), and have revealed no evidence of harm to the fetus due to bupropion. There are no adequate and well-controlled studies in pregnant women. Because animal reproduction studies are not always predictive of human response, this drug should be used during pregnancy only if clearly needed.

To monitor fetal outcomes of pregnant women exposed to WELLBUTRIN XL, GlaxoSmithKline maintains a Bupropion Pregnancy Registry. Health care providers are encouraged to register patients by calling (800) 336-2176.

Labor and Delivery: The effect of WELLBUTRIN XL Tablets on labor and delivery in humans is unknown.

Nursing Mothers: Like many other drugs, bupropion and its metabolites are secreted in human milk. Because of the potential for serious adverse reactions in nursing infants from WELLBUTRIN XL Tablets, a decision should be made whether to discontinue nursing or to discontinue the drug, taking into account the importance of the drug to the mother.

Pediatric Use: The safety and effectiveness of WELLBUTRIN XL Tablets in pediatric patients below 18 years old have not been established. The immediate-release formulation of bupropion was studied in 104 pediatric patients (age range, 6 to 16) in clinical trials of the drug for other indications. Although generally well tolerated, the limited exposure is insufficient to assess the safety of bupropion in pediatric patients **(see WARNINGS—Clinical Worsening and Suicide Risk).**

Geriatric Use: Of the approximately 6,000 patients who participated in clinical trials with bupropion sustained-release tablets (depression and smoking cessation studies), 275 were ≥65 years old and 47 were ≥75 years old. In addition, several hundred patients 65 and over participated in clinical trials using the immediate-release formulation of bupropion (depression studies). No overall differences in safety or effectiveness were observed between these subjects and younger subjects. Reported clinical experience has not identified differences in responses between the elderly and younger patients, but greater sensitivity of some older individuals cannot be ruled out.

A single-dose pharmacokinetic study demonstrated that the disposition of bupropion and its metabolites in elderly subjects was similar to that of younger subjects; however, another pharmacokinetic study, single and multiple dose, has suggested that the elderly are at increased risk for accumulation of bupropion and its metabolites (see CLINICAL PHARMACOLOGY).

Bupropion is extensively metabolized in the liver to active metabolites, which are further metabolized and excreted by the kidneys. The risk of toxic reaction to this drug may be greater in patients with impaired renal function. Because elderly patients are more likely to have decreased renal function, care should be taken in dose selection, and it may be useful to monitor renal function (see PRECAUTIONS: Renal Impairment and DOSAGE AND ADMINISTRATION).

ADVERSE REACTIONS (See also WARNINGS and PRECAUTIONS.)

WELLBUTRIN XL has been demonstrated to have similar bioavailability to the immediate-release formulation of bupropion (see CLINICAL PHARMACOLOGY). The information included under the Incidence in Controlled Trials subsection of ADVERSE REACTIONS is based primarily on data from controlled clinical trials with WELLBUTRIN SR Tablets, the sustained-release formulation of bupropion. WELLBUTRIN XL has not been studied in placebo-controlled trials, although it has been studied in non-placebo-controlled clinical bioavailability studies. Information on additional adverse events associated with the sustained-release formulation of bupropion in smoking cessation trials, as well as the immediate-release formulation of bupropion, is included in a separate section (see Other Events Observed During the Clinical Development and Postmarketing Experience of Bupropion).

Incidence in Controlled Trials With Bupropion: ***Adverse Events Associated With Discontinuation of Treatment Among Patients Treated With Bupropion:*** In placebo-controlled clinical trials, 9% and 11% of patients treated with 300 and 400 mg/day, respectively, of the sustained-release formulation of bupropion and 4% of patients treated with placebo discontinued treatment due to adverse events. The specific adverse events in these trials that led to discontinuation in at least 1% of patients treated with either 300 mg/day or 400 mg/day of WELLBUTRIN SR, the sustained-release formulation of bupropion, and at a rate at least twice the placebo rate are listed in Table 3.

[See table 3 below]

In clinical trials with the immediate-release formulation of bupropion, 10% of patients and volunteers discontinued due to an adverse event. Events resulting in discontinuation, in addition to those listed above for the sustained-release formulation of bupropion, include vomiting, seizures, and sleep disturbances.

Adverse Events Occurring at an Incidence of 1% or More Among Patients Treated With Bupropion: Table 4 enumerates treatment-emergent adverse events that occurred among patients treated with 300 and 400 mg/day of the sustained-release formulation of bupropion and with placebo in controlled trials. Events that occurred in either the 300- or 400-mg/day group at an incidence of 1% or more and were more frequent than in the placebo group are included. Reported adverse events were classified using a COSTART-based dictionary.

Accurate estimates of the incidence of adverse events associated with the use of any drug are difficult to obtain. Estimates are influenced by drug dose, detection technique, setting, physician judgments, etc. The figures cited cannot be used to predict precisely the incidence of untoward events in the course of usual medical practice where patient characteristics and other factors differ from those that prevailed in the clinical trials. These incidence figures also cannot be compared with those obtained from other clinical studies involving related drug products as each group of drug trials is conducted under a different set of conditions.

Finally, it is important to emphasize that the tabulation does not reflect the relative severity and/or clinical importance of the events. A better perspective on the serious adverse events associated with the use of bupropion is provided in the WARNINGS and PRECAUTIONS sections.

[See table 4 at top of next page]

Additional events to those listed in Table 4 that occurred at an incidence of at least 1% in controlled clinical trials of the immediate-release formulation of bupropion (300 to 600 mg/day) and that were numerically more frequent than placebo were: cardiac arrhythmias (5% vs 4%), hypertension (4% vs 2%), hypotension (3% vs 2%), tachycardia (11% vs 9%), appetite increase (4% vs 2%), dyspepsia (3% vs 2%), menstrual complaints (5% vs 1%), akathisia (2% vs 1%), impaired sleep quality (4% vs 2%), sensory disturbance (4% vs 3%), confusion (8% vs 5%), decreased libido (3% vs 2%), hostility (6% vs 4%), auditory disturbance (5% vs 3%), and gustatory disturbance (3% vs 1%).

Incidence of Commonly Observed Adverse Events in Controlled Clinical Trials: Adverse events from Table 4 occurring in at least 5% of patients treated with the sustained-release formulation of bupropion and at a rate at least twice the placebo rate are listed below for the 300- and 400-mg/day dose groups.

300 mg/day of the Sustained-Release Formulation: Anorexia, dry mouth, rash, sweating, tinnitus, and tremor.

400 mg/day of the Sustained-Release Formulation: Abdominal pain, agitation, anxiety, dizziness, dry mouth, insomnia, myalgia, nausea, palpitation, pharyngitis, sweating, tinnitus, and urinary frequency.

Other Events Observed During the Clinical Development and Postmarketing Experience of Bupropion: In addition to the adverse events noted above, the following events have been reported in clinical trials and postmarketing experience with the sustained-release formulation of bupropion in depressed patients and in nondepressed smokers, as well as in clinical trials and postmarketing clinical experience with the immediate-release formulation of bupropion.

Adverse events for which frequencies are provided below occurred in clinical trials with the sustained-release formulation of bupropion. The frequencies represent the proportion of patients who experienced a treatment-emergent adverse event on at least one occasion in placebo-controlled studies for depression (n = 987) or smoking cessation (n = 1,013), or patients who experienced an adverse event requiring discontinuation of treatment in an open-label surveillance study with the sustained-release formulation of bupropion (n = 3,100). All treatment-emergent adverse events are included except those listed in Tables 1 through 4, those events listed in other safety-related sections, those adverse events subsumed under COSTART terms that are either overly general or excessively specific so as to be uninformative, those events not reasonably associated with the use of the drug, and those events that were not serious and occurred in fewer than 2 patients. Events of major clinical importance are described in the WARNINGS and PRECAUTIONS sections of the labeling.

Events are further categorized by body system and listed in order of decreasing frequency according to the following definitions of frequency: Frequent adverse events are defined as those occurring in at least 1/100 patients. Infrequent adverse events are those occurring in 1/100 to 1/1,000 patients, while rare events are those occurring in less than 1/1,000 patients.

Adverse events for which frequencies are not provided occurred in clinical trials or postmarketing experience with bupropion. Only those adverse events not previously listed

Table 3. Treatment Discontinuations Due to Adverse Events in Placebo-Controlled Trials

Adverse Event Term	WELLBUTRIN SR 300 mg/day (n = 376)	WELLBUTRIN SR 400 mg/day (n = 114)	Placebo (n = 385)
Rash	2.4%	0.9%	0.0%
Nausea	0.8%	1.8%	0.3%
Agitation	0.3%	1.8%	0.3%
Migraine	0.0%	1.8%	0.3%

for sustained-release bupropion are included. The extent to which these events may be associated with WELLBUTRIN XL is unknown.

Body (General): Infrequent were chills, facial edema, musculoskeletal chest pain, and photosensitivity. Rare was malaise. Also observed were arthralgia, myalgia, and fever with rash and other symptoms suggestive of delayed hypersensitivity. These symptoms may resemble serum sickness (see PRECAUTIONS).

Cardiovascular: Infrequent were postural hypotension, stroke, tachycardia, and vasodilation. Rare was syncope. Also observed were complete atrioventricular block, extrasystoles, hypotension, hypertension (in some cases severe, see PRECAUTIONS), myocardial infarction, phlebitis, and pulmonary embolism.

Digestive: Infrequent were abnormal liver function, bruxism, gastric reflux, gingivitis, glossitis, increased salivation, jaundice, mouth ulcers, stomatitis, and thirst. Rare was edema of tongue. Also observed were colitis, esophagitis, gastrointestinal hemorrhage, gum hemorrhage, hepatitis, intestinal perforation, liver damage, pancreatitis, and stomach ulcer.

Endocrine: Also observed were hyperglycemia, hypoglycemia, and syndrome of inappropriate antidiuretic hormone.

Hemic and Lymphatic: Infrequent was ecchymosis. Also observed were anemia, leukocytosis, leukopenia, lymphadenopathy, pancytopenia, and thrombocytopenia. Altered PT and/or INR, infrequently associated with hemorrhagic or thrombotic complications, were observed when bupropion was coadministered with warfarin.

Metabolic and Nutritional: Infrequent were edema and peripheral edema. Also observed was glycosuria.

Musculoskeletal: Infrequent were leg cramps. Also observed were muscle rigidity/fever/rhabdomyolysis and muscle weakness.

Nervous System: Infrequent were abnormal coordination, decreased libido, depersonalization, dysphoria, emotional lability, hostility, hyperkinesia, hypertonia, hypesthesia, suicidal ideation, and vertigo. Rare were amnesia, ataxia, derealization, and hypomania. Also observed were abnormal electroencephalogram (EEG), akinesia, aphasia, coma, delirium, dysarthria, dyskinesia, dystonia, euphoria, extrapyramidal syndrome, hallucinations, hypokinesia, increased libido, manic reaction, neuralgia, neuropathy, paranoid reaction, and unmasking tardive dyskinesia.

Respiratory: Rare was bronchospasm. Also observed was pneumonia.

Skin: Rare was maculopapular rash. Also observed were alopecia, angioedema, exfoliative dermatitis, and hirsutism.

Special Senses: Infrequent were accommodation abnormality and dry eye. Also observed were deafness, diplopia, and mydriasis.

Urogenital: Infrequent were impotence, polyuria, and prostate disorder. Also observed were abnormal ejaculation, cystitis, dyspareunia, dysuria, gynecomastia, menopause, painful erection, salpingitis, urinary incontinence, urinary retention, and vaginitis.

DRUG ABUSE AND DEPENDENCE

Controlled Substance Class: Bupropion is not a controlled substance.

Humans: Controlled clinical studies of bupropion (immediate-release formulation) conducted in normal volunteers, in subjects with a history of multiple drug abuse, and in depressed patients showed some increase in motor activity and agitation/excitement.

In a population of individuals experienced with drugs of abuse, a single dose of 400 mg of bupropion produced mild amphetamine-like activity as compared to placebo on the Morphine-Benzedrine Subscale of the Addiction Research Center Inventories (ARCI), and a score intermediate between placebo and amphetamine on the Liking Scale of the ARCI. These scales measure general feelings of euphoria and drug desirability.

Findings in clinical trials, however, are not known to reliably predict the abuse potential of drugs. Nonetheless, evidence from single-dose studies does suggest that the recommended daily dosage of bupropion when administered in divided doses is not likely to be especially reinforcing to amphetamine or stimulant abusers. However, higher doses that could not be tested because of the risk of seizure might be modestly attractive to those who abuse stimulant drugs.

Animals: Studies in rodents and primates have shown that bupropion exhibits some pharmacologic actions common to psychostimulants. In rodents, it has been shown to increase locomotor activity, elicit a mild stereotyped behavioral response, and increase rates of responding in several schedule-controlled behavior paradigms. In primate models to assess the positive reinforcing effects of psychoactive drugs, bupropion was self-administered intravenously. In rats, bupropion produced amphetamine-like and cocaine-like discriminative stimulus effects in drug discrimination paradigms used to characterize the subjective effects of psychoactive drugs.

OVERDOSAGE

Human Overdose Experience: There has been very limited experience with overdosage of the sustained-release formulation of bupropion (WELLBUTRIN SR Tablets); 3 cases were reported during clinical trials. One patient ingested 3,000 mg of the sustained-release formulation of bupropion and vomited quickly after the overdose; the patient experienced blurred vision and lightheadedness. A second patient ingested a "handful" of WELLBUTRIN SR Tablets (the sustained-release formulation) and experienced confusion, lethargy, nausea, jitteriness, and seizure. A third patient ingested 3,600 mg of the sustained-release formulation of bupropion and a bottle of wine; the patient experienced nausea, visual hallucinations, and "grogginess." None of the patients experienced further sequelae.

Table 4. Treatment-Emergent Adverse Events in Placebo-Controlled Trials*

Body System/ Adverse Event	WELLBUTRIN SR 300 mg/day (n = 376)	WELLBUTRIN SR 400 mg/day (n = 114)	Placebo (n = 385)
Body (General)			
Headache	26%	25%	23%
Infection	8%	9%	6%
Abdominal pain	3%	9%	2%
Asthenia	2%	4%	2%
Chest pain	3%	4%	1%
Pain	2%	3%	2%
Fever	1%	2%	—
Cardiovascular			
Palpitation	2%	6%	2%
Flushing	1%	4%	—
Migraine	1%	4%	1%
Hot flashes	1%	3%	1%
Digestive			
Dry mouth	17%	24%	7%
Nausea	13%	18%	8%
Constipation	10%	5%	7%
Diarrhea	5%	7%	6%
Anorexia	5%	3%	2%
Vomiting	4%	2%	2%
Dysphagia	0%	2%	0%
Musculoskeletal			
Myalgia	2%	6%	3%
Arthralgia	1%	4%	1%
Arthritis	0%	2%	0%
Twitch	1%	2%	—
Nervous system			
Insomnia	11%	16%	6%
Dizziness	7%	11%	5%
Agitation	3%	9%	2%
Anxiety	5%	6%	3%
Tremor	6%	3%	1%
Nervousness	5%	3%	3%
Somnolence	2%	3%	2%
Irritability	3%	2%	2%
Memory decreased	—	3%	1%
Paresthesia	1%	2%	1%
Central nervous system stimulation	2%	1%	1%
Respiratory			
Pharyngitis	3%	11%	2%
Sinusitis	3%	1%	2%
Increased cough	1%	2%	1%
Skin			
Sweating	6%	5%	2%
Rash	5%	4%	1%
Pruritus	2%	4%	2%
Urticaria	2%	1%	0%
Special senses			
Tinnitus	6%	6%	2%
Taste perversion	2%	4%	—
Amblyopia	3%	2%	2%
Urogenital			
Urinary frequency	2%	5%	2%
Urinary urgency	—	2%	0%
Vaginal hemorrhage†	0%	2%	—
Urinary tract infection	1%	0%	—

*Adverse events that occurred in at least 1% of patients treated with either 300 or 400 mg/day of the sustained-release formulation of bupropion, but equally or more frequently in the placebo group, were: abnormal dreams, accidental injury, acne, appetite increased, back pain, bronchitis, dysmenorrhea, dyspepsia, flatulence, flu syndrome, hypertension, neck pain, respiratory disorder, rhinitis, and tooth disorder.

† Incidence based on the number of female patients.

— Hyphen denotes adverse events occurring in greater than 0 but less than 0.5% of patients.

There has been extensive experience with overdosage of the immediate-release formulation of bupropion. Thirteen overdoses occurred during clinical trials. Twelve patients ingested 850 to 4,200 mg and recovered without significant sequelae. Another patient who ingested 9,000 mg of the immediate-release formulation of bupropion and 300 mg of tranylcypromine experienced a grand mal seizure and recovered without further sequelae.

Since introduction, overdoses of up to 17,500 mg of the immediate-release formulation of bupropion have been reported. Seizure was reported in approximately one third of all cases. Other serious reactions reported with overdoses of the immediate-release formulation of bupropion alone included hallucinations, loss of consciousness, and sinus tachycardia. Fever, muscle rigidity, rhabdomyolysis, hypotension, stupor, coma, and respiratory failure have been reported when the immediate-release formulation of bupropion was part of multiple drug overdoses.

Although most patients recovered without sequelae, deaths associated with overdoses of the immediate-release formulation of bupropion alone have been reported rarely in patients ingesting massive doses of the drug. Multiple uncontrolled seizures, bradycardia, cardiac failure, and cardiac arrest prior to death were reported in these patients.

Overdosage Management: Ensure an adequate airway, oxygenation, and ventilation. Monitor cardiac rhythm and vital signs. EEG monitoring is also recommended for the first 48 hours post-ingestion. General supportive and symptomatic measures are also recommended. Induction of emesis is not recommended. Gastric lavage with a large-bore orogastric tube with appropriate airway protection, if needed, may be indicated if performed soon after ingestion or in symptomatic patients.

Activated charcoal should be administered. There is no experience with the use of forced diuresis, dialysis, hemoperfusion, or exchange transfusion in the management of bupropion overdoses. No specific antidotes for bupropion are known.

Continued on next page

Product information on these pages is effective as of August 2004. Further information is available at: GlaxoSmithKline, PO Box 13398, Research Triangle Park, NC 27709. 1-888-825-5249. Corporate Web Site: www.gsk.com

Wellbutrin XL—Cont.

Due to the dose-related risk of seizures with WELLBUTRIN XL, hospitalization following suspected overdose should be considered. Based on studies in animals, it is recommended that seizures be treated with intravenous benzodiazepine administration and other supportive measures, as appropriate.

In managing overdosage, consider the possibility of multiple drug involvement. The physician should consider contacting a poison control center for additional information on the treatment of any overdose. Telephone numbers for certified poison control centers are listed in the *Physicians' Desk Reference* (PDR).

DOSAGE AND ADMINISTRATION

General Dosing Considerations: It is particularly important to administer WELLBUTRIN XL Tablets in a manner most likely to minimize the risk of seizure (see WARNINGS). Gradual escalation in dosage is also important if agitation, motor restlessness, and insomnia, often seen during the initial days of treatment, are to be minimized. If necessary, these effects may be managed by temporary reduction of dose or the short-term administration of an intermediate to long-acting sedative hypnotic. A sedative hypnotic usually is not required beyond the first week of treatment. Insomnia may also be minimized by avoiding bedtime doses. If distressing, untoward effects supervene, dose escalation should be stopped. WELLBUTRIN XL should be swallowed whole and not crushed, divided, or chewed. WELLBUTRIN XL may be taken without regard to meals.

Initial Treatment: The usual adult target dose for WELLBUTRIN XL Tablets is 300 mg/day, given once daily in the morning. Dosing with WELLBUTRIN XL Tablets should begin at 150 mg/day given as a single daily dose in the morning. If the 150-mg initial dose is adequately tolerated, an increase to the 300-mg/day target dose, given as once daily, may be made as early as day 4 of dosing. There should be an interval of at least 24 hours between successive doses.

Increasing the Dosage Above 300 mg/day: As with other antidepressants, the full antidepressant effect of WELLBUTRIN XL Tablets may not be evident until 4 weeks of treatment or longer. An increase in dosage to the maximum of 450 mg/day, given as a single dose, may be considered for patients in whom no clinical improvement is noted after several weeks of treatment at 300 mg/day.

Switching Patients from WELLBUTRIN Tablets or from WELLBUTRIN SR Sustained-Release Tablets: When switching patients from WELLBUTRIN Tablets to WELLBUTRIN XL or from WELLBUTRIN SR Sustained-Release Tablets to WELLBUTRIN XL, give the same total daily dose when possible. Patients who are currently being treated with WELLBUTRIN Tablets at 300 mg/day (for example, 100 mg 3 times a day) may be switched to WELLBUTRIN XL 300 mg once daily. Patients who are currently being treated with WELLBUTRIN SR Sustained-Release Tablets at 300 mg/day (for example, 150 mg twice daily) may be switched to WELLBUTRIN XL 300 mg once daily.

Maintenance Treatment: It is generally agreed that acute episodes of depression require several months or longer of sustained pharmacological therapy beyond response to the acute episode. It is unknown whether or not the dose of WELLBUTRIN XL needed for maintenance treatment is identical to the dose needed to achieve an initial response. Patients should be periodically reassessed to determine the need for maintenance treatment and the appropriate dose for such treatment.

Dosage Adjustment for Patients With Impaired Hepatic Function: WELLBUTRIN XL should be used with extreme caution in patients with severe hepatic cirrhosis. The dose should not exceed 150 mg every other day in these patients. WELLBUTRIN XL should be used with caution in patients with hepatic impairment (including mild to moderate hepatic cirrhosis) and a reduced frequency and/or dose should be considered in patients with mild to moderate hepatic cirrhosis (see CLINICAL PHARMACOLOGY, WARNINGS, and PRECAUTIONS).

Dosage Adjustment for Patients With Impaired Renal Function: WELLBUTRIN XL should be used with caution in patients with renal impairment and a reduced frequency and/or dose should be considered (see CLINICAL PHARMACOLOGY and PRECAUTIONS).

HOW SUPPLIED

WELLBUTRIN XL Extended-Release Tablets, 150 mg of bupropion hydrochloride, are creamy-white to pale yellow, round, tablets printed with "WELLBUTRIN XL 150" in bottles of 30 tablets (NDC 0173-0730-01).

WELLBUTRIN XL Extended-Release Tablets, 300 mg of bupropion hydrochloride, are creamy-white to pale yellow, round, tablets printed with "WELLBUTRIN XL 300" in bottles of 30 tablets (NDC 0173-0731-01).

Store at 25°C (77°F); excursions permitted to 15–30°C (59–86°F) [see USP Controlled Room Temperature].

Manufactured by: Biovail Corporation
Mississauga, ON L5N 8M5, Canada
for GlaxoSmithKline, Research Triangle Park, NC 27709

April 2004/RL-2074

Shown in Product Identification Guide, page 318

ZANTAC® ℞
[zan 'tak]
(ranitidine hydrochloride)
Injection

ZANTAC® ℞
(ranitidine hydrochloride)
Injection Premixed

DESCRIPTION

The active ingredient in ZANTAC Injection and ZANTAC Injection Premixed is ranitidine hydrochloride (HCl), a histamine H_2-receptor antagonist. Chemically it is N[2-[[[5-[(dimethylamino)methyl]-2-furanyl]methyl]thio]ethyl]-N′-methyl-2-nitro-1,1-ethenediamine, hydrochloride.

The empirical formula is $C_{13}H_{22}N_4O_3S \bullet HCl$, representing a molecular weight of 350.87.

Ranitidine HCl is a white to pale yellow, granular substance that is soluble in water.

ZANTAC Injection is a clear, colorless to yellow, nonpyrogenic liquid. The yellow color of the liquid tends to intensify without adversely affecting potency. The pH of the injection solution is 6.7 to 7.3.

Sterile Injection for Intramuscular or Intravenous Administration: Each 1 mL of aqueous solution contains ranitidine 25 mg (as the hydrochloride); phenol 5 mg as preservative; and 0.96 mg of monobasic potassium phosphate and 2.4 mg of dibasic sodium phosphate as buffers.

A pharmacy bulk package is a container of a sterile preparation for parenteral use that contains many single doses. The contents are intended for use in a pharmacy admixture program and are restricted to the preparation of admixtures for intravenous (IV) infusion.

Sterile, Premixed Solution for Intravenous Administration in Single-Dose, Flexible Plastic Containers: Each 50 mL contains ranitidine HCl equivalent to 50 mg of ranitidine, sodium chloride 225 mg, and citric acid 15 mg and dibasic sodium phosphate 90 mg as buffers in water for injection. It contains no preservatives. The osmolarity of this solution is 180 mOsm/L (approx.), and the pH is 6.7 to 7.3.

The flexible plastic container is fabricated from a specially formulated, nonplasticized, thermoplastic co-polyester (CR3). Water can permeate from inside the container into the overwrap but not in amounts sufficient to affect the solution significantly. Solutions inside the plastic container also can leach out certain of the chemical components in very small amounts before the expiration period is attained. However, the safety of the plastic has been confirmed by tests in animals according to USP biological standards for plastic containers.

CLINICAL PHARMACOLOGY

ZANTAC is a competitive, reversible inhibitor of the action of histamine at the histamine H_2-receptors, including receptors on the gastric cells. ZANTAC does not lower serum Ca^{++} in hypercalcemic states. ZANTAC is not an anticholinergic agent.

Pharmacokinetics: ***Absorption:*** ZANTAC is absorbed very rapidly after intramuscular (IM) injection. Mean peak levels of 576 ng/mL occur within 15 minutes or less following a 50-mg IM dose. Absorption from IM sites is virtually complete, with a bioavailability of 90% to 100% compared with intravenous (IV) administration. Following oral administration, the bioavailability of ZANTAC Tablets is 50%.

Distribution: The volume of distribution is about 1.4 L/kg. Serum protein binding averages 15%.

Metabolism: In humans, the N-oxide is the principal metabolite in the urine; however, this amounts to <4% of the dose. Other metabolites are the S-oxide (1%) and the desmethyl ranitidine (1%). The remainder of the administered dose is found in the stool. Studies in patients with hepatic dysfunction (compensated cirrhosis) indicate that there are minor, but clinically insignificant, alterations in ranitidine half-life, distribution, clearance, and bioavailability.

Excretion: Following IV injection, approximately 70% of the dose is recovered in the urine as unchanged drug. Renal clearance averages 530 mL/min, with a total clearance of 760 mL/min. The elimination half-life is 2.0 to 2.5 hours. Four patients with clinically significant renal function impairment (creatinine clearance 25 to 35 mL/min) administered 50 mg of ranitidine intravenously had an average plasma half-life of 4.8 hours, a ranitidine clearance of 29 mL/min, and a volume of distribution of 1.76 L/kg. In general, these parameters appear to be altered in proportion to creatinine clearance (see DOSAGE AND ADMINISTRATION).

Geriatrics: The plasma half-life is prolonged and total clearance is reduced in the elderly population due to a decrease in renal function. The elimination half-life is 3.1 hours (see PRECAUTIONS: Geriatric Use and DOSAGE AND ADMINISTRATION: Dosage Adjustment for Patients with Impaired Renal Function).

Pediatrics: There are no significant differences in the pharmacokinetic parameter values for ranitidine in pediatric patients (from 1 month up to 16 years of age) and healthy adults when correction is made for body weight. The pharmacokinetics of ZANTAC in pediatric patients are summarized in Table 1.

[See table 1 below]

Plasma clearance in neonatal patients (less than 1 month of age) receiving ECMO was considerably lower (3 to 4 mL/min/kg) than observed in children or adults. The elimination half-life in neonates averages 6.6 hours as compared to approximately 2 hours in adults and pediatric patients.

Pharmacodynamics: Serum concentrations necessary to inhibit 50% of stimulated gastric acid secretion are estimated to be 36 to 94 ng/mL. Following single IV or IM 50-mg doses, serum concentrations of ZANTAC are in this range for 6 to 8 hours.

Antisecretory Activity: ***1. Effects on Acid Secretion:*** ZANTAC Injection inhibits basal gastric acid secretion as well as gastric acid secretion stimulated by betazole and pentagastrin, as shown in Table 2.

[See table 2 below]

In a group of 10 known hypersecretors, ranitidine plasma levels of 71, 180, and 376 ng/mL inhibited basal acid secretion by 76%, 90%, and 99.5%, respectively.

It appears that basal- and betazole-stimulated secretions are most sensitive to inhibition by ZANTAC, while pentagastrin-stimulated secretion is more difficult to suppress.

2. Effects on Other Gastrointestinal Secretions:

Pepsin: ZANTAC does not affect pepsin secretion. Total pepsin output is reduced in proportion to the decrease in volume of gastric juice.

Intrinsic Factor: ZANTAC has no significant effect on pentagastrin-stimulated intrinsic factor secretion.

Serum Gastrin: ZANTAC has little or no effect on fasting or postprandial serum gastrin.

Other Pharmacologic Actions:

a. Gastric bacterial flora—increase in nitrate-reducing organisms, significance not known.

b. Prolactin levels—no effect in recommended oral or intravenous (IV) dosage, but small, transient, dose-related increases in serum prolactin have been reported after IV bolus injections of 100 mg or more.

c. Other pituitary hormones—no effect on serum gonadotropins, TSH, or GH. Possible impairment of vasopressin release.

d. No change in cortisol, aldosterone, androgen, or estrogen levels.

e. No antiandrogenic action.

f. No effect on count, motility, or morphology of sperm.

Table 1. Ranitidine Pharmacokinetics in Pediatric Patients Following IV Dosing

Population (age)	n	Dose (mg/kg)	$T_{1/2}$ (hours)	Vd (L/kg)	CLp (mL/min/kg)
Peptic ulcer disease					
(<6 years)	6	1.25 or 2.5	2.2	1.29	11.41
(6–11.9 years)	11	1.25 or 2.5	2.1	1.14	8.96
(>12 years)	6	1.25 or 2.5	1.7	0.98	9.89
Adults	6	2.5	1.9	1.04	8.77
Peptic ulcer disease (3.5–16 years)	12	0.13–0.80	1.8	2.3	795 mL/min/ $1.73/m^2$
Children in intensive care (1 day–12.6 years)	17	1.0	2.4	2	11.7
Neonates receiving ECMO	12	2	6.6	1.8	4.3

$T_{1/2}$ = Terminal half-life; CLp = Plasma clearance of ranitidine.
ECMO = extracorporeal membrane oxygenation.

Table 2. Effect of Intravenous ZANTAC on Gastric Acid Secretion

	Time After Dose, h	% Inhibition of Gastric Acid Output by Intravenous Dose, mg		
		20 mg	60 mg	100 mg
Betazole	Up to 2	93	99	99
Pentagastrin	Up to 3	47	66	77

Pediatrics: The ranitidine concentration necessary to suppress basal acid secretion by at least 90% has been reported to be 40 to 60 ng/mL in pediatric patients with duodenal or gastric ulcers.
In a study of 20 critically ill pediatric patients receiving ranitidine IV at 1 mg/kg every 6 hours, 10 patients with a baseline pH≥4 maintained this baseline throughout the study. Eight of the remaining 10 patients with a baseline of pH≤2 achieved pH≥4 throughout varying periods after dosing. It should be noted, however, that because these pharmacodynamic parameters were assessed in critically ill pediatric patients, the data should be interpreted with caution when dosing recommendations are made for a less seriously ill pediatric population.
In another small study of neonatal patients (n=5) receiving ECMO, gastric pH<4 pretreatment increased to >4 after a 2 mg/kg dose and remained above 4 for at least 15 hours.
Clinical Trials: ***Active Duodenal Ulcer:*** In a multicenter, double-blind, controlled, US study of endoscopically diagnosed duodenal ulcers, earlier healing was seen in the patients treated with oral ZANTAC as shown in Table 3.
[See table 3 at right]
In these studies, patients treated with oral ZANTAC reported a reduction in both daytime and nocturnal pain, and they also consumed less antacid than the placebo-treated patients.
[See table 4 at right]
Pathological Hypersecretory Conditions (such as Zollinger-Ellison syndrome): ZANTAC inhibits gastric acid secretion and reduces occurrence of diarrhea, anorexia, and pain in patients with pathological hypersecretion associated with Zollinger-Ellison syndrome, systemic mastocytosis, and other pathological hypersecretory conditions (e.g., postoperative, "short-gut" syndrome, idiopathic). Use of oral ZANTAC was followed by healing of ulcers in 8 of 19 (42%) patients who were intractable to previous therapy.
In a retrospective review of 52 Zollinger-Ellison patients given ZANTAC as a continuous IV infusion for up to 15 days, no patients developed complications of acid-peptic disease such as bleeding or perforation. Acid output was controlled to ≤10 mEq/h.

INDICATIONS AND USAGE

ZANTAC Injection and ZANTAC Injection Premixed are indicated in some hospitalized patients with pathological hypersecretory conditions or intractable duodenal ulcers, or as an alternative to the oral dosage form for short-term use in patients who are unable to take oral medication.

CONTRAINDICATIONS

ZANTAC Injection and ZANTAC Injection Premixed are contraindicated for patients known to have hypersensitivity to the drug.

PRECAUTIONS

General: 1. Symptomatic response to therapy with ZANTAC does not preclude the presence of gastric malignancy.
2. Since ZANTAC is excreted primarily by the kidney, dosage should be adjusted in patients with impaired renal function (see DOSAGE AND ADMINISTRATION). Caution should be observed in patients with hepatic dysfunction since ZANTAC is metabolized in the liver.
3. In controlled studies in normal volunteers, elevations in SGPT have been observed when H_2-antagonists have been administered intravenously at greater than recommended dosages for 5 days or longer. Therefore, it seems prudent in patients receiving IV ranitidine at dosages ≥100 mg q.i.d. for periods of 5 days or longer to monitor SGPT daily (from day 5) for the remainder of IV therapy.
4. Bradycardia in association with rapid administration of ZANTAC Injection has been reported rarely, usually in patients with factors predisposing to cardiac rhythm disturbances. Recommended rates of administration should not be exceeded (see DOSAGE AND ADMINISTRATION).
5. Rare reports suggest that ZANTAC may precipitate acute porphyric attacks in patients with acute porphyria. ZANTAC should therefore be avoided in patients with a history of acute porphyria.
Laboratory Tests: False-positive tests for urine protein with MULTISTIX® may occur during therapy with ZANTAC and therefore testing with sulfosalicylic acid is recommended.
Drug Interactions: Although ZANTAC has been reported to bind weakly to cytochrome P-450 *in vitro*, recommended doses of the drug do not inhibit the action of the cytochrome P-450–linked oxygenase enzymes in the liver. However, there have been isolated reports of drug interactions that suggest that ZANTAC may affect the bioavailability of certain drugs by some mechanism as yet unidentified (e.g., a pH-dependent effect on absorption or a change in volume of distribution).
Increased or decreased prothrombin times have been reported during concurrent use of ranitidine and warfarin. However, in human pharmacokinetic studies with dosages of ranitidine up to 400 mg/day, no interaction occurred; ranitidine had no effect on warfarin clearance or prothrombin time. The possibility of an interaction with warfarin at dosages of ranitidine higher than 400 mg/day has not been investigated.
In a ranitidine-triazolam drug-drug interaction study, triazolam plasma concentrations were higher during b.i.d. dosing of ranitidine than triazolam given alone. The mean area under the triazolam concentration-time curve (AUC) values, in 18- to 60-year-old subjects were 10% and 28% higher following administration of 75-mg and 150-mg ranitidine tablets, respectively, than triazolam given alone. In subjects older than 60 years of age, the mean AUC values were approximately 30% higher following administration of 75-mg and 150-mg ranitidine tablets. It appears that there were no changes in pharmacokinetics of triazolam and α-hydroxytriazolam, a major metabolite, and in their elimination. Reduced gastric acidity due to ranitidine may have resulted in an increase in the availability of triazolam. The clinical significance of this triazolam and ranitidine pharmacokinetic interaction is unknown.
Carcinogenesis, Mutagenesis, Impairment of Fertility: There was no indication of tumorigenic or carcinogenic effects in life-span studies in mice and rats at oral dosages up to 2,000 mg/kg per day.
Ranitidine was not mutagenic in standard bacterial tests *(Salmonella, Escherichia coli)* for mutagenicity at concentrations up to the maximum recommended for these assays. In a dominant lethal assay, a single oral dose of 1,000 mg/kg to male rats was without effect on the outcome of two matings per week for the next 9 weeks.
Pregnancy: ***Teratogenic Effects:*** Pregnancy Category B. Reproduction studies have been performed in rats and rabbits at oral doses up to 160 times the human oral dose and have revealed no evidence of impaired fertility or harm to the fetus due to ZANTAC. There are, however, no adequate and well-controlled studies in pregnant women. Because animal reproduction studies are not always predictive of human response, this drug should be used during pregnancy only if clearly needed.
Nursing Mothers: ZANTAC is secreted in human milk. Caution should be exercised when ZANTAC is administered to a nursing mother.
Pediatric Use: The safety and effectiveness of ZANTAC Injection have been established in the age-group of 1 month to 16 years for the treatment of duodenal ulcer. Use of ZANTAC in this age-group is supported by adequate and well-controlled studies in adults, as well as additional pharmacokinetic data in pediatric patients, and an analysis of the published literature.
Safety and effectiveness in pediatric patients for the treatment of pathological hypersecretory conditions have not been established.
Limited data in neonatal patients (less than one month of age) receiving ECMO suggest that ZANTAC may be useful and safe for increasing gastric pH for patients at risk of gastrointestinal hemorrhage.
Geriatric Use: Clinical studies of ZANTAC Injection did not include sufficient numbers of subjects aged 65 and over to determine whether they responded differently from younger subjects. However, in clinical studies of oral formulations of ZANTAC, of the total number of subjects enrolled in US and foreign controlled clinical trials, for which there were subgroup analyses, 4,197 were 65 and over, while 899 were 75 and over. No overall differences in safety or effectiveness were observed between these subjects and younger subjects, and other reported clinical experience has not identified differences in responses between the elderly and younger patients, but greater sensitivity of some older individuals cannot be ruled out.
This drug is known to be substantially excreted by the kidney and the risk of toxic reactions to this drug may be greater in patients with impaired renal function. Because elderly patients are more likely to have decreased renal function, caution should be exercised in dose selection, and it may be useful to monitor renal function (see CLINICAL PHARMACOLOGY: Pharmacokinetics: Geriatric Use and DOSAGE AND ADMINISTRATION: Dosage Adjustment for Patients with Impaired Renal Function).

ADVERSE REACTIONS

Transient pain at the site of IM injection has been reported. Transient local burning or itching has been reported with IV administration of ZANTAC.
The following have been reported as events in clinical trials or in the routine management of patients treated with oral or parenteral ZANTAC. The relationship to therapy with ZANTAC has been unclear in many cases. Headache, sometimes severe, seems to be related to administration of ZANTAC.

Table 3. Duodenal Ulcer Patient Healing Rates

	Oral ZANTAC*		Oral Placebo*	
	Number Entered	Healed/ Evaluable	Number Entered	Healed/ Evaluable
Outpatients				
Week 2	195	69/182 (38%)[†]	188	31/164 (19%)
Week 4		137/187 (73%)[†]		76/168 (45%)

*All patients were permitted p.r.n. antacids for relief of pain.
[†]$P<0.0001$.

Table 4. Mean Daily Doses of Antacid

	Ulcer Healed	Ulcer Not Healed
Oral ZANTAC	0.06	0.71
Oral placebo	0.71	1.43

Central Nervous System: Rarely, malaise, dizziness, somnolence, insomnia, and vertigo. Rare cases of reversible mental confusion, agitation, depression, and hallucinations have been reported, predominantly in severely ill elderly patients. Rare cases of reversible blurred vision suggestive of a change in accommodation have been reported. Rare reports of reversible involuntary motor disturbances have been received.
Cardiovascular: As with other H_2-blockers, rare reports of arrhythmias such as tachycardia, bradycardia, asystole, atrioventricular block, and premature ventricular beats.
Gastrointestinal: Constipation, diarrhea, nausea/vomiting, abdominal discomfort/pain, and rare reports of pancreatitis.
Hepatic: In normal volunteers, SGPT values were increased to at least twice the pretreatment levels in 6 of 12 subjects receiving 100 mg q.i.d. intravenously for 7 days, and in 4 of 24 subjects receiving 50 mg q.i.d. intravenously for 5 days. There have been occasional reports of hepatocellular, cholestatic, or mixed hepatitis, with or without jaundice. In such circumstances, ranitidine should be immediately discontinued. These events are usually reversible, but in rare circumstances death has occurred. Rare cases of hepatic failure have also been reported.
Musculoskeletal: Rare reports of arthralgias and myalgias.
Hematologic: Blood count changes (leukopenia, granulocytopenia, and thrombocytopenia) have occurred in a few patients. These were usually reversible. Rare cases of agranulocytosis, pancytopenia, sometimes with marrow hypoplasia, and aplastic anemia and exceedingly rare cases of acquired immune hemolytic anemia have been reported.
Endocrine: Controlled studies in animals and humans have shown no stimulation of any pituitary hormone by ZANTAC and no antiandrogenic activity, and cimetidine-induced gynecomastia and impotence in hypersecretory patients have resolved when ZANTAC has been substituted. However, occasional cases of gynecomastia, impotence, and loss of libido have been reported in male patients receiving ZANTAC, but the incidence did not differ from that in the general population.
Integumentary: Rash, including rare cases of erythema multiforme. Rare cases of alopecia and vasculitis.
Other: Rare cases of hypersensitivity reactions (e.g., bronchospasm, fever, rash, eosinophilia), anaphylaxis, angioneurotic edema, and small increases in serum creatinine.

OVERDOSAGE

There has been virtually no experience with overdosage with ZANTAC Injection and limited experience with oral doses of ranitidine. Reported acute ingestions of up to 18 g orally have been associated with transient adverse effects similar to those encountered in normal clinical experience (see ADVERSE REACTIONS). In addition, abnormalities of gait and hypotension have been reported.
When overdosage occurs, clinical monitoring and supportive therapy should be employed.
Studies in dogs receiving dosages of ZANTAC in excess of 225 mg/kg per day have shown muscular tremors, vomiting, and rapid respiration. Single oral doses of 1,000 mg/kg in mice and rats were not lethal. Intravenous LD_{50} values in mice and rats were 77 and 83 mg/kg, respectively.

DOSAGE AND ADMINISTRATION

Parenteral Administration: In some hospitalized patients with pathological hypersecretory conditions or intractable duodenal ulcers, or in patients who are unable to take oral medication, ZANTAC may be administered parenterally according to the following recommendations:
Intramuscular Injection: 50 mg (2 mL) every 6 to 8 hours. (No dilution necessary.)

Continued on next page

Product information on these pages is effective as of August 2004. Further information is available at: GlaxoSmithKline, PO Box 13398, Research Triangle Park, NC 27709. 1-888-825-5249. Corporate Web Site: www.gsk.com

Zantac Injection—Cont.

Intermittent Intravenous Injection:

a. Intermittent Bolus: 50 mg (2 mL) every 6 to 8 hours. Dilute ZANTAC Injection, 50 mg, in 0.9% sodium chloride injection or other compatible IV solution (see Stability) to a concentration no greater than 2.5 mg/mL (20 mL). Inject at a rate no greater than 4 mL/min (5 minutes).

b. Intermittent Infusion: 50 mg (2 mL) every 6 to 8 hours. Dilute ZANTAC Injection, 50 mg, in 5% dextrose injection or other compatible IV solution (see Stability) to a concentration no greater than 0.5 mg/mL (100 mL). Infuse at a rate no greater than 5 to 7 mL/min (15 to 20 minutes).

ZANTAC Injection Premixed solution, 50 mg, in 0.45% sodium chloride, 50 mL, requires no dilution and should be infused over 15 to 20 minutes.

In some patients it may be necessary to increase dosage. When this is necessary, the increases should be made by more frequent administration of the dose, but generally should not exceed 400 mg/day.

Continuous Intravenous Infusion: Add ZANTAC Injection to 5% dextrose injection or other compatible IV solution (see Stability). Deliver at a rate of 6.25 mg/h (e.g., 150 mg [6 mL] of ZANTAC Injection in 250 mL of 5% dextrose injection at 10.7 mL/h).

For Zollinger-Ellison patients, dilute ZANTAC Injection in 5% dextrose injection or other compatible IV solution (see Stability) to a concentration no greater than 2.5 mg/mL. Start the infusion at a rate of 1.0 mg/kg per hour. If after 4 hours either a measured gastric acid output is >10 mEq/h or the patient becomes symptomatic, the dose should be adjusted upward in 0.5-mg/kg per hour increments, and the acid output should be remeasured. Dosages up to 2.5 mg/kg per hour and infusion rates as high as 220 mg/h have been used.

Pediatric Use: While limited data exist on the administration of IV ranitidine to children, the recommended dose in pediatric patients is for a total daily dose of 2 to 4 mg/kg, to be divided and administered every 6 to 8 hours, up to a maximum of 50 mg given every 6 to 8 hours. This recommendation is derived from adult clinical studies and pharmacokinetic data in pediatric patients. Limited data in neonatal patients (less than one month of age) receiving ECMO have shown that a dose of 2 mg/kg is usually sufficient to increase gastric pH to >4 for at least 15 hours. Therefore, doses of 2 mg/kg given every 12 to 24 hours or as a continuous infusion should be considered.

ZANTAC Injection Premixed in Flexible Plastic Containers:

Instructions for Use: ***To Open:*** Tear outer wrap at notch and remove solution container. Check for minute leaks by squeezing container firmly. If leaks are found, discard unit as sterility may be impaired.

Preparation for Administration: Use aseptic technique.

1. Close flow control clamp of administration set.
2. Remove cover from outlet port at bottom of container.
3. Insert piercing pin of administration set into port with a twisting motion until the pin is firmly seated. NOTE: See full directions on administration set carton.
4. Suspend container from hanger.
5. Squeeze and release drip chamber to establish proper fluid level in chamber during infusion of ZANTAC Injection Premixed.
6. Open flow control clamp to expel air from set. Close clamp.
7. Attach set to venipuncture device. If device is not indwelling, prime and make venipuncture.
8. Perform venipuncture.
9. Regulate rate of administration with flow control clamp.

Caution: ZANTAC Injection Premixed in flexible plastic containers is to be administered by slow IV drip infusion only. **Additives should not be introduced into this solution.** If used with a primary IV fluid system, the primary solution should be discontinued during ZANTAC Injection Premixed infusion.

Do not administer unless solution is clear and container is undamaged.

Warning: Do not use flexible plastic container in series connections.

Dosage Adjustment for Patients With Impaired Renal Function: The administration of ranitidine as a continuous infusion has not been evaluated in patients with impaired renal function. On the basis of experience with a group of subjects with severely impaired renal function treated with ZANTAC, the recommended dosage in patients with a creatinine clearance <50 mL/min is 50 mg every 18 to 24 hours. Should the patient's condition require, the frequency of dosing may be increased to every 12 hours or even further with caution. Hemodialysis reduces the level of circulating ranitidine. Ideally, the dosing schedule should be adjusted so that the timing of a scheduled dose coincides with the end of hemodialysis.

Elderly patients are more likely to have decreased renal function, therefore caution should be exercised in dose selection, and it may be useful to monitor renal function (see CLINICAL PHARMACOLOGY: Pharmacokinetics: Geriatric Use and PRECAUTIONS: Geriatric Use).

Stability: Undiluted, ZANTAC Injection tends to exhibit a yellow color that may intensify over time without adversely affecting potency. ZANTAC Injection is stable for 48 hours at room temperature when added to or diluted with most commonly used IV solutions, e.g., 0.9% sodium chloride injection, 5% dextrose injection, 10% dextrose injection, lactated ringer's injection, or 5% sodium bicarbonate injection. ZANTAC Injection Premixed in flexible plastic containers is sterile through the expiration date on the label when stored under recommended conditions.

Note: Parenteral drug products should be inspected visually for particulate matter and discoloration before administration whenever solution and container permit.

Directions for Dispensing: ***Pharmacy Bulk Package—Not for Direct Infusion:*** The pharmacy bulk package is for use in a pharmacy admixture service only under a laminar flow hood. The closure should be penetrated only once with a sterile transfer set or other sterile dispensing device, which allows measured distribution of the contents, and the contents dispensed in aliquots using aseptic technique. CONTENTS SHOULD BE USED AS SOON AS POSSIBLE FOLLOWING INITIAL CLOSURE PUNCTURE. DISCARD ANY UNUSED PORTION WITHIN 24 HOURS OF FIRST ENTRY. Following closure puncture, container should be maintained below 30°C (86°F) under a laminar flow hood until contents are dispensed.

HOW SUPPLIED

ZANTAC Injection, 25 mg/mL, containing phenol 0.5% as preservative, is available as follows:

NDC 0173-0362-38, 2-mL single-dose vials (Tray of 10)
NDC 0173-0363-01, 6-mL multidose vials (Singles)
NDC 0173-0363-00, 40-mL pharmacy bulk packages (Singles)

Store between 4° and 25°C (39° and 77°F); excursions permitted to 30°C (86°F). Protect from light. Store pharmacy bulk vial in carton until time of use.

ZANTAC Injection Premixed, 50 mg/50 mL, in 0.45% sodium chloride, is available as a sterile, premixed solution for IV administration in single-dose, flexible plastic containers (NDC 0173-0441-00) (case of 24). It contains no preservatives.

Store between 2° and 25°C (36° and 77°F). Protect from light.

Exposure of pharmaceutical products to heat should be minimized. Avoid excessive heat; however, brief exposure up to 40°C does not adversely affect the product. Protect from freezing.

ZANTAC® Injection:
GlaxoSmithKline, Research Triangle Park, NC 27709
ZANTAC® Injection Premixed:
Manufactured for GlaxoSmithKline
Research Triangle Park, NC 27709
by Abbott Laboratories, North Chicago, IL 60064
ZANTAC is a registered trademark of
Warner-Lambert Company, used under license.

December 2002/RL-1158-1159

Shown in Product Identification Guide, page 318

ZANTAC® 150 ℞
[*zan'tak*]
(ranitidine hydrochloride)
Tablets, USP

ZANTAC® 300 ℞
(ranitidine hydrochloride)
Tablets, USP

ZANTAC® 25 ℞
(ranitidine hydrochloride effervescent)
EFFERdose® Tablets

ZANTAC® 150 ℞
(ranitidine hydrochloride effervescent)
EFFERdose® Tablets

ZANTAC® ℞
(ranitidine hydrochloride)
Syrup, USP

DESCRIPTION

The active ingredient in ZANTAC 150 Tablets, ZANTAC 300 Tablets, ZANTAC 25 EFFERdose Tablets, ZANTAC 150 EFFERdose Tablets, and ZANTAC Syrup is ranitidine hydrochloride (HCl), USP, a histamine H_2-receptor antagonist. Chemically it is N[2-[[[5-[(dimethylamino)methyl]-2-furanyl]methyl]thio]ethyl]-N′-methyl-2-nitro-1,1-ethenediamine, HCl.

The empirical formula is $C_{13}H_{22}N_4O_3S \bullet HCl$, representing a molecular weight of 350.87.

Ranitidine HCl is a white to pale yellow, granular substance that is soluble in water. It has a slightly bitter taste and sulfurlike odor.

Each ZANTAC 150 Tablet for oral administration contains 168 mg of ranitidine HCl equivalent to 150 mg of ranitidine. Each tablet also contains the inactive ingredients FD&C Yellow No. 6 Aluminum Lake, hypromellose, magnesium stearate, microcrystalline cellulose, titanium dioxide, triacetin, and yellow iron oxide.

Each ZANTAC 300 Tablet for oral administration contains 336 mg of ranitidine HCl equivalent to 300 mg of ranitidine. Each tablet also contains the inactive ingredients croscarmellose sodium, D&C Yellow No. 10 Aluminum Lake, hypromellose, magnesium stearate, microcrystalline cellulose, titanium dioxide, and triacetin.

ZANTAC 25 EFFERdose Tablets for oral administration is an effervescent formulation of ranitidine that must be dissolved in water before use. Each individual tablet contains 28 mg of ranitidine HCl equivalent to 25 mg of ranitidine and the following inactive ingredients: aspartame, monosodium citrate anhydrous, povidone, and sodium bicarbonate. Each tablet also contains sodium benzoate. The total sodium content of each tablet is 30.52 mg (1.33 mEq) per 25 mg of ranitidine.

ZANTAC 150 EFFERdose Tablets for oral administration is an effervescent formulation of ranitidine that must be dissolved in water before use. Each individual tablet contains 168 mg of ranitidine HCl equivalent to 150 mg of ranitidine and the following inactive ingredients: aspartame, monosodium citrate anhydrous, povidone, and sodium bicarbonate. Each tablet also contains sodium benzoate. The total sodium content of each tablet is 183.12 mg (7.96 mEq) per 150 mg of ranitidine.

Each 1 mL of ZANTAC Syrup contains 16.8 mg of ranitidine HCl equivalent to 15 mg of ranitidine. ZANTAC Syrup also contains the inactive ingredients alcohol (7.5%), butylparaben, dibasic sodium phosphate, hypromellose, peppermint flavor, monobasic potassium phosphate, propylparaben, purified water, saccharin sodium, sodium chloride, and sorbitol.

CLINICAL PHARMACOLOGY

ZANTAC is a competitive, reversible inhibitor of the action of histamine at the histamine H_2-receptors, including receptors on the gastric cells. ZANTAC does not lower serum Ca^{++} in hypercalcemic states. ZANTAC is not an anticholinergic agent.

Pharmacokinetics:

Absorption: ZANTAC is 50% absorbed after oral administration, compared to an intravenous (IV) injection with mean peak levels of 440 to 545 ng/mL occurring 2 to 3 hours after a 150-mg dose. The syrup and EFFERdose formulations are bioequivalent to the tablets. Absorption is not significantly impaired by the administration of food or antacids. Propantheline slightly delays and increases peak blood levels of ZANTAC, probably by delaying gastric emptying and transit time. In one study, simultaneous administration of high-potency antacid (150 mmol) in fasting subjects has been reported to decrease the absorption of ZANTAC.

Distribution: The volume of distribution is about 1.4 L/kg. Serum protein binding averages 15%.

Metabolism: In humans, the N-oxide is the principal metabolite in the urine; however, this amounts to <4% of the dose. Other metabolites are the S-oxide (1%) and the desmethyl ranitidine (1%). The remainder of the administered dose is found in the stool. Studies in patients with hepatic dysfunction (compensated cirrhosis) indicate that there are minor, but clinically insignificant, alterations in ranitidine half-life, distribution, clearance, and bioavailability.

Excretion: The principal route of excretion is the urine, with approximately 30% of the orally administered dose collected in the urine as unchanged drug in 24 hours. Renal clearance is about 410 mL/min, indicating active tubular excretion. The elimination half-life is 2.5 to 3 hours. Four patients with clinically significant renal function impairment (creatinine clearance 25 to 35 mL/min) administered 50 mg of ranitidine intravenously had an average plasma half-life of 4.8 hours, a ranitidine clearance of 29 mL/min, and a volume of distribution of 1.76 L/kg. In general, these parameters appear to be altered in proportion to creatinine clearance (see DOSAGE AND ADMINISTRATION).

Geriatrics: The plasma half-life is prolonged and total clearance is reduced in the elderly population due to a decrease in renal function. The elimination half-life is 3 to 4 hours. Peak levels average 526 ng/mL following a 150-mg twice daily dose and occur in about 3 hours (see PRECAUTIONS: Geriatric Use and DOSAGE AND ADMINISTRATION: Dosage Adjustment for Patients With Impaired Renal Function).

Pediatrics: There are no significant differences in the pharmacokinetic parameter values for ranitidine in pediatric patients (from 1 month up to 16 years of age) and healthy adults when correction is made for body weight. The average bioavailability of ranitidine given orally to pediatric patients is 48% which is comparable to the bioavailability of ranitidine in the adult population. All other pharmacokinetic parameter values ($t_{1/2}$, Vd, and CL) are similar to those observed with intravenous ranitidine use in pediatric patients. Estimates of C_{max} and T_{max} are displayed in Table 1.

[See table 1 at top of next page]

Plasma clearance measured in 2 neonatal patients (less than 1 month of age) was considerably lower (3 mL/min/kg) than children or adults and is likely due to reduced renal function observed in this population (see PRECAUTIONS: Pediatric Use and DOSAGE AND ADMINISTRATION: Pediatric Use).

Pharmacodynamics: Serum concentrations necessary to inhibit 50% of stimulated gastric acid secretion are estimated to be 36 to 94 ng/mL. Following a single oral dose of 150 mg, serum concentrations of ZANTAC are in this range up to 12 hours. However, blood levels bear no consistent relationship to dose or degree of acid inhibition.

In a pharmacodynamic comparison of the EFFERdose with the ZANTAC Tablets, during the first hour after administration, the EFFERdose tablet formulation gave a significantly higher intragastric pH, by approximately 1 pH unit, compared to the ZANTAC tablets.

Antisecretory Activity: ***1. Effects on Acid Secretion:*** ZANTAC inhibits both daytime and nocturnal basal gastric acid secretions as well as gastric acid secretion stimulated by food, betazole, and pentagastrin, as shown in Table 2.

Table 2. Effect of Oral ZANTAC on Gastric Acid Secretion

	Time After Dose, h	% Inhibition of Gastric Acid Output by Dose, mg			
		75-80	100	150	200
Basal	Up to 4		99	95	
Nocturnal	Up to 13	95	96	92	
Betazole	Up to 3		97	99	
Pentagastrin	Up to 5	58	72	72	80
Meal	Up to 3		73	79	95

It appears that basal-, nocturnal-, and betazole-stimulated secretions are most sensitive to inhibition by ZANTAC, responding almost completely to doses of 100 mg or less, while pentagastrin- and food-stimulated secretions are more difficult to suppress.

2. Effects on Other Gastrointestinal Secretions:

Pepsin: Oral ZANTAC does not affect pepsin secretion. Total pepsin output is reduced in proportion to the decrease in volume of gastric juice.

Intrinsic Factor: Oral ZANTAC has no significant effect on pentagastrin-stimulated intrinsic factor secretion.

Serum Gastrin: ZANTAC has little or no effect on fasting or postprandial serum gastrin.

Other Pharmacologic Actions:

a. Gastric bacterial flora—increase in nitrate-reducing organisms, significance not known.

b. Prolactin levels—no effect in recommended oral or intravenous (IV) dosage, but small, transient, dose-related increases in serum prolactin have been reported after IV bolus injections of 100 mg or more.

c. Other pituitary hormones—no effect on serum gonadotropins, TSH, or GH. Possible impairment of vasopressin release.

d. No change in cortisol, aldosterone, androgen, or estrogen levels.

e. No antiandrogenic action.

f. No effect on count, motility, or morphology of sperm.

Pediatrics: Oral doses of 6 to 10 mg/kg per day in 2 or 3 divided doses maintain gastric pH>4 throughout most of the dosing interval.

Clinical Trials: ***Active Duodenal Ulcer:*** In a multicenter, double-blind, controlled, US study of endoscopically diagnosed duodenal ulcers, earlier healing was seen in the patients treated with ZANTAC as shown in Table 3.

[See table 3 above]

In these studies, patients treated with ZANTAC reported a reduction in both daytime and nocturnal pain, and they also consumed less antacid than the placebo-treated patients.

Table 4. Mean Daily Doses of Antacid

	Ulcer Healed	Ulcer Not Healed
ZANTAC	0.06	0.71
Placebo	0.71	1.43

Foreign studies have shown that patients heal equally well with 150 mg b.i.d. and 300 mg h.s. (85% versus 84%, respectively) during a usual 4-week course of therapy. If patients require extended therapy of 8 weeks, the healing rate may be higher for 150 mg b.i.d. as compared to 300 mg h.s. (92% versus 87%, respectively).

Studies have been limited to short-term treatment of acute duodenal ulcer. Patients whose ulcers healed during therapy had recurrences of ulcers at the usual rates.

Maintenance Therapy in Duodenal Ulcer: Ranitidine has been found to be effective as maintenance therapy for patients following healing of acute duodenal ulcers. In 2 independent, double-blind, multicenter, controlled trials, the number of duodenal ulcers observed was significantly less in patients treated with ZANTAC (150 mg h.s.) than in patients treated with placebo over a 12-month period.

Table 5. Duodenal Ulcer Prevalence

Double-Blind, Multicenter, Placebo-Controlled Trials					
Multicenter Trial	Drug	Duodenal Ulcer Prevalence			No. of Patients
		0-4 Months	0-8 Months	0-12 Months	
USA	RAN	20%*	24%*	35%*	138
	PLC	44%	54%	59%	139
Foreign	RAN	12%*	21%*	28%*	174
	PLC	56%	64%	68%	165

% = Life table estimate.
* = $P<0.05$ (ZANTAC versus comparator).
RAN = ranitidine (ZANTAC).
PLC = placebo.

As with other H_2-antagonists, the factors responsible for the significant reduction in the prevalence of duodenal ulcers include prevention of recurrence of ulcers, more rapid healing of ulcers that may occur during maintenance therapy, or both.

Table 1. Ranitidine Pharmacokinetics in Pediatric Patients Following Oral Dosing

Population (age)	n	Dosage Form (dose)	C_{max} (ng/mL)	T_{max} (hours)
Gastric or duodenal ulcer (3.5 to 16 years)	12	Tablets (1 to 2 mg/kg)	54 to 492	2.0
Otherwise healthy requiring ZANTAC (0.7 to 14 years, Single dose)	10	Syrup (2 mg/kg)	244	1.61
Otherwise healthy requiring ZANTAC (0.7 to 14 years, Multiple dose)	10	Syrup (2 mg/kg)	320	1.66

Table 3. Duodenal Ulcer Patient Healing Rates

	ZANTAC*		Placebo*	
	Number Entered	Healed/ Evaluable	Number Entered	Healed/ Evaluable
Outpatients Week 2	195	69/182 (38%)†	188	31/164 (19%)
Week 4		137/187 (73%)†		76/168 (45%)

*All patients were permitted p.r.n. antacids for relief of pain.
†$P<0.0001$.

Gastric Ulcer: In a multicenter, double-blind, controlled, US study of endoscopically diagnosed gastric ulcers, earlier healing was seen in the patients treated with ZANTAC as shown in Table 6.

Table 6. Gastric Ulcer Patient Healing Rates

	ZANTAC*		Placebo*	
	Number Entered	Healed/ Evaluable	Number Entered	Healed/ Evaluable
Outpatients Week 2	92	16/83 (19%)	94	10/83 (12%)
Week 6		50/73 (68%)†		35/69 (51%)

*All patients were permitted p.r.n. antacids for relief of pain.
†$P = 0.009$.

In this multicenter trial, significantly more patients treated with ZANTAC became pain free during therapy.

Maintenance of Healing of Gastric Ulcers: In 2 multicenter, double-blind, randomized, placebo-controlled, 12-month trials conducted in patients whose gastric ulcers had been previously healed, ZANTAC 150 mg h.s. was significantly more effective than placebo in maintaining healing of gastric ulcers.

Pathological Hypersecretory Conditions (such as Zollinger-Ellison syndrome): ZANTAC inhibits gastric acid secretion and reduces occurrence of diarrhea, anorexia, and pain in patients with pathological hypersecretion associated with Zollinger-Ellison syndrome, systemic mastocytosis, and other pathological hypersecretory conditions (e.g., postoperative, "short-gut" syndrome, idiopathic). Use of ZANTAC was followed by healing of ulcers in 8 of 19 (42%) patients who were intractable to previous therapy.

Gastroesophageal Reflux Disease (GERD): In 2 multicenter, double-blind, placebo-controlled, 6-week trials performed in the United States and Europe, ZANTAC 150 mg b.i.d. was more effective than placebo for the relief of heartburn and other symptoms associated with GERD. Ranitidine-treated patients consumed significantly less antacid than did placebo-treated patients.

The US trial indicated that ZANTAC 150 mg b.i.d. significantly reduced the frequency of heartburn attacks and severity of heartburn pain within 1 to 2 weeks after starting therapy. The improvement was maintained throughout the 6-week trial period. Moreover, patient response rates demonstrated that the effect on heartburn extends through both the day and night time periods.

In 2 additional US multicenter, double-blind, placebo-controlled, 2-week trials, ZANTAC 150 mg b.i.d. was shown to provide relief of heartburn pain within 24 hours of initiating therapy and a reduction in the frequency of severity of heartburn. In these trials, ZANTAC EFFERdose Tablets were shown to provide heartburn relief within 45 minutes of dosing.

Erosive Esophagitis: In 2 multicenter, double-blind, randomized, placebo-controlled, 12-week trials performed in the United States, ZANTAC 150 mg q.i.d. was significantly more effective than placebo in healing endoscopically diagnosed erosive esophagitis and in relieving associated heartburn. The erosive esophagitis healing rates were as follows:

Table 7. Erosive Esophagitis Patient Healing Rates

	Healed/Evaluable	
	Placebo* n = 229	ZANTAC 150 mg q.i.d.* n = 215
Week 4	43/198 (22%)	96/206 (47%)†
Week 8	63/176 (36%)	142/200 (71%)†
Week 12	92/159 (58%)	162/192 (84%)†

*All patients were permitted p.r.n. antacids for relief of pain.
†$P<0.001$ versus placebo.

No additional benefit in healing of esophagitis or in relief of heartburn was seen with a ranitidine dose of 300 mg q.i.d.

Maintenance of Healing of Erosive Esophagitis: In 2 multicenter, double-blind, randomized, placebo-controlled, 48-week trials conducted in patients whose erosive esophagitis had been previously healed, ZANTAC 150 mg b.i.d. was significantly more effective than placebo in maintaining healing of erosive esophagitis.

INDICATIONS AND USAGE

ZANTAC is indicated in:

1. Short-term treatment of active duodenal ulcer. Most patients heal within 4 weeks. Studies available to date have not assessed the safety of ranitidine in uncomplicated duodenal ulcer for periods of more than 8 weeks.
2. Maintenance therapy for duodenal ulcer patients at reduced dosage after healing of acute ulcers. No placebo-controlled comparative studies have been carried out for periods of longer than 1 year.
3. The treatment of pathological hypersecretory conditions (e.g., Zollinger-Ellison syndrome and systemic mastocytosis).
4. Short-term treatment of active, benign gastric ulcer. Most patients heal within 6 weeks and the usefulness of further treatment has not been demonstrated. Studies available to date have not assessed the safety of ranitidine in uncomplicated, benign gastric ulcer for periods of more than 6 weeks.
5. Maintenance therapy for gastric ulcer patients at reduced dosage after healing of acute ulcers. Placebo-controlled studies have been carried out for 1 year.
6. Treatment of GERD. Symptomatic relief commonly occurs within 24 hours after starting therapy with ZANTAC 150 mg b.i.d.
7. Treatment of endoscopically diagnosed erosive esophagitis. Symptomatic relief of heartburn commonly occurs within 24 hours of therapy initiation with ZANTAC 150 mg q.i.d.
8. Maintenance of healing of erosive esophagitis. Placebo-controlled trials have been carried out for 48 weeks.

Concomitant antacids should be given as needed for pain relief to patients with active duodenal ulcer; active, benign gastric ulcer; hypersecretory states; GERD; and erosive esophagitis.

CONTRAINDICATIONS

ZANTAC is contraindicated for patients known to have hypersensitivity to the drug or any of the ingredients (see PRECAUTIONS).

Continued on next page

Product information on these pages is effective as of August 2004. Further information is available at: GlaxoSmithKline, PO Box 13398, Research Triangle Park, NC 27709. 1-888-825-5249. Corporate Web Site: www.gsk.com

Zantac Tablets/Syrup—Cont.

PRECAUTIONS

General: 1. Symptomatic response to therapy with ZANTAC does not preclude the presence of gastric malignancy.

2. Since ZANTAC is excreted primarily by the kidney, dosage should be adjusted in patients with impaired renal function (see DOSAGE AND ADMINISTRATION). Caution should be observed in patients with hepatic dysfunction since ZANTAC is metabolized in the liver.

3. Rare reports suggest that ZANTAC may precipitate acute porphyric attacks in patients with acute porphyria. ZANTAC should therefore be avoided in patients with a history of acute porphyria.

Information for Patients: ***Phenylketonurics:*** ZANTAC 25 EFFERdose Tablets contain phenylalanine 2.81 mg per 25 mg of ranitidine. ZANTAC 150 EFFERdose Tablets contain phenylalanine 16.84 mg per 150 mg of ranitidine.

Laboratory Tests: False-positive tests for urine protein with MULTISTIX® may occur during ZANTAC therapy, and therefore testing with sulfosalicylic acid is recommended.

Drug Interactions: Although ZANTAC has been reported to bind weakly to cytochrome P-450 in vitro, recommended doses of the drug do not inhibit the action of the cytochrome P-450–linked oxygenase enzymes in the liver. However, there have been isolated reports of drug interactions that suggest that ZANTAC may affect the bioavailability of certain drugs by some mechanism as yet unidentified (e.g., a pH-dependent effect on absorption or a change in volume of distribution).

Increased or decreased prothrombin times have been reported during concurrent use of ranitidine and warfarin. However, in human pharmacokinetic studies with dosages of ranitidine up to 400 mg/day, no interaction occurred; ranitidine had no effect on warfarin clearance or prothrombin time. The possibility of an interaction with warfarin at dosages of ranitidine higher than 400 mg/day has not been investigated.

In a ranitidine-triazolam drug-drug interaction study, triazolam plasma concentrations were higher during b.i.d. dosing of ranitidine than triazolam given alone. The mean area under the triazolam concentration-time curve (AUC) values in 18- to 60-year-old subjects were 10% and 28% higher following administration of 75-mg and 150-mg ranitidine tablets, respectively, than triazolam given alone. In subjects older than 60 years of age, the mean AUC values were approximately 30% higher following administration of 75-mg and 150-mg ranitidine tablets. It appears that there were no changes in pharmacokinetics of triazolam and α-hydroxytriazolam, a major metabolite, and in their elimination. Reduced gastric acidity due to ranitidine may have resulted in an increase in the availability of triazolam. The clinical significance of this triazolam and ranitidine pharmacokinetic interaction is unknown.

Carcinogenesis, Mutagenesis, Impairment of Fertility: There was no indication of tumorigenic or carcinogenic effects in life-span studies in mice and rats at dosages up to 2,000 mg/kg per day.

Ranitidine was not mutagenic in standard bacterial tests *(Salmonella, Escherichia coli)* for mutagenicity at concentrations up to the maximum recommended for these assays. In a dominant lethal assay, a single oral dose of 1,000 mg/kg to male rats was without effect on the outcome of 2 matings per week for the next 9 weeks.

Pregnancy: ***Teratogenic Effects:*** Pregnancy Category B. Reproduction studies have been performed in rats and rabbits at doses up to 160 times the human dose and have revealed no evidence of impaired fertility or harm to the fetus due to ZANTAC. There are, however, no adequate and well-controlled studies in pregnant women. Because animal reproduction studies are not always predictive of human response, this drug should be used during pregnancy only if clearly needed.

Nursing Mothers: ZANTAC is secreted in human milk. Caution should be exercised when ZANTAC is administered to a nursing mother.

Pediatric Use: The safety and effectiveness of ZANTAC have been established in the age-group of 1 month to 16 years for the treatment of duodenal and gastric ulcers, gastroesophageal reflux disease and erosive esophagitis, and the maintenance of healed duodenal and gastric ulcer. Use of ZANTAC in this age-group is supported by adequate and well-controlled studies in adults, as well as additional pharmacokinetic data in pediatric patients and an analysis of the published literature (see CLINICAL PHARMACOLOGY: Pediatrics and DOSAGE AND ADMINISTRATION: Pediatric Use).

Safety and effectiveness in pediatric patients for the treatment of pathological hypersecretory conditions or the maintenance of healing of erosive esophagitis have not been established.

Safety and effectiveness in neonates (less than 1 month of age) have not been established (see CLINICAL PHARMACOLOGY: Pediatrics).

Geriatric Use: Of the total number of subjects enrolled in US and foreign controlled clinical trials of oral formulations of ZANTAC, for which there were subgroup analyses, 4,197 were 65 and over, while 899 were 75 and over. No overall differences in safety or effectiveness were observed between these subjects and younger subjects, and other reported clinical experience has not identified differences in responses between the elderly and younger patients, but greater sensitivity of some older individuals cannot be ruled out.

This drug is known to be substantially excreted by the kidney and the risk of toxic reactions to this drug may be greater in patients with impaired renal function. Because elderly patients are more likely to have decreased renal function, caution should be exercised in dose selection, and it may be useful to monitor renal function (see CLINICAL PHARMACOLOGY: Pharmacokinetics: Geriatrics and DOSAGE AND ADMINISTRATION: Dosage Adjustment for Patients With Impaired Renal Function).

ADVERSE REACTIONS

The following have been reported as events in clinical trials or in the routine management of patients treated with ZANTAC. The relationship to therapy with ZANTAC has been unclear in many cases. Headache, sometimes severe, seems to be related to administration of ZANTAC.

Central Nervous System: Rarely, malaise, dizziness, somnolence, insomnia, and vertigo. Rare cases of reversible mental confusion, agitation, depression, and hallucinations have been reported, predominantly in severely ill elderly patients. Rare cases of reversible blurred vision suggestive of a change in accommodation have been reported. Rare reports of reversible involuntary motor disturbances have been received.

Cardiovascular: As with other H_2-blockers, rare reports of arrhythmias such as tachycardia, bradycardia, atrioventricular block, and premature ventricular beats.

Gastrointestinal: Constipation, diarrhea, nausea/vomiting, abdominal discomfort/pain, and rare reports of pancreatitis.

Hepatic: There have been occasional reports of hepatocellular, cholestatic, or mixed hepatitis, with or without jaundice. In such circumstances, ranitidine should be immediately discontinued. These events are usually reversible, but in rare circumstances death has occurred. Rare cases of hepatic failure have also been reported. In normal volunteers, SGPT values were increased to at least twice the pretreatment levels in 6 of 12 subjects receiving 100 mg q.i.d. intravenously for 7 days, and in 4 of 24 subjects receiving 50 mg q.i.d. intravenously for 5 days.

Musculoskeletal: Rare reports of arthralgias and myalgias.

Hematologic: Blood count changes (leukopenia, granulocytopenia, and thrombocytopenia) have occurred in a few patients. These were usually reversible. Rare cases of agranulocytosis, pancytopenia, sometimes with marrow hypoplasia, and aplastic anemia and exceedingly rare cases of acquired immune hemolytic anemia have been reported.

Endocrine: Controlled studies in animals and man have shown no stimulation of any pituitary hormone by ZANTAC and no antiandrogenic activity, and cimetidine-induced gynecomastia and impotence in hypersecretory patients have resolved when ZANTAC has been substituted. However, occasional cases of gynecomastia, impotence, and loss of libido have been reported in male patients receiving ZANTAC, but the incidence did not differ from that in the general population.

Integumentary: Rash, including rare cases of erythema multiforme. Rare cases of alopecia and vasculitis.

Other: Rare cases of hypersensitivity reactions (e.g., bronchospasm, fever, rash, eosinophilia), anaphylaxis, angioneurotic edema, and small increases in serum creatinine.

OVERDOSAGE

There has been limited experience with overdosage. Reported acute ingestions of up to 18 g orally have been associated with transient adverse effects similar to those encountered in normal clinical experience (see ADVERSE REACTIONS). In addition, abnormalities of gait and hypotension have been reported.

When overdosage occurs, the usual measures to remove unabsorbed material from the gastrointestinal tract, clinical monitoring, and supportive therapy should be employed.

Studies in dogs receiving dosages of ZANTAC in excess of 225 mg/kg per day have shown muscular tremors, vomiting, and rapid respiration. Single oral doses of 1,000 mg/kg in mice and rats were not lethal. Intravenous LD_{50} values in mice and rats were 77 and 83 mg/kg, respectively.

DOSAGE AND ADMINISTRATION

Active Duodenal Ulcer: The current recommended adult oral dosage of ZANTAC for duodenal ulcer is 150 mg or 10 mL of syrup (2 teaspoonfuls of syrup equivalent to 150 mg of ranitidine) twice daily. An alternative dosage of 300 mg or 20 mL of syrup (4 teaspoonfuls of syrup equivalent to 300 mg of ranitidine) once daily after the evening meal or at bedtime can be used for patients in whom dosing convenience is important. The advantages of one treatment regimen compared to the other in a particular patient population have yet to be demonstrated (see Clinical Trials: *Active Duodenal Ulcer*). Smaller doses have been shown to be equally effective in inhibiting gastric acid secretion in US studies, and several foreign trials have shown that 100 mg twice daily is as effective as the 150-mg dose.

Antacid should be given as needed for relief of pain (see CLINICAL PHARMACOLOGY: Pharmacokinetics).

Maintenance of Healing of Duodenal Ulcers: The current recommended adult oral dosage is 150 mg or 10 mL of syrup (2 teaspoonfuls of syrup equivalent to 150 mg of ranitidine) at bedtime.

Pathological Hypersecretory Conditions (such as Zollinger-Ellison syndrome): The current recommended adult oral dosage is 150 mg or 10 mL of syrup (2 teaspoonfuls of syrup equivalent to 150 mg of ranitidine) twice a day. In some patients it may be necessary to administer ZANTAC 150-mg doses more frequently. Dosages should be adjusted to individual patient needs, and should continue as long as clinically indicated. Dosages up to 6 g/day have been employed in patients with severe disease.

Benign Gastric Ulcer: The current recommended adult oral dosage is 150 mg or 10 mL of syrup (2 teaspoonfuls of syrup equivalent to 150 mg of ranitidine) twice a day.

Maintenance of Healing of Gastric Ulcers: The current recommended adult oral dosage is 150 mg or 10 mL of syrup (2 teaspoonfuls of syrup equivalent to 150 mg of ranitidine) at bedtime.

GERD: The current recommended adult oral dosage is 150 mg or 10 mL of syrup (2 teaspoonfuls of syrup equivalent to 150 mg of ranitidine) twice a day.

Erosive Esophagitis: The current recommended adult oral dosage is 150 mg or 10 mL of syrup (2 teaspoonfuls of syrup equivalent to 150 mg of ranitidine) 4 times a day.

Maintenance of Healing of Erosive Esophagitis: The current recommended adult oral dosage is 150 mg or 10 mL of syrup (2 teaspoonfuls of syrup equivalent to 150 mg of ranitidine) twice a day.

Pediatric Use: The safety and effectiveness of ZANTAC have been established in the age-group of 1 month to 16 years. There is insufficient information about the pharmacokinetics of ZANTAC in neonatal patients (less than 1 month of age) to make dosing recommendations.

The following 3 subsections provide dosing information for each of the pediatric indications. Also, see the subsection of Preparation of ZANTAC 25 EFFERdose Tablets, below.

Treatment of Duodenal and Gastric Ulcers: The recommended oral dose for the treatment of active duodenal and gastric ulcers is 2 to 4 mg/kg twice daily to a maximum of 300 mg/day. This recommendation is derived from adult clinical studies and pharmacokinetic data in pediatric patients.

Maintenance of Healing of Duodenal and Gastric Ulcers: The recommended oral dose for the maintenance of healing of duodenal and gastric ulcers is 2 to 4 mg/kg once daily to a maximum of 150 mg/day. This recommendation is derived from adult clinical studies and pharmacokinetic data in pediatric patients.

Treatment of GERD and Erosive Esophagitis: Although limited data exist for these conditions in pediatric patients, published literature supports a dosage of 5 to 10 mg/kg per day, usually given as 2 divided doses.

Dosage Adjustment for Patients With Impaired Renal Function: On the basis of experience with a group of subjects with severely impaired renal function treated with ZANTAC, the recommended dosage in patients with a creatinine clearance <50 mL/min is 150 mg or 10 mL of syrup (2 teaspoonfuls of syrup equivalent to 150 mg of ranitidine) every 24 hours. Should the patient's condition require, the frequency of dosing may be increased to every 12 hours or even further with caution. Hemodialysis reduces the level of circulating ranitidine. Ideally, the dosing schedule should be adjusted so that the timing of a scheduled dose coincides with the end of hemodialysis.

Elderly patients are more likely to have decreased renal function, therefore caution should be exercised in dose selection, and it may be useful to monitor renal function (see CLINICAL PHARMACOLOGY: Pharmacokinetics: Geriatrics and PRECAUTIONS: Geriatric Use).

Preparation of ZANTAC 25 EFFERdose Tablets: Dissolve 1 tablet in no less than 5 mL (1 teaspoonful) of water in an appropriate measuring cup. Wait until the tablet is completely dissolved before administering the solution to the infant/child. The solution may be administered by medicine dropper for infants.

Preparation of ZANTAC 150 EFFERdose Tablets: Dissolve each dose in approximately 6 to 8 oz of water before drinking.

HOW SUPPLIED

ZANTAC 150 Tablets (ranitidine HCl equivalent to 150 mg of ranitidine) are peach, film-coated, 5-sided tablets embossed with "ZANTAC 150" on one side and "Glaxo" on the other. They are available in bottles of 60 (NDC 0173-0344-42), 180 (NDC 0173-0344-17), 500 (NDC 0173-0344-14), and 1,000 (NDC 0173-0344-12) tablets and unit dose packs of 100 (NDC 0173-0344-47) tablets.

ZANTAC 300 Tablets (ranitidine HCl equivalent to 300 mg of ranitidine) are yellow, film-coated, capsule-shaped tablets embossed with "ZANTAC 300" on one side and "Glaxo" on the other. They are available in bottles of 30 (NDC 0173-0393-40) and 250 (NDC 0173-0393-06) tablets and unit dose packs of 100 (NDC 0173-0393-47) tablets.

Store between 15° and 30°C (59° and 86°F) in a dry place. Protect from light. Replace cap securely after each opening.

ZANTAC 25 EFFERdose Tablets (ranitidine HCl equivalent to 25 mg of ranitidine) are white to pale yellow, round, flat-faced, bevel-edged tablets embossed with "GS" on one side and "25C" on the other side. They are packaged in foil strips and are available in a carton of 60 (NDC 0173-0734-00) tablets.

ZANTAC 150 EFFERdose Tablets (ranitidine HCl equivalent to 150 mg of ranitidine) are white to pale yellow, round, flat-faced, bevel-edged tablets embossed with "ZANTAC 150" on one side and "427" on the other. They are packaged individually in foil and are available in a carton of 60 (NDC 0173-0427-02) tablets.

Store between 2° and 30°C (36° and 86°F).

ZANTAC Syrup, a clear, peppermint-flavored liquid, contains 16.8 mg of ranitidine HCl equivalent to 15 mg of ranitidine per 1 mL (75 mg/5 mL) in bottles of 16 fluid ounces (one pint) (NDC 0173-0383-54).

Store between 4° and 25°C (39° and 77°F). Dispense in tight, light-resistant containers as defined in the USP/NF.

GlaxoSmithKline, Research Triangle Park, NC 27709

ZANTAC and EFFERdose are registered trademarks of Warner-Lambert Company, used under license.

April 2004/RL-2080

Shown in Product Identification Guide, page 318

ZIAGEN® ℞

[zi'ə-jin]

(abacavir sulfate)

Tablets

ZIAGEN® ℞

(abacavir sulfate)

Oral Solution

> **WARNING**
> **FATAL HYPERSENSITIVITY REACTIONS HAVE BEEN ASSOCIATED WITH THERAPY WITH ZIAGEN. PATIENTS DEVELOPING SIGNS OR SYMPTOMS OF HYPERSENSITIVITY (WHICH INCLUDE FEVER; SKIN RASH; FATIGUE; GASTROINTESTINAL SYMPTOMS SUCH AS NAUSEA, VOMITING, DIARRHEA, OR ABDOMINAL PAIN; AND RESPIRATORY SYMPTOMS SUCH AS PHARYNGITIS, DYSPNEA, OR COUGH) SHOULD DISCONTINUE ZIAGEN AS SOON AS A HYPERSENSITIVITY REACTION IS SUSPECTED. TO AVOID A DELAY IN DIAGNOSIS AND MINIMIZE THE RISK OF A LIFE-THREATENING HYPERSENSITIVITY REACTION, ZIAGEN SHOULD BE PERMANENTLY DISCONTINUED IF HYPERSENSITIVITY CANNOT BE RULED OUT, EVEN WHEN OTHER DIAGNOSES ARE POSSIBLE (E.G., ACUTE ONSET RESPIRATORY DISEASES, GASTROENTERITIS, OR REACTIONS TO OTHER MEDICATIONS).**
> **ZIAGEN SHOULD NOT BE RESTARTED FOLLOWING A HYPERSENSITIVITY REACTION BECAUSE MORE SEVERE SYMPTOMS WILL RECUR WITHIN HOURS AND MAY INCLUDE LIFE-THREATENING HYPOTENSION AND DEATH.**
> **SEVERE OR FATAL HYPERSENSITIVITY REACTIONS CAN OCCUR WITHIN HOURS AFTER REINTRODUCTION OF ZIAGEN IN PATIENTS WHO HAVE NO IDENTIFIED HISTORY OR UNRECOGNIZED SYMPTOMS OF HYPERSENSITIVITY TO ABACAVIR THERAPY (SEE WARNINGS, PRECAUTIONS: INFORMATION FOR PATIENTS, AND ADVERSE REACTIONS).**
> **LACTIC ACIDOSIS AND SEVERE HEPATOMEGALY WITH STEATOSIS, INCLUDING FATAL CASES, HAVE BEEN REPORTED WITH THE USE OF NUCLEOSIDE ANALOGUES ALONE OR IN COMBINATION, INCLUDING ZIAGEN AND OTHER ANTIRETROVIRALS (SEE WARNINGS).**

DESCRIPTION

ZIAGEN is the brand name for abacavir sulfate, a synthetic carbocyclic nucleoside analogue with inhibitory activity against HIV. The chemical name of abacavir sulfate is *(1S,cis)*-4-[2-amino-6-(cyclopropylamino)-9*H*-purin-9-yl]-2-cyclopentene-1-methanol sulfate (salt) (2:1). Abacavir sulfate is the enantiomer with *1S, 4R* absolute configuration on the cyclopentene ring. It has a molecular formula of $(C_{14}H_{18}N_6O)_2 \bullet H_2SO_4$ and a molecular weight of 670.76 daltons.

Abacavir sulfate is a white to off-white solid with a solubility of approximately 77 mg/mL in distilled water at 25°C. It has an octanol/water (pH 7.1 to 7.3) partition coefficient (log *P*) of approximately 1.20 at 25°C.

ZIAGEN Tablets are for oral administration. Each tablet contains abacavir sulfate equivalent to 300 mg of abacavir and the inactive ingredients colloidal silicon dioxide, magnesium stearate, microcrystalline cellulose, and sodium starch glycolate. The tablets are coated with a film that is made of hypromellose, polysorbate 80, synthetic yellow iron oxide, titanium dioxide, and triacetin.

ZIAGEN Oral Solution is for oral administration. One milliliter (1 mL) of ZIAGEN Oral Solution contains abacavir sulfate equivalent to 20 mg of abacavir (20 mg/mL) in an aqueous solution and the inactive ingredients artificial strawberry and banana flavors, citric acid (anhydrous), methylparaben and propylparaben (added as preservatives), propylene glycol, saccharin sodium, sodium citrate (dihydrate), and sorbitol solution.

In vivo, abacavir sulfate dissociates to its free base, abacavir. In this insert, all dosages for ZIAGEN are expressed in terms of abacavir.

MICROBIOLOGY

Mechanism of Action: Abacavir is a carbocyclic synthetic nucleoside analogue. Intracellularly, abacavir is converted by cellular enzymes to the active metabolite carbovir triphosphate, an analogue of deoxyguanosine-5′-triphosphate (dGTP). Carbovir triphosphate inhibits the activity of HIV-1 reverse transcriptase (RT) both by competing with the natural substrate dGTP and by its incorporation into viral DNA. The lack of a 3′-OH group in the incorporated nucleoside analogue prevents the formation of the 5′ to 3′ phosphodiester linkage essential for DNA chain elongation, and therefore, the viral DNA growth is terminated. Abacavir is a weak inhibitor of cellular DNA polymerases α, β, and γ.

Antiviral Activity: The in vitro anti-HIV-1 activity of abacavir was evaluated against a T-cell tropic laboratory strain HIV-1_{IIIB} in lymphoblastic cell lines, a monocyte/macrophage tropic laboratory strain HIV-1_{BaL} in primary monocytes/macrophages, and clinical isolates in peripheral blood mononuclear cells. The concentration of drug necessary to inhibit viral replication by 50 percent (IC_{50}) ranged from 3.7 to 5.8 μM against HIV-1_{IIIB}, and was 0.26 ± 0.18 μM (1 μM = 0.28 mcg/mL) against 8 clinical isolates. The IC_{50} value of abacavir against HIV-1_{BaL} varied from 0.07 to 1.0 μM. Abacavir had synergistic activity in vitro in combination with amprenavir, nevirapine, and zidovudine, and additive activity in combination with didanosine, lamivudine, stavudine, and zalcitabine.

Resistance: HIV-1 isolates with reduced sensitivity to abacavir have been selected in vitro and were also obtained from patients treated with abacavir. Genetic analysis of isolates from abacavir-treated patients showed point mutations in the reverse transcriptase gene that resulted in K65R, L74V, Y115F, and M184V amino acid substitutions. HIV-1 isolates from virologic failure antiretroviral-naive patients treated with abacavir alone (n = 67) contained the M184V mutation (n = 27), often in combination with the L74V mutation (n = 18). In some patients, the M184V mutation was also detected in combination with K65R and/or Y115F. Genetic analysis of isolates from virologic failure antiretroviral-naive patients treated with abacavir in combination with other antiretrovirals (n = 55) also showed that many isolates contained the M184V mutation (n = 26) alone, and, sometimes in combination with L74V (n = 2). In a clinical study of treatment-naive patients (CNA30024, n = 649) comparing ZIAGEN to zidovudine both in combination with efavirenz and lamivudine, 34 patients experienced virologic failure (plasma HIV-1 RNA >50 copies/mL, see CLINICAL STUDIES). Four patients in each treatment arm had viral isolates containing resistance-associated mutations including M184V and non-nucleoside reverse transcriptase inhibitor (NNRTI) mutations.

Cross-Resistance: Cross-resistance has been observed among nucleoside reverse transcriptase inhibitors. Recombinant laboratory strains of HIV-1_{HXB2} containing multiple abacavir resistance-associated mutations, namely, K65R, L74V, M184V, and Y115F, exhibited cross-resistance to didanosine, emtricitabine, lamivudine, tenofovir, and zalcitabine in vitro. The K65R mutation may also confer resistance to stavudine. An increasing number of thymidine analogue mutations (TAMs) (M41L, D67N, K70R, L210W, T215Y/F, K219E/R/H/Q/N) is associated with a progressive reduction in abacavir susceptibility.

CLINICAL PHARMACOLOGY

Pharmacokinetics in Adults: The pharmacokinetic properties of abacavir have been studied in asymptomatic, HIV-infected adult patients after administration of a single intravenous (IV) dose of 150 mg and after single and multiple oral doses. The pharmacokinetic properties of abacavir were independent of dose over the range of 300 to 1,200 mg/day.

Absorption and Bioavailability: Abacavir was rapidly and extensively absorbed after oral administration. The geometric mean absolute bioavailability of the tablet was 83%. After oral administration of 300 mg twice daily in 20 patients, the steady-state peak serum abacavir concentration (C_{max}) was 3.0 ± 0.89 mcg/mL (mean ± SD) and $AUC_{(0-12\ hr)}$ was 6.02 ± 1.73 mcg•hr/mL. Bioavailability of abacavir tablets was assessed in the fasting and fed states. There was no significant difference in systemic exposure (AUC_∞) in the fed and fasting states; therefore, ZIAGEN Tablets may be administered with or without food. Systemic exposure to abacavir was comparable after administration of ZIAGEN Oral Solution and ZIAGEN Tablets. Therefore, these products may be used interchangeably.

Distribution: The apparent volume of distribution after IV administration of abacavir was 0.86 ± 0.15 L/kg, suggesting that abacavir distributes into extravascular space. In 3 subjects, the CSF $AUC_{(0-6\ hr)}$ to plasma abacavir $AUC_{(0-6\ hr)}$ ratio ranged from 27% to 33%.

Binding of abacavir to human plasma proteins is approximately 50%. Binding of abacavir to plasma proteins was independent of concentration. Total blood and plasma drug-related radioactivity concentrations are identical, demonstrating that abacavir readily distributes into erythrocytes.

Metabolism: In humans, abacavir is not significantly metabolized by cytochrome P450 enzymes. The primary routes of elimination of abacavir are metabolism by alcohol dehydrogenase (to form the 5′-carboxylic acid) and glucuronyl transferase (to form the 5′-glucuronide). The metabolites do not have antiviral activity. In vitro experiments reveal that abacavir does not inhibit human CYP3A4, CYP2D6, or CYP2C9 activity at clinically relevant concentrations.

Elimination: Elimination of abacavir was quantified in a mass balance study following administration of a 600-mg dose of ^{14}C-abacavir: 99% of the radioactivity was recovered, 1.2% was excreted in the urine as abacavir, 30% as the 5′-carboxylic acid metabolite, 36% as the 5′-glucuronide metabolite, and 15% as unidentified minor metabolites in the urine. Fecal elimination accounted for 16% of the dose.

In single-dose studies, the observed elimination half-life ($t_{1/2}$) was 1.54 ± 0.63 hours. After intravenous administration, total clearance was 0.80 ± 0.24 L/hr/kg (mean ± SD).

Special Populations: ***Adults With Impaired Renal Function:*** The pharmacokinetic properties of ZIAGEN have not been determined in patients with impaired renal function. Renal excretion of unchanged abacavir is a minor route of elimination in humans.

Adults with Impaired Hepatic Function: The pharmacokinetics of abacavir have been studied in patients with mild hepatic impairment (Child-Pugh score 5 to 6). Results showed that there was a mean increase of 89% in the abacavir AUC, and an increase of 58% in the half-life of abacavir after a single dose of 600 mg of abacavir. The AUCs of the metabolites were not modified by mild liver disease; however, the rates of formation and elimination of the metabolites were decreased. A dose of 200 mg (provided by 10 mL of ZIAGEN Oral Solution) administered twice daily is recommended for patients with mild liver disease. The safety, efficacy, and pharmacokinetics of abacavir have not been studied in patients with moderate or severe hepatic impairment, therefore ZIAGEN is contraindicated in these patients.

Pediatric Patients: The pharmacokinetics of abacavir have been studied after either single or repeat doses of ZIAGEN in 68 pediatric patients. Following multiple-dose administration of ZIAGEN 8 mg/kg twice daily, steady-state $AUC_{(0-12\ hr)}$ and C_{max} were 9.8 ± 4.56 mcg•hr/mL and 3.71 ± 1.36 mcg/mL (mean ± SD), respectively (see PRECAUTIONS: Pediatric Use).

Geriatric Patients: The pharmacokinetics of ZIAGEN have not been studied in patients over 65 years of age.

Gender: The pharmacokinetics of ZIAGEN with respect to gender have not been determined.

Race: The pharmacokinetics of ZIAGEN with respect to race have not been determined.

Drug Interactions: In human liver microsomes, abacavir did not inhibit cytochrome P450 isoforms (2C9, 2D6, 3A4). Based on these data, it is unlikely that clinically significant drug interactions will occur between abacavir and drugs metabolized through these pathways.

Due to their common metabolic pathways via glucuronyl transferase with zidovudine, 15 HIV-infected patients were enrolled in a crossover study evaluating single doses of abacavir (600 mg), lamivudine (150 mg), and zidovudine (300 mg) alone or in combination. Analysis showed no clinically relevant changes in the pharmacokinetics of abacavir with the addition of lamivudine or zidovudine or the combination of lamivudine and zidovudine. Lamivudine exposure (AUC decreased 15%) and zidovudine exposure (AUC increased 10%) did not show clinically relevant changes with concurrent abacavir.

Due to their common metabolic pathways via alcohol dehydrogenase, the pharmacokinetic interaction between abacavir and ethanol was studied in 24 HIV-infected male patients. Each patient received the following treatments on separate occasions: a single 600-mg dose of abacavir, 0.7 g/kg ethanol (equivalent to 5 alcoholic drinks), and abacavir 600 mg plus 0.7 g/kg ethanol. Coadministration of ethanol and abacavir resulted in a 41% increase in abacavir AUC_∞ and a 26% increase in abacavir $t_{1/2}$. In males, abacavir had no effect on the pharmacokinetic properties of ethanol, so no clinically significant interaction is expected in men. This interaction has not been studied in females.

Methadone: In a study of 11 HIV-infected patients receiving methadone-maintenance therapy (40 mg and 90 mg daily), with 600 mg of ZIAGEN twice daily (twice the currently recommended dose), oral methadone clearance increased 22% (90% CI 6% to 42%). This alteration will not result in a methadone dose modification in the majority of patients; however, an increased methadone dose may be required in a small number of patients.

INDICATIONS AND USAGE

ZIAGEN Tablets and Oral Solution, in combination with other antiretroviral agents, are indicated for the treatment of HIV-1 infection.

Description of Clinical Studies: ***Therapy-Naive Adults:*** **CNA30024** was a multicenter, double-blind, controlled study in which 649 HIV-infected, therapy-naive adults were randomized and received either ZIAGEN (300 mg twice daily), lamivudine (150 mg twice daily), and efavirenz (600 mg once daily) or zidovudine (300 mg twice daily), lamivduine (150 mg twice daily), and efavirenz (600 mg once daily). The duration of double-blind treatment was at least 48 weeks. Study participants were: male (81%), Caucasian (51%), black (21%), and Hispanic (26%). The median age was 35 years, the median pretreatment CD4+ cell count was 264 cells/mm^3, and median plasma HIV-1 RNA was 4.79 $\log_{10}$ copies/mL. The outcomes of randomized treatment are provided in Table 1.

[See table 1 at top of next page]

After 48 weeks of therapy, the median CD4+ cell count increases from baseline were 209 cells/mm^3 in the group receiving ZIAGEN and 155 cells/mm^3 in the zidovudine group. Through Week 48, 8 subjects (2%) in the group receiving ZIAGEN (5 CDC classification C events and 3

Continued on next page

Product information on these pages is effective as of August 2004. Further information is available at: GlaxoSmithKline, PO Box 13398, Research Triangle Park, NC 27709. 1-888-825-5249. Corporate Web Site: www.gsk.com

Ziagen—Cont.

deaths) and 5 subjects (2%) on the zidovudine arm (3 CDC classification C events and 2 deaths) experienced clinical disease progression.

CNA3005 was a multicenter, double-blind, controlled study in which 562 HIV-infected, therapy-naive adults with a pre-entry plasma HIV-1 RNA >10,000 copies/mL were randomized to receive either ZIAGEN (300 mg twice daily) plus COMBIVIR (lamivudine 150 mg/zidovudine 300 mg twice daily), or indinavir (800 mg 3 times a day) plus COMBIVIR twice daily. Study participants were male (87%), Caucasian (73%), black (15%), and Hispanic (9%). At baseline the median age was 36 years, the median pretreatment CD4+ cell count was 360 cells/mm^3, and median plasma HIV-1 RNA was 4.8 $\log_{10}$ copies/mL. Proportions of patients with plasma HIV-1 RNA <400 copies/mL (using Roche Amplicor HIV-1 MONITOR Test) through 48 weeks of treatment are summarized in Table 2.

[See table 2 at right]

Through Week 48, an overall mean increase in CD4+ cell count of about 150 cells/mm^3 was observed in both treatment arms.

Table 1. Outcomes of Randomized Treatment Through Week 48 (CNA30024)

Outcome	ZIAGEN plus Lamivudine plus Efavirenz (n = 324)	Zidovudine plus Lamivudine plus Efavirenz (n = 325)
Responder*	69% (73%)	69% (71%)
Virologic failures†	6%	4%
Discontinued due to adverse reactions	14%	16%
Discontinued due to other reasons‡	10%	11%

*Patients achieved and maintained confirmed HIV-1 RNA ≤50 copies/mL (<400 copies/mL through Week 48 (Roche® AMPLICOR Ultrasensitive HIV-1 MONITOR standard test 1.0 PCR).
† Includes viral rebound, insufficient viral response according to the investigator, and failure to achieve confirmed ≤50 copies/mL by Week 48.
‡ Includes consent withdrawn, lost to follow up, protocol violations, those with missing data, clinical progression, and other.

Table 2. Outcomes of Randomized Treatment Through Week 48 (CNA3005)

Outcome	ZIAGEN plus Lamivudine/Zidovudine (n = 282)	Indinavir plus Lamivudine/Zidovudine (n = 280)
HIV-1 RNA <400 copies/mL	46%	47%
HIV-1 RNA ≥400 copies/mL*	29%	28%
Discontinued due to adverse reactions	10%	13%
Discontinued due to other reasons†	8%	8%
Randomized but never initiated treatment	7%	5%

*Includes viral rebound and failure to achieve confirmed <400 copies/mL by Week 48.
† Includes consent withdrawn, lost to follow up, protocol violations, those with missing data, clinical progression, and other.

CONTRAINDICATIONS

Abacavir sulfate has been associated with fatal hypersensitivity reactions. ZIAGEN SHOULD NOT BE RESTARTED FOLLOWING A HYPERSENSITIVITY REACTION TO ABACAVIR (see WARNINGS, PRECAUTIONS, and ADVERSE REACTIONS).

ZIAGEN Tablets and Oral Solution are contraindicated in patients with previously demonstrated hypersensitivity to any of the components of the products (see WARNINGS).

ZIAGEN Tablets and Oral Solution are contraindicated in patients with moderate or severe hepatic impairment.

WARNINGS

Hypersensitivity Reaction: Fatal hypersensitivity reactions have been associated with therapy with ZIAGEN. Patients developing signs or symptoms of hypersensitivity (which include fever; skin rash; fatigue; gastrointestinal symptoms such as nausea, vomiting, diarrhea, or abdominal pain; and respiratory symptoms such as pharyngitis, dyspnea, or cough) should discontinue ZIAGEN as soon as a hypersensitivity reaction is first suspected, and should seek medical evaluation immediately. To avoid a delay in diagnosis and minimize the risk of a life-threatening hypersensitivity reaction, ZIAGEN should be permanently discontinued if hypersensitivity cannot be ruled out, even when other diagnoses are possible (e.g., acute onset respiratory diseases, gastroenteritis, or reactions to other medications).

ZIAGEN SHOULD NOT be restarted following a hypersensitivity reaction because more severe symptoms will recur within hours and may include life-threatening hypotension and death.

Severe or fatal hypersensitivity reactions can occur within hours after reintroduction of ZIAGEN in patients who have no identified history or unrecognized symptoms of hypersensitivity to abacavir therapy.

When therapy with ZIAGEN has been discontinued for reasons other than symptoms of a hypersensitivity reaction, and if reinitiation of therapy is under consideration, the reason for discontinuation should be evaluated to ensure that the patient did not have symptoms of a hypersensitivity reaction. If hypersensitivity cannot be ruled out, abacavir should **NOT** be reintroduced. If symptoms consistent with hypersensitivity are not identified, reintroduction can be undertaken with continued monitoring for symptoms of a hypersensitivity reaction. Patients should be made aware that a hypersensitivity reaction can occur with reintroduction of abacavir, and that abacavir reintroduction should be undertaken only if medical care can be readily accessed by the patient or others (see ADVERSE REACTIONS).

In clinical trials, hypersensitivity reactions have been reported in approximately 5% of adult and pediatric patients receiving abacavir. Symptoms usually appear within the first 6 weeks of treatment with ZIAGEN although these reactions may occur at any time during therapy (see PRECAUTIONS: Information for Patients and ADVERSE REACTIONS).

Abacavir Hypersensitivity Reaction Registry: To facilitate reporting of hypersensitivity reactions and collection of information on each case, an Abacavir Hypersensitivity Registry has been established. Physicians should register patients by calling 1-800-270-0425.

Lactic Acidosis/Severe Hepatomegaly with Steatosis: Lactic acidosis and severe hepatomegaly with steatosis, including fatal cases, have been reported with the use of nucleoside analogues alone or in combination, including abacavir and other antiretrovirals. A majority of these cases have been in women. Obesity and prolonged nucleoside exposure may be risk factors. Particular caution should be exercised when administering ZIAGEN to any patient with known risk factors for liver disease; however, cases have also been reported in patients with no known risk factors. Treatment with ZIAGEN should be suspended in any patient who develops clinical or laboratory findings suggestive of lactic acidosis or pronounced hepatotoxicity (which may include hepatomegaly and steatosis even in the absence of marked transaminase elevations).

PRECAUTIONS

General: Abacavir should always be used in combination with other antiretroviral agents. Abacavir should not be added as a single agent when antiretroviral regimens are changed due to loss of virologic response.

Therapy-Experienced Patients: In clinical trials, patients with prolonged prior nucleoside reverse transcriptase inhibitor (NRTI) exposure or who had HIV-1 isolates that contained multiple mutations conferring resistance to NRTIs had limited response to abacavir. The potential for cross-resistance between abacavir and other NRTIs should be considered when choosing new therapeutic regimens in therapy-experienced patients (see MICROBIOLOGY: Cross-Resistance).

Fat Redistribution: Redistribution/accumulation of body fat including central obesity, dorsocervical fat enlargement (buffalo hump), peripheral wasting, facial wasting, breast enlargement, and "cushingoid appearance" have been observed in patients receiving antiretroviral therapy. The mechanism and long-term consequences of these events are currently unknown. A causal relationship has not been established.

Information for Patients: PATIENTS SHOULD BE ADVISED THAT A MEDICATION GUIDE AND WARNING CARD SUMMARIZING THE SYMPTOMS OF ABACAVIR HYPERSENSITIVITY REACTIONS SHOULD BE DISPENSED BY THE PHARMACIST WITH EACH NEW PRESCRIPTION AND REFILL OF ZIAGEN. THE COMPLETE TEXT OF THE MEDICATION GUIDE IS REPRINTED AT THE END OF THIS DOCUMENT. PATIENTS SHOULD BE INSTRUCTED TO CARRY THE WARNING CARD WITH THEM.

Patients should be advised of the possibility of a hypersensitivity reaction to ZIAGEN that may result in death. Patients developing signs or symptoms of hypersensitivity (which include fever; skin rash; fatigue; gastrointestinal symptoms such as nausea, vomiting, diarrhea, or abdominal pain; and respiratory symptoms such as sore throat, shortness of breath, or cough) should discontinue treatment with ZIAGEN and seek medical evaluation immediately. **ZIAGEN SHOULD NOT be restarted following a hypersensitivity reaction because more severe symptoms will recur within hours and may include life-threatening hypotension and death.** Patients who have interrupted ZIAGEN for reasons other than symptoms of hypersensitivity (for example, those who have an interruption in drug supply) should be made aware that a severe or fatal hypersensitivity reaction can occur with reintroduction of abacavir. Patients should be instructed not to reintroduce abacavir without medical consultation and that reintroduction of abacavir should be undertaken only if medical care can be readily accessed by the patient or others (see ADVERSE REACTIONS and WARNINGS).

ZIAGEN is not a cure for HIV infection and patients may continue to experience illnesses associated with HIV infection, including opportunistic infections. Patients should remain under the care of a physician when using ZIAGEN. Patients should be advised that the use of ZIAGEN has not been shown to reduce the risk of transmission of HIV to others through sexual contact or blood contamination.

Patients should be informed that redistribution or accumulation of body fat may occur in patients receiving antiretroviral therapy and that the cause and long-term health effects of these conditions are not known at this time.

ZIAGEN Tablets and Oral Solution are for oral ingestion only.

Patients should be advised of the importance of taking ZIAGEN exactly as it is prescribed.

Drug Interactions: Pharmacokinetic properties of abacavir were not altered by the addition of either lamivudine or zidovudine or the combination of lamivudine and zidovudine. No clinically significant changes to lamivudine or zidovudine pharmacokinetics were observed following concomitant administration of abacavir.

Abacavir has no effect on the pharmacokinetic properties of ethanol. Ethanol decreases the elimination of abacavir causing an increase in overall exposure (see CLINICAL PHARMACOLOGY: Drug Interactions).

The addition of methadone has no clinically significant effect on the pharmacokinetic properties of abacavir. In a study of 11 HIV-infected patients receiving methadone-maintenance therapy (40 mg and 90 mg daily) with 600 mg of ZIAGEN twice daily (twice the currently recommended dose), oral methadone clearance increased 22% (90% CI 6% to 42%). This alteration will not result in a methadone dose modification in the majority of patients; however, an increased methadone dose may be required in a small number of patients.

Carcinogenesis, Mutagenesis, and Impairment of Fertility: Abacavir was administered orally at 3 dosage levels to separate groups of mice (60 females and 60 males per group) and rats (56 females and 56 males in each group) in carcinogenicity studies. Single doses were 55, 110, and 330 mg/kg/day in mice and 30, 120, and 600 mg/kg/day in rats. Results showed an increase in the incidence of malignant and non-malignant tumors. Malignant tumors occurred in the preputial gland of males and the clitoral gland of females of both species, and in the liver of female rats. In addition, non-malignant tumors also occurred in the liver and thyroid gland of female rats. These observations were made at systemic exposures in the range of 6 to 32 times the human exposure at the recommended dose (300 mg twice daily). It is not known how predictive the results of rodent carcinogenicity studies may be for humans.

Abacavir induced chromosomal aberrations both in the presence and absence of metabolic activation in an in vitro cytogenetic study in human lymphocytes. Abacavir was mutagenic in the absence of metabolic activation, although it was not mutagenic in the presence of metabolic activation in an L5178Y mouse lymphoma assay. At systemic exposures approximately 9 times higher than that in humans at the therapeutic dose, abacavir was clastogenic in males and not clastogenic in females in an in vivo mouse bone marrow micronucleus assay.

Abacavir was not mutagenic in bacterial mutagenicity assays in the presence and absence of metabolic activation.

Abacavir had no adverse effects on the mating performance or fertility of male and female rats at doses of up to 500 mg/kg/day, a dose expected to produce exposures approximately 8-fold higher than that in humans at the therapeutic dose based on body surface area comparisons.

Pregnancy: Pregnancy Category C. Studies in pregnant rats showed that abacavir is transferred to the fetus through the placenta. Developmental toxicity (depressed fetal body weight and reduced crown-rump length) and increased incidences of fetal anasarca and skeletal malformations were observed when rats were treated with abacavir at doses of 1,000 mg/kg during organogenesis. This dose produced 35 times the human exposure, based on AUC. In a fertility study, evidence of toxicity to the developing embryo and fetuses (increased resorptions, decreased fetal body weights) occurred only at 500 mg/kg/day. The offspring of female rats treated with abacavir at 500 mg/kg/day (beginning at embryo implantation and ending at weaning) showed increased incidence of stillbirth and lower body weights throughout life. In the rabbit, there was no evidence of drug-related developmental toxicity and no increases in fetal malformations at doses up to 700 mg/kg (8.5 times the human exposure at the recommended dose, based on AUC).

There are no adequate and well-controlled studies in pregnant women. ZIAGEN should be used during pregnancy only if the potential benefits outweigh the risk.

Antiretroviral Pregnancy Registry: To monitor maternal-fetal outcomes of pregnant women exposed to ZIAGEN, an Antiretroviral Pregnancy Registry has been established. Physicians are encouraged to register patients by calling 1-800-258-4263.

Nursing Mothers: The Centers for Disease Control and Prevention recommend that HIV-infected mothers not breastfeed their infants to avoid risking postnatal transmission of HIV infection.

Although it is not known if abacavir is excreted in human milk, abacavir is secreted into the milk of lactating rats. Because of both the potential for HIV transmission and the potential for serious adverse reactions in nursing infants, **mothers should be instructed not to breastfeed if they are receiving ZIAGEN.**

Pediatric Use: The safety and effectiveness of ZIAGEN have been established in pediatric patients aged 3 months to 13 years. Use of ZIAGEN in these age groups is supported by pharmacokinetic studies and evidence from adequate and well-controlled studies of ZIAGEN in adults and pediatric patients (see CLINICAL PHARMACOLOGY: Pharmacokinetics: Special Populations: Pediatric Patients, INDICATIONS AND USAGE: Description of Clinical Studies, WARNINGS, ADVERSE REACTIONS, and DOSAGE AND ADMINISTRATION).

CNA3006 was a randomized, double-blind study comparing ZIAGEN 8 mg/kg twice daily plus lamivudine 4 mg/kg twice daily plus zidovudine 180 mg/m^2 twice daily versus lamivudine 4 mg/kg twice daily plus zidovudine 180 mg/m^2 twice daily. Two hundred and five **therapy-experienced pediatric patients** were enrolled: female (56%), Caucasian (17%), black (50%), Hispanic (30%), median age of 5.4 years, baseline CD4+ cell percent >15% (median = 27%), and median baseline plasma HIV-1 RNA of 4.6 $\log_{10}$ copies/mL. Eighty percent and 55% of patients had prior therapy with zidovudine and lamivudine, respectively, most often in combination. The median duration of prior nucleoside analogue therapy was 2 years. At 16 weeks the proportion of patients responding based on plasma HIV-1 RNA ≤400 copies/mL was significantly higher in patients receiving ZIAGEN plus lamivudine plus zidovudine compared with patients receiving lamivudine plus zidovudine, (13% versus 2%), respectively. Median plasma HIV-1 RNA changes from baseline were -0.53 $\log_{10}$ copies/mL in the group receiving ZIAGEN plus lamivudine plus zidovudine compared with -0.21 $\log_{10}$ copies/mL in the group receiving lamivudine plus zidovudine. Median CD4+ cell count increases from baseline were 69 cells/mm^3 in the group receiving ZIAGEN plus lamivudine plus zidovudine and 9 cells/mm^3 in the group receiving lamivudine plus zidovudine.

Geriatric Use: Clinical studies of ZIAGEN did not include sufficient numbers of patients aged 65 and over to determine whether they respond differently from younger patients. In general, dose selection for an elderly patient should be cautious, reflecting the greater frequency of decreased hepatic, renal, or cardiac function, and of concomitant disease or other drug therapy.

ADVERSE REACTIONS

Hypersensitivity Reaction: Fatal hypersensitivity reactions have been associated with therapy with ZIAGEN. Therapy with ZIAGEN SHOULD NOT be restarted following a hypersensitivity reaction because more severe symptoms will recur within hours and may include life-threatening hypotension and death. Patients developing signs or symptoms of hypersensitivity should discontinue treatment as soon as a hypersensitivity reaction is first suspected, and should seek medical evaluation immediately. To avoid a delay in diagnosis and minimize the risk of a life-threatening hypersensitivity reaction, ZIAGEN should be permanently discontinued if hypersensitivity cannot be ruled out, even when other diagnoses are possible (e.g., acute onset respiratory diseases, gastroenteritis, or reactions to other medications).

Severe or fatal hypersensitivity reactions can occur within hours after reintroduction of ZIAGEN in patients who have no identified history or unrecognized symptoms of hypersensitivity to abacavir therapy (see WARNINGS and PRECAUTIONS: Information for Patients).

When therapy with ZIAGEN has been discontinued for reasons other than symptoms of a hypersensitivity reaction, and if reinitiation of therapy is under consideration, the reason for discontinuation should be evaluated to ensure that the patient did not have symptoms of a hypersensitivity reaction. If hypersensitivity cannot be ruled out, abacavir should **NOT** be reintroduced. If symptoms consistent with hypersensitivity are not identified, reintroduction can be undertaken with continued monitoring for symptoms of hypersensitivity reaction. Patients should be made aware that a hypersensitivity reaction can occur with reintroduction of abacavir, and that abacavir reintroduction should be undertaken only if medical care can be readily accessed by the patient or others (see WARNINGS).

In clinical studies, approximately 5% of adult and pediatric patients receiving ZIAGEN developed a hypersensitivity reaction. This reaction is characterized by the appearance of symptoms indicating multi-organ/body system involvement. Symptoms usually appear within the first 6 weeks of treatment with ZIAGEN, although these reactions may occur at any time during therapy. Frequently observed signs and symptoms include fever, skin rash, fatigue, and gastrointestinal symptoms such as nausea, vomiting, diarrhea, or abdominal pain. Other signs and symptoms include malaise, lethargy, myalgia, myolysis, arthralgia, edema, pharyngitis, cough, abnormal chest x-ray findings (predominantly infiltrates, which can be localized), dyspnea, headache, and paresthesia. Some patients who experienced a hypersensitivity reaction were initially thought to have acute onset or worsening respiratory disease. The diagnosis of hypersensitivity reaction should be carefully considered for patients presenting with symptoms of acute onset respiratory diseases, even if alternative respiratory diagnoses (pneumonia, bronchitis, pharyngitis, or flu-like illness) are possible.

Physical findings include lymphadenopathy, mucous membrane lesions (conjunctivitis and mouth ulcerations), and rash. The rash usually appears maculopapular or urticarial but may be variable in appearance. There have been reports of erythema multiforme. Hypersensitivity reactions have occurred without rash.

Laboratory abnormalities include elevated liver function tests, increased creatine phosphokinase or creatinine, and lymphopenia. Anaphylaxis, liver failure, renal failure, hypotension, adult respiratory distress syndrome, respiratory failure, and death have occurred in association with hypersensitivity reactions. Symptoms worsen with continued therapy but often resolve upon discontinuation of ZIAGEN.

Risk factors that may predict the occurrence or severity of hypersensitivity to abacavir have not been identified.

Therapy-Naive Adults: Treatment-emergent clinical adverse reactions (rated by the investigator as moderate or severe) with a ≥5% frequency during therapy with ZIAGEN 300 mg twice daily, lamivudine 150 mg twice daily, and efavirenz 600 mg daily compared with zidovudine 300 mg twice daily, lamivudine 150 mg twice daily, and efavirenz 600 mg daily from CNA30024 are listed in Table 3.

[See table 3 above]

Table 3. Treatment-Emergent (All Causality) Adverse Reactions of at Least Moderate Intensity (Grades 2-4, ≥5% Frequency) in Therapy-Naive Adults (CNA30024) Through 48 Weeks of Treatment

Adverse Reaction	ZIAGEN plus Lamivudine plus Efavirenz (n = 324)	Zidovudine plus Lamivudine plus Efavirenz (n = 325)
Dreams/sleep disorders	10%	10%
Drug hypersensitivity	9%	<1%
Headaches/migraine	7%	11%
Nausea	7%	11%
Fatigue/malaise	7%	10%
Diarrhea	7%	6%
Rashes	6%	12%
Abdominal pain/gastritis gastrointestinal signs and symptoms	6%	8%
Depressive disorders	6%	6%
Dizziness	6%	6%
Musculoskeletal pain	6%	5%
Bronchitis	4%	5%
Vomiting	2%	9%

Treatment-emergent clinical adverse reactions (rated by the investigator as moderate or severe) with a ≥5% frequency during therapy with ZIAGEN 300 mg twice daily, lamivudine 150 mg twice daily, and zidovudine 300 mg twice daily compared with indinavir 800 mg 3 times daily, lamivudine 150 mg twice daily, and zidovudine 300 mg twice daily from CNA3005 are listed in Table 4.

[See table 4 above]

Table 4. Treatment-Emergent (All Causality) Adverse Reactions of at Least Moderate Intensity (Grades 2-4, ≥5% Frequency) in Therapy-Naive Adults (CNA3005) Through 48 Weeks of Treatment

Adverse Reaction	ZIAGEN plus Lamivudine/Zidovudine (n = 262)	Indinavir plus Lamivudine/Zidovudine (n = 264)
Nausea	19%	17%
Headache	13%	9%
Malaise and fatigue	12%	12%
Nausea and vomiting	10%	10%
Diarrhea	7%	5%
Fever and/or chills	6%	3%
Depressive disorders	6%	4%
Musculoskeletal pain	5%	7%
Skin rashes	5%	4%
Ear/nose/throat infections	5%	4%
Viral respiratory infections	5%	5%
Anxiety	5%	3%
Renal sign/symptoms	<1%	5%
Pain (non-site-specific)	<1%	5%

Five patients receiving ZIAGEN in Study CNA3005 experienced worsening of pre-existing depression compared to none in the indinavir arm. The background rates of pre-existing depression were similar in the 2 treatment arms.

Therapy-Experienced Pediatric Patients: Treatment-emergent clinical adverse reactions (rated by the investigator as moderate or severe) with a ≥5% frequency during therapy with ZIAGEN 8 mg/kg twice daily, lamivudine 4 mg/kg twice daily, and zidovudine 180 mg/m^2 twice daily compared with lamivudine 4 mg/kg twice daily and zidovudine 180 mg/m^2 twice daily from CNA3006 are listed in Table 5.

[See table 5 at top of next page]

Laboratory Abnormalities: Laboratory abnormalities (Grades 3-4) in therapy-naive adults during therapy with ZIAGEN 300 mg twice daily, lamivudine 150 mg twice daily, and efavirenz 600 mg daily compared with zidovudine 300 mg twice daily, lamivudine 150 mg twice daily, and efavirenz 600 mg daily from CNA30024 are listed in Table 6.

[See table 6 at top of next page]

In another study of therapy-naive adults (CNA3005), hyperglycemia and disorders of lipid metabolism occurred with similar frequency in patients treated with ZIAGEN and patients treated with indinavir.

In a study of therapy-experienced pediatric patients (CNA3006), laboratory abnormalities (anemia, neutropenia, liver function test abnormalities, and CPK elevations) were observed with similar frequencies as in a study of therapy-naive adults (CNA30024). Mild elevations of blood glucose were more frequent in pediatric patients receiving ZIAGEN (CNA3006) as compared to adult patients (CNA30024).

Other Adverse Events: In addition to adverse reactions in Tables 3, 4, 5, and 6, other adverse events observed in the expanded access program were pancreatitis and increased GGT.

Observed During Clinical Practice: In addition to adverse reactions reported from clinical trials, the following events have been identified during use of abacavir in clinical practice. Because they are reported voluntarily from a population of unknown size, estimates of frequency cannot be made. These events have been chosen for inclusion due to either their seriousness, frequency of reporting, potential causal connection to abacavir, or a combination of these factors.

Body as a Whole: Redistribution/accumulation of body fat (see PRECAUTIONS: Fat Redistribution).

Skin: Suspected Stevens-Johnson syndrome (SJS) and toxic epidermal necrolysis (TEN) have been reported in patients receiving abacavir primarily in combination with medications known to be associated with SJS and TEN, respectively. Because of the overlap of clinical signs and symptoms between hypersensitivity to abacavir and SJS and TEN, and the possibility of multiple drug sensitivities in some patients, abacavir should be discontinued and not restarted in such cases.

There have also been reports of erythema multiforme with abacavir use.

OVERDOSAGE

There is no known antidote for ZIAGEN. It is not known whether abacavir can be removed by peritoneal dialysis or hemodialysis.

DOSAGE AND ADMINISTRATION

A Medication Guide and Warning Card that provide information about recognition of hypersensitivity reactions should be dispensed with each new prescription and refill.

Continued on next page

Product information on these pages is effective as of August 2004. Further information is available at: GlaxoSmithKline, PO Box 13398, Research Triangle Park, NC 27709. 1-888-825-5249. Corporate Web Site: www.gsk.com

Ziagen—Cont.

To facilitate reporting of hypersensitivity reactions and collection of information on each case, an Abacavir Hypersensitivity Registry has been established. Physicians should register patients by calling 1-800-270-0425.

ZIAGEN may be taken with or without food.

Adults: The recommended oral dose of ZIAGEN for adults is 300 mg twice daily in combination with other antiretroviral agents.

Adolescents and Pediatric Patients: The recommended oral dose of ZIAGEN for adolescents and pediatric patients 3 months to up to 16 years of age is 8 mg/kg twice daily (up to a maximum of 300 mg twice daily) in combination with other antiretroviral agents.

Dose Adjustment in Hepatic Impairment: The recommended dose of ZIAGEN in patients with mild hepatic impairment (Child-Pugh score 5 to 6) is 200 mg twice daily. To enable dose reduction, ZIAGEN Oral Solution (10 mL twice daily) should be used for the treatment of these patients. The safety, efficacy, and pharmacokinetic properties of abacavir have not been established in patients with moderate to severe hepatic impairment, therefore ZIAGEN is contraindicated in these patients.

HOW SUPPLIED

ZIAGEN is available as tablets and oral solution.

ZIAGEN Tablets: Each tablet contains abacavir sulfate equivalent to 300 mg abacavir. The tablets are yellow, biconvex, capsule-shaped, film-coated, and imprinted with "GX 623" on one side with no marking on the reverse side. They are packaged as follows:

Bottles of 60 tablets (NDC 0173-0661-01).

Unit dose blister packs of 60 tablets (NDC 0173-0661-00). Each pack contains 6 blister cards of 10 tablets each.

Store at controlled room temperature of 20° to 25°C (68° to 77°F) (see USP).

ZIAGEN Oral Solution: It is a clear to opalescent, yellowish, strawberry-banana-flavored liquid. Each mL of the solution contains abacavir sulfate equivalent to 20 mg of abacavir. It is packaged in plastic bottles as follows:

Bottles of 240 mL (NDC 0173-0664-00) with child-resistant closure. This product does not require reconstitution.

Store at controlled room temperature of 20° to 25°C (68° to 77°F) (see USP). DO NOT FREEZE. May be refrigerated.

ANIMAL TOXICOLOGY

Myocardial degeneration was found in mice and rats following administration of abacavir for 2 years. The systemic exposures were equivalent to 7 to 24 times the expected systemic exposure in humans. The clinical relevance of this finding has not been determined.

GlaxoSmithKline, Research Triangle Park, NC 27709

April 2004/RL-2086

MEDICATION GUIDE

ZIAGEN® (z-EYE-uh-jen) (abacavir sulfate) Tablets and Oral Solution

Generic name: abacavir (uh-BACK-ah-veer) sulfate tablets and oral solution

Read the Medication Guide you get each time you fill your prescription for Ziagen. There may be new information since you filled your last prescription.

What is the most important information I should know about Ziagen?

About 1 in 20 patients (5%) who take Ziagen will have a **serious allergic reaction** (hypersensitivity reaction) **that may cause death if the drug is not stopped right away.**

You may be having this reaction if:

(1) you get a skin rash, or

(2) you get 1 or more symptoms from at least 2 of the following groups:

- **Fever**
- **Nausea, vomiting, diarrhea, abdominal (stomach area) pain**
- **Extreme tiredness, achiness, generally ill feeling**
- **Sore throat, shortness of breath, cough**

If you think you may be having a reaction, **STOP taking Ziagen and call your doctor right away.**

If you stop treatment with Ziagen because of this serious reaction, **NEVER take Ziagen (abacavir) again.** If you take Ziagen again after you have had this serious reaction, **you could die within hours.**

Some patients who have stopped taking Ziagen (abacavir) and who have then started taking Ziagen (abacavir) again have had serious or life-threatening allergic (hypersensitivity) reactions. If you must stop treatment with Ziagen for reasons other than symptoms of hypersensitivity, do not begin taking it again without talking to your health care provider. If your health care provider decides that you may begin taking Ziagen again, you should do so only in a setting with other people to get access to a doctor if needed.

A written list of these symptoms is on the Warning Card your pharmacist gives you. Carry this Warning Card with you.

Ziagen can have other serious side effects. Be sure to read the section below entitled "What are the possible side effects of Ziagen?"

Table 5. Treatment-Emergent (All Causality) Adverse Reactions of at Least Moderate Intensity (Grades 2-4, ≥5% Frequency) in Therapy-Experienced Pediatric Patients (CNA3006) Through 16 Weeks of Treatment

Adverse Reaction	ZIAGEN plus Lamivudine plus Zidovudine (n = 102)	Lamivudine plus Zidovudine (n = 103)
Fever and/or chills	9%	7%
Nausea and vomiting	9%	2%
Skin rashes	7%	1%
Ear/nose/throat infections	5%	1%
Pneumonia	4%	5%
Headache	1%	5%

Table 6. Laboratory Abnormalities (Grades 3-4) in Therapy-Naive Adults (CNA30024) Through 48 Weeks of Treatment

Grade 3/4 Laboratory Abnormalities	ZIAGEN plus Lamivudine plus Efavirenz (n = 324)	Zidovudine plus Lamivudine plus Efavirenz (n = 325)
Elevated CPK (>4 X ULN)	8%	8%
Elevated ALT (>5 X ULN)	6%	6%
Elevated AST (>5 X ULN)	6%	5%
Hypertriglyceridemia (>750 mg/dL)	6%	5%
Hyperamylasemia (>2 X ULN)	4%	5%
Neutropenia (ANC <750/mm^3)	2%	4%
Anemia (Hgb ≤6.9 gm/dL)	<1%	2%
Thrombocytopenia (Plt <50,000/mm^3)	1%	<1%
Leukopenia (WBC ≤1,500/mm^3)	<1%	2%

What is Ziagen?

Ziagen is a medication used to treat HIV infection. Ziagen is taken by mouth as a tablet or a strawberry-banana-flavored liquid. Ziagen is a medicine called a nucleoside analogue reverse transcriptase inhibitor (NRTI). Ziagen is only proven to work when taken in combination with other anti-HIV medications. When used in combination with these other medications, Ziagen helps lower the amount of HIV found in your blood. This helps to keep your immune system as healthy as possible so that it can help fight infection.

Ziagen does not cure HIV infection or AIDS. Ziagen has not been studied long enough to know if it will help you live longer or have fewer of the medical problems that are associated with HIV infection or AIDS. Therefore, you must see your health care provider regularly.

Who should not take Ziagen?

Do not take Ziagen if you have ever had a serious allergic reaction (a hypersensitivity reaction) to abacavir (as Ziagen or Trizivir® [abacavir, lamivudine, and zidovudine] Tablets). If you have had such a reaction, return all of your unused Ziagen to your doctor or pharmacist.

Talk to your doctor if you have liver problems, as some patients with liver disease should not take Ziagen.

How should I take Ziagen?

To help make sure that your anti-HIV therapy is as effective as possible, take your Ziagen exactly as your doctor prescribes it. Do not skip any doses.

The usual dosage for adults (at least 16 years of age) is one 300-mg tablet twice a day. You can take Ziagen with food or on an empty stomach.

Adolescents and children 3 months and older can also take Ziagen. Your doctor will tell you if the oral solution or tablet is best for your child. Also, your child's doctor will decide the right dose based on your child's weight and age. Ziagen has not been studied in children under 3 months of age.

If you miss a dose of Ziagen, take the missed dose right away. Then, take the next dose at the usual scheduled time. Do not let your Ziagen run out. The amount of virus in your blood may increase if your anti-HIV drugs are stopped, even for a short time. Also, the virus in your body may become harder to treat.

What should I avoid while taking Ziagen?

Practice safe sex while using Ziagen. Do not use or share dirty needles. Ziagen does not reduce the risk of passing HIV to others through sexual contact or blood contamination.

Talk to your doctor if you are pregnant or if you become pregnant while taking Ziagen. Ziagen has not been studied in pregnant women. It is not known whether Ziagen will harm the unborn child.

Mothers with HIV should not breastfeed their babies because HIV is passed to the baby in breast milk. Also Ziagen can be passed to babies in breast milk and could cause the child to have side effects.

What are the possible side effects of Ziagen?

Life-threatening allergic reaction. Ziagen has caused some people to have a life-threatening reaction (hypersensitivity reaction) that can cause death. How to recognize a possible reaction, and what to do are discussed in "What is the most important information I should know about Ziagen?" at the beginning of this Medication Guide.

Lactic Acidosis and severe liver problems. Ziagen can cause a serious condition called lactic acidosis and, in some cases, this condition can cause death. Nausea and tiredness that don't get better may be symptoms of lactic acidosis. Women are more likely than men to get this rare but serious side effect.

Ziagen can cause other side effects. In studies, the most common side effects with Ziagen were nausea, vomiting, malaise or fatigue, headache, diarrhea, and loss of appetite. Most of these side effects did not cause people to stop taking Ziagen.

Changes in body fat have been seen in some patients taking antiretroviral therapy. These changes may include increased amount of fat in the upper back and neck ("buffalo hump"), breast, and around the trunk. Loss of fat from the legs, arms, and face may also happen. The cause and long-term health effects of these conditions are not known at this time.

This listing of side effects is not complete. Your doctor or pharmacist can discuss with you a more complete list of side effects with Ziagen.

Ask a health care professional about any concerns about Ziagen. If you want more information, ask your doctor or pharmacist for the labeling for Ziagen that was written for health care professionals.

Do not use Ziagen for a condition for which it was not prescribed. Do not give Ziagen to other persons.

GlaxoSmithKline, Research Triangle Park, NC 27709

July 2003/MG-019

This Medication Guide has been approved by the US Food and Drug Administration.

Shown in Product Identification Guide, page 318

ZINACEF® ℞

[zin'a-sef]

(cefuroxime for injection)

ZINACEF® ℞

(cefuroxime injection)

To reduce the development of drug-resistant bacteria and maintain the effectiveness of ZINACEF and other antibacterial drugs, ZINACEF should be used only to treat or prevent infections that are proven or strongly suspected to be caused by bacteria.

DESCRIPTION

Cefuroxime is a semisynthetic, broad-spectrum, cephalosporin antibiotic for parenteral administration. It is the sodium salt of (6R,7R)-3-carbamoyloxymethyl-7-[Z-2-methoxyimino-2-(fur-2-yl)acetamido]ceph-3-em-4-carboxylate.

The empirical formula is $C_{16}H_{15}N_4NaO_8S$, representing a molecular weight of 446.4.

ZINACEF contains approximately 54.2 mg (2.4 mEq) of sodium per gram of cefuroxime activity.

ZINACEF in sterile crystalline form is supplied in vials equivalent to 750 mg, 1.5 g, or 7.5 g of cefuroxime as cefuroxime sodium and in ADD-Vantage® vials equivalent to 750 mg or 1.5 g of cefuroxime as cefuroxime sodium. Solutions of ZINACEF range in color from light yellow to amber, depending on the concentration and diluent used. The pH of freshly constituted solutions usually ranges from 6 to 8.5.

ZINACEF is available as a frozen, iso-osmotic, sterile, nonpyrogenic solution with 750 mg or 1.5 g of cefuroxime as cefuroxime sodium. Approximately 1.4 g of Dextrose Hydrous, USP has been added to the 750-mg dose to adjust the osmolality. Sodium Citrate Hydrous, USP has been added as a buffer (300 mg and 600 mg to the 750-mg and 1.5-g doses, respectively). ZINACEF contains approximately 111 mg (4.8 mEq) and 222 mg (9.7 mEq) of sodium in the 750-mg and 1.5-g doses, respectively. The pH has been adjusted with hydrochloric acid and may have been adjusted with sodium hydroxide. Solutions of premixed ZINACEF range in color from light yellow to amber. The solution is intended for intravenous (IV) use after thawing to room temperature. The osmolality of the solution is approximately 300 mOsmol/kg, and the pH of thawed solutions ranges from 5 to 7.5.

The plastic container for the frozen solution is fabricated from a specially designed multilayer plastic, PL 2040. Solutions are in contact with the polyethylene layer of this container and can leach out certain chemical components of the plastic in very small amounts within the expiration period. The suitability of the plastic has been confirmed in tests in animals according to USP biological tests for plastic containers as well as by tissue culture toxicity studies.

CLINICAL PHARMACOLOGY

After intramuscular (IM) injection of a 750-mg dose of cefuroxime to normal volunteers, the mean peak serum concentration was 27 mcg/mL. The peak occurred at approximately 45 minutes (range, 15 to 60 minutes). Following IV doses of 750 mg and 1.5 g, serum concentrations were approximately 50 and 100 mcg/mL, respectively, at 15 minutes. Therapeutic serum concentrations of approximately 2 mcg/mL or more were maintained for 5.3 hours and 8 hours or more, respectively. There was no evidence of accumulation of cefuroxime in the serum following IV administration of 1.5-g doses every 8 hours to normal volunteers. The serum half-life after either IM or IV injections is approximately 80 minutes.

Approximately 89% of a dose of cefuroxime is excreted by the kidneys over an 8-hour period, resulting in high urinary concentrations.

Following the IM administration of a 750-mg single dose, urinary concentrations averaged 1,300 mcg/mL during the first 8 hours. Intravenous doses of 750 mg and 1.5 g produced urinary levels averaging 1,150 and 2,500 mcg/mL, respectively, during the first 8-hour period.

The concomitant oral administration of probenecid with cefuroxime slows tubular secretion, decreases renal clearance by approximately 40%, increases the peak serum level by approximately 30%, and increases the serum half-life by approximately 30%. Cefuroxime is detectable in therapeutic concentrations in pleural fluid, joint fluid, bile, sputum, bone, and aqueous humor.

Cefuroxime is detectable in therapeutic concentrations in cerebrospinal fluid (CSF) of adults and pediatric patients with meningitis. The following table shows the concentrations of cefuroxime achieved in cerebrospinal fluid during multiple dosing of patients with meningitis.

[See table 1 above]

Table 1. Concentrations of Cefuroxime Achieved in Cerebrospinal Fluid During Multiple Dosing of Patients With Meningitis

Patients	Dose	Number of Patients	Mean (Range) CSF Cefuroxime Concentrations (mcg/mL) Achieved Within 8 Hours Post Dose
Pediatric patients (4 weeks to 6.5 years)	200 mg/kg/day, divided q 6 hours	5	6.6 (0.9-17.3)
Pediatric patients (7 months to 9 years)	200 to 230 mg/kg/day, divided q 8 hours	6	8.3 (<2-22.5)
Adults	1.5 grams q 8 hours	2	5.2 (2.7-8.9)
Adults	1.5 grams q 6 hours	10	6.0 (1.5-13.5)

Cefuroxime is approximately 50% bound to serum protein.

Microbiology: Cefuroxime has in vitro activity against a wide range of gram-positive and gram-negative organisms, and it is highly stable in the presence of beta-lactamases of certain gram-negative bacteria. The bactericidal action of cefuroxime results from inhibition of cell-wall synthesis.

Cefuroxime is usually active against the following organisms in vitro.

Aerobes, Gram-positive: *Staphylococcus aureus, Staphylococcus epidermidis, Streptococcus pneumoniae,* and *Streptococcus pyogenes* (and other streptococci).

NOTE: Most strains of enterococci, e.g., *Enterococcus faecalis* (formerly *Streptococcus faecalis*), are resistant to cefuroxime. Methicillin-resistant staphylococci and *Listeria monocytogenes* are resistant to cefuroxime.

Aerobes, Gram-negative: *Citrobacter* spp., *Enterobacter* spp., *Escherichia coli, Haemophilus influenzae* (including ampicillin-resistant strains), *Haemophilus parainfluenzae, Klebsiella* spp. (including *Klebsiella pneumoniae*), *Moraxella (Branhamella) catarrhalis* (including ampicillin- and cephalothin-resistant strains), *Morganella morganii* (formerly *Proteus morganii*), *Neisseria gonorrhoeae* (including penicillinase- and non–penicillinase-producing strains), *Neisseria meningitidis, Proteus mirabilis, Providencia rettgeri* (formerly *Proteus rettgeri*), *Salmonella* spp., and *Shigella* spp.

NOTE: Some strains of *Morganella morganii, Enterobacter cloacae,* and *Citrobacter* spp. have been shown by in vitro tests to be resistant to cefuroxime and other cephalosporins. *Pseudomonas* and *Campylobacter* spp., *Acinetobacter calcoaceticus,* and most strains of *Serratia* spp. and *Proteus vulgaris* are resistant to most first- and second-generation cephalosporins.

Anaerobes: Gram-positive and gram-negative cocci (including *Peptococcus* and *Peptostreptococcus* spp.), gram-positive bacilli (including *Clostridium* spp.), and gram-negative bacilli (including *Bacteroides* and *Fusobacterium* spp.).

NOTE: *Clostridium difficile* and most strains of *Bacteroides fragilis* are resistant to cefuroxime.

Susceptibility Tests: *Diffusion Techniques:* Quantitative methods that require measurement of zone diameters give an estimate of antibiotic susceptibility. One such standard procedure[1] that has been recommended for use with disks to test susceptibility of organisms to cefuroxime uses the 30-mcg cefuroxime disk. Interpretation involves the correlation of the diameters obtained in the disk test with the minimum inhibitory concentration (MIC) for cefuroxime.

A report of "Susceptible" indicates that the pathogen is likely to be inhibited by generally achievable blood levels. A report of "Moderately Susceptible" suggests that the organism would be susceptible if high dosage is used or if the infection is confined to tissues and fluids in which high antibiotic levels are attained. A report of "Intermediate" suggests an equivocable or indeterminate result. A report of "Resistant" indicates that achievable concentrations of the antibiotic are unlikely to be inhibitory and other therapy should be selected.

Reports from the laboratory giving results of the standard single-disk susceptibility test for organisms other than *Haemophilus* spp. and *Neisseria gonorrhoeae* with a 30-mcg cefuroxime disk should be interpreted according to the following criteria:

Zone Diameter (mm)	Interpretation
≥18	(S) Susceptible
15-17	(MS) Moderately Susceptible
≤14	(R) Resistant

Results for *Haemophilus* spp. should be interpreted according to the following criteria:

Zone Diameter (mm)	Interpretation
≥24	(S) Susceptible
21-23	(I) Intermediate
≤20	(R) Resistant

Results for *Neisseria gonorrhoeae* should be interpreted according to the following criteria:

Zone Diameter (mm)	Interpretation
≥31	(S) Susceptible
26-30	(MS) Moderately Susceptible
≤25	(R) Resistant

Organisms should be tested with the cefuroxime disk since cefuroxime has been shown by in vitro tests to be active against certain strains found resistant when other beta-lactam disks are used. The cefuroxime disk should not be used for testing susceptibility to other cephalosporins.

Standardized procedures require the use of laboratory control organisms. The 30-mcg cefuroxime disk should give the following zone diameters.

1. Testing for organisms other than *Haemophilus* spp. and *Neisseria gonorrhoeae:*

Organism	Zone Diameter (mm)
Staphylococcus aureus ATCC 25923	27-35
Escherichia coli ATCC 25922	20-26

2. Testing for *Haemophilus* spp.:

Organism	Zone Diameter (mm)
Haemophilus influenzae ATCC 49766	28-36

3. Testing for *Neisseria gonorrhoeae:*

Organism	Zone Diameter (mm)
Neisseria gonorrhoeae ATCC 49226	33-41
Staphylococcus aureus ATCC 25923	29-33

Dilution Techniques: Use a standardized dilution method[1] (broth, agar, microdilution) or equivalent with cefuroxime powder. The MIC values obtained for bacterial isolates other than *Haemophilus* spp. and *Neisseria gonorrhoeae* should be interpreted according to the following criteria:

MIC (mcg/mL)	Interpretation
≤8	(S) Susceptible
16	(MS) Moderately Susceptible
≥32	(R) Resistant

MIC values obtained for *Haemophilus* spp. should be interpreted according to the following criteria:

MIC (mcg/mL)	Interpretation
≤4	(S) Susceptible
8	(I) Intermediate
≥16	(R) Resistant

MIC values obtained for *Neisseria gonorrhoeae* should be interpreted according to the following criteria:

MIC (mcg/mL)	Interpretation
≤1	(S) Susceptible
2	(MS) Moderately Susceptible
≥4	(R) Resistant

As with standard diffusion techniques, dilution methods require the use of laboratory control organisms. Standard cefuroxime powder should provide the following MIC values.

1. For organisms other than *Haemophilus* spp. and *Neisseria gonorrhoeae:*

Organism	MIC (mcg/mL)
Staphylococcus aureus ATCC 29213	0.5-2.0
Escherichia coli ATCC 25922	2.0-8.0

2. For *Haemophilus* spp.:

Organism	MIC (mcg/mL)
Haemophilus influenzae ATCC 49766	0.25-1.0

3. For *Neisseria gonorrhoeae:*

Organism	MIC (mcg/mL)
Neisseria gonorrhoeae ATCC 49226	0.25-1.0
Staphylococcus aureus ATCC 29213	0.25-1.0

INDICATIONS AND USAGE

ZINACEF is indicated for the treatment of patients with infections caused by susceptible strains of the designated organisms in the following diseases:

1. **Lower Respiratory Tract Infections,** including pneumonia, caused by *Streptococcus pneumoniae, Haemophilus influenzae* (including ampicillin-resistant strains), *Klebsiella* spp., *Staphylococcus aureus* (penicillinase- and non–penicillinase-producing strains), *Streptococcus pyogenes,* and *Escherichia coli.*
2. **Urinary Tract Infections** caused by *Escherichia coli* and *Klebsiella* spp.
3. **Skin and Skin-Structure Infections** caused by *Staphylococcus aureus* (penicillinase- and non–penicillinase-producing strains), *Streptococcus pyogenes, Escherichia coli, Klebsiella* spp., and *Enterobacter* spp.
4. **Septicemia** caused by *Staphylococcus aureus* (penicillinase- and non–penicillinase-producing strains), *Streptococcus pneumoniae, Escherichia coli, Haemophilus influenzae* (including ampicillin-resistant strains), and *Klebsiella* spp.
5. **Meningitis** caused by *Streptococcus pneumoniae, Haemophilus influenzae* (including ampicillin-resistant strains), *Neisseria meningitidis,* and *Staphylococcus aureus* (penicillinase- and non–penicillinase-producing strains).
6. **Gonorrhea:** Uncomplicated and disseminated gonococcal infections due to *Neisseria gonorrhoeae* (penicillinase- and non–penicillinase-producing strains) in both males and females.
7. **Bone and Joint Infections** caused by *Staphylococcus aureus* (penicillinase- and non–penicillinase-producing strains).

Clinical microbiological studies in skin and skin-structure infections frequently reveal the growth of susceptible strains of both aerobic and anaerobic organisms. ZINACEF has been used successfully in these mixed infections in which several organisms have been isolated.

In certain cases of confirmed or suspected gram-positive or gram-negative sepsis or in patients with other serious infections in which the causative organism has not been identified, ZINACEF may be used concomitantly with an aminoglycoside (see PRECAUTIONS). The recommended doses of both antibiotics may be given depending on the severity of the infection and the patient's condition.

To reduce the development of drug-resistant bacteria and maintain the effectiveness of ZINACEF and other antibacterial drugs. ZINACEF should be used only to treat or prevent infections that are proven or strongly suspected to be caused by susceptible bacteria. When culture and susceptibility information are available, they should be considered in selecting or modifying antibacterial therapy. In the absence of such data, local epidemiology and susceptibility patterns may contribute to the empiric selection of therapy.

Prevention: The preoperative prophylactic administration of ZINACEF may prevent the growth of susceptible disease-causing bacteria and thereby may reduce the incidence of certain postoperative infections in patients undergoing surgical procedures (e.g., vaginal hysterectomy) that are classified as clean-contaminated or potentially contaminated procedures. Effective prophylactic use of antibiotics in surgery depends on the time of administration. ZINACEF should usually be given one-half to 1 hour before the operation to allow sufficient time to achieve effective antibiotic concentrations in the wound tissues during the procedure. The dose should be repeated intraoperatively if the surgical procedure is lengthy.

Continued on next page

Product information on these pages is effective as of August 2004. Further information is available at: GlaxoSmithKline, PO Box 13398, Research Triangle Park, NC 27709. 1-888-825-5249. Corporate Web Site: www.gsk.com

Zinacef—Cont.

Prophylactic administration is usually not required after the surgical procedure ends and should be stopped within 24 hours. In the majority of surgical procedures, continuing prophylactic administration of any antibiotic does not reduce the incidence of subsequent infections but will increase the possibility of adverse reactions and the development of bacterial resistance.

The perioperative use of ZINACEF has also been effective during open heart surgery for surgical patients in whom infections at the operative site would present a serious risk. For these patients it is recommended that therapy with ZINACEF be continued for at least 48 hours after the surgical procedure ends. If an infection is present, specimens for culture should be obtained for the identification of the causative organism, and appropriate antimicrobial therapy should be instituted.

CONTRAINDICATIONS

ZINACEF is contraindicated in patients with known allergy to the cephalosporin group of antibiotics.

WARNINGS

BEFORE THERAPY WITH ZINACEF IS INSTITUTED, CAREFUL INQUIRY SHOULD BE MADE TO DETERMINE WHETHER THE PATIENT HAS HAD PREVIOUS HYPERSENSITIVITY REACTIONS TO CEPHALOSPORINS, PENICILLINS, OR OTHER DRUGS. THIS PRODUCT SHOULD BE GIVEN CAUTIOUSLY TO PENICILLIN-SENSITIVE PATIENTS. ANTIBIOTICS SHOULD BE ADMINISTERED WITH CAUTION TO ANY PATIENT WHO HAS DEMONSTRATED SOME FORM OF ALLERGY, PARTICULARLY TO DRUGS. IF AN ALLERGIC REACTION TO ZINACEF OCCURS, DISCONTINUE THE DRUG. SERIOUS ACUTE HYPERSENSITIVITY REACTIONS MAY REQUIRE EPINEPHRINE AND OTHER EMERGENCY MEASURES.

Pseudomembranous colitis has been reported with nearly all antibacterial agents, including cefuroxime, and may range in severity from mild to life threatening. Therefore, it is important to consider this diagnosis in patients who present with diarrhea subsequent to the administration of antibacterial agents.

Treatment with antibacterial agents alters the normal flora of the colon and may permit overgrowth of clostridia. Studies indicate that a toxin produced by *Clostridium difficile* is one primary cause of "antibiotic-associated colitis."

After the diagnosis of pseudomembranous colitis has been established, appropriate therapeutic measures should be initiated. Mild cases of pseudomembranous colitis usually respond to drug discontinuation alone. In moderate to severe cases, consideration should be given to management with fluids and electrolytes, protein supplementation, and treatment with an antibacterial drug clinically effective against *Clostridium difficile* colitis.

When the colitis is not relieved by drug discontinuation or when it is severe, oral vancomycin is the treatment of choice for antibiotic-associated pseudomembranous colitis produced by *Clostridium difficile*. Other causes of colitis should also be considered.

PRECAUTIONS

General: Although ZINACEF rarely produces alterations in kidney function, evaluation of renal status during therapy is recommended, especially in seriously ill patients receiving the maximum doses. Cephalosporins should be given with caution to patients receiving concurrent treatment with potent diuretics as these regimens are suspected of adversely affecting renal function.

The total daily dose of ZINACEF should be reduced in patients with transient or persistent renal insufficiency (see DOSAGE AND ADMINISTRATION), because high and prolonged serum antibiotic concentrations can occur in such individuals from usual doses.

As with other antibiotics, prolonged use of ZINACEF may result in overgrowth of nonsusceptible organisms. Careful observation of the patient is essential. If superinfection occurs during therapy, appropriate measures should be taken. Broad-spectrum antibiotics should be prescribed with caution in individuals with a history of gastrointestinal disease, particularly colitis.

Nephrotoxicity has been reported following concomitant administration of aminoglycoside antibiotics and cephalosporins.

As with other therapeutic regimens used in the treatment of meningitis, mild-to-moderate hearing loss has been reported in a few pediatric patients treated with cefuroxime. Persistence of positive CSF (cerebrospinal fluid) cultures at 18 to 36 hours has also been noted with cefuroxime injection, as well as with other antibiotic therapies; however, the clinical relevance of this is unknown.

Cephalosporins may be associated with a fall in prothrombin activity. Those at risk include patients with renal or hepatic impairment, or poor nutritional state, as well as patients receiving a protracted course of antimicrobial therapy, and patients previously stabilized on anticoagulant therapy. Prothrombin time should be monitored in patients at risk and exogenous Vitamin K administered as indicated.

Prescribing ZINACEF in the absence of a proven or strongly suspected bacterial infection or a prophylactic indication is unlikely to provide benefit to the patient and increases the risk of the development of drug-resistant bacteria.

Information for Patients: Patients should be counseled that antibacterial drugs, including ZINACEF, should only be used to treat bacterial infections. They do not treat viral infections (e.g., the common cold). When ZINACEF is prescribed to treat a bacterial infection, patients should be told that although it is common to feel better early in the course of therapy, the medication should be taken exactly as directed. Skipping doses or not completing the full course of therapy may: (1) decrease the effectiveness of the immediate treatment, and (2) increase the likelihood that bacteria will develop resistance and will not be treatable by ZINACEF or other antibacterial drugs in the future.

Drug/Laboratory Test Interactions: A false-positive reaction for glucose in the urine may occur with copper reduction tests (Benedict's or Fehling's solution or with CLINITEST® tablets) but not with enzyme-based tests for glycosuria. As a false-negative result may occur in the ferricyanide test, it is recommended that either the glucose oxidase or hexokinase method be used to determine blood plasma glucose levels in patients receiving ZINACEF.

Cefuroxime does not interfere with the assay of serum and urine creatinine by the alkaline picrate method.

Carcinogenesis, Mutagenesis, Impairment of Fertility: Although lifetime studies in animals have not been performed to evaluate carcinogenic potential, no mutagenic activity was found for cefuroxime in the mouse lymphoma assay and a battery of bacterial mutation tests. Positive results were obtained in an in vitro chromosome aberration assay, however, negative results were found in an in vivo micronucleus test at doses up to 10 g/kg. Reproduction studies in mice at doses up to 3,200 mg/kg/day (3.1 times the recommended maximum human dose based on mg/m^2) have revealed no impairment of fertility.

Reproductive studies revealed no impairment of fertility in animals.

Pregnancy: ***Teratogenic Effects:*** Pregnancy Category B. Reproduction studies have been performed in mice at doses up to 6,400 mg/kg/day (6.3 times the recommended maximum human dose based on mg/m^2) and rabbits at doses up to 400 mg/kg/day (2.1 times the recommended maximum human dose based on mg/m^2) and have revealed no evidence of impaired fertility or harm to the fetus due to cefuroxime. There are, however, no adequate and well-controlled studies in pregnant women. Because animal reproduction studies are not always predictive of human response, this drug should be used during pregnancy only if clearly needed.

Nursing Mothers: Since cefuroxime is excreted in human milk, caution should be exercised when ZINACEF is administered to a nursing woman.

Pediatric Use: Safety and effectiveness in pediatric patients below 3 months of age have not been established. Accumulation of other members of the cephalosporin class in newborn infants (with resulting prolongation of drug half-life) has been reported.

Geriatric Use: Of the 1,914 subjects who received cefuroxime in 24 clinical studies of ZINACEF, 901 (47%) were 65 and over while 421 (22%) were 75 and over. No overall differences in safety or effectiveness were observed between these subjects and younger subjects, and other reported clinical experience has not identified differences in responses between the elderly and younger patients, but greater susceptibility of some older individuals to drug effects cannot be ruled out. This drug is known to be substantially excreted by the kidney, and the risk of toxic reactions to this drug may be greater in patients with impaired renal function. Because elderly patients are more likely to have decreased renal function, care should be taken in dose selection, and it may be useful to monitor renal function (see DOSAGE AND ADMINISTRATION).

ADVERSE REACTIONS

ZINACEF is generally well tolerated. The most common adverse effects have been local reactions following IV administration. Other adverse reactions have been encountered only rarely.

Local Reactions: Thrombophlebitis has occurred with IV administration in 1 in 60 patients.

Gastrointestinal: Gastrointestinal symptoms occurred in 1 in 150 patients and included diarrhea (1 in 220 patients) and nausea (1 in 440 patients). The onset of pseudomembranous colitis may occur during or after antibacterial treatment (see WARNINGS).

Hypersensitivity Reactions: Hypersensitivity reactions have been reported in fewer than 1% of the patients treated with ZINACEF and include rash (1 in 125). Pruritus, urticaria, and positive Coombs' test each occurred in fewer than 1 in 250 patients, and, as with other cephalosporins, rare cases of anaphylaxis, drug fever, erythema multiforme, interstitial nephritis, toxic epidermal necrolysis, and Stevens-Johnson syndrome have occurred.

Blood: A decrease in hemoglobin and hematocrit has been observed in 1 in 10 patients and transient eosinophilia in 1 in 14 patients. Less common reactions seen were transient neutropenia (fewer than 1 in 100 patients) and leukopenia (1 in 750 patients). A similar pattern and incidence were seen with other cephalosporins used in controlled studies. As with other cephalosporins, there have been rare reports of thrombocytopenia.

Hepatic: Transient rise in SGOT and SGPT (1 in 25 patients), alkaline phosphatase (1 in 50 patients), LDH (1 in 75 patients), and bilirubin (1 in 500 patients) levels has been noted.

Kidney: Elevations in serum creatinine and/or blood urea nitrogen and a decreased creatinine clearance have been observed, but their relationship to cefuroxime is unknown.

Postmarketing Experience with ZINACEF Products: In addition to the adverse events reported during clinical trials, the following events have been observed during clinical practice in patients treated with ZINACEF and were reported spontaneously. Data are generally insufficient to allow an estimate of incidence or to establish causation.

Neurologic: Seizure.

Non-site specific: Angioedema.

Cephalosporin-class Adverse Reactions: In addition to the adverse reactions listed above that have been observed in patients treated with cefuroxime, the following adverse reactions and altered laboratory tests have been reported for cephalosporin-class antibiotics:

Adverse Reactions: Vomiting, abdominal pain, colitis, vaginitis including vaginal candidiasis, toxic nephropathy, hepatic dysfunction including cholestasis, aplastic anemia, hemolytic anemia, hemorrhage.

Several cephalosporins, including ZINACEF, have been implicated in triggering seizures, particularly in patients with renal impairment when the dosage was not reduced (see DOSAGE AND ADMINISTRATION). If seizures associated with drug therapy should occur, the drug should be discontinued. Anticonvulsant therapy can be given if clinically indicated.

Altered Laboratory Tests: Prolonged prothrombin time, pancytopenia, agranulocytosis.

OVERDOSAGE

Overdosage of cephalosporins can cause cerebral irritation leading to convulsions. Serum levels of cefuroxime can be reduced by hemodialysis and peritoneal dialysis.

DOSAGE AND ADMINISTRATION

Dosage: ***Adults:*** The usual adult dosage range for ZINACEF is 750 mg to 1.5 grams every 8 hours, usually for 5 to 10 days. In uncomplicated urinary tract infections, skin and skin-structure infections, disseminated gonococcal infections, and uncomplicated pneumonia, a 750-mg dose every 8 hours is recommended. In severe or complicated infections, a 1.5-gram dose every 8 hours is recommended.

In bone and joint infections, a 1.5-gram dose every 8 hours is recommended. In clinical trials, surgical intervention was performed when indicated as an adjunct to therapy with ZINACEF. A course of oral antibiotics was administered when appropriate following the completion of parenteral administration of ZINACEF.

In life-threatening infections or infections due to less susceptible organisms, 1.5 grams every 6 hours may be required. In bacterial meningitis, the dosage should not exceed 3 grams every 8 hours. The recommended dosage for uncomplicated gonococcal infection is 1.5 grams given intramuscularly as a single dose at 2 different sites together with 1 gram of oral probenecid. For preventive use for clean-contaminated or potentially contaminated surgical procedures, a 1.5-gram dose administered intravenously just before surgery (approximately one-half to 1 hour before the initial incision) is recommended. Thereafter, give 750 mg intravenously or intramuscularly every 8 hours when the procedure is prolonged.

For preventive use during open heart surgery, a 1.5-gram dose administered intravenously at the induction of anesthesia and every 12 hours thereafter for a total of 6 grams is recommended.

Impaired Renal Function: A reduced dosage must be employed when renal function is impaired. Dosage should be determined by the degree of renal impairment and the susceptibility of the causative organism (see Table 2).

Table 2. Dosage of ZINACEF in Adults With Reduced Renal Function

Creatinine Clearance (mL/min)	Dose	Frequency
>20	750 mg-1.5 grams	q8h
10-20	750 mg	q12h
<10	750 mg	q24h*

* Since ZINACEF is dialyzable, patients on hemodialysis should be given a further dose at the end of the dialysis.

When only serum creatinine is available, the following formula[2] (based on sex, weight, and age of the patient) may be used to convert this value into creatinine clearance. The serum creatinine should represent a steady state of renal function.

Males: $$\text{Creatinine clearance (mL/min)} = \frac{\text{Weight (kg)} \times (140 - \text{age})}{72 \times \text{serum creatinine (mg/dL)}}$$

Females: $0.85 \times$ male value

Note: As with antibiotic therapy in general, administration of ZINACEF should be continued for a minimum of 48 to 72 hours after the patient becomes asymptomatic or after evidence of bacterial eradication has been obtained; a minimum of 10 days of treatment is recommended in infections caused by *Streptococcus pyogenes* in order to guard against the risk of rheumatic fever or glomerulonephritis; frequent bacteriologic and clinical appraisal is necessary during therapy of chronic urinary tract infection and may be required for several months after therapy has been completed; persistent infections may require treatment for several weeks;

and doses smaller than those indicated above should not be used. In staphylococcal and other infections involving a collection of pus, surgical drainage should be carried out where indicated.

Pediatric Patients Above 3 Months of Age: Administration of 50 to 100 mg/kg/day in equally divided doses every 6 to 8 hours has been successful for most infections susceptible to cefuroxime. The higher dosage of 100 mg/kg/day (not to exceed the maximum adult dosage) should be used for the more severe or serious infections.

In bone and joint infections, 150 mg/kg/day (not to exceed the maximum adult dosage) is recommended in equally divided doses every 8 hours. In clinical trials, a course of oral antibiotics was administered to pediatric patients following the completion of parenteral administration of ZINACEF.

In cases of bacterial meningitis, a larger dosage of ZINACEF is recommended, 200 to 240 mg/kg/day intravenously in divided doses every 6 to 8 hours.

In pediatric patients with renal insufficiency, the frequency of dosing should be modified consistent with the recommendations for adults.

Preparation of Solution and Suspension: The directions for preparing ZINACEF for both IV and IM use are summarized in Table 3.

For Intramuscular Use: Each 750-mg vial of ZINACEF should be constituted with 3.0 mL of Sterile Water for Injection. Shake gently to disperse and withdraw completely the resulting suspension for injection.

For Intravenous Use: Each 750-mg vial should be constituted with 8.0 mL of Sterile Water for Injection. Withdraw completely the resulting solution for injection.

Each 1.5-gram vial should be constituted with 16.0 mL of Sterile Water for Injection, and the solution should be completely withdrawn for injection.

The 7.5-gram pharmacy bulk vial should be constituted with 77 mL of Sterile Water for Injection; each 8 mL of the resulting solution contains 750 mg of cefuroxime.

Each 750-mg and 1.5-gram infusion pack should be constituted with 100 mL of Sterile Water for Injection, 5% Dextrose Injection, 0.9% Sodium Chloride Injection, or any of the solutions listed under the Intravenous portion of the COMPATIBILITY AND STABILITY section.

[See table 3 above]

Administration: After constitution, ZINACEF may be given intravenously or by deep IM injection into a large muscle mass (such as the gluteus or lateral part of the thigh). Before injecting intramuscularly, aspiration is necessary to avoid inadvertent injection into a blood vessel.

Intravenous Administration: The IV route may be preferable for patients with bacterial septicemia or other severe or life-threatening infections or for patients who may be poor risks because of lowered resistance, particularly if shock is present or impending.

For direct intermittent IV administration, slowly inject the solution into a vein over a period of 3 to 5 minutes or give it through the tubing system by which the patient is also receiving other IV solutions.

For intermittent IV infusion with a Y-type administration set, dosing can be accomplished through the tubing system by which the patient may be receiving other IV solutions. However, during infusion of the solution containing ZINACEF, it is advisable to temporarily discontinue administration of any other solutions at the same site.

ADD-Vantage vials are to be constituted only with 50 or 100 mL of 5% Dextrose Injection, 0.9% Sodium Chloride Injection, or 0.45% Sodium Chloride Injection in Abbott ADD-Vantage flexible diluent containers (see Instructions for Constitution). ADD-Vantage vials that have been joined to Abbott ADD-Vantage diluent containers and activated to dissolve the drug are stable for 24 hours at room temperature or for 7 days under refrigeration. Joined vials that have not been activated may be used within a 14-day period; this period corresponds to that for use of Abbott ADD-Vantage containers following removal of the outer packaging (overwrap).

Freezing solutions of ZINACEF in the ADD-Vantage system is not recommended.

For continuous IV infusion, a solution of ZINACEF may be added to an IV infusion pack containing one of the following fluids: 0.9% Sodium Chloride Injection; 5% Dextrose Injection; 10% Dextrose Injection; 5% Dextrose and 0.9% Sodium Chloride Injection; 5% Dextrose and 0.45% Sodium Chloride Injection; or 1/6 M Sodium Lactate Injection.

Solutions of ZINACEF, like those of most beta-lactam antibiotics, should not be added to solutions of aminoglycoside antibiotics because of potential interaction.

However, if concurrent therapy with ZINACEF and an aminoglycoside is indicated, each of these antibiotics can be administered separately to the same patient.

Directions for Use of ZINACEF Frozen in GALAXY® Plastic Containers: ZINACEF supplied as a frozen, sterile, iso-osmotic, nonpyrogenic solution in plastic containers is to be administered after thawing either as a continuous or intermittent IV infusion. The thawed solution of the premixed product is stable for 28 days if stored under refrigeration (5°C) or for 24 hours if stored at room temperature (25°C).

Do not refreeze.

Thaw container at room temperature (25°C) or under refrigeration (5°C). Do not force thaw by immersion in water baths or by microwave irradiation. Components of the solution may precipitate in the frozen state and will dissolve upon reaching room temperature with little or no agitation. Potency is not affected. Mix after solution has reached room temperature. Check for minute leaks by squeezing bag firmly. Discard bag if leaks are found as sterility may be impaired. Do not add supplementary medication. Do not use unless solution is clear and seal is intact.

Table 3. Preparation of Solution and Suspension

Strength	Amount of Diluent to Be Added (mL)	Volume to Be Withdrawn	Approximate Cefuroxime Concentration (mg/mL)
750-mg Vial	3.0 (IM)	Total*	220
750-mg Vial	8.0 (IV)	Total	90
1.5-gram Vial	16.0 (IV)	Total	90
750-mg Infusion pack	100 (IV)	—	7.5
1.5-gram Infusion pack	100 (IV)	—	15
7.5-gram Pharmacy bulk package	77 (IV)	Amount Needed†	95

***Note:** ZINACEF is a suspension at IM concentrations.
†8 mL of solution contains 750 mg of cefuroxime; 16 mL of solution contains 1.5 grams of cefuroxime.

Use sterile equipment.

Caution: Do not use plastic containers in series connections. Such use could result in air embolism due to residual air being drawn from the primary container before administration of the fluid from the secondary container is complete.

Preparation for Administration:

1. Suspend container from eyelet support.
2. Remove protector from outlet port at bottom of container.
3. Attach administration set. Refer to complete directions accompanying set.

COMPATIBILITY AND STABILITY

Intramuscular: When constituted as directed with Sterile Water for Injection, suspensions of ZINACEF for IM injection maintain satisfactory potency for 24 hours at room temperature and for 48 hours under refrigeration (5°C).

After the periods mentioned above any unused suspensions should be discarded.

Intravenous: When the 750-mg, 1.5-g, and 7.5-g pharmacy bulk vials are constituted as directed with Sterile Water for Injection, the solutions of ZINACEF for IV administration maintain satisfactory potency for 24 hours at room temperature and for 48 hours (750-mg and 1.5-g vials) or for 7 days (7.5-g pharmacy bulk vial) under refrigeration (5°C). More dilute solutions, such as 750 mg or 1.5 g plus 100 mL of Sterile Water for Injection, 5% Dextrose Injection, or 0.9% Sodium Chloride Injection, also maintain satisfactory potency for 24 hours at room temperature and for 7 days under refrigeration.

These solutions may be further diluted to concentrations of between 1 and 30 mg/mL in the following solutions and will lose not more than 10% activity for 24 hours at room temperature or for at least 7 days under refrigeration: 0.9% Sodium Chloride Injection; 1/6 M Sodium Lactate Injection; Ringer's Injection, USP; Lactated Ringer's Injection, USP; 5% Dextrose and 0.9% Sodium Chloride Injection; 5% Dextrose Injection; 5% Dextrose and 0.45% Sodium Chloride Injection; 5% Dextrose and 0.225% Sodium Chloride Injection; 10% Dextrose Injection; and 10% Invert Sugar in Water for Injection.

Unused solutions should be discarded after the time periods mentioned above.

ZINACEF has also been found compatible for 24 hours at room temperature when admixed in IV infusion with heparin (10 and 50 U/mL) in 0.9% Sodium Chloride Injection and Potassium Chloride (10 and 40 mEq/L) in 0.9% Sodium Chloride Injection. Sodium Bicarbonate Injection, USP is not recommended for the dilution of ZINACEF.

The 750-mg and 1.5-g ZINACEF ADD-Vantage vials, when diluted in 50 or 100 mL of 5% Dextrose Injection, 0.9% Sodium Chloride Injection, or 0.45% Sodium Chloride Injection, may be stored for up to 24 hours at room temperature or for 7 days under refrigeration.

Frozen Stability: Constitute the 750-mg, 1.5-g, or 7.5-g vial as directed for IV administration in Table 3. Immediately withdraw the total contents of the 750-mg or 1.5-g vial or 8 or 16 mL from the 7.5-g bulk vial and add to a Baxter VIAFLEX® MINI-BAG™ containing 50 or 100 mL of 0.9% Sodium Chloride Injection or 5% Dextrose Injection and freeze. Frozen solutions are stable for 6 months when stored at -20°C. Frozen solutions should be thawed at room temperature and not refrozen. Do not force thaw by immersion in water baths or by microwave irradiation. Thawed solutions may be stored for up to 24 hours at room temperature or for 7 days in a refrigerator.

Note: Parenteral drug products should be inspected visually for particulate matter and discoloration before administration whenever solution and container permit.

As with other cephalosporins, ZINACEF powder as well as solutions and suspensions tend to darken, depending on storage conditions, without adversely affecting product potency.

Directions for Dispensing: *Pharmacy Bulk Package—Not for Direct Infusion:* The pharmacy bulk package is for use in a pharmacy admixture service only under a laminar flow hood. Entry into the vial must be made with a sterile transfer set or other sterile dispensing device, and the contents dispensed in aliquots using aseptic technique. The use of syringe and needle is not recommended as it may cause leakage (see DOSAGE AND ADMINISTRATION). AFTER INITIAL WITHDRAWAL USE ENTIRE CONTENTS OF VIAL PROMPTLY. ANY UNUSED PORTION MUST BE DISCARDED WITHIN 24 HOURS.

HOW SUPPLIED

ZINACEF in the dry state should be stored between 15° and 30°C (59° and 86°F) and protected from light. ZINACEF is a dry, white to off-white powder supplied in vials and infusion packs as follows:

NDC 0173-0352-31 750-mg* Vial (Tray of 25)
NDC 0173-0354-35 1.5-g* Vial (Tray of 25)
NDC 0173-0353-32 750-mg* Infusion Pack (Tray of 10)
NDC 0173-0356-32 1.5-g* Infusion Pack (Tray of 10)
NDC 0173-0400-00 7.5-g* Pharmacy Bulk Package (Tray of 6)
NDC 0173-0436-00 750-mg ADD-Vantage Vial (Tray of 25)
NDC 0173-0437-00 1.5-g ADD-Vantage Vial (Tray of 10)

(The above ADD-Vantage vials are to be used only with Abbott ADD-Vantage diluent containers.)

ZINACEF frozen as a premixed solution of cefuroxime injection should not be stored above -20°C. ZINACEF is supplied frozen in 50-mL, single-dose, plastic containers as follows:

NDC 0173-0424-00 750-mg* Plastic Container (Carton of 24)
NDC 0173-0425-00 1.5-g* Plastic Container (Carton of 24)

*Equivalent to cefuroxime.

REFERENCES

1. National Committee for Clinical Laboratory Standards. *Performance Standards for Antimicrobial Susceptibility Testing.* Third Informational Supplement. NCCLS Document M100-S3, Vol. 11, No. 17. Villanova, Pa: NCCLS; 1991.
2. Cockcroft DW, Gault MH. Prediction of creatinine clearance from serum creatinine. *Nephron.* 1976;16:31-41.

ZINACEF® (cefuroxime for injection):
GlaxoSmithKline, Research Triangle Park, NC 27709
ZINACEF® (cefuroxime injection):
Manufactured for GlaxoSmithKline
Research Triangle Park, NC 27709
by Baxter Healthcare Corporation, Deerfield, IL 60015
ZINACEF is a registered trademark of
GlaxoSmithKline.
ADD-Vantage is a registered trademark of
Abbott Laboratories.
CLINITEST is a registered trademark of
Ames Division, Miles Laboratories, Inc.
GALAXY and VIAFLEX are registered trademarks
of Baxter International Inc.
October 2003/RL-2045

Shown in Product Identification Guide, page 318

ZOFRAN® ℞
[*zō' fran*]
(ondansetron hydrochloride)
Injection
ZOFRAN® ℞
(ondansetron hydrochloride)
Injection Premixed

DESCRIPTION

The active ingredient in ZOFRAN Injection and ZOFRAN Injection Premixed is ondansetron hydrochloride (HCl), the racemic form of ondansetron and a selective blocking agent of the serotonin 5-HT_3 receptor type. Chemically it is (±) 1, 2, 3, 9-tetrahydro-9-methyl-3-[(2-methyl-1H-imidazol-1-yl) methyl]-4H-carbazol-4-one, monohydrochloride, dihydrate. The empirical formula is $C_{18}H_{19}N_3O \bullet HCl \bullet 2H_2O$, representing a molecular weight of 365.9.

Ondansetron HCl is a white to off-white powder that is soluble in water and normal saline.

Sterile Injection for Intravenous (I.V.) or Intramuscular (I.M.) Administration: Each 1 mL of aqueous solution in the 2-mL single-dose vial contains 2 mg of ondansetron as

Continued on next page

Product information on these pages is effective as of August 2004. Further information is available at: GlaxoSmithKline, PO Box 13398, Research Triangle Park, NC 27709. 1-888-825-5249. Corporate Web Site: www.gsk.com

Zofran Injection—Cont.

the hydrochloride dihydrate; 9.0 mg of sodium chloride, USP; and 0.5 mg of citric acid monohydrate, USP and 0.25 mg of sodium citrate dihydrate, USP as buffers in Water for Injection, USP.

Each 1 mL of aqueous solution in the 20-mL multidose vial contains 2 mg of ondansetron as the hydrochloride dihydrate; 8.3 mg of sodium chloride, USP; 0.5 mg of citric acid monohydrate, USP and 0.25 mg of sodium citrate dihydrate, USP as buffers; and 1.2 mg of methylparaben, NF and 0.15 mg of propylparaben, NF as preservatives in Water for Injection, USP.

ZOFRAN Injection is a clear, colorless, nonpyrogenic, sterile solution. The pH of the injection solution is 3.3 to 4.0.

Sterile, Premixed Solution for Intravenous Administration in Single-Dose, Flexible Plastic Containers: Each 50 mL contains ondansetron 32 mg (as the hydrochloride dihydrate); dextrose 2,500 mg; and citric acid 26 mg and sodium citrate 11.5 mg as buffers in Water for Injection, USP. It contains no preservatives. The osmolarity of this solution is 270 mOsm/L (approx.), and the pH is 3.0 to 4.0.

The flexible plastic container is fabricated from a specially formulated, nonplasticized, thermoplastic co-polyester (CR3). Water can permeate from inside the container into the overwrap but not in amounts sufficient to affect the solution significantly. Solutions inside the plastic container also can leach out certain of the chemical components in very small amounts before the expiration period is attained. However, the safety of the plastic has been confirmed by tests in animals according to USP biological standards for plastic containers.

CLINICAL PHARMACOLOGY

Pharmacodynamics: Ondansetron is a selective 5-HT_3 receptor antagonist. While ondansetron's mechanism of action has not been fully characterized, it is not a dopamine-receptor antagonist. Serotonin receptors of the 5-HT_3 type are present both peripherally on vagal nerve terminals and centrally in the chemoreceptor trigger zone of the area postrema. It is not certain whether ondansetron's antiemetic action in chemotherapy-induced emesis is mediated centrally, peripherally, or in both sites. However, cytotoxic chemotherapy appears to be associated with release of serotonin from the enterochromaffin cells of the small intestine. In humans, urinary 5-HIAA (5-hydroxyindoleacetic acid) excretion increases after cisplatin administration in parallel with the onset of emesis. The released serotonin may stimulate the vagal afferents through the 5-HT_3 receptors and initiate the vomiting reflex.

In animals, the emetic response to cisplatin can be prevented by pretreatment with an inhibitor of serotonin synthesis, bilateral abdominal vagotomy and greater splanchnic nerve section, or pretreatment with a serotonin 5-HT_3 receptor antagonist.

In normal volunteers, single I.V. doses of 0.15 mg/kg of ondansetron had no effect on esophageal motility, gastric motility, lower esophageal sphincter pressure, or small intestinal transit time. In another study in six normal male volunteers, a 16-mg dose infused over 5 minutes showed no effect of the drug on cardiac output, heart rate, stroke volume, blood pressure, or electrocardiogram (ECG). Multiday administration of ondansetron has been shown to slow colonic transit in normal volunteers. Ondansetron has no effect on plasma prolactin concentrations.

In a gender-balanced pharmacodynamic study (n = 56), ondansetron 4 mg administered intravenously or intramuscularly was dynamically similar in the prevention of emesis and nausea using the ipecacuanha model of emesis. Both treatments were well tolerated.

Ondansetron does not alter the respiratory depressant effects produced by alfentanil or the degree of neuromuscular blockade produced by atracurium. Interactions with general or local anesthetics have not been studied.

Pharmacokinetics: Ondansetron is extensively metabolized in humans, with approximately 5% of a radiolabeled dose recovered as the parent compound from the urine. The primary metabolic pathway is hydroxylation on the indole ring followed by glucuronide or sulfate conjugation.

Although some nonconjugated metabolites have pharmacologic activity, these are not found in plasma at concentrations likely to significantly contribute to the biological activity of ondansetron.

In vitro metabolism studies have shown that ondansetron is a substrate for human hepatic cytochrome P-450 enzymes, including CYP1A2, CYP2D6, and CYP3A4. In terms of overall ondansetron turnover, CYP3A4 played the predominant role. Because of the multiplicity of metabolic enzymes capable of metabolizing ondansetron, it is likely that inhibition or loss of one enzyme (e.g., CYP2D6 genetic deficiency) will be compensated by others and may result in little change in overall rates of ondansetron elimination. Ondansetron elimination may be affected by cytochrome P-450 inducers. In a pharmacokinetic study of 16 epileptic patients maintained chronically on CYP3A4 inducers, carbamazepine, or phenytoin, reduction in AUC, C_{max}, and $T_{½}$ of ondansetron was observed.[1] This resulted in a significant increase in clearance. However, on the basis of available data, no dosage adjustment for ondansetron is recommended (see PRECAUTIONS: Drug Interactions).

In humans, carmustine, etoposide, and cisplatin do not affect the pharmacokinetics of ondansetron.

Table 1. Pharmacokinetics in Normal Volunteers

Age-group	n	Peak Plasma Concentration (ng/mL)	Mean Elimination Half-life (h)	Plasma Clearance (L/h/kg)
19–40	11	102	3.5	0.381
61–74	12	106	4.7	0.319
≥75	11	170	5.5	0.262

Table 2. Prevention of Chemotherapy-Induced Nausea and Emesis in Single-Day Cisplatin Therapy*

	ZOFRAN Injection	Placebo	*P* Value†
Number of patients	14	14	
Treatment response			
0 Emetic episodes	2 (14%)	0 (0%)	
1-2 Emetic episodes	8 (57%)	0 (0%)	
3-5 Emetic episodes	2 (14%)	1 (7%)	
More than 5 emetic episodes/rescued	2 (14%)	13 (93%)	0.001
Median number of emetic episodes	1.5	Undefined‡	
Median time to first emetic episode (h)	11.6	2.8	0.001
Median nausea scores (0–100)§	3	59	0.034
Global satisfaction with control of nausea and vomiting (0–100)‖	96	10.5	0.009

* Chemotherapy was high dose (100 and 120 mg/m²; ZOFRAN Injection n = 6, placebo n = 5) or moderate dose (50 and 80 mg/m²; ZOFRAN Injection n = 8, placebo n = 9). Other chemotherapeutic agents included fluorouracil, doxorubicin, and cyclophosphamide. There was no difference between treatments in the types of chemotherapy that would account for differences in response.

† Efficacy based on "all patients treated" analysis.

‡ Median undefined since at least 50% of the patients were rescued or had more than five emetic episodes.

§ Visual analog scale assessment of nausea: 0 = no nausea, 100 = nausea as bad as it can be.

‖ Visual analog scale assessment of satisfaction: 0 = not at all satisfied, 100 = totally satisfied.

In normal volunteers, the following mean pharmacokinetic data have been determined following a single 0.15-mg/kg I.V. dose.

[See table 1 above]

A reduction in clearance and increase in elimination half-life are seen in patients over 75 years of age. In clinical trials with cancer patients, safety and efficacy were similar in patients over 65 years of age and those under 65 years of age; there was an insufficient number of patients over 75 years of age to permit conclusions in that age-group. No dose adjustment is recommended in the elderly.

In patients with mild-to-moderate hepatic impairment, clearance is reduced twofold and mean half-life is increased to 11.6 hours compared to 5.7 hours in normals. In patients with severe hepatic impairment (Child-Pugh score[2] of 10 or greater), clearance is reduced twofold to threefold and apparent volume of distribution is increased with a resultant increase in half-life to 20 hours. In patients with severe hepatic impairment, a total daily dose of 8 mg should not be exceeded.

Due to the very small contribution (5%) of renal clearance to the overall clearance, renal impairment was not expected to significantly influence the total clearance of ondansetron. However, ondansetron mean plasma clearance was reduced by about 41% in patients with severe renal impairment (creatinine clearance <30 mL/min). This reduction in clearance is variable and was not consistent with an increase in half-life. No reduction in dose or dosing frequency in these patients is warranted.

In adult cancer patients, the mean elimination half-life was 4.0 hours, and there was no difference in the multidose pharmacokinetics over a 4-day period. In a study of 21 pediatric cancer patients (aged 4 to 18 years) who received three I.V. doses of 0.15 mg/kg of ondansetron at 4-hour intervals, patients older than 15 years of age exhibited ondansetron pharmacokinetic parameters similar to those of adults. Patients aged 4 to 12 years generally showed higher clearance and somewhat larger volume of distribution than adults. Most pediatric patients younger than 15 years of age with cancer had a shorter (2.4 hours) ondansetron plasma half-life than patients older than 15 years of age. It is not known whether these differences in ondansetron plasma half-life may result in differences in efficacy between adults and some young pediatric patients (see CLINICAL TRIALS: Pediatric Studies).

In a study of 21 pediatric patients (aged 3 to 12 years) who were undergoing surgery requiring anesthesia for a duration of 45 minutes to 2 hours, a single I.V. dose of ondansetron, 2 mg (3 to 7 years) or 4 mg (8 to 12 years), was administered immediately prior to anesthesia induction. Mean weight-normalized clearance and volume of distribution values in these pediatric surgical patients were similar to those previously reported for young adults. Mean terminal half-life was slightly reduced in pediatric patients (range, 2.5 to 3 hours) in comparison with adults (range, 3 to 3.5 hours).

In normal volunteers (19 to 39 years old, n = 23), the peak plasma concentration was 264 ng/mL following a single 32-mg dose administered as a 15-minute I.V. infusion. The mean elimination half-life was 4.1 hours. Systemic exposure to 32 mg of ondansetron was not proportional to dose as measured by comparing dose-normalized AUC values to an 8-mg dose. This is consistent with a small decrease in systemic clearance with increasing plasma concentrations.

A study was performed in normal volunteers (n = 56) to evaluate the pharmacokinetics of a single 4-mg dose administered as a 5-minute infusion compared to a single intramuscular injection. Systemic exposure as measured by mean AUC was equivalent, with values of 156 [95% CI 136, 180] and 161 [95% CI 137, 190] ng•h/mL for I.V. and I.M. groups, respectively. Mean peak plasma concentrations were 42.9 [95% CI 33.8, 54.4] ng/mL at 10 minutes after I.V. infusion and 31.9 [95% CI 26.3, 38.6] ng/mL at 41 minutes after I.M. injection. The mean elimination half-life was not affected by route of administration.

Plasma protein binding of ondansetron as measured in vitro was 70% to 76%, with binding constant over the pharmacologic concentration range (10 to 500 ng/mL). Circulating drug also distributes into erythrocytes.

A positive lymphoblast transformation test to ondansetron has been reported, which suggests immunologic sensitivity to ondansetron.

CLINICAL TRIALS

Chemotherapy-Induced Nausea and Vomiting: In a double-blind study of three different dosing regimens of ZOFRAN Injection, 0.015 mg/kg, 0.15 mg/kg, and 0.30 mg/kg, each given three times during the course of cancer chemotherapy, the 0.15-mg/kg dosing regimen was more effective than the 0.015-mg/kg dosing regimen. The 0.30-mg/kg dosing regimen was not shown to be more effective than the 0.15-mg/kg dosing regimen.

Cisplatin-Based Chemotherapy: In a double-blind study in 28 patients, ZOFRAN Injection (three 0.15-mg/kg doses) was significantly more effective than placebo in preventing nausea and vomiting induced by cisplatin-based chemotherapy. Treatment response was as shown in Table 2.

[See table 2 above]

Ondansetron was compared with metoclopramide in a single-blind trial in 307 patients receiving cisplatin ≥100 mg/m² with or without other chemotherapeutic agents. Patients received the first dose of ondansetron or metoclopramide 30 minutes before cisplatin. Two additional ondansetron doses were administered 4 and 8 hours later, or five additional metoclopramide doses were administered 2, 4, 7, 10, and 13 hours later. Cisplatin was administered over a period of 3 hours or less. Episodes of vomiting and retching were tabulated over the period of 24 hours after cisplatin. The results of this study are summarized in Table 3.

[See table 3 at top of next page]

In a stratified, randomized, double-blind, parallel-group, multicenter study, a single 32-mg dose of ondansetron was compared with three 0.15-mg/kg doses in patients receiving cisplatin doses of either 50 to 70 mg/m² or ≥100 mg/m². Patients received the first ondansetron dose 30 minutes before cisplatin. Two additional ondansetron doses were administered 4 and 8 hours later to the group receiving three 0.15-mg/kg doses. In both strata, significantly fewer patients on the single 32-mg dose than those receiving the three-dose regimen failed.

[See table 4 on next page]

Table 3. Prevention of Emesis Induced by Cisplatin (≥100 mg/m²) Single-Day Therapy*

	ZOFRAN Injection	Metoclopramide	*P* Value
Dose	0.15 mg/kg × 3	2 mg/kg × 6	
Number of patients in efficacy population	136	138	
Treatment response			
0 Emetic episodes	54 (40%)	41 (30%)	
1-2 Emetic episodes	34 (25%)	30 (22%)	
3-5 Emetic episodes	19 (14%)	18 (13%)	
More than 5 emetic episodes/rescued	29 (21%)	49 (36%)	
Comparison of treatments with respect to			
0 Emetic episodes	54/136	41/138	0.083
More than 5 emetic episodes/rescued	29/136	49/138	0.009
Median number of emetic episodes	1	2	0.005
Median time to first emetic episode (h)	20.5	4.3	<0.001
Global satisfaction with control of nausea and vomiting (0-100)†	85	63	0.001
Acute dystonic reactions	0	8	0.005
Akathisia	0	10	0.002

* In addition to cisplatin, 68% of patients received other chemotherapeutic agents, including cyclophosphamide, etoposide, and fluorouracil. There was no difference between treatments in the types of chemotherapy that would account for differences in response.
† Visual analog scale assessment: 0 = not at all satisfied, 100 = totally satisfied.

Table 4. Prevention of Chemotherapy-Induced Nausea and Emesis in Single-Dose Therapy

	Ondansetron Dose		
	0.15 mg/kg x 3	32 mg x 1	*P* Value
High-dose cisplatin (≥100 mg/m²)			
Number of patients	100	102	
Treatment response			
0 Emetic episodes	41 (41%)	49 (48%)	0.315
1-2 Emetic episodes	19 (19%)	25 (25%)	
3-5 Emetic episodes	4 (4%)	8 (8%)	
More than 5 emetic episodes/rescued	36 (36%)	20 (20%)	0.009
Median time to first emetic episode (h)	21.7	23	0.173
Median nausea scores (0–100)*	28	13	0.004
Medium-dose cisplatin (50-70 mg/m²)			
Number of patients	101	93	
Treatment response			
0 Emetic episodes	62 (61%)	68 (73%)	0.083
1-2 Emetic episodes	11 (11%)	14 (15%)	
3-5 Emetic episodes	6 (6%)	3 (3%)	
More than 5 emetic episodes/rescued	22 (22%)	8 (9%)	0.011
Median time to first emetic episode (h)	Undefined†	Undefined	
Median nausea scores (0-100)*	9	3	0.131

* Visual analog scale assessment: 0 = no nausea, 100 = nausea as bad as it can be.
† Median undefined since at least 50% of patients did not have any emetic episodes.

Table 5. Prevention of Chemotherapy-Induced Nausea and Emesis in Single-Day Cyclophosphamide Therapy*

	ZOFRAN Injection	Placebo	*P* Value†
Number of patients	10	10	
Treatment response			
0 Emetic episodes	7 (70%)	0 (0%)	0.001
1-2 Emetic episodes	0 (0%)	2 (20%)	
3-5 Emetic episodes	2 (20%)	4 (40%)	
More than 5 emetic episodes/rescued	1 (10%)	4 (40%)	0.131
Median number of emetic episodes	0	4	0.008
Median time to first emetic episode (h)	Undefined‡	8.79	
Median nausea scores (0-100)§	0	60	0.001
Global satisfaction with control of nausea and vomiting (0-100)‖	100	52	0.008

* Chemotherapy consisted of cyclophosphamide in all patients, plus other agents, including fluorouracil, doxorubicin, methotrexate, and vincristine. There was no difference between treatments in the type of chemotherapy that would account for differences in response.
† Efficacy based on "all patients treated" analysis.
‡ Median undefined since at least 50% of patients did not have any emetic episodes.
§ Visual analog scale assessment of nausea: 0 = no nausea, 100 = nausea as bad as it can be.
‖ Visual analog scale assessment of satisfaction: 0 = not at all satisfied, 100 = totally satisfied.

Cyclophosphamide-Based Chemotherapy: In a double-blind, placebo-controlled study of ZOFRAN Injection (three 0.15-mg/kg doses) in 20 patients receiving cyclophosphamide (500 to 600 mg/m²) chemotherapy, ZOFRAN Injection was significantly more effective than placebo in preventing nausea and vomiting. The results are summarized in Table 5.

[See table 5 above]

Re-treatment: In uncontrolled trials, 127 patients receiving cisplatin (median dose, 100 mg/m²) and ondansetron who had two or fewer emetic episodes were re-treated with ondansetron and chemotherapy, mainly cisplatin, for a total of 269 re-treatment courses (median, 2; range, 1 to 10). No emetic episodes occurred in 160 (59%), and two or fewer emetic episodes occurred in 217 (81%) re-treatment courses.

Pediatric Studies: Four open-label, noncomparative (one US, three foreign) trials have been performed with 209 pediatric cancer patients aged 4 to 18 years given a variety of cisplatin or noncisplatin regimens. In the three foreign trials, the initial ZOFRAN Injection dose ranged from 0.04 to 0.87 mg/kg for a total dose of 2.16 to 12 mg. This was followed by the oral administration of ondansetron ranging from 4 to 24 mg daily for 3 days. In the US trial, ZOFRAN was administered intravenously (only) in three doses of 0.15 mg/kg each for a total daily dose of 7.2 to 39 mg. In these studies, 58% of the 196 evaluable patients had a complete response (no emetic episodes) on day 1. Thus, prevention of emesis in these pediatric patients was essentially the same as for patients older than 18 years of age. Overall, ZOFRAN Injection was well tolerated in these pediatric patients.

Postoperative Nausea and Vomiting: ***Prevention of Postoperative Nausea and Vomiting:*** Adult surgical patients who received ondansetron immediately before the induction of general balanced anesthesia (barbiturate: thiopental, methohexital, or thiamylal; opioid: alfentanil or fentanyl; nitrous oxide; neuromuscular blockade: succinylcholine/curare and/or vecuronium or atracurium; and supplemental isoflurane) were evaluated in two double-blind US studies involving 554 patients. ZOFRAN Injection (4 mg) I.V. given over 2 to 5 minutes was significantly more effective than placebo. The results of these studies are summarized in Table 6.

[See table 6 at top of next page]

The study populations in Table 6 consisted mainly of females undergoing laparoscopic procedures.

In a placebo-controlled study conducted in 468 males undergoing outpatient procedures, a single 4 mg I.V. ondansetron dose prevented postoperative vomiting over a 24-hour study period in 79% of males receiving drug compared to 63% of males receiving placebo (*P*<0.001).

Two other placebo-controlled studies were conducted in 2,792 patients undergoing major abdominal or gynecological surgeries to evaluate a single 4-mg or 8-mg I.V. ondansetron dose for prevention of postoperative nausea and vomiting over a 24-hour study period. At the 4-mg dosage, 59% of patients receiving ondansetron versus 45% receiving placebo in the first study (*P*<0.001) and 41% of patients receiving ondansetron versus 30% receiving placebo in the second study (*P*=0.001) experienced no emetic episodes. No additional benefit was observed in patients who received I.V. ondansetron 8 mg compared to patients who received I.V. ondansetron 4 mg.

Pediatric Studies: Three double-blind, placebo-controlled studies have been performed (one US, two foreign) in 1,049 male and female patients (2 to 12 years of age) undergoing general anesthesia with nitrous oxide. The surgical procedures included tonsillectomy with or without adenoidectomy, strabismus surgery, herniorrhaphy, and orchidopexy. Patients were randomized to either single I.V. doses of ondansetron (0.1 mg/kg for pediatric patients weighing 40 kg or less, 4 mg for pediatric patients weighing more than 40 kg) or placebo. Study drug was administered over at least 30 seconds, immediately prior to or following anesthesia induction. Ondansetron was significantly more effective than placebo in preventing nausea and vomiting. The results of these studies are summarized in Table 7.

[See table 7 on next page]

Prevention of Further Postoperative Nausea and Vomiting: Adult surgical patients receiving general balanced anesthesia (barbiturate: thiopental, methohexital, or thiamylal; opioid: alfentanil or fentanyl; nitrous oxide; neuromuscular blockade: succinylcholine/curare and/or vecuronium or atracurium; and supplemental isoflurane) who received no prophylactic antiemetics and who experienced nausea and/or vomiting within 2 hours postoperatively were evaluated in two double-blind US studies involving 441 patients. Patients who experienced an episode of postoperative nausea and/or vomiting were given ZOFRAN Injection (4 mg) I.V. over 2 to 5 minutes, and this was significantly more effective than placebo. The results of these studies are summarized in Table 8.

[See table 8 on next page]

The study populations in Table 8 consisted mainly of women undergoing laparoscopic procedures.

Pediatric Studies: One double-blind, placebo-controlled, US study was performed in 351 male and female outpatients (2 to 12 years of age) who received general anesthesia with nitrous oxide and no prophylactic antiemetics. Surgical procedures were unrestricted. Patients who experienced two or more emetic episodes within 2 hours following discontinuation of nitrous oxide were randomized to either single I.V. doses of ondansetron (0.1 mg/kg for pediatric patients weighing 40 kg or less, 4 mg for pediatric patients weighing more than 40 kg) or placebo administered over at

Continued on next page

Product information on these pages is effective as of August 2004. Further information is available at: GlaxoSmithKline, PO Box 13398, Research Triangle Park, NC 27709. 1-888-825-5249. Corporate Web Site: www.gsk.com

Zofran Injection—Cont.

least 30 seconds. Ondansetron was significantly more effective than placebo in preventing further episodes of nausea and vomiting. The results of the study are summarized in Table 9.

[See table 9 at top of next page]

Repeat Dosing in Adults: In patients who do not achieve adequate control of postoperative nausea and vomiting following a single, prophylactic, preinduction, I.V. dose of ondansetron 4 mg, administration of a second I.V. dose of ondansetron 4 mg postoperatively does not provide additional control of nausea and vomiting.

INDICATIONS AND USAGE

1. Prevention of nausea and vomiting associated with initial and repeat courses of emetogenic cancer chemotherapy, including high-dose cisplatin. Efficacy of the 32-mg single dose beyond 24 hours in these patients has not been established.
2. Prevention of postoperative nausea and/or vomiting. As with other antiemetics, routine prophylaxis is not recommended for patients in whom there is little expectation that nausea and/or vomiting will occur postoperatively. In patients where nausea and/or vomiting must be avoided postoperatively, ZOFRAN Injection is recommended even where the incidence of postoperative nausea and/or vomiting is low. For patients who do not receive prophylactic ZOFRAN Injection and experience nausea and/or vomiting postoperatively, ZOFRAN Injection may be given to prevent further episodes (see CLINICAL TRIALS).

CONTRAINDICATIONS

ZOFRAN Injection and ZOFRAN Injection Premixed are contraindicated for patients known to have hypersensitivity to the drug.

WARNINGS

Hypersensitivity reactions have been reported in patients who have exhibited hypersensitivity to other selective 5-HT_3 receptor antagonists.

PRECAUTIONS

Ondansetron is not a drug that stimulates gastric or intestinal peristalsis. It should not be used instead of nasogastric suction. The use of ondansetron in patients following abdominal surgery or in patients with chemotherapy-induced nausea and vomiting may mask a progressive ileus and/or gastric distention.

Drug Interactions: Ondansetron does not itself appear to induce or inhibit the cytochrome P-450 drug-metabolizing enzyme system of the liver (see CLINICAL PHARMACOLOGY, Pharmacokinetics). Because ondansetron is metabolized by hepatic cytochrome P-450 drug-metabolizing enzymes (CYP3A4, CYP2D6, CYP1A2), inducers or inhibitors of these enzymes may change the clearance and, hence, the half-life of ondansetron. On the basis of limited available data, no dosage adjustment is recommended for patients on these drugs.

Phenytoin, Carbamazepine, and Rifampicin: In patients treated with potent inducers of CYP3A4 (i.e., phenytoin, carbamazepine, and rifampicin), the clearance of ondansetron was significantly increased and ondansetron blood concentrations were decreased. However, on the basis of available data, no dosage adjustment for ondansetron is recommended for patients on these drugs.[1,3]

Tramadol: Although no pharmacokinetic drug interaction between ondansetron and tramadol has been observed, data from 2 small studies indicate that ondansetron may be associated with an increase in patient controlled administration of tramadol.[4,5]

Chemotherapy: Tumor response to chemotherapy in the P 388 mouse leukemia model is not affected by ondansetron. In humans, carmustine, etoposide, and cisplatin do not affect the pharmacokinetics of ondansetron.

In a crossover study in 76 pediatric patients, I.V. ondansetron did not increase blood levels of high-dose methotrexate.

Carcinogenesis, Mutagenesis, Impairment of Fertility: Carcinogenic effects were not seen in 2-year studies in rats and mice with oral ondansetron doses up to 10 and 30 mg/kg per day, respectively. Ondansetron was not mutagenic in standard tests for mutagenicity. Oral administration of ondansetron up to 15 mg/kg per day did not affect fertility or general reproductive performance of male and female rats.

Pregnancy: ***Teratogenic Effects:*** Pregnancy Category B. Reproduction studies have been performed in pregnant rats and rabbits at I.V. doses up to 4 mg/kg per day and have revealed no evidence of impaired fertility or harm to the fetus due to ondansetron. There are, however, no adequate and well-controlled studies in pregnant women. Because animal reproduction studies are not always predictive of human response, this drug should be used during pregnancy only if clearly needed.

Nursing Mothers: Ondansetron is excreted in the breast milk of rats. It is not known whether ondansetron is excreted in human milk. Because many drugs are excreted in human milk, caution should be exercised when ondansetron is administered to a nursing woman.

Pediatric Use: Little information is available about dosage in pediatric patients under 2 years of age (see DOSAGE AND ADMINISTRATION section for use in pediatric patients 4 to 18 years of age receiving cancer chemotherapy or for use in pediatric patients 2 to 12 years of age receiving general anesthesia).

Geriatric Use: Of the total number of subjects enrolled in cancer chemotherapy-induced and postoperative nausea and vomiting in US- and foreign-controlled clinical trials, 862 were 65 years of age and over. No overall differences in safety or effectiveness were observed between these subjects and younger subjects, and other reported clinical experience has not identified differences in responses between the elderly and younger patients, but greater sensitivity of some older individuals cannot be ruled out. Dosage adjustment is not needed in patients over the age of 65 (see CLINICAL PHARMACOLOGY).

ADVERSE REACTIONS

Chemotherapy-Induced Nausea and Vomiting: The adverse events in Table 10 have been reported in individuals

Table 6. Prevention of Postoperative Nausea and Vomiting in Adult Patients

	Ondansetron 4 mg I.V.	Placebo	*P* Value
Study 1			
Emetic episodes:			
Number of patients	136	139	
Treatment response over 24-h postoperative period			
0 Emetic episodes	103 (76%)	64 (46%)	<0.001
1 Emetic episode	13 (10%)	17 (12%)	
More than 1 emetic episode/rescued	20 (15%)	58 (42%)	
Nausea assessments:			
Number of patients	134	136	
No nausea over 24-h postoperative period	56 (42%)	39 (29%)	
Study 2			
Emetic episodes:			
Number of patients	136	143	
Treatment response over 24-h postoperative period			
0 Emetic episodes	85 (63%)	63 (44%)	0.002
1 Emetic episode	16 (12%)	29 (20%)	
More than 1 emetic episode/rescued	35 (26%)	51 (36%)	
Nausea assessments:			
Number of patients	125	133	
No nausea over 24-h postoperative period	48 (38%)	42 (32%)	

Table 7. Prevention of Postoperative Nausea and Vomiting in Pediatric Patients

Treatment Response Over 24 Hours	Ondansetron n (%)	Placebo n (%)	*P* Value
Study 1			
Number of patients	205	210	
0 Emetic episodes	140 (68%)	82 (39%)	≤0.001
Failure*	65 (32%)	128 (61%)	
Study 2			
Number of patients	112	110	
0 Emetic episodes	68 (61%)	38 (35%)	≤0.001
Failure*	44 (39%)	72 (65%)	
Study 3			
Number of patients	206	206	
0 Emetic episodes	123 (60%)	96 (47%)	≤0.01
Failure*	83 (40%)	110 (53%)	
Nausea assessments†:			
Number of patients	185	191	
None	119 (64%)	99 (52%)	≤0.01

* Failure was one or more emetic episodes, rescued, or withdrawn.
† Nausea measured as none, mild, or severe.

Table 8. Prevention of Further Postoperative Nausea and Vomiting in Adult Patients

	Ondansetron 4 mg I.V.	Placebo	*P* Value
Study 1			
Emetic episodes:			
Number of patients	104	117	
Treatment response 24 h after study drug			
0 Emetic episodes	49 (47%)	19 (16%)	<0.001
1 Emetic episode	12 (12%)	9 (8%)	
More than 1 emetic episode/rescued	43 (41%)	89 (76%)	
Median time to first emetic episode (min)*	55.0	43.0	
Nausea assessments:			
Number of patients	98	102	
Mean nausea score over 24-h postoperative period†	1.7	3.1	
Study 2			
Emetic episodes:			
Number of patients	112	108	
Treatment response 24 h after study drug			
0 Emetic episodes	49 (44%)	28 (26%)	0.006
1 Emetic episode	14 (13%)	3 (3%)	
More than 1 emetic episode/rescued	49 (44%)	77 (71%)	
Median time to first emetic episode (min)*	60.5	34.0	
Nausea assessments:			
Number of patients	105	85	
Mean nausea score over 24-h postoperative period†	1.9	2.9	

* After administration of study drug.
† Nausea measured on a scale of 0-10 with 0 = no nausea, 10 = nausea as bad as it can be.

receiving ondansetron at a dosage of three 0.15-mg/kg doses or as a single 32-mg dose in clinical trials. These patients were receiving concomitant chemotherapy, primarily cisplatin, and I.V. fluids. Most were receiving a diuretic.

[See table 10 at right]

The following have been reported during controlled clinical trials:

Cardiovascular: Rare cases of angina (chest pain), electrocardiographic alterations, hypotension, and tachycardia have been reported. In many cases, the relationship to ZOFRAN Injection was unclear.

Gastrointestinal: Constipation has been reported in 11% of chemotherapy patients receiving multiday ondansetron.

Hepatic: In comparative trials in cisplatin chemotherapy patients with normal baseline values of aspartate transaminase (AST) and alanine transaminase (ALT), these enzymes have been reported to exceed twice the upper limit of normal in approximately 5% of patients. The increases were transient and did not appear to be related to dose or duration of therapy. On repeat exposure, similar transient elevations in transaminase values occurred in some courses, but symptomatic hepatic disease did not occur.

Integumentary: Rash has occurred in approximately 1% of patients receiving ondansetron.

Neurological: There have been rare reports consistent with, but not diagnostic of, extrapyramidal reactions in patients receiving ZOFRAN Injection, and rare cases of grand mal seizure. The relationship to ZOFRAN was unclear.

Other: Rare cases of hypokalemia have been reported. The relationship to ZOFRAN Injection was unclear.

Postoperative Nausea and Vomiting: The adverse events in Table 11 have been reported in ≥2% of adults receiving ondansetron at a dosage of 4 mg I.V. over 2 to 5 minutes in clinical trials. Rates of these events were not significantly different in the ondansetron and placebo groups. These patients were receiving multiple concomitant perioperative and postoperative medications.

[See table 11 at right]

Pediatric Use: The adverse events in Table 12 were the most commonly reported adverse events in pediatric patients receiving ondansetron (a single 0.1-mg/kg dose for pediatric patients weighing 40 kg or less, or 4 mg for pediatric patients weighing more than 40 kg) administered intravenously over at least 30 seconds. Rates of these events were not significantly different in the ondansetron and placebo groups. These patients were receiving multiple concomitant perioperative and postoperative medications.

[See table 12 at top of next page]

Observed During Clinical Practice: In addition to adverse events reported from clinical trials, the following events have been identified during post-approval use of intravenous formulations of ZOFRAN. Because they are reported voluntarily from a population of unknown size, estimates of frequency cannot be made. The events have been chosen for inclusion due to a combination of their seriousness, frequency of reporting, or potential causal connection to ZOFRAN.

Cardiovascular: Arrhythmias (including ventricular and supraventricular tachycardia, premature ventricular contractions, and atrial fibrillation), bradycardia, electrocardiographic alterations (including second-degree heart block and ST segment depression), palpitations, and syncope.

General: Flushing. Rare cases of hypersensitivity reactions, sometimes severe (e.g., anaphylaxis/anaphylactoid reactions, angioedema, bronchospasm, cardiopulmonary arrest, hypotension, laryngeal edema, laryngospasm, shock, shortness of breath, stridor) have also been reported.

Hepatobiliary: Liver enzyme abnormalities have been reported. Liver failure and death have been reported in patients with cancer receiving concurrent medications including potentially hepatotoxic cytotoxic chemotherapy and antibiotics. The etiology of the liver failure is unclear.

Local Reactions: Pain, redness, and burning at site of injection.

Lower Respiratory: Hiccups

Neurological: Oculogyric crisis, appearing alone, as well as with other dystonic reactions.

Skin: Urticaria

Special Senses: Transient blurred vision, in some cases associated with abnormalities of accommodation, and transient dizziness during or shortly after I.V. infusion.

DRUG ABUSE AND DEPENDENCE

Animal studies have shown that ondansetron is not discriminated as a benzodiazepine nor does it substitute for benzodiazepines in direct addiction studies.

OVERDOSAGE

There is no specific antidote for ondansetron overdose. Patients should be managed with appropriate supportive therapy. Individual doses as large as 150 mg and total daily dosages (three doses) as large as 252 mg have been administered intravenously without significant adverse events. These doses are more than 10 times the recommended daily dose.

In addition to the adverse events listed above, the following events have been described in the setting of ondansetron overdose: "Sudden blindness" (amaurosis) of 2 to 3 minutes' duration plus severe constipation occurred in one patient that was administered 72 mg of ondansetron intravenously as a single dose. Hypotension (and faintness) occurred in another patient that took 48 mg of oral ondansetron. Following infusion of 32 mg over only a 4-minute period, a vasovagal episode with transient second-degree heart block was observed. In all instances, the events resolved completely.

Table 9. Prevention of Further Postoperative Nausea and Vomiting in Pediatric Patients

Treatment Response Over 24 Hours	Ondansetron n (%)	Placebo n (%)	*P* Value
Number of patients	180	171	
0 Emetic episodes	96 (53%)	29 (17%)	≤0.001
Failure*	84 (47%)	142 (83%)	

* Failure was one or more emetic episodes, rescued, or withdrawn.

Table 10. Principal Adverse Events in Comparative Trials

	Number of Patients With Event			
	ZOFRAN Injection 0.15 mg/kg × 3 n = 419	ZOFRAN Injection 32 mg × 1 n = 220	Metoclopramide n = 156	Placebo n = 34
Diarrhea	16%	8%	44%	18%
Headache	17%	25%	7%	15%
Fever	8%	7%	5%	3%
Akathisia	0%	0%	6%	0%
Acute dystonic reactions*	0%	0%	5%	0%

* See Neurological.

Table 11. Adverse Events in ≥2% of Adults Receiving Ondansetron at a Dosage of 4 mg I.V. over 2 to 5 Minutes in Clinical Trials

	ZOFRAN Injection 4 mg I.V. n = 547 patients	Placebo n = 547 patients
Headache	92 (17%)	77 (14%)
Dizziness	67 (12%)	88 (16%)
Musculoskeletal pain	57 (10%)	59 (11%)
Drowsiness/sedation	44 (8%)	37 (7%)
Shivers	38 (7%)	39 (7%)
Malaise/fatigue	25 (5%)	30 (5%)
Injection site reaction	21 (4%)	18 (3%)
Urinary retention	17 (3%)	15 (3%)
Postoperative CO_2-related pain*	12 (2%)	16 (3%)
Chest pain (unspecified)	12 (2%)	15 (3%)
Anxiety/agitation	11 (2%)	16 (3%)
Dysuria	11 (2%)	9 (2%)
Hypotension	10 (2%)	12 (2%)
Fever	10 (2%)	6 (1%)
Cold sensation	9 (2%)	8 (1%)
Pruritus	9 (2%)	3 (<1%)
Paresthesia	9 (2%)	2 (<1%)

*Sites of pain included abdomen, stomach, joints, rib cage, shoulder.

DOSAGE AND ADMINISTRATION

Prevention of Chemotherapy-Induced Nausea and Vomiting: The recommended I.V. dosage of ZOFRAN is a single 32-mg dose or three 0.15-mg/kg doses. A single 32-mg dose is infused over 15 minutes beginning 30 minutes before the start of emetogenic chemotherapy. The recommended infusion rate should not be exceeded (see OVERDOSAGE). With the three-dose (0.15-mg/kg) regimen, the first dose is infused over 15 minutes beginning 30 minutes before the start of emetogenic chemotherapy. Subsequent doses (0.15 mg/kg) are administered 4 and 8 hours after the first dose of ZOFRAN.

ZOFRAN Injection should not be mixed with solutions for which physical and chemical compatibility have not been established. In particular, this applies to alkaline solutions as a precipitate may form.

Vial: **DILUTE BEFORE USE.** ZOFRAN Injection should be diluted in 50 mL of 5% Dextrose Injection or 0.9% Sodium Chloride Injection before administration.

Flexible Plastic Container: ZOFRAN Injection Premixed, 32 mg in 5% Dextrose, 50 mL, **REQUIRES NO DILUTION.**

Pediatric Use: On the basis of the limited available information (see CLINICAL TRIALS: Pediatric Studies and CLINICAL PHARMACOLOGY: Pharmacokinetics), the dosage in pediatric patients 4 to 18 years of age should be three 0.15-mg/kg doses (see above). Little information is available about dosage in pediatric patients 3 years of age and younger.

Geriatric Use: The dosage recommendation is the same as for the general population.

Prevention of Postoperative Nausea and Vomiting: The recommended I.V. dosage of ZOFRAN for adults is 4 mg **undiluted** administered intravenously in not less than 30 seconds, preferably over 2 to 5 minutes, immediately before induction of anesthesia, or postoperatively if the patient experiences nausea and/or vomiting occurring shortly after surgery. Alternatively, 4 mg **undiluted** may be administered intramuscularly as a single injection for adults. While recommended as a fixed dose for patients weighing more than 40 kg, few patients above 80 kg have been studied. In patients who do not achieve adequate control of postoperative nausea and vomiting following a single, prophylactic, preinduction, I.V. dose of ondansetron 4 mg, administration of a second I.V. dose of 4 mg ondansetron postoperatively does not provide additional control of nausea and vomiting.

Vial: ZOFRAN Injection **REQUIRES NO DILUTION FOR ADMINISTRATION FOR POSTOPERATIVE NAUSEA AND VOMITING.**

Continued on next page

Product information on these pages is effective as of August 2004. Further information is available at: GlaxoSmithKline, PO Box 13398, Research Triangle Park, NC 27709. 1-888-825-5249. Corporate Web Site: www.gsk.com

Table 12. Frequency of Adverse Events From Controlled Studies in Pediatric Patients

Adverse Event	Ondansetron n = 755 Patients	Placebo n = 731 Patients
Wound problem	80 (11%)	86 (12%)
Anxiety/agitation	49 (6%)	47 (6%)
Headache	44 (6%)	43 (6%)
Drowsiness/sedation	41 (5%)	56 (8%)
Pyrexia	32 (4%)	41 (6%)

Zofran Injection—Cont.

Pediatric Use: The recommended I.V. dosage of ZOFRAN for pediatric patients (2 to 12 years of age) is a single 0.1-mg/kg dose for pediatric patients weighing 40 kg or less, or a single 4-mg dose for pediatric patients weighing more than 40 kg. The rate of administration should not be less than 30 seconds, preferably over 2 to 5 minutes. Little information is available about dosage in pediatric patients younger than 2 years of age.

Geriatric Use: The dosage recommendation is the same as for the general population.

Dosage Adjustment for Patients With Impaired Renal Function: The dosage recommendation is the same as for the general population. There is no experience beyond first-day administration of ondansetron.

Dosage Adjustment for Patients With Impaired Hepatic Function: In patients with severe hepatic impairment (Child-Pugh[2] score of 10 or greater), a single maximal daily dose of 8 mg to be infused over 15 minutes beginning 30 minutes before the start of the emetogenic chemotherapy is recommended. There is no experience beyond first-day administration of ondansetron.

ZOFRAN Injection Premixed in Flexible Plastic Containers:

Instructions for Use: ***To Open:*** Tear outer wrap at notch and remove solution container. Check for minute leaks by squeezing container firmly. If leaks are found, discard unit as sterility may be impaired.

Preparation for Administration: Use aseptic technique.

1. Close flow control clamp of administration set.
2. Remove cover from outlet port at bottom of container.
3. Insert piercing pin of administration set into port with a twisting motion until the pin is firmly seated. NOTE: See full directions on administration set carton.
4. Suspend container from hanger.
5. Squeeze and release drip chamber to establish proper fluid level in chamber during infusion of ZOFRAN Injection Premixed.
6. Open flow control clamp to expel air from set. Close clamp.
7. Attach set to venipuncture device. If device is not indwelling, prime and make venipuncture.
8. Perform venipuncture.
9. Regulate rate of administration with flow control clamp.

Caution: ZOFRAN Injection Premixed in flexible plastic containers is to be administered by I.V. drip infusion only. ZOFRAN Injection Premixed should not be mixed with solutions for which physical and chemical compatibility have not been established. In particular, this applies to alkaline solutions as a precipitate may form. If used with a primary I.V. fluid system, the primary solution should be discontinued during ZOFRAN Injection Premixed infusion.

Do not administer unless solution is clear and container is undamaged.

Warning: Do not use flexible plastic container in series connections.

Stability: ZOFRAN Injection is stable at room temperature under normal lighting conditions for 48 hours after dilution with the following I.V. fluids: 0.9% Sodium Chloride Injection, 5% Dextrose Injection, 5% Dextrose and 0.9% Sodium Chloride Injection, 5% Dextrose and 0.45% Sodium Chloride Injection, and 3% Sodium Chloride Injection.

Although ZOFRAN Injection is chemically and physically stable when diluted as recommended, sterile precautions should be observed because diluents generally do not contain preservative. After dilution, do not use beyond 24 hours.

Note: Parenteral drug products should be inspected visually for particulate matter and discoloration before administration whenever solution and container permit.

Precaution: Occasionally, ondansetron precipitates at the stopper/vial interface in vials stored upright. Potency and safety are not affected. If a precipitate is observed, resolubilize by shaking the vial vigorously.

HOW SUPPLIED

ZOFRAN Injection, 2 mg/mL, is supplied as follows:

NDC 0173-0442-02 2-mL single-dose vials (Carton of 5)
NDC 0173-0442-00 20-mL multidose vials (Singles)

Store between 2° and 30°C (36° and 86°F). Protect from light.

ZOFRAN Injection Premixed, 32 mg/50 mL, in 5% Dextrose, contains no preservatives and is supplied as a sterile, premixed solution for I.V. administration in single-dose, flexible plastic containers (NDC 0173-0461-00) (case of 6).

Store between 2° and 30°C (36° and 86°F). Protect from light. Avoid excessive heat. Protect from freezing.

REFERENCES

1. Britto MR, Hussey EK, Mydlow P, et al. Effect of enzyme inducers on ondansetron (OND) metabolism in humans. *Clin Pharmacol Ther.* 1997;61:228.
2. Pugh RNH, Murray-Lyon IM, Dawson JL, Pietroni MC, Williams R. Transection of the oesophagus for bleeding oesophageal varices. *Brit J Surg.* 1973;60:646-649.
3. Villikka K, Kivisto KT, Neuvonen PJ. The effect of rifampin on the pharmacokinetics of oral and intravenous ondansetron. *Clin Pharmacol Ther* 1999;65:377-381.
4. De Witte JL, Schoenmaekers B, Sessler DI, et al. *Anesth Analg.* 2001;92:1319-1321.
5. Arcioni R, della Rocca M, Romanò R, et al. *Anesth Analg.* 2002;94:1553-1557.

ZOFRAN® Injection Premixed:
Manufactured for GlaxoSmithKline
Research Triangle Park, NC 27709
by Abbott Laboratories, North Chicago, IL 60064

May 2004/RL-2083

Shown in Product Identification Guide, page 318

ZOFRAN® ℞
[*zō' fran*]
(ondansetron hydrochloride)
Tablets

ZOFRAN ODT® ℞
(ondansetron)
Orally Disintegrating Tablets

ZOFRAN® ℞
(ondansetron hydrochloride)
Oral Solution

DESCRIPTION

The active ingredient in ZOFRAN Tablets and ZOFRAN Oral Solution is ondansetron hydrochloride (HCl) as the dihydrate, the racemic form of ondansetron and a selective blocking agent of the serotonin 5-HT_3 receptor type. Chemically it is (±) 1, 2, 3, 9-tetrahydro-9-methyl-3-[(2-methyl-1H-imidazol-1-yl)methyl]-4H-carbazol-4-one, monohydrochloride, dihydrate.

The empirical formula is $C_{18}H_{19}N_3O \bullet HCl \bullet 2H_2O$, representing a molecular weight of 365.9.

Ondansetron HCl dihydrate is a white to off-white powder that is soluble in water and normal saline.

The active ingredient in ZOFRAN ODT Orally Disintegrating Tablets is ondansetron base, the racemic form of ondansetron, and a selective blocking agent of the serotonin 5-HT_3 receptor type. Chemically it is (±) 1, 2, 3, 9-tetrahydro-9-methyl-3-[(2-methyl-1H-imidazol-1-yl)methyl]-4H-carbazol-4-one.

The empirical formula is $C_{18}H_{19}N_3O$ representing a molecular weight of 293.4.

Each 4-mg ZOFRAN Tablet for oral administration contains ondansetron HCl dihydrate equivalent to 4 mg of ondansetron. Each 8-mg ZOFRAN Tablet for oral administration contains ondansetron HCl dihydrate equivalent to 8 mg of ondansetron. Each 24-mg ZOFRAN Tablet for oral administration contains ondansetron HCl dihydrate equivalent to 24 mg of ondansetron. Each tablet also contains the inactive ingredients lactose, microcrystalline cellulose, pregelatinized starch, hypromellose, magnesium stearate, titanium dioxide, triacetin, iron oxide yellow (8-mg tablet only), and iron oxide red (24-mg tablet only).

Each 4-mg ZOFRAN ODT Orally Disintegrating Tablet for oral administration contains 4 mg ondansetron base. Each 8-mg ZOFRAN ODT Orally Disintegrating Tablet for oral administration contains 8 mg ondansetron base. Each ZOFRAN ODT Tablet also contains the inactive ingredients aspartame, gelatin, mannitol, methylparaben sodium, propylparaben sodium, and strawberry flavor. ZOFRAN ODT Tablets are a freeze-dried, orally administered formulation of ondansetron which rapidly disintegrates on the tongue and does not require water to aid dissolution or swallowing.

Each 5 mL of ZOFRAN Oral Solution contains 5 mg of ondansetron HCl dihydrate equivalent to 4 mg of ondansetron. ZOFRAN Oral Solution contains the inactive ingredients citric acid anhydrous, purified water, sodium benzoate, sodium citrate, sorbitol, and strawberry flavor.

CLINICAL PHARMACOLOGY

Pharmacodynamics: Ondansetron is a selective 5-HT_3 receptor antagonist. While its mechanism of action has not been fully characterized, ondansetron is not a dopamine-receptor antagonist. Serotonin receptors of the 5-HT_3 type are present both peripherally on vagal nerve terminals and centrally in the chemoreceptor trigger zone of the area postrema. It is not certain whether ondansetron's antiemetic action is mediated centrally, peripherally, or in both sites. However, cytotoxic chemotherapy appears to be associated with release of serotonin from the enterochromaffin cells of the small intestine. In humans, urinary 5-HIAA (5-hydroxyindoleacetic acid) excretion increases after cisplatin administration in parallel with the onset of emesis. The released serotonin may stimulate the vagal afferents through the 5-HT_3 receptors and initiate the vomiting reflex.

In animals, the emetic response to cisplatin can be prevented by pretreatment with an inhibitor of serotonin synthesis, bilateral abdominal vagotomy and greater splanchnic nerve section, or pretreatment with a serotonin 5-HT_3 receptor antagonist.

In normal volunteers, single intravenous doses of 0.15 mg/kg of ondansetron had no effect on esophageal motility, gastric motility, lower esophageal sphincter pressure, or small intestinal transit time. Multiday administration of ondansetron has been shown to slow colonic transit in normal volunteers. Ondansetron has no effect on plasma prolactin concentrations.

Ondansetron does not alter the respiratory depressant effects produced by alfentanil or the degree of neuromuscular blockade produced by atracurium. Interactions with general or local anesthetics have not been studied.

Pharmacokinetics: Ondansetron is well absorbed from the gastrointestinal tract and undergoes some first-pass metabolism. Mean bioavailability in healthy subjects, following administration of a single 8-mg tablet, is approximately 56%.

Ondansetron systemic exposure does not increase proportionately to dose. AUC from a 16-mg tablet was 24% greater than predicted from an 8-mg tablet dose. This may reflect some reduction of first-pass metabolism at higher oral doses. Bioavailability is also slightly enhanced by the presence of food but unaffected by antacids.

Ondansetron is extensively metabolized in humans, with approximately 5% of a radiolabeled dose recovered from the urine as the parent compound. The primary metabolic pathway is hydroxylation on the indole ring followed by subsequent glucuronide or sulfate conjugation. Although some nonconjugated metabolites have pharmacologic activity, these are not found in plasma at concentrations likely to significantly contribute to the biological activity of ondansetron.

In vitro metabolism studies have shown that ondansetron is a substrate for human hepatic cytochrome P-450 enzymes, including CYP1A2, CYP2D6, and CYP3A4. In terms of overall ondansetron turnover, CYP3A4 played the predominant role. Because of the multiplicity of metabolic enzymes capable of metabolizing ondansetron, it is likely that inhibition or loss of one enzyme (e.g., CYP2D6 genetic deficiency) will be compensated by others and may result in little change in overall rates of ondansetron elimination. Ondansetron elimination may be affected by cytochrome P-450 inducers. In a pharmacokinetic study of 16 epileptic patients maintained chronically on CYP3A4 inducers, carbamazepine, or phenytoin, reduction in AUC, C_{max}, and $T_{1/2}$ of ondansetron was observed.[1] This resulted in a significant increase in clearance. However, on the basis of available data, no dosage adjustment for ondansetron is recommended (see PRECAUTIONS: Drug Interactions).

In humans, carmustine, etoposide, and cisplatin do not affect the pharmacokinetics of ondansetron.

Gender differences were shown in the disposition of ondansetron given as a single dose. The extent and rate of ondansetron's absorption is greater in women than men. Slower clearance in women, a smaller apparent volume of distribution (adjusted for weight), and higher absolute bioavailability resulted in higher plasma ondansetron levels. These higher plasma levels may in part be explained by differences in body weight between men and women. It is not known whether these gender-related differences were clinically important. More detailed pharmacokinetic information is contained in Tables 1 and 2 taken from 2 studies.

[See table 1 at top of next page]

[See table 2 at top of next page]

A reduction in clearance and increase in elimination half-life are seen in patients over 75 years of age. In clinical trials with cancer patients, safety and efficacy was similar in patients over 65 years of age and those under 65 years of age; there was an insufficient number of patients over 75 years of age to permit conclusions in that age-group. No dosage adjustment is recommended in the elderly.

In patients with mild-to-moderate hepatic impairment, clearance is reduced 2-fold and mean half-life is increased to 11.6 hours compared to 5.7 hours in normals. In patients with severe hepatic impairment (Child-Pugh[2] score of 10 or greater), clearance is reduced 2-fold to 3-fold and apparent volume of distribution is increased with a resultant increase in half-life to 20 hours. In patients with severe hepatic impairment, a total daily dose of 8 mg should not be exceeded.

Due to the very small contribution (5%) of renal clearance to the overall clearance, renal impairment was not expected to significantly influence the total clearance of ondansetron. However, ondansetron oral mean plasma clearance was reduced by about 50% in patients with severe renal impairment (creatinine clearance <30 mL/min). This reduction in clearance is variable and was not consistent with an increase in half-life. No reduction in dose or dosing frequency in these patients is warranted.

Plasma protein binding of ondansetron as measured in vitro was 70% to 76% over the concentration range of 10 to 500 ng/mL. Circulating drug also distributes into erythrocytes.

Four- and 8-mg doses of either ZOFRAN Oral Solution or ZOFRAN ODT Orally Disintegrating Tablets are bioequivalent to corresponding doses of ZOFRAN Tablets and may be used interchangeably. One 24-mg ZOFRAN Tablet is bioequivalent to and interchangeable with three 8-mg ZOFRAN Tablets.

CLINICAL TRIALS

Chemotherapy-Induced Nausea and Vomiting: ***Highly Emetogenic Chemotherapy:*** In 2 randomized, double-blind, monotherapy trials, a single 24-mg ZOFRAN Tablet was superior to a relevant historical placebo control in the prevention of nausea and vomiting associated with highly emetogenic cancer chemotherapy, including cisplatin ≥50 mg/m². Steroid administration was excluded from these clinical trials. More than 90% of patients receiving a cisplatin dose ≥50 mg/m² in the historical placebo comparator experienced vomiting in the absence of antiemetic therapy.

The first trial compared oral doses of ondansetron 24 mg once a day, 8 mg twice a day, and 32 mg once a day in 357 adult cancer patients receiving chemotherapy regimens containing cisplatin ≥50 mg/m². A total of 66% of patients in the ondansetron 24-mg once a day group, 55% in the ondansetron 8-mg twice a day group, and 55% in the ondansetron 32-mg once a day group completed the 24-hour study period with 0 emetic episodes and no rescue antiemetic medications, the primary endpoint of efficacy. Each of the 3 treatment groups was shown to be statistically significantly superior to a historical placebo control.

In the same trial, 56% of patients receiving oral ondansetron 24 mg once a day experienced no nausea during the 24-hour study period, compared with 36% of patients in the oral ondansetron 8-mg twice a day group (p = 0.001) and 50% in the oral ondansetron 32-mg once a day group.

In a second trial, efficacy of the oral ondansetron 24 mg once a day regimen in the prevention of nausea and vomiting associated with highly emetogenic cancer chemotherapy, including cisplatin ≥50 mg/m², was confirmed.

Moderately Emetogenic Chemotherapy: In 1 double-blind US study in 67 patients, ZOFRAN Tablets 8 mg administered twice a day were significantly more effective than placebo in preventing vomiting induced by cyclophosphamide-based chemotherapy containing doxorubicin. Treatment response is based on the total number of emetic episodes over the 3-day study period. The results of this study are summarized in Table 3:

[See table 3 at right]

In 1 double-blind US study in 336 patients, ZOFRAN Tablets 8 mg administered twice a day were as effective as ZOFRAN Tablets 8 mg administered 3 times a day in preventing nausea and vomiting induced by cyclophosphamide-based chemotherapy containing either methotrexate or doxorubicin. Treatment response is based on the total number of emetic episodes over the 3-day study period. The results of this study are summarized in Table 4:

[See table 4 at right]

Re-treatment: In uncontrolled trials, 148 patients receiving cyclophosphamide-based chemotherapy were re-treated with ZOFRAN Tablets 8 mg 3 times daily of oral ondansetron during subsequent chemotherapy for a total of 396 re-treatment courses. No emetic episodes occurred in 314 (79%) of the re-treatment courses, and only 1 to 2 emetic episodes occurred in 43 (11%) of the re-treatment courses.

Pediatric Studies: Three open-label, uncontrolled, foreign trials have been performed with 182 pediatric patients 4 to 18 years old with cancer who were given a variety of cisplatin or noncisplatin regimens. In these foreign trials, the initial dose of ZOFRAN® (ondansetron HCl) Injection ranged from 0.04 to 0.87 mg/kg for a total dose of 2.16 to 12 mg. This was followed by the administration of ZOFRAN Tablets ranging from 4 to 24 mg daily for 3 days. In these studies, 58% of the 170 evaluable patients had a complete response (no emetic episodes) on day 1. Two studies showed the response rates for patients less than 12 years of age who received ZOFRAN Tablets 4 mg 3 times a day to be similar to those in patients 12 to 18 years of age who received ZOFRAN Tablets 8 mg 3 times daily. Thus, prevention of emesis in these pediatric patients was essentially the same as for patients older than 18 years of age. Overall, ZOFRAN Tablets were well tolerated in these pediatric patients.

Radiation-Induced Nausea and Vomiting: ***Total Body Irradiation:*** In a randomized, double-blind study in 20 patients, ZOFRAN Tablets (8 mg given 1.5 hours before each fraction of radiotherapy for 4 days) were significantly more effective than placebo in preventing vomiting induced by total body irradiation. Total body irradiation consisted of 11 fractions (120 cGy per fraction) over 4 days for a total of 1,320 cGy. Patients received 3 fractions for 3 days, then 2 fractions on day 4.

Single High-Dose Fraction Radiotherapy: Ondansetron was significantly more effective than metoclopramide with respect to complete control of emesis (0 emetic episodes) in a double-blind trial in 105 patients receiving single high-dose radiotherapy (800 to 1,000 cGy) over an anterior or posterior field size of ≥80 cm² to the abdomen. Patients received the first dose of ZOFRAN Tablets (8 mg) or metoclopramide (10 mg) 1 to 2 hours before radiotherapy. If radiotherapy was given in the morning, 2 additional doses of study treatment were given (1 tablet late afternoon and 1 tablet before bedtime). If radiotherapy was given in the afternoon, patients took only 1 further tablet that day before bedtime. Patients continued the oral medication on a 3 times a day basis for 3 days.

Daily Fractionated Radiotherapy: Ondansetron was significantly more effective than prochlorperazine with respect to complete control of emesis (0 emetic episodes) in a double-blind trial in 135 patients receiving a 1- to 4-week course of fractionated radiotherapy (180 cGy doses) over a field size of ≥100 cm² to the abdomen. Patients received the first dose of ZOFRAN Tablets (8 mg) or prochlorperazine (10 mg) 1 to 2 hours before the patient received the first daily radiotherapy fraction, with 2 subsequent doses on a 3 times a day basis. Patients continued the oral medication on a 3 times a day basis on each day of radiotherapy.

Postoperative Nausea and Vomiting: Surgical patients who received ondansetron 1 hour before the induction of general balanced anesthesia (barbiturate: thiopental, methohexital, or thiamylal; opioid: alfentanil, sufentanil, morphine, or fentanyl; nitrous oxide; neuromuscular blockade: succinylcholine/curare or gallamine and/or vecuronium, pancuronium, or atracurium; and supplemental isoflurane or enflurane) were evaluated in 2 double-blind studies (1 US study, 1 foreign) involving 865 patients. ZOFRAN Tablets (16 mg) were significantly more effective than placebo in preventing postoperative nausea and vomiting.

The study populations in all trials thus far consisted of women undergoing inpatient surgical procedures. No studies have been performed in males. No controlled clinical study comparing ZOFRAN Tablets to ZOFRAN Injection has been performed.

Table 1. Pharmacokinetics in Normal Volunteers: Single 8-mg ZOFRAN Tablet Dose

Age-group (years)	Mean Weight (kg)	n	Peak Plasma Concentration (ng/mL)	Time of Peak Plasma Concentration (h)	Mean Elimination Half-life (h)	Systemic Plasma Clearance L/h/kg	Absolute Bioavailability
18-40 M	69.0	6	26.2	2.0	3.1	0.403	0.483
F	62.7	5	42.7	1.7	3.5	0.354	0.663
61-74 M	77.5	6	24.1	2.1	4.1	0.384	0.585
F	60.2	6	52.4	1.9	4.9	0.255	0.643
≥75 M	78.0	5	37.0	2.2	4.5	0.277	0.619
F	67.6	6	46.1	2.1	6.2	0.249	0.747

Table 2. Pharmacokinetics in Normal Volunteers: Single 24-mg ZOFRAN Tablet Dose

Age-group (years)	Mean Weight (kg)	n	Peak Plasma Concentration (ng/mL)	Time of Peak Plasma Concentration (h)	Mean Elimination Half-life (h)
18-43 M	84.1	8	125.8	1.9	4.7
F	71.8	8	194.4	1.6	5.8

Table 3. Emetic Episodes: Treatment Response

	Ondansetron 8-mg b.i.d. ZOFRAN Tablets*	Placebo	p Value
Number of patients	33	34	
Treatment response			
0 Emetic episodes	20 (61%)	2 (6%)	<0.001
1-2 Emetic episodes	6 (18%)	8 (24%)	
More than 2 emetic episodes/withdrawn	7 (21%)	24 (71%)	<0.001
Median number of emetic episodes	0.0	Undefined†	
Median time to first emetic episode (h)	Undefined‡	6.5	

*The first dose was administered 30 minutes before the start of emetogenic chemotherapy, with a subsequent dose 8 hours after the first dose. An 8-mg ZOFRAN Tablet was administered twice a day for 2 days after completion of chemotherapy.

† Median undefined since at least 50% of the patients were withdrawn or had more than 2 emetic episodes.

‡ Median undefined since at least 50% of patients did not have any emetic episodes.

Table 4. Emetic Episodes: Treatment Response

	Ondansetron	
	8-mg b.i.d. ZOFRAN Tablets*	8-mg t.i.d. ZOFRAN Tablets†
Number of patients	165	171
Treatment response		
0 Emetic episodes	101 (61%)	99 (58%)
1-2 Emetic episodes	16 (10%)	17 (10%)
More than 2 emetic episodes/withdrawn	48 (29%)	55 (32%)
Median number of emetic episodes	0.0	0.0
Median time to first emetic episode (h)	Undefined‡	Undefined‡
Median nausea scores (0-100)§	6	6

*The first dose was administered 30 minutes before the start of emetogenic chemotherapy, with a subsequent dose 8 hours after the first dose. An 8-mg ZOFRAN Tablet was administered twice a day for 2 days after completion of chemotherapy.

† The first dose was administered 30 minutes before the start of emetogenic chemotherapy, with subsequent doses 4 and 8 hours after the first dose. An 8-mg ZOFRAN Tablet was administered 3 times a day for 2 days after completion of chemotherapy.

‡ Median undefined since at least 50% of patients did not have any emetic episodes.

§ Visual analog scale assessment: 0 = no nausea, 100 = nausea as bad as it can be.

Continued on next page

Product information on these pages is effective as of August 2004. Further information is available at: GlaxoSmithKline, PO Box 13398, Research Triangle Park, NC 27709. 1-888-825-5249. Corporate Web Site: www.gsk.com

Zofran Tabs/ODT/O.S.—Cont.

INDICATIONS AND USAGE

1. Prevention of nausea and vomiting associated with highly emetogenic cancer chemotherapy, including cisplatin ≥50 mg/m².
2. Prevention of nausea and vomiting associated with initial and repeat courses of moderately emetogenic cancer chemotherapy.
3. Prevention of nausea and vomiting associated with radiotherapy in patients receiving either total body irradiation, single high-dose fraction to the abdomen, or daily fractions to the abdomen.
4. Prevention of postoperative nausea and/or vomiting. As with other antiemetics, routine prophylaxis is not recommended for patients in whom there is little expectation that nausea and/or vomiting will occur postoperatively. In patients where nausea and/or vomiting must be avoided postoperatively, ZOFRAN Tablets, ZOFRAN ODT Orally Disintegrating Tablets, and ZOFRAN Oral Solution are recommended even where the incidence of postoperative nausea and/or vomiting is low.

CONTRAINDICATIONS

ZOFRAN Tablets, ZOFRAN ODT Orally Disintegrating Tablets, and ZOFRAN Oral Solution are contraindicated for patients known to have hypersensitivity to the drug.

WARNINGS

Hypersensitivity reactions have been reported in patients who have exhibited hypersensitivity to other selective 5-HT$_3$ receptor antagonists.

PRECAUTIONS

Ondansetron is not a drug that stimulates gastric or intestinal peristalsis. It should not be used instead of nasogastric suction. The use of ondansetron in patients following abdominal surgery or in patients with chemotherapy-induced nausea and vomiting may mask a progressive ileus and/or gastric distension.

Information for Patients: ***Phenylketonurics:*** Phenylketonuric patients should be informed that ZOFRAN ODT Orally Disintegrating Tablets contain phenylalanine (a component of aspartame). Each 4-mg and 8-mg orally disintegrating tablet contains <0.03 mg phenylalanine.

Patients should be instructed not to remove ZOFRAN ODT Tablets from the blister until just prior to dosing. The tablet should not be pushed through the foil. With dry hands, the blister backing should be peeled completely off the blister. The tablet should be gently removed and immediately placed on the tongue to dissolve and be swallowed with the saliva. Peelable illustrated stickers are affixed to the product carton that can be provided with the prescription to ensure proper use and handling of the product.

Drug Interactions: Ondansetron does not itself appear to induce or inhibit the cytochrome P-450 drug-metabolizing enzyme system of the liver (see CLINICAL PHARMACOLOGY, Pharmacokinetics). Because ondansetron is metabolized by hepatic cytochrome P-450 drug-metabolizing enzymes (CYP3A4, CYP2D6, CYP1A2), inducers or inhibitors of these enzymes may change the clearance and, hence, the half-life of ondansetron. On the basis of available data, no dosage adjustment is recommended for patients on these drugs.

Phenytoin, Carbamazepine, and Rifampicin: In patients treated with potent inducers of CYP3A4 (i.e., phenytoin, carbamazepine, and rifampicin), the clearance of ondansetron was significantly increased and ondansetron blood concentrations were decreased. However, on the basis of available data, no dosage adjustment for ondansetron is recommended for patients on these drugs.[1,3]

Tramadol: Although no pharmacokinetic drug interaction between ondansetron and tramadol has been observed, data from 2 small studies indicate that ondansetron may be associated with an increase in patient controlled administration of tramadol.[4,5]

Chemotherapy: Tumor response to chemotherapy in the P-388 mouse leukemia model is not affected by ondansetron. In humans, carmustine, etoposide, and cisplatin do not affect the pharmacokinetics of ondansetron.

In a crossover study in 76 pediatric patients, I.V. ondansetron did not increase blood levels of high-dose methotrexate.

Use in Surgical Patients: The coadministration of ondansetron had no effect on the pharmacokinetics and pharmacodynamics of temazepam.

Carcinogenesis, Mutagenesis, Impairment of Fertility: Carcinogenic effects were not seen in 2-year studies in rats and mice with oral ondansetron doses up to 10 and 30 mg/kg/day, respectively. Ondansetron was not mutagenic in standard tests for mutagenicity. Oral administration of ondansetron up to 15 mg/kg/day did not affect fertility or general reproductive performance of male and female rats.

Pregnancy: ***Teratogenic Effects:*** Pregnancy Category B. Reproduction studies have been performed in pregnant rats and rabbits at daily oral doses up to 15 and 30 mg/kg/day, respectively, and have revealed no evidence of impaired fertility or harm to the fetus due to ondansetron. There are, however, no adequate and well-controlled studies in pregnant women. Because animal reproduction studies are not always predictive of human response, this drug should be used during pregnancy only if clearly needed.

Nursing Mothers: Ondansetron is excreted in the breast milk of rats. It is not known whether ondansetron is excreted in human milk. Because many drugs are excreted in human milk, caution should be exercised when ondansetron is administered to a nursing woman.

Table 5. Principal Adverse Events in US Trials: Single Day Therapy With 24-mg ZOFRAN Tablets (Highly Emetogenic Chemotherapy)

Event	Ondansetron 24 mg q.d. n = 300	Ondansetron 8 mg b.i.d. n = 124	Ondansetron 32 mg q.d. n = 117
Headache	33 (11%)	16 (13%)	17 (15%)
Diarrhea	13 (4%)	9 (7%)	3 (3%)

Table 6. Principal Adverse Events in US Trials: 3 Days of Therapy With 8 mg ZOFRAN Tablets (Moderately Emetogenic Chemotherapy)

Event	Ondansetron 8 mg b.i.d. n = 242	Ondansetron 8 mg t.i.d. n = 415	Placebo n = 262
Headache	58 (24%)	113 (27%)	34 (13%)
Malaise/fatigue	32 (13%)	37 (9%)	6 (2%)
Constipation	22 (9%)	26 (6%)	1 (<1%)
Diarrhea	15 (6%)	16 (4%)	10 (4%)
Dizziness	13 (5%)	18 (4%)	12 (5%)

Table 7. Frequency of Adverse Events From Controlled Studies With ZOFRAN Tablets (Postoperative Nausea and Vomiting)

Adverse Event	Ondansetron 16 mg (n = 550)	Placebo (n = 531)
Wound problem	152 (28%)	162 (31%)
Drowsiness/sedation	112 (20%)	122 (23%)
Headache	49 (9%)	27 (5%)
Hypoxia	49 (9%)	35 (7%)
Pyrexia	45 (8%)	34 (6%)
Dizziness	36 (7%)	34 (6%)
Gynecological disorder	36 (7%)	33 (6%)
Anxiety/agitation	33 (6%)	29 (5%)
Bradycardia	32 (6%)	30 (6%)
Shiver(s)	28 (5%)	30 (6%)
Urinary retention	28 (5%)	18 (3%)
Hypotension	27 (5%)	32 (6%)
Pruritus	27 (5%)	20 (4%)

Pediatric Use: Little information is available about dosage in pediatric patients 4 years of age or younger (see CLINICAL PHARMACOLOGY and DOSAGE AND ADMINISTRATION sections for use in pediatric patients 4 to 18 years of age).

Geriatric Use: Of the total number of subjects enrolled in cancer chemotherapy-induced and postoperative nausea and vomiting in US- and foreign-controlled clinical trials, for which there were subgroup analyses, 938 were 65 years of age and over. No overall differences in safety or effectiveness were observed between these subjects and younger subjects, and other reported clinical experience has not identified differences in responses between the elderly and younger patients, but greater sensitivity of some older individuals cannot be ruled out. Dosage adjustment is not needed in patients over the age of 65 (see CLINICAL PHARMACOLOGY).

ADVERSE REACTIONS

The following have been reported as adverse events in clinical trials of patients treated with ondansetron, the active ingredient of ZOFRAN. A causal relationship to therapy with ZOFRAN has been unclear in many cases.

Chemotherapy-Induced Nausea and Vomiting: The adverse events in Table 5 have been reported in ≥5% of adult patients receiving a single 24-mg ZOFRAN Tablet in 2 trials. These patients were receiving concurrent highly emetogenic cisplatin-based chemotherapy regimens (cisplatin dose ≥50 mg/m²).

[See table 5 above]

The adverse events in Table 6 have been reported in ≥5% of adults receiving either 8 mg of ZOFRAN Tablets 2 or 3 times a day for 3 days or placebo in 4 trials. These patients were receiving concurrent moderately emetogenic chemotherapy, primarily cyclophosphamide-based regimens.

[See table 6 above]

Central Nervous System: There have been rare reports consistent with, but not diagnostic of, extrapyramidal reactions in patients receiving ondansetron.

Hepatic: In 723 patients receiving cyclophosphamide-based chemotherapy in US clinical trials, AST and/or ALT values have been reported to exceed twice the upper limit of normal in approximately 1% to 2% of patients receiving ZOFRAN Tablets. The increases were transient and did not appear to be related to dose or duration of therapy. On repeat exposure, similar transient elevations in transaminase values occurred in some courses, but symptomatic hepatic disease did not occur. The role of cancer chemotherapy in these biochemical changes cannot be clearly determined.

There have been reports of liver failure and death in patients with cancer receiving concurrent medications including potentially hepatotoxic cytotoxic chemotherapy and antibiotics. The etiology of the liver failure is unclear.

Integumentary: Rash has occurred in approximately 1% of patients receiving ondansetron.

Other: Rare cases of anaphylaxis, bronchospasm, tachycardia, angina (chest pain), hypokalemia, electrocardiographic alterations, vascular occlusive events, and grand mal seizures have been reported. Except for bronchospasm and anaphylaxis, the relationship to ZOFRAN was unclear.

Radiation-Induced Nausea and Vomiting: The adverse events reported in patients receiving ZOFRAN Tablets and concurrent radiotherapy were similar to those reported in patients receiving ZOFRAN Tablets and concurrent chemotherapy. The most frequently reported adverse events were headache, constipation, and diarrhea.

Postoperative Nausea and Vomiting: The adverse events in Table 7 have been reported in ≥5% of patients receiving ZOFRAN Tablets at a dosage of 16 mg orally in clinical trials. With the exception of headache, rates of these events were not significantly different in the ondansetron and placebo groups. These patients were receiving multiple concomitant perioperative and postoperative medications.

[See table 7 above]

Preliminary observations in a small number of subjects suggest a higher incidence of headache when ZOFRAN ODT Orally Disintegrating Tablets are taken with water, when compared to without water.

Observed During Clinical Practice: In addition to adverse events reported from clinical trials, the following events have been identified during post-approval use of oral formulations of ZOFRAN. Because they are reported voluntarily from a population of unknown size, estimates of frequency cannot be made. The events have been chosen for inclusion due to a combination of their seriousness, frequency of reporting, or potential causal connection to ZOFRAN.

General: Flushing. Rare cases of hypersensitivity reactions, sometimes severe (e.g., anaphylaxis/anaphylactoid reactions, angioedema, bronchospasm, shortness of breath, hypotension, laryngeal edema, stridor) have also been reported. Laryngospasm, shock, and cardiopulmonary arrest have occurred during allergic reactions in patients receiving injectable ondansetron.

Hepatobiliary: Liver enzyme abnormalities

Lower Respiratory: Hiccups

Neurology: Oculogyric crisis, appearing alone, as well as with other dystonic reactions

Skin: Urticaria

DRUG ABUSE AND DEPENDENCE

Animal studies have shown that ondansetron is not discriminated as a benzodiazepine nor does it substitute for benzodiazepines in direct addiction studies.

OVERDOSAGE

There is no specific antidote for ondansetron overdose. Patients should be managed with appropriate supportive therapy. Individual intravenous doses as large as 150 mg and total daily intravenous doses as large as 252 mg have been inadvertently administered without significant adverse events. These doses are more than 10 times the recommended daily dose.

In addition to the adverse events listed above, the following events have been described in the setting of ondansetron overdose: "Sudden blindness" (amaurosis) of 2 to 3 minutes' duration plus severe constipation occurred in 1 patient that was administered 72 mg of ondansetron intravenously as a single dose. Hypotension (and faintness) occurred in a patient that took 48 mg of ZOFRAN Tablets. Following infusion of 32 mg over only a 4-minute period, a vasovagal episode with transient second-degree heart block was observed. In all instances, the events resolved completely.

DOSAGE AND ADMINISTRATION

Instructions for Use/Handling ZOFRAN ODT Orally Disintegrating Tablets: Do not attempt to push ZOFRAN ODT Tablets through the foil backing. With dry hands, PEEL BACK the foil backing of 1 blister and GENTLY remove the tablet. IMMEDIATELY place the ZOFRAN ODT Tablet on top of the tongue where it will dissolve in seconds, then swallow with saliva. Administration with liquid is not necessary.

Prevention of Nausea and Vomiting Associated With Highly Emetogenic Cancer Chemotherapy: The recommended adult oral dosage of ZOFRAN is a single 24-mg tablet administered 30 minutes before the start of single-day highly emetogenic chemotherapy, including cisplatin $\geq$50 mg/m^2. Multiday, single-dose administration of ZOFRAN 24-mg Tablets has not been studied.

Pediatric Use: There is no experience with the use of 24-mg ZOFRAN Tablets in pediatric patients.

Geriatric Use: The dosage recommendation is the same as for the general population.

Prevention of Nausea and Vomiting Associated With Moderately Emetogenic Cancer Chemotherapy: The recommended adult oral dosage is one 8-mg ZOFRAN Tablet or one 8-mg ZOFRAN ODT Tablet or 10 mL (2 teaspoonfuls equivalent to 8 mg of ondansetron) of ZOFRAN Oral Solution given twice a day. The first dose should be administered 30 minutes before the start of emetogenic chemotherapy, with a subsequent dose 8 hours after the first dose. One 8-mg ZOFRAN Tablet or one 8-mg ZOFRAN ODT Tablet or 10 mL (2 teaspoonfuls equivalent to 8 mg of ondansetron) of ZOFRAN Oral Solution should be administered twice a day (every 12 hours) for 1 to 2 days after completion of chemotherapy.

Pediatric Use: For pediatric patients 12 years of age and older, the dosage is the same as for adults. For pediatric patients 4 through 11 years of age, the dosage is one 4-mg ZOFRAN Tablet or one 4-mg ZOFRAN ODT Tablet or 5 mL (1 teaspoonful equivalent to 4 mg of ondansetron) of ZOFRAN Oral Solution given 3 times a day. The first dose should be administered 30 minutes before the start of emetogenic chemotherapy, with subsequent doses 4 and 8 hours after the first dose. One 4-mg ZOFRAN Tablet or one 4-mg ZOFRAN ODT Tablet or 5 mL (1 teaspoonful equivalent to 4 mg of ondansetron) of ZOFRAN Oral Solution should be administered 3 times a day (every 8 hours) for 1 to 2 days after completion of chemotherapy.

Geriatric Use: The dosage is the same as for the general population.

Prevention of Nausea and Vomiting Associated With Radiotherapy, Either Total Body Irradiation, or Single High-Dose Fraction or Daily Fractions to the Abdomen:

The recommended oral dosage is one 8-mg ZOFRAN Tablet or one 8-mg ZOFRAN ODT Tablet or 10 mL (2 teaspoonfuls equivalent to 8 mg of ondansetron) of ZOFRAN Oral Solution given 3 times a day.

For total body irradiation, one 8-mg ZOFRAN Tablet or one 8-mg ZOFRAN ODT Tablet or 10 mL (2 teaspoonfuls equivalent to 8 mg of ondansetron) of ZOFRAN Oral Solution should be administered 1 to 2 hours before each fraction of radiotherapy administered each day.

For single high-dose fraction radiotherapy to the abdomen, one 8-mg ZOFRAN Tablet or one 8-mg ZOFRAN ODT Tablet or 10 mL (2 teaspoonfuls equivalent to 8 mg of ondansetron) of ZOFRAN Oral Solution should be administered 1 to 2 hours before radiotherapy, with subsequent doses every 8 hours after the first dose for 1 to 2 days after completion of radiotherapy.

For daily fractionated radiotherapy to the abdomen, one 8-mg ZOFRAN Tablet or one 8-mg ZOFRAN ODT Tablet or 10 mL (2 teaspoonfuls equivalent to 8 mg of ondansetron) of ZOFRAN Oral Solution should be administered 1 to 2 hours before radiotherapy, with subsequent doses every 8 hours after the first dose for each day radiotherapy is given.

Pediatric Use: There is no experience with the use of ZOFRAN Tablets, ZOFRAN ODT Tablets, or ZOFRAN Oral Solution in the prevention of radiation-induced nausea and vomiting in pediatric patients.

Geriatric Use: The dosage recommendation is the same as for the general population.

Postoperative Nausea and Vomiting: The recommended dosage is 16 mg given as two 8-mg ZOFRAN Tablets or two 8-mg ZOFRAN ODT Tablets or 20 mL (4 teaspoonfuls equivalent to 16 mg of ondansetron) of ZOFRAN Oral Solution 1 hour before induction of anesthesia.

Pediatric Use: There is no experience with the use of ZOFRAN Tablets, ZOFRAN ODT Tablets, or ZOFRAN Oral Solution in the prevention of postoperative nausea and vomiting in pediatric patients.

Geriatric Use: The dosage is the same as for the general population.

Dosage Adjustment for Patients With Impaired Renal Function: The dosage recommendation is the same as for the general population. There is no experience beyond first-day administration of ondansetron.

Dosage Adjustment for Patients With Impaired Hepatic Function: In patients with severe hepatic impairment (Child-Pugh[2] score of 10 or greater), clearance is reduced and apparent volume of distribution is increased with a resultant increase in plasma half-life. In such patients, a total daily dose of 8 mg should not be exceeded.

HOW SUPPLIED

ZOFRAN Tablets, 4 mg (ondansetron HCl dihydrate equivalent to 4 mg of ondansetron), are white, oval, film-coated tablets engraved with "Zofran" on one side and "4" on the other in daily unit dose packs of 3 tablets (NDC 0173-0446-04), bottles of 30 tablets (NDC 0173-0446-00), and unit dose packs of 100 tablets (NDC 0173-0446-02).

ZOFRAN Tablets, 8 mg (ondansetron HCl dihydrate equivalent to 8 mg of ondansetron), are yellow, oval, film-coated tablets engraved with "Zofran" on one side and "8" on the other in daily unit dose packs of 3 tablets (NDC 0173-0447-04), bottles of 30 tablets (NDC 0173-0447-00), and unit dose packs of 100 tablets (NDC 0173-0447-02).

Bottles: Store between 2° and 30°C (36° and 86°F). Protect from light. Dispense in tight, light-resistant container as defined in the USP.

Unit Dose Packs: Store between 2° and 30°C (36° and 86°F). Protect from light. Store blisters in cartons.

ZOFRAN Tablets, 24 mg (ondansetron HCl dihydrate equivalent to 24 mg of ondansetron), are pink, oval, film-coated tablets engraved with "GX CF7" on one side and "24" on the other in daily unit dose packs of 1 tablet (NDC 0173-0680-00).

Store between 2° and 30°C (36° and 86°F).

ZOFRAN ODT Orally Disintegrating Tablets, 4 mg (as 4 mg ondansetron base) are white, round and plano-convex tablets debossed with a "Z4" on one side in unit dose packs of 30 tablets (NDC 0173-0569-00).

ZOFRAN ODT Orally Disintegrating Tablets, 8 mg (as 8 mg ondansetron base) are white, round and plano-convex tablets debossed with a "Z8" on one side in unit dose packs of 10 tablets (NDC 0173-0570-04) and 30 tablets (NDC 0173-0570-00).

Store between 2° and 30°C (36° and 86°F).

ZOFRAN Oral Solution, a clear, colorless to light yellow liquid with a characteristic strawberry odor, contains 5 mg of ondansetron HCl dihydrate equivalent to 4 mg of ondansetron per 5 mL in amber glass bottles of 50 mL with child-resistant closures (NDC 0173-0489-00).

Store upright between 15° and 30°C (59° and 86°F). Protect from light. Store bottles upright in cartons.

REFERENCES

1. Britto MR, Hussey EK, Mydlow P, et al. Effect of enzyme inducers on ondansetron (OND) metabolism in humans. *Clin Pharmacol Ther* 1997;61:228.
2. Pugh RNH, Murray-Lyon IM, Dawson JL, Pietroni MC, Williams R. Transection of the oesophagus for bleeding oesophageal varices. *Brit J Surg* 1973;60:646-649.
3. Villikka K, Kivisto KT, Neuvonen PJ. The effect of rifampin on the pharmacokinetics of oral and intravenous ondansetron. *Clin Pharmacol Ther* 1999;65:377-381.
4. De Witte JL, Schoenmaekers B, Sessler DI, et al. *Anesth Analg* 2001;92:1319-1321.
5. Arcioni R, della Rocca M, Romanò R, et al. *Anesth Analg* 2002;94:1553-1557.

ZOFRAN Tablets and Oral Solution:
GlaxoSmithKline, Research Triangle Park, NC 27709
ZOFRAN ODT Orally Disintegrating Tablets:
Manufactured for GlaxoSmithKline
Research Triangle Park, NC 27709
by Cardinal Health
Blagrove, Swindon, Wiltshire, UK SN5 8RU

May 2004/RL-2082

Shown in Product Identification Guide, page 318

ZOVIRAX® ℞
[zō-vī′rax]
(acyclovir)
Capsules

ZOVIRAX® ℞
(acyclovir)
Tablets

ZOVIRAX® ℞
(acyclovir)
Suspension

DESCRIPTION

ZOVIRAX is the brand name for acyclovir, a synthetic nucleoside analogue active against herpesviruses. ZOVIRAX Capsules, Tablets, and Suspension are formulations for oral administration. Each capsule of ZOVIRAX contains 200 mg of acyclovir and the inactive ingredients corn starch, lactose, magnesium stearate, and sodium lauryl sulfate. The capsule shell consists of gelatin, FD&C Blue No. 2, and titanium dioxide. May contain one or more parabens. Printed with edible black ink.

Each 800-mg tablet of ZOVIRAX contains 800 mg of acyclovir and the inactive ingredients FD&C Blue No. 2, magnesium stearate, microcrystalline cellulose, povidone, and sodium starch glycolate.

Each 400-mg tablet of ZOVIRAX contains 400 mg of acyclovir and the inactive ingredients magnesium stearate, microcrystalline cellulose, povidone, and sodium starch glycolate.

Each teaspoonful (5 mL) of ZOVIRAX Suspension contains 200 mg of acyclovir and the inactive ingredients methylparaben 0.1% and propylparaben 0.02% (added as preservatives), carboxymethylcellulose sodium, flavor, glycerin, microcrystalline cellulose, and sorbitol.

Acyclovir is a white, crystalline powder with the molecular formula $C_8H_{11}N_5O_3$ and a molecular weight of 225. The maximum solubility in water at 37°C is 2.5 mg/mL. The pka's of acyclovir are 2.27 and 9.25.

The chemical name of acyclovir is 2-amino-1,9-dihydro-9-[(2-hydroxyethoxy)methyl]-6*H*-purin-6-one.

VIROLOGY

Mechanism of Antiviral Action: Acyclovir is a synthetic purine nucleoside analogue with in vitro and in vivo inhibitory activity against herpes simplex virus types 1 (HSV-1), 2 (HSV-2), and varicella-zoster virus (VZV). The inhibitory activity of acyclovir is highly selective due to its affinity for the enzyme thymidine kinase (TK) encoded by HSV and VZV. This viral enzyme converts acyclovir into acyclovir monophosphate, a nucleotide analogue. The monophosphate is further converted into diphosphate by cellular guanylate kinase and into triphosphate by a number of cellular enzymes. In vitro, acyclovir triphosphate stops replication of herpes viral DNA. This is accomplished in 3 ways: 1) competitive inhibition of viral DNA polymerase, 2) incorporation into and termination of the growing viral DNA chain, and 3) inactivation of the viral DNA polymerase. The greater antiviral activity of acyclovir against HSV compared to VZV is due to its more efficient phosphorylation by the viral TK.

Antiviral Activities: The quantitative relationship between the in vitro susceptibility of herpes viruses to antivirals and the clinical response to therapy has not been established in humans, and virus sensitivity testing has not been standardized. Sensitivity testing results, expressed as the concentration of drug required to inhibit by 50% the growth of virus in cell culture (IC_{50}), vary greatly depending upon a number of factors. Using plaque-reduction assays, the IC_{50} against herpes simplex virus isolates ranges from 0.02 to 13.5 mcg/mL for HSV-1 and from 0.01 to 9.9 mcg/mL for HSV-2. The IC_{50} for acyclovir against most laboratory strains and clinical isolates of VZV ranges from 0.12 to 10.8 mcg/mL. Acyclovir also demonstrates activity against the Oka vaccine strain of VZV with a mean IC_{50} of 1.35 mcg/mL.

Drug Resistance: Resistance of HSV and VZV to acyclovir can result from qualitative and quantitative changes in the viral TK and/or DNA polymerase. Clinical isolates of HSV and VZV with reduced susceptibility to acyclovir have been recovered from immunocompromised patients, especially with advanced HIV infection. While most of the acyclovir-resistant mutants isolated thus far from immunocompromised patients have been found to be TK-deficient mutants, other mutants involving the viral TK gene (TK partial and TK altered) and DNA polymerase have been isolated. TK-negative mutants may cause severe disease in infants and immunocompromised adults. The possibility of viral resistance to acyclovir should be considered in patients who show poor clinical response during therapy.

CLINICAL PHARMACOLOGY

Pharmacokinetics: The pharmacokinetics of acyclovir after oral administration have been evaluated in healthy volunteers and in immunocompromised patients with herpes simplex or varicella-zoster virus infection. Acyclovir pharmacokinetic parameters are summarized in Table 1.

Continued on next page

Product information on these pages is effective as of August 2004. Further information is available at: GlaxoSmithKline, PO Box 13398, Research Triangle Park, NC 27709. 1-888-825-5249. Corporate Web Site: www.gsk.com

Zovirax Caps/Tabs/Susp.—Cont.

Table 1. Acyclovir Pharmacokinetic Characteristics (Range)

Parameter	Range
Plasma protein binding	9% to 33%
Plasma elimination half-life	2.5 to 3.3 hr
Average oral bioavailability	10% to 20%*

*Bioavailability decreases with increasing dose.

In one multiple-dose, crossover study in healthy subjects (n = 23), it was shown that increases in plasma acyclovir concentrations were less than dose proportional with increasing dose, as shown in Table 2. The decrease in bioavailability is a function of the dose and not the dosage form.

Table 2. Acyclovir Peak and Trough Concentrations at Steady State

Parameter	200 mg	400 mg	800 mg
C^{SS}_{max}	0.83 mcg/mL	1.21 mcg/mL	1.61 mcg/mL
C^{SS}_{trough}	0.46 mcg/mL	0.63 mcg/mL	0.83 mcg/mL

There was no effect of food on the absorption of acyclovir (n = 6); therefore, ZOVIRAX Capsules, Tablets, and Suspension may be administered with or without food.

The only known urinary metabolite is 9-[(carboxymethoxy)methyl]guanine.

Special Populations: ***Adults with Impaired Renal Function:*** The half-life and total body clearance of acyclovir are dependent on renal function. A dosage adjustment is recommended for patients with reduced renal function (see DOSAGE AND ADMINISTRATION).

Geriatrics: Acyclovir plasma concentrations are higher in geriatric patients compared to younger adults, in part due to age-related changes in renal function. Dosage reduction may be required in geriatric patients with underlying renal impairment (see PRECAUTIONS: Geriatric Use).

Pediatrics: In general, the pharmacokinetics of acyclovir in pediatric patients is similar to that of adults. Mean half-life after oral doses of 300 mg/m^2 and 600 mg/m^2 in pediatric patients aged 7 months to 7 years was 2.6 hours (range 1.59 to 3.74 hours).

Drug Interactions: Coadministration of probenecid with intravenous acyclovir has been shown to increase the mean acyclovir half-life and the area under the concentration-time curve. Urinary excretion and renal clearance were correspondingly reduced.

Clinical Trials: ***Initial Genital Herpes:*** Double-blind, placebo-controlled studies have demonstrated that orally administered ZOVIRAX significantly reduced the duration of acute infection and duration of lesion healing. The duration of pain and new lesion formation was decreased in some patient groups.

Recurrent Genital Herpes: Double-blind, placebo-controlled studies in patients with frequent recurrences (6 or more episodes per year) have shown that orally administered ZOVIRAX given daily for 4 months to 10 years prevented or reduced the frequency and/or severity of recurrences in greater than 95% of patients.

In a study of patients who received ZOVIRAX 400 mg twice daily for 3 years, 45%, 52%, and 63% of patients remained free of recurrences in the first, second, and third years, respectively. Serial analyses of the 3-month recurrence rates for the patients showed that 71% to 87% were recurrence free in each quarter.

Herpes Zoster Infections: In a double-blind, placebo-controlled study of immunocompetent patients with localized cutaneous zoster infection, ZOVIRAX (800 mg 5 times daily for 10 days) shortened the times to lesion scabbing, healing, and complete cessation of pain, and reduced the duration of viral shedding and the duration of new lesion formation.

In a similar double-blind, placebo-controlled study, ZOVIRAX (800 mg 5 times daily for 7 days) shortened the times to complete lesion scabbing, healing, and cessation of pain; reduced the duration of new lesion formation; and reduced the prevalence of localized zoster-associated neurologic symptoms (paresthesia, dysesthesia, or hyperesthesia).

Treatment was begun within 72 hours of rash onset and was most effective if started within the first 48 hours.

Adults greater than 50 years of age showed greater benefit.

Chickenpox: Three randomized, double-blind, placebo-controlled trials were conducted in 993 pediatric patients aged 2 to 18 years with chickenpox. All patients were treated within 24 hours after the onset of rash. In 2 trials, ZOVIRAX was administered at 20 mg/kg 4 times daily (up to 3,200 mg per day) for 5 days. In the third trial, doses of 10, 15, or 20 mg/kg were administered 4 times daily for 5 to 7 days. Treatment with ZOVIRAX shortened the time to 50% healing; reduced the maximum number of lesions; reduced the median number of vesicles; decreased the median number of residual lesions on day 28; and decreased the proportion of patients with fever, anorexia, and lethargy by day 2. Treatment with ZOVIRAX did not affect varicella-zoster virus-specific humoral or cellular immune responses at 1 month or 1 year following treatment.

INDICATIONS AND USAGE

Herpes Zoster Infections: ZOVIRAX is indicated for the acute treatment of herpes zoster (shingles).

Genital Herpes: ZOVIRAX is indicated for the treatment of initial episodes and the management of recurrent episodes of genital herpes.

Chickenpox: ZOVIRAX is indicated for the treatment of chickenpox (varicella).

CONTRAINDICATIONS

ZOVIRAX is contraindicated for patients who develop hypersensitivity to acyclovir or valacyclovir.

WARNINGS

ZOVIRAX Capsules, Tablets, and Suspension are intended for oral ingestion only. Renal failure, in some cases resulting in death, has been observed with acyclovir therapy (see ADVERSE REACTIONS: Observed During Clinical Practice and OVERDOSAGE). Thrombotic thrombocytopenic purpura/hemolytic uremic syndrome (TTP/HUS), which has resulted in death, has occurred in immunocompromised patients receiving acyclovir therapy.

PRECAUTIONS

Dosage adjustment is recommended when administering ZOVIRAX to patients with renal impairment (see DOSAGE AND ADMINISTRATION). Caution should also be exercised when administering ZOVIRAX to patients receiving potentially nephrotoxic agents since this may increase the risk of renal dysfunction and/or the risk of reversible central nervous system symptoms such as those that have been reported in patients treated with intravenous acyclovir.

Information for Patients: Patients are instructed to consult with their physician if they experience severe or troublesome adverse reactions, they become pregnant or intend to become pregnant, they intend to breastfeed while taking orally administered ZOVIRAX, or they have any other questions.

Herpes Zoster: There are no data on treatment initiated more than 72 hours after onset of the zoster rash. Patients should be advised to initiate treatment as soon as possible after a diagnosis of herpes zoster.

Genital Herpes Infections: Patients should be informed that ZOVIRAX is not a cure for genital herpes. There are no data evaluating whether ZOVIRAX will prevent transmission of infection to others. Because genital herpes is a sexually transmitted disease, patients should avoid contact with lesions or intercourse when lesions and/or symptoms are present to avoid infecting partners. Genital herpes can also be transmitted in the absence of symptoms through asymptomatic viral shedding. If medical management of a genital herpes recurrence is indicated, patients should be advised to initiate therapy at the first sign or symptom of an episode.

Chickenpox: Chickenpox in otherwise healthy children is usually a self-limited disease of mild to moderate severity. Adolescents and adults tend to have more severe disease. Treatment was initiated within 24 hours of the typical chickenpox rash in the controlled studies, and there is no information regarding the effects of treatment begun later in the disease course.

Drug Interactions: See CLINICAL PHARMACOLOGY: Pharmacokinetics.

Carcinogenesis, Mutagenesis, Impairment of Fertility: The data presented below include references to peak steady-state plasma acyclovir concentrations observed in humans treated with 800 mg given orally 5 times a day (dosing appropriate for treatment of herpes zoster) or 200 mg given orally 5 times a day (dosing appropriate for treatment of genital herpes). Plasma drug concentrations in animal studies are expressed as multiples of human exposure to acyclovir at the higher and lower dosing schedules (see CLINICAL PHARMACOLOGY: Pharmacokinetics).

Acyclovir was tested in lifetime bioassays in rats and mice at single daily doses of up to 450 mg/kg administered by gavage. There was no statistically significant difference in the incidence of tumors between treated and control animals, nor did acyclovir shorten the latency of tumors. Maximum plasma concentrations were 3 to 6 times human levels in the mouse bioassay and 1 to 2 times human levels in the rat bioassay.

Acyclovir was tested in 16 in vitro and in vivo genetic toxicity assays. Acyclovir was positive in 5 of the assays.

Acyclovir did not impair fertility or reproduction in mice (450 mg/kg/day, p.o.) or in rats (25 mg/kg/day, s.c.). In the mouse study, plasma levels were 9 to 18 times human levels, while in the rat study, they were 8 to 15 times human levels. At higher doses (50 mg/kg/day, s.c.) in rats and rabbits (11 to 22 and 16 to 31 times human levels, respectively) implantation efficacy, but not litter size, was decreased. In a rat peri- and post-natal study at 50 mg/kg/day, s.c., there was a statistically significant decrease in group mean numbers of corpora lutea, total implantation sites, and live fetuses.

No testicular abnormalities were seen in dogs given 50 mg/kg/day, IV for 1 month (21 to 41 times human levels) or in dogs given 60 mg/kg/day orally for 1 year (6 to 12 times human levels). Testicular atrophy and aspermatogenesis were observed in rats and dogs at higher dose levels.

Pregnancy: ***Teratogenic Effects:*** Pregnancy Category B. Acyclovir administered during organogenesis was not teratogenic in the mouse (450 mg/kg/day, p.o.), rabbit (50 mg/kg/day, s.c. and IV), or rat (50 mg/kg/day, s.c.). These exposures resulted in plasma levels 9 and 18, 16 and 106, and 11 and 22 times, respectively, human levels.

There are no adequate and well-controlled studies in pregnant women. A prospective epidemiologic registry of acyclovir use during pregnancy was established in 1984 and completed in April 1999. There were 749 pregnancies followed in women exposed to systemic acyclovir during the first trimester of pregnancy resulting in 756 outcomes. The occurrence rate of birth defects approximates that found in the general population. However, the small size of the registry is insufficient to evaluate the risk for less common defects or to permit reliable or definitive conclusions regarding the safety of acyclovir in pregnant women and their developing fetuses. Acyclovir should be used during pregnancy only if the potential benefit justifies the potential risk to the fetus.

Nursing Mothers: Acyclovir concentrations have been documented in breast milk in 2 women following oral administration of ZOVIRAX and ranged from 0.6 to 4.1 times corresponding plasma levels. These concentrations would potentially expose the nursing infant to a dose of acyclovir up to 0.3 mg/kg/day. ZOVIRAX should be administered to a nursing mother with caution and only when indicated.

Pediatric Use: Safety and effectiveness of oral formulations of acyclovir in pediatric patients younger than 2 years of age have not been established.

Geriatric Use: Of 376 subjects who received ZOVIRAX in a clinical study of herpes zoster treatment in immunocompetent subjects ≥50 years of age, 244 were 65 and over while 111 were 75 and over. No overall differences in effectiveness for time to cessation of new lesion formation or time to healing were reported between geriatric subjects and younger adult subjects. The duration of pain after healing was longer in patients 65 and over. Nausea, vomiting, and dizziness were reported more frequently in elderly subjects. Elderly patients are more likely to have reduced renal function and require dose reduction. Elderly patients are also more likely to have renal or CNS adverse events. With respect to CNS adverse events observed during clinical practice, somnolence, hallucinations, confusion, and coma were reported more frequently in elderly patients (see CLINICAL PHARMACOLOGY, ADVERSE REACTIONS: Observed During Clinical Practice, and DOSAGE AND ADMINISTRATION).

ADVERSE REACTIONS

Herpes Simplex: ***Short-Term Administration:*** The most frequent adverse events reported during clinical trials of treatment of genital herpes with ZOVIRAX 200 mg administered orally 5 times daily every 4 hours for 10 days were nausea and/or vomiting in 8 of 298 patient treatments (2.7%). Nausea and/or vomiting occurred in 2 of 287 (0.7%) patients who received placebo.

Long-Term Administration: The most frequent adverse events reported in a clinical trial for the prevention of recurrences with continuous administration of 400 mg (two 200-mg capsules) 2 times daily for 1 year in 586 patients treated with ZOVIRAX were nausea (4.8%) and diarrhea (2.4%). The 589 control patients receiving intermittent treatment of recurrences with ZOVIRAX for 1 year reported diarrhea (2.7%), nausea (2.4%), and headache (2.2%).

Herpes Zoster: The most frequent adverse event reported during 3 clinical trials of treatment of herpes zoster (shingles) with 800 mg of oral ZOVIRAX 5 times daily for 7 to 10 days in 323 patients was malaise (11.5%). The 323 placebo recipients reported malaise (11.1%).

Chickenpox: The most frequent adverse event reported during 3 clinical trials of treatment of chickenpox with oral ZOVIRAX at doses of 10 to 20 mg/kg 4 times daily for 5 to 7 days or 800 mg 4 times daily for 5 days in 495 patients was diarrhea (3.2%). The 498 patients receiving placebo reported diarrhea (2.2%).

Observed During Clinical Practice: In addition to adverse events reported from clinical trials, the following events have been identified during post-approval use of ZOVIRAX. Because they are reported voluntarily from a population of unknown size, estimates of frequency cannot be made. These events have been chosen for inclusion due to either their seriousness, frequency of reporting, potential causal connection to ZOVIRAX, or a combination of these factors.

General: Anaphylaxis, angioedema, fever, headache, pain, peripheral edema.

Nervous: Aggressive behavior, agitation, ataxia, coma, confusion, decreased consciousness, delirium, dizziness, dysarthria, encephalopathy, hallucinations, paresthesia, psychosis, seizure, somnolence, tremors and dysarthria. These symptoms may be marked, particularly in older adults or in patients with renal impairment (see PRECAUTIONS).

Digestive: Diarrhea, gastrointestinal distress, nausea.

Hematologic and Lymphatic: Anemia, leukocytoclastic vasculitis, leukopenia, lymphadenopathy, thrombocytopenia.

Hepatobiliary Tract and Pancreas: Elevated liver function tests, hepatitis, hyperbilirubinemia, jaundice.

Musculoskeletal: Myalgia.

Skin: Alopecia, erythema multiforme, photosensitive rash, pruritus, rash, Stevens-Johnson syndrome, toxic epidermal necrolysis, urticaria.

Special Senses: Visual abnormalities.

Urogenital: Renal failure, elevated blood urea nitrogen, elevated creatinine, hematuria (see WARNINGS).

Table 3. Dosage Modification for Renal Impairment

Normal Dosage Regimen	Creatinine Clearance (mL/min/1.73 m^2)	Adjusted Dosage Regimen: Dose (mg)	Adjusted Dosage Regimen: Dosing Interval
200 mg every 4 hours	>10 0-10	200 200	every 4 hours, 5x daily every 12 hours
400 mg every 12 hours	>10 0-10	400 200	every 12 hours every 12 hours
800 mg every 4 hours	>25 10-25 0-10	800 800 800	every 4 hours, 5x daily every 8 hours every 12 hours

OVERDOSAGE

Overdoses involving ingestion of up to 100 capsules (20 g) have been reported. Adverse events that have been reported in association with overdosage include agitation, coma, seizures, and lethargy. Precipitation of acyclovir in renal tubules may occur when the solubility (2.5 mg/mL) is exceeded in the intratubular fluid. Overdosage has been reported following bolus injections or inappropriately high doses and in patients whose fluid and electrolyte balance were not properly monitored. This has resulted in elevated BUN and serum creatinine and subsequent renal failure. In the event of acute renal failure and anuria, the patient may benefit from hemodialysis until renal function is restored (see DOSAGE AND ADMINISTRATION).

DOSAGE AND ADMINISTRATION

Acute Treatment of Herpes Zoster: 800 mg every 4 hours orally, 5 times daily for 7 to 10 days.

Genital Herpes: ***Treatment of Initial Genital Herpes:*** 200 mg every 4 hours, 5 times daily for 10 days.

Chronic Suppressive Therapy for Recurrent Disease: 400 mg 2 times daily for up to 12 months, followed by re-evaluation. Alternative regimens have included doses ranging from 200 mg 3 times daily to 200 mg 5 times daily.

The frequency and severity of episodes of untreated genital herpes may change over time. After 1 year of therapy, the frequency and severity of the patient's genital herpes infection should be re-evaluated to assess the need for continuation of therapy with ZOVIRAX.

Intermittent Therapy: 200 mg every 4 hours, 5 times daily for 5 days. Therapy should be initiated at the earliest sign or symptom (prodrome) of recurrence.

Treatment of Chickenpox: *Children (2 years of age and older):* 20 mg/kg **per dose** orally 4 times daily (80 mg/kg/day) for 5 days. Children over 40 kg should receive the adult dose for chickenpox.

Adults and Children over 40 kg: 800 mg 4 times daily for 5 days.

Intravenous ZOVIRAX is indicated for the treatment of varicella-zoster infections in immunocompromised patients.

When therapy is indicated, it should be initiated at the earliest sign or symptom of chickenpox. There is no information about the efficacy of therapy initiated more than 24 hours after onset of signs and symptoms.

Patients With Acute or Chronic Renal Impairment: In patients with renal impairment, the dose of ZOVIRAX Capsules, Tablets, or Suspension should be modified as shown in Table 3:

[See table 3 above]

Hemodialysis: For patients who require hemodialysis, the mean plasma half-life of acyclovir during hemodialysis is approximately 5 hours. This results in a 60% decrease in plasma concentrations following a 6-hour dialysis period. Therefore, the patient's dosing schedule should be adjusted so that an additional dose is administered after each dialysis.

Peritoneal Dialysis: No supplemental dose appears to be necessary after adjustment of the dosing interval.

Bioequivalence of Dosage Forms: ZOVIRAX Suspension was shown to be bioequivalent to ZOVIRAX Capsules (n = 20) and 1 ZOVIRAX 800-mg tablet was shown to be bioequivalent to 4 ZOVIRAX 200-mg capsules (n = 24).

HOW SUPPLIED

ZOVIRAX Capsules (blue, opaque cap and body) containing 200 mg acyclovir and printed with "Wellcome ZOVIRAX 200."

Bottle of 100 (NDC 0173-0991-55).

Unit dose pack of 100 (NDC 0173-0991-56).

Store at 15° to 25°C (59° to 77°F) and protect from moisture.

ZOVIRAX Tablets (light blue, oval) containing 800 mg acyclovir and engraved with "ZOVIRAX 800."

Bottle of 100 (NDC 0173-0945-55).

Store at 15° to 25°C (59° to 77°F) and protect from moisture.

ZOVIRAX Tablets (white, shield-shaped) containing 400 mg acyclovir and engraved with "ZOVIRAX" on one side and a triangle on the other side.

Bottle of 100 (NDC 0173-0949-55).

Store at 15° to 25°C (59° to 77°F) and protect from moisture.

ZOVIRAX Suspension (off-white, banana-flavored) containing 200 mg acyclovir in each teaspoonful (5 mL) – Bottle of 1 pint (473 mL) (NDC 0173-0953-96).

Store at 15° to 25°C (59° to 77°F).

GlaxoSmithKline, Research Triangle Park, NC 27709

November 2003/RL-2049

Shown in Product Identification Guide, page 318

ZOVIRAX® ℞

[zō-vī′rax]

(acyclovir sodium)

for Injection

FOR INTRAVENOUS INFUSION ONLY

DESCRIPTION

ZOVIRAX is the brand name for acyclovir, a synthetic nucleoside analog active against herpesviruses. Acyclovir sodium for injection is a sterile lyophilized powder for intravenous administration only. Each 500-mg vial contains 500 mg of acyclovir and 49 mg of sodium, and each 1,000-mg vial contains 1,000 mg acyclovir and 98 mg of sodium. Reconstitution of the 500-mg or 1,000-mg vials with 10 mL or 20 mL, respectively, of Sterile Water for Injection, USP results in a solution containing 50 mg/mL of acyclovir. The pH of the reconstituted solution is approximately 11. Further dilution in any appropriate intravenous solution must be performed before infusion (see DOSAGE AND ADMINISTRATION: Method of Preparation and Administration).

Acyclovir sodium is a white, crystalline powder with the molecular formula $C_8H_{10}N_5NaO_3$ and a molecular weight of 247.19. The maximum solubility in water at 25°C exceeds 100 mg/mL. At physiologic pH, acyclovir sodium exists as the un-ionized form with a molecular weight of 225 and a maximum solubility in water at 37°C of 2.5 mg/mL. The pka's of acyclovir are 2.27 and 9.25.

The chemical name of acyclovir sodium is 2-amino-1,9-dihydro-9-[(2-hydroxyethoxy)methyl]-6*H*-purin-6-one monosodium salt.

VIROLOGY

Mechanism of Antiviral Action: Acyclovir is a synthetic purine nucleoside analogue with in vitro and in vivo inhibitory activity against herpes simplex virus types 1 (HSV-1), 2 (HSV-2), and varicella-zoster virus (VZV).

The inhibitory activity of acyclovir is highly selective due to its affinity for the enzyme thymidine kinase (TK) encoded by HSV and VZV. This viral enzyme converts acyclovir into acyclovir monophosphate, a nucleotide analogue. The monophosphate is further converted into diphosphate by cellular guanylate kinase and into triphosphate by a number of cellular enzymes. In vitro, acyclovir triphosphate stops replication of herpes viral DNA. This is accomplished in 3 ways: 1) competitive inhibition of viral DNA polymerase, 2) incorporation into and termination of the growing viral DNA chain, and 3) inactivation of the viral DNA polymerase. The greater antiviral activity of acyclovir against HSV compared to VZV is due to its more efficient phosphorylation by the viral TK.

Antiviral Activities: The quantitative relationship between the in vitro susceptibility of herpes viruses to antivirals and the clinical response to therapy has not been established in humans, and virus sensitivity testing has not been standardized. Sensitivity testing results, expressed as the concentration of drug required to inhibit by 50% the growth of virus in cell culture (IC_{50}), vary greatly depending upon a number of factors. Using plaque-reduction assays, the IC_{50} against herpes simplex virus isolates ranges from 0.02 to 13.5 mcg/mL for HSV-1 and from 0.01 to 9.9 mcg/mL for HSV-2. The IC_{50} for acyclovir against most laboratory strains and clinical isolates of VZV ranges from 0.12 to 10.8 mcg/mL. Acyclovir also demonstrates activity against the Oka vaccine strain of VZV with a mean IC_{50} of 1.35 mcg/mL.

Drug Resistance: Resistance of HSV and VZV to acyclovir can result from qualitative and quantitative changes in the viral TK and/or DNA polymerase. Clinical isolates of HSV and VZV with reduced susceptibility to acyclovir have been recovered from immunocompromised patients, especially with advanced HIV infection. While most of the acyclovir-resistant mutants isolated thus far from such patients have been found to be TK-deficient mutants, other mutants involving the viral TK gene (TK partial and TK altered) and DNA polymerase have been isolated. TK-negative mutants may cause severe disease in infants and immunocompromised adults. The possibility of viral resistance to acyclovir should be considered in patients who show poor clinical response during therapy.

CLINICAL PHARMACOLOGY

Pharmacokinetics: The pharmacokinetics of acyclovir after intravenous administration have been evaluated in adult patients with normal renal function during Phase 1/2 studies after single doses ranging from 0.5 to 15 mg/kg and after multiple doses ranging from 2.5 to 15 mg/kg every 8 hours. Proportionality between dose and plasma levels is seen after single doses or at steady state after multiple dosing. Average steady-state peak and trough concentrations from 1-hour infusions administered every 8 hours are given in Table 1.

Table 1. Acyclovir Peak and Trough Concentrations at Steady State

Dosage Regimen	C^{ss}_{max}	C^{ss}_{trough}
5 mg/kg q 8 h (n = 8)	9.8 mcg/mL range: 5.5 to 13.8	0.7 mcg/mL range: 0.2 to 1.0
10 mg/kg q 8 h (n = 7)	22.9 mcg/mL range: 14.1 to 44.1	1.9 mcg/mL range: 0.5 to 2.9

Concentrations achieved in the cerebrospinal fluid are approximately 50% of plasma values. Plasma protein binding is relatively low (9% to 33%) and drug interactions involving binding site displacement are not anticipated.

Renal excretion of unchanged drug is the major route of acyclovir elimination accounting for 62% to 91% of the dose. The only major urinary metabolite detected is 9-carboxymethoxymethylguanine accounting for up to 14.1% of the dose in patients with normal renal function.

The half-life and total body clearance of acyclovir are dependent on renal function as shown in Table 2.

[See table 2 at top of next page]

Special Populations: ***Adults With Impaired Renal Function:*** ZOVIRAX was administered at a dose of 2.5 mg/kg to 6 adult patients with severe renal failure. The peak and trough plasma levels during the 47 hours preceding hemodialysis were 8.5 mcg/mL and 0.7 mcg/mL, respectively.

Consult DOSAGE AND ADMINISTRATION section for recommended adjustments in dosing based upon creatinine clearance.

Pediatrics: Acyclovir pharmacokinetics were determined in 16 pediatric patients with normal renal function ranging in age from 3 months to 16 years at doses of approximately 10 mg/kg and 20 mg/kg every 8 hours (Table 3). Concentrations achieved at these regimens are similar to those in adults receiving 5 mg/kg and 10 mg/kg every 8 hours, respectively (Table 1). Acyclovir pharmacokinetics were determined in 12 patients ranging in age from birth to 3 months at doses of 5 mg/kg, 10 mg/kg, and 15 mg/kg every 8 hours (Table 3).

[See table 3 at top of next page]

Geriatrics: Acyclovir plasma concentrations are higher in geriatric patients compared to younger adults, in part due to age-related changes in renal function. Dosage reduction may be required in geriatric patients with underlying renal impairment (see PRECAUTIONS: Geriatric Use).

Drug Interactions: Coadministration of probenecid with acyclovir has been shown to increase the mean acyclovir half-life and the area under the concentration-time curve. Urinary excretion and renal clearance were correspondingly reduced.

Clinical Trials: ***Herpes Simplex Infections in Immunocompromised Patients:*** A multicenter trial of ZOVIRAX for Injection at a dose of 250 mg/m^2 every 8 hours (750 mg/m^2/day) for 7 days was conducted in 98 immunocompromised patients (73 adults and 25 children) with orofacial, esophageal, genital, and other localized infections (52 treated with ZOVIRAX and 46 with placebo). ZOVIRAX decreased virus excretion, reduced pain, and promoted healing of lesions.

Initial Episodes of Herpes Genitalis: In placebo-controlled trials, 58 patients with initial genital herpes were treated with intravenous ZOVIRAX 5 mg/kg or placebo (27 patients treated with ZOVIRAX and 31 treated with placebo) every 8 hours for 5 days. ZOVIRAX decreased the duration of viral excretion, new lesion formation, duration of vesicles, and promoted healing of lesions.

Herpes Simplex Encephalitis: Sixty-two patients ages 6 months to 79 years with brain biopsy-proven herpes simplex encephalitis were randomized to receive either ZOVIRAX (10 mg/kg every 8 hours) or vidarabine (15 mg/kg/day) for 10 days (28 were treated with ZOVIRAX and 34 with vidarabine). Overall mortality at 12 months for patients treated with ZOVIRAX was 25% compared to 59% for patients treated with vidarabine. The proportion of patients treated with ZOVIRAX functioning normally or with only mild sequelae (e.g., decreased attention span) was 32% compared to 12% of patients treated with vidarabine.

Patients less than 30 years of age and those who had the least severe neurologic involvement at time of entry into

Continued on next page

Product information on these pages is effective as of August 2004. Further information is available at: GlaxoSmithKline, PO Box 13398, Research Triangle Park, NC 27709. 1-888-825-5249. Corporate Web Site: www.gsk.com

Zovirax Injection—Cont.

study had the best outcome with treatment with ZOVIRAX. An additional controlled study performed in Europe demonstrated similar findings.

Neonatal Herpes Simplex Virus Infection: Two hundred and two infants with neonatal herpes simplex infections were randomized to receive either ZOVIRAX 10 mg/kg every 8 hours (n = 107) or vidarabine 30 mg/kg/day (n = 95) for 10 days. Outcomes are presented in Table 4.

Table 4. Mortality at 1 Year

HSV Disease Classification	Treatment Group	
	Acyclovir (n = 107)	Vidarabine (n = 95)
SEM* (n = 85)	0/54	0/31
CNS† (n = 71)	5/35	5/36
DISS‡ (n = 46)	11/18	14/28

*SEM refers to localized infection with disease limited to skin, eye, and/or mouth.
†CNS refers to infection of the central nervous system with compatible neurologic and CSF findings.
‡DISS refers to visceral organ involvement such as hepatitis or pneumonitis with or without CNS involvement.

Rates of neurologic sequelae at 1 year were comparable between the treatment groups.

Varicella-Zoster Infections in Immunocompromised Patients: A multicenter trial of ZOVIRAX for Injection at a dose of 500 mg/m^2 every 8 hours for 7 days was conducted in immunocompromised patients with zoster infections (shingles). Ninety-four (94) patients were evaluated (52 patients were treated with ZOVIRAX and 42 with placebo). ZOVIRAX was superior to placebo as measured by reductions in cutaneous dissemination and visceral dissemination.

Table 2. Acyclovir Half-life and Total Body Clearance

Creatinine Clearance (mL/min per 1.73 m^2)	Half-life (hr)	Total Body Clearance	
		(mL/min per 1.73 m^2)	(mL/min per kg)
>80	2.5	327	5.1
50 - 80	3.0	248	3.9
15 - 50	3.5	190	3.4
0 (Anuric)	19.5	29	0.5

Table 3. Acyclovir Pharmacokinetics in Pediatric Patients (Mean ± SD)

Parameter	Birth to 3 Months of Age (n = 12)	3 Months to 12 Years of Age (n = 16)
CL (mL/min/kg)	4.46 ± 1.61	8.44 ± 2.92
VDSS (L/kg)	1.08 ± 0.35	1.01 ± 0.28
Elimination half-life (hr)	3.80 ± 1.19	2.36 ± 0.97

INDICATIONS AND USAGE

Herpes Simplex Infections in Immunocompromised Patients: ZOVIRAX for Injection is indicated for the treatment of initial and recurrent mucosal and cutaneous herpes simplex (HSV-1 and HSV-2) in immunocompromised patients.

Initial Episodes of Herpes Genitalis: ZOVIRAX for Injection is indicated for the treatment of severe initial clinical episodes of herpes genitalis in immunocompetent patients.

Herpes Simplex Encephalitis: ZOVIRAX for Injection is indicated for the treatment of herpes simplex encephalitis.

Neonatal Herpes Simplex Virus Infection: ZOVIRAX for Injection is indicated for the treatment of neonatal herpes infections.

Varicella-Zoster Infections in Immunocompromised Patients: ZOVIRAX for Injection is indicated for the treatment of varicella-zoster (shingles) infections in immunocompromised patients.

CONTRAINDICATIONS

ZOVIRAX for Injection is contraindicated for patients who develop hypersensitivity to acyclovir or valacyclovir.

WARNINGS

ZOVIRAX for Injection is intended for intravenous infusion only, and should not be administered topically, intramuscularly, orally, subcutaneously, or in the eye. Intravenous infusions must be given over a period of at least 1 hour to reduce the risk of renal tubular damage (see PRECAUTIONS and DOSAGE AND ADMINISTRATION).

Renal failure, in some cases resulting in death, has been observed with acyclovir therapy (see ADVERSE REACTIONS: Observed During Clinical Practice and OVERDOSAGE).

Thrombotic thrombocytopenic purpura/hemolytic uremic syndrome (TTP/HUS), which has resulted in death, has occurred in immunocompromised patients receiving acyclovir therapy.

PRECAUTIONS

General: Precipitation of acyclovir crystals in renal tubules can occur if the maximum solubility of free acyclovir (2.5 mg/mL at 37°C in water) is exceeded or if the drug is administered by bolus injection. Ensuing renal tubular damage can produce acute renal failure.

Abnormal renal function (decreased creatinine clearance) can occur as a result of acyclovir administration and depends on the state of the patient's hydration, other treatments, and the rate of drug administration. Concomitant use of other nephrotoxic drugs, pre-existing renal disease, and dehydration make further renal impairment with acyclovir more likely.

Administration of ZOVIRAX by intravenous infusion must be accompanied by adequate hydration.

When dosage adjustments are required, they should be based on estimated creatinine clearance (see DOSAGE AND ADMINISTRATION).

Approximately 1% of patients receiving intravenous acyclovir have manifested encephalopathic changes characterized by either lethargy, obtundation, tremors, confusion, hallucinations, agitation, seizures, or coma. ZOVIRAX should be used with caution in those patients who have underlying neurologic abnormalities and those with serious renal, hepatic, or electrolyte abnormalities, or significant hypoxia.

Drug Interactions: See CLINICAL PHARMACOLOGY: Pharmacokinetics.

Carcinogenesis, Mutagenesis, Impairment of Fertility: The data presented below include references to peak steady-state plasma acyclovir concentrations observed in humans treated with 30 mg/kg per day (10 mg/kg every 8 hours, dosing appropriate for treatment of herpes zoster or herpes encephalitis), or 15 mg/kg per day (5 mg/kg every 8 hours, dosing appropriate for treatment of primary genital herpes or herpes simplex infections in immunocompromised patients). Plasma drug concentrations in animal studies are expressed as multiples of human exposure to acyclovir at the higher and lower dosing schedules (see CLINICAL PHARMACOLOGY: Pharmacokinetics).

Acyclovir was tested in lifetime bioassays in rats and mice at single daily doses of up to 450 mg/kg administered by gavage. There was no statistically significant difference in the incidence of tumors between treated and control animals, nor did acyclovir shorten the latency of tumors. At 450 mg/kg per day, plasma concentrations in both the mouse and rat bioassay were lower than concentrations in humans.

Acyclovir was tested in 16 in vitro and in vivo genetic toxicity assays. Acyclovir was positive in 5 of the assays.

Acyclovir did not impair fertility or reproduction in mice (450 mg/kg/day, p.o.) or in rats (25 mg/kg/day, s.c.). In the mouse study, plasma levels were the same as human levels, while in the rat study, they were 1 to 2 times human levels. At higher doses (50 mg/kg/day, s.c.) in rats and rabbits (1 to 2 and 1 to 3 times human levels, respectively) implantation efficacy, but not litter size, was decreased. In a rat peri- and post-natal study at 50 mg/kg/day, s.c., there was a statistically significant decrease in group mean numbers of corpora lutea, total implantation sites, and live fetuses.

No testicular abnormalities were seen in dogs given 50 mg/kg/day, IV for 1 month (1 to 3 times human levels) or in dogs given 60 mg/kg/day orally for 1 year (the same as human levels). Testicular atrophy and aspermatogenesis were observed in rats and dogs at higher dose levels.

Pregnancy: ***Teratogenic Effects:*** Pregnancy Category B. Acyclovir administered during organogenesis was not teratogenic in the mouse (450 mg/kg/day, p.o.), rabbit (50 mg/kg/day, s.c. and IV), or rat (50 mg/kg/day, s.c.). These exposures resulted in plasma levels the same as, 4 and 9, and 1 and 2 times, respectively, human levels.

There are no adequate and well-controlled studies in pregnant women. A prospective epidemiologic registry of acyclovir use during pregnancy was established in 1984 and completed in April 1999. There were 749 pregnancies followed in women exposed to systemic acyclovir during the first trimester of pregnancy resulting in 756 outcomes. The occurrence rate of birth defects approximates that found in the general population. However, the small size of the registry is insufficient to evaluate the risk for less common defects or to permit reliable or definitive conclusions regarding the safety of acyclovir in pregnant women and their developing fetuses. Acyclovir should be used during pregnancy only if the potential benefit justifies the potential risk to the fetus.

Nursing Mothers: Acyclovir concentrations have been documented in breast milk in 2 women following oral administration of ZOVIRAX and ranged from 0.6 to 4.1 times corresponding plasma levels. These concentrations would potentially expose the nursing infant to a dose of acyclovir up to 0.3 mg/kg/day. ZOVIRAX should be administered to a nursing mother with caution and only when indicated.

Pediatric Use: See DOSAGE AND ADMINISTRATION.

Geriatric Use: Clinical studies of ZOVIRAX for Injection did not include sufficient numbers of patients aged 65 and over to determine whether they respond differently from younger patients. Other reported clinical experience has identified differences in the severity of CNS adverse events between elderly and younger patients (see ADVERSE REACTIONS: Observed During Clinical Practice). In general, dose selection for an elderly patient should be cautious, reflecting the greater frequency of decreased renal function, and of concomitant disease or other drug therapy. This drug is known to be substantially excreted by the kidney, and the risk of toxic reactions to this drug may be greater in patients with impaired renal function. Because elderly patients are more likely to have decreased renal function, care should be taken in dose selection, and it may be useful to monitor renal function.

ADVERSE REACTIONS

The adverse reactions listed below have been observed in controlled and uncontrolled clinical trials in approximately 700 patients who received ZOVIRAX at ~5 mg/kg (250 mg/m^2) 3 times daily, and approximately 300 patients who received ~10 mg/kg (500 mg/m^2) 3 times daily.

The most frequent adverse reactions reported during administration of ZOVIRAX were inflammation or phlebitis at the injection site in approximately 9% of the patients, and transient elevations of serum creatinine or BUN in 5% to 10% (the higher incidence occurred usually following rapid [less than 10 minutes] intravenous infusion). Nausea and/or vomiting occurred in approximately 7% of the patients (the majority occurring in nonhospitalized patients who received 10 mg/kg). Itching, rash, or hives occurred in approximately 2% of patients. Elevation of transaminases occurred in 1% to 2% of patients.

The following hematologic abnormalities occurred at a frequency of less than 1%: anemia, neutropenia, thrombocytopenia, thrombocytosis, leukocytosis, and neutrophilia. In addition, anorexia and hematuria were observed.

Observed During Clinical Practice: In addition to adverse events reported from clinical trials, the following events have been identified during post-approval use of ZOVIRAX for Injection in clinical practice. Because they are reported voluntarily from a population of unknown size, estimates of frequency cannot be made. These events have been chosen for inclusion due to either their seriousness, frequency of reporting, potential causal connection to ZOVIRAX, or a combination of these factors.

General: Anaphylaxis, angioedema, fatigue, fever, headache, pain, peripheral edema, fatigue.

Digestive: Abdominal pain, diarrhea, gastrointestinal distress, nausea.

Cardiovascular: Hypotension.

Hematologic and Lymphatic: Disseminated intravascular coagulation, hemolysis, leukocytoclastic vasculitis, leukopenia, lymphadenopathy.

Hepatobiliary Tract and Pancreas: Elevated liver function tests, hepatitis, hyperbilirubinemia, jaundice.

Musculoskeletal: Myalgia.

Nervous: Aggressive behavior, agitation, ataxia, coma, confusion, delirium, dizziness, dysarthria, encephalopathy, hallucinations, obtundation, paresthesia, psychosis, seizure, somnolence, tremor. These symptoms may be marked, particularly in older adults (see PRECAUTIONS).

Skin: Alopecia, erythema multiforme, photosensitive rash, pruritus, rash, Stevens-Johnson syndrome, toxic epidermal necrolysis, urticaria. Severe local inflammatory reactions, including tissue necrosis, have occurred following infusion of ZOVIRAX into extravascular tissues.

Special Senses: Visual abnormalities.

Urogenital: Renal failure, elevated blood urea nitrogen, elevated creatinine (see WARNINGS).

OVERDOSAGE

Overdoses involving ingestions of up to 20 g have been reported. Adverse events that have been reported in association with overdosage include agitation, coma, seizures, and lethargy. Precipitation of acyclovir in renal tubules may occur when the solubility (2.5 mg/mL) is exceeded in the intratubular fluid. Overdosage has been reported following bolus injections or inappropriately high doses, and in patients whose fluid and electrolyte balance were not properly monitored. This has resulted in elevated BUN and serum creatinine, and subsequent renal failure. In the event of acute renal failure and anuria, the patient may benefit from hemodialysis until renal function is restored (see DOSAGE AND ADMINISTRATION).

DOSAGE AND ADMINISTRATION

CAUTION—RAPID OR BOLUS INTRAVENOUS INJECTION MUST BE AVOIDED (see WARNINGS and PRECAUTIONS).

INTRAMUSCULAR OR SUBCUTANEOUS INJECTION MUST BE AVOIDED (see WARNINGS).

Therapy should be initiated as early as possible following onset of signs and symptoms of herpes infections.

A maximum dose equivalent to 20 mg/kg every 8 hours should not be exceeded for any patient.

Dosage: ***Herpes Simplex Infections: Mucosal and Cutaneous Herpes Simplex (HSV-1 and HSV-2) Infections in Immunocompromised Patients:***

Adults and Adolescents (12 years of age and older): 5 mg/kg infused at a constant rate over 1 hour, every 8 hours for 7 days.

Pediatrics (Under 12 years of age): 10 mg/kg infused at a constant rate over 1 hour, every 8 hours for 7 days.

Severe Initial Clinical Episodes of Herpes Genitalis:

Adults and Adolescents (12 years of age and older): 5 mg/kg infused at a constant rate over 1 hour, every 8 hours for 5 days.

Herpes Simplex Encephalitis:

Adults and Adolescents (12 years of age and older): 10 mg/kg infused at a constant rate over 1 hour, every 8 hours for 10 days.

Pediatrics (3 months to 12 years of age): 20 mg/kg infused at a constant rate over 1 hour, every 8 hours for 10 days.

Neonatal Herpes Simplex Virus Infections (Birth to 3 months): 10 mg/kg infused at a constant rate over 1 hour, every 8 hours for 10 days. In neonatal herpes simplex infections, doses of 15 mg/kg or 20 mg/kg (infused at a constant rate over 1 hour every 8 hours) have been used; the safety and efficacy of these doses are not known.

Varicella Zoster Infections: Zoster in Immunocompromised Patients:

Adults and Adolescents (12 years of age and older): 10 mg/kg infused at a constant rate over 1 hour, every 8 hours for 7 days.

Pediatrics (Under 12 years of age): 20 mg/kg infused at a constant rate over 1 hour, every 8 hours for 7 days.

Obese Patients: Obese patients should be dosed at the recommended adult dose using Ideal Body Weight.

Patients with Acute or Chronic Renal Impairment: Refer to DOSAGE AND ADMINISTRATION section for recommended doses, and adjust the dosing interval as indicated in Table 5.

Table 5. Dosage Adjustments for Patients with Renal Impairment

Creatinine Clearance (mL/min per 1.73 m^2)	Percent of Recommended Dose	Dosing Interval (hours)
>50	100%	8
25 - 50	100%	12
10 - 25	100%	24
0 - 10	50%	24

Hemodialysis: For patients who require dialysis, the mean plasma half-life of acyclovir during hemodialysis is approximately 5 hours. This results in a 60% decrease in plasma concentrations following a 6-hour dialysis period. Therefore, the patient's dosing schedule should be adjusted so that an additional dose is administered after each dialysis.

Peritoneal Dialysis: No supplemental dose appears to be necessary after adjustment of the dosing interval.

Method of Preparation: Each 10-mL vial contains acyclovir sodium equivalent to 500 mg of acyclovir. Each 20-mL vial contains acyclovir sodium equivalent to 1,000 mg of acyclovir. The contents of the vial should be dissolved in Sterile Water for Injection as follows:

Contents of Vial	Amount of Diluent
500 mg	10 mL
1,000 mg	20 mL

The resulting solution in each case contains 50 mg acyclovir per mL (pH approximately 11). Shake the vial well to assure complete dissolution before measuring and transferring each individual dose. The reconstituted solution should be used within 12 hours. Refrigeration of reconstituted solution may result in the formation of a precipitate which will redissolve at room temperature.

DO NOT USE BACTERIOSTATIC WATER FOR INJECTION CONTAINING BENZYL ALCOHOL OR PARABENS.

Administration: The calculated dose should then be removed and added to any appropriate intravenous solution at a volume selected for administration during each 1-hour infusion. Infusion concentrations of approximately 7 mg/mL or lower are recommended. In clinical studies, the average 70-kg adult received between 60 and 150 mL of fluid per dose. Higher concentrations (e.g., 10 mg/mL) may produce phlebitis or inflammation at the injection site upon inadvertent extravasation. Standard, commercially available electrolyte and glucose solutions are suitable for intravenous administration; biologic or colloidal fluids (e.g., blood products, protein solutions, etc.) are not recommended.

Once diluted for administration, each dose should be used within 24 hours.

HOW SUPPLIED

10-mL sterile vials, each containing acyclovir sodium equivalent to 500 mg of acyclovir. Tray of 10 (NDC 0173-0995-01).

20-mL sterile vials, each containing acyclovir sodium equivalent to 1,000 mg of acyclovir. Tray of 10 (NDC 0173-0952-01).

Store at 15° to 25°C (59° to 77°F).

Manufactured by DSM Pharmaceuticals, Inc.
Greenville, NC 27834
for GlaxoSmithKline, Research Triangle Park, NC 27709

November 2003/RL-2050

Shown in Product Identification Guide, page 318

ZYBAN® ℞

[zī' ban]
(bupropion hydrochloride)
Sustained-Release Tablets

DESCRIPTION

ZYBAN (bupropion hydrochloride) Sustained-Release Tablets are a non-nicotine aid to smoking cessation. ZYBAN is chemically unrelated to nicotine or other agents currently used in the treatment of nicotine addiction. Initially developed and marketed as an antidepressant (WELLBUTRIN® [bupropion hydrochloride] Tablets and WELLBUTRIN SR® [bupropion hydrochloride] Sustained-Release Tablets), ZYBAN is also chemically unrelated to tricyclic, tetracyclic, selective serotonin re-uptake inhibitor, or other known antidepressant agents. Its structure closely resembles that of diethylpropion; it is related to phenylethylamines. It is (±)-1-(3-chlorophenyl)-2-[(1,1-dimethylethyl)amino]-1-propanone hydrochloride. The molecular weight is 276.2. The molecular formula is $C_{13}H_{18}ClNO•HCl$. Bupropion hydrochloride powder is white, crystalline, and highly soluble in water. It has a bitter taste and produces the sensation of local anesthesia on the oral mucosa.

ZYBAN is supplied for oral administration as 150-mg (purple), film-coated, sustained-release tablets. Each tablet contains the labeled amount of bupropion hydrochloride and the inactive ingredients carnauba wax, cysteine hydrochloride, hypromellose, magnesium stearate, microcrystalline cellulose, polyethylene glycol, polysorbate 80 and titanium dioxide and is printed with edible black ink. In addition, the 150-mg tablet contains FD&C Blue No. 2 Lake and FD&C Red No. 40 Lake.

CLINICAL PHARMACOLOGY

Pharmacodynamics: Bupropion is a relatively weak inhibitor of the neuronal uptake of norepinephrine, serotonin, and dopamine, and does not inhibit monoamine oxidase. The mechanism by which ZYBAN enhances the ability of patients to abstain from smoking is unknown. However, it is presumed that this action is mediated by noradrenergic and/or dopaminergic mechanisms.

Pharmacokinetics: Bupropion is a racemic mixture. The pharmacologic activity and pharmacokinetics of the individual enantiomers have not been studied. Bupropion follows biphasic pharmacokinetics best described by a 2-compartment model. The terminal phase has a mean half-life (±%CV) of about 21 hours (±20%), while the distribution phase has a mean half-life of 3 to 4 hours.

Absorption: Bupropion has not been administered intravenously to humans; therefore, the absolute bioavailability of ZYBAN Sustained-Release Tablets in humans has not been determined. In rat and dog studies, the bioavailability of bupropion ranged from 5% to 20%.

Following oral administration of ZYBAN to healthy volunteers, peak plasma concentrations of bupropion are achieved within 3 hours. The mean peak concentration (C_{max}) values were 91 and 143 ng/mL from 2 single-dose (150-mg) studies. At steady state, the mean C_{max} following a 150-mg dose every 12 hours is 136 ng/mL.

In a single-dose study, food increased the C_{max} of bupropion by 11% and the extent of absorption as defined by area under the plasma concentration-time curve (AUC) by 17%. The mean time to peak concentration (T_{max}) was prolonged by 1 hour. This effect was of no clinical significance.

Distribution: In vitro tests show that bupropion is 84% bound to human plasma proteins at concentrations up to 200 mcg/mL. The extent of protein binding of the hydroxybupropion metabolite is similar to that for bupropion, whereas the extent of protein binding of the threohydrobupropion metabolite is about half that seen with bupropion. The volume of distribution (V_{ss}/F) estimated from a single 150-mg dose given to 17 subjects is 1,950 L (20% CV).

Metabolism: Bupropion is extensively metabolized in humans. Three metabolites have been shown to be active: hydroxybupropion, which is formed via hydroxylation of the *tert*-butyl group of bupropion, and the amino-alcohol isomers threohydrobupropion and erythrohydrobupropion, which are formed via reduction of the carbonyl group. In vitro findings suggest that cytochrome P450IIB6 (CYP2B6) is the principal isoenzyme involved in the formation of hydroxybupropion, while cytochrome P450 isoenzymes are not involved in the formation of threohydrobupropion. Oxidation of the bupropion side chain results in the formation of a glycine conjugate of meta-chlorobenzoic acid, which is then excreted as the major urinary metabolite. The potency and toxicity of the metabolites relative to bupropion have not been fully characterized. However, it has been demonstrated in an antidepressant screening test in mice that hydroxybupropion is one half as potent as bupropion, while threohydrobupropion and erythrohydrobupropion are 5-fold less potent than bupropion. This may be of clinical importance because the plasma concentrations of the metabolites are as high or higher than those of bupropion.

Because bupropion is extensively metabolized, there is the potential for drug-drug interactions, particularly with those agents that are metabolized by the cytochrome P450IIB6 (CYP2B6) isoenzyme. Although bupropion is not metabolized by cytochrome P450IID6 (CYP2D6), there is the potential for drug-drug interactions when bupropion is co-administered with drugs metabolized by this isoenzyme (see PRECAUTIONS: Drug Interactions).

Following a single dose in humans, peak plasma concentrations of hydroxybupropion occur approximately 6 hours after administration of ZYBAN Tablets. Peak plasma concentrations of hydroxybupropion are approximately 10 times the peak level of the parent drug at steady state. The elimination half-life of hydroxybupropion is approximately 20 (±5) hours, and its AUC at steady state is about 17 times that of bupropion. The times to peak concentrations for the erythrohydrobupropion and threohydrobupropion metabolites are similar to that of the hydroxybupropion metabolite; however, their elimination half-lives are longer, 33 (±10) and 37 (±13) hours, respectively, and steady-state AUCs are 1.5 and 7 times that of bupropion, respectively.

Bupropion and its metabolites exhibit linear kinetics following chronic administration of 300 to 450 mg/day.

Elimination: The mean (±%CV) apparent clearance (Cl/F) estimated from 2 single-dose (150-mg) studies are 135 (±20%) and 209 L/hr (±21%). Following chronic dosing of 150 mg of ZYBAN every 12 hours for 14 days (n=34), the mean Cl/F at steady state was 160 L/hr (±23%). The mean elimination half-life of bupropion estimated from a series of studies is approximately 21 hours. Estimates of the half-lives of the metabolites determined from a multiple-dose study were 20 hours (±25%) for hydroxybupropion, 37 hours (±35%) for threohydrobupropion, and 33 hours (±30%) for erythrohydrobupropion. Steady-state plasma concentrations of bupropion and metabolites are reached within 5 and 8 days, respectively.

Following oral administration of 200 mg of ^{14}C-bupropion in humans, 87% and 10% of the radioactive dose were recovered in the urine and feces, respectively. The fraction of the oral dose of bupropion excreted unchanged was only 0.5%.

The effects of cigarette smoking on the pharmacokinetics of bupropion were studied in 34 healthy male and female volunteers; 17 were chronic cigarette smokers and 17 were nonsmokers. Following oral administration of a single 150-mg dose of ZYBAN, there was no statistically significant difference in C_{max}, half-life, T_{max}, AUC, or clearance of bupropion or its major metabolites between smokers and nonsmokers.

In a study comparing the treatment combination of ZYBAN and nicotine transdermal system (NTS) versus ZYBAN alone, no statistically significant differences were observed between the 2 treatment groups of combination ZYBAN and NTS (n=197) and ZYBAN alone (n=193) in the plasma concentrations of bupropion or its active metabolites at weeks 3 and 6.

Population Subgroups: Factors or conditions altering metabolic capacity (e.g., liver disease, congestive heart failure, age, concomitant medications, etc.) or elimination may be expected to influence the degree and extent of accumulation of the active metabolites of bupropion. The elimination of the major metabolites of bupropion may be affected by reduced renal or hepatic function because they are moderately polar compounds and are likely to undergo further metabolism or conjugation in the liver prior to urinary excretion.

Hepatic: The effect of hepatic impairment on the pharmacokinetics of bupropion was characterized in 2 single-dose studies, one in patients with alcoholic liver disease and one in patients with mild to severe cirrhosis.

The first study showed that the half-life of hydroxybupropion was significantly longer in 8 patients with alcoholic liver disease than in 8 healthy volunteers (32±14 hours versus 21±5 hours, respectively). Although not statistically significant, the AUCs for bupropion and hydroxybupropion were more variable and tended to be greater (by 53% to 57%) in patients with alcoholic liver disease. The differences in half-life for bupropion and the other metabolites in the 2 patient groups were minimal.

The second study showed that there were no statistically significant differences in the pharmacokinetics of bupropion and its active metabolites in 9 patients with mild to moderate hepatic cirrhosis compared to 8 healthy volunteers. However, more variability was observed in some of the pharmacokinetic parameters for bupropion (AUC, C_{max}, and T_{max}) and its active metabolites ($t_{1/2}$) in patients with mild to moderate hepatic cirrhosis. In addition, in patients with severe hepatic cirrhosis, the bupropion C_{max} and AUC were

Continued on next page

Product information on these pages is effective as of August 2004. Further information is available at: GlaxoSmithKline, PO Box 13398, Research Triangle Park, NC 27709. 1-888-825-5249. Corporate Web Site: www.gsk.com

Zyban—Cont.

substantially increased (mean difference: by approximately 70% and 3-fold, respectively) and more variable when compared to values in healthy volunteers; the mean bupropion half-life was also longer (29 hours in patients with severe hepatic cirrhosis vs. 19 hours in healthy subjects). For the metabolites hydroxybupropion, the mean C_{max} was approximately 69% lower.

For the combined amino-alcohol isomers threohydrobupropion and erythrohydrobupropion, the mean C_{max} was approximately 31% lower. The mean AUC increased by 28% for hydroxybupropion and 50% for threo/erythrohydrobupropion.

The median T_{max} was observed 19 hours later for hydroxybupropion and 21 hours later for threo/erythrohydrobupropion. The mean half-lives for hydroxybupropion and threo/erythrohydrobupropion were increased 2- and 4-fold, respectively, in patients with severe hepatic cirrhosis compared to healthy volunteers (see WARNINGS, PRECAUTIONS, and DOSAGE AND ADMINISTRATION).

Renal: The effect of renal disease on the pharmacokinetics of bupropion has not been studied. The elimination of the major metabolites of bupropion may be affected by reduced renal function.

Left Ventricular Dysfunction: During a chronic dosing study with bupropion in 14 depressed patients with left ventricular dysfunction (history of congestive heart failure [CHF] or an enlarged heart on x-ray), no apparent effect on the pharmacokinetics of bupropion or its metabolites, compared to healthy normal volunteers, was revealed.

Age: The effects of age on the pharmacokinetics of bupropion and its metabolites have not been fully characterized, but an exploration of steady-state bupropion concentrations from several depression efficacy studies involving patients dosed in a range of 300 to 750 mg/day, on a 3 times a day schedule, revealed no relationship between age (18 to 83 years) and plasma concentration of bupropion. A single-dose pharmacokinetic study demonstrated that the disposition of bupropion and its metabolites in elderly subjects was similar to that of younger subjects. These data suggest there is no prominent effect of age on bupropion concentration; however, another pharmacokinetic study, single and multiple dose, has suggested that the elderly are at increased risk for accumulation of bupropion and its metabolites (see PRECAUTIONS: Geriatric Use).

Gender: A single-dose study involving 12 healthy male and 12 healthy female volunteers revealed no sex-related differences in the pharmacokinetic parameters of bupropion.

CLINICAL TRIALS

The efficacy of ZYBAN as an aid to smoking cessation was demonstrated in 3 placebo-controlled, double-blind trials in nondepressed chronic cigarette smokers (n=1,940, ≥15 cigarettes per day). In these studies, ZYBAN was used in conjunction with individual smoking cessation counseling.

The first study was a dose-response trial conducted at 3 clinical centers. Patients in this study were treated for 7 weeks with 1 of 3 doses of ZYBAN (100, 150, or 300 mg/day) or placebo; quitting was defined as total abstinence during the last 4 weeks of treatment (weeks 4 through 7). Abstinence was determined by patient daily diaries and verified by carbon monoxide levels in expired air.

Results of this dose-response trial with ZYBAN demonstrated a dose-dependent increase in the percentage of patients able to achieve 4-week abstinence (weeks 4 through 7). Treatment with ZYBAN at both 150 and 300 mg/day was significantly more effective than placebo in this study.

Table 1 presents quit rates over time in the multicenter trial by treatment group. The quit rates are the proportions of all persons initially enrolled (i.e., intent to treat analysis) who abstained from week 4 of the study through the specified week. Treatment with ZYBAN (150 or 300 mg/day) was more effective than placebo in helping patients achieve 4-week abstinence. In addition, treatment with ZYBAN (7 weeks at 300 mg/day) was more effective than placebo in helping patients maintain continuous abstinence through week 26 (6 months) of the study.

[See table 1 above]

Table 1. Dose-Response Trial: Quit Rates by Treatment Group

	Treatment Groups			
Abstinence From Week 4 Through Specified Week	Placebo (n = 151) % (95% CI)	ZYBAN 100 mg/day (n = 153) % (95% CI)	ZYBAN 150 mg/day (n = 153) % (95% CI)	ZYBAN 300 mg/day (n = 156) % (95% CI)
Week 7 (4-week quit)	17% (11-23)	22% (15-28)	27%* (20-35)	36%* (28-43)
Week 12	14% (8-19)	20% (13-26)	20% (14-27)	25%* (18-32)
Week 26	11% (6-16)	16% (11-22)	18% (12-24)	19%* (13-25)

* Significantly different from placebo ($p \leq 0.05$).

The second study was a comparative trial conducted at 4 clinical centers. Four treatments were evaluated: ZYBAN 300 mg/day, nicotine transdermal system (NTS) 21 mg/day, combination of ZYBAN 300 mg/day plus NTS 21 mg/day, and placebo. Patients were treated for 9 weeks. Treatment with ZYBAN was initiated at 150 mg/day while the patient was still smoking and was increased after 3 days to 300 mg/day given as 150 mg twice daily. NTS 21 mg/day was added to treatment with ZYBAN after approximately 1 week when the patient reached the target quit date. During weeks 8 and 9 of the study, NTS was tapered to 14 and 7 mg/day, respectively. Quitting, defined as total abstinence during weeks 4 through 7, was determined by patient daily diaries and verified by expired air carbon monoxide levels. In this study, patients treated with any of the 3 treatments achieved greater 4-week abstinence rates than patients treated with placebo.

Table 2 presents quit rates over time by treatment group for the comparative trial.

[See table 2 above]

Table 2. Comparative Trial: Quit Rates by Treatment Group

	Treatment Groups			
Abstinence From Week 4 Through Specified Week	Placebo (n = 160) % (95% CI)	Nicotine Transdermal System (NTS) 21 mg/day (n = 244) % (95% CI)	ZYBAN 300 mg/day (n = 244) % (95% CI)	ZYBAN 300 mg/day and NTS 21 mg/day (n = 245) % (95% CI)
Week 7 (4-week quit)	23% (17-30)	36% (30-42)	49% (43-56)	58% (51-64)
Week 10	20% (14-26)	32% (26-37)	46% (39-52)	51% (45-58)

When patients in this study were followed out to one year, the superiority of ZYBAN and the combination of ZYBAN and NTS over placebo in helping patients to achieve abstinence from smoking was maintained. The continuous abstinence rate was 30% (95% CI 24-35) in the ZYBAN treated patients, and 33% (95% CI 27-39) for patients treated with the combination at 26 weeks compared with 13% (95% CI 7-18) in the placebo group. At 52 weeks, the continuous abstinence rate was 23% (95% CI 18-28) in the ZYBAN treated patients, and 28% (95% CI 23-34) for patients treated with the combination, compared with 8% (95% CI 3-12) in the placebo group. Although the treatment combination of ZYBAN and NTS displayed the highest rates of continuous abstinence throughout the study, the quit rates for the combination were not significantly higher ($p > 0.05$) than for ZYBAN alone.

The comparisons between ZYBAN, NTS, and combination treatment in this study have not been replicated, and, therefore should not be interpreted as demonstrating the superiority of any of the active treatment arms over any other.

The third study was a long-term maintenance trial conducted at 5 clinical centers. Patients in this study received open-label ZYBAN 300 mg/day for 7 weeks. Patients who quit smoking while receiving ZYBAN (n = 432) were then randomized to ZYBAN 300 mg/day or placebo for a total study duration of 1 year. Abstinence from smoking was determined by patient self-report and verified by expired air carbon monoxide levels. This trial demonstrated that at 6 months, continuous abstinence rates were significantly higher for patients continuing to receive ZYBAN than for those switched to placebo ($p<0.05$; 55% versus 44%).

Quit rates in clinical trials are influenced by the population selected. Quit rates in an unselected population may be lower than the above rates. Quit rates for ZYBAN were similar in patients with and without prior quit attempts using nicotine replacement therapy.

Treatment with ZYBAN reduced withdrawal symptoms compared to placebo. Reductions on the following withdrawal symptoms were most pronounced: irritability, frustration, or anger; anxiety; difficulty concentrating; restlessness; and depressed mood or negative affect. Depending on the study and the measure used, treatment with ZYBAN showed evidence of reduction in craving for cigarettes or urge to smoke compared to placebo.

Use In Patients With Chronic Obstructive Pulmonary Disease (COPD): ZYBAN was evaluated in a randomized, double-blind, comparative study of 404 patients with mild-to-moderate COPD, defined as $FEV_1 \geq 35\%$, $FEV_1/FVC \leq 70\%$ and a diagnosis of chronic bronchitis, emphysema and/or small airways disease. Patients aged 36 to 76 years were randomized to ZYBAN 300 mg/day (n = 204) or placebo (n = 200) and treated for 12 weeks. Treatment with ZYBAN was initiated at 150 mg/day for 3 days while the patient was still smoking and increased to 150 mg twice daily for the remaining treatment period. Abstinence from smoking was determined by patient daily diaries and verified by carbon monoxide levels in expired air. Quitters are defined as subjects who were abstinent during the last 4 weeks of treatment. Table 3 shows quit rates in the COPD Trial.

Table 3. COPD Trial: Quit Rates by Treatment Group

	Treatment Groups	
4-Week Abstinence Period	Placebo (n = 200) % (95% CI)	ZYBAN 300 mg/day (n = 204) % (95% CI)
Weeks 9 through 12	12% (8-16)	22%* (17-27)

*Significantly different from placebo ($p<0.05$).

INDICATIONS AND USAGE

ZYBAN is indicated as an aid to smoking cessation treatment.

CONTRAINDICATIONS

ZYBAN is contraindicated in patients with a seizure disorder.

ZYBAN is contraindicated in patients treated with WELLBUTRIN, WELLBUTRIN SR, WELLBUTRIN XL, or any other medications that contain bupropion because the incidence of seizure is dose dependent.

ZYBAN is contraindicated in patients with a current or prior diagnosis of bulimia or anorexia nervosa because of a higher incidence of seizures noted in patients treated for bulimia with the immediate-release formulation of bupropion.

ZYBAN is contraindicated in patients undergoing abrupt discontinuation of alcohol or sedatives (including benzodiazepines).

The concurrent administration of ZYBAN and a monoamine oxidase (MAO) inhibitor is contraindicated. At least 14 days should elapse between discontinuation of an MAO inhibitor and initiation of treatment with ZYBAN.

ZYBAN is contraindicated in patients who have shown an allergic response to bupropion or the other ingredients that make up ZYBAN.

WARNINGS

Patients should be made aware that ZYBAN contains the same active ingredient found in WELLBUTRIN, WELLBUTRIN SR, and WELLBUTRIN XL used to treat depression, and that ZYBAN should not be used in combination with WELLBUTRIN, WELLBUTRIN SR, WELLBUTRIN XL, or any other medications that contain bupropion.

Because the use of bupropion is associated with a dose-dependent risk of seizures, *clinicians should not prescribe doses over 300 mg/day for smoking cessation.* The risk of seizures is also related to patient factors, clinical situation, and concurrent medications, which must be considered in selection of patients for therapy with ZYBAN. ZYBAN should be discontinued and not restarted in patients who experience a seizure while on treatment.

- **Dose: *For smoking cessation, doses above 300 mg/day should not be used.* The seizure rate associated with doses of sustained-release bupropion up to 300 mg/day is approximately 0.1% (1/1,000). This incidence was prospectively determined during an 8-week treatment exposure in approximately 3,100 depressed patients. Data for the immediate-release formulation of bupropion re-**

vealed a seizure incidence of approximately 0.4% (4/1,000) in depressed patients treated at doses in a range of 300 to 450 mg/day. In addition, the estimated seizure incidence increases almost tenfold between 450 and 600 mg/day.

- **Patient factors: Predisposing factors that may increase the risk of seizure with bupropion use include history of head trauma or prior seizure, central nervous system (CNS) tumor, the presence of severe hepatic cirrhosis, and concomitant medications that lower seizure threshold.**
- **Clinical situations: Circumstances associated with an increased seizure risk include, among others, excessive use of alcohol or sedatives (including benzodiazepines); addiction to opiates, cocaine, or stimulants; use of over-the-counter stimulants and anorectics; and diabetes treated with oral hypoglycemics or insulin.**
- **Concomitant medications: Many medications (e.g., antipsychotics, antidepressants, theophylline, systemic steroids) are known to lower seizure threshold.**

Recommendations for Reducing the Risk of Seizure: Retrospective analysis of clinical experience gained during the development of bupropion suggests that the risk of seizure may be minimized if

- **the total daily dose of ZYBAN does *not* exceed 300 mg (the maximum recommended dose for smoking cessation), and**
- **the recommended daily dose for most patients (300 mg/day) is administered in divided doses (150 mg twice daily).**
- **No single dose should exceed 150 mg to avoid high peak concentrations of bupropion and/or its metabolites.**

ZYBAN should be administered with extreme caution to patients with a history of seizure, cranial trauma, or other predisposition(s) toward seizure, or patients treated with other agents (e.g., antipsychotics, antidepressants, theophylline, systemic steroids, etc.) that lower seizure threshold.

Hepatic Impairment: ZYBAN should be used with extreme caution in patients with severe hepatic cirrhosis. In these patients a reduced frequency of dosing is required, as peak bupropion levels are substantially increased and accumulation is likely to occur in such patients to a greater extent than usual. The dose should not exceed 150 mg every other day in these patients (see CLINICAL PHARMACOLOGY, PRECAUTIONS, and DOSAGE AND ADMINISTRATION).

Potential for Hepatotoxicity: In rats receiving large doses of bupropion chronically, there was an increase in incidence of hepatic hyperplastic nodules and hepatocellular hypertrophy. In dogs receiving large doses of bupropion chronically, various histologic changes were seen in the liver, and laboratory tests suggesting mild hepatocellular injury were noted.

Clinical Worsening and Suicide Risk: Although ZYBAN is not indicated for treatment of depression, it contains the same active ingredient as WELLBUTRIN, WELLBUTRIN SR, and WELLBUTRIN XL, antidepressant medications. Therefore, clinicians should be aware of the following information.

Patients with major depressive disorder, both adult and pediatric, may experience worsening of their depression and/or the emergence of suicidal ideation and behavior (suicidality), whether or not they are taking antidepressant medications, and this risk may persist until significant remission occurs. Although there has been a long-standing concern that antidepressants may have a role in inducing worsening of depression and the emergence of suicidality in certain patients, a causal role for antidepressants in inducing such behaviors has not been established. **Nevertheless, patients being treated with antidepressants should be observed closely for clinical worsening and suicidality, especially at the beginning of a course of drug therapy, or at the time of dose changes, either increases or decreases.** Consideration should be given to changing the therapeutic regimen, including possibly discontinuing the medication in patients whose depression is persistently worse or whose emergent suicidality is severe, abrupt in onset, or was not part of the patient's presenting symptoms.

Because of the possibility of co-morbidity between major depressive disorder and other psychiatric and nonpsychiatric disorders, the same precautions observed when treating patients with major depressive disorder should be observed when treating patients with other psychiatric and nonpsychiatric disorders.

The following symptoms, anxiety, agitation, panic attacks, insomnia, irritability, hostility (aggressiveness), impulsivity, akathisia (psychomotor restlessness), hypomania, and mania, have been reported in adult and pediatric patients being treated with antidepressants for major depressive disorder as well as for other indications, both psychiatric and nonpsychiatric. Although a causal link between the emergence of such symptoms and either the worsening of depression and/or the emergence of suicidal impulses has not been established, consideration should be given to changing the therapeutic regimen, including possibly discontinuing the medication in patients for whom such symptoms are severe, abrupt in onset, or were not part of the patient's presenting symptoms.

Families and caregivers of patients being treated with antidepressants for major depressive disorder or other indications, both psychiatric and nonpsychiatric, should be alerted about the need to monitor patients for the emergence of agitation, irritability, and the other symptoms described above, as well as the emergence of suicidality, and to report such symptoms immediately to health care providers. Prescriptions for ZYBAN should be written for the smallest quantity of tablets consistent with good patient management, in order to reduce the risk of overdose.

It should be noted that ZYBAN is not approved for use in treating any indications in the pediatric population.

A major depressive episode may be the initial presentation of bipolar disorder. It is generally believed (although not established in controlled trials) that treating such an episode with an antidepressant alone may increase the likelihood of precipitation of a mixed/manic episode in patients at risk for bipolar disorder. Whether any of the symptoms described above represent such a conversion is unknown. However, prior to initiating treatment with an antidepressant, patients should be adequately screened to determine if they are at risk for bipolar disorder; such screening should include a detailed psychiatric history, including a family history of suicide, bipolar disorder, and depression. It should be noted that ZYBAN is not approved for use in treating bipolar depression.

PRECAUTIONS

General: ***Allergic Reactions:*** Anaphylactoid/anaphylactic reactions characterized by symptoms such as pruritus, urticaria, angioedema, and dyspnea requiring medical treatment have been reported at a rate of about 1 to 3 per thousand in clinical trials of ZYBAN. In addition, there have been rare spontaneous postmarketing reports of erythema multiforme, Stevens-Johnson syndrome, and anaphylactic shock associated with bupropion. A patient should stop taking ZYBAN and consult a doctor if experiencing allergic or anaphylactoid/anaphylactic reactions (e.g., skin rash, pruritus, hives, chest pain, edema, and shortness of breath) during treatment.

Arthralgia, myalgia, and fever with rash and other symptoms suggestive of delayed hypersensitivity have been reported in association with bupropion. These symptoms may resemble serum sickness.

Insomnia: In the dose-response smoking cessation trial, 29% of patients treated with 150 mg/day of ZYBAN and 35% of patients treated with 300 mg/day of ZYBAN experienced insomnia, compared to 21% of placebo-treated patients. Symptoms were sufficiently severe to require discontinuation of treatment in 0.6% of patients treated with ZYBAN and none of the patients treated with placebo.

In the comparative trial, 40% of the patients treated with 300 mg/day of ZYBAN, 28% of the patients treated with 21 mg/day of NTS, and 45% of the patients treated with the combination of ZYBAN and NTS experienced insomnia compared to 18% of placebo-treated patients. Symptoms were sufficiently severe to require discontinuation of treatment in 0.8% of patients treated with ZYBAN and none of the patients in the other 3 treatment groups.

Insomnia may be minimized by avoiding bedtime doses and, if necessary, reduction in dose.

Psychosis, Confusion, and Other Neuropsychiatric Phenomena: In clinical trials with ZYBAN conducted in nondepressed smokers, the incidence of neuropsychiatric side effects was generally comparable to placebo. Depressed patients treated with bupropion in depression trials have been reported to show a variety of neuropsychiatric signs and symptoms including delusions, hallucinations, psychosis, concentration disturbance, paranoia, and confusion. In some cases, these symptoms abated upon dose reduction and/or withdrawal of treatment.

Activation of Psychosis and/or Mania: Antidepressants can precipitate manic episodes in bipolar disorder patients during the depressed phase of their illness and may activate latent psychosis in other susceptible individuals. The sustained-release formulation of bupropion is expected to pose similar risks. There were no reports of activation of psychosis or mania in clinical trials with ZYBAN conducted in nondepressed smokers.

Depression and Nicotine Withdrawal: Depressed mood may be a symptom of nicotine withdrawal. Depression, rarely including suicidal ideation, has been reported in patients undergoing a smoking cessation attempt **(see WARNINGS—Clinical Worsening and Suicide Risk)**.

Cardiovascular Effects: In clinical practice, hypertension, in some cases severe, requiring acute treatment, has been reported in patients receiving bupropion alone and in combination with nicotine replacement therapy. These events have been observed in both patients with and without evidence of preexisting hypertension.

Data from a comparative study of ZYBAN, nicotine transdermal system (NTS), the combination of sustained-release bupropion plus NTS, and placebo as an aid to smoking cessation suggest a higher incidence of treatment-emergent hypertension in patients treated with the combination of ZYBAN and NTS. In this study, 6.1% of patients treated with the combination of ZYBAN and NTS had treatment-emergent hypertension compared to 2.5%, 1.6%, and 3.1% of patients treated with ZYBAN, NTS, and placebo, respectively. The majority of these patients had evidence of preexisting hypertension. Three patients (1.2%) treated with the combination of ZYBAN and NTS and one patient (0.4%) treated with NTS had study medication discontinued due to hypertension compared to none of the patients treated with ZYBAN or placebo. Monitoring of blood pressure is recommended in patients who receive the combination of bupropion and nicotine replacement.

There is no clinical experience establishing the safety of ZYBAN in patients with a recent history of myocardial infarction or unstable heart disease. Therefore, care should be exercised if it is used in these groups. Bupropion was well tolerated in depressed patients who had previously developed orthostatic hypotension while receiving tricyclic antidepressants, and was also generally well tolerated in a group of 36 depressed inpatients with stable congestive heart failure (CHF). However, bupropion was associated with a rise in supine blood pressure in the study of patients with CHF, resulting in discontinuation of treatment in 2 patients for exacerbation of baseline hypertension.

Hepatic Impairment: ZYBAN should be used with extreme caution in patients with severe hepatic cirrhosis. In these patients, a reduced frequency of dosing is required. ZYBAN should be used with caution in patients with hepatic impairment (including mild to moderate hepatic cirrhosis) and reduced frequency of dosing should be considered in patients with mild to moderate hepatic cirrhosis.

All patients with hepatic impairment should be closely monitored for possible adverse effects that could indicate high drug and metabolite levels (see CLINICAL PHARMACOLOGY, WARNINGS, and DOSAGE AND ADMINISTRATION).

Renal Impairment: No studies have been conducted in patients with renal impairment. Bupropion is extensively metabolized in the liver to active metabolites, which are further metabolized and excreted by the kidneys. ZYBAN should be used with caution in patients with renal impairment and a reduced frequency of dosing should be considered as bupropion and its metabolites may accumulate in such patients to a greater extent than usual. The patient should be closely monitored for possible adverse effects that could indicate high drug or metabolite levels.

Information for Patients: See PATIENT INFORMATION at the end of this labeling for the text of the tear-off leaflet provided for patients. Physicians are advised to review the leaflet with their patients and to emphasize that ZYBAN contains the same active ingredient found in WELLBUTRIN, WELLBUTRIN SR, and WELLBUTRIN XL used to treat depression and that ZYBAN should not be used in conjunction with WELLBUTRIN, WELLBUTRIN SR, WELLBUTRIN XL, or any other medications that contain bupropion hydrochloride.

Although ZYBAN is not indicated for treatment of depression, it contains the same active ingredient as WELLBUTRIN, WELLBUTRIN SR, and WELLBUTRIN XL, antidepressant medications. Therefore, patients should be aware of the following information.

Patients and their families should be encouraged to be alert to the emergence of anxiety, agitation, panic attacks, insomnia, irritability, hostility, impulsivity, akathisia, hypomania, mania, worsening of depression, and suicidal ideation, especially early during antidepressant treatment. Such symptoms should be reported to the patient's physician, especially if they are severe, abrupt in onset, or were not part of the patient's presenting symptoms.

Laboratory Tests: There are no specific laboratory tests recommended.

Drug Interactions: In vitro studies indicate that bupropion is primarily metabolized to hydroxybupropion by the cytochrome P450IIB6 (CYP2B6) isoenzyme. Therefore, the potential exists for a drug interaction between ZYBAN and drugs that affect the CYP2B6 isoenzyme (e.g., orphenadrine and cyclophosphamide). The threohydrobupropion metabolite of bupropion does not appear to be produced by the cytochrome P450 isoenzymes. Few systemic data have been collected on the metabolism of ZYBAN following concomitant administration with other drugs or, alternatively, the effect of concomitant administration of ZYBAN on the metabolism of other drugs.

Animal data indicated that bupropion may be an inducer of drug-metabolizing enzymes in humans. However, following chronic administration of bupropion, 100 mg t.i.d. to 8 healthy male volunteers for 14 days, there was no evidence of induction of its own metabolism. Because bupropion is extensively metabolized, the coadministration of other drugs may affect its clinical activity. In particular, certain drugs may induce the metabolism of bupropion (e.g., carbamazepine, phenobarbital, phenytoin), while other drugs may inhibit the metabolism of bupropion (e.g., cimetidine). The effects of concomitant administration of cimetidine on the pharmacokinetics of bupropion and its active metabolites were studied in 24 healthy young male volunteers. Following oral administration of two 150-mg ZYBAN tablets with and without 800 mg of cimetidine, the pharmacokinetics of bupropion and its hydroxy metabolite were unaffected. However, there were 16% and 32% increases, respectively, in the AUC and C_{max} of the combined moieties of threohydro- and erythrohydro- bupropion.

Drugs Metabolized by Cytochrome P450IID6 (CYP2D6): Many drugs, including most antidepressants (SSRIs, many tricyclics), beta-blockers, antiarrhythmics, and antipsychotics are metabolized by the CYP2D6 isoenzyme. Although bupropion is not metabolized by this isoenzyme, bupropion and hydroxybupropion are inhibitors of the CYP2D6 isoenzyme in vitro. In a study of 15 male subjects

Continued on next page

Product information on these pages is effective as of August 2004. Further information is available at: GlaxoSmithKline, PO Box 13398, Research Triangle Park, NC 27709. 1-888-825-5249. Corporate Web Site: www.gsk.com

Zyban—Cont.

(ages 19 to 35 years) who were extensive metabolizers of the CYP2D6 isoenzyme, daily doses of bupropion given as 150 mg twice daily followed by a single dose of 50 mg desipramine increased the C_{max}, AUC, and $t_{1/2}$ of desipramine by an average of approximately 2-, 5- and 2-fold, respectively. The effect was present for at least 7 days after the last dose of bupropion. Concomitant use of bupropion with other drugs metabolized by CYP2D6 has not been formally studied.

Therefore, co-administration of bupropion with drugs that are metabolized by CYP2D6 isoenzyme including certain antidepressants (e.g., nortriptyline, imipramine, desipramine, paroxetine, fluoxetine, sertraline), antipsychotics (e.g., haloperidol, risperidone, thioridazine), beta-blockers (e.g., metoprolol), and Type 1C antiarrhythmics (e.g., propafenone, flecainide), should be approached with caution and should be initiated at the lower end of the dose range of the concomitant medication. If bupropion is added to the treatment regimen of a patient already receiving a drug metabolized by CYP2D6, the need to decrease the dose of the original medication should be considered, particularly for those concomitant medications with a narrow therapeutic index.

MAO Inhibitors: Studies in animals demonstrate that the acute toxicity of bupropion is enhanced by the MAO inhibitor phenelzine (see CONTRAINDICATIONS).

Levodopa and Amantadine: Limited clinical data suggest a higher incidence of adverse experiences in patients receiving bupropion concurrently with either levodopa or amantadine. Administration of ZYBAN to patients receiving either levodopa or amantadine concurrently should be undertaken with caution, using small initial doses and gradual dose increases.

Drugs that Lower Seizure Threshold: Concurrent administration of ZYBAN and agents (e.g., antipsychotics, antidepressants, theophylline, systemic steroids, etc.) that lower seizure threshold should be undertaken only with extreme caution (see WARNINGS).

Nicotine Transdermal System: (see PRECAUTIONS: Cardiovascular Effects).

Smoking Cessation: Physiological changes resulting from smoking cessation itself, with or without treatment with ZYBAN, may alter the pharmacokinetics of some concomitant medications, which may require dosage adjustment. Blood concentrations of concomitant medications that are extensively metabolized, such as theophylline and warfarin, may be expected to increase following smoking cessation due to de-induction of hepatic enzymes.

Alcohol: In post-marketing experience, there have been rare reports of adverse neuropsychiatric events or reduced alcohol tolerance in patients who were drinking alcohol during treatment with ZYBAN. The consumption of alcohol during treatment with ZYBAN should be minimized or avoided (also see CONTRAINDICATIONS).

Carcinogenesis, Mutagenesis, Impairment of Fertility: Lifetime carcinogenicity studies were performed in rats and mice at doses up to 300 and 150 mg/kg per day, respectively. These doses are approximately 10 and 2 times the maximum recommended human dose (MRHD), respectively, on a mg/m² basis. In the rat study, there was an increase in nodular proliferative lesions of the liver at doses of 100 to 300 mg/kg per day (approximately 3 to 10 times the MRHD on a mg/m² basis); lower doses were not tested. The question of whether or not such lesions may be precursors of neoplasms of the liver is currently unresolved. Similar liver lesions were not seen in the mouse study, and no increase in malignant tumors of the liver and other organs was seen in either study.

Bupropion produced a positive response (2 to 3 times control mutation rate) in 2 of 5 strains in the Ames bacterial mutagenicity test and an increase in chromosomal aberrations in 1 of 3 in vivo rat bone marrow cytogenic studies.

A fertility study in rats at doses up to 300 mg/kg revealed no evidence of impaired fertility.

Pregnancy: ***Teratogenic Effects:*** Pregnancy Category B: Teratology studies have been performed at doses up to 450 mg/kg in rats (approximately 14 times the MRHD on a mg/m² basis), and at doses up to 150 mg/kg in rabbits (approximately 10 times the MRHD on a mg/m² basis). There is no evidence of impaired fertility or harm to the fetus due to bupropion. There are no adequate and well-controlled studies in pregnant women. Because animal reproduction studies are not always predictive of human response, this drug should be used during pregnancy only if clearly needed. Pregnant smokers should be encouraged to attempt cessation using educational and behavioral interventions before pharmacological approaches are used.

To monitor fetal outcomes of pregnant women exposed to ZYBAN, GlaxoSmithKline maintains a Bupropion Pregnancy Registry. Health care providers are encouraged to register patients by calling (800) 336-2176.

Labor and Delivery: The effect of ZYBAN on labor and delivery in humans is unknown.

Nursing Mothers: Bupropion and its metabolites are secreted in human milk. Because of the potential for serious adverse reactions in nursing infants from ZYBAN, a decision should be made whether to discontinue nursing or to discontinue the drug, taking into account the importance of the drug to the mother.

Pediatric Use: Clinical trials with ZYBAN did not include individuals under the age of 18. Therefore, the safety and efficacy in a pediatric smoking population have not been established. The immediate-release formulation of bupropion was studied in 104 pediatric patients (age range, 6 to 16) in clinical trials of the drug for other indications. Although generally well tolerated, the limited exposure is insufficient to assess the safety of bupropion in pediatric patients **(see WARNINGS—Clinical Worsening and Suicide Risk).**

Geriatric Use: Of the approximately 6,000 patients who participated in clinical trials with bupropion sustained-release tablets (depression and smoking cessation studies), 275 were 65 and over and 47 were 75 and over. In addition, several hundred patients 65 and over participated in clinical trials using the immediate-release formulation of bupropion (depression studies). No overall differences in safety or effectiveness were observed between these subjects and younger subjects, and other reported clinical experience has not identified differences in responses between the elderly and younger patients, but greater sensitivity of some older individuals cannot be ruled out.

A single-dose pharmacokinetic study demonstrated that the disposition of bupropion and its metabolites in elderly subjects was similar to that of younger subjects; however, another pharmacokinetic study, single and multiple dose, has suggested that the elderly are at increased risk for accumulation of bupropion and its metabolites (see CLINICAL PHARMACOLOGY).

Bupropion is extensively metabolized in the liver to active metabolites, which are further metabolized and excreted by the kidneys. The risk of toxic reaction to this drug may be greater in patients with impaired renal function. Because elderly patients are more likely to have decreased renal function, care should be taken in dose selection, and it may be useful to monitor renal function (see PRECAUTIONS: Renal Impairment and DOSAGE AND ADMINISTRATION).

ADVERSE REACTIONS (see also WARNINGS and PRECAUTIONS)

The information included under ADVERSE REACTIONS is based primarily on data from the dose-response trial and the comparative trial that evaluated ZYBAN for smoking cessation (see CLINICAL TRIALS). Information on additional adverse events associated with the sustained-release formulation of bupropion in depression trials, as well as the immediate-release formulation of bupropion, is included in a separate section (see Other Events Observed During the Clinical Development and Postmarketing Experience of Bupropion).

Adverse Events Associated With the Discontinuation of Treatment: Adverse events were sufficiently troublesome to cause discontinuation of treatment in 8% of the 706 patients treated with ZYBAN and 5% of the 313 patients treated with placebo. The more common events leading to discontinuation of treatment with ZYBAN included nervous system disturbances (3.4%), primarily tremors, and skin disorders (2.4%), primarily rashes.

Incidence of Commonly Observed Adverse Events: The most commonly observed adverse events consistently associated with the use of ZYBAN were dry mouth and insomnia. The most commonly observed adverse events were defined as those that consistently occurred at a rate of 5 percentage points greater than that for placebo across clinical studies.

Dose Dependency of Adverse Events: The incidence of dry mouth and insomnia may be related to the dose of ZYBAN. The occurrence of these adverse events may be minimized by reducing the dose of ZYBAN. In addition, insomnia may be minimized by avoiding bedtime doses.

Adverse Events Occurring at an Incidence of 1% or More Among Patients Treated With ZYBAN: Table 4 enumerates selected treatment-emergent adverse events from the dose-response trial that occurred at an incidence of 1% or more and were more common in patients treated with ZYBAN compared to those treated with placebo. Table 5 enumerates selected treatment-emergent adverse events from the comparative trial that occurred at an incidence of 1% or more and were more common in patients treated with ZYBAN, NTS, or the combination of ZYBAN and NTS compared to those treated with placebo. Reported adverse events were classified using a COSTART-based dictionary.

[See table 4 at left]

[See table 5 at top of next page]

ZYBAN was well-tolerated in the long-term maintenance trial, that evaluated chronic administration of ZYBAN for up to 1 year and in the COPD trial that evaluated patients with mild-to-moderate COPD for a 12-week period. Adverse events in both studies were quantitatively and qualitatively similar to those observed in the dose-response and comparative trials.

Other Events Observed During the Clinical Development and Postmarketing Experience of Bupropion: In addition to the adverse events noted above, the following events have been reported in clinical trials and postmarketing experience with the sustained-release formulation of bupropion in depressed patients and in nondepressed smokers, as well as in clinical trials and postmarketing clinical experience with the immediate-release formulation of bupropion.

Adverse events for which frequencies are provided below occurred in clinical trials with bupropion sustained-release. The frequencies represent the proportion of patients who experienced a treatment-emergent adverse event on at least one occasion in placebo-controlled studies for depression (n = 987) or smoking cessation (n = 1,013), or patients who experienced an adverse event requiring discontinuation of treatment in an open-label surveillance study with bupropion sustained-release tablets (n = 3,100). All treatment-emergent adverse events are included except those listed in Tables 4 and 5, those events listed in other safety-related sections of the insert, those adverse events subsumed under COSTART terms that are either overly general or excessively specified so as to be uninformative, those events not reasonably associated with the use of the drug, and those events that were not serious and occurred in fewer than 2 patients.

Events are further categorized by body system and listed in order of decreasing frequency according to the following

Table 4. Treatment-Emergent Adverse Event Incidence in the Dose-Response Trial*

Body System/ Adverse Experience	ZYBAN 100 to 300 mg/day (n = 461) %	Placebo (n = 150) %
Body (General)		
Neck pain	2	<1
Allergic reaction	1	0
Cardiovascular		
Hot flashes	1	0
Hypertension	1	<1
Digestive		
Dry mouth	11	5
Increased appetite	2	<1
Anorexia	1	<1
Musculoskeletal		
Arthralgia	4	3
Myalgia	2	1
Nervous system		
Insomnia	31	21
Dizziness	8	7
Tremor	2	1
Somnolence	2	1
Thinking abnormality	1	0
Respiratory		
Bronchitis	2	0
Skin		
Pruritus	3	<1
Rash	3	<1
Dry skin	2	0
Urticaria	1	0
Special senses		
Taste perversion	2	<1

*Selected adverse events with an incidence of at least 1% of patients treated with ZYBAN and more frequent than in the placebo group.

definitions of frequency: Frequent adverse events are defined as those occurring in at least 1/100 patients. Infrequent adverse events are those occurring in 1/100 to 1/1,000 patients, while rare events are those occurring in less than 1/1,000 patients.

Adverse events for which frequencies are not provided occurred in clinical trials or postmarketing experience with bupropion. Only those adverse events not previously listed for sustained-release bupropion are included. The extent to which these events may be associated with ZYBAN is unknown.

Body (General): Frequent were asthenia, fever, and headache. Infrequent were back pain, chills, inguinal hernia, musculoskeletal chest pain, pain, and photosensitivity. Rare was malaise. Also observed were arthralgia, myalgia, and fever with rash and other symptoms suggestive of delayed hypersensitivity. These symptoms may resemble serum sickness (see PRECAUTIONS).

Cardiovascular: Infrequent were flushing, migraine, postural hypotension, stroke, tachycardia, and vasodilation. Rare was syncope. Also observed were cardiovascular disorder, complete AV block, extrasystoles, hypotension, hypertension (in some cases severe, see PRECAUTIONS), myocardial infarction, phlebitis, and pulmonary embolism.

Digestive: Frequent were dyspepsia, flatulence, and vomiting. Infrequent were abnormal liver function, bruxism, dysphagia, gastric reflux, gingivitis, glossitis, jaundice, and stomatitis. Rare was edema of tongue. Also observed were colitis, esophagitis, gastrointestinal hemorrhage, gum hemorrhage, hepatitis, increased salivation, intestinal perforation, liver damage, pancreatitis, stomach ulcer, and stool abnormality.

Endocrine: Also observed were hyperglycemia, hypoglycemia, and syndrome of inappropriate antidiuretic hormone.

Hemic and Lymphatic: Infrequent was ecchymosis. Also observed were anemia, leukocytosis, leukopenia, lymphadenopathy, pancytopenia, and thrombocytopenia. Altered PT and/or INR, infrequently associated with hemorrhagic or thrombotic complications, were observed when bupropion was co-administered with warfarin.

Metabolic and Nutritional: Infrequent were edema, increased weight, and peripheral edema. Also observed was glycosuria.

Musculoskeletal: Infrequent were leg cramps and twitching. Also observed were arthritis and muscle rigidity/fever/rhabdomyolysis, and muscle weakness.

Nervous System: Frequent were agitation, depression, and irritability. Infrequent were abnormal coordination, CNS stimulation, confusion, decreased libido, decreased memory, depersonalization, emotional lability, hostility, hyperkinesia, hypertonia, hypesthesia, paresthesia, suicidal ideation, and vertigo. Rare were amnesia, ataxia, derealization, and hypomania. Also observed were abnormal electroencephalogram (EEG), akinesia, aphasia, coma, delirium, delusions, dysarthria, dyskinesia, dystonia, euphoria, extrapyramidal syndrome, hallucinations, hypokinesia, increased libido, manic reaction, neuralgia, neuropathy, paranoid reaction, and unmasking tardive dyskinesia.

Respiratory: Rare was bronchospasm. Also observed was pneumonia.

Skin: Frequent was sweating. Infrequent was acne and dry skin. Rare was maculopapular rash. Also observed were alopecia, angioedema, exfoliative dermatitis, and hirsutism.

Special Senses: Frequent was amblyopia. Infrequent were accommodation abnormality and dry eye. Also observed were deafness, diplopia, and mydriasis.

Urogenital: Frequent was urinary frequency. Infrequent were impotence, polyuria, and urinary urgency. Also observed were abnormal ejaculation, cystitis, dyspareunia, dysuria, gynecomastia, menopause, painful erection, prostate disorder, salpingitis, urinary incontinence, urinary retention, urinary tract disorder, and vaginitis.

DRUG ABUSE AND DEPENDENCE

ZYBAN is likely to have a low abuse potential.

Humans: There have been few reported cases of drug dependence and withdrawal symptoms associated with the immediate-release formulation of bupropion. In human studies of abuse liability, individuals experienced with drugs of abuse reported that bupropion produced a feeling of euphoria and desirability. In these subjects, a single dose of 400 mg (1.33 times the recommended daily dose) of bupropion produced mild amphetamine-like effects compared to placebo on the Morphine-Benzedrine Subscale of the Addiction Research Center Inventories (ARCI), which is indicative of euphorigenic properties and a score intermediate between placebo and amphetamine on the Liking Scale of the ARCI.

Animals: Studies in rodents and primates have shown that bupropion exhibits some pharmacologic actions common to psychostimulants. In rodents, it has been shown to increase locomotor activity, elicit a mild stereotyped behavioral response, and increase rates of responding in several schedule-controlled behavior paradigms. In primate models to assess the positive reinforcing effects of psychoactive drugs, bupropion was self-administered intravenously. In rats, bupropion produced amphetamine- and cocaine-like discriminative stimulus effects in drug discrimination paradigms used to characterize the subjective effects of psychoactive drugs.

The possibility that bupropion may induce dependence should be kept in mind when evaluating the desirability of including the drug in smoking cessation programs of individual patients.

Table 5. Treatment-Emergent Adverse Event Incidence in the Comparative Trial*

Adverse Experience (COSTART Term)	ZYBAN 300 mg/day (n = 243) %	Nicotine Transdermal System (NTS) 21 mg/day (n = 243) %	ZYBAN and NTS (n = 244) %	Placebo (n = 159) %
Body				
Abdominal pain	3	4	1	1
Accidental injury	2	2	1	1
Chest pain	<1	1	3	1
Neck pain	2	1	<1	0
Facial edema	<1	0	1	0
Cardiovascular				
Hypertension	1	<1	2	0
Palpitations	2	0	1	0
Digestive				
Nausea	9	7	11	4
Dry mouth	10	4	9	4
Constipation	8	4	9	3
Diarrhea	4	4	3	1
Anorexia	3	1	5	1
Mouth ulcer	2	1	1	1
Thirst	<1	<1	2	0
Musculoskeletal				
Myalgia	4	3	5	3
Arthralgia	5	3	3	2
Nervous system				
Insomnia	40	28	45	18
Dream abnormality	5	18	13	3
Anxiety	8	6	9	6
Disturbed concentration	9	3	9	4
Dizziness	10	2	8	6
Nervousness	4	<1	2	2
Tremor	1	<1	2	0
Dysphoria	<1	1	2	1
Respiratory				
Rhinitis	12	11	9	8
Increased cough	3	5	<1	1
Pharyngitis	3	2	3	0
Sinusitis	2	2	2	1
Dyspnea	1	0	2	1
Epistaxis	2	1	1	0
Skin				
Application site reaction†	11	17	15	7
Rash	4	3	3	2
Pruritus	3	1	5	1
Urticaria	2	0	2	0
Special senses				
Taste perversion	3	1	3	2
Tinnitus	1	0	<1	0

*Selected adverse events with an incidence of at least 1% of patients treated with either ZYBAN, NTS, or the combination of ZYBAN and NTS and more frequent than in the placebo group.

†Patients randomized to ZYBAN or placebo received placebo patches.

OVERDOSAGE

Human Overdose Experience: There has been very limited experience with overdosage of the sustained-release formulation of bupropion; 3 such cases were reported during clinical trials in depressed patients. One patient ingested 3,000 mg of bupropion sustained-release tablets and vomited quickly after the overdose; the patient experienced blurred vision and lightheadedness. A second patient ingested a "handful" of bupropion sustained-release tablets and experienced confusion, lethargy, nausea, jitteriness, and seizure. A third patient ingested 3,600 mg of bupropion sustained-release tablets and a bottle of wine; the patient experienced nausea, visual hallucinations, and "grogginess." None of the patients experienced further sequelae.

There has been extensive experience with overdosages of the immediate-release formulation of bupropion. Thirteen overdoses occurred during clinical trials in depressed patients. Twelve patients ingested 850 to 4,200 mg and recovered without significant sequelae. Another patient who ingested 9,000 mg of the immediate-release formulation of bupropion and 300 mg of tranylcypromine experienced a grand mal seizure and recovered without further sequelae. Since introduction, overdoses of up to 17,500 mg of the immediate-release formulation of bupropion have been reported. Seizure was reported in approximately one third of all cases. Other serious reactions reported with overdoses of the immediate-release formulation of bupropion alone included hallucinations, loss of consciousness, and sinus tachycardia. Fever, muscle rigidity, rhabdomyolysis, hypotension, stupor, coma, and respiratory failure have been reported when the immediate-release formulation of bupropion was part of multiple drug overdoses.

Although most patients recovered without sequelae, deaths associated with overdoses of the immediate-release formulation of bupropion alone have been reported rarely in patients ingesting massive doses of the drug. Multiple uncontrolled seizures, bradycardia, cardiac failure, and cardiac arrest prior to death were reported in these patients.

Overdosage Management: Ensure an adequate airway, oxygenation, and ventilation. Monitor cardiac rhythm and vital signs. EEG monitoring is also recommended for the first 48 hours post-ingestion. General supportive and symptomatic measures are also recommended. Induction of emesis is not recommended. Gastric lavage with a large-bore orogastric tube with appropriate airway protection, if needed, may be indicated if performed soon after ingestion or in symptomatic patients.

Activated charcoal should be administered. There is no experience with the use of forced diuresis, dialysis, hemoperfusion, or exchange transfusion in the management of bupropion overdoses. No specific antidotes for bupropion are known.

Due to the dose-related risk of seizures with ZYBAN, hospitalization following suspected overdose should be considered. Based on studies in animals, it is recommended that seizures be treated with intravenous benzodiazepine administration and other supportive measures, as appropriate.

In managing overdosage, consider the possibility of multiple drug involvement. The physician should consider contacting a poison control center for additional information on the treatment of any overdose. Telephone numbers for certified poison control centers are listed in the *Physicians' Desk Reference* (PDR).

DOSAGE AND ADMINISTRATION

ZYBAN: ***Usual Dosage for Adults:*** The recommended and maximum dose of ZYBAN is 300 mg/day, given as 150 mg twice daily. Dosing should begin at 150 mg/day given every day for the first 3 days, followed by a dose increase for most patients to the recommended usual dose of 300 mg/day. There should be an interval of at least 8 hours between successive doses. Doses above 300 mg/day should not be used

Continued on next page

Product information on these pages is effective as of August 2004. Further information is available at: GlaxoSmithKline, PO Box 13398, Research Triangle Park, NC 27709. 1-888-825-5249. Corporate Web Site: www.gsk.com

Zyban—Cont.

(see WARNINGS). ZYBAN should be swallowed whole and not crushed, divided, or chewed. Treatment with ZYBAN should be initiated **while the patient is still smoking,** since approximately 1 week of treatment is required to achieve steady-state blood levels of bupropion. Patients should set a "target quit date" within the first 2 weeks of treatment with ZYBAN, generally in the second week. Treatment with ZYBAN should be continued for 7 to 12 weeks; longer treatment should be guided by the relative benefits and risks for individual patients. If a patient has not made significant progress towards abstinence by the seventh week of therapy with ZYBAN, it is unlikely that he or she will quit during that attempt, and treatment should probably be discontinued. Conversely, a patient who successfully quits after 7 to 12 weeks of treatment should be considered for ongoing therapy with ZYBAN. Dose tapering of ZYBAN is not required when discontinuing treatment. It is important that patients continue to receive counseling and support throughout treatment with ZYBAN, and for a period of time thereafter.

Individualization of Therapy: Patients are more likely to quit smoking and remain abstinent if they are seen frequently and receive support from their physicians or other health care professionals. It is important to ensure that patients read the instructions provided to them and have their questions answered. Physicians should review the patient's overall smoking cessation program that includes treatment with ZYBAN. Patients should be advised of the importance of participating in the behavioral interventions, counseling, and/or support services to be used in conjunction with ZYBAN. See information for patients at the end of the package insert.

The goal of therapy with ZYBAN is complete abstinence. If a patient has not made significant progress towards abstinence by the seventh week of therapy with ZYBAN, it is unlikely that he or she will quit during that attempt, and treatment should probably be discontinued.

Patients who fail to quit smoking during an attempt may benefit from interventions to improve their chances for success on subsequent attempts. Patients who are unsuccessful should be evaluated to determine why they failed. A new quit attempt should be encouraged when factors that contributed to failure can be eliminated or reduced, and conditions are more favorable.

Maintenance: Nicotine dependence is a chronic condition. Some patients may need continuous treatment. Systematic evaluation of ZYBAN 300 mg/day for maintenance therapy demonstrated that treatment for up to 6 months was efficacious. Whether to continue treatment with ZYBAN for periods longer than 12 weeks for smoking cessation must be determined for individual patients.

Combination Treatment With ZYBAN and a Nicotine Transdermal System (NTS): Combination treatment with ZYBAN and NTS may be prescribed for smoking cessation. The prescriber should review the complete prescribing information for both ZYBAN and NTS before using combination treatment. See also CLINICAL TRIALS for methods and dosing used in the ZYBAN and NTS combination trial. Monitoring for treatment-emergent hypertension in patients treated with the combination of ZYBAN and NTS is recommended.

Dosage Adjustment for Patients with Impaired Hepatic Function: ZYBAN should be used with extreme caution in patients with severe hepatic cirrhosis. The dose should not exceed 150 mg every other day in these patients. ZYBAN should be used with caution in patients with hepatic impairment (including mild to moderate hepatic cirrhosis) and a reduced frequency of dosing should be considered in patients with mild to moderate hepatic cirrhosis (see CLINICAL PHARMACOLOGY, WARNINGS, and PRECAUTIONS).

Dosage Adjustment for Patients with Impaired Renal Function: ZYBAN should be used with caution in patients with renal impairment and a reduced frequency of dosing should be considered (see CLINICAL PHARMACOLOGY and PRECAUTIONS).

HOW SUPPLIED

ZYBAN Sustained-Release Tablets, 150 mg of bupropion hydrochloride, are purple, round, biconvex, film-coated tablets printed with "ZYBAN 150" in bottles of 60 (NDC 0173-0556-02) tablets and the ZYBAN Advantage Pack® containing 1 bottle of 60 (NDC 0173-0556-01) tablets.

Store at controlled room temperature, 20° to 25°C (68° to 77°F) (see USP). Dispense in tight, light-resistant containers as defined in the USP.

PATIENT INFORMATION

The following wording is contained in a tear-off leaflet provided for patients.

Information for the Patient

ZYBAN® (bupropion hydrochloride) Sustained-Release Tablets

Please read this information before you start taking ZYBAN. Also read this leaflet each time you renew your prescription, in case anything has changed. This information is not intended to take the place of discussions between you and your doctor. You and your doctor should discuss ZYBAN as part of your plan to stop smoking. Your doctor has prescribed ZYBAN for your use only. Do not let anyone else use your ZYBAN.

IMPORTANT WARNING:

There is a chance that approximately 1 out of every 1,000 people taking bupropion hydrochloride, the active ingredient in ZYBAN, will have a seizure. The chance of this happening increases if you:

- have or have had a seizure disorder (for example, epilepsy);
- have or have had an eating disorder (for example, bulimia or anorexia nervosa);
- are abruptly discontinuing use of alcohol or sedatives (including benzodiazepines);
- take more than the recommended amount of ZYBAN; or
- take other medicines with the same active ingredient that is in ZYBAN, such as WELLBUTRIN® (bupropion hydrochloride) Tablets, WELLBUTRIN SR® (bupropion hydrochloride) Sustained-Release Tablets, and WELLBUTRIN XL (bupropion hydrochloride extended-release tablets). (These medicines are used to treat depression.)

You can reduce the chance of experiencing a seizure by following your doctor's directions on how to take ZYBAN. If you experience a seizure while taking ZYBAN, stop taking the tablets immediately, contact your doctor, and do not restart ZYBAN. In addition, tell your doctor if you have or have had other medical conditions. You should also discuss with your doctor whether ZYBAN is right for you.

Important information I should know and share with my family about taking antidepressants.

Although ZYBAN is not a treatment for depression, it contains the same active ingredient as WELLBUTRIN, WELLBUTRIN SR, and WELLBUTRIN XL that are used for depression. Therefore, you should be aware of the following information. Patients taking antidepressants, and their families, should watch out for worsening depression or thoughts of suicide. Also watch out for sudden or severe changes in feelings such as feeling anxious, agitated, panicky, irritable, hostile, aggressive, impulsive, severely restless, overly excited and hyperactive, or not being able to sleep. If this happens, especially at the beginning of antidepressant treatment or after a change in dose, call your doctor.

1. What is ZYBAN?

ZYBAN is a prescription medicine to help people quit smoking. Studies have shown that more than one third of people quit smoking for at least 1 month while taking ZYBAN and participating in a patient support program. For many patients, ZYBAN reduces withdrawal symptoms and the urge to smoke. ZYBAN should be used with a patient support program. It is important to participate in the behavioral program, counseling, or other support program your health care professional recommends.

2. Who should not take ZYBAN?

You should not take ZYBAN if you:

- have or have had a seizure disorder (for example, epilepsy);
- are already taking WELLBUTRIN, WELLBUTRIN SR, WELLBUTRIN XL, or any other medicines that contain bupropion hydrochloride;
- have or have had an eating disorder (for example, bulimia or anorexia nervosa);
- are abruptly discontinuing use of alcohol or sedatives (including benzodiazepines);
- are currently taking or have recently taken a monoamine oxidase inhibitor (MAOI); or
- are allergic to bupropion.

3. Can I take ZYBAN if I have mild-to-moderate chronic bronchitis and/or emphysema (also called chronic obstructive pulmonary disease or COPD)?

Yes, ZYBAN combined with a behavior modification program has been shown to help people with COPD quit smoking. It is important to participate in the behavior program, counseling, or other support program your health care professional recommends.

4. Are there special concerns for women?

ZYBAN is not recommended for women who are pregnant or breastfeeding. Women should notify their doctor if they become pregnant or intend to become pregnant while taking ZYBAN.

5. Are there any concerns for patients with liver or kidney problems?

If you have liver or kidney problems, tell your doctor before taking ZYBAN. Depending on the severity of your condition, your doctor may need to adjust your dosage.

6. How should I take ZYBAN?

- You should take ZYBAN as directed by your doctor. The usual recommended dosing is to take one 150-mg tablet in the morning for the first 3 days. On the fourth day, begin taking one 150-mg tablet in the morning and one 150-mg tablet in the early evening. Doses should be taken at least 8 hours apart.
- **Never take an "extra" dose of ZYBAN.** If you forget to take a dose, do not take an extra tablet to "catch up" for the dose you forgot. Wait and take your next tablet at the regular time. Do not take more tablets than your doctor prescribed. This is important so you do not increase your chance of having a seizure.
- It is important to swallow ZYBAN Tablets whole. Do not chew, divide, or crush tablets.

7. How long should I take ZYBAN?

Most people should take ZYBAN for at least 7 to 12 weeks. Some people may need to take ZYBAN for a longer period of time to assist in their smoking cessation efforts. Follow your doctor's instructions.

8. When should I stop smoking?

It takes about 1 week for ZYBAN to reach the right levels in your body to be effective. So, to maximize your chance of quitting, you should not stop smoking until you have been taking ZYBAN for 1 week. You should set a date to stop smoking during the second week you're taking ZYBAN.

9. Can I smoke while taking ZYBAN?

It is not physically dangerous to smoke and use ZYBAN at the same time. However, continuing to smoke after the date you set to stop smoking will seriously reduce your chance of breaking your smoking habit.

10. Can ZYBAN be used at the same time as nicotine patches?

Yes, ZYBAN and nicotine patches can be used at the same time but should only be used together under the supervision of your doctor. Using ZYBAN and nicotine patches together may raise your blood pressure, sometimes severely. Tell your doctor if you are planning to use nicotine replacement therapy because your doctor will probably want to check your blood pressure regularly to make sure that it stays within acceptable levels.

DO NOT SMOKE AT ANY TIME if you are using a nicotine patch or any other nicotine product along with ZYBAN. It is possible to get too much nicotine and have serious side effects.

11. What are possible side effects of ZYBAN?

Like all medicines, ZYBAN may cause side effects. Do not rely on this summary alone for information about side effects. Your doctor can discuss with you a more complete list of side effects that may be relevant to you.

- Hypertension (high blood pressure), in some cases severe, has been reported in patients taking ZYBAN alone and in combination with nicotine replacement therapy (for example, a nicotine patch, see Question #10).
- The most common side effects include dry mouth and difficulty sleeping. These side effects are generally mild and often disappear after a few weeks. If you have difficulty sleeping, avoid taking your medicine too close to bedtime.
- The most common side effects that caused people to stop taking ZYBAN during clinical studies were shakiness and skin rash.
- Stop taking ZYBAN and contact your doctor or health care professional if you have signs of an allergic reaction such as a rash, hives, or difficulty in breathing. It is not possible to predict whether a mild rash will develop into a more serious reaction. Therefore, if you experience a skin rash, hives, fever, swollen lymph glands, painful sores in the mouth or around the eyes, or swelling of lips or tongue, tell a doctor immediately, since these symptoms may be the first signs of a serious reaction. Discuss any other troublesome side effects with your doctor.
- Use caution before driving a car or operating complex, hazardous machinery until you know if ZYBAN affects your ability to perform these tasks.

12. Can I drink alcohol while I am taking ZYBAN?

It is best to not drink alcohol at all or to drink very little while taking ZYBAN. If you drink a lot of alcohol and suddenly stop, you may increase your chance of having a seizure. Some people have reported lower alcohol tolerance during treatment with ZYBAN. Therefore, it is important to discuss your use of alcohol with your doctor before you begin taking ZYBAN.

13. Will ZYBAN affect other medicines I am taking?

ZYBAN may affect other medicines you're taking. It is important not to take medicines that may increase the chance for you to have a seizure. Therefore, you should make sure that your doctor knows about all medicines—prescription or over-the-counter—you are taking or plan to take.

14. Do ZYBAN Tablets have a characteristic odor?

ZYBAN Tablets may have a characteristic odor. If present, this odor is normal.

15. How should I store ZYBAN?

- Store ZYBAN at room temperature, out of direct sunlight.
- Keep ZYBAN in a tightly closed container.
- Keep ZYBAN out of the reach of children.

This summary provides important information about ZYBAN. This summary cannot replace the more detailed information that you need from your doctor. If you have any questions or concerns about either ZYBAN or smoking cessation, talk to your doctor or other health care professional.

Manufactured by DSM Pharmaceuticals, Inc.
Greenville, NC 27834 for
GlaxoSmithKline, Research Triangle Park, NC 27709

April 2004/RL-2078

Shown in Product Identification Guide, page 318

GlaxoSmithKline Consumer Healthcare, L.P.
POST OFFICE BOX 1467
1000 GSK DRIVE
MOON TOWNSHIP, PA 15108

Direct Inquiries to:
1-800-245-1040 weekdays

COMMIT® **OTC**
[ko-mĭt]
nicotine polacrilex lozenge

DRUG FACTS

ACTIVE INGREDIENT *Purpose*
(in each lozenge)
Nicotine polacrilex, 2mg and 4mg .... Stop smoking aid

USE
- reduces withdrawal symptoms, including nicotine craving, associated with quitting smoking

WARNINGS

If you are pregnant or breast-feeding, only use this medicine on the advice of your health care provider. Smoking can seriously harm your child. Try to stop smoking without using any nicotine replacement medicine. This medicine is believed to be safer than smoking. However, the risks to your child from this medicine are not fully known.

Do not use
- If you continue to smoke, chew tobacco, use snuff, or use a nicotine patch or other nicotine containing products

Ask a doctor before use if you have
- heart disease, recent heart attack, or irregular heartbeat. Nicotine can increase your heart rate.
- high blood pressure not controlled with medication. Nicotine can increase your blood pressure.
- stomach ulcer or diabetes

Ask a doctor or pharmacist before use if you are
- using a non-nicotine stop smoking drug
- taking prescription medicine for depression or asthma. Your prescription dose may need to be adjusted.

Stop use and ask a doctor if
- mouth problems occur
- persistent indigestion or severe sore throat occurs
- irregular heartbeat or palpitations occur
- you get symptoms of nicotine overdose such as nausea, vomiting, dizziness, diarrhea, weakness and rapid heartbeat

Keep out of reach of children and pets. Nicotine lozenges may have enough nicotine to make children and pets sick. If you need to remove the lozenge, wrap it in paper and throw away in the trash. In case of overdose, get medical help or contact a Poison Control Center right away.

DIRECTIONS
- **if you are under 18 years of age, ask a doctor before use**
- before using this product, read the enclosed User's Guide for complete directions and other important information
- stop smoking completely when you begin using the lozenge

For Commit® 2mg
- **if you smoke your first cigarette within 30 minutes of waking up,** use 4 mg nicotine lozenge
- **if you smoke your first cigarette more than 30 minutes after waking up,** use 2mg nicotine lozenge according to the 12 week schedule below.

For Commit® 4mg
- **If you smoke your first cigarette within 30 minutes of waking up,** use 4mg nicotine lozenge according to the following 12 week schedule:

Weeks 1 to 6	Weeks 7 to 9	Weeks 10 to 12
1 lozenge every 1 to 2 hours	1 lozenge every 2 to 4 hours	1 lozenge every 4 to 8 hours

- **nicotine lozenge is a medicine and must be used a certain way to get the best results**
- place the lozenge in your mouth and allow the lozenge to slowly dissolve (about 20-30 minutes). Minimize swallowing. **Do not chew or swallow lozenge.**
- you may feel a warm or tingling sensation
- occasionally move the lozenge from one side of your mouth to the other until completely dissolved (about 20-30 minutes)
- do not eat or drink 15 minutes before using or while the lozenge is in your mouth
- to improve your chances of quitting, use at least 9 lozenges per day for the first 6 weeks
- do not use more than one lozenge at a time or continuously use one lozenge after another since this may cause you hiccups, heartburn, nausea or other side effects
- **do not use more than 5 lozenges in 6 hours. Do not use more than 20 lozenges per day.**
- stop using the nicotine lozenge at the end of 12 weeks. If you still feel the need to use nicotine lozenges, talk to your doctor.

OTHER INFORMATION
- Phenylketonurics: Contains Phenylalanine 3.4 mg per lozenge
- store at 20 - 25 °C (68 - 77°F)
- protect from light

INACTIVE INGREDIENTS
aspartame, calcium polycarbophil, flavor, magnesium stearate, mannitol, potassium bicarbonate, sodium alginate, sodium carbonate, xanthan gum

Questions or comments? call weekdays 1-888-569-1743 (10:00am - 4:30pm EST)

INCREASE YOUR SUCCESS IN QUITTING:
1. You must be motivated to quit.
2. **Use Enough** - Use **at least 9 lozenges** of Commit per day during the first six weeks.
3. **Use Long Enough** - Use Commit for the full 12 weeks.
4. **Use With a Support Program** as directed in the enclosed User's Guide.

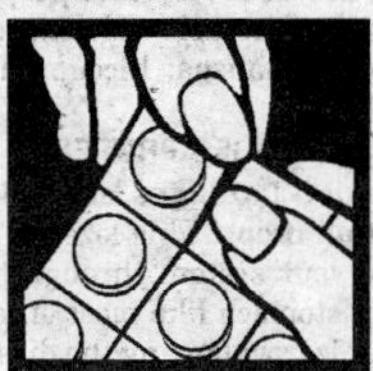

To remove the lozenge, tear off single unit.

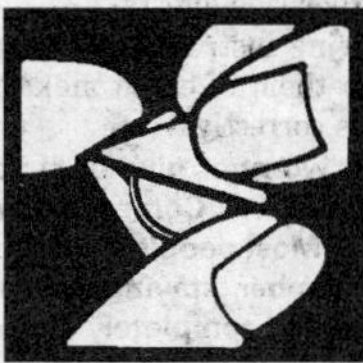

Peel off backing starting at corner with loose edge.

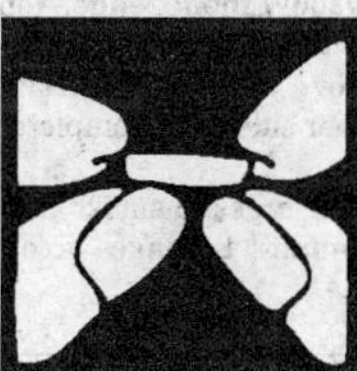

Push lozenge through foil.

*The American Cancer Society supports the use of stop smoking aids and counseling as effective tools when quitting smoking but does not endorse any specific product. GlaxoSmithKline pays a fee to the American Cancer Society for the use of its logo.

Distributed By:
GlaxoSmithKline Consumer Healthcare, L.P.
Moon Township, PA 15108, Made in the U.S.A.

Commit®
nicotine polacrilex lozenge
2mg and 4mg User's Guide

How to Use Commit® Lozenges and Tips to Help You Quit Smoking.
- **Not for sale to those under 18 years of age.**
- **Proof of age required.**
- **Not for sale in vending machines or from any source where proof of age cannot be verified.**

WALLET CARD
My most important reasons to quit smoking are:

____
____
____
____
____

WALLET CARD
WHERE TO CALL FOR HELP:
American Lung Association
1-800-586-4872
American Cancer Society
1-800-227-2345
American Heart Association
1-800-242-8721
Quitting Buddy or Friend who has Quit
_ _ _ _ _ _ _ _ _ _ _ _ _ _ _ _ _

PLANNING YOUR SUCCESS
1) The key to accomplishing anything important is commitment. When it comes to quitting smoking, that is especially true. **Commit®** Lozenges can help if you really want to quit. **Commit®** Lozenges help reduce withdrawal symptoms including nicotine craving associated with quitting smoking.
2) Your chances of staying off cigarettes are much better if you start with at least 9 **Commit®** Lozenges daily. For best results, use the lozenges on a regular schedule (as outlined in this User's Guide).
3) Stop smoking completely when you start using **Commit®** Lozenges. Even a single cigarette is likely to put you right back to square one.
4) This User's Guide outlines a 12-week plan for **Commit®** Lozenges. Even though you may feel confident about your non-smoking status after a few weeks, it's important to stick with the plan to help you remain smoke free.
5) **Commit®** Lozenges work best when used together with a support plan. See insert between pages 8 and 9 for instructions on enrollment in the Committed Quitters Personalized Stop Smoking Plan.
6) After the first six weeks, start using fewer **Commit®** Lozenges, as directed in the instructions, so you can become smoke-and nicotine-free by the end of the 12 week plan.
7) If you have questions about using **Commit®** Lozenges, call 1-888-569-1743 weekdays (10:00am–4:30pm EST), or talk to your pharmacist or family doctor.

YES! YOU WANT TO QUIT.
Wonderful. You've made the most important decision of all, to stop smoking. And by choosing **Commit®** Lozenges to help you, you're starting on the right path. Now remember, using **Commit®** doesn't just mean taking a **Commit®** Lozenge. It means setting and following a program like the one we suggest in this User's Guide.
Your own success depends on your effort, your level of addiction to tobacco, and your commitment to following your program.

LET'S FACE IT.
Quitting smoking isn't easy! You or someone you know may have tried unsuccessfully. That's okay. It's hard to stop smoking the first time you try. The important part is to learn from your previous attempts, consider what went wrong and keep trying to quit until you succeed.
Look to this User's Guide for support as you undergo this terrific task. The guide includes important information on how to use **Commit®** Lozenges and also gives you tips to help you stop smoking. Refer back to it often for advice, answers, and encouragement to help you stay on track.

GET MOTIVATED. STAY MOTIVATED.
Everyone has a reason for quitting—whether you're concerned about your health, your appearance, family or peer pressure, or the effect of secondhand smoke on your loved ones—all of the above, or something else entirely. Whatever your reasons, write them down. There's a wallet card inside the back cover of this User's Guide. Write your reasons on the card and carry it with you. When you have an urge to smoke or experience a difficult moment it can help you focus on your reasons for quitting. Lots of people quit with a co-worker, spouse or friend and use them as a quitting buddy. You can help each other out by providing extra encouragement in tough moments.
There may be support groups in your area for people trying to quit. Call your local chapter of the American Lung Association, American Cancer Society or American Heart Association for further information. Toll free phone numbers are printed on the wallet card on the back cover of this User's Guide.

UNDERSTANDING THE DOUBLE-EDGED SWORD.
Smoking has two addictive components, a physical and a mental need for the nicotine in tobacco. You need to conquer both to succeed. **Commit®** Lozenges can ease your physical nicotine addiction. But your readiness and resolve are necessary to help overcome the mental side of your cigarette dependence. So once you're ready, it's time to begin. But first, read and consider the following important warnings.

IMPORTANT WARNINGS
This product is only for those who want to stop smoking.
If you are pregnant or breast-feeding, only use this medicine on the advice of your health care provider. Smoking can seriously harm your child. Try to stop smoking without using any nicotine replacement medicine. This medicine is believed to be safer than smoking. However, the risks to your child from this medicine are not fully known.

Do not use
- if you continue to smoke, chew tobacco, use snuff, or use a nicotine patch or other nicotine containing products.

Ask a doctor before use if you have
- heart disease, recent heart attack or irregular heartbeat. Nicotine can increase your heart rate.
- high blood pressure not controlled with medication. Nicotine can increase your blood pressure.
- stomach ulcers or diabetes.

Ask a doctor or pharmacist before use if you are
- using a non-nicotine stop smoking drug
- taking prescription medicine for depression or asthma. Your prescription dose may need to be adjusted.

Continued on next page

Product information on these pages is effective as of August 2004. Further information is available at: GlaxoSmithKline, PO Box 13398, Research Triangle Park, NC 27709. 1-888-825-5249. Corporate Web Site: www.gsk.com

Commit—Cont.

Stop use and ask a doctor if

- mouth problems occur
- persistent indigestion or severe sore throat occurs
- irregular heartbeat or palpitations occur
- you get symptoms of nicotine overdose such as nausea, vomiting, dizziness, diarrhea, weakness and rapid heartbeat

Keep out of reach of children and pets.

Nicotine lozenges may have enough nicotine to make children and pets sick. If you need to remove the lozenge, wrap it in paper and throw away in the trash. In case of overdose, get medical help or contact a Poison Control Center right away.

YOU'RE READY TO START.

Okay, you're ready. To become a non- smoker, start today. Now before you do anything else, you have a bit of planning to do. Read this User's Guide all the way through. You want to make sure you bought the right dose to start. If you typically smoke **your first cigarette within 30 minutes of waking up,** use the 4mg **Commit®** Lozenges. If you smoke your **first cigarette more than 30 minutes after waking up,** use the 2mg **Commit®** Lozenges. Next, plan your quitting schedule. Get a calendar to follow your progress and mark the following four important dates (see the stickers in the middle of this booklet).

THE PROGRAM

STEP 1. (Weeks 1-6) Starting on your quit date it's best to use at least 9 Commit® Lozenges each day, one every 1-2 hours.

First choose the day you plan to quit (make it soon). Place the Step 1 sticker on this date. That's the day you will stop smoking cigarettes completely and start using **Commit®** Lozenges to calm your cravings for nicotine and help you stay smoke free. Prior to the quit date, get rid of all your cigarettes to remove temptations and make it more difficult to start smoking again.

Use a **Commit®** Lozenge every 1 to 2 hours and at least 9 lozenges each day for the first 6 weeks to help prevent unexpected cravings and improve your chances of quitting. **These aren't ordinary lozenges.** Place the lozenge in your mouth and allow the lozenge to slowly dissolve (about 20-30 minutes). Minimize swallowing. **Do not chew or swallow the lozenge.** You may feel a warm or tingling sensation. Occasionally move the lozenge from one side of your mouth to the other until completely dissolved (about 20 to 30 minutes). **Remember to read the instructions on page 7 before you take your first Commit® Lozenge.**

STEP 2. (The next three weeks, that is weeks 7-9). At the beginning of week 7 start using fewer Commit® Lozenges, one every 2-4 hours.

After six weeks, you should wait a little longer between lozenges, one lozenge every two to four hours. This will help you gradually use fewer **Commit®** Lozenges. Put the Step 2 sticker on the first day of week 7 to help remind you when to start reducing the number of **Commit®** Lozenges you take.

STEP 3. (The last three weeks, that is weeks 10-12). At the beginning of week 10, reduce Commit® Lozenge use even further, one every 4-8 hours.

At the beginning of week 10 further decrease the number of **Commit®** Lozenges you use each day to reduce the amount of nicotine you get. You should do this by using one lozenge every 4 to 8 hours. Put the Step 3 sticker on the first day of week 10 so you know when you should be starting this last step to becoming smoke and nicotine-free.

END. At the end of week 12 stop using Commit® Lozenges to become both cigarette and nicotine-free.

Put the "EX-SMOKER" sticker on your calendar on the date 12 weeks after the day you stopped smoking and started using **Commit®** Lozenges. You should not use **Commit®** Lozenges beyond this date.

BE PREPARED.

Since smoking is an addiction, it is hard to quit. Even after you stop, there will be times when you WANT a cigarette, sometimes strongly. (See also section on "Challenges To Watch For"). The best defense is to be prepared. Plan now for handling tough times so you don't give in. For example: think about situations when you usually get a craving for cigarettes or where you think you might experience strong cravings. Try to avoid these situations where you can (for example, avoid spending time with smokers, or drinking alcohol, if those things tempt you to smoke).

Change your habits. For example, take your coffee break somewhere else. Take a walk. In other words, break the association between your usual habits and cigarettes.

If you do encounter a situation where you feel a strong craving, fight it! Take a break from the situation; keep yourself busy or distracted with other activities. Remind yourself why you want to quit, and above all, remind yourself that having "just one" really will hurt your goal of quitting!

To prepare for tough situations, assemble a "survival package"—items that can keep you distracted in case you get a craving. For example, you may include cinnamon gum or hard candy, relaxing music, and things to keep your hands busy like a smooth stone, paper clips, or a rubber ball.

Track your progress as you quit. Keep a journal. Write down how many pieces of **Commit®** Lozenges you use each day. Note if and when you get a craving. If you slip and have a cigarette, don't give up. Stop smoking again and get back on your program with **Commit®** Lozenges.

Establish your support network. Keep friends' and family members' phone numbers ready to get the moral support you need. Before quitting, ask friends and family to support and encourage you. Think of specific ways they can help.

Reward yourself. Set aside little gifts to yourself such as a CD or video, which you can earn by overcoming difficult hurdles.

HOW Commit® LOZENGES WORK.

Commit® Lozenges are a form of Nicotine Replacement Therapy. They deliver nicotine to your body, temporarily relieving craving and nicotine withdrawal symptoms when you quit smoking. But unlike cigarettes, **Commit®** Lozenges deliver a lower, steady level of nicotine to your blood. When used as directed, **Commit®** Lozenges help you regulate, control, and gradually reduce your body's craving for nicotine.

The good news is that **Commit®** Lozenges contain no tar or carbon monoxide, and therefore don't present the same medical risks as cigarettes.

However, the lozenges still deliver nicotine, the addictive ingredient in cigarettes. And for some people the nicotine in **Commit®** Lozenges can occasionally cause mouth or throat irritation, headaches, nausea, hiccups, upset stomach or dizziness.

USING Commit® LOZENGES PROPERLY.

Remember, **Commit® Lozenges aren't like ordinary lozenges such as cough drops.** This lozenge is designed to deliver nicotine into your system through the lining of your mouth, not in your stomach like most other medicines. It is important to minimize swallowing the dissolved medicine in these lozenges so that it can be properly absorbed in your mouth.

Do not use more than one lozenge at a time, or many lozenges one after another since this can cause hiccups, heartburn, nausea or other side effects.

Read all the following instructions before using **Commit®** Lozenges. Refer to them often to make sure you're using **Commit®** Lozenges correctly.

IMPORTANT: Don't worry or give up if you do not like the taste of the lozenge at first. Commit® Lozenges are a medication, not a candy. Most people get used to the taste after a day or two. Remember, staying with the plan will help you quit. Stop smoking completely before you start using Commit® Lozenges.

1) Remove the **Commit®** Lozenge from the blister. Place the lozenge in your mouth and allow the lozenge to slowly dissolve (about 20–30 minutes). Minimize swallowing. **Do not chew or swallow the lozenge.** You may feel a warm or tingling sensation.
2) Occasionally move the lozenge from one side of your mouth to the other side until completely dissolved (about 20-30 minutes).

To reduce cravings or urges to smoke and other withdrawal symptoms, use **Commit®** Lozenges according to the following dosage schedule.

Weeks 1 through 6	Weeks 7 through 9	Weeks 10 through 12
1 lozenge every 1 to 2 hours	1 lozenge every 2 to 4 hours	1 lozenge every 4 to 8 hours

Do not use more than 5 lozenges in 6 hours. Do not use more than 20 lozenges per day. Stop using the lozenge at the end of 12 weeks (3 months).

FOR THE BEST CHANCE OF QUITTING, use **Commit®** Lozenges on a regular schedule, using at least 9 lozenges a day during the first 6 weeks. That will help your body better adjust to the lack of cigarettes and better help prevent cravings. Some people may need more lozenges to reduce their cravings. Do not exceed the recommended maximum daily dosage of 20 lozenges per day. Do not continuously use one lozenge after another, since this may cause you hiccups, heartburn, nausea or other side effects.

Do not eat or drink 15 minutes before using or while the lozenge is in your mouth.

CUTTING BACK ON YOUR Commit® LOZENGE USAGE.

The whole reason for using **Commit®** Lozenges is to decrease and slowly eliminate your need for nicotine, while you control cravings. So, as the above schedule indicates, you should gradually reduce the amount of **Commit®** Lozenges you take per day. Some people find it easier to reduce by substituting ordinary sweets or sugar free candy for some of the **Commit®** Lozenges they would normally use. As time goes on, you can increase the number of pieces of candy as you further reduce your use of **Commit®** Lozenges. **Stop using Commit® Lozenge at the end of week 12.** If you still feel the need to use **Commit®** Lozenge after week 12, talk with your doctor.

MAKE QUITTING EASIER ON YOURSELF.

Soon after your quit date, parties, bars, celebrations, and socializing may all tempt you to smoke. Please remember these tips to help you resist those urges and stay smoke-free.

The Day You Quit Smoking:

- Look to your family and friends for support. Let them know what to do or avoid doing to help you quit.
- Throw away ALL cigarettes, ashtrays, matches, lighters. You don't need them. You don't want them and you want to make it difficult to go back.
- Keep yourself occupied. Take a walk. See a movie. See friends. Do anything to keep your mind off cigarettes.
- Calculate all the money you'll save by not buying cigarettes. Probably well over $1,000 a year! $1,000 a year? Think of what you can spend it on!
- Know what situations are going to make you want to smoke. Plan now how you'll avoid them or deal with them so you don't smoke.
- Keep **Commit®** Lozenges next to your bed so you're prepared when you get up. A lot of people get cravings first thing in the morning.
- Make an appointment to see your dentist and get the tobacco stains cleaned off. While you're getting rid of the evidence of cigarettes in the house, do the same for your teeth. Have clothes or drapes that smell of smoking cleaned.
- Now that your house is smoke-free, try to spend most of your time in smoke-free environments.
- If you usually smoked with coffee or alcohol, try to keep away from them for now. Remember you are also trying to break a habit.
- Smoking is a "hands-on" habit. So use something else to occupy your hands: a rubber band or a pen.
- Now's a good time to get active. Find activities to take your mind off cigarettes and relax. Take up jogging, swimming, or walking.
- Don't stress out about gaining weight. Dieting now may weaken your efforts to quit smoking. Eat sensibly and exercise daily; drink large quantities of water and fruit juices; this can help your chances of staying smoke-free.
- Laugh. Watch a sitcom. Read a comic book. It really helps.

REMEMBER: Urges to smoke are temporary. They'll pass, even if you don't smoke.

WHAT YOU CAN EXPECT.

As you are successful at staying smoke-free, initially you will probably notice a few of the following typical withdrawal symptoms, so don't be surprised. Use of **Commit®** Lozenges reduces these symptoms, but may not eliminate them entirely. They will go away with time. Stay focused on your goal of becoming an ex-smoker. Research shows that if you manage to avoid all smoking in the first week (that means not having a single puff), your chances of success increase dramatically.

The First Few Days. You may feel nervous or irritable or have difficulty concentrating during the first few days after you quit smoking. Your body needs time to regain balance. Initially, you might feel a little out of sorts, get headaches, feel light-headed, or have trouble sleeping. Your smoker's cough may get worse before it improves. But fear not, it's a positive sign. Coughing helps clean your lungs of the tar residue you got from smoking.

After a Couple of Weeks. Your confidence and ability to cope with urges to smoke should be getting stronger. But don't be over-confident and think you can smoke just one cigarette. Even now, having even a single puff can lead to a return to smoking cigarettes regularly. Be prepared, and remember why you wanted to stop smoking.

Have you noticed that your sense of taste and smell has improved? You are probably coughing less and finding it easier to breathe. You've also probably noticed your withdrawal symptoms are subsiding (though don't worry if they're still there: they last longer for some people). These are all positive signs that your body is getting used to your success at stopping smoking.

By The End of The First Month. You are less likely to have cravings for cigarettes as often. However sudden cravings may still happen, and when they do, be on your guard, as they can be strong and seem to come out of the blue. Be prepared for these challenging times. The key is do what you can so these unexpected cravings can't beat you. Keep focused on the ways non-smokers are more attractive than smokers. Their breath smells better. Their clothes and hair are fresher. Their teeth are cleaner and brighter. Their skin is less likely to wrinkle. Not smoking around children and your friends is also healthier for them too.

What If You Do Slip And Smoke?

"What if I relapse?" One cigarette is a slip-up, but it's not the end of the quit effort. Everybody slips at something. The key is this: forgive yourself and stop at that one cigarette. Don't let this slip ruin your good intentions, keep at your quit attempt. So, throw out your cigarettes and continue with your quit attempt, keeping in mind what went wrong and led to the slip.

If you do go back to smoking, certainly don't throw out your **Commit®** Lozenges. Keep them for the next time you're ready to quit. In fact research says that even if you are back to smoking regularly the best thing you can do is learn and try again.

Try to understand the reason you had those cigarettes that made you slip. That's important, because now you can plan better to deal with these moments next time. It's true you stumbled, but don't think of yourself as having failed. Encourage yourself by treating the last attempt as a learning experience, even a "trial run" for the real thing.

Take a look at the usage instructions and check that you used the **Commit®** Lozenges correctly and for the full 12 weeks of the program. When you try again make sure you use enough and the right way. That way you'll be best equipped to deal with the unexpected cravings.

Don't forget; quitting isn't easy and it takes practice to do anything. Stopping smoking is no different.

YOU'VE MADE IT.

Once your twelve week quitting program is over, you've taken your last **Commit®** Lozenge. Now you are both cigarette and nicotine-free. Get up and give yourself a standing ovation. We mean it. Do you realize that you have just done a really difficult thing?

Now's a good time to think back on the process. Think of all your reasons for quitting smoking. Think of your goals. Think of how they're going to be a reality now.

Think of what you're going to do with your newly liberated cigarette money. The places you can now go smoke-free.

Think of the extra time you may have added to your life and what you can do with it. And although you may still experience the occasional temptation, and cigarettes still want you back, think positively. Think forward. And consider yourself a proud non-smoker.

FREQUENTLY ASKED QUESTIONS.

1. When I stop smoking and start using Commit® Lozenges how will I feel? Commit® Lozenges help reduce cravings, but be prepared for some nicotine withdrawal symptoms. After you stop smoking they can begin almost at once and are normally at their strongest during the first three or four days. For some people, any of the following may occur:

- unexpected craving or urges for cigarettes
- anxiety, irritability, restlessness, mood changes, nervousness
- drowsiness
- trouble concentrating
- increased appetite and weight gain
- headaches, muscular pain, constipation, fatigue

Commit® Lozenges are designed to reduce the craving for nicotine you used to satisfy with cigarettes. **Commit®** Lozenges can also help provide relief from other withdrawal symptoms such as irritability and nervousness.

2. Are Commit® Lozenges just swapping one type of nicotine addiction for another?

Commit® Lozenges do contain nicotine, however there is probably less nicotine in your daily dose of lozenges than in your cigarettes. **Commit®** Lozenges give you enough nicotine to help you combat the physical withdrawal symptoms so you can cope with the mental side of stopping smoking. Also, since the nicotine from the lozenges goes into your blood stream more slowly, it produces less of the effects of nicotine that people find rewarding. In fact, when used as directed in the 12 week program, **Commit®** Lozenges gradually wean you off your dependence for both nicotine and cigarettes. Remember, don't use **Commit®** Lozenges together with nicotine patches or other nicotine containing products.

3. Can Commit® Lozenges do any harm?

Some people with conditions like heart disease or people taking prescription medicine for asthma or depression should not use this product without talking to their doctor – check the IMPORTANT WARNINGS on page 3. You may also experience side effects such as hiccups, mouth or throat irritation, heartburn or other stomach problems such as nausea especially if **Commit®** Lozenges are chewed or swallowed. In any case, **Commit®** Lozenges do not contain the tar, carbon monoxide, and other toxins present in cigarette smoke.

4. Will I put on weight?

In the first couple of months after quitting smoking, some people do put on a few pounds. But think of it this way. Overall, you'll be healthier and look better. You can always tackle your weight by changing your diet and increasing the amount you exercise once you have gotten through the difficult part of stopping smoking.

5. Does taking Commit® Lozenges cost more than smoking?

If you normally smoke a pack and a half a day, your total cost of using **Commit®** Lozenges during the 12-week period is about the same as smoking. But guess what? After you've finished the **Commit®** Lozenge program all that money you used to spend on cigarettes is now savings. And think of the health issues you'll hopefully be able to avoid.

6. What if I have a cigarette and start smoking?

Don't panic. First, don't think badly of yourself. Throw away your cigarettes and forgive yourself. Then think about what went wrong and get back on track. In fact people who have already tried to stop smoking are more likely to be successful the next time.

CHALLENGES TO WATCH FOR.

Once you quit smoking, you are likely to experience periodic, and sometimes intense, temptations to smoke. Certain situations present special challenges. Some common ones include:

Stress and upset.

When you are feeling stressed or upset, you may think a cigarette will make everything better. It won't. Find other ways to relax and unwind.

The blues.

You may be especially vulnerable when you feel bored or blue. Remember that having a cigarette will just make you feel worse.

Smoking cues.

Seeing cigarettes or watching other people smoke can trigger temptation. Remember that you choose not to smoke anymore.

Alcohol.

Drinking and smoking seem to go together, and alcoholic beverages may weaken your resolve, making drinking dangerous to your quit effort. Avoid drinking early in your quit effort, and try to drink with non-smokers.

Automatic slips.

Sometimes you may find yourself preparing to smoke without even realizing it. Watch out for those moments when your hand seems to 'automatically' reach for a cigarette.

Watch out for these situations: they can trigger a relapse. You probably know which one (s) are most dangerous for you; plan ahead to deal with the situation effectively. Always remember that you're trying to break a habit, and the most important thing is to do some- thing to combat the urge in these situations.

COPING AFTER QUITTING.

The key to staying smoke-free is to prepare for and cope with challenges as they occur. If you find yourself tempted to smoke, do something! Here are some things to consider.

- Escape. Leave the situation, even for a few minutes. Most temptations don't last long.
- Distract yourself. Get your mind off smoking. Think of something else or get busy with something.
- Relax. Don't let stress get to you. Think of pleasant, relaxing things; breathe slowly and regularly. Let the stress drain out of you.
- Talk yourself out of it. What you say to yourself matters. So, remind yourself how important it is for you to quit; remind yourself you can't have just one; or just command yourself to STOP.

DEBROX® Drops OTC

[de 'brox]

Ear Wax Removal Aid

(See PDR For Nonprescription Drugs.)

ECOTRIN OTC

Enteric-Coated Aspirin

Antiarthritic, Antiplatelet

COMPREHENSIVE PRESCRIBING INFORMATION

DESCRIPTION

Ecotrin enteric coated aspirin (acetylsalicylic acid) tablets available in 81mg, 325mg and 500 mg tablets for oral administration. The 325 mg and 500 mg tablets contain the following inactive ingredients: Carnuba Wax, Colloidal Silicon Dioxide, FD&C Yellow No. 6, Hypromellose, Methacrylic Acid Copolymer, Microcrystalline Cellulose, Pregelatinized Starch, Propylene Glycol, Simethicone, Sodium Starch Glycolate, Stearic Acid, Talc, Titanium Dioxide, and Triethyl Citrate. The 81 mg tablets contain Carnuba Wax, Corn Starch, D&C Yellow No. 10, FD&C Yellow No. 6, Hypromellose, Methacrylic Acid Copolymer, Microcrystalline Cellulose, Propylene Glycol, Simethicone, Stearic Acid, Talc and Triethyl Citrate.

Aspirin is an odorless white, needle-like crystalline or powdery substance. When exposed to moisture, aspirin hydrolyzes into salicylic and acetic acids, and gives off a vinegary-odor. It is highly lipid soluble and slightly soluble in water.

CLINICAL PHARMACOLOGY

Mechanism of Action: Aspirin is a more potent inhibitor of both prostaglandin synthesis and platelet aggregation than other salicylic acid derivatives. The differences in activity between aspirin and salicylic acid are thought to be due to the acetyl group on the aspirin molecule. This acetyl group is responsible for the inactivation of cyclo-oxygenase via acetylation.

PHARMACOKINETICS

Absorption: In general, immediate release aspirin is well and completely absorbed from the gastrointestinal (GI) tract. Following absorption, aspirin is hydrolyzed to salicylic acid with peak plasma levels of salicylic acid occurring within 1–2 hours of dosing (see Pharmacokinetics—Metabolism). The rate of absorption from the GI tract is dependent upon the dosage form, the presence or absence of food, gastric pH (the presence or absence of GI antacids or buffering agents), and other physiologic factors. Enteric coated aspirin products are erratically absorbed from the GI tract.

Distribution: Salicylic acid is widely distibuted to all tissues and fluids in the body including the central nervous system (CNS), breast milk, and fetal tissues. The highest concentrations are found in the plasma, liver, renal cortex, heart, and lungs. The protein binding of salicylate is concentration-dependent, i.e., non-linear. At low concentrations (< 100 mcg/mL) approximately 90 percent of plasma salicylate is bound to albumin while at higher concentrations (> 400 mcg/mL), only about 75 percent is bound. The early signs of salicylic overdose (salicylism), including tinnitus (ringing in the ears), occur at plasma concentrations approximating 200 mcg/mL. Severe toxic effects are associated with levels > 400 mcg/mL (See Adverse Reactions and Overdosage.)

Metabolism: Aspirin is rapidly hydrolyzed in the plasma to salicylic acid such that plasma levels of aspirin are essentially undetectable 1–2 hours after dosing. Salicylic acid is primarily conjugated in the liver to form salicyluric acid, a phenolic glucuronide, an acyl glucuronide, and a number of minor metabolites. Salicylic acid has a plasma half-life of approximately 6 hours. Salicylate metabolism is saturable and total body clearance decreases at higher serum concentrations due to the limited ability of the liver to form both salicyluric acid and phenolic glucuronide. Following toxic doses (10–20 grams (g)), the plasma half-life may be increased to over 20 hours.

Elimination: The elimination of salicylic acid follows zero order pharmacokinetics; (i.e., the rate of drug elimination is constant in relation to plasma concentration). Renal excretion of unchanged drug depends upon urine pH. As urinary pH rises above 6.5, the renal clearance of free salicylate increases from < 5 percent to > 80 percent. Alkalinization of the urine is a key concept in the management of salicylate overdose. (See Overdosage.) Following therapeutic doses, approximately 10 percent is found excreted in the urine as salicylic acid, 75 percent as salicyluric acid, and 10 percent phenolic and 5 percent acyl glucoronides of salicylic acid.

Pharmacodynamics: Aspirin affects platelet aggregation by irreversibly inhibiting prostaglandin cyclo-oxygenase. This effect lasts for the life of the platelet and prevents the formation of the platelet aggregating factor thromboxane A2. Non-acetylated salicylates do not inhibit this enzyme and have no effect on platelet aggregation. At somewhat higher doses, aspirin reversibly inhibits the formation of prostaglandin I_2 (prostacyclin), which is an arterial vasodilator and inhibits platelet aggregation.

At higher doses aspirin is an effective anti-inflammatory agent, partially due to inhibition of inflammatory mediators via cyclooxygenase inhibition in peripheral tissues. In vitro studies suggest that other mediators of inflammation may also be suppressed by aspirin administration, although the precise mechanism of action has not been elucidated. It is this non-specific suppression of cyclooxygenase activity in peripheral tissues following large doses that leads to its primary side effect of gastric irritation. (See Adverse Reactions.)

CLINICAL STUDIES

Ischemic Stroke and Transient Ischemic Attack (TIA): In clinical trials of subjects with TIA's due to fibrin platelet emboli or ischemic stroke, aspirin has been shown to significantly reduce the risk of the combined endpoint of stroke or death and the combined endpoint of TIA, stroke, or death by about 13–18 percent.

Suspect Acute Myocardial Infarction (MI): In a large, multi-center study of aspirin, streptokinase, and the combination of aspirin and streptokinase in 17,187 patients with suspected acute MI, aspirin treatment produced a 23-percent reduction in the risk of vascular mortality. Aspirin was also shown to have an additional benefit in patients given a thrombolytic agent.

Prevention of Recurrent MI and Unstable Angina Pectoris: These indications are supported by the results of six large, randomized, multi-center, placebo-controlled trials of predominantly male post-MI subjects and one randomized placebo-controlled study of men with unstable angina pectoris. Aspirin therapy in MI subjects was associated with a significant reduction (about 20 percent) in the risk of the combination endpoint of subsequent death and/or nonfatal reinfarction in these patients. In aspirin-treated unstable angina patients the event rate was reduced to 5 percent from the 10 percent rate in the placebo group.

Chronic Stable Angina Pectoris: In a randomized, multicenter, double-blind trial designed to assess the role of aspirin for prevention of MI in patients with chronic stable angina pectoris, aspirin significantly reduced the primary combined endpoint of nonfatal MI, fatal MI, and sudden death by 34 percent. The secondary endpoint for vascular events (first occurrence of MI, stroke, or vascular death) was also significantly reduced (32 percent).

Revascularization Procedures: Most patients who undergo coronary artery revascularization procedures have already had symptomatic coronary artery disease for which aspirin is indicated. Similarly, patients with lesions of the carotid bifurcation sufficient to require carotid endarterectomy are likely to have had a precedent event. Aspirin is recommended for patients who undergo revascularization procedures if there is a preexisting condition for which aspirin is already indicated.

Rheumatologic Diseases: In clinical studies in patients with rheumatoid arthritis, juvenile rheumatoid arthritis, ankylosing spondylitis and osteoarthritis, aspirin has been shown to be effective in controlling various indices of clinical disease activity.

ANIMAL TOXICOLOGY

The acute oral 50 percent lethal dose in rats is about 1.5 g/kg and in mice 1.1 g/kg. Renal papillary necrosis and decreased urinary concentrating ability occur in rodents chronically administered high doses. Dose-dependent gastric mucosal injury occurs in rats and humans. Mammals may develop aspirin toxicosis associated with GI symptoms, circulatory effects, and central nervous system depression. (See Overdosage.)

INDICATIONS AND USAGE

Vascular Indications (Ischemic Stroke, TIA, Acute MI, Prevention of Recurrent MI, Unstable Angina Pectoris, and Chronic Stable Angina Pectoris): Aspirin is indicated to: (1) Reduce the combined risk of death and nonfatal stroke in patients who have had ischemic stroke or transient ischemia of the brain due to fibrin platelet emboli, (2) reduce the risk of vascular mortality in patients with a suspected acute MI, (3) reduce the combined risk of death and nonfatal MI

Continued on next page

Product information on these pages is effective as of August 2004. Further information is available at: GlaxoSmithKline, PO Box 13398, Research Triangle Park, NC 27709. 1-888-825-5249. Corporate Web Site: www.gsk.com

Ecotrin—Cont.

in patients with a previous MI or unstable angina pectoris, and (4) reduce the combined risk of MI and sudden death in patients with chronic stable angina pectoris.

Revascularization Procedures (Coronary Artery Bypass Graft (CABG), Percutaneous Transluminal Coronary Angioplasty (PTCA), and Carotid Endarterectomy): Aspirin is indicated in patients who have undergone revascularization procedures (i.e., CABG, PTCA, or carotid endarterectomy) when there is a preexisting condition for which aspirin is already indicated.

Rheumatologic Disease Indications (Rheumatoid Arthritis, Juvenile Rheumatoid Arthritis, Spondyloarthropathies, Osteoarthritis, and the Arthritis and Pleurisy of Systemic Lupus Erythematosus (SLE)): Aspirin is indicated for the relief of the signs and symptoms of rheumatoid arthritis, juvenile rheumatoid arthritis, osteoarthritis, spondyloarthropathies, and arthritis and pleurisy associated with SLE.

CONTRAINDICATIONS

Allergy: Aspirin is contraindicated in patients with known allergy to nonsteroidal anti-inflammatory drug products and in patients with the syndrome of asthma, rhinitis, and nasal polyps. Aspirin may cause severe urticaria, angioedema, or bronchospasm (asthma).

Reye's Syndrome: Aspirin should not be used in children or teenagers for viral infections, with or without fever, because of the risk of Reye's syndrome with concomitant use of aspirin in certain viral illnesses.

WARNINGS

Alcohol Warning: Patients who consume three or more alcoholic drinks every day should be counseled about the bleeding risks involved with chronic, heavy alcohol use while taking aspirin.

Coagulation Abnormalities: Even low doses of aspirin can inhibit platelet function leading to an increase in bleeding time. This can adversely affect patients with inherited (hemophilia) or acquired (liver disease or vitamin K deficiency) bleeding disorders.

GI Side Effects: GI side effects include stomach pain, heartburn, nausea, vomiting, and gross GI bleeding. Although minor upper GI symptoms, such as dyspepsia, are common and can occur anytime during therapy, physicians should remain alert for signs of ulceration and bleeding, even in the absence of previous GI symptoms. Physicians should inform patients about the signs and symptoms of GI side effects and what steps to take if they occur.

Peptic Ulcer Disease: Patients with a history of active peptic ulcer disease should avoid using aspirin, which can cause gastric mucosal irritation and bleeding.

PRECAUTIONS

General

Renal Failure: Avoid aspirin in patients with severe renal failure (glomerular filtration rate less than 10 mL/minute).

Hepatic Insufficiency: Avoid aspirin in patients with severe hepatic insufficiency.

Sodium Restricted Diets: Patients with sodium-retaining states, such as congestive heart failure or renal failure, should avoid sodium-containing buffered aspirin preparations because of their high sodium content.

Laboratory Tests: Aspirin has been associated with elevated hepatic enzymes, blood urea nitrogen and serum creatinine, hyperkalemia, proteinuria, and prolonged bleeding time.

Drug Interactions

Angiotensin Converting Enzyme (ACE) Inhibitors: The hyponatremic and hypotensive effects of ACE inhibitors may be diminished by the concomitant administration of aspirin due to its direct effect on the renin-angiotensin conversion pathway.

Acetazolamide: Concurrent use of aspirin and acetazolamide can lead to high serum concentrations of acetazolamide (and toxicity) due to competition at the renal tubule for secretion.

Anticoagulant Therapy (Heparin and Warfarin): Patients on anticoagulation therapy are at increased risk for bleeding because of drug-drug interactions and the effect on platelets. Aspirin can displace warfarin from protein binding sites, leading to prolongation of both the prothrombin time and the bleeding time. Aspirin can increase the anticoagulant activity of heparin, increasing bleeding risk.

Anticonvulsants: Salicylate can displace protein-bound phenytoin and valproic acid, leading to a decrease in the total concentration of phenytoin and an increase in serum valproic acid levels.

Beta Blockers: The hypotensive effects of beta blockers may be diminished by the concomitant administration of aspirin due to inhibition of renal prostaglandins, leading to decreased renal blood flow, and salt and fluid retention.

Diuretics: The effectiveness of diuretics in patients with underlying renal or cardiovascular disease may be diminished by the concomitant administration of aspirin due to inhibition of renal prostaglandins, leading to decreased renal blood flow and salt and fluid retention.

Methotrexate: Salicylate can inhibit renal clearance of methotrexate, leading to bone marrow toxicity, especially in the elderly or renal impaired.

Nonsteroidal Anti-inflammatory Drugs (NSAID's): The concurrent use of aspirin with other NSAID's should be avoided because this may increase bleeding or lead to decreased renal function.

Oral Hypoglycemics: Moderate doses of aspirin may increase the effectiveness of oral hypoglycemic drugs, leading to hypoglycemia.

Uricosuric Agents (Probenecid and Sulfinpyrazone): Salicylates antagonize the uricosuric action of uricosuric agents.

Carcinogenesis, Mutagenesis, Impairment of Fertility: Administration of aspirin for 68 weeks at 0.5 percent in the feed of rats was not carcinogenic. In the Ames Salmonella assay, aspirin was not mutagenic; however, aspirin did induce chromosome aberrations in cultured human fibroblasts. Aspirin inhibits ovulation in rats. (See Pregnancy.)

Pregnancy: Pregnant women should only take aspirin if clearly needed. Because of the known effects of NSAID's on the fetal cardiovascular system (closure of the ductus arteriosus), use during the third trimester of pregnancy should be avoided. Salicylate products have also been associated with alterations in maternal and neonatal hemostasis mechanisms, decreased birth weight, and with perinatal mortality.

Labor and Delivery: Aspirin should be avoided 1 week prior to and during labor and delivery because it can result in excessive blood loss at delivery. Prolonged gestation and prolonged labor due to prostaglandin inhibition have been reported.

Nursing Mothers: Nursing mothers should avoid using aspirin because salicylate is excreted in breast milk. Use of high doses may lead to rashes, platelet abnormalities, and bleeding in nursing infants.

Pediatric Use: Pediatric dosing recommendations for juvenile rheumatoid arthritis are based on well-controlled clinical studies. An initial dose of 90–130 mg/kg/day in divided doses, with an increase as needed for anti-inflammatory efficacy (target plasma salicylate levels of 150–300 mcg/mL) are effective. At high doses (i.e., plasma levels of greater than 200 mg/mL), the incidence of toxicity increases.

ADVERSE REACTIONS

Many adverse reactions due to aspirin ingestion are dose-related. The following is a list of adverse reactions that have been reported in the literature. (See Warnings.)

Body as a Whole: Fever, hypothermia, thirst.

Cardiovascular: Dysrhythmias, hypotension, tachycardia.

Central Nervous System: Agitation, cerebral edema, coma, confusion, dizziness, headache, subdural or intracranial hemorrhage, lethargy, seizures.

Fluid and Electrolyte: Dehydration, hyperkalemia, metabolic acidosis, respiratory alkalosis.

Gastrointestinal: Dyspepsia, GI bleeding, ulceration and perforation, nausea, vomiting, transient elevations of hepatic enzymes, hepatitis, Reye's Syndrome, pancreatitis.

Hematologic: Prolongation of the prothrombin time, disseminated intravascular coagulation, coagulopathy, thrombocytopenia.

Hypersensitivity: Acute anaphylaxis, angioedema, asthma, bronchospasm, laryngeal edema, urticaria.

Musculoskeletal: Rhabdomyolysis.

Metabolism: Hypoglycemia (in children), hyperglycemia.

Reproductive: Prolonged pregnancy and labor, stillbirths, lower birth weight infants, antepartum and postpartum bleeding.

Respiratory: Hyperpnea, pulmonary edema, tachypnea.

Special Senses: Hearing loss, tinnitus. Patients with high frequency hearing loss may have difficulty perceiving tinnitus. In these patients, tinnitus cannot be used as a clinical indicator of salicylism.

Urogenital: Interstitial nephritis, papillary necrosis, proteinuria, renal insufficiency and failure.

DRUG ABUSE AND DEPENDENCE

Aspirin is non-narcotic. There is no known potential for addiction associated with the use of aspirin.

OVERDOSAGE

Salicylate toxicity may result from acute ingestion (overdose) or chronic intoxication. The early signs of salicylic overdose (salicylism), including tinnitus (ringing in the ears), occur at plasma concentrations approaching 200 mcg/mL. Plasma concentrations of aspirin above 300 mcg/mL are clearly toxic. Severe toxic effects are associated with levels above 400 mcg/mL. (See Clinical Pharmacology.) A single lethal dose of aspirin in adults is not known with certainty but death may be expected at 30 g. For real or suspected overdose, a Poison Control Center should be contacted immediately. Careful medical management is essential.

Signs and Symptoms: In acute overdose, severe acid-base and electrolyte disturbances may occur and are complicated by hyperthermia and dehydration. Respiratory alkalosis occurs early while hyperventilation is present, but is quickly followed by metabolic acidosis.

Treatment: Treatment consists primarily of supporting vital functions, increasing salicylate elimination, and correcting the acid-base disturbance. Gastric emptying and/or lavage is recommended as soon as possible after ingestion, even if the patient has vomited spontaneously. After lavage and/or emesis, administration of activated charcoal, as a slurry, is beneficial, if less than 3 hours have passed since ingestion. Charcoal adsorption should not be employed prior to emesis and lavage.

Severity of aspirin intoxication is determined by measuring the blood salicylate level. Acid-base status should be closely followed with serial blood gas and serum pH measurements. Fluid and electrolyte balance should be maintained.

In severe cases, hyperthermia and hypovolemia are the major immediate threats to life. Children should be sponged with tepid water. Replacement fluid should be administered intravenously and augmented with correction of acidosis. Plasma electrolytes and pH should be monitored to promote alkaline diuresis of salicylate if renal function is normal. Infusion of glucose may be required to control hypoglycemia. Hemodialysis and peritoneal dialysis can be performed to reduce the body drug content. In patients with renal insufficiency or in cases of life-threatening intoxication, dialysis is usually required. Exchange transfusion may be indicated in infants and young children.

DOSAGE AND ADMINISTRATION

Each dose of aspirin should be taken with a full glass of water unless patient is fluid restricted. Anti-inflammatory and analgesic dosages should be individualized. When aspirin is used in high doses, the development of tinnitus may be used as a clinical sign of elevated plasma salicylate levels except in patients with high frequency hearing loss.

Ischemic Stroke and TIA: 50–325 mg once a day. Continue therapy indefinitely.

Suspected Acute MI: The initial dose of 160–162.5 mg is administered as soon as an MI is suspected. The maintenance dose of 160–162.5 mg a day is continued for 30 days post infarction. After 30 days, consider further therapy based on dosage and administration for prevention of recurrent MI.

Prevention of Recurrent MI: 75–325 mg once a day. Continue therapy indefinitely.

Unstable Angina Pectoris: 75–325 mg once a day. Continue therapy indefinitely.

Chronic Stable Angina Pectoris: 75–325 mg once a day. Continue therapy indefinitely.

CABG: 325 mg daily starting 6 hours post-procedure. Continue therapy for 1 year post-procedure.

PTCA: The initial dose of 325 mg should be given 2 hours pre-surgery. Maintenance dose is 160–325 mg daily. Continue therapy indefinitely.

Carotid Endarterectomy: Doses of 80 mg once daily to 650 mg twice daily, started presurgery, are recommended. Continue therapy indefinitely.

Rheumatoid Arthritis: The initial dose is 3 g a day in divided doses. Increase as needed for anti-inflammatory efficacy with target plasma salicylate levels of 150–300 mcg/mL. At high doses (i.e., plasma levels of greater than 200 mg/mL), the incidence of toxicity increases.

Juvenile Rheumatoid Arthritis: Initial dose is 90–130 mg/kg/day in divided doses. Increase as needed for anti-inflammatory efficacy with target plasma salicylate levels of 150–300 mcg/mL. At high doses (i.e., plasma levels of greater than 200 mg/mL), the incidence of toxicity increases.

Spondyloarthropathies: Up to 4 g per day in divided doses.

Osteoarthritis: Up to 3 g per day in divided doses.

Arthritis and Pleurisy of SLE: The initial dose is 3 g a day in divided doses. Increase as needed for anti-inflammatory efficacy with target plasma salicylate levels of 150–300 mcg/mL. At high doses (i.e., plasma levels of greater than 200 mg/mL), the incidence of toxicity increases.

HOW SUPPLIED

81 mg convex orange film coated tablet with ECOTRIN LOW printed in black ink on one side of the tablet. Available as follows

NDC 0108-0117-82 Bottle of 36 tablets
NDC 0108-0117-83 Bottle of 120 tablets

325 mg convex orange film coated tablet with ECOTRIN REG printed in black ink on one side of the tablet. Available as follows:

NDC 0108-0014-26 Bottle of 100 tablets
NDC 0108-0014-29 Bottle of 250 tablets

500 mg convex orange film coated tablet with ECOTRIN MAX printed in black ink on one side of the tablet. Available as follows:

NDC 0108-0016-23 Bottle of 60 tablets
NDC 0108-0016-27 Bottle of 150 tablets

Store in a tight container at 25°C (77° F); excursions permitted to 15–30° C (59–86° F).

FEOSOL® CAPLETS OTC

Hematinic
Iron Supplement

DESCRIPTION

FEOSOL Caplets contain pure iron micro particles called carbonyl iron. This advanced formula is specially designed to be well absorbed and gentle on the stomach. Each FEOSOL carbonyl iron caplet delivers 45 mg of pure elemental iron, the same amount of elemental iron contained in the 225 mg ferrous sulfate capsule. At equivalent doses, carbonyl iron and ferrous sulfate were shown to be equally efficacious in correcting hemoglobin, hematocrit and serum iron levels in iron-deficient patients[1].

SAFETY

According to the American Association of Poison Control Centers, iron containing supplements are the leading cause of pediatric poisoning deaths for children under six in the United States[2]. Widely used as a food additive, carbonyl iron must be gastrically solubilized before it can be absorbed, giving it lower toxicity and enhancing its safety versus any of the ferrous salts[3]. As a result, carbonyl iron presents less chance of harm from accidental overdose. In addition, at equivalent doses, carbonyl iron side effects are no greater than those experienced with ferrous sulfate[4].

WARNINGS

Do not exceed recommended dosage. The treatment of any anemic condition should be under the advice and supervision of a physician. Since oral iron products interfere with absorption of oral tetracycline antibiotics, these products should not be taken within two hours of each other. Occasional gastrointestinal discomfort (such as nausea) may be minimized by taking with meals. Iron containing medication may occasionally cause constipation or diarrhea.
If you are pregnant or nursing a baby, seek the advice of a health professional before using this product.
WARNING: Accidental overdose of iron-containing products is a leading cause of fatal poisoning in children under 6. Keep this product out of reach of children. In case of accidental overdose, call a doctor or poison control center immediately.

SUPPLEMENT FACTS

Serving Size: 1 Caplet

Amount per Caplet	% Daily Value
Iron 45 mg	250%

INGREDIENTS

Lactose, Sorbitol, Carbonyl Iron, Hypromellose. Contains 1% or less of the following ingredients: Carnauba Wax, Crospovidone, FD&C Blue #2 Al Lake, FD&C Red #40 Al Lake, FD&C Yellow #6 Al Lake, Magnesium Stearate, Polydextrose, Polyethylene Glycol, Polyethylene Glycol 8000 (Powder), Stearic Acid, Titanium Dioxide, Triacetin.

DIRECTIONS

Adults—one caplet daily or as directed by a physician. Children under 12 years: Consult a physician.

TAMPER-EVIDENT FEATURE

Each caplet is encased in a plastic cell with a foil back; do not use if cell or foil is broken.

REFERENCES

[1]Devasthali SD, Gordeuk VR, Brittenham GM, et al, "Bioavailability of Carbonyl Iron: A randomized, double-blind study." Eur J Haematology, 1991; 46:272–278.
[2]FDA Consumer; March 1996:7
[3]Heubers, JA, Brittenham GM, Csiba E and Finch CA. "Absorption of carbonyl iron." J Lab Clin Med 1986; 108:473–78.
[4]Devasthali SD, Gordeuk VR, Brittenham GM, et al, "Bioavailability of a Carbonyl Iron: A randomized, double-blind study." Eur J Haematology, 1991; 46:272–278.

Store at room temperature, avoid excessive heat (greater than 100°F) or humidity.

HOW SUPPLIED

Boxes of 30 and 60 caplets in blisters. Also available in single unit packages of 100 caplets intended for institutional use
Also Available: Feosol Tablets.
Comments or Questions? Call Toll-Free 1-800-245-1040 Weekdays.
GlaxoSmithKline Consumer Healthcare, L.P.
Moon Township, PA 15108 Made in USA

FEOSOL® TABLETS OTC

Hematinic
Iron Supplement

DESCRIPTION

Feosol tablets provide the body with ferrous sulfate—an iron supplement for iron deficiency and iron deficiency anemia when the need for such therapy has been determined by a physician.

Supplement Facts

Serving Size: 1 Tablet

Amount per Tablet	% Daily Value
Iron 65 mg	360%

INGREDIENTS

Dried ferrous sulfate 200 mg (65 mg of elemental iron) equivalent to 325 mg of ferrous sulfate, per tablet, Lactose, Sorbitol, Cospovidone, Magnesium Stearate, Carnauba Wax. Contains 2% or less of the following ingredients: FD&C Blue #1, FD&C Yellow #6, Hypromellose, Polydextrose, Polyethylene Glycol, Titanium Dioxide, Triacetin.

DIRECTIONS

Adults and children 12 years and over—One tablet daily or as directed by a physician. Children under 12 years—Consult a physician.

TAMPER-EVIDENT FEATURES:

Each tablet is encased in a plastic cell with a foil back; do not use if cell or foil is broken.

WARNINGS

Do not exceed recommended dosage. The treatment of any anemic condition should be under the advice and supervision of a physician. Since oral iron products interfere with absorption of certain antibiotics, these products should not be taken within two hours of each other. Occassional gastrointestinal discomfort (such as nausea) may be minimized by taking with meals. Iron containing medication may occassionally cause constipation or diarrhea.
If you are pregnant or nursing a baby, seek the advice of a health professional before using this product.
WARNING: Accidental overdose of iron-contraining products is a leading cause of fatal poisoning in children under 6. Keep this product out of reach of children. In case of accidental overdose, call a doctor, or poison control center immediately.
Store at room temperature (59°–86° F).
Not USP for dissolution.

HOW SUPPLIED

Cartons of 100 tablets in child-resistant blisters.
Previously packaged in bottles.
Also available in caplets.
Comments or Questions?
Call Toll-Free 1-800-245-1040 Weekdays
GlaxoSmithKline Consumer Healthcare, L.P.
Moon Township, PA 15108
Made in USA

GAVISCON® REGULAR AND EXTRA STRENGTH TABLETS OTC

Antacid Tablets

GAVISCON® REGULAR AND EXTRA STRENGTH LIQUID ANTACID

[*gav 'is-kon*]

(See PDR For Nonprescription Drugs.)

NICODERM® CQ® OTC

[*nĭc ō dərm*]

Nicotine Transdermal System/Stop Smoking Aid

Formerly available only by prescription
Available as:

Step 1 - 21 mg/24 hours
Step 2 - 14 mg/24 hours
Step 3 - 7 mg/24 hours

If you smoke:
More than 10 cigarettes per Day: Start with Step 1
10 Cigarettes a Day or Less: Start with Step 2

WHAT IS THE NICODERM CQ PATCH AND HOW IS IT USED?

NicoDerm CQ is a small, nicotine containing patch. When you put on a NicoDerm CQ patch, nicotine passes through the skin and into your body. NicoDerm CQ is very thin and uses special material to control how fast nicotine passes through the skin. Unlike the sudden jolts of nicotine delivered by cigarettes, the amount of nicotine you receive remains relatively smooth throughout the 24 or 16 hour period you wear the NicoDerm CQ patch. This helps to reduce cravings you may have for nicotine.

ACTIVE INGREDIENT

Nicotine

PURPOSE

Stop Smoking Aid

USE

To reduce withdrawal symptoms, including nicotine craving, associated with quitting smoking

WARNINGS

- **If you are pregnant or breast-feeding, only use this medicine on the advice of your health care provider.** Smoking can seriously harm your child. Try to stop smoking without using any nicotine replacement medicine. This medicine is believed to be safer than smoking. However, the risks to your child from this medicine are not fully known.
- **Keep out of reach of children and pets.** Used patches have enough nicotine to poison children and pets. For accidental overdose, seek medical help or contact a Poison Control Center right away. Dispose of the used patches by folding sticky ends together and inserting in disposal tray in this box.
- Do not smoke even when not wearing the patch. The nicotine in your skin will still be entering your bloodstream for several hours after you take off the patch.
- If you have vivid dreams or other sleep disturbances remove this patch at bedtime.

Do Not Use

- if you continue to smoke, chew tobacco, use snuff, or use a nicotine gum or other nicotine containing products

Ask a doctor before use if you

- are under 18 years of age
- have heart disease, recent heart attack, or irregular heartbeat. Nicotine can increase your heart rate.
- have high blood pressure not controlled with medication. Nicotine can increase your blood pressure.
- are allergic to adhesive tape or have skin problems because you are more likely to get rashes
- using a non-nicotine stop smoking drug
- take a prescription medication for depression or asthma. Your prescription dose may need to be adjusted.

Stop use and ask a doctor if you have

- skin redness caused by the patch that does not go away after four days, or if skin swells, or you get a rash
- irregular heartbeat or palpitations
- symptoms of nicotine overdose such as nausea, vomiting, dizziness, weakness and rapid heartbeat

DIRECTIONS

- **stop smoking completely when you begin using NicoDerm CQ.**
- before using this product, read the enclosed user's guide for complete directions and other information
- stop smoking completely when you begin using the patch
- **if you smoke more than 10 cigarettes per day,** use according to the following 10 week schedule:

STEP 1 (21 mg)	STEP 2 (14 mg)	STEP 3 (7 mg)
Initial Treatment Period	Step Down Treatment Period	Step Down Treatment Period
Weeks 1–6	Weeks 7–8	Weeks 9–10

- if you smoke 10 cigarettes or less per day, do not use **STEP 1 (21 mg).** Start with **STEP 2 (14 mg)** for 6 weeks, then **STEP 3 (7 mg)** for two weeks and then stop.
- steps 2 and 3 allow you to gradually reduce your level of nicotine. Completing the full program will increase your chances of quitting successfully.
- apply one new patch every 24 hours on skin that is dry, clean and hairless
- remove backing from patch and immediately press onto skin. Hold for 10 seconds.
- wash hands after applying or removing patch. Throw away the patch in the enclosed disposal tray. See enclosed user's guide for safety and handling.
- you may wear the patch for 16 or 24 hours
- if you crave cigarettes when you wake up, wear the patch for 24 hours
- if you have vivid dreams or other sleep disturbances, you may remove the patch at bedtime and apply a new one in the morning
- the used patch should be removed and a new one applied to a different skin site at the same time each day
- do not wear more than one patch at a time
- do not cut patch in half or into smaller pieces
- do not leave patch on for more than 24 hours because it may irritate your skin and loses strength after 24 hours
- stop using the patch at the end of 10 weeks. If you started with **STEP 2**, stop using the patch at the end of 8 weeks. If you still feel the need to use the patch talk to your doctor.

READ THE LABEL

Read the carton and the User's Guide before using this product. Keep the carton and User's Guide. They contain important information.

INACTIVE INGREDIENTS

Ethylene vinyl acetate-copolymer, polyisobutylene and high density polyethylene between pigmented and clear polyester backings.
Store at 20–25°C (68–77°F)

TO INCREASE YOUR SUCCESS IN QUITTING:

1. You must be motivated to quit.
2. Complete the full treatment program, applying a new patch every day.
3. Use with a support program as described in the Users Guide.

NicoDerm CQ User's Guide

KEYS TO SUCCESS

1) You must really want to quit smoking for **NicoDerm® CQ®** to help you.
2) Complete the full program, applying a new patch every day.
3) **NicoDerm CQ** works best when used together with a support program: See page 3 for details.
4) If you have trouble using **NicoDerm CQ**, ask your doctor or pharmacist or call GlaxoSmithKline at 1-800-834-5895 weekdays (10:00 am 4:30 pm EST).

SO, YOU'VE DECIDED TO QUIT.

Congratulations. Your decision to stop smoking is one of the most important things you can do to improve your health. Quitting smoking is a two-part process that involves:
1) overcoming your physical need for nicotine, and
2) breaking your smoking habit.
NicoDerm CQ helps smokers quit by reducing nicotine withdrawal symptoms.
Many NicoDerm CQ users will be able to stop smoking for a few days but often will start smoking again. Most smokers have to try to quit several times before they completely stop. Your own chances of quitting smoking depend on how strongly you are addicted to nicotine, how much you want to quit, and how closely you follow a quitting plan like the one that comes with NicoDerm CQ.

QUITTING SMOKING IS HARD!

If you find you cannot stop or if you start smoking again after using NicoDerm CQ please talk to a health care professional who can help you find a program that may work better for you. Breaking this addiction doesn't happen overnight.

Continued on next page

Product information on these pages is effective as of August 2004. Further information is available at: GlaxoSmithKline, PO Box 13398, Research Triangle Park, NC 27709. 1-888-825-5249. Corporate Web Site: www.gsk.com

NicoDerm CQ—Cont.

Because NicoDerm CQ provides some nicotine, the NicoDerm CQ patch will help you stop smoking by reducing nicotine withdrawal symptoms such as nicotine craving, nervousness and irritability.
This User's Guide will give you support as you become a non-smoker. It will answer common questions about NicoDerm CQ and give tips to help you stop smoking, and should be referred to often.

WHERE TO GET HELP.
You are more likely to stop smoking by using NicoDerm CQ with a support program that helps you break your smoking habit. There may be support groups in your area for people trying to quit. Call your local chapter of the American Lung Association, American Cancer Society or American Heart Association for further information. Toll free phone numbers are printed on the wallet card on the back cover of this User's Guide.
If you find you cannot stop smoking or if you start smoking again after using NicoDerm CQ, remember breaking this addiction doesn't happen overnight. You may want to talk to a health care professional who can help you improve your chances of quitting the next time you try NicoDerm CQ or another method.

LET'S GET ORGANIZED.
Your reason for quitting may be a combination of concerns about health, the effect of smoking on your appearance, and pressure from your family and friends to stop smoking. Or maybe you're concerned about the dangerous effect of second-hand smoke on the people you care about.
All of these are good reasons. You probably have others. Decide your most important reasons, and write them down on the wallet card inside the back cover of this User's Guide. Carry this card with you. In difficult moments, when you want to smoke, the card will remind you why you are quitting.

WHAT YOU'RE UP AGAINST.
Smoking is addictive in two ways. Your need for nicotine has become both physical and mental. You must overcome both addictions to stop smoking. So while NicoDerm CQ will lessen your body's craving for nicotine, you've got to want to quit smoking to overcome the mental dependence on cigarettes. Once you've decided that you're going to quit, it's time to get started. But first, there are some important cautions you should consider.

SOME IMPORTANT WARNINGS.
This product is only for those who want to stop smoking.
If you are pregnant or breast-feeding, only use this medicine on the advice of your health care provider. Smoking can seriously harm your child. Try to stop smoking without using any nicotine replacement medicine. This medicine is believed to be safer than smoking. However, the risks to your child from this medicine are not fully known.

Do not use
- if you continue to smoke, chew tobacco, use snuff or use a nicotine gum or other nicotine products. You may get a nicotine overdose.

Ask a doctor before use if you have
- heart disease, recent heart attack, or irregular heartbeat. Nicotine can increase your heart rate.
- high blood pressure not controlled with medication. Nicotine can increase your blood pressure.

Ask a doctor or pharmacist before use if you are
- an allergic to adhesive tape or have skin problems because you are more likely to get rashes
- taking a prescription medication for asthma or depression. Your prescription dose may need to be adjusted.
- using a non-nicotine stop smoking drug.

When using this product
- Do not smoke even when not wearing the patch. The nicotine in your skin will still be entering your blood stream for several hours after you take off the patch.
- If you have vivid dreams or other sleep disturbances remove this patch at bedtime.

Stop use and ask a doctor if
- skin redness caused by the patch does not go away after four days, or if your skin swells or you get a rash.
- irregular heartbeat or palpitations occur
- you get symptoms of nicotine overdose, such as nausea, vomiting, dizziness, weakness and rapid heartbeat.

Keep out of reach of children and pets. Used patches have enough nicotine to poison children and pets. If swallowed, get medical help or contact a poison control center right away. Dispose of the used patches by folding sticky ends together and inserting in disposal tray in this box.

LET'S GET STARTED.
If you are under 18 years of age, ask a doctor before use.
Becoming a non-smoker starts today. Your first step is to read through this entire User's Guide carefully.
First, check that you bought the right starting dose.
If you smoke more than 10 cigarettes a day, begin with Step 1 (21 mg). As the carton indicates, people who smoke 10 or less cigarettes per day should not use Step 1 (21 mg). They should start with Step 2 (14 mg). Throughout this User's Guide we will give specific instructions for people who smoke 10 or less cigarettes per day.
Next, set your personalized quitting schedule.
Take out a calendar that you can use to track your progress. Pick a quit date, and mark this on your calendar using the stickers inside the front cover of this User's Guide, as described below.

DIRECTIONS: FOR PEOPLE WHO SMOKE OVER 10 CIGARETTES PER DAY
STEP 1. (Weeks 1–6). Your Quit Date (and the day you'll start using NicoDerm CQ patch).
Choose your quit date (it should be soon).
This is the day you will quit smoking cigarettes entirely and begin using NicoDerm CQ to reduce your cravings for nicotine. Place the Step 1 sticker on this date. For the first six weeks, you'll use the highest-strength (21 mg) NicoDerm CQ patches. Be sure to follow the directions on page 10.
Completing the full program will increase your chances of quitting successfully. This is done by changing over to the Step 2 (14mg) patch for 2 weeks followed by a final 2 weeks with the Step 3 (7mg) patch. The Step 2 and Step 3 treatment periods allow you to gradually reduce the amount of nicotine you get, rather than stopping suddenly, and will increase your chances of quitting.
STEP 2. (Weeks 7–8). The day you'll start reducing your use of NicoDerm CQ patch.
Switching to Step 2 (14mg) patches after 6 weeks begins to gradually reduce your nicotine usage. Place the Step 2 sticker on this date (the first day of week seven). Use the 14mg patches for two weeks.
STEP 3. (Weeks 9–10). The day you'll further start reducing your use of NicoDerm CQ patch.
After eight weeks, nicotine intake is further reduced by moving down to Step 3 (7mg) patches. Place the Step 3 sticker on this date (the first day of week nine). Use the 7 mg patches for two weeks.

THE NICODERM CQ PROGRAM

STEP 1 (21 mg)	STEP 2 (14 mg)	STEP 3 (7 mg)
Initial Treatment Period	Step Down Treatment Period	
Weeks 1–6	Weeks 7–8	Weeks 9–10

STOP USING NicoDerm CQ AT THE END OF WEEK 10. If you still feel the need to use the patch after Week 10, talk with your doctor or health professional.
DIRECTIONS: For people who smoke 10 or less cigarettes per day.
Do not use Step 1 (21 mg).
Begin with STEP 2 – Initial Treatment Period (Weeks 1–6): 14mg patches.
Choose our quit date (it should be soon). This is the Day you will quit smoking cigarettes entirely and begin using NicoDerm CQ to reduce your cravings for nicotine. Place the Step 2 sticker on this date. For the first six weeks, you'll use the Step 2 (14mg) NicoDerm CQ patches. Be sure to follow the directions on page 10.
Continue with STEP 3 – Step Down Treatment Period (Weeks 7–8): 7mg patches.
Completing the full program will increase your chances of quitting successfully. This is done by changing over to the Step 3 (7mg) patches for 2 weeks. The two week step down treatment period allows you to gradually reduce the amount of nicotine you get, rather than stopping suddenly, and will increase your chances of quitting. Place the Step 3 sticker on the first day of week seven. Use the 7mg patches for two weeks.
People who smoke 10 or less cigarettes per day should not use NicoDerm CQ for longer than 8 weeks. If you still feel the need to use NicoDerm CQ after 8 weeks, talk with your doctor.

PLAN AHEAD.
Because smoking is an addiction, it is not easy to stop. After you've given up nicotine, you may still have a strong urge to smoke. Plan ahead NOW for these times, so you're not tempted to start smoking again in a moment of weakness. The following tips may help:
- Keep the phone numbers of supportive friends and family members handy.
- Keep a record of your quitting process. Track whether you feel a craving for cigarettes. In the event that you slip, immediately stop smoking and resume your quit attempt with the NicoDerm CQ patch. If you smoke at all, write down what you think caused the slip.
- Put together an Emergency Kit that includes items that will help take your mind off occasional urges to smoke. You might include cinnamon gum or lemon drops to suck on, a relaxing cassette tape, and something for your hands to play with, like a smooth rock, rubber band or small metal balls.
- Set aside some small rewards, like a new magazine or a gift certificate from your favorite store, which you'll "give" yourself after passing difficult hurdles.
- Think now about the times when you most often want a cigarette, and then plan what else you might do instead of smoking. For instance, you might plan to take your coffee break in a new location, or take a walk right after dinner, so you won't be tempted to smoke.

HOW NICODERM CQ WORKS.
NicoDerm CQ patches provide nicotine to your system. They work as a temporary aid to help you quit smoking by reducing nicotine withdrawal symptoms, including nicotine craving. NicoDerm CQ provides a lower level of nicotine to your blood than cigarettes, and allows you to gradually do away with your body's need for nicotine.
Because NicoDerm CQ does not contain the tar or carbon monoxide of cigarette smoke, it does not have the same health dangers as tobacco. However, it still delivers nicotine, the addictive part of cigarette smoke. Nicotine can cause side effects such as headache, nausea, upset stomach, and dizziness.

HOW TO USE NICODERM CQ PATCHES.
Read all the following instructions, and the instructions on the outer carton, before using NicoDerm CQ. Refer to them often to make sure you're using NicoDerm CQ correctly. Please refer to the compact disc for additional help.
1) Stop smoking completely before you start using NicoDerm CQ.
2) To reduce nicotine craving and other withdrawal symptoms, use NicoDerm CQ according to the directions on pages 6–8.
3) Insert used NicoDerm CQ patches in the child resistant disposal tray provided in the box – safely away from children and pets.

When to apply and remove NicoDerm CQ patches.
Each day apply a new patch to a different place on skin that is dry, clean and hairless. **You can wear a NicoDerm CQ patch for either 16 or 24 hours.** If you crave cigarettes when you wake up, wear the patch for 24 hours. If you begin to have vivid dreams or other disruptions of your sleep while wearing the patch 24 hours, try taking the patch off at bedtime (after about 16 hours) and putting on a new one when you get up the next day.

PLACE THESE STICKERS ON YOUR CALENDAR

STEP 1	**STEP 2**
A new 21 mg patch every day AT THE BEGINNING OF WEEK #1 (QUIT DAY)	A new 14 mg patch every day AT THE BEGINNING OF WEEK #7

For people who smoke 10 or less cigarettes per day: Do not use STEP 1 (21 mg). Use STEP 2 (14 mg) at the beginning of week #1 and STEP 3 (7 mg) at the beginning of week #7.

PLACE THESE STICKERS ON YOUR CALENDAR

STEP 3	**EX-SMOKER**
A new 7 mg patch every day AT THE BEGINNING OF WEEK #9	WHEN YOU HAVE COMPLETED YOUR QUITTING PROGRAM

Do not smoke even when you are not wearing the patch.
Remove the used patch and put on a new patch at the same time every day. Applying the patch at about the same time each day (first thing in the morning, for instance) will help you remember when to put on a new patch. Do not leave the same NicoDerm CQ patch on for more than 24 hours because it may irritate your skin and because it loses strength after 24 hours.
Do not use NicoDerm CQ continuously for more than 10 weeks (8 weeks for people who smoke 10 or less cigarettes per day).

How to apply a NicoDerm CQ patch.
1. Do not remove the NicoDerm CQ patch from its sealed protective pouch until you are ready to use it. NicoDerm CQ patches will lose nicotine to the air if you store them out of the pouch.
2. Choose a non-hairy, clean, dry area of skin. Do not put a NicoDerm CQ patch on skin that is burned, broken out, cut, or irritated in any way. Make sure your skin is free of lotion and soap before applying a patch.
3. A clear, protective liner covers the sticky back side of the NicoDerm CQ patch—the side that will be put on your skin. The liner has a slit down the middle to help you remove it from the patch. With the sticky back side facing you, pull half the liner away from the NicoDerm CQ patch starting at the middle slit, as shown in the illustration above. Hold the NicoDerm CQ patch at one of the outside edges (touch the sticky side as little as possible), and pull off the other half of the protective liner.
Place this liner in the slot in the disposable tray provided in the NicoDerm CQ package where it will be out of reach of children and pets.
4. Immediately apply the sticky side of the NicoDerm CQ patch to your skin. **Press the patch firmly on your skin with the heel of your hand for at least 10 seconds.** Make sure it sticks well to your skin, especially around the edges.
5. Wash your hands when you have finished applying the NicoDerm CQ patch. Nicotine on your hands could get into your eyes and nose, and cause stinging, redness, or more serious problems.
6. After 24 or 16 hours, remove the patch you have been wearing. Fold the used NicoDerm CQ patch in half with the sticky side together. Carefully dispose of the used patch in the slot of the disposal tray provided in the NicoDerm CQ package where it will be out of the reach of children and pets. Even used patches have enough nicotine to poison children and pets. Wash your hands.
7. Chose a different place on your skin to apply the next NicoDerm CQ patch and repeat Steps 1 to 6. Do not apply a new patch to a previously used skin site for at least one week.

If your NicoDerm CQ patch gets wet during wearing.
Water will not harm the NicoDerm CQ patch you are wearing if applied properly. You can bathe, swim, or shower for short periods while you are wearing the NicoDerm CQ patch.

If your NicoDerm CQ patch comes off while wearing.
NicoDerm CQ patches generally stick well to most people's skin. However, a patch may occasionally come off. If your NicoDerm CQ patch falls off during the day, put on a new patch, making sure you select a non-hairy, non-irritated area of the skin that is clean and dry.
If the soap you use has lanolin or moisturizers, the patch may not stick well. Using a different soap may help. Body creams, lotions and sunscreens can also cause problems with keeping your patch on. Do not apply creams or lotions to the place on your skin where you will put the patch.
If you have followed the directions and the patch still does not stick to you, try using medical adhesive tape over the patch.
Disposing of NicoDerm CQ patches.
Fold the used patch in half with the sticky side together. Carefully dispose of the patch in the disposal slot of the tray provided in the NicoDerm CQ package where it will be out of the reach of children and pets. Small amounts of nicotine, even from a used patch, can poison children and pets. **Keep all nicotine patches away from children and pets.** Wash your hands after disposing of the patch.
If your skin reacts to the NicoDerm CQ patch.
When you first put on a NicoDerm CQ patch, mild itching, burning, or tingling is normal and should go away within an hour. After you remove a NicoDerm CQ patch, the skin under the patch might be somewhat red. Your skin should not stay red for more than a day after removing the patch. **Stop use and ask a doctor if skin redness caused by the patch does not go away after four days, or if your skin swells, or you get a rash. Do not put on a new patch.**
Storage Instructions
Keep each NicoDerm CQ patch in its protective pouch, unopened, until you are ready to use it, because the patch will lose nicotine to the air if it's outside the pouch.
Do not store NicoDerm CQ patches at 20–25°C (68–77°F) because they are sensitive to heat. Remember, the inside of your car can reach temperatures much higher than this. A slight yellowing of the sticky side of the patch is normal. Do not use NicoDerm CQ patches stored in pouches that are open or torn.
TIPS TO MAKE QUITTING EASIER.
Within the first few weeks of giving up smoking, you may be tempted to smoke for pleasure, particularly after completing a difficult task, or at a party or bar. Hear are some tips to help get you through the important first stages of becoming a nonsmoker:
On Your Quit Date:
- Ask your family, friends and co-workers to support you in your efforts to stop smoking.
- Throw away all your cigarettes, matches, lighters, ashtrays, etc.
- Keep busy on your quit day. Exercise. Go to a movie. Take a walk. Get together with friends.
- Figure out how much money you'll save by not smoking. Most ex-smokers can save more than $1,000 a year on the price of cigarettes alone.
- Write down what you will do with the money you save.
- Know your high risk situations and plan ahead how you will deal with them.
- Visit your dentist and have your teeth cleaned to get rid of the tobacco stains.

Right after Quitting:
- During the first few days after you've stopped smoking, spend as much time as possible at places where smoking is not allowed.
- Drink large quantities of water and fruit juices.
- Try to avoid alcohol, coffee and other beverages you associate with smoking.
- Remember that temporary urges to smoke will pass, even if you don't smoke a cigarette.
- Keep your hands busy with something like a pencil or a paper clip.
- Find other activities that help you relax without cigarettes. Swim, jog, take a walk, play basketball.
- Don't worry too much about gaining weight. Watch what you eat, take time for daily exercise, and change your eating habits if you need to.
- Laughter helps. Watch or read something funny

WHAT TO EXPECT.
The First Few Days.
Your body is now coming back into balance. During the first few days after you stop smoking, you might feel edgy and nervous and have trouble concentrating. You might get headaches, feel dizzy and a little out of sorts, feel sweaty or have stomach upsets. You might even have trouble sleeping at first. These are typical nicotine withdrawal symptoms that will go away with time. Your smoker's cough will get worse before it gets better. But don't worry, that's a good sign. Coughing helps clear the tar deposits out of your lungs.
After A Week Or Two.
By now you should be feeling more confident that you can handle those smoking urges. Many of your nicotine withdrawal symptoms have left by now, and you should be noticing some positive signs: less coughing, better breathing and an improved sense of taste and smell, to name a few.
After A Month.
You probably have the urge to smoke much less often now. But urges may still occur, and when they do, they are likely to be powerful ones that come out of nowhere. Don't let them catch you off guard. Plan ahead for these difficult times. Concentrate on the ways non-smokers are more attractive than smokers. Their skin is less likely to wrinkle. Their teeth are whiter, cleaner. Their breath is fresher.
Their hair and clothes smell better. That cough that seems to make even a laugh sound more like a rattle is a thing of the past. Their children and others around them are healthier, too.
What To Do About Relapse.
What should you do if you slip and start smoking again? The answer is simple. A lapse of one or two or even a few cigarettes should not spoil your efforts! Throw away your cigarettes, forgive yourself and continue with the program. Listen to the Audio Tape again and re-read the User's Guide to ensure that you're using NicoDerm CQ correctly and following the other important tips for dealing with the mental and social dependence on nicotine. Your doctor, pharmacist or other health professional can also provide useful counseling on the importance of stopping smoking. You should consider them partners in your quit attempt.
What To Do About Relapse After a Successful Quit Attempt.
If you have taken up regular smoking again, don't be discouraged. Research shows that the best thing you can do is try again, since several quitting attempts may be needed before you're successful. And your chances of quitting successfully increase with each quit attempt.
The important thing is to learn from your last attempt.
- Admit that you've slipped, but don't treat yourself as a failure.
- Try to identify the "trigger" that caused you to slip, and prepare a better plan for dealing with this problem next time.
- Talk positively to yourself – tell yourself that you have learned something from this experience.
- Make sure you used NicoDerm CQ patches correctly
- Remember that it takes practice to do anything, and quitting smoking is no exception.

WHEN THE STRUGGLE IS OVER.
Once you've stopped smoking, take a second and pat yourself on your back. Now do it again. You deserve it. Remember now why you decided to stop smoking in the first place. Look at your list of reasons. Read them again. And smile. Now think about all the money you are saving and what you'll do with it. All the non-smoking places you can go, and what you might do there. All those years you may have added to your life, and what you'll do with them. Remember that temptation may not be gone forever. However, the hard part is behind you so look forward with a positive attitude, and enjoy your new life as a non-smoker.
QUESTIONS & ANSWERS
1. How will I feel when I stop smoking and start using NicoDerm CQ?
You'll need to prepare yourself for some nicotine withdrawal symptoms. These begin almost immediately after you stop smoking, and are usually at their worst during the first three or four days. Understand that any of the following is possible:
- craving for nicotine
- anxiety, irritability, restlessness, mood changes, nervousness
- disruptions of your sleep
- drowsiness
- trouble concentrating
- increased appetite and weight gain, headaches, muscular pain, constipation, fatigue.

NicoDerm CQ reduces nicotine withdrawal symptoms such as irritability and nervousness, as well as the craving for nicotine you used to satisfy by having a cigarette.
2. Is NicoDerm CQ just substituting one form of nicotine for another?
NicoDerm CQ does contain nicotine. The purpose of NicoDerm CQ is to provide you with enough nicotine to reduce the physical withdrawal symptoms so you can deal with the mental aspects of quitting.
3. Can I be hurt by using NicoDerm CQ?
For most adults, the amount of nicotine delivered from the patch is less than from smoking. If you believe you may be sensitive to even this amount of nicotine, you should not use this product without advice from your doctor. There are also some important warnings in this User's Guide (See page 4).
4. Will I gain weight?
Many people do tend to gain a few pounds the first 8–10 weeks after they stop smoking. This is a very small price to pay for the enormous gains that you will make in your overall health and attractiveness. If you continue to gain weight after the first two months, try to analyze what you're doing differently. Reduce your fat intake, choose healthy snacks, and increase your physical activity to burn off the extra calories. Drink lots of water. This is good for your body and skin, and also helps to reduce the amount you eat.
5. Is NicoDerm CQ more expensive than smoking?
The total cost of NicoDerm CQ program is similar to what a person who smokes one and a half packs of cigarettes a day would spend on cigarettes for the same period of time. Also, use of NicoDerm CQ is only a short-term cost, while the cost of smoking is a long-term cost, including the health problems smoking causes.
6. What if I slip up?
Discard your cigarettes, forgive yourself and then get back on track. Don't consider yourself a failure or punish yourself. In fact, people who have already tried to quit are more likely to be successful the next time.
GOOD LUCK!

WALLET CARD
My most important reasons to quit smoking are:
WALLET CARD
Where to call for Help:

American Lung Association	American Cancer Society	American Heart Association
800-586-4872	800-227-2345	800-242-8721

For people who smoke more than 10 cigarettes per day:

STEP 1	STEP 2	STEP 3
Use one 21 mg patch/day	Use one 14 mg patch/day	Use one 7 mg patch/day
Weeks 1–6	Weeks 7–8	Weeks 9–10

People who smoke 10 or less cigarettes per day. Do not use STEP 1 (21 mg). Use STEP 2 (14 mg) for six weeks and STEP 3 (7 mg) for two weeks and then stop.

For your family's protection, NicoDerm CQ patches are supplied in child resistant pouches. Do not use if individual pouch is open or torn.
Manufactured by ALZA Corporation, Mountain View, CA 94043 for GlaxoSmithKline Consumer Healthcare, L.P.
Comments or Questions? Call 1–800–834–5895 Weekdays. (10 a.m.–4:30 p.m. EST).
- **Not for sale to those under 18 years of age.**
- **Proof of age required.**
- **Not for sale in vending machines or from any source where proof of age cannot be verified.**

Available as
NicoDerm CQ Step 1 (21 mg/24 hours)–7 Patches*
NicoDerm CQ Step 1 (21 mg/24 hours)–14 Patches*
Clear NicoDerm CQ Step 1 (21 mg/24 hours)–7 Patches*
Clear NicoDerm CQ Step 1 (21 mg/24 hours)–14 Patches*
Clear NicoDerm CQ Step 1 (21 mg/24 hours)–21 Patches*
NicoDerm CQ Step 2 (14 mg/24 hours)–7 Patches*
NicoDerm CQ Step 2 (14 mg/24 hours)–14 Patches*
Clear NicoDerm CQ Step 2 (14 mg/24 hours)–14 Patches*
NicoDerm CQ Step 3 (7 mg/24 hours)–7 Patches**
NicoDerm CQ Step 3 (7 mg/24 hours)–14 Patches**
Clear NicoDerm CQ Step 3 (7 mg/24 hours)–14 Patches**
* User's Guide, Compact Disk & Child Resistant Disposal Tray
** User's Guide, & Child Resistant Disposal Tray

NICORETTE® OTC

Nicotine Polacrilex Gum/Stop Smoking Aid
Available in Original 2mg and 4mg Strengths and Mint 2mg and 4mg Strengths and Orange 2mg and 4mg Strengths

IF YOU SMOKE LESS THAN 25 CIGARETTES A DAY: Use 2 mg
IF YOU SMOKE 25 OR MORE CIGARETTES A DAY: Use 4 mg
Active Ingredient: Nicotine Polacrilex
Purpose: Stop Smoking Aid
USE
- reduces withdrawal symptoms, including nicotine craving, associated with quitting smoking

WARNINGS
If you are pregnant or breast-feeding, only use this medicine on the advice of your health care provider. Smoking can seriously harm your child. Try to stop smoking without using any nicotine replacement medicine. This medicine is believed to be safer than smoking. However, the risks to your child from this medicine are not fully known.
DO NOT USE
- if you continue to smoke, chew tobacco, use snuff, or use a nicotine patch or other nicotine containing products

ASK YOUR DOCTOR BEFORE USE IF YOU HAVE
- heart disease, recent heart attack, or irregular heartbeat. Nicotine can increase your heart rate.
- high blood pressure not controlled with medication. Nicotine can increase blood pressure.
- stomach ulcer or diabetes

ASK A DOCTOR OR PHARMACIST BEFORE USE IF YOU ARE
- using a non-nicotine stop smoking drug
- taking prescription medicine for depression or asthma. Your prescription dose may need to be adjusted.

STOP USE AND ASK A DOCTOR IF
- mouth, teeth or jaw problems occur
- irregular heartbeat or palpitations occur
- you get symptoms of nicotine overdose such as nausea, vomiting, dizziness, diarrhea, weakness and rapid heartbeat.

Keep out of reach of children and pets. Pieces of nicotine gum may have enough nicotine to make children and pets sick. Wrap used pieces of gum in paper and throw away in the trash. In case of overdose, get medical help or contact a Poison Control Center right away.

Continued on next page

Product information on these pages is effective as of August 2004. Further information is available at: GlaxoSmithKline, PO Box 13398, Research Triangle Park, NC 27709. 1-888-825-5249. Corporate Web Site: www.gsk.com

Nicorette—Cont.

DIRECTIONS

- **if you are under 18 years of age, ask doctor before use**
- before using this product, read the enclosed User's Guide for complete directions and other important information
- stop smoking completely when you begin using the gum
- **if you smoke 25 or more cigarettes a day;** use 4 mg nicotine gum
- **if you smoke less than 25 cigarettes a day;** use 2 mg nicotine gum

Use according to the following 12 week schedule:

Weeks 1 to 6	Weeks 7 to 9	Weeks 10 to 12
1 piece every 1 to 2 hours	1 piece every 2 to 4 hours	1 piece every 4 to 8 hours

- nicotine gum is a medicine and must be used a certain way to get the best results
- chew the gum slowly until it tingles. Then park it between your cheek & gum. When the tingle is gone, begin chewing again, until the tingle returns.
- repeat this process until most of the tingle is gone (about 30 minutes)
- do not eat or drink for 15 minutes before chewing the nicotine gum, or while chewing a piece
- to improve your chances of quitting, use at least 9 pieces per day for the first 6 weeks
- if you experience strong or frequent cravings, you may use a second piece within the hour. However, do not continuously use one piece after another since this may cause you hiccups, heartburn, nausea or other side effects.
- do not use more than 24 pieces a day
- stop using the nicotine gum at the end of week 12. If you still feel the need for nicotine gum, talk to your doctor.

OTHER INFORMATION

- store at 20–25°C (68–77°F)
- protect from light

INACTIVE INGREDIENTS

Original [2 mg] Inactive Ingredients: flavors, glycerin, gum base, sodium carbonate, sorbitol, sodium bicarbonate

Original [4 mg] Inactive Ingredients: flavors, glycerin, gum base, sodium carbonate, sorbitol, D&C yellow #10

Mint 2 mg Inactive Ingredients: gum base, magnesium oxide, menthol, peppermint oil, sodium bicarbonate, sodium carbonate, xylitol

Mint 4 mg Inactive Ingredients: gum base, magnesium oxide, menthol, peppermint oil, sodium carbonate, xylitol, D&C yellow #10. Al. Lake

Orange (2 mg) Inactive Ingredients: flavor, gum base, magnesium oxide, sodium bicarbonate, sodium carbonate, xylitol

Orange (4 mg) Inactive Ingredients: flavor, gum base, magnesium oxide, sodium carbonate, xylitol, D&C yellow #10. Al. Lake

TO INCREASE YOUR SUCCESS IN QUITTING:

1. You must be motivated to quit.
2. **Use Enough**—Chew **at least 9 pieces** of Nicorette per day during the first six weeks.
3. **Use long enough**—Use Nicorette for the full 12 weeks.
4. **Use with a support program** as directed in the enclosed User's Guide.*

*The American Cancer Society supports the use of a stop smoking aid and counseling as effective tools when quitting smoking but does not endorse any specific product. GlaxoSmithKline pays a fee to the American Cancer Society for the use of its logo.

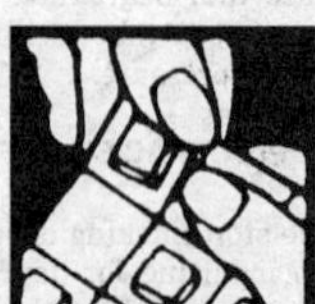

To remove the gum, tear off single unit.

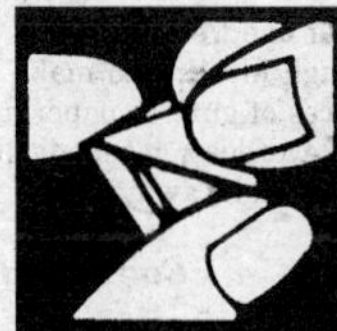

Peel off backing starting at corner with loose edge.

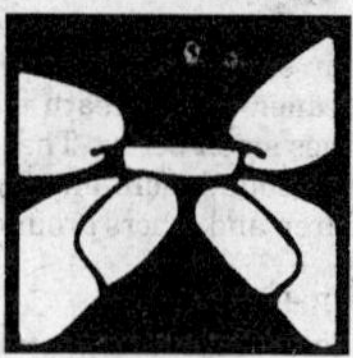

Push gum through foil.

Blister packaged for your protection. **Do not use if individual seals are open or torn.**

- **not for sale to those under 18 years of age**
- **proof of age required**
- **not for sale in vending machines or from any source where proof of age cannot be verified**

HOW SUPPLIED

Nicorette Original and Mint are available in:
2 mg or 4 mg Starter kit*—110 pieces
2 mg or 4 mg Refill—48 pieces, 168 pieces or 192 pieces
Nicorette Orange is available in:
2 mg or 4 mg Starter kit*—110 pieces
2 mg or 4 mg Refill—48 pieces
*User's Guide and CD included in kit

Questions or Comments? Call 1-800-419-4766 weekdays. (10 a.m.–4:30 p.m. EST).

Manufactured by Pharmacia AB, Stockholm, Sweden for **GlaxoSmithKline** Consumer Healthcare, L.P. Moon Township, PA 15108

USER'S GUIDE

HOW TO USE NICORETTE TO HELP YOU QUIT SMOKING.

KEYS TO SUCCESS:

1) You must really want to quit smoking for **Nicorette®** to help you.
2) You can greatly increase your chances for success by using at least 9 to 12 pieces every day when you start using **Nicorette**. See page 11 of User's Guide.
3) You should continue to use **Nicorette** as explained in the User's Guide for 12 full weeks.
4) **Nicorette** works best when used together with a support program—See page 3 of User's Guide for details.
5) If you have trouble using **Nicorette**, ask your doctor or pharmacist or call GlaxoSmithKline at 1-800-419-4766 weekdays (10:00am–4:30pm EST).

SO YOU DECIDED TO QUIT

Congratulations. Your decision to stop smoking is an important one. That's why you've made the right choice in choosing **Nicorette** gum. Your own chances of quitting smoking depend on how much you want to quit, how strongly you are addicted to tobacco, and how closely you follow a quitting program like the one that comes with **Nicorette**.

QUITTING SMOKING IS HARD!

If you've tried to quit before and haven't succeeded, don't be discouraged! Quitting isn't easy. It takes time, and most people try a few times before they are successful. The important thing is to try again until you succeed. This User's Guide will give you support as you become a non-smoker. It will answer common questions about **Nicorette** and give tips to help you stop smoking, and should be referred to often.

WHERE TO GET HELP

You are more likely to stop smoking by using **Nicorette** with a support program that helps you break your smoking habit. There may be support groups in your area for people trying to quit. Call your local chapter of the American Lung Association (1-800-586-4872), American Cancer Society (1-800-227-2345) or American Heart Association (1-800-242-8721) for further information. If you find you cannot stop smoking or if you start smoking again after using **Nicorette**, remember breaking this addiction doesn't happen overnight. You may want to talk to a health care professional who can help you improve your chances of quitting the next time you try **Nicorette** or another method.

LET'S GET ORGANIZED

Your reason for quitting may be a combination of concerns about health, the effect of smoking on your appearance, and pressure from your family and friends to stop smoking. Or maybe you're concerned about the dangerous effect of second-hand smoke on the people you care about. All of these are good reasons. You probably have others. Decide your most important reasons, and write them down on the wallet card inside the back cover of the User's Guide. Carry this card with you. In difficult moments, when you want to smoke, the card will remind you why you are quitting.

WHAT YOU'RE UP AGAINST

Smoking is addictive in two ways. Your need for nicotine has become both physical and mental. You must overcome both addictions to stop smoking. So while **Nicorette** will lessen your body's physical addition to nicotine, you've got to want to quit smoking to overcome the mental dependence on cigarettes. Once you've decided that you're going to quit, it's time to get started. But first, there are some important warnings you should consider.

SOME IMPORTANT WARNINGS.

This product is only for those who want to stop smoking. **If you are pregnant or breast-feeding, only use this medicine on the advice of your health care provider.** Smoking can seriously harm your child. Try to stop smoking without using any nicotine replacement medicine. This medicine is believed to be safer than smoking. However, the risks to your child from this medicine are not fully known.

Do not use

- if you continue to smoke, chew tobacco, use snuff, or use a nicotine patch or other nicotine containing products

Ask a doctor before use if you have

- heart disease, recent heart attack, or irregular heartbeat. Nicotine can increase your heart rate.
- high blood pressure not controlled with medication. Nicotine can increase your blood pressure.
- stomach ulcer or diabetes

Ask a doctor or pharmacist before use if you are

- using a non-nicotine stop smoking drug
- taking a prescription medicine for depression or asthma. Your prescription dose may need to be adjusted.

Stop use and ask a doctor if

- mouth, teeth or jaw problems occur
- irregular heartbeat or palpitations occur
- you get symptoms of nicotine overdose such as nausea, vomiting, dizziness, diarrhea, weakness and rapid heartbeat

Keep out of reach of children and pets. Pieces of nicotine gum may have enough nicotine to make children and pets sick. Wrap used pieces of gum in paper and throw away in trash. In case of overdose, get medical help or contact a Poison Control Center right away.

LET'S GET STARTED

Becoming a non-smoker starts today. First, check that you bought the right starting dose. **If you smoke 25 or more cigarettes a day,** use 4 mg nicotine gum. **If you smoke less than 25 cigarettes a day,** use 2 mg nicotine gum. Next, read through the entire User's Guide carefully. Then, set your personalized quitting schedule. Take out a calendar that you can use to track your progress, and identify four dates, using the stickers in the User's Guide.

STEP 1 (Weeks 1–6): Your quit date (and the day you'll start using Nicorette gum). Choose your quit date (it should be soon). This is the day you will quit smoking cigarettes entirely and begin using **Nicorette** to satisfy your cravings for nicotine. For the first six weeks, you'll use a piece of **Nicorette** every hour or two. Be sure to follow the directions on pages 9 and 11 of the User's Guide. Place the Step 1 sticker on this date.

STEP 2 (Weeks 7–9): The day you'll start reducing your use of Nicorette. After six weeks, you'll begin gradually reducing your **Nicorette** usage to one piece every two to four hours. Place the Step 2 sticker on this date (the first day of week seven).

STEP 3 (Weeks 10–12): The day you'll further reduce your use of Nicorette. Nine weeks after you begin using **Nicorette**, you will further reduce your nicotine intake by using one piece every four to eight hours. Place the Step 3 sticker on this date (the first day of week ten). For the next three weeks, you'll use a piece of **Nicorette** every four to eight hours.

End of treatment: The day you'll complete Nicorette therapy. Nicorette should not be used for longer than twelve weeks. Identify the date thirteen weeks after the date you chose in Step 1 and place the "EX-Smoker" sticker on your calendar.

PLAN AHEAD

Because smoking is an addiction, it is not easy to stop. After you've given up cigarettes, you will still have a strong urge to smoke. Plan ahead NOW for these times, so you're not defeated in a moment of weakness. The following tips may help:

- Keep the phone numbers of supportive friends and family members handy.
- Keep a record of your quitting process. Track the number of **Nicorette** pieces you use each day, and whether you feel a craving for cigarettes. In the event that you slip, immediately stop smoking and resume your quit attempt with the **Nicorette** program.
- Put together an Emergency Kit that includes items that will help take your mind off occasional urges to smoke. Include cinnamon gum or lemon drops to suck on, a relaxing cassette tape and something for your hands to play with, like a smooth rock, rubber band or small metal balls.
- Set aside some small rewards, like a new magazine or a gift certificate from your favorite store, which you'll 'give' yourself after passing difficult hurdles.
- Think now about the times when you most often want a cigarette, and then plan what else you might do instead of smoking. For instance, you might plan to take your coffee break in a new location, or take a walk right after dinner, so you won't be tempted to smoke.

HOW NICORETTE GUM WORKS

Nicorette's sugar-free chewing pieces provide nicotine to your system—they work as a temporary aid to help you quit smoking by reducing nicotine withdrawal symptoms. **Nicorette** provides a lower level of nicotine to your blood than cigarettes, and allows you to gradually do away with your body's need for nicotine. Because **Nicorette** does not contain the tar or carbon monoxide of cigarette smoke, it does not have the same health dangers as tobacco. However, it still delivers nicotine, the addictive part of cigarette smoke. Nicotine can cause side effects such as headache, nausea, upset stomach and dizziness.

HOW TO USE NICORETTE GUM

If you are under 18 years of age, ask a doctor before use. Before you can use **Nicorette** correctly, you have to practice! That sounds silly, but it isn't.

Nicorette isn't like ordinary chewing gum. It's a medicine, and must be chewed a certain way to work right. Chewed like ordinary gum, **Nicorette** won't work well and can cause side effects. An overdose can occur if you chew more than one piece of **Nicorette** at the same time, or if you chew many pieces one after another. Read all the following instructions before using **Nicorette**. Refer to them often to make sure you're using **Nicorette** gum correctly. If you chew too fast, or do not chew correctly, you may get hiccups, heartburn, or other stomach problems. Don't eat or drink for 15 minutes before using **Nicorette** or while chewing a piece. The effectiveness of **Nicorette** may be reduced by some foods and drinks, such as coffee, juices, wine or soft drinks.

1. Stop smoking completely before you start using **Nicorette**.
2. To reduce craving and other withdrawal symptoms, use **Nicorette** according to the dosage schedule on page 11 of the User's Guide.
3. Chew each **Nicorette** piece very slowly several times.
4. Stop chewing when you notice a peppery taste, or a slight tingling in your mouth. (This usually happens after about 15 chews, but may vary from person to person.)
5. "PARK" the **Nicorette** piece between your cheek and gum and leave it there.
6. When the peppery taste or tingle is almost gone (in about a minute), start to chew a few times slowly again. When the taste or tingle returns, stop again.
7. Park the **Nicorette** piece again (in a different place in your mouth).
8. Repeat steps 3 to 7 (chew, chew, park) until most of the nicotine is gone from the **Nicorette** piece (usually happens in about half an hour; the peppery taste or tingle won't return).
9. Wrap the used **Nicorette** piece in paper and throw away in the trash.

See the chart in the **"DIRECTIONS"** section above for the recommended usage schedule for **Nicorette**.

To improve your chances of quitting, use at least 9 pieces of **Nicorette** a day. If you experience strong or frequent cravings, you may use a second piece within the hour. However, do not continuously use one piece after another, since this may cause you hiccups, heartburn, nausea, or other side effects.

HOW TO REDUCE YOUR NICORETTE USAGE

The goal of using **Nicorette** is to slowly reduce your dependence on nicotine. The schedule for using **Nicorette** will help you reduce your nicotine craving gradually. Here are some tips to help you cut back during each step:

- After a while, start chewing each **Nicorette** piece for only 10 to 15 minutes, instead of half an hour. Then, gradually begin to reduce the number of pieces used.
- Or, try chewing each piece for longer than half an hour, but reduce the number of pieces you use each day.
- Substitute ordinary chewing gum for some of the **Nicorette** pieces you would normally use. Increase the number of pieces of ordinary gum as you cut back on the **Nicorette** pieces.

STOP USING NICORETTE AT THE END OF WEEK 12. If you still feel the need to use **Nicorette** after Week 12, talk with your doctor.

TIPS TO MAKE QUITTING EASIER

Within the first few weeks of giving up smoking, you may be tempted to smoke for pleasure, particularly after completing a difficult task, or at a party or bar. Here are some tips to help get you through the important first stages of becoming a non-smoker:

On your Quit Date:

- Ask your family, friends, and co-workers to support you in your efforts to stop smoking.
- Throw away all your cigarettes, matches, lighters, ashtrays, etc.
- Keep busy on your quit day. Exercise. Go to a movie. Take a walk. Get together with friends.
- Figure out how much money you'll save by not smoking. Most ex-smokers can save more than $1,000 a year.
- Write down what you will do with the money you save.
- Know your high risk situations and plan ahead how you will deal with them.
- Keep **Nicorette** gum near your bed, so you'll be prepared for any nicotine cravings when you wake up in the morning.
- Visit your dentist and have your teeth cleaned to get rid of the tobacco stains.

Right after Quitting:

- During the first few days after you've stopped smoking, spend as much time as possible at places where smoking is not allowed.
- Drink large quantities of water and fruit juices.
- Try to avoid alcohol, coffee and other beverages you associate with smoking.
- Remember that temporary urges to smoke will pass, even if you don't smoke a cigarette.
- Keep your hands busy with something like a pencil or a paper clip.
- Find other activities which help you relax without cigarettes.
- Swim, jog, take a walk, play basketball.
- Don't worry too much about gaining weight. Watch what you eat, take time for daily exercise, and change your eating habits if you need to.
- Laughter helps. Watch or read something funny.

WHAT TO EXPECT

Your body is now coming back into balance. During the first few days after you stop smoking, you might feel edgy and nervous and have trouble concentrating. You might get headaches, feel dizzy and a little out of sorts, feel sweaty or have stomach upsets. You might even have trouble sleeping at first. These are typical withdrawal symptoms that will go away with time. Your smoker's cough will get worse before it gets better. But don't worry, that's a good sign. Coughing helps clear the tar deposits out of your lungs.

After a Week or Two.

By now you should be feeling more confident that you can handle those smoking urges. Many of your withdrawal symptoms have left by now, and you should be noticing some positive signs: less coughing, better breathing and an improved sense of taste and smell, to name a few.

After a Month.

You probably have the urge to smoke much less often now. But urges may still occur, and when they do, they are likely to be powerful ones that come out of nowhere. Don't let them catch you off guard. Plan ahead for these difficult times. Concentrate on the ways non-smokers are more attractive than smokers. Their skin is less likely to wrinkle. Their teeth are whiter, cleaner. Their breath is fresher. Their hair and clothes smell better. That cough that seems to make even a laugh sound more like a rattle is a thing of the past. Their children and others around them are healthier, too.

What To Do About Relapse.

What should you do if you slip and start smoking again? The answer is simple. A lapse of one or two or even a few cigarettes has not spoiled your efforts! Discard your cigarettes, forgive yourself and try again. If you start smoking again, keep your box of **Nicorette** for your next quit attempt. If you have taken up regular smoking again, don't be discouraged. Research shows that the best thing you can do is to try again. The important thing is to learn from your last attempt.

- Admit that you've slipped, but don't treat yourself as a failure.
- Try to identify the 'trigger' that caused you to slip, and prepare a better plan for dealing with this problem next time.
- Talk positively to yourself—tell yourself that you have learned something from this experience.
- Make sure you used **Nicorette** gum correctly over the full 12 weeks to reduce your craving for nicotine.
- Remember that it takes practice to do anything, and quitting smoking is no exception.

WHEN THE STRUGGLE IS OVER

Once you've stopped smoking, take a second and pat yourself on the back. Now do it again. You deserve it. Remember now why you decided to stop smoking in the first place. Look at your list of reasons. Read them again. And smile. Now think about all the money you are saving and what you'll do with it. All the non-smoking places you can go, and what you might do there. All those years you may have added to your life, and what you'll do with them. Remember that temptation may not be gone forever. However, the hard part is behind you, so look forward with a positive attitude, and enjoy your new life as a non-smoker.

QUESTIONS & ANSWERS

1. How will I feel when I stop smoking and start using Nicorette? You'll need to prepare yourself for some nicotine withdrawal symptoms. These begin almost immediately after you stop smoking, and are usually at their worst during the first three to four days. Understand that any of the following is possible:

- craving for cigarettes
- anxiety, irritability, restlessness, mood changes, nervousness
- drowsiness
- trouble concentrating
- increased appetite and weight gain
- headaches, muscular pain, constipation, fatigue.

Nicorette can help provide relief from withdrawal symptoms such as irritability and nervousness, as well as the craving for nicotine you used to satisfy by having a cigarette.

2. Is Nicorette just substuting one form of nicotine for another? Nicorette does contain nicotine. The purpose of **Nicorette** is to provide you with enough nicotine to help control the physical withdrawal symptoms so you can deal with the mental aspects of quitting. During the 12 week program, you will gradually reduce your nicotine intake by switching to fewer pieces each day. Remember, don't use **Nicorette** together with nicotine patches or other nicotine containing products.

3. Can I be hurt by using Nicorette? For most adults, the amount of nicotine in the gum is less than from smoking. Some people will be sensitive to even this amount of nicotine and should not use this product without advice from their doctor. (See page 4 of User's Guide). Because **Nicorette** is a gum-based product, chewing it can cause dental fillings to loosen and aggravate other mouth, tooth and jaw problems. **Nicorette** can also cause hiccups, heartburn and other stomach problems especially if chewed too quickly or not chewed correctly.

4. Will I gain weight? Many people do tend to gain a few pounds in the first 8–10 weeks after they stop smoking. This is a very small price to pay for the enormous gains that you will make in your overall health and attractiveness. If you continue to gain weight after the first two months, try to analyze what you're doing differently. Reduce your fat intake, choose healthy snacks, and increase your physical activity to burn off the extra calories.

5. Is Nicorette more expensive than smoking? The total cost of **Nicorette** for the twelve week program is about equal to what a person who smokes one and a half packs of cigarettes a day would spend on cigarettes for the same period of time. Also, use of **Nicorette** is only a short-term cost, while the cost of smoking is a long-term cost, because of the health problems smoking causes.

6. What if I slip up? Discard your cigarettes, forgive yourself and then get back on track. Don't consider yourself a failure or punish yourself. In fact, people who have already tried to quit are more likely to be successful the next time. **GOOD LUCK!**

[End User's Guide]

OS-CAL® 500+D
calcium & vitamin D supplement

OS-CAL® 500 and 500 Chewable Tablets
calcium supplement
[ahs 'kal]

(See PDR For Dietary Supplements.)

TAGAMET HB 200® OTC
Cimetidine Tablets 200 mg/Acid Reducer

(See PDR For Nonprescription Drugs)

TUMS® REGULAR, TUMS E-X®, & TUMS ULTRA® OTC
Antacid/Calcium Supplement Tablets

(See PDR For Nonprescription Drugs.)

Glenwood

111 CEDAR LANE
ENGLEWOOD, NJ 07631

Direct Inquiries to:
Professional Services Department
201 569-0050
800 542-0772

For Medical Information Contact:
In Emergencies:
Professional Services Department
201 569-0050
800 542-0772

POTABA® ℞
Aminobenzoate Potassium, USP
Systemic ANTIFIBROSIS THERAPY

PRODUCT OVERVIEW

KEY FACTS

Potaba® (Aminobenzoate Potassium, USP) is considered a member of the vitamin B complex. It has been suggested that the antifibrotic action of Potaba® is due to its mediation of increased oxygen uptake at the tissue level.

MAJOR USES

Potaba® offers a means of treatment of serious and often chronic entities, such as scleroderma and Peyronie's Disease.

SAFETY INFORMATION

Contraindicated in patients taking sulfonamides. Anorexia, nausea, fever and rash have occurred infrequently and subside with omission of the drug. Often, desensitization can be accomplished and treatment resumed.

PRESCRIBING INFORMATION

POTABA® ℞
Aminobenzoate Potassium, USP
Systemic ANTIFIBROSIS THERAPY

FORMULA

POTABA® is chemically pure potassium p-aminobenzoate

INDICATIONS

Based on a review of this drug by the National Academy of Sciences-National Research Council and/or other information, FDA has classified the indications as follows:

"Possibly" effective: Potassium aminobenzoate is possibly effective in the treatment of scleroderma, dermatomyositis, morphea, linear scleroderma, pemphigus, and Peyronie's disease.

Final classification of the less-than-effective indications requires further investigation.

Continued on next page

Potaba—Cont.

ADVANTAGES

POTABA® offers a means of treatment of serious and often chronic entities involving fibrosis and nonsuppurative inflammation.

PHARMACOLOGY

P-Aminobenzoate is considered a member of the vitamin B complex. Small amounts are found in cereal, eggs, milk and meats. Detectable amounts are normally present in human blood, spinal fluid, urine, and sweat. PABA is a component of several biologically important systems, and it participates in a number of fundamental biological processes.

It has been suggested that the antifibrosis action of POTABA® is due to its mediation of increased oxygen uptake at the tissue level. Fibrosis is believed to occur from either too much serotonin or too little monoamine oxidase (MAO) activity over a period of time. Monoamine oxidase requires an adequate supply of oxygen to function properly. By increasing oxygen supply at the tissue level POTABA® may enhance MAO activity and prevent or bring about regression of fibrosis.

CLINICAL USES

PEYRONIE'S DISEASE: 21 patients with Peyronie's disease were placed on POTABA® therapy for periods ranging from 3 months to 2 years. Pain disappeared from 16 of 16 cases in which it had been present. There was objective improvement in penile deformity in 10 of 17 patients, and decrease in plaque size in 16 of 21. The authors suggest that this medication offers no hazard of further local injury as may result from other therapy. There were no significant untoward effects encountered on long term POTABA® therapy.

SCLERODERMA: Of 135 patients with diffuse systemic sclerosis treated with POTABA® every patient but one has shown softening of the involved skin if treatment has been continued for 3 months or longer. The responses have been reported in a number of publications. The treatment program consists of systemic antifibrosis therapy with POTABA®, physical therapy, including deep breathing exercises and dynamic traction splints where indicated, and bethanechol chloride for relief of dysphagia as well as small doses of reserpine for amelioration of Raynaud's phenomena.

DERMATOMYOSITIS: Five patients with scleroderma and 2 with dermatomyositis were treated with POTABA®. There was striking clinical improvement in each patient. Doses of 15-20 grams per day were well tolerated, and patients were easily able to take these doses.

MORPHEA and LINEAR SCLERODERMA: All 14 patients with localized forms of scleroderma placed on long-term POTABA® treatment showed softening of the sclerotic component of their disorder. Treatment is particularly indicated in patients where persistent compressive sclerosis may contribute even greater disfigurement or functional embarrassment from secondary pressure atrophy.

DOSAGE AND ADMINISTRATION

The average adult daily dose of POTABA® is 12 grams, usually given in four to six divided doses. Tablets and capsules 0.5 gram are given at the rate of 4 tablets or capsules 6 times daily, or 6 given four times daily, usually with meals, and at bedtime with a snack. Tablets must be taken with an adequate amount of liquid to prevent gastrointestinal upset.

POTABA® Envules contain 2 grams pure drug each. 6 Envules are given for a total of 12 grams POTABA® daily. Children are given 1 gram POTABA® daily in divided doses for each 10 lbs. of body weight. Envules must be dissolved in an adequate amount of liquid to prevent gastrointestinal upset.

SIDE EFFECTS

Anorexia, nausea, fever and rash have occurred infrequently and subside with omission of the drug. Desensitization can be accomplished and treatment resumed.

USAGE IN PREGNANCY

Safety for use in pregnancy or during lactation has not been established.

PRECAUTIONS

Should anorexia or nausea occur, therapy is interrupted until the patient is eating normally again. This permits prompt subsidence of symptoms and also avoids the possible development of hypoglycemia. Give cautiously to patients with renal disease. If a hypersensitivity reaction should occur, POTABA® should be stopped.

CONTRAINDICATIONS

POTABA® should not be administered to patients taking sulfonamides.

HOW SUPPLIED

POTABA Capsules—0.5 gm.
NDC 0516-0051-25 Bottle of 250
NDC 0516-0051-10 Bottle of 1000
POTABA Tablets—0.5 gm.
NDC 0516-0054-01 Bottle of 100
NDC 0516-0054-10 Bottle of 1000
POTABA Powder—2.0 gm Envules
NDC 0516-0052-50 Box of 50 × 2.0 gm
Rx only

Shown in Product Identification Guide, page 318

Gordon Laboratories

**6801 LUDLOW STREET
UPPER DARBY, PA 19082**

Direct inquiries to:
Customer Service
(610) 734-2011
Fax (610) 734-2049
Website: http://www.gordonlabs.com
E-mail: gordonlabs@worldnet.att.net
For medical emergencies contact:
David Dercher (610) 734-2011
Fax (610) 734-2049

GORDOCHOM™ Solution OTC

[*gōrdō'kōm*]

DESCRIPTION

Gordochom is an antifungal solution for topical use containing 25% Undecylenic Acid and 3% Chloroxylenol as its active ingredients in a penetrating oil base. Undecylenic Acid is chemically 10 hendecenoic acid having the empirical formula $C_{11}H_{20}O_2$ and the chemical bond structure CH_2=CH $(CH_2)8$ CO_2H.

Undecylenic Acid is a colorless to pale yellow liquid. It is insoluble in water and soluble in alcohol, chloroform and ether.

Chloroxylenol is chemically 2-chloro-5-hydroxy-1,3-dimethylbenzene having the empirical formula C_8H_9 ClO.

CLINICAL PHARMACOLOGY

Undecylenic Acid is a fungistatic agent employed in the treatment of tinea pedis, ringworm and dermatophytosis.

Chloroxylenol is a topical antiseptic, germicide and antifungal agent effective against a wide variety of causative fungi and yeast organisms. Among those affected by chloroxylenol are candida albicans, aspergillus niger, aspergillus flavus, trichophyton rubrum, trichophyton mentagrophytes, penicillum luteum and epidermophyton floccosum.

The penetrating oil base vehicle serves as a delivery system, enhancing the impregnation of Undecylenic Acid and Chloroxylenol as antimicrobial agents.

INDICATIONS

Cures athlete's foot (tinea pedis), and ringworm (tinea corporis).

CONTRAINDICATIONS

Gordochom is contraindicated in patients who are sensitive to Undecylenic Acid or Chloroxylenol.

WARNINGS

FOR EXTERNAL USE ONLY. Not for opthalmic or optic use. Avoid inhaling and contact with eyes or other mucous membranes. Not to be applied over blistered, raw or oozing areas of skin or over deep puncture wounds.

PRECAUTIONS

If a reaction suggesting sensitivity or chemical irritation should occur with the use of Gordochom, treatment should be discontinued. Use of Gordochom in pregnancy has not been established.

ADVERSE REACTIONS

No significant adverse reactions have been reported. However, attention should be paid to localized hypersensitivity.

DOSAGE AND ADMINISTRATION

Cleanse and dry affected areas. Apply a thin application twice a day (morning and night) to the affected area, or as recommended by your physician. Supervise children in the use of this product. For athlete's foot, pay special attention to the spaces between the toes; wear well-fitting, ventilated shoes, and change shoes and socks at least once daily. For athlete's foot and ringworm, use daily for 4 weeks. If condition persists longer, consult a physician. This product has not been proven effective on the scalp or nails.

HOW SUPPLIED

Gordochom is available in 1 oz. bottles with special brush applicator. (NDC 10481-8010-2)
Store at controlled room temperatures (59°–86°F).
For external use only.
Keep out of reach of children.

For EMERGENCY telephone numbers, consult the **Manufacturers' Index**.

Grifols Biologicals Inc.

**5555 VALLEY BOULEVARD
LOS ANGELES, CA 90032**

Direct Inquiries to:
CONTACTS:
All services, incl. 24 hr. ordering 888 Grifols (474-3657)
Direct Inquiries: (323) 225-2221
Fax: (323) 227-7613
Website www.grifolsusa.com

HUMAN ALBUMIN GRIFOLS® 20% ℞

Albumin (Human), USP, 20% Solution

DESCRIPTION

Albumin (Human), Human Albumin Grifols® 20% is a sterile aqueous solution for single dose intravenous administration containing 20% human albumin (weight/volume). Human Albumin Grifols® 20% is prepared by a cold alcohol fractionation method from pooled human plasma obtained from venous blood. The product is stabilized with 0.08 millimole sodium caprylate and 0.08 millimole sodium acetyltryptophanate per gram of protein. Human Albumin Grifols® 20% is osmotically equivalent to four times its volume of normal citrated plasma.

A liter of Human Albumin Grifols® 20% solution contains 130–160 milliequivalents of sodium ion. The product contains no preservatives.

Human Albumin Grifols® 20% is heated at 60°C for ten hours. No positive assertion can be made, however, that this heat treatment completely destroys the causative agents of viral hepatitis. There are no known cases of viral hepatitis, which have resulted from the administration of Human Albumin Grifols® 20%.

HOW SUPPLIED

Albumin (Human), Human Albumin Grifols® 20% is supplied in 50 ml vial.
NDC 61953-0001-1 May 1998

HUMAN ALBUMIN GRIFOLS 25%

Albumin (Human), USP, 25% Solution

10 vials per case
NDC 61953-0002-01 50 ml vial
NDC 61953-0002-02 100 ml vial

ALBUTEIN® 5% ℞

Albumin (Human), USP, 5% Solution

10 vials per case.
250mL vial NDC 68516-5211-01
500mL vial NDC 68516-5211-02

ALBUTEIN® 25% ℞

Albumin (Human), USP, 25% Solution

10 vials per case.
50mL vial NDC 68516-5213-02
100mL vial NDC 68516-5213-03

ALPHANATE® ℞

Antihemophilic Factor, (Human) Solvent Detergent/Heat Treated

DESCRIPTION

Alphanate® Antihemophilic Factor (Human) Solvent Detergent/Heat Treated is a highly purified Factor VIII/VWF product for the treatment of Hemophilia A and acquired Factor VIII deficiency. It is intended for intravenous administration. The product is purified by column chromatography and utilizes a solvent detergent treatment and heat treatment for viral inactivation.

HOW SUPPLIED

The product is available in the following potencies:

Factor VIII Activity	Diluent	NDC Number
250 i.u.	5 mL	68516-4600-01
500 i.u.	5 mL	68516-4600-01
1000 i.u.	10 mL	68516-4600-02
1500 i.u.	10 mL	68516-4600-02

Each carton contains a single dose vial of concentrate, sterile water for injection, a double ended transfer needle and microaggragate filter, and a package insert with full prescribing information. 12 vials per case.

ALPHANINE® SD ℞

Coagulation Factor IX (Human)
Solvent Detergent Treated/Virus Filtered

DESCRIPTION

AlphaNine® SD, Coagulation Factor IX (Human) is a highly purified Factor IX product for the treatment of Hemophilia B. It is intended for intravenous administration. The product is purified by a dual affinity column process and includes both solvent detergent treatment and virus filtration for added safeguards.

HOW SUPPLIED

The product is available in the following potencies:

Factor IX Activity	Diluent	NDC Number
500 IU	10 mL	68516-3600-02
1000 IU	10 mL	68516-3600-02
1500 IU	10 mL	68516-3600-02

Each carton contains a single dose vial of concentrate, sterile water for injection, a double-ended transfer needle, microaggregate filter, and a package insert with full prescribing information. 12 vials per case.

FLEBOGAMMA® 5% ℞

[flĕb-ō-gă-mă]
Immune Globulin Intravenous (Human)
Rx only

DESCRIPTION

Immune Globulin Intravenous (Human), Flebogamma® 5% (IGIV) is a sterile, clear or slightly opalescent and colorless to pale yellow, liquid pasteurized preparation of highly purified immunoglobulin (IgG) obtained from human plasma pools. The purification process includes cold alcohol fractionation, polyethylene glycol precipitation, and ion exchange chromatography.

Flebogamma® 5% is a highly purified (≥ 99% IgG), unmodified, human IgG that contains the antibody specificities found in the donor population, IgG subclasses are fully represented with the following approximate percents of total IgG: IgG_1 is 70.3%, IgG_2, 24.7%, IgG_3, 3.1%, and IgG_4, 1.9% (1). The IgA content is < 0.05 mg/mL and IgM is present in trace amounts.

In the final formulation, Flebogamma® 5% contains 50 mg IgG per mL, 50 mg D-sorbitol per mL, and ≤ 6 mg/mL polyethylene glycol. There is no preservative in the formulation. The pH of the solution ranges from 5 to 6 and the osmolarity from 240 to 350 mOsm/L.

All Source Plasma used in the manufacture of this product was tested by FDA-licensed serological tests for HBsAg, antibodies to HCV and HIV and Nucleic Acid Test (NAT) for HCV and HIV-1 and found to be nonreactive (negative).

WARNINGS

Immune Globulin Intravenous (Human) (IGIV) products have been reported to be associated with renal dysfunction, acute renal failure, osmotic nephrosis, and death (6). Patients predisposed to acute renal failure include patients witn any degree of pre-existing renal insufficiency, diabetes mellitus, age greater than 65, volume depletion, sepsis, paraproteinemia, or patients receiving known nephrotoxic drugs. Especially in such patients, IGIV products should be administered at the minimum concentration available and the minimum rate of infusion practicable. While these reports of renal dysfunction and acute renal failure have been associated with the use of many of the licensed IGIV products, those containing sucrose as a stabilizer accounted for a disproportionate share of the total number. Flebogamma® 5% does not contain sucrose.

See PRECAUTIONS and DOSAGE AND ADMINISTRATION sections for important information intended to reduce the risk of acute renal failure.

HOW SUPPLIED

Flebogamma® 5% is supplied in the following vial sizes:

NDC Number	Size	Grams IgG
61953-0003-01	10 mL	0.5
61953-0003-02	50 mL	2.5
61953-0003-03	100 mL	5
61953-0003-04	200 mL	10

STORAGE

Store at +2 to +25 °C (36 to 77 °F). Do not freeze. Discard after expiration date.

PROFILNINE® SD ℞

Factor IX Complex
Solvent Detergent Treated

DESCRIPTION

Profilnine® SD, Factor IX Complex, Solvent Detergent Treated is a lyophilized concentrate containing factors II, IX, and X plus low levels of factor VII. The product is available in single dose vials of Factor IX for the treatment of Hemophilia B (Factor IX deficiency).

HOW SUPPLIED

The product is available in the following potencies:

Factor IX Activity	Diluent	NDC Number
500 i.u.	5 mL	68516-3200-02
1000 i.u.	10 mL	68516-3200-03
1500 i.u.	10 mL	68516-3200-03

Each individual carton contains a single dose vial of Factor IX, sterile water for injection, transfer needle, microaggregate filter, and a package insert with full prescribing information. 12 vials per case.

EDUCATIONAL MATERIAL

Scientific publications, monographs, product literature, brochures and formulary kits available upon request.

Guardian Laboratories

a division of United-Guardian, Inc.
P.O. Box 18050
HAUPPAUGE, NY 11788

For Medical Information Contact:
Director of Medical Research
(631) 273-0900
(800) 645-5566

CLORPACTIN® WCS-90 OTC

[klor-pak 'tin]
(brand of sodium oxychlorosene)

COMPOSITION

Stabilized organic derivative of hypochlorous acid. A white, water soluble powder with a characteristic smell of hypochlorous acid. Active chlorine derived from calcium hypochlorite: 3–4%.

ACTION AND USES

For use as a topical antiseptic for treating localized infections, particularly when resistant organisms are present. Complete spectrum (bacteria, fungi, viruses, mold, yeast and spores); effective in cases of antibiotic resistance; nontoxic and non-allergenic in use concentrations.

ADMINISTRATION AND DOSAGE

Applied by irrigation, instillations, spray, soaks or wet compresses, preferably thoroughly cleansing with gravity flow irrigation or syringe to provide copious quantities of fresh solution to remove the organic wastes and debris from the site of the involvement. Also for preoperative skin preparation and postoperative protection. Generally applied as the 0.4% solution in water, or isotonic saline, but as the 0.1% to 0.2% in Urology and Ophthalmology.

CONTRAINDICATIONS

The use of this product is contraindicated where the site of the infection is not exposed to the direct contact with the solution. Not for systemic use.

HOW SUPPLIED

In boxes containing 5 x 2 gram bottles. NDC: 0327-0001-10 Store under refrigeration.

RENACIDIN® ℞

(Citric Acid, Glucono-delta-lactone, and Magnesium Carbonate)
Irrigation

DESCRIPTION

Renacidin® (Citric Acid, Glucono-delta-lactone, and Magnesium Carbonate) Irrigation is a sterile, non-pyrogenic irrigation for use within the urinary tract in the prevention and dissolution of calculi.

Each 100 ml. of Renacidin Irrigation contains:

Active ingredients:

Citric Acid (anhydrous), U.S.P. $C_6H_8O_7$	6.602 grams
Glucono-delta-lactone $C_6H_{10}O_6$	0.198 grams
Magnesium Carbonate, U.S.P. $(MgCO_3)_4 \cdot Mg(OH)_2 \cdot 3H_2O$	3.177 grams

Citric Acid

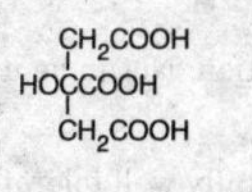

Glucono-delta-lactone

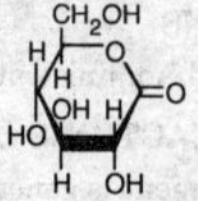

Magnesium Carbonate

$(MgCO_3)_4 \cdot Mg(OH)_2 \cdot 3H_2O$

Inert ingredients:

Benzoic Acid, U.S.P.	0.023 grams

Solution pH: 3.85 (3.50–4.20)

HOW SUPPLIED

Renacidin Irrigation is available as a sterile, non-pyrogenic solution in 500 ml containers, packaged in cartons of six. Exposure of Renacidin Irrigation to heat or cold should be minimized. Renacidin Irrigation should be stored at controlled room temperature, 59° to 86°F (15° to 30°C). Avoid excessive heat or cold (keep from freezing). Brief exposure to temperatures of up to 40°C or temperatures down to 5°C does not adversely affect the product.
NDC: 0327-0011-05
PRODUCT CODE: RN500

Healthpoint, Ltd.

3909 HULEN STREET
FORT WORTH, TX 76107

Direct Inquiries to:
800-441-8227

ACCUZYME® Ointment ℞

[ă-kew-zīm]
NDC 0064-1000-01 (30g tube)
NDC 0064-1000-07 (6g tube)
Papain, Urea
Rx ONLY

DESCRIPTION

ACCUZYME enzymatic debriding ointment contains papain, USP (8.3×10^5 USP units of activity per gram) and urea, USP 10% in a hydrophilic ointment base composed of emulsifying wax, fragrance, glycerin, isopropyl palmitate, lactose, methylparaben, potassium phosphate monobasic, propylparaben, and purified water.

CLINICAL PHARMACOLOGY

Papain, the proteolytic enzyme from the fruit of carica papaya, is a potent digestant of nonviable protein matter but is harmless to viable tissue. It is active over a pH range of 3 to 12. Papain is relatively ineffective when used alone as a debriding agent and requires the presence of activators to stimulate its digestive potency. In ACCUZYME Ointment, papain is combined with urea, a denaturant of proteins, to bring about two supplemental chemical actions: (1) to expose by solvent action the activators of papain, and (2) to denature the nonviable protein matter in lesions and thereby render it more susceptible to enzymatic digestion. Pharmacologic studies have shown that the combination of papain and urea result in twice as much digestive activity as papain alone.

INDICATIONS AND USAGE

ACCUZYME Ointment is indicated for debridement of necrotic tissue and liquefaction of slough in acute and chronic lesions such as pressure ulcers, varicose and diabetic ulcers, burns, postoperative wounds, pilonidal cyst wounds, carbuncles and miscellaneous traumatic or infected wounds.

CONTRAINDICATIONS

Do not use if you are allergic to or have known or suspected hypersensitivity to any ingredient in this product.

PRECAUTIONS

See Dosage and Administration. Not to be used in eyes.

ADVERSE REACTIONS

ACCUZYME Ointment is generally well-tolerated and nonirritating. A transient "burning" sensation may be experienced by a small percentage of patients upon applying ACCUZYME Ointment. Occasionally, the profuse exudate from enzymatic digestion may irritate the skin. In such cases, more frequent dressing changes will alleviate discomfort until exudate decreases.

DOSAGE AND ADMINISTRATION

Cleanse the wound with ALLCLENZ® Wound Cleanser or saline. Avoid cleansing with hydrogen peroxide solution as it may inactivate the papain. Apply ACCUZYME Ointment directly to the wound, cover with appropriate dressing, and secure into place. Daily or twice daily applications are preferred. Irrigate the wound at each redressing to remove any accumulation of liquefied necrotic material. NOTE: Papain may also be inactivated by the salts of heavy metals such as lead, silver and mercury. Contact with medications containing these metals should be avoided.

HOW SUPPLIED

30g tube, 6g tube. Store in a cool place 8°-15°C (46°-59°F). Do not refrigerate.

ACCUZYME Ointment is a registered trademark of Healthpoint, Ltd.

ALLCLENZ Wound Cleanser is a registered trademark of Healthpoint, Ltd.

Continued on next page

Accuzyme Ointment—Cont.

Marketed by:
HEALTHPOINT
Healthpoint, Ltd.
Fort Worth, Texas 76107
1-800-441-8227
www.healthpoint.com
Manufactured by:
DPT Laboratories, Ltd.
San Antonio, Texas 78215
REORDER NO. 0064-1000-01 (30g tube)
0064-1000-07 (6g tube)
128027-0304
Shown in Product Identification Guide, page 318

ACCUZYME® SPRAY ℞

[ăk'yoo-zīm]
(Papain, Urea)
NDC 0064-1001-33
Rx only

DESCRIPTION

ACCUZYME enzymatic debrinding spray contains papain, USP (8.3×10^5 USP units of activity per gram) and urea, USP 10% in a base composed of anhydrous lactose, cetearyl alcohol & ceteth-20 phosphate & dicetyl phosphate, fragrance, glycerin, methylparaben, mineral oil, potassium phosphate monobasic, propylparaben, purified water, and sodium hydroxide.

CLINICAL PHARMACOLOGY

Papain, the proteolytic enzyme from the fruit of carica papaya, is a potent digestant of nonviable protein matter but is harmless to viable tissue. It is active over a pH range of 3 to 12. Papain is relatively ineffective when used alone as a debriding agent and requires the presence of activators to stimulate its digestive potency. In ACCUZYME Spray, papain is combined with urea, a denaturant of proteins, to bring about two supplemental chemical actions: (1) to expose by solvent action the activators of papain, and (2) to denature the nonviable protein matter in lesions and thereby render it more susceptible to enzymatic digestion. Pharmacologic studies have shown that the combination of papain and urea result in twice as much digestive activity a papain alone.

INDICATIONS AND USES

ACCUZYME Spray is indicated for debridement of necrotic tissue and liquefaction of slough in acute and chronic lesions such as pressure ulcers, varicose and diabetic ulcers, burns, postoperative wounds, pilonidal cyst wounds, carbuncles and miscellaneous traumatic or infected wounds.

CONTRAINDICATIONS

ACCUZYME Spray is contraindicated in patients who have shown sensitivity to papain or any other components of this preparation.

PRECAUTIONS

See Dosage and Administration. Not to be used in eyes.

ADVERSE REACTIONS

ACCUZYME Spray is generally well-tolerated and nonirritating. A transient "burning" sensation may be experienced by a small percentage of patients upon applying ACCUZYME Spray. Occasionally, the profuse exudate from enzymatic digestion may irritate the skin. In such cases, more frequent dressing changes will alleviate discomfort until exudate decreases.

DOSAGE AND ADMINISTRATION

Cleanse the wound with ALLCLENZ® Wound Cleanser or saline. Avoid cleansing with hydrogen peroxide solution as it may inactivate the papain. NOTE: Papain may also be inactivated by the salts of heavy metals such as lead, silver and mercury. Contact with medications containing these metals should be avoided. In accordance with good wound care practices, protect the periwound with a skin protectant of choice to prevent and/or reduce maceration and irritation due to drainage from the wound. When practicable, daily or twice-daily changes of dressings are preferred. Longer intervals between redressings (two or three days) have proved satisfactory, and ACCUZYME Spray may be applied under pressure dressings.
If eschar is present, it may be necessary to consult a qualified practitioner in the use of a #10 blade to cross-hatch the eschar prior to application of ACCUZYME Spray in order to improve penetration of the product. Prior to cross-hatching, moisten the eschar with saline or a suitable wound cleanser such as ALLCLENZ Wound Cleanser.

INSTRUCTION FOR USE

Shake well before use.
Prime Container: Upon initial use only, the user will need to prime the non-aerosol ACCUZYME Spray pump. Begin first time use by holding ACCUZYME Spray upright directly over the wound, and prime the pump 6-8 times.
Once the pump has been primed, hold the ACCUZYME Spray bottle approximately 1″ from the wound and use even, firm, and consistent pressure to dispense product. When sprayed from the appropriate distance of 1″, the spray should appear in a nickel-sized diameter.
Completely cover the wound site with the ACCUZYME Spray. The wound should not be visible under the product. Cover wound with appropriate dressing of choice (saline-moistened gauze or semi-occlusive dressings are appropriate), and secure into place.
ACCUZYME Spray is designed to be used at an angle; however, as the product is dispensed, it may be necessary to hold the ACCUZYME Spray bottle in an upright position to achieve a full pump.

HOW SUPPLIED

33 mL spray bottle. Store upright in a cool place 8-15°C (46–59°F). Do not regfrigerate.
Marketed by:
HEALTHPOINT®
Healthpoint Ltd.
Fort Worth, Texas 76107
1-800-441-8227
www.healthpoint.com
Manufactured by:
DPT Laboratories, Ltd.
San Antonio, Texas 78215
REORDER NO. 0064-1001-33 (33 mL spray)
128028-0304
ACCUZYME is a registered trademark of Healthpoint, Ltd.
ALLCLENZ is a registered trademark of Healthpoint, Ltd.
Shown in Product Identification Guide, page 319

PANAFIL® Ointment ℞

[păn-ă-fĭl]
NDC 0064-3410-30 (30g tube)
NDC 0064-3410-07 (6g tube)
Papain, Urea, Chlorophyllin Copper Complex Sodium
Rx ONLY

DESCRIPTION

PANAFIL Ointment is an enzymatic healing-debriding ointment which contains papain, USP (not less than 521,700 USP units of activity per gram); urea, USP 10%; and chlorophyllin copper complex sodium, USP 0.5% in a hydrophilic base composed of boric acid, chlorobutanol (anhydrous) as a preservative, polyoxyl 40 stearate, propylene glycol, purified water, sodium borate, sorbitan monostearate, stearyl alcohol, and white petrolatum.

CLINICAL PHARMACOLOGY

Papain, the proteolytic enzyme derived from the fruit of carica papaya, is a potent digestant of nonviable protein matter, but is harmless to viable tissue. It has the unique advantage of being active over a wide pH range, 3 to 12. Despite its recognized value as a digestive agent, papain is relatively ineffective when used alone as a debriding agent, primarily because it requires the presence of activators to exert its digestive function. Urea is combined with papain to provide two supplementary chemical actions: 1) to expose by solvent action the activators of papain (sulfhydryl groups) which are always present, but not necessarily accessible, in the nonviable tissue or debris of lesions, and 2) to denature the nonviable protein matter in lesions and thereby render it more susceptible to enzymatic digestion. In pharmacologic studies involving digestion of beef powder, Miller[1] showed that the combination of papain and urea produced twice as much digestion as papain alone.
Chlorophyllin Copper Complex Sodium adds healing action to the cleansing action of the proteolytic papain-urea combination. The basic wound-healing properties of Chlorophyllin Copper Complex Sodium are promotion of healthy granulations, control of local inflammation and reduction of wound odors.[2] Specifically, Chlorophyllin Copper Complex Sodium inhibits the hemagglutinating and inflammatory properties of protein degradation products in the wound, including the products of enzymatic digestion, thus providing an additional protective factor.[1,3] The incorporation of Chlorophyllin Copper Complex Sodium in PANAFIL Ointment permits its continuous use for as long as desired to help produce and then maintain a clean wound base and to promote healing.

INDICATIONS AND USES

PANAFIL Ointment is suggested for treatment of acute and chronic lesions such as varicose, diabetic and decubitus ulcers, burns, postoperative wounds, pilonidal cyst wounds, carbuncles and miscellaneous traumatic or infected wounds.
PANAFIL Ointment is applied continuously throughout treatment of these conditions (1) for enzymatic debridement of necrotic tissue and liquefaction of fibrinous, purulent debris, (2) to keep the wound clean, and simultaneously (3) to promote normal healing.

CONTRAINDICATIONS

Do not use if you are allergic to or have known or suspected hypersensitivity to any ingredient in this product.

PRECAUTIONS

See Dosage and Administration. Not to be used in eyes.

ADVERSE REACTIONS

PANAFIL Ointment is generally well tolerated and nonirritating. A small percentage of patients may experience a transient "burning" sensation on application of the ointment. Occasionally, the profuse exudate resulting from enzymatic digestion may cause irritation. In such cases, more frequent changes of dressings until exudate diminishes will alleviate discomfort.

DOSAGE AND ADMINISTRATION

Cleanse the wound with ALLCLENZ® Wound Cleanser or saline. Avoid cleansing with hydrogen peroxide solution as it may inactivate the papain. Apply PANAFIL Ointment directly to the wound, cover with appropriate dressing, and secure into place. Note: Papain may also be inactivated by the salts of heavy metals such as lead, silver and mercury. Contact with medications containing these metals should be avoided. When practicable, daily or twice daily changes of dressings are preferred. Longer intervals between redressings (two or three days) have proved satisfactory, and PANAFIL Ointment may be applied under pressure dressings.

HOW SUPPLIED

30g tube, 6g tube. Store at controlled room temperature 20°-25°C, (68°-77°F).

REFERENCES

1. Miller, J.M.: The Interaction of Papain, Urea and Water-Soluble Chlorophyll in a Proteolytic Ointment for Infected Wounds, Surgery 43:939, 1958.
2. Smith, L.W.: The Present Status of Topical Chlorophyll Therapy, New York J. Med. 55:2041, 1955.
3. Barnard, R.D.: Elucidation of Chemically Defined Haptens For Competitive Inhibition of Aggressin Activity, Immunol. 8:78, 1954.

PANAFIL Ointment is a registered trademark of Healthpoint, Ltd.
ALLCLENZ Wound Cleanser is a registered trademark of Healthpoint, Ltd.
Marketed by:
Healthpoint,
Healthpoint, Ltd.
Fort Worth, Texas 76107
1-800-441-8227
www.healthpoint.com
Manufactured by:
DPT Laboratories, Ltd.
San Antonio, Texas 78215
REORDER NO. 0064-3410-30 (30g tube)
0064-3410-07 (6g tube)
128024-0304
Shown in Product Identification Guide, page 319

PANAFIL® SPRAY ℞

[pă-nă-fĭl]
HEALING, DEBRIDING AND DEODORIZING SPRAY
NDC 0064-3510-33
Papain-Urea-Chlorophyllin Copper Complex Sodium
Patent Pending

DESCRIPTION

PANAFIL® Spray is an enzymatic healing-debriding spray which contains standardized Papain, USP (not less than 521,700 USP units per gram of spray), Urea, USP 10% and Chlorophyllin Copper Complex Sodium, USP 0.5% in a base composed of Purified Water, USP; Glycerin, USP; Cetearyl Alcohol & Ceteth-20 Phosphate & Dicetyl Phosphate; Mineral Oil, USP; Lactose, Anhydrous; Sodium Hydroxide, NF; Methylparaben, NF; Propylparaben, NF.

CLINICAL PHARMACOLOGY

Papain, the proteolytic enzyme derived from the fruit of carica papaya, is a potent digestant of nonviable protein matter, but is harmless to viable tissue. It has the unique advantage of being active over a wide pH range, 3 to 12. Despite its recognized value as a digestive agent, papain is relatively ineffective when used alone as a debriding agent, primarily because it requires the presence of activators to exert its digestive function. Urea is combined with papain to provide two supplementary chemical actions: (1) to expose by solvent action the activators of papain (sulfhydryl groups) which are always present, but not necessarily accessible, in the nonviable tissue or debris of lesions, and (2) to denature the nonviable protein matter in lesions and thereby render it more susceptible to enzymatic digestion. In pharmacologic studies involving digestion of beef powder, Miller[1] showed that the combination of papain and urea produced twice as much digestion as papain alone. Chlorophyllin Copper Complex Sodium adds healing action to the cleansing action of the proteolytic papain-urea combination. The basic wound-healing properties of Chlorophyllin Copper Complex Sodium are promotion of healthy granulations, control of local inflammation and reduction of wound odors.[2] Specifically, Chlorophyllin Copper Complex Sodium inhibits the hemagglutinating and inflammatory properties of protein degradation products in the wound, including the products of enzymatic digestion, thus providing an additional protective factor.[1,3] The incorporation of Chlorophyllin Copper Complex Sodium in PANAFIL® Spray permits its continuous use for as long as desired to help produce and then maintain a clean wound base and to promote healing.

INDICATIONS AND USES

PANAFIL® Spray is suggested for treatment of acute and chronic lesions such as varicose, diabetic and decubitus ulcers, burns, postoperative wounds, pilonidal cyst wounds, carbuncles and miscellaneous traumatic or infected wounds.

PANAFIL® Spray is applied continuously throughout treatment of these conditions (1) for enzymatic debridement of necrotic tissue and liquefaction of fibrinous, purulent debris, (2) to keep the wound clean, and simultaneously (3) to promote normal healing.

CONTRAINDICATIONS

None known.

PRECAUTIONS

See Dosage and Administration. Not to be used in eyes.

ADVERSE REACTIONS

PANAFIL® Spray is generally well tolerated and nonirritating. A small percentage of patients may experience a transient "burning" sensation on application of the spray. Occasionally, the profuse exudate resulting from enzymatic digestion may cause irritation. In such cases, more frequent changes of dressings until exudate diminishes will alleviate discomfort.

DOSAGE AND ADMINISTRATION

Cleanse the wound with ALLCLENZ® Wound Cleanser or saline. Avoid cleansing with hydrogen peroxide solution as it may inactivate the papain. Note: Papain may also be inactivated by the salts of heavy metals such as lead, silver and mercury. Contact with medications containing these metals should be avoided. In accordance with good wound care practices, protect the periwound with a skin protectant of choice to prevent and/or reduce maceration and irritation due to drainage from the wound. When practicable, daily or twice daily changes of dressings are preferred. Longer intervals between redressings (two or three days) have proved satisfactory, and PANAFIL® Spray may be applied under pressure dressings.

INSTRUCTIONS FOR USE

Shake well before use.

Prime Container: Upon initial use only, the user will need to prime the non-aerosol PANAFIL® Spray pump. Begin first time use by holding PANAFIL® Spray upright directly over the wound, and prime the pump 6–8 times.

Once the pump has been primed, hold the PANAFIL® Spray bottle approximately 1″ from the wound and use even, firm, and consistent pressure to dispense product. When sprayed from the appropriate distance of 1″, the spray should appear in a nickel-sized diameter.

Completely cover the wound site with the PANAFIL® Spray. The wound should not be visible under the product. Cover wound with appropriate dressing of choice (saline-moistened gauze or semi-occlusive dressings are appropriate), and secure into place.

PANAFIL® Spray is designed to be used at an angle; however, as the product is dispensed, it may be necessary to hold the PANAFIL® Spray bottle in an upright position to achieve a full pump.

HOW SUPPLIED

33 mL spray bottle. Store upright at controlled room temperature 20–25°C (68–77°F).

Rx ONLY

REFERENCES

1. Miller, J.M.: The Interaction of Papain, Urea and Water-Soluble Chlorophyll in a Proteolytic Ointment for Infected Wounds, Surgery 43:939, 1958.

2. Smith, L.W.: The Present Status of Topical Chlorophyll Therapy, New York J. Med. 55:2041, 1955.

3. Barnard, R.D.: Elucidation of Chemically Defined Haptens For Competitive Inhibition of Aggressin Activity, Immunol. 8:78, 1954.

Manufactured by:
DPT Laboratories, Ltd.
San Antonio, Texas 78215
Marketed by:
Healthpoint, Ltd.
www.healthpoint.com
REORDER NO. 0064-3510-33 (33 mL spray)
128019-1203

Shown in Product Identification Guide, page 319

PRUDOXIN® Cream ℞

[prū 'dock-çĭn]

(Doxepin Hydrochloride Cream), 5%

NDC 0064-3600-45

For Topical Dermatologic Use Only—

Not For Ophthalmic, Oral, or Intravaginal Use.

Brief Summary: See full prescribing information for complete product information

DESCRIPTION

PRUDOXIN® Cream (doxepin hydrochloride cream) is a topical antipuritic cream. Each gram contains: 50 mg of doxepin hydrochloride (equivalent to 44.3 mg of doxepin). Doxepin hydrochloride is one of a class of agents known as dibenzoxepin tricyclic compounds. It is an isomeric mixture of N,N-Dimethyldibenz [*b,e*] oxepin-$\Delta^{11(6H)}$-propylamine hydrochloride. Doxepin hydrochloride has an empirical formula of $C_{19}H_{21}NO \bullet HCl$ and a molecular weight of 316. The base is a cream of pH 3.5 to 5.5 that includes the inactive ingredients: sorbitol, cetyl alcohol, isopropyl myristate, glyceryl stearate, PEG-100 stearate, petrolatum, benzyl alcohol, titanium dioxide and purified water.

HOW SUPPLIED

PRUDOXIN® Cream is available in a 45 g (NDC 0064-3600-45) aluminum tube. Store at or below 27°C (80°F).

Rx ONLY

Distributed by:
HEALTHPOINT®
Healthpoint, Ltd.
Ft. Worth, TX 76107
1-800-441-8227
Manufactured by:
DPT Laboratories, Ltd.
San Antonio, Texas 78215

Shown in Product Identification Guide, page 319

XENADERM™ Ointment ℞

[zen'ə-dŭrm]

(Balsam Peru, Castor Oil USP/NF, Trypsin USP)

FOR EXTERNAL USE ONLY

Rx ONLY

PAT. NO. 6,479,060

ACTIVE INGREDIENTS

Each gram contains Trypsin USP NLT 90 USP units, Balsam Peru 87.0 mg, Castor Oil USP/NF 788.0 mg.

INACTIVE INGREDIENTS

Safflower Oil, Aluminum Magnesium Hydroxide Stearate.

ACTION

Balsam Peru is an effective capillary bed stimulant used to increase circulation in the wound site area. Also, Balsam Peru has a mildly bactericidal action. Castor Oil is used to improve epithelialization by reducing premature epithelial desiccation and cornification. Also, it can act as a protective covering and aids in the reduction of pain. Trypsin is intended for debridement of eschar and other necrotic tissue. It appears that in many instances removal of wound debris strengthens humoral defense mechanisms sufficiently to retard proliferation of local pathogens.

INDICATIONS

To promote wound healing and for the treatment of decubitus ulcers, varicose ulcers and dehiscent wounds.

USES

XENADERM™ Ointment is easy to apply and quickly reduces odor frequently accompanying a decubitus ulcer. The wound may be left open or appropriate dressing applied. As a suggestion, keep in mind wounds heal poorly in the presence of hemoglobin or zinc deficiency.

WARNING

Do not apply to fresh arterial clots. Avoid contact with eyes. Keep out of reach of children. Use only as directed. When applied to a sensitive area, a temporary stinging sensation may be noted.

DOSAGE

Apply a thin film of XENADERM™ Ointment a minimum of twice daily or as often as necessary. Wound may be left unbandaged or appropriate dressing applied. To remove, wash gently with appropriate cleanser.

HOW SUPPLIED

XENADERM™ Ointment is supplied in 60 gram tubes.
NDC 0064-3900-60
Store XENADERM™ Ointment between 15° and 30°C (59° and 86°F). Avoid freezing.

Distributed by:
HEALTHPOINT®
Healthpoint, Ltd.
Fort Worth, TX 76107
1-800-441-8227
www.healthpoint.com
Manufactured by:
DPT Laboratories, Ltd.
San Antonio, TX 78215
127826-0502

Shown in Product Identification Guide, page 319

Heel Inc.

10421 RESEARCH RD. SE
ALBUQUERQUE, NM 87123

Direct Inquiries to:
Medical Department
800-621-7644
(505) 293-3843
Fax: (800) 217-6934
www.HeelUSA.com

TRAUMEEL® Gel OTC
Anti-inflammatory

TRAUMEEL® Tablets OTC
Anti-inflammatory

TRAUMEEL® Ointment OTC
Anti-inflammatory

TRAUMEEL® Oral Drops OTC
Anti-inflammatory

TRAUMEEL® Oral Liquid in Vials OTC
Anti-inflammatory

TRAUMEEL® Injection Solution ℞

DESCRIPTION

TRAUMEEL® Injection Solution is an anti-inflammatory, anti-edematous, anti-exudative combination formulation of 12 botanical substances and 1 mineral substance. TRAUMEEL® Injection Solution is officially classified as a homeopathic combination remedy (1).

1. Botanical ingredients:
   - Arnica montana, radix (mountain arnica)
   - Calendula officinalis (marigold)
   - Hamamelis virginiana (witch hazel)
   - Millefolium (milfoil)
   - Belladonna (deadly nightshade)
   - Aconitum napellus (monkshood)
   - Chamomilla (chamomile)
   - Symphytum officinale (comfrey)
   - Bellis perennis (daisy)
   - Echinacea angustifolia (narrow-leafed cone flower)
   - Echinacea purpurea (purple cone flower)
   - Hypericum perforatum (St. John's wort)
2. Mineral ingredients:
   - Hepar sulphuris calcareum (calcium sulfide)

Injection Solution: Each 2.0 ml ampule contains as active ingredients: Hepar sulphuris calcareum 8X 200.0 µl; Belladonna 3X 20.0 µl; Calendula officinalis 3X 20.0 µl; Chamomilla 4X 20.0 µl; Millefolium 4X 20.0 µl; Aconitum napellus 3X 12.0 µl; Bellis perennis 3X 10.0 µl; Hypericum perforatum 3X 6.0 µl; Echinacea angustifolia 3X 5.0 µl; Echinacea purpurea 3X 5.0 µl; Arnica montana, radix 2X 2.0 µl; Hamamelis virginiana 2X 2.0 µl; Symphytum officinale 6X 2.0 µl. Each 2.0 ml ampule contains as an inactive ingredient: Sterile isotonic sodium chloride solution.

CLINICAL PHARMACOLOGY

The exact mechanism of action of TRAUMEEL® Injection Solution is not fully understood. Various cellular and biochemical pathways appear to be modulated by the product ingredients. The mechanism of action of TRAUMEEL® Injection Solution does not appear to be the result of cyclooxygenase or lipoxygenase enzyme inhibition, as is the case with nonsteroidal anti-inflammatory drugs (NSAIDs). TRAUMEEL® Injection Solution does not inhibit the arachidonic acid pathway of prostaglandin synthesis. Instead, the mechanism of action of TRAUMEEL® Injection Solution appears to be the result of modulation of the release of oxygen radicals from activated neutrophils, and inhibition of the release of inflammatory mediators (possibly interleukin-1 from activated macrophages) and neuropeptides (2).

In vitro studies show that the ingredients in TRAUMEEL® Injection Solution are noncytotoxic to granulocytes, lymphocytes, platelets, and endothelia, which indicates that the defensive functions of these cells are preserved during treatment with TRAUMEEL® Injection Solution (3).

The anti-inflammatory, anti-edematous, and anti-exudative effects of TRAUMEEL® Injection Solution have been demonstrated in clinical trials as well as in *in vivo* experimental models including the carrageenin-induced edema test and the adjuvant arthritis test (3).

INDICATIONS AND USAGE

TRAUMEEL® Injection Solution is indicated for the treatment of symptoms associated with inflammatory, exudative, and degenerative processes due to acute trauma (such as contusions, lacerations, fractures, sprains, post-operative wounds, etc.), repetitive or overuse injuries (such as tendonitis, bursitis, epicondylitis, etc.), and for minor aches and pains associated with such conditions. TRAUMEEL® Injection Solution is also indicated for the treatment of minor aches and pains associated with backache, muscular aches, and the minor pain from rheumatoid arthritis, osteoarthritis, gouty arthritis, and ankylosing spondylitis.

Continued on next page

Traumeel Injection—Cont.

CONTRAINDICATIONS

TRAUMEEL® Injection Solution is contraindicated in patients with a known hypersensitivity to TRAUMEEL® Injection Solution or any of its ingredients (see **ADVERSE REACTIONS**).

WARNINGS

If pain persists or worsens, if new symptoms occur, or if redness or swelling is present, the patient should be carefully re-evaluated because these could be signs of a serious condition.

PRECAUTIONS

General:
Adverse effects with TRAUMEEL® Injection Solution are extremely rare. TRAUMEEL® Injection Solution exhibits no known adverse renal, hepatic, cardiovascular, gastrointestinal or central nervous system effects.

Information for Patients:
No harmful or potentially hazardous side effects such as central nervous system depression are known. TRAUMEEL® Injection Solution is generally well-tolerated. However, if symptoms persist or worsen, a physician should be consulted (see **WARNINGS**).

Drug Interactions:
TRAUMEEL® Injection Solution is not known to interact with other medications. Furthermore, the administration of TRAUMEEL® Injection Solution can be safely augmented by the application of a topical dosage form of TRAUMEEL®.

Drug/Laboratory Test Interactions:
TRAUMEEL® Injection Solution is not known to interact with any laboratory tests.

Carcinogenesis:
No studies have been performed to evaluate the carcinogenicity of TRAUMEEL® Injection Solution. In world-wide post-marketing surveillance studies no evidence of carcinogenicity has been found (2).

Pregnancy:
Pregnancy Category C. In general, medications such as TRAUMEEL® Injection Solution that are classified as homeopathic are not known to cause direct or indirect harm to the fetus. However, animal reproduction studies have not been performed and there are no well-controlled studies in pregnant women. In cases of pregnancy or suspected pregnancy, TRAUMEEL® Injection Solution should be used only if potential benefits justify potential risks to the fetus.

Nursing Mothers:
It is not known whether any of the ingredients in TRAUMEEL® Injection Solution are excreted in human milk. However, because many drugs are excreted in human milk, TRAUMEEL® Injection Solution should be administered with caution to nursing mothers.

Pediatric Use:
TRAUMEEL® Injection Solution can be safely administered to children as young as 2 years (see **DOSAGE AND ADMINISTRATION**).

ADVERSE REACTIONS

In rare cases, patients with hypersensitivity to botanicals of the Compositae family may experience an allergic reaction after the administration of TRAUMEEL® Injection Solution including anaphylactic reaction. TRAUMEEL® Injection Solution ingredients of the Compositae family are:

- Arnica montana, radix (mountain arnica)
- Calendula officinalis (marigold)
- Millefolium (milfoil)
- Chamomilla (chamomile)
- Bellis perennis (daisy)
- Echinacea angustifolia (narrow-leafed cone flower)
- Echinacea purpurea (purple cone flower)

OVERDOSAGE

Due to the low concentration of active ingredients in homeopathic preparations such as TRAUMEEL® Injection Solution, adverse reactions following overdosage are extremely unlikely. However, care must be taken not to exceed the recommended dosage.

DOSAGE AND ADMINISTRATION

The dosage schedules listed below can be used as a general guide for the administration of TRAUMEEL® Injection Solution. TRAUMEEL® Injection Solution shows individual differences in clinical response. Therefore, the dosage for each patient should be individualized according to the patient's response to therapy. For best results, treatment with TRAUMEEL® Injection Solution should be initiated immediately following injury or at the first sign of symptoms. TRAUMEEL® Injection Solution may be administered until symptoms disappear.

TRAUMEEL® Injection Solution:
Adults and children above 6 years: 1 ampule daily for acute disorders, or 1 to 2 ampules 1 to 3 times weekly.
Children (2 to 6 years): Half the adult dosage. Discard unused solution.

TRAUMEEL® Injection Solution may be administered intravenously, intramuscularly, subcutaneously or intradermally. TRAUMEEL® Injection Solution is indicated for peri-articular administration, and for intra-articular aseptic conditions. If administration with a local anesthetic is desired, TRAUMEEL® Injection Solution may be mixed in a 1:1 ratio with 1% or 2% lidocaine hydrochloride. Similar local anesthetics may also be used. The required dose of TRAUMEEL® Injection Solution is first withdrawn from the ampule into the syringe. The local anesthetic is then withdrawn into the syringe, and the syringe is then shaken briefly. Normally, about 0.5 to 1.0 milliliters of each drug is withdrawn into the syringe.

TRAUMEEL® Injection Solution should be administered using a narrow gauge needle (e.g., 22 to 30 gauge). **Note:** Parenteral drug products like TRAUMEEL® Injection Solution should be inspected visually for particulate matter and discoloration prior to administration whenever solution and container permit. TRAUMEEL® Injection Solution is a clear, colorless solution. Discolored solutions should be discarded.

HOW SUPPLIED

TRAUMEEL® Injection Solution in 2.0 ml ampules:
Packs of 10: NDC 50114-7000-1.
Avoid freezing and excessive heat. Store at room temperature. Protect from light.
CAUTION: Rx only.

REFERENCES

(1) The Homeopathic Pharmacopoeia of the United States (HPUS), 8th edition, Falls Church, Virginia, 1979; and the Homeopathic Pharmacopoeia of the United States Revision Service (HPRS), 1988.
(2) Data on file, Heel GmbH, Baden-Baden, Germany.
(3) Conforti A, *et al.* Experimental Studies on the Anti-inflammatory Activity of a Homeopathic Preparation. *Biomedical Therapy XV* No.1:28-31, 1997.

This full prescribing information has been compiled in accordance with the Code of Federal Regulations (CFR), 21 sections 201.56 and 201.57.

Hemispherx Biopharma, Inc.

ONE PENN CENTER
1617 JFK BOULEVARD
PHILADELPHIA, PA 19103-1806

Direct Inquiries to:
Alferon Access Program™
Phone 1 888 ALFERON
Fax 1 888 FAXX AFN
website: www.hemispherx.net

ALFERON N INJECTION® ℞

Interferon alfa-n3
(human leukocyte derived)

This product is now manufactured and distributed by HEMISPHERX BIOPHARMA, Inc., Philadelphia, PA 19103-1806.

DESCRIPTION

Alferon N Injection® [Interferon alfa-n3 (human leukocyte derived)] is a sterile aqueous formulation of purified, natural, human interferon alpha proteins for use by injection. Alferon N Injection® consists of interferon alpha proteins comprising approximately 166 amino acids ranging in molecular weights from 16,000 to 27,000 daltons. The specific activity of Interferon alfa-n3 is approximately equal to, or greater than, 2×10^8 IU/mg of protein.

Alferon N Injection® is manufactured from pooled units of human leukocytes which have been induced by incomplete infection with a murine virus (Sendai virus) to produce Interferon alfa-n3. The manufacturing process includes immunoaffinity chromatography with a murine monoclonal antibody, acidification (pH 2) for 5 days at 4°C, and gel filtration chromatography.

Since Alferon N Injection® is manufactured using source leukocytes, human donor screening is performed to minimize the risk that the leukocytes could contain infectious agents. In addition, the manufacturing process contains steps which have been shown to inactivate known viruses. There has been no evidence of infection transmission to recipients in clinical trials (See WARNINGS).

The Alferon N Injection® manufacturing process was evaluated for quantitative removal or inactivation of model pathogenic viruses. The viruses were deliberately added to the leukocytes in amounts far exceeding those present in contaminated blood, i.e., $\geq 10^9$ infectious units per milliliter. The manufacturing process yielded a cumulative reduction of $\geq 10^{14}$ of infectious HIV-1, i.e., $\geq 10^{6.5}$ removal by acid inactivation and $\geq 10^{7.9}$ removal by the purification process. In the validation studies, there was 10^8 reduction in the titer of hepatitis B virus as determined by HBsAg assay, and a 10^9 reduction in the infectious titer of herpes simplex virus 1 (HSV-1). Cultivation of Alferon N Injection® [Interferon alfa-n3 (human leukocyte derived)] Purified Drug Concentrate with human indicator cells, i.e., MRC-5 cells, peripheral blood leukocytes in the presence of Cyclosporin A, and fetal cord blood cells, did not detect the presence of infectious viruses.

As part of a validation study, Alferon N Injection® was examined for the presence of the following viruses; Sendai virus (SV), HIV-1, HTLV-1, HBV, HSV-1, CMV, and EBV. Alferon N Injection® contained no detectable quantities of these viruses. In addition, other studies, i.e., Polymerase Chain Reaction (PCR) and Dot Blot Hybridization (DBH), have shown no detectable genetic material from these viruses in Alferon N Injection®. The sensitivity of the PCR was 10 copies for HIV-1 (env gene probe) and 10 copies for HBV (S/P gene probe). The sensitivity of the DBH was 1 pg for EBV, < 10 pg for CMV, < 10 pg for HSV-1, and < 2 pg for SV. Furthermore, sera from 105 patients treated with Alferon N Injection® (95 with condylomata acuminata and 10 with cancer) were tested for antibody to HIV-1 and HIV p24 antigen. There was no evidence to suggest transmission of HIV-1 by Alferon N Injection®. Sera from 135 patients with condylomata acuminata treated with Alferon N Injection® were tested to determine abnormal SGOT laboratory values. There was no evidence to suggest transmission of hepatitis by Alferon N Injection® based on both SGOT results and patient data collected during clinical trials.

Alferon N Injection® has been extensively purified using immunoaffinity chromatography with a murine monoclonal antibody, acidification (pH 2) for 5 days at 4°C, and gel filtration chromatography. Alferon N Injection® has been subjected to the acid treatment for five days during its manufacture in order to reduce the risk of viral transmission. Subsequent analyses of the Alferon N Injection® [Interferon alfa-n3 (human leukocyte derived)] Purified Drug Concentrate confirm the absence of detectable infectious or non-infectious viral particles.

The leukocyte nutrient medium contains the antibiotic neomycin sulfate at a concentration of 35 mg/L; however, neomycin sulfate is not detectable in the final product, i.e., < 0.64 μg/ml.

Murine immunoglobulin (IgG) is detected in the Alferon N Injection® Purified Drug Concentrate at levels below 0.15% of the Interferon alfa-n3 protein. This equates to levels less than 8 ng of murine IgG per million of IU Interferon alfa-n3 (range of 0.9 to 5.6 ng typically found).

Alferon N Injection® is available in an injectable solution containing 5 million IU Interferon alfa-n3 per vial for intralesional injection. The solution is clear and colorless. Each milliliter (ml) contains five million IU of Interferon alfa-n3 in phosphate-buffered saline (8.0 mg sodium chloride, 1.74 mg sodium phosphate dibasic, 0.20 mg potassium phosphate monobasic, and 0.20 mg potassium chloride) containing 3.3 mg phenol as a preservative and 1 mg Albumin (Human) as a stabilizer.

CLINICAL PHARMACOLOGY

General—Interferons are naturally occurring proteins with antiviral, antiproliferative, and immunoregulatory properties. They are produced and secreted in response to viral infections and to a variety of other synthetic and biological inducers. Four major families of interferons have been identified: alpha, beta, gamma, and omega. The interferon alpha family contains 13 different non-allelic molecular species. Their molecular weights range from 16,000 to 27,000 daltons.

Interferons bind to specific membrane receptors on cell surfaces. Interferon alfa-n3 has been shown to bind to the same receptors as Interferon alfa-2b. The receptors have a high degree of selectivity for the binding of human but not mouse interferon. This correlates with the high species specificity found in laboratory studies.

Binding of interferon to membrane receptors initiates a series of events including induction of protein synthesis. These actions are followed by a variety of cellular responses, including inhibition of virus replication and suppression of cell proliferation. Immunomodulation, including enhancement of phagocytosis by macrophages, augmentation of the cytotoxicity of lymphocytes and enhancement of human leukocyte antigen expression occurs in response to exposure to interferons. One or more of these activities may contribute to the therapeutic effect of interferon.

Pharmacokinetics—In a study of intralesional use of Alferon N Injection® [Interferon alfa-n3 (human leukocyte derived)] for the treatment of condylomata acuminata, plasma concentrations of interferon were below the detection limit of the assay, i.e., ≤ 3 IU/ml. Minor systemic effects (e.g., myalgias, fever, and headaches) were noted, indicating that some of the injected interferon entered the systemic circulation (See ADVERSE REACTIONS).

Condylomata Acuminata—Condylomata acuminata (venereal or genital warts) are associated with infections of human papilloma virus (HPV), especially HPV type-6 and possibly type-11. Given the antiviral and antiproliferative activities of interferons and the viral etiology of condylomata, a placebo-controlled clinical trial was conducted to evaluate the safety and efficacy of intralesional injection of Alferon N Injection® in the treatment of condylomata acuminata.

In a multicenter, randomized, double-blind, placebo-controlled, clinical trial, intralesional administration of Alferon N Injection® was an effective treatment for condylomata acuminata.[1–4] One hundred fifty-six (156) patients were evaluable for efficacy (81 Alferon N Injection® patients and 75 placebo patients). Patients had a mean of five warts (range was 2-14) and all warts were treated. Patients were injected intralesionally with a mean of 225,000 IU of Alferon N Injection® per wart 2 times a week for up to 8 weeks.

Overall, 80% ($^{65}/_{81}$) of patients treated with Alferon N Injection® had a complete or partial resolution of warts compared with 44% ($^{33}/_{75}$) of placebo-treated patients ($p < 0.001$). Alferon N Injection® was significantly more effective than placebo in producing a complete resolution of warts ($p < 0.001$), as shown by Table 1.

[See table 1 at top of next page]

Of the patients who had a complete resolution of warts, approximately half ($^{21}/_{44}$) the patients had complete resolution of warts by the end of treatment, and half $(^{23}/_{44})$ had complete resolution of warts during the three months after the cessation of treatment. Patients with complete resolution of warts were followed for a median of 48 weeks. Overall, 76% $(^{31}/_{41})$ of Alferon N Injection® [Interferon alfa-n3 (human leukocyte derived)]-treated patients who achieved complete resolution of warts remained clear of all treated lesions during follow-up, while 79% $(^{11}/_{14})$ of the placebo-treated patients remained clear of all treated lesions during follow-up. A total of 762 evaluable warts were injected in this trial. Of the 407 Alferon N Injection®-treated warts, 73% $(^{297}/_{407})$ completely resolved, as compared to 35% $(^{125}/_{355})$ of the placebo-treated warts ($p < 0.0001$). Alferon N Injection® was effective in treating lesions of all sizes, and there was no difference in resolution for perianal, penile, or vulvar lesions.

There was no difference in resolution for patients who had received prior treatment of their warts and for those who had not. Among patients with recalcitrant warts (i.e., warts that were refractory to previous treatment or recurring), 82% $(^{58}/_{71})$ of the evaluable patients had complete or partial resolution of warts due to intralesional administration of Alferon N Injection® as compared to 43% $(^{29}/_{67})$ of placebo patients ($p < 0.001$). Fifty-four percent $(^{38}/_{71})$ of the evaluable Alferon N Injection® patients had complete resolution of warts as compared to 18% $(^{12}/_{67})$ of placebo patients ($p < 0.001$). Patients with primary occurrence of genital warts (i.e., no prior treatment of warts) had a similar resolution rate compared to the patients with recalcitrant warts: 70% $(^{7}/_{10})$ had complete or partial resolution of warts due to Alferon N Injection® [Interferon alfa-n3 (human leukocyte derived)] treatment and 60% $(^{6}/_{10})$ had complete resolution of warts, as compared to 50% $(^{4}/_{8})$ of placebo recipients who had complete or partial resolution of warts and 38% $(^{3}/_{8})$ who had complete resolution. Overall, 83% $(^{5}/_{6})$ of Alferon N Injection®-treated patients with primary occurrence, who achieved complete resolution of warts, remained clear of all treated lesions during a median follow-up of 52 weeks. Because the number of patients with primary occurrence of warts was small (10 Alferon N Injection® recipients and 8 placebo recipients), the difference between Alferon N Injection® and placebo treatment was not statistically significant. However, when the resolution of primary warts was examined, 75% $(^{33}/_{44})$ of the Alferon N Injection®-treated primary warts resolved completely as compared to 39% $(^{11}/_{28})$ of the placebo-treated primary warts ($p = 0.003$).

In an open clinical trial using a once-a-week treatment schedule for up to 16 weeks, 28 patients were evaluable for efficacy. Eighty-nine percent $(^{25}/_{28})$ of patients had a complete or partial resolution of warts following treatment with Alferon N Injection®. The condylomata acuminata resolved completely in 46% $(^{13}/_{28})$ of the patients. Of the 154 warts treated, 77% $(^{118}/_{154})$ resolved completely.

After injections of Alferon N Injection®, side effects were minor and transient. After 4 weeks of treatment, the frequency of adverse reactions was similar in Alferon N Injection® and placebo treatment groups. The most frequent side effects were myalgias, fever, and headache (See ADVERSE REACTIONS).

Antigenicity

1. Alferon N Injection®
   One hundred five (105) patients treated with Alferon N Injection® [Interferon alfa-n3 (human leukocyte derived)] during clinical trials were tested for the presence of anti-interferon antibodies using three different antibody assays: Immunoradiometric Assay (IRMA), Enzyme Linked Immunosorbent Assay (ELISA), and neutralization by the Cytopathic Effect Assay (CPE). To date, no antibodies to Interferon alfa-n3 have been detected in any of the patients.
2. Mouse Proteins
   No hypersensitivity reactions to the components in Alferon N Injection® have been observed. Alferon N Injection® uses a murine monoclonal antibody in one of the purification procedures. A possibility exists that patients treated with Alferon N Injection® may develop hypersensitivity to the mouse proteins. However, none of the patients receiving Alferon N Injection® during clinical trials developed antibodies or hypersensitivity to mouse proteins (See CONTRAINDICATIONS).
3. Egg Protein
   The initial stage in the manufacture of Alferon N Injection® uses Sendai virus which was grown in chicken-embryonated eggs as the specific Interferon alfa-n3 inducer. Although no egg protein (ovalbumin) has been detected in the initial stage of interferon manufacture using an ELISA (sensitivity of 16 ng/ml), a possibility exists that patients treated with Alferon N Injection® may develop hypersensitivity to egg protein (See CONTRAINDICATIONS).

INDICATIONS AND USAGE

Alferon N Injection® is indicated for the intralesional treatment of refractory or recurring external condylomata acuminata.

CONTRAINDICATIONS

Alferon N Injection® [Interferon alfa-n3 (human leukocyte derived)] is contraindicated in patients with known hypersensitivity to human interferon alpha proteins or any component of the product. The product is also contraindicated in patients who have anaphylactic sensitivity to mouse immunoglobulin (IgG), egg protein or neomycin.

Table 1
Degree of Resolution as Measured By Total Wart Volume per Patient

	Percent of Patients with:			
	Complete Resolution	Partial Resolution (≥50% resolution)	Minor Resolution (<50% resolution)	Progression/ No change
Alferon (n = 81)	54%	26%	15%	5%
Placebo (n = 75)	20%	24%	13%	43%

WARNINGS

Because of the fever and other "flu-like" symptoms associated with Alferon N Injection® (See ADVERSE REACTIONS), it should be used cautiously in patients with debilitating medical conditions such as cardiovascular disease (e.g., unstable angina and uncontrolled congestive heart failure), severe pulmonary disease (e.g., chronic obstructive pulmonary disease), or diabetes mellitus with ketoacidosis. Alferon N Injection® should be used cautiously in patients with coagulation disorders (e.g., thrombophlebitis, pulmonary embolism and hemophilia), severe myelosuppression, or seizure disorders. Acute, serious hypersensitivity reactions (e.g., urticaria, angioedema, bronchoconstriction, and anaphylaxis) have not been observed in patients receiving Alferon N Injection®. However, if such reactions develop, drug administration should be discontinued immediately and appropriate medical therapy should be instituted.

Because this product is made from human blood, it may carry a risk of transmitting infectious agents, e.g., viruses, and theoretically, the Creutzfeldt Jakob disease (CJD) agent.

PRECAUTIONS

General—Patients being treated with Alferon N Injection® should be informed of the benefits and risks associated with the treatment. Because the manufacturing process, strength, and type of interferon (e.g., natural, human leukocyte interferon versus single-species recombinant interferon) may vary for different interferon formulations, changing brands may require a change in dosage. Therefore, physicians are cautioned not to change from one interferon product to another without considering these factors.

The physician should select patients for treatment with Alferon N Injection® after consideration of the locations and sizes of the lesions, response to previous treatment, and the patient's ability to comply with the treatment regimen. Data on Alferon N Injection® as initial treatment are limited. There are no data on a second course of Alferon N Injection® treatment. The mean number of warts treated in one treatment cycle was five.

Information for Patients—Patients should be informed of the early signs of hypersensitivity reactions including hives, generalized urticaria, tightness of the chest, wheezing, hypotension, and anaphylaxis, and should be advised to contact their physician if these symptoms occur.

Patients being treated with Alferon N Injection® [Interferon alfa-n3 (human leukocyte derived)] should be informed of benefits and risks associated with treatment.

Patients should be cautioned not to change brands of interferon without medical consultation, as a change in dosage may occur.

Carcinogenesis, Mutagenesis, Impairment of Fertility—Studies with Alferon N Injection® have not been performed to determine carcinogenicity, mutagenicity, or the effect on fertility. In studies with adult females, interferon alpha has been shown to affect the menstrual cycle and decrease serum estradiol and progesterone levels[5].

Alferon N Injection® should be used with caution in fertile men. Fertile women should be cautioned to use effective contraception while being treated with Alferon N Injection®.

Changes in the menstrual cycle and abortions have been reported to occur in non-human primates given extremely high doses of recombinant interferon alpha[6]. In these studies, Macaca mulatta (rhesus monkeys) were given interferon daily by intramuscular injection. When given at daily intramuscular doses 326 times the average intralesional dose of Alferon N Injection® (120 times the maximum recommended dose), this recombinant interferon formulation produced menstrual cycle changes in the monkeys.

In human clinical trials with Alferon N Injection®, menstrual cycle data were reported by 51 patients (36 Alferon N Injection® and 15 placebo). There was no significant difference between Alferon N Injection® and placebo treatment groups with regard to menstrual cycle changes.

PREGNANCY Pregnancy Category C—Animal reproduction studies have not been conducted with Alferon N Injection®. It is also not known whether Alferon N Injection® [Interferon alfa-n3 (human leukocyte derived)] can cause fetal harm when administered to a pregnant woman or can affect reproductive capacity. Alferon N Injection® should be given to a pregnant woman only if clearly needed.

Changes in the menstrual cycle and abortions have been reported to occur in non-human primates given extremely high doses of recombinant interferon alpha. In these studies, Macaca mulatta (rhesus monkeys) were given interferon daily by intramuscular injection. Abortifacient effects were noted when the recombinant interferon alpha was given daily during early to mid-gestation at intramuscular doses of 978 times the average intralesional dose of Alferon N Injection® (360 times the maximum recommended dose).

Nursing Mothers—It is not known whether Alferon N Injection® is excreted in human milk. Studies in mice have shown that mouse interferons are excreted in milk[7]. Because many drugs are excreted in human milk and because of the potential for serious adverse reactions in nursing infants, a decision should be made whether to discontinue nursing or to not initiate drug treatment, taking into account the importance of the drug to the mother and the potential risks to the infant.

Pediatric Use—There have been no studies with this product in adolescents.

ADVERSE REACTIONS

Adverse reactions were evaluated in 202 patients with condylomata acuminata receiving Alferon N Injection® by intralesional administration and in 31 patients with cancer receiving Alferon N Injection® by systemic administration. In the double-blind efficacy trial for the treatment of condylomata acuminata, 104 patients were treated with doses of Alferon N Injection® of 0.05 million to 2.5 million IU per treatment session (average dose = 0.92 million IU per treatment session) by intralesional injection. In open trials, an additional 98 patients received a dose range of 0.05 to 4.6 million IU of Alferon N Injection® per treatment session (average dose = 1.12 million IU per treatment session). Patients with cancer were given doses of Alferon N Injection® [Interferon alfa-n3 (human leukocyte derived)] of 3 million, 9 million, or 15 million IU per day for ten days by intramuscular injection.

Adverse Reactions in Patients with Condylomata Acuminata—A total of 104 patients with condylomata acuminata was treated with Alferon N Injection® during the double-blind clinical trial. Adverse reactions were reported to be likely, unlikely, or not known to be related to Alferon N Injection®. Adverse reactions consisted primarily of "flu-like" symptoms (myalgias, fever, and/or headache) which were in most cases mild or moderate, and transient, and did not interfere with treatment.

The "flu-like" adverse reactions, consisting of fever, myalgias, and/or headache, occurred primarily after the first treatment session and were reported by 30% of the patients. The frequency of "flu-like" adverse reactions abated with repeated dosing of Alferon N Injection® so that the incidences due to Alferon N Injection® and placebo were similar after three to four weeks of treatment (after six to eight treatment sessions). "Flu-like" symptoms were relieved by administration of acetaminophen.

Adverse reactions were reported at least once during the course of treatment in the following percentages of patients in each treatment group:

Table 2
Percent of Patients with Adverse Reactions

Adverse Reactions:	Alferon (n = 104)	Placebo (n = 85)
Autonomic Nervous System		
Sweating	2%	1%
Vasovagal Reaction	2%	0%
Body as a Whole		
Fever	40%	19%
Chills	14%	2%
Fatigue	14%	6%
Malaise	9%	9%
Skin		
Generalized Pruritus	2%	0%
Central & Peripheral Nervous System		
Dizziness	9%	4%
Insomnia	2%	1%
Gastrointestinal System		
Nausea	4%	7%
Vomiting	3%	0%
Dyspepsia/Heartburn	3%	1%
Diarrhea	2%	2%

Continued on next page

Alferon N—Cont.

Musculoskeletal System		
Arthralgia	5%	1%
Back Pain	4%	1%
Myalgias	45%	15%
Headache	31%	15%
Psychiatric Disorders		
Depression	2%	1%
Nasopharyngeal		
Nose/sinus drainage	2%	2%

Most of the systemic adverse reactions were mild or moderate. Severe systemic adverse reactions were reported by 18% of Alferon N Injection® [Interferon alfa-n3 (human leukocyte derived)]-treated patients and 13% of placebo-treated patients (not a statistically significant difference). Most of the severe systemic adverse reactions reported were "flu-like". Other severe systemic adverse reactions included back pain, insomnia, and sensitivity to allergens. Those adverse reactions which were reported by 1% of patients treated with Alferon N Injection® in the double-blind trial include: left groin lymph node swelling, tongue hyperaesthesia, thirst, tingling of legs/feet, hot sensation on bottom of feet, strange taste in mouth, increased salivation, heat intolerance, visual disturbances, pharyngitis, sensitivity to allergens, muscle cramps, nosebleed, throat tightness, and papular rash on neck. Additional adverse reactions which were reported by 1% of patients treated with placebo include: pharyngitis, oral pain, penile discharge, cold, knuckle stiffness, herpes outbreak, cough, disorientation, and weight/appetite loss.

Additional adverse reactions which occurred only in open clinical trials of intralesional use of Alferon N Injection® [Interferon alfa-n3 (human leukocyte derived)] for treatment of condylomata acuminata were herpes labialis, hot flashes, nervousness, decrease in concentration, dysuria, photosensitivity, and swollen lymph nodes. These reactions occurred in 1% of the patients. One patient with a history of epilepsy, who was not taking anticonvulsant medication, had a grand mal seizure while being treated with Alferon N Injection®; this seizure was judged to be unrelated to Alferon N Injection® administration.

Application Site Disorders—The frequency of application site disorders (such as itching and pain) for patients treated with Alferon N Injection® was significantly less than that reported with placebo (12% versus 26%). No severe application site disorders were reported by patients treated with Alferon N Injection®, while 7% of placebo-treated patients reported severe disorders.

Laboratory Test Values—Abnormalities were seen with statistically equivalent frequencies in both the Alferon N Injection® and placebo groups. None of the laboratory abnormalities were considered clinically significant. The abnormalities in the Alferon N Injection®-treated patients consisted primarily of decreased WBC (11%). Decreases also occurred in 4% of the placebo patients (not a statistically significant difference). The abnormalities in Alferon N Injection®-treated patients involved increases of only one WHO grade.

Adverse Reactions in Patients with Cancer—Thirty-one (31) patients with cancer were treated with a maximum of ten intramuscular injections of Alferon N Injection® in doses of 3 million IU, 9 million IU, or 15 million IU per treatment session. The occurrence of adverse reactions was judged to be unrelated to the dose of Alferon N Injection®. The following adverse reactions were reported at least once (the percentage of patients experiencing the reaction is indicated in parentheses): chills (87%), fever (81%), anorexia (68%), malaise (65%), nausea (48%), vomiting (29%), myalgias (16%), arthralgia (10%), chest pains (10%), soreness at injection site (10%), sleepiness (10%), headache (10%), diarrhea (6%), fatigue (6%), low blood pressure (6%), sore mouth/stomatitis (6%), and blurred vision (6%). Those adverse reactions which were each reported by only one patient treated with Alferon N Injection® [Interferon alfa-n3 (human leukocyte derived)] include: stiff shoulders, flushed face, edema, dry mouth, mucositis, coughing, numbness, numbness in hands, numbness in fingers, pain on ocular rotation, shakes/shivers, ringing in ears, cramps, constipation, muscle soreness, confusion, light-headedness, depression, upset stomach, and sweating. The following adverse reactions were reported as severe by at least one patient (the percentage of patients experiencing the reaction is indicated in parentheses): fever (55%), malaise (54%), anorexia (45%), chills (45%), nausea (16%), myalgias (13%), vomiting (10%), fatigue (6%), low blood pressure (6%), chest pains (6%), sore mouth/stomatitis (6%), headache (3%), diarrhea (3%), sleepiness (3%), arthralgia (3%), blurred vision (3%), stiff shoulders (3%), numbness (3%), pain on ocular rotation (3%), muscle soreness (3%), confusion (3%), light-headedness (3%), depression (3%), and sweating (3%).

The number and percentage of patients with cancer who experienced a significant abnormal laboratory test value (values that changed from WHO Grades 0, 1, or 2 at baseline to WHO Grades 3 or 4 during or after treatment) at least once during the trials are shown in the following table:

Table 3
Abnormal Laboratory Test Values

	Cancer (n = 31)
Hemoglobin Level	2 (7%)
White Blood Cell Count	1 (3%)
Platelet Count	1 (3%)
GGT	1 (6%)
SGOT	1 (3%)
Alkaline Phosphatase	2 (8%)
Total Bilirubin	1 (4%)

DOSAGE AND ADMINISTRATION

The recommended dose of Alferon N Injection® for the treatment of condylomata acuminata is 0.05 ml (250,000 IU) per wart. Alferon N Injection® should be administered twice weekly for up to 8 weeks. The maximum recommended dose per treatment session is 0.5 ml (2.5 million IU). Alferon N Injection® [Interferon alfa-n3 (human leukocyte derived)] should be injected into the base of each wart, preferably using a 30 gauge needle. For large warts, Alferon N Injection® may be injected at several points around the periphery of the wart, using a total dose of 0.05 ml per wart. The minimum effective dose of Alferon N Injection® for the treatment of condylomata acuminata has not been established. Moderate to severe adverse experiences may require modification of the dosage regimen or, in some cases, termination of therapy with Alferon N Injection®.

Genital warts usually begin to disappear after several weeks of treatment with Alferon N Injection®. Treatment should continue for a maximum of 8 weeks. In clinical trials with Alferon N Injection®, many patients who had partial resolution of warts during treatment experienced further resolution of their warts after cessation of treatment. Of the patients who had complete resolution of warts due to treatment, half the patients had complete resolution of warts by the end of the treatment and half had complete resolution of warts during the 3 months after cessation of treatment. Thus, it is recommended that no further therapy (Alferon N Injection® or conventional therapy) be administered for 3 months after the initial 8-week course of treatment unless the warts enlarge or new warts appear. Studies to determine the safety and efficacy of a second course of treatment with Alferon N Injection® have not been conducted.

Parenteral drug products should be inspected visually for particulate matter and discoloration prior to administration, whenever solution and container permit.

HOW SUPPLIED

Injectable Solution: Each vial contains 1 ml of Alferon N Injection®. Each ml of Alferon N Injection® contains 5 million IU of Interferon alfa-n3, 3.3 mg of phenol, and 1 mg of Albumin (Human) in a pH 7.4 phosphate-buffered saline solution (8.0 mg/ml sodium chloride, 1.74 mg/ml sodium phosphate dibasic, 0.20 mg/ml potassium phosphate monobasic, and 0.20 mg/ml potassium chloride). One vial per box. (NDC 54746-001-01).

STORAGE

Alferon N Injection® [Interferon alfa-n3 (human leukocyte derived)] should be stored at 2° to 8°C (36° to 46°F). Do not freeze. Do not shake.

℞ Only

REFERENCES

1. Friedman-Kien, AE; Eron, LJ; Conant, M; et al., *JAMA* 1988; *259:* 533–538.
2. Kirby, P; (editorial comment), *JAMA* 1988; *259:* 570–572.
3. Friedman-Kien, AE; Plasse, TF; et al., *Papilloma Viruses: Molecular and Clinical Aspects* [Howley, PM, Broker, TR (eds)], New York, Alan R. Liss, Inc.; 1986; 217–233.
4. Geffen, JR; Klein, RJ; Friedman-Kien, AE; *J. Infect. Dis.* 1984; *150:* 612–615.
5. Kauppila, A; et al., *Int. J. Cancer* 1982; *29:* 291–294.
6. Trown, PW; et al., *Cancer* 1986; *57 (Suppl):* 1648–1656.
7. Schafer, TW; et al., *Science* 1972; *176:* 1326–1327.

Manufactured and Distributed by:
Hemispherx Biopharma, Inc.
One Penn Center
1617 JFK Boulevard
Philadelphia, PA 19103-1806
U.S. Lic. 1703

07/04

Shown in Product Identification Guide, page 319

High Chemical Co.

3901-A NEBRASKA ST.
LEVITTOWN, PA 19056

Direct Inquiries to:
800-447-8792
877–SARAPIN

SARAPIN® ℞

DESCRIPTION

A sterile aqueous solution of soluble salts of the volatile bases from Sarraceniaceae (Pitcher Plant). Benzyl Alcohol 0.75%.

ACTIONS

The painful syndromes most commonly encountered in general practice which are relieved by SARAPIN® treatment are as follows:
Sciatic Pain
Intercostal Neuralgia
Alcoholic Neuritis
Occipital Neuritis
Brachial Plexus Neuralgia
Meralgia Paresthetica
Lumbar Neuralgia
Trigeminal Neuralgia

ADMINISTRATION

These and allied conditions may be treated with success in a majority of cases by nerve block or local infiltration:
Paravertebral—Careful localization of the zone of tenderness permits a determination of the corresponding trunk levels to be injected.
Perineural—In some instances, as in sciatica, the affected nerve can be injected at a site distant from its origin.
Local Infiltration—Multiple injections throughout an area of tenderness provide for diffusion into all the affected parts.

DOSAGE

Paravertebral Injections

Cervical	2–3 ml
Dorsal	5–10 ml
Lumbar	5–10 ml
Sacral	3–5 ml
Caudal Canal	10 ml
Sciatic Nerve	10 ml
Local Infiltration	5–10 ml

WARNINGS

Withdraw plunger of syringe to make sure the needle point is not in a blood vessel.

PRECAUTIONS

Procedure should be gentle and unhurried.
SARAPIN® is intended only for professional use. Its successful employment depends upon a thorough knowledge of the anatomy involved.

ADVERSE REACTIONS

Patients should be maintained in a recumbent position for 10 to 15 minutes following injection. A local sensation is to be expected, limited to the distribution of the nerve injected, and usually appearing as a temporary feeling of heaviness, although some cases will feel heat or a transitory aggravation of symptoms.

CONTRAINDICATIONS

SARAPIN® is non-toxic, has no side effects other than above and is contraindicated only in areas of local infection.

HOW SUPPLIED

50 ml Multiple Dose Vial.
NDC-10541-492-50
Store at room temperature (59°-86°F)
CAUTION: Federal law prohibits dispensing without prescription.

HIGH CHEMICAL COMPANY
3901-A Nebraska Street
Levittown, PA 19056-3333
800-447-8792

NOTICE
Before prescribing or administering any product described in PHYSICIANS' DESK REFERENCE check the **PDR Supplements** for revised information.

Hill Dermaceuticals, Inc.

2650 SO. MELLONVILLE AVE.
SANFORD, FL 32773

Direct Inquiries to:
Rosario G. Ramirez, MD
(407) 323-1887
FAX: (407) 649-9213

DERMA-SMOOTHE/FS TOPICAL OIL ℞
Fluocinolone acetonide, 0.01%, Topical Oil

ICN Pharmaceuticals, Inc.

Please see Valeant Pharmaceuticals International

IDEC Pharmaceuticals Corp

Please see Biogen Idec

Immunotec Research Ltd.

292 ADRIEN PATENAUDE
VAUDREUIL-DORION (QUEBEC)
CANADA J7V 5V5

For Direct Inquiries Contact:
1-800-440-6250

IMMUNOCAL® OTC
2003
NUTRACEUTICAL
(Bonded cysteine supplement)
Powder Sachets

DESCRIPTION and CLINICAL PHARMACOLOGY

IMMUNOCAL® is a U.S. patented natural food protein concentrate in the FDA category of GRAS (generally recognized as safe) which assists the body in maintaining optimal concentrations of glutathione (GSH) by supplying the precursors required for intracellular glutathione synthesis. It is clinically proven to raise glutathione values (Lands et al, 1999).

Glutathione is a tripeptide made intracellularly from its constituent amino acids L-glutamate, L-cysteine and glycine. The sulfhydryl (thiol) group (SH) of cysteine serves as a proton donor and is responsible for the biological activity of glutathione. Provision of this amino acid is the rate-limiting factor in glutathione synthesis by the cells since cysteine is relatively rare in foodstuffs and furthermore, if released as the free amino acid, is toxic and spontaneously catabolized in the gastrointestinal tract and blood plasma.

Immunocal® is a bovine whey protein isolate specially prepared so as to provide a rich source of bioavailable cysteine. Following digestion, the cysteine remains as the stable form cystine (2 molecules of cysteine linked by disulfide bond) and glutamylcystine. After absorption, these dipeptides travel safely in the blood stream and readily enter the cells to release free cysteine for intracellular glutathione synthesis. Immunocal® can thus be viewed as a cysteine delivery system.

The disulphide bond in cystine is pepsin and trypsin resistant but may be split by heat, low pH or mechanical stress releasing free cysteine. When subject to heat or shearing forces (inherent in most extraction processes), the fragile disulfide bonds within the peptides are broken and the bioavailablility of cysteine is greatly diminished.

Glutathione is a tightly regulated intracellular constituent and is limited in its production by negative feedback inhibition of its own synthesis through the enzyme gamma-glutamylcysteine synthetase, thus greatly minimizing any possibility of overdosage.

Glutathione has multiple functions:

1. It is the major endogenous antioxidant produced by the cells, participating directly in the neutralization of free radicals and reactive oxygen compounds, as well as maintaining exogenous antioxidants such as vitamins C and E in their reduced (active) forms.
2. Through direct conjugation, it detoxifies many xenobiotics (foreign compounds) and carcinogens, both organic and inorganic.
3. It is essential for the immune system to exert its full potential, e.g. (1) modulating antigen presentation to lymphocytes, thereby influencing cytokine production and type of response (cellular or humoral) that develops, (2) enhancing proliferation of lymphocytes thereby increasing magnitude of response, (3) enhancing killing activity of cytotoxic T cells and NK cells, and (4) regulating apoptosis, thereby maintaining control of the immune response.
4. It plays a fundamental role in numerous metabolic and biochemical reactions such as DNA synthesis and repair, protein synthesis, prostaglandin synthesis, amino acid transport and enzyme activation. Thus, every system in the body can be affected by the state of the glutathione system, especially the immune system, the nervous system, the gastrointestinal system and the lungs.

INDICATIONS AND USAGE

IMMUNOCAL® is a natural food supplement and as such is limited from stating medical claims per se. Statements have not been evaluated by the FDA. As such, this product is thus not intended to diagnose, cure, prevent or treat any disease.

Glutathione augmentation is a strategy developed to address states of glutathione deficiency, high oxidative stress, immune deficiency, and xenobiotic overload in which glutathione plays a part in the detoxification of the xenobiotic in question. Glutathione deficiency states include, but are not limited to: HIV/AIDS, chemical and infectious hepatitis, prostate and other cancers, cataracts, Alzheimer's, Parkinsons, chronic obstructive pulmonary disease, asthma, radiation poisoning, malnutritive states, arduous physical stress, aging, and has been associated with suboptimal immune response. Many clinical pathologies are associated with oxidative stress and are elaborated upon in numerous medical references.

Low glutathione is also strongly implicated in wasting and negative nitrogen balance (Droge and Holm, 1997), notably as seen in cancer, AIDS, sepsis, trauma, burns and even athletic overtraining. Glutathione supplementation can oppose this process and in AIDS, for example, result in improved survival rates (Herzenberg et al, 1997).

CONTRAINDICATIONS

IMMUNOCAL® is contraindicated in individuals who develop or have known hypersensitivity to specific milk proteins.

PRECAUTIONS

Each sachet of IMMUNOCAL® contains nine grams of protein. Patients on a protein-restricted diet need to take this into account when calculating their daily protein load. Although a bovine milk derivative, IMMUNOCAL® contains less than 1% lactose and therefore is generally well tolerated by lactose-intolerant individuals.

WARNINGS

Patients undergoing immunosuppressive therapy should discuss the use of this product with their health professional.

ADVERSE REACTIONS

Gastrointestinal bloating and cramps if not sufficiently rehydrated. Transient urticarial-like rash in rare individuals undergoing severe detoxification reaction. Rash abates when product intake stopped or reduced.

OVERDOSAGE

Overdosing on IMMUNOCAL® has not been reported.

DOSAGE AND ADMINISTRATION

For mild to moderate health challenges, 20 grams per day is recommended. Clinical trials in patients with AIDS, COPD, cancer and chronic fatigue syndrome have used 30–40 grams per day without ill effect. IMMUNOCAL® is best administered on an empty stomach or with a light meal. Concomitant intake of another high protein load may adversely affect absorption.

RECONSTITUTION

IMMUNOCAL® is a dehydrated powdered protein isolate. It must be appropriately rehydrated before use. Remains bioactive up to 12 hours after mixing. DO NOT heat or use a hot liquid to rehydrate the product. DO NOT use a high-speed blender for reconstitution. These methods will decrease the activity of the product.

Proper mixing is imperative. Consult instructions included in packaging.

HOW SUPPLIED

10 grams of bovine milk protein isolate powder per sachet. 30 sachets per box.

STORAGE

Store in a cool dry environment. Refrigeration is not necessary.

Patent no.'s: 5,230,902 - 5,290,571 - 5,456,924 - 5,451,412 - 5,888,552

REFERENCES

1. Baruchel S, Viau G, Olivier R. et al. Nutraceutical modulation of glutathione with a humanized native milk serum protein isolate, Immunocal®: application in AIDS and cancer. In: Oxidative Stress in Cancer, AIDS and Neurodegenerative Diseases. Ed.; Montagnier L, Olivier R, Pasquier C. Marcel Dekker Inc. New York, 447–461, 1998
2. Bounous G, Kongshavn P. Influence of protein type in nutritionally adequate diets on the development of immunity. *In* Absorption and Utilization of Amino Acids Vol.II. Ed. M. Friedman. CRC Press, Inc., Fla. 2:219–32, 1989
3. Bounous G, Gold P. The biological activity of undenatured whey proteins: role of glutathione. Clin Invest Med 14:296–309, 1991
4. Bounous G, Baruchel S, Falutz J. Gold P. Whey proteins as a food supplement in HIV-seropositive individuals. Clin Invest Med. 16:3; 204–209, 1992
5. Bounous G. Whey protein concentrate (WPC) and glutathione modulation in cancer treatment. Anticancer Res. 20:4785–4792,2000
6. Bounous G. Immunoenhancing properties of undenatured milk serum protein isolate in HIV patients. Int. Diary Fed: Whey: 293–305, 1998
7. Droge W, Holm E. Role of cysteine and glutathione in HIV infection and other diseases associated with muscle wasting and immunological dysfunction. FASEB J: 11(13):1077–1089, 1997
8. Herzenberg LA, De Rosa SC, Dubs JG et al. Glutathione deficiency is associated with impaired survival in HIV disease. Proc Natl Acad Sci 94:1967–72,1997
9. Kennedy R, Konok G, Bounous G et al.. The use of a whey protein concentrate in the treatment of patients with metastatic carcinoma: A phase 1-II clinical study. Anticancer Res. 15:2643–50,1995
10. Lands LC, Grey VL, Smountas AA. Effect of supplementation with a cysteine donor on muscular performance. J. Appl. Physiol. 87:1381–1385, 1999
11. Locigno R, Castronovo V. Reduced glutathione System: Role in cancer development, prevention and treatment. International Journal of Oncology 19:221–236, 2001
12. Lomaestro B, Malone M. Glutathione in health and disease: pharmacotherapeutic issues. Ann Pharmacother 29: 1263–73,1995
13. Lothian B, Grey V, Kimoff RJ, Lands. Treatment of obstructive airway disease with a cysteine donor protein supplement: a case report. Chest 117:914–916, 2000
14. Meister A. Glutathione. Ann Rev Biochem 52:711–60,1983
15. Peterson JD, Herzenberg LA, Vasquez KK, Waltenbaugh C. Glutathione levels in antigen-presenting cells modulate Th1 versus Th2 response patterns. Proc.Natl. Acad. Sci. 95:3071–3076, 1998
16. Watanabe A, Higachi K, Yasumura S. et al. Nutritional modulation of glutathione level and cellular immunity in chronic hepatitis B and C. Hepatology. 24:597A, 1996

Manufactured by Immunotec Research, Ltd. and Immunotec Medical Corp.
Distributed by AmmunoMed, LLC and NuMedTec
Tel: 877-687-2277
www.immunocal.com

PRONUTRA OTC
[*prō-new-tră*]
Cystine-Rich Protein Supplement

DESCRIPTION

ProNutra is a dietary protein supplement containing Immunocal which is prepared using a proprietary microfiltration process to produce a highly undenatured whey protein product. ProNutra furnishes all of the amino acids and is a good source of nitrogen for replacing nitrogen losses that occur in patients with pressure ulcers. This process of preparation also ensures that ProNutra contains a rich source of bioavailable cystine[1] (two molecules of cysteine linked by a disulfide bond – "bonded cysteine") to promote positive nitrogen balance for minimizing muscle breakdown and rebuilding lean body mass (LBM). Cystine is required to synthesize glutathione which (1) is the cell's major antioxidant and (2) plays a vital role in many cell cycle related events that are needed during tissue repair such as DNA synthesis, protein synthesis and production of growth factors. Glutathione is also vital for maintaining normal functioning of the immune system

PHARMACOLOGY

- The bioactive protein component of ProNutra is Immunocal, a highly undenatured whey protein isolate. Whey protein isolates have the highest biological value (BV), greatest protein efficiency ratio (PER), and highest amino acid score (AAS) of all proteins [2]. ProNutra provides all of the essential amino acids as well as those such as arginine, cystine and glutamine that are essential in stressed patients who cannot synthesize sufficient amounts to meet demands.
- ProNutra is rich in cystine (bonded cysteine). It is rare in foodstuffs.
- ProNutra is clinically proven to raise intracellular glutathione [3].
- Animal experiments have shown that ProNutra enhances the response of the immune system and exerts an anticancer effect [1].
- ProNutra is clinically proven to increase body weight[4,5].
- ProNutra has a significant quantity of branch chain amino acids (BCAA) (leucine, isoleucine and valine) [6].
- ProNutra contains zinc, omega 3 & 6 fatty acids, vitamins A, C & E.

INDICATIONS AND USAGE

ProNutra is designed for individuals with, or at risk for developing, pressure ulcers, and for individuals who are malnourished and/or have protein energy malnutrition.

CONTRAINDICATIONS

ProNutra® is contraindicated in individuals who develop or have known hypersensitivity to specific milk proteins.

Continued on next page

ProNutra—Cont.

PRECAUTIONS

Each bottle of ProNutra® contains 18 grams of protein. Physicians may need to consider this fact when calculating their daily protein intake for patients on a protein-restricted diet. Because ProNutra contains less than .07% lactose, lactose-intolerant individuals tolerate ProNutra well. When used long term, physicians should note that ProNutra contains 9 mg of zinc per serving.

WARNINGS

Patients undergoing immunosuppressive therapy should discuss the use of ProNutra with their health professional.

ADVERSE REACTIONS

Gastrointestinal bloating and cramps may occur if ProNutra is not sufficiently rehydrated. Transient urticarial-like rash may occur in rare individuals undergoing severe detoxification reaction. Rash abates when ProNutra intake is stopped or reduced.

OVER DOSAGE

None Reported.

DOSAGE AND ADMINISTRATION

For high risk patients susceptible to muscle wasting, stage I & II pressure ulcers, PEM, protein malabsorption, or compromised immune systems: 1 serving (1 bottle) per day is recommended. Stage III & IV pressure ulcers or patients with severe PEM: 2 servings (2 bottles) per day are recommended. For long term maintenance: 1 serving (1 bottle) 2 or 3 times per week according to patient response. ProNutra may be added to oral and tube-administered enteral products.

Reconstitution

ProNutra® is a powder with a pleasant citrus flavor, designed to mix with water. **DO NOT** heat or use a hot liquid to rehydrate the product or use a high-speed blender for reconstitution. If refrigerated after mixing, it will remain bioactive for up to 12 hours after mixing.

HOW SUPPLIED

ProNutra comes in individual, disposable, plastic bottles containing 37 grams per serving.

REFERENCES:

1. Bounous G. Whey protein concentrate (WPC) and glutathione modulation in cancer treatment. Anticancer Res. 2000;20(6C):4785-92.
2. Reference Manual for U.S. Whey Products, 2nd ed., U.S. Diary Export Council, 1999.
3. Lands LC, Grey VL, Smountas AA. Effect of supplementation with a cysteine donor on muscular performance. J Appl Physiol.1999;87:1381-5.
4. Bounous G, Baruchel B, Gold P. Whey Proteins as a food supplement in HIV-seropositive individuals. Clin Invest Med 1993; 16: 204-209.
5. Pacheco L, Goldart J, Guilford T, Kwyer T, Kongshavn, PAL. Bioactive, cysteine-rich dietary supplement alleviates gastrointestinal side-effects, with associated weight gain and marked improvement in HAART adherence in AIDS patients. Presented at 2002 International Meeting of the Institute of Human Virology, September 9-13, 2002, Baltimore, Maryland.
6. Ha E, Zemel, MB. Functional properties of whey, whey components, and essential amino acids: mechanisms underlying health benefits for active people. J Nutr Biochem 2003;14:251-258.
7. Clarke RH et al. Nutritional treatment for acquired immunodeficiency virus-associated wasting using beta-hydroxy-beta-methylbutyrate, glutamine and arginine: a randomized, double-blind, placebo-controlled study. JPEN 2000; 133-139.
8. Stechmiller JK. Roundtable 107, Wound healing and arginine. A.S.P.E.N. Nutrition Week, Las Vegas, February 9, 2004.

Integrity Pharmaceutical Corporation

Please see Xanodyne Pharmaceuticals, Inc.

IDENTIFICATION PROBLEM?
Turn to the **Product Identification Guide**, where you'll find more than 1600 products pictured in actual size and full color.

InterCure, Inc.

PARKER PLAZA
400 KELBY ST.
FORT LEE, NJ 07024

Direct Inquiries to:
RESPeRATE support center
(877) 988-9388
www.resperate.com/md
supportmd@resperate.com

RESPeRATE® OTC

[*rĕs-pər-āt*]
Therapeutic device for hypertension

DESCRIPTION

RESPeRATE is a medical device indicated for the adjunctive treatment of hypertension. The device utilizes a patented *Interactive Respiratory-Pacing* technology to reduce sympathetic neural activity and relax the muscles surrounding the small blood vessels, leading to a sustained reduction in blood pressure.

Pooled data from 6 separate clinical studies show an average high blood pressure reduction of 14/9 mmHg within 8 weeks of using the device. There were no side effects and no interactions with existing medications. The reductions were significant over control (P<0.005/0.002) and were in addition to those achieved through other hypertension therapies, including medications.

Please note: Although RESPeRATE does not require a prescription, it should only be used as part of the patient's overall health program for achieving goal blood pressure, as recommended by a physician.

For complete clinical information including journal reprints, and information about the Take Control Sample Program, see www.resperate.com/md or call 877-988-9388.

InterCure, Inc.
Parker Plaza
400 Kelby St.
Fort Lee, NJ 07024
Phone: 201-720-7750
www.intercure.com
Direct Inquiries to:
RESPeRATE support center
(877) 988-9388 or supportmd@resperate.com

InterMune Inc.

3280 BAYSHORE BOULEVARD
BRISBANE, CA 94005

For Direct Inquiries Contact:
For Medical Information Contact:
(888) 486-6411
Corporate Offices:
(415) 466-2200
Corporate Fax:
(415) 466-2300

ACTIMMUNE® ℞

(Interferon gamma-1b)

DESCRIPTION

ACTIMMUNE® (Interferon gamma-1b), a biologic response modifier, is a single-chain polypeptide containing 140 amino acids. Production of *ACTIMMUNE* is achieved by fermentation of a genetically engineered Escherichia coli bacterium containing the DNA which encodes for the human protein. Purification of the product is achieved by conventional column chromatography. *ACTIMMUNE* is a highly purified sterile solution consisting of non-covalent dimers of two identical 16,465 dalton monomers; with a specific activity of 20 million International Units (IU)/mg (2×10^6 IU per 0.5 mL) which is equivalent to 30 million units/mg.

ACTIMMUNE is a sterile, clear, colorless solution filled in a single-dose vial for subcutaneous injection. Each 0.5 mL of *ACTIMMUNE* contains: **100 mcg (2 million IU)** of Interferon gamma-1b formulated in 20 mg mannitol, 0.36 mg sodium succinate, 0.05 mg polysorbate 20 and Sterile Water for Injection. *Note that the above activity is expressed in International Units (1 million IU/50mcg). This is equivalent to what was previously expressed as units (1.5 million U/50mcg).*

CLINICAL PHARMACOLOGY

General

Interferons are a family of functionally related, species-specific, proteins synthesized by eukaryotic cells in response to viruses and a variety of natural and synthetic stimuli. The most striking differences between interferon-gamma and other classes of interferon concern the immunomodulatory properties of this molecule. While gamma, alpha and beta interferons share certain properties, interferon-gamma has potent phagocyte-activating effects not seen with other interferon preparations. These effects include the generation of toxic oxygen metabolites within phagocytes *in vitro*, which are capable of mediating the intracellular killing of selected microorganisms such as *Staphylococcus aureus, Toxoplasma gondii, Leishmania donovani, Listeria monocytogenes,* and *Mycobacterium avium intracellulare.*

Clinical studies in patients using interferon-gamma, have revealed a broad range of biological activities including the enhancement of the oxidative metabolism of tissue macrophages, enhancement of antibody-dependent cellular cytotoxicity (ADCC) and natural killer (NK) cell activity. Additionally, effects on Fc receptor expression on monocytes and major histocompatibility antigen expression have been noted.[1,2]

To the extent that interferon-gamma is produced by antigen-stimulated T lymphocytes and regulates the activity of immune cells, it is appropriate to characterize interferon-gamma as a lymphokine of the interleukin type. There is growing evidence that interferon-gamma interacts functionally with other interleukin molecules such as interleukin-2 and that all of the interleukins form part of a complex, lymphokine regulatory network.[3] For example, interferon-gamma and interleukin-4 appear to reciprocally interact to regulate murine IgE levels; interferon-gamma can suppress IgE levels in humans.[4,5] Interferon-gamma also inhibits the production of collagen at the transcription level in human systems.[6]

With respect to Chronic Granulomatous Disease (an inherited disorder characterized by deficient phagocyte oxidative metabolism), pilot clinical trials of the systemic administration of *ACTIMMUNE* in patients with Chronic Granulomatous Disease provided evidence for a treatment-related enhancement of phagocyte function including elevation of superoxide levels and improved killing of *Staphylococcus aureus.*[7,8]

In severe, malignant osteopetrosis (another inherited disorder characterized by an osteoclast defect leading to bone overgrowth and deficient phagocyte oxidative metabolism),[9] a treatment-related enhancement of superoxide production by phagocytes was observed *in situ.*[10] *ACTIMMUNE* was found to enhance osteoclast function *in vitro.*[11,12]

Pharmacokinetics

The intravenous, intramuscular, and subcutaneous pharmacokinetics of *ACTIMMUNE* have been investigated in 24 healthy male subjects following single-dose administration of 100 mcg/m^2. *ACTIMMUNE* is rapidly cleared after intravenous administration (1.4 liters/minute) and slowly absorbed after intramuscular or subcutaneous injection. After intramuscular or subcutaneous injection, the apparent fraction of dose absorbed was greater than 89%. The mean elimination half-life after intravenous administration of 100 mcg/m^2 in healthy male subjects was 38 minutes. The mean elimination half-lives for intramuscular and subcutaneous dosing with 100 mcg/m^2 were 2.9 and 5.9 hours, respectively. Peak plasma concentrations, determined by ELISA, occurred approximately 4 hours (1.5 ng/mL) after intramuscular dosing and 7 hours (0.6 ng/mL) after subcutaneous dosing. Multiple dose subcutaneous pharmacokinetic studies were conducted in 38 healthy male subjects. There was no accumulation of *ACTIMMUNE* after 12 consecutive daily injections of 100 mcg/m^2. Pharmacokinetic studies in patients with Chronic Granulomatous Disease have not been performed.

Trace amounts of interferon-gamma were detected in the urine of squirrel monkeys following intravenous administration of 500 mcg/kg. Interferon-gamma was not detected in the urine of healthy human volunteers following administration of 100 mcg/m^2 of *ACTIMMUNE* by the intravenous, intramuscular and subcutaneous routes. *In vitro* perfusion studies utilizing rabbit livers and kidneys demonstrate that these organs are capable of clearing interferon-gamma from perfusate. Studies of the administration of interferon-gamma to nephrectomized mice and squirrel monkeys demonstrate a reduction in clearance of interferon-gamma from blood; however, prior nephrectomy did not prevent elimination.

Effects in Chronic Granulomatous Disease

A randomized, double-blind, placebo-controlled study of *ACTIMMUNE* (Interferon gamma-1b) in patients with Chronic Granulomatous Disease (CGD), was performed to determine whether *ACTIMMUNE* administered subcutaneously on a three times weekly schedule could decrease the incidence of serious infectious episodes and improve existing infectious and inflammatory conditions in patients with Chronic Granulomatous Disease. One hundred twenty-eight eligible patients were enrolled on this study including patients with different patterns of inheritance. Most patients received prophylactic antibiotics. Patients ranged in age from 1 to 44 years with the mean age being 14.6 years. The study was terminated early following demonstration of a highly statistically significant benefit of *ACTIMMUNE* therapy compared to placebo with respect to time to serious infection (p=0.0036), the primary endpoint of the investigation. Serious infection was defined as a clinical event requiring hospitalization and the use of parenteral antibiotics. The final analysis provided further support for the primary endpoint (p=0.0006). There was a 67 percent reduction in relative risk of serious infection in patients receiving *ACTIMMUNE* (n=63) compared to placebo (n=65). Additional supportive evidence of treatment benefit included a twofold reduction in the number of primary serious infections in the *ACTIMMUNE* group (30 on placebo versus 14 on *ACTIMMUNE*, p=0.002) and the total number and rate of serious infections including recurrent events (56 on placebo versus 20 on *ACTIMMUNE*, p=<0.0001). Moreover, the length of hospitalization for the treatment of all clinical events provided evidence highly supportive of an *ACTIMMUNE* treatment benefit. Placebo patients required three times as many inpatient hospitalization days for treatment of clinical events compared to patients receiving *ACTIMMUNE* (1493 versus 497 total days, p=0.02). An *ACTIMMUNE* treatment benefit with respect to time to serious infection was consistently demonstrated in all subgroup analyses according to stratification factors, including pattern of inheritance, use of prophylactic antibiotics, as well as age. There was a 67 percent reduction in relative risk of serious infection in patients receiving *ACTIMMUNE* compared to placebo across all groups. The beneficial effect of *ACTIMMUNE* therapy was observed throughout the entire study, in which the mean duration of *ACTIMMUNE* administration was 8.9 months/patient.

Effects in Osteopetrosis

A controlled, randomized study in patients with severe, malignant osteopetrosis was conducted with *ACTIMMUNE* administered subcutaneously three times weekly. Sixteen patients were randomized to receive either *ACTIMMUNE* plus calcitriol (n=11), or calcitriol alone (n=5). Patients ranged in age from 1 month to 8 years, mean 1.5 years. Treatment failure was considered to be disease progression as defined by 1) death, 2) significant reduction in hemoglobin or platelet counts, 3) a serious bacterial infection requiring antibiotics, or 4) a 50 dB decrease in hearing or progressive optic atrophy. The median time to disease progression was significantly delayed in the *ACTIMMUNE* plus calcitriol arm versus calcitriol alone. In the treatment arm, the median was not reached. Based on the observed data, however, the median time to progression in this arm was at least 165 days versus a median of 65 days in the calcitriol alone arm. In an analysis which combined data from a second study, 19 of 24 patients treated with *ACTIMMUNE* plus or minus calcitriol for at least 6 months had reduced trabecular bone volume compared to baseline.

INDICATIONS AND USAGE

ACTIMMUNE is indicated for reducing the frequency and severity of serious infections associated with Chronic Granulomatous Disease.

ACTIMMUNE is indicated for delaying time to disease progression in patients with severe, malignant osteopetrosis.

CONTRAINDICATIONS

ACTIMMUNE is contraindicated in patients who develop or have known hypersensitivity to interferon-gamma, *E. coli* derived products, or any component of the product.

WARNINGS

Cardiovascular Disorders

Acute and transient "flu-like" symptoms such as fever and chills induced by *ACTIMMUNE* at doses of 250 mcg/m^2/day (greater than 10 times the weekly recommended dose) or higher may exacerbate pre-existing cardiac conditions. *ACTIMMUNE* should be used with caution in patients with pre-existing cardiac conditions, including ischemia, congestive heart failure or arrhythmia.

Neurologic Disorders

Decreased mental status, gait disturbance and dizziness have been observed, particularly in patients receiving *ACTIMMUNE* doses greater than 250 mcg/m^2/day (greater than 10 times the weekly recommended dose). Most of these abnormalities were mild and reversible within a few days upon dose reduction or discontinuation of therapy. Caution should be exercised when administering *ACTIMMUNE* to patients with seizure disorders or compromised central nervous system function.

Bone Marrow Toxicity

Reversible neutropenia and thrombocytopenia that can be severe and may be dose related have been observed during *ACTIMMUNE* therapy. Caution should be exercised when administering *ACTIMMUNE* to patients with myelosuppression.

Hepatic Toxicity

Elevations of AST and/or ALT (up to 25-fold) have been observed during *ACTIMMUNE* therapy. The incidence appeared to be higher in patients less than 1 year of age compared to older children. The transaminase elevations were reversible with reduction in dosage or interruption of *ACTIMMUNE* treatment. Patients begun on Actimmune before age one year should receive monthly assessments of liver function. If severe hepatic enzyme elevations develop, *ACTIMMUNE* dosage should be modified (See **DOSAGE AND ADMINISTRATION: Dose Modification**).

PRECAUTIONS

General

Acute serious hypersensitivity reactions have not been observed in patients receiving *ACTIMMUNE*, however, if such an acute reaction develops the drug should be discontinued immediately and appropriate medical therapy instituted. Transient cutaneous rashes have occurred in some patients following injection but have rarely necessitated treatment interruption.

Information for Patients

Patients being treated with *ACTIMMUNE* and/or their parents should be informed regarding the potential benefits and risks associated with treatment. If home use is determined to be desirable by the physician, instructions on appropriate use should be given, including review of the contents of the Patient Information Insert. This information is intended to aid in the safe and effective use of the medication. It is not a disclosure of all possible adverse or intended effects.

If home use is prescribed, a puncture resistant container for the disposal of used syringes and needles should be supplied to the patient. Patients should be thoroughly instructed in the importance of proper disposal and cautioned against any reuse of needles and syringes. The full container should be disposed of according to the directions provided by the physician (see Patient Information Insert).

The most common adverse experiences occurring with *ACTIMMUNE* therapy are "flu-like" or constitutional symptoms such as fever, headache, chills, myalgia or fatigue (see ADVERSE REACTIONS Section) which may decrease in severity as treatment continues. Some of the "flu-like" symptoms may be minimized by bedtime administration. Acetaminophen may be used to prevent or partially alleviate the fever and headache.

Laboratory Tests

In addition to those tests normally required for monitoring patients with Chronic Granulomatous Disease and osteopetrosis, the following laboratory tests are recommended for all patients on *ACTIMMUNE*® (Interferon gamma-1b) therapy prior to the beginning of and at three month intervals during treatment. (See **WARNINGS: Bone Marrow** and **Hepatic Toxicity**).

- Hematologic tests—including complete blood counts, differential and platelet counts
- Blood chemistries—including renal and liver function tests. In patients less than 1 year of age, liver function tests should be measured monthly (See **ADVERSE REACTIONS: Post Marketing Experience**).
- Urinalysis

Drug Interactions

Interactions between *ACTIMMUNE* and other drugs have not been fully evaluated. Caution should be exercised when administering *ACTIMMUNE* in combination with other potentially myelosuppressive agents (see WARNINGS).

Preclinical studies in rodents using species-specific interferon-gamma have demonstrated a decrease in hepatic microsomal cytochrome P-450 concentrations. This could potentially lead to a depression of the hepatic metabolism of certain drugs that utilize this degradative pathway.

Carcinogenesis, Mutagenesis and Impairment of Fertility

Carcinogenesis: *ACTIMMUNE* has not been tested for its carcinogenic potential.

Mutagenesis: Ames tests using five different tester strains of bacteria with and without metabolic activation revealed no evidence of mutagenic potential. *ACTIMMUNE* was tested in a micronucleus assay for its ability to induce chromosomal damage in bone marrow cells of mice following two intravenous doses of 20 mg/kg. No evidence of chromosomal damage was noted.

Impairment of Fertility: Female cynomolgus monkeys treated with daily subcutaneous doses of 30 or 150 mcg/kg *ACTIMMUNE* (approximately 20 and 100 times the human dose) exhibited irregular menstrual cycles or absence of cyclicity during treatment. Similar findings were not observed in animals treated with 3 mcg/kg *ACTIMMUNE*.

Female mice receiving recombinant murine IFN-gamma (rmuIFN-gamma) at 32 times the maximum recommended clinical dose of ACTIMMUNE for 4 weeks via intramuscular injection exhibited an increased incidence of atretic ovarian follicles.

Male cynomolgus monkeys treated intravenously for 4 weeks with 8 times the maximum recommended clinical dose of ACTIMMUNE exhibited decreased spermatogenesis. The impact of this finding on fertility is not known. Male mice receiving rmuIFN-gamma at 32 times the maximum recommended clinical dose of ACTIMMUNE for 4 weeks via intramuscular injection exhibited decreased spermatogenesis.

Male mice treated subcutaneously with rmuIFN-gamma from shortly after birth through puberty, with 280 times the maximum recommended clinical dose of ACTIMMUNE exhibited profound yet reversible decreases in sperm counts and fertility, and an increase in the number of abnormal sperm.

The clinical significance of these findings observed following treatment of mice with rmuIFN-gamma is uncertain.

Pregnancy

Teratogenic Effects: Pregnancy Category C. *ACTIMMUNE* has shown an increased incidence of abortions in primates when given in doses approximately 100 times the human dose. A study in pregnant primates treated with subcutaneous doses 2–100 times the human dose failed to demonstrate teratogenic activity for *ACTIMMUNE*.

Female mice treated subcutaneously with rmuIFN-gamma at 280 times the maximum recommended clinical dose of ACTIMMUNE from shortly after birth through puberty but not during pregnancy had offspring which exhibited decreased body weight during the lactation period. The clinical significance of this finding observed following treatment of mice with rmuIFN-gamma is uncertain.

There are no adequate and well-controlled studies in pregnant women. *ACTIMMUNE* should be used during pregnancy only if the potential benefit justifies the potential risk to the fetus

Nursing Mothers

It is not known whether *ACTIMMUNE* is excreted in human milk. Because many drugs are excreted in human milk and because of the potential for serious adverse reactions in nursing infants from *ACTIMMUNE*, a decision should be made whether to discontinue nursing or to discontinue the drug, dependent upon the importance of the drug to the mother.

ADVERSE REACTIONS

The following data on adverse reactions are based on the subcutaneous administration of *ACTIMMUNE* at a dose of 50 mcg/m^2, three times weekly, in patients with Chronic Granulomatous Disease (CGD) during an investigational trial in the United States and Europe.

The most common adverse events observed in patients with CGD are shown in the following table:

Clinical Toxicity	Percent of Patients *ACTIMMUNE* CGD(n=63)	Placebo CGD(n=65)
Fever	52	28
Headache	33	9
Rash	17	6
Chills	14	0
Injection site erythema or tenderness	14	2
Fatigue	14	11
Diarrhea	14	12
Vomiting	13	5
Nausea	10	2
Myalgia	6	0
Arthralgia	2	0
Injection site pain	0	2

Miscellaneous adverse events which occurred infrequently in patients with CGD and may have been related to underlying disease included back pain (2 percent versus 0 percent), abdominal pain (8 percent versus 3 percent) and depression (3 percent versus 0 percent) for *ACTIMMUNE* and placebo treated patients, respectively.

Similar safety data were observed in 34 patients with severe malignant osteopetrosis.

ACTIMMUNE has also been evaluated in additional disease states in studies in which patients have generally received higher doses (>100 mcg/m^2/day) administered by intramuscular injection or intravenous infusion. All of the previously described adverse reactions which occurred in patients with Chronic Granulomatous Disease have also been observed in patients receiving higher doses. Adverse reactions not observed in patients with Chronic Granulomatous Disease receiving doses less than 100 mcg/m^2/day but seen rarely in patients receiving *ACTIMMUNE* (Interferon gamma-1b) in other studies include: *Cardiovascular*—hypotension, syncope, tachyarrhythmia, heart block, heart failure, and myocardial infarction. *Central Nervous System*—confusion, disorientation, gait disturbance, Parkinsonian symptoms, seizure, hallucinations, and transient ischemic attacks. *Gastrointestinal*—hepatic insufficiency, gastrointestinal bleeding, and pancreatitis. *Renal*—reversible renal insufficiency. *Hematologic*—deep venous thrombosis and pulmonary embolism. *Pulmonary*—tachypnea, bronchospasm, and interstitial pneumonitis. *Metabolic*—hyponatremia and hyperglycemia. *Other*—exacerbation of dermatomyositis.

Abnormal Laboratory Test Values: Elevations of ALT and AST, neutropenia, thrombocytopenia, and proteinuria have been observed (See **WARNINGS and PRECAUTIONS: Laboratory Tests**).

No neutralizing antibodies to *ACTIMMUNE* have been detected in any Chronic Granulomatous Disease patients receiving *ACTIMMUNE*.

Post-Marketing Experience

Children with CGD less than 3 years of age

Data on the safety and activity of *ACTIMMUNE* in 37 patients under the age of 3 years was pooled from four uncontrolled post-marketing studies. The rate of serious infections per patient-year in this uncontrolled group was similar to the rate observed in the *ACTIMMUNE* treatment groups in controlled trials. Developmental parameters (height, weight and endocrine maturation) for this uncontrolled group conformed to national normative scales before and during *ACTIMMUNE* therapy.

In 6 of the 10 patients receiving *ACTIMMUNE* therapy before age one year 2-fold to 25-fold elevations from baseline of AST and/or ALT were observed. These elevations occurred as early as 7 days after starting treatment. Treatment with *ACTIMMUNE* was interrupted in all 6 of these patients and was restarted at a reduced dosage in 4. Liver transaminase values returned to baseline in all patients and transaminase elevation recurred in one patient upon *ACTIMMUNE* rechallenge. An 11-fold alkaline phosphatase elevation and hypokalemia in one patient and neutropenia (ANC= 525 cells/mm^3) in another patient resolved with interruption of *ACTIMMUNE* treatment and did not recur with rechallenge.

In the post-marketing safety database clinically significant adverse events observed during *ACTIMMUNE* therapy in children under the age of three years (n=14) included: two cases of hepatomegaly, and one case each of Stevens-Johnson syndrome, granulomatous colitis, urticaria, and atopic dermatitis.

DOSAGE AND ADMINISTRATION

The recommended dosage of *ACTIMMUNE* for the treatment of patients with Chronic Granulomatous Disease and severe, malignant osteopetrosis is 50 mcg/m^2 (1 million IU/m^2) for patients whose body surface area is greater than 0.5

Continued on next page

Actimmune—Cont.

m^2 and 1.5 mcg/kg/dose for patients whose body surface area is equal to or less than 0.5 m^2. *Note that the above activity is expressed in International Units (1 million IU/50mcg). This is equivalent to what was previously expressed as units (1.5 million U/50mcg).* Injections should be administered subcutaneously three times weekly (for example, Monday, Wednesday, Friday). The optimum sites of injection are the right and left deltoid and anterior thigh. *ACTIMMUNE* can be administered by a physician, nurse, family member or patient when trained in the administration of subcutaneous injections. Parenteral drug products should be inspected visually for particulate matter and discoloration prior to administration, whenever solution and container permit.

The formulation does not contain a preservative. A vial of *ACTIMMUNE* is suitable for a single dose only. The unused portion of any vial should be discarded.

Higher doses are not recommended. Safety and efficacy has not been established for *ACTIMMUNE* given in doses greater or less than the recommended dose of 50 mcg/m^2. The minimum effective dose of *ACTIMMUNE* has not been established.

Dose Modification

If severe reactions occur, the dosage should be modified (50 percent reduction) or therapy should be discontinued until the adverse reaction abates.

ACTIMMUNE may be administered using either sterilized glass or plastic disposable syringes.

HOW SUPPLIED

ACTIMMUNE (Interferon gamma-1b) is a sterile, clear, colorless solution filled in a single-dose vial for subcutaneous injection. Each 0.5 mL of *ACTIMMUNE* contains: **100 mcg (2 million IU)** of Interferon gamma-1b, formulated in 20 mg mannitol, 0.36 mg sodium succinate, 0.05 mg polysorbate 20 and Sterile Water for Injection.

Single vial (NDC 64116-011-01)

Cartons of 12 (NDC 64116-011-12)

Stability and Storage

Vials of *ACTIMMUNE* must be placed in a 2–8°C (36–46°F) refrigerator immediately upon receipt to insure optimal retention of physical and biochemical integrity. DO NOT FREEZE. Avoid excessive or vigorous agitation. DO NOT SHAKE. An unentered vial of *ACTIMMUNE* should not be left at room temperature for a total time exceeding 12 hours prior to use. Vials exceeding this time period should not be returned to the refrigerator; such vials should be discarded. Do not use beyond the expiration date stamped on the vial.

REFERENCES

1. Maluish AE, Urba WJ, Longo DL, *et al*: The determination of an immunologically active dose of interferon gamma in patients with melanoma. J Clin Onc *6*: 434–445, 1988.
2. Nathan CF, Kaplan G, Levis W, et al: Local and systemic effects of intradermal recombinant interferon gamma in patients with lepromatous leprosy. NEJM *315*: 6–11, 1986.
3. Fauci AS, Rosenberg SA, Sherwin SA, *et al*: Immunomodulators in clinical medicine. Ann Internal Med *106*: 421–433, 1987.
4. Snapper CM, Paul WE: Interferon-gamma and B cell stimulatory factor-1 reciprocally regulate Ig isotype production. Science *236*: 944–947, 1987.
5. King CL, Gallin JI, Malech HL, *et al*: Regulation of immunoglobulin production in hyperimmunoglobulin E recurrent-infection syndrome by interferon gamma. PNAS USA *86*:10085–10089, 1989.
6. Rosenbloom J, Feldman G, Freundlich B, Jimenez SA: Inhibition of excessive scleroderma fibroblast collagen production by recombinant gamma-interferon. Arth Rheum *29*: 851–856, 1986.
7. Ezekowitz RAB, Dinauer MC, Jaffe HS, *et al*: Partial correction of the phagocyte defect in patients with X-linked chronic granulomatous disease by subcutaneous interferon gamma. NEJM *319*: 146–151, 1988.
8. Sechler JMG, Malech HL, White CJ, Gallin JI: Recombinant human interferon-gamma reconstitutes defective phagocyte function in patients with chronic granulomatous disease of childhood. PNAS USA *85*:4874–4878, 1988.
9. Shapiro F: Osteopetrosis, current clinical considerations. Clin Orth & Rel Res *296*: 34–44, 1993.
10. Beard CJ, Key L, Newburger PE, Ezekowitz RAB, *et al*: Neutrophil defect associated with malignant infantile osteopetrosis. J Lab Clin Med *108*: 498–505, 1986.
11. Shankar L, Gerritsen EJA, and Key LL: Osteopetrosis: pathogenesis and rationale for the use of interferon-γ-1b. Biodrugs *1*: 23–29, 1997.
12. Key LL, Rodriguiz RM, Willi SM: Long-term treatment of osteopetrosis with recombinant human interferon gamma. NEJM *24*: 1594–1599, 1995.

Manufactured by:
InterMune, Inc.
Brisbane, CA 94005
U.S. License No. 1626
Revised March 2004 (A102)

PH01017.00

Shown in Product Identification Guide, page 319

INFERGEN® ℞

[ĭn-fər-jĕn]

(Interferon alfacon-1)

> **Alpha interferons, including Interferon alfacon-1, cause or aggravate fatal or life-threatening neuropsychiatric, autoimmune, ischemic, and infectious disorders. Patients should be monitored closely with periodic clinical and laboratory evaluations. Patients with persistently severe or worsening symptoms of these conditions should be withdrawn from therapy. In many but not all cases, these disorders resolve after stopping Interferon alfacon-1 therapy.**
> **See WARNINGS, and ADVERSE REACTIONS.**

DESCRIPTION

Interferon alfacon-1 is a recombinant non-naturally occurring type-I interferon. The 166-amino acid sequence of Interferon alfacon-1 was derived by scanning the sequences of several natural interferon alpha subtypes and assigning the most frequently observed amino acid in each corresponding position.[1] Four additional amino acid changes were made to facilitate the molecular construction, and a corresponding synthetic DNA sequence was constructed using chemical synthesis methodology. Interferon alfacon-1 differs from interferon alfa-2b at 20/166 amino acids (88% homology), and comparison with interferon-beta shows identity at over 30% of the amino acid positions. Interferon alfacon-1 is produced in *Escherichia coli (E. coli)* cells that have been genetically altered by insertion of a synthetically constructed sequence that codes for Interferon alfacon-1. Prior to final purification, Interferon alfacon-1 is allowed to oxidize to its native state, and its final purity is achieved by sequential passage over a series of chromatography columns. This protein has a molecular weight of 19,434 daltons.

INFERGEN is a sterile, clear, colorless, preservative-free liquid formulated with 100 mM sodium chloride and 25 mM sodium phosphate at pH 7.0 ± 0.2. The product is available in single-use vials containing 9 mcg and 15 mcg Interferon alfacon-1 at a fill volume of 0.3 mL and 0.5 mL, respectively. INFERGEN vials contain 0.03 mg/mL Interferon alfacon-1, 5.9 mg/mL sodium chloride, and 3.8 mg/mL sodium phosphate in Water for Injection, USP. INFERGEN is to be administered undiluted by subcutaneous (SC) injection.

CLINICAL PHARMACOLOGY

General

Interferons are a family of naturally occurring, small protein molecules with molecular weights of 15,000 to 21,000 daltons that are produced and secreted by cells in response to viral infections or to various synthetic and biological inducers. Two major classes of interferons have been identified (i.e., type-I and type-II). Type-I interferons include a family of more than 25 alpha interferons as well as beta interferon and omega interferon. While all alpha interferons have similar biological effects, not all the activities are shared by each alpha interferon and, in many cases, the extent of activity varies substantially for each interferon subtype.

All type-I interferons share common biological activities generated by binding of interferon to the cell-surface receptor, leading to the production of several interferon-stimulated gene products. Type-I interferons induce pleiotropic biologic responses which include antiviral, antiproliferative, and immunomodulatory effects, regulation of cell surface major histocompatibility antigen (HLA class I and class II) expression and regulation of cytokine expression. Examples of interferon-stimulated gene products include 2′5′ oligoadenylate synthetase (2′5′OAS) and β-2 microglobulin.

The antiviral, antiproliferative, natural killer (NK) cell activation, and gene-induction activities of INFERGEN have been compared with other recombinant alpha interferons in *in vitro* assays and have demonstrated similar ranges of activity. INFERGEN exhibited at least five times higher specific activity *in vitro* than Interferon alfa-2a and Interferon alfa-2b.[2] Comparison of INFERGEN with a WHO international potency standard for recombinant alpha interferon (83/514) revealed that the specific activity of INFERGEN in both an *in vitro* antiviral cytopathic effect assay and an antiproliferative assay was 1×10^9 U/mg. However, correlation between *in vitro* activity and clinical activity of any interferon is unknown.

Pharmacokinetics and Pharmacodynamics

The pharmacokinetic properties of INFERGEN have not been evaluated in patients with chronic hepatitis C. Pharmacokinetic profiles were evaluated in normal, healthy volunteer subjects after SC injection of 1, 3, or 9 mcg INFERGEN. Plasma levels of INFERGEN after SC administration of any dose were too low to be detected by either enzyme-linked immunosorbent assay (ELISA) or by inhibition of viral cytopathic effect. However, analysis of INFERGEN-induced cellular products (induction of 2′5′ OAS and β-2 microglobulin) after treatment in these subjects revealed a statistically significant, dose-related increase in the area under the curve (AUC) for the levels of 2′5′ OAS or β-2 microglobulin induced over time ($p < 0.001$ for all comparisons). Concentrations of 2′5′ OAS were maximal at 24 hours after dosing, while serum levels of β-2 microglobulin appeared to reach a maximum 24 to 36 hours after dosing. The dose-response relationships observed for 2′5′ OAS and β-2 microglobulin were indicative of biological activity after SC administration of 1 to 9 mcg INFERGEN.

Preclinical Experience

All interferons have been shown to be highly species-specific. Antiviral activity of INFERGEN was observed in the rhesus monkey LLC cell line and golden Syrian hamster BHK cell line. Antiviral activity of INFERGEN in the golden Syrian hamster was confirmed further *in vivo*.[3] Pharmacokinetic studies of INFERGEN in golden Syrian hamsters and rhesus monkeys demonstrated rapid absorption following SC injection. Peak serum concentrations of INFERGEN were observed at 1 hour and 4 hours in golden Syrian hamsters and in rhesus monkeys, respectively. Subcutaneous bioavailability was high in both species, averaging 99% in golden Syrian hamsters and 83% to 104% in rhesus monkeys. Clearance of INFERGEN, averaging 1.99 mL/minute/kg in golden Syrian hamsters and 0.71 to 0.92 mL/minute/kg in rhesus monkeys, was due predominantly to catabolism and excretion by the kidneys. The terminal half-life of INFERGEN following SC dosing was 1.3 hours in golden Syrian hamsters and 3.4 hours in rhesus monkeys. Upon 7-day multiple SC dosing, no accumulation of serum levels was observed in golden Syrian hamsters.

In preclinical toxicology studies in golden Syrian hamsters and rhesus monkeys, administration of INFERGEN at doses of up to 100 mcg/kg/day was associated with decreased body weight, decreased food consumption, and bone marrow suppression. High-dose chronic exposure at doses of 10 to 100 mcg/kg/day (50- to 500-fold higher than the maximum clinical dose given daily) in rhesus monkeys was not tolerated for greater than 1 month, due to the development of vascular leak syndrome.

Reproductive toxicity studies in pregnant rhesus monkeys and golden Syrian hamsters demonstrated an increase in fetal loss in hamsters treated with INFERGEN at doses of > 150 mcg/kg/day, and in rhesus monkeys at doses of 3 and 10 mcg/kg/day. The INFERGEN toxicity profile described is consistent with the known toxicity profile of other alpha interferons.[4]

CLINICAL EXPERIENCE: RESPONSE TO INFERGEN®

Initial Treatment

INFERGEN was studied in an open-label dose escalation study using 3, 6, 9, 12, or 15 mcg administered three times per week (TIW) to patients with compensated liver disease secondary to chronic hepatitis C virus (HCV) infection. The 15 mcg dose was the maximum tolerated dose. All doses demonstrated an acceptable safety profile and preliminary evidence of efficacy.

The efficacy of 3 and 9 mcg doses of INFERGEN in the treatment of chronic HCV infection was examined in a randomized, double-blind clinical trial involving 704 patients previously untreated with alpha interferon.[5] Patients were 18 years or older, had compensated liver disease, tested positive for HCV RNA, and had elevated serum alanine aminotransferase (ALT) averaging greater than 1.5 times the upper limit of normal. Staging of chronic liver disease was confirmed by a liver biopsy taken within 1 year prior to enrollment. Other causes of chronic liver disease were ruled out prior to randomization. Notable exclusion criteria were decompensated liver disease, thyroid abnormality, or history of depression.

Efficacy of INFERGEN therapy was assessed on an intent-to-treat basis and was determined by measurement of serum ALT at the end of therapy (24 weeks) and following 24 weeks of observation after the end of treatment (sustained response rate). Serum HCV RNA was also assessed using a research-based quantitative reverse transcriptase polymerase chain reaction (RT-PCR) assay with a lower limit of sensitivity of 100 copies/mL. Liver histology was assessed by comparing the histology activity index (HAI) score[6] of a pretreatment biopsy specimen with the HAI score from a specimen obtained 24 weeks after cessation of interferon therapy.

Patients enrolled in the study were randomized to 1 of 3 treatment groups: INFERGEN at a dose of 3 mcg (n = 232), INFERGEN at a dose of 9 mcg (n = 232), or Interferon alfa-2b recombinant [IFN α-2b, Intron® A (Intron® is a registered trademark of the Schering Corporation)] at a dose of 3 million international units (mIU) (approximately 15 mcg) (n = 240). All patients were scheduled to receive their respective interferons SC TIW for 24 weeks (end of treatment). Following treatment, patients were observed for an additional 24 weeks to assess durability of ALT normalization (end of posttreatment observation). In all patients, a complete response was defined as a decrease in serum ALT to at or below the upper limit of normal (48 U/L) at the end of the posttreatment observation period, even if ALT normalization had not been observed at the end of treatment. Complete response was dependent on 2 consecutive normal serum ALT values determined 4 weeks apart. Reduction of HCV RNA to less than 100 copies/mL was measured as a secondary efficacy endpoint (2 consecutive measurements).

Sustained response rates by ALT normalization and HCV RNA reductions to below detectable limits for patients who received initial treatment are included in Table 1. Among the INFERGEN treatment groups in this study, the 9 mcg dosage arm demonstrated a similar efficacy profile when compared to the IFN α-2b dosage arm. The 3 mcg INFERGEN dosage arm had lesser efficacy; 3% of patients receiving 3 mcg INFERGEN had sustained reductions in their ALT to within the normal range and 3% had sustained reductions in HCV RNA to below detectable limits.

[See table 1 at top of next page]

In this study, liver biopsies were taken at baseline and at the end of posttreatment observation. Similar improvement in liver histology, assessed by HAI score, was observed in the 9 mcg INFERGEN (68%), 3 mcg INFERGEN (63%), and IFN α-2b (65%) dosage arms.

Subsequent Treatment

Subsequent treatment with 15 mcg of INFERGEN for 24 and 48 weeks was evaluated in an open-label clinical trial in 208 patients who had failed initial therapy for 24 weeks with either 9 mcg INFERGEN or 3 mIU (approximately 15 mcg) IFN α-2b.[7] Of these patients, 133/208 had failed to normalize ALT during the initial treatment period. Seventy-five of 208 achieved normal ALT during initial treatment, but experienced relapse (return of abnormal ALT) during posttreatment observation. Patients were assessed for normalization of ALT (ALT response rate) and HCV RNA reduction to less than 100 copies/mL (HCV response rate) at the end of 24 weeks of observation following discontinuation of therapy. Sustained response rates measured by ALT normalization and HCV RNA reductions to below detectable limits for patients who received subsequent treatment with 15 mcg of INFERGEN are included in Table 2.

Patients who received 48 weeks of interferon therapy were more likely to experience a sustained response than were those who received 24 weeks of therapy. Similarly, patients who normalized their serum ALT but subsequently relapsed following initial therapy were more likely to experience a sustained response than those who were refractory to initial therapy.

[See table 2 at right]

Serum antibody levels were measured in all patients using both an INFERGEN-binding radioimmunoassay and an IFN α-2b-binding ELISA. A patient was considered to have developed binding antibodies if, using serum samples from 2 consecutive time points, a positive response was detected in either assay. The number of patients developing positive binding antibody responses in either assay was similar in the 9 mcg INFERGEN (11%) and 3 mIU IFN α-2b groups (15%). The titer of neutralizing antibodies to interferon was not measured. Sustained ALT response rates in patients treated with INFERGEN who developed binding antibodies (4/25) were similar to sustained ALT response rates in patients who did not develop detectable antibody titers (40/195). The most frequently observed time to first antibody response was week 16 of interferon treatment. Following cessation of interferon therapy, the number of patients with a positive antibody response declined during posttreatment observation.

Table 1. Rates (95% CI[a]) of ALT Normalization and HCV RNA Reductions to Below Detectable Limits in Previously Untreated Patients

	End of 24-week Treatment		End of Observation (Sustained Response Rate)	
	INFERGEN 9 mcg n=232	IFN α-2b 3 MIU[b] n=240	INFERGEN 9 mcg n=232	IFN α-2b 3 MIU[b] n=240
Normalized ALT	39% (33%, 46%)	35% (29%, 41%)	17% (12%, 22%)	17% (13%, 22%)
HCV RNA Negative	33% (27%, 39%)	25% (19%, 31%)	9% (6%, 14%)	8% (5%, 13%)

[a] CI = Confidence Interval.
[b] 3 MIU IFN α-2b is equivalent to approximately 15 mcg IFN α-2b.

Table 2. Sustained Response Rates (95% CI) of ALT Normalization and HCV RNA Reductions to Below Detectable Limits After Subsequent Treatment[b] with 15 mcg INFERGEN

	All Patients 24 Weeks n = 107	All Patients 48 Weeks n = 101	Prior Nonresponders 24 Weeks n = 74	Prior Nonresponders 48 Weeks n = 59	Prior Relapsers 24 Weeks n = 33	Prior Relapsers 48 Weeks n = 42
End of Observation Normalized ALT	13% (7.3%, 21.0%)	19% (11.7%, 27.8%)	7% (2.2%, 15.1%)	7% (1.9%, 16.5%)	27% (13.3%, 45.5%)	36% (21.6%, 52.0%)
End of Observation HCV RNA Negative	9% (4.6%, 16.7%)	22%[a] (13.4%, 30.0%)	4% (0.9%, 11.5%)	12% (4.9%, 22.9%)	21% (9.0%, 38.9%)	36% (21.6%, 52.0%)

[a] P value = 0.01.
[b] Subsequent treatment data are presented for patients initially treated with 9 mcg INFERGEN or 3 MIU IFN α-2b in the initial treatment study; patients initially treated with 3 mcg INFERGEN were excluded from this analysis.

INDICATIONS AND USAGE

INFERGEN is indicated for the treatment of chronic HCV infection in patients 18 years of age or older with compensated liver disease who have anti-HCV serum antibodies and/or the presence of HCV RNA. Other causes of hepatitis, such as viral hepatitis B or autoimmune hepatitis, should be ruled out prior to initiation of therapy with INFERGEN. In some patients with chronic HCV infection, INFERGEN normalizes serum ALT, reduces serum HCV RNA concentrations to undetectable quantities (< 100 copies/mL), and improves liver histology.

CONTRAINDICATIONS

INFERGEN is contraindicated in patients with known hypersensitivity to alpha interferons, to *E. coli*-derived products, or to any component of the product.

WARNINGS

Treatment with INFERGEN should be administered under the guidance of a qualified physician, and may lead to moderate-to-severe adverse experiences requiring dose reduction, temporary dose cessation, or discontinuation of further therapy.

Withdrawal from study for adverse events occurred in 7% of patients initially treated with 9 mcg INFERGEN (including 4% due to psychiatric events). Withdrawal from study due to adverse events occurred in 5% of patients subsequently treated with 15 mcg INFERGEN for 24 weeks and 11% of patients subsequently treated with 15 mcg INFERGEN for 48 weeks.

SEVERE PSYCHIATRIC ADVERSE EVENTS MAY MANIFEST IN PATIENTS RECEIVING THERAPY WITH ALPHA INTERFERONS, INCLUDING INFERGEN. DEPRESSION, SUICIDAL IDEATION, AND SUICIDE ATTEMPT MAY OCCUR. The incidence of psychiatric events of suicidal ideation and attempts was small (1%) for patients treated with 9 mcg INFERGEN compared to the overall incidence (55%) of psychiatric events. INFERGEN should be used with caution in patients who report a history of depression and physicians should monitor all patients for evidence of depression. Physicians should inform patients of the possible development of depression prior to initiation of INFERGEN therapy, and patients should report any sign or symptom of depression immediately. Other prominent psychiatric adverse events may also occur, including nervousness, anxiety, emotional lability, abnormal thinking, agitation, or apathy (see PRECAUTIONS).

INFERGEN SHOULD BE ADMINISTERED WITH CAUTION TO PATIENTS WITH PRE-EXISTING CARDIAC DISEASE. Hypertension and supraventricular arrhythmias, chest pain, and myocardial infarction have been associated with alpha interferon therapies.[8]

No studies with INFERGEN have been conducted in patients with decompensated hepatic disease. Patients with decompensated hepatic disease should not be treated with INFERGEN, and patients who develop symptoms of hepatic decompensation, such as jaundice, ascites, coagulopathy, or decreased serum albumin, should halt further interferon therapy.

Bone Marrow Toxicity: Alpha interferons suppress bone marrow function and may result in severe cytopenias including very rare events of aplastic anemia. It is advised that complete blood counts be obtained pretreatment and monitored routinely during therapy. Alpha interferon therapy should be discontinued in patients who develop severe decreases in neutrophil ($< 0.5 \times 10^9$/L) or platelet counts ($< 50 \times 10^9$/L).

Ophthalmologic Disorders: Decrease or loss of vision, retinopathy including macular edema, retinal artery or vein thrombosis, retinal hemorrhages and cotton wool spots; optic neuritis, and papilledema are induced or aggravated by treatment with Interferon alfacon-1 or other alpha interferons. All patients should receive an eye examination at baseline. Patients with preexisting ophthalmologic disorders (e.g., diabetic or hypertensive retinopathy) should receive periodic ophthalmologic exams during interferon alpha treatment. Any patient who develops ocular symptoms should receive a prompt and complete eye examination. Interferon alfacon-1 therapy should be discontinued in patients who develop new or worsening ophthalmologic disorders.

PRECAUTIONS

General

Since the use of type-I interferons has been associated with depression, INFERGEN therapy should not be used in patients with a history of severe psychiatric disorders and should be discontinued in patients developing severe depression, suicidal ideation, or other severe psychiatric disorders (see WARNINGS).

INFERGEN should be used with caution in patients with a history of cardiac disease. Hypertension (5%), tachycardia (4%), and palpitation (3%) were the most common cardiovascular adverse events reported for 9 mcg INFERGEN therapy, with 1% of patients reporting tachyarrhythmias which were dose-limiting (see WARNINGS).

INFERGEN should be used cautiously in patients with abnormally low peripheral blood cell counts or who are receiving agents that are known to cause myelosuppression. Transplantation patients, or other chronically immunosuppressed patients, should receive alfa interferon therapy with caution.

Serious acute hypersensitivity reactions have been reported in rare instances following treatment with alpha interferons.[8] If hypersensitivity reactions occur (e.g., urticaria, angioedema, bronchoconstriction, anaphylaxis), the drug should be discontinued immediately and appropriate medical treatment instituted.

INFERGEN should be administered with caution to patients with a history of endocrine disorders. Abnormal thyroid stimulating hormone (TSH) and free thyroxine (T_4) with hypothyroidism occurred in 4% of patients administered 9 mcg INFERGEN, and thyroid supplements were required in approximately two-thirds of those patients.

Exacerbation of autoimmune disease has been reported in patients receiving type-I interferon therapy.[8] INFERGEN should not be used in patients with autoimmune hepatitis and be used with caution in patients with other autoimmune disorders.

While fever may be related to the flu-like symptoms reported in patients treated with INFERGEN, when fever occurs, other possible causes of persistent fever should be ruled out.

Information for Patients

If home use is determined to be desirable by the physician, instructions on appropriate use should be given by a health care professional. The patient must be instructed as to the proper dosage and administration. Information included in the **MEDICATION GUIDE** should be fully reviewed with the patient; it is not a disclosure of all, or possible, adverse effects. The most common adverse reactions occurring with INFERGEN therapy are flu-like symptoms including fatigue, fever, rigors, headache, arthralgia, myalgia, and increased sweating. Non-narcotic analgesics and bedtime administration of INFERGEN may be used to prevent or lessen some of these symptoms. Additionally, patients must be thoroughly instructed in the importance of proper disposal procedures and cautioned against the reuse of needles, syringes, or re-entry of the drug product. A puncture-resistant container for the disposal of used syringes and needles should be used by the patient and should be disposed of according to the directions provided by the health care provider (see MEDICATION GUIDE).

Laboratory Tests

Laboratory tests are recommended for all patients on INFERGEN therapy, prior to beginning treatment (baseline), 2 weeks after initiation of therapy, and periodically thereafter during the 24 or 48 weeks of therapy at the discretion of the physician. Following completion of INFERGEN therapy, any abnormal test values should be monitored periodically. The entrance criteria that were used for the clinical study of INFERGEN may be considered as a guideline to acceptable baseline values for initiation of treatment:

- Platelet count $\geq 75 \times 10^9$/L
- Hemoglobin concentration ≥ 100 g/L
- ANC $\geq 1500 \times 10^6$/L
- Serum creatinine concentration < 180 μmol/L (< 2.0 mg/dL) or creatinine clearance > 0.83 mL/second (> 50 mL/minute)
- Serum albumin concentration ≥ 25 g/L
- Bilirubin within normal limits
- TSH and T_4 within normal limits

Neutropenia, thrombocytopenia, hypertriglyceridemia, and thyroid disorders have been reported with administration of INFERGEN (see ADVERSE REACTIONS). Therefore, these laboratory parameters should be monitored closely.

Drug Interactions

No formal drug interaction studies have been conducted with INFERGEN. INFERGEN should be used cautiously in patients who are receiving agents that are known to cause myelosuppression or with agents known to be metabolized via the cytochrome P-450 pathway.[9] Patients taking drugs that are metabolized by this pathway should be monitored closely for changes in the therapeutic and/or toxic levels of concomitant drugs.

Carcinogenesis, Mutagenesis, Impairment of Fertility

Carcinogenesis: No carcinogenicity data for INFERGEN are available in animals or humans.

Mutagenesis: INFERGEN was not mutagenic when tested in several *in vitro* assays, including the Ames bacterial mutagenicity assay and an *in vitro* cytogenetic assay in human lymphocytes, either in the presence or absence of metabolic activation.

Impairment of Fertility: INFERGEN at doses as high as 100 mcg/kg did not selectively affect reproductive performance or the development of the offspring when adminis-

Continued on next page

Infergen—Cont.

tered SC to male and female golden Syrian hamsters for 70 and 14 days before mating, respectively, and then through mating and to day 7 of pregnancy.

Pregnancy Category C

INFERGEN has been shown to have embryolethal or abortifacient effects in golden Syrian hamsters when given at 135 times the human dose and in cynomolgus and rhesus monkeys when given at 9 to 81 times (based on body surface area) the human dose. There are no adequate and well-controlled studies in pregnant women. INFERGEN should not be used during pregnancy. If a woman becomes pregnant or plans to become pregnant while taking INFERGEN, she should be informed of the potential hazards to the fetus. Males and females treated with INFERGEN should be advised to use effective contraception.

Nursing Mothers

It is not known whether INFERGEN is excreted in human milk. Because many drugs are excreted in human milk, caution should be exercised if INFERGEN is administered to a nursing woman. The effect on the nursing neonate of orally-ingested INFERGEN in breast milk has not been evaluated.

Pediatric Use

The safety and effectiveness of INFERGEN have not been established in patients below the age of 18 years. INFERGEN therapy is not recommended in pediatric patients.

Table 3. Patient Incidence of Adverse Events in Phase 3 Clinical Trials Regardless of Attribution[a]

	Initial Treatment[b]		Subsequent Treatment[b]	
	INFERGEN 9 mcg (n = 231)	IFN α-2b (n = 236)	INFERGEN 15 mcg 24 wks (n = 165)	INFERGEN 15 mcg 48 wks (n = 168)
Body System/Preferred Term	% of Patients		% of Patients	
APPLICATION SITE				
Injection Site Erythema	23	15	17	22
Injection Site Pain	9	3	8	11
Injection Site Ecchymosis	6	7	5	5
BODY AS A WHOLE				
Fatigue	69	67	65	71
Fever	61	45	58	55
Rigors	57	45	62	66
Body Pain	54	45	39	51
Influenza-like Symptoms[c]	15	11	8	8
Pain Chest	13	14	5	9
Hot Flushes	13	7	7	4
Malaise	11	10	2	5
Asthenia	9	11	10	7
Edema Peripheral	9	8	4	3
Access Pain	8	9	1	1
Allergic Reaction	7	5	3	4
Weight Decrease	5	7	5	2
CARDIOVASCULAR				
Hypertension	5	3	2	4
Palpitation	3	6	5	2
CNS/PNS				
Headache	82	83	78	80
Insomnia	39	30	24	28
Dizziness	22	25	18	25
Paresthesia	13	10	9	9
Hypoesthesia	10	8	8	10
Amnesia	10	6	2	5
Hypertonia	7	10	6	6
Somnolence	4	8	6	7
Confusion	4	6	4	5
Hyperesthesia	1	1	1	5
ENDOCRINE DISORDERS				
Thyroid Test Abnormal	9	5	4	6
GASTROINTESTINAL				
Abdominal Pain	41	40	24	32
Nausea	40	36	30	36
Diarrhea	29	24	24	22
Anorexia	24	17	21	14
Dyspepsia	21	18	12	10
Vomiting	12	11	13	11
Constipation	9	6	5	6
Flatulence	8	9	6	5
Tooth Ache	7	7	3	7
Saliva Decreased	6	7	4	1
Hemorrhoids	6	3	1	2
Stomatitis Ulcerative	3	4	2	6
Gingivitis	2	3	1	5
HEARING/VESTIBULAR				
Tinnitus	6	4	4	2
Earache	5	7	5	5
Otitis	2	5	1	3
HEMATOLOGIC				
Granulocytopenia	23	25	42	39
Thrombocytopenia	19	16	18	18
Leukopenia	15	13	19	28
Lymphadenopathy	0	0	4	4
Ecchymosis	6	4	4	2
Lymphocytosis	5	7	11	5
PT Increased	3	5	1	0
Anemia	2	3	2	6
LIVER AND BILIARY				
Liver Tender	5	3	6	2
Hepatomegaly	3	5	5	2
METABOLIC/NUTRITION				
Hypertriglyceridemia	6	7	5	5
MUSCULO-SKELETAL				
Myalgia	58	56	51	55
Arthralgia	51	44	43	46
Back Pain	42	37	29	23
Limb Pain	26	25	13	23
Skeletal Pain	14	14	10	12
Neck Pain	14	13	8	5
Musculo-skeletal Disorder	4	4	7	4

(Table continued on next page)

Geriatric Use

Clinical studies of INFERGEN did not include sufficient numbers of subjects aged 65 and over to determine whether they respond differently than younger subjects. Other reported clinical experience has not identified differences in responses between the elderly and younger patients. However, treatment with interferons, including INFERGEN, is associated with psychiatric, cardiac, and systemic (flu-like) adverse effects. Since decreased hepatic, renal or cardiac function, concomitant disease and the use of other drug therapies in elderly patients may produce adverse reactions of greater severity, caution should be exercised in the use of INFERGEN in this population.

ADVERSE REACTIONS

Adverse experiences that were reported, regardless of attribution to treatment, in at least 5% of patients in the 9 mcg INFERGEN or 3 MIU IFN α-2b groups of the pivotal study are presented in Table 3, listed in decreasing order by the 9 mcg INFERGEN group. The incidence of adverse events is expressed based on the number of patients experiencing each event at least once during treatment or during post-treatment observation.

Most adverse events were mild-to-moderate in severity and abated with cessation of therapy. Flu-like symptoms (ie, headache, fatigue, fever, rigors, myalgia, sweating increased, and arthralgia) were the most frequently reported treatment-related adverse reactions. Most were short-lived and could be treated symptomatically.

Depression, usually mild-to-moderate in severity, was reported in 26% of patients who received 9 mcg INFERGEN and was the most common adverse event resulting in study drug discontinuation.

In patients who had tolerated previous interferon therapy (9 mcg INFERGEN or 3 MIU IFN α-2b) and failed to normalize ALT, or who had achieved normalization of ALT during the treatment period but who relapsed during the post-treatment observation period, subsequent treatment with 15 mcg TIW of INFERGEN for 24 or 48 weeks was generally tolerated. Adverse experiences of patients receiving subsequent treatment, regardless of attribution to treatment, are reported in Table 3. The higher dose of INFERGEN used in these patients was associated with a greater incidence of leukopenia and granulocytopenia. One or more dose reductions for all causes were required in up to 36% of patients. Patients who do not tolerate initial standard interferon therapy should not receive therapy with 15 mcg TIW of INFERGEN.

[See table 3 at left and on next page]

Laboratory Values

The following laboratory values were found to be affected by therapy with INFERGEN in the 231 patients who received treatment with 9 mcg INFERGEN.

Hemoglobin and Hematocrit: Treatment with INFERGEN was associated with gradual decreases in mean values for hemoglobin and hematocrit, which were 4% and 5% below baseline at the end of treatment. Decreases from baseline of 20% or more in hemoglobin or hematocrit were seen in 1% of patients or less.

White Blood Cells: INFERGEN treatment was associated with decreases in mean values for both total white blood cell (WBC) count and ANC within the first 2 weeks of treatment. By the end of treatment, mean decreases from baseline of 19% for WBCs and 23% for ANC were observed. These effects reversed during the posttreatment observation period. In 2 INFERGEN-treated patients in the phase 3 trial, decreases in ANC to levels below 500×10^6 cells/L were seen. In both cases, the ANC returned to clinically acceptable levels with reduction of the dose of INFERGEN, and these transient decreases in neutrophils were not associated with infections.

Platelets: INFERGEN treatment was associated with alterations in platelet count. Decreases in mean platelet count of 16% compared to baseline were seen by the end of treatment. These decreases were reversed during the posttreatment observation period. Values below normal were common during treatment with 3% of patients developing values less than 50×10^9 cells/L, usually necessitating dose reduction.

Triglycerides: Mean values for serum triglyceride increased shortly after the start of administration of INFERGEN, with increases of 41%, compared with baseline, at the end of the treatment period. Seven percent of the patients developed values which were at least 3 times above pretreatment levels during treatment. This effect was promptly reversed after discontinuation of treatment.

Thyroid Function: INFERGEN treatment was associated with biochemical changes consistent with hypothyroidism including increases in TSH and decreases in T_4 mean values. Increases in TSH to greater than 7 mU/L were seen in 10% of 9 mcg INFERGEN-treated patients either during the treatment period or the 24-week posttreatment observation period. Thyroid supplements were instituted in approximately one-third of these patients.

Laboratory Values for Subsequent Treatment: From a database of 165 patients receiving subsequent treatment with 15 mcg of INFERGEN for 24 weeks, and 168 patients receiving subsequent treatment with 15 mcg of INFERGEN for 48 weeks after failing initial interferon therapy, similar changes in the laboratory values as outlined above were observed. Mean decreases from baseline up to 23% for WBCs and up to 27% for ANC were observed for patients subsequently treated with interferon, which was greater than during initial treatment. Two patients in the 24-week group experienced reversible reductions in ANC to less than 500 × 10^6 cells/L, which were not associated with infectious complications. No patients discontinued as a result of hematologic toxicity.

OVERDOSAGE

In INFERGEN trials, the maximum overdose reported was a dose of 150 mcg INFERGEN administered SC in a patient enrolled in a phase 1 advanced malignancy trial. The patient received 10 times the prescribed dosage for 3 days. The patient experienced a mild increase in anorexia, chills, fever, and myalgia. Increases in ALT (15 to 127 IU/L), aspartate transaminase (AST) (15 to 164 IU/L), and lactic dehydrogenase (LDH) (183 to 281 IU/L) were reported. These laboratory values returned to normal or to the patient's baseline values within 30 days.

DOSAGE AND ADMINISTRATION

The recommended dose of INFERGEN® for treatment of chronic HCV infection is 9 mcg TIW administered SC as a single injection for 24 weeks. At least 48 hours should elapse between doses of INFERGEN. (See illustrated MEDICATION GUIDE for instructions.)

Patients who tolerated previous interferon therapy and did not respond or relapsed following its discontinuation may be subsequently treated with 15 mcg of INFERGEN TIW administered SC as a single injection for up to 48 weeks. (See illustrated MEDICATION GUIDE for instructions.)

There are significant differences in specific activities among interferons. Health care providers should be aware that changes in interferon brand may require adjustments of dosage and/or change in route of administration. Patients should be warned not to change brands of interferon without medical consultation. Patients should also be instructed by their physician not to reduce the dosage of INFERGEN prior to medical consultation.

Dose Reduction

For patients who experience a severe adverse reaction on INFERGEN, dosage should be withheld temporarily. If the adverse reaction does not become tolerable, therapy should be discontinued. Dose reduction to 7.5 mcg may be necessary following an intolerable adverse event. In the pivotal study, 11% of patients (26/231) who initially received INFERGEN at a dose of 9 mcg (0.3 mL) were dose-reduced to 7.5 mcg (0.25 mL).

If adverse reactions continue to occur at the reduced dosage, the physician may discontinue treatment or reduce dosage further. However, decreased efficacy may result from continued treatment at dosages below 7.5 mcg.

During subsequent treatment for 48 weeks with 15 mcg of INFERGEN, up to 36% of patients required dose reductions in 3 mcg increments.

Administration of INFERGEN

If home use is determined to be desirable by the physician, instructions on appropriate use should be given by a health care professional. After administration of INFERGEN, it is essential to follow the procedure for proper disposal of syringes and needles. See the MEDICATION GUIDE for detailed instructions.

Storage

Just prior to injection, INFERGEN may be allowed to reach room temperature.

Parenteral drug products should be inspected visually for particulate matter and discoloration prior to administration; if particulates or discoloration are observed, the container should not be used.

HOW SUPPLIED

Use only one dose per vial; do not re-enter the vial. Discard unused portions. Do not save unused drug for later administration.

Single-dose, preservative-free vials containing 9 mcg (0.3 mL) of Interferon alfacon-1 are available in dispensing packs of 6 vials (NDC 64116-039-06).

Single-dose, preservative-free vials containing 15 mcg (0.5 mL) of Interferon alfacon-1 are available in dispensing packs of 6 vials (NDC 64116-031-06).

INFERGEN should be stored in the refrigerator at 2° to 8°C (36° to 46°F). Do not freeze. Avoid vigorous shaking and exposure to direct sunlight.

REFERENCES

1. Alton K, Stabinsky Y, Richards R, et al. Production, characterization and biological effects of recombinant DNA derived human IFN-α and IFN-γ analogs. In: De Maeyer E, Schellekens H, eds. *The Biology of the Interferon System 1983*. Elsevier Science Publishers: Amsterdam. 1983;119-128.
2. Blatt LM, Davis J, Klein SB, Taylor MW. The biologic activity and molecular characterization of a novel synthetic interferon-alpha species, consensus interferon. *J Interferon Cytokine Res*. 1996;16:489-499.
3. Fish EN, Banerjee K, Levine HL, Stebbing N. Antiherpetic effects of a human alpha interferon analog, IFN-alpha Con_1, in hamsters. *Antimicrob Agents Chemother*. 1986;30:52-56.
4. Trown PW, Willis RJ, Kamm JJ. The preclinical development of Roferon®-A. *Cancer*. 1986;57:1648-1656.
5. Tong MJ, Reddy KR, Lee WM, et al. Treatment of chronic hepatitis C with consensus interferon: a multicenter, randomized, controlled trial. *Hepatology*. 1997;26:747-754.
6. Knodell RG, Ishak KG, Black WC, et al. Formulation and application of a numerical scoring system for assessing histological activity in asymptomatic chronic active hepatitis. *Hepatology*. 1981;1:431-435.
7. Heathcote E, Keeffe E, Lee S, et al. Retreatment of chronic hepatitis C with consensus interferon. *Hepatology*. 1997;27:1136-1143.
8. Vial T, Descotes J. Clinical toxicity of interferons. *Drug Safety*. 1994;10:115-150.
9. Horsmans Y, Brenard R, Geubel AP. Short report: interferon-α decreases ^{14}C-aminopyrine breath test values in patients with chronic hepatitis C. *Aliment Pharmacol Ther.* 1994;8:353-355.

This product and its use are covered by the following US Patent Nos.: 4,695,623; 5,372,808; 5,541,293; 5,980,884.

INTERMUNE®

InterMune, Inc.
Brisbane, CA 94005
U.S. License No. 1626

FDA Approval November 2002 (B101)
Revised February 2003
LB-2007.2
3265701

Shown in Product Identification Guide, page 319

Table 3 *(cont.)*. Patient Incidence of Adverse Events in Phase 3 Clinical Trials Regardless of Attribution[a]

	Initial Treatment[b]		Subsequent Treatment[b]	
	INFERGEN 9 mcg (n = 231)	IFN α-2b (n = 236)	INFERGEN 15 mcg 24 wks (n = 165)	INFERGEN 15 mcg 48 wks (n = 168)
Body System/Preferred Term	% of Patients		% of Patients	
PSYCHIATRIC DISORDER				
Nervousness	31	29	16	22
Depression	26	25	18	19
Anxiety	19	18	9	14
Emotional Lability	12	11	6	3
Thinking Abnormal	8	12	10	20
Agitation	6	6	4	4
Libido Decreased	5	5	5	4
Apathy	2	3	4	5
REPRODUCTIVE (FEMALE)				
Dysmenorrhea	9	9	2	7
Vaginitis	8	2	5	5
Menstrual Disorder	6	5	2	5
Menorrhagia	3	0	2	5
Moniliasis Genital	2	6	2	0
Breast Mass	0	3	0	5
Pain Breast	0	5	2	0
RESISTANCE MECHANISM				
Infection	3	5	2	6
RESPIRATORY				
Pharyngitis	34	31	17	21
Infection Upper Respiratory	31	34	16	18
Cough	22	17	12	11
Sinusitis	17	22	12	16
Rhinitis	13	16	7	9
Respiratory Tract Congestion	12	7	4	9
Upper Respiratory Tract Congestion	10	14	7	9
Epistaxis	8	12	6	6
Dyspnea	7	12	8	7
Bronchitis	6	6	2	1
SKIN AND APPENDAGES				
Alopecia	14	25	10	13
Pruritus	14	14	11	10
Rash	13	15	13	10
Sweating Increased	12	11	13	11
Erythema	6	6	7	9
Skin Dry	6	5	2	5
Wound	4	7	3	4
SPECIAL SENSES				
Taste Perversion	3	6	3	5
VISION DISORDERS				
Conjunctivitis	8	8	4	6
Pain Eye	5	6	4	2
Vision Abnormal	3	5	5	5

[a] Only events that occurred at a frequency of ≥ 5% in any treatment group are included. Patients can appear more than once in Table 3. Because the 2 studies were conducted at different times with nonidentical patient groups, the adverse events profile for the subsequent treatment study is not directly comparable to the initial treatment study.

[b] Adverse events reported in patients during treatment or posttreatment observation in the pivotal initial treatment and subsequent treatment studies are listed regardless of attribution to treatment.

[c] Influenza-like Symptoms: presumed viral etiology.

International Nutrition Research Center, Inc.

**7900 LOS PINOS CIRCLE
CORAL GABLES, FL 33143**

Direct Inquiries to:
phone (305) 740-7480
fax (305) 740-7478

SON FORMULA® TABLETS — OTC

[(Master Amino Acid Pattern (MAP®)]
A safe and effective substitute for dietary proteins

DESCRIPTION

SON Formula® (MAP®) is a patented dietary proteins substitute, which provides a unique pattern of essential amino acids, in a highly purified, free, crystalline form. After oral ingestion, SON Formula® is rapidly utilized. SON Formula® does not require the aid of peptidases and therefore, it is absorbed, within 23 minutes, through the first 100 cm of functional small intestine. SON Formula® does not provide any fecal residue. SON Formula® is amphoteric. SON Formula® is supplied in tablets of 1,000 mg for oral administration. Each tablet of SON Formula®, in addition to the active ingredient MAP®, contains no inactive ingredients.

COMPOSITION

SON Formula®, in a dose of 10 g, provides the following essential amino acids profile:

L-Leucine	1.964 g
L-Valine	1.657 g
L-Isoleucine	1.483 g
L-Lysine	1.429 g
L-Phenylalanine	1.289 g
L-Threonine	1.111 g
L-Methionine	0.699 g
L-Tryptophan	0.368 g

CLINICAL STUDIES

The results of a comparative, double-blind, triple crossover Net Nitrogen Utilization (NNU) clinical study have shown that the subjects, while taking MAP®, as a dietary proteins substitute, achieved a body's 99% NNU. This means that 99% of MAP's constituent amino acids followed the anabolic pathway, thus acting as precursor of body's protein synthesis. By comparison, dietary proteins only provide between 16 to 48% NNU. This fact evidences that MAP is more nutritious than dietary proteins. This has been confirmed by the fact that during the study, each subject body's nitrogen balance was maintained in equilibrium by taking MAP, as a sole and total substitute of dietary proteins, in a dosage of only 400 mg/kg/day, which provided less than 2 kcal/day (1g

Continued on next page

SON Formula® Vs Dietary Proteins

Characteristics	SON Formula®	Dietary Proteins
Net Nitrogen Utilization (NNU)	99%	16%– 48%
Nitrogen Catabolites	1%	52%–84%
Body's Protein Synthesis	10g	Approx. 350g
Energy	0.04 Kcal/g	4 Kcal/g
Digestion	Approx. 23 minutes	3–5 hours
Contraindications	None	Renal Failure or Hepatic Failure
Adverse Reactions	None	Food Sensitivities
Shelf-Life	3 years	1–4 days
Refrigeration	Not needed	Needed
Volume	Approx. 30cc.	500–1000cc.

Son Formula—Cont.

MAP= 0.04 Kcal). The study results have also shown that 1% of MAP's constituent amino acids followed the catabolic pathway, thus releasing only 1% of nitrogen catabolites and energy. By comparison dietary proteins release between 52% to 84% nitrogen catabolites and energy. This fact evidences that MAP is safer than dietary proteins, and that provides the lowest amount of energy in comparison to any dietary protein.
To illustrate: when a dietary protein is digested, it releases its constituent amino acids into the small intestine, where they are absorbed. Then, those amino acids can follow either the *anabolic pathway* or the *catabolic pathway* (Fig. I).

Figure I. Dietary Protein Metabolism

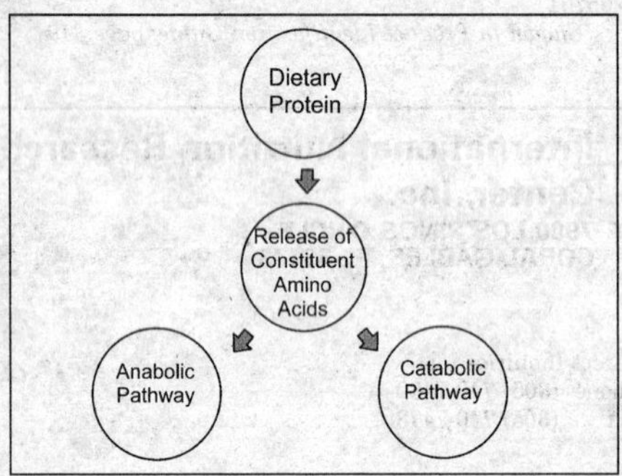

When dietary amino acids follow the *anabolic pathway*, they act as precursors for the body's protein synthesis, thus becoming the body's constituent proteins. Throughout the *anabolic pathway*, amino acids do not release any nitrogen catabolites or energy (Fig. II).

Figure II. The Protein Metabolism Anabolic Pathway

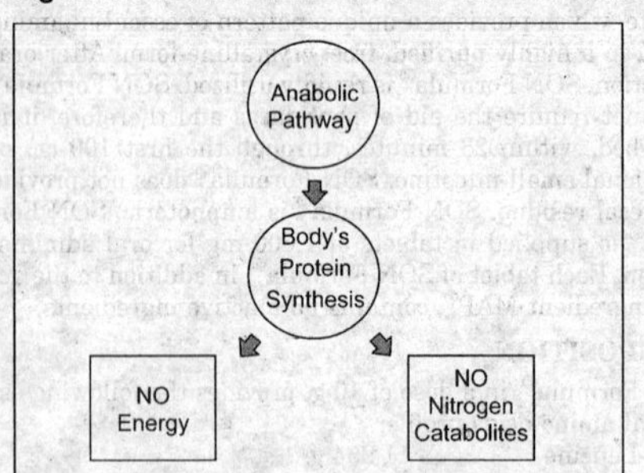

On the other hand, when dietary amino acids follow the *catabolic pathway*, they act only as a source of energy and not as precursors of body's proteins synthesis. Throughout the *catabolic pathway*, amino acids do release nitrogen catabolites and energy (Fig. III).

Figure III. The Protein Metabolism Catabolic Pathway

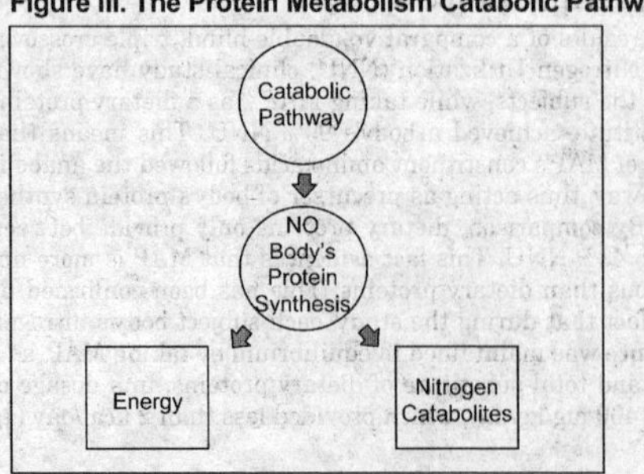

INDICATIONS AND USAGE

SON Formula® is indicated as a safe and effective substitute for dietary proteins.
[See table above]

ADVERSE REACTIONS

No adverse reactions have been reported.

OVERDOSAGE

No adverse reactions have been reported.

DOSAGE AND ADMINISTRATION

SON Formula® should be administered with food. SON Formula® in a dosage of 400mg/kg/day has been shown to be adequate, as a sole and total substitute of dietary proteins, to maintain the body's nitrogen balance in equilibrium. To calculate the SON Formula® dosage necessary to substitute dietary proteins, apply the following:

SON Formula® dosage = (Dietary Protein × 0.4) g

For instance: to calculate the dosage of SON Formula® necessary to substitute 10 g of dietary proteins, proceed as follows:

a. SON Formula® dosage = (Dietary Proteins × 0.4) g
b. SON Formula® dosage = (10 × 0.4) g
c. SON Formula® dosage = 4 g

Therefore, 4 g of SON Formula® provide a body's protein synthesis equivalent to that provided by 10 g of high biological value dietary proteins.

SUPPLY INFORMATION

SON Formula®, is available in bottles of 100 tablets of 1,000 mg, for oral administration.
Additional professional information on SON Formula® is available thorough the International Nutritional Research Center, Inc.
Patent No. 5,132,113

IVAX Laboratories, Inc.

4400 BISCAYNE BLVD., 9TH FLOOR
MIAMI, FL 33137

Direct Inquiries to:
IVAX Laboratories, Inc.
888-IVAX-LAB
305-575-6221 fax

NASAREL® ℞

(flunisolide)
Nasal Spray, 29 mcg

For Intranasal Use Only
℞ Only

DESCRIPTION

Flunisolide, the active component of NASAREL nasal spray, is an anti-inflammatory glucocorticosteroid with the chemical name: 6α-fluoro-11β,16α,17,21 tetrahydroxypregna-1,4-diene-3,20-dione cyclic 16,17-acetal with acetone, hemihydrate. It has the following chemical structure:

Flunisolide is a white to creamy white crystalline powder with a molecular weight of 443.51 and molecular formula of $C_{24}H_{31}FO_6$. It is soluble in acetone, sparingly soluble in chloroform, slightly soluble in methanol, and practically insoluble in water. It has a melting point of about 245°C. The octanol:water partition coefficient is 2.17 at neutral pH.
NASAREL is a metered dose manual pump spray unit containing 0.025% w/w flunisolide in an aqueous medium containing benzalkonium chloride, butylated hydroxytoluene, citric acid, edetate disodium, polyethylene glycol 400, polysorbate 20, propylene glycol, sodium citrate dihydrate, sorbitol and purified water. Sodium hydroxide and/or hydrochloric acid may be added to adjust the pH to a target of 5.2. Each 25 mL spray bottle contains 6.25 mg of flunisolide.
After initial priming (5 to 6 sprays), each spray of the pump spray unit delivers a metered spray of 100 mg formulation containing 29 mcg of flunisolide. The size of 99.5% of the droplets produced by the unit is greater than 8 microns. The contents of one nasal spray bottle delivers 200 sprays in addition to the priming sprays.

CLINICAL PHARMACOLOGY

General Pharmacology: Flunisolide nasal spray has demonstrated potent glucocorticoid and weak mineralocorticoid activity in classical animal test systems. As a glucocorticoid it was 180 times more potent than the cortisol standard in a rat anti-granuloma assay.
Pharmacokinetics: Flunisolide is well absorbed and is rapidly converted by the liver to the much less active primary metabolite and to glucuronide and sulfate conjugates. The primary metabolite results from the loss of the 6α fluorine and addition of a 6β hydroxy group. Following administration of radiolabeled flunisolide to man, approximately half of the label is recovered in the urine and half in the stool. The primary metabolite accounts for 65% to 70% of the amount recovered in the urine. Due to first-pass liver metabolism, only 20% of an oral flunisolide dose reaches the systemic circulation unmetabolized as compared to 50% of an intranasal dose. The plasma half-life of flunisolide is 1 to 2 hours.
In a pharmacokinetic study comparing NASAREL with NASALIDE®, the original formulation, the two formulations were not bioequivalent. The total absorption of NASAREL was 25% less than that of NASALIDE, and the peak plasma concentration was 30% lower. The clinical significance of these differences is likely to be small, particularly since clinical efficacy is attributable to a local effect on nasal mucosa (see Pharmacodynamics).
Pharmacodynamics: A study in approximately 100 patients compared control of hay fever symptoms by the recommended dose of flunisolide as NASALIDE (200 mcg/day), with control by an oral dose of flunisolide providing equivalent plasma levels. The results demonstrated that the clinical effectiveness was due to the direct topical effect of flunisolide and not to an indirect effect through systemic absorption.
The effects of flunisolide on hypothalamic-pituitary-adrenal (HPA) axis function have been studied in adult volunteers. Flunisolide as NASALIDE, the original nasal formulation, was administered to 20 subjects intranasally in average total daily doses ranging from approximately 350 mcg to 2200 mcg (equivalent to about 14 to 88 sprays per day) for 4 to 10 days. Early morning plasma cortisol concentrations and 24-hour urinary 17-ketogenic steroids were measured daily. There was no consistent effect on endogenous cortisol production, although evidence of mild adrenal suppression was seen in some subjects.
Controlled studies evaluated adult patients receiving average total daily doses ranging from approximately 50 to 400 mcg (equivalent to about 2 to 16 sprays per day) of NASALIDE, the original flunisolide nasal spray, for periods as long as 3 months. Three hundred and thirty-nine patients from these studies were entered into a long-term open label study. Morning plasma cortisol levels were available for 182 patients at baseline, 129 after 6 months, and 36 after 12 months of continuous treatment with flunisolide. No effect of flunisolide on cortisol production was detected.
The mechanisms responsible for anti-inflammatory action of corticosteroids and for their effect on the nasal mucosa are not completely understood.

CLINICAL TRIALS

The effectiveness of NASAREL was tested in 289 patients for up to 6 weeks at doses up to 300 mcg per day. NASAREL was shown to be effective in treating the symptoms of allergic rhinitis, including rhinorrhea, nasal congestion and sneezing.
A pivotal, 3-center trial involved 196 patients with seasonal allergic rhinitis randomized to NASALIDE, the vehicle of NASALIDE, NASAREL and the vehicle of NASAREL. Both active treatments were statistically significantly more effective than the vehicles. There was not statistically significant difference in efficacy between NASALIDE and NASAREL.
The two formulations do differ in the nature and incidence of adverse complaints. There were more reports of nasal burning and stinging with NASALIDE and more problems related to taste, such as aftertaste, with NASAREL, owing to the differences in their respective vehicles. Some patients may prefer one formulation to the other.
INDIVIDUALIZATION OF DOSAGE: The therapeutic effects of corticosteroid nasal sprays, unlike those of decongestants, are not immediate. This should be explained to the patient in advance in order to ensure cooperation and continuation of treatment with the prescribed dosage regimen. Full therapeutic benefit requires regular use and is usually evident

within a few days. A longer period of therapy may be required for some patients. However, NASAREL should not be continued beyond 3 weeks in the absence of significant symptomatic improvement (see PRECAUTIONS, WARNINGS, *Information for Patients* and ADVERSE REACTIONS sections).
A starting dose of 2 sprays in each nostril twice daily is recommended. If greater control of symptoms is needed, the dose may be increased to 2 sprays in each nostril 3 times a day. For adults, maximum total daily doses should not exceed 8 sprays in each nostril per day (400 mcg/day).
After the desired clinical effect is obtained, the maintenance dose should be reduced to the smallest amount necessary to control the symptoms. Some patients with perennial rhinitis may be maintained on as little as 1 spray in each nostril per day. It is always desirable to titrate an individual patient to the minimum effective dose to reduce the possibility of side effects.
NASAREL and NASALIDE should not be considered to be identical. Physicians should consider the observed differences in the mean responses in terms of side effects (see ADVERSE REACTIONS) and flunisolide absorption (see *Pharmacokinetics*) in treating individual patients.
For pediatric patients 6 to 14 years of age, the recommended starting dose of NASAREL is one spray (29 mcg) in each nostril 3 times a day (total dose 174 mcg/day) or 2 sprays (58 mcg) in each nostril 2 times a day (total dose 232 mcg/day). Maximum daily doses should not exceed 4 sprays in each nostril per day (total dose 232 mcg/day) as the safety and efficacy of higher doses have not been established. NASAREL is not recommended for use in pediatric patients less than 6 years of age as the safety and efficacy have not been assessed in this age group.

INDICATIONS AND USAGE

NASAREL is indicated for the management of the nasal symptoms of seasonal or perennial rhinitis.

CONTRAINDICATIONS

Hypersensitivity to any of the ingredients. NASAREL should not be used in the presence of untreated localized infection involving the nasal mucosa.

WARNINGS

The replacement of a systemic corticosteroid with topical corticoid can be accompanied by signs of adrenal insufficiency, and in addition some patients may experience symptoms of withdrawal, e.g., joint and/or muscular pain, lassitude and depression. Patients previously treated for prolonged periods with systemic corticosteroids and transferred to NASAREL should be carefully monitored to avoid acute adrenal insufficiency in response to stress.
Careful attention must also be given to patients who have associated asthma or other clinical conditions where too rapid a decrease in systemic corticosteroids may exacerbate their symptoms.
The use of NASAREL with systemic prednisone as alternate day therapy or with daily doses of less than 7.5 mg could increase the likelihood of hypothalamic-pituitary-adrenal axis suppression compared to a therapeutic dose of either one alone. Therefore, NASAREL treatment should be used with caution in patients already on prednisone regimens for any disease.
Persons who are on drugs which suppress the immune system are more susceptible to infections than healthy individuals. Chicken pox and measles, for example, can have a more serious or even fatal course in nonimmune pediatric patients or adults on corticosteroids. In such pediatric patients or adults who have not had these diseases, particular care should be taken to avoid exposure. How the dose, route and duration of corticosteroid administration affects the risk of developing a disseminated infection is not known. The contribution of underlying disease and/or prior corticosteroid treatment to the risk is also not known. If a nonimmune patient is exposed to chicken pox, prophylaxis with varicella zoster immune globulin (VZIG) may be indicated. If exposed to measles, prophylaxis with pooled intramuscular immunoglobulin (IG) may be indicated. (See the respective package insert for complete VZIG and IG prescribing information). If chicken pox develops, treatment with antiviral agents may be considered.

PRECAUTIONS

General: Intranasal corticosteroids may also cause a reduction in growth velocity when administered to pediatric patients (see **PRECAUTIONS, Pediatric Use** section).
Symptomatic relief may not occur in some patients for as long as 2 weeks. Although systemic effects are minimal at recommended doses, NASAREL should not be continued beyond 3 weeks in the absence of significant symptomatic improvement. In clinical studies with flunisolide administered intranasally, the development of localized infections of the nose and pharynx with *Candida albicans* has occurred only rarely. When such an infection develops it may require treatment with appropriate local therapy or discontinuance of treatment with NASAREL. Since there is no evidence that exceeding the maximum recommended dose of NASAREL is more effective, higher doses should be avoided.
Patients should be advised to clear their nasal passages of secretions prior to use. NASAREL should not be used in the presence of untreated local infection involving the nasal mucosa. Flunisolide should be used with caution, if at all, in patients with active or quiescent tuberculosis infection, fungal, bacterial or systemic viral infections or ocular herpes simplex.
As with other nasally inhaled corticosteroids, nasal septal perforations have been reported in rare instances with the use of flunisolide nasal sprays. Temporary or permanent loss of the sense of smell and taste have also been reported with the use of flunisolide nasal sprays.
Because of the inhibitory effect of corticosteroids on wound healing, a nasal corticosteroid should be used with caution in patients who have experienced recent nasal septal ulcers, recurrent epistaxis, nasal surgery or trauma, until healing has occurred.
Although systemic corticoid effects typical of Cushing's syndrome are minimal with recommended doses of topical steroids, this potential increases with excessive doses. If recommended doses are exceeded with long-term use, or if individuals are particularly sensitive, symptoms of hypercorticism could occur including suppression of hypothalamic-pituitary-adrenal function and/or retardation of growth in pediatric patients. Therefore, larger than recommended doses of NASAREL should be avoided.
Information for Patients: Patients should use NASAREL at regular intervals since its effectiveness depends on its regular use. Patients should take the medication as directed and should not exceed the prescribed dose. A decrease in symptoms can be expected to occur within a few days of initiating therapy in allergic rhinitis patients. Patients should contact their physician if the condition worsens, if sneezing or nasal irritation occurs, or if symptoms do not improve by 3 weeks.
Persons taking immunosuppressant doses of corticosteroids should be warned to avoid exposure to chicken pox or measles. Patients should also be advised that if they are exposed, medical advice should be sought without delay.
For proper use of this unit and to attain maximum improvement, the patient should read and follow the accompanying Patient Instructions carefully.
Carcinogenesis: Long-term studies were conducted in mice and rats using oral administration to evaluate the carcinogenic potential of the drug. Flunisolide was administered to mice at doses of 5, 50 and 500 mcg/kg/day (15, 150 and 1500 mcg/m^2 respectively), and to rats at doses of 0.5, 1 and 2.5 mcg/kg/day (3.0, 5.9 and 14.8 mcg/m^2 respectively). There was an increase in the incidence of benign pulmonary adenomas in mice, but not in rats. Female rats receiving the highest oral dose had an increased incidence of mammary adenocarcinoma compared to control rats. An increased incidence of this tumor type has been reported for other corticosteroids.
Impairment of Fertility: Female rats receiving high doses of flunisolide (200 mcg/kg/day or 1180 mcg/m^2 body surface area) showed some evidence of impaired fertility. Reproductive performance in the low (8 mcg/kg/day or 47.2 mcg/m^2) and mid-dose (40 mcg/kg/day or 236 mcg/m^2) groups was comparable to controls.
Pregnancy: Pregnancy Category C. As with other corticosteroids, flunisolide has been shown to be teratogenic and fetotoxic in rabbits and rats at oral doses of 40 and 200 mcg/kg/day (480 mcg/m^2 and 1180 mcg/m^2) respectively. There are no adequate and well-controlled studies in pregnant women. Flunisolide should be used during pregnancy only if the potential benefit justifies the potential risk to the fetus.
Nursing Mothers: It is not known whether this drug is excreted in human milk. Because other corticosteroids are excreted in human milk, caution should be exercised when flunisolide is administered to nursing women.
Pediatric Use: NASAREL is not recommended for use in pediatric patients less than 6 years of age as safety and efficacy have not been assessed in this age group. For pediatric patients 6 years of age and over, recommended maximum daily doses should not be exceeded in order to minimize the risk of systemic corticoid effects, including potential growth retardation. (See INDIVIDUALIZATION OF DOSAGE and DOSAGE AND ADMINISTRATION.) Controlled clinical studies have shown that intranasal corticosteroids may cause a reduction in growth velocity in pediatric patients. This effect has been observed in the absence of laboratory evidence of hypothalamic-pituitary-adrenal (HPA) axis suppression, suggesting that growth velocity is a more sensitive indicator of systemic corticosteroid exposure in pediatric patients than some commonly used tests of HPA axis function. The long-term effects of this reduction in growth velocity associated with intranasal corticosteroids, including the impact on final adult height, are unknown. The potential for "catch up" growth following discontinuation of treatment with intranasal corticosteroids has not been adequately studied. The growth of pediatric patients receiving intranasal corticosteroids, including NASAREL, should be monitored routinely (e.g., via stadiometry). The potential growth effects of prolonged treatment should be weighed against clinical benefits obtained and the availability of safe and effective noncorticosteroid treatment alternatives. To minimize the systemic effects of intranasal corticosteroids, including NASAREL, each patient should be titrated to the lowest dose that effectively controls his/her symptoms.
Geriatric Use: Clinical studies of NASAREL did not include sufficient numbers of subjects aged 65 and over to determine whether they respond differently from younger subjects. Other reported clinical experience has not identified differences in responses between the elderly and younger patients. In general, dose selection for an elderly patient should be cautious, usually starting at the low end of the dosing range, reflecting the greater frequency of decreased hepatic, renal, or cardiac function, and of concomitant disease or other drug therapy.

ADVERSE REACTIONS

The adverse events rates listed below are based on symptoms spontaneously reported in multidose controlled clinical trials in comparing NASAREL and NASALIDE for treatment of allergic rhinitis. In patients receiving NASAREL the most common adverse events were transient aftertaste (17%) and transient nasal burning and stinging (13%). These symptoms did not usually interfere with treatment.
Adverse Event Rates for NASAREL:
Incidence Greater than 1% (probably causally related)
Respiratory: Nasal burning/stinging (13%), epistaxis*, nasal dryness, pharyngitis, cough increased
Gastrointestinal: Nausea
Special Senses: Aftertaste (17%)
Incidence 1% or Less (probably causally related)
Respiratory: Hoarseness
Special Senses: Abnormal sense of smell
Incidence 1% or Less (causal relationship unknown)[†]
Respiratory: Sinusitis
Adverse Event Rates for NASALIDE:
Incidence Greater than 1% (probably causally related)
Respiratory: Nasal burning/stinging (44%), epistaxis*, nasal dryness*, pharyngitis*, cough increased
Gastrointestinal: Nausea
Special Senses: Aftertaste (8%)
Incidence 1% or Less (probably causally related)
Respiratory: Hoarseness, nasal ulcer
Incidence 1% or Less (causal relationship unknown)[†]
Respiratory: Sinusitis

*Incidence of reported reaction between 3% and 9%. Those reactions occurring in less than 3% of the patients are unmarked.
[†]Reactions occurred under circumstances where the causal relationship has not been clearly established; they are presented as alerting information for physicians.

Cases of growth suppression have been reported for intranasal corticosteroids (including NASAREL) (see **PRECAUTIONS, Pediatric Use** section).

OVERDOSAGE

In mice, rats and dogs, intravenous flunisolide at doses up to 4 mg/kg showed no effect. One spray bottle contains 6.25 mg of flunisolide; therefore, acute overdosage is unlikely.

DOSAGE AND ADMINISTRATION

For adults, the recommended starting dose of NASAREL is 2 sprays (58 mcg) in each nostril 2 times a day (total dose 232 mcg/day): the effect should be assessed in 4 to 7 days (see INDIVIDUALIZATION OF DOSAGE section). Some relief can be expected in approximately two-thirds of patients within that time. This dose may be increased to 2 sprays in each nostril 3 times a day (total dose 348 mcg/day) if greater effect is needed. For adults, maximum total daily doses should not exceed 8 sprays in each nostril per day (464 mcg/day). After the desired clinical effect is obtained, the maintenance dose should be reduced to the smallest amount necessary to control the symptoms (See INDIVIDUALIZATION OF DOSAGE section).
For pediatric patients 6 to 14 years of age, the recommended starting dose of NASAREL is one spray, (29 mcg) in each nostril 3 times a day (total dose 174 mcg/day) or 2 sprays (58 mcg) in each nostril 2 times a day (total dose 232 mcg/day). For pediatric patients 6 to 14 years of age, maximum daily doses should not exceed 4 sprays in each nostril per day (total dose 232 mcg/day) as the safety and efficacy of higher doses have not been established. NASAREL is not recommended for use in pediatric patients less than 6 years of age as safety and efficacy, including possible adverse effects on growth, have not been assessed in this age group.
For priming and repriming of nasal spray unit after storage: The patient should remove the protective cap. Put two fingers on the "shoulders" and thumb on the bottom of the bottle. Push the bottle with your thumb FIRMLY and QUICKLY 5–6 times or until a fine mist appears. Now your preset pump is primed. The patient must prime the present pump unit again if it has not been used for 5 days or more, or if it has been disassembled for cleaning. NASAREL and NASALIDE should not be considered to be identical products. Physicians should consider the observed differences in the mean responses in terms of side effects (see ADVERSE REACTIONS) and flunisolide absorption (see Pharmacokinetics) in treating individual patients.
DIRECTIONS FOR USE: A patient leaflet of instructions accompanies each package of NASAREL Nasal Spray.

WARNING

Do not spray in eyes.

HOW SUPPLIED

Each 25 mL of NASAREL 0.025% nasal spray (6.25 mg flunisolide) is supplied in a white, HDPE, spray bottle fitted with a meter pump, nasal adapter and a protective cap (NDC 59310-037-25). The unit contains 200 metered sprays and comes with a patient instruction leaflet. Store at 15° to 30°C (59° to 86°F).
CONTENTS MADE IN CANADA.
Manufactured for: **IVAX LABORATORIES INC.**
Miami, FL 33137
By: **PATHEON INC.**
Mississauga, Ontario
Canada L5N 7K9
IN-5124/S
Rev. 10/02)

Continued on next page

QVAR® 40 mcg ℞
(beclomethasone dipropionate HFA, 40 mcg)
INHALATION AEROSOL
For Oral Inhalation Only

QVAR® 80 mcg ℞
(beclomethasone dipropionate HFA, 80 mcg)
INHALATION AEROSOL
For Oral Inhalation Only

DESCRIPTION

The active component of QVAR 40 mcg Inhalation Aerosol and QVAR 80 mcg Inhalation Aerosol is beclomethasone dipropionate, USP, an anti-inflammatory corticosteroid having the chemical name 9-chloro-11β,17,21-trihydroxy-16β-methylpregna-1,4-diene-3,20-dione 17,21-dipropionate. Beclomethasone dipropionate is a diester of beclomethasone, a synthetic corticosteroid chemically related to dexamethasone. Beclomethasone differs from dexamethasone in having a chlorine at the 9-alpha carbon in place of a fluorine, and in having a 16 beta-methyl group instead of a 16 alpha-methyl group. Beclomethasone dipropionate is a white to creamy white, odorless powder with a molecular formula of $C_{28}H_{37}ClO_7$ and a molecular weight of 521.1. Its chemical structure is:

Beclomethasone dipropionate is slightly soluble in water, very soluble in chloroform and freely soluble in acetone and in alcohol.

QVAR is a pressurized, metered-dose aerosol intended for oral inhalation only. Each unit contains a solution of beclomethasone dipropionate in propellant HFA-134a (1,1,1,2 tetrafluoroethane) and ethanol. QVAR 40 mcg delivers 40 mcg of beclomethasone dipropionate from the actuator and 50 mcg from the valve. QVAR 80 mcg delivers 80 mcg of beclomethasone dipropionate from the actuator and 100 mcg from the valve. This product delivers 50 microliters (59 milligrams) of solution formulation from the valve with each actuation. Each canister provides 100 inhalations. QVAR should be "primed" or actuated twice prior to taking the first dose from a new canister, or when the inhaler has not been used for more than ten days. Avoid spraying in the eyes or face while priming QVAR.

This product does not contain chlorofluorocarbons (CFCs).

CLINICAL PHARMACOLOGY

Airway inflammation is known to be an important component in the pathogenesis of asthma. Inflammation occurs in both large and small airways. Corticosteroids have multiple anti-inflammatory effects, inhibiting both inflammatory cells and release of inflammatory mediators. It is presumed that these anti-inflammatory actions play an important role in the efficacy of beclomethasone dipropionate in controlling symptoms and improving lung function in asthma. Inhaled beclomethasone dipropionate probably acts topically at the site of deposition in the bronchial tree after inhalation.

Pharmacokinetics

Bioavailability information on beclomethasone dipropionate (BDP) after inhaled administration is not available in adults. BDP undergoes rapid and extensive conversion to beclomethasone-17-monopropionate (17-BMP) during absorption. The pharmacokinetics of 17-BMP has been studied in asthmatics given single doses.

Absorption: The mean peak plasma concentration (C_{max}) of BDP was 88 pg/ml at 0.5 hour after inhalation of 320 mcg using QVAR (four actuations of the 80 mcg/actuation strength). The mean peak plasma concentration of the major and most active metabolite, 17-BMP, was 1419 pg/ml at 0.7 hour after inhalation of 320 mcg of QVAR. When the same nominal dose is provided by the two QVAR strengths (40 and 80 mcg/actuation), equivalent systemic pharmacokinetics can be expected. The C_{max} of 17-BMP increased dose proportionally in the dose range of 80 and 320 mcg.

Metabolism: Three major metabolites are formed via cytochrome P450 3A catalyzed biotransformation - beclomethasone-17-monopropionate (17-BMP), beclomethasone-21-monopropionate (21-BMP) and beclomethasone (BOH). Lung slices metabolize BDP rapidly to 17-BMP and more slowly to BOH. 17-BMP is the most active metabolite.

Distribution: There is no evidence of tissue storage of BDP or its metabolites.

Elimination: The major route of elimination of inhaled BDP appears to be via metabolism. More than 90% of inhaled BDP is found as 17-BMP in the systemic circulation. The mean elimination half-life of 17-BMP is 2.8 hours. Irrespective of the route of administration (injection, oral or inhalation), BDP and its metabolites are mainly excreted in the feces. Less than 10% of the drug and its metabolites are excreted in the urine.

Special Populations: Formal pharmacokinetic studies using QVAR were not conducted in any special populations.

Pediatrics: The pharmacokinetics of 17-BMP, including dose and strength proportionalities, is similar in children and adults, although the exposure is highly variable. In 17 children (mean age 10 years), the Cmax of 17-BMP was 787 pg/ml at 0.6 hour after inhalation of 160 mcg (four actuations of the 40 mcg/actuation strength of HFA beclomethasone dipropionate). The systemic exposure to 17-BMP from 160 mcg of HFA-BDP administered without a spacer was comparable to the systemic exposure to 17-BMP from 336 mcg CFC-BDP administered with a large volume spacer in 14 children (mean age 12 years).

This implies that approximately twice the systemic exposure to 17-BMP would be expected for comparable mg doses of HFA-BDP without a spacer and CFC-BDP with a large volume spacer.

Pharmacodynamics

Improvement in asthma control following inhalation can occur within 24 hours of beginning treatment in some patients, although maximum benefit may not be achieved for 1 to 2 weeks, or longer. The effects of QVAR on the hypothalamic-pituitary-adrenal (HPA) axis were studied in 40 corticosteroid naive patients. QVAR, at doses of 80, 160 or 320 mcg twice daily was compared with placebo and 336 mcg twice daily of beclomethasone dipropionate in a CFC propellant based formulation (CFC-BDP). Active treatment groups showed an expected dose-related reduction in 24-hour urinary free cortisol (a sensitive marker of adrenal production of cortisol). Patients treated with the highest recommended dose of QVAR (320 mcg twice daily) had a 37.3% reduction in 24-hour urinary free cortisol compared to a reduction of 47.3% produced by treatment with 336 mcg twice daily of CFC-BDP. There was a 12.2% reduction in 24 hour urinary free cortisol seen in the group of patients that received 80 mcg twice daily of QVAR and a 24.6% reduction in the group of patients that received 160 mcg twice daily. An open label study of 354 asthma patients given QVAR at recommended doses for one year assessed the effect of QVAR treatment on the HPA axis (as measured by both morning and stimulated plasma cortisol). Less than 1% of patients treated for one year with QVAR had an abnormal response (peak less than 18 mcg/dL) to short-cosyntropin test.

CLINICAL TRIALS

Blinded, randomized, parallel, placebo-controlled and active-controlled clinical studies were conducted in 940 adult asthma patients to assess the efficacy and safety of QVAR in the treatment of asthma. Fixed doses ranging from 40 mcg to 160 mcg twice daily were compared to placebo, and doses ranging from 40 mcg to 320 mcg twice daily were compared with doses of 42 mcg to 336 mcg twice daily of an active CFC-BDP comparator. These studies provided information about appropriate dosing through a range of asthma severity. In all adult efficacy trials, at the doses studied, measures of pulmonary function [forced expiratory volume in 1 second (FEV_1) and morning peak expiratory flow (AM PEF)] and asthma symptoms were significantly improved with QVAR treatment when compared to placebo. A blinded, randomized, parallel, placebo-controlled study was conducted in 353 pediatric patients (age 5-12 years) to assess the efficacy and safety of HFA beclomethasone dipropionate in the treatment of asthma. Fixed doses of 40 mcg and 80 mcg twice daily were compared with placebo in this study.

In controlled clinical trials with adult patients not adequately controlled with beta-agonist alone, QVAR was effective at improving asthma control at doses as low as 40 mcg twice daily (80 mcg/day). Comparable asthma control was achieved at lower daily doses of QVAR than with CFC-BDP. Treatment with increasing doses of both QVAR and CFC-BDP generally resulted in increased improvement in FEV_1. In this trial the improvement in FEV_1 across doses was greater for QVAR than for CFC-BDP, indicating a shift in the dose response curve for QVAR. For this reason, when considering QVAR dosing selection for patients currently using CFC-BDP, it is important to consult the dosing recommendations specifically for QVAR (see DOSAGE AND ADMINISTRATION).

Patients Not Previously Receiving Corticosteroid Therapy

In a 6 week clinical trial, 270 steroid naive patients with symptomatic asthma being treated with as-needed beta-agonist bronchodilators, were randomized to receive either 40 mcg twice daily of QVAR, 80 mcg twice daily of QVAR, or placebo. Both doses of QVAR were effective in improving asthma control with significantly greater improvements in FEV_1, AM PEF, and asthma symptoms than with placebo. Shown below is the change from baseline in AM PEF during this trial.

A 6-Week Clinical Trial in Patients with Mild to Moderate Asthma Not on Corticosteroid Therapy Prior to Study Entry: Mean Change in AM PEF

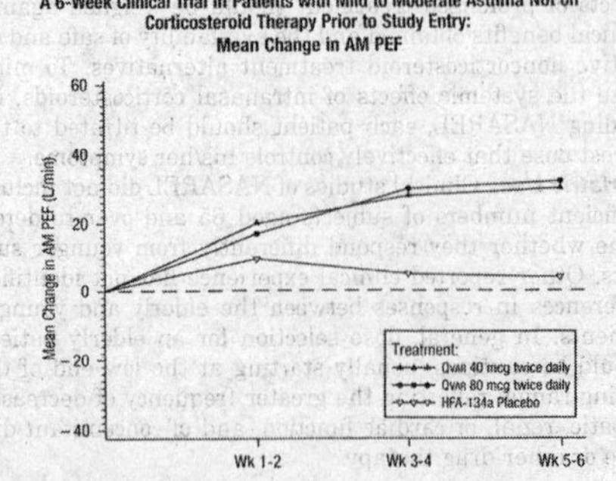

In a 6-week clinical trial, 256 patients with symptomatic asthma being treated with as-needed beta-agonist bronchodilators, were randomized to receive either 160 mcg twice daily of QVAR (delivered as either 40 mcg/actuation or 80 mcg/actuation) or placebo. Treatment with QVAR significantly improved asthma control, as assessed by FEV_1 AM PEF, and asthma symptoms, when compared to treatment with placebo. Comparable improvement in AM PEF was seen for patients receiving 160 mcg twice daily QVAR from the 40 mcg and 80 mcg strength products.

Patients Responsive to a Short Course of Oral Corticosteroids

In another clinical trial, 347 patients with symptomatic asthma, being treated with as-needed inhaled beta-agonist bronchodilators and, in some cases, inhaled corticosteroids, were given a 7-12 day course of oral corticosteroids and then randomized to receive either 320 mcg daily of QVAR, 672 mcg of CFC-BDP, or placebo. Patients treated with either QVAR or CFC-BDP had significantly better asthma control, as assessed by AM PEF, FEV_1 and asthma symptoms, and fewer study withdrawals due to asthma symptoms, than those treated with placebo over 12 weeks of treatment. A daily dose of 320 mcg QVAR administered in divided doses provided comparable control of AM PEF and FEV_1 as 672 mcg of CFC-BDP. Shown below are the mean AM PEF results from this trial.

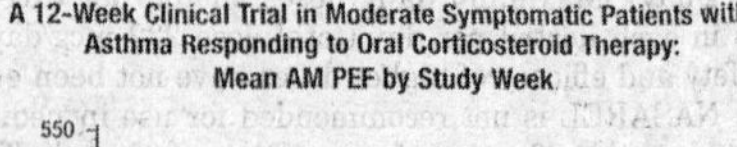
A 12-Week Clinical Trial in Moderate Symptomatic Patients with Asthma Responding to Oral Corticosteroid Therapy: Mean AM PEF by Study Week

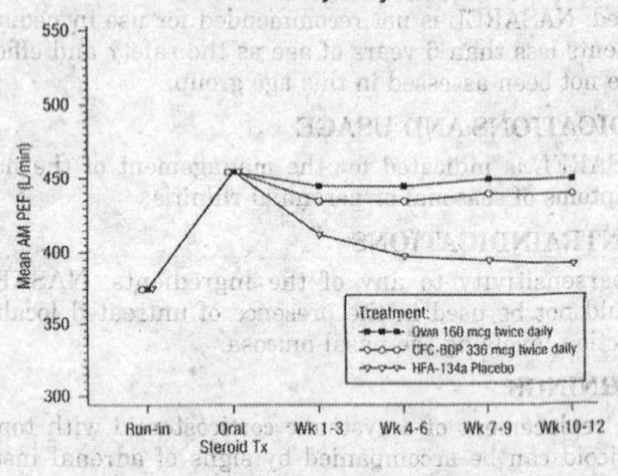

Patients Previously on Inhaled Corticosteroids

In a 6-week clinical trial, 323 patients, who exhibited a deterioration in asthma control during an inhaled corticosteroid washout period, were randomized to daily treatment with either 40, 160, or 320 mcg twice daily QVAR or 42, 168, or 336 mcg twice daily CFC-BDP. Treatment with increasing doses of both QVAR and CFC-BDP resulted in increased improvement in FEV_1, $FEF_{<None>}$ (forced expiratory flow over 25-75% of the vital capacity), and asthma symptoms. Shown below is the change from baseline in FEV_1 as percent predicted after 6 weeks of treatment.

A 6-Week Dose Response Clinical Trial in Patients with Inhaled Corticosteroid Dependent Asthma: Mean Change in FEV_1 as Percent of Predicted

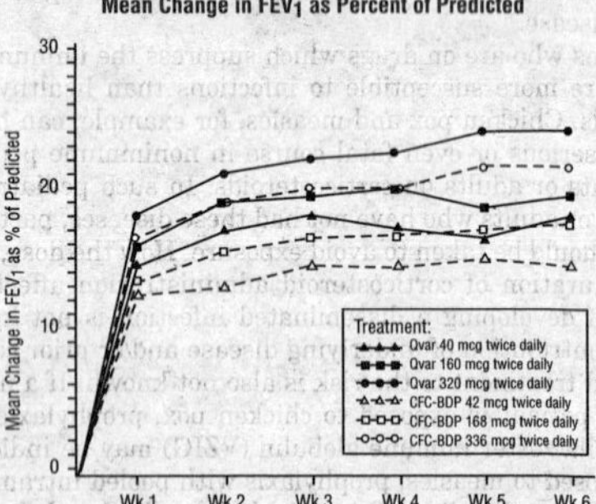

Patients Previously Maintained on Oral Corticosteroids

Clinical experience has shown that some patients with asthma who require oral corticosteroid therapy for control of symptoms can be partially or completely withdrawn from oral corticosteroids if therapy with beclomethasone dipropionate aerosol is substituted. Inhaled corticosteroids may not be effective for all patients with asthma or at all stages of the disease in a given patient.

Pediatric Experience: In one 12-week clinical trial, pediatric patients (age 5-12 years) with symptomatic asthma (N=353) being treated with as-needed beta-agonist bronchodilators were randomized to receive either 40 mcg or 80 mcg twice daily of HFA beclomethasone dipropionate or placebo. Both doses were effective in improving asthma control with significantly greater improvements in FEV_1 (9% and 10% predicted change from baseline at week 12 in FEV_1 percent predicted, respectively) than with placebo (4% predicted change).

INDICATIONS AND USAGE

QVAR is indicated in the maintenance treatment of asthma as prophylactic therapy in patients 5 years of age and older. QVAR is also indicated for asthma patients who require systemic corticosteroid administration, where adding QVAR may reduce or eliminate the need for the systemic corticosteroids.

Beclomethasone dipropionate is NOT indicated for the relief of acute bronchospasm.

Adverse Events Reported by at Least 3% of the Patients for Either QVAR or CFC-BDP by Treatment and Daily Dose

Adverse Events		QVAR				CFC-BDP			
	80–160 Placebo (N=289) %	320 Total (N=624) %	640 mcg (N=233) %	mcg (N=335) %	84 mcg (N=56) %	336 Total (N=283) %	672 mcg (N=59) %	mcg (N=55) %	mcg (N=169) %
HEADACHE	9	12	15	8	25	15	14	11	17
PHARYNGITIS	4	8	6	5	27	10	12	9	10
UPPER RESP TRACT INFECTION	11	9	7	11	5	12	3	9	17
RHINITIS	9	6	8	3	7	11	15	9	10
INCREASED ASTHMA SYMPTOMS	18	3	2	4	0	8	14	5	7
ORAL SYMPTOMS INHALATION ROUTE	2	3	3	3	2	6	7	5	5
SINUSITIS	2	3	3	3	0	4	7	2	4
PAIN	<1	2	1	2	5	3	3	5	2
BACK PAIN	1	1	2	<1	4	4	2	4	4
NAUSEA	0	1	<1	1	2	3	5	5	1
DYSPHONIA	2	<1	1	0	4	4	0	0	6

CONTRAINDICATIONS

QVAR is contraindicated in the primary treatment of status asthmaticus or other acute episodes of asthma where intensive measures are required.

Hypersensitivity to any of the ingredients of this preparation contraindicates its use.

WARNINGS

Particular care is needed in patients who are transferred from systemically active corticosteroids to QVAR because deaths due to adrenal insufficiency have occurred in asthmatic patients during and after transfer from systemic corticosteroids to less systemically available inhaled corticosteroids. After withdrawal from systemic corticosteroids, a number of months are required for recovery of hypothalamic-pituitary-adrenal (HPA) function.

Patients who have been previously maintained on 20 mg or more per day of prednisone (or its equivalent) may be most susceptible, particularly when their systemic corticosteroids have been almost completely withdrawn. During this period of HPA suppression, patients may exhibit signs and symptoms of adrenal insufficiency when exposed to trauma, surgery, or infections (particularly gastroenteritis) or other conditions with severe electrolyte loss. Although QVAR may provide control of asthmatic symptoms during these episodes, in recommended doses it supplies less than normal physiological amounts of glucocorticoid systemically and does NOT provide the mineralocorticoid that is necessary for coping with these emergencies.

During periods of stress or a severe asthmatic attack, patients who have been withdrawn from systemic corticosteroids should be instructed to resume oral corticosteroids (in large doses) immediately and to contact their physician for further instruction. These patients should also be instructed to carry a warning card indicating that they may need supplementary systemic steroids during periods of stress or a severe asthma attack.

Transfer of patients from systemic steroid therapy to QVAR may unmask allergic conditions previously suppressed by the systemic steroid therapy, e.g., rhinitis, conjunctivitis, and eczema.

Persons who are on drugs which suppress the immune system are more susceptible to infections than healthy individuals. Chickenpox and measles, for example, can have a more serious or even fatal course in non-immune children or adults on corticosteroids. In such children or adults who have not had these diseases or been properly immunized, particular care should be taken to avoid exposure. It is not known how the dose, route and duration of corticosteroid administration affects the risk of developing a disseminated infection. Nor is the contribution of the underlying disease and/or prior corticosteroid treatment known. If exposed to chickenpox, prophylaxis with varicella-zoster immune globulin (VZIG) may be indicated. If exposed to measles, prophylaxis with pooled intramuscular immunoglobulin (IG) may be indicated. (See the respective package inserts for complete VZIG and IG prescribing information.) If chickenpox develops, treatment with antiviral agents may be considered. QVAR is not a bronchodilator and is not indicated for rapid relief of bronchospasm.

As with other inhaled asthma medications, bronchospasm, with an immediate increase in wheezing, may occur after dosing. If bronchospasm occurs following dosing with QVAR, it should be treated immediately with a short acting inhaled bronchodilator. Treatment with QVAR should be discontinued and alternate therapy instituted. Patients should be instructed to contact their physician immediately when episodes of asthma, which are not responsive to bronchodilators, occur during the course of treatment with QVAR. During such episodes, patients may require therapy with oral corticosteroids.

PRECAUTIONS

General: During withdrawal from oral corticosteroids, some patients may experience symptoms of systemically active corticosteroid withdrawal, e.g., joint and/or muscular pain, lassitude and depression, despite maintenance or even improvement of respiratory function. Although suppression of HPA function below the clinical normal range did not occur with doses of QVAR up to and including 640 mcg/day, a dose dependent reduction of adrenal cortisol production was observed. Since inhaled beclomethasone dipropionate is absorbed into the circulation and can be systemically active, HPA axis suppression by QVAR could occur when recommended doses are exceeded or in particularly sensitive individuals. Since individual sensitivity to effects on cortisol production exist, physicians should consider this information when prescribing QVAR.

Because of the possibility of systemic absorption of inhaled corticosteroids, patients treated with these drugs should be observed carefully for any evidence of systemic corticosteroid effect. Particular care should be taken in observing patients postoperatively or during periods of stress for evidence of inadequate adrenal response.

It is possible that systemic corticosteroid effects, such as hypercorticism and adrenal suppression, may appear in a small number of patients, particularly at higher doses. If such changes occur, QVAR should be reduced slowly, consistent with accepted procedures for management of asthma symptoms and for tapering of systemic steroids.

A 12 month randomized controlled clinical trial evaluated the effects of HFA beclomethasone dipropionate without spacer versus CFC beclomethasone dipropionate with large volume spacer on growth in children age 5-11. A total of 520 patients were enrolled, of whom 394 received HFA-BDP (100 - 400 mcg/day ex-valve) and 126 received CFC-BDP (200 - 800 mcg/day ex-valve). Similar control of asthma was noted in each treatment arm. When comparing results at month 12 to baseline, the mean growth velocity in children treated with HFA-BDP was approximately 0.5 cm/year less than that noted with children treated with CFC-BDP via large volume spacer.

A reduction in growth velocity in growing children may occur as a result of inadequate control of chronic diseases such as asthma or from use of corticosteroids for treatment. Physicians should closely follow the growth of all pediatric patients taking corticosteroids by any route and weigh the benefits of corticosteroid therapy and asthma control against the possibility of growth suppression.

The long-term and systemic effects of QVAR in humans are still not fully known. In particular, the effects resulting from chronic use of the agent on developmental or immunologic processes in the mouth, pharynx, trachea, and lung are unknown.

Inhaled corticosteroids should be used with caution, if at all, in patients with active or quiescent tuberculosis infection of the respiratory tract; untreated systemic fungal, bacterial, parasitic or viral infections; or ocular herpes simplex.

Rare instances of glaucoma, increased intraocular pressure, and cataracts have been reported following the inhaled administration of corticosteroids.

Information for Patients: Patients being treated with QVAR should receive the following information and instructions. This information is intended to aid them in the safe and effective use of this medication. It is not a disclosure of all possible adverse or intended effects.

Persons who are on immunosuppressant doses of corticosteroids should be warned to avoid exposure to chickenpox or measles. Patients should also be advised that if they are exposed to these diseases, medical advice should be sought without delay. Patients should use QVAR at regular intervals as directed. Results of clinical trials indicated significant improvements may occur within the first 24 hours of treatment in some patients; however, the full benefit may not be achieved until treatment has been administered for 1 to 2 weeks, or longer. The patient should not increase the prescribed dosage but should contact their physician if symptoms do not improve or if the condition worsens.

Patients should be advised that QVAR is not intended for use in the treatment of acute asthma. The patient should be instructed to contact their physician immediately if there is any deterioration of their asthma.

Patients should be instructed on the proper use of their inhaler. Patients may wish to rinse their mouth after QVAR use. The patient should also be advised that QVAR may have a different taste and inhalation sensation than that of an inhaler containing CFC propellant.

QVAR use should not be stopped abruptly. The patient should contact their physician immediately if use of QVAR is discontinued.

For the proper use of QVAR, the patient should read and carefully follow the accompanying Patient's Instructions.

Carcinogenesis, Mutagenesis, Impairment of Fertility: The carcinogenicity of beclomethasone dipropionate was evaluated in rats which were exposed for a total of 95 weeks, 13 weeks at inhalation doses up to 0.4 mg/kg/day and the remaining 82 weeks at combined oral and inhalation doses up to 2.4 mg/kg/day. There was no evidence of carcinogenicity in this study at the highest dose, which is approximately 30 and 55 times the maximum recommended daily inhalation dose in adults and children, respectively, on a mg/m^2 basis.

Beclomethasone dipropionate did not induce gene mutation in the bacterial cells or mammalian Chinese Hamster ovary (CHO) cells *in vitro*. No significant clastogenic effect was seen in cultured CHO cells *in vitro* or in the mouse micronucleus test *in vivo*.

In rats, beclomethasone dipropionate caused decreased conception rates at an oral dose of 16 mg/kg/day (approximately 200 times the maximum recommended daily inhalation dose in adults on a mg/m^2 basis). Impairment of fertility, as evidenced by inhibition of the estrous cycle in dogs, was observed following treatment by the oral route at a dose of 0.5 mg/kg/day (approximately 20 times the maximum recommended daily inhalation dose in adults on a mg/m^2 basis). No inhibition of the estrous cycle in dogs was seen following 12 months of exposure to beclomethasone dipropionate by the inhalation route at an estimated daily dose of 0.33 mg/kg (approximately 15 times the maximum recommended daily inhalation dose in adults on a mg/m^2 basis).

Pregnancy: Teratogenic Effects: Pregnancy Category C: Like other corticosteroids, parenteral (subcutaneous) beclomethasone dipropionate was teratogenic and embryocidal in the mouse and rabbit when given at a dose of 0.1 mg/kg/day in mice or at a dose of 0.025 mg/kg/day in rabbits. These doses in mice and rabbits were approximately one-half the maximum recommended daily inhalation dose in adults on a mg/m^2 basis. No teratogenicity or embryocidal effects were seen in rats when exposed to an inhalation dose of 15 mg/kg/day (approximately 190 times the maximum recommended daily inhalation dose in adults on a mg/m^2 basis). There are no adequate and well controlled studies in pregnant women. Beclomethasone dipropionate should be used during pregnancy only if the potential benefit justifies the potential risk to the fetus.

Non-teratogenic Effects: Findings of drug-related adrenal toxicity in fetuses following administration of beclomethasone dipropionate to rats suggest that infants born of mothers receiving substantial doses of QVAR during pregnancy should be observed for adrenal suppression.

Nursing Mothers: Corticosteroids are secreted in human milk. Because of the potential for serious adverse reactions in nursing infants from QVAR, a decision should be made whether to discontinue nursing or to discontinue the drug, taking into account the importance of the drug to the mother.

Pediatric Use: Eight-hundred and thirty-four children between the ages of 5 and 12 were treated with HFA beclomethasone dipropionate (HPA BDP) in clinical trials. The safety and effectiveness of QVAR in children below 5 years of age have not been established. Oral corticosteroids have been shown to cause a reduction in growth velocity in children and teenagers with extended use. If a child or teenager on any corticosteroid appears to have growth suppression, the possibility that they are particularly sensitive to this effect of corticosteroids should be considered (see PRECAUTIONS, General).

Geriatric Use: Clinical studies of QVAR did not include sufficient numbers of subjects aged 65 and over to determine whether they respond differently from younger subjects. Other reported clinical experience has not identified differences in response between the elderly and younger patients. In general, dose selection for an elderly patient should be cautious, usually starting at the low end of the dosing range, reflecting the greater frequency of decreased hepatic, renal, or cardiac function, and of concomitant disease or other drug therapy.

ADVERSE REACTIONS

The following reporting rates of common adverse experiences are based upon four clinical trials in which 1196 Patients (671 female and 525 male adults previously treated with as-needed bronchodilators and/or inhaled corticosteroids) were treated with QVAR (doses of 40, 80, 160, or 320 mcg twice daily) or CFC-BDP (doses of 42, 168, or 336 mcg twice daily) or placebo. The table below includes all events reported by patients taking QVAR (whether considered drug related or not) that occurred at a rate over 3% for either QVAR or CFC-BDP. In considering these data, difference in average duration of exposure and clinical trial design should be taken into account.

[See table above]

Other adverse events that occurred in these clinical trials using QVAR with an incidence of 1% to 3% and which occurred at a greater incidence than placebo were: dysphonia, dysmenorrhea and coughing.

No patients treated with QVAR in the clinical development program developed symptomatic oropharyngeal candidiasis. If such an infection develops, treatment with appropriate antifungal therapy or discontinuance of treatment with QVAR may be required.

Continued on next page

Recommended Dosage for QVAR:

Previous Therapy	Recommended Starting Dose	Highest Recommended Dose
Adults and Adolescents:		
Bronchodilators Alone	40 to 80 mcg twice daily	320 mcg twice daily
Inhaled Corticosteroids	40 to 160 mcg twice daily	320 mcg twice daily
Children 5 to 11 years:		
Bronchodilators Alone	40 mcg twice daily	80 mcg twice daily
Inhaled Corticosteroids	40 mcg twice daily	80 mcg twice daily

Qvar—Cont.

Pediatric Studies: In two 12-week placebo controlled studies in steroid naïve pediatric patients 5 to 12 years of age, no clinically relevant differences were found in the pattern, severity, or frequency of adverse events compared with those reported in adults, with the exception of conditions which are more prevalent in a pediatric population generally.

Adverse Event Reports from Other Sources: Rare cases of immediate and delayed hypersensitivity reactions, including urticaria, angioedema, rash, and bronchospasm, have been reported following the oral and intranasal inhalation of beclomethasone dipropionate.

OVERDOSAGE

There were no deaths over 15 days following the oral administration of a single dose of 3000 mg/kg in mice, 2000 mg/kg in rats, and 1000 mg/kg in rabbits. The doses in mice, rats, and rabbits were 19,000, 25,000, and 25,000 times, respectively, the maximum recommended daily inhalation in adults or 36,000, 48,000, and 48,000 times, respectively the maximum recommended daily inhalation dose in children on a mg/m^2 basis.

DOSAGE AND ADMINISTRATION

Patients should prime QVAR by actuating into the air twice before using for the first time or if QVAR has not been used for over ten days. Avoid spraying in the eyes or face when priming QVAR. QVAR is a solution aerosol, which does not require shaking. Consistent dose delivery is achieved, whether using the 40 or 80 mcg strengths, due to proportionality of the two products (i.e., two actuations of 40 mcg strength should provide a dose comparable to one actuation of the 80 mcg strength.)

QVAR should be administered by the oral inhaled route in patients 5 years of age and older. The onset and degree of symptom relief will vary in individual patients. Improvement in asthma symptoms should be expected within the first or second week of starting treatment, but maximum benefit should not be expected until 3-4 weeks of therapy. For patients who do not respond adequately to the starting dose after 3-4 weeks of therapy, higher doses may provide additional asthma control. The safety and efficacy of QVAR when administered in excess of recommended doses has not been established.

[See table above]

The recommended dosage of QVAR relative to CFC-based beclomethasone dipropionate (CFC-BDP) inhalation aerosols is lower due to differences in delivery characteristics between the products. Recognizing that a definitive comparative therapeutic ratio between QVAR and CFC-BDP has not been demonstrated, any patient who is switched from CFC-BDP to QVAR should be dosed appropriately, taking into account the dosing recommendations above, and should be monitored to ensure that the dose of QVAR selected is safe and efficacious. As with any inhaled corticosteroid, physicians are advised to titrate the dose of QVAR downward over time to the lowest level that maintains proper asthma control. This is particularly important in children since a controlled study has shown that QVAR has the potential to affect growth in children.

Patients should be instructed on the proper use of their inhaler. Patients should be advised that QVAR may have a different taste and inhalation sensation than that of an inhaler containing CFC propellant.

Patients Not Receiving Systemic Corticosteroids

Patients who require maintenance therapy of their asthma may benefit from treatment with QVAR at the doses recommended above. In patients who respond to QVAR, improvement in pulmonary function is usually apparent within 1 to 4 weeks after the start of therapy. Once the desired effect is achieved, consideration should be given to tapering to the lowest effective dose.

Patients Maintained on Systemic Corticosteroids

QVAR may be effective in the management of asthmatics maintained on systemic corticosteroids and may permit replacement or significant reduction in the dosage of systemic corticosteroids.

The patient's asthma should be reasonably stable before treatment with QVAR is started. Initially, QVAR should be used concurrently with the patient's usual maintenance dose of systemic corticosteroids. After approximately one week, gradual withdrawal of the systemic corticosteroids is started by reducing the daily or alternate daily dose. Reductions may be made after an interval of one or two weeks, depending on the response of the patient. A slow rate of withdrawal is strongly recommended. Generally these decrements should not exceed 2.5 mg of prednisone or its equivalent. During withdrawal, some patients may experience symptoms of systemic corticosteroid withdrawal, e.g. joint and/or muscular pain, lassitude and depression, despite maintenance or even improvement in pulmonary function. Such patients should be encouraged to continue with the inhaler but should be monitored for objective signs of adrenal insufficiency. If evidence of adrenal insufficiency occurs, the systemic corticosteroid doses should be increased temporarily and thereafter withdrawal should continue more slowly. During periods of stress or a severe asthma attack, transfer patients may require supplementary treatment with systemic corticosteroids.

DIRECTIONS FOR USE

Illustrated Patient's Instructions for proper use accompany each package of QVAR.

HOW SUPPLIED

QVAR is supplied in two strengths:

QVAR 40 mcg is supplied in a 7.3 g canister containing 100 actuations with a beige plastic actuator and gray dust cap, and Patient's Instructions; box of one;
100 Actuations – NDC 59310-175-40

QVAR 80 mcg is supplied in a 7.3 g canister containing 100 actuations with a dark mauve plastic actuator and gray dust cap, and Patient's Instructions; box of one;
100 Actuations – NDC 59310-177-80

The correct amount of medication in each inhalation cannot be assured after 100 actuations from the 7.3 g canister even though the canister is not completely empty. The canister should be discarded when the labeled number of actuations have been used.

Store QVAR Inhalation Aerosol when not being used, so that the product rests on the concave end of the canister with the plastic actuator on top.

Store at 25°C (77°F).

Excursions between 15° and 30°C (59° and 86°F) are permitted (see USP). For optimal results, the canister should be at room temperature when used. QVAR Inhalation Aerosol canister should only be used with the QVAR Inhalation Aerosol actuator and the actuator should not be used with any other inhalation drug product.

CONTENTS UNDER PRESSURE

Do not puncture. Do not use store near heat or open flame. Exposure to temperatures above 49°C (120°F) may cause bursting. Never throw container into fire or incinerator.

Keep out of reach of children.

Rx only

Distributed by:
IVAX Laboratories, Inc.
Miami, FL 33137
Developed and Manufactured by:
3M Pharmaceuticals
Northridge, CA 91324
OR
3M Health Care, Ltd.
Loughborough, UK
AUGUST 2003

QVAR® is a registered trademark of 3M through its subsidiary, Riker Labs., Inc. and is used under license.

628102
Rev. 08/03

Jacobus Pharmaceutical Co., Inc.

37 CLEVELAND LANE
P.O. BOX 5290
PRINCETON, NJ 08540

Direct Inquiries to:
Professional Services
(609) 921-7447
FAX: (609) 799-1176

For Medical Information Contact:
In Emergencies:
Medical Department
(609) 921-7447
FAX: (609) 799-1176

DAPSONE TABLETS USP ℞

[dap 'sōne]
25 mg. & 100 mg.

PRODUCT OVERVIEW

KEY FACTS

Dapsone is a sulfone for the primary treatment of Dermatitis herpetiformis and an antibacterial drug for susceptible cases of leprosy.

MAJOR USES

Dapsone is used to control the dermatologic symptoms of Dermatitis herpetiformis. Dapsone is used alone or in combination with other anti-leprosy drugs for leprosy.

SAFETY INFORMATION

Dapsone is contraindicated in patients with Dapsone hypersensitivity. Complete blood counts and laboratory monitoring should be done frequently. See labeling.

PRODUCT INFORMATION

DAPSONE TABLETS USP ℞

[dap 'sōne]
25 mg. & 100 mg.

DESCRIPTION

Dapsone-USP, 4,4′-diaminodiphenylsulfone (DDS) is a primary treatment for Dermatitis herpetiformis. It is an antibacterial drug for susceptible cases of leprosy. It is a white, odorless crystalline powder, practically insoluble in water and insoluble in fixed and vegetable oils.

Dapsone is issued on prescription in tablets of 25 and 100 mg. for oral use.

NH_2–C_6H_4–SO_2–C_6H_4–NH_2

Inactive Ingredients: Colloidal silicone dioxide, magnesium stearate, microcrystalline cellulose, and corn starch.

CLINICAL PHARMACOLOGY

Actions: The mechanism of action in Dermatitis herpetiformis has not been established. By the kinetic method in mice, Dapsone is bactericidal as well as bacteriostatic against *Mycobacterium leprae.*

Absorption and Excretion: Dapsone, when given orally, is rapidly and almost completely absorbed. About 85 percent of the daily intake is recoverable from the urine mainly in the form of water-soluble metabolites. Excretion of the drug is slow and a constant blood level can be maintained with the usual dosage.

Blood Levels: Detected a few minutes after ingestion, the drug reaches peak concentration in 4–8 hours. Daily administration for at least eight days is necessary to achieve a plateau level. With doses of 200 mg. daily, this level averaged 2.3 μg/ml with a range of 0.1–7.0 μg/ml. The half-life in the plasma in different individuals varies from ten hours to fifty hours and averages twenty-eight hours. Repeat tests in the same individual are constant. Daily administration (50–100 mg.) in leprosy patients will provide blood levels in excess of the usual minimum inhibitory concentration even for patients with a short Dapsone half-life.

INDICATIONS AND USAGE

Dermatitis herpetiformis: (D.H.)

Leprosy: All forms of leprosy except for cases of proven Dapsone resistance.

CONTRAINDICATION

Hypersensitivity to Dapsone and/or its derivatives.

WARNINGS

The patient should be warned to respond to the presence of clinical signs such as sore throat, fever, pallor, purpura or jaundice. Deaths associated with the administration of Dapsone have been reported from agranulocytosis, aplastic anemia and other blood dyscrasias. Complete blood counts should be done frequently in patients receiving Dapsone. The FDA Dermatology Advisory Committee recommended that, when feasible counts should be done weekly for the first month, monthly for six months and semi-annually thereafter. If a significant reduction in leucocytes, platelets or hemopoiesis is noted, Dapsone should be discontinued and the patient followed intensively. Folic acid antagonists have similar effects and may increase the incidence of hematologic reactions; if co-administered with Dapsone the patient should be monitored more frequently. Patients on weekly Pyrimethamine and Dapsone have developed agranulocytosis during the second and third month of therapy.

Severe anemia should be treated prior to initiation of therapy and hemoglobin monitored. Hemolysis and methemoglobin may be poorly tolerated by patients with severe cardio-pulmonary disease.

Cutaneous reactions, especially bullous, include exfoliative dermatitis and are probably one of the most serious, though rare, complications of sulfone therapy. They are directly due to drug sensitization. Such reactions include toxic erythema, erythema multiforme, toxic epidermal necrolysis, morbilliform and scarlatiniform reactions, urticaria and erythema nodosum. If new or toxic dermatologic reactions occur, sulfone therapy must be promptly discontinued and appropriate therapy instituted.

Leprosy reactional states, including cutaneous, are not hypersensitivity reactions to Dapsone and do not require discontinuation. See special section.

PRECAUTIONS

General: Hemolysis and Heinz body formation may be exaggerated in individuals with a glucose-6-phosphate dehydrogenase (G6PD) deficiency, or methemoglobin reductase deficiency, or hemoglobin M. This reaction is frequently dose-related. Dapsone should be given with caution to these patients or if the patient is exposed to other agents or conditions such as infection or diabetic ketosis capable of producing hemolysis. Drugs or chemicals which have produced significant hemolysis in G6PD or methemoglobin reductase deficient patients include Dapsone, sulfanilamide, nitrite, aniline, phenylhydrazine, napthalene, niridazole, nitrofurantoin and 8-amino-antimalarials such as primaquine.

Toxic hepatitis and cholestatic jaundice have been reported early in therapy. Hyperbilirubinemia may occur more often in G6PD deficient patients. When feasible, baseline and subsequent monitoring of liver function is recommended. If abnormal, Dapsone should be discontinued until the source of the abnormality is established.

Drug Interactions: Rifampin lowers Dapsone levels 7 to 10-fold by accelerating plasma clearance; in leprosy this reduction has not required a change in dosage.

Folic acid antagonists such as pyrimethamine may increase the likelihood of hematologic reactions.

A modest interaction has been reported for patients receiving 100 mg Dapsone od in combination with trimethoprim 5 mg/kg q6h. On Day 7, the serum Dapsone levels averaged 2.1 ± 1.0 μg/mL in comparison to 1.5 ± 0.5 μg/mL for Dapsone alone. On Day 7, trimethoprim levels averaged 18.4 ± 5.2 μg/mL in comparison to 12.4 ± 4.5 μg/mL for patients not receiving Dapsone. Thus, there is a mutual interaction between Dapsone and trimethoprim in which each raises the level of the other about 1.5 times.

Carcinogenesis, mutagenesis: Dapsone has been found carcinogenic (sarcomagenic) for male rats and female mice causing mesenchymal tumors in the spleen and peritoneum, and thyroid carcinoma in female rats. Dapsone is not mutagenic with or without microsomal activation in *S. typhimurium* tester strains 1535, 1537, 1538, 98, or 100.

Pregnancy Category C: Animal reproduction studies have not been conducted with Dapsone. Extensive, but uncontrolled experience and two published surveys on the use of Dapsone in pregnant women have not shown that Dapsone increases the risk of fetal abnormalities if administered during all trimesters of pregnancy or can affect reproduction capacity. Because of the lack of animal studies or controlled human experience, Dapsone should be given to a pregnant woman only if clearly needed. In general, for leprosy, USPHS at Carville recommends maintenance of Dapsone. Dapsone has been important for the management of some pregnant D.H. patients.

Nursing Mothers: Dapsone is excreted in breast milk in substantial amounts. Hemolytic reactions can occur in neonates. See section on hemolysis. Because of the potential for tumorgenicity shown for Dapsone in animal studies a decision should be made whether to discontinue nursing or discontinue the drug taking into account the importance of the drug to the mother.

Pediatric Use: Children are treated on the same schedule as adults but with correspondingly smaller doses. Dapsone is generally not considered to have an effect on the later growth, development and functional development of the child.

ADVERSE REACTIONS

In addition to the warnings listed above, the following syndromes and serious reactions have been reported in patients on Dapsone.

Hematologic Effects: Dose-related hemolysis is the most common adverse effect and is seen in patients with or without G6PD deficiency. Almost all patients demonstrate the interrelated changes of a loss of 1–2g of HB, an increase in the reticulocytes (2–12%), a shortened red cell life span and a rise in methemoglobin. G6PD deficient patients have greater responses.

Nervous System Effects: Peripheral neuropathy is a definite but unusual complication of Dapsone therapy in non-leprosy patients. Motor loss is predominent. If muscle weakness appears, Dapsone should be withdrawn. Recovery on withdrawal is usually substantially complete. The mechanism of recovery is reportedly by axonal regeneration. Some recovered patients have tolerated retreatment at reduced dosage. In leprosy this complication may be difficult to distinguish from a leprosy reactional state.

Body As A Whole: In addition to the warnings and adverse effects reported above, additional adverse reactions include: nausea, vomiting, abdominal pains, pancreatitis, vertigo, blurred vision, tinnitus, insomnia, fever, headache, psychosis, phototoxicity, pulmonary eosinophilia, tachycardia, albuminuria, the nephrotic syndrome, hypoalbuminemia without proteinuria, renal papillary necrosis, male infertility, drug-induced Lupus erythematosus and an infectious mononucleosis-like syndrome. In general, with the exception of the complications of severe anoxia from overdosage (retinal and optic nerve damage, etc.) these adverse reactions have regressed off drug.

OVERDOSAGE

Nausea, vomiting, hyperexcitability can appear a few minutes up to 24 hours after ingestion of an overdose. Methemoglobin induced depression, convulsions and severe cyanosis requires prompt treatment. In normal and methemoglobin reductase deficient patients, methylene blue, 1–2 mg/kg of body weight, given slowly intravenously is the treatment of choice. The effect is complete in 30 minutes, but may have to be repeated if methemoglobin reaccumulates. For non-emergencies, if treatment is needed, methylene blue may be given orally in doses of 3–5 mg/kg every 4–6 hours.

Methylene blue reduction depends on G6PD and should not be given to fully expressed G6PD deficient patients.

DOSAGE AND ADMINISTRATION

Dermatitis herpetiformis: The dosage should be individually titrated starting in adults with 50 mg. daily and correspondingly smaller doses in children. If full control is not achieved within the range of 50–300 mg. daily, higher doses may be tried. Dosage should be reduced to a minimum maintenance level as soon as possible. In responsive patients there is a prompt reduction in pruritus followed by clearance of skin lesions. There is no effect on the gastrointestinal component of the disease.

Dapsone levels are influenced by acetylation rates. Patients with high acetylation rates, or who are receiving treatment affecting acetylation may require an adjustment in dosage. A strict gluten free diet is an option for the patient to elect, permitting many to reduce or eliminate the need for Dapsone; the average time for dosage reduction is 8 months with a range of 4 months to $2^1/_2$ years and for dosage elimination 29 months with a range of 6 months to 9 years.

Leprosy: In order to reduce secondary Dapsone resistance, the WHO Expert Committee on Leprosy and the USPHS at Carville, LA, recommend that Dapsone should be commenced in combination with one or more anti-leprosy drugs. In the multi-drug program Dapsone should be maintained at the full dosage of 100 mg. daily without interruption (with correspondingly smaller doses for children) and provided to all patients who have sensitive organisms with new or recrudescent disease or who have not yet completed a two year course of Dapsone monotherapy. For advice and other drugs, the USPHS at Carville, LA, (1 800-642-2477) should be contacted. Before using other drugs consult appropriate product labeling.

In bacteriologically negative tuberculoid and indeterminate disease, the recommendation is the coadministration of Dapsone 100 mg. daily with six months of Rifampin 600 mg. daily. Under WHO, daily Rifampin may be replaced by 600 mg. Rifampin monthly, if supervised. The Dapsone is continued until all signs of clinical activity are controlled—usually after an additional six months. Then Dapsone should be continued for an additional three years for tuberculoid and indeterminate patients and for five years for borderline tuberculoid patients.

In lepromatous and borderline lepromatous patients, the recommendation is the coadministration of Dapsone 100 mg. daily with two years of Rifampin 600 mg. daily. Under WHO, daily Rifampin may be replaced by 600 mg. Rifampin monthly, if supervised. One may elect the concurrent administration of a third anti-leprosy drug, usually either Clofazamine 50–100mg. daily or Ethionamide 250–500 mg. daily. Dapsone 100 mg. daily is continued 3–10 years until all signs of clinical activity are controlled with skin scrapings and biopsies negative for one year. Dapsone should then be continued for an additional 10 years for borderline patients and for life for lepromatous patients.

Secondary Dapsone resistance should be suspected whenever a lepromatous or borderline lepromatous patient receiving Dapsone treatment relapses clinically and bacteriologically, solid staining bacilli being found in the smears taken from the new active lesions. If such cases show no response to regular and supervised Dapsone therapy within three to six months or good compliance for the past 3–6 months can be assured, Dapsone resistance should be considered confirmed clinically. Determination of drug sensitivity using the mouse footpad method is recommended and, after prior arrangement, is available without charge from the USPHS, Carville, LA. Patients with proven Dapsone resistance should be treated with other drugs.

LEPROSY REACTIONAL STATES

Abrupt changes in clinical activity occur in leprosy with any effective treatment and are known as reactional states. The majority can be classified into two groups.

The "Reversal" reaction (Type 1) may occur in borderline or tuberculoid leprosy patients often soon after chemotherapy is started. The mechanism is presumed to result from a reduction in the antigenic load: the patient is able to mount an enhanced delayed hypersensitivity response to residual infection leading to swelling ("Reversal") of existing skin and nerve lesions. If severe, or if neuritis is present, large doses of steroids should always be used. If severe, the patient should be hospitalized. In general anti-leprosy treatment is continued and therapy to suppress the reaction is indicated such as analgesics, steroids, or surgical decompression of swollen nerve trunks. USPHS at Carville, LA should be contacted for advice in management.

Erythema nodosum leprosum (ENL) (lepromatous reaction) (Type 2 reaction) occurs mainly in lepromatous patients and small numbers of borderline patients. Approximately 50% of treated patients show this reaction in the first year. The principal clinical features are fever and tender erythematous skin nodules sometimes associated with malaise, neuritis, orchitis, albuminuria, joint swelling, iritis, epistaxis or depression. Skin lesions can become pustular and/or ulcerate. Histologically there is a vasculitis with an intense polymorphonuclear infiltrate. Elevated circulating immune complexes are considered to be the mechanism of reaction. If severe, patients should be hospitalized. In general, anti-leprosy treatment is continued. Analgesics, steroids, and other agents available from USPHS, Carville, LA, are used to suppress the reaction.

HOW SUPPLIED

Rx: Dapsone 25 mg, round white scored tablet, debossed "25" above and "102" below the score and on the obverse "Jacobus" in light and child-resistant bottles, of 100, NDC 49938-102-01.

Dapsone 100 mg, round white scored tablet, debossed "100" above and "101" below the score and on the obverse "Jacobus" in light and child-resistant bottles of 100, NDC 49938-101-01.

Store at controlled room temperature, 20°–25°C (68°–77°F). Protect from light.

CAUTION: Federal law prohibits dispensing without prescription.

Dispense this product in a well-closed child-resistant container.

JACOBUS PHARMACEUTICAL CO., INC.
P.O. Box 5290
Princeton, NJ 08540

9J JUNE, 1997

PASER® GRANULES ℞
(aminosalicylic acid granules)

DESCRIPTION

PASER granules are a delayed release granule preparation of aminosalicylic acid (p-aminosalicylic acid: 4–aminosalicylic acid) for use with other anti-tuberculosis drugs for the treatment of all forms of active tuberculosis due to susceptible strains of tubercle bacilli. The granules are designed for gradual release to avoid high peak levels not useful (and perhaps toxic) with bacteriostatic drugs. Aminosalicylic acid is rapidly degraded in acid media; the protective acid-resistant outer coating is rapidly dissolved in neutral media so a mildly acidic food such as orange, apple or tomato juice, yogurt or apple sauce should be used.

Aminosalicylic acid (p-aminosalicylic acid) is 4–Amino-2-hydroxybenzoic acid. PASER granules are the free base of aminosalicylic acid and do NOT contain sodium or a sugar. The molecular formula is $C_7H_7NO_3$ with a molecular weight of 153.14. With heat p-aminosalicylic acid is decarboxylated to produce CO_2 and m-aminophenol. If the airtight packets are swollen, storage has been improper. DO NOT USE if packets are swollen or the granules have lost their tan color and are dark brown or purple.

The structural formula is:

PASER granules are supplied as off-white tan colored granules with an average diameter of 1.5 mm and an average content of 60% aminosalicylic acid by weight. The acid resistant outer coating will be completely removed by a few minutes at a neutral pH. The inert ingredients are:

colloidal silicon dioxide
dibutyl sebacate
hydroxypropyl methyl cellulose
methacrylic acid copolymer
microcystalline cellulose
talc

The packets contain 4 grams of aminosalicylic acid for oral administration three times a day by sprinkling an apple sauce or yogurt to be eaten without chewing. Suspension in an acidic fruit drink such as orange juice or tomato juice will protect the coating for at least 2 hours. Swirling the juice in the glass will help resuspend the granules if they sink.

CLINICAL PHARMACOLOGY

Mechanism of Action: Aminosalicylic acid is bacteriostatic against Mycobacterium tuberculosis. It inhibits the onset of bacterial resistance to streptomycin and isoniazid. The mechanism of action has been postulated to be inhibition of folic acid synthesis (but without potentiation with antifolic compounds) and/or inhibition of synthesis of the cell wall component, mycobactin, thus reducing iron uptake by M. tuberculosis.

Characteristics: The two major considerations in the clinical pharmacology of aminosalicylic acid are the prompt production of a toxic inactive metabolite under acid conditions and the short serum half life of one hour for the free drug. Both are discussed below.

After two hours in simulated gastric fluid, 10% of unprotected aminosalicylic acid is decarboxylated to form meta-aminophenol, a known hepatotoxin. The acid-resistant coating of the PASER granules protects against degradation in the stomach. The small granules are designed to escape the usual restriction on gastric emptying of large particles. Under neutral conditions such as are found in the small intestine or in neutral foods, the acid-resistant coating is dissolved within one minute. Care must be taken in the administration of these granules to protect the acid-resistant coating by maintaining the granules in an acidic food during dosage administration. Patients who have neutralized gastric acid with antacids will not need to protect the acid resistant coating with an acidic food since no acid is present to spoil the drug. Antacids may influence the absorption of other medications and are not necessary for PASER consumed with an acidic food.

Because PASER granules are protected by an enteric coating absorption does not commence until they leave the stomach; the soft skeletons of the granules remain and may be seen in the stool.

Absorption and excretion: In a single 4 gram pharmacokinetic study with food in normal volunteers the initial time to a 2 μg/mL serum level of aminosalicylic acid was 2 hours with a range of 45 minutes to 24 hours; the median time to

Continued on next page

Paser—Cont.

peak was 6 hours with a range of 1.5 to 24 hours; the mean peak level was 20 µg/mL with a range of 9 to 35 µg/mL; a level of 2 µg/mL was maintained for an average of 7.9 hours with a range of 5 to 9; a level of 1 µg/mL was maintained for an average of 8.8 hours with a range of 6 to 11.5 hours. The recommended schedule is 4 grams every 8 hours.

80% of aminosalicylic acid is excreted in the urine, with 50% or more of the dosage excreted in acetylated form. The acetylation process is not genetically determined as is the case for isoniazid. Aminosalicylic acid is excreted by glomerular filtration; although previously reported otherwise, probenecid, a tubular blocking agent, does not enhance plasma concentration. In a 1954 study thyroxine synthesis but not iodide uptake was reported reduced about 40% when the sodium salt (not PASER granules) of aminosalicylic acid was administered one hour before radio-iodine; the sodium salt typically produces a serum level over 120 µg/mL at one hour lasting one hour. Occasional goiter development can be prevented by the administration of thyroxine but not iodide. Penetration into the cerebrospinal fluid occurs only if the meninges are inflamed.

Approximately 50–60% of aminosalicylic acid is protein bound; binding is reported to be reduced 50% in kwashiorkor.

Microbiology: The aminosalicylic acid MIC for M. tuberculosis in 7H11 agar was less than 1.0 µg/mL for nine strains including three multidrug resistant strains, but 4 and 8 µg/mL for two other multidrug resistant strains. The 90% inhibition in 7H12 broth (Bactec) showed little dose response but was interpreted as being less than or equal to 0.12–0.25 µg/mL for eight strains of which three were multiresistant, 0.50 µg/mL for one resistant strain, questionable for four nonresistant strains and greater than 1 µg/mL for one non-resistant and three resistant strains. Aminosalicylic acid is not active in vitro against M. avium.

INDICATIONS AND USAGE

PASER is indicated for the treatment of tuberculosis in combination with other active agents. It is most commonly used in patients with Multi-drug Resistant TB (MDR-TB) or in situations when therapy with isoniazid and rifampin is not possible due to a combination of resistance and/or intolerance. When PASER is added to the treatment regimen in patients with proven or suspected drug resistance, it should be accompanied by at least one and preferably two other new agents to which the patient's organism is known or expected to be susceptible.

CONTRAINDICATIONS

Hypersensitivity to any component of this medication.

Severe renal disease.

Patients with severe renal disease will accumulate aminosalicylic acid and its acetyl metabolite but will continue to acetylate, thus leading exclusively to the inactive acetylated form; deacetylation, if any, is not significant.

The half life of free aminosalicylic acid in renal disease is 30.8 minutes in comparison to 26.4 minutes in normal volunteers, but the half life of the inactive metabolite is 309 minutes in uremic patients in comparison to 51 minutes in normal volunteers. Although aminosalicylic acid passes dialysis membranes, the frequency of dialysis usually is not comparable to the half-life of 50 minutes for the free acid. Patients with end stage renal disease should not receive aminosalicylic acid.

WARNINGS

Liver Function

In one retrospective study of 7492 patients on rapidly absorbed aminosalicylic acid preparations, drug-induced hepatitis occurred in 38 patients (0.5%); in these 38 the first symptom usually appeared within three months of the start of therapy with a rash as the most common event followed by fever and much less frequently by GI disturbances of anorexia, nausea or diarrhea. Only one patient was diagnosed on routine biochemistry.

Premonitory symptoms in 90% of these 38 patients preceded jaundice by a few days to several weeks with the mean time of onset 33 days with a range of 7–90 days. Half of the adverse reactions occurred during the third, fourth or fifth weeks. When aminosalicylic acid-induced hepatitis was diagnosed, hepatomegaly was invariably present with lymphadenopathy in 46%, leucocytosis in 79%, and eosinophilia in 55%. Prompt recognition with discontinuation led to the recovery of all 38 patients. If recognized in the premonitory stage, the reaction is reported to "settle" in 24 hours and no jaundice ensues. From other reported studies failure to recognize the reaction can result in a mortality of up to 21%. The patient must be monitored carefully during the first three months of therapy and treatment must be discontinued immediately at the first sign of a rash, fever or other premonitory signs of intolerance.

PRECAUTIONS

(1) General:

All drugs should be stopped at the first sign suggesting a hypersensitivity reaction. They may be restarted one at a time in very small but gradually increasing doses to determine whether the manifestations are drug-induced and, if so, which drug is responsible.

Desensitization has been accomplished successfully in 15 of 17 patients starting with 10 mg aminosalicylic acid given as a single dose. The dosage is doubled every 2 days until reaching a total of 1 gram after which the dosage is divided to follow the regular schedule of administration. If a mild temperature rise or skin reaction develops, the increment is to be dropped back one level or the progression held for one cycle. Reactions are rare after a total dosage of 1.5 grams. Patients with hepatic disease may not tolerate aminosalicylic acid as well as normal patients, even though the metabolism in patients with hepatic disease has been reported to be comparable to that in normal volunteers.

(2) Information for Patients:

The patient should be advised that the first signs of hypersensitivity include a rash, often followed by fever, and much less frequently, GI disturbances of anorexia, nausea or diarrhea. If such symptoms develop, the patient should immediately cease taking the medication and arrange for a prompt clinical visit.

Patients should be advised that poor compliance in taking anti-TB medication often leads to treatment failure, and, not infrequently, to the development of resistance of the organisms in the individual patient.

Patients should be advised that the skeleton of the granules may be seen in the stool.

The coating to protect the PASER granules dissolves promptly under neutral conditions; the granules therefore should be administered by sprinkling on acidic foods such as apple sauce or yogurt or by suspension in a fruit drink which will protect the coating, but the granules sink and will have to be swirled. The coating will last at least 2 hours in either system. All juices tested to date have been satisfactory; tested are: tomato, orange, grapefruit, grape, cranberry, apple, "fruit punch".

Patients should be advised to store PASER in a refrigerator or freezer. PASER packets may be stored at room temperature for short periods of time.

Patients should be advised NOT to use if the packets are swollen or the granules have lost their tan color and are dark brown or purple. The patient should inform the pharmacist or physician immediately and return the medication.

(3) Laboratory Tests:

Aminosalicylic acid has been reported to interfere technically with the serum determinations of albumin by dye-binding. SGOT by the azoene dye method and with qualitative urine tests for ketones, bilirubin, urobilinogen or porphobilinogen.

(4) Drug Interactions:

Aminosalicytic acid at a dosage of 12 grams in a rapidly available form has been reported to produce a 20 percent reduction in the acetylation of isoniazid, especially in patients who are rapid acetylators; INH serum levels, half lives and excretions in fast acetylators still remain half of the levels seen in slow acetylators with or without p-aminosalicylic acid. The effect is dose related and, while it has not been studied with the current delayed release preparation, the lower serum levels with this preparation will result in a reduced effect on the acetylation of INH.

Aminosalicylic acid has previously been reported to block the absorption of rifampin. A subsequent report has shown that this blockade was due to an excipient not included in PASER granules. Oral administration of a solution containing both aminosalicylic acid and rifampin showed full absorption of each product.

As a result of competition, Vitamin B_{12} absorption has been reduced 55% by 5 grams of aminosalicylic acid with clinically significant erythrocyte abnormalities developing after depletion; patients on therapy of more than one month should be considered for maintenance B_{12}.

A malabsorption syndrome can develop in patients on aminosalicylic acid but is usually not complete. The complete syndrome includes steatorrhea, an abnormal small bowel pattern on x-ray, villus atrophy, depressed cholesterol, reduced D-xylose and iron absorption. Triglyceride absorption always is normal.

In one literature report 8 hours after the last dosage of aminosalicylic acid at 2 gm qid serum digoxin levels were reduced 40% in two of ten patients but not changed in the remaining eight.

(5) Carcinogenesis, mutagenesis, impairment of fertility:

Sodium aminosalicylate produced an occipital bone defect, probably with a dose response, when administered to ten pregnant Wistar rats at five doses from 3.85 to 385 mg/kg from days 6 to 14. There were no significant changes from controls in any group in corpora lutea, early resorptions, total resorptions, fetal death, litter size, or hematomas. For all except the 77 mg/kg group, fetal weights were significantly greater than controls. Chinchilla rabbits on 5 mg/kg from days 7 to 14 did not show any significant differences as compared to controls for the same parameters studied.

Sodium aminosalicylic acid was not mutagenic in Ames tester strain TA 100. In human lymphocyte cultures in-vitro clastogenic effects of achromatic, chromatid, isochromatic breaks or chromatid translocations were not seen at 153 or 600 µg/mL. At 1500 and 3000 µg/mL there was a dose related increase in chromatid aberrations.

Patients on isoniazid and aminosalicylic acid have been reported to have an increased number of chromosomal aberrations as compared to controls.

(6) Pregnancy: Pregnancy Category C:

Aminosalicylic acid has been reported to produce occipital malformations in rats when given at doses within the human dose range. Although there probably is a dose response, the frequency of abnormalities was comparable to controls at the highest level tested (two times the human dosage). When administered to rabbits at 5 mg/kg, throughout all three trimesters, no teratologic embryocidal effects were seen. Literature reports on aminosalicylic acid in pregnant women always report coadministration of other medications. Because there are no adequate and well controlled studies of aminosalicylic acid in humans, PASER granules should be given to a pregnant woman only if clearly needed.

(8) Nursing mothers:

After administration of a different preparation of aminosalicylic acid to one patient, the maximum concentration in the milk was 1 µg/mL at 3 hours with a half-life of 2.5 hours; the maximum maternal plasma concentration was 70 µg/mL at two hours.

ADVERSE EFFECTS

The most common side effect is gastrointestinal intolerance manifested by nausea, vomiting, diarrhea, and abdominal pain.

Hypersensitivity reactions: Fever, skin eruptions of various types, including exfoliative dermatitis, infectious mononucleosis-like, or lymphoma-like syndrome, leucopenia, agranulocytosis, thrombocytopenia, Coombs' positive hemolytic anemia, jaundice, hepatitis, pericarditis, hypoglycemia, optic neuritis, encephalopathy, Leoffler's syndrome, and vasculitis and a reduction in prothrombin.

Crystalluria may be prevented by the maintenance of urine at a neutral or an alkaline pH.

OVERDOSAGE

Overdosage has not been reported.

DOSAGE AND ADMINISTRATION

PASER granules should be administered with other drugs to which the organism is known or expected to be susceptible. It is most commonly administered to patients with Multi-drug Resistant TB (MDR-TB) or in other situations in which therapy with isoniazid or rifampin is not possible due to a combination of resistance and/or tolerance. The adult dosage of four grams (one packet) three times per day or correspondingly smaller doses in children should be given by sprinking on apple sauce or yogurt or by swirling in the glass to suspend the granules in an acidic drink such as tomato or orange juice.

DO NOT USE if the packet is swollen or the granules have lost their tan color, turning dark brown or purple.

HOW SUPPLIED

Carton of 30 PASER packets (NDC 49938-107-04).

Each packet contains four grams aminosalicylic acid.

PASER granules are supplied in packets containing 4 grams of aminosalicylic acid for administration three times a day by suspension in an acidic drink or food with a pH less than 5. Examples include apple sauce, yogurt, tomato or orange juice.

Distributors and Pharmacists: Store below 59°F (15°C) (in a refrigerator or freezer).

Patients are urged to store PASER in a refrigerator or freezer. PASER packets may be stored at room temperature for short periods of time.

AVOID EXCESSIVE HEAT. DO NOT USE if packet is swollen or the granules have lost their tan color, turning dark brown or purple.

Caution: Federal, law prohibits dispensing without prescription.

JACOBUS PHARMACEUTICAL CO. INC.
P.O. Box 5290
Princeton, NJ 08540

2A JULY, 1996

Janssen Pharmaceutica Products, L.P.

1125 TRENTON-HARBOURTON ROAD
P.O. BOX 200
TITUSVILLE, NJ 08560-0200

For Medical Information Monday through Friday
9 am-5 pm EST Contact:
(800) JANSSEN
FAX: (609) 730-3138
After Hours and Weekends:
(800) JANSSEN

ACIPHEX® ℞

[ˈa-sə-ˌfeks]
(rabeprazole sodium)
Delayed-Release Tablets

DESCRIPTION

The active ingredient in ACIPHEX® Delayed-Release Tablets is rabeprazole sodium, a substituted benzimidazole that inhibits gastric acid secretion. Rabeprazole sodium is known chemically as 2-[[[4-(3-methoxypropoxy)-3-methyl-2-pyridinyl]-methyl]sulfinyl]-1*H*-benzimidazole sodium salt. It has an empirical formula of $C_{18}H_{20}N_3NaO_3S$ and a molecular weight of 381.43. Rabeprazole sodium is a white to slightly yellowish-white solid. It is very soluble in water and methanol, freely soluble in ethanol, chloroform and ethyl acetate and insoluble in ether and n-hexane. The stability of rabeprazole sodium is a function of pH; it is rapidly degraded in acid media, and is more stable under alkaline conditions. The structural formula is:

RABEPRAZOLE SODIUM

ACIPHEX® is available for oral administration as delayed-release, enteric-coated tablets containing 20 mg of rabeprazole sodium. Inactive ingredients are carnauba wax, crospovidone, diacetylated monoglycerides, ethylcellulose, hydroxypropyl cellulose, hypromellose phthalate, magnesium stearate, mannitol, sodium hydroxide, sodium stearyl fumarate, talc, titanium dioxide, and yellow ferric oxide as a coloring agent.

CLINICAL PHARMACOLOGY

Pharmacokinetics and Metabolism

ACIPHEX® delayed-release tablets are enteric-coated to allow rabeprazole sodium, which is acid labile, to pass through the stomach relatively intact. After oral administration of 20 mg ACIPHEX®, peak plasma concentrations (C_{max}) of rabeprazole occur over a range of 2.0 to 5.0 hours (T_{max}). The rabeprazole C_{max} and AUC are linear over an oral dose range of 10 mg to 40 mg. There is no appreciable accumulation when doses of 10 mg to 40 mg are administered every 24 hours; the pharmacokinetics of rabeprazole are not altered by multiple dosing. The plasma half-life ranges from 1 to 2 hours.

Absorption: Absolute bioavailability for a 20 mg oral tablet of rabeprazole (compared to intravenous administration) is approximately 52%. When rabeprazole is administered with a high fat meal, its T_{max} is variable and may delay its absorption up to 4 hours or longer, however, the C_{max} and the extent of rabeprazole absorption (AUC) are not significantly altered. Thus rabeprazole may be taken without regard to timing of meals.

Distribution: Rabeprazole is 96.3% bound to human plasma proteins.

Metabolism: Rabeprazole is extensively metabolized. The thioether and sulphone are the primary metabolites measured in human plasma. These metabolites were not observed to have significant antisecretory activity. *In vitro* studies have demonstrated that rabeprazole is metabolized in the liver primarily by cytochromes P450 3A (CYP3A) to a sulphone metabolite and cytochrome P450 2C19 (CYP2C19) to desmethyl rabeprazole. The thioether metabolite is formed non-enzymatically by reduction of rabeprazole. CYP2C19 exhibits a known genetic polymorphism due to its deficiency in some sub-populations (e.g. 3 to 5% of Caucasians and 17 to 20% of Asians). Rabeprazole metabolism is slow in these sub-populations, therefore, they are referred to as poor metabolizers of the drug.

Elimination: Following a single 20 mg oral dose of ^{14}C-labeled rabeprazole, approximately 90% of the drug was eliminated in the urine, primarily as thioether carboxylic acid; its glucuronide, and mercapturic acid metabolites. The remainder of the dose was recovered in the feces. Total recovery of radioactivity was 99.8%. No unchanged rabeprazole was recovered in the urine or feces.

Special Populations

Geriatric: In 20 healthy elderly subjects administered 20 mg rabeprazole once daily for seven days, AUC values approximately doubled and the C_{max} increased by 60% compared to values in a parallel younger control group. There was no evidence of drug accumulation after once daily administration. (see PRECAUTIONS).

Pediatric: The pharmacokinetics of rabeprazole in pediatric patients under the age of 18 years have not been studied.

Gender and Race: In analyses adjusted for body mass and height, rabeprazole pharmacokinetics showed no clinically significant differences between male and female subjects. In studies that used different formulations of rabeprazole, $AUC_{0-\infty}$ values for healthy Japanese men were approximately 50–60% greater than values derived from pooled data from healthy men in the United States.

Renal Disease: In 10 patients with stable end-stage renal disease requiring maintenance hemodialysis (creatinine clearance ≤5 mL/min/1.73 m^2), no clinically significant differences were observed in the pharmacokinetics of rabeprazole after a single 20 mg oral dose when compared to 10 healthy volunteers.

Hepatic Disease: In a single dose study of 10 patients with chronic mild to moderate compensated cirrhosis of the liver who were administered a 20 mg dose of rabeprazole, AUC_{0-24} was approximately doubled, the elimination half-life was 2- to 3-fold higher, and total body clearance was decreased to less than half compared to values in healthy men.

In a multiple dose study of 12 patients with mild to moderate hepatic impairment administered 20 mg rabeprazole once daily for eight days, $AUC_{0-\infty}$ and C_{max} values increased approximately 20% compared to values in healthy age- and gender-matched subjects. These increases were not statistically significant.

No information exists on rabeprazole disposition in patients with severe hepatic impairment. Please refer to the DOSAGE AND ADMINISTRATION section for information on dosage adjustment in patients with hepatic impairment.

Combined Administration with Antimicrobials: Sixteen healthy volunteers genotyped as extensive metabolizers with respect to CYP2C19 were given 20 mg rabeprazole sodium, 1000 mg amoxicillin, 500 mg clarithromycin, or all 3 drugs in a four-way crossover study. Each of the four regimens was administered twice daily for 6 days. The AUC and C_{max} for clarithromycin and amoxicillin were not different following combined administration compared to values following single administration. However, the rabeprazole AUC and C_{max} increased by 11% and 34%, respectively, following combined administration. The AUC and C_{max} for 14-hydroxyclarithromycin (active metabolite of clarithromycin) also increased by 42% and 46%, respectively. This increase in exposure to rabeprazole and 14-hydroxyclarithromycin is not expected to produce safety concerns.

PHARMACODYNAMICS

Mechanism of Action

Rabeprazole belongs to a class of antisecretory compounds (substituted benzimidazole proton-pump inhibitors) that do not exhibit anticholinergic or histamine H_2-receptor antagonist properties, but suppress gastric acid secretion by inhibiting the gastric H^+, K^+ATPase at the secretory surface of the gastric parietal cell. Because this enzyme is regarded as the acid (proton) pump within the parietal cell, rabeprazole has been characterized as a gastric proton-pump inhibitor. Rabeprazole blocks the final step of gastric acid secretion.

In gastric parietal cells, rabeprazole is protonated, accumulates, and is transformed to an active sulfenamide. When studied *in vitro*, rabeprazole is chemically activated at pH 1.2 with a half-life of 78 seconds. It inhibits acid transport in porcine gastric vesicles with a half-life of 90 seconds.

Antisecretory Activity

The anti-secretory effect begins within one hour after oral administration of 20 mg ACIPHEX®. The median inhibitory effect of ACIPHEX® on 24 hour gastric acidity is 88% of maximal after the first dose. ACIPHEX® 20 mg inhibits basal and peptone meal-stimulated acid secretion versus placebo by 86% and 95%, respectively, and increases the percent of a 24-hour period that the gastric pH>3 from 10% to 65% (see table below). This relatively prolonged pharmacodynamic action compared to the short pharmacokinetic half-life (1–2 hours) reflects the sustained inactivation of the H^+, K^+ATPase.

Gastric Acid Parameters ACIPHEX® Versus Placebo After 7 Days of Once Daily Dosing

Parameter	ACIPHEX® (20 mg QD)	Placebo
Basal Acid Output (mmol/hr)	0.4*	2.8
Stimulated Acid Output (mmol/hr)	0.6*	13.3
% Time Gastric pH>3	65*	10

* (p<0.01 versus placebo)

Compared to placebo, ACIPHEX®, 10 mg, 20 mg, and 40 mg, administered once daily for 7 days significantly decreased intragastric acidity with all doses for each of four meal-related intervals and the 24-hour time period overall. In this study, there were no statistically significant differences between doses; however, there was a significant dose-related decrease in intragastric acidity. The ability of rabeprazole to cause a dose-related decrease in mean intragastric acidity is illustrated below.

[See first table above]

AUC Acidity (mmol•hr/L) ACIPHEX® Versus Placebo on Day 7 of Once Daily Dosing (mean ± SD)

	Treatment			
AUC Interval (hrs)	10 mg RBP (N=24)	20 mg RBP (N=24)	40 mg RBP (N=24)	Placebo (N=24)
08:00 – 13:00	19.6±21.5*	12.9±23*	7.6±14.7*	91.1±39.7
13:00 – 19:00	5.6±9.7*	8.3±29.8*	1.3±5.2*	95.5±48.7
19:00 – 22:00	0.1±0.1*	0.1±0.06*	0.0±0.02*	11.9±12.5
22:00 – 08:00	129.2±84*	109.6±67.2*	76.9±58.4*	479.9±165
AUC 0–24 hours	155.5±90.6*	130.9±81*	85.8±64.3*	678.5±216

*(p<0.001 versus placebo)

After administration of 20 mg ACIPHEX® once daily for eight days, the mean percent of time that gastric pH>3 or gastric pH>4 after a single dose (Day 1) and multiple doses (Day 8) was significantly greater than placebo (see table below). The decrease in gastric acidity and the increase in gastric pH observed with 20 mg ACIPHEX® administered once daily for eight days were compared to the same parameters for placebo, as illustrated below:

[See second table above]

Gastric Acid Parameters ACIPHEX® Once Daily Dosing Versus Placebo on Day 1 and Day 8

	ACIPHEX® 20 mg QD		Placebo	
Parameter	Day 1	Day 8	Day 1	Day 8
Mean AUC_{0-24} Acidity	340.8*	176.9*	925.5	862.4
Median trough pH (23-hr)[a]	3.77	3.51	1.27	1.38
% Time Gastric pH>3[b]	54.6*	68.7*	19.1	21.7
% Time Gastric pH>4[b]	44.1*	60.3*	7.6	11.0

[a] No inferential statistics conducted for this parameter.
* (p<0.001 versus placebo)
[b] Gastric pH was measured every hour over a 24-hour period.

Effects on Esophageal Acid Exposure

In patients with gastroesophageal reflux disease (GERD) and moderate to severe esophageal acid exposure, ACIPHEX® 20 mg and 40 mg per day decreased 24-hour esophageal acid exposure. After seven days of treatment, the percentage of time that esophageal pH<4 decreased from baselines of 24.7% for 20 mg and 23.7% for 40 mg, to 5.1% and 2.0%, respectively. Normalization of 24-hour intraesophageal acid exposure was correlated to gastric pH>4 for at least 35% of the 24-hour period; this level was achieved in 90% of subjects receiving ACIPHEX® 20 mg and in 100% of subjects receiving ACIPHEX® 40 mg. With ACIPHEX® 20 mg and 40 mg per day, significant effects on gastric and esophageal pH were noted after one day of treatment, and more pronounced after seven days of treatment.

Effects on Serum Gastrin

In patients given daily doses of ACIPHEX® for up to eight weeks to treat ulcerative or erosive esophagitis and in patients treated for up to 52 weeks to prevent recurrence of disease the median fasting gastrin level increased in a dose-related manner. The group median values stayed within the normal range.

In a group of subjects treated daily with ACIPHEX® 20 mg for 4 weeks a doubling of mean serum gastrin concentrations were observed. Approximately 35% of these treated subjects developed serum gastrin concentrations above the upper limit of normal. In a study of CYP2C19 genotyped subjects in Japan, poor metabolizers developed statistically significantly higher serum gastrin concentrations than extensive metabolizers.

Effects on Enterochromaffin-like (ECL) Cells

Increased serum gastrin secondary to antisecretory agents stimulates proliferation of gastric ECL cells which, over time, may result in ECL cell hyperplasia in rats and mice and gastric carcinoids in rats, especially in females (see Carcinogenesis, Mutagenesis, Impairment of Fertility).

In over 400 patients treated with ACIPHEX® (10 or 20 mg/day) for up to one year, the incidence of ECL cell hyperplasia increased with time and dose, which is consistent with the pharmacological action of the proton-pump inhibitor. No patient developed the adenomatoid, dysplastic or neoplastic changes of ECL cells in the gastric mucosa. No patient developed the carcinoid tumors observed in rats.

Endocrine Effects

Studies in humans for up to one year have not revealed clinically significant effects on the endocrine system. In healthy male volunteers treated with ACIPHEX® for 13 days, no clinically relevant changes have been detected in the following endocrine parameters examined: 17 β-estradiol, thyroid stimulating hormone, tri-iodothyronine, thyroxine, thyroxine-binding protein, parathyroid hormone, insulin,

Continued on next page

Aciphex—Cont.

glucagon, renin, aldosterone, follicle-stimulating hormone, luteotrophic hormone, prolactin, somatotrophic hormone, dehydroepiandrosterone, cortisol-binding globulin, and urinary 6β-hydroxycortisol, serum testosterone and circadian cortisol profile.

Other Effects

In humans treated with ACIPHEX® for up to one year, no systemic effects have been observed on the central nervous, lymphoid, hematopoietic, renal, hepatic, cardiovascular, or respiratory systems. No data are available on long-term treatment with ACIPHEX® and ocular effects.

Microbiology

Rabeprazole sodium, amoxicillin and clarithromycin as a three drug regimen has been shown to be active against most strains of *Helicobacter pylori* in vitro and in clinical infections as described in the **CLINICAL STUDIES** and **INDICATIONS AND USAGE** sections.

Helicobacter pylori

Susceptibility testing of *H. pylori* isolates was performed for amoxicillin and clarithromycin using agar dilution methodology[1], and minimum inhibitory concentrations (MICs) were determined. The clarithromycin and amoxicillin MIC values should be interpreted according to the following criteria:

Clarithromycin MIC (µg/mL)[a]	Interpretation
≤ 0.25	Susceptible (S)
0.5	Intermediate (I)
≥ 1.0	Resistant (R)

Amoxicillin MIC (µg/mL)[a,b]	Interpretation
≤ 0.25	Susceptible (S)

[a] These are breakpoints for the agar dilution methodology and they should not be used to interpret results using alternative methods.

[b] There were not enough organisms with MICs > 0.25 µg/mL to determine a resistance breakpoint.

Standardized susceptibility test procedures require the use of laboratory control microorganisms to control the technical aspects of the laboratory procedures. Standard clarithromycin and amoxicillin powders should provide the following MIC values:

Microorganism	Antimicrobial Agent	MIC (µg/mL)[a]
H. pylori ATCC 43504	Clarithromycin	0.015–0.12 µg/mL
H. pylori ATCC 43504	Amoxicillin	0.015–0.12 µg/mL

[a] These are quality control ranges for the agar dilution methodology and they should not be used to control test results obtained using alternative methods.

Incidence of Antibiotic-Resistant Organisms Among Clinical Isolates

Pretreatment Resistance: Clarithromycin pretreatment resistance rate (MIC ≥ 1 µg/mL) to *H. pylori* was 9% (51/560) at baseline in all treatment groups combined. A total of > 99% (558/560) of patients had *H. pylori* isolates which were considered to be susceptible (MIC ≤ 0.25 µg/mL) to amoxicillin at baseline. Two patients had baseline *H. pylori* isolates with an amoxicillin MIC of 0.5 µg/mL.

Clarithromycin Susceptibility Test Results and Clinical/Bacteriologic Outcomes: For the U.S. multi-center study, the baseline *H. pylori* clarithromycin susceptibility results and the *H. pylori* eradication results post-treatment are shown in the table below:

[See first table above]

Patients with persistent *H. pylori* infection following rabeprazole, amoxicillin, and clarithromycin therapy will likely have clarithromycin resistant clinical isolates. Therefore, clarithromycin susceptibility testing should be done when possible. If resistance to clarithromycin is demonstrated or susceptibility testing is not possible, alternative antimicrobial therapy should be instituted.

Amoxicillin Susceptibility Test Results and Clinical/Bacteriological Outcomes: In the U.S. multicenter study, a total of >99% (558/560) of patients had *H. pylori* isolates which were considered to be susceptible (MIC ≤ 0.25 µg/mL) to amoxicillin at baseline. The other 2 patients had baseline *H. pylori* isolates with an amoxicillin MIC of 0.5 µg/mL, and both isolates were clarithromycin-resistant at baseline; in one case the *H. pylori* was eradicated. In the 7- and 10-day treatment groups 75% (107/145) and 79% (112/142), respectively, of the patients who had pretreatment amoxicillin susceptible MICs (≤ 0.25 µg/mL) were eradicated of *H. pylori*. No patients developed amoxicillin-resistant *H. pylori* during therapy.

CLINICAL STUDIES

Healing of Erosive or Ulcerative Gastroesophageal Reflux Disease (GERD)

In a U.S., multicenter, randomized, double-blind, placebo-controlled study, 103 patients were treated for up to eight weeks with placebo, 10 mg, 20 mg or 40 mg ACIPHEX® QD. For this and all studies of GERD healing, only patients with GERD symptoms and at least grade 2 esophagitis (modified Hetzel-Dent grading scale) were eligible for entry. Endoscopic healing was defined as grade 0 or 1. Each rabeprazole dose was significantly superior to placebo in producing endoscopic healing after four and eight weeks of treatment. The percentage of patients demonstrating endoscopic healing was as follows:

[See second table above]

In addition, there was a statistically significant difference in favor of the ACIPHEX® 10 mg, 20 mg, and 40 mg doses compared to placebo at Weeks 4 and 8 regarding complete resolution of GERD heartburn frequency (p≤0.026). All ACIPHEX® groups reported significantly greater rates of complete resolution of GERD daytime heartburn severity compared to placebo at Weeks 4 and 8 (p≤0.036). Mean reductions from baseline in daily antacid dose were statistically significant for all ACIPHEX® groups when compared to placebo at both Weeks 4 and 8 (p≤0.007).

In a North American multicenter, randomized, double-blind, active-controlled study of 336 patients, ACIPHEX® was statistically superior to ranitidine with respect to the percentage of patients healed at endoscopy after four and eight weeks of treatment (see table below):

Clarithromycin Susceptibility Test Results and Clinical/Bacteriologic Outcomes[a] for a Three Drug Regimen (Rabeprazole 20 mg twice daily, amoxicillin 1000 mg twice daily, and clarithromycin 500 mg twice daily for 7 or 10 days)

Days of RAC Therapy	Clarithromycin Pretreatment Results	Total Number	*H. pylori* Negative (Eradicated)	*H. pylori* Positive (Persistent) Post-Treatment Susceptibility Results			
				S[b]	I[b]	R[b]	No MIC
7	Susceptible[b]	129	103	2	0	1	23
7	Intermediate[b]	0	0	0	0	0	0
7	Resistant[b]	16	5	2	1	4	4
10	Susceptible[b]	133	111	3	1	2	16
10	Intermediate[b]	0	0	0	0	0	0
10	Resistant[b]	9	1	0	0	5	3

[a]Includes only patients with pretreatment and post-treatment clarithromycin susceptibility test results.

[b]Susceptible (S) MIC ≤ 0.25 µg/mL, Intermediate (I) MIC = 0.5 µg/mL, Resistant (R) MIC ≥ 1 µg/mL

Healing of Erosive or Ulcerative Gastroesophageal Reflux Disease (GERD) Percentage of Patients Healed

Week	10 mg ACIPHEX® QD N=27	20 mg ACIPHEX® QD N=25	40 mg ACIPHEX® QD N=26	Placebo N=25
4	63%*	56%*	54%*	0%
8	93%*	84%*	85%*	12%

*(p<0.001 versus placebo)

Long-term Maintenance of Healing of Erosive or Ulcerative Gastroesophageal Reflux Disease (GERD Maintenance) Percent of Patients in Endoscopic Remission

	ACIPHEX® 10 mg	ACIPHEX® 20 mg	Placebo
Study 1	N=66	N=67	N=70
Week 4	83%*	96%*	44%
Week 13	79%*	93%*	39%
Week 26	77%*	93%*	31%
Week 39	76%*	91%*	30%
Week 52	73%*	90%*	29%
Study 2	N=93	N=93	N=99
Week 4	89%*	94%*	40%
Week 13	86%*	91%*	33%
Week 26	85%*	89%*	30%
Week 39	84%*	88%*	29%
Week 52	77%*	86%*	29%
COMBINED STUDIES	N=159	N=160	N=169
Week 4	87%*	94%*	42%
Week 13	83%*	92%*	36%
Week 26	82%*	91%*	31%
Week 39	81%*	89%*	30%
Week 52	75%*	87%*	29%

*(p<0.001 versus placebo)

Healing of Erosive or Ulcerative Gastroesophageal Reflux Disease (GERD) Percentage of Patients Healed

Week	ACIPHEX® 20 mg QD N=167	Ranitidine 150 mg QID N=169
4	59%*	36%
8	87%*	66%

*(p<0.001 versus ranitidine)

ACIPHEX® 20 mg once daily was significantly more effective than ranitidine 150 mg QID in the percentage of patients with complete resolution of heartburn at Weeks 4 and 8 (p<0.001). ACIPHEX® 20 mg once daily was also more effective in complete resolution of daytime heartburn (p≤0.025), and nighttime heartburn (p≤0.012) at both Weeks 4 and 8, with significant differences by the end of the first week of the study.

Long-term Maintenance of Healing of Erosive or Ulcerative Gastroesophageal Reflux Disease (GERD Maintenance)

The long-term maintenance of healing in patients with erosive or ulcerative GERD previously healed with gastric antisecretory therapy was assessed in two U.S., multicenter,

randomized, double-blind, placebo-controlled studies of identical design of 52 weeks duration. The two studies randomized 209 and 285 patients, respectively, to receive either 10 mg or 20 mg of ACIPHEX® QD or placebo. As demonstrated in the tables below, ACIPHEX® was significantly superior to placebo in both studies with respect to the maintenance of healing of GERD and the proportions of patients remaining free of heartburn symptoms at 52 weeks:
[See third table on previous page]
[See first table at right]

Symptomatic Gastroesophageal Reflux Disease (GERD)
Two U.S., multicenter, double-blind, placebo controlled studies were conducted in 316 patients with daytime and nighttime heartburn. Patients reported 5 or more periods of moderate to very severe heartburn during the placebo treatment phase the week prior to randomization. Patients were confirmed by endoscopy to have no esophageal erosions.
The percentage of heartburn-free daytime and/or nighttime periods was greater with ACIPHEX® 20 mg compared to placebo over the 4 weeks of study in Study RAB-USA-2 (47% vs. 23%) and Study RAB-USA-3 (52% vs. 28%). The mean decreases from baseline in average daytime and nighttime heartburn scores were significantly greater for ACIPHEX® 20 mg as compared to placebo at week 4. Graphical displays depicting the daily mean daytime and nighttime scores are provided in Figures 1 to 4.

Figure 1: Mean Daytime heartburn scores RAB - USA - 2

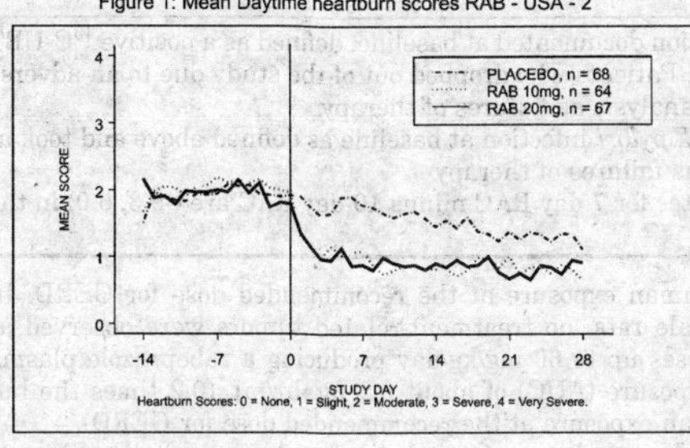

Figure 2: Mean Nighttime heartburn scores RAB - USA - 2

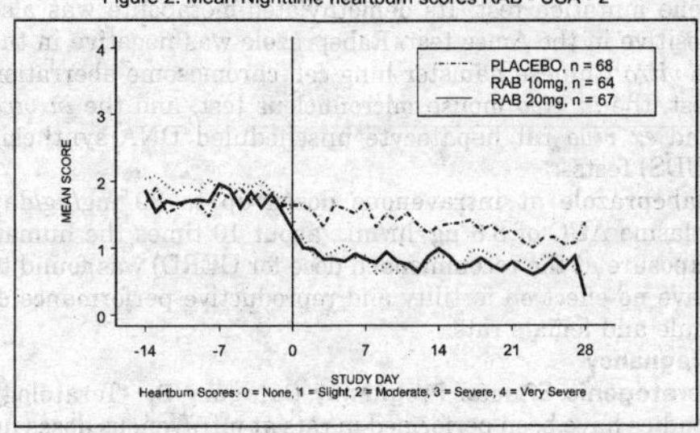

Figure 3: Mean Daytime heartburn scores RAB - USA - 3

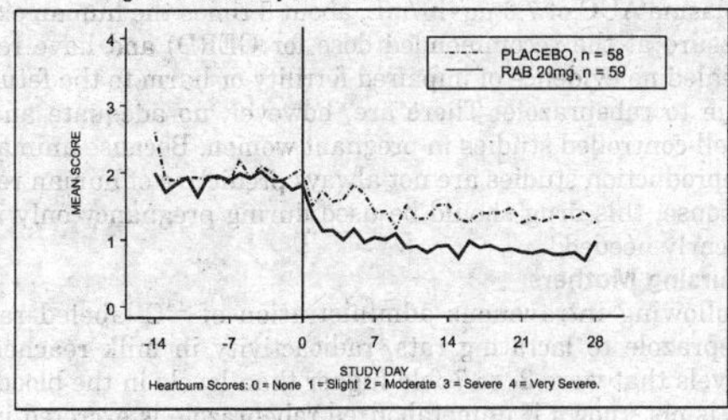

Figure 4: Mean Nighttime heartburn scores RAB - USA - 3

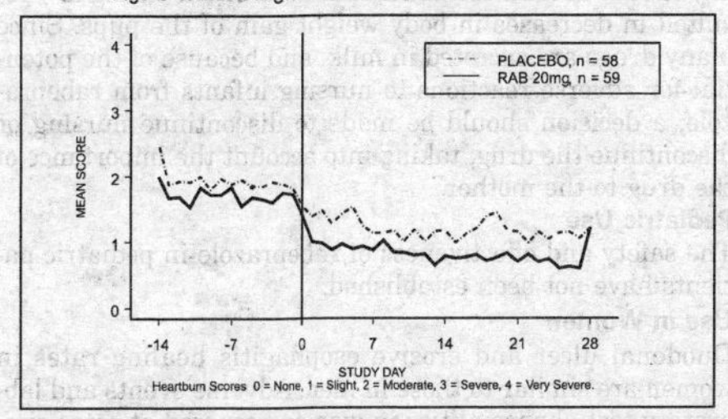

ACIPHEX® 20 mg also significantly reduced daily antacid consumption versus placebo over 4 weeks ($p<0.001$).

Healing of Duodenal Ulcers
In a U.S., randomized, double-blind, multi-center study assessing the effectiveness of 20 mg and 40 mg of ACIPHEX® QD versus placebo for healing endoscopically-defined duodenal ulcers, 100 patients were treated for up to four weeks. ACIPHEX® was significantly superior to placebo in producing healing of duodenal ulcers. The percentages of patients with endoscopic healing are presented below:
[See second table above]
At Weeks 2 and 4, significantly more patients in the ACIPHEX® 20 and 40 mg groups reported complete resolution of ulcer pain frequency ($p \leq 0.018$), daytime pain severity ($p \leq 0.023$), and nighttime pain severity ($p \leq 0.035$) compared with placebo patients. The only exception was the ACIPHEX® 40 mg group versus placebo at Week 2 for duodenal ulcer pain frequency (p=0.094). Significant differences in resolution of daytime and nighttime pain were noted in both ACIPHEX® groups relative to placebo by the end of the first week of the study. Significant reductions in daily antacid use were also noted in both ACIPHEX® groups compared to placebo at Weeks 2 and 4 ($p<0.001$).
An international randomized, double-blind, active-controlled trial was conducted in 205 patients comparing 20 mg ACIPHEX® QD with 20 mg omeprazole QD. The study was designed to provide at least 80% power to exclude a difference of at least 10% between ACIPHEX® and omeprazole, assuming four-week healing response rates of 93% for both groups. In patients with endoscopically-defined duodenal ulcers treated for up to four weeks, ACIPHEX® was comparable to omeprazole in producing healing of duodenal ulcers. The percentages of patients with endoscopic healing at two and four weeks are presented below:
[See third table above]
ACIPHEX® and omeprazole were comparable in providing complete resolution of symptoms.

***Helicobacter pylori* Eradication in Patients with Peptic Ulcer Disease or Symptomatic Non-Ulcer Disease**
The U.S. multicenter study was a double-blind, parallel group comparison of rabeprazole, amoxicillin, and clarithromycin for 3, 7, or 10 days vs. omeprazole, amoxicillin and clarithromycin for 10 days. Therapy consisted of rabeprazole 20 mg twice daily, amoxicillin 1000 mg twice daily, and clarithromycin 500 mg twice daily (RAC) or omeprazole 20 mg twice daily, amoxicillin 1000 mg twice daily, and clarithromycin 500 mg twice daily (OAC). Patients with *H. pylori* infection were stratified in a 1:1 ratio for those with peptic ulcer disease (active or a history of ulcer in the past five years) [PUD] and those who were symptomatic but without peptic ulcer disease [NPUD], as determined by upper gastrointestinal endoscopy. The overall *H. pylori* eradication rates, defined as negative ^{13}C-UBT for *H. pylori* ≥ 6 weeks from the end of the treatment are shown in the following table. The eradication rates in the 7-day and 10-day RAC regimens were found to be similar to 10-day OAC regimen using either the Intent-to-Treat (ITT) or Per-Protocol (PP) populations. Eradication rates in the RAC 3-day regimen were inferior to the other regimens.
[See table at top of next page]

Pathological Hypersecretory Conditions Including Zollinger-Ellison Syndrome
Twelve patients with idiopathic gastric hypersecretion or Zollinger-Ellison syndrome have been treated successfully with ACIPHEX® at doses from 20 to 120 mg for up to 12 months. ACIPHEX® produced satisfactory inhibition of gastric acid secretion in all patients and complete resolution of signs and symptoms of acid-peptic disease where present. ACIPHEX® also prevented recurrence of gastric hypersecretion and manifestations of acid-peptic disease in all patients. The high doses of ACIPHEX® used to treat this small cohort of patients with gastric hypersecretion were well tolerated.

Long-term Maintenance of Healing of Erosive or Ulcerative Gastroesophageal Reflux Disease (GERD Maintenance): Percent of Patients Without Relapse in Heartburn Frequency and Daytime and Nighttime Heartburn Severity at Week 52

	ACIPHEX® 10 mg	ACIPHEX® 20 mg	Placebo
Heartburn Frequency			
Study 1	46/55 (84%)*	48/52 (92%)*	17/45 (38%)
Study 2	50/72 (69%)*	57/72 (79%)*	22/79 (28%)
Daytime Heartburn Severity			
Study 1	61/64 (95%)*	60/62 (97%)*	42/61 (69%)
Study 2	73/84 (87%)†	82/87 (94%)*	67/90 (74%)
Nighttime Heartburn Severity			
Study 1	57/61 (93%)*	60/61 (98%)*	37/56 (66%)
Study 2	67/80 (84%)	79/87 (91%)†	64/87 (74%)

*$p \leq 0.001$ versus placebo
†$0.001<p<0.05$ versus placebo

Healing of Duodenal Ulcers—Percentage of Patients Healed

Week	ACIPHEX® 20 mg QD N=34	ACIPHEX® 40 mg QD N=33	Placebo N=33
2	44%	42%	21%
4	79%*	91%*	39%

*$p \leq 0.001$ versus placebo

Healing of Duodenal Ulcers—Percentage of Patients Healed

Week	ACIPHEX® 20 mg QD N=102	Omeprazole 20 mg QD N=103	95% Confidence Interval for the Treatment Difference (ACIPHEX®–Omeprazole)
2	69%	61%	(−6%, 22%)
4	98%	93%	(−3%, 15%)

INDICATIONS AND USAGE

Healing of Erosive or Ulcerative Gastroesophageal Reflux Disease (GERD)
ACIPHEX® is indicated for short-term (4 to 8 weeks) treatment in the healing and symptomatic relief of erosive or ulcerative gastroesophageal reflux disease (GERD). For those patients who have not healed after 8 weeks of treatment, an additional 8-week course of ACIPHEX® may be considered.

Maintenance of Healing of Erosive or Ulcerative Gastroesophageal Reflux Disease (GERD)
ACIPHEX® is indicated for maintaining healing and reduction in relapse rates of heartburn symptoms in patients with erosive or ulcerative gastroesophageal reflux disease (GERD Maintenance). Controlled studies do not extend beyond 12 months.

Treatment of Symptomatic Gastroesophageal Reflux Disease (GERD)
ACIPHEX® is indicated for the treatment of daytime and nighttime heartburn and other symptoms associated with GERD.

Healing of Duodenal Ulcers
ACIPHEX® is indicated for short-term (up to four weeks) treatment in the healing and symptomatic relief of duodenal ulcers. Most patients heal within four weeks.

***Helicobacter pylori* Eradication to Reduce the Risk of Duodenal Ulcer recurrence**
ACIPHEX® in combination with amoxicillin and clarithromycin as a three-drug regimen, is indicated for the treatment of patients with *H. pylori* infection and duodenal ulcer disease (active or history within the past 5 years) to eradicate *H. pylori*. Eradication of *H. pylori* has been shown to reduce the risk of duodenal ulcer recurrence. (See **CLINICAL STUDIES** and **DOSAGE AND ADMINISTRATION**.)
In patients who fail therapy, susceptibility testing should be done. If resistance to clarithromycin is demonstrated or susceptibility testing is not possible, alternative antimicrobial therapy should be instituted. (See **CLINICAL PHARMACOLOGY, Microbiology** and the clarithromycin package insert, **CLINICAL PHARMACOLOGY, Microbiology**.)

Treatment of Pathological Hypersecretory Conditions, Including Zollinger-Ellison Syndrome
ACIPHEX® is indicated for the long-term treatment of pathological hypersecretory conditions, including Zollinger-Ellison syndrome.

CONTRAINDICATIONS

Rabeprazole is contraindicated in patients with known hypersensitivity to rabeprazole, substituted benzimidazoles or to any component of the formulation.

Continued on next page

Aciphex—Cont.

Clarithromycin is contraindicated in patients with known hypersensitivity to any macrolide antibiotic.
Concomitant administration of clarithromycin with pimozide and cisapride is contraindicated. There have been post-marketing reports of drug interactions when clarithromycin and/or erythromycin are co-administered with pimozide resulting in cardiac arrhythmias (QT prolongation, ventricular tachycardia, ventricular fibrillation, and torsade de pointes) most likely due to inhibition of hepatic metabolism of pimozide by erythromycin and clarithromycin. Fatalities have been reported. (Please refer to full prescribing information for clarithromycin.)
Amoxicillin is contraindicated in patients with a known hypersensitivity to any penicillin. (Please refer to full prescribing information for amoxicillin.)

WARNINGS

CLARITHROMYCIN SHOULD NOT BE USED IN PREGNANT WOMEN EXCEPT IN CLINICAL CIRCUMSTANCES WHERE NO ALTERNATIVE THERAPY IS APPROPRIATE. If pregnancy occurs while taking clarithromycin, the patient should be apprised of the potential hazard to the fetus. (See WARNINGS in prescribing information for clarithromycin.)
Amoxicillin: Serious and occasionally fatal hypersensitivity (anaphylactic) reactions have been reported in patients on penicillin therapy. These reactions are more likely to occur in individuals with a history of penicillin hypersensitivity and/or a history of sensitivity to multiple allergens.
There have been well-documented reports of individuals with a history of penicillin hypersensitivity reactions who have experienced severe hypersensitivity reactions when treated with a cephalosporin. Before initiating therapy with any penicillin, careful inquiry should be made concerning previous hypersensitivity reactions to penicillin, cephalosporin, and other allergens. If an allergic reaction occurs, amoxicillin should be discontinued and the appropriate therapy instituted. (See WARNINGS in prescribing information for amoxicillin.)
SERIOUS ANAPHYLACTIC REACTIONS REQUIRE IMMEDIATE EMERGENCY TREATMENT WITH EPINEPHRINE. OXYGEN, INTRAVENOUS STEROIDS, AND AIRWAY MANAGEMENT, INCLUDING INTUBATION, SHOULD ALSO BE ADMINISTERED AS INDICATED.
Pseudomembranous colitis has been reported with nearly all antibacterial agents, including clarithromycin and amoxicillin, and may range in severity from mild to life threatening. Therefore, it is important to consider this diagnosis in patients who present with diarrhea subsequent to the administration of antibacterial agents.
Treatment with antibacterial agents alters the normal flora of the colon and may permit overgrowth of clostridia. Studies indicate that a toxin produced by *Clostridium difficile* is a primary cause of "antibiotic-associated colitis".
After the diagnosis of pseudomembranous colitis has been established, therapeutic measures should be initiated. Mild cases of pseudomembranous colitis usually respond to discontinuation of the drug alone. In moderate to severe cases, consideration should be given to management with fluid and electrolytes, protein supplementation, and treatment with an antibacterial drug clinically effective against *Clostridium difficile colitis.*

PRECAUTIONS

General
Symptomatic response to therapy with rabeprazole does not preclude the presence of gastric malignancy.
Patients with healed GERD were treated for up to 40 months with rabeprazole and monitored with serial gastric biopsies. Patients without *H. pylori* infection (221 of 326 patients) had no clinically important pathologic changes in the gastric mucosa. Patients with *H. pylori* infection at baseline (105 of 326 patients) had mild or moderate inflammation in the gastric body or mild inflammation in the gastric antrum. Patients with mild grades of infection or inflammation in the gastric body tended to change to moderate, whereas those graded moderate at baseline tended to remain stable. Patients with mild grades of infection or inflammation in the gastric antrum tended to remain stable. At baseline 8% of patients had atrophy of glands in the gastric body and 15% had atrophy in the gastric antrum. At endpoint, 15% of patients had atrophy of glands in the gastric body and 11% had atrophy in the gastric antrum. Approximately 4% of patients had intestinal metaplasia at some point during follow-up, but no consistent changes were seen.
Steady-state interactions of rabeprazole and warfarin have not been adequately evaluated in patients. There have been reports of increased INR and prothrombin time in patients receiving a proton pump inhibitor and warfarin concomitantly. Increases in INR and prothrombin time may lead to abnormal bleeding and even death. Patients treated with a proton pump inhibitor and warfarin concomitantly may need to be monitored for increases in INR and prothrombin time.
Information for Patients
Patients should be cautioned that ACIPHEX® delayed-release tablets should be swallowed whole. The tablets should not be chewed, crushed, or split. ACIPHEX® can be taken with or without food.
Drug Interactions
Rabeprazole is metabolized by the cytochrome P450 (CYP450) drug metabolizing enzyme system. Studies in healthy subjects have shown that rabeprazole does not have clinically significant interactions with other drugs metabolized by the CYP450 system, such as warfarin and theophylline given as single oral doses, diazepam as a single intravenous dose, and phenytoin given as a single intravenous dose (with supplemental oral dosing). Steady-state interactions of rabeprazole and other drugs metabolized by this enzyme system have not been studied in patients. There have been reports of increased INR and prothrombin time in patients receiving proton pump inhibitors, including rabeprazole, and warfarin concomitantly. Increases in INR and prothrombin time may lead to abnormal bleeding and even death.

Helicobacter pylori Eradication at ≥ 6 Weeks After The End of Treatment

	Treatment Group - Percent (%) of Patients Cured (Number of Patients)		Difference - (RAC – OAC) [95% Confidence Interval]
	7-day RAC*	**10-day OAC**	
Per Protocol[a]	84.3% (N=166)	81.6% (N=179)	2.8 [-5.2, 10.7]
Intent-to-Treat[b]	77.3% (N=194)	73.3% (N=206)	4.0 [-4.4, 12.5]
	10-day RAC*	**10-day OAC**	
Per Protocol[a]	86.0% (N=171)	81.6% (N=179)	4.4 [-3.3, 12.1]
Intent-to-Treat[b]	78.1% (N=196)	73.3% (N=206)	4.8 [-3.6, 13.2]
	3-day RAC	**10-day OAC**	
Per Protocol[a]	29.9% (N=167)	81.6% (N=179)	-51.6 [-60.6, -42.6]
Intent-to-Treat[b]	27.3% (N=187)	73.3% (N=206)	-46.0 [-54.8, -37.2]

[a] Patients were included in the analysis if they had *H. pylori* infection documented at baseline, defined as a positive ^{13}C-UBT plus rapid urease test or culture and were not protocol violators. Patients who dropped out of the study due to an adverse event related to the study drug were included in the evaluable analysis as failures of therapy.
[b] Patients were included in the analysis if they had documented *H. pylori* infection at baseline as defined above and took at least one dose of study medication. All dropouts were included as failures of therapy.
*The 95% confidence intervals for the difference in eradication rates for 7-day RAC minus 10-day RAC are (-9.3, 6.0) in the PP population and (-9.0, 7.5) in the ITT population.

In vitro incubations employing human liver microsomes indicated that rabeprazole inhibited cyclosporine metabolism with an IC_{50} of 62 micromolar, a concentration that is over 50 times higher than the C_{max} in healthy volunteers following 14 days of dosing with 20 mg of rabeprazole. This degree of inhibition is similar to that by omeprazole at equivalent concentrations.
Rabeprazole produces sustained inhibition of gastric acid secretion. An interaction with compounds which are dependent on gastric pH for absorption may occur due to the magnitude of acid suppression observed with rabeprazole. For example, in normal subjects, co-administration of rabeprazole 20 mg QD resulted in an approximately 30% decrease in the bioavailability of ketoconazole and increases in the AUC and C_{max} for digoxin of 19% and 29%, respectively. Therefore, patients may need to be monitored when such drugs are taken concomitantly with rabeprazole. Co-administration of rabeprazole and antacids produced no clinically relevant changes in plasma rabeprazole concentrations.
In a clinical study in Japan evaluating rabeprazole in patients categorized by CYP2C19 genotype (n=6 per genotype category), gastric acid suppression was higher in poor metabolizers as compared to extensive metabolizers. This could be due to higher rabeprazole plasma levels in poor metabolizers. Whether or not interactions of rabeprazole sodium with other drugs metabolized by CYP2C19 would be different between extensive metabolizers and poor metabolizers has not been studied.
Combined Administration with Clarithromycin
Combined administration consisting of rabeprazole, amoxicillin, and clarithromycin resulted in increases in plasma concentrations of rabeprazole and 14-hydroxyclarithromycin. (See **CLINICAL PHARMACOLOGY, Combination Therapy with Antimicrobials.**)
Concomitant administration of clarithromycin with pimozide and cisapride is contraindicated. (See **PRECAUTIONS** in prescribing information for clarithromycin.) (See **PRECAUTIONS** in prescribing information for amoxicillin.)
Carcinogenesis, Mutagenesis, Impairment of Fertility
In a 88/104-week carcinogenicity study in CD-1 mice, rabeprazole at oral doses up to 100 mg/kg/day did not produce any increased tumor occurrence. The highest tested dose produced a systemic exposure to rabeprazole (AUC) of 1.40 µg•hr/mL which is 1.6 times the human exposure (plasma $AUC_{0-\infty}$ = 0.88 µg•hr/mL) at the recommended dose for GERD (20 mg/day). In a 104-week carcinogenicity study in Sprague-Dawley rats, males were treated with oral doses of 5, 15, 30 and 60 mg/kg/day and females with 5, 15, 30, 60 and 120 mg/kg/day. Rabeprazole produced gastric enterochromaffin-like (ECL) cell hyperplasia in male and female rats and ECL cell carcinoid tumors in female rats at all doses including the lowest tested dose. The lowest dose (5 mg/kg/day) produced a systemic exposure to rabeprazole (AUC) of about 0.1 µg•hr/mL which is about 0.1 times the human exposure at the recommended dose for GERD. In male rats, no treatment-related tumors were observed at doses up to 60 mg/kg/day producing a rabeprazole plasma exposure (AUC) of about 0.2 µg•hr/mL (0.2 times the human exposure at the recommended dose for GERD).
Rabeprazole was positive in the Ames test, the Chinese hamster ovary cell (CHO/HGPRT) forward gene mutation test and the mouse lymphoma cell (L5178Y/TK+/−) forward gene mutation test. Its demethylated-metabolite was also positive in the Ames test. Rabeprazole was negative in the *in vitro* Chinese hamster lung cell chromosome aberration test, the *in vivo* mouse micronucleus test, and the *in vivo* and *ex vivo* rat hepatocyte unscheduled DNA synthesis (UDS) tests.
Rabeprazole at intravenous doses up to 30 mg/kg/day (plasma AUC of 8.8 µg•hr/mL, about 10 times the human exposure at the recommended dose for GERD) was found to have no effect on fertility and reproductive performance of male and female rats.
Pregnancy
Teratogenic Effects. Pregnancy Category B: Teratology studies have been performed in rats at intravenous doses up to 50 mg/kg/day (plasma AUC of 11.8 µg•hr/mL, about 13 times the human exposure at the recommended dose for GERD) and rabbits at intravenous doses up to 30 mg/kg/day (plasma AUC of 7.3 µg•hr/mL, about 8 times the human exposure at the recommended dose for GERD) and have revealed no evidence of impaired fertility or harm to the fetus due to rabeprazole. There are, however, no adequate and well-controlled studies in pregnant women. Because animal reproduction studies are not always predictive of human response, this drug should be used during pregnancy only if clearly needed.
Nursing Mothers
Following intravenous administration of ^{14}C-labeled rabeprazole to lactating rats, radioactivity in milk reached levels that were 2- to 7-fold higher than levels in the blood. It is not known if unmetabolized rabeprazole is excreted in human breast milk. Administration of rabeprazole to rats in late gestation and during lactation at doses of 400 mg/kg/day (about 195-times the human dose based on mg/m^2) resulted in decreases in body weight gain of the pups. Since many drugs are excreted in milk, and because of the potential for adverse reactions to nursing infants from rabeprazole, a decision should be made to discontinue nursing or discontinue the drug, taking into account the importance of the drug to the mother.
Pediatric Use
The safety and effectiveness of rabeprazole in pediatric patients have not been established.
Use in Women
Duodenal ulcer and erosive esophagitis healing rates in women are similar to those in men. Adverse events and laboratory test abnormalities in women occurred at rates similar to those in men.
Geriatric Use
Of the total number of subjects in clinical studies of ACIPHEX®, 19% were 65 years and over, while 4% were 75 years and over. No overall differences in safety or effectiveness were observed between these subjects and younger subjects, and other reported clinical experience has not identified differences in responses between the elderly and younger patients, but greater sensitivity of some older individuals cannot be ruled out.

ADVERSE REACTIONS

Worldwide, over 2900 patients have been treated with rabeprazole in Phase II-III clinical trials involving various dosages and durations of treatment. In general, rabeprazole treatment has been well-tolerated in both short-term and long-term trials. The adverse events rates were generally similar between the 10 and 20 mg doses.

Incidence in Controlled North American and European Clinical Trials

In an analysis of adverse events assessed as possibly or probably related to treatment appearing in greater than 1% of ACIPHEX® patients and appearing with greater frequency than placebo in controlled North American and European trials, the incidence of headache was 2.4% (n=1552) for ACIPHEX® versus 1.6% (n=258) for placebo.

In short and long-term studies, the following adverse events, regardless of causality, were reported in ACIPHEX®-treated patients. Rare events are those reported in ≤1/1000 patients.

Body as a Whole: asthenia, fever, allergic reaction, chills, malaise, chest pain substernal, neck rigidity, photosensitivity reaction. Rare: abdomen enlarged, face edema, hangover effect. *Cardiovascular System:* hypertension, myocardial infarct, electrocardiogram abnormal, migraine, syncope, angina pectoris, bundle branch block, palpitation, sinus bradycardia, tachycardia. Rare: bradycardia, pulmonary embolus, supraventricular tachycardia, thrombophlebitis, vasodilation, QTC prolongation and ventricular tachycardia. *Digestive System:* diarrhea, nausea, abdominal pain, vomiting, dyspepsia, flatulence, constipation, dry mouth, eructation, gastroenteritis, rectal hemorrhage, melena, anorexia, cholelithiasis, mouth ulceration, stomatitis, dysphagia, gingivitis, cholecystitis, increased appetite, abnormal stools, colitis, esophagitis, glossitis, pancreatitis, proctitis. Rare: bloody diarrhea, cholangitis, duodenitis, gastrointestinal hemorrhage, hepatic encephalopathy, hepatitis, hepatoma, liver fatty deposit, salivary gland enlargement, thirst. *Endocrine System:* hyperthyroidism, hypothyroidism. *Hemic & Lymphatic System:* anemia, ecchymosis, lymphadenopathy, hypochromic anemia. *Metabolic & Nutritional Disorders:* peripheral edema, edema, weight gain, gout, dehydration, weight loss. *Musculo-Skeletal System:* myalgia, arthritis, leg cramps, bone pain, arthrosis, bursitis. Rare: twitching. *Nervous System:* insomnia, anxiety, dizziness, depression, nervousness, somnolence, hypertonia, neuralgia, vertigo, convulsion, abnormal dreams, libido decreased, neuropathy, paresthesia, tremor. Rare: agitation, amnesia, confusion, extrapyramidal syndrome, hyperkinesia. *Respiratory System:* dyspnea, asthma, epistaxis, laryngitis, hiccup, hyperventilation. Rare: apnea, hypoventilation. *Skin and Appendages:* rash, pruritus, sweating, urticaria, alopecia. Rare: dry skin, herpes zoster, psoriasis, skin discoloration. *Special Senses:* cataract, amblyopia, glaucoma, dry eyes, abnormal vision, tinnitus, otitis media. Rare: corneal opacity, blurry vision, diplopia, deafness, eye pain, retinal degeneration, strabismus. *Urogenital System:* cystitis, urinary frequency, dysmenorrhea, dysuria, kidney calculus, metrorrhagia, polyuria. Rare: breast enlargement, hematuria, impotence, leukorrhea, menorrhagia, orchitis, urinary incontinence.

Laboratory Values: The following changes in laboratory parameters were reported as adverse events: abnormal platelets, albuminuria, creatine phosphokinase increased, erythrocytes abnormal, hypercholesteremia, hyperglycemia, hyperlipemia, hypokalemia, hyponatremia, leukocytosis, leukorrhea, liver function tests abnormal, prostatic specific antigen increase, SGPT increased, urine abnormality, WBC abnormal.

In controlled clinical studies, 3/1456 (0.2%) patients treated with rabeprazole and 2/237 (0.8%) patients treated with placebo developed treatment-emergent abnormalities (which were either new on study or present at study entry with an increase of 1.25 × baseline value) in SGOT (AST), SGPT (ALT), or both. None of the three rabeprazole patients experienced chills, fever, right upper quadrant pain, nausea or jaundice.

Combination Treatment with Amoxicillin and Clarithromycin: In clinical trials using combination therapy with rabeprazole plus amoxicillin and clarithromycin (RAC), no adverse events unique to this drug combination were observed. In the U.S. multicenter study, the most frequently reported drug related adverse events for patients who received RAC therapy for 7 or 10 days were diarrhea (8% and 7%) and taste perversion (6% and 10%), respectively.

No clinically significant laboratory abnormalities particular to the drug combinations were observed.

For more information on adverse events or laboratory changes with amoxicillin or clarithromycin, refer to their respective package prescribing information, **ADVERSE REACTIONS** section.

Post-Marketing Adverse Events: Additional adverse events reported from worldwide marketing experience with rabeprazole sodium are: sudden death, coma and hyperammonemia, jaundice, rhabdomyolysis, disorientation and delirium, anaphylaxis, angioedema, bullous and other drug eruptions of the skin, interstitial pneumonia, interstitial nephritis, and TSH elevations. In most instances, the relationship to rabeprazole sodium was unclear. In addition, agranulocytosis, hemolytic anemia, leukopenia, pancytopenia, and thrombocytopenia have been reported. Increases in prothrombin time/INR in patients treated with concomitant warfarin have been reported.

OVERDOSAGE

Because strategies for the management of overdose are continually evolving, it is advisable to contact a Poison Control Center to determine the latest recommendations for the management of an overdose of any drug. There has been no experience with large overdoses with rabeprazole. Seven reports of accidental overdosage with rabeprazole have been received. The maximum reported overdose was 80 mg. There were no clinical signs or symptoms associated with any reported overdose. Patients with Zollinger-Ellison syndrome have been treated with up to 120 mg rabeprazole QD. No specific antidote for rabeprazole is known. Rabeprazole is extensively protein bound and is not readily dialyzable. In the event of overdosage, treatment should be symptomatic and supportive.

Single oral doses of rabeprazole at 786 mg/kg and 1024 mg/kg were lethal to mice and rats, respectively. The single oral dose of 2000 mg/kg was not lethal to dogs. The major symptoms of acute toxicity were hypoactivity, labored respiration, lateral or prone position and convulsion in mice and rats and watery diarrhea, tremor, convulsion and coma in dogs.

DOSAGE AND ADMINISTRATION

Healing of Erosive or Ulcerative Gastroesophageal Reflux Disease (GERD)

The recommended adult oral dose is one ACIPHEX® 20 mg delayed-release tablet to be taken once daily for four to eight weeks. (See **INDICATIONS AND USAGE**). For those patients who have not healed after 8 weeks of treatment, an additional 8-week course of ACIPHEX® may be considered.

Maintenance of Healing of Erosive or Ulcerative Gastroesophageal Reflux Disease (GERD Maintenance)

The recommended adult oral dose is one ACIPHEX® 20 mg delayed-release tablet to be taken once daily. (See **INDICATIONS AND USAGE**).

Treatment of Symptomatic Gastroesophageal Reflux Disease (GERD)

The recommended adult oral dose is one ACIPHEX® 20 mg delayed-release tablet to be taken once daily for 4 weeks. (See **INDICATIONS AND USAGE**). If symptoms do not resolve completely after 4 weeks, an additional course of treatment may be considered.

Healing of Duodenal Ulcers

The recommended adult oral dose is one ACIPHEX® 20 mg delayed-release tablet to be taken once daily after the morning meal for a period up to four weeks. (See **INDICATIONS AND USAGE**). Most patients with duodenal ulcer heal within four weeks. A few patients may require additional therapy to achieve healing.

Helicobacter pylori **Eradication to Reduce the Risk of Duodenal Ulcer Recurrence**

Three-Drug Regimen[a]:

ACIPHEX	20 mg	Twice Daily for 7 Days
Amoxicillin	1000 mg	Twice Daily for 7 Days
Clarithromycin	500 mg	Twice Daily for 7 Days

All three medications should be taken twice daily with the morning and evening meals.

[a] It is important that patients comply with the full 7-day regimen. (See **CLINICAL STUDIES** section.)

Treatment of Pathological Hypersecretory Conditions Including Zollinger-Ellison Syndrome

The dosage of ACIPHEX® in patients with pathologic hypersecretory conditions varies with the individual patient. The recommended adult oral starting dose is 60 mg once a day. Doses should be adjusted to individual patient needs and should continue for as long as clinically indicated. Some patients may require divided doses. Doses up to 100 mg QD and 60 mg BID have been administered. Some patients with Zollinger-Ellison syndrome have been treated continuously with ACIPHEX® for up to one year.

No dosage adjustment is necessary in elderly patients, in patients with renal disease or in patients with mild to moderate hepatic impairment. Administration of rabeprazole to patients with mild to moderate liver impairment resulted in increased exposure and decreased elimination. Due to the lack of clinical data on rabeprazole in patients with severe hepatic impairment, caution should be exercised in those patients.

ACIPHEX® tablets should be swallowed whole. The tablets should not be chewed, crushed, or split. ACIPHEX® can be taken with or without food.

HOW SUPPLIED

ACIPHEX® 20 mg is supplied as delayed-release light yellow enteric-coated tablets. The name and strength, in mg, (ACIPHEX 20) is imprinted on one side.

Bottles of 30 (NDC#62856-243-30)

Bottles of 90 (NDC#62856-243-90)

Unit Dose Blisters Package of 100 (10 × 10) (NDC#62856-243-41)

Store at 25°C (77°F); excursions permitted to 15–30°C (59-86°F).

Protect from moisture.

REFERENCES

1. National Committee for Clinical Laboratory Standards. *Methods for Dilution Antimicrobial Susceptibility Tests for Bacteria That Grow Aerobically*—Fifth Edition. Approved Standard NCCLS Document M7-A5, Vol. 20, No. 2, NCCLS, Wayne, PA, January 2000.

200268

AX-PI42

Shown in Product Identification Guide, page 319

DURAGESIC® Ⓒ℞

[*Dər 'ă-jēsĭk*]

(fentanyl transdermal system)

Full Prescribing Information

BECAUSE SERIOUS OR LIFE-THREATENING HYPOVENTILATION COULD OCCUR, DURAGESIC® (FENTANYL TRANSDERMAL SYSTEM) IS CONTRAINDICATED:

- **In the management of acute or post-operative pain, including use in out-patient surgeries**
- **In the management of mild or intermittent pain responsive to PRN or non-opioid therapy**
- **In doses exceeding 25 μg/h at the initiation of opioid therapy**

(See CONTRAINDICATIONS for further information.)

SAFETY OF DURAGESIC® HAS NOT BEEN ESTABLISHED IN CHILDREN UNDER 2 YEARS OF AGE. DURAGESIC® SHOULD BE ADMINISTERED TO CHILDREN ONLY IF THEY ARE OPIOID-TOLERANT AND AGE 2 YEARS OR OLDER (See PRECAUTIONS—Pediatric Use).

DURAGESIC® is indicated for treatment of chronic pain (such as that of malignancy) that:

- **Cannot be managed by lesser means such as acetaminophen-opioid combinations, non-steroidal analgesics, or PRN dosing with short-acting opioids and**
- **Requires continuous opioid administration.**

The 50, 75, and 100 μg/h dosages should ONLY be used in patients who are already on and are tolerant to opioid therapy.

DESCRIPTION

DURAGESIC® (fentanyl transdermal system) is a transdermal system providing continuous systemic delivery of fentanyl, a potent opioid analgesic, for 72 hours. The chemical name is N-Phenyl-N-(1-2-phenylethyl-4-piperidyl) propanamide. The structural formula is:

CH_3CH_2CON—[piperidyl]—$N—CH_2CH_2$—[phenyl]

The molecular weight of fentanyl base is 336.5, and the empirical formula is $C_{22}H_{28}N_2O$. The n-octanol:water partition coefficient is 860:1. The pKa is 8.4.

System Components and Structure

The amount of fentanyl released from each system per hour is proportional to the surface area (25 μg/h per 10 cm^2). The composition per unit area of all system sizes is identical. Each system also contains 0.1 mL of alcohol USP per 10 cm^2.

Dose* (μg/h)	Size (cm^2)	Fentanyl Content (mg)
25	10	2.5
50**	20	5
75**	30	7.5
100**	40	10

* Nominal delivery rate per hour

** FOR USE ONLY IN OPIOID TOLERANT PATIENTS

DURAGESIC® is a rectangular transparent unit comprising a protective liner and four functional layers. Proceeding from the outer surface toward the surface adhering to skin, these layers are:

1) a backing layer of polyester film; 2) a drug reservoir of fentanyl and alcohol usp gelled with hydroxyethyl cellulose; 3) an ethylene-vinyl acetate copolymer membrane that controls the rate of fentanyl delivery to the skin surface; and 4) a fentanyl containing silicone adhesive. Before use, a protective liner covering the adhesive layer is removed and discarded.

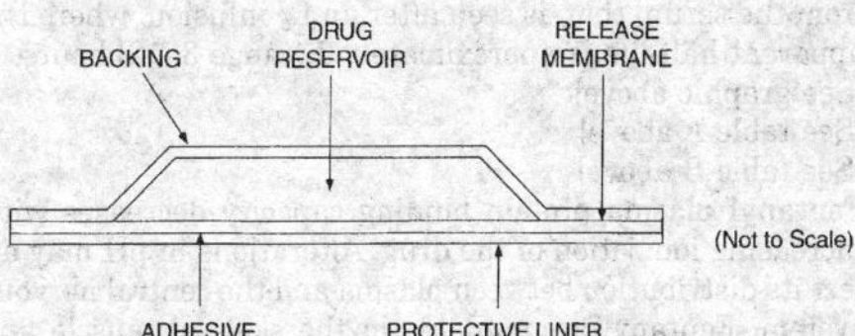

The active component of the system is fentanyl. The remaining components are pharmacologically inactive. Less than 0.2 mL of alcohol is also released from the system during use.

Do not cut or damage DURAGESIC®. If the DURAGESIC® system is cut or damaged, controlled drug delivery will not be possible.

CLINICAL PHARMACOLOGY

Pharmacology

Fentanyl is an opioid analgesic. Fentanyl interacts predominantly with the opioid μ-receptor. These μ-binding sites are discretely distributed in the human brain, spinal cord and other tissues.

Continued on next page

Duragesic—Cont.

In clinical settings, fentanyl exerts its principal pharmacologic effects on the central nervous system. Its primary actions of therapeutic value are analgesia and sedation. Fentanyl may increase the patient's tolerance for pain and decrease the perception of suffering, although the presence of the pain itself may still be recognized.

In addition to analgesia, alterations in mood, euphoria and dysphoria, and drowsiness commonly occur. Fentanyl depresses the respiratory centers, depresses the cough reflex, and constricts the pupils. Analgesic blood levels of fentanyl may cause nausea and vomiting directly by stimulating the chemoreceptor trigger zone, but nausea and vomiting are significantly more common in ambulatory than in recumbent patients, as is postural syncope.

Opioids increase the tone and decrease the propulsive contractions of the smooth muscle of the gastrointestinal tract. The resultant prolongation in gastrointestinal transit time may be responsible for the constipating effect of fentanyl. Because opioids may increase biliary tract pressure, some patients with biliary colic may experience worsening rather than relief of pain.

While opioids generally increase the tone of urinary tract smooth muscle, the net effect tends to be variable, in some cases producing urinary urgency, in others, difficulty in urination.

At therapeutic dosages, fentanyl usually does not exert major effects on the cardiovascular system. However, some patients may exhibit orthostatic hypotension and fainting.

Histamine assays and skin wheal testing in man indicate that clinically significant histamine release rarely occurs with fentanyl administration. Assays in man show no clinically significant histamine release in dosages up to 50 µg/kg.

Pharmacokinetics (see graph and tables)

DURAGESIC® (fentanyl transdermal system) releases fentanyl from the reservoir at a nearly constant amount per unit time. The concentration gradient existing between the saturated solution of drug in the reservoir and the lower concentration in the skin drives drug release. Fentanyl moves in the direction of the lower concentration at a rate determined by the copolymer release membrane and the diffusion of fentanyl through the skin layers. While the actual rate of fentanyl delivery to the skin varies over the 72 hour application period, each system is labeled with a nominal flux which represents the average amount of drug delivered to the systemic circulation per hour across average skin.

While there is variation in dose delivered among patients, the nominal flux of the systems (25, 50, 75, and 100 µg of fentanyl per hour) is sufficiently accurate as to allow individual titration of dosage for a given patient. The small amount of alcohol which has been incorporated into the system enhances the rate of drug flux through the rate-limiting copolymer membrane and increases the permeability of the skin to fentanyl.

Following DURAGESIC® application, the skin under the system absorbs fentanyl, and a depot of fentanyl concentrates in the upper skin layers. Fentanyl then becomes available to the systemic circulation. Serum fentanyl concentrations increase gradually following initial DURAGESIC® application, generally leveling off between 12 and 24 hours and remaining relatively constant, with some fluctuation, for the remainder of the 72 hour application period. Peak serum concentrations of fentanyl generally occurred between 24 and 72 hours after initial application (see Table A). Serum fentanyl concentrations achieved are proportional to the DURAGESIC® delivery rate. With continuous use, serum fentanyl concentrations continue to rise for the first few system applications. After several sequential 72-hour applications, patients reach and maintain a steady-state serum concentration that is determined by individual variation in skin permeability and body clearance of fentanyl (see graph and Table B).

After system removal, serum fentanyl concentrations decline gradually, falling about 50% in approximately 17 (range 13-22) hours. Continued absorption of fentanyl from the skin accounts for a slower disappearance of the drug from the serum than is seen after an IV infusion, where the apparent half-life is approximately 7 (range 3–12) hours.

[See graphic above]

[See table A above]

[See table B above]

Fentanyl plasma protein binding capacity decreases with increasing ionization of the drug. Alterations in pH may affect its distribution between plasma and the central nervous system. Fentanyl accumulates in the skeletal muscle and fat and is released slowly into the blood. The average volume of distribution for fentanyl is 6 L/kg (range 3–8; N=8). In 1.5–5 year old non-opioid-tolerant pediatric patients, the fentanyl plasma levels were approximately twice as high as that of the adult patients. In older pediatric age patients, the pharmacokinetic parameters were similar to that of adults. However, these findings have been taken into consideration in determining the dosing recommendations for pediatric patients. For pediatric dosing information, refer to the DOSAGE and ADMINISTRATION section.

The kinetics of fentanyl in geriatric patients has not been well studied, but in geriatric patients the clearance of IV fentanyl may be reduced and the terminal half-life greatly prolonged (see PRECAUTIONS).

Fentanyl is metabolized primarily via human cytochrome P450 3A4 isoenzyme system. In humans the drug appears

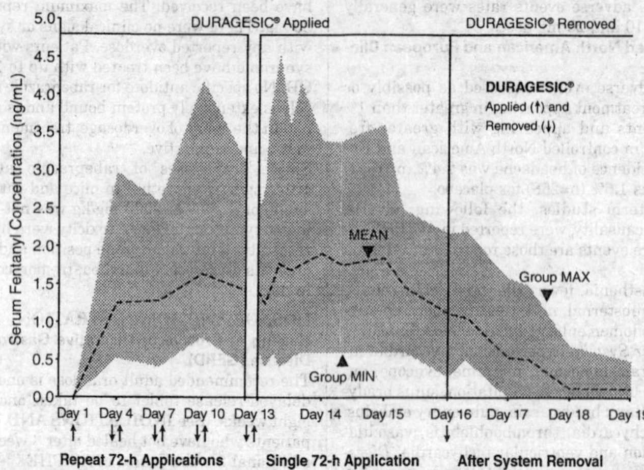

TABLE A
FENTANYL PHARMACOKINETIC PARAMETERS FOLLOWING FIRST 72-HOUR APPLICATION OF DURAGESIC®

Dose	Mean (SD) Time to Maximal Concentration T_{max} (h)	Mean (SD) Maximal Concentration C_{max} (ng/mL)
DURAGESIC® 25 µg/h	38.1 (18.0)	0.6 (0.3)
DURAGESIC® 50 µg/h	34.8 (15.4)	1.4 (0.5)
DURAGESIC® 75 µg/h	33.5 (14.5)	1.7 (0.7)
DURAGESIC® 100 µg/h	36.8 (15.7)	2.5 (1.2)

NOTE: After system removal there is continued systemic absorption from residual fentanyl in the skin so that serum concentrations fall 50%, on average, in 17 hours

TABLE B
RANGE OF PHARMACOKINETIC PARAMETERS OF INTRAVENOUS FENTANYL IN PATIENTS

	Clearance (L/h) Range [70 kg]	Volume of Distribution V_{ss} (L/kg) Range	Half-Life $t_{½}$ (h) Range
Surgical Patients	27-75	3-8	3-12
Hepatically Impaired Patients	3-80⁺	0.8-8⁺	4-12⁺
Renally Impaired Patients	30-78	—	—

⁺Estimated

NOTE: Information on volume of distribution and half-life not available for renally impaired patients.

to be metabolized primarily by oxidative N-dealkylation to norfentanyl and other inactive metabolites that do not contribute materially to the observed activity of the drug. Within 72 hours of IV fentanyl administration, approximately 75% of the dose is excreted in urine, mostly as metabolites with less than 10% representing unchanged drug. Approximately 9% of the dose is recovered in the feces, primarily as metabolites. Mean values for unbound fractions of fentanyl in plasma are estimated to be between 13 and 21%. Skin does not appear to metabolize fentanyl delivered transdermally. This was determined in a human keratinocyte cell assay and in clinical studies in which 92% of the dose delivered from the system was accounted for as unchanged fentanyl that appeared in the systemic circulation.

Pharmacodynamics

Analgesia

DURAGESIC® is a strong opioid analgesic. In controlled clinical trials in non-opioid-tolerant patients, 60 mg/day IM morphine was considered to provide analgesia approximately equivalent to DURAGESIC® 100 µg/h in an acute pain model.

Minimum effective analgesic serum concentrations of fentanyl in opioid-naive adult patients range from 0.2 to 1.2 ng/mL; side effects increase in frequency at serum levels above 2 ng/mL. Both the minimum effective concentration and the concentration at which toxicity occurs rise with increasing tolerance. The rate of development of tolerance varies widely among individuals.

Ventilatory Effects

At equivalent analgesic serum concentrations, fentanyl and morphine produce a similar degree of hypoventilation. A small number of patients have experienced clinically significant hypoventilation with DURAGESIC®. Hypoventilation was manifested by respiratory rates of less than 8 breaths/minute or a pCO_2 greater than 55 mm Hg. In clinical trials of 357 postoperative (acute pain) patients treated with DURAGESIC®, 13 patients experienced hypoventilation. In these studies the incidence of hypoventilation was higher in nontolerant women (10) than in men (3) and in patients weighing less than 63 kg (9 of 13). Although patients with impaired respiration were not common in the trials, they had higher rates of hypoventilation. In addition, postmarketing reports have been received of opioid-naive postoperative patients who have experienced clinically significant hypoventilation with DURAGESIC®. DURAGESIC® is contraindicated in the treatment of postoperative and acute pain.

While most adult and pediatric patients using DURAGESIC® chronically develop tolerance to fentanyl induced hypoventilation, episodes of slowed respirations may occur at any time during therapy; medical intervention generally was not required in these instances.

Hypoventilation can occur throughout the therapeutic range of fentanyl serum concentrations. However, in non-opioid-tolerant patients the risk of hypoventilation increases at serum fentanyl concentrations greater than 2 ng/mL, especially for patients who have an underlying pulmonary condition or who receive usual doses of opioids or other CNS drugs associated with hypoventilation in addition to DURAGESIC®. The use of initial doses in adults exceeding 25 µg/h is contraindicated in patients who are not tolerant to opioid therapy. DURAGESIC® should be administered to children only if they are opioid-tolerant and age 2 years or older.

The use of DURAGESIC® should be monitored by clinical evaluation. As with other drug level measurements, serum fentanyl concentrations may be useful clinically, although they do not reflect patient sensitivity to fentanyl and should not be used by physicians as a sole indicator of effectiveness or toxicity.

See BOX WARNING, CONTRAINDICATIONS, WARNINGS, PRECAUTIONS, ADVERSE REACTIONS and OVERDOSAGE for additional information on hypoventilation.

Cardiovascular Effects

Fentanyl may infrequently produce bradycardia. The incidence of bradycardia in clinical trials with DURAGESIC® was less than 1%.

CNS Effects

In opioid-naive patients, central nervous system effects increase when serum fentanyl concentrations are greater than 3 ng/mL.

CLINICAL TRIALS

Adults

DURAGESIC® (fentanyl transdermal system) was studied in patients with acute and chronic pain (postoperative and cancer pain models); however, DURAGESIC® is contraindicated for postoperative analgesia.

The analgesic efficacy of DURAGESIC® was demonstrated in an acute pain model with surgical procedures expected to produce various intensities of pain (eg, hysterectomy, major orthopedic surgery). Clinical use and safety was evaluated in patients experiencing chronic pain due to malignancy. Based on the results of these trials, DURAGESIC® was determined to be effective in both populations, but safe only for use in patients with chronic pain. Because of the risk of hypoventilation (4% incidence) in postoperative patients with acute pain, DURAGESIC® is contraindicated for postoperative analgesia (See BOX WARNING CLINICAL PHARMACOLOGY-Ventilatory Effects, and CONTRAINDICATIONS).

DURAGESIC® as therapy for pain due to cancer has been studied in 153 patients. In this patient population, DURAGESIC® has been administered in doses of 25 µg/h to 600 µg/h. Individual patients have used DURAGESIC® continuously for up to 866 days. At one month after initiation of DURAGESIC® therapy, patients generally reported lower pain intensity scores as compared to a prestudy analgesic regimen of oral morphine (see graph).

Visual Analogue Score of Pain Intensity Ratings at Entry in the Study and After One Month of DURAGESIC® Use

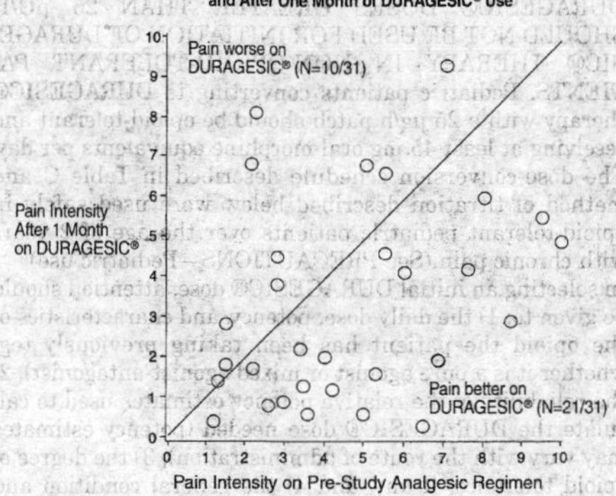

Pediatrics

The safety of DURAGESIC® was evaluated in three open-label trials in 291 pediatric patients, 2 years through 18 years of age, with chronic pain. Starting doses of 25µg/h and higher were used by 181 patients. Approximately 90% of the total daily opioid requirement (DURAGESIC® plus rescue medication) was provided by DURAGESIC®.

INDICATIONS AND USAGE

DURAGESIC® (fentanyl transdermal system) is indicated in the management of chronic pain in patients who require continuous opioid analgesia for pain that cannot be managed by lesser means such as acetaminophen-opioid combinations, non-steroidal analgesics, or PRN dosing with short-acting opioids.

DURAGESIC® should not be used in the management of acute or postoperative pain because serious or life-threatening hypoventilation could result. (See BOX WARNING and CONTRAINDICATIONS.)

In patients with chronic pain, it is possible to individually titrate the dose of the transdermal system to minimize the risk of adverse effects while providing analgesia. In properly selected patients, DURAGESIC® is a safe and effective alternative to other opioid regimens. (See DOSAGE AND ADMINISTRATION.)

CONTRAINDICATIONS

BECAUSE SERIOUS OR LIFE-THREATENING HYPOVENTILATION COULD OCCUR, DURAGESIC® (FENTANYL TRANSDERMAL SYSTEM) IS CONTRAINDICATED:

- **In the management of acute or post-operative pain, including use in out-patient surgeries because there is no opportunity for proper dose titration (See CLINICAL PHARMACOLOGY and DOSAGE AND ADMINISTRATION),**
- **In the management of mild or intermittent pain that can otherwise be managed by lesser means such as acetaminophen-opioid combinations, non-steroidal analgesics, or PRN dosing with short-acting opioids, and**
- **In doses exceeding 25 µg/h at the initiation of opioid therapy because of the need to individualize dosing by titrating to the desired analgesic effect.**

DURAGESIC® is also contraindicated in patients with known hypersensitivity to fentanyl or adhesives.

WARNINGS

The safety of DURAGESIC® (fentanyl transdermal system) has not been established in children under 2 years of age. DURAGESIC® SHOULD BE ADMINISTERED TO CHILDREN ONLY IF THEY ARE OPIOID-TOLERANT AND AGE 2 YEARS OR OLDER **(See PRECAUTIONS-Pediatric Use.)**

PATIENTS WHO HAVE EXPERIENCED ADVERSE EVENTS SHOULD BE MONITORED FOR AT LEAST 12 HOURS AFTER DURAGESIC® REMOVAL SINCE SERUM FENTANYL CONCENTRATIONS DECLINE GRADUALLY AND REACH AN APPROXIMATE 50% REDUCTION IN SERUM CONCENTRATIONS 17 HOURS AFTER SYSTEM REMOVAL.

DURAGESIC® SHOULD BE PRESCRIBED ONLY BY PERSONS KNOWLEDGEABLE IN THE CONTINUOUS ADMINISTRATION OF POTENT OPIOIDS, IN THE MANAGEMENT OF PATIENTS RECEIVING POTENT OPIOIDS FOR TREATMENT OF PAIN, AND IN THE DETECTION AND MANAGEMENT OF HYPOVENTILATION INCLUDING THE USE OF OPIOID ANTAGONISTS.

THE CONCOMITANT USE OF OTHER CENTRAL NERVOUS SYSTEM DEPRESSANTS, INCLUDING OTHER OPIOIDS, SEDATIVES OR HYPNOTICS, GENERAL ANESTHETICS, PHENOTHIAZINES, TRANQUILIZERS, SKELETAL MUSCLE RELAXANTS, SEDATING ANTIHISTAMINES, AND ALCOHOLIC BEVERAGES MAY PRODUCE ADDITIVE DEPRESSANT EFFECTS, HYPOVENTILATION, HYPOTENSION AND PROFOUND SEDATION OR COMA MAY OCCUR. WHEN SUCH COMBINED THERAPY IS CONTEMPLATED, THE DOSE OF ONE OR BOTH AGENTS SHOULD BE REDUCED BY AT LEAST 50%.

ALL PATIENTS AND THEIR CAREGIVERS SHOULD BE ADVISED TO AVOID EXPOSING THE DURAGESIC® APPLICATION SITE TO DIRECT EXTERNAL HEAT SOURCES, SUCH AS HEATING PADS OR ELECTRIC BLANKETS, HEAT LAMPS, SAUNAS, HOT TUBS, AND HEATED WATER BEDS, ETC., WHILE WEARING THE SYSTEM. THERE IS A POTENTIAL FOR TEMPERATURE-DEPENDENT INCREASES IN FENTANYL RELEASE FROM THE SYSTEM. (See PRECAUTIONS—Patients with Fever/External Heat.)

PRECAUTIONS

General

DURAGESIC® (fentanyl transdermal system) doses greater than 25 µg/h are too high for initiation of therapy in non-opioid-tolerant patients and should not be used to begin DURAGESIC® therapy in these patients. Children converting to DURAGESIC® should be opioid-tolerant (See BOX WARNING).

DURAGESIC® may impair mental and/or physical ability required for the performance of potentially hazardous tasks (eg, driving, operating machinery). Patients who have been given DURAGESIC® should not drive or operate dangerous machinery unless they are tolerant to the side effects of the drug.

Patients and their caregivers should be instructed to keep both used and unused systems out of the reach of children. Used systems should be folded so that the adhesive side of the system adheres to itself and flushed down the toilet immediately upon removal. Patients should be advised to dispose of any systems remaining from a prescription as soon as they are no longer needed. Unused systems should be removed from their pouch and flushed down the toilet.

Hypoventilation (Respiratory Depression)

Hypoventilation may occur at any time during the use of DURAGESIC®.

Because significant amounts of fentanyl are absorbed from the skin for 17 hours or more after the system is removed, hypoventilation may persist beyond the removal of DURAGESIC®. Consequently, patients with hypoventilation should be carefully observed for degree of sedation and their respiratory rate monitored until respiration has stabilized.

The use of concomitant CNS active drugs requires special patient care and observation. (See WARNINGS.)

Chronic Pulmonary Disease

Because potent opioids can cause hypoventilation, DURAGESIC® should be administered with caution to patients with pre-existing medical conditions predisposing them to hypoventilation. In such patients, normal analgesic doses of opioids may further decrease respiratory drive to the point of respiratory failure.

Head Injuries and Increased Intracranial Pressure

DURAGESIC® should not be used in patients who may be particularly susceptible to the intracranial effects of CO_2 retention such as those with evidence of increased intracranial pressure, impaired consciousness, or coma. Opioids may obscure the clinical course of patients with head injury. DURAGESIC® should be used with caution in patients with brain tumors.

Cardiac Disease

Fentanyl may produce bradycardia. Fentanyl should be administered with caution to patients with bradyarrhythmias.

Hepatic or Renal Disease

At the present time insufficient information exists to make recommendations regarding the use of DURAGESIC® in patients with impaired renal or hepatic function. If the drug is used in these patients, it should be used with caution because of the hepatic metabolism and renal excretion of fentanyl.

Patients with Fever/External Heat

Based on a pharmacokinetic model, serum fentanyl concentrations could theoretically increase by approximately one-third for patients with a body temperature of 40°C (104°F) due to temperature-dependent increases in fentanyl release from the system and increased skin permeability. Therefore, patients wearing DURAGESIC® systems who develop fever should be monitored for opioid side effects and the DURAGESIC® dose should be adjusted if necessary.

ALL PATIENTS AND THEIR CAREGIVERS SHOULD BE ADVISED TO AVOID EXPOSING THE DURAGESIC® APPLICATION SITE TO DIRECT EXTERNAL HEAT SOURCES, SUCH AS HEATING PADS OR ELECTRIC BLANKETS, HEAT LAMPS, SAUNAS, HOT TUBS, AND HEATED WATER BEDS, ETC., WHILE WEARING THE SYSTEM. THERE IS A POTENTIAL FOR TEMPERATURE-DEPENDENT INCREASES IN FENTANYL RELEASE FROM THE SYSTEM.

Drug Interactions

Central Nervous System Depressants

When patients are receiving DURAGESIC®, the dose of additional opioids or other CNS depressant drugs (including benzodiazepines) should be reduced by at least 50%. With the concomitant use of CNS depressants, hypotension may occur.

Agents Affecting Cytochrome P450 3A4 Isoenzyme System

CYP3A4 Inhibitors: Since the metabolism of fentanyl is mediated by the CYP3A4 isozyme, coadministration of drugs that inhibit CYP3A4 activity may cause decreased clearance of fentanyl. The expected clinical results would be increased or prolonged opioid effects. Thus patients coadministered with inhibitors of CYP3A4 such as macrolide antibiotics (e.g., erythromycin), azole antifungal agents (e.g., ketoconazole), and protease inhibitors (e.g., ritanovir) while receiving DURAGESIC® should be carefully monitored and dosage adjustment made if warranted.

CYP3A4 Inducers: Cytochrome P450 inducers, such as rifampin, carbamazepine, and phenytoin, induce metabolism and as such may cause increased clearance of fentanyl. Caution is advised when administering DURAGESIC® to patients receiving these medications and if necessary dose adjustments should be considered.

Drug or Alcohol Dependence

Use of DURAGESIC® in combination with alcoholic beverages and/or other CNS depressants can result in increased risk to the patient. DURAGESIC® should be used with caution in individuals who have a history of drug or alcohol abuse, especially if they are outside a medically controlled environment.

Ambulatory Patients

Strong opioid analgesics impair the mental or physical abilities required for the performance of potentially dangerous tasks such as driving a car or operating machinery. Patients who have been given DURAGESIC® should not drive or operate dangerous machinery unless they are tolerant to the effects of the drug.

Carcinogenesis, Mutagenesis, and Impairment of Fertility

Because long-term animal studies have not been conducted, the potential carcinogenic effects of DURAGESIC® are unknown. There was no evidence of mutagenicity in the Ames *Salmonella typhimurium* assay, the primary rat hepatocyte unscheduled DNA synthesis assay, the BALB/c-3T3 transformation test, the mouse lymphoma assay, the human lymphocyte and CHO chromosomal aberration in-vitro assays, or the in-vivo micronucleus test.

Pregnancy—Pregnancy Category C

Fentanyl has been shown to impair fertility and to have an embryocidal effect in rats when given in intravenous doses 0.3 times the human dose for a period of 12 days. No evidence of teratogenic effects has been observed after administration of fentanyl to rats. There are no adequate and well-controlled studies in pregnant women. DURAGESIC® should be used during pregnancy only if the potential benefit justifies the potential risk to the fetus.

Labor and Delivery

DURAGESIC® is not recommended for analgesia during labor and delivery.

Nursing Mothers

Fentanyl is excreted in human milk; therefore DURAGESIC® is not recommended for use in nursing women because of the possibility of effects in their infants.

Pediatric Use

DURAGESIC® was not studied in children under 2 years of age. DURAGESIC® should be administered to children only if they are opioid tolerant and age 2 years or older. (See DOSAGE AND ADMINISTRATION and BOX WARNING).

To guard against accidental ingestion by children, use caution when choosing the application site for DURAGESIC® (See DOSAGE and ADMINISTRATION) and monitor adhesion of the system closely.

Geriatric Use

Information from a pilot study of the pharmacokinetics of IV fentanyl in geriatric patients indicates that the clearance of fentanyl may be greatly decreased in the population above the age of 60. The relevance of these findings to transdermal fentanyl is unknown at this time.

Since elderly, cachectic, or debilitated patients may have altered pharmacokinetics due to poor fat stores, muscle wasting, or altered clearance, they should not be started on DURAGESIC® doses higher than 25 µg/h unless they are already taking more than 135 mg of oral morphine a day or an equivalent dose of another opioid (see DOSAGE AND ADMINISTRATION).

Information for Patients

A patient instruction sheet is included in the package of DURAGESIC® systems dispensed to the patient.

Disposal of DURAGESIC®

DURAGESIC® should be kept out of the reach of children. DURAGESIC® systems should be folded so that the adhesive side of the system adheres to itself, then the system should be flushed down the toilet immediately upon removal. Patients should dispose of any systems remaining

Continued on next page

Duragesic—Cont.

from a prescription as soon as they are no longer needed. Unused systems should be removed from their pouches and flushed down the toilet.

IF THE GEL FROM THE DRUG RESERVOIR ACCIDENTALLY CONTACTS THE SKIN, THE AREA SHOULD BE WASHED WITH CLEAR WATER.

ADVERSE REACTIONS

In post-marketing experience, deaths from hypoventilation due to inappropriate use of DURAGESIC® (fentanyl transdermal system) have been reported. (See BOX WARNING and CONTRAINDICATIONS.)

Pre-marketing Clinical Trial Experience:

In adults, the safety of DURAGESIC® has been evaluated in 357 postoperative patients and 153 cancer patients for a total of 510 patients. Patients with acute pain used DURAGESIC® for 1 to 3 days. The duration of DURAGESIC® use varied in cancer patients; 56% of patients used DURAGESIC® for over 30 days, 28% continued treatment for more than 4 months, and 10% used DURAGESIC® for more than 1 year.

Hypoventilation was the most serious adverse reaction observed in 13 (4%) postoperative patients and in 3 (2%) of the cancer patients. Hypotension and hypertension were observed in 11 (3%) and 4 (1%) of the opioid-naive patients.

Various adverse events were reported; a causal relationship to DURAGESIC® was not always determined. The frequencies presented here reflect the actual frequency of each adverse effect in patients who received DURAGESIC®. There has been no attempt to correct for a placebo effect, concomitant use of other opioids, or to subtract the frequencies reported by placebo-treated patients in controlled trials.

Adverse reactions reported in 153 cancer patients at a frequency of 1% or greater are presented in Table 1; similar reactions were seen in the 357 postoperative patients studied.

In the pediatric population, the safety of DURAGESIC® has been evaluated in 291 patients ages 2-18 years with chronic pain. The duration of DURAGESIC® use varied; 20% of pediatric patients were treated for ≤ 15 days; 46% for 16-30 days; 16% for 31-60 days; and 17% for at least 61 days. Twenty-five patients were treated with DURAGESIC® for at least 4 months and 9 patients for more than 9 months.

There was no apparent pediatric-specific risk associated with DURAGESIC® use in children as young as 2 years old when used as directed.

The most common adverse events were fever (35%), vomiting (33%), and nausea (24%).

Adverse events reported in pediatric patients at a rate of ≥ 1% are presented in Table 1.

[See table 1 below]

The following adverse effects have been reported in less than 1% of the 510 adult postoperative and cancer patients studied; the association between these events and DURAGESIC® administration is unknown. This information is listed to serve as alerting information for the physician.

Cardiovascular: bradycardia

Digestive: abdominal distention

Nervous: aphasia, hypertonia, vertigo, stupor, hypotonia, depersonalization, hostility

Respiratory: stertorous breathing, asthma, respiratory disorder

Skin and Appendages, General: exfoliative dermatitis, pustules

Special Senses: amblyopia

Urogenital: bladder pain, oliguria, urinary frequency

Post-Marketing Experience—Adults:

The following adverse reactions reported to have been observed in association with the use of DURAGESIC® and not reported in the pre-marketing adverse reactions section above include:

Body as a Whole: edema

Cardiovascular: tachycardia

Metabolic and Nutritional: weight loss

Special Senses: blurred vision

DRUG ABUSE AND DEPENDENCE

Fentanyl is a Schedule II controlled substance and can produce drug dependence similar to that produced by morphine. DURAGESIC® (fentanyl transdermal system) therefore has the potential for abuse. Tolerance, physical and psychological dependence may develop upon repeated administration of opioids. Iatrogenic addiction following opioid administration is relatively rare. Physicians should not let concerns of physical dependence deter them from using adequate amounts of opioids in the management of severe pain when such use is indicated.

OVERDOSAGE

Clinical Presentation

The manifestations of fentanyl overdosage are an extension of its pharmacologic actions with the most serious significant effect being hypoventilation.

Treatment

For the management of hypoventilation immediate countermeasures include removing the DURAGESIC® (fentanyl transdermal system) system and physically or verbally stimulating the patient. These actions can be followed by administration of a specific narcotic antagonist such as naloxone. The duration of hypoventilation following an overdose may be longer than the effects of the narcotic antagonist's action (the half-life of naloxone ranges from 30 to 81 minutes). The interval between IV antagonist doses should be carefully chosen because of the possibility of re-narcotization after system removal; repeated administration of naloxone may be necessary. Reversal of the narcotic effect may result in acute onset of pain and the release of catecholamines.

If the clinical situation warrants, ensure a patent airway is established and maintained, administer oxygen and assist or control respiration as indicated and use an oropharyngeal airway or endotracheal tube if necessary. Adequate body temperature and fluid intake should be maintained.

If severe or persistent hypotension occurs, the possibility of hypovolemia should be considered and managed with appropriate parenteral fluid therapy.

DOSAGE AND ADMINISTRATION

With all opioids, the safety of patients using the products is dependent on health care practitioners prescribing them in strict conformity with their approved labeling with respect to patient selection, dosing, and proper conditions for use.

As with all opioids, dosage should be individualized. The most important factor to be considered in determining the appropriate dose is the extent of pre-existing opioid tolerance. (See BOX WARNING and CONTRAINDICATIONS.) Initial doses should be reduced in elderly or debilitated patients (see PRECAUTIONS).

DURAGESIC® (fentanyl transdermal system) should be applied to non-irritated and non-irradiated skin on a flat surface such as chest, back, flank or upper arm. In young children, adhesion should be monitored and the upper back is the preferred location to minimize the potential of the child removing the patch. Hair at the application site should be clipped (not shaved) prior to system application. If the site of DURAGESIC® application must be cleansed prior to application of the system, do so with clear water. Do not use soaps, oils, lotions, alcohol, or any other agents that might irritate the skin or alter its characteristics. Allow the skin to dry completely prior to system application.

DURAGESIC® should be applied immediately upon removal from the sealed package. Do not alter the system (eg, cut) in any way prior to application.

The transdermal system should be pressed firmly in place with the palm of the hand for 30 seconds, making sure the contact is complete, especially around the edges.

Each DURAGESIC® may be worn continuously for 72 hours. If analgesia for more than 72 hours is required, a new system should be applied to a different skin site after removal of the previous transdermal system.

DURAGESIC® should be kept out of the reach of children. Used systems should be folded so that the adhesive side of the system adheres to itself, then the system should be flushed down the toilet immediately upon removal. Patients should dispose of any systems remaining from a prescription as soon as they are no longer needed. Unused systems should be removed from their pouches and flushed down the toilet.

Dose Selection

DOSES MUST BE INDIVIDUALIZED BASED UPON THE STATE OF EACH PATIENT AND SHOULD BE ASSESSED AT REGULAR INTERVALS AFTER DURAGESIC® APPLICATION. REDUCED DOSES OF DURAGESIC® ARE SUGGESTED FOR THE ELDERLY AND OTHER GROUPS DISCUSSED IN PRECAUTIONS.

DURAGESIC® DOSES GREATER THAN 25 µG/H SHOULD NOT BE USED FOR INITIATION OF DURAGESIC® THERAPY IN NON-OPIOID-TOLERANT PATIENTS. Pediatric patients converting to DURAGESIC® therapy with a 25 µg/h patch should be opioid-tolerant and receiving at least 45 mg oral morphine equivalents per day. The dose-conversion schedule described in Table C and method of titration described below were used safely in opioid-tolerant pediatric patients over the age of 2 years with chronic pain (See PRECAUTIONS—Pediatric use)

In selecting an initial DURAGESIC® dose, attention should be given to: 1) the daily dose, potency, and characteristics of the opioid the patient has been taking previously (eg, whether it is a pure agonist or mixed agonist-antagonist), 2) the reliability of the relative potency estimates used to calculate the DURAGESIC® dose needed (potency estimates may vary with the route of administration), 3) the degree of opioid tolerance, if any, and 4) the general condition and medical status of the patient. Each patient should be maintained at the lowest dose providing acceptable pain control.

Initial DURAGESIC® Dose Selection

There has been no systematic evaluation of DURAGESIC® as an initial opioid analgesic in the management of chronic pain, since most patients in the clinical trials were converted to DURAGESIC® from other narcotics. Therefore, unless the patient has pre-existing opioid tolerance, the lowest DURAGESIC® dose, 25 µg/h, should be used as the initial dose.

To convert adult and pediatric patients from oral or parenteral opioids to DURAGESIC® use the following methodology:

1. Calculate the previous 24-hour analgesic requirement.
2. Convert this amount to the equianalgesic oral morphine dose using Table C.
3. Table D displays the range of 24-hour oral morphine doses that are recommended for conversion to each DURAGESIC® dose. Use this table to find the calculated 24-hour morphine dose and the corresponding DURAGESIC® dose. Initiate DURAGESIC® treatment using the recommended dose and titrate patients upwards (no more frequently than every 3 days after the initial dose or than every 6 days thereafter) until analgesic efficacy is attained. The recommended starting dose when converting from other opioids to DURAGESIC® is likely too low for 50% of patients. This starting dose is recommended to minimize the potential for overdosing patients with the first dose. For delivery rates in excess of 100 µg/h, multiple systems may be used.

TABLE C[a]
EQUIANALGESIC POTENCY CONVERSION

Name	Equianalgesic Dose (mg) IM[b,c]	PO
Morphine	10	60 (30)[d]
Hydromorphone (Dilaudid®)	1.5	7.5
Methadone (Dolophine®)	10	20
Oxycodone	15	30
Levorphanol (Levo-Dromoran®)	2	4
Oxymorphone (Numorphan®)	1	10 (PR)
Meperidine (Demerol®)	75	—
Codeine	130	200

[a] All IM and PO doses in this chart are considered equivalent to 10 mg of IM morphine in analgesic effect. IM denotes intramuscular, PO oral, and PR rectal.

[b] Based on single-dose studies in which an intramuscular dose of each drug listed was compared with morphine to establish the relative potency. Oral doses are those rec-

TABLE 1: ADVERSE EVENTS (at rate of ≥ 1%)
Adult (N = 153) and Pediatric (N = 291) Pre-Marketing Clinical Trial Experience

Body System	Adults	Pediatrics
Body as a Whole	Abdominal pain*, headache*	Pain*, headache*, fever, syncope, abdominal pain, allergic reaction, flushing
Cardiovascular	Arrhythmia, chest pain	Hypertension, tachycardia
Digestive	Nausea**, vomiting**, constipation**, dry mouth**, anorexia*, diarrhea*, dyspepsia*, flatulence	Nausea**, vomiting**, constipation*, dry mouth, diarrhea
Nervous	Somnolence**, confusion**, asthenia**, dizziness*, nervousness*, hallucinations*, anxiety*, depression*, euphoria*, tremor, abnormal coordination, speech disorder, abnormal thinking, abnormal gait, abnormal dreams, agitation, paresthesia, amnesia, syncope, paranoid reaction	Somnolence*, nervousness*, insomnia*, asthenia*, hallucinations, anxiety, depression, convulsions, dizziness, tremor, speech disorder, agitation, stupor, confusion, paranoid reaction
Respiratory	Dyspnea*, hypoventilation*, hemoptysis, pharyngitis, hiccups	Dyspnea, respiratory depression, rhinitis, coughing
Skin and Appendages	Sweating**, pruritus*, rash, application site reaction—erythema, papules, itching, edema	Pruritus*, application site reaction*, sweating increased, rash, rash erythematous, skin reaction localized
Urogenital	Urinary retention*	Urinary retention

*Reactions occurring in 3%-10% of DURAGESIC® patients
**Reactions occurring in 10% or more of DURAGESIC® patients

ommended when changing from parenteral to an oral route. Reference: Foley, K.M. (1985) The treatment of cancer pain. NEJM 313(2):84-95.

[c] Although controlled studies are not available, in clinical practice it is customary to consider the doses of opioid given IM, IV or subcutaneously to be equivalent. There may be some differences in pharmacokinetic parameters such as C_{max} and T_{max}.

[d] The conversion ratio of 10 mg parenteral morphine = 30 mg oral morphine is based on clinical experience in patients with chronic pain. The conversion ratio of 10 mg parenteral morphine = 60 mg oral morphine is based on a potency study in acute pain. Reference: Ashburn and Lipman (1993) Management of pain in the cancer patient. Anesth Analg 76:402-416.

TABLE D[1]
RECOMMENDED INITIAL DURAGESIC® DOSE BASED UPON DAILY ORAL MORPHINE DOSE

Oral 24-hour Morphine (mg/day)	DURAGESIC® Dose (μg/h)
45-134[2]	25
135-224	50
225-314	75
315-404	100
405-494	125
495-584	150
585-674	175
675-764	200
765-854	225
855-944	250
945-1034	275
1035-1124	300

NOTE: In clinical trials these ranges of daily oral morphine doses were used as a basis for conversion to DURAGESIC®.

[1] THIS TABLE SHOULD NOT BE USED TO CONVERT FROM DURAGESIC® TO OTHER THERAPIES, BECAUSE THIS CONVERSION TO DURAGESIC® IS CONSERVATIVE. USE OF TABLE D FOR CONVERSION TO OTHER ANALGESIC THERAPIES CAN OVERESTIMATE THE DOSE OF THE NEW AGENT. OVERDOSAGE OF THE NEW ANALGESIC AGENT IS POSSIBLE. (See DOSAGE AND ADMINISTRATION—Discontinuation of DURAGESIC®.)

[2] PEDIATRIC PATIENTS INITIATING THERAPY ON A 25 μG/H DURAGESIC® SYSTEM SHOULD BE OPIOID-TOLERANT AND RECEIVING AT LEAST 45 MG ORAL MORPHINE EQUIVALENTS PER DAY.

The majority of patients are adequately maintained with DURAGESIC® administered every 72 hours. A small number of patients may not achieve adequate analgesia using this dosing interval and may require systems to be applied every 48 hours rather than every 72 hours. An increase in the DURAGESIC® dose should be evaluated before changing dosing intervals in order to maintain patients on a 72-hour regimen. Dosing intervals less than every 72 hours were not studied in children and adolescents and are not recommended.

Because of the increase in serum fentanyl concentration over the first 24 hours following initial system application, the initial evaluation of the maximum analgesic effect of DURAGESIC® cannot be made before 24 hours of wearing. The initial DURAGESIC® dosage may be increased after 3 days (see Dose Titration).

During the initial application of DURAGESIC®, patients should use short-acting analgesics as needed until analgesic efficacy with DURAGESIC® is attained. Thereafter, some patients still may require periodic supplemental doses of other short-acting analgesics for 'breakthrough' pain.

Dose Titration

The recommended initial DURAGESIC® dose based upon the daily oral morphine dose is conservative, and 50% of patients are likely to require a dose increase after initial application of DURAGESIC®. The initial DURAGESIC® dosage may be increased after 3 days based on the daily dose of supplemental analgesics required by the patient in the second or third day of the initial application.

Physicians are advised that it may take up to 6 days after increasing the dose of DURAGESIC® for the patient to reach equilibrium on the new dose (see graph in CLINICAL PHARMACOLOGY). Therefore, patients should wear a higher dose through two applications before any further increase in dosage is made on the basis of the average daily use of a supplemental analgesic.

Appropriate dosage increments should be based on the daily dose of supplementary opioids, using the ratio of 90 mg/24 hours of oral morphine to a 25 μg/h increase in DURAGESIC® dose.

Discontinuation of DURAGESIC®

To convert patients to another opioid, remove DURAGESIC® and titrate the dose of the new analgesic based upon the patient's report of pain until adequate analgesia has been attained. Upon system removal, 17 hours or more are required for a 50% decrease in serum fentanyl concentrations. Opioid withdrawal symptoms (such as nausea, vomiting, diarrhea, anxiety, and shivering) are possible in some patients after conversion or dose adjustment. For patients requiring discontinuation of opioids, a gradual downward titration is recommended since it is not known at what dose level the opioid may be discontinued without producing the signs and symptoms of abrupt withdrawal.

TABLE D SHOULD NOT BE USED TO CONVERT FROM DURAGESIC® TO OTHER THERAPIES. BECAUSE THE CONVERSION TO DURAGESIC® IS CONSERVATIVE, USE OF TABLE D FOR CONVERSION TO OTHER ANALGESIC THERAPIES CAN OVERESTIMATE THE DOSE OF THE NEW AGENT. OVERDOSAGE OF THE NEW ANALGESIC AGENT IS POSSIBLE.

HOW SUPPLIED

DURAGESIC® (fentanyl transdermal system) is supplied in cartons containing 5 individually packaged systems. See chart for information regarding individual systems.

DURAGESIC® Dose (μg/h)	System Size (cm^2)	Fentanyl Content (mg)	NDC Number
DURAGESIC®-25	10	2.5	50458-033-05
DURAGESIC®-50*	20	5	50458-034-05
DURAGESIC®-75*	30	7.5	50458-035-05
DURAGESIC®-100*	40	10	50458-036-05

* FOR USE ONLY IN OPIOID TOLERANT PATIENTS.

Safety and Handling

DURAGESIC® is supplied in sealed transdermal systems which pose little risk of exposure to health care workers. If the gel from the drug reservoir accidentally contacts the skin, the area should be washed with copious amounts of water. Do not use soap, alcohol, or other solvents to remove the gel because they may enhance the drug's ability to penetrate the skin. Do not cut or damage DURAGESIC®. If the DURAGESIC® system is cut or damaged, controlled drug delivery will not be possible.

KEEP DURAGESIC® OUT OF THE REACH OF CHILDREN

Do not store above 77°F (25°C). Apply immediately after removal from individually sealed package. Do not use if the seal is broken. **For transdermal use only.**

Rx only

DEA order form required. A schedule CII narcotic.

Manufactured by: 7500316
ALZA Corporation, Revised May 2003
Mountain View, CA 94043 © Janssen 2003

Distributed by:
Janssen Pharmaceutica Products, L.P.
Titusville, NJ 08560

Shown in Product Identification Guide, page 319

NIZORAL® ℞

[*nī 'zōr-ăl*]
(ketoconazole)
Tablets

WARNING: When used orally, ketoconazole has been associated with hepatic toxicity, including some fatalities. Patients receiving this drug should be informed by the physician of the risk and should be closely monitored. See WARNINGS and PRECAUTIONS sections.

Coadministration of terfenadine with ketoconazole tablets is contraindicated. Rare cases of serious cardiovascular adverse events, including death, ventricular tachycardia and torsades de pointes have been observed in patients taking ketoconazole tablets concomitantly with terfenadine, due to increased terfenadine concentrations induced by ketoconazole tablets. See CONTRAINDICATIONS, WARNINGS, and PRECAUTIONS sections.

Pharmacokinetic data indicate that oral ketoconazole inhibits the metabolism of astemizole, resulting in elevated plasma levels of astemizole and its active metabolite desmethylastemizole which may prolong QT intervals. Coadministration of astemizole with ketoconazole tablets is therefore contraindicated. See CONTRAINDICATIONS, WARNINGS, and PRECAUTIONS sections.

Coadministration of cisapride with ketoconazole is contraindicated. Serious cardiovascular adverse events including ventricular tachycardia, ventricular fibrillation and torsades de pointes have occurred in patients taking ketoconazole concomitantly with cisapride. See CONTRAINDICATIONS, WARNINGS, and PRECAUTIONS sections.

DESCRIPTION

NIZORAL® (ketoconazole) is a synthetic broad-spectrum antifungal agent available in scored white tablets, each containing 200 mg ketoconazole base for oral administration. Inactive ingredients are colloidal silicon dioxide, corn starch, lactose, magnesium stearate, microcrystalline cellulose, and povidone. Ketoconazole is cis-1-acetyl-4-[4-[[2-(2,4-dichlorophenyl)-2-(1H-imidazol-1-ylmethyl)-1,3-dioxolan-4-yl] methoxyl]phenyl] piperazine and has the following structural formula:.

Ketoconazole is a white to slightly beige, odorless powder, soluble in acids, with a molecular weight of 531.44.

CLINICAL PHARMACOLOGY

Mean peak plasma levels of approximately 3.5 μg/mL are reached within 1 to 2 hours, following oral administration of a single 200 mg dose taken with a meal. Subsequent plasma elimination is biphasic with a half-life of 2 hours during the first 10 hours and 8 hours thereafter. Following absorption from the gastrointestinal tract, NIZORAL® (ketoconazole) is converted into several inactive metabolites. The major identified metabolic pathways are oxidation and degradation of the imidazole and piperazine rings, oxidative O-dealkylation and aromatic hydroxylation. About 13% of the dose is excreted in the urine, of which 2 to 4% is unchanged drug. The major route of excretion is through the bile into the intestinal tract. *In vitro*, the plasma protein binding is about 99% mainly to the albumin fraction. Only a negligible proportion of ketoconazole reaches the cerebral-spinal fluid. Ketoconazole is a weak dibasic agent and thus requires acidity for dissolution and absorption.

NIZORAL® Tablets are active against clinical infections with *Blastomyces dermatitidis, Candida spp., Coccidioides immitis, Histoplasma capsulatum, Paracoccidioides brasiliensis,* and *Phialophora spp.* NIZORAL® Tablets are also active against *Trichophyton spp., Epidermophyton spp.,* and *Microsporum spp.* Ketoconazole is also active *in vitro* against a variety of fungi and yeast. In animal models, activity has been demonstrated against *Candida spp., Blastomyces dermatitidis, Histoplasma capsulatum, Malassezia furfur, Coccidioides immitis,* and *Cryptococcus neoformans.*

Mode of Action: *In vitro* studies suggest that ketoconazole impairs the synthesis of ergosterol, which is a vital component of fungal cell membranes.

INDICATIONS AND USAGE

NIZORAL® (ketoconazole) Tablets are indicated for the treatment of the following systemic fungal infections: candidiasis, chronic mucocutaneous candidiasis, oral thrush, candiduria, blastomycosis, coccidioidomycosis, histoplasmosis, chromomycosis, and paracoccidioidomycosis. NIZORAL® Tablets should not be used for fungal meningitis because it penetrates poorly into the cerebral-spinal fluid.

NIZORAL® Tablets are also indicated for the treatment of patients with severe recalcitrant cutaneous dermatophyte infections who have not responded to topical therapy or oral griseofulvin, or who are unable to take griseofulvin.

CONTRAINDICATIONS

Coadministration of terfenadine or astemizole with ketoconazole tablets is contraindicated. (See BOX WARNING, WARNINGS, and PRECAUTIONS sections.)

Concomitant administration of NIZORAL® Tablets with cisapride is contraindicated. (See BOX WARNING, WARNINGS, and PRECAUTIONS sections.)

Concomitant administration of NIZORAL® Tablets with oral triazolam is contraindicated. (See PRECAUTIONS section.)

NIZORAL® is contraindicated in patients who have shown hypersensitivity to the drug.

WARNINGS

Hepatotoxicity, primarily of the hepatocellular type, has been associated with the use of NIZORAL® (ketoconazole) Tablets, including rare fatalities. The reported incidence of hepatotoxicity has been about 1:10,000 exposed patients, but this probably represents some degree of under-reporting, as is the case for most reported adverse reactions to drugs. The median duration of NIZORAL® Tablet therapy in patients who developed symptomatic hepatotoxicity was about 28 days, although the range extended to as low as 3 days. The hepatic injury has usually, but not always, been reversible upon discontinuation of NIZORAL® Tablet treatment. Several cases of hepatitis have been reported in children.

Prompt recognition of liver injury is essential. Liver function tests (such as SGGT, alkaline phosphatase, SGPT, SGOT and bilirubin) should be measured before starting treatment and at frequent intervals during treatment. Patients receiving NIZORAL® Tablets concurrently with other potentially hepatotoxic drugs should be carefully monitored, particularly those patients requiring prolonged therapy or those who have had a history of liver disease.

Most of the reported cases of hepatic toxicity have to date been in patients treated for onychomycosis. Of 180 patients worldwide developing idiosyncratic liver dysfunction during NIZORAL® Tablet therapy, 61.3% had onychomycosis and 16.8% had chronic recalcitrant dermatophytoses.

Transient minor elevations in liver enzymes have occurred during treatment with NIZORAL® Tablets. The drug should be discontinued if these persist, if the abnormalities worsen, or if the abnormalities become accompanied by symptoms of possible liver injury.

Continued on next page

Nizoral—Cont.

In rare cases anaphylaxis has been reported after the first dose. Several cases of hypersensitivity reactions including urticaria have also been reported.
Coadministration of ketoconazole tablets and terfenadine has led to elevated plasma concentrations of terfenadine which may prolong QT intervals, sometimes resulting in life-threatening cardiac dysrhythmias. Cases of torsades de pointes and other serious ventricular dysrhythmias, in rare cases leading to fatality, have been reported among patients taking terfenadine concurrently with ketoconazole tablets. Coadministration of ketoconazole tablets and terfenadine is contraindicated.
Coadministration of astemizole with ketoconazole tablets is contraindicated. (See BOX WARNING, CONTRAINDICATIONS, and PRECAUTIONS sections.)
Concomitant administration of NIZORAL® Tablets with cisapride is contraindicated because it has resulted in markedly elevated cisapride plasma concentrations and prolonged QT interval, and has rarely been associated with ventricular arrhythmias and torsades de pointes. (See BOX WARNINGS, CONTRAINDICATIONS and PRECAUTIONS sections.)
In European clinical trials involving 350 patients with metastatic prostatic cancer, eleven deaths were reported within two weeks of starting treatment with high doses of ketoconazole tablets (1200 mg/day). It is not possible to ascertain from the information available whether death was related to ketoconazole therapy in these patients with serious underlying disease. However, high doses of ketoconazole tablets are known to suppress adrenal corticosteroid secretion.
In female rats treated three to six months with ketoconazole at dose levels of 80 mg/kg and higher, increased fragility of long bones, in some cases leading to fracture, was seen. The maximum "no-effect" dose level in these studies was 20 mg/kg (2.5 times the maximum recommended human dose). The mechanism responsible for this phenomenon is obscure. Limited studies in dogs failed to demonstrate such an effect on the metacarpals and ribs.

PRECAUTIONS

General: NIZORAL® (ketoconazole) Tablets have been demonstrated to lower serum testosterone. Once therapy with NIZORAL® Tablets has been discontinued, serum testosterone levels return to baseline values. Testosterone levels are impaired with doses of 800 mg per day and abolished by 1600 mg per day. NIZORAL® Tablets also decrease ACTH induced corticosteroid serum levels at similar high doses. The recommended dose of 200 mg–400 mg daily should be followed closely.
In four subjects with drug-induced achlorhydria, a marked reduction in ketoconazole absorption was observed. NIZORAL® Tablets require acidity for dissolution. If concomitant antacids, anticholinergics, and H_2-blockers are needed, they should be given at least two hours after administration of NIZORAL® Tablets. In cases of achlorhydria, the patients should be instructed to dissolve each tablet in 4 mL aqueous solution of 0.2 N HCl. For ingesting the resulting mixture, they should use a drinking straw so as to avoid contact with the teeth. This administration should be followed with a cup of tap water.
Information for Patients: Patients should be instructed to report any signs and symptoms which may suggest liver dysfunction so that appropriate biochemical testing can be done. Such signs and symptoms may include unusual fatigue, anorexia, nausea and/or vomiting, jaundice, dark urine or pale stools (see WARNINGS section).
Drug Interactions: Ketoconazole is a potent inhibitor of the cytochrome P450 3A4 enzyme system. Coadministration of NIZORAL® Tablets and drugs primarily metabolized by the cytochrome P450 3A4 enzyme system may result in increased plasma concentrations of the drugs that could increase or prolong both therapeutic and adverse effects. Therefore, unless otherwise specified, appropriate dosage adjustments may be necessary. The following drug interactions have been identified involving NIZORAL® Tablets and other drugs metabolized by the cytochrome P450 3A4 enzyme system.
Ketoconazole tablets inhibit the metabolism of terfenadine, resulting in an increased plasma concentration of terfenadine and a delay in the elimination of its acid metabolite. The increased plasma concentration of terfenadine or its metabolite may result in prolonged QT intervals. (See BOX WARNING, CONTRAINDICATIONS, and WARNINGS sections.)
Pharmacokinetic data indicate that oral ketoconazole inhibits the metabolism of astemizole, resulting in elevated plasma levels of astemizole and its active metabolite desmethylastemizole which may prolong QT intervals. Coadministration of astemizole with ketoconazole tablets is therefore contraindicated. (See BOX WARNING, CONTRAINDICATIONS, and WARNINGS sections.)
Human pharmacokinetics data indicate that oral ketoconazole potently inhibits the metabolism of cisapride resulting in a mean eight-fold increase in AUC of cisapride. Data suggest that coadministration of oral ketoconazole and cisapride can result in prolongation of the QT interval on the ECG. Therefore concomitant administration of ketoconazole tablets with cisapride is contraindicated. (See BOX WARNING, CONTRAINDICATIONS, and WARNINGS sections.)
Ketoconazole tablets may alter the metabolism of cyclosporine, tacrolimus, and methylprednisolone, resulting in elevated plasma concentrations of the latter drugs. Dosage adjustment may be required if cyclosporine, tacrolimus, or methylprednisolone are given concomitantly with NIZORAL® Tablets.
Coadministration of NIZORAL® Tablets with midazolam or triazolam has resulted in elevated plasma concentrations of the latter two drugs. This may potentiate and prolong hypnotic and sedative effects, especially with repeated dosing or chronic administration of these agents. These agents should not be used in patients treated with NIZORAL® Tablets. If midazolam is administered parenterally, special precaution is required since the sedative effect may be prolonged.
Rare cases of elevated plasma concentrations of digoxin have been reported. It is not clear whether this was due to the combination of therapy. It is, therefore, advisable to monitor digoxin concentrations in patients receiving ketoconazole.
When taken orally, imidazole compounds like ketoconazole may enhance the anticoagulant effect of coumarin-like drugs. In simultaneous treatment with imidazole drugs and coumarin drugs, the anticoagulant effect should be carefully titrated and monitored.
Because severe hypoglycemia has been reported in patients concomitantly receiving oral miconazole (an imidazole) and oral hypoglycemic agents, such a potential interaction involving the latter agents when used concomitantly with ketoconazole tablets (an imidazole) cannot be ruled out.
Concomitant administration of ketoconazole tablets with phenytoin may alter the metabolism of one or both of the drugs. It is suggested to monitor both ketoconazole and phenytoin.
Concomitant administration of rifampin with ketoconazole tablets reduces the blood levels of the latter. INH (Isoniazid) is also reported to affect ketoconazole concentrations adversely. These drugs should not be given concomitantly.
After the coadministration of 200 mg oral ketoconazole twice daily and one 20 mg dose of loratadine to 11 subjects, the AUC and C_{max} of loratadine averaged 302% (± 142 S.D.) and 251% (± 68 S.D.), respectively, of those obtained after co-treatment with placebo. The AUC and C_{max} of descarboethoxyloratadine, an active metabolite, averaged 155% (± 27 S.D.) and 141% (± 35 S.D.), respectively. However, no related changes were noted in the QT_c on ECG taken at 2, 6, and 24 hours after the coadministration. Also, there were no clinically significant differences in adverse events when loratadine was administered with or without ketoconazole.
Rare cases of a disulfiram-like reaction to alcohol have been reported. These experiences have been characterized by flushing, rash, peripheral edema, nausea, and headache. Symptoms resolved within a few hours.
Carcinogenesis, Mutagenesis, Impairment of Fertility: The dominant lethal mutation test in male and female mice revealed that single oral doses of ketoconazole as high as 80 mg/kg produced no mutation in any stage of germ cell development. The *Ames Salmonella* microsomal activator assay was also negative. A long term feeding study in Swiss Albino mice and in Wistar rats showed no evidence of oncogenic activity.
Pregnancy: Teratogenic effects: *Pregnancy Category C:* Ketoconazole has been shown to be teratogenic (syndactylia and oligodactylia) in the rat when given in the diet at 80 mg/kg/day (10 times the maximum recommended human dose). However, these effects may be related to maternal toxicity, evidence of which also was seen at this and higher dose levels.
There are no adequate and well controlled studies in pregnant women. NIZORAL® Tablets should be used during pregnancy only if the potential benefit justifies the potential risk to the fetus.
Nonteratogenic Effects: Ketoconazole has also been found to be embryotoxic in the rat when given in the diet at doses higher than 80 mg/kg during the first trimester of gestation. In addition, dystocia (difficult labor) was noted in rats administered oral ketoconazole during the third trimester of gestation. This occurred when ketoconazole was administered at doses higher than 10 mg/kg (higher than 1.25 times the maximum human dose).
It is likely that both the malformations and the embryotoxicity resulting from the administration of oral ketoconazole during gestation are a reflection of the particular sensitivity of the female rat to this drug. For example, the oral LD_{50} of ketoconazole given by gavage to the female rat is 166 mg/kg whereas in the male rat the oral LD_{50} is 287 mg/kg.
Nursing Mothers: Since ketoconazole is probably excreted in the milk, mothers who are under treatment should not breast feed.
Pediatric Use: NIZORAL® (ketoconazole) Tablets have not been systematically studied in children of any age, and essentially no information is available on children under 2 years. NIZORAL® Tablets should not be used in pediatric patients unless the potential benefit outweighs the risks.

ADVERSE REACTIONS

In rare cases, anaphylaxis has been reported after the first dose. Several cases of hypersensitivity reactions including urticaria have also been reported. However, the most frequent adverse reactions were nausea and/or vomiting in approximately 3%, abdominal pain in 1.2%, pruritus in 1.5%, and the following in less than 1% of the patients: headache, dizziness, somnolence, fever and chills, photophobia, diarrhea, gynecomastia, impotence, thrombocytopenia, leukopenia, hemolytic anemia, and bulging fontanelles. Oligospermia has been reported in investigational studies with the drug at dosages above those currently approved. Oligospermia has not been reported at dosages up to 400 mg daily, however sperm counts have been obtained infrequently in patients treated with these dosages. Most of these reactions were mild and transient and rarely required discontinuation of NIZORAL® (ketoconazole) Tablets. In contrast, the rare occurrences of hepatic dysfunction require special attention (see WARNINGS section).
In worldwide postmarketing experience with NIZORAL® Tablets there have been rare reports of alopecia, paresthesia, and signs of increased intracranial pressure including bulging fontanelles and papilledema. Hypertriglyceridemia has also been reported but a causal association with NIZORAL® Tablets is uncertain.
Neuropsychiatric disturbances, including suicidal tendencies and severe depression, have occurred rarely in patients using NIZORAL® Tablets.
Ventricular dysrhythmias (prolonged QT intervals) have occurred with the concomitant use of terfenadine with ketoconazole tablets. (See BOX WARNING, CONTRAINDICATIONS, and WARNINGS sections.) Data suggest that coadministration of ketoconazole tablets and cisapride can result in prolongation of the QT interval and has rarely been associated with ventricular arrhythmias. (See CONTRAINDICATIONS, WARNINGS, and PRECAUTIONS sections.)

OVERDOSAGE

In the event of accidental overdosage, supportive measures, including gastric lavage with sodium bicarbonate, should be employed.

DOSAGE AND ADMINISTRATION

Adults: The recommended starting dose of NIZORAL® (ketoconazole) Tablets is a single daily administration of 200 mg (one tablet). In very serious infections or if clinical responsiveness is insufficient within the expected time, the dose of NIZORAL® Tablets may be increased to 400 mg (two tablets) once daily.
Children: In small numbers of children over 2 years of age, a single daily dose of 3.3 to 6.6 mg/kg has been used. NIZORAL® Tablets have not been studied in children under 2 years of age.
There should be laboratory as well as clinical documentation of infection prior to starting ketoconazole therapy. Treatment should be continued until tests indicate that active fungal infection has subsided. Inadequate periods of treatment may yield poor response and lead to early recurrence of clinical symptoms. Minimum treatment for candidiasis is one or two weeks. Patients with chronic mucocutaneous candidiasis usually require maintenance therapy. Minimum treatment for the other indicated systemic mycoses is six months.
Minimum treatment for recalcitrant dermatophyte infections is four weeks in cases involving glabrous skin. Palmar and plantar infections may respond more slowly. Apparent cures may subsequently recur after discontinuation of therapy in some cases.

HOW SUPPLIED

NIZORAL® (ketoconazole) is available as white, scored tablets containing 200 mg of ketoconazole debossed "JANSSEN" and on the reverse side debossed "NIZORAL". They are supplied in bottles of 100 tablets (NDC 50458-220-10).
Store at controlled room temperature
15°–25°C(59°–77°F). Protect from moisture.
U.S. Patent 4,335,125
Rev. March 1997, July 1998
JANSSEN PHARMACEUTICA
Titusville, NJ 08560-0200
Shown in Product Identification Guide, page 319

REMINYL® ℞
[rĕm ĭ-nĭl]
(GALANTAMINE HBr)
TABLETS AND ORAL SOLUTION

DESCRIPTION

REMINYL® (galantamine hydrobromide) is a reversible, competitive acetylcholinesterase inhibitor. It is known chemically as (4a*S*,6*R*,8a*S*)-4a,5,9,10,11,12-hexahydro-3-methoxy-11-methyl-6*H*-benzofuro[3a,3,2-*ef*][2]benzazepin-6-ol hydrobromide. It has an empirical formula of $C_{17}H_{21}NO_3 \cdot HBr$ and a molecular weight of 368.27. Galantamine hydrobromide is a white to almost white powder and is sparingly soluble in water. The structural formula for galantamine hydrobromide is:

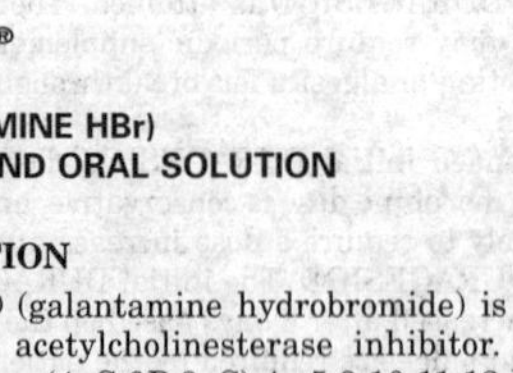

REMINYL® for oral use is available in circular biconvex film-coated tablets of 4 mg (off-white), 8 mg (pink), and 12 mg (orange-brown). Each 4, 8, and 12 mg (base equivalent) tablet contains 5.126, 10.253, and 15.379 mg of galan-

tamine hydrobromide, respectively. Inactive ingredients include colloidal silicon dioxide, crospovidone, hydroxypropyl methylcellulose, lactose monohydrate, magnesium stearate, microcrystalline cellulose, propylene glycol, talc, and titanium dioxide. The 4 mg tablets contain yellow ferric oxide. The 8 mg tablets contain red ferric oxide. The 12 mg tablets contain red ferric oxide and FD&C yellow #6 aluminum lake.
REMINYL® is also available as a 4 mg/mL oral solution. The inactive ingredients for this solution are methyl parahydroxybenzoate, propyl parahydroxybenzoate, sodium saccharin, sodium hydroxide and purified water.

CLINICAL PHARMACOLOGY

Mechanism of Action

Although the etiology of cognitive impairment in Alzheimer's disease (AD) is not fully understood, it has been reported that acetylcholine-producing neurons degenerate in the brains of patients with Alzheimer's disease. The degree of this cholinergic loss has been correlated with degree of cognitive impairment and density of amyloid plaques (a neuropathological hallmark of Alzheimer's disease).
Galantamine, a tertiary alkaloid, is a competitive and reversible inhibitor of acetylcholinesterase. While the precise mechanism of galantamine's action is unknown, it is postulated to exert its therapeutic effect by enhancing cholinergic function. This is accomplished by increasing the concentration of acetylcholine through reversible inhibition of its hydrolysis by cholinesterase. If this mechanism is correct, galantamine's effect may lessen as the disease process advances and fewer cholinergic neurons remain functionally intact. There is no evidence that galantamine alters the course of the underlying dementing process.

Pharmacokinetics

Galantamine is well absorbed with absolute oral bioavailability of about 90%. It has a terminal elimination half-life of about 7 hours and pharmacokinetics are linear over the range of 8-32 mg /day.
The maximum inhibition of anticholinesterase activity of about 40% was achieved about one hour after a single oral dose of 8 mg galantamine in healthy male subjects.

Absorption and Distribution

Galantamine is rapidly and completely absorbed with time to peak concentration about 1 hour. Bioavailability of the tablet was the same as the bioavailability of an oral solution. Food did not affect the AUC of galantamine but C_{max} decreased by 25% and T_{max} was delayed by 1.5 hours. The mean volume of distribution of galantamine is 175 L.
The plasma protein binding of galantamine is 18% at therapeutically relevant concentrations. In whole blood, galantamine is mainly distributed to blood cells (52.7%). The blood to plasma concentration ratio of galantamine is 1.2.

Metabolism and Elimination

Galantamine is metabolized by hepatic cytochrome P450 enzymes, glucuronidated, and excreted unchanged in the urine. *In vitro* studies indicate that cytochrome CYP2D6 and CYP3A4 were the major cytochrome P450 isoenzymes involved in the metabolism of galantamine, and inhibitors of both pathways increase oral bioavailability of galantamine modestly (see **PRECAUTIONS**, **Drug-Drug Interactions**). O-demethylation, mediated by CYP2D6 was greater in extensive metabolizers of CYP2D6 than in poor metabolizers. In plasma from both poor and extensive metabolizers, however, unchanged galantamine and its glucuronide accounted for most of the sample radioactivity.
In studies of oral ^{3}H-galantamine, unchanged galantamine and its glucuronide, accounted for most plasma radioactivity in poor and extensive CYP2D6 metabolizers. Up to 8 hours post-dose, unchanged galantamine accounted for 39-77% of the total radioactivity in the plasma, and galantamine glucuronide for 14-24%. By 7 days, 93-99% of the radioactivity had been recovered, with about 95% in urine and about 5% in the feces. Total urinary recovery of unchanged galantamine accounted for, on average, 32% of the dose and that of galantamine glucuronide for another 12% on average.
After i.v. or oral administration, about 20% of the dose was excreted as unchanged galantamine in the urine in 24 hours, representing a renal clearance of about 65 mL/min, about 20-25% of the total plasma clearance of about 300 mL/min.

Special Populations

CYP2D6 poor metabolizers

Approximately 7% of the normal population has a genetic variation that leads to reduced levels of activity of CYP2D6 isozyme. Such individuals have been referred to as poor metabolizers. After a single oral dose of 4 mg or 8 mg galantamine, CYP2D6 poor metabolizers demonstrated a similar C_{max} and about 35% AUC_{∞} increase of unchanged galantamine compared to extensive metabolizers.
A total of 356 patients with Alzheimer's disease enrolled in two phase 3 studies were genotyped with respect to CYP2D6 (n=210 hetero-extensive metabolizers, 126 homo-extensive metabolizers, and 20 poor metabolizers). Population pharmacokinetic analysis indicated that there was a 25% decrease in median clearance in poor metabolizers compared to extensive metabolizers. Dosage adjustment is not necessary in patients identified as poor metabolizers as the dose of drug is individually titrated to tolerability.
Hepatic Impairment: Following a single 4 mg dose of galantamine, the pharmacokinetics of galantamine in subjects with mild hepatic impairment (n=8; Child-Pugh score of 5-6) were similar to those in healthy subjects. In patients with moderate hepatic impairment (n=8; Child-Pugh score of 7-9), galantamine clearance was decreased by about 25% compared to normal volunteers. Exposure would be expected to increase further with increasing degree of hepatic impairment (see **PRECAUTIONS** and **DOSAGE AND ADMINISTRATION**).
Renal Impairment: Following a single 8 mg dose of galantamine, AUC increased by 37% and 67% in moderate and severely renal-impaired patients compared to normal volunteers (see **PRECAUTIONS** and **DOSAGE AND ADMINISTRATION**).
Elderly: Data from clinical trials in patients with Alzheimer's disease indicate that galantamine concentrations are 30-40% higher than in healthy young subjects.
Gender and Race: No specific pharmacokinetic study was conducted to investigate the effect of gender and race on the disposition of REMINYL® (galantamine hydrobromide), but a population pharmacokinetic analysis indicates (n= 539 males and 550 females) that galantamine clearance is about 20% lower in females than in males (explained by lower body weight in females) and race (n=1029 White, 24 Black, 13 Asian and 23 other) did not affect the clearance of REMINYL®.

Drug-Drug Interactions

Multiple metabolic pathways and renal excretion are involved in the elimination of galantamine so no single pathway appears predominant. Based on *in vitro* studies, CYP2D6 and CYP3A4 were the major enzymes involved in the metabolism of galantamine. CYP2D6 was involved in the formation of O-desmethyl-galantamine, whereas CYP3A4 mediated the formation of galantamine-N-oxide. Galantamine is also glucuronidated and excreted unchanged in urine.

(A) Effect of other drugs on the metabolism of REMINYL®: Drugs that are potent inhibitors for CYP2D6 or CYP3A4 may increase the AUC of galantamine. Multiple dose pharmacokinetic studies demonstrated that the AUC of galantamine increased 30% and 40%, respectively, during coadministration of ketoconazole and paroxetine. As coadministered with erythromycin, another CYP3A4 inhibitor, the galantamine AUC increased only 10%. Population PK analysis with a database of 852 patients with Alzheimer's disease showed that the clearance of galantamine was decreased about 25-33% by concurrent administration of amitriptyline (n=17), fluoxetine (n=48), fluvoxamine (n=14), and quinidine (n=7), known inhibitors of CYP2D6.
Concurrent administration of H_2-antagonists demonstrated that ranitidine did not affect the pharmacokinetics of galantamine, and cimetidine increased the galantamine AUC by approximately 16%.

(B) Effect of REMINYL® on the metabolism of other drugs: *In vitro* studies show that galantamine did not inhibit the metabolic pathways catalyzed by CYP1A2, CYP2A6, CYP3A4, CYP4A, CYP2C, CYP2D6 and CYP2E1. This indicated that the inhibitory potential of galantamine towards the major forms of cytochrome P450 is very low. Multiple doses of galantamine (24 mg/day) had no effect on the pharmacokinetics of digoxin and warfarin (R- and S-forms). Galantamine had no effect on the increased prothrombin time induced by warfarin.

CLINICAL TRIALS

The effectiveness of REMINYL® (galantamine hydrobromide) as a treatment for Alzheimer's disease is demonstrated by the results of 4 randomized, double-blind, placebo-controlled clinical investigations in patients with probable Alzheimer's disease [diagnosed by NINCDS-ADRDA criteria, with Mini-Mental State Examination scores that were ≥10 and ≤24]. Doses studied were 8-32 mg/day given as twice daily doses. In 3 of the 4 studies patients were started on a low dose of 8 mg, then titrated weekly by 8 mg/day to 24 or 32 mg as assigned. In the fourth study (USA 4-week Dose-Escalation Fixed-Dose Study) dose escalation of 8 mg/day occurred over 4 week intervals. The mean age of patients participating in the 4 REMINYL® trials was 75 years with a range of 41 to 100. Approximately 62% of patients were women and 38% were men. The racial distribution was White 94%, Black 3% and other races 3%. Two other studies examined a three times daily dosing regimen; these also showed or suggested benefit but did not suggest an advantage over twice daily dosing.
Study Outcome Measures: In each study, the primary effectiveness of REMINYL® was evaluated using a dual outcome assessment strategy as measured by the Alzheimer's Disease Assessment Scale (ADAS-cog) and the Clinician's Interview Based Impression of Change (CIBIC-plus).
The ability of REMINYL® to improve cognitive performance was assessed with the cognitive sub-scale of the Alzheimer's Disease Assessment Scale (ADAS-cog), a multi-item instrument that has been extensively validated in longitudinal cohorts of Alzheimer's disease patients. The ADAS-cog examines selected aspects of cognitive performance including elements of memory, orientation, attention, reasoning, language and praxis. The ADAS-cog scoring range is from 0 to 70, with higher scores indicating greater cognitive impairment. Elderly normal adults may score as low as 0 or 1, but it is not unusual for non-demented adults to score slightly higher.
The patients recruited as participants in each study had mean scores on ADAS-cog of approximately 27 units, with a range from 5 to 69. Experience gained in longitudinal studies of ambulatory patients with mild to moderate Alzheimer's disease suggests that they gain 6 to 12 units a year on the ADAS-cog. Lesser degrees of change, however, are seen in patients with very mild or very advanced disease because the ADAS-cog is not uniformly sensitive to change over the course of the disease. The annualized rate of decline in the placebo patients participating in REMINYL® trials was approximately 4.5 units per year.
The ability of REMINYL® to produce an overall clinical effect was assessed using a Clinician's Interview Based Impression of Change that required the use of caregiver information, the CIBIC-plus. The CIBIC-plus is not a single instrument and is not a standardized instrument like the ADAS-cog. Clinical trials for investigational drugs have used a variety of CIBIC formats, each different in terms of depth and structure. As such, results from a CIBIC-plus reflect clinical experience from the trial or trials in which it was used and can not be compared directly with the results of CIBIC-plus evaluations from other clinical trials. The CIBIC-plus used in the trials was a semi-structured instrument based on a comprehensive evaluation at baseline and subsequent time-points of 4 major areas of patient function: general, cognitive, behavioral and activities of daily living. It represents the assessment of a skilled clinician based on his/her observation at an interview with the patient, in combination with information supplied by a caregiver familiar with the behavior of the patient over the interval rated. The CIBIC-plus is scored as a seven point categorical rating, ranging from a score of 1, indicating "markedly improved," to a score of 4, indicating "no change" to a score of 7, indicating "marked worsening." The CIBIC-plus has not been systematically compared directly to assessments not using information from caregivers (CIBIC) or other global methods.

U.S. Twenty-One-Week Fixed-Dose Study

In a study of 21 weeks duration, 978 patients were randomized to doses of 8, 16, or 24 mg of REMINYL® per day, or to placebo, each given in 2 divided doses. Treatment was initiated at 8 mg/day for all patients randomized to REMINYL®, and increased by 8 mg/day every 4 weeks. Therefore, the maximum titration phase was 8 weeks and the minimum maintenance phase was 13 weeks (in patients randomized to 24 mg/day of REMINYL®).
Effects on the ADAS-cog: Figure 1 illustrates the time course for the change from baseline in ADAS-cog scores for all four dose groups over the 21 weeks of the study. At 21 weeks of treatment, the mean differences in the ADAS-cog change scores for the REMINYL®-treated patients compared to the patients on placebo were 1.7, 3.3, and 3.6 units for the 8, 16 and 24 mg/day treatments, respectively. The 16 mg/day and 24 mg/day treatments were statistically significantly superior to placebo and to the 8 mg/day treatment. There was no statistically significant difference between the 16 mg/day and 24 mg/day dose groups.

Figure 1: Time-course of the Change from Baseline in ADAS-cog Score for Patients Completing 21 Weeks (5 Months) of Treatment

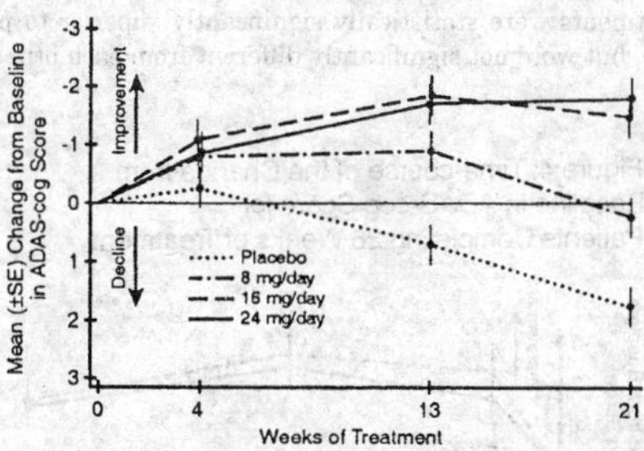

Figure 2 illustrates the cumulative percentages of patients from each of the four treatment groups who had attained at least the measure of improvement in ADAS-cog score shown on the X axis. Three change scores (10-point, 7-point and 4-point reductions) and no change in score from baseline have been identified for illustrative purposes, and the percent of patients in each group achieving that result is shown in the inset table.
The curves demonstrate that both patients assigned to galantamine and placebo have a wide range of responses, but that the REMINYL® groups are more likely to show the greater improvements.
[See figure 2 at top of next column]
Effects on the CIBIC-plus: Figure 3 is a histogram of the percentage distribution of CIBIC-plus scores attained by patients assigned to each of the four treatment groups who completed 21 weeks of treatment. The REMINYL®-placebo differences for these groups of patients in mean rating were 0.15, 0.41 and 0.44 units for the 8, 16 and 24 mg/day treatments, respectively. The 16 mg/day and 24 mg/day treatments were statistically significantly superior to placebo. The differences vs. the 8 mg/day treatment for the 16 and 24 mg/day treatments were 0.26 and 0.29, respectively. There were no statistically significant differences between the 16 mg/day and 24 mg/day dose groups.
[See figure 3 at top of next column]

U.S. Twenty-Six-Week Fixed-Dose Study

In a study of 26 weeks duration, 636 patients were randomized to either a dose of 24 mg or 32 mg of REMINYL® per day, or to placebo, each given in two divided doses. The 26-week study was divided into a 3-week dose titration phase and a 23-week maintenance phase.

Continued on next page

Reminyl—Cont.

Figure 2: Cumulative Percentage of Patients Completing 21 Weeks of Double-blind Treatment with Specified Changes from Baseline in ADAS-cog Scores.
The Percentages of Randomized Patients who Completed the Study were: Placebo 84%, 8 mg/day 77%, 16 mg/day 78% and 24 mg/day 78%.

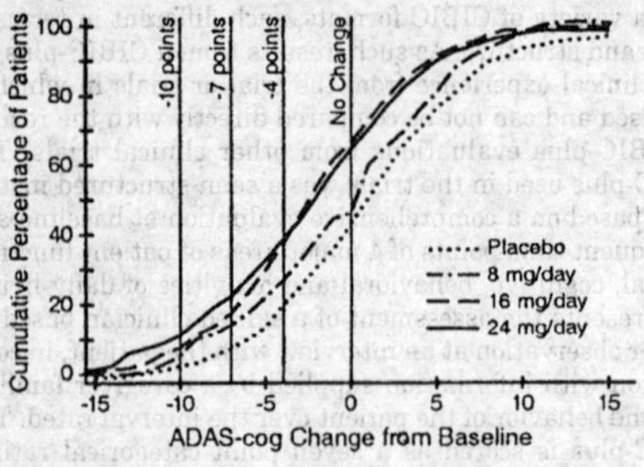

	Change in ADAS-cog			
Treatment	-10	-7	-4	0
Placebo	3.6%	7.6%	19.6%	41.8%
8 mg/day	5.9%	13.9%	25.7%	46.5%
16 mg/day	7.2%	15.9%	35.6%	65.4%
24 mg/day	10.4%	22.3%	37.0%	64.9%

Figure 3: Distribution of CIBIC-plus Ratings at Week 21

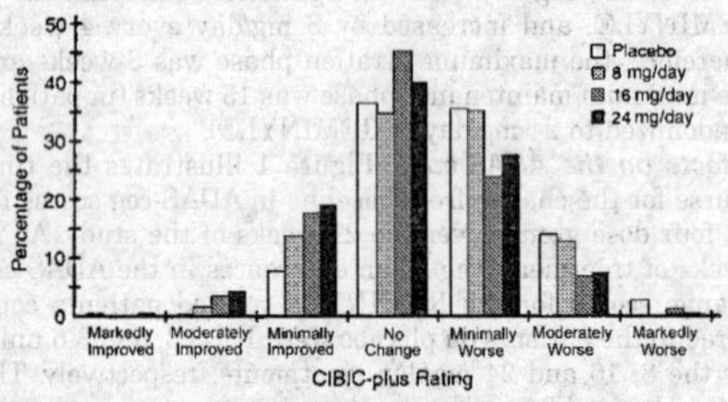

Effects on the ADAS-cog: Figure 4 illustrates the time course for the change from baseline in ADAS-cog scores for all three dose groups over the 26 weeks of the study. At 26 weeks of treatment, the mean differences in the ADAS-cog change scores for the REMINYL®-treated patients compared to the patients on placebo were 3.9 and 3.8 units for the 24 mg/day and 32 mg/day treatments, respectively. Both treatments were statistically significantly superior to placebo, but were not significantly different from each other.

Figure 4: Time-course of the Change from Baseline in ADAS-cog Score for Patients Completing 26 Weeks of Treatment

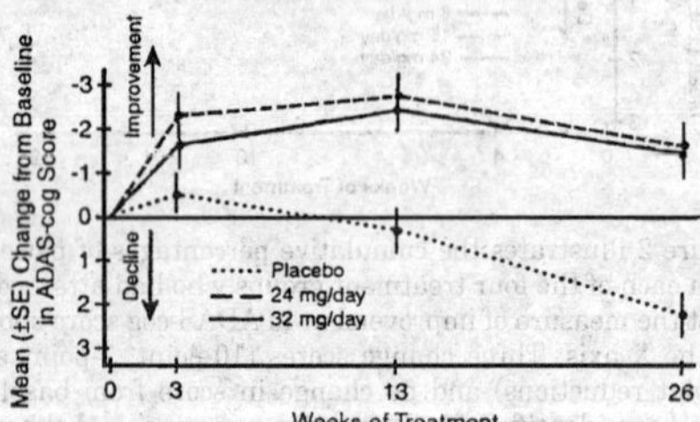

Figure 5 illustrates the cumulative percentages of patients from each of the three treatment groups who had attained at least the measure of improvement in ADAS-cog score shown on the X axis. Three change scores (10-point, 7-point and 4-point reductions) and no change in score from baseline have been identified for illustrative purposes, and the percent of patients in each group achieving that result is shown in the inset table.

The curves demonstrate that both patients assigned to REMINYL® and placebo have a wide range of responses, but that the REMINYL® groups are more likely to show the greater improvements. A curve for an effective treatment would be shifted to the left of the curve for placebo, while an ineffective or deleterious treatment would be superimposed upon, or shifted to the right of the curve for placebo, respectively.

[See figure 5 at top of next column]

Effects on the CIBIC-plus: Figure 6 is a histogram of the percentage distribution of CIBIC-plus scores attained by patients assigned to each of the three treatment groups who completed 26 weeks of treatment. The mean REMINYL®-placebo differences for these groups of patients in the mean rating were 0.28 and 0.29 units for 24 and 32 mg/day of REMINYL®, respectively. The mean ratings for both groups were statistically significantly superior to placebo, but were not significantly different from each other.

Figure 5: Cumulative Percentage of Patients Completing 26 Weeks of Double-blind Treatment with Specified Changes from Baseline in ADAS-cog Scores.
The Percentages of Randomized Patients who Completed the Study were: Placebo 81%, 24 mg/day 68%, and 32 mg/day 58%.

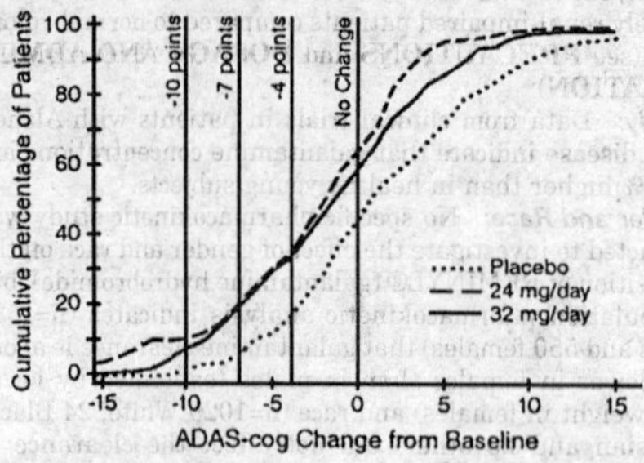

	Change in ADAS-cog			
Treatment	-10	-7	-4	0
Placebo	2.1%	5.7%	16.6%	43.9%
24 mg/day	7.6%	18.3%	33.6%	64.1%
32 mg/day	11.1%	19.7%	33.3%	58.1%

Figure 6: Distribution of CIBIC-plus Ratings at Week 26

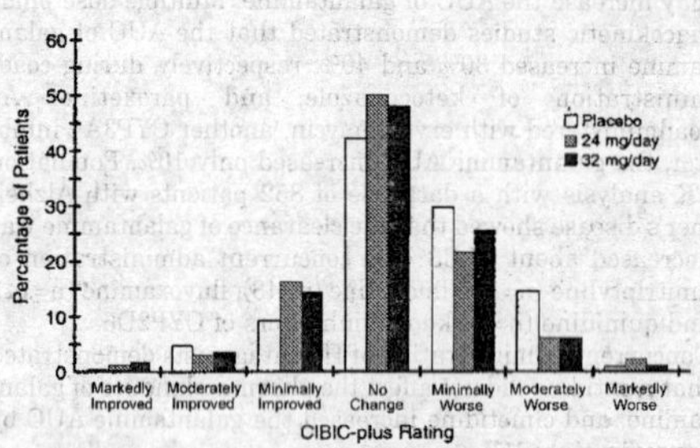

International Twenty-Six-Week Fixed-Dose Study

In a study of 26 weeks duration identical in design to the USA 26-Week Fixed-Dose Study, 653 patients were randomized to either a dose of 24 mg or 32 mg of REMINYL® per day, or to placebo, each given in two divided doses. The 26-week study was divided into a 3-week dose titration phase and a 23-week maintenance phase.

Effects on the ADAS-cog: Figure 7 illustrates the time course for the change from baseline in ADAS-cog scores for all three dose groups over the 26 weeks of the study. At 26 weeks of treatment, the mean differences in the ADAS-cog change scores for the REMINYL®-treated patients compared to the patients on placebo were 3.1 and 4.1 units for the 24 mg/day and 32 mg/day treatments, respectively. Both treatments were statistically significantly superior to placebo, but were not significantly different from each other.

Figure 7: Time-course of the Change from Baseline in ADAS-cog Score for Patients Completing 26 Weeks of Treatment

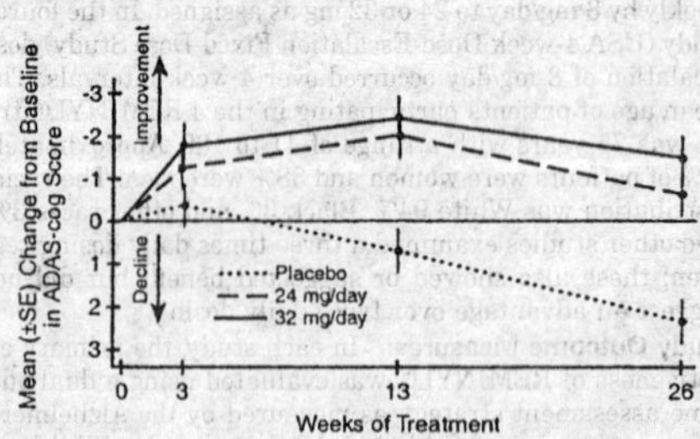

Figure 8 illustrates the cumulative percentages of patients from each of the three treatment groups who had attained at least the measure of improvement in ADAS-cog score shown on the X axis. Three change scores (10-point, 7-point and 4-point reductions) and no change in score from baseline have been identified for illustrative purposes, and the percent of patients in each group achieving that result is shown in the inset table.

The curves demonstrate that both patients assigned to REMINYL® and placebo have a wide range of responses, but that the REMINYL® groups are more likely to show the greater improvements.

[See figure 8 at top of next column]

Effects on the CIBIC-plus: Figure 9 is a histogram of the percentage distribution of CIBIC-plus scores attained by patients assigned to each of the three treatment groups who completed 26 weeks of treatment. The mean REMINYL®-placebo differences for these groups of patients in the mean rating of change from baseline were 0.34 and 0.47 for 24 and 32 mg/day of REMINYL®, respectively. The mean ratings for the REMINYL® groups were statistically significantly superior to placebo, but were not significantly different from each other.

Figure 8: Cumulative Percentage of Patients Completing 26 Weeks of Double-blind Treatment with Specified Changes from Baseline in ADAS-cog Scores.
The Percentages of Randomized Patients who Completed the Study were: Placebo 87%, 24 mg/day 80%, and 32 mg/day 75%.

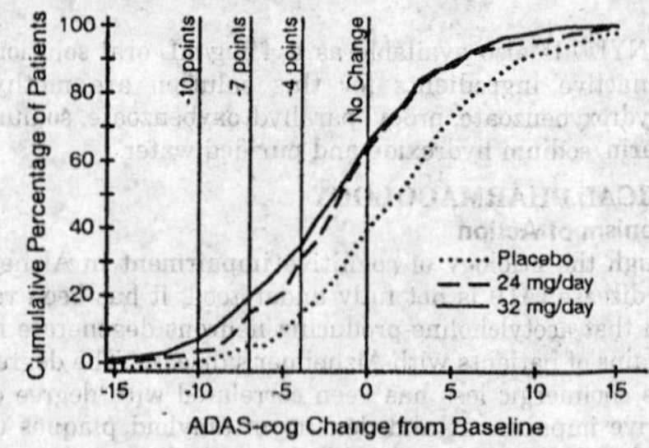

	Change in ADAS-cog			
Treatment	-10	-7	-4	0
Placebo	1.2%	5.8%	15.2%	39.8%
24 mg/day	4.5%	15.4%	30.8%	65.4%
32 mg/day	7.9%	19.7%	34.9%	63.8%

Figure 9: Distribution of CIBIC-plus Rating at Week 26

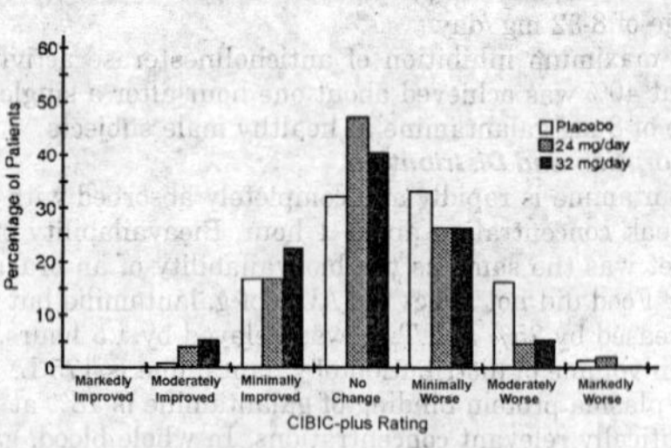

International Thirteen-Week Flexible-Dose Study

In a study of 13 weeks duration, 386 patients were randomized to either a flexible dose of 24-32 mg/day of REMINYL® or to placebo, each given in two divided doses. The 13-week study was divided into a 3-week dose titration phase and a 10-week maintenance phase. The patients in the active treatment arm of the study were maintained at either 24 mg/day or 32 mg/day at the discretion of the investigator.

Effects on the ADAS-cog: Figure 10 illustrates the time course for the change from baseline in ADAS-cog scores for both dose groups over the 13 weeks of the study. At 13 weeks of treatment, the mean difference in the ADAS-cog change scores for the treated patients compared to the patients on placebo was 1.9. REMINYL® at a dose of 24-32 mg/day was statistically significantly superior to placebo.

Figure 10: Time-course of the Change from Baseline in ADAS-cog Score for Patients Completing 13 Weeks of Treatment

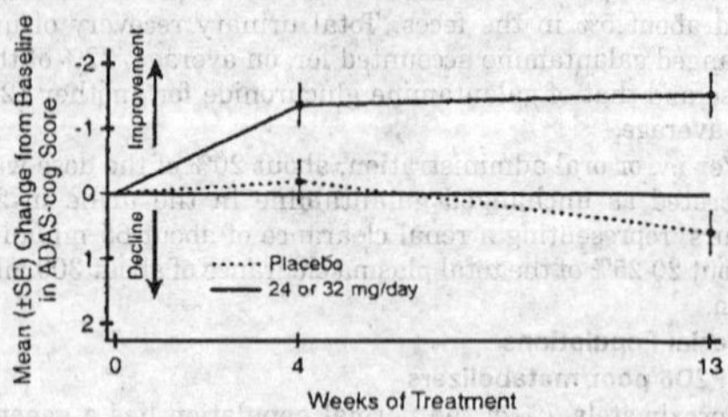

Figure 11 illustrates the cumulative percentages of patients from each of the two treatment groups who had attained at least the measure of improvement in ADAS-cog score shown on the X axis. Three change scores (10-point, 7-point and 4-point reductions) and no change in score from baseline have been identified for illustrative purposes, and the percent of patients in each group achieving that result is shown in the inset table.

The curves demonstrate that both patients assigned to REMINYL® and placebo have a wide range of responses, but that the REMINYL® group is more likely to show the greater improvement.

[See figure 11 at top of next column]

Effects on the CIBIC-plus: Figure 12 is a histogram of the percentage distribution of CIBIC-plus scores attained by patients assigned to each of the two treatment groups who completed 13 weeks of treatment. The mean REMINYL®-placebo differences for the group of patients in the mean rating of change from baseline was 0.37 units. The mean rating

Figure 11: Cumulative Percentage of Patients Completing 13 Weeks of Double-blind Treatment with Specified Changes from Baseline in ADAS-cog Scores. The Percentages of Randomized Patients who Completed the Study were: Placebo 90%, 24-32 mg/day 67%.

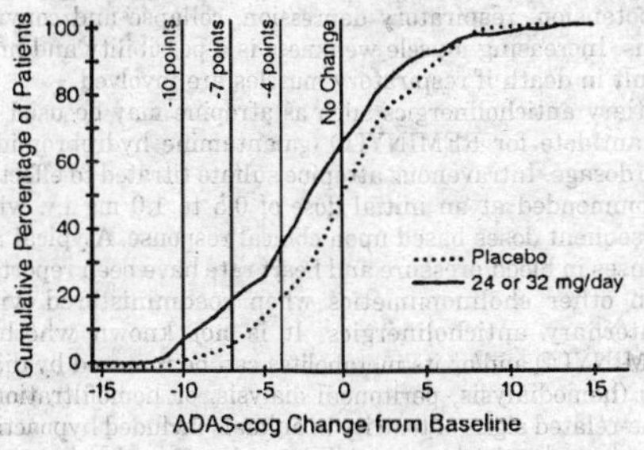

	Change in ADAS-cog			
Treatment	-10	-7	-4	0
Placebo	1.9%	5.6%	19.4%	50.0%
24 or 32 mg/day	7.1%	18.8%	32.9%	65.3%

for the 24-32 mg/day group was statistically significantly superior to placebo.

Figure 12: Distribution of CIBIC-plus Ratings at Week 13

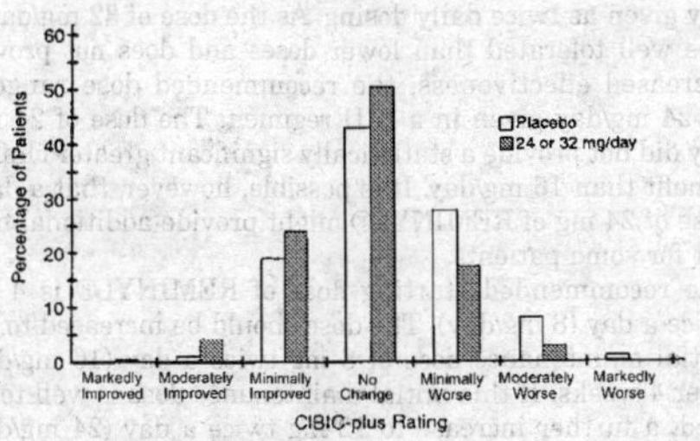

Age, Gender and Race: Patient's age, gender, or race did not predict clinical outcome of treatment.

INDICATIONS AND USAGE

REMINYL® (galantamine hydrobromide) is indicated for the treatment of mild to moderate dementia of the Alzheimer's type.

CONTRAINDICATIONS

REMINYL® (galantamine hydrobromide) is contraindicated in patients with known hypersensitivity to galantamine hydrobromide or to any excipients used in the formulation.

WARNINGS

Anesthesia

Galantamine, as a cholinesterase inhibitor, is likely to exaggerate the neuromuscular blocking effects of succinylcholine-type and similar neuromuscular blocking agents during anesthesia.

Cardiovascular Conditions

Because of their pharmacological action, cholinesterase inhibitors have vagotonic effects on the sinoatrial and atrioventricular nodes, leading to bradycardia and AV block. These actions may be particularly important to patients with supraventricular cardiac conduction disorders or to patients taking other drugs concomitantly that significantly slow heart rate. Postmarketing surveillance of marketed anticholinesterase inhibitors has shown, however, that bradycardia and all types of heart block have been reported in patients both with and without known underlying cardiac conduction abnormalities. Therefore all patients should be considered at risk for adverse effects on cardiac conduction.

In randomized controlled trials, bradycardia was reported more frequently in galantamine-treated patients than in placebo-treated patients, but rarely led to treatment discontinuation. The overall frequency of this event was 2-3% for galantamine doses up to 24 mg/day compared with <1% for placebo. No increased incidence of heart block was observed at the recommended doses.

Patients treated with galantamine up to 24 mg/day using the recommended dosing schedule showed a dose-related increase in risk of syncope (placebo 0.7% [2/286]; 4 mg BID 0.4% [3/692]; 8 mg BID 1.3% [7/552]; 12 mg BID 2.2% [6/273]).

Gastrointestinal Conditions

Through their primary action, cholinomimetics may be expected to increase gastric acid secretion due to increased cholinergic activity. Therefore, patients should be monitored closely for symptoms of active or occult gastrointestinal bleeding, especially those with an increased risk for developing ulcers, e.g., those with a history of ulcer disease or patients using concurrent nonsteroidal anti-inflammatory drugs (NSAIDS). Clinical studies of REMINYL® (galantamine hydrobromide) have shown no increase, relative to placebo, in the incidence of either peptic ulcer disease or gastrointestinal bleeding.

REMINYL®, as a predictable consequence of its pharmacological properties, has been shown to produce nausea, vomiting, diarrhea, anorexia, and weight loss (see ADVERSE REACTIONS).

Genitourinary

Although this was not observed in clinical trials with REMINYL®, cholinomimetics may cause bladder outflow obstruction.

Neurological Conditions

Seizures: Cholinesterase inhibitors are believed to have some potential to cause generalized convulsions. However, seizure activity may also be a manifestation of Alzheimer's disease. In clinical trials, there was no increase in the incidence of convulsions with REMINYL® compared to placebo.

Pulmonary Conditions

Because of its cholinomimetic action, galantamine should be prescribed with care to patients with a history of severe asthma or obstructive pulmonary disease.

PRECAUTIONS

Information for Patients and Caregivers: Caregivers should be instructed in the recommended administration (twice per day, preferably with morning and evening meal) and dose escalation (dose increases should follow minimum of four weeks at prior dose).

Patients and caregivers should be advised that the most frequent adverse events associated with use of the drug can be minimized by following the recommended dosage and administration.

Patients and caregivers should be advised to ensure adequate fluid intake during treatment. If therapy has been interrupted for several days or longer, the patient should be restarted at the lowest dose and the dose escalated to the current dose.

Caregivers should be instructed in the correct procedure for administering REMINYL® (galantamine hydrobromide) Oral Solution. In addition, they should be informed of the existence of an Instruction Sheet (included with the product) describing how the solution is to be administered. They should be urged to read this sheet prior to administering REMINYL® Oral Solution. Caregivers should direct questions about the administration of the solution to either their physician or pharmacist.

Special Populations

Hepatic Impairment

In patients with moderately impaired hepatic function, dose titration should proceed cautiously (see **CLINICAL PHARMACOLOGY** and **DOSAGE AND ADMINISTRATION**). The use of REMINYL® in patients with severe hepatic impairment is not recommended.

Renal Impairment

In patients with moderately impaired renal function, dose titration should proceed cautiously (see **CLINICAL PHARMACOLOGY** and **DOSAGE AND ADMINISTRATION**). In patients with severely impaired renal function (CL_{cr} < 9 mL/min) the use of REMINYL® is not recommended.

Drug-Drug Interactions

Use With Anticholinergics

REMINYL® has the potential to interfere with the activity of anticholinergic medications.

Use With Cholinomimetics and Other Cholinesterase Inhibitors

A synergistic effect is expected when cholinesterase inhibitors are given concurrently with succinylcholine, other cholinesterase inhibitors, similar neuromuscular blocking agents or cholinergic agonists such as bethanechol.

A) Effect of Other Drugs on Galantamine

In vitro

CYP3A4 and CYP2D6 are the major enzymes involved in the metabolism of galantamine. CYP3A4 mediates the formation of galantamine-N-oxide; CYP2D6 leads to the formation of O-desmethyl-galantamine. Because galantamine is also glucuronidated and excreted unchanged, no single pathway appears predominant.

In vivo

Cimetidine and Ranitidine: Galantamine was administered as a single dose of 4 mg on day 2 of a 3-day treatment with either cimetidine (800 mg daily) or ranitidine (300 mg daily). Cimetidine increased the bioavailability of galantamine by approximately 16%. Ranitidine had no effect on the PK of galantamine.

Ketoconazole: Ketoconazole, a strong inhibitor of CYP3A4 and an inhibitor of CYP2D6, at a dose of 200 mg BID for 4 days, increased the AUC of galantamine by 30%.

Erythromycin: Erythromycin, a moderate inhibitor of CYP3A4, at a dose of 500 mg QID for 4 days, affected the AUC of galantamine minimally (10% increase).

Paroxetine: Paroxetine, a strong inhibitor of CYP2D6, at 20 mg/day for 16 days, increased the oral bioavailability of galantamine by about 40%.

B) Effect of Galantamine on Other Drugs

In vitro

Galantamine did not inhibit the metabolic pathways catalyzed by CYP1A2, CYP2A6, CYP3A4, CYP4A, CYP2C, CYP2D6 or CYP2E1. This indicates that the inhibitory potential of galantamine towards the major forms of cytochrome P450 is very low.

In vivo

Warfarin: Galantamine at 24 mg/day had no effect on the pharmacokinetics of R-and-S-warfarin (25 mg single dose) or on the prothrombin time. The protein binding of warfarin was unaffected by galantamine.

Digoxin: Galantamine at 24 mg/day had no effect on the steady-state pharmacokinetics of digoxin (0.375 mg once daily) when they were coadministered. In this study, however, one healthy subject was hospitalized for 2nd and 3rd degree heart block and bradycardia.

Carcinogenesis, Mutagenesis and Impairment of Fertility

In a 24-month oral carcinogenicity study in rats, a slight increase in endometrial adenocarcinomas was observed at 10 mg/kg/day (4 times the Maximum Recommended Human Dose [MRHD] on a mg/m^2 basis or 6 times on an exposure [AUC] basis and 30 mg/kg/day (12 times MRHD on a mg/m^2 basis or 19 times on an AUC basis). No increase in neoplastic changes was observed in females at 2.5 mg/kg/day (equivalent to the MRHD on a mg/m^2 basis or 2 times on an AUC basis) or in males up to the highest dose tested of 30 mg/kg/day (12 times the MRHD on a mg/m^2 and AUC basis).

Galantamine was not carcinogenic in a 6-month oral carcinogenicity study in transgenic (P 53-deficient) mice up to 20 mg/kg/day, or in a 24-month oral carcinogenicity study in male and female mice up to 10 mg/kg/day (2 times the MRHD on a mg/m^2 basis and equivalent on an AUC basis).

Galantamine produced no evidence of genotoxic potential when evaluated in the *in vitro* Ames *S. typhimurium* or *E. coli* reverse mutation assay, *in vitro* mouse lymphoma assay, *in vivo* micronucleus test in mice, or *in vitro* chromosome aberration assay in Chinese hamster ovary cells.

No impairment of fertility was seen in rats given up to 16 mg/kg/day (7 times the MRHD on a mg/m^2 basis) for 14 days prior to mating in females and for 60 days prior to mating in males.

Pregnancy

Pregnancy Category B: In a study in which rats were dosed from day 14 (females) or day 60 (males) prior to mating through the period of organogenesis, a slightly increased incidence of skeletal variations was observed at doses of 8 mg/kg/day (3 times the Maximum Recommended Human Dose [MRHD] on a mg/m^2 basis) and 16 mg/kg/day. In a study in which pregnant rats were dosed from the beginning of organogenesis through day 21 post-partum, pup weights were decreased at 8 and 16 mg/kg/day, but no adverse effects on other postnatal developmental parameters were seen. The doses causing the above effects in rats produced slight maternal toxicity. No major malformations were caused in rats given up to 16 mg/kg/day. No drug related teratogenic effects were observed in rabbits given up to 40 mg/kg/day (32 times the MRHD on a mg/m^2 basis) during the period of organogenesis.

There are no adequate and well-controlled studies of REMINYL® in pregnant women. REMINYL® should be used during pregnancy only if the potential benefit justifies the potential risk to the fetus.

Nursing Mothers

It is not known whether galantamine is excreted in human breast milk. REMINYL® has no indication for use in nursing mothers.

Pediatric Use

There are no adequate and well-controlled trials documenting the safety and efficacy of galantamine in any illness occurring in children. Therefore, use of REMINYL® in children is not recommended.

ADVERSE REACTIONS

Pre-Marketing Clinical Trial Experience:

Adverse Events Leading to Discontinuation: In two large scale, placebo-controlled trials of 6 months duration, in which patients were titrated weekly from 8 to 16 to 24, and to 32 mg/day, the risk of discontinuation because of an adverse event in the galantamine group exceeded that in the placebo group by about threefold. In contrast, in a 5-month trial with escalation of the dose by 8 mg/day every 4 weeks, the overall risk of discontinuation because of an adverse event was 7%, 7%, and 10% for the placebo, galantamine 16 mg/day, and galantamine 24 mg/day groups, respectively, with gastrointestinal adverse effects the principle reason for discontinuing galantamine. Table 1 shows the most frequent adverse events leading to discontinuation in this study.

Table 1: Most Frequent Adverse Events Leading to Discontinuation in a Placebo-Controlled, Double-Blind Trial With a 4-Week Dose Escalation Schedule

	4-Week Escalation		
	Placebo	16 mg/day	24 mg/day
Adverse Event	N=286	N=279	N=273
Nausea	<1%	2%	4%
Vomiting	0%	1%	3%
Anorexia	<1%	1%	<1%
Dizziness	<1%	2%	1%
Syncope	0%	0%	1%

Adverse Events Reported in Controlled Trials: The reported adverse events in REMINYL® (galantamine hydrobromide) trials reflect experience gained under closely monitored conditions in a highly selected patient population. In actual practice or in other clinical trials, these frequency es-

Continued on next page

Reminyl—Cont.

timates may not apply, as the conditions of use, reporting behavior and the types of patients treated may differ.
The majority of these adverse events occurred during the dose-escalation period. In those patients who experienced the most frequent adverse event, nausea, the median duration of the nausea was 5-7 days.
Administration of REMINYL® with food, the use of antiemetic medication, and ensuring adequate fluid intake may reduce the impact of these events.
The most frequent adverse events, defined as those occurring at a frequency of at least 5% and at least twice the rate on placebo with the recommended maintenance dose of either 16 or 24 mg/day of REMINYL® under conditions of every 4 week dose-escalation for each dose increment of 8 mg/day, are shown in Table 2. These events were primarily gastrointestinal and tended to be less frequent with the 16 mg/day recommended initial maintenance dose.

Table 2: The Most Frequent Adverse Events in the Placebo-Controlled Trial With Dose Escalation Every 4 Weeks Occurring in at Least 5% of Patients Receiving REMINYL® and at Least Twice the Rate on Placebo.

	Placebo	REMINYL® 16 mg/day	REMINYL® 24 mg/day
Adverse Event	N=286	N=279	N=273
Nausea	5%	13%	17%
Vomiting	1%	6%	10%
Diarrhea	6%	12%	6%
Anorexia	3%	7%	9%
Weight decrease	1%	5%	5%

Table 3: The most common adverse events (adverse events occurring with an incidence of at least 2% with REMINYL® treatment and in which the incidence was greater than with placebo treatment) are listed in Table 3 for four placebo-controlled trials for patients treated with 16 or 24 mg/day of REMINYL®.

Table 3: Adverse Events Reported in at Least 2% of Patients With Alzheimer's Disease Administered REMINYL® and at a Frequency Greater Than With Placebo

Body System Adverse Event	Placebo (N=801)	REMINYL®[a] (N=1040)
Body as a whole – general disorders		
Fatigue	3%	5%
Syncope	1%	2%
Central & peripheral nervous system disorders		
Dizziness	6%	9%
Headache	5%	8%
Tremor	2%	3%
Gastrointestinal system disorders		
Nausea	9%	24%
Vomiting	4%	13%
Diarrhea	7%	9%
Abdominal pain	4%	5%
Dyspepsia	2%	5%
Heart rate and rhythm disorders		
Bradycardia	1%	2%
Metabolic and nutritional disorders		
Weight decrease	2%	7%
Psychiatric disorders		
Anorexia	3%	9%
Depression	5%	7%
Insomnia	4%	5%
Somnolence	3%	4%
Red blood cell disorders		
Anemia	2%	3%
Respiratory system disorders		
Rhinitis	3%	4%
Urinary system disorders		
Urinary tract infection	7%	8%
Hematuria	2%	3%

a: Adverse events in patients treated with 16 or 24 mg/day of REMINYL® in four placebo-controlled trials are included.

Adverse events occurring with an incidence of at least 2% in placebo-treated patients that was either equal to or greater than with REMINYL® treatment were constipation, agitation, confusion, anxiety, hallucination, injury, back pain, peripheral edema, asthenia, chest pain, urinary incontinence, upper respiratory tract infection, bronchitis, coughing, hypertension, fall, and purpura.
There were no important differences in adverse event rate related to dose or sex. There were too few non-Caucasian patients to assess the effects of race on adverse event rates. No clinically relevant abnormalities in laboratory values were observed.

Other Adverse Events Observed During Clinical Trials
REMINYL® was administered to 3055 patients with Alzheimer's disease. A total of 2357 patients received galantamine in placebo-controlled trials and 761 patients with Alzheimer's disease received galantamine 24 mg/day, the maximum recommended maintenance dose. About 1000 patients received galantamine for at least one year and approximately 200 patients received galantamine for two years.
To establish the rate of adverse events, data from all patients receiving any dose of galantamine in 8 placebo-controlled trials and 6 open-label extension trials were pooled. The methodology to gather and codify these adverse events was standardized across trials, using WHO terminology. All adverse events occurring in approximately 0.1% are included, except for those already listed elsewhere in labeling, WHO terms too general to be informative, or events unlikely to be drug caused. Events are classified by body system and listed using the following definitions: frequent adverse events – those occurring in at least 1/100 patients; infrequent adverse events – those occurring in 1/100 to 1/1000 patients; rare adverse events – those occurring in fewer than 1/1000 patients. These adverse events are not necessarily related to REMINYL® treatment and in most cases were observed at a similar frequency in placebo-treated patients in the controlled studies.
Body As a Whole – General Disorders: *Frequent:* chest pain
Cardiovascular System Disorders: *Infrequent:* postural hypotension, hypotension, dependent edema, cardiac failure
Central & Peripheral Nervous System Disorders *Infrequent:* vertigo, hypertonia, convulsions, involuntary muscle contractions, paresthesia, ataxia, hypokinesia, hyperkinesia, apraxia, aphasia
Gastrointestinal System Disorders: *Frequent:* flatulence; Infrequent: gastritis, melena, dysphagia, rectal hemorrhage, dry mouth, saliva increased, diverticulitis, gastroenteritis, hiccup; rare: esophageal perforation
Heart Rate & Rhythm Disorders: *Infrequent:* AV block, palpitation, atrial fibrillation, QT prolonged, bundle branch block, supraventricular tachycardia, T-wave inversion, ventricular tachycardia
Metabolic & Nutritional Disorders: *Infrequent:* hyperglycemia, alkaline phosphatase increased
Platelet, Bleeding & Clotting Disorders: *Infrequent:* purpura, epistaxis, thrombocytopenia
Psychiatric Disorders: *Infrequent:* apathy, paroniria, paranoid reaction, libido increased, delirium
Urinary System Disorders: *Frequent:* incontinence; *Infrequent:* hematuria, micturition frequency, cystitis, urinary retention, nocturia, renal calculi
Post-Marketing Experience:
Other adverse events from post-approval controlled and uncontrolled clinical trials and post-marketing experience observed in patients treated with REMINYL® include:
Body as a Whole – General Disorders: dehydration (including rare, severe cases leading to renal insufficiency and renal failure)
Central & Peripheral Nervous System Disorders: aggression
Gastrointestinal System Disorders: upper and lower GI bleeding
Metabolic & Nutritional Disorders: hypokalemia
These adverse events may or may not be causally related to the drug.

OVERDOSAGE

Because strategies for the management of overdose are continually evolving, it is advisable to contact a poison control center to determine the latest recommendations for the management of an overdose of any drug.
As in any case of overdose, general supportive measures should be utilized. Signs and symptoms of significant overdosing of galantamine are predicted to be similar to those of overdosing of other cholinomimetics. These effects generally involve the central nervous system, the parasympathetic nervous system, and the neuromuscular junction. In addition to muscle weakness or fasciculations, some or all of the following signs of cholinergic crisis may develop: severe nausea, vomiting, gastrointestinal cramping, salivation, lacrimation, urination, defecation, sweating, bradycardia, hypotension, respiratory depression, collapse and convulsions. Increasing muscle weakness is a possibility and may result in death if respiratory muscles are involved.
Tertiary anticholinergics such as atropine may be used as an antidote for REMINYL® (galantamine hydrobromide) overdosage. Intravenous atropine sulfate titrated to effect is recommended at an initial dose of 0.5 to 1.0 mg i.v. with subsequent doses based upon clinical response. Atypical responses in blood pressure and heart rate have been reported with other cholinomimetics when coadministered with quaternary anticholinergics. It is not known whether REMINYL® and/or its metabolites can be removed by dialysis (hemodialysis, peritoneal dialysis, or hemofiltration).
Dose-related signs of toxicity in animals included hypoactivity, tremors, clonic convulsions, salivation, lacrimation, chromodacryorrhea, mucoid feces, and dyspnea.
In a postmarketing report, one patient who had been taking 4 mg of galantamine daily for a week inadvertently ingested eight 4 mg tablets (32 mg total) on a single day. Subsequently, she developed bradycardia, QT prolongation, ventricular tachycardia and torsades de pointes accompanied by a brief loss of consciousness for which she required hospital treatment.

DOSAGE AND ADMINISTRATION

The dosage of REMINYL® (galantamine hydrobromide) shown to be effective in controlled clinical trials is 16-32 mg/day given as twice daily dosing. As the dose of 32 mg/day is less well tolerated than lower doses and does not provide increased effectiveness, the recommended dose range is 16-24 mg/day given in a BID regimen. The dose of 24 mg/day did not provide a statistically significant greater clinical benefit than 16 mg/day. It is possible, however, that a daily dose of 24 mg of REMINYL® might provide additional benefit for some patients.
The recommended starting dose of REMINYL® is 4 mg twice a day (8 mg/day). The dose should be increased to the initial maintenance dose of 8 mg twice a day (16 mg/day) after 4 weeks. If this initial maintenance dose is well tolerated, a further increase to 12 mg twice a day (24 mg/day) should be attempted only after a minimum of 4 weeks at 8 mg twice a day (16 mg/day). Dose increases should be based upon assessment of clinical benefit and tolerability of the previous dose.
REMINYL® should be administered twice a day, preferably with morning and evening meals.
Patients and caregivers should be advised to ensure adequate fluid intake during treatment. If therapy has been interrupted for several days or longer, the patient should be restarted at the lowest dose and the dose escalated to the current dose.
Caregivers should be instructed in the correct procedure for administering REMINYL® Oral Solution. In addition, they should be informed of the existence of an Instruction Sheet (included with the product) describing how the solution is to be administered. They should be urged to read this sheet prior to administering REMINYL® Oral Solution. Caregivers should direct questions about the administration of the solution to either their physician or pharmacist.
The abrupt withdrawal of REMINYL® in those patients who had been receiving doses in the effective range was not associated with an increased frequency of adverse events in comparison with those continuing to receive the same doses of that drug. The beneficial effects of REMINYL® are lost, however, when the drug is discontinued.

Doses in Special Populations
Galantamine plasma concentrations may be increased in patients with moderate to severe hepatic impairment. In patients with moderately impaired hepatic function (Child-Pugh score of 7-9), the dose should generally not exceed 16 mg/day. The use of REMINYL® in patients with severe hepatic impairment (Child-Pugh score of 10-15) is not recommended.
For patients with moderate renal impairment the dose should generally not exceed 16 mg/day. In patients with severe renal impairment (creatinine clearance < 9 mL/min), the use of REMINYL® is not recommended.

HOW SUPPLIED

REMINYL® (galantamine hydrobromide) tablets are imprinted "JANSSEN" on one side, and "G" and the strength "4", "8", or "12" on the other.
4 mg off-white tablet: bottles of 60 NDC 50458-390-60
8 mg pink tablet: bottles of 60 NDC 50458-391-60
12 mg orange-brown tablet: bottles of 60 NDC 50458-392-60
REMINYL® (galantamine hydrobromide) 4 mg/mL oral solution (NDC 50458-399-10) is a clear colorless solution supplied in 100 mL bottles with a calibrated (in milligrams and milliliters) pipette. The minimum calibrated volume is 0.5 mL, while the maximum calibrated volume is 4 mL.

Storage and Handling
REMINYL® tablets should be stored at 25°C (77°F); excursions permitted to 15-30°C (59-86°F) [see USP Controlled Room Temperature].
REMINYL® oral solution should be stored at 25°C (77°F); excursions permitted to 15-30°C (59-86°F) [see USP Controlled Room Temperature]. DO NOT FREEZE.
Keep out of reach of children.

7519003
247170
March 2003
US Patent No. 4,663,318

REMINYL® tablets are manufactured by:
JOLLC, Gurabo, Puerto Rico or
Janssen-Cilag SpA Latina, Italy
REMINYL® oral solution is manufactured by:
Janssen Pharmaceutica N.V.
Beerse, Belgium
REMINYL® tablets and oral solution are distributed by:
Janssen Pharmaceutica Products, L.P.
Titusville, NJ 08560

USING YOUR REMINYL® DISPENSING-PIPETTE AND BOTTLE

Follow the directions below to use your REMINYL® Dispensing-Pipette and bottle, unless your doctor gave you different directions.

IMPORTANT: Read these instructions before using REMINYL® oral solution.

To open the bottle and use the pipette (plastic tube)

The bottle comes with a child-proof cap. Here is how to open it:

1. Push the plastic cap on the bottle down while turning the cap counter-clockwise (to the left) (Figure 1). Remove the unscrewed cap.

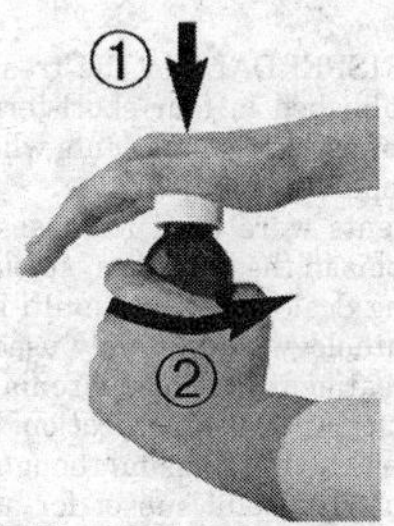

FIG.1

2. Pull the pipette out of its case. The pipette is a tube that you use to measure your dose of REMINYL®. Place the pipette fully into the bottle of REMINYL®. (Figures 2a-2b)

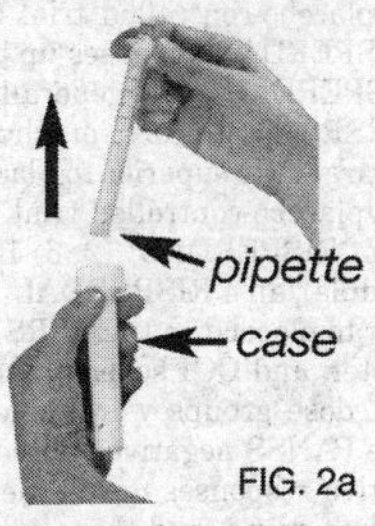

FIG. 2a

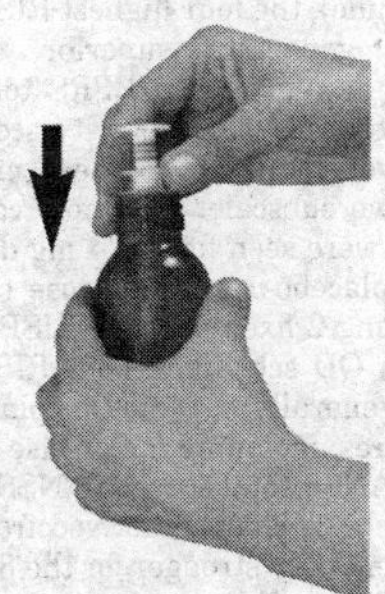
FIG. 2b

3. While holding the bottom ring of the pipette, pull the pipette plunger up to the level that equals the dose prescribed by your doctor. Use the markings on the pipette to guide you. This will draw the medicine into the pipette. (Figures 3a-3b)

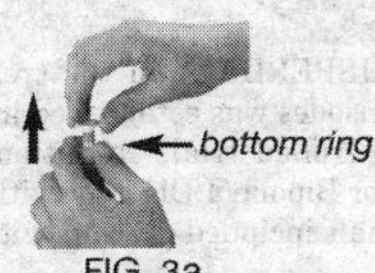

FIG. 3a

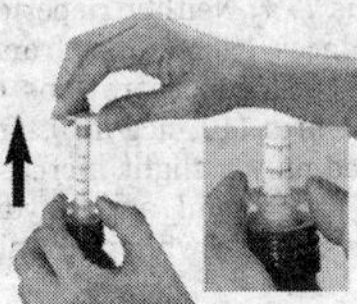
FIG. 3b

4. Be careful not to push the plunger in during this step. Hold the bottom ring of the pipette. Remove the entire pipette from the bottle. (Figures 4a-4b)

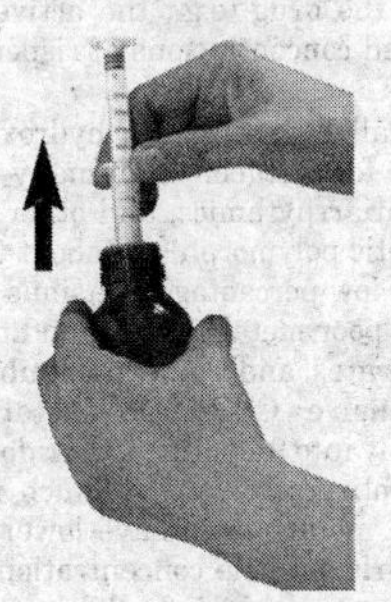
FIG. 4a

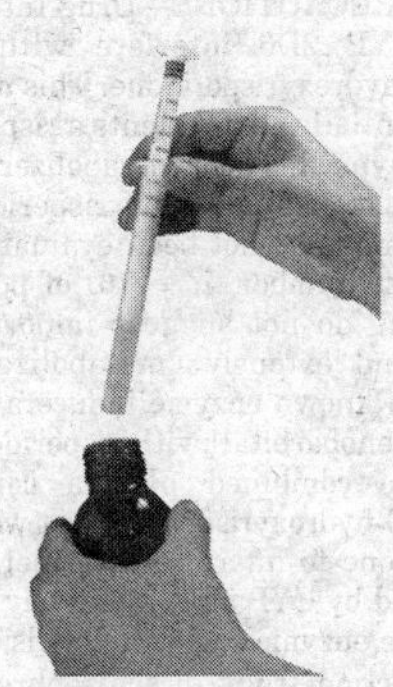
FIG. 4b

5. Empty all the medicine in the pipette into 3–4 ounces (100 mL) of any non-alcoholic drink. To do this, push the plunger all the way in. (Figures 5a-5b)

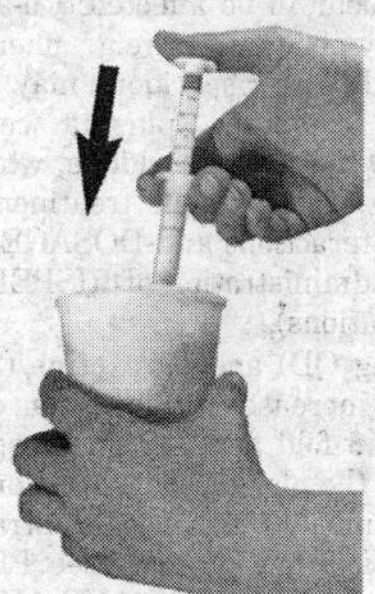
FIG. 5a

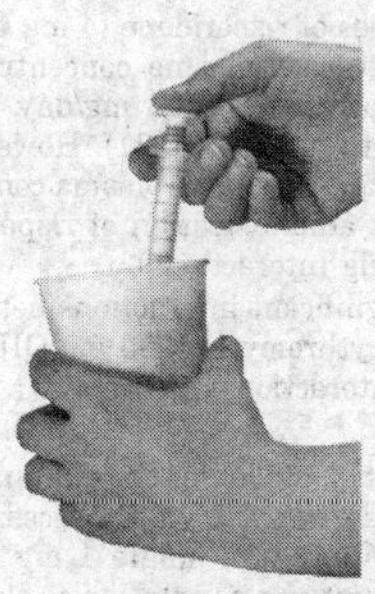
FIG. 5b

6. Stir the drink well (Figure 6). Drink all of the mixture right away.

[See figure 6 at top of next column]

7. Replace the plastic cap on the bottle by turning it clockwise (to the right). (Figure 7)

[See figure 7 at top of next column]

8. Rinse the empty pipette by inserting the open end of the pipette into a glass of water, pulling the plunger out, and pushing the plunger in to remove the water. (Figures 8a-8b)

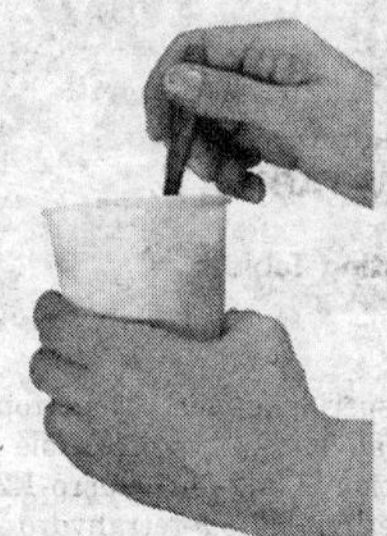
FIG. 6

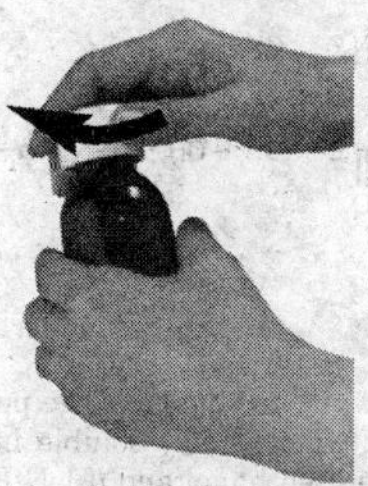
FIG. 7

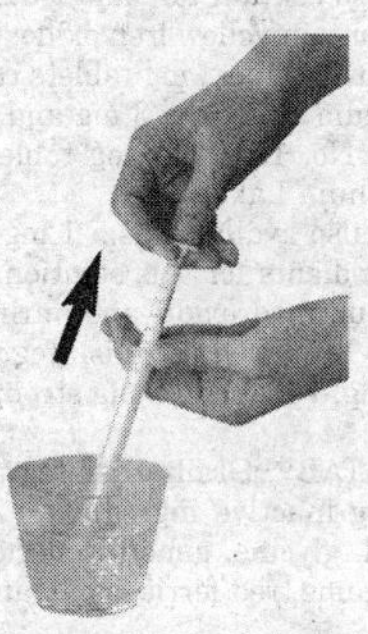
FIG. 8a

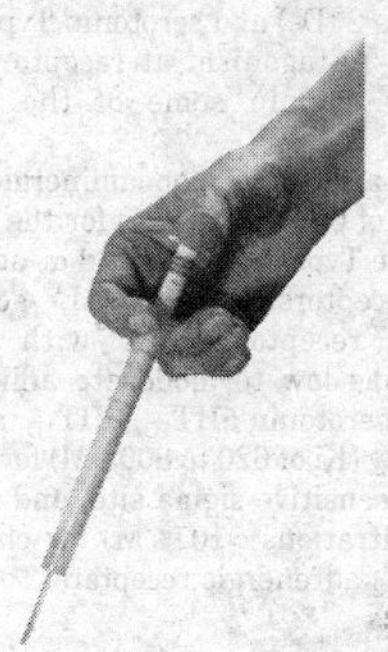
FIG. 8b

For more information about REMINYL®, see the leaflet that came with the package.

STORAGE: REMINYL® oral solution should be stored at 25°C (77°F); excursions permitted to 15–30°C (59–86°F) [see USP Controlled Room Temperature]. DO NOT FREEZE

NDC 50458-399-10 100 mL
REMINYL®
(galantamine hydrobromide)
Oral Solution
4 mg/mL

Each 1 mL contains: 4 mg of galantamine hydrobromide in an aqueous solution.

7519003
March 2003
US Patent No. 4,663,318

Manufactured by:
Janssen Pharmaceutica N.V.
Beerse, Belgium
Distributed by:
Janssen Pharmaceutica Products, L.P.
Titusville, NJ 08560

Shown in Product Identification Guide, page 319

Continued on next page

RISPERDAL® ℞
[rĭs-pər-dăl]
(risperidone)
Tablets/Oral Solution
RISPERDAL® M-TAB™
(risperidone)
Orally Disintegrating Tablets

DESCRIPTION

RISPERDAL® (risperidone) is a psychotropic agent belonging to the chemical class of benzisoxazole derivatives. The chemical designation is 3-[2-[4-(6-fluoro-1,2-benzisoxazol-3-yl)-1-piperidinyl]ethyl]-6,7,8,9-tetrahydro-2-methyl-4H-pyrido[1,2-a]pyrimidin-4-one. Its molecular formula is $C_{23}H_{27}FN_4O_2$ and its molecular weight is 410.49. The structural formula is:

Risperidone is a white to slightly beige powder. It is practically insoluble in water, freely soluble in methylene chloride, and soluble in methanol and 0.1 N HCl.
RISPERDAL® tablets are available in 0.25 mg (dark yellow), 0.5 mg (red-brown), 1 mg (white), 2 mg (orange), 3 mg (yellow), and 4 mg (green) strengths. Inactive ingredients are colloidal silicon dioxide, hypromellose, lactose, magnesium stearate, microcrystalline cellulose, propylene glycol, sodium lauryl sulfate, and starch (corn). Tablets of 0.25, 0.5, 2, 3, and 4 mg also contain talc and titanium dioxide. The 0.25 mg tablets contain yellow iron oxide; the 0.5 mg tablets contain red iron oxide; the 2 mg tablets contain FD&C Yellow No. 6 Aluminum Lake; the 3 mg and 4 mg tablets contain D&C Yellow No. 10; the 4 mg tablets contain FD&C Blue No. 2 Aluminum Lake.
RISPERDAL® is also available as a 1 mg/mL oral solution. The inactive ingredients for this solution are tartaric acid, benzoic acid, sodium hydroxide, and purified water.
RISPERDAL® M-TAB™ Orally Disintegrating Tablets are available in 0.5 mg, 1 mg, and 2 mg strengths and are light coral in color.
RISPERDAL® M-TAB™ Orally Disintegrating Tablets contain the following inactive ingredients: Amberlite® resin, gelatin, mannitol, glycine, simethicone, carbomer, sodium hydroxide, aspartame, red ferric oxide, and peppermint oil.

CLINICAL PHARMACOLOGY

Pharmacodynamics
The mechanism of action of RISPERDAL® (risperidone), as with other drugs used to treat schizophrenia, is unknown. However, it has been proposed that the drug's therapeutic activity in schizophrenia is mediated through a combination of dopamine Type 2 (D_2) and serotonin Type 2 ($5HT_2$) receptor antagonism. Antagonism at receptors other than D_2 and $5HT_2$ may explain some of the other effects of RISPERDAL®.
RISPERDAL® is a selective monoaminergic antagonist with high affinity (Ki of 0.12 to 7.3 nM) for the serotonin Type 2 ($5HT_2$), dopamine Type 2 (D_2), α_1 and α_2 adrenergic, and H_1 histaminergic receptors. RISPERDAL® acts as an antagonist at other receptors, but with lower potency. RISPERDAL® has low to moderate affinity (Ki of 47 to 253 nM) for the serotonin $5HT_{1C}$, $5HT_{1D}$, and $5HT_{1A}$ receptors, weak affinity (Ki of 620 to 800 nM) for the dopamine D_1 and haloperidol-sensitive sigma site, and no affinity (when tested at concentrations $>10^{-5}$ M) for cholinergic muscarinic or β_1 and β_2 adrenergic receptors.
Pharmacokinetics
Absorption
Risperidone is well absorbed. The absolute oral bioavailability of risperidone is 70% (CV=25%). The relative oral bioavailability of risperidone from a tablet is 94% (CV=10%) when compared to a solution.
Pharmacokinetic studies showed that RISPERDAL® M-TAB™ Orally Disintegrating Tablets and RISPERDAL® Oral Solution are bioequivalent to RISPERDAL® Tablets.
Plasma concentrations of risperidone, its major metabolite, 9-hydroxyrisperidone, and risperidone plus 9-hydroxyrisperidone are dose proportional over the dosing range of 1 to 16 mg daily (0.5 to 8 mg BID). Following oral administration of solution or tablet, mean peak plasma concentrations of risperidone occurred at about 1 hour. Peak concentrations of 9-hydroxyrisperidone occurred at about 3 hours in extensive metabolizers, and 17 hours in poor metabolizers. Steady-state concentrations of risperidone are reached in 1 day in extensive metabolizers and would be expected to reach steady-state in about 5 days in poor metabolizers. Steady-state concentrations of 9-hydroxyrisperidone are reached in 5–6 days (measured in extensive metabolizers).
Food Effect
Food does not affect either the rate or extent of absorption of risperidone. Thus, risperidone can be given with or without meals.
Distribution
Risperidone is rapidly distributed. The volume of distribution is 1–2 L/kg. In plasma, risperidone is bound to albumin and α_1-acid glycoprotein. The plasma protein binding of risperidone is 90%, and that of its major metabolite, 9-hydroxyrisperidone, is 77%. Neither risperidone nor 9-hydroxyrisperidone displaces each other from plasma binding sites. High therapeutic concentrations of sulfamethazine (100 mcg/mL), warfarin (10 mcg/mL), and carbamazepine (10 mcg/mL) caused only a slight increase in the free fraction of risperidone at 10 ng/mL and 9-hydroxyrisperidone at 50 ng/mL, changes of unknown clinical significance.
Metabolism
Risperidone is extensively metabolized in the liver. The main metabolic pathway is through hydroxylation of risperidone to 9-hydroxyrisperidone by the enzyme, CYP 2D6. A minor metabolic pathway is through *N*-dealkylation. The main metabolite, 9-hydroxyrisperidone, has similar pharmacological activity as risperidone. Consequently, the clinical effect of the drug (e.g., the active moiety) results from the combined concentrations of risperidone plus 9-hydroxyrisperidone.
CYP 2D6, also called debrisoquin hydroxylase, is the enzyme responsible for metabolism of many neuroleptics, antidepressants, antiarrhythmics, and other drugs. CYP 2D6 is subject to genetic polymorphism (about 6%–8% of Caucasians, and a very low percentage of Asians, have little or no activity and are "poor metabolizers") and to inhibition by a variety of substrates and some non-substrates, notably quinidine. Extensive CYP 2D6 metabolizers convert risperidone rapidly into 9-hydroxyrisperidone, whereas poor CYP 2D6 metabolizers convert it much more slowly. Although extensive metabolizers have lower risperidone and higher 9-hydroxyrisperidone concentrations than poor metabolizers, the pharmacokinetics of the active moiety, after single and multiple doses, are similar in extensive and poor metabolizers.
Risperidone could be subject to two kinds of drug-drug interactions (see PRECAUTIONS—Drug Interactions). First, inhibitors of CYP 2D6 interfere with conversion of risperidone to 9-hydroxyrisperidone. This occurs with quinidine, giving essentially all recipients a risperidone pharmacokinetic profile typical of poor metabolizers. The therapeutic benefits and adverse effects of risperidone in patients receiving quinidine have not been evaluated, but observations in a modest number (n ≅ 70) of poor metabolizers given risperidone do not suggest important differences between poor and extensive metabolizers. Second, coadministration of known enzyme inducers (e.g., phenytoin, rifampin, and phenobarbital) with risperidone may cause a decrease in the combined plasma concentrations of risperidone and 9-hydroxyrisperidone. It would also be possible for risperidone to interfere with metabolism of other drugs metabolized by CYP 2D6. Relatively weak binding of risperidone to the enzyme suggests this is unlikely.
In a drug interaction study in schizophrenic patients, 11 subjects received risperidone titrated to 6 mg/day for 3 weeks, followed by concurrent administration of carbamazepine for an additional 3 weeks. During co-administration, the plasma concentrations of risperidone and its pharmacologically active metabolite, 9-hydroxyrisperidone, were decreased by about 50%. Plasma concentrations of carbamazepine did not appear to be affected. Co-administration of other known enzyme inducers (e.g., phenytoin, rifampin, and phenobarbital) with risperidone may cause similar decreases in the combined plasma concentrations of risperidone and 9-hydroxyrisperidone, which could lead to decreased efficacy of risperidone treatment (see PRECAUTIONS – Drug Interactions and DOSAGE AND ADMINISTRATION – Co-Administration of RISPERDAL® with Certain Other Medications).
Fluoxetine (20 mg QD) and paroxetine (20 mg QD) have been shown to increase the plasma concentration of risperidone 2.5–2.8 fold and 3–9 fold respectively. Fluoxetine did not affect the plasma concentration of 9-hydroxyrisperidone. Paroxetine lowered the concentration of 9-hydroxyrisperidone an average of 13% (see PRECAUTIONS – Drug Interactions and DOSAGE AND ADMINISTRATION – Co-Administration of RISPERDAL® with Certain Other Medications).
Repeated oral doses of risperidone (3 mg BID) did not affect the exposure (AUC) or peak plasma concentrations (C_{max}) of lithium (n=13) (see PRECAUTIONS – Drug Interactions).
Repeated oral doses of risperidone (4 mg QD) did not affect the pre-dose or average plasma concentrations and exposure (AUC) of valproate (1000 mg/day in three divided doses) compared to placebo (n=21). However, there was a 20% increase in valproate peak plasma concentration (C_{max}) after concomitant administration of risperidone (see PRECAUTIONS – Drug Interactions).
There were no significant interactions between risperidone (1 mg QD) and erythromycin (500 mg QID) (see PRECAUTIONS – Drug Interactions).
Excretion
Risperidone and its metabolites are eliminated via the urine and, to a much lesser extent, via the feces. As illustrated by a mass balance study of a single 1 mg oral dose of ^{14}C-risperidone administered as solution to three healthy male volunteers, total recovery of radioactivity at 1 week was 84%, including 70% in the urine and 14% in the feces.
The apparent half-life of risperidone was 3 hours (CV=30%) in extensive metabolizers and 20 hours (CV=40%) in poor metabolizers. The apparent half-life of 9-hydroxyrisperidone was about 21 hours (CV=20%) in extensive metabolizers and 30 hours (CV=25%) in poor metabolizers. The pharmacokinetics of the active moiety, after single and multiple doses, were similar in extensive and poor metabolizers, with an overall mean elimination half-life of about 20 hours.
Special Populations
Renal Impairment
In patients with moderate to severe renal disease, clearance of the sum of risperidone and its active metabolite decreased by 60% compared to young healthy subjects. RISPERDAL® doses should be reduced in patients with renal disease (see PRECAUTIONS and DOSAGE AND ADMINISTRATION).
Hepatic Impairment
While the pharmacokinetics of risperidone in subjects with liver disease were comparable to those in young healthy subjects, the mean free fraction of risperidone in plasma was increased by about 35% because of the diminished concentration of both albumin and α_1-acid glycoprotein. RISPERDAL® doses should be reduced in patients with liver disease (see PRECAUTIONS and DOSAGE AND ADMINISTRATION).
Elderly
In healthy elderly subjects, renal clearance of both risperidone and 9-hydroxyrisperidone was decreased, and elimination half-lives were prolonged compared to young healthy subjects. Dosing should be modified accordingly in the elderly patients (see DOSAGE AND ADMINISTRATION).
Race and Gender Effects
No specific pharmacokinetic study was conducted to investigate race and gender effects, but a population pharmacokinetic analysis did not identify important differences in the disposition of risperidone due to gender (whether corrected for body weight or not) or race.
Clinical Trials
Schizophrenia
Short-Term Efficacy
The efficacy of RISPERDAL® in the treatment of schizophrenia was established in four short-term (4- to 8-week) controlled trials of psychotic inpatients who met DSM-III-R criteria for schizophrenia.
Several instruments were used for assessing psychiatric signs and symptoms in these studies, among them the Brief Psychiatric Rating Scale (BPRS), a multi-item inventory of general psychopathology traditionally used to evaluate the effects of drug treatment in schizophrenia. The BPRS psychosis cluster (conceptual disorganization, hallucinatory behavior, suspiciousness, and unusual thought content) is considered a particularly useful subset for assessing actively psychotic schizophrenic patients. A second traditional assessment, the Clinical Global Impression (CGI), reflects the impression of a skilled observer, fully familiar with the manifestations of schizophrenia, about the overall clinical state of the patient. In addition, the Positive and Negative Syndrome Scale (PANSS) and the Scale for Assessing Negative Symptoms (SANS) were employed.
The results of the trials follow:
(1) In a 6-week, placebo-controlled trial (n=160) involving titration of RISPERDAL® in doses up to 10 mg/day (BID schedule), RISPERDAL® was generally superior to placebo on the BPRS total score, on the BPRS psychosis cluster, and marginally superior to placebo on the SANS.
(2) In an 8-week, placebo-controlled trial (n=513) involving 4 fixed doses of RISPERDAL® (2, 6, 10, and 16 mg/day, on a BID schedule), all 4 RISPERDAL® groups were generally superior to placebo on the BPRS total score, BPRS psychosis cluster, and CGI severity score; the 3 highest RISPERDAL® dose groups were generally superior to placebo on the PANSS negative subscale. The most consistently positive responses on all measures were seen for the 6 mg dose group, and there was no suggestion of increased benefit from larger doses.
(3) In an 8-week, dose comparison trial (n=1356) involving 5 fixed doses of RISPERDAL® (1, 4, 8, 12, and 16 mg/day, on a BID schedule), the four highest RISPERDAL® dose groups were generally superior to the 1 mg RISPERDAL® dose group on BPRS total score, BPRS psychosis cluster, and CGI severity score. None of the dose groups were superior to the 1 mg group on the PANSS negative subscale. The most consistently positive responses were seen for the 4 mg dose group.
(4) In a 4-week, placebo-controlled dose comparison trial (n=246) involving 2 fixed doses of RISPERDAL® (4 and 8 mg/day on a QD schedule), both RISPERDAL® dose groups were generally superior to placebo on several PANSS measures, including a response measure (> 20% reduction in PANSS total score), PANSS total score, and the BPRS psychosis cluster (derived from PANSS). The results were generally stronger for the 8 mg than for the 4 mg dose group.

Long-Term Efficacy
In a longer-term trial, 365 adult outpatients predominantly meeting DSM-IV criteria for schizophrenia and who had been clinically stable for at least 4 weeks on an antipsychotic medication were randomized to RISPERDAL® (2–8 mg/day) or to an active comparator, for 1 to 2 years of observation for relapse. Patients receiving RISPERDAL® experienced a significantly longer time to relapse over this time period compared to those receiving the active comparator.
Bipolar Mania
Monotherapy
The efficacy of RISPERDAL® in the treatment of acute manic or mixed episodes was established in 2 short-term (3-week) placebo-controlled trials in patients who met the DSM-IV criteria for Bipolar I Disorder with manic or mixed episodes. These trials included patients with or without psychotic features.

The primary rating instrument used for assessing manic symptoms in these trials was the Young Mania Rating Scale (Y-MRS), an 11-item clinician-rated scale traditionally used to assess the degree of manic symptomatology (irritability, disruptive/aggressive behavior, sleep, elevated mood, speech, increased activity, sexual interest, language/thought disorder, thought content, appearance, and insight) in a range from 0 (no manic features) to 60 (maximum score). The primary outcome in these trials was change from baseline in the Y-MRS total score. The results of the trials follow:

(1) In one 3-week placebo-controlled trial (n=246), limited to patients with manic episodes, which involved a dose range of RISPERDAL® 1–6 mg/day, once daily, starting at 3 mg/day (mean modal dose was 4.1 mg/day), RISPERDAL® was superior to placebo in the reduction of Y-MRS total score.

(2) In another 3-week placebo-controlled trial (n=286), which involved a dose range of 1–6 mg/day, once daily, starting at 3 mg/day (mean modal dose was 5.6 mg/day), RISPERDAL® was superior to placebo in the reduction of Y-MRS total score.

Combination Therapy

The efficacy of risperidone with concomitant lithium or valproate in the treatment of acute manic or mixed episodes was established in one controlled trial in patients who met the DSM-IV criteria for Bipolar I Disorder. This trial included patients with or without psychotic features and with or without a rapid-cycling course.

(1) In this 3-week placebo-controlled combination trial, 148 in- or outpatients on lithium or valproate therapy with inadequately controlled manic or mixed symptoms were randomized to receive RISPERDAL®, placebo, or an active comparator, in combination with their original therapy. RISPERDAL®, in a dose range of 1–6 mg/day, once daily, starting at 2 mg/day (mean modal dose of 3.8 mg/day), combined with lithium or valproate (in a therapeutic range of 0.6 mEq/L to 1.4 mEq/L or 50 mcg/mL to 120 mcg/mL, respectively) was superior to lithium or valproate alone in the reduction of Y-MRS total score.

(2) In a second 3-week placebo-controlled combination trial, 142 in- or outpatients on lithium, valproate, or carbamazepine therapy with inadequately controlled manic or mixed symptoms were randomized to receive RISPERDAL® or placebo, in combination with their original therapy. RISPERDAL®, in a dose range of 1-6 mg/day, once daily, starting at 2 mg/day (mean modal dose of 3.7 mg/day), combined with lithium, valproate, or carbamazepine (in therapeutic ranges of 0.6 mEq/L to 1.4 mEq/L for lithium, 50 mcg/mL to 125 mcg/mL for valproate, or 4–12 mcg/mL for carbamazepine, respectively) was not superior to lithium, valproate, or carbamazepine alone in the reduction of Y-MRS total score. A possible explanation for the failure of this trial was induction of risperidone and 9-hydroxyrisperidone clearance by carbamazepine, leading to subtherapeutic levels of risperidone and 9-hydroxyrisperidone.

INDICATIONS AND USAGE

Schizophrenia

RISPERDAL® (risperidone) is indicated for the treatment of schizophrenia.

The efficacy of RISPERDAL® in schizophrenia was established in short-term (6- to 8-weeks) controlled trials of schizophrenic inpatients (see CLINICAL PHARMACOLOGY).

The efficacy of RISPERDAL® in delaying relapse was demonstrated in schizophrenic patients who had been clinically stable for at least 4 weeks before initiation of treatment with RISPERDAL® or an active comparator and who were then observed for relapse during a period of 1 to 2 years (see CLINICAL PHARMACOLOGY – Clinical Trials). Nevertheless, the physician who elects to use RISPERDAL® for extended periods should periodically re-evaluate the long-term usefulness of the drug for the individual patient (see DOSAGE AND ADMINISTRATION).

Bipolar Mania

Monotherapy

RISPERDAL® is indicated for the short-term treatment of acute manic or mixed episodes associated with Bipolar I Disorder.

The efficacy of RISPERDAL® was established in two placebo-controlled trials (3-week) with patients meeting DSM-IV criteria for Bipolar I Disorder who currently displayed an acute manic or mixed episode with or without psychotic features (see CLINICAL PHARMACOLOGY).

Combination Therapy

The combination of RISPERDAL® with lithium or valproate is indicated for the short-term treatment of acute manic or mixed episodes associated with Bipolar I Disorder.

The efficacy of RISPERDAL® in combination with lithium or valproate was established in one placebo-controlled (3-week) trial with patients meeting DSM-IV criteria for Bipolar I Disorder who currently displayed an acute manic or mixed episode with or without psychotic features (see CLINICAL PHARMACOLOGY).

The effectiveness of RISPERDAL® for longer-term use, that is, for more than 3 weeks of treatment of an acute episode, and for prophylactic use in mania, has not been systematically evaluated in controlled clinical trials. Therefore, physicians who elect to use RISPERDAL® for extended periods should periodically re-evaluate the long-term risks and benefits of the drug for the individual patient (see DOSAGE AND ADMINISTRATION).

CONTRAINDICATIONS

RISPERDAL® (risperidone) is contraindicated in patients with a known hypersensitivity to the product.

WARNINGS

Neuroleptic Malignant Syndrome (NMS)

A potentially fatal symptom complex sometimes referred to as Neuroleptic Malignant Syndrome (NMS) has been reported in association with antipsychotic drugs. Clinical manifestations of NMS are hyperpyrexia, muscle rigidity, altered mental status, and evidence of autonomic instability (irregular pulse or blood pressure, tachycardia, diaphoresis, and cardiac dysrhythmia). Additional signs may include elevated creatinine phosphokinase, myoglobinuria (rhabdomyolysis), and acute renal failure.

The diagnostic evaluation of patients with this syndrome is complicated. In arriving at a diagnosis, it is important to identify cases in which the clinical presentation includes both serious medical illness (e.g., pneumonia, systemic infection, etc.) and untreated or inadequately treated extrapyramidal signs and symptoms (EPS). Other important considerations in the differential diagnosis include central anticholinergic toxicity, heat stroke, drug fever, and primary central nervous system pathology.

The management of NMS should include: (1) immediate discontinuation of antipsychotic drugs and other drugs not essential to concurrent therapy; (2) intensive symptomatic treatment and medical monitoring; and (3) treatment of any concomitant serious medical problems for which specific treatments are available. There is no general agreement about specific pharmacological treatment regimens for uncomplicated NMS.

If a patient requires antipsychotic drug treatment after recovery from NMS, the potential reintroduction of drug therapy should be carefully considered. The patient should be carefully monitored, since recurrences of NMS have been reported.

Tardive Dyskinesia

A syndrome of potentially irreversible, involuntary, dyskinetic movements may develop in patients treated with antipsychotic drugs. Although the prevalence of the syndrome appears to be highest among the elderly, especially elderly women, it is impossible to rely upon prevalence estimates to predict, at the inception of antipsychotic treatment, which patients are likely to develop the syndrome. Whether antipsychotic drug products differ in their potential to cause tardive dyskinesia is unknown.

The risk of developing tardive dyskinesia and the likelihood that it will become irreversible are believed to increase as the duration of treatment and the total cumulative dose of antipsychotic drugs administered to the patient increase. However, the syndrome can develop, although much less commonly, after relatively brief treatment periods at low doses.

There is no known treatment for established cases of tardive dyskinesia, although the syndrome may remit, partially or completely, if antipsychotic treatment is withdrawn. Antipsychotic treatment, itself, however, may suppress (or partially suppress) the signs and symptoms of the syndrome and thereby may possibly mask the underlying process. The effect that symptomatic suppression has upon the long-term course of the syndrome is unknown.

Given these considerations, RISPERDAL® (risperidone) should be prescribed in a manner that is most likely to minimize the occurrence of tardive dyskinesia. Chronic antipsychotic treatment should generally be reserved for patients who suffer from a chronic illness that (1) is known to respond to antipsychotic drugs, and (2) for whom alternative, equally effective, but potentially less harmful treatments are not available or appropriate. In patients who do require chronic treatment, the smallest dose and the shortest duration of treatment producing a satisfactory clinical response should be sought. The need for continued treatment should be reassessed periodically.

If signs and symptoms of tardive dyskinesia appear in a patient treated on RISPERDAL®, drug discontinuation should be considered. However, some patients may require treatment with RISPERDAL® despite the presence of the syndrome.

Cerebrovascular Adverse Events, Including Stroke, in Elderly Patients With Dementia

Cerebrovascular adverse events (e.g., stroke, transient ischemic attack), including fatalities, were reported in patients (mean age 85 years; range 73–97) in trials of risperidone in elderly patients with dementia-related psychosis. In placebo-controlled trials, there was a significantly higher incidence of cerebrovascular adverse events in patients treated with risperidone compared to patients treated with placebo. RISPERDAL® is not approved for the treatment of patients with dementia-related psychosis.

Hyperglycemia and Diabetes Mellitus

Hyperglycemia, in some cases extreme and associated with ketoacidosis or hyperosmolar coma or death, has been reported in patients treated with atypical antipsychotics including RISPERDAL®. Assessment of the relationship between atypical antipsychotic use and glucose abnormalities is complicated by the possibility of an increased background risk of diabetes mellitus in patients with schizophrenia and the increasing incidence of diabetes mellitus in the general population. Given these confounders, the relationship between atypical antipsychotic use and hyperglycemia-related adverse events is not completely understood. However, epidemiological studies suggest an increased risk of treatment-emergent hyperglycemia-related adverse events in patients treated with the atypical antipsychotics. Precise risk estimates for hyperglycemia-related adverse events in patients treated with atypical antipsychotics are not available.

Patients with an established diagnosis of diabetes mellitus who are started on atypical antipsychotics should be monitored regularly for worsening of glucose control. Patients with risk factors for diabetes mellitus (e.g., obesity, family history of diabetes) who are starting treatment with atypical antipsychotics should undergo fasting blood glucose testing at the beginning of treatment and periodically during treatment. Any patient treated with atypical antipsychotics should be monitored for symptoms of hyperglycemia including polydipsia, polyuria, polyphagia, and weakness. Patients who develop symptoms of hyperglycemia during treatment with atypical antipsychotics should undergo fasting blood glucose testing. In some cases, hyperglycemia has resolved when the atypical antipsychotic was discontinued; however, some patients required continuation of anti-diabetic treatment despite discontinuation of the suspect drug.

PRECAUTIONS

General

Orthostatic Hypotension

RISPERDAL® (risperidone) may induce orthostatic hypotension associated with dizziness, tachycardia, and in some patients, syncope, especially during the initial dose-titration period, probably reflecting its alpha-adrenergic antagonistic properties. Syncope was reported in 0.2% (6/2607) of RISPERDAL®-treated patients in Phase 2 and 3 studies. The risk of orthostatic hypotension and syncope may be minimized by limiting the initial dose to 2 mg total (either QD or 1 mg BID) in normal adults and 0.5 mg BID in the elderly and patients with renal or hepatic impairment (see DOSAGE AND ADMINISTRATION). Monitoring of orthostatic vital signs should be considered in patients for whom this is of concern. A dose reduction should be considered if hypotension occurs. RISPERDAL® should be used with particular caution in patients with known cardiovascular disease (history of myocardial infarction or ischemia, heart failure, or conduction abnormalities), cerebrovascular disease, and conditions which would predispose patients to hypotension, e.g., dehydration and hypovolemia. Clinically significant hypotension has been observed with concomitant use of RISPERDAL® and antihypertensive medication.

Seizures

During premarketing testing, seizures occurred in 0.3% (9/2607) of RISPERDAL®-treated patients, two in association with hyponatremia. RISPERDAL® should be used cautiously in patients with a history of seizures.

Dysphagia

Esophageal dysmotility and aspiration have been associated with antipsychotic drug use. Aspiration pneumonia is a common cause of morbidity and mortality in patients with advanced Alzheimer's dementia. RISPERDAL® and other antipsychotic drugs should be used cautiously in patients at risk for aspiration pneumonia.

Hyperprolactinemia

As with other drugs that antagonize dopamine D_2 receptors, risperidone elevates prolactin levels and the elevation persists during chronic administration. Tissue culture experiments indicate that approximately one-third of human breast cancers are prolactin dependent *in vitro*, a factor of potential importance if the prescription of these drugs is contemplated in a patient with previously detected breast cancer. Although disturbances such as galactorrhea, amenorrhea, gynecomastia, and impotence have been reported with prolactin-elevating compounds, the clinical significance of elevated serum prolactin levels is unknown for most patients. As is common with compounds which increase prolactin release, an increase in pituitary gland, mammary gland, and pancreatic islet cell hyperplasia and/or neoplasia was observed in the risperidone carcinogenicity studies conducted in mice and rats (see PRECAUTIONS – Carcinogenesis, Mutagenesis, Impairment of Fertility). However, neither clinical studies nor epidemiologic studies conducted to date have shown an association between chronic administration of this class of drugs and tumorigenesis in humans; the available evidence is considered too limited to be conclusive at this time.

Potential for Cognitive and Motor Impairment

Somnolence was a commonly reported adverse event associated with RISPERDAL® treatment, especially when ascertained by direct questioning of patients. This adverse event is dose-related, and in a study utilizing a checklist to detect adverse events, 41% of the high-dose patients (RISPERDAL® 16 mg/day) reported somnolence compared to 16% of placebo patients. Direct questioning is more sensitive for detecting adverse events than spontaneous reporting, by which 8% of RISPERDAL® 16 mg/day patients and 1% of placebo patients reported somnolence as an adverse event. Since RISPERDAL® has the potential to impair judgment, thinking, or motor skills, patients should be cautioned about operating hazardous machinery, including automobiles, until they are reasonably certain that RISPERDAL® therapy does not affect them adversely.

Priapism

Rare cases of priapism have been reported. While the relationship of the events to RISPERDAL® use has not been established, other drugs with alpha-adrenergic blocking effects have been reported to induce priapism, and it is possible that RISPERDAL® may share this capacity. Severe priapism may require surgical intervention.

Continued on next page

Risperdal—Cont.

Thrombotic Thrombocytopenic Purpura (TTP)
A single case of TTP was reported in a 28 year-old female patient receiving RISPERDAL® in a large, open premarketing experience (approximately 1300 patients). She experienced jaundice, fever, and bruising, but eventually recovered after receiving plasmapheresis. The relationship to RISPERDAL® therapy is unknown.

Antiemetic Effect
Risperidone has an antiemetic effect in animals; this effect may also occur in humans, and may mask signs and symptoms of overdosage with certain drugs or of conditions such as intestinal obstruction, Reye's syndrome, and brain tumor.

Body Temperature Regulation
Disruption of body temperature regulation has been attributed to antipsychotic agents. Both hyperthermia and hypothermia have been reported in association with oral RISPERDAL® use. Caution is advised when prescribing for patients who will be exposed to temperature extremes.

Suicide
The possibility of a suicide attempt is inherent in schizophrenia, and close supervision of high-risk patients should accompany drug therapy. Prescriptions for RISPERDAL® should be written for the smallest quantity of tablets, consistent with good patient management, in order to reduce the risk of overdose.

Use in Patients With Concomitant Illness
Clinical experience with RISPERDAL® in patients with certain concomitant systemic illnesses is limited. Caution is advisable in using RISPERDAL® in patients with diseases or conditions that could affect metabolism or hemodynamic responses.
RISPERDAL® has not been evaluated or used to any appreciable extent in patients with a recent history of myocardial infarction or unstable heart disease. Patients with these diagnoses were excluded from clinical studies during the product's premarket testing.
Increased plasma concentrations of risperidone and 9-hydroxyrisperidone occur in patients with severe renal impairment (creatinine clearance <30 mL/min/1.73 m^2), and an increase in the free fraction of risperidone is seen in patients with severe hepatic impairment. A lower starting dose should be used in such patients (see DOSAGE AND ADMINISTRATION).

Information for Patients
Physicians are advised to discuss the following issues with patients for whom they prescribe RISPERDAL®:

Orthostatic Hypotension
Patients should be advised of the risk of orthostatic hypotension, especially during the period of initial dose titration.

Interference With Cognitive and Motor Performance
Since RISPERDAL® has the potential to impair judgment, thinking, or motor skills, patients should be cautioned about operating hazardous machinery, including automobiles, until they are reasonably certain that RISPERDAL® therapy does not affect them adversely.

Pregnancy
Patients should be advised to notify their physician if they become pregnant or intend to become pregnant during therapy.

Nursing
Patients should be advised not to breast-feed an infant if they are taking RISPERDAL®.

Concomitant Medication
Patients should be advised to inform their physicians if they are taking, or plan to take, any prescription or over-the-counter drugs, since there is a potential for interactions.

Alcohol
Patients should be advised to avoid alcohol while taking RISPERDAL®.

Phenylketonurics
Phenylalanine is a component of aspartame. Each 2 mg RISPERDAL® M-TAB™ Orally Disintegrating Tablet contains 0.56 mg phenylalanine; each 1 mg RISPERDAL® M-TAB™ Orally Disintegrating Tablet contains 0.28 mg phenylalanine; and each 0.5 mg RISPERDAL® M-TAB™ Orally Disintegrating Tablet contains 0.14 mg phenylalanine.

Laboratory Tests
No specific laboratory tests are recommended.

Drug Interactions
The interactions of RISPERDAL® and other drugs have not been systematically evaluated. Given the primary CNS effects of risperidone, caution should be used when RISPERDAL® is taken in combination with other centrally acting drugs and alcohol.
Because of its potential for inducing hypotension, RISPERDAL® may enhance the hypotensive effects of other therapeutic agents with this potential.
RISPERDAL® may antagonize the effects of levodopa and dopamine agonists.
Amytriptyline does not affect the pharmacokinetics of risperidone or the active antipsychotic fraction. Cimetidine and ranitidine increased the bioavailability of risperidone, but only marginally increased the plasma concentration of the active antipsychotic fraction.
Chronic administration of clozapine with risperidone may decrease the clearance of risperidone.

Carbamazepine and Other Enzyme Inducers
In a drug interaction study in schizophrenic patients, 11 subjects received risperidone titrated to 6 mg/day for 3 weeks, followed by concurrent administration of carbamazepine for an additional 3 weeks. During co-administration, the plasma concentrations of risperidone and its pharmacologically active metabolite, 9-hydroxyrisperidone, were decreased by about 50%. Plasma concentrations of carbamazepine did not appear to be affected. The dose of risperidone may need to be titrated accordingly for patients receiving carbamazepine, particularly during initiation or discontinuation of carbamazepine therapy. Co-administration of other known enzyme inducers (e.g., phenytoin, rifampin, and phenobarbital) with risperidone may cause similar decreases in the combined plasma concentrations of risperidone and 9-hydroxyrisperidone, which could lead to decreased efficacy of risperidone treatment.

Fluoxetine and Paroxetine
Fluoxetine (20 mg QD) and paroxetine (20 mg QD) have been shown to increase the plasma concentration of risperidone 2.5–2.8 fold and 3-9 fold respectively. Fluoxetine did not affect the plasma concentration of 9-hydroxyrisperidone. Paroxetine lowered the concentration of 9-hydroxyrisperidone an average of 13%. When either concomitant fluoxetine or paroxetine is initiated or discontinued, the physician should re-evaluate the dosing of RISPERDAL®. The effects of discontinuation of concomitant fluoxetine or paroxetine therapy on the pharmacokinetics of risperidone and 9-hydroxyrisperidone have not been studied.

Lithium
Repeated oral doses of risperidone (3 mg BID) did not affect the exposure (AUC) or peak plasma concentrations (C_{max}) of lithium (n=13).

Valproate
Repeated oral doses of risperidone (4 mg QD) did not affect the pre-dose or average plasma concentrations and exposure (AUC) of valproate (1000 mg/day in three divided doses) compared to placebo (n=21). However, there was a 20% increase in valproate peak plasma concentration (C_{max}) after concomitant administration of risperidone.

Digoxin
RISPERDAL® (0.25 mg BID) did not show a clinically relevant effect on the pharmacokinetics of digoxin.

Drugs That Inhibit CYP 2D6 and Other CYP Isozymes
Risperidone is metabolized to 9-hydroxyrisperidone by CYP 2D6, an enzyme that is polymorphic in the population and that can be inhibited by a variety of psychotropic and other drugs (see CLINICAL PHARMACOLOGY). Drug interactions that reduce the metabolism of risperidone to 9-hydroxyrisperidone would increase the plasma concentrations of risperidone and lower the concentrations of 9-hydroxyrisperidone. Analysis of clinical studies involving a modest number of poor metabolizers ($n \cong 70$) does not suggest that poor and extensive metabolizers have different rates of adverse effects. No comparison of effectiveness in the two groups has been made.
In vitro studies showed that drugs metabolized by other CYP isozymes, including 1A1, 1A2, 2C9, 2C19, and 3A4, are only weak inhibitors of risperidone metabolism.
There were no significant interactions between risperidone and erythromycin (see CLINICAL PHARMACOLOGY).

Drugs Metabolized by CYP 2D6
In vitro studies indicate that risperidone is a relatively weak inhibitor of CYP 2D6. Therefore, RISPERDAL® is not expected to substantially inhibit the clearance of drugs that are metabolized by this enzymatic pathway. In drug interaction studies, risperidone did not significantly affect the pharmacokinetics of donepezil and galantamine, which are metabolized by CYP 2D6.

Carcinogenesis, Mutagenesis, Impairment of Fertility
Carcinogenesis
Carcinogenicity studies were conducted in Swiss albino mice and Wistar rats. Risperidone was administered in the diet at doses of 0.63, 2.5, and 10 mg/kg for 18 months to mice and for 25 months to rats. These doses are equivalent to 2.4, 9.4, and 37.5 times the maximum recommended human dose (MRHD) (16 mg/day) on a mg/kg basis or 0.2, 0.75, and 3 times the MRHD (mice) or 0.4, 1.5, and 6 times the MRHD (rats) on a mg/m^2 basis. A maximum tolerated dose was not achieved in male mice. There were statistically significant increases in pituitary gland adenomas, endocrine pancreas adenomas, and mammary gland adenocarcinomas. The following table summarizes the multiples of the human dose on a mg/m^2 (mg/kg) basis at which these tumors occurred.
[See table below]

Tumor Type	Species	Sex	Multiples of Maximum Human Dose in mg/m^2 (mg/kg): Lowest Effect Level	Highest No-Effect Level
Pituitary adenomas	mouse	female	0.75 (9.4)	0.2 (2.4)
Endocrine pancreas adenomas	rat	male	1.5 (9.4)	0.4 (2.4)
Mammary gland adenocarcinomas	mouse	female	0.2 (2.4)	none
	rat	female	0.4 (2.4)	none
	rat	male	6.0 (37.5)	1.5 (9.4)
Mammary gland neoplasms, Total	rat	male	1.5 (9.4)	0.4 (2.4)

Antipsychotic drugs have been shown to chronically elevate prolactin levels in rodents. Serum prolactin levels were not measured during the risperidone carcinogenicity studies; however, measurements during subchronic toxicity studies showed that risperidone elevated serum prolactin levels 5–6 fold in mice and rats at the same doses used in the carcinogenicity studies. An increase in mammary, pituitary, and endocrine pancreas neoplasms has been found in rodents after chronic administration of other antipsychotic drugs and is considered to be prolactin-mediated. The relevance for human risk of the findings of prolactin-mediated endocrine tumors in rodents is unknown (see PRECAUTIONS, General—Hyperprolactinemia).

Mutagenesis
No evidence of mutagenic potential for risperidone was found in the Ames reverse mutation test, mouse lymphoma assay, in vitro rat hepatocyte DNA-repair assay, in vivo micronucleus test in mice, the sex-linked recessive lethal test in Drosophila, or the chromosomal aberration test in human lymphocytes or Chinese hamster cells.

Impairment of Fertility
Risperidone (0.16 to 5 mg/kg) was shown to impair mating, but not fertility, in Wistar rats in three reproductive studies (two Segment I and a multigenerational study) at doses 0.1 to 3 times the maximum recommended human dose (MRHD) on a mg/m^2 basis. The effect appeared to be in females, since impaired mating behavior was not noted in the Segment I study in which males only were treated. In a subchronic study in Beagle dogs in which risperidone was administered at doses of 0.31 to 5 mg/kg, sperm motility and concentration were decreased at doses 0.6 to 10 times the MRHD on a mg/m^2 basis. Dose-related decreases were also noted in serum testosterone at the same doses. Serum testosterone and sperm parameters partially recovered, but remained decreased after treatment was discontinued. No no-effect doses were noted in either rat or dog.

Pregnancy
Pregnancy Category C
The teratogenic potential of risperidone was studied in three Segment II studies in Sprague-Dawley and Wistar rats (0.63–10 mg/kg or 0.4 to 6 times the maximum recommended human dose [MRHD] on a mg/m^2 basis) and in one Segment II study in New Zealand rabbits (0.31–5 mg/kg or 0.4 to 6 times the MRHD on a mg/m^2 basis). The incidence of malformations was not increased compared to control in offspring of rats or rabbits given 0.4 to 6 times the MRHD on a mg/m^2 basis. In three reproductive studies in rats (two Segment III and a multigenerational study), there was an increase in pup deaths during the first 4 days of lactation at doses of 0.16–5 mg/kg or 0.1 to 3 times the MRHD on a mg/m^2 basis. It is not known whether these deaths were due to a direct effect on the fetuses or pups or to effects on the dams.
There was no no-effect dose for increased rat pup mortality. In one Segment III study, there was an increase in stillborn rat pups at a dose of 2.5 mg/kg or 1.5 times the MRHD on a mg/m^2 basis. In a cross-fostering study in Wistar rats, toxic effects on the fetus or pups, as evidenced by a decrease in the number of live pups and an increase in the number of dead pups at birth (Day 0), and a decrease in birth weight in pups of drug-treated dams were observed. In addition, there was an increase in deaths by Day 1 among pups of drug-treated dams, regardless of whether or not the pups were cross-fostered. Risperidone also appeared to impair maternal behavior in that pup body weight gain and survival (from Day 1 to 4 of lactation) were reduced in pups born to control but reared by drug-treated dams. These effects were all noted at the one dose of risperidone tested, i.e., 5 mg/kg or 3 times the MRHD on a mg/m^2 basis.
Placental transfer of risperidone occurs in rat pups. There are no adequate and well-controlled studies in pregnant women. However, there was one report of a case of agenesis of the corpus callosum in an infant exposed to risperidone *in utero*. The causal relationship to RISPERDAL® therapy is unknown.
RISPERDAL® should be used during pregnancy only if the potential benefit justifies the potential risk to the fetus.

Labor and Delivery
The effect of RISPERDAL® on labor and delivery in humans is unknown.

Nursing Mothers
In animal studies, risperidone and 9-hydroxyrisperidone are excreted in milk. Risperidone and 9-hydroxyrisperidone are also excreted in human breast milk. Therefore, women receiving risperidone should not breast-feed.

Pediatric Use
Safety and effectiveness in children have not been established.

Geriatric Use
Clinical studies of RISPERDAL® did not include sufficient numbers of patients aged 65 and over to determine whether or not they respond differently than younger patients. Other reported clinical experience has not identified differences in responses between elderly and younger patients. In general, a lower starting dose is recommended for an elderly patient, reflecting a decreased pharmacokinetic clearance in the elderly, as well as a greater frequency of decreased hepatic, renal, or cardiac function, and of concomitant disease or other drug therapy (see CLINICAL PHARMACOLOGY and DOSAGE AND ADMINISTRATION). While elderly patients exhibit a greater tendency to orthostatic hypotension, its risk in the elderly may be minimized by limiting the initial dose to 0.5 mg BID followed by careful titration (see PRECAUTIONS). Monitoring of orthostatic vital signs should be considered in patients for whom this is of concern.

This drug is substantially excreted by the kidneys, and the risk of toxic reactions to this drug may be greater in patients with impaired renal function. Because elderly patients are more likely to have decreased renal function, care should be taken in dose selection, and it may be useful to monitor renal function (see DOSAGE AND ADMINISTRATION).

ADVERSE REACTIONS

The following findings are based on the short-term, placebo-controlled, North American, premarketing trials for schizophrenia and acute bipolar mania. In patients with Bipolar I Disorder, treatment-emergent adverse events are presented separately for risperidone as monotherapy and as adjunctive therapy to mood stabilizers.

Certain portions of the discussion below relating to objective or numeric safety parameters, namely dose-dependent adverse events, vital sign changes, weight gain, laboratory changes, and ECG changes are derived from studies in patients with schizophrenia. However, this information is also generally applicable to bipolar mania.

Associated With Discontinuation of Treatment

Schizophrenia

Approximately 9% (244/2607) of RISPERDAL® (risperidone)-treated patients in Phase 2 and 3 studies discontinued treatment due to an adverse event, compared with about 7% on placebo and 10% on active control drugs. The more common events (≥0.3%) associated with discontinuation and considered to be possibly or probably drug-related included:

Adverse Event	RISPERDAL®	Placebo
Extrapyramidal symptoms	2.1%	0%
Dizziness	0.7%	0%
Hyperkinesia	0.6%	0%
Somnolence	0.5%	0%
Nausea	0.3%	0%

Suicide attempt was associated with discontinuation in 1.2% of RISPERDAL®-treated patients compared to 0.6% of placebo patients, but, given the almost 40-fold greater exposure time in RISPERDAL® compared to placebo patients, it is unlikely that suicide attempt is a RISPERDAL®-related adverse event (see PRECAUTIONS). Discontinuation for extrapyramidal symptoms was 0% in placebo patients, but 3.8% in active-control patients in the Phase 2 and 3 trials.

Bipolar Mania

In the US placebo-controlled trial with risperidone as monotherapy, approximately 8% (10/134) of RISPERDAL®-treated patients discontinued treatment due to an adverse event, compared with approximately 6% (7/125) of placebo-treated patients. The adverse events associated with discontinuation and considered to be possibly, probably, or very likely drug-related included paroniria, somnolence, dizziness, extrapyramidal disorder, and muscle contractions involuntary. Each of these events occurred in one RISPERDAL®-treated patient (0.7%) and in no placebo-treated patients (0%).

In the US placebo-controlled trial with risperidone as adjunctive therapy to mood stabilizers, there was no overall difference in the incidence of discontinuation due to adverse events (4% for RISPERDAL® vs. 4% for placebo).

Incidence in Controlled Trials

Commonly Observed Adverse Events in Controlled Clinical Trials

Schizophrenia

In two 6- to 8-week placebo-controlled trials, spontaneously-reported, treatment-emergent adverse events with an incidence of 5% or greater in at least one of the RISPERDAL® groups and at least twice that of placebo were anxiety, somnolence, extra-pyramidal symptoms, dizziness, constipation, nausea, dyspepsia, rhinitis, rash, and tachycardia.

Adverse events were also elicited in one of these two trials (i.e., in the fixed-dose trial comparing RISPERDAL® at doses of 2, 6, 10, and 16 mg/day with placebo) utilizing a checklist for detecting adverse events, a method that is more sensitive than spontaneous reporting. By this method, the following additional common and drug-related adverse events occurred at an incidence of at least 5% and twice the rate of placebo: increased dream activity, increased duration of sleep, accommodation disturbances, reduced salivation, micturition disturbances, diarrhea, weight gain, menorrhagia, diminished sexual desire, erectile dysfunction, ejaculatory dysfunction, and orgastic dysfunction.

Bipolar Mania

In the US placebo-controlled trial with risperidone as monotherapy, the most commonly observed adverse events associated with the use of RISPERDAL® (incidence of 5% or greater and at least twice that of placebo) were somnolence, dystonia, akathisia, dyspepsia, nausea, parkinsonism, vision abnormal, and saliva increased. In the US placebo-controlled trial with risperidone as adjunctive therapy to mood stabilizers, the most commonly observed adverse events associated with the use of RISPERDAL® were somnolence, dizziness, parkinsonism, saliva increased, akathisia, abdominal pain, and urinary incontinence.

Adverse Events Occurring at an Incidence of 1% or More Among RISPERDAL®-Treated Patients - Schizophrenia

The table that follows enumerates adverse events that occurred at an incidence of 1% or more, and were more frequent among RISPERDAL®-treated patients treated at doses of ≤ 10 mg/day than among placebo-treated patients in the pooled results of two 6- to 8-week controlled trials. Patients received RISPERDAL® doses of 2, 6, 10, or 16 mg/day in the dose comparison trial, or up to a maximum dose of 10 mg/day in the titration study. This table shows the percentage of patients in each dose group (≤ 10 mg/day or 16 mg/day) who spontaneously reported at least one episode of an event at some time during their treatment. Patients given doses of 2, 6, or 10 mg did not differ materially in these rates. Reported adverse events were classified using the World Health Organization preferred terms.

The prescriber should be aware that these figures cannot be used to predict the incidence of side effects in the course of usual medical practice where patient characteristics and other factors differ from those which prevailed in this clinical trial. Similarly, the cited frequencies cannot be compared with figures obtained from other clinical investigations involving different treatments, uses, and investigators. The cited figures, however, do provide the prescribing physician with some basis for estimating the relative contribution of drug and non-drug factors to the side effect incidence rate in the population studied.

Table 1. Incidence of Treatment-Emergent Adverse Events in 6- to 8-Week Controlled Clinical Trials[1]

Body System/ Preferred Term	RISPERDAL® ≤10 mg/day (N=324)	RISPERDAL® 16 mg/day (N=77)	Placebo (N=142)
Psychiatric			
Insomnia	26%	23%	19%
Agitation	22%	26%	20%
Anxiety	12%	20%	9%
Somnolence	3%	8%	1%
Aggressive reaction	1%	3%	1%
Central & peripheral nervous system			
Extrapyramidal symptoms[2]	17%	34%	16%
Headache	14%	12%	12%
Dizziness	4%	7%	1%
Gastrointestinal			
Constipation	7%	13%	3%
Nausea	6%	4%	3%
Dyspepsia	5%	10%	4%
Vomiting	5%	7%	4%
Abdominal pain	4%	1%	0%
Saliva increased	2%	0%	1%
Toothache	2%	0%	0%
Respiratory system			
Rhinitis	10%	8%	4%
Coughing	3%	3%	1%
Sinusitis	2%	1%	1%
Pharyngitis	2%	3%	0%
Dyspnea	1%	0%	0%
Body as a whole-general			
Back pain	2%	0%	1%
Chest pain	2%	3%	1%
Fever	2%	3%	0%
Dermatological			
Rash	2%	5%	1%
Dry skin	2%	4%	0%
Seborrhea	1%	0%	0%
Infections			
Upper respiratory	3%	3%	1%
Visual			
Abnormal vision	2%	1%	1%
Musculo-Skeletal			
Arthralgia	2%	3%	0%
Cardiovascular			
Tachycardia	3%	5%	0%

[1] Events reported by at least 1% of patients treated with RISPERDAL® ≤ 10 mg/day are included, and are rounded to the nearest %. Comparative rates for RISPERDAL® 16 mg/day and placebo are provided as well. Events for which the RISPERDAL® incidence (in both dose groups) was equal to or less than placebo are not listed in the table, but included the following: nervousness, injury, and fungal infection.

[2] Includes tremor, dystonia, hypokinesia, hypertonia, hyperkinesia, oculogyric crisis, ataxia, abnormal gait, involuntary muscle contractions, hyporeflexia, akathisia, and extrapyramidal disorders. Although the incidence of 'extrapyramidal symptoms' does not appear to differ for the '10 mg/day' group and placebo, the data for individual dose groups in fixed dose trials do suggest a dose/response relationship (see ADVERSE REACTIONS – Dose Dependency of Adverse Events).

Adverse Events Occurring at an Incidence of 2% or More Among RISPERDAL®-Treated Patients - Bipolar Mania

Tables 2 and 3 display adverse events that occurred at an incidence of 2% or more, and were more frequent among patients treated with flexible doses of RISPERDAL® (1–6 mg daily as monotherapy and as adjunctive therapy to mood stabilizers, respectively) than among patients treated with placebo. Reported adverse events were classified using the World Health Organization preferred terms.

Table 2. Incidence of Treatment-Emergent Adverse Events in a 3-Week, Placebo-Controlled Trial - Monotherapy in Bipolar Mania[1]

Body System/ Preferred Term	RISPERDAL® (N=134)	Placebo (N=125)
Central & peripheral nervous system		
Dystonia	18%	6%
Akathisia	16%	6%
Dizziness	11%	9%
Parkinsonism	6%	3%
Hypoaesthesia	2%	1%
Psychiatric		
Somnolence	28%	7%
Agitation	8%	6%
Manic reaction	8%	6%
Anxiety	4%	2%
Concentration impaired	2%	1%
Gastrointestinal system		
Dyspepsia	11%	6%
Nausea	11%	2%
Saliva increased	5%	1%
Mouth dry	3%	2%
Body as a whole - general		
Pain	5%	3%
Fatigue	4%	2%
Injury	2%	0%
Respiratory system		
Sinusitis	4%	1%
Rhinitis	3%	2%
Coughing	2%	2%
Skin and appendages		
Acne	2%	0%
Pruritus	2%	1%
Musculo-Skeletal		
Myalgia	5%	2%
Skeletal pain	2%	1%
Metabolic and nutritional		
Weight increase	2%	0%
Vision disorders		
Vision abnormal	6%	2%
Cardiovascular, general		
Hypertension	3%	1%
Hypotension	2%	0%
Heart rate and rhythm		
Tachycardia	3%	2%

[1] Events reported by at least 2% of patients treated with RISPERDAL® are included and are rounded to the nearest %. Events reported by at least 2% of patients treated with RISPERDAL® that were less than the incidence reported by patients treated with placebo are not listed in the table, but included the following: headache, tremor, insomnia, constipation, back pain, upper respiratory tract infection, pharyngitis, and arthralgia.

Table 3. Incidence of Treatment-Emergent Adverse Events in a 3-Week, Placebo-Controlled Trial - Adjunctive in Bipolar Mania[1]

Body System/ Preferred Term	RISPERDAL® + Mood Stabilizer (N=152)	Placebo + Mood Stabilizer (N=51)
Gastrointestinal system		
Saliva increased	10%	0%
Diarrhea	8%	4%
Abdominal pain	6%	0%
Constipation	6%	4%
Mouth dry	6%	4%
Tooth ache	4%	0%
Tooth disorder	4%	0%
Central & peripheral nervous sytem		
Dizziness	14%	2%
Parkinsonism	14%	4%
Akathisia	8%	0%
Dystonia	6%	4%
Psychiatric		
Somnolence	25%	12%
Anxiety	6%	4%
Confusion	4%	0%
Respiratory system		
Rhinitis	8%	4%
Pharyngitis	6%	4%
Coughing	4%	0%
Body as a whole - general		
Asthenia	4%	2%

Continued on next page

Risperdal—Cont.

Urinary system		
Urinary incontinence	6%	2%
Heart rate and rhythm		
Tachycardia	4%	2%
Metabolic and nutritional		
Weight increase	4%	2%
Skin and appendages		
Rash	4%	2%

[1] Events reported by at least 2% of patients treated with RISPERDAL® are included and are rounded to the nearest %. Events reported by at least 2% of patients treated with RISPERDAL® that were less than the incidence reported by patients treated with placebo are not listed in the table, but included the following: dyspepsia, nausea, vomiting, headache, tremor, insomnia, chest pain, fatigue, pain, skeletal pain, hypertension, and vision abnormal.

Dose Dependency of Adverse Events

Extrapyramidal Symptoms

Data from two fixed-dose trials provided evidence of dose-relatedness for extrapyramidal symptoms associated with risperidone treatment.

Two methods were used to measure extrapyramidal symptoms (EPS) in an 8-week trial comparing 4 fixed doses of risperidone (2, 6, 10, and 16 mg/day), including (1) a parkinsonism score (mean change from baseline) from the Extrapyramidal Symptom Rating Scale, and (2) incidence of spontaneous complaints of EPS:

Dose Groups	Placebo	Ris 2	Ris 6	Ris 10	Ris 16
Parkinsonism	1.2	0.9	1.8	2.4	2.6
EPS Incidence	13%	13%	16%	20%	31%

Similar methods were used to measure extrapyramidal symptoms (EPS) in an 8-week trial comparing 5 fixed doses of risperidone (1, 4, 8, 12, and 16 mg/day):

Dose Groups	Ris 1	Ris 4	Ris 8	Ris 12	Ris 16
Parkinsonism	0.6	1.7	2.4	2.9	4.1
EPS Incidence	7%	12%	18%	18%	21%

Other Adverse Events

Adverse event data elicited by a checklist for side effects from a large study comparing 5 fixed doses of RISPERDAL® (1, 4, 8, 12, and 16 mg/day) were explored for dose-relatedness of adverse events. A Cochran-Armitage Test for trend in these data revealed a positive trend ($p<0.05$) for the following adverse events: sleepiness, increased duration of sleep, accommodation disturbances, orthostatic dizziness, palpitations, weight gain, erectile dysfunction, ejaculatory dysfunction, orgastic dysfunction, asthenia/lassitude/increased fatigability, and increased pigmentation.

Vital Sign Changes

RISPERDAL® is associated with orthostatic hypotension and tachycardia (see PRECAUTIONS).

Weight Changes

The proportions of RISPERDAL® and placebo-treated patients meeting a weight gain criterion of ≥7% of body weight were compared in a pool of 6- to 8-week, placebo-controlled trials, revealing a statistically significantly greater incidence of weight gain for RISPERDAL® (18%) compared to placebo (9%).

Laboratory Changes

A between-group comparison for 6- to 8-week placebo-controlled trials revealed no statistically significant RISPERDAL®/placebo differences in the proportions of patients experiencing potentially important changes in routine serum chemistry, hematology, or urinalysis parameters. Similarly, there were no RISPERDAL®/placebo differences in the incidence of discontinuations for changes in serum chemistry, hematology, or urinalysis. However, RISPERDAL® administration was associated with increases in serum prolactin (see PRECAUTIONS).

ECG Changes

Between-group comparisons for pooled placebo-controlled trials revealed no statistically significant differences between risperidone and placebo in mean changes from baseline in ECG parameters, including QT, QTc, and PR intervals, and heart rate. When all RISPERDAL® doses were pooled from randomized controlled trials in several indications, there was a mean increase in heart rate of 1 beat per minute compared to no change for placebo patients. In short-term schizophrenia trials, higher doses of risperidone (8–16 mg/day) were associated with a higher mean increase in heart rate compared to placebo (4–6 beats per minute).

Other Events Observed During the Premarketing Evaluation of RISPERDAL®

During its premarketing assessment, multiple doses of RISPERDAL® were administered to 2607 patients in Phase 2 and 3 studies. The conditions and duration of exposure to RISPERDAL® varied greatly, and included (in overlapping categories) open-label and double-blind studies, uncontrolled and controlled studies, inpatient and outpatient studies, fixed-dose and titration studies, and short-term or longer-term exposure. In most studies, untoward events associated with this exposure were obtained by spontaneous report and recorded by clinical investigators using terminology of their own choosing. Consequently, it is not possible to provide a meaningful estimate of the proportion of individuals experiencing adverse events without first grouping similar types of untoward events into a smaller number of standardized event categories. In two large studies, adverse events were also elicited utilizing the UKU (direct questioning) side effect rating scale, and these events were not further categorized using standard terminology. (Note: These events are marked with an asterisk in the listings that follow.)

In the listings that follow, spontaneously reported adverse events were classified using World Health Organization (WHO) preferred terms. The frequencies presented, therefore, represent the proportion of the 2607 patients exposed to multiple doses of RISPERDAL® who experienced an event of the type cited on at least one occasion while receiving RISPERDAL®. All reported events are included, except those already listed in Table 1, those events for which a drug cause was remote, and those event terms which were so general as to be uninformative. It is important to emphasize that, although the events reported occurred during treatment with RISPERDAL®, they were not necessarily caused by it.

Events are further categorized by body system and listed in order of decreasing frequency according to the following definitions: frequent adverse events are those occurring in at least 1/100 patients (only those not already listed in the tabulated results from placebo-controlled trials appear in this listing); infrequent adverse events are those occurring in 1/100 to 1/1000 patients; rare events are those occurring in fewer than 1/1000 patients.

Psychiatric Disorders

Frequent: increased dream activity*, diminished sexual desire*, nervousness. *Infrequent*: impaired concentration, depression, apathy, catatonic reaction, euphoria, increased libido, amnesia. *Rare*: emotional lability, nightmares, delirium, withdrawal syndrome, yawning.

Central and Peripheral Nervous System Disorders

Frequent: increased sleep duration*. *Infrequent*: dysarthria, vertigo, stupor, paraesthesia, confusion. *Rare*: aphasia, cholinergic syndrome, hypoesthesia, tongue paralysis, leg cramps, torticollis, hypotonia, coma, migraine, hyperreflexia, choreoathetosis.

Gastrointestinal Disorders

Frequent: anorexia, reduced salivation*. *Infrequent*: flatulence, diarrhea, increased appetite, stomatitis, melena, dysphagia, hemorrhoids, gastritis. *Rare*: fecal incontinence, eructation, gastroesophageal reflux, gastroenteritis, esophagitis, tongue discoloration, cholelithiasis, tongue edema, diverticulitis, gingivitis, discolored feces, GI hemorrhage, hematemesis.

Body as a Whole/General Disorders

Frequent: fatigue. *Infrequent*: edema, rigors, malaise, influenza-like symptoms. *Rare*: pallor, enlarged abdomen, allergic reaction, ascites, sarcoidosis, flushing.

Respiratory System Disorders

Infrequent: hyperventilation, bronchospasm, pneumonia, stridor. *Rare*: asthma, increased sputum, aspiration.

Skin and Appendage Disorders

Frequent: increased pigmentation*, photosensitivity*. *Infrequent*: increased sweating, acne, decreased sweating, alopecia, hyperkeratosis, pruritus, skin exfoliation. *Rare*: bullous eruption, skin ulceration, aggravated psoriasis, furunculosis, verruca, dermatitis lichenoid, hypertrichosis, genital pruritus, urticaria.

Cardiovascular Disorders

Infrequent: palpitation, hypertension, hypotension, AV block, myocardial infarction. *Rare*: ventricular tachycardia, angina pectoris, premature atrial contractions, T wave inversions, ventricular extrasystoles, ST depression, myocarditis.

Vision Disorders

Infrequent: abnormal accommodation, xerophthalmia. *Rare*: diplopia, eye pain, blepharitis, photopsia, photophobia, abnormal lacrimation.

Metabolic and Nutritional Disorders

Infrequent: hyponatremia, weight increase, creatinine phosphokinase increase, thirst, weight decrease, diabetes mellitus. *Rare*: decreased serum iron, cachexia, dehydration, hypokalemia, hypoproteinemia, hyperphosphatemia, hypertriglyceridemia, hyperuricemia, hypoglycemia.

Urinary System Disorders

Frequent: polyuria/polydipsia*. *Infrequent*: urinary incontinence, hematuria, dysuria. *Rare*: urinary retention, cystitis, renal insufficiency.

Musculo-Skeletal System Disorders

Infrequent: myalgia. *Rare*: arthrosis, synostosis, bursitis, arthritis, skeletal pain.

Reproductive Disorders, Female

Frequent: menorrhagia*, orgastic dysfunction*, dry vagina*. *Infrequent*: nonpuerperal lactation, amenorrhea, female breast pain, leukorrhea, mastitis, dysmenorrhea, female perineal pain, intermenstrual bleeding, vaginal hemorrhage.

Liver and Biliary System Disorders

Infrequent: increased SGOT, increased SGPT. *Rare*: hepatic failure, cholestatic hepatitis, cholecystitis, cholelithiasis, hepatitis, hepatocellular damage.

Platelet, Bleeding, and Clotting Disorders

Infrequent: epistaxis, purpura. *Rare*: hemorrhage, superficial phlebitis, thrombophlebitis, thrombocytopenia.

Hearing and Vestibular Disorders

Rare: tinnitus, hyperacusis, decreased hearing.

Red Blood Cell Disorders

Infrequent: anemia, hypochromic anemia. *Rare*: normocytic anemia.

Reproductive Disorders, Male

Frequent: erectile dysfunction*. *Infrequent*: ejaculation failure.

White Cell and Resistance Disorders

Rare: leukocytosis, lymphadenopathy, leucopenia, Pelger-Huet anomaly.

Endocrine Disorders

Rare: gynecomastia, male breast pain, antidiuretic hormone disorder.

Special Senses

Rare: bitter taste.

* Incidence based on elicited reports.

Postintroduction Reports

Adverse events reported since market introduction which were temporally (but not necessarily causally) related to RISPERDAL® therapy, include the following: anaphylactic reaction, angioedema, apnea, atrial fibrillation, cerebrovascular disorder, including cerebrovascular accident, hyperglycemia, diabetes mellitus aggravated, including diabetic ketoacidosis, intestinal obstruction, jaundice, mania, pancreatitis, Parkinson's disease aggravated, pulmonary embolism. There have been rare reports of sudden death and/or cardiopulmonary arrest in patients receiving RISPERDAL®. A causal relationship with RISPERDAL® has not been established. It is important to note that sudden and unexpected death may occur in psychotic patients whether they remain untreated or whether they are treated with other antipsychotic drugs.

DRUG ABUSE AND DEPENDENCE

Controlled Substance Class

RISPERDAL® (risperidone) is not a controlled substance.

Physical and Psychological Dependence

RISPERDAL® has not been systematically studied in animals or humans for its potential for abuse, tolerance, or physical dependence. While the clinical trials did not reveal any tendency for any drug-seeking behavior, these observations were not systematic and it is not possible to predict on the basis of this limited experience the extent to which a CNS-active drug will be misused, diverted, and/or abused once marketed. Consequently, patients should be evaluated carefully for a history of drug abuse, and such patients should be observed closely for signs of RISPERDAL® misuse or abuse (e.g., development of tolerance, increases in dose, drug-seeking behavior).

OVERDOSAGE

Human Experience

Premarketing experience included eight reports of acute RISPERDAL® (risperidone) overdosage with estimated doses ranging from 20 to 300 mg and no fatalities. In general, reported signs and symptoms were those resulting from an exaggeration of the drug's known pharmacological effects, i.e., drowsiness and sedation, tachycardia and hypotension, and extrapyramidal symptoms. One case, involving an estimated overdose of 240 mg, was associated with hyponatremia, hypokalemia, prolonged QT, and widened QRS. Another case, involving an estimated overdose of 36 mg, was associated with a seizure.

Postmarketing experience includes reports of acute RISPERDAL® overdosage, with estimated doses of up to 360 mg. In general, the most frequently reported signs and symptoms are those resulting from an exaggeration of the drug's known pharmacological effects, i.e., drowsiness, sedation, tachycardia, hypotension, and extrapyramidal symptoms. Other adverse events reported since market introduction which were temporally (but not necessarily causally) related to RISPERDAL® overdose, include torsade de pointes, prolonged QT interval, convulsions, cardiopulmonary arrest, and rare fatality associated with multiple drug overdose.

Management of Overdosage

In case of acute overdosage, establish and maintain an airway and ensure adequate oxygenation and ventilation. Gastric lavage (after intubation, if patient is unconscious) and administration of activated charcoal together with a laxative should be considered. Because of the rapid disintegration of RISPERDAL® M-TAB™ Orally Disintegrating Tablets, pill fragments may not appear in gastric contents obtained with lavage.

The possibility of obtundation, seizures, or dystonic reaction of the head and neck following overdose may create a risk of aspiration with induced emesis. Cardiovascular monitoring should commence immediately and should include continuous electrocardiographic monitoring to detect possible arrhythmias. If antiarrhythmic therapy is administered, disopyramide, procainamide, and quinidine carry a theoretical hazard of QT-prolonging effects that might be additive to those of risperidone. Similarly, it is reasonable to expect that the alpha-blocking properties of bretylium might be additive to those of risperidone, resulting in problematic hypotension.

There is no specific antidote to RISPERDAL®. Therefore, appropriate supportive measures should be instituted. The possibility of multiple drug involvement should be considered. Hypotension and circulatory collapse should be treated with appropriate measures, such as intravenous fluids and/or sympathomimetic agents (epinephrine and dopamine should not be used, since beta stimulation may worsen hypotension in the setting of risperidone-induced alpha blockade). In cases of severe extrapyramidal symptoms, anticholinergic medication should be administered. Close medical supervision and monitoring should continue until the patient recovers.

DOSAGE AND ADMINISTRATION

Schizophrenia

Usual Initial Dose

RISPERDAL® (risperidone) can be administered on either a BID or a QD schedule. In early clinical trials, RISPERDAL® was generally administered at 1 mg BID initially, with increases in increments of 1 mg BID on the second and third day, as tolerated, to a target dose of 3 mg BID by the third day. Subsequent controlled trials have indicated that total daily risperidone doses of up to 8 mg on a QD regimen are also safe and effective. However, regardless of which regimen is employed, in some patients a slower titration may be medically appropriate. Further dosage adjustments, if indicated, should generally occur at intervals of not less than 1 week, since steady state for the active metabolite would not be achieved for approximately 1 week in the typical patient. When dosage adjustments are necessary, small dose increments/decrements of 1–2 mg are recommended.

Efficacy in schizophrenia was demonstrated in a dose range of 4 to 16 mg/day in the clinical trials supporting effectiveness of RISPERDAL®; however, maximal effect was generally seen in a range of 4 to 8 mg/day. Doses above 6 mg/day for BID dosing were not demonstrated to be more efficacious than lower doses, were associated with more extrapyramidal symptoms and other adverse effects, and are not generally recommended. In a single study supporting QD dosing, the efficacy results were generally stronger for 8 mg than for 4 mg. The safety of doses above 16 mg/day has not been evaluated in clinical trials.

Maintenance Therapy

While there is no body of evidence available to answer the question of how long the schizophrenic patient treated with RISPERDAL® should remain on it, the effectiveness of RISPERDAL® 2 mg/day to 8 mg/day at delaying relapse was demonstrated in a controlled trial in patients who had been clinically stable for at least 4 weeks and were then followed for a period of 1 to 2 years. In this trial, RISPERDAL® was administered on a QD schedule, at 1 mg QD initially, with increases to 2 mg QD on the second day, and to a target dose of 4 mg QD on the third day (see CLINICAL PHARMACOLOGY – Clinical Trials). Nevertheless, patients should be periodically reassessed to determine the need for maintenance treatment with an appropriate dose.

Reinitiation of Treatment in Patients Previously Discontinued

Although there are no data to specifically address reinitiation of treatment, it is recommended that when restarting patients who have had an interval off RISPERDAL®, the initial titration schedule should be followed.

Switching From Other Antipsychotics

There are no systematically collected data to specifically address switching schizophrenic patients from other antipsychotics to RISPERDAL®, or concerning concomitant administration with other antipsychotics. While immediate discontinuation of the previous antipsychotic treatment may be acceptable for some schizophrenic patients, more gradual discontinuation may be most appropriate for others. In all cases, the period of overlapping antipsychotic administration should be minimized. When switching schizophrenic patients from depot antipsychotics, if medically appropriate, initiate RISPERDAL® therapy in place of the next scheduled injection. The need for continuing existing EPS medication should be re-evaluated periodically.

Bipolar Mania

Usual Dose

Risperidone should be administered on a once daily schedule, starting with 2 mg to 3 mg per day. Dosage adjustments, if indicated, should occur at intervals of not less than 24 hours and in dosage increments/decrements of 1 mg per day, as studied in the short-term, placebo-controlled trials. In these trials, short-term (3 week) anti-manic efficacy was demonstrated in a flexible dosage range of 1-6 mg per day (see CLINICAL PHARMACOLOGY – Clinical Trials). RISPERDAL® doses higher than 6 mg per day were not studied.

Maintenance Therapy

There is no body of evidence available from controlled trials to guide a clinician in the longer-term management of a patient who improves during treatment of an acute manic episode with risperidone. While it is generally agreed that pharmacological treatment beyond an acute response in mania is desirable, both for maintenance of the initial response and for prevention of new manic episodes, there are no systematically obtained data to support the use of risperidone in such longer-term treatment (i.e., beyond 3 weeks).

Pediatric Use

Safety and effectiveness of RISPERDAL® in pediatric patients with schizophrenia or acute mania associated with Bipolar I Disorder have not been established.

Dosage in Special Populations

The recommended initial dose is 0.5 mg BID in patients who are elderly or debilitated, patients with severe renal or hepatic impairment, and patients either predisposed to hypotension or for whom hypotension would pose a risk. Dosage increases in these patients should be in increments of no more than 0.5 mg BID. Increases to dosages above 1.5 mg BID should generally occur at intervals of at least 1 week. In some patients, slower titration may be medically appropriate.

Elderly or debilitated patients, and patients with renal impairment, may have less ability to eliminate RISPERDAL® than normal adults. Patients with impaired hepatic function may have increases in the free fraction of risperidone, possibly resulting in an enhanced effect (see CLINICAL PHARMACOLOGY). Patients with a predisposition to hypotensive reactions or for whom such reactions would pose a particular risk likewise need to be titrated cautiously and carefully monitored (see PRECAUTIONS). If a once-a-day dosing regimen in the elderly or debilitated patient is being considered, it is recommended that the patient be titrated on a twice-a-day regimen for 2–3 days at the target dose. Subsequent switches to a once-a-day dosing regimen can be done thereafter.

Co-Administration of RISPERDAL® with Certain Other Medications

Co-administration of carbamazepine and other enzyme inducers (e.g., phenytoin, rifampin, phenobarbital) with risperidone would be expected to cause decreases in the plasma concentrations of active moiety (the sum of risperidone and 9-hydroxyrisperidone), which could lead to decreased efficacy of risperidone treatment. The dose of risperidone needs to be titrated accordingly for patients receiving these enzyme inducers, especially during initiation or discontinuation of therapy with these inducers (see CLINICAL PHARMACOLOGY and PRECAUTIONS).

Fluoxetine and paroxetine have been shown to increase the plasma concentration of risperidone 2.5–2.8 fold and 3–9 fold respectively. Fluoxetine did not affect the plasma concentration of 9-hydroxyrisperidone. Paroxetine lowered the concentration of 9-hydroxyrisperidone an average of 13%. The dose of risperidone needs to be titrated accordingly when fluoxetine or paroxetine is co-administered (see CLINICAL PHARMACOLOGY and PRECAUTIONS).

Directions for Use of RISPERDAL® M-TAB™ Orally Disintegrating Tablets

RISPERDAL® M-TAB™ Orally Disintegrating Tablets are supplied in blister packs of 4 tablet units each.

Tablet Accessing

Do not open the blister until ready to administer. For single tablet removal, separate one of the four blister units by tearing apart at the perforations. Bend the corner where indicated. Peel back foil to expose the tablet. DO NOT push the tablet through the foil because this could damage the tablet.

Tablet Administration

Using dry hands, remove the tablet from the blister unit and immediately place the entire RISPERDAL® M-TAB™ Orally Disintegrating Tablet on the tongue. The RISPERDAL® M-TAB™ Orally Disintegrating Tablet should be consumed immediately, as the tablet cannot be stored once removed from the blister unit. RISPERDAL® M-TAB™ Orally Disintegrating Tablets disintegrate in the mouth within seconds and can be swallowed subsequently with or without liquid. Patients should not attempt to split or to chew the tablet.

HOW SUPPLIED

RISPERDAL® (risperidone) tablets are imprinted "JANSSEN", and either "Ris" and the strength "0.25", "0.5", or "R" and the strength "1", "2", "3", or "4".

0.25 mg dark yellow tablet: bottles of 60 NDC 50458-301-04, bottles of 500 NDC 50458-301-50, hospital unit dose packs of 100 NDC 50458-301-01.

0.5 mg red-brown tablet: bottles of 60 NDC 50458-302-06, bottles of 500 NDC 50458-302-50, hospital unit dose packs of 100 NDC 50458-302-01.

1 mg white tablet: bottles of 60 NDC 50458-300-06, blister pack of 100 NDC 50458-300-01, bottles of 500 NDC 50458-300-50.

2 mg orange tablet: bottles of 60 NDC 50458-320-06, blister pack of 100 NDC 50458-320-01, bottles of 500 NDC 50458-320-50.

3 mg yellow tablet: bottles of 60 NDC 50458-330-06, blister pack of 100 NDC 50458-330-01, bottles of 500 NDC 50458-330-50.

4 mg green tablet: bottles of 60 NDC 50458-350-06, blister pack of 100 NDC 50458-350-01.

RISPERDAL® (risperidone) 1 mg/mL oral solution (NDC 50458-305-03) is supplied in 30 mL bottles with a calibrated (in milligrams and milliliters) pipette. The minimum calibrated volume is 0.25 mL, while the maximum calibrated volume is 3 mL.

Tests indicate that RISPERDAL® (risperidone) oral solution is compatible in the following beverages: water, coffee, orange juice, and low-fat milk; it is NOT compatible with either cola or tea, however.

RISPERDAL® M-TAB™ (risperidone) Orally Disintegrating Tablets are etched on one side with "R0.5", "R1", and "R2", respectively, and are packaged in blister packs of 4 (2 × 2) tablets.

0.5 mg light coral, round, biconvex tablets: 7 blister packages per box, NDC 50458-395-28, long-term care packaging of 30 tablets NDC 50458-395-30.

1 mg light coral, square, biconvex tablets: 7 blister packages per box, NDC 50458-315-28, long-term care packaging of 30 tablets NDC 50458-315-30.

2 mg light coral, round, biconvex tablets: 7 blister packages per box, NDC 50458-325-28.

Storage and Handling

RISPERDAL® tablets should be stored at controlled room temperature 15°–25°C (59°–77°F). Protect from light and moisture.

Keep out of reach of children.

RISPERDAL® 1 mg/mL oral solution should be stored at controlled room temperature 15°–25°C (59°–77°F). Protect from light and freezing.

Keep out of reach of children.

RISPERDAL® M-TAB™ Orally Disintegrating Tablets should be stored at controlled room temperature 15°–25°C (59°–77°F).

Keep out of reach of children.

7503226
US Patent 4,804,663
December 2003

RISPERDAL® tablets are manufactured by:
JOLLC, Gurabo, Puerto Rico or
Janssen-Cilag, SpA, Latina, Italy

RISPERDAL® oral solution is manufactured by:
Janssen Pharmaceutica N.V.
Beerse, Belgium

RISPERDAL® M-TAB™ Orally Disintegrating Tablets are manufactured by:
JOLLC, Gurabo, Puerto Rico

RISPERDAL® tablets, RISPERDAL® M-TAB™ Orally Disintegrating Tablets, and oral solution are distributed by:
Janssen Pharmaceutica Products, L.P.
Titusville, NJ 08560

JANSSEN
PHARMACEUTICA PRODUCTS, L.P.

Shown in Product Identification Guide, page 319

RISPERDAL® CONSTA™ ℞

[rĭs-pər-dăl cŏn-stă]
(RISPERIDONE)
LONG-ACTING INJECTION

Rx Only

DESCRIPTION

RISPERDAL® (risperidone) is a psychotropic agent belonging to the chemical class of benzisoxazole derivatives. The chemical designation is 3-[2-[4-(6-fluoro-1,2-benzisoxazol-3-yl)-1-piperidinyl]ethyl]-6,7,8,9-tetrahydro-2-methyl-4H-pyrido[1,2-a]pyrimidin-4-one. Its molecular formula is $C_{23}H_{27}FN_4O_2$ and its molecular weight is 410.49. The structural formula is:

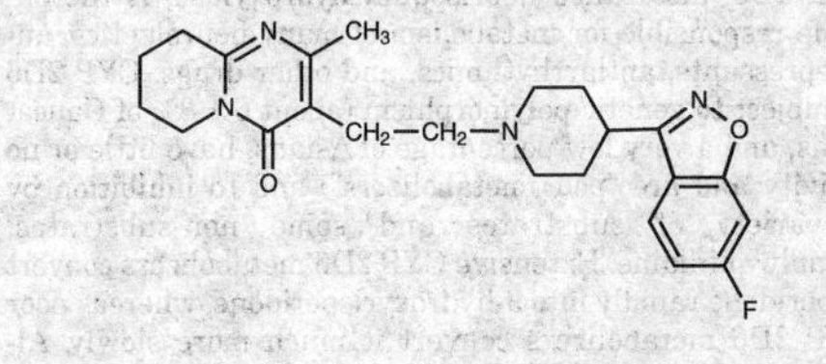

Risperidone is practically insoluble in water, freely soluble in methylene chloride, and soluble in methanol and 0.1 N HCl.

RISPERDAL® CONSTA™ (risperidone) Long-Acting Injection is a combination of extended release microspheres for injection and diluent for parenteral use.

The extended release microspheres formulation is a white to off-white, free-flowing powder that is available in dosage strengths of 25, 37.5, or 50 mg risperidone per vial. Risperidone is micro-encapsulated in 7525 polylactide-co-glycolide (PLG) at a concentration of 381 mg risperidone per gram of microspheres.

The diluent for parenteral use is a clear, colorless solution. Composition of the diluent includes polysorbate 20, sodium carboxymethyl cellulose, disodium hydrogen phosphate dihydrate, citric acid anhydrous, sodium chloride, sodium hydroxide, and water for injection. The microspheres are suspended in the diluent prior to injection.

RISPERDAL® CONSTA™ is provided as a dose pack, consisting of a vial containing the microspheres, a pre-filled syringe containing the diluent, a SmartSite® Needle-Free Vial Access Device, and one Needle-Pro® 20 G TW safety needle.

CLINICAL PHARMACOLOGY

Pharmacodynamics

The mechanism of action of RISPERDAL® (risperidone), as with other drugs used to treat schizophrenia, is unknown. However, it has been proposed that the drug's therapeutic activity in schizophrenia is mediated through a combination of dopamine Type 2 (D_2) and serotonin Type 2 ($5HT_2$) receptor antagonism. Antagonism at receptors other than D_2 and $5HT_2$ may explain some of the other effects of RISPERDAL®.

RISPERDAL® is a selective monoaminergic antagonist with high affinity (Ki of 0.12 to 7.3 nM) for the serotonin Type 2 ($5HT_2$), dopamine Type 2 (D_2), α_1 and α_2 adrenergic, and H_1 histaminergic receptors. RISPERDAL® acts as an antagonist at other receptors, but with lower potency. RISPERDAL® has low to moderate affinity (Ki of 47 to 253 nM) for the serotonin $5HT_{1C}$, $5HT_{1D}$, and $5HT_{1A}$ receptors, weak affinity (Ki of 620 to 800 nM) for the dopamine D_1 and

Continued on next page

Risperdal Consta—Cont.

haloperidol-sensitive sigma site, and no affinity (when tested at concentrations $>10^{-5}$ M) for cholinergic muscarinic or β_1 and β_2 adrenergic receptors.

Pharmacokinetics

Absorption

After a single intramuscular (gluteal) injection of RISPERDAL® CONSTA™ (risperidone), there is a small initial release of the drug (<about 1% of the dose), followed by a lag time of 3 weeks. The main release of the drug starts from 3 weeks onward, is maintained from 4 to 6 weeks, and subsides by 7 weeks following the intramuscular (IM) injection. Therefore, oral antipsychotic supplementation should be given during the first 3 weeks of treatment with RISPERDAL® CONSTA™ to maintain therapeutic levels until the main release of risperidone from the injection site has begun (see DOSAGE AND ADMINISTRATION).

The combination of the release profile and the dosage regimen (IM injections every 2 weeks) of RISPERDAL® CONSTA™ results in sustained therapeutic concentrations. Steady-state plasma concentrations are reached after 4 injections and are maintained for 4 to 6 weeks after the last injection. Plasma concentrations of risperidone, 9-hydroxyrisperidone (the major metabolite), and risperidone plus 9-hydroxyrisperidone are linear over the dosing range of 25 mg to 50 mg.

Distribution

Once absorbed, risperidone is rapidly distributed. The volume of distribution is 1-2 L/kg. In plasma, risperidone is bound to albumin and α_1-acid glycoprotein. The plasma protein binding of risperidone is approximately 90%, and that of its major metabolite, 9-hydroxyrisperidone, is 77%. Neither risperidone nor 9-hydroxyrisperidone displaces each other from plasma binding sites. High therapeutic concentrations of sulfamethazine (100 mcg/mL), warfarin (10 mcg/mL), and carbamazepine (10 mcg/mL) caused only a slight increase in the free fraction of risperidone at 10 ng/mL and of 9-hydroxyrisperidone at 50 ng/mL, changes of unknown clinical significance.

Metabolism

Risperidone is extensively metabolized in the liver. The main metabolic pathway is through hydroxylation of risperidone to 9-hydroxyrisperidone by the enzyme, CYP 2D6. A minor metabolic pathway is through N-dealkylation. The main metabolite, 9-hydroxyrisperidone, has similar pharmacological activity as risperidone. Consequently, the clinical effect of the drug (i.e., the active moiety) results from the combined concentrations of risperidone plus 9-hydroxyrisperidone.

CYP 2D6, also called debrisoquin hydroxylase, is the enzyme responsible for metabolism of many neuroleptics, antidepressants, antiarrhythmics, and other drugs. CYP 2D6 is subject to genetic polymorphism (about 6%-8% of Caucasians, and a very low percentage of Asians, have little or no activity and are "poor metabolizers") and to inhibition by a variety of substrates and some non-substrates, notably quinidine. Extensive CYP 2D6 metabolizers convert risperidone rapidly into 9-hydroxyrisperidone, whereas poor CYP 2D6 metabolizers convert it much more slowly. Although extensive metabolizers have lower risperidone and higher 9-hydroxyrisperidone concentrations than poor metabolizers, the pharmacokinetics of the active moiety, after single and multiple doses, are similar in extensive and poor metabolizers.

The interactions of RISPERDAL® CONSTA™ and other drugs have not been systematically evaluated in human subjects. Risperidone could be subject to two kinds of drug-drug interactions (see PRECAUTIONS – Drug Interactions). First, inhibitors of CYP 2D6 interfere with conversion of risperidone to 9-hydroxyrisperidone. This occurs with quinidine, giving essentially all recipients a risperidone pharmacokinetic profile typical of poor metabolizers. The therapeutic benefits and adverse effects of risperidone in patients receiving quinidine have not been evaluated, but observations in a modest number (n≅70) of poor metabolizers given risperidone do not suggest important differences between poor and extensive metabolizers. Second, co-administration of carbamazepine and other known enzyme inducers (e.g., phenytoin, rifampin, and phenobarbital) with risperidone cause a decrease in the combined plasma concentrations of risperidone and 9-hydroxyrisperidone (see PRECAUTIONS – Drug Interactions). It would also be possible for risperidone to interfere with metabolism of other drugs metabolized by CYP 2D6. Relatively weak binding of risperidone to the enzyme suggests this is unlikely.

In a drug interaction study in schizophrenic patients, 11 subjects received oral risperidone titrated to 6 mg/day for 3 weeks, followed by concurrent administration of carbamazepine for an additional 3 weeks. During co-administration, the plasma concentrations of risperidone and its pharmacologically active metabolite, 9-hydroxyrisperidone, were decreased by about 50%. Plasma concentrations of carbamazepine did not appear to be affected. Co-administration of other known enzyme inducers (e.g., phenytoin, rifampin, and phenobarbital) with risperidone may cause similar decreases in the combined plasma concentrations of risperidone and 9-hydroxyrisperidone, which could lead to decreased efficacy of risperidone treatment (see PRECAUTIONS – Drug Interactions and DOSAGE AND ADMINISTRATION – Co-Administration of RISPERDAL® CONSTA™ with Certain Other Medications).

Fluoxetine (20 mg QD) and paroxetine (20 mg QD) have been shown to increase the plasma concentration of risperidone 2.5–2.8 fold and 3–9 fold respectively. Fluoxetine did not affect the plasma concentration of 9-hydroxyrisperidone. Paroxetine lowered the concentration of 9-hydroxyrisperidone an average of 13% (see PRECAUTIONS – Drug Interactions and DOSAGE AND ADMINISTRATION – Co-Administration of RISPERDAL® CONSTA™ with Certain Other Medications).

Repeated oral doses of risperidone (3 mg BID) did not affect the exposure (AUC) or peak plasma concentrations (C_{max}) of lithium (n=13) (see PRECAUTIONS – Drug Interactions).

Repeated oral doses of risperidone (4 mg QD) did not affect the pre-dose or average plasma concentrations and exposure (AUC) of valproate (1000 mg/day in three divided doses) compared to placebo (n=21). However, there was a 20% increase in valproate peak plasma concentration (C_{max}) after concomitant administration of risperidone (see PRECAUTIONS – Drug Interactions).

There were no significant interactions between oral risperidone (1 mg QD) and erythromycin (500 mg QID) (see PRECAUTIONS – Drug Interactions).

Excretion

Risperidone and its metabolites are eliminated via the urine and, to a much lesser extent, via the feces. As illustrated by a mass balance study of a single 1 mg oral dose of ^{14}C-risperidone administered as solution to three healthy male volunteers, total recovery of radioactivity at 1 week was 84%, including 70% in the urine and 14% in the feces.

The apparent half-life of risperidone plus 9-hydroxyrisperidone following RISPERDAL® CONSTA™ administration is 3 to 6 days, and is associated with a monoexponential decline in plasma concentrations. This half-life of 3-6 days is related to the erosion of the microspheres and subsequent absorption of risperidone. The clearance of risperidone and risperidone plus 9-hydroxyrisperidone was 13.7 L/h and 5.0 L/h in extensive CYP 2D6 metabolizers, and 3.3 L/h and 3.2 L/h in poor CYP 2D6 metabolizers, respectively. No accumulation of risperidone was observed during long-term use (up to 12 months) in patients treated every 2 weeks with 25 mg or 50 mg RISPERDAL® CONSTA™. The elimination phase is complete approximately 7 to 8 weeks after the last injection.

Special Populations

Renal Impairment

In patients with moderate to severe renal disease treated with oral RISPERDAL®, clearance of the sum of risperidone and its active metabolite decreased by 60% compared with young healthy subjects. Although patients with renal impairment were not studied with RISPERDAL® CONSTA™, it is recommended that patients with renal impairment be carefully titrated on oral RISPERDAL® before treatment with RISPERDAL® CONSTA™ is initiated (see PRECAUTIONS and DOSAGE AND ADMINISTRATION).

Hepatic Impairment

While the pharmacokinetics of oral RISPERDAL® in subjects with liver disease were comparable to those in young healthy subjects, the mean free fraction of risperidone in plasma was increased by about 35% because of the diminished concentration of both albumin and α_1-acid glycoprotein. Although patients with hepatic impairment were not studied with RISPERDAL® CONSTA™, it is recommended that patients with hepatic impairment be carefully titrated on oral RISPERDAL® before treatment with RISPERDAL® CONSTA™ is initiated (see PRECAUTIONS and DOSAGE AND ADMINISTRATION).

Elderly

In an open-label trial, steady-state concentrations of risperidone plus 9-hydroxyrisperidone in otherwise healthy elderly patients (≥65 years old) treated with RISPERDAL® CONSTA™ for up to 12 months fell within the range of values observed in otherwise healthy nonelderly patients. Dosing recommendations are the same for otherwise healthy elderly patients and nonelderly patients (see DOSAGE AND ADMINISTRATION).

Race and Gender Effects

No specific pharmacokinetic study was conducted to investigate race and gender effects, but a population pharmacokinetic analysis did not identify important differences in the disposition of risperidone due to gender (whether or not corrected for body weight) or race.

Clinical Trials

The effectiveness of RISPERDAL® CONSTA™ (risperidone) in the treatment of schizophrenia was established, in part, on the basis of extrapolation from the established effectiveness of the oral formulation of risperidone. In addition, the effectiveness of RISPERDAL® CONSTA™ in the treatment of schizophrenia was established in a 12-week, placebo-controlled trial in adult psychotic inpatients and outpatients who met the DSM-IV criteria for schizophrenia.

Efficacy data were obtained from 400 patients with schizophrenia who were randomized to receive injections of 25, 50, or 75 mg RISPERDAL® CONSTA™ or placebo every 2 weeks. During a 1-week run-in period, patients were discontinued from other antipsychotics and were titrated to a dose of 4 mg oral RISPERDAL®. Patients who received RISPERDAL® CONSTA™ were given doses of oral RISPERDAL® (2 mg for patients in the 25-mg group, 4 mg for patients in the 50-mg group, and 6 mg for patients in the 75-mg group) for the 3 weeks after the first injection to provide therapeutic plasma concentrations until the main release phase of risperidone from the injection site had begun. Patients who received placebo injections were given placebo tablets.

Efficacy was evaluated using the Positive and Negative Syndrome Scale (PANSS), a validated, multi-item inventory, composed of five subscales to evaluate positive symptoms, negative symptoms, disorganized thoughts, uncontrolled hostility/excitement, and anxiety/depression.

The primary efficacy variable in this trial was change from baseline to endpoint in the total PANSS score. The mean total PANSS score at baseline for schizophrenic patients in this study was 81.5.

Total PANSS scores showed significant improvement in the change from baseline to endpoint in schizophrenic patients treated with each dose of RISPERDAL® CONSTA™ (25 mg, 50 mg, or 75 mg) compared with patients treated with placebo. While there were no statistically significant differences between the treatment effects for the three dose groups, the effect size for the 75 mg dose group was actually numerically less than that observed for the 50 mg dose group.

Subgroup analyses did not indicate any differences in treatment outcome as a function of age, race, or gender.

INDICATIONS AND USAGE

RISPERDAL® CONSTA™ (risperidone) is indicated for the treatment of schizophrenia.

The efficacy of RISPERDAL® CONSTA™ is based in part on a 12-week, placebo-controlled trial in schizophrenic inpatients or outpatients, along with extrapolation from the established efficacy of oral RISPERDAL® in this population.

The effectiveness of RISPERDAL® CONSTA™ in longer-term use, that is, more than 12 weeks, has not been systematically evaluated in controlled trials. However, oral risperidone has been shown to be effective in delaying time to relapse in longer-term use. Patients should be periodically reassessed to determine the need for continued treatment (see DOSAGE AND ADMINISTRATION).

CONTRAINDICATIONS

RISPERDAL® CONSTA™ (risperidone) is contraindicated in patients with a known hypersensitivity to the product or any of its components.

WARNINGS

Neuroleptic Malignant Syndrome (NMS)

A potentially fatal symptom complex sometimes referred to as Neuroleptic Malignant Syndrome (NMS) has been reported in association with antipsychotic drugs. Clinical manifestations of NMS are hyperpyrexia, muscle rigidity, altered mental status, and evidence of autonomic instability (irregular pulse or blood pressure, tachycardia, diaphoresis, and cardiac dysrhythmia). Additional signs may include elevated creatine phosphokinase, myoglobinuria (rhabdomyolysis), and acute renal failure.

The diagnostic evaluation of patients with this syndrome is complicated. In arriving at a diagnosis, it is important to identify cases in which the clinical presentation includes both serious medical illness (e.g., pneumonia, systemic infection, etc.) and untreated or inadequately treated extrapyramidal signs and symptoms (EPS). Other important considerations in the differential diagnosis include central anticholinergic toxicity, heat stroke, drug fever, and primary central nervous system pathology.

The management of NMS should include: (1) immediate discontinuation of antipsychotic drugs and other drugs not essential to concurrent therapy; (2) intensive symptomatic treatment and medical monitoring; and (3) treatment of any concomitant serious medical problems for which specific treatments are available. There is no general agreement about specific pharmacological treatment regimens for uncomplicated NMS.

If a patient requires antipsychotic drug treatment after recovery from NMS, the potential reintroduction of drug therapy should be carefully considered. The patient should be carefully monitored, since recurrences of NMS have been reported.

Tardive Dyskinesia

A syndrome of potentially irreversible, involuntary, dyskinetic movements may develop in patients treated with antipsychotic drugs. Although the prevalence of the syndrome appears to be highest among the elderly, especially elderly women, it is impossible to rely upon prevalence estimates to predict, at the inception of antipsychotic treatment, which patients are likely to develop the syndrome. Whether antipsychotic drug products differ in their potential to cause tardive dyskinesia is unknown.

The risk of developing tardive dyskinesia and the likelihood that it will become irreversible are believed to increase as the duration of treatment and the total cumulative dose of antipsychotic drugs administered to the patient increase. However, the syndrome can develop, although much less commonly, after relatively brief treatment periods at low doses.

There is no known treatment for established cases of tardive dyskinesia, although the syndrome may remit, partially or completely, if antipsychotic treatment is withdrawn. Antipsychotic treatment, itself, however, may suppress (or partially suppress) the signs and symptoms of the syndrome and thereby may possibly mask the underlying process. The effect that symptomatic suppression has upon the long-term course of the syndrome is unknown.

Given these considerations, RISPERDAL® CONSTA™ should be prescribed in a manner that is most likely to minimize the occurrence of tardive dyskinesia. Chronic antipsychotic treatment should generally be reserved for patients who suffer from a chronic illness that (1) is known to respond to antipsychotic drugs, and (2) for whom alternative, equally effective, but potentially less harmful treatments are not available or appropriate. In patients who do require chronic treatment, the smallest dose and the shortest duration of treatment producing a satisfactory clinical response should be sought. The need for continued treatment should be reassessed periodically.

If signs and symptoms of tardive dyskinesia appear in a patient treated with RISPERDAL® CONSTA™, drug discontinuation should be considered. However, some patients may require treatment with RISPERDAL® CONSTA™ despite the presence of the syndrome.

Cerebrovascular Adverse Events, Including Stroke, in Elderly Patients with Dementia

Cerebrovascular adverse events (e.g., stroke, transient ischemic attack), including fatalities, were reported in patients (mean age 85 years; range 73-97) in trials of oral risperidone in elderly patients with dementia-related psychosis. In placebo-controlled trials, there was a significantly higher incidence of cerebrovascular adverse events in patients treated with oral risperidone compared to patients treated with placebo. RISPERDAL® CONSTA™ is not approved for the treatment of patients with dementia-related psychosis.

Hyperglycemia and Diabetes Mellitus

Hyperglycemia, in some cases extreme and associated with ketoacidosis or hyperosmolar coma or death, has been reported in patients treated with atypical antipsychotics including RISPERDAL®. Assessment of the relationship between atypical antipsychotic use and glucose abnormalities is complicated by the possibility of an increased background risk of diabetes mellitus in patients with schizophrenia and the increasing incidence of diabetes mellitus in the general population. Given these confounders, the relationship between atypical antipsychotic use and hyperglycemia-related adverse events is not completely understood. However, epidemiological studies suggest an increased risk of treatment-emergent hyperglycemia-related adverse events in patients treated with the atypical antipsychotics. Precise risk estimates for hyperglycemia-related adverse events in patients treated with atypical antipsychotics are not available.

Patients with an established diagnosis of diabetes mellitus who are started on atypical antipsychotics should be monitored regularly for worsening of glucose control. Patients with risk factors for diabetes mellitus (e.g., obesity, family history of diabetes) who are starting treatment with atypical antipsychotics should undergo fasting blood glucose testing at the beginning of treatment and periodically during treatment. Any patient treated with atypical antipsychotics should be monitored for symptoms of hyperglycemia including polydipsia, polyuria, polyphagia, and weakness. Patients who develop symptoms of hyperglycemia during treatment with atypical antipsychotics should undergo fasting blood glucose testing. In some cases, hyperglycemia has resolved when the atypical antipsychotic was discontinued; however, some patients required continuation of anti-diabetic treatment despite discontinuation of the suspect drug.

PRECAUTIONS

General

Orthostatic Hypotension

RISPERDAL® CONSTA™ (risperidone) may induce orthostatic hypotension associated with dizziness, tachycardia, and in some patients, syncope, probably reflecting its alpha-adrenergic antagonistic properties. Syncope was reported in 0.8% (12/1499 patients) of patients treated with RISPERDAL® CONSTA™ in multiple-dose studies. Patients should be instructed in nonpharmacologic interventions that help to reduce the occurrence of orthostatic hypotension (e.g., sitting on the edge of the bed for several minutes before attempting to stand in the morning and slowly rising from a seated position).

RISPERDAL® CONSTA™ should be used with particular caution in (1) patients with known cardiovascular disease (history of myocardial infarction or ischemia, heart failure, or conduction abnormalities), cerebrovascular disease, and conditions which would predispose patients to hypotension, e.g., dehydration and hypovolemia, and (2) in the elderly and patients with renal or hepatic impairment. Monitoring of orthostatic vital signs should be considered in all such patients, and a dose reduction should be considered if hypotension occurs. Clinically significant hypotension has been observed with concomitant use of oral RISPERDAL® and antihypertensive medication.

Seizures

During premarketing testing, seizures occurred in 0.3% (5/1499 patients) of patients treated with RISPERDAL® CONSTA™. Therefore, RISPERDAL® CONSTA™ should be used cautiously in patients with a history of seizures.

Dysphagia

Esophageal dysmotility and aspiration have been associated with antipsychotic drug use. Aspiration pneumonia is a common cause of morbidity and mortality in patients with advanced Alzheimer's dementia. RISPERDAL® CONSTA™ and other antipsychotic drugs should be used cautiously in patients at risk for aspiration pneumonia.

Osteodystrophy and Tumors in Animals

RISPERDAL® CONSTA™ produced osteodystrophy in male and female rats in a 1-year toxicity study and a 2-year carcinogenicity study at a dose of 40 mg/kg administered IM every 2 weeks.

RISPERDAL® CONSTA™ produced renal tubular tumors (adenoma, adenocarcinoma) and adrenomedullary pheochromocytomas in male rats in the 2-year carcinogenicity study at 40 mg/kg administered IM every 2 weeks. In addition, RISPERDAL® CONSTA™ produced an increase in a marker of cellular proliferation in renal tissue in males in the 1-year toxicity study and in renal tumor-bearing males in the 2-year carcinogenicity study at 40 mg/kg administered IM every 2 weeks. (Cellular proliferation was not measured at the low dose or in females in either study.)

The effect dose for osteodystrophy and the tumor findings is 8 times the IM maximum recommended human dose (MRHD) (50 mg) on a mg/m^2 basis and is associated with a plasma exposure (AUC) 2 times the expected plasma exposure (AUC) at the IM MRHD. The no-effect dose for these findings was 5 mg/kg (equal to the IM MRHD on a mg/m^2 basis). Plasma exposure (AUC) at the no-effect dose was one third the expected plasma exposure (AUC) at the IM MRHD.

Neither the renal or adrenal tumors, nor osteodystrophy, were seen in studies of orally administered risperidone. Osteodystrophy was not observed in dogs at doses up to 14 times (based on AUC) the IM MRHD in a 1-year toxicity study.

The renal tubular and adrenomedullary tumors in male rats and other tumor findings are described in more detail under PRECAUTIONS, Carcinogenicity, Mutagenesis, Impairment of Fertility.

The relevance of these findings to human risk is unknown.

Hyperprolactinemia

As with other drugs that antagonize dopamine D_2 receptors, risperidone elevates prolactin levels and the elevation persists during chronic administration. Tissue culture experiments indicate that approximately one-third of human breast cancers are prolactin-dependent *in vitro*, a factor of potential importance if the prescription of these drugs is contemplated in a patient with previously detected breast cancer. Although disturbances such as galactorrhea, amenorrhea, gynecomastia, and impotence have been reported with prolactin-elevating compounds, the clinical significance of elevated serum prolactin levels is unknown for most patients.

As has been observed with other compounds that increase prolactin release, an increase in the incidence of pituitary gland, mammary gland, and endocrine pancreatic islet cell hyperplasias and/or neoplasias, was observed in rodent carcinogenicity studies with RISPERDAL® Tablets and RISPERDAL® CONSTA™ (see PRECAUTIONS – Carcinogenicity, Mutagenesis, Impairment of Fertility). Neither clinical studies nor epidemiologic studies conducted to date have shown an association between chronic administration of this class of drugs and tumorigenesis in humans; the available evidence is considered too limited to be conclusive at this time.

Potential for Cognitive and Motor Impairment

Somnolence was reported by 5% of patients treated with RISPERDAL® CONSTA™ in multiple-dose trials. Since risperidone has the potential to impair judgment, thinking, or motor skills, patients should be cautioned about operating hazardous machinery, including automobiles, until they are reasonably certain that treatment with RISPERDAL® CONSTA™ does not affect them adversely.

Priapism

No cases of priapism have been reported in patients treated with RISPERDAL® CONSTA™. However, rare cases of priapism have been reported in patients treated with oral RISPERDAL®. While the relationship of these events to oral RISPERDAL® use has not been established, other drugs with alpha-adrenergic blocking effects have been reported to induce priapism, and it is possible that RISPERDAL® may share this capacity. Severe priapism may require surgical intervention.

Thrombotic Thrombocytopenic Purpura (TTP)

A single case of TTP was reported in a 28 year-old female patient receiving oral RISPERDAL® in a large, open premarketing experience (approximately 1300 patients). She experienced jaundice, fever, and bruising, but eventually recovered after receiving plasmapheresis. The relationship to RISPERDAL® therapy is unknown.

Antiemetic Effect

Risperidone has an antiemetic effect in animals; this effect may also occur in humans, and may mask signs and symptoms of overdosage with certain drugs or of conditions such as intestinal obstruction, Reye's syndrome, and brain tumor.

Body Temperature Regulation

Disruption of body temperature regulation has been attributed to antipsychotic agents. Both hyperthermia and hypothermia have been reported in association with oral RISPERDAL® use. Caution is advised when prescribing RISPERDAL® CONSTA™ for patients who will be exposed to temperature extremes.

Suicide

The possibility of a suicide attempt is inherent in schizophrenia, and close supervision of high-risk patients should accompany drug therapy. RISPERDAL® CONSTA™ is to be administered by a health care professional (see DOSAGE and ADMINISTRATION); therefore, suicide due to an overdose is unlikely.

Use in Patients with Concomitant Illness

Clinical experience with RISPERDAL® CONSTA™ in patients with certain concomitant systemic illnesses is limited. Caution is advisable when using RISPERDAL® CONSTA™ in patients with diseases or conditions that could affect metabolism or hemodynamic responses.

RISPERDAL® CONSTA™ has not been evaluated or used to any appreciable extent in patients with a recent history of myocardial infarction or unstable heart disease. Patients with these diagnoses were excluded from clinical studies during the product's premarket testing.

Increased plasma concentrations of risperidone and 9-hydroxyrisperidone occur in patients with severe renal impairment (creatinine clearance <30 mL/min/1.73 m^2) treated with oral RISPERDAL®; an increase in the free fraction of risperidone is also seen in patients with severe hepatic impairment. Patients with renal or hepatic impairment should be carefully titrated on oral RISPERDAL® before treatment with RISPERDAL® CONSTA™ is initiated (see DOSAGE AND ADMINISTRATION).

Information for Patients

Physicians are advised to discuss the following issues with patients for whom they prescribe RISPERDAL® CONSTA™.

Orthostatic Hypotension

Patients should be advised of the risk of orthostatic hypotension and instructed in nonpharmacologic interventions that help to reduce the occurrence of orthostatic hypotension (e.g., sitting on the edge of the bed for several minutes before attempting to stand in the morning and slowly rising from a seated position).

Interference With Cognitive and Motor Performance

Because RISPERDAL® CONSTA™ has the potential to impair judgment, thinking, or motor skills, patients should be cautioned about operating hazardous machinery, including automobiles, until they are reasonably certain that treatment with RISPERDAL® CONSTA™ does not affect them adversely.

Pregnancy

Patients should be advised to notify their physician if they become pregnant or intend to become pregnant during therapy and for at least 12 weeks after the last injection of RISPERDAL® CONSTA™.

Nursing

Patients should be advised not to breast-feed an infant during treatment and for at least 12 weeks after the last injection of RISPERDAL® CONSTA™.

Concomitant Medication

Patients should be advised to inform their physicians if they are taking, or plan to take, any prescription or over-the-counter drugs, since there is a potential for interactions.

Alcohol

Patients should be advised to avoid alcohol during treatment with RISPERDAL® CONSTA™.

Laboratory Tests

No specific laboratory tests are recommended.

Drug Interactions

The interactions of RISPERDAL® CONSTA™ and other drugs have not been systematically evaluated. Given the primary CNS effects of risperidone, caution should be used when RISPERDAL® CONSTA™ is administered in combination with other centrally-acting drugs or alcohol.

Because of its potential for inducing hypotension, RISPERDAL® CONSTA™ may enhance the hypotensive effects of other therapeutic agents with this potential.

RISPERDAL® CONSTA™ may antagonize the effects of levodopa and dopamine agonists.

Amytriptyline does not affect the pharmacokinetics of risperidone or the active antipsychotic fraction. Cimetidine and ranitidine increased the bioavailability of risperidone, but only marginally increased the plasma concentration of the active antipsychotic fraction.

Chronic administration of clozapine with risperidone may decrease the clearance of risperidone.

Carbamazepine and Other Enzyme Inducers

In a drug interaction study in schizophrenic patients, 11 subjects received oral risperidone titrated to 6 mg/day for 3 weeks, followed by concurrent administration of carbamazepine for an additional 3 weeks. During co-administration, the plasma concentrations of risperidone and its pharmacologically active metabolite, 9-hydroxyrisperidone, were decreased by about 50%. Plasma concentrations of carbamazepine did not appear to be affected. Co-administration of other known enzyme inducers (e.g., phenytoin, rifampin, and phenobarbital) with risperidone may cause similar decreases in the combined plasma concentrations of risperidone and 9-hydroxyrisperidone, which could lead to decreased efficacy of risperidone treatment. At the initiation of therapy with carbamazepine or other known hepatic enzyme inducers, patients should be closely monitored during the first 4-8 weeks, since the dose of RISPERDAL® CONSTA™ may need to be adjusted. A dose increase, or additional oral RISPERDAL®, may need to be considered. On discontinuation of carbamazepine or other hepatic enzyme inducers, the dosage of RISPERDAL® CONSTA™ should be re-evaluated and, if necessary, decreased. Patients may be placed on a lower dose of RISPERDAL® CONSTA™ between 2 to 4 weeks before the planned discontinuation of carbamazepine therapy to adjust for the expected increase in plasma concentrations of risperidone plus 9-hydroxyrisperidone. For patients treated with the lowest available dose (25 mg) of RISPERDAL® CONSTA™, it is recommended to continue treatment with the 25-mg dose unless clinical judgment necessitates interruption of treatment with RISPERDAL® CONSTA™.

Fluoxetine and Paroxetine

Fluoxetine (20 mg QD) and paroxetine (20 mg QD), which inhibit CYP 2D6, have been shown to increase the plasma concentration of risperidone 2.5-2.8 fold and 3-9 fold respectively. Fluoxetine did not affect the plasma concentration of

Continued on next page

Risperdal Consta—Cont.

9-hydroxyrisperidone. Paroxetine lowered the concentration of 9-hydroxyrisperidone an average of 13%. When either concomitant fluoxetine or paroxetine is initiated or discontinued, the physician should re-evaluate the dosage of RISPERDAL® CONSTA™. When initiation of fluoxetine or paroxetine is considered, patients may be placed on a lower dose of RISPERDAL® CONSTA™ between 2 to 4 weeks before the planned start of fluoxetine or paroxetine therapy to adjust for the expected increase in plasma concentrations of risperidone. For patients treated with the lowest available dose (25 mg), it is recommended to continue treatment with the 25-mg dose unless clinical judgment necessitates interruption of treatment with RISPERDAL® CONSTA™. The effects of discontinuation of concomitant fluoxetine or paroxetine therapy on the pharmacokinetics of risperidone and 9-hydroxyrisperidone have not been studied.

Lithium

Repeated oral doses of risperidone (3 mg BID) did not affect the exposure (AUC) or peak plasma concentrations (C_{max}) of lithium (n=13).

Valproate

Repeated oral doses of risperidone (4 mg QD) did not affect the pre-dose or average plasma concentrations and exposure (AUC) of valproate (1000 mg/day in three divided doses) compared to placebo (n=21). However, there was a 20% increase in valproate peak plasma concentration (C_{max}) after concomitant administration of risperidone.

Digoxin

RISPERDAL® (0.25 mg BID) did not show a clinically relevant effect on the pharmacokinetics of digoxin.

Drugs that Inhibit CYP 2D6 and Other CYP Isozymes

Risperidone is metabolized to 9-hydroxyrisperidone by CYP 2D6, an enzyme that is polymorphic in the population and that can be inhibited by a variety of psychotropic and other drugs (see CLINICAL PHARMACOLOGY). Drug interactions that reduce the metabolism of risperidone to 9-hydroxyrisperidone would increase the plasma concentrations of risperidone and lower the concentrations of 9-hydroxyrisperidone. Analysis of clinical studies involving a modest number of poor metabolizers (n≅70 patients) does not suggest that poor and extensive metabolizers have different rates of adverse effects. No comparison of effectiveness in the two groups has been made.

In vitro studies showed that drugs metabolized by other CYP isozymes, including 1A1, 1A2, 2C9, 2C19, and 3A4, are only weak inhibitors of risperidone metabolism.

There were no significant interactions between risperidone and erythromycin (see CLINICAL PHARMACOLOGY).

Drugs Metabolized by CYP 2D6

In vitro studies indicate that risperidone is a relatively weak inhibitor of CYP 2D6. Therefore, RISPERDAL® CONSTA™ is not expected to substantially inhibit the clearance of drugs that are metabolized by this enzymatic pathway. In drug interaction studies, oral risperidone did not significantly affect the pharmacokinetics of donepezil and galantamine, which are metabolized by CYP 2D6.

Carcinogenesis, Mutagenesis, Impairment of Fertility

Carcinogenesis - Oral

Carcinogenicity studies were conducted in Swiss albino mice and Wistar rats. Risperidone was administered in the diet at doses of 0.63, 2.5, and 10 mg/kg for 18 months to mice and for 25 months to rats. These doses are equivalent to 2.4, 9.4, and 37.5 times the oral maximum recommended human dose (MRHD) (16 mg/day) on a mg/kg basis, or 0.2, 0.75, and 3 times the oral MRHD (mice) or 0.4, 1.5, and 6 times the oral MRHD (rats) on a mg/m^2 basis. A maximum tolerated dose was not achieved in male mice. There was a significant increase in pituitary gland adenomas in female mice at doses 0.75 and 3 times the oral MRHD on a mg/m^2 basis. There was a significant increase in endocrine pancreatic adenomas in male rats at doses 1.5 and 6 times the oral MRHD on a mg/m^2 basis. Mammary gland adenocarcinomas were significantly increased in female mice at all doses tested (0.2, 0.75, and 3 times the oral MRHD on a mg/m^2 basis), in female rats at all doses tested (0.4, 1.5, and 6 times the oral MRHD on a mg/m^2 basis), and in male rats at a dose 6 times the oral MRHD on a mg/m^2 basis.

Carcinogenesis - IM

RISPERDAL® CONSTA™ was evaluated in a 24-month carcinogenicity study in which SPF Wistar rats were treated every 2 weeks with IM injections of either 5 mg/kg or 40 mg/kg of risperidone. These doses are 1 and 8 times the MRHD (50 mg) on a mg/m^2 basis. A control group received injections of 0.9% NaCl, and a vehicle control group was injected with placebo microspheres. There was a significant increase in pituitary gland adenomas, endocrine pancreas adenomas, and adrenomedullary pheochromocytomas at 8 times the IM MRHD on a mg/m^2 basis. The incidence of mammary gland adenocarcinomas was significantly increased in female rats at both doses (1 and 8 times the IM MRHD on a mg/m^2 basis). A significant increase in renal tubular tumors (adenoma, adenocarcinomas) was observed in male rats at 8 times the IM MRHD on a mg/m^2 basis. Plasma exposures (AUC) in rats were 0.3 and 2 times (at 5 and 40 mg/kg, respectively) the expected plasma exposure (AUC) at the IM MRHD.

Dopamine D_2 receptor antagonists have been shown to chronically elevate prolactin levels in rodents. Serum prolactin levels were not measured during the carcinogenicity studies of oral risperidone; however, measurements taken during subchronic toxicity studies showed that oral risperidone elevated serum prolactin levels 5- to 6-fold in mice and rats at the same doses used in the oral carcinogenicity studies. Serum prolactin levels increased in a dose-dependent manner up to 6- and 1.5-fold in male and female rats, respectively, at the end of the 24-month treatment with RISPERDAL® CONSTA™ every 2 weeks. Increases in the incidence of pituitary gland, endocrine pancreas, and mammary gland neoplasms have been found in rodents after chronic administration of other antipsychotic drugs and may be prolactin-mediated.

The relevance for human risk of the findings of prolactin-mediated endocrine tumors in rodents is unknown (see PRECAUTIONS - Hyperprolactinemia).

Mutagenesis

No evidence of mutagenic potential for oral risperidone was found in the *in vitro* Ames reverse mutation test, *in vitro* mouse lymphoma assay, *in vitro* rat hepatocyte DNA-repair assay, *in vivo* oral micronucleus test in mice, the sex-linked recessive lethal test in *Drosophila*, or the *in vitro* chromosomal aberration test in human lymphocytes or in Chinese hamster cells.

In addition, no evidence of mutagenic potential was found in the *in vitro* Ames reverse mutation test for RISPERDAL® CONSTA™.

Impairment of Fertility

Oral risperidone (0.16 to 5 mg/kg) was shown to impair mating, but not fertility, in Wistar rats in three reproductive studies (two mating and fertility studies and a multigenerational study) at doses 0.1 to 3 times the oral maximum recommended human dose (MRHD) (16 mg/day) on a mg/m^2 basis. The effect appeared to be in females, since impaired mating behavior was not noted in the mating and fertility study in which males only were treated. In a subchronic study in Beagle dogs in which oral risperidone was administered at doses of 0.31 to 5 mg/kg, sperm motility and concentration were decreased at doses 0.6 to 10 times the oral MRHD on a mg/m^2 basis. Dose-related decreases were also noted in serum testosterone at the same doses. Serum testosterone and sperm values partially recovered, but remained decreased after treatment was discontinued. No no-effect doses were noted in either rat or dog.

No mating and fertility studies were conducted with RISPERDAL® CONSTA™.

Pregnancy

Pregnancy Category C

The teratogenic potential of oral risperidone was studied in three embryofetal development studies in Sprague-Dawley and Wistar rats (0.63-10 mg/kg or 0.4 to 6 times the oral maximum recommended human dose [MRHD] on a mg/m^2 basis) and in one embryofetal development study in New Zealand rabbits (0.31-5 mg/kg or 0.4 to 6 times the oral MRHD on a mg/m^2 basis). The incidence of malformations was not increased compared to control in offspring of rats or rabbits given 0.4 to 6 times the oral MRHD on a mg/m^2 basis. In three reproductive studies in rats (two peri/postnatal development studies and a multigenerational study), there was an increase in pup deaths during the first 4 days of lactation at doses of 0.16-5 mg/kg or 0.1 to 3 times the oral MRHD on a mg/m^2 basis. It is not known whether these deaths were due to a direct effect on the fetuses or pups or to effects on the dams.

There was no no-effect dose for increased rat pup mortality. In one peri/post-natal development study, there was an increase in stillborn rat pups at a dose of 2.5 mg/kg or 1.5 times the oral MRHD on a mg/m^2 basis. In a cross-fostering study in Wistar rats, toxic effects on the fetus or pups, as evidenced by a decrease in the number of live pups and an increase in the number of dead pups at birth (Day 0), and a decrease in birth weight in pups of drug-treated dams were observed. In addition, there was an increase in deaths by Day 1 among pups of drug-treated dams, regardless of whether or not the pups were cross-fostered. Risperidone also appeared to impair maternal behavior in that pup body weight gain and survival (from Days 1 to 4 of lactation) were reduced in pups born to control but reared by drug-treated dams. These effects were all noted at the one dose of risperidone tested, i.e., 5 mg/kg or 3 times the oral MRHD on a mg/m^2 basis.

No studies were conducted with RISPERDAL® CONSTA™. Placental transfer of risperidone occurs in rat pups. There are no adequate and well-controlled studies in pregnant women. However, there was one report of a case of agenesis of the corpus callosum in an infant exposed to risperidone *in utero*. The causal relationship to oral RISPERDAL® therapy is unknown.

RISPERDAL® CONSTA™ should be used during pregnancy only if the potential benefit justifies the potential risk to the fetus.

Labor and Delivery

The effect of RISPERDAL® CONSTA™ on labor and delivery in humans is unknown.

Nursing Mothers

In animal studies, risperidone and 9-hydroxyrisperidone are excreted in milk. Risperidone and 9-hydroxyrisperidone are also excreted in human breast milk. Therefore, women should not breast-feed during treatment with RISPERDAL® CONSTA™ and for at least 12 weeks after the last injection.

Pediatric Use

RISPERDAL® CONSTA™ has not been studied in children younger than 18 years old.

Geriatric Use

In an open-label study, 57 clinically stable, elderly patients (≥65 years old) with schizophrenia or schizoaffective disorder received RISPERDAL® CONSTA™ every 2 weeks for up to 12 months. In general, no differences in the tolerability of RISPERDAL® CONSTA™ were observed between otherwise healthy elderly and nonelderly patients. Therefore, dosing recommendations for otherwise healthy elderly patients are the same as for nonelderly patients. Because elderly patients exhibit a greater tendency to orthostatic hypotension than nonelderly patients, elderly patients should be instructed in nonpharmacologic interventions that help to reduce the occurrence of orthostatic hypotension (e.g., sitting on the edge of the bed for several minutes before attempting to stand in the morning and slowly rising from a seated position). In addition, monitoring of orthostatic vital signs should be considered in elderly patients for whom orthostatic hypotension is of concern (see CLINICAL PHARMACOLOGY, PRECAUTIONS, and DOSAGE AND ADMINISTRATION).

ADVERSE REACTIONS

Adverse findings were assessed by spontaneous reports of adverse events, laboratory tests, vital signs, body weight, and ECGs. Adverse events were classified using the World Health Organization preferred terms. Treatment-emergent adverse events were defined as those events with an onset between the first dose and 49 days after the last dose.

The prescriber should be aware that these figures cannot be used to predict the incidence of side effects in the course of usual medical practice where patient characteristics and other factors differ from those which prevailed in this clinical trial. Similarly, the cited frequencies cannot be compared with figures obtained from other clinical investigations involving different treatments, uses, and investigators. The cited figures, however, do provide the prescribing physician with some basis for estimating the relative contribution of drug and nondrug factors to the side effect incidence rate in the population studied.

Associated with Discontinuation of Treatment

In the 12-week, placebo-controlled trial, the incidence of schizophrenic patients who discontinued treatment due to an adverse event was lower with RISPERDAL® CONSTA™ (11%; 22/202 patients) than with placebo (13%; 13/98 patients).

Incidence in Controlled Trials

The incidence of adverse reactions in the placebo-controlled trial was based on 202 schizophrenic patients treated with 25 or 50 mg RISPERDAL® CONSTA™ and 98 schizophrenic patients treated with placebo for up to 12 weeks.

Commonly Observed Adverse Events in Controlled Clinical Trials

Spontaneously reported, treatment-emergent adverse events with an incidence of 5% or greater in at least one of the RISPERDAL® CONSTA™ groups (25 mg or 50 mg) and at least twice that of placebo were: somnolence, akathisia, parkinsonism, dyspepsia, constipation, dry mouth, fatigue, weight increase.

Adverse Events Occurring at an Incidence of 2% or More in Patients Treated with RISPERDAL® CONSTA™:

Table 1 enumerates adverse events that occurred at an incidence of 2% or more, and were at least as frequent among patients treated with 25 mg or 50 mg RISPERDAL® CONSTA™ as patients treated with placebo in the 12-week, placebo-controlled trial. This table shows the percentage of patients in each dose group who spontaneously reported at least one episode of an event at some time during double-blind treatment. All patients were titrated to a dose of 4 mg oral RISPERDAL® during a 1-week run-in period. Patients who received RISPERDAL® CONSTA™ were given doses of oral RISPERDAL® (2 mg for patients in the 25-mg group, and 4 mg for patients in the 50-mg group) during the 3 weeks after the first injection to provide therapeutic levels until the main release phase of risperidone from the injection site had begun. Patients who received placebo injections were given placebo tablets.

Table 1. Incidence (% of Patients) of Treatment-Emergent Adverse Events in a 12-Week, Placebo-Controlled Clinical Trial

WHO Body System Disorder/ Preferred Term	RISPERDAL® CONSTA™ 25 mg (N=99)	RISPERDAL® CONSTA™ 50 mg (N=103)	Placebo (N=98)
Psychiatric			
Insomnia	16	13	14
Hallucination	7	6	5
Somnolence	5	6	3
Suicide attempt	1	4	3
Abnormal thinking	0	3	2
Abnormal dreaming	2	0	0
Central & peripheral nervous system			
Headache	15	22	12
Dizziness	8	11	6
Akathisia	2	9	4
Parkinsonism[a]	4	10	3
Tremor	0	3	0
Hypoaesthesia	2	0	0
Gastrointestinal			
Dyspepsia	7	7	2
Constipation	5	7	1
Mouth dry	0	7	1
Toothache	1	3	0
Saliva increased	6	2	1

Tooth disorder	4	2	0
Diarrhea	5	1	3
Body as a whole - general			
Fatigue	3	7	0
Pain	10	3	4
Peripheral edema	2	3	1
Leg pain	4	1	1
Fever	2	1	0
Syncope	2	0	0
Respiratory system			
Rhinitis	14	4	8
Coughing	5	2	4
Sinusitis	3	1	0
Upper respiratory tract infection	2	0	1
Metabolic & nutritional			
Weight increase	5	4	2
Weight decrease	4	1	1
Cardiovascular			
Hypertension	3	3	2
Hearing & vestibular			
Ear disorder (NOS)	0	3	0
Vision			
Vision abnormal	2	3	0
Skin & appendage			
Acne	2	2	0
Skin dry	2	0	0
Musculo-Skeletal			
Myalgia	4	2	1

[a] Includes adverse events of bradykinesia, extrapyramidal disorder, and hypokinesia.

Dose Dependency of Adverse Events

Extrapyramidal Symptoms:

Two methods were used to measure extrapyramidal symptoms (EPS) in the 12-week, placebo-controlled trial comparing three doses of RISPERDAL® CONSTA™ (25 mg, 50 mg, and 75 mg) with placebo, including: (1) the incidence of spontaneous reports of EPS symptoms; and (2) the change from baseline to endpoint on the total score (sum of the subscale scores for parkinsonism, dystonia, and dyskinesia) of the Extrapyramidal Symptom Rating Scale (ESRS).

As shown in Table 1, the overall incidence of EPS-related adverse events (akathisia, dystonia, parkinsonism, and tremor) in patients treated with 25 mg RISPERDAL® CONSTA™ was comparable to that of patients treated with placebo; the incidence of EPS-related adverse events was higher in patients treated with 50 mg RISPERDAL® CONSTA™.

The median change from baseline to endpoint in total ESRS score showed no worsening in patients treated with RISPERDAL® CONSTA™ compared with patients treated with placebo: 0 (placebo group); -1 (25-mg group, significantly less than the placebo group); and 0 (50-mg group).

Vital Sign Changes:

RISPERDAL® is associated with orthostatic hypotension and tachycardia (see PRECAUTIONS). In the placebo-controlled trial, orthostatic hypotension was observed in 2% of patients treated with 25 mg or 50 mg RISPERDAL® CONSTA™ (see PRECAUTIONS).

Weight Changes:

In the 12-week, placebo-controlled trial, 9% of patients treated with RISPERDAL® CONSTA™, compared with 6% of patients treated with placebo, experienced a weight gain of >7% of body weight at endpoint.

Laboratory Changes:

The percentage of patients treated with RISPERDAL® CONSTA™ who experienced potentially important changes in routine serum chemistry, hematology, or urinalysis parameters was similar to or less than that of placebo patients. Additionally, no patients discontinued treatment due to changes in serum chemistry, hematology, or urinalysis parameters.

ECG Changes:

The electrocardiograms of 202 schizophrenic patients treated with 25 mg or 50 mg RISPERDAL® CONSTA™ and 98 schizophrenic patients treated with placebo in a 12-week, double-blind, placebo-controlled trial were evaluated. Compared with placebo, there were no statistically significant differences in QTc intervals (using Fridericia's and linear correction factors) during treatment with RISPERDAL® CONSTA™.

Between-group comparisons for pooled placebo-controlled trials with oral RISPERDAL® revealed no statistically significant differences between risperidone and placebo in mean changes from baseline in ECG parameters, including QT, QTc, and PR intervals, and heart rate. When all oral RISPERDAL® doses were pooled from randomized controlled trials in several indications, there was a mean increase in heart rate of 1 beat per minute compared to no change for placebo patients. In short-term schizophrenia trials, higher doses of oral risperidone (8-16 mg/day) were associated with a higher mean increase in heart rate compared to placebo (4-6 beats per minute).

Pain assessment and local injection site reactions:

The mean intensity of injection pain reported by patients using a visual analog scale (0 = no pain to 100 = unbearably painful) decreased in all treatment groups from the first to the last injection (placebo: 16.7 to 12.6; 25 mg: 12.0 to 9.0; 50 mg: 18.2 to 11.8). After the sixth injection (Week 10), investigator ratings indicated that 1% of patients treated with 25 mg or 50 mg RISPERDAL® CONSTA™ experienced redness, swelling, or induration at the injection site.

Other Events Observed During the Premarketing Evaluation of RISPERDAL® CONSTA™

During its premarketing assessment, RISPERDAL® CONSTA™ was administered to 1499 patients in multiple-dose studies. The conditions and duration of exposure to RISPERDAL® CONSTA™ varied greatly, and included (in overlapping categories) open-label and double-blind studies, uncontrolled and controlled studies, inpatient and outpatient studies, fixed-dose and titration studies, and short-term and long-term exposure studies. In all studies, untoward events associated with this exposure were obtained by spontaneous report and were recorded by clinical investigators using terminology of their own choosing. Consequently, it is not possible to provide a meaningful estimate of the proportion of individuals experiencing adverse events without first grouping similar types of untoward events into a smaller number of standardized event categories.

In the listings that follow, spontaneously reported adverse events were classified using World Health Organization (WHO) preferred terms. The frequencies presented, therefore, represent the proportion of the 1499 patients exposed to multiple doses of RISPERDAL® CONSTA™ who experienced an event of the type cited on at least one occasion while receiving RISPERDAL® CONSTA™. All reported events are included except those already listed in Table 1, those events for which a drug cause was remote, those event terms which were so general as to be uninformative, and those events reported only once which did not have a substantial probability of being acutely life-threatening. It is important to emphasize that, although the reported events occurred during treatment with RISPERDAL® CONSTA™, they were not necessarily caused by it.

Events are further categorized by body system and listed in order of decreasing frequency according to the following definitions: frequent adverse events are those occurring in at least 1/100 patients (only those not already listed in the tabulated results from the placebo-controlled trial appear in this listing); infrequent adverse events are those occurring in 1/100 to 1/1000 patients; and rare events are those occurring in fewer than 1/1000 patients.

Psychiatric Disorders

Frequent: anxiety, psychosis, depression, agitation, nervousness, paranoid reaction, delusion, apathy. *Infrequent:* anorexia, impaired concentration, impotence, emotional lability, manic reaction, decreased libido, increased appetite, amnesia, confusion, euphoria, depersonalization, paroniria, delirium, psychotic depression.

Central and Peripheral Nervous System Disorders

Frequent: hypertonia, dystonia. *Infrequent:* dyskinesia, vertigo, leg cramps, tardive dyskinesia[a], involuntary muscle contractions, paraesthesia, abnormal gait, bradykinesia, convulsions, hypokinesia, ataxia, fecal incontinence, oculogyric crisis, tetany, apraxia, dementia, migraine. *Rare:* neuroleptic malignant syndrome.

[a] In the integrated database of multiple-dose studies (1499 patients with schizophrenia or schizoaffective disorder), 9 patients (0.6%) treated with RISPERDAL® CONSTA™ (all dosages combined) experienced an adverse event of tardive dyskinesia.

Body as a Whole/General Disorders

Frequent: back pain, chest pain, asthenia. *Infrequent:* malaise, choking.

Gastrointestinal Disorders

Frequent: nausea, vomiting, abdominal pain. *Infrequent:* gastritis, gastroesophageal reflux, flatulence, hemorrhoids, melena, dysphagia, rectal hemorrhage, stomatitis, colitis, gastric ulcer, gingivitis, irritable bowel syndrome, ulcerative stomatitis.

Respiratory System Disorders

Frequent: dyspnea. *Infrequent:* pneumonia, stridor, hemoptysis. *Rare:* pulmonary edema.

Skin and Appendage Disorders

Frequent: rash. *Infrequent:* eczema, pruritus, erythematous rash, dermatitis, alopecia, seborrhea, photosensitivity reaction, increased sweating.

Metabolic and Nutritional Disorders

Infrequent: hyperuricemia, hyperglycemia, hyperlipemia, hypokalemia, glycosuria, hypercholesterolemia, obesity, dehydration, diabetes mellitus, hyponatremia.

Musculo-Skeletal System Disorders

Frequent: arthralgia, skeletal pain. *Infrequent:* torticollis, arthrosis, muscle weakness, tendinitis, arthritis, arthropathy.

Heart Rate and Rhythm Disorders

Frequent: tachycardia. *Infrequent:* bradycardia, AV block, palpitation, bundle branch block. *Rare:* T-wave inversion.

Cardiovascular Disorders

Frequent: hypotension. *Infrequent:* postural hypotension.

Urinary System Disorders

Frequent: urinary incontinence. *Infrequent:* hematuria, micturition frequency, renal pain, urinary retention.

Vision Disorders

Infrequent: conjunctivitis, eye pain, abnormal accommodation.

Reproductive Disorders, Female

Frequent: amenorrhea. *Infrequent:* nonpuerperal lactation, vaginitis, dysmenorrhea, breast pain, leukorrhea.

Resistance Mechanism Disorders

Infrequent: abscess.

Liver and Biliary System Disorders

Frequent: increased hepatic enzymes. *Infrequent:* hepatomegaly, increased SGPT. *Rare:* bilirubinemia, increased GGT, hepatitis, hepatocellular damage, jaundice, fatty liver, increased SGOT.

Reproductive Disorders, Male

Infrequent: ejaculation failure.

Application Site Disorders

Frequent: injection site pain. *Infrequent:* injection site reaction.

Hearing and Vestibular Disorders

Infrequent: earache, deafness, hearing decreased.

Red Blood Cell Disorders

Frequent: anemia.

White Cell and Resistance Disorders

Infrequent: lymphadenopathy, leucopenia, cervical lymphadenopathy.

Rare: granulocytopenia, leukocytosis, lymphopenia.

Endocrine Disorders

Infrequent: hyperprolactinemia, gynecomastia, hypothyroidism.

Platelet, Bleeding and Clotting Disorders

Infrequent: purpura, epistaxis. *Rare:* pulmonary embolism, hematoma, thrombocytopenia.

Myo-, Endo-, and Pericardial and Valve Disorders

Infrequent: myocardial ischemia, angina pectoris, myocardial infarction.

Vascular (Extracardiac) Disorders

Infrequent: phlebitis. *Rare:* intermittent claudication, flushing, thrombophlebitis.

Postintroduction Reports

Adverse events reported since market introduction which were temporally (but not necessarily causally) related to oral RISPERDAL® therapy include the following: anaphylactic reaction, angioedema, apnea, atrial fibrillation, cerebrovascular disorder, including cerebrovascular accident, hyperglycemia, diabetes mellitus aggravated, including diabetic ketoacidosis, intestinal obstruction, jaundice, mania, pancreatitis, Parkinson's disease aggravated, pulmonary embolism. There have been rare reports of sudden death and/or cardiopulmonary arrest in patients receiving oral RISPERDAL®. A causal relationship with oral RISPERDAL® has not been established. It is important to note that sudden and unexpected death may occur in psychotic patients whether they remain untreated or whether they are treated with other antipsychotic drugs.

DRUG ABUSE AND DEPENDENCE

Controlled Substance Class

RISPERDAL® CONSTA™ (risperidone) is not a controlled substance.

Physical and Psychological Dependence

RISPERDAL® CONSTA™ has not been systematically studied in animals or humans for its potential for abuse, tolerance, or physical dependence. Because RISPERDAL® CONSTA™ is to be administered by health care professionals, the potential for misuse or abuse by patients is low.

OVERDOSAGE

Human Experience

No cases of overdose were reported in premarketing studies with RISPERDAL® CONSTA™ (risperidone). Because RISPERDAL® CONSTA™ is to be administered by health care professionals, the potential for overdosage by patients is low.

In premarketing experience with oral RISPERDAL® (risperidone), there were eight reports of acute RISPERDAL® overdosage, with estimated doses ranging from 20 to 300 mg and no fatalities. In general, reported signs and symptoms were those resulting from an exaggeration of the drug's known pharmacological effects, i.e., drowsiness and sedation, tachycardia and hypotension, and extrapyramidal symptoms. One case, involving an estimated overdose of 240 mg, was associated with hyponatremia, hypokalemia, prolonged QT, and widened QRS. Another case, involving an estimated overdose of 36 mg, was associated with a seizure.

Postmarketing experience with oral RISPERDAL® includes reports of acute overdose, with estimated doses of up to 360 mg. In general, the most frequently reported signs and symptoms are those resulting from an exaggeration of the drug's known pharmacological effects, i.e., drowsiness, sedation, tachycardia, hypotension, and extrapyramidal symptoms. Other adverse events reported since market introduction which were temporally (but not necessarily causally) related to oral RISPERDAL® overdose include torsades de pointes, prolonged QT interval, convulsions, cardiopulmonary arrest, and rare fatality associated with multiple drug overdose.

Management of Overdosage

In case of acute overdosage, establish and maintain an airway and ensure adequate oxygenation and ventilation. Cardiovascular monitoring should commence immediately and should include continuous electrocardiographic monitoring to detect possible arrhythmias. If antiarrhythmic therapy is administered, disopyramide, procainamide, and quinidine carry a theoretical hazard of QT prolonging effects that might be additive to those of risperidone. Similarly, it is reasonable to expect that the alpha-blocking properties of bretylium might be additive to those of risperidone, resulting in problematic hypotension.

There is no specific antidote to oral RISPERDAL®. Therefore, appropriate supportive measures should be instituted. The possibility of multiple drug involvement should be considered. Hypotension and circulatory collapse should be treated with appropriate measures, such as intravenous flu-

Continued on next page

Risperdal Consta—Cont.

ids and/or sympathomimetic agents (epinephrine and dopamine should not be used, since beta stimulation may worsen hypotension in the setting of risperidone-induced alpha blockade). In cases of severe extrapyramidal symptoms, anticholinergic medication should be administered. Close medical supervision and monitoring should continue until the patient recovers.

DOSAGE AND ADMINISTRATION

For patients who have never taken oral RISPERDAL®, it is recommended to establish tolerability with oral RISPERDAL® prior to initiating treatment with RISPERDAL® CONSTA™ (risperidone).

RISPERDAL® CONSTA™ should be administered every 2 weeks by deep intramuscular (IM) gluteal injection. Each injection should be administered by a health care professional using the enclosed safety needle (see HOW SUPPLIED). Injections should alternate between the two buttocks. Do not administer intravenously.

The recommended dose is 25 mg IM every 2 weeks. Although dose response for effectiveness has not been established for RISPERDAL® CONSTA™, some patients not responding to 25 mg may benefit from a higher dose of 37.5 mg or 50 mg. The maximum dose should not exceed 50 mg RISPERDAL® CONSTA™ every 2 weeks. No additional benefit was observed with dosages greater than 50 mg RISPERDAL® CONSTA™; however, a higher incidence of adverse effects was observed.

Oral RISPERDAL® (or another antipsychotic medication) should be given with the first injection of RISPERDAL® CONSTA™ and continued for 3 weeks (and then discontinued) to ensure that adequate therapeutic plasma concentrations are maintained prior to the main release phase of risperidone from the injection site (see CLINICAL PHARMACOLOGY).

Upward dosage adjustment should not be made more frequently than every 4 weeks. The clinical effects of this dose adjustment should not be anticipated earlier than 3 weeks after the first injection with the higher dose.

Do not combine two different dosage strengths of RISPERDAL® CONSTA™ in a single administration.

Pediatric Use

RISPERDAL® CONSTA™ has not been studied in children younger than 18 years old.

Dosage in Special Populations

For elderly patients treated with RISPERDAL® CONSTA™, the recommended dosage is 25 mg IM every 2 weeks. Oral RISPERDAL® (or another antipsychotic medication) should be given with the first injection of RISPERDAL® CONSTA™ and should be continued for 3 weeks to ensure that adequate therapeutic plasma concentrations are maintained prior to the main release phase of risperidone from the injection site (see CLINICAL PHARMACOLOGY).

Patients with renal or hepatic impairment should be treated with titrated doses of oral RISPERDAL® prior to initiating treatment with RISPERDAL® CONSTA™. The recommended starting dose is 0.5 mg oral RISPERDAL® b.i.d. during the first week, which can be increased to 1 mg b.i.d. or 2 mg once daily during the second week. If a dose of at least 2 mg oral RISPERDAL® is well tolerated, an injection of 25 mg RISPERDAL® CONSTA™ can be administered every 2 weeks. Oral supplementation should be continued for 3 weeks after the first injection until the main release of risperidone from the injection site has begun. In some patients, slower titration may be medically appropriate.

Patients with renal impairment may have less ability to eliminate risperidone than normal adults. Patients with impaired hepatic function may have an increase in the free fraction of the risperidone, possibly resulting in an enhanced effect (see CLINICAL PHARMACOLOGY). Elderly patients and patients with a predisposition to hypotensive reactions or for whom such reactions would pose a particular risk should be instructed in nonpharmacologic interventions that help to reduce the occurrence of orthostatic hypotension (e.g., sitting on the edge of the bed for several minutes before attempting to stand in the morning and slowly rising from a seated position). These patients should avoid sodium depletion or dehydration, and circumstances that accentuate hypotension (alcohol intake, high ambient temperature, etc.). Monitoring of orthostatic vital signs should be considered (see PRECAUTIONS).

Maintenance Therapy

Although no controlled studies have been conducted to answer the question of how long patients should be treated with RISPERDAL® CONSTA™, oral risperidone has been shown to be effective in delaying time to relapse in longer-term use. It is recommended that responding patients be continued on treatment with RISPERDAL® CONSTA™ at the lowest dose needed. Patients should be periodically reassessed to determine the need for continued treatment.

Reinitiation of Treatment in Patients Previously Discontinued

There are no data to specifically address reinitiation of treatment. When restarting patients who have had an interval off treatment with RISPERDAL® CONSTA™, supplementation with oral RISPERDAL® (or another antipsychotic medication) should be administered.

Switching from Other Antipsychotics

There are no systematically collected data to specifically address switching schizophrenic patients from other antipsychotics to RISPERDAL® CONSTA™, or concerning concomitant administration with other antipsychotics. Previous antipsychotics should be continued for 3 weeks after the first injection of RISPERDAL® CONSTA™ to ensure that therapeutic concentrations are maintained until the main release phase of risperidone from the injection site has begun (see CLINICAL PHARMACOLOGY). For schizophrenic patients who have never taken oral RISPERDAL®, it is recommended to establish tolerability with oral RISPERDAL® prior to initiating treatment with RISPERDAL® CONSTA™. As recommended with other antipsychotic medications, the need for continuing existing EPS medication should be re-evaluated periodically.

Co-Administration of RISPERDAL® CONSTA™ with Certain Other Medications

Co-administration of carbamazepine and other enzyme inducers (e.g., phenytoin, rifampin, phenobarbital) with risperidone would be expected to cause decreases in the plasma concentrations of active moiety (the sum of risperidone and 9-hydroxyrisperidone), which could lead to decreased efficacy of risperidone treatment. The dose of risperidone needs to be titrated accordingly for patients receiving these enzyme inducers, especially during initiation or discontinuation of therapy with these inducers (see CLINICAL PHARMACOLOGY and PRECAUTIONS). At the initiation of therapy with carbamazepine or other known hepatic enzyme inducers, patients should be closely monitored during the first 4-8 weeks, since the dose of RISPERDAL® CONSTA™ may need to be adjusted. A dose increase, or additional oral RISPERDAL®, may need to be considered. On discontinuation of carbamazepine or other hepatic enzyme inducers, the dosage of RISPERDAL® CONSTA™ should be re-evaluated and, if necessary, decreased. Patients may be placed on a lower dose of RISPERDAL® CONSTA™ between 2 to 4 weeks before the planned discontinuation of carbamazepine therapy to adjust for the expected increase in plasma concentrations of risperidone plus 9-hydroxyrisperidone. For patients treated with the lowest available dose (25 mg) of RISPERDAL® CONSTA™, it is recommended to continue treatment with the 25-mg dose unless clinical judgment necessitates interruption of treatment with RISPERDAL® CONSTA™.

Fluoxetine and paroxetine have been shown to increase the plasma concentration of risperidone 2.5-2.8 fold and 3-9 fold respectively. Fluoxetine did not affect the plasma concentration of 9-hydroxyrisperidone. Paroxetine lowered the concentration of 9-hydroxyrisperidone an average of 13%. The dose of risperidone needs to be titrated accordingly when fluoxetine or paroxetine is co-administered. When either concomitant fluoxetine or paroxetine is initiated or discontinued, the physician should re-evaluate the dosage of RISPERDAL® CONSTA™. When initiation of fluoxetine or paroxetine is considered, patients may be placed on a lower dose of RISPERDAL® CONSTA™ between 2 to 4 weeks before the planned start of fluoxetine or paroxetine therapy to adjust for the expected increase in plasma concentrations of risperidone. For patients treated with the lowest available dose (25 mg), it is recommended to continue treatment with the 25-mg dose unless clinical judgment necessitates interruption of treatment with RISPERDAL® CONSTA™. The effects of discontinuation of concomitant fluoxetine or paroxetine therapy on the pharmacokinetics of risperidone and 9-hydroxyrisperidone have not been studied.

Instructions for Use

RISPERDAL® CONSTA™ must be suspended **only** in the diluent supplied in the dose pack, and must be administered with the needle supplied in the dose pack. All components are required for administration. Do not substitute any components of the dose pack.

[See graphic below]

Remove the dose pack of RISPERDAL® CONSTA™ from the refrigerator and allow it to come to room temperature prior to reconstitution.

1. Flip off the plastic colored cap from the vial.

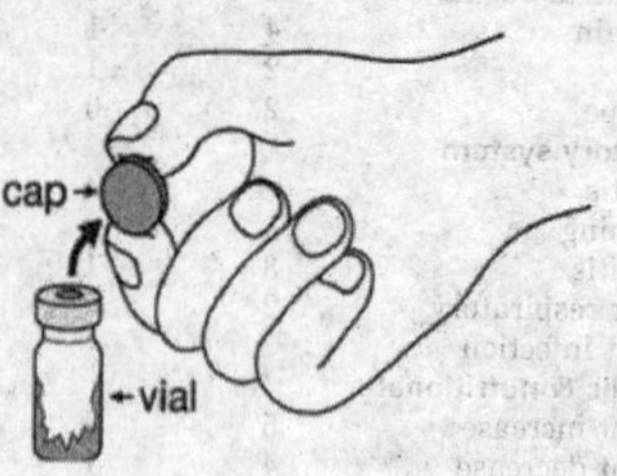

2. Peel back the blister pouch and remove the SmartSite® Needle-Free Vial Access Device by holding the white luer cap. Do **not** touch the spike tip of the access device at any time.

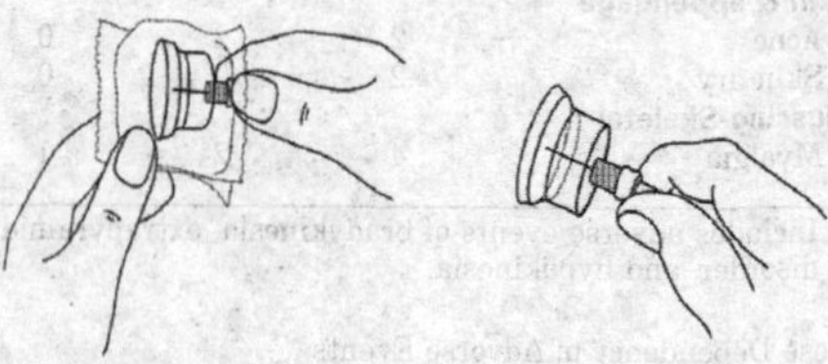

3. Press the spike tip of the SmartSite® Access Device through the vial's rubber stopper until the device clicks into place.

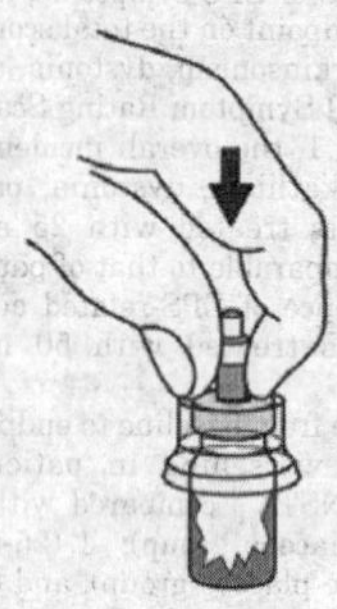

4. Swab the syringe connection point (blue circle) of the SmartSite® Access Device with preferred antiseptic prior to attaching the syringe to the SmartSite® Access Device.

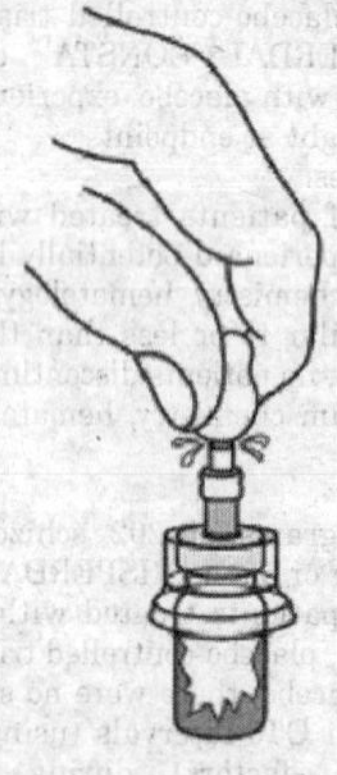

5. Twist off the white cap from the pre-filled syringe and remove together with the rubber tip cap inside.

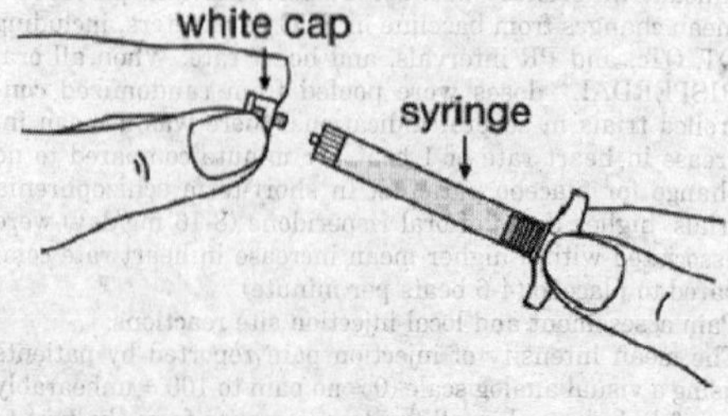

6. **Press** the syringe tip into the blue circle of the SmartSite® Access Device and **Twist** in a clockwise motion to ensure that the syringe is securely attached to the white luer cap of the access device. Keep the syringe and SmartSite® Access Device aligned, and hold the

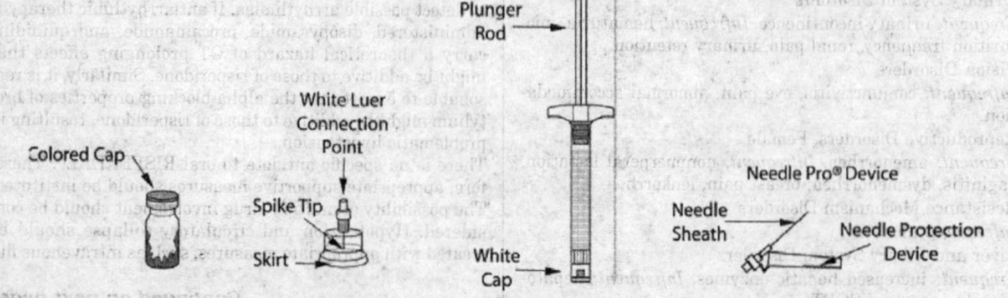

skirt of the access device during attachment to prevent spinning.

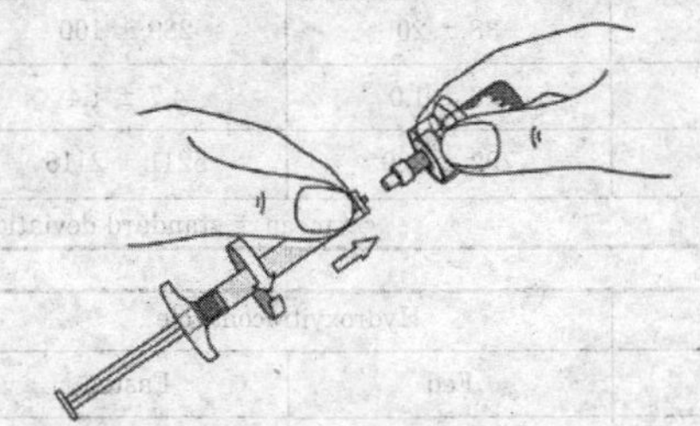

7. Inject the entire contents of the syringe containing the diluent into the vial.

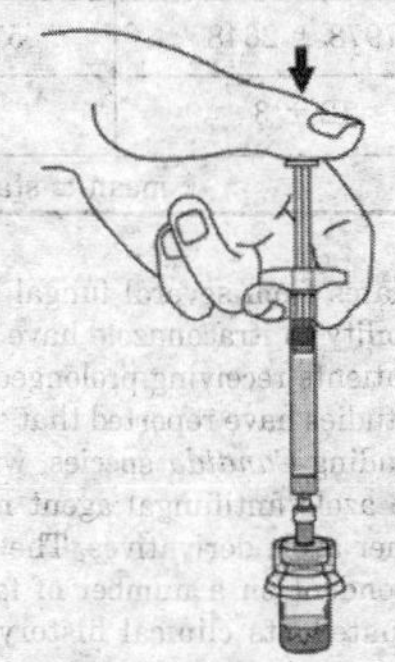

8. Shake the vial vigorously while holding the plunger rod down with the thumb for a minimum of 10 seconds to ensure a homogeneous suspension. When properly mixed, the suspension appears uniform, thick, and milky in color. The particles will be visible in liquid, but no dry particles remain.

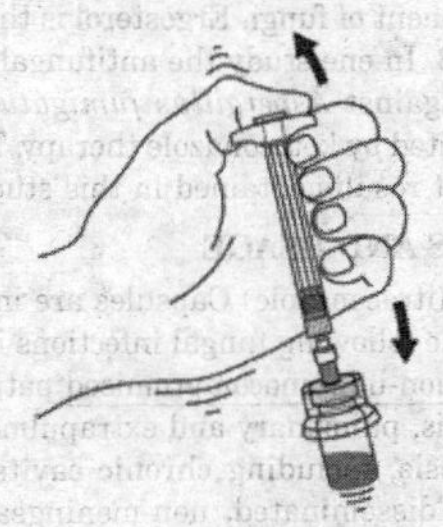

9. Do not store the vial after reconstitution or the suspension may settle. *If 2 minutes pass before injection, reconstitute by shaking vigorously.*
10. Invert the vial completely and slowly withdraw the suspension from the vial. Tear section of the vial label at the perforation and apply detached label to syringe for identification purposes.

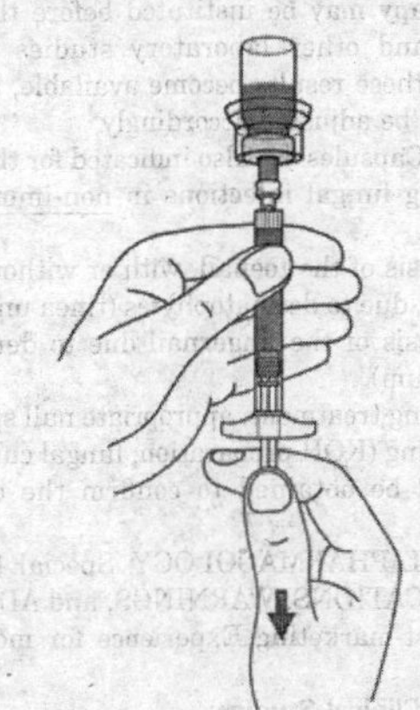

11. Unscrew the syringe from the SmartSite® access device and discard both the vial and access device appropriately.

[See figure at top of next column]

12. Peel the blister pouch of the Needle-Pro® device open halfway. Grasp sheath using the plastic peel pouch.

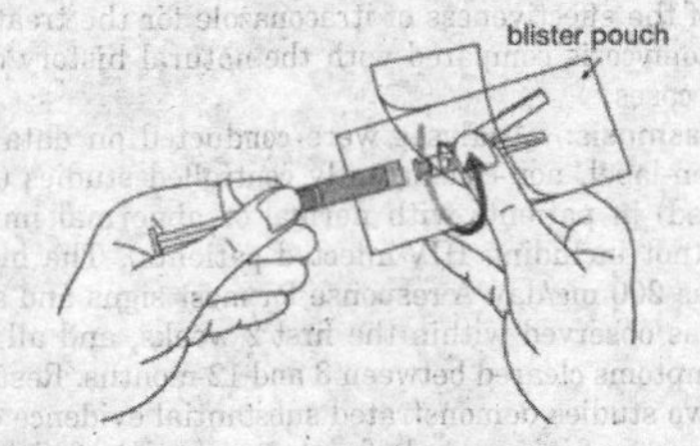

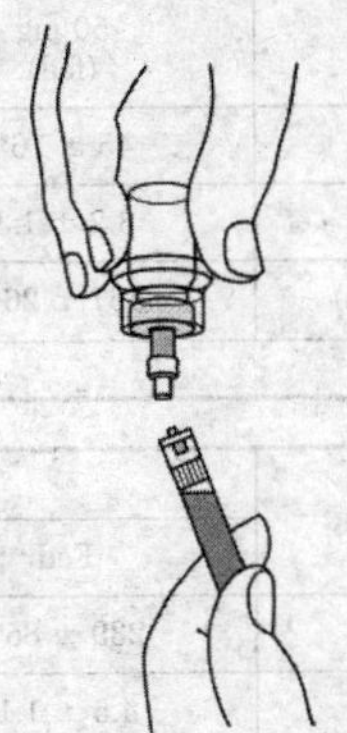

13. Attach the luer connection of the Needle-Pro® device to the syringe with an easy clockwise twisting motion. Seat the needle firmly on the Needle-Pro® device with a push and clockwise twist.
14. *If 2 minutes pass before injection, reconstitute by shaking vigorously.*
15. Pull sheath away from the needle. Do not twist sheath, as needle may be loosened from Needle-Pro® device. Tap the syringe gently to make any air bubbles rise to the top. De-aerate syringe by moving plunger rod carefully forward, with needle in an upward position. Inject entire contents intramuscularly (IM) into the upper-outer quadrant of the gluteal area within 2 minutes to avoid settling. **DO NOT ADMINISTER INTRAVENOUSLY.**

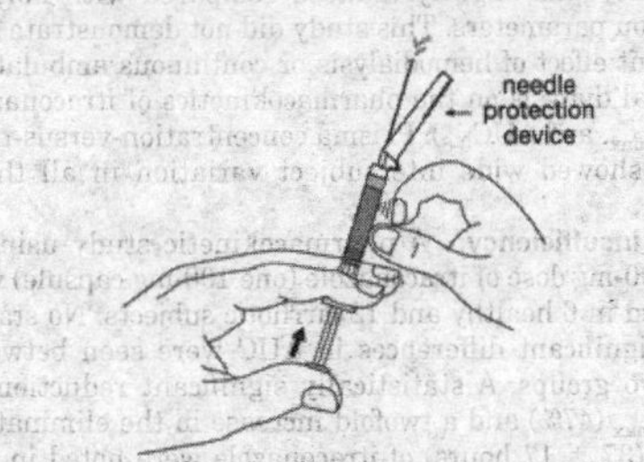

WARNING: To avoid a needle stick injury with a contaminated needle, do not:

- intentionally disengage the Needle-Pro® device
- attempt to straighten the needle or engage Needle-Pro® device if the needle is bent or damaged
- mishandle the needle protection device which could lead to protrusion of the needle from the needle protector sheath

16. After injection is complete, use only one hand and tabletop or other hard surface to snap needle into the orange safety guard before discarding. Discard needle appropriately.

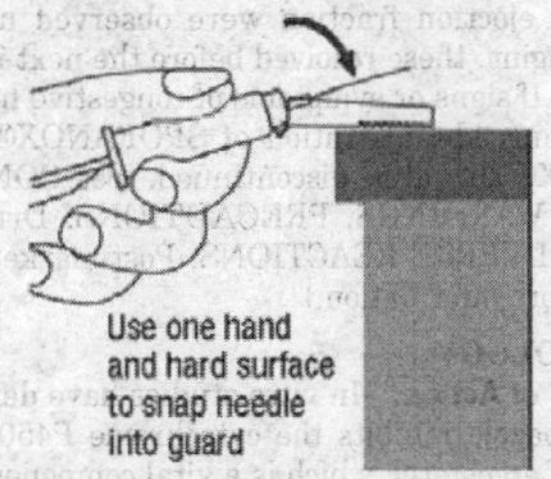

Upon suspension in the diluent, it is recommended to use RISPERDAL® CONSTA™ immediately. RISPERDAL® CONSTA™ must be used within 6 hours of suspension. Resuspension of RISPERDAL® CONSTA™ will be necessary prior to administration, as settling will occur over time once the product is in suspension. Keeping the vial upright, shake vigorously back and forth for as long as it takes to resuspend the microspheres. Once in suspension, the product should not be exposed to temperatures above 77°F (25°C).

Parenteral drug products should be inspected visually for particulate matter and discoloration prior to administration, whenever solution and container permit.

HOW SUPPLIED

RISPERDAL® CONSTA™ (risperidone) is available in dosage strengths of 25, 37.5, or 50 mg risperidone. It is provided as a dose pack, consisting of a vial containing the risperidone microspheres, a pre-filled syringe containing 2 mL of diluent for RISPERDAL® CONSTA™, a SmartSite® Needle-Free Vial Access Device, and one Needle-Pro® safety needle for intramuscular injection (20 G TW needle with needle protection device).

25-mg vial/kit (NDC 50458-306-11): 25 mg of a white to off-white powder provided in a vial with a pink flip-off cap (NDC 50458-306-01).

37.5-mg vial/kit (NDC 50458-307-11): 37.5 mg of a white to off-white powder provided in a vial with a green flip-off cap (NDC 50458-307-01).

50-mg vial/kit (NDC 50458-308-11): 50 mg of a white to off-white powder provided in a vial with a blue flip-off cap (NDC 50458-308-01).

Storage and Handling

The entire dose pack should be stored in the refrigerator (36°-46°F; 2°-8°C) and protected from light.

If refrigeration is unavailable, RISPERDAL® CONSTA™ can be stored at temperatures not exceeding 77°F (25°C) for no more than 7 days prior to administration. Do not expose unrefrigerated product to temperatures above 77°F (25°C).

Keep out of reach of children.

7519501
US Patent 4,804,663
January 2004

Risperidone is manufactured by:
Janssen Pharmaceutical Ltd.
Wallingstown, Little Island, County Cork, Ireland
Microspheres are manufactured by:
Alkermes Controlled Therapeutics II
Wilmington, Ohio
Diluent is manufactured by:
Vetter Pharma Fertigung GmbH & Co. KG
Ravensburg, Germany
RISPERDAL® CONSTA™ is distributed by:
Janssen Pharmaceutica Products, L.P.
Titusville, NJ 08560

Shown in Product Identification Guide, page 319

SPORANOX® CAPSULES ℞
itraconazole

Congestive Heart Failure

SPORANOX® (itraconazole) Capsules should not be administered for the treatment of onychomycosis in patients with evidence of ventricular dysfunction such as congestive heart failure (CHF) or a history of CHF. If signs or symptoms of congestive heart failure occur during administration of SPORANOX® Capsules, discontinue administration. When itraconazole was administered intravenously to dogs and healthy human volunteers, negative inotropic effects were seen. (See CLINICAL PHARMACOLOGY: Special Populations, CONTRAINDICATIONS, WARNINGS, PRECAUTIONS: Drug Interactions and ADVERSE REACTIONS: Post-marketing Experience for more information.)

Drug Interactions: Coadministration of cisapride, pimozide, quinidine, dofetilide, or levacetylmethadol (levomethadyl) with SPORANOX® (itraconazole) Capsules, Injection or Oral Solution is contraindicated. SPORANOX®, a potent cytochrome P450 3A4 isoenzyme system (CYP3A4) inhibitor, may increase plasma concentrations of drugs metabolized by this pathway. Serious cardiovascular events, including QT prolongation, torsades de pointes, ventricular tachycardia, cardiac arrest, and/or sudden death have occurred in patients using cisapride, pimozide, levacetylmethadol (levomethadyl), or quinidine concomitantly with SPORANOX® and/or other CYP3A4 inhibitors. See CONTRAINDICATIONS, WARNINGS, and PRECAUTIONS: Drug Interactions for more information.

DESCRIPTION

SPORANOX® is the brand name for itraconazole, a synthetic triazole antifungal agent. Itraconazole is a 1:1:1:1 racemic mixture of four diastereomers (two enantiomeric pairs), each possessing three chiral centers. It may be represented by the following structural formula and nomenclature:

(±)-1-[(R*)-sec-butyl]-4-[p-[4-[p-[[(2R*,4S*)-2-(2,4-dichlorophenyl)-2-(1H-1,2,4-triazol-1-ylmethyl)-1,3-dioxolan-4-yl]methoxy] phenyl]-1-piperazinyl]phenyl]-Δ²-1,2,4-triazolin-5-one mixture with (±)-1-[(R*)-sec-butyl]-4-[p-[4-[p-[[(2S*,4R*)-2-(2,4-dichlorophenyl)-2-(1H-1,2,4-triazol-1-ylmethyl)-1,3-dioxolan-4-yl]methoxy]phenyl]-1-piperazinyl] phenyl]-Δ²-1,2,4-triazolin-5-one

or

(±)-1-[(RS)-sec-butyl]-4-[p-[4-[p-[[(2R,4S)-2-(2,4-dichlorophenyl)-2-(1H-1,2,4-triazol-1-ylmethyl)-1,3-dioxolan-4-yl] methoxy] phenyl]-1-piperazinyl]phenyl]-Δ²-1,2,4-triazolin-5-one

Itraconazole has a molecular formula of $C_{35}H_{38}Cl_2N_8O_4$ and a molecular weight of 705.64. It is a white to slightly yellowish powder. It is insoluble in water, very slightly soluble in alcohols, and freely soluble in dichloromethane. It has a pKa of 3.70 (based on extrapolation of values obtained from methanolic solutions) and a log (n-octanol/water) partition coefficient of 5.66 at pH 8.1.

SPORANOX® Capsules contain 100 mg of itraconazole coated on sugar spheres. Inactive ingredients are gelatin, hypromellose, polyethylene glycol (PEG) 20,000, starch, sucrose, titanium dioxide, FD&C Blue No. 1, FD&C Blue No. 2, D&C Red No. 22 and D&C Red No. 28.

Continued on next page

Sporanox Capsules—Cont.

CLINICAL PHARMACOLOGY

Pharmacokinetics and Metabolism: NOTE: The plasma concentrations reported below were measured by high-performance liquid chromatography (HPLC) specific for itraconazole. When itraconazole in plasma is measured by a bioassay, values reported are approximately 3.3 times higher than those obtained by HPLC due to the presence of the bioactive metabolite, hydroxyitraconazole. (See MICROBIOLOGY.)

The pharmacokinetics of itraconazole after intravenous administration and its absolute oral bioavailability from an oral solution were studied in a randomized crossover study in 6 healthy male volunteers. The observed absolute oral bioavailability of itraconazole was 55%.

The oral bioavailability of itraconazole is maximal when SPORANOX® (itraconazole) Capsules are taken with a full meal. The pharmacokinetics of itraconazole were studied in 6 healthy male volunteers who received, in a crossover design, single 100-mg doses of itraconazole as a polyethylene glycol capsule, with or without a full meal. The same 6 volunteers also received 50 mg or 200 mg with a full meal in a crossover design. In this study, only itraconazole plasma concentrations were measured. The respective pharmacokinetic parameters for itraconazole are presented in the table below:

[See first table above]

	50 mg (fed)	100 mg (fed)	100 mg (fasted)	200 mg (fed)
C_{max} (ng/mL)	45 ± 16*	132 ± 67	38 ± 20	289 ± 100
T_{max} (hours)	3.2 ± 1.3	4.0 ± 1.1	3.3 ± 1.0	4.7 ± 1.4
$AUC_{0-\infty}$ (ng•h/mL)	567 ± 264	1899 ± 838	722 ± 289	5211 ± 2116

* mean ± standard deviation

Doubling the SPORANOX® dose results in approximately a three-fold increase in the itraconazole plasma concentrations.

Values given in the table below represent data from a crossover pharmacokinetics study in which 27 healthy male volunteers each took a single 200-mg dose of SPORANOX® Capsules with or without a full meal:

[See second table above]

	Itraconazole		Hydroxyitraconazole	
	Fed	Fasted	Fed	Fasted
C_{max} (ng/mL)	239 ± 85*	140 ± 65	397 ± 103	286 ± 101
T_{max} (hours)	4.5 ± 1.1	3.9 ± 1.0	5.1 ± 1.6	4.5 ± 1.1
$AUC_{0-\infty}$ (ng•h/mL)	3423 ± 1154	2094 ± 905	7978 ± 2648	5191 ± 2489
$t_{1/2}$ (hours)	21 ± 5	21 ± 7	12 ± 3	12 ± 3

* mean ± standard deviation

Absorption of itraconazole under fasted conditions in individuals with relative or absolute achlorhydria, such as patients with AIDS or volunteers taking gastric acid secretion suppressors (e.g., H_2 receptor antagonists), was increased when SPORANOX® Capsules were administered with a cola beverage. Eighteen men with AIDS received single 200-mg doses of SPORANOX® Capsules under fasted conditions with 8 ounces of water or 8 ounces of a cola beverage in a crossover design. The absorption of itraconazole was increased when SPORANOX® Capsules were coadministered with a cola beverage, with AUC_{0-24} and C_{max} increasing 75% ± 121% and 95% ± 128%, respectively.

Thirty healthy men received single 200-mg doses of SPORANOX® Capsules under fasted conditions either 1) with water; 2) with water, after ranitidine 150 mg b.i.d. for 3 days; or 3) with cola, after ranitidine 150 mg b.i.d. for 3 days. When SPORANOX® Capsules were administered after ranitidine pretreatment, itraconazole was absorbed to a lesser extent than when SPORANOX® Capsules were administered alone, with decreases in AUC_{0-24} and C_{max} of 39% ± 37% and 42% ± 39%, respectively. When SPORANOX® Capsules were administered with cola after ranitidine pretreatment, itraconazole absorption was comparable to that observed when SPORANOX® Capsules were administered alone. (See PRECAUTIONS: Drug Interactions.)

Steady-state concentrations were reached within 15 days following oral doses of 50 mg to 400 mg daily. Values given in the table below are data at steady-state from a pharmacokinetics study in which 27 healthy male volunteers took 200-mg SPORANOX® Capsules b.i.d.(with a full meal) for 15 days:

	Itraconazole	Hydroxyitraconazole
C_{max} (ng/mL)	2282 ± 514*	3488 ± 742
C_{min} (ng/mL)	1855 ± 535	3349 ± 761
T_{max} (hours)	4.6 ± 1.8	3.4 ± 3.4
AUC_{0-12h} (ng•h/mL)	22569 ± 5375	38572 ± 8450
$t_{1/2}$ (hours)	64 ± 32	56 ± 24

* mean ± standard deviation

The plasma protein binding of itraconazole is 99.8% and that of hydroxyitraconazole is 99.5%. Following intravenous administration, the volume of distribution of itraconazole averaged 796 ± 185 liters.

Itraconazole is metabolized predominately by the cytochrome P450 3A4 isoenzyme system (CYP3A4), resulting in the formation of several metabolites, including hydroxyitraconazole, the major metabolite. Results of a pharmacokinetics study suggest that itraconazole may undergo saturable metabolism with multiple dosing. Fecal excretion of the parent drug varies between 3–18% of the dose. Renal excretion of the parent drug is less than 0.03% of the dose. About 40% of the dose is excreted as inactive metabolites in the urine. No single excreted metabolite represents more than 5% of a dose. Itraconazole total plasma clearance averaged 381 ± 95 mL/minute following intravenous administration. (See CONTRAINDICATIONS and PRECAUTIONS: Drug Interactions for more information.)

Special Populations:

Renal Insufficiency: A pharmacokinetic study using a single 200-mg dose of itraconazole (four 50-mg capsules) was conducted in three groups of patients with renal impairment (uremia: n=7; hemodialysis: n=7; and continuous ambulatory peritoneal dialysis: n=5). In uremic subjects with a mean creatinine clearance of 13 mL/min. x 1.73 m^2, the bioavailability was slightly reduced compared with normal population parameters. This study did not demonstrate any significant effect of hemodialysis or continuous ambulatory peritoneal dialysis on the pharmacokinetics of itraconazole (T_{max}, C_{max}, and AUC_{0-8}). Plasma concentration-versus-time profiles showed wide intersubject variation in all three groups.

Hepatic Insufficiency: A pharmacokinetic study using a single 100-mg dose of itraconazole (one 100-mg capsule) was conducted in 6 healthy and 12 cirrhotic subjects. No statistically significant differences in AUC were seen between these two groups. A statistically significant reduction in mean C_{max} (47%) and a twofold increase in the elimination half-life (37 ± 17 hours) of itraconazole were noted in cirrhotic subjects compared with healthy subjects. Patients with impaired hepatic function should be carefully monitored when taking itraconazole. The prolonged elimination half-life of itraconazole observed in cirrhotic patients should be considered when deciding to initiate therapy with other medications metabolized by CYP3A4. (See BOX WARNING, CONTRAINDICATIONS, and PRECAUTIONS: Drug Interactions.)

Decreased Cardiac Contractility: When itraconazole was administered intravenously to anesthetized dogs, a dose-related negative inotropic effect was documented. In a healthy volunteer study of SPORANOX® Injection (intravenous infusion), transient, asymptomatic decreases in left ventricular ejection fraction were observed using gated SPECT imaging; these resolved before the next infusion, 12 hours later. If signs or symptoms of congestive heart failure appear during administration of SPORANOX® Capsules, SPORANOX® should be discontinued. (See CONTRAINDICATIONS, WARNINGS, PRECAUTIONS: Drug Interactions and ADVERSE REACTIONS: Post-marketing Experience for more information.)

MICROBIOLOGY

Mechanism of Action: In vitro studies have demonstrated that itraconazole inhibits the cytochrome P450-dependent synthesis of ergosterol, which is a vital component of fungal cell membranes.

Activity In Vitro and In Vivo: Itraconazole exhibits in vitro activity against *Blastomyces dermatitidis, Histoplasma capsulatum, Histoplasma duboisii, Aspergillus flavus, Aspergillus fumigatus, Candida albicans,* and *Cryptococcus neoformans*. Itraconazole also exhibits varying in vitro activity against *Sporothrix schenckii, Trichophyton species, Candida krusei,* and other *Candida* species. The bioactive metabolite, hydroxyitraconazole, has not been evaluated against *Histoplasma capsulatum* and *Blastomyces dermatitidis*. Correlation between minimum inhibitory concentration (MIC) results in vitro and clinical outcome has yet to be established for azole antifungal agents.

Itraconazole administered orally was active in a variety of animal models of fungal infection using standard laboratory strains of fungi. Fungistatic activity has been demonstrated against disseminated fungal infections caused by *Blastomyces dermatitidis, Histoplasma duboisii, Aspergillus fumigatus, Coccidioides immitis, Cryptococcus neoformans, Paracoccidioides brasiliensis, Sporothrix schenckii, Trichophyton rubrum,* and *Trichophyton mentagrophytes.*

Itraconazole administered at 2.5 mg/kg and 5 mg/kg via the oral and parenteral routes increased survival rates and sterilized organ systems in normal and immunosuppressed guinea pigs with disseminated *Aspergillus fumigatus* infections. Oral itraconazole administered daily at 40 mg/kg and 80 mg/kg increased survival rates in normal rabbits with disseminated disease and in immunosuppressed rats with pulmonary *Aspergillus fumigatus* infection, respectively. Itraconazole has demonstrated antifungal activity in a variety of animal models infected with *Candida albicans* and other *Candida* species.

Resistance: Isolates from several fungal species with decreased susceptibility to itraconazole have been isolated in vitro and from patients receiving prolonged therapy.

Several in vitro studies have reported that some fungal clinical isolates, including *Candida* species, with reduced susceptibility to one azole antifungal agent may also be less susceptible to other azole derivatives. The finding of cross-resistance is dependent on a number of factors, including the species evaluated, its clinical history, the particular azole compounds compared, and the type of susceptibility test that is performed. The relevance of these in vitro susceptibility data to clinical outcome remains to be elucidated. Studies (both in vitro and in vivo) suggest that the activity of amphotericin B may be suppressed by prior azole antifungal therapy. As with other azoles, itraconazole inhibits the ^{14}C-demethylation step in the synthesis of ergosterol, a cell wall component of fungi. Ergosterol is the active site for amphotericin B. In one study the antifungal activity of amphotericin B against *Aspergillus fumigatus* infections in mice was inhibited by ketoconazole therapy. The clinical significance of test results obtained in this study is unknown.

INDICATIONS AND USAGE

SPORANOX® (itraconazole) Capsules are indicated for the treatment of the following fungal infections in immunocompromised and non-immunocompromised patients:

1. Blastomycosis, pulmonary and extrapulmonary
2. Histoplasmosis, including chronic cavitary pulmonary disease and disseminated, non-meningeal histoplasmosis, and
3. Aspergillosis, pulmonary and extrapulmonary, in patients who are intolerant of or who are refractory to amphotericin B therapy.

Specimens for fungal cultures and other relevant laboratory studies (wet mount, histopathology, serology) should be obtained before therapy to isolate and identify causative organisms. Therapy may be instituted before the results of the cultures and other laboratory studies are known; however, once these results become available, antiinfective therapy should be adjusted accordingly.

SPORANOX® Capsules are also indicated for the treatment of the following fungal infections in non-immunocompromised patients:

1. Onychomycosis of the toenail, with or without fingernail involvement, due to dermatophytes (tinea unguium), and
2. Onychomycosis of the fingernail due to dermatophytes (tinea unguium).

Prior to initiating treatment, appropriate nail specimens for laboratory testing (KOH preparation, fungal culture, or nail biopsy) should be obtained to confirm the diagnosis of onychomycosis.

(See CLINICAL PHARMACOLOGY: Special Populations, CONTRAINDICATIONS, WARNINGS, and ADVERSE REACTIONS: Post-marketing Experience for more information.)

Description of Clinical Studies:

Blastomycosis: Analyses were conducted on data from two open-label, non-concurrently controlled studies (N=73 combined) in patients with normal or abnormal immune status. The median dose was 200 mg/day. A response for most signs and symptoms was observed within the first 2 weeks, and all signs and symptoms cleared between 3 and 6 months. Results of these two studies demonstrated substantial evidence of the effectiveness of itraconazole for the treatment of blastomycosis compared with the natural history of untreated cases.

Histoplasmosis: Analyses were conducted on data from two open-label, non-concurrently controlled studies (N=34 combined) in patients with normal or abnormal immune status (not including HIV-infected patients). The median dose was 200 mg/day. A response for most signs and symptoms was observed within the first 2 weeks, and all signs and symptoms cleared between 3 and 12 months. Results of these two studies demonstrated substantial evidence of the effectiveness of itraconazole for the treatment of histoplasmosis, compared with the natural history of untreated cases.

Histoplasmosis in HIV-infected patients: Data from a small number of HIV-infected patients suggested that the response rate of histoplasmosis in HIV-infected patients is similar to that of non-HIV-infected patients. The clinical course of histoplasmosis in HIV-infected patients is more severe and usually requires maintenance therapy to prevent relapse.

Aspergillosis: Analyses were conducted on data from an open-label, "single-patient-use" protocol designed to make itraconazole available in the U.S. for patients who either failed or were intolerant of amphotericin B therapy (N=190). The findings were corroborated by two smaller open-label studies (N=31 combined) in the same patient population. Most adult patients were treated with a daily dose of 200 to 400 mg, with a median duration of 3 months. Results of these studies demonstrated substantial evidence of effectiveness of itraconazole as a second-line therapy for the treatment of aspergillosis compared with the natural history of the disease in patients who either failed or were intolerant of amphotericin B therapy.

Onychomycosis of the toenail: Analyses were conducted on data from three double-blind, placebo-controlled studies (N=214 total; 110 given SPORANOX® Capsules) in which patients with onychomycosis of the toenails received 200 mg of SPORANOX® Capsules once daily for 12 consecutive weeks. Results of these studies demonstrated mycologic cure, defined as simultaneous occurrence of negative KOH plus negative culture, in 54% of patients. Thirty-five percent (35%) of patients were considered an overall success (mycologic cure plus clear or minimal nail involvement with significantly decreased signs) and 14% of patients demonstrated mycologic cure plus clinical cure (clearance of all signs, with or without residual nail deformity). The mean time to overall success was approximately 10 months. Twenty-one percent (21%) of the overall success group had a relapse (worsening of the global score or conversion of KOH or culture from negative to positive).

Onychomycosis of the fingernail: Analyses were conducted on data from a double-blind, placebo-controlled study (N=73 total; 37 given SPORANOX® Capsules) in which patients with onychomycosis of the fingernails received a 1-week course (pulse) of 200 mg of SPORANOX® Capsules b.i.d., followed by a 3-week period without SPORANOX®, which was followed by a second 1-week pulse of 200 mg of SPORANOX® Capsules b.i.d. Results demonstrated mycologic cure in 61% of patients. Fifty-six percent (56%) of patients were considered an overall success and 47% of patients demonstrated mycologic cure plus clinical cure. The mean time to overall success was approximately 5 months. None of the patients who achieved overall success relapsed.

CONTRAINDICATIONS

Congestive Heart Failure: SPORANOX® (itraconazole) Capsules should not be administered for the treatment of onychomycosis in patients with evidence of ventricular dysfunction such as congestive heart failure (CHF) or a history of CHF. (See CLINICAL PHARMACOLOGY: Special Populations, WARNINGS, PRECAUTIONS: Drug Interactions-Calcium Channel Blockers, and ADVERSE REACTIONS: Post-marketing Experience.)

Drug Interactions: Concomitant administration of SPORANOX® (itraconazole) Capsules, Injection, or Oral Solution and certain drugs metabolized by the cytochrome P450 3A4 isoenzyme system (CYP3A4) may result in increased plasma concentrations of those drugs, leading to potentially serious and/or life-threatening adverse events. Cisapride, oral midazolam, pimozide, quinidine, dofetilide, triazolam and levacetylmethadol (levomethadyl) are contraindicated with SPORANOX®. HMG CoA-reductase inhibitors metabolized by CYP3A4, such as lovastatin and simvastatin, are also contraindicated with SPORANOX®. Ergot alkaloids metabolized by CYP3A4 such as dihydroergotamine, ergometrine (ergonovine), ergotamine and methylergometrine (methylergonovine) are contraindicated with SPORANOX®. (See BOX WARNING, and PRECAUTIONS: Drug Interactions.)

SPORANOX® should not be administered for the treatment of onychomycosis to pregnant patients or to women contemplating pregnancy.

SPORANOX® is contraindicated for patients who have shown hypersensitivity to itraconazole or its excipients. There is no information regarding cross-hypersensitivity between itraconazole and other azole antifungal agents. Caution should be used when prescribing SPORANOX® to patients with hypersensitivity to other azoles.

WARNINGS

SPORANOX® (itraconazole) Capsules and SPORANOX® Oral Solution should not be used interchangeably. This is because drug exposure is greater with the Oral Solution than with the Capsules when the same dose of drug is given. In addition, the topical effects of mucosal exposure may be different between the two formulations. Only the Oral Solution has been demonstrated effective for oral and/or esophageal candidiasis.

Hepatic Effects: SPORANOX® has been associated with rare cases of serious hepatotoxicity, including liver failure and death. Some of these cases had neither pre-existing liver disease nor a serious underlying medical condition, and some of these cases developed within the first week of treatment. If clinical signs or symptoms develop that are consistent with liver disease, treatment should be discontinued and liver function testing performed. Continued SPORANOX® use or reinstitution of treatment with SPORANOX® is strongly discouraged unless there is a serious or life threatening situation where the expected benefit exceeds the risk. (See PRECAUTIONS: Information for Patients and ADVERSE REACTIONS.)

Cardiac Dysrhythmias: Life-threatening cardiac dysrhythmias and/or sudden death have occurred in patients using cisapride, pimozide, levacetylmethadol (levomethadyl), or quinidine concomitantly with SPORANOX® and/or other CYP3A4 inhibitors. Concomitant administration of these drugs with SPORANOX® is contraindicated. (See BOX WARNING, CONTRAINDICATIONS, and PRECAUTIONS: Drug Interactions.)

Cardiac Disease: SPORANOX® Capsules should not be administered for the treatment of onychomycosis in patients with evidence of ventricular dysfunction such as congestive heart failure (CHF) or a history of CHF. SPORANOX® Capsules should not be used for other indications in patients with evidence of ventricular dysfunction unless the benefit clearly outweighs the risk.

For patients with risk factors for congestive heart failure, physicians should carefully review the risks and benefits of SPORANOX® therapy. These risk factors include cardiac disease such as ischemic and valvular disease; significant pulmonary disease such as chronic obstructive pulmonary disease; and renal failure and other edematous disorders. Such patients should be informed of the signs and symptoms of CHF, should be treated with caution, and should be monitored for signs and symptoms of CHF during treatment. If signs or symptoms of CHF appear during administration of SPORANOX® Capsules, discontinue administration.

When itraconazole was administered intravenously to anesthetized dogs, a dose-related negative inotropic effect was documented. In a healthy volunteer study of SPORANOX® Injection (intravenous infusion), transient, asymptomatic decreases in left ventricular ejection fraction were observed using gated SPECT imaging; these resolved before the next infusion, 12 hours later.

Cases of CHF, peripheral edema, and pulmonary edema have been reported in the post-marketing period among patients being treated for onychomycosis and/or systemic fungal infections. (See CLINICAL PHARMACOLOGY: Special Populations, CONTRAINDICATIONS, PRECAUTIONS: Drug Interactions, and ADVERSE REACTIONS: Post-marketing Experience for more information.)

PRECAUTIONS

General: Rare cases of serious hepatotoxicity have been observed with SPORANOX® treatment, including some cases within the first week. In patients with elevated or abnormal liver enzymes or active liver disease, or who have experienced liver toxicity with other drugs, treatment with SPORANOX® is strongly discouraged unless there is a serious or life threatening situation where the expected benefit exceeds the risk. Liver function monitoring should be done in patients with pre-existing hepatic function abnormalities or those who have experienced liver toxicity with other medications and should be considered in all patients receiving SPORANOX®. Treatment should be stopped immediately and liver function testing should be conducted in patients who develop signs and symptoms suggestive of liver dysfunction.

If neuropathy occurs that may be attributable to SPORANOX® Capsules, the treatment should be discontinued.

SPORANOX® (itraconazole) Capsules should be administered after a full meal. (See CLINICAL PHARMACOLOGY: Pharmacokinetics and Metabolism.)

Under fasted conditions, itraconazole absorption was decreased in the presence of decreased gastric acidity. The absorption of itraconazole may be decreased with the concomitant administration of antacids or gastric acid secretion suppressors. Studies conducted under fasted conditions demonstrated that administration with 8 ounces of a cola beverage resulted in increased absorption of itraconazole in AIDS patients with relative or absolute achlorhydria. This increase relative to the effects of a full meal is unknown. (See CLINICAL PHARMACOLOGY: Pharmacokinetics and Metabolism.)

Information for Patients:

- The topical effects of mucosal exposure may be different between the SPORANOX® Capsules and Oral Solution. Only the Oral Solution has been demonstrated effective for oral and/or esophageal candidiasis. SPORANOX® Capsules should not be used interchangeably with SPORANOX® Oral Solution.
- Instruct patients to take SPORANOX® Capsules with a full meal.
- Instruct patients about the signs and symptoms of congestive heart failure, and if these signs or symptoms occur during SPORANOX® administration, they should discontinue SPORANOX® and contact their healthcare provider immediately.
- Instruct patients to stop SPORANOX® treatment immediately and contact their healthcare provider if any signs and symptoms suggestive of liver dysfunction develop. Such signs and symptoms may include unusual fatigue, anorexia, nausea and/or vomiting, jaundice, dark urine, or pale stools.
- Instruct patients to contact their physician before taking any concomitant medications with itraconazole to ensure there are no potential drug interactions.

Drug Interactions: Itraconazole and its major metabolite, hydroxyitraconazole, are inhibitors of CYP3A4. Therefore, the following drug interactions may occur (See Table 1 below and the following drug class subheadings that follow):

1. SPORANOX® may decrease the elimination of drugs metabolized by CYP3A4, resulting in increased plasma concentrations of these drugs when they are administered with SPORANOX®. These elevated plasma concentrations may increase or prolong both therapeutic and adverse effects of these drugs. Whenever possible, plasma concentrations of these drugs should be monitored, and dosage adjustments made after concomitant SPORANOX® therapy is initiated. When appropriate, clinical monitoring for signs or symptoms of increased or prolonged pharmacologic effects is advised. Upon discontinuation, depending on the dose and duration of treatment, itraconazole plasma concentrations decline gradually (especially in patients with hepatic cirrhosis or in those receiving CYP3A4 inhibitors). This is particularly important when initiating therapy with drugs whose metabolism is affected by itraconazole.
2. Inducers of CYP3A4 may decrease the plasma concentrations of itraconazole. SPORANOX® may not be effective in patients concomitantly taking SPORANOX® and one of these drugs. Therefore, administration of these drugs with SPORANOX® is not recommended.
3. Other inhibitors of CYP3A4 may increase the plasma concentrations of itraconazole. Patients who must take SPORANOX® concomitantly with one of these drugs should be monitored closely for signs or symptoms of increased or prolonged pharmacologic effects of SPORANOX®.

Table 1. Selected Drugs that are predicted to alter the plasma concentration of itraconazole or have their plasma concentration altered by SPORANOX®[1]

Drug plasma concentration increased by itraconazole	
Antiarrhythmics	digoxin, dofetilide,[2] quinidine[2], disopyramide
Anticonvulsants	carbamazepine
Antimycobacterials	rifabutin
Antineoplastics	busulfan, docetaxel, vinca alkaloids
Antipsychotics	pimozide[2]
Benzodiazepines	alprazolam, diazepam, midazolam,[2,3] triazolam[2]
Calcium Channel Blockers	dihydropyridines, verapamil
Gastrointestinal Motility Agents	cisapride[2]
HMG CoA-Reductase Inhibitors	atorvastatin, cerivastatin, lovastatin,[2] simvastatin[2]
Immunosuppressants	cyclosporine, tacrolimus, sirolimus
Oral Hypoglycemics	oral hypoglycemics
Protease Inhibitors	indinavir, ritonavir, saquinavir
Other	levacetylmethadol (levomethadyl), ergot alkaloids, halofantrine, alfentanil, buspirone, methylprednisolone, budesonide, dexamethasone, trimetrexate, warfarin, cilostazol, eletriptan
Decrease plasma concentration of itraconazole	
Anticonvulsants	carbamazepine, phenobarbital, phenytoin
Antimycobacterials	isoniazid, rifabutin, rifampin
Gastric Acid Suppressors/ Neutralizers	antacids, H_2-receptor antagonists, proton pump inhibitors
Non-nucleoside Reverse Transcriptase Inhibitors	nevirapine
Increase plasma concentration of itraconazole	
Macrolide Antibiotics	clarithromycin, erythromycin
Protease Inhibitors	indinavir, ritonavir

[1] This list is not all-inclusive.

[2] Contraindicated with SPORANOX® based on clinical and/or pharmacokinetics studies. (See WARNINGS and below.)

Continued on next page

Sporanox Capsules—Cont.

[3] For information on parenterally administered midazolam, see the Benzodiazepine paragraph below.

Antiarrhythmics: The class IA antiarrhythmic quinidine and class III antiarrhythmic dofetilide are known to prolong the QT interval. Coadministration of quinidine or dofetilide with SPORANOX® may increase plasma concentrations of quinidine or dofetilide which could result in serious cardiovascular events. Therefore, concomitant administration of SPORANOX® and quinidine or dofetilide is contraindicated. (See BOX WARNING, CONTRAINDICATIONS, and WARNINGS.)

The class IA antiarrhythmic disopyramide has the potential to increase the QT interval at high plasma concentrations. Caution is advised when SPORANOX® and disopyramide are administered concomitantly.

Concomitant administration of digoxin and SPORANOX® has led to increased plasma concentrations of digoxin.

Anticonvulsants: Reduced plasma concentrations of itraconazole were reported when SPORANOX® was administered concomitantly with phenytoin. Carbamazepine, phenobarbital, and phenytoin are all inducers of CYP3A4. Although interactions with carbamazepine and phenobarbital have not been studied, concomitant administration of SPORANOX® and these drugs would be expected to result in decreased plasma concentrations of itraconazole. In addition, in vivo studies have demonstrated an increase in plasma carbamazepine concentrations in subjects concomitantly receiving ketoconazole. Although there are no data regarding the effect of itraconazole on carbamazepine metabolism, because of the similarities between ketoconazole and itraconazole, concomitant administration of SPORANOX® and carbamazepine may inhibit the metabolism of carbamazepine.

Antimycobacterials: Drug interaction studies have demonstrated that plasma concentrations of azole antifungal agents and their metabolites, including itraconazole and hydroxyitraconazole, were significantly decreased when these agents were given concomitantly with rifabutin or rifampin. In vivo data suggest that rifabutin is metabolized in part by CYP3A4. SPORANOX® may inhibit the metabolism of rifabutin. Although no formal study data are available for isoniazid, similar effects should be anticipated. Therefore, the efficacy of SPORANOX® could be substantially reduced if given concomitantly with one of these agents. Coadministration is not recommended.

Antineoplastics: SPORANOX® may inhibit the metabolism of busulfan, docetaxel, and vinca alkaloids.

Antipsychotics: Pimozide is known to prolong the QT interval and is partially metabolized by CYP3A4. Coadministration of pimozide with SPORANOX® could result in serious cardiovascular events. Therefore, concomitant administration of SPORANOX® and pimozide is contraindicated. (See BOX WARNING, CONTRAINDICATIONS, and WARNINGS.)

Benzodiazepines: Concomitant administration of SPORANOX® and alprazolam, diazepam, oral midazolam, or triazolam could lead to increased plasma concentrations of these benzodiazepines. Increased plasma concentrations could potentiate and prolong hypnotic and sedative effects. Concomitant administration of SPORANOX® and oral midazolam or triazolam is contraindicated. (See CONTRAINDICATIONS and WARNINGS.) If midazolam is administered parenterally, special precaution and patient monitoring is required since the sedative effect may be prolonged.

Calcium Channel Blockers: Edema has been reported in patients concomitantly receiving SPORANOX® and dihydropyridine calcium channel blockers. Appropriate dosage adjustment may be necessary.

Calcium channel blockers can have a negative inotropic effect which may be additive to those of itraconazole; itraconazole can inhibit the metabolism of calcium channel blockers such as dihydropyridines (e.g., nifedipine and felodipine) and verapamil. Therefore, caution should be used when co-administering itraconazole and calcium channel blockers. (See CLINICAL PHARMACOLOGY: Special Populations, CONTRAINDICATIONS, WARNINGS, and ADVERSE REACTIONS: Post-marketing Experience for more information).

Gastric Acid Suppressors/Neutralizers: Reduced plasma concentrations of itraconazole were reported when SPORANOX® Capsules were administered concomitantly with H_2-receptor antagonists. Studies have shown that absorption of itraconazole is impaired when gastric acid production is decreased. Therefore, SPORANOX® should be administered with a cola beverage if the patient has achlorhydria or is taking H_2-receptor antagonists or other gastric acid suppressors. Antacids should be administered at least 1 hour before or 2 hours after administration of SPORANOX® Capsules. In a clinical study, when SPORANOX® Capsules were administered with omeprazole (a proton pump inhibitor), the bioavailability of itraconazole was significantly reduced.

Gastrointestinal Motility Agents: Coadministration of SPORANOX® with cisapride can elevate plasma cisapride concentrations which could result in serious cardiovascular events. Therefore, concomitant administration of SPORANOX® with cisapride is contraindicated. (See BOX WARNING, CONTRAINDICATIONS, and WARNINGS.)

HMG CoA-Reductase Inhibitors: Human pharmacokinetic data suggest that SPORANOX® inhibits the metabolism of atorvastatin, cerivastatin, lovastatin, and simvastatin, which may increase the risk of skeletal muscle toxicity, including rhabdomyolysis. Concomitant administration of SPORANOX® with HMG CoA-reductase inhibitors, such as lovastatin and simvastatin, is contraindicated. (See CONTRAINDICATIONS and WARNINGS.)

Immunosuppressants: Concomitant administration of SPORANOX® and cyclosporine or tacrolimus has led to increased plasma concentrations of these immunosuppressants. Concomitant administration of SPORANOX® and sirolimus could increase plasma concentrations of sirolimus.

Macrolide Antibiotics: Erythromycin and clarithromycin are known inhibitors of CYP3A4 (See Table 1) and may increase plasma concentrations of itraconazole. In a small pharmacokinetic study involving HIV infected patients, clarithromycin was shown to increase plasma concentrations of itraconazole. Similarly, following administration of 1 gram of erythromycin ethyl succinate and 200 mg itraconazole as single doses, the mean C_{max} and $AUC_{0-\infty}$ of itraconazole increased by 44% (90% CI: 119-175%) and 36% (90% CI: 108-171%), respectively.

Non-nucleoside Reverse Transcriptase Inhibitors: Nevirapine is an inducer of CYP3A4. In vivo studies have shown that nevirapine induces the metabolism of ketoconazole, significantly reducing the bioavailability of ketoconazole. Studies involving nevirapine and itraconazole have not been conducted. However, because of the similarities between ketoconazole and itraconazole, concomitant administration of SPORANOX® and nevirapine is not recommended.

In a clinical study, when 8 HIV-infected subjects were treated concomitantly with SPORANOX® Capsules 100 mg twice daily and the nucleoside reverse transcriptase inhibitor zidovudine 8 ± 0.4 mg/kg/day, the pharmacokinetics of zidovudine were not affected. Other nucleoside reverse transcriptase inhibitors have not been studied.

Oral Hypoglycemic Agents: Severe hypoglycemia has been reported in patients concomitantly receiving azole antifungal agents and oral hypoglycemic agents. Blood glucose concentrations should be carefully monitored when SPORANOX® and oral hypoglycemic agents are co-administered.

Polyenes: Prior treatment with itraconazole, like other azoles, may reduce or inhibit the activity of polyenes such as amphotericin B. However, the clinical significance of this drug effect has not been clearly defined.

Protease Inhibitors: Concomitant administration of SPORANOX® and protease inhibitors metabolized by CYP3A4, such as indinavir, ritonavir, and saquinavir, may increase plasma concentrations of these protease inhibitors. In addition, concomitant administration of SPORANOX® and indinavir and ritonavir (but not saquinavir) may increase plasma concentrations of itraconazole. Caution is advised when SPORANOX® and protease inhibitors must be given concomitantly.

Other:

- Levacetylmethadol (levomethadyl) is known to prolong the QT interval and is metabolized by CYP3A4. Coadministration of levacetylmethadol with SPORANOX® could result in serious cardiovascular events. Therefore, concomitant administration of SPORANOX® and levacetylmethadol is contraindicated.
- Elevated concentrations of ergot alkaloids can cause ergotism, ie. a risk for vasospasm potentially leading to cerebral ischemia and/or ischemia of the extremities. Concomitant administration of ergot alkaloids such as dihydroergotamine, ergometrine (ergonovine), ergotamine and methylergometrine (methylergonovine) with SPORANOX® is contraindicated.
- Halofantrine has the potential to prolong the QT interval at high plasma concentrations. Caution is advised when SPORANOX® and halofantrine are administered concomitantly.
- In vitro data suggest that alfentanil is metabolized by CYP3A4. Administration with SPORANOX® may increase plasma concentrations of alfentanil.
- Human pharmacokinetic data suggest that concomitant administration of SPORANOX® and buspirone results in significant increases in plasma concentrations of buspirone.
- SPORANOX® may inhibit the metabolism of certain glucocorticosteroids such as budesonide, dexamethasone and methylprednisolone.
- In vitro data suggest that trimetrexate is extensively metabolized by CYP3A4. In vitro animal models have demonstrated that ketoconazole potently inhibits the metabolism of trimetrexate. Although there are no data regarding the effect of itraconazole on trimetrexate metabolism, because of the similarities between ketoconazole and itraconazole, concomitant administration of SPORANOX® and trimetrexate may inhibit the metabolism of trimetrexate.
- SPORANOX® enhances the anticoagulant effect of coumarin-like drugs, such as warfarin.
- Cilostazol and eletriptan are CYP3A4 metabolized drugs that should be used with caution when co-administered with SPORANOX®.

Carcinogenesis, Mutagenesis, and Impairment of Fertility: Itraconazole showed no evidence of carcinogenicity potential in mice treated orally for 23 months at dosage levels up to 80 mg/kg/day (approximately 10x the maximum recommended human dose [MRHD]). Male rats treated with 25 mg/kg/day (3.1× MRHD) had a slightly increased incidence of soft tissue sarcoma. These sarcomas may have been a consequence of hypercholesterolemia, which is a response of rats, but not dogs or humans, to chronic itraconazole administration. Female rats treated with 50 mg/kg/day (6.25× MRHD) had an increased incidence of squamous cell carcinoma of the lung (2/50) as compared to the untreated group. Although the occurrence of squamous cell carcinoma in the lung is extremely uncommon in untreated rats, the increase in this study was not statistically significant.

Itraconazole produced no mutagenic effects when assayed in DNA repair test (unscheduled DNA synthesis) in primary rat hepatocytes, in Ames tests with *Salmonella typhimurium* (6 strains) and *Escherichia coli*, in the mouse lymphoma gene mutation tests, in a sex-linked recessive lethal mutation (*Drosophila melanogaster*) test, in chromosome aberration tests in human lymphocytes, in a cell transformation test with C3H/10T½ C18 mouse embryo fibroblasts cells, in a dominant lethal mutation test in male and female mice, and in micronucleus tests in mice and rats.

Itraconazole did not affect the fertility of male or female rats treated orally with dosage levels of up to 40 mg/kg/day (5× MRHD), even though parental toxicity was present at this dosage level. More severe signs of parental toxicity, including death, were present in the next higher dosage level, 160 mg/kg/day (20× MRHD).

Pregnancy: Teratogenic effects. Pregnancy Category C: Itraconazole was found to cause a dose-related increase in maternal toxicity, embryotoxicity, and teratogenicity in rats at dosage levels of approximately 40–160 mg/kg/day (5–20× MRHD), and in mice at dosage levels of approximately 80 mg/kg/day (10× MRHD). In rats, the teratogenicity consisted of major skeletal defects; in mice, it consisted of encephaloceles and/or macroglossia.

There are no studies in pregnant women. SPORANOX® should be used for the treatment of systemic fungal infections in pregnancy only if the benefit outweighs the potential risk. SPORANOX® should not be administered for the treatment of onychomycosis to pregnant patients or to women contemplating pregnancy. SPORANOX® should not be administered to women of childbearing potential for the treatment of onychomycosis unless they are using effective measures to prevent pregnancy and they begin therapy on the second or third day following the onset of menses. Effective contraception should be continued throughout SPORANOX® therapy and for 2 months following the end of treatment.

During post-marketing experience, cases of congenital abnormalities have been reported. (See ADVERSE REACTIONS, Post-marketing Experience.)

Nursing Mothers: Itraconazole is excreted in human milk; therefore, the expected benefits of SPORANOX® therapy for the mother should be weighed against the potential risk from exposure of itraconazole to the infant. The U.S. Public Health Service Centers for Disease Control and Prevention advises HIV-infected women not to breast-feed to avoid potential transmission of HIV to uninfected infants.

Pediatric Use: The efficacy and safety of SPORANOX® have not been established in pediatric patients. No pharmacokinetic data on SPORANOX® Capsules are available in children. A small number of patients ages 3 to 16 years have been treated with 100 mg/day of itraconazole capsules for systemic fungal infections, and no serious unexpected adverse events have been reported. SPORANOX® Oral Solution (5 mg/kg/day) has been administered to pediatric patients (N=26; ages 6 months to 12 years) for 2 weeks and no serious unexpected adverse events were reported.

The long-term effects of itraconazole on bone growth in children are unknown. In three toxicology studies using rats, itraconazole induced bone defects at dosage levels as low as 20 mg/kg/day (2.5× MRHD). The induced defects included reduced bone plate activity, thinning of the zona compacta of the large bones, and increased bone fragility. At a dosage level of 80 mg/kg/day (10× MRHD) over 1 year or 160 mg/kg/day (20× MRHD) for 6 months, itraconazole induced small tooth pulp with hypocellular appearance in some rats. No such bone toxicity has been reported in adult patients.

HIV-Infected Patients: Because hypochlorhydria has been reported in HIV-infected individuals, the absorption of itraconazole in these patients may be decreased.

ADVERSE REACTIONS

SPORANOX® has been associated with rare cases of serious hepatotoxicity, including liver failure and death. Some of these cases had neither pre-existing liver disease nor a serious underlying medical condition. If clinical signs or symptoms develop that are consistent with liver disease, treatment should be discontinued and liver function testing performed. The risks and benefits of SPORANOX® use should be reassessed. (See WARNINGS: Hepatic Effects and PRECAUTIONS: General and Information for Patients.)

Adverse Events in the Treatment of Systemic Fungal Infections

Adverse event data were derived from 602 patients treated for systemic fungal disease in U.S. clinical trials who were immunocompromised or receiving multiple concomitant medications. Treatment was discontinued in 10.5% of patients due to adverse events. The median duration before discontinuation of therapy was 81 days (range: 2 to 776 days). The table lists adverse events reported by at least 1% of patients.

Clinical Trials of Systemic Fungal Infections: Adverse Events Occurring with an Incidence of Greater than or Equal to 1%

Body System/Adverse Event	Incidence (%) (N=602)
Gastrointestinal	
Nausea	11
Vomiting	5
Diarrhea	3
Abdominal Pain	2
Anorexia	1
Body as a Whole	
Edema	4
Fatigue	3
Fever	3
Malaise	1
Skin and Appendages	
Rash*	9
Pruritus	3
Central/Peripheral Nervous System	
Headache	4
Dizziness	2
Psychiatric	
Libido Decreased	1
Somnolence	1
Cardiovascular	
Hypertension	3
Metabolic/Nutritional	
Hypokalemia	2
Urinary System	
Albuminuria	1
Liver and Biliary System	
Hepatic Function Abnormal	3
Reproductive System, Male	
Impotence	1

*Rash tends to occur more frequently in immunocompromised patients receiving immunosuppressive medications.

Adverse events infrequently reported in all studies included constipation, gastritis, depression, insomnia, tinnitus, menstrual disorder, adrenal insufficiency, gynecomastia, and male breast pain.

Adverse Events Reported in Toenail Onychomycosis Clinical Trials

Patients in these trials were on a continuous dosing regimen of 200 mg once daily for 12 consecutive weeks.

The following adverse events led to temporary or permanent discontinuation of therapy.

Clinical Trials of Onychomycosis of the Toenail: Adverse Events Leading to Temporary or Permanent Discontinuation of Therapy

Adverse Event	Incidence (%) Itraconazole (N=112)
Elevated Liver Enzymes (greater than twice the upper limit of normal)	4
Gastrointestinal Disorders	4
Rash	3
Hypertension	2
Orthostatic Hypotension	1
Headache	1
Malaise	1
Myalgia	1
Vasculitis	1
Vertigo	1

The following adverse events occurred with an incidence of greater than or equal to 1% (N=112): headache: 10%; rhinitis: 9%; upper respiratory tract infection: 8%; sinusitis, injury: 7%; diarrhea, dyspepsia, flatulence, abdominal pain, dizziness, rash: 4%; cystitis, urinary tract infection, liver function abnormality, myalgia, nausea: 3%; appetite increased, constipation, gastritis, gastroenteritis, pharyngitis, asthenia, fever, pain, tremor, herpes zoster, abnormal dreaming: 2%.

Adverse Events Reported in Fingernail Onychomycosis Clinical Trials

Patients in these trials were on a pulse regimen consisting of two 1-week treatment periods of 200 mg twice daily, separated by a 3-week period without drug.

The following adverse events led to temporary or permanent discontinuation of therapy.

Clinical Trials of Onychomycosis of the Fingernail: Adverse Events Leading to Temporary or Permanent Discontinuation of Therapy

Adverse Event	Incidence (%) Itraconazole (N=37)
Rash/Pruritus	3
Hypertriglyceridemia	3

The following adverse events occurred with an incidence of greater than or equal to 1% (N=37): headache: 8%; pruritus, nausea, rhinitis: 5%; rash, bursitis, anxiety, depression, constipation, abdominal pain, dyspepsia, ulcerative stomatitis, gingivitis, hypertriglyceridemia, sinusitis, fatigue, malaise, pain, injury: 3%.

Post-marketing Experience

Worldwide post-marketing experiences with the use of SPORANOX® include adverse events of gastrointestinal origin, such as dyspepsia, nausea, vomiting, diarrhea, abdominal pain and constipation. Other reported adverse events include peripheral edema, congestive heart failure and pulmonary edema, headache, dizziness, peripheral neuropathy, menstrual disorders, reversible increases in hepatic enzymes, hepatitis, liver failure, hypokalemia, hypertriglyceridemia, alopecia, allergic reactions (such as pruritus, rash, urticaria, angioedema, anaphylaxis), Stevens-Johnson syndrome, anaphylactic, anaphylactoid and allergic reactions, photosensitivity and neutropenia. There is limited information on the use of SPORANOX® during pregnancy. Cases of congenital abnormalities including skeletal, genitourinary tract, cardiovascular and ophthalmic malformations as well as chromosomal and multiple malformations have been reported during post-marketing experience. A causal relationship with SPORANOX® has not been established. (See CLINICAL PHARMACOLOGY: Special Populations, CONTRAINDICATIONS, WARNINGS, and PRECAUTIONS: Drug Interactions for more information).

OVERDOSAGE

Itraconazole is not removed by dialysis. In the event of accidental overdosage, supportive measures, including gastric lavage with sodium bicarbonate, should be employed.

Limited data exist on the outcomes of patients ingesting high doses of itraconazole. In patients taking either 1000 mg of SPORANOX® (itraconazole) Oral Solution or up to 3000 mg of SPORANOX® (itraconazole) Capsules, the adverse event profile was similar to that observed at recommended doses.

DOSAGE AND ADMINISTRATION

SPORANOX® (itraconazole) Capsules should be taken with a full meal to ensure maximal absorption.

SPORANOX® Capsules is a different preparation than SPORANOX® Oral Solution and should not be used interchangeably.

Treatment of Blastomycosis and Histoplasmosis: The recommended dose is 200 mg once daily (2 capsules). If there is no obvious improvement, or there is evidence of progressive fungal disease, the dose should be increased in 100-mg increments to a maximum of 400 mg daily. Doses above 200 mg/day should be given in two divided doses.

Treatment of Aspergillosis: A daily dose of 200 to 400 mg is recommended.

Treatment in Life-Threatening Situations: In life-threatening situations, a loading dose should be used whether given as oral capsules or intravenously.

- IV Injection: the recommended intravenous dose is 200 mg b.i.d. for four consecutive doses, followed by 200 mg once daily thereafter. Each intravenous dose should be infused over 1 hour. The safety and efficacy of SPORANOX® Injection administered for greater than 14 days is not known. See complete prescribing information for SPORANOX® (itraconazole) Injection.
- Capsules: although clinical studies did not provide for a loading dose, it is recommended, based on pharmacokinetic data, that a loading dose of 200 mg (2 capsules) three times daily (600 mg/day) be given for the first 3 days of treatment.

Treatment should be continued for a minimum of three months and until clinical parameters and laboratory tests indicate that the active fungal infection has subsided. An inadequate period of treatment may lead to recurrence of active infection.

SPORANOX® Capsules and SPORANOX® Oral Solution should not be used interchangeably. Only the oral solution has been demonstrated effective for oral and/or esophageal candidiasis.

Treatment of Onychomycosis: Toenails with or without fingernail involvement: The recommended dose is 200 mg (2 capsules) once daily for 12 consecutive weeks.

Treatment of Onychomycosis: Fingernails only: The recommended dosing regimen is 2 treatment pulses, each consisting of 200 mg (2 capsules) b.i.d. (400 mg/day) for 1 week. The pulses are separated by a 3-week period without SPORANOX®.

HOW SUPPLIED

SPORANOX® (itraconazole) Capsules are available containing 100 mg of itraconazole, with a blue opaque cap and pink transparent body, imprinted with "JANSSEN" and "SPORANOX 100." The capsules are supplied in unit-dose blister packs of 3 × 10 capsules (NDC 50458-290-01), bottles of 30 capsules (NDC 50458-290-04) and in the PulsePak® containing 7 blister packs × 4 capsules each (NDC 50458-290-28).

Store at controlled room temperature 15°-25°C (59°-77°F). Protect from light and moisture.

Keep out of reach of children.

 7501622

U.S. Patent Nos. 4,267,179; 5,633,015

Revised January 2004

Distributed by:

JANSSEN PHARMACEUTICA PRODUCTS, L.P.

Titusville, New Jersey 08560, USA

Capsule contents manufactured by:

JANSSEN PHARMACEUTICA N.V.

Beerse, Belgium

Shown in Product Identification Guide, page 319

SPORANOX IV® ℞

itraconazole

Congestive Heart Failure: When itraconazole was administered intravenously to dogs and healthy human volunteers, negative inotropic effects were seen. If signs or symptoms of congestive heart failure occur during administration of SPORANOX® (itraconazole) Injection, continued SPORANOX® use should be reassessed. (See CLINICAL PHARMACOLOGY: Special Populations, CONTRAINDICATIONS, WARNINGS, PRECAUTIONS: Drug Interactions and ADVERSE REACTIONS: Post-marketing Experience for more information.)

Drug Interactions: Coadministration of cisapride, pimozide, quinidine, dofetilide, or levacetylmethadol (levomethadyl) with SPORANOX® (itraconazole) Capsules, Injection or Oral Solution is contraindicated. SPORANOX®, a potent cytochrome P450 3A4 isoenzyme system (CYP3A4) inhibitor, may increase plasma concentrations of drugs metabolized by this pathway. Serious cardiovascular events, including QT prolongation, torsades de pointes, ventricular tachycardia, cardiac arrest, and/or sudden death have occurred in patients using cisapride, pimozide, levacetylmethadol (levomethadyl), or quinidine concomitantly with SPORANOX® and/or other CYP3A4 inhibitors. (See CONTRAINDICATIONS, WARNINGS, and PRECAUTIONS: Drug Interactions for more information.)

DESCRIPTION

For intravenous infusion (NOT FOR IV BOLUS INJECTION)

SPORANOX® is the brand name for itraconazole, a synthetic triazole antifungal agent. Itraconazole is a 1:1:1:1 racemic mixture of four diastereomers (two enantiomeric pairs), each possessing three chiral centers. It may be represented by the following structural formula and nomenclature:

(±)-1-[(R*)-sec-butyl]-4-[p-[4-[p-[[(2R*,4S*)-2-(2,4-dichlorophenyl)-2-(1H-1,2,4-triazol-1-ylmethyl)-1,3-dioxolan-4-yl]methoxy]phenyl]-1-piperazinyl]phenyl]-Δ²-1,2,4-triazolin-5-one mixture with (±)-1-[(R*)-sec-butyl]-4-[p-[4-[p-[[(2S*,4R*)-2-(2,4-dichlorophenyl)-2-(1H-1,2,4-triazol-1-ylmethyl)-1,3-dioxolan-4-yl]methoxy] phenyl]-1-piperazinyl]phenyl]-Δ²-1,2,4-triazolin-5-one.

or

(±)-1-[(RS)-sec-butyl]-4-[p-[4-[p-[[(2R,4S)-2-(2,4-dichlorophenyl)-2-(1H-1,2,4-triazol-1-ylmethyl)-1,3-dioxolan-4-yl]methoxy]phenyl]-1-piperazinyl]phenyl]-Δ²-1,2,4-triazolin-5-one.

Itraconazole has a molecular formula of $C_{35}H_{38}Cl_2N_8O_4$ and a molecular weight of 705.64. It is a white to slightly yellowish powder. It is insoluble in water, very slightly soluble in alcohols, and freely soluble in dichloromethane. It has a pKa of 3.70 (based on extrapolation of values obtained from methanolic solutions) and a log (n-octanol/water) partition coefficient of 5.66 at pH 8.1.

SPORANOX® (itraconazole) Injection is a sterile pyrogen-free clear, colorless to slightly yellow solution for intravenous infusion. Each mL contains 10 mg of itraconazole, solubilized by hydroxypropyl-cyclodextrin (400 mg) as a molecular inclusion complex, with 3.8 µL hydrochloric acid, 25 µL propylene glycol, and sodium hydroxide for pH ad-

Continued on next page

Sporanox IV—Cont.

justment to 4.5, in water for injection. SPORANOX® Injection is packaged in 25 mL colorless glass ampules, containing 250 mg of itraconazole, contents of which are diluted in 50 mL 0.9% Sodium Chloride Injection, USP (Normal Saline) prior to infusion. When properly administered, contents of one ampule will supply 200 mg of itraconazole.

CLINICAL PHARMACOLOGY

Pharmacokinetics and Metabolism: NOTE: The plasma concentrations reported below were measured by high-performance liquid chromatography (HPLC) specific for itraconazole. When itraconazole in plasma is measured by a bioassay, values reported may be higher than those obtained by HPLC due to the presence of the bioactive metabolite, hydroxyitraconazole. (See MICROBIOLOGY.)

The pharmacokinetics of SPORANOX® (itraconazole) Injection (200 mg b.i.d. for two days, then 200 mg q.d. for five days) followed by oral dosing of SPORANOX® Capsules were studied in patients with advanced HIV infection. Steady-state plasma concentrations were reached after the fourth dose for itraconazole and by the seventh dose for hydroxyitraconazole. Steady-state plasma concentrations were maintained by administration of SPORANOX® Capsules, 200 mg b.i.d. Pharmacokinetic parameters for itraconazole and hydroxyitraconazole are presented in the table below:

[See first table above]

Parameter	Injection Day 7 n=29		Capsules, 200 mg b.i.d. Day 36 n=12	
	itraconazole	hydroxyitraconazole	itraconazole	hydroxyitraconazole
C_{max} (ng/mL)	2856 ± 866*	1906 ± 612	2010 ± 1420	2614 ± 1703
t_{max} (hr)	1.08 ± 0.14	8.53 ± 6.36	3.92 ± 1.83	5.92 ± 6.14
$AUC_{0\text{-}12h}$ (ng•h/mL)	—	—	18768 ± 13933	28516 ± 19149
$AUC_{0\text{-}24h}$ (ng•h/mL)	30605 ± 8961	42445 ± 13282	—	—

*mean ± standard deviation

The estimated mean ±SD half-life at steady-state of itraconazole after intravenous infusion was 35.4 ± 29.4 hours. In previous studies, the mean elimination half-life for itraconazole at steady-state after daily oral administration of 100 to 400 mg was 30-40 hours. Approximately 93-101% of hydroxypropyl-β-cyclodextrin was excreted unchanged in the urine within 12 hours after dosing.

The plasma protein binding of itraconazole is 99.8% and that of hydroxyitraconazole is 99.5%. Following intravenous administration, the volume of distribution of itraconazole averaged 796 ± 185 L.

Itraconazole is metabolized predominately by the cytochrome P450 3A4 isoenzyme system (CYP3A4), resulting in the formation of several metabolites, including hydroxyitraconazole, the major metabolite. Results of a pharmacokinetics study suggest that itraconazole may undergo saturable metabolism with multiple dosing. Fecal excretion of the parent drug varies between 3-18% of the dose. Renal excretion of the parent drug is less than 0.03% of the dose. About 40% of the dose is excreted as inactive metabolites in the urine. No single excreted metabolite represents more than 5% of a dose. Itraconazole total plasma clearance averaged 381 ± 95 mL/min following intravenous administration. Approximately 80–90% of hydroxypropyl-β-cyclodextrin is eliminated through the kidneys. (See CONTRAINDICATIONS and PRECAUTIONS: Drug Interactions for more information.)

Special Populations

Renal Insufficiency: Plasma concentrations of itraconazole in patients with mild to moderate renal insufficiency were comparable to those obtained in healthy subjects. The majority of the 8-gram dose of hydroxypropyl-β-cyclodextrin was eliminated in the urine during the 120-hour collection period in normal subjects and in patients with mild to severe renal insufficiency. Following a single intravenous dose of 200 mg to subjects with severe renal impairment (creatinine clearance ≤ 19 mL/minute), clearance of hydroxypropyl-β-cyclodextrin was reduced six-fold compared with subjects with normal renal function. SPORANOX® Injection should not be used in patients with creatinine clearance < 30 mL/min.

In patients with mild to moderate renal impairment, SPORANOX® Injection should be used with caution. Serum creatinine levels should be closely monitored and, if renal toxicity is suspected, consideration should be given to changing to SPORANOX® Capsules.

Hepatic Insufficiency: Patients with impaired hepatic function should be carefully monitored when taking itraconazole. The prolonged elimination half-life of itraconazole observed in a clinical trial with itraconazole capsules in cirrhotic patients should be considered when deciding to initiate therapy with other medications metabolized by CYP3A4. (See BOX WARNING, CONTRAINDICATIONS, and PRECAUTIONS: Drug Interactions.)

Decreased Cardiac Contractility: When itraconazole was administered intravenously to anesthetized dogs, a dose-related negative inotropic effect was documented. In a healthy volunteer study of SPORANOX® Injection (intravenous infusion), transient, asymptomatic decreases in left ventricular ejection fraction were observed using gated SPECT imaging; these resolved before the next infusion, 12 hours later. If signs or symptoms of congestive heart failure appear during administration of SPORANOX® Injection, monitor carefully and consider other treatment alternatives which may include discontinuation of SPORANOX® Injection administration. (See WARNINGS, PRECAUTIONS: Drug Interactions and ADVERSE REACTIONS: Post-marketing Experience for more information.)

MICROBIOLOGY

Mechanism of Action: In vitro studies have demonstrated that itraconazole inhibits the cytochrome P450-dependent synthesis of ergosterol, which is a vital component of fungal cell membranes.

Activity In Vitro and In Vivo: Itraconazole exhibits in vitro activity against *Blastomyces dermatitidis, Histoplasma capsulatum, Histoplasma duboisii, Aspergillus flavus, Aspergillus fumigatus, Candida albicans,* and *Cryptococcus neoformans.* Itraconazole also exhibits varying in vitro activity against *Sporothrix schenckii, Trichophyton* species, *Candida krusei,* and other *Candida* species. The bioactive metabolite, hydroxyitraconazole, has not been evaluated against *Histoplasma capsulatum* and *Blastomyces dermatitidis.* Correlation between minimum inhibitory concentration (MIC) results in vitro and clinical outcome has yet to be established for azole antifungal agents.

Itraconazole administered orally was active in a variety of animal models of fungal infection using standard laboratory strains of fungi. Fungistatic activity has been demonstrated against disseminated fungal infections caused by *Blastomyces dermatitidis, Histoplasma duboisii, Aspergillus fumigatus, Coccidioides immitis, Cryptococcus neoformans, Paracoccidioides brasiliensis, Sporothrix schenckii, Trichophyton rubrum,* and *Trichophyton mentagrophytes.*

Itraconazole administered at 2.5 mg/kg and 5 mg/kg via the oral and parenteral routes increased survival rates and sterilized organ systems in normal and immunosuppressed guinea pigs with disseminated *Aspergillus fumigatus* infections. Oral itraconazole administered daily at 40 mg/kg and 80 mg/kg increased survival rates in normal rabbits with disseminated disease and in immunosuppressed rats with pulmonary *Aspergillus fumigatus* infection, respectively. Itraconazole has demonstrated antifungal activity in a variety of animal models infected with *Candida albicans* and other *Candida* species.

Resistance: Isolates from several fungal species with decreased susceptibility to itraconazole have been isolated in vitro and from patients receiving prolonged therapy.

Several in vitro studies have reported that some fungal clinical isolates, including *Candida* species, with reduced susceptibility to one azole antifungal agent may also be less susceptible to other azole derivatives. The finding of cross-resistance is dependent on a number of factors, including the species evaluated, its clinical history, the particular azole compounds compared, and the type of susceptibility test that is performed. The relevance of these in vitro susceptibility data to clinical outcome remains to be elucidated.

Studies (both in vitro and in vivo) suggest that the activity of amphotericin B may be suppressed by prior azole antifungal therapy. As with other azoles, itraconazole inhibits the ^{14}C-demethylation step in the synthesis of ergosterol, a cell wall component of fungi. Ergosterol is the active site for amphotericin B. In one study the anti-fungal activity of amphotericin B against *Aspergillus fumigatus* infections in mice was inhibited by ketoconazole therapy. The clinical significance of test results obtained in this study is unknown.

CLINICAL STUDIES

Empiric Therapy in Febrile Neutropenic Patients: An open randomized trial compared the efficacy and safety of itraconazole (intravenous followed by oral solution) with amphotericin B for empiric therapy in 384 febrile, neutropenic patients with hematologic malignancies who had suspected fungal infections. Patients received either itraconazole (injection, 200 mg b.i.d. for 2 days followed by 200 mg once daily for up to 14 days, followed by oral solution, 200 mg b.i.d.) or amphotericin B (total daily dose of 0.7-1.0 mg/kg body weight). The longest treatment duration was 28 days. An outcome assignment of "success" required (a) patient survival with resolution of fever and neutropenia within 28 days of treatment, (b) absence of emergent fungal infections, (c) no discontinuation of therapy due to toxicity or lack of efficacy, and (d) treatment for three or more days. The success rate using an intent-to-treat analysis was 47% for the itraconazole group and 38% for the amphotericin B arm.

[See second table above]

Overview of Efficacy (Intent-to-Treat Population)

Efficacy Parameters	SPORANOX® N=179 (%)	Amphotericin B N=181 (%)
Success	84 (47%)	68 (38%)
Unevaluable*	24 (13%)	44 (24%)
Failure	71 (40%)	69 (38%)
Reason for Failure		
Intolerance after > 3 days of antifungal medication	12	37
Persistent fever	20	7
Change in antifungal medication due to fever	13	1
Emergent fungal infection	10	9
Documented bacterial or viral infection	7	8
Insufficient response	6	5
Deterioration of signs and symptoms	2	0
Death after > 3 days antifungal medication	1	2
Resolution of fever	131 (73%)	127 (70%)
Survival	161 (90%)	156 (86%)

* Treatment duration ≤ 3 days (including patients who died within 3 days, withdrew because of adverse events or were deemed ineligible due to a confirmed pre-treatment infection).

INDICATIONS AND USAGE

SPORANOX® (itraconazole) Injection/Oral Solution is indicated for empiric therapy of febrile neutropenic patients with suspected fungal infections. (NOTE: In a comparative trial, the overall response rate for itraconazole-treated subjects was higher than for amphotericin B-treated subjects. However, compared to amphotericin B-treated subjects, a larger number of itraconazole-treated subjects discontinued treatment due to persistent fever and a change in antifungal medication due to fever. Whereas, a larger number of amphotericin B-treated subjects discontinued due to drug intolerance. (See CLINICAL STUDIES section.)

SPORANOX® (itraconazole) Injection is also indicated for the treatment of the following fungal infections in immunocompromised and non-immunocompromised patients:

1. Blastomycosis, pulmonary and extrapulmonary;
2. Histoplasmosis, including chronic cavitary pulmonary disease and disseminated, non-meningeal histoplasmosis; and
3. Aspergillosis, pulmonary and extrapulmonary, in patients who are intolerant of or who are refractory to amphotericin B therapy.

Specimens for fungal cultures and other relevant laboratory studies (wet mount, histopathology, serology) should be obtained prior to therapy to isolate and identify causative organisms. Therapy may be instituted before the results of the cultures and other laboratory studies are known; however, once these results become available, anti-infective therapy should be adjusted accordingly.
(See CLINICAL PHARMACOLOGY: Special Populations, WARNINGS, and ADVERSE REACTIONS: Post-marketing Experience for more information).

CONTRAINDICATIONS

Drug Interactions: Concomitant administration of SPORANOX® (itraconazole) Capsules, Injection, or Oral Solution and certain drugs metabolized by the cytochrome P450 3A4 isoenzyme system (CYP3A4) may result in increased plasma concentrations of those drugs, leading to potentially serious and/or life-threatening adverse events. Cisapride, oral midazolam, pimozide, quinidine, dofetilide, triazolam and levacetylmethadol (levomethadyl) are contraindicated with SPORANOX®. HMG CoA-reductase inhibitors metabolized by CYP3A4, such as lovastatin and simvastatin, are also contraindicated with SPORANOX®. Ergot alkaloids metabolized by CYP3A4 such as dihydroergotamine, ergometrine (ergonovine), ergotamine and methylergometrine (methylergonovine) are contraindicated with SPORANOX®. (See BOX WARNING, and PRECAUTIONS: Drug Interactions.)

SPORANOX® is contraindicated for patients who have shown hypersensitivity to itraconazole or its excipients. There is no information regarding cross-hypersensitivity between itraconazole and other azole antifungal agents. Caution should be used when prescribing SPORANOX® to patients with hypersensitivity to other azoles.

WARNINGS

SPORANOX® (itraconazole) Injection contains the excipient hydroxypropyl-β-cyclodextrin which produced pancreatic adenocarcinomas in a rat carcinogenicity study. These findings were not observed in a similar mouse carcinogenicity study. The clinical relevance of these findings is unknown. (See PRECAUTIONS: Carcinogenesis, Mutagenesis, and Impairment of Fertility.)

Hepatic Effects: SPORANOX® has been associated with rare cases of serious hepatotoxicity, including liver failure and death. Some of these cases had neither pre-existing liver disease nor a serious underlying medical condition, and some of these cases developed within the first week of treatment. If clinical signs or symptoms develop that are consistent with liver disease, treatment should be discontinued and liver function testing performed. Continued SPORANOX® use or reinstitution of treatment with SPORANOX® is strongly discouraged unless there is a serious or life threatening situation where the expected benefit exceeds the risk. (See PRECAUTIONS: Information for Patients and ADVERSE REACTIONS.)

Cardiac Dysrhythmias: Life-threatening cardiac dysrhythmias and/or sudden death have occurred in patients using cisapride, pimozide, levacetylmethadol (levomethadyl), or quinidine concomitantly with SPORANOX® and/or other CYP3A4 inhibitors. Concomitant administration of these drugs with SPORANOX® is contraindicated. (See BOX WARNING, CONTRAINDICATIONS, and PRECAUTIONS: Drug Interactions.)

Cardiac Disease: SPORANOX® Injection should not be used in patients with evidence of ventricular dysfunction unless the benefit clearly outweighs the risk. For patients with risk factors for congestive heart failure, physicians should carefully review the risks and benefits of SPORANOX® therapy. These risk factors include cardiac disease such as ischemic and valvular disease; significant pulmonary disease such as chronic obstructive pulmonary disease; and renal failure and other edematous disorders. Such patients should be informed of the signs and symptoms of CHF, should be treated with caution, and should be monitored for signs and symptoms of CHF during treatment. If signs or symptoms of CHF appear during administration of SPORANOX® Injection, monitor carefully and consider other treatment alternatives which may include discontinuation of SPORANOX® Injection administration.

When itraconazole was administered intravenously to anesthetized dogs, a dose-related negative inotropic effect was documented. In a healthy volunteer study of SPORANOX® Injection (intravenous infusion), transient, asymptomatic decreases in left ventricular ejection fraction were observed using gated SPECT imaging; these resolved before the next infusion, 12 hours later.

Cases of CHF, peripheral edema, and pulmonary edema have been reported in the post-marketing period among patients being treated for onychomycosis and/or systemic fungal infections. (See CLINICAL PHARMACOLOGY: Special Populations, PRECAUTIONS: Drug Interactions, and ADVERSE REACTIONS: Post-marketing Experience for more information.)

PRECAUTIONS

General: Rare cases of serious hepatotoxicity have been observed with SPORANOX® treatment, including some cases within the first week. In patients with elevated or abnormal liver enzymes or active liver disease, or who have experienced liver toxicity with other drugs, treatment with SPORANOX® is strongly discouraged unless there is a serious or life threatening situation where the expected benefit exceeds the risk. Liver function monitoring should be done in patients with pre-existing hepatic function abnormalities or those who have experienced liver toxicity with other medications and should be considered in all patients receiving SPORANOX®. Treatment should be stopped immediately and liver function testing should be conducted in patients who develop signs and symptoms suggestive of liver dysfunction.

If neuropathy occurs that may be attributable to SPORANOX® Injection, the treatment should be discontinued.

As severe renal impairment prolongs the elimination rate of hydroxypropyl-β-cyclodextrin, SPORANOX® (itraconazole) Injection should not be used in patients with severe renal dysfunction (creatinine clearance < 30 mL/min). (See CLINICAL PHARMACOLOGY: Special Populations.)

Information for Patients: SPORANOX® Injection contains the excipient hydroxypropyl-β-cyclodextrin which produced pancreatic adenocarcinomas in a rat carcinogenicity study. These findings were not observed in a similar mouse carcinogenicity study. The clinical relevance of these findings is unknown. (See PRECAUTIONS: Carcinogenesis, Mutagenesis, and Impairment of Fertility.)

Drug Interactions: Itraconazole and its major metabolite, hydroxyitraconazole, are inhibitors of CYP3A4. Therefore, the following drug interactions may occur (See Table 1 below and the following drug class subheadings that follow):

1. SPORANOX® may decrease the elimination of drugs metabolized by CYP3A4, resulting in increased plasma concentrations of these drugs when they are administered with SPORANOX®. These elevated plasma concentrations may increase or prolong both therapeutic and adverse effects of these drugs. Whenever possible, plasma concentrations of these drugs should be monitored, and dosage adjustments made after concomitant SPORANOX® therapy is initiated. When appropriate, clinical monitoring for signs or symptoms of increased or prolonged pharmacologic effects is advised. Upon discontinuation, depending on the dose and duration of treatment, itraconazole plasma concentrations decline gradually (especially in patients with hepatic cirrhosis or in those receiving CYP3A4 inhibitors). This is particularly important when initiating therapy with drugs whose metabolism is affected by itraconazole.
2. Inducers of CYP3A4 may decrease the plasma concentrations of itraconazole. SPORANOX® may not be effective in patients concomitantly taking SPORANOX® and one of these drugs. Therefore, administration of these drugs with SPORANOX® is not recommended.
3. Other inhibitors of CYP3A4 may increase the plasma concentrations of itraconazole. Patients who must take SPORANOX® concomitantly with one of these drugs should be monitored closely for signs or symptoms of increased or prolonged pharmacologic effects of SPORANOX®.

[See table 1 above]

Table 1. Selected Drugs that are predicted to alter the plasma concentration of itraconazole or have their plasma concentration altered by SPORANOX®[1]

Drug plasma concentration increased by itraconazole	
Antiarrhythmics	digoxin, dofetilide[2], quinidine disopyramide
Anticonvulsants	carbamazepine
Antimycobacterials	rifabutin
Antineoplastics	busulfan, docetaxel, vinca alkaloids
Antipsychotics	pimozide[2]
Benzodiazepines	alprazolam, diazepam, midazolam,[2,3] triazolam[2]
Calcium Channel Blockers	dihydropyridines, verapamil
Gastrointestinal Motility Agents	cisapride[2]
HMG CoA-Reductase Inhibitors	atorvastatin, cerivastatin, lovastatin,[2] simvastatin[2]
Immunosuppressants	cyclosporine, tacrolimus, sirolimus
Oral Hypoglycemics	oral hypoglycemics
Protease Inhibitors	indinavir, ritonavir, saquinavir
Other	levacetylmethadol (levomethadyl), ergot alkaloids, halofantrine, alfentanil, buspirone, methylprednisolone, budesonide, dexamethasone trimetrexate, warfarin, cilostazol, eletripan
Decrease plasma concentration of itraconazole	
Anticonvulsants	carbamazepine, phenobarbital, phenytoin
Antimycobacterials	isoniazid, rifabutin, rifampin
Reverse Transcriptase Inhibitors	nevirapine
Increase plasma concentration of itraconazole	
Macrolide Antibiotics	clarithromycin, erythromycin
Protease Inhibitors	indinavir, ritonavir

[1] This list is not all-inclusive.
[2] Contraindicated with SPORANOX® based on clinical and/or pharmacokinetics studies. (See WARNINGS and below.)
[3] For information on parenterally administered midazolam, see the Benzodiazepine paragraph below.

Antiarrhythmics: The class IA antiarrhythmic quinidine and class III antiarrhythmic dofetilide are known to prolong the QT interval. Coadministration of quinidine or dofetilide with SPORANOX® may increase plasma concentrations of quinidine or dofetilide which could result in serious cardiovascular events. Therefore, concomitant administration of SPORANOX® and quinidine or dofetilide is contraindicated. (See BOX WARNING, CONTRAINDICATIONS, and WARNINGS.)

The class IA antiarrhythmic disopyramide has the potential to increase the QT interval at high plasma concentrations. Caution is advised when SPORANOX® and disopyramide are administered concomitantly.

Concomitant administration of digoxin and SPORANOX® has led to increased plasma concentrations of digoxin.

Anticonvulsants: Reduced plasma concentrations of itraconazole were reported when SPORANOX® was administered concomitantly with phenytoin. Carbamazepine, phenobarbital, and phenytoin are all inducers of CYP3A4. Although interactions with carbamazepine and phenobarbital have not been studied, concomitant administration of SPORANOX® and these drugs would be expected to result in decreased plasma concentrations of itraconazole. In addition, in vivo studies have demonstrated an increase in plasma carbamazepine concentrations in subjects concomitantly receiving ketoconazole. Although there are no data regarding the effect of itraconazole on carbamazepine metabolism, because of the similarities between ketoconazole and itraconazole, concomitant administration of SPORANOX® and carbamazepine may inhibit the metabolism of carbamazepine.

Antimycobacterials: Drug interaction studies have demonstrated that plasma concentrations of azole antifungal agents and their metabolites, including itraconazole and hydroxyitraconazole, were significantly decreased when these agents were given concomitantly with rifabutin or rifampin. In vivo data suggest that rifabutin is metabolized in part by CYP3A4. SPORANOX® may inhibit the metabolism of rifabutin. Although no formal study data are available for isoniazid, similar effects should be anticipated. Therefore, the efficacy of SPORANOX® could be substantially reduced if given concomitantly with one of these agents. Coadministration is not recommended.

Antineoplastics: SPORANOX® may inhibit the metabolism of busulfan, docetaxel, and vinca alkaloids.

Continued on next page

Sporanox IV—Cont.

Antipsychotics: Pimozide is known to prolong the QT interval and is partially metabolized by CYP3A4. Coadministration of pimozide with SPORANOX® could result in serious cardiovascular events. Therefore, concomitant administration of SPORANOX® and pimozide is contraindicated. (See BOX WARNING, CONTRAINDICATIONS, and WARNINGS.)
Benzodiazepines: Concomitant administration of SPORANOX® and alprazolam, diazepam, oral midazolam, or triazolam could lead to increased plasma concentrations of these benzodiazepines. Increased plasma concentrations could potentiate and prolong hypnotic and sedative effects. Concomitant administration of SPORANOX® and oral midazolam or triazolam is contraindicated. (See CONTRAINDICATIONS and WARNINGS.) If midazolam is administered parenterally, special precaution and patient monitoring is required since the sedative effect may be prolonged.
Calcium Channel Blockers: Edema has been reported in patients concomitantly receiving SPORANOX® and dihydropyridine calcium channel blockers. Appropriate dosage adjustment may be necessary.
Calcium channel blockers can have a negative inotropic effect which may be additive to those of itraconazole; itraconazole can inhibit the metabolism of calcium channel blockers such as dihydropyridines (e.g., nifedipine and felodipine) and verapamil. Therefore, caution should be used when co-administering itraconazole and calcium channel blockers. (See CLINICAL PHARMACOLOGY: Special Populations, WARNINGS, and ADVERSE REACTIONS: Post-marketing Experience for more information.)
Gastrointestinal Motility Agents: Coadministration of SPORANOX® with cisapride can elevate plasma cisapride concentrations which could result in serious cardiovascular events. Therefore, concomitant administration of SPORANOX® with cisapride is contraindicated. (See BOX WARNING, CONTRAINDICATIONS, and WARNINGS.)
HMG CoA-Reductase Inhibitors: Human pharmacokinetic data suggest that SPORANOX® inhibits the metabolism of atorvastatin, cerivastatin, lovastatin, and simvastatin, which may increase the risk of skeletal muscle toxicity, including rhabdomyolysis. Concomitant administration of SPORANOX® with HMG CoA-reductase inhibitors, such as lovastatin and simvastatin, is contraindicated. (See CONTRAINDICATIONS, and WARNINGS.)
Immunosuppressants: Concomitant administration of SPORANOX® and cyclosporine or tacrolimus has led to increased plasma concentrations of these immunosuppressants. Concomitant administration of SPORANOX® and sirolimus could increase plasma concentrations of sirolimus.
Macrolide Antibiotics: Erythromycin and clarithromycin are known inhibitors of CYP3A4 (See Table 1) and may increase plasma concentrations of itraconazole. In a small pharmacokinetic study involving HIV infected patients, clarithromycin was shown to increase plasma concentrations of itraconazole. Similarly, following administration of 1 gram of erythromycin ethyl succinate and 200 mg itraconazole as single doses, the mean C_{max} and $AUC_{0-\infty}$ of itraconazole increased by 44% (90% CI: 119-175%) and 36% (90% CI: 108-171%), respectively.
Oral Hypoglycemic Agents: Severe hypoglycemia has been reported in patients concomitantly receiving azole antifungal agents and oral hypoglycemic agents. Blood glucose concentrations should be carefully monitored when SPORANOX® and oral hypoglycemic agents are coadministered.
Polyenes: Prior treatment with itraconazole, like other azoles, may reduce or inhibit the activity of polyenes such as amphotericin B. However, the clinical significance of this drug effect has not been clearly defined.
Protease Inhibitors: Concomitant administration of SPORANOX® and protease inhibitors metabolized by CYP3A4, such as indinavir, ritonavir, and saquinavir, may increase plasma concentrations of these protease inhibitors. In addition, concomitant administration of SPORANOX® and indinavir and ritonavir (but not saquinavir) may increase plasma concentrations of itraconazole. Caution is advised when SPORANOX® and protease inhibitors must be given concomitantly.
Reverse Transcriptase Inhibitors: Nevirapine is an inducer of CYP3A4. In vivo studies have shown that nevirapine induces the metabolism of ketoconazole, significantly reducing the bioavailability of ketoconazole. Studies involving nevirapine and itraconazole have not been conducted. However, because of the similarities between ketoconazole and itraconazole, concomitant administration of SPORANOX® and nevirapine is not recommended. In a clinical study, when 8 HIV-infected subjects were treated concomitantly with SPORANOX® Capsules 100 mg twice daily and the nucleoside reverse transcriptase inhibitor zidovudine 8 ± 0.4 mg/kg/day, the pharmacokinetics of zidovudine were not affected. Other nucleoside reverse transcriptase inhibitors have not been studied.
Other:

- Levacetylmethadol (levomethadyl) is known to prolong the QT interval and is metabolized by CYP3A4. Coadministration of levacetylmethadol with SPORANOX® could result in serious cardiovascular events. Therefore, concomitant administration of SPORANOX® and levacetylmethadol is contraindicated.
- Elevated concentrations of ergot alkaloids can cause ergotism, ie. a risk for vasospasm potentially leading to cerebral ischemia and/or ischemia of the extremities. Concomitant administration of ergot alkaloids such as dihydroergotamine, ergometrine (ergonovine), ergotamine and methylergometrine (methylergonovine) with SPORANOX® is contraindicated.
- Halofantrine has the potential to prolong the QT interval at high plasma concentrations. Caution is advised when SPORANOX® and halofantrine are administered concomitantly.
- In vitro data suggest that alfentanil is metabolized by CYP3A4. Administration with SPORANOX® may increase plasma concentrations of alfentanil.
- Human pharmacokinetic data suggest that concomitant administration of SPORANOX® and buspirone results in significant increases in plasma concentrations of buspirone.
- SPORANOX® may inhibit the metabolism of certain glucocorticosteroids such as budesonide, dexamethasone and methylprednisolone.
- In vitro data suggest that trimetrexate is extensively metabolized by CYP3A4. In vitro animal models have demonstrated that ketoconazole potently inhibits the metabolism of trimetrexate. Although there are no data regarding the effect of itraconazole on trimetrexate metabolism, because of the similarities between ketoconazole and itraconazole, concomitant administration of SPORANOX® and trimetrexate may inhibit the metabolism of trimetrexate.
- Cilostazol and eletriptan are CYP3A4 metabolized drugs that should be used with caution when co-administered with SPORANOX®.
- SPORANOX® enhances the anticoagulant effect of coumarin-like drugs, such as warfarin.

Carcinogenesis, Mutagenesis and Impairment of Fertility: Itraconazole showed no evidence of carcinogenicity potential in mice treated orally for 23 months at dosage levels up to 80 mg/kg/day (approximately 10× the maximum recommended human dose [MRHD]). Male rats treated with 25 mg/kg/day (3.1× MRHD) had a slightly increased incidence of soft tissue sarcoma. These sarcomas may have been a consequence of hypercholesterolemia, which is a response of rats, but not dogs or humans, to chronic itraconazole administration. Female rats treated with 50 mg/kg/day (6.25× MRHD) had an increased incidence of squamous cell carcinoma of the lung (2/50) as compared to the untreated group. Although the occurrence of squamous cell carcinoma in the lung is extremely uncommon in untreated rats, the increase in this study was not statistically significant.
Hydroxypropyl-β-cyclodextrin (HP-β-CD), the solubilizing excipient used in SPORANOX® Injection and Oral Solution, was found to produce pancreatic exocrine hyperplasia and neoplasia when administered orally to rats at doses of 500, 2000 or 5000 mg/kg/day for 25 months. Adenocarcinomas of the exocrine pancreas produced in the treated animals were not seen in the untreated group and are not reported in the historical controls. Development of these tumors may be related to a mitogenic action of cholecystokinin. This finding was not observed in the mouse carcinogenicity study at doses of 500, 2000 or 5000 mg/kg/day for 22-23 months; however, the clinical relevance of these findings is unknown. Based on body surface area comparisons, the exposure to humans of HP-β-CD at the recommended clinical dose of SPORANOX® Oral Solution, is approximately equivalent to 1.7 times the exposure at the lowest dose in the rat study. The relevance of the findings with orally administered HP-β-CD to potential carcinogenic effects for SPORANOX® Injection is uncertain.
Itraconazole produced no mutagenic effects when assayed in a DNA repair test (unscheduled DNA synthesis) in primary rat hepatocytes, in Ames tests with *Salmonella typhimurium* (6 strains) and *Escherichia coli*, in the mouse lymphoma gene mutation tests, in a sex-linked recessive lethal mutation (*Drosophila melanogaster*) test, in chromosome aberration tests in human lymphocytes, in a cell transformation test with C3H/10T½ C18 mouse embryo fibroblasts cells, in a dominant lethal mutation test in male and female mice, and in micronucleus tests in mice and rats.
Itraconazole did not affect the fertility of male or female rats treated orally with dosage levels of up to 40 mg/kg/day (5× MRHD), even though parental toxicity was present at this dosage level. More severe signs of parental toxicity, including death, were present in the next higher dosage level, 160 mg/kg/day (20× MRHD).
Pregnancy: Teratogenic Effects. Pregnancy Category C: Itraconazole was found to cause a dose-related increase in maternal toxicity, embryotoxicity, and teratogenicity in rats at dosage levels of approximately 40-160 mg/kg/day (5-20× MRHD), and in mice at dosage levels of approximately 80 mg/kg/day (10× MRHD). In rats, the teratogenicity consisted of major skeletal defects; in mice, it consisted of encephaloceles and/or macroglossia.
There are no studies in pregnant women. SPORANOX® should be used for the treatment of systemic fungal infections in pregnancy only if the benefit outweighs the potential risk.
During post-marketing experience, cases of congenital abnormalities have been reported. (See ADVERSE REACTIONS, Post-marketing Experience.)
Nursing Mothers: Itraconazole is excreted in human milk; therefore, the expected benefits of SPORANOX® therapy for the mother should be weighed against the potential risk from exposure of itraconazole to the infant. The U.S. Public Health Service Centers for Disease Control and Prevention advises HIV-infected women not to breast-feed to avoid potential transmission of HIV to uninfected infants.
Pediatric Use: The efficacy and safety of SPORANOX® have not been established in pediatric patients. No pharmacokinetic data on SPORANOX® Capsules or Injection are available in children. A small number of patients ages 3 to 16 years have been treated with 100 mg/day of itraconazole capsules for systemic fungal infections, and no serious unexpected adverse effects have been reported. SPORANOX® Oral Solution (5 mg/kg/day) has been administered to pediatric patients (N=26, ages 6 months to 12 years) for 2 weeks and no serious unexpected adverse events were reported.
The long-term effects of itraconazole on bone growth in children are unknown. In three toxicology studies using rats, itraconazole induced bone defects at dosage levels as low as 20 mg/kg/day (2.5× MRHD). The induced defects included reduced bone plate activity, thinning of the zona compacta of the large bones, and increased bone fragility. At a dosage level of 80 mg/kg/day (10× MRHD) over 1 year or 160 mg/kg/day (20× MRHD) for 6 months, itraconazole induced small tooth pulp with hypocellular appearance in some rats. No such bone toxicity has been reported in adult patients.
Geriatric Use: Clinical studies of SPORANOX® Injection did not include sufficient numbers of subjects aged 65 and over to determine whether they respond differently from younger subjects. Other reported clinical experience has not identified differences in responses between the elderly and younger patients. In general, dose selection for an elderly patient should be cautious, reflecting the greater frequency of decreased hepatic, renal, or cardiac function, and of concomitant disease or other drug therapy.

ADVERSE REACTIONS

SPORANOX® has been associated with rare cases of serious hepatotoxicity, including liver failure and death. Some of these cases had neither pre-existing liver disease nor a serious underlying medical condition. If clinical signs or symptoms develop that are consistent with liver disease, treatment should be discontinued and liver function testing performed. The risks and benefits of SPORANOX® use should be reassessed. (See WARNINGS: Hepatic Effects and PRECAUTIONS: General and Information for Patients.)
Adverse Events Reported in Trials in Patients with SPORANOX® Injection
Adverse events considered at least possibly drug related are shown in Table 2 and are based on the experience of 360 patients treated with SPORANOX® Injection in four pharmacokinetic, one uncontrolled and four active controlled studies where the control was amphotericin B or fluconazole. Nearly all patients were neutropenic or were otherwise immunocompromised and were treated empirically for febrile episodes, for documented systemic fungal infections, or in trials to determine pharmacokinetics. The dose of SPORANOX® Injection was 200 mg twice daily for the first two days followed by a single daily dose of 200 mg for the remainder of the intravenous treatment period. The majority of patients received between 7 and 14 days of SPORANOX® Injection.
[See table 2 at bottom of next page]
The following adverse events occurred in less than 2% of patients in clinical trials of SPORANOX® Injection: LDH increased, edema, albuminuria, hyperglycemia, and hepatitis.
Post-marketing Experience
Worldwide post-marketing experiences with the use of SPORANOX® include adverse events of gastrointestinal origin, such as dyspepsia, nausea, vomiting, diarrhea, abdominal pain and constipation. Other reported adverse events include peripheral edema, congestive heart failure and pulmonary edema, headache, dizziness, peripheral neuropathy, menstrual disorders, reversible increases in hepatic enzymes, hepatitis, liver failure, hypokalemia, hypertriglyceridemia, alopecia, allergic reactions (such as pruritus, rash, urticaria, angioedema, anaphylaxis), Stevens-Johnson syndrome, anaphylactic, anaphylactoid and allergic reactions, photosensitivity and neutropenia. There is limited information on the use of SPORANOX® during pregnancy. Cases of congenital abnormalities including skeletal, genitourinary tract, cardiovascular and ophthalmic malformations as well as chromosomal and multiple malformations have been reported during post-marketing experience. A causal relationship with SPORANOX® has not been established. (See CLINICAL PHARMACOLOGY: Special Populations, CONTRAINDICATIONS, WARNINGS, and PRECAUTIONS: Drug Interactions for more information.)

OVERDOSAGE

Itraconazole is not removed by dialysis.
There are limited data on the outcomes of patients ingesting high doses of itraconazole. In patients taking either 1000 mg of SPORANOX® (itraconazole) Oral Solution or up to 3000 mg of SPORANOX® Capsules, or b.i.d. dosing for four days with SPORANOX® Injection, the adverse event profile was similar to that observed at recommended doses.

DOSAGE AND ADMINISTRATION

Use only the components [SPORANOX® (itraconazole) Injection ampule, 0.9% Sodium Chloride Injection, USP (Normal Saline) bag and filtered infusion set] provided in the kit: **DO NOT SUBSTITUTE.**

SPORANOX® Injection should not be diluted with 5% Dextrose Injection, USP, or with Lactated Ringer's Injection, USP, alone or in combination with any other diluent. The compatibility of SPORANOX® Injection with diluents other than 0.9% Sodium Chloride Injection, USP (Normal Saline) is not known. **NOT FOR IV BOLUS INJECTION.**

NOTE: After reconstitution, the diluted SPORANOX® Injection may be stored refrigerated (2-8°C) or at room temperature (15-25°C) for up to 48 hours, when protected from direct light. During administration, exposure to normal room light is acceptable.

NOTE: Use only a dedicated infusion line for administration of SPORANOX® Injection. Do not introduce concomitant medication in the same bag nor through the same line as SPORANOX® Injection. Other medications may be administered after flushing the line/catheter with 0.9% Sodium Chloride Injection, USP, as described below, and removing and replacing the entire infusion line. Alternatively, utilize another lumen, in the case of a multi-lumen catheter.

Correct preparation and administration of SPORANOX® Injection are necessary to ensure maximal efficacy and safety. A precise mixing ratio is required in order to obtain a stable admixture. It is critical to maintain a 3.33 mg/mL itraconazole:diluent ratio. Failure to maintain this concentration will lead to the formation of a precipitate.

Add the full contents (25 mL) of the SPORANOX® Injection ampule into the infusion bag provided, which contains 50 mL of 0.9% Sodium Chloride Injection, USP (Normal Saline). Mix gently after the solution is completely transferred. Withdraw and discard 15 mL of the solution before administering to the patient. Using a flow control device, infuse 60 mL of the dilute solution (3.33 mg/mL = 200 mg itraconazole, pH apx. 4.8) intravenously over 60 minutes, using an extension line and the infusion set provided. After administration, flush the infusion set with 15-20 mL of 0.9% Sodium Chloride Injection, USP, over 30 seconds-15 minutes, via the two-way stopcock. Do not use Bacteriostatic Sodium Chloride Injection, USP. The compatibility of SPORANOX® Injection with flush solutions other than 0.9% Sodium Chloride Injection, USP (Normal Saline) is not known. Discard the entire infusion line.

Parenteral drug products should be inspected visually for particulate matter and discoloration prior to administration, whenever solution and container permit.

Empiric Therapy in Febrile, Neutropenic Patients with Suspected Fungal Infections (ETFN): The recommended dose of SPORANOX® Injection is 200 mg b.i.d. for four doses, followed by 200 mg once daily for up to 14 days. Each intravenous dose should be infused over 1 hour. Treatment should be continued with SPORANOX® Oral Solution 200 mg (20 mL) b.i.d. until resolution of clinically significant neutropenia. The safety and efficacy of SPORANOX® use exceeding 28 days in ETFN is not known.

Treatment of Blastomycosis, Histoplasmosis and Aspergillosis: The recommended intravenous dose is 200 mg b.i.d. for four doses, followed by 200 mg q.d. Each intravenous dose should be infused over 1 hour.

For the treatment of blastomycosis, histoplasmosis and aspergillosis, SPORANOX® can be given as oral capsules or intravenously. The safety and efficacy of SPORANOX® Injection administered for greater than 14 days is not known. Total itraconazole therapy (SPORANOX® Injection followed by SPORANOX® Capsules) should be continued for a minimum of 3 months and until clinical parameters and laboratory tests indicate that the active fungal infection has subsided. An inadequate period of treatment may lead to recurrence of active infection.

SPORANOX® Injection should not be used in patients with creatinine clearance <30 mL/min.

Table 2. Summary of Possibly or Definitely Drug-Related Adverse Events Reported by ≥2% of Subjects

Adverse Event	Total SPORANOX® Injection (N=360) %	Comparative Studies		
		SPORANOX® Injection (N=234) %	Intravenous Fluconazole (N=32) %	Intravenous Amphotericin B (N=202) %
Gastrointestinal system disorders				
Nausea	8	9	0	15
Diarrhea	6	6	3	9
Vomiting	4	6	0	10
Abdominal pain	2	2	0	3
Constipation	0	1	3	0
Metabolic and nutritional disorders				
Hypokalemia	5	8	0	29
Alkaline phosphatase increased	1	2	3	2
Serum creatinine increased	2	2	3	26
Hypomagnesemia	1	1	0	5
Blood urea nitrogen increased	0	1	0	7
Fluid overload	0	0	0	3
Hypocalcemia	0	0	0	3
Liver and biliary system disorders				
Bilirubinemia	4	6	9	3
SGPT/ALT increased	2	3	3	1
Hepatic function abnormal	1	2	0	2
Jaundice	1	2	0	0
SGOT/AST increased	1	2	0	0
Body as a whole – General disorders				
Pain	1	2	0	0
Rigors	0	0	0	34
Fever	0	0	0	6
Skin and appendages disorders				
Rash	3	3	3	3
Sweating increased	1	2	0	0
Respiratory system disorder				
Dyspnea	0	0	0	3
Central and peripheral nervous system disorders				
Dizziness	1	2	0	1
Headache	2	2	0	3
Urinary system disorders				
Renal function abnormal	1	1	0	11
Application site disorder				
Application site reaction	4	0	0	0
Cardiovascular disorders, general				
Hypotension	0	0	0	3
Hypertension	0	0	0	2
Heart rate and rhythm disorders				
Tachycardia	0	1	0	3
Vascular (extracardiac) disorders				
Vein disorder	3	0	0	0

HOW SUPPLIED

SPORANOX® (itraconazole) Injection for intravenous infusion is supplied as a kit (NDC 50458-298-01), containing one 25 mL colorless glass ampule of itraconazole 10 mg/mL sterile, pyrogen-free solution (NDC 50458-297-10), one 50 mL bag (100 mL capacity) of 0.9% Sodium Chloride Injection, USP (Normal Saline) and one filtered infusion set. Store at or below 25°C (77°F). Protect from light and freezing.

SPORANOX®
(ITRACONAZOLE)
INJECTION

Manufactured by:
Abbott Laboratories, Inc.
North Chicago, IL 60064
631-10-938-7
Distributed by:
Ortho Biotech Products, L.P.
Raritan, NJ 08869
ORTHO BIOTECH
U.S. Patent 4,727,064
58-7309-R7
Revised January 2004

SPORANOX® ℞
(itraconazole)
ORAL SOLUTION

Congestive Heart Failure: When itraconazole was administered intravenously to dogs and healthy human volunteers, negative inotropic effects were seen. If signs or symptoms of congestive heart failure occur during administration of SPORANOX® (itraconazole) Oral Solution, continued SPORANOX® use should be reassessed. (See CLINICAL PHARMACOLOGY: Special Populations, CONTRAINDICATIONS, WARNINGS, PRECAUTIONS: Drug Interactions and ADVERSE REACTIONS: Post-marketing Experience for more information.)

Drug Interactions: Coadministration of cisapride, pimozide, quinidine, dofetilide, or levacetylmethadol (levomethadyl) with SPORANOX® (itraconazole) Capsules, Injection or Oral Solution is contraindicated. SPORANOX®, a potent cytochrome P450 3A4 isoenzyme system (CYP3A4) inhibitor, may increase plasma concentrations of drugs metabolized by this pathway. Serious cardiovascular events, including QT prolongation, torsades de pointes, ventricular tachycardia, cardiac arrest, and/or sudden death have occurred in patients using cisapride, pimozide, levacetylmethadol (levomethadyl), or quinidine concomitantly with SPORANOX® and/or other CYP3A4 inhibitors. (See CONTRAINDICATIONS, WARNINGS, and PRECAUTIONS: Drug Interactions for more information.)

DESCRIPTION

SPORANOX® is the brand name for itraconazole, a synthetic triazole antifungal agent. Itraconazole is a 1:1:1:1 racemic mixture of four diastereomers (two enantiomeric pairs), each possessing three chiral centers. It may be represented by the following structural formula and nomenclature:

(±)-1-[(R*)-sec-butyl]-4-[p-[4-[p-[[(2R*,4S*)-2-(2,4-dichlorophenyl)-2-(1H-1,2,4-triazol-1-ylmethyl)-1,3-dioxolan-4-yl] methoxy]phenyl]-1-piperazinyl] phenyl]-Δ^2-1,2,4-triazolin-5-one mixture with (±)-1-[(R*)-sec-butyl]-4-[p-[4-[p-[[(2S*, 4R*)-2-(2,4-dichlorophenyl)-2-(1H-1,2,4-triazol-1-ylmethyl)-1,3-dioxolan-4-yl]methoxy]phenyl]-1-piperazinyl]phenyl]-Δ^2-1,2,4-triazolin-5-one

or

(±)-1-[(RS)-sec-butyl]-4-[p-[4-[p-[[(2R,4S)-2-(2,4-dichlorophenyl)-2-(1H-1,2,4-triazol-1-ylmethyl)-1,3-dioxolan-4-yl] methoxy]phenyl]-1-piperazinyl] phenyl]-Δ^2-1,2,4-triazolin-5-one.

Itraconazole has a molecular formula of $C_{35}H_{38}Cl_2N_8O_4$ and a molecular weight of 705.64. It is a white to slightly yellowish powder. It is insoluble in water, very slightly soluble in alcohols, and freely soluble in dichloromethane. It has a pKa of 3.70 (based on extrapolation of values obtained from methanolic solutions) and a log (n-octanol/water) partition coefficient of 5.66 at pH 8.1.

SPORANOX® (itraconazole) Oral Solution contains 10 mg of itraconazole per mL, solubilized by hydroxypropyl-β-cyclodextrin (400 mg/mL) as a molecular inclusion complex. SPORANOX® Oral Solution is clear and yellowish in color with a target pH of 2. Other ingredients are hydrochloric

Continued on next page

Sporanox Oral Solution—Cont.

acid, propylene glycol, purified water, sodium hydroxide, sodium saccharin, sorbitol, cherry flavor 1, cherry flavor 2 and caramel flavor.

CLINICAL PHARMACOLOGY

Pharmacokinetics and Metabolism: NOTE: The plasma concentrations reported below were measured by high-performance liquid chromatography (HPLC) specific for itraconazole. When itraconazole in plasma is measured by a bioassay, values reported may be higher than those obtained by HPLC due to the presence of the bioactive metabolite, hydroxyitraconazole. (See MICROBIOLOGY.)

The absolute bioavailability of itraconazole administered as a non-marketed solution formulation under fed conditions was 55% in 6 healthy male volunteers. However, the bioavailability of SPORANOX® (itraconazole) Oral Solution is increased under fasted conditions reaching higher maximum plasma concentrations (C_{max}) in a shorter period of time. In 27 healthy male volunteers, the steady-state area under the plasma concentration versus time curve (AUC_{0-24h}) of itraconazole (SPORANOX® Oral Solution, 200 mg daily for 15 days) under fasted conditions was 131 ± 30% of that obtained under fed conditions. Therefore, unlike SPORANOX® Capsules, it is recommended that SPORANOX® Oral Solution be administered without food. Presented in the table below are the steady-state (Day 15) pharmacokinetic parameters for itraconazole and hydroxyitraconazole (SPORANOX® Oral Solution) under fasted and fed conditions:

[See first table at right]

The bioavailability of SPORANOX® Oral Solution relative to SPORANOX® Capsules was studied in 30 healthy male volunteers who received 200 mg of itraconazole as the oral solution and capsules under fed conditions. The $AUC_{0-\infty}$ from SPORANOX® Oral Solution was 149 ± 68% of that obtained from SPORANOX® Capsules; a similar increase was observed for hydroxyitraconazole. In addition, a cross study comparison of itraconazole and hydroxyitraconazole pharmacokinetics following the administration of single 200 mg doses of SPORANOX® Oral Solution (under fasted conditions) or SPORANOX® Capsules (under fed conditions) indicates that when these two formulations are administered under conditions which optimize their systemic absorption, the bioavailability of the solution relative to capsules is expected to be increased further. Therefore, it is recommended that SPORANOX® Oral Solution and SPORANOX® Capsules not be used interchangeably. The following table contains pharmacokinetic parameters for itraconazole and hydroxyitraconazole following single 200 mg doses of SPORANOX® Oral Solution (n=27) or SPORANOX® Capsules (n=30) administered to healthy male volunteers under fasted and fed conditions, respectively:

[See second table above]

The plasma protein binding of itraconazole is 99.8% and that of hydroxyitraconazole is 99.5%. Following intravenous administration, the volume of distribution of itraconazole averaged 796 ± 185 L.

Itraconazole is metabolized predominately by the cytochrome P450 3A4 isoenzyme system (CYP3A4), resulting in the formation of several metabolites, including hydroxyitraconazole, the major metabolite. Results of a pharmacokinetics study suggest that itraconazole may undergo saturable metabolism with multiple dosing. Fecal excretion of the parent drug varies between 3-18% of the dose. Renal excretion of the parent drug is less than 0.03% of the dose. About 40% of the dose is excreted as inactive metabolites in the urine. No single excreted metabolite represents more than 5% of a dose. Itraconazole total plasma clearance averaged 381 ± 95 mL/minute following intravenous administration. (See CONTRAINDICATIONS and PRECAUTIONS: Drug Interactions for more information.)

Special Populations:

Pediatrics: The pharmacokinetics of SPORANOX® Oral Solution were studied in 26 pediatric patients requiring systemic antifungal therapy. Patients were stratified by age: 6 months to 2 years (n=8), 2 to 5 years (n=7) and 5 to 12 years (n=11), and received itraconazole oral solution 5 mg/kg once daily for 14 days. Pharmacokinetic parameters at steady-state (Day 14) were not significantly different among the age strata and are summarized in the table below for all 26 patients:

	Itraconazole	Hydroxyitraconazole
C_{max} (ng/mL)	582.5 ± 382.4*	692.4 ± 355.0
C_{min} (ng/mL)	187.5 ± 161.4	403.8 ± 336.1
AUC_{0-24h} (ng·h/mL)	7706.7 ± 5245.2	13356.4 ± 8942.4
$t_{1/2}$ (hours)	35.8 ± 35.6	17.7 ± 13.0

*mean ± standard deviation

Renal Insufficiency: A pharmacokinetic study using a single 200-mg dose of itraconazole (four 50-mg capsules) was conducted in three groups of patients with renal impairment (uremia: n=7; hemodialysis: n=7; and continuous ambulatory peritoneal dialysis: n=5). In uremic subjects with a mean creatinine clearance of 13 mL/min. × 1.73 m², the bioavailability was slightly reduced compared with normal population parameters. This study did not demonstrate any significant effect of hemodialysis or continuous ambulatory peritoneal dialysis on the pharmacokinetics of itraconazole (T_{max}, C_{max}, and AUC_{0-8}). Plasma concentration-versus-time profiles showed wide intersubject variation in all three groups.

Hepatic Insufficiency: Patients with impaired hepatic function should be carefully monitored when taking itraconazole. The prolonged elimination half-life of itraconazole observed in cirrhotic patients should be considered when deciding to initiate therapy with other medications metabolized by CYP3A4. (See BOX WARNING, CONTRAINDICATIONS, and PRECAUTIONS: Drug Interactions.)

Decreased Cardiac Contractility: When itraconazole was administered intravenously to anesthetized dogs, a dose-related negative inotropic effect was documented. In a healthy volunteer study of SPORANOX® Injection (intravenous infusion), transient, asymptomatic decreases in left ventricular ejection fraction were observed using gated SPECT imaging; these resolved before the next infusion, 12 hours later. If signs or symptoms of congestive heart failure appear during administration of SPORANOX® Oral Solution, monitor carefully and consider other treatment alternatives which may include discontinuation of SPORANOX® Oral Solution administration. (See WARNINGS, PRECAUTIONS: Drug Interactions and ADVERSE REACTIONS: Post-marketing Experience for more information.)

Cystic Fibrosis: Seventeen cystic fibrosis patients, ages 7 to 28 years old, were administered itraconazole oral solution 2.5 mg/kg bid for 14 days in a pharmacokinetic study. Sixteen patients completed the study. Steady state trough concentrations >250ng/mL were achieved in 6 out of 11 patients ≥16 years of age but in none of the 5 patients <16 years of age. Large variability was observed in the pharmacokinetic data (%CV for trough concentrations = 98% and 70% for ≥16 and <16 years, respectively; %CV for AUC = 75% and 58% for ≥16 and <16 years, respectively). If a patient with cystic fibrosis does not respond to SPORANOX® Oral Solution, consideration should be given to switching to alternative therapy.

MICROBIOLOGY

Mechanism of Action: In vitro studies have demonstrated that itraconazole inhibits the cytochrome P450-dependent synthesis of ergosterol, which is a vital component of fungal cell membranes.

Activity In Vitro and In Vivo: Itraconazole exhibits in vitro activity against *Blastomyces dermatitidis, Histoplasma capsulatum, Histoplasma duboisii, Aspergillus flavus, Aspergillus fumigatus, Candida albicans,* and *Cryptococcus neoformans.* Itraconazole also exhibits varying in vitro activity against *Sporothrix schenckii, Trichophyton* species, *Candida krusei,* and other *Candida* species. The bioactive metabolite, hydroxyitraconazole, has not been evaluated against *Histoplasma capsulatum* and *Blastomyces dermatitidis.* Correlation between minimum inhibitory concentration (MIC) results in vitro and clinical outcome has yet to be established for azole antifungal agents.

Itraconazole administered orally was active in a variety of animal models of fungal infection using standard laboratory strains of fungi. Fungistatic activity has been demonstrated against disseminated fungal infections caused by *Blastomyces dermatitidis, Histoplasma duboisii, Aspergillus fumigatus, Coccidioides immitis, Cryptococcus neoformans, Paracoccidioides brasiliensis, Sporothrix schenckii, Trichophyton rubrum,* and *Trichophyton mentagrophytes.*

Itraconazole administered at 2.5 mg/kg and 5 mg/kg via the oral and parenteral routes increased survival rates and sterilized organ systems in normal and immunosuppressed guinea pigs with disseminated *Aspergillus fumigatus* infections. Oral itraconazole administered daily at 40 mg/kg and 80 mg/kg increased survival rates in normal rabbits with disseminated disease and in immunosuppressed rats with pulmonary *Aspergillus fumigatus* infection, respectively. Itraconazole has demonstrated antifungal activity in a variety of animal models infected with *Candida albicans* and other *Candida* species.

	Itraconazole		Hydroxyitraconazole	
	Fasted	Fed	Fasted	Fed
C_{max} (ng/mL)	1963 ± 601*	1435 ± 477	2055 ± 487	1781 ± 397
T_{max} (hours)	2.5 ± 0.8	4.4 ± 0.7	5.3 ± 4.3	4.3 ± 1.2
AUC_{0-24h} (ng·h/mL)	29271 ± 10285	22815 ± 7098	45184 ± 10981	38823 ± 8907
$t_{1/2}$ (hours)	39.7 ± 13	37.4 ± 13	27.3 ± 13	26.1 ± 10

*mean ± standard deviation

	Itraconazole		Hydroxyitraconazole	
	Oral Solution fasted	Capsules fed	Oral Solution fasted	Capsules fed
C_{max} (ng/mL)	544 ± 213*	302 ± 119	622 ± 116	504 ± 132
T_{max} (hours)	2.2 ± 0.8	5 ± 0.8	3.5 ± 1.2	5 ± 1
AUC_{0-24h} (ng·h/mL)	4505 ± 1670	2682 ± 1084	9552 ± 1835	7293 ± 2144

*mean ± standard deviation

Overview of Efficacy (Intent-to-Treat Population)

Efficacy Parameters	SPORANOX® N=179 (%)	Amphotericin B N=181 (%)
Success	84 (47%)	68 (38%)
Unevaluable*	24 (13%)	44 (24%)
Failure	71 (40%)	69 (38%)
Reason for Failure		
Intolerance after > 3 days of antifungal medication	12	37
Persistent fever	20	7
Change in antifungal medication due to fever	13	1
Emergent fungal infection	10	9
Documented bacterial or viral infection	7	8
Insufficient response	6	5
Deterioration of signs and symptoms	2	0
Death after > 3 days antifungal medication	1	2
Resolution of fever	131 (73%)	127 (70%)
Survival	161 (90%)	156 (86%)

*Treatment duration ≤ 3 days (including patients who died within 3 days, withdrew because of adverse events or were deemed ineligible due to a confirmed pre-treatment infection).

Resistance: Isolates from several fungal species with decreased susceptibility to itraconazole have been isolated in vitro and from patients receiving prolonged therapy.

Several in vitro studies have reported that some fungal clinical isolates, including *Candida* species, with reduced susceptibility to one azole antifungal agent may also be less susceptible to other azole derivatives. The finding of cross-resistance is dependent on a number of factors, including the species evaluated, its clinical history, the particular azole compounds compared, and the type of susceptibility test that is performed. The relevance of these in vitro susceptibility data to clinical outcome remains to be elucidated.

Studies (both in vitro and in vivo) suggest that the activity of amphotericin B may be suppressed by prior azole antifungal therapy. As with other azoles, itraconazole inhibits the ^{14}C-demethylation step in the synthesis of ergosterol, a cell wall component of fungi. Ergosterol is the active site for amphotericin B. In one study the antifungal activity of amphotericin B against *Aspergillus fumigatus* infections in mice was inhibited by ketoconazole therapy. The clinical significance of test results obtained in this study is unknown.

CLINICAL STUDIES

Empiric Therapy in Febrile Neutropenic Patients: An open randomized trial compared the efficacy and safety of itraconazole (intravenous followed by oral solution) with amphotericin B for empiric therapy in 384 febrile, neutropenic patients with hematologic malignancies who had suspected fungal infections. Patients received either itraconazole (injection, 200 mg b.i.d. for 2 days followed by 200 mg once daily for up to 14 days, followed by oral solution, 200 mg b.i.d.) or amphotericin B (total daily dose of 0.7-1.0 mg/kg body weight). The longest treatment duration was 28 days. An outcome assignment of "success" required (a) patient survival with resolution of fever and neutropenia within 28 days of treatment, (b) absence of emergent fungal infections, (c) no discontinuation of therapy due to toxicity or lack of efficacy, and (d) treatment for three or more days. The success rate using an intent-to-treat analysis was 47% for the itraconazole group and 38% for the amphotericin B arm.

[See third table on previous page]

Oropharyngeal Candidiasis: Two randomized, controlled studies for the treatment of oropharyngeal candidiasis have been conducted (total n=344). In one trial, clinical response to either 7 or 14 days of itraconazole oral solution, 200 mg/day, was similar to fluconazole tablets and averaged 84% across all arms. Clinical response in this study was defined as cured or improved (only minimal signs and symptoms with no visible lesions). Approximately 5% of subjects were lost to follow-up before any evaluations could be performed. Response to 14 days therapy of itraconazole oral solution was associated with a lower relapse rate than 7 days of itraconazole therapy. In another trial, the clinical response rate (defined as cured or improved) for itraconazole oral solution was similar to clotrimazole troches and averaged approximately 71% across both arms, with approximately 3% of subjects lost to follow-up before any evaluations could be performed. Ninety-two percent of the patients in these studies were HIV seropositive.

In an uncontrolled, open-label study of selected patients clinically unresponsive to fluconazole tablets (n=74, all patients HIV seropositive), patients were treated with itraconazole oral solution 100 mg b.i.d. (Clinically unresponsive to fluconazole in this study was defined as having received a dose of fluconazole tablets at least 200 mg/day for a minimum of 14 days.) Treatment duration was 14-28 days based on response. Approximately 55% of patients had complete resolution of oral lesions. Of patients who responded and then entered a follow-up phase (n=22), all relapsed within 1 month (median 14 days) when treatment was discontinued. Although baseline endoscopies had not been performed, several patients in this study developed symptoms of esophageal candidiasis while receiving therapy with itraconazole oral solution. Itraconazole oral solution has not been directly compared to other agents in a controlled trial of similar patients.

Esophageal Candidiasis: A double-blind randomized study (n=119, 111 of whom were HIV seropositive) compared itraconazole oral solution (100 mg/day) to fluconazole tablets (100 mg/day). The dose of each was increased to 200 mg/day for patients not responding initially. Treatment continued for 2 weeks following resolution of symptoms, for a total duration of treatment of 3-8 weeks. Clinical response (a global assessment of cured or improved) was not significantly different between the two study arms, and averaged approximately 86% with 8% lost to follow-up. Six of 53 (11%) itraconazole-treated patients and 12/57 (21%) fluconazole-treated patients were escalated to the 200 mg dose in this trial. Of the subgroup of patients who responded and entered a follow-up phase (n=88), approximately 23% relapsed across both arms within 4 weeks.

INDICATIONS AND USAGE

SPORANOX® (itraconazole) Injection/Oral Solution is indicated for empiric therapy of febrile neutropenic patients with suspected fungal infections. (NOTE: In a comparative trial, the overall response rate for itraconazole-treated subjects was higher than for amphotericin B-treated subjects. However, compared to amphotericin B-treated subjects, a larger number of itraconazole-treated subjects discontinued treatment due to persistent fever and a change in antifungal medication due to fever. Whereas, a larger number of amphotericin B-treated subjects discontinued due to drug intolerance. (See CLINICAL STUDIES section.)

Table 1. Selected Drugs that are predicted to alter the plasma concentration of itraconazole or have their plasma concentration altered by SPORANOX®[1]

Drug plasma concentration increased by itraconazole	
Antiarrhythmics	digoxin, dofetilide[2], quinidine[2], disopyramide
Anticoagulants	Warfarin
Anticonvulsants	Carbamazepine
Antimycobacterials	Rifabutin
Antineoplastics	busulfan, docetaxel, vinca alkaloids
Antipsychotics	pimozide[2],
Benzodiazepines	alprazolam, diazepam, midazolam,[2,3] triazolam[2]
Calcium Channel Blockers	dihydropyridines, verapamil
Gastrointestinal Motility Agents	cisapride[2]
HMG CoA-Reductase Inhibitors	atorvastatin, cerivastatin, lovastatin,[2] simvastatin[2]
Immunosuppressants	cyclosporine, tacrolimus, sirolimus
Oral Hypoglycemics	oral hypoglycemics
Protease Inhibitors	indinavir, ritonavir, saquinavir
Other	levacetylmethadol, (levomethadyl), ergot alkaloids, halofantrine, alfentanil, buspirone, methylprednisolone, budesonide, dexamethasone, trimetrexate, warfarin, cilostazol, eletriptan
Decrease plasma concentration of itraconazole	
Anticonvulsants	carbamazepine, phenobarbital, phenytoin
Antimycobacterials	isoniazid, rifabutin, rifampin
Gastric Acid Suppressors/Neutralizers	antacids, H_2-receptor antagonists, proton pump inhibitors
Reverse Transcriptase Inhibitors	Nevirapine
Increase plasma concentration of itraconazole	
Macrolide Antibiotics	clarithromycin, erythromycin
Protease Inhibitors	indinavir, ritonavir

[1]This list is not all-inclusive.
[2]Contraindicated with SPORANOX® based on clinical and/or pharmacokinetics studies. (See WARNINGS and below.)
[3]For information on parenterally administered midazolam, see the Benzodiazepine paragraph below.

SPORANOX® (itraconazole) Oral Solution is also indicated for the treatment of oropharyngeal and esophageal candidiasis.

(See CLINICAL PHARMACOLOGY: Special Populations, WARNINGS, and ADVERSE REACTIONS: Post-marketing Experience for more information.)

CONTRAINDICATIONS

Drug Interactions: Concomitant administration of SPORANOX® (itraconazole) Capsules, Injection, or Oral Solution and certain drugs metabolized by the cytochrome P450 3A4 isoenzyme system (CYP3A4) may result in increased plasma concentrations of those drugs, leading to potentially serious and/or life-threatening adverse events. Cisapride, oral midazolam, pimozide, quinidine, dofetilide, triazolam and levacetylmethadol (levomethadyl) are contraindicated with SPORANOX®. HMG CoA-reductase inhibitors metabolized by CYP3A4, such as lovastatin and simvastatin, are also contraindicated with SPORANOX®. Ergot alkaloids metabolized by CYP3A4 such as dihydroergotamine, ergometrine (ergonovine), ergotamine and methylergometrine (methylergonovine) are contraindicated with SPORANOX®. (See BOX WARNING, and PRECAUTIONS: Drug Interactions.)

SPORANOX® is contraindicated for patients who have shown hypersensitivity to itraconazole or its excipients. There is no information regarding cross-hypersensitivity between itraconazole and other azole antifungal agents. Caution should be used when prescribing SPORANOX® to patients with hypersensitivity to other azoles.

WARNINGS

SPORANOX® (itraconazole) Oral Solution and SPORANOX® Capsules should not be used interchangeably. Only SPORANOX® Oral Solution has been demonstrated effective for oral and/or esophageal candidiasis. SPORANOX® Oral Solution contains the excipient hydroxypropyl-β-cyclodextrin which produced pancreatic adenocarcinomas in a rat carcinogenicity study. These findings were not observed in a similar mouse carcinogenicity study. The clinical relevance of these findings is unknown. (See Carcinogenesis, Mutagenesis, and Impairment of Fertility.)

Hepatic Effects: SPORANOX® has been associated with rare cases of serious hepatotoxicity, including liver failure and death. Some of these cases had neither pre-existing liver disease nor a serious underlying medical condition and some of these cases developed within the first week of treatment. If clinical signs or symptoms develop that are consistent with liver disease, treatment should be discontinued and liver function testing performed. Continued SPORANOX® use or reinstitution of treatment with SPORANOX® is strongly discouraged unless there is a serious or life threatening situation where the expected benefit exceeds the risk. (See PRECAUTIONS: Information for Patients and ADVERSE REACTIONS.)

Cardiac Dysrhythmias: Life-threatening cardiac dysrhythmias and/or sudden death have occurred in patients using cisapride, pimozide, levacetylmethadol (levomethadyl), or quinidine concomitantly with SPORANOX® and/or other CYP3A4 inhibitors. Concomitant administration of these drugs with SPORANOX® is contraindicated. (See BOX WARNING, CONTRAINDICATIONS, and PRECAUTIONS: Drug Interactions.)

Cardiac Disease: SPORANOX® Oral Solution should not be used in patients with evidence of ventricular dysfunction unless the benefit clearly outweighs the risk. For patients with risk factors for congestive heart failure, physicians should carefully review the risks and benefits of SPORANOX® therapy. These risk factors include cardiac disease such as ischemic and valvular disease; significant pulmonary disease such as chronic obstructive pulmonary disease; and renal failure and other edematous disorders. Such patients should be informed of the signs and symptoms of CHF, should be treated with caution, and should be monitored for signs and symptoms of CHF during treatment. If signs or symptoms of CHF appear during administration of SPORANOX® Oral Solution, monitor carefully and consider other treatment alternatives which may include discontinuation of SPORANOX® Oral Solution administration.

When itraconazole was administered intravenously to anesthetized dogs, a dose-related negative inotropic effect was documented. In a healthy volunteer study of SPORANOX® Injection (intravenous infusion), transient, asymptomatic decreases in left ventricular ejection fraction were observed using gated SPECT imaging; these resolved before the next infusion, 12 hours later.

Cases of CHF, peripheral edema, and pulmonary edema have been reported in the post-marketing period among patients being treated for onychomycosis and/or systemic fungal infections. (See CLINICAL PHARMACOLOGY: Special Populations, PRECAUTIONS: Drug Interactions, and ADVERSE REACTIONS: Post-marketing Experience for more information.)

Cystic Fibrosis: If a patient with cystic fibrosis does not respond to SPORANOX® Oral Solution, consideration should be given to switching to alternative therapy (see CLINICAL PHARMACOLOGY/Special Populations).

Treatment of Severely Neutropenic Patients: SPORANOX® Oral Solution as treatment for oropharyngeal and/or esophageal candidiasis was not investigated in se-

Continued on next page

Sporanox Oral Solution—Cont.

verely neutropenic patients. Due to its pharmacokinetic properties, SPORANOX® Oral Solution is not recommended for initiation of treatment in patients at immediate risk of systemic candidiasis.

PRECAUTIONS

General: Rare cases of serious hepatotoxicity have been observed with SPORANOX® treatment, including some cases within the first week. In patients with elevated or abnormal liver enzymes or active liver disease, or who have experienced liver toxicity with other drugs, treatment with SPORANOX® is strongly discouraged unless there is a serious or life threatening situation where the expected benefit exceeds the risk. Liver function monitoring should be done in patients with pre-existing hepatic function abnormalities or those who have experienced liver toxicity with other medications and should be considered in all patients receiving SPORANOX®. Treatment should be stopped immediately and liver function testing should be conducted in patients who develop signs and symptoms suggestive of liver dysfunction.

If neuropathy occurs that may be attributable to SPORANOX® Oral Solution, the treatment should be discontinued.

Information for Patients:

- Only SPORANOX® Oral Solution has been demonstrated effective for oral and/or esophageal candidiasis. SPORANOX® Oral Solution contains the excipient hydroxypropyl-β-cyclodextrin which produced pancreatic adenocarcinomas in a rat carcinogenicity study. These findings were not observed in a similar mouse carcinogenicity study. The clinical relevance of these findings is unknown. (See Carcinogenesis, Mutagenesis, and Impairment of Fertility.)
- Taking SPORANOX® Oral Solution under fasted conditions improves the systemic availability of itraconazole. Instruct patients to take SPORANOX® Oral Solution without food, if possible.
- SPORANOX® Oral Solution should not be used interchangeably with SPORANOX® Capsules.
- Instruct patients about the signs and symptoms of congestive heart failure, and if these signs or symptoms occur during SPORANOX® administration, they should discontinue SPORANOX® and contact their healthcare provider immediately.
- Instruct patients to stop SPORANOX® treatment immediately and contact their healthcare provider if any signs and symptoms suggestive of liver dysfunction develop. Such signs and symptoms may include unusual fatigue, anorexia, nausea and/or vomiting, jaundice, dark urine or pale stools.
- Instruct patients to contact their physician before taking any concomitant medications with itraconazole to ensure there are no potential drug interactions.

Drug Interactions: Itraconazole and its major metabolite, hydroxyitraconazole, are inhibitors of CYP3A4. Therefore, the following drug interactions may occur (See Table 1 below and the following drug class subheadings that follow):

1. SPORANOX® may decrease the elimination of drugs metabolized by CYP3A4, resulting in increased plasma concentrations of these drugs when they are administered with SPORANOX®. These elevated plasma concentrations may increase or prolong both therapeutic and adverse effects of these drugs. Whenever possible, plasma concentrations of these drugs should be monitored, and dosage adjustments made after concomitant SPORANOX® therapy is initiated. When appropriate, clinical monitoring for signs or symptoms of increased or prolonged pharmacologic effects is advised. Upon discontinuation, depending on the dose and duration of treatment, itraconazole plasma concentrations decline gradually (especially in patients with hepatic cirrhosis or in those receiving CYP3A4 inhibitors). This is particularly important when initiating therapy with drugs whose metabolism is affected by itraconazole.
2. Inducers of CYP3A4 may decrease the plasma concentrations of itraconazole. SPORANOX® may not be effective in patients concomitantly taking SPORANOX® and one of these drugs. Therefore, administration of these drugs with SPORANOX® is not recommended.
3. Other inhibitors of CYP3A4 may increase the plasma concentrations of itraconazole. Patients who must take SPORANOX® concomitantly with one of these drugs should be monitored closely for signs or symptoms of increased or prolonged pharmacologic effects of SPORANOX®.

[See table 1 at top of previous page]

Antiarrhythmics: The class IA antiarrhythmic quinidine and class III antiarrhythmic dofetilide are known to prolong the QT interval. Coadministration of quinidine or dofetilide with SPORANOX® may increase plasma concentrations of quinidine or dofetilide which could result in serious cardiovascular events. Therefore, concomitant administration of SPORANOX® and quinidine or dofetilide is contraindicated. (See BOX WARNING, CONTRAINDICATIONS, and WARNINGS.)

The class IA antiarrhythmic disopyramide has the potential to increase the QT interval at high plasma concentrations. Caution is advised when SPORANOX® and disopyramide are administered concomitantly.

Table 2: Summary of possibly or definitely drug-related adverse events reported in ≥ 2% of subjects (Empiric Therapy Trial in Febrile Neutropenic Patients)

Adverse Event	SPORANOX® (N=192) %	Amphotericin B (N=192) %
Gastrointestinal system disorders		
Nausea	11	15
Diarrhea	10	9
Vomiting	7	10
Abdominal pain	3	3
Metabolic and nutritional disorders		
Hypokalemia	9	28
Serum creatinine increased	3	25
LDH increased	2	0
Alkaline phosphatase increased	2	2
Hypomagnesemia	2	4
Blood urea nitrogen increased	1	6
Fluid overload	1	3
Hypocalcemia	1	2
Liver and biliary system disorders		
Bilirubinemia	6	3
Hepatic function abnormal	3	2
SGPT/ALT increased	3	1
Jaundice	2	1
SGOT/AST increased	2	1
Skin and appendage disorders		
Rash	5	3
Sweating increased	2	1
CNS and peripheral nervous system		
Headache	2	2
Body as a whole		
Edema	2	2
Rigors	1	34
Fever	0	7
Respiratory system disorder		
Dyspnea	1	3
Urinary system disorder		
Renal function abnormal	1	12
Cardiovascular disorders, general		
Hypotension	1	3
Hypertension	0	2
Heart rate and rhythm disorders		
Tachycardia	1	3

Concomitant administration of digoxin and SPORANOX® has led to increased plasma concentrations of digoxin.

Anticoagulants: SPORANOX® enhances the anticoagulant effect of coumarin-like drugs, such as warfarin.

Anticonvulsants: Reduced plasma concentrations of itraconazole were reported when SPORANOX® was administered concomitantly with phenytoin. Carbamazepine, phenobarbital, and phenytoin are all inducers of CYP3A4. Although interactions with carbamazepine and phenobarbital have not been studied, concomitant administration of SPORANOX® and these drugs would be expected to result in decreased plasma concentrations of itraconazole. In addition, in vivo studies have demonstrated an increase in plasma carbamazepine concentrations in subjects concomitantly receiving ketoconazole. Although there are no data regarding the effect of itraconazole on carbamazepine metabolism, because of the similarities between ketoconazole and itraconazole, concomitant administration of SPORANOX® and carbamazepine may inhibit the metabolism of carbamazepine.

Antimycobacterials: Drug interaction studies have demonstrated that plasma concentrations of azole antifungal agents and their metabolites, including itraconazole and hydroxyitraconazole, were significantly decreased when these agents were given concomitantly with rifabutin or rifampin. In vivo data suggest that rifabutin is metabolized in part by CYP3A4. SPORANOX® may inhibit the metabolism of rifabutin. Although no formal study data are available for isoniazid, similar effects should be anticipated. Therefore, the efficacy of SPORANOX® could be substantially reduced if given concomitantly with one of these agents. Coadministration is not recommended.

Antineoplastics: SPORANOX® may inhibit the metabolism of busulfan, docetaxel, and vinca alkaloids.

Antipsychotics: Pimozide is known to prolong the QT interval and is partially metabolized by CYP3A4. Coadministration of pimozide with SPORANOX® could result in serious cardiovascular events. Therefore, concomitant administration of SPORANOX® and pimozide is contraindicated. (See BOX WARNING, CONTRAINDICATIONS, and WARNINGS.)

Benzodiazepines: Concomitant administration of SPORANOX® and alprazolam, diazepam, oral midazolam, or triazolam could lead to increased plasma concentrations of these benzodiazepines. Increased plasma concentrations could potentiate and prolong hypnotic and sedative effects. Concomitant administration of SPORANOX® and oral midazolam or triazolam is contraindicated. (See CONTRAINDI-

CATIONS and WARNINGS.) If midazolam is administered parenterally, special precaution and patient monitoring is required since the sedative effect may be prolonged.

Calcium Channel Blockers: Edema has been reported in patients concomitantly receiving SPORANOX® and dihydropyridine calcium channel blockers. Appropriate dosage adjustment may be necessary.

Calcium channel blockers can have a negative inotropic effect which may be additive to those of itraconazole; itraconazole can inhibit the metabolism of calcium channel blockers such as dihydropyridines (e.g., nifedipine and felodipine) and verapamil. Therefore, caution should be used when co-administering itraconazole and calcium channel blockers. (See CLINICAL PHARMACOLOGY: Special Populations, WARNINGS, and ADVERSE REACTIONS: Post-marketing Experience for more information.)

Gastric Acid Suppressors/Neutralizers: Reduced plasma concentrations of itraconazole were reported when SPORANOX® Capsules were administered concomitantly with H_2-receptor antagonists. Studies have shown that absorption of itraconazole is impaired when gastric acid production is decreased. Therefore, SPORANOX® should be administered with a cola beverage if the patient has achlorhydria or is taking H_2-receptor antagonists or other gastric acid suppressors. Antacids should be administered at least 1 hour before or 2 hours after administration of SPORANOX® Capsules. In a clinical study, when SPORANOX® Capsules were administered with omeprazole (a proton pump inhibitor), the bioavailability of itraconazole was significantly reduced. However, as itraconazole is already dissolved in SPORANOX® Oral Solution, the effect of H_2 antagonists is expected to be substantially less than with the capsules. Nevertheless, caution is advised when the two drugs are co-administered.

Gastrointestinal Motility Agents: Coadministration of SPORANOX® with cisapride can elevate plasma cisapride concentrations which could result in serious cardiovascular events. Therefore, concomitant administration of SPORANOX® with cisapride is contraindicated. (See BOX WARNING, CONTRAINDICATIONS, and WARNINGS.)

HMG CoA-Reductase Inhibitors: Human pharmacokinetic data suggest that SPORANOX® inhibits the metabolism of atorvastatin, cerivastatin, lovastatin, and simvastatin, which may increase the risk of skeletal muscle toxicity, including rhabdomyolysis. Concomitant administration of SPORANOX® with HMG CoA-reductase inhibitors, such as lovastatin or simvastatin is contraindicated. (See CONTRAINDICATIONS and WARNINGS.)

Immunosuppressants: Concomitant administration of SPORANOX® and cyclosporine or tacrolimus has led to increased plasma concentrations of these immunosuppressants. Concomitant administration of SPORANOX® and sirolimus could increase plasma concentrations of sirolimus.

Macrolide Antibiotics: Erythromycin and clarithromycin are known inhibitors of CYP3A4 (See Table 1) and may increase plasma concentrations of itraconazole. In a small pharmacokinetic study involving HIV infected patients, clarithromycin was shown to increase plasma concentrations of itraconazole. Similarly, following administration of 1 gram of erythromycin ethyl succinate and 200 mg itraconazole as single doses, the mean C_{max} and $AUC_{0-\infty}$ of itraconazole increased by 44% (90% CI: 119-175%) and 36% (90% CI: 108-171%), respectively.

Oral Hypoglycemic Agents: Severe hypoglycemia has been reported in patients concomitantly receiving azole antifungal agents and oral hypoglycemic agents. Blood glucose concentrations should be carefully monitored when SPORANOX® and oral hypoglycemic agents are coadministered.

Polyenes: Prior treatment with itraconazole, like other azoles, may reduce or inhibit the activity of polyenes such as amphotericin B. However, the clinical significance of this drug effect has not been clearly defined.

Protease Inhibitors: Concomitant administration of SPORANOX® and protease inhibitors metabolized by CYP3A4, such as indinavir, ritonavir, and saquinavir, may increase plasma concentrations of these protease inhibitors. In addition, concomitant administration of SPORANOX® and indinavir and ritonavir (but not saquinavir) may increase plasma concentrations of itraconazole. Caution is advised when SPORANOX® and protease inhibitors must be given concomitantly.

Reverse Transcriptase Inhibitors: Nevirapine is an inducer of CYP3A4. In vivo studies have shown that nevirapine induces the metabolism of ketoconazole, significantly reducing the bioavailability of ketoconazole. Studies involving nevirapine and itraconazole have not been conducted. However, because of the similarities between ketoconazole and itraconazole, concomitant administration of SPORANOX® and nevirapine is not recommended. In a clinical study, when 8 HIV-infected subjects were treated concomitantly with SPORANOX® Capsules 100 mg twice daily and the nucleoside reverse transcriptase inhibitor zidovudine 8 ± 0.4 mg/kg/day, the pharmacokinetics of zidovudine were not affected. Other nucleoside reverse transcriptase inhibitors have not been studied.

Other:

- Levacetylmethadol (levomethadyl) is known to prolong the QT interval and is metabolized by CYP3A4. Co-administration of levacetylmethadol with SPORANOX® could result in serious cardiovascular events. Therefore, concomitant administration of SPORANOX® and levacetylmethadol is contraindicated.

Table 3: Summary of Adverse Events Reported by ≥2% of SPORANOX® Treated Patients in U.S. Clinical Trials (Total)

Body System/Adverse Event	Itraconazole		Clotrimazole (n=125**)%	(n=81***)%
	All Total (n=350*)%	Fluconazole controlled studies (n=272)%		
Gastrointestinal disorders				
Nausea	11	10	11	5
Diarrhea	11	10	10	4
Vomiting	7	6	8	1
Abdominal pain	6	4	7	7
Constipation	2	2	1	0
Body as a whole				
Fever	7	6	8	5
Chest pain	3	3	2	0
Pain	2	2	4	0
Fatigue	2	1	2	0
Respiratory disorders				
Coughing	4	4	10	0
Dyspnea	2	3	5	1
Pneumonia	2	2	0	0
Sinusitis	2	2	4	0
Sputum increased	2	3	3	1
Skin and appendages disorders				
Rash	4	5	4	6
Increased sweating	4	4	6	1
Skin disorder, unspecified	2	2	2	1
Central/peripheral nervous system				
Headache	4	4	6	6
Dizziness	2	2	4	1
Resistance mechanism disorders				
Pneumocystis carinii infection	2	2	2	0
Psychiatric disorders				
Depression	2	1	0	1

* Of the 350 patients, 209 were treated for oropharyngeal candidiasis in controlled studies, 63 were treated for esophageal candidiasis in controlled studies and 78 were treated for oropharyngeal candidiasis in an open study.

** Of the 125 patients, 62 were treated for oropharyngeal candidiasis and 63 were treated for esophageal candidiasis.

*** All 81 patients were treated for oropharyngeal candidiasis.

- Elevated concentrations of ergot alkaloids can cause ergotism, ie. a risk for vasospasm potentially leading to cerebral ischemia and/or ischemia of the extremities. Concomitant administration of ergot alkaloids such as dihydroergotamine, ergometrine (ergonovine), ergotamine and methylergometrine (methylergonovine) with SPORANOX® is contraindicated.
- Halofantrine has the potential to prolong the QT interval at high plasma concentrations. Caution is advised when SPORANOX® and halofantrine are administered concomitantly.
- In vitro data suggest that alfentanil is metabolized by CYP3A4. Administration with SPORANOX® may increase plasma concentrations of alfentanil.
- Human pharmacokinetic data suggest that concomitant administration of SPORANOX® and buspirone results in significant increases in plasma concentrations of buspirone.
- SPORANOX® may inhibit the metabolism of certain glucocorticosteroids such as budesonide, dexamethasone and methylprednisolone.
- In vitro data suggest that trimetrexate is extensively metabolized by CYP3A4. In vitro animal models have demonstrated that ketoconazole potently inhibits the metabolism of trimetrexate. Although there are no data regarding the effect of itraconazole on trimetrexate metabolism, because of the similarities between ketoconazole and itraconazole, concomitant administration of SPORANOX® and trimetrexate may inhibit the metabolism of trimetrexate.
- Cilostazol and eletriptan are CYP3A4 metabolized drugs that should be used with caution when co-administered with SPORANOX®.

Carcinogenesis, Mutagenesis, and Impairment of Fertility: Itraconazole showed no evidence of carcinogenicity potential in mice treated orally for 23 months at dosage levels up to 80 mg/kg/day (approximately 10x the maximum recommended human dose [MRHD]). Male rats treated with 25 mg/kg/day (3.1× MRHD) had a slightly increased incidence of soft tissue sarcoma. These sarcomas may have been a consequence of hypercholesterolemia, which is a response of rats, but not dogs or humans, to chronic itraconazole administration. Female rats treated with 50 mg/kg/day (6.25× MRHD) had an increased incidence of squamous cell carcinoma of the lung (2/50) as compared to the untreated group. Although the occurrence of squamous cell carcinoma in the lung is extremely uncommon in untreated rats, the increase in this study was not statistically significant.

Hydroxypropyl-β-cyclodextrin (HP-β-CD), the solubilizing excipient used in SPORANOX® Oral Solution, was found to produce pancreatic exocrine hyperplasia and neoplasia when administered orally to rats at doses of 500, 2000 or 5000 mg/kg/day for 25 months. Adenocarcinomas of the exocrine pancreas produced in the treated animals were not seen in the untreated group and are not reported in the historical controls. Development of these tumors may be related to a mitogenic action of cholecystokinin. This finding was not observed in the mouse carcinogenicity study at doses of 500, 2000 or 5000 mg/kg/day for 22-23 months; however, the clinical relevance of these findings is unknown. Based on body surface area comparisons, the exposure to humans of HP-β-CD at the recommended clinical dose of SPORANOX® Oral Solution, is approximately equivalent to 1.7 times the exposure at the lowest dose in the rat study.

Itraconazole produced no mutagenic effects when assayed in a DNA repair test (unscheduled DNA synthesis) in primary rat hepatocytes, in Ames tests with *Salmonella typhimurium* (6 strains) and *Escherichia coli*, in the mouse lymphoma gene mutation tests, in a sex-linked recessive lethal mutation (*Drosophila melanogaster*) test, in chromosome aberration tests in human lymphocytes, in a cell transformation test with C3H/10T½ C18 mouse embryo fibroblasts cells, in a dominant lethal mutation test in male and female mice, and in micronucleus tests in mice and rats.

Itraconazole did not affect the fertility of male or female rats treated orally with dosage levels of up to 40 mg/kg/day (5× MRHD), even though parental toxicity was present at this dosage level. More severe signs of parental toxicity, including death, were present in the next higher dosage level, 160 mg/kg/day (20× MRHD).

Pregnancy: Teratogenic Effects. Pregnancy Category C: Itraconazole was found to cause a dose-related increase in maternal toxicity, embryotoxicity, and teratogenicity in rats at dosage levels of approximately 40-160 mg/kg/day (5-20× MRHD), and in mice at dosage levels of approximately 80 mg/kg/day (10× MRHD). In rats, the teratogenicity consisted of major skeletal defects; in mice, it consisted of encephaloceles and/or macroglossia.

There are no studies in pregnant women. SPORANOX® should be used in pregnancy only if the benefit outweighs the potential risk.

During post-marketing experience, cases of congenital abnormalities have been reported. (See ADVERSE REACTIONS, Post-marketing Experience.)

Nursing Mothers: Itraconazole is excreted in human milk; therefore, the expected benefits of SPORANOX® therapy for the mother should be weighed against the potential risk from exposure of itraconazole to the infant. The U.S. Public Health Service Centers for Disease Control and Prevention advises HIV-infected women not to breast-feed to avoid potential transmission of HIV to uninfected infants.

Pediatric Use: The efficacy and safety of SPORANOX® have not been established in pediatric patients. A pharmacokinetic study was conducted with SPORANOX® Oral Solution in 26 pediatric patients, ages 6 months to 12 years, requiring systemic antifungal treatment. Itraconazole was dosed at 5 mg/kg once daily for two weeks and no serious

Continued on next page

Sporanox Oral Solution—Cont.

unexpected adverse events were reported. (See CLINICAL PHARMACOLOGY.)

The long-term effects of itraconazole on bone growth in children are unknown. In three toxicology studies using rats, itraconazole induced bone defects at dosage levels as low as 20 mg/kg/day (2.5× MRHD). The induced defects included reduced bone plate activity, thinning of the zona compacta of the large bones, and increased bone fragility. At a dosage level of 80 mg/kg/day (10× MRHD) over 1 year or 160 mg/kg/day (20× MRHD) for 6 months, itraconazole induced small tooth pulp with hypocellular appearance in some rats. No such bone toxicity has been reported in adult patients.

ADVERSE REACTIONS

SPORANOX® has been associated with rare cases of serious hepatotoxicity, including liver failure and death. Some of these cases had neither pre-existing liver disease nor a serious underlying medical condition. If clinical signs or symptoms develop that are consistent with liver disease, treatment should be discontinued and liver function testing performed. The risks and benefits of SPORANOX® use should be reassessed. (See WARNINGS: Hepatic Effects and PRECAUTIONS: General and Information for Patients.)

Adverse Events Reported in Empiric Therapy in Febrile Neutropenic (ETFN) Patients

Adverse events considered at least possibly drug related in a clinical trial of empiric therapy in 384 febrile, neutropenic patients (192 treated with SPORANOX® and 192 with amphotericin B) with suspected fungal infections are listed in Table 2 below. Patients received a regimen of SPORANOX® Injection followed by SPORANOX® Oral Solution. The dose of SPORANOX® Injection was 200 mg twice daily for the first two days followed by a single daily dose of 200 mg for the remainder of the intravenous treatment period. The majority of patients received between 7 and 14 days of SPORANOX® Injection. The dose of SPORANOX® Oral Solution was 200 mg (20 mL) b.i.d. for the remainder of therapy.

[See table 2 at top of page 1764]

The following additional adverse events considered at least possibly related occurred in between 1 and 2% of patients who received SPORANOX® Injection and Oral Solution: constipation, hypophosphatemia, gamma-GT increased, erythematous rash, pruritus, dizziness, tremor, and pulmonary infiltration.

Adverse Events Reported in Oropharyngeal or Esophageal Candidiasis Trials

U.S. adverse experience data are derived from 350 immunocompromised patients (332 HIV seropositive/AIDS) treated for oropharyngeal or esophageal candidiasis. Table 3 below lists adverse events reported by at least 2% of patients treated with SPORANOX® Oral Solution in U.S. clinical trials. Data on patients receiving comparator agents in these trials are included for comparison.

[See table 3 at top of previous page]

Adverse events reported by less than 2% of patients in U.S. clinical trials with SPORANOX® included: adrenal insufficiency, asthenia, back pain, dehydration, dyspepsia, dysphagia, flatulence, gynecomastia, hematuria, hemorrhoids, hot flushes, implantation complication, infection unspecified, injury, insomnia, male breast pain, myalgia, pharyngitis, pruritus, rhinitis, rigors, stomatitis ulcerative, taste perversion, tinnitus, upper respiratory tract infection, vision abnormal, and weight decrease. Edema, hypokalemia and menstrual disorders have been reported in clinical trials with itraconazole capsules.

Post-marketing Experience

Worldwide post-marketing experiences with the use of SPORANOX® include adverse events of gastrointestinal origin, such as dyspepsia, nausea, vomiting, diarrhea, abdominal pain and constipation. Other reported adverse events include peripheral edema, congestive heart failure and pulmonary edema, headache, dizziness, peripheral neuropathy, menstrual disorders, reversible increases in hepatic enzymes, hepatitis, liver failure, hypokalemia, hypertriglyceridemia, alopecia, allergic reactions (such as pruritus, rash, urticaria, angioedema, anaphylaxis), Stevens-Johnson syndrome, anaphylactic, anaphylactoid and allergic reactions, photosensitivity and neutropenia. There is limited information on the use of SPORANOX® during pregnancy. Cases of congenital abnormalities including skeletal, genitourinary tract, cardiovascular and ophthalmic malformations as well as chromosomal and multiple malformations have been reported during post-marketing experience. A causal relationship with SPORANOX® has not been established. (See CLINICAL PHARMACOLOGY: Special Populations, CONTRAINDICATIONS, WARNINGS, and PRECAUTIONS: Drug Interactions for more information.)

OVERDOSAGE

Itraconazole is not removed by dialysis. In the event of accidental overdosage, supportive measures, including gastric lavage with sodium bicarbonate, should be employed.

There are limited data on the outcomes of patients ingesting high doses of itraconazole. In patients taking either 1000 mg of SPORANOX® (itraconazole) Oral Solution or up to 3000 mg of SPORANOX® Capsules, the adverse event profile was similar to that observed at recommended doses.

DOSAGE AND ADMINISTRATION

Empiric Therapy in Febrile, Neutropenic Patients with Suspected Fungal Infections (ETFN): The recommended dose of SPORANOX® Injection is 200 mg b.i.d. for four doses, followed by 200 mg once daily for up to 14 days. Each intravenous dose should be infused over 1 hour. Treatment should be continued with SPORANOX® Oral Solution 200 mg (20 mL) b.i.d. until resolution of clinically significant neutropenia. The safety and efficacy of SPORANOX® use exceeding 28 days in ETFN is not known.

SPORANOX® Oral Solution is a different preparation than SPORANOX® Capsules and should not be used interchangeably.

Treatment of Oropharyngeal and Esophageal Candidiasis: The solution should be vigorously swished in the mouth (10 mL at a time) for several seconds and swallowed.

The recommended dosage of SPORANOX® (itraconazole) Oral Solution for oropharyngeal candidiasis is 200 mg (20 mL) daily for 1 to 2 weeks. Clinical signs and symptoms of oropharyngeal candidiasis generally resolve within several days.

For patients with oropharyngeal candidiasis unresponsive/refractory to treatment with fluconazole tablets, the recommended dose is 100 mg (10 mL) b.i.d. For patients responding to therapy, clinical response will be seen in 2 to 4 weeks. Patients may be expected to relapse shortly after discontinuing therapy. Limited data on the safety of long-term use (>6 months) of SPORANOX® Oral Solution are available at this time.

The recommended dosage of SPORANOX® Oral Solution for esophageal candidiasis is 100 mg (10 mL) daily for a minimum treatment of three weeks. Treatment should continue for 2 weeks following resolution of symptoms. Doses up to 200 mg (20 mL) per day may be used based on medical judgement of the patient's response to therapy.

SPORANOX® Oral Solution and SPORANOX® Capsules should not be used interchangeably. Patients should be instructed to take SPORANOX® Oral Solution without food, if possible. Only SPORANOX® Oral Solution has been demonstrated effective for oral and/or esophageal candidiasis.

HOW SUPPLIED

SPORANOX® (itraconazole) Oral Solution is available in 150 mL amber glass bottles (NDC 50458-295-15) containing 10 mg of itraconazole per mL.

Store at or below 25°C (77°F). Do not freeze.

Keep out of reach of children.

U.S. Patent No. 4,267,179; 5,707,975; 4,727,064

Revised January 2004 631-10-939-6

Manufactured by:
Janssen Pharmaceutica N.V.
Beerse, Belgium
Distributed by:
Ortho Biotech Products, L.P.
Raritan, NJ 08869
ORTHO BIOTECH

Johnson & Johnson • MERCK

Consumer Pharmaceuticals Co.
CAMP HILL ROAD
FORT WASHINGTON, PA 19034

Direct Inquiries to:
Consumer Relationship Center
Fort Washington, PA 19034
1-800-469-5268
For Medical Information Contact:
In Emergencies:
1-800-469-5268

PEPCID AC® OTC
TABLETS, CHEWABLE TABLETS AND GELCAPS
Maximum Strength PEPCID AC Tablets
SOI-acid reducer

DESCRIPTION (PEPCID AC)

Each Pepcid AC Tablet, Chewable tablet, and gelcap contain famotidine 10 mg as an active ingredient.

Each Maximum Strength Pepcid AC Tablet contains famotidine 20 mg as an active ingredient.

INACTIVE INGREDIENTS

TABLETS: Hydroxypropyl cellulose, hypromellose, red iron oxide, magnesium stearate, microcrystalline cellulose red iron oxide*, starch, talc, titanium dioxide.

CHEWABLE TABLETS: aspartame, cellulose acetate, flavors, hydroxypropyl cellulose, hypromellose, lactose, magnesium stearate, mannitol, microcrystalline cellulose, red ferric oxide.

GELCAPS: benzyl alcohol, black iron oxide, butylparaben, castor oil, edetate calcium disodium, FD&C red #40, gelatin, hypromellose, magnesium stearate, methylparaben, microcrystalline cellulose, pregelatinized corn starch, propylene glycol, propylparaben, sodium lauryl sulfate, sodium propionate, talc, titanium dioxide.

INACTIVE INGREDIENTS (Max. Strength Pepcid AC.)

carnauba wax, hydroxypropyl cellulose, hypromellose, magnesium stearate, microcrystalline cellulose, pregelatinized starch, talc, titanium dioxide.

Product Benefits:

- **1 Tablet, Chewable Tablet or Gelcap** relieves heartburn associated with acid indigestion and sour stomach.
- prevents heartburn associated with acid indigestion and sour stomach brought on by eating or drinking certain food and beverages.

It contains famotidine, a prescription-proven medicine.

The ingredient in PEPCID AC and Maximum Strength Pepcid AC, famotidine, has been prescribed by doctors for years to treat millions of patients safely and effectively. The active ingredient in PEPCID AC and Maximum Strength Pepcid AC has been taken safely with many frequently prescribed medications.

ACTION

It is normal for the stomach to produce acid, especially after consuming food and beverages. However, acid in the wrong place (the esophagus), or too much acid, can cause burning pain and discomfort that interfere with everyday activities.

- **Heartburn—Caused by acid in the esophagus**

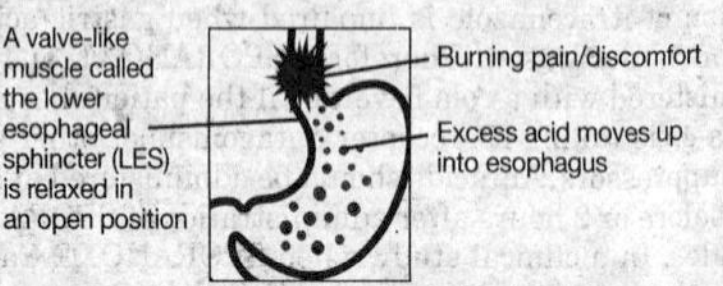

In clinical studies, PEPCID AC and Maximum Strength Pepcid AC film-coated tablets were significantly better than placebo tablet (tablets without the medicine) in relieving and preventing heartburn. Pepcid AC and Maximum Strength Pepcid AC chewables contain the same active ingredient.

Percent of heartburn episodes completely relieved

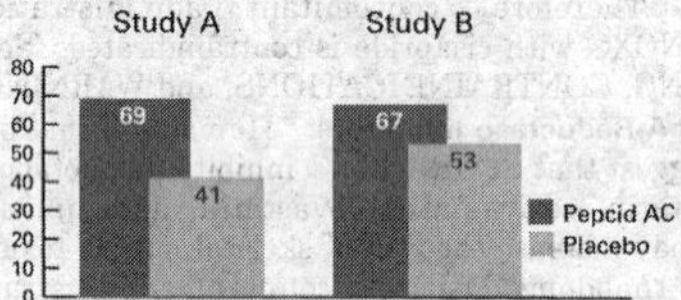

Percent of patients with prevention or reduction of heartburn symptoms

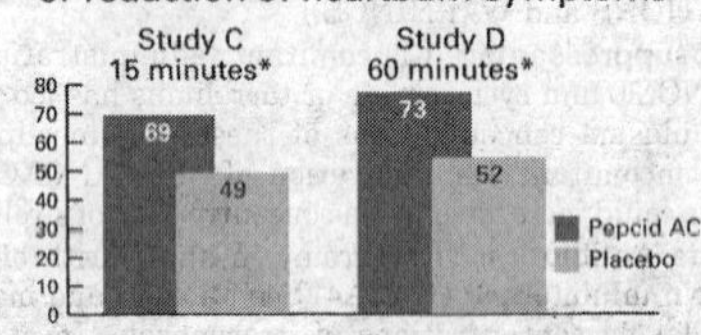

*Time taken before eating a meal that is expected to cause symptoms.

USES

- **Relieves heartburn, associated with acid indigestion and sour stomach;**
- **Prevents of heartburn associated with acid indigestion and sour stomach brought on by eating or drinking certain food and beverages.**

Tips for Managing Heartburn:

- Do not lie flat or bend over soon after eating.
- Do not eat late at night, or just before bedtime.
- Certain foods or drinks are more likely to cause heartburn, such as rich, spicy, fatty, and fried foods, chocolate, caffeine, alcohol, and even some fruits and vegetables.
- Eat slowly and do not eat big meals.
- If you are overweight, lose weight.
- If you smoke, quit smoking.
- Raise the head of your bed.
- Wear loose fitting clothing around your stomach.

WARNINGS

Allergy alert Do not use if you are allergic to famotidine or other acid reducers

Do not use:

- if you have trouble swallowing
- with other acid reducers
- if you have kidney disease, except under the advice and supervision of a doctor (for Maximum Strength Pepcid AC)

Stop use and ask a doctor if:

- stomach pain continues
- you need to take this product for more than 14 days

If pregnant or breast-feeding, ask a health professional before use.

Keep out of reach of children. In case of overdose, get medical help or contact a Poison Control Center right away.

DIRECTIONS

Pepcid AC:

- Adults and children 12 years and over:
- Tablet: To **relieve** symptoms, swallow 1 tablet with a glass of water.

  Chewable Tablet: **Do not swallow tablet whole: chew completely.** To **relieve** symptoms, **chew** one tablet before swallowing.

  Gelcap: To **relieve** symptoms, swallow one gelcap with a glass of water.

In clinical studies, PEPCID COMPLETE was significantly better than placebo pills tablets (without medicine) in relieving heartburn.

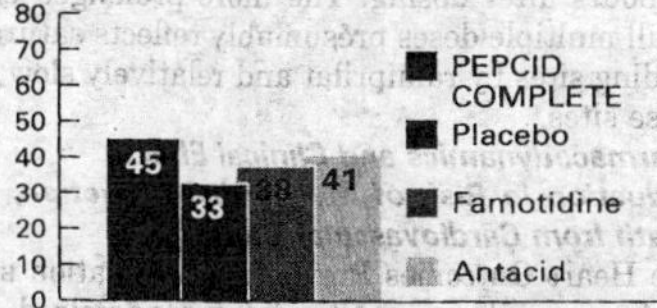

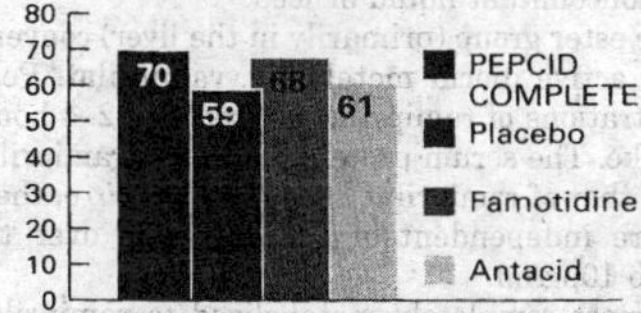

- Tablet & Gelcap: To prevent symptoms, swallow 1 tablet or gelcap with a glass of water at any time from **15 to 60 minutes before** eating food or drinking beverages that cause heartburn.
- Chewable Tablet: To **prevent** symptoms, **chew** one chewable tablet with a glass of water at any time from **15 to 60 minutes before** eating food or drinking beverages that cause heartburn.
- Do not use more than 2 tablets, chewable tablets or gelcaps in 24 hours.
- Children under 12 years: ask a doctor.

Maximum Strength Pepcid AC:
- adults and children 12 years and over:
  - to **relieve** symptoms, swallow 1 tablet with a glass of water
  - to **prevent** symptoms, swallow 1 tablet with a glass of water at any time from **15 to 60 minutes before** eating food or drinking beverages that cause heartburn.
  - do not use more than 2 tablets in 24 hours
- children under 12 years: ask a doctor

OTHER INFORMATION
- read the directions and warnings before use
- store at 25°–30°C (77°–86°F)
- keep the carton and package insert. They contain important information
- protect from moisture

in addition to the above the following also applies to the chewable tablet
- phenylketonurics: Contains Phenylalanine 1.4 mg per chewable tablet

HOW SUPPLIED

Pepcid AC Tablet is available as a rose-colored tablet identified as 'PEPCID AC'. NDC 16837-872

Pepcid AC Gelcap is available as a rose and white gelatin coated, capsule shaped tablet identified as 'PEPCID AC'. NDC 16837-856

Pepcid AC Chewable Tablet is available as a rose-colored chewable tablet identified as 'PEPCID AC'. NDC 16837-873

Maximum Strength Pepcid AC Tablet is a white, "D" shaped, film coated tablet identified as "PAC 20." NDC 16837 855

Shown in Product Identification Guide, page 319

PEPCID® COMPLETE — OTC

Acid Reducer + Antacid with DUAL ACTION Reduces and Neutralizes Acid

DESCRIPTION

ACTIVE INGREDIENTS (in each chewablet tablet) — **Purpose:**

Ingredient	Purpose
famotidine 10mg	Acid Reducer
calcium carbonate 800 mg	Antacid
magnesium hydroxide 165 mg	Antacid

INACTIVE INGREDIENTS

Mint flavor: cellulose acetate, corn starch, dextrates, flavors, hydroxypropyl cellulose, hypromellose, lactose, magnesium stearate, pregelatinized starch, red iron oxide, sodium lauryl sulfate, sugar

Berry flavor: cellulose acetate, corn starch, D&C red #7, dextrates, FD&C blue #1, FD&C red #40, flavors, hydropropyl cellulose, hypromellose, lactose, magnesium stearate, pregelatinized starch, sodium lauryl sulfate, sugar

Sodium Content:

Each chewable tablet contains 0.5 mg of sodium.

Acid Neutralizing Capacity:

Each chewable tablet contains 21.7 mEq of acid neutralizing capacity.

Product Benefits: Pepcid Complete combines an acid reducer (famotidine) with antacids (calcium carbonate and magnesium hydroxide) to relieve heartburn in two different ways: Acid reducers decrease the production of new stomach acid; antacids neutralize acid that is already in the stomach. The active ingredients in PEPCID COMPLETE have been used for years to treat acid-related problems in millions of people safely and effectively.

USES

Relives heartburn associated with acid indigestion and sour stomach.

ACTION

It is normal for the stomach to produce acid, especially after consuming food and beverages. However, acid in the stomach may move up into the wrong place (the esophagus), causing burning pain and discomfort that interfere with everyday activities.

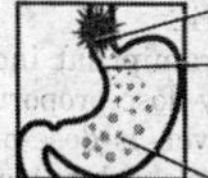

Tips For Managing Heartburn
- Do not lie flat or bend over soon after eating.
- Do not eat late at night, or just before bedtime.
- Certain foods or drinks are more likely to cause heartburn, such as rich, spicy, fatty, and fried foods, chocolate, caffeine, alcohol, and even some fruits and vegetables.
- Eat slowly and do not eat big meals.
- If you are overweight, lose weight.
- If you smoke, quit smoking.
- Raise the head of your bed.
- Wear loose fitting clothing around your stomach.

PROVEN EFFECTIVE IN CLINICAL STUDIES

[See graphic above]

WARNINGS
- **Allergy alert:** Do not use if you are allergic to famotidine or other acid reducers.
- **Do not use:** if you have trouble swallowing.
- With other famotidine products or acid reducers.
- **Ask a doctor or pharmacist before use if you are presently** taking a prescription drug. Antacids may interact with certain prescription drugs.
- **Stop use and ask a doctor if** stomach pain continues
- You need to take this product for more than 14 days.
- **If pregnant or breast-feeding,** ask a health professional before use.
- **Keep out of reach of children.** In case of overdose, get medical help or contact a Poison Control Center right away.

DIRECTIONS
- Adults and children 12 years and over:
  - **do not swallow tablet whole; chew completely.**
  - to relieve symptoms, **chew** 1 tablet before swallowing.
  - do not use more than 2 chewable tablets in 24 hours.
- Children under 12 years: ask a doctor.

OTHER INFORMATION
- read the directions and warnings before use.
- keep the carton and package insert booklet. They contain important information.
- store at 25°–30°C (77–86 F).
- protect from moisture.

HOW SUPPLIED

Pepcid Complete is available as a rose-colored chewable tablet identified by *'P'*. NDC 16837-888 – Mint flavor

Pepcid Complete Berry flavor

NDC 16837-291

Shown in Product Identification Guide, page 319

IDENTIFICATION PROBLEM?

Turn to the **Product Identification Guide,** where you'll find more than 1600 products pictured in actual size and full color.

Jones Pharma Inc.

Please see King Pharmaceuticals, Inc.

Key Pharmaceuticals, Inc.

GALLOPING HILL ROAD
KENILWORTH, NJ 07033

(For product information, please see Schering Corporation.)

King Pharmaceuticals, Inc.

501 FIFTH STREET
BRISTOL, TN 37620

Direct Inquiries to:
Customer Service:
800-776-3637
Fax:
423-989-6279
To report an Adverse Drug Experience:
(800) 546-4905
Fax: (423) 990-0519

ADRENALIN® CHLORIDE SOLUTION — ℞

(Epinephrine Injection, USP), 1:1000

DESCRIPTION

A sterile solution intended for subcutaneous or intramuscular injection. When diluted, it may also be administered intracardially or intravenously. Each milliliter contains 1 mg Adrenalin (epinephrine) as the hydrochloride dissolved in Water for Injection, USP, with sodium chloride added for isotonicity. The ampoules contain not more than 0.1% sodium bisulfite as an antioxidant, and the air in the ampoule has been displaced by nitrogen. The Steri-Vials® contain 0.5% Chlorobutanol (chloroform derivative) as a preservative and not more than 0.15% sodium bisulfite as an antioxidant. Epinephrine is the active principle of the adrenal medulla, chemically described as (—)-3,4-Dihydroxy-alpha-[(methylamino) methyl] benzyl alcohol, and has the following structural formula:

HO, OH, CH-CH$_2$-NHCH$_3$, OH

HOW SUPPLIED

NDC 61570-418-81 (Amp 88) Sterile solution containing 1 mg Adrenalin (epinephrine) as the hydrochloride in each 1-mL ampoule (1:1000). For intramuscular or subcutaneous use. When diluted, it may also be administered intracardially, intravenously, or intraspinally. Supplied in packages of ten.

NDC 61570-401-11 (S.V. 11) Sterile solution containing 1 mg Adrenalin (epinephrine) as the hydrochloride (1:1000). For intramuscular or subcutaneous use. When diluted, it may also be administered intracardially or intravenously. Supplied in a 30-mL Steri-Vial® (rubber-diaphragm-capped vial).

Store between 15° and 25°C (59° and 77°F).
Protect from light and freezing.
Rx Only.

Manufactured for:
Monarch Pharmaceuticals, Inc., Bristol, TN 37620
By: Parkedale Pharmaceuticals, Inc.
Rochester, MI 48307
418G031
238

ALTACE® CAPSULES — ℞

[ôl' tās]
(ramipril)

Prescribing Information as of April 2004

USE IN PREGNANCY

When used in pregnancy during the second and third trimesters, ACE inhibitors can cause injury and even death to the developing fetus. When pregnancy is detected, ALTACE® should be discontinued as soon as possible. **See WARNINGS: Fetal/neonatal morbidity and mortality.**

DESCRIPTION

Ramipril is a 2-aza-bicyclo [3.3.0]-octane-3-carboxylic acid derivative. It is a white, crystalline substance soluble in polar organic solvents and buffered aqueous solutions. Ramipril melts between 105°C and 112°C.

Continued on next page

Altace—Cont.

The CAS Registry Number is 87333-19-5. Ramipril's chemical name is (2*S*,3a*S*,6a*S*)-1[(*S*)-N-[(*S*)-1-Carboxy-3-phenylpropyl] alanyl] octahydrocyclopenta [*b*]pyrrole-2-carboxylic acid, 1-ethyl ester; its structural formula is:

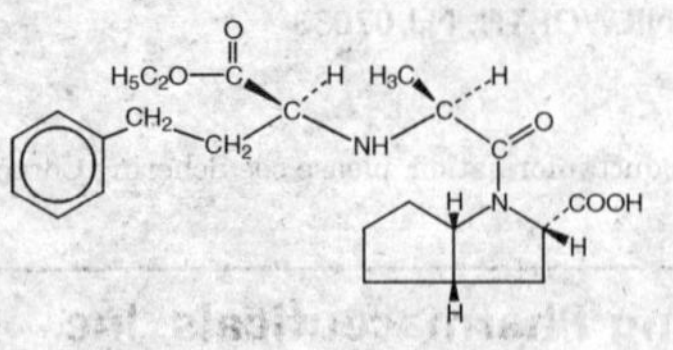

Its empiric formula is $C_{23}H_{32}N_2O_5$, and its molecular weight is 416.5.

Ramiprilat, the diacid metabolite of ramipril, is a non-sulfhydryl angiotensin converting enzyme inhibitor. Ramipril is converted to ramiprilat by hepatic cleavage of the ester group.

ALTACE (ramipril) is supplied as hard shell capsules for oral administration containing 1.25 mg, 2.5 mg, 5 mg, and 10 mg of ramipril. The inactive ingredients present are pregelatinized starch NF, gelatin, and titanium dioxide. The 1.25 mg capsule shell contains yellow iron oxide, the 2.5 mg capsule shell contains D&C yellow #10 and FD&C red #40, the 5 mg capsule shell contains FD&C blue #1 and FD&C red #40, and the 10 mg capsule shell contains FD&C blue #1.

CLINICAL PHARMACOLOGY

Mechanism of Action

Ramipril and ramiprilat inhibit angiotensin-converting enzyme (ACE) in human subjects and animals. ACE is a peptidyl dipeptidase that catalyzes the conversion of angiotensin I to the vasoconstrictor substance, angiotensin II. Angiotensin II also stimulates aldosterone secretion by the adrenal cortex. Inhibition of ACE results in decreased plasma angiotensin II, which leads to decreased vasopressor activity and to decreased aldosterone secretion. The latter decrease may result in a small increase of serum potassium. In hypertensive patients with normal renal function treated with ALTACE alone for up to 56 weeks, approximately 4% of patients during the trial had an abnormally high serum potassium and an increase from baseline greater than 0.75 mEq/L, and none of the patients had an abnormally low potassium and a decrease from baseline greater than 0.75 mEq/L. In the same study, approximately 2% of patients treated with ALTACE and hydrochlorothiazide for up to 56 weeks had abnormally high potassium values and an increase from baseline of 0.75 mEq/L or greater, and approximately 2% had abnormally low values and decreases from baseline of 0.75 mEq/L or greater. (See **PRECAUTIONS**.) Removal of angiotensin II negative feedback on renin secretion leads to increased plasma renin activity.

The effect of ramipril on hypertension appears to result at least in part from inhibition of both tissue and circulating ACE activity, thereby reducing angiotensin II formation in tissue and plasma.

ACE is identical to kininase, an enzyme that degrades bradykinin. Whether increased levels of bradykinin, a potent vasodepressor peptide, play a role in the therapeutic effects of ALTACE remains to be elucidated.

While the mechanism through which ALTACE lowers blood pressure is believed to be primarily suppression of the renin-angiotensin-aldosterone system, ALTACE has an antihypertensive effect even in patients with low-renin hypertension. Although ALTACE was antihypertensive in all races studied, black hypertensive patients (usually a low-renin hypertensive population) had a smaller average response to monotherapy than non-black patients.

Pharmacokinetics and Metabolism

Following oral administration of ALTACE, peak plasma concentrations of ramipril are reached within one hour. The extent of absorption is at least 50–60% and is not significantly influenced by the presence of food in the GI tract, although the rate of absorption is reduced.

In a trial in which subjects received ALTACE capsules or the contents of identical capsules dissolved in water, dissolved in apple juice, or suspended in apple sauce, serum ramiprilat levels were essentially unrelated to the use or nonuse of the concomitant liquid or food.

Cleavage of the ester group (primarily in the liver) converts ramipril to its active diacid metabolite, ramiprilat. Peak plasma concentrations of ramiprilat are reached 2–4 hours after drug intake. The serum protein binding of ramipril is about 73% and that of ramiprilat about 56%; *in vitro*, these percentages are independent of concentration over the range of 0.01 to 10µg/ml.

Ramipril is almost completely metabolized to ramiprilat, which has about 6 times the ACE inhibitory activity of ramipril, and to the diketopiperazine ester, the diketopiperazine acid, and the glucuronides of ramipril and ramiprilat, all of which are inactive. After oral administration of ramipril, about 60% of the parent drug and its metabolites is eliminated in the urine, and about 40% is found in the feces. Drug recovered in the feces may represent both biliary excretion of metabolites and/or unabsorbed drug, however the proportion of a dose eliminated by the bile has not been determined. Less than 2% of the administered dose is recovered in urine as unchanged ramipril.

Blood concentrations of ramipril and ramiprilat increase with increased dose, but are not strictly dose-proportional. The 24-hour AUC for ramiprilat, however, is dose-proportional over the 2.5–20 mg dose range. The absolute bioavailabilities of ramipril and ramiprilat were 28% and 44%, respectively, when 5 mg of oral ramipril was compared with the same dose of ramipril given intravenously.

Plasma concentrations of ramiprilat decline in a triphasic manner (initial rapid decline, apparent elimination phase, terminal elimination phase). The initial rapid decline, which represents distribution of the drug into a large peripheral compartment and subsequent binding to both plasma and tissue ACE, has a half-life of 2–4 hours. Because of its potent binding to ACE and slow dissociation from the enzyme, ramiprilat shows two elimination phases. The apparent elimination phase corresponds to the clearance of free ramiprilat and has a half-life of 9–18 hours. The terminal elimination phase has a prolonged half-life (>50 hours) and probably represents the binding/dissociation kinetics of the ramiprilat/ACE complex. It does not contribute to the accumulation of the drug. After multiple daily doses of ramipril 5–10 mg, the half-life of ramiprilat concentrations within the therapeutic range was 13–17 hours.

After once-daily dosing, steady-state plasma concentrations of ramiprilat are reached by the fourth dose. Steady-state concentrations of ramiprilat are somewhat higher than those seen after the first dose of ALTACE, especially at low doses (2.5 mg), but the difference is clinically insignificant.

In patients with creatinine clearance less than 40 ml/min/1.73m^2 peak levels of ramiprilat are approximately doubled, and trough levels may be as much as quintupled. In multiple-dose regimens, the total exposure to ramiprilat (AUC) in these patients is 3–4 times as large as it is in patients with normal renal function who receive similar doses.

The urinary excretion of ramipril, ramiprilat, and their metabolites is reduced in patients with impaired renal function. Compared to normal subjects, patients with creatinine clearance less than 40 ml/min/1.73m^2 had higher peak and trough ramiprilat levels and slightly longer times to peak concentrations. (See **DOSAGE AND ADMINISTRATION**.)

In patients with impaired liver function, the metabolism of ramipril to ramiprilat appears to be slowed, possibly because of diminished activity of hepatic esterases, and plasma ramipril levels in these patients are increased about 3-fold. Peak concentrations of ramiprilat in these patients, however, are not different from those seen in subjects with normal hepatic function, and the effect of a given dose on plasma ACE activity does not vary with hepatic function.

Pharmacodynamics

Single doses of ramipril of 2.5–20 mg produce approximately 60–80% inhibition of ACE activity 4 hours after dosing with approximately 40–60% inhibition after 24 hours. Multiple oral doses of ramipril of 2.0 mg or more cause plasma ACE activity to fall by more than 90% 4 hours after dosing, with over 80% inhibition of ACE activity remaining 24 hours after dosing. The more prolonged effect of even small multiple doses presumably reflects saturation of ACE binding sites by ramiprilat and relatively slow release from those sites.

Pharmacodynamics and Clinical Effects

Reduction in Risk of Myocardial Infarction, Stroke, and Death from Cardiovascular Causes

The Heart Outcomes Prevention Evaluation study (HOPE study) was a large, multi-center, randomized, placebo controlled, 2×2 factorial design, double-blind study conducted in 9,541 patients (4,645 on ALTACE) who were 55 years or older and considered at high risk of developing a major cardiovascular event because of a history of coronary artery disease, stroke, peripheral vascular disease, or diabetes that was accompanied by at least one other cardiovascular risk factor (hypertension, elevated total cholesterol levels, low HDL levels, cigarette smoking, or documented microalbuminuria). Patients were either normotensive or under treatment with other antihypertensive agents. Patients were excluded if they had clinical heart failure or were known to have a low ejection fraction (<0.40). This study was designed to examine the long-term (mean of five years) effects of ALTACE (10 mg orally once a day) on the combined endpoint of myocardial infarction, stroke or death from cardiovascular causes.

The HOPE study results showed that ALTACE (10 mg/day) significantly reduced the rate of myocardial infarction, stroke or death from cardiovascular causes (651/4645 vs. 826/4652, relative risk 0.78), as well as the rates of the 3 components of the combined endpoint.

[See first table below]

This effect was evident after about one year of treatment.

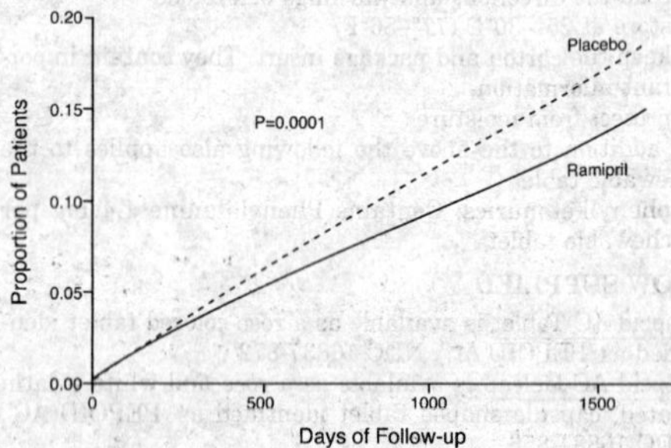

Figure 1: *Kaplan-Meier Estimates of the composite outcome of MI, Stroke, or Death from CV causes in the Ramipril Group and the Placebo Group. The relative risk of the composite outcomes in the Ramipril Group as compared with the Placebo Group was 0.78% (95% confidence interval, 0.70–0.86).*

Ramipril was effective in different demographic subgroups, (i.e., gender, age), subgroups defined by underlying disease (e.g., cardiovascular disease, hypertension), and subgroups defined by concomitant medication. There were insufficient data to determine whether or not ramipril was equally effective in ethnic subgroups.

This study was designed with a prespecified substudy in diabetics with at least one other cardiovascular risk factor. Effects of ramipril on the combined endpoint and its components were similar in diabetics (n=3,577) to those in the overall study population.

[See second table at left]

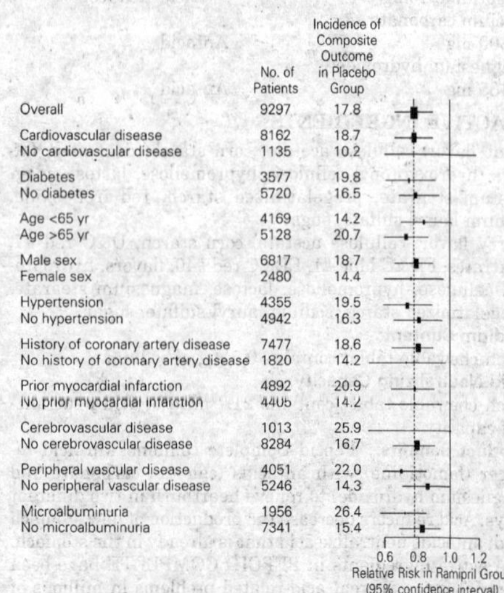

Figure 2. *The Beneficial Effect of Treatment with Ramipril on the Composite Outcome of Myocardial Infarction, Stroke, or Death from Cardiovascular Causes Overall and in Various Subgroups. Cerebrovascular disease was defined as*

Outcome	Altace (N=4645)	Placebo (N=4652)	Relative Risk (95% CI) P value
	no. (%)		
Combined End-point			
(MI, stroke, or death from CV cause)	651 (14.0%)	826 (17.8%)	0.78 (0.70–0.86), P=0.0001
Component End-point			
Death from Cardiovascular Causes	282 (6.1%)	377 (8.1%)	0.74 (0.64–0.87), P=0.0002
Myocardial infarction	459 (9.9%)	570 (12.3%)	0.80 (0.70–0.90), P=0.0003
Stroke	156 (3.4%)	226 (4.9%)	0.68 (0.56–0.84), P=0.0002
Overall Mortality			
(Death from any Cause)	482 (10.4%)	569 (12.2%)	0.84 (0.75–0.95), P=0.005

Outcome	Altace (N=1808)	Placebo (N=1769)	Relative Risk Reduction (95% CI)
	no. (%)		
Combined End-point			
(MI, stroke, or death from CV cause)	277 (15.3%)	351 (19.8%)	0.25 (0.12–0.36), P=0.0004
Component End-point			
Death from Cardiovascular Causes	112 (6.2%)	172 (9.7%)	0.37 (0.21–0.51), P=0.0001
Myocardial infarction	185 (10.2%)	229 (12.9%)	0.22 (0.60–0.36), P=0.01
Stroke	76 (4.2%)	108 (6.1%)	0.33 (0.10–0.50), P=0.007

stroke or transient ischemic attacks. The size of each symbol is proportional to the number of patients in each group. The dashed line indicates overall relative risk.

The benefits of Altace were observed among patients who were taking aspirin or other anti-platelet agents, beta-blockers, and lipid-lowering agents as well as diuretics and calcium channel blockers.

Hypertension

Administration of ALTACE to patients with mild to moderate hypertension results in a reduction of both supine and standing blood pressure to about the same extent with no compensatory tachycardia. Symptomatic postural hypotension is infrequent, although it can occur in patients who are salt- and/or volume-depleted. (See **WARNINGS** Use of ALTACE in combination with thiazide diuretics gives a blood pressure lowering effect greater than that seen with either agent alone.

In single-dose studies, doses of 5–20 mg of ALTACE lowered blood pressure within 1–2 hours, with peak reductions achieved 3–6 hours after dosing. The antihypertensive effect of a single dose persisted for 24 hours. In longer term (4–12 weeks) controlled studies, once-daily doses of 2.5–10 mg were similar in their effect, lowering supine or standing systolic and diastolic blood pressures 24 hours after dosing by about 6/4 mm Hg more than placebo. In comparisons of peak vs. trough effect, the trough effect represented about 50–60% of the peak response. In a titration study comparing divided (bid) vs. qd treatment, the divided regimen was superior, indicating that for some patients the antihypertensive effect with once-daily dosing is not adequately maintained. (See **DOSAGE AND ADMINISTRATION**.)

In most trials, the antihypertensive effect of ALTACE increased during the first several weeks of repeated measurements. The antihypertensive effect of ALTACE has been shown to continue during long-term therapy for at least 2 years. Abrupt withdrawal of ALTACE has not resulted in a rapid increase in blood pressure.

ALTACE has been compared with other ACE inhibitors, beta-blockers, and thiazide diuretics. It was approximately as effective as other ACE inhibitors and as atenolol. In both caucasians and blacks, hydrochlorothiazide (25 or 50 mg) was significantly more effective than ramipril.

Except for thiazides, no formal interaction studies of ramipril with other antihypertensive agents have been carried out. Limited experience in controlled and uncontrolled trials combining ramipril with a calcium channel blocker, a loop diuretic, or triple therapy (beta-blocker, vasodilator, and a diuretic) indicate no unusual drug-drug interactions. Other ACE inhibitors have had less than additive effects with beta adrenergic blockers, presumably because both drugs lower blood pressure by inhibiting parts of the renin-angiotensin system.

ALTACE was less effective in blacks than in caucasians. The effectiveness of ALTACE was not influenced by age, sex, or weight.

In a baseline controlled study of 10 patients with mild essential hypertension, blood pressure reduction was accompanied by a 15% increase in renal blood flow. In healthy volunteers, glomerular filtration rate was unchanged.

Heart Failure Post Myocardial Infarction

ALTACE was studied in the Acute Infarction Ramipril Efficacy (AIRE) trial. This was a multinational (mainly European) 161-center, 2006-patient, double-blind, randomized, parallel-group study comparing ALTACE to placebo in stable patients, 2–9 days after an acute myocardial infarction (MI), who had shown clinical signs of congestive heart failure (CHF) at any time after the MI. Patients in severe (NYHA class IV) heart failure, patients with unstable angina, patients with heart failure of congenital or valvular etiology, and patients with contraindications to ACE inhibitors were all excluded. The majority of patients had received thrombolytic therapy at the time of the index infarction, and the average time between infarction and initiation of treatment was 5 days.

Patients randomized to ramipril treatment were given an initial dose of 2.5 mg twice daily. If the initial regimen caused undue hypotension, the dose was reduced to 1.25 mg, but in either event doses were titrated upward (as tolerated) to a target regimen (achieved in 77% of patients randomized to ramipril) of 5 mg twice daily. Patients were then followed for an average of 15 months (range 6–46).

The use of ALTACE was associated with a 27% reduction (p=0.002), in the risk of death from any cause; about 90% of the deaths that occurred were cardiovascular, mainly sudden death. The risks of progression to severe heart failure and of CHF-related hospitalization were also reduced, by 23% (p=0.017) and 26% (p=0.011), respectively. The benefits of ALTACE therapy were seen in both genders, and they were not affected by the exact timing of the initiation of therapy, but older patients may have had a greater benefit than those under 65. The benefits were seen in patients on, and not on, various concomitant medications; at the time of randomization these included aspirin (about 80% of patients), diuretics (about 60%), organic nitrates (about 55%), beta-blockers (about 20%), calcium channel blockers (about 15%), and digoxin (about 12%).

INDICATIONS AND USAGE

Reduction in Risk of Myocardial Infarction, Stroke, and Death from Cardiovascular Causes

Altace is indicated in patients 55 years or older at high risk of developing a major cardiovascular event because of a history of coronary artery disease, stroke, peripheral vascular disease, or diabetes that is accompanied by at least one other cardiovascular risk factor (hypertension, elevated total cholesterol levels, low HDL levels, cigarette smoking, or documented microalbuminuria), to reduce the risk of myocardial infarction, stroke, or death from cardiovascular causes. Altace can be used in addition to other needed treatment (such as antihypertensive, antiplatelet or lipid-lowering therapy).

Hypertension

ALTACE is indicated for the treatment of hypertension. It may be used alone or in combination with thiazide diuretics.

In using ALTACE, consideration should be given to the fact that another angiotensin converting enzyme inhibitor, captopril, has caused agranulocytosis, particularly in patients with renal impairment or collagen-vascular disease. Available data are insufficient to show that ALTACE does not have a similar risk. (See **WARNINGS**.)

In considering use of ALTACE, it should be noted that in controlled trials ACE inhibitors have an effect on blood pressure that is less in black patients than in non-blacks. In addition, ACE inhibitors (for which adequate data are available) cause a higher rate of angioedema in black than in non-black patients. (See **WARNINGS, Angioedema**.)

Heart Failure Post Myocardial Infarction

Ramipril is indicated in stable patients who have demonstrated clinical signs of congestive heart failure within the first few days after sustaining acute myocardial infarction. Administration of ramipril to such patients has been shown to decrease the risk of death (principally cardiovascular death) and to decrease the risks of failure-related hospitalization and progression to severe/resistant heart failure. (See **CLINICAL PHARMACOLOGY, Heart Failure Post Myocardial Infarction** for details and limitations of the survival trial.)

CONTRAINDICATIONS

ALTACE is contraindicated in patients who are hypersensitive to this product or any other angiotensin converting enzyme inhibitor (e.g., a patient who has experienced angioedema during therapy with any other ACE inhibitor).

WARNINGS

Anaphylactoid and Possibly Related Reactions

Presumably because angiotensin-converting enzyme inhibitors affect the metabolism of eicosanoids and polypeptides, including endogenous bradykinin, patients receiving ACE inhibitors (including ALTACE) may be subject to a variety of adverse reactions, some of them serious.

Head and Neck Angioedema

Patients with a history of angioedema unrelated to ACE inhibitor therapy may be at increased risk of angioedema while receiving an ACE inhibitor. (See also **CONTRAINDICATIONS**.)

Angioedema of the face, extremities, lips, tongue, glottis, and larynx has been reported in patients treated with angiotensin converting enzyme inhibitors. Angioedema associated with laryngeal edema can be fatal. If laryngeal stridor or angioedema of the face, tongue, or glottis occurs, treatment with ALTACE should be discontinued and appropriate therapy instituted immediately. **Where there is involvement of the tongue, glottis, or larynx, likely to cause airway obstruction, appropriate therapy, e.g., subcutaneous epinephrine solution 1:1,000 (0.3 ml to 0.5 ml) should be promptly administered.** (See **ADVERSE REACTIONS**.)

Intestinal Angioedema

Intestinal angioedema has been reported in patients treated with ACE inhibitors. These patients presented with abdominal pain (with or without nausea or vomiting); in some cases there was no prior history of facial angioedema and C-1 esterase levels were normal. The angioedema was diagnosed by procedures including abdominal CT scan or ultrasound, or at surgery, and symptoms resolved after stopping the ACE inhibitor. Intestinal angioedema should be included in the differential diagnosis of patients on ACE inhibitors presenting with abdominal pain.

In a large U.S. postmarketing study, angioedema (defined as reports of angio, face, larynx, tongue, or throat edema) was reported in 3/1523 (0.20%) of black patients and in 8/8680 (0.09%) of white patients. These rates were not different statistically.

Anaphylactoid reactions during desensitization: Two patients undergoing desensitizing treatment with hymenoptera venom while receiving ACE inhibitors sustained life-threatening anaphylactoid reactions. In the same patients, these reactions were avoided when ACE inhibitors were temporarily withheld, but they reappeared upon inadvertent rechallenge.

Anaphylactoid reactions during membrane exposure: Anaphylactoid reactions have been reported in patients dialyzed with high-flux membranes and treated concomitantly with an ACE inhibitor. Anaphylactoid reactions have also been reported in patients undergoing low-density lipoprotein apheresis with dextran sulfate absorption.

Hypotension

ALTACE can cause symptomatic hypotension, after either the initial dose or a later dose when the dosage has been increased. Like other ACE inhibitors, ramipril has been only rarely associated with hypotension in uncomplicated hypertensive patients. Symptomatic hypotension is most likely to occur in patients who have been volume- and/or salt-depleted as a result of prolonged diuretic therapy, dietary salt restriction, dialysis, diarrhea, or vomiting. Volume and/or salt depletion should be corrected before initiating therapy with ALTACE.

In patients with congestive heart failure, with or without associated renal insufficiency, ACE inhibitor therapy may cause excessive hypotension, which may be associated with oliguria or azotemia and, rarely, with acute renal failure and death. In such patients, ALTACE therapy should be started under close medical supervision; they should be followed closely for the first 2 weeks of treatment and whenever the dose of ramipril or diuretic is increased.

If hypotension occurs, the patient should be placed in a supine position and, if necessary, treated with intravenous infusion of physiological saline. ALTACE treatment usually can be continued following restoration of blood pressure and volume.

Hepatic Failure

Rarely, ACE inhibitors have been associated with a syndrome that starts with cholestatic jaundice and progresses to fulminant hepatic necrosis and (sometimes) death. The mechanism of this syndrome is not understood. Patients receiving ACE inhibitors who develop jaundice or marked elevations of hepatic enzymes should discontinue the ACE inhibitor and receive appropriate medical follow-up.

Neutropenia/Agranulocytosis

As with other ACE inhibitors, rarely, a mild – in isolated cases severe – reduction in the red blood cell count and hemoglobin content, white blood cell or platelet count may develop. In isolated cases, agranulocytosis, pancytopenia, and bone marrow depression may occur. Hematological reactions to ACE inhibitors are more likely to occur in patients with collagen vascular disease (e.g. systemic lupus erythematosus, scleroderma) and renal impairment. Monitoring of white blood cell counts should be considered in patients with collagen-vascular disease, especially if the disease is associated with impaired renal function.

Fetal/Neonatal Morbidity and Mortality

ACE inhibitors can cause fetal and neonatal morbidity and death when administered to pregnant women. Several dozen cases have been reported in the world literature. When pregnancy is detected, ACE inhibitors should be discontinued as soon as possible.

The use of ACE inhibitors during the second and third trimesters of pregnancy has been associated with fetal and neonatal injury, including hypotension, neonatal skull hypoplasia, anuria, reversible or irreversible renal failure, and death. Oligohydramnios has also been reported, presumably resulting from decreased fetal renal function; oligohydramnios in this setting has been associated with fetal limb contractures, craniofacial deformation, and hypoplastic lung development. Prematurity, intrauterine growth retardation, and patent ductus arteriosus have also been reported, although it is not clear whether these occurrences were due to the ACE inhibitor exposure.

These adverse effects do not appear to have resulted from intrauterine ACE inhibitor exposure that has been limited to the first trimester. Mothers whose embryos and fetuses are exposed to ACE inhibitors only during the first trimester should be so informed. Nonetheless, when patients become pregnant, physicians should make every effort to discontinue the use of ALTACE as soon as possible.

Rarely (probably less often than once in every thousand pregnancies), no alternative to ACE inhibitors will be found. In these rare cases, the mothers should be apprised of the potential hazards to their fetuses, and serial ultrasound examinations should be performed to assess the intraamniotic environment.

If oligohydramnios is observed, ALTACE should be discontinued unless it is considered life-saving for the mother. Contraction stress testing (CST), a non-stress test (NST), or biophysical profiling (BPP) may be appropriate, depending upon the week of pregnancy. Patients and physicians should be aware, however, that oligohydramnios may not appear until after the fetus has sustained irreversible injury.

Infants with histories of *in utero* exposure to ACE inhibitors should be closely observed for hypotension, oliguria, and hyperkalemia. If oliguria occurs, attention should be directed toward support of blood pressure and renal perfusion. Exchange transfusion or dialysis may be required as means of reversing hypotension and/or substituting for disordered renal function. ALTACE which crosses the placenta can be removed from the neonatal circulation by these means, but limited experience has not shown that such removal is central to the treatment of these infants.

No teratogenic effects of ALTACE were seen in studies of pregnant rats, rabbits, and cynomolgus monkeys. On a body surface area basis, the doses used were up to approximately 400 times (in rats and monkeys) and 2 times (in rabbits) the recommended human dose.

PRECAUTIONS

Impaired Renal Function: As a consequence of inhibiting the renin-angiotensin-aldosterone system, changes in renal function may be anticipated in susceptible individuals. In patients with severe congestive heart failure whose renal function may depend on the activity of the renin-angiotensin-aldosterone system, treatment with angiotensin converting enzyme inhibitors, including ALTACE, may be associated with oliguria and/or progressive azotemia and (rarely) with acute renal failure and/or death.

In hypertensive patients with unilateral or bilateral renal artery stenosis, increases in blood urea nitrogen and serum creatinine may occur. Experience with another angiotensin converting enzyme inhibitor suggests that these increases are usually reversible upon discontinuation of ALTACE and/or diuretic therapy. In such patients renal function should be monitored during the first few weeks of therapy.

Continued on next page

Altace—Cont.

Some hypertensive patients with no apparent pre-existing renal vascular disease have developed increases in blood urea nitrogen and serum creatinine, usually minor and transient, especially when ALTACE has been given concomitantly with a diuretic. This is more likely to occur in patients with pre-existing renal impairment. Dosage reduction of ALTACE and/or discontinuation of the diuretic may be required.

Evaluation of the hypertensive patient should always include assessment of renal function. (See **DOSAGE AND ADMINISTRATION.**)

Hyperkalemia: In clinical trials, hyperkalemia (serum potassium greater than 5.7 mEq/L) occurred in approximately 1% of hypertensive patients receiving ALTACE (ramipril). In most cases, these were isolated values, which resolved despite continued therapy. None of these patients was discontinued from the trials because of hyperkalemia. Risk factors for the development of hyperkalemia include renal insufficiency, diabetes mellitus, and the concomitant use of potassium-sparing diuretics, potassium supplements, and/or potassium-containing salt substitutes, which should be used cautiously, if at all, with ALTACE. (See **Drug Interactions.**)

Cough: Presumably due to the inhibition of the degradation of endogenous bradykinin, persistent nonproductive cough has been reported with all ACE inhibitors, always resolving after discontinuation of therapy. ACE inhibitor-induced cough should be considered in the differential diagnosis of cough.

Impaired Liver Function: Since ramipril is primarily metabolized by hepatic esterases to its active moiety, ramiprilat, patients with impaired liver function could develop markedly elevated plasma levels of ramipril. No formal pharmacokinetic studies have been carried out in hypertensive patients with impaired liver function. However, since the renin-angiotensin system may be activated in patients with severe liver cirrhosis and/or ascites, particular caution should be exercised in treating these patients.

Surgery/Anesthesia: In patients undergoing surgery or during anesthesia with agents that produce hypotension, ramipril may block angiotensin II formation that would otherwise occur secondary to compensatory renin release. Hypotension that occurs as a result of this mechanism can be corrected by volume expansion.

Information for Patients

Pregnancy: Female patients of childbearing age should be told about the consequences of second- and third-trimester exposure to ACE inhibitors, and they should also be told that these consequences do not appear to have resulted from intrauterine ACE inhibitor exposure that has been limited to the first trimester. These patients should be asked to report pregnancies to their physicians as soon as possible.

Angioedema: Angioedema, including laryngeal edema, can occur with treatment with ACE inhibitors, especially following the first dose. Patients should be so advised and told to report immediately any signs or symptoms suggesting angioedema (swelling of face, eyes, lips, or tongue, or difficulty in breathing) and to take no more drug until they have consulted with the prescribing physician.

Symptomatic Hypotension: Patients should be cautioned that lightheadedness can occur, especially during the first days of therapy, and it should be reported. Patients should be told that if syncope occurs, ALTACE should be discontinued until the physician has been consulted.

All patients should be cautioned that inadequate fluid intake or excessive perspiration, diarrhea, or vomiting can lead to an excessive fall in blood pressure, with the same consequences of lightheadedness and possible syncope.

Hyperkalemia: Patients should be told not to use salt substitutes containing potassium without consulting their physician.

Neutropenia: Patients should be told to promptly report any indication of infection (e.g., sore throat, fever), which could be a sign of neutropenia.

Drug Interactions

With nonsteroidal anti-inflammatory agents: Rarely, concomitant treatment with ACE inhibitors and nonsteroidal anti-inflammatory agents have been associated with worsening of renal failure and an increase in serum potassium.

With diuretics: Patients on diuretics, especially those in whom diuretic therapy was recently instituted, may occasionally experience an excessive reduction of blood pressure after initiation of therapy with ALTACE. The possibility of hypotensive effects with ALTACE can be minimized by either discontinuing the diuretic or increasing the salt intake prior to initiation of treatment with ALTACE. If this is not possible, the starting dose should be reduced. (See **DOSAGE AND ADMINISTRATION.**)

With potassium supplements and potassium-sparing diuretics: ALTACE can attenuate potassium loss caused by thiazide diuretics. Potassium-sparing diuretics (spironolactone, amiloride, triamterene, and others) or potassium supplements can increase the risk of hyperkalemia. Therefore, if concomitant use of such agents is indicated, they should be given with caution, and the patient's serum potassium should be monitored frequently.

With lithium: Increased serum lithium levels and symptoms of lithium toxicity have been reported in patients receiving ACE inhibitors during therapy with lithium. These drugs should be coadministered with caution, and frequent monitoring of serum lithium levels is recommended. If a diuretic is also used, the risk of lithium toxicity may be increased.

Other: Neither ALTACE nor its metabolites have been found to interact with food, digoxin, antacid, furosemide, cimetidine, indomethacin, and simvastatin. The combination of ALTACE and propranolol showed no adverse effects on dynamic parameters (blood pressure and heart rate). The co-administration of ALTACE and warfarin did not adversely affect the anticoagulant effects of the latter drug. Additionally, co-administration of ALTACE with phenprocoumon did not affect minimum phenprocoumon levels or interfere with the subjects' state of anti-coagulation.

Carcinogenesis, Mutagenesis, Impairment of Fertility

No evidence of a tumorigenic effect was found when ramipril was given by gavage to rats for up to 24 months at doses of up to 500 mg/kg/day or to mice for up to 18 months at doses of up to 1000 mg/kg/day. (For either species, these doses are about 200 times the maximum recommended human dose when compared on the basis of body surface area.) No mutagenic activity was detected in the Ames test in bacteria, the micronucleus test in mice, unscheduled DNA synthesis in a human cell line, or a forward gene-mutation assay in a Chinese hamster ovary cell line. Several metabolites and degradation products of ramipril were also negative in the Ames test. A study in rats with dosages as great as 500 mg/kg/day did not produce adverse effects on fertility.

Pregnancy

Pregnancy Categories C (first trimester) and D (second and third trimesters). See **WARNINGS: Fetal/Neonatal Morbidity and Mortality.**

Nursing Mothers

Ingestion of single 10 mg oral dose of ALTACE resulted in undetectable amounts of ramipril and its metabolites in breast milk. However, because multiple doses may produce low milk concentrations that are not predictable from single doses, women receiving ALTACE should not breast feed.

Geriatric Use

Of the total number of patients who received ramipril in US clinical studies of ALTACE 11.0% were 65 and over while 0.2% were 75 and over. No overall differences in effectiveness or safety were observed between these patients and younger patients, and other reported clinical experience has not identified differences in responses between the elderly and younger patients, but greater sensitivity of some older individuals cannot be ruled out.

One pharmacokinetic study conducted in hospitalized elderly patients indicated that peak ramiprilat levels and area under the plasma concentration time curve (AUC) for ramiprilat are higher in older patients.

Pediatric Use

Safety and effectiveness in pediatric patients have not been established. Irreversible kidney damae has been observed in very young rats given a single dose of rampipril.

ADVERSE REACTIONS

Hypertension

ALTACE has been evaluated for safety in over 4,000 patients with hypertension; of these, 1,230 patients were studied in US controlled trials, and 1,107 were studied in foreign controlled trials. Almost 700 of these patients were treated for at least one year. The overall incidence of reported adverse events was similar in ALTACE and placebo patients. The most frequent clinical side effects (possibly or probably related to study drug) reported by patients receiving ALTACE in US placebo-controlled trials were: headache (5.4%), "dizziness" (2.2%) and fatigue or asthenia (2.0%), but only the last was more common in ALTACE patients than in patients given placebo. Generally, the side effects were mild and transient, and there was no relation to total dosage within the range of 1.25 to 20 mg. Discontinuation of therapy because of a side effect was required in approximately 3% of US patients treated with ALTACE. The most common reasons for discontinuation were: cough (1.0%), "dizziness" (0.5%), and impotence (0.4%).

Of observed side effects considered possibly or probably related to study drug that occurred in US placebo-controlled trials in more than 1% of patients treated with ALTACE, only asthenia (fatigue) was more common on Altace than placebo (2% vs. 1%).

PATIENTS IN US PLACEBO CONTROLLED STUDIES

	ALTACE (n=651)		Placebo (n=286)	
	n	%	n	%
Asthenia (Fatigue)	13	2	2	1

In placebo-controlled trials, there was also an excess of upper respiratory infection and flu syndrome in the ramipril group, not attributed at that time to ramipril. As these studies were carried out before the relationship of cough to ACE inhibitors was recognized, some of these events may represent ramipril-induced cough. In a later 1-year study, increased cough was seen in almost 12% of ramipril patients, with about 4% of patients requiring discontinuation of treatment.

Heart Failure Post Myocardial Infarction

Adverse reactions (except laboratory abnormalities) considered possibly/probably related to study drug that occurred in more than one percent of patients and more frequently on ramipril are shown below. The incidences represent the experiences from the AIRE study. The follow-up time was between 6 and 46 months for this study.

Percentage of Patients with Adverse Events Possibly/ Probably Related to Study Drug
Placebo-Controlled (AIRE) Mortality Study

Adverse Event	Ramipril (n=1004)	Placebo (n=982)
Hypotension	11	5
Cough Increased	8	4
Dizziness	4	3
Angina Pectoris	3	2
Nausea	2	1
Postural Hypotension	2	1
Syncope	2	1
Vomiting	2	0.5
Vertigo	2	0.7
Abnormal Kidney Function	1	0.5
Diarrhea	1	0.4

HOPE Study:

Safety data in the HOPE trial were collected as reasons for discontinuation or temporary interruption of treatment. The incidence of cough was similar to that seen in the AIRE trial. The rate of angioedema was the same as in previous clinical trials (see **WARNINGS**).

	RAMIPRIL (N=4645)	PLACEBO (N=4652)
	%	%
Discontinuation at any time	34	32
Permanent discontinuation	29	28
Reasons for stopping Cough	7	2
Hypotension or Dizziness	1.9	1.5
Angioedema	0.3	0.1

Other adverse experiences reported in controlled clinical trials (in less than 1% of ramipril patients), or rarer events seen in postmarketing experience, include the following (in some, a causal relationship to drug use is uncertain):

Body As a Whole: Anaphylactoid reactions. (See **WARNINGS.**)

Cardiovascular: Symptomatic hypotension (reported in 0.5% of patients in US trials) (See **WARNINGS** and **PRECAUTIONS**), syncope and palpitations.

Hematologic: hemolytic anemia and thrombocytopenia.

Renal: Some hypertensive patients with no apparent pre-existing renal disease have developed minor, usually transient, increases in blood urea nitrogen and serum creatinine when taking ALTACE, particularly when ALTACE was given concomitantly with a diuretic. (See **WARNINGS.**) Acute renal failure.

Angioneurotic Edema: Angioneurotic edema has been reported in 0.3% of patients in US clinical trials. (See **WARNINGS.**)

Gastrointestinal: Pancreatitis, abdominal pain (sometimes with enzyme changes suggesting pancreatitis), anorexia, constipation, diarrhea, dry mouth, dyspepsia, dysphagia, gastroenteritis, hepatitis, increased salivation and taste disturbance.

Dermatologic: Apparent hypersensitivity reactions (manifested by urticaria, pruritus, or rash, with or without fever), photosensitivity, purpura, onycholysis, pemphigus, pemphigoid, erythema multiforme, toxic epidermal necrolysis, and Stevens-Johnson syndrome.

Neurologic and Psychiatric: Anxiety, amnesia, convulsions, depression, hearing loss, insomnia, nervousness, neuralgia, neuropathy, paresthesia, somnolence, tinnitus, tremor, vertigo, and vision disturbances.

Miscellaneous: As with other ACE inhibitors, a symptom complex has been reported which may include a positive ANA, an elevated erythrocyte sedimentation rate, arthralgia/arthritis, myalgia, fever, vasculitis, eosinophilia, photosensitivity, rash and other dermatologic manifestations. Additionally, as with other ACE inhibitors, eosinophilic pneumonitis has been reported.

Fetal/Neonatal Morbidity and Mortality. See **WARNINGS: Fetal/Neonatal Morbidity and Mortality.**

Other: arthralgia, arthritis, dyspnea, edema, epistaxis, (see **PRECAUTIONS, Drug Interactions**), impotence, increased sweating, malaise, myalgia, and weight gain.

Clinical Laboratory Test Findings:

Creatinine and Blood Urea Nitrogen: Increases in creatinine levels occurred in 1.2% of patients receiving ALTACE alone, and in 1.5% of patients receiving ALTACE and a diuretic. Increases in blood urea nitrogen levels occurred in 0.5% of patients receiving ALTACE alone and in 3% of patients receiving ALTACE with a diuretic. None of these increases required discontinuation of treatment. Increases in these laboratory values are more likely to occur in patients with renal insufficiency or those pretreated with a diuretic and, based on experience with other ACE inhibitors, would be expected to be especially likely in patients with renal artery stenosis. (See **WARNINGS** and **PRECAUTIONS.**)

Since ramipril decreases aldosterone secretion, elevation of serum potassium can occur. Potassium supplements and potassium-sparing diuretics should be given with caution, and the patient's serum potassium should be monitored frequently. (See **WARNINGS** and **PRECAUTIONS.**)

Hemoglobin and Hematocrit: Decreases in hemoglobin or hematocrit (a low value and a decrease of 5 g/dl or 5% respectively) were rare, occurring in 0.4% of patients receiving ALTACE alone and in 1.5% of patients receiving ALTACE plus a diuretic. No US patients discontinued treatment because of decreases in hemoglobin or hematocrit.

Other (causal relationships unknown): Clinically important changes in standard laboratory tests were rarely associated with ALTACE administration. Elevations of liver enzymes, serum bilirubin, uric acid, and blood glucose have been reported, as have cases of hyponatremia and scattered incidents of leukopenia, eosinophilia, and proteinuria. In US trials, less than 0.2% of patients discontinued treatment for laboratory abnormalities; all of these were cases of proteinuria or abnormal liver-function tests.

OVERDOSAGE

Single oral doses in rats and mice of 10–11 g/kg resulted in significant lethality. In dogs, oral doses as high as 1 g/kg induced only mild gastrointestinal distress. Limited data on human overdosage are available. The most likely clinical manifestations would be symptoms attributable to hypotension.

Laboratory determinations of serum levels of ramipril and its metabolites are not widely available, and such determinations have, in any event, no established role in the management of ramipril overdose.

No data are available to suggest physiological maneuvers (e.g., maneuvers to change the pH of the urine) that might accelerate elimination of ramipril and its metabolites. Similarly, it is not known which, if any, of these substances can be usefully removed from the body by hemodialysis.

Angiotensin II could presumably serve as a specific antagonist-antidote in the setting of ramipril overdose, but angiotensin II is essentially unavailable outside of scattered research facilities. Because the hypotensive effect of ramipril is achieved through vasodilation and effective hypovolemia, it is reasonable to treat ramipril overdose by infusion of normal saline solution.

DOSAGE AND ADMINISTRATION

Blood pressure decreases associated with any dose of ALTACE depend, in part, on the presence or absence of volume depletion (e.g., past and current diuretic use) or the presence or absence of renal artery stenosis. If such circumstances are suspected to be present, the initial starting dose should be 1.25 mg once daily.

Reduction in Risk of Myocardial Infarction, Stroke, and Death from Cardiovascular Causes

ALTACE should be given at an initial dose of 2.5 mg, once a day for 1 week, 5 mg, once a day for the next 3 weeks, and then increased as tolerated, to a maintenance dose of 10 mg, once a day. If the patient is hypertensive or recently post myocardial infarction, it can also be given as a divided dose.

Hypertension

The recommended initial dose for patients not receiving a diuretic is 2.5 mg once a day. Dosage should be adjusted according to the blood pressure response. The usual maintenance dosage range is 2.5 to 20 mg per day administered as a single dose or in two equally divided doses. In some patients treated once daily, the antihypertensive effect may diminish toward the end of the dosing interval. In such patients, an increase in dosage or twice daily administration should be considered. If blood pressure is not controlled with ALTACE alone, a diuretic can be added.

Heart Failure Post Myocardial Infarction

For the treatment of post-infarction patients who have shown signs of congestive failure, the recommended starting dose of ALTACE is 2.5 mg twice daily (5 mg per day). A patient who becomes hypotensive at this dose may be switched to 1.25 mg twice daily, and after one week at the starting dose, patients should then be titrated (if tolerated) toward a target dose of 5 mg twice daily, with dosage increases being about 3 weeks apart.

After the initial dose of ALTACE, the patient should be observed under medical supervision for at least two hours and until blood pressure has stabilized for at least an additional hour. (See **WARNINGS** and **PRECAUTIONS, Drug Interactions**.) If possible, the dose of any concomitant diuretic should be reduced which may diminish the likelihood of hypotension. The appearance of hypotension after the initial dose of ALTACE does not preclude subsequent careful dose titration with the drug, following effective management of the hypotension.

The ALTACE Capsule is usually swallowed whole. The ALTACE Capsule can also be opened and the contents sprinkled on a small amount (about 4 oz.) of apple sauce or mixed in 4 oz. (120 ml) of water or apple juice. To be sure that ramipril is not lost when such a mixture is used, the mixture should be consumed in its entirety. The described mixtures can be pre-prepared and stored for up to 24 hours at room temperature or up to 48 hours under refrigeration.

Concomitant administration of ALTACE with potassium supplements, potassium salt substitutes, or potassium-sparing diuretics can lead to increases of serum potassium. (See **PRECAUTIONS**.)

In patients who are currently being treated with a diuretic, symptomatic hypotension occasionally can occur following the initial dose of ALTACE. To reduce the likelihood of hypotension, the diuretic should, if possible, be discontinued two to three days prior to beginning therapy with ALTACE. (See **WARNINGS**.) Then, if blood pressure is not controlled with ALTACE alone, diuretic therapy should be resumed.

If the diuretic cannot be discontinued, an initial dose of 1.25 mg ALTACE should be used to avoid excess hypotension.

Dosage Adjustment in Renal Impairment

In patients with creatinine clearance <40 ml/min/1.73m^2 (serum creatinine approximately >2.5 mg/dl) doses only 25% of those normally used should be expected to induce full therapeutic levels of ramiprilat. (See **CLINICAL PHARMACOLOGY**.)

Hypertension: For patients with hypertension and renal impairment, the recommended initial dose is 1.25 mg ALTACE once daily. Dosage may be titrated upward until blood pressure is controlled or to a maximum total daily dose of 5 mg.

Heart Failure Post Myocardial Infarction: For patients with heart failure and renal impairment, the recommended initial dose is 1.25 mg ALTACE once daily. The dose may be increased to 1.25 mg b.i.d. and up to a maximum dose of 2.5 mg b.i.d. depending upon clinical response and tolerability.

HOW SUPPLIED

ALTACE is available in potencies of 1.25 mg, 2.5 mg, 5 mg, and 10 mg in hard gelatin capsules.

ALTACE 1.25 mg capsules are supplied as yellow, hard gelatin capsules in bottles of 100 (NDC 61570-110-01), and Unit Dose packs of 100 (NDC 61570-110-56).

ALTACE 2.5 mg capsules are supplied as orange, hard gelatin capsules in bottles of 100 (NDC 61570-111-01), 500 (NDC 61570-111-05), 1000 (NDC 61570-111-10) and Unit Dose packs of 100 (NDC 61570-111-56), and Bulk pack of 5000's (NDC 61570-111-50).

ALTACE 5 mg capsules are supplied as red, hard gelatin capsules in bottles of 100 (NDC 61570-112-01), 500 (NDC 61570-112-05), 1000 (NDC 61570-112-10) and Unit Dose packs of 100 (NDC 61570-112-56), and Bulk pack of 5000's (NDC 61570-112-50).

ALTACE 10 mg capsules are supplied as Process Blue, hard gelatin capsules in bottles of 100 (NDC 61570-120-01), 500 (NDC 61570-120-05), 1000 (NDC 61570-120-10).

Dispense in well-closed container with safety closure.

Store at controlled room temperature (59° to 86°F).

℞ only.

Prescribing information as of April 2004.

Monarch Pharmaceuticals®

Distributed by: Monarch Pharmaceuticals, Inc., Bristol, TN 37620

(A wholly owned subsidiary of King Pharmaceuticals, Inc.)

Manufactured by: King Pharmaceuticals, Inc., Bristol, TN 37620

3000246

Shown in Product Identification Guide, page 319

APLISOL® ℞

[*ăp' lĭsōl*]

(Tuberculin Purified Protein Derivative, Diluted [Stabilized Solution])
Diagnostic Antigen
For Intradermal Injection Only

DESCRIPTION

Aplisol (tuberculin PPD, diluted) is a sterile aqueous solution of a purified protein fraction for intradermal administration as an aid in the diagnosis of tuberculosis. The solution is stabilized with polysorbate (Tween) 80, buffered with potassium and sodium phosphates and contains approximately 0.35% phenol as a preservative. This product is ready for immediate use without further dilution.

The purified protein fraction is isolated from culture media filtrates of a human strain of *Mycobacterium tuberculosis* by the method of F.B. Seibert.[1,2] Tuberculin PPD, diluted, is prepared from Tuberculin PPD Powder Master Lot 154616 which is clinically bioequivalent in potency to the standard PPD-S* (5 TU** per 0.1mL) of the U.S. Public Health Service, National Centers for Disease Control. This product is made from a single master lot (No. 154616) to eliminate lot to lot variation inherent in manufacturing.

The potency of each lot of tuberculin PPD, diluted is determined in sensitized guinea pigs.

CLINICAL PHARMACOLOGY

In the United States, the prevalence of *Mycobacterium tuberculosis* infection and active disease varies for different segments of the population; however, the risk for *M. tuberculosis* infection in the overall population is low. Tuberculosis (TB) case rates declined steadily for decades in the United States. However, in 1985 the TB case rate stabilized and subsequently increased through 1992, accompanied by a 14% increase in the TB mortality rate in 1988. This has been attributed to several complex social and medical factors, including the human immunodeficiency virus (HIV) epidemic, the occurrence of TB in foreign-born persons from countries that have a high prevalence of TB, the emergence of drug-resistant strains of TB, and the transmission of *M. tuberculosis* in congregate settings. (e.g., health-care facilities, correctional facilities, drug-treatment centers, and homeless shelters). Because the overall risk of acquiring M. tuberculosis is low for the total U.S. population, the primary strategy for preventing and controlling TB in the United States is to minimize the risk of transmission by the early identification and treatment of patients who have active infectious TB, finding and screening persons who have been in contact with active infectious TB patients and screening high-risk populations.

Tuberculin PPD is recommended by the American Lung Association as an aid in the detection of infection with *Mycobacterium tuberculosis*.[3,4] After a person becomes infected with mycobacteria, T lymphocytes proliferate and become sensitized. These sensitized T cells enter the bloodstream and circulate for months or years. This sensitization process occurs principally in the regional lymph nodes and may take 2–10 weeks to develop following infection. Once acquired, tuberculin sensitivity tends to persist, although it often wanes with time and advancing age. The injection of tuberculin into the skin stimulates the lymphocytes and activates the series of events leading to a delayed-type hypersensitivity (DTH) response. This response is called "delayed" because the reaction becomes evident hours after injection. Dermal reactivity involves vasodilation, edema, and the infiltration of lymphocytes, basophils, monocytes, and neutrophils into the site of antigen injection. Antigen-specific T lymphocytes proliferate and release lymphokines, which mediate the accumulation of other cells at the site. The area of induration reflects DTH activity.[5] In most tuberculin-sensitive individuals, the delayed hypersensitivity reaction is evident 5–6 hours after administration of a tuberculin skin test and is maximal 48–72 hours. In geriatric patients or in patients receiving a tuberculin skin test for the first time, the reaction may develop more slowly and may not be maximal until after 72 hours.[6] Because their immune systems are immature, many neonates and infants < 6 weeks of age, who are infected with *M. tuberculosis*, do not react at all to tuberculin tests.[5]

Immediate erythematous or other hypersensitivity reactions to tuberculin or the constituents of the diluent may occur at the injection site.

A possible decrease in responsiveness to skin testing may occur in the presence of tuberculous infections including viral infections, live virus vaccination, overwhelming tuberculosis, other bacterial infections, drugs and malignancy.

Tuberculin skin-test results are also less reliable as CD4 counts decline in HIV infected individuals.[3]

The 5TU dose of Tuberculin PPD intradermally (Mantoux) is recommended as the standard tuberculin test, and Tuberculin PPD is recommended by the American Lung Association as an aid in the detection of infection with *Mycobacterium tuberculosis*. Reactions to the Mantoux test are interpreted on the basis of a quantitative measurement of the response to a specific dose (5 TU PPD-S or equivalent) of Tuberculin PPD.[7]

To determine that Tuberculin PPD Master Lot 154616 is clinically bioequivalent in potency to standard 5TU PPD-S*, 3 dose-response studies were conducted in the following populations (1) persons with a history of bacteriologically confirmed TB; (2) healthy volunteers in a geographical region of low endemicity of atypical mycobacterial infection; and (3) healthy volunteers in a geographical location of high endemicity of atypical mycobacterial infection.

INDICATIONS AND USAGE

Tuberculin PPD is recommended by the American Lung Association as an aid in the detection of infection with *Mycobacterium tuberculosis*. The standard tuberculin test recommended employs the intradermal (Mantoux) test using a 5 TU dose of tuberculin PPD.[7] The 0.1 mL test dose of Aplisol (tuberculin PPD, diluted) is equivalent to the 5 TU dose recommended as clinically established and standardized with PPD-S. Tuberculin skin testing is not contraindicated for persons who have been vaccinated with BCG and the skin-test results of such persons are used to support or exclude the diagnosis of *M. tuberculosis* infections.[4] HIV infection is a strong risk factor for the development of TB disease in persons having TB infection. All HIV-infected persons should receive a PPD-tuberculin skin test.[3]

CONTRAINDICATIONS

Aplisol is contraindicated in patients with known hypersensitivity or allergy to Aplisol or any of its components. Aplisol should not be administered to persons who have previously experienced a severe reaction (e.g., vesiculation, ulceration, or necrosis) because of the severity of reactions that may occur at the test site.

WARNINGS

Aplisol should not be administered to persons who previously experienced a severe reaction (e.g., vesiculation, ulceration, or necrosis) because of the severity of reactions that may occur at the test site (see **CONTRAINDICATIONS**).

Not all infected persons will have a delayed hypersensitivity reaction to a tuberculin test. A number of factors have been reported to cause a decreased ability to respond to the tuberculin test, such as the presence of tuberculous infection or viral infections (measles, mumps, chickenpox, and HIV), live virus vaccination (measles, mumps, rubella, oral polio and yellow fever), overwhelming tuberculosis, other bacterial infections, drugs (corticosteroids and other immunosuppressive agents) and malignancy.[8,9]

Any condition that impairs or attenuates cell mediated immunity potentially can cause a false negative reaction.

Tuberculin skin test results are less reliable in HIV-infected individuals as CD4 counts decline (see **CLINICAL PHARMACOLOGY**).[3]

Avoid injecting tuberculin subcutaneously. If this occurs, no local reaction develops, but a general febrile reaction and/or acute inflammation around old tuberculous lesions may occur in highly sensitive individuals.

PRECAUTIONS

General

The predictive value of the tuberculin skin test depends on the prevalence of infection with *M. tuberculosis* and the relative prevalence of cross-reactions with nontuberculous mycobacteria.[9,10]

Continued on next page

Aplisol—Cont.

A separate, sterile, single-use disposable syringe and needle should be used for each individual patient to prevent possible transmission of serum hepatitis virus and other infectious agents from one person to another.
Special care should be taken to ensure that the product is injected intradermally and not into a blood vessel.
Before administration of Aplisol, a review of the patient's history with respect to possible immediate-type hypersensitivity to the product, determination of previous use of Aplisol and the presence of any contraindication to the test should be made (see **CONTRAINDICATIONS**).
As with any biological product, epinephrine should be immediately available in case an anaphylactoid or acute hypersensitivity reaction occurs.
Failure to store and handle Aplisol as recommended may result in a loss of potency and inaccurate test results.[11,8]
Reactivity to the test may be depressed or suppressed for as long as 5–6 weeks in individuals following immunization with certain live viral vaccines, viral infections or discontinuation of corticosteroids or immunosuppressive agents.[8,9]

Information to Patients
Patients should be instructed to report adverse events such as vesiculation, ulceration or necrosis which may occur at the test site in highly sensitive individuals. Patients should be informed that pain, pruritus and discomfort may occur at injection site.
Patient should be informed of the need to return to their physician or health care provider for the reading of the test and of the need to keep and maintain a personal immunization record.

Drug Interactions
In patients who are receiving corticosteroids or immunosuppressive agents, reactivity to the test may be depressed or suppressed. This reduced reactivity may be present for as long as 5–6 weeks after discontinuation of therapy (see **PRECAUTIONS—General**).[9]
The reactivity to PPD may be temporarily depressed by certain live virus vaccines. Therefore, if a tuberculin test is to be performed, it should be administered either before or simultaneously with the use of oral polio and/or injection of measles, mumps and rubella vaccines in combined form or as separate antigens, or testing should be postponed for 4–6 weeks.[10]

Carcinogenesis, Mutagenesis, Impairment of Fertility
No long term studies have been conducted in animals or in humans to evaluate carcinogenic or mutagenic potential or effects on fertility with Aplisol.

Pregnancy
Teratogenic effects: Pregnancy Category C. Animal reproduction studies have not been conducted with Aplisol. It is also not known whether Aplisol can cause fetal harm when administered to a pregnant woman or can affect the reproduction capacity. Aplisol should be given to a pregnant woman only if clearly needed.
However, the risk of unrecognized tuberculosis and the postpartum contact between a mother with active disease and an infant leaves the infant in grave danger of tuberculosis and complications such as tuberculous meningitis. Although there have not been any reported adverse effects upon the fetus recognized as being due to tuberculosis skin testing, the prescribing physician will want to consider if the potential benefits outweigh the possible risks for performing the tuberculin test on a pregnant woman or a woman of childbearing age, particularly in certain high risk populations.
Tuberculin skin testing is considered valid and safe throughout pregnancy.[3]

ADVERSE REACTIONS

In highly sensitive individuals, strongly positive reactions including vesiculation, ulceration or necrosis may occur at the test site; however, there were no reports of these reactions for the period 1995 through 1998. Cold packs or topical steroid preparations may be employed for symptomatic relief of the associated pain, pruritus and discomfort.
Strongly positive test reactions may result in scarring at the test site.
Immediate erythematous or other reactions may occur at the injection site.

DOSAGE AND ADMINISTRATION

Aplisol vials should be inspected visually for both particulate matter and discoloration prior to administration and discarded if either is seen. Vials in use for more than 30 days should be discarded.

Standard Method (Mantoux Test)
The Mantoux test is performed by **intradermally** injecting with a syringe and needle exactly 0.1mL of Aplisol. The result is read 48 to 72 hours later and **induration only is considered in interpreting the test.** Induration is a hard, raised area with clearly defined margins at and around the injection site. Erythema may develop at the injection site but has no diagnostic value. The standard test is performed as follows:

1. The site of the test is usually the flexor or dorsal surface of the forearm about 4″ below the elbow. Other skin sites may be used, but the flexor surface of the forearm is preferred. The use of a skin area free of lesions and away from any veins is recommended.[7]
2. The skin at the injection site is cleansed with 70% alcohol and allowed to dry.
3. The test material is administered with a tuberculin syringe (0.5 or 1.0mL) fitted with a short (1/2″) 26 or 27 gauge needle.
4. A separate, sterile, single-use disposable syringe and needle should be used for each individual patient.
5. The diaphragm of the vial-stopper should be wiped with 70% alcohol.
6. The needle is inserted through the stopper diaphragm of the inverted vial. Exactly 0.1mL is filled into the syringe with care being taken to exclude air bubbles and to maintain the lumen of the needle filled.
7. The point of the needle is inserted into the most superficial layers of the skin with the needle bevel pointed upward. **As the Tuberculin solution is injected, a pale bleb 6 to 10mm in size (1/3″) will rise over the point of the needle.** This is quickly absorbed and no dressing is required.

In the event the injection is delivered subcutaneously (i.e., no bleb will form), or if a significant part of the dose leaks from the injection site, the test should be repeated immediately at another site at least 5 cm (2″) removed.
The Mantoux test is the standard of comparison for all other tuberculin tests.

Interpretation of Tuberculin Reaction
Readings of Mantoux reactions should be made during the period from 48 to 72 hours after the injection. **Induration only should be considered in interpreting the test.** The diameter of induration should be measured transversely to the long axis of the forearm and recorded in millimeters. Erythema has no diagnostic value and should be disregarded. The presence and size of necrosis and edema if present should be recorded although not used in the interpretation of the test. In the absence of induration, an area of erythema greater than 10 mm is diameter may indicate the injection was made too deeply and retesting is indicated.

Reactions should be interpreted as follows:
Positive—A positive reaction to the tuberculin skin test may not be seen until 2–10 weeks after the infection.[7] Based in current guidelines,[3,12] interpretation of positive reactions (depending on the age, immune status or risk factors of the persons tested) is:

1. An induration of >5 mm is classified as positive in the following:
   - Persons who have had recent close contact with persons who have active TB;
   - Persons who have human immunodeficiency virus (HIV) infection or risk factors for HIV infection but unknown HIV status;
   - Persons who have fibrotic chest radiographs consistent with healed TB.
2. An induration of >10 mm is classified as positive in all persons who do not meet any of the above criteria, but who belong to one or more of the following groups at high risk for TB:
   - Injecting-drug users known to be HIV seronegative;
   - Persons who have other medical conditions that have been reported to increase the risk for progressing from latent TB infection to active TB. These medical conditions include diabetes mellitus, conditions requiring prolonged high-dose corticosteroid therapy and other immunosuppressive therapy (including bone marrow and organ transplantation), chronic renal failure, some hematologic disorders (e.g., leukemias and lymphomas), other specific malignancies (e.g., carcinoma of the head or neck), weight loss of >10% below ideal body weight, silicosis, gastrectomy, jejunileal bypass;
   - Residents and employees of high-risk congregate settings; prisons and jails, nursing homes and other long-term facilities for the elderly, health-care facilities (including some residential mental health facilities), and homeless shelters;
   - Foreign-born persons recently arrived (i.e., within the last 5 years) from countries having a high prevalence or incidence of TB;
   - Some medically underserved, low-income populations, including migrant farm workers and homeless persons;
   - High-risk racial or ethnic minority populations, as defined locally;
   - Children <4 years of age or infants, children and adolescents exposed to adults in high-risk categories.
3. An induration of > 15mm is classified as positive in persons who do not meet any of the above criteria.

Negative—Induration of less than 5 mm. This indicates a lack of hypersensitivity to tuberculoprotein and tuberculous infection is highly unlikely.
Booster Effect—Infection of an individual with tubercle bacilli or other mycobacteria or BCG vaccination results in a delayed hypersensitivity response to tuberculin which is demonstrated by the skin test. The delayed hypersensitivity response may gradually wane over a period of years. If a person receives a tuberculin test at this time, a significant reaction may not be detected. However, the stimulus of the test may boost or increase the size of the reaction to a second test, sometimes causing an apparent conversion or development of sensitivity. This booster effect can be seen on a second test done one week after the initial stimulating test and can persist for a year, and perhaps longer. When routine periodic tuberculin testing of adults is done, initially two-stage testing should be considered to minimize the likelihood of interpreting a boosted reaction as a conversion.[13,14]
It should be noted that reactivity to tuberculin may be depressed or suppressed for as long as 5–6 weeks by viral infections, live virus vaccines (i.e., measles, smallpox, polio, rubella and mumps), or after discontinuation of therapy with corticosteroids or immunosuppressive agents. Malnutrition may also have a similar effect. When of diagnostic importance, a negative test should be accepted as proof that hypersensitivity is absent only after normal reactivity to non-specific irritants has been demonstrated. A primary injection of tuberculin may possibly have a boosting effect on subsequent tuberculin reactions. A pediatric patient who is known to have been exposed to a person with tuberculosis must not be adjudged free of infection until that patient has a negative tuberculin reaction at least ten weeks after contact with tuberculous person has ceased.[15] Annual testing is generally recommended for pediatric patients in high risk populations, such as persons from countries with a high prevalence of tuberculosis and low-income groups.[16]
A positive tuberculin reaction does not necessarily signify the presence of active disease. Further diagnostic procedures (e.g., chest radiograph, sputum smear and/or culture examination) should be carried out before a diagnosis of tuberculosis is made. A small percentage of responders may not have been infected with *M. tuberculosis* but by some other mycobacterium. The negative tuberculin skin test should never be used to exclude the possibility of active tuberculosis among persons for whom the diagnosis is being considered (symptoms compatible with tuberculosis).

HOW SUPPLIED

Tuberculin PPD-Aplisol bioequivalent to 5US units (TU) PPD-S per test dose (0.1mL) is available in the following presentations:
NDC 64029-4525-1 (Bio. 1525)
1 mL (10 tests) – rubber-diaphragm-capped vial
NDC 64029-4525-2 (Bio. 1607)
5 mL (50 tests) – rubber-diaphragm-capped vial
This product is ready for use without further dilution.

Storage
DO NOT FREEZE
This product should be stored at 2°–8°C (36°–46°F) and protected from light.
Vials in use more than 30 days should be discarded due to possible oxidation and degradation which may affect potency.

REFERENCES

1 Seibert, F.B.: Am Rev Tuberc, 30:713, 1934
2 Seibert, F.B., and Glenn, J.T.: Am Rev Tuberc, 44:9, 1941
3 MMWR, 1995:44 RR-11
4 MMWR, 1996:45 RR-4
5 Huebner RE, Shein MF, Bass JB, The Tuberculin Skin Test, *Clin Infect Dis*, 1993;17:968–75
6 AHFS Drug Information, 1997, 36:84 pp 1962–1968
7 American Thoracic Society: Diagnostic Standards and classification of tuberculosis, 1990 Am Rev Respir Dis, 142:725–735
8 Am Rev Respir Dis, 1985;886
9 Brickman HF et.Al., The Timing of Tuberculin Tests in Relation to Immunization with Live Viral Vaccines, *Pediatrics*; 1975;55:392
10 Red Book Report of the Committee on Infectious Disease, (1994)
11 Landi S, Held HR, Stability of a dilute solution of tuberculin purified derivative at extreme temperatures, *J Biol Stand*, 1981; 9:195
12 Diagnosis of TB Infection and TB Disease, Centers For Disease Control and Prevention(CDC), March 21, 1996, Doc# 2250102
13 Sewell E.M., O'Hare, D., and Kendig, E.L., Jr.: The Tuberculin Test, Pediatrics, Vol.54, No. 5, Nov.1974.
14 Advisory Committee of Elimination of Tuberculosis (ACET/CDC: Prevention and control of tuberculosis in facilities providing long-term care to the elderly, 1990. MMWR 39(10): 7–13,15.
15 ACET(CDC): The use of preventative therapy for tuberculosis infection in the United States, 1990. MMWR 39(8):9–12.
16 ACET(CDC): Screening for tuberculosis and tuberculosis infection in high risk populations. Recommendations of the ACET, 1990, MMWR 39(8):1–7.

℞ only.
Prescribing Information as of May 2002
PARKEDALE PHARMACEUTICALS
Manufactured by:
Parkedale Pharmaceuticals, Inc.
Rochester, MI 48307

4525G320

Shown in Product Identification Guide, page 319

BICILLIN® L-A ℞

[*bī-sil 'in*]
(penicillin G benzathine suspension)
INJECTION
FOR DEEP IM INJECTION ONLY

DESCRIPTION

Bicillin L-A (penicillin G benzathine suspension) is prepared by the reaction of dibenzylethylene diamine with two molecules of penicillin G. It is chemically designated as (2*S*, 5*R*, 6*R*) 3,3-Dimethyl-7-oxo -6- (2-phenylacetamido) -4-thia-1-azabicyclo[3.2.0]heptane-2-carboxylic acid compound with *N,N* '-dibenzylethylenediamine (2:1), tetrahydrate.
It is available for deep intramuscular injection. It contains penicillin G benzathine in aqueous suspension with sodium

citrate buffer and, as w/v, approximately 0.5% lecithin, 0.6% carboxymethylcellulose, 0.6% povidone, 0.1% methylparaben, and 0.01% propylparaben. It occurs as a white, crystalline powder and is very slightly soluble in water and sparingly soluble in alcohol.

Bicillin L-A suspension in the multiple-dose vial formulation, disposable syringe formulation and **TUBEX** formulation is viscous and opaque. The multiple-dose vial formulation contains the equivalent of 300,000 units per mL of penicillin G as the benzathine salt. The disposable syringe formulation is available in a 4 mL size containing the equivalent of 2,400,000 units of penicillin G as the benzathine salt. The **TUBEX** formulation is available in 1 mL and 2 mL **TUBEX** Sterile Cartridge-Needle Units containing the equivalent of 600,000 units and 1,200,000 units respectively of penicillin G as the benzathine salt. Read **CONTRAINDICATIONS, WARNINGS, PRECAUTIONS**, and **DOSAGE AND ADMINISTRATION** sections prior to use.

CLINICAL PHARMACOLOGY

General

Penicillin G benzathine has an extremely low solubility and, thus, the drug is slowly released from intramuscular injection sites. The drug is hydrolyzed to penicillin G. This combination of hydrolysis and slow absorption results in blood serum levels much lower but much more prolonged than other parenteral penicillins.

Intramuscular administration of 300,000 units of penicillin G benzathine in adults results in blood levels of 0.03 to 0.05 units per mL, which are maintained for 4 to 5 days. Similar blood levels may persist for 10 days following administration of 600,000 units and for 14 days following administration of 1,200,000 units. Blood concentrations of 0.003 units per mL may still be detectable 4 weeks following administration of 1,200,000 units.

Approximately 60% of penicillin G is bound to serum protein. The drug is distributed throughout the body tissues in widely varying amounts. Highest levels are found in the kidneys with lesser amounts in the liver, skin, and intestines. Penicillin G penetrates into all other tissues and the spinal fluid to a lesser degree. With normal kidney function, the drug is excreted rapidly by tubular excretion. In neonates and young infants and in individuals with impaired kidney function, excretion is considerably delayed.

Microbiology

Penicillin G exerts a bactericidal action against penicillin-susceptible microorganisms during the stage of active multiplication. It acts through the inhibition of biosynthesis of cell-wall mucopeptide. It is not active against the penicillinase-producing bacteria, which include many strains of staphylococci.

The following *in vitro* data are available, but their clinical significance is unknown. Penicillin G exerts high *in vitro* activity against staphylococci (except penicillinase-producing strains), streptococci (Groups A, C, G, H, L, and M), and pneumococci. Other organisms susceptible to penicillin G are *Neisseria gonorrhoeae, Corynebacterium diphtheriae, Bacillus anthracis,* Clostridia species, *Actinomyces bovis, Streptobacillus moniliformis, Listeria monocytogenes,* and Leptospira species. *Treponema pallidum* is extremely susceptible to the bactericidal action of penicillin G.

Susceptibility Test: If the Kirby-Bauer method of disc susceptibility is used, a 20-unit penicillin disc should give a zone greater than 28 mm when tested against a penicillin-susceptible bacterial strain.

INDICATIONS AND USAGE

Intramuscular penicillin G benzathine is indicated in the treatment of infections due to penicillin-G-sensitive microorganisms that are susceptible to the low and very prolonged serum levels common to this particular dosage form. Therapy should be guided by bacteriological studies (including sensitivity tests) and by clinical response.

The following infections will usually respond to adequate dosage of intramuscular penicillin G benzathine:

Mild-to-moderate infections of the upper respiratory tract due to susceptible streptococci.

Venereal infections —Syphilis, yaws, bejel, and pinta.

Medical Conditions in which Penicillin G Benzathine Therapy is Indicated as Prophylaxis:

Rheumatic fever and/or chorea—Prophylaxis with penicillin G benzathine has proven effective in preventing recurrence of these conditions. It has also been used as follow-up prophylactic therapy for rheumatic heart disease and acute glomerulonephritis.

CONTRAINDICATIONS

A history of a previous hypersensitivity reaction to any of the penicillins is a contraindication.

Do not inject into or near an artery or nerve.

WARNINGS

Penicillin G benzathine should only be prescribed for the indications listed in this insert.

SERIOUS AND OCCASIONALLY FATAL HYPERSENSITIVITY (ANAPHYLACTIC) REACTIONS HAVE BEEN REPORTED IN PATIENTS ON PENICILLIN THERAPY. THESE REACTIONS ARE MORE LIKELY TO OCCUR IN INDIVIDUALS WITH A HISTORY OF PENICILLIN HYPERSENSITIVITY AND/OR A HISTORY OF SENSITIVITY TO MULTIPLE ALLERGENS. THERE HAVE BEEN REPORTS OF INDIVIDUALS WITH A HISTORY OF PENICILLIN HYPERSENSITIVITY WHO HAVE EXPERIENCED SEVERE REACTIONS WHEN TREATED WITH CEPHALOSPORINS. BEFORE INITIATING THERAPY WITH BICILLIN L-A, CAREFUL INQUIRY SHOULD BE MADE CONCERNING PREVIOUS HYPERSENSITIVITY REACTIONS TO PENICILLINS, CEPHALOSPORINS AND OTHER ALLERGENS. IF AN ALLERGIC REACTION OCCURS, BICILLIN L-A SHOULD BE DISCONTINUED AND APPROPRIATE THERAPY INSTITUTED. **SERIOUS ANAPHYLACTIC REACTIONS REQUIRE IMMEDIATE EMERGENCY TREATMENT WITH EPINEPHRINE, OXYGEN, INTRAVENOUS STEROIDS AND AIRWAY MANAGEMENT, INCLUDING INTUBATION, SHOULD ALSO BE ADMINISTERED AS INDICATED.**

Pseudomembranous colitis has been reported with nearly all antibacterial agents, including penicillin, and may range in severity from mild to life-threatening. Therefore, it is important to consider this diagnosis in patients who present with diarrhea subsequent to the administration of any antibacterial agent.

Treatment with antibacterial agents alter the normal flora of the colon and may permit overgrowth of clostridia. Studies indicate that a toxin produced by *Clostridium difficile* is one primary cause of "antibiotic-associated colitis".

After the diagnosis of pseudomembranous colitis has been established, appropriate therapeutic measures should be initiated. Mild cases of pseudomembranous colitis usually respond to drug discontinuation alone. In moderate to severe cases, consideration should be given to management with fluids and electrolytes, protein supplementation, and treatment with an antibacterial drug clinically effective against *C. difficile* colitis.

Inadvertent intravascular administration, including inadvertent direct intra-arterial injection or injection immediately adjacent to arteries, of Bicillin L-A and other penicillin preparations has resulted in severe neurovascular damage, including transverse myelitis with permanent paralysis, gangrene requiring amputation of digits and more proximal portions of extremities, and necrosis and sloughing at and surrounding the injection site. Such severe effects have been reported following injections into the buttock, thigh, and deltoid areas. Other serious complications of suspected intravascular administration which have been reported include immediate pallor, mottling, or cyanosis of the extremity both distal and proximal to the injection site, followed by bleb formation; severe edema requiring anterior and/or posterior compartment fasciotomy in the lower extremity. The above-described severe effects and complications have most often occurred in infants and small children. Prompt consultation with an appropriate specialist is indicated if any evidence of compromise of the blood supply occurs at, proximal to, or distal to the site of injection.[1–9] See **CONTRAINDICATIONS, PRECAUTIONS**, and **DOSAGE AND ADMINISTRATION** sections.

Quadriceps femoris fibrosis and atrophy have been reported following repeated intramuscular injections of penicillin preparations into the anterolateral thigh.

Injection into or near a nerve may result in permanent neurological damage.

PRECAUTIONS

General

Penicillin should be used with caution in individuals with histories of significant allergies and/or asthma.

Care should be taken to avoid intravenous or intra-arterial administration, or injection into or near major peripheral nerves or blood vessels, since such injection may produce neurovascular damage. See **CONTRAINDICATIONS, WARNINGS**, and **DOSAGE AND ADMINISTRATION** sections.

Prolonged use of antibiotics may promote the overgrowth of nonsusceptible organisms, including fungi. Should superinfection occur, appropriate measures should be taken.

Laboratory Tests

In streptococcal infections, therapy must be sufficient to eliminate the organism; otherwise, the sequelae of streptococcal disease may occur. Cultures should be taken following completion of treatment to determine whether streptococci have been eradicated.

Drug Interactions

Tetracycline, a bacteriostatic antibiotic, may antagonize the bactericidal effect of penicillin, and concurrent use of these drugs should be avoided.

Concurrent administration of penicillin and probenecid increases and prolongs serum penicillin levels by decreasing the apparent volume of distribution and slowing the rate of excretion by competitively inhibiting renal tubular secretion of penicillin.

Pregnancy Category B

Reproduction studies performed in the mouse, rat, and rabbit have revealed no evidence of impaired fertility or harm to the fetus due to penicillin G. Human experience with the penicillins during pregnancy has not shown any positive evidence of adverse effects on the fetus. There are, however, no adequate and well-controlled studies in pregnant women showing conclusively that harmful effects of these drugs on the fetus can be excluded. Because animal reproduction studies are not always predictive of human response, this drug should be used during pregnancy only if clearly needed.

Nursing Mothers

Soluble penicillin G is excreted in breast milk. Caution should be exercised when penicillin G benzathine is administered to a nursing woman.

Carcinogenesis, Mutagenesis, Impairment Of Fertility

No long-term animal studies have been conducted with this drug.

Pediatric Use

See **INDICATIONS AND USAGE** and **DOSAGE AND ADMINISTRATION**.

ADVERSE REACTIONS

As with other penicillins, untoward reactions of the sensitivity phenomena are likely to occur, particularly in individuals who have previously demonstrated hypersensitivity to penicillins or in those with a history of allergy, asthma, hay fever, or urticaria.

As with other treatments for syphilis, the Jarisch-Herxheimer reaction has been reported.

The following have been reported with parenteral penicillin G:

General: Hypersensitivity reactions including the following: skin eruptions (maculopapular to exfoliative dermatitis), urticaria, laryngeal edema, fever, eosinophilia; other serum sickness-like reactions (including chills, fever, edema, arthralgia, and prostration); and anaphylaxis including shock and death. Note: Urticaria, other skin rashes, and serum sickness-like reactions may be controlled with antihistamines and, if necessary, systemic corticosteroids. Whenever such reactions occur, penicillin G should be discontinued unless, in the opinion of the physician, the condition being treated is life-threatening and amenable only to therapy with penicillin G. Serious anaphylactic reactions require immediate emergency treatment with epinephrine. Oxygen, intravenous steroids, and airway management, including intubation, should also be administered as indicated.

Gastrointestinal: Pseudomembranous colitis. Onset of pseudomembranous colitis symptoms may occur during or after antibacterial treatment. See **WARNINGS**.

Hematologic: Hemolytic anemia, leukopenia, thrombocytopenia.

Neurologic: Neuropathy.

Urogenital: Nephropathy.

The following adverse events have been temporally associated with parenteral administration of penicillin G benzathine:

Body as a Whole: Hypersensitivity reactions including allergic vasculitis, pruritus, fatigue, asthenia, and pain; aggravation of existing disorder; headache.

Cardiovascular: Cardiac arrest; hypotension; tachycardia; palpitations; pulmonary hypertension; pulmonary embolism; vasodilatation; vasovagal reaction; cerebrovascular accident; syncope.

Gastrointestinal: Nausea, vomiting; blood in stool; intestinal necrosis.

Hemic and Lymphatic: Lymphadenopathy.

Injection Site: Injection site reactions including pain, inflammation, lump, abscess, necrosis, edema, hemorrhage, cellulitis, hypersensitivity, atrophy, ecchymosis, and skin ulcer. Neurovascular reactions including warmth, vasospasm, pallor, mottling, gangrene, numbness of the extremities, and neurovascular damage.

Metabolic: Elevated BUN, creatinine, and SGOT.

Musculoskeletal: Joint disorder; periostitis; exacerbation of arthritis; myoglobinura; rhabdomyolysis.

Nervous System: Nervousness; tremors; dizziness; somnolence; confusion; anxiety; euphoria; transverse myelitis; seizures; coma. A syndrome manifested by a variety of CNS symptoms such as severe agitation with confusion, visual and auditory hallucinations, and a fear of impending death (Hoigne's syndrome), has been reported after administration of penicillin G procaine and, less commonly, after injection of the combination of penicillin G benzathine and penicillin G procaine. Other symptoms associated with this syndrome, such as psychosis, seizures, dizziness, tinnitus, cyanosis, palpitations, tachycardia, and/or abnormal perception in taste, also may occur.

Respiratory: Hypoxia; apnea; dyspnea.

Skin: Diaphoresis.

Special Senses: Blurred vision; blindness.

Urogenital: Neurogenic bladder; hematuria; proteinuria; renal failure; impotence; priapism.

OVERDOSAGE

Penicillin in overdosage has the potential to cause neuromuscular hyperirritability or convulsive seizures.

DOSAGE AND ADMINISTRATION

Due to the viscous nature of this medication, a 23 gauge or larger bore needle should be used to withdraw medication from the vial and for patient administration. A smaller bore needle, such as a 24 or 25 gauge, is not recommended.

Streptococcal (Group A) Upper-respiratory infections (for example, pharyngitis)

Adults—a single injection of 1,200,000 units; older pediatric patients—a single injection of 900,000 units; infants and pediatric patients under 60 lbs.—300,000 to 600,000 units.

Syphilis

Primary, secondary, and latent—2,400,000 units (1 dose). Late (tertiary and neurosyphilis)—2,400,000 units at 7-day intervals for three doses.

Congenital—under 2 years of age: 50,000 units/kg/body weight; ages 2 to 12 years: adjust dosage based on adult dosage schedule.

Yaws, Bejel, and Pinta—1,200,000 units (1 injection).

Prophylaxis—for rheumatic fever and glomerulonephritis. Following an acute attack, penicillin G benzathine (parenteral) may be given in doses of 1,200,000 units once a month or 600,000 units every 2 weeks.

Continued on next page

Bicillin L-A—Cont.

Administer by DEEP INTRAMUSCULAR INJECTION in the upper, outer quadrant of the buttock. In neonates, infants and small children, the midlateral aspect of the thigh may be preferable. When doses are repeated, vary the injection site.

When using the multiple-dose vial:

After selection of the proper site and insertion of the needle into the selected muscle, aspirate by pulling back on the plunger. While maintaining negative pressure for 2 to 3 seconds, carefully observe the barrel of the syringe immediately proximal to the needle hub for appearance of blood or any discoloration. Blood or "typical blood color" may *not* be seen if a blood vessel has been entered—only a mixture of blood and Bicillin L-A. The appearance of any discoloration is reason to withdraw the needle and discard the syringe. If it is elected to inject at another site, a new syringe and needle should be used. If no blood or discoloration appears, inject the contents of the syringe slowly. Discontinue delivery of the dose if the subject complains of severe immediate pain at the injection site or if, especially in neonates, infants and young children symptoms or signs occur suggesting onset of severe pain.

Because of the high concentration of suspended material in this product, the needle may be blocked if the injection is not made at a slow, steady rate.

When using the **TUBEX** cartridge:

The Wyeth-Ayerst **TUBEX®** cartridge for this product incorporates several features that are designed to facilitate the visualization of blood on aspiration if a blood vessel is inadvertently entered.

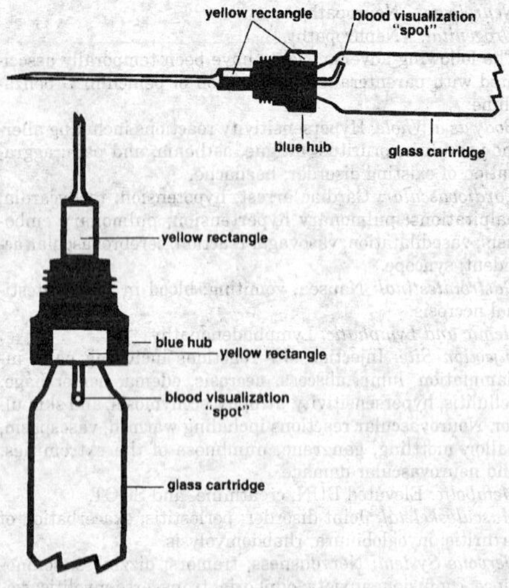

The design of this cartridge is such that blood which enters its needle will be quickly visualized as a red or dark-colored "spot." This "spot" will appear on the barrel of the glass cartridge immediately proximal to the blue hub. The **TUBEX** is designed with two orientation marks, in order to determine where the "spot" can be seen. First insert and secure the cartridge in the **TUBEX** injector in the usual fashion. Locate the yellow rectangle at the base of the blue hub. This yellow rectangle is aligned with the blood visualization "spot." An imaginary straight line, drawn from this yellow rectangle to the shoulder of the glass cartridge, will point to the area on the cartridge where the "spot" can be visualized. When the needle cover is removed, a second yellow rectangle will be visible. The second yellow rectangle is also aligned with the blood visualization "spot" to assist the operator in locating this "spot." If the 2 mL metal or plastic syringe is used, the glass cartridge should be rotated by turning the plunger of the syringe clockwise until the yellow rectangle is visualized. If the 1 mL metal syringe is used, it will not be possible to continue to rotate the glass cartridge clockwise once it is properly engaged and fully threaded; it can, however, then be rotated counterclockwise as far as necessary to properly orient the yellow rectangles and locate the observation area. (In this same area in some cartridges, a dark spot may sometimes be visualized prior to injection. This is the proximal end of the needle and does not represent a foreign body in, or other abnormality of, the suspension.)

Thus, before the needle is inserted into the selected muscle, it is important for the operator to orient the yellow rectangle so that any blood which may enter after needle insertion and during aspiration can be visualized in the area on the cartridge where it will appear and not be obscured by any obstructions.

After selection of the proper site and insertion of the needle into the selected muscle, aspirate by pulling back on the plunger. While maintaining negative pressure for 2 to 3 seconds, carefully observe the barrel of the cartridge in the area previously identified (see above) for the appearance of a red or dark-colored "spot."

Blood or "typical blood color" may not be seen if a blood vessel has been entered—only a mixture of blood and Bicillin L-A. The appearance of any discoloration is reason to withdraw the needle and discard the glass **TUBEX** cartridge. If it is elected to inject at another site, a new cartridge should be used. If no blood or discoloration appears, inject the contents of the cartridge slowly. Discontinue delivery of the dose if the subject complains of severe immediate pain at the injection site or if, especially in infants and young children, symptoms or signs occur suggesting onset of severe pain.

Some **TUBEX** cartridges may contain a small air bubble which may be disregarded, since it does not affect administration of the product.

DO NOT clear any air bubbles from the cartridge or needle as this may interfere with the visualization of any blood or discoloration during aspiration.

Because of the high concentration of suspended material in this product, the needle may be blocked if the injection is not made at a slow, steady rate.

When using the disposable syringe:

The Wyeth-Ayerst disposable syringe for this product incorporates several features that are designed to facilitate its use.

A single, small indentation, or "dot," has been punched into the metal ring that surrounds the neck of the syringe near the base of the needle. It is important that this "dot" be placed in a position so that it can be easily visualized by the operator following the intramuscular insertion of the syringe needle.

After selection of the proper site and insertion of the needle into the selected muscle, aspirate by pulling back on the plunger. While maintaining negative pressure for 2 to 3 seconds, carefully observe the barrel of the syringe immediately proximal to the location of the "dot" for appearance of blood or any discoloration. Blood or "typical blood color" may *not* be seen if a blood vessel has been entered—only a mixture of blood and Bicillin L-A. The appearance of any discoloration is reason to withdraw the needle and discard the syringe. If it is elected to inject at another site, a new syringe should be used. If no blood or discoloration appears, inject the contents of the syringe slowly. Discontinue delivery of the dose if the subject complains of severe immediate pain at the injection site or if, especially in neonates, infants and young children, symptoms or signs occur suggesting onset of severe pain.

Some disposable syringes may contain a small air bubble which may be disregarded, since it does not affect administration of the product. DO NOT clear any air bubbles from the disposable syringe or needle as this may interfere with the visualization of any blood or discoloration during aspiration.

Because of the high concentration of suspended material in this product, the needle may be blocked if the injection is not made at a slow, steady rate.

Parenteral drug products should be inspected visually for particulate matter and discoloration prior to administration whenever solution and container permit.

HOW SUPPLIED

Bicillin® L-A (penicillin G benzathine suspension) is supplied in packages of 10 **TUBEX®** Sterile Cartridge-Needle Units as follows:

1 mL size, containing 600,000 units per **TUBEX®** (21 gauge, thin-wall 1 inch needle for pediatric use), NDC 61570-146-10.

2 mL size, containing 1,200,000 units per **TUBEX®** (21 gauge, thin-wall 1–1/4 inch needle), NDC 61570-147-10.

Store in a refrigerator.

Keep from freezing.

ALSO AVAILABLE

Bicillin L-A (penicillin G benzathine suspension) is also available in packages of 10 disposable syringes as follows:

4 mL size, containing 2,400,000 units per syringe (18 gauge × 2 inch needle), NDC 61570-148-10

Store in a refrigerator.

Keep from freezing.

Shake multiple-dose vials well before using.

REFERENCES

1. SHAW, E.: Transverse myelitis from injection of penicillin. *Am. J. Dis. Child., 111:* 548, 1966.

2. KNOWLES, J.: Accidental intra-arterial injection of penicillin. *Am. J. Dis. Child., 111:* 552, 1966.

3. DARBY, C., et al: Ischemia following an intragluteal injection of benzathine-procaine penicillin G mixture in a one-year-old boy. *Clin. Pediatrics, 12:* 485, 1973.

4. BROWN, L. & NELSON, A.: Postinfectious intravascular thrombosis with gangrene. *Arch. Surg., 94:* 652, 1967.

5. BORENSTINE, J.: Transverse myelitis and penicillin (Correspondence). *Am. J. Dis. Child., 112:* 166, 1966.

6. ATKINSON, J.: Transverse myelopathy secondary to penicillin injection. *J. Pediatrics, 75:* 867, 1969.

7. TALBERT, J. et al: Gangrene of the foot following intramuscular injection in the lateral thigh: A case report with recommendations for prevention. *J. Pediatrics, 70:* 110, 1967.

8. FISHER, T.: Medicolegal affairs. *Canad. Med. Assoc. J., 112:* 395, 1975.

9. SCHANZER, H. et al: Accidental intra-arterial injection of penicillin G. *JAMA, 242:* 1289, 1979.

Manufactured by:
Wyeth Laboratories
A Wyeth-Ayerst Company
Philadelphia, PA 19101
Distributed by:
Monarch Pharmaceuticals, Inc.
Bristol, TN 37620

Refer to the Tubex® Closed Injection System instructions in the Wyeth-Ayerst section of the 2002 PDR®.

Revised March 14, 2001 CI 4656-4

BREVITAL® SODIUM ℂ ℞

[*brĕ-vĭ-tŏl*]

METHOHEXITAL SODIUM FOR INJECTION, USP
For Intravenous Use in Adults
For Rectal and Intramuscular Use Only in Pediatric Patients

Prescribing information as of November 2003. **3000870 242**

WARNING

Brevital should be used only in hospital or ambulatory care settings that provide for continuous monitoring of respiratory (e.g. pulse oximetry) and cardiac function. Immediate availability of resuscitative drugs and age- and size-appropriate equipment for bag/valve/mask ventilation and intubation and personnel trained in their use and skilled in airway management should be assured. For deeply sedated patients, a designated individual other than the practitioner performing the procedure should be present to continuously monitor the patient. (See WARNINGS)

DESCRIPTION

Brevital® Sodium (Methohexital Sodium for Injection, USP) is 2,4,6 (*1H, 3H, 5H*)-Pyrimidinetrione, 1-methyl-5-(1-methyl-2-pentynyl)-5-(2-propenyl)-, (±)-, monosodium salt and has the empirical formula $C_{14}H_{17}N_2NaO_3$. Its molecular weight is 284.29.

The structural formula is as follows:

Methohexital sodium is a rapid, ultrashort-acting barbiturate anesthetic. Methohexital sodium for injection is a freeze-dried, sterile, nonpyrogenic mixture of methohexital sodium with 6% anhydrous sodium carbonate added as a buffer. It contains not less than 90% and not more than 110% of the labeled amount of methohexital sodium. It occurs as a white, freeze-dried plug that is freely soluble in water.

This product is oxygen sensitive. The pH of the 1% solution is between 10 and 11; the pH of the 0.2% solution in 5% dextrose is between 9.5 and 10.5.

Methohexital sodium may be administered by direct intravenous injection or continuous intravenous drip, intramuscular or rectal routes (see **PRECAUTIONS**—*Pediatric Use*). Reconstituting instructions vary depending on the route of administration (see **DOSAGE AND ADMINISTRATION**).

CLINICAL PHARMACOLOGY

Compared with thiamylal and thiopental, methohexital is at least twice as potent on a weight basis, and its duration of action is only about half as long. Although the metabolic fate of methohexital in the body is not clear, the drug does not appear to concentrate in fat depots to the extent that other barbiturate anesthetics do. Thus, cumulative effects are fewer and recovery is more rapid with methohexital than with thiobarbiturates. In experimental animals, the drug cannot be detected in the blood 24 hours after administration.

Methohexital differs chemically from the established barbiturate anesthetics in that it contains no sulfur. Little analgesia is conferred by barbiturates; their use in the presence of pain may result in excitation.

Intravenous administration of methohexital results in rapid uptake by the brain (within 30 seconds) and rapid induction of sleep.

Following intramuscular administration to pediatric patients, the onset of sleep occurs in 2 to 10 minutes. A plasma concentration of 3 µg/mL was achieved in pediatric patients 15 minutes after an intramuscular dose (10 mg/kg) of a 5% solution. Following rectal administration to pediatric patients, the onset of sleep occurs in 5 to 15 minutes. Plasma methohexital concentrations achieved following rectal administration tend to increase both with dose and with the use of more dilute solution concentrations when using the same dose. A 25 mg/kg dose of a 1% methohexital solution yielded plasma concentrations of 6.9 to 7.9 µg/mL 15 minutes after dosing. The absolute bioavailability of rectal methohexital sodium is 17%.

With single doses, the rate of redistribution determines duration of pharmacologic effect. Metabolism occurs in the liver through demethylation and oxidation. Side-chain oxidation is the most important biotransformation involved in termination of biologic activity. Excretion occurs via the kidneys through glomerular filtration.

INDICATIONS AND USAGE

Brevital Sodium can be used in adults as follows:

1. For *intravenous* induction of anesthesia prior to the use of other general anesthetic agents.

2. For *intravenous* induction of anesthesia and as an adjunct to subpotent inhalational anesthetic agents (such as nitrous oxide in oxygen) for short surgical procedures; Brevital Sodium may be given by infusion or intermittent injection.
3. For use along with other parenteral agents, usually narcotic analgesics, to supplement subpotent inhalational anesthetic agents (such as nitrous oxide in oxygen) for longer surgical procedures.
4. As *intravenous* anesthesia for short surgical, diagnostic, or therapeutic procedures associated with minimal painful stimuli (see **WARNINGS**).
5. As an agent for inducing a hypnotic state.

Brevital Sodium can be used in pediatric patients older than 1 month as follows:

1. For *rectal* or *intramuscular* induction of anesthesia prior to the use of other general anesthetic agents.
2. For *rectal* or *intramuscular* induction of anesthesia and as an adjunct to subpotent inhalational anesthetic agents for short surgical procedures.
3. As *rectal* or *intramuscular* anesthesia for short surgical, diagnostic, or therapeutic procedures associated with minimal painful stimuli.

CONTRAINDICATIONS

Brevital Sodium is contraindicated in patients in whom general anesthesia is contraindicated, in those with latent or manifest porphyria, or in patients with a known hypersensitivity to barbiturates.

WARNINGS

See boxed Warning.

As with all potent anesthetic agents and adjuncts, Brevital should be used only in hospital or ambulatory care settings that provide for continuous monitoring of respiratory (e.g. pulse oximetry) and cardiac function. Immediate availability of resuscitative drugs and age- and size-appropriate equipment for bag/valve/mask ventilation and intubation and personnel trained in their use and skilled in airway management should be assured. For deeply sedated patients, a designated individual other than the practitioner performing the procedure should be present to continuously monitor the patient.

Maintenance of a patent airway and adequacy of ventilation must be ensured during induction and maintenance of anesthesia with methohexital sodium solution. Laryngospasm is common during induction with all barbiturates and may be due to a combination of secretions and accentuated reflexes following induction or may result from painful stimuli during light anesthesia. Apnea/hypoventilation may be noted during induction, which may impair pulmonary ventilation; the duration of apnea may be longer than that produced by other barbiturate anesthetics. Cardiorespiratory arrest may occur.

This prescribing information describes intravenous use of methohexital sodium in adults. It also discusses intramuscular and rectal administration in pediatric patients older than one month. Although the published literature discusses intravenous administration in pediatric patients, the safety and effectiveness of intravenous administration of methohexital sodium in pediatric patients have not been established in well-controlled, prospective studies. (See **PRECAUTIONS**—*Pediatric Use*)

Seizures may be elicited in subjects with a previous history of convulsive activity, especially partial seizure disorders.

Because the liver is involved in demethylation and oxidation of methohexital and because barbiturates may enhance preexisting circulatory depression, severe hepatic dysfunction, severe cardiovascular instability, or a shock-like condition may be reason for selecting another induction agent.

Prolonged administration may result in cumulative effects, including extended somnolence, protracted unconsciousness, and respiratory and cardiovascular depression. Respiratory depression in the presence of an impaired airway may lead to hypoxia, cardiac arrest, and death.

The CNS-depressant effect of Brevital Sodium may be additive with that of other CNS depressants, including ethyl alcohol and propylene glycol.

DANGER OF INTRA-ARTERIAL INJECTION—Unintended intra-arterial injection of barbiturate solutions may be followed by the production of platelet aggregates and thrombosis, starting in arterioles distal to the site of injection. The resulting necrosis may lead to gangrene, which may require amputation. The first sign in conscious patients may be a complaint of fiery burning that roughly follows the distribution path of the injected artery; if noted, the injection should be stopped immediately and the situation reevaluated. Transient blanching may or may not be noted very early; blotchy cyanosis and dark discoloration may then be the first sign in anesthetized patients. There is no established treatment other than prevention. The following should be considered prior to injection:

1. The extent of injury is related to concentration. Concentrations of 1% methohexital will usually suffice; higher concentrations should ordinarily be avoided.
2. Check the infusion to ensure that the catheter is in the lumen of a vein before injection. Injection through a running intravenous infusion may enhance the possibility of detecting arterial placement; however, it should be remembered that the characteristic bright-red color of arterial blood is often altered by contact with drugs. The possibility of aberrant arteries should always be considered.

Postinjury arterial injection of vasodilators and/or arterial infusion of parenteral fluids are generally regarded to be of no value in altering outcome. Animal experiments and published individual case reports concerned with a variety of arteriolar irritants, including barbiturates, suggest that 1 or more of the following may be of benefit in reducing the area of necrosis:

1. Arterial injection of heparin at the site of injury, followed by systemic anticoagulation.
2. Sympathetic blockade (or brachial plexus blockade in the arm).
3. Intra-arterial glucocorticoid injection at the site of injury, followed by systemic steroids.
4. A case report (nonbarbiturate injury) suggests that intra-arterial urokinase may promote fibrinolysis, even if administered late in treatment.

If extravasation is noted during injection of methohexital, the injection should be discontinued until the situation is remedied. Local irritation may result from extravasation; subcutaneous swelling may also serve as a sign of arterial or periarterial placement of the catheter.

PRECAUTIONS

General—All routes of administration of Brevital Sodium are often associated with hiccups, coughing, and/or muscle twitching, which may also impair pulmonary ventilation.

Following induction, temporary hypotension and tachycardia may occur.

Recovery from methohexital anesthesia is rapid and smooth. The incidence of postoperative nausea and vomiting is low if the drug is administered to fasting patients. Postanesthetic shivering has occurred in a few instances.

The usual precautions taken with any barbiturate anesthetic should be observed with Brevital Sodium. The drug should be used with caution in patients with asthma, obstructive pulmonary disease, severe hypertension or hypotension, myocardial disease, congestive heart failure, severe anemia, or extreme obesity.

Methohexital sodium should be used with extreme caution in patients in status asthmaticus.

Caution should be exercised in debilitated patients or in those with impaired function of respiratory, circulatory, renal, hepatic, or endocrine systems.

Information for Patients—When appropriate, patients should be instructed as to the hazards of drowsiness that may follow use of Brevital Sodium. Outpatients should be released in the company of another individual, and no skilled activities, such as operating machinery or driving a motor vehicle, should be engaged in for 8 to 12 hours.

Laboratory Tests—BSP and liver function studies may be influenced by administration of a single dose of barbiturates.

Drug Interactions—Prior chronic administration of barbiturates or phenytoin (e.g. for seizure disorder) appears to reduce the effectiveness of Brevital Sodium. Barbiturates may influence the absorption and elimination of other concomitantly used drugs, such as phenytoin, halothane, anticoagulants, corticosteroids, ethyl alcohol, and propylene glycol-containing solutions.

Carcinogenesis, Mutagenesis, Impairment of Fertility—Studies in animals to evaluate the carcinogenic and mutagenic potential of Brevital Sodium have not been conducted. Reproduction studies in animals have revealed no evidence of impaired fertility.

Usage in Pregnancy—Pregnancy Category B—Reproduction studies have been performed in rabbits and rats at doses up to 4 and 7 times the human dose respectively and have revealed no evidence of harm to the fetus due to methohexital sodium. There are, however, no adequate and well-controlled studies in pregnant women. Because animal reproduction studies are not always predictive of human response, this drug should be used during pregnancy only if clearly needed.

Labor and Delivery—Brevital Sodium has been used in cesarean section delivery but, because of its solubility and lack of protein binding, it readily and rapidly traverses the placenta.

Nursing Mothers—Caution should be exercised when Brevital Sodium is administered to a nursing woman.

Pediatric Use—The safety and effectiveness of methohexital sodium in pediatric patients below the age of 1 month have not been established. Seizures may be elicited in subjects with a previous history of convulsive activity, especially partial seizure disorders. Apnea has been reported following dosing with methohexital regardless of the route of administration used. Studies using methohexital sodium intravenously in pediatric patients have been reported in the published literature. This literature is not adequate to establish the safety and effectiveness of intravenous administration of methohexital sodium in pediatric patients. Due to a variety of limitations such as study design, biopharmaceutic issues, and the wide range of effects observed with similar doses of intravenous methohexital, additional studies of intravenous methohexital in pediatric patients are necessary before this route can be recommended in pediatric patients. (See **WARNINGS**)

ADVERSE REACTIONS

Side effects associated with Brevital Sodium are extensions of pharmacologic effects and include:

Cardiovascular—Circulatory depression, thrombophlebitis, hypotension, tachycardia, peripheral vascular collapse, and convulsions in association with cardiorespiratory arrest

Respiratory—Respiratory depression (including apnea), cardiorespiratory arrest, laryngospasm, bronchospasm, hiccups, and dyspnea

Neurologic—Skeletal muscle hyperactivity (twitching), injury to nerves adjacent to injection site, and seizures

Psychiatric—Emergence delirium, restlessness, and anxiety may occur, especially in the presence of postoperative pain

Gastrointestinal—Nausea, emesis, abdominal pain, and liver function tests abnormal

Allergic—Erythema, pruritus, urticaria, and cases of anaphylaxis have been reported rarely

Other—Other adverse reactions include pain at injection site, salivation, headache, and rhinitis

DRUG ABUSE AND DEPENDENCE

Controlled Substance—Brevital Sodium is a Schedule IV drug.

Brevital Sodium may be habit-forming.

OVERDOSAGE

Signs and Symptoms—The onset of toxicity following an overdose of intravenously administered methohexital will be within seconds of the infusion. If methohexital is administered rectally or is ingested, the onset of toxicity may be delayed. The manifestations of an ultrashort-acting barbiturate in overdose include central nervous system depression, respiratory depression, hypotension, loss of peripheral vascular resistance, and muscular hyperactivity ranging from twitching to convulsive-like movements. Other findings may include convulsions and allergic reactions. Following massive exposure to any barbiturate, pulmonary edema, circulatory collapse with loss of peripheral vascular tone, and cardiac arrest may occur.

Treatment—To obtain up-to-date information about the treatment of overdose, a good resource is your certified Regional Poison Control Center. Telephone numbers of certified poison control centers are listed in the *Physicians' Desk Reference (PDR)*. In managing overdosage, consider the possibility of multiple drug overdoses, interaction among drugs, and unusual drug kinetics in your patient.

Establish an airway and ensure oxygenation and ventilation. Resuscitative measures should be initiated promptly. For hypotension, intravenous fluids should be administered and the patient's legs raised. If desirable increase in blood pressure is not obtained, vasopressor and/or inotropic drugs may be used as dictated by the clinical situation.

For convulsions, diazepam intravenously and phenytoin may be required. If the seizures are refractory to diazepam and phenytoin, general anesthesia and paralysis with a neuromuscular blocking agent may be necessary.

Protect the patient's airway and support ventilation and perfusion. Meticulously monitor and maintain, within acceptable limits, the patient's vital signs, blood gases, serum electrolytes, etc. Absorption of drugs from the gastrointestinal tract may be decreased by giving activated charcoal, which, in many cases, is more effective than emesis or lavage; consider charcoal instead of or in addition to gastric emptying. Repeated doses of charcoal over time may hasten elimination of some drugs that have been absorbed. Safeguard the patient's airway when employing gastric emptying or charcoal.

DOSAGE AND ADMINISTRATION

Facilities for assisting ventilation and administering oxygen are necessary adjuncts for all routes of administration of anesthesia. Since cardiorespiratory arrest may occur, patients should be observed carefully during and after use of Brevital Sodium. Age- and size-appropriate resuscitative equipment (ie, intubation and cardioversion equipment, oxygen, suction, and a secure intravenous line) and personnel qualified in its use must be immediately available.

Preanesthetic medication is generally advisable. Brevital Sodium may be used with any of the recognized preanesthetic medications.

Preparation of Solution—FOLLOW DILUTING INSTRUCTIONS EXACTLY.

Solutions of Brevital Sodium should be freshly prepared and used promptly. Reconstituted solutions of Brevital Sodium are chemically stable at room temperature for 24 hours.

Diluents—DO NOT USE DILUENTS CONTAINING BACTERIOSTATS.

Preferred diluent: Sterile Water for Injection
Acceptable diluents: 5% Dextrose Injection, 0.9% Sodium Chloride Injection
Incompatible diluents: Lactated Ringer's Injection

Dilution Instructions—1% solutions (10 mg/mL) should be prepared for intravenous use. Contents of vials should be diluted as follows:

Strength	Amount of Diluent to Be Added to the Contents of the Vial	For 1% solution
500 mg	50 mL	no further dilution needed
2.5 g	15 mL	add to 235 mL for 250 mL total volume

When the first dilution is made with the 2.5 g, the solution in the vial will be yellow. When further diluted to make a 1% solution, it must be *clear and colorless* or should not be used.

Continued on next page

Active Ingredient	Potency per mL	Volume Used	Physical Change Immediate	15 min	30 min	1 h
Brevital Sodium	10 mg	10 mL			CONTROL	
Atropine Sulfate	1/150 gr	1 mL	None	Haze		
Atropine Sulfate	1/100 gr	1 mL	None	Ppt	Ppt	
Succinylcholine chloride	0.5 mg	4 mL	None	None	Haze	
Succinylcholine chloride	1 mg	4 mL	None	None	Haze	
Metocurine iodide	0.5 mg	4 mL	None	None	Ppt	
Metocurine iodide	1 mg	4 mL	None	None	Ppt	
Scopolamine hydrobromide	1/120 gr	1 mL	None	None	None	Haze
Tubocurarine chloride	3 mg	4 mL	None	Haze		

Brevital Sodium—Cont.

For continuous drip anesthesia, prepare a 0.2% solution by adding 500 mg of Brevital Sodium to 250 mL of diluent. For this dilution, either 5% glucose solution or isotonic (0.9%) sodium chloride solution is recommended instead of distilled water in order to avoid extreme hypotonicity.
For *intramuscular* administration, contents of the vials should be diluted as follows:

FOR INTRAMUSCULAR ADMINISTRATION

Strength	Amount of Diluent to Be Added to the Contents of the Vial	Concentration after Dilution
500 mg vial	10 mL	5% Solution (50 mg/mL)
2.5 g vial	50 mL	5% Solution (50 mg/mL)

For *rectal* administration, contents of the vials should be diluted as follows:

FOR RECTAL ADMINISTRATION

Strength	Amount of Diluent to Be Added to the Contents of the Vial	Concentration after Dilution
500 mg vial	50 mL	1% Solution (10 mg/mL)
2.5 g vial (larger vial needed)	250 mL	1% Solution (10 mg/mL)

Administration—Dosage is highly individualized; the drug should be administered only by those completely familiar with its quantitative differences from other barbiturate anesthetics.
Adults—Brevital Sodium is administered intravenously in a concentration of no higher than 1%. Higher concentrations markedly increase the incidence of muscular movements and irregularities in respiration and blood pressure.
Induction of anesthesia—For induction of anesthesia, a 1% solution is administered at a rate of about 1 mL/5 seconds. Gaseous anesthetics and/or skeletal muscle relaxants may be administered concomitantly. The dose required for induction may range from 50 to 120 mg or more but averages about 70 mg. The usual dosage in adults ranges from 1 to 1.5 mg/kg. The induction dose usually provides anesthesia for 5 to 7 minutes.
Maintenance of anesthesia—Maintenance of anesthesia may be accomplished by intermittent injections of the 1% solution or, more easily, by continuous intravenous drip of a 0.2% solution. Intermittent injections of about 20 to 40 mg (2 to 4 mL of a 1% solution) may be given as required, usually every 4 to 7 minutes. For continuous drip, the average rate of administration is about 3 mL of a 0.2% solution/minute (1 drop/second). The rate of flow must be individualized for each patient. For longer surgical procedures, gradual reduction in the rate of administration is recommended (see discussion of prolonged administration in **WARNINGS**). Other parenteral agents, usually narcotic analgesics, are ordinarily employed along with Brevital Sodium during longer procedures.
Pediatric Patients—Brevital Sodium is administered intramuscularly in a 5% concentration and administered rectally as a 1% solution.
Induction of anesthesia—For the induction of anesthesia by the *intramuscular* route of administration, the usual dose ranges from 6.6 to 10 mg/kg of the 5% concentration. For *rectal* administration, the usual dose for induction is 25 mg/kg using the 1% solution.
Parenteral drug products should be inspected visually for particulate matter and discoloration prior to administration, whenever solution and container permit.

COMPATIBILITY INFORMATION

Solutions of Brevital Sodium should not be mixed in the same syringe or administered simultaneously during intravenous infusion through the same needle with acid solutions, such as atropine sulfate, metocurine iodide, and succinylcholine chloride. Alteration of pH may cause free barbituric acid to be precipitated. Solubility of the soluble sodium salts of barbiturates, including Brevital Sodium, is maintained only at a relatively high (basic) pH.
Because of numerous requests from anesthesiologists for information regarding the chemical compatibility of these mixtures, the following chart contains information obtained from compatibility studies in which a 1% solution of Brevital Sodium was mixed with therapeutic amounts of agents whose solutions have a low (acid) pH.
[See table above]

HOW SUPPLIED

Store at controlled room temperature (20° to 25°C) (68° to 77°F) [see USP].
The expiration period for the vials is 2 years.
Brevital® Sodium Vials*:
500 mg (with 30 mg anhydrous sodium carbonate) are available as follows:
50-mL size, multiple dose—1's (NDC 61570-095-01)
50-mL size, multiple dose—25's (NDC 61570-095-25)
The 2.5 g vials (with 150 mg anhydrous sodium carbonate) are available as follows:
50-mL size, multiple dose—25's (NDC 61570-096-25)

*In crystalline form.
Prescribing Information as of September 2003.
Monarch Pharmaceuticals®
Distributed for:
Monarch Pharmaceuticals, Inc.
Bristol, TN 37620
(A wholly owned subsidiary of King Pharmaceuticals, Inc.)
Manufactured by:
King Pharmaceuticals, Inc.
Bristol, TN 37620 3000870
242

COLY-MYCIN® M PARENTERAL ℞

[cōlē-mīsin]
(Colistimethate for Injection, USP)
FOR INTRAMUSCULAR AND INTRAVENOUS USE

DESCRIPTION

Coly-Mycin® M Parenteral (Colistimethate for Injection, USP) is a sterile parenteral antibiotic product which, when reconstituted (see **Reconstitution**), is suitable for intramuscular or intravenous administration.
Each vial contains colistimethate sodium or pentasodium colistinmethanesulfonate (150 mg colistin base activity). Colistimethate sodium is a polypeptide antibiotic with an approximate molecular weight of 1750. The empirical formula is $C_{58}H_{105}N_{16}Na_5O_{28}S_5$ and the structural formula is represented below:

R–C(=O)–L-Dbu–L-Thr–L-Dbu–L-Dbu(Nγ)–L-Dbu–D-Leu–L-Leu–L-Dbu–L-Dbu–L-Thr (ring closed between Thr and Nγ of the fourth residue); side chains on L-Dbu: Nγ–CH_2–S(=O)(=O)–ONa

Dbu is 2, 4-diaminobutanoic acid; R is 5-methylheptyl in colistin A and 5-methylhexyl in colistin B

CLINICAL PHARMACOLOGY

Typical serum and urine levels following a single 150 mg dose of Coly-Mycin M Parenteral IM or IV in normal adult subjects are shown in Figure 1.
Higher serum levels were obtained at10 minutes following IV administration. Serum concentration declined with a half-life of 2–3 hours following either intravenous or intramuscular administration in adults and in the pediatric population, including premature infants.
Average urine levels ranged from about 270 mcg/mL at 2 hours to about 15 mcg/mL at 8 hours after intravenous administration and from 200 to about 25 mcg/mL during a similar period following intramuscular administration.
[See figure 1 at top of next column]
Microbiology: Colistimethate sodium is a surface active agent which penetrates into and disrupts the bacterial cell membrane. It has been shown to have bactericidal activity against most strains of the following microorganisms, both *in vitro* and in clinical infections as described in the **INDICATIONS AND USAGE** section:
Aerobic gram-negative microorganisms: *Enterobacter aerogenes, Escherichia coli, Klebsiella pneumoniae*, and *Pseudomonas aeruginosa*.
Susceptibility Tests: Colistimethate sodium is no longer listed as an antimicrobial for routine testing and reporting by clinical microbiology laboratories.

INDICATIONS AND USAGE

Coly-Mycin M Parenteral is indicated for the treatment of acute or chronic infections due to sensitive strains of certain gram-negative bacilli. It is particularly indicated when the infection is caused by sensitive strains of *Pseudomonas aeruginosa*. This antibiotic is not indicated for infections due to *Proteus* or *Neisseria*. Coly-Mycin M Parenteral has proven clinically effective in treatment of infections due to the following gram-negative organisms: *Enterobacter aerogenes, Escherichia coli, Klebsiella pneumoniae*, and *Pseudomonas aeruginosa*.
Coly-Mycin M Parenteral may be used to initiate therapy in serious infections that are suspected to be due to gram-negative organisms and in the treatment of infections due to susceptible gram-negative pathogenic bacilli.

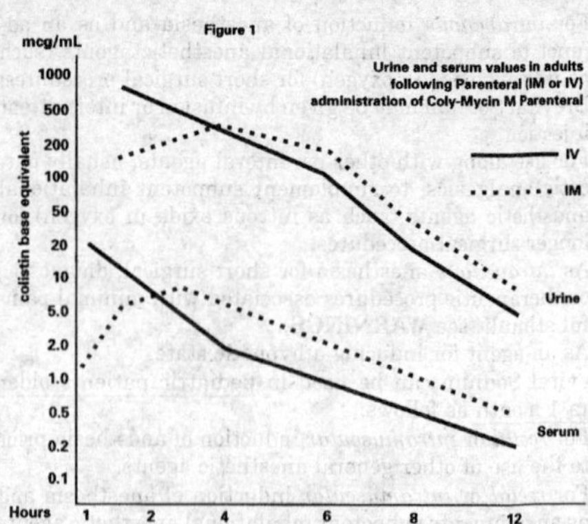

CONTRAINDICATIONS

The use of Coly-Mycin M Parenteral is contraindicated for patients with a history of sensitivity to the drug or any of its components.

WARNINGS

Maximum daily dose should not exceed 5 mg/kg/day (2.3 mg/lb) with normal renal function.
Transient neurological disturbances may occur. These include circumoral paresthesia or numbness, tingling or formication of the extremities, generalized pruritus, vertigo, dizziness, and slurring of speech. For these reasons, patients should be warned not to drive vehicles or use hazardous machinery while on therapy. Reduction of dosage may alleviate symptoms. Therapy need not be discontinued, but such patients should be observed with particular care.
Nephrotoxicity can occur and is probably a dose-dependent effect of colistimethate sodium. These manifestations of nephrotoxicity are reversible following discontinuation of the antibiotic.
Overdosage can result in renal insufficiency, muscle weakness, and apnea (see **OVERDOSAGE** section). See **PRECAUTIONS, Drug Interactions** subsection for use concomitantly with other antibiotics and curariform drugs.
Respiratory arrest has been reported following intramuscular administration of colistimethate sodium. Impaired renal function increases the possibility of apnea and neuromuscular blockade following administration of colistimethate sodium. Therefore, it is important to follow recommended dosing guidelines. See **DOSAGE AND ADMINISTRATION** section for use in renal impairment.
Pseudomembranous colitis has been reported with nearly all antimicrobial agents, and may range in severity from mild to life-threatening. Therefore, it is important to consider this diagnosis in patients who present with diarrhea subsequent to the administration of antibacterial agents.
Treatment with antibacterial agents alters the normal flora of the colon and may permit overgrowth of clostridia. Studies indicate that a toxin produced by *Clostridium difficile* is a primary cause of "antibiotic-associated colitis."
After the diagnosis of pseudomembranous colitis has been established, appropriate therapeutic measures should be initiated. Mild cases of pseudomembranous colitis usually respond to drug discontinuation alone. In moderate-to-severe cases, consideration should be given to management with fluids and electrolytes, protein supplementation, and treatment with an antibacterial drug clinically effective against *Clostridium difficile* colitis.

PRECAUTIONS

General

Since Coly-Mycin M Parenteral is eliminated mainly by renal excretion, it should be used with caution when the possibility of impaired renal function exists. The decline in renal function with advanced age should be considered.
When actual renal impairment is present, Coly-Mycin M Parenteral may be used, but the greatest caution should be exercised and the dosage should be reduced in proportion to the extent of the impairment. Administration of amounts of Coly-Mycin M Parenteral in excess of renal excretory capacity will lead to high serum levels and can result in further impairment of renal function, initiating a cycle which, if not recognized, can lead to acute renal insufficiency, renal shutdown, and further concentration of the antibiotic to toxic levels in the body. At this point, interference of nerve transmission at neuromuscular junctions may occur and result in muscle weakness and apnea (see **OVERDOSAGE** section).
Signs indicating the development of impaired renal function include: diminishing urine output, rising BUN and serum creatinine and decreased creatinine clearance. Therapy with Coly-Mycin M Parenteral should be discontinued immediately if signs of impaired renal function occur. How-

TABLE 1. Suggested Modification of Dosage Schedules of Coly-Mycin M Parenteral for Adults with Impaired Renal Function

Renal Function	Degree of Impairment			
	Normal	Mild	Moderate	Considerable
Plasma creatinine, mg/100 mL	0.7–1.2	1.3–1.5	1.6–2.5	2.6–4.0
Urea clearance, % of normal	80–100	40–70	25–40	10–25
Dosage				
Unit dose of Coly-Mycin M, mg	100–150	75–115	66–150	100–150
Frequency, times/day	4 to 2	2	2 or 1	every 36 hr
Total daily dose, mg	300	150–230	133–150	100
Approximate daily dose, mg/kg/day	5.0	2.5–3.8	2.5	1.5

Note: The suggested unit dose is 2.5–5 mg/kg; however, the time INTERVAL between injections should be increased in the presence of impaired renal function.

ever, if it is necessary to reinstate the drug, dosing should be adjusted accordingly after drug plasma levels have fallen (see **DOSAGE AND ADMINISTRATION** section).

Drug Interactions
Certain other antibiotics (aminoglycosides and polymyxin) have also been reported to interfere with the nerve transmission at the neuromuscular junction. Based on this reported activity, they should not be given concomitantly with Coly-Mycin M Parenteral except with the greatest caution. Curariform muscle relaxants (e.g., tubocurarine) and other drugs, including ether, succinylcholine, gallamine, decamethonium and sodium citrate, potentiate the neuromuscular blocking effect and should be used with extreme caution in patients being treated with Coly-Mycin M Parenteral.
Sodium cephalothin may enhance the nephrotoxicity of Coly-Mycin M Parenteral. The concomitant use of sodium cephalothin and Coly-Mycin M Parenteral should be avoided.

Carcinogenesis, Mutagenesis, Impairment of Fertility
Long-term animal carcinogenicity studies and genetic toxicology studies have not been performed with colistimethate sodium. There were no adverse effects on fertility or reproduction in rats at doses of 9.3 mg/kg/day (0.30 times the maximum daily human dose when based on mg/m^2).

Pregnancy—Teratogenic Effects
Pregnancy Category C: Colistimethate sodium given intramuscularly during organogenesis to rabbits at 4.15 and 9.3 mg/kg resulted in talipes varus in 2.6% and 2.9% of fetuses, respectively. These doses are 0.25 and 0.55 times the maximum daily human dose based on mg/m^2. In addition, increased resorption occurred at 9.3 mg/kg. Colistimethate sodium was not teratogenic in rats at 4.15 or 9.3 mg/kg. These doses are 0.13 and 0.30 times the maximum daily human dose based on mg/m^2. There are no adequate and well-controlled studies in pregnant women. Since colistimethate sodium is transferred across the placental barrier in humans, it should be used during pregnancy only if the potential benefit justifies the potential risk to the fetus.

Nursing Mothers
It is not known whether colistimethate sodium is excreted in human breast milk. However, colistin sulphate is excreted in human breast milk. Therefore, caution should be exercised when colistimethate sodium is administered to nursing women.

Geriatric Use
Clinical studies of colistemethate sodium did not include sufficient numbers of subjects aged 65 and over to determine whether they respond differently from younger subjects. Other reported clinical experience has not identified differences in responses between the elderly and younger patients. In general, dose selection for an elderly patient should be cautious, usually starting at the low end of the dosing range, reflecting the greater frequency of decreased hepatic, renal, or cardiac function, and of concomitant disease or other drug therapy. This drug is known to be substantially excreted by the kidney, and the risk of toxic reactions to this drug may be greater in patients with impaired renal function. Because elderly patients are more likely to have decreased renal function, care should be taken in dose selection, and it may be useful to monitor renal function.

Pediatric Use
In clinical studies, colistimethate sodium was administered to the pediatric population (neonates, infants, children and adolescents). Although adverse reactions appear to be similar in the adult and pediatric populations, subjective symptoms of toxicity may not be reported by pediatric patients. Close clinical monitoring of pediatric patients is recommended.

ADVERSE REACTIONS

The following adverse reactions have been reported:
Gastrointestinal: gastrointestinal upset
Nervous System: tingling of extremities and tongue, slurred speech, dizziness, vertigo and paresthesia
Integumentary: generalized itching, urticaria and rash
Body as a Whole: fever
Laboratory Deviations: increased blood urea nitrogen (BUN), elevated creatinine and decreased creatinine clearance
Respiratory System: respiratory distress and apnea
Renal System: nephrotoxicity and decreased urine output

OVERDOSAGE

Overdosage with colistimethate sodium can cause neuromuscular blockade characterized by paresthesia, lethargy, confusion, dizziness, ataxia, nystagmus, disorders of speech and apnea. Respiratory muscle paralysis may lead to apnea, respiratory arrest and death. Overdosage with the drug can also cause acute renal failure, manifested as decreased urine output and increases in serum concentrations of BUN and creatinine.
As in any case of overdose, colistimethate sodium therapy should be discontinued and general supportive measures should be utilized.
It is unknown whether colistimethate sodium can be removed by hemodialysis or peritoneal dialysis in overdose cases.

DOSAGE AND ADMINISTRATION

Important: Coly-Mycin M Parenteral is supplied in vials containing colistimethate sodium equivalent to 150 mg colistin base activity per vial.
Reconstitution: The **150 mg** vial should be reconstituted with **2.0 mL** Sterile Water for Injection, USP. The reconstituted solution provides colistimethate sodium at a concentration equivalent to 75 mg/mL colistin base activity.
During reconstitution swirl **gently** to avoid frothing.
Parenteral drug products should be inspected visually for particulate matter and discoloration prior to administration, whenever solution and container permit. If these conditions are observed, the product should not be used.

Dosage
Adults and pediatric patients—Intravenous or Intramuscular Administration: Coly-Mycin M Parenteral should be given in 2 to 4 divided doses at dose levels of 2.5 to 5 mg/kg per day for patients with normal renal function, depending on the severity of the infection.
In obese individuals, dosage should be based on ideal body weight.
The daily dose should be reduced in the presence of renal impairment. Modifications of dosage in the presence of renal impairment are presented in Table 1.
[See table 1 above]

INTRAVENOUS ADMINISTRATION

1. Direct Intermittent Administration—Slowly inject one-half of the total daily dose over a period of 3 to 5 minutes every 12 hours.
2. Continuous Infusion—Slowly inject one-half of the total daily dose over 3 to 5 minutes. Add the remaining half of the total daily dose of Coly-Mycin M Parenteral to one of the following:
   - 0.9% NaCI
   - 5% dextrose in 0.9% NaCI
   - 5% dextrose in water
   - 5% dextrose in 0.45% NaCI
   - 5% dextrose in 0.225% NaCI
   - lactated Ringer's solution
   - 10% invert sugar solution

There are not sufficient data to recommend usage of Coly-Mycin M Parenteral with other drugs or other than the above listed infusion solutions.
Administer the second half of the total daily dose by slow intravenous infusion, starting 1 to 2 hours after the initial dose, over the next 22 to 23 hours. In the presence of impaired renal function, reduce the infusion rate depending on the degree of renal impairment.
The choice of intravenous solution and the volume to be employed are dictated by the requirements of fluid and electrolyte management.
Any infusion solution containing colistimethate sodium should be freshly prepared and used for no longer than 24 hours.

HOW SUPPLIED

Coly-Mycin M Parenteral is supplied in vials containing colistimethate sodium (equivalent to 150 mg colistin base activity per vial) as a white to slightly yellow lyophilized cake and is available as one vial per carton (NDC 61570-414-51)
Store between 20°–25°C (68°–77°F). (See USP controlled room temperature.)
Store reconstituted solution in refrigerator 2°–8°C (36°–46°F) or between 20°–25°C (68°–77°F) and use within 7 days.
Rx only.
Prescribing Information as of February 2004.
Distributed by:
Monarch Pharmaceuticals, Inc.
Bristol, TN 37620
(A wholly owned subsidiary of King Pharmaceuticals, Inc.)
Manufactured by:
Parkedale Pharmaceuticals, Inc.
Rochester, MI 48307
3000818
Shown in Product Identification Guide, page 319

CORTISPORIN® Cream ℞

[*cŏr 'tĭ-spŏrin*]
(neomycin and polymyxin B sulfates and hydrocortisone acetate cream, USP)

DESCRIPTION

CORTISPORIN Cream (neomycin and polymyxin B sulfates and hydrocortisone acetate cream, USP) is a topical antibacterial cream. Each gram contains: neomycin sulfate equivalent to 3.5 mg neomycin base, polymyxin B sulfate equivalent to 10,000 polymyxin B units, and hydrocortisone acetate 5 mg (0.5%). The inactive ingredients are liquid petrolatum, white petrolatum, propylene glycol, polyoxyethylene polyoxypropylene compound, emulsifying wax, purified water, and 0.25% methylparaben added as a preservative. Sodium hydroxide or sulfuric acid may be added to adjust pH.
Neomycin sulfate is the sulfate salt of neomycin B and C, which are produced by the growth of *Streptomyces fradiae* Waksman (Fam. Streptomycetaceae). It has a potency equivalent of not less than 600 µg of neomycin standard per mg, calculated on an anhydrous basis. The structural formulae are:

Neomycin B (R_1=H, R_2=CH_2NH_2)
Neomycin C (R_1=CH_2NH_2, R_2=H)

Polymyxin B sulfate is the sulfate salt of polymyxin B_1 and B_2, which are produced by the growth of *Bacillus polymyxa* (Prazmowski) Migula (Fam. Bacillaceae). It has a potency of not less than 6,000 polymyxin B units per mg, calculated on an anhydrous basis. The structural formulae are:

Polymyxin B_1 (R=CH_3)
Polymyxin B_2 (R=H)
DAB=α,γ-diaminobutyric acid

Hydrocortisone acetate is the acetate ester of hydrocortisone, an anti-inflammatory hormone. Its chemical name is 21-(acetyloxy)-11β,17-dihydroxypregn-4-ene-3,20-dione. Its structural formula is:

The base is a smooth vanishing cream with a pH of approximately 5.0.

CLINICAL PHARMACOLOGY

Corticoids suppress the inflammatory response to a variety of agents and they may delay healing. Since corticoids may inhibit the body's defense mechanism against infection, a concomitant antimicrobial drug may be used when this inhibition is considered to be clinically significant in a particular case.
The anti-infective components in the combination are included to provide action against specific organisms susceptible to them. Polymyxin B sulfate and neomycin sulfate together are considered active against the following microorganisms: *Staphylococcus aureus, Escherichia coli, Haemophilus influenzae, Klebsiella-Enterobacter* species, *Neisseria* species, and *Pseudomonas aeruginosa*. The product does not provide adequate coverage against *Serratia marcescens* and streptococci, including *Streptococcus pneumoniae*.
The relative potency of corticosteroids depends on the molecular structure, concentration, and release from the vehicle.
The acid pH helps restore normal cutaneous acidity. Owing to its excellent spreading and penetrating properties, the cream facilitates treatment of hairy and intertriginous areas. It may also be of value in selective cases where the lesions are moist.

Continued on next page

Cortisporin—Cont.

INDICATIONS AND USAGE

For the treatment of corticosteroid-responsive dermatoses with secondary infection. It has not been demonstrated that this steroid-antibiotic combination provides greater benefit than the steroid component alone after 7 days of treatment (see **WARNINGS**).

CONTRAINDICATIONS

Not for use in the eyes or in the external ear canal if the eardrum is perforated. This product is contraindicated in tuberculous, fungal, or viral lesions of the skin (herpes simplex, vaccinia, and varicella). This product is contraindicated in those individuals who have shown hypersensitivity to any of its components.

WARNINGS

Because of the concern of nephrotoxicity and ototoxicity associated with neomycin, this combination should not be used over a wide area or for extended periods of time.

PRECAUTIONS

General: As with any antibacterial preparation, prolonged use may result in overgrowth of nonsusceptible organisms, including fungi. Appropriate measures should be taken if this occurs. Use of steroids on infected areas should be supervised with care as anti-inflammatory steroids may encourage spread of infection. If this occurs, steroid therapy should be stopped and appropriate antibacterial drugs used. Generalized dermatological conditions may require systemic corticosteroid therapy.

Signs and symptoms of exogenous hyperadrenocorticism can occur with the use of topical corticosteroids, including adrenal suppression. Systemic absorption of topically applied steroids will be increased if extensive body surface areas are treated or if occlusive dressings are used. Under these circumstances, suitable precautions should be taken when long-term use is anticipated.

Specifically, sufficient percutaneous absorption of hydrocortisone can occur in pediatric patients during prolonged use to cause cessation of growth, as well as other systemic signs and symptoms of hyperadrenocorticism.

Information for Patients: If redness, irritation, swelling or pain persists or increases, discontinue use and notify physician. Do not use in the eyes.

Laboratory Tests: Systemic effects of excessive levels of hydrocortisone may include a reduction in the number of circulating eosinophils and a decrease in urinary excretion of 17-hydroxycorticosteroids.

Carcinogenesis, Mutagenesis, Impairment of Fertility: Long-term studies in animals (rats, rabbits, mice) showed no evidence of carcinogenicity attributable to oral administration of corticosteroids.

Pregnancy: ***Teratogenic Effects:*** Pregnancy Category C. Corticosteroids have been shown to be teratogenic in rabbits when applied topically at concentrations of 0.5% on days 6 to 18 of gestation and in mice when applied topically at a concentration of 15% on days 10 to 13 of gestation. There are no adequate and well-controlled studies in pregnant women.

Corticosteroids should be used during pregnancy only if the potential benefit justifies the potential risk to the fetus.

Nursing Mothers: Hydrocortisone acetate appears in human milk following oral administration of the drug. Since systemic absorption of hydrocortisone may occur when applied topically, caution should be exercised when CORTISPORIN Cream is used by a nursing woman.

Geriatric Use: Clinical studies of Cortisporin Cream did not include sufficient numbers of subjects aged 65 and over to determine whether they respond differently from younger subjects. Other reported clinical experience has not identified differences in responses between the elderly and younger patients. In general, dose selection for an elderly patient should be cautious, usually starting at the low end of the dosing range, reflecting the greater frequency of decreased hepatic, renal, or cardiac function, and of concomitant disease or other drug therapy.

Pediatric Use: Safety and effectiveness in pediatric patients have not been established (see **PRECAUTIONS: General**).

ADVERSE REACTIONS

Neomycin occasionally causes skin sensitization. Ototoxicity and nephrotoxicity have also been reported (see **WARNINGS**). Adverse reactions have occurred with topical use of antibiotic combinations including neomycin and polymyxin B. Exact incidence figures are not available since no denominator of treated patients is available. The reaction occurring most often is allergic sensitization. In one clinical study, using a 20% neomycin patch, neomycin-induced allergic skin reactions occurred in two of 2,175 (0.09%) individuals in the general population.[1] In another study, the incidence was found to be approximately 1%.[2]

The following local adverse reactions have been reported with topical corticosteroids, especially under occlusive dressings: burning, itching, irritation, dryness, folliculitis, hypertrichosis, acneiform eruptions, hypopigmentation, perioral dermatitis, allergic contact dermatitis, maceration of the skin, secondary infection, skin atrophy, striae, and miliaria.

When steroid preparations are used for long periods of time in intertriginous areas or over extensive body areas, with or without occlusive non-permeable dressings, striae may occur; also there exists the possibility of systemic side effects when steroid preparations are used over large areas or for a long period of time.

DOSAGE AND ADMINISTRATION

A small quantity of the cream should be applied 2 to 4 times daily, as required. The cream should, if conditions permit, be gently rubbed into the affected areas.

HOW SUPPLIED

Tube of 7.5 g (NDC 61570-032-75).
Store at 15° to 25°C (59° to 77°F).

REFERENCES

1. Leyden JJ, Kligman AM. Contact dermatitis to neomycin sulfate. *JAMA*. 1979;242:1276–1278.
2. Prystowsky SD, Allen AM, Smith RW, et al. Allergic contact hypersensitivity to nickel, neomycin, ethylenediamine, and benzocaine. *Arch Dermatol*. 1979;115:959–962.

Prescribing Information as of November 2003.
Distributed by: Monarch Pharmaceuticals, Inc., Bristol, TN 37620
(A wholly owned subsidiary of King Pharmaceuticals, Inc.)
Manufactured by: King Pharmaceuticals, Inc., Bristol, TN 37620
MONARCH
Pharmaceuticals®
3000212-A

CORTISPORIN®-TC Otic Suspension ℞

[*cōr 'ti -spōr-ĭn*]

with Neomycin and Hydrocortisone

(colistin sulfate — neomycin sulfate — thonzonium bromide— hydrocortisone acetate otic suspension)

DESCRIPTION

Cortisporin®-TC Otic Suspension with Neomycin and Hydrocortisone (colistin sulfate—neomycin sulfate—thonzonium bromide—hydrocortisone acetate otic suspension) is a sterile antibacterial and anti-inflammatory aqueous suspension containing in each mL: Colistin base activity, 3 mg (as the sulfate); Neomycin base activity, 3.3 mg (as the sulfate); Hydrocortisone acetate, 10 mg (1%); Thonzonium bromide, 0.5 mg (0.05%); Polysorbate 80, acetic acid, and sodium acetate in a buffered aqueous vehicle. Thimerosal (mercury derivative), 0.002%, is added as a preservative. It is a nonviscous liquid, buffered at pH 5, for instillation into the canal of the external ear or direct application to the affected aural skin.

The structural formulas of colistin sulfate (mixture of Colistin A & B), neomycin sulfate (mixture of neomycin A, B & C), hydrocortisone acetate ((11β)-21-(acetyloxy)-11,17-dihydroxypregn)methyl]-2 pyrim- idinylamino] ethyl]-N,N-dimethyl-1-hexadecanaminium, bromide) are represented below:

Thonzonium Bromide

RC(O)—Dbu - Thr - Dbu - Dbu - Dbu - DLeu - Leu - Dbu - DbuThr • 2.5 H_2SO_4

Dbu is L - α, γ -diaminobuyric acid; R is 5- methylhoptyl in Colistin A and 5-methylhexyl in Colistin B

Colistin sulfate

Neomycin A

Neomycin B Sulfate

Hydrocortisone Acetate

Neomycin C Sulfate

CLINICAL PHARMACOLOGY

Colistin sulfate is a polypeptide antibiotic which penetrates into and disrupts the bacterial cell membrane. Neomycin sulfate is an aminoglycoside antibiotic which inhibits protein synthesis, disrupting the normal cycle of ribosomal function. Hydrocortisone acetate is a corticosteroid hormone which is thought to act by regulating the rate of protein synthesis; it controls inflammation, edema, pruritus and other dermal reactions. Cortiscosteroids suppress the inflammatory response to a variety of agents and they may delay healing. Since corticoids may inhibit the body's defense mechanism against infection, a concomitant antimicrobial drug may be used when this inhibition is considered to be clinically significant in a particular case.

The relative potency of corticosteroids depends on the molecular structure, concentration, and release from the vehicle.

Thonzonium bromide is a surface-active agent that promotes tissue contact by dispersion and penetration of the cellular debris and exudate.

Microbiology:

Together, colistin sulfate and neomycin sulfate have bactericidal activity against most strains of the following microorganisms, both *in vitro* and in clinical infections as described in the INDICATIONS AND USAGE section.

Aerobic gram-positive microorganisms:
Staphylococcus aureus.

Aerobic gram-negative microorganisms:
Enterobacter aerogenes
Escherichia coli
Klebsiella pneumoniae
Pseudomonas aeruginosa.

Susceptibility Tests: It is not recommended that colistin sulfate or neomycin sulfate be routinely tested and reported by clinical microbiology laboratories.[1]

INDICATIONS AND USAGE

Cortisporin®-TC Otic Suspension is indicated for the treatment of superficial bacterial infections of the external auditory canal, caused by organisms susceptible to the action of the antibiotics; and for the treatment of infections of mastoidectomy and fenestration cavities, caused by organisms susceptible to the antibiotics.

CONTRAINDICATIONS

This product is contraindicated in those individuals who have shown hypersensitivity to any of its components.

This product should not be used if the external auditory canal disorder is suspected or known to be due to cutaneous viral infection (e.g., herpes simplex virus or varicella zoster virus).

WARNINGS

Neomycin can induce permanent sensorineural hearing loss due to cochlear damage, mainly destruction of hair cells in the organ of Corti. The risk is greater with prolonged use. Therapy should be limited to 10 consecutive days. (See PRECAUTIONS-General.) Patients being treated with eardrops containing neomycin should be under close clinical observation. Cortisporin®-TC Otic Suspension should be used cautiously in any patient with a perforated tympanic membrane.

Neomycin sulfate may cause cutaneous sensitization. A precise incidence of hypersensitivity reactions (primarily skin rash) due to topical neomycin is not known. Discontinue promptly if sensitivity or irritation occurs.

When using neomycin-containing products to control secondary infection in the chronic dermatoses, such as chronic otitis externa or stasis dermatitis, it should be borne in mind that the skin in these conditions is more liable than is normal skin to become sensitized to many substances, including neomycin. The manifestation of sensitization to neomycin is usually a low-grade reddening with swelling, dry scaling, and itching; it may be manifest simply as a failure to heal. Periodic examination for such signs is advisable, and the patient should be told to discontinue the product if they are observed. These symptoms regress quickly on withdrawing the medication. Neomycin-containing applications should be avoided for the patient thereafter.

PRECAUTIONS

General

As with any other antibiotic preparation, prolonged treatment may result in overgrowth of nonsusceptible organisms and fungi. If the infection is not improved after one week, cultures should be repeated to verify the identity of the organism and to determine whether therapy should be changed.

Treatment should not be continued for longer than ten days. Allergic cross-reactions may occur which could prevent the use of any or all of the aminoglycoside antibiotics for the treatment of future infections.

Information for Patients

Avoid contaminating the dropper with material from the ear, fingers, or other source. This caution is necessary if the sterility of the drops is to be preserved.

If sensitization or irritation occurs, discontinue use immediately and contact your physician.

Do not use in the eyes.

If you prefer to warm the medication before using it, do not heat the suspension above body temperature in order to avoid loss of potency.

SHAKE WELL BEFORE USING.

Laboratory Tests

Systemic effects of excessive levels of hydrocortisone may include a reduction in the number of circulating eosinophils and a decrease in urinary excretion of 17-hydroxycorticosteroids.

Carcinogenesis, Mutagenesis, Impairment of Fertility

Long-term animal carcinogenicity studies have not been performed with colistin or neomycin, or Cortisporin®-TC Otic Suspension. An increased incidence of chromosome aberrations in human lymphocytes has been reported following *in vitro* exposure to colistin or neomycin.

Fertility studies have not been performed with neomycin, but reports from the scientific literature suggest that it may decrease spermatogenesis in rats. No adverse effects on fertility were observed in male or female rats given intramuscular doses of colistimethate sodium, the methanesulfonate salt of colistin, up to 20 mg/kg (equivalent to 9.3 mg/kg of colistin base). This is approximately 30 times the clinical daily dose based on body surface area, assuming 100% absorption from the ear; however, significant systemic levels of colistin or neomycin would not be anticipated in humans when Cortisporin®-TC Otic Suspension is used as directed.

Long term studies in rodents showed no evidence of carcinogenicity attributable to oral administration of corticosteroids. Mutagenicity studies with hydrocortisone were negative. Studies have not been performed to evaluate the effect on fertility of topical corticosteroids.

Pregnancy-Teratogenic Effects

Pregnancy Category C – There are no adequate and well controlled studies of Cortisporin®-TC Otic Suspension in pregnant women. It is not known whether Cortisporin®-TC Otic Suspension can cause fetal harm when administered to a pregnant woman.

Colistimethate sodium, the methanesulfonate salt of colistin, was not teratogenic in rats or rabbits given intramuscular doses up to 20 mg/kg (equivalent to 9.3 mg/kg of colisitin base, approximately 30 times (rats) or 55 times (rabbits) the clinical daily dose based on body suface area and assuming 100% absorption from the ear). Increased resorptions were observed in rabbits at 20 mg/kg, but not 10 mg/kg (equivalent to 4.15 mg/kg of colistin base). Decreased pup survival at weaning was observed in rats at 20 mg/kg, a maternally toxic dose of colistin, but not 10 mg/kg. Colistin has not been shown to have any adverse effects on the developing embryo or fetus at doses relevant to the amount that will be delivered ototopically at the recommended clinical doses.

Although aminoglycosides can cause congenital deafness in humans if administered during pregnancy, significant systemic levels of neomycin would not be anticipated when Cortisporin®-TC Otic Suspension is used as directed.

Corticosteroids are generally teratogenic in laboratory animals when administered systemically at relatively low dosage levels. The more potent corticosteroids have been shown to be teratogenic after dermal application in laboratory animals.

Cortisporin®-TC Otic Suspension should be used during pregnancy only if the potential benefit justifies the potential risk to the fetus.

Nursing Mothers:

Hydrocortisone and colistin sulfate appear in human milk following oral administration of the drugs. Since systemic absorption of these drugs may occur when they are used topically, caution should be exercised when Cortisporin®-TC Otic Suspension is used by a nursing woman.

Pediatric Use: See **DOSAGE AND ADMINISTRATION**.

ADVERSE REACTIONS

Neomycin occasionally causes skin sensitization.

Ototoxicity (see WARNINGS section) and nephrotoxicity have also been reported. Adverse reactions have occurred with topical use of antibiotic combinations. Exact incidence figures are not available since no denominator of treated patients is available. The reaction occurring most often is allergic sensitization. In one clinical study, using a 20% neomycin patch, neomycin-induced allergic skin reactions occurred in two of 2,175 (0.09%) individuals in the general populaton.[2] In another study the incidence was found to be approximately 1%.[3]

The following local adverse events have been reported with topical corticosteroids, especially under occlusive dressings: burning, itching, irritation, dryness, folliculitis, hypertrichosis, acneiform eruptions, hypopigmentation, perioral dermatitis, allergic contact dermatitis, maceration of the skin, secondary infection, skin atrophy, striae, and miliaria.

DOSAGE AND ADMINISTRATION

Therapy with this product should be limited to 10 days. (See WARNINGS.)

The external auditory canal should be thoroughly cleansed and dried with a sterile cotton applicator.

When using the calibrated dropper:

For adults, 5 drops of the suspension should be instilled into the affected ear 3 or 4 times daily using the provided dropper. For pediatric patients, 4 drops (using the provided dropper) are suggested because of the smaller capacity of the ear canal.

The patient should lie with the affected ear upward and then the drops should be instilled. This position should be maintained for 5 minutes to facilitate penetration of the drops into the ear canal. Repeat, if necessary, for the opposite ear.

If preferred, a cotton wick may be inserted into the canal and then the cotton may be saturated with the suspension. This wick should be kept moist by adding further solution every 4 hours. The wick should be replaced at least once every 24 hours.

HOW SUPPLIED

Cortisporin®-TC Otic Suspension is supplied as: NDC 61570-090-10 .... 10 mL bottle with dropper

Each mL contains: Colistin sulfate equivalent to 3 mg of colistin base activity, Neomycin sulfate equivalent to 3.3 mg neomycin base activity, Hydrocortisone acetate 10 mg (1%), Thonzonium bromide 0.5 mg (0.05%), and Polysorbate 80 in an aqueous vehicle buffered with acetic acid and sodium acetate. Thimerosal (mercury derivative) 0.002% is added as a preservative.

A sterilized dropper-cap assembly for use on the bottle of suspension is included in the package.

Shake well before using.

Store at 20°–25°C (68°–77°F). (See USP controlled room temperature.)

Rx only.

REFERENCES

1. National Committee for Clinical Laboratory Standards, Suggested Groupings of U.S. FDA Approved Antimicrobial Agents That Should be Considered for Routine Testing and Reporting on Nonfastidious Organisms by Clinical Microbiology Laboratories, Table 1-M2-A6 (M100-S7), NCCLS Vol. 17, No. 1, Wayne, PA, 1997.
2. Leyden JJ, Kligman AM. Contact dermatitis to neomycin sulfate. *JAMA* 1979; 242 (12): 1276–1278.
3. Prystowsky SD, Allen AM, Smith RW, et al. Allergic contact hypersensitivity to nickel, neomycin, ethylenediamine, and benzocaine; relationship between age, sex, history of exposure, and reactivity to standard patch tests and use tests in a general populaton. *Arch Dermatol* 1979; 115:959–962.

Monarch Pharmaceuticals®

Distributed by: Monarch Pharmaceuticals, Inc., Bristol, TN 37620

Manufactured by: Parkedale Pharmaceuticals, Inc., Rochester, MI 48307

Prescribing Information as of April 2002

Shown in Product Identification Guide, page 319

CORZIDE® 40/5 ℞

CORZIDE® 80/5

[*kōr-zīd*]

(Nadolol and Bendroflumethiazide) Tablets

℞ **only**

DESCRIPTION

CORZIDE (Nadolol and Bendroflumethiazide Tablets) for oral administration combines two antihypertensive agents: CORGARD® (nadolol), a nonselective beta-adrenergic blocking agent, and NATURETIN® (bendroflumethiazide), a thiazide diuretic-antihypertensive. Formulations: 40 mg and 80 mg nadolol per tablet combined with 5 mg bendroflumethiazide. Inactive ingredients: cellulose, colorant (FD&C Blue No. 2), lactose, magnesium stearate, povidone, sodium starch glycolate, and starch.

Nadolol

Nadolol is a white crystalline powder. It is freely soluble in ethanol, soluble in hydrochloric acid, slightly soluble in water and in chloroform, and very slightly soluble in sodium hydroxide.

Nadolol is designated chemically as 1-(tert-butylamino)-3-[(5,6,7,8-tetrahydro-*cis*-6,7-dihydroxy-1-naphthyl)oxy]-2-propanol. Structural formula:

[See chemical structure at top of next column]

Bendroflumethiazide

Bendroflumethiazide is a white crystalline powder. It is soluble in alcohol and in sodium hydroxide, and insoluble in hydrochloric acid, water, and chloroform.

OH H H OH

$OCH_2CHCH_2NHC(CH_3)_3$

OH

$C_{17}H_{27}NO_4$ MW 309.40 CAS-42200-33-9

Bendroflumethiazide is designated chemically as 3-benzyl-3,4-dihydro-6-(trifluoromethyl)-2H-1,2,4-benzothiadiazine-7-sulfonamide 1,1-dioxide. Structural formula:

NH_2SO_2 O S O NH CF_3 N H CH_2

$C_{15}H_{14}F_3N_3O_4S_2$ MW 421.41 CAS-73-48-3

CLINICAL PHARMACOLOGY

Nadolol

Nadolol is a nonselective beta-adrenergic receptor blocking agent. Clinical pharmacology studies have demonstrated beta-blocking activity by showing (1) reduction in heart rate and cardiac output at rest and on exercise, (2) reduction of systolic and diastolic blood pressure at rest and on exercise, (3) inhibition of isoproterenol-induced tachycardia, and (4) reduction of reflex orthostatic tachycardia.

Nadolol specifically competes with beta-adrenergic receptor agonists for available beta receptor sites; it inhibits both the $beta_1$ receptors located chiefly in cardiac muscle and the $beta_2$ receptors located chiefly in the bronchial and vascular musculature, inhibiting the chronotropic, inotropic, and vasodilator responses to beta-adrenergic stimulation proportionately. Nadolol has no intrinsic sympathomimetic activity and, unlike some other beta-adrenergic blocking agents, nadolol has little direct myocardial depressant activity and does not have an anesthetic-like membrane-stabilizing action. Animal and human studies show that nadolol slows the sinus rate and depresses AV conduction. In dogs, only minimal amounts of nadolol were detected in the brain relative to amounts in blood and other organs and tissues. Nadolol has low lipophilicity as determined by octanol/water partition coefficient, a characteristic of certain beta-blocking agents that has been correlated with the limited extent to which these agents cross the blood-brain barrier, their low concentration in the brain, and low incidence of CNS-related side effects.

In controlled clinical studies, nadolol at doses of 40 to 320 mg/day has been shown to decrease both standing and supine blood pressure, the effect persisting for approximately 24 hours after dosing.

The mechanism of the antihypertensive effects of beta-adrenergic receptor blocking agents has not been established; however, factors that may be involved include (1) competitive antagonism of catecholamines at peripheral (non-CNS) adrenergic neuron sites (especially cardiac) leading to decreased cardiac output, (2) a central effect leading to reduced tonic-sympathetic nerve outflow to the periphery, and (3) suppression of renin secretion by blockade of the beta-adrenergic receptors responsible for renin release from the kidneys.

While cardiac output and arterial pressure are reduced by nadolol therapy, renal hemodynamics are stable, with preservation of renal blood flow and glomerular filtration rate. By blocking catecholamine-induced increases in heart rate, velocity and extent of myocardial contraction, and blood pressure, nadolol generally reduces the oxygen requirements of the heart at any given level of effort, making it useful for many patients in the long-term management of angina pectoris. On the other hand, nadolol can increase oxygen requirements by increasing left ventricular fiber length and end diastolic pressure, particularly in patients with heart failure.

Although beta-adrenergic receptor blockade is useful in treatment of angina and hypertension, there are also situations in which sympathetic stimulation is vital. For example, in patients with severely damaged hearts, adequate ventricular function may depend on sympathetic drive. Beta-adrenergic blockade may worsen AV block by preventing the necessary facilitating effects of sympathetic activity on conduction. $Beta_2$-adrenergic blockade results in passive bronchial constriction by interfering with endogenous adrenergic bronchodilator activity in patients subject to bronchospasm and may also interfere with exogenous bronchodilators in such patients.

Absorption of nadolol after oral dosing is variable, averaging about 30 percent. Peak serum concentrations of nadolol usually occur in three to four hours after oral administration and the presence of food in the gastrointestinal tract does not affect the rate or extent of nadolol absorption. Approximately 30 percent of the nadolol present in serum is reversibly bound to plasma protein.

Unlike many other beta-adrenergic blocking agents, nadolol is not metabolized by the liver and is excreted unchanged, principally by the kidneys.

The half-life of therapeutic doses of nadolol is about 20 to 24 hours, permitting once-daily dosage. Because nadolol is excreted predominantly in the urine, its half-life increases in renal failure (see **PRECAUTIONS, General,** and **DOSAGE AND ADMINISTRATION**). Steady state serum concentra-

Continued on next page

Corzide—Cont.

tions of nadolol are attained in six to nine days with once-daily dosage in persons with normal renal function. Because of variable absorption and different individual responsiveness, the proper dosage must be determined by titration.
Exacerbation of angina and, in some cases, myocardial infarction and ventricular dysrhythmias have been reported after abrupt discontinuation of therapy with beta-adrenergic blocking agents in patients with coronary artery disease. Abrupt withdrawal of these agents in patients without coronary artery disease has resulted in transient symptoms, including tremulousness, sweating, palpitation, headache, and malaise. Several mechanisms have been proposed to explain these phenomena, among them increased sensitivity to catecholamines because of increased numbers of beta receptors.

Bendroflumethiazide
The mechanism of action of bendroflumethiazide results in an interference with the renal tubular mechanism of electrolyte reabsorption. At maximal therapeutic dosage all thiazides are approximately equal in their diuretic potency.
Thiazides increase excretion of sodium and chloride in approximately equivalent amounts. Natriuresis causes a secondary loss of potassium and bicarbonate.
The mechanism of the antihypertensive effect of thiazides is unknown. Thiazides do not affect normal blood pressure.
Onset of action of thiazides occurs in two hours and the peak effect at about four hours. Duration of action persists for approximately six to 12 hours. Thiazides are eliminated rapidly by the kidney.

INDICATIONS

CORZIDE (Nadolol and Bendroflumethiazide Tablets) is indicated in the management of hypertension.
This fixed combination drug is not indicated for initial therapy of hypertension. If the fixed combination represents the dose titrated to the individual patient's needs, it may be more convenient than the separate components.

CONTRAINDICATIONS

Nadolol
Nadolol is contraindicated in bronchial asthma, sinus bradycardia and greater than first degree conduction block, cardiogenic shock, and overt cardiac failure (see **WARNINGS**).
Bendroflumethiazide
Bendroflumethiazide is contraindicated in anuria. It is also contraindicated in patients who have previously demonstrated hypersensitivity to bendroflumethiazide or other sulfonamide-derived drugs.

WARNINGS

Nadolol
Cardiac Failure—Sympathetic stimulation may be a vital component supporting circulatory function in patients with congestive heart failure, and its inhibition by beta-blockade may precipitate more severe failure. Although beta-blockers should be avoided in overt congestive heart failure, if necessary, they can be used with caution in patients with a history of failure who are well compensated, usually with digitalis and diuretics. Beta-adrenergic blocking agents do not abolish the inotropic action of digitalis on heart muscle.
IN PATIENTS WITHOUT A HISTORY OF HEART FAILURE, continued use of beta-blockers can, in some cases, lead to cardiac failure. Therefore, at the first sign or symptom of heart failure, the patient should be digitalized and/or treated with diuretics, and the response observed closely, or nadolol should be discontinued (gradually, if possible).

> **Exacerbation of Ischemic Heart Disease Following Abrupt Withdrawal**—Hypersensitivity to catecholamines has been observed in patients withdrawn from beta-blocker therapy; exacerbation of angina and, in some cases, myocardial infarction have occurred after abrupt discontinuation of such therapy. When discontinuing chronically administered nadolol, particularly in patients with ischemic heart disease, the dosage should be gradually reduced over a period of one to two weeks and the patient should be carefully monitored. If angina markedly worsens or acute coronary insufficiency develops, nadolol administration should be reinstituted promptly, at least temporarily, and other measures appropriate for the management of unstable angina should be taken. Patients should be warned against interruption or discontinuation of therapy without the physician's advice. Because coronary artery disease is common and may be unrecognized, it may be prudent not to discontinue nadolol therapy abruptly even in patients treated only for hypertension.

Nonallergic Bronchospasm (e.g., chronic bronchitis, emphysema)—PATIENTS WITH BRONCHOSPASTIC DISEASES SHOULD IN GENERAL NOT RECEIVE BETA-BLOCKERS. Nadolol should be administered with caution since it may block bronchodilation produced by endogenous or exogenous catecholamine stimulation of $beta_2$ receptors.
Major Surgery—Because beta-blockade impairs the ability of the heart to respond to reflex stimuli and may increase the risks of general anesthesia and surgical procedures, resulting in protracted hypotension or low cardiac output, it has generally been suggested that such therapy should be withdrawn several days prior to surgery. Recognition of the increased sensitivity to catecholamines of patients recently withdrawn from beta-blocker therapy, however, has made this recommendation controversial. If possible, beta-blockers should be withdrawn well before surgery takes place. In the event of emergency surgery, the anesthesiologist should be informed that the patient is on beta-blocker therapy. The effects of nadolol can be reversed by administration of beta-receptor agonists such as isoproterenol, dopamine, dobutamine, or levarterenol. Difficulty in restarting and maintaining the heart beat has also been reported with beta-adrenergic receptor blocking agents.
Diabetes and Hypoglycemia—Beta-adrenergic blockade may prevent the appearance of premonitory signs and symptoms (e.g., tachycardia and blood pressure changes) of acute hypoglycemia. This is especially important with labile diabetics. Beta-blockade also reduces the release of insulin in response to hyperglycemia; therefore, it may be necessary to adjust the dose of antidiabetic drugs.
Thyrotoxicosis—Beta-adrenergic blockade may mask certain clinical signs (e.g., tachycardia) of hyperthyroidism. Patients suspected of developing thyrotoxicosis should be managed carefully to avoid abrupt withdrawal of beta-adrenergic blockade which might precipitate a thyroid storm.
Bendroflumethiazide
Thiazides should be used with caution in severe renal disease. In patients with renal disease, thiazides may precipitate azotemia. Cumulative effects of the drug may develop in patients with impaired renal function.
Thiazides should be used with caution in patients with impaired hepatic function or progressive liver disease, since minor alterations of fluid and electrolyte balance may precipitate hepatic coma.
Sensitivity reactions may occur in patients with or without a history of allergy or bronchial asthma.
The possibility of exacerbation or activation of systemic lupus erythematosus has been reported.
Lithium generally should not be given with diuretics; diuretic agents reduce the renal clearance of lithium and add a high risk of lithium toxicity. Refer to the package insert for lithium preparations before use of such concomitant therapy.

PRECAUTIONS

General
Nadolol
Nadolol should be used with caution in patients with impaired renal function (see **DOSAGE AND ADMINISTRATION**).
Bendroflumethiazide
Periodic determination of serum electrolytes to detect possible electrolyte imbalance should be performed at appropriate intervals.
All patients receiving thiazide therapy should be observed for clinical signs of fluid or electrolyte imbalance, namely: hyponatremia, hypochloremic alkalosis, and hypokalemia. Serum and urine electrolyte determinations are particularly important when the patient is vomiting excessively or receiving parenteral fluids. Warning signs or symptoms of fluid and electrolyte imbalance may include: dryness of the mouth, thirst, weakness, lethargy, drowsiness, restlessness, muscle pains or cramps, muscular fatigue, hypotension, oliguria, tachycardia, and gastrointestinal disturbances, such as nausea and vomiting.
Hypokalemia may develop, especially with brisk diuresis or when severe cirrhosis is present.
Interference with adequate oral electrolyte intake will also contribute to hypokalemia. Hypokalemia can sensitize or exaggerate the response of the heart to the toxic effects of digitalis (e.g., increased ventricular irritability). Concurrent administration of a potassium-sparing diuretic or potassium supplements may be indicated in these patients.
Any chloride deficit is generally mild and usually does not require specific treatment except under extraordinary circumstances (as in liver disease or renal disease). Dilutional hyponatremia may occur in edematous patients in hot weather; appropriate therapy is water restriction, rather than administration of salt, except in rare instances when the hyponatremia is life-threatening. In actual salt depletion, appropriate replacement is the therapy of choice.
Hyperuricemia may occur or frank gout may be precipitated in certain patients receiving thiazide therapy.
Latent diabetes mellitus may become manifest during thiazide administration.
The antihypertensive effect of thiazide diuretics may be enhanced in the postsympathectomy patient.
If progressive renal impairment becomes evident, as indicated by a rising nonprotein nitrogen or blood urea nitrogen (BUN), a careful reappraisal of therapy is necessary with consideration given to withholding or discontinuing diuretic therapy.
Thiazides may decrease serum PBI levels without signs of thyroid disturbance.
Calcium excretion is decreased by thiazides. Pathological changes in the parathyroid gland with hypercalcemia and hypophosphatemia have been observed in a few patients on prolonged thiazide therapy. The common complications of hyperparathyroidism such as renal lithiasis, bone resorption, and peptic ulceration have not been seen. Thiazides should be discontinued before carrying out tests for parathyroid function.
Thiazides have been shown to increase the urinary excretion of magnesium; this may result in hypomagnesemia.

Information for Patients
Patients, especially those with evidence of coronary artery insufficiency, should be warned against interruption or discontinuation of therapy without the physician's advice. Although cardiac failure rarely occurs in properly selected patients, patients being treated with beta-adrenergic blocking agents should be advised to consult the physician at the first sign or symptom of impending failure.
The patient should also be advised of a proper course in the event of an inadvertently missed dose.
The patient should be informed of symptoms that would suggest potential adverse effects and told to report them promptly.
Laboratory Tests
Serum electrolyte levels should be regularly monitored (see **WARNINGS, Bendroflumethiazide**, also **PRECAUTIONS, General, Bendroflumethiazide**).
Drug Interactions
Nadolol
When administered concurrently the following drugs may interact with beta-adrenergic receptor blocking agents:
Anesthetics, general—exaggeration of the hypotension induced by general anesthetics (see **WARNINGS, Nadolol, Major Surgery**).
Antidiabetic drugs (oral agents and insulin)—hypoglycemia or hyperglycemia; adjust dosage of antidiabetic drug accordingly (see **WARNINGS, Nadolol, Diabetes and Hypoglycemia**).
Catecholamine-depleting drugs (e.g., reserpine)—additive effect; monitor closely for evidence of hypotension and/or excessive bradycardia (e.g., vertigo, syncope, postural hypotension).
Response to Treatment for Anaphylactic Reaction—While taking beta-blockers, patients with a history of severe anaphylactic reaction to a variety of allergens may be more reactive to repeated challenge, either accidental, diagnostic, or therapeutic. Such patients may be unresponsive to the usual doses of epinephrine used to treat allergic reaction.
Bendroflumethiazide
When administered concurrently the following drugs may interact with thiazide diuretics:
Alcohol, barbiturates, or narcotics—potentiation of orthostatic hypotension may occur.
Amphotericin B, corticosteroids, or corticotropin (ACTH)—may intensify electrolyte imbalance, particularly hypokalemia. Monitor potassium levels; use potassium replacements if necessary.
Anticoagulants (oral)—dosage adjustments of anticoagulant medication may be necessary since bendroflumethiazide may decrease their effects.
Antigout medications—dosage adjustments of antigout medication may be necessary since bendroflumethiazide may raise the level of blood uric acid.
Other antihypertensive medications (e.g., ganglionic or peripheral adrenergic blocking agents)—dosage adjustments may be necessary since bendroflumethiazide may potentiate their effects.
Antidiabetic drugs (oral agents and insulin)—since thiazides may elevate blood glucose levels, dosage adjustments of antidiabetic agents may be necessary.
Calcium salts—increased serum calcium levels due to decreased excretion may occur. If calcium must be prescribed monitor serum calcium levels and adjust calcium dosage accordingly.
Cardiac glycosides—enhanced possibility of digitalis toxicity associated with hypokalemia. Monitor potassium levels; use potassium replacement if necessary.
Cholestyramine resin and colestipol HCl—may delay or decrease absorption of bendroflumethiazide. Sulfonamide diuretics should be taken at least one hour before or four to six hours after these medications.
Diazoxide—enhanced hyperglycemic, hyperuricemic, and antihypertensive effects. Be cognizant of possible interaction; monitor blood glucose and serum uric acid levels.
Lithium salts—may enhance lithium toxicity due to reduced renal clearance. Avoid concurrent use; if lithium must be prescribed monitor serum lithium levels and adjust lithium dosage accordingly. (See **WARNINGS**.)
MAO inhibitors—dosage adjustments of one or both agents may be necessary since hypotensive effects are enhanced.
Nondepolarizing muscle relaxants, preanesthetics and anesthetics used in surgery (e.g., tubocurarine chloride and gallamine triethiodide)—effects of these agents may be potentiated; dosage adjustments may be required. Monitor and correct any fluid and electrolyte imbalances prior to surgery if feasible.
Nonsteroidal anti-inflammatory agents—in some patients, the administration of a nonsteroidal anti-inflammatory agent can reduce the diuretic, natriuretic, and antihypertensive effect of loop, potassium-sparing or thiazide diuretics. Therefore, when bendroflumethiazide and nonsteroidal anti-inflammatory agents are used concomitantly, the patient should be observed closely to determine if the desired effect of the diuretic is obtained.
Methenamine—possible decreased effectiveness due to alkalinization of the urine.
Pressor amines (e.g., norepinephrine)—decreased arterial responsiveness, but not sufficient to preclude effectiveness of the pressor agent for therapeutic use. Use caution in patients taking both medications who undergo surgery. Administer preanesthetic and anesthetic agents in reduced dosage, and if possible, discontinue bendroflumethiazide one week prior to surgery.

Probenecid or sulfinpyrazone—increased dosage of these agents may be necessary since bendroflumethiazide may have hyperuricemic effects.

Drug/Laboratory Test Interactions

Bendroflumethiazide may produce false-negative results with the phentolamine and tyramine tests; may interfere with the phenosulfonphthalein test due to decreased excretion; and it may cause diagnostic interference of serum electrolyte levels, blood and urine glucose levels, and a decrease in serum PBI levels without signs of thyroid disturbance.

Carcinogenesis, Mutagenesis, Impairment of Fertility

Nadolol

In chronic oral toxicologic studies (one to two years) in mice, rats, and dogs, nadolol did not produce any significant toxic effects. In two-year oral carcinogenicity studies in rats and mice, nadolol did not produce any neoplastic, preneoplastic, or nonneoplastic pathologic lesions. In fertility and general reproductive performance studies in rats, nadolol caused no adverse effect.

Bendroflumethiazide

Studies have not been performed to evaluate carcinogenic potential, mutagenesis, or whether this drug adversely affects fertility in males or females.

Pregnancy—Teratogenic Effects

Nadolol

Category C. In animal reproduction studies with nadolol, evidence of embryo- and fetotoxicity was found in rabbits, but not in rats or hamsters, at doses 5 to 10 times greater (on a mg/kg basis) than the maximum indicated human dose. No teratogenic potential was observed in any of these species.

There are no adequate and well-controlled studies in pregnant women. Nadolol should be used during pregnancy only if the potential benefit justifies the potential risk to the fetus. Neonates whose mothers are receiving nadolol at parturition have exhibited bradycardia, hypoglycemia, and associated symptoms.

Bendroflumethiazide

Category C. Animal reproduction studies have not been conducted with bendroflumethiazide. It is also not known whether this drug can cause fetal harm when administered to a pregnant woman or can affect reproduction capacity. Bendroflumethiazide should be given to a pregnant woman only if clearly needed.

Pregnancy—Nonteratogenic Effects

Thiazides cross the placental barrier and appear in cord blood. The use of thiazides in pregnant women requires that the anticipated benefit be weighed against possible hazards to the fetus. These hazards include fetal or neonatal jaundice, thrombocytopenia, and possibly other adverse reactions which have occurred in the adult.

Nursing Mothers

Both nadolol and bendroflumethiazide are excreted in human milk. Because of the potential for serious adverse reactions in nursing infants from both drugs, a decision should be made whether to discontinue nursing or to discontinue therapy taking into account the importance of CORZIDE (Nadolol and Bendroflumethiazide Tablets) to the mother.

Pediatric Use

Safety and effectiveness in pediatric patients have not been established.

Geriatric Use

Clinical studies of Corzide did not include sufficient numbers of subjects aged 65 and over to determine whether they respond differently from younger subjects. Other reported clinical experience has not identified differences in responses between the elderly and younger patients. In general, dose selection for an elderly patient should be cautious, usually starting at the low end of the dosing range, reflecting the greater frequency of hepatic, renal, or cardiac function, and of concomitant disease or other drug therapy. This drug is known to be substantially excreted by the kidney, and the risk of toxic reaction to this drug may be greater in patients with impaired function. Because elderly patients are more likely to have decreased renal function, care should be taken in dose selection, and it may be useful to monitor renal function.

ADVERSE REACTIONS

Nadolol

Most adverse effects have been mild and transient and have rarely required withdrawal of therapy.

Cardiovascular—Bradycardia with heart rates of less than 60 beats per minute occurs commonly, and heart rates below 40 beats per minute and/or symptomatic bradycardia were seen in about 2 of 100 patients. Symptoms of peripheral vascular insufficiency, usually of the Raynaud type, have occurred in approximately 2 of 100 patients. Cardiac failure, hypotension, and rhythm/conduction disturbances have each occurred in about 1 of 100 patients. Single instances of first degree and third degree heart block have been reported; intensification of AV block is a known effect of beta-blockers (see also **CONTRAINDICATIONS, WARNINGS**, and **PRECAUTIONS**).

Central Nervous System—Dizziness or fatigue has been reported in approximately 2 of 100 patients; paresthesias, sedation, and change in behavior have each been reported in approximately 6 of 1000 patients.

Respiratory—Bronchospasm has been reported in approximately 1 of 1000 patients (see **CONTRAINDICATIONS** and **WARNINGS**).

Gastrointestinal—Nausea, diarrhea, abdominal discomfort, constipation, vomiting, indigestion, anorexia, bloating, and flatulence have been reported in 1 to 5 of 1000 patients.

Miscellaneous—Each of the following has been reported in 1 to 5 of 1000 patients: rash; pruritus; headache; dry mouth, eyes, or skin; impotence or decreased libido; facial swelling; weight gain; slurred speech; cough; nasal stuffiness; sweating; tinnitus; blurred vision. Reversible alopecia has been reported infrequently.

The following adverse reactions have been reported in patients taking nadolol and/or other beta-adrenergic blocking agents, but no causal relationship to nadolol has been established.

Central Nervous System—Reversible mental depression progressing to catatonia; visual disturbances; hallucinations; an acute reversible syndrome characterized by disorientation for time and place, short-term memory loss, emotional lability with slightly clouded sensorium, and decreased performance on neuropsychometrics.

Gastrointestinal—Mesenteric arterial thrombosis; ischemic colitis; elevated liver enzymes.

Hematologic—Agranulocytosis; thrombocytopenic or nonthrombocytopenic purpura.

Allergic—Fever combined with aching and sore throat; laryngospasm; respiratory distress.

Miscellaneous—Pemphigoid rash; hypertensive reaction in patients with pheochromocytoma; sleep disturbances; Peyronie's disease.

The oculomucocutaneous syndrome associated with the beta-blocker practolol has not been reported with nadolol.

Bendroflumethiazide

Gastrointestinal—Nausea, vomiting, cramping and anorexia are not uncommon; diarrhea, constipation, gastric irritation, abdominal bloating, jaundice (intrahepatic cholestatic jaundice), hepatitis, and sialadenitis occasionally occur; and pancreatitis has been reported.

Central Nervous System—Dizziness, vertigo, paresthesia, headache, and xanthopsia occasionally occur.

Hematologic—Leukopenia, agranulocytosis, thrombocytopenia, agranulocytosis, thrombocytopenia, hemolytic anemia, and aplastic anemia have been reported.

Dermatologic-Hypersensitivity—Purpura, exfoliative dermatitis, pruritus, ecchymosis, urticaria, necrotizing angiitis (vasculitis, cutaneous vasculitis), respiratory distress including pneumonitis, fever, and anaphylactic reactions occasionally occur; photosensitivity and rash have been reported.

Cardiovascular—Orthostatic hypotension may occur and may be potentiated by coadministration with certain other drugs (e.g., alcohol, barbiturates, narcotics, other antihypertensive medications, etc.; see **PRECAUTIONS, Drug Interactions**).

Other—Muscle spasm, weakness, or restlessness is not uncommon; hyperglycemia, glycosuria, metabolic acidosis in diabetic patients, hyperuricemia, allergic glomerulonephritis, and transient blurred vision occasionally occur.

Whenever adverse reactions are moderate or severe, thiazide dosage should be reduced or therapy withdrawn.

OVERDOSAGE

In the event of overdosage, nadolol may cause excessive bradycardia, cardiac failure, hypotension, or bronchospasm. In addition to the expected diuresis, overdosage of bendroflumethiazide may produce varying degrees of lethargy which may progress to coma with minimal depression of respiration and cardiovascular function and without significant serum electrolyte changes or dehydration. The mechanism of thiazide-induced CNS depression is unknown. Gastrointestinal irritation may occur. Transitory increase in BUN has been reported, and serum electrolyte changes may occur, especially in patients with impaired renal function.

Treatment

Nadolol can be removed from the general circulation by hemodialysis. In determining the duration of corrective therapy, note must be taken of the long duration of the effect of nadolol. In addition to gastric lavage, the following measures should be employed, as appropriate.

Excessive Bradycardia—Administer atropine (0.25 to 1.0 mg). If there is no response to vagal blockade, administer isoproterenol cautiously.

Cardiac Failure—Administer a digitalis glycoside and diuretic. It has been reported that glucagon may also be useful in this situation.

Hypotension—Administer vasopressors, e.g., epinephrine or levarterenol. (There is evidence that epinephrine may be the drug of choice.)

Bronchospasm—Administer a beta$_2$-stimulating agent and/or a theophylline derivative.

Stupor or Coma—Supportive therapy as warranted.

Gastrointestinal Effects—Symptomatic treatment as needed.

BUN and/or Serum Electrolyte Abnormalities—Institute supportive measures as required to maintain hydration, electrolyte balance, respiration, and cardiovascular and renal function.

DOSAGE AND ADMINISTRATION

DOSAGE MUST BE INDIVIDUALIZED (SEE **INDICATIONS**). CORZIDE MAY BE ADMINISTERED WITHOUT REGARD TO MEALS.

Bendroflumethiazide is usually given at a dose of 5 mg daily. The usual initial dose of nadolol is 40 mg once daily whether used alone or in combination with a diuretic. Bendroflumethiazide in CORZIDE is 30 percent more bioavailable than that of 5 mg Naturetin tablets. Conversion from 5 mg NATURETIN to CORZIDE represents a 30 percent increase in dose of bendroflumethiazide.

The initial dose of CORZIDE (Nadolol and Bendroflumethiazide Tablets) may therefore be the 40 mg/5 mg tablet once daily. When the antihypertensive response is not satisfactory, the dose may be increased by administering the 80 mg/5 mg tablet once daily.

When necessary, another antihypertensive agent may be added gradually beginning with 50 percent of the usual recommended starting dose to avoid an excessive fall in blood pressure.

Dosage Adjustment in Renal Failure—Absorbed nadolol is excreted principally by the kidneys and, although nonrenal elimination does occur, dosage adjustments are necessary in patients with renal impairment. The following dose intervals are recommended:

Creatinine Clearance (mL/min/1.73 m^2)	Dosage Interval (hours)
>50	24
31–50	24–36
10–30	24–48
<10	40–60

HOW SUPPLIED

CORZIDE (Nadolol and Bendroflumethiazide Tablets)

- **40 mg nadolol combined with 5 mg bendroflumethiazide** in bottles of 100 tablets (NDC 61570-175-01).
- **80 mg nadolol combined with 5 mg bendroflumethiazide** in bottles of 100 tablets (NDC 61570-176-01).

Round, biconvex tablets are white to bluish white with dark blue specks. Each tablet has a full bisect bar. Tablet identification numbers: 40 mg/5 mg combination, **283**; 80 mg/5 mg combination, **284**.

Storage

Keep bottle tightly closed. Store at room temperature; avoid excessive heat.

Distributed by:
Monarch Pharmaceuticals, Inc., Bristol, TN 37620
Manufactured by:
Bristol-Myers Squibb Company, Princeton, NJ 08543 USA
Prescribing Information as of March 2002 1131064A2

CYTOMEL® ℞

[sī'tō-mĕl]

brand of (liothyronine sodium) tablets

DESCRIPTION

Thyroid hormone drugs are natural or synthetic preparations containing tetraiodothyronine (T_4, levothyroxine) sodium or triiodothyronine (T_3, liothyronine) sodium or both. T_4 and T_3 are produced in the human thyroid gland by the iodination and coupling of the amino acid tyrosine. T_4 contains four iodine atoms and is formed by the coupling of two molecules of diiodotyrosine (DIT). T_3 contains three atoms of iodine and is formed by the coupling of one molecule of DIT with one molecule of monoiodotyrosine (MIT). Both hormones are stored in the thyroid colloid as thyroglobulin.

Thyroid hormone preparations belong to two categories: (1) natural hormonal preparations derived from animal thyroid, and (2) synthetic preparations. Natural preparations include desiccated thyroid and thyroglobulin. Desiccated thyroid is derived from domesticated animals that are used for food by man (either beef or hog thyroid), and thyroglobulin is derived from thyroid glands of the hog. The United States Pharmacopeia (USP) has standardized the total iodine content of natural preparations. Thyroid USP contains not less than (NLT) 0.17 percent and not more than (NMT) 0.23 percent iodine, and thyroglobulin contains not less than (NLT) 0.7 percent of organically bound iodine. Iodine content is only an indirect indicator of true hormonal biologic activity.

Cytomel (liothyronine sodium) Tablets contain liothyronine (L-triiodothyronine or LT_3), a synthetic form of a natural thyroid hormone, and is available as the sodium salt.

The structural and empirical formulas and molecular weight of liothyronine sodium are given below.

Liothyronine Sodium

$C_{15}H_{11}I_3NNaO_4$ M.W.672.96

L-Tyrosine, *O*-(4-hydroxy-3-iodophenyl)-3,5-diiodo-, monosodium salt

Twenty-five mcg of liothyronine is equivalent to approximately 1 grain of desiccated thyroid or thyroglobulin and 0.1 mg of L-thyroxine.

Each round, white to off-white Cytomel (liothyronine sodium) tablet contains liothyronine sodium equivalent to liothyronine as follows: 5 mcg debossed JMI and D14; 25 mcg scored and debossed JMI and D16; 50 mcg scored

Continued on next page

Cytomel—Cont.

and debossed JMI and D17. Inactive ingredients consist of calcium sulfate, gelatin, starch, stearic acid, sucrose and talc.

CLINICAL PHARMACOLOGY

The mechanisms by which thyroid hormones exert their physiologic action are not well understood. These hormones enhance oxygen consumption by most tissues of the body, increase the basal metabolic rate and the metabolism of carbohydrates, lipids and proteins. Thus, they exert a profound influence on every organ system in the body and are of particular importance in the development of the central nervous system.

Pharmacokinetics

Since liothyronine sodium (T_3) is not firmly bound to serum protein, it is readily available to body tissues. The onset of activity of liothyronine sodium is rapid, occurring within a few hours. Maximum pharmacologic response occurs within 2 or 3 days, providing early clinical response. The biological half-life is about 2-½ days.

T_3 is almost totally absorbed, 95 percent in 4 hours. The hormones contained in the natural preparations are absorbed in a manner similar to the synthetic hormones.

Liothyronine sodium has a rapid cutoff of activity which permits quick dosage adjustment and facilitates control of the effects of overdosage, should they occur.

The higher affinity of levothyroxine (T_4) for both thyroid-binding globulin and thyroid-binding prealbumin as compared to triiodothyronine (T_3) partially explains the higher serum levels and longer half-life of the former hormone. Both protein-bound hormones exist in reverse equilibrium with minute amounts of free hormone, the latter accounting for the metabolic activity.

INDICATIONS AND USAGE

Thyroid hormone drugs are indicated:

1. As replacement or supplemental therapy in patients with hypothyroidism of any etiology, except transient hypothyroidism during the recovery phase of subacute thyroiditis. This category includes cretinism, myxedema and ordinary hypothyroidism in patients of any age (pediatric patients, adults, the elderly), or state (including pregnancy); primary hypothyroidism resulting from functional deficiency, primary atrophy, partial or total absence of thyroid gland, or the effects of surgery, radiation, or drugs, with or without the presence of goiter; and secondary (pituitary) or tertiary (hypothalamic) hypothyroidism (see WARNINGS).
2. As pituitary thyroid-stimulating hormone (TSH) suppressants, in the treatment or prevention of various types of euthyroid goiters, including thyroid nodules, subacute or chronic lymphocytic thyroiditis (Hashimoto's) and multinodular goiter.
3. As diagnostic agents in suppression tests to differentiate suspected mild hyperthyroidism or thyroid gland autonomy.

Cytomel (liothyronine sodium) Tablets can be used in patients allergic to desiccated thyroid or thyroid extract derived from pork or beef.

CONTRAINDICATIONS

Thyroid hormone preparations are generally contraindicated in patients with diagnosed but as yet uncorrected adrenal cortical insufficiency, untreated thyrotoxicosis and apparent hypersensitivity to any of their active or extraneous constituents. There is no well-documented evidence from the literature, however, of true allergic or idiosyncratic reactions to thyroid hormone.

WARNINGS

> Drugs with thyroid hormone activity, alone or together with other therapeutic agents, have been used for the treatment of obesity. In euthyroid patients, doses within the range of daily hormonal requirements are ineffective for weight reduction. Larger doses may produce serious or even life-threatening manifestations of toxicity, particularly when given in association with sympathomimetic amines such as those used for their anorectic effects.

The use of thyroid hormones in the therapy of obesity, alone or combined with other drugs, is unjustified and has been shown to be ineffective. Neither is their use justified for the treatment of male or female infertility unless this condition is accompanied by hypothyroidism.

Thyroid hormones should be used with great caution in a number of circumstances where the integrity of the cardiovascular system, particularly the coronary arteries, is suspected. These include patients with angina pectoris or the elderly, in whom there is a greater likelihood of occult cardiac disease. In these patients, liothyronine sodium therapy should be initiated with low doses, with due consideration for its relatively rapid onset of action. Starting dosage of Cytomel (liothyronine sodium) Tablets is 5 mcg daily, and should be increased by no more than 5 mcg increments at 2-week intervals. When, in such patients, a euthyroid state can only be reached at the expense of an aggravation of the cardiovascular disease, thyroid hormone dosage should be reduced.

Morphologic hypogonadism and nephrosis should be ruled out before the drug is administered. If hypopituitarism is present, the adrenal deficiency must be corrected prior to starting the drug.

Myxedematous patients are very sensitive to thyroid; dosage should be started at a very low level and increased gradually.

Severe and prolonged hypothyroidism can lead to a decreased level of adrenocortical activity commensurate with the lowered metabolic state. When thyroid-replacement therapy is administered, the metabolism increases at a greater rate than adrenocortical activity. This can precipitate adrenocortical insufficiency. Therefore, in severe and prolonged hypothyroidism, supplemental adrenocortical steroids may be necessary. In rare instances the administration of thyroid hormone may precipitate a hyperthyroid state or may aggravate existing hyperthyroidism.

PRECAUTIONS

General – Thyroid hormone therapy in patients with concomitant diabetes mellitus or insipidus or adrenal cortical insufficiency aggravates the intensity of their symptoms. Appropriate adjustments of the various therapeutic measures directed at these concomitant endocrine diseases are required.

The therapy of myxedema coma requires simultaneous administration of glucocorticoids.

Hypothyroidism decreases and hyperthyroidism increases the sensitivity to oral anticoagulants. Prothrombin time should be closely monitored in thyroid-treated patients on oral anticoagulants and dosage of the latter agents adjusted on the basis of frequent prothrombin time determinations.

In infants, excessive doses of thyroid hormone preparations may produce craniosynostosis.

Information for the Patient – Patients on thyroid hormone preparations and parents of pediatric patients on thyroid therapy should be informed that:

1. Replacement therapy is to be taken essentially for life, with the exception of cases of transient hypothyroidism, usually associated with thyroiditis, and in those patients receiving a therapeutic trial of the drug.
2. They should immediately report during the course of therapy any signs or symptoms of thyroid hormone toxicity, e.g., chest pain, increased pulse rate, palpitations, excessive sweating, heat intolerance, nervousness, or any other unusual event.
3. In case of concomitant diabetes mellitus, the daily dosage of antidiabetic medication may need readjustment as thyroid hormone replacement is achieved. If thyroid medication is stopped, a downward readjustment of the dosage of insulin or oral hypoglycemic agent may be necessary to avoid hypoglycemia. At all times, close monitoring of urinary glucose levels is mandatory in such patients.
4. In case of concomitant oral anticoagulant therapy, the prothrombin time should be measured frequently to determine if the dosage of oral anticoagulants is to be readjusted.
5. Partial loss of hair may be experienced by pediatric patients in the first few months of thyroid therapy, but this is usually a transient phenomenon and later recovery is usually the rule.

Laboratory Tests – Treatment of patients with thyroid hormones requires the periodic assessment of thyroid status by means of appropriate laboratory tests besides the full clinical evaluation. The TSH suppression test can be used to test the effectiveness of any thyroid preparation, bearing in mind the relative insensitivity of the infant pituitary to the negative feedback effect of thyroid hormones. Serum T_4 levels can be used to test the effectiveness of all thyroid medications except products containing liothyronine sodium. When the total serum T_4 is low but TSH is normal, a test specific to assess unbound (free) T_4 levels is warranted. Specific measurements of T_4 and T_3 by competitive protein binding or radioimmunoassay are not influenced by blood levels of organic or inorganic iodine and have essentially replaced older tests of thyroid hormone measurements, i.e., PBI, BEI and T_4 by column.

Drug Interactions

Oral Anticoagulants – Thyroid hormones appear to increase catabolism of vitamin K-dependent clotting factors. If oral anticoagulants are also being given, compensatory increases in clotting factor synthesis are impaired. Patients stabilized on oral anticoagulants who are found to require thyroid replacement therapy should be watched very closely when thyroid is started. If a patient is truly hypothyroid, it is likely that a reduction in anticoagulant dosage will be required. No special precautions appear to be necessary when oral anticoagulant therapy is begun in a patient already stabilized on maintenance thyroid replacement therapy.

Insulin or Oral Hypoglycemics – thyroid replacement therapy may cause increases in insulin or oral hypoglycemic requirements. The effects seen are poorly understood and depend upon a variety of factors such as dose and type of thyroid preparations and endocrine status of the patient. Patients receiving insulin or oral hypoglycemics should be closely watched during initiation of thyroid replacement therapy.

Cholestyramine – Cholestyramine binds both T_4 and T_3 in the intestine, thus impairing absorption of these thyroid hormones. *In vitro* studies indicate that the binding is not easily removed. Therefore, 4 to 5 hours should elapse between administration of cholestyramine and thyroid hormones.

Estrogen, Oral Contraceptives – Estrogens tend to increase serum thyroxine-binding globulin (TBg). In a patient with a nonfunctioning thyroid gland who is receiving thyroid replacement therapy, free levothyroxine may be decreased when estrogens are started thus increasing thyroid requirements. However, if the patient's thyroid gland has sufficient function, the decreased free thyroxine will result in a compensatory increase in thyroxine output by the thyroid. Therefore, patients without a functioning thyroid gland who are on thyroid replacement therapy may need to increase their thyroid dose if estrogens or estrogen-containing oral contraceptives are given.

Tricyclic Antidepressants – Use of thyroid products with imipramine and other tricyclic antidepressants may increase receptor sensitivity and enhance antidepressant activity; transient cardiac arrhythmias have been observed. Thyroid hormone activity may also be enhanced.

Digitalis – Thyroid preparations may potentiate the toxic effects of digitalis. Thyroid hormonal replacement increases metabolic rate, which requires an increase in digitalis dosage.

Ketamine – When administered to patients on a thyroid preparation, this parenteral anesthetic may cause hypertension and tachycardia. Use with caution and be prepared to treat hypertension, if necessary.

Vasopressors – Thyroxine increases the adrenergic effect of catecholamines such as epinephrine and norepinephrine. Therefore, injection of these agents into patients receiving thyroid preparations increases the risk of precipitating coronary insufficiency, especially in patients with coronary artery disease. Careful observation is required.

Drug/Laboratory Test Interactions – The following drugs or moieties are known to interfere with laboratory tests performed in patients on thyroid hormone therapy: androgens, corticosteroids, estrogens, oral contraceptives containing estrogens, iodine-containing preparations and the numerous preparations containing salicylates.

1. Changes in TBg concentration should be taken into consideration in the interpretation of T_4 and T_3 values. In such cases, the unbound (free) hormone should be measured. Pregnancy, estrogens and estrogen-containing oral contraceptives increase TBg concentrations. TBg may also be increased during infectious hepatitis. Decreases in TBg concentrations are observed in nephrosis, acromegaly and after androgen or corticosteroid therapy. Familial hyper- or hypo-thyroxine-binding-globulinemias have been described. The incidence of TBg deficiency approximates 1 in 9000. The binding of thyroxine by thyroxine-binding prealbumin (TBPA) is inhibited by salicylates.
2. Medicinal or dietary iodine interferes with all *in vivo* tests of radioiodine uptake, producing low uptakes which may not be reflective of a true decrease in hormone synthesis.
3. The persistence of clinical and laboratory evidence of hypothyroidism in spite of adequate dosage replacement indicates either poor patient compliance, poor absorption, excessive fecal loss, or inactivity of the preparation. Intracellular resistance to thyroid hormone is quite rare.

Carcinogenesis, Mutagenesis and Impairment of Fertility – A reportedly apparent association between prolonged thyroid therapy and breast cancer has not been confirmed and patients on thyroid for established indications should not discontinue therapy. No confirmatory long-term studies in animals have been performed to evaluate carcinogenic potential, mutagenicity, or impairment of fertility in either males or females.

Pregnancy – Category A. Thyroid hormones do not readily cross the placental barrier. The clinical experience to date does not indicate any adverse effect on fetuses when thyroid hormones are administered to pregnant women. On the basis of current knowledge, thyroid replacement therapy to hypothyroid women should not be discontinued during pregnancy.

Nursing Mothers – Minimal amounts of thyroid hormones are excreted in human milk. Thyroid is not associated with serious adverse reactions and does not have a known tumorigenic potential. However, caution should be exercised when thyroid is administered to a nursing woman.

Geriatric Use – Clinical studies of liothyronine sodium did not include sufficient numbers of subjects aged 65 and over to determine whether they respond differently from younger subjects. Other reported clinical experience has not identified differences in responses between the elderly and younger patients. In general, dose selection for an elderly patient should be cautious, usually starting at the low end of the dosing range, reflecting the greater frequency of decreased hepatic, renal, or cardiac function, and of concomitant disease or other drug therapy. This drug is known to be substantially excreted by the kidney, and the risk of toxic reactions to this drug may be greater in patients with impaired renal function. Because elderly patients are more likely to have decreased renal function, care should be taken in dose selection, and it may be useful to monitor renal function.

Pediatric Use – Pregnant mothers provide little or no thyroid hormone to the fetus. The incidence of congenital hypothyroidism is relatively high (1:4000) and the hypothyroid fetus would not derive any benefit from the small amounts of hormone crossing the placental barrier. Routine determinations of serum T_4 and/or TSH is strongly advised in neonates in view of the deleterious effects of thyroid deficiency on growth and development.

Treatment should be initiated immediately upon diagnosis and maintained for life, unless transient hypothyroidism is suspected, in which case, therapy may be interrupted for 2 to 8 weeks after the age of 3 years to reassess the condition. Cessation of therapy is justified in patients who have maintained a normal TSH during those 2 to 8 weeks.

ADVERSE REACTIONS

Adverse reactions, other than those indicative of hyperthyroidism because of therapeutic overdosage, either initially or during the maintenance period are rare (see OVERDOSAGE).

In rare instances, allergic skin reactions have been reported with Cytomel (liothyronine sodium) Tablets.

OVERDOSAGE

Signs and Symptoms – Headache, irritability, nervousness, sweating, arrhythmia (including tachycardia), increased bowel motility and menstrual irregularities. Angina pectoris or congestive heart failure may be induced or aggravated. Shock may also develop. Massive overdosage may result in symptoms resembling thyroid storm. Chronic excessive dosage will produce the signs and symptoms of hyperthyroidism.

Treatment Of Overdosage – Dosage should be reduced or therapy temporarily discontinued if signs and symptoms of overdosage appear. Treatment may be reinstituted at a lower dosage. In normal individuals, normal hypothalamic-pituitary-thyroid axis function is restored in 6 to 8 weeks after thyroid suppression.

Treatment of acute massive thyroid hormone overdosage is aimed at reducing gastrointestinal absorption of the drugs and counteracting central and peripheral effects, mainly those of increased sympathetic activity. Vomiting may be induced initially if further gastrointestinal absorption can reasonably be prevented and barring contraindications such as coma, convulsions, or loss of the gagging reflex. Treatment is symptomatic and supportive. Oxygen may be administered and ventilation maintained. Cardiac glycosides may be indicated if congestive heart failure develops. Measures to control fever, hypoglycemia, or fluid loss should be instituted if needed. Antiadrenergic agents, particularly propranolol, have been used advantageously in the treatment of increased sympathetic activity. Propranolol may be administered intravenously at a dosage of 1 to 3 mg over a 10-minute period or orally, 80 to 160 mg/day, especially when no contraindications exist for its use.

DOSAGE AND ADMINISTRATION

The dosage of thyroid hormones is determined by the indication and must in every case be individualized according to patient response and laboratory findings.

Cytomel (liothyronine sodium) Tablets are intended for oral administration; once-a-day dosage is recommended. Although liothyronine sodium has a rapid cutoff, its metabolic effects persist for a few days following discontinuance.

Mild Hypothyroidism: Recommended starting dosage is 25 mcg daily. Daily dosage then may be increased by up to 25 mcg every 1 or 2 weeks. Usual maintenance dose is 25 to 75mcg daily.

The rapid onset and dissipation of action of liothyronine sodium (T_3), as compared with levothyroxine sodium (T_4), has led some clinicians to prefer its use in patients who might be more susceptible to the untoward effects of thyroid medication. However, the wide swings in serum T_3 levels that follow its administration and the possibility of more pronounced cardiovascular side effects tend to counterbalance the stated advantages.

Cytomel (liothyronine sodium) Tablets may be used in preference to levothyroxine (T_4) during radioisotope scanning procedures, since induction of hypothyroidism in those cases is more abrupt and can be of shorter duration. It may also be preferred when impairment of peripheral conversion of T_4 to T_3 is suspected.

Myxedema: Recommended starting dosage is 5 mcg daily. This may be increased by 5 to 10 mcg daily every 1 or 2 weeks. When 25 mcg daily is reached, dosage may be increased by 5 to 25 mcg every 1 or 2 weeks until a satisfactory therapeutic response is attained. Usual maintenance dose is 50 to 100 mcg daily.

Myxedema Coma: Myxedema coma is usually precipitated in the hypothyroid patient of long standing by intercurrent illness or drugs such as sedatives and anesthetics and should be considered a medical emergency.

An intravenous preparation of liothyronine sodium is marketed by JONES PHARMA INCORPORATED, under the trade name Triostat® for use in myxedema coma/precoma.

Congenital Hypothyroidism: Recommended starting dosage is 5 mcg daily, with a 5 mcg increment every 3 to 4 days until the desired response is achieved. Infants a few months old may require only 20 mcg daily for maintenance. At 1 year, 50 mcg daily may be required. Above 3 years, full adult dosage may be necessary (see PRECAUTIONS, Pediatric Use).

Simple (non-toxic) Goiter: Recommended starting dosage is 5 mcg daily. This dosage may be increased by 5 to 10 mcg daily every 1 or 2 weeks. When 25 mcg daily is reached, dosage may be increased every week or two by 12.5 or 25 mcg. Usual maintenance dosage is 75 mcg daily.

In the elderly or in pediatric patients, therapy should be started with 5 mcg daily and increased only by 5 mcg increments at the recommended intervals.

When switching a patient to Cytomel (liothyronine sodium) Tablets from thyroid, L-thyroxine or thyroglobulin, discontinue the other medication, initiate *Cytomel* at a low dosage, and increase gradually according to the patient's response. When selecting a starting dosage, bear in mind that this drug has a rapid onset of action, and that residual effects of the other thyroid preparation may persist for the first several weeks of therapy.

Thyroid Suppression Therapy: Administration of thyroid hormone in doses higher than those produced physiologically by the gland results in suppression of the production of endogenous hormone. This is the basis for the thyroid suppression test and is used as an aid in the diagnosis of patients with signs of mild hyperthyroidism in whom baseline laboratory tests appear normal or to demonstrate thyroid gland autonomy in patients with Graves' ophthalmopathy. ^{131}I uptake is determined before and after the administration of the exogenous hormone. A 50% or greater suppression of uptake indicates a normal thyroid-pituitary axis and thus rules out thyroid gland autonomy.

Cytomel (liothyronine sodium) Tablets are given in doses of 75 to 100 mcg/day for 7 days, and radioactive iodine uptake is determined before and after administration of the hormone. If thyroid function is under normal control, the radioiodine uptake will drop significantly after treatment. Cytomel (liothyronine sodium) Tablets should be administered cautiously to patients in whom there is a strong suspicion of thyroid gland autonomy, in view of the fact that the exogenous hormone effects will be additive to the endogenous source.

HOW SUPPLIED

Cytomel (liothyronine sodium) Tablets: 5 mcg in bottles of 100; 25 mcg in bottles of 100; and 50 mcg in bottles of 100.

5 mcg 100's: NDC 52604-3414-1

25 mcg 100's: NDC 52604-3416-1

50 mcg 100's: NDC 52604-3417-1

Store between 15° and 30°C (59° and 86°F).

DATE OF ISSUANCE November 2001

Manufactured by Schering Canada, Inc., 3535 Trans-Canada Highway,

Pointe Claire, Quebec H9R 1B4 Canada

Distributed by: Jones Pharma Inc.

(A wholly owned subsidiary of King Pharmaceuticals, Inc.)

St. Louis, MO 63146

S83-481651

Rev. 07/02

Shown in Product Identification Guide, page 319

INTAL® Inhaler ℞

[in-tăl]

(cromolyn sodium inhalation aerosol)

For Oral Inhalation Only

Rx only

DESCRIPTION

The active ingredient of **Intal** Inhaler is cromolyn sodium, USP. It is an inhaled anti-inflammatory agent for the preventive management of asthma. Cromolyn sodium is disodium 5,5′-[(2-hydroxytrimethylene)dioxy]bis[4-oxo-4*H*-1-benzopyran-2-carboxylate]. The empirical formula is $C_{23}H_{14}Na_2O_{11}$; the molecular weight is 512.34. Cromolyn sodium is a water soluble, odorless, white, hydrated crystalline powder. It is tasteless at first, but leaves a slightly bitter aftertaste. The molecular structure of cromolyn sodium is:

NaOOC COONa OH O OCH_2CHCH_2O O

Intal Inhaler (cromolyn sodium inhalation aerosol) is a metered dose aerosol unit for oral inhalation containing micronized cromolyn sodium, sorbitan trioleate with dichlorotetrafluoroethane and dichlorodifluoromethane as propellants. Each actuation delivers approximately 1 mg cromolyn sodium from the valve and 800 mcg cromolyn sodium through the mouthpiece to the patient. Each 8.1 g canister delivers at least 112 metered inhalations (56 doses); each 14.2 g canister delivers at least 200 metered inhalations (100 doses).

CLINICAL PHARMACOLOGY

In vitro and *in vivo* animal studies have shown that cromolyn sodium inhibits sensitized mast cell degranulation which occurs after exposure to specific antigens. Cromolyn sodium acts by inhibiting the release of mediators from mast cells. Studies show that cromolyn sodium indirectly blocks calcium ions from entering the mast cell, thereby preventing mediator release.

Cromolyn sodium inhibits both the immediate and non-immediate bronchoconstrictive reactions to inhaled antigen. Cromolyn sodium also attenuates bronchospasm caused by exercise, toluene diisocyanate, aspirin, cold air, sulfur dioxide, and environmental pollutants, at least in some patients.

Cromolyn sodium has no intrinsic bronchodilator or antihistamine activity.

After administration of cromolyn sodium capsules by inhalation, approximately 8% of the total dose administered is absorbed and rapidly excreted unchanged, approximately equally divided between urine and bile. The remainder of the dose is either exhaled or deposited in the oropharynx, swallowed, and excreted via the alimentary tract.

INDICATIONS AND USAGE

Intal Inhaler is a prophylactic agent indicated in the management of patients with bronchial asthma.

In patients whose symptoms are sufficiently frequent to require a continuous program of medication, **Intal** Inhaler is given by inhalation on a regular daily basis. (See **DOSAGE AND ADMINISTRATION.**) The effect of **Intal** Inhaler is usually evident after several weeks of treatment, although some patients show an almost immediate response.

If improvement occurs, it will ordinarily occur within the first 4 weeks of administration as manifested by a decrease in the severity of clinical symptoms of asthma, or in the need for concomitant therapy, or both.

In patients who develop acute bronchoconstriction in response to exposure to exercise, toluene diisocyanate, environmental pollutants, known antigens, etc., **Intal** Inhaler should be used shortly before exposure to the precipitating factor, i.e., within 10 to 15 minutes but not more than 60 minutes. (See **DOSAGE AND ADMINISTRATION.**) **Intal** Inhaler may be effective in relieving bronchospasm in some, but not all, patients with exercise induced bronchospasm.

CONTRAINDICATIONS

Intal Inhaler is contraindicated in those patients who have shown hypersensitivity to cromolyn sodium or other ingredients in this preparation.

WARNINGS

Intal Inhaler has no role in the treatment of an acute attack of asthma, especially status asthmaticus. Severe anaphylactic reactions can occur after cromolyn sodium administration. The recommended dosage should be decreased in patients with decreased renal or hepatic function. Intal Inhaler should be discontinued if the patient develops eosinophilic pneumonia (or pulmonary infiltrates with eosinophilia). Because of the propellants in this preparation, it should be used with caution in patients with coronary artery disease or a history of cardiac arrhythmias.

PRECAUTIONS

General: In view of the biliary and renal routes of excretion for cromolyn sodium, consideration should be given to decreasing the dosage or discontinuing the administration of the drug in patients with impaired renal or hepatic function.

Occasionally, patients may experience cough and/or bronchospasm following cromolyn sodium inhalation. At times, patients who develop bronchospasm may not be able to continue administration despite prior bronchodilator administration. Rarely, very severe bronchospasm has been encountered.

Carcinogenesis, Mutagenesis, and Impairment of Fertility: Long-term studies of cromolyn sodium in mice (12 months intraperitoneal administration at doses up to 150 mg/kg/day three days per week), hamsters (intraperitoneal administration at doses up to 53 mg/kg/day three days per week for 15 weeks followed by 17.5 mg/kg/day three days per week for 37 weeks), and rats (18 months subcutaneous treatment at doses up to 75 mg/kg/day six days per week) showed no neoplastic effects. These doses in mice, hamsters, and rats correspond to approximately 40, 10, and 80 times, respectively, the maximum recommended daily inhalation dose in adults on a mg/m^2 basis, or, approximately 20, 5, and 40 times, respectively, the maximum recommended daily inhalation dose in children on a mg/m^2 basis.

Cromolyn sodium showed no mutagenic potential in Ames Salmonella/microsome plate assays, mitotic gene conversion in *Saccharomyces cerevisiae*, and in an *in vitro* cytogenetic study in human peripheral lymphocytes.

No evidence of impaired fertility was shown in laboratory reproduction studies conducted subcutaneously in rats at the highest doses tested, 175 mg/kg/day in males and 100 mg/kg/day in females. These doses are approximately 220 and 130 times, respectively, the maximum recommended daily inhalation dose in adults on a mg/m^2 basis.

Pregnancy: *Pregnancy Category B:* Reproduction studies with cromolyn sodium administered subcutaneously to pregnant mice and rats at maximum daily doses of 540 mg/kg/day and 160 mg/kg/day, respectively, and intravenously to rabbits at a maximum daily dose of 485 mg/kg/day produced no evidence of fetal malformations. These doses represent approximately 340, 210, and 1,200 times, respectively, the maximum recommended daily inhalation dose in adults on a mg/m^2 basis. Adverse fetal effects (increased resorption and decreased fetal weight) were noted only at the very high parenteral doses that produced maternal toxicity. There are, however, no adequate and well-controlled studies in pregnant women.

Because animal reproduction studies are not always predictive of human response, **Intal** Inhaler should be used during pregnancy only if clearly needed.

Drug Interaction During Pregnancy: Cromolyn sodium and isoproterenol were studied following subcutaneous injections in pregnant mice. Cromolyn sodium alone in doses up to 540 mg/kg/day (approximately 340 times the maximum recommended daily inhalation dose in adults on a mg/m^2 basis) did not cause significant increases in resorptions or major malformations. Isoproterenol alone at a dose of 2.7 mg/kg/day (approximately 7 times the maximum recommended daily inhalation dose in adults on a mg/m^2 basis) increased both resorptions and malformations. The addition of 540 mg/kg/day of cromolyn sodium (approximately 340 times the maximum recommended daily inhalation dose in adults on a mg/m^2 basis) to 2.7 mg/kg/day of isoproterenol (approximately 7 times the maximum recommended daily inhalation dose in adults on a mg/m^2 basis) appears to have increased the incidence of both resorptions and malformations.

Continued on next page

Intal—Cont.

Nursing Mothers: It is not known whether this drug is excreted in human milk, therefore, caution should be exercised when **Intal** Inhaler is administered to a nursing woman and the attending physician must make a benefit/risk assessment in regard to its use in this situation.

Pediatric Use: Safety and effectiveness in pediatric patients below the age of 5 years have not been established. For young pediatric patients unable to utilize the Inhaler, **Intal** Nebulizer Solution (cromolyn sodium inhalation solution, USP) is recommended. Because of the possibility that adverse effects of this drug could become apparent only after many years, a benefit/risk consideration of the long-term use of **Intal** Inhaler is particularly important in pediatric patients.

ADVERSE REACTIONS

In controlled clinical studies of Intal Inhaler, the most frequently reported adverse reactions attributed to cromolyn sodium treatment were:

Throat irritation or dryness
Bad taste
Cough
Wheeze
Nausea

The most frequently reported adverse reactions attributed to other forms of cromolyn sodium (on the basis of reoccurrence following readministration) involve the respiratory tract and are: bronchospasm [sometimes severe, associated with a precipitous fall in pulmonary function (FEV_1)], cough, laryngeal edema (rare), nasal congestion (sometimes severe), pharyngeal irritation, and wheezing.

Adverse reactions which occur infrequently and are associated with administration of the drug are: anaphylaxis, angioedema, dizziness, dysuria and urinary frequency, joint swelling and pain, lacrimation, nausea and headache, rash, swollen parotid gland, urticaria, pulmonary infiltrates with eosinophilia, substernal burning, and myopathy.

The following adverse reactions have been reported as rare events and it is unclear whether they are attributable to the drug: anemia, exfoliative dermatitis, hemoptysis, hoarseness, myalgia, nephrosis, periarteritic vasculitis, pericarditis, peripheral neuritis, photodermatitis, sneezing, drowsiness, nasal itching, nasal bleeding, nasal burning, serum sickness, stomachache, polymyositis, vertigo, and liver disease.

OVERDOSAGE

There is no clinical syndrome associated with an overdosage of cromolyn sodium. In several animal species acute toxicity with cromolyn sodium occurs only with very high exposure levels. No deaths occurred at the highest oral doses tested in mice, 8000 mg/kg (approximately 5100 and 2700 times the maximum recommended daily inhalation doses in adults and children, respectively, on a mg/m² basis) or in rats, 8000 mg/kg (approximately 10,000 and 5400 times the maximum recommended daily inhalation doses in adults and children, respectively, on a mg/m² basis).

DOSAGE AND ADMINISTRATION

For management of bronchial asthma in adults and pediatric patients (5 years of age and over) who are able to use the Inhaler, the usual starting dosage is two metered inhalations four times daily at regular intervals. This dose should not be exceeded. Not all patients will respond to the recommended dose and there is evidence to suggest, at least in younger patients, that a lower dose may provide efficacy.

Patients with chronic asthma should be advised that the effect of **Intal** Inhaler therapy is dependent upon its administration at regular intervals, as directed. **Intal** Inhaler should be introduced into the patient's therapeutic regimen when the acute episode has been controlled, the airway has been cleared, and the patient is able to inhale adequately.

For the prevention of acute bronchospasm which follows exercise, exposure to cold, dry air, or environmental agents, the usual dose is two metered inhalations shortly before exposure to the precipitating factor, i.e., within 10 to 15 minutes but not more than 60 minutes.

Intal Inhaler Therapy in Relation to Other Treatments for Asthma: *Non-steroidal agents:* **Intal** Inhaler should be *added* to the patient's existing treatment regimen (e.g., bronchodilators). When a clinical response to **Intal** Inhaler is evident, usually within two to four weeks, and if the asthma is under good control, an attempt may be made to decrease concomitant medication usage gradually.

If concomitant medications are eliminated or required on no more than a prn basis, the frequency of administration of **Intal** Inhaler may be titrated downward to the lowest level consistent with the desired effect. The usual decrease is from two metered inhalations four times daily to three times daily to twice daily. It is important that the dosage be reduced gradually to avoid exacerbation of asthma. It is emphasized that in patients whose dosage has been titrated to fewer than four inhalations per day, an increase in the dosage of **Intal** Inhaler and the introduction of, or increase in, symptomatic medications may be needed if the patient's clinical condition deteriorates.

Corticosteroids: In patients chronically receiving corticosteroids for the management of bronchial asthma, the dosage should be maintained following the introduction of **Intal** Inhaler. If the patient improves, an attempt to decrease corticosteroids should be made. Even if the corticosteroid-dependent patient fails to show symptomatic improvement following **Intal** Inhaler administration, the potential to reduce corticosteroids may nonetheless be present. Thus, gradual tapering of corticosteroid dosage may be attempted. It is important that the dose be reduced slowly, maintaining close supervision of the patient to avoid an exacerbation of asthma.

It should be borne in mind that prolonged corticosteroid therapy frequently causes an impairment in the activity of the hypothalamic-pituitary-adrenal axis and a reduction in the size of the adrenal cortex. A potentially critical degree of impairment or insufficiency may persist asymptomatically for some time even after gradual discontinuation of adrenocortical steroids. Therefore, if a patient is subjected to significant stress, such as a severe asthmatic attack, surgery, trauma, or severe illness while being treated or within one year (occasionally up to two years) after corticosteroid treatment has been terminated, consideration should be given to reinstituting corticosteroid therapy. When respiratory function is impaired, as may occur in severe exacerbation of asthma, a temporary increase in the amount of corticosteroids may be required to regain control of the patient's asthma.

It is particularly important that great care be exercised if for any reason cromolyn sodium is withdrawn in cases where its use has permitted a reduction in the maintenance dose of corticosteroids. In such cases, continued close supervision of the patient is essential since there may be sudden reappearance of severe manifestations of asthma which will require immediate therapy and possible reintroduction of corticosteroids.

For best results, the canister should be at room temperature before use.

HOW SUPPLIED

Intal Inhaler is supplied as an aerosol canister which provides 112 metered dose actuations from the 8.1 gram inhaler and 200 metered dose actuations from the 14.2 gram inhaler. The correct amount of medication in each inhalation cannot be assured after 112 actuations from the 8.1 gram canister or 200 actuations from the 14.2 gram canister even though the canister may not feel completely empty. The canister should be discarded when the labeled number of actuations have been used.

Each actuation delivers 1 mg cromolyn sodium through the valve and 800 mcg through the mouthpiece to the patient. The **Intal** Inhaler canister and accompanying mouthpiece are designed to be used together. The **Intal** Inhaler canister should not be used with other mouthpieces and the supplied mouthpiece should not be used with other products' canisters. **Intal** Inhaler is supplied with a white plastic mouthpiece with blue dust cap and patient instructions.

NDC 60793-011-14 .... 14.2 g canister
NDC 60793-011-08 .... 8.1 g canister

Store between 15° to 30°C (59° to 86°F). Contents under pressure. Do not puncture, incinerate, or place near sources of heat. Exposure to temperatures above 120°F may cause bursting. **Avoid spraying in eyes. Keep out of the reach of children.**

Note: The indented statement below is required by the Federal government's Clean Air Act for all products containing or manufactured with chlorofluorocarbons (CFCs).

> WARNING: Contains CFC-12 (dichlorodifluoromethane) and CFC-114 (dichlorotetrafluoroethane), substances which harm public health and the environment by destroying ozone in the upper atmosphere.

A notice similar to the above WARNING has been placed in the "Information For The Patient" portion of this package insert under the Environmental Protection Agency's (EPA's) regulations. The patient's warning states that the patient should consult his or her physician if there are questions about alternatives.

Rx only

Intal® is a registered trademark of Fisons, PLC and licensed to King Pharmaceuticals™.

KING™

Distributed by: King Pharmaceuticals, Inc., Bristol, TN 37620

Manufactured by: Health Care Specialties Division, 3M Health Care Limited, Loughborough, England LE11 1EP

Prescribing Information as of August 2003.

PHARMACIST—DETACH HERE AND GIVE INSTRUCTIONS TO PATIENT

Information For The Patient

INTAL® INHALER (cromolyn sodium inhalation aerosol)
Metered Dose Inhaler
For Oral Inhalation Only

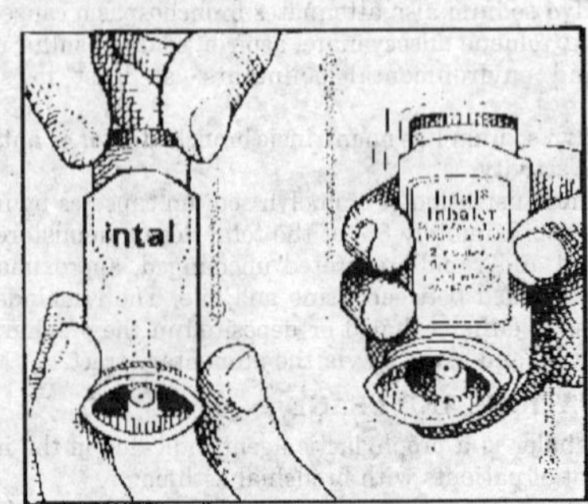

1. Make sure the canister is properly inserted into the Inhaler unit. Take the cover off the mouthpiece. **Shake the Inhaler gently.** If the mouthpiece cover is not present, the Inhaler should be inspected for the presence of foreign objects.

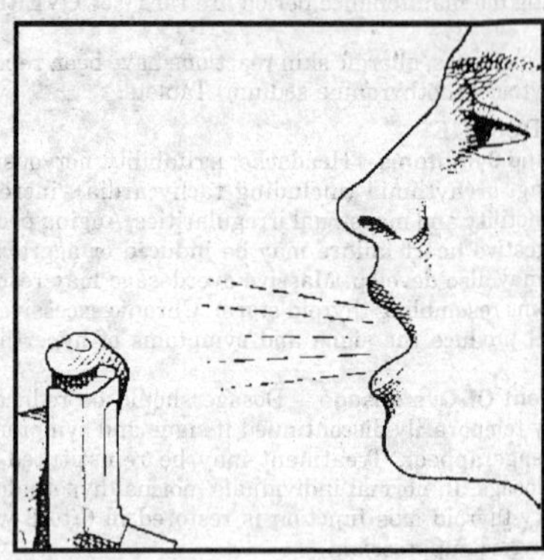

2. Hold Inhaler and breathe out slowly and fully, expelling as much air as possible. **Do not breathe into the Inhaler** – it could clog the Inhaler valve.
3. **Avoid spraying in eyes.**

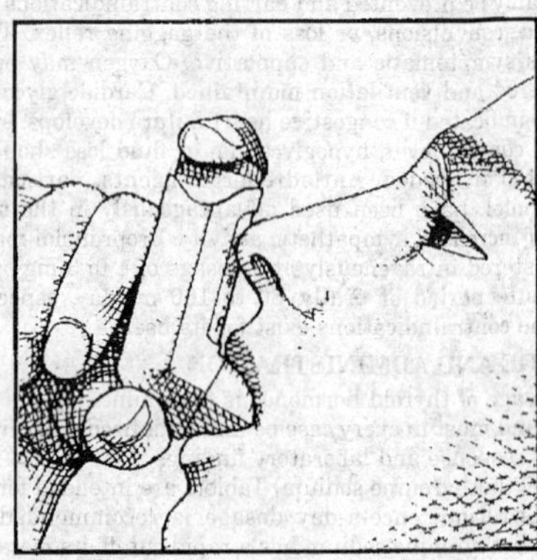

4. Place the mouthpiece into your mouth, close your lips around it, and tilt your head back. Keep your tongue below the opening of the Inhaler.

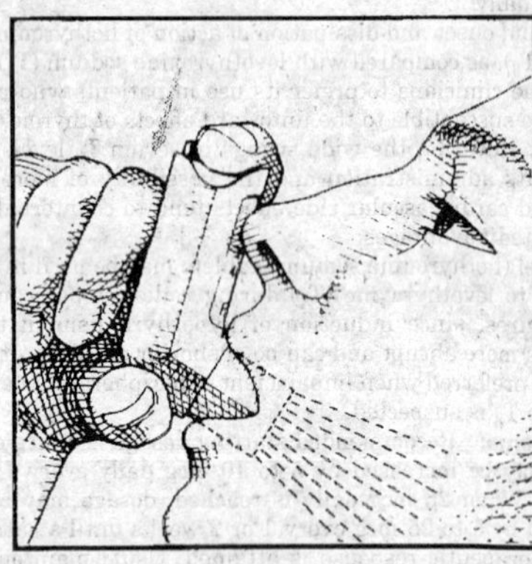

5. While breathing in deeply and slowly through the mouth, fully depress the top of the metal canister with your index finger.

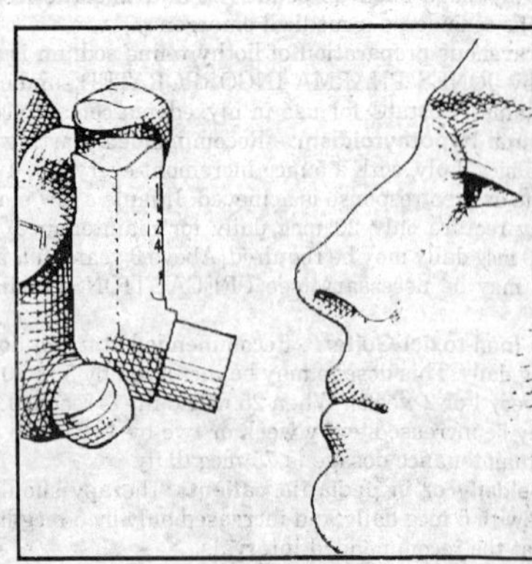

6. Remove the Inhaler from your mouth. Hold your breath for several seconds, then breathe out slowly. This step is very important. It allows the **Intal** to spread throughout your lungs. Repeat steps 2-5, then replace the mouthpiece cover.

FOR BEST RESULTS:

1. Before using the Inhaler for the first time, or if it has not been used for a while, it's a good idea to test it. Just give the canister one press.

2. It is essential that the canister be pressed at exactly the same time as you breathe in, so it's worth some time practicing this.
3. The dose delivered from the Inhaler can be seen as a fine white mist. If any of this can be seen escaping from your mouth or nose, then you are not using the Inhaler correctly.
4. To keep your Inhaler in good working order, do not exhale into mouthpiece.
5. Keep the cap on the Inhaler while not in use so that dirt can't get into it. You can clean the Inhaler by removing the metal canister and rinsing the plastic mouthpiece in warm water. (See **CLEANING** Instructions.)
6. The correct amount of medication in each inhalation cannot be assured after 112 actuations from the 8.1 gram canister or 200 actuations from the 14.2 gram canister even though the canister may not feel completely empty. You should keep track of the number of actuations used from each canister of **Intal** Inhaler and discard the canister after 112 actuations from the 8.1 gram canister or 200 actuations from the 14.2 gram canister. Before you reach the specified number of actuations, you should consult your physician to determine whether a refill is needed. Just as you should not take extra doses without consulting your physician, you also should not stop using **Intal** Inhaler without consulting your physician.
7. For optimal results, the canister should be at room temperature before use.

HOW TO CHECK CONTENTS OF YOUR CANISTER

Shaking the canister will NOT give you a good estimate of how much medication is left. We have included a convenient check-off chart to assist you in keeping track of medication inhalations used. This will help assure that you receive the labeled number of inhalations present.

Each 8.1 gram Inhaler delivers 112 metered inhalations
Each 14.2 gram Inhaler delivers 200 metered inhalations

Intal® Inhaler Check-Off Chart

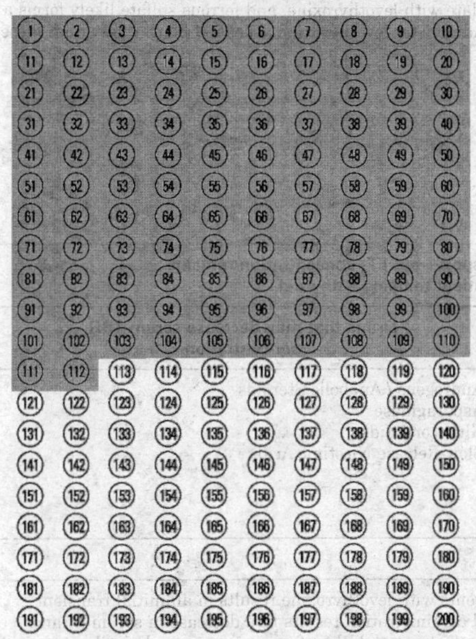

1	2	3	4	5	6	7	8	9	10
11	12	13	14	15	16	17	18	19	20
21	22	23	24	25	26	27	28	29	30
31	32	33	34	35	36	37	38	39	40
41	42	43	44	45	46	47	48	49	50
51	52	53	54	55	56	57	58	59	60
61	62	63	64	65	66	67	68	69	70
71	72	73	74	75	76	77	78	79	80
81	82	83	84	85	86	87	88	89	90
91	92	93	94	95	96	97	98	99	100
101	102	103	104	105	106	107	108	109	110
111	112	113	114	115	116	117	118	119	120
121	122	123	124	125	126	127	128	129	130
131	132	133	134	135	136	137	138	139	140
141	142	143	144	145	146	147	148	149	150
151	152	153	154	155	156	157	158	159	160
161	162	163	164	165	166	167	168	169	170
171	172	173	174	175	176	177	178	179	180
181	182	183	184	185	186	187	188	189	190
191	192	193	194	195	196	197	198	199	200

— Retain with medication or affix to convenient location.
— Starting with inhalation #1, check off one circle for each inhalation used.
— DISCARD MEDICATION AFTER THE LABELED NUMBER OF INHALATIONS HAVE BEEN USED
— NEVER IMMERSE THE METAL CANISTER IN WATER

IMPORTANT: Remember — a little time spent taking Intal correctly and regularly can save you from countless attacks of asthma and the upheaval they cause.

It must be used every day as directed by your doctor. Do not stop the treatment or even reduce the dose without consulting your doctor.

The **Intal** Inhaler canister and accompanying mouthpiece are designed to be used together. The **Intal** Inhaler canister should not be used with other mouthpieces and the supplied mouthpiece should not be used with other products' canisters.

DOSAGE: For management of bronchial asthma in adults and children 5 years of age and older, the usual starting dosage is two metered inhalations four times a day at regular intervals. When asthma symptoms are well controlled, your doctor may reduce the dose to three times a day, and sometimes two times a day.

For prevention of acute bronchospasm which follows exercise, exposure to cold, dry air, or environmental agents, the usual dosage is two metered inhalations shortly **before exposure** to the offending factor.

Use as directed by your physician.

CLEANING: Twice a week, remove the metal canister from the plastic mouthpiece. Wash the mouthpiece in warm water and **dry thoroughly** before replacing the metal canister. **Never immerse the metal canister in water.**

STORAGE: Store between 15° to 30°C (59° to 86°F). Contents under pressure. Do not puncture, incinerate, or place near sources of heat. Exposure to temperatures above 120°F may cause bursting. **Keep out of the reach of children. Avoid spraying in eyes.**

Note: The indented statement below is required by the Federal Government's Clean Air Act for all products containing or manufactured with chlorofluorocarbons (CFCs).

> This product contains CFC-12 (dichlorodifluoromethane) and CFC-114 (dichlorotetrafluoroethane), substances which harm the environment by destroying ozone in the upper atmosphere.

Your physician has determined that this product is likely to help your personal health. USE THIS PRODUCT AS DIRECTED, UNLESS INSTRUCTED TO DO OTHERWISE BY YOUR PHYSICIAN. If you have any questions about alternatives, consult with your physician.

Intal® is a registered trademark of Fisons, PLC and licensed to King Pharmaceuticals™.

KING™
Distributed by:
King Pharmaceuticals, Inc., Bristol, TN 37620
Manufactured by:
Health Care Specialties Division, 3M Health Care Limited
Loughborough, England LE11 1EP
Prescribing Information as of August 2003.

Shown in Product Identification Guide, page 319

LEVOXYL® ℞

[lĕ-vŏks-əl]
(levothyroxine sodium tablets, USP)

DESCRIPTION

—LEVOXYL® (levothyroxine sodium tablets, USP) contain synthetic crystalline L-3,3′,5,5′-tetraiodothyronine sodium salt [levothyroxine (T_4) sodium]. Synthetic T_4 is identical to that produced in the human thyroid gland. Levothyroxine (T_4) sodium has an empirical formula of $C_{15}H_{10}I_4N\ NaO_4 \bullet H_2O$, molecular weight of 798.86 g/mol (anhydrous), and structural formula as shown:

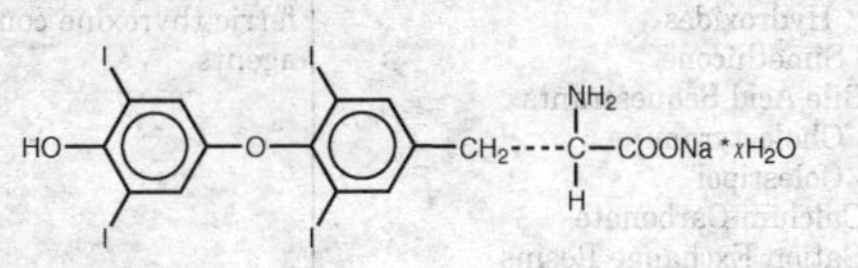

Inactive Ingredients

Microcrystalline cellulose, croscarmellose sodium and magnesium stearate. The following are the coloring additives per tablet strength:

Strength (mcg)	Color additive(s)
25	FD&C Yellow No. 6 Aluminum Lake
50	None
75	FD&C Blue No. 1 Aluminum Lake, D&C Red No. 30 Aluminum Lake
88	FD&C Yellow No. 6 Aluminum Lake, FD&C Blue No. 1 Aluminum Lake, D&C Yellow No. 10 Aluminum Lake
100	FD&C Yellow No. 6 Aluminum Lake, D&C Yellow No. 10 Aluminum Lake
112	FD&C Yellow No. 6 Aluminum Lake, FD&C Red No. 40 Aluminum Lake, D&C Red No. 30 Aluminum Lake
125	FD&C Red No. 40 Aluminum Lake, D&C Yellow No. 10 Aluminum Lake
137	FD&C Blue No. 1 Aluminum Lake
150	FD&C Blue No. 1 Aluminum Lake, D&C Red No. 30 Aluminum Lake
175	FD&C Blue No. 1 Aluminum Lake, D&C Yellow No. 10 Aluminum Lake
200	D&C Red No. 30 Aluminum Lake, D&C Yellow No. 10 Aluminum Lake
300	FD&C Yellow No. 6 Aluminum Lake, FD&C Blue No. 1 Aluminum Lake, D&C Yellow No. 10 Aluminum Lake

CLINICAL PHARMACOLOGY

Thyroid hormone synthesis and secretion is regulated by the hypothalamic-pituitary-thyroid axis. Thyrotropin-releasing hormone (TRH) released from the hypothalamus stimulates secretion of thyrotropin-stimulating hormone, TSH, from the anterior pituitary. TSH, in turn, is the physiologic stimulus for the synthesis and secretion of thyroid hormones, L-thyroxine (T_4) and L-triiodothyronine (T_3), by the thyroid gland. Circulating serum T_3 and T_4 levels exert a feedback effect on both TRH and TSH secretion. When serum T_3 and T_4 levels increase, TRH and TSH secretion decrease. When thyroid hormone levels decrease, TRH and TSH secretion increase.

The mechanisms by which thyroid hormones exert their physiologic actions are not completely understood, but it is thought that their principal effects are exerted through control of DNA transcription and protein synthesis. T_3 and T_4 diffuse into the cell nucleus and bind to thyroid receptor proteins attached to DNA. This hormone nuclear receptor complex activates gene transcription and synthesis of messenger RNA and cytoplasmic proteins.

Thyroid hormones regulate multiple metabolic processes and play an essential role in normal growth and development, and normal maturation of the central nervous system and bone. The metabolic actions of thyroid hormones include augmentation of cellular respiration and thermogenesis, as well as metabolism of proteins, carbohydrates and lipids. The protein anabolic effects of thyroid hormones are essential to normal growth and development.

The physiologic actions of thyroid hormones are produced predominately by T_3, the majority of which (approximately 80%) is derived from T_4 by deiodination in peripheral tissues.

Levothyroxine, at doses individualized according to patient response, is effective as replacement or supplemental therapy in hypothyroidism of any etiology, except transient hypothyroidism during the recovery phase of subacute thyroiditis.

Levothyroxine is also effective in the suppression of pituitary TSH secretion in the treatment or prevention of various types of euthyroid goiters, including thyroid nodules, Hashimoto's thyroiditis, multinodular goiter and, as adjunctive therapy in the management of thyrotropin-dependent well-differentiated thyroid cancer (see **INDICATIONS AND USAGE, PRECAUTIONS, DOSAGE AND ADMINISTRATION**).

Pharmacokinetics

Absorption – Absorption of orally administered T_4 from the gastrointestinal (GI) tract ranges from 40% to 80%. The majority of the levothyroxine dose is absorbed from the jejunum and upper ileum. The relative bioavailability of LEVOXYL® tablets, compared to an equal nominal dose of oral levothyroxine sodium solution, is approximately 98%. T_4 absorption is increased by fasting, and decreased in malabsorption syndromes and by certain foods such as soybean infant formula. Dietary fiber decreases bioavailability of T_4. Absorption may also decrease with age. In addition, many drugs and foods affect T_4 absorption (see **PRECAUTIONS, Drug Interactions and Drug-Food Interactions**).

Distribution – Circulating thyroid hormones are greater than 99% bound to plasma proteins, including thyroxine-binding globulin (TBG), thyroxine-binding prealbumin (TBPA), and albumin (TBA), whose capacities and affinities vary for each hormone. The higher affinity of both TBG and TBPA for T_4 partially explains the higher serum levels, slower metabolic clearance, and longer half-life of T_4 compared to T_3. Protein-bound thyroid hormones exist in reverse equilibrium with small amounts of free hormone. Only unbound hormone is metabolically active. Many drugs and physiologic conditions affect the binding of thyroid hormones to serum proteins (see **PRECAUTIONS, Drug Interactions and Drug-Laboratory Test Interactions**). Thyroid hormones do not readily cross the placental barrier (see **PRECAUTIONS, Pregnancy**).

Metabolism – T_4 is slowly eliminated (see **TABLE 1**). The major pathway of thyroid hormone metabolism is through sequential deiodination. Approximately eighty-percent of circulating T_3 is derived from peripheral T_4 by monodeiodination. The liver is the major site of degradation for both T_4 and T_3, with T_4 deiodination also occurring at a number of additional sites, including the kidney and other tissues. Approximately 80% of the daily dose of T_4 is deiodinated to yield equal amounts of T_3 and reverse T_3 (rT_3). T_3 and rT_3 are further deiodinated to diiodothyronine. Thyroid hormones are also metabolized via conjugation with glucuronides and sulfates and excreted directly into the bile and gut where they undergo enterohepatic recirculation.

Elimination – Thyroid hormones are primarily eliminated by the kidneys. A portion of the conjugated hormone reaches the colon unchanged and is eliminated in the feces. Approximately 20% of T_4 is eliminated in the stool. Urinary excretion of T_4 decreases with age.

[See table 1 below]

INDICATIONS AND USAGE

Levothyroxine sodium is used for the following indications:

Hypothyroidism – As replacement or supplemental therapy in congenital or acquired hypothyroidism of any etiology, ex-

Continued on next page

Table 1: Pharmacokinetic Parameters of Thyroid Hormones in Euthyroid Patients

Hormone	Ratio in Thyroglobulin	Biologic Potency	$t_{1/2}$ (days)	Protein Binding (%)[2]
Levothyroxine (T_4)	10–20	1	6–7[1]	99.96
Liothyronine (T_3)	1	4	≤ 2	99.5

[1] 3 to 4 days in hyperthyroidism, 9 to 10 days in hypothyroidism; [2] Includes TBG, TBPA, and TBA

Levoxyl—Cont.

cept transient hypothyroidism during the recovery phase of subacute thyroiditis. Specific indications include: primary (thyroidal), secondary (pituitary), and tertiary (hypothalamic) hypothyroidism and subclinical hypothyroidism. Primary hypothyroidism may result from functional deficiency, primary atrophy, partial or total congenital absence of the thyroid gland, or from the effects of surgery, radiation, or drugs, with or without the presence of goiter.

Pituitary TSH Suppression – In the treatment or prevention of various types of euthyroid goiters (see **WARNINGS** and **PRECAUTIONS**), including thyroid nodules (see **WARNINGS** and **PRECAUTIONS**), subacute or chronic lymphocytic thyroiditis (Hashimoto's thyroiditis), multinodular goiter (see **WARNINGS** and **PRECAUTIONS**) and, as an adjunct to surgery and radioiodine therapy in the management of thyrotropin-dependent well-differentiated thyroid cancer.

CONTRAINDICATIONS

Levothyroxine is contraindicated in patients with untreated subclinical (suppressed serum TSH level with normal T_3 and T_4 levels) or overt thyrotoxicosis of any etiology and in patients with acute myocardial infarction. Levothyroxine is contraindicated in patients with uncorrected adrenal insufficiency since thyroid hormones may precipitate an acute adrenal crisis by increasing the metabolic clearance of glucocorticoids (see **PRECAUTIONS**). LEVOXYL® is contraindicated in patients with hypersensitivity to any of the inactive ingredients in LEVOXYL® tablets (see **DESCRIPTION, Inactive Ingredients.**)

WARNINGS

WARNING: Thyroid hormones, including LEVOXYL®, either alone or with other therapeutic agents, should not be used for the treatment of obesity or for weight loss. In euthyroid patients, doses within the range of daily hormonal requirements are ineffective for weight reduction. Larger doses may produce serious or even life threatening manifestations of toxicity, particularly when given in association with sympathomimetic amines such as those used for their anorectic effects.

Levothyroxine sodium should not be used in the treatment of male or female infertility unless this condition is associated with hypothyroidism.

In patients with nontoxic diffuse goiter or nodular thyroid disease, particularly the elderly or those with underlying cardiovascular disease, levothyroxine sodium therapy is contraindicated if the serum TSH level is already suppressed due to the risk of precipitating overt thyrotoxicosis (see **CONTRAINDICATIONS**). If the serum TSH level is not suppressed, LEVOXYL® should be used with caution in conjunction with careful monitoring of thyroid function for evidence of hyperthyroidism and clinical monitoring for potential associated adverse cardiovascular signs and symptoms of hyperthyroidism.

PRECAUTIONS

General

Levothyroxine has a narrow therapeutic index. Regardless of the indication for use, careful dosage titration is necessary to avoid the consequences of over- or under-treatment. These consequences include, among others, effects on growth and development, cardiovascular function, bone metabolism, reproductive function, cognitive function, emotional state, gastrointestinal function, and on glucose and lipid metabolism. Many drugs interact with levothyroxine sodium necessitating adjustments in dosing to maintain therapeutic response (see **Drug Interactions**).

Effects on bone mineral density – In women, long-term levothyroxine sodium therapy has been associated with decreased bone mineral density, especially in postmenopausal women on greater than replacement doses or in women who are receiving suppressive doses of levothyroxine sodium. Therefore, it is recommended that patients receiving levothyroxine sodium be given the minimum dose necessary to achieve the desired clinical and biochemical response.

Patients with underlying cardiovascular disease – Exercise caution when administering levothyroxine to patients with cardiovascular disorders and to the elderly in whom there is an increased risk of occult cardiac disease. In these patients, levothyroxine therapy should be initiated at lower doses than those recommended in younger individuals or in patients without cardiac disease (see **WARNINGS; PRECAUTIONS, Geriatric Use;** and **DOSAGE AND ADMINISTRATION**). If cardiac symptoms develop or worsen, the levothyroxine dose should be reduced or withheld for one week and then cautiously restarted at a lower dose. Overtreatment with levothyroxine sodium may have adverse cardiovascular effects such as an increase in heart rate, cardiac wall thickness, and cardiac contractility and may precipitate angina or arrhythmias. Patients with coronary artery disease who are receiving levothyroxine therapy should be monitored closely during surgical procedures, since the possibility of precipitating cardiac arrhythmias may be greater in those treated with levothyroxine. Concomitant administration of levothyroxine and sympathomimetic agents to patients with coronary artery disease may precipitate coronary insufficiency.

Patients with nontoxic diffuse goiter or nodular thyroid disease – Exercise caution when administering levothyroxine to patients with nontoxic diffuse goiter or nodular thyroid disease in order to prevent precipitation of thyrotoxicosis (see **WARNINGS**). If the serum TSH is already suppressed, levothyroxine sodium should not be administered (see **Contraindications**).

Associated endocrine disorders

Hypothalamic/pituitary hormone deficiencies – In patients with secondary or tertiary hypothyroidism, additional hypothalamic/pituitary hormone deficiencies should be considered, and, if diagnosed, treated (see **PRECAUTIONS, Autoimmune polyglandular syndrome**) for adrenal insufficiency.

Autoimmune polyglandular syndrome – Occasionally, chronic autoimmune thyroiditis may occur in association with other autoimmune disorders such as adrenal insufficiency, pernicious anemia, and insulin-dependent diabetes mellitus. Patients with concomitant adrenal insufficiency should be treated with replacement glucocorticoids prior to initiation of treatment with levothyroxine sodium. Failure to do so may precipitate an acute adrenal crisis when thyroid hormone therapy is initiated, due to increased metabolic clearance of glucocorticoids by thyroid hormone. Patients with diabetes mellitus may require upward adjustments of their antidiabetic therapeutic regimens when treated with levothyroxine (see **PRECAUTIONS, Drug Interactions**).

Other associated medical conditions

Infants with congenital hypothyroidism appear to be at increased risk for other congenital anomalies, with cardiovascular anomalies (pulmonary stenosis, atrial septal defect, and ventricular septal defect,) being the most common association.

Information for Patients

Patients should be informed of the following information to aid in the safe and effective use of LEVOXYL®:

1. Notify your physician if you are allergic to any foods or medicines, are pregnant or intend to become pregnant, are breast-feeding or are taking any other medications, including prescription and over-the-counter preparations.
2. Notify your physician of any other medical conditions you may have, particularly heart disease, diabetes, clotting disorders, and adrenal or pituitary gland problems. Your dose of medications used to control these other conditions may need to be adjusted while you are taking LEVOXYL®. If you have diabetes, monitor your blood and/or urinary glucose levels as directed by your physician and immediately report any changes to your physician. If you are taking anticoagulants (blood thinners), your clotting status should be checked frequently.

Table 2: Drug-Thyroidal Axis Interactions

Drug or Drug Class	Effect
Drugs that may reduce TSH secretion—the reduction is not sustained; therefore, hypothyroidism does not occur	
Dopamine/Dopamine Agonists Glucocorticoids Octreotide	Use of these agents may result in a transient reduction in TSH secretion when administered at the following doses: Dopamine (≥ 1 mcg/kg/min); Glucocorticoids (hydrocortisone ≥ 100 mg/day or equivalent); Octreotide (> 100 mcg/day).
Drugs that alter thyroid hormone secretion	
Drugs that may decrease thyroid hormone secretion, which may result in hypothyroidism	
Aminoglutethimide Amiodarone Iodine (including iodine-Containing Radiographic contrast agents) Lithium Methimazole Propylthiouracil (PTU) Sulfonamides Tolbutamide	Long-term lithium therapy can result in goiter in up to 50% of patients, and either subclinical or overt hypothyroidism, each in up to 20% of patients. The fetus, neonate, elderly and euthyroid patients with underlying thyroid disease (e.g., Hashimoto's thyroiditis or with Grave's disease previously treated with radioiodine or surgery) are among those individuals who are particularly susceptible to iodine-induced hypothyroidism. Oral cholecystographic agents and amiodarone are slowly excreted, producing more prolonged hypothyroidism than parenterally administered iodinated contrast agents. Long-term aminoglutethimide therapy may minimally decrease T_4 and T_3 levels and increase TSH, although all values remain within normal limits in most patients.
Drugs that may increase thyroid hormone secretion, which may result in hyperthyroidism	
Amiodarone Iodide (including iodine-containing Radiographic contrast agents)	Iodide and drugs that contain pharmacologic amounts of iodide may cause hyperthyroidism in euthyroid patients with Grave's disease previously treated with antithyroid drugs or in euthyroid patients with thyroid autonomy (e.g., multinodular goiter or hyperfunctioning thyroid adenoma). Hyperthyroidism may develop over several weeks and may persist for several months after therapy discontinuation. Amiodarone may induce hyperthyroidism by causing thyroiditis.
Drugs that may decrease T_4 absorption, which may result in hypothyroidism	
Antacids - Aluminum & Magnesium Hydroxides - Simethicone Bile Acid Sequestrants - Cholestyramine - Colestipol Calcium Carbonate Cation Exchange Resins - Kayexalate Ferrous Sulfate Sucralfate	Concurrent use may reduce the efficacy of levothyroxine by binding and delaying or preventing absorption, potentially resulting in hypothyroidism. Calcium carbonate may form an insoluble chelate with levothyroxine, and ferrous sulfate likely forms a ferric-thyroxine complex. Administer levothyroxine at least 4 hours apart from these agents.
Drugs that may alter T_4 and T_3 serum transport—but FT_4 concentration remains normal; and, therefore, the patient remains euthyroid	
Drugs that may increase serum TBG concentration	**Drugs that may decrease serum TBG concentration**
Clofibrate Estrogen-containing oral contraceptives Estrogens (oral) Heroin / Methadone 5-Fluorouracil Mitotane Tamoxifen	Androgens / Anabolic Steroids Asparaginase Glucocorticoids Slow-Release Nicotinic Acid
Drugs that may cause protein-binding site displacement	
Furosemide (> 80 mg IV) Heparin Hydantoins Non Steroidal Anti-Inflammatory Drugs -Fenamates -Phenylbutazone Salicylates (> 2 g/day)	Administration of these agents with levothyroxine results in an initial transient increase in FT_4. Continued administration results in a decrease in serum T_4 and normal FT_4 and TSH concentrations and, therefore, patients are clinically euthyroid. Salicylates inhibit binding of T_4 and T_3 to TBG and transthyretin. An initial increase in serum FT_4 is followed by return of FT_4 to normal levels with sustained therapeutic serum salicylate concentrations, although total-T_4 levels may decrease by as much as 30%.

(Table continued on next page)

3. Use LEVOXYL® only as prescribed by your physician. Do not discontinue or change the amount you take or how often you take it, unless directed to do so by your physician.
4. The levothyroxine in LEVOXYL® is intended to replace a hormone that is normally produced by your thyroid gland. Generally, replacement therapy is to be taken for life, except in cases of transient hypothyroidism, which is usually associated with an inflammation of the thyroid gland (thyroiditis).
5. Take LEVOXYL® in the morning on an empty stomach, at least one-half hour before eating any food.
6. It may take several weeks before you notice an improvement in your symptoms.
7. Notify your physician if you experience any of the following symptoms: rapid or irregular heartbeat, chest pain, shortness of breath, leg cramps, headache, nervousness, irritability, sleeplessness, tremors, change in appetite, weight gain or loss, vomiting, diarrhea, excessive sweating, heat intolerance, fever, changes in menstrual periods, hives or skin rash, or any other unusual medical event.
8. Notify your physician if you become pregnant while taking LEVOXYL®. It is likely that your dose of LEVOXYL® will need to be increased while you are pregnant.
9. Notify your physician or dentist that you are taking LEVOXYL® prior to any surgery.
10. Partial hair loss may occur rarely during the first few months of LEVOXYL® therapy, but this is usually temporary.
11. LEVOXYL® should not be used as a primary or adjunctive therapy in a weight control program.
12. Keep LEVOXYL® out of the reach of children. Store LEVOXYL® away from heat, moisture, and light.

Laboratory Tests

General

The diagnosis of hypothyroidism is confirmed by measuring TSH levels using a sensitive assay (second generation assay sensitivity ≤ 0.1 mIU/L or third generation assay sensitivity ≤ 0.01 mIU/L) and measurement of free-T_4.

The adequacy of therapy is determined by periodic assessment of appropriate laboratory tests and clinical evaluation. The choice of laboratory tests depends on various factors including the etiology of the underlying thyroid disease, the presence of concomitant medical conditions, including pregnancy, and the use of concomitant medications (see **PRECAUTIONS, Drug Interactions** and **Drug-Laboratory Test Interactions**). Persistent clinical and laboratory evidence of hypothyroidism despite an apparent adequate replacement dose of LEVOXYL® may be evidence of inadequate absorption, poor compliance, drug interactions, or decreased T_4 potency of the drug product.

Adults

In adult patients with primary (thyroidal) hypothyroidism, serum TSH levels (using a sensitive assay) alone may be used to monitor therapy. The frequency of TSH monitoring during levothyroxine dose titration depends on the clinical situation but it is generally recommended at 6–8 week intervals until normalization. For patients who have recently initiated levothyroxine therapy and whose serum TSH has normalized or in patients who have had their dosage or brand of levothyroxine changed, the serum TSH concentration should be measured after 8–12 weeks. When the optimum replacement dose has been attained, clinical (physical examination) and biochemical monitoring may be performed every 6–12 months, depending on the clinical situation, and whenever there is a change in the patient's status. It is recommended that a physical examination and a serum TSH measurement be performed at least annually in patients receiving LEVOXYL® (see **WARNINGS, PRECAUTIONS,** and **DOSAGE AND ADMINISTRATION**).

Pediatrics

In patients with congenital hypothyroidism, the adequacy of replacement therapy should be assessed by measuring both serum TSH (using a sensitive assay) and total- or free-T_4. During the first three years of life, the serum total- or free-T_4 should be maintained at all times in the upper half of the normal range. While the aim of therapy is to also normalize the serum TSH level, this is not always possible in a small percentage of patients, particularly in the first few months of therapy. TSH may not normalize due to a resetting of the pituitary-thyroid feedback threshold as a result of *in utero* hypothyroidism. Failure of the serum T_4 to increase into the upper half of the normal range within 2 weeks of initiation of LEVOXYL® therapy and/or of the serum TSH to decrease below 20 mU/L within 4 weeks should alert the physician to the possibility that the child is not receiving adequate therapy. Careful inquiry should then be made regarding compliance, dose of medication administered, and method of administration prior to raising the dose of LEVOXYL®.

The recommended frequency of monitoring of TSH and total or free T_4 in children is as follows: at 2 and 4 weeks after the initiation of treatment; every 1–2 months during the first year of life; every 2–3 months between 1 and 3 years of age; and every 3 to 12 months thereafter until growth is completed. More frequent intervals of monitoring may be necessary if poor compliance is suspected or abnormal values are obtained. It is recommended that TSH and T_4 levels, and a physical examination, if indicated, be performed 2 weeks after any change in LEVOXYL® dosage. Routine clinical examination, including assessment of mental and physical growth and development, and bone maturation, should be performed at regular intervals (see **PRECAUTIONS, Pediatric Use** and **DOSAGE AND ADMINISTRATION**).

Table 2 *(cont.)*: Drug-Thyroidal Axis Interactions

Drug or Drug Class	Effect
Drugs that may alter T_4 and T_3 metabolism	
Drugs that may increase hepatic metabolism, which may result in hypothyroidism	
Carbamazepine Hydantoins Phenobarbital Rifampin	Stimulation of hepatic microsomal drug-metabolizing enzyme activity may cause increased hepatic degradation of levothyroxine, resulting in increased levothyroxine requirements. Phenytoin and carbamazepine reduce serum protein binding of levothyroxine, and total- and free-T_4 may be reduced by 20% to 40%, but most patients have normal serum TSH levels and are clinically euthyroid.
Drugs that may decrease T_4 5′-deiodinase activity	
Amiodarone Beta-adrenergic antagonists - (e.g., Propranolol > 160 mg/day) Glucocorticoids - (e.g., Dexamethasone > 4 mg/day) Propylthiouracil (PTU)	Administration of these enzyme inhibitors decreases the peripheral conversion of T_4 to T_3, leading to decreased T_3 levels. However, serum T_4 levels are usually normal but may occasionally be slightly increased. In patients treated with large doses of propranolol (> 160 mg/day), T_3 and T_4 levels change slightly, TSH levels remain normal, and patients are clinically euthyroid. It should be noted that actions of particular beta-adrenergic antagonists may be impaired when the hypothyroid patient is converted to the euthyroid state. Short-term administration of large doses of glucocorticoids may decrease serum T_3 concentrations by 30% with minimal change in serum T_4 levels. However, long-term glucocorticoid therapy may result in slightly decreased T_3 and T_4 levels due to decreased TBG production (see above).
Miscellaneous	
Anticoagulants (oral) - Coumarin Derivatives - Indandione Derivatives	Thyroid hormones appear to increase the catabolism of vitamin K-dependent clotting factors, thereby increasing the anticoagulant activity of oral anticoagulants. Concomitant use of these agents impairs the compensatory increases in clotting factor synthesis. Prothrombin time should be carefully monitored in patients taking levothyroxine and oral anticoagulants and the dose of anticoagulant therapy adjusted accordingly.
Antidepressants - Tricyclics (e.g., Amitriptyline) - Tetracyclics (e.g., Maprotiline) - Selective Serotonin Reuptake Inhibitors (SSRIs; e.g., Sertraline)	Concurrent use of tri/tetracyclic antidepressants and levothyroxine may increase the therapeutic and toxic effects of both drugs, possibly due to increased receptor sensitivity to catecholamines. Toxic effects may include increased risk of cardiac arrhythmias and CNS stimulation; onset of action of tricyclics may be accelerated. Administration of sertraline in patients stabilized on levothyroxine may result in increased levothyroxine requirements.
Antidiabetic Agents - Biguanides - Meglitinides - Sulfonylureas - Thiazolidediones - Insulin	Addition of levothyroxine to antidiabetic or insulin therapy may result in increased antidiabetic agent or insulin requirements. Careful monitoring of diabetic control is recommended, especially when thyroid therapy is started, changed, or discontinued.
Cardiac Glycosides	Serum digitalis glycoside levels may be reduced in hyperthyroidism or when the hypothyroid patient is converted to the euthyroid state. Therapeutic effect of digitalis glycosides may be reduced.
Cytokines - Interferon-α - Interleukin-2	Therapy with interferon-α has been associated with the development of antithyroid microsomal antibodies in 20% of patients and some have transient hypothyroidism, hyperthyroidism, or both. Patients who have antithyroid antibodies before treatment are at higher risk for thyroid dysfunction during treatment. Interleukin-2 has been associated with transient painless thyroiditis in 20% of patients. Interferon-β and -γ have not been reported to cause thyroid dysfunction.
Growth Hormones - Somatrem - Somatropin	Excessive use of thyroid hormones with growth hormones may accelerate epiphyseal closure. However, untreated hypothyroidism may interfere with growth response to growth hormone.
Ketamine	Concurrent use may produce marked hypertension and tachycardia; cautious administration to patients receiving thyroid hormone therapy is recommended.
Methylxanthine Bronchodilators - (e.g., Theophylline)	Decreased theophylline clearance may occur in hypothyroid patients; clearance returns to normal when the euthyroid state is achieved.
Radiographic Agents	Thyroid hormones may reduce the uptake of ^{123}I, ^{131}I, and ^{99m}Tc.
Sympathomimetics	Concurrent use may increase the effects of sympathomimetics or thyroid hormone. Thyroid hormones may increase the risk of coronary insufficiency when sympathomimetic agents are administered to patients with coronary artery disease.
Choral Hydrate Diazepam Ethionamide Lovastatin Metoclopramide 6-Mercaptopurine Nitroprusside Para-aminosalicylate sodium Perphenazine Resorcinol (excessive topical use) Thiazide Diuretics	These agents have been associated with thyroid hormone and / or TSH level alterations by various mechanisms.

Secondary (pituitary) and tertiary (hypothalamic) hypothyroidism

Adequacy of therapy should be assessed by measuring serum free-T_4 levels, which should be maintained in the upper half of the normal range in these patients.

Drug Interactions

Many drugs affect thyroid hormone pharmacokinetics and metabolism (e.g., absorption, synthesis, secretion, catabolism, protein binding, and target tissue response) and may alter the therapeutic response to LEVOXYL®. In addition, thyroid hormones and thyroid status have varied effects on the pharmacokinetics and action of other drugs. A listing of drug-thyroidal axis interactions is contained in Table 2.

The list of drug-thyroidal axis interactions in Table 2 may not be comprehensive due to the introduction of new drugs that interact with the thyroidal axis or the discovery of previously unknown interactions. The prescriber should be aware of this fact and should consult appropriate reference sources. (e.g., package inserts of newly approved drugs, medical literature) for additional information if a drug-drug interaction with levothyroxine is suspected.

[See table 2 on previous page and above]

Oral anticoagulants – Levothyroxine increases the response to oral anticoagulant therapy. Therefore, a decrease in the dose of anticoagulant may be warranted with correction of the hypothyroid state or when the LEVOXYL® dose is increased. Prothrombin time should be closely monitored to

Continued on next page

Levoxyl—Cont.

permit appropriate and timely dosage adjustments (see **Table 2**).

Digitalis glycosides – The therapeutic effects of digitalis glycosides may be reduced by levothyroxine. Serum digitalis glycoside levels may be decreased when a hypothyroid patient becomes euthyroid, necessitating an increase in the dose of digitalis glycosides (see **Table 2**).

Drug-Food Interactions – Consumption of certain foods may affect levothyroxine absorption thereby necessitating adjustments in dosing. Soybean flour (infant formula), cotton seed meal, walnuts, and dietary fiber may bind and decrease the absorption of levothyroxine sodium from the GI tract.

Drug-Laboratory Test Interactions – Changes in TBG concentration must be considered when interpreting T_4 and T_3 values, which necessitates measurement and evaluation of unbound (free) hormone and/or determination of the free T_4 index (FT_4I). Pregnancy, infectious hepatitis, estrogens, estrogen-containing oral contraceptives, and acute intermittent porphyria increase TBG concentrations. Decreases in TBG concentrations are observed in nephrosis, severe hypoproteinemia, severe liver disease, acromegaly, and after androgen or corticosteroid therapy (see also **Table 2**). Familial hyper- or hypo-thyroxine binding globulinemias have been described, with the incidence of TBG deficiency approximating 1 in 9000.

Carcinogenesis, Mutagenesis, and Impairment of Fertility – Animal studies have not been performed to evaluate the carcinogenic potential, mutagenic potential or effects on fertility of levothyroxine. The synthetic T_4 in LEVOXYL® is identical to that produced naturally by the human thyroid gland. Although there has been a reported association between prolonged thyroid hormone therapy and breast cancer, this has not been confirmed. Patients receiving LEVOXYL® for appropriate clinical indications should be titrated to the lowest effective replacement dose.

Pregnancy – Category A – Studies in women taking levothyroxine sodium during pregnancy have not shown an increased risk of congenital abnormalities. Therefore, the possibility of fetal harm appears remote. LEVOXYL® should not be discontinued during pregnancy and hypothyroidism diagnosed during pregnancy should be promptly treated.

Hypothyroidism during pregnancy is associated with a higher rate of complications, including spontaneous abortion, pre-eclampsia, stillbirth and premature delivery. Maternal hypothyroidism may have an adverse effect on fetal and childhood growth and development. During pregnancy, serum T_4 levels may decrease and serum TSH levels increase to values outside the normal range. Since elevations in serum TSH may occur as early as 4 weeks gestation, pregnant women taking LEVOXYL® should have their TSH measured during each trimester. An elevated serum TSH level should be corrected by an increase in the dose of LEVOXYL®. Since postpartum TSH levels are similar to preconception values, the LEVOXYL® dosage should return to the pre-pregnancy dose immediately after delivery. A serum TSH level should be obtained 6–8 weeks postpartum.

Thyroid hormones do not readily cross the placental barrier; however, some transfer does occur as evidenced by levels in cord blood of athyreotic fetuses being approximately one-third maternal levels. Transfer of thyroid hormone from the mother to the fetus, however, may not be adequate to prevent in utero hypothyroidism.

Nursing Mothers – Although thyroid hormones are excreted only minimally in human milk, caution should be exercised when LEVOXYL® is administered to a nursing woman. However, adequate replacement doses of levothyroxine are generally needed to maintain normal lactation.

Pediatric Use

General

The goal of treatment in pediatric patients with hypothyroidism is to achieve and maintain normal intellectual and physical growth and development.

The initial dose of levothyroxine varies with age and body weight (see **DOSAGE AND ADMINISTRATION, Table 3**). Dosing adjustments are based on an assessment of the individual patient's clinical and laboratory parameters (see **PRECAUTIONS, Laboratory Tests**).

In children in whom a diagnosis of permanent hypothyroidism has not been established, it is recommended that levothyroxine administration be discontinued for a 30-day trial period, but only after the child is at least 3 years of age. Serum T_4 and TSH levels should then be obtained. If the T_4 is low and the TSH high, the diagnosis of permanent hypothyroidism is established, and levothyroxine therapy should be reinstituted. If the T_4 and TSH levels are normal, euthyroidism may be assumed and, therefore, the hypothyroidism can be considered to have been transient. In this instance, however, the physician should carefully monitor the child and repeat the thyroid function tests if any signs or symptoms of hypothyroidism develop. In this setting, the clinician should have a high index of suspicion of relapse. If the results of the levothyroxine withdrawal test are inconclusive, careful follow-up and subsequent testing will be necessary.

Since some more severely affected children may become clinically hypothyroid when treatment is discontinued for 30 days, an alternate approach is to reduce the replacement dose of levothyroxine by half during the 30-day trial period. If, after 30 days, the serum TSH is elevated above 20 mU/L, the diagnosis of permanent hypothyroidism is confirmed, and full replacement therapy should be resumed. However, if the serum TSH has not risen to greater than 20mU/L, levothyroxine treatment should be discontinued for another 30-day trial period followed by repeat serum T_4 and TSH.

The presence of concomitant medical conditions should be considered in certain clinical circumstances and, if present, appropriately treated (see **PRECAUTIONS**).

Congenital Hypothyroidism (see **PRECAUTIONS, Laboratory Tests** and **DOSAGE and ADMINISTRATION**)

Rapid restoration of normal serum T_4 concentrations is essential for preventing the adverse effects of congenital hypothyroidism on intellectual development as well as on overall physical growth and maturation. Therefore, LEVOXYL® therapy should be initiated immediately upon diagnosis and is generally continued for life.

During the first 2 weeks of LEVOXYL® therapy, infants should be closely monitored for cardiac overload, arrhythmias, and aspiration from avid suckling.

The patient should be monitored closely to avoid undertreatment or overtreatment. Undertreatment may have deleterious effects on intellectual development and linear growth. Overtreatment has been associated with craniosynostosis in infants, and may adversely affect the tempo of brain maturation and accelerate the bone age with resultant premature closure of the epiphyses and compromised adult stature.

Acquired Hypothyroidism in Pediatric Patients

The patient should be monitored closely to avoid undertreatment and overtreatment. Undertreatment may result in poor school performance due to impaired concentration and slowed mentation and in reduced adult height. Overtreatment may accelerate the bone age and result in premature epiphyseal closure and compromised adult stature.

Treated children may manifest a period of catch-up growth, which may be adequate in some cases to normalize adult height. In children with severe or prolonged hypothyroidism, catch-up growth may not be adequate to normalize adult height.

Geriatric Use

Because of the increased prevalence of cardiovascular disease among the elderly, levothyroxine therapy should not be initiated at the full replacement dose (see **WARNINGS, PRECAUTIONS,** and **DOSAGE AND ADMINISTRATION**).

ADVERSE REACTIONS

Adverse reactions associated with levothyroxine therapy are primarily those of hyperthyroidism due to therapeutic overdosage. They include the following:

General: fatigue, increased appetite, weight loss, heat intolerance, fever, excessive sweating;

Central nervous system: headache, hyperactivity, nervousness, anxiety, irritability, emotional lability, insomnia;

Musculoskeletal: tremors, muscle weakness;

Cardiac: palpitations, tachycardia, arrhythmias, increased pulse and blood pressure, heart failure, angina, myocardial infarction, cardiac arrest;

Pulmonary: dyspnea;

GI: diarrhea, vomiting, abdominal cramps;

Dermatologic: hair loss, flushing;

Reproductive: menstrual irregularities, impaired fertility.

Pseudotumor cerebri and slipped capital femoral epiphysis have been reported in children receiving levothyroxine therapy. Overtreatment may result in craniosynostosis in infants and premature closure of the epiphyses in children with resultant compromised adult height.

Seizures have been reported rarely with the institution of levothyroxine therapy.

Inadequate levothyroxine dosage will produce or fail to ameliorate the signs and symptoms of hypothyroidism.

Hypersensitivity reactions to inactive ingredients have occurred in patients treated with thyroid hormone products. These include urticaria, pruritus, skin rash, flushing, angioedema, various GI symptoms (abdominal pain, nausea, vomiting and diarrhea), fever, arthralgia, serum sickness and wheezing. Hypersensitivity to levothyroxine itself is not known to occur.

OVERDOSAGE

The signs and symptoms of overdosage are those of hyperthyroidism (see **PRECAUTIONS** and **ADVERSE REACTIONS**). In addition, confusion and disorientation may occur. Cerebral embolism, shock, coma, and death have been reported. Seizures have occurred in a child ingesting approximately 20 mg of levothyroxine. Symptoms may not necessarily be evident or may not appear until several days after ingestion of levothyroxine sodium.

Treatment of Overdosage

Levothyroxine sodium should be reduced in dose or temporarily discontinued if signs or symptoms of overdosage occur.

Acute Massive Overdosage – This may be a life-threatening emergency, therefore, symptomatic and supportive therapy should be instituted immediately. If not contraindicated (e.g., by seizures, coma, or loss of the gag reflex), the stomach should be emptied by emesis or gastric lavage to decrease gastrointestinal absorption. Activated charcoal or cholestyramine may also be used to decrease absorption. Central and peripheral increased sympathetic activity may be treated by administering B-receptor antagonists, e.g., propranolol (1 to 3 mg intravenously over a 10-minute period, or orally, 80 to 160 mg/day). Provide respiratory support as needed; control congestive heart failure; control fever, hypoglycemia, and fluid loss as necessary. Glucocorticoids may be given to inhibit the conversion of T_4 to T_3. Because T_4 is highly protein bound, very little drug will be removed by dialysis.

DOSAGE AND ADMINISTRATION

General Principles:

The goal of replacement therapy is to achieve and maintain a clinical and biochemical euthyroid state. The goal of suppressive therapy is to inhibit growth and/or function of abnormal thyroid tissue. The dose of LEVOXYL® that is adequate to achieve these goals depends on a variety of factors including the patient's age, body weight, cardiovascular status, concomitant medical conditions, including pregnancy, concomitant medications, and the specific nature of the condition being treated (see **WARNINGS** and **PRECAUTIONS**). Hence, the following recommendations serve only as dosing guidelines. Dosing must be individualized and adjustments made based on periodic assessment of the patient's clinical response and laboratory parameters (see **PRECAUTIONS, Laboratory Tests**).

The LEVOXYL® should be taken in the morning on an empty stomach, at least one-half hour before any food is eaten. LEVOXYL® should be taken at least 4 hours apart from drugs that are known to interfere with its absorption (see **PRECAUTIONS, Drug Interactions**).

Due to the long half-life of levothyroxine, the peak therapeutic effect at a given dose of levothyroxine sodium may not be attained for 4–6 weeks.

Caution should be exercised when administering LEVOXYL® to patients with underlying cardiovascular disease, to the elderly, and to those with concomitant adrenal insufficiency (see **PRECAUTIONS**).

Specific Patient Populations:

Hypothyroidism in Adults and in Children in Whom Growth and Puberty are Complete (see **WARNINGS** and **PRECAUTIONS, Laboratory Tests**)

Therapy may begin at full replacement doses in otherwise healthy individuals less than 50 years old and in those older than 50 years who have been recently treated for hyperthyroidism or who have been hypothyroid for only a short time (such as a few months). The average full replacement dose of levothyroxine sodium is approximately 1.7 mcg/kg/day (e.g., **100–125 mcg/day** for a 70 kg adult). Older patients may require less than 1 mcg/kg/day. Levothyroxine sodium doses greater than 200 mcg/day are seldom required. An inadequate response to daily doses ≥ 300 mcg/day is rare and may indicate poor compliance, malabsorption, and/or drug interactions.

For most patients older than 50 years or for patients under 50 years of age with underlying cardiac disease, an initial starting dose of **25–50 mcg/day** of levothyroxine sodium is recommended, with gradual increments in dose at 6–8 week

Strength (mcg)	Color	NDC # for bottles of 100	NDC # for bottles of 1000	NDC # for Unit Dose Cartons of 100
25	Orange	NDC 52604-5025-1	NDC 52604-5025-2	NDC 52604-5025-5
50	White	NDC 52604-5050-1	NDC 52604-5050-2	NDC 52604-5050-5
75	Purple	NDC 52604-5075-1	NDC 52604-5075-2	NDC 52604-5075-5
88	Olive	NDC 52604-5088-1	NDC 52604-5088-2	NDC 52604-5088-5
100	Yellow	NDC 52604-5100-1	NDC 52604-5100-2	NDC 52604-5100-5
112	Rose	NDC 52604-5112-1	NDC 52604-5112-2	NDC 52604-5112-5
125	Brown	NDC 52604-5125-1	NDC 52604-5125-2	NDC 52604-5125-5
137	Dark Blue	NDC 52604-5137-1	NDC 52604-5137-2	NDC 52604-5137-5
150	Blue	NDC 52604-5150-1	NDC 52604-5150-2	NDC 52604-5150-5
175	Turquoise	NDC 52604-5175-1	NDC 52604-5175-2	NDC 52604-5175-5
200	Pink	NDC 52604-5200-1	NDC 52604-5200-2	NDC 52604-5200-5
300	Green	NDC 52604-5300-1	NDC 52604-5300-2	NDC 52604-5300-5

intervals, as needed. The recommended starting dose of levothyroxine sodium in elderly patients with cardiac disease is **12.5–25 mcg/day**, with gradual dose increments at 4–6 week intervals. The levothyroxine sodium dose is generally adjusted in 12.5–25 mcg increments until the patient with primary hypothyroidism is clinically euthyroid and the serum TSH has normalized.

In patients with severe hypothyroidism, the recommended initial levothyroxine sodium dose is **12.5–25 mcg/day** with increases of 25 mcg/day every 2–4 weeks, accompanied by clinical and laboratory assessment, until the TSH level is normalized.

In patients with secondary (pituitary) or tertiary (hypothalamic) hypothyroidism, the levothyroxine sodium dose should be titrated until the patient is clinically euthyroid and the serum free-T_4 level is restored to the upper half of the normal range.

Pediatric Dosage – Congenital or Acquired Hypothyroidism (see **PRECAUTIONS, Laboratory Tests**)

General Principles

In general, levothyroxine therapy should be instituted at full replacement doses as soon as possible. Delays in diagnosis and institution of therapy may have deleterious effects on the child's intellectual and physical growth and development.

Undertreatment and overtreatment should be avoided (see **PRECAUTIONS, Pediatric Use**).

LEVOXYL® may be administered to infants and children who cannot swallow intact tablets by crushing the tablet and suspending the freshly crushed tablet in a small amount (5–10 mL or 1–2 teaspoons) of water. This suspension can be administered by spoon or dropper. **DO NOT STORE THE SUSPENSION.** Foods that decrease absorption of levothyroxine, such as soybean infant formula, should not be used for administering levothyroxine sodium tablets. (see **PRECAUTIONS, Drug-Food Interactions**).

Newborns

The recommended starting dose of levothyroxine sodium in newborn infants is **10–15 mcg/kg/day**. A lower starting dose (e.g., 25 mcg/day) should be considered in infants at risk for cardiac failure, and the dose should be increased in 4–6 weeks as needed based on clinical and laboratory response to treatment. In infants with very low (< 5 mcg/dL) or undetectable serum T_4 concentrations, the recommended initial starting dose is **50 mcg/day** of levothyroxine sodium.

Infants and Children

Levothyroxine therapy is usually initiated at full replacement doses, with the recommended dose per body weight decreasing with age (see **TABLE 3**). However, in children with chronic or severe hypothyroidism, an initial dose of **25 mcg/day** of levothyroxine sodium is recommended with increments of 25 mcg every 2–4 weeks until the desired effect is achieved.

Hyperactivity in an older child can be minimized if the starting dose is one-fourth of the recommended full replacement dose, and the dose is then increased on a weekly basis by an amount equal to one-fourth the full-recommended replacement dose until the full recommended replacement dose is reached.

Table 3: Levothyroxine Sodium Dosing Guidelines for Pediatric Hypothyroidism

AGE	Daily Dose Per Kg Body Weight[a]
0–3 months	10–15 mcg/kg/day
3–6 months	8–10 mcg/kg/day
6–12 months	6–8 mcg/kg/day
1–5 years	5–6 mcg/kg/day
6–12 years	4–5 mcg/kg/day
>12 years	2–3 mcg/kg/day
Growth and puberty complete	1.7 mcg/kg/day

[a] – The dose should be adjusted based on clinical response and laboratory parameters (see **PRECAUTIONS, Laboratory Tests and Pediatric Use**).

Pregnancy–Pregnancy may increase levothyroxine requirements (see **PREGNANCY**).

Subclinical Hypothyroidism – If this condition is treated, a lower levothyroxine sodium dose (e.g., **1 mcg/kg/day**) than that used for full replacement may be adequate to normalize the serum TSH level. Patients who are not treated should be monitored yearly for changes in clinical status and thyroid laboratory parameters.

TSH Suppression in Well-differentiated Thyroid Cancer and Thyroid Nodules – The target level for TSH suppression in these conditions has not been established with controlled studies. In addition, the efficacy of TSH suppression for benign nodular disease is controversial. Therefore, the dose of LEVOXYL® used for TSH suppression should be individualized based on the specific disease and the patient being treated.

In the treatment of well differentiated (papillary and follicular) thyroid cancer, levothyroxine is used as an adjunct to surgery and radioiodine therapy. Generally, TSH is suppressed to <0.1 mU/L, and this usually requires a levothyroxine sodium dose of **greater than 2 mcg/kg/day**. However, in patients with high-risk tumors, the target level for TSH suppression may be <0.01 mU/L.

In the treatment of benign nodules and nontoxic multinodular goiter, TSH is generally suppressed to a higher target (e.g., 0.1–0.5 mU/L for nodules and 0.5–1.0 mU/L for multinodular goiter) than that used for the treatment of thyroid cancer. Levothyroxine sodium is contraindicated if the serum TSH is already suppressed due to the risk of precipitating overt thyrotoxicosis (see **CONTRAINDICATIONS, WARNINGS** and **PRECAUTIONS**).

Myxedema Coma – Myxedema coma is a life-threatening emergency characterized by poor circulation and hypometabolism, and may result in unpredictable absorption of levothyroxine sodium from the gastrointestinal tract. Therefore, oral thyroid hormone drug products are not recommended to treat this condition. Thyroid hormone products formulated for intravenous administration should be administered.

HOW SUPPLIED

—LEVOXYL® (levothyroxine sodium tablets, USP) are supplied as oval, color-coded, potency marked tablets in 12 strengths:

[See table at top of previous page]

STORAGE CONDITIONS

20–25°C (68–77°F) with excursions permitted between 15–30°C (59–86°F)

Meets USP Dissolution Tests 1 and 2.

Rx ONLY

MANUFACTURER

JONES PHARMA INCORPORATED

(A wholly owned subsidiary of King Pharmaceuticals, Inc.)

St. Louis, MO 63146

Prescribing Information as of August 2003

3000000-A

Shown in Product Identification Guide, page 319

NEOSPORIN® G.U. Irrigant Sterile ℞

[*nē "ō-spor 'in*]

(neomycin sulfate-polymyxin B sulfate solution for irrigation)

NOT FOR INJECTION

DESCRIPTION

NEOSPORIN G.U. Irrigant is a concentrated sterile antibiotic solution to be diluted for urinary bladder irrigation. Each mL contains neomycin sulfate equivalent to 40 mg neomycin base, 200,000 units polymyxin B sulfate, and Water for Injection. The 20-mL multiple-dose vial contains, in addition to the above, 1 mg methylparaben (0.1%) added as a preservative.

Neomycin sulfate, an antibiotic of the aminoglycoside group, is the sulfate salt of neomycin B and C produced by *Streptomyces fradiae*. It has a potency equivalent to not less than 600 µg of neomycin per mg. The structural formulae are:

Neomycin B (R_1=H, R_2=CH_2NH_2)

Neomycin C (R_1=CH_2NH_2, R_2=H)

Polymyxin B sulfate, a polypeptide antibiotic, is the sulfate salt of polymyxin B_1 and B_2 produced by the growth of *Bacillus polymyxa*. It has a potency of not less than 6,000 polymyxin B units per mg. The structural formulae are:

Polymyxin B_1 (R=CH_3)

Polymyxin B_2 (R=H)

DAB=α,γ-diaminobutyric acid

CLINICAL PHARMACOLOGY

After prophylactic irrigation of the intact urinary bladder, neomycin and polymyxin B are absorbed in clinically insignificant quantities. A neomycin serum level of 0.1 µg/mL was observed in three of 33 patients receiving the rinse solution. This level is well below that which has been associated with neomycin-induced toxicity.

When used topically, polymyxin B sulfate and neomycin are rarely irritating.

Microbiology: The prepared NEOSPORIN G.U. Irrigant Sterile solution is bactericidal. The aminoglycosides act by inhibiting normal protein synthesis in susceptible microorganisms. Polymyxins increase the permeability of bacterial cell wall membranes. The solution is active in vitro against

Escherichia coli
Staphylococcus aureus
Haemophilus influenzae
Klebsiella and *Enterobacter* species
Neisseria species, and
Pseudomonas aeruginosa.

It is not active in vitro against *Serratia marcescens* and streptococci.

Bacterial resistance may develop following the use of the antibiotics in the catheter-rinse solution.

INDICATIONS AND USAGE

NEOSPORIN G.U. Irrigant is indicated for short-term use (up to 10 days) as a continuous irrigant or rinse in the urinary bladder of abacteriuric patients to help prevent bacteriuria and gram-negative rod septicemia associated with the use of indwelling catheters.

Since organisms gain entrance to the bladder by way of, through, and around the catheter, significant bacteriuria is induced by bacterial multiplication in the bladder urine, in the mucoid film often present between catheter and urethra, and in other sites. Urinary tract infection may result from the repeated presence in the urine of large numbers of pathogenic bacteria. The use of closed systems with indwelling catheters has been shown to reduce the risk of infection. A three-way closed catheter system with constant neomycin-polymyxin B bladder rinse is indicated to prevent the development of infection while using indwelling catheters.

If uropathogens are isolated, they should be identified and tested for susceptibility so that appropriate antimicrobial therapy for systemic use can be initiated.

CONTRAINDICATIONS

Hypersensitivity to neomycin, the polymyxins, or any ingredient in the solution is a contraindication to its use. A history of hypersensitivity or serious toxic reaction to an aminoglycoside may also contraindicate the use of any other aminoglycoside because of the known cross-sensitivity of patients to drugs of this class.

WARNINGS

PROPHYLACTIC BLADDER CARE WITH NEOSPORIN G.U. IRRIGANT STERILE SHOULD NOT BE GIVEN WHERE THERE IS A POSSIBILITY OF SYSTEMIC ABSORPTION. NEOSPORIN G.U. IRRIGANT STERILE SHOULD NOT BE USED FOR IRRIGATION OTHER THAN FOR THE URINARY BLADDER. Systemic absorption after topical application of neomycin to open wounds, burns, and granulating surfaces is significant and serum concentrations comparable to and often higher than those attained following oral and parenteral therapy have been reported. Absorption of neomycin from the denuded bladder surface has been reported.

However, the likelihood of toxicity following topical irrigation of the intact urinary bladder with NEOSPORIN G.U. Irrigant Sterile is low since no appreciable amounts of these antibiotics enter the systemic circulation by this route if irrigation does not exceed 10 days.

NEOSPORIN G.U. Irrigant is intended for continuous prophylactic irrigation of the lumen of the intact urinary bladder of patients with indwelling catheters. Patients should be under constant supervision by a physician. Irrigation should be avoided in patients with defects in the bladder mucosa or bladder wall, such as vesical rupture, or in association with operative procedures on the bladder wall, because of the risk of toxicity due to systemic absorption following diffusion into absorptive tissues and spaces. When absorbed, neomycin and polymyxin B are nephrotoxic antibiotics, and the nephrotoxic potentials are additive. In addition, both antibiotics, when absorbed, are neurotoxins: neomycin can destroy fibers of the acoustic nerve causing permanent bilateral deafness; neomycin and polymyxin B are additive in their neuromuscular blocking effects, not only in terms of potency and duration, but also in terms of characteristics of the blocks produced.

Aminoglycosides, when absorbed, can cause fetal harm when administered to a pregnant woman. Aminoglycoside antibiotics cross the placenta and there have been several reports of total, irreversible, bilateral, congenital deafness in children whose mothers received streptomycin during pregnancy. Although serious side effects have not been reported in the treatment of pregnant women with other aminoglycosides, the potential for harm exists. If NEOSPORIN G.U. Irrigant Sterile is used during pregnancy, the patient should be apprised of the potential hazard to the fetus (see **PRECAUTIONS**).

PRECAUTIONS

General: Ototoxicity, nephrotoxicity, and neuromuscular blockade may occur if NEOSPORIN G.U. Irrigant ingredients are systemically absorbed (see **WARNINGS**). Absorption of neomycin from the denuded bladder surface has been reported. Patients with impaired renal function, infants, dehydrated patients, elderly patients, and patients receiving high doses of prolonged treatment are especially at risk for the development of toxicity.

Irrigation of the bladder with NEOSPORIN G.U. Irrigant may result in overgrowth of nonsusceptible organisms, including fungi. Appropriate measures should be taken if this occurs. The safety and effectiveness of the preparation for use in the care of patients with recent lower urinary tract surgery have not been established.

Continued on next page

Neosporin G.U. Irrigant—Cont.

Urine specimens should be collected during prophylactic bladder care for urinalysis, culture, and susceptibility testing. Positive cultures suggest the presence of organisms which are resistant to the bladder rinse antibiotics.

Pregnancy: ***Teratogenic Effects:*** Pregnancy Category D. See **WARNINGS** section.

Pediatric Use: Safety and effectiveness in pediatric patients have not been established.

ADVERSE REACTIONS

Neomycin occasionally causes skin sensitization when applied topically; however, topical application to mucus membranes rarely results in local or systemic hypersensitivity reactions.

Irritation of the urinary bladder mucosa has been reported. Signs of ototoxicity and nephrotoxicity have been reported following parenteral use of these drugs and following the oral and topical use of neomycin (see **WARNINGS**).

DOSAGE AND ADMINISTRATION

This preparation is specifically designed for use with "three-way" catheters or with other catheter systems permitting **continuous** irrigation of the urinary bladder. The usual irrigation dose is one 1-mL ampul a day for up to 10 days.

Using strict aseptic techniques, the contents of one 1-mL ampul of NEOSPORIN G.U. Irrigant Sterile (neomycin sulfate-polymyxin B sulfate solution for irrigation) should be added to a 1,000-mL container of isotonic saline solution. This container should then be connected to the inflow lumen of the "three-way" catheter which has been inserted with full aseptic precautions; use of a sterile lubricant is recommended during insertion of the catheter. The outflow lumen should be connected, via a sterile disposable plastic tube, to a disposable plastic collection bag. Stringent procedures, such as taping the inflow and outflow junction at the catheter, should be observed when necessary to insure the junctional integrity of the system.

For most patients, the inflow rate of the 1,000-mL saline solution of neomycin and polymyxin B should be adjusted to a slow drip to deliver about 1,000 mL every 24 hours. If the patient's urine output exceeds 2 liters per day, it is recommended that the inflow rate be adjusted to deliver 2,000 mL of the solution in a 24-hour period.

It is important that the rinse of the bladder be **continuous**; the inflow or rinse solution should not be interrupted for more than a few minutes.

Preparation of the irrigation solution should be performed with strict aseptic techniques. The prepared solution should be stored at 4°C, and should be used within 48 hours following preparation to reduce the risk of contamination with resistant microorganisms.

HOW SUPPLIED

1-mL ampuls, boxes of 10 (61570-047-10) and 50 ampuls (61570-047-50); 20-mL multi-dose vial (NDC 61570-048-20).

Store at 2° to 8°C (36° to 46°F).

RX ONLY.

Prescribing Information as of May 2003.

Distributed by: Monarch Pharmaceuticals, Inc.
Bristol, TN 37620
Manufactured by: DSM Pharmaceuticals, Inc.
Greenville, NC 27834
Monarch Pharmaceuticals®

561074

SEPTRA® Tablets ℞
[*sĕp tra*]
SEPTRA® DS (Double Strength) Tablets ℞
SEPTRA® Suspension ℞
SEPTRA® Grape Suspension ℞
(trimethoprim and sulfamethoxazole)
PRODUCT INFORMATION

DESCRIPTION

SEPTRA (trimethoprim and sulfamethoxazole) is a synthetic antibacterial combination product. Each SEPTRA Tablet contains 80 mg trimethoprim and 400 mg sulfamethoxazole and the inactive ingredients docusate sodium (0.4 mg per tablet), FD&C Red No. 40, magnesium stearate, povidone, and sodium starch glycolate.

Each SEPTRA DS (double strength) Tablet contains 160 mg trimethoprim and 800 mg sulfamethoxazole and the inactive ingredients docusate sodium (0.8 mg per tablet), FD&C Red No. 40, magnesium stearate, povidone, and sodium starch glycolate.

Each teaspoonful (5 mL) of SEPTRA Suspension contains 40 mg trimethoprim and 200 mg sulfamethoxazole and the inactive ingredients alcohol 0.26%, methylparaben 0.1% and sodium benzoate 0.1% (added as preservatives), carboxymethylcellulose sodium, citric acid, FD&C Red No. 40 and Yellow No. 6, flavor, glycerin, microcrystalline cellulose, polysorbate 80, saccharin sodium, and sorbitol. Each teaspoonful (5 mL) of SEPTRA Grape Suspension contains 40 mg trimethoprim and 200 mg sulfamethoxazole and the inactive ingredients alcohol 0.26%, methylparaben 0.1%, and sodium benzoate 0.1% (added as preservatives), carboxymethylcellulose sodium, citric acid, FD&C Red No. 40 and Blue No. 1, flavor, glycerin, microcrystalline cellulose, polysorbate 80, saccharin sodium, and sorbitol. Both tablet and suspension forms are for oral administration.

REPRESENTATIVE MINIMUM INHIBITORY CONCENTRATION VALUES FOR ORGANISMS SUSCEPTIBLE TO SEPTRA (MIC-μg/mL)

Bacteria	TMP Alone	SMX Alone	TMP/SMX (1:19) TMP	TMP/SMX (1:19) SMX
Escherichia coli	0.05–1.5	1.0–245	0.05–0.5	0.95–9.5
Escherichia coli (enterotoxigenic strains)	0.015–0.15	0.285–>950	0.005–0.15	0.095–2.85
Proteus species (indole positive)	0.5–5.0	7.35–300	0.05–1.5	0.95–28.5
Morganella morganii	0.5–5.0	7.35–300	0.05–1.5	0.95–28.5
Proteus mirabilis	0.5–1.5	7.35–30	0.05–0.15	0.95–2.85
Klebsiella species	0.15–5.0	2.45–245	0.05–1.5	0.95–28.5
Enterobacter species	0.15–5.0	2.45–245	0.05–1.5	0.95–28.5
Haemophilus influenzae	0.15–1.5	2.85–95	0.015–0.15	0.285–2.85
Streptococcus pneumonia	0.15–1.5	7.35–24.5	0.05–0.15	0.95–2.85
*Shigella flexneri**	<0.01–0.04	<0.16–>320	<0.002–0.03	0.04–0.625
*Shigella sonnei**	0.02–0.08	0.625–>320	0.004–0.06	0.08–1.25

TMP=trimethoprim SMX=sulfamethoxazole
*Rudoy RC, Nelson JD, Haltalin KC. *Antimicrobial Agents and Chemotherapy.* 1974;5:439–443.

Trimethoprim is 5-[(3,4,5-trimethoxyphenyl)methyl]-2,4-pyrimidinediamine. It is a white to light yellow, odorless, bitter compound with a molecular weight of 290.32, and the molecular formula $C_{14}H_{18}N_4O_3$. The structural formula is:

Sulfamethoxazole is 4-amino-*N*-(5-methyl-3-isoxazolyl)benzenesulfonamide. It is an almost white, odorless, tasteless compound with a molecular weight of 253.28, and the molecular formula $C_{10}H_{11}N_3O_3S$. The structural formula is:

CLINICAL PHARMACOLOGY

SEPTRA is rapidly absorbed following oral administration. Both sulfamethoxazole and trimethoprim exist in the blood as unbound, protein-bound, and metabolized forms; sulfamethoxazole also exists as the conjugated form. The metabolism of sulfamethoxazole occurs predominately by N_4-acetylation although the glucuronide conjugate has been identified. The principal metabolites of trimethoprim are the 1- and 3-oxides and the 3'- and 4'-hydroxy derivatives. The free forms of sulfamethoxazole and trimethoprim are considered to be the therapeutically active forms. Approximately 44% of trimethoprim and 70% of sulfamethoxazole are bound to plasma proteins. The presence of 10 mg percent sulfamethoxazole in plasma decreases the protein binding of trimethoprim by an insignificant degree; trimethoprim does not influence the protein binding of sulfamethoxazole.

Peak blood levels for the individual components occur 1 to 4 hours after oral administration. The mean serum half-lives of sulfamethoxazole and trimethoprim are 10 and 8 to 10 hours, respectively. However, patients with severely impaired renal function exhibit an increase in the half-lives of both components, requiring dosage regimen adjustment (see DOSAGE AND ADMINISTRATION). Detectable amounts of trimethoprim and sulfamethoxazole are present in the blood 24 hours after drug administration. During administration of 160 mg trimethoprim and 800 mg sulfamethoxazole b.i.d., the mean steady-state plasma concentration of trimethoprim was 1.72 mcg/mL. The steady-state minimal levels of free and total sulfamethoxazole were 57.4 mcg/mL and 68.0 mcg/mL, respectively. These steady-state levels were achieved after 3 days of drug administration.[1]

Excretion of sulfamethoxazole and trimethoprim is primarily by the kidneys through both glomerular filtration and tubular secretion. Urine concentrations of both sulfamethoxazole and trimethoprim are considerably higher than are the concentrations in the blood. The average percentage of the dose recovered in urine from 0 to 72 hours after a single oral dose if 84.5% for total sulfonamide and 66.8% for free trimethoprim. Thirty percent of the total sulfonamide is excreted as free sulfamethoxazole, with the remaining as N_4-acetylated metabolite.[2] When administered together as SEPTRA, neither sulfamethoxazole nor trimethoprim affects the urinary excretion pattern of the other.

Both trimethoprim and sulfamethoxazole distribute to sputum, vaginal fluid, and middle ear fluid; trimethoprim also distributes to bronchial secretions, and both pass the placental barrier and are excreted in human milk.

Microbiology: Sulfamethoxazole inhibits bacterial synthesis of dihydrofolic acid by competing with *para*-aminobenzoic acid (PABA). Trimethoprim blocks the production of tetrahydrofolic acid from dihydrofolic acid by binding to and reversibly inhibiting the required enzyme, dihydrofolate reductase. Thus, SEPTRA blocks two consecutive steps in the biosynthesis of nucleic acids and proteins essential to many bacteria.

In vitro studies have shown that bacterial resistance develops more slowly with SEPTRA than with either trimethoprim or sulfamethoxazole alone.

In vitro serial dilution tests have shown that the spectrum of antibacterial activity of SEPTRA includes the common urinary tract pathogens with the exception of *Pseudomonas aeruginosa*. The following organisms are usually susceptible: *Escherichia coli, Klebsiella* species, *Enterobacter* species, *Morganella morganii, Proteus mirabilis,* and indole-positive *Proteus* species including *Proteus vulgaris.*

The usual spectrum of antimicrobial activity of SEPTRA includes bacterial pathogens isolated from middle ear exudate and from bronchial secretions (*Haemophilus influenzae*, including ampicillin-resistant strains, and *Streptococcus pneumoniae*), and enterotoxigenic strains of *Escherichia coli* (ETEC) causing bacterial gastroenteritis. *Shigella flexneri* and *Shigella sonnei* are also usually susceptible.

[See table above]

Susceptibility Testing: The recommended quantitative disc susceptibility method may be used for estimating the susceptibility of bacteria of SEPTRA.[3,4] With this procedure, a report from the laboratory of "Susceptible to trimethoprim and sulfamethoxazole" indicates that the infection is likely to respond to therapy with SEPTRA. If the infection is confined to the urine, a report of "Intermediate susceptibility to trimethoprim and sulfamethoxazole" also indicates that the infection is likely to respond. A report of "Resistant to trimethoprim and sulfamethoxazole" indicates that the infection is unlikely to respond to therapy with SEPTRA.

INDICATIONS AND USAGE

Urinary Tract Infections: For the treatment of urinary tract infections due to susceptible strains of the following organisms: *Escherichia coli, Kelbsiella* species, *Enterobacter* species, *Morganella morganii, Proteus mirabilis,* and *Proteus vulgaris.* It is recommended that initial episodes of uncomplicated urinary tract infections be treated with a single effective antibacterial agent rather than the combination.

Acute Otitis Media: For the treatment of acute otitis media in pediatric patients due to susceptible strains of *Streptococcus pneumoniae* or *Haemophilus influenzae* when, in the judgment of the physician, SEPTRA offers some advantage over the use of other antimicrobial agents. To date, there are limited data on the safety of repeated use of SEPTRA in pediatric patients under two years of age. SEPTRA is not indicated for prophylactic or prolonged administration in otitis media at any age.

Acute Exacerbations of Chronic Bronchitis in Adults: For the treatment of acute exacerbations of chronic bronchitis due to susceptible strains of *Streptococcus pneumoniae* or *Haemophilus influenzae* when, in the judgment of the physician, SEPTRA offers some advantage over the use of a single antimicrobial agent.

Travelers' Diarrhea in Adults: For the treatment of travelers' diarrhea due to susceptible strains of enterotoxigenic *E. coli.* Shigellosis: For the treatment of enteritis caused by susceptible strains of *Shigella flexneri* and *Shigella sonnei* when antibacterial therapy is indicated.

***Pneumocystis Carinii* Pneumonia:** For the treatment of documented *Pneumocystis carinii* pneumonia. For prophylaxis against *Pneumocystis carinii* pneumonia in individuals who are immunosuppressed and considered to be at an increased risk of developing *Pneumocystis carinii* pneumonia.

CONTRAINDICATIONS

SEPTRA is contraindicated in patients with a known hypersensitivity to trimethoprim or sulfonamides and in patients with documented megaloblastic anemia due to folate deficiency. SEPTRA is also contraindicated in pregnant patients at term and in nursing mothers, because sulfonamides pass the placenta and are excreted in the milk and may cause kernicterus. SEPTRA is contraindicated in pediatric patients less than 2 months of age.

WARNINGS:

FATALITIES ASSOCIATED WITH THE ADMINISTRATION OF SULFONAMIDES, ALTHOUGH RARE, HAVE OCCURRED DUE TO SEVERE REACTIONS, INCLUDING STEVENS-JOHNSON SYNDROME, TOXIC EPIDERMAL NECROLYSIS, FULMINANT HEPATIC NECROSIS, AGRANULOCYTOSIS, APLASTIC ANEMIA, AND OTHER BLOOD DYSCRASIAS.

SULFONAMIDES, INCLUDING SULFONAMIDE-CONTAINING PRODUCTS SUCH AS TRIMETHOPRIM/SULFAMETHOXAZOLE, SHOULD BE DISCONTINUED AT THE FIRST APPEARANCE OF SKIN RASH OR ANY SIGN OF ADVERSE REACTION. In rare instances, a skin rash may be followed by a more severe reaction, such as Stevens-Johnson syndrome, toxic epidermal necrolysis, hepatic necrosis, and serious blood disorder (see PRECAUTIONS).

Clinical signs, such as rash, sore throat, fever, arthralgia, pallor, purpura, or jaundice may be early indications of serious reactions.

Cough, shortness of breath, and pulmonary infiltrates are hypersensitivity reactions of the respiratory tract that have been reported in association with sulfonamide treatment.

The sulfonamides should not be used for the treatment of group A beta-hemolytic streptococcal infections. In an established infection, they will not eradicate the streptococcus and, therefore, will not prevent sequelae such as rheumatic fever.

Pseudomembranous colitis has been reported with nearly all antibacterial agents, including trimethoprim/sulfamethoxazole, and may range in severity from mild to life-threatening. Therefore, it is important to consider this diagnosis in patients who present with diarrhea subsequent to the administration of antibacterial agents.

Treatment with antibacterial agents alters the normal flora of the colon and may permit overgrowth of clostridia. Studies indicate that a toxin produced by Clostridium difficile is one primary cause of "antibiotic-associated colitis."

After the diagnosis of pseudomembranous colitis has been established, therapeutic measures should be initiated. Mild cases of pseudomembranous colitis usually respond to drug discomtinuation alone. In moderate to severe cases, consideration should be given to management with fluids and electrolytes, protein supplementation, and treatment with an antibacterial drug effective against *C. difficile*.

PRECAUTIONS

General: SEPTRA should be given with caution to patients with impaired renal or hepatic function, to those with possible folate deficiency (e.g., the elderly, chronic alcoholics, patients receiving anticonvulsant therapy, patients with malabsorption syndrome, and patients in malnutrition states), and to those with severe allergy or bronchial asthma. In glucose-6-phosphate dehydrognase-deficient individuals, hemolysis may occur. This reaction is frequently dose-related (see CLINICAL PHARMACOLOGY and DOSAGE AND ADMINISTRATION).

Use in the Elderly: There may be an increased risk of severe adverse reactions in elderly patients, particularly when complicating conditions exist, e.g, impaired kidney and/or liver function, or concomitant use of other drugs. Severe skin reactions, or generalized bone marrow suppression (see WARNINGS and ADVERSE REACTIONS), or a specific decrease in platelets (with or without purpura) are the most frequently reported severe adverse reactions in elderly patients. In those concurrently receiving certain diuretics, primarily thiazides, an increased incidence of thrombocytopenia with purpura has been reported. Appropriate dosage adjustments should be made for patients with impaired kidney function (see DOSAGE AND ADMINISTRATION).

Use in the Treatment of and Prophylaxis for *Pneumocystis carinii* Pneumonia in Patients with Acquired Immunodeficiency Syndrome (AIDS): The incidence of side effects, particularly rash, fever, leukopenia, and elevated aminotransferase (transaminase) values in AIDS patients who are being treated with SEPTRA for *Pneumocystis carinii* pneumonia has been reported to be greatly increased compared with the incidence normally associated with the use of SEPTRA in non-AIDS patients. The incidence of hyperkalemia and hyponatremia appears to be increased in AIDS patients receiving SEPTRA. Adverse effects are generally less severe in patients receiving SEPTRA for prophylaxis. A history of mild intolerance to SEPTRA in AIDS patients does not appear to predict intolerance of subsequent secondary prophylaxis. However, if a patient develops skin rash or any sign of adverse reaction, therapy with SEPTRA should be re-evaluated (see WARNINGS).

The concomitant use of leucovorin with trimethoprim-sulfamethoxazole for the acute treatment of *Pneumocystis carinii* pneumonia in patients with HIV infection was associated with increased rates of treatment failure and morbidity in a placebo-controlled study.

Information for Patients: Patients should be instructed to maintain an adequate fluid intake in order to prevent crystalluria and stone formation.

Laboratory Tests: Complete blood counts should be done frequently in patients receiving SEPTRA; if a significant reduction in the count of any formed blood element is noted, SEPTRA should be discontinued. Urinalyses with careful microscopic examination and renal function tests should be performed during therapy, particularly for those patients with impaired renal function.

Drug Interactions: In elderly patients concurrently receiving certain diuretics, primarily thiazides, an increased incidence of thrombocytopenia with purpura has been reported. It has been reported that SEPTRA may prolong the prothrombin time in patients who are receiving the anticoagulant warfarin. This interaction should be kept in mind when SEPTRA is given to patients already on anticoagulant therapy, and the coagulation time should be reassessed.

SEPTRA may inhibit the hepatic metabolism of phenytoin. SEPTRA, given at a common clinical dosage, increased the phenytoin half-life by 39% and decreased the phenytoin metabolic clearance rate by 27%. When administering these drugs concurrently, one should be alert for possible excessive phenytoin effect.

Sulfonamides can also displace methotrexate from plasma protein binding sites, thus increasing free methotrexate concentrations.

Drug/Laboratory Test Interactions: SEPTRA, specifically the trimethoprim component, can interfere with a serum methotrexate assay as determined by the competitive binding protein technique (CBPA) when a bacterial dihydrofolate reductase is used as the binding protein. No interference occurs, however, if methotrexate is measured by a radioimmunoassay (RIA).

The presence of trimethoprim and sulfamethoxazole may also interfere with the Jaffé alkaline picrate reaction assay for creatinine, resulting in overestimations of about 10% in the range of normal values.

Carcinogenesis, Mutagenesis, Impairment of Fertility:

Carcinogenesis: Long-term studies in animals to evaluate carcinogenic potential have not been conducted with SEPTRA.

Mutagenesis: Bacterial mutagenic studies have not been performed with sulfamethoxazole and trimethoprim in combination. Trimethoprim was demonstrated to be non-mutagenic in the Ames assay. In studies at two laboratories, no chromosomal damage was detected in cultured Chinese hamster ovary cells at concentrations approximately 500 times human plasma levels; at concentrations approximately 1,000 times human plasma levels in these same cells, a low level of chromosomal damage was induced at one of the laboratories. No chormosomal abnormalities were observed in cultured human leukocytes at concentrations of trimethoprim up to 20 times human steady-state plasma levels. No chromosomal effects were detected in peripheral lympocytes of human subjects receiving 320 mg of trimethoprim in combination with up to 1,600 mg of sulfamethoxazole per day for as long as 112 weeks.

Impairment of Fertility: No adverse effects on fertility or general reproductive performance were observed in rats given oral dosages as high as 70 mg/kg/day trimethoprim plus 350 mg/kg/day sulfamethoxazole.

Pregnancy:

Teratogenic Effects: Pregnancy Category C. In rats, oral doses of 533 mg/kg sulfamethoxazole or 200 mg/kg trimethoprim produced teratological effects manifested mainly as cleft palates. The highest dose which did not cause cleft palates in rats was 512 mg/kg sulfamethoxazole or 192 mg/kg trimethoprim when administered separately. In two studies in rats, no teratogenicity was observed when 512 mg/kg of sulfamethoxazole was used in combination with 128 mg/kg of trimethoprim. In one study, however, cleft palates were observed in one litter out of nine when 355 mg/kg of sulfamethoxazole was used in combination with 88 mg/kg of trimethoprim.

In some rabbit studies, an overall increase in fetal loss (dead and resorbed and malformed conceptuses) was associated with doses of trimethoprim six times the human therapeutic dose.

While there are no large, well-controlled studies in the use of trimethoprim and sulfamethoxazole in pregnant women, Brumfitt and Pursell,[5] in a retrospective study, reported the outcome of 186 pregnancies during which the mother received either placebo or trimethoprim and sulfamethoxazole. The incidence of congenital abnormalities was 4.5% (3 of 66) in those who received placebo and 3.3% (4 of 120) in those receiving trimethoprim and sulfamethoxazole. There were no abnormalities in the 10 children whose mothers received the drug during the first trimester. In a separate survey, Brumfitt and Pursell also found no congenital abnormalities in 35 children whose mothers had received oral trimethoprim and sulfamethoxazole at the time of conception or shortly thereafter.

Because trimethoprim and sulfamethoxazole may interfere with folic acid metabolism, SEPTRA should be used during pregnancy only if the potential benefit justifies the potential risk to the fetus.

Nonteratogenic Effects: See CONTRAINDICATIONS section.

Nursing Mothers: See CONTRAINDICATIONS section.

Pediatric Use: SEPTRA is not indicated for pediatric patients younger than 2 months of age (see INDICATIONS AND USAGE and CONTRAINDICATIONS).

ADVERSE REACTIONS

The most common adverse effects are gastrointestinal disturbances (nausea, vomiting, anorexia) and allergic skin reactions (such as rash and urticaria). **FATALITIES ASSOCIATED WITH THE ADMINISTRATION OF SULFONAMIDES, ALTHOUGH RARE, HAVE OCCURRED DUE TO SEVERE REACTIONS, INCLUDING STEVENS-JOHNSON SYNDROME, TOXIC EPIDERMAL NECROLYSIS, FLUMINANT HEPATIC NECROSIS, AGRANULOCYTOSIS, APLASTIC ANEMIA, OTHER BLOOD DYSCRASIAS, AND HYPERSENSITIVITY OF THE RESPIRATORY TRACT (SEE WARNINGS).**

Hematologic: Agranulocytosis, aplastic anemia, thrombocytopenia, leukopenia, neutropenia, hemolytic anemia, megaloblastic anemia, hypoprothrombinemia, methemoglobinemia, eosinophilia.

Allergic: Stevens-Johnson syndrome, toxic epidermal necrolysis, anaphylaxis, allergic myocarditis, erythema multiforme, exfoliative dermatitis, angioedema, drug fever, chills, Henoch-Schönlein purpura, serum sickness-like syndrome, generalized allergic reactions, generalized skin eruptions, photosensitivity, conjunctival and scleral injection, pruritus, urticaria, and rash. In addition, periarteritis nodosa and systemic lupus erythematosus have been reported.

Gastrointestinal: Hepatitis, including cholestatic jaundice and hepatic necrosis, elevation of serum transaminase and bilirubin, pseudomembranous enterocolitis, pancreatitis, stomatitis, glossitis, nausea, emesis, abdominal pain, diarrhea, anorexia.

Genitourinary: Renal failure, interstitial nephritis, BUN and serum creatinine elevation, toxic nephrosis with oliguria and anuria, and crystalluria.

Metabolic: Hyperkalemia, hyponatremia.

Neurologic: Aseptic meningitis, convulsions, peripheral neuritis, ataxia, vertigo, tinnitus, headache.

Psychiatric: Hallucinations, depression, apathy, nervousness.

Endocrine: The sulfonamides bear certain chemical similarities to some goitrogens, diuretics (acetazolamide and the thiazides), and oral hypoglycemic agents. Cross-sensitivity may exist with these agents. Diuresis and hypoglycemia have occurred rarely in patients receiving sulfonamides.

Musculoskeletal: Arthralgia and myalgia.

Respiratory System: Cough, shortness of breath, and pulmonary infiltrates (see WARNINGS).

Miscellaneous: Weakness, fatigue, insomnia.

OVERDOSAGE

Acute: The amount of a single dose of SEPTRA that is either associated with symptoms of overdosage or is likely to be life-threatening has not been reported. Signs and symptoms of overdosage reported with sulfonamides include anorexia, colic, nausea, vomiting, dizziness, headache, drowsiness, and unconsciousness. Pyrexia, hematuria, and crystalluria may be noted. Blood dyscrasias and jaundice are potential late manifestations of overdosage. Signs of acute overdosage with trimethoprim include nausea, vomiting, dizziness, headache, mental depression, confusion, and bone marrow depression.

General principles of treatment include the institution of gastric lavage or emesis; forcing oral fluids; and the administration of intravenous fluids if urine output is low and renal function is normal. Acidification of the urine will increase renal elimination of trimethoprim. The patient should be monitored with blood counts and appropriate blood chemistries, including electrolytes. If a significant blood dyscrasia or jaundice occurs, specific therapy should be instituted for these complications. Peritoneal dialysis is not effective and hemodialysis is only moderately effective in eliminating trimethoprim and sulfamethoxazole.

Chronic: Use of SEPTRA at high doses and/or for extended periods of time may cause bone marrow depression manifested as thrombocytopenia, leukopenia, and/or megaloblastic anemia. If signs of bone marrow depression occur, the patient should be given leucovorin; 5 to 15 mg leucovorin daily has been recommended by some investigators.

DOSAGE AND ADMINISTRATION

Contraindicated in pediatric patients less than 2 months of age.

Urinary Tract Infections And Shigellosis In Adults And Pediatric Patients and Acute Otitis Media in Pediatric Patients:

Adults: The usual adult dosage in the treatment of urinary tract infections is one SEPTRA DS (double strength) tablet, two SEPTRA tablets, or four teaspoonfuls (20 mL) SEPTRA Suspension every 12 hours for 10 to 14 days. An identical daily dosage is used for 5 days in the treatment of shigellosis.

Pediatric Patients: The recommended dose for pediatric patients with urinary tract infections or acute otitis media is 8 mg/kg trimethoprim and 40 mg/kg sulfamethoxazole per 24 hours, given in two divided doses every 12 hours for 10 days. An identical dosage is used for 5 days in the treatment of shigellosis. The following table is a guideline for the attainment of this dosage:

Continued on next page

Septra/Septra DS—Cont.

Pediatric Patients: Two Months of Age or Older

Weight		Dose – Every 12 Hours	
lb	kg	Teaspoonfuls	Tablets
22	10	1 (5 mL)	
44	20	2 (10 mL)	1
66	30	3 (15 mL)	$1^1/_2$
88	40	4 (20 mL)	2 (or 1 DS Tablet)

For Patients With Impaired Renal Function: When renal function is impaired, a reduced dosage should be employed using the following table:

Creatinine Clearance (mL/min)	Recommended Dosage Regimen
Above 30	Use Standard Regimen
15–30	$^1/_2$ the Usual Regimen
Below 15	Use Not Recommended

Acute Exacerbations of Chronic Bronchitis in Adults: The usual adult dosage in the treatment of acute exacerbations of chronic bronchitis is one SEPTRA DS (double strength) tablet, two SEPTRA tablets, or four teaspoonfuls (20 mL) SEPTRA Suspension every 12 hours for 14 days.

Travelers' Diarrhea in Adults: For the treatment of travelers' diarrhea, the usual adult dosage is one SEPTRA DS (double strength) tablet, two SEPTRA tablets, or four teaspoonfuls (20 mL) of SEPTRA Suspension every 12 hours for 5 days.

Pneumocystis Carinii Pneumonia: Treatment:

Adults and Pediatric Patients:

The recommended dosage for treatment of patients with documented *Pneumocystis carinii* pneumonia is 15 to 20 mg/kg trimethoprim and 75 to 100 mg/kg sulfamethoxazole per 24 hours given in equally divided doses every 6 hours for 14 to 21 days. The following table is a guideline for the upper limit of this dosage:

Weight		Dose – Every 6 Hours	
lb	kg	Teaspoonfuls	Tablets
18	8	1 (5 mL)	
35	16	2 (10 mL)	1
53	24	3 (15 mL)	$1^1/_2$
70	32	4 (20 mL)	2 (or 1 DS Tablet)
88	40	5 (25 mL)	$2^1/_2$
106	48	6 (30 mL)	3 (or $1^1/_2$ DS Tablets)
141	64	8 (40 mL)	4 (or 2 DS Tablets)
176	80	10 (50 mL)	5 (or $2^1/_2$ DS Tablets)

For the lower limit dose (15 mg/kg trimethoprim and 75 mg/kg sulfamethoxazole per 24 hours) administer 75% of the dose in the above table.

Prophylaxis:

Adults:

The recommended dosage for prophylaxis in adults is one SEPTRA DS (double strength) tablet daily.

Pediatric Patients:

For pediatric patients, the recommended dose is 150 mg/m²/day trimethoprim with 750 mg/m²/day sulfamethoxazole given orally in equally divided doses twice a day, on 3 consecutive days per week. The total daily dose should not exceed 320 mg trimethoprim and 1,600 mg sulfamethoxazole. The following table is a guideline for the attainment of this dosage in pediatric patients:

Body Surface Area (m^2)	Dose – every 12 hours Teaspoonfuls	Tablets
0.26	$^1/_2$ (2.5 mL)	
0.53	1 (5 mL)	$^1/_2$
1.06	2 (10 mL)	1

HOW SUPPLIED

TABLETS (pink, scored, round-shaped) containing 80 mg trimethoprim and 400 mg sulfamethoxazole: Bottles of 100 (NDC 61570-052-01). Imprint on tablets "M052".

DS (DOUBLE STRENGTH) TABLETS (pink, scored, oval-shaped) containing 160 mg trimethoprim and 800 mg sulfamethoxazole: Bottles of 20 (NDC 61570-053-20), 100 (NDC 61570-053-01), 250 (NDC 61570-053-52) and 500 (NDC 61570-053-05). Imprint on tablets "M053".

ORAL SUSPENSIONS (pink, cherry-flavored) containing 40 mg trimethoprim and 200 mg sulfamethoxazole in each teaspoonful (5 mL): Bottle of 1 pint (473 mL) (NDC 61570-050-16) and 100 mL–package of 6 (NDC 61570-050-11); and (purple, grape-flavored) containing 40 mg trimethoprim and 200 mg sulfamethoxazole in each teaspoonful (5 mL): Bottle of 1 pint (473 mL) (NDC 61570-051-16).

Tablets should be stored at 15° to 25°C (59° to 77°F) in a dry place and protected from light.

Suspensions should be stored at 15° to 25°C (59° to 77°F) and protected from light.

Also available:

SEPTRA I.V. Infusion: 5 mL vials, containing 80 mg trimethoprim (16 mg/mL) and 400 mg sulfamethoxazole (80 mg/mL), tray of 10;

10 mL multiple dose vials containing 160 mg trimethoprim (16 mg/mL) and 800 mg sulfamethoxazole (80 mg/mL), tray of 10;

20 mL multiple dose vials containing 320 mg trimethoprim (16 mg/mL) and 1600 mg sulfamethoxazole (80 mg/mL), tray of 10.

REFERENCES

1. Kremers P, Duvivier J, Heusghem C. Pharmacokinetic studies of co-trimoxazole in man after single and repeated doses. *J Clin Pharmacol.* 1974;14:112–117.
2. Kaplan SA, Weinfeld RE, Abruzzo CW, McFaden K, Jack ML, Weissman L. Pharmacokinetic profile of trimethoprim-sulfamethoxazole in man. *J Infect Dis.* 1973;128(suppl):S547–S555.
3. Antibiotic susceptibility discs: certification procedure. *Federal Register.* 1972;37:20527–20529.
4. Bauer AW, Kirby WMM, Sherris JC, Turck M. Antibiotic susceptibility testing by standardized single disk method. *Am J Clin Pathol.* 1966;45:493–496.
5. Brumfitt W, Pursell R. Trimethoprim-sulfamethoxazole in the treatment of bacteriuria in women. *J Infect Dis.* 1973;128(suppl):S657–S663.

Manufactured for: Monarch Pharmaceuticals, Inc., Bristol, TN 37620

By: King Pharmaceuticals, Inc., Bristol, TN 37620

0934075
Rev. 2/00

SILVADENE® CREAM 1% ℞

[*sĭl-vă-dēn*]

(silver sulfadiazine)

DESCRIPTION

SILVADENE Cream 1% is a soft, white, water-miscible cream containing the antimicrobial agent silver sulfadiazine in micronized form, which has the following structural formula:

Each gram of SILVADENE Cream 1% contains 10 mg of micronized silver sulfadiazine. The cream vehicle consists of white petrolatum, stearyl alcohol, isopropyl myristate, sorbitan monooleate, polyoxyl 40 stearate, propylene glycol, and water, with methylparaben 0.3% as a preservative. SILVADENE Cream 1% (silver sulfadiazine) spreads easily and can be washed off readily with water.

CLINICAL PHARMACOLOGY

Silver sulfadiazine has broad antimicrobial activity. It is bactericidal for many gram-negative and gram-positive bacteria as well as being effective against yeast. Results from *in vitro* testing are listed below.

Sufficient data have been obtained to demonstrate that silver sulfadiazine will inhibit bacteria that are resistant to other antimicrobial agents and that the compound is superior to sulfadiazine.

Studies utilizing radioactive micronized silver sulfadiazine, electron microscopy, and biochemical techniques have revealed that the mechanism of action of silver sulfadiazine on bacteria differs from silver nitrate and sodium sulfadiazine. Silver sulfadiazine acts only on the cell membrane and cell wall to produce its bactericidal effect.

Results of *In Vitro* Testing with SILVADENE® Cream 1% (silver sulfadiazine) Concentration of Silver Sulfadiazine Number of Sensitive Strains/Total Number of Strains Tested

Genus & Species	50 μg/mL	100 μg/mL
Pseudomonas aeruginosa	130/130	130/130
Xanthomonas (Pseudomonas) maltophilia	7/7	7/7
Enterobacter species	48/50	50/50
Enterobacter cloacae	24/24	24/24
Klebsiella species	53/54	54/54
Escherichia coli	63/63	63/63
Serratia species	27/28	28/28
Proteus mirabilis	53/53	53/53
Morganella morganii	10/10	10/10
Providencia rettgeri	2/2	2/2
Providencia species	1/1	1/1
Proteus vulgaris	2/2	2/2
Citrobacter species	10/10	10/10
Acinetobacter calcoaceticus	10/11	11/11
Staphylococcus aureus	100/101	100/101
Staphylococcus epidermidis	51/51	51/51
β-Hemolytic *Streptococcus*	4/4	4/4
Enterococcus species	52/53	53/53
Corynebacterium diphtheriae	2/2	2/2
Clostridium perfringens	0/2	2/2
Candida albicans	43/50	50/50

Silver sulfadiazine is not a carbonic anhydrase inhibitor and may be useful in situations where such agents are contraindicated.

INDICATIONS AND USAGE

SILVADENE Cream 1% (silver sulfadiazine) is a topical antimicrobial drug indicated as an adjunct for the prevention and treatment of wound sepsis in patients with second- and third-degree burns.

CONTRAINDICATIONS

SILVADENE Cream 1% (silver sulfadiazine) is contraindicated in patients who are hypersensitive to silver sulfadiazine or any of the other ingredients in the preparation.

Because sulfonamide therapy is known to increase the possibility of kernicterus, SILVADENE Cream 1% should not be used on pregnant women approaching or at term, on premature infants, or on newborn infants during the first 2 months of life.

WARNINGS

There is potential cross-sensitivity between silver sulfadiazine and other sulfonamides. If allergic reactions attributable to treatment with silver sulfadiazine occur, continuation of therapy must be weighed against the potential hazards of the particular allergic reaction.

Fungal proliferation in and below the eschar may occur. However, the incidence of clinically reported fungal superinfection is low.

The use of SILVADENE Cream 1% (silver sulfadiazine) in some cases of glucose-6-phosphate dehydrogenase-deficient individuals may be hazardous, as hemolysis may occur.

PRECAUTIONS

General

If hepatic and renal functions become impaired and elimination of drug decreases, accumulation may occur and discontinuation of SILVADENE Cream 1% (silver sulfadiazine) should be weighed against the therapeutic benefit being achieved.

In considering the use of topical proteolytic enzymes in conjunction with SILVADENE Cream 1%, the possibility should be noted that silver may inactivate such enzymes.

Laboratory Tests

In the treatment of burn wounds involving extensive areas of the body, the serum sulfa concentrations may approach adult therapeutic levels (8 mg% to 12 mg%). Therefore, in these patients it would be advisable to monitor serum sulfa concentrations. Renal function should be carefully monitored and the urine should be checked for sulfa crystals. Absorption of the pro-pylene glycol vehicle has been reported to affect serum osmolality, which may affect the interpretation of laboratory tests.

Carcinogenesis, Mutagenesis, Impairment of Fertility

Long-term dermal toxicity studies of 24 months' duration in rats and 18 months' in mice with concentrations of silver sulfadiazine three to ten times the concentration in SILVADENE Cream 1% revealed no evidence of carcinogenicity.

Pregnancy

Teratogenic Effects.

Pregnancy Category B. A reproductive study has been performed in rabbits at doses up to three to ten times the concentration of silver sulfadiazine in SILVADENE Cream 1% and has revealed no evidence of harm to the fetus due to silver sulfadiazine. There are, however, no adequate and well-controlled studies in pregnant women. Because animal reproduction studies are not always predictive of human response, this drug should be used during pregnancy only if clearly justified, especially in pregnant women approaching or at term. (See **CONTRAINDICATIONS.**)

Nursing Mothers

It is not known whether silver sulfadiazine is excreted in human milk. However, sulfonamides are known to be excreted in human milk, and all sulfonamide derivatives are known to increase the possibility of kernicterus. Because of the possibility for serious adverse reactions in nursing infants from sulfonamides, a decision should be made whether to discontinue nursing or to discontinue the drug, taking into account the importance of the drug to the mother.

Geriatric Use

Of the total number of subjects in clinical studies of Silvadene Cream 1%, seven percent were 65 years of age and over. No overall differences in safety or effectiveness were observed between these subjects and younger subjects, and other reported clinical experience has not identified differences in responses between the elderly and younger patients, but greater sensitivity of some older individuals cannot be ruled out.

Pediatric Use

Safety and effectiveness in pediatric patients have not been established. (See **CONTRAINDICATIONS.**)

ADVERSE REACTIONS

Several cases of transient leukopenia have been reported in patients receiving silver sulfadiazine therapy.[1,2,3] Leukopenia associated with silver sulfadiazine administration is primarily characterized by decreased neutrophil count. Maximal white blood cell depression occurs within 2 to 4 days of initiation of therapy. Rebound to normal leukocyte levels follows onset within 2 to 3 days. Recovery is not influenced by continuation of silver sulfadiazine therapy. An increased incidence of leukopenia has been reported in patients treated concurrently with cimetidine.

Other infrequently occurring events include skin necrosis, erythema multiforme, skin discoloration, burning sensation, rashes, and interstitial nephritis.

Reduction in bacterial growth after application of topical antibacterial agents has been reported to permit spontaneous healing of deep partial-thickness burns by preventing conversion of the partial thickness to full thickness by sep-

sis. However, reduction in bacterial colonization has caused delayed separation, in some cases necessitating escharotomy in order to prevent contracture.
Absorption of silver sulfadiazine varies depending upon the percent of body surface area and the extent of the tissue damage. Although few have been reported, it is possible that any adverse reaction associated with sulfonamides may occur. Some of the reactions, which have been associated with sulfonamides, are as follows: blood dyscrasias including agranulocytosis, aplastic anemia, thrombocytopenia, leukopenia, and hemolytic anemia; dermatologic and allergic reactions, including Stevens-Johnson syndrome and exfoliative dermatitis; gastrointestinal reactions; hepatitis and hepatocellular necrosis; CNS reactions; and toxic nephrosis.

DOSAGE AND ADMINISTRATION

Prompt institution of appropriate regimens for care of the burned patient is of prime importance and includes the control of shock and pain. The burn wounds are then cleansed and debrided, and SILVADENE Cream 1% (silver sulfadiazine) is applied under sterile conditions. The burn areas should be covered with SILVADENE Cream 1% at all times. The cream should be applied once to twice daily to a thickness of approximately 1/16 inch. Whenever necessary, the cream should be reapplied to any areas from which it has been removed by patient activity. Administration may be accomplished in minimal time because dressings are not required. However, if individual patient requirements make dressings necessary, they may be used.
Reapply immediately after hydrotherapy.
Treatment with SILVADENE Cream 1% should be continued until satisfactory healing has occurred, or until the burn site is ready for grafting. The drug should not be withdrawn from the therapeutic regimen while there remains the possibility of infection except if a significant adverse reaction occurs.

HOW SUPPLIED

SILVADENE Cream 1% (silver sulfadiazine) is available in jars containing 50 g (NDC 61570-131-50), 400 g (NDC 61570-131-40), and 1000 g (NDC 61570-131-98) and tubes containing 20 g (NDC 61570-131-20) and 85 g (NDC 61570-131-85).

REFERENCES

1. Caffee F, Bingham H. Leukopenia and silver sulfadiazine. *J Trauma.* 1982;22:586–587.
2. Jarret F, Ellerbe S, Demling R. Acute leukopenia during topical burn therapy with silver sulfadiazine. *Amer J Surg.* 1978;135:818–819.
3. Kiker RG, Carvajal HF, Micak RP, Larson DL. A controlled study of the effects of silver sulfadiazine on white blood cell counts in burned children. *J Trauma.* 1977;17:835–836.

Prescribing Information as of July 2003.
Monarch Pharmaceuticals®
Distributed by:
Monarch Pharmaceuticals, Inc.
Bristol, TN 37620
(A wholly owned subsidiary of King Pharmaceuticals, Inc.)
Manufactured by:
King Pharmaceuticals, Inc.
Bristol, TN 37620

3000247-B

SKELAXIN® ℞
[*skĕ-lăks-ĭn*]
(Metaxalone)

DESCRIPTION

SKELAXIN® (metaxalone) has the following chemical structure and name:

5-[(3,5-dimethylphenoxy)methyl]-2-oxazolidinone
SKELAXIN (metaxalone) is available as a 400 mg round, pale rose tablet and an 800 mg oval, pink scored tablet.

CLINICAL PHARMACOLOGY

The mechanism of action of metaxalone in humans has not been established, but may be due to general central nervous system depression. It has no direct action on the contractile mechanism of striated muscle, the motor end plate or the nerve fiber.
Pharmacokinetics: In a single center randomized, two-period crossover study in 42 healthy volunteers (31 males, 11 females), a single 400 mg SKELAXIN (metaxalone) tablet was administered under both fasted and fed conditions. Under fasted conditions, the back calculated geometric mean of metaxalone peak plasma concentrations (C_{max}) of 865.3 ng/mL were achieved within 3.3 +/- 1.2 hours (S.D.) after dosing (T_{max}). Metaxalone concentrations declined with a mean terminal half-life ($t_{1/2}$) of 9.2 +/- 4.8 hours. The mean apparent oral clearance (CL/F) of metaxalone was 68 +/- 34 L/h.
In the same study, following a standardized high fat meal, food statistically significantly increased the rate (C_{max}) and extent of absorption (AUC_{0-t}, AUC_{inf}) of metaxalone from SKELAXIN tablets. Relative to the fasted treatment the observed increases were 177.5%, 123.5%, and 115.4%, respectively. The mean T_{max} was also increased to 4.3 +/- 2.3 hours, whereas the mean $t_{1/2}$ was decreased to 2.4 +/- 1.2 hours. This decrease in half-life over that seen in the fasted subjects is felt to be due to the more complete absorption of metaxalone in the presence of a meal resulting in a better estimate of half-life. The mean apparent oral clearance (CL/F) of metaxalone was relatively unchanged relative to fasted administration (59 +/- 29 L/hr). Although a higher C_{max} and AUC were observed after the administration of SKELAXIN (metaxalone) with a standardized high fat meal, the clinical relevance of these effects is unknown.
In another single center, randomized four-period crossover study in 59 healthy volunteers (37 males, 22 females), the rate and extent of metaxalone absorption were determined after the administration of SKELAXIN tablets under both fasted and fed conditions.
Under fasted conditions, following administration of two SKELAXIN 400 mg tablets, the resulting back calculated geometric mean peak plasma metaxalone concentrations (C_{max}) of 1653 ng/mL were achieved within 3.0 +/- 1.2 hours after dosing (T_{max}). Metaxalone concentrations declined with mean terminal half-life ($t_{1/2}$) of 8.0 +/- 4.6 hours. The mean apparent oral clearance (CL/F) of metaxalone was 66 +/- 34 L/hr. Except for a 17% decrease in mean C_{max}, these values were not statistically different from those after the administration of one SKELAXIN 800 mg tablet.
In the same study, the administration of two SKELAXIN 400mg tablets following a standardized high fat meal showed an increase in the mean C_{max}, and the area under the curve (AUC_{0-inf}) of metaxalone by 194% and 142%, respectively. A high fat meal also increased the mean T_{max} to 4.9 +/- 2.3 hours but decreased the mean $t_{1/2}$ to 4.2 +/– 2.5 hr. The effect of a high fat meal on the absorption of metaxalone from one SKELAXIN 800 mg tablet was very similar to that on the absorption from two SKELAXIN 400 mg tablets in quality and quantity. The clinical relevance of these effects is unknown.
The absolute bioavailability of metaxalone from SKELAXIN tablets is not known. Metaxalone is metabolized by the liver and excreted in the urine as unidentified metabolites. The impact of age, gender, hepatic, and renal disease on the pharmacokinetics of SKELAXIN (metaxalone) has not been determined. In the absence of such information, SKELAXIN should be used with caution in patients with hepatic and/or renal impairment and in the elderly.

INDICATIONS AND USAGE

SKELAXIN (metaxalone) is indicated as an adjunct to rest, physical therapy, and other measures for the relief of discomforts associated with acute, painful musculoskeletal conditions. The mode of action of this drug has not been clearly identified, but may be related to its sedative properties. Metaxalone does not directly relax tense skeletal muscles in man.

CONTRAINDICATIONS

Known hypersensitiviy to any components of this product. Known tendency to drug induced, hemolytic, or other anemias.
Significantly impaired renal or hepatic function.

WARNINGS

SKELAXIN may enhance the effects of alcohol and other CNS depressants.

PRECAUTIONS

Metaxalone should be administered with great care to patients with pre-existing liver damage. Serial liver function studies should be performed in these patients.
False-positive Benedict's tests, due to an unknown reducing substance, have been noted. A glucose-specific test will differentiate findings.

Information for Patients

SKELAXIN may impair mental and/or physical abilities required for performance of hazardous tasks, such as operating machinery or driving a motor vehicle, especially when used with alcohol or other CNS depressants.

Drug Interactions

SKELAXIN may enhance the effects of alcohol, barbiturates and other CNS depressants.

Carcinogenesis, Mutagenesis, Impairment of Fertility

The carcinogenic potential of metaxalone has not been determined.

Pregnancy

Reproduction studies in rats have not revealed evidence of impaired fertility or harm to the fetus due to metaxalone. Post marketing experience has not revealed evidence of fetal injury, but such experience cannot exclude the possibility of infrequent or subtle damage to the human fetus. Safe use of metaxalone has not been established with regard to possible adverse effects upon fetal development. Therefore, metaxalone tablets should not be used in women who are or may become pregnant and particularly during early pregnancy unless in the judgement of the physician the potential benefits outweigh the possible hazards.

Nursing Mothers

It is not known whether this drug is secreted in human milk. As a general rule, nursing should not be undertaken while a patient is on a drug since many drugs are excreted in human milk.

Pediatric Use

Safety and effectiveness in children 12 years of age and below have not been established.

ADVERSE REACTIONS

The most frequent reactions to metaxalone include:
CNS: drowsiness, dizziness, headache, and nervousness or "irritability";
Digestive: nause, vomiting, gastrointestinal upset.
Other adverse reactions are:
Immune System: hypersensitivity reaction, rash with or without pruritus;
Hematologic: leukopenia; hemolytic anemia;
Hepatobiliary: jaundice.
Though rare, anaphylactoid reactions have been reported with metaxalone.

OVERDOSAGE

Deaths by deliberate or accidental overdose have occurred with this class of drugs, particularly in combination with antidepressants and/or alcohol.
When determining the LD_{50} in rats and mice, progressive sedation, hypnosis and finally respiratory failure were noted as the dosage increased. In dogs, no LD_{50} could be determined as the higher doses produced an emetic action in 15 to 30 minutes.
Treatment—Gastric lavage and supportive therapy. Consultation with a regional poison control center is recommended.

DOSAGE AND ADMINISTRATION

The recommended dose for adults and children over 12 years of age is two 400 mg tablets (800 mg) or one 800 mg tablet three to four times a day.

HOW SUPPLIED

SKELAXIN (metaxalone) is available as a 400 mg pale rose tablet, inscribed with 8662 on the scored side and "C" on the other. Available in bottles of 100 (NDC 60793-135-01) and in bottles of 500 (NDC 60793-135-05).
SKELAXIN (metaxalone) is also available as an 800 mg oval, scored pink tablet inscribed with 8667 on the scored side and "S" on the other. Available in bottles of 100 (NDC 60793-136-01) and in bottles of 500 (60793-136-05).
Store at Controlled Room Temperature, between 15°C and 30°C (59°F and 86°F).
Rx Only
KING™
Distributed by:
King Pharmaceuticals, Inc., Bristol, TN 37620
Manufactured by:
Mallinckrodt Inc., Hobart, NY 13788
Prescribing Information as of August 2003.

Shown in Product Identification Guide, page 320

SONATA® Ⓒ℞
[*sō-nă-tă*]
(zaleplon)
Capsules
℞ only

DESCRIPTION

Zaleplon is a nonbenzodiazepine hypnotic from the pyrazolopyrimidine class. The chemical name of zaleplon is N-[3-(3-cyanopyrazolo[1,5-a]pyrimidin-7-yl)phenyl]-N-ethylacetamide. Its empirical formula is $C_{17}H_{15}N_5O$, and its molecular weight is 305.34. The structural formula is shown below.

ZALEPLON

Zaleplon is a white to off-white powder that is practically insoluble in water and sparingly soluble in alcohol or propylene glycol. Its partition coefficient in octanol/water is constant (log PC = 1.23) over the pH range of 1 to 7.
Sonata® capsules contain zaleplon as the active ingredient. Inactive ingredients consist of microcrystalline cellulose, pregelatinized starch, silicon dioxide, sodium lauryl sulfate, magnesium stearate, lactose, gelatin, titanium dioxide, D&C yellow #10, FD&C blue #1, FD&C green #3, and FD&C yellow #5.

CLINICAL PHARMACOLOGY

Pharmacodynamics and Mechanism of Action

While Sonata (zaleplon) is a hypnotic agent with a chemical structure unrelated to benzodiazepines, barbiturates, or other drugs with known hypnotic properties, it interacts with the gamma-aminobutyric acid-benzodiazepine (GABA-BZ) receptor complex. Subunit modulation of the

Continued on next page

Sonata—Cont.

GABA-BZ receptor chloride channel macromolecular complex is hypothesized to be responsible for some of the pharmacological properties of benzodiazepines, which include sedative, anxiolytic, muscle relaxant, and anticonvulsive effects in animal models.

Other nonclinical studies have also shown that zaleplon binds selectively to the brain omega-1 receptor situated on the alpha subunit of the $GABA_A$/chloride ion channel receptor complex and potentiates t-butyl-bicyclophosphorothionate (TBPS) binding. Studies of binding of zaleplon to recombinant $GABA_A$ receptors ($\alpha_1\beta_1\gamma_2$ [omega-1] and $\alpha_2\beta_1\gamma_2$ [omega-2]) have shown that zaleplon has a low affinity for these receptors, with preferential binding to the omega-1 receptor.

Pharmacokinetics

The pharmacokinetics of zaleplon have been investigated in more than 500 healthy subjects (young and elderly), nursing mothers, and patients with hepatic disease or renal disease. In healthy subjects, the pharmacokinetic profile has been examined after single doses of up to 60 mg and once-daily administration at 15 mg and 30 mg for 10 days. Zaleplon was rapidly absorbed with a time to peak concentration (t_{max}) of approximately 1 hour and a terminal-phase elimination half-life ($t_{1/2}$) of approximately 1 hour. Zaleplon does not accumulate with once-daily administration and its pharmacokinetics are dose proportional in the therapeutic range.

Absorption

Zaleplon is rapidly and almost completely absorbed following oral administration. Peak plasma concentrations are attained within approximately 1 hour after oral administration. Although zaleplon is well absorbed, its absolute bioavailability is approximately 30% because it undergoes significant presystemic metabolism.

Distribution

Zaleplon is a lipophilic compound with a volume of distribution of approximately 1.4 L/kg following intravenous (IV) administration, indicating substantial distribution into extravascular tissues. The in vitro plasma protein binding is approximately 60%±15% and is independent of zaleplon concentration over the range of 10 ng/mL to 1000 ng/mL. This suggests that zaleplon disposition should not be sensitive to alterations in protein binding. The blood to plasma ratio for zaleplon is approximately 1, indicating that zaleplon is uniformly distributed throughout the blood with no extensive distribution into red blood cells.

Metabolism

After oral administration, zaleplon is extensively metabolized, with less than 1% of the dose excreted unchanged in urine. Zaleplon is primarily metabolized by aldehyde oxidase to form 5-oxo-zaleplon. Zaleplon is metabolized to a lesser extent by cytochrome P_{450} (CYP) 3A4 to form desethylzaleplon, which is quickly converted, presumably by aldehyde oxidase, to 5-oxo-desethylzaleplon. These oxidative metabolites are then converted to glucuronides and eliminated in urine. All of zaleplon's metabolites are pharmacologically inactive.

Elimination

After either oral or IV administration, zaleplon is rapidly eliminated with a mean $t_{1/2}$ of approximately 1 hour. The oral-dose plasma clearance of zaleplon is about 3 L/h/kg and the IV zaleplon plasma clearance is approximately 1 L/h/kg. Assuming normal hepatic blood flow and negligible renal clearance of zaleplon, the estimated hepatic extraction ratio of zaleplon is approximately 0.7, indicating that zaleplon is subject to high first-pass metabolism.

After administration of a radiolabeled dose of zaleplon, 70% of the administered dose is recovered in urine within 48 hours (71% recovered within 6 days), almost all as zaleplon metabolites and their glucuronides. An additional 17% is recovered in feces within 6 days, most as 5-oxo-zaleplon.

Effect of Food

In healthy adults a high-fat/heavy meal prolonged the absorption of zaleplon compared to the fasted state, delaying t_{max} by approximately 2 hours and reducing C_{max} by approximately 35%. Zaleplon AUC and elimination half-life were not significantly affected. These results suggest that the effects of Sonata on sleep onset may be reduced if it is taken with or immediately after a high-fat/heavy meal.

Special Populations

Age: The pharmacokinetics of Sonata (zaleplon) have been investigated in three studies with elderly men and women ranging in age from 65 to 85 years. The pharmacokinetics of Sonata in elderly subjects, including those over 75 years of age, are not significantly different from those in young healthy subjects.

Gender: There is no significant difference in the pharmacokinetics of Sonata in men and women.

Race: The pharmacokinetics of zaleplon have been studied in Japanese subjects as representative of Asian populations. For this group, C_{max} and AUC were increased 37% and 64%, respectively. This finding can likely be attributed to differences in body weight, or alternatively, may represent differences in enzyme activities resulting from differences in diet, environment, or other factors. The effects of race on pharmacokinetic characteristics in other ethnic groups have not been well characterized.

Hepatic impairment: Zaleplon is metabolized primarily by the liver and undergoes significant presystemic metabolism. Consequently, the oral clearance of zaleplon was reduced by 70% and 87% in compensated and decompensated cirrhotic patients, respectively, leading to marked increases in mean C_{max} and AUC (up to 4-fold and 7-fold in compensated and decompensated patients, respectively), in comparison with healthy subjects. The dose of Sonata should therefore be reduced in patients with mild to moderate hepatic impairment (see **DOSAGE AND ADMINISTRATION**). Sonata is not recommended for use in patients with severe hepatic impairment.

Renal impairment: Because renal excretion of unchanged zaleplon accounts for less than 1% of the administered dose, the pharmacokinetics of zaleplon are not altered in patients with renal insufficiency. No dose adjustment is necessary in patients with mild to moderate renal impairment. Sonata has not been adequately studied in patients with severe renal impairment.

Drug-Drug Interactions

Because zaleplon is primarily metabolized by aldehyde oxidase, and to a lesser extent by CYP3A4, inhibitors of these enzymes might be expected to decrease zaleplon's clearance and inducers of these enzymes might be expected to increase its clearance. Zaleplon has been shown to have minimal effects on the kinetics of warfarin (both R- and S-forms), imipramine, ethanol, ibuprofen, diphenhydramine, thioridazine, and digoxin. However, the effects of zaleplon on inhibition of enzymes involved in the metabolism of other drugs have not been studied. (See **Drug Interactions** under **PRECAUTIONS**.)

Clinical Trials

Controlled Trials Supporting Effectiveness

Sonata (typically administered in doses of 5 mg, 10 mg, or 20 mg) has been studied in patients with chronic insomnia (n = 3,435) in 12 placebo- and active-drug-controlled trials. Three of the trials were in elderly patients (n = 1,019). It has also been studied in transient insomnia (n = 264). Because of its very short half-life, studies focused on decreasing sleep latency, with less attention to duration of sleep and number of awakenings, for which consistent differences from placebo were not demonstrated. Studies were also carried out to examine the time course of effects on memory and psychomotor function, and to examine withdrawal phenomena.

Transient Insomnia

Normal adults experiencing transient insomnia during the first night in a sleep laboratory were evaluated in a double-blind, parallel-group trial comparing the effects of two doses of Sonata (5 mg and 10 mg) with placebo. Sonata 10 mg, but not 5 mg, was superior to placebo in decreasing latency to persistent sleep (LPS), a polysomnographic measure of time to onset of sleep.

Chronic Insomnia

Non-elderly patients:

Adult outpatients with chronic insomnia were evaluated in three double-blind, parallel-group outpatient studies, one of 2 weeks duration and two of 4 weeks duration, that compared the effects of Sonata at doses of 5 mg (in two studies), 10 mg, and 20 mg with placebo on a subjective measure of time to sleep onset (TSO). Sonata 10 mg and 20 mg were consistently superior to placebo for TSO, generally for the full duration of all three studies. Although both doses were effective, the effect was greater and more consistent for the 20-mg dose. The 5-mg dose was less consistently effective than were the 10-mg and 20-mg doses. Sleep latency with Sonata 10 mg and 20 mg was on the order of 10-20 minutes (15%-30%) less than with placebo in these studies.

Adult outpatients with chronic insomnia were evaluated in six double-blind, parallel-group sleep laboratory studies that varied in duration from a single night up to 35 nights. Overall, these studies demonstrated a superiority of Sonata 10 mg and 20 mg over placebo in reducing LPS on the first 2 nights of treatment. At later time points in 5-, 14-, and 28-night studies, a reduction in LPS from baseline was observed for all treatment groups, including the placebo group, and thus, a significant difference between Sonata and placebo was not seen beyond 2 nights. In a 35-night study, Sonata 10 mg was significantly more effective than placebo in reducing LPS at the primary efficacy endpoint on nights 29 and 30.

Elderly patients:

Elderly outpatients with chronic insomnia were evaluated in two 2-week, double-blind, parallel-group outpatient studies that compared the effects of Sonata 5 mg and 10 mg with placebo on a subjective measure of time to sleep onset (TSO). Sonata at both doses was superior to placebo on TSO, generally for the full duration of both studies, with an effect size generally similar to that seen in younger persons. The 10-mg dose tended to have a greater effect in reducing TSO.

Elderly outpatients with chronic insomnia were also evaluated in a 2-night sleep laboratory study involving doses of 5 mg and 10 mg. Both 5-mg and 10-mg doses of Sonata were superior to placebo in reducing latency to persistent sleep (LPS).

Generally in these studies, there was a slight increase in sleep duration, compared to baseline, for all treatment groups, including placebo, and thus, a significant difference from placebo on sleep duration was not demonstrated.

Studies Pertinent to Safety Concerns for Sedative/Hypnotic Drugs

Memory Impairment

Studies involving the exposure of normal subjects to single fixed doses of Sonata (10 mg or 20 mg) with structured assessments of short-term memory at fixed times after dosing (eg, 1, 2, 3, 4, 5, 8, and 10 hours) generally revealed the expected impairment of short-term memory at 1 hour, the time of peak exposure to zaleplon, for both doses, with a tendency for the effect to be greater after 20 mg. Consistent with the rapid clearance of zaleplon, memory impairment was no longer present as early as 2 hours post dosing in one study, and in none of the studies after 3-4 hours. Nevertheless, spontaneous reporting of adverse events in larger premarketing clinical trials revealed a difference between Sonata and placebo in the risk of next-day amnesia (3% vs 1%), and an apparent dose-dependency for this event (see **ADVERSE REACTIONS**).

Sedative/Psychomotor Effects

Studies involving the exposure of normal subjects to single fixed doses of Sonata (zaleplon) (10 mg or 20 mg) with structured assessments of sedation and psychomotor function (eg, reaction time and subjective ratings of alertness) at fixed times after dosing (eg, 1, 2, 3, 4, 5, 8, and 10 hours) generally revealed the expected sedation and impairment of psychomotor function at 1 hour, the time of peak exposure to zaleplon, for both doses. Consistent with the rapid clearance of zaleplon, impairment of psychomotor function was no longer present as early as 2 hours post dosing in one study, and in none of the studies after 3-4 hours. Spontaneous reporting of adverse events in larger premarketing clinical trials did not suggest a difference between Sonata and placebo in the risk of next-day somnolence (see **ADVERSE REACTIONS**).

Withdrawal-Emergent Anxiety and Insomnia

During nightly use for an extended period, pharmacodynamic tolerance or adaptation to some effects of hypnotics may develop. If the drug has a short elimination half-life, it is possible that a relative deficiency of the drug or its active metabolites (ie, in relationship to the receptor site) may occur at some point in the interval between each night's use. This sequence of events is believed to be responsible for two clinical findings reported to occur after several weeks of nightly use of other rapidly eliminated hypnotics: increased wakefulness during the last quarter of the night and the appearance of increased signs of daytime anxiety.

Zaleplon has a short half-life and no active metabolites. At the primary efficacy endpoint (nights 29 and 30) in a 35-night sleep laboratory study, polysomnographic recordings showed that wakefulness was not significantly longer with Sonata than with placebo during the last quarter of the night. No increase in the signs of daytime anxiety was observed in clinical trials with Sonata. In two sleep laboratory studies involving 14- and 28-nightly doses of Sonata (5 mg and 10 mg in one study and 10 mg and 20 mg in the second) and structured assessments of daytime anxiety, no increases in daytime anxiety were detected. Similarly, in a pooled analysis (all the parallel-group, placebo-controlled studies) of spontaneously reported daytime anxiety, no difference was observed between Sonata and placebo.

Rebound insomnia, defined as a dose-dependent temporary worsening in sleep parameters (latency, total sleep time, and number of awakenings) compared to baseline following discontinuation of treatment, is observed with short- and intermediate-acting hypnotics. Rebound insomnia following discontinuation of Sonata relative to baseline was examined at both nights 1 and 2 following discontinuation in three sleep laboratory studies (14, 28, and 35 nights) and five outpatient studies utilizing patient diaries (14 and 28 nights). Overall, the data suggest that rebound insomnia may be dose dependent. At 20 mg, there appeared to be both objective (polysomnographic) and subjective (diary) evidence of rebound insomnia on the first night after discontinuation of treatment with Sonata. At 5 mg and 10 mg, there was no objective and minimal subjective evidence of rebound insomnia on the first night after discontinuation of treatment with Sonata. At all doses, the rebound effect appeared to resolve by the second night following withdrawal. In the 35-night study, there was a worsening in sleep on the first night off for both the 10-mg and 20-mg groups compared to placebo, but not to baseline. This discontinuation-emergent effect was mild, had the characteristics of the return of the symptoms of chronic insomnia, and appeared to resolve by the second night after zaleplon discontinuation.

Other Withdrawal-Emergent Phenomena

The potential for other withdrawal phenomena was also assessed in 14- to 28-night studies, including both the sleep laboratory studies and the outpatient studies, and in open-label studies of 6- and 12-month durations. The Benzodiazepine Withdrawal Symptom Questionnaire was used in several of these studies, both at baseline and then during days 1 and 2 following discontinuation. Withdrawal was operationally defined as the emergence of 3 or more new symptoms after discontinuation. Sonata was not distinguishable from placebo at doses of 5 mg, 10 mg, or 20 mg on this measure, nor was Sonata distinguishable from placebo on spontaneously reported withdrawal-emergent adverse events. There were no instances of withdrawal delirium, withdrawal associated hallucinations, or any other manifestations of severe sedative/hypnotic withdrawal.

INDICATIONS AND USAGE

Sonata is indicated for the short-term treatment of insomnia. Sonata has been shown to decrease the time to sleep onset for up to 30 days in controlled clinical studies (see **Clinical Trials** under **CLINICAL PHARMACOLOGY**). It has not been shown to increase total sleep time or decrease the number of awakenings.

Hypnotics should generally be limited to 7 to 10 days of use, and reevaluation of the patient is recommended if they are to be taken for more than 2 to 3 weeks. Sonata should not be prescribed in quantities exceeding a 1-month supply (see **WARNINGS**).

CONTRAINDICATIONS

Hypersensitivity to zaleplon or any excipients in the formulation (see also **PRECAUTIONS**).

WARNINGS

Because sleep disturbances may be the presenting manifestation of a physical and/or psychiatric disorder, symptomatic treatment of insomnia should be initiated only after a careful evaluation of the patient. The failure of insomnia to remit after 7 to 10 days of treatment may indicate the presence of a primary psychiatric and/or medical illness that should be evaluated. Worsening of insomnia or the emergence of new thinking or behavior abnormalities may be the consequence of an unrecognized psychiatric or physical disorder. Such findings have emerged during the course of treatment with sedative/hypnotic drugs, including Sonata. Because some of the important adverse effects of Sonata appear to be dose-related, it is important to use the lowest possible effective dose, especially in the elderly (see **DOSAGE AND ADMINISTRATION**).

A variety of abnormal thinking and behavior changes have been reported to occur in association with the use of sedative/hypnotics. Some of these changes may be characterized by decreased inhibition (eg, aggressiveness and extroversion that seem out of character), similar to effects produced by alcohol and other CNS depressants. Other reported behavioral changes have included bizarre behavior, agitation, hallucinations, and depersonalization. Amnesia and other neuropsychiatric symptoms may occur unpredictably. In primarily depressed patients, worsening of depression, including suicidal thinking, has been reported in association with the use of sedative/hypnotics.

It can rarely be determined with certainty whether a particular instance of the abnormal behaviors listed above is drug induced, spontaneous in origin, or a result of an underlying psychiatric or physical disorder. Nonetheless, the emergence of any new behavioral sign or symptom of concern requires careful and immediate evaluation.

Following rapid dose decrease or abrupt discontinuation of the use of sedative/hypnotics, there have been reports of signs and symptoms similar to those associated with withdrawal from other CNS-depressant drugs (see **DRUG ABUSE AND DEPENDENCE**).

Sonata, like other hypnotics, has CNS-depressant effects. Because of the rapid onset of action, Sonata should only be ingested immediately prior to going to bed or after the patient has gone to bed and has experienced difficulty falling asleep. Patients receiving Sonata should be cautioned against engaging in hazardous occupations requiring complete mental alertness or motor coordination (eg, operating machinery or driving a motor vehicle) after ingesting the drug, including potential impairment of the performance of such activities that may occur the day following ingestion of Sonata. Sonata, as well as other hypnotics, may produce additive CNS-depressant effects when coadministered with other psychotropic medications, anticonvulsants, antihistamines, narcotic analgesics, anesthetics, ethanol, and other drugs that themselves produce CNS depression. Sonata should not be taken with alcohol. Dosage adjustment may be necessary when Sonata is administered with other CNS-depressant agents because of the potentially additive effects.

PRECAUTIONS

General

Timing of Drug Administration

Sonata should be taken immediately before bedtime or after the patient has gone to bed and has experienced difficulty falling asleep. As with all sedative/hypnotics, taking Sonata while still up and about may result in short-term memory impairment, hallucinations, impaired coordination, dizziness, and lightheadedness.

Use in the elderly and/or debilitated patients

Impaired motor and/or cognitive performance after repeated exposure or unusual sensitivity to sedative/hypnotic drugs is a concern in the treatment of elderly and/or debilitated patients. A dose of 5 mg is recommended for elderly patients to decrease the possibility of side effects (see **DOSAGE AND ADMINISTRATION**). Elderly and/or debilitated patients should be monitored closely.

Use in patients with concomitant illness

Clinical experience with Sonata in patients with concomitant systemic illness is limited. Sonata should be used with caution in patients with diseases or conditions that could affect metabolism or hemodynamic responses.

Although preliminary studies did not reveal respiratory depressant effects at hypnotic doses of Sonata in normal subjects, caution should be observed if Sonata (zaleplon) is prescribed to patients with compromised respiratory function, because sedative/hypnotics have the capacity to depress respiratory drive. Controlled trials of acute administration of Sonata 10 mg in patients with mild to moderate chronic obstructive pulmonary disease or moderate obstructive sleep apnea showed no evidence of alterations in blood gases or apnea/hypopnea index, respectively. However, patients with compromised respiration due to preexisting illness should be monitored carefully.

The dose of Sonata should be reduced to 5 mg in patients with mild to moderate hepatic impairment (see **DOSAGE AND ADMINISTRATION**). It is not recommended for use in patients with severe hepatic impairment.

No dose adjustment is necessary in patients with mild to moderate renal impairment. Sonata has not been adequately studied in patients with severe renal impairment.

Use in patients with depression

As with other sedative/hypnotic drugs, Sonata should be administered with caution to patients exhibiting signs or symptoms of depression. Suicidal tendencies may be present in such patients and protective measures may be required. Intentional overdosage is more common in this group of patients (see **OVERDOSAGE**); therefore, the least amount of drug that is feasible should be prescribed for the patient at any one time.

This product contains FD&C Yellow No. 5 (tartrazine) which may cause allergic-type reactions (including bronchial asthma) in certain susceptible persons. Although the overall incidence of FD&C Yellow No. 5 (tartrazine) sensitivity in the general population is low, it is frequently seen in patients who also have aspirin hypersensitivity.

Information for Patients

Patient information is printed at the end of this insert. To assure safe and effective use of Sonata, the information and instructions provided in the patient information section should be discussed with patients.

Laboratory Tests

There are no specific laboratory tests recommended.

Drug Interactions

As with all drugs, the potential exists for interaction with other drugs by a variety of mechanisms.

CNS-Active Drugs

Ethanol: Sonata 10 mg potentiated the CNS-impairing effects of ethanol 0.75 g/kg on balance testing and reaction time for 1 hour after ethanol administration and on the digit symbol substitution test (DSST), symbol copying test, and the variability component of the divided attention test for 2.5 hours after ethanol administration. The potentiation resulted from a CNS pharmacodynamic interaction; zaleplon did not affect the pharmacokinetics of ethanol.

Imipramine: Coadministration of single doses of Sonata 20 mg and imipramine 75 mg produced additive effects on decreased alertness and impaired psychomotor performance for 2 to 4 hours after administration. The interaction was pharmacodynamic with no alteration of the pharmacokinetics of either drug.

Paroxetine Coadministration of a single dose of Sonata 20 mg and paroxetine 20 mg daily for 7 days did not produce any interaction on psychomotor performance. Additionally, paroxetine did not alter the pharmacokinetics of Sonata, reflecting the absence of a role of CYP2D6 in zaleplon's metabolism.

Thioridazine: Coadministration of single doses of Sonata 20 mg and thioridazine 50 mg produced additive effects on decreased alertness and impaired psychomotor performance for 2 to 4 hours after administration. The interaction was pharmacodynamic with no alteration of the pharmacokinetics of either drug.

Venlafaxine: Coadministration of multiple doses of zaleplon 10 mg and venlafaxine ER (extended release) 75 mg or 150 mg did not produce any interaction on psychomotor performance. Additionally, there was no pharmacokinetic interaction between zaleplon and venlafaxine ER.

Promethazine: There was no pharmacokinetic interaction between zaleplon and promethazine following the administration of a single dose (10 and 25 mg, respectively) of each drug.

Drugs That Induce CYP3A4

Rifampin: CYP3A4 is ordinarily a minor metabolizing enzyme of zaleplon. Multiple-dose administration of the potent CYP3A4 inducer rifampin (600 mg every 24 hours, q24h, for 14 days), however, reduced zaleplon C_{max} and AUC by approximately 80%. The coadministration of a potent CYP3A4 enzyme inducer, although not posing a safety concern, thus could lead to ineffectiveness of zaleplon. An alternative non-CYP3A4 substrate hypnotic agent may be considered in patients taking CYP3A4 inducers such as rifampin, phenytoin, carbamazepine, and phenobarbital.

Drugs That Inhibit CYP3A4

CYP3A4 is a minor metabolic pathway for the elimination of zaleplon because the sum of desethylzaleplon (formed via CYP3A4 in vitro) and its metabolites, 5-oxo-desethylzaleplon and 5-oxo-desethylzaleplon glucuronide, account for only 9% of the urinary recovery of a zaleplon dose. Coadministration of zaleplon with erythromycin, a strong, selective CYP3A4 inhibitor, produced a 34% increase in zaleplon's plasma concentrations. Similar increases would be expected with other strong, selective CYP3A4 inhibitors, such as ketoconazole. A routine dosage adjustment of zaleplon is not considered necessary.

Drugs That Inhibit Aldehyde Oxidase

The aldehyde oxidase enzyme system is less well studied than the cytochrome P450 enzyme system.

Diphenhydramine: Diphenhydramine is reported to be a weak inhibitor of aldehyde oxidase in rat liver, but its inhibitory effects in human liver are not known. There is no pharmacokinetic interaction between zaleplon and diphenhydramine following the administration of a single dose (10 mg and 50 mg, respectively) of each drug. However, because both of these compounds have CNS effects, an additive pharmacodynamic effect is possible.

Drugs That Inhibit Both Aldehyde Oxidase and CYP3A4

Cimetidine: Cimetidine inhibits both aldehyde oxidase (in vitro) and CYP3A4 (in vitro and in vivo), the primary and secondary enzymes, respectively, responsible for zaleplon metabolism. Concomitant administration of Sonata (10 mg) and cimetidine (800 mg) produced an 85% increase in the mean C_{max} and AUC of zaleplon. An initial dose of 5 mg should be given to patients who are concomitantly being treated with cimetidine (see **DOSAGE AND ADMINISTRATION**).

Drugs Highly Bound to Plasma Protein

Zaleplon is not highly bound to plasma proteins (fraction bound 60%±15%); therefore, the disposition of zaleplon is not expected to be sensitive to alterations in protein binding. In addition, administration of Sonata to a patient taking another drug that is highly protein bound should not cause transient increase in free concentrations of the other drug.

Drugs with a Narrow Therapeutic Index

Digoxin: Sonata (10 mg) did not affect the pharmacokinetic or pharmacodynamic profile of digoxin (0.375 mg q24h for 8 days).

Warfarin: Multiple oral doses of Sonata (20 mg q24h for 13 days) did not affect the pharmacokinetics of warfarin (R+)- or (S-)-enantiomers or the pharmacodynamics (prothrombin time) following a single 25-mg oral dose of warfarin.

Drugs That Alter Renal Excretion

Ibuprofen: Ibuprofen is known to affect renal function and, consequently, alter the renal excretion of other drugs. There was no apparent pharmacokinetic interaction between zaleplon and ibuprofen following single dose administration (10 mg and 600 mg, respectively) of each drug. This was expected because zaleplon is primarily metabolized and renal excretion of unchanged zaleplon accounts for less than 1% of the administered dose.

Carcinogenesis, Mutagenesis, and Impairment of Fertility

Carcinogenesis

Lifetime carcinogenicity studies of zaleplon were conducted in mice and rats. Mice received doses of 25 mg/kg/day, 50 mg/kg/day, 100 mg/kg/day, and 200 mg/kg/day in the diet for two years. These doses are equivalent to 6 to 49 times the maximum recommended human dose (MRHD) of 20 mg on a mg/m^2 basis. There was a significant increase in the incidence of hepatocellular adenomas in female mice in the high dose group. Rats received doses of 1 mg/kg/day, 10 mg/kg/day, and 20 mg/kg/day in the diet for two years. These doses are equivalent to 0.5 to 10 times the maximum recommended human dose (MRHD) of 20 mg on a mg/m^2 basis. Zaleplon was not carcinogenic in rats.

Mutagenesis

Zaleplon was clastogenic, both in the presence and absence of metabolic activation, causing structural and numerical aberrations (polyploidy and endoreduplication), when tested for chromosomal aberrations in the in vitro Chinese hamster ovary cell assay. In the in vitro human lymphocyte assay, zaleplon caused numerical, but not structural, aberrations only in the presence of metabolic activation at the highest concentrations tested. In other in vitro assays, zaleplon was not mutagenic in the Ames bacterial gene mutation assay or the Chinese hamster ovary HGPRT gene mutation assay. Zaleplon was not clastogenic in two in vivo assays, the mouse bone marrow micronucleus assay and the rat bone marrow chromosomal aberration assay, and did not cause DNA damage in the rat hepatocyte unscheduled DNA synthesis assay.

Impairment of Fertility

In a fertility and reproductive performance study in rats, mortality and decreased fertility were associated with administration of an oral dose of zaleplon of 100 mg/kg/day to males and females prior to and during mating. This dose is equivalent to 49 times the maximum recommended human dose (MRHD) of 20 mg on a mg/m^2 basis. Follow-up studies indicated that impaired fertility was due to an effect on the female.

Pregnancy: Pregnancy Category C

In embryofetal development studies in rats and rabbits, oral administration of up to 100 mg/kg/day and 50 mg/kg/day, respectively, to pregnant animals throughout organogenesis produced no evidence of teratogenicity. These doses are equivalent to 49 (rat) and 48 (rabbit) times the maximum recommended human dose (MRHD) of 20 mg on a mg/m^2 basis. In rats, pre- and postnatal growth was reduced in the offspring of dams receiving 100 mg/kg/day. This dose was also maternally toxic, as evidenced by clinical signs and decreased maternal body weight gain during gestation. The no-effect dose for rat offspring growth reduction was 10 mg/kg (a dose equivalent to 5 times the MRHD of 20 mg on a mg/m^2 basis). No adverse effects on embryofetal development were observed in rabbits at the doses examined.

In a pre- and postnatal development study in rats, increased stillbirth and postnatal mortality, and decreased growth and physical development, were observed in the offspring of females treated with doses of 7 mg/kg/day or greater during the latter part of gestation and throughout lactation. There was no evidence of maternal toxicity at this dose. The no-effect dose for offspring development was 1 mg/kg/day (a dose equivalent to 0.5 times the MRHD of 20 mg on a mg/m^2 basis). When the adverse effects on offspring viability and growth were examined in a cross-fostering study, they appeared to result from both *in utero* and lactational exposure to the drug.

Continued on next page

Sonata—Cont.

There are no studies of zaleplon in pregnant women; therefore, Sonata® (zaleplon) is not recommended for use in women during pregnancy.

Labor and Delivery

Sonata has no established use in labor and delivery.

Nursing Mothers

A study in lactating mothers indicated that the clearance and half-life of zaleplon is similar to that in young normal subjects. A small amount of zaleplon is excreted in breast milk, with the highest excreted amount occurring during a feeding at approximately 1 hour after Sonata administration. Since the small amount of the drug from breast milk may result in potentially important concentrations in infants, and because the effects of zaleplon on a nursing infant are not known, it is recommended that nursing mothers not take Sonata.

Pediatric Use

The safety and effectiveness of Sonata in pediatric patients have not been established.

Geriatric Use

A total of 628 patients in double-blind, placebo-controlled, parallel-group clinical trials who received Sonata were at least 65 years of age; of these, 311 received 5 mg and 317 received 10 mg. In both sleep laboratory and outpatient studies, elderly patients with insomnia responded to a 5 mg dose with a reduced sleep latency, and thus 5 mg is the recommended dose in this population. During short-term treatment (14 night studies) of elderly patients with Sonata, no adverse event with a frequency of at least 1% occurred at a significantly higher rate with either 5 mg or 10 mg Sonata than with placebo.

ADVERSE REACTIONS

The premarketing development program for Sonata included zaleplon exposures in patients and/or normal subjects from 2 different groups of studies: approximately 900 normal subjects in clinical pharmacology/pharmacokinetic studies; and approximately 2,900 exposures from patients in placebo-controlled clinical effectiveness studies, corresponding to approximately 450 patient exposure years. The conditions and duration of treatment with Sonata varied greatly and included (in overlapping categories) open-label and double-blind phases of studies, inpatients and outpatients, and short-term or longer-term exposure. Adverse reactions were assessed by collecting adverse events, results of physical examinations, vital signs, weights, laboratory analyses, and ECGs.

Adverse events during exposure were obtained primarily by general inquiry and recorded by clinical investigators using terminology of their own choosing. Consequently, it is not possible to provide a meaningful estimate of the proportion of individuals experiencing adverse events without first grouping similar types of events into a smaller number of standardized event categories. In the tables and tabulations that follow, COSTART terminology has been used to classify reported adverse events.

The stated frequencies of adverse events represent the proportion of individuals who experienced, at least once, a treatment-emergent adverse event of the type listed. An event was considered treatment-emergent if it occurred for the first time or worsened while receiving therapy following baseline evaluation.

Adverse Findings Observed in Short-Term, Placebo-Controlled Trials

Adverse Events Associated With Discontinuation of Treatment

In premarketing placebo-controlled, parallel-group phase 2 and phase 3 clinical trials, 3.1% of 744 patients who received placebo and 3.7% of 2,149 patients who received Sonata discontinued treatment because of an adverse clinical event. This difference was not statistically significant. No event that resulted in discontinuation occurred at a rate of ≥ 1%.

Adverse Events Occurring at an Incidence of 1% or More Among Sonata 20 mg-Treated Patients

Table 1 enumerates the incidence of treatment-emergent adverse events for a pool of three 28-night and one 35-night placebo-controlled studies of Sonata at doses of 5 mg or 10 mg and 20 mg. The table includes only those events that occurred in 1% or more of patients treated with Sonata 20 mg and that had a higher incidence in patients treated with Sonata 20 mg than in placebo-treated patients.

The prescriber should be aware that these figures cannot be used to predict the incidence of adverse events in the course of usual medical practice where patient characteristics and other factors differ from those which prevailed in the clinical trials. Similarly, the cited frequencies cannot be compared with figures obtained from other clinical investigations involving different treatments, uses, and investigators. The cited figures, however, do provide the prescribing physician with some basis for estimating the relative contribution of drug and non-drug factors to the adverse event incidence rate in the population studied.

[See table 1 below]

Other Adverse Events Observed During the Premarketing Evaluation of Sonata

Listed below are COSTART terms that reflect treatment-emergent adverse events as defined in the introduction to the **ADVERSE REACTIONS** section. These events were reported by patients treated with Sonata (zaleplon) at doses in a range of 5 mg/day to 20 mg/day during premarketing phase 2 and phase 3 clinical trials throughout the United States, Canada, and Europe, including approximately 2,900 patients. All reported events are included except those already listed in Table 1 or elsewhere in labeling, those events for which a drug cause was remote, and those event terms that were so general as to be uninformative. It is important to emphasize that although the events reported occurred during treatment with Sonata, they were not necessarily caused by it.

Events are further categorized by body system and listed in order of decreasing frequency according to the following definitions: **frequent** adverse events are those occurring on one or more occasions in at least 1/100 patients; **infrequent** adverse events are those occurring in less than 1/100 patients but at least 1/1,000 patients; **rare** events are those occurring in fewer than 1/1,000 patients.

Body as a whole - **Frequent**: back pain, chest pain, fever; **Infrequent**: chest pain substernal, chills, face edema, generalized edema, hangover effect, neck rigidity.

Cardiovascular system - **Frequent**: migraine; **Infrequent**: angina pectoris, bundle branch block, hypertension, hypotension, palpitation, syncope, tachycardia, vasodilatation, ventricular extrasystoles; **Rare**: bigeminy, cerebral ischemia, cyanosis, pericardial effusion, postural hypotension, pulmonary embolus, sinus bradycardia, thrombophlebitis, ventricular tachycardia.

Digestive system - **Frequent**: constipation, dry mouth, dyspepsia; **Infrequent**: eructation, esophagitis, flatulence, gastritis, gastroenteritis, gingivitis, glossitis, increased appetite, melena, mouth ulceration, rectal hemorrhage, stomatitis; **Rare**: aphthous stomatitis, biliary pain, bruxism, cardiospasm, cheilitis, cholelithiasis, duodenal ulcer, dysphagia, enteritis, gum hemorrhage, increased salivation, intestinal obstruction, abnormal liver function tests, peptic ulcer, tongue discoloration, tongue edema, ulcerative stomatitis.

Endocrine system - **Rare**: diabetes mellitus, goiter, hypothyroidism.

Hemic and lymphatic system - **Infrequent**: anemia, ecchymosis, lymphadenopathy; **Rare**: eosinophilia, leukocytosis, lymphocytosis, purpura.

Metabolic and nutritional - **Infrequent**: edema, gout, hypercholesteremia, thirst, weight gain; **Rare**: bilirubinemia, hyperglycemia, hyperuricemia, hypoglycemia, hypoglycemic reaction, ketosis, lactose intolerance, AST (SGOT) increased, ALT (SGPT) increased, weight loss.

Musculoskeletal system - **Frequent**: arthralgia, arthritis, myalgia; **Infrequent**: arthrosis, bursitis, joint disorder (mainly swelling, stiffness, and pain), myasthenia, tenosynovitis; **Rare**: myositis, osteoporosis.

Nervous system - **Frequent**: anxiety, depression, nervousness, thinking abnormal (mainly difficulty concentrating); **Infrequent**: abnormal gait, agitation, apathy, ataxia, circumoral paresthesia, emotional lability, euphoria, hyperesthesia, hyperkinesia, hypotonia, incoordination, insomnia, libido decreased, neuralgia, nystagmus; **Rare**: CNS stimulation, delusions, dysarthria, dystonia, facial paralysis, hostility, hypokinesia, myoclonus, neuropathy, psychomotor retardation, ptosis, reflexes decreased, reflexes increased, sleep talking, sleep walking, slurred speech, stupor, trismus.

Respiratory system - **Frequent**: bronchitis; **Infrequent**: asthma, dyspnea, laryngitis, pneumonia, snoring, voice alteration; **Rare**: apnea, hiccup, hyperventilation, pleural effusion, sputum increased.

Skin and appendages - **Frequent**: pruritus, rash; **Infrequent**: acne, alopecia, contact dermatitis, dry skin, eczema, maculopapular rash, skin hypertrophy, sweating, urticaria, vesiculobullous rash; **Rare**: melanosis, psoriasis, pustular rash, skin discoloration.

Special senses - **Frequent**: conjunctivitis, taste perversion; **Infrequent**: diplopia, dry eyes, photophobia, tinnitus, watery eyes; **Rare**: abnormality of accommodation, blepharitis, cataract specified, corneal erosion, deafness, eye hemorrhage, glaucoma, labyrinthitis, retinal detachment, taste loss, visual field defect.

Urogenital system - **Infrequent**: bladder pain, breast pain, cystitis, decreased urine stream, dysuria, hematuria, impotence, kidney calculus, kidney pain, menorrhagia, metrorrhagia, urinary frequency, urinary incontinence, urinary urgency, vaginitis; **Rare**: albuminuria, delayed menstrual period, leukorrhea, menopause, urethritis, urinary retention, vaginal hemorrhage.

Postmarketing Reports

Anaphylactic/anaphylactoid reactions, including severe reactions.

DRUG ABUSE AND DEPENDENCE

Controlled Substance Class

Sonata is classified as a Schedule IV controlled substance by federal regulation.

Abuse, Dependence, and Tolerance

Abuse

Two studies assessed the abuse liability of Sonata at doses of 25 mg, 50 mg, and 75 mg in subjects with known histories of sedative drug abuse. The results of these studies indicate that Sonata has an abuse potential similar to benzodiazepine and benzodiazepine-like hypnotics.

Dependence

The potential for developing physical dependence on Sonata and a subsequent withdrawal syndrome was assessed in controlled studies of 14-, 28-, and 35-night durations and in open-label studies of 6- and 12-month durations by examining for the emergence of rebound insomnia following drug discontinuation. Some patients (mostly those treated with 20 mg) experienced a mild rebound insomnia on the first night following withdrawal that appeared to be resolved by the second night. The use of the Benzodiazepine Withdrawal Symptom Questionnaire and examination of any other withdrawal-emergent events did not detect any other evidence for a withdrawal syndrome following abrupt discontinuation of Sonata therapy in pre-marketing studies.

However, available data cannot provide a reliable estimate of the incidence of dependence during treatment at recommended doses of Sonata. Other sedative/hypnotics have been associated with various signs and symptoms following abrupt discontinuation, ranging from mild dysphoria and

Table 1
Incidence (%) of Treatment-Emergent Adverse Events in Long-Term (28 and 35 Nights) Placebo-Controlled Clinical Trials of Sonata[1]

Body System Preferred Term	Placebo (n = 344)	Sonata 5 mg or 10 mg (n = 569)	Sonata 20 mg (n = 297)
Body as a whole			
Abdominal pain	3	6	6
Asthenia	5	5	7
Headache	35	30	42
Malaise	<1	<1	2
Photosensitivity reaction	<1	<1	1
Digestive system			
Anorexia	<1	<1	2
Colitis	0	0	1
Nausea	7	6	8
Metabolic and nutritional			
Peripheral edema	<1	<1	1
Nervous system			
Amnesia	1	2	4
Confusion	<1	<1	1
Depersonalization	<1	<1	2
Dizziness	7	7	9
Hallucinations	<1	<1	1
Hypertonia	<1	1	1
Hypesthesia	<1	<1	2
Paresthesia	1	3	3
Somnolence	4	5	6
Tremor	1	2	2
Vertigo	<1	<1	1
Respiratory system			
Epistaxis	<1	<1	1
Special senses			
Abnormal vision	<1	<1	2
Ear pain	0	<1	1
Eye pain	2	4	3
Hyperacusis	<1	1	2
Parosmia	<1	<1	2
Urogenital system			
Dysmenorrhea	2	3	4

1: Events for which the incidence for Sonata 20 mg-treated patients was at least 1% and greater than the incidence among placebo-treated patients. Incidence greater than 1% has been rounded to the nearest whole number.

insomnia to a withdrawal syndrome that may include abdominal and muscle cramps, vomiting, sweating, tremors, and convulsions. Seizures have been observed in two patients, one of which had a prior seizure, in clinical trials with Sonata. Seizures and death have been seen following the withdrawal of zaleplon from animals at doses many times higher than those proposed for human use. Because individuals with a history of addiction to, or abuse of, drugs or alcohol are at risk of habituation and dependence, they should be under careful surveillance when receiving Sonata or any other hypnotic.

Tolerance

Possible tolerance to the hypnotic effects of Sonata 10 mg and 20 mg was assessed by evaluating time to sleep onset for Sonata compared with placebo in two 28-night placebo-controlled studies and latency to persistent sleep in one 35-night placebo-controlled study where tolerance was evaluated on nights 29 and 30. No development of tolerance to Sonata was observed for time to sleep onset over 4 weeks.

OVERDOSAGE

There is limited pre-marketing clinical experience with the effects of an overdosage of Sonata. Two cases of overdose were reported. One was the accidental ingestion by a 2½ year old boy of 20 mg to 40 mg of zaleplon. The second was a 20 year old man who took 100 mg zaleplon plus 2.25 mg of triazolam. Both were treated and recovered uneventfully.

Signs and Symptoms

Signs and symptoms of overdose effects of CNS depressants can be expected to present as exaggerations of the pharmacological effects noted in preclinical testing. Overdose is usually manifested by degrees of central nervous system depression ranging from drowsiness to coma. In mild cases, symptoms include drowsiness, mental confusion, and lethargy; in more serious cases, symptoms may include ataxia, hypotonia, hypotension, respiratory depression, rarely coma, and very rarely death.

Recommended Treatment

General symptomatic and supportive measures should be used along with immediate gastric lavage where appropriate. Intravenous fluids should be administered as needed. Animal studies suggest that flumazenil is an antagonist to zaleplon. However, there is no pre-marketing clinical experience with the use of flumazenil as an antidote to a Sonata overdose. As in all cases of drug overdose, respiration, pulse, blood pressure, and other appropriate signs should be monitored and general supportive measures employed. Hypotension and CNS depression should be monitored and treated by appropriate medical intervention.

Poison Control Center

As with the management of all overdosage, the possibility of multiple drug ingestion should be considered. The physician may wish to consider contacting a poison control center for up-to-date information on the management of hypnotic drug product overdosage.

DOSAGE AND ADMINISTRATION

The dose of Sonata should be individualized. The recommended dose of Sonata for most nonelderly adults is 10 mg. For certain low weight individuals, 5 mg may be a sufficient dose. Although the risk of certain adverse events associated with the use of Sonata appears to be dose dependent, the 20 mg dose has been shown to be adequately tolerated and may be considered for the occasional patient who does not benefit from a trial of a lower dose. Doses above 20 mg have not been adequately evaluated and are not recommended.

Sonata should be taken immediately before bedtime or after the patient has gone to bed and has experienced difficulty falling asleep (see **PRECAUTIONS**). Taking Sonata with or immediately after a heavy, high-fat meal results in slower absorption and would be expected to reduce the effect of Sonata on sleep latency (see **Pharmacokinetics** under **CLINICAL PHARMACOLOGY**).

Special Populations

Elderly patients and debilitated patients appear to be more sensitive to the effects of hypnotics, and respond to 5 mg of Sonata. The recommended dose for these patients is therefore 5 mg. Doses over 10 mg are not recommended.

Hepatic insufficiency: Patients with mild to moderate hepatic impairment should be treated with Sonata 5 mg because clearance is reduced in this population. Sonata is not recommended for use in patients with severe hepatic impairment.

Renal insufficiency: No dose adjustment is necessary in patients with mild to moderate renal impairment. Sonata has not been adequately studied in patients with severe renal impairment.

An initial dose of 5 mg should be given to patients concomitantly taking cimetidine because zaleplon clearance is reduced in this population (see **Drug Interactions** under **PRECAUTIONS**).

HOW SUPPLIED

Sonata (zaleplon) capsules are available in bottles of 100 capsules in the following dosage strengths:

5 mg, NDC 0008-0925, opaque green cap and opaque pale green body with "5 mg" on the cap and "SONATA" on the body.

10 mg, NDC 0008-0926, opaque green cap and opaque light green body with "10 mg" on the cap and "SONATA" on the body.

The appearance of these capsules is a trademark of Wyeth Pharmaceuticals.

STORAGE CONDITIONS

Store at controlled room temperature, 20°C to 25°C (68°F to 77°F).

Dispense in a light-resistant container as defined in the USP.

INFORMATION FOR PATIENTS TAKING SONATA

Your doctor has prescribed Sonata to help you sleep. The following information is intended to guide you in the safe use of this medicine. It is not meant to take the place of your doctor's instructions. If you have any questions about Sonata capsules, be sure to ask your doctor or pharmacist.

Sonata is used to treat difficulty in falling asleep. Sonata works very quickly and has its effect during the first part of the night, since it is rapidly eliminated by the body. You should take Sonata immediately before going to bed or after you have gone to bed and are having difficulty falling asleep. If your principal sleep difficulty is awakening prematurely after falling asleep, there is no evidence that Sonata will be helpful to you. For Sonata to help you fall asleep you should not take it with or immediately after a high-fat/heavy meal.

Sonata belongs to a group of medicines known as the "hypnotics", or simply, sleep medicines. There are many different sleep medicines available to help people sleep better. Sleep problems are usually temporary, requiring treatment for only a short time, usually 1 or 2 days up to 1 or 2 weeks. Some people have chronic sleep problems that may require more prolonged use of sleep medicine. However, you should not use these medicines for long periods without talking with your doctor about the risks and benefits of prolonged use.

Who should not take Sonata

Do not take Sonata if you are hypersensitive to its active substance, zaleplon, or to any of its inactive ingredients, including tartrazine (FD&C Yellow No. 5).

This product contains FD&C Yellow No. 5 (tartrazine) which may cause allergic-type reactions (including bronchial asthma) in certain susceptible persons. Although the overall incidence of FD&C Yellow No. 5 (tartrazine) sensitivity in the general population is low, it is frequently seen in patients who also have aspirin hypersensitivity.

Side Effects

All medicines have side effects. The most common side effects of sleep medicines are:

- Drowsiness
- Dizziness
- Lightheadedness
- Difficulty with coordination

These side effects with Sonata occur most often within an hour after taking it, so it is especially important to take it only when you are about to go to bed or are already in bed. Severe allergic reactions, sometimes with difficulty in breathing and possibly life threatening, have been reported and may require immediate medical care.

Sleep medicines can make you sleepy during the day. How drowsy you feel depends upon how your body reacts to the medicine, which sleep medicine you are taking, and how large a dose your doctor has prescribed. Daytime drowsiness is best avoided by taking the lowest dose possible that will still help you sleep at night. Your doctor will work with you to find the dose of Sonata that is best for you. Sonata generally does not cause next-day sleepiness but a few people have reported this.

To manage these side effects while you are taking this medicine:

— When you first start taking Sonata or any other sleep medicine, until you know whether the medicine will still have some carryover effect in you the next day, use extreme care while doing anything that requires complete alertness, such as driving a car, operating machinery, or piloting an aircraft.

— NEVER drink alcohol while you are being treated with Sonata or any sleep medicine. Alcohol can increase the side effects of Sonata or any other sleep medicine.

— Do not take any other medicines without asking your doctor first. This includes medicines you can buy without a prescription. Some medicines can cause drowsiness and are best avoided while taking Sonata.

— Always take the exact dose of Sonata prescribed by your doctor. Never change your dose without talking to your doctor first.

Special Concerns

There are some special problems that may occur while taking sleep medicines.

Memory Problems

Sleep medicines may cause a special type of memory loss or "amnesia." When this occurs, a person may not remember what has happened for several hours after taking the medicine. This is usually not a problem since most people fall asleep after taking the medicine. Memory loss can be a problem, however, when sleep medicines are taken while traveling, such as during an airplane flight and the person wakes up before the effect of the medicine is gone. This has been called "traveler's amnesia." Memory problems are not common while taking Sonata. In most instances memory problems can be avoided if you take Sonata only when you are able to get 4 or more hours of sleep before you need to be active again. Be sure to talk to your doctor if you think you are having memory problems.

Tolerance

When sleep medicines are used every night for more than a few weeks, they may lose their effectiveness to help you sleep. This is known as "tolerance." Development of tolerance to Sonata has not been observed in outpatient clinical studies of up to 4 weeks in duration; however, it is unknown if the benefits of Sonata in falling asleep more quickly persist beyond 4 weeks. Sleep medicines should, in most cases, be used only for short periods of time, such as 1 or 2 days and generally no longer than 1 or 2 weeks. If your sleep problems continue, consult your doctor, who will determine whether other measures are needed to overcome your sleep problems.

Dependence

Sleep medicines can cause dependence, especially when these medicines are used regularly for longer than a few weeks or at high doses. Some people develop a need to continue taking their medicines. This is known as dependence or "addiction."

When people develop dependence, they may have difficulty stopping the sleep medicine. If the medicine is suddenly stopped, the body is not able to function normally and unpleasant symptoms (see *Withdrawal*) may occur. They may find they have to keep taking the medicine either at the prescribed dose or at increasing doses just to avoid withdrawal symptoms.

All people taking sleep medicines have some risk of becoming dependent on the medicine. However, people who have been dependent on alcohol or other drugs in the past may have a higher chance of becoming addicted to sleep medicines. This possibility must be considered before using these medicines for more than a few weeks. If you have been addicted to alcohol or drugs in the past, it is important to tell your doctor before starting Sonata or any sleep medicine.

Withdrawal

Withdrawal symptoms may occur when sleep medicines are stopped suddenly after being used daily for a long time. In some cases, these symptoms can occur even if the medicine has been used for only a week or two. In mild cases, withdrawal symptoms may include unpleasant feelings. In more severe cases, abdominal and muscle cramps, vomiting, sweating, shakiness, and rarely, seizures may occur. These more severe withdrawal symptoms are very uncommon. Although withdrawal symptoms have not been observed in the relatively limited controlled trials experience with Sonata, there is, nevertheless, the risk of such events in association with the use of any sleep medicines.

Another problem that may occur when sleep medicines are stopped is known as "rebound insomnia." This means that a person may have more trouble sleeping the first few nights after the medicine is stopped than before starting the medicine. If you should experience rebound insomnia, do not get discouraged. This problem usually goes away on its own after 1 or 2 nights.

If you have been taking Sonata or any other sleep medicine for more than 1 or 2 weeks, do not stop taking it on your own. Always follow your doctor's directions.

Changes In Behavior and Thinking

Some people using sleep medicines have experienced unusual changes in their thinking and/or behavior. These effects are not common. However, they have included:

— more outgoing or aggressive behavior than normal
— loss of personal identity
— confusion
— strange behavior
— agitation
— hallucinations
— worsening of depression
— suicidal thoughts

How often these effects occur depends on several factors, such as a person's general health, the use of other medicines, and which sleep medicine is being used. Clinical experience with Sonata (zaleplon) suggests that it is uncommonly associated with these behavior changes.

It is also important to realize that it is rarely clear whether these behavior changes are caused by the medicine, an illness, or occur on their own. In fact, sleep problems that do not improve may be due to illnesses that were present before the medicine was used. If you or your family notice any changes in your behavior, or if you have any unusual or disturbing thoughts, call your doctor immediately.

Pregnancy and Breastfeeding

Sleep medicines may cause sedation or other potential effects in the unborn baby when used during the last weeks of pregnancy.

Therefore, Sonata is not recommended for use during pregnancy. Be sure to tell your doctor if you are pregnant, if you are planning to become pregnant, or if you become pregnant while taking Sonata.

In addition, a very small amount of Sonata may be present in breast milk after use of the medication. The effects of very small amounts of Sonata on an infant are not known; therefore, as with all other hypnotics, it is recommended that you not take Sonata if you are breastfeeding a baby.

Safe Use of Sleeping Medicines

To ensure the safe and effective use of Sonata or any other sleep medicine, you should observe the following cautions:

1. Sonata is a prescription medicine and should be used ONLY as directed by your doctor. Follow your doctor's instructions about how to take, when to take, and how long to take Sonata.
2. Never use Sonata or any other sleep medicine for longer than directed by your doctor.
3. If you notice any unusual and/or disturbing thoughts or behavior during treatment with Sonata or any other sleep medicine, contact your doctor.

Continued on next page

Sonata—Cont.

4. Tell your doctor about any medicines you may be taking, including medicines you may buy without a prescription. You should also tell your doctor if you drink alcohol. DO NOT use alcohol while taking Sonata or any other sleep medicine.
5. Do not take Sonata unless you are able to get 4 or more hours of sleep before you must be active again.
6. Do not increase the prescribed dose of Sonata or any other sleep medicine unless instructed by your doctor.
7. When you first start taking Sonata or any other sleep medicine, until you know whether the medicine will still have some carryover effect in you the next day, use extreme care while doing anything that requires complete alertness, such as driving a car, operating machinery, or piloting an aircraft.
8. Be aware that you may have more sleeping problems the first night or two after stopping any sleep medicine.
9. Be sure to tell your doctor if you are pregnant, if you are planning to become pregnant, if you become pregnant, or are breastfeeding a baby while taking Sonata.
10. As with all prescription medicines, never share Sonata or any other sleep medicine with anyone else. Always store Sonata or any other sleep medicine in the original container and out of reach of children.
11. Be sure to tell your physician if you suffer from depression.
12. Sonata works very quickly. You should only take Sonata immediately before going to bed or after you have gone to bed and are having difficulty falling asleep.
13. For Sonata to work best, you should not take Sonata with or immediately after a high-fat/heavy meal.
14. Some people should start with the lowest dose (5 mg) of Sonata; these include the elderly (ie, ages 65 and over) and people with liver disease.

Distributed by:
King Pharmaceuticals, Inc.,
Bristol, TN 37620

Revised October 2, 2002

Shown in Product Identification Guide, page 320

SYNERCID® I.V. ℞

[sī-nər-sĕd]

quinupristin and
dalfopristin for injection
Prescribing Information as of July 2003
℞ only

One of **Synercid's** approved indications is for the treatment of patients with serious or life-threatening infections associated with vancomycin-resistant Enterococcus faecium (VREF) bacteremia. **Synercid** has been approved for marketing in the United States for this indication under FDA's accelerated approval regulations that allow marketing of products for use in life-threatening conditions when other therapies are not available. Approval of drugs for marketing under these regulations is based upon a demonstrated effect on a surrogate endpoint that is likely to predict clinical benefit.
Approval of this indication is based upon **Synercid's** ability to clear VREF from the bloodstream, with clearance of bacteremia considered to be a surrogate endpoint. There are no results from well-controlled clinical studies that confirm the validity of this surrogate marker. However, a study to verify the clinical benefit of therapy with **Synercid** on traditional clinical endpoints (such as cure of the underlying infection) is presently underway.

DESCRIPTION

Synercid® (quinupristin and dalfopristin powder for injection) I.V., a streptogramin antibacterial agent for intravenous administration, is a sterile lyophilized formulation of two semisynthetic pristinamycin derivatives, quinupristin (derived from pristinamycin I) and dalfopristin (derived from pristinamycin IIA) in the ratio of 30:70 (w/w).
Quinupristin is a white to very slightly yellow, hygroscopic powder. It is a combination of three peptide macrolactones. The main component of quinupristin (>88.0%) has the following chemical name: N-[(6*R*,9*S*,10*R*,13*S*,15a*S*,18*R*,22*S*,24a*S*)-22-[*p*-(dimethylamino)benzyl]-6-ethyldocosahydro-10,23-dimethyl-5,8,12,15,17,21,24-heptaoxo-13-phenyl-18-[[(3*S*)-3-quinuclidinylthio] methyl]-12*H*-pyrido[2,1-f]pyrrolo-[2,1-l][1,4,7,10,13,16] oxapentaazacyclononadecin-9-yl]-3-hydroxypicolinamide.
The main component of quinupristin has an empirical formula of $C_{53}H_{67}N_9O_{10}S$, a molecular weight of 1022.24 and the following structural formula:

Dalfopristin is a slightly yellow to yellow, hygroscopic, powder. The chemical name for dalfopristin is: (3*R*,4*R*,10*E*,12*E*,14*S*,26*R*,26a*S*)-26-[[2-(diethylamino)-ethyl]sulfonyl]-8,9,14,15,24, 25,26,26a-octahydro-14-hydroxy-3-isopropyl-4,12-dimethyl-3*H*-21,18-nitrilo-1*H*,22*H*-pyrrolo[2,1-c][1,8,4,19]-dioxadiazacyclotetracosine-1,7,16,22 (4*H*,17*H*)-tetrone.
Dalfopristin has an empirical formula of $C_{34}H_{50}N_4O_9S$, a molecular weight of 690.85 and the following structural formula:

CLINICAL PHARMACOLOGY

Pharmacokinetics: Quinupristin and dalfopristin are the main active components circulating in plasma in human subjects. Quinupristin and dalfopristin are converted to several active major metabolites: two conjugated metabolites for quinupristin (one with glutathione and one with cysteine) and one non-conjugated metabolite for dalfopristin (formed by drug hydrolysis).
Pharmacokinetic profiles of quinupristin and dalfopristin in combination with their metabolites were determined using a bioassay following multiple 60-minute infusions of **Synercid** in two groups of healthy young adult male volunteers. Each group received 7.5 mg/kg of **Synercid** intravenously q12h or q8h for a total of 9 or 10 doses, respectively. The pharmacokinetic parameters were proportional with q12h and q8h dosing; those of the q8h regimen are shown in the following table:
[See table below]
The clearances of unchanged quinupristin and dalfopristin are similar (0.72 L/h/kg), and the steady-state volume of distribution for quinupristin is 0.45 L/kg and for dalfopristin is 0.24 L/kg. The elimination half-life of quinupristin and dalfopristin is approximately 0.85 and 0.70 hours, respectively.
The protein binding of **Synercid** is moderate.
Penetration of unchanged quinupristin and dalfopristin in noninflammatory blister fluid corresponds to about 19% and 11% of that estimated in plasma, respectively. The penetration into blister fluid of quinupristin and dalfopristin in combination with their major metabolites was in total approximately 40% compared to that in plasma.
In vitro, the transformation of the parent drugs into their major active metabolites occurs by non-enzymatic reactions and is not dependent on cytochrome-P450 or glutathione-transferase enzyme activities.
Synercid has been shown to be a major inhibitor (in vitro inhibits 70% cyclosporin A biotransformation at 10 µg/mL of **Synercid**) of the activity of cytochrome P450 3A4 isoenzyme. (See **Warnings**.)
Synercid can interfere with the metabolism of other drug products that are associated with QTc prolongation. However, electrophysiologic studies confirm that **Synercid** does not itself induce QTc prolongation. (See **Warnings**.)
Fecal excretion constitutes the main elimination route for both parent drugs and their metabolites (75 to 77% of dose). Urinary excretion accounts for approximately 15% of the quinupristin and 19% of the dalfopristin dose. Preclinical data in rats have demonstrated that approximately 80% of the dose is excreted in the bile and suggest that in man, biliary excretion is probably the principal route for fecal elimination.

Special Populations
Elderly: The pharmacokinetics of quinupristin and dalfopristin were studied in a population of elderly individuals (range 69 to 74 years). The pharmacokinetics of the drug products were not modified in these subjects.
Gender: The pharmacokinetics of quinupristin and dalfopristin are not modified by gender.
Renal Insufficiency: In patients with creatinine clearance 6 to 28 mL/min, the AUC of quinupristin and dalfopristin in combination with their major metabolites increased about 40% and 30%, respectively.
In patients undergoing Continuous Ambulatory Peritoneal Dialysis, dialysis clearance for quinupristin, dalfopristin and their metabolites is negligible. The plasma AUC of unchanged quinupristin and dalfopristin increased about 20% and 30%, respectively. The high molecular weight of both components of **Synercid** suggests that it is unlikely to be removed by hemodialysis.
Hepatic Insufficiency: In patients with hepatic dysfunction (Child-Pugh scores A and B), the terminal half-life of quinupristin and dalfopristin was not modified. However, the AUC of quinupristin and dalfopristin in combination with their major metabolites increased about 180% and 50%, respectively. (See **Dosage and Administration** and **Precautions**.)
Obesity (body mass index ≥30): In obese patients the C_{max} and AUC of quinupristin increased about 30% and those of dalfopristin about 40%.
Pediatric Patients: The pharmacokinetics of **Synercid** in patients less than 16 years of age have not been studied.

Microbiology: The streptogramin components of **Synercid**, quinupristin and dalfopristin, are present in a ratio of 30 parts quinupristin to 70 parts dalfopristin. These two components act synergistically so that **Synercid's** microbiologic in vitro activity is greater than that of the components individually. Quinupristin's and dalfopristin's metabolites also contribute to the antimicrobial activity of **Synercid**. In vitro synergism of the major metabolites with the complementary parent compound has been demonstrated.
Synercid is bacteriostatic against *Enterococcus faecium* and bactericidal against strains of methicillin susceptible and methicillin-resistant staphylococci.
The site of action of quinupristin and dalfopristin is the bacterial ribosome. Dalfopristin has been shown to inhibit the early phase of protein synthesis while quinupristin inhibits the late phase of protein synthesis.
In vitro combination testing of **Synercid** with aztreonam, cefotaxime, ciprofloxacin, and gentamicin against *Enterobacteriaceae* and *Pseudomonas aeruginosa* did not show antagonism.
In vitro combination testing of **Synercid** with prototype drugs of the following classes: aminoglycosides (gentamicin), β-lactams (cefepime, ampicillin, and amoxicillin), glycopeptides (vancomycin), quinolones (ciprofloxacin), tetracyclines (doxycycline) and also chloramphenicol against enterococci and staphylococci did not show antagonism.
The mode of action differs from that of other classes of antibacterial agents such as β-lactams aminoglycosides, glycopeptides, quinolones, macrolides, lincosamides and tetracyclines. There is no cross resistance between **Synercid** and these agents when tested by the minimum inhibitory concentration (MIC) method.
In non-comparative studies, emerging resistance to **Synercid** during treatment of VREF infections occurred. Resistance to **Synercid** is associated with resistance to both components (i.e., quinupristin and dalfopristin).
Synercid has been shown to be active against most strains of the following microorganisms, both in vitro and in clinical infections, as described in the **Indications and Usage** section.

Aerobic Gram-Positive Microorganisms
Enterococcus faecium (Vancomycin-resistant and multi-drug resistant strains only)
Staphylococcus aureus (methicillin-susceptible strains only)
Streptococcus pyogenes

Note: **Synercid** is not active against Enterococcus faecalis. Differentiation of enterococcal species is important to avoid misidentification of Enterococcus faecalis as Enterococcus faecium.
The following in vitro data are available, **but their clinical significance is unknown.**
The combination of quinupristin and dalfopristin (**Synercid**) exhibits in vitro minimum inhibitory concentrations (MIC's) of ≤1.0 µg/mL against most (≥90%) isolates of the following microorganisms; however, the safety and effectiveness of **Synercid** in treating clinical infections due to these microorganisms have not been established in adequate and well-controlled clinical trials.

Aerobic gram-positive microorganisms
Corynebacterium jeikeium
Staphylococcus aureus (methicillin-resistant strains)
Staphylococcus epidermidis (including methicillin-resistant strains)
Streptococcus agalactiae

Susceptibility Testing
Dilution Techniques
Quantitative methods are used to determine antimicrobial minimum inhibitory concentrations (MICs). These MICs provide estimates of the susceptibility of microorganisms to antimicrobial compounds. The MICs should be determined

Mean Steady-State Pharmacokinetic Parameters of Quinupristin and Dalfopristin in Combination with their Metabolites (± SD[1]) (dose = 7.5 mg/kg q8h; n=10)

	C_{max}[2] (µg/mL)	AUC[3] (µg.h/mL)	$t_{1/2}$[4] (hr)
Quinupristin and metabolites	3.20 ± 0.67	7.20 ± 1.24	3.07 ± 0.51
Dalfopristin and metabolite	7.96 ± 1.30	10.57 ± 2.24	1.04 ± 0.20

[1] SD= Standard Deviation
[2] C_{max} = Maximum drug plasma concentration
[3] AUC = Area under the drug plasma concentration-time curve
[4] $t_{1/2}$ = Half-life

using a standardized procedure. Standardized procedures are based on a dilution[1] method (broth or agar) or equivalent using standardized inoculum concentrations, and standardized concentrations of quinupristin/dalfopristin (**Synercid**) in a 30:70 ratio made from powder of known potency. The MIC values should be interpreted according to the following criteria:

For Susceptibility Testing of Enterococcus faecium, Staphylococcus spp., and Streptococcus spp. (excluding Streptococcus pneumoniae)[a]

MIC (μg/mL)	Interpretation
≤1.0	Susceptible (S)
2.0	Intermediate (I)
≥4.0	Resistant (R)

[a] These interpretive values for Streptococcus spp. are applicable only to broth microdilution susceptibility testing using cation-adjusted Mueller-Hinton broth with 2 to 5% lysed horse blood.

A report of "Susceptible" indicates that the pathogen is likely to be inhibited if the concentration of the antimicrobial compound in the blood reaches usually achievable levels. A report of "Intermediate" indicates that the result should be considered equivocal, and if the microorganism is not fully susceptible to alternative, clinically feasible drugs, the test should be repeated. This category implies possible clinical applicability in body sites where the drug is physiologically concentrated or in situations where high dosage of drug can be used. This category provides a buffer zone which prevents small uncontrolled technical factors from causing major discrepancies in interpretation. A report of "Resistant" indicates that the pathogen is not likely to be inhibited if the antimicrobial compound in the blood reaches the concentrations usually achievable; other therapy should be selected.

Quality Control

A standardized susceptibility test procedure requires the use of laboratory control organisms to control the technical aspects of the laboratory procedures. Standard quinupristin/dalfopristin powder in a 30:70 ratio should provide the following MIC values with the indicated quality control strains:

Microorganism (ATCC®#)	MIC (μg/mL)
Enterococcus faecalis (29212)	2.0 to 8.0
Staphylococcus aureus (29213)	0.25 to 1.0

Diffusion Techniques

Quantitative methods that require measurement of zone diameters also provide reproducible estimates of the susceptibility of bacteria to antimicrobial compounds. One such standardized procedure[2] requires the use of standardized inoculum concentrations. This procedure uses paper disks impregnated with 15 μg quinupristin/dalfopristin in a ratio of 30:70 (**Synercid**) to test the susceptibility of microorganisms to quinupristin/dalfopristin. Reports from the laboratory providing results of the standard single-disk susceptibility test with a 15 μg quinupristin/dalfopristin disk should be interpreted according to the following criteria:

For Susceptibility Testing of Enterococcus faecium, Staphylococcus spp., and Streptococcus spp. (excluding Streptococcus pneumoniae)[b]

Zone Diameter (mm)	Interpretation
≥19	Susceptible (S)
16 to 18	Intermediate (I)
≤15	Resistant (R)

[b] The zone diameter for Streptococcus spp. are applicable only to tests performed using Mueller-Hinton agar supplemented with 5% sheep blood when incubated in 5% CO_2.

Interpretation should be as stated above for results using dilution techniques. Interpretation involves correlation of the diameter obtained in the disk test with the MIC for quinupristin/dalfopristin.

Quality Control

As with standardized dilution techniques, diffusion methods require the use of laboratory control microorganisms that are used to control the technical aspects of the laboratory procedures. For the diffusion technique, the 15 μg quinupristin/dalfopristin (30:70 ratio) disk should provide the following zone diameter with the quality control strain listed below:

Microorganism (ATCC®#)	Zone Diameter Range (mm)
Staphylococcus aureus (25923)	21 to 28

ATCC® is a registered trademark of the American Type Culture Collection

INDICATIONS AND USAGE

Synercid is indicated in adults for the treatment of the following infections when caused by susceptible strains of the designated microorganisms.

Vancomycin-resistant Enterococcus faecium **(VREF)**

Synercid is indicated for the treatment of patients with serious or life-threatening infections associated with vancomycin-resistant Enterococcus faecium (VREF) bacteremia. (See **Clinical Studies**.)

One of **Synercid's** approved indications is for the treatment of patients with serious or life-threatening infections associated with vancomycin-resistant Enterococcus faecium (VREF) bacteremia. **Synercid** has been approved for marketing in the United States for this indication under FDA's accelerated approval regulations that allow marketing of products for use in life-threatening conditions when other therapies are not available. Approval of drugs for marketing under these regulations is based upon a demonstrated effect on a surrogate endpoint that is likely to predict clinical benefit.

Approval of this indication is based upon **Synercid's** ability to clear VREF from the bloodstream, with clearance of bacteremia considered to be a surrogate endpoint. There are no results from well-controlled clinical studies that confirm the validity of this surrogate marker. However, a study to verify the clinical benefit of therapy with **Synercid** on traditional clinical endpoints (such as cure of the underlying infection) is presently underway.

Complicated skin and skin structure infections caused by Staphylococcus aureus (methicillin susceptible) or Streptococcus pyogenes. (See CLINICAL STUDIES.)

CONTRAINDICATIONS

Synercid is contraindicated in patients with known hypersensitivity to **Synercid**, or with prior hypersensitivity to other streptogramins (e.g., pristinamycin or virginiamycin).

WARNINGS

Drug Interactions: In vitro drug interaction studies have demonstrated that **Synercid** significantly inhibits cytochrome P450 3A4 metabolism of cyclosporin A, midazolam, nifedipine and terfenadine. In addition, 24 subjects given **Synercid** 7.5 mg/kg q8h for 2 days and 300 mg of cyclosporine on day 3 showed an increase of 63% in the AUC of cyclosporine, an increase of 30% in the C_{max} of cyclosporine, a 77% increase in the $t_{1/2}$ of cyclosporine, and, a decrease of 34% in the clearance of cyclosporine. **Therapeutic level monitoring of cyclosporine should be performed when cyclosporine must be used concomitantly with Synercid.**

It is reasonable to expect that the concomitant administration of Synercid and other drugs primarily metabolized by the cytochrome P450 3A4 enzyme system may likely result in increased plasma concentrations of these drugs that could increase or prolong their therapeutic effect and/or increase adverse reactions. (See Table below.) Therefore, coadministration of Synercid with drugs which are cytochrome P450 3A4 substrates and possess a narrow therapeutic window requires caution and monitoring of these drugs (e.g., cyclosporine), whenever possible. Concomitant medications metabolized by the cytochrome P450 3A4 enzyme system that may prolong the QTc interval should be avoided.

Concomitant administration of **Synercid** and nifedipine (repeated oral doses) and midazolam (intravenous bolus dose) in healthy volunteers led to elevated plasma concentrations of these drugs. The C_{max} increased by 18% and 14% (median values) and the AUC increased by 44% and 33% for nifedipine and midazolam, respectively.

Table of Selected Drugs That Are Predicted to Have Plasma Concentrations Increased by **Synercid** +

Antihistamines: astemizole, terfenadine
Anti-HIV (NNRTIs and Protease inhibitors): delavirdine, nevirapine, indinavir, ritonavir
Antineoplastic agents: vinca alkaloids (e.g., vinblastine), docetaxel, paclitaxel
Benzodiazepines: midazolam, diazepam
Calcium channel blockers: dihydropyridines (e.g., nifedipine), verapamil, diltiazem
Cholesterol-lowering agents: HMG-CoA reductase inhibitors (e.g., lovastatin)
GI motility agents: cisapride
Immunosuppressive agents: cyclosporine, tacrolimus
Steroids: methylprednisolone
Other: carbamazepine, quinidine, lidocaine, disopyramide

+ This list of drugs is not all inclusive.

Pseudomembranous colitis has been reported with nearly all antibacterial agents, including Synercid, and may range in severity from mild to life-threatening. Therefore, it is important to consider this diagnosis in patients who present with diarrhea subsequent to the administration of antibacterial agents.

Treatment with antibacterial agents alters the normal flora of the colon and may permit overgrowth of clostridia. Studies indicate that a toxin produced by Clostridium difficile is one primary cause of "antibiotic-associated colitis".

After the diagnosis of pseudomembranous colitis has been established, therapeutic measures should be initiated. Mild cases usually respond to drug discontinuation alone. In moderate to severe cases, consideration should be given to management with fluids and electrolytes, protein supplementation and treatment with an antibacterial drug clinically effective against C. difficile colitis.

PRECAUTIONS

General: Venous Irritation: Following completion of a peripheral infusion, the vein should be flushed with 5% Dextrose in Water solution to minimize venous irritation. **DO NOT FLUSH** with saline or heparin **after Synercid** administration because of incompatibility concerns.

If moderate to severe venous irritation occurs following peripheral administration of **Synercid** diluted in 250 mL of Dextrose 5% in water, consideration should be given to increasing the infusion volume to 500 or 750 mL, changing the infusion site, or infusing by a peripherally inserted central catheter (PICC) or a central venous catheter. In clinical trials, concomitant administration of hydrocortisone or diphenhydramine did not appear to alleviate venous pain or inflammation.

Rate of Infusion: In animal studies toxicity was higher when **Synercid** was administered as a bolus compared to slow infusion. However, the safety of an intravenous bolus of **Synercid** has not been studied in humans. Clinical trial experience has been exclusively with an intravenous duration of 60 minutes and, thus, other infusion rates cannot be recommended.

Arthralgias/Myalgias: Episodes of arthralgia and myalgia, some severe, have been reported in patients treated with **Synercid**. In some patients, improvement has been noted with a reduction in dose frequency to q12h. In those patients available for follow-up, treatment discontinuation has been followed by resolution of symptoms. The etiology of these myalgias and arthralgias is under investigation.

Superinfections: The use of antibiotics may promote the overgrowth of nonsusceptible organisms. Should superinfection occur during therapy, appropriate measures should be taken.

Hyperbilirubinemia: Elevations of total bilirubin greater than 5 times the upper limit of normal were noted in approximately 25% of patients in the non-comparative studies. (See **Clinical Studies**: **Non-Comparative Trials**.) In some patients, isolated hyperbilirubinemia (primarily conjugated) can occur during treatment, possibly resulting from competition between **Synercid** and bilirubin for excretion. Of note, in the comparative trials, elevations in ALT and AST occurred at a similar frequency in both the **Synercid** and comparator groups.

Drug Interactions: In vitro drug interaction studies have shown that **Synercid** significantly inhibits cytochrome P450 3A4. (See **Warnings**.)

Synercid does not significantly inhibit human cytochrome P450 1A2, 2A6, 2C9, 2C19, 2D6, or 2E1. Therefore, clinical interactions with drugs metabolized by these cytochrome P450 isoenzymes are not expected.

A drug interaction between **Synercid** and digoxin cannot be excluded but is unlikely to occur via CYP3A4 enzyme inhibition. **Synercid** has shown in vitro activity (MICs of 0.25 mcg/mL when tested on two strains) against Eubacterium lentum. Digoxin is metabolized in part by bacteria in the gut and as such, a drug interaction based on **Synercid's** inhibition of digoxin's gut metabolism (by Eubacterium lentum) may be possible.

In vitro combination testing of **Synercid** with aztreonam, ceftotaxime, ciprofloxacin, and gentamicin, against Enterobacteriaceae and Pseudomonas aeruginosa did not show antagonism.

In vitro combination testing of **Synercid** with prototype drugs of the following classes: aminoglycosides (gentamicin), β-lactams (cefepime, ampicillin, and amoxicillin), glycopeptides (vancomycin), quinolones (ciprofloxacin), tetracyclines (doxycycline) and also chloramphenicol against enterococci and staphylococci did not show antagonism.

Carcinogenesis, Mutagenesis, Impairment of Fertility: Long-term carcinogenicity studies in animals have not been conducted with **Synercid**. Five genetic toxicity tests were performed. **Synercid**, dalfopristin, and quinupristin were tested in the bacterial reverse mutation assay, the Chinese hamster ovary cell HGPRT gene mutation assay, the unscheduled DNA synthesis assay in rat hepatocytes, the Chinese hamster ovary cell chromosome aberration assay, and the mouse micronucleus assay in bone marrow. Dalfopristin was associated with the production of structural chromosome aberrations when tested in the Chinese hamster ovary cell chromosome aberration assay. **Synercid** and quinupristin were negative in this assay. **Synercid**, dalfopristin, and quinupristin were all negative in the other four genetic toxicity assays.

No impairment of fertility or perinatal/postnatal development was observed in rats at doses up to 12 to 18 mg/kg (approximately 0.3 to 0.4 times the human dose based on body-surface area).

Pregnancy: Teratogenic Effects: Pregnancy Category B: Reproductive studies have been performed in mice at doses up to 40 mg/kg/day (approximately half the human dose based on body-surface area), in rats at doses up to 120 mg/kg/day (approximately 2.5 times the human dose based on body-surface area), and in rabbits at doses up to 12 mg/kg/day (approximately half the human dose based on body-surface area) and have revealed no evidence of impaired fertility or harm to the fetus due to **Synercid**.

There are, however, no adequate and well-controlled studies with **Synercid** in pregnant women. Because animal reproduction studies are not always predictive of the human response, this drug should be used during pregnancy only if clearly needed.

Nursing Mothers: In lactating rats, **Synercid** was excreted in milk. It is not known whether **Synercid** is excreted in human breast milk. Because many drugs are excreted in human milk, caution should be exercised when **Synercid** is administered to a nursing woman.

Hepatic Insufficiency: Following a single 1-hour infusion of **Synercid** (7.5 mg/kg) to patients with hepatic insufficiency, plasma concentrations were significantly increased. (See **Clinical Pharmacology**: **Special Populations**.) However, the effect of dose reduction or increase in dosing interval on the pharmacokinetics of **Synercid** in these patients has not

Continued on next page

Synercid—Cont.

been studied. Therefore, no recommendations can be made at this time regarding the appropriate dose modification.

Pediatric Use: **Synercid** has been used in a limited number of pediatric patients under emergency-use conditions at a dose of 7.5 mg/kg q8h or q12h. However, the safety and effectiveness of **Synercid** in patients under 16 years of age have not been established.

Geriatric Use: In phase 3 comparative trials of **Synercid**, 37% of patients (n=404) were ≥65 years of age, of which 145 were ≥75 years of age. In the phase 3 non-comparative trials, 29% of patients (n=346) were ≥65 years of age, of which 112 were ≥75 years of age. There were no apparent differences in the frequency, type, or severity of related adverse reactions including cardiovascular events between elderly and younger individuals.

ADVERSE REACTIONS

The safety of **Synercid** was evaluated in 1099 patients enrolled in 5 comparative clinical trials. Additionally, 4 non-comparative clinical trials (3 prospective and 1 retrospective in design) were conducted in which 1199 patients received **Synercid** for infections due to Gram-positive pathogens for which no other treatment option was available. In non-comparative trials, the patients were severely ill, often with multiple co-morbidities or physiological impairments, and may have been intolerant to or failed other antibacterial therapies.

Comparative Trials

Adverse Reaction Summary—All Comparative Studies

Safety data are available from five comparative clinical studies (n= 1099 **Synercid**; n= 1095 comparator). One of the deaths in the comparative studies was assessed as possibly related to **Synercid**. The most frequent reasons for discontinuation due to drug-related adverse reactions were as follows:

Type	% Of Patients Discontinuing Therapy By Reaction Type	
	Synercid	Comparator
Venous	9.2	2.0
Non-venous	9.6	4.3
-Rash	1.0	0.5
-Nausea	0.9	0.6
-Vomiting	0.5	0.5
-Pain	0.5	0.0
-Pruritus	0.5	0.3

Clinical Reactions—All Comparative Studies

Adverse reactions with an incidence of ≥1% and possibly or probably related to **Synercid** administration include:

Adverse Reactions	% of patients with adverse reactions	
	Synercid	Comparator
Inflammation at infusion site	42.0	25.0
Pain at infusion site	40.0	23.7
Edema at infusion site	17.3	9.5
Infusion site reaction	13.4	10.1
Nausea	4.6	7.2
Thrombophlebitis	2.4	0.3
Diarrhea	2.7	3.2
Vomiting	2.7	3.8
Rash	2.5	1.4
Headache	1.6	0.9
Pruritus	1.5	1.1
Pain	1.5	0.1

Additional adverse reactions that were possibly or probably related to **Synercid** with an incidence less than 1% within each body system are listed below:

Body as a Whole: abdominal pain, worsening of underlying illness, allergic reaction, chest pain, fever, infection;

Cardiovascular: palpitation, phlebitis;

Digestive: constipation, dyspepsia, oral moniliasis, pancreatitis, pseudomembranous enterocolitis, stomatitis;

Metabolic: gout, peripheral edema;

Musculoskeletal: arthralgia, myalgia, myasthenia;

Nervous: anxiety, confusion, dizziness, hypertonia, insomnia, leg cramps, paresthesia, vasodilation;

Respiratory: dyspnea, pleural effusion;

Skin and Appendages: maculopapular rash, sweating, urticaria;

Urogenital: hematuria, vaginitis

Clinical Reactions—Skin And Skin Structure Studies

In two of the five comparative clinical trials **Synercid** (n=450) and comparator regimens (e.g., oxacillin/vancomycin or cefazolin/vancomycin; n=443) were studied for safety and efficacy in the treatment of complicated skin and skin structure infections. The adverse event profile seen in the **Synercid** patients in these two studies differed significantly from that seen in the other comparative studies. What follows is safety data from these two studies.

Discontinuation of therapy was most frequently due to the following drug related events:

Type	% of patients discontinuing therapy by reaction type	
	Synercid	Comparator
Venous	12.0	2.0
Non-venous	11.8	4.0
-Rash	2.0	0.9
-Nausea	1.1	0.0
-Vomiting	0.9	0.0
-Pain	0.9	0.0
-Pruritus	0.9	0.5

Venous adverse events were seen predominately in patients who had peripheral infusions. The most frequently reported venous and non-venous adverse reactions possibly or probably related to study drug were:

	% of patients with adverse reactions	
	Synercid	Comparator
Venous	68.0	32.7
-Pain at infusion site	44.7	17.8
-Inflammation at infusion site	38.2	14.7
-Edema at infusion site	18.0	7.2
-Infusion site reaction	11.6	3.6
Non-venous	24.7	13.1
-Nausea	4.0	2.0
-Vomiting	3.7	1.0
-Rash	3.1	1.3
-Pain	3.1	0.2

There were eight (1.7%) episodes of thrombus or thrombophlebitis in the **Synercid** arms and none in the comparator arms.

Laboratory Events—All Comparative Studies

The following table shows the number (%) of patients exhibiting laboratory values above or below the clinically relevant "critical" values during treatment phase (with an incidence of 0.1% or greater in either treatment group).

[See table below]

Non-Comparative Trials

Clinical Adverse Reactions

Approximately one-third of patients discontinued therapy in these trials due to adverse events. However, the discontinuation rate due to adverse reactions assessed by the investigator as possibly or probably related to **Synercid** therapy was approximately 5.0%.

There were three prospectively designed non-comparative clinical trials in patients (n = 972) treated with **Synercid**. One of these studies (301), had more complete documentation than the other two (398A and 398B). The most common events probably or possibly related to therapy were:

Adverse Reactions	% of patients with adverse reaction		
	Study 301	Study 398A	Study 398B
Arthralgia	7.8	5.2	4.3
Myalgia	5.1	0.95	3.1
Arthralgia and Myalgia	7.4	3.3	6.8
Nausea	3.8	2.8	4.9

The percentage of patients who experienced severe related arthralgia and myalgia was 3.3% and 3.1%, respectively. The percentage of patients who discontinued treatment due to related arthralgia and myalgia was 2.3% and 1.8%, respectively.

Laboratory Events

The most frequently observed abnormalities in laboratory studies were in total and conjugated bilirubin, with increases greater than 5 times upper limit of normal, irrespective of relationship to **Synercid**, reported in 25.0% and 34.6% of patients, respectively. The percentage of patients who discontinued treatment due to increased total and conjugated bilirubin was 2.7% and 2.3%, respectively. Of note, 46.5% and 59.0% of patients had high baseline total and conjugated bilirubin levels before study entry.

Other

Serious adverse reactions in clinical trials, including non-comparative studies, considered possibly or probably related to **Synercid** administration with an incidence <0.1% include: acidosis, anaphylactoid reaction, apnea, arrhythmia, bone pain, cerebral hemorrhage, cerebrovascular accident, coagulation disorder, convulsion, dysautonomia, encephalopathy, grand mal convulsion, hemolysis, hemolytic anemia, heart arrest, hepatitis, hypoglycemia, hyponatremia, hypoplastic anemia, hypoventilation, hypovolemia, hypoxia, jaundice, mesenteric arterial occlusion, neck rigidity, neuropathy, pancytopenia, paraplegia, pericardial effusion, pericarditis, respiratory distress syndrome, shock, skin ulcer, supraventricular tachycardia, syncope, tremor, ventricular extrasystoles and ventricular fibrillation. Cases of hypotension and gastrointestinal hemorrhage were reported in less than 0.2% of patients.

Post-marketing Experiences: In addition to adverse events reported from clinical trials, reports of angioedema and anaphylactic shock have been identified during post approval use of **Synercid**.

OVERDOSAGE

There are four reports of patients receiving **Synercid** doses at up to three times that recommended (7.5 mg/kg). No adverse events were considered possibly or probably related to **Synercid** overdose. Signs of acute overdosage may include dyspnea, emesis, tremors, and ataxia as seen in animals given extremely high doses (50 mg/kg) of **Synercid**. Patients who receive an overdose should be carefully observed and given supportive treatment. **Synercid** is not removed by peritoneal dialysis or by hemodialysis.

DOSAGE AND ADMINISTRATION

Synercid should be administered by intravenous infusion in 5% Dextrose in Water solution over a 60-minute period. (See **Warnings**.) The recommended dosage for the treatment of infections is described in the table below. An infusion pump or device may be used to control the rate of infusion. If necessary, central venous access (e.g., PICC) can be used to administer **Synercid** to decrease the incidence of venous irritation.

	Dose
Vancomycin-Resistant Enterococcus faecium	7.5 mg/kg q8h
Complicated Skin and Skin Structure Infection	7.5 mg/kg q12h

The minimum recommended treatment duration for Complicated Skin and Skin Structure Infections is seven days. For Vancomycin-Resistant Enterococcus faecium infection, the treatment duration should be determined based on the site and severity of the infection.

Special Populations: Elderly: No dosage adjustment of **Synercid** is required for use in the elderly. (See **Clinical Pharmacology: Pharmacokinetics and Precautions: Geriatric Use.**)

Renal Insuffiency: No dosage adjustment of **Synercid** is required for use in patients with renal impairment or patients undergoing peritoneal dialysis. (See **Clinical Pharmacology: Pharmacokinetics.**)

Hepatic Insuffiency: Data from clinical trials of **Synercid** suggest that the incidence of adverse effects in patients with chronic liver insufficiency or cirrhosis was comparable to that in patients with normal hepatic function. Pharmacokinetic data in patients with hepatic cirrhosis (Child Pugh A or B) suggest that dosage reduction may be necessary but exact recommendations cannot be made at this time. (See **Clinical Pharmacology: Special Populations** and **Precautions: General:** *Hepatic Insufficiency* sections.)

Pediatric Patients (less than 16 years of age): Based on a limited number of pediatric patients treated under emergency-use conditions, no dosage adjustment of **Synercid** is required. (See **Precautions: Pediatric Use.**)

Preparation and Administration of Solution:

1. Reconstitute the 500 mg single dose vial by slowly adding 5 mL of 5% Dextrose in Water or Sterile Water for injection. Reconstitute the 600 mg single dose vial by slowly adding

Parameter	Critically High or Low Value	Synercid Critically High or Low	Comparator Critically High or Low
AST	> 10 × ULN	9 (0.9)	2 (0.2)
ALT	> 10 × ULN	4 (0.4)	4 (0.4)
Total Bilirubin	> 5 × ULN	9 (0.9)	2 (0.2)
Conjugated Bilirubin	> 5 × ULN	29 (3.1)	12 (1.3)
LDH	> 5 × ULN	10 (2.6)	8 (2.1)
Alk Phosphatase	> 5 × ULN	3 (0.3)	7 (0.7)
Gamma-GT	> 10 × ULN	19 (1.9)	10 (1.0)
CPK	> 10 × ULN	6 (1.6)	5 (1.4)
Creatinine	≥ 440 μmol/L	1 (0.1)	1 (0.1)
BUN	≥ 35.5 mmol/L	2 (0.3)	9 (1.2)
Blood Glucose	> 22.2 mmol/L	11 (1.3)	11 (1.3)
	< 2.2 mmol/L	1 (0.1)	1 (0.1)
Bicarbonates	> 40 mmol/L	2 (0.3)	3 (0.5)
	< 10 mmol/L	3 (0.5)	3 (0.5)
CO_2	> 50 mmol/L	0 (0.0)	0 (0.0)
	< 15 mmol/L	1 (0.2)	0 (0.0)
Sodium	> 160 mmol/L	0 (0.0)	0 (0.0)
	< 120 mmol/L	5 (0.5)	3 (0.3)
Potassium	> 6.0 mmol/L	3 (0.3)	6 (0.6)
	< 2.0 mmol/L	0 (0.0)	1 (0.1)
Hemoglobin	< 8 g/dL	25 (2.6)	16 (1.6)
Hematocrit	> 60%	2 (0.2)	0 (0.0)
Platelets	> 1,000,000/mm³	2 (0.2)	2 (0.2)
	< 50,000/mm³	6 (0.6)	7 (0.7)

Y-Site Injection Compatibility of Synercid at 2 mg/mL Concentration

Admixture and Concentration	IV Infusion Solutions for Admixture
Aztreonam 20 mg/mL	D5W
Ciprofloxacin 1 mg/mL	D5W
Fluconazole 2 mg/mL	Used as the undiluted solution
Haloperidol 0.2 mg/mL	D5W
Metoclopramide 5 mg/mL	D5W
Potassium Chloride 40 mEq/L	D5W

D5W = 5% Dextrose Injection

NDC 61570-260-10	**Synercid** IV 500 mg	150 mg quinupristin and 350 mg dalfoptistin	10 vials
NDC 61570-261-10	**Synercid** IV 600 mg	180 mg quinupristin and 420 mg dalfoptistin	10 vials

6 mL of 5% Dextrose in Water or Sterile Water for injection.
2. **GENTLY** swirl the vial by manual rotation without shaking to ensure dissolution of contents while **LIMITING FOAM FORMATION.**
3. Allow the solution to sit for a few minutes until all the foam has disappeared. The resulting solution should be clear. Vials reconstituted in this manner will give a solution of 100 mg/mL **CAUTION: FURTHER DILUTION REQUIRED BEFORE INFUSION.**
4. According to the patient's weight, the reconstituted **Synercid solution** should be added to 250 mL of 5% Dextrose solution. An infusion volume of 100 mL may be used for central line infusions.
5. If moderate to severe venous irritation occurs following peripheral administration of **Synercid** diluted in 250 mL of Dextrose 5% in water, consideration should be given to increasing the infusion volume to 500 or 750 mL, changing the infusion site, or infusing by a peripherally inserted central catheter (PICC) or a central venous catheter.
6. The desired dose should be administered by intravenous infusion over 60 minutes.

NOTE: As for other parenteral drug products, **Synercid** should be inspected visually for particulate matter prior to administration.

COMPATIBILITY:

Do Not Dilute With Saline Solutions Because Synercid Is Not Compatible With These Agents. Synercid should not be mixed with, or physically added to, other drugs except for the following drugs where compatibility by Y-site injection has been established:
[See first table above]

If **Synercid** is to be given concomitantly with another drug, each drug should be given separately in accordance with the recommended dosage and route of administration for each drug.

With intermittent infusion of **Synercid** and other drugs through a common intravenous line, the line should be flushed before and after administration with 5% Dextrose in Water solution.

Stability and Storage: Before Reconstitution: The unopened vials should be stored in a refrigerator at 2 to 8°C (36 to 46°F).

Reconstituted and Infusions Solutions: Because **Synercid** contains no antibacterial preservative, it should be reconstituted under strict aseptic conditions (e.g., Laminar Air Flow Hood). The reconstituted solution should be diluted within 30 minutes. Vials are for single use. The storage time of the diluted solution should be as short as possible to minimize the risk of microbial contamination. Stability of the diluted solution prior to the infusion is established as 5 hours at room temperature or 54 hours if stored under refrigeration 2 to 8°C (36 to 46°F). The solution should not be frozen.

HOW SUPPLIED

Synercid is supplied as a sterile lyophilized pyrogen-free preparation in single-dose 10 mL type I glass vials with gray elastomeric closure, and aluminum seal with a dark blue flip-off cap for the 500 mg vial and a red flip-offcap for the 600 mg vial.
[See second table above]

CLINICAL STUDIES

Non-Comparative Trials

In the non-comparative trials, patients often presented with multiple co-morbidities and/or physiologic impairments, and may have been intolerant to or failed other antibacterial therapies.

Vancomycin-Resistant Enterococcus Faecium

Results are available from four non-comparative studies of **Synercid** (7.5 mg/kg q8h) for the treatment of vancomycin-resistant Enterococcus faecium (VREF) (N=1222). Three of these studies were prospective, the fourth consisted of a collection of individual emergency-use requests.

Of the 1222 patients, 27% did not have a specific site of infection identified, but presented with pure growth of VREF in two or more blood cultures. Ninety percent (90%) of these patients had clearance of their VREF bacteremia within the first 48 to 72 hours of therapy.

Because of the emergency use nature of the VREF trials and the variability in data collection in these severely ill patients, the percentage of patients found to be evaluable was 24.4%. The overall efficacy rate (defined as clinical success and eradication of the initial pathogen) in the evaluable patients (n=298) was 52.3%. The most common sites of infection included intra-abdominal, skin and skin structure, and the urinary tract. In these subgroups, the efficacy rates for the evaluable patients having the most complete documentation were 46.3% (n=67), 66.7% (n=15), and 73.9% (n=23), respectively.

The most common adverse reactions considered related to **Synercid** use were myalgias and arthralgias. (See **ADVERSE REACTIONS**.) All-cause mortality in the 4 studies ranged from 49.5% to 54.0%.

Comparative Trials

Complicated Skin and Skin Structure Infections

Two randomized, open-label, controlled clinical trials of **Synercid** (7.5 mg/kg q12h intravenously [iv]) in the treatment of complicated skin and skin structure infections were performed. The comparator drug was oxacillin (2g q6h iv) in the first study (JRV 304) and cefazolin (1g q8h iv) in the second study (JRV 305); however, in both studies vancomycin (1g q12h iv) could be substituted for the specified comparator if the causative pathogen was suspected or confirmed methicillin-resistant staphylococcus or if the patient was allergic to penicillins, cephalosporins or carbapenems. Study JRV 304 enrolled 450 patients (n = 229 **Synercid**; n= 221 Comparator) and Study JRV 305 enrolled 443 patients (n = 221 **Synercid**; n = 222 Comparator).

In the first study, 105 patients (45.9%) and 106 patients (48.0%) in the **Synercid** and Comparator arms, respectively, were found to be clinically evaluable. For the second study, these values were 113 (51.1%) and 120 (54.1%) patients in the **Synercid** and Comparator arms, respectively. Patients were found not to be clinically evaluable for reasons such as: wrong diagnosis, lower extremity infection in patients with diabetes or peripheral vascular disease since these infections were assumed to include aerobic gram-negative and anaerobic organisms, no specimen for culture obtained, insufficient therapy, no test of cure assessment, etc.

For the patients found to be clinically evaluable, in Study JRV 304 the success rate was 49.5% in the **Synercid** arm and 51.9% in the Comparator arm. In Study JRV 305, the success rates were 66.4% and 64.2% in the **Synercid** and Comparator arms, respectively.

The following table shows the clinical success rate (combined results from two clinical trials) in the clinically evaluable population. Due to the small numbers of patients in the subsets, statistical conclusions could not be reached.

Infection Type	Cured or Improved Synercid (n/N) (%)	Cured or Improved Comparator (n/N) (%)
Erysipelas (cellulitis)	52/82 (63.4)	43/77 (55.8)
Post-operative infections	14/38 (36.8)	24/42 (57.1)
Traumatic wound infection	33/55 (60.0)	33/55 (60.0)

Safety

Discontinuations of therapy because of adverse reactions which were probably or possibly due to drug therapy occurred more than four times as often in the **Synercid** group than in the comparator group. Approximately half of the discontinuations in the **Synercid** arm were due to venous adverse events. (See **ADVERSE REACTIONS: Clinical Reactions: Skin and Skin Structure Studies.**)

Keep out of the reach of children.

REFERENCES

1. National Committee for Clinical Laboratory Standards, Methods for Dilution Antimicrobial Susceptibility Tests for Bacteria that Grow Aerobically - Fourth Edition; Approved Standard. NCCLS Document M7-A4 (ISBN 1-56238-309-4). NCCLS, 940 West Valley Road, Suite 1400, Wayne, PA 19087-1898, 1997.
2. National Committee for Clinical Laboratory Standards, Performance Standards for Antimicrobial Disk Susceptibility Tests - Sixth Edition; Approved Standard. NCCLS document M2-A6 (ISBN 1-56238-308-6). NCCLS, 940 West Valley Road, Suite 1400, Wayne, PA 19087-1898, 1997.

Monarch Pharmaceuticals®

Distributed by: Monarch Pharmaceuticals, Inc., Bristol, TN 37620

Manufactured by: DSM Pharmaceuticals, Inc., Greenville, NC 27834

595454 Prescribing Information as of July 2003

Shown in Product Identification Guide, page 320

THROMBIN, TOPICAL U.S.P. ℞

(BOVINE ORIGIN)

[thrŏm-bĭn]

THROMBIN-JMI®

Thrombin, Topical (Bovine) must not be injected! Apply on the surface of bleeding tissue.

DESCRIPTION

The thrombin in Thrombin, Topical (Bovine Origin) THROMBIN-JMI® is a protein substance produced through a conversion reaction in which prothrombin of bovine origin is activated by tissue thromboplastin of bovine origin in the presence of calcium chloride. It is supplied as a sterile powder that has been freeze-dried in the final container. Also contained in the preparation are mannitol and sodium chloride. Mannitol is included to make the dried product friable and more readily soluble. The material contains no preservative.

THROMBIN-JMI® has been chromatographically purified.

CLINICAL PHARMACOLOGY

THROMBIN-JMI® requires no intermediate physiological agent for its action. It clots the fibrinogen of the blood directly. Failure to clot blood occurs in the rare case where the primary clotting defect is the absence of fibrinogen itself. The speed with which thrombin clots blood is dependent upon the concentration of both thrombin and fibrinogen.

INDICATIONS AND USAGE

THROMBIN-JMI® is indicated as an aid to hemostasis whenever oozing blood and minor bleeding from capillaries and small venules is accessible.

In various types of surgery, solutions of THROMBIN-JMI® may be used in conjunction with an Absorbable Gelatin Sponge, USP for hemostasis, or any medical device approved by FDA for an indicated use with a specified, approved dosage of Thrombin, Topical (Bovine Origin).

CONTRAINDICATIONS

THROMBIN-JMI® is contraindicated in persons known to be sensitive to any of its components and/or to material of bovine origin.

WARNING

The use of topical bovine thrombin preparations has occasionally been associated with abnormalities in hemostasis ranging from asymptomatic alterations in laboratory determinations, such as prothrombin time (PT) and partial thromboplastin time (PTT), to severe bleeding or thrombosis which rarely have been fatal. These hemostatic effects appear to be related to the formation of antibodies against bovine thrombin and/or factor V which in some cases may cross react with human factor V, potentially resulting in factor V deficency. Repeated clinical applications of topical bovine thrombin increase the likelihood that antibodies against thrombin and/or factor V may be formed. Consultation with an expert in coagulation disorders is recommended if a patient exhibits abnormal coagulation laboratory values, abnormal bleeding, or abnormal thrombosis following the use of topical thrombin. Any interventions should consider the immunologic basis of this condition. Patients with antibodies to bovine thrombin preparations should not be re-exposed to these products.

Because of its action in the clotting mechanism, THROMBIN-JMI® must not be injected or otherwise allowed to enter large blood vessels. Extensive intravascular clotting and even death may result.

PRECAUTIONS

General—Consult the Absorbable Gelatin Sponge, USP labeling for complete information for use prior to utilizing the thrombin saturated sponge procedure.

Pregnancy—Category C—Animal reproduction studies have not been conducted with THROMBIN-JMI®. It is also not known whether THROMBIN-JMI® can cause fetal harm when administered to a pregnant woman or can affect reproduction capacity. THROMBIN-JMI® should be given to a pregnant woman only if clearly indicated.

Pediatric Use—Safety and effectiveness in children have not been established.

ADVERSE REACTIONS

Allergic reactions may be encountered in persons known to be sensitive to bovine materials. Inhibitory antibodies which interfere with hemostasis may develop in a small percentage of patients. See Warning.

DOSAGE AND ADMINISTRATION

Solutions of Thrombin, Topical (Bovine Origin), USP, THROMBIN-JMI® may be reconstituted with sterile isotonic saline at a recommended concentration of 1,000 to 2,000 U.S. units/mL. Where bleeding is profuse, as from abraided surfaces of liver or spleen, concentrations of 1,000 U.S. units per mL may be required. For general use in plastic surgery, dental extractions, skin grafting, etc. solutions containing approximately 100 U.S. units/mL are frequently used. Intermediate strengths to suit the needs of the case may be prepared by diluting the contents of the THROMBIN-JMI® container with an appropriate volume of sterile isotonic saline. In many situations, it may be advantageous to use THROMBIN-JMI® in a dry form on oozing surfaces.

In instances where a concentration of approximately 1,000 units/mL is desired, the contents of the vial of sterile isotonic saline diluent may be transferred into the

Continued on next page

Thrombin/Thrombin-JMI—Cont.

THROMBIN-JMI® container with a sterile syringe or sterile transfer needle. If the transfer needle is used for reconstitution, transfer the diluent in the following manner.
1. Remove the plastic cap off of the diluent vial.
2. Twist the clear plastic cover on the transfer needle and remove.
3. Insert the exposed needle into the diaphragm of the diluent vial.
4. Flip the plastic cover up on the THROMBIN-JMI® container. DO NOT REMOVE THE COVER AND ALUMINUM SEAL.
5. Remove the pink plastic cap from the transfer needle exposing the needle.
6. Invert the vial of diluent and insert the exposed needle into the diaphragm of the THROMBIN-JMI® container.

THROMBIN-JMI® SPRAY KIT
Each spray kit contains one vial of THROMBIN-JMI® and one spray pump and actuator.
1. Remove the outer lid by pulling up at the indicated edge. The inner tray is sterile and suitable for introduction into any operating field.
2. Remove the cover on inner tray to expose sterile contents.
3. Reconstitute the THROMBIN-JMI® to desired potency by introducing sterile isotonic saline with a sterile syringe or a sterile transfer needle. If the transfer needle is used, follow the previously described procedure.
4. When the THROMBIN-JMI® is completely dissolved, open vial by flipping up metal and tearing counterclockwise.
5. Remove the rubber diaphragm from vial. Remove pump with protective cap from tray and snap onto vial. Remove protective cap and attach actuator.
6. To spray, hold vial upright or at a slight angle. Several strokes of the pump will be required to expel the solution.
7. Discard unused contents and pump: DO NOT TRANSFER SPRAY PUMP TO ANOTHER VIAL.

THROMBIN-JMI® SYRINGE SPRAY KIT
Each syringe kit contains one vial of THROMBIN-JMI® and one spray tip and syringe.
1. Remove the outer lid by pulling up at the indicated edge. The inner tray is sterile and suitable for introduction into any operating field.
2. Remove the cover on the inner tray to expose sterile contents.
3. Using the sterile syringe equipped with a needle, draw the desired amount of saline diluent from the vial into the syringe.
4. Inject the saline diluent into the THROMBIN-JMI® thrombin vial from the syringe to reconstitute the THROMBIN-JMI® thrombin powder.
5. When the THROMBIN-JMI® powder is completely dissolved, draw the THROMBIN-JMI® Thrombin solution into the syringe.
6. Replace the needle guard.
7. Turn needle guard counterclockwise and remove and discard the needle.
8. Affix spray tip by pushing down and turning clockwise until the spray tip locks in place.
9. To spray, depress the syringe plunger in a normal fashion to dispense the THROMBIN-JMI® Thrombin solution through the tip in a fine spray.
10. Discard unused contents and syringe.

CAUTION: Solutions should be used promptly upon removal from the container. However, the solution may be refrigerated at 2–8°C for up to three hours.
The following techniques are suggested for the topical application of THROMBIN-JMI®.
1. The recipient surface should be sponged (not wiped) free of blood before THROMBIN-JMI® is applied.
2. A spray may be used or the surface may be flooded using a sterile syringe and small gauge needle. The most effective hemostasis results occur when the THROMBIN-JMI® mixes freely with the blood as soon as it reaches the surface.
3. Sponging of the treated surfaces should be avoided to assure that the clot remains securely in place.

THROMBIN-JMI® may be used in conjunction with Absorbable Gelatin Sponge, USP as follows:
1. Prepare THROMBIN-JMI® solution to desired strength.
2. Immerse sponge strips of the desired size in THROMBIN-JMI® solution. Knead the sponge strips vigorously with moistened, gloved fingers to remove trapped air, thereby facilitating saturation of the sponge.
3. Apply saturated sponge to bleeding area. Hold in place with a pledget of cotton or a small gauze sponge until hemostasis occurs.

HOW SUPPLIED
THROMBIN-JMI® is supplied in the following packages:
NDC 052604-7100-1
1,000 U.S. unit vial.
NDC 052604-7102-1
5,000 U.S. unit vial with 5 mL diluent.
NDC 052604-7104-3
10,000 U.S. unit vial with 10 mL diluent.
NDC 052604-7105-3
20,000 U.S. unit vial with 20 mL diluent.
NDC 052604-7106-1
50,000 U.S. unit vial.
THROMBIN-JMI® Spray Kit is supplied in the following packages:
NDC 052604-7102-2
5,000 U.S. unit vial with 5 mL diluent, spray pump and actuator.
NDC 052604-7104-2
10,000 U.S. unit vial with 10 mL diluent, spray pump and actuator.
NDC 052604-7105-2
20,000 U.S. unit vial with 20 mL diluent, spray pump and actuator.
THROMBIN-JMI® Syringe Spray Kit is supplied in the following packages:
NDC 052604-7354-2
10,000 U.S. unit vial with 10 mL diluent, spray tip and syringe.
NDC 052604-7355-2
20,000 U.S. unit vial with 20 mL diluent, spray tip and syringe.

STORAGE
Store 1,000 unit vial THROMBIN, TOPICAL (Bovine) THROMBIN-JMI® at 2–8°C (36–46°F). Store 5,000, 10,000, 20,000 and 50,000 unit/vial sizes of THROMBIN-JMI® at 2–25°C (36–77°F).

Distributed By:
JONES PHARMA INCORPORATED
(a wholly owned subsidiary of King Pharmaceuticals, Inc.)
St. Louis, MO
Manufactured by:
GenTrac, Incorporated
Middleton, Wisconsin 53562
U.S. License No. 977
Rev. 9/00

Shown in Product Identification Guide, page 320

TRIOSTAT® ℞
[trī-ō-stăt]
brand of liothyronine sodium injection (T_3)

DESCRIPTION
Thyroid hormone drugs are natural or synthetic preparations containing tetraiodothyronine (T_4, levothyroxine) sodium or triiodothyronine (T_3, liothyronine) sodium or both. T_4 and T_3 are produced in the human thyroid gland by the iodination and coupling of the amino acid tyrosine. T_4 contains four iodine atoms and is formed by the coupling of two molecules of diiodotyrosine (DIT). T_3 contains three atoms of iodine and is formed by the coupling of one molecule of DIT with one molecule of monoiodotyrosine (MIT). Both hormones are stored in the thyroid colloid as thyroglobulin and released into the circulation. The major source of T_3 has been shown to be peripheral deiodination of T_4. T_3 is bound less firmly than T_4 in the serum, enters peripheral tissues more readily, and binds to specific nuclear receptor(s) to initiate hormonal, metabolic effects. T_4 is the prohormone which is deiodinated to T_3 for hormone activity.
Thyroid hormone preparations belong to two categories: (1) natural hormonal preparations derived from animal thyroid, and (2) synthetic preparations. Natural preparations include desiccated thyroid and thyroglobulin. Desiccated thyroid is derived from domesticated animals that are used for food by man (either beef or hog thyroid), and thyroglobulin is derived from thyroid glands of the hog.
Triostat (liothyronine sodium injection) (T_3) contains liothyronine (L-triiodothyronine or L-T_3), a synthetic form of a natural thyroid hormone, as the sodium salt.
The structural and empirical formulas and molecular weight of liothyronine sodium are given below.

Liothyronine Sodium

$C_{15}H_{11}I_3NNaO_4$ M.W. 672.96

L-Tyrosine, *O*-(4-hydroxy-3-iodophenyl)-3,5-diiodo-, monosodium salt

In euthyroid patients, 25 mcg of liothyronine is equivalent to approximately 1 grain of desiccated thyroid or thyroglobulin and 0.1 mg of L-thyroxine.
Each mL of *Triostat* in amber-glass vials contains, in sterile non-pyrogenic aqueous solution, liothyronine sodium equivalent to 10 mcg of liothyronine; alcohol, 6.8% by volume; anhydrous citric acid, 0.175 mg; ammonia, 2.19 mg, as ammonium hydroxide.

CLINICAL PHARMACOLOGY
Thyroid hormones enhance oxygen consumption by most tissues of the body and increase the basal metabolic rate and the metabolism of carbohydrates, lipids and proteins. In vitro studies indicate that T_3 increases aerobic mitochondrial function, thereby increasing the rates of synthesis and utilization of myocardial high-energy phosphates. This, in turn, stimulates myosin ATPase and reduces tissue lactic acidosis. Thus, thyroid hormones exert a profound influence on virtually every organ system in the body and are of particular importance in the development of the central nervous system.
While the source of levothyroxine (T_4) and some triiodothyronine (T_3) is via secretion from the thyroid gland, it is now well-established that approximately 80% of circulating T_3 arises predominantly by way of the extrathyroidal conversion of T_4. The membrane-bound enzyme responsible for this reaction is iodothyronine 5′-deiodinase. Activity of the enzyme is greatest in the liver and kidney. A second pathway of T_4 to T_3 conversion occurs via a PTU-insensitive 5′-deiodinase located primarily in the pituitary and central nervous system.
The prohormone T_4 must be converted to T_3 in the body before it can exert biological effects. During periods of illness or stress, this conversion is often inhibited and can be diverted to the inactive reverse T_3 (rT_3) moiety. Therefore, correction of the hypothyroid condition in patients with myxedema coma is facilitated by the parenteral administration of triiodothyronine (T_3). T_3 is bound much less firmly to serum binding proteins and therefore penetrates into the cells much more rapidly than T_4. Also, the binding of T_3 to a nuclear thyroid hormone receptor seems to initiate most of the effects of thyroid hormone in tissues. Although most thyroid hormone analogs, both natural and synthetic, will bind to this protein, the affinity of T_3 for this receptor is roughly 10-fold higher than that of T_4. Thus, T_3 is the biologically active thyroid hormone.

Pharmacodynamics
The clinical features of myxedema coma include depression of the cardiovascular, respiratory, gastrointestinal and central nervous systems, impaired diuresis, and hypothermia. Administration of thyroid hormones reverses or attenuates these conditions. Thyroid hormones increase heart rate, ventricular contractility and cardiac output, as well as decrease total systemic vascular resistance. They also increase the rate and depth of respiration, motility of the gastrointestinal tract, rapidity of cerebration, and vasodilatation. Thyroid hormones correct hypothermia by markedly increasing the basal metabolic rate, as well as the number and activity of mitochondria in almost all cells of the body.

Pharmacokinetics
Since liothyronine sodium (T_3) is not firmly bound to serum protein, it is readily available to body tissues.
Liothyronine sodium has a rapid cutoff of activity which permits quick dosage adjustment and facilitates control of the effects of overdosage, should they occur.
The higher affinity of levothyroxine (T_4) as compared to triiodothyronine (T_3) for both thyroid-binding globulin and thyroid-binding prealbumin partially explains the higher serum levels and longer half-life of the former hormone. Both protein-bound hormones exist in reverse equilibrium with minute amounts of free hormone, the latter accounting for the metabolic activity. T_4 is deiodinated to T_3.
A single dose of liothyronine sodium administered intravenously produces a detectable metabolic response in as little as two to four hours and a maximum therapeutic response within two days. However, no pharmacokinetic studies have been performed with intravenous liothyronine (T_3) in myxedema coma or precoma patients.

INDICATIONS AND USAGE
Triostat (liothyronine sodium injection) (T_3) is indicated in the treatment of myxedema coma/precoma.
Triostat can be used in patients allergic to desiccated thyroid or thyroid extract derived from pork or beef.

CONTRAINDICATIONS
Thyroid hormone preparations are generally contraindicated in patients with diagnosed but as yet uncorrected adrenal cortical insufficiency or untreated thyrotoxicosis. Thyroid hormone preparations are also generally contraindicated in patients with hypersensitivity to any of the active or extraneous constituents of these preparations; however, there is no well-documented evidence in the literature of true allergic or idiosyncratic reactions to thyroid hormone.
Concomitant use of *Triostat* and artificial rewarming of patients is contraindicated. (See **PRECAUTIONS**.)

WARNINGS
Drugs with thyroid hormone activity, alone or together with other therapeutic agents, have been used for the treatment of obesity. In euthyroid patients, doses within the range of daily hormonal requirements are ineffective for weight reduction. Larger doses may produce serious or even life-threatening manifestations of toxicity, particularly when given in association with sympathomimetic amines such as those used for their anorectic effects.

The use of thyroid hormones in the therapy of obesity, alone or combined with other drugs, is unjustified and has been shown to be ineffective. Neither is their use justified for the treatment of male or female infertility unless this condition is accompanied by hypothyroidism.
Thyroid hormones should be used with great caution in a number of circumstances where the integrity of the cardiovascular system, particularly the coronary arteries, is suspect. These include patients with angina pectoris or the elderly, in whom there is a greater likelihood of occult cardiac disease. Therefore, in patients with compromised cardiac function, use thyroid hormones in conjunction with careful cardiac monitoring. Although the specific dosage of *Triostat* depends upon individual circumstances, in patients with known or suspected cardiovascular disease the extremely

rapid onset of action of *Triostat* may warrant initiating therapy at a dose of 10 mcg to 20 mcg. (See **DOSAGE AND ADMINISTRATION**.)
Myxedematous patients are very sensitive to thyroid hormones; dosage should be started at a low level and increased gradually as acute changes may precipitate adverse cardiovascular events.
Severe and prolonged hypothyroidism can lead to a decreased level of adrenocortical activity commensurate with the lowered metabolic state. When thyroid-replacement therapy is administered, the metabolism increases at a greater rate than adrenocortical activity. This can precipitate adrenocortical insufficiency. Therefore, in severe and prolonged hypothyroidism, supplemental adrenocortical steroids may be necessary.
In rare instances, the administration of thyroid hormone may precipitate a hyperthyroid state or may aggravate existing hyperthyroidism.
Extreme caution is advised when administering thyroid hormones with digitalis or vasopressors. (See **PRECAUTIONS–Drug Interactions**.)
Fluid therapy should be administered with great care to prevent cardiac decompensation. (See **PRECAUTIONS–Adjunctive Therapy**.)

PRECAUTIONS

General
Thyroid hormone therapy in patients with concomitant diabetes mellitus (see **PRECAUTIONS–Drug Interactions, *Insulin or Oral Hypoglycemics*** regarding interaction and dose adjustment with insulin) or insipidus or adrenal cortical insufficiency may aggravate the intensity of their symptoms. Appropriate adjustments of the various therapeutic measures directed at these concomitant endocrine diseases are required.
The therapy of myxedema coma requires simultaneous administration of glucocorticoids. (See **PRECAUTIONS–Adjunctive Therapy**).
Hypothyroidism decreases and hyperthyroidism increases the sensitivity to anticoagulants. Prothrombin time should be closely monitored in thyroid-treated patients on anticoagulants and dosage of the latter agents adjusted on the basis of frequent prothrombin time determinations.
Oral therapy should be resumed as soon as the clinical situation has been stabilized and the patient is able to take oral medication. If L-thyroxine rather than liothyronine sodium is used in initiating oral therapy, the physician should bear in mind that there is a delay of several days in the onset of L-thyroxine activity and that intravenous therapy should be discontinued gradually.

Adjunctive Therapy
Many investigators recommend that corticosteroids be administered routinely in the initial emergency treatment of all patients with myxedema coma. Patients with pituitary myxedema should receive adrenocortical hormone replacement therapy at or before the start of *Triostat* therapy. Similarly, patients with primary myxedema may also require adrenocortical hormone replacement therapy since a rapid return to normal body metabolism from a severely hypothyroid state may result in acute adrenocortical insufficiency and shock.
In considering the need to elevate blood pressure, it should be kept in mind that tissue metabolic requirements are markedly reduced in the hypothyroid patient. Because arrhythmias and circulatory collapse have infrequently occurred following the concomitant administration of thyroid hormones and vasopressor therapies, use caution when administering these therapies concomitantly. (See **PRECAUTIONS–Drug Interactions, Vasopressors**.)
Hyponatremia is frequently present in myxedema coma, but usually resolves without specific therapy as the metabolic status of the patient is improved with thyroid hormone treatment. Fluid therapy should be administered with great care to prevent cardiac decompensation. In addition, some patients with myxedema have inappropriate secretion of ADH and are susceptible to water intoxication.
In some patients, respiratory depression has been a significant factor in the development or persistence of the comatose state. Decreased oxygen saturation and elevated CO_2 levels respond quickly to artificial respiration.
Infection is often present in myxedema coma and should be looked for and treated appropriately.
Concomitant use of *Triostat* and artificial rewarming of patients is contraindicated. Although patients in myxedema coma are often hypothermic, most investigators believe that artificial rewarming is of little value or may be harmful. The peripheral vasodilation produced by external heat serves to further decrease circulation to vital internal organs and to increase shock if present. It has been reported that the administration of liothyronine sodium will restore a normal body temperature in 24 to 48 hours if heat loss is prevented by keeping the patient covered with blankets in a warm room.

Laboratory Tests
Treatment of patients with thyroid hormones requires the periodic assessment of thyroid status by means of appropriate laboratory tests besides the full clinical evaluation. Serum T_3 and TSH levels should be monitored to assess dosage adequacy and biologic effectiveness.

Drug Interactions
Oral Anticoagulants: Thyroid hormones appear to increase catabolism of vitamin K-dependent clotting factors. If oral anticoagulants are also being given, compensatory increases in clotting factor synthesis are impaired. Patients stabilized on oral anticoagulants who are found to require thyroid replacement therapy should be watched very closely when thyroid is started. If a patient is truly hypothyroid, it is likely that a reduction in anticoagulant dosage will be required. No special precautions appear to be necessary when oral anticoagulant therapy is begun in a patient already stabilized on maintenance thyroid replacement therapy.
Insulin or Oral Hypoglycemics: Initiating thyroid replacement therapy may cause increases in insulin or oral hypoglycemic requirements. The effects seen are poorly understood and depend upon a variety of factors such as dose and type of thyroid preparations and endocrine status of the patient. Patients receiving insulin or oral hypoglycemics should be closely watched during initiation of thyroid replacement therapy.
Estrogen, Oral Contraceptives: Estrogens tend to increase serum thyroxine-binding globulin (TBG). In a patient with a nonfunctioning thyroid gland who is receiving thyroid replacement therapy, free levothyroxine may be decreased when estrogens are started thus increasing thyroid requirements. However, if the patient's thyroid gland has sufficient function, the decreased free thyroxine will result in a compensatory increase in thyroxine output by the thyroid. Therefore, patients without a functioning thyroid gland who are on thyroid replacement therapy may need to increase their thyroid dose if estrogens or estrogen-containing oral contraceptives are given.
Tricyclic Antidepressants: Use of thyroid products with imipramine and other tricyclic antidepressants may increase receptor sensitivity and enhance antidepressant activity; transient cardiac arrhythmias have been observed. Thyroid hormone activity may also be enhanced.
Digitalis: Thyroid preparations may potentiate the toxic effects of digitalis. Thyroid hormonal replacement increases metabolic rate, which requires an increase in digitalis dosage.
Ketamine: When administered to patients on a thyroid preparation, this parenteral anesthetic may cause hypertension and tachycardia. Use with caution and be prepared to treat hypertension, if necessary.
Vasopressors: Thyroid hormones increase the adrenergic effect of catecholamines such as epinephrine and norepinephrine. Therefore, use of vasopressors in patients receiving thyroid hormone preparations may increase the risk of precipitating coronary insufficiency, especially in patients with coronary artery disease. Therefore, use caution when administering vasopressors with liothyronine (T_3).

Drug/Laboratory Test Interactions
The following drugs or moieties are known to interfere with laboratory tests performed in patients on thyroid hormone therapy: androgens, corticosteroids, estrogens, oral contraceptives containing estrogens, iodine-containing preparations and the numerous preparations containing salicylates.

1. Changes in TBG concentration should be taken into consideration in the interpretation of T_4 and T_3 values. In such cases, the unbound (free) hormone should be measured. Pregnancy, estrogens and estrogen-containing oral contraceptives increase TBG concentrations. TBG may also be increased during infectious hepatitis. Decreases in TBG concentrations are observed in nephrosis, acromegaly and after androgen or corticosteroid therapy. Familial hyper- or hypothyroxine-binding globulinemias have been described. The incidence of TBG deficiency approximates 1 in 9000. The binding of thyroxine by thyroxine-binding prealbumin (TBPA) is inhibited by salicylates.
2. Medicinal or dietary iodine interferes with all in vivo tests of radioiodine uptake, producing low uptakes which may not be reflective of a true decrease in hormone synthesis.

Carcinogenesis, Mutagenesis and Impairment of Fertility
A reportedly apparent association between prolonged thyroid therapy and breast cancer has not been confirmed and patients on thyroid for established indications should not discontinue therapy. No confirmatory long-term studies in animals have been performed to evaluate carcinogenic potential, mutagenicity, or impairment of fertility in either males or females.

Pregnancy
Pregnancy Category A: Thyroid hormones do not readily cross the placental barrier. The clinical experience to date does not indicate any adverse effect on fetuses when thyroid hormones are administered to pregnant women. On the basis of current knowledge, thyroid replacement therapy to hypothyroid women should not be discontinued during pregnancy.

Nursing Mothers
Minimal amounts of thyroid hormones are excreted in human milk. Thyroid hormones are not associated with serious adverse reactions and do not have a known tumorigenic potential. However, caution should be exercised when thyroid hormones are administered to a nursing woman.

Geriatric Use
Clinical studies of liothyronine sodium did not include sufficient numbers of subjects aged 65 and over to determine whether they respond differently from younger subjects. Other reported clinical experience has not identified differences in responses between the elderly and younger patients. In general, dose selection for an elderly patient should be cautious, usually starting at the low end of the dosing range, reflecting the greater frequency of decreased hepatic, renal, or cardiac function, and of concomitant disease or other drug therapy. This drug is known to be substantially excreted by the kidney, and the risk of toxic reactions to this drug may be greater in patients with impaired renal function. Because elderly patients are more likely to have decreased renal function, care should be taken in dose selection, and it may be useful to monitor renal function.

Pediatric Use
There is limited experience with *Triostat* in the pediatric population. Safety and effectiveness in pediatric patients have not been established.

ADVERSE REACTIONS

The most frequently reported adverse events were arrhythmia (6% of patients) and tachycardia (3%). Cardiopulmonary arrest, hypotension and myocardial infarction occurred in approximately 2% of patients. The following events occurred in approximately 1% or fewer of patients: angina, congestive heart failure, fever, hypertension, phlebitis and twitching.
In rare instances, allergic skin reactions have been reported with liothyronine sodium tablets.

OVERDOSAGE

Signs and Symptoms: Headache, irritability, nervousness, tremor, sweating, increased bowel motility and menstrual irregularities. Angina pectoris, arrhythmia, tachycardia, acute myocardial infarction or congestive heart failure may be induced or aggravated. Shock may also develop if there is untreated pituitary or adrenocortical failure. Massive overdosage may result in symptoms resembling thyroid storm.
Treatment of Overdosage: Dosage should be reduced or therapy temporarily discontinued if signs and symptoms of overdosage appear. Treatment may be reinstituted at a lower dosage. In normal individuals, normal hypothalamic-pituitary-thyroid axis function is restored in six to eight weeks after cessation of therapy following thyroid suppression.
Treatment is symptomatic and supportive. Oxygen may be administered and ventilation maintained. Cardiac glycosides may be indicated if congestive heart failure develops. Beta-adrenergic antagonists have been used advantageously in the treatment of increased sympathetic activity. Measures to control fever, hypoglycemia or fluid loss should be instituted if needed.

DOSAGE AND ADMINISTRATION

Adults
Myxedema coma is usually precipitated in the hypothyroid patient of long standing by intercurrent illness or drugs such as sedatives and anesthetics and should be considered a medical emergency. Therapy should be directed at the correction of electrolyte disturbances, possible infection, or other intercurrent illness in addition to the administration of intravenous liothyronine (T_3). Simultaneous glucocorticosteroids are required.
Triostat (liothyronine sodium injection) (T_3) is for intravenous administration only. It should not be given intramuscularly or subcutaneously.

- Prompt administration of an adequate dose of intravenous liothyronine (T_3) is important in determining clinical outcome.
- Initial and subsequent doses of *Triostat* should be based on continuous monitoring of the patient's clinical status and response to therapy.
- *Triostat* doses should normally be administered at least four hours–and not more than 12 hours–apart.
- Administration of at least 65 mcg/day of intravenous liothyronine (T_3) in the initial days of therapy was associated with lower mortality.
- There is limited clinical experience with intravenous liothyronine (T_3) at total daily doses exceeding 100 mcg/day.

No controlled clinical studies have been done with *Triostat*. The following dosing guidelines have been derived from data analysis of myxedema coma/precoma case reports collected by SmithKline Beecham Pharmaceuticals since 1963 and from scientific literature since 1956.
An initial intravenous *Triostat* dose ranging from 25 mcg to 50 mcg is recommended in the emergency treatment of myxedema coma/precoma in adults. In patients with known or suspected cardiovascular disease, an initial dose of 10 mcg to 20 mcg is suggested (see **WARNINGS**). However, both the initial dose and subsequent doses should be determined on the basis of continuous monitoring of the patient's clinical condition and response to *Triostat* therapy. Normally at least four hours should be allowed between doses to adequately assess therapeutic response and no more than 12 hours should elapse between doses to avoid fluctuations in hormone levels. Caution should be exercised in adjusting the dose due to the potential of large changes to precipitate adverse cardiovascular events. Review of the myxedema case reports indicates decreased mortality in patients receiving at least 65 mcg/day in the initial days of treatment. However, there is limited clinical experience at total daily doses above 100 mcg. See **PRECAUTIONS–Drug Interactions** for potential interactions between thyroid hormones and digitalis and vasopressors.

Pediatric Use
There is limited experience with *Triostat* in the pediatric population. Safety and effectiveness in pediatric patients have not been established.

Switching to Oral Therapy
Oral therapy should be resumed as soon as the clinical situation has been stabilized and the patient is able to take oral medication. When switching a patient to liothyronine

Continued on next page

Triostat—Cont.

sodium tablets from *Triostat*, discontinue *Triostat*, initiate oral therapy at a low dosage, and increase gradually according to the patient's response.
If L-thyroxine rather than liothyronine sodium is used in initiating oral therapy, the physician should bear in mind that there is a delay of several days in the onset of L-thyroxine activity and that intravenous therapy should be discontinued gradually.

HOW SUPPLIED

In packages of six 1 mL vials at a concentration of 10 mcg/mL.
NDC 52604-5210-6
Store between 2° and 8°C (35° and 46°F).
Prescribing Information as of September 2002.
Manufactured for:
Jones Pharma Incorporated
(A wholly owned subsidiary of King Pharmaceuticals, Inc.)
St. Louis, MO 63146
Manufactured by:
Parkedale Pharmaceuticals, Inc.
Rochester, MI 48307
5210G030
Shown in Product Identification Guide, page 320

Knoll Laboratories/ Pharmaceuticals

Due to the acquisition of Knoll Laboratories, Knoll Pharmaceutical Company, by Abbott Laboratories, please refer to ABBOTT LABORATORIES for product information.

Kos Pharmaceuticals, Inc.

1 CEDAR BROOK DRIVE
CRANBURY, NJ 08512

For medical information contact:
Drug Information Services
1-888-454-7437

ADVICOR® ℞

[ad' vĭ kor"]
(niacin extended-release/lovastatin tablets)
℞ Only

DESCRIPTION

ADVICOR contains niacin extended-release and lovastatin in combination. Niacin, a B-complex vitamin, and lovastatin, an inhibitor of 3-hydroxy-3-methylglutaryl-coenzyme A (HMG-CoA) reductase, are both lipid-altering agents.
Niacin is nicotinic acid, or 3-pyridinecarboxylic acid. Niacin is a white, nonhygroscopic crystalline powder that is very soluble in water, boiling ethanol and propylene glycol. It is insoluble in ethyl ether. The empirical formula of niacin is $C_6H_5NO_2$ and its molecular weight is 123.11. Niacin has the following structural formula:

N COOH

Lovastatin is [1S -[1(alpha)(R *), 3(alpha), 7(beta), 8(beta)(2S *, 4S *), 8a(beta)]]-1,2,3, 7,8,8a-hexahydro-3,7-dimethyl-8-[2-(tetrahydro-4-hydroxy-6-oxo-2H-pyran-2-yl) ethyl]-1-naphthalenyl 2-methylbutanoate. Lovastatin is a white, nonhygroscopic crystalline powder that is insoluble in water and sparingly soluble in ethanol, methanol, and acetonitrile. The empirical formula of lovastatin is $C_{24}H_{36}O_5$ and its molecular weight is 404.55. Lovastatin has the following structural formula:

ADVICOR tablets contain the labeled amount of niacin and lovastatin and have the following inactive ingredients: hypromellose, povidone, stearic acid, polyethylene glycol, titanium dioxide, polysorbate 80. The individual tablet strengths (expressed in terms of mg niacin/mg lovastatin) contain the following coloring agents:

ADVICOR 500 mg/20 mg - synthetic red and yellow iron oxides.
ADVICOR 1000 mg/20 mg - synthetic red, yellow, and black iron oxides.

CLINICAL PHARMACOLOGY

A variety of clinical studies have demonstrated that elevated levels of total cholesterol (TC), low-density lipoprotein cholesterol (LDL-C), and apolipoprotein B-100 (Apo B) promote human atherosclerosis. Similarly, decreased levels of high-density lipoprotein cholesterol (HDL-C) are associated with the development of atherosclerosis. Epidemiological investigations have established that cardiovascular morbidity and mortality vary directly with the level of TC and LDL-C, and inversely with the level of HDL-C.
Cholesterol-enriched triglyceride-rich lipoproteins, including very low-density lipoproteins (VLDL), intermediate-density lipoproteins (IDL), and their remnants, can also promote atherosclerosis. Elevated plasma triglycerides (TG) are frequently found in a triad with low HDL-C levels and small LDL particles, as well as in association with non-lipid metabolic risk factors for coronary heart disease (CHD). As such, total plasma TG have not consistently been shown to be an independent risk factor for CHD.
As an adjunct to diet, the efficacy of niacin and lovastatin in improving lipid profiles (either individually, or in combination with each other, or niacin in combination with other statins) for the treatment of dyslipidemia has been well documented. The effect of combined therapy with niacin and lovastatin on cardiovascular morbidity and mortality has not been determined.

Effects on Lipids
ADVICOR
ADVICOR reduces LDL-C, TC, and TG, and increases HDL-C due to the individual actions of niacin and lovastatin. The magnitude of individual lipid and lipoprotein responses may be influenced by the severity and type of underlying lipid abnormality.
Niacin
Niacin functions in the body after conversion to nicotinamide adenine dinucleotide (NAD) in the NAD coenzyme system. Niacin (but not nicotinamide) in gram doses reduces LDL-C, Apo B, Lp(a), TG, and TC, and increases HDL-C. The increase in HDL-C is associated with an increase in apolipoprotein A-I (Apo A-I) and a shift in the distribution of HDL subfractions. These shifts include an increase in the HDL_2:HDL_3 ratio, and an elevation in lipoprotein A-I (Lp A-I, an HDL-C particle containing only Apo A-I). In addition, preliminary reports suggest that niacin causes favorable LDL particle size transformations, although the clinical relevance of this effect is not yet clear.
Lovastatin
Lovastatin has been shown to reduce both normal and elevated LDL-C concentrations. Apo B also falls substantially during treatment with lovastatin. Since each LDL-C particle contains one molecule of Apo B, and since little Apo B is found in other lipoproteins, this strongly suggests that lovastatin does not merely cause cholesterol to be lost from LDL-C, but also reduces the concentration of circulating LDL particles. In addition, lovastatin can produce increases of variable magnitude in HDL-C, and modestly reduces VLDL-C and plasma TG. The effects of lovastatin on Lp(a), fibrinogen, and certain other independent biochemical risk markers for coronary heart disease are not well characterized.

Mechanism of Action
Niacin
The mechanism by which niacin alters lipid profiles is not completely understood and may involve several actions, including partial inhibition of release of free fatty acids from adipose tissue, and increased lipoprotein lipase activity (which may increase the rate of chylomicron triglyceride removal from plasma). Niacin decreases the rate of hepatic synthesis of VLDL-C and LDL-C, and does not appear to affect fecal excretion of fats, sterols, or bile acids.
Lovastatin
Lovastatin is a specific inhibitor of 3-hydroxy-3-methylglutaryl-coenzyme A (HMG-CoA) reductase, the enzyme that catalyzes the conversion of HMG-CoA to mevalonate. The conversion of HMG-CoA to mevalonate is an early step in the biosynthetic pathway for cholesterol. Lovastatin is a prodrug and has little, if any, activity until hydrolyzed to its active beta-hydroxyacid form, lovastatin acid. The mechanism of the LDL-lowering effect of lovastatin may involve both reduction of VLDL-C concentration and induction of the LDL receptor, leading to reduced production and/or increased catabolism of LDL-C.

Pharmacokinetics
Absorption and Bioavailability
ADVICOR
In single-dose studies of ADVICOR, rate and extent of niacin and lovastatin absorption were bioequivalent under fed conditions to that from NIASPAN® (niacin extended-release tablets) and Mevacor® (lovastatin) tablets, respectively. After administration of two ADVICOR 1000 mg/20 mg tablets, peak niacin concentrations averaged about 18 mcg/mL and occurred about 5 hours after dosing; about 72% of the niacin dose was absorbed according to the urinary excretion data. Peak lovastatin concentrations averaged about 11 ng/mL and occurred about 2 hours after dosing.
The extent of niacin absorption from ADVICOR was increased by administration with food. The administration of two ADVICOR 1000 mg/20 mg tablets under low-fat or high-fat conditions resulted in a 22 to 30% increase in niacin bioavailability relative to dosing under fasting conditions. Lovastatin bioavailability is affected by food. Lovastatin Cmax was increased 48% and 21% after a high- and a low-fat meal, respectively, but the lovastatin AUC was decreased 26% and 24% after a high- and a low-fat meal, respectively, compared to those under fasting conditions.
Niacin
Due to extensive and saturable first-pass metabolism, niacin concentrations in the general circulation are dose dependent and highly variable. Peak steady-state niacin concentrations were 0.6, 4.9, and 15.5 mcg/mL after doses of 1000, 1500, and 2000 mg NIASPAN once daily (given as two 500 mg, two 750 mg, and two 1000 mg tablets, respectively).
Lovastatin
Lovastatin appears to be incompletely absorbed after oral administration. Because of extensive hepatic extraction, the amount of lovastatin reaching the systemic circulation as active inhibitors after oral administration is low (<5%) and shows considerable inter-individual variation. Peak concentrations of active and total inhibitors occur within 2 to 4 hours after Mevacor® administration.
Lovastatin absorption appears to be increased by at least 30% by grapefruit juice; however, the effect is dependent on the amount of grapefruit juice consumed and the interval between grapefruit juice and lovastatin ingestion.
With a once-a-day dosing regimen, plasma concentrations of total inhibitors over a dosing interval achieved a steady-state between the second and third days of therapy and were about 1.5 times those following a single dose of Mevacor®.

Distribution
Niacin
Niacin is less than 20% bound to human serum proteins and distributes into milk. Studies using radiolabeled niacin in mice show that niacin and its metabolites concentrate in the liver, kidney, and adipose tissue.
Lovastatin
Both lovastatin and its beta-hydroxyacid metabolite are highly bound (>95%) to human plasma proteins. Distribution of lovastatin or its metabolites into human milk is unknown; however, lovastatin distributes into milk in rats. In animal studies, lovastatin concentrated in the liver, and crossed the blood-brain and placental barriers.

Metabolism
Niacin
Niacin undergoes rapid and extensive first-pass metabolism that is dose-rate specific and, at the doses used to treat dyslipidemia, saturable. In humans, one pathway is through a simple conjugation step with glycine to form nicotinuric acid (NUA). NUA is then excreted, although there may be a small amount of reversible metabolism back to niacin. The other pathway results in the formation of NAD. It is unclear whether nicotinamide is formed as a precursor to, or following the synthesis of, NAD. Nicotinamide is further metabolized to at least N-methylnicotinamide (MNA) and nicotinamide-N-oxide (NNO). MNA is further metabolized to two other compounds, N-methyl-2-pyridone-5-carboxamide (2PY) and N-methyl-4-pyridone-5-carboxamide (4PY). The formation of 2PY appears to predominate over 4PY in humans.
Lovastatin
Lovastatin undergoes extensive first-pass extraction and metabolism by cytochrome P450 3A4 in the liver, its primary site of action. The major active metabolites present in human plasma are the beta-hydroxyacid of lovastatin (lovastatin acid), its 6'-hydroxy derivative, and two additional metabolites.

Elimination
ADVICOR
Niacin is primarily excreted in urine mainly as metabolites. After a single dose of ADVICOR, at least 60% of the niacin dose was recovered in urine as unchanged niacin and its metabolites. The plasma half-life for lovastatin was about 4.5 hours in single-dose studies.
Niacin
The plasma half-life for niacin is about 20 to 48 minutes after oral administration and dependent on dose administered. Following multiple oral doses of NIASPAN, up to 12% of the dose was recovered in urine as unchanged niacin depending on dose administered. The ratio of metabolites recovered in the urine was also dependent on the dose administered.
Lovastatin
Lovastatin is excreted in urine and bile, based on studies of Mevacor®. Following an oral dose of radiolabeled lovastatin in man, 10% of the dose was excreted in urine and 83% in feces. The latter represents absorbed drug equivalents excreted in bile, as well as any unabsorbed drug.

Special Populations
Hepatic
No pharmacokinetic studies have been conducted in patients with hepatic insufficiency for either niacin or lovastatin (see **WARNINGS, Liver Dysfunction**).
Renal
No information is available on the pharmacokinetics of niacin in patients with renal insufficiency.
In a study of patients with severe renal insufficiency (creatinine clearance 10 to 30 mL/min), the plasma concentrations of total inhibitors after a single dose of lovastatin were approximately two-fold higher than those in healthy volunteers.
ADVICOR should be used with caution in patients with renal disease.

Gender

Plasma concentrations of niacin and metabolites after single- or multiple-dose administration of niacin are generally higher in women than in men, with the magnitude of the difference varying with dose and metabolite. Recovery of niacin and metabolites in urine, however, is generally similar for men and women, indicating similar absorption for both genders. The gender differences observed in plasma niacin and metabolite levels may be due to gender-specific differences in metabolic rate or volume of distribution. Data from clinical trials suggest that women have a greater hypolipidemic response than men at equivalent doses of NIASPAN and ADVICOR.

In a multiple-dose study, plasma concentrations of active and total HMG-CoA reductase inhibitors were 20 to 50% higher in women than in men. In two single-dose studies with ADVICOR, lovastatin concentrations were about 30% higher in women than men, and total HMG-CoA reductase inhibitor concentrations were about 20 to 25% greater in women.

In a multi-center, randomized, double-blind, active-comparator study in patients with Type IIa and IIb hyperlipidemia, ADVICOR was compared to single-agent treatment (NIASPAN and lovastatin). The treatment effects of ADVICOR compared to lovastatin and NIASPAN differed for males and females with a significantly larger treatment effect seen for females. The mean percent change from baseline at endpoint for LDL-C, TG, and HDL-C by gender are as follows (Table 1):

Table 1. Mean percent change from baseline at endpoint for LDL-C, HDL-C and TG by gender

	ADVICOR 2000 mg/40 mg		NIASPAN 2000 mg		Lovastatin 40 mg	
	Women (n=22)	Men (n=30)	Women (n=28)	Men (n=28)	Women (n=21)	Men (n=38)
LDL-C	-47%	-34%	-12%	-9%	-31%	-31%
HDL-C	+33%	+24%	+22%	+15%	+3%	+7%
TG	-48%	-35%	-25%	-15%	-15%	-23%

Clinical Studies

In a multi-center, randomized, double-blind, parallel, 28-week, active-comparator study in patients with Type IIa and IIb hyperlipidemia, ADVICOR was compared to each of its components (NIASPAN and lovastatin). Using a forced dose-escalation study design, patients received each dose for at least 4 weeks. Patients randomized to treatment with ADVICOR initially received 500 mg/20 mg. The dose was increased at 4-week intervals to a maximum of 1000 mg/20 mg in one-half of the patients and 2000 mg/40 mg in the other half. The NIASPAN monotherapy group underwent a similar titration from 500 mg to 2000 mg. The patients randomized to lovastatin monotherapy received 20 mg for 12 weeks titrated to 40 mg for up to 16 weeks. Up to a third of the patients randomized to ADVICOR or NIASPAN discontinued prior to Week 28. In this study, ADVICOR decreased LDL-C, TG and Lp(a), and increased HDL-C in a dose-dependent fashion (Tables 2, 3, 4 and 5 below). Results from this study for LDL-C mean percent change from baseline (the primary efficacy variable) showed that:

1) LDL-lowering with ADVICOR was significantly greater than that achieved with lovastatin 40 mg only after 28 weeks of titration to a dose of 2000 mg/40 mg ($p<.0001$)
2) ADVICOR at doses of 1000 mg/20 mg or higher achieved greater LDL-lowering than NIASPAN ($p<.0001$)

The LDL-C results are summarized in Table 2.

[See table 2 above]

ADVICOR achieved significantly greater HDL-raising compared to lovastatin and NIASPAN monotherapy at all doses (Table 3).

[See table 3 above]

In addition, ADVICOR achieved significantly greater TG-lowering at doses of 1000 mg/20 mg or greater compared to lovastatin and NIASPAN monotherapy (Table 4).

[See table 4 above]

The Lp(a) lowering effects of ADVICOR and NIASPAN were similar, and both were superior to lovastatin (Table 5). The independent effect of lowering Lp(a) with NIASPAN or ADVICOR on the risk of coronary and cardiovascular morbidity and mortality has not been determined.

[See table 5 above]

ADVICOR Long-Term Study

A total of 814 patients were enrolled in a long-term (52-week), open-label, single-arm study of ADVICOR. Patients were force dose-titrated to 2000 mg/40 mg over 16 weeks. After titration, patients were maintained on the maximum tolerated dose of ADVICOR for a total of 52 weeks. Five hundred-fifty (550) patients (68%) completed the study, and fifty-six percent (56%) of all patients were able to maintain a dose of 2000 mg/40 mg for the 52 weeks of treatment. The lipid-altering effects of ADVICOR peaked after 4 weeks on the maximum tolerated dose, and were maintained for the duration of treatment. These effects were comparable to what was observed in the double-blind study of ADVICOR (Tables 2-4).

Table 2. LDL-C mean percent change from baseline

Week	ADVICOR			NIASPAN			Lovastatin		
	n*	Dose (mg/mg)	LDL	n*	Dose (mg)	LDL	n*	Dose (mg)	LDL
Baseline	57	-	190.9 mg/dL	61	-	189.7 mg/dL	61	-	185.6 mg/dL
12	47	1000/20	-30%	46	1000	-3%	56	20	-29%
16	45	1000/40	-36%	44	1000	-6%	56	40	-31%
20	42	1500/40	-37%	43	1500	-12%	54	40	-34%
28	42	2000/40	-42%	41	2000	-14%	53	40	-32%

*n = number of patients remaining in the trial at each timepoint

Table 3. HDL-C mean percent change from baseline

Week	ADVICOR			NIASPAN			Lovastatin		
	n*	Dose (mg/mg)	HDL	n*	Dose (mg)	HDL	n*	Dose (mg)	HDL
Baseline	57	-	45 mg/dL	61	-	47 mg/dL	61	-	43 mg/dL
12	47	1000/20	+20%	46	1000	+14%	56	20	+3%
16	45	1000/40	+20%	44	1000	+15%	56	40	+5%
20	42	1500/40	+27%	43	1500	+22%	54	40	+6%
28	42	2000/40	+30%	41	2000	+24%	53	40	+6%

*n = number of patients remaining in the trial at each timepoint

Table 4. TG median percent change from baseline

Week	ADVICOR			NIASPAN			Lovastatin		
	n*	Dose (mg/mg)	TG	n*	Dose (mg)	TG	n*	Dose (mg)	TG
Baseline	57	-	174 mg/dL	61	-	186 mg/dL	61	-	171 mg/dL
12	47	1000/20	-32%	46	1000	-22%	56	20	-20%
16	45	1000/40	-39%	44	1000	-23%	56	40	-17%
20	42	1500/40	-44%	43	1500	-31%	54	40	-21%
28	42	2000/40	-44%	41	2000	-31%	53	40	-20%

*n = number of patients remaining in the trial at each timepoint

Table 5. Lp(a) median percent change from baseline

Week	ADVICOR			NIASPAN			Lovastatin		
	n*	Dose (mg/mg)	Lp(a)	n*	Dose (mg)	Lp(a)	n*	Dose (mg)	Lp(a)
Baseline	57	-	34 mg/dL	61	-	41 mg/dL	60	-	42 mg/dL
12	47	1000/20	-9%	46	1000	-8%	55	20	+8%
16	45	1000/40	-9%	44	1000	-12%	55	40	+8%
20	42	1500/40	-17%	43	1500	-22%	53	40	+6%
28	42	2000/40	-22%	41	2000	-32%	52	40	0%

*n = number of patients remaining in the trial at each timepoint

INDICATIONS AND USAGE

ADVICOR is a fixed-dose combination product and is not indicated for initial therapy (see **DOSAGE AND ADMINISTRATION**). Therapy with lipid-altering agents should be only one component of multiple risk-factor intervention in individuals at significantly increased risk for atherosclerotic vascular disease due to hypercholesterolemia. Initial medical therapy is indicated with a single agent as an adjunct to diet when the response to a diet restricted in saturated fat and cholesterol and other nonpharmacologic measures alone has been inadequate (see also Table 7 and the NCEP treatment guidelines[1]).

ADVICOR is indicated for the treatment of primary hypercholesterolemia (heterozygous familial and nonfamilial) and mixed dyslipidemia (Frederickson Types IIa and IIb; Table 6) in:

- Patients treated with lovastatin who require further TG-lowering or HDL-raising who may benefit from having niacin added to their regimen
- Patients treated with niacin who require further LDL-lowering who may benefit from having lovastatin added to their regimen

Table 6. Classification of Hyperlipoproteinemias

Type	Lipoproteins Elevated	Lipid Elevations	
		Major	Minor
I (rare)	Chylomicrons	TG	↑→TC
IIa	LDL	TC	
IIb	LDL, VLDL	TC	TG
III (rare)	IDL	TC/TG	
IV	VLDL	TG	↑→TC
V (rare)	Chylomicrons, VLDL	TG	↑→TC

TC = total cholesterol; TG = triglycerides; LDL = low-density lipoprotein; VLDL = very low-density lipoprotein; IDL = intermediate-density lipoprotein

↑→ = increased or no change

General Recommendations

Prior to initiating therapy with a lipid-lowering agent, secondary causes for hypercholesterolemia (e.g., poorly controlled diabetes mellitus, hypothyroidism, nephrotic syndrome, dysproteinemias, obstructive liver disease, other drug therapy, alcoholism) should be excluded, and a lipid profile performed to measure TC, HDL-C, and TG. For patients with TG < 400 mg/dL, LDL-C can be estimated using the following equation:

$$LDL\text{-}C = TC - [(0.20 \times TG) + HDL\text{-}C]$$

For TG levels > 400 mg/dL, this equation is less accurate and LDL-C concentrations should be determined by ultracentrifugation. Lipid determinations should be performed at intervals of no less than 4 weeks and dosage adjusted according to the patient's response to therapy. The NCEP Treatment Guidelines are summarized in Table 7.

[See table 7 at top of next page]

After the LDL-C goal has been achieved, if the TG is still ≥ 200 mg/dL, non-HDL-C (TC minus HDL-C) becomes a secondary target of therapy. Non-HDL-C goals are set 30 mg/dL higher than LDL-C goals for each risk category.

CONTRAINDICATIONS

ADVICOR is contraindicated in patients with a known hypersensitivity to niacin, lovastatin or any component of this medication, active liver disease or unexplained persistent elevations in serum transaminases (see **WARNINGS**), active peptic ulcer disease, or arterial bleeding.

Pregnancy and lactation—Atherosclerosis is a chronic process and the discontinuation of lipid-lowering drugs during pregnancy should have little impact on the outcome of long-term therapy of primary hypercholesterolemia. Moreover, cholesterol and other products of the cholesterol biosynthesis pathway are essential components for fetal development, including synthesis of steroids and cell membranes. Because of the ability of inhibitors of HMG-CoA reductase, such as lovastatin, to decrease the synthesis of cholesterol and possibly other products of the cholesterol biosynthesis pathway, ADVICOR is contraindicated in women who are pregnant and in lactating mothers. ADVICOR may cause fetal harm when administered to pregnant women. **ADVICOR should be administered to women of childbearing age only when such patients are highly unlikely to conceive.** If the patient becomes pregnant while taking this drug, ADVICOR should be discontinued immediately and the patient should be apprised of the potential hazard to the fetus (see **PRECAUTIONS**, **Pregnancy**).

WARNINGS

ADVICOR should not be substituted for equivalent doses of immediate-release (crystalline) niacin. For patients switch-

Continued on next page

Advicor—Cont.

ing from immediate-release niacin to NIASPAN, therapy with NIASPAN should be initiated with low doses (i.e., 500 mg once daily at bedtime) and the NIASPAN dose should then be titrated to the desired therapeutic response (see DOSAGE AND ADMINISTRATION).

Liver Dysfunction

Cases of severe hepatic toxicity, including fulminant hepatic necrosis, have occurred in patients who have substituted sustained-release (modified-release, timed-release) niacin products for immediate-release (crystalline) niacin at equivalent doses.

ADVICOR should be used with caution in patients who consume substantial quantities of alcohol and/or have a past history of liver disease. Active liver disease or unexplained transaminase elevations are contraindications to the use of ADVICOR.

Niacin preparations and lovastatin preparations have been associated with abnormal liver tests. In studies using NIASPAN alone, 0.8% of patients were discontinued for transaminase elevations. In studies using lovastatin alone, 0.2% of patients were discontinued for transaminase elevations.[2] In three safety and efficacy studies involving titration to final daily ADVICOR doses ranging from 500 mg/10 mg to 2500 mg/40 mg, ten of 1028 patients (1.0%) experienced reversible elevations in AST/ALT to more than 3 times the upper limit of normal (ULN). Three of ten elevations occurred at doses outside the recommended dosing limit of 2000 mg/40 mg; no patient receiving 1000 mg/20 mg had 3-fold elevations in AST/ALT.

In clinical studies with ADVICOR, elevations in transaminases did not appear to be related to treatment duration; elevations in AST and ALT levels did appear to be dose related. Transaminase elevations were reversible upon discontinuation of ADVICOR.

Liver function tests should be performed on all patients during therapy with ADVICOR. Serum transaminase levels, including AST and ALT (SGOT and SGPT), should be monitored before treatment begins, every 6 to 12 weeks for the first 6 months, and periodically thereafter (e.g., at approximately 6-month intervals). Special attention should be paid to patients who develop elevated serum transaminase levels, and in these patients, measurements should be repeated promptly and, if confirmed, then performed more frequently. If the transaminase levels show evidence of progression, particularly if they rise to 3 times ULN and are persistent, or if they are associated with symptoms of nausea, fever, and/or malaise, the drug should be discontinued.

Skeletal Muscle

Lovastatin

Lovastatin and other inhibitors of HMG-CoA reductase occasionally cause myopathy, which is manifested as muscle pain or weakness associated with grossly elevated creatine kinase (> 10 times ULN).

Rhabdomyolysis, with or without acute renal failure secondary to myoglobinuria, has been reported rarely and can occur at any time. In a large, long-term, clinical safety and efficacy study (the EXCEL study)[3,4] with lovastatin, myopathy occurred in up to 0.2% of patients treated with lovastatin 20 to 80 mg for up to 2 years. When drug treatment was interrupted or discontinued in these patients, muscle symptoms and creatine kinase (CK) increases promptly resolved. The risk of myopathy is increased by concomitant therapy with certain drugs, some of which were excluded by the EXCEL study design.

The risk of myopathy appears to be increased by high levels of HMG-CoA reductase inhibitory activity in plasma. Lovastatin is metabolized by the cytochrome P450 isoform 3A4. Certain drugs which share this metabolic pathway can raise the plasma levels of lovastatin and may increase the risk of myopathy. These include cyclosporine, itraconazole, ketoconazole and other antifungal azoles, the macrolide antibiotics erythromycin and clarithromycin, HIV protease inhibitors, the antidepressant nefazodone, or large quantities of grapefruit juice (>1 quart daily).

ADVICOR

Myopathy and/or rhabdomyolysis have been reported when lovastatin is used in combination with lipid-altering doses (≥1g/day) of niacin. Physicians contemplating the use of ADVICOR, a combination of lovastatin and niacin, should weigh the potential benefits and risks, and should carefully monitor patients for any signs and symptoms of muscle pain, tenderness, or weakness, particularly during the initial month of treatment or during any period of upward dosage titration of either drug. Periodic CK determinations may be considered in such situations, but there is no assurance that such monitoring will prevent myopathy.

In clinical studies, no cases of rhabdomyolysis and one suspected case of myopathy have been reported in 1079 patients who were treated with ADVICOR at doses up to 2000 mg/40 mg for periods up to 2 years.

Patients starting therapy with ADVICOR should be advised of the risk of myopathy, and told to report promptly unexplained muscle pain, tenderness, or weakness. A CK level above 10 times ULN in a patient with unexplained muscle symptoms indicates myopathy. ADVICOR therapy should be discontinued if myopathy is diagnosed or suspected.

In patients with complicated medical histories predisposing to rhabdomyolysis, such as preexisting renal insufficiency, dose escalation requires caution. Also, as there are no known adverse consequences of brief interruption of therapy, treatment with ADVICOR should be stopped for a few days before elective major surgery and when any major acute medical or surgical condition supervenes.

Table 7. NCEP Treatment Guidelines: LDL-C Goals and Cutpoints for Therapeutic Lifestyle Changes and Drug Therapy in Different Risk Categories

Risk Category	LDL Goal (mg/dL)	LDL Level at Which to Initiate Therapeutic Lifestyle Changes (mg/dL)	LDL Level at Which to Consider Drug Therapy (mg/dL)
CHD† or CHD risk equivalents (10-year risk >20%)	<100	≥100	≥130 (100-129: drug optional)††
2+ Risk factors (10-year risk ≤20%)	<130	≥130	10-year risk 10%-20%:≥130 10-year risk <10%:≥160
0-1 Risk factor†††	<160	≥160	≥190 (160-189: LDL-lowering drug optional)

†CHD, coronary heart disease

††Some authorities recommend use of LDL-lowering drugs in this category if an LDL-C level of <100 mg/dL cannot be achieved by therapeutic lifestyle changes. Others prefer use of drugs that primarily modify triglycerides and HDL-C, e.g., nicotinic acid or fibrate. Clinical judgement also may call for deferring drug therapy in this subcategory.

†††Almost all people with 0-1 risk factor have 10-year risk <10%; thus, 10-year risk assessment in people with 0-1 risk factor is not necessary.

Use of ADVICOR with other Drugs

The incidence and severity of myopathy may be increased by concomitant administration of ADVICOR with drugs that can cause myopathy when given alone, such as gemfibrozil and other fibrates.

The use of ADVICOR in combination with fibrates should be avoided unless the benefit of further alterations in lipid levels is likely to outweigh the increased risk of this drug combination. In patients taking concomitant cyclosporine or fibrates, the dose of ADVICOR should generally not exceed 1000 mg/20 mg (see DOSAGE AND ADMINISTRATION), as the risk of myopathy may increase at higher doses. Interruption of ADVICOR therapy during a course of treatment with a systemic antifungal azole or a macrolide antibiotic should be considered.

PRECAUTIONS

General

Before instituting therapy with a lipid-altering medication, an attempt should be made to control dyslipidemia with appropriate diet, exercise, and weight reduction in obese patients, and to treat other underlying medical problems (see **INDICATIONS AND USAGE**).

Patients with a past history of jaundice, hepatobiliary disease, or peptic ulcer should be observed closely during ADVICOR therapy. Frequent monitoring of liver function tests and blood glucose should be performed to ascertain that the drug is producing no adverse effects on these organ systems.

Diabetic patients may experience a dose-related rise in fasting blood sugar (FBS). In three clinical studies, which included 1028 patients exposed to ADVICOR (6 to 22% of whom had diabetes type II at baseline), increases in FBS above normal occurred in 46 to 65% of patients at any time during study treatment with ADVICOR. Fourteen patients (1.4%) were discontinued from study treatment: 3 patients for worsening diabetes, 10 patients for hyperglycemia and 1 patient for a new diagnosis of diabetes. In the studies in which lovastatin and NIASPAN were used as active controls, 24 to 41% of patients receiving lovastatin and 43 to 58% of patients receiving NIASPAN also had increases in FBS above normal. One patient (1.1%) receiving lovastatin was discontinued for hyperglycemia. Diabetic or potentially diabetic patients should be observed closely during treatment with ADVICOR, and adjustment of diet and/or hypoglycemic therapy may be necessary.

In one long-term study of 106 patients treated with ADVICOR, elevations in prothrombin time (PT) >3 times ULN occurred in 2 patients (2%) during study drug treatment. In a long-term study of 814 patients treated with ADVICOR, 7 patients were noted to have platelet counts <100,000 during study drug treatment. Four of these patients were discontinued, and one patient with a platelet count <100,000 had prolonged bleeding after a tooth extraction. Prior studies have shown that NIASPAN can be associated with dose-related reductions in platelet count (mean of -11% with 2000 mg) and increases of PT (mean of approximately +4%). Accordingly, patients undergoing surgery should be carefully evaluated. In controlled studies, ADVICOR has been associated with small but statistically significant dose-related reductions in phosphorus levels (mean of -10% with 2000 mg/40 mg). Phosphorus levels should be monitored periodically in patients at risk for hypophosphatemia. In clinical studies with ADVICOR, hypophosphatemia was more common in males than in females. The clinical relevance of hypophosphatemia in this population is not known.

Niacin

Caution should also be used when ADVICOR is used in patients with unstable angina or in the acute phase of MI, particularly when such patients are also receiving vasoactive drugs such as nitrates, calcium channel blockers, or adrenergic blocking agents.

Elevated uric acid levels have occurred with niacin therapy; therefore, in patients predisposed to gout, niacin therapy should be used with caution. Niacin is rapidly metabolized by the liver, and excreted through the kidneys. ADVICOR is contraindicated in patients with significant or unexplained hepatic dysfunction (see **CONTRAINDICATIONS** and **WARNINGS**) and should be used with caution in patients with renal dysfunction.

Lovastatin

Lovastatin may elevate creatine phosphokinase and transaminase levels (see **WARNINGS** and **ADVERSE REACTIONS**). This should be considered in the differential diagnosis of chest pain in a patient on therapy with lovastatin.

Endocrine function—HMG-CoA reductase inhibitors interfere with cholesterol synthesis and as such might theoretically blunt adrenal and/or gonadal steroid production. Results of clinical studies with drugs in this class have been inconsistent with regard to drug effects on basal and reserve steroid levels. However, clinical studies have shown that lovastatin does not reduce basal plasma cortisol concentration or impair adrenal reserve, and does not reduce basal plasma testosterone concentration. Another HMG-CoA reductase inhibitor has been shown to reduce the plasma testosterone response to human chorionic gonadotropin (HCG). In the same study, the mean testosterone response to HCG was slightly but not significantly reduced after treatment with lovastatin 40 mg daily for 16 weeks in 21 men. The effects of HMG-CoA reductase inhibitors on male fertility have not been studied in adequate numbers of male patients. The effects, if any, on the pituitary-gonadal axis in premenopausal women are unknown. Patients treated with lovastatin who develop clinical evidence of endocrine dysfunction should be evaluated appropriately. Caution should also be exercised if an HMG-CoA reductase inhibitor or other agent used to lower cholesterol levels is administered to patients also receiving other drugs (e.g., ketoconazole, spironolactone, cimetidine) that may decrease the levels or activity of endogenous steroid hormones.

CNS toxicity—Lovastatin produced optic nerve degeneration (Wallerian degeneration of retinogeniculate fibers) in clinically normal dogs in a dose-dependent fashion starting at 60 mg/kg/day, a dose that produced mean plasma drug levels about 30 times higher than the mean drug level in humans taking the highest recommended dose (as measured by total enzyme inhibitory activity). Vestibulocochlear Wallerian-like degeneration and retinal ganglion cell chromatolysis were also seen in dogs treated for 14 weeks at 180 mg/kg/day, a dose which resulted in a mean plasma drug level (Cmax) similar to that seen with the 60 mg/kg/day dose.

CNS vascular lesions, characterized by perivascular hemorrhage and edema, mononuclear cell infiltration of perivascular spaces, perivascular fibrin deposits and necrosis of small vessels, were seen in dogs treated with lovastatin at a dose of 180 mg/kg/day, a dose which produced plasma drug levels (Cmax) which were about 30 times higher than the mean values in humans taking 80 mg/day.

Similar optic nerve and CNS vascular lesions have been observed with other drugs of this class.

Cataracts were seen in dogs treated with lovastatin for 11 and 28 weeks at 180 mg/kg/day and 1 year at 60 mg/kg/day.

Information for Patients

Patients should be advised of the following:

— to report promptly unexplained muscle pain, tenderness, or weakness (see **WARNINGS**, **Skeletal Muscle**);

— to take ADVICOR at bedtime, with a low-fat snack. Administration on an empty stomach is not recommended;

— to carefully follow the prescribed dosing regimen (see **DOSAGE AND ADMINISTRATION**);

— that flushing is a common side effect of niacin therapy that usually subsides after several weeks of consistent niacin use. Flushing may last for several hours after dosing, may vary in severity, and will, by taking ADVICOR at bedtime, most likely occur during sleep. If awakened by flushing, especially if taking antihypertensives, rise slowly to minimize the potential for dizziness and/or syncope;

— that taking aspirin (up to approximately 30 minutes before taking ADVICOR) or another non-steroidal anti-inflammatory drug (e.g., ibuprofen) may minimize flushing;
— to avoid ingestion of alcohol or hot drinks around the time of ADVICOR administration, to minimize flushing;
— should not be administered with grapefruit juice;
— that if ADVICOR therapy is discontinued for an extended length of time, their physician should be contacted prior to re-starting therapy; re-titration is recommended (see **DOSAGE AND ADMINISTRATION**);
— to notify their physician if they are taking vitamins or other nutritional supplements containing niacin or related compounds such as nicotinamide (see **Drug Interactions**);
— to notify their physician if symptoms of dizziness occur;
— if diabetic, to notify their physician of changes in blood glucose;
— that ADVICOR tablets should not be broken, crushed, or chewed, but should be swallowed whole.

Drug Interactions

Niacin

Antihypertensive Therapy—Niacin may potentiate the effects of ganglionic blocking agents and vasoactive drugs resulting in postural hypotension.

Aspirin: Concomitant aspirin may decrease the metabolic clearance of niacin. The clinical relevance of this finding is unclear.

Bile Acid Sequestrants—An *in vitro* study was carried out investigating the niacin-binding capacity of colestipol and cholestyramine. About 98% of available niacin was bound to colestipol, with 10 to 30% binding to cholestyramine. These results suggest that 4 to 6 hours, or as great an interval as possible, should elapse between the ingestion of bile acid-binding resins and the administration of ADVICOR.

Other—Concomitant alcohol or hot drinks may increase the side effects of flushing and pruritus and should be avoided around the time of ADVICOR ingestion. Vitamins or other nutritional supplements containing large doses of niacin or related compounds such as nicotinamide may potentiate the adverse effects of ADVICOR.

Lovastatin

Serious skeletal muscle disorders, e.g., rhabdomyolysis, have been reported during concomitant therapy of lovastatin or other HMG-CoA reductase inhibitors with cyclosporine, itraconazole, ketoconazole, gemfibrozil, niacin, erythromycin, clarithromycin, nefazodone or HIV protease inhibitors. (See **WARNINGS, Skeletal Muscle**).

Coumarin Anticoagulants—In a small clinical study in which lovastatin was administered to warfarin-treated patients, no effect on PT was detected. However, another HMG-CoA reductase inhibitor has been found to produce a less than two seconds increase in PT in healthy volunteers receiving low doses of warfarin. Also, bleeding and/or increased PT have been reported in a few patients taking coumarin anticoagulants concomitantly with lovastatin. It is recommended that in patients taking anticoagulants, PT be determined before starting ADVICOR and frequently enough during early therapy to insure that no significant alteration of PT occurs. Once a stable PT has been documented, PT can be monitored at the intervals usually recommended for patients on coumarin anticoagulants. If the dose of ADVICOR is changed, the same procedure should be repeated.

Antipyrine—Lovastatin had no effect on the pharmacokinetics of antipyrine or its metabolites. However, since lovastatin is metabolized by the cytochrome P450 isoform 3A4 enzyme system, this does not preclude an interaction with other drugs metabolized by the same isoform.

Propranolol—In normal volunteers, there was no clinically significant pharmacokinetic or pharmacodynamic interaction with concomitant administration of single doses of lovastatin and propranolol.

Digoxin—In patients with hypercholesterolemia, concomitant administration of lovastatin and digoxin resulted in no effect on digoxin plasma concentrations.

Oral Hypoglycemic Agents—In pharmacokinetic studies of lovastatin in hypercholesterolemic, non-insulin dependent diabetic patients, there was no drug interaction with glipizide or with chlorpropamide.

Drug/Laboratory Test Interactions

Niacin may produce false elevations in some fluorometric determinations of plasma or urinary catecholamines. Niacin may also give false-positive reactions with cupric sulfate solution (Benedict's reagent) in urine glucose tests.

Carcinogenesis, Mutagenesis, Impairment of Fertility

No studies have been conducted with ADVICOR regarding carcinogenesis, mutagenesis, or impairment of fertility.

Niacin

Niacin, administered to mice for a lifetime as a 1% solution in drinking water, was not carcinogenic. The mice in this study received approximately 6 to 8 times a human dose of 3000 mg/day as determined on a mg/m^2 basis. Niacin was negative for mutagenicity in the Ames test. No studies on impairment of fertility have been performed.

Lovastatin

In a 21-month carcinogenic study in mice, there was a statistically significant increase in the incidence of hepatocellular carcinomas and adenomas in both males and females at 500 mg/kg/day. This dose produced a total plasma drug exposure 3 to 4 times that of humans given the highest recommended dose of lovastatin (drug exposure was measured as total HMG-CoA reductase inhibitory activity in extracted plasma). Tumor increases were not seen at 20 and 100 mg/kg/day, doses that produced drug exposures of 0.3 to 2 times that of humans at the 80 mg/day dose. A statistically significant increase in pulmonary adenomas was seen in female mice at approximately 4 times the human drug exposure. (Although mice were given 300 times the human dose on a mg/kg body weight basis, plasma levels of total inhibitory activity were only 4 times higher in mice than in humans given 80 mg of lovastatin.)

There was an increase in incidence of papilloma in the non-glandular mucosa of the stomach of mice beginning at exposures of 1 to 2 times that of humans. The glandular mucosa was not affected. The human stomach contains only glandular mucosa.

In a 24-month carcinogenicity study in rats, there was a positive dose-response relationship for hepatocellular carcinogenicity in males at drug exposures between 2 to 7 times that of human exposure at 80 mg/day (doses in rats were 5, 30, and 180 mg/kg/day).

An increased incidence of thyroid neoplasms in rats appears to be a response that has been seen with other HMG-CoA reductase inhibitors.

A drug in this class chemically similar to lovastatin was administered to mice for 72 weeks at 25, 100, and 400 mg/kg body weight, which resulted in mean serum drug levels approximately 3, 15, and 33 times higher than the mean human serum drug concentration (as total inhibitory activity) after a 40 mg oral dose. Liver carcinomas were significantly increased in high-dose females and mid- and high-dose males, with a maximum incidence of 90% in males. The incidence of adenomas of the liver was significantly increased in mid- and high-dose females. Drug treatment also significantly increased the incidence of lung adenomas in mid- and high-dose males and females. Adenomas of the Harderian gland (a gland of the eye of rodents) were significantly higher in high-dose mice than in controls.

No evidence of mutagenicity was observed in a microbial mutagen test using mutant strains of *Salmonella typhimurium* with or without rat or mouse liver metabolic activation. In addition, no evidence of damage to genetic material was noted in an *in vitro* alkaline elution assay using rat or mouse hepatocytes, a V-79 mammalian cell forward mutation study, an *in vitro* chromosome aberration study in CHO cells, or an *in vivo* chromosomal aberration assay in mouse bone marrow.

Drug-related testicular atrophy, decreased spermatogenesis, spermatocytic degeneration and giant cell formation were seen in dogs starting at 20 mg/kg/day. Similar findings were seen with another drug in this class. No drug-related effects on fertility were found in studies with lovastatin in rats. However, in studies with a similar drug in this class, there was decreased fertility in male rats treated for 34 weeks at 25 mg/kg body weight, although this effect was not observed in a subsequent fertility study when this same dose was administered for 11 weeks (the entire cycle of spermatogenesis, including epididymal maturation). In rats treated with this same reductase inhibitor at 180 mg/kg/day, seminiferous tubule degeneration (necrosis and loss of spermatogenic epithelium) was observed. No microscopic changes were observed in the testes from rats of either study. The clinical significance of these findings is unclear.

Pregnancy

Pregnancy Category X—See **CONTRAINDICATIONS**.

ADVICOR should be administered to women of childbearing potential only when such patients are highly unlikely to conceive and have been informed of the potential hazard. Safety in pregnant women has not been established and there is no apparent benefit to therapy with ADVICOR during pregnancy (see **CONTRAINDICATIONS**). Treatment should be immediately discontinued as soon as pregnancy is recognized.

Niacin

Animal reproduction studies have not been conducted with niacin or with ADVICOR. It is also not known whether niacin at doses typically used for lipid disorders can cause fetal harm when administered to pregnant women or whether it can affect reproductive capacity. If a woman receiving niacin or ADVICOR for primary hypercholesterolemia (Types IIa or IIb) becomes pregnant, the drug should be discontinued.

Lovastatin

Rare reports of congenital anomalies have been received following intrauterine exposure to HMG-CoA reductase inhibitors. In a review[5] of approximately 100 prospectively followed pregnancies in women exposed to lovastatin or another structurally related HMG-CoA reductase inhibitor, the incidences of congenital anomalies, spontaneous abortions and fetal deaths/stillbirths did not exceed what would be expected in the general population. The number of cases is adequate only to exclude a 3- to 4-fold increase in congenital anomalies over the background incidence. In 89% of the prospectively followed pregnancies, drug treatment was initiated prior to pregnancy and was discontinued at some point in the first trimester when pregnancy was identified. Lovastatin has been shown to produce skeletal malformations at plasma levels 40 times the human exposure (for mouse fetus) and 80 times the human exposure (for rat fetus) based on mg/m^2 surface area (doses were 800 mg/kg/day). No drug-induced changes were seen in either species at multiples of 8 times (rat) or 4 times (mouse) based on surface area. No evidence of malformations was noted in rabbits at exposures up to 3 times the human exposure (dose of 15 mg/kg/day, highest tolerated dose).

Labor and Delivery

No studies have been conducted on the effect of ADVICOR, niacin or lovastatin on the mother or the fetus during labor or delivery, on the duration of labor or delivery, or on the growth, development, and functional maturation of the child.

Nursing Mothers

No studies have been conducted with ADVICOR in nursing mothers.

Because of the potential for serious adverse reactions in nursing infants from lipid-altering doses of niacin and lovastatin (see **CONTRAINDICATIONS**), ADVICOR should not be taken while a woman is breastfeeding.

Niacin has been reported to be excreted in human milk. It is not known whether lovastatin is excreted in human milk. A small amount of another drug in this class is excreted in human breast milk.

Pediatric use

No studies in patients under 18 years-of-age have been conducted with ADVICOR. Because pediatric patients are not likely to benefit from cholesterol lowering for at least a decade and because experience with this drug or its active ingredients is limited, treatment of pediatric patients with ADVICOR is not recommended at this time.

Geriatric Use

Of the 214 patients who received ADVICOR in double-blind clinical studies, 37.4% were 65 years-of-age and older, and of the 814 patients who received ADVICOR in open-label clinical studies, 36.2% were 65 years-of-age and older. Responses in LDL-C, HDL-C, and TG were similar in geriatric patients. No overall differences in the percentage of patients with adverse events were observed between older and younger patients. No overall differences were observed in selected chemistry values between the two groups except for amylase which was higher in older patients.

ADVERSE REACTIONS

Overview

In controlled clinical studies, 40/214 (19%) of patients randomized to ADVICOR discontinued therapy prior to study completion, 18/214 (8%) of discontinuations being due to flushing. In the same controlled studies, 9/94 (10%) of patients randomized to lovastatin and 19/92 (21%) of patients randomized to NIASPAN also discontinued treatment prior to study completion secondary to adverse events. Flushing episodes (i.e., warmth, redness, itching and/or tingling) were the most common treatment-emergent adverse events, and occurred in 53% to 83% of patients treated with ADVICOR. Spontaneous reports with NIASPAN and clinical studies with ADVICOR suggest that flushing may also be accompanied by symptoms of dizziness or syncope, tachycardia, palpitations, shortness of breath, sweating, chills, and/or edema.

Adverse Reactions Information

Because clinical studies are conducted under widely varying conditions, adverse reaction rates observed in clinical studies of a drug cannot be directly compared to rates in the clinical studies of another drug and may not reflect the rates observed in clinical practice. The adverse reaction information from clinical studies does, however provide a basis for identifying the adverse events that appear to be related to drug use and for approximating rates.

The data described in this section reflect the exposure to ADVICOR in two double-blind, controlled clinical studies of 400 patients. The population was 28 to 86 years-of-age, 54% male, 85% Caucasian, 9% Black, and 7% Other, and had mixed dyslipidemia (Frederickson Types IIa and IIb).

In addition to flushing, other adverse events occurring in 5% or greater of patients treated with ADVICOR are shown in Table 8 below.

[See table 8 at top of next page]

The following adverse events have also been reported with niacin, lovastatin, and/or other HMG-CoA reductase inhibitors, but not necessarily with ADVICOR, either during clinical studies or in routine patient management.

Body as a Whole:	chest pain; abdominal pain; edema; chills; malaise
Cardiovascular:	atrial fibrillation; tachycardia; palpitations, and other cardiac arrhythmias; orthostasis; hypotension; syncope
Eye:	toxic amblyopia; cystoid macular edema; ophthalmoplegia; eye irritation
Gastrointestinal:	activation of peptic ulcers and peptic ulceration; dyspepsia; vomiting; anorexia; constipation; flatulence, pancreatitis; hepatitis; fatty change in liver; jaundice; and rarely, cirrhosis, fulminant hepatic necrosis, and hepatoma
Metabolic:	gout
Musculoskeletal:	muscle cramps; myopathy; rhabdomyolysis; arthralgia
Nervous:	dizziness; insomnia; dry mouth; paresthesia; anxiety; tremor; vertigo; memory loss; peripheral neuropathy; psychic disturbances; dysfunction of certain cranial nerves
Skin:	hyper-pigmentation; acanthosis nigricans; urticaria; alopecia; dry skin; sweating; and a variety of skin changes (e.g.,

Continued on next page

Table 8. Treatment-Emergent Adverse Events in ≥ 5% of Patients
(Events Irrespective of Causality; Data from Controlled, Double-Blind Studies)

Adverse Event	ADVICOR	NIASPAN	Lovastatin
Total Number of Patients	214	92	94
Cardiovascular	**163 (76%)**	**66 (72%)**	**24 (26%)**
Flushing	152 (71%)	60 (65%)	17 (18%)
Body as a Whole	**104 (49%)**	**50 (54%)**	**42 (45%)**
Asthenia	10 (5%)	6 (7%)	5 (5%)
Flu Syndrome	12 (6%)	7 (8%)	4 (4%)
Headache	20 (9%)	12 (13%)	5 (5%)
Infection	43 (20%)	14 (15%)	19 (20%)
Pain	18 (8%)	3 (3%)	9 (10%)
Pain, Abdominal	9 (4%)	1 (1%)	6 (6%)
Pain, Back	10 (5%)	5 (5%)	5 (5%)
Digestive System	**51 (24%)**	**26 (28%)**	**16 (17%)**
Diarrhea	13 (6%)	8 (9%)	2 (2%)
Dyspepsia	6 (3%)	5 (5%)	4 (4%)
Nausea	14 (7%)	11 (12%)	2 (2%)
Vomiting	7 (3%)	5 (5%)	0
Metabolic and Nutrit. System	**37 (17%)**	**18 (20%)**	**13 (14%)**
Hyperglycemia	8 (4%)	6 (7%)	6 (6%)
Musculoskeletal System	**19 (9%)**	**9 (10%)**	**17 (18%)**
Myalgia	6 (3%)	5 (5%)	8 (9%)
Skin and Appendages	**3 (2%)**	**19 (21%)**	**11 (12%)**
Pruritus	14 (7%)	7 (8%)	3 (3%)
Rash	11 (5%)	11 (12%)	3 (3%)

Note: Percentages are calculated from the total number of patients in each column.

Advicor—Cont.

	nodules, discoloration, dryness of mucous membranes, changes to hair/nails)
Respiratory:	dyspnea; rhinitis
Urogenital:	gynecomastia; loss of libido; erectile dysfunction
Hypersensitivity reactions:	An apparent hypersensitivity syndrome has been reported rarely, which has included one or more of the following features: anaphylaxis, angioedema, lupus erythematous-like syndrome, polymyalgia rheumatica, vasculitis, purpura, thrombocytopenia, leukopenia, hemolytic anemia, positive ANA, ESR increase, eosinophilia, arthritis, arthralgia, urticaria, asthenia, photosensitivity, fever, chills, flushing, malaise, dyspnea, toxic epidermal necrolysis, erythema multiforme, including Stevens-Johnson syndrome.
Other:	migraine

Clinical Laboratory Abnormalities

Chemistry

Elevations in serum transaminases (see **WARNINGS - Liver Dysfunction**), CPK and fasting glucose, and reductions in phosphorus. Niacin extended-release tablets have been associated with slight elevations in LDH, uric acid, total bilirubin, and amylase. Lovastatin and/or HMG-CoA reductase inhibitors have been associated with elevations in alkaline phosphatase, γ-glutamyl transpeptidase and bilirubin, and thyroid function abnormalities.

Hematology

Niacin extended-release tablets have been associated with slight reductions in platelet counts and prolongation in PT (see **WARNINGS**).

DRUG ABUSE AND DEPENDENCE

Neither niacin nor lovastatin is a narcotic drug. ADVICOR has no known addiction potential in humans.

OVERDOSAGE

Information on acute overdose with ADVICOR in humans is limited. Until further experience is obtained, no specific treatment of overdose with ADVICOR can be recommended. The patient should be carefully observed and given supportive treatment.

Niacin

The s.c. LD50 of niacin is 5 g/kg in rats.

The signs and symptoms of an acute overdose of niacin can be anticipated to be those of excessive pharmacologic effect: severe flushing, nausea/vomiting, diarrhea, dyspepsia, dizziness, syncope, hypotension, possibly cardiac arrhythmias and clinical laboratory abnormalities. Insufficient information is available on the potential for the dialyzability of niacin.

Lovastatin

After oral administration of lovastatin to mice the median lethal dose observed was >15 g/m^2.

Five healthy human volunteers have received up to 200 mg of lovastatin as a single dose without clinically significant adverse experiences. A few cases of accidental overdose have been reported; no patients had any specific symptoms, and all patients recovered without sequelae. The maximum dose taken was 5 to 6 g. The dialyzability of lovastatin and its metabolites in man is not known at present.

DOSAGE AND ADMINISTRATION

The usual recommended starting dose for NIASPAN is 500 mg qhs. NIASPAN must be titrated and the dose should not be increased by more than 500 mg every 4 weeks up to a maximum dose of 2000 mg a day, to reduce the incidence and severity of side effects. Patients already receiving a stable dose of NIASPAN may be switched directly to a niacin-equivalent dose of ADVICOR.

The usual recommended starting dose of lovastatin is 20 mg once a day. Dose adjustments should be made at intervals of 4 weeks or more. Patients already receiving a stable dose of lovastatin may receive concomitant dosage titration with NIASPAN, and switch to ADVICOR once a stable dose of NIASPAN has been reached.

Flushing of the skin (see **ADVERSE REACTIONS**) may be reduced in frequency or severity by pretreatment with aspirin (taken up to approximately 30 minutes prior to ADVICOR dose) or other non-steroidal anti-inflammatory drugs. Flushing, pruritus, and gastrointestinal distress are also greatly reduced by slowly increasing the dose of niacin and avoiding administration on an empty stomach.

Equivalent doses of ADVICOR may be substituted for equivalent doses of NIASPAN but should not be substituted for other modified-release (sustained-release or time-release) niacin preparations or immediate-release (crystalline) niacin preparations (see WARNINGS). Patients previously receiving niacin products other than NIASPAN should be started on NIASPAN with the recommended NIASPAN titration schedule, and the dose should subsequently be individualized based on patient response.

ADVICOR should be taken at bedtime, with a low-fat snack. ADVICOR tablets should be taken whole and should not be broken, crushed, or chewed before swalowing. The lowest initial ADVICOR dose is a single 500 mg/20 mg tablet once daily at bedtime. The dose of ADVICOR should not be increased by more than 500 mg daily (based on the NIASPAN component) every 4 weeks. The dose of ADVICOR should be individualized based on targeted goals for cholesterol and triglycerides, and on patient response. Doses of ADVICOR greater than 2000 mg/40 mg daily are not recommended. **If ADVICOR therapy is discontinued for an extended period (>7 days), reinstitution of therapy should begin with the lowest dose of ADVICOR.**

HOW SUPPLIED

ADVICOR is an unscored, capsule-shaped tablet containing either 500 or 1000 mg of niacin in an extended-release formulation and 20 mg of lovastatin in an immediate-release formulation. Tablets are color-coated and debossed with "KOS" on one side and the tablet strength code on the other side. ADVICOR 500 mg/20 mg tablets are light yellow, code "502". ADVICOR 1000 mg/20 mg tablets are dark pink/light purple, code "1002". Tablets are supplied in bottles of 90 tablets as shown below.

500 mg/20 mg tablets: bottles of 90 - NDC# 60598-006-90
1000 mg/20 mg tablets: bottles of 90 - NDC# 60598-008-90

Store at room temperature (20° to 25°C or 68° to 77°F).

Niaspan is a registered trademark of Kos Pharmaceuticals, Inc. and Mevacor is a registered trademark of Merck & Co., Inc.

REFERENCES

1. Executive Summary of the Third Report of the National Cholesterol Education Program (NCEP) Expert Panel on Detection, Evaluation, and Treatment of High Blood Cholesterol in Adults (Adult Treatment Panel III). *JAMA* 2001; 285:2486-2497.
2. Downs JR, et al. *JAMA* 1998; 279:1615-1622.
3. Bradford RH, et al. *Arch Intern Med* 1991;151:43-49.
4. Bradford RH, et al. *Am J Cardiol* 1994; 74:667-673.
5. Manson JM, et al. *Reprod Toxicol* 1996; 10(6): 439-446.

Mfr. by:
Kos Pharmaceuticals, Inc.
Miami, FL 33131

400161/0604

Shown in Product Identification Guide, page 320

AZMACORT® ℞

[*ăz 'ma-kort*]
(triamcinolone acetonide)
Inhalation Aerosol

Rx only
For Oral Inhalation Only
Shake Well Before Using
Prescribing Information as of March 2003

DESCRIPTION

Triamcinolone acetonide, USP, the active ingredient in **Azmacort®** Inhalation Aerosol, is a corticosteroid with a molecular weight of 434.5 and with the chemical designation 9-Fluoro-11β,16α,17,21-tetrahydroxypregna-1,4-diene-3,20-dione cyclic 16,17-acetal with acetone. ($C_{24}H_{31}FO_6$).

Azmacort Inhalation Aerosol is a metered-dose aerosol unit containing a microcrystalline suspension of triamcinolone acetonide in the propellant dichlorodifluoromethane and dehydrated alcohol USP 1% w/w. Each canister contains 60 mg triamcinolone acetonide. The canister must be primed prior to the first use. After an initial priming of 2 actuations, each actuation delivers 200 mcg triamcinolone acetonide from the valve and 100 mcg from the spacer-mouthpiece under defined *in vitro* test conditions. The canister will remain primed for 3 days. If the canister is not used for more than 3 days, then it should be reprimed with 2 actuations. There are at least 240 actuations in one **Azmacort** Inhalation Aerosol canister. **After 240 actuations, the amount delivered per actuation may not be consistent and the unit should be discarded.**

CLINICAL PHARMACOLOGY

Triamcinolone acetonide is a more potent derivative of triamcinolone. Although triamcinolone itself is approximately one to two times as potent as prednisone in animal models of inflammation, triamcinolone acetonide is approximately 8 times more potent than prednisone.

The precise mechanism of the action of glucocorticoids in asthma is unknown. However, the inhaled route makes it possible to provide effective local anti-inflammatory activity with reduced systemic corticosteroid effects. Though highly effective for asthma, glucocorticoids do not affect asthma symptoms immediately. While improvement in asthma may occur as soon as one week after initiation of **Azmacort** Inhalation Aerosol therapy, maximum improvement may not be achieved for 2 weeks or longer.

Based upon intravenous dosing of triamcinolone acetonide phosphate ester, the half-life of triamcinolone acetonide was reported to be 88 minutes. The volume of distribution (Vd) reported was 99.5 L (SD ± 27.5) and clearance was 45.2 L/hour (SD ± 9.1) for triamcinolone acetonide. The plasma half-life of glucocorticoids does not correlate well with the biologic half-life.

The pharmacokinetics of radiolabeled triamcinolone acetonide [^{14}C] were evaluated following a single oral dose of 800 mcg to healthy male volunteers. Radiolabeled triamcinolone acetonide was found to undergo relatively rapid absorption following oral administration with maximum plasma triamcinolone acetonide and [^{14}C]-derived radioactivity occurring between 1.5 and 2 hours. Plasma protein binding of triamcinolone acetonide appears to be relatively low and consistent over a wide plasma triamcinolone acetonide concentration range as a function of time. The overall mean percent fraction bound was approximately 68%.

The metabolism and excretion of triamcinolone acetonide were both rapid and extensive with no parent compound being detected in the plasma after 24 hours post-dose and a low ratio (10.6%) of parent compound $AUC_{0-\infty}$ to total [^{14}C] radioactivity $AUC_{0-\infty}$. Greater than 90% of the oral [^{14}C]-radioactive dose was recovered within 5 days after administration in 5 out of the 6 subjects in the study. Of the recovered [^{14}C]-radioactivity, approximately 40% and 60% were found in the urine and feces, respectively.

Three metabolites of triamcinolone acetonide have been identified. They are 6β-hydroxytriamcinolone acetonide, 21-carboxytriamcinolone acetonide and 21-carboxy-6β-hydroxytriamcinolone acetonide. All three metabolites are expected to be substantially less active than the parent compound due to (a) the dependence of anti-inflammatory activity on the presence of a 21-hydroxyl group, (b) the decreased activity observed upon 6-hydroxylation, and (c) the markedly increased water solubility favoring rapid elimination. There appeared to be some quantitative differences in the metabolites among species. No differences were detected in metabolic pattern as a function of route of administration.

CLINICAL TRIALS

Double-blind, placebo controlled efficacy and safety studies have been conducted in asthma patients with a range of asthma severities, from those patients with mild disease to those with severe disease requiring oral steroid therapy.

The efficacy and safety of **Azmacort** Inhalation Aerosol given twice daily was demonstrated in two placebo-controlled clinical trials. In two separate studies, 222 asthmatic patients were randomized to receive either **Azmacort** Inhalation Aerosol 400 mcg twice daily or matching placebo for a treatment period of 6 weeks. Patients were adult asthmatics who were using inhaled beta$_2$-agonists on more than an occasional basis (at least three times weekly), either without or with inhaled corticosteroids, for control of their asthma symptoms. For the combined studies, 48% (52/109) patients randomized to placebo and 41% (46/113) patients randomized to **Azmacort** Inhalation Aerosol treatment were previously treated with inhaled corticosteroids.

Results of weekly lung function tests (FEV$_1$) from one of these trials is presented graphically below. Results of the second study are presented in tabular form as the changes in asthma measures from baseline to the end of the treatment period.

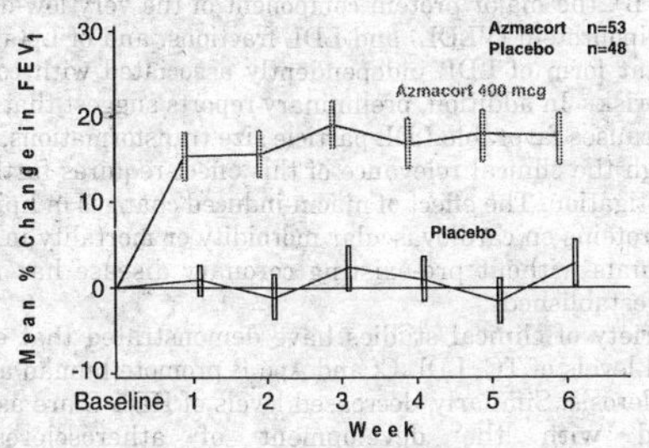

Mean Changes in Asthma Measures from Baseline to Endpoint[a]
All-Treated Patients
Results from a Placebo-Controlled, 6 Week Study

Asthma Measure	Placebo (N=61)	Azmacort 400 mcg bid (N=60)
Percent Change in FEV$_1$(%)	2.8%	17.5%
Increase in Morning Peak Flow Rate (L/min)	6.7	45.9
Decrease in Albuterol Use (puffs/day)	0.6	3.4
Decrease in Daily Asthma Symptom Score (units/day)[b]	0.5	2.3

[a] Endpoint results are obtained from the last evaluable data, regardless of whether the patient completed 6 weeks of treatment.

[b] Scale (0–6) with 0 = no symptom: Maximum Score (AM + PM) = 12

In both studies, treatment with **Azmacort** Inhalation Aerosol (400 mcg twice daily) resulted in significant improvements in all clinical asthma measures (lung functions, asthma symptoms, use of as-needed beta$_2$-agonist medications) when compared to placebo.

INDICATIONS

Azmacort Inhalation Aerosol is indicated in the maintenance treatment of asthma as prophylactic therapy. **Azmacort** Inhalation Aerosol is also indicated for asthma patients who require systemic corticosteroid administration, where adding **Azmacort** may reduce or eliminate the need for the systemic corticosteroids.

Azmacort Inhalation Aerosol is NOT indicated for the relief of acute bronchospasm.

CONTRAINDICATIONS

Azmacort Inhalation Aerosol is contraindicated in the primary treatment of status asthmaticus or other acute episodes of asthma where intensive measures are required.

Hypersensitivity to triamcinolone acetonide or any of the other ingredients in this preparation contraindicates its use.

WARNINGS

Particular care is needed in patients who are transferred from systemically active corticosteroids to **Azmacort** Inhalation Aerosol because deaths due to adrenal insufficiency have occurred in asthmatic patients during and after transfer from systemic corticosteroids to aerosolized steroids in recommended doses. After withdrawal from systemic corticosteroids, a number of months is usually required for recovery of hypothalamic-pituitary-adrenal (HPA) function. For some patients who have received large doses of oral steroids for long periods of time before therapy with **Azmacort** Inhalation Aerosol is initiated, recovery may be delayed for one year or longer. During this period of HPA suppression, patients may exhibit signs and symptoms of adrenal insufficiency when exposed to trauma, surgery, or infections, particularly gastroenteritis or other conditions with acute electrolyte loss. Although **Azmacort** Inhalation Aerosol may provide control of asthmatic symptoms during these episodes, in recommended doses it supplies only normal physiological amounts of corticosteroid systemically and does NOT provide the increased systemic steroid which is necessary for coping with these emergencies.

During periods of stress or a severe asthmatic attack, patients who have been recently withdrawn from systemic corticosteroids should be instructed to resume systemic steroids (in large doses) immediately and to contact their physician for further instruction. These patients should also be instructed to carry a warning card indicating that they may need supplementary systemic steroids during periods of stress or a severe asthma attack.

Localized infections with *Candida albicans* have occurred infrequently in the mouth and pharynx. These areas should be examined by the treating physician at each patient visit. The percentage of positive mouth and throat cultures for *Candida albicans* did not change during a year of continuous therapy. The incidence of clinically apparent infection is low (2.5%). These infections may disappear spontaneously or may require treatment with appropriate antifungal therapy or discontinuance of treatment with **Azmacort** Inhalation Aerosol.

Children who are on immunosuppressant drugs are more susceptible to infections than healthy children. Chickenpox and measles, for example, can have a more serious or even fatal course in children on immunosuppressant doses of corticosteroids. In such children, or in adults who have not had these diseases, particular care should be taken to avoid exposure. If exposed, therapy with varicella zoster immune globulin (VZIG) or pooled intravenous immunoglobulin (IVIG), as appropriate, may be indicated. If chickenpox develops, treatment with antiviral agents may be considered.

Azmacort Inhalation Aerosol is not to be regarded as a bronchodilator and is not indicated for rapid relief of bronchospasm.

As with other inhaled asthma medications, bronchospasm may occur with an immediate increase in wheezing following dosing. If bronchospasm occurs following use of **Azmacort** Inhalation Aerosol, it should be treated immediately with a fast-acting inhaled bronchodilator. Treatment with **Azmacort** Inhalation Aerosol should be discontinued and alternative treatment should be instituted.

Patients should be instructed to contact their physician immediately when episodes of asthma which are not responsive to bronchodilators occur during the course of treatment with **Azmacort** Inhalation Aerosol. During such episodes, patients may require therapy with systemic corticosteroids.

The use of **Azmacort** Inhalation Aerosol with systemic prednisone, dosed either daily or on alternate days, could increase the likelihood of HPA suppression compared to a therapeutic dose of either one alone. Therefore, **Azmacort** Inhalation Aerosol should be used with caution in patients already receiving prednisone treatment for any disease.

Transfer of patients from systemic steroid therapy to **Azmacort** Inhalation Aerosol may unmask allergic conditions previously suppressed by the systemic steroid therapy, *e.g.*, rhinitis, conjunctivitis, and eczema.

PRECAUTIONS

During withdrawal from oral steroids, some patients may experience symptoms of systemically active steroid withdrawal, *e.g.*, joint and/or muscular pain, lassitude, and depression, despite maintenance or even improvement of respiratory function. (See **DOSAGE AND ADMINISTRATION**.) Although steroid withdrawal effects are usually transient and not severe, severe and even fatal exacerbation of asthma can occur if the previous daily oral corticosteroid requirement had significantly exceeded 10 mg/day of prednisone or equivalent.

In responsive patients, inhaled corticosteroids will often permit control of asthmatic symptoms with less suppression of HPA function than therapeutically equivalent oral doses of prednisone. Since triamcinolone acetonide is absorbed into the circulation and can be systemically active, the beneficial effects of **Azmacort** Inhalation Aerosol in minimizing or preventing HPA dysfunction may be expected only when recommended dosages are not exceeded.

Suppression of HPA function has been reported in volunteers who received 4000 mcg daily of triamcinolone acetonide by oral inhalation. In addition, suppression of HPA function has been reported in some patients who have received recommended doses for as little as 6 to 12 weeks. Since the response of HPA function to inhaled corticosteroids is highly individualized, the physician should consider this information when treating patients.

When used at excessive doses or at recommended doses in a small number of susceptible individuals, systemic corticosteroid effects such as hypercorticoidism and adrenal suppression may appear. If such changes occur, **Azmacort** Inhalation Aerosol should be discontinued slowly, consistent with accepted procedures for reducing systemic steroid therapy and for management of asthma symptoms.

Azmacort Inhalation Aerosol should be used with caution, if at all, in patients with active or quiescent tuberculosis infection of the respiratory tract; untreated systemic fungal, bacterial, parasitic, or viral infections; or ocular herpes simplex.

The long-term local and systemic effects of **Azmacort** Inhalation Aerosol in human subjects are still not fully known. While there has been no clinical evidence of adverse experiences, the effects resulting from chronic use of **Azmacort** Inhalation Aerosol on developmental or immunologic processes in the mouth, pharynx, trachea, and lung are unknown.

Because of the possibility of systemic absorption of inhaled corticosteroids, patients treated with these drugs should be observed carefully for any evidence of systemic corticosteroid effects including suppression of growth in children. Particular care should be taken in observing patients postoperatively or during periods of stress for evidence of a decrease in adrenal function.

Information for Patients: Patients being treated with **Azmacort** Inhalation Aerosol should receive the following information and instructions. This information is intended to aid them in the safe and effective use of this medication. It is not a complete disclosure of all possible adverse or intended effects.

Patients should use **Azmacort** Inhalation Aerosol at regular intervals as directed. Results of clinical trials indicate that significant improvement in asthma may occur by 1 week, but maximum benefit may not be achieved for 2 weeks or more. The patient should not increase the prescribed dosage but should contact the physician if symptoms do not improve or if the condition worsens.

In clinical studies and post-marketing experience with **Azmacort** Inhalation Aerosol, local infections of the oropharynx with *Candida albicans* have occurred. When such an infection develops, it should be treated with appropriate local or systemic (*i.e.*, oral antifungal) therapy while remaining on treatment with **Azmacort** Inhalation Aerosol. However, at times therapy with **Azmacort** Inhalation Aerosol may need to be interrupted.

Patients should be instructed to track their use of **Azmacort** Inhalation Aerosol and to dispose of the canister after 240 actuations since reliable dose delivery cannot be assured after 240 doses.

Patients who are on immunosuppressant doses of corticosteroids should be warned to avoid exposure to chickenpox or measles and, if exposed, to obtain medical advice.

Carcinogenesis, Mutagenesis, Impairment of Fertility: No evidence of treatment-related carcinogenicity was demonstrated after two years of once daily gavage of triamcinolone acetonide at doses of 0.05, 0.2, and 1.0 mcg/kg (approximately 0.02, 0.07, and 0.4% of the maximum recommended human daily inhalation dose on a mcg/m^2 basis) in the rat and 0.1, 0.6, and 3.0 mcg/kg (approximately 0.02, 0.1, and 0.6% of the maximum recommended human daily inhalation dose on a mcg/m^2 basis) in a mouse.

Mutagenesis studies with triamcinolone acetonide have not been carried out.

No evidence of impaired fertility was manifested when oral doses of up to 15.0 mcg/kg (8% of the maximum recommended human daily inhalation dose on a mcg/m^2 basis) were administered to female and male rats. However, triamcinolone acetonide at oral doses of 8 mcg/kg (approximately 4% of the maximum recommended human daily inhalation dose on a mcg/m^2 basis) caused dystocia and prolonged delivery and at oral doses of 5.0 mcg/kg (approximately 2.5% of the maximum recommended human daily inhalation dose on a mcg/m^2 basis) and above caused increases in fetal resorptions and stillbirths and decreases in pup body weight and survival. At a lower dose of 1.0 mcg/kg (approximately 0.5% of the maximum recommended human daily inhalation dose on a mcg/m^2 basis) it did not induce the above mentioned effects.

Pregnancy: Pregnancy Category C. Triamcinolone acetonide has been shown to be teratogenic at inhalational doses of 20, 40, and 80 mcg/kg in rats (approximately 0.1, 0.2, and 0.4 times the maximum recommended human daily inhalation dose on a mcg/m^2 basis, respectively), in rabbits at the same doses (approximately 0.2, 0.4, and 0.8 times the maximum recommended human daily inhalation dose on a mcg/m^2 basis, respectively) and in monkeys, at an inhalational dose of 500 mcg/kg (approximately 5 times the maximum recommended human daily inhalation dose on a mcg/m^2 basis). Dose related teratogenic effects in rats and rabbits included cleft palate and/or internal hydrocephaly and axial skeletal defects whereas the teratogenic effects observed in the monkey were CNS and/or cranial malformations. There are no adequate and well controlled studies in pregnant women. Triamcinolone acetonide should be used during pregnancy only if the potential benefit justifies the potential risk to the fetus.

Experience with oral glucocorticoids since their introduction in pharmacologic as opposed to physiologic doses suggests that rodents are more prone to teratogenic effects from glucocorticoids than humans. In addition, because there is a natural increase in glucocorticoid production during pregnancy, most women will require a lower exogenous steroid dose and many will not need glucocorticoid treatment during pregnancy.

Nonteratogenic Effects: Hypoadrenalism may occur in infants born of mothers receiving corticosteroids during pregnancy. Such infants should be carefully observed.

Nursing Mothers: It is not known whether triamcinolone acetonide is excreted in human milk. Because other corticosteroids are excreted in human milk, caution should be exercised when **Azmacort** Inhalation Aerosol is administered to nursing women.

Continued on next page

Azmacort—Cont.

Pediatric Use: Safety and effectiveness have not been established in pediatric patients below the age of 6. Oral corticosteroids have been shown to cause growth suppression in children and teenagers, particularly with higher doses over extended periods. If a child or teenager on any corticosteroid appears to have growth suppression, the possibility that they are particularly sensitive to this effect of steroids should be considered.

Geriatric Use: Clinical studies of **Azmacort** Inhalation Aerosol did not include sufficient numbers of subjects aged 65 and over to determine whether they respond differently from younger subjects. Other reported clinical experience has not identified differences in responses between the elderly and younger patients. In general, dose selection for an elderly patient should be cautious, usually starting at the low end of the dosing range, reflecting the greater frequency of decreased hepatic, renal, or cardiac function, and of concomitant disease or other drug therapy.

ADVERSE REACTIONS

The table below describes the incidence of common adverse experiences based upon three placebo-controlled, multicenter US clinical trials of 507 patients (297 female and 210 male adults (age range 18-64)). These trials included asthma patients who had previously received inhaled beta$_2$-agonists alone, as well as those who previously required inhaled corticosteroid therapy for the control of their asthma. The patients were treated with **Azmacort** Inhalation Aerosol (including doses ranging from 200 to 800 mcg twice daily for 6 weeks) or placebo.

Adverse Events Occurring at an Incidence of Greater Than 3% and Greater Than Placebo

Adverse Event	Azmacort Dose 200 mcg bid (n=57)	Azmacort Dose 400 mcg bid (n=170)	Azmacort Dose 800 mcg bid (n=57)	Placebo (n=167)
Sinusitis	5 (9%)	7 (4%)	1 (2%)	6 (4%)
Pharyngitis	4 (7%)	42 (25%)	10 (18%)	19 (11%)
Headache	4 (7%)	35 (21%)	7 (12%)	24 (14%)
Flu Syndrome	2 (4%)	8 (5%)	1 (2%)	5 (3%)
Back Pain	2 (4%)	3 (2%)	2 (4%)	3 (2%)

Adverse events that occurred at an incidence of 1-3% in the overall **Azmacort** Inhalation Aerosol treatment group and greater than placebo included:

Body as a whole: facial edema, pain, abdominal pain, photosensitivity
Digestive system: diarrhea, oral monilia, toothache, vomiting
Metabolic and Nutrition: weight gain
Musculoskeletal system: bursitis, myalgia, tenosynovitis
Nervous system: dry mouth
Organs of special sense: rash
Respiratory system: chest congestion, voice alteration
Urogenital system: cystitis, urinary tract infection, vaginal monilia

In older controlled clinical trials of steroid dependent asthmatics, urticaria was reported rarely. Anaphylaxis was not reported in these controlled trials. Typical steroid withdrawal effects including muscle aches, joint aches, and fatigue were noted in clinical trials when patients were transferred from oral steroid therapy to **Azmacort** Inhalation Aerosol. Easy bruisability was also noted in these trials. Hoarseness, dry throat, irritated throat, dry mouth, facial edema, increased wheezing, and cough have been reported. These adverse effects have generally been mild and transient. Cases of oral candidiasis occurring with clinical use have been reported. (See **WARNINGS.**)

Post Marketing: In addition to adverse events reported from clinical trials, the following events have been reported post marketing: anaphylaxis, cataracts, and glaucoma.

OVERDOSAGE

There are no data available on the effects of acute or chronic overdose. However, acute overdosing with **Azmacort** Inhalation Aerosol is unlikely in view of the total amount of active ingredient present and the route of administration. The maximum total daily dose (1600 mcg) has been well tolerated when administered as a single dose of 16 consecutive inhalations to adult asthmatics in a controlled clinical trial. Chronic overdosage may result in signs/symptoms of hypercorticoidism. (See **PRECAUTIONS.**) The risk of candidiasis could also be increased.

DOSAGE AND ADMINISTRATION

Adults: The usual recommended dosage is two inhalations (200 mcg) given three to four times a day or four inhalations (400 mcg) given twice daily. The maximal daily intake should not exceed 16 inhalations (1600 mcg) in adults. Higher initial doses (12 to 16 inhalations per day) may be considered in patients with more severe asthma.

Children 6 to 12 Years of Age: The usual recommended dosage is one or two inhalations (100 to 200 mcg) given three to four times a day or two to four inhalations (200 to 400 mcg) given twice daily. The maximal daily intake should not exceed 12 inhalations (1200 mcg) in children 6 to 12 years of age. Insufficient clinical data exist with respect to the safety and efficacy of the administration of **Azmacort** Inhalation Aerosol to children below the age of 6. The long-term effects of inhaled steroids, including **Azmacort** Inhalation Aerosol, on growth are still not fully known.

Rinsing the mouth after inhalation is advised.

Different considerations must be given to the following groups of patients in order to obtain the full therapeutic benefit of **Azmacort** Inhalation Aerosol:

Note: In all patients, it is desirable to titrate to the lowest effective dose once asthma stability has been achieved.

Patients Not Receiving Systemic Corticosteroids: Patients who require maintenance therapy of their asthma may benefit from treatment with **Azmacort** Inhalation Aerosol at the doses recommended above. In patients who respond to **Azmacort** Inhalation Aerosol, improvement in pulmonary function is usually apparent within one to two weeks after the initiation of therapy.

Patients Maintained on Systemic Corticosteroids: Clinical studies have shown that **Azmacort** Inhalation Aerosol may be effective in the management of asthmatics dependent or maintained on systemic corticosteroids and may permit replacement or significant reduction in the dosage of systemic corticosteroids.

The patient's asthma should be reasonably stable before treatment with **Azmacort** Inhalation Aerosol is started. Initially, **Azmacort** Inhalation Aerosol should be used concurrently with the patient's usual maintenance dose of systemic corticosteroid. After approximately one week, gradual withdrawal of the systemic corticosteroid is started by reducing the daily or alternate daily dose. Reductions may be made after an interval of one or two weeks, depending on the response of the patient. A slow rate of withdrawal is strongly recommended. Generally, these decrements should not exceed 2.5 mg of prednisone or its equivalent. During withdrawal, some patients may experience symptoms of systemic corticosteroid withdrawal, *e.g.,* joint and/or muscular pain, lassitude, and depression, despite maintenance or even improvement in pulmonary function. Such patients should be encouraged to continue with the inhaler but should be monitored for objective signs of adrenal insufficiency. If evidence of adrenal insufficiency occurs, the systemic corticosteroid doses should be increased temporarily and thereafter withdrawal should continue more slowly. Inhaled corticosteroids should be used with caution when used chronically in patients receiving prednisone regimens, either daily or alternate day. (See **WARNINGS.**)

During periods of stress or a severe asthma attack, transfer patients may require supplementary treatment with systemic corticosteroids.

Directions for Use: An illustrated leaflet of patient instructions for proper use accompanies each package of **Azmacort** Inhalation Aerosol.

HOW SUPPLIED

Azmacort Inhalation Aerosol contains 60 mg triamcinolone acetonide in a 20 gram package which delivers at least 240 actuations. It is supplied with a white plastic actuator, a white plastic spacer-mouthpiece and patient's leaflet of instructions: box of one. NDC 60598-061-60. Each actuation delivers 200 mcg triamcinolone acetonide from the valve and 100 mcg from the spacer-mouthpiece under defined *in vitro* test conditions.

Avoid spraying in eyes.

For best results, the canister should be at room temperature before use.

Shake well before using.

CONTENTS UNDER PRESSURE. Do not puncture. Do not use or store near heat or open flame. Exposure to temperatures above 120°F may cause bursting. Never throw canister into fire or incinerator. Keep out of reach of children unless otherwise prescribed. Store at Controlled Room Temperature 20 to 25°C (68 to 77°F) [see USP].

Note: The indented statement below is required by the Federal government's Clean Air Act for all products containing or manufactured with chlorofluorocarbons (CFCs):

> WARNING: Contains CFC-12, a substance which harms public health and the environment by destroying ozone in the upper atmosphere.

A notice similar to the above WARNING has been placed in the "Information For The Patient" portion of this package insert under the Environmental Protection Agency's (EPA's) regulations. The patient's warning states that the patient should consult his or her physician if there are questions about alternatives.

Azmacort is a registered trademark

Manufactured for: Kos Pharmaceuticals, Inc.
Cranbury, NJ 08512
400201/0604
Rev. June 2004
50072141

Shown in Product Identification Guide, page 320

NIASPAN® ℞

[niă-span]
(niacin extended-release tablets)
℞ Only

DESCRIPTION

NIASPAN® (niacin extended-release tablets), contain niacin, a B-complex vitamin and antihyperlipidemic agent. Niacin (nicotinic acid, or 3-pyridinecarboxylic acid) is a white, crystalline powder, very soluble in water, with the following structural formula:

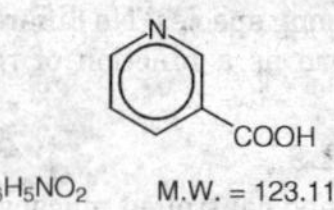

$C_6H_5NO_2$ M.W. = 123.11

NIASPAN is an unscored, off-white tablet for oral administration that contains no color additives and is available in three tablet strengths containing 500, 750, and 1000mg niacin. NIASPAN tablets also contain the inactive ingredients hypromellose, povidone, and stearic acid.

CLINICAL PHARMACOLOGY

Niacin functions in the body after conversion to nicotinamide adenine dinucleotide (NAD) in the NAD coenzyme system. Niacin (but not nicotinamide) in gram doses reduces total cholesterol (TC), low-density lipoprotein cholesterol (LDL-C) and triglycerides (TG), and increases high-density lipoprotein cholesterol (HDL-C). The magnitude of the individual lipid and lipoprotein responses may be influenced by the severity and type of underlying lipid abnormality. The increase in total HDL-C is associated with an increase in apolipoprotein A-I (Apo A-I) and a shift in the distribution of HDL subfractions. These shifts include an increase in the HDL_2:HDL_3 ratio, and an elevation in lipoprotein A-I (Lp A-I, an HDL particle containing only Apo A-I). Niacin treatment also decreases serum levels of apolipoprotein B-100 (Apo B), the major protein component of the very low-density lipoprotein (VLDL) and LDL fractions, and of Lp(a), a variant form of LDL independently associated with coronary risk.[1] In addition, preliminary reports suggest that niacin causes favorable LDL particle size transformations, although the clinical relevance of this effect requires further investigation. The effect of niacin-induced changes in lipids/lipoproteins on cardiovascular morbidity or mortality in individuals without pre-existing coronary disease has not been established.

A variety of clinical studies have demonstrated that elevated levels of TC, LDL-C, and Apo B promote human atherosclerosis. Similarly, decreased levels of HDL-C are associated with the development of atherosclerosis. Epidemiological investigations have established that cardiovascular morbidity and mortality vary directly with the level of TC and LDL-C, and inversely with the level of HDL-C.

Like LDL, cholesterol-enriched triglyceride-rich lipoproteins, including VLDL, intermediate-density lipoprotein (IDL), and remnants, can also promote atherosclerosis. Elevated plasma TG are frequently found in a triad with low HDL-C levels and small LDL particles, as well as in association with non-lipid metabolic risk factors for coronary heart disease (CHD). As such total plasma TG has not consistently been shown to be an independent risk factor for CHD. Furthermore, the independent effect of raising HDL-C or lowering TG on the risk of coronary and cardiovascular morbidity and mortality has not been determined.

Mechanism of Action

The mechanism by which niacin alters lipid profiles has not been well defined. It may involve several actions including partial inhibition of release of free fatty acids from adipose tissue, and increased lipoprotein lipase activity, which may increase the rate of chylomicron triglyceride removal from plasma. Niacin decreases the rate of hepatic synthesis of VLDL and LDL, and does not appear to affect fecal excretion of fats, sterols, or bile acids.

Pharmacokinetics/Metabolism

Absorption

Niacin is rapidly and extensively absorbed (at least 60 to 76% of dose) when administered orally. To maximize bioavailability and reduce the risk of gastrointestinal (GI) upset, administration of NIASPAN with a low-fat meal or snack is recommended.

Single-dose bioavailability studies have demonstrated that NIASPAN tablet strengths are not interchangeable.

Distribution

Studies using radiolabeled niacin in mice show that niacin and its metabolites concentrate in the liver, kidney and adipose tissue.

Metabolism

The pharmacokinetic profile of niacin is complicated due to rapid and extensive first-pass metabolism, which is species and dose-rate specific. In humans, one pathway is through a simple conjugation step with glycine to form nicotinuric acid (NUA). NUA is then excreted in the urine, although there may be a small amount of reversible metabolism back to niacin. The other pathway results in the formation of nicotinamide adenine dinucleotide (NAD). It is unclear whether nicotinamide is formed as a precursor to, or following the synthesis of, NAD. Nicotinamide is further metabolized to at least N-methylnicotinamide (MNA) and nicotinamide-N-oxide (NNO). MNA is further metabolized to two other compounds, N-methyl-2-pyridone-5-carboxamide (2PY) and N-methyl-4-pyridone-5-carboxamide (4PY). The formation of 2PY appears to predominate over 4PY in humans. At the doses used to treat hyperlipidemia, these metabolic pathways are saturable, which explains the nonlinear relationship between niacin dose and plasma concentrations following multiple-dose NIASPAN administration (Table 1).

Nicotinamide does not have hypolipidemic activity; the activity of the other metabolites is unknown.

Table 1. Mean Steady-State Pharmacokinetic Parameters for Plasma Niacin

NIASPAN dose/day	Niacin given as	Peak Concentration (µg/mL)	Time to Peak (hrs)
1000mg	2×500mg	0.6	5
1500mg	2×750mg	4.9	4
2000mg	2×1000mg	15.5	5

Elimination
Niacin and its metabolites are rapidly eliminated in the urine. Following single and multiple doses, approximately 60 to 76% of the niacin dose administered as NIASPAN was recovered in urine as niacin and metabolites; up to 12% was recovered as unchanged niacin after multiple dosing. The ratio of metabolites recovered in the urine was dependent on the dose administered.

Special Populations
Hepatic
No studies have been performed. NIASPAN should be used with caution in patients with a past history of liver disease, who consume substantial quantities of alcohol, or have unexplained transaminase elevations. NIASPAN is contraindicated in patients with active liver disease (see WARNINGS).
Renal
There are no data in this population. NIASPAN should be used with caution in patients with renal disease (see PRECAUTIONS).
Gender
Steady-state plasma concentrations of niacin and metabolites after administration of NIASPAN are generally higher in women than in men, with the magnitude of the difference varying with dose and metabolite. Recovery of niacin and metabolites in urine, however, is generally similar for men and women, indicating that absorption is similar for both genders. The gender differences observed in plasma levels of niacin and its metabolites may be due to gender-specific differences in metabolic rate or volume of distribution. Data from the clinical trials suggest that women have a greater hypolipidemic response than men at equivalent doses of NIASPAN.

Niacin Clinical Studies
The role of LDL-C in atherogenesis is supported by pathological observations, clinical studies, and many animal experiments. Observational epidemiological studies have clearly established that high TC or LDL-C and low HDL-C are risk factors for CHD. Additionally, elevated levels of Lp(a) have been shown to be independently associated with CHD risk.[1] The efficacy of niacin in improving lipoprotein lipid profiles, either alone or in combination with other lipid-altering drugs, as an adjunct to diet therapy in the treatment of hyperlipoproteinemia has been well documented.
Niacin's ability to reduce mortality and the risk of definite, nonfatal myocardial infarction (MI) has also been assessed in long-term studies. The Coronary Drug Project,[2] completed in 1975, was designed to assess the safety and efficacy of niacin and other lipid-altering drugs in men 30 to 64 years old with a history of MI. Over an observation period of 5 years, niacin treatment was associated with a statistically significant reduction in nonfatal, recurrent MI. The incidence of definite, nonfatal MI was 8.9% for the 1,119 patients randomized to nicotinic acid versus 12.2% for the 2,789 patients who received placebo ($p<0.004$). Total mortality was similar in the two groups at 5 years (24.4% with nicotinic acid versus 25.4% with placebo; p=N.S.). At the time of a 15-year follow-up, there were 11% (69) fewer deaths in the niacin group compared to the placebo cohort (52.0% versus 58.2%; $p=0.0004$).[3] However, mortality at 15 years was not an original endpoint of the Coronary Drug Project. In addition, patients had not received niacin for approximately 9 years, and confounding variables such as concomitant medication use and medical or surgical treatments were not controlled.
The Cholesterol-Lowering Atherosclerosis Study (CLAS) was a randomized, placebo-controlled, angiographic trial testing combined colestipol and niacin therapy in 162 non-smoking males with previous coronary bypass surgery.[4] The primary, per-subject cardiac endpoint was global coronary artery change score. After 2 years, 61% of patients in the placebo cohort showed disease progression by global change score (n=82), compared with only 38.8% of drug-treated subjects (n=80), when both native arteries and grafts were considered ($p<0.005$); disease regression also occurred more frequently in the drug-treated group (16.2% versus 2.4%; $p=0.002$). In a follow-up to this trial in a subgroup of 103 patients treated for 4 years, again, significantly fewer patients in the drug-treated group demonstrated progression than in the placebo cohort (48% versus 85%, respectively; $p<0.0001$).[5]
The Familial Atherosclerosis Treatment Study (FATS) in 146 men ages 62 and younger with Apo B levels ≥125 mg/dL, established coronary artery disease, and family histories of vascular disease, assessed change in severity of disease in the proximal coronary arteries by quantitative arteriography.[6] Patients were given dietary counseling and randomized to treatment with either conventional therapy with double placebo (or placebo plus colestipol if the LDL-C was elevated); lovastatin plus colestipol; or niacin plus colestipol. In the conventional therapy group, 46% of patients had disease progression (and no regression) in at least one of nine proximal coronary segments; regression was the only change in 11%. In contrast, progression (as the only change) was seen in only 25% in the niacin plus colestipol group, while regression was observed in 39%. Though not an original endpoint of the trial, clinical events (death, MI, or revascularization for worsening angina) occurred in 10 of 52 patients who received conventional therapy, compared with 2 of 48 who received niacin plus colestipol.
The Harvard Atherosclerosis Reversibility Project (HARP) was a randomized placebo-controlled, 2.5-year study of the effect of a stepped-care antihyperlipidemic drug regimen on 91 patients (80 men and 11 women) with CHD and average baseline TC levels less than 250 mg/dL and ratios of TC to HDL-C greater than 4.0.[7] Drug treatment consisted of an HMG-CoA reductase inhibitor administered alone as initial therapy followed by addition of varying dosages of either a slow-release nicotinic acid, cholestyramine, or gemfibrozil. Addition of nicotinic acid to the HMG-CoA reductase inhibitor resulted in further statistically significant mean reductions in TC, LDL-C, and TG, as well as a further increase in HDL-C in a majority of patients (40 of 44 patients). The ratios of TC to HDL-C and LDL-C to HDL-C were also significantly reduced by this combination drug regimen (see WARNINGS, *Skeletal Muscle*).

NIASPAN Clinical Studies
Placebo-Controlled Clinical Studies in Patients with Primary Hypercholesterolemia and Mixed Dyslipidemia: In two randomized, double-blind, parallel, multi-center, placebo-controlled trials, NIASPAN dosed at 1000, 1500 or 2000mg daily at bedtime with a low-fat snack for 16 weeks (including 4 weeks of dose escalation) favorably altered lipid profiles compared to placebo (Table 2). Women appeared to have a greater response than men at each NIASPAN dose level (see *Gender Effect*, below).

Table 2. Lipid Response to NIASPAN Therapy

Treatment	n	Mean Percent Change from Baseline to Week 16* TC	LDL-C	HDL-C	TC/HDL-C	TG	Lp(a)	Apo B	Apo A-1
NIASPAN 1000mg qhs	41	−3	−5	+18	−17	−21	−13	−6	+9
NIASPAN 2000mg qhs	41	−10	−14	+22	−25	−28	−27	−16	+8
Placebo	40	0	−1	+4	−3	0	0	+1	+3
NIASPAN 1500mg qhs	76	−8	−12	+20	−20	−13	−15	−12	+8
Placebo	73	+2	+1	+2	+1	+12	+2	+1	+2

n = number of patients at baseline;
* Mean percent change from baseline for all NIASPAN doses was significantly different ($p<0.05$) from placebo for all lipid parameters shown except Apo A-1 at 2000mg.

Table 3. Lipid Response in Dose-Escalation Study

Treatment	n	Mean Percent Change from Baseline* TC	LDL-C	HDL-C	TC/HDL-C	TG	Lp(a)	Apo B	Apo A-1
Placebo‡	44	−2	−1	+5	−7	−6	−5	−2	+4
NIASPAN	87								
500mg qhs		−2	−3	+10	−10	−5	−3	−2	+5
1000mg qhs		−5	−9	+15	−17	−11	−12	−7	+8
1500mg qhs		−11	−14	+22	−26	−28	−20	−15	+10
2000mg qhs		−12	−17	+26	−29	−35	−24	−16	+12

n = number of patients enrolled;
‡ Placebo data shown are after 24 weeks of placebo treatment.
* For all NIASPAN doses except 500mg, mean percent change from baseline was significantly different ($p<0.05$) from placebo for all lipid parameters shown except Lp(a) and Apo A-1 which were significantly different from placebo starting with 1500mg and 2000mg, respectively.

Table 4. Selected Lipid Response to NIASPAN in Placebo-Controlled Clinical Studies*

NIASPAN Dose	n	Mean Baseline and Median Percent Change from Baseline (25th, 75th Percentiles) LDL-C	HDL-C	TG
1000mg qhs	104			
Baseline (mg/dL)		218	45	172
Percent Change		−7 (−15, 0)	+14 (+7,+23)	−16 (−34,+3)
1500mg qhs	120			
Baseline (mg/dL)		212	46	171
Percent Change		−13 (−21,−4)	+19 (+9,+31)	−25 (−45,−2)
2000mg qhs	85			
Baseline (mg/dL)		220	44	160
Percent Change		−16 (−26,−7)	+22 (+15,+34)	−38 (−52,−14)

* Represents pooled analyses of results; minimum duration on therapy at each dose was 4 weeks.

Table 5. Effect of Gender on NIASPAN Dose Response

NIASPAN Dose	n (M/F)	Mean Percent Change from Baseline LDL-C M	LDL-C F	HDL-C M	HDL-C F	TG M	TG F	Apo B M	Apo B F
500mg qhs	50/37	−2	−5	+11	+8	−3	−9	−1	−5
1000mg qhs	76/52	−6*	−11*	+14	+20	−10	−20	−5*	−10*
1500mg qhs	104/59	−12	−16	+19	+24	−17	−28	−13	−15
2000mg qhs	75/53	−15	−18	+23	+26	−30	−36	−16	−16

n = number of male/female patients enrolled.
* Percent change significantly different between genders ($p<0.05$).

Table 6. Lipid Response to NIASPAN in Patients with Low HDL-C

	n	Mean Baseline and Mean Percent Change from Baseline TC	LDL-C	HDL-C	TC/HDL-C	TG	Lp(a)†	Apo B†	Apo A-I†	Lp A-I‡
Baseline (mg/dL)	88	190	120	31	6	194	8	106	105	32
Week 19 (% Change)	71	−3	0	+26	−22	−30	−20	−9	+11	+20

n = number of patients enrolled
* Mean percent change from baseline was significantly different ($p<0.05$) for all lipid parameters shown except LDL-C.
†n=72 at baseline and 69 at week 19.
‡n=30 at baseline and week 19.

Continued on next page

Niaspan—Cont.

[See table 2 at top of previous page]
In a double-blind, multi-center, forced dose-escalation study, monthly 500mg increases in NIASPAN dose resulted in incremental reductions of approximately 5% in LDL-C and Apo B levels in the daily dose range of 500mg through 2000mg (Table 3). Women again tended to have a greater response to NIASPAN than men (see *Gender Effect*, below).
[See table 3 at top of previous page]
Pooled results for major lipids from these three placebo-controlled studies are shown below (Table 4).
[See table 4 on previous page]
Gender Effect: Combined data from the three placebo-controlled NIASPAN studies in patients with primary hypercholesterolemia and mixed dyslipidemia suggest that, at each NIASPAN dose level studied, changes in lipid concentrations are greater for women than for men (Table 5).
[See table 5 on previous page]
Other Patient Populations: In a double-blind, multi-center, 19-week study the lipid-altering effects of NIASPAN (forced titration to 2000mg qhs) were compared to baseline in patients whose primary lipid abnormality was a low level of HDL-C (HDL-C ≤40 mg/dL, TG ≤400 mg/dL, and LDL-C ≤160, or <130 mg/dL in the presence of CHD). Results are shown below (Table 6).
[See table 6 on previous page]
At NIASPAN 2000 mg/day, median changes from baseline (25th, 75th percentiles) for LDL-C, HDL-C, and TG were −3% (−14, +12%), +27% (+13, +38%), and −33% (−50, −19%), respectively.
Combination NIASPAN and Lovastatin Study: In a multi-center, randomized, double-blind, parallel, 28-week study, a combination tablet of NIASPAN and lovastatin was compared to each individual component in patients with Type IIa and IIb hyperlipidemia. Using a forced dose-escalation study design, patients received each dose for at least 4 weeks. Patients randomized to treatment with the combination tablet of NIASPAN and lovastatin initially received 500mg/20mg (expressed as mg of niacin/mg of lovastatin) once daily before bedtime. The dose was increased by 500mg at 4-week intervals (based on the NIASPAN component) to a maximum dose of 1000mg/20mg in one-half of the patients and 2000mg/40mg in the other half. The NIASPAN monotherapy group underwent a similar titration from 500mg to 2000mg. The patients randomized to lovastatin monotherapy received 20mg for 12 weeks titrated to 40mg for up to 16 weeks. Up to a third of the patients randomized to the combination tablet of NIASPAN and lovastatin or NIASPAN monotherapy discontinued prior to Week 28. Results from this study showed that combination therapy decreased LDL-C, TG and Lp(a), and increased HDL-C in a dose-dependent fashion (Tables 7, 8, 9, and 10). Results from this study for LDL-C mean percent change from baseline (the primary efficacy variable) showed that:

1) LDL-lowering with the combination tablet of NIASPAN and lovastatin was significantly greater than that achieved with lovastatin 40mg only after 28 weeks of titration to a dose of 2000mg/40mg ($p<0.0001$)
2) The combination tablet of NIASPAN and lovastatin at doses of 1000mg/20mg or higher achieved greater LDL-lowering NIASPAN ($p<0.0001$)

The LDL-C results are sumarized in Table 7.
[See table 7 above]
Combination therapy achieved significantly greater HDL-raising compared to lovastatin and NIASPAN monotherapy at all doses (Table 8).
[See table 8 above]
In addition, combination therapy achieved significantly greater TG-lowering at doses of 1000mg/20mg or greater compared to lovastatin and NIASPAN monotherapy (Table 9).
[See table 9 at right]
The Lp(a)-lowering effects of combination therapy and NIASPAN monotherapy were similar, and both were superior to lovastatin (Table 10). The independent effect of lowering Lp(a) with NIASPAN or combination therapy on the risk of coronary and cardiovascular morbidity and mortality has not been determined.
[See table 10 at right]

Table 7. LDL-C mean percent change from baseline

Week	Combination tablet of NIASPAN and lovastatin			NIASPAN			Lovastatin		
	n*	Dose (mg/mg)	LDL	n*	Dose (mg)	LDL	n*	Dose (mg)	LDL
Baseline	57	-	190.9 mg/dL	61	-	189.7 mg/dL	61	-	185.6 mg/dL
12	47	1000/20	−30%	46	1000	−3%	56	20	−29%
16	45	1000/40	−36%	44	1000	−6%	56	40	−31%
20	42	1500/40	−37%	43	1500	−12%	54	40	−34%
28	42	2000/40	−42%	41	2000	−14%	53	40	−32%

*n = number of patients remaining in trial at each time point.

Table 8. HDL-C mean percent change from baseline

Week	Combination tablet of NIASPAN and lovastatin			NIASPAN			Lovastatin		
	n*	Dose (mg/mg)	HDL	n*	Dose (mg)	HDL	n*	Dose (mg)	HDL
Baseline	57	-	45 mg/dL	61	-	47 mg/dL	61	-	43 mg/dL
12	47	1000/20	+20%	46	1000	+14%	56	20	+3%
16	45	1000/40	+20%	44	1000	+15%	56	40	+5%
20	42	1500/40	+27%	43	1500	+22%	54	40	+6%
28	42	2000/40	+30%	41	2000	+24%	53	40	+6%

*n = number of patients remaining in trial at each time point.

Table 9. TG median percent change from baseline

Week	Combination tablet of NIASPAN and lovastatin			NIASPAN			Lovastatin		
	n*	Dose (mg/mg)	TG	n*	Dose (mg)	TG	n*	Dose (mg)	TG
Baseline	57	-	174 mg/dL	61	-	186 mg/dL	61	-	171 mg/dL
12	47	1000/20	−32%	46	1000	−22%	56	20	−20%
16	45	1000/40	−39%	44	1000	−23%	56	40	−17%
20	42	1500/40	−44%	43	1500	−31%	54	40	−21%
28	42	2000/40	−44%	41	2000	−31%	53	40	−20%

*n = number of patients remaining in trial at each time point.

Table 10. Lp(a) median percent change from baseline

Week	Combination tablet of NIASPAN and lovastatin			NIASPAN			Lovastatin		
	n*	Dose (mg/mg)	Lp(a)	n*	Dose (mg)	Lp(a)	n*	Dose (mg)	Lp(a)
Baseline	57	-	34 mg/dL	61	-	41 mg/dL	60	-	42 mg/dL
12	47	1000/20	−9%	46	1000	−8%	55	20	+8%
16	45	1000/40	−9%	44	1000	−12%	55	40	+8%
20	42	1500/40	−17%	43	1500	−22%	53	40	+6%
28	42	2000/40	−22%	41	2000	−32%	52	40	0%

*n = number of patients remaining in trial at each time point.

Table 11. NCEP Treatment Guidelines: LDL-C Goals and Cutpoints for Therapeutic Lifestyle Changes and Drug Therapy in Different Risk Categories

Risk Category	LDL Goal (mg/dL)	LDL Level at Which to Initiate Therapeutic Lifestyle Changes (mg/dL)	LDL Level at Which to Consider Drug Therapy (mg/dL)
CHD† or CHD risk equivalents (10-year risk >20%)	<100	≥100	≥130 (100–129: drug optional)††
2+ Risk factors (10-year risk ≤20%)	<130	≥130	10-year risk 10%–20%: ≥130 10-year risk <10%: ≥160
0–1 Risk factor†††	<160	≥160	≥190 (160–189: LDL-lowering drug optional)

†CHD, coronary heart disease
††Some authorities recommend use of LDL-lowering drugs in this category if an LDL-C level of <100 mg/dL cannot be achieved by therapeutic lifestyle changes. Others prefer use of drugs that primarily modify triglycerides and HDL-C, e.g., nicotinic acid or fibrate. Clinical judgment also may call for deferring drug therapy in this subcategory.
†††Almost all people with 0–1 risk factor have 10-year risk <10%; thus, 10-year risk assessment in people with 0–1 risk factor is not necessary.

INDICATIONS AND USAGE

Therapy with lipid-altering agents should be only one component of multiple risk factor intervention in individuals at significantly increased risk for atherosclerotic vascular disease due to hypercholesterolemia. Niacin therapy is indicated as an adjunct to diet when the response to a diet restricted in saturated fat and cholesterol and other nonpharmacologic measures alone has been inadequate (see also the NCEP treatment guideline[8]; Table 11). Prior to initiating therapy with niacin, secondary causes for hypercholesterolemia (e.g., poorly controlled diabetes mellitus, hypothyroidism, nephrotic syndrome, dysproteinemias, obstructive liver disease, other drug therapy, alcoholism) should be excluded, and a lipid profile obtained to measure TC, HDL-C, and TG.

1. NIASPAN is indicated as an adjunct to diet for reduction of elevated TC, LDL-C, Apo B and TG levels, and to increase HDL-C in patients with primary hypercholesterolemia (heterozygous familial and nonfamilial) and mixed dyslipidemia (Frederickson Types IIa and IIb; Table 12), when the response to an appropriate diet has been inadequate.
2. NIASPAN in combination with lovastatin is indicated for the treatment of primary hypercholesterolemia (heterozygous familial and nonfamilial) and mixed dyslipidemia (Frederickson Types IIa and IIb; Table 12) in:
   - Patients treated with lovastatin who require further TG-lowering or HDL-raising who may benefit from having niacin added to their regimen
   - Patients treated with niacin who require further LDL-lowering who may benefit from having lovastatin added to their regimen

   Combination therapy is not indicated as initial therapy. (See DOSAGE AND ADMINISTRATION.)
3. In patients with a history of myocardial infarction and hypercholesterolemia, niacin is indicated to reduce the risk of recurrent nonfatal myocardial infarction.
4. In patients with a history of coronary artery disease (CAD) and hypercholesterolemia, niacin, in combination with a bile acid binding resin, is indicated to slow progression or promote regression of atherosclerotic disease.
5. NIASPAN in combination with a bile acid binding resin is indicated as an adjunct to diet for reduction of elevated TC and LDL-C levels in adult patients with primary hy-

percholesterolemia (Type IIa; Table 12), when the response to an appropriate diet, or diet plus monotherapy, has been inadequate.

6. Niacin is also indicated as adjunctive therapy for treatment of adult patients with very high serum triglyceride levels (Types IV and V hyperlipidemia; Table 12) who present a risk of pancreatitis and who do not respond adequately to a determined dietary effort to control them. Such patients typically have serum TG levels over 2000 mg/dL and have elevations of VLDL-C as well as fasting chylomicrons (Type V hyperlipidemia; Table 12). Patients who consistently have total serum or plasma TG below 1000 mg/dL are unlikely to develop pancreatitis. Therapy with niacin may be considered for those patients with TG elevations between 1000 and 2000 mg/dL who have a history of pancreatitis or of recurrent abdominal pain typical of pancreatitis. Some Type IV patients with TG under 1000 mg/dL may, through dietary or alcohol indiscretion, convert to a Type V pattern with massive TG elevations accompanying fasting chylomicronemia, but the influence of niacin therapy on risk of pancreatitis in such situations has not been adequately studied. Drug therapy is not indicated for patients with Type I hyperlipoproteinemia, who have elevations of chylomicrons and plasma TG, but who have normal levels of VLDL-C. Inspection of plasma refrigerated for 14 hours is helpful in distinguishing Types I, IV, and V hyperlipoproteinemia.[9]

[See table 11 on previous page]

After the LDL-C goal has been achieved, if the TG is still ≥200 mg/dL, non-HDL-C (TC minus HDL-C) becomes a secondary target of therapy. Non-HDL-C goals are set 30 mg/dL higher than LDL-C goals for each risk therapy.

Table 12.[1] Classification of Hyperlipoproteinemias

Type	Lipoproteins Elevated	Lipid Elevations Major	Minor
I (rare)	chylomicrons	TG	↑→TC
IIa	LDL	TC	-
IIb	LDL, VLDL	TC	TG
III (rare)	IDL	TC/TG	
IV	VLDL	TG	↑→TC
V (rare)	chylomicrons, VLDL	TG	↑→TC

TC = total cholesterol; TG = triglycerides; LDL = low-density lipoprotein; VLDL = very low-density lipoprotein; IDL = intermediate-density lipoprotein
↑→ = increased or no change

CONTRAINDICATIONS

NIASPAN is contraindicated in patients with a known hypersensitivity to niacin or any component of this medication, significant or unexplained hepatic dysfunction, active peptic ulcer disease, or arterial bleeding.

WARNINGS

NIASPAN preparations should not be substituted for equivalent doses of immediate-release (crystalline) niacin. For patients switching from immediate-release niacin to NIASPAN, therapy with NIASPAN should be initiated with low doses (i.e., 500 mg qhs) and the NIASPAN dose should then be titrated to the desired therapeutic response (see DOSAGE AND ADMINISTRATION).

Liver Dysfunction

Cases of severe hepatic toxicity, including fulminant hepatic necrosis, have occurred in patients who have substituted sustained-release (modified-release, timed-release) niacin products for immediate-release (crystalline) niacin at equivalent doses.

NIASPAN should be used with caution in patients who consume substantial quantities of alcohol and/or have a past history of liver disease. Active liver diseases or unexplained transaminase elevations are contraindications to the use of NIASPAN.

Niacin preparations, like some other lipid-lowering therapies, have been associated with abnormal liver tests. In three placebo-controlled clinical trials involving titration to final daily NIASPAN doses ranging from 500 to 3000mg, 245 patients received NIASPAN for a mean duration of 17 weeks. No patient with normal serum transaminase levels (AST, ALT) at baseline experienced elevations to more than 3 times the upper limit of normal (ULN) during treatment with NIASPAN. In these studies, fewer than 1% (2/245) of NIASPAN patients discontinued due to transaminase elevations greater than 2 times the ULN.

In three safety and efficacy studies with a combination tablet of NIASPAN and lovastatin involving titration to final daily doses (expressed as mg of NIASPAN/mg of lovastatin) 500mg/10mg to 2500mg/40mg, ten of 1028 patients (1.0%) experienced reversible elevations in AST/ALT to more than 3 times the upper limit of normal (ULN). Three of ten elevations occurred at doses outside the recommended dosing limit of 2000mg/40mg; no patient receiving 1000mg/20mg had 3-fold elevations in AST/ALT.

In the placebo-controlled clinical trials and the long-term extension study, elevations in transaminases did not appear to be related to treatment duration; elevations in AST levels did appear to be dose related. Transaminase elevations were reversible upon discontinuation of NIASPAN.

Liver tests should be performed on all patients during therapy with NIASPAN. Serum transaminase levels, including AST and ALT (SGOT and SGPT), should be monitored before treatment begins, every 6 weeks to 12 weeks for the

Table 13 Treatment-Emergent Adverse Events by Dose Level in ≥5% of Patients; Events Considered At Least Remotely Related to Study Medication

	Placebo-Controlled Studies NIASPAN Treatment†						
			Recommended Daily Maintenance Doses			Greater Than Recommended Daily Doses	
	Placebo (n=157) %	500mg‡ (n=87) %	1000mg (n=110) %	1500mg (n=136) %	2000mg (n=95) %	2500mg‡ (n=49) %	3000mg‡ (n=46) %
Headache	15	5*	9	11	8	4*	4
Pain	3	1	2	5	3	0	2
Pain, Abdominal	3	3	2	3	5	0	0
Diarrhea	8	6	7	6	8	10	11
Dyspepsia	8	2	4	5	5	6	0
Nausea	4	2	5	3	8	10	4
Vomiting	2	0	2	3	8*	8	2
Rhinitis	7	2	5	4	3	0	0
Pruritus	1	6	<1	3	1	0	0
Rash	<1	5	5	4	0	0	0

Note: Percentages are calculated from the total number of patients in each column. AEs are reported at the lowest dose where they occurred.
†Pooled results from placebo-controlled studies; for NIASPAN, n=245 and mean treatment duration = 17 weeks. Number of NIASPAN patients (n) are not additive across doses.
‡The 500mg, 2500mg and 3000mg/day doses are outside the recommended daily maintenance dosing range; see DOSAGE AND ADMINISTRATION.
* Significantly different from placebo at $p \leq 0.05$; Chi-square test (cell size>5), Fisher's Exact test (cell sizes≤5).
In general, the incidence of adverse events was higher in women compared to men.

first year, and periodically thereafter (e.g., at approximately 6-month intervals). Special attention should be paid to patients who develop elevated serum transaminase levels, and in these patients, measurements should be repeated promptly and then performed more frequently. If the transaminase levels show evidence of progression, particularly if they rise to 3 times the ULN and are persistent, or if they are associated with symptoms of nausea, fever, and/or malaise, the drug should be discontinued.

Skeletal Muscle

Rare cases of rhabdomyolysis have been associated with concomitant administration of lipid-altering doses (≥1 g/day) of niacin and HMG-CoA reductase inhibitors. In clinical studies with a combination tablet of NIASPAN and lovastatin, no cases of rhabdomyolysis and one suspected case of myopathy have been reported in 1079 patients who were treated with doses up to 2000mg of NIASPAN and 40mg of lovastatin daily for periods up to 2 years. Physicians contemplating combined therapy with HMG-CoA reductase inhibitors and NIASPAN should carefully weigh the potential benefits and risks and should carefully monitor patients for any signs and symptoms of muscle pain, tenderness, or weakness, particularly during the initial months of therapy and during any periods of upward dosage titration of either drug. Periodic serum creatine phosphokinase (CPK) and potassium determinations should be considered in such situations, but there is no assurance that such monitoring will prevent the occurrence of severe myopathy.

PRECAUTIONS

General

Before instituting therapy with NIASPAN, an attempt should be made to control hyperlipidemia with appropriate diet, exercise, and weight reduction in obese patients, and to treat other underlying medical problems (see INDICATIONS AND USAGE).

Patients with a past history of jaundice, hepatobiliary disease, or peptic ulcer should be observed closely during NIASPAN therapy. Frequent monitoring of liver function tests and blood glucose should be performed to ascertain that the drug is producing no adverse effects on these organ systems. Diabetic patients may experience a dose-related rise in glucose intolerance, the clinical significance of which is unclear. Diabetic or potentially diabetic patients should be observed closely. Adjustment of diet and/or hypoglycemic therapy may be necessary.

Caution should also be used when NIASPAN is used in patients with unstable angina or in the acute phase of MI, particularly when such patients are also receiving vasoactive drugs such as nitrates, calcium channel blockers, or adrenergic blocking agents.

Elevated uric acid levels have occurred with niacin therapy, therefore use with caution in patients predisposed to gout.

NIASPAN has been associated with small but statistically significant dose-related reductions in platelet count (mean of -11% with 2000mg). In addition, NIASPAN has been associated with small but statistically significant increases in prothrombin time (mean of approximately +4%); accordingly, patients undergoing surgery should be carefully evaluated. Caution should be observed when NIASPAN is administered concomitantly with anticoagulants; prothrombin time and platelet counts should be monitored closely in such patients.

In placebo-controlled trials, NIASPAN has been associated with small but statistically significant, dose-related reductions in phosphorus levels (mean of −13% with 2000mg). Although these reductions were transient, phosphorus levels should be monitored periodically in patients at risk for hypophosphatemia.

Niacin is rapidly metabolized by the liver, and excreted through the kidneys. NIASPAN is contraindicated in patients with significant or unexplained hepatic dysfunction (see CONTRAINDICATIONS and WARNINGS) and should be used with caution in patients with renal dysfunction.

Information for Patients

Patients should be advised:

— to take NIASPAN at bedtime, after a low-fat snack. Administration on an empty stomach is not recommended;
— to carefully follow the prescribed dosing regimen, including the recommended titration schedule, in order to minimize side effects (see DOSAGE AND ADMINISTRATION);
— that flushing is a common side effect of niacin therapy that usually subsides after several weeks of consistent niacin use. Flushing may vary in severity, may last for several hours after dosing, and will, by taking NIASPAN at bedtime, most likely occur during sleep; however, if awakened by flushing at night, to get up slowly, especially if feeling dizzy, feeling faint, or taking blood pressure medications;
— that taking aspirin (approximately 30 minutes before taking NIASPAN) or a non-steroidal anti-inflammatory drug (e.g., ibuprofen) may minimize flushing;
— to avoid ingestion of alcohol or hot drinks around the time of NIASPAN administration, to minimize flushing;
— that if NIASPAN therapy is discontinued for an extended length of time, their physician should be contacted prior to re-starting therapy; re-titration is recommended (see DOSAGE AND ADMINISTRATION; Table 14);
— to notify their physician if they are taking vitamins or other nutritional supplements containing niacin or related compounds such as nicotinamide (see Drug Interactions);
— to notify their physician if symptoms of dizziness occur;
— if diabetic, to notify their physician of changes in blood glucose;
— that NIASPAN tablets should not be broken, crushed or chewed, but should be swallowed whole.

Drug Interactions

HMG-CoA Reductase Inhibitors: See WARNINGS, *Skeletal Muscle.*

Antihypertensive Therapy: Niacin may potentiate the effects of ganglionic blocking agents and vasoactive drugs resulting in postural hypotension.

Aspirin: Concomitant aspirin may decrease the metabolic clearance of nicotinic acid. The clinical relevance of this finding is unclear.

Bile Acid Sequestrants: An *in vitro* study was carried out investigating the niacin-binding capacity of colestipol and cholestyramine. About 98% of available niacin was bound to colestipol, with 10 to 30% binding to cholestyramine. These results suggest that 4 to 6 hours, or as great an interval as possible, should elapse between the ingestion of bile acid-binding resins and the administration of NIASPAN.

Other: Concomitant alcohol or hot drinks may increase the side effects of flushing and pruritus and should be avoided around the time of NIASPAN ingestion. Vitamins or other nutritional supplements containing large doses of niacin or related compounds such as nicotinamide may potentiate the adverse effects of NIASPAN.

Drug/Laboratory Test Interactions

Niacin may produce false elevations in some fluorometric determinations of plasma or urinary catecholamines. Niacin may also give false-positive reactions with cupric sulfate solution (Benedict's reagent) in urine glucose tests.

Carcinogenesis, Mutagenesis, Impairment of Fertility

Niacin administered to mice for a lifetime as a 1% solution in drinking water was not carcinogenic. The mice in this study received approximately 6 to 8 times a human dose of 3000 mg/day as determined on a mg/m^2 basis. Niacin was

Continued on next page

Niaspan—Cont.

negative for mutagenicity in the Ames test. No studies on impairment of fertility have been performed. No studies have been conducted with NIASPAN regarding carcinogenesis, mutagenesis, or impairment of fertility.

Pregnancy

Pregnancy Category C.

Animal reproduction studies have not been conducted with niacin or with NIASPAN. It is also not known whether niacin at doses typically used for lipid disorders can cause fetal harm when administered to pregnant women or whether it can affect reproductive capacity. If a woman receiving niacin for primary hypercholesterolemia (Types IIa or IIb) becomes pregnant, the drug should be discontinued. If a woman being treated with niacin for hypertriglyceridemia (Types IV or V) conceives, the benefits and risks of continued therapy should be assessed on an individual basis.

Nursing Mothers

Niacin has been reported to be excreted in human milk. Because of the potential for serious adverse reactions in nursing infants from lipid-altering doses of nicotinic acid, a decision should be made whether to discontinue nursing or to discontinue the drug, taking into account the importance of the drug to the mother. No studies have been conducted with NIASPAN in nursing mothers.

Pediatric Use

Safety and effectiveness of niacin therapy in pediatric patients (≤16 years) have not been established. No studies in patients under 21 years of age have been conducted with NIASPAN.

ADVERSE REACTIONS

NIASPAN is generally well tolerated; adverse reactions have been mild and transient. In the placebo-controlled clinical trials, flushing episodes (i.e., warmth, redness, itching and/or tingling) were the most common treatment-emergent adverse events (reported by as many as 88% of patients) for NIASPAN. Spontaneous reports suggest that flushing may also be accompanied by symptoms of dizziness, tachycardia, palpitations, shortness of breath, sweating, chills, and/or edema, which in rare cases may lead to syncope. In pivotal studies, fewer that 6% (14/245) of NIASPAN patients discontinued due to flushing. In comparisons of immediate-release (IR) niacin and NIASPAN, although the proportion of patients who flushed was similar, fewer flushing episodes were reported by patients who received NIASPAN. Following 4 weeks of maintenance therapy at daily doses of 1500mg, the incidence of flushing over the 4-week period averaged 8.56 events per patient for IR niacin versus 1.88 following NIASPAN.

Other adverse events occurring in 5% or greater of patients treated with NIASPAN, at least remotely related to NIASPAN, are shown in Table 13 below.

[See table 13 at top of previous page]

The following adverse events have also been reported with niacin products, either during clinical trials or in routine patient management.

Body as a Whole: edema, asthenia, chills

Cardiovascular: atrial fibrillation, and other cardiac arrhythmias; tachycardia, palpitations; orthostasis; syncope; hypotension

Eye: toxic amblyopia, crystoid macular edema

Gastrointestinal: activation of peptic ulcers and peptic ulceration; jaundice

Metabolic: decreased glucose tolerance; gout

Musculoskeletal: myalgia

Nervous: dizziness, insomnia

Skin: hyper-pigmentation; acanthosis nigricans; maculopapular rash; urticaria; dry skin; sweating

Other: migraine

Clinical Laboratory Abnormalities

Chemistry: Elevations in serum transaminases (see WARNINGS - *Liver Dysfunction*), LDH, fasting glucose, uric acid, total bilirubin, and amylase; reductions in phosphorus

Hematology: Slight reductions in platelet counts and prolongation in prothrombin time (see WARNINGS)

DRUG ABUSE AND DEPENDENCE

Niacin is a non-narcotic drug. It has no known addiction potential in humans.

OVERDOSE

Supportive measures should be undertaken in the event of an overdosage.

DOSAGE AND ADMINISTRATION

NIASPAN should be taken at bedtime, after a low-fat snack, and doses should be individualized according to patient response. Therapy with NIASPAN must be initiated at 500mg qhs in order to reduce the incidence and severity of side effects which may occur during early therapy. The recommended dose escalation is shown in Table 14 below.

[See table 14 below]

Maintenance Dose:

The daily dosage of NIASPAN should not be increased by more than 500mg in any 4-week period. The recommended maintenance dose is 1000mg (two 500mg tablets) to 2000mg (two 1000mg tablets or four 500mg tablets) once daily at bedtime. Doses greater than 2000mg daily are not recommended. Women may respond at lower NIASPAN doses than men (see CLINICAL PHARMACOLOGY, *Gender Effect*).

If lipid response to NIASPAN alone is insufficient (see NCEP treatment guidelines; Table 11), or if higher doses of NIASPAN are not well tolerated, some patients may benefit from combination therapy with a bile acid binding resin or an HMG-CoA reductase inhibitor (See WARNINGS, PRECAUTIONS, Drug Interactions, Concomitant Therapy below, and CLINICAL PHARMACOLOGY, NIASPAN Clinical Studies)

Flushing of the skin (see ADVERSE REACTIONS) may be reduced in frequency or severity by pretreatment with aspirin (taken 30 minutes prior to NIASPAN dose) or non-steroidal anti-inflammatory drugs. Tolerance to this flushing develops rapidly over the course of several weeks. Flushing, pruritus, and gastrointestinal distress are also greatly reduced by slowly increasing the dose of niacin and avoiding administration on an empty stomach.

Equivalent doses of NIASPAN should **not** be substituted for sustained-release (modified-release, timed-release) niacin preparations or immediate-release (crystalline) niacin (see WARNINGS). Patients previously receiving other niacin products should be started with the recommended NIASPAN titration schedule (see Table 14), and the dose should subsequently be individualized based on patient response. Single-dose bioavailability studies have demonstrated that NIASPAN tablet strengths are not interchangeable.

If NIASPAN therapy is discontinued for an extended period, reinstitution of therapy should include a titration phase (see Table 14).

NIASPAN tablets should be taken whole and should not be broken, crushed or chewed before swallowing.

Concomitant Therapy

Concomitant Therapy with Lovastatin

Patients already receiving a stable dose of lovastatin who require TG-lowering or HDL-raising (e.g., to achieve NCEP non-HDL-C goals), may receive concomitant dosage titration with NIASPAN per NIASPAN recommended initial titration schedule (see Table 14, DOSAGE AND ADMINISTRATION section). For patients already receiving a stable dose of NIASPAN who require further LDL-lowering (e.g., to achieve NCEP LDL-C goals; Table 11), the usual recommended starting dose of lovastatin is 20mg once a day. Dose adjustments should be made at intervals of 4 weeks or more. Combination therapy with NIASPAN and lovastatin should not exceed doses of 2000mg and 40mg daily, respectively.

Dosage in Patients with Renal or Hepatic Insufficiency

Use of NIASPAN in patients with renal or hepatic insufficiency has not be studied. NIASPAN is contraindicated in patients with significant or unexplained hepatic dysfunction. NIASPAN should be used with caution in patients with renal insufficiency (see WARNINGS, PRECAUTIONS).

Table 14. Recommended Dosing

		Week(s)	Daily Dose	NIASPAN Dosage
INITIAL	TITRATION SCHEDULE	1 to 4	500mg	1 NIASPAN 500mg tablet at bedtime
		5 to 8	1000mg	2 NIASPAN 500mg tablets at bedtime
		*	1500mg	2 NIASPAN 750mg tablets or 3 NIASPAN 500mg tablets at bedtime
		*	2000mg	2 NIASPAN 1000mg tablets or 4 NIASPAN 500mg tablets at bedtime

* After Week 8, titrate to patient response and tolerance. If response to 1000mg daily is inadequate, increase dose to 1500mg daily; may subsequently increase dose to 2000mg daily. Daily dose should not be increased more than 500mg in a 4-week period, and doses above 2000mg daily are not recommended. Women may respond at lower doses than men.

HOW SUPPLIED

NIASPAN is supplied as unscored, off-white capsule-shaped tablets containing 500, 750 or 1000mg of niacin in an extended-release formulation. Tablets are debossed KOS on one side and the tablet strength (500, 750 or 1000) on the other side. Tablets are supplied in bottles of 100 as shown below.

500mg tablets: bottles of 100 - NDC# 60598-001-01
750mg tablets: bottles of 100 - NDC# 60598-002-01
1000mg tablets: bottles of 100 - NDC# 60598-003-01

Store at room temperature (20 to 25°C or 68 to 77°F).

REFERENCES

1. Bostom AG et al. *JAMA.* 1996; 276:544–548.
2. The Coronary Drug Project Research Group. *JAMA.* 1975; 231:360–381.
3. Canner PL et al. *J Am Coll Cardiol.* 1986; 8(6):1245–1255.
4. Blankenhorn DH et al. *JAMA.* 1987; 257(23):3233–3240.
5. Cashin-Hemphill L et al. *JAMA.* 1990; 264(23):3013–3017.
6. Brown G et al. *N Engl J Med.* 1990; 323:1289–1298.
7. Pasternak RC et al. *Annals Int Med.* 1996; 125:529–540.
8. Executive Summary of the Third Report of the National Cholesterol Education Program (NCEP) Expert Panel on Detection, Evaluation, and Treatment of High Blood Cholesterol in Adults (Adult Treatment Panel III), *JAMA* 2001;285:2486–2497.
9. Nikkila EA, In: *The Metabolic Basis of Inherited Disease.* 5th ed. Chap. 30: 622–642. 1983.

Manufactured by:
Kos Pharmaceuticals, Inc.
Miami, FL 33131

U.S. Patent Nos. 6,080,428; 6,129,930; 6,406,715 B1, and other patents pending.

Shown in Product Identification Guide, page 320

Kyowa Engineering-Sundory

6-964 NAKAMOZU-CHO, SAKAI-CITY, OSAKA, JAPAN

Direct Inquiries to:
Consumer Relations
Tel: 81-72-257-8568
Osaka
Fax: 81-722-57-8655
URL:http://www.Sundory.co.jp

SEN-SEI-RO LIQUID GOLD™

Kyowa's *Agaricus blazei* Murill Mushroom Extract
100 ml liquid
Dietary Supplement

SEN-SEI-RO LIQUID ROYAL™

Kyowa's *Agaricus blazei* Murill Mushroom Extract
50ml liquid (2 x concentrate of Liquid Gold, v/v)
Dietary Supplement

DESCRIPTION

Sen-Sei-Ro Liquid Gold™, a dietary supplement containing an exclusive all-natural, standardized extract of the Kyowa's cultured *Agaricus blazei* Murill mushroom is primarily used to reduce symptoms of fatigue, to promote vitality, overall well-being, and to support immune functions.[†] Normal immune function can decline with age, and are necessary for maintenance of vitality, energy, good health, and quality of life. A few major biomarkers for decreased immune functions are decreased natural killer cell (NK) activity, and the number of lymphocytes and macrophage cells. These cells, primarily attack diseased cells and thereby, maintain body homeostasis, promote health and quality of life. For the past half a century in Brazil and other countries, *Agaricus blazei* Murill mushroom has been used to restore vitality, and energy, and to serve as a potent tonic conducive to general health and aging concerns.[†]

CLINICAL TRIALS

The effectiveness of ABMK22 in Sen-Sei-Ro Gold™ and Sen-Sei-Ro Royal™ for health benefits were tested in several controlled pre- and clinical trials in animals and in humans.[†] Recent studies in Japan led researchers to report that in humans, ABMK22 in Sen-Sei-Ro Gold™ and Sen-Sei-Ro Royal™ enhanced NK cell activity, promoted maturation and activation of dendritic cells indicated by increased cell kill, elevated expression of CD80 and CD83 expressions (Biotherapy 15(4): 503–507, 2001), increased the number of macrophage (Anticancer Research 17(1A): 274–284, 1997; Japanese Association of Cancer Research, no. 2268, 1999) and tumor necrosis factor α (TNF-α)(Japanese Association of Cancer Research, no. 1406, 1999; Japanese J. Veterinary Clin. Medicine 17(2):31–42, 1998).[†] Further clinical studies with Sen-Sei-Ro Gold™ and Sen-Sei-Ro Royal™ among 100 cancer patients undergoing chemotherapy in Korea have shown that NK cell activity were significantly enhanced, while NK cell activity in the placebo group was markedly diminished (Int. J. Gynecol.

Cancer 14: 589–594, 2004).† Earlier and recent both pre- and clinical studies in Japan, and Korea, led researchers to report that Kyowa's *Agaricus blazei* Murill mushroom extract can be part of an effective treatment for supporting the immune systems of cancer patients by stimulating host defense system (Biotherapy 15(4): 503–507, 2001; Carbohydrate Res. 186(2): 267–273, 1989; Japanese J. Pharmacology 662: 265–271, 1994; Agricultural and Biological Chemistry 54: 2889–2905, 1990).†

INGREDIENTS

Each 100ml heat-treated high pressure pack of all natural Kyowa's *Agaricus blazei* Murill water extract is scientifically standardized to contain 300mg% carbohydrate, 700mg% protein, 0mg% fat,; 1.4mg% sodium, 0% food quality cellulose, and 4 Kcal energy.

Molecular weights of polysaccharopeptides ranges between 600~8,000. Water: 99.2g%,; includes a variety of amino acids and vitamins (arginine 12mg%, lysine 6mg%, histidine 2mg%, phenylalanine 4mg%, tyrosine 4mg%, leucine 5mg%, isoleucine 3mg%, methionine 1mg%, valine 5mg%, alanine 13mg%, glycine 7mg%, proline 13mg%, glutamic acid 53mg%, serine 6mg%, threonine 5mg%, and asparagine 10mg%.

RECOMMENDED USE

As a dietary supplement, take 1~3 packs per day. Pour the liquid content into a cup or drink directly from the pack. Do not heat the pack either in a microwave oven or heating range or leave the pack open since the product does not contain any preservatives. If warming is necessary, place the pack in warm to mildly hot water for desired length of time. Once the pack is open, drink immediately.

ADVERSE REACTIONS

No subjects have reported any side effects since the dietary supplement was placed for consumers in Japan, and Korea for the past 10, and 5 years, respectively. The use of this dietary supplements (Sen-Sei-Ro Gold™, Royal™, and ABMK22) is generally safe based on FDA's INDA required tripartite genotoxicities, and 28-day subacute toxicity involving a comprehensive microscopic pathology of rats and dogs. In addition, two-year chronic toxicity studies of the product carried out by the Good Laboratory Practice (GLP) and American Association of Accreditation of Laboratory Animal Certification (AAALAC) certified Toxicology Research Center. Toxicity evaluation of general, CNS, reproductive and developmental, cardiovascular, immunology, and the two-year bioassay for carcinogenicity was negative. Recent clinical studies with 100 cancer patients undergoing chemotherapy in Korea have shown no known side effects or contraindications (Int. J. Gynecol. Cancer 14: 589–594, 2004).†

WARNINGS

Sen-Sei-Ro Liquid Gold™ and Sen-Sei-Ro Liquid Royal™ have not been evaluated in pregnant and breast feeding mothers or children and should consult a physician prior to use. Also consult a physician prior to use if taking a prescription medication. **Keep this product out of the reach of children. Do not use if you are pregnant, can become pregnant or breast feeding.**

HOW SUPPLIED

Sen-Sei-Ro Liquid Gold™ 100ml, and Sen-Sei-Ro Liquid Royal™ 50ml in water extract are high pressure heat sealed. A box contains 30, 100ml packs, and can be purchased directly from company representatives, health food stores, and independent pharmacies. Storage condition keep at room temperature and avoid any direct heat or sun light.

†These statements have not been evaluated by the Food and Drug Administration. These products are not intended to diagnose, treat, cure or prevent any disease.

SEN-SEI-RO POWDER GOLD™

KYOWA'S *Agaricus blazei* Murill Mushroom
1800mg standard granulated powder
Dietary Supplement

DESCRIPTION

Sen-Sei-Ro Powder Gold™ slim pack, a dietary supplement containing an exclusively all natural and prepared from Kyowa's *Agaricus blazei* Murill mushroom is primarily used to reduce symptoms of fatigue, to promote vitality, overall well-being, and to support immune functions.† Normal immune function can decline with age, and are necessary for maintenance of vitality, energy, good health, and quality of life. A few major biomarkers for decreased immune functions are decreased natural killer cell (NK) activity, and the number of lymphocytes and macrophage cells. These cells, primarily attack diseased cells and thereby, maintain body homeostasis, promote health and quality of life. For the past half a century in Brazil and other countries, *Agaricus blazei* Murill mushroom has been used to restore vitality, and energy, and to serve as a potent tonic conducive to general health and aging concerns.†

CLINICAL TRIALS

The effectiveness of Sen-Sei-Ro Powder Gold™ for health benefits were tested in several controlled pre- and clinical trials in animals and in humans.† Recent studies in Japan, and Korea led researcher to report that in humans, Sen-Sei-Ro Powder Gold™ enhanced NK cell activity, increased the number of macrophage cells (Anticancer Research 17 (1A): 274–284, 1997; Japanese Association of Cancer Research, no. 2268, 1999) and tumor necrosis factor α (TNF-α)(Japanese Association of Cancer Research, no. 1406, 1999).† Antitumor effects of Sen-Sei-Ro against various murine and dog tumors were thought to be mediated by stimulation of NK cell activity, increased number of macrophage cells, and increased activity of tumor necrosis factor α (TNF-α)(Japanese J. Veterinary Clin. Medicine 17(2):31–42, 1998).† Recent clinical studies in Japan, and Korea, led researchers to report that *Agaricus blazei* Murill mushroom extract can be part of an effective treatment for supporting the immune systems of cancer patients by stimulating host defense system (Biotherapy 15(4): 503–507, 2001; Carbohydrate Res. 186(2): 267–273, 1989; Japanese J. Pharmacology 662: 265–271, 1994; Agricultural and Biological Chemistry 54: 2889–2905, 1990).†

INGREDIENTS

Each 1800mg granulated powder in a slim pack contains 488 mg protein, 820 mg carbohydrate, 47 mg fat, 0.19 mg Sodium; 284 mg food grade cellulose; 5.7 kcal energy.

Water: 68mg, includes 0.1 mg Fe, 0.24 mg Ca, 37 mg K, 0.01mg thiamine, 0.04mg ergosterol, 0.59mg niacin.

RECOMMENDED USE

As a dietary supplement, take 1~3 packs per day. Pour the content into a cup containing warm water or other desirable beverage and mix and drink. Do not heat the pack either in a microwave oven or heating range or leave the pack open since the product does not contain any preservatives. Once the pack is open, drink immediately.

ADVERSE REACTIONS

No subjects have reported any side effects since the dietary supplement was placed for consumers in Japan and Korea for the past 8, and 3 years, respectively. The use of this dietary supplement is generally safe based on two-year chronic toxicity studies of the product by the Good Laboratory Practice (GLP) and American Association of Accreditation of Laboratory Animal Certification (AAALAC) certified Toxicology Research Center. Toxicity evaluation of general, CNS, reproductive and developmental, cardiovascular, immunology, and the two-year bioassay for carcinogenicity was negative.†

WARNINGS

Sen-Sei-Ro Powder Gold™ has not been evaluated in pregnant and breast feeding mothers or children and should consult a physician prior to use. Also consult a physician prior to use if taking a prescription medications.. **Keep this product out of the reach of children. Do not use if you are pregnant, can become pregnant or breast feeding.** Quality of the dietary supplement is guaranteed for 2 years from the manufactured date, but for more information, please write or call 81-72-257-8568 or 81-3-3512-5032.

HOW SUPPLIED

Sen-Sei-Ro Powder Gold™ is high pressure heat sealed. A box contains 30 slim packs of each with 1800mg per pack, and can be purchased directly from company representatives, health food stores, and independent pharmacies. Storage condition keep at room temperature and avoid any direct heat or sun light.

†These statements have not been evaluated by the Food and Drug Administration. These products are not intended to diagnose, treat, cure or prevent any disease.

Lane Labs USA, Inc.

25 COMMERCE DRIVE
ALLENDALE, NJ 07401

Direct Inquiries to:
phone 800-526-3001

NATURE'S LINING™ OTC

Strengthens the Stomach Wall*
Light Mint Flavor
60 Chewable Tablets
Stomach Wall Dietary Supplement*

DESCRIPTION

Nature's Lining has the unique ability to travel through the digestive tract, "seek out" and attach itself to thinning areas in the stomach lining. Once attached, its patented formula actually strengthens the stomach wall. The dramatic activity of safe, natural Nature's Lining has been proven in human clinical trials and widely recommended by doctors since 1994.

RECOMMENDED USE

Directions: Always take with food. Chew 1 tablet twice daily (morning and evening) for eight weeks. Continue using 1–2 tablets daily thereafter for ongoing stomach lining support.

Store in a cool, dry place. Keep out of reach of children. Do not use if bottle seal is broken or missing.

Supplement Facts

Serving Size: 1 Tablet — Servings Per Container: 60

Amount Per Serving		**% Daily Value**
Zinc (from PepZin GI™ Zinc-Camosine)	8 mg	53%
L-Camosine (from PepZin GI™ Zinc-Camosine)	29.5 mg	*

*Daily Value Not Established.

Other Ingredients

Fructose, Guar Gum, Microcrystalline Cellulose, Magnesium Stearate, Corn Starch and Peppermint Oil.

Distributed by LaneLabs-USA, Inc., Allendale, NJ 07401 USA ©

For more information, call **1-800-526-3001**
www.lanelabs.com

***These statements have not been evaluated by the Food & Drug Administration. This product is not intended to diagnose, treat, cure or prevent any disease.**

Ligand Pharmaceuticals Incorporated

10275 SCIENCE CENTER DRIVE
SAN DIEGO, CA 92121

Direct Inquiries to:
(858) 550-7500
Internet: http://www.ligand.com
Customer Service
(877) 454-4263
Medical Information
(800) 964-5836
Reimbursement Support
(877) 654-4263

AVINZA® Ⓒ ℞

[*ā-vĭn-ză*]
(morphine sulfate extended-release capsules)
30 mg, 60 mg, 90 mg, 120 mg
℞ Only

WARNING:
AVINZA capsules are a modified-release formulation of morphine sulfate indicated for once daily administration for the relief of moderate to severe pain requiring continuous, around-the-clock opioid therapy for an extended period of time. AVINZA CAPSULES ARE TO BE SWALLOWED WHOLE OR THE CONTENTS OF THE CAPSULES SPRINKLED ON APPLESAUCE. THE CAPSULE BEADS ARE NOT TO BE CHEWED, CRUSHED, OR DISSOLVED DUE TO THE RISK OF RAPID RELEASE AND ABSORPTION OF A POTENTIALLY FATAL DOSE OF MORPHINE.

DESCRIPTION

AVINZA (morphine sulfate extended-release capsules) 30, 60, 90, and 120 mg contain both immediate release and extended release beads of morphine sulfate for once daily oral administration.

Chemically, morphine sulfate is 7,8-didehydro-4,5 alpha-epoxy-17-methyl-morphinan-3,6 alpha-diol sulfate (2:1) (salt) pentahydrate with a molecular weight of 758. Morphine sulfate occurs as white, feathery, silky crystals; cubical masses of crystal; or white crystalline powder. It is soluble in water and slightly soluble in alcohol, but is practically insoluble in chloroform or ether. The octanol: water partition coefficient of morphine is 1.42 at physiologic pH and the pK_a is 7.9 for the tertiary nitrogen (the majority is ionized at pH 7.4).

Each AVINZA Capsule contains either 30, 60, 90, or 120 mg of morphine sulfate, USP and the following inactive ingredients: ammonio-methacrylate copolymers, NF, fumaric acid, NF, povidone, USP, sodium lauryl sulfate, NF, sugar starch spheres, NF, and talc, USP. The capsule shell contains black ink, gelatin, titanium dioxide, D&C yellow No. 10 (30 mg), FC&C green No. 3 (60 mg), FD&C red No. 40 (90 mg), FD&C red No. 3 (120 mg), and FD&C blue No. 1 (120 mg).

Structure:

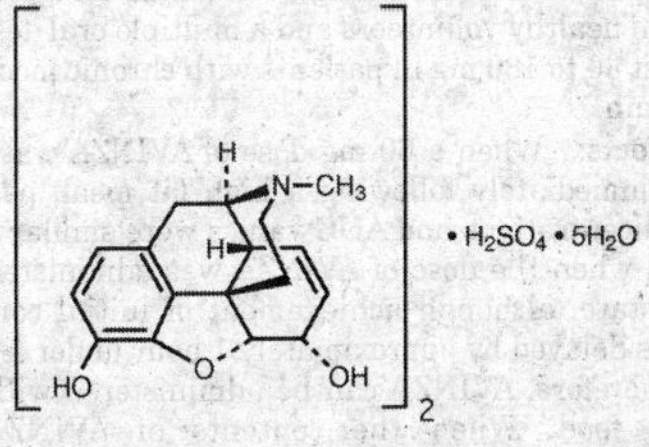

Continued on next page

Avinza—Cont.

AVINZA uses the proprietary SODAS™ (Spheroidal Oral Drug Absorption System) technology to produce the extended release component of AVINZA, which combined with an immediate release component achieves the desired release profile characteristics of AVINZA capsules. Within the gastrointestinal tract, due to the permeability of the ammonio-methacrylate copolymers of the beads, fluid enters the beads and solubilizes the drug. This is mediated by fumaric acid, which acts as an osmotic agent and a local pH modifier. The resultant solution then diffuses out in a predetermined manner which prolongs the *in vivo* dissolution and absorption phases. (see **Pharmacokinetics**)

CLINICAL PHARMACOLOGY

Morphine, a pure opioid agonist, is relatively selective for the mu receptor, although it can interact with other opioid receptors at higher doses. In addition to analgesia, the widely diverse effects of morphine include drowsiness, changes in mood, respiratory depression, decreased gastrointestinal motility, nausea, vomiting, and alterations of the endocrine and autonomic nervous system.

Effects on the Central Nervous System (CNS): The principal therapeutic action of morphine is analgesia. Other therapeutic effects of morphine include anxiolysis, euphoria and feelings of relaxation. Although the precise mechanism of the analgesic action is unknown, specific CNS opiate receptors and endogenous compounds with morphine-like activity have been identified throughout the brain and spinal cord and are likely to play a role in the expression and perception of analgesic effects. In common with other opioids, morphine causes respiratory depression, in part by a direct effect on the brainstem respiratory centers. Morphine and related opioids depress the cough reflex by direct effect on the cough center in the medulla. Antitussive effects may occur with doses lower than those usually required for analgesia. Morphine causes miosis, even in total darkness. Pinpoint pupils are a sign of opioid overdose; however, when asphyxia is present during opioid overdose, marked mydriasis occurs.

Effects on the Gastrointestinal Tract and on Other Smooth Muscle: Gastric, biliary and pancreatic secretions are decreased by morphine. Morphine causes a reduction in motility and is associated with an increase in tone in the antrum of the stomach and duodenum. Digestion of food in the small intestine is delayed and propulsive contractions are decreased. Propulsive peristaltic waves in the colon are decreased, while tone is increased to the point of spasm. The end result may be constipation. Morphine can cause a marked increase in biliary tract pressure as a result of spasm of the sphincter of Oddi. Morphine may also cause spasm of the sphincter of the urinary bladder.

Effects on the Cardiovascular System: In therapeutic doses, morphine does not usually exert major effects on the cardiovascular system. Morphine produces peripheral vasodilation which may result in orthostatic hypotension and fainting. Release of histamine can occur, which may play a role in opioid-induced hypotension. Manifestations of histamine release and/or peripheral vasodilation may include pruritus, flushing, red eyes and sweating.

Pharmacodynamics

Morphine concentrations are not predictive of analgesic response, especially in patients previously treated with opioids. The minimum effective concentration varies widely and is influenced by a variety of factors, including the extent of previous opioid use, age, and general medical condition. Effective doses in tolerant patients may be significantly higher than in opioid-naïve patients.

In all patients, the dose of morphine should be titrated on the basis of clinical evaluation of the patient and to achieve a balance between therapeutic and adverse effects.

Pharmacokinetics

AVINZA consists of two components, an immediate release component that rapidly achieves plateau morphine plasma concentrations and an extended release component that maintains plasma concentrations throughout the 24-hour dosing interval. The amount of morphine absorbed from AVINZA following oral administration is similar to that absorbed from other oral morphine formulations.

The oral bioavailability of morphine is less than 40% and shows large inter-individual variability due to extensive pre-systemic metabolism.

Absorption

Following single-dose oral administration of a 60 mg dose of AVINZA under fasting conditions, morphine concentrations of approximately 3 to 6 ng/ml were achieved within 30 minutes after dosing and maintained for the 24-hour dosing interval. The pharmacokinetics of AVINZA were shown to be dose-proportional over a single oral dose range of 30 to 120 mg in healthy volunteers and a multiple oral dose range of at least 30 to 180 mg in patients with chronic moderate to severe pain.

Food Effects: When a 60 mg dose of AVINZA was administered immediately following a high fat meal, peak morphine concentrations and AUC values were similar to those observed when the dose of AVINZA was administered in a fasting state, although achievement of initial concentrations was delayed by approximately 1 hour under fed conditions. Therefore, AVINZA can be administered without regard to food. When the contents of AVINZA were administered by sprinkling on applesauce, the rate and extent of morphine absorption were found to be bioequivalent to the same dose when administered as an intact capsule.

Steady-State: When dosed once-daily, AVINZA steady-state pharmacokinetics are characterized by a plateau-like plasma concentration profile. Steady-state plasma concentrations of morphine are achieved 2 to 3 days after initiation of once-daily administration of AVINZA.

AVINZA 60 mg Capsules (once-daily) and 10 mg morphine oral solution (6 times daily) were equally bioavailable.

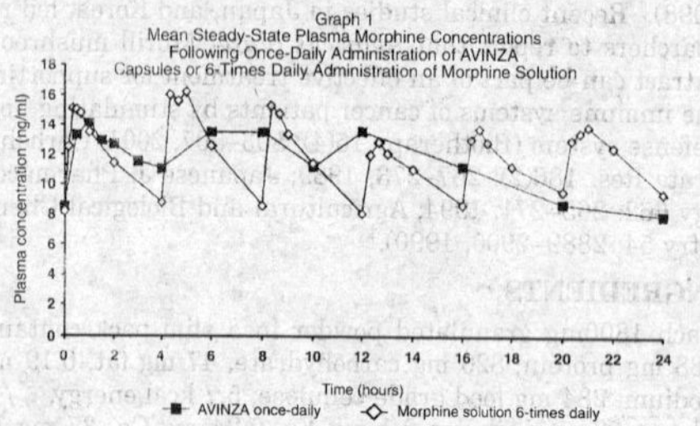

A once-daily dose of AVINZA provided similar C_{max}, C_{min}, and AUC values and peak-trough fluctuations (% FL, C_{max}-C_{min}/C_{av}) compared to 6-times daily administration of the same total daily dose of morphine oral solution (Table 1).

Table 1
Pharmacokinetic Data
Mean ± SD

Parameter	AVINZA Capsules Once-Daily	Morphine Oral Solution 6-Times Daily
AUC (ng/ml.h)	273.25 ± 81.24	279.11 ± 63.00
C_{max} (ng/ml)	18.65 ± 7.13	19.96 ± 4.82
C_{min} (ng/ml)	6.98 ± 2.44	6.61 ± 2.15
% FL	106.38 ± 78.14	116.22 ± 26.67

Distribution

Once absorbed, morphine is distributed to skeletal muscle, kidneys, liver, intestinal tract, lungs, spleen and brain. Although the primary site of action is the CNS, only small quantities cross the blood-brain barrier. Morphine also crosses the placental membranes and has been found in breast milk. The volume of distribution of morphine is approximately 1 to 6 L/kg, and morphine is 20 to 35% reversibly bound to plasma proteins.

Metabolism

The major pathway of morphine detoxification is conjugation, either with D-glucuronic acid to produce glucuronides or with sulfuric acid to produce morphine-3-etheral sulfate. While a small fraction (less than 5%) of morphine is demethylated, virtually all morphine is converted by hepatic metabolism to the 3- and 6-glucuronide metabolites (M3G and M6G; about 50% and 15%, respectively). M6G has been shown to have analgesic activity but crosses the blood-brain barrier poorly, while M3G has no significant analgesic activity.

Excretion

Most of a dose of morphine is excreted in urine as M3G and M6G, with elimination of morphine occurring primarily as renal excretion of M3G. Approximately 10% of the dose is excreted unchanged in urine. A small amount of the glucuronide conjugates are excreted in bile, with minor enterohepatic recycling. Seven to 10% of administered morphine is excreted in the feces.

The mean adult plasma clearance is approximately 20 to 30 ml/min/kg. The effective terminal half-life of morphine after IV administration is reported to be approximately 2 hours. In some studies involving longer periods of plasma sampling, a longer terminal half-life of morphine of about 15 hours was reported.

Special Populations

Geriatric: Elderly patients (aged 65 years or older) may have increased sensitivity to morphine. AVINZA pharmacokinetics have not been studied specifically in elderly patients.

Nursing Mothers: Low levels of morphine sulfate have been detected in maternal milk. The milk:plasma morphine AUC ratio is about 2.5:1. The amount of morphine delivered to the infant depends on the plasma concentration of the mother, the amount of milk ingested by the infant, and the extent of first-pass metabolism.

Pediatric: The pharmacokinetics of AVINZA have not been studied in pediatric patients below the age of 18. The range of dose strengths available may not be appropriate for treatment of very young pediatric patients. Sprinkling on applesauce is **NOT** a suitable alternative for these patients.

Gender: A gender analysis of pharmacokinetic data from healthy subjects taking AVINZA indicated that morphine concentrations were similar in males and females.

Race: There may be some pharmacokinetic differences associated with race. In one published study, Chinese subjects given intravenous morphine had a higher clearance when compared to Caucasian subjects (1852 +/- 116 ml/min compared to 1495 +/- 80 ml/min).

Hepatic Failure: Morphine pharmacokinetics have been reported to be significantly altered in patients with cirrhosis. Clearance was found to decrease with a corresponding increase in half-life. The M3G and M6G to morphine plasma AUC ratios also decreased in these subjects, indicating diminished metabolic activity.

Renal Insufficiency: Morphine pharmacokinetics are altered in patients with renal failure. Clearance is decreased and the metabolites, M3G and M6G, may accumulate to much higher plasma levels in patients with renal failure as compared to patients with normal renal function.

Drug-Drug Interactions: Known drug-drug interactions involving morphine are pharmacodynamic, not pharmacokinetic. (see **PRECAUTIONS, Drug Interactions**)

Clinical Studies

AVINZA was studied in over 140 healthy volunteers and 560 patients with chronic, moderate to severe pain who participated in 6 pharmacokinetic studies, 4 clinical studies and 3 studies which provided both pharmacokinetic and clinical data. The patient population included those who were either receiving chronic opioid therapy or had a prior suboptimal response to acetaminophen and/or NSAID therapy, as well as patients who previously received intermittent opioid analgesic therapy. In the controlled clinical studies, patients were followed from 7 days to up to 4 weeks, and in the open label studies, patients were followed for up to 6 to 12 months.

AVINZA was studied in a double-blind, placebo-controlled, fixed-dose, parallel group trial in 295 patients with moderate to severe pain due to osteoarthritis. These patients had either a prior sub-optimal response to acetaminophen, NSAID therapy, or previously received intermittent opioid analgesic therapy. Thirty-milligrams AVINZA capsules administered once-daily, either in the morning or the evening, were more effective than placebo in reducing pain.

Table 2
Change from Baseline in WOMAC OA Index Pain VAS Subscale Score

Overall	Placebo	AVINZA QAM	AVINZA QPM
LS Mean	-36.23	-75.26*	-75.39*
Std. Error	11.482	11.305	11.747

*P<0.05; REPEATED MEASURES ANALYSIS

This study was not designed to assess the effects of AVINZA on the course of the osteoarthritis.

INDICATIONS AND USAGE

AVINZA capsules are a modified-release formulation of morphine sulfate intended for once daily administration indicated for the relief of moderate to severe pain requiring continuous, around-the-clock opioid therapy for an extended period of time.

AVINZA is **NOT** intended for use as a prn analgesic.

The safety and efficacy of using AVINZA in the postoperative setting has not been evaluated. AVINZA is not indicated for postoperative use. If the patient has been receiving the drug prior to surgery, resumption of the pre-surgical dose may be appropriate once the patient is able to take the drug by mouth. Physicians should individualize treatment, moving from parenteral to oral analgesics as appropriate. (see American Pain Society guidelines)

CONTRAINDICATIONS

AVINZA is contraindicated in patients with known hypersensitivity to morphine, morphine salts, or any components of the product. AVINZA, like all opioids, is contraindicated in patients with respiratory depression in the absence of resuscitative equipment and in patients with acute or severe bronchial asthma.

AVINZA, like all opioids, is contraindicated in any patient who has or is suspected of having paralytic ileus.

WARNINGS

AVINZA must be swallowed whole (not chewed, crushed, or dissolved) or AVINZA may be opened and the entire bead contents sprinkled on a small amount of applesauce immediately prior to ingestion. **THE CAPSULES MUST NOT BE CHEWED, CRUSHED, OR DISSOLVED DUE TO THE RISK OF RAPID RELEASE AND ABSORPTION OF A POTENTIALLY FATAL DOSE OF MORPHINE.** (see **BOX WARNING, CLINICAL PHARMACOLOGY**)

THE DAILY DOSE OF AVINZA MUST BE LIMITED TO A MAXIMUM OF 1600 MG/DAY. AVINZA DOSES OF OVER 1600 MG/DAY CONTAIN A QUANTITY OF FUMARIC ACID THAT HAS NOT BEEN DEMONSTRATED TO BE SAFE, AND WHICH MAY RESULT IN SERIOUS RENAL TOXICITY.

Misuse, Abuse and Diversion of Opioids

Morphine is an opioid agonist and a Schedule II controlled substance. Such drugs are sought by drug abusers and people with addiction disorders. Diversion of Schedule II products is an act subject to criminal penalty.

Morphine can be abused in a manner similar to other opioid agonists, legal or illicit. This should be considered when prescribing or dispensing AVINZA in situations where the physican or pharmacist is concerned about an increased risk of misuse, abuse, or diversion.

Abuse of AVINZA by crushing, chewing, snorting, or injecting the dissolved product will result in the immediate release of the entire daily dose of the opioid and pose a significant risk to the abuser that could result in overdose and death. Intravenous abuse of a water extract of AVINZA may lead to serious pulmonary complications due to the extraction of talc along with morphine sulfate. (see **DRUG ABUSE AND ADDICTION**)

Concerns about abuse, addiction, and diversion should not prevent the proper management of pain. Healthcare professionals should contact their State Professional Licensing Board, or State Controlled Substances Authority for information on how to prevent and detect abuse or diversion of this product.

Interactions with Alcohol and Drugs of Abuse

Morphine may be expected to have additive effects when used in conjunction with alcohol, other opioids, or illicit drugs that cause central nervous system depression.

Impaired Respiration

Respiratory depression is the chief hazard of all morphine preparations. Respiratory depression occurs more frequently in elderly or debilitated patients and in those suffering from conditions accompanied by hypoxia, hypercapnia, or upper airway obstruction, in whom even moderate therapeutic doses may significantly decrease pulmonary ventilation.

Morphine should be used with extreme caution in patients with chronic obstructive pulmonary disease or cor pulmonale and in patients having a substantially decreased respiratory reserve (e.g., severe kyphoscoliosis), hypoxia, hypercapnia, or pre-existing respiratory depression. In such patients, even usual therapeutic doses of morphine may increase airway resistance and decrease respiratory drive to the point of apnea.

Head Injury and Increased Intracranial Pressure

The respiratory depressant effects of morphine with carbon dioxide retention and secondary elevation of cerebrospinal fluid pressure may be markedly exaggerated in the presence of head injury, other intracranial lesions, or a pre-existing increase in intracranial pressure. Morphine produces effects which may obscure neurologic signs of further increases in intracranial pressure in patients with head injuries. Morphine should only be administered under such circumstances when considered essential and then with extreme care.

Hypotensive Effect

AVINZA, like all morphine products, may cause severe hypotension in an individual whose ability to maintain blood pressure has already been compromised by a depleted blood volume or concurrent administration of drugs such as phenothiazines or general anesthetics. (see also **PRECAUTIONS, Drug Interactions**) AVINZA may produce orthostatic hypotension and syncope in ambulatory patients.

AVINZA is an opioid analgesic which should be administered with caution to patients in circulatory shock, as vasodilation produced by the drug may further reduce cardiac output and blood pressure.

Gastrointestinal Obstruction

AVINZA should not be administered to patients with gastrointestinal obstruction, especially paralytic ileus because AVINZA, like all morphine preparations, diminishes propulsive peristaltic waves in the gastrointestinal tract and may prolong the obstruction.

PRECAUTIONS

General

AVINZA is intended for use in patients requiring continuous around-the-clock treatment with an opioid analgesic. It is not appropriate as a prn treatment for pain. As with any opioid, it is critical to adjust the dose of AVINZA for each individual patient, taking into account the patient's prior experience with analgesics. (see **DOSAGE AND ADMINISTRATION**)

Use in Pancreatic/Biliary Tract Disease

AVINZA should be used with caution in patients with biliary tract disease, including acute pancreatitis, as morphine may cause spasm of the sphincter of Oddi and diminish biliary and pancreatic secretions.

Special Risk Groups

AVINZA should be administered cautiously and in reduced dosages in patients with severe renal or hepatic insufficiency, Addison's disease, hypothyroidism, prostatic hypertrophy, or urethral stricture, and in elderly or debilitated patients. (see **Geriatric Use** and **CLINICAL PHARMACOLOGY, Special Populations**)

Caution should be exercised in the administration of morphine to patients with CNS depression, toxic psychosis, acute alcoholism and delirium tremens, and seizure disorders.

Driving and Operating Machinery

Patients should be cautioned that AVINZA could impair the mental and/or physical abilities needed to perform potentially hazardous activities such as driving a car or operating machinery.

Patients should also be cautioned about the potential combined effects of AVINZA with other CNS depressants, including other opioids, phenothiazines, sedative/hypnotics and alcohol. (see **PRECAUTIONS, Drug Interactions**)

Tolerance and Physical Dependence

Tolerance is the need for increasing doses of opioids to maintain a defined effect such as analgesia (in the absence of disease progression or other external factors). Physical dependence is manifested by withdrawal symptoms after abrupt discontinuation of a drug or upon administration of an antagonist. Physical dependence and tolerance are not unusual during chronic opioid therapy.

The opioid abstinence or withdrawal syndrome is characterized by some or all of the following: restlessness, lacrimation, rhinorrhea, yawning, perspiration, chills, myalgia, and mydriasis. Other symptoms also may develop, including irritability, anxiety, backache, joint pain, weakness, abdominal cramps, insomnia, nausea, anorexia, vomiting, diarrhea, or increased blood pressure, respiratory rate, or heart rate.

In general, opioids should not be abruptly discontinued (see **DOSAGE AND ADMINISTRATION, Cessation of Therapy**).

Information for Patients

Patients receiving AVINZA (morphine sulfate extended-release capsules) should be given the following instructions by the physician:

1. Patients should be advised that AVINZA capsules contain morphine and should be taken once daily.
2. AVINZA must be swallowed whole (not chewed, crushed, or dissolved) or AVINZA may be opened and the entire bead contents sprinkled on a small amount of applesauce immediately prior to ingestion. **The beads must NOT be chewed, crushed, or dissolved due to the risk of exposure to a potentially toxic dose of morphine.**
3. The dose of AVINZA should not be adjusted without consulting with a physician or other healthcare professional.
4. Patients should be advised that AVINZA may impair mental and/or physical ability required for the performance of potentially hazardous tasks (e.g., driving, operating machinery). Patients started on AVINZA or patients whose dose has been adjusted should refrain from any potentially dangerous activity until it is established that they are not adversely affected.
5. Patients should be advised that AVINZA should not be combined with alcohol or other CNS depressants (e.g., sleep medications, tranquilizers). A physician should be consulted if other medications are currently being used or are added in the future.
6. Women of childbearing potential who become or are planning to become pregnant should consult a physician prior to initiating or continuing therapy with AVINZA.
7. If patients have been receiving treatment with AVINZA for more than a few weeks and cessation of therapy is indicated, they should be counseled on the importance of safely tapering the dose and that abruptly discontinuing the medication could precipitate withdrawal symptoms. The physician should provide a dose schedule to accomplish a gradual discontinuation of the medication.
8. Patients should be advised that AVINZA is a potential drug of abuse. They should protect it from theft. It should never be given to anyone other than the individual for whom it was prescribed.
9. Patients should be instructed to keep AVINZA in a secure place out of the reach of children. When AVINZA is no longer needed, the unused capsules should be destroyed by flushing down the toilet.

As with other opioids, patients taking AVINZA should be advised of the potential for severe constipation; appropriate laxatives, and/or stool softeners as well as other appropriate treatments should be initiated from the onset of opioid therapy.

Drug Interactions

CNS Depressants: The concurrent use of other central nervous system (CNS) depressants including sedatives, hypnotics, general anesthetics, antiemetics, phenothiazines, or other tranquilizers or alcohol increases the risk of respiratory depression, hypotension, profound sedation, or coma. Use with caution and in reduced dosages in patients taking these agents.

Muscle Relaxants: Morphine may enhance the neuromuscular blocking action of skeletal muscle relaxants and produce an increased degree of respiratory depression.

Mixed Agonist/Antagonist Opioid Analgesics: Mixed agonist/antagonist analgesics (i.e., pentazocine, nalbuphine and butorphanol) should NOT be administered to patients who have received or are receiving a course of therapy with a pure opioid agonist analgesic. In these patients, mixed agonist/antagonist analgesics may reduce the analgesic effect and/or may precipitate withdrawal symptoms.

Monoamine Oxidase Inhibitors (MAOIs): MAOIs markedly potentiate the action of morphine. AVINZA should not be used in patients taking MAOIs or within 14 days of stopping such treatment.

Cimetidine: Concomitant administration of morphine and cimetidine has been reported to precipitate apnea, confusion and muscle twitching in an isolated report. Patients should be monitored for increased respiratory and CNS depression when receiving cimetidine concomitantly with AVINZA.

Food: AVINZA can be administered without regard to food. (see **CLINICAL PHARMACOLOGY, Food Effects**)

Carcinogenicity/Mutagenicity/Impairment of Fertility

Studies in animals to evaluate the carcinogenic potential of morphine sulfate have not been conducted. No formal studies to assess the mutagenic potential of morphine have been conducted. In the published literature, the results of *in vitro* studies showed that morphine is non-mutagenic in the *Drosophila melanogaster* lethal mutation assay and produced no evidence of chromosomal aberrations when incubated with murine splenocytes. Contrary to these results, morphine was found to increase DNA fragmentation when incubated *in vitro* with a human lymphoma cell line. *In vivo,* morphine has been reported to produce an increase in the frequency of micronuclei in bone marrow cells and immature red blood cells in the mouse micronucleus test and to induce chromosomal aberrations in murine lymphocytes and spermatids. Some of the *in vivo* clastogenic effects reported with morphine in mice may be directly related to increases in glucocorticoid levels produced by morphine in this species.

Pregnancy

Teratogenic Effects (Pregnancy Category C)

No formal studies to assess the teratogenic effects of morphine in animals have been performed. Several literature reports indicate that morphine administered subcutaneously during the early gestational period in mice and hamsters produced neurological, soft tissue and skeletal abnormalities. With one exception, the effects that have been reported were following doses that were maternally toxic and the abnormalities noted were characteristic of those observed when maternal toxicity is present. In one study, following subcutaneous infusion of doses greater than or equal to 0.15 mg/kg to mice, exencephaly, hydronephrosis, intestinal hemorrhage, split supraoccipital, malformed sternebrae, and malformed xiphoid were noted in the absence of maternal toxicity. In the hamster, morphine sulfate given subcutaneously on gestation day 8 produced exencephaly and cranioschisis. Morphine was not a significant teratogen in the rat at exposure levels significantly beyond that normally encountered in clinical practice. In one study however, decreased litter size and viability were observed in the offspring of male rats administered morphine at doses approximately 3-fold the maximum recommended human daily dose (MRHDD) for 10 days prior to mating. In two studies performed in the rabbit, no evidence of teratogenicity was reported at subcutaneous doses up to 100 mg/kg.

In humans, the frequency of congenital anomalies has been reported to be no greater than expected among the children of 70 women who were treated with morphine during the first four months of pregnancy or in 448 women treated with this drug anytime during pregnancy. Furthermore, no malformations were observed in the infant of a woman who attempted suicide by taking an overdose of morphine and other medication during the first trimester of pregnancy.

Nonteratogenic Effects

Published literature has reported that exposure to morphine during pregnancy is associated with reduction in growth and a host of behavioral abnormalities in the offspring of animals. Morphine treatment during gestational periods of organogenesis in rats, hamsters, guinea pigs and rabbits resulted in the following treatment-related embryotoxicity and neonatal toxicity in one or more studies: decreased litter size, embryo-fetal viability, fetal and neonatal body weights, absolute brain and cerebellar weights, lengths or widths at birth and during the neonatal period, delayed motor and sexual maturation, and increased neonatal mortality, cyanosis and hypothermia. Decreased fertility in female offspring, and decreased plasma and testicular levels of luteinizing hormone and testosterone, decreased testes weights, seminiferous tubule shrinkage, germinal cell aplasia, and decreased spermatogenesis in male offspring were also observed. Behavioral abnormalities resulting from chronic morphine exposure of fetal animals included altered reflex and motor skill development, mild withdrawal, and altered responsiveness to morphine persisting into adulthood.

Controlled studies of chronic *in utero* morphine exposure in pregnant women have not been conducted. Infants born to mothers who have taken opioids chronically may exhibit withdrawal symptoms, reversible reduction in brain volume, small size, decreased ventilatory response to CO_2 and increased risk of sudden infant death syndrome. Morphine sulfate should be used by a pregnant woman only if the need for opioid analgesia clearly outweighs the potential risks to the fetus.

Labor and Delivery

Opioids cross the placenta and may produce respiratory depression and psycho-physiologic effects in neonates. AVINZA is not recommended for use in women during and immediately prior to labor, when use of shorter acting analgesics or other analgesic techniques are more appropriate. Occasionally, opioid analgesics may prolong labor through actions which temporarily reduce the strength, duration and frequency of uterine contractions. However this effect is not consistent and may be offset by an increased rate of cervical dilatation, which tends to shorten labor. Neonates whose mothers received opioid analgesics during labor should be observed closely for signs of respiratory depression. A specific opioid antagonist, such as naloxone or nalmefene, should be available for reversal of opioid-induced respiratory depression in the neonate.

Neonatal Withdrawal Syndrome

Chronic maternal use of opioids during pregnancy may cause newborns to suffer from neonatal withdrawal syndrome (NWS) following birth. Manifestations of this syndrome include irritability, hyperactivity, abnormal sleep pattern, high-pitched cry, tremor, vomiting, diarrhea, weight loss, and failure to gain weight. The time and amount of the mother's last dose, and the rate of elimination of the drug from the newborn may affect the onset, duration, and severity of the disorder. When severe symptoms occur, pharmacologic intervention may be required.

Nursing Mothers

Low levels of morphine sulfate have been detected in human milk. Breast-feeding infants might experience withdrawal symptoms upon cessation of AVINZA administration to the mother. Because of the potential for nursing infants to experience adverse reactions, a decision should be made whether to discontinue nursing or discontinue AVINZA, taking into account the benefit of the drug to the mother.

Continued on next page

Avinza—Cont.

Pediatric Use
Safety and effectiveness of AVINZA in pediatric patients below the age of 18 have not been established. The range of dose strengths available may not be appropriate for treatment of very young pediatric patients. Sprinkling on applesauce is **NOT** a suitable alternative for these patients.
Geriatric Use
Of the total number of subjects in clinical studies of AVINZA, there were 168 patients age 65 and over, including 64 patients over the age of 74, 100 of whom were treated with AVINZA. Subgroup analyses comparing efficacy were not possible given the small number of subjects in each treatment group. No overall differences in safety were observed between these subjects and younger subjects. In general, caution should be exercised in the selection of the starting dose of AVINZA for an elderly patient, usually starting at the low end of the dosing range. As with all opioids, the starting dose should be reduced in debilitated and non-tolerant patients. (see **CLINICAL PHARMACOLOGY, Special Populations, Geriatric** and **PRECAUTIONS, Special Risk Groups**)

ADVERSE REACTIONS

In controlled and open label clinical studies, 560 patients with chronic malignant or non-malignant pain were treated with AVINZA. The most common serious adverse events reported with administration of AVINZA were vomiting, nausea, death, dehydration, dyspnea, and sepsis. (Deaths occurred in patients treated for pain due to underlying malignancy.) Serious adverse events caused by morphine include respiratory depression, apnea, and to a lesser degree, circulatory depression, respiratory arrest, shock and cardiac arrest.
Adverse Events
The common adverse events seen on initiation of therapy with morphine are dose-dependent and are typical opioid-related side effects. The most frequent of these include constipation, nausea and somnolence. The frequency of these events depends upon several factors including the clinical setting, the patient's level of opioid tolerance, and host factors specific to the individual. These events should be anticipated and managed as part of opioid analgesia therapy.
The most common adverse events (seen in greater than 10%) reported by patients treated with AVINZA during the clinical trials at least once during therapy were constipation, nausea, somnolence, vomiting, and headache. Adverse events occurring in 5-10% of study patients were peripheral edema, diarrhea, abdominal pain, infection, urinary tract infection, accidental injury, flu syndrome, back pain, rash, sweating, fever, insomnia, depression, paresthesia, anorexia, dry mouth, asthenia and dyspnea. Other less common side effects expected from opioid analgesics, including morphine, or seen in fewer than 5% of patients taking AVINZA in the clinical trials were:
Body as a Whole: malaise, withdrawal syndrome.
Cardiovascular System: bradycardia, hypertension, hypotension, palpitations, syncope, tachycardia.
Digestive System: biliary pain, dyspepsia, dysphagia, gastroenteritis, abnormal liver function tests, rectal disorder, thirst.
Hemic and Lymphatic System: anemia, thrombocytopenia.
Metabolic and Nutritional Disorders: edema, weight loss.
Musculoskeletal: skeletal muscle rigidity.
Nervous System: abnormal dreams, abnormal gait, agitation, amnesia, anxiety, ataxia, confusion, convulsions, coma, delirium, euphoria, hallucinations, lethargy, nervousness, abnormal thinking, tremor, vasodilation, vertigo.
Respiratory System: hiccup, hypoventilation, voice alteration.
Skin and Appendages: dry skin, urticaria.
Special Senses: amblyopia, eye pain, taste perversion.
Urogenital System: abnormal ejaculation, dysuria, impotence, decreased libido, oliguria, urinary retention.

DRUG ABUSE AND ADDICTION

AVINZA is a mu-agonist opioid and is a Schedule II controlled substance. Morphine, like other opioids used in analgesia, can be abused and is subject to criminal diversion.
Drug addiction is characterized by compulsive use, use for non-medical purposes, and continued use despite harm or risk of harm. Drug addiction is a treatable disease, utilizing a multi-disciplinary approach, but relapse is common.
"Drug-seeking" behavior is very common in addicts and drug abusers. Drug-seeking tactics include emergency calls or visits near the end of office hours, refusal to undergo appropriate examination, testing or referral, repeated "loss" of prescriptions, tampering with prescriptions and reluctance to provide prior medical records or contact information for other treating physician(s). "Doctor shopping" to obtain additional prescriptions is common among drug abusers and people suffering from untreated addiction.
Abuse and addiction are separate and distinct from physical dependence and tolerance. Physicians should be aware that addiction may not be accompanied by concurrent tolerance and symptoms of physical dependence. The converse is also true. In addition, abuse of opioids can occur in the absence of true addiction and is characterized by misuse for non-medical purposes, often in combination with other psychoactive substances. Careful record-keeping of prescribing information, including quantity, frequency, and renewal requests is strongly advised.
Proper assessment of the patient, proper prescribing practices, periodic re-evaluation of therapy, and proper dispensing and storage are appropriate measures that help to limit abuse of opioid drugs.
AVINZA is intended for oral use only. Abuse of the crushed capsule poses a hazard of overdose and death. This risk is increased with concurrent abuse of alcohol and other substances. With parenteral abuse, the capsule excipients, especially talc, can be expected to result in local tissue necrosis, infection, pulmonary granulomas, and increased risk of endocarditis and valvular heart injury. Parenteral drug abuse is commonly associated with transmission of infectious diseases such as hepatitis and HIV.

AVINZA OVERDOSAGE

Symptoms
Acute overdosage with morphine is manifested by respiratory depression, somnolence progressing to stupor or coma, skeletal muscle flaccidity, cold and clammy skin, constricted pupils, and, in some cases, pulmonary edema, bradycardia, hypotension, and death.
Treatment
Primary attention should be given to re-establishment of a patent airway and institution of assisted or controlled ventilation when overdose of an extended-release formulation such as AVINZA has been ingested. Elimination or evacuation of gastric contents may be necessary in order to eliminate unabsorbed drug. Before attempting treatment by gastric emptying or activated charcoal, care should be taken to secure the airway. Pure opioid antagonists, naloxone or nalmefene, are specific antidotes to respiratory depression resulting from opioid overdose. Since the duration of reversal is expected to be less than the duration of action of AVINZA, the patient must be carefully monitored until spontaneous respiration is reliably re-established. AVINZA, as with other controlled delivery preparations in overdose situations, may continue to release morphine for 36 to 48 hours or longer following ingestion, and management of an overdose should be monitored accordingly. If the response to opioid antagonists is sub-optimal or only brief in nature, additional antagonist should be administered as directed by the manufacturer of the product.
Opioid antagonists should not be administered in the absence of clinically significant respiratory or circulatory depression secondary to morphine overdose. Such agents should be administered cautiously to persons who are known, or suspected to be physically dependent on AVINZA. In such cases, an abrupt or complete reversal of opioid effects may precipitate an acute abstinence syndrome.
Opioid-Tolerant Individuals: In an individual physically dependent on opioids, administration of the usual dose of the antagonist will precipitate an acute withdrawal syndrome. The severity of the withdrawal symptoms experienced will depend on the degree of physical dependence and the dose of the antagonist administered. Use of an opioid antagonist should be reserved for cases where such treatment is clearly needed. If it is necessary to treat serious respiratory depression in the physically dependent patient, administration of the antagonist should be initiated with care and titrated with smaller than usual doses.
Supportive measures (including oxygen, vasopressors) should be employed in the managment of circulatory shock and pulmonary edema as indicated. Cardiac arrest or arrhythmias may require cardiac massage or defibrillation.

DOSAGE AND ADMINISTRATION

AVINZA MUST BE SWALLOWED WHOLE (NOT CHEWED, CRUSHED, OR DISSOLVED) OR AVINZA MAY BE OPENED AND THE ENTIRE BEAD CONTENTS SPRINKLED ON A SMALL AMOUNT OF APPLESAUCE IMMEDIATELY PRIOR TO INGESTION. THE BEADS MUST NOT BE CHEWED, CRUSHED, OR DISSOLVED DUE TO RISK OF ACUTE OVERDOSE. INGESTING CHEWED OR CRUSHED AVINZA BEADS WILL LEAD TO THE RAPID RELEASE AND ABSORPTION OF A POTENTIALLY TOXIC DOSE OF MORPHINE.
The daily dose of AVINZA must be limited to a maximum of 1600 mg/day. AVINZA doses of over 1600 mg/day contain a quantity of fumaric acid that has not been demonstrated to be safe, and which may result in serious renal toxicity. (see **WARNINGS**)
The 60, 90, and 120 mg capsules are for use only in opioid-tolerant patients.
All doses are intended to be administered once daily. As with any opioid drug product, it is necessary to adjust the dosing regimen for each patient individually, taking into account the patient's prior analgesic treatment experience. In the selection of the initial dose of AVINZA, attention should be given to the following:
1. the total daily dose, potency and specific characteristics of the opioid the patient has been taking previously;
2. the reliability of the relative potency estimate used to calculate the equivalent morphine dose needed;
3. the patient's degree of opioid tolerance;
4. the general condition and medical status of the patient;
5. concurrent medications;
6. the type and severity of the patient's pain.

The following dosing recommendations, therefore, can only be considered suggested approaches to what is actually a series of clinical decisions over time in the management of the pain of each individual patient.
Conversion from Other Oral Morphine Formulations to AVINZA
Patients receiving other oral morphine formulations may be converted to AVINZA by administering the patient's total daily oral morphine dose as AVINZA once-daily. AVINZA should not be given more frequently than every 24 hours. As with conversion from any oral morphine formulation to another, supplemental pain medication may be required until the response to the patient's daily AVINZA dosage has stabilized (up to 4 days).
Conversion from Parenteral Morphine or Other Non-Morphine Opioids (Parenteral or Oral) to AVINZA
There is inter-patient variability in the potency of opioid drugs and opioid formulations. Therefore, a conservative approach is advised when determining the total daily dose of AVINZA. It is better to underestimate a patient's 24-hour oral morphine dose and make available rescue medication than to overestimate the 24-hour oral morphine dose and manage an adverse experience or overdose. The following general points should be considered regarding opioid conversions.
Parenteral to oral morphine ratio: Anywhere from 3 to 6 mg of oral morphine may be required to provide pain relief equivalent to 1 mg of parenteral morphine. Based on this rationale, a reasonable starting dose of AVINZA would be approximately three times the previous daily parenteral morphine requirement.
Other parenteral or oral non-morphine opioids to oral morphine sulfate: Physicians and other healthcare professionals are advised to refer to published relative potency information, keeping in mind that conversion ratios are only approximate. In general, it is safest to administer half of the estimated daily morphine requirement as the initial AVINZA dose once per day and then manage insufficient pain relief by supplementation with immediate-release morphine or other short-acting analgesics. (see **Individualization of Dosage**)
Individualization of Dosage
Physicians should individualize treatment using a progressive plan of pain management such as outlined by the World Health Organization, the American Pain Society and the Federation of State Medical Boards Model Guidelines. Healthcare professionals should follow appropriate pain management principles of careful assessment and ongoing monitoring. AVINZA (morphine sulfate) is on the third step of the WHO three step analgesic ladder and is of most benefit when a constant level of opioid analgesia is used as a platform from which break-through pain is managed. Once acceptable pain relief is no longer achieved from combinations of non-opioid medications (NSAIDs and acetaminophen) and intermittent usage of moderate or strong opioids, conversion to a 24-hour oral morphine equivalent is warranted.
The dose may be titrated as frequently as every other day to control analgesia. In the event that break-through pain occurs, AVINZA may be supplemented with a small dose (5-15% of the total daily dose of morphine) of a short-acting analgesic.
When AVINZA is chosen as the initial opioid for patients who do not have a proven tolerance to opioids, patients should be treated initially at a dose of 30 mg once-daily (at 24-hour intervals). For opioid-naïve patients, the dose should be increased conservatively. For such patients, it is recommended that the dose of AVINZA be adjusted in increments not greater than 30 mg every 4 days. Some degree of tolerance may occur, requiring dosage adjustment until the achievement of a balance between analgesia and opioid side effects. When necessary, the total dose of AVINZA should be increased until pain relief is reached or clinically significant opioid-related adverse reactions occur.
Alternative Methods of Administration
AVINZA beads sprinkled over applesauce were found to be bioequivalent to AVINZA capsules swallowed whole under fasting conditions in a study of healthy volunteers. Absorption of the beads sprinkled on other foods has not been tested. This method of administration may be beneficial for patients who have difficulty swallowing whole capsules or tablets.
1. Sprinkle the entire contents of the capsule(s) onto a small amount of applesauce. The applesauce should be at room temperature or cooler. Use immediately. (see also **CLINICAL PHARMACOLOGY, Food Effects**)
2. Swallow mixture without chewing or crushing beads.
3. Rinse mouth and swallow to ensure all beads have been ingested.
4. Patients should consume the entire portion and should not divide applesauce into separate doses.

Conversion from AVINZA to Other Pain Control Therapies
It is important to remember that the persistence of AVINZA-derived plasma morphine concentrations may be in excess of 36 hours when making a conversion to other pain control therapies.
Conversion from AVINZA to Other Controlled-Release Oral Morphine Formulations
For a given dose, the same total amount of morphine is available from AVINZA as from oral morphine solution or controlled-release morphine tablets. The extended duration of release of morphine from AVINZA results in reduced maximum and increased minimum plasma morphine concentrations than with shorter acting morphine products. Conversion from AVINZA to the same total daily dose of another controlled-release morphine formulation could lead to either excessive sedation at peak serum levels or inadequate analgesia at trough serum levels. Dosage adjustment with close observation is recommended.
Conversion from AVINZA to Parenteral Opioids
When converting from AVINZA to parenteral opioids, it is best to calculate an equivalent parenteral dose and then initiate treatment at half of this calculated value. As an exam-

ple, an estimated total 24-hour parenteral morphine requirement of a patient receiving AVINZA is one-third of the dose of AVINZA. This is because the oral bioavailability of morphine is one-third that of parenteral morphine. This estimated dose should then be divided in half, and this last calculated dose is the total daily dose. This value should be further divided by six if the desire is to dose with parenteral morphine every four hours.

Consider a patient taking 360 mg of AVINZA daily. First, divide by 3, to account for differences in bioavailability between oral and parenteral morphine. This new figure, 120 mg, is the estimated total 24-hour requirement of parenteral morphine. Dividing by 2, the result gives the total daily dose of 60 mg. If it is decided to administer the drug at four-hour intervals, then administer 10 mg (60 divided by 6) every four hours.

Although this approach may require a dosage increase in the first 24 hours for many patients, this method is recommended, as it is less likely to result in overdose. Overdose is more likely to occur when administering an equivalent dose of parenteral morphine without titration. Provision for break-through pain should be made.

Cessation of Therapy

When the patient no longer requires therapy with AVINZA capsules, doses should be tapered gradually to prevent signs and symptoms of withdrawal in the physically dependent patient.

SAFETY AND HANDLING

AVINZA consists of hard gelatin capsules containing polymer-coated morphine sulfate beads that pose no known risk of handling to healthcare workers. All opioids are liable to diversion and misuse both by the general public and healthcare workers and should be handled accordingly.

HOW SUPPLIED

30 mg Capsule: size 3 capsule, yellow cap imprinted [logo] and white, opaque body imprinted 30 mg and 505.
NDC 64365-505-03: Bottles of 100 capsules.

60 mg Capsule: size 3 capsule, bluish-green cap imprinted [logo] and white, opaque body imprinted 60 mg and 506.
NDC 64365-506-03: Bottles of 100 capsules.

90 mg Capsule: size 1 capsule, red cap imprinted [logo] and white, opaque body imprinted 90 mg and 507.
NDC 64365-507-02: Bottles of 100 capsules.

120 mg Capsule: size 1 capsule, blue-violet cap imprinted [logo] and white, opaque body imprinted 120 mg and 508.
NDC 64365-508-02: Bottles of 100 capsules.

Store at 25°C (77°F); excursions permitted to 15-30°C (59-86°F). [see USP Controlled Room Temperature]

Protect from light and moisture.

Dispense in a tight, light-resistant container as defined in USP.

CAUTION: DEA Order Form Required.

Rx Only.

Manufactured for:
LIGAND®
PHARMACEUTICALS
Ligand Pharmaceuticals Incorporated
San Diego, CA 92121
AVINZA Information Service: 1-888-8-AVINZA
By:
élan
Elan Holdings, Inc.
Gainesville, GA 30504
Rev. 02/03

AVINZA® is a registered trademark of Ligand® Pharmaceuticals Inc.
SODAS™ is a trademark of Elan Corporation, plc.
U.S. Patent No.: 6,066,339

Shown in Product Identification Guide, page 320

ONTAK® ℞

[*ŏn-tăk*]
(denileukin diftitox)
Rx Only

> **WARNING:** Only physicians experienced in the use of antineoplastic therapy and management of patients with cancer should use ONTAK (denileukin diftitox). Patients treated with denileukin diftitox must be managed in a facility equipped and staffed for cardiopulmonary resuscitation and where the patient can be closely monitored for an appropriate period based on his or her health status.

DESCRIPTION

ONTAK® (denileukin diftitox), a recombinant DNA-derived cytotoxic protein composed of the amino acid sequences for diphtheria toxin fragments A and B (Met_1-Thr_{387})-His followed by the sequences for interleukin-2 (IL-2; Ala_1-Thr_{133}), is produced in an *E. coli* expression system. ONTAK has a molecular weight of 58 kD. Neomycin is used in the fermentation process but is undetectable in the final product. The product is purified using reverse phase chromatography followed by a multistep diafiltration process.

ONTAK is supplied in single use vials as a sterile, frozen solution intended for intravenous (IV) administration. Each 2 mL vial of ONTAK contains 300 mcg of recombinant denileukin diftitox in a sterile solution of citric acid (20 mM), EDTA (0.05 mM) and polysorbate 20 (<1%) in Water for Injection, USP. The solution has a pH of 6.9 to 7.2.

CLINICAL PHARMACOLOGY

General: Denileukin diftitox is a fusion protein designed to direct the cytocidal action of diphtheria toxin to cells which express the IL-2 receptor. The human IL-2 receptor exists in three forms, low (CD25), intermediate (CD122/CD132) and high (CD25/CD122/CD132) affinity. The high affinity form of this receptor is usually found only on activated T lymphocytes, activated B lymphocytes and activated macrophages. Malignant cells expressing one or more of the subunits of the IL-2 receptor are found in certain leukemias and lymphomas including cutaneous T-cell lymphoma (CTCL)[1]. *Ex vivo* studies suggest that denileukin diftitox interacts with the high affinity IL-2 receptor on the cell surface and inhibits cellular protein synthesis, resulting in cell death within hours.

The biodistribution and excretion of radiolabeled denileukin diftitox were evaluated over 48 hours in rats. The liver and kidneys were the primary sites of distribution and accumulation of radiolabeled material outside of the vasculature. Denileukin diftitox was metabolized by proteolytic degradation. Excreted material was less than 25% of the total injected dose and consisted of low molecular weight breakdown products.

Pharmacokinetics: Pharmacokinetic parameters associated with denileukin diftitox were determined over a range of doses (3 to 31 mcg/kg/day) in patients with lymphoma. Denileukin diftitox was administered as an IV infusion following the schedule used in the clinical trials. Following the first dose, denileukin diftitox displayed 2-compartment behavior with a distribution phase (half-life approximately 2 to 5 minutes) and a terminal phase (half-life approximately 70 to 80 minutes). Systemic exposure was variable but proportional to dose. Clearance was approximately 1.5 to 2.0 mL/min/kg and the volume of distribution was similar to that of circulating blood (0.06 to 0.08 L/kg). No accumulation was evident between the first and fifth doses. Development of antibodies to denileukin diftitox has been shown to significantly impact clearance rates (see **PRECAUTIONS**, Immunogenicity). Gender, age, and race were introduced into a multivariate analysis with various pharmacokinetic parameters. The limited available data revealed no statistical relationships between these variables.

CLINICAL STUDIES

A randomized, double-blind study was conducted to evaluate doses of 9 or 18 mcg/kg/day in 71 patients with recurrent or persistent, Stage Ib to IVa CTCL. Entry to this study required demonstration of CD25 expression on at least 20% of the cells in any relevant tumor tissue sample (skin biopsy) or circulating cells. Tumor biopsies were not evaluated for expression of other IL-2 receptor subunit components (CD122/CD132). ONTAK was administered as an IV infusion daily for 5 days every 3 weeks. Patients received a median of 6 courses of ONTAK therapy (range 1 to 11). The study population had received a median of 5 prior therapies (range 1 to 12) with 63% of patients entering the trial with Stage IIb or more advanced stage disease. Overall, 30% (95% CI: 18-41%) of patients treated with ONTAK experienced an objective tumor response (50% reduction in tumor burden which was sustained for ≥ 6 weeks; Table 1). Seven patients (10%) achieved a complete response and 14 patients (20%) achieved a partial response. The overall median duration of response, measured from first day of response, was 4 months with a median duration for complete response of 9 months and for partial response of 4 months.

In a Phase I/II dose-escalation study, 35 patients with Stage Ia to IVb CTCL were treated. ONTAK was administered as an IV infusion at doses ranging from 3 to 31 mcg/kg/day, daily for 5 days every 3 weeks. The overall response rate in patients with CTCL who expressed CD25 was 38% (12 of 32 patients); the complete response rate was 16% and the partial response rate was 22%. There were no responses in 21 patients with Hodgkin's Disease.

Table 1
Response in the Phase III Double-Blind Study
Patients with CTCL

Clinical Response	9 mcg/kg/day N = 35	18 mcg/kg/day N = 36
Complete Response	3 (9%)	4 (11%)
95% Confidence Interval	2-23%	3-26%
Partial Response	5 (14%)	9 (25%)
95% Confidence Interval	5-30%	12-42%
Overall Response	8 (23%)	13 (36%)
95% Confidence Interval	10-40%	21-54%

INDICATIONS

ONTAK is indicated for the treatment of patients with persistent or recurrent cutaneous T-cell lymphoma whose malignant cells express the CD25 component of the IL-2 receptor (See **PRECAUTIONS**, Laboratory Tests, for CD25 expression testing). The safety and efficacy of denileukin diftitox in patients with CTCL whose malignant cells do not express the CD25 component of the IL-2 receptor have not been examined.

CONTRAINDICATIONS

ONTAK is contraindicated for use in patients with a known hypersensitivity to denileukin diftitox or any of its components: diphtheria toxin, interleukin-2, or excipients.

WARNINGS

Acute Hypersensitivity-type Reactions: Acute hypersensitivity reactions were reported in 98 of 143 patients (69%) during or within 24 hours of ONTAK infusion; approximately half of the events occurred on the first day of dosing regardless of the treatment cycle. The constellation of symptoms included one or more of the following, defined as the incidence (%) in these 98 patients: hypotension (50%), back pain (30%), dyspnea (28%), vasodilation (28%), rash (25%), chest pain or tightness (24%), tachycardia (12%), dysphagia or laryngismus (5%), syncope (3%), allergic reaction (1%) or anaphylaxis (1%). These events were severe in 2% of patients. Death during infusion has been reported. Management consists of interruption or a decrease in the rate of infusion (depending on the severity of the reaction); 3% of infusions were terminated prematurely and reduction in rate occurred in 4% of the infusions during the clinical trials. The administration of IV antihistamines, corticosteroids, and epinephrine may also be required; two subjects received epinephrine and 18 (13%) received systemic corticosteroids in the clinical studies. These drugs and resuscitative equipment should be readily available during ONTAK administration.

Vascular Leak Syndrome: This syndrome, characterized by 2 or more of the following 3 symptoms (hypotension, edema, hypoalbuminemia) was reported in 27% (38/143) of patients in the clinical studies. Six percent (8/143) of patients were hospitalized for the management of these symptoms. The onset of symptoms in patients with vascular leak syndrome was delayed, usually occurring within the first two weeks of infusion; symptoms may persist or worsen after the cessation of denileukin diftitox. Cases of vascular (capillary) leak with a fatal outcome have been reported. Special caution should be taken in patients with preexisting cardiovascular disease (See **ADVERSE REACTIONS**, Cardiovascular System).

Weight, edema, blood pressure and serum albumin levels should be carefully monitored on an outpatient basis. This syndrome is usually self-limited and treatment should be used only if clinically indicated. The type of treatment will depend on whether edema or hypotension is the primary clinical problem. Pre-existing low serum albumin levels appear to predict and may predispose patients to the syndrome (see **PRECAUTIONS**, Laboratory Tests).

PRECAUTIONS

General: Patients should be monitored carefully for infection since patients with CTCL have a predisposition to cutaneous infection. Also, the binding of denileukin diftitox to activated lymphocytes and macrophages can lead to cell death and may impair immune function in patients.

Immunogenicity: The immunogenicity data reflect the percentage of patients whose test results were considered positive for antibody to denileukin diftitox in ELISA assays and in a functional cellular assay. These results are highly dependent on the sensitivity and the specificity of the assays. Additionally, the observed incidence of the antibody positivity may be influenced by several factors including sample handling, concomitant medication, and underlying disease. For these reasons, the comparison of the incidence of antibodies to denileukin diftitox with the incidence of antibodies to other products may be misleading. Patients who develop a hypersensitivity to denileukin diftitox may have allergic or hypersensitivity reactions to other products produced in *E. coli* expression systems and to vaccines against diphtheria.

An immune response to denileukin diftitox was assessed using two enzyme-linked immunoassays (ELISA), one measuring reactivity directed against the intact DAB_{389}IL-2 and the other against the IL-2 portion of the protein. An additional *in vitro* cell-based assay that measured the ability of antibodies in serum to protect a human IL-2R-expressing cell line from toxicity by DAB_{389}IL-2, was used to detect the presence of antibodies which inhibited functional activity. A total of 131 patients were assessed for an immune response by ELISA prior to treatment. Of these, 51 patients (39%) had antibodies to the intact fusion protein and 24 (18%) had antibodies that were directed against the IL-2 portion of the molecule. Among the 60 patients assessed prior to treatment, 27 (45%) had evidence of an immune response inhibiting activity in the cellular assay. After one cycle of treatment, 76% of the patients tested had an antibody response against DAB_{389}IL-2 and 35% against the IL-2 portion by ELISA; 73% of patients had a positive immune response in the cellular assay. After 3 cycles of treatment, 97% of patients tested had an immune response to DAB_{389}IL-2 in both the ELISA and the cellular assay.

The development of antibodies was correlated with a significant increase (two- to three-fold) in clearance. The increased clearance resulted in a decrease in mean systemic exposure of approximately 75%. The presence of antibodies did not correlate with risk of immediate hypersensitivity-type infusional adverse events.

Laboratory Tests: Prior to administration of this product, the patient's malignant cells should be tested for CD25 expression. A testing service for the assay of CD25 on skin biopsy samples is available. For information on this service call 800-964-5836.

A complete blood count and a blood chemistry panel, including liver and renal function and serum albumin levels, should be performed prior to initiation of ONTAK treatment and weekly during therapy.

Continued on next page

Ontak—Cont.

Eighty-three percent (118/143) of patients with lymphoma experienced hypoalbuminemia, which was considered moderate or severe in 17% (20/118) of the affected patients. For most patients, the nadir for hypoalbuminemia occurs one to two weeks after ONTAK administration. Serum albumin levels should be monitored prior to the initiation of each treatment course. Administration of ONTAK should be delayed until serum albumin levels are at least 3.0 g/dL (see **WARNINGS**).

Drug Interactions: No clinical drug interaction studies have been conducted. However, in a single *in vivo* rodent study denileukin diftitox had no effect on P450 levels.

Carcinogenesis, Mutagenesis, Impairment of Fertility: There have been no studies to assess the carcinogenic potential of denileukin diftitox. Denileukin diftitox showed no evidence of mutagenicity in the Ames test and the chromosomal aberration assay. There have been no studies to assess the effect of denileukin diftitox on fertility.

Pregnancy Category C: Animal reproduction studies have not been conducted with ONTAK. It is also not known whether ONTAK can cause fetal harm when administered to a pregnant woman or affect reproductive capacity. ONTAK should be given to a pregnant woman only if clearly needed.

Nursing Mothers: It is not known whether this drug is excreted in human milk. Because many drugs are excreted in human milk, and because of the potential for serious adverse reactions in nursing infants, patients receiving ONTAK should discontinue nursing.

Pediatric Use: Safety and effectiveness in pediatric patients have not been established.

Geriatric Use: Forty-nine percent (35/71) of the patients enrolled in the randomized two dose study were 65 years of age or older, and those patients had response rates similar to those seen in younger patients. The following adverse events (regardless of causality) tended to be more frequent and/or more severe in lymphoma patients who were 65 years of age or older: anorexia, hypotension, anemia, confusion, rash, nausea and/or vomiting.

ADVERSE REACTIONS

Adverse reactions are presented in Table 2. These data are based on adverse reactions observed in two clinical studies of 143 patients with lymphoma, including 105 patients with CTCL, treated at doses ranging from 3 to 31 mcg/kg/day. All patients experienced one or more adverse events. Twenty-one percent (30/143) of patients required hospitalization for drug-related adverse events; the most common reasons were evaluation of fever, management of vascular leak syndrome or dehydration secondary to gastrointestinal toxicity. Five percent of clinical adverse reactions were severe or life-threatening. The occurrence of adverse events tended to diminish in frequency after the first two courses, possibly related to antibody development.

[See table 2 below]

Hypersensitivity: (see **WARNINGS**)

Vascular Leak Syndrome: (see **WARNINGS**)

Table 2
Adverse Reactions Occurring in Lymphoma Patients
(Frequency ≥ 5% of Patients)
N = 143 patients

Body System	Combined Term	All Grades n (%)	Grades 3 and 4 n (%)
Body as a Whole			
	Chills/fever	116 (81)	31 (22)
	Asthenia	95 (66)	31 (22)
	Infection	69 (48)	34 (24)
	Pain	69 (48)	19 (13)
	Headache	37 (26)	5 (3)
	Chest pain	34 (24)	8 (6)
	Flu-like syndrome	11 (8)	0
	Injection site reaction	11 (8)	1 (1)
Cardiovascular			
	Hypotension	52 (36)	11 (8)
	Vasodilation	31 (22)	1 (1)
	Tachycardia	17 (12)	2 (1)
	Thrombotic events	10 (7)	6 (4)
	Hypertension	9 (6)	0
	Arrhythmia	8 (6)	5 (3)
Digestive			
	Nausea/vomiting	91 (64)	20 (14)
	Anorexia	51 (36)	12 (8)
	Diarrhea	42 (29)	5 (3)
	Constipation	13 (9)	2 (1)
	Dyspepsia	10 (7)	0
	Dysphagia	9 (6)	2 (1)
Hematologic and Lymphatic			
	Anemia	26 (18)	9 (6)
	Thrombocytopenia	12 (8)	3 (2)
	Leukopenia	9 (6)	4 (3)
Metabolic and Nutritional			
	Hypoalbuminemia	118 (83)	20 (14)
	Transaminase increase	87 (61)	22 (15)
	Edema	67 (47)	22 (15)
	Hypocalcemia	24 (17)	4 (3)
	Weight decrease	20 (14)	6 (4)
	Dehydration	13 (9)	10 (7)
	Hypokalemia	9 (6)	0
Musculoskeletal			
	Myalgia	25 (17)	3 (2)
	Arthralgia	11 (8)	2 (1)
Nervous			
	Dizziness	31 (22)	1 (1)
	Paresthesia	19 (13)	2 (1)
	Nervousness	16 (11)	2 (1)
	Confusion	11 (8)	8 (6)
	Insomnia	13 (9)	4 (3)
Respiratory			
	Dyspnea	42 (29)	20 (14)
	Cough increase	37 (26)	3 (2)
	Pharyngitis	25 (17)	0
	Rhinitis	19 (13)	2 (1)
	Lung disorder	11 (8)	0
Skin and Appendages			
	Rash	48 (34)	18 (13)
	Pruritus	29 (20)	5 (3)
	Sweating	15 (10)	1 (1)
Urogenital			
	Hematuria	15 (10)	5 (3)
	Albuminuria	14 (10)	1 (1)
	Pyuria	14 (10)	1 (1)
	Creatinine increase	10 (7)	1 (1)

Hypoalbuminemia: (see **PRECAUTIONS**, Laboratory Tests)

Infectious Complications: Infections of various types were reported by 48% (69/143) of the study population, of which 23% (16/69) were considered severe. Six of the 143 patients (4%) discontinued ONTAK therapy because of infections. Decreased lymphocyte counts (<900 cells/µL) occurred in 34% of lymphoma patients. In general, lymphocyte counts dropped during the dosing period (Days 1 to 5) and then returned to normal by Day 15. Smaller changes and more rapid recoveries were observed with subsequent courses.

Infusion-associated Reactions: (see **WARNINGS**) There are two distinct clinical syndromes associated with ONTAK infusion, an acute hypersensitivity-type symptom complex and a flu-like symptom complex. Overall, 69% of patients had infusion-related, hypersensitivity-type symptoms; for additional information, see **WARNINGS**. A flu-like syndrome was experienced by 91% of patients within several hours to days after ONTAK infusion. The symptom complex consists of one or more of the following: fever and/or chills (81%), asthenia (66%), digestive (64%), myalgia (17%) and arthralgia (8%). In the majority of patients, these symptoms were mild to moderate and responded to treatment with antipyretics and/or anti-emetics. Antipyretics and/or anti-emetics were used to relieve flu-like symptoms; however, the usefulness of these agents in ameliorating these toxicities or as prophylactic agents to decrease the incidence of the acute, flu-like toxicities has not been prospectively studied.

Gastrointestinal: Diarrhea was reported in 29% (42/143) of the study population. The onset of diarrhea may be delayed and the duration can be prolonged. Dehydration, usually concurrent with vomiting or anorexia, occurred in 9% (13/143) of the patients. The majority of transient hepatic transaminase elevations occurred during the first course of ONTAK, were self-limited and resolved within two weeks.

Rash: Generalized maculopapular, petechial, vesicular bullous, urticarial and/or eczematous rashes with both acute and delayed onset, have been reported in 34% (48/143) of patients. Antihistamines may be effective in relieving the symptoms, but more severe rashes may require the use of topical and/or oral corticosteroids.

Cardiovascular System: Two patients, both of whom had known or suspected pre-existing coronary artery disease, sustained acute myocardial infarctions while on study. Ten additional patients (7%) experienced thrombotic events. Two patients with progressive disease and multiple medical problems experienced deep vein thrombosis. Another patient sustained a deep vein thrombosis and pulmonary embolus during hospitalization for management of congestive heart failure and vascular leak syndrome. One patient with a history of severe peripheral vascular disease sustained an arterial thrombosis. Six patients experienced less severe superficial thrombophlebitis. Thrombotic events were also observed in preclinical animal studies.

Infrequent Serious Adverse Events: The following serious adverse events occurred at an incidence of less than 5%: pancreatitis, acute renal insufficiency, microscopic hematuria, oral ulcer, hyperthyroidism including thyroiditis and thyrotoxicosis, and hypothyroidism.

OVERDOSAGE

There is no clinical experience with accidental ONTAK overdosage and no known antidote. At a dose of 31 mcg/kg/day, the dose-limiting toxicities were moderate-to-severe nausea, vomiting, fever, chills and/or persistent asthenia. Doses greater than 31 mcg/kg/day have not been evaluated in humans. If overdose occurs, hepatic and renal function and overall fluid balance should be closely monitored.

DOSAGE AND ADMINISTRATION

ONTAK is for intravenous (IV) use only. The recommended treatment regimen (one treatment cycle) is 9 or 18 mcg/kg/day administered intravenously for five consecutive days every 21 days. ONTAK should be infused over at least 15 minutes. If infusional adverse reactions occur (see **ADVERSE REACTIONS**), the infusion should be discontinued or the rate should be reduced depending on the severity of the reaction. There is no clinical experience with prolonged infusion times (> 80 minutes).

The optimal duration of therapy has not been determined; however, only 2% (1/51) of patients who did not demonstrate at least a 25% decrease in tumor burden prior to the fourth course of treatment subsequently responded.

Special Handling:

- ONTAK must be brought to room temperature, up to 25°C (77°F), before preparing the dose. The vials may be thawed in the refrigerator at 2 to 8°C (36 to 46°F) for not more than 24 hours or at room temperature for 1 to 2 hours. **ONTAK MUST NOT BE HEATED.**
- The solution in the vial may be mixed by gentle swirling; **DO NOT VIGOROUSLY SHAKE ONTAK SOLUTION.**
- After thawing, a haze may be visible. This haze should clear when the solution is at room temperature.
- ONTAK solution must not be used unless the solution is clear, colorless and without visible particulate matter.
- **ONTAK MUST NOT BE REFROZEN.**

Preparation and Administration:

- **USE APPROPRIATE ASEPTIC TECHNIQUE IN DILUTION AND ADMINISTRATION OF ONTAK.**
- Prepare and hold diluted ONTAK in plastic syringes or soft plastic IV bags. **DO NOT USE A GLASS CONTAINER** because adsorption to glass may occur in the dilute state.
- The concentration of ONTAK must be at least 15 mcg/mL during all steps in the preparation of the solution for IV

Continued on next page

infusion. This is best accomplished by withdrawing the calculated dose from the vial(s) and injecting it into an empty IV infusion bag. **FOR EACH 1 ML OF ONTAK FROM THE VIAL(S), NO MORE THAN 9 ML OF STERILE SALINE WITHOUT PRESERVATIVE SHOULD THEN BE ADDED TO THE IV BAG.**

- The ONTAK dose should be infused over at least 15 minutes.
- **ONTAK SHOULD NOT BE ADMINISTERED AS A BOLUS INJECTION.**
- Do not physically mix ONTAK with other drugs.
- **DO NOT ADMINISTER ONTAK THROUGH AN IN-LINE FILTER.**
- Prepared solutions of ONTAK should be administered within 6 hours, using a syringe pump or IV infusion bag.
- Unused portions of ONTAK should be discarded immediately.

HOW SUPPLIED

ONTAK is supplied as:
150 mcg/mL sterile, frozen solution (300 mcg in 2 mL) in a sterile, single-use vial
NDC 64365-503-01, 6 vials in a package.
Store frozen at or below -10°C (14°F).

REFERENCES

1. Nakase K, Kita K, Nasu K, Ueda T, Tanaka I, Shirakawa S and Tsudo M. Differential expression of interleukin-2 receptor (α and β chain) in mature lymphoid neoplasms. Amer. J. Hematol. 1994; 46: 179-183.

Revised February 2002
Manufactured by:
Seragen, Incorporated
San Diego, CA 92121
US License No. 1258
Distributed by:
Ligand Pharmaceuticals Incorporated
San Diego, CA 92121

PANRETIN® ℞

[*păn-rĕtĭn*]
(alitretinoin) gel 0.1%
(For topical use only)

DESCRIPTION

Panretin® gel 0.1% contains alitretinoin and is intended for topical application only. The chemical name is 9-*cis*-retinoic acid and the structural formula is as follows:

[structural formula: H_3C, CH_3, CH_3, CH_3, H_3C, COOH]

Chemically, alitretinoin is related to vitamin A. It is a yellow powder with a molecular weight of 300.44 and a molecular formula of $C_{20}H_{28}O_2$. It is slightly soluble in ethanol (7.01 mg/g at 25°C) and insoluble in water. Panretin® gel is a clear, yellow gel containing 0.1% (w/w) alitretinoin in a base of dehydrated alcohol USP, polyethylene glycol 400 NF, hydroxypropyl cellulose NF, and butylated hydroxytoluene NF.

HOW SUPPLIED

Panretin® gel is available in tubes containing 60 grams. Store at 25° C (77° F); excursions permitted to 15–30° C (59–86° F) [see USP Controlled Room Temperature].
Manufactured for: Ligand Pharmaceuticals Incorporated
San Diego, CA 92121
by: Bristol-Myers Squibb Company
Princeton, NJ 08543 USA
NDC 64365-501-01
Ligand Part #3000153 (Rev. 1001)

TARGRETIN® ℞

[*tahr-greh'-tən*]
(bexarotene)
Capsules, 75 mg
Rx only.

Targretin® capsules are a member of the retinoid class of drugs that is associated with birth defects in humans. Targretin® capsules also caused birth defects when administered orally to pregnant rats. Targretin® capsules must not be administered to a pregnant woman. See CONTRAINDICATIONS.

DESCRIPTION

Targretin® (bexarotene) is a member of a subclass of retinoids that selectively activate retinoid X receptors (RXRs). These retinoid receptors have biologic activity distinct from that of retinoic acid receptors (RARs). Each soft gelatin capsule for oral administration contains 75 mg of bexarotene. The chemical name is 4-[1-(5,6,7,8-tetrahydro-3,5,5,8,8-pentamethyl-2-naphthalenyl) ethenyl] benzoic acid, and the structural formula is as follows:

[structural formula: H_3C, CH_3, CH_2, CH_3, COOH, H_3C, CH_3]

Bexarotene is an off-white to white powder with a molecular weight of 348.48 and a molecular formula of $C_{24}H_{28}O_2$. It is insoluble in water and slightly soluble in vegetable oils and ethanol, USP.
Each Targretin® (bexarotene) capsule also contains the following inactive ingredients: polyethylene glycol 400, NF, polysorbate 20, NF, povidone, USP, and butylated hydroxyanisole, NF. The capsule shell contains gelatin, NF, sorbitol special-glycerin blend, and titanium dioxide, USP.

CLINICAL PHARMACOLOGY

Mechanism of Action

Bexarotene selectively binds and activates retinoid X receptor subtypes (RXRα, RXRβ, RXRγ). RXRs can form heterodimers with various receptor partners such as retinoic acid receptors (RARs), vitamin D receptor, thyroid receptor, and peroxisome proliferator activator receptors (PPARs). Once activated, these receptors function as transcription factors that regulate the expression of genes that control cellular differentiation and proliferation. Bexarotene inhibits the growth *in vitro* of some tumor cell lines of hematopoietic and squamous cell origin. It also induces tumor regression *in vivo* in some animal models. The exact mechanism of action of bexarotene in the treatment of cutaneous T-cell lymphoma (CTCL) is unknown.

Pharmacokinetics

General

After oral administration of Targretin® capsules, bexarotene is absorbed with a T_{max} of about two hours. Terminal half-life of bexarotene is about seven hours. Studies in patients with advanced malignancies show approximate single dose linearity within the therapeutic range and low accumulation with multiple doses. Plasma bexarotene AUC and C_{max} values resulting from a 75 to 300 mg dose were 35% and 48% higher, respectively, after a fat-containing meal than after a glucose solution (see **PRECAUTIONS**: ***Drug-Food Interaction*** and **DOSAGE AND ADMINISTRATION**). Bexarotene is highly bound (>99%) to plasma proteins. The plasma proteins to which bexarotene binds have not been elucidated, and the ability of bexarotene to displace drugs bound to plasma proteins and the ability of drugs to displace bexarotene binding have not been studied (see **PRECAUTIONS**: ***Protein Binding***). The uptake of bexarotene by organs or tissues has not been evaluated.

Metabolism

Four bexarotene metabolites have been identified in plasma: 6- and 7-hydroxy-bexarotene and 6- and 7-oxo-bexarotene. *In vitro* studies suggest that cytochrome P450 3A4 is the major cytochrome P450 responsible for formation of the oxidative metabolites and that the oxidative metabolites may be glucuronidated. The oxidative metabolites are active in *in vitro* assays of retinoid receptor activation, but the relative contribution of the parent and any metabolites to the efficacy and safety of Targretin® capsules is unknown.

Elimination

The renal elimination of bexarotene and its metabolites was examined in patients with Type 2 diabetes mellitus. Neither bexarotene nor its metabolites were excreted in urine in appreciable amounts. Bexarotene is thought to be eliminated primarily through the hepatobiliary system.

Special Populations

Elderly: Bexarotene C_{max} and AUC were similar in advanced cancer patients <60 years old and in patients >60 years old, including a subset of patients >70 years old.
Pediatric: Studies to evaluate bexarotene pharmacokinetics in the pediatric population have not been conducted (see **PRECAUTIONS**: ***Pediatric Use***).
Gender: The pharmacokinetics of bexarotene were similar in male and female patients with advanced cancer.
Ethnic Origin: The effect of ethnic origin on bexarotene pharmacokinetics is unknown.
Renal Insufficiency: No formal studies have been conducted with Targretin® capsules in patients with renal insufficiency. Urinary elimination of bexarotene and its known metabolites is a minor excretory pathway (<1% of administered dose), but because renal insufficiency can result in significant protein binding changes, pharmacokinetics may be altered in patients with renal insufficiency (see **PRECAUTIONS**: ***Renal Insufficiency***).
Hepatic Insufficiency: No specific studies have been conducted with Targretin® capsules in patients with hepatic insufficiency. Because less than 1% of the dose is excreted in the urine unchanged and there is *in vitro* evidence of extensive hepatic contribution to bexarotene elimination, hepatic impairment would be expected to lead to greatly decreased clearance (see **WARNINGS**: *Hepatic insufficiency*).

Drug-Drug Interactions

No specific studies to evaluate drug interactions with bexarotene have been conducted. Bexarotene oxidative metabolites appear to be formed by cytochrome P450 3A4.
Because bexarotene is metabolized by cytochrome P450 3A4, ketoconazole, itraconazole, erythromycin, gemfibrozil, grapefruit juice, and other inhibitors of cytochrome P450 3A4 would be expected to lead to an increase in plasma bexarotene concentrations. Furthermore, rifampin, phenytoin, phenobarbital and other inducers of cytochrome P450 3A4 may cause a reduction in plasma bexarotene concentrations.
Concomitant administration of Targretin® capsules and gemfibrozil resulted in substantial increases in plasma concentrations of bexarotene, probably at least partially related to cytochrome P450 3A4 inhibition by gemfibrozil. Under similar conditions, bexarotene concentrations were not affected by concomitant atorvastatin administration. Concomitant administration of gemfibrozil with Targretin® capsules is not recommended (see **PRECAUTIONS**: ***Drug-Drug Interactions***).
Based on interim data, concomitant administration of Targretin® capsules and tamoxifen resulted in approximately a 35% decrease in plasma concentrations of tamoxifen, possibly through an induction of cytochrome P450 3A4. Based on this known interaction, bexarotene may theoretically increase the rate of metabolism and reduce plasma concentrations of other substrates metabolized by cytochrome P450 3A4, including oral or other systemic hormonal contraceptives (see **CONTRAINDICATIONS**: ***Pregnancy*: Category X** and **PRECAUTIONS**: ***Drug-Drug Interactions***).

Clinical Studies

Targretin® capsules were evaluated in 152 patients with advanced and early stage cutaneous T-cell lymphoma (CTCL) in two multicenter, open-label, historically-controlled clinical studies conducted in the U.S., Canada, Europe, and Australia.
The advanced disease patients had disease refractory to at least one prior systemic therapy (median of two, range one to six prior systemic therapies) and had been treated with a median of five (range 1 to 11) prior systemic, irradiation, and/or topical therapies. Early disease patients were intolerant to, had disease that was refractory to, or had reached a response plateau of six months on, at least two prior therapies. The patients entered had been treated with a median of 3.5 (range 2 to 12) therapies (systemic, irradiation, and/or topical).
The two clinical studies enrolled a total of 152 patients, 102 of whom had disease refractory to at least one prior systemic therapy, 90 with advanced disease and 12 with early disease. This is the patient population for whom Targretin® capsules are indicated.
Patients were initially treated with a starting dose of 650 mg/m²/day with a subsequent reduction of starting dose to 500 mg/m²/day. Neither of these starting doses was tolerated, and the starting dose was then reduced to 300 mg/m²/day. If, however, a patient on 300 mg/m²/day of Targretin® capsules showed no response after eight or more weeks of therapy, the dose could be increased to 400 mg/m²/day.
Tumor response was assessed in both studies by observation of up to five baseline-defined index lesions using a Composite Assessment of Index Lesion Disease Severity (CA). This endpoint was based on a summation of the grades, for all index lesions, of erythema, scaling, plaque elevation, hypopigmentation or hyperpigmentation, and area of involvement. Also considered in response assessment was the presence or absence of cutaneous tumors and extracutaneous disease manifestations.
All tumor responses required confirmation over at least two assessments separated by at least four weeks. A partial response was defined as an improvement of at least 50% in the index lesions without worsening, or development of new cutaneous tumors or non-cutaneous manifestations. A complete clinical response required complete disappearance of all manifestations of disease, but did not require confirmation by biopsy.
At the initial dose of 300 mg/m²/day, 1/62 (1.6%) of patients had a complete clinical tumor response and 19/62 (30%) of patients had a partial tumor response. The rate of relapse (25% increase in CA or worsening of other aspects of disease) in the 20 patients who had a tumor response was 6/20 (30%) over a median duration of observation of 21 weeks, and the median duration of tumor response had not been reached. Responses were seen as early as 4 weeks and new responses continued to be seen at later visits.

INDICATIONS AND USAGE

Targretin® (bexarotene) capsules are indicated for the treatment of cutaneous manifestations of cutaneous T-cell lymphoma in patients who are refractory to at least one prior systemic therapy.

CONTRAINDICATIONS

Targretin® capsules are contraindicated in patients with a known hypersensitivity to bexarotene or other components of the product.

Pregnancy: Category X

Targretin® (bexarotene) capsules may cause fetal harm when administered to a pregnant woman. Targretin® capsules must not be given to a pregnant woman or a woman who intends to become pregnant. If a woman becomes pregnant while taking Targretin® capsules, Targretin® capsules must be stopped immediately and the woman given appropriate counseling.
Bexarotene caused malformations when administered orally to pregnant rats during days 7–17 of gestation. Developmental abnormalities included incomplete ossification at 4 mg/kg/day and cleft palate, depressed eye bulge/microphthalmia, and small ears at 16 mg/kg/day. The plasma AUC of bexarotene in rats at 4 mg/kg/day is approximately one third the AUC in humans at the recommended daily dose. At doses greater than 10 mg/kg/day, bexarotene caused developmental mortality. The no effect dose for fetal

Continued on next page

Targretin Capsules—Cont.

effects in rats was 1 mg/kg/day (producing an AUC approximately one sixth of the AUC at the recommended human daily dose).

Women of child-bearing potential should be advised to avoid becoming pregnant when Targretin® capsules are used. The possibility that a woman of child-bearing potential is pregnant at the time therapy is instituted should be considered. A negative pregnancy test (e.g., serum beta-human chorionic gonadotropin, beta-HCG) with a sensitivity of at least 50 mIU/L should be obtained within one week prior to Targretin® capsules therapy, and the pregnancy test must be repeated at monthly intervals while the patient remains on Targretin® capsules. Effective contraception must be used for one month prior to the initiation of therapy, during therapy and for at least one month following discontinuation of therapy; it is recommended that two reliable forms of contraception be used simultaneously unless abstinence is the chosen method. Bexarotene can potentially induce metabolic enzymes and thereby theoretically reduce the plasma concentrations of oral or other systemic hormonal contraceptives (see **CLINICAL PHARMACOLOGY**: ***Drug-Drug Interactions*** and **PRECAUTIONS**: ***Drug-Drug Interactions***). Thus, if treatment with Targretin® capsules is intended in a woman with child-bearing potential, it is strongly recommended that one of the two reliable forms of contraception should be non-hormonal. Male patients with sexual partners who are pregnant, possibly pregnant, or who could become pregnant must use condoms during sexual intercourse while taking Targretin® capsules and for at least one month after the last dose of drug. Targretin® capsules therapy should be initiated on the second or third day of a normal menstrual period. No more than a one month supply of Targretin® capsules should be given to the patient so that the results of pregnancy testing can be assessed and counseling regarding avoidance of pregnancy and birth defects can be reinforced.

WARNINGS

Lipid abnormalities: Targretin® capsules induce major lipid abnormalities in most patients. These must be monitored and treated during long-term therapy. About 70% of patients with CTCL who received an initial dose of ≥300 mg/m²/day of Targretin® capsules had fasting triglyceride levels greater than 2.5 times the upper limit of normal. About 55% had values over 800 mg/dL with a median of about 1200 mg/dL in those patients. Cholesterol elevations above 300 mg/dL occurred in approximately 60% and 75% of patients with CTCL who received an initial dose of 300 mg/m²/day or greater than 300 mg/m²/day, respectively. Decreases in high density lipoprotein (HDL) cholesterol to less than 25 mg/dL were seen in about 55% and 90% of patients receiving an initial dose of 300 mg/m²/day or greater than 300 mg/m²/day, respectively, of Targretin® capsules. The effects on triglycerides, HDL cholesterol, and total cholesterol were reversible with cessation of therapy, and could generally be mitigated by dose reduction or concomitant antilipemic therapy.

Fasting blood lipid determinations should be performed before Targretin® capsules therapy is initiated and weekly until the lipid response to Targretin® capsules is established, which usually occurs within two to four weeks, and at eight week intervals thereafter. Fasting triglycerides should be normal or normalized with appropriate intervention prior to initiating Targretin® capsules therapy. Attempts should be made to maintain triglyceride levels below 400 mg/dL to reduce the risk of clinical sequelae (see **WARNINGS**: *Pancreatitis*). If fasting triglycerides are elevated or become elevated during treatment, antilipemic therapy should be instituted, and if necessary, the dose of Targretin® capsules reduced or suspended. In the 300 mg/m²/day initial dose group, 60% of patients were given lipid lowering drugs. Atorvastatin was used in 48% (73/152) of patients with CTCL. Because of a potential drug-drug interaction (see **PRECAUTIONS**: ***Drug-Drug Interactions***), gemfibrozil is not recommended for use with Targretin® capsules.

Pancreatitis: Acute pancreatitis has been reported in four patients with CTCL and in six patients with non-CTCL cancers treated with Targretin® capsules; the cases were associated with marked elevations of fasting serum triglycerides, the lowest being 770 mg/dL in one patient. One patient with advanced non-CTCL cancer died of pancreatitis. Patients with CTCL who have risk factors for pancreatitis (e.g., prior pancreatitis, uncontrolled hyperlipidemia, excessive alcohol consumption, uncontrolled diabetes mellitus, biliary tract disease, and medications known to increase triglyceride levels or to be associated with pancreatic toxicity) should generally not be treated with Targretin® capsules (see **WARNINGS**: *Lipids abnormalities* and **PRECAUTIONS**: ***Laboratory Tests***).

Liver function test abnormalities: For patients with CTCL receiving an initial dose of 300 mg/m²/day of Targretin® capsules, elevations in liver function tests (LFTs) have been observed in 5% (SGOT/AST), 2% (SGPT/ALT), and 0% (bilirubin). In contrast, with an initial dose greater than 300 mg/m²/day of Targretin® capsules, the incidence of LFT elevations was higher at 7% (SGOT/AST), 9% (SGPT/ALT), and 6% (bilirubin). Two patients developed cholestasis, including one patient who died of liver failure. In clinical trials, elevation of LFTs resolved within one month in 80% of patients following a decrease in dose or discontinuation of

Table 1. Adverse Events with Incidence ≥10% in CTCL Trials

Body System Adverse Event[1,2]	Initial Assigned Dose Group (mg/m²/day) 300 N=84 N (%)	>300 N=53 N (%)
METABOLIC AND NUTRITIONAL DISORDERS		
Hyperlipemia	66 (78.6)	42 (79.2)
Hypercholesteremia	27 (32.1)	33 (62.3)
Lactic dehydrogenase increased	6 (7.1)	7 (13.2)
BODY AS A WHOLE		
Headache	25 (29.8)	22 (41.5)
Asthenia	17 (20.2)	24 (45.3)
Infection	11 (13.1)	12 (22.6)
Abdominal pain	9 (10.7)	2 (3.8)
Chills	8 (9.5)	7 (13.2)
Fever	4 (4.8)	9 (17.0)
Flu syndrome	3 (3.6)	7 (13.2)
Back pain	2 (2.4)	6 (11.3)
Infection bacterial	1 (1.2)	7 (13.2)
ENDOCRINE		
Hypothyroidism	24 (28.6)	28 (52.8)
SKIN AND APPENDAGES		
Rash	14 (16.7)	12 (22.6)
Dry skin	9 (10.7)	5 (9.4)
Exfoliative dermatitis	8 (9.5)	15 (28.3)
Alopecia	3 (3.6)	6 (11.3)
HEMIC AND LYMPHATIC SYSTEM		
Leukopenia	14 (16.7)	25 (47.2)
Anemia	5 (6.0)	13 (24.5)
Hypochromic anemia	3 (3.6)	7 (13.2)
DIGESTIVE SYSTEM		
Nausea	13 (15.5)	4 (7.5)
Diarrhea	6 (7.1)	22 (41.5)
Vomiting	3 (3.6)	7 (13.2)
Anorexia	2 (2.4)	12 (22.6)
CARDIOVASCULAR SYSTEM		
Peripheral edema	11 (13.1)	6 (11.3)
NERVOUS SYSTEM		
Insomnia	4 (4.8)	6 (11.3)

[1] Preferred English term coded according to Ligand-modified COSTART 5 Dictionary.
[2] Patients are counted at most once in each AE category.

therapy. Baseline LFTs should be obtained, and LFTs should be carefully monitored after one, two and four weeks of treatment initiation, and if stable, at least every eight weeks thereafter during treatment. Consideration should be given to a suspension or discontinuation of Targretin® capsules if test results reach greater than three times the upper limit of normal values for SGOT/AST, SGPT/ALT, or bilirubin.

Hepatic insufficiency: No specific studies have been conducted with Targretin® capsules in patients with hepatic insufficiency. Because less than 1% of the dose is excreted in the urine unchanged and there is *in vitro* evidence of extensive hepatic contribution to bexarotene elimination, hepatic impairment would be expected to lead to greatly decreased clearance. Targretin® capsules should be used only with great caution in this population.

Thyroid axis alterations: Targretin® capsules induce biochemical evidence of or clinical hypothyroidism in about half of all patients treated, causing a reversible reduction in thyroid hormone (total thyroxine [total T4]) and thyroid-stimulating hormone (TSH) levels. The incidence of decreases in TSH and total T4 were about 60% and 45%, respectively, in patients with CTCL receiving an initial dose of 300 mg/m²/day. Hypothyroidism was reported as an adverse event in 29% of patients. Treatment with thyroid hormone supplements should be considered in patients with laboratory evidence of hypothyroidism. In the 300 mg/m²/day initial dose group, 37% of patients were treated with thyroid hormone replacement. Baseline thyroid function tests should be obtained and patients monitored during treatment.

Leukopenia: A total of 18% of patients with CTCL receiving an initial dose of 300 mg/m²/day of Targretin® capsules had reversible leukopenia in the range of 1000 to <3000 WBC/mm³. Patients receiving an initial dose greater than 300 mg/m²/day of Targretin® capsules had an incidence of leukopenia of 43%. No patient with CTCL treated with Targretin® capsules developed leukopenia of less than 1000 WBC/mm³. The time to onset of leukopenia was generally four to eight weeks. The leukopenia observed in most patients was explained by neutropenia. In the 300 mg/m²/day initial dose group, the incidence of NCI Grade 3 and Grade 4 neutropenia, respectively, was 12% and 4%. The leukopenia and neutropenia experienced during Targretin® capsules therapy resolved after dose reduction or discontinuation of treatment, on average within 30 days in 93% of the patients with CTCL and 82% of patients with non-CTCL cancers. Leukopenia and neutropenia were rarely associated with severe sequelae or serious adverse events. Determination of WBC with differential should be obtained at baseline and periodically during treatment.

Cataracts: Posterior subcapsular cataracts were observed in preclinical toxicity studies in rats and dogs administered bexarotene daily for 6 months. In 15 of 79 patients who had serial slit lamp examinations, new cataracts or worsening of previous cataracts were found. Because of the high prevalence and rate of cataract formation in older patient populations, the relationship of Targretin® capsules and cataracts cannot be determined in the absence of an appropriate control group. Patients treated with Targretin® capsules who experience visual difficulties should have an appropriate ophthalmologic evaluation.

PRECAUTIONS

Pregnancy: **Category X.** See **CONTRAINDICATIONS**.

General: Targretin® capsules should be used with caution in patients with a known hypersensitivity to retinoids. Clinical instances of cross-reactivity have not been noted.

Vitamin A Supplementation: In clinical studies, patients were advised to limit vitamin A intake to ≤15,000 IU/day. Because of the relationship of bexarotene to vitamin A, patients should be advised to limit vitamin A supplements to avoid potential additive toxic effects.

Patients with Diabetes Mellitus: Caution should be used when administering Targretin® capsules in patients using insulin, agents enhancing insulin secretion (e.g., sulfonylureas), or insulin-sensitizers (e.g., thiazolidinedione class). Based on the mechanism of action, Targretin® capsules could enhance the action of these agents, resulting in hypoglycemia. Hypoglycemia has not been associated with the use of Targretin® capsules as monotherapy.

Photosensitivity: Retinoids as a class have been associated with photosensitivity. *In vitro* assays indicate that bexarotene is a potential photosensitizing agent. Mild phototoxicity manifested as sunburn and skin sensitivity to sunlight was observed in patients who were exposed to direct sunlight while receiving Targretin® capsules. Patients should be advised to minimize exposure to sunlight and artificial ultraviolet light while receiving Targretin® capsules.

Laboratory Tests

Blood lipid determinations should be performed before Targretin® capsules are given. Fasting triglycerides should be normal or normalized with appropriate intervention prior to therapy. Hyperlipidemia usually occurs within the initial two to four weeks. Therefore, weekly lipid determinations are recommended during this interval. Subsequently, in patients not hyperlipidemic, determinations can be performed less frequently (see **WARNINGS**: *Lipid abnormalities*).

A white blood cell count with differential should be obtained at baseline and periodically during treatment. Baseline liver function tests should be obtained and should be carefully monitored after one, two and four weeks of treatment initiation, and if stable, periodically thereafter during treatment. Baseline thyroid function tests should be obtained and then monitored during treatment as indicated (see **WARNINGS**: *Leukopenia, Liver function test abnormalities, and Thyroid axis alterations*).

Drug-Food Interaction

In all clinical trials, patients were instructed to take Targretin® capsules with or immediately following a meal. In one clinical study, plasma bexarotene AUC and C_{max} values were substantially higher following a fat-containing meal versus those following the administration of a glucose solution. Because safety and efficacy data are based upon administration with food, it is recommended that Targretin® capsules be administered with food (see **CLINICAL PHARMACOLOGY: Pharmacokinetics** and **DOSAGE AND ADMINISTRATION**).

Drug-Drug Interactions

No formal studies to evaluate drug interactions with bexarotene have been conducted. Bexarotene oxidative metabolites appear to be formed by cytochrome P450 3A4.

On the basis of the metabolism of bexarotene by cytochrome P450 3A4, ketoconazole, itraconazole, erythromycin, gemfibrozil, grapefruit juice, and other inhibitors of cytochrome P450 3A4 would be expected to lead to an increase in plasma bexarotene concentrations. Furthermore, rifampin, phenytoin, phenobarbital, and other inducers of cytochrome P450 3A4 may cause a reduction in plasma bexarotene concentrations.

Concomitant administration of Targretin® capsules and gemfibrozil resulted in substantial increases in plasma concentrations of bexarotene, probably at least partially related to cytochrome P450 3A4 inhibition by gemfibrozil. Under similar conditions, bexarotene concentrations were not affected by concomitant atorvastatin administration. Concomitant administration of gemfibrozil with Targretin® capsules is not recommended.

Based on interim data, concomitant administration of Targretin® capsules and tamoxifen resulted in approximately a 35% decrease in plasma concentrations of tamoxifen, possibly through an induction of cytochrome P450 3A4. Based on this known interaction, bexarotene may theoretically increase the rate of metabolism and reduce plasma concentrations of other substrates metabolized by cytochrome P450 3A4, including oral or other systemic hormonal contraceptives (see **CLINICAL PHARMACOLOGY**: ***Drug-Drug Interactions*** and **CONTRAINDICATIONS**: ***Pregnancy: Category X***). Thus, if treatment with Targretin® capsules is intended in a woman with child-bearing potential, it is strongly recommended that two reliable forms of contraception be used concurrently, one of which should be non-hormonal.

Renal Insufficiency

No formal studies have been conducted with Targretin® capsules in patients with renal insufficiency. Urinary elimination of bexarotene and its known metabolites is a minor excretory pathway for bexarotene (<1% of administered dose), but because renal insufficiency can result in significant protein binding changes, and bexarotene is >99% protein bound, pharmacokinetics may be altered in patients with renal insufficiency.

Protein Binding

Bexarotene is highly bound (>99%) to plasma proteins. The plasma proteins to which bexarotene binds have not been elucidated, and the ability of bexarotene to displace drugs bound to plasma proteins and the ability of drugs to displace bexarotene binding have not been studied.

Drug/Laboratory Test Interactions

CA125 assay values in patients with ovarian cancer may be increased by Targretin® capsule therapy.

Carcinogenesis, Mutagenesis, Impairment of Fertility

Long-term studies in animals to assess the carcinogenic potential of bexarotene have not been conducted. Bexarotene is not mutagenic to bacteria (Ames assay) or mammalian cells (mouse lymphoma assay). Bexarotene was not clastogenic *in vivo* (micronucleus test in mice). No formal fertility studies were conducted with bexarotene. Bexarotene caused testicular degeneration when oral doses of 1.5 mg/kg/day were given to dogs for 91 days (producing an AUC of approximately one fifth the AUC at the recommended human daily dose).

Use in Nursing Mothers

It is not known whether bexarotene is excreted in human milk. Because many drugs are excreted in human milk and because of the potential for serious adverse reactions in nursing infants from bexarotene, a decision should be made whether to discontinue nursing or to discontinue the drug, taking into account the importance of the drug to the mother.

Pediatric Use

Safety and effectiveness in pediatric patients have not been established.

Geriatric Use

Of the total patients with CTCL in clinical studies of Targretin® capsules, 64% were 60 years or older, while 33% were 70 years or older. No overall differences in safety were observed between patients 70 years or older and younger patients, but greater sensitivity of some older individuals to Targretin® capsules cannot be ruled out. Responses to Targretin® capsules were observed across all age group decades, without preference for any individual age group decade.

ADVERSE REACTIONS

The safety of Targretin® capsules has been evaluated in clinical studies of 152 patients with CTCL who received Targretin® capsules for up to 97 weeks and in 352 patients in other studies. The mean duration of therapy for the 152 patients with CTCL was 166 days. The most common adverse events reported with an incidence of at least 10% in patients with CTCL treated at an initial dose of 300 mg/m²/day of Targretin® capsules are shown in Table 1. The events at least possibly related to treatment are lipid abnormalities (elevated triglycerides, elevated total and LDL cholesterol and decreased HDL cholesterol), hypothyroidism, headache, asthenia, rash, leukopenia, anemia, nausea, infection, peripheral edema, abdominal pain, and dry skin. Most adverse events occurred at a higher incidence in patients treated at starting doses of greater than 300 mg/m²/day (see Table 1).

Adverse events leading to dose reduction or study drug discontinuation in at least two patients were hyperlipemia, neutropenia/leukopenia, diarrhea, fatigue/lethargy, hypothyroidism, headache, liver function test abnormalities, rash, pancreatitis, nausea, anemia, allergic reaction, muscle spasm, pneumonia, and confusion.

The moderately severe (NCI Grade 3) and severe (NCI Grade 4) adverse events reported in two or more patients with CTCL treated at an initial dose of 300 mg/m²/day of Targretin® capsules (see Table 2) were hypertriglyceridemia, pruritus, headache, peripheral edema, leukopenia, rash, and hypercholesteremia. Most of these moderately severe or severe adverse events occurred at a higher rate in patients treated at starting doses of greater than 300 mg/m²/day than in patients treated at a starting dose of 300 mg/m²/day.

As shown in Table 3, in patients with CTCL receiving an initial dose of 300 mg/m²/day, the incidence of NCI Grade 3 or 4 elevations in triglycerides and total cholesterol was 28% and 25%, respectively. In contrast, in patients with CTCL receiving greater than 300 mg/m²/day, the incidence of NCI Grade 3 or 4 elevated triglycerides and total cholesterol was 45% and 45%, respectively. Other Grade 3 and 4 laboratory abnormalities are shown in Table 3.

In addition to the 152 patients enrolled in the two CTCL studies, 352 patients received Targretin® capsules as monotherapy for various advanced malignancies at doses from 5 mg/m²/day to 1000 mg/m²/day. The common adverse events (incidence greater than 10%) were similar to those seen in patients with CTCL.

In the 504 patients (CTCL and non-CTCL) who received Targretin® capsules as monotherapy, drug-related serious adverse events that were fatal, in one patient each, were acute pancreatitis, subdural hematoma, and liver failure.

In the patients with CTCL receiving an initial dose of 300 mg/m²/day of Targretin® capsules, adverse events reported at an incidence of less than 10% and not included in Tables 1–3 or discussed in other parts of labeling and possibly related to treatment were as follows:

Body as a Whole: chills, cellulitis, chest pain, sepsis, and monilia.

Cardiovascular: hemorrhage, hypertension, angina pectoris, right heart failure, syncope, and tachycardia.

Digestive: constipation, dry mouth, flatulence, colitis, dyspepsia, cheilitis, gastroenteritis, gingivitis, liver failure, and melena.

Hemic and Lymphatic: eosinophilia, thrombocythemia, coagulation time increased, lymphocytosis, and thrombocytopenia.

Table 2. Incidence of Moderately Severe and Severe Adverse Events Reported in at Least Two Patients (CTCL Trials)

	Initial Assigned Dose Group (mg/m²/day)			
	300 (N=84)		>300 (N=53)	
	Mod Sev	Severe	Mod Sev	Severe
Body System Adverse Event[1,2]	N (%)	N (%)	N (%)	N (%)
BODY AS A WHOLE				
Asthenia	1 (1.2)	0 (0.0)	11 (20.8)	0 (0.0)
Headache	3 (3.6)	0 (0.0)	5 (9.4)	1 (1.9)
Infection bacterial	1 (1.2)	0 (0.0)	0 (0.0)	2 (3.8)
CARDIOVASCULAR SYS.				
Peripheral edema	2 (2.4)	1 (1.2)	0 (0.0)	0 (0.0)
DIGESTIVE SYSTEM				
Anorexia	0 (0.0)	0 (0.0)	3 (5.7)	0 (0.0)
Diarrhea	1 (1.2)	1 (1.2)	2 (3.8)	1 (1.9)
Pancreatitis	1 (1.2)	0 (0.0)	3 (5.7)	0 (0.0)
Vomiting	0 (0.0)	0 (0.0)	2 (3.8)	0 (0.0)
ENDOCRINE				
Hypothyroidism	1 (1.2)	1 (1.2)	2 (3.8)	0 (0.0)
HEM. & LYMPH. SYS.				
Leukopenia	3 (3.6)	0 (0.0)	6 (11.3)	1 (1.9)
META. AND NUTR. DIS.				
Bilirubinemia	0 (0.0)	1 (1.2)	2 (3.8)	0 (0.0)
Hypercholesteremia	2 (2.4)	0 (0.0)	5 (9.4)	0 (0.0)
Hyperlipemia	16 (19.0)	6 (7.1)	17 (32.1)	5 (9.4)
SGOT/AST increased	0 (0.0)	0 (0.0)	2 (3.8)	0 (0.0)
SGPT/ALT increased	0 (0.0)	0 (0.0)	2 (3.8)	0 (0.0)
RESPIRATORY SYSTEM				
Pneumonia	0 (0.0)	0 (0.0)	2 (3.8)	2 (3.8)
SKIN AND APPENDAGES				
Exfoliative dermatitis	0 (0.0)	1 (1.2)	3 (5.7)	1 (1.9)
Rash	1 (1.2)	2 (2.4)	1 (1.9)	0 (0.0)

[1] Preferred English term coded according to Ligand-modified COSTART 5 Dictionary.
[2] Patients are counted at most once in each AE category. Patients are classified by the highest severity within each row.

Table 3. Treatment-Emergent Abnormal Laboratory Values in CTCL Trials

	Initial Assigned Dose (mg/m²/day)			
	300		>300	
	N=83[1]		N=53[1]	
Analyte	Grade 3[2] (%)	Grade 4[2] (%)	Grade 3 (%)	Grade 4 (%)
Triglycerides[3]	21.3	6.7	31.8	13.6
Total Cholesterol[3]	18.7	6.7	15.9	29.5
Alkaline Phosphatase	1.2	0.0	0.0	1.9
Hyperglycemia	1.2	0.0	5.7	0.0
Hypocalcemia	1.2	0.0	0.0	0.0
Hyponatremia	1.2	0.0	9.4	0.0
SGPT/ALT	1.2	0.0	1.9	1.9
Hyperkalemia	0.0	0.0	1.9	0.0
Hypernatremia	0.0	1.2	0.0	0.0
SGOT/AST	0.0	0.0	1.9	1.9
Total Bilirubin	0.0	0.0	0.0	1.9
ANC	12.0	3.6	18.9	7.5
ALC	7.2	0.0	15.1	0.0
WBC	3.6	0.0	11.3	0.0
Hemoglobin	0.0	0.0	1.9	0.0

[1] Number of patients with at least one analyte value post-baseline.
[2] Adapted from NCI Common Toxicity Criteria, Grade 3 and 4, Version 2.0. Patients are considered to have had a Grade 3 or 4 value if either of the following occurred: a) Value becomes Grade 3 or 4 during the study; b) Value is abnormal at baseline and worsens to Grade 3 or 4 on study, including all values beyond study drug discontinuation, as defined in data handling conventions.
[3] The denominator used to calculate the incidence rates for fasting Total Cholesterol and Triglycerides were N=75 for the 300 mg/m²/day initial dose group and N=44 for the >300 mg/m²/day initial dose group.

Continued on next page

Targretin Capsules—Cont.

Metabolic and Nutritional: LDH increased, creatinine increased, hypoproteinemia, hyperglycemia, weight decreased, weight increased, and amylase increased.
Musculoskeletal: arthralgia, myalgia, bone pain, myasthenia, and arthrosis.
Nervous: depression, agitation, ataxia, cerebrovascular accident, confusion, dizziness, hyperesthesia, hypesthesia, and neuropathy.
Respiratory: pharyngitis, rhinitis, dyspnea, pleural effusion, bronchitis, cough increased, lung edema, hemoptysis, and hypoxia.
Skin and Appendages: skin ulcer, acne, alopecia, skin nodule, macular papular rash, pustular rash, serous drainage, and vesicular bullous rash.
Special Senses: dry eyes, conjunctivitis, ear pain, blepharitis, corneal lesion, keratitis, otitis externa, and visual field defect.
Urogenital: albuminuria, hematuria, urinary incontinence, urinary tract infection, urinary urgency, dysuria, kidney function abnormal, and breast pain.
[See table 1 at top of page 1822]
[See table 2 on previous page]
[See table 3 on previous page]

OVERDOSAGE

Doses up to 1000 mg/m²/day of Targretin® capsules have been administered in short-term studies in patients with advanced cancer without acute toxic effects. Single doses of 1500 mg/kg and 720 mg/kg were tolerated without significant toxicity in rats and dogs, respectively. These doses are approximately 30 and 50 times, respectively, the recommended human dose on a mg/m² basis.
No clinical experience with an overdose of Targretin® capsules has been reported. Any overdose with Targretin® capsules should be treated with supportive care for the signs and symptoms exhibited by the patient.

DOSAGE AND ADMINISTRATION

The recommended initial dose of Targretin® capsules is 300 mg/m²/day. (See Table 4.) Targretin® capsules should be taken as a single oral daily dose with a meal. See **CONTRAINDICATIONS**: ***Pregnancy: Category X*** section for precautions to prevent pregnancy and birth defects in women of child-bearing potential.

Table 4. Targretin® Capsule Initial Dose Calculation According to Body Surface Area

Initial Dose Level (300 mg/m²/day)		Number of 75 mg Targretin® Capsules
Body Surface Area (m²)	Total Daily Dose (mg/day)	
0.88–1.12	300	4
1.13–1.37	375	5
1.38–1.62	450	6
1.63–1.87	525	7
1.88–2.12	600	8
2.13–2.37	675	9
2.38–2.62	750	10

Dose Modification Guidelines: The 300 mg/m²/day dose level of Targretin® capsules may be adjusted to 200 mg/m²/day then to 100 mg/m²/day, or temporarily suspended, if necessitated by toxicity. When toxicity is controlled, doses may be carefully readjusted upward. If there is no tumor response after eight weeks of treatment and if the initial dose of 300 mg/m²/day is well tolerated, the dose may be escalated to 400 mg/m²/day with careful monitoring.
Duration of Therapy: In clinical trials in CTCL, Targretin® capsules were administered for up to 97 weeks. Targretin® capsules should be continued as long as the patient is deriving benefit.

HOW SUPPLIED

Targretin® capsules are supplied as 75 mg off-white, oblong soft gelatin capsules, imprinted with "Targretin", in high density polyethylene bottles with child-resistant closures.
Bottles of 100 capsules .... NDC 64365-502-01
Store at 2°–25°C (36°–77°F). Avoid exposing to high temperatures and humidity after the bottle is opened. Protect from light.
LIGAND Pharmaceuticals
Manufactured for: Ligand Pharmaceuticals Incorporated
San Diego, CA 92121
Medical Information Telephone Number: (800) 964-5836
Manufactured by: Cardinal Health
St. Petersburg, FL 33716
"Ligand", the Ligand logo and Targretin® are registered trademarks of Ligand Pharmaceuticals Inc.
U.S. Patent Nos. 5,466,861, 5,780,676, and 5,962,731
Ligand Part #3000207 (Rev. 0403)
Anderson Part #5422101-03
Shown in Product Identification Guide, page 320

TARGRETIN® ℞

[*tahr-greh' tən*]
(bexarotene) gel 1%
Rx only.

DESCRIPTION

Targretin® (bexarotene) gel 1% contains bexarotene and is intended for topical application only. Bexarotene is a member of a subclass of retinoids that selectively activate retinoid X receptors (RXRs). These retinoid receptors have biologic activity distinct from that of retinoic acid receptors (RARs).
The chemical name is 4-[1-(5,6,7,8-tetrahydro-3,5,5,8,8-pentamethyl-2-naphthalenyl)ethenyl] benzoic acid, and the structural formula is as follows:

[Structural formula: H_3C, CH_3, CH_2, CH_3, COOH, H_3C, CH_3]

Bexarotene is an off-white to white powder with a molecular weight of 348.48 and a molecular formula of $C_{24}H_{28}O_2$. It is insoluble in water and slightly soluble in vegetable oils and ethanol, USP.
Targretin® gel is a clear gelled solution containing 1.0% (w/w) bexarotene in a base of dehydrated alcohol, USP, polyethylene glycol 400, NF, hydroxypropyl cellulose, NF, and butylated hydroxytoluene, NF.

HOW SUPPLIED

Targretin® gel is supplied in tubes containing 60 g (600 mg active bexarotene).
60 g tube .... NDC 64365-504-01
Store at 25°C (77°F); with excursions permitted to 15°–30°C (59°–86°F) [see USP]. Avoid exposing to high temperatures and humidity after the tube is opened. Protect from light.
Manufactured for: Ligand Pharmaceuticals Incorporated
San Diego, CA 92121
by: Bristol-Myers Squibb Company
Princeton, NJ 08543 USA
Ligand Part #3000204 (Rev. 0101)

Eli Lilly and Company

LILLY CORPORATE CENTER
INDIANAPOLIS, IN 46285

Direct Inquiries to:
Lilly Corporate Center
Indianapolis, IN 46285
(317) 276-2000
www.lilly.com
For Medical Information Contact:
Lilly Research Laboratories
Lilly Corporate Center
Indianapolis, IN 46285
(800) 545-5979

ALIMTA® ℞

[*ă-lĭm-tă*]
pemetrexed for injection

DESCRIPTION

ALIMTA®, pemetrexed for injection, is an antifolate antineoplastic agent that exerts its action by disrupting folate-dependent metabolic processes essential for cell replication.
Pemetrexed disodium heptahydrate has the chemical name L-Glutamic acid, *N*-[4-[2-(2-amino-4,7-dihydro-4-oxo-1*H*-pyrrolo[2,3-*d*]pyrimidin-5-yl)ethyl]benzoyl]-, disodium salt, heptahydrate. It is a white to almost-white solid with a molecular formula of $C_{20}H_{19}N_5Na_2O_6 \bullet 7H_2O$ and a molecular weight of 597.49. The structural formula is as follows:

[Structural formula: O, CO_2^- Na^+, N, H, •$7H_2O$, O, HN, CO_2^- Na^+, H_2N, N, N, H]

ALIMTA is supplied as a sterile lyophilized powder for intravenous infusion available in single-dose vials. The product is a white to either light yellow or green-yellow lyophilized solid. Each 500-mg vial of ALIMTA contains pemetrexed disodium equivalent to 500 mg pemetrexed and 500 mg of mannitol. Hydrochloric acid and/or sodium hydroxide may have been added to adjust pH.

CLINICAL PHARMACOLOGY

Pharmacodynamics
Pemetrexed is an antifolate containing the pyrrolopyrimidine-based nucleus that exerts its antineoplastic activity by disrupting folate-dependent metabolic processes essential for cell replication. In vitro studies have shown that pemetrexed inhibits thymidylate synthase (TS), dihydrofolate reductase (DHFR), and glycinamide ribonucleotide formyltransferase (GARFT), all folate-dependent enzymes involved in the de novo biosynthesis of thymidine and purine nucleotides. Pemetrexed is transported into cells by both the reduced folate carrier and membrane folate binding protein transport systems. Once in the cell, pemetrexed is converted to polyglutamate forms by the enzyme folyl polyglutamate synthase. The polyglutamate forms are retained in cells and are inhibitors of TS and GARFT. Polyglutamation is a time- and concentration-dependent process that occurs in tumor cells and, to a lesser extent, in normal tissues. Polyglutamated metabolites have an increased intracellular half-life resulting in prolonged drug action in malignant cells.
Preclinical studies have shown that pemetrexed inhibits the in vitro growth of mesothelioma cell lines (MSTO-211H, NCI-H2052). Studies with the MSTO-211H mesothelioma cell line showed synergistic effects when pemetrexed was combined concurrently with cisplatin.
Absolute neutrophil counts (ANC) following single-agent administration of pemetrexed to patients not receiving folic acid and vitamin B_{12} supplementation were characterized using population pharmacodynamic analyses. Severity of hematologic toxicity, as measured by the depth of the ANC nadir, is inversely proportional to the systemic exposure of ALIMTA. It was also observed that lower ANC nadirs occurred in patients with elevated baseline cystathionine or homocysteine concentrations. The levels of these substances can be reduced by folic acid and vitamin B_{12} supplementation. There is no cumulative effect of pemetrexed exposure on ANC nadir over multiple treatment cycles.
Time to ANC nadir with pemetrexed systemic exposure (AUC), varied between 8 to 9.6 days over a range of exposures from 38.3 to 316.8 µg•hr/mL. Return to baseline ANC occurred 4.2 to 7.5 days after the nadir over the same range of exposures.

Pharmacokinetics
The pharmacokinetics of pemetrexed administered as a single agent in doses ranging from 0.2 to 838 mg/m² infused over a 10-minute period have been evaluated in 426 cancer patients with a variety of solid tumors. Pemetrexed is not metabolized to an appreciable extent and is primarily eliminated in the urine, with 70% to 90% of the dose recovered unchanged within the first 24 hours following administration. The total systemic clearance of pemetrexed is 91.8 mL/min and the elimination half-life of pemetrexed is 3.5 hours in patients with normal renal function (creatinine clearance of 90 mL/min). The clearance decreases, and exposure (AUC) increases, as renal function decreases. Pemetrexed total systemic exposure (AUC) and maximum plasma concentration (C_{max}) increase proportionally with dose. The pharmacokinetics of pemetrexed do not change over multiple treatment cycles. Pemetrexed has a steady-state volume of distribution of 16.1 liters. In vitro studies indicate that pemetrexed is approximately 81% bound to plasma proteins. Binding is not affected by degree of renal impairment.

Drug Interactions
Chemotherapeutic Agents—Cisplatin does not affect the pharmacokinetics of pemetrexed and the pharmacokinetics of total platinum are unaltered by pemetrexed.
Vitamins—Coadministration of oral folic acid or intramuscular vitamin B_{12} does not affect the pharmacokinetics of pemetrexed.
Drugs Metabolized by Cytochrome P450 Enzymes—Results from in vitro studies with human liver microsomes predict that pemetrexed would not cause clinically significant inhibition of metabolic clearance of drugs metabolized by CYP3A, CYP2D6, CYP2C9, and CYP1A2. No studies were conducted to determine the cytochrome P450 isozyme induction potential of pemetrexed, because ALIMTA used as recommended (once every 21 days) would not be expected to cause any significant enzyme induction.
Aspirin—Aspirin, administered in low to moderate doses (325 mg every 6 hours), does not affect the pharmacokinetics of pemetrexed. The effect of greater doses of aspirin on pemetrexed pharmacokinetics is unknown.
Ibuprofen—Daily ibuprofen doses of 400 mg qid reduce pemetrexed's clearance by about 20% (and increase AUC by 20%) in patients with normal renal function. The effect of greater doses of ibuprofen on pemetrexed pharmacokinetics is unknown (*see* **Drug Interactions** *under* **PRECAUTIONS**).

Special Populations
The pharmacokinetics of pemetrexed in special populations were examined in about 400 patients in controlled and single arm studies.
Geriatric—No effect of age on the pharmacokinetics of pemetrexed was observed over a range of 26 to 80 years.
Pediatric—Pediatric patients were not included in clinical trials.
Gender—The pharmacokinetics of pemetrexed were not different in male and female patients.
Race—The pharmacokinetics of pemetrexed were similar in Caucasians and patients of African descent. Insufficient data are available to compare pharmacokinetics for other ethnic groups.
Hepatic Insufficiency—There was no effect of elevated AST (SGOT), ALT (SGPT), or total bilirubin on the pharmacokinetics of pemetrexed. However, studies of hepatically impaired patients have not been conducted (*see* **PRECAUTIONS**).
Renal Insufficiency—Pharmacokinetic analyses of pemetrexed included 127 patients with reduced renal function. Plasma clearance of pemetrexed in the presence of cisplatin decreases as renal function decreases, with increase

in systemic exposure. Patients with creatinine clearances of 45, 50, and 80 mL/min had 65%, 54%, and 13% increases, respectively in pemetrexed total systemic exposure (AUC) compared to patients with creatinine clearance of 100 mL/min (*see* **WARNINGS** *and* **DOSAGE AND ADMINISTRATION**).

CLINICAL STUDIES

Malignant Pleural Mesothelioma—The safety and efficacy of ALIMTA have been evaluated in chemonaive patients with malignant pleural mesothelioma (MPM) in combination with cisplatin.

Randomized Trial: A multi-center, randomized, single-blind study in 448 chemonaive patients with MPM compared survival in patients treated with ALIMTA in combination with cisplatin to survival in patients receiving cisplatin alone. ALIMTA was administered intravenously over 10 minutes at a dose of 500 mg/m^2 and cisplatin was administered intravenously over 2 hours at a dose of 75 mg/m^2 beginning approximately 30 minutes after the end of administration of ALIMTA. Both drugs were given on Day 1 of each 21-day cycle. After 112 patients were treated, white cell and GI toxicity led to a change in protocol whereby all patients were given folic acid and vitamin B_{12} supplementation.

The primary analysis of this study was performed on the population of all patients randomly assigned to treatment who received study drug (randomized and treated). An analysis was also performed on patients who received folic acid and vitamin B_{12} supplementation during the entire course of study therapy (fully supplemented), as supplementation is recommended (*see* **DOSAGE AND ADMINISTRATION**). Results in all patients and those fully supplemented were similar. Patient demographics are shown in Table 1.

[See table 1 at right]

Table 2 summarizes the survival results for all randomized and treated patients regardless of vitamin supplementation status and those patients receiving vitamin supplementation from the time of enrollment in the trial.

[See table 2 at right]

Similar results were seen in the analysis of patients (N=303) with confirmed histologic diagnosis of malignant pleural mesothelioma. Exploratory demographic analyses showed no apparent differences in patients over or under 65. There were too few non-white patients to assess possible ethnic differences. The effect in women (median survival 15.7 months with the combination vs. 7.5 months on cisplatin alone), however, was larger than the effect in males (median survival 11 vs. 9.4 respectively). As with any exploratory analysis, it is not clear whether this difference is real or is a chance finding.

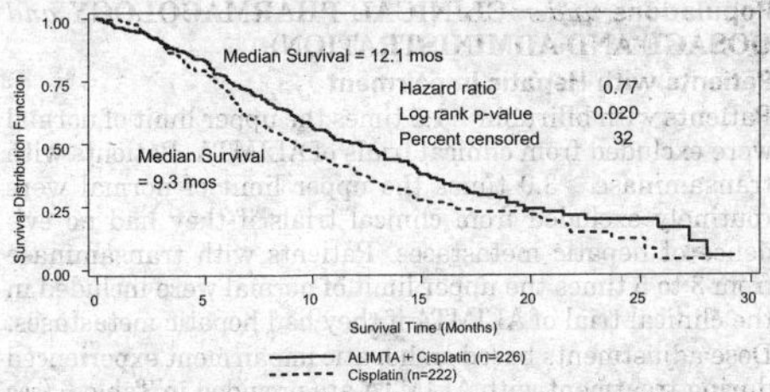

Figure 1: Kaplan-Meier Estimates of Survival Time for ALIMTA plus Cisplatin and Cisplatin Alone in all Randomized and Treated Patients.

Objective tumor response for malignant pleural mesothelioma is difficult to measure and response criteria are not universally agreed upon. However, based upon prospectively defined criteria, the objective tumor response rate for ALIMTA plus cisplatin was greater than the objective tumor response rate for cisplatin alone. There was also improvement in lung function (forced vital capacity) in the ALIMTA plus cisplatin arm compared to the control arm.

Patients who received full supplementation with folic acid and vitamin B_{12} during study therapy received a median of 6 and 4 cycles in the ALIMTA/cisplatin (N=168) and cisplatin (N=163) arms, respectively. Patients who never received folic acid and vitamin B_{12} during study therapy received a median of 2 cycles in both treatment arms (N=32 and N=38 for the ALIMTA/cisplatin and cisplatin arm, respectively). Patients receiving ALIMTA in the fully supplemented group received a relative dose intensity of 93% of the protocol specified ALIMTA dose intensity; patients treated with cisplatin in the same group received 94% of the projected dose intensity. Patients treated with cisplatin alone had a dose intensity of 96%.

INDICATIONS AND USAGE

ALIMTA in combination with cisplatin is indicated for the treatment of patients with malignant pleural mesothelioma whose disease is unresectable or who are otherwise not candidates for curative surgery.

CONTRAINDICATIONS

ALIMTA is contraindicated in patients who have a history of severe hypersensitivity reaction to pemetrexed or to any other ingredient used in the formulation.

WARNINGS

Decreased Renal Function

ALIMTA is primarily eliminated unchanged by renal excretion. No dosage adjustment is needed in patients with creatinine clearance ≥45 mL/min. Insufficient numbers of patients have been studied with creatinine clearance <45 mL/min to give a dose recommendation. Therefore, ALIMTA should not be administered to patients whose creatinine clearance is <45 mL/min (*see* **Dose Reduction Recommendations** *under* **DOSAGE AND ADMINISTRATION**).

One patient with severe renal impairment (creatinine clearance 19 mL/min) who did not receive folic acid and vitamin B_{12} died of drug-related toxicity following administration of ALIMTA alone.

Bone Marrow Suppression

ALIMTA can suppress bone marrow function, manifested by neutropenia, thrombocytopenia, and anemia (*see* **ADVERSE REACTIONS**); myelosuppression is usually the dose-limiting toxicity. Dose reductions for subsequent cycles are based on nadir ANC, platelet count, and maximum nonhematologic toxicity seen in the previous cycle (*see* **Dose Reduction Recommendations** *under* **DOSAGE AND ADMINISTRATION**).

Need for Folate and Vitamin B_{12} Supplementation

Patients treated with ALIMTA must be instructed to take folic acid and vitamin B_{12} as a prophylactic measure to reduce treatment-related hematologic and GI toxicity (*see* **DOSAGE AND ADMINISTRATION**). In clinical studies, less overall toxicity and reductions in Grade 3/4 hematologic and nonhematologic toxicities such as neutropenia, febrile neutropenia, and infection with Grade 3/4 neutropenia were reported when pretreatment with folic acid and vitamin B_{12} was administered.

Pregnancy Category D

ALIMTA may cause fetal harm when administered to a pregnant woman. Pemetrexed was fetotoxic and teratogenic in mice at i.v. doses of 0.2 mg/kg (0.6 mg/m^2) or 5 mg/kg (15 mg/m^2) when given on gestation days 6 through 15. Pemetrexed caused fetal malformations (incomplete ossification of talus and skull bone) at 0.2 mg/kg (about 1/833 the recommended i.v. human dose on a mg/m^2 basis), and cleft palate at 5 mg/kg (about 1/33 the recommended i.v. human dose on a mg/m^2 basis). Embryotoxicity was characterized by increased embryo-fetal deaths and reduced litter sizes. There are no studies of ALIMTA in pregnant women. Patients should be advised to avoid becoming pregnant. If ALIMTA is used during pregnancy, or if the patient becomes pregnant while taking ALIMTA, the patient should be apprised of the potential hazard to the fetus.

PRECAUTIONS

General

ALIMTA should be administered under the supervision of a qualified physician experienced in the use of antineoplastic agents. Appropriate management of complications is possible only when adequate diagnostic and treatment facilities are readily available. Treatment-related adverse events of ALIMTA seen in clinical trials have been reversible. Skin rash has been reported more frequently in patients not pretreated with a corticosteroid in clinical trials. Pretreatment with dexamethasone (or equivalent) reduces the incidence and severity of cutaneous reaction (*see* **DOSAGE AND ADMINISTRATION**).

The effect of third space fluid, such as pleural effusion and ascites, on ALIMTA is unknown. In patients with clinically

Continued on next page

Table 1: Summary of Patient Characteristics

Patient characteristic	Randomized and Treated Patients		Fully Supplemented Patients	
	ALIMTA/cis (N=226)	Cisplatin (N=222)	ALIMTA/cis (N=168)	Cisplatin (N=163)
Age (yrs)				
Median (range)	61 (29-85)	60 (19-84)	60 (29-85)	60 (19–82)
Gender (%)				
Male	184 (81.4)	181 (81.5)	136 (81.0)	134 (82.2)
Female	42 (18.6)	41 (18.5)	32 (19.0)	29 (17.8)
Origin (%)				
Caucasian	204 (90.3)	206 (92.8)	150 (89.3)	153 (93.9)
Hispanic	11 (4.9)	12 (5.4)	10 (6.0)	7 (4.3)
Asian	10 (4.4)	4 (1.9)	7 (4.2)	3 (1.8)
African descent	1 (0.4)	0	1 (0.6)	0
Stage at Entry (%)				
I	16 (7.1)	14 (6.3)	15 (8.9)	12 (7.4)
II	35 (15.6)	33 (15.0)	27 (16.2)	27 (16.8)
III	73 (32.4)	68 (30.6)	51 (30.5)	49 (30.4)
IV	101 (44.9)	105 (47.2)	74 (44.3)	73 (45.3)
Unspecified	1 (0.4)	2 (0.9)	1 (0.6)	2 (1.2)
Diagnosis/Histology[a] (%)				
Epithelial	154 (68.1)	152 (68.5)	117 (69.6)	113 (69.3)
Mixed	37 (16.4)	36 (16.2)	25 (14.9)	25 (15.3)
Sarcomatoid	18 (8.0)	25 (11.3)	14 (8.3)	17 (10.4)
Other	17 (7.5)	9 (4.1)	12 (7.1)	8 (4.9)
Baseline KPS[b] (%)				
70-80	109 (48.2)	97 (43.7)	83 (49.4)	69 (42.3)
90-100	117 (51.8)	125 (56.3)	85 (50.6)	94 (57.7)

[a] Only 67% of the patients had the histologic diagnosis of malignant mesothelioma confirmed by independent review.
[b] Karnofsky Performance Scale.

Table 2: Efficacy of ALIMTA plus Cisplatin vs. Cisplatin in Malignant Pleural Mesothelioma

Efficacy Parameter	Randomized and Treated Patients		Fully Supplemented Patients	
	ALIMTA/cis (N=226)	Cisplatin (N=222)	ALIMTA/cis (N=168)	Cisplatin (N=163)
Median overall survival (95% CI)	12.1 mos (10.0-14.4)	9.3 mos (7.8-10.7)	13.3 mos (11.4-14.9)	10.0 mos (8.4-11.9)
Hazard ratio	0.77		0.75	
Log rank p-value*	0.020		0.051	

* p-value refers to comparison between arms.

*** Identi-Code® symbol. This product information was prepared in June 2004. Current information on these and other products of Eli Lilly and Company may be obtained by direct inquiry to Lilly Research Laboratories, Lilly Corporate Center, Indianapolis, Indiana 46285, (800) 545-5979.**

Alimta—Cont.

significant third space fluid, consideration should be given to draining the effusion prior to ALIMTA administration.

Laboratory Tests

Complete blood cell counts, including platelet counts and periodic chemistry tests, should be performed on all patients receiving ALIMTA. Patients should be monitored for nadir and recovery, which were tested in the clinical study before each dose and on days 8 and 15 of each cycle. Patients should not begin a new cycle of treatment unless the ANC is ≥1500 cells/mm^3, the platelet count is ≥100,000 cells/mm^3, and creatinine clearance is ≥45 mL/min.

Drug Interactions

ALIMTA is primarily eliminated unchanged renally as a result of glomerular filtration and tubular secretion. Concomitant administration of nephrotoxic drugs could result in delayed clearance of ALIMTA. Concomitant administration of substances that are also tubularly secreted (e.g., probenecid) could potentially result in delayed clearance of ALIMTA.

Although ibuprofen (400 mg qid) can be administered with ALIMTA in patients with normal renal function (creatinine clearance ≥80 mL/min), caution should be used when administering ibuprofen concurrently with ALIMTA to patients with mild to moderate renal insufficiency (creatinine clearance from 45 to 79 mL/min). Patients with mild to moderate renal insufficiency should avoid taking NSAIDs with short elimination half-lives for a period of 2 days before, the day of, and 2 days following administration of ALIMTA.

In the absence of data regarding potential interaction between ALIMTA and NSAIDs with longer half-lives, all patients taking these NSAIDs should interrupt dosing for at least 5 days before, the day of, and 2 days following ALIMTA administration. If concomitant administration of an NSAID is necessary, patients should be monitored closely for toxicity, especially myelosuppression, renal, and gastrointestinal toxicity.

Drug/Laboratory Test Interactions

None known.

Carcinogenesis, Mutagenesis, Impairment of Fertility

No carcinogenicity studies have been conducted with pemetrexed. Pemetrexed was clastogenic in the in vivo micronucleus assay in mouse bone marrow but was not mutagenic in multiple in vitro tests (Ames assay, CHO cell assay). Pemetrexed administered at i.v. doses of 0.1 mg/kg/day or greater to male mice (about 1/1666 the recommended human dose on a mg/m^2 basis) resulted in reduced fertility, hypospermia, and testicular atrophy.

Pregnancy

Pregnancy Category D (*see* **WARNINGS**).

Nursing Mothers

It is not known whether ALIMTA or its metabolites are excreted in human milk. Because many drugs are excreted in human milk, and because of the potential for serious adverse reactions in nursing infants from ALIMTA, it is recommended that nursing be discontinued if the mother is treated with ALIMTA.

Pediatric Use

The safety and effectiveness of ALIMTA in pediatric patients have not been established.

Geriatric Use

Dose adjustments based on age other than those recommended for all patients have not been necessary (*see* **Special Populations** *under* **CLINICAL PHARMACOLOGY** *and* **DOSAGE AND ADMINISTRATION**).

Gender

Dose adjustments based on gender other than those recommended for all patients have not been necessary (*see* **Special Populations** *under* **CLINICAL PHARMACOLOGY** *and* **DOSAGE AND ADMINISTRATION**).

Patients with Hepatic Impairment

Patients with bilirubin >1.5 times the upper limit of normal were excluded from clinical trials of ALIMTA. Patients with transaminase >3.0 times the upper limit of normal were routinely excluded from clinical trials if they had no evidence of hepatic metastases. Patients with transaminase from 3 to 5 times the upper limit of normal were included in the clinical trial of ALIMTA if they had hepatic metastases. Dose adjustments based on hepatic impairment experienced during treatment with ALIMTA are provided in Table 6 (*see* **Special Populations** *under* **CLINICAL PHARMACOLOGY** *and* **DOSAGE AND ADMINISTRATION**).

Patients with Renal Impairment

ALIMTA is known to be primarily excreted by the kidney. Decreased renal function will result in reduced clearance and greater exposure (AUC) to ALIMTA compared with patients with normal renal function. Cisplatin coadministration with ALIMTA has not been studied in patients with moderate renal impairment (*see* **Special Populations** *under* **CLINICAL PHARMACOLOGY**).

ADVERSE REACTIONS

In Table 3 adverse events occurring in at least 5% of patients are shown along with important effects (renal failure, infection) occurring at lower rates. Adverse events equally or more common in the cisplatin group are not included. The adverse effects more common in the ALIMTA group were primarily hematologic effects, fever and infection, stomatitis/pharyngitis, and rash/desquamation.

[See table 3 at left]

Table 3: Adverse Events* in Fully Supplemented Patients Receiving ALIMTA plus Cisplatin in MPM CTC Grades (% incidence)

	All Reported Adverse Events Regardless of Causality					
	ALIMTA/cis (N=168)			Cisplatin (N=163)		
	All Grades	Grade 3	Grade 4	All Grades	Grade 3	Grade 4
Laboratory						
Hematologic						
Neutropenia	58	19	5	16	3	1
Leukopenia	55	14	2	20	1	0
Anemia	33	5	1	14	0	0
Thrombocytopenia	27	4	1	10	0	0
Renal						
Creatinine elevation	16	1	0	12	1	0
Renal failure	2	0	1	1	0	0
Clinical						
Constitutional Symptoms						
Fatigue	80	17	0	74	12	1
Fever	17	0	0	9	0	0
Other constitutional symptoms	11	2	1	8	1	1
Cardiovascular General						
Thrombosis/embolism	7	4	2	4	3	1
Gastrointestinal						
Nausea	84	11	1	79	6	0
Vomiting	58	10	1	52	4	1
Constipation	44	2	1	39	1	0
Anorexia	35	2	0	25	1	0
Stomatitis/pharyngitis	28	2	1	9	0	0
Diarrhea without colostomy	26	4	0	16	1	0
Dehydration	7	3	1	1	1	0
Dysphagia/esophagitis/ odynophagia	6	1	0	6	0	0
Pulmonary						
Dyspnea	66	10	1	62	5	2
Pain						
Chest pain	40	8	1	30	5	1
Neurology						
Neuropathy/sensory	17	0	0	15	1	0
Mood alteration/depression	14	1	0	9	1	0
Infection/Febrile Neutropenia						
Infection without neutropenia	11	1	1	4	0	0
Infection with Grade 3 or Grade 4 neutropenia	6	1	0	4	0	0
Infection/febrile neutropenia-other	3	1	0	2	0	0
Febrile neutropenia	1	1	0	1	0	0
Immune						
Allergic reaction/hypersensitivity	2	0	0	1	0	0
Dermatology/Skin						
Rash/desquamation	22	1	0	9	0	0

* Refer to NCI CTC Version 2.0.

Table 4 compares the incidence (percentage of patients) of CTC Grade 3/4 toxicities in patients who received vitamin supplementation with daily folic acid and vitamin B_{12} from the time of enrollment in the study (fully supplemented) with the incidence in patients who never received vitamin supplementation (never supplemented) during the study in the ALIMTA plus cisplatin arm.

Table 4: Selected Grade 3/4 Adverse Events Comparing Fully Supplemented versus Never Supplemented Patients in the ALIMTA plus Cisplatin arm (% incidence)

Adverse Event Regardless of Causality[a](%)	Fully Supplemented Patients (N=168)	Never Supplemented Patients (N=32)
Neutropenia	24	38
Thrombocytopenia	5	9

Nausea	12	31
Vomiting	11	34
Anorexia	2	9
Diarrhea without colostomy	4	9
Dehydration	4	9
Fever	0	6
Febrile neutropenia	1	9
Infection with Grade 3/4 neutropenia	1	6
Fatigue	17	25

[a] Refer to NCI CTC criteria for lab and non-laboratory values for each grade of toxicity (Version 2.0).

The following adverse events were greater in the fully supplemented group compared to the never supplemented group: hypertension (11%, 3%), chest pain (8%, 6%), and thrombosis/embolism (6%, 3%).

For fully supplemented patients treated with ALIMTA plus cisplatin, the incidence of CTC Grade 3/4 fatigue, leukopenia, neutropenia, and thrombocytopenia were greater in patients 65 years or older as compared to patients younger than 65. No relevant effect for ALIMTA safety due to gender or race was identified, except an increased incidence of rash in men (24%) compared to women (16%).

OVERDOSAGE

There have been few cases of ALIMTA overdose. Reported toxicities included neutropenia, anemia, thrombocytopenia, mucositis, and rash. Anticipated complications of overdose include bone marrow suppression as manifested by neutropenia, thrombocytopenia, and anemia. In addition, infection with or without fever, diarrhea, and mucositis may be seen. If an overdose occurs, general supportive measures should be instituted as deemed necessary by the treating physician.

In clinical trials, leucovorin was permitted for CTC Grade 4 leukopenia lasting ≥3 days, CTC Grade 4 neutropenia lasting ≥3 days, and immediately for CTC Grade 4 thrombocytopenia, bleeding associated with Grade 3 thrombocytopenia, or Grade 3 or 4 mucositis. The following intravenous doses and schedules of leucovorin were recommended for intravenous use: 100 mg/m^2, intravenously once, followed by leucovorin, 50 mg/m^2, intravenously every 6 hours for 8 days.

The ability of ALIMTA to be dialyzed is unknown.

DOSAGE AND ADMINISTRATION

ALIMTA is for Intravenous Infusion Only

Combination Use With Cisplatin

Malignant Pleural Mesothelioma—The recommended dose of ALIMTA is 500 mg/m^2 administered as an intravenous infusion over 10 minutes on Day 1 of each 21-day cycle. The recommended dose of cisplatin is 75 mg/m^2 infused over 2 hours beginning approximately 30 minutes after the end of ALIMTA administration. Patients should receive hydration consistent with local practice prior to and/or after receiving cisplatin. See cisplatin package insert for more information.

Premedication Regimen

Corticosteroid—Skin rash has been reported more frequently in patients not pretreated with a corticosteroid. Pretreatment with dexamethasone (or equivalent) reduces the incidence and severity of cutaneous reaction. In clinical trials, dexamethasone 4 mg was given by mouth twice daily the day before, the day of, and the day after ALIMTA administration.

Vitamin Supplementation—To reduce toxicity, patients treated with ALIMTA must be instructed to take a low-dose oral folic acid preparation or multivitamin with folic acid on a daily basis. At least 5 daily doses of folic acid must be taken during the 7-day period preceding the first dose of ALIMTA; and dosing should continue during the full course of therapy and for 21 days after the last dose of ALIMTA. Patients must also receive one (1) intramuscular injection of vitamin B_{12} during the week preceding the first dose of ALIMTA and every 3 cycles thereafter. Subsequent vitamin B_{12} injections may be given the same day as ALIMTA. In clinical trials, the dose of folic acid studied ranged from 350 to 1000 µg, and the dose of vitamin B_{12} was 1000 µg. The most commonly used dose of oral folic acid in clinical trials was 400 µg (*see* **WARNINGS**).

Laboratory Monitoring and Dose Reduction Recommendations

Monitoring—Complete blood cell counts, including platelet counts, should be performed on all patients receiving ALIMTA. Patients should be monitored for nadir and recovery, which were tested in the clinical study before each dose and on days 8 and 15 of each cycle. Patients should not begin a new cycle of treatment unless the ANC is ≥1500 cells/mm^3, the platelet count is ≥100,000 cells/mm^3, and creatinine clearance is ≥45 mL/min. Periodic chemistry tests should be performed to evaluate renal and hepatic function.

Dose Reduction Recommendations—Dose adjustments at the start of a subsequent cycle should be based on nadir hematologic counts or maximum nonhematologic toxicity from the preceding cycle of therapy. Treatment may be delayed to allow sufficient time for recovery. Upon recovery, patients should be retreated using the guidelines in Tables 5–7.

$$\text{Males: } \frac{[140 - \text{Age in years}] \times \text{Actual Body Weight (kg)}}{72 \times \text{Serum Creatinine (mg/dL)}} = \text{mL/min}$$

Females: Estimated creatinine clearance for males × 0.85

Table 5: Dose Reduction for ALIMTA and Cisplatin - Hematologic Toxicities

Nadir ANC <500/mm^3 and nadir platelets ≥50,000/mm^3.	75% of previous dose (both drugs).
Nadir platelets <50,000/mm^3 regardless of nadir ANC.	50% of previous dose (both drugs).

If patients develop nonhematologic toxicities (excluding neurotoxicity) ≥Grade 3 (except Grade 3 transaminase elevations), ALIMTA should be withheld until resolution to less than or equal to the patient's pre-therapy value. Treatment should be resumed according to guidelines in Table 6.

Table 6: Dose Reduction - Nonhematologic Toxicities[a,b]

	Dose of ALIMTA (mg/m^2)	Dose of Cisplatin (mg/m^2)
Any Grade 3[c] or 4 toxicities except mucositis	75% of previous dose	75% of previous dose
Any diarrhea requiring hospitalization	75% of previous dose	75% of previous dose
Grade 3 or 4 mucositis	50% of previous dose	100% of previous dose

[a] NCI Common Toxicity Criteria (CTC).
[b] Excluding neurotoxicity.
[c] Except Grade 3 transaminase elevation.

In the event of neurotoxicity, the recommended dose adjustments for ALIMTA and cisplatin are described in Table 7. Patients should discontinue therapy if Grade 3 or 4 neurotoxicity is experienced.

Table 7: Dose Reduction for ALIMTA and Cisplatin - Neurotoxicity

CTC Grade	Dose of ALIMTA (mg/m^2)	Dose of Cisplatin (mg/m^2)
0-1	100% of previous dose	100% of previous dose
2	100% of previous dose	50% of previous dose

ALIMTA therapy should be discontinued if a patient experiences any hematologic or nonhematologic Grade 3 or 4 toxicity after 2 dose reductions (except Grade 3 transaminase elevations) or immediately if Grade 3 or 4 neurotoxicity is observed.

Elderly Patients—No dose reductions other than those recommended for all patients are necessary for patients ≥65 years of age.

Children—ALIMTA is not recommended for use in children, as safety and efficacy have not been established in children.

Renally Impaired Patients—In clinical studies, patients with creatinine clearance ≥45 mL/min required no dose adjustments other than those recommended for all patients. Insufficient numbers of patients with creatinine clearance below 45 mL/min have been treated to make dosage recommendations for this group of patients. Therefore, ALIMTA should not be administered to patients whose creatinine clearance is <45 mL/min using the standard Cockcroft and Gault formula (below) or GFR measured by Tc99m-DPTA serum clearance method:

[See table above]

Caution should be exercised when administering ALIMTA concurrently with NSAIDs to patients whose creatinine clearance is <80 mL/min (*see* **Drug Interactions** *under* **PRECAUTIONS**).

Hepatically Impaired Patients—ALIMTA is not extensively metabolized by the liver. Dose adjustments based on hepatic impairment experienced during treatment with ALIMTA are provided in Table 6 (*see* **Patients with Hepatic Impairment** *under* **PRECAUTIONS**).

Preparation and Administration Precautions

As with other potentially toxic anticancer agents, care should be exercised in the handling and preparation of infusion solutions of ALIMTA. The use of gloves is recommended. If a solution of ALIMTA contacts the skin, wash the skin immediately and thoroughly with soap and water. If ALIMTA contacts the mucous membranes, flush thoroughly with water. Several published guidelines for handling and disposal of anticancer agents are available.[1–8] There is no general agreement that all of the procedures recommended in the guidelines are necessary or appropriate.

ALIMTA is not a vesicant. There is no specific antidote for extravasation of ALIMTA. To date, there have been few reported cases of ALIMTA extravasation, which were not assessed as serious by the investigator. ALIMTA extravasation should be managed with local standard practice for extravasation as with other non-vesicants.

Preparation for Intravenous Infusion Administration

1. Use aseptic technique during the reconstitution and further dilution of ALIMTA for intravenous infusion administration.
2. Calculate the dose and the number of ALIMTA vials needed. Each vial contains 500 mg of ALIMTA. The vial contains an excess of ALIMTA to facilitate delivery of label amount.
3. Reconstitute 500-mg vials with 20 mL of 0.9% Sodium Chloride Injection (preservative free) to give a solution containing 25 mg/mL ALIMTA. Gently swirl each vial until the powder is completely dissolved. The resulting solution is clear and ranges in color from colorless to yellow or green-yellow without adversely affecting product quality. The pH of the reconstituted ALIMTA solution is between 6.6 and 7.8. FURTHER DILUTION IS REQUIRED.
4. Parenteral drug products should be inspected visually for particulate matter and discoloration prior to administration. If particulate matter is observed, do not administer.
5. The appropriate volume of reconstituted ALIMTA solution should be further diluted to 100 mL with 0.9% Sodium Chloride Injection (preservative free) and administered as an intravenous infusion over 10 minutes.
6. Chemical and physical stability of reconstituted and infusion solutions of ALIMTA were demonstrated for up to 24 hours following initial reconstitution, when stored at refrigerated or ambient room temperature [see USP Controlled Room Temperature] and lighting. When prepared as directed, reconstitution and infusion solutions of ALIMTA contain no antimicrobial preservatives. Discard any unused portion.

Reconstitution and further dilution prior to intravenous infusion is only recommended with 0.9% Sodium Chloride Injection (preservative free). ALIMTA is physically incompatible with diluents containing calcium, including Lactated Ringer's Injection, USP and Ringer's Injection, USP and therefore these should not be used. Coadministration of ALIMTA with other drugs and diluents has not been studied, and therefore is not recommended.

HOW SUPPLIED

ALIMTA®, pemetrexed for injection is available in sterile single-use vials containing 500 mg pemetrexed.

NDC 0002-7623-01 (VL7623): single-use vial with flip-off cap individually packaged in a carton.

Storage

ALIMTA, pemetrexed for injection, should be stored at 25°C (77°F); excursions permitted to 15-30°C (59-86°F) [see USP Controlled Room Temperature].

Chemical and physical stability of reconstituted and infusion solutions of ALIMTA were demonstrated for up to 24 hours following initial reconstitution, when stored refrigerated, 2-8°C (36-46°F), or at 25°C (77°F), excursions permitted to 15-30°C (59-86°F) [see USP Controlled Room Temperature]. When prepared as directed, reconstituted and infusion solutions of ALIMTA contain no antimicrobial preservatives. Discard unused portion.

ALIMTA is not light sensitive.

REFERENCES

1. ONS Clinical Practice Committee. Cancer Chemotherapy Guidelines and Recommendations for Practice. Pittsburgh, PA: Oncology Nursing Society; 1999:32-41.
2. Recommendations for the Safe Handling of Parenteral Antineoplastic Drugs. Washington, DC: Division of Safety, Clinical Center Pharmacy Department and Cancer Nursing Services, National Institutes of Health; 1992. US Dept of Health and Human Services, Public Health Service Publication NIH 92-2621.
3. AMA Council on Scientific Affairs. Guidelines for Handling Parenteral Antineoplastics. *JAMA*. 1985;253:1590-1591.
4. National Study Commission on Cytotoxic Exposure-Recommendations for Handling Cytotoxic Agents. 1987. Available from Louis P. Jeffrey, ScD, Chairman, National Study Commission on Cytotoxic Exposure. Massachusetts College of Pharmacy and Allied Health Sciences, 179 Longwood Avenue, Boston, MA 02115.
5. Clinical Oncological Society of Australia. Guidelines and Recommendations for Safe Handling of Antineoplastic Agents. *Med J Australia*. 1983;1:426-428.
6. Jones RB, Frank R, Mass T. Safe Handling of Chemotherapeutic Agents: A Report from the Mount Sinai Medical Center. CA — *A Cancer J for Clin*. 1983;33:258-263.
7. American Society of Hospital Pharmacists. ASHP Technical Assistance Bulletin on Handling Cytotoxic and Hazardous Drugs. *Am J Hosp Pharm*. 1990;47:1033-1049.

Continued on next page

*** Identi-Code® symbol. This product information was prepared in June 2004. Current information on these and other products of Eli Lilly and Company may be obtained by direct inquiry to Lilly Research Laboratories, Lilly Corporate Center, Indianapolis, Indiana 46285, (800) 545-5979.**

Alimta—Cont.

8. Controlling Occupational Exposure to Hazardous Drugs. (OSHA Work-Practice Guidelines). *Am J Health-Syst Pharm.* 1996;53:1669-1685.

Literature issued February 5, 2004
Manufactured by Lilly France S.A.S.
F-67640 Fegersheim, France
for Eli Lilly and Company
Indianapolis, IN 46285, USA
www.ALIMTA.com
PA 9301 FSAMP

INFORMATION FOR PATIENTS AND CAREGIVERS

ALIMTA® (uh-LIM-tuh)
(pemetrexed for injection)
Read the Patient Information that comes with ALIMTA before you start treatment and each time you get treated with ALIMTA. There may be new information. This leaflet does not take the place of talking to your doctor about your medical condition or treatment. Talk to your doctor if you have any questions about ALIMTA.

What is ALIMTA?
ALIMTA is a treatment for a type of cancer called malignant pleural mesothelioma. This cancer affects the inside lining of the chest cavity. ALIMTA is given with cisplatin, another anti-cancer medicine (chemotherapy). **To lower your chances of side effects of ALIMTA, you must also take folic acid and vitamin B_{12} prior to and during your treatment with ALIMTA.** Your doctor will prescribe a medicine called a "corticosteroid" to take for 3 days during your treatment with ALIMTA. Corticosteroid medicines lower your chances of getting skin reactions with ALIMTA.
ALIMTA has not been studied in children.

What should I tell my doctor before taking ALIMTA?
Tell your doctor about all of your medical conditions, including if you:

- **are pregnant or planning to become pregnant.** ALIMTA may harm your unborn baby.
- **are breastfeeding.** It is not known if ALIMTA passes into breast milk. You should stop breastfeeding once you start treatment with ALIMTA.
- **are taking other medicines,** including prescription and nonprescription medicines, vitamins, and herbal supplements. ALIMTA and other medicines may affect each other causing serious side effects. Especially, tell your doctor if you are taking medicines called "nonsteroidal anti-inflammatory drugs" (NSAIDs) for pain or swelling. There are many NSAID medicines. If you are not sure, ask your doctor or pharmacist if any of your medicines are NSAIDs.

How is ALIMTA given?

- ALIMTA is slowly infused (injected) into a vein. The injection or infusion will last about 10 minutes. You will usually receive ALIMTA once every 21 days (3 weeks).
- Cisplatin is infused in your vein for about 2 hours starting about 30 minutes after your treatment with ALIMTA.
- Your doctor will prescribe a medicine called a "corticosteroid" to take for 3 days during your treatment with ALIMTA. Corticosteroid medicines lower your chances for getting skin reactions with ALIMTA.
- **It is very important to take folic acid and vitamin B_{12} during your treatment with ALIMTA to lower your chances of harmful side effects.** You must start taking 350–1000 micrograms of folic acid every day for at least 5 days out of the 7 days before your first dose of ALIMTA. You must keep taking folic acid every day during the time you are getting treatment with ALIMTA, and for 21 days after your last treatment. You can get folic acid vitamins over-the-counter. Folic acid is also found in many multivitamin pills. Ask your doctor or pharmacist for help if you are not sure how to choose a folic acid product. Your doctor will give you vitamin B_{12} injections while you are getting treatment with ALIMTA. You will get your first vitamin B_{12} injection during the week before your first dose of ALIMTA, and then about every 9 weeks during treatment.
- You will have regular blood tests before and during your treatment with ALIMTA. Your doctor may adjust your dose of ALIMTA or delay treatment based on the results of your blood tests and on your general condition.

What should I avoid while taking ALIMTA?

- **Women who can become pregnant should not become pregnant during treatment with ALIMTA.** ALIMTA may harm the unborn baby.
- **Ask your doctor before taking medicines called NSAIDs.** There are many NSAID medicines. If you are not sure, ask your doctor or pharmacist if any of your medicines are NSAIDs.

What are the possible side effects of ALIMTA?
Most patients taking ALIMTA will have side effects. Sometimes it is not always possible to tell whether ALIMTA, another medicine, or the cancer itself is causing these side effects. **Call your doctor right away if you have a fever, chills, diarrhea, or mouth sores.** These symptoms could mean you have an infection.
The most common side effects of ALIMTA when taken with cisplatin are:

- **Stomach upset, including nausea, vomiting, and diarrhea.** You can obtain medicines to help control some of these symptoms. Call your doctor if you get any of these symptoms.
- **Low blood cell counts:**
  - **Low red blood cells.** Low red blood cells may make you feel tired, get tired easily, appear pale, and become short of breath.
  - **Low white blood cells.** Low white blood cells may give you a greater chance for infection. If you have a fever (temperature above 100.4°F) or other signs of infection, call your doctor right away.
  - **Low platelets.** Low platelets give you a greater chance for bleeding. Your doctor will do blood tests to check your blood counts before and during treatment with ALIMTA.
- **Tiredness.** You may feel tired or weak for a few days after your ALIMTA treatments. If you have severe weakness or tiredness, call your doctor.
- **Mouth, throat, or lip sores** (stomatitis, pharyngitis). You may get redness or sores in your mouth, throat, or on your lips. These symptoms may happen a few days after ALIMTA treatment. Talk with your doctor about proper mouth and throat care.
- **Loss of appetite.** You may lose your appetite and lose weight during your treatment. Talk to your doctor if this is a problem for you.
- **Rash.** You may get a rash or itching during treatment. These usually appear between treatments with ALIMTA and usually go away before the next treatment. Call your doctor if you get a severe rash or itching.

Talk with your doctor, nurse or pharmacist about any side effect that bothers you or that doesn't go away.
These are not all the side effects of ALIMTA. For more information, ask your doctor, nurse or pharmacist.

General information about ALIMTA
Medicines are sometimes prescribed for conditions other than those listed in patient information leaflets. ALIMTA was prescribed for your medical condition.
This leaflet summarizes the most important information about ALIMTA. If you would like more information, talk with your doctor. You can ask your doctor or pharmacist for information about ALIMTA that is written for health professionals. You can also call 1-800-LILLY-RX (1-800-545-5979) or visit www.ALIMTA.com.
Literature issued February 5, 2004
Manufactured by Lilly France S.A.S.
F-67640 Fegersheim, France
for Eli Lilly and Company
Indianapolis, IN 46285, USA
www.ALIMTA.com
PA 9301 FSAMP

CAPASTAT® SULFATE ℞

CAPREOMYCIN FOR INJECTION, USP
FOR INTRAMUSCULAR AND INTRAVENOUS INFUSION ONLY
NOT FOR PEDIATRIC USE

WARNINGS

The use of Capastat® Sulfate (Capreomycin for Injection, USP) in patients with renal insufficiency or preexisting auditory impairment must be undertaken with great caution, and the risk of additional cranial nerve VIII impairment or renal injury should be weighed against the benefits to be derived from therapy.
Refer to ANIMAL PHARMACOLOGY *for additional information.*
Since other parenteral antituberculosis agents (streptomycin, viomycin) also have similar and sometimes irreversible toxic effects, particularly on cranial nerve VIII and renal function, simultaneous administration of these agents with Capastat Sulfate is not recommended. Use with nonantituberculosis drugs (polymyxin A sulfate, colistin sulfate, amikacin, gentamicin, tobramycin, vancomycin, kanamycin, and neomycin) having ototoxic or nephrotoxic potential should be undertaken only with great caution.
Usage in Pregnancy: The safety of the use of Capastat Sulfate in pregnancy has not been determined.
Pediatric Usage: Safety and effectiveness in pediatric patients have not been established.

DESCRIPTION

Capastat Sulfate is a polypeptide antibiotic isolated from *Streptomyces capreolus*. It is a complex of 4 microbiologically active components which have been characterized in part; however, complete structural determination of all the components has not been established.
Capreomycin is supplied as the disulfate salt and is soluble in water. In complete solution, it is almost colorless.
Each vial contains the equivalent of 1 g capreomycin activity.
The structural formula is as follows:
[See chemical structure at top of next column]

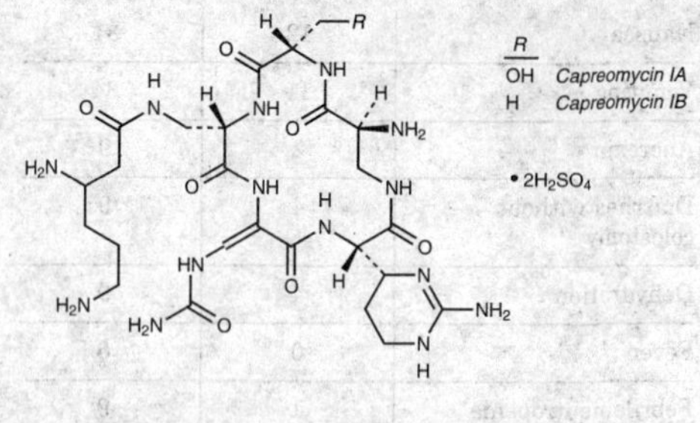

CLINICAL PHARMACOLOGY

Human Pharmacology
Capreomycin is not absorbed in significant quantities from the gastrointestinal tract and must be administered parenterally. In 2 studies of 10 patients each, peak serum concentrations following 1 g of capreomycin given intramuscularly were achieved 1 to 2 hours after administration, and average peak levels reached were 28 and 32 µg/mL respectively (range, 20 to 47 µg/mL). Low serum concentrations were present at 24 hours. However, 1 g of capreomycin daily for 30 days or more produced no significant accumulation in subjects with normal renal function. Two patients with marked reduction of renal function had high serum concentrations 24 hours after administration of the drug. When a 1-g dose of capreomycin was given intramuscularly to normal volunteers, 52% was excreted in the urine within 12 hours.
Lehmann, et al, examined the pharmacokinetics of single dose capreomycin (1.0 g) administered intramuscularly and by intravenous infusion (1 hour) in 6 healthy volunteers. The area under the serum concentration versus time curve was similar for the two routes of administration. Capreomycin peak concentrations after intravenous infusion were 30 ± 47% higher than after intramuscular administration.[1, 2]
Paper chromatographic studies indicated that capreomycin is excreted essentially unaltered. Urine concentrations averaged 1.68 mg/mL (average urine volume, 228 mL) during the 6 hours following a 1-g dose.

Microbiology
Capreomycin is active against strains of *Mycobacterium tuberculosis* found in humans.

Susceptibility Tests
The *in vitro* susceptibility of strains of *M. tuberculosis* to capreomycin varies with the media and techniques employed. In general, the minimum inhibitory concentrations for *M. tuberculosis* are lowest in liquid media that are free of egg protein (7H10 or Dubos) and range from 1 to 5 µg/mL when the indirect method is used. Comparable inhibitory concentrations are obtained when 7H10 agar is used for direct susceptibility testing. When indirect susceptibility tests are performed on standard tube slants with 7H10 media, susceptible strains are inhibited by 10 to 25 µg/mL capreomycin. Egg-containing media, such as Löwenstein-Jensen or ATS, require concentrations of 25 to 50 µg/mL to inhibit susceptible strains.

Cross-Resistance
Frequent cross-resistance occurs between capreomycin and viomycin. Varying degrees of cross-resistance between capreomycin and kanamycin and neomycin have been reported. No cross-resistance has been observed between capreomycin and isoniazid, aminosalicylic acid, cycloserine, streptomycin, ethionamide, or ethambutol.

INDICATIONS AND USAGE

Capastat Sulfate, which is to be used concomitantly with other appropriate antituberculosis agents, is indicated in pulmonary infections caused by capreomycin-susceptible strains of *M. tuberculosis* when the primary agents (isoniazid, rifampin, ethambutol, aminosalicylic acid, and streptomycin) have been ineffective or cannot be used because of toxicity or the presence of resistant tubercle bacilli.
Susceptibility studies should be performed to determine the presence of a capreomycin- susceptible strain of *M. tuberculosis*.

CONTRAINDICATION

Capastat Sulfate is contraindicated in patients who are hypersensitive to capreomycin.

PRECAUTIONS

General
Audiometric measurements and assessment of vestibular function should be performed prior to initiation of therapy with Capastat Sulfate and at regular intervals during treatment.
Renal injury, with tubular necrosis, elevation of the blood urea nitrogen (BUN) or serum creatinine, and abnormal urinary sediment, has been noted. Slight elevation of the BUN and serum creatinine has been observed in a significant number of patients receiving prolonged therapy. The appearance of casts, red cells, and white cells in the urine has been noted in a high percentage of these cases. Elevation of the BUN above 30 mg/100 mL or any other evidence of decreasing renal function with or without a rise in BUN levels calls for careful evaluation of the patient, and the dosage should be reduced or the drug completely withdrawn. The clinical significance of abnormal urine sediment and slight elevation in the BUN (or serum creatinine) observed during long-term therapy with Capastat Sulfate has not been established.
The peripheral neuromuscular blocking action that has been attributed to other polypeptide antibiotics (colistin sulfate, polymyxin A sulfate, paromomycin, and viomycin) and to aminoglycoside antibiotics (streptomycin, dihydrostreptomycin, neomycin, and kanamycin) has been studied

with Capastat Sulfate. A partial neuromuscular blockade was demonstrated after large intravenous doses of Capastat Sulfate. This action was enhanced by ether anesthesia (as has been reported for neomycin) and was antagonized by neostigmine.

Caution should be exercised in the administration of antibiotics, including Capastat Sulfate, to any patient who has demonstrated some form of allergy, particularly to drugs.

Laboratory Tests

Regular tests of renal function should be made throughout the period of treatment, and reduced dosage should be employed in patients with known or suspected renal impairment.

Renal function studies should be made both before therapy with Capastat Sulfate is started and on a weekly basis during treatment.

Since hypokalemia may occur during therapy, serum potassium levels should be determined frequently.

Drug Interactions

For neuromuscular blocking action of this drug, *see* PRECAUTIONS, GENERAL.

Carcinogenesis, Mutagenesis, Impairment of Fertility

Studies have not been performed to determine potential for carcinogenicity, mutagenicity, or impairment of fertility.

Usage in Pregnancy — Pregnancy Category C

Capastat Sulfate has been shown to be teratogenic in rats when given in doses 3 1/2 times the human dose. There are no adequate and well-controlled studies in pregnant women. Capastat Sulfate should be used during pregnancy only if the potential benefit justifies the potential risk to the fetus (*see boxed* WARNINGS *and* ANIMAL PHARMACOLOGY).

Nursing Mothers

It is not known whether this drug is excreted in human milk. Because many drugs are excreted in human milk, caution should be exercised when Capastat Sulfate is administered to a nursing woman.

Pediatric Use

Safety and effectiveness in pediatric patients have not been established (*see boxed* WARNINGS).

Geriatric Use

Clinical studies of Capastat Sulfate did not analyze the safety and efficacy of patients aged 65 and over to determine whether they respond differently from younger patients. Other reported clinical experience has not identified differences in responses between the elderly and younger patients. In general, dose selection for an elderly patient should be cautious, usually starting at the low end of the dosing range, reflecting the greater frequency of decreased hepatic, renal, or cardiac function, and of concomitant disease or other drug therapy.

Capastat Sulfate is known to be substantially excreted by the kidney (*see* CLINICAL PHARMACOLOGY), and the risk of toxic reactions to this drug may be greater in patients with impaired renal function. Because elderly patients are more likely to have decreased renal function, care should be taken in dose selection, and it may be useful to monitor renal function (*see* PRECAUTIONS, Laboratory Tests). Patients with reduced renal function should have dosage reduction based on creatinine clearance using the guidelines included in Table 1 (*see* DOSAGE AND ADMINISTRATION).

The geriatric population is also more likely to have impaired hearing at baseline. Audiometric measurements and assessment of vestibular function should be performed prior to initiation of therapy with Capastat Sulfate and at regular intervals during treatment (*see* PRECAUTIONS, General).

ADVERSE REACTIONS

Nephrotoxicity: In 36% of 722 patients treated with Capastat Sulfate, elevation of the BUN above 20 mg/100 mL has been observed. In many instances, there was also depression of PSP excretion and abnormal urine sediment. In 10% of this series, the BUN elevation exceeded 30 mg/100 mL.

Toxic nephritis was reported in 1 patient with tuberculosis and portal cirrhosis who was treated with Capastat Sulfate (1 g) and aminosalicylic acid daily for 1 month. This patient developed renal insufficiency and oliguria and died. Autopsy showed subsiding acute tubular necrosis.

Electrolyte disturbances resembling Bartter's syndrome have been reported in 1 patient.

Ototoxicity: Subclinical auditory loss was noted in approximately 11% of 722 patients undergoing treatment with Capastat Sulfate. This was a 5- to 10-decibel loss in the 4000- to 8000-CPS range. Clinically apparent hearing loss occurred in 3% of the 722 subjects. Some audiometric changes were reversible. Other cases with permanent loss were not progressive following withdrawal of Capastat Sulfate.

Tinnitus and vertigo have occurred.

Liver: Serial tests of liver function have demonstrated a decrease in BSP excretion without change in AST (SGOT) or ALT (SGPT) in the presence of preexisting liver disease. Abnormal results in liver function tests have occurred in many persons receiving Capastat Sulfate in combination with other antituberculosis agents that also are known to cause changes in hepatic function. The role of Capastat Sulfate in producing these abnormalities is not clear; however, periodic determinations of liver function are recommended.

Blood: Leukocytosis and leukopenia have been observed. The majority of patients treated have had eosinophilia exceeding 5% while receiving daily injections of Capastat Sulfate. This has subsided with reduction of the Capastat Sulfate dosage to 2 or 3 g weekly.

Pain and induration at the injection site have been observed. Excessive bleeding at the injection site has been reported. Sterile abscesses have been noted. Rare cases of thrombocytopenia have been reported.

Hypersensitivity: Urticaria and maculopapular skin rashes associated in some cases with febrile reactions have been reported when Capastat Sulfate and other antituberculosis drugs were given concomitantly.

OVERDOSAGE

Signs and Symptoms

Nephrotoxicity following the parenteral administration of Capastat Sulfate is most closely related to the area under the curve of the serum concentration versus time graph. The elderly patient, patients with abnormal renal function or dehydration, and patients receiving other nephrotoxic drugs are at much greater risk for developing acute tubular necrosis.

Damage to the auditory and vestibular divisions of cranial nerve VIII has been associated with Capastat Sulfate given to patients with abnormal renal function or dehydration and in those receiving medications with additive auditory toxicities. These patients often experience dizziness, tinnitus, vertigo, and a loss of high-tone acuity.

Neuromuscular blockage or respiratory paralysis may occur following rapid intravenous infusion.

If capreomycin is ingested, toxicity would be unlikely because it is poorly absorbed (less than 1%) from an intact gastrointestinal system.

Hypokalemia, hypocalcemia, hypomagnesemia, and an electrolyte disturbance resembling Bartter's syndrome have been reported to occur in patients with capreomycin toxicity.

The subcutaneous median lethal dose in mice was 514 mg/kg.

Treatment

To obtain up-to-date information about the treatment of overdose, a good resource is your certified Regional Poison Control Center. Telephone numbers of certified poison control centers are listed in the *Physicians' Desk Reference (PDR)*. In managing overdosage, consider the possibility of multiple drug overdoses, interaction among drugs, and unusual drug kinetics in your patient.

Protect the patient's airway and support ventilation and perfusion. Meticulously monitor and maintain, within acceptable limits, the patient's vital signs, blood gases, serum electrolytes, etc. Absorption of drugs from the gastrointestinal tract may be decreased by giving activated charcoal, which, in many cases, is more effective than emesis or lavage; consider charcoal instead of or in addition to gastric emptying. Repeated doses of charcoal over time may hasten elimination of some drugs that have been absorbed. Safeguard the patient's airway when employing gastric emptying or charcoal.

Patients who have received an overdose of capreomycin and have normal renal function should be carefully hydrated to maintain a urine output of 3 to 5 mL/kg/h. Fluid balance, electrolytes, and creatinine clearance should be carefully monitored.

Hemodialysis may be effectively used to remove capreomycin in patients with significant renal disease.

DOSAGE AND ADMINISTRATION

Capastat Sulfate may be administered intramuscularly or intravenously following reconstitution. Reconstitution is achieved by dissolving the vial contents (1 g) in 2 mL of 0.9% Sodium Chloride Injection or Sterile Water for Injection. Two to 3 minutes should be allowed for complete dissolution.

Intravenously — For intravenous infusion, reconstituted Capastat Sulfate should be diluted in 100 mL of 0.9% Sodium Chloride Injection and administered over 60 minutes.

Intramuscularly — Reconstituted Capastat Sulfate should be given by deep intramuscular injection into a large muscle mass, since superficial injection may be associated with increased pain and the development of sterile abscesses.

For administration of a 1-g dose, the entire contents of the vial should be given. For doses lower than 1 g, the following dilution table may be used.

DILUTION TABLE

Diluent Added to 1-g, 10-mL Vial	Volume of Capastat Sulfate Solution	Concentration (Approx)
2.15 mL	2.85 mL	370 mg*/mL
2.63 mL	3.33 mL	315 mg*/mL
3.3 mL	4 mL	260 mg*/mL
4.3 mL	5 mL	210 mg*/mL

*Equivalent to capreomycin activity. Approximated concentration takes into account the retention volume.

The solution may acquire a pale straw color and darken with time, but this is not associated with loss of potency or the development of toxicity. After reconstitution, all solutions of Capastat Sulfate may be stored for up to 24 hours under refrigeration.

Capreomycin is always administered in combination with at least 1 other antituberculosis agent to which the patient's strain of tubercle bacilli is susceptible. The usual dose is 1 g daily (not to exceed 20 mg/kg/day) given intramuscularly or intravenously for 60 to 120 days, followed by 1 g by either route 2 or 3 times weekly. (Note — Therapy for tuberculosis should be maintained for 12 to 24 months. If facilities for administering injectable medication are not available, a change to appropriate oral therapy is indicated on the patient's release from the hospital.)

Patients with reduced renal function should have dosage reduction based on creatinine clearance using the guidelines included in Table 1. These dosages are designed to achieve a mean steady-state capreomycin level of 10 µg/mL.

Table 1. Estimated Dosages to Attain Mean Steady-State Serum Capreomycin Concentration of 10 µg/mL (Based on Creatinine Clearance)

CrCl (mL/min)	Capreomycin Clearance (L/kg/h × 10^{-2})	Half-life (hours)	Dose[a](mg/kg) for the Following Dosing Intervals 24 h	48 h	72 h
0	0.54	55.5	1.29	2.58	3.87
10	1.01	29.4	2.43	4.87	7.30
20	1.49	20.0	3.58	7.16	10.7
30	1.97	15.1	4.72	9.45	14.2
40	2.45	12.2	5.87	11.7	
50	2.92	10.2	7.01	14.0	
60	3.40	8.8	8.16		
80	4.35	6.8	10.4[b]		
100	5.31	5.6	12.7[b]		
110	5.78	5.2	13.9[b]		

[a] For patients with renal impairment, initial maintenance dose estimates are given for optional dosing intervals; longer dosing intervals are expected to provide greater peak and lower trough serum capreomycin levels than shorter dosing intervals.

[b] The usual dosage for patients with normal renal function is 1000 mg daily, not to exceed 20 mg/kg/day, for 60 to 120 days, then 1000 mg 2 to 3 times weekly.

Parenteral drug products should be inspected visually for particulate matter and discoloration prior to administration, whenever solution and container permit.

HOW SUPPLIED

Capastat® Sulfate, Capreomycin for Injection, USP, is available in:

Vials: 1 g*, 10 mL size (No. 718) (1s) NDC 0002-1485-01

*Equivalent to capreomycin activity.

Store at controlled room temperature 15° to 30°C (59° to 86°F) prior to reconstitution.

ANIMAL PHARMACOLOGY

In addition to renal and cranial nerve VIII toxicity demonstrated in animal toxicology studies, cataracts developed in 2 dogs on doses of 62 mg/kg and 100 mg/kg for prolonged periods.

In teratology studies, a low incidence of "wavy ribs" was noted in litters of female rats treated with daily doses of 50 mg/kg or more of capreomycin.

REFERENCES

1. Lehmann CR, Garrett LE, Winn RE, Springberg PD, Vicks S, Porter DK, Pierson WP, Wolny JD, Brier GL, Black HR. Capreomycin kinetics in renal impairment and clearance by hemodialysis. Am Rev Respir Dis 1988;138/5:1312–3.
2. Unpublished data on file at Lilly.

Literature revised December 8, 2003
Eli Lilly and Company
Indianapolis, IN 46285, USA
PV 4800 AMP PRINTED IN USA

CECLOR® ℞

[*sē 'klôr*]

CEFACLOR, USP

To reduce the development of drug-resistant bacteria and maintain the effectiveness of Ceclor and other antibacterial drugs, Ceclor should be used only to treat or prevent infections that are proven or strongly suspected to be caused by bacteria.

DESCRIPTION

Ceclor® (Cefaclor, USP) is a semisynthetic cephalosporin antibiotic for oral administration. It is chemically designated as 3-chloro-7-D-(2-phenylglycinamido)-3-cephem-4-carboxylic acid monohydrate. The chemical formula for

Continued on next page

*** Identi-Code® symbol. This product information was prepared in June 2004. Current information on these and other products of Eli Lilly and Company may be obtained by direct inquiry to Lilly Research Laboratories, Lilly Corporate Center, Indianapolis, Indiana 46285, (800) 545-5979.**

Ceclor—Cont.

cefaclor is $C_{15}H_{14}ClN_3O_4S \bullet H_2O$ and the molecular weight is 385.82.

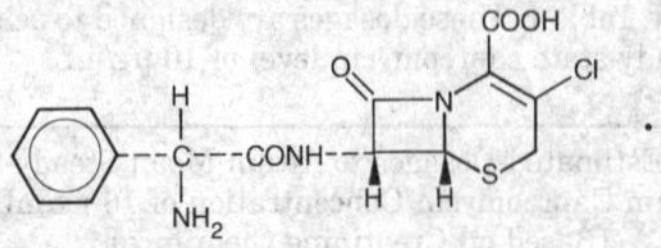

Each Pulvule® contains cefaclor monohydrate equivalent to 250 mg (0.68 mmol) or 500 mg (1.36 mmol) anhydrous cefaclor. The Pulvules also contain cornstarch, F D & C Blue No. 1, F D & C Red No. 40, gelatin, magnesium stearate, silicone, titanium dioxide, and other inactive ingredients. The 500-mg Pulvule also contains iron oxide.

After mixing, each 5 mL of Ceclor for Oral Suspension will contain cefaclor monohydrate equivalent to 125 mg (0.34 mmol), 187 mg (0.51 mmol), 250 mg (0.68 mmol), or 375 mg (1.0 mmol) anhydrous cefaclor. The suspensions also contain cellulose, cornstarch, F D & C Red No. 40, flavors, silicone, sodium lauryl sulfate, sucrose, and xanthan gum.

CLINICAL PHARMACOLOGY

Cefaclor is well absorbed after oral administration to fasting subjects. Total absorption is the same whether the drug is given with or without food; however, when it is taken with food, the peak concentration achieved is 50% to 75% of that observed when the drug is administered to fasting subjects and generally appears from three fourths to 1 hour later. Following administration of 250-mg, 500-mg, and 1-g doses to fasting subjects, average peak serum levels of approximately 7, 13, and 23 μg/mL respectively were obtained within 30 to 60 minutes. Approximately 60% to 85% of the drug is excreted unchanged in the urine within 8 hours, the greater portion being excreted within the first 2 hours. During this 8-hour period, peak urine concentrations following the 250-mg, 500-mg, and 1-g doses were approximately 600, 900, and 1900 μg/mL, respectively. The serum half-life in normal subjects is 0.6 to 0.9 hour. In patients with reduced renal function, the serum half-life of cefaclor is slightly prolonged. In those with complete absence of renal function, the plasma half-life of the intact molecule is 2.3 to 2.8 hours. Excretion pathways in patients with markedly impaired renal function have not been determined. Hemodialysis shortens the half-life by 25% to 30%.

Microbiology

In vitro tests demonstrate that the bactericidal action of the cephalosporins results from inhibition of cell-wall synthesis. Cefaclor has been shown to be active against most strains of the following microorganisms, both *in vitro* and in clinical infections as described in the INDICATIONS AND USAGE section.

Aerobes, Gram-positive
- Staphylococci, including coagulase-positive, coagulase-negative, and penicillinase-producing strains
- *Streptococcus pneumoniae*
- *Streptococcus pyogenes* (group A β-hemolytic streptococci)

Aerobes, Gram-negative
- *Escherichia coli*
- *Haemophilus influenzae*, excluding β-lactamase-negative ampicillin-resistant strains
- *Klebsiella* spp.
- *Proteus mirabilis*

The following *in vitro* data are available, **but their clinical significance is unknown.**

Cefaclor exhibits *in vitro* minimal inhibitory concentrations (MICs) of ≤8 μg/mL against most (≥90%) strains of the following microorganisms; however, the safety and effectiveness of cefaclor in treating clinical infections due to these microorganisms have not been established in adequate and well-controlled clinical trials.

Aerobes, Gram-negative
- *Citrobacter diversus*
- *Moraxella (Branhamella) catarrhalis*
- *Neisseria gonorrhoeae*

Anaerobes, Gram-positive
- *Bacteroides* spp. (excluding *Bacteroides fragilis*)
- *Peptococcus*
- *Peptostreptococcus*
- *Propionibacterium acnes*

Note: Pseudomonas spp., *Acinetobacter calcoaceticus* and most strains of enterococci (*Enterococcus faecalis*, group D streptococci), *Enterobacter* spp., indole-positive *Proteus, Morganella morganii* (formerly *Proteus morganii*), *Providencia rettgeri* (formerly *Proteus rettgeri*), and *Serratia* spp. are resistant to cefaclor. When tested by *in vitro* methods, staphylococci exhibit cross-resistance between cefaclor and methicillin-type antibiotics.

Susceptibility Testing

Dilution Techniques—Quantitative methods that are used to determine minimum inhibitory concentrations (MIC) provide reproducible estimates of the susceptibility of bacteria to antimicrobial compounds. One such standardized procedure that has been recommended for use with cefaclor powder uses a standardized dilution method[1] (broth, agar, or microdilution). The MIC values obtained should be interpreted according to the following criteria:

MIC (μg/mL)	Interpretation*
≤8	Susceptible (S)
16	Intermediate (I)
≥32	Resistant (R)

*When testing *H. influenzae* spp. these interpretive standards are applicable only to broth microdilution method using Haemophilus Test Medium (HTM)[1]

Note: β-lactamase-negative, ampicillin-resistant strains of *H. influenzae* should be considered resistant to cefaclor despite apparent *in vitro* susceptibility to this agent.

A report of "Susceptible" indicates that the pathogen is likely to be inhibited by usually achievable concentrations of the antimicrobial compound in blood. A report of "Intermediate" indicates that the result should be considered equivocal, and, if the microorganism is not fully susceptible to alternative, clinically feasible drugs, the test should be repeated. This category implies possible clinical applicability in body sites where the drug is physiologically concentrated or in situations where high dosage of drug can be used. This category also provides a buffer zone that prevents small uncontrolled technical factors from causing major discrepancies in interpretation. A report of "Resistant" indicates that usually achievable concentrations of the antimicrobial compound in the blood are unlikely to be inhibitory and that other therapy should be selected.

Standardized susceptibility test procedures require the use of laboratory control microorganisms. Standard cefaclor powder should provide the following MIC values:

Microorganism		MIC (μg/mL)
E. coli	ATCC 25922	1-4
E. faecalis	ATCC 29212	>32
S. aureus	ATCC 29213	1-4
When testing *H. influenzae**		
Microorganism		MIC (μg/mL)
H. influenzae	ATCC 49766	1-4

*Broth microdilution test performed using Haemophilus Test Medium (HTM)[1]

Diffusion Techniques—Quantitative methods that require measurement of zone diameters provide reproducible estimates of the susceptibility of bacteria to antimicrobial compounds. One such standardized procedure[2] that has been recommended for use with disks to test the susceptibility of microorganisms to cefaclor uses the 30-μg cefaclor disk. Interpretation involves correlation of the diameter obtained in the disk test with the MIC for cefaclor. Reports from the laboratory providing results of the standard single-disk susceptibility test with a 30-μg cefaclor disk should be interpreted according to the following criteria:

When Testing Organisms Other Than *Haemophilus* spp. and Streptococci

Zone Diameter (mm)	Interpretation
≥18	Susceptible (S)
15-17	Intermediate (I)
≤14	Resistant (R)
When testing *H. influenzae**	
Zone Diameter (mm)	Interpretation
≥20	Susceptible (S)
17-19	Intermediate (I)
≤16	Resistant (R)

*Disk susceptibility test performed using Haemophilus Test Medium (HTM)[2]

Note: β-lactamase-negative, ampicillin-resistant strains of *H. influenzae* should be considered resistant to cefaclor despite apparent *in vitro* susceptibility to this agent.

Interpretation should be as stated above for results using dilution techniques.

As with standard dilution techniques, diffusion methods require the use of laboratory control microorganisms. The 30-μg cefaclor disk should provide the following zone diameters in these laboratory test quality control strains:

Microorganisms		Zone Diameter (mm)
E. coli	ATCC 25922	23-27
S. aureus	ATCC 25923	27-31
When testing *H. influenzae**		
Microorganisms		Zone Diameter (mm)
H. influenzae	ATCC 49766	25-31

*Disk susceptibility test performed using Haemophilus Test Medium (HTM)[2]

INDICATIONS AND USAGE

Ceclor is indicated in the treatment of the following infections when caused by susceptible strains of the designated microorganisms:

Otitis media caused by *Streptococcus pneumoniae, Haemophilus influenzae*, staphylococci, and *Streptococcus pyogenes*

Note: β-lactamase-negative, ampicillin-resistant (BLNAR) strains of *Haemophilus influenzae* should be considered resistant to cefaclor despite apparent *in vitro* susceptibility of some BLNAR strains.

Lower respiratory tract infections, including pneumonia, caused by *Streptococcus pneumoniae, Haemophilus influenzae*, and *Streptococcus pyogenes*

Note: β-lactamase-negative, ampicillin-resistant (BLNAR) strains of *Haemophilus influenzae* should be considered resistant to cefaclor despite apparent *in vitro* susceptibility of some BLNAR strains.

Pharyngitis and Tonsillitis, caused by *Streptococcus pyogenes*

Note: Penicillin is the usual drug of choice in the treatment and prevention of streptococcal infections, including the prophylaxis of rheumatic fever. Ceclor is generally effective in the eradication of streptococci from the nasopharynx; however, substantial data establishing the efficacy of Ceclor in the subsequent prevention of rheumatic fever are not available at present.

Urinary tract infections, including pyelonephritis and cystitis, caused by *Escherichia coli, Proteus mirabilis, Klebsiella* spp., and coagulase-negative staphylococci

Skin and skin structure infections caused by *Staphylococcus aureus* and *Streptococcus pyogenes*

Appropriate culture and susceptibility studies should be performed to determine susceptibility of the causative organism to cefaclor.

To reduce the development of drug-resistant bacteria and maintain the effectiveness of Ceclor and other antibacterial drugs, Ceclor should be used only to treat or prevent infections that are proven or strongly suspected to be caused by susceptible bacteria. When culture and susceptibility information are available, they should be considered in selecting or modifying antibacterial therapy. In the absence of such data, local epidemiology and susceptibility patterns may contribute to the empiric selection of therapy.

CONTRAINDICATION

Ceclor is contraindicated in patients with known allergy to the cephalosporin group of antibiotics.

WARNINGS

BEFORE THERAPY WITH CECLOR IS INSTITUTED, CAREFUL INQUIRY SHOULD BE MADE TO DETERMINE WHETHER THE PATIENT HAS HAD PREVIOUS HYPERSENSITIVITY REACTIONS TO CEFACLOR, CEPHALOSPORINS, PENICILLINS, OR OTHER DRUGS. IF THIS PRODUCT IS TO BE GIVEN TO PENICILLIN-SENSITIVE PATIENTS, CAUTION SHOULD BE EXERCISED BECAUSE CROSS-HYPERSENSITIVITY AMONG β-LACTAM ANTIBIOTICS HAS BEEN CLEARLY DOCUMENTED AND MAY OCCUR IN UP TO 10% OF PATIENTS WITH A HISTORY OF PENICILLIN ALLERGY.

IF AN ALLERGIC REACTION TO CECLOR OCCURS, DISCONTINUE THE DRUG. SERIOUS ACUTE HYPERSENSITIVITY REACTIONS MAY REQUIRE TREATMENT WITH EPINEPHRINE AND OTHER EMERGENCY MEASURES, INCLUDING OXYGEN, INTRAVENOUS FLUIDS, INTRAVENOUS ANTIHISTAMINES, CORTICOSTEROIDS, PRESSOR AMINES, AND AIRWAY MANAGEMENT, AS CLINICALLY INDICATED.

Antibiotics, including Ceclor, should be administered cautiously to any patient who has demonstrated some form of allergy, particularly to drugs.

Pseudomembranous colitis has been reported with nearly all antibacterial agents, including cefaclor, and has ranged in severity from mild to life-threatening. Therefore, it is important to consider this diagnosis in patients who present with diarrhea subsequent to the administration of antibacterial agents.

Treatment with antibacterial agents alters the normal flora of the colon and may permit overgrowth of clostridia. Studies indicate that a toxin produced by *Clostridium difficile* is one primary cause of antibiotic-associated colitis.

After the diagnosis of pseudomembranous colitis has been established, therapeutic measures should be initiated. Mild cases of pseudomembranous colitis usually respond to drug discontinuation alone. In moderate to severe cases, consideration should be given to management with fluids and electrolytes, protein supplementation and treatment with an antibacterial drug effective against *C. difficile*.

PRECAUTIONS

General

Prescribing Ceclor in the absence of a proven or strongly suspected bacterial infection or a prophylactic indication is unlikely to provide benefit to the patient and increases the risk of the development of drug-resistant bacteria.

Prolonged use of Ceclor may result in the overgrowth of nonsusceptible organisms. Careful observation of the patient is essential. If superinfection occurs during therapy, appropriate measures should be taken.

Positive direct Coombs' tests have been reported during treatment with the cephalosporin antibiotics. It should be recognized that a positive Coombs' test may be due to the drug, e.g., in hematologic studies or in transfusion cross-matching procedures when antiglobulin tests are performed on the minor side or in Coombs' testing of newborns whose mothers have received cephalosporin antibiotics before parturition.

Ceclor should be administered with caution in the presence of markedly impaired renal function. Since the half-life of cefaclor in anuria is 2.3 to 2.8 hours, dosage adjustments for patients with moderate or severe renal impairment are usually not required. Clinical experience with cefaclor under such conditions is limited; therefore, careful clinical observation and laboratory studies should be made.

As with other β-lactam antibiotics, the renal excretion of cefaclor is inhibited by probenecid.

Antibiotics, including cephalosporins, should be prescribed with caution in individuals with a history of gastrointestinal disease, particularly colitis.

Information for Patients

Patients should be counseled that antibacterial drugs including Ceclor should only be used to treat bacterial infections. They do not treat viral infections (e.g., the common cold). When Ceclor is prescribed to treat a bacterial infection, patients should be told that although it is common to feel better early in the course of therapy, the medication should be taken exactly as directed. Skipping doses or not completing the full course of therapy may (1) decrease the effectiveness of the immediate treatment and (2) increase the likelihood that bacteria will develop resistance and will not be treatable by Ceclor or other antibacterial drugs in the future.

Drug / Laboratory Test Interactions

Patients receiving Ceclor may show a false-positive reaction for glucose in the urine with tests that use Benedict's and Fehling's solutions and also with Clinitest® tablets.

There have been reports of increased anticoagulant effect when Ceclor and oral anticoagulants were administered concomitantly.

Carcinogenesis, Mutagenesis, Impairment of Fertility

Studies have not been performed to determine potential for carcinogenicity, mutagenicity, or impairment of fertility.

Pregnancy

Teratogenic Effects—Pregnancy Category B—Reproduction studies have been performed in mice and rats at doses up to 12 times the human dose and in ferrets given 3 times the maximum human dose and have revealed no harm to the fetus due to Ceclor. There are, however, no adequate and well-controlled studies in pregnant women. Because animal reproduction studies are not always predictive of human response, this drug should be used during pregnancy only if clearly needed.

Labor and Delivery

The effect of Ceclor on labor and delivery is unknown.

Nursing Mothers

Small amounts of Ceclor have been detected in mother's milk following administration of single 500-mg doses. Average levels were 0.18, 0.20, 0.21, and 0.16 μg/mL at 2, 3, 4, and 5 hours respectively. Trace amounts were detected at 1 hour. The effect on nursing infants is not known. Caution should be exercised when Ceclor is administered to a nursing woman.

Pediatric Use

Safety and effectiveness of this product for use in infants less than 1 month of age have not been established.

Geriatric Use

Of the 3703 patients in clinical studies of Ceclor, 594 (16.0%) were 65 and older. No overall differences in safety or effectiveness were observed between these subjects and younger subjects. Other reported clinical experience has not identified differences in responses between the elderly and younger patients, but greater sensitivity of some older individuals cannot be ruled out.

This drug is known to be substantially excreted by the kidney (*see* **CLINICAL PHARMACOLOGY**), and the risk of toxic reactions to this drug may be greater in patients with impaired renal function. Because elderly patients are more likely to have decreased renal function, care should be taken in dose selection, and it may be useful to monitor renal function (*see* **DOSAGE AND ADMINISTRATION**).

ADVERSE REACTIONS

Adverse effects considered to be related to therapy with Ceclor are listed below:

Hypersensitivity reactions have been reported in about 1.5% of patients and include morbilliform eruptions (1 in 100). Pruritus, urticaria, and positive Coombs' tests each occur in less than 1 in 200 patients.

Cases of **serum-sickness-like** reactions have been reported with the use of Ceclor. These are characterized by findings of erythema multiforme, rashes, and other skin manifestations accompanied by arthritis/arthralgia, with or without fever, and differ from classic serum sickness in that there is infrequently associated lymphadenopathy and proteinuria, no circulating immune complexes, and no evidence to date of sequelae of the reaction. Occasionally, solitary symptoms may occur, but do not represent a **serum-sickness-like** reaction. While further investigation is ongoing, **serum-sickness-like** reactions appear to be due to hypersensitivity and more often occur during or following a second (or subsequent) course of therapy with Ceclor. Such reactions have been reported more frequently in pediatric patients than in adults with an overall occurrence ranging from 1 in 200 (0.5%) in one focused trial to 2 in 8346 (0.024%) in overall clinical trials (with an incidence in pediatric patients in clinical trials of 0.055%) to 1 in 38,000 (0.003%) in spontaneous event reports. Signs and symptoms usually occur a few days after initiation of therapy and subside within a few days after cessation of therapy; occasionally these reactions have resulted in hospitalization, usually of short duration (median hospitalization = 2 to 3 days, based on postmarketing surveillance studies). In those requiring hospitalization, the symptoms have ranged from mild to severe at the time of admission with more of the severe reactions occurring in pediatric patients. Antihistamines and glucocorticoids appear to enhance resolution of the signs and symptoms. No serious sequelae have been reported.

More severe hypersensitivity reactions, including Stevens-Johnson syndrome, toxic epidermal necrolysis, and anaphylaxis have been reported rarely. Anaphylactoid events may be manifested by solitary symptoms, including angioedema, asthenia, edema (including face and limbs), dyspnea, paresthesias, syncope, hypotension, or vasodilatation. Anaphylaxis may be more common in patients with a history of penicillin allergy.

Rarely, hypersensitivity symptoms may persist for several months.

Gastrointestinal symptoms occur in about 2.5% of patients and include diarrhea (1 in 70).

Onset of pseudomembranous colitis symptoms may occur during or after antibiotic treatment (*see* **WARNINGS**). Nausea and vomiting have been reported rarely. As with some penicillins and some other cephalosporins, transient hepatitis and cholestatic jaundice have been reported rarely.

Other effects considered related to therapy included eosinophilia (1 in 50 patients), genital pruritus, moniliasis or vaginitis (about 1 in 50 patients), and, rarely, thrombocytopenia or reversible interstitial nephritis.

Causal Relationship Uncertain—

CNS—Rarely, reversible hyperactivity, agitation, nervousness, insomnia, confusion, hypertonia, dizziness, hallucinations, and somnolence have been reported.

Transitory abnormalities in clinical laboratory test results have been reported. Although they were of uncertain etiology, they are listed below to serve as alerting information for the physician.

Hepatic—Slight elevations of AST, ALT, or alkaline phosphatase values (1 in 40).

Hematopoietic—As has also been reported with other β-lactam antibiotics, transient lymphocytosis, leukopenia, and, rarely, hemolytic anemia, aplastic anemia, agranulocytosis, and reversible neutropenia of possible clinical significance.

There have been rare reports of increased prothrombin time with or without clinical bleeding in patients receiving Ceclor and Coumadin® concomitantly.

Renal—Slight elevations in BUN or serum creatinine (less than 1 in 500) or abnormal urinalysis (less than 1 in 200).

Cephalosporin-class Adverse Reactions

In addition to the adverse reactions listed above that have been observed in patients treated with cefaclor, the following adverse reactions and altered laboratory tests have been reported for cephalosporin-class antibiotics: fever, abdominal pain, superinfection, renal dysfunction, toxic nephropathy, hemorrhage, false positive test for urinary glucose, elevated bilirubin, elevated LDH, and pancytopenia.

Several cephalosporins have been implicated in triggering seizures, particularly in patients with renal impairment when the dosage was not reduced. If seizures associated with drug therapy occur, the drug should be discontinued. Anticonvulsant therapy can be given if clinically indicated (*see* **DOSAGE AND ADMINISTRATION** *and* **OVERDOSAGE** sections).

OVERDOSAGE

Signs and Symptoms—The toxic symptoms following an overdose of cefaclor may include nausea, vomiting, epigastric distress, and diarrhea. The severity of the epigastric distress and the diarrhea are dose related. If other symptoms are present, it is probable that they are secondary to an underlying disease state, an allergic reaction, or the effects of other intoxication.

Treatment—To obtain up-to-date information about the treatment of overdose, a good resource is your certified Regional Poison Control Center. Telephone numbers of certified poison control centers are listed in the *Physicians' Desk Reference (PDR)*. In managing overdosage, consider the possibility of multiple drug overdoses, interaction among drugs, and unusual drug kinetics in your patient.

Unless 5 times the normal dose of cefaclor has been ingested, gastrointestinal decontamination will not be necessary.

Protect the patient's airway and support ventilation and perfusion. Meticulously monitor and maintain, within acceptable limits, the patient's vital signs, blood gases, serum electrolytes, etc. Absorption of drugs from the gastrointestinal tract may be decreased by giving activated charcoal, which, in many cases, is more effective than emesis or lavage; consider charcoal instead of or in addition to gastric emptying. Repeated doses of charcoal over time may hasten elimination of some drugs that have been absorbed. Safeguard the patient's airway when employing gastric emptying or charcoal.

Forced diuresis, peritoneal dialysis, hemodialysis, or charcoal hemoperfusion have not been established as beneficial for an overdose of cefaclor.

DOSAGE AND ADMINISTRATION

Ceclor is administered orally.

Adults—The usual adult dosage is 250 mg every 8 hours. For more severe infections (such as pneumonia) or those caused by less susceptible organisms, doses may be doubled.

Pediatric patients—The usual recommended daily dosage for pediatric patients is 20 mg/kg/day in divided doses every 8 hours. In more serious infections, otitis media, and infections caused by less susceptible organisms, 40 mg/kg/day are recommended, with a maximum dosage of 1 g/day.

Ceclor Suspension

Weight	125 mg/5 mL	250 mg/5 mL
20 mg/kg/day		
9 kg	1/2 tsp t.i.d.	
18 kg	1 tsp t.i.d.	1/2 tsp t.i.d.
40 mg/kg/day		
9 kg	1 tsp t.i.d.	1/2 tsp t.i.d.
18 kg		1 tsp t.i.d.

B.I.D. Treatment Option—For the treatment of otitis media and pharyngitis, the total daily dosage may be divided and administered every 12 hours.

Ceclor Suspension

Weight	187 mg/5 mL	375 mg/5 mL
20 mg/kg/day (Pharyngitis)		
9 kg	1/2 tsp b.i.d.	
18 kg	1 tsp b.i.d	1/2 tsp b.i.d.
40 mg/kg/day (Otitis Media)		
9 kg	1 tsp b.i.d.	1/2 tsp b.i.d.
18 kg		1 tsp b.i.d.

Ceclor may be administered in the presence of impaired renal function. Under such a condition, the dosage usually is unchanged (*see* **PRECAUTIONS**).

In the treatment of β-hemolytic streptococcal infections, a therapeutic dosage of Ceclor should be administered for at least 10 days.

HOW SUPPLIED

Pulvules:

250 mg, purple and white (No. 3061)—(RxPak* of 15) NDC 0002-3061-15; (100s) NDC 0002-3061-02; (ID†100) NDC 0002-3061-33

500 mg, purple and gray (No. 3062)—(RxPak of 15) NDC 0002-3062-15

For Oral Suspension:

125 mg/5 mL, strawberry flavor (M-5057‡)—(150-mL size) NDC 0002-5057-68

187 mg/5 mL, strawberry flavor (M-5130‡)—(100-mL size) NDC 0002-5130-48

250 mg/5 mL, strawberry flavor (M-5058‡)—(75-mL size) NDC 0002-5058-18; (150-mL size) NDC 0002-5058-68

375 mg/5 mL, strawberry flavor (M-5132‡)—(100-mL size) NDC 0002-5132-48

*All RxPaks (prescription packages, Lilly) have safety closures.

†Identi-Dose® (unit dose medication, Lilly).

‡After mixing, store in a refrigerator. Shake well before using. Keep tightly closed. The mixture may be kept for 14 days without significant loss of potency. Discard unused portion after 14 days.

Store at 25°C (77°F); excursions permitted to 15-30°C (59-86°F) [see USP Controlled Room Temperature]

REFERENCES

1. National Committee for Clinical Laboratory Standards. Methods for Dilution Antimicrobial Susceptibility Tests for Bacteria that Grow Aerobically—Fourth Edition. Approved Standard NCCLS Document M7-A4, Vol. 17, No. 2, NCCLS, Wayne, PA, January, 1997.
2. National Committee for Clinical Laboratory Standards. Performance Standards for Antimicrobial Disk Susceptibility Tests—Sixth Edition. Approved Standard NCCLS Document M2-A6, Vol. 17, No. 1, NCCLS, Wayne, PA, January, 1997.

Literature revised March 28, 2003

Manufactured by Eli Lilly Italia, S.p.A.
Sesto Fiorentino (Firenze), Italy
for Eli Lilly and Company
Indianapolis, IN 46285, USA

IT 0083 ITAMP

CIALIS® ℞
[*See-AL-iss*]
(tadalafil) tablets

For full prescribing information see listing under LILLY ICOS LLC.

CYMBALTA® ℞
[*sĭm-băl-tă*]
(duloxetine hydrochloride)

DESCRIPTION

Cymbalta® (duloxetine hydrochloride) is a selective serotonin and norepinephrine reuptake inhibitor (SSNRI) for oral administration. Its chemical designation is (+)-(*S*)-*N*-methyl-γ-(1-naphthyloxy)-2-thiophenepropylamine hydrochloride. The empirical formula is $C_{18}H_{19}NOS \cdot HCl$, which cor-

Continued on next page

*** Identi-Code® symbol. This product information was prepared in June 2004. Current information on these and other products of Eli Lilly and Company may be obtained by direct inquiry to Lilly Research Laboratories, Lilly Corporate Center, Indianapolis, Indiana 46285, (800) 545-5979.**

Cymbalta—Cont.

responds to a molecular weight of 333.88. The structural formula is:

Duloxetine hydrochloride is a white to slightly brownish white solid, which is slightly soluble in water.
Each capsule contains enteric-coated pellets of 22.4, 33.7, or 67.3 mg of duloxetine hydrochloride equivalent to 20, 30, or 60 mg of duloxetine, respectively. These enteric-coated pellets are designed to prevent degradation of the drug in the acidic environment of the stomach. Inactive ingredients include FD&C Blue No. 2, gelatin, hypromellose, hydroxypropyl methylcellulose acetate succinate, sodium lauryl sulfate, sucrose, sugar spheres, talc, titanium dioxide, and triethyl citrate. The 20 and 60 mg capsules also contain iron oxide yellow.

CLINICAL PHARMACOLOGY

Pharmacodynamics
Although the mechanism of the antidepressant action of duloxetine in humans is unknown, it is believed to be related to its potentiation of serotonergic and noradrenergic activity in the CNS. Preclinical studies have shown that duloxetine is a potent inhibitor of neuronal serotonin and norepinephrine reuptake and a less potent inhibitor of dopamine reuptake. Duloxetine has no significant affinity for dopaminergic, adrenergic, cholinergic or histaminergic receptors *in vitro*. Duloxetine does not inhibit monoamine oxidase (MAO). Duloxetine undergoes extensive metabolism, but the major circulating metabolites have not been shown to contribute significantly to the pharmacologic activity of duloxetine.

Pharmacokinetics
Duloxetine has an elimination half-life of about 12 hours (range 8 to 17 hours) and its pharmacokinetics are dose proportional over the therapeutic range. Steady-state plasma concentrations are typically achieved after 3 days of dosing. Elimination of duloxetine is mainly through hepatic metabolism involving two P450 isozymes, CYP2D6 and CYP1A2.
Absorption and Distribution—Orally administered duloxetine hydrochloride is well absorbed. There is a median 2-hour lag until absorption begins (T_{lag}), with maximal plasma concentrations (C_{max}) of duloxetine occurring 6 hours post dose. Food does not affect the C_{max} of duloxetine, but delays the time to reach peak concentration from 6 to 10 hours and it marginally decreases the extent of absorption (AUC) by about 10%. There is a 3-hour delay in absorption and a one-third increase in apparent clearance of duloxetine after an evening dose as compared to a morning dose.
The apparent volume of distribution averages about 1640 L. Duloxetine is highly bound (>90%) to proteins in human plasma, binding primarily to albumin and α_1-acid glycoprotein. Plasma protein binding of duloxetine is not affected by renal or hepatic impairment.
Metabolism and Elimination—Biotransformation and disposition of duloxetine in humans have been determined following oral administration of ^{14}C-labeled duloxetine. Duloxetine comprises about 3% of the total radiolabeled material in the plasma, indicating that it undergoes extensive metabolism to numerous metabolites. The major biotransformation pathways for duloxetine involve oxidation of the naphthyl ring followed by conjugation and further oxidation. Both CYP2D6 and CYP1A2 catalyze the oxidation of the naphthyl ring *in vitro*. Metabolites found in plasma include 4-hydroxy duloxetine glucuronide and 5-hydroxy, 6-methoxy duloxetine sulfate. Many additional metabolites have been identified in urine, some representing only minor pathways of elimination. Only trace (<1% of the dose) amounts of unchanged duloxetine are present in the urine. Most (about 70%) of the duloxetine dose appears in the urine as metabolites of duloxetine; about 20% is excreted in the feces.

Special Populations
Gender—Duloxetine's half-life is similar in men and women. Dosage adjustment based on gender is not necessary.
Age—The pharmacokinetics of duloxetine after a single dose of 40 mg were compared in healthy elderly females (65 to 77 years) and healthy middle-age females (32 to 50 years). There was no difference in the C_{max}, but the AUC of duloxetine was somewhat (about 25%) higher and the half-life about 4 hours longer in the elderly females. Population pharmacokinetic analyses suggest that the typical values for clearance decrease by approximately 1% for each year of age between 25 to 75 years of age; but age as a predictive factor only accounts for a small percentage of between-patient variability. Dosage adjustment based on the age of the patient is not necessary (*see* DOSAGE AND ADMINISTRATION).
Smoking Status—Duloxetine bioavailability (AUC) appears to be reduced by about one-third in smokers. Dosage modifications are not recommended for smokers.
Race—No specific pharmacokinetic study was conducted to investigate the effects of race.
Renal Insufficiency—Limited data are available on the effects of duloxetine in patients with end stage renal disease (ESRD). After a single 60-mg dose of duloxetine, C_{max} and AUC values were approximately 100% greater in patients with end stage renal disease receiving chronic intermittent hemodialysis than in subjects with normal renal function. The elimination half-life, however, was similar in both groups. The AUCs of the major circulating metabolites, 4-hydroxy duloxetine glucuronide and 5-hydroxy, 6-methoxy duloxetine sulfate, largely excreted in urine, were approximately 7- to 9-fold higher and would be expected to increase further with multiple dosing. For this reason, duloxetine is not recommended for patients with ESRD (*see* DOSAGE AND ADMINISTRATION). Studies have not been conducted in patients with a moderate degree of renal dysfunction, but population PK analyses suggest that mild renal dysfunction has no significant effect on duloxetine apparent clearance.
Hepatic Insufficiency—Patients with clinically evident hepatic insufficiency have decreased duloxetine metabolism and elimination. After a single 20-mg dose of duloxetine, 6 cirrhotic patients with moderate liver impairment (Child-Pugh Class B) had a mean plasma duloxetine clearance about 15% that of age- and gender-matched healthy subjects, with a 5-fold increase in mean exposure (AUC). Although C_{max} was similar to normals in the cirrhotic patients, the half-life was about 3 times longer (*see* PRECAUTIONS). It is recommended that duloxetine not be administered to patients with any hepatic insufficiency (*see* DOSAGE AND ADMINISTRATION).

Drug-Drug Interactions (also *see* PRECAUTIONS, Drug Interactions)
Potential for Other Drugs to Affect Duloxetine
Both CYP1A2 and CYP2D6 are responsible for duloxetine metabolism.
Inhibitors of CYP1A2—When duloxetine was co-administered with fluvoxamine, a potent CYP1A2 inhibitor, to male subjects (n=14) the AUC was increased over 5-fold, the C_{max} was increased about 2.5-fold, and duloxetine $t_{1/2}$ was increased approximately 3-fold. Other drugs that inhibit CYP1A2 metabolism include cimetidine and quinolone antimicrobials such as ciprofloxacin and enoxacin.
Inhibitors of CYP2D6—Because CYP2D6 is involved in duloxetine metabolism, concomitant use of duloxetine with potent inhibitors of CYP2D6 would be expected to, and does, result in higher concentrations of duloxetine (*see* PRECAUTIONS, Drug Interactions).
Studies with Benzodiazepines
Lorazepam—Under steady-state conditions for duloxetine (60 mg Q 12 hours) and lorazepam (2 mg Q 12 hours), the pharmacokinetics of duloxetine were not affected by co-administration.
Temazepam—Under steady-state conditions for duloxetine (20 mg qhs) and temazepam (30 mg qhs), the pharmacokinetics of duloxetine were not affected by co-administration.
Potential for Duloxetine to Affect Other Drugs
Drugs Metabolized by CYP1A2—*In vitro* drug interaction studies demonstrate that duloxetine does not induce CYP1A2 activity. Therefore, an increase in the metabolism of CYP1A2 substrates (e.g., theophylline, caffeine) resulting from induction is not anticipated, although clinical studies of induction have not been performed. Although duloxetine is an inhibitor of the CYP1A2 isoform in *in vitro* studies, the pharmacokinetics of theophylline, a CYP1A2 substrate, were not significantly affected by co-administration with duloxetine (60 mg BID). Duloxetine is thus unlikely to have a clinically significant effect on the metabolism of CYP1A2 substrates.
Drugs Metabolized by CYP2D6—Duloxetine is a moderate inhibitor of CYP2D6 and increases the AUC and C_{max} of drugs metabolized by CYP2D6 (*see* PRECAUTIONS). Therefore, co-administration of duloxetine with other drugs that are extensively metabolized by this isozyme and that have a narrow therapeutic index should be approached with caution (*see* PRECAUTIONS, Drug Interactions).
Drugs Metabolized by CYP2C9—Duloxetine does not inhibit the *in vitro* enzyme activity of CYP2C9. Inhibition of the metabolism of CYP2C9 substrates is therefore not anticipated, although clinical studies have not been performed.
Drugs Metabolized by CYP3A—Results of *in vitro* studies demonstrate that duloxetine does not inhibit or induce CYP3A activity. Therefore, an increase or decrease in the metabolism of CYP3A substrates (e.g., oral contraceptives and other steroidal agents) resulting from induction or inhibition is not anticipated, although clinical studies have not been performed.
Studies with Benzodiazepines
Lorazepam—Under steady-state conditions for duloxetine (60 mg Q 12 hours) and lorazepam (2 mg Q 12 hours), the pharmacokinetics of lorazepam were not affected by co-administration.
Temazepam—Under steady-state conditions for duloxetine (20 mg qhs) and temazepam (30 mg qhs), the pharmacokinetics of temazepam were not affected by co-administration.
Drugs Highly Bound to Plasma Protein—Because duloxetine is highly bound to plasma protein, administration of duloxetine to a patient taking another drug that is highly protein bound may cause increased free concentrations of the other drug, potentially resulting in adverse events.

CLINICAL STUDIES

The efficacy of Cymbalta as a treatment for depression was established in 4 randomized, double-blind, placebo-controlled, fixed-dose studies in adult outpatients (18 to 83 years) meeting DSM-IV criteria for major depression. In 2 studies, patients were randomized to Cymbalta 60 mg once daily (N=123 and N=128, respectively) or placebo (N=122 and N=139, respectively) for 9 weeks; in the third study, patients were randomized to Cymbalta 20 or 40 mg twice daily (N=86 and N=91, respectively) or placebo (N=89) for 8 weeks; in the fourth study, patients were randomized to Cymbalta 40 or 60 mg twice daily (N=95 and N=93, respectively) or placebo (N=93) for 8 weeks. There is no evidence that doses greater than 60 mg/day confer any additional benefit.
In all 4 studies, Cymbalta demonstrated superiority over placebo as measured by improvement in the 17-item Hamilton Depression Rating Scale (HAMD-17) total score.
Analyses of the relationship between treatment outcome and age, gender, and race did not suggest any differential responsiveness on the basis of these patient characteristics.

INDICATIONS AND USAGE

Cymbalta is indicated for the treatment of major depressive disorder (MDD).
The efficacy of Cymbalta has been established in 8- and 9-week placebo-controlled trials of outpatients who met DSM-IV diagnostic criteria for major depressive disorder (*see* CLINICAL STUDIES).
A major depressive episode (DSM-IV) implies a prominent and relatively persistent (nearly every day for at least 2 weeks) depressed or dysphoric mood that usually interferes with daily functioning, and includes at least 5 of the following 9 symptoms: depressed mood, loss of interest in usual activities, significant change in weight and/or appetite, insomnia or hypersomnia, psychomotor agitation or retardation, increased fatigue, feelings of guilt or worthlessness, slowed thinking or impaired concentration, or a suicide attempt or suicidal ideation.
The effectiveness of Cymbalta in hospitalized patients with major depressive disorder has not been studied.
The effectiveness of Cymbalta in long-term use for major depressive disorder, that is, for more than 9 weeks, has not been systematically evaluated in controlled trials. The physician who elects to use Cymbalta for extended periods should periodically evaluate the long-term usefulness of the drug for the individual patient.

CONTRAINDICATIONS

Hypersensitivity
Duloxetine is contraindicated in patients with a known hypersensitivity to the product.

Monoamine Oxidase Inhibitors
Concomitant use in patients taking monoamine oxidase inhibitors (MAOIs) is contraindicated (*see* WARNINGS).

Uncontrolled Narrow-Angle Glaucoma
In clinical trials, duloxetine use was associated with an increased risk of mydriasis; therefore, its use should be avoided in patients with uncontrolled narrow-angle glaucoma.

WARNINGS

Clinical Worsening and Suicide Risk—Patients with major depressive disorder, both adult and pediatric, may experience worsening of their depression and/or the emergence of suicidal ideation and behavior (suicidality), whether or not they are taking antidepressant medications, and this risk may persist until significant remission occurs. Although there has been a long-standing concern that antidepressants may have a role in inducing worsening of depression and the emergence of suicidality in certain patients, a causal role for antidepressants in inducing such behaviors has not been established. **Nevertheless, patients being treated with antidepressants should be observed closely for clinical worsening and suicidality, especially at the beginning of a course of drug therapy, or at the time of dose changes, either increases or decreases.** Consideration should be given to changing the therapeutic regimen, including possibly discontinuing the medication, in patients whose depression is persistently worse or whose emergent suicidality is severe, abrupt in onset, or was not part of the patient's presenting symptoms.
Because of the possibility of co-morbidity between major depressive disorder and other psychiatric and nonpsychiatric disorders, the same precautions observed when treating patients with major depressive disorder should be observed when treating patients with other psychiatric and nonpsychiatric disorders.
The following symptoms - anxiety, agitation, panic attacks, insomnia, irritability, hostility (aggressiveness), impulsivity, akathisia (psychomotor restlessness), hypomania, and mania - have been reported in adult and pediatric patients being treated with antidepressants for major depressive disorder as well as for other indications, both psychiatric and nonpsychiatric. Although a causal link between the emergence of such symptoms and either the worsening of depression and/or the emergence of suicidal impulses has not been established, consideration should be given to changing the therapeutic regimen, including possibly discontinuing the medication, in patients for whom such symptoms are severe, abrupt in onset, or were not part of the patient's presenting symptoms.
Families and caregivers of patients being treated with antidepressants for major depressive disorder or other indications, both psychiatric and nonpsychiatric, should be alerted about the need to monitor patients for the emergence of agitation, irritability, and the other symptoms described above, as well as the emergence of suicidality, and to report such symptoms immediately to health care pro-

viders. Prescriptions for Cymbalta should be written for the smallest quantity of capsules consistent with good patient management, in order to reduce the risk of overdose.

If the decision has been made to discontinue treatment, medication should be tapered, as rapidly as is feasible, but with recognition that abrupt discontinuation can be associated with certain symptoms (*see* PRECAUTIONS *and* DOSAGE AND ADMINISTRATION, Discontinuing Cymbalta (duloxetine hydrochloride), for a description of the risks of discontinuation of Cymbalta).

A major depressive episode may be the initial presentation of bipolar disorder. It is generally believed (though not established in controlled trials) that treating such an episode with an antidepressant alone may increase the likelihood of precipitation of a mixed/manic episode in patients at risk for bipolar disorder. Whether any of the symptoms described above represent such a conversion is unknown. However, prior to initiating treatment with an antidepressant, patients should be adequately screened to determine if they are at risk for bipolar disorder; such screening should include a detailed psychiatric history, including a family history of suicide, bipolar disorder, and depression. It should be noted that Cymbalta is not approved for use in treating bipolar depression.

Monoamine Oxidase Inhibitors (MAOI)—In patients receiving a serotonin reuptake inhibitor in combination with a monoamine oxidase inhibitor, there have been reports of serious, sometimes fatal, reactions including hyperthermia, rigidity, myoclonus, autonomic instability with possible rapid fluctuations of vital signs, and mental status changes that include extreme agitation progressing to delirium and coma. These reactions have also been reported in patients who have recently discontinued serotonin reuptake inhibitors and are then started on an MAOI. Some cases presented with features resembling neuroleptic malignant syndrome. The effects of combined use of duloxetine and MAOIs have not been evaluated in humans or animals. Therefore, because duloxetine is an inhibitor of both serotonin and norepinephrine reuptake, it is recommended that duloxetine not be used in combination with an MAOI, or within at least 14 days of discontinuing treatment with an MAOI. Based on the half-life of duloxetine, at least 5 days should be allowed after stopping duloxetine before starting an MAOI.

PRECAUTIONS

General

Hepatotoxicity—Duloxetine increases the risk of elevation of serum transaminase levels. Liver transaminase elevations resulted in the discontinuation of 0.3% (27/8454) of duloxetine-treated patients. In these patients, the median time to detection of the transaminase elevation was about two months. In controlled trials in MDD, elevations of alanine transaminase (ALT) to >3 times the upper limit of normal occurred in 0.9% (8/930) of duloxetine-treated patients and in 0.3% (2/652) placebo-treated patients. In the full cohort of placebo-controlled trials in any indication, 1% (39/3732) of duloxetine-treated patients had a >3 times the upper limit of normal elevation of ALT compared to 0.2% (6/2568) of placebo-treated patients. In placebo-controlled studies using a fixed-dose design, there was evidence of a dose-response relationship for ALT and AST elevation of >3 times the upper limit of normal and >5 times the upper limit of normal, respectively.

The combination of transaminase elevations and elevated bilirubin, without evidence of obstruction, is generally recognized as an important predictor of severe liver injury. Three duloxetine patients had elevations of transaminases and bilirubin, but also had elevation of alkaline phosphatase, suggesting an obstructive process; in these patients, there was evidence of heavy alcohol use and this may have contributed to the abnormalities seen. Two placebo-treated patients also had transaminase elevations with elevated bilirubin. Because it is possible that duloxetine and alcohol may interact to cause liver injury, duloxetine should ordinarily not be prescribed to patients with substantial alcohol use.

Effect on Blood Pressure—In clinical trials, duloxetine treatment was associated with mean increases in blood pressure, averaging 2 mm Hg systolic and 0.5 mm Hg diastolic and an increase in the incidence of at least one measurement of systolic blood pressure over 140 mm Hg compared to placebo. Blood pressure should be measured prior to initiating treatment and periodically measured throughout treatment (*see* ADVERSE REACTIONS, Vital Sign Changes).

Activation of Mania/Hypomania—In placebo-controlled trials in patients with major depressive disorder, activation of mania or hypomania was reported in 0.1% (1/1139) of duloxetine-treated patients and 0.1% (1/777) of placebo-treated patients. Activation of mania/hypomania has been reported in a small proportion of patients with mood disorders who were treated with other marketed drugs effective in the treatment of major depressive disorder. As with these other agents, duloxetine should be used cautiously in patients with a history of mania.

Seizures—Duloxetine has not been systematically evaluated in patients with a seizure disorder, and such patients were excluded from clinical studies. In placebo-controlled clinical trials in patients with major depressive disorder, seizures occurred in 0.1% (1/1139) of patients treated with duloxetine and 0% (0/777) of patients treated with placebo. Like other drugs effective in the treatment of major depressive disorder, duloxetine should be prescribed with care in patients with a history of a seizure disorder.

Controlled Narrow-Angle Glaucoma—In clinical trials, duloxetine was associated with an increased risk of mydriasis; therefore, it should be used cautiously in patients with controlled narrow-angle glaucoma (*see* CONTRAINDICATIONS, Uncontrolled Narrow-Angle Glaucoma).

Discontinuation of Treatment with Cymbalta—Discontinuation symptoms have been systematically evaluated in patients taking Cymbalta. Following abrupt discontinuation in placebo-controlled clinical trials of up to 9-weeks duration, the following symptoms occurred at a rate greater than or equal to 2% and at a significantly higher rate in duloxetine-treated patients compared to those discontinuing from placebo: dizziness; nausea; headache; paresthesia; vomiting; irritability; and nightmare.

During marketing of other SSRIs and SNRIs (serotonin and norepinephrine reuptake inhibitors), there have been spontaneous reports of adverse events occurring upon discontinuation of these drugs, particularly when abrupt, including the following: dysphoric mood, irritability, agitation, dizziness, sensory disturbances (e.g., paresthesias such as electric shock sensations), anxiety, confusion, headache, lethargy, emotional lability, insomnia, hypomania, tinnitus, and seizures. Although these events are generally self-limiting, some have been reported to be severe.

Patients should be monitored for these symptoms when discontinuing treatment with Cymbalta. A gradual reduction in the dose rather than abrupt cessation is recommended whenever possible. If intolerable symptoms occur following a decrease in the dose or upon discontinuation of treatment, then resuming the previously prescribed dose may be considered. Subsequently, the physician may continue decreasing the dose but at a more gradual rate (*see* DOSAGE AND ADMINISTRATION).

Use in Patients with Concomitant Illness—Clinical experience with duloxetine in patients with concomitant systemic illnesses is limited. There is no information on the effect that alterations in gastric motility may have on the stability of duloxetine's enteric coating. As duloxetine is rapidly hydrolyzed in acidic media to naphthol, caution is advised in using duloxetine in patients with conditions that may slow gastric emptying.

Duloxetine has not been systematically evaluated in patients with a recent history of myocardial infarction or unstable coronary artery disease. Patients with these diagnoses were generally excluded from clinical studies during the product's premarketing testing. However, the electrocardiograms of 321 patients who received duloxetine in placebo-controlled clinical trials and had qualitatively normal ECGs at baseline were evaluated; duloxetine was not associated with the development of clinically significant ECG abnormalities (*see* ADVERSE REACTIONS, Electrocardiogram Changes).

Increased plasma concentrations of duloxetine, and especially of its metabolites, occur in patients with ESRD and severe renal impairment (creatinine clearance <30 mL/min). For this reason, duloxetine is not recommended for patients with ESRD (*see* CLINICAL PHARMACOLOGY *and* DOSAGE AND ADMINISTRATION).

Markedly increased exposure to duloxetine occurs in patients with hepatic insufficiency and duloxetine should not be administered to these patients (*see* CLINICAL PHARMACOLOGY *and* DOSAGE AND ADMINISTRATION).

Information for Patients

Physicians are advised to discuss the following issues with patients for whom they prescribe Cymbalta.

Patients and their families should be encouraged to be alert to the emergence of anxiety, agitation, panic attacks, insomnia, irritability, hostility, impulsivity, akathisia, hypomania, mania, worsening of depression, and suicidal ideation, especially early during antidepressant treatment. Such symptoms should be reported to the patient's physician, especially if they are severe, abrupt in onset, or were not part of the patient's presenting symptoms.

Duloxetine should be swallowed whole and should not be chewed or crushed, nor should the contents be sprinkled on food or mixed with liquids. All of these might affect the enteric coating.

Any psychoactive drug may impair judgment, thinking, or motor skills. Although in controlled studies duloxetine has not been shown to impair psychomotor performance, cognitive function, or memory, it may be associated with sedation. Therefore, patients should be cautioned about operating hazardous machinery including automobiles, until they are reasonably certain that duloxetine therapy does not affect their ability to engage in such activities.

Patients should be advised to inform their physicians if they are taking, or plan to take, any prescription or over-the-counter medications, since there is a potential for interactions.

Although duloxetine does not increase the impairment of mental and motor skills caused by alcohol, use of duloxetine concomitantly with heavy alcohol intake may be associated with severe liver injury. For this reason, duloxetine should ordinarily not be prescribed for patients with substantial alcohol use.

Patients should be advised to notify their physician if they become pregnant or intend to become pregnant during therapy.

Patients should be advised to notify their physician if they are breast-feeding.

While patients may notice improvement with duloxetine therapy in 1 to 4 weeks, they should be advised to continue therapy as directed.

Laboratory Tests

No specific laboratory tests are recommended.

Drug Interactions (also *see* CLINICAL PHARMACOLOGY, Drug-Drug Interactions)

Potential for Other Drugs to Affect Duloxetine

Both CYP1A2 and CYP2D6 are responsible for duloxetine metabolism.

Inhibitors of CYP1A2—Concomitant use of duloxetine with fluvoxamine, an inhibitor of CYP1A2, results in approximately a 6-fold increase in AUC and about a 2.5-fold increase in C_{max} of duloxetine. Some quinolone antibiotics would be expected to have similar effects and these combinations should be avoided.

Inhibitors of CYP2D6—Because CYP2D6 is involved in duloxetine metabolism, concomitant use of duloxetine with potent inhibitors of CYP2D6 may result in higher concentrations of duloxetine. Paroxetine (20 mg QD) increased the concentration of duloxetine (40 mg QD) by about 60%, and greater degrees of inhibition are expected with higher doses of paroxetine. Similar effects would be expected with other potent CYP2D6 inhibitors (e.g., fluoxetine, quinidine).

Potential for Duloxetine to Affect Other Drugs

Drugs Metabolized by CYP1A2 —*In vitro* drug interaction studies demonstrate that duloxetine does not induce CYP1A2 activity, and it is unlikely to have a clinically significant effect on the metabolism of CYP1A2 substrates (*see* CLINICAL PHARMACOLOGY, Drug Interactions).

Drugs Metabolized by CYP2D6—Duloxetine is a moderate inhibitor of CYP2D6. When duloxetine was administered (at a dose of 60 mg BID) in conjunction with a single 50-mg dose of desipramine, a CYP2D6 substrate, the AUC of desipramine increased 3-fold. Therefore, co-administration of duloxetine with other drugs that are extensively metabolized by this isozyme and which have a narrow therapeutic index, including certain antidepressants (tricyclic antidepressants [TCAs], such as nortriptyline, amitriptyline, and imipramine), phenothiazines and Type 1C antiarrhythmics (e.g., propafenone, flecainide), should be approached with caution. Plasma TCA concentrations may need to be monitored and the dose of the TCA may need to be reduced if a TCA is co-administered with duloxetine. Because of the risk of serious ventricular arrhythmias and sudden death potentially associated with elevated plasma levels of thioridazine, duloxetine and thioridazine should not be co-administered.

Drugs Metabolized by CYP3A—Results of *in vitro* studies demonstrate that duloxetine does not inhibit or induce CYP3A activity (*see* CLINICAL PHARMACOLOGY, Drug Interactions).

Duloxetine May Have a Clinically Important Interaction with the Following Other Drugs:

Alcohol—When duloxetine and ethanol were administered several hours apart so that peak concentrations of each would coincide, duloxetine did not increase the impairment of mental and motor skills caused by alcohol.

In the duloxetine clinical trials database, three duloxetine-treated patients had liver injury as manifested by ALT and total bilirubin elevations, with evidence of obstruction. Substantial intercurrent ethanol use was present in each of these cases, and this may have contributed to the abnormalities seen (*see* PRECAUTIONS, Hepatotoxicity).

CNS Acting Drugs—Given the primary CNS effects of duloxetine, it should be used with caution when it is taken in combination with or substituted for other centrally acting drugs, including those with a similar mechanism of action.

Potential for Interaction with Drugs that Affect Gastric Acidity—Duloxetine has an enteric coating that resists dissolution until reaching a segment of the gastrointestinal tract where the pH exceeds 5.5. In extremely acidic conditions, duloxetine, unprotected by the enteric coating, may undergo hydrolysis to form naphthol. Drugs that raise the gastrointestinal pH may lead to an earlier release of duloxetine. However, co-administration of duloxetine with aluminum- and magnesium-containing antacids (51 mEq) or duloxetine with famotidine, had no significant effect on the rate or extent of duloxetine absorption after administration of a 40-mg oral dose. It is unknown whether the concomitant administration of proton pump inhibitors affects duloxetine absorption.

Monoamine Oxidase Inhibitors—*See* CONTRAINDICATIONS *and* WARNINGS.

Carcinogenesis, Mutagenesis, Impairment of Fertility

Carcinogenesis—Duloxetine was administered in the diet to mice and rats for 2 years.

In female mice receiving duloxetine at dietary doses of approximately 140 mg/kg/day (11 times the maximum recommended human dose [MRHD] of 60 mg/day on a mg/m^2 basis), there was an increased incidence of hepatocellular adenomas and carcinomas; the no-effect level was approximately 50 mg/kg (4 times the MRHD on a mg/m^2 basis). Tumor incidence was not increased in male mice receiving duloxetine at dietary doses up to approximately 100 mg/kg/day (8 times the MRHD on a mg/m^2 basis).

In rats, dietary doses of duloxetine up to approximately 27 mg/kg/day in females (4 times the MRHD on a mg/m^2

Continued on next page

*** Identi-Code® symbol. This product information was prepared in June 2004. Current information on these and other products of Eli Lilly and Company may be obtained by direct inquiry to Lilly Research Laboratories, Lilly Corporate Center, Indianapolis, Indiana 46285, (800) 545-5979.**

Cymbalta—Cont.

basis) or approximately 36 mg/kg/day in males (6 times the MRHD on a mg/m^2 basis) did not increase the incidence of tumors.

Mutagenesis—Duloxetine was not mutagenic in the *in vitro* bacterial reverse mutation assay (Ames test) and was not clastogenic in an *in vivo* chromosomal aberration test in mouse bone marrow cells. Additionally, duloxetine was not genotoxic in an *in vitro* mammalian forward gene mutation assay in mouse lymphoma cells or in an *in vitro* unscheduled DNA synthesis (UDS) assay in primary rat hepatocytes, and did not induce sister chromatid exchange in Chinese hamster bone marrow *in vivo*.

Impairment of Fertility—Duloxetine administered orally to either male or female rats prior to and throughout mating at daily doses up to 45 mg/kg (7 times the maximum recommended human dose [MRHD] on a mg/m^2 basis) did not alter mating or fertility.

Pregnancy

Pregnancy-Nonteratogenic Effects—Neonates exposed to SSRIs or serotonin and norepinephrine reuptake inhibitors (SNRIs), late in the third trimester have developed complications requiring prolonged hospitalization, respiratory support, and tube feeding. Such complications can arise immediately upon delivery. Reported clinical findings have included respiratory distress, cyanosis, apnea, seizures, temperature instability, feeding difficulty, vomiting, hypoglycemia, hypotonia, hypertonia, hyperreflexia, tremor, jitteriness, irritability, and constant crying. These features are consistent with either a direct toxic effect of SSRIs and SNRIs or, possibly, a drug discontinuation syndrome. It should be noted that, in some cases, the clinical picture is consistent with serotonin syndrome (*see* WARNINGS, Monoamine Oxidase Inhibitors). When treating a pregnant woman with Cymbalta during the third trimester, the physician should carefully consider the potential risks and benefits of treatment (*see* DOSAGE AND ADMINISTRATION).

Pregnancy Category C —In animal reproduction studies, duloxetine has been shown to have adverse effects on embryo/fetal and postnatal development.

When duloxetine was administered orally to pregnant rats and rabbits during the period of organogenesis, there was no evidence of teratogenicity at doses up to 45 mg/kg/day (7 and 15 times the maximum recommended human dose [MRHD] on a mg/m^2 basis, in rats and rabbits, respectively). However, fetal weights were decreased at this dose, with a no-effect level of 10 mg/kg (2 and 3 times the MRHD on a mg/m^2 basis, in rats and rabbits, respectively).

When duloxetine was administered orally to pregnant rats throughout gestation and lactation, the survival of pups to 1 day postpartum and pup body weights at birth and during the lactation period were decreased following maternal exposure to 30 mg/kg/day (5 times the MRHD on a mg/m^2 basis), with a no-effect level of 10 mg/kg. Furthermore, behaviors consistent with increased reactivity, such as increased startle response to noise and decreased habituation of locomotor activity, were observed in pups following maternal exposure to 30 mg/kg/day. Post-weaning growth and reproductive performance of the progeny were not affected adversely by maternal duloxetine treatment.

There are no adequate and well-controlled studies in pregnant women; therefore, duloxetine should be used during pregnancy only if the potential benefit justifies the potential risk to the fetus.

Labor and Delivery

The effect of duloxetine on labor and delivery in humans is unknown. Duloxetine should be used during labor and delivery only if the potential benefit justifies the potential risk to the fetus.

Nursing Mothers

Duloxetine and/or its metabolites are excreted into the milk of lactating rats. It is unknown whether or not duloxetine and/or its metabolites are excreted into human milk, but nursing while on duloxetine is not recommended.

Pediatric Use

Safety and efficacy in pediatric patients have not been established (*see* WARNINGS, Clinical Worsening and Suicide Risk).

Geriatric Use

Of the 2418 patients in clinical studies of duloxetine, 5.9% (143) were 65 years of age or over. No overall differences in safety or effectiveness were observed between these subjects and younger subjects, and other reported clinical experience has not identified differences in responses between the elderly and younger patients, but greater sensitivity of some older individuals cannot be ruled out.

ADVERSE REACTIONS

Duloxetine has been evaluated for safety in 2418 patients diagnosed with major depressive disorder who participated in multiple-dose premarketing trials, representing 1099 patient-years of exposure. Among these 2418 duloxetine-treated patients, 1139 patients participated in eight 8- or 9-week, placebo-controlled trials at doses ranging from 40 to 120 mg/day, while the remaining 1279 patients were followed for up to 1 year in an open-label safety study using flexible doses from 80 to 120 mg/day. Two placebo-controlled studies with doses of 80 and 120 mg/day had 6-month maintenance extensions. Of these 2418 patients, 993 duloxetine-treated patients were exposed for at least 180 days and 445 duloxetine-treated patients were exposed for at least 1 year.

Adverse reactions were assessed by collecting adverse events, results of physical examinations, vital signs, weights, laboratory analyses, and ECGs.

Clinical investigators recorded adverse events using descriptive terminology of their own choosing. To provide a meaningful estimate of the proportion of individuals experiencing adverse events, grouping similar types of events into a smaller number of standardized event categories is necessary. In the tables and tabulations that follow, MedDRA terminology has been used to classify reported adverse events.

The stated frequencies of adverse events represent the proportion of individuals who experienced, at least once, a treatment-emergent adverse event of the type listed. An event was considered treatment-emergent if it occurred for the first time or worsened while receiving therapy following baseline evaluation. Events reported during the studies were not necessarily caused by the therapy, and the frequencies do not reflect investigator impression (assessment) of causality.

The cited figures provide the prescriber with some basis for estimating the relative contribution of drug and non-drug factors to the adverse event incidence rate in the population studied. The prescriber should be aware that the figures in the tables and tabulations cannot be used to predict the incidence of adverse events in the course of usual medical practice where patient characteristics and other factors differ from those that prevailed in the clinical trials. Similarly, the cited frequencies cannot be compared with figures obtained from other clinical investigations involving different treatments, uses, and investigators.

Adverse Events Reported as Reasons for Discontinuation of Treatment in Placebo-Controlled Trials

Approximately 10% of the 1139 patients who received duloxetine in the placebo-controlled trials discontinued treatment due to an adverse event, compared with 4% of the 777 patients receiving placebo. Nausea (duloxetine 1.4%, placebo 0.1%) was the only common adverse event reported as reason for discontinuation and considered to be drug-related (i.e., discontinuation occurring in at least 1% of the duloxetine-treated patients and at a rate of at least twice that of placebo).

Adverse Events Occurring at an Incidence of 2% or More Among Duloxetine-Treated Patients in Placebo-Controlled Trials

Table 1 gives the incidence of treatment-emergent adverse events that occurred in 2% or more of patients treated with duloxetine in the acute phase of MDD placebo-controlled trials and with an incidence greater than placebo. The most commonly observed adverse events in duloxetine-treated MDD patients (incidence of 5% or greater and at least twice the incidence in placebo patients) were: nausea; dry mouth; constipation; decreased appetite; fatigue; somnolence; and increased sweating (*see* Table 1).

[See table 1 at left]

Table 1: Treatment-Emergent Adverse Events Incidence in Placebo-Controlled Trials[1]

System Organ Class / Adverse Event	Percentage of Patients Reporting Event	
	Duloxetine (N=1139)	Placebo (N=777)
Gastrointestinal Disorders		
Nausea	20	7
Dry mouth	15	6
Constipation	11	4
Diarrhea	8	6
Vomiting	5	3
Metabolism and Nutrition Disorders		
Appetite decreased[2]	8	2
Investigations		
Weight decreased	2	1
General Disorders and Administration Site Conditions		
Fatigue	8	4
Nervous System Disorders		
Dizziness	9	5
Somnolence	7	3
Tremor	3	1
Skin and Subcutaneous Tissue Disorders		
Sweating increased	6	2
Vascular Disorders		
Hot flushes	2	1
Eye Disorders		
Vision blurred	4	1
Psychiatric Disorders		
Insomnia[3]	11	6
Anxiety	3	2
Libido decreased	3	1
Orgasm abnormal[4]	3	1
Reproductive System and Breast Disorders		
Erectile dysfunction[5]	4	1
Ejaculation delayed[5]	3	1
Ejaculatory dysfunction[5,6]	3	1

[1] Events reported by at least 2% of patients treated with duloxetine and more often with placebo. The following events were reported by at least 2% of patients treated with duloxetine and had an incidence equal to or less than placebo: upper abdominal pain, palpitations, dyspepsia, back pain, arthralgia, headache, pharyngitis, cough, nasopharyngitis, and upper respiratory tract infection.

[2] Term includes anorexia.

[3] Term includes middle insomnia.

[4] Term includes anorgasmia.

[5] Male patients only.

[6] Term includes ejaculation disorder and ejaculation failure.

Adverse events seen in men and women were generally similar except for effects on sexual function (described below). Clinical studies of Cymbalta did not suggest a difference in adverse event rates in people over or under 65 years of age. There were too few non-Caucasian patients studied to determine if these patients responded differently from Caucasian patients.

Effects on Male and Female Sexual Function

Although changes in sexual desire, sexual performance and sexual satisfaction often occur as manifestations of a psychiatric disorder, they may also be a consequence of pharmacologic treatment. Reliable estimates of the incidence and severity of untoward experiences involving sexual desire, performance and satisfaction are difficult to obtain, however, in part because patients and physicians may be reluctant to discuss them. Accordingly, estimates of the incidence of untoward sexual experience and performance cited in product labeling are likely to underestimate their actual incidence. Table 2 displays the incidence of sexual side effects spontaneously reported by at least 2% of either male or female patients taking duloxetine in placebo-controlled trials.

[See table 2 at top of next page]

Because adverse sexual events are presumed to be voluntarily underreported, the Arizona Sexual Experience Scale (ASEX), a validated measure designed to identify sexual side effects, was used prospectively in 4 placebo-controlled trials. In these trials, as shown in Table 3 below, patients treated with duloxetine experienced significantly more sexual dysfunction, as measured by the total score on the ASEX, than did patients treated with placebo. Gender analysis showed that this difference occurred only in males. Males treated with duloxetine experienced more difficulty with ability to reach orgasm (ASEX Item 4) than males treated with placebo. Females did not experience more sexual dysfunction on duloxetine than on placebo as measured by ASEX total score. These studies did not, however, include an active control drug with known effects on female sexual dysfunction, so that there is no evidence that its effects differ from other antidepressants. Negative numbers signify

an improvement from a baseline level of dysfunction, which is commonly seen in depressed patients. Physicians should routinely inquire about possible sexual side effects.
[See table 3 at right]

Urinary Hesitation
Duloxetine is in a class of drugs known to affect urethral resistance. If symptoms of urinary hesitation develop during treatment with duloxetine, consideration should be given to the possibility that they might be drug-related.

Laboratory Changes
Duloxetine treatment, for up to 9-weeks in placebo-controlled clinical trials, was associated with small mean increases from baseline to endpoint in ALT, AST, CPK, and alkaline phosphatase; infrequent, modest, transient, abnormal values were observed for these analytes in duloxetine-treated patients when compared with placebo-treated patients (*see* PRECAUTIONS).

Vital Sign Changes
Duloxetine treatment, for up to 9-weeks in placebo-controlled clinical trials of 40 to 120 mg daily doses caused increases in blood pressure, averaging 2 mm Hg systolic and 0.5 mm Hg diastolic compared to placebo and an increase in the incidence of at least one measurement of systolic blood pressure over 140 mm Hg (*see* PRECAUTIONS).
Duloxetine treatment, for up to 9-weeks in placebo-controlled clinical trials caused a small increase in heart rate compared to placebo of about 2 beats per minute.

Weight Changes
In placebo-controlled clinical trials, patients treated with duloxetine for up to 9-weeks experienced a mean weight loss of approximately 0.5 kg, compared with a mean weight gain of approximately 0.2 kg in placebo-treated patients.

Electrocardiogram Changes
Electrocardiograms were obtained from 321 duloxetine-treated patients with major depressive disorder and 169 placebo-treated patients in clinical trials lasting up to 8-weeks. The rate-corrected QT (QTc) interval in duloxetine-treated patients did not differ from that seen in placebo-treated patients. No clinically significant differences were observed for QT, PR, and QRS intervals between duloxetine-treated and placebo-treated patients.

Other Adverse Events Observed During the Premarketing Evaluation of Duloxetine
Following is a list of modified MedDRA terms that reflect treatment-emergent adverse events as defined in the introduction to the ADVERSE REACTIONS section reported by patients treated with duloxetine at multiple doses throughout the dose range studied during any phase of a trial within the premarketing database. The events included are those not already listed elsewhere in ADVERSE REACTIONS and not considered in the WARNINGS and PRECAUTIONS sections, that were reported with an incidence of greater than or equal to 0.05%, are not common as background events and were considered possibly drug related (e.g., because of the drug's pharmacology) or potentially important.
It is important to emphasize that, although the events reported occurred during treatment with duloxetine, they were not necessarily caused by it. Events are further categorized by body system and listed in order of decreasing frequency according to the following definitions: frequent adverse events are those occurring in at least 1/100 patients (only those not already listed in the tabulated results from placebo-controlled trials appear in this listing); infrequent adverse events are those occurring in 1/100 to 1/1000 patients; rare events are those occurring in fewer than 1/1000 patients.

Blood and Lymphatic System Disorders—*Infrequent:* anemia, leukopenia, increased white blood cell count, lymphadenopathy, and thrombocytopenia.

Gastrointestinal Disorders—*Frequent:* gastritis; *Infrequent:* blood in stool, colitis, dysphagia, esophageal stenosis acquired, gastric ulcer, gingivitis, irritable bowel syndrome, and lower abdominal pain.

Psychiatric Disorders—*Frequent:* initial insomnia, irritability, lethargy, nervousness, nightmare, restlessness, and sleep disorder; *Infrequent:* completed suicide, mania, mood swings, pressure of speech, sluggishness, and suicide attempt.

Renal and Urinary Disorders—*Frequent:* dysuria; *Infrequent:* micturition urgency, urinary hesitation, urinary incontinence, urinary retention, and urine flow decreased.

Skin and Subcutaneous Tissue Disorders—*Frequent:* night sweats, pruritus, and rash; *Infrequent:* acne, alopecia, cold sweat, ecchymosis, eczema, erythema, face edema, increased tendency to bruise, and photosensitivity reaction.

Vascular Disorders—*Infrequent:* peripheral edema and phlebitis.

DRUG ABUSE AND DEPENDENCE

Controlled Substance Class
Duloxetine is not a controlled substance.

Physical and Psychological Dependence
In animal studies, duloxetine did not demonstrate barbiturate-like (depressant) abuse potential. In drug dependence studies, duloxetine did not demonstrate dependence-producing potential in rats.
While duloxetine has not been systematically studied in humans for its potential for abuse, there was no indication of drug-seeking behavior in the clinical trials. However, it is not possible to predict on the basis of premarketing experience the extent to which a CNS active drug will be misused, diverted, and/or abused once marketed. Consequently, physicians should carefully evaluate patients for a history of drug abuse and follow such patients closely, observing them for signs of misuse or abuse of duloxetine (e.g., development of tolerance, incrementation of dose, drug-seeking behavior).

Table 2: Treatment-Emergent Sexual Dysfunction-Related Adverse Events Incidence in Placebo-Controlled Trials[1]

Adverse Event	Percentage of Patients Reporting Event			
	% Male Patients		% Female Patients	
	Duloxetine (N=378)	Placebo (N=247)	Duloxetine (N=761)	Placebo (N=530)
Orgasm abnormal[2]	4	1	2	0
Ejaculatory dysfunction[3]	3	1	NA	NA
Libido decreased	6	2	1	0
Erectile dysfunction	4	1	NA	NA
Ejaculation delayed	3	1	NA	NA

[1] Events reported by at least 2% of patients treated with duloxetine and more often than with placebo.
[2] Term includes anorgasmia.
[3] Term includes ejaculation disorder and ejaculation failure.
NA=Not applicable.

Table 3: Mean Change in ASEX Scores by Gender in Placebo-Controlled Trials

Adverse Event	Male Patients		Female Patients	
	Duloxetine (n=175)	Placebo (n=83)	Duloxetine (n=241)	Placebo (n=126)
ASEX Total (Items 1–5)	0.56*	-1.07	-1.15	-1.07
Item 1—Sex drive	-0.07	-0.12	-0.32	-0.24
Item 2—Arousal	0.01	-0.26	-0.21	-0.18
Item 3—Ability to achieve erection (men); Lubrication (women)	0.03	-0.25	-0.17	-0.18
Item 4—Ease of reaching orgasm	0.40**	-0.24	-0.09	-0.13
Item 5—Orgasm satisfaction	0.09	-0.13	-0.11	-0.17

n=Number of patients with non-missing change score for ASEX total.
* p=0.013 versus placebo.
**p<0.001 versus placebo.

OVERDOSAGE

There is limited clinical experience with duloxetine overdose in humans. In premarketing clinical trials, as of November 2002, no cases of fatal acute overdose of duloxetine have been reported. Four non-fatal acute ingestions of duloxetine (300 to 1400 mg), alone or in combination with other drugs, have been reported.

Management of Overdose
There is no specific antidote to duloxetine. In case of acute overdose, treatment should consist of those general measures employed in the management of overdose with any drug effective in the treatment of major depressive disorder. An adequate airway, oxygenation, and ventilation should be assured, and cardiac rhythm and vital signs should be monitored. Induction of emesis is not recommended. Gastric lavage with a large-bore orogastric tube with appropriate airway protection, if needed, may be indicated if performed soon after ingestion or in symptomatic patients.
Activated charcoal may be useful in limiting absorption of duloxetine from the gastrointestinal tract. Administration of activated charcoal has been shown to decrease AUC and C_{max} by an average of one-third, although some subjects had a limited effect of activated charcoal. Due to the large volume of distribution of this drug, forced diuresis, dialysis, hemoperfusion, and exchange transfusion are unlikely to be beneficial.
In managing overdose, the possibility of multiple drug involvement should be considered. A specific caution involves patients who are taking or have recently taken duloxetine and might ingest excessive quantities of a TCA. In such a case, decreased clearance of the parent tricyclic and/or its active metabolite may increase the possibility of clinically significant sequelae and extend the time needed for close medical observation (*see* PRECAUTIONS, Drug Interactions). The physician should consider contacting a poison control center for additional information on the treatment of any overdose. Telephone numbers for certified poison control centers are listed in the *Physicians' Desk Reference* (PDR).

DOSAGE AND ADMINISTRATION

Initial Treatment
Cymbalta should be administered at a total dose of 40 mg/day (given as 20 mg BID) to 60 mg/day (given either once a day or as 30 mg BID) without regard to meals.
There is no evidence that doses greater than 60 mg/day confer any additional benefits.

Maintenance/Continuation/Extended Treatment
It is generally agreed that acute episodes of major depression require several months or longer of sustained pharmacologic therapy. There is insufficient evidence available to answer the question of how long a patient should continue to be treated with Cymbalta. Patients should be periodically reassessed to determine the need for maintenance treatment and the appropriate dose for such treatment.

Special Populations
Dosage for Renally Impaired Patients—Cymbalta is not recommended for patients with end stage renal disease (ESRD) (*see* CLINICAL PHARMACOLOGY).
Dosage for Hepatically Impaired Patients—It is recommended that Cymbalta not be administered to patients with any hepatic insufficiency (*see* CLINICAL PHARMACOLOGY *and* PRECAUTIONS).
Dosage for Elderly Patients—No dose adjustment is recommended for elderly patients on the basis of age. As with any drugs effective in the treatment of major depressive disorder, however, caution should be exercised in treating the elderly. When individualizing the dosage, extra care should be taken when increasing the dose.
Treatment of Pregnant Women During the Third Trimester—Neonates exposed to SSRIs or SNRIs, late in the third trimester have developed complications requiring prolonged hospitalization, respiratory support, and tube feeding (*see* PRECAUTIONS). When treating pregnant women with Cymbalta during the third trimester, the physician should carefully consider the potential risks and benefits of treatment. The physician may consider tapering Cymbalta in the third trimester.

Discontinuing Cymbalta (duloxetine hydrochloride)
Symptoms associated with discontinuation of Cymbalta and other SSRIs and SNRIs have been reported (*see* PRECAUTIONS). Patients should be monitored for these symptoms when discontinuing treatment. A gradual reduction in the dose rather than abrupt cessation is recommended whenever possible. If intolerable symptoms occur following a decrease in the dose or upon discontinuation of treatment, then resuming the previously prescribed dose may be considered. Subsequently, the physician may continue decreasing the dose but at a more gradual rate.

Switching Patients to or from a Monoamine Oxidase Inhibitor
At least 14 days should elapse between discontinuation of an MAOI and initiation of therapy with Cymbalta. In addition, at least 5 days should be allowed after stopping Cymbalta before starting an MAOI (*see* CONTRAINDICATIONS *and* WARNINGS).

HOW SUPPLIED

Cymbalta® (duloxetine hydrochloride) capsules are available in 20, 30, and 60 mg strengths.
The 20 mg* capsule has an opaque green body and cap, and is imprinted with "20 mg" on the body and "LILLY 3235" on the cap:
NDC 0002-3235-60 (PU3235)—Bottles of 60
NDC 0002-3235-33 (PU3235)—(ID† 100) Blisters
The 30 mg* capsule has an opaque white body and opaque blue cap, and is imprinted with "30 mg" on the body and "LILLY 3240" on the cap:
NDC 0002-3240-30 (PU3240)—Bottles of 30
NDC 0002-3240-90 (PU3240)—Bottles of 90
NDC 0002-3240-04 (PU3240)—Bottles of 1000
NDC 0002-3240-33 (PU3240)—(ID†100) Blisters
The 60 mg* capsule has an opaque green body and opaque blue cap, and is imprinted with "60 mg" on the body and "LILLY 3237" on the cap:

Continued on next page

*** Identi-Code® symbol. This product information was prepared in June 2004. Current information on these and other products of Eli Lilly and Company may be obtained by direct inquiry to Lilly Research Laboratories, Lilly Corporate Center, Indianapolis, Indiana 46285, (800) 545-5979.**

Cymbalta—Cont.

NDC 0002-3237-30 (PU3237)—Bottles of 30
NDC 0002-3237-90 (PU3237)—Bottles of 90
NDC 0002-3237-04 (PU3237)—Bottles of 1000
NDC 0002-3237-33 (PU3237)—(ID† 100) Blisters

*equivalent to duloxetine base.
†Identi-Dose® (unit dose medication, Lilly).
Store at 25°C (77°F); excursions permitted to 15–30°C (59–86°F) [see USP Controlled Room Temperature].
Literature issued August 3, 2004
Eli Lilly and Company
Indianapolis, IN 46285, USA
www.Cymbalta.com
PV 3600 AMP PRINTED IN USA

Shown in Product Identification Guide, page 320

EVISTA® ℞
[*ē-vĭs-tă*]
(Raloxifene Hydrochloride)
60 mg Tablets

DESCRIPTION
EVISTA® (raloxifene hydrochloride) is a selective estrogen receptor modulator (SERM) that belongs to the benzothiophene class of compounds. The chemical structure is:

The chemical designation is methanone, [6-hydroxy-2-(4-hydroxyphenyl)benzo[*b*]thien-3-yl]-[4-[2-(1-piperidinyl) ethoxy]phenyl]-, hydrochloride. Raloxifene hydrochloride (HCl) has the empirical formula $C_{28}H_{27}NO_4S \cdot HCl$, which corresponds to a molecular weight of 510.05. Raloxifene HCl is an off-white to pale-yellow solid that is very slightly soluble in water.
EVISTA is supplied in a tablet dosage form for oral administration. Each EVISTA tablet contains 60 mg of raloxifene HCl, which is the molar equivalent of 55.71 mg of free base. Inactive ingredients include anhydrous lactose, carnauba wax, crospovidone, FD&C Blue No. 2 aluminum lake, hypromellose, lactose monohydrate, magnesium stearate, modified pharmaceutical glaze, polyethylene glycol, polysorbate 80, povidone, propylene glycol, and titanium dioxide.

CLINICAL PHARMACOLOGY
Mechanism of Action
Decreases in estrogen levels after oophorectomy or menopause lead to increases in bone resorption and accelerated bone loss. Bone is initially lost rapidly because the compensatory increase in bone formation is inadequate to offset resorptive losses. In addition to loss of estrogen, this imbalance between resorption and formation may be due to age-related impairment of osteoblasts or their precursors. In some women, these changes will eventually lead to decreased bone mass, osteoporosis, and increased risk for fractures, particularly of the spine, hip, and wrist. Vertebral fractures are the most common type of osteoporotic fracture in postmenopausal women.
The biological actions of raloxifene are largely mediated through binding to estrogen receptors. This binding results in activation of certain estrogenic pathways and blockade of others. Thus, raloxifene is a SERM.
Raloxifene decreases resorption of bone and reduces biochemical markers of bone turnover to the premenopausal range. These effects on bone are manifested as reductions in the serum and urine levels of bone turnover markers, decreases in bone resorption based on radiocalcium kinetics studies, increases in bone mineral density (BMD), and decreases in incidence of fractures. Raloxifene also has effects on lipid metabolism. Raloxifene decreases total and LDL cholesterol levels but does not increase triglyceride levels (*see* PRECAUTIONS). It does not change total HDL cholesterol levels. Preclinical data demonstrate that raloxifene is an estrogen antagonist in uterine and breast tissues. Clinical trial data (through a median of 42 months) suggest that EVISTA lacks estrogen-like effects on the uterus and breast tissue.

Pharmacokinetics
The disposition of raloxifene has been evaluated in more than 3000 postmenopausal women in selected raloxifene osteoporosis treatment and prevention clinical trials using a population approach. Pharmacokinetic data were also obtained in conventional pharmacology studies in 292 postmenopausal women. Raloxifene exhibits high within-subject variability (approximately 30% coefficient of variation) of most pharmacokinetic parameters. Table 1 summarizes the pharmacokinetic parameters of raloxifene.
Absorption
Raloxifene is absorbed rapidly after oral administration. Approximately 60% of an oral dose is absorbed, but presystemic glucuronide conjugation is extensive. Absolute bioavailability of raloxifene is 2.0%. The time to reach average maximum plasma concentration and bioavailability are functions of systemic interconversion and enterohepatic cycling of raloxifene and its glucuronide metabolites.
Administration of raloxifene HCl with a standardized, high-fat meal increases the absorption of raloxifene (C_{max} 28% and AUC 16%), but does not lead to clinically meaningful changes in systemic exposure. EVISTA can be administered without regard to meals.
Distribution
Following oral administration of single doses ranging from 30 to 150 mg of raloxifene HCl, the apparent volume of distribution is 2348 L/kg and is not dose dependent.
Raloxifene and the monoglucuronide conjugates are highly (95%) bound to plasma proteins. Raloxifene binds to both albumin and α1-acid glycoprotein, but not to sex-steroid binding globulin.
Metabolism
Biotransformation and disposition of raloxifene in humans have been determined following oral administration of ^{14}C-labeled raloxifene. Raloxifene undergoes extensive first-pass metabolism to the glucuronide conjugates: raloxifene-4′-glucuronide, raloxifene-6-glucuronide, and raloxifene-6, 4′-diglucuronide. No other metabolites have been detected, providing strong evidence that raloxifene is not metabolized by cytochrome P450 pathways. Unconjugated raloxifene comprises less than 1% of the total radiolabeled material in plasma. The terminal log-linear portions of the plasma concentration curves for raloxifene and the glucuronides are generally parallel. This is consistent with interconversion of raloxifene and the glucuronide metabolites.
Following intravenous administration, raloxifene is cleared at a rate approximating hepatic blood flow. Apparent oral clearance is 44.1 L/kg•hr. Raloxifene and its glucuronide conjugates are interconverted by reversible systemic metabolism and enterohepatic cycling, thereby prolonging its plasma elimination half-life to 27.7 hours after oral dosing.
Results from single oral doses of raloxifene predict multiple-dose pharmacokinetics. Following chronic dosing, clearance ranges from 40 to 60 L/kg•hr. Increasing doses of raloxifene HCl (ranging from 30 to 150 mg) result in slightly less than a proportional increase in the area under the plasma time concentration curve (AUC).
Excretion
Raloxifene is primarily excreted in feces, and less than 0.2% is excreted unchanged in urine. Less than 6% of the raloxifene dose is eliminated in urine as glucuronide conjugates.
[See table 1 below]

Special Populations
Geriatric—No differences in raloxifene pharmacokinetics were detected with regard to age (range 42 to 84 years).
Pediatric—The pharmacokinetics of raloxifene have not been evaluated in a pediatric population.
Gender—Total extent of exposure and oral clearance, normalized for lean body weight, are not significantly different between age-matched female and male volunteers.
Race—Pharmacokinetic differences due to race have been studied in 1712 women including 97.5% Caucasian, 1.0% Asian, 0.7% Hispanic, and 0.5% Black in the osteoporosis treatment trial and in 1053 women including 93.5% Caucasian, 4.3% Hispanic, 1.2% Asian, and 0.5% Black in the osteoporosis prevention trials. There were no discernible differences in raloxifene plasma concentrations among these groups; however, the influence of race cannot be conclusively determined.
Renal Insufficiency—Since negligible amounts of raloxifene are eliminated in urine, a study in patients with renal insufficiency was not conducted. In the osteoporosis treatment and prevention trials, raloxifene and metabolite concentrations in women with estimated creatinine clearance as low as 21 mL/min are similar to women with normal creatinine clearance.
Hepatic Dysfunction—Raloxifene was studied, as a single dose, in Child-Pugh Class A patients with cirrhosis and total serum bilirubin ranging from 0.6 to 2.0 mg/dL. Plasma raloxifene concentrations were approximately 2.5 times higher than in controls and correlated with bilirubin concentrations. Safety and efficacy have not been evaluated further in patients with hepatic insufficiency (*see* WARNINGS).

Drug-Drug Interactions
Clinically significant drug-drug interactions are discussed in PRECAUTIONS.
Ampicillin and Amoxicillin—Peak concentrations of raloxifene and the overall extent of absorption are reduced 28% and 14%, respectively, with co-administration of ampicillin. These reductions are consistent with decreased enterohepatic cycling associated with antibiotic reduction of enteric bacteria. However, the systemic exposure and the elimination rate of raloxifene were not affected. Therefore, EVISTA can be concurrently administered with ampicillin. In the osteoporosis treatment trial, co-administration of amoxicillin had no discernible differences in plasma raloxifene concentrations.
Antacids—Concurrent administration of calcium carbonate or aluminum and magnesium hydroxide-containing antacids does not affect the systemic exposure of raloxifene.
Corticosteroids—The chronic administration of raloxifene in postmenopausal women has no effect on the pharmacokinetics of methylprednisolone given as a single oral dose.
Cholestyramine—See PRECAUTIONS.
Cyclosporine—The co-administration of EVISTA with cyclosporine has not been evaluated.
Digoxin—Raloxifene has no effect on the pharmacokinetics of digoxin.
Warfarin—See PRECAUTIONS.

ANIMAL PHARMACOLOGY
The skeletal effects of raloxifene treatment were assessed in ovariectomized rats and monkeys. In rats, raloxifene prevented increased bone resorption and bone loss after ovariectomy. There were positive effects of raloxifene on bone strength, but the effects varied with time. Cynomolgus monkeys were treated with raloxifene or conjugated estrogens for 2 years. In terms of bone cycles, this is equivalent to approximately 6 years in humans. Raloxifene and estrogen suppressed bone turnover, and increased BMD in the lumbar spine and in the central cancellous bone of the proximal tibia. In this animal model, there was a positive correlation between vertebral compressive breaking force and BMD of the lumbar spine.
Histologic examination of bone from rats and monkeys treated with raloxifene showed no evidence of woven bone, marrow fibrosis, or mineralization defects.
These results are consistent with data from human studies of radiocalcium kinetics and markers of bone metabolism, and are consistent with the action of EVISTA as a skeletal antiresorptive agent.

CLINICAL STUDIES
In postmenopausal women with osteoporosis, EVISTA reduced the risk of vertebral fractures. EVISTA also increased BMD of the spine, hip, and total body. Similarly, in early postmenopausal women without osteoporosis (women with normal or low BMD without fracture), EVISTA increased spine, hip, and total body BMD relative to calcium alone at 24 months. The effect on hip bone mass was similar to that for the spine.

Treatment of Osteoporosis
The effects of EVISTA on fracture incidence and BMD in postmenopausal women with osteoporosis were examined at 3 years in a large randomized, placebo-controlled, double-blind multinational osteoporosis treatment trial. All vertebral fractures were diagnosed radiographically; some of these fractures also were associated with symptoms (i.e., clinical fractures). The study population consisted of 7705 postmenopausal women with osteoporosis as defined by: a) low BMD (vertebral or hip BMD at least 2.5 standard deviations below the mean value for healthy young women) without baseline vertebral fractures, or b) one or more baseline vertebral fractures. Women enrolled in this study had a median age of 67 years (range 31 to 80) and a median time since menopause of 19 years.
EVISTA, 60 mg administered once daily, increased spine and hip BMD by 2 to 3%. EVISTA decreased the incidence of the first vertebral fracture from 4.3% for placebo to 1.9% for EVISTA (relative risk reduction = 55%) and subsequent vertebral fractures from 20.2% for placebo to 14.1% for EVISTA (relative risk reduction = 30%) (Table 2). All women in the study received calcium (500 mg/day) and vitamin D (400 to 600 IU/day). EVISTA reduced the incidence of vertebral fractures whether or not patients had a vertebral fracture upon study entry. The decrease in incidence of vertebral fracture was greater than could be accounted for by increase in BMD alone.
[See table 2 at top of next page]

Table 1. Summary of Raloxifene Pharmacokinetic Parameters in the Healthy Postmenopausal Woman

	C_{max}[a] (ng/mL)/(mg/kg)	$t_{1/2}$ (hr)	$AUC_{0-\infty}$[a] (ng•hr/mL)/(mg/kg)	CL/F (L/kg•hr)	V/F (L/kg)
Single Dose					
Mean	0.50	27.7	27.2	44.1	2348
CV (%)	52	10.7 to 273[b]	44	46	52
Multiple Dose					
Mean	1.36	32.5	24.2	47.4	2853
CV (%)	37	15.8 to 86.6[b]	36	41	56

Abbreviations: C_{max} = maximum plasma concentration, $t_{1/2}$ = half-life, AUC = area under the curve, CL = clearance, V = volume of distribution, F = bioavailability, CV= coefficient of variation.
[a] Data normalized for dose in mg and body weight in kg.
[b] Range of observed half-life.

The mean percentage change in BMD from baseline for EVISTA was statistically significantly greater than for placebo at each skeletal site (Table 3).

Table 3. EVISTA (60 mg Once Daily) Related Increases in BMD for the Osteoporosis Treatment Study Expressed as Mean Percentage Increase vs. Placebo[ab]

	Time		
Site	12 Months %	24 Months %	36 Months %
Lumbar Spine	2.0	2.6	2.6
Femoral Neck	1.3	1.9	2.1
Ultradistal Radius	ND	2.2	ND
Distal Radius	ND	0.9	ND
Total Body	ND	1.1	ND

Note: all BMD increases were significant ($p<0.001$)
[a] Intent-to-treat analysis; last observation carried forward.
[b] All patients received calcium and vitamin D.
ND= not done (total body and radius BMD were measured only at 24 months)

Discontinuation from the study was required when excessive bone loss or multiple incident vertebral fractures occurred. Such discontinuation was statistically significantly more frequent in the placebo group (3.7%) than in the EVISTA group (1.1%).

Prevention of Osteoporosis

The effects of EVISTA on BMD in postmenopausal women were examined in three randomized, placebo-controlled, double-blind osteoporosis prevention trials: (1) a North American trial enrolled 544 women; (2) a European trial, 601 women; and (3) an international trial, 619 women who had undergone hysterectomy. In these trials, all women received calcium supplementation (400 to 600 mg/day). Women enrolled in these studies had a median age of 54 years and a median time since menopause of 5 years (less than 1 year up to 15 years postmenopause). The majority of the women were Caucasian (93.5%). Women were included if they had spine BMD between 2.5 standard deviations below and 2 standard deviations above the mean value for healthy young women. The mean T scores (number of standard deviations above or below the mean in healthy young women) for the three studies ranged from −1.01 to −0.74 for spine BMD and included women both with normal and low BMD. EVISTA, 60 mg administered once daily, produced increases in bone mass vs. calcium supplementation alone, as reflected by dual-energy x-ray absorptiometric (DXA) measurements of hip, spine, and total body BMD. Compared with placebo, the increases in BMD for each of the three studies were statistically significant at 12 months and were maintained at 24 months (Table 4). The placebo groups lost approximately 1% of BMD over 24 months.

Table 4. EVISTA (60 mg Once Daily) Related Increases in BMD for the Three Osteoporosis Prevention Studies Expressed as Mean Percentage Increase vs. Placebo[a] at 24 Months[b]

	Study		
Site	NA %	EU %	INT[c] %
Total Hip	2.0	2.4	1.3
Femoral Neck	2.1	2.5	1.6
Trochanter	2.2	2.7	1.3
Intertrochanter	2.3	2.4	1.3
Lumbar Spine	2.0	2.4	1.8

Abbreviations: NA = North American, EU = European, INT = International. Note: all BMD increases were significant ($p\leq0.001$)
[a] All patients received calcium.
[b] Intent-to-treat analysis; last observation carried forward.
[c] All women in the study had previously undergone hysterectomy.

EVISTA also increased BMD compared with placebo in the total body by 1.3% to 2.0% and in Ward's Triangle (hip) by 3.1% to 4.0%. The effects of EVISTA on forearm BMD were inconsistent between studies. In Study EU, EVISTA prevented bone loss at the ultradistal radius, whereas in Study NA, it did not.

Total hip mean percentage change from baseline All placebo and EVISTA subjects 24-month data from Studies NA and EU[a]

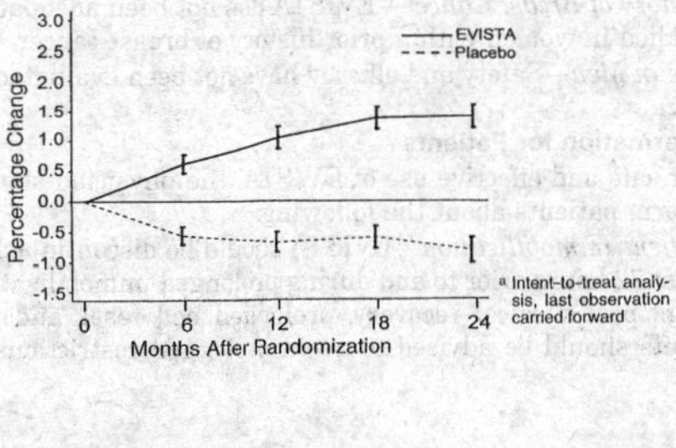

Table 2. Effect of EVISTA on Risk of Vertebral Fractures

	Number of Patients EVISTA	Number of Patients Placebo	Absolute Risk Reduction	Relative Risk Reduction (95% CI)
Fractures diagnosed radiographically				
Patients with no baseline fracture[a]	n=1401	n=1457		
Number (%) of patients with ≥1 new vertebral fracture	27 (1.9%)	62 (4.3%)	2.4%	55% (29%, 71%)
Patients with ≥1 baseline fracture[a]	n=858	n=835		
Number (%) of patients with ≥1 new vertebral fracture	121 (14.1%)	169 (20.2%)	6.1%	30% (14%, 44%)
Symptomatic vertebral fractures				
All randomized patients	n=2557	n=2576		
Number (%) of patients with ≥1 new clinical (painful) vertebral fracture	47 (1.8%)	81 (3.1%)	1.3%	41% (17%, 59%)

[a] Includes all patients with baseline and at least one follow-up radiograph.

Total hip mean percentage change from baseline All placebo, EVISTA, and CE subjects 24-month data from Study INT (hysterectomized women)[a]

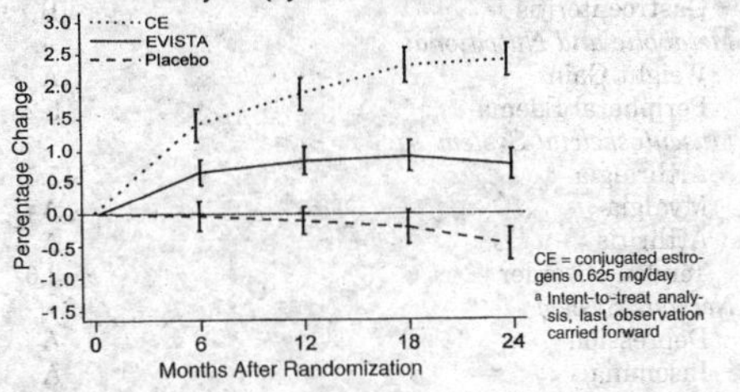

Assessments of Bone Turnover

In a 31-week, open-label, radiocalcium kinetics study, 33 early postmenopausal women were randomized to treatment with once-daily EVISTA 60 mg, cyclic estrogen/progestin (0.625 mg conjugated estrogens daily with 5 mg medroxyprogesterone acetate daily for the first 2 weeks of each month [HRT]), or no treatment. Treatment with either EVISTA or HRT was associated with reduced bone resorption and a positive shift in calcium balance (−82 mg Ca/day and +60 mg Ca/day, respectively, for EVISTA and −162 mg Ca/day and +91 mg Ca/day, respectively, for HRT).

In both the osteoporosis treatment and prevention trials, EVISTA therapy resulted in consistent, statistically significant suppression of bone resorption and bone formation, as reflected by changes in serum and urine markers of bone turnover (e.g., bone-specific alkaline phosphatase, osteocalcin, and collagen breakdown products). The suppression of bone turnover markers was evident by 3 months and persisted throughout the 36-month and 24-month observation periods.

Bone Histomorphometry

In the treatment study, bone biopsies for qualitative and quantitative histomorphometry were obtained at baseline and after 2 years of treatment. There were 56 paired biopsies evaluable for all indices. In EVISTA-treated patients, there were statistically significant decreases in bone formation rate per tissue volume, consistent with a reduction in bone turnover. Normal bone quality was maintained; specifically, there was no evidence of osteomalacia, marrow fibrosis, cellular toxicity, or woven bone after 2 years of treatment.

The tissue- and cellular-level effects of raloxifene were assessed by histomorphometric evaluation of human iliac crest bone biopsies taken after administration of a fluorochrome substance to label areas of mineralizing bone. The effects of EVISTA on bone histomorphometry were determined by pre- and post-treatment biopsies in a 6-month study of Caucasian postmenopausal women who received once-daily doses of EVISTA 60 mg or 0.625 mg conjugated estrogens. Ten raloxifene-treated and eight estrogen-treated women had evaluable bone biopsies at baseline and after 6 months of therapy. Bone formation rate/bone volume and activation frequency, the primary efficacy parameters, decreased to a greater extent with conjugated estrogen treatment vs. EVISTA treatment, although the differences were not statistically significant. Bone in EVISTA- and estrogen-treated women showed no evidence of mineralization defects, woven bone, or marrow fibrosis.

Effects on Lipid Metabolism

The effects of EVISTA on selected lipid fractions and clotting factors were evaluated in a 6-month study of 390 postmenopausal women. EVISTA was compared with oral continuous combined estrogen/progestin (0.625 mg conjugated estrogens plus 2.5 mg medroxyprogesterone acetate, [HRT]) and placebo (Table 5). EVISTA decreased serum total and LDL cholesterol without effects on serum total HDL cholesterol or triglycerides. In addition, EVISTA statistically significantly decreased serum fibrinogen and lipoprotein (a).

Table 5. EVISTA (60 mg Once Daily) and Oral HRT Effects on Selected Lipid Fractions and Clotting Factors in a 6-Month Study—Median Percentage Change from Baseline

	Treatment Group		
Endpoint	EVISTA (N=95) %	HRT (N=96) %	PLACEBO (N=98) %
Total Cholesterol	−6.6[a]	−4.4[a]	0.9
LDL Cholesterol	−10.9[a]	−12.7[a]	1.0
HDL Cholesterol	0.7[b]	10.6[a]	0.9
HDL-2 Cholesterol	15.4[b]	33.3[a]	0.0
HDL-3 Cholesterol	−2.5[ab]	2.7	0.0
Fibrinogen	−12.2[ab]	−2.8	−2.1
Lipoprotein (a)	−4.1[ab]	−16.3[a]	3.3
Triglycerides	−4.1[b]	20.0[a]	−0.3
Plasminogen Activator Inhibitor-1	−2.1[b]	−29.0[a]	−9.4

Abbreviations: HRT = continuous combined estrogen/progestin (0.625 mg conjugated estrogens plus 2.5 mg medroxyprogesterone acetate).
[a] Significantly different from placebo ($p<0.05$).
[b] Significantly different from HRT ($p<0.05$).

Consistent with results from the 6-month study, in the osteoporosis treatment (36 months) and prevention (24 months) studies, EVISTA statistically significantly decreased serum total and LDL cholesterol by 5% to 6% and 8% to 10%, respectively, compared to placebo. EVISTA did not affect HDL cholesterol or triglyceride levels. The effect of EVISTA-induced reductions in total and LDL cholesterol on risk for cardiovascular disease is currently under study.

Effects on the Uterus

In the osteoporosis treatment trial, endometrial thickness was evaluated annually in a subset of the study population (1781 patients) for 3 years. Placebo-treated women had a 0.27 mm mean decrease from baseline in endometrial thickness over 3 years, whereas the EVISTA-treated women had a 0.06 mm mean increase. Patients in the osteoporosis treatment study were not screened at baseline or excluded for pre-existing endometrial or uterine disease. This study was not specifically designed to detect endometrial polyps. Over the 36 months of the study, clinically or histologically benign endometrial polyps were reported in 17 of 1999 placebo-treated women, 37 of 1948 EVISTA-treated women, and in 31 of 2010 women treated with raloxifene HCl 120 mg/day.

There was no difference between EVISTA- and placebo-treated women in the incidences of endometrial carcinoma, vaginal bleeding, or vaginal discharge.

In placebo-controlled osteoporosis prevention trials, endometrial thickness was evaluated every 6 months (for 24 months) by transvaginal ultrasonography (TVU). A total of 2978 TVU measurements were collected from 831 women in all dose groups. Placebo-treated women had a 0.04 mm mean increase from baseline in endometrial thickness over 2 years, whereas the EVISTA-treated women had a 0.09 mm mean increase. Endometrial thickness measurements in raloxifene-treated women were indistinguishable from placebo. There were no differences between the raloxifene and placebo groups with respect to the incidence of reported vaginal bleeding.

In a 6-month study of 18 postmenopausal women that compared EVISTA to conjugated estrogens (0.625 mg/day [ERT]), endpoint endometrial biopsies demonstrated stimulatory effects of ERT, which were not observed for EVISTA. All samples from EVISTA-treated women showed nonproliferative endometria.

Continued on next page

*** Identi-Code® symbol. This product information was prepared in June 2004. Current information on these and other products of Eli Lilly and Company may be obtained by direct inquiry to Lilly Research Laboratories, Lilly Corporate Center, Indianapolis, Indiana 46285, (800) 545-5979.**

Evista—Cont.

Table 6. Adverse Events Occurring in Placebo-Controlled Osteoporosis Clinical Trials at a Frequency ≥2.0% and in more Evista-Treated (60 mg Once Daily) Women than Placebo-Treated Women

	Treatment		Prevention	
Body System	**EVISTA N=2557 %**	**Placebo N=2576 %**	**EVISTA N=581 %**	**Placebo N=584 %**
Body as a Whole				
Infection	A	A	15.1	14.6
Flu Syndrome	13.5	11.4	14.6	13.5
Headache	9.2	8.5	A	A
Leg Cramps	7.0	3.7	5.9	1.9
Chest Pain	A	A	4.0	3.6
Fever	3.9	3.8	3.1	2.6
Cardiovascular System				
Hot Flashes	9.7	6.4	24.6	18.3
Migraine	A	A	2.4	2.1
Syncope	2.3	2.1	B	B
Varicose Vein	2.2	1.5	A	A
Digestive System				
Nausea	8.3	7.8	8.8	8.6
Diarrhea	7.2	6.9	A	A
Dyspepsia	A	A	5.9	5.8
Vomiting	4.8	4.3	3.4	3.3
Flatulence	A	A	3.1	2.4
Gastrointestinal Disorder	A	A	3.3	2.1
Gastroenteritis	B	B	2.6	2.1
Metabolic and Nutritional				
Weight Gain	A	A	8.8	6.8
Peripheral Edema	5.2	4.4	3.3	1.9
Musculoskeletal System				
Arthralgia	15.5	14.0	10.7	10.1
Myalgia	A	A	7.7	6.2
Arthritis	A	A	4.0	3.6
Tendon Disorder	3.6	3.1	A	A
Nervous System				
Depression	A	A	6.4	6.0
Insomnia	A	A	5.5	4.3
Vertigo	4.1	3.7	A	A
Neuralgia	2.4	1.9	B	B
Hypesthesia	2.1	2.0	B	B
Respiratory System				
Sinusitis	7.9	7.5	10.3	6.5
Rhinitis	10.2	10.1	A	A
Bronchitis	9.5	8.6	A	A
Pharyngitis	5.3	5.1	7.6	7.2
Cough Increased	9.3	9.2	6.0	5.7
Pneumonia	A	A	2.6	1.5
Laryngitis	B	B	2.2	1.4
Skin and Appendages				
Rash	A	A	5.5	3.8
Sweating	2.5	2.0	3.1	1.7
Special Senses				
Conjunctivitis	2.2	1.7	A	A
Urogenital System				
Vaginitis	A	A	4.3	3.6
Urinary Tract Infection	A	A	4.0	3.9
Cystitis	4.6	4.5	3.3	3.1
Leukorrhea	A	A	3.3	1.7
Uterine Disorder[a,b]	3.3	2.3	A	A
Endometrial Disorder[a]	B	B	3.1	1.9
Vaginal Hemorrhage	2.5	2.4	A	A
Urinary Tract Disorder	2.5	2.1	A	A

A Placebo incidence greater than or equal to EVISTA incidence.
B Less than 2% incidence and more frequent with EVISTA.
[a] Treatment-emergent, uterine-related adverse event, including only patients with an intact uterus: Prevention Trials: EVISTA, n=354, Placebo, n=364; Treatment Trial: EVISTA, n=1948, Placebo, n=1999.
[b] Actual terms most frequently referred to endometrial fluid.

A 12-month study of uterine effects compared a higher dose of raloxifene HCl (150 mg/day) with HRT. At baseline, 43 raloxifene-treated postmenopausal women and 37 HRT-treated women had a nonproliferative endometrium. At study completion, endometria in all of the raloxifene-treated women remained nonproliferative whereas 13 HRT-treated women had developed proliferative changes. Also, HRT significantly increased uterine volume; raloxifene did not increase uterine volume. Thus, no stimulatory effect of raloxifene on the endometrium was detected at more than twice the recommended dose.

Compared to placebo, EVISTA did not increase the risk of ovarian carcinoma.

Effects on the Breast

Across all placebo-controlled trials, EVISTA was indistinguishable from placebo with regard to frequency and severity of breast pain and tenderness. EVISTA was associated with significantly less breast pain and tenderness than reported by women receiving estrogens with or without added progestin (*see* ADVERSE REACTIONS *and* Table 6).

Mammograms were routinely performed on an annual or biennial basis in all placebo-controlled clinical trials lasting at least 12 months. Independent review has determined that 25 cases (raloxifene and placebo combined) represented newly-diagnosed invasive breast cancer. Among 7108 women randomized to raloxifene, there were 10 cases of invasive breast cancer per 19,381 person-years of follow-up (0.52 per 1000). Among 3467 women randomized to placebo, there were 15 cases of invasive breast cancer per 9250 person-years of follow-up (1.62 per 1000). The effectiveness of raloxifene in reducing the risk of breast cancer has not been established.

INDICATIONS AND USAGE

EVISTA is indicated for the treatment and prevention of osteoporosis in postmenopausal women.

For either osteoporosis treatment or prevention, supplemental calcium and/or vitamin D should be added to the diet if daily intake is inadequate.

Postmenopausal osteoporosis may be diagnosed by history or radiographic documentation of osteoporotic fracture, bone mineral densitometry, or physical signs of vertebral crush fractures (e.g., height loss, dorsal kyphosis).

No single clinical finding or test result can quantify risk of postmenopausal osteoporosis with certainty. However, clinical assessment can help to identify women at increased risk. Widely accepted risk factors include Caucasian or Asian descent, slender body build, early estrogen deficiency, smoking, alcohol consumption, low calcium diet, sedentary lifestyle, and family history of osteoporosis. Evidence of increased bone turnover from serum and urine markers and low bone mass (e.g., at least 1 standard deviation below the mean for healthy, young adult women) as determined by densitometric techniques are also predictive. The greater the number of clinical risk factors, the greater the probability of developing postmenopausal osteoporosis.

CONTRAINDICATIONS

EVISTA is contraindicated in lactating women or women who are or may become pregnant. EVISTA may cause fetal harm when administered to a pregnant woman. In rabbit studies, abortion and a low rate of fetal heart anomalies (ventricular septal defects) occurred in rabbits at doses ≥0.1 mg/kg (≥0.04 times the human dose based on surface area, mg/m^2), and hydrocephaly was observed in fetuses at doses ≥10 mg/kg (≥4 times the human dose based on surface area, mg/m). In rat studies, retardation of fetal development and developmental abnormalities (wavy ribs, kidney cavitation) occurred at doses ≥1 mg/kg (≥0.2 times the human dose based on surface area, mg/m^2). Treatment of rats at doses of 0.1 to 10 mg/kg (0.02 to 1.6 times the human dose based on surface area, mg/m^2) during gestation and lactation produced effects that included delayed and disrupted parturition; decreased neonatal survival and altered physical development; sex- and age-specific reductions in growth and changes in pituitary hormone content; and decreased lymphoid compartment size in offspring. At 10 mg/kg, raloxifene disrupted parturition which resulted in maternal and progeny death and morbidity. Effects in adult offspring (4 months of age) included uterine hypoplasia and reduced fertility; however, no ovarian or vaginal pathology was observed. The patient should be apprised of the potential hazard to the fetus if this drug is used during pregnancy, or if the patient becomes pregnant while taking this drug.

EVISTA is contraindicated in women with active or past history of venous thromboembolic events, including deep vein thrombosis, pulmonary embolism, and retinal vein thrombosis.

EVISTA is contraindicated in women known to be hypersensitive to raloxifene or other constituents of the tablets.

WARNINGS

Venous Thromboembolism—In clinical trials, EVISTA-treated women had an increased risk of venous thromboembolism (deep vein thrombosis and pulmonary embolism). Other venous thromboembolic events could also occur. A less serious event, superficial thrombophlebitis, also has been reported more frequently with EVISTA. The greatest risk for deep vein thrombosis and pulmonary embolism occurs during the first 4 months of treatment, and the magnitude of risk appears to be similar to the reported risk associated with use of hormone replacement therapy. Because immobilization increases the risk for venous thromboembolic events independent of therapy, EVISTA should be discontinued at least 72 hours prior to and during prolonged immobilization (e.g., post-surgical recovery, prolonged bed rest), and EVISTA therapy should be resumed only after the patient is fully ambulatory. In addition, women taking EVISTA should be advised to move about periodically during prolonged travel. The risk-benefit balance should be considered in women at risk of thromboembolic disease for other reasons, such as congestive heart failure, superficial thrombophlebitis, and active malignancy.

Premenopausal Use—There is no indication for premenopausal use of EVISTA. Safety of EVISTA in premenopausal women has not been established and its use is not recommended (*see* CONTRAINDICATIONS).

Hepatic Dysfunction—Raloxifene was studied, as a single dose, in Child-Pugh Class A patients with cirrhosis and serum total bilirubin ranging from 0.6 to 2.0 mg/dL. Plasma raloxifene concentrations were approximately 2.5 times higher than in controls and correlated with total bilirubin concentrations. Safety and efficacy have not been evaluated further in patients with severe hepatic insufficiency.

PRECAUTIONS

General

Concurrent Estrogen Therapy—The concurrent use of EVISTA and systemic estrogen or hormone replacement therapy (ERT or HRT) has not been studied in prospective clinical trials and therefore concomitant use of EVISTA with systemic estrogens is not recommended.

Lipid Metabolism—EVISTA lowers serum total and LDL cholesterol by 6% to 11%, but does not affect serum concentrations of total HDL cholesterol or triglycerides. These effects should be taken into account in therapeutic decisions for patients who may require therapy for hyperlipidemia.

Limited clinical data suggest that some women with a history of marked hypertriglyceridemia (>5.6 mmol/L or >500 mg/dL) in response to treatment with oral estrogen or estrogen plus progestin may develop increased levels of triglycerides when treated with EVISTA. Women with this medical history should have serum triglycerides monitored when taking EVISTA.

Concurrent use of EVISTA and lipid-lowering agents has not been studied.

Endometrium—EVISTA has not been associated with endometrial proliferation (*see* Clinical Studies *and* ADVERSE REACTIONS). Unexplained uterine bleeding should be investigated as clinically indicated.

Breast—EVISTA has not been associated with breast enlargement, breast pain, or an increased risk of breast cancer (*see* Clinical Studies *and* ADVERSE REACTIONS). Any unexplained breast abnormality occurring during EVISTA therapy should be investigated.

History of Breast Cancer—EVISTA has not been adequately studied in women with a prior history of breast cancer.

Use in Men—Safety and efficacy have not been evaluated in men.

Information for Patients

For safe and effective use of EVISTA, the physician should inform patients about the following:

Patient Immobilization—EVISTA should be discontinued at least 72 hours prior to and during prolonged immobilization (e.g., post-surgical recovery, prolonged bed rest), and patients should be advised to avoid prolonged restrictions of movement during travel because of the increased risk of venous thromboembolic events.

Hot Flashes or Flushes—EVISTA may increase the incidence of hot flashes and is not effective in reducing hot flashes or flushes associated with estrogen deficiency. In some asymptomatic patients, hot flashes may occur upon beginning EVISTA therapy.

Other Osteoporosis Treatment and Prevention Measures—Patients should be instructed to take supplemental calcium and/or vitamin D, if daily dietary intake is inadequate. Weight-bearing exercise should be considered along with the modification of certain behavioral factors, such as cigarette smoking, and/or alcohol consumption, if these factors exist.

Physicians should instruct their patients to read the patient package insert before starting therapy with EVISTA and to re-read it each time the prescription is renewed.

Drug Interactions

Cholestyramine—Cholestyramine, an anion exchange resin, causes a 60% reduction in the absorption and enterohepatic cycling of raloxifene after a single dose. Co-administration of cholestyramine with EVISTA is not recommended. Although not specifically studied, it is anticipated that other anion exchange resins would have a similar effect.

Warfarin—In vitro, raloxifene did not interact with the binding of warfarin. The co-administration of EVISTA and warfarin, a coumarin derivative, has been assessed in a single-dose study. In this study, raloxifene had no effect on the pharmacokinetics of warfarin. However, a 10% decrease in prothrombin time was observed in the single-dose study. If EVISTA is given concurrently with warfarin or other coumarin derivatives, prothrombin time should be monitored more closely when starting or stopping therapy with EVISTA. In the osteoporosis treatment trial, there were no clinically relevant effects of warfarin co-administration on plasma concentrations of raloxifene.

Other Highly Protein-Bound Drugs—Raloxifene is more than 95% bound to plasma proteins. Other highly protein-bound drugs should not cause clinically relevant changes in EVISTA plasma concentrations. Furthermore, in the osteoporosis treatment trial, there were no clinically relevant effects of co-administration of other highly protein-bound drugs (e.g., gemfibrozil) on plasma concentrations of raloxifene. In vitro, raloxifene did not interact with the binding of phenytoin, tamoxifen, or warfarin (see above). Although not examined, EVISTA might affect the protein binding of other drugs and should be used with caution with certain other highly protein-bound drugs such as diazepam, diazoxide, and lidocaine.

Carcinogenesis, Mutagenesis, and Impairment of Fertility

Carcinogenesis—In a 21-month carcinogenicity study in mice, there was an increased incidence of ovarian tumors in female animals given 9 to 242 mg/kg, which included benign and malignant tumors of granulosa/theca cell origin and benign tumors of epithelial cell origin. Systemic exposure (AUC) of raloxifene in this group was 0.3 to 34 times that in postmenopausal women administered a 60-mg dose. There was also an increased incidence of testicular interstitial cell tumors and prostatic adenomas and adenocarcinomas in male mice given 41 or 210 mg/kg (4.7 or 24 times the AUC in humans), and prostatic leiomyoblastoma in male mice given 210 mg/kg.

In a 2-year carcinogenicity study in rats, an increased incidence in ovarian tumors of granulosa/theca cell origin was observed in female rats given 279 mg/kg (approximately 400 times the AUC in humans). The female rodents in these studies were treated during their reproductive lives when their ovaries were functional and responsive to hormonal stimulation.

Mutagenesis—Raloxifene HCl was not genotoxic in any of the following test systems: the Ames test for bacterial mutagenesis with and without metabolic activation, the unscheduled DNA synthesis assay in rat hepatocytes, the mouse lymphoma assay for mammalian cell mutation, the chromosomal aberration assay in Chinese hamster ovary cells, the in vivo sister chromatid exchange assay in Chinese hamsters, and the in vivo micronucleus test in mice.

Impairment of Fertility—When male and female rats were given daily doses ≥5 mg/kg (≥0.8 times the human dose based on surface area, mg/m^2) prior to and during mating, no pregnancies occurred. In male rats, daily doses up to 100 mg/kg (16 times the human dose based on surface area, mg/m^2) for at least 2 weeks did not affect sperm production or quality, or reproductive performance. In female rats, at doses of 0.1 to 10 mg/kg/day (0.02 to 1.6 times the human dose based on surface area, mg/m^2), raloxifene disrupted estrous cycles and inhibited ovulation. These effects of raloxifene were reversible. In another study in rats in which raloxifene was given during the preimplantation period at doses ≥0.1 mg/kg (≥0.02 times the human dose based on surface area, mg/m^2), raloxifene delayed and disrupted embryo implantation resulting in prolonged gestation and reduced litter size. The reproductive and developmental effects observed in animals are consistent with the estrogen receptor activity of raloxifene.

Pregnancy Category X

EVISTA should not be used in women who are or may become pregnant (*see* CONTRAINDICATIONS).

Nursing Mothers

EVISTA should not be used by lactating women (*see* CONTRAINDICATIONS). It is not known whether raloxifene is excreted in human milk.

Pediatric Use

EVISTA should not be used in pediatric patients.

Table 7. Adverse Events reported in the Clinical Trials for Osteoporosis Prevention with EVISTA (60 mg Once Daily) and Continuous Combined or Cyclic Estrogen Plus Progestin (HRT) at an Incidence ≥2.0% in any Treatment Group[a]

Adverse Event	EVISTA (N=317) %	HRT-Continuous Combined (N=96) %	HRT-Cyclic (N=219) %
Urogenital			
Breast Pain	4.4	37.5	29.7
Vaginal Bleeding[b]	6.2	64.2	88.5
Digestive			
Flatulence	1.6	12.5	6.4
Cardiovascular			
Hot Flashes	28.7	3.1	5.9
Body as a Whole			
Infection	11.0	0	6.8
Abdominal Pain	6.6	10.4	18.7
Chest Pain	2.8	0	0.5

[a] These data are from both blinded and open-label studies.

[b] Treatment-emergent, uterine-related adverse event, including only patients with an intact uterus: EVISTA, n=290; HRT-Continuous Combined, n=67; HRT-Cyclic, n=217.

Continuous Combined HRT = 0.625 mg conjugated estrogens plus 2.5 mg medroxyprogesterone acetate.

Cyclic HRT = 0.625 mg conjugated estrogens for 28 days with concomitant 5 mg medroxyprogesterone acetate or 0.15 mg norgestrel on Days 1 through 14 or 17 through 28.

Geriatric Use

In the osteoporosis treatment trial of 7705 postmenopausal women, 4621 women were considered geriatric (greater than 65 years old). Of these, 845 women were greater than 75 years old. Safety and efficacy in older and younger postmenopausal women in the osteoporosis treatment trial appeared to be comparable.

ADVERSE REACTIONS

Adverse Events in the Osteoporosis Treatment Clinical Trial

The safety of raloxifene in the treatment of osteoporosis was assessed in a large (7705 patients) multinational, placebo-controlled trial. Duration of treatment was 36 months and 5129 postmenopausal women were exposed to raloxifene (2557 received 60 mg/day and 2572 received 120 mg/day).

The majority of adverse events occurring during the study were mild and generally did not require discontinuation of therapy.

Therapy was discontinued due to an adverse event in 10.9% of EVISTA-treated women and 8.8% of placebo-treated women. Common adverse events considered to be related to EVISTA therapy were hot flashes and leg cramps. Hot flashes were most commonly reported during the first 6 months of treatment and were not different from placebo thereafter.

Adverse Events in Placebo-Controlled Clinical Trials to Support the Osteoporosis Prevention Indication

The safety of raloxifene has been assessed primarily in 12 Phase 2 and Phase 3 studies with placebo, estrogen, and estrogen-progestin replacement therapy (HRT) control groups. The duration of treatment ranged from 2 to 30 months and 2036 women were exposed to raloxifene (371 patients received 10 to 50 mg/day, 828 received 60 mg/day, and 837 received from 120 to 600 mg/day).

The majority of adverse events occurring during clinical trials were mild and generally did not require discontinuation of therapy.

Therapy was discontinued due to an adverse event in 11.4% of 581 EVISTA-treated women and 12.2% of 584 placebo-treated women. Common adverse events considered to be drug-related were hot flashes and leg cramps (*see* Table 6). The first occurrence of hot flashes was most commonly reported during the first 6 months of treatment. Discontinuation rates due to hot flashes did not differ significantly between EVISTA and placebo groups (1.7% and 2.2%, respectively).

Table 6 lists adverse events occurring in either the osteoporosis treatment or the prevention placebo-controlled clinical trial databases at a frequency ≥2.0% in either group and in more EVISTA-treated women than in placebo-treated women. Adverse events are shown without attribution of causality.

[See table 6 at top of previous page]

Comparison of EVISTA and Hormone Replacement Therapy Adverse Events

EVISTA was compared with estrogen-progestin replacement therapy (HRT) in three clinical trials for prevention of osteoporosis. Table 7 shows adverse events occurring more frequently in one treatment group and at an incidence ≥2.0% in any group. Adverse events are shown without attribution of causality.

[See table 7 above]

Laboratory Changes

The following changes in analyte concentrations are commonly observed during EVISTA therapy: increased apolipoprotein A1; and reduced serum total cholesterol, LDL cholesterol, fibrinogen, apolipoprotein B, and lipoprotein (a). EVISTA modestly increases hormone-binding globulin concentrations, including sex steroid-binding globulin, thyroxine-binding globulin, and corticosteroid-binding globulin with corresponding increases in measured total hormone concentrations. There is no evidence that these changes in hormone-binding globulin concentrations affect concentrations of the corresponding free hormones.

There were small decreases in serum total calcium, inorganic phosphate, total protein, and albumin which were generally of lesser magnitude than decreases observed during ERT/HRT. Platelet count was also decreased slightly and was not different from ERT.

Additional Safety Information

Incidences of estrogen-dependent carcinoma of the endometrium and breast are being evaluated across all completed and ongoing clinical trials involving 17,151 patients, of which at least 10,850 women have received at least one dose of raloxifene. These trials provided over 21,000 person-years of raloxifene exposure with a maximum exposure of 58 months.

Endometrium—Compared to placebo, raloxifene did not increase the risk of endometrial cancer.

Breast—Compared to placebo, raloxifene did not increase the risk of breast cancer (*see* CLINICAL PHARMACOLOGY, Effects on the Breast).

Postintroduction Reports

Adverse events reported since market introduction include: very rarely—retinal vein occlusion.

OVERDOSAGE

Incidents of overdose in humans have not been reported. In an 8-week study of 63 postmenopausal women, a dose of raloxifene HCl 600 mg/day was safely tolerated. No mortality was seen after a single oral dose in rats or mice at 5000 mg/kg (810 times the human dose for rats and 405 times the human dose for mice based on surface area, mg/m^2) or in monkeys at 1000 mg/kg (80 times the AUC in humans). There is no specific antidote for raloxifene.

DOSAGE AND ADMINISTRATION

The recommended dosage is one 60-mg EVISTA tablet daily which may be administered any time of day without regard to meals.

HOW SUPPLIED

EVISTA 60-mg tablets are white, elliptical, and film coated. They are imprinted on one side with LILLY and the tablet code 4165 in edible blue ink. They are available as follows:

Bottle (count)	NDC Number
30 (unit of use)	NDC—0002-4165-30
100 (unit of use)	NDC—0002-4165-02
2000	NDC—0002-4165-07

Store at controlled room temperature, 20° to 25°C (68° to 77°F) [*see* USP]. The USP defines controlled room temperature as a temperature maintained thermostatically that encompasses the usual and customary working environment of 20° to 25°C (68° to 77°F); that results in a mean kinetic temperature calculated to be not more than 25°C; and that allows for excursions between 15° and 30°C (59° and 86°F) that are experienced in pharmacies, hospitals, and warehouses.

Literature revised July 11, 2003

Eli Lilly and Company, Indianapolis, IN 46285, USA

www.lilly.com

PV 3086 AMP PRINTED IN USA

Shown in Product Identification Guide, page 320

Continued on next page

*** Identi-Code® symbol. This product information was prepared in June 2004. Current information on these and other products of Eli Lilly and Company may be obtained by direct inquiry to Lilly Research Laboratories, Lilly Corporate Center, Indianapolis, Indiana 46285, (800) 545-5979.**

FORTEO™ ℞
[for-tay-o]
teriparatide (rDNA origin)
injection 750 mcg/3 mL

WARNING
In male and female rats, teriparatide caused an increase in the incidence of osteosarcoma (a malignant bone tumor) that was dependent on dose and treatment duration. The effect was observed at systemic exposures to teriparatide ranging from 3 to 60 times the exposure in humans given a 20-mcg dose. Because of the uncertain relevance of the rat osteosarcoma finding to humans, teriparatide should be prescribed only to patients for whom the potential benefits are considered to outweigh the potential risk. Teriparatide should not be prescribed for patients who are at increased baseline risk for osteosarcoma (including those with Paget's disease of bone or unexplained elevations of alkaline phosphatase, open epiphyses, or prior radiation therapy involving the skeleton) (*see* WARNINGS *and* PRECAUTIONS, Carcinogenesis).

DESCRIPTION

FORTEO™ [teriparatide (rDNA origin) injection] contains recombinant human parathyroid hormone (1-34), [rhPTH (1-34)], which has an identical sequence to the 34 N-terminal amino acids (the biologically active region) of the 84-amino acid human parathyroid hormone.

Teriparatide has a molecular weight of 4117.8 daltons and its amino acid sequence is shown below:

1 5 10
H-(Ser)(Val)(Ser)(Glu)(Ile)(Gln)(Leu)(Met)(His)(Asn)
(Leu)
20 15 (Gly)
(Trp)(Glu)(Val)(Arg)(Glu)(Met)(Ser)(Asn)(Leu)(His)(Lys)
(Leu)
(Arg)(Lys)(Lys)(Leu)(Gln)(Asp)(Val)(His)(Asn)(Phe)-OH
25 30

Teriparatide (rDNA origin) is manufactured by Eli Lilly and Company using a strain of *Escherichia coli* modified by recombinant DNA technology. FORTEO is supplied as a sterile, colorless, clear, isotonic solution in a glass cartridge which is pre-assembled into a disposable pen device for subcutaneous injection. Each prefilled delivery device is filled with 3.3 mL to deliver 3 mL. Each mL contains 250 mcg teriparatide (corrected for acetate, chloride, and water content), 0.41 mg glacial acetic acid, 0.10 mg sodium acetate (anhydrous), 45.4 mg mannitol, 3.0 mg Metacresol, and Water for Injection. In addition, hydrochloric acid solution 10% and/or sodium hydroxide solution 10% may have been added to adjust the product to pH 4.

Each cartridge pre-assembled into a pen device delivers 20 mcg of teriparatide per dose each day for up to 28 days.

See accompanying User Manual: Instructions for Use.

CLINICAL PHARMACOLOGY

Mechanism of Action—Endogenous 84-amino-acid parathyroid hormone (PTH) is the primary regulator of calcium and phosphate metabolism in bone and kidney. Physiological actions of PTH include regulation of bone metabolism, renal tubular reabsorption of calcium and phosphate, and intestinal calcium absorption. The biological actions of PTH and teriparatide are mediated through binding to specific high-affinity cell-surface receptors. Teriparatide and the 34 N-terminal amino acids of PTH bind to these receptors with the same affinity and have the same physiological actions on bone and kidney. Teriparatide is not expected to accumulate in bone or other tissues.

The skeletal effects of teriparatide depend upon the pattern of systemic exposure. Once-daily administration of teriparatide stimulates new bone formation on trabecular and cortical (periosteal and/or endosteal) bone surfaces by preferential stimulation of osteoblastic activity over osteoclastic activity. In monkey studies, teriparatide improved trabecular microarchitecture and increased bone mass and strength by stimulating new bone formation in both cancellous and cortical bone. In humans, the anabolic effects of teriparatide are manifest as an increase in skeletal mass, an increase in markers of bone formation and resorption, and an increase in bone strength. By contrast, continuous excess of endogenous PTH, as occurs in hyperparathyroidism, may be detrimental to the skeleton because bone resorption may be stimulated more than bone formation.

Human Pharmacokinetics—Teriparatide is extensively absorbed after subcutaneous injection; the absolute bioavailability is approximately 95% based on pooled data from 20-, 40-, and 80-mcg doses. The rates of absorption and elimination are rapid. The peptide reaches peak serum concentrations about 30 minutes after subcutaneous injection of a 20-mcg dose and declines to non-quantifiable concentrations within 3 hours.

Systemic clearance of teriparatide (approximately 62 L/hr in women and 94 L/hr in men) exceeds the rate of normal liver plasma flow, consistent with both hepatic and extrahepatic clearance. Volume of distribution, following intravenous injection, is approximately 0.12 L/kg. Intersubject

Table 1. Effect of FORTEO on Risk of Vertebral Fractures in Postmenopausal Women with Osteoporosis

	Percent of Women With Fracture			
	FORTEO (N=444)	Placebo (N=448)	Absolute Risk Reduction (%, 95% CI)	Relative Risk Reduction (%, 95% CI)
New fracture (≥1)	5.0[a]	14.3	9.3 (5.5-13.1)	65 (45-78)
1 fracture	3.8	9.4		
2 fractures	0.9	2.9		
≥3 fractures	0.2	2.0		

[a]$p \leq 0.001$ compared with placebo

variability in systemic clearance and volume of distribution is 25% to 50%. The half-life of teriparatide in serum is 5 minutes when administered by intravenous injection and approximately 1 hour when administered by subcutaneous injection. The longer half-life following subcutaneous administration reflects the time required for absorption from the injection site.

No metabolism or excretion studies have been performed with teriparatide. However, the mechanisms of metabolism and elimination of PTH(1-34) and intact PTH have been extensively described in published literature. Peripheral metabolism of PTH is believed to occur by non-specific enzymatic mechanisms in the liver followed by excretion via the kidneys.

Special Populations—Pediatric—Pharmacokinetic data in pediatric patients are not available (*see* WARNINGS).

Geriatric—No age-related differences in teriparatide pharmacokinetics were detected (range 31 to 85 years).

Gender—Although systemic exposure to teriparatide was approximately 20% to 30% lower in men than women, the recommended dose for both genders is 20 mcg/day.

Race—The populations included in the pharmacokinetic analyses were 98.5% Caucasian. The influence of race has not been determined.

Renal insufficiency—No pharmacokinetic differences were identified in 11 patients with mild or moderate renal insufficiency [creatinine clearance (CrCl) 30 to 72 mL/min] administered a single dose of teriparatide. in 5 patients with severe renal insufficiency (CrCl < 30 mL/min), the AUC and T1/2 of teriparatide were increased by 73% and 77%, respectively. Maximum serum concentration of teriparatide was not increased. No studies have been performed in patients undergoing dialysis for chronic renal failure (*see* PRECAUTIONS).

Heart failure—No clinically relevant pharmacokinetic, blood pressure, or pulse rate differences were identified in 13 patients with stable New York Heart Association Class I to III heart failure after the administration of two 20-mcg doses of teriparatide.

Hepatic insufficiency—Non-specific proteolytic enzymes in the liver (possibly Kupffer cells) cleave PTH(1-34) and PTH(1-84) into fragments that are cleared from the circulation mainly by the kidney. No studies have been performed in patients with hepatic impairment.

Drug Interactions—Hydrochlorothiazide—In a study of 20 healthy people, the coadministration of hydrochlorothiazide 25 mg with teriparatide did not affect the serum calcium response to teriparatide 40 mcg. The 24-hour urine excretion of calcium was reduced by a clinically unimportant amount (15%). The effect of coadministration of a higher dose of hydrochlorothiazide with teriparatide on serum calcium levels has not been studied.

Furosemide—In a study of 9 healthy people and 17 patients with mild, moderate, or severe renal insufficiency (CrCl 13 to 72 mL/min), coadministration of intravenous furosemide (20 to 100 mg) with teriparatide 40 mcg resulted in small increases in the serum calcium (2%) and 24-hour urine calcium (37%) responses to teriparatide that did not appear to be clinically important.

Human Pharmacodynamics—Effects on mineral metabolism—Teriparatide affects calcium and phosphorus metabolism in a pattern consistent with the known actions of endogenous PTH (eg, increases serum calcium and decreases serum phosphorus).

Serum calcium concentrations—When teriparatide 20 mcg is administered once daily, the serum calcium concentration increases transiently, beginning approximately 2 hours after dosing and reaching a maximum concentration between 4 and 6 hours (median increase, 0.4 mg/dL). The serum calcium concentration begins to decline approximately 6 hours after dosing and returns to baseline by 16 to 24 hours after each dose.

In a clinical study of postmenopausal women with osteoporosis, the median peak serum calcium concentration measured 4 to 6 hours after dosing with FORTEO (teriparatide 20 mcg) was 2.42 mmol/L (9.68 mg/dL) at 12 months. The peak serum calcium remained below 2.76 mmol/L (11.0 mg/dL) in >99% of women at each visit. Sustained hypercalcemia was not observed.

In this study, 11.1% of women treated with FORTEO had at least 1 serum calcium value above the upper limit of normal [2.64 mmol/L (10.6 mg/dL)] compared with 1.5% of women treated with placebo. The percentage of women treated with FORTEO whose serum calcium was above the upper limit of normal on consecutive 4- to 6-hour post-dose measurements was 3.0% compared with 0.2% of women treated with placebo. In these women, calcium supplements and/or FORTEO doses were reduced. The timing of these dose reductions was at the discretion of the investigator. FORTEO dose adjustments were made at varying intervals after the first observation of increased serum calcium (median 21 weeks). During these intervals, there was no evidence of progressive increases in serum calcium.

In a clinical study of men with either primary or hypogonadal osteoporosis, the effects on serum calcium were similar to those observed in postmenopausal women. The median peak serum calcium concentration measured 4 to 6 hours after dosing with FORTEO was 2.35 mmol/L (9.44 mg/dL) at 12 months. The peak serum calcium remained below 2.76 mmol/L (11.0 mg/dL) in 98% of men at each visit. Sustained hypercalcemia was not observed.

In this study, 6.0% of men treated with FORTEO daily had at least 1 serum calcium value above the upper limit of normal [2.64 mmol/L (10.6 mg/dL)] compared with none of the men treated with placebo. The percentage of men treated with FORTEO whose serum calcium was above the upper limit of normal on consecutive measurements was 1.3% (2 men) compared with none of the men treated with placebo. Although calcium supplements and/or FORTEO doses could have been reduced in these men, only calcium supplementation was reduced (*see* PRECAUTIONS *and* ADVERSE EVENTS).

In a clinical study of women previously treated for 18 to 39 months with raloxifene (n=26) or alendronate (n=33), mean serum calcium >12 hours after FORTEO injection was increased by 0.09 to 0.14 mmol/L (0.36 to 0.56 mg/dL), after 1 to 6 months of FORTEO treatment compared with baseline. Of the women pretreated with raloxifene, 3 (11.5%) had a serum calcium >2.76 mmol/L (11.0 mg/dL), and of those pretreated with alendronate, 3 (9.1%) had a serum calcium >2.76 mmol/L (11.0 mg/dL). The highest serum calcium reported was 3.12 mmol/L (12.5 mg/dL). None of the women had symptoms of hypercalcemia. There were no placebo controls in this study.

Urinary calcium excretion—In a clinical study of postmenopausal women with osteoporosis who received 1000 mg of supplemental calcium and at least 400 IU of vitamin D, daily FORTEO increased urinary calcium excretion. The median urinary excretion of calcium was 4.8 mmol/day (190 mg/day) at 6 months and 4.2 mmol/day (170 mg/day) at 12 months. These levels were 0.76 mmol/day (30 mg/day) and 0.30 mmol/day (12 mg/day) higher, respectively, than in women treated with placebo. The incidence of hypercalciuria (>7.5 mmol Ca/day or 300 mg/day) was similar in the women treated with FORTEO or placebo.

In a clinical study of men with either primary or hypogonadal osteoporosis who received 1000 mg of supplemental calcium and at least 400 IU of vitamin D, daily FORTEO had inconsistent effects on urinary calcium excretion. The median urinary excretion of calcium was 5.6 mmol/day (220 mg/day) at 1 month and 5.3 mmol/day (210 mg/day) at 6 months. These levels were 0.50 mmol/day (20 mg/day) higher and 0.20 mmol/day (8.0 mg/day) lower, respectively, than in men treated with placebo. The incidence of hypercalciuria (>7.5 mmol Ca/day or 300 mg/day) was similar in the men treated with FORTEO or placebo.

Phosphorus and vitamin D—In single-dose studies, teriparatide produced transient phosphaturia and mild transient reductions in serum phosphorus concentration. However, hypophosphatemia (<0.74 mmol/L or 2.4 mg/dL) was not observed in clinical trials with FORTEO.

In clinical trials of daily FORTEO, the median serum concentration of 1,25-dihydroxyvitamin D was increased at 12 months by 19% in women and 14% in men, compared with baseline. In the placebo group, this concentration decreased by 2% in women and increased by 5% in men. The median serum 25-hydroxyvitamin D concentration at 12 months was decreased by 19% in women and 10% in men compared with baseline. In the placebo group, this concentration was unchanged in women and increased by 1% in men.

Effects on markers of bone turnover—Daily administration of FORTEO to men and postmenopausal women with osteoporosis in clinical studies stimulated bone formation, as shown by increases in the formation markers serum bone-specific alkaline phosphatase (BSAP) and procollagen I carboxy-terminal propeptide (PICP). Data on biochemical markers of bone turnover were available for the first 12 months of treatment. Peak concentrations of PICP at 1 month of treatment were approximately 41% above baseline, followed by a decline to near-baseline values by 12 months. BSAP concentrations increased by 1 month of treatment and continued to rise more slowly from 6 through

12 months. The maximum increases of BSAP were 45% above baseline in women and 23% in men. After discontinuation of therapy, BSAP concentrations returned toward baseline. The increases in formation markers were accompanied by secondary increases in the markers of bone resorption: urinary N-telopeptide (NTX) and urinary deoxypyridinoline (DPD), consistent with the physiological coupling of bone formation and resorption in skeletal remodeling. Changes in BSAP, NTX, and DPD were lower in men than in women, possibly because of lower systemic exposure to teriparatide in men.

CLINICAL STUDIES

Treatment of Osteoporosis in Postmenopausal Women—The safety and efficacy of once-daily FORTEO, median exposure of 19 months, were examined in a double-blind, placebo-controlled clinical study of 1637 postmenopausal women with osteoporosis (FORTEO 20 mcg, n = 541).

This multicenter study was performed in the US and 16 other countries. All women received 1000 mg of calcium per day and at least 400 IU of vitamin D per day. Baseline and endpoint spinal radiographs were evaluated using the semiquantitative scoring method of Genant et al [*J Bone Miner Res* 1993;8(9):1137–48]. Ninety percent of the women in the study had 1 or more radiographically diagnosed vertebral fractures at baseline. The primary efficacy endpoint was the occurrence of new radiographically diagnosed vertebral fractures defined as changes in the height of previously undeformed vertebrae. Such fractures are not necessarily symptomatic.

Effect on fracture incidence—New vertebral fractures—FORTEO, when taken with calcium and vitamin D and compared with calcium and vitamin D alone, reduced the risk of 1 or more new vertebral fractures from 14.3% of women in the placebo group to 5.0% in the FORTEO group. This difference was statistically significant ($p<0.001$); the absolute reduction in risk was 9.3% and the relative reduction was 65%. FORTEO was effective in reducing the risk for vertebral fractures regardless of age, baseline rate of bone turnover, or baseline BMD.

[See table 1 at top of previous page]

New nonvertebral osteoporotic fractures—Table 2 shows the effect of FORTEO on the risk of nonvertebral fractures. FORTEO significantly reduced the risk of any nonvertebral fracture from 5.5% in the placebo group to 2.6% in the FORTEO group ($p<0.05$). The absolute reduction in risk was 2.9% and the relative reduction was 53%.

Table 2. Effects of FORTEO on Risk of New Nonvertebral Fractures in Postmenopausal Women with Osteoporosis

Skeletal site	FORTEO[a] N=541	Placebo[a] N=544
Wrist	2 (0.4%)	7 (1.3%)
Ribs	3 (0.6%)	5 (0.9%)
Hip	1 (0.2%)	4 (0.7%)
Ankle/Foot	1 (0.2%)	4 (0.7%)
Humerus	2 (0.4%)	2 (0.4%)
Pelvis	0	3 (0.6%)
Other	6 (1.1%)	8 (1.5%)
Total	14 (2.6%)[b]	30 (5.5%)

[a]Data shown as number (%) of women with fractures.
[b]$p<0.05$ compared with placebo.

The cumulative percentage of postmenopausal women with osteoporosis who sustained new nonvertebral fractures was lower in women treated with FORTEO than in women treated with placebo (*see* Figure 1).

Figure 1. Cumulative percentage of postmenopausal women with osteoporosis sustaining new nonvertebral osteoporotic fractures.*

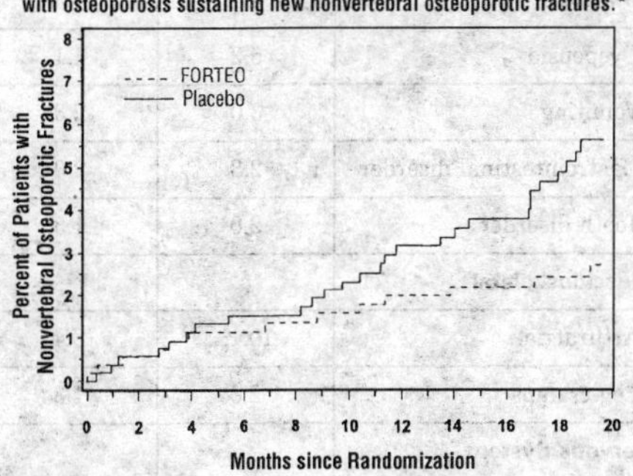

*This graph includes all fractures listed above in Table 2.

Effect on bone mineral density (BMD)—FORTEO increased lumbar spine BMD in postmenopausal women with osteoporosis. Statistically significant increases were seen at 3 months and continued throughout the treatment period, as shown in Figure 2.

Figure 2. Time course of change in lumbar spine BMD in postmenopausal women with osteoporosis treated with FORTEO vs placebo (women with data available at all time points). ($p<0.001$ for FORTEO compared with placebo at each post-baseline time point)

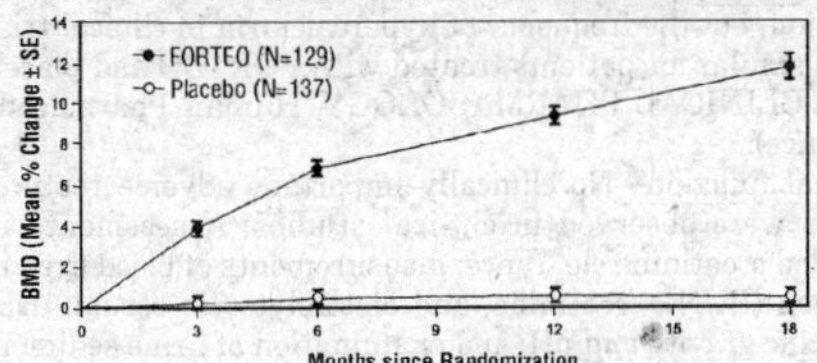

Postmenopausal women with osteoporosis who were treated with FORTEO also had statistically significant increases in BMD at the femoral neck, total hip, and total body (*see* Table 3).

Table 3. Mean Percent Change in BMD from Baseline to Endpoint* in Postmenopausal Women with Osteoporosis, Treated with FORTEO or Placebo

	FORTEO N=541	Placebo N=544
Lumber spine BMD	9.7[a]	1.1
Femoral neck BMD	2.8[b]	-0.7
Total hip BMD	2.6[b]	-1.0
Trochanter BMD	3.5[b]	-0.2
Intertrochanter BMD	2.6[b]	-1.3
Ward's triangle BMD	4.2[b]	-0.8
Total body BMD	0.6[b]	-0.5
Distal 1/3 radius BMD	-2.1	-1.3
Ultradistal radius BMD	-0.1	-1.6

*Intent-to-treat analysis, last observation carried forward.
[a]$p<0.001$ compared with placebo.
[b]$p<0.05$ compared with placebo.

Figure 3 shows the cumulative distribution of the percentage change from baseline of lumbar spine BMD for the FORTEO and placebo groups. FORTEO treatment increased lumbar spine BMD from baseline in 96% of postmenopausal women treated (*see* Figure 3). Seventy-two percent of patients treated with FORTEO achieved at least a 5% increase in spine BMD, and 44% gained 10% or more.

Figure 3. Percent of postmenopausal women with osteoporosis attaining a lumbar spine BMD percent change from baseline at least as great as the value on the x-axis (median duration of treatment 19 months).

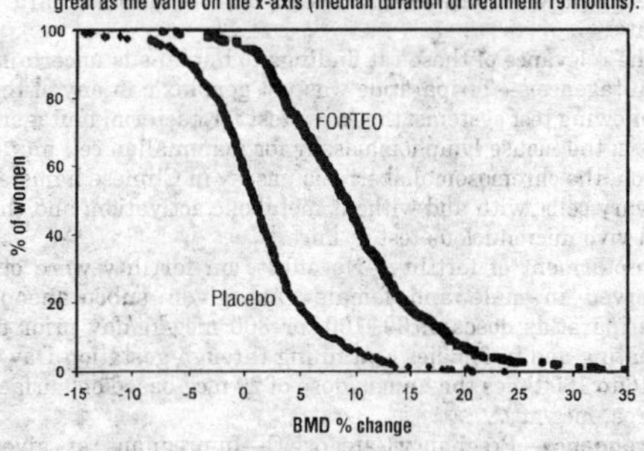

Both treatment groups lost height during the trial. The mean decreases were 3.61 and 2.81 mm in the placebo and FORTEO groups, respectively.

Bone histology—The effects of teriparatide on bone histology were evaluated in iliac crest biopsies of 35 postmenopausal women treated for 12 to 24 months with calcium and vitamin D and teriparatide 20 or 40 mcg/day. Normal mineralization was observed with no evidence of cellular toxicity. The new bone formed with teriparatide was of normal quality (as evidenced by the absence of woven bone and marrow fibrosis).

Treatment to increase bone mass in men with primary or hypogonadal osteoporosis—The safety and efficacy of once-daily FORTEO, median exposure of 10 months, were examined in a double-blind, placebo-controlled clinical study of 437 men with either primary (idiopathic) or hypogonadal osteoporosis (FORTEO 20 mcg, n = 151). This multicenter efficacy study was performed in the US and 10 other countries. All men received 1000 mg of calcium per day and at least 400 IU of vitamin D per day. The primary efficacy endpoint was change in lumbar spine BMD.

FORTEO increased lumbar spine BMD in men with primary or hypogonadal osteoporosis. Statistically significant increases were seen at 3 months and continued throughout the treatment period. FORTEO was effective in increasing lumbar spine BMD regardless of age, baseline rate of bone turnover, and baseline BMD. The effects of FORTEO at additional skeletal sites are shown in table 4.

Table 4. Mean Percent Change in BMD from Baseline to Endpoint* in Men with Primary or Hypogonadal Osteoporosis, Treated with FORTEO or Placebo for a Median of 10 Months

	FORTEO N=151	Placebo N=147
Lumber spine BMD	5.9[a]	0.5
Femoral neck BMD	1.5[b]	0.3
Total hip BMD	1.2	0.5
Trochanter BMD	1.3	1.1
Intertrochanter BMD	1.2	0.6
Ward's triangle BMD	2.8	1.1
Total body BMD	0.4	-0.4
Distal 1/3 radius BMD	-0.5	-0.2
Ultradistal radius BMD	-0.5	-0.3

*Intent-to-treat analysis, last observation carried forward.
[a]$p<0.001$ compared with placebo.
[b]$p<0.05$ compared with placebo.

Figure 4 shows the cumulative distribution of the percentage change from baseline of lumbar spine BMD for the FORTEO and placebo groups. FORTEO treatment for a median of 10 months increased lumbar spine BMD from baseline in 94% of men treated. Fifty-three percent of patients treated with FORTEO achieved at least a 5% increase in spine BMD, and 14% gained 10% or more.

Figure 4. Percent of men with primary or hypogonadal osteoporosis attaining a lumbar spine BMD percent change from baseline at least as great as the value on the x-axis (median duration of treatment 10 months).

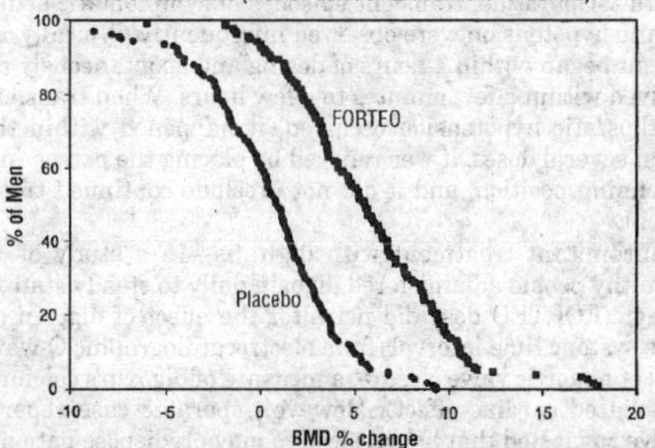

INDICATIONS AND USAGE

FORTEO is indicated for the treatment of postmenopausal women with osteoporosis who are at high risk for fracture. These include women with a history of osteoporotic fracture, or who have multiple risk factors for fracture, or who have failed or are intolerant of previous osteoporosis therapy, based upon physician assessment (*see* BLACK BOX WARNING). In postmenopausal women with osteoporosis, FORTEO increases BMD and reduces the risk of vertebral and nonvertebral fractures.

FORTEO is indicated to increase bone mass in men with primary or hypogonadal osteoporosis who are at high risk for fracture. These include men with a history of osteoporotic fracture, or who have multiple risk factors for fracture, or who have failed or are intolerant to previous osteoporosis therapy, based upon physician assessment (*see* BLACK BOX WARNING). In men with primary or hypogonadal osteoporosis, FORTEO increases BMD. The effects of FORTEO on risk for fracture in men have not been studied.

- FORTEO reduces the risk of vertebral fractures in postmenopausal women with osteoporosis.
- FORTEO reduces the risk of nonvertebral fractures in postmenopausal women with osteoporosis.
- FORTEO increases vertebral and femoral neck BMD in postmenopausal women with osteoporosis and in men with primary or hypogonadal osteoporosis.
- The effects of FORTEO on fracture risk have not been studied in men.

CONTRAINDICATIONS

FORTEO should not be given to patients with hypersensitivity to teriparatide or to any of its excipients.

WARNINGS

In male and female rats, teriparatide caused an increase in the incidence of osteosarcoma (a malignant bone tumor) that was dependent on dose and treatment duration (*see* BLACK BOX WARNING *and* PRECAUTIONS; Carcinogenesis).

Continued on next page

*** Identi-Code® symbol. This product information was prepared in June 2004. Current information on these and other products of Eli Lilly and Company may be obtained by direct inquiry to Lilly Research Laboratories, Lilly Corporate Center, Indianapolis, Indiana 46285, (800) 545-5979.**

Forteo—Cont.

The following categories of patients have increased baseline risk of osteosarcoma and therefore should not be treated with FORTEO:

- Paget's disease of bone. FORTEO should not be given to patients with Paget's disease of bone. Unexplained elevations of alkaline phosphatase may indicate Paget's disease of bone.
- Pediatric populations. FORTEO has not been studied in pediatric populations. FORTEO should not be used in pediatric patients or young adults with open epiphyses.
- Prior radiation therapy. Patients with a prior history of radiation therapy involving the skeleton should be excluded from treatment with FORTEO.

Patients with bone metastases or a history of skeletal malignancies should be excluded from treatment with FORTEO.

Patients with metabolic bone diseases other than osteoporosis should be excluded from treatment with FORTEO.

FORTEO has not been studied in patients with pre-existing hypercalcemia. These patients should be excluded from treatment with FORTEO because of the possibility of exacerbating hypercalcemia.

PRECAUTIONS

General—The safety and efficacy of FORTEO have not been evaluated beyond 2 years of treatment. Consequently, use of the drug for more than 2 years is not recommended.

In clinical trials, the frequency of urolithiasis was similar in patients treated with FORTEO and placebo. However, FORTEO has not been studied in patients with active urolithiasis. If active urolithiasis or pre-existing hypercalciuria are suspected, measurement of urinary calcium excretion should be considered. FORTEO should be used with caution in patients with active or recent urolithiasis because of the potential to exacerbate this condition.

Hypotension—In short-term clinical pharmacology studies with teriparatide, transient episodes of symptomatic orthostatic hypotension were observed infrequently. Typically, an event began within 4 hours of dosing and spontaneously resolved within a few minutes to a few hours. When transient orthostatic hypotension occurred, it happened within the first several doses, it was relieved by placing the person in a reclining position, and it did not preclude continued treatment.

Concomitant treatment with digitalis—In a study of 15 healthy people administered digoxin daily to steady state, a single FORTEO dose did not alter the effect of digoxin on the systolic time interval (from electrocardiographic Q-wave onset to aortic valve closure, a measure of digoxin's calcium-mediated cardiac effect). However, sporadic case reports have suggested that hypercalcemia may predispose patients to digitalis toxicity. Because FORTEO transiently increases serum calcium, FORTEO should be used with caution in patients taking digitalis.

Hepatic, renal, and cardiac—Limited information is available to evaluate safety in patients with hepatic, renal, and cardiac disease.

Information for Patients—For safe and effective use of FORTEO, the physician should inform patients about the following:

General—Patients should read the *Medication Guide* and pen *User Manual* before starting therapy with FORTEO and re-read them each time the prescription is renewed.

Osteosarcomas in rats—Patients should be made aware that FORTEO caused osteosarcomas in rats and that the clinical relevance of these findings is unknown.

Orthostatic hypotension—FORTEO should be administered initially under circumstances where the patient can immediately sit or lie down if symptoms occur. Patients should be instructed that if they feel lightheaded or have palpitations after the injection, they should sit or lie down until the symptoms resolve. If symptoms persist or worsen, patients should be instructed to consult a physician before continuing treatment (*see* PRECAUTIONS, General).

Hypercalcemia—Although symptomatic hypercalcemia was not observed in clinical trials, physicians should instruct patients to contact a health care provider if they develop persistent symptoms of hypercalcemia (ie, nausea, vomiting, constipation, lethargy, muscle weakness).

Use of the pen—Patients should be instructed on how to properly use the delivery device (refer to *User Manual*), properly dispose of needles, and be advised not to share their pens with other patients.

Other osteoporosis treatments—Patients should be informed regarding the roles of supplemental calcium and/or vitamin D, weight-bearing exercise, and modification of certain behavioral factors such as cigarette smoking and/or alcohol consumption.

Laboratory Tests—Serum calcium—FORTEO transiently increases serum calcium, with the maximal effect observed at approximately 4 to 6 hours post-dose. By 16 hours post-dose, serum calcium generally has returned to or near baseline. These effects should be kept in mind because serum calcium concentrations observed within 16 hours after a dose may reflect the pharmacologic effect of teriparatide. Persistent hypercalcemia was not observed in clinical trials with FORTEO. If persistent hypercalcemia is detected, treatment with FORTEO should be discontinued pending further evaluation of the cause of hypercalcemia.

Patients known to have an underlying hypercalcemic disorder, such as primary hyperparathyroidism, should not be treated with FORTEO (*see* WARNINGS).

Urinary calcium—FORTEO increases urinary calcium excretion, but the frequency of hypercalciuria in clinical trials was similar for patients treated with FORTEO and placebo (*see* CLINICAL PHARMACOLOGY, Human Pharmacodynamics).

Renal function—No clinically important adverse renal effects were observed in clinical studies. Assessments included creatinine clearance; measurements of blood urea nitrogen (BUN), creatinine, and electrolytes in serum; urine specific gravity and pH; and examination of urine sediment. Long-term evaluation of patients with severe renal insufficiency, patients undergoing acute or chronic dialysis, or patients who have functioning renal transplants has not been performed.

Serum uric acid—FORTEO increases serum uric acid concentrations. In clinical trials, 2.8% of FORTEO patients had serum uric acid concentrations above the upper limit of normal compared with 0.7% of placebo patients. However, the hyperuricemia did not result in an increase in gout, arthralgia, or urolithiasis.

Carcinogenesis, Mutagenesis, Impairment of Fertility—Carcinogenesis—Two carcinogenicity bioassays were conducted in Fischer 344 rats. In the first study, male and female rats were given daily subcutaneous teriparatide injections of 5, 30, or 75 mcg/kg/day for 24 months from 2 months of age. These doses resulted in systemic exposures that were, respectively, 3, 20, and 60 times higher than the systemic exposure observed in humans following a subcutaneous dose of 20 mcg (based on AUC comparison). Teriparatide treatment resulted in a marked dose-related increase in the incidence of osteosarcoma, a rare malignant bone tumor, in both male and female rats. Osteosarcomas were observed at all doses and the incidence reached 40% to 50% in the high-dose groups. Teriparatide also caused a dose-related increase in osteoblastoma and osteoma in both sexes. No osteosarcomas, osteoblastomas or osteomas were observed in untreated control rats. The bone tumors in rats occurred in association with a large increase in bone mass and focal osteoblast hyperplasia.

The second 2-year study was carried out in order to determine the effect of treatment duration and animal age on the development of bone tumors. Female rats were treated for different periods between 2 and 26 months of age with subcutaneous doses and 5 and 30 mcg/kg (equivalent to 3 and 20 times the human exposure at the 20-mcg dose, based on AUC comparison). The study showed that the occurrence of osteosarcoma, osteoblastoma and osteoma was dependent upon dose and duration of exposure. Bone tumors were observed when immature 2-month old rats were treated with 30 mcg/kg/day for 24 months or with 5 or 30 mcg/kg/day for 6 months. Bone tumors were also observed when mature 6-month old rats were treated with 30 mcg/kg/day for 6 or 20 months. Tumors were not detected when mature 6-month old rats were treated with 5 mcg/kg/day for 6 or 20 months. The results did not demonstrate a difference in susceptibility to bone tumor formation, associated with teriparatide treatment, between mature and immature rats.

The relevance of these rat findings to humans is uncertain.

Mutagenesis—Teriparatide was not genotoxic in any of the following test systems: the Ames test for bacterial mutagenesis; the mouse lymphoma assay for mammalian cell mutation, the chromosomal aberration assay in Chinese hamster ovary cells, with and without metabolic activation; and the in vivo micronucleus test in mice.

Impairment of fertility—No effects on fertility were observed in male and female rats given subcutaneous teriparatide doses of 30, 100, or 300 mcg/kg/day prior to mating and in females continuing through gestation Day 6 (16 to 160 times the human dose of 20 mcg based on surface area, mcg/m^2).

Pregnancy—Pregnancy Category C—In pregnant rats given subcutaneous teriparatide doses up to 1000 mcg/kg/day, there were no findings. In pregnant mice given subcutaneous doses of 225 or 1000 mcg/kg/day (≥60 times the human dose based on surface area, mcg/m^2) from gestation Day 6 through 15, the fetuses showed an increased incidence of skeletal deviations or variations (interrupted rib, extra vertebra or rib).

Developmental effects in a perinatal/postnatal study in pregnant rats given subcutaneous doses of teriparatide from gestation Day 6 through postpartum Day 20 included mild growth retardation in female offspring at doses ≥225 mcg/kg/day (≥120 times the human dose based on surface area, mcg/m^2), and in male offspring at 1000 mcg/kg/day (540 times the human dose based on surface area, mcg/m^2). There was also reduced motor activity in both male and female offspring at 1000 mcg/kg/day. There were no developmental or reproductive effects in mice or rats at a dose of 30 mcg/kg (8 or 16 times the human dose based on surface area, mcg/m^2). The effect of teriparatide treatment on human fetal development has not been studied. FORTEO is not indicated for use in pregnancy.

Nursing Mothers—Because FORTEO is indicated for the treatment of osteoporosis in postmenopausal women, it should not be administered to women who are nursing their children. There have been no clinical studies to determine if teriparatide is secreted into breast milk.

Pediatric Use—The safety and efficacy of FORTEO have not been established in pediatric populations. FORTEO is not indicated for use in pediatric patients (*see* WARNINGS).

Geriatric Use—Of the patients receiving FORTEO in the osteoporosis trial of 1637 postmenopausal women, 75% were 65 years of age and over and 23% were 75 years of age and over. Of the patients receiving FORTEO in the osteoporosis trial of 437 men, 39% were 65 years of age and over and 13% were 75 years of age and over. No significant differences in bone response or adverse reactions were seen in geriatric patients receiving FORTEO as compared with younger patients. Nonetheless, as with many medications, elderly patients may have greater sensitivity to the adverse effects of FORTEO.

ADVERSE EVENTS

The safety of teriparatide has been evaluated in 24 clinical trials that enrolled over 2800 women and men. Four long-term Phase 3 clinical trials included 1 large placebo-controlled, double-blind, multinational trial with 1637 postmenopausal women; 1 placebo-controlled, double-blind, multinational trial with 437 men; and 2 active-controlled trials including 393 postmenopausal women. Teriparatide doses ranged from 5 to 100 mcg/day in short-term trials and 20 to 40 mcg/day in the other trials. A total of 1943 of the patients studied received teriparatide, including 815 patients at 20 mcg/day and 1107 patients at 40 mcg/day. In the clinical trials, a total of 1432 patients were treated with teriparatide for 3 months to 2 years, of whom 1137 were treated for greater than 1 year (500 at 20 mcg/day and 637 at 40 mcg/day). The maximum duration of treatment was 2 years. Adverse events associated with FORTEO usually were mild and generally did not require discontinuation of therapy.

In the two Phase 3, placebo-controlled clinical trials in men and postmenopausal women, early discontinuation due to adverse events occurred in 5.6% of patients assigned to placebo and 7.1% of patients assigned to FORTEO. Reported adverse events that appeared to be increased by FORTEO treatment were dizziness and leg cramps.

Table 5 lists adverse events that occurred in the two Phase 3, placebo-controlled clinical trials in men and postmenopausal women at a frequency ≥2.0% in the FORTEO groups and in more FORTEO-treated patients than in placebo-treated patients, without attribution of causality.

Table 5. Percentage of Patients with Adverse Events Reported by at Least 2% of FORTEO-Treated Patients and in More FORTEO-Treated Patients than Placebo-Treated Patients from the Two Principal Osteoporosis Trials in Women and Men
Adverse events are shown without attribution of causality.

	FORTEO	Placebo
	N=691	N=691
Event Classification	(%)	(%)
Body as a Whole		
Pain	21.3	20.5
Headache	7.5	7.4
Asthenia	8.7	6.8
Neck pain	3.0	2.7
Cardiovascular		
Hypertension	7.1	6.8
Angina pectoris	2.5	1.6
Syncope	2.6	1.4
Digestive System		
Nausea	8.5	6.7
Constipation	5.4	4.5
Diarrhea	5.1	4.6
Dyspepsia	5.2	4.1
Vomiting	3.0	2.3
Gastrointestinal disorder	2.3	2.0
Tooth disorder	2.0	1.3
Musculoskeletal		
Arthralgia	10.1	8.4
Leg cramps	2.6	1.3
Nervous System		
Dizziness	8.0	5.4
Depression	4.1	2.7
Insomnia	4.3	3.6
Vertigo	3.8	2.7

Respiratory System		
Rhinitis	9.6	8.8
Cough increased	6.4	5.5
Pharyngitis	5.5	4.8
Dyspnea	3.6	2.6
Pneumonia	3.9	3.3
Skin and Appendages		
Rash	4.9	4.5
Sweating	2.2	1.7

Serum calcium—FORTEO transiently increases serum calcium, with the maximal effect observed at approximately 4 to 6 hours post-dose. Serum calcium measured at least 16 hours post-dose was not different from pretreatment levels. In clinical trials, the frequency of at least 1 episode of transient hypercalcemia in the 4 to 6 hours after FORTEO administration was increased from 1.5% of women and none of the men treated with placebo to 11.1% of women and 6.0% of men treated with FORTEO. The number of patients treated with FORTEO whose transient hypercalcemia was verified on consecutive measurements was 3.0% of women and 1.3% of men.

Immunogenicity—In a large clinical trial, antibodies that cross-reacted with teriparatide were detected in 2.8% of women receiving FORTEO. Generally, antibodies were first detected following 12 months of treatment and diminished after withdrawal of therapy. There was no evidence of hypersensitivity reactions, allergic reactions, effects on serum calcium, or effects on BMD response.

OVERDOSAGE

Incidents of overdose in humans have not been reported in clinical trials. Teriparatide has been administered in single doses of up to 100 mcg and in repeated doses of up to 60 mcg/day for 6 weeks. The effects of overdose that might be expected include a delayed hypercalcemic effect and risk of orthostatic hypotension. Nausea, vomiting, dizziness, and headache might also occur.

In single-dose rodent studies using subcutaneous injection of teriparatide, no mortality was seen in rats given doses of 1000 mcg/kg (540 times the human dose based on surface area, mcg/m^2) or in mice given 10,000 mcg/kg (2700 times the human dose based on surface area, mcg/m^2).

Overdose management—There is no specific antidote for teriparatide. Treatment of suspected overdose should include discontinuation of FORTEO, monitoring of serum calcium and phosphorus, and implementation of appropriate supportive measures, such as hydration.

DOSAGE AND ADMINISTRATION

FORTEO should be administered as a subcutaneous injection into the thigh or abdominal wall. The recommended dosage is 20 mcg once a day.

FORTEO should be administered initially under circumstances in which the patient can sit or lie down if symptoms of orthostatic hypotension occur (*see* PRECAUTIONS, Information for the Patient).

FORTEO is a clear and colorless liquid. Do not use if solid particles appear or if the solution is cloudy or colored. The FORTEO pen should not be used past the stated expiration date.

No data are available on the safety or efficacy of intravenous or intramuscular injection of FORTEO.

The safety and efficacy of FORTEO have not been evaluated beyond 2 years of treatment. Consequently, use of the drug for more than 2 years is not recommended.

INSTRUCTIONS FOR PEN USE

Patients and caregivers who administer FORTEO should receive appropriate training and instruction on the proper use of the FORTEO pen from a qualified health professional. It is important to read, understand, and follow the instructions in the FORTEO pen User Manual for priming the pen and dosing. Failure to do so may result in inaccurate dosing. Each FORTEO pen can be used for up to 28 days after the first injection. After the 28-day use period, discard the FORTEO pen, even if it still contains some unused solution. Never share a FORTEO pen.

STORAGE

The FORTEO pen should be stored under refrigeration at 2° to 8°C (36° to 46°F) at all times. Recap the pen when not in use to protect the cartridge from physical damage and light. During the use period, time out of the refrigerator should be minimized; the dose may be delivered immediately following removal from the refrigerator.

Do not freeze. Do not use FORTEO if it has been frozen.

HOW SUPPLIED

The FORTEO pen is available in the following package size:

One 3 mL prefilled pen delivery device NDC 0002-8971-01 (MS8971)

Literature issued November 2002
Manufactured by Lilly France S.A.S.
F-67640 Fegersheim, France
for Eli Lilly and Company
Indianapolis, IN 46285, USA
www.lilly.com

Medication Guide
FORTEO™

Generic name: teriparatide (rDNA origin) injection

Read this information carefully before you start taking FORTEO (for-TAY-o) to learn about the benefits and risks of FORTEO. Before beginning therapy, read the FORTEO pen User Manual for information on how to use the pen to inject your medicine. Read the information you get with FORTEO each time you get a refill, in case something has changed. Talk with your health care provider if there is something you do not understand or if you want to learn more about FORTEO.

What is the most important information I should know about FORTEO?

As part of drug testing, teriparatide, the active ingredient in FORTEO, was given to rats for a significant part of their lifetime. **In these studies, teriparatide caused some rats to develop osteosarcoma, a bone cancer.** Osteosarcoma in humans is a serious but very rare cancer. Osteosarcoma occurs in about 4 out of every million older adults each year. **It is not known if humans treated with FORTEO also have a higher chance of getting osteosarcoma.**

FORTEO is approved for use in both men and postmenopausal (after the "change of life") women with osteoporosis who are at high risk for having broken bones (fractures) from osteoporosis.

Before starting treatment, talk with your doctor about the possible benefits and risks of FORTEO so you can decide if it is right for you.

What is Osteoporosis?

Osteoporosis is a disease in which the bones become thin and weak, increasing the chance of having a broken bone. Osteoporosis usually causes no symptoms until a fracture happens. The most common fractures are in the spine (backbone). They can shorten height, even without causing pain. Over time, the spine can become curved or deformed and the body bent over. Fractures from osteoporosis can also happen in almost any bone in the body, for example, the wrist, rib, or hip. Once you have had a fracture, the chance for more fractures greatly increases.

The following risk factors increase your chance of getting fractures from osteoporosis:

- past broken bones from osteoporosis
- very low bone mineral density (BMD)
- frequent falls
- limited movement, such as using a wheelchair
- medical conditions likely to cause bone loss, such as some kinds of arthritis
- medicines that may cause bone loss, for example: seizure medicines (such as phenytoin), blood thinners (such as heparin), steroids (such as prednisone), or high doses of vitamins A or D.

What is FORTEO?

FORTEO is a prescription medicine used to treat osteoporosis by forming new bone. FORTEO is the brand name for teriparatide, which is the same as the active part of a natural hormone called parathyroid hormone or "PTH." FORTEO forms new bone, increases bone mineral density and bone strength, and as a result, reduces the chance of getting a fracture. In a study of postmenopausal (after the "change of life") women with osteoporosis, FORTEO reduced the number of fractures of the spine and other bones. The effect on fractures has not been studied in men.

FORTEO is approved for use in both men and postmenopausal women with osteoporosis who are at high risk for having fractures. FORTEO can be used by people who have had a fracture related to osteoporosis, or who have multiple risk factors for fracture (See "What is osteoporosis?"), or who cannot use other osteoporosis treatments.

Who should not use FORTEO?

Do not use FORTEO if you:

- have Paget's disease of the bone
- have unexplained high levels of alkaline phosphatase in your blood, which means you might have Paget's disease. If you are not sure, ask your doctor.
- are a child or growing adult
- have ever been diagnosed with bone cancer or other cancers that have spread (metastasized) to your bones
- have had radiation therapy involving your bones
- have certain bone diseases. If you have a bone disease, tell your doctor.
- have too much calcium in your blood (hypercalcemia)
- are pregnant or nursing
- have had an allergic reaction to FORTEO or one of its ingredients (See the ingredients section at the end of this Medication Guide)
- have trouble injecting yourself and do not have someone who can help you.

FORTEO should not be used to prevent osteoporosis or to treat patients who are not considered to be at high risk for fracture.

Tell your health care provider and pharmacist about all the medicines you are taking when you start taking FORTEO, and if you start taking a new medicine after you start FORTEO treatment. Tell them about all medicines you get with prescriptions and without prescriptions, as well as herbal or natural remedies. Your doctor and pharmacist need this information to help keep you from taking a combination of products that may harm you.

How should I take FORTEO?

- Take FORTEO once a day for as long as your doctor prescribes it for you. Use of FORTEO for more than 2 years is not recommended. Your health care professional (doctor, nurse, or pharmacist) should teach you how to use the FORTEO pen (prefilled delivery device). (See the User Manual for written instructions on how to use the FORTEO pen.)
- Some patients get dizzy or get a fast heartbeat after the first few doses. For the first few doses, inject FORTEO where you can sit or lie down right away if you get dizzy.
- Inject FORTEO once each day in your thigh or abdomen (lower stomach area).
- You can take FORTEO with or without food or drink.
- You can take FORTEO at any time of the day. To help you remember to take FORTEO, take it at about the same time each day.
- Do not use FORTEO if it has solid particles in it, or if it is cloudy or colored. It should be clear and colorless.
- Do not use FORTEO after the expiration date printed on the pen and pen packaging.
- Throw away any FORTEO pen that you started using more than 28 days earlier, even if it still has medicine in it (See the User Manual).
- Inject FORTEO shortly after you take the pen out of the refrigerator. Recap the pen and put it back into the refrigerator right after use (See the User Manual).
- If you forget or are unable to take FORTEO at your usual time, take it as soon as possible on that day. Do not take more than one injection in the same day.
- Talk with your health care provider about other ways you can help your osteoporosis, such as exercise, diet, supplements, and reducing or stopping your use of tobacco and alcohol. If your health care provider recommends calcium and vitamin D supplements, you can take them at the same time as FORTEO.

What are the possible side effects of FORTEO?

Most side effects are mild and include dizziness and leg cramps. If you become lightheaded or have fast heartbeats after your injection, sit or lie down until you feel better. If you do not feel better, call your health care provider before continuing treatment.

Contact your health care provider if you have continuing nausea, vomiting, constipation, low energy, or muscle weakness. These may be signs there is too much calcium in your blood.

These are not all the possible side effects of FORTEO. For more information, ask your health care provider or pharmacist.

Your health care provider may take samples of blood and urine during treatment to check your response to FORTEO. Also, your health care provider may ask you to have follow-up tests of bone mineral density.

How should I store FORTEO?

- Keep your FORTEO pen in the refrigerator at 36° to 46°F (2° to 8°C).
- Do not freeze the pen. Do not use FORTEO if it has been frozen.
- You can use your FORTEO pen for up to 28 days after the first injection from the pen.
- Throw away the pen properly (See the User Manual) after 28 days of use, even if it is not completely empty.
- Recap the pen after each use (See the User Manual) to protect from physical damage.

General information about using FORTEO safely and effectively

Medicines are sometimes prescribed for conditions that are not mentioned in Medication Guides. Do not use FORTEO for a condition for which it was not prescribed. Do not give FORTEO to other people, even if they have the same condition you have.

This Medication Guide summarizes the most important information about FORTEO. If you would like more information, talk with your doctor, nurse, or pharmacist. You can ask your pharmacist or health care provider for information about FORTEO that is written for health care professionals. You can also call Lilly toll free at 1-866-4FORTEO (1-866-436-7836).

Ingredients

In addition to the active ingredient teriparatide, inactive ingredients are glacial acetic acid, sodium acetate (anhydrous), mannitol, Metacresol, and Water for Injection. In addition, hydrochloric acid solution 10% and/or sodium hydroxide solution 10% may have been added to adjust product pH.

This Medication Guide has been approved by the US Food and Drug Administration.

Literature issued November 2002
Manufactured by Lilly France S.A.S.
F-67640 Fegersheim, France
for Eli Lilly and Company
Indianapolis, IN 46285, USA
www.lilly.com

Continued on next page

*** Identi-Code® symbol. This product information was prepared in June 2004. Current information on these and other products of Eli Lilly and Company may be obtained by direct inquiry to Lilly Research Laboratories, Lilly Corporate Center, Indianapolis, Indiana 46285, (800) 545-5979.**

Forteo—Cont.

PA 9241 FSAMP

Shown in Product Identification Guide, page 320

GEMZAR® ℞
[jĕm-zar]
(GEMCITABINE HCl)
FOR INJECTION

DESCRIPTION

Gemzar® (gemcitabine HCl) is a nucleoside analogue that exhibits antitumor activity. Gemcitabine HCl is 2′-deoxy-2′,2′-difluorocytidine monohydrochloride (β-isomer). The structural formula is as follows:

[structural formula: NH₂ • HCl, HO, N, O, F, H, OH]

The empirical formula for gemcitabine HCl is $C_9H_{11}F_2N_3O_4$ • HCl. It has a molecular weight of 299.66.
Gemcitabine HCl is a white to off-white solid. It is soluble in water, slightly soluble in methanol, and practically insoluble in ethanol and polar organic solvents.
The clinical formulation is supplied in a sterile form for intravenous use only. Vials of Gemzar contain either 200 mg or 1 g of gemcitabine HCl (expressed as free base) formulated with mannitol (200 mg or 1 g, respectively) and sodium acetate (12.5 mg or 62.5 mg, respectively) as a sterile lyophilized powder. Hydrochloric acid and/or sodium hydroxide may have been added for pH adjustment.

CLINICAL PHARMACOLOGY

Gemcitabine exhibits cell phase specificity, primarily killing cells undergoing DNA synthesis (S-phase) and also blocking the progression of cells through the G1/S-phase boundary. Gemcitabine is metabolized intracellularly by nucleoside kinases to the active diphosphate (dFdCDP) and triphosphate (dFdCTP) nucleosides. The cytotoxic effect of gemcitabine is attributed to a combination of two actions of the diphosphate and the triphosphate nucleosides, which leads to inhibition of DNA synthesis. First, gemcitabine diphosphate inhibits ribonucleotide reductase, which is responsible for catalyzing the reactions that generate the deoxynucleoside triphosphates for DNA synthesis. Inhibition of this enzyme by the diphosphate nucleoside causes a reduction in the concentrations of deoxynucleotides, including dCTP. Second, gemcitabine triphosphate competes with dCTP for incorporation into DNA. The reduction in the intracellular concentration of dCTP (by the action of the diphosphate) enhances the incorporation of gemcitabine triphosphate into DNA (self-potentiation). After the gemcitabine nucleotide is incorporated into DNA, only one additional nucleotide is added to the growing DNA strands. After this addition, there is inhibition of further DNA synthesis. DNA polymerase epsilon is unable to remove the gemcitabine nucleotide and repair the growing DNA strands (masked chain termination). In CEM T lymphoblastoid cells, gemcitabine induces internucleosomal DNA fragmentation, one of the characteristics of programmed cell death.
Gemcitabine demonstrated dose-dependent synergistic activity with cisplatin *in vitro*. No effect of cisplatin on gemcitabine triphosphate accumulation or DNA double-strand breaks was observed. *In vivo*, gemcitabine showed activity in combination with cisplatin against the LX-1 and CALU-6 human lung xenografts, but minimal activity was seen with the NCI-H460 or NCI-H520 xenografts. Gemcitabine was synergistic with cisplatin in the Lewis lung murine xenograft. Sequential exposure to gemcitabine 4 hours before cisplatin produced the greatest interaction.
Human Pharmacokinetics — Gemcitabine disposition was studied in 5 patients who received a single 1000 mg/m²/30 minute infusion of radiolabeled drug. Within one (1) week, 92% to 98% of the dose was recovered, almost entirely in the urine. Gemcitabine (<10%) and the inactive uracil metabolite, 2′-deoxy-2′,2′-difluorouridine (dFdU), accounted for 99% of the excreted dose. The metabolite dFdU is also found in plasma. Gemcitabine plasma protein binding is negligible.
The pharmacokinetics of gemcitabine were examined in 353 patients, about 2/3 men, with various solid tumors. Pharmacokinetic parameters were derived using data from patients treated for varying durations of therapy given weekly with periodic rest weeks and using both short infusions (<70 minutes) and long infusions (70 to 285 minutes). The total Gemzar dose varied from 500 to 3600 mg/m².
Gemcitabine pharmacokinetics are linear and are described by a 2-compartment model. Population pharmacokinetic analyses of combined single and multiple dose studies showed that the volume of distribution of gemcitabine was significantly influenced by duration of infusion and gender. Clearance was affected by age and gender. Differences in either clearance or volume of distribution based on patient characteristics or the duration of infusion result in changes in half-life and plasma concentrations. Table 1 shows plasma clearance and half-life of gemcitabine following short infusions for typical patients by age and gender.

Table 1: Gemcitabine Clearance and Half-Life for the "Typical" Patient

Age	Clearance Men (L/hr/m²)	Clearance Women (L/hr/m²)	Half-Life[a] Men (min)	Half-Life[a] Women (min)
29	92.2	69.4	42	49
45	75.7	57.0	48	57
65	55.1	41.5	61	73
79	40.7	30.7	79	94

[a] Half-life for patients receiving a short infusion (<70 min).

Gemcitabine half-life for short infusions ranged from 32 to 94 minutes, and the value for long infusions varied from 245 to 638 minutes, depending on age and gender, reflecting a greatly increased volume of distribution with longer infusions. The lower clearance in women and the elderly results in higher concentrations of gemcitabine for any given dose. The volume of distribution was increased with infusion length. Volume of distribution of gemcitabine was 50 L/m² following infusions lasting <70 minutes, indicating that gemcitabine, after short infusions, is not extensively distributed into tissues. For long infusions, the volume of distribution rose to 370 L/m², reflecting slow equilibration of gemcitabine within the tissue compartment.
The maximum plasma concentrations of dFdU (inactive metabolite) were achieved up to 30 minutes after discontinuation of the infusions and the metabolite is excreted in urine without undergoing further biotransformation. The metabolite did not accumulate with weekly dosing, but its elimination is dependent on renal excretion, and could accumulate with decreased renal function.
The effects of significant renal or hepatic insufficiency on the disposition of gemcitabine have not been assessed.
The active metabolite, gemcitabine triphosphate, can be extracted from peripheral blood mononuclear cells. The half-life of the terminal phase for gemcitabine triphosphate from mononuclear cells ranges from 1.7 to 19.4 hours.
Drug Interactions — When Gemzar (1250 mg/m² on Days 1 and 8) and cisplatin (75 mg/m² on Day 1) were administered in NSCLC patients, the clearance of gemcitabine on Day 1 was 128 L/hr/m² and on Day 8 was 107 L/hr/m². The clearance of cisplatin in the same study was reported to be 3.94 mL/min/m² with a corresponding half-life of 134 hours (*see Drug Interactions under* **PRECAUTIONS**).

CLINICAL STUDIES

Breast Cancer — Data from a multi-national, randomized Phase 3 study (529 patients) support the use of Gemzar in combination with paclitaxel for treatment of breast cancer patients who have received prior adjuvant/neoadjuvant anthracycline chemotherapy unless clinically contraindicated. Gemzar 1250 mg/m² was administered on Days 1 and 8 of a 21-day cycle with paclitaxel 175 mg/m² administered prior to Gemzar on Day 1 of each cycle. Single-agent paclitaxel 175 mg/m² was administered on Day 1 of each 21-day cycle as the control arm.
The addition of Gemzar to paclitaxel resulted in statistically significant improvement in time to documented disease progression and overall response rate compared to monotherapy with paclitaxel as shown in Table 2 and Figure 1. Further, there was a strong trend toward improved survival for the group given Gemzar based on an interim survival analysis.
[See table 2 below]

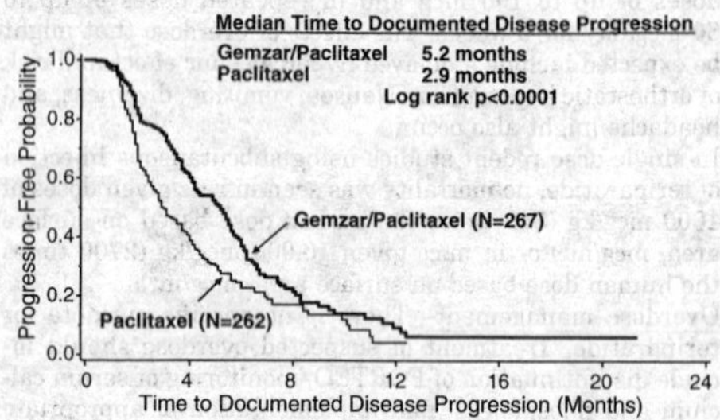

Figure 1: Kaplan-Meier Curve of Time to Documented Disease Progression in Gemzar plus Paclitaxel versus Paclitaxel Breast Cancer Study (N=529).

Non-Small Cell Lung Cancer (NSCLC) — Data from 2 randomized clinical studies (657 patients) support the use of Gemzar in combination with cisplatin for the first-line treatment of patients with locally advanced or metastatic NSCLC.
Gemzar plus cisplatin versus cisplatin: This study was conducted in Europe, the US, and Canada in 522 patients with inoperable Stage IIIA, IIIB, or IV NSCLC who had not received prior chemotherapy. Gemzar 1000 mg/m² was administered on Days 1, 8, and 15 of a 28-day cycle with cisplatin 100 mg/m² administered on Day 1 of each cycle. Single-agent cisplatin 100 mg/m² was administered on Day 1 of each 28-day cycle. The primary endpoint was survival. Patient demographics are shown in Table 3. An imbalance with regard to histology was observed with 48% of patients on the cisplatin arm and 37% of patients on the Gemzar plus cisplatin arm having adenocarcinoma.
The Kaplan-Meier survival curve is shown in Figure 2. Median survival time on the Gemzar plus cisplatin arm was 9.0 months compared to 7.6 months on the single-agent cisplatin arm (Logrank p=0.008, two-sided). Median time to disease progression was 5.2 months on the Gemzar plus cisplatin arm compared to 3.7 months on the cisplatin arm (Logrank p=0.009, two-sided). The objective response rate on the Gemzar plus cisplatin arm was 26% compared to 10% with cisplatin (Fisher's Exact p<0.0001, two-sided). No difference between treatment arms with regard to duration of response was observed.
Gemzar plus cisplatin versus etoposide plus cisplatin: A second, multi-center, study in Stage IIIB or IV NSCLC randomized 135 patients to Gemzar 1250 mg/m² on Days 1 and 8, and cisplatin 100 mg/m² on Day 1 of a 21-day cycle or to etoposide 100 mg/m² I.V. on Days 1, 2, and 3 and cisplatin 100 mg/m² on Day 1 on a 21-day cycle (Table 3).
There was no significant difference in survival between the two treatment arms (Logrank p=0.18, two-sided). The median survival was 8.7 months for the Gemzar plus cisplatin arm versus 7.0 months for the etoposide plus cisplatin arm. Median time to disease progression for the Gemzar plus cisplatin arm was 5.0 months compared to 4.1 months on the etoposide plus cisplatin arm (Logrank p=0.015, two-sided).

Table 2: Gemzar Plus Paclitaxel Versus Paclitaxel in Breast Cancer

	Gemzar/Paclitaxel	Paclitaxel	
Number of patients	267	262	
Median age, years	53	52	
Range	26 to 83	26 to 75	
Metastatic disease	97.0%	96.9%	
Baseline KPS[a] ≥90	70.4%	74.4%	
Number of tumor sites			
1-2	56.6%	58.8%	
≥3	43.4%	41.2%	
Visceral disease	73.4%	72.9%	
Prior anthracycline	96.6%	95.8%	
Time to Documented Disease Progression[b]			p<0.0001
Median (95%, C.I.), months	5.2 (4.2, 5.6)	2.9 (2.6, 3.7)	
Hazard Ratio (95% C.I.)	0.650 (0.524, 0.805)		p<0.0001
Overall Response Rate[b] (95%, C.I.)	40.8% (34.9, 46.7)	22.1% (17.1, 27.2)	p<0.0001

[a] Karnofsky Performance Status.
[b] These represent reconciliation of investigator and Independent Review Committee assessments according to a predefined algorithm.

The objective response rate for the Gemzar plus cisplatin arm was 33% compared to 14% on the etoposide plus cisplatin arm (Fisher's Exact p=0.01, two-sided).

Quality of Life (QOL): QOL was a secondary endpoint in both randomized studies. In the Gemzar plus cisplatin versus cisplatin study, QOL was measured using the FACT-L, which assessed physical, social, emotional and functional well-being, and lung cancer symptoms. In the study of Gemzar plus cisplatin versus etoposide plus cisplatin, QOL was measured using the EORTC QLQ-C30 and LC13, which assessed physical and psychological functioning and symptoms related to both lung cancer and its treatment. In both studies no significant differences were observed in QOL between the Gemzar plus cisplatin arm and the comparator arm.

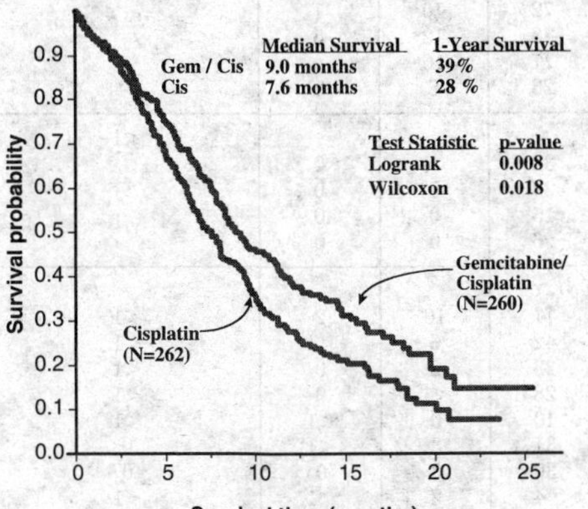

Figure 2: Kaplan-Meier Survival Curve in Gemzar plus Cisplatin versus Cisplatin NSCLC Study (N=522).

[See table 3 at right]

Pancreatic Cancer — Data from 2 clinical trials evaluated the use of Gemzar in patients with locally advanced or metastatic pancreatic cancer. The first trial compared Gemzar to 5-Fluorouracil (5-FU) in patients who had received no prior chemotherapy. A second trial studied the use of Gemzar in pancreatic cancer patients previously treated with 5-FU or a 5-FU-containing regimen. In both studies, the first cycle of Gemzar was administered intravenously at a dose of 1000 mg/m^2 over 30 minutes once weekly for up to 7 weeks (or until toxicity necessitated holding a dose) followed by a week of rest from treatment with Gemzar. Subsequent cycles consisted of injections once weekly for 3 consecutive weeks out of every 4 weeks.

The primary efficacy parameter in these studies was "clinical benefit response," which is a measure of clinical improvement based on analgesic consumption, pain intensity, performance status, and weight change. Definitions for improvement in these variables were formulated prospectively during the design of the 2 trials. A patient was considered a clinical benefit responder if either:

i) the patient showed a ≥50% reduction in pain intensity (Memorial Pain Assessment Card) or analgesic consumption, or a 20-point or greater improvement in performance status (Karnofsky Performance Scale) for a period of at least 4 consecutive weeks, without showing any sustained worsening in any of the other parameters. Sustained worsening was defined as 4 consecutive weeks with either any increase in pain intensity or analgesic consumption or a 20-point decrease in performance status occurring during the first 12 weeks of therapy.

OR:

ii) the patient was stable on all of the aforementioned parameters, and showed a marked, sustained weight gain (≥7% increase maintained for ≥4 weeks) not due to fluid accumulation.

The first study was a multi-center (17 sites in US and Canada), prospective, single-blinded, two-arm, randomized, comparison of Gemzar and 5-FU in patients with locally advanced or metastatic pancreatic cancer who had received no prior treatment with chemotherapy. 5-FU was administered intravenously at a weekly dose of 600 mg/m^2 for 30 minutes. The results from this randomized trial are shown in Table 4. Patients treated with Gemzar had statistically significant increases in clinical benefit response, survival, and time to disease progression compared to 5-FU. The Kaplan-Meier curve for survival is shown in Figure 3. No confirmed objective tumor responses were observed with either treatment.

[See table 4 at right]

Clinical benefit response was achieved by 14 patients treated with Gemzar and 3 patients treated with 5-FU. One patient on the Gemzar arm showed improvement in all 3 primary parameters (pain intensity, analgesic consumption, and performance status). Eleven patients on the Gemzar arm and 2 patients on the 5-FU arm showed improvement in analgesic consumption and/or pain intensity with stable performance status. Two patients on the Gemzar arm showed improvement in analgesic consumption or pain intensity with improvement in performance status. One patient on the 5-FU arm was stable with regard to pain intensity and analgesic consumption with improvement in performance status. No patient on either arm achieved a clinical benefit response based on weight gain.

[See figure at top of next page]

The second trial was a multi-center (17 US and Canadian centers), open-label study of Gemzar in 63 patients with advanced pancreatic cancer previously treated with 5-FU or a 5-FU-containing regimen. The study showed a clinical benefit response rate of 27% and median survival of 3.9 months.

Other Clinical Studies — When Gemzar was administered more frequently than once weekly or with infusions longer than 60 minutes, increased toxicity was observed. Results of a Phase 1 study of Gemzar to assess the maximum tolerated dose (MTD) on a daily x 5 schedule showed that patients developed significant hypotension and severe flu-like symptoms that were intolerable at doses above 10 mg/m^2. The incidence and severity of these events were dose-related. Other Phase 1 studies using a twice-weekly schedule reached MTDs of only 65 mg/m^2 (30-minute infusion) and 150 mg/m^2 (5-minute bolus). The dose-limiting toxicities were thrombocytopenia and flu-like symptoms, particularly asthenia. In a Phase 1 study to assess the maximum tolerated infusion time, clinically significant toxicity, defined as myelosuppression, was seen with weekly doses of 300 mg/m^2 at or above a 270-minute infusion time. The half-life of gemcitabine is influenced by the length of the infusion (*see* **CLINICAL PHARMACOLOGY**) and the toxicity appears to be increased if Gemzar is administered more frequently than once weekly or with infusions longer than 60 minutes (*see* **WARNINGS**).

Table 3: Randomized Trials of Combination Therapy with Gemzar plus Cisplatin in NSCLC

Trial	28-day Schedule[a]			21-day Schedule[b]		
Treatment Arm	Gemzar/ Cisplatin	Cisplatin		Gemzar/ Cisplatin	Cisplatin/ Etoposide	
Number of patients	260	262		69	66	
Male	182	186		64	61	
Female	78	76		5	5	
Median age, years	62	63		58	60	
Range	36 to 88	35 to 79		33 to 76	35 to 75	
Stage IIIA	7%	7%		N/A	N/A	
Stage IIIB	26%	23%		48%	52%	
Stage IV	67%	70%		52%	49%	
Baseline KPS[c] 70 to 80	41%	44%		45%	52%	
Baseline KPS[c] 90 to 100	57%	55%		55%	49%	
Survival			p=0.008			p=0.18
Median, months	9.0	7.6		8.7	7.0	
(95%, C.I.) months	8.2, 11.0	6.6, 8.8		7.8, 10.1	6.0, 9.7	
Time to Disease Progression			p=0.009			p=0.015
Median, months	5.2	3.7		5.0	4.1	
(95%, C.I.) months	4.2, 5.7	3.0, 4.3		4.2, 6.4	2.4, 4.5	
Tumor Response	26%	10%	p<0.0001[d]	33%	14%	p=0.01[d]

[a] 28-day schedule—Gemzar plus cisplatin: Gemzar 1000 mg/m^2 on Days 1, 8, and 15 and cisplatin 100 mg/m^2 on Day 1 every 28 days; Single-agent cisplatin: cisplatin 100 mg/m^2 on Day 1 every 28 days.

[b] 21-day schedule—Gemzar plus cisplatin: Gemzar 1250 mg/m^2 on Days 1 and 8 and cisplatin 100 mg/m^2 on Day 1 every 21 days; Etoposide plus Cisplatin: cisplatin 100 mg/m^2 on Day 1 and I.V. etoposide 100 mg/m^2 on Days 1, 2, and 3 every 21 days.

[c] Karnofsky Performance Status.

[d] p-value for tumor response was calculated using the two-sided Fisher's exact test for difference in binomial proportions. All other p-values were calculated using the Logrank test for difference in overall time to an event.

N/A Not applicable.

Table 4: Gemzar Versus 5-FU in Pancreatic Cancer

	Gemzar	5-FU	
Number of patients	63	63	
Male	34	34	
Female	29	29	
Median age	62 years	61 years	
Range	37 to 79	36 to 77	
Stage IV disease	71.4%	76.2%	
Baseline KPS[a] ≤70	69.8%	68.3%	
Clinical benefit response	22.2% (N[c]=14)	4.8% (N=3)	p=0.004
Survival			p=0.0009
Median	5.7 months	4.2 months	
6-month probability[b]	(N=30) 46%	(N=19) 29%	
9-month probability[b]	(N = 14) 24%	(N = 4) 5%	
1-year probability[b]	(N = 9) 18%	(N = 2) 2%	
Range	0.2 to 18.6 months	0.4 to 15.1+ months	
95% C.I. of the median	4.7 to 6.9 months	3.1 to 5.1 months	
Time to Disease Progression			p = 0.0013
Median	2.1 months	0.9 months	
Range	0.1+ to 9.4 months	0.1 to 12.0+ months	
95% C.I. of the median	1.9 to 3.4 months	0.9 to 1.1 months	

[a] Karnofsky Performance Status.

[b] Kaplan-Meier estimates.

[c] N=number of patients.

\+ No progression at last visit; remains alive.

The p-value for clinical benefit response was calculated using the two-sided test for difference in binomial proportions. All other p-values were calculated using the Logrank test for difference in overall time to an event.

INDICATIONS AND USAGE

Therapeutic Indications

Breast Cancer — Gemzar in combination with paclitaxel is indicated for the first-line treatment of patients with meta-

Continued on next page

*** Identi-Code® symbol. This product information was prepared in June 2004. Current information on these and other products of Eli Lilly and Company may be obtained by direct inquiry to Lilly Research Laboratories, Lilly Corporate Center, Indianapolis, Indiana 46285, (800) 545-5979.**

Gemzar—Cont.

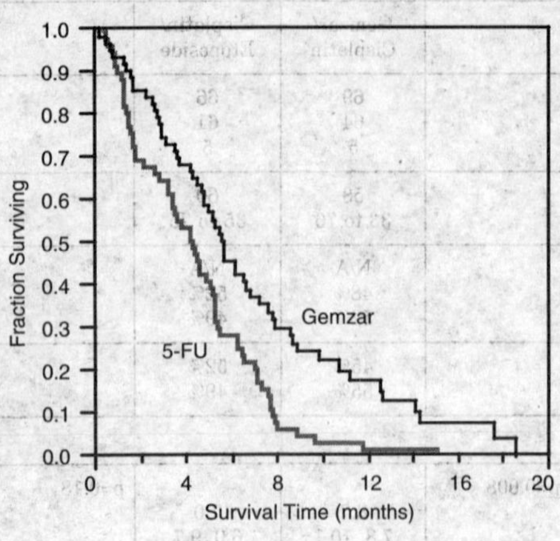

Figure 3: Kaplan-Meier Survival Curve.

static breast cancer after failure of prior anthracycline-containing adjuvant chemotherapy, unless anthracyclines were clinically contraindicated.

Non-Small Cell Lung Cancer — Gemzar is indicated in combination with cisplatin for the first-line treatment of patients with inoperable, locally advanced (Stage IIIA or IIIB), or metastatic (Stage IV) non-small cell lung cancer.

Pancreatic Cancer — Gemzar is indicated as first-line treatment for patients with locally advanced (nonresectable Stage II or Stage III) or metastatic (Stage IV) adenocarcinoma of the pancreas. Gemzar is indicated for patients previously treated with 5-FU.

CONTRAINDICATION

Gemzar is contraindicated in those patients with a known hypersensitivity to the drug (*see Allergic under* **ADVERSE REACTIONS**).

WARNINGS

Caution — Prolongation of the infusion time beyond 60 minutes and more frequent than weekly dosing have been shown to increase toxicity (*see* **CLINICAL STUDIES**).

Hematology — Gemzar can suppress bone marrow function as manifested by leukopenia, thrombocytopenia, and anemia (*see* **ADVERSE REACTIONS**), and myelosuppression is usually the dose-limiting toxicity. Patients should be monitored for myelosuppression during therapy. *See* **DOSAGE AND ADMINISTRATION** for recommended dose adjustments.

Pulmonary — Pulmonary toxicity has been reported with the use of Gemzar. In cases of severe lung toxicity, Gemzar therapy should be discontinued immediately and appropriate supportive care measures instituted (*see Pulmonary under* **Single-Agent Use** *and under* **Post-marketing experience** in **ADVERSE REACTIONS** section).

Renal — Hemolytic Uremic Syndrome (HUS) and/or renal failure have been reported following one or more doses of Gemzar. Renal failure leading to death or requiring dialysis, despite discontinuation of therapy, has been rarely reported. The majority of the cases of renal failure leading to death were due to HUS (*see Renal under* **Single-Agent Use** *and under* **Post-marketing experience** in **ADVERSE REACTIONS** section).

Hepatic — Serious hepatotoxicity, including liver failure and death, has been reported very rarely in patients receiving Gemzar alone or in combination with other potentially hepatotoxic drugs (*see Hepatic under* **Single-Agent Use** *and under* **Post-marketing experience** in **ADVERSE REACTIONS** section).

Pregnancy — Pregnancy Category D. Gemzar can cause fetal harm when administered to a pregnant woman. Gemcitabine is embryotoxic causing fetal malformations (cleft palate, incomplete ossification) at doses of 1.5 mg/kg/day in mice (about 1/200 the recommended human dose on a mg/m^2 basis). Gemcitabine is fetotoxic causing fetal malformations (fused pulmonary artery, absence of gall bladder) at doses of 0.1 mg/kg/day in rabbits (about 1/600 the recommended human dose on a mg/m^2 basis). Embryotoxicity was characterized by decreased fetal viability, reduced live litter sizes, and developmental delays. There are no studies of Gemzar in pregnant women. If Gemzar is used during pregnancy, or if the patient becomes pregnant while taking Gemzar, the patient should be apprised of the potential hazard to the fetus.

PRECAUTIONS

General — Patients receiving therapy with Gemzar should be monitored closely by a physician experienced in the use of cancer chemotherapeutic agents. Most adverse events are reversible and do not need to result in discontinuation, although doses may need to be withheld or reduced. There was a greater tendency in women, especially older women, not to proceed to the next cycle.

Laboratory Tests — Patients receiving Gemzar should be monitored prior to each dose with a complete blood count (CBC), including differential and platelet count. Suspension or modification of therapy should be considered when marrow suppression is detected (*see* **DOSAGE AND ADMINISTRATION**).

Laboratory evaluation of renal and hepatic function should be performed prior to initiation of therapy and periodically thereafter (*see* **WARNINGS**).

Table 5: Selected WHO-Graded Adverse Events in Patients Receiving Single-Agent Gemzar
WHO Grades (% incidence)

	All Patients[a]			Pancreatic Cancer Patients[b]			Discontinuations (%)[c]
	All Grades	Grade 3	Grade 4	All Grades	Grade 3	Grade 4	All Patients
Laboratory[d]							
Hematologic							
Anemia	68	7	1	73	8	2	<1
Leukopenia	62	9	<1	64	8	1	<1
Neutropenia	63	19	6	61	17	7	
Thrombocytopenia	24	4	1	36	7	<1	<1
Hepatic							<1
ALT	68	8	2	72	10	1	
AST	67	6	2	78	12	5	
Alkaline Phosphatase	55	7	2	77	16	4	
Bilirubin	13	2	<1	26	6	2	
Renal							<1
Proteinuria	45	<1	0	32	<1	0	
Hematuria	35	<1	0	23	0	0	
BUN	16	0	0	15	0	0	
Creatinine	8	<1	0	6	0	0	
Non-laboratory[e]							
Nausea and Vomiting	69	13	1	71	10	2	<1
Pain	48	9	<1	42	6	<1	<1
Fever	41	2	0	38	2	0	<1
Rash	30	<1	0	28	<1	0	<1
Dyspnea	23	3	<1	10	0	<1	<1
Constipation	23	1	<1	31	3	<1	0
Diarrhea	19	1	0	30	3	0	0
Hemorrhage	17	<1	<1	4	2	<1	<1
Infection	16	1	<1	10	2	<1	<1
Alopecia	15	<1	0	16	0	0	0
Stomatitis	11	<1	0	10	<1	0	<1
Somnolence	11	<1	<1	11	2	<1	<1
Paresthesias	10	<1	0	10	<1	0	0

Grade based on criteria from the World Health Organization (WHO).
[a] N=699-974; all patients with laboratory or non-laboratory data.
[b] N=161-241; all pancreatic cancer patients with laboratory or non-laboratory data.
[c] N=979.
[d] Regardless of causality.
[e] Table includes non-laboratory data with incidence for all patients ≥10%. For approximately 60% of the patients, non-laboratory events were graded only if assessed to be possibly drug-related.

Table 6: Selected WHO-Graded Adverse Events from Comparative Trial of Gemzar and 5-FU in Pancreatic Cancer
WHO Grades (% incidence)

	Gemzar[a]			5-FU[b]		
	All Grades	Grade 3	Grade 4	All Grades	Grade 3	Grade 4
Laboratory[c]						
Hematologic						
Anemia	65	7	3	45	0	0
Leukopenia	71	10	0	15	2	0
Neutropenia	62	19	7	18	2	3
Thrombocytopenia	47	10	0	15	2	0
Hepatic						
ALT	72	8	2	38	0	0
AST	72	10	2	52	2	0
Alkaline Phosphatase	71	16	0	64	10	3
Bilirubin	16	2	2	25	6	3
Renal						
Proteinuria	10	0	0	2	0	0
Hematuria	13	0	0	0	0	0
BUN	8	0	0	10	0	0
Creatinine	2	0	0	0	0	0
Non-laboratory[d]						
Nausea and Vomiting	64	10	3	58	5	0
Pain	10	2	0	7	0	0
Fever	30	0	0	16	0	0
Rash	24	0	0	13	0	0
Dyspnea	6	0	0	3	0	0
Constipation	10	3	0	11	2	0
Diarrhea	24	2	0	31	5	0
Hemorrhage	0	0	0	2	0	0
Infection	8	0	0	3	2	0
Alopecia	18	0	0	16	0	0
Stomatitis	14	0	0	15	0	0
Somnolence	5	2	0	7	2	0
Paresthesias	2	0	0	2	0	0

Grade based on criteria from the World Health Organization (WHO).
[a] N=58-63; all Gemzar patients with laboratory or non-laboratory data.
[b] N=61-63; all 5-FU patients with laboratory or non-laboratory data.
[c] Regardless of causality.
[d] Non-laboratory events were graded only if assessed to be possibly drug-related.

Carcinogenesis, Mutagenesis, Impairment of Fertility — Long-term animal studies to evaluate the carcinogenic potential of Gemzar have not been conducted. Gemcitabine induced forward mutations *in vitro* in a mouse lymphoma (L5178Y) assay and was clastogenic in an *in vivo* mouse micronucleus assay. Gemcitabine was negative when tested using the Ames, *in vivo* sister chromatid exchange, and *in vitro* chromosomal aberration assays, and did not cause unscheduled DNA synthesis *in vitro*. Gemcitabine I.P. doses of 0.5 mg/kg/day (about 1/700 the human dose on a mg/m^2 basis) in male mice had an effect on fertility with moderate to severe hypospermatogenesis, decreased fertility, and decreased implantations. In female mice, fertility was not affected but maternal toxicities were observed at 1.5 mg/kg/day I.V. (about 1/200 the human dose on a mg/m^2 basis) and fetotoxicity or embryolethality was observed at 0.25 mg/kg/day I.V. (about 1/1300 the human dose on a mg/m^2 basis).

Pregnancy — Category D. *See* **WARNINGS**.

Nursing Mothers — It is not known whether Gemzar or its metabolites are excreted in human milk. Because many drugs are excreted in human milk and because of the potential for serious adverse reactions from Gemzar in nursing infants, the mother should be warned and a decision should be made whether to discontinue nursing or to discontinue the drug, taking into account the importance of the drug to the mother and the potential risk to the infant.

Elderly Patients — Gemzar clearance is affected by age (*see* **CLINICAL PHARMACOLOGY**). There is no evidence, however, that unusual dose adjustments, (i.e., other than those already recommended in the **DOSAGE AND ADMINISTRATION** section) are necessary in patients over 65, and in general, adverse reaction rates in the single-agent safety database of 979 patients were similar in patients above and below 65. Grade 3/4 thrombocytopenia was more common in the elderly.

Gender — Gemzar clearance is affected by gender (*see* **CLINICAL PHARMACOLOGY**). In the single-agent safety database (N=979 patients), however, there is no evidence that unusual dose adjustments (i.e., other than those already recommended in the **DOSAGE AND ADMINISTRATION** section) are necessary in women. In general, in single-agent studies of Gemzar, adverse reaction rates were similar in men and women, but women, especially older women, were more likely not to proceed to a subsequent cycle and to experience Grade 3/4 neutropenia and thrombocytopenia.

Pediatric Patients — Gemzar has not been studied in pediatric patients. Safety and effectiveness in pediatric patients have not been established.

Patients with Renal or Hepatic Impairment — Gemzar should be used with caution in patients with preexisting renal impairment or hepatic insufficiency. Gemzar has not been studied in patients with significant renal or hepatic impairment.

Drug Interactions — No specific drug interaction studies have been conducted. For information on the pharmacokinetics of Gemzar and cisplatin in combination, *see Drug Interactions under* **CLINICAL PHARMACOLOGY** section.

Radiation Therapy — Safe and effective regimens for the administration of Gemzar with therapeutic doses of radiation have not yet been determined.

ADVERSE REACTIONS

Gemzar has been used in a wide variety of malignancies, both as a single-agent and in combination with other cytotoxic drugs.

Single-Agent Use: Myelosuppression is the principal dose-limiting toxicity with Gemzar therapy. Dosage adjustments for hematologic toxicity are frequently needed and are described in the **DOSAGE AND ADMINISTRATION** section.

The data in Table 5 are based on 979 patients receiving Gemzar as a single-agent administered weekly as a 30-minute infusion for treatment of a wide variety of malignancies. The Gemzar starting doses ranged from 800 to 1250 mg/m^2. Data are also shown for the subset of patients with pancreatic cancer treated in 5 clinical studies. The frequency of all grades and severe (WHO Grade 3 or 4) adverse events were generally similar in the single-agent safety database of 979 patients and the subset of patients with pancreatic cancer. Adverse reactions reported in the single-agent safety database resulted in discontinuation of Gemzar therapy in about 10% of patients. In the comparative trial in pancreatic cancer, the discontinuation rate for adverse reactions was 14.3% for the gemcitabine arm and 4.8% for the 5-FU arm.

All WHO-graded laboratory events are listed in Table 5, regardless of causality. Non-laboratory adverse events listed in Table 5 or discussed below were those reported, regardless of causality, for at least 10% of all patients, except the categories of Extravasation, Allergic, and Cardiovascular and certain specific events under the Renal, Pulmonary, and Infection categories. Table 6 presents the data from the comparative trial of Gemzar and 5-FU in pancreatic cancer for the same adverse events as those in Table 5, regardless of incidence.

[See table 5 at top of previous page]

[See table 6 on previous page]

Hematologic — In studies in pancreatic cancer myelosuppression is the dose-limiting toxicity with Gemzar, but <1% of patients discontinued therapy for either anemia, leukopenia, or thrombocytopenia. Red blood cell transfusions were required by 19% of patients. The incidence of sepsis was less than 1%. Petechiae or mild blood loss (hemorrhage), from any cause, was reported in 16% of patients; less than 1% of patients required platelet transfusions. Patients should be monitored for myelosuppression during Gemzar therapy and dosage modified or suspended according to the degree of hematologic toxicity (*see* **DOSAGE AND ADMINISTRATION**).

Table 7: Selected CTC-Graded Adverse Events from Comparative Trial of Gemzar plus Cisplatin versus Single-Agent Cisplatin in NSCLC
CTC Grades (% incidence)

	Gemzar plus Cisplatin[a]			Cisplatin[b]		
	All Grades	Grade 3	Grade 4	All Grades	Grade 3	Grade 4
Laboratory[c]						
Hematologic						
Anemia	89	22	3	67	6	1
RBC Transfusion[d]	39			13		
Leukopenia	82	35	11	25	2	1
Neutropenia	79	22	35	20	3	1
Thrombocytopenia	85	25	25	13	3	1
Platelet Transfusions[d]	21			<1		
Lymphocytes	75	25	18	51	12	5
Hepatic						
Transaminase	22	2	1	10	1	0
Alkaline Phosphatase	19	1	0	13	0	0
Renal						
Proteinuria	23	0	0	18	0	0
Hematuria	15	0	0	13	0	0
Creatinine	38	4	<1	31	2	<1
Other Laboratory						
Hyperglycemia	30	4	0	23	3	0
Hypomagnesemia	30	4	3	17	2	0
Hypocalcemia	18	2	0	7	0	<1
Non-laboratory[e]						
Nausea	93	25	2	87	20	<1
Vomiting	78	11	12	71	10	9
Alopecia	53	1	0	33	0	0
Neuro Motor	35	12	0	15	3	0
Constipation	28	3	0	21	0	0
Neuro Hearing	25	6	0	21	6	0
Diarrhea	24	2	2	13	0	0
Neuro Sensory	23	1	0	18	1	0
Infection	18	3	2	12	1	0
Fever	16	0	0	5	0	0
Neuro Cortical	16	3	1	9	1	0
Neuro Mood	16	1	0	10	1	0
Local	15	0	0	6	0	0
Neuro Headache	14	0	0	7	0	0
Stomatitis	14	1	0	5	0	0
Hemorrhage	14	1	0	4	0	0
Dyspnea	12	4	3	11	3	2
Hypotension	12	1	0	7	1	0
Rash	11	0	0	3	0	0

Grade based on Common Toxicity Criteria (CTC). Table includes data for adverse events with incidence ≥10% in either arm.
[a] N=217-253; all Gemzar plus cisplatin patients with laboratory or non-laboratory data. Gemzar at 1000 mg/m^2 on Days 1, 8, and 15 and cisplatin at 100 mg/m^2 on Day 1 every 28 days.
[b] N=213-248; all cisplatin patients with laboratory or non-laboratory data. Cisplatin at 100 mg/m^2 on Day 1 every 28 days.
[c] Regardless of causality.
[d] Percent of patients receiving transfusions. Percent transfusions are not CTC-graded events.
[e] Non-laboratory events were graded only if assessed to be possibly drug-related.

Gastrointestinal — Nausea and vomiting were commonly reported (69%) but were usually of mild to moderate severity. Severe nausea and vomiting (WHO Grade 3/4) occurred in <15% of patients. Diarrhea was reported by 19% of patients, and stomatitis by 11% of patients.

Hepatic — In clinical trials, Gemzar was associated with transient elevations of one or both serum transaminases in approximately 70% of patients, but there was no evidence of increasing hepatic toxicity with either longer duration of exposure to Gemzar or with greater total cumulative dose. Serious hepatotoxicity, including liver failure and death, has been reported very rarely in patients receiving Gemzar alone or in combination with other potentially hepatotoxic drugs (*see Hepatic under* **Post-marketing experience**).

Renal — In clinical trials, mild proteinuria and hematuria were commonly reported. Clinical findings consistent with the Hemolytic Uremic Syndrome (HUS) were reported in 6 of 2429 patients (0.25%) receiving Gemzar in clinical trials. Four patients developed HUS on Gemzar therapy, 2 immediately post-therapy. The diagnosis of HUS should be considered if the patient develops anemia with evidence of microangiopathic hemolysis, elevation of bilirubin or LDH, reticulocytosis, severe thrombocytopenia, and/or evidence of renal failure (elevation of serum creatinine or BUN). Gemzar therapy should be discontinued immediately. Renal failure may not be reversible even with discontinuation of therapy and dialysis may be required (*see Renal under* **Post-marketing experience**).

Fever — The overall incidence of fever was 41%. This is in contrast to the incidence of infection (16%) and indicates that Gemzar may cause fever in the absence of clinical infection. Fever was frequently associated with other flu-like symptoms and was usually mild and clinically manageable.

Rash — Rash was reported in 30% of patients. The rash was typically a macular or finely granular maculopapular pruritic eruption of mild to moderate severity involving the trunk and extremities. Pruritus was reported for 13% of patients.

Pulmonary — In clinical trials, dyspnea, unrelated to underlying disease, has been reported in association with Gemzar therapy. Dyspnea was occasionally accompanied by bronchospasm. Pulmonary toxicity has been reported with the use of Gemzar (*see Pulmonary under* **Post-marketing experience**). The etiology of these effects is unknown. If such effects develop, Gemzar should be discontinued. Early use of supportive care measures may help ameliorate these conditions.

Edema — Edema (13%), peripheral edema (20%), and generalized edema (<1%) were reported. Less than 1% of patients discontinued due to edema.

Flu-like Symptoms — "Flu syndrome" was reported for 19% of patients. Individual symptoms of fever, asthenia, anorexia, headache, cough, chills, and myalgia were commonly reported. Fever and asthenia were also reported frequently as isolated symptoms. Insomnia, rhinitis, sweating, and malaise were reported infrequently. Less than 1% of patients discontinued due to flu-like symptoms.

Infection — Infections were reported for 16% of patients. Sepsis was rarely reported (<1%).

Alopecia — Hair loss, usually minimal, was reported by 15% of patients.

Neurotoxicity — There was a 10% incidence of mild paresthesias and a <1% rate of severe paresthesias.

Extravasation — Injection-site related events were reported for 4% of patients. There were no reports of injection site necrosis. Gemzar is not a vesicant.

Allergic — Bronchospasm was reported for less than 2% of patients. Anaphylactoid reaction has been reported rarely. Gemzar should not be administered to patients with a known hypersensitivity to this drug (*see* **CONTRAINDICATION**).

Cardiovascular — During clinical trials, 2% of patients discontinued therapy with Gemzar due to cardiovascular

Continued on next page

*** Identi-Code® symbol. This product information was prepared in June 2004. Current information on these and other products of Eli Lilly and Company may be obtained by direct inquiry to Lilly Research Laboratories, Lilly Corporate Center, Indianapolis, Indiana 46285, (800) 545-5979.**

Gemzar—Cont.

events such as myocardial infarction, cerebrovascular accident, arrhythmia, and hypertension. Many of these patients had a prior history of cardiovascular disease (*see Cardiovascular under* **Post-marketing experience**).

Combination Use in Non-Small Cell Lung Cancer: In the Gemzar plus cisplatin vs. cisplatin study, dose adjustments occurred with 35% of Gemzar injections and 17% of cisplatin injections on the combination arm, versus 6% on the cisplatin-only arm. Dose adjustments were required in greater than 90% of patients on the combination, versus 16% on cisplatin. Study discontinuations for possibly drug-related adverse events occurred in 15% of patients on the combination arm and 8% of patients on the cisplatin arm. With a median of 4 cycles of Gemzar plus cisplatin treatment, 94 of 262 patients (36%) experienced a total of 149 hospitalizations due to possibly treatment-related adverse events. With a median of 2 cycles of cisplatin treatment, 61 of 260 patients (23%) experienced 78 hospitalizations due to possibly treatment-related adverse events.

In the Gemzar plus cisplatin vs. etoposide plus cisplatin study, dose adjustments occurred with 20% of Gemzar injections and 16% of cisplatin injections in the Gemzar plus cisplatin arm compared with 20% of etoposide injections and 15% of cisplatin injections in the etoposide plus cisplatin arm. With a median of 5 cycles of Gemzar plus cisplatin treatment, 15 of 69 patients (22%) experienced 15 hospitalizations due to possibly treatment-related adverse events. With a median of 4 cycles of etoposide plus cisplatin treatment, 18 of 66 patients (27%) experienced 22 hospitalizations due to possibly treatment-related adverse events. In patients who completed more than one cycle, dose adjustments were reported in 81% of the Gemzar plus cisplatin patients, compared with 68% on the etoposide plus cisplatin arm. Study discontinuations for possibly drug-related adverse events occurred in 14% of patients on the Gemzar plus cisplatin arm and in 8% of patients on the etoposide plus cisplatin arm. The incidence of myelosuppression was increased in frequency with Gemzar plus cisplatin treatment (∼90%) compared to that with the Gemzar monotherapy (∼60%). With combination therapy Gemzar dosage adjustments for hematologic toxicity were required more often while cisplatin dose adjustments were less frequently required.

Table 7 presents the safety data from the Gemzar plus cisplatin vs. cisplatin study in non-small cell lung cancer. The NCI Common Toxicity Criteria (CTC) were used. The two-drug combination was more myelosuppressive with 4 (1.5%) possibly treatment-related deaths, including 3 resulting from myelosuppression with infection and 1 case of renal failure associated with pancytopenia and infection. No deaths due to treatment were reported on the cisplatin arm. Nine cases of febrile neutropenia were reported on the combination therapy arm compared to 2 on the cisplatin arm. More patients required RBC and platelet transfusions on the Gemzar plus cisplatin arm.

Myelosuppression occurred more frequently on the combination arm, and in 4 possibly treatment-related deaths myelosuppression was observed. Sepsis was reported in 4% of patients on the Gemzar plus cisplatin arm compared to 1% on the cisplatin arm. Platelet transfusions were required in 21% of patients on the combination arm and <1% of patients on the cisplatin arm. Hemorrhagic events occurred in 14% of patients on the combination arm and 4% on the cisplatin arm. However, severe hemorrhagic events were rare. Red blood cell transfusions were required in 39% of the patients on the Gemzar plus cisplatin arm, versus 13% on the cisplatin arm. The data suggest cumulative anemia with continued Gemzar plus cisplatin use.

Nausea and vomiting despite the use of antiemetics occurred slightly more often with Gemzar plus cisplatin therapy (78%) than with cisplatin alone (71%). In studies with single-agent Gemzar, a lower incidence of nausea and vomiting (58% to 69%) was reported. Renal function abnormalities, hypomagnesemia, neuromotor, neurocortical, and neurocerebellar toxicity occurred more often with Gemzar plus cisplatin than with cisplatin monotherapy. Neurohearing toxicity was similar on both arms.

Cardiac dysrrhythmias of Grade 3 or greater were reported in 7 (3%) patients treated with Gemzar plus cisplatin compared to one (<1%) Grade 3 dysrrhythmia reported with cisplatin therapy. Hypomagnesemia and hypokalemia were associated with one Grade 4 arrhythmia on the Gemzar plus cisplatin combination arm.

Table 8 presents data from the randomized study of Gemzar plus cisplatin versus etoposide plus cisplatin in 135 patients with NSCLC for the same WHO graded adverse events as those in Table 6. One death (1.5%) was reported on the Gemzar plus cisplatin arm due to febrile neutropenia associated with renal failure which was possibly treatment-related. No deaths related to treatment occurred on the etoposide plus cisplatin arm. The overall incidence of Grade 4 neutropenia on the Gemzar plus cisplatin arm was less than on the etoposide plus cisplatin arm (28% vs. 56%). Sepsis was experienced by 2% of patients on both treatment arms. Grade 3 anemia and Grade 3/4 thrombocytopenia were more common on the Gemzar plus cisplatin arm. RBC transfusions were given to 29% of the patients who received Gemzar plus cisplatin vs. 21% of patients who received etoposide plus cisplatin. Platelet transfusions were given to 3% of the patients who received Gemzar plus cisplatin vs. 8% of patients who received etoposide plus cisplatin. Grade 3/4 nausea and vomiting were also more common on the Gemzar plus cisplatin arm. On the Gemzar plus cisplatin arm, 7% of participants were hospitalized due to febrile neutropenia compared to 12% on the etoposide plus cisplatin arm. More than twice as many patients had dose reductions or omissions of a scheduled dose of Gemzar as compared to etoposide, which may explain the differences in the incidence of neutropenia and febrile neutropenia between treatment arms. Flu syndrome was reported by 3% of patients on the Gemzar plus cisplatin arm with none reported on the comparator arm. Eight patients (12%) on the Gemzar plus cisplatin arm reported edema compared to 1 patient (2%) on the etoposide plus cisplatin arm.

Table 8: Selected WHO-Graded Adverse Events from Comparative Trial of Gemzar plus Cisplatin versus Etoposide plus Cisplatin in NSCLC
WHO Grades (% incidence)

	Gemzar plus Cisplatin[a]			Etoposide plus Cisplatin[b]		
	All Grades	Grade 3	Grade 4	All Grades	Grade 3	Grade 4
Laboratory[c]						
Hematologic						
Anemia	88	22	0	77	13	2
RBC Transfusions[d]	29			21		
Leukopenia	86	26	3	87	36	7
Neutropenia	88	36	28	87	20	56
Thrombocytopenia	81	39	16	45	8	5
Platelet Transfusions[d]	3			8		
Hepatic						
ALT	6	0	0	12	0	0
AST	3	0	0	11	0	0
Alkaline Phosphatase	16	0	0	11	0	0
Bilirubin	0	0	0	0	0	0
Renal						
Proteinuria	12	0	0	5	0	0
Hematuria	22	0	0	10	0	0
BUN	6	0	0	4	0	0
Creatinine	2	0	0	2	0	0
Non-laboratory[e,f]						
Nausea and Vomiting	96	35	4	86	19	7
Fever	6	0	0	3	0	0
Rash	10	0	0	3	0	0
Dyspnea	1	0	1	3	0	0
Constipation	17	0	0	15	0	0
Diarrhea	14	1	1	13	0	2
Hemorrhage	9	0	3	3	0	3
Infection	28	3	1	21	8	0
Alopecia	77	13	0	92	51	0
Stomatitis	20	4	0	18	2	0
Somnolence	3	0	0	3	2	0
Paresthesias	38	0	0	16	2	0

Grade based on criteria from the World Health Organization (WHO).
[a] N=67-69; all Gemzar plus cisplatin patients with laboratory or non-laboratory data. Gemzar at 1250 mg/m^2 on Days 1 and 8 and cisplatin at 100 mg/m^2 on Day 1 every 21 days.
[b] N=57-63; all cisplatin plus etoposide patients with laboratory or non-laboratory data. Cisplatin at 100 mg/m^2 on Day 1 and I.V. etoposide at 100 mg/m^2 on Days 1, 2, and 3 every 21 days.
[c] Regardless of causality.
[d] Percent of patients receiving transfusions. Percent transfusions are not WHO-graded events.
[e] Non-laboratory events were graded only if assessed to be possibly drug-related.
[f] Pain data were not collected.

Table 9: Adverse Events from Comparative Trial of Gemzar plus Paclitaxel versus Single-Agent Paclitaxel in Breast Cancer[a]
CTC Grades (% incidence)

	Gemzar plus Paclitaxel (N=262)			Paclitaxel (N=259)		
	All Grades	Grade 3	Grade 4	All Grades	Grade 3	Grade 4
Laboratory[b]						
Hematologic						
Anemia	69	6	1	51	3	<1
Neutropenia	69	31	17	31	4	7
Thrombocytopenia	26	5	<1	7	<1	<1
Leukopenia	21	10	1	12	2	0
Hepatobiliary						
ALT	18	5	<1	6	<1	0
AST	16	2	0	5	<1	0
Non-laboratory[c]						
Alopecia	90	14	4	92	19	3
Neuropathy-sensory	64	5	<1	58	3	0
Nausea	50	1	0	31	2	0
Fatigue	40	6	<1	28	1	<1
Myalgia	33	4	0	33	3	<1
Vomiting	29	2	0	15	2	0
Arthralgia	24	3	0	22	2	<1
Diarrhea	20	3	0	13	2	0
Anorexia	17	0	0	12	<1	0
Neuropathy-motor	15	2	<1	10	<1	0
Stomatitis/pharyngitis	13	1	<1	8	<1	0
Fever	13	<1	0	3	0	0
Constipation	11	<1	0	12	0	0
Bone pain	11	2	0	10	<1	0
Pain-other	11	<1	0	8	<1	0
Rash/desquamation	11	<1	<1	5	0	0

[a] Grade based on Common Toxicity Criteria (CTC) Version 2.0 (all grades ≥10%).
[b] Regardless of causality.
[c] Non-laboratory events were graded only if assessed to be possibly drug-related.

[See table 7 at top of previous page]
[See table 8 above]

Combination Use in Breast Cancer: In the Gemzar plus paclitaxel versus paclitaxel study, dose reductions occurred with 8% of Gemzar injections and 5% of paclitaxel injections on the combination arm, versus 2% on the paclitaxel arm. On the combination arm, 7% of Gemzar doses were omitted and <1% of paclitaxel doses were omitted, compared to <1% of paclitaxel doses on the paclitaxel arm. A total of 18 patients (7%) on the Gemzar plus paclitaxel arm and 12 (5%) on the paclitaxel arm discontinued the study because of adverse events. There were two deaths on study or within 30 days after study drug discontinuation that were possibly drug-related, one on each arm.

Table 9 presents the safety data occurrences of ≥10% (all grades) from the Gemzar plus paclitaxel versus paclitaxel study in breast cancer.

[See table 9 on previous page]

The following are the clinically relevant adverse events that occurred in >1% and <10% (all grades) of patients on either arm. In parentheses are the incidences of Grade 3 and 4 adverse events (Gemzar plus paclitaxel versus paclitaxel): febrile neutropenia (5.0% versus 1.2%), infection (0.8% versus 0.8%), dyspnea (1.9% versus 0), and allergic reaction/hypersensitivity (0 versus 0.8%).

No differences in the incidence of laboratory and non-laboratory events were observed in patients 65 years or older, as compared to patients younger than 65.

Post-marketing experience: The following adverse events have been identified during post-approval use of Gemzar. These events have occurred after Gemzar single-agent use and Gemzar in combination with other cytotoxic agents. Decisions to include these events are based on the seriousness of the event, frequency of reporting, or potential causal connection to Gemzar.

Cardiovascular — Congestive heart failure and myocardial infarction have been reported very rarely with the use of Gemzar. Arrhythmias, predominantly supraventricular in nature, have been reported very rarely.

Vascular Disorders — Vascular toxicity reported with Gemzar includes clinical signs of vasculitis, which has been reported very rarely. Gangrene has also been reported very rarely.

Skin — Cellulitis and non-serious injection site reactions in the absence of extravasation have been rarely reported.

Hepatic — Serious hepatotoxicity including liver failure and death has been reported very rarely in patients receiving Gemzar alone or in combination with other potentially hepatotoxic drugs.

Pulmonary — Parenchymal toxicity, including interstitial pneumonitis, pulmonary fibrosis, pulmonary edema, and adult respiratory distress syndrome (ARDS), has been reported rarely following one or more doses of Gemzar administered to patients with various malignancies. Some patients experienced the onset of pulmonary symptoms up to 2 weeks after the last Gemzar dose. Respiratory failure and death occurred very rarely in some patients despite discontinuation of therapy.

Renal — Hemolytic-Uremic Syndrome (HUS) and/or renal failure have been reported following one or more doses of Gemzar. Renal failure leading to death or requiring dialysis, despite discontinuation of therapy, has been rarely reported. The majority of the cases of renal failure leading to death were due to HUS.

OVERDOSAGE

There is no known antidote for overdoses of Gemzar. Myelosuppression, paresthesias, and severe rash were the principal toxicities seen when a single dose as high as 5700 mg/m^2 was administered by I.V. infusion over 30 minutes every 2 weeks to several patients in a Phase 1 study. In the event of suspected overdose, the patient should be monitored with appropriate blood counts and should receive supportive therapy, as necessary.

DOSAGE AND ADMINISTRATION

Gemzar is for intravenous use only.

Adults

Single-Agent Use:

Pancreatic Cancer — Gemzar should be administered by intravenous infusion at a dose of 1000 mg/m^2 over 30 minutes once weekly for up to 7 weeks (or until toxicity necessitates reducing or holding a dose), followed by a week of rest from treatment. Subsequent cycles should consist of infusions once weekly for 3 consecutive weeks out of every 4 weeks.

Dose Modifications — Dosage adjustment is based upon the degree of hematologic toxicity experienced by the patient (*see* **WARNINGS**). Clearance in women and the elderly is reduced and women were somewhat less able to progress to subsequent cycles (*see Human Pharmacokinetics under* **CLINICAL PHARMACOLOGY** *and* **PRECAUTIONS**).

Patients receiving Gemzar should be monitored prior to each dose with a complete blood count (CBC), including differential and platelet count. If marrow suppression is detected, therapy should be modified or suspended according to the guidelines in Table 10.

Table 10: Dosage Reduction Guidelines

Absolute granulocyte count (× 10^6/L)		Platelet count (× 10^6/L)	% of full dose
≥1000	and	≥100,000	100
500-999	or	50,000-99,000	75
<500	or	<50,000	Hold

Laboratory evaluation of renal and hepatic function, including transaminases and serum creatinine, should be performed prior to initiation of therapy and periodically thereafter. Gemzar should be administered with caution in patients with evidence of significant renal or hepatic impairment.

Patients treated with Gemzar who complete an entire cycle of therapy may have the dose for subsequent cycles increased by 25%, provided that the absolute granulocyte count (AGC) and platelet nadirs exceed 1500 x 10^6/L and 100,000 x 10^6/L, respectively, and if non-hematologic toxicity has not been greater than WHO Grade 1. If patients tolerate the subsequent course of Gemzar at the increased dose, the dose for the next cycle can be further increased by 20%, provided again that the AGC and platelet nadirs exceed 1500 x 10^6/L and 100,000 x 10^6/L, respectively, and that non-hematologic toxicity has not been greater than WHO Grade 1.

Combination Use:

Non-Small Cell Lung Cancer — Two schedules have been investigated and the optimum schedule has not been determined (*see* **CLINICAL STUDIES**). With the 4-week schedule, Gemzar should be administered intravenously at 1000 mg/m^2 over 30 minutes on Days 1, 8, and 15 of each 28-day cycle. Cisplatin should be administered intravenously at 100 mg/m^2 on Day 1 after the infusion of Gemzar. With the 3-week schedule, Gemzar should be administered intravenously at 1250 mg/m^2 over 30 minutes on Days 1 and 8 of each 21-day cycle. Cisplatin at a dose of 100 mg/m^2 should be administered intravenously after the infusion of Gemzar on Day 1. See prescribing information for cisplatin administration and hydration guidelines.

Dose Modifications — Dosage adjustments for hematologic toxicity may be required for Gemzar and for cisplatin. Gemzar dosage adjustment for hematological toxicity is based on the granulocyte and platelet counts taken on the day of therapy. Patients receiving Gemzar should be monitored prior to each dose with a complete blood count (CBC), including differential and platelet counts. If marrow suppression is detected, therapy should be modified or suspended according to the guidelines in Table 10. For cisplatin dosage adjustment, see manufacturer's prescribing information.

In general, for severe (Grade 3 or 4) non-hematological toxicity, except alopecia and nausea/vomiting, therapy with Gemzar plus cisplatin should be held or decreased by 50% depending on the judgment of the treating physician. During combination therapy with cisplatin, serum creatinine, serum potassium, serum calcium, and serum magnesium should be carefully monitored (Grade 3/4 serum creatinine toxicity for Gemzar plus cisplatin was 5% versus 2% for cisplatin alone).

Breast Cancer — Gemzar should be administered intravenously at a dose of 1250 mg/m^2 over 30 minutes on Days 1 and 8 of each 21-day cycle. Paclitaxel should be administered at 175 mg/m^2 on Day 1 as a 3-hour intravenous infusion before Gemzar administration. Patients should be monitored prior to each dose with a complete blood count, including differential counts. Patients should have an absolute granulocyte count ≥1500 x 10^6/L and a platelet count ≥100,000 x 10^6/L prior to each cycle.

Dose Modifications — Gemzar dosage adjustments for hematological toxicity is based on the granulocyte and platelet counts taken on Day 8 of therapy. If marrow suppression is detected, Gemzar dosage should be modified according to the guidelines in Table 11.

Table 11: Day 8 Dosage Reduction Guidelines for Gemzar in Combination with Paclitaxel

Absolute granulocyte count (× 10^6/L)		Platelet count (× 10^6/L)	% of full dose
≥1200	and	>75,000	100
1000-1199	or	50,000-75,000	75
700-999	and	≥50,000	50
<700	or	<50,000	Hold

In general, for severe (Grade 3 or 4) non-hematological toxicity, except alopecia and nausea/vomiting, therapy with Gemzar should be held or decreased by 50% depending on the judgment of the treating physician. For paclitaxel dosage adjustment, see manufacturer's prescribing information.

Gemzar may be administered on an outpatient basis.

Instructions for Use/Handling — The recommended diluent for reconstitution of Gemzar is 0.9% Sodium Chloride Injection without preservatives. Due to solubility considerations, the maximum concentration for Gemzar upon reconstitution is 40 mg/mL. Reconstitution at concentrations greater than 40 mg/mL may result in incomplete dissolution, and should be avoided.

To reconstitute, add 5 mL of 0.9% Sodium Chloride Injection to the 200-mg vial or 25 mL of 0.9% Sodium Chloride Injection to the 1-g vial. Shake to dissolve. These dilutions each yield a gemcitabine concentration of 38 mg/mL which includes accounting for the displacement volume of the lyophilized powder (0.26 mL for the 200-mg vial or 1.3 mL for the 1-g vial). The total volume upon reconstitution will be 5.26 mL or 26.3 mL, respectively. Complete withdrawal of the vial contents will provide 200 mg or 1 g of gemcitabine, respectively. The appropriate amount of drug may be administered as prepared or further diluted with 0.9% Sodium Chloride Injection to concentrations as low as 0.1 mg/mL.

Reconstituted Gemzar is a clear, colorless to light straw-colored solution. After reconstitution with 0.9% Sodium Chloride Injection, the pH of the resulting solution lies in the range of 2.7 to 3.3. The solution should be inspected visually for particulate matter and discoloration, prior to administration, whenever solution or container permit. If particulate matter or discoloration is found, do not administer. When prepared as directed, Gemzar solutions are stable for 24 hours at controlled room temperature 20° to 25°C (68° to 77°F) [*See* USP]. Discard unused portion. Solutions of reconstituted Gemzar should not be refrigerated, as crystallization may occur.

The compatibility of Gemzar with other drugs has not been studied. No incompatibilities have been observed with infusion bottles or polyvinyl chloride bags and administration sets.

Unopened vials of Gemzar are stable until the expiration date indicated on the package when stored at controlled room temperature 20° to 25°C (68° to 77°F) [*See* USP].

Caution should be exercised in handling and preparing Gemzar solutions. The use of gloves is recommended. If Gemzar solution contacts the skin or mucosa, immediately wash the skin thoroughly with soap and water or rinse the mucosa with copious amounts of water. Although acute dermal irritation has not been observed in animal studies, 2 of 3 rabbits exhibited drug-related systemic toxicities (death, hypoactivity, nasal discharge, shallow breathing) due to dermal absorption.

Procedures for proper handling and disposal of anti-cancer drugs should be considered. Several guidelines on this subject have been published.[1-8] There is no general agreement that all of the procedures recommended in the guidelines are necessary or appropriate.

HOW SUPPLIED

Vials:

200 mg white, lyophilized powder in a 10-mL size sterile single use vial (No. 7501) NDC 0002-7501-01

1 g white, lyophilized powder in a 50-mL size sterile single use vial (No. 7502) NDC 0002-7502-01

Store at controlled room temperature (20° to 25°C) (68° to 77°F). The USP has defined controlled room temperature as "A temperature maintained thermostatically that encompasses the usual and customary working environment of 20° to 25°C (68° to 77°F); that results in a mean kinetic temperature calculated to be not more than 25°C; and that allows for excursions between 15° and 30°C (59° and 86°F) that are experienced in pharmacies, hospitals, and warehouses."

REFERENCES

1. Recommendations for the safe handling of parenteral antineoplastic drugs. NIH publication No. 83-2621. US Government Printing Office, Washington, DC 20402.
2. Council on Scientific Affairs: Guidelines for handling parenteral antineoplastics. *JAMA* 1985;253:1590.
3. National Study Commission on Cytotoxic Exposure — Recommendations for handling cytotoxic agents, 1987. Available from Louis P Jeffrey, ScD, Director of Pharmacy Services, Rhode Island Hospital, 593 Eddy Street, Providence, Rhode Island 02902.
4. Clinical Oncological Society of Australia: Guidelines and recommendations for safe handling of antineoplastic agents. *Med J Aust* 1983;1:426.
5. Jones RB, et al. Safe handling of chemotherapeutic agents: A report from the Mount Sinai Medical Center. *CA* 1983;33(Sept/Oct):258.
6. American Society of Hospital Pharmacists: Technical assistance bulletin on handling cytotoxic drugs in hospitals. *Am J Hosp Pharm* 1990;47:1033.
7. Controlling Occupational Exposure to Hazardous Drugs, OSHA Work Practice Guidelines. *Am J Health-Sys Pharm* 1996;53:1669-1685.
8. ONS Clinical Practice Committee. Cancer Chemotherapy Guidelines and Recommendations for Practice. Pittsburg, PA: Oncology Nursing Society; 1999:32-41.

Literature revised May 19, 2004
Eli Lilly and Company
Indianapolis, IN 46285, USA
PV 4062 AMP PRINTED IN USA

GLUCAGON ℞

[*glōō 'ka-gŏn*]
FOR INJECTION
(rDNA ORIGIN)

INFORMATION FOR THE PHYSICIAN

DESCRIPTION

Glucagon for Injection (rDNA origin) is a polypeptide hormone identical to human glucagon that increases blood glucose and relaxes smooth muscle of the gastrointestinal tract. Glucagon is synthesized in a special non-pathogenic

Continued on next page

*** Identi-Code® symbol. This product information was prepared in June 2004. Current information on these and other products of Eli Lilly and Company may be obtained by direct inquiry to Lilly Research Laboratories, Lilly Corporate Center, Indianapolis, Indiana 46285, (800) 545-5979.**

Glucagon—Cont.

laboratory strain of *Escherichia coli* bacteria that has been genetically altered by the addition of the gene for glucagon. Glucagon is a single-chain polypeptide that contains 29 amino acid residues and has a molecular weight of 3,483. The empirical formula is $C_{153}H_{225}N_{43}O_{49}S$. The primary sequence of glucagon is shown below.

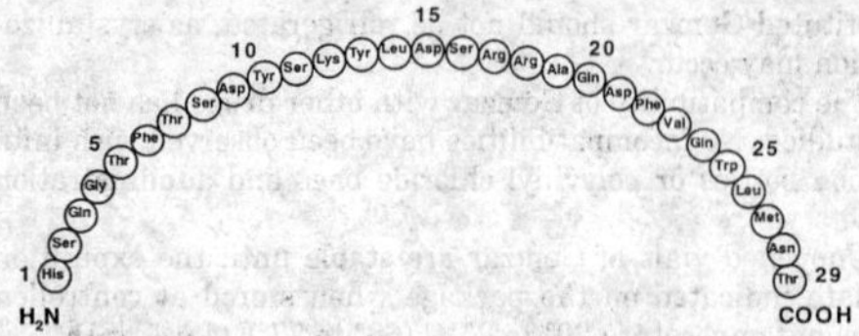

Crystalline glucagon is a white to off-white powder. It is relatively insoluble in water but is soluble at a pH of less than 3 or more than 9.5.

Glucagon is available for use intravenously, intramuscularly, or subcutaneously in a kit that contains a vial of sterile glucagon and a syringe of sterile diluent. The vial contains 1 mg (1 unit) of glucagon and 49 mg of lactose. Hydrochloric acid may have been added during manufacture to adjust the pH of the glucagon. One International Unit of glucagon is equivalent to 1 mg of glucagon.[1] The diluent syringe contains 12 mg/mL of glycerin, water for injection, and hydrochloric acid.

CLINICAL PHARMACOLOGY

Glucagon increases blood glucose concentration and is used in the treatment of hypoglycemia. Glucagon acts only on liver glycogen, converting it to glucose.

Glucagon administered through a parenteral route relaxes smooth muscle of the stomach, duodenum, small bowel, and colon.

Pharmacokinetics

Glucagon has been studied following intramuscular, subcutaneous, and intravenous administration in adult volunteers. Administration of the intravenous glucagon showed dose proportionality of the pharmacokinetics between 0.25 and 2.0 mg. Calculations from a 1 mg dose showed a small volume of distribution (mean, 0.25 L/kg) and a moderate clearance (mean, 13.5 mL/min/kg). The half-life was short, ranging from 8 to 18 minutes.

Maximum plasma concentrations of 7.9 ng/mL were achieved approximately 20 minutes after subcutaneous administration (*see* Figure 1A). With intramuscular dosing, maximum plasma concentrations of 6.9 ng/mL were attained approximately 13 minutes after dosing.

Glucagon is extensively degraded in liver, kidney, and plasma. Urinary excretion of intact glucagon has not been measured.

Pharmacodynamics

In a study of 25 volunteers, a subcutaneous dose of 1 mg glucagon resulted in a mean peak glucose concentration of 136 mg/dL 30 minutes after injection (*see* Figure 1B). Similarly, following intramuscular injection, the mean peak glucose level was 138 mg/dL, which occurred at 26 minutes after injection. No difference in maximum blood glucose concentration between animal-sourced and rDNA glucagon was observed after subcutaneous and intramuscular injection.

Figure 1
Mean (±SE) serum glucagon and blood glucose levels after subcutaneous injection of glucagon (1mg) in 25 normal volunteers

A

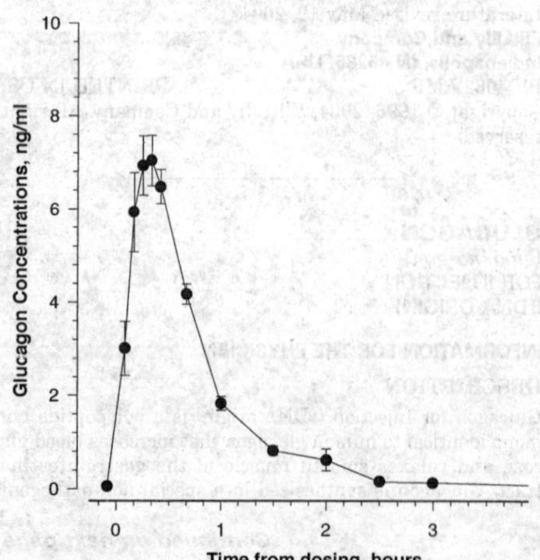

[See figure B at top of next column]

INDICATIONS AND USAGE

For the treatment of hypoglycemia:

Glucagon is indicated as a treatment for severe hypoglycemia.

B

Blood Glucose Concentrations, mg/dL
Time, hours

Because patients with type 1 diabetes may have less of an increase in blood glucose levels compared with a stable type 2 patient, supplementary carbohydrate should be given as soon as possible, especially to a pediatric patient.

For use as a diagnostic aid:

Glucagon is indicated as a diagnostic aid in the radiologic examination of the stomach, duodenum, small bowel, and colon when diminished intestinal motility would be advantageous.

Glucagon is as effective for this examination as are the anticholinergic drugs. However, the addition of the anticholinergic agent may result in increased side effects.

CONTRAINDICATIONS

Glucagon is contraindicated in patients with known hypersensitivity to it or in patients with known pheochromocytoma.

WARNINGS

Glucagon should be administered cautiously to patients with a history suggestive of insulinoma, pheochromocytoma, or both. In patients with insulinoma, intravenous administration of glucagon may produce an initial increase in blood glucose; however, because of glucagon's hyperglycemic effect the insulinoma may release insulin and cause subsequent hypoglycemia. A patient developing symptoms of hypoglycemia after a dose of glucagon should be given glucose orally, intravenously, or by gavage, whichever is most appropriate.

Exogenous glucagon also stimulates the release of catecholamines. In the presence of pheochromocytoma, glucagon can cause the tumor to release catecholamines, which may result in a sudden and marked increase in blood pressure. If a patient develops a sudden increase in blood pressure, 5 to 10 mg of phentolamine mesylate may be administered intravenously in an attempt to control the blood pressure.

Generalized allergic reactions, including urticaria, respiratory distress, and hypotension, have been reported in patients who received glucagon by injection.

PRECAUTIONS

General—Glucagon is effective in treating hypoglycemia only if sufficient liver glycogen is present. Because glucagon is of little or no help in states of starvation, adrenal insufficiency, or chronic hypoglycemia, hypoglycemia in these conditions should be treated with glucose.

Information for Patients—Refer patients and family members to the attached Information for the User for instructions describing the method of preparing and injecting glucagon. Advise the patient and family members to become familiar with the technique of preparing glucagon before an emergency arises. Instruct patients to use 1 mg (1 unit) for adults and 1/2 the adult dose (0.5 mg) [0.5 unit] for pediatric patients weighing less than 44 lb (20 kg).

Patients and family members should be informed of the following measures to prevent hypoglycemic reactions due to insulin:

1. Reasonable uniformity from day to day with regard to diet, insulin, and exercise.
2. Careful adjustment of the insulin program so that the type (or types) of insulin, dose, and time (or times) of administration are suited to the individual patient.
3. Frequent testing of the blood or urine for glucose so that a change in insulin requirements can be foreseen.
4. Routine carrying of sugar, candy, or other readily absorbable carbohydrate by the patient so that it may be taken at the first warning of an oncoming reaction.

To prevent severe hypoglycemia, patients and family members should be informed of the symptoms of mild hypoglycemia and how to treat it appropriately.

Family members should be informed to arouse the patient as quickly as possible because prolonged hypoglycemia may result in damage to the central nervous system. Glucagon or intravenous glucose should awaken the patient sufficiently so that oral carbohydrates may be taken.

Patients should be advised to inform their physician when hypoglycemic reactions occur so that the treatment regimen may be adjusted if necessary.

Laboratory Tests—Blood glucose determinations should be obtained to follow the patient with hypoglycemia until patient is asymptomatic.

Carcinogenesis, Mutagenesis, Impairment of Fertility—Because glucagon is usually given in a single dose and has a very short half-life, no studies have been done regarding carcinogenesis. In a series of studies examining effects on the bacterial mutagenesis (Ames) assay, it was determined that *an increase* in colony counts was related to technical difficulties in running this assay with peptides and was not due to mutagenic activities of the glucagon.

Reproduction studies have been performed in rats at doses up to 2 mg/kg glucagon administered two times a day (up to 40 times the human dose based on body surface area, mg/m^2) and have revealed no evidence of impaired fertility.

Pregnancy—Pregnancy Category B—Reproduction studies have not been performed with recombinant glucagon. However, studies with animal-sourced glucagon were performed in rats at doses up to 2 mg/kg glucagon administered two times a day (up to 40 times the human dose based on body surface area, mg/m^2), and have revealed no evidence of impaired fertility or harm to the fetus due to glucagon. There are, however, no adequate and well-controlled studies in pregnant women. Because animal reproduction studies are not always predictive of human response, this drug should be used during pregnancy only if clearly needed.

Nursing Mothers—It is not known whether this drug is excreted in human milk. Because many drugs are excreted in human milk, caution should be exercised when glucagon is administered to a nursing woman. If the drug is excreted in human milk during its short half-life, it will be hydrolyzed and absorbed like any other polypeptide. Glucagon is not active when taken orally because it is destroyed in the gastrointestinal tract before it can be absorbed.

Pediatric Use—For the treatment of hypoglycemia: The use of glucagon in pediatric patients has been reported to be safe and effective.[2-6]

For use as a diagnostic aid: Effectiveness has not been established in pediatric patients.

ADVERSE REACTIONS

Severe adverse reactions are very rare, although nausea and vomiting may occur occasionally. These reactions may also occur with hypoglycemia. Generalized allergic reactions have been reported (*see* WARNINGS). In a three month controlled study of 75 volunteers comparing animal-sourced glucagon with glucagon manufactured through rDNA technology, no glucagon-specific antibodies were detected in either treatment group.

OVERDOSAGE

Signs and Symptoms—If overdosage occurs, nausea, vomiting, gastric hypotonicity, and diarrhea would be expected without causing consequential toxicity.

Intravenous administration of glucagon has been shown to have positive inotropic and chronotropic effects. A transient increase in both blood pressure and pulse rate may occur following the administration of glucagon. Patients taking β-blockers might be expected to have a greater increase in both pulse and blood pressure, an increase of which will be transient because of glucagon's short half-life. The increase in blood pressure and pulse rate may require therapy in patients with pheochromocytoma or coronary artery disease.

When glucagon was given in large doses to patients with cardiac disease, investigators reported a positive inotropic effect. These investigators administered glucagon in doses of 0.5 to 16 mg/hour by continuous infusion for periods of 5 to 166 hours. Total doses ranged from 25 to 996 mg, and a 21-month-old infant received approximately 8.25 mg in 165 hours. Side effects included nausea, vomiting, and decreasing serum potassium concentration. Serum potassium concentration could be maintained within normal limits with supplemental potassium.

The intravenous median lethal dose for glucagon in mice and rats is approximately 300 mg/kg and 38.6 mg/kg, respectively.

Because glucagon is a polypeptide, it would be rapidly destroyed in the gastrointestinal tract if it were to be accidentally ingested.

Treatment—To obtain up-to-date information about the treatment of overdose, a good resource is your certified Regional Poison Control Center. Telephone numbers of certified poison control centers are listed in the *Physicians' Desk Reference (PDR)*. In managing overdosage, consider the possibility of multiple drug overdoses, interaction among drugs, and unusual drug kinetics in your patient.

In view of the extremely short half-life of glucagon and its prompt destruction and excretion, the treatment of overdosage is symptomatic, primarily for nausea, vomiting, and possible hypokalemia.

If the patient develops a dramatic increase in blood pressure, 5 to 10 mg of phentolamine mesylate has been shown to be effective in lowering blood pressure for the short time that control would be needed.

Forced diuresis, peritoneal dialysis, hemodialysis, or charcoal hemoperfusion have not been established as beneficial for an overdose of glucagon; it is extremely unlikely that one of these procedures would ever be indicated.

DOSAGE AND ADMINISTRATION

General Instructions for Use:

- The diluent is provided for use only in the preparation of glucagon for parenteral injection and for no other use.
- Glucagon should not be used at concentrations greater than 1 mg/mL (1 unit/mL).
- Reconstituted glucagon should be used immediately. **Discard any unused portion.**
- Reconstituted glucagon solutions should be used only if they are clear and of a water-like consistency.
- Parenteral drug products should be inspected visually for particulate matter and discoloration prior to administration.

Directions for Treatment of Severe Hypoglycemia:

Severe hypoglycemia should be treated initially with intravenous glucose, if possible.

1. If parenteral glucose can not be used, dissolve the lyophilized glucagon using the accompanying diluting solution and use immediately.
2. For adults and for pediatric patients weighing more than 44 lb (20 kg), give 1 mg (1 unit) by subcutaneous, intramuscular, or intravenous injection.
3. For pediatric patients weighing less than 44 lb (20 kg), give 0.5 mg (0.5 unit) or a dose equivalent to 20-30 µg/kg.[2–6]
4. **Discard any unused portion.**
5. An unconscious patient will usually awaken within 15 minutes following the glucagon injection. If the response is delayed, there is no contraindication to the administration of an additional dose of glucagon; however, in view of the deleterious effects of cerebral hypoglycemia emergency aid should be sought so that parenteral glucose can be given.
6. After the patient responds, supplemental carbohydrate should be given to restore liver glycogen and to prevent secondary hypoglycemia.

Directions for Use as a Diagnostic Aid:

Dissolve the lyophilized glucagon using the accompanying diluting solution and use immediately. **Discard any unused portion.**

The doses in the following table may be administered for relaxation of the stomach, duodenum, and small bowel, depending on the onset and duration of effect required for the examination. Since the stomach is less sensitive to the effect of glucagon, 0.5 mg (0.5 units) IV or 2 mg (2 units) IM are recommended.

[See table above]

For examination of the colon, it is recommended that a 2 mg (2 units) dose be administered intramuscularly approximately 10 minutes prior to the procedure. Colon relaxation and reduction of patient discomfort may allow the radiologist to perform a more satisfactory examination.

Dose	Route of Administration	Time of Onset of Action	Approximate Duration of Effect
0.25–0.5 mg (0.25–0.5 units)	IV	1 minute	9–17 minutes
1 mg (1 unit)	IM	8–10 minutes	12–27 minutes
2 mg* (2 units)	IV	1 minute	22–25 minutes
2 mg* (2 units)	IM	4–7 minutes	21–32 minutes

*Administration of 2 mg (2 units) doses produces a higher incidence of nausea and vomiting than do lower doses.

HOW SUPPLIED

Glucagon Emergency Kit for Low Blood Sugar (Glucagon for Injection [rDNA origin]) (MS8031):
1 mg (1 unit)—(VL7529), with 1 mL of diluting solution (Hyporet®* HY7530) (1s)
NDC 0002-8031-01

Glucagon Diagnostic Kit (Glucagon for Injection [rDNA origin]) (MS8085):
1 mg (1 unit)—(VL7529), with 1 mL of diluting solution (Hyporet®* HY7530) (1s)
NDC 0002-8085-01 (available in US market only).

*Hyporet® (disposable syringe, Lilly).

Stability and Storage:

Before Reconstitution—Vials of Glucagon, as well as the Diluting Solution for Glucagon, may be stored at controlled room temperature 20° to 25°C (68° to 77°F)[see USP].

The USP defines controlled room temperature by the following: A temperature maintained thermostatically that encompasses the usual and customary working environment of 20° to 25°C (68° to 77°F); that results in a mean kinetic temperature calculated to be not more than 25°C; and that allows for excursions between 15° and 30°C (59° and 86°F) that are experienced in pharmacies, hospitals, and warehouses.

After Reconstitution—Glucagon for Injection (rDNA origin) should be used immediately. **Discard any unused portion.**

REFERENCES

1. *Drug Information for the Health Care Professional.* 18th ed. Rockville, Maryland: The United States Pharmacopeial Convention, Inc; 1998; I:1512.
2. Gibbs et al: Use of glucagon to terminate insulin reactions in diabetic children. *Nebr Med J* 1958;43:56–57.
3. Cornblath M, et al: Studies of carbohydrate metabolism in the newborn: Effect of glucagon on concentration of sugar in capillary blood of newborn infant. *Pediatrics* 1958;21:885–892.
4. Carson MJ, Koch R: Clinical studies with glucagon in children. *J Pediatr* 1955;47:161–170.
5. Shipp JC, et al: Treatment of insulin hypoglycemia in diabetic campers. *Diabetes* 1964;13:645–648.
6. Aman J, Wranne L: Hypoglycemia in childhood diabetes II: Effect of subcutaneous or intramuscular injection of different doses of glucagon. *Acta Pediatr Scand* 1988;77: 548–553.

Literature revised April 27, 2001
PA 2282 AMP

INFORMATION FOR THE USER

GLUCAGON FOR INJECTION (rDNA ORIGIN)

BECOME FAMILIAR WITH THE FOLLOWING INSTRUCTIONS BEFORE AN EMERGENCY ARISES. DO NOT USE THIS KIT AFTER DATE STAMPED ON THE BOTTLE LABEL. IF YOU HAVE QUESTIONS CONCERNING THE USE OF THIS PRODUCT, CONSULT A DOCTOR, NURSE OR PHARMACIST.

Make sure that your relatives or close friends know that if you become unconscious, medical assistance must always be sought. Glucagon may have been prescribed so that members of your household can give the injection if you become hypoglycemic and are unable to take sugar by mouth. If you are unconscious, glucagon can be given while awaiting medical assistance.

Show your family members and others where you keep this kit and how to use it. They need to know how to use it before you need it. They can practice giving a shot by giving you your normal insulin shots. It is important that they practice. A person who has never given a shot probably will not be able to do it in an emergency.

IMPORTANT

- Act quickly. Prolonged unconsciousness may be harmful.
- These simple instructions will help you give glucagon successfully.
- Turn patient on his/her side to prevent patient from choking.
- The contents of the syringe are inactive. You must mix the contents of the syringe with the glucagon in the accompanying bottle before giving injection. (See DIRECTIONS FOR USE below.)
- Do not prepare Glucagon for Injection until you are ready to use it.

WARNING: THE PATIENT MAY BE IN A COMA FROM SEVERE HYPERGLYCEMIA (HIGH BLOOD GLUCOSE) RATHER THAN HYPOGLYCEMIA. IN SUCH A CASE, THE PATIENT WILL **NOT** RESPOND TO GLUCAGON AND REQUIRES IMMEDIATE MEDICAL ATTENTION.

INDICATIONS FOR USE

Use glucagon to treat insulin coma or insulin reaction resulting from severe hypoglycemia (low blood sugar). Symptoms of severe hypoglycemia include disorientation, unconsciousness, and seizures or convulsions. Give glucagon if (1) the patient is unconscious (2) the patient is unable to eat sugar or a sugar-sweetened product (3) the patient is having a seizure, or (4) repeated administration of sugar or a sugar-sweetened product such as a regular soft drink or fruit juice does not improve the patient's condition. Milder cases of hypoglycemia should be treated promptly by eating sugar or a sugar-sweetened product. (See INFORMATION ON HYPOGLYCEMIA below for more information on the symptoms of hypoglycemia.) Glucagon is not active when taken orally.

DIRECTIONS FOR USE

TO PREPARE GLUCAGON FOR INJECTION

1. Remove the flip-off seal from the bottle of glucagon. Wipe rubber stopper on bottle with alcohol swab.

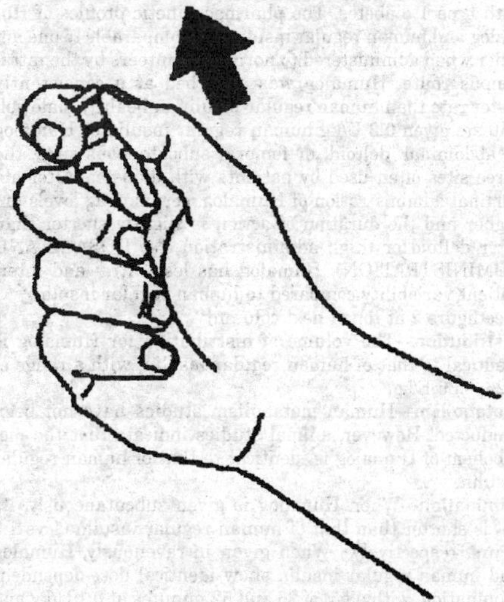

2. Remove the needle protector from the syringe, and inject the entire contents of the syringe into the bottle of glucagon. DO NOT REMOVE THE PLASTIC CLIP FROM THE SYRINGE. Remove syringe from the bottle.

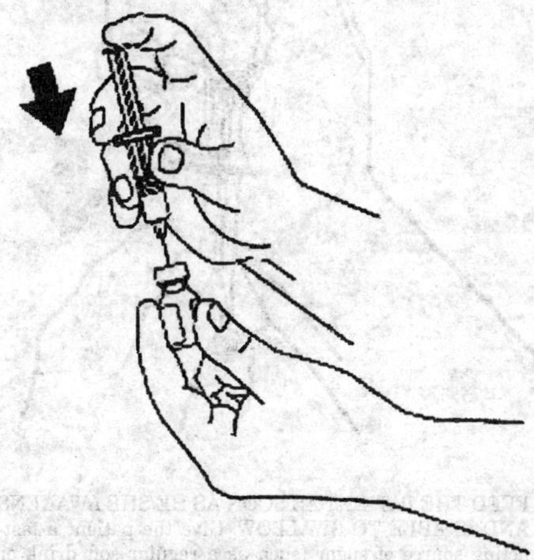

3. Swirl bottle gently until glucagon dissolves completely. GLUCAGON SHOULD NOT BE USED UNLESS THE SOLUTION IS CLEAR AND OF A WATER-LIKE CONSISTENCY.

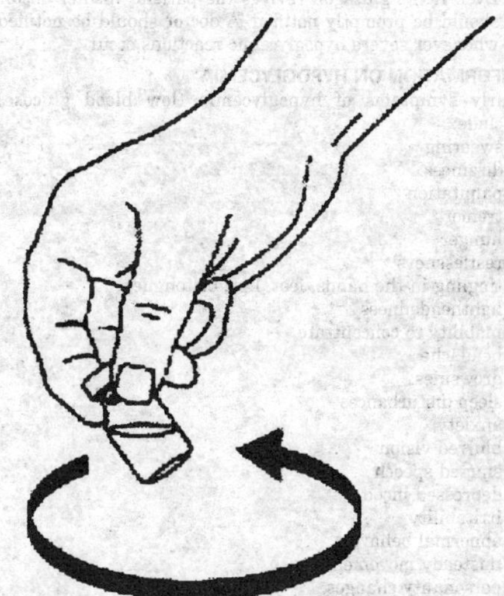

TO INJECT GLUCAGON

Use Same Technique as for Injecting Insulin

4. Using the same syringe, hold bottle upside down and, making sure the needle tip remains in solution, gently withdraw all of the solution (1 mg mark on syringe) from bottle. The plastic clip on the syringe will prevent the rubber stopper from being pulled out of the syringe; however, if the plastic plunger rod separates from the rubber stopper, simply reinsert the rod by turning it clockwise. The usual adult dose is 1 mg (1 unit). For children weighing less than 44 lb (20 kg), give 1/2 adult dose (0.5 mg). For children, withdraw 1/2 of the solution from the bottle (0.5 mg mark on syringe). DISCARD UNUSED PORTION.

[See figure at top of next column]

USING THE FOLLOWING DIRECTIONS, INJECT GLUCAGON IMMEDIATELY AFTER MIXING.

5. Cleanse injection site on buttock, arm, or thigh with alcohol swab.
6. Insert the needle into the loose tissue under the cleansed injection site, and inject all (or ½ for children weighing less than 44 lb) of the glucagon solution. THERE IS NO DANGER OF OVERDOSE. Apply light pressure at the injection site, and withdraw the needle. Press an alcohol swab against the injection site.
7. Turn the patient on his/her side. When an unconscious person awakens, he/she may vomit. Turning the patient on his/her side will prevent him/her from choking.

Continued on next page

*** Identi-Code® symbol. This product information was prepared in June 2004. Current information on these and other products of Eli Lilly and Company may be obtained by direct inquiry to Lilly Research Laboratories, Lilly Corporate Center, Indianapolis, Indiana 46285, (800) 545-5979.**

Glucagon—Cont.

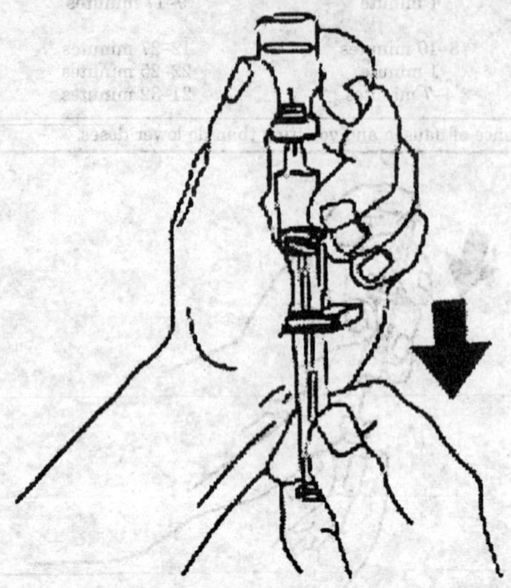

8. FEED THE PATIENT AS SOON AS HE/SHE AWAKENS AND IS ABLE TO SWALLOW. Give the patient a fast-acting source of sugar (such as a regular soft drink or fruit juice) and a long-acting source of sugar (such as crackers and cheese or a meat sandwich). If the patient does not awaken within 15 minutes, give another dose of glucagon and INFORM A DOCTOR OR EMERGENCY SERVICES IMMEDIATELY.
9. Even if the glucagon revives the patient, his/her doctor should be promptly notified. A doctor should be notified whenever severe hypoglycemic reactions occur.

INFORMATION ON HYPOGLYCEMIA

Early symptoms of hypoglycemia (low blood glucose) include:

- sweating
- dizziness
- palpitation
- tremor
- hunger
- restlessness
- tingling in the hands, feet, lips, or tongue
- lightheadedness
- inability to concentrate
- headache
- drowsiness
- sleep disturbances
- anxiety
- blurred vision
- slurred speech
- depressed mood
- irritability
- abnormal behavior
- unsteady movement
- personality changes

If not treated, the patient may progress to severe hypoglycemia that can include:

- disorientation
- unconsciousness
- seizures
- death

The occurrence of early symptoms calls for prompt and, if necessary, repeated administration of some form of carbohydrate. Patients should always carry a quick source of sugar, such as candy mints or glucose tablets. The prompt treatment of mild hypoglycemic symptoms can prevent severe hypoglycemic reactions. If the patient does not improve or if administration of carbohydrate is impossible, glucagon should be given or the patient should be treated with intravenous glucose at a medical facility. Glucagon, a naturally occurring substance produced by the pancreas, is helpful because it enables the patient to produce his/her own blood glucose to correct the hypoglycemia.

POSSIBLE PROBLEMS WITH GLUCAGON TREATMENT

Severe side effects are very rare, although nausea and vomiting may occur occasionally.

A few people may be allergic to glucagon or to one of the inactive ingredients in glucagon, or may experience rapid heart beat for a short while.

If you experience any other reactions which are likely to have been caused by glucagon, please contact your doctor.

STORAGE

Before dissolving glucagon with diluting solution—Store the kit at controlled room temperature between 20° to 25°C (68° to 77°F).

After dissolving glucagon with diluting solution—Should be used immediately. **Discard any unused portion.** Solutions should be clear and of a water-like consistency at time of use.

Literature revised April 27, 2001

PA 2282 AMP

HUMALOG® ℞

[*hū'mă-lōg*]

(INSULIN LISPRO INJECTION (rDNA ORIGIN))

DESCRIPTION

Humalog® (insulin lispro, rDNA origin) is a human insulin analog that is a rapid-acting, parenteral blood glucose-lowering agent. Chemically, it is Lys(B28), Pro(B29) human insulin analog, created when the amino acids at positions 28 and 29 on the insulin B-chain are reversed. Humalog is synthesized in a special non-pathogenic laboratory strain of *Escherichia coli* bacteria that has been genetically altered by the addition of the gene for insulin lispro.

Humalog has the following primary structure:

Figure 1

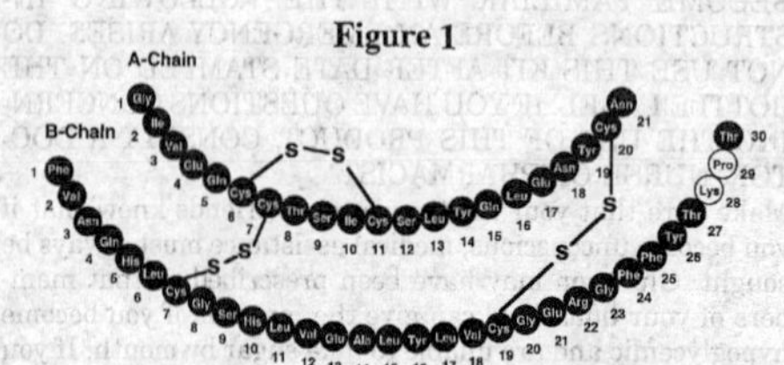

Insulin lispro has the empirical formula $C_{257}H_{383}N_{65}O_{77}S_6$ and a molecular weight of 5808, both identical to that of human insulin.

The vials and cartridges contain a sterile solution of Humalog for use as an injection. Humalog injection consists of zinc-insulin lispro crystals dissolved in a clear aqueous fluid.

Each milliliter of Humalog injection contains insulin lispro 100 Units, 16 mg glycerin, 1.88 mg dibasic sodium phosphate, 3.15 mg *m*-cresol, zinc oxide content adjusted to provide 0.0197 mg zinc ion, trace amounts of phenol, and water for injection. Insulin lispro has a pH of 7.0–7.8. Hydrochloric acid 10% and/or sodium hydroxide 10% may be added to adjust pH.

CLINICAL PHARMACOLOGY

Antidiabetic Activity—The primary activity of insulin, including Humalog, is the regulation of glucose metabolism. In addition, all insulins have several anabolic and anti-catabolic actions on many tissues in the body. In muscle and other tissues (except the brain), insulin causes rapid transport of glucose and amino acids intracellularly, promotes anabolism, and inhibits protein catabolism. In the liver, insulin promotes the uptake and storage of glucose in the form of glycogen, inhibits gluconeogenesis, and promotes the conversion of excess glucose into fat.

Humalog has been shown to be equipotent to human insulin on a molar basis. One unit of Humalog has the same glucose-lowering effect as one unit of human regular insulin, but its effect is more rapid and of shorter duration. The glucose-lowering activity of Humalog and human regular insulin is comparable when administered to normal volunteers by the intravenous route.

Pharmacokinetics-

Absorption and Bioavailability—Humalog is as bioavailable as human regular insulin, with absolute bioavailability ranging between 55%–77% with doses between 0.1–0.2 U/kg, inclusive. Studies in normal volunteers and patients with type 1 (insulin-dependent) diabetes demonstrated that Humalog is absorbed faster than human regular insulin (U-100) (Figure 2). In normal volunteers given subcutaneous doses of Humalog ranging from 0.1–0.4 U/kg, peak serum levels were seen 30–90 minutes after dosing. When normal volunteers received equivalent doses of human regular insulin, peak insulin levels occurred between 50–120 minutes after dosing. Similar results were seen in patients with type 1 diabetes. The pharmacokinetic profiles of Humalog and human regular insulin are comparable to one another when administered to normal volunteers by the intravenous route. Humalog was absorbed at a consistently faster rate than human regular insulin in healthy male volunteers given 0.2 U/kg human regular insulin or Humalog at abdominal, deltoid, or femoral subcutaneous sites, the three sites often used by patients with diabetes. After abdominal administration of Humalog, serum drug levels are higher and the duration of action is slightly shorter than after deltoid or thigh administration (*see* DOSAGE AND ADMINISTRATION). Humalog has less intra- and inter-patient variability compared to human regular insulin.

[See figure 2 at top of next column]

Distribution—The volume of distribution for Humalog is identical to that of human regular insulin, with a range of 0.26–0.36 L/kg.

Metabolism—Human metabolism studies have not been conducted. However, animal studies indicate that the metabolism of Humalog is identical to that of human regular insulin.

Elimination—When Humalog is given subcutaneously, its $t_{1/2}$ is shorter than that of human regular insulin (1 vs 1.5 hours, respectively). When given intravenously, Humalog and human regular insulin show identical dose-dependent elimination, with a $t_{1/2}$ of 26 and 52 minutes at 0.1 U/kg and 0.2 U/kg, respectively.

Pharmacodynamics—Studies in normal volunteers and patients with diabetes demonstrated that Humalog has a more rapid onset of glucose-lowering activity, an earlier peak for glucose lowering, and a shorter duration of glucose-

Figure 2

Serum Humalog and Insulin levels after subcutaneous injection of human regular insulin or Humalog (0.2 U/kg) immediately before a high carbohydrate meal in 10 patients with type 1 diabetes.*

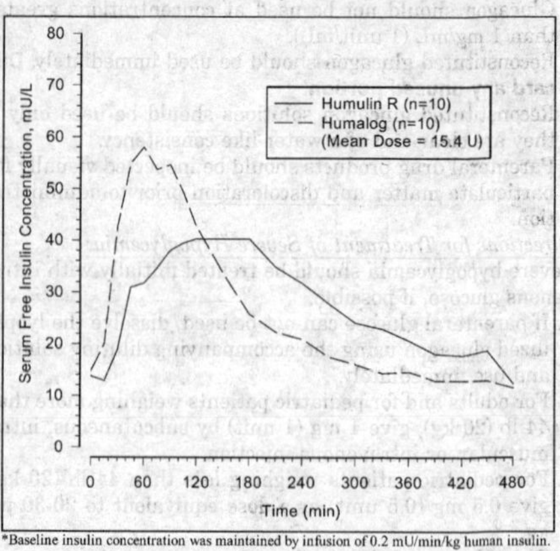

*Baseline insulin concentration was maintained by infusion of 0.2 mU/min/kg human insulin.

lowering activity than human regular insulin (Figure 3). The earlier onset of activity of Humalog is directly related to its more rapid rate of absorption. The time course of action of insulin and insulin analogs such as Humalog may vary considerably in different individuals or within the same individual. The parameters of Humalog activity (time of onset, peak time, and duration) as designated in Figure 3 should be considered only as general guidelines. The rate of insulin absorption and consequently the onset of activity is known to be affected by the site of injection, exercise, and other variables (*see* PRECAUTIONS, *General*).

Figure 3

Blood glucose levels after subcutaneous injection of human regular insulin or Humalog (0.2 U/kg) immediately before a high carbohydrate meal in 10 patients with type 1 diabetes.*

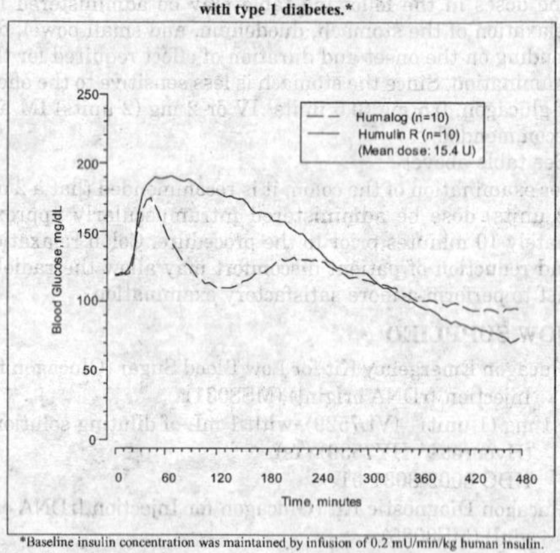

*Baseline insulin concentration was maintained by infusion of 0.2 mU/min/kg human insulin.

In open-label, crossover studies of 1008 patients with type 1 diabetes and 722 patients with type 2 (non-insulin-dependent) diabetes, Humalog reduced postprandial glucose compared with human regular insulin (*see* Table 1). The clinical significance of improvement in postprandial hyperglycemia has not been established.

Table 1

Comparison of Means of Glycemic Parameters at the End of Combined Treatment Periods. All Randomized Patients in Cross-over Studies (3 months for each treatment)

Type 1, N=1008 Glycemic Parameter, (mg/dL)	Humalog[a]	Humulin® R[a]*
Fasting Blood Glucose	209.5 ± 91.6	204.1 ± 89.3
1-Hour Postprandial	232.4 ± 97.7	250.0 ± 96.7
2-Hour Postprandial	200.9 ± 95.4	231.7 ± 103.9
HbA_{1c} (%)	8.2 ± 1.5	8.2 ± 1.5
Type 2, N=722 Glycemic Parameter, (mg/dL)	**Humalog[a]**	**Humulin R[a]**
Fasting Blood Glucose	192.1 ± 67.9	183.1 ± 66.1
1-Hour Postprandial	238.1 ± 79.7	250.0 ± 75.2
2-Hour Postprandial	217.4 ± 83.2	236.5 ± 80.6
HbA_{1c} (%)	8.2 ± 1.3	8.2 ± 1.4

[a]Mean ± Standard Deviation

*Humulin® R (human insulin [rDNA origin] injection)

In 12-month parallel studies in patients with type 1 and type 2 diabetes, HbA_{1c} did not differ between patients treated with human regular insulin and those treated with Humalog.

Hypoglycemia—While the overall rate of hypoglycemia did not differ between patients with type 1 and type 2 diabetes treated with Humalog compared with human regular insulin, patients with type 1 diabetes treated with Humalog had fewer hypoglycemic episodes between midnight and 6 a.m.

The lower rate of hypoglycemia in the Humalog-treated group may have been related to higher nocturnal blood glucose levels, as reflected by a small increase in mean fasting blood glucose levels.

Humalog in Combination with Sulfonylurea Agents—In a two-month study in patients with fasting hyperglycemia despite maximal dosing with sulfonylureas (SU), patients were randomized to one of three treatment regimens; Humulin NPH at bedtime plus SU, Humalog three times a day before meals plus SU, or Humalog three times a day before meals and Humulin NPH at bedtime. The combination of Humalog and SU resulted in an improvement in HbA_{1c} accompanied by a weight gain (*see* Table 2).

Table 2

Results of a Two-Month Study in Which Humalog Was Added to Sulfonylurea Therapy in Patients Not Adequately Controlled on Sulfonylurea Alone.

	Humulin® N h.s. + SU	Humalog a.c. + SU	Humalog a.c.+ Humulin® N h.s.
Randomized (n)	135	139	149
HbA_{1c} (%) at baseline	9.9	10.0	10.0
HbA_{1c} (%) at 2-months	8.7	8.4	8.5
HbA_{1c} (%) change from baseline	−1.2	−1.6	−1.4
Weight gain at 2-months (kg)	0.6	1.2	1.5
Hypoglycemia* (events/mo)	0.11	0.03	0.09
Number of injections	1	3	4
Total insulin dose (U/kg) at 2-months	0.23	0.33	0.52

a.c.-three times a day before meals, h.s.-at bedtime, SU-oral sulfonylurea agent

*blood glucose ≤ 36mg/dL or needing assistance from third party

Special Populations—

Age and Gender—Information on the effect of age and gender on the pharmacokinetics of Humalog is unavailable. However, in large clinical trials, subgroup analysis based on age and gender did not indicate any difference in postprandial glucose parameters between Humalog and human regular insulin.

Smoking—The effect of smoking on the pharmacokinetics and glucodynamics of Humalog has not been studied.

Pregnancy—The effect of pregnancy on the pharmacokinetics and glucodynamics of Humalog has not been studied.

Obesity—The effect of obesity and/or subcutaneous fat thickness on the pharmacokinetics and glucodynamics of Humalog has not been studied. In large clinical trials, which included patients with Body Mass Index up to and including 35 kg/m^2 no consistent differences were seen between Humalog and Humulin R with respect to postprandial glucose parameters.

Renal Impairment—Some studies with human insulin have shown increased circulating levels of insulin in patients with renal failure. In a study of 25 patients with type 2 diabetes and a wide range of renal function, the pharmacokinetic differences between Humalog and human regular insulin were generally maintained. However, the sensitivity of the patients to insulin did change, with an increased response to insulin as the renal function declined. Careful glucose monitoring and dose adjustments of insulin, including Humalog, may be necessary in patients with renal dysfunction.

Hepatic Impairment—Some studies with human insulin have shown increased circulating levels of insulin in patients with hepatic failure. In a study of 22 patients with type 2 diabetes, impaired hepatic function did not affect the subcutaneous absorption or general disposition of Humalog when compared to patients with no history of hepatic dysfunction. In that study, Humalog maintained its more rapid absorption and elimination when compared to human regular insulin. Careful glucose monitoring and dose adjustments of insulin, including Humalog, may be necessary in patients with hepatic dysfunction.

INDICATIONS AND USAGE

Humalog is an insulin analog that is indicated in the treatment of patients with diabetes mellitus for the control of hyperglycemia. Humalog has a more rapid onset and a shorter duration of action than human regular insulin. Therefore, in patients with type 1 diabetes, Humalog should be used in regimens that include a longer-acting insulin. However, in patients with type 2 diabetes, Humalog may be used without a longer-acting insulin when used in combination therapy with sulfonylurea agents.

CONTRAINDICATIONS

Humalog is contraindicated during episodes of hypoglycemia and in patients sensitive to Humalog or one of its excipients.

WARNINGS

This human insulin analog differs from human regular insulin by its rapid onset of action as well as a shorter duration of activity. When used as a mealtime insulin, the dose of Humalog should be given within 15 minutes before or immediately after the meal. Because of the short duration of action of Humalog, patients with type 1 diabetes also require a longer-acting insulin to maintain glucose control. Hypoglycemia is the most common adverse effect associated with insulins, including Humalog. As with all insulins, the timing of hypoglycemia may differ among various insulin formulations. Glucose monitoring is recommended for all patients with diabetes.

Any change of insulin should be made cautiously and only under medical supervision. Changes in insulin strength, manufacturer, type (e.g., regular, NPH, analog), species (animal, human), or method of manufacture (rDNA versus animal-source insulin) may result in the need for a change in dosage.

PRECAUTIONS

General—Hypoglycemia and hypokalemia are among the potential clinical adverse effects associated with the use of all insulins. Because of differences in the action of Humalog and other insulins, care should be taken in patients in whom such potential side effects might be clinically relevant (e.g., patients who are fasting, have autonomic neuropathy, or are using potassium-lowering drugs or patients taking drugs sensitive to serum potassium level). Lipodystrophy and hypersensitivity are among other potential clinical adverse effects associated with the use of all insulins.

As with all insulin preparations, the time course of Humalog action may vary in different individuals or at different times in the same individual and is dependent on site of injection, blood supply, temperature, and physical activity.

Adjustment of dosage of any insulin may be necessary if patients change their physical activity or their usual meal plan. Insulin requirements may be altered during illness, emotional disturbances, or other stresses.

Hypoglycemia—As with all insulin preparations, hypoglycemic reactions may be associated with the administration of Humalog. Rapid changes in serum glucose levels may induce symptoms of hypoglycemia in persons with diabetes, regardless of the glucose value. Early warning symptoms of hypoglycemia may be different or less pronounced under certain conditions, such as long duration of diabetes, diabetic nerve disease, use of medications such as beta-blockers, or intensified diabetes control.

Renal Impairment—The requirements for insulin may be reduced in patients with renal impairment.

Hepatic Impairment—Although impaired hepatic function does not affect the absorption or disposition of Humalog, careful glucose mointoring and dose adjustments of insulin, including Humalog, may be necessary.

Allergy—Local Allergy—As with any insulin therapy, patients may experience redness, swelling, or itching at the site of injection. These minor reactions usually resolve in a few days to a few weeks. In some instances, these reactions may be related to factors other than insulin, such as irritants in a skin cleansing agent or poor injection technique.

Systemic Allergy—Less common, but potentially more serious, is generalized allergy to insulin, which may cause rash (including pruritus) over the whole body, shortness of breath, wheezing, reduction in blood pressure, rapid pulse, or sweating. Severe cases of generalized allergy, including anaphylactic reaction, may be life threatening. In controlled clinical trials, pruritus (with or without rash) was seen in 17 patients receiving Humulin R (N=2969) and 30 patients receiving Humalog (N=2944) (p=.053). Localized reactions and generalized myalgias have been reported with the use of cresol as an injectable excipient.

Antibody Production—In large clinical trials, antibodies that cross react with human insulin and insulin lispro were observed in both Humulin R- and Humalog-treatment groups. As expected, the largest increase in the antibody levels during the 12-month clinical trials was observed with patients new to insulin therapy.

Information for Patients—Patients should be informed of the potential risks and advantages of Humalog and alternative therapies. Patients should also be informed about the importance of proper insulin storage, injection technique, timing of dosage, adherence to meal planning, regular physical activity, regular blood glucose monitoring, periodic glycosylated hemoglobin testing, recognition and management of hypo- and hyperglycemia, and periodic assessment for diabetes complications.

Patients should be advised to inform their physician if they are pregnant or intend to become pregnant.

Refer patients to the Information for the Patient circular for information on proper injection technique, timing of Humalog dosing (≤ 15 minutes before or immediately after a meal), storing and mixing insulin, and common adverse effects.

Use of the Humalog Pen: Patients should read the "Information for the Patient" insert and the "Disposable Insulin Delivery Device User Manual" before starting therapy with a Humalog Pen and re-read them each time the prescription is renewed. Patients should be instructed on how to properly use the delivery device (refer to "Disposable Insulin Delivery Device User Manual"), prime the pen, and properly dispose of needles. Patients should be advised not to share their pens with others.

Laboratory Tests—As with all insulins, the therapeutic response to Humalog should be monitored by periodic blood glucose tests. Periodic measurement of glycosylated hemoglobin is recommended for the monitoring of long-term glycemic control.

Drug Interactions—(*see* CLINICAL PHARMACOLOGY) Insulin requirements may be increased by medications with hyperglycemic activity such as corticosteroids, isoniazid, certain lipid-lowering drugs (e.g., niacin), estrogens, oral contraceptives, phenothiazines, and thyroid replacement therapy.

Insulin requirements may be decreased in the presence of drugs with hypoglycemic activity, such as oral hypoglycemic agents, salicylates, sulfa antibiotics, and certain antidepressants (monoamine oxidase inhibitors), certain angiotensin-converting-enzyme inhibitors, beta-adrenergic blockers, inhibitors of pancreatic function (e.g., octreotide), and alcohol. Beta-adrenergic blockers may mask the symptoms of hypoglycemia in some patients.

Mixing of Insulins—Care should be taken when mixing all insulins as a change in peak action may occur. The American Diabetes Association warns in its Position Statement on Insulin Administration, "On mixing, physiochemical changes in the mixture may occur (either immediately or over time). As a result, the physiological response to the insulin mixture may differ from that of the injection of the insulins separately." Mixing Humalog with Humulin N or Humulin U does not decrease the absorption rate or the total bioavailability of Humalog. Given alone or mixed with Humulin N, Humalog results in a more rapid absorption and glucose-lowering effect compared with human regular insulin.

The effects of mixing Humalog with insulins of animal source or insulin preparations produced by other manufacturers have not been studied (*see* WARNINGS).

If Humalog is mixed with a longer-acting insulin, such as Humulin N or Humulin U, Humalog should be drawn into the syringe first to prevent clouding of the Humalog by the longer-acting insulin. Injection should be made immediately after mixing. Mixtures should not be administered intravenously.

Carcinogenesis, Mutagenesis, Impairment of Fertility—Long-term studies in animals have not been performed to evaluate the carcinogenic potential of Humalog. Humalog was not mutagenic in a battery of *in vitro* and *in vivo* genetic toxicity assays (bacterial mutation tests, unscheduled DNA synthesis, mouse lymphoma assay, chromosomal aberration tests, and a micronucleus test). There is no evidence from animal studies of Humalog-induced impairment of fertility.

Pregnancy—Teratogenic Effects—Pregnancy Category B—Reproduction studies have been performed in pregnant rats and rabbits at parenteral doses up to 4 and 0.3 times, respectively, the average human dose (40 units/day) based on body surface area. The results have revealed no evidence of impaired fertility or harm to the fetus due to Humalog. There are, however, no adequate and well-controlled studies in pregnant women. Because animal reproduction studies are not always predictive of human response, this drug should be used during pregnancy only if clearly needed.

Published studies with human insulins suggest that optimizing overall glycemic control, including postprandial control, before conception and during pregnancy improves fetal outcome. Although the fetal complications of maternal hyperglycemia have been well documented, fetal toxicity also has been reported with maternal hypoglycemia. Insulin requirements usually fall during the first trimester and increase during the second and third trimesters. Careful monitoring of the patient is required throughout pregnancy. During the perinatal period, careful monitoring of infants born to mothers with diabetes is warranted.

Nursing Mothers—It is unknown whether Humalog is excreted in significant amounts in human milk. Many drugs, including human insulin, are excreted in human milk. For this reason, caution should be exercised when Humalog is administered to a nursing woman. Patients with diabetes who are lactating may require adjustments in Humalog dose, meal plan, or both.

Pediatric Use—In a 9-month, cross-over study of prepubescent children (n=60), aged 3 to 11 years, comparable glycemic control as measured by HbA_{1c} was achieved regardless of treatment group: human regular insulin 30 minutes before meals 8.4%, Humalog immediately before meals 8.4%, and Humalog immediately after meals 8.5%. In an 8-month, cross-over study of adolescents (n=463), aged 9 to 19 years, comparable glycemic control as measured by HbA_{1c} was achieved regardless of treatment group; human regular insulin 30 to 45 minutes before meals 8.7% and Humalog immediately before meals 8.7%. The incidence of hypoglycemia was similar for all three treatment regimens. Adjustment of basal insulin may be required. To improve accuracy in dosing in pediatric patients, a diluent may be used. If the diluent is added directly to the Humalog vial, the shelf-life may be reduced (*see* DOSAGE AND ADMINISTRATION).

Continued on next page

*** Identi-Code® symbol. This product information was prepared in June 2004. Current information on these and other products of Eli Lilly and Company may be obtained by direct inquiry to Lilly Research Laboratories, Lilly Corporate Center, Indianapolis, Indiana 46285, (800) 545-5979.**

Humalog—Cont.

Geriatric Use—Of the total number of subjects (n=2,834) in eight clinical studies of Humalog, twelve percent (n=338) were 65 years of age or over. The majority of these were type 2 patients. HbA_{1c} values and hypoglycemia rates did not differ by age. Pharmacokinetic/pharmacodynamic studies to assess the effect of age on the onset of Humalog action have not been performed.

ADVERSE REACTIONS

Clinical studies comparing Humalog with human regular insulin did not demonstrate a difference in frequency of adverse events between the two treatments.

Adverse events commonly associated with human insulin therapy include the following:

Body as a Whole— reactions (*see* PRECAUTIONS)

Skin and Appendages—injection site reaction, lipodystrophy, pruritus, rash

Other—hypoglycemia (*see* WARNINGS *and* PRECAUTIONS)

OVERDOSAGE

Hypoglycemia may occur as a result of an excess of insulin relative to food intake, energy expenditure, or both. Mild episodes of hypoglycemia usually can be treated with oral glucose. Adjustments in drug dosage, meal patterns, or exercise, may be needed. More severe episodes with coma, seizure, or neurologic impairment may be treated with intramuscular/subcutaneous glucagon or concentrated intravenous glucose. Sustained carbohydrate intake and observation may be necessary because hypoglycemia may recur after apparent clinical recovery.

DOSAGE AND ADMINISTRATION

Humalog is intended for subcutaneous administration. Dosage regimens of Humalog will vary among patients and should be determined by the health care professional familiar with the patient's metabolic needs, eating habits, and other lifestyle variables. Pharmacokinetic and pharmacodynamic studies showed Humalog to be equipotent to human regular insulin (i.e., one unit of Humalog has the same glucose-lowering capability as one unit of human regular insulin), but with more rapid activity. The quicker glucose-lowering effect of Humalog is related to the more rapid absorption rate from subcutaneous tissue. An adjustment of dose or schedule of basal insulin may be needed when a patient changes from other insulins to Humalog, particularly to prevent pre-meal hyperglycemia.

When used as a meal-time insulin, Humalog should be given within 15 minutes before or immediately after a meal. Human regular insulin is best given 30–60 minutes before a meal. To achieve optimal glucose control, the amount of longer-acting insulin being given may need to be adjusted when using Humalog.

The rate of insulin absorption and consequently the onset of activity is known to be affected by the site of injection, exercise, and other variables. Humalog was absorbed at a consistently faster rate than human regular insulin in healthy male volunteers given 0.2 U/kg human regular insulin or Humalog at abdominal, deltoid, or femoral sites, the three sites often used by patients with diabetes. When not mixed in the same syringe with other insulins, Humalog maintains its rapid onset of action and has less variability in its onset of action among injection sites compared with human regular insulin (*see* PRECAUTIONS). After abdominal administration, Humalog concentrations are higher than those following deltoid or thigh injections. Also, the duration of action of Humalog is slightly shorter following abdominal injection, compared with deltoid and femoral injections. As with all insulin preparations, the time course of action of Humalog may vary considerably in different individuals or within the same individual. Patients must be educated to use proper injection techniques.

Humalog may be diluted with STERILE DILUENT for Humalog®, Humulin® N, Humulin® 50/50, Humulin® 70/30, and NPH Iletin® to a concentration of 1:10 (equivalent to U-10) or 1:2 (equivalent to U-50). Diluted Humalog may remain in patient use for 28 days when stored at 5°C (41°F) and for 14 days when stored at 30°C (86°F).

Parenteral drug products should be inspected visually prior to administration whenever the solution and the container permit. If the solution is cloudy, contains particulate matter, is thickened, or is discolored, the contents must not be injected. Humalog should not be used after its expiration date.

HOW SUPPLIED

Humalog (insulin lispro injection, rDNA origin) vials are available in the following package size:

100 units per mL (U-100)

10 mL vials NDC 0002-7510-01 (VL-7510)

Humalog (insulin lispro injection, rDNA origin) cartridges are available in the following package sizes:

5 × 1.5 mL cartridges* NDC 0002-7515-59 (VL-7515)

5 × 3 mL cartridges** NDC 0002-7516-59 (VL-7516)

Humalog (insulin lispro injection, rDNA origin) Pen, disposable insulin delivery device, is available in the following package size:

5 × 3 mL disposable insulin delivery devices NDC 0002-8725-59 (HP-8725)

* 1.5 mL cartridges are for use in Becton Dickinson and Company's B-D®† Pen and Novo Nordisk A/S's NovoPen®‡ NovolinPen®‡, and NovoPen®‡ 1.5 insulin delivery devices.

** 3 mL cartridge is for use in Owen Mumford, Ltd.'s Autopen®§ 3 mL insulin delivery device.

† B-D® is a registered trademark of Becton Dickinson and Company.

‡ NovolinPen® and NovoPen® are registered trademarks of Novo Nordisk A/S.

§ Autopen® is a registered trademark of Owen Mumford, Ltd.

Storage—Humalog should be stored in a refrigerator (2° to 8°C [36° to 46°F]), but not in the freezer. If refrigeration is impossible, the vial or cartridge of Humalog in use can be unrefrigerated for up to 28 days, as long as it is kept as cool as possible (not greater than 30°C [86°F]) and away from direct heat and light. Unrefrigerated vials and cartridges must be used within this time period or be discarded. Do not use Humalog if it has been frozen.

Literature revised May 31, 2002

Manufactured by Lilly France S.A.S.
F-67640 Fegersheim, France
for Eli Lilly and Company
Indianapolis, IN 46285, USA

PA 9164 FSAMP

Shown in Product Identification Guide, page 320

HUMALOG® MIX75/25™ ℞

[*hū-mă-lŏg*]

75% INSULIN LISPRO PROTAMINE SUSPENSION AND 25% INSULIN LISPRO INJECTION (rDNA ORIGIN)

DESCRIPTION

Humalog® Mix75/25™ [75% insulin lispro protamine suspension and 25% insulin lispro injection, (rDNA origin)] is a mixture of insulin lispro solution, a rapid-acting blood glucose-lowering agent and insulin lispro protamine suspension, an intermediate-acting blood glucose-lowering agent. Chemically, insulin lispro is Lys(B28), Pro(B29) human insulin analog, created when the amino acids at positions 28 and 29 on the insulin B-chain are reversed. Insulin lispro is synthesized in a special non-pathogenic laboratory strain of *Escherichia coli* bacteria that has been genetically altered by the addition of the gene for insulin lispro. Insulin lispro protamine suspension (NPL component) is a suspension of crystals produced from combining insulin lispro and protamine sulfate under appropriate conditions for crystal formation.

Insulin lispro has the following primary structure:

Figure 1

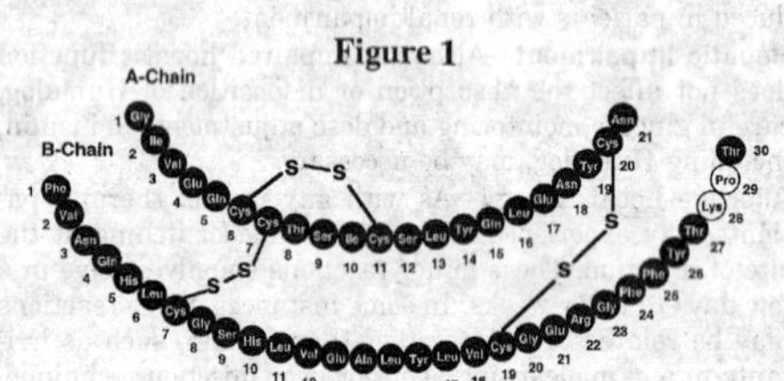

Insulin lispro has the empirical formula $C_{257}H_{383}N_{65}O_{77}S_6$ and a molecular weight of 5808, both identical to that of human insulin.

Humalog Mix75/25 disposable insulin delivery devices contain a sterile suspension of insulin lispro protamine suspension mixed with soluble insulin lispro for use as an injection.

Each milliliter of Humalog Mix75/25 injection contains insulin lispro 100 Units, 0.28 mg protamine sulfate, 16 mg glycerin, 3.78 mg dibasic sodium phosphate, 1.76 mg *m*-cresol, zinc oxide content adjusted to provide 0.025 mg zinc ion, 0.715 mg phenol, and water for injection. Humalog Mix75/25 has a pH of 7.0-7.8. Hydrochloric acid 10% and/or sodium hydroxide 10% may have been added to adjust pH.

CLINICAL PHARMACOLOGY

Antidiabetic Activity—The primary activity of insulin, including Humalog Mix75/25, is the regulation of glucose metabolism. In addition, all insulins have several anabolic and anti-catabolic actions on many tissues in the body. In muscle and other tissues (except the brain), insulin causes rapid transport of glucose and amino acids intracellularly, promotes anabolism, and inhibits protein catabolism. In the liver, insulin promotes the uptake and storage of glucose in the form of glycogen, inhibits gluconeogenesis, and promotes the conversion of excess glucose into fat.

Insulin lispro, the rapid-acting component of Humalog Mix75/25, has been shown to be equipotent to regular human insulin on a molar basis. One unit of Humalog® has the same glucose-lowering effect as one unit of regular human insulin, but its effect is more rapid and of shorter duration. Humalog Mix75/25 has a similar glucose-lowering effect as compared to Humulin® 70/30 on a unit for unit basis.

Pharmacokinetics—

Absorption—Studies in nondiabetic subjects and patients with type 1 (insulin-dependent) diabetes demonstrated that Humalog, the rapid-acting component of Humalog Mix75/25, is absorbed faster than regular human insulin (U-100). In nondiabetic subjects given subcutaneous doses of Humalog ranging from 0.1-0.4 U/kg, peak serum concentrations were observed 30-90 minutes after dosing. When nondiabetic subjects received equivalent doses of regular human insulin, peak insulin concentrations occurred 50-120 minutes after dosing. Similar results were found in patients with type 1 diabetes.

Figure 2
Serum immunoreactive insulin (IRI) concentrations, after subcutaneous injection of Humalog Mix75/25 or Humulin 70/30 in healthy nondiabetic subjects.

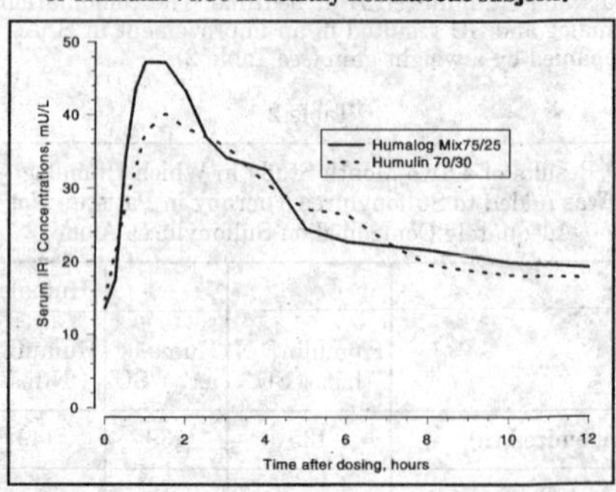

Humalog Mix75/25 has two phases of absorption. The early phase represents insulin lispro and its distinct characteristics of rapid onset. The late phase represents the prolonged action of insulin lispro protamine suspension. In 30 nondiabetic subjects given subcutaneous doses (0.3 U/kg) of Humalog Mix75/25, peak serum concentrations were observed 30 to 240 minutes (median, 60 minutes) after dosing (Figure 2). Identical results were found in patients with type 1 diabetes. The rapid absorption characteristics of Humalog are maintained with Humalog Mix75/25 (Figure 2).

Figure 2 represents serum insulin concentration versus time curves of Humalog Mix75/25 and Humulin 70/30. Humalog Mix75/25 has a more rapid absorption than Humulin 70/30, which has been confirmed in patients with type 1 diabetes.

Distribution—radiolabeled distribution studies of Humalog Mix75/25 have not been conducted. However, the volume of distribution following injection of Humalog is identical to that of regular human insulin, with a range of 0.26–0.36 L/kg.

Metabolism—Human metabolism studies of Humalog Mix75/25 have not been conducted. Studies in animals indicate that the metabolism of Humalog, the rapid-acting component of Humalog Mix75/25, is identical to that of regular human insulin.

Elimination—Humalog Mix75/25 has two absorption phases, a rapid and a prolonged phase, representative of the insulin lispro and insulin lispro protamine suspension components of the mixture. As with other intermediate-acting insulins, a meaningful terminal phase half-life cannot be calculated after administration of Humalog Mix75/25 because of the prolonged insulin lispro protamine suspension absorption.

Pharmacodynamics—Studies in nondiabetic subjects and patients with diabetes demonstrated that Humalog has a more rapid onset of glucose-lowering activity, an earlier peak for glucose lowering, and a shorter duration of glucose-lowering activity than regular human insulin. The early onset of activity of Humalog Mix75/25 is directly related to the rapid absorption of Humalog. The time course of action of insulin and insulin analogs such as Humalog (and hence Humalog Mix75/25) may vary considerably in different individuals or within the same individual. The parameters of Humalog Mix75/25 activity (time of onset, peak time, and duration) as presented in Figures 2, 3, and 4 should be considered only as general guidelines. The rate of insulin absorption and consequently the onset of activity is known to be affected by the site of injection, exercise, and other variables (*see* General *under* PRECAUTIONS).

In a glucose clamp study performed in 30 nondiabetic subjects, the onset of action and glucose-lowering activity of Humalog, Humalog Mix75/25, Humalog® Mix50/50™ and insulin lispro protamine suspension were compared (Figure 3). Graphs of mean glucose infusion rate versus time showed a distinct insulin activity profile for each formulation. The rapid onset of glucose-lowering activity characteristic of Humalog was maintained in Humalog Mix75/25.

In separate glucose clamp studies performed in nondiabetic subjects, glucodynamics of Humalog Mix75/25 and Humulin 70/30 were assessed and are presented in Figure 4. Humalog Mix75/25 has a duration of activity similar to that of Humulin 70/30.

[See figure 3 at top of next column]

[See figure 4 at bottom of next page]

Figures 3 and 4 represent insulin activity profiles as measured by glucose clamp studies in healthy nondiabetic subjects.

Figure 3 shows the time activity profiles of Humalog, Humalog Mix75/25, Humalog Mix50/50, and insulin lispro protamine suspension (NPL component).

Figure 4 is a comparison of the time activity profiles of Humalog Mix75/25 (Figure 4a) and of Humulin 70/30 (Figure 4b) from two different studies.

Special Populations—

Age and Gender—Information on the effect of age on the pharmacokinetics of Humalog Mix75/25 is unavailable.

Figure 3
Insulin activity after injection of Humalog, Humalog Mix50/50, Humalog Mix75/25, or insulin lispro protamine suspension (NPL component) in 30 nondiabetic subjects.

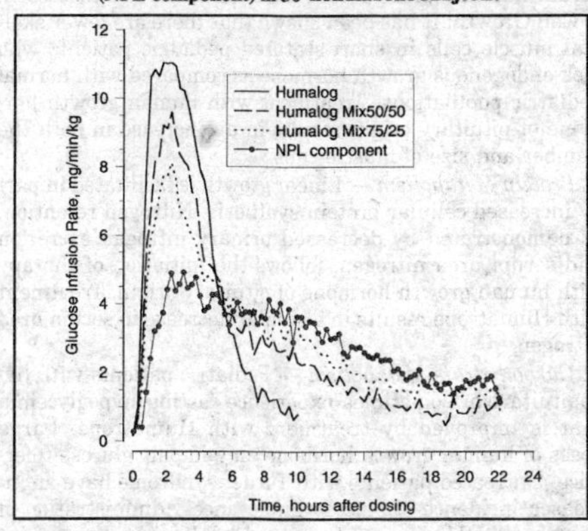

Pharmacokinetic and pharmacodynamic comparisons between men and women administered Humalog Mix75/25 showed no gender differences. In large Humalog clinical trials, subgroup analyses based upon age and gender demonstrated that differences between Humalog and regular human insulin in postprandial glucose parameters are maintained across sub-groups.

Smoking—The effect of smoking on the pharmacokinetics and glucodynamics of Humalog Mix75/25 has not been studied.

Pregnancy—The effect of pregnancy on the pharmacokinetics and glucodynamics of Humalog Mix75/25 has not been studied.

Obesity—The effect of obesity and/or subcutaneous fat thickness on the pharmacokinetics and glucodynamics of Humalog Mix75/25 has not been studied. In large clinical trials, which included patients with Body-Mass-Index up to and including 35 kg/m^2, no consistent differences were observed between Humalog and Humulin R with respect to postprandial glucose parameters.

Renal Impairment—The effect of renal impairment on the pharmacokinetics and glucodynamics of Humalog Mix75/25 has not been studied. In a study of 25 patients with type 2 diabetes and a wide range of renal function, the pharmacokinetic differences between Humalog and human regular insulin were generally maintained. However, the sensitivity of the patients to insulin did change, with an increased response to insulin as the renal function declined. Careful glucose monitoring and dose reductions of insulin, including Humalog Mix75/25, may be necessary in patients with renal dysfunction.

Hepatic Impairment—Some studies with human insulin have shown increased circulating levels of insulin in patients with hepatic failure. The effect of hepatic impairment on the pharmacokinetics and glucodynamics of Humalog Mix75/25 has not been studied. However, in a study of 22 patients with type 2 diabetes, impaired hepatic function did not affect the subcutaneous absorption or general disposition of Humalog when compared to patients with no history of hepatic dysfunction. In that study, Humalog maintained its more rapid absorption and elimination when compared to regular human insulin. Careful glucose monitoring and dose adjustments of insulin, including Humalog Mix75/25, may be necessary in patients with hepatic dysfunction.

INDICATIONS AND USAGE

Humalog Mix75/25, a mixture of 75% insulin lispro protamine suspension and 25% insulin lispro, is indicated in the treatment of patients with diabetes mellitus for the control of hyperglycemia. Humalog Mix75/25 has a more rapid onset of glucose-lowering activity compared to Humulin 70/30 while having a similar duration of action. This profile is achieved by combining the rapid onset of Humalog with the intermediate action of insulin lispro protamine suspension.

CONTRAINDICATIONS

Humalog Mix75/25 is contraindicated during episodes of hypoglycemia and in patients sensitive to insulin lispro or any of the excipients contained in the formulation.

WARNINGS

Humalog differs from regular human insulin by its rapid onset of action as well as a shorter duration of activity. Therefore, the dose of Humalog Mix75/25 should be given within 15 minutes before a meal.

Hypoglycemia is the most common adverse effect associated with the use of insulins, including Humalog Mix75/25. As with all insulins, the timing of hypoglycemia may differ among various insulin formulations. Glucose monitoring is recommended for all patients with diabetes.

Any change of insulin should be made cautiously and only under medical supervision. Changes in insulin strength, manufacturer, type (e.g., regular, NPH, analog), species (animal, human), or method of manufacture (rDNA versus animal-source insulin) may result in the need for a change in dosage.

PRECAUTIONS

General—Hypoglycemia and hypokalemia are among the potential clinical adverse effects associated with the use of all insulins. Because of differences in the action of Humalog Mix75/25 and other insulins, care should be taken in patients in whom such potential side effects might be clinically relevant (e.g., patients who are fasting, have autonomic neuropathy, or are using potassium-lowering drugs or patients taking drugs sensitive to serum potassium level). Lipodystrophy and hypersensitivity are among other potential clinical adverse effects associated with the use of all insulins.

As with all insulin preparations, the time course of action of Humalog Mix75/25 may vary in different individuals or at different times in the same individual and is dependent on site of injection, blood supply, temperature, and physical activity.

Adjustment of dosage of any insulin may be necessary if patients change their physical activity or their usual meal plan. Insulin requirements may be altered during illness, emotional disturbances, or other stress.

Hypoglycemia—As with all insulin preparations, hypoglycemic reactions may be associated with the administration of Humalog Mix75/25. Rapid changes in serum glucose concentrations may induce symptoms of hypoglycemia in persons with diabetes, regardless of the glucose value. Early warning symptoms of hypoglycemia may be different or less pronounced under certain conditions, such as long duration of diabetes, diabetic nerve disease, use of medications such as beta-blockers, or intensified diabetes control.

Renal Impairment—As with other insulins, the requirements for Humalog Mix75/25 may be reduced in patients with renal impairment.

Hepatic Impairment—Although impaired hepatic function does not affect the absorption or disposition of Humalog, careful glucose monitoring and dose adjustments of insulin, including Humalog Mix75/25, may be necessary.

Allergy—Local Allergy—As with any insulin therapy, patients may experience redness, swelling, or itching at the site of injection. These minor reactions usually resolve in a few days to a few weeks. In some instances, these reactions may be related to factors other than insulin, such as irritants in the skin cleansing agent or poor injection technique.

Systemic Allergy—Less common, but potentially more serious, is generalized allergy to insulin, which may cause rash (including pruritus) over the whole body, shortness of breath, wheezing, reduction in blood pressure, rapid pulse, or sweating. Severe cases of generalized allergy, including anaphylactic reaction, may be life threatening. Localized reactions and generalized myalgias have been reported with the use of cresol as an injectable excipient.

Antibody Production—In clinical trials, antibodies that cross react with human insulin and insulin lispro were observed in both human insulin mixtures and insulin lispro mixtures treatment groups.

Information for Patients—Patients should be informed of the potential risks and advantages of Humalog Mix75/25 and alternative therapies. Patients should not mix Humalog Mix75/25 with any other insulin. They should also be informed about the importance of proper insulin storage, injection technique, timing of dosage, adherence to meal planning, regular physical activity, regular blood glucose monitoring, periodic glycosylated hemoglobin testing, recognition and management of hypo- and hyperglycemia, and periodic assessment for diabetes complications.

Patients should be advised to inform their physician if they are pregnant or intend to become pregnant.

Refer patients to the Information for the Patient insert for information on normal appearance, proper resuspension and injection techniques, timing of dosing (within 15 minutes before a meal), storing, and common adverse effects.

Use of the Humalog Pen: Patients should read the "Information for the Patient" insert and the "Disposable Insulin Delivery Device User Manual" before starting therapy with a Humalog Pen and re-read them each time the prescription is renewed. Patients should be instructed on how to properly use the delivery device (refer to "Disposable Insulin Delivery Device User Manual"), prime the pen, and properly dispose of needles. Patients should be advised not to share their pens with others.

Laboratory Tests—As with all insulins, the therapeutic response to Humalog Mix75/25 should be monitored by periodic blood glucose tests. Periodic measurement of glycosylated hemoglobin is recommended for the monitoring of long-term glycemic control.

Drug Interactions—Insulin requirements may be increased by medications with hyperglycemic activity such as corticosteroids, isoniazid, certain lipid-lowering drugs (e.g., niacin), estrogens, oral contraceptives, phenothiazines, and thyroid replacement therapy.

Insulin requirements may be decreased in the presence of drugs with hypoglycemic activity, such as oral antidiabetic agents, salicylates, sulfa antibiotics, certain antidepressants (monoamine oxidase inhibitors), certain angiotensin-converting-enzyme inhibitors, beta-adrenergic blockers, inhibitors of pancreatic function (e.g., octreotide), and alcohol. Beta-adrenergic blockers may mask the symptoms of hypoglycemia in some patients.

Carcinogenesis, Mutagenesis, Impairment of Fertility—Long-term studies in animals have not been performed to evaluate the carcinogenic potential of Humalog or Humalog Mix75/25. Insulin lispro was not mutagenic in a battery of *in vitro* and *in vivo* genetic toxicity assays (bacterial mutation tests, unscheduled DNA synthesis, mouse lymphoma assay, chromosomal aberration tests, and a micronucleus test). There is no evidence from animal studies of impairment of fertility induced by insulin lispro.

Pregnancy—Teratogenic Effects—Pregnancy Category B—Reproduction studies with insulin lispro have been performed in pregnant rats and rabbits at parenteral doses up to 4 and 0.3 times, respectively, the average human dose (40 units/day) based on body surface area. The results have revealed no evidence of impaired fertility or harm to the fetus due to insulin lispro. There are, however, no adequate and well-controlled studies with Humalog or Humalog Mix75/25 in pregnant women. Because animal reproduction studies are not always predictive of human response, this drug should be used during pregnancy only if clearly needed.

Nursing Mothers—It is unknown whether insulin lispro is excreted in significant amounts in human milk. Many drugs, including human insulin, are excreted in human milk. For this reason, caution should be exercised when Humalog Mix75/25 is administered to a nursing woman. Patients with diabetes who are lactating may require adjustments in Humalog Mix75/25 dose, meal plan, or both.

Pediatric Use—Safety and effectiveness of Humalog Mix75/25 in patients less than 18 years of age have not been established.

Geriatric Use—Clinical studies of Humalog Mix75/25 did not include sufficient numbers of patients aged 65 and over to determine whether they respond differently than younger patients. In general, dose selection for an elderly patient should take into consideration the greater frequency of decreased hepatic, renal, or cardiac function, and of concomitant disease or other drug therapy in this population.

ADVERSE REACTIONS

Clinical studies comparing Humalog Mix75/25 with human insulin mixtures did not demonstrate a difference in frequency of adverse events between the two treatments.

Adverse events commonly associated with human insulin therapy include the following:

Body as a Whole—allergic reactions (*see* PRECAUTIONS)

Skin and Appendages—injection site reaction, lipodystrophy, pruritus, rash

Other—hypoglycemia (*see* WARNINGS *and* PRECAUTIONS)

OVERDOSAGE

Hypoglycemia may occur as a result of an excess of insulin relative to food intake, energy expenditure, or both. Mild episodes of hypoglycemia usually can be treated with oral

Continued on next page

Figure 4
Insulin activity after injection of Humalog Mix75/25 and Humulin 70/30 in nondiabetic subjects.

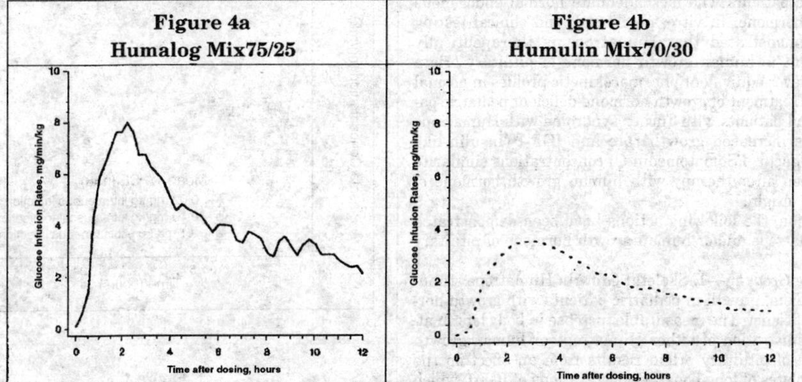

*** Identi-Code® symbol. This product information was prepared in June 2004. Current information on these and other products of Eli Lilly and Company may be obtained by direct inquiry to Lilly Research Laboratories, Lilly Corporate Center, Indianapolis, Indiana 46285, (800) 545-5979.**

Table 1*
Summary of glucodynamic properties of insulin products (pooled cross-study comparison)

Insulin Products	Dose, U/kg	Time of peak activity, hours after dosing	Percent of total activity occurring in the first 4 hours
Humalog	0.3	2.4 (0.8–4.3)	70% (49–89%)
Humulin R	0.32 (0.26–0.37)	4.4 (4.0–5.5)	54% (38–65%)
Humalog Mix75/25	0.3	2.6 (1.0–6.5)	35% (21–56%)
Humulin 70/30	0.3	4.4 (1.5–16)	32% (14–60%)
Humalog Mix50/50	0.3	2.3 (0.8–4.8)	45% (27–69%)
Humulin 50/50	0.3	3.3 (2.0–5.5)	44% (21–60%)
NPH	0.32 (0.27–0.40)	5.5 (3.5–9.5)	14% (3.0–48%)
NPL component	0.3	5.8 (1.3–18.3)	22% (6.3–40%)

*The information supplied in Table 1 indicates when peak insulin activity can be expected and the percent of the total insulin activity occurring during the first 4 hours. The information was derived from 3 separate glucose clamp studies in nondiabetic subjects. Values represent means, with ranges provided in parentheses.

Humalog Mix 75/25—Cont.

glucose. Adjustments in drug dosage, meal patterns, or exercise, may be needed. More severe episodes with coma, seizure, or neurologic impairment may be treated with intramuscular/subcutaneous glucagon or concentrated intravenous glucose. Sustained carbohydrate intake and observation may be necessary because hypoglycemia may recur after apparent clinical recovery.

DOSAGE AND ADMINISTRATION

[See table 1 above]

Humalog Mix75/25 is intended only for subcutaneous administration. Humalog Mix75/25 should not be administered intravenously. Dosage regimens of Humalog Mix75/25 will vary among patients and should be determined by the health care professional familiar with the patient's metabolic needs, eating habits, and other lifestyle variables. Humalog has been shown to be equipotent to regular human insulin on a molar basis. One unit of Humalog has the same glucose-lowering effect as one unit of regular human insulin, but its effect is more rapid and of shorter duration. Humalog Mix75/25 has a similar glucose-lowering effect as compared to Humulin 70/30 on a unit for unit basis. The quicker glucose-lowering effect of Humalog is related to the more rapid absorption rate of insulin lispro from subcutaneous tissue.

Humalog Mix75/25 starts lowering blood glucose more quickly than regular human insulin, allowing for convenient dosing immediately before a meal (within 15 minutes). In contrast, mixtures containing regular human insulin should be given 30-60 minutes before a meal.

The rate of insulin absorption and consequently the onset of activity are known to be affected by the site of injection, exercise, and other variables. As with all insulin preparations, the time course of action of Humalog Mix75/25 may vary considerably in different individuals or within the same individual. Patients must be educated to use proper injection techniques.

Humalog Mix75/25 should be inspected visually before use. Humalog Mix75/25 should be used only if it appears uniformly cloudy after mixing. Humalog Mix75/25 should not be used after its expiration date.

HOW SUPPLIED

Humalog Mix75/25 vials are available in the following package size:

100 units per mL (U-100)
10 mL vials
NDC 0002-7511-01 (VL-7511)

Humalog Mix75/25 Pen, a disposable insulin delivery device, is available in the following package size:

5 × 3 mL disposable insulin delivery devices
NDC 0002-8794-59 (HP-8794)

Storage—Humalog Mix75/25 should be stored in a refrigerator (2° to 8°C [36° to 46°F]) before use, but not in the freezer. However, vials of Humalog Mix75/25 in use can be kept unrefrigerated at room temperature for up to 28 days, as long as they are kept as cool as possible and away from direct heat and light. Humalog Mix 75/25 Pens in use can be kept unrefrigerated at room temperature for up to 10 days, as long as they are kept as cool as possible and away from direct heat and light. Unrefrigerated vials and Pens must be used within the specified time period or be discarded. Do not use Humalog Mix 75/25 if it has been frozen.

Literature revised May 31, 2002
Manufactured by Lilly France S.A.S.
F-67640 Fegersheim, France
for Eli Lilly and Company
Indianapolis, IN 46285, USA

PA 9223 FSAMP

Shown in Product Identification Guide, page 320

HUMATROPE® ℞

[hew-mă-trōp]

SOMATROPIN (rDNA ORIGIN) FOR INJECTION VIALS and CARTRIDGES FOR USE WITH THE HumatroPen™ INJECTION DEVICE

DESCRIPTION

Humatrope® (Somatropin, rDNA Origin, for Injection) is a polypeptide hormone of recombinant DNA origin. Humatrope has 191 amino acid residues and a molecular weight of about 22,125 daltons. The amino acid sequence of the product is identical to that of human growth hormone of pituitary origin. Humatrope is synthesized in a strain of *Escherichia coli* that has been modified by the addition of the gene for human growth hormone.

Humatrope is a sterile, white, lyophilized powder intended for subcutaneous or intramuscular administration after reconstitution. Humatrope is a highly purified preparation. Phosphoric acid and/or sodium hydroxide may have been added to adjust the pH. Reconstituted solutions have a pH of approximately 7.5. This product is oxygen sensitive.

VIAL — Each vial of Humatrope contains 5 mg somatropin (15 IU or 225 nanomoles); 25 mg mannitol; 5 mg glycine; and 1.13 mg dibasic sodium phosphate. Each vial is supplied in a combination package with an accompanying 5-mL vial of diluting solution. The diluent contains Water for Injection with 0.3% Metacresol as a preservative and 1.7% glycerin.

CARTRIDGE — The cartridges of somatropin contain either 6 mg (18 IU), 12 mg (36 IU), or 24 mg (72 IU) of somatropin. The 6, 12, and 24 mg cartridges contain respectively: mannitol 18, 36, and 72 mg; glycine 6, 12, and 24 mg; dibasic sodium phosphate 1.36, 2.72, and 5.43 mg. Each cartridge is supplied in a combination package with an accompanying syringe containing approximately 3 mL of diluting solution. The diluent contains Water for Injection; 0.3% Metacresol as a preservative; and 1.7%, 0.29%, and 0.29% glycerin in the 6, 12, and 24 mg cartridges, respectively.

CLINICAL PHARMACOLOGY

General

Linear Growth — Humatrope stimulates linear growth in pediatric patients who lack adequate normal endogenous growth hormone. In vitro, preclinical, and clinical testing have demonstrated that Humatrope is therapeutically equivalent to human growth hormone of pituitary origin and achieves equivalent pharmacokinetic profiles in normal adults. Treatment of growth hormone-deficient pediatric patients and patients with Turner syndrome with Humatrope produces increased growth rate and IGF-I (Insulin-like Growth Factor-I/Somatomedin-C) concentrations similar to those seen after therapy with human growth hormone of pituitary origin.

In addition, the following actions have been demonstrated for Humatrope and/or human growth hormone of pituitary origin.

A. *Tissue Growth* — 1. Skeletal Growth: Humatrope stimulates skeletal growth in pediatric patients with growth hormone deficiency. The measurable increase in body length after administration of either Humatrope or human growth hormone of pituitary origin results from an effect on the growth plates of long bones. Concentrations of IGF-I, which may play a role in skeletal growth, are low in the serum of growth hormone-deficient pediatric patients but increase during treatment with Humatrope. Elevations in mean serum alkaline phosphatase concentrations are also seen. 2. Cell Growth: It has been shown that there are fewer skeletal muscle cells in short-statured pediatric patients who lack endogenous growth hormone as compared with normal pediatric populations. Treatment with human growth hormone of pituitary origin results in an increase in both the number and size of muscle cells.

B. *Protein Metabolism* — Linear growth is facilitated in part by increased cellular protein synthesis. Nitrogen retention, as demonstrated by decreased urinary nitrogen excretion and serum urea nitrogen, follows the initiation of therapy with human growth hormone of pituitary origin. Treatment with Humatrope results in a similar decrease in serum urea nitrogen.

C. *Carbohydrate Metabolism* — Pediatric patients with hypopituitarism sometimes experience fasting hypoglycemia that is improved by treatment with Humatrope. Large doses of human growth hormone may impair glucose tolerance. Untreated patients with Turner syndrome have an increased incidence of glucose intolerance. Administration of human growth hormone to normal adults or patients with Turner syndrome resulted in increases in mean serum fasting and postprandial insulin levels although mean values remained in the normal range. In addition, mean fasting and postprandial glucose and hemoglobin A_{1c} levels remained in the normal range.

D. *Lipid Metabolism* — In growth hormone-deficient patients, administration of human growth hormone of pituitary origin has resulted in lipid mobilization, reduction in body fat stores, and increased plasma fatty acids.

E. *Mineral Metabolism* — Retention of sodium, potassium, and phosphorus is induced by human growth hormone of pituitary origin. Serum concentrations of inorganic phosphate increased in patients with growth hormone deficiency after therapy with Humatrope or human growth hormone of pituitary origin. Serum calcium is not significantly altered in patients treated with either human growth hormone of pituitary origin or Humatrope.

Pharmacokinetics

Absorption — Humatrope has been studied following intramuscular, subcutaneous, and intravenous administration in adult volunteers. The absolute bioavailability of somatropin is 75% and 63% after subcutaneous and intramuscular administration, respectively.

Distribution — The volume of distribution of somatropin after intravenous injection is about 0.07 L/kg.

Metabolism — Extensive metabolism studies have not been conducted. The metabolic fate of somatropin involves classical protein catabolism in both the liver and kidneys. In renal cells, at least a portion of the breakdown products of growth hormone is returned to the systemic circulation. In normal volunteers, mean clearance is 0.14 L/hr/kg. The mean half-life of intravenous somatropin is 0.36 hours, whereas subcutaneously and intramuscularly administered somatropin have mean half-lives of 3.8 and 4.9 hours, respectively. The longer half-life observed after subcutaneous or intramuscular administration is due to slow absorption from the injection site.

Excretion — Urinary excretion of intact Humatrope has not been measured. Small amounts of somatropin have been detected in the urine of pediatric patients following replacement therapy.

Special Populations

Geriatric — The pharmacokinetics of Humatrope has not been studied in patients greater than 65 years of age.

Pediatric — The pharmacokinetics of Humatrope in pediatric patients is similar to adults.

Gender — No studies have been performed with Humatrope. The available literature indicates that the pharmacokinetics of growth hormone is similar in both men and women.

Race — No data are available.

Renal, Hepatic insufficiency — No studies have been performed with Humatrope.

[See table 1 at top of next page]

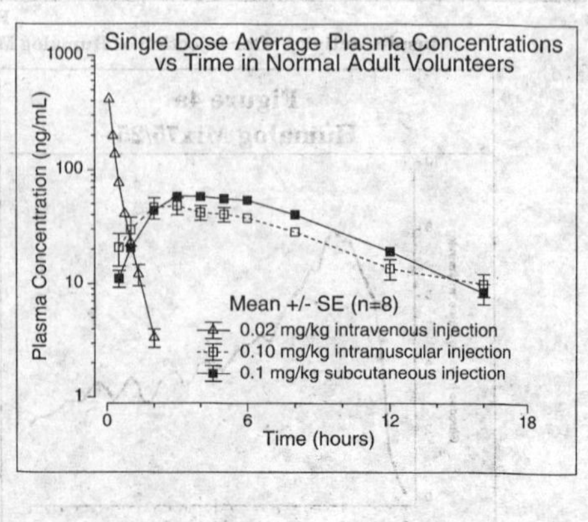

Figure 1

CLINICAL TRIALS

Effects of Humatrope Treatment in Adults with Growth Hormone Deficiency

Two multicenter trials in adult-onset growth hormone deficiency (n=98) and two studies in childhood-onset growth hormone deficiency (n=67) were designed to assess the effects of replacement therapy with Humatrope. The primary efficacy measures were body composition (lean body mass and fat mass), lipid parameters, and the Nottingham Health Profile. The Nottingham Health Profile is a general health-related quality of life questionnaire. These four studies each included a 6-month randomized, blinded, placebo-controlled phase followed by 12 months of open-label therapy for all patients. The Humatrope dosages for all studies were identical: 1 month of therapy at 0.00625 mg/kg/day followed by the proposed maintenance dose of 0.0125 mg/kg/day. Adult-onset patients and childhood-onset patients differed by diagnosis (organic vs. idiopathic pituitary disease), body size (normal vs. small for mean height and weight), and age (mean=44 vs. 29 years). Lean body mass was determined by bioelectrical impedance analysis (BIA), validated with potassium 40. Body fat was assessed by BIA and sum of skinfold thickness. Lipid subfractions were analyzed by standard assay methods in a central laboratory.

Humatrope-treated adult-onset patients, as compared to placebo, experienced an increase in lean body mass (2.59 vs. -0.22 kg, $p<0.001$) and a decrease in body fat (-3.27 vs. 0.56 kg, $p<0.001$). Similar changes were seen in childhood-onset growth hormone-deficient patients. These significant changes in lean body mass persisted throughout the 18-month period as compared to baseline for both groups, and for fat mass in the childhood-onset group. Total cholesterol decreased short-term (first 3 months) although the changes did not persist. However, the low HDL cholesterol levels observed at baseline (mean=30.1 mg/mL and 33.9 mg/mL in adult-onset and childhood-onset patients) normalized by the end of 18 months of therapy (a change of 13.7 and 11.1 mg/dL for the adult-onset and childhood-onset groups, $p<0.001$). Adult-onset patients reported significant improvements as compared to placebo in the following two of six possible health-related domains: physical mobility and social isolation (Table 2). Patients with childhood-onset disease failed to demonstrate improvements in Nottingham Health Profile outcomes.

Two additional studies on the effect of Humatrope on exercise capacity were also conducted. Improved physical function was documented by increased exercise capacity (VO_2 max, $p<0.005$) and work performance (Watts, $p<0.01$) (J Clin Endocrinol Metab 1995; 80:552-557).

Table 2
Changes[a] in Nottingham Health Profile Scores[b] in Adult-Onset Growth Hormone-Deficient Patients

Outcome Measure	Placebo (6 Months)	Humatrope Therapy (6 Months)	Significance
Energy level	-11.4	-15.5	NS
Physical mobility	-3.1	-10.5	p<0.01
Social isolation	0.5	-4.7	p<0.01
Emotional reactions	-4.5	-5.4	NS
Sleep	-6.4	-3.7	NS
Pain	-2.8	-2.9	NS

[a] An improvement in score is indicated by a more negative change in the score.
[b] To account for multiple analyses, appropriate statistical methods were applied and the required level of significance is 0.01.
NS = not significant.

Effects of Growth Hormone Treatment in Patients with Turner Syndrome

One long-term, randomized, open-label multicenter concurrently controlled study, two long-term, open-label multicenter, historically controlled studies and one long-term, randomized, dose-response study were conducted to evaluate the efficacy of growth hormone for the treatment of patients with short stature due to Turner syndrome.

In the randomized study, GDCT, comparing growth hormone-treated patients to a concurrent control group who received no growth hormone, the growth hormone-treated patients who received a dose of 0.3 mg/kg/wk given 6 times per week from a mean age of 11.7 years for a mean duration of 4.7 years attained a mean near final height of 146.0 ± 6.2 cm (n=27, mean ± SD) as compared to the control group who attained a near final height of 142.1 ± 4.8 cm (n=19). By analysis of covariance*, the effect of growth hormone therapy was a mean height increase of 5.4 cm (p=0.001).

*Analysis of covariance includes adjustments for baseline height relative to age and for mid-parental height.

Table 1
Summary of Somatropin Parameters in the Normal Population

	C_{max} (ng/mL)	$t_{½}$ (hr)	$AUC_{0-\infty}$ (ng•hr/mL)	Cls (L/kg•hr)	Vβ (L/kg)
0.02 mg (0.05 IU*)/kg iv					
MEAN	415	0.363	156	0.135	0.0703
SD	75	0.053	33	0.029	0.0173
0.1 mg (0.27 IU*)/kg im					
MEAN	53.2	4.93	495	0.215	1.55
SD	25.9	2.66	106	0.047	0.91
0.1 mg (0.27 IU*)/kg sc					
MEAN	63.3	3.81	585	0.179	0.957
SD	18.2	1.40	90	0.028	0.301

Abbreviations: C_{max}=maximum concentration; $t_{½}$=half-life; $AUC_{0-\infty}$=area under the curve; Cls=systemic clearance; Vβ=volume distribution; iv=intravenous; SD=standard deviation; im=intramuscular; sc=subcutaneous.
*Based on previous International Standard of 2.7 IU=1 mg.

Table 3
Summary Table of Efficacy Results

Study/ Group	Study Design[a]	N at Adult Height	GH Age (yr)	Estrogen Age (yr)	GH Duration (yr)	Adult Height Gain (cm)[b]
GDCT	RCT	27	11.7	13	4.7	5.4
85-023	MHT	17	9.1	15.2	7.6	7.4
85-044: A*	MHT	29	9.4	15	6.1	8.3
B*		26	9.6	12.3	5.6	5.9
C*		51	12.7	13.7	3.8	5
GDCI	RDT	31	11.1	8-13.5	5.3	~5[c]

[a] RCT: randomized controlled trial; MHT: matched historical controlled trial; RDT: randomized dose-response trial.
[b] Analysis of covariance vs. controls.
[c] Compared with historical data.
*A: GH age <11 yr, estrogen age 15 yr.
B: GH age <11 yr, estrogen age 12 yr.
C: GH age >11 yr, estrogen at month 12.

In two of the studies (85-023 and 85-044), the effect of long-term growth hormone treatment (0.375 mg/kg/wk given either 3 times per week or daily) on adult height was determined by comparing adult heights in the treated patients with those of age-matched historical controls with Turner syndrome who never received any growth-promoting therapy. The greatest improvement in adult height was observed in patients who received early growth hormone treatment and estrogen after age 14 years. In Study 85-023, this resulted in a mean adult height gain of 7.4 cm (mean duration of GH therapy of 7.6 years) vs. matched historical controls by analysis of covariance.

In Study 85-044, patients treated with early growth hormone therapy were randomized to receive estrogen replacement therapy (conjugated estrogens, 0.3 mg escalating to 0.625 mg daily) at either age 12 or 15 years. Compared with matched historical controls, early GH therapy (mean duration of GH therapy 5.6 years) combined with estrogen replacement at age 12 years resulted in an adult height gain of 5.9 cm (n=26), whereas patients who initiated estrogen at age 15 years (mean duration of GH therapy 6.1 years) had a mean adult height gain of 8.3 cm (n=29). Patients who initiated GH therapy after age 11 (mean age 12.7 years; mean duration of GH therapy 3.8 years) had a mean adult height gain of 5.0 cm (n=51).

In a randomized blinded dose-response study, GDCI, patients were treated from a mean age of 11.1 years for a mean duration of 5.3 years with a weekly dose of either 0.27 mg/kg or 0.36 mg/kg administered 3 or 6 times weekly. The mean near final height of patients receiving growth hormone was 148.7 ± 6.5 cm (n=31). When compared to historical control data, the mean gain in adult height was approximately 5 cm.

In some studies, Turner syndrome patients (n=181) treated to final adult height achieved statistically significant average height gains ranging from 5.0 to 8.3 cm.

[See table 3 above]

Effect of Humatrope Treatment in Pediatric Patients with Idiopathic Short Stature

Two randomized, multicenter trials, 1 placebo-controlled and 1 dose-response, were conducted in pediatric patients with idiopathic short stature, also called non-growth hormone-deficient short stature. The diagnosis of idiopathic short stature was made after excluding other known causes of short stature, as well as growth hormone deficiency. Limited safety and efficacy data are available below the age of 7 years. No specific studies have been conducted in pediatric patients with familial short stature or who were born small for gestational age (SGA).

The placebo-controlled study enrolled 71 pediatric patients (55 males, 16 females) 9 to 15 years old (mean age 12.38 ± 1.51 years), with short stature, 68 of whom received study drug. Patients were predominately Tanner I (45.1%) and Tanner II (46.5%) at baseline.

In this double-blind trial, patients received subcutaneous injections of either Humatrope 0.222 mg/kg/wk or placebo. Study drug was given in divided doses 3 times per week until height velocity decreased to ≤1.5 cm/year ("final height"). Thirty-three subjects (22 Humatrope, 11 placebo) had final height measurements after a mean treatment duration of 4.4 years (range 0.11-9.08 years).

The Humatrope group achieved a mean final height Standard Deviation Score (SDS) of -1.8 (Table 4). Placebo-treated patients had a mean final height SDS of -2.3 (mean treatment difference = 0.51, p=0.017). Height gain across the duration of the study and final height SDS minus baseline predicted height SDS were also significantly greater in Humatrope-treated patients than in placebo-treated patients (Table 4 and 5). In addition, the number of patients who achieved a final height above the 5th percentile of the general population for age and sex was significantly greater in the Humatrope group than the placebo group (41% vs. 0%, $p<0.05$), as was the number of patients who gained at least 1 SDS unit in height across the duration of the study (50% vs. 0%, $p<0.05$).

[See table 4 at top of next page]

The dose-response study included 239 pediatric patients (158 males, 81 females), 5 to 15 years old, (mean age 9.8 ± 2.3 years). Mean baseline characteristics included: a height SDS of -3.21 (±0.70), a predicted adult height SDS of -2.63 (±1.08), and a height velocity SDS of -1.09 (±1.15). All but 3 patients were Tanner I. Patients were randomized to one of three Humatrope treatment groups: 0.24 mg/kg/wk; 0.24 mg/kg/wk for 1 year, followed by 0.37 mg/kg/wk; and 0.37 mg/kg/wk.

The primary hypothesis of this study was that treatment with Humatrope would increase height velocity during the first 2 years of therapy in a dose-dependent manner. Additionally, after completing the initial 2-year dose-response phase of the study, 50 patients were followed to final height. Patients receiving 0.37 mg/kg/wk had a significantly greater increase in mean height velocity after 2 years of treatment than patients receiving 0.24 mg/kg/wk (4.04 vs. 3.27 cm/year, p=0.003). The mean difference between final height and baseline predicted height was 7.2 cm for patients receiving 0.37 mg/kg/wk and 5.4 cm for patients receiving 0.24 mg/kg/wk (Table 5). While no patient had height above the 5th percentile in any dose group at baseline, 82% of the patients receiving 0.37 mg/kg/wk and 47% of the patients receiving 0.24 mg/kg/wk achieved a final height above the 5th percentile of the general population height standards (p=NS).

[See table 5 at top of next page]

INDICATIONS AND USAGE

Pediatric Patients — Humatrope is indicated for the long-term treatment of pediatric patients who have growth failure due to an inadequate secretion of normal endogenous growth hormone.

Humatrope is indicated for the treatment of short stature associated with Turner syndrome in patients whose epiphyses are not closed.

Continued on next page

*** Identi-Code® symbol. This product information was prepared in June 2004. Current information on these and other products of Eli Lilly and Company may be obtained by direct inquiry to Lilly Research Laboratories, Lilly Corporate Center, Indianapolis, Indiana 46285, (800) 545-5979.**

Humatrope—Cont.

Humatrope is indicated for the long-term treatment of idiopathic short stature, also called non-growth hormone-deficient short stature, defined by height SDS ≤-2.25, and associated with growth rates unlikely to permit attainment of adult height in the normal range, in pediatric patients whose epiphyses are not closed and for whom diagnostic evaluation excludes other causes associated with short stature that should be observed or treated by other means.

Adult Patients — Humatrope is indicated for replacement of endogenous growth hormone in adults with growth hormone deficiency who meet either of the following two criteria:

1. Adult Onset: Patients who have growth hormone deficiency either alone, or with multiple hormone deficiencies (hypopituitarism), as a result of pituitary disease, hypothalamic disease, surgery, radiation therapy, or trauma;

or

2. Childhood Onset: Patients who were growth hormone-deficient during childhood who have growth hormone deficiency confirmed as an adult before replacement therapy with Humatrope is started.

CONTRAINDICATIONS

Humatrope should not be used for growth promotion in pediatric patients with closed epiphyses.

Humatrope should not be used or should be discontinued when there is any evidence of active malignancy. Antimalignancy treatment must be complete with evidence of remission prior to the institution of therapy.

Humatrope should **not** be reconstituted with the supplied Diluent for Humatrope for use by patients with a known sensitivity to either Metacresol or glycerin.

Growth hormone should not be initiated to treat patients with acute critical illness due to complications following open heart or abdominal surgery, multiple accidental trauma or to patients having acute respiratory failure. Two placebo-controlled clinical trials in non-growth hormone-deficient adult patients (n=522) with these conditions revealed a significant increase in mortality (41.9% vs. 19.3%) among somatropin-treated patients (doses 5.3 to 8 mg/day) compared to those receiving placebo (*see* WARNINGS).

Growth hormone is contraindicated in patients with Prader-Willi syndrome who are severely obese or have severe respiratory impairment (*see* WARNINGS). Unless patients with Prader-Willi syndrome also have a diagnosis of growth hormone deficiency, Humatrope is not indicated for the long term treatment of pediatric patients who have growth failure due to genetically confirmed Prader-Willi syndrome.

WARNINGS

If sensitivity to the diluent should occur, the **vials** may be reconstituted with Bacteriostatic Water for Injection, USP or, Sterile Water for Injection, USP. When Humatrope is used with Bacteriostatic Water (Benzyl Alcohol preserved), the solution should be kept refrigerated at 2° to 8°C (36° to 46°F) and used within 14 days. **Benzyl alcohol as a preservative in Bacteriostatic Water for Injection, USP has been associated with toxicity in newborns.** When administering Humatrope to newborns, use the Humatrope diluent provided or if the patient is sensitive to the diluent, use Sterile Water for Injection, USP. When Humatrope is reconstituted with Sterile Water for Injection, USP in this manner, use only one dose per Humatrope vial and discard the unused portion. If the solution is not used immediately, it must be refrigerated [2° to 8°C (36° to 46°F)] and used within 24 hours.

Cartridges should be reconstituted only with the supplied diluent. Cartridges should not be reconstituted with the Diluent for Humatrope provided with Humatrope Vials, or with any other solution. Cartridges should not be used if the patient is allergic to Metacresol or glycerin.

See CONTRAINDICATIONS for information on increased mortality in patients with acute critical illnesses in intensive care units due to complications following open heart or abdominal surgery, multiple accidental trauma or with acute respiratory failure. The safety of continuing growth hormone treatment in patients receiving replacement doses for approved indications who concurrently develop these illnesses has not been established. Therefore, the potential benefit of treatment continuation with growth hormone in patients having acute critical illnesses should be weighed against the potential risk.

There have been reports of fatalities after initiating therapy with growth hormone in pediatric patients with Prader-Willi syndrome who had one or more of the following risk factors: severe obesity, history of upper airway obstruction or sleep apnea, or unidentified respiratory infection. Male patients with one or more of these factors may be at greater risk than females. Patients with Prader-Willi syndrome should be evaluated for signs of upper airway obstruction and sleep apnea before initiation of treatment with growth hormone. If, during treatment with growth hormone, patients show signs of upper airway obstruction (including onset of or increased snoring) and/or new onset sleep apnea, treatment should be interrupted. All patients with Prader-Willi syndrome treated with growth hormone should also have effective weight control and be monitored for signs of respiratory infection, which should be diagnosed as early as possible and treated aggressively (*see* CONTRAINDICATIONS). Unless patients with Prader-Willi syndrome also have a diagnosis of growth hormone deficiency, Humatrope is not indicated for the long term treatment of pediatric patients who have growth failure due to genetically confirmed Prader-Willi syndrome.

Table 4
Baseline Height Characteristics and Effect of Humatrope on Final Height[a]

	Humatrope (n=22) Mean (SD)	Placebo (n=11) Mean (SD)	Treatment Effect Mean (95% CI)	p-value
Baseline height SDS	-2.7 (0.6)	-2.75 (0.6)		0.77
BPH SDS	-2.1 (0.7)	-2.3 (0.8)		0.53
Final height SDS[b]	-1.8 (0.8)	-2.3 (0.6)	0.51 (0.10, 0.92)	0.017
FH SDS - baseline height SDS	0.9 (0.7)	0.4 (0.2)	0.51 (0.04, 0.97)	0.034
FH SDS - BPH SDS	0.3 (0.6)	-0.1 (0.6)	0.46 (0.02, 0.89)	0.043

[a] For final height population.
[b] Between-group comparison was performed using analysis of covariance with baseline predicted height SDS as the covariant. Treatment effect is expressed as least squares mean (95% CI).
Abbreviations: FH=final height; SDS=standard deviation score; BPH=baseline predicted height; CI=confidence interval.

Table 5
Final Height Minus Baseline Predicted Height: Idiopathic Short Stature Trials

	Placebo-controlled Trial 3× per week dosing		Dose Response Trial 6× per week dosing		
	Placebo (n=10)	Humatrope 0.22 mg/kg (n=22)	Humatrope 0.24 mg/kg (n=13)	Humatrope 0.24/0.37 mg/kg (n=13)	Humatrope 0.37 mg/kg (n=13)
FH – Baseline PH					
Mean cm	-0.7	+2.2	+5.4	+6.7	+7.2
(95% CI)	(-3.6, 2.3)	(0.4, 3.9)	(2.8, 7.9)	(4.1, 9.2)	(4.6, 9.8)
Mean inches	-0.3	+0.8	+2.1	+2.6	+2.8
(95% CI)	(-1.4, 0.9)	(0.2, 1.5)	(1.1, 3.1)	(1.6, 3.6)	(1.8, 3.9)

Abbreviations: PH=predicted height; FH=final height; CI=confidence interval.

PRECAUTIONS

General — Therapy with Humatrope should be directed by physicians who are experienced in the diagnosis and management of patients with growth hormone deficiency, Turner syndrome, idiopathic short stature, or adult patients with either childhood-onset or adult-onset growth hormone deficiency.

Patients with preexisting tumors or with growth hormone deficiency secondary to an intracranial lesion should be examined routinely for progression or recurrence of the underlying disease process. In pediatric patients, clinical literature has demonstrated no relationship between somatropin replacement therapy and CNS tumor recurrence. In adults, it is unknown whether there is any relationship between somatropin replacement therapy and CNS tumor recurrence. Patients should be monitored carefully for any malignant transformation of skin lesions.

For patients with diabetes mellitus, the insulin dose may require adjustment when somatropin therapy is instituted. Because human growth hormone may induce a state of insulin resistance, patients should be observed for evidence of glucose intolerance. Patients with diabetes or glucose intolerance should be monitored closely during somatropin therapy.

In patients with hypopituitarism (multiple hormonal deficiencies) standard hormonal replacement therapy should be monitored closely when somatropin therapy is administered. Hypothyroidism may develop during treatment with somatropin and inadequate treatment of hypothyroidism may prevent optimal response to somatropin.

Pediatric Patients (*see* General Precautions) — Pediatric patients with endocrine disorders, including growth hormone deficiency, may develop slipped capital epiphyses more frequently. Any pediatric patient with the onset of a limp during growth hormone therapy should be evaluated.

Growth hormone has not been shown to increase the incidence of scoliosis. Progression of scoliosis can occur in children who experience rapid growth. Because growth hormone increases growth rate, patients with a history of scoliosis who are treated with growth hormone should be monitored for progression of scoliosis. Skeletal abnormalities including scoliosis are commonly seen in untreated Turner syndrome patients.

Patients with Turner syndrome should be evaluated carefully for otitis media and other ear disorders since these patients have an increased risk of ear or hearing disorders (*see* Adverse Reactions). Patients with Turner syndrome are at risk for cardiovascular disorders (e.g., stroke, aortic aneurysm, hypertension) and these conditions should be monitored closely.

Patients with Turner syndrome have an inherently increased risk of developing autoimmune thyroid disease. Therefore, patients should have periodic thyroid function tests and be treated as indicated (*see* General Precautions).

Intracranial hypertension (IH) with papilledema, visual changes, headache, nausea and/or vomiting has been reported in a small number of pediatric patients treated with growth hormone products. Symptoms usually occurred within the first 8 weeks of the initiation of growth hormone therapy. In all reported cases, IH-associated signs and symptoms resolved after termination of therapy or a reduction of the growth hormone dose. Funduscopic examination of patients is recommended at the initiation and periodically during the course of growth hormone therapy. Patients with Turner syndrome may be at increased risk for development of IH.

Adult Patients (*see* General Precautions) — Patients with epiphyseal closure who were treated with growth hormone replacement therapy in childhood should be re-evaluated according to the criteria in *INDICATIONS AND USAGE* before continuation of somatropin therapy at the reduced dose level recommended for growth hormone-deficient adults. Experience with prolonged treatment in adults is limited.

Geriatric Use — The safety and effectiveness of Humatrope in patients aged 65 and over has not been evaluated in clinical studies. Elderly patients may be more sensitive to the action of Humatrope and may be more prone to develop adverse reactions.

Drug Interactions — Excessive glucocorticoid therapy may prevent optimal response to somatropin. If glucocorticoid replacement therapy is required, the glucocorticoid dosage and compliance should be monitored carefully to avoid either adrenal insufficiency or inhibition of growth promoting effects.

Limited published data indicate that growth hormone (GH) treatment increases cytochrome P450 (CP450) mediated antipyrine clearance in man. These data suggest that GH administration may alter the clearance of compounds known to be metabolized by CP450 liver enzymes (e.g., corticosteroids, sex steroids, anticonvulsants, cyclosporin). Careful monitoring is advisable when GH is administered in combination with other drugs known to be metabolized by CP450 liver enzymes.

Carcinogenesis, Mutagenesis, Impairment of Fertility — Long-term animal studies for carcinogenicity and impairment of fertility with this human growth hormone (Humatrope) have not been performed. There has been no evidence to date of Humatrope-induced mutagenicity.

Pregnancy — Pregnancy Category C — Animal reproduction studies have not been conducted with Humatrope. It is not known whether Humatrope can cause fetal harm when administered to a pregnant woman or can affect reproductive capacity. Humatrope should be given to a pregnant woman only if clearly needed.

Nursing Mothers — There have been no studies conducted with Humatrope in nursing mothers. It is not known whether this drug is excreted in human milk. Because many drugs are excreted in human milk, caution should be exercised when Humatrope is administered to a nursing woman.

Information for Patients — Patients being treated with growth hormone and/or their parents should be informed of the potential risks and benefits associated with treatment. Instructions on appropriate use should be given, including a review of the contents of the patient information insert. This information is intended to aid in the safe and effective administration of the medication. It is not a disclosure of all possible adverse or intended effects.

Patients and/or parents should be thoroughly instructed in the importance of proper needle disposal. A puncture resistant container should be used for the disposal of used needles and/or syringes (consistent with applicable state requirements). Needles and syringes must not be reused (*see* Information for the Patient insert).

ADVERSE REACTIONS

Growth Hormone-Deficient Pediatric Patients

As with all protein pharmaceuticals, a small percentage of patients may develop antibodies to the protein. During the first 6 months of Humatrope therapy in 314 naive patients, only 1.6% developed specific antibodies to Humatrope (binding capacity ≥0.02 mg/L). None had antibody concentrations which exceeded 2 mg/L. Throughout 8 years of this same study, two patients (0.6%) had binding capacity >2 mg/L. Neither patient demonstrated a decrease in growth velocity at or near the time of increased antibody production. It has been reported that growth attenuation from pituitary-derived growth hormone may occur when antibody concentrations are >1.5 mg/L.

In addition to an evaluation of compliance with the treatment program and of thyroid status, testing for antibodies to human growth hormone should be carried out in any patient who fails to respond to therapy.

In studies with growth hormone-deficient pediatric patients, injection site pain was reported infrequently. A mild and transient edema, which appeared in 2.5% of patients, was observed early during the course of treatment.

Leukemia has been reported in a small number of pediatric patients who have been treated with growth hormone, including growth hormone of pituitary origin as well as of recombinant DNA origin (somatrem and somatropin). The relationship, if any, between leukemia and growth hormone therapy is uncertain.

Turner Syndrome Patients

In a randomized, concurrent controlled trial, there was a statistically significant increase in the occurrence of otitis media (43% vs. 26%), ear disorders (18% vs. 5%) and surgical procedures (45% vs. 27%) in patients receiving Humatrope compared with untreated control patients (Table 6). Other adverse events of special interest to Turner syndrome patients were not significantly different between treatment groups (Table 6). A similar increase in otitis media was observed in an 18-month placebo-controlled trial.

[See table 6 at right]

Patients with Idiopathic Short Stature

In the placebo-controlled study, the adverse events associated with Humatrope therapy were similar to those observed in other pediatric populations treated with Humatrope (Table 7). Mean serum glucose level did not change during Humatrope treatment. Mean fasting serum insulin levels increased 10% in the Humatrope treatment group at the end of treatment relative to baseline values but remained within the normal reference range. For the same duration of treatment the mean fasting serum insulin levels decreased by 2% in the placebo group. The incidence of above-range values for glucose, insulin, and HbA_{1c} were similar in the growth hormone and placebo-treated groups. No patient developed diabetes mellitus. Consistent with the known mechanism of growth hormone action, Humatrope-treated patients had greater mean increases, relative to baseline, in serum insulin-like growth factor-I (IGF-I) than placebo-treated patients at each study observation. However, there was no significant difference between the Humatrope and placebo treatment groups in the proportion of patients who had at least one serum IGF-I concentration more than 2.0 SD above the age- and gender-appropriate mean (Humatrope: 9 of 35 patients [26%]; placebo: 7 of 28 patients [25%]).

Table 7
Nonserious Clinically Significant Treatment-Emergent Adverse Events by Treatment Group in Idiopathic Short Stature

Adverse Event	Treatment Group Humatrope	Placebo
Total Number of Patients	37	31
Scoliosis	7 (18.9%)	4 (12.9%)
Otitis media	6 (16.2%)	2 (6.5%)
Hyperlipidemia	3 (8.1%)	1 (3.2%)
Gynecomastia	2 (5.4%)	1 (3.2%)
Hypothyroidism	0	2 (6.5%)
Aching joints	0	1 (3.2%)
Hip pain	1 (2.7%)	0
Arthralgia	4 (10.8%)	1 (3.2%)
Arthrosis	4 (10.8%)	2 (6.5%)
Myalgia	9 (24.3%)	4 (12.9%)
Hypertension	1 (2.7%)	0

The adverse events observed in the dose-response study (239 patients treated for 2 years) did not indicate a pattern suggestive of a growth hormone dose effect. Among Humatrope dose groups, mean fasting blood glucose, mean glycosylated hemoglobin, and the incidence of elevated fasting blood glucose concentrations were similar. One patient developed abnormalities of carbohydrate metabolism (glucose intolerance and high serum HbA_{1c}) on treatment.

Adult Patients — In clinical studies in which high doses of Humatrope were administered to healthy adult volunteers, the following events occurred infrequently: headache, localized muscle pain, weakness, mild hyperglycemia, and glucosuria.

In the first 6 months of controlled blinded trials during which patients received either Humatrope or placebo, adult-onset growth hormone-deficient adults who received Humatrope experienced a statistically significant increase in edema (Humatrope 17.3% vs. placebo 4.4%, p=0.043) and peripheral edema (11.5% vs. 0%, respectively, p=0.017). In patients with adult-onset growth hormone deficiency, edema, muscle pain, joint pain, and joint disorder were reported early in therapy and tended to be transient or responsive to dosage titration.

Table 6
Treatment-Emergent Events of Special Interest by Treatment Group in Turner Syndrome

Adverse Event	Overall	Treatment Group hGH[1]	Untreated[2]	Significance
Total Number of Patients	136	74	62	
Surgical procedure	50 (36.8%)	33 (44.6%)	17 (27.4%)	p≤0.05
Otitis media	48 (35.3%)	32 (43.2%)	16 (25.8%)	p≤0.05
Ear disorders	16 (11.8%)	13 (17.6%)	3 (4.8%)	p≤0.05
Bone disorder	13 (9.6%)	6 (8.1%)	7 (11.3%)	NS
Edema				
Conjunctival	1 (0.7%)	0	1 (1.6%)	NS
Non-specific	3 (2.2%)	2 (2.7%)	1 (1.6%)	NS
Facial	1 (0.7%)	1 (1.4%)	0	NS
Peripheral	6 (4.4%)	5 (6.8%)	1 (1.6%)	NS
Hyperglycemia	0	0	0	NS
Hypothyroidism	15 (11.0%)	10 (13.5%)	5 (8.1%)	NS
Increased nevi[3]	10 (7.4%)	8 (10.8%)	2 (3.2%)	NS
Lymphedema	0	0	0	NS

[1] Dose=0.3 mg/kg/wk.
[2] Open-label study.
[3] Includes any nevi coded to the following preferred terms: melanosis, skin hypertrophy, or skin benign neoplasm.
NS=not significant.

Table 8
Treatment-Emergent Adverse Events with ≥5% Overall Incidence in Adult-Onset Growth Hormone-Deficient Patients Treated with Humatrope for 18 Months as Compared with 6-Month Placebo and 12-Month Humatrope Exposure

	18 Months Exposure [Placebo (6 Months)/hGH (12 Months)] (N=46)		18 Months hGH Exposure (N=52)	
Adverse Event	n	%	n	%
Edema[a]	7	15.2	11	21.2
Arthralgia	7	15.2	9	17.3
Paresthesia	6	13.0	9	17.3
Myalgia	6	13.0	7	13.5
Pain	6	13.0	7	13.5
Rhinitis	5	10.9	7	13.5
Peripheral edema[b]	8	17.4	6	11.5
Back pain	5	10.9	5	9.6
Headache	5	10.9	4	7.7
Hypertension	2	4.3	4	7.7
Acne	0	0	3	5.8
Joint disorder	1	2.2	3	5.8
Surgical procedure	1	2.2	3	5.8
Flu syndrome	3	6.5	2	3.9

Abbreviations: hGH=Humatrope; N=number of patients receiving treatment in the period stated; n=number of patients reporting each treatment-emergent adverse event.
[a] p=0.04 as compared to placebo (6 months).
[b] p=0.02 as compared to placebo (6 months).

Table 9
Treatment-Emergent Adverse Events with ≥5% Overall Incidence in Childhood-Onset Growth Hormone-Deficient Patients Treated with Humatrope for 18 Months as Compared with 6-Month Placebo and 12-Month Humatrope Exposure

	18 Months Exposure [Placebo (6 Months)/hGH (12 Months)] (N=35)		18 Months hGH Exposure (N=32)	
Adverse Event	n	%	n	%
Flu sndrome	8	22.9	5	15.6
AST icreased[a]	2	5.7	4	12.5
Headache	4	11.4	3	9.4
Asthenia	1	2.9	2	6.3
Cough increased	0	0	2	6.3
Edema	3	8.6	2	6.3
Hypesthesia	0	0	2	6.3
Myalgia	2	5.7	2	6.3
Pain	3	8.6	2	6.3
Rhinitis	2	5.7	2	6.3
ALT increased	2	5.7	2	6.3
Respiratory disorder	2	5.7	1	3.1
Gastritis	2	5.7	0	0
Pharyngitis	5	14.3	1	3.1

Abbreviations: hGH=Humatrope; N=number of patients receiving treatment in the period stated; n=number of patients reporting each treatment-emergent adverse event; ALT=alanine amino transferase, formerly SGPT; AST=aspartate amino transferase, formerly SGOT.
[a] p=0.03 as compared to placebo (6 months)

Two of 113 adult-onset patients developed carpal tunnel syndrome after beginning maintenance therapy without a low dose (0.00625 mg/kg/day) lead-in phase. Symptoms abated in these patients after dosage reduction.

All treatment-emergent adverse events with ≥5% overall incidence during 12 or 18 months of replacement therapy with Humatrope are shown in Table 8 (adult-onset patients) and in Table 9 (childhood-onset patients).

Adult patients treated with Humatrope who had been diagnosed with growth hormone deficiency in childhood reported side effects less frequently than those with adult-onset growth hormone deficiency.

[See table 8 above]
[See table 9 above]

Other adverse drug events that have been reported in growth hormone-treated patients include the following:

1) Metabolic: Infrequent, mild and transient peripheral or generalized edema.
2) Musculoskeletal: Rare carpal tunnel syndrome.
3) Skin: Rare increased growth of pre-existing nevi. Patients should be monitored carefully for malignant transformation.
4) Endocrine: Rare gynecomastia. Rare pancreatitis.

Continued on next page

*** Identi-Code® symbol. This product information was prepared in June 2004. Current information on these and other products of Eli Lilly and Company may be obtained by direct inquiry to Lilly Research Laboratories, Lilly Corporate Center, Indianapolis, Indiana 46285, (800) 545-5979.**

Table 10
Concentration of Reconstituted Humatrope Solutions, Incremental Dosage and Maximum Injectable Dose for Each Cartridge

Cartridge	Somatropin Concentration	Dose Per Click of Dosage Knob	Maximum Injectable Dose
6 mg	2.08 mg/mL	0.1 mg	1.2 mg
12 mg	4.17 mg/mL	0.2 mg	2.4 mg
24 mg	8.33 mg/mL	0.4 mg	4.8 mg

Humatrope—Cont.

OVERDOSAGE

Acute overdosage could lead initially to hypoglycemia and subsequently to hyperglycemia. Long-term overdosage could result in signs and symptoms of gigantism/acromegaly consistent with the known effects of excess human growth hormone. (See recommended and maximal dosage instructions given below.)

DOSAGE AND ADMINISTRATION

Pediatric Patients

The Humatrope dosage and administration schedule should be individualized for each patient. Therapy should not be continued if epiphyseal fusion has occurred. Response to growth hormone therapy tends to decrease with time. However, failure to increase growth rate, particularly during the first year of therapy, should prompt close assessment of compliance and evaluation of other causes of growth failure such as hypothyroidism, under-nutrition and advanced bone age.

Growth hormone-deficient pediatric patients — The recommended weekly dosage is 0.18 mg/kg (0.54 IU/kg) of body weight. The maximal replacement weekly dosage is 0.3 mg/kg (0.90 IU/kg) of body weight. It should be divided into equal doses given either on 3 alternate days, 6 times per week or daily. The subcutaneous route of administration is preferable; intramuscular injection is also acceptable. The dosage and administration schedule for Humatrope should be individualized for each patient.

Turner Syndrome — A weekly dosage of up to 0.375 mg/kg (1.125 IU/kg) of body weight administered by subcutaneous injection is recommended. It should be divided into equal doses given either daily or on 3 alternate days.

Patients with idiopathic short stature — A weekly dosage of up to 0.37 mg/kg of body weight administered by subcutaneous injection is recommended. It should be divided into equal doses given 6 to 7 times per week.

Adult Patients

Growth hormone-deficient adult patients — The recommended dosage at the start of therapy is not more than 0.006 mg/kg/day (0.018 IU/kg/day) given as a daily subcutaneous injection. The dose may be increased according to individual patient requirements to a maximum of 0.0125 mg/kg/day (0.0375 IU/kg/day).

During therapy, dosage should be titrated if required by the occurrence of side effects or to maintain the IGF-I response below the upper limit of normal IGF-I levels, matched for age and sex. To minimize the occurrence of adverse events in patients with increasing age or excessive body weight, dose reductions may be necessary.

Reconstitution

Vial — Each 5-mg vial of Humatrope should be reconstituted with 1.5 to 5 mL of Diluent for Humatrope. The diluent should be injected into the vial of Humatrope by aiming the stream of liquid against the glass wall. Following reconstitution, the vial should be swirled with a GENTLE rotary motion until the contents are completely dissolved. DO NOT SHAKE. The resulting solution should be inspected for clarity. It should be clear. If the solution is cloudy or contains particulate matter, the contents MUST NOT be injected.

Before and after injection, the septum of the vial should be wiped with rubbing alcohol or an alcoholic antiseptic solution to prevent contamination of the contents by repeated needle insertions. Sterile disposable syringes and needles should be used for administration of Humatrope. The volume of the syringe should be small enough so that the prescribed dose can be withdrawn from the vial with reasonable accuracy.

Cartridge — Each cartridge of Humatrope should only be reconstituted using the diluent syringe and the diluent connector which accompany the cartridge **and should not be reconstituted with the Diluent for Humatrope provided with Humatrope Vials.** (*See* WARNINGS section.) **See the HumatroPen™ User Guide for comprehensive directions on Humatrope cartridge reconstitution.**

The reconstituted solution should be inspected for clarity. It should be clear. If the solution is cloudy or contains particulate matter, the contents MUST NOT be injected.

The HumatroPen allows the somatropin dosage volume to be dialed in increments of 0.048 mL per click of dosage knob, and the maximum dosage volume that can be injected is 0.576 mL (based on a 12-click maximum). (See Table 10 for additional information.)

[See table 10 above]

This cartridge has been designed for use only with the HumatroPen. A sterile disposable needle should be used for each administration of Humatrope.

STABILITY AND STORAGE

Vials

Before Reconstitution — Vials of Humatrope and Diluent for Humatrope are stable when refrigerated [2° to 8°C (36° to 46°F)]. Avoid freezing Diluent for Humatrope. Expiration dates are stated on the labels.

After Reconstitution — Vials of Humatrope are stable for up to 14 days when reconstituted with Diluent for Humatrope or Bacteriostatic Water for Injection, USP and stored in a refrigerator at 2° to 8°C (36° to 46°F). Avoid freezing the reconstituted vial of Humatrope.

After Reconstitution with Sterile Water, USP — Use only one dose per Humatrope vial and discard the unused portion. If the solution is not used immediately, it must be refrigerated [2° to 8°C (36° to 46°F)] and used within 24 hours.

Cartridges

Before Reconstitution — Cartridges of Humatrope and Diluent for Humatrope are stable when refrigerated [2° to 8°C (36° to 46°F)]. Avoid freezing Diluent for Humatrope. Expiration dates are stated on the labels.

After Reconstitution — Cartridges of Humatrope are stable for up to 28 days when reconstituted with Diluent for Humatrope and stored in a refrigerator at 2° to 8°C (36° to 46°F). Store the HumatroPen without the needle attached. Avoid freezing the reconstituted cartridge of Humatrope.

HOW SUPPLIED

Vials

5 mg (No. 7335) — (6s) NDC 0002-7335-16, and 5-mL vials of Diluent for Humatrope (No. 7336)

Cartridges

Cartridge Kit (MS8089) NDC 0002-8089-01
6 mg cartridge (VL7554), and prefilled syringe of Diluent for Humatrope (VL7557)
Cartridge Kit (MS8090) NDC 0002-8090-01
12 mg cartridge (VL7555), and prefilled syringe of Diluent for Humatrope (VL7558)
Cartridge Kit (MS8091) NDC 0002-8091-01
24 mg cartridge (VL7556), and prefilled syringe of Diluent for Humatrope (VL7558)

Literature revised March 17, 2004
Eli Lilly and Company, Indianapolis, IN 46285, USA
www.lilly.com
PA 1643 AMP PRINTED IN USA

HUMULIN® 50/50 OTC

[*hū ′mū-lin*]

50% HUMAN INSULIN ISOPHANE SUSPENSION AND 50% HUMAN INSULIN INJECTION (rDNA ORIGIN)

INFORMATION FOR THE PATIENT

WARNINGS

THIS LILLY HUMAN INSULIN PRODUCT DIFFERS FROM ANIMAL-SOURCE INSULINS BECAUSE IT IS STRUCTURALLY IDENTICAL TO THE INSULIN PRODUCED BY YOUR BODY'S PANCREAS AND BECAUSE OF ITS UNIQUE MANUFACTURING PROCESS.

ANY CHANGE OF INSULIN SHOULD BE MADE CAUTIOUSLY AND ONLY UNDER MEDICAL SUPERVISION. CHANGES IN STRENGTH, MANUFACTURER, TYPE (E.G., REGULAR, NPH, LENTE®), SPECIES (BEEF, PORK, BEEF-PORK, HUMAN), OR METHOD OF MANUFACTURE (rDNA VERSUS ANIMAL-SOURCE INSULIN) MAY RESULT IN THE NEED FOR A CHANGE IN DOSAGE.

SOME PATIENTS TAKING HUMULIN® (HUMAN INSULIN, rDNA ORIGIN) MAY REQUIRE A CHANGE IN DOSAGE FROM THAT USED WITH ANIMAL-SOURCE INSULINS. IF AN ADJUSTMENT IS NEEDED, IT MAY OCCUR WITH THE FIRST DOSE OR DURING THE FIRST SEVERAL WEEKS OR MONTHS.

DIABETES

Insulin is a hormone produced by the pancreas, a large gland that lies near the stomach. This hormone is necessary for the body's correct use of food, especially sugar. Diabetes occurs when the pancreas does not make enough insulin to meet your body's needs.

To control your diabetes, your doctor has prescribed injections of insulin products to keep your blood glucose at a near-normal level. You have been instructed to test your blood and/or your urine regularly for glucose. Studies have shown that some chronic complications of diabetes such as eye disease, kidney disease, and nerve disease can be significantly reduced if the blood sugar is maintained as close to normal as possible. The American Diabetes Association recommends that if your premeal glucose levels are consistently above 140 mg/dL or your hemoglobin A_{1c} (HbA_{1c}) is more than 8%, consult your doctor. A change in your diabetes therapy may be needed. If your blood tests consistently show below-normal glucose levels you should also let your doctor know. Proper control of your diabetes requires close and constant cooperation with your doctor. Despite diabetes, you can lead an active and healthy life if you eat a balanced diet, exercise regularly, and take your insulin injections as prescribed.

Always keep an extra supply of insulin as well as a spare syringe and needle on hand. Always wear diabetic identification so that appropriate treatment can be given if complications occur away from home.

50/50 HUMAN INSULIN

Description

Humulin is synthesized in a non-disease-producing special laboratory strain of *Escherichia coli* bacteria that has been genetically altered by the addition of the gene for human insulin production. Humulin 50/50 is a mixture of 50% Human Insulin Isophane Suspension and 50% Human Insulin Injection. It is an intermediate-acting insulin combined with the more rapid onset of action of regular insulin. The duration of activity may last up to 24 hours following injection. The time course of action of any insulin may vary considerably in different individuals or at different times in the same individual. As with all insulin preparations, the duration of action of Humulin 50/50 is dependent on dose, site of injection, blood supply, temperature, and physical activity. Humulin 50/50 is a sterile suspension and is for subcutaneous injection only. It should not be used intravenously or intramuscularly. The concentration of Humulin 50/50 is 100 units/mL (U-100).

Identification

Human insulin manufactured by Eli Lilly and Company has the trademark Humulin and is available in 6 formulations—Regular (**R**), NPH (**N**), Lente (**L**), Ultralente® (**U**), 50% Human Insulin Isophane Suspension [NPH]/50% Human Insulin Injection [buffered regular] (**50/50**) and 70% Human Insulin Isophane Suspension [NPH]/30% Human Insulin Injection [buffered regular] (**70/30**). Your doctor has prescribed the type of insulin that he/she believes is best for you. **DO NOT USE ANY OTHER INSULIN EXCEPT ON HIS/HER ADVICE AND DIRECTION.**

Always check the carton and the bottle label for the name and letter designation of the insulin you receive from your pharmacy to make sure it is the same as that your doctor has prescribed.

Always examine the appearance of your bottle of insulin before withdrawing each dose. A bottle of Humulin 50/50 must be carefully shaken or rotated before each injection so that the contents are uniformly mixed. Humulin 50/50 should look uniformly cloudy or milky after mixing. Do not use it if the insulin substance (the white material) remains at the bottom of the bottle after mixing. Do not use a bottle of Humulin 50/50 if there are clumps in the insulin after mixing. Do not use a bottle of Humulin 50/50 if solid white particles stick to the bottom or wall of the bottle, giving it a frosted appearance. Always check the appearance of your bottle of insulin before using, and if you note anything unusual in the appearance of your insulin or notice your insulin requirements changing markedly, consult your doctor.

Storage

Insulin should be stored in a refrigerator but not in the freezer. If refrigeration is not possible, the bottle of insulin that you are currently using can be kept unrefrigerated as long as it is kept as cool as possible (below 86°F [30°C]) and away from heat and light. Do not use insulin if it has been frozen. Do not use a bottle of insulin after the expiration date stamped on the label.

INJECTION PROCEDURES

Correct Syringe

Doses of insulin are measured in **units.** U-100 insulin contains 100 units/mL (1 mL = 1 cc). With Humulin 50/50, it is important to use a syringe that is marked for U-100 insulin preparations. Failure to use the proper syringe can lead to a mistake in dosage, causing serious problems for you, such as a blood glucose level that is too low or too high.

Syringe Use

To help avoid contamination and possible infection, follow these instructions exactly.

Disposable syringes and needles should be used only once and then discarded. **NEEDLES AND SYRINGES MUST NOT BE SHARED.**

Reusable syringes and needles must be sterilized before each injection. **Follow the package directions supplied with your syringe.** Described below are 2 methods of sterilizing.

Boiling

1. Put syringe, plunger, and needle in strainer, place in saucepan, and cover with water. Boil for 5 minutes.
2. Remove articles from water. When they have cooled, insert plunger into barrel, and fasten needle to syringe with a slight twist.
3. Push plunger in and out several times until water is completely removed.

Isopropyl Alcohol

If the syringe, plunger, and needle cannot be boiled, as when you are traveling, they may be sterilized by immersion for at least 5 minutes in Isopropyl Alcohol, 91%. Do not use bathing, rubbing, or medicated alcohol for this sterilization. If the syringe is sterilized with alcohol, it must be absolutely dry before use.

Preparing the Dose

1. Wash your hands.
2. Carefully shake or rotate the insulin bottle several times to completely mix the insulin.

3. Inspect the insulin. Humulin 50/50 should look uniformly cloudy or milky. Do not use it if you notice anything unusual in the appearance.
4. If using a new bottle, flip off the plastic protective cap, but **do not** remove the stopper. When using a new bottle, wipe the top of the bottle with an alcohol swab.
5. Draw air into the syringe equal to your insulin dose. Put the needle through rubber top of the insulin bottle and inject the air into the bottle.
6. Turn the bottle and syringe upside down. Hold the bottle and syringe firmly in 1 hand and shake gently.
7. Making sure the tip of the needle is in the insulin, withdraw the correct dose of insulin into the syringe.
8. Before removing the needle from the bottle, check your syringe for air bubbles which reduce the amount of insulin in it. If bubbles are present, hold the syringe straight up and tap its side until the bubbles float to the top. Push them out with the plunger and withdraw the correct dose.
9. Remove the needle from the bottle and lay the syringe down so that the needle does not touch anything.

Injection

Cleanse the skin with alcohol where the injection is to be made. Stabilize the skin by spreading it or pinching up a large area. Insert the needle as instructed by your doctor. Push the plunger in as far as it will go. Pull the needle out and apply gentle pressure over the injection site for several seconds. **Do not rub the area.** To avoid tissue damage, give the next injection at a site at least 1/2″ from the previous site.

DOSAGE

Your doctor has told you which insulin to use, how much, and when and how often to inject it. Because each patient's case of diabetes is different, this schedule has been individualized for you.

Your usual insulin dose may be affected by changes in your food, activity, or work schedule. Carefully follow your doctor's instructions to allow for these changes. Other things that may affect your insulin dose are:

Illness

Illness, especially with nausea and vomiting, may cause your insulin requirements to change. Even if you are not eating, you will still require insulin. You and your doctor should establish a sick day plan for you to use in case of illness. When you are sick, test your blood/urine frequently and call your doctor as instructed.

Pregnancy

Good control of diabetes is especially important for you and your unborn baby. Pregnancy may make managing your diabetes more difficult. If you are planning to have a baby, are pregnant, or are nursing a baby, consult your doctor.

Medication

Insulin requirements may be increased if you are taking other drugs with hyperglycemic activity, such as oral contraceptives, corticosteroids, or thyroid replacement therapy. Insulin requirements may be reduced in the presence of drugs with hypoglycemic activity, such as oral hypoglycemics, salicylates (for example, aspirin), sulfa antibiotics, and certain antidepressants. Always discuss any medications you are taking with your doctor.

Exercise

Exercise may lower your body's need for insulin during and for some time after the activity. Exercise may also speed up the effect of an insulin dose, especially if the exercise involves the area of injection site (for example, the leg should not be used for injection just prior to running). Discuss with your doctor how you should adjust your regimen to accommodate exercise.

Travel

Persons traveling across more than 2 time zones should consult their doctor concerning adjustments in their insulin schedule.

COMMON PROBLEMS OF DIABETES

Hypoglycemia (Insulin Reaction)

Hypoglycemia (too little glucose in the blood) is one of the most frequent adverse events experienced by insulin users. It can be brought about by:
1. Taking too much insulin
2. Missing or delaying meals
3. Exercising or working more than usual
4. An infection or illness (especially with diarrhea or vomiting)
5. A change in the body's need for insulin
6. Diseases of the adrenal, pituitary, or thyroid gland, or progression of kidney or liver disease
7. Interactions with other drugs that lower blood glucose, such as oral hypoglycemics, salicylates (for example, aspirin), sulfa antibiotics, and certain antidepressants
8. Consumption of alcoholic beverages

Symptoms of mild to moderate hypoglycemia may occur suddenly and can include:
- sweating
- dizziness
- palpitation
- tremor
- hunger
- restlessness
- tingling in the hands, feet, lips, or tongue
- lightheadedness
- inability to concentrate
- headache
- drowsiness
- sleep disturbances
- anxiety
- blurred vision
- slurred speech
- depressed mood
- irritability
- abnormal behavior
- unsteady movement
- personality changes

Signs of severe hypoglycemia can include:
- disorientation
- unconsciousness
- seizures
- death

Therefore, it is important that assistance be obtained immediately.

Early warning symptoms of hypoglycemia may be different or less pronounced under certain conditions, such as long duration of diabetes, diabetic nerve disease, medications such as beta-blockers, change in insulin preparations, or intensified control (3 or more insulin injections per day) of diabetes.

A few patients who have experienced hypoglycemic reactions after transfer from animal-source insulin to human insulin have reported that the early warning symptoms of hypoglycemia were less pronounced or different from those experienced with their previous insulin.

Without recognition of early warning symptoms, you may not be able to take steps to avoid more serious hypoglycemia. Be alert for all of the various types of symptoms that may indicate hypoglycemia. Patients who experience hypoglycemia without early warning symptoms should monitor their blood glucose frequently, especially prior to activities such as driving. If the blood glucose is below your normal fasting glucose, you should consider eating or drinking sugar-containing foods to treat your hypoglycemia.

Mild to moderate hypoglycemia may be treated by eating foods or drinks that contain sugar. Patients should always carry a quick source of sugar, such as candy mints or glucose tablets. More severe hypoglycemia may require the assistance of another person. Patients who are unable to take sugar orally or who are unconscious require an injection of glucagon or should be treated with intravenous administration of glucose at a medical facility.

You should learn to recognize your own symptoms of hypoglycemia. If you are uncertain about these symptoms, you should monitor your blood glucose frequently to help you learn to recognize the symptoms that you experience with hypoglycemia.

If you have frequent episodes of hypoglycemia or experience difficulty in recognizing the symptoms, you should consult your doctor to discuss possible changes in therapy, meal plans, and/or exercise programs to help you avoid hypoglycemia.

Hyperglycemia and Diabetic Acidosis

Hyperglycemia (too much glucose in the blood) may develop if your body has too little insulin. Hyperglycemia can be brought about by:
1. Omitting your insulin or taking less than the doctor has prescribed
2. Eating significantly more than your meal plan suggests
3. Developing a fever, infection, or other significant stressful situation

In patients with insulin-dependent diabetes, prolonged hyperglycemia can result in diabetic acidosis. The first symptoms of diabetic acidosis usually come on gradually, over a period of hours or days, and include a drowsy feeling, flushed face, thirst, loss of appetite, and fruity odor on the breath. With acidosis, urine tests show large amounts of glucose and acetone. Heavy breathing and a rapid pulse are more severe symptoms. If uncorrected, prolonged hyperglycemia or diabetic acidosis can lead to nausea, vomiting, dehydration, loss of consciousness or death. Therefore, it is important that you obtain medical assistance immediately.

Lipodystrophy

Rarely, administration of insulin subcutaneously can result in lipoatrophy (depression in the skin) or lipohypertrophy (enlargement or thickening of tissue). If you notice either of these conditions, consult your doctor. A change in your injection technique may help alleviate the problem.

Allergy to Insulin

Local Allergy—Patients occasionally experience redness, swelling, and itching at the site of injection of insulin. This condition, called local allergy, usually clears up in a few days to a few weeks. In some instances, this condition may be related to factors other than insulin, such as irritants in the skin cleansing agent or poor injection technique. If you have local reactions, contact your doctor.

Systemic Allergy—Less common, but potentially more serious, is generalized allergy to insulin, which may cause rash over the whole body, shortness of breath, wheezing, reduction in blood pressure, fast pulse, or sweating. Severe cases of generalized allergy may be life threatening. If you think you are having a generalized allergic reaction to insulin, notify a doctor immediately.

ADDITIONAL INFORMATION

Additional information about diabetes may be obtained from your diabetes educator.

DIABETES FORECAST is a national magazine designed especially for patients with diabetes and their families and is available by subscription from the American Diabetes Association, National Service Center, 1660 Duke Street, Alexandria, Virginia 22314, 1-800-DIABETES (1-800-342-2383).

Another publication, **DIABETES COUNTDOWN**, is available from the Juvenile Diabetes Foundation International (JDF), 120 Wall Street, 19th Floor, New York, New York 10005, 1-800-JDF-CURE (1-800-533-2873).

Additional information about Humulin can be obtained by calling 1-888-88-LILLY (1-888-885-4559).

Literature revised August 3, 2000

PA 6054 AMP

HUMULIN® 70/30 Pen ℞

[*hū'mŭ-lĭn*]

70% HUMAN INSULIN ISOPHANE SUSPENSION AND 30% HUMAN INSULIN INJECTION (rDNA ORIGIN)

INFORMATION FOR THE PATIENT
3 ML DISPOSABLE INSULIN DELIVERY DEVICE

WARNINGS

THIS LILLY HUMAN INSULIN PRODUCT DIFFERS FROM ANIMAL-SOURCE INSULINS BECAUSE IT IS STRUCTURALLY IDENTICAL TO THE INSULIN PRODUCED BY YOUR BODY'S PANCREAS AND BECAUSE OF ITS UNIQUE MANUFACTURING PROCESS.

ANY CHANGE OF INSULIN SHOULD BE MADE CAUTIOUSLY AND ONLY UNDER MEDICAL SUPERVISION. CHANGES IN STRENGTH, MANUFACTURER, TYPE (E.G., REGULAR, NPH, LENTE, ETC), SPECIES (BEEF, PORK, BEEF-PORK, HUMAN), OR METHOD OF MANUFACTURE (rDNA VERSUS ANIMAL-SOURCE INSULIN) MAY RESULT IN THE NEED FOR A CHANGE IN DOSAGE.

SOME PATIENTS TAKING HUMULIN® (HUMAN INSULIN, rDNA ORIGIN) MAY REQUIRE A CHANGE IN DOSAGE FROM THAT USED WITH ANIMAL-SOURCE INSULINS. IF AN ADJUSTMENT IS NEEDED, IT MAY OCCUR WITH THE FIRST DOSE OR DURING THE FIRST SEVERAL WEEKS OR MONTHS.

TO OBTAIN AN ACCURATE DOSE, CAREFULLY READ AND FOLLOW THE "DISPOSABLE INSULIN DELIVERY DEVICE USER MANUAL" AND THIS INFORMATION FOR THE PATIENT INSERT BEFORE USING THIS PRODUCT. BEFORE EACH INJECTION, YOU SHOULD PRIME THE PEN, A NECESSARY STEP TO MAKE SURE THE PEN IS READY TO DOSE. PRIMING THE PEN IS IMPORTANT TO CONFIRM THAT INSULIN COMES OUT WHEN YOU PUSH THE INJECTION BUTTON AND TO REMOVE AIR THAT MAY COLLECT IN THE INSULIN CARTRIDGE DURING NORMAL USE. IF YOU DO NOT PRIME, YOU MAY RECEIVE TOO MUCH OR TOO LITTLE INSULIN (*see also* INSTRUCTIONS FOR PEN USE section.)

DIABETES

Insulin is a hormone produced by the pancreas, a large gland that lies near the stomach. This hormone is necessary for the body's correct use of food, especially sugar. Diabetes occurs when the pancreas does not make enough insulin to meet your body's needs.

To control your diabetes, your doctor has prescribed injections of insulin products to keep your blood glucose at a near-normal level. You have been instructed to test your blood and/or your urine regularly for glucose. Studies have shown that some chronic complications of diabetes such as eye disease, kidney disease, and nerve disease can be significantly reduced if the blood sugar is maintained as close to normal as possible. The American Diabetes Association recommends that if your premeal glucose levels are consistently above 140 mg/dL or your hemoglobin A_{1c} (HbA_{1c}) is more than 8%, consult your doctor. A change in your diabetes therapy may be needed. If your blood tests consistently show below-normal glucose levels, you should also let your doctor know. Proper control of your diabetes requires close and constant cooperation with your doctor. Despite diabetes, you can lead an active and healthy life if you eat a balanced diet, exercise regularly, and take your insulin injections as prescribed.

Always keep an extra supply of insulin as well as a spare syringe and needle on hand. Always wear diabetic identification so that appropriate treatment can be given if complications occur away from home.

70/30 HUMAN INSULIN

Description

Humulin is synthesized in a non-disease-producing special laboratory strain of *Escherichia coli* bacteria that has been genetically altered by the addition of the human gene for insulin production. Humulin® 70/30 is a mixture of 70% Human Insulin Isophane Suspension and 30% Human Insulin Injection. It is an intermediate-acting insulin combined with the more rapid onset of action of regular insulin. The duration of activity may last up to 24 hours following injection. The time course of action of any insulin may vary

Continued on next page

*** Identi-Code® symbol. This product information was prepared in June 2004. Current information on these and other products of Eli Lilly and Company may be obtained by direct inquiry to Lilly Research Laboratories, Lilly Corporate Center, Indianapolis, Indiana 46285, (800) 545-5979.**

Humulin 70/30 Pen—Cont.

considerably in different individuals or at different times in the same individual. As with all insulin preparations, the duration of action of Humulin 70/30 is dependent on dose, site of injection, blood supply, temperature, and physical activity. Humulin 70/30 is a sterile suspension and is for subcutaneous injection only. It should not be used intravenously or intramuscularly. The concentration of Humulin 70/30 in the Humulin 70/30 Pen is 100 units/mL (U-100).

Identification

Humulin disposable insulin delivery devices, manufactured by Eli Lilly and Company, are available in 2 formulations—NPH and 70/30.

Your doctor has prescribed the type of insulin that he/she believes is best for you. **DO NOT USE ANY OTHER INSULIN EXCEPT ON HIS/HER ADVICE AND DIRECTION.**

The Humulin 70/30 Pen is available in boxes of 5 disposable insulin delivery devices ("insulin pens"). The Humulin 70/30 Pen is not designed to allow any other insulin to be mixed in its cartridge, or for the cartridge to be removed.

Always examine the appearance of Humulin 70/30 suspension in the insulin pen before administering a dose. A cartridge of Humulin 70/30 contains a small glass bead to assist in mixing. Humulin 70/30 Pen must be rolled between the palms 10 times and inverted 180° 10 times before each injection so that the contents are uniformly mixed (*see* Figures 1 and 2). Inspect the Humulin 70/30 suspension for uniform mixing and repeat the above steps as necessary.

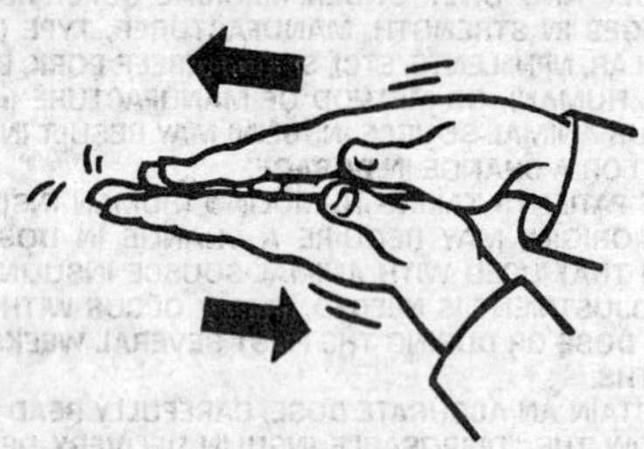

Figure 1.

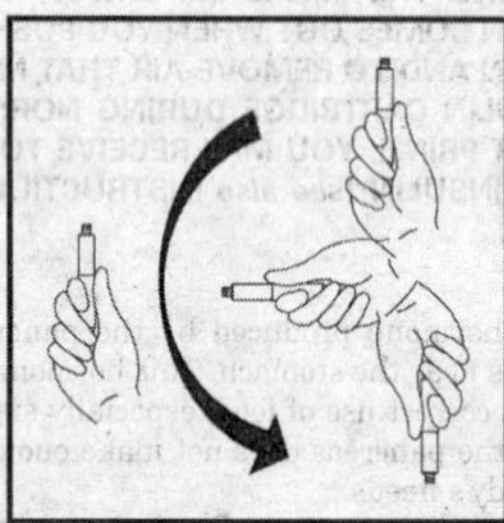

Figure 2.

Humulin 70/30 should look uniformly cloudy or milky after mixing. Do not use if the insulin substance (the white material) remains visibly separated from the liquid after mixing. Do not use the Humulin 70/30 Pen if there are clumps in the insulin after mixing. Do not use the Humulin 70/30 Pen if solid white particles stick to the walls of the cartridge, giving it a frosted appearance.

Always check the appearance of the Humulin 70/30 suspension in the insulin pen before using, and if you note anything unusual in the appearance of Humulin 70/30 suspension or notice your insulin requirements changing markedly, consult your doctor.

Never attempt to remove the cartridge from the Humulin 70/30 Pen. Inspect the cartridge through the clear cartridge holder.

Storage

Humulin 70/30 Pens should be stored in a refrigerator but not in the freezer. The Humulin 70/30 Pen that you are currently using should not be refrigerated but should be kept as cool as possible (below 86°F [30°C]) and away from heat and light. Do not use an insulin pen if it has been frozen. Unrefrigerated Humulin 70/30 Pens **must be discarded after 10 days**, even if they still contain insulin. Do not use Humulin 70/30 Pens after the expiration date stamped on the label.

INSTRUCTIONS FOR PEN USE

It is important to read, understand, and follow the instructions in the "Disposable Insulin Delivery Device User Manual" before using. Failure to follow instructions may result in getting too much or too little insulin. The needle must be changed and the pen must be primed before each injection to make sure the pen is ready to dose. These steps are important to confirm that insulin comes out when you push the injection button, and to remove air that may collect in the insulin cartridge during normal use.

Every time you inject:

- **Use a new needle**
- **Prime to make sure the pen is ready to dose**
- **Make sure you got a full dose.**

NEVER SHARE INSULIN PENS, CARTRIDGES, OR NEEDLES.

PREPARING THE PEN FOR INJECTION

1. Always check the appearance of the Humulin 70/30 suspension in the insulin pen before using.
2. Roll the Humulin 70/30 Pen between the palms 10 times (*see* Figure 1 above).
3. Holding the Humulin 70/30 Pen by one end, invert it 180° slowly 10 times to allow the glass bead to travel the full length of the cartridge with each inversion (*see* Figure 2 above). The cartridge is contained in the clear cartridge holder of the Humulin 70/30 Pen.
4. Inspect the appearance of the Humulin 70/30 suspension to make sure the contents look uniformly cloudy or milky. If not, repeat the above steps until the contents are mixed. Do not use a Humulin 70/30 Pen if there are clumps in the insulin or if solid white particles stick to the walls of the cartridge.
5. Follow the instructions in the "Disposable Insulin Delivery Device User Manual" for these steps:

- Preparing the Pen
- Attaching the Needle. **Use a new needle for each injection.**
- Priming the Pen. **The pen must be primed before each injection to make sure the pen is ready to dose.** Performing the priming step is important to confirm that insulin comes out when you push the injection button, and to remove air that may collect in the insulin cartridge during normal use.
- Setting (Dialing) a Dose
- Injecting the Dose. **To make sure you have received your dose, you must push the injection button all the way down until you see a diamond (◆) or an arrow (→) in the center of the dose window.**
- Following an Injection

PREPARING FOR INJECTION

1. Wash your hands.
2. To avoid tissue damage, choose a site for each injection that is at least 1/2 inch from the previous injection site. The usual sites of injection are abdomen, thighs, and arms.
3. Cleanse the skin with alcohol where the injection is to be made.
4. With one hand, stabilize the skin by spreading it or pinching up a large area.
5. Inject the dose as instructed by your doctor.
6. After dispensing a dose, pull the needle out and apply gentle pressure over the injection site for several seconds. Do not rub the area.
7. Immediately after an injection, remove the needle from the Humulin 70/30 Pen. Doing so will guard against contamination, leakage, reentry of air, and needle clogs. Do not reuse needles. Dispose of needles in a responsible manner.

DOSAGE

Your doctor has told you which insulin to use, how much, and when and how often to inject it. Because each patient's case of diabetes is different, this schedule has been individualized for you.

Your usual insulin dose may be affected by changes in your food, activity, or work schedule. Carefully follow your doctor's instructions to allow for these changes. Other things that may affect your insulin dose are:

Illness

Illness, especially with nausea and vomiting, may cause your insulin requirements to change. Even if you are not eating, you will still require insulin. You and your doctor should establish a sick day plan for you to use in case of illness. When you are sick, test your blood glucose/urine glucose and ketones frequently and call your doctor as instructed.

Pregnancy

Good control of diabetes is especially important for you and your unborn baby. Pregnancy may make managing your diabetes more difficult. If you are planning to have a baby, are pregnant, or are nursing a baby, consult your doctor.

Medication

Insulin requirements may be increased if you are taking other drugs with hyperglycemic activity, such as oral contraceptives, corticosteroids, or thyroid replacement therapy. Insulin requirements may be reduced in the presence of drugs with hypoglycemic activity, such as oral hypoglycemics, salicylates (for example, aspirin), sulfa antibiotics, and certain antidepressants. Always discuss any medications you are taking with your doctor.

Exercise

Exercise may lower your body's need for insulin during and for some time after the activity. Exercise may also speed up the effect of an insulin dose, especially if the exercise involves the area of injection site (for example, the leg should not be used for injection just prior to running). Discuss with your doctor how you should adjust your regimen to accommodate exercise.

Travel

Persons traveling across more than 2 time zones should consult their doctor concerning adjustments in their insulin schedule.

COMMON PROBLEMS OF DIABETES

Hypoglycemia (Insulin Reaction)

Hypoglycemia (too little glucose in the blood) is one of the most frequent adverse events experienced by insulin users. It can be brought about by:

1. Taking too much insulin
2. Missing or delaying meals
3. Exercising or working more than usual
4. An infection or illness (especially with diarrhea or vomiting)
5. A change in the body's need for insulin
6. Diseases of the adrenal, pituitary or thyroid gland, or progression of kidney or liver disease
7. Interactions with other drugs that lower blood glucose, such as oral hypoglycemics, salicylates (for example, aspirin), sulfa antibiotics, and certain antidepressants
8. Consumption of alcoholic beverages

Symptoms of mild to moderate hypoglycemia may occur suddenly and can include:

- sweating
- dizziness
- palpitation
- tremor
- hunger
- restlessness
- tingling in the hands, feet, lips, or tongue
- lightheadedness
- inability to concentrate
- headache
- drowsiness
- sleep disturbances
- anxiety
- blurred vision
- slurred speech
- depressed mood
- irritability
- abnormal behavior
- unsteady movement
- personality changes

Signs of severe hypoglycemia can include:

- disorientation
- unconsciousness
- seizures
- death

Therefore, it is important that assistance be obtained immediately.

Early warning symptoms of hypoglycemia may be different or less pronounced under certain conditions, such as long duration of diabetes, diabetic nerve disease, medications such as beta-blockers, change in insulin preparations, or intensified control (3 or more insulin injections per day) of diabetes.

A few patients who have experienced hypoglycemic reactions after transfer from animal-source insulin to human insulin have reported that the early warning symptoms of hypoglycemia were less pronounced or different from those experienced with their previous insulin.

Without recognition of early warning symptoms, you may not be able to take steps to avoid more serious hypoglycemia. Be alert for all of the various types of symptoms that may indicate hypoglycemia. Patients who experience hypoglycemia without early warning symptoms should monitor their blood glucose frequently, especially prior to activities such as driving. If the blood glucose is below your normal fasting glucose, you should consider eating or drinking sugar-containing foods to treat your hypoglycemia.

Mild to moderate hypoglycemia may be treated by eating foods or drinks that contain sugar. Patients should always carry a quick source of sugar, such as candy mints or glucose tablets. More severe hypoglycemia may require the assistance of another person. Patients who are unable to take sugar orally or who are unconscious require an injection of glucagon or should be treated with intravenous administration of glucose at a medical facility.

You should learn to recognize your own symptoms of hypoglycemia. If you are uncertain about these symptoms, you should monitor your blood glucose frequently to help you learn to recognize the symptoms that you experience with hypoglycemia.

If you have frequent episodes of hypoglycemia or experience difficulty in recognizing the symptoms, you should consult your doctor to discuss possible changes in therapy, meal plans, and/or exercise programs to help you avoid hypoglycemia.

Hyperglycemia and Diabetic Acidosis

Hyperglycemia (too much glucose in the blood) may develop if your body has too little insulin. Hyperglycemia can be brought about by:

1. Omitting your insulin or taking less than the doctor has prescribed
2. Eating significantly more than your meal plan suggests
3. Developing a fever, infection, or other significant stressful situation

In patients with insulin-dependent diabetes, prolonged hyperglycemia can result in diabetic acidosis. The first symptoms of diabetic acidosis usually come on gradually, over a period of hours or days, and include a drowsy feeling, flushed face, thirst, loss of appetite, and fruity odor on the breath. With acidosis, urine tests show large amounts of glucose and acetone. Heavy breathing and a rapid pulse are more severe symptoms. If uncorrected, prolonged hyperglycemia or diabetic acidosis can lead to nausea, vomiting, dehydration, loss of consciousness or death. Therefore, it is important that you obtain medical assistance immediately.

Lipodystrophy

Rarely, administration of insulin subcutaneously can result in lipoatrophy (depression in the skin) or lipohypertrophy (enlargement or thickening of tissue). If you notice either of these conditions, consult your doctor. A change in your injection technique may help alleviate the problem.

Allergy to Insulin

Local Allergy—Patients occasionally experience redness, swelling, and itching at the site of injection of insulin. This condition, called local allergy, usually clears up in a few days to a few weeks. In some instances, this condition may be related to factors other than insulin, such as irritants in the skin cleansing agent or poor injection technique. If you have local reactions, contact your doctor.

Systemic Allergy—Less common, but potentially more serious, is generalized allergy to insulin, which may cause rash over the whole body, shortness of breath, wheezing, reduction in blood pressure, fast pulse, or sweating. Severe cases of generalized allergy may be life threatening. If you think you are having a generalized allergic reaction to insulin, notify a doctor immediately.

ADDITIONAL INFORMATION

Additional information about diabetes may be obtained from your diabetes educator.

DIABETES FORECAST is a national magazine designed especially for patients with diabetes and their families and is available on subscription from the American Diabetes Association, National Service Center, 1660 Duke Street, Alexandria, Virginia 22314, 1-800-DIABETES (1-800-342-2383).

Another publication, **DIABETES COUNTDOWN**, is available from the Juvenile Diabetes Foundation, 120 Wall Street 19th Floor, New York, New York 10005-4001, 1-800-JDF-CURE (1-800-533-2873).

Additional information about Humulin and Humulin 70/30 Pen can be obtained by calling 1-888-88-LILLY (1-888-885-4559).

Literature revised October 8, 2003

Manufactured by Lilly France S.A.S.
F-67640 Fegersheim, France
for Eli Lilly and Company
Indianapolis, IN 46285, USA

PA 9144 FSAMP

HUMULIN® L **OTC**

[hū 'mū-lĭn ĕl]

LENTE®

(HUMAN INSULIN [rDNA ORIGIN]
ZINC SUSPENSION)

INFORMATION FOR THE PATIENT

WARNINGS

THIS LILLY HUMAN INSULIN PRODUCT DIFFERS FROM ANIMAL-SOURCE INSULINS BECAUSE IT IS STRUCTURALLY IDENTICAL TO THE INSULIN PRODUCED BY YOUR BODY'S PANCREAS AND BECAUSE OF ITS UNIQUE MANUFACTURING PROCESS.

ANY CHANGE OF INSULIN SHOULD BE MADE CAUTIOUSLY AND ONLY UNDER MEDICAL SUPERVISION. CHANGES IN STRENGTH, MANUFACTURER, TYPE (E.G., REGULAR, NPH, LENTE®), SPECIES (BEEF, PORK, BEEF-PORK, HUMAN), OR METHOD OF MANUFACTURE (rDNA VERSUS ANIMAL-SOURCE INSULIN) MAY RESULT IN THE NEED FOR A CHANGE IN DOSAGE.

SOME PATIENTS TAKING HUMULIN® (HUMAN INSULIN, rDNA ORIGIN) MAY REQUIRE A CHANGE IN DOSAGE FROM THAT USED WITH ANIMAL-SOURCE INSULINS. IF AN ADJUSTMENT IS NEEDED, IT MAY OCCUR WITH THE FIRST DOSE OR DURING THE FIRST SEVERAL WEEKS OR MONTHS.

DIABETES

Insulin is a hormone produced by the pancreas, a large gland that lies near the stomach. This hormone is necessary for the body's correct use of food, especially sugar. Diabetes occurs when the pancreas does not make enough insulin to meet your body's needs.

To control your diabetes, your doctor has prescribed injections of insulin products to keep your blood glucose at a near-normal level. You have been instructed to test your blood and/or your urine regularly for glucose. Studies have shown that some chronic complications of diabetes such as eye disease, kidney disease, and nerve disease can be significantly reduced if the blood sugar is maintained as close to normal as possible. The American Diabetes Association recommends that if your premeal glucose levels are consistently above 140 mg/dL or your hemoglobin A_{1c} (HbA_{1c}) is more than 8%, consult your doctor. A change in your diabetes therapy may be needed. If your blood tests consistently show below-normal glucose levels, you should also let your doctor know. Proper control of your diabetes requires close and constant cooperation with your doctor. Despite diabetes, you can lead an active and healthy life if you eat a balanced diet, exercise regularly, and take your insulin injections as prescribed.

Always keep an extra supply of insulin as well as a spare syringe and needle on hand. Always wear diabetic identification so that appropriate treatment can be given if complications occur away from home.

LENTE HUMAN INSULIN

Description

Humulin is synthesized in a special non-disease-producing laboratory strain of *Escherichia coli* bacteria that has been genetically altered by the addition of the gene for human insulin production. Humulin L is an amorphous and crystalline suspension of human insulin with zinc providing an intermediate-acting insulin with a slower onset and a longer duration of activity (up to 24 hours) than regular insulin. The time course of action of any insulin may vary considerably in different individuals or at different times in the same individual. As with all insulin preparations, the duration of action of Humulin L is dependent on dose, site of injection, blood supply, temperature, and physical activity. Humulin L is a sterile suspension and is for subcutaneous injection only. It should not be used intravenously or intramuscularly. The concentration of Humulin L is 100 units/mL (U-100).

Identification

Human insulin manufactured by Eli Lilly and Company has the trademark Humulin and is available in 6 formulations—Regular (**R**), NPH (**N**), Lente (**L**), Ultralente® (**U**), 50% Human Insulin Isophane Suspension [NPH]/50% Human Insulin Injection [buffered regular] (**50/50**), and 70% Human Insulin Isophane Suspension [NPH]/30% Human Insulin Injection [buffered regular] (**70/30**). Your doctor has prescribed the type of insulin that he/she believes is best for you. **DO NOT USE ANY OTHER INSULIN EXCEPT ON HIS/HER ADVICE AND DIRECTION.**

Always check the carton and the bottle label for the name and letter designation of the insulin you receive from your pharmacy to make sure it is the same as that your doctor has prescribed.

Always examine the appearance of your bottle of insulin before withdrawing each dose. A bottle of Humulin L must be carefully shaken or rotated before each injection so that the contents are uniformly mixed. Humulin L should look uniformly cloudy or milky after mixing. Do not use it if the insulin substance (the white material) remains at the bottom of the bottle after mixing. Do not use a bottle of Humulin L if there are clumps in the insulin after mixing. Always check the appearance of your bottle of insulin before using, and if you note anything unusual in the appearance of your insulin or notice your insulin requirements changing markedly, consult your doctor.

Storage

Insulin should be stored in a refrigerator but not in the freezer. If refrigeration is not possible, the bottle of insulin that you are currently using can be kept unrefrigerated as long as it is kept as cool as possible (below 86°F [30°C]) and away from heat and light. Do not use insulin if it has been frozen. Do not use a bottle of insulin after the expiration date stamped on the label.

INJECTION PROCEDURES

Correct Syringe

Doses of insulin are measured in **units**. U-100 insulin contains 100 units/mL (1 mL = 1 cc). With Humulin L, it is important to use a syringe that is marked for U-100 insulin preparations. Failure to use the proper syringe can lead to a mistake in dosage, causing serious problems for you, such as a blood glucose level that is too low or too high.

Syringe Use

To help avoid contamination and possible infection, follow these instructions exactly.

Disposable syringes and needles should be used only once and then discarded. **NEEDLES AND SYRINGES MUST NOT BE SHARED.**

Reusable syringes and needles must be sterilized before each injection. **Follow the package directions supplied with your syringe.** Described below are 2 methods of sterilizing.

Boiling

1. Put syringe, plunger, and needle in strainer, place in saucepan, and cover with water. Boil for 5 minutes.
2. Remove articles from water. When they have cooled, insert plunger into barrel, and fasten needle to syringe with a slight twist.
3. Push plunger in and out several times until water is completely removed.

Isopropyl Alcohol

If the syringe, plunger, and needle cannot be boiled, as when you are traveling, they may be sterilized by immersion for at least 5 minutes in Isopropyl Alcohol, 91%. Do not use bathing, rubbing, or medicated alcohol for this sterilization. If the syringe is sterilized with alcohol, it must be absolutely dry before use.

Preparing the Dose

1. Wash your hands.
2. Carefully shake or rotate the insulin bottle several times to completely mix the insulin.
3. Inspect the insulin. Humulin L should look uniformly cloudy or milky. Do not use it if you notice anything unusual in the appearance.
4. If using a new bottle, flip off the plastic protective cap, but **do not** remove the stopper. When using a new bottle, wipe the top of the bottle with an alcohol swab.
5. If you are mixing insulins, refer to the instructions for mixing that follow.
6. Draw air into the syringe equal to your insulin dose. Put the needle through rubber top of the insulin bottle and inject the air into the bottle.
7. Turn the bottle and syringe upside down. Hold the bottle and syringe firmly in 1 hand and shake gently.
8. Making sure the tip of the needle is in the insulin, withdraw the correct dose of insulin into the syringe.
9. Before removing the needle from the bottle, check your syringe for air bubbles which reduce the amount of insulin in it. If bubbles are present, hold the syringe straight up and tap its side until the bubbles float to the top. Push them out with the plunger and withdraw the correct dose.
10. Remove the needle from the bottle and lay the syringe down so that the needle does not touch anything.

Mixing Humulin L with Regular or Ultralente Human Insulin

1. Lente human insulin should be mixed with regular or Ultralente human insulin only on the advice of your doctor.
2. Draw air into your syringe equal to the amount of Humulin L you are taking. Insert the needle into the Humulin L bottle and inject the air. Withdraw the needle.
3. Now inject air into your regular or Ultralente human insulin bottle in the same manner, but **do not** withdraw the needle.
4. Turn the bottle and syringe upside down.
5. Making sure the tip of the needle is in the insulin, withdraw the correct dose of regular or Ultralente insulin into the syringe.
6. Before removing the needle from the bottle, check your syringe for air bubbles which reduce the amount of insulin in it. If bubbles are present, hold the syringe straight up and tap its side until the bubbles float to the top. Push them out with the plunger and withdraw the correct dose.
7. Remove the needle from the bottle of regular or Ultralente insulin and insert it into the bottle of Humulin L. Turn the bottle and syringe upside down. Hold the bottle and syringe firmly in 1 hand and shake gently. Making sure the tip of the needle is in the insulin, withdraw your dose of Humulin L.
8. Remove the needle and lay the syringe down so that the needle does not touch anything.

Follow your doctor's instructions on whether to mix your insulins ahead of time or just before giving your injection. It is important to be consistent in your method.

Syringes from different manufacturers may vary in the amount of space between the bottom line and the needle. Because of this, do not change:

- the sequence of mixing, or
- the model and brand of syringe or needle that the doctor has prescribed.

Injection

Cleanse the skin with alcohol where the injection is to be made. Stabilize the skin by spreading it or pinching up a large area. Insert the needle as instructed by your doctor. Push the plunger in as far as it will go. Pull the needle out and apply gentle pressure over the injection site for several seconds. **Do not rub the area.** To avoid tissue damage, give the next injection at a site at least 1/2" from the previous site.

DOSAGE

Your doctor has told you which insulin to use, how much, and when and how often to inject it. Because each patient's case of diabetes is different, this schedule has been individualized for you.

Your usual insulin dose may be affected by changes in your food, activity, or work schedule. Carefully follow your doctor's instructions to allow for these changes. Other things that may affect your insulin dose are:

Illness

Illness, especially with nausea and vomiting, may cause your insulin requirements to change. Even if you are not eating, you will still require insulin. You and your doctor should establish a sick day plan for you to use in case of illness. When you are sick, test your blood/urine frequently and call your doctor as instructed.

Pregnancy

Good control of diabetes is especially important for you and your unborn baby. Pregnancy may make managing your diabetes more difficult. If you are planning to have a baby, are pregnant, or are nursing a baby, consult your doctor.

Medication

Insulin requirements may be increased if you are taking other drugs with hyperglycemic activity, such as oral contraceptives, corticosteroids, or thyroid replacement therapy. Insulin requirements may be reduced in the presence of drugs with hypoglycemic activity, such as oral hypoglycemics, salicylates (for example, aspirin), sulfa antibiotics, and certain antidepressants. Always discuss any medications you are taking with your doctor.

Exercise

Exercise may lower your body's need for insulin during and for some time after the activity. Exercise may also speed up the effect of an insulin dose, especially if the exercise involves the area of injection site (for example, the leg should not be used for injection just prior to running). Discuss with your doctor how you should adjust your regimen to accommodate exercise.

Travel

Persons traveling across more than 2 time zones should consult their doctor concerning adjustments in their insulin schedule.

Continued on next page

*** Identi-Code® symbol. This product information was prepared in June 2004. Current information on these and other products of Eli Lilly and Company may be obtained by direct inquiry to Lilly Research Laboratories, Lilly Corporate Center, Indianapolis, Indiana 46285, (800) 545-5979.**

Humulin L—Cont.

COMMON PROBLEMS OF DIABETES

Hypoglycemia (Insulin Reaction)

Hypoglycemia (too little glucose in the blood) is one of the most frequent adverse events experienced by insulin users. It can be brought about by:

1. Taking too much insulin
2. Missing or delaying meals
3. Exercising or working more than usual
4. An infection or illness (especially with diarrhea or vomiting)
5. A change in the body's need for insulin
6. Diseases of the adrenal, pituitary, or thyroid gland, or progression of kidney or liver disease
7. Interactions with other drugs that lower blood glucose, such as oral hypoglycemics, salicylates (for example, aspirin), sulfa antibiotics, and certain antidepressants
8. Consumption of alcoholic beverages

Symptoms of mild to moderate hypoglycemia may occur suddenly and can include:

- sweating
- dizziness
- palpitation
- tremor
- hunger
- restlessness
- tingling in the hands, feet, lips, or tongue
- lightheadedness
- inability to concentrate
- headache
- drowsiness
- sleep disturbances
- anxiety
- blurred vision
- slurred speech
- depressed mood
- irritability
- abnormal behavior
- unsteady movement
- personality changes

Signs of severe hypoglycemia can include:

- disorientation
- unconsciousness
- seizures
- death

Therefore, it is important that assistance be obtained immediately.

Early warning symptoms of hypoglycemia may be different or less pronounced under certain conditions, such as long duration of diabetes, diabetic nerve disease, medications such as beta-blockers, change in insulin preparations, or intensified control (3 or more insulin injections per day) of diabetes.

A few patients who have experienced hypoglycemic reactions after transfer from animal-source insulin to human insulin have reported that the early warning symptoms of hypoglycemia were less pronounced or different from those experienced with their previous insulin.

Without recognition of early warning symptoms, you may not be able to take steps to avoid more serious hypoglycemia. Be alert for all of the various types of symptoms that may indicate hypoglycemia. Patients who experience hypoglycemia without early warning symptoms should monitor their blood glucose frequently, especially prior to activities such as driving. If the blood glucose is below your normal fasting glucose, you should consider eating or drinking sugar-containing foods to treat your hypoglycemia.

Mild to moderate hypoglycemia may be treated by eating foods or drinks that contain sugar. Patients should always carry a quick source of sugar, such as candy mints or glucose tablets. More severe hypoglycemia may require the assistance of another person. Patients who are unable to take sugar orally or who are unconscious require an injection of glucagon or should be treated with intravenous administration of glucose at a medical facility.

You should learn to recognize your own symptoms of hypoglycemia. If you are uncertain about these symptoms, you should monitor your blood glucose frequently to help you learn to recognize the symptoms that you experience with hypoglycemia.

If you have frequent episodes of hypoglycemia or experience difficulty in recognizing the symptoms, you should consult your doctor to discuss possible changes in therapy, meal plans, and/or exercise programs to help you avoid hypoglycemia.

Hyperglycemia and Diabetic Acidosis

Hyperglycemia (too much glucose in the blood) may develop if your body has too little insulin. Hyperglycemia can be brought about by:

1. Omitting your insulin or taking less than the doctor has prescribed
2. Eating significantly more than your meal plan suggests
3. Developing a fever, infection, or other significant stressful situation

In patients with insulin-dependent diabetes, prolonged hyperglycemia can result in diabetic acidosis. The first symptoms of diabetic acidosis usually come on gradually, over a period of hours or days, and include a drowsy feeling, flushed face, thirst, loss of appetite, and fruity odor on the breath. With acidosis, urine tests show large amounts of glucose and acetone. Heavy breathing and a rapid pulse are more severe symptoms. If uncorrected, prolonged hyperglycemia or diabetic acidosis can lead to nausea, vomiting, dehydration, loss of consciousness or death. Therefore, it is important that you obtain medical assistance immediately.

Lipodystrophy

Rarely, administration of insulin subcutaneously can result in lipoatrophy (depression in the skin) or lipohypertrophy (enlargement or thickening of tissue). If you notice either of these conditions, consult your doctor. A change in your injection technique may help alleviate the problem.

Allergy to Insulin

Local Allergy—Patients occasionally experience redness, swelling, and itching at the site of injection of insulin. This condition, called local allergy, usually clears up in a few days to a few weeks. In some instances, this condition may be related to factors other than insulin, such as irritants in the skin cleansing agent or poor injection technique. If you have local reactions, contact your doctor.

Systemic Allergy—Less common, but potentially more serious, is generalized allergy to insulin, which may cause rash over the whole body, shortness of breath, wheezing, reduction in blood pressure, fast pulse, or sweating. Severe cases of generalized allergy may be life threatening. If you think you are having a generalized allergic reaction to insulin, notify a doctor immediately.

ADDITIONAL INFORMATION

Additional information about diabetes may be obtained from your diabetes educator.

DIABETES FORECAST is a national magazine designed especially for patients with diabetes and their families and is available by subscription from the American Diabetes Association, National Service Center, 1660 Duke Street, Alexandria, Virginia 22314, 1-800-DIABETES (1-800-342-2383). Another publication, **DIABETES COUNTDOWN**, is available from the Juvenile Diabetes Foundation International (JDF), 120 Wall Street, 19th Floor, New York, New York 10005, 1-800-JDF-CURE (1-800-533-2873).

Additional information about Humulin can be obtained by calling 1-888-88-LILLY (1-888-885-4559).

Literature revised August 3, 2000

PA 6356 AMP

HUMULIN® N OTC

[*hū 'mū-lĭn ĕn*]

NPH

HUMAN INSULIN (rDNA ORIGIN)

ISOPHANE SUSPENSION

INFORMATION FOR THE PATIENT

WARNINGS

THIS LILLY HUMAN INSULIN PRODUCT DIFFERS FROM ANIMAL-SOURCE INSULINS BECAUSE IT IS STRUCTURALLY IDENTICAL TO THE INSULIN PRODUCED BY YOUR BODY'S PANCREAS AND BECAUSE OF ITS UNIQUE MANUFACTURING PROCESS.

ANY CHANGE OF INSULIN SHOULD BE MADE CAUTIOUSLY AND ONLY UNDER MEDICAL SUPERVISION. CHANGES IN STRENGTH, MANUFACTURER, TYPE (E.G., REGULAR, NPH, LENTE®), SPECIES (BEEF, PORK, BEEF-PORK, HUMAN), OR METHOD OF MANUFACTURE (rDNA VERSUS ANIMAL-SOURCE INSULIN) MAY RESULT IN THE NEED FOR A CHANGE IN DOSAGE.

SOME PATIENTS TAKING HUMULIN® (HUMAN INSULIN, rDNA ORIGIN) MAY REQUIRE A CHANGE IN DOSAGE FROM THAT USED WITH ANIMAL-SOURCE INSULINS. IF AN ADJUSTMENT IS NEEDED, IT MAY OCCUR WITH THE FIRST DOSE OR DURING THE FIRST SEVERAL WEEKS OR MONTHS.

DIABETES

Insulin is a hormone produced by the pancreas, a large gland that lies near the stomach. This hormone is necessary for the body's correct use of food, especially sugar. Diabetes occurs when the pancreas does not make enough insulin to meet your body's needs.

To control your diabetes, your doctor has prescribed injections of insulin products to keep your blood glucose at a near-normal level. You have been instructed to test your blood and/or your urine regularly for glucose. Studies have shown that some chronic complications of diabetes such as eye disease, kidney disease, and nerve disease can be significantly reduced if the blood sugar is maintained as close to normal as possible. The American Diabetes Association recommends that if your premeal glucose levels are consistently above 140 mg/dL or your hemoglobin A_{1c} (HbA_{1c}) is more than 8%, consult your doctor. A change in your diabetes therapy may be needed. If your blood tests consistently show below-normal glucose levels you should also let your doctor know. Proper control of your diabetes requires close and constant cooperation with your doctor. Despite diabetes, you can lead an active and healthy life if you eat a balanced diet, exercise regularly, and take your insulin injections as prescribed.

Always keep an extra supply of insulin as well as a spare syringe and needle on hand. Always wear diabetic identification so that appropriate treatment can be given if complications occur away from home.

NPH HUMAN INSULIN

Description

Humulin is synthesized in a special non-disease-producing laboratory strain of *Escherichia coli* bacteria that has been genetically altered by the addition of the gene for human insulin production. Humulin N is a crystalline suspension of human insulin with protamine and zinc providing an intermediate-acting insulin with a slower onset of action and a longer duration of activity (up to 24 hours) than that of regular insulin. The time course of action of any insulin may vary considerably in different individuals or at different times in the same individual. As with all insulin preparations, the duration of action of Humulin N is dependent on dose, site of injection, blood supply, temperature, and physical activity. Humulin N is a sterile suspension and is for subcutaneous injection only. It should not be used intravenously or intramuscularly. The concentration of Humulin N is 100 units/mL (U-100).

Identification

Human insulin manufactured by Eli Lilly and Company has the trademark Humulin and is available in 6 formulations—Regular (**R**), NPH (**N**), Lente (**L**), Ultralente® (**U**), 50% Human Insulin Isophane Suspension [NPH]/50% Human Insulin Injection [buffered regular] (**50/50**), and 70% Human Insulin Isophane Suspension [NPH]/30% Human Insulin Injection [buffered regular] (**70/30**). Your doctor has prescribed the type of insulin that he/she believes is best for you. **DO NOT USE ANY OTHER INSULIN EXCEPT ON HIS/HER ADVICE AND DIRECTION.**

Always check the carton and the bottle label for the name and letter designation of the insulin you receive from your pharmacy to make sure it is the same as that your doctor has prescribed.

Always examine the appearance of your bottle of insulin before withdrawing each dose. A bottle of Humulin N must be carefully shaken or rotated before each injection so that the contents are uniformly mixed. Humulin N should look uniformly cloudy or milky after mixing. Do not use it if the insulin substance (the white material) remains at the bottom of the bottle after mixing. Do not use a bottle of Humulin N if there are clumps in the insulin after mixing. Do not use a bottle of Humulin N if solid white particles stick to the bottom or wall of the bottle, giving it a frosted appearance. Always check the appearance of your bottle of insulin before using, and if you note anything unusual in the appearance of your insulin or notice your insulin requirements changing markedly, consult your doctor.

Storage

Insulin should be stored in a refrigerator but not in the freezer. If refrigeration is not possible, the bottle of insulin that you are currently using can be kept unrefrigerated as long as it is kept as cool as possible (below 86°F [30°C]) and away from heat and light. Do not use insulin if it has been frozen. Do not use a bottle of insulin after the expiration date stamped on the label.

INJECTION PROCEDURES

Correct Syringe

Doses of insulin are measured in **units.** U-100 insulin contains 100 units/mL (1 mL = 1 cc). With Humulin N, it is important to use a syringe that is marked for U-100 insulin preparations. Failure to use the proper syringe can lead to a mistake in dosage, causing serious problems for you, such as a blood glucose level that is too low or too high.

Syringe Use

To help avoid contamination and possible infection, follow these instructions exactly.

Disposable syringes and needles should be used only once and then discarded. **NEEDLES AND SYRINGES MUST NOT BE SHARED.**

Reusable syringes and needles must be sterilized before each injection. **Follow the package directions supplied with your syringe.** Described below are 2 methods of sterilizing.

Boiling

1. Put syringe, plunger, and needle in strainer, place in saucepan, and cover with water. Boil for 5 minutes.
2. Remove articles from water. When they have cooled, insert plunger into barrel, and fasten needle to syringe with a slight twist.
3. Push plunger in and out several times until water is completely removed.

Isopropyl Alcohol

If the syringe, plunger, and needle cannot be boiled, as when you are traveling, they may be sterilized by immersion for at least 5 minutes in Isopropyl Alcohol, 91%. Do not use bathing, rubbing, or medicated alcohol for this sterilization. If the syringe is sterilized with alcohol, it must be absolutely dry before use.

Preparing the Dose

1. Wash your hands.
2. Carefully shake or rotate the insulin bottle several times to completely mix the insulin.
3. Inspect the insulin. Humulin N should look uniformly cloudy or milky. Do not use it if you notice anything unusual in the appearance.
4. If using a new bottle, flip off the plastic protective cap, but **do not** remove the stopper. When using a new bottle, wipe the top of the bottle with an alcohol swab.
5. If you are mixing insulins, refer to the instructions for mixing that follow.
6. Draw air into the syringe equal to your insulin dose. Put the needle through rubber top of the insulin bottle and inject the air into the bottle.
7. Turn the bottle and syringe upside down. Hold the bottle and syringe firmly in 1 hand and shake gently.
8. Making sure the tip of the needle is in the insulin, withdraw the correct dose of insulin into the syringe.
9. Before removing the needle from the bottle, check your syringe for air bubbles which reduce the amount of insulin in it. If bubbles are present, hold the syringe

straight up and tap its side until the bubbles float to the top. Push them out with the plunger and withdraw the correct dose.
10. Remove the needle from the bottle and lay the syringe down so that the needle does not touch anything.

Mixing Humulin N and Regular Human Insulin

1. NPH human insulin should be mixed only with regular human insulin.
2. Draw air into your syringe equal to the amount of Humulin N you are taking. Insert the needle into the Humulin N bottle and inject the air. Withdraw the needle.
3. Now inject air into your regular human insulin bottle in the same manner, but **do not** withdraw the needle.
4. Turn the bottle and syringe upside down.
5. Making sure the tip of the needle is in the insulin, withdraw the correct dose of regular insulin into the syringe.
6. Before removing the needle from the bottle, check your syringe for air bubbles which reduce the amount of insulin in it. If bubbles are present, hold the syringe straight up and tap its side until the bubbles float to the top. Push them out with the plunger and withdraw the correct dose.
7. Remove needle from the bottle of regular insulin and insert it into the bottle of Humulin N. Turn the bottle and syringe upside down. Hold the bottle and syringe firmly in 1 hand and shake gently. Making sure the tip of the needle is in the insulin, withdraw your dose of Humulin N.
8. Remove the needle and lay the syringe down so that the needle does not touch anything.

Follow your doctor's instructions on whether to mix your insulins ahead of time or just before giving your injection. It is important to be consistent in your method.

Syringes from different manufacturers may vary in the amount of space between the bottom line and the needle. Because of this, do not change:

- the sequence of mixing, or
- the model and brand of syringe or needle that the doctor has prescribed.

Injection

Cleanse the skin with alcohol where the injection is to be made. Stabilize the skin by spreading it or pinching up a large area. Insert the needle as instructed by your doctor. Push the plunger in as far as it will go. Pull the needle out and apply gentle pressure over the injection site for several seconds. **Do not rub the area.** To avoid tissue damage, give the next injection at a site at least ½″ from the previous site.

DOSAGE

Your doctor has told you which insulin to use, how much, and when and how often to inject it. Because each patient's case of diabetes is different, this schedule has been individualized for you.

Your usual insulin dose may be affected by changes in your food, activity, or work schedule. Carefully follow your doctor's instructions to allow for these changes. Other things that may affect your insulin dose are:

Illness

Illness, especially with nausea and vomiting, may cause your insulin requirements to change. Even if you are not eating, you will still require insulin. You and your doctor should establish a sick day plan for you to use in case of illness. When you are sick, test your blood/urine frequently and call your doctor as instructed.

Pregnancy

Good control of diabetes is especially important for you and your unborn baby. Pregnancy may make managing your diabetes more difficult. If you are planning to have a baby, are pregnant, or are nursing a baby, consult your doctor.

Medication

Insulin requirements may be increased if you are taking other drugs with hyperglycemic activity, such as oral contraceptives, corticosteroids, or thyroid replacement therapy. Insulin requirements may be reduced in the presence of drugs with hypoglycemic activity, such as oral hypoglycemics, salicylates (for example, aspirin), sulfa antibiotics, and certain antidepressants. Always discuss any medications you are taking with your doctor.

Exercise

Exercise may lower your body's need for insulin during and for some time after the activity. Exercise may also speed up the effect of an insulin dose, especially if the exercise involves the area of injection site (for example, the leg should not be used for injection just prior to running). Discuss with your doctor how you should adjust your regimen to accomodate exercise.

Travel

Persons traveling across more than 2 time zones should consult their doctor concerning adjustments in their insulin schedule.

COMMON PROBLEMS OF DIABETES

Hypoglycemia (Insulin Reaction)

Hypoglycemia (too little glucose in the blood) is one of the most frequent adverse events experienced by insulin users. It can be brought about by:

1. Taking too much insulin
2. Missing or delaying meals
3. Exercising or working more than usual
4. An infection or illness (especially with diarrhea or vomiting)
5. A change in the body's need for insulin
6. Diseases of the adrenal, pituitary, or thyroid gland, or progression of kidney or liver disease
7. Interactions with other drugs that lower blood glucose, such as oral hypoglycemics, salicylates (for example, aspirin), sulfa antibiotics, and certain antidepressants
8. Consumption alcoholic beverages

Symptoms of mild to moderate hypoglycemia may occur suddenly and can include:

- sweating
- dizziness
- palpitation
- tremor
- hunger
- restlessness
- tingling in the hands, feet, lips, or tongue
- lightheadedness
- inability to concentrate
- headache
- drowsiness
- sleep disturbances
- anxiety
- blurred vision
- slurred speech
- depressed mood
- irritability
- abnormal behavior
- unsteady movement
- personality changes

Signs of severe hypoglycemia can include:

- disorientation
- unconsciousness
- seizures
- death

Therefore, it is important that assistance be obtained immediately.

Early warning symptoms of hypoglycemia may be different or less pronounced under certain conditions, such as long duration of diabetes, diabetic nerve disease, medications such as beta-blockers, change in insulin preparations, or intensified control (3 or more insulin injections per day) of diabetes.

A few patients who have experienced hypoglycemic reactions after transfer from animal-source insulin to human insulin have reported that the early warning symptoms of hypoglycemia were less pronounced or different from those experienced with their previous insulin.

Without recognition of early warning symptoms, you may not be able to take steps to avoid more serious hypoglycemia. Be alert for all of the various types of symptoms that may indicate hypoglycemia. Patients who experience hypoglycemia without early warning symptoms should monitor their blood glucose frequently, especially prior to activities such as driving. If the blood glucose is below your normal fasting glucose, you should consider eating or drinking sugar-containing foods to treat your hypoglycemia.

Mild to moderate hypoglycemia may be treated by eating foods or drinks that contain sugar. Patients should always carry a quick source of sugar, such as candy mints or glucose tablets. More severe hypoglycemia may require the assistance of another person. Patients who are unable to take sugar orally or who are unconscious require an injection of glucagon or should be treated with intravenous administration of glucose at a medical facility.

You should learn to recognize your own symptoms of hypoglycemia. If you are uncertain about these symptoms, you should monitor your blood glucose frequently to help you learn to recognize the symptoms that you experience with hypoglycemia.

If you have frequent episodes of hypoglycemia or experience difficulty in recognizing the symptoms, you should consult your doctor to discuss possible changes in therapy, meal plans, and/or exercise programs to help you avoid hypoglycemia.

Hyperglycemia and Diabetic Acidosis

Hyperglycemia (too much glucose in the blood) may develop if your body has too little insulin. Hyperglycemia can be brought about by:

1. Omitting your insulin or taking less than the doctor has prescribed
2. Eating significantly more than your meal plan suggests
3. Developing a fever, infection, or other significant stressful situation

In patients with insulin-dependent diabetes, prolonged hyperglycemia can result in diabetic acidosis. The first symptoms of diabetic acidosis usually come on gradually, over a period of hours or days, and include a drowsy feeling, flushed face, thirst, loss of appetite, and fruity odor on the breath. With acidosis, urine tests show large amounts of glucose and acetone. Heavy breathing and a rapid pulse are more severe symptoms. If uncorrected, prolonged hyperglycemia or diabetic acidosis can lead to nausea, vomiting, dehydration, loss of consciousness or death. Therefore, it is important that you obtain medical assistance immediately.

Lipodystrophy

Rarely, administration of insulin subcutaneously can result in lipoatrophy (depression in the skin) or lipohypertrophy (enlargement or thickening of tissue). If you notice either of these conditions, consult your doctor. A change in your injection technique may help alleviate the problem.

Allergy to Insulin

Local Allergy—Patients occasionally experience redness, swelling, and itching at the site of injection of insulin. This condition, called local allergy, usually clears up in a few days to a few weeks. In some instances, this condition may be related to factors other than insulin, such as irritants in the skin cleansing agent or poor injection technique. If you have local reactions, contact your doctor.

Systemic Allergy—Less common, but potentially more serious, is generalized allergy to insulin, which may cause rash over the whole body, shortness of breath, wheezing, reduction in blood pressure, fast pulse, or sweating. Severe cases of generalized allergy may be life threatening. If you think you are having a generalized allergic reaction to insulin, notify a doctor immediately.

ADDITIONAL INFORMATION

Additional information about diabetes may be obtained from your diabetes educator.

DIABETES FORECAST is a national magazine designed especially for patients with diabetes and their families and is available by subscription from the American Diabetes Association, National Service Center, 1660 Duke Street, Alexandria, Virginia 22314, 1-800-DIABETES (1-800-342-2383).

Another publication, **DIABETES COUNTDOWN**, is available from the Juvenile Diabetes Foundation International (JDF), 120 Wall Street, 19th Floor, New York, New York 10005, 1-800-JDF-CURE (1-800-533-2873).

Additional information about Humulin can be obtained by calling 1-888-88-LILLY (1-888-885-4559).

Literature revised August 3, 2000

PA 6347 AMP

HUMULIN® N Pen ℞

[*hū ′mū-lĭn ĕn*]

NPH HUMAN INSULIN (rDNA ORIGIN) ISOPHANE SUSPENSION

INFORMATION FOR THE PATIENT
3 ML DISPOSABLE INSULIN DELIVERY DEVICE

WARNINGS

THIS LILLY HUMAN INSULIN PRODUCT DIFFERS FROM ANIMAL-SOURCE INSULINS BECAUSE IT IS STRUCTURALLY IDENTICAL TO THE INSULIN PRODUCED BY YOUR BODY'S PANCREAS AND BECAUSE OF ITS UNIQUE MANUFACTURING PROCESS.

ANY CHANGE OF INSULIN SHOULD BE MADE CAUTIOUSLY AND ONLY UNDER MEDICAL SUPERVISION. CHANGES IN STRENGTH, MANUFACTURER, TYPE (E.G., REGULAR, NPH, LENTE, ETC), SPECIES (BEEF, PORK, BEEF-PORK, HUMAN), OR METHOD OF MANUFACTURE (rDNA VERSUS ANIMAL-SOURCE INSULIN) MAY RESULT IN THE NEED FOR A CHANGE IN DOSAGE.

SOME PATIENTS TAKING HUMULIN® (HUMAN INSULIN, rDNA ORIGIN) MAY REQUIRE A CHANGE IN DOSAGE FROM THAT USED WITH ANIMAL-SOURCE INSULINS. IF AN ADJUSTMENT IS NEEDED, IT MAY OCCUR WITH THE FIRST DOSE OR DURING THE FIRST SEVERAL WEEKS OR MONTHS.

TO OBTAIN AN ACCURATE DOSE, CAREFULLY READ AND FOLLOW THE "DISPOSABLE INSULIN DELIVERY DEVICE USER MANUAL" AND THIS INFORMATION FOR THE PATIENT INSERT BEFORE USING THIS PRODUCT. BEFORE EACH INJECTION, YOU SHOULD PRIME THE PEN, A NECESSARY STEP TO MAKE SURE THE PEN IS READY TO DOSE. PRIMING THE PEN IS IMPORTANT TO CONFIRM THAT INSULIN COMES OUT WHEN YOU PUSH THE INJECTION BUTTON AND TO REMOVE AIR THAT MAY COLLECT IN THE INSULIN CARTRIDGE DURING NORMAL USE. IF YOU DO NOT PRIME, YOU MAY RECEIVE TOO MUCH OR TOO LITTLE INSULIN (*see also* INSTRUCTIONS FOR PEN USE section.)

DIABETES

Insulin is a hormone produced by the pancreas, a large gland that lies near the stomach. This hormone is necessary for the body's correct use of food, especially sugar. Diabetes occurs when the pancreas does not make enough insulin to meet your body's needs.

To control your diabetes, your doctor has prescribed injections of insulin products to keep your blood glucose at a near-normal level. You have been instructed to test your blood and/or your urine regularly for glucose. Studies have shown that some chronic complications of diabetes such as eye disease, kidney disease, and nerve disease can be significantly reduced if the blood sugar is maintained as close to normal as possible. The American Diabetes Association recommends that if your premeal glucose levels are consistently above 140 mg/dL or your hemoglobin A_{1c} (HbA_{1c}) is more than 8%, consult your doctor. A change in your diabetes therapy may be needed. If your blood tests consistently show below-normal glucose levels, you should also let your doctor know. Proper control of your diabetes requires close and constant cooperation with your doctor. Despite diabetes, you can lead an active and healthy life if you eat a balanced diet, exercise regularly, and take your insulin injections as prescribed.

Continued on next page

*** Identi-Code® symbol. This product information was prepared in June 2004. Current information on these and other products of Eli Lilly and Company may be obtained by direct inquiry to Lilly Research Laboratories, Lilly Corporate Center, Indianapolis, Indiana 46285, (800) 545-5979.**

Humulin N Pen—Cont.

Always keep an extra supply of insulin as well as a spare syringe and needle on hand. Always wear diabetic identification so that appropriate treatment can be given if complications occur away from home.

NPH HUMAN INSULIN

DESCRIPTION

Humulin is synthesized in a non-disease-producing special laboratory strain of *Escherichia coli* bacteria that has been genetically altered by the addition of the human gene for insulin production. Humulin® N is a crystalline suspension of human insulin with protamine and zinc providing an intermediate-acting insulin with a slower onset of action and a longer duration of activity (up to 24 hours) than that of regular insulin. The time course of action of any insulin may vary considerably in different individuals or at different times in the same individual. As with all insulin preparations, the duration of action of Humulin N is dependent on dose, site of injection, blood supply, temperature, and physical activity. Humulin N is a sterile suspension and is for subcutaneous injection only. It should not be used intravenously or intramuscularly. The concentration of Humulin N in Humulin N Pen is 100 units/mL (U-100).

Identification

Humulin disposable insulin delivery devices, manufactured by Eli Lilly and Company, are available in 2 formulations—NPH and 70/30.

Your doctor has prescribed the type of insulin that he/she believes is best for you. **DO NOT USE ANY OTHER INSULIN EXCEPT ON HIS/HER ADVICE AND DIRECTION.**

The Humulin N Pen is available in boxes of 5 disposable insulin delivery devices ("insulin pens"). The Humulin N Pen is not designed to allow any other insulin to be mixed in its cartridge, or for the cartridge to be removed.

Always examine the appearance of Humulin N suspension in the insulin pen before administering a dose. A cartridge of Humulin N contains a small glass bead to assist in mixing. Humulin N Pen must be rolled between the palms 10 times and inverted 180° 10 times before each injection so that the contents are uniformly mixed (*see* Figures 1 and 2). Inspect the Humulin N suspension for uniform mixing and repeat the above steps as necessary.

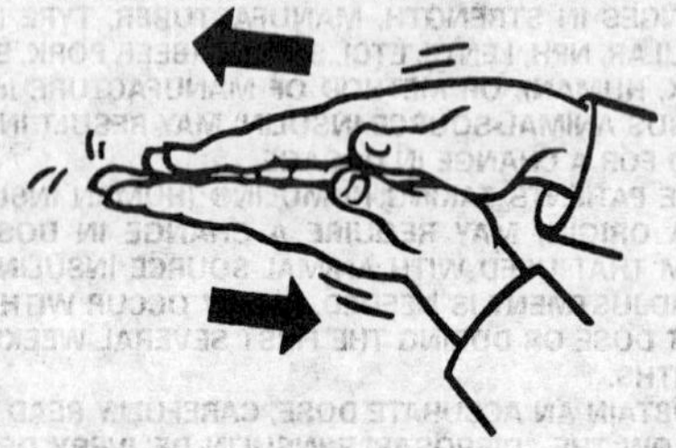

Figure 1.

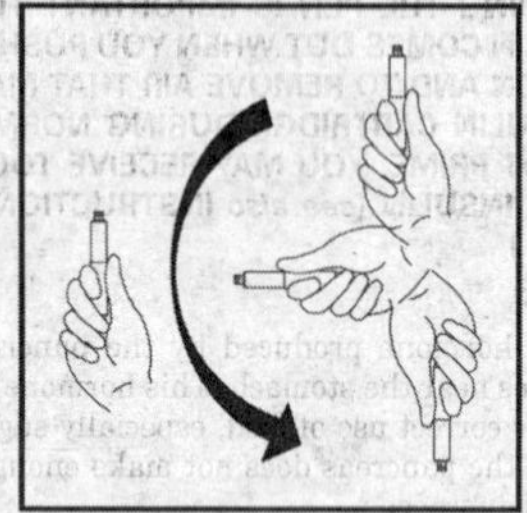

Figure 2.

Humulin N should look uniformly cloudy or milky after mixing. Do not use if the insulin substance (the white material) remains visibly separated from the liquid after mixing. Do not use the Humulin N Pen if there are clumps in the insulin after mixing. Do not use the Humulin N Pen if solid white particles stick to the walls of the cartridge, giving it a frosted appearance.

Always check the appearance of the Humulin N suspension in the insulin pen before using, and if you note anything unusual in the appearance of Humulin N suspension or notice your insulin requirements changing markedly, consult your doctor.

Never attempt to remove the cartridge from the Humulin N Pen. Inspect the cartridge through the clear cartridge holder.

Storage

Humulin N Pens should be stored in a refrigerator but not in the freezer. The Humulin N Pen that you are currently using should not be refrigerated but should be kept as cool as possible (below 86°F [30°C]) and away from heat and light. Do not use an insulin pen if it has been frozen. Unrefrigerated Humulin N Pens **must be discarded after 2 weeks,** even if they still contain insulin. Do not use Humulin N Pens after the expiration date stamped on the label.

INSTRUCTIONS FOR PEN USE

It is important to read, understand, and follow the instructions in the "Disposable Insulin Delivery Device User Manual" before using. Failure to follow instructions may result in getting too much or too little insulin. The needle must be changed and the pen must be primed before each injection to make sure the pen is ready to dose. These steps are important to confirm that insulin comes out when you push the injection button, and to remove air that may collect in the insulin cartridge during normal use.

Every time you inject:

- **Use a new needle**
- **Prime to make sure the pen is ready to dose**
- **Make sure you got a full dose.**

NEVER SHARE INSULIN PENS, CARTRIDGES, OR NEEDLES.

PREPARING THE PEN FOR INJECTION

1. Always check the appearance of the Humulin N suspension in the insulin pen before using.
2. Roll the Humulin N Pen between the palms 10 times (*see* Figure 1 above).
3. Holding the Humulin N Pen by one end, invert it 180° slowly 10 times to allow the glass bead to travel the full length of the cartridge with each inversion (*see* Figure 2 above). The cartridge is contained in the clear cartridge holder of the Humulin N Pen.
4. Inspect the appearance of the Humulin N suspension to make sure the contents look uniformly cloudy or milky. If not, repeat the above steps until the contents are mixed. Do not use a Humulin N Pen if there are clumps in the insulin or if solid white particles stick to the walls of the cartridge.
5. Follow the instructions in the "Disposable Insulin Delivery Device User Manual" for these steps:
   - Preparing the Pen
   - Attaching the Needle. **Use a new needle for each injection.**
   - Priming the Pen. **The pen must be primed before each injection to make sure the pen is ready to dose.** Performing the priming step is important to confirm that insulin comes out when you push the injection button, and to remove air that may collect in the insulin cartridge during normal use.
   - Setting (Dialing) a Dose
   - Injecting the Dose. **To make sure you have received your dose, you must push the injection button all the way down until you see a diamond (◆) or an arrow (→) in the center of the dose window.**
   - Following an Injection

PREPARING FOR INJECTION

1. Wash your hands.
2. To avoid tissue damage, choose a site for each injection that is at least ½ inch from the previous injection site. The usual sites of injection are abdomen, thighs, and arms.
3. Cleanse the skin with alcohol where the injection is to be made.
4. With one hand, stabilize the skin by spreading it or pinching up a large area.
5. Inject the dose as instructed by your doctor.
6. After dispensing a dose, pull the needle out and apply gentle pressure over the injection site for several seconds. Do not rub the area.
7. Immediately after an injection, remove the needle from the Humulin N Pen. Doing so will guard against contamination, leakage, reentry of air, and needle clogs. Do not reuse needles. Dispose of needles in a responsible manner.

DOSAGE

Your doctor has told you which insulin to use, how much, and when and how often to inject it. Because each patient's case of diabetes is different, this schedule has been individualized for you.

Your usual insulin dose may be affected by changes in your food, activity, or work schedule. Carefully follow your doctor's instructions to allow for these changes. Other things that may affect your insulin dose are:

Illness

Illness, especially with nausea and vomiting, may cause your insulin requirements to change. Even if you are not eating, you will still require insulin. You and your doctor should establish a sick day plan for you to use in case of illness. When you are sick, test your blood glucose/urine glucose and ketones frequently and call your doctor as instructed.

Pregnancy

Good control of diabetes is especially important for you and your unborn baby. Pregnancy may make managing your diabetes more difficult. If you are planning to have a baby, are pregnant, or are nursing a baby, consult your doctor.

Medication

Insulin requirements may be increased if you are taking other drugs with hyperglycemic activity, such as oral contraceptives, corticosteroids, or thyroid replacement therapy. Insulin requirements may be reduced in the presence of drugs with hypoglycemic activity, such as oral hypoglycemics, salicylates (for example, aspirin), sulfa antibiotics, and certain antidepressants. Always discuss any medications you are taking with your doctor.

Exercise

Exercise may lower your body's need for insulin during and for some time after the activity. Exercise may also speed up the effect of an insulin dose, especially if the exercise involves the area of injection site (for example, the leg should not be used for injection just prior to running). Discuss with your doctor how you should adjust your regimen to accommodate exercise.

Travel

Persons traveling across more than 2 time zones should consult their doctor concerning adjustments in their insulin schedule.

COMMON PROBLEMS OF DIABETES

Hypoglycemia (Insulin Reaction)

Hypoglycemia (too little glucose in the blood) is one of the most frequent adverse events experienced by insulin users. It can be brought about by:

1. Taking too much insulin
2. Missing or delaying meals
3. Exercising or working more than usual
4. An infection or illness (especially with diarrhea or vomiting)
5. A change in the body's need for insulin
6. Diseases of the adrenal, pituitary or thyroid gland, or progression of kidney or liver disease
7. Interactions with other drugs that lower blood glucose, such as oral hypoglycemics, salicylates (for example, aspirin), sulfa antibiotics, and certain antidepressants
8. Consumption of alcoholic beverages

Symptoms of mild to moderate hypoglycemia may occur suddenly and can include:

- sweating
- dizziness
- palpitation
- tremor
- hunger
- restlessness
- tingling in the hands, feet, lips, or tongue
- lightheadedness
- inability to concentrate
- headache
- drowsiness
- sleep disturbances
- anxiety
- blurred vision
- slurred speech
- depressed mood
- irritability
- abnormal behavior
- unsteady movement
- personality changes

Signs of severe hypoglycemia can include:

- disorientation
- unconsciousness
- seizures
- death

Therefore, it is important that assistance be obtained immediately.

Early warning symptoms of hypoglycemia may be different or less pronounced under certain conditions, such as long duration of diabetes, diabetic nerve disease, medications such as beta-blockers, change in insulin preparations, or intensified control (3 or more insulin injections per day) of diabetes.

A few patients who have experienced hypoglycemic reactions after transfer from animal-source insulin to human insulin have reported that the early warning symptoms of hypoglycemia were less pronounced or different from those experienced with their previous insulin.

Without recognition of early warning symptoms, you may not be able to take steps to avoid more serious hypoglycemia. Be alert for all of the various types of symptoms that may indicate hypoglycemia. Patients who experience hypoglycemia without early warning symptoms should monitor their blood glucose frequently, especially prior to activities such as driving. If the blood glucose is below your normal fasting glucose, you should consider eating or drinking sugar-containing foods to treat your hypoglycemia.

Mild to moderate hypoglycemia may be treated by eating foods or drinks that contain sugar. Patients should always carry a quick source of sugar, such as candy mints or glucose tablets. More severe hypoglycemia may require the assistance of another person. Patients who are unable to take sugar orally or who are unconscious require an injection of glucagon or should be treated with intravenous administration of glucose at a medical facility.

You should learn to recognize your own symptoms of hypoglycemia. If you are uncertain about these symptoms, you should monitor your blood glucose frequently to help you learn to recognize the symptoms that you experience with hypoglycemia.

If you have frequent episodes of hypoglycemia or experience difficulty in recognizing the symptoms, you should consult your doctor to discuss possible changes in therapy, meal plans, and/or exercise programs to help you avoid hypoglycemia.

Hyperglycemia and Diabetic Acidosis

Hyperglycemia (too much glucose in the blood) may develop if your body has too little insulin. Hyperglycemia can be brought about by:

1. Omitting your insulin or taking less than the doctor has prescribed
2. Eating significantly more than your meal plan suggests
3. Developing a fever, infection, or other significant stressful situation

In patients with insulin-dependent diabetes, prolonged hyperglycemia can result in diabetic acidosis. The first symptoms of diabetic acidosis usually come on gradually, over a period of hours or days, and include a drowsy feeling, flushed face, thirst, loss of appetite, and fruity odor on the breath. With acidosis, urine tests show large amounts of glucose and acetone. Heavy breathing and a rapid pulse are more severe symptoms. If uncorrected, prolonged hyperglycemia or diabetic acidosis can lead to nausea, vomiting, dehydration, loss of consciousness or death. Therefore, it is important that you obtain medical assistance immediately.

Lipodystrophy

Rarely, administration of insulin subcutaneously can result in lipoatrophy (depression in the skin) or lipohypertrophy (enlargement or thickening of tissue). If you notice either of these conditions, consult your doctor. A change in your injection technique may help alleviate the problem.

Allergy to Insulin

Local Allergy—Patients occasionally experience redness, swelling, and itching at the site of injection of insulin. This condition, called local allergy, usually clears up in a few days to a few weeks. In some instances, this condition may be related to factors other than insulin, such as irritants in the skin cleansing agent or poor injection technique. If you have local reactions, contact your doctor.

Systemic Allergy—Less common, but potentially more serious, is generalized allergy to insulin, which may cause rash over the whole body, shortness of breath, wheezing, reduction in blood pressure, fast pulse, or sweating. Severe cases of generalized allergy may be life threatening. If you think you are having a generalized allergic reaction to insulin, notify a doctor immediately.

ADDITIONAL INFORMATION

Additional information about diabetes may be obtained from your diabetes educator.

DIABETES FORECAST is a national magazine designed especially for patients with diabetes and their families and is available on subscription from the American Diabetes Association, National Service Center, 1660 Duke Street, Alexandria, Virginia 22314, 1-800-DIABETES (1-800-342-2383).

Another publication, **DIABETES COUNTDOWN**, is available from the Juvenile Diabetes Foundation, 120 Wall Street 19th Floor, New York, New York 10005-4001, 1-800-JDF-CURE (1-800-533-2873).

Additional information about Humulin and Humulin N Pen can be obtained by calling 1-888-88-LILLY (1-888-885-4559).

Literature revised October 8, 2003

Manufactured by Lilly France S.A.S.
F-67640 Fegersheim, France
for Eli Lilly and Company
Indianapolis, IN 46285, USA

PA 9134FSAMP

HUMULIN® R OTC

[hū'mū-lĭn är]

REGULAR

INSULIN HUMAN INJECTION, USP (rDNA ORIGIN)

INFORMATION FOR THE PATIENT

WARNINGS

THIS LILLY HUMAN INSULIN PRODUCT DIFFERS FROM ANIMAL-SOURCE INSULINS BECAUSE IT IS STRUCTURALLY IDENTICAL TO THE INSULIN PRODUCED BY YOUR BODY'S PANCREAS AND BECAUSE OF ITS UNIQUE MANUFACTURING PROCESS.

ANY CHANGE OF INSULIN SHOULD BE MADE CAUTIOUSLY AND ONLY UNDER MEDICAL SUPERVISION. CHANGES IN STRENGTH, MANUFACTURER, TYPE (E.G., REGULAR, NPH, LENTE®), SPECIES (BEEF, PORK, BEEF-PORK, HUMAN), OR METHOD OF MANUFACTURE (rDNA VERSUS ANIMAL-SOURCE INSULIN) MAY RESULT IN THE NEED FOR A CHANGE IN DOSAGE.

SOME PATIENTS TAKING HUMULIN® (HUMAN INSULIN, rDNA ORIGIN) MAY REQUIRE A CHANGE IN DOSAGE FROM THAT USED WITH ANIMAL-SOURCE INSULINS. IF AN ADJUSTMENT IS NEEDED, IT MAY OCCUR WITH THE FIRST DOSE OR DURING THE FIRST SEVERAL WEEKS OR MONTHS.

DIABETES

Insulin is a hormone produced by the pancreas, a large gland that lies near the stomach. This hormone is necessary for the body's correct use of food, especially sugar. Diabetes occurs when the pancreas does not make enough insulin to meet your body's needs.

To control your diabetes, your doctor has prescribed injections of insulin products to keep your blood glucose at a near-normal level. You have been instructed to test your blood and/or your urine regularly for glucose. Studies have shown that some chronic complications of diabetes such as eye disease, kidney disease, and nerve disease can be significantly reduced if the blood sugar is maintained as close to normal as possible. The American Diabetes Association recommends that if your premeal glucose levels are consistently above 140 mg/dL or your hemoglobin A_{1c} (HbA_{1c}) is more than 8%, consult your doctor. A change in your diabetes therapy may be needed. If your blood tests consistently show below-normal glucose levels you should also let your doctor know. Proper control of your diabetes requires close and constant cooperation with your doctor. Despite diabetes, you can lead an active and healthy life if you eat a balanced diet, exercise regularly, and take your insulin injections as prescribed.

Always keep an extra supply of insulin as well as a spare syringe and needle on hand. Always wear diabetic identification so that appropriate treatment can be given if complications occur away from home.

REGULAR HUMAN INSULIN

Description

Humulin is synthesized in a special non-disease-producing laboratory strain of *Escherichia coli* bacteria that has been genetically altered by the addition of the gene for human insulin production. Humulin R consists of zinc-insulin crystals dissolved in a clear fluid. Humulin R has had nothing added to change the speed or length of its action. It takes effect rapidly and has a relatively short duration of activity (4 to 12 hours) as compared with other insulins. The time course of action of any insulin may vary considerably in different individuals or at different times in the same individual. As with all insulin preparations, the duration of action of Humulin R is dependent on dose, site of injection, blood supply, temperature, and physical activity. Humulin R is a sterile solution and is for subcutaneous injection. It should not be used intramuscularly. The concentration of Humulin R is 100 units/mL (U-100).

Identification

Human insulin manufactured by Eli Lilly and Company has the trademark Humulin and is available in 6 formulations—Regular (**R**), NPH (**N**), Lente (**L**), Ultralente® (**U**), 50% Human Insulin Isophane Suspension [NPH]/50% Human Insulin Injection [buffered regular] (**50/50**), and 70% Human Insulin Isophane Suspension [NPH]/30% Human Insulin Injection [buffered regular] (**70/30**). Your doctor has prescribed the type of insulin that he/she believes is best for you. **DO NOT USE ANY OTHER INSULIN EXCEPT ON HIS/HER ADVICE AND DIRECTION.**

Always check the carton and the bottle label for the name and letter designation of the insulin you receive from your pharmacy to make sure it is the same as that your doctor has prescribed.

Always examine the appearance of your bottle of insulin before withdrawing each dose. Humulin R is a clear and colorless liquid with a water-like appearance and consistency. Do not use if it appears cloudy, thickened, or slightly colored or if solid particles are visible. Always check the appearance of your bottle of insulin before using, and if you note anything unusual in the appearance of your insulin or notice your insulin requirements changing markedly, consult your doctor.

Storage

Insulin should be stored in a refrigerator but not in the freezer. If refrigeration is not possible, the bottle of insulin that you are currently using can be kept unrefrigerated as long as it is kept as cool as possible (below 86°F [30°C]) and away from heat and light. Do not use insulin if it has been frozen. Do not use a bottle of insulin after the expiration date stamped on the label.

INJECTION PROCEDURES

Correct Syringe

Doses of insulin are measured in **units**. U-100 insulin contains 100 units/mL (1 mL = 1 cc). With Humulin R, it is important to use a syringe that is marked for U-100 insulin preparations. Failure to use the proper syringe can lead to a mistake in dosage, causing serious problems for you, such as a blood glucose level that is too low or too high.

Syringe Use

To help avoid contamination and possible infection, follow these instructions exactly.

Disposable syringes and needles should be used only once and then discarded. **NEEDLES AND SYRINGES MUST NOT BE SHARED.**

Reusable syringes and needles must be sterilized before each injection. **Follow the package directions supplied with your syringe.** Described below are 2 methods of sterilizing.

Boiling

1. Put syringe, plunger, and needle in strainer, place in saucepan, and cover with water. Boil for 5 minutes.
2. Remove articles from water. When they have cooled, insert plunger into barrel, and fasten needle to syringe with a slight twist.
3. Push plunger in and out several times until water is completely removed.

Isopropyl Alcohol

If the syringe, plunger, and needle cannot be boiled, as when you are traveling, they may be sterilized by immersion for at least 5 minutes in Isopropyl Alcohol, 91%. Do not use bathing, rubbing, or medicated alcohol for this sterilization. If the syringe is sterilized with alcohol, it must be absolutely dry before use.

Preparing the Dose

1. Wash your hands.
2. Inspect the insulin. Humulin R should look clear and colorless. Do not use Humulin R if it appears cloudy, thickened, or slightly colored or if solid particles are visible.
3. If using a new bottle, flip off the plastic protective cap, but **do not** remove the stopper. When using a new bottle, wipe the top of the bottle with an alcohol swab.
4. If you are mixing insulins, refer to the instructions for mixing that follow.
5. Draw air into the syringe equal to your insulin dose. Put the needle through rubber top of the insulin bottle and inject the air into the bottle.
6. Turn the bottle and syringe upside down. Hold the bottle and syringe firmly in 1 hand.
7. Making sure the tip of the needle is in the insulin, withdraw the correct dose of insulin into the syringe.
8. Before removing the needle from the bottle, check your syringe for air bubbles which reduce the amount of insulin in it. If bubbles are present, hold the syringe straight up and tap its side until the bubbles float to the top. Push them out with the plunger and withdraw the correct dose.
9. Remove the needle from the bottle and lay the syringe down so that the needle does not touch anything.

Mixing Humulin R with Longer-acting Human Insulins

1. Regular human insulin should be mixed with longer-acting human insulins only on the advice of your doctor.
2. Draw air into your syringe equal to the amount of longer-acting insulin you are taking. Insert the needle into the longer-acting insulin bottle and inject the air. Withdraw the needle.
3. Now inject air into your regular human insulin bottle in the same manner, but **do not** withdraw the needle.
4. Turn the bottle and syringe upside down.
5. Making sure the tip of the needle is in the insulin, withdraw the correct dose of regular insulin into the syringe.
6. Before removing the needle from the bottle, check your syringe for air bubbles which reduce the amount of insulin in it. If bubbles are present, hold the syringe straight up and tap its side until the bubbles float to the top. Push them out with the plunger and withdraw the correct dose.
7. Remove the needle from the bottle of regular insulin and insert it into the bottle of the longer-acting insulin. Turn the bottle and syringe upside down. Hold the bottle and syringe firmly in 1 hand and shake gently. Making sure the tip of the needle is in the insulin, withdraw your dose of longer-acting insulin.
8. Remove the needle and lay the syringe down so that the needle does not touch anything.

Follow your doctor's instructions on whether to mix your insulins ahead of time or just before giving your injection. It is important to be consistent in your method.

Syringes from different manufacturers may vary in the amount of space between the bottom line and the needle. Because of this, do not change:

- the sequence of mixing, or
- the model and brand of syringe or needle that the doctor has prescribed.

Injection

Cleanse the skin with alcohol where the injection is to be made. Stabilize the skin by spreading it or pinching up a large area. Insert the needle as instructed by your doctor. Push the plunger in as far as it will go. Pull the needle out and apply gentle pressure over the injection site for several seconds. **Do not rub the area.** To avoid tissue damage, give the next injection at a site at least 1/2" from the previous site.

DOSAGE

Your doctor has told you which insulin to use, how much, and when and how often to inject it. Because each patient's case of diabetes is different, this schedule has been individualized for you.

Your usual insulin dose may be affected by changes in your food, activity, or work schedule. Carefully follow your doctor's instructions to allow for these changes. Other things that may affect your insulin dose are:

Illness

Illness, especially with nausea and vomiting, may cause your insulin requirements to change. Even if you are not eating, you will still require insulin. You and your doctor should establish a sick day plan for you to use in case of illness. When you are sick, test your blood/urine frequently and call your doctor as instructed.

Pregnancy

Good control of diabetes is especially important for you and your unborn baby. Pregnancy may make managing your diabetes more difficult. If you are planning to have a baby, are pregnant, or are nursing a baby, consult your doctor.

Medication

Insulin requirements may be increased if you are taking other drugs with hyperglycemic activity, such as oral contraceptives, corticosteroids, or thyroid replacement therapy. Insulin requirements may be reduced in the presence of drugs with hypoglycemic activity, such as oral hypoglycemics, salicylates (for example, aspirin), sulfa antibiotics, and certain antidepressants. Always discuss any medications you are taking with your doctor.

Exercise

Exercise may lower your body's need for insulin during and for some time after the activity. Exercise may also speed up the effect of an insulin dose, especially if the exercise involves the area of injection site (for example, the leg should not be used for injection just prior to running). Discuss with your doctor how you should adjust your regimen to accommodate exercise.

Continued on next page

*** Identi-Code® symbol. This product information was prepared in June 2004. Current information on these and other products of Eli Lilly and Company may be obtained by direct inquiry to Lilly Research Laboratories, Lilly Corporate Center, Indianapolis, Indiana 46285, (800) 545-5979.**

Humulin R—Cont.

Travel
Persons traveling across more than 2 time zones should consult their doctor concerning adjustments in their insulin schedule.

COMMON PROBLEMS OF DIABETES

Hypoglycemia (Insulin Reaction)
Hypoglycemia (too little glucose in the blood) is one of the most frequent adverse events experienced by insulin users. It can be brought about by:
1. Taking too much insulin
2. Missing or delaying meals
3. Exercising or working more than usual
4. An infection or illness (especially with diarrhea or vomiting)
5. A change in the body's need for insulin
6. Diseases of the adrenal, pituitary, or thyroid gland, or progression of kidney or liver disease
7. Interactions with other drugs that lower blood glucose, such as oral hypoglycemics, salicylates (for example, aspirin), sulfa antibiotics, and certain antidepressants
8. Consumption of alcoholic beverages

Symptoms of mild to moderate hypoglycemia may occur suddenly and can include:
- sweating
- dizziness
- palpitation
- tremor
- hunger
- restlessness
- tingling in the hands, feet, lips, or tongue
- lightheadedness
- inability to concentrate
- headache
- drowsiness
- sleep disturbances
- anxiety
- blurred vision
- slurred speech
- depressed mood
- irritability
- abnormal behavior
- unsteady movement
- personality changes

Signs of severe hypoglycemia can include:
- disorientation
- unconsciousness
- seizures
- death

Therefore, it is important that assistance be obtained immediately.
Early warning symptoms of hypoglycemia may be different or less pronounced under certain conditions, such as long duration of diabetes, diabetic nerve disease, medications such as beta-blockers, change in insulin preparations, or intensified control (3 or more insulin injections per day) of diabetes.
A few patients who have experienced hypoglycemic reactions after transfer from animal-source insulin to human insulin have reported that the early warning symptoms of hypoglycemia were less pronounced or different from those experienced with their previous insulin.
Without recognition of early warning symptoms, you may not be able to take steps to avoid more serious hypoglycemia. Be alert for all of the various types of symptoms that may indicate hypoglycemia. Patients who experience hypoglycemia without early warning symptoms should monitor their blood glucose frequently, especially prior to activities such as driving. If the blood glucose is below your normal fasting glucose, you should consider eating or drinking sugar-containing foods to treat your hypoglycemia.
Mild to moderate hypoglycemia may be treated by eating foods or drinks that contain sugar. Patients should always carry a quick source of sugar, such as candy mints or glucose tablets. More severe hypoglycemia may require the assistance of another person. Patients who are unable to take sugar orally or who are unconscious require an injection of glucagon or should be treated with intravenous administration of glucose at a medical facility.
You should learn to recognize your own symptoms of hypoglycemia. If you are uncertain about these symptoms, you should monitor your blood glucose frequently to help you learn to recognize the symptoms that you experience with hypoglycemia.
If you have frequent episodes of hypoglycemia or experience difficulty in recognizing the symptoms, you should consult your doctor to discuss possible changes in therapy, meal plans, and/or exercise programs to help you avoid hypoglycemia.

Hyperglycemia and Diabetic Acidosis
Hyperglycemia (too much glucose in the blood) may develop if your body has too little insulin. Hyperglycemia can be brought about by:
1. Omitting your insulin or taking less than the doctor has prescribed
2. Eating significantly more than your meal plan suggests
3. Developing a fever, infection, or other significant stressful situation

In patients with insulin-dependent diabetes, prolonged hyperglycemia can result in diabetic acidosis. The first symptoms of diabetic acidosis usually come on gradually, over a period of hours or days, and include a drowsy feeling, flushed face, thirst, loss of appetite, and fruity odor on the breath. With acidosis, urine tests show large amounts of glucose and acetone. Heavy breathing and a rapid pulse are more severe symptoms. If uncorrected, prolonged hyperglycemia or diabetic acidosis can lead to nausea, vomiting, dehydration, loss of consciousness or death. Therefore, it is important that you obtain medical assistance immediately.

Lipodystrophy
Rarely, administration of insulin subcutaneously can result in lipoatrophy (depression in the skin) or lipohypertrophy (enlargement or thickening of tissue). If you notice either of these conditions, consult your doctor. A change in your injection technique may help alleviate the problem.

Allergy to Insulin
Local Allergy—Patients occasionally experience redness, swelling, and itching at the site of injection of insulin. This condition, called local allergy, usually clears up in a few days to a few weeks. In some instances, this condition may be related to factors other than insulin, such as irritants in the skin cleansing agent or poor injection technique. If you have local reactions, contact your doctor.
Systemic Allergy—Less common, but potentially more serious, is generalized allergy to insulin, which may cause rash over the whole body, shortness of breath, wheezing, reduction in blood pressure, fast pulse, or sweating. Severe cases of generalized allergy may be life threatening. If you think you are having a generalized allergic reaction to insulin, notify a doctor immediately.

ADDITIONAL INFORMATION
Additional information about diabetes may be obtained from your diabetes educator.
DIABETES FORECAST is a national magazine designed especially for patients with diabetes and their families and is available by subscription from the American Diabetes Association, National Service Center, 1660 Duke Street, Alexandria, Virginia 22314, 1-800-DIABETES (1-800-342-2383).
Another publication, **DIABETES COUNTDOWN**, is available from the Juvenile Diabetes Foundation International (JDF), 120 Wall Street, 19th Floor, New York, New York 10005, 1-800-JDF-CURE (1-800-533-2873).
Additional information about Humulin can be obtained by calling 1-888-88-LILLY (1-888-885-4559).
Literature revised August 3, 2000
PA 6327 AMP

HUMULIN® R ℞
[*hū 'mū-lĭn är*]
REGULAR U-500 (CONCENTRATED)
INSULIN HUMAN INJECTION, USP
(rDNA ORIGINAL)

INFORMATION FOR THE PHYSICIAN

WARNINGS
THIS LILLY HUMAN INSULIN PRODUCT DIFFERS FROM ANIMAL-SOURCE INSULINS BECAUSE IT IS STRUCTURALLY IDENTICAL TO THE INSULIN PRODUCED BY YOUR BODY'S PANCREAS AND BECAUSE OF ITS UNIQUE MANUFACTURING PROCESS.
ANY CHANGE OF INSULIN SHOULD BE MADE CAUTIOUSLY AND ONLY UNDER MEDICAL SUPERVISION. CHANGES IN PURITY, STRENGTH, BRAND (MANUFACTURER), TYPE (REGULAR, NPH, LENTE®, ETC), SPECIES (BEEF, PORK, BEEF-PORK, HUMAN), AND/OR METHOD OF MANUFACTURE (rDNA VERSUS ANIMAL-SOURCE INSULIN) MAY RESULT IN THE NEED FOR A CHANGE IN DOSAGE.
SOME PATIENTS TAKING HUMULIN® (HUMAN INSULIN, rDNA ORIGIN, LILLY) MAY REQUIRE A CHANGE IN DOSAGE FROM THAT USED WITH ANIMAL-SOURCE INSULINS. IF AN ADJUSTMENT IS NEEDED, IT MAY OCCUR WITH THE FIRST DOSE OR DURING THE FIRST SEVERAL WEEKS OR MONTHS.
This insulin preparation contains 500 units of insulin in each milliliter. Extreme caution must be observed in the measurement of dosage because inadvertent overdose may result in irreversible insulin shock. Serious consequences may result if it is used other than under constant medical supervision.

DESCRIPTION
Humulin is synthesized in a special non-disease-producing laboratory strain of *Escherichia coli* bacteria that has been genetically altered by the addition of the gene for human insulin production. Humulin R (U-500) consists of zinc-insulin crystals dissolved in a clear fluid. Humulin R (U-500) is a sterile solution and is for subcutaneous injection. It should not be used intravenously or intramuscularly. The concentration of Humulin R (U-500) is 500 units/mL. Each milliliter contains 500 units of biosynthetic human insulin, 16 mg glycerin, 2.5 mg *m*-cresol as a preservative, and zinc-oxide calculated to supplement endogenous zinc to obtain a total zinc content of 0.017 mg/100 units. Sodium hydroxide and/or hydrochloric acid may be added during manufacture to adjust the pH.

CLINICAL PHARMACOLOGY
Adequate insulin dosage permits the diabetic patient to utilize carbohydrates and fats in a comparatively satisfactory manner. Regardless of concentration, the action of insulin is basically the same: to enable carbohydrate metabolism to occur and thus to prevent the production of ketone bodies by the liver. Although, under usual circumstances, diabetes can be controlled with doses in the vicinity of 40 to 60 units or less, an occasional patient develops such resistance or becomes so unresponsive to the effect of insulin that daily doses of several hundred, or even several thousand, units are required. Patients who require doses in excess of 300 to 500 units daily usually have impaired insulin receptor function.
Occasionally, a cause of the insulin resistance can be found (such as hemochromatosis, cirrhosis of the liver, some complicating disease of the endocrine glands other than the pancreas, allergy, or infection), but in other cases, no cause of the high insulin requirement can be determined.
Humulin R (U-500) is unmodified by any agent that might prolong its action; however, clinical experience has shown that it frequently has a time action similar to a repository insulin preparation. It takes effect rapidly but has a relatively long duration of activity following a single dose (up to 24 hours) as compared with other Regular insulins. This effect has been credited to the high concentration of the preparation. The time course of action of any insulin may vary considerably in different individuals or at different times in the same individual. As with all insulin preparations, the duration of action of Humulin R (U-500) is dependent on dose, site of injection, blood supply, temperature, and physical activity.

INDICATIONS AND USAGE
Humulin R (U-500) is especially useful for the treatment of diabetic patients with marked insulin resistance (daily requirements more than 200 units), since a large dose may be administered subcutaneously in a reasonable volume.

CONTRAINDICATIONS
Humulin R (U-500) is contraindicated in hypoglycemia.

PRECAUTIONS
General—Every patient exhibiting insulin resistance who requires Humulin R (U-500) for control of diabetes should be under close observation until appropriate dosage is established. The response will vary among patients. Some patients can be controlled with a single dose daily; others may require 2 or 3 injections per day. Most patients will show a "tolerance" to insulin, so that minor variations in dosage can occur without the development of untoward symptoms of insulin shock.
Insulin resistance is frequently self-limited; after several weeks or months during which high dosage is required, responsiveness to the pharmacologic effect of insulin may be regained and dosage can be reduced.
Information for Patients—Patients should be instructed regarding their dosage and should be reminded that this formulation requires the administration of a smaller volume of solution than is the case with less concentrated formulations.
Laboratory Tests—Blood and urine glucose, glycohemoglobin, and urine ketones should be monitored frequently.
Drug Interactions—The concurrent use of oral hypoglycemic agents with Humulin R (U-500) is not recommended since there are no data to support such use.
Pregnancy-Teratogenic Effects—No reproduction studies have been conducted in animals, and there are no adequate and well-controlled studies in pregnant women. It would be anticipated that the benefits of this insulin preparation would outweigh any risk to the developing fetus.
Nonteratogenic Effects—Insulin does not cross the placenta as does glucose.
Labor and Delivery—Careful monitoring of the patient is required, since the insulin requirement may decrease following delivery.
Nursing Mothers—It is not known whether insulin is excreted in significant amounts in human milk. Because many drugs are excreted in human milk, caution should be exercised when Humulin R (U-500) insulin injection is administered to a nursing woman.
Pediatric Use—There are no special precautions relating to the use of this insulin formulation in the pediatric age group.

ADVERSE REACTIONS
As with other human insulin preparations, hypoglycemic reactions may be associated with the administration of Humulin R (U-500). However, deep secondary hypoglycemic reactions may develop 18 to 24 hours after the original injection of Humulin R (U-500). Consequently, patients should be carefully observed, and prompt treatment of such reactions should be initiated with glucagon injections and/or with glucose by intravenous injection or gavage.

Hypoglycemia
Hypoglycemia is one of the most frequent adverse events experienced by insulin users.
Symptoms of mild to moderate hypoglycemia may occur suddenly and can include:
- sweating
- dizziness
- palpitation
- tremor
- hunger
- restlessness
- tingling in the hands, feet, lips, or tongue
- lightheadedness
- inability to concentrate
- headache
- drowsiness
- sleep disturbances

- anxiety
- blurred vision
- slurred speech
- depressive mood
- irritability
- abnormal behavior
- unsteady movement
- personality changes

Signs of severe hypoglycemia can include:

- disorientation
- unconsciousness
- seizures
- death

Early warning symptoms of hypoglycemia may be different or less pronounced under certain conditions, such as long duration of diabetes, diabetic nerve disease, medications such as beta-blockers, change in insulin preparations, or intensified control (3 or more insulin injections per day) of diabetes.

A few patients who have experienced hypoglycemic reactions after transfer from animal-source insulin to human insulin have reported that the early warning symptoms of hypoglycemia were less pronounced or different from those experienced with their previous insulin.

Without recognition of early warning symptoms, the patient may not be able to take steps to avoid more serious hypoglycemia. Patients who experience hypoglycemia without early warning symptoms should monitor their blood glucose frequently, especially prior to activities such as driving. Mild to moderate hypoglycemia may be treated by eating foods or taking drinks that contain sugar. Patients should always carry a quick source of sugar, such as candy mints or glucose tablets.

Hypoglycemia when using Humulin R (U-500) can be prolonged and severe.

Lipodystrophy

Rarely, administration of insulin subcutaneously can result in lipoatrophy (depression in the skin) or lipohypertrophy (enlargement or thickening of tissue).

Allergy to Insulin

Local Allergy—Patients occasionally experience erythema, local edema, and pruritus at the site of injection of insulin. This condition usually is self-limiting. In some instances, this condition may be related to factors other than insulin, such as irritants in the skin cleansing agent or poor injection technique.

Systemic Allergy—Less common, but potentially more serious, is generalized allergy to insulin, which may cause rash over the whole body, shortness of breath, wheezing, reduction in blood pressure, fast pulse, or sweating. Severe cases of generalized allergy (anaphylaxis) may be life threatening.

DOSAGE AND ADMINISTRATION

Humulin R (U-500) should only be administered subcutaneously. It is inadvisable to inject Humulin R (U-500) intravenously because of possible inadvertent overdosage.

It is recommended that an insulin syringe or tuberculin-type syringe be used for the measurement of dosage. Variations in dosage are frequently possible in the insulin-resistant patient, since the individual is unresponsive to the pharmacologic effect of the insulin. Nevertheless, accuracy of measurement is to be encouraged because of the potential danger of the preparation.

STORAGE

Insulin should be kept in a cold place, preferably in a refrigerator, but must not be frozen.

Do not inject insulin that is not water-clear. Discoloration, turbidity, or unusual viscosity indicates deterioration or contamination.

Use of a package of insulin should not be started after the expiration date stamped on it.

HOW SUPPLIED

Vials, 500 units/mL, 20 mL (HI-500) (1s), NDC 0002-8501-01

Literature issued August 15, 2000

PA 3050 AMP

HUMULIN® R
REGULAR
U-500 (CONCENTRATED)
INSULIN HUMAN INJECTION, USP
(rDNA ORIGIN)
INFORMATION FOR THE PATIENT

WARNINGS

THIS LILLY HUMAN INSULIN PRODUCT DIFFERS FROM ANIMAL-SOURCE INSULINS BECAUSE IT IS STRUCTURALLY IDENTICAL TO THE INSULIN PRODUCED BY YOUR BODY'S PANCREAS AND BECAUSE OF ITS UNIQUE MANUFACTURING PROCESS.

ANY CHANGE OF INSULIN SHOULD BE MADE CAUTIOUSLY AND ONLY UNDER MEDICAL SUPERVISION. CHANGES IN PURITY, STRENGTH, BRAND (MANUFACTURER), TYPE (REGULAR, NPH, LENTE®, ETC), SPECIES (BEEF, PORK, BEEF-PORK, HUMAN), AND/OR METHOD OF MANUFACTURE (rDNA VERSUS ANIMAL-SOURCE INSULIN) MAY RESULT IN THE NEED FOR A CHANGE IN DOSAGE.

SOME PATIENTS TAKING HUMULIN® (HUMAN INSULIN, rDNA ORIGIN, LILLY) MAY REQUIRE A CHANGE IN DOSAGE FROM THAT USED WITH ANIMAL-SOURCE INSULINS. IF AN ADJUSTMENT IS NEEDED, IT MAY OCCUR WITH THE FIRST DOSE OR DURING THE FIRST SEVERAL WEEKS OR MONTHS.

This insulin preparation contains 500 units of insulin in each milliliter. Extreme caution must be observed in the measurement of dosage because inadvertent overdose may result in irreversible insulin shock. Serious consequences may result if it is used other than under constant medical supervision.

DIABETES

Insulin is a hormone produced by the pancreas, a large gland that lies near the stomach. This hormone is necessary for the body's correct use of food, especially sugar. Diabetes occurs when the pancreas does not make enough insulin to meet your body's needs.

To control your diabetes, your doctor has prescribed injections of insulin products to keep your blood glucose at a near-normal level. You have been instructed to test your blood and/or your urine regularly for glucose. Studies have shown that some chronic complications of diabetes such as eye disease, kidney disease, and nerve disease can be significantly reduced if the blood sugar is maintained as close to normal as possible. The American Diabetes Association recommends that if your premeal glucose levels are consistently above 140 mg/dL or your hemoglobin A_{1c} (HbA_{1c}) is more than 8%, consult your doctor. A change in your diabetes therapy may be needed. If your blood tests consistently show below-normal glucose levels you should also let your doctor know. Proper control of your diabetes requires close and constant cooperation with your doctor. Despite diabetes, you can lead an active and healthy life if you eat a balanced diet, exercise regularly, and take your insulin injections as prescribed.

Always keep an extra supply of insulin as well as a spare syringe and needle on hand. Always wear diabetic identification so that appropriate treatment can be given if complications occur away from home.

REGULAR HUMAN INSULIN

Description

Humulin is synthesized in a special non-disease-producing laboratory strain of *Escherichia coli* bacteria that has been genetically altered by the addition of the gene for human insulin production. Humulin R (U-500) consists of zinc-insulin crystals dissolved in a clear fluid. Humulin R (U-500) has had nothing added to change the speed or length of its action. It takes effect rapidly but has a relatively long duration of activity (up to 24 hours) as compared with other Regular insulins. The time course of action of any insulin may vary considerably in different individuals or at different times in the same individual. As with all insulin preparations, the duration of action of Humulin R (U-500) is dependent on dose, site of injection, blood supply, temperature, and physical activity. Humulin R (U- 500), is a sterile solution and should only be administered subcutaneously. It should not be used intravenously or intramuscularly. The concentration of Humulin R (U-500) is 500 units/mL.

Identification

Human insulin manufactured by Eli Lilly and Company has the trademark Humulin and is available in 6 formulations—Regular (**R**), NPH (**N**), Lente (**L**), Ultralente® (**U**), 50% Human Insulin Isophane Suspension [NPH]/50% Human Insulin Injection [buffered regular] (**50/50**), and 70% Human Insulin Isophane Suspension [NPH]/30% Human Insulin Injection [buffered regular] (**70/30**). Humulin R (U-500) is the only human insulin manufactured by Eli Lilly and Company that has a concentration of 500 units/mL. Your doctor has prescribed this type of insulin because he/she believes it is best for you. **DO NOT USE ANY OTHER INSULIN EXCEPT ON HIS/HER ADVICE AND DIRECTION.**

Always check the carton and the bottle label for the name and letter designation of the insulin you receive from your pharmacy to make sure it is the same as that your doctor has prescribed.

Always examine the appearance of your bottle of insulin before withdrawing each dose. Humulin R (U-500) is a clear and colorless liquid with a water-like appearance and consistency. Do not use if it appears cloudy, thickened, or slightly colored or if solid particles are visible. Always check the appearance of your bottle of insulin before using, and if you note anything unusual in the appearance of your insulin or notice your insulin requirements changing markedly, consult your doctor.

Storage

Insulin should be stored in a refrigerator but not in the freezer. If refrigeration is not possible, the bottle of insulin that you are currently using can be kept unrefrigerated as long as it is kept as cool as possible (below 86°F [30°C]) and away from heat and light. Do not use insulin if it has been frozen. Do not use a bottle of insulin after the expiration date stamped on the label.

INJECTION PROCEDURES

Correct Syringe

Doses of insulin are measured in **units**. U-500 insulin contains 500 units/mL (1 mL = 1 cc). With Humulin R (U-500), it is important to use a tuberculin (or similar) syringe as instructed by your doctor. Failure to use the syringe properly can lead to a mistake in dosage, potentially causing serious problems for you, such as a blood glucose level that is too low or too high.

Syringe Use

To help avoid contamination and possible spread of infection, follow these instructions exactly.

Disposable syringes and needles should be used only once and then discarded. **NEEDLES AND SYRINGES MUST NOT BE SHARED.**

Reusable syringes and needles must be sterilized before each injection. **Follow the package directions supplied with your syringe.** Described below are 2 methods of sterilizing.

Boiling

1. Put syringe, plunger, and needle in strainer, place in saucepan, and cover with water. Boil for 5 minutes.
2. Remove articles from water. When they have cooled, insert plunger into barrel, and fasten needle to syringe with a slight twist.
3. Push plunger in and out several times until water is completely removed.

Isopropyl Alcohol

If the syringe, plunger, and needle cannot be boiled, as when you are traveling, they may be sterilized by immersion for at least 5 minutes in Isopropyl Alcohol, 91%. Do not use bathing, rubbing, or medicated alcohol for this sterilization. If the syringe is sterilized with alcohol, it must be absolutely dry before use.

Preparing the Dose

1. Wash your hands.
2. Inspect the insulin. Humulin R (U-500) should look clear and colorless. Do not use Humulin R (U-500) if it appears cloudy, thickened, or slightly colored or if solid particles are visible.
3. If using a new bottle, flip off the plastic protective cap, but **do not** remove the stopper. When using a new bottle, wipe the top of the bottle with an alcohol swab.
4. Draw air into the syringe equal to your insulin dose. Put the needle through the rubber top of the insulin bottle and inject the air into the bottle.
5. Turn the bottle and syringe upside down. Hold the bottle and syringe firmly in 1 hand.
6. Making sure the tip of the needle is in the insulin, withdraw the correct dose of insulin into the syringe.
7. Before removing the needle from the bottle, check your syringe for air bubbles which reduce the amount of insulin in it. If bubbles are present, hold the syringe straight up and tap its side until the bubbles float to the top. Push them out with the plunger and withdraw the correct dose.
8. Remove the needle from the bottle and lay the syringe down so that the needle does not touch anything.

Injection

Cleanse the skin with alcohol where the injection is to be made. Stabilize the skin by spreading it or pinching up a large area. Insert the needle as instructed by your doctor. Push the plunger in as far as it will go. Pull the needle out and apply gentle pressure over the injection site for several seconds. **Do not rub the area.** To avoid tissue damage, give the next injection at a site at least 1/2″ from the previous site.

DOSAGE

Your doctor has told you which insulin to use, how much, and when and how often to inject it. Because each patient's case of diabetes is different, this schedule has been individualized for you.

Your usual insulin dose may be affected by changes in your food, activity, or work schedule. Carefully follow your doctor's instructions to allow for these changes. Other things that may affect your insulin dose are:

Illness

Illness, especially with nausea and vomiting, may cause your insulin requirements to change. Even if you are not eating, you will still require insulin. You and your doctor should establish a sick day plan for you to use in case of illness. When you are sick, test your blood/urine frequently and call your doctor as instructed.

Pregnancy

Good control of diabetes is especially important for you and your unborn baby. Pregnancy may make managing your diabetes more difficult. If you are planning to have a baby, are pregnant, or are nursing a baby, consult your doctor.

Medication

Insulin requirements may be increased if you are taking other drugs with hyperglycemic activity, such as oral contraceptives, corticosteroids, or thyroid replacement therapy. Insulin requirements may be reduced in the presence of drugs with hypoglycemic activity, such as oral hypoglycemics, salicylates (for example, aspirin), sulfa antibiotics, and certain antidepressants. Always discuss any medications you are taking with your doctor.

Exercise

Exercise may lower your body's need for insulin during and for some time after the activity. Exercise may also speed up the effect of an insulin dose, especially if the exercise involves the area of injection site (for example, the leg should not be used for injection just prior to running). Discuss with your doctor how you should adjust your regimen to accommodate exercise.

Continued on next page

*** Identi-Code® symbol. This product information was prepared in June 2004. Current information on these and other products of Eli Lilly and Company may be obtained by direct inquiry to Lilly Research Laboratories, Lilly Corporate Center, Indianapolis, Indiana 46285, (800) 545-5979.**

Humulin R U-500—Cont.

Travel
Persons traveling across more than 2 time zones should consult their doctor concerning adjustments in their insulin schedule.

COMMON PROBLEMS OF DIABETES

Hypoglycemia (Insulin Reaction)
Hypoglycemia (too little glucose in the blood) is one of the most frequent adverse events experienced by insulin users. It can be brought about by:

1. Taking too much insulin
2. Missing or delaying meals
3. Exercising or working more than usual
4. An infection or illness (especially with diarrhea or vomiting)
5. A change in the body's need for insulin
6. Diseases of the adrenal, pituitary, or thyroid gland, or progression of kidney or liver disease
7. Interactions with other drugs that lower blood glucose, such as oral hypoglycemics, salicylates (for example, aspirin), sulfa antibiotics, and certain antidepressants
8. Consumption of alcoholic beverages

Symptoms of mild to moderate hypoglycemia may occur suddenly and can include:

- sweating
- dizziness
- palpitation
- tremor
- hunger
- restlessness
- tingling in the hands, feet, lips, or tongue
- lightheadedness
- inability to concentrate
- headache
- drowsiness
- sleep disturbances
- anxiety
- blurred vision
- slurred speech
- depressive mood
- irritability
- abnormal behavior
- unsteady movement
- personality changes

Signs of severe hypoglycemia can include:

- disorientation
- unconsciousness
- seizures
- death

Therefore, it is important that assistance be obtained immediately.

Early warning symptoms of hypoglycemia may be different or less pronounced under certain conditions, such as long duration of diabetes, diabetic nerve disease, medications such as beta-blockers, change in insulin preparations, or intensified control (3 or more insulin injections per day) of diabetes.

A few patients who have experienced hypoglycemic reactions after transfer from animal-source insulin to human insulin have reported that the early warning symptoms of hypoglycemia were less pronounced or different from those experienced with their previous insulin.

Without recognition of early warning symptoms, you may not be able to take steps to avoid more serious hypoglycemia. Be alert for all of the various types of symptoms that may indicate hypoglycemia. Patients who experience hypoglycemia without early warning symptoms should monitor their blood glucose frequently, especially prior to activities such as driving. If the blood glucose is below your normal fasting glucose, you should consider eating or drinking sugar-containing foods to treat your hypoglycemia.

Mild to moderate hypoglycemia may be treated by eating foods or taking drinks that contain sugar. Patients should always carry a quick source of sugar, such as candy mints or glucose tablets. More severe hypoglycemia may require the assistance of another person. Patients who are unable to take sugar orally or who are unconscious require an injection of glucagon or should be treated with intravenous administration of glucose at a medical facility.

Hypoglycemia when using Humulin R (U-500) can be prolonged and severe. All hypoglycemic episodes should be reported to your doctor.

You should learn to recognize your own symptoms of hypoglycemia. If you are uncertain about these symptoms, you should monitor your blood glucose frequently to help you learn to recognize the symptoms that you experience with hypoglycemia.

If you have frequent episodes of hypoglycemia or experience difficulty in recognizing the symptoms, you should consult your doctor to discuss possible changes in therapy, meal plans, and/or exercise programs to help you avoid hypoglycemia.

Hyperglycemia and Diabetic Acidosis
Hyperglycemia (too much glucose in the blood) may develop if your body has too little insulin. Hyperglycemia can be brought about by:

1. Omitting your insulin or taking less than the doctor has prescribed
2. Eating significantly more than your meal plan suggests
3. Developing a fever, infection, or other significant stressful situation

In patients with insulin-dependent diabetes, prolonged hyperglycemia can result in diabetic acidosis. The first symptoms of diabetic acidosis usually come on gradually, over a period of hours or days, and include a drowsy feeling, flushed face, thirst, loss of appetite, and fruity odor on the breath. With acidosis, urine tests show large amounts of glucose and acetone. Heavy breathing and a rapid pulse are more severe symptoms. If uncorrected, prolonged hyperglycemia or diabetic acidosis can lead to nausea, vomiting, dehydration, loss of consciousness or death. Therefore, it is important that you obtain medical assistance immediately.

Lipodystrophy
Rarely, administration of insulin subcutaneously can result in lipoatrophy (depression in the skin) or lipohypertrophy (enlargement or thickening of tissue). If you notice either of these conditions, consult your doctor. A change in your injection technique may help alleviate the problem.

Allergy to Insulin
Local Allergy—Patients occasionally experience redness, swelling, and itching at the site of injection of insulin. This condition, called local allergy, usually clears up in a few days to a few weeks. In some instances, this condition may be related to factors other than insulin, such as irritants in the skin cleansing agent or poor injection technique. If you have local reactions, contact your doctor.

Systemic Allergy—Less common, but potentially more serious, is generalized allergy to insulin, which may cause rash over the whole body, shortness of breath, wheezing, reduction in blood pressure, fast pulse, or sweating. Severe cases of generalized allergy may be life threatening. If you think you are having a generalized allergic reaction to insulin, notify a doctor immediately.

ADDITIONAL INFORMATION
Additional information about diabetes may be obtained from your diabetes educator.

DIABETES FORECAST is a national magazine designed especially for patients with diabetes and their families and is available by subscription from the American Diabetes Association, National Service Center, 1660 Duke Street, Alexandria, Virginia 22314.

Another publication, **DIABETES COUNTDOWN**, is available from the Juvenile Diabetes Foundation International (JDF), 120 Wall Street, 19th Floor, New York, New York 10005, 1-800-JDF-CURE (1-800-533-2873).

Additional information about Humulin can be obtained by calling 1-888-88-LILLY (1-888-885-4559).

Literature issued August 15, 2000
PA 3050 AMP

HUMULIN® U ULTRALENTE® OTC

[*hū 'mū-lĭn ū*]
HUMAN INSULIN (rDNA ORIGIN)
EXTENDED ZINC SUSPENSION

INFORMATION FOR THE PATIENT

WARNINGS

THIS LILLY HUMAN INSULIN PRODUCT DIFFERS FROM ANIMAL-SOURCE INSULINS BECAUSE IT IS STRUCTURALLY IDENTICAL TO THE INSULIN PRODUCED BY YOUR BODY'S PANCREAS AND BECAUSE OF ITS UNIQUE MANUFACTURING PROCESS.

ANY CHANGE OF INSULIN SHOULD BE MADE CAUTIOUSLY AND ONLY UNDER MEDICAL SUPERVISION. CHANGES IN STRENGTH, MANUFACTURER, TYPE (E.G., REGULAR, NPH, LENTE®), SPECIES (BEEF, PORK, BEEF-PORK, HUMAN), OR METHOD OF MANUFACTURE (rDNA VERSUS ANIMAL-SOURCE INSULIN) MAY RESULT IN THE NEED FOR A CHANGE IN DOSAGE.

SOME PATIENTS TAKING HUMULIN® (HUMAN INSULIN, rDNA ORIGIN) MAY REQUIRE A CHANGE IN DOSAGE FROM THAT USED WITH ANIMAL-SOURCE INSULINS. IF AN ADJUSTMENT IS NEEDED, IT MAY OCCUR WITH THE FIRST DOSE OR DURING THE FIRST SEVERAL WEEKS OR MONTHS.

DIABETES
Insulin is a hormone produced by the pancreas, a large gland that lies near the stomach. This hormone is necessary for the body's correct use of food, especially sugar. Diabetes occurs when the pancreas does not make enough insulin to meet your body's needs.

To control your diabetes, your doctor has prescribed injections of insulin products to keep your blood glucose at a near-normal level. You have been instructed to test your blood and/or your urine regularly for glucose. Studies have shown that some chronic complications of diabetes such as eye disease, kidney disease, and nerve disease can be significantly reduced if the blood sugar is maintained as close to normal as possible. The American Diabetes Association recommends that if your premeal glucose levels are consistently above 140 mg/dL or your hemoglobin A_{1c} (HbA_{1c}) is more than 8%, consult your doctor. A change in your diabetes therapy may be needed. If your blood tests consistently show below-normal glucose levels, you should also let your doctor know. Proper control of your diabetes requires close and constant cooperation with your doctor. Despite diabetes, you can lead an active and healthy life if you eat a balanced diet, exercise regularly, and take your insulin injections as prescribed.

Always keep an extra supply of insulin as well as a spare syringe and needle on hand. Always wear diabetic identification so that appropriate treatment can be given if complications occur away from home.

ULTRALENTE HUMAN INSULIN

Description
Humulin is synthesized in a special non-disease-producing laboratory strain of *Escherichia coli* bacteria that has been genetically altered by the addition of the gene for human insulin production. Humulin U is a crystalline suspension of human insulin with zinc providing a slower onset and a longer and less intense duration of activity (up to 28 hours) than regular insulin or the intermediate-acting insulins (NPH and Lente). The time course of action of any insulin may vary considerably in different individuals or at different times in the same individual. As with all insulin preparations, the duration of action of Humulin U is dependent on dose, site of injection, blood supply, temperature, and physical activity. Humulin U is a sterile suspension and is for subcutaneous injection only. It should not be used intravenously or intramuscularly. The concentration of Humulin U is 100 units/mL (U-100).

Identification
Human insulin manufactured by Eli Lilly and Company has the trademark Humulin and is available in 6 formulations—Regular (**R**), NPH (**N**), Lente (**L**), Ultralente (**U**), 50% Human Insulin Isophane Suspension [NPH]/50% Human Insulin Injection [buffered regular] (**50/50**), and 70% Human Insulin Isophane Suspension [NPH]/30% Human Insulin Injection [buffered regular] (**70/30**). Your doctor has prescribed the type of insulin that he/she believes is best for you. **DO NOT USE ANY OTHER INSULIN EXCEPT ON HIS/HER ADVICE AND DIRECTION.**

Always check the carton and the bottle label for the name and letter designation of the insulin you receive from your pharmacy to make sure it is the same as that your doctor has prescribed.

Always examine the appearance of your bottle of insulin before withdrawing each dose. A bottle of Humulin U must be carefully shaken or rotated before each injection so that the contents are uniformly mixed. Humulin U should look uniformly cloudy or milky after mixing. Do not use it if the insulin substance (the white material) remains at the bottom of the bottle after mixing. Do not use a bottle of Humulin U if there are clumps in the insulin after mixing. Always check the appearance of your bottle of insulin before using, and if you note anything unusual in the appearance of your insulin or notice your insulin requirements changing markedly, consult your doctor.

Storage
Insulin should be stored in a refrigerator but not in the freezer. If refrigeration is not possible, the bottle of insulin that you are currently using can be kept unrefrigerated as long as it is kept as cool as possible (below 86°F [30°C]) and away from heat and light. Do not use insulin if it has been frozen. Do not use a bottle of insulin after the expiration date stamped on the label.

INJECTION PROCEDURES

Correct Syringe
Doses of insulin are measured in **units**. U-100 insulin contains 100 units/mL (1 mL = 1 cc). With Humulin U, it is important to use a syringe that is marked for U-100 insulin preparations. Failure to use the proper syringe can lead to a mistake in dosage, causing serious problems for you, such as a blood glucose level that is too low or too high.

Syringe Use
To help avoid contamination and possible infection, follow these instructions exactly.

Disposable syringes and needles should be used only once and then discarded. **NEEDLES AND SYRINGES MUST NOT BE SHARED.**

Reusable syringes and needles must be sterilized before each injection. **Follow the package directions supplied with your syringe.** Described below are 2 methods of sterilizing.

Boiling

1. Put syringe, plunger, and needle in strainer, place in saucepan, and cover with water. Boil for 5 minutes.
2. Remove articles from water. When they have cooled, insert plunger into barrel, and fasten needle to syringe with a slight twist.
3. Push plunger in and out several times until water is completely removed.

Isopropyl Alcohol
If the syringe, plunger, and needle cannot be boiled, as when you are traveling, they may be sterilized by immersion for at least 5 minutes in Isopropyl Alcohol, 91%. Do not use bathing, rubbing, or medicated alcohol for this sterilization. If the syringe is sterilized with alcohol, it must be absolutely dry before use.

Preparing the Dose

1. Wash your hands.
2. Carefully shake or rotate the insulin bottle several times to completely mix the insulin.
3. Inspect the insulin. Humulin U should look uniformly cloudy or milky. Do not use it if you notice anything unusual in the appearance.
4. If using a new bottle, flip off the plastic protective cap, but **do not** remove the stopper. When using a new bottle, wipe the top of the bottle with an alcohol swab.
5. If you are mixing insulins, refer to the instructions for mixing that follow.
6. Draw air into the syringe equal to your insulin dose. Put the needle through rubber top of the insulin bottle and inject the air into the bottle.

7. Turn the bottle and syringe upside down. Hold the bottle and syringe firmly in 1 hand and shake gently.
8. Making sure the tip of the needle is in the insulin, withdraw the correct dose of insulin into the syringe.
9. Before removing the needle from the bottle, check your syringe for air bubbles which reduce the amount of insulin in it. If bubbles are present, hold the syringe straight up and tap its side until the bubbles float to the top. Push them out with the plunger and withdraw the correct dose.
10. Remove the needle from the bottle and lay the syringe down so that the needle does not touch anything.

Mixing Humulin U with Regular or Lente Human Insulin

1. Ultralente human insulin should be mixed with regular or Lente human insulin only on the advice of your doctor.
2. Draw air into your syringe equal to the amount of Humulin U you are taking. Insert the needle into the Humulin U bottle and inject the air. Withdraw the needle.
3. Now inject air into your regular or Lente human insulin bottle in the same manner, but **do not** withdraw the needle.
4. Turn the bottle and syringe upside down.
5. Making sure the tip of the needle is in the insulin, withdraw the correct dose of regular or Lente insulin into the syringe.
6. Before removing the needle from the bottle, check your syringe for air bubbles which reduce the amount of insulin in it. If bubbles are present, hold the syringe straight up and tap its side until the bubbles float to the top. Push them out with the plunger and withdraw the correct dose.
7. Remove the needle from the bottle of regular or Lente insulin and insert it into the bottle of Humulin U. Turn the bottle and syringe upside down. Hold the bottle and syringe firmly in 1 hand and shake gently. Making sure the tip of the needle is in the insulin, withdraw your dose of Humulin U.
8. Remove the needle and lay the syringe down so that the needle does not touch anything.

Follow your doctor's instructions on whether to mix your insulins ahead of time or just before giving your injection. It is important to be consistent in your method.

Syringes from different manufacturers may vary in the amount of space between the bottom line and the needle. Because of this, do not change:

- the sequence of mixing, or
- the model and brand of syringe or needle that the doctor has prescribed.

Injection

Cleanse the skin with alcohol where the injection is to be made. Stabilize the skin by spreading it or pinching up a large area. Insert the needle as instructed by your doctor. Push the plunger in as far as it will go. Pull the needle out and apply gentle pressure over the injection site for several seconds. **Do not rub the area.** To avoid tissue damage, give the next injection at a site at least 1/2″ from the previous site.

DOSAGE

Your doctor has told you which insulin to use, how much, and when and how often to inject it. Because each patient's case of diabetes is different, this schedule has been individualized for you.

Your usual insulin dose may be affected by changes in your food, activity, or work schedule. Carefully follow your doctor's instructions to allow for these changes. Other things that may affect your insulin dose are:

Illness

Illness, especially with nausea and vomiting, may cause your insulin requirements to change. Even if you are not eating, you will still require insulin. You and your doctor should establish a sick day plan for you to use in case of illness. When you are sick, test your blood/urine frequently and call your doctor as instructed.

Pregnancy

Good control of diabetes is especially important for you and your unborn baby. Pregnancy may make managing your diabetes more difficult. If you are planning to have a baby, are pregnant, or are nursing a baby, consult your doctor.

Medication

Insulin requirements may be increased if you are taking other drugs with hyperglycemic activity, such as oral contraceptives, corticosteroids, or thyroid replacement therapy. Insulin requirements may be reduced in the presence of drugs with hypoglycemic activity, such as oral hypoglycemics, salicylates (for example, aspirin), sulfa antibiotics, and certain antidepressants. Always discuss any medications you are taking with your doctor.

Exercise

Exercise may lower your body's need for insulin during and for some time after the activity. Exercise may also speed up the effect of an insulin dose, especially if the exercise involves the area of injection site (for example, the leg should not be used for injection just prior to running). Discuss with your doctor how you should adjust your regimen to accommodate exercise.

Travel

Persons traveling across more than 2 time zones should consult their doctor concerning adjustments in their insulin schedule.

COMMON PROBLEMS OF DIABETES

Hypoglycemia (Insulin Reaction)

Hypoglycemia (too little glucose in the blood) is one of the most frequent adverse events experienced by insulin users. It can be brought about by:

1. Taking too much insulin
2. Missing or delaying meals
3. Exercising or working more than usual
4. An infection or illness (especially with diarrhea or vomiting)
5. A change in the body's need for insulin
6. Diseases of the adrenal, pituitary, or thyroid gland, or progression of kidney or liver disease
7. Interactions with other drugs that lower blood glucose, such as oral hypoglycemics, salicylates (for example, aspirin), sulfa antibiotics, and certain antidepressants
8. Consumption of alcoholic beverages

Symptoms of mild to moderate hypoglycemia may occur suddenly and can include:

- sweating
- dizziness
- palpitation
- tremor
- hunger
- restlessness
- tingling in the hands, feet, lips, or tongue
- lightheadedness
- inability to concentrate
- headache
- drowsiness
- sleep disturbances
- anxiety
- blurred vision
- slurred speech
- depressed mood
- irritability
- abnormal behavior
- unsteady movement
- personality changes

Signs of severe hypoglycemia can include:

- disorientation
- unconsciousness
- seizures
- death

Therefore, it is important that assistance be obtained immediately.

Early warning symptoms of hypoglycemia may be different or less pronounced under certain conditions, such as long duration of diabetes, diabetic nerve disease, medications such as beta-blockers, change in insulin preparations, or intensified control (3 or more insulin injections per day) of diabetes.

A few patients who have experienced hypoglycemic reactions after transfer from animal-source insulin to human insulin have reported that the early warning symptoms of hypoglycemia were less pronounced or different from those experienced with their previous insulin.

Without recognition of early warning symptoms, you may not be able to take steps to avoid more serious hypoglycemia. Be alert for all of the various types of symptoms that may indicate hypoglycemia. Patients who experience hypoglycemia without early warning symptoms should monitor their blood glucose frequently, especially prior to activities such as driving. If the blood glucose is below your normal fasting glucose, you should consider eating or drinking sugar-containing foods to treat your hypoglycemia.

Mild to moderate hypoglycemia may be treated by eating foods or drinks that contain sugar. Patients should always carry a quick source of sugar, such as candy mints or glucose tablets. More severe hypoglycemia may require the assistance of another person. Patients who are unable to take sugar orally or who are unconscious require an injection of glucagon or should be treated with intravenous administration of glucose at a medical facility.

You should learn to recognize your own symptoms of hypoglycemia. If you are uncertain about these symptoms, you should monitor your blood glucose frequently to help you learn to recognize the symptoms that you experience with hypoglycemia.

If you have frequent episodes of hypoglycemia or experience difficulty in recognizing the symptoms, you should consult your doctor to discuss possible changes in therapy, meal plans, and/or exercise programs to help you avoid hypoglycemia.

Hyperglycemia and Diabetic Acidosis

Hyperglycemia (too much glucose in the blood) may develop if your body has too little insulin. Hyperglycemia can be brought about by:

1. Omitting your insulin or taking less than the doctor has prescribed
2. Eating significantly more than your meal plan suggests
3. Developing a fever, infection, or other significant stressful situation

In patients with insulin-dependent diabetes, prolonged hyperglycemia can result in diabetic acidosis. The first symptoms of diabetic acidosis usually come on gradually, over a period of hours or days, and include a drowsy feeling, flushed face, thirst, loss of appetite, and fruity odor on the breath. With acidosis, urine tests show large amounts of glucose and acetone. Heavy breathing and a rapid pulse are more severe symptoms. If uncorrected, prolonged hyperglycemia or diabetic acidosis can lead to nausea, vomiting, dehydration, loss of consciousness or death. Therefore, it is important that you obtain medical assistance immediately.

Lipodystrophy

Rarely, administration of insulin subcutaneously can result in lipoatrophy (depression in the skin) or lipohypertrophy (enlargement or thickening of tissue). If you notice either of these conditions, consult your doctor. A change in your injection technique may help alleviate the problem.

Allergy to Insulin

Local Allergy—Patients occasionally experience redness, swelling, and itching at the site of injection of insulin. This condition, called local allergy, usually clears up in a few days to a few weeks. In some instances, this condition may be related to factors other than insulin, such as irritants in the skin cleansing agent or poor injection technique. If you have local reactions, contact your doctor.

Systemic Allergy—Less common, but potentially more serious, is generalized allergy to insulin, which may cause rash over the whole body, shortness of breath, wheezing, reduction in blood pressure, fast pulse, or sweating. Severe cases of generalized allergy may be life threatening. If you think you are having a generalized allergic reaction to insulin, notify a doctor immediately.

ADDITIONAL INFORMATION

Additional information about diabetes may be obtained from your diabetes educator.

DIABETES FORECAST is a national magazine designed especially for patients with diabetes and their families and is available by subscription from the American Diabetes Association, National Service Center, 1660 Duke Street, Alexandria, Virginia 22314, 1-800-DIABETES (1-800-342-2383).

Another publication, **DIABETES COUNTDOWN**, is available from the Juvenile Diabetes Foundation International (JDF), 120 Wall Street, 19th Floor, New York, New York 10005, 1-800-JDF-CURE (1-800-533-2873).

Additional information about Humulin can be obtained by calling 1-888-88-LILLY (1-888-885-4559).

Literature revised August 3, 2000

PA 6366 AMP

KEFLEX® ℞

[kē′flěks]

CEPHALEXIN CAPSULES, USP

To reduce the development of drug-resistant bacteria and maintain the effectiveness of Keflex and other antibacterial drugs, Keflex should be used only to treat or prevent infections that are proven or strongly suspected to be caused by bacteria.

DESCRIPTION

Keflex® (Cephalexin Capsules, USP) is a semisynthetic cephalosporin antibiotic intended for oral administration. It is 7-(D-α-Amino-α-phenylacetamido)-3-methyl-3-cephem-4-carboxylic acid monohydrate. Cephalexin has the molecular formula $C_{16}H_{17}N_3O_4S \cdot H_2O$ and the molecular weight is 365.41.

Cephalexin has the following structural formula:

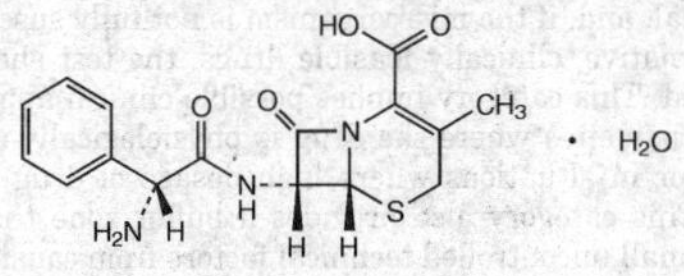

The nucleus of cephalexin is related to that of other cephalosporin antibiotics. The compound is a zwitterion; i.e., the molecule contains both a basic and an acidic group. The isoelectric point of cephalexin in water is approximately 4.5 to 5.

The crystalline form of cephalexin which is available is a monohydrate. It is a white crystalline solid having a bitter taste. Solubility in water is low at room temperature; 1 or 2 mg/mL may be dissolved readily, but higher concentrations are obtained with increasing difficulty.

The cephalosporins differ from penicillins in the structure of the bicyclic ring system. Cephalexin has a *D*-phenylglycyl group as substituent at the 7-amino position and an unsubstituted methyl group at the 3-position.

Each Pulvule® contains cephalexin monohydrate equivalent to 250 mg (720 μmol) or 500 mg (1439 μmol) of cephalexin. The Pulvules also contain cellulose, D & C Yellow No. 10, F D & C Blue No. 1, F D & C Yellow No. 6, gelatin, magnesium stearate, silicone, titanium dioxide, and other inactive ingredients.

CLINICAL PHARMACOLOGY

Human Pharmacology

Keflex is acid stable and may be given without regard to meals. It is rapidly absorbed after oral administration. Following doses of 250 mg, 500 mg, and 1 g, average peak serum levels of approximately 9, 18, and 32 μg/mL respectively were obtained at 1 hour. Measurable levels were pres-

Continued on next page

*** Identi-Code® symbol. This product information was prepared in June 2004. Current information on these and other products of Eli Lilly and Company may be obtained by direct inquiry to Lilly Research Laboratories, Lilly Corporate Center, Indianapolis, Indiana 46285, (800) 545-5979.**

Keflex—Cont.

ent 6 hours after administration. Cephalexin is excreted in the urine by glomerular filtration and tubular secretion. Studies showed that over 90% of the drug was excreted unchanged in the urine within 8 hours. During this period, peak urine concentrations following the 250-mg, 500-mg, and 1-g doses were approximately 1000, 2200, and 5000 μg/mL respectively.

Microbiology

In vitro tests demonstrate that the cephalosporins are bactericidal because of their inhibition of cell-wall synthesis. Cephalexin has been shown to be active against most strains of the following microorganisms both *in vitro* and in clinical infections as described in the INDICATIONS AND USAGE section.

Aerobes, Gram-positive:
Staphylococcus aureus (including penicillinase-producing strains)
Staphylococcus epidermidis (penicillin-susceptible strains)
Streptococcus pneumoniae
Streptococcus pyogenes

Aerobes, Gram-negative:
Escherichia coli
Haemophilus influenzae
Klebsiella pneumoniae
Moraxella (Branhamella) catarrhalis
Proteus mirabilis

Note—Methicillin-resistant staphylococci and most strains of enterococci (*Enterococcus faecalis* [formerly *Streptococcus faecalis*]) are resistant to cephalosporins, including cephalexin. It is not active against most strains of *Enterobacter* spp., *Morganella morganii*, and *Proteus vulgaris*. It has no activity against *Pseudomonas* spp. or *Acinetobacter calcoaceticus*.

Susceptibility Tests

Diffusion techniques—Quantitative methods that require measurement of zone diameters provide reproducible estimates of the susceptibility of bacteria to antimicrobial compounds. One such standardized procedure[1] that has been recommended for use with disks to test the susceptibility of microorganisms to cephalexin uses the 30-μg cephalothin disk. Interpretation involves correlation of the diameter obtained in the disk test with the minimal inhibitory concentration (MIC) for cephalexin.

Reports from the laboratory providing results of the standard single-disk susceptibility test with a 30-μg cephalothin disk should be interpreted according to the following criteria:

Zone Diameter (mm)	Interpretation
≥18	(S) Susceptible
15-17	(I) Intermediate
≤14	(R) Resistant

A report of "Susceptible" indicates that the pathogen is likely to be inhibited by usually achievable concentrations of the antimicrobial compound in blood. A report of "Intermediate" indicates that the result should be considered equivocal, and, if the microorganism is not fully susceptible to alternative, clinically feasible drugs, the test should be repeated. This category implies possible clinical applicability in body sites where the drug is physiologically concentrated or in situations where high dosage of drug can be used. This category also provides a buffer zone that prevents small uncontrolled technical factors from causing major discrepancies in interpretation. A report of "Resistant" indicates that usually achievable concentrations of the antimicrobial compound in the blood are unlikely to be inhibitory and that other therapy should be selected.

Measurement of MIC or MBC and achieved antimicrobial compound concentrations may be appropriate to guide therapy in some infections. (See CLINICAL PHARMACOLOGY section for information on drug concentrations achieved in infected body sites and other pharmacokinetic properties of this antimicrobial drug product.)

Standardized susceptibility test procedures require the use of laboratory control microorganisms. The 30-μg cephalothin disk should provide the following zone diameters in these laboratory test quality control strains:

Microorganism	Zone Diameter (mm)
E. coli ATCC 25922	15-21
S. aureus ATCC 25923	29-37

Dilution techniques—Quantitative methods that are used to determine MICs provide reproducible estimates of the susceptibility of bacteria to antimicrobial compounds. One such standardized procedure uses a standardized dilution method[2] (broth, agar, microdilution) or equivalent with cephalothin powder. The MIC values obtained should be interpreted according to the following criteria:

MIC (μg/mL)	Interpretation
≤8	(S) Susceptible
16	(I) Intermediate
≥32	(R) Resistant

Interpretation should be as stated above for results using diffusion techniques.

As with standard diffusion techniques, dilution methods require the use of laboratory control microorganisms. Standard cephalothin powder should provide the following MIC values:

Microorganism	MIC (μg/mL)
E. coli ATCC 25922	4-16
S. aureus ATCC 29213	0.12-0.5

INDICATIONS AND USAGE

Keflex is indicated for the treatment of the following infections when caused by susceptible strains of the designated microorganisms:

Respiratory tract infections caused by *S. pneumoniae* and *S. pyogenes* (Penicillin is the usual drug of choice in the treatment and prevention of streptococcal infections, including the prophylaxis of rheumatic fever. Keflex is generally effective in the eradication of streptococci from the nasopharynx; however, substantial data establishing the efficacy of Keflex in the subsequent prevention of rheumatic fever are not available at present.)

Otitis media due to *S. pneumoniae, H. influenzae*, staphylococci, streptococci, and *M. catarrhalis*

Skin and skin structure infections caused by staphylococci and/or streptococci

Bone infections caused by staphylococci and/or *P. mirabilis*

Genitourinary tract infections, including acute prostatitis, caused by *E. coli, P. mirabilis*, and *K. pneumoniae*

Note—Culture and susceptibility tests should be initiated prior to and during therapy. Renal function studies should be performed when indicated.

To reduce the development of drug-resistant bacteria and maintain the effectiveness of Keflex and other antibacterial drugs, Keflex should be used only to treat or prevent infections that are proven or strongly suspected to be caused by susceptible bacteria. When culture and susceptibility information are available, they should be considered in selecting or modifying antibacterial therapy. In the absence of such data, local epidemiology and susceptibility patterns may contribute to the empiric selection of therapy.

CONTRAINDICATIONS

Keflex is contraindicated in patients with known allergy to the cephalosporin group of antibiotics.

WARNINGS

BEFORE CEPHALEXIN THERAPY IS INSTITUTED, CAREFUL INQUIRY SHOULD BE MADE CONCERNING PREVIOUS HYPERSENSITIVITY REACTIONS TO CEPHALOSPORINS AND PENICILLIN. CEPHALOSPORIN C DERIVATIVES SHOULD BE GIVEN CAUTIOUSLY TO PENICILLIN-SENSITIVE PATIENTS.

SERIOUS ACUTE HYPERSENSITIVITY REACTIONS MAY REQUIRE EPINEPHRINE AND OTHER EMERGENCY MEASURES.

There is some clinical and laboratory evidence of partial cross-allergenicity of the penicillins and the cephalosporins. Patients have been reported to have had severe reactions (including anaphylaxis) to both drugs.

Any patient who has demonstrated some form of allergy, particularly to drugs, should receive antibiotics cautiously. No exception should be made with regard to Keflex.

Pseudomembranous colitis has been reported with nearly all antibacterial agents, including cephalexin, and may range from mild to life threatening. Therefore, it is important to consider this diagnosis in patients with diarrhea subsequent to the administration of antibacterial agents.

Treatment with antibacterial agents alters the normal flora of the colon and may permit overgrowth of clostridia. Studies indicate that a toxin produced by *Clostridium difficile* is one primary cause of antibiotic-associated colitis.

After the diagnosis of pseudomembranous colitis has been established, appropriate therapeutic measures should be initiated. Mild cases of pseudomembranous colitis usually respond to drug discontinuation alone. In moderate to severe cases, consideration should be given to management with fluids and electrolytes, protein supplementation, and treatment with an antibacterial drug clinically effective against *Clostridium difficile* colitis.

Usage in Pregnancy—Safety of this product for use during pregnancy has not been established.

PRECAUTIONS

General

Prescribing Keflex in the absence of a proven or strongly suspected bacterial infection or a prophylactic indication is unlikely to provide benefit to the patient and increases the risk of the development of drug-resistant bacteria.

Patients should be followed carefully so that any side effects or unusual manifestations of drug idiosyncrasy may be detected. If an allergic reaction to Keflex occurs, the drug should be discontinued and the patient treated with the usual agents (e.g., epinephrine or other pressor amines, antihistamines, or corticosteroids).

Prolonged use of Keflex may result in the overgrowth of nonsusceptible organisms. Careful observation of the patient is essential. If superinfection occurs during therapy, appropriate measures should be taken.

Positive direct Coombs' tests have been reported during treatment with the cephalosporin antibiotics. In hematologic studies or in transfusion cross-matching procedures when antiglobulin tests are performed on the minor side or in Coombs' testing of newborns whose mothers have received cephalosporin antibiotics before parturition, it should be recognized that a positive Coombs' test may be due to the drug.

Keflex should be administered with caution in the presence of markedly impaired renal function. Under such conditions, careful clinical observation and laboratory studies should be made because safe dosage may be lower than that usually recommended.

Indicated surgical procedures should be performed in conjunction with antibiotic therapy.

As a result of administration of Keflex, a false-positive reaction for glucose in the urine may occur. This has been observed with Benedict's and Fehling's solutions and also with Clinitest® tablets.

In healthy subjects given single 500 mg doses of cephalexin and metformin, plasma metformin C_{max} and AUC increased by an average of 34% and 24%, respectively, and metformin renal clearance decreased by an average of 14%. No information is available about the interaction of cephalexin and metformin following multiple dose administration.

As with other β-lactams, the renal excretion of cephalexin is inhibited by probenecid.

Broad-spectrum antibiotics should be prescribed with caution in individuals with a history of gastrointestinal disease, particularly colitis.

Information for Patients

Patients should be counseled that antibacterial drugs including Keflex should only be used to treat bacterial infections. They do not treat viral infections (e.g., the common cold). When Keflex is prescribed to treat a bacterial infection, patients should be told that although it is common to feel better early in the course of therapy, the medication should be taken exactly as directed. Skipping doses or not completing the full course of therapy may (1) decrease the effectiveness of the immediate treatment and (2) increase the likelihood that bacteria will develop resistance and will not be treatable by Keflex or other antibacterial drugs in the future.

Usage in Pregnancy

Pregnancy Category B—The daily oral administration of cephalexin to rats in doses of 250 or 500 mg/kg prior to and during pregnancy, or to rats and mice during the period of organogenesis only, had no adverse effect on fertility, fetal viability, fetal weight, or litter size. Note that the safety of cephalexin during pregnancy in humans has not been established.

Cephalexin showed no enhanced toxicity in weanling and newborn rats as compared with adult animals. Nevertheless, because the studies in humans cannot rule out the possibility of harm, Keflex should be used during pregnancy only if clearly needed.

Nursing Mothers

The excretion of cephalexin in the milk increased up to 4 hours after a 500-mg dose; the drug reached a maximum level of 4 μg/mL, then decreased gradually, and had disappeared 8 hours after administration. Caution should be exercised when Keflex is administered to a nursing woman.

Geriatric Use

Of the 701 subjects in 3 published clinical studies of cephalexin, 433 (62%) were 65 and over. No overall differences in safety or effectiveness were observed between these subjects and younger subjects, and other reported clinical experience has not identified differences in responses between the elderly and younger patients, but greater sensitivity of some older individuals cannot be ruled out.

This drug is known to be substantially excreted by the kidney, and the risk of toxic reactions to this drug may be greater in patients with impaired renal function. Because elderly patients are more likely to have decreased renal function, care should be taken in dose selection, and it may be useful to monitor renal function (*see* **PRECAUTIONS, General**).

ADVERSE REACTIONS

Gastrointestinal—Symptoms of pseudomembranous colitis may appear either during or after antibiotic treatment. Nausea and vomiting have been reported rarely. The most frequent side effect has been diarrhea. It was very rarely severe enough to warrant cessation of therapy. Dyspepsia, gastritis, and abdominal pain have also occurred. As with some penicillins and some other cephalosporins, transient hepatitis and cholestatic jaundice have been reported rarely.

Hypersensitivity—Allergic reactions in the form of rash, urticaria, angioedema, and, rarely, erythema multiforme, Stevens-Johnson syndrome, or toxic epidermal necrolysis have been observed. These reactions usually subsided upon discontinuation of the drug. In some of these reactions, supportive therapy may be necessary. Anaphylaxis has also been reported.

Other reactions have included genital and anal pruritus, genital moniliasis, vaginitis and vaginal discharge, dizziness, fatigue, headache, agitation, confusion, hallucinations, arthralgia, arthritis, and joint disorder. Reversible interstitial nephritis has been reported rarely. Eosinophilia, neutropenia, thrombocytopenia, and slight elevations in AST and ALT have been reported.

OVERDOSAGE

Signs and Symptoms—Symptoms of oral overdose may include nausea, vomiting, epigastric distress, diarrhea, and hematuria. If other symptoms are present, it is probably secondary to an underlying disease state, an allergic reaction, or toxicity due to ingestion of a second medication.

Treatment—To obtain up-to-date information about the treatment of overdose, a good resource is your certified Regional Poison Control Center. Telephone numbers of certified poison control centers are listed in the *Physicians' Desk Reference (PDR)*. In managing overdosage, consider the possibility of multiple drug overdoses, interaction among drugs, and unusual drug kinetics in your patient.

Unless 5 to 10 times the normal dose of cephalexin has been ingested, gastrointestinal decontamination should not be necessary.

Protect the patient's airway and support ventilation and perfusion. Meticulously monitor and maintain, within acceptable limits, the patient's vital signs, blood gases, serum electrolytes, etc. Absorption of drugs from the gastrointestinal tract may be decreased by giving activated charcoal, which, in many cases, is more effective than emesis or lavage; consider charcoal instead of or in addition to gastric emptying. Repeated doses of charcoal over time may hasten elimination of some drugs that have been absorbed. Safeguard the patient's airway when employing gastric emptying or charcoal.

Forced diuresis, peritoneal dialysis, hemodialysis, or charcoal hemoperfusion have not been established as beneficial for an overdose of cephalexin; however, it would be extremely unlikely that one of these procedures would be indicated.

The oral median lethal dose of cephalexin in rats is >5000 mg/kg.

DOSAGE AND ADMINISTRATION

Keflex is administered orally.

Adults—The adult dosage ranges from 1 to 4 g daily in divided doses. The usual adult dose is 250 mg every 6 hours. For the following infections, a dosage of 500 mg may be administered every 12 hours: streptococcal pharyngitis, skin and skin structure infections, and uncomplicated cystitis in patients over 15 years of age. Cystitis therapy should be continued for 7 to 14 days. For more severe infections or those caused by less susceptible organisms, larger doses may be needed. If daily doses of Keflex greater than 4 g are required, parenteral cephalosporins, in appropriate doses, should be considered.

Pediatric Patients—The usual recommended daily dosage for pediatric patients is 25 to 50 mg/kg in divided doses. For streptococcal pharyngitis in patients over 1 year of age and for skin and skin structure infections, the total daily dose may be divided and administered every 12 hours.

In severe infections, the dosage may be doubled.

In the therapy of otitis media, clinical studies have shown that a dosage of 75 to 100 mg/kg/day in 4 divided doses is required.

In the treatment of β-hemolytic streptococcal infections, a therapeutic dosage of Keflex should be administered for at least 10 days.

HOW SUPPLIED

Keflex® (Cephalexin Capsules, USP), are available in:

The 250 mg Pulvules® are a white powder filled into size 2 Posilok® Caps (opaque white and opaque dark green) that are imprinted with "Dista" and identity code "H69" on the green cap, and Keflex 250 mg on the white body in edible black ink. They are available as follows:

Bottles of 20 NDC 0777-0869-20 (PU402)
Bottles of 100 NDC 0777-0869-02 (PU402)

The 500 mg Pulvules are a white powder filled into an elongated, size 0 Posilok Caps (opaque light green and opaque dark green) that are imprinted with "Dista" and identity code "H71" on the dark green cap, and Keflex 500 mg on the light green body in edible black ink. They are available as follows:

Bottles of 20 NDC 0777-0871-20 (PU403)
Bottles of 100 NDC 0777-0871-02 (PU403)

Store at 25°C (77°F); excursions permitted to 15-30°C (59-86°F) [see USP Controlled Room Temperature].

REFERENCES

1. National Committee for Clinical Laboratory Standards: Performance standards for antimicrobial disk susceptibility tests — 5th ed. Approved Standard NCCLS Document M2-A5, Vol. 13, No. 24, NCCLS, Villanova, PA, 1993.
2. National Committee for Clinical Laboratory Standards: Methods for dilution antimicrobial susceptibility tests for bacteria that grow aerobically — 3rd ed. Approved Standard NCCLS Document M7-A3, Vol. 13, No. 25, NCCLS, Villanova, PA, 1993.

Literature revised January 15, 2004
Manufactured by Eli Lilly Italia S.p.A.
Sesto Fiorentino (Firenze), Italy
for **DISTA PRODUCTS COMPANY**
Division of Eli Lilly and Company
Indianapolis, IN 46285, USA
IT 0243 ITAMP

PROZAC® ℞

[prō-zăk]

FLUOXETINE HYDROCHLORIDE

DESCRIPTION

Prozac® (fluoxetine hydrochloride) is a psychotropic drug for oral administration. It is also marketed for the treatment of premenstrual dysphoric disorder (Sarafem®, fluoxetine hydrochloride). It is designated (±)-N-methyl-3-phenyl-3-[(α,α,α-trifluoro-p-tolyl)oxy]propylamine hydrochloride and has the empirical formula of $C_{17}H_{18}F_3NO \bullet HCl$. Its molecular weight is 345.79. The structural formula is:

F_3C—(benzene ring)—O—$CHCH_2CH_2NHCH_3$ • HCl (with phenyl on CH)

Fluoxetine hydrochloride is a white to off-white crystalline solid with a solubility of 14 mg/mL in water.

Each Pulvule® contains fluoxetine hydrochloride equivalent to 10 mg (32.3 μmol), 20 mg (64.7 μmol), or 40 mg (129.3 μmol) of fluoxetine. The Pulvules also contain starch, gelatin, silicone, titanium dioxide, iron oxide, and other inactive ingredients. The 10- and 20-mg Pulvules also contain FD&C Blue No. 1, and the 40-mg Pulvule also contains FD&C Blue No. 1 and FD&C Yellow No. 6.

Each tablet contains fluoxetine hydrochloride equivalent to 10 mg (32.3 μmol) of fluoxetine. The tablets also contain microcrystalline cellulose, magnesium stearate, crospovidone, hypromellose, titanium dioxide, polyethylene glycol, and yellow iron oxide. In addition to the above ingredients, the 10-mg tablet contains FD&C Blue No. 1 aluminum lake and polysorbate 80.

The oral solution contains fluoxetine hydrochloride equivalent to 20 mg/5 mL (64.7 μmol) of fluoxetine. It also contains alcohol 0.23%, benzoic acid, flavoring agent, glycerin, purified water, and sucrose.

Prozac Weekly™ capsules, a delayed-release formulation, contain enteric-coated pellets of fluoxetine hydrochloride equivalent to 90 mg (291 μmol) of fluoxetine. The capsules also contain D&C Yellow No. 10, FD&C Blue No. 2, gelatin, hypromellose, hydroxypropyl methylcellulose acetate succinate, sodium lauryl sulfate, sucrose, sugar spheres, talc, titanium dioxide, triethyl citrate, and other inactive ingredients.

CLINICAL PHARMACOLOGY

Pharmacodynamics

The antidepressant, antiobsessive-compulsive, and antibulimic actions of fluoxetine are presumed to be linked to its inhibition of CNS neuronal uptake of serotonin. Studies at clinically relevant doses in man have demonstrated that fluoxetine blocks the uptake of serotonin into human platelets. Studies in animals also suggest that fluoxetine is a much more potent uptake inhibitor of serotonin than of norepinephrine.

Antagonism of muscarinic, histaminergic, and α_1-adrenergic receptors has been hypothesized to be associated with various anticholinergic, sedative, and cardiovascular effects of classical tricyclic antidepressant (TCA) drugs. Fluoxetine binds to these and other membrane receptors from brain tissue much less potently in vitro than do the tricyclic drugs.

Absorption, Distribution, Metabolism, and Excretion

Systemic bioavailability—In man, following a single oral 40-mg dose, peak plasma concentrations of fluoxetine from 15 to 55 ng/mL are observed after 6 to 8 hours.

The Pulvule, tablet, oral solution, and Prozac Weekly capsule dosage forms of fluoxetine are bioequivalent. Food does not appear to affect the systemic bioavailability of fluoxetine, although it may delay its absorption by 1 to 2 hours, which is probably not clinically significant. Thus, fluoxetine may be administered with or without food. Prozac Weekly capsules, a delayed-release formulation, contain enteric-coated pellets that resist dissolution until reaching a segment of the gastrointestinal tract where the pH exceeds 5.5. The enteric coating delays the onset of absorption of fluoxetine 1 to 2 hours relative to the immediate-release formulations.

Protein binding—Over the concentration range from 200 to 1000 ng/mL, approximately 94.5% of fluoxetine is bound in vitro to human serum proteins, including albumin and α_1-glycoprotein. The interaction between fluoxetine and other highly protein-bound drugs has not been fully evaluated, but may be important (*see* PRECAUTIONS).

Enantiomers—Fluoxetine is a racemic mixture (50/50) of *R*-fluoxetine and *S*-fluoxetine enantiomers. In animal models, both enantiomers are specific and potent serotonin uptake inhibitors with essentially equivalent pharmacologic activity. The *S*-fluoxetine enantiomer is eliminated more slowly and is the predominant enantiomer present in plasma at steady state.

Metabolism—Fluoxetine is extensively metabolized in the liver to norfluoxetine and a number of other unidentified metabolites. The only identified active metabolite, norfluoxetine, is formed by demethylation of fluoxetine. In animal models, *S*-norfluoxetine is a potent and selective inhibitor of serotonin uptake and has activity essentially equivalent to *R*- or *S*-fluoxetine. *R*-norfluoxetine is significantly less potent than the parent drug in the inhibition of serotonin uptake. The primary route of elimination appears to be hepatic metabolism to inactive metabolites excreted by the kidney.

Clinical issues related to metabolism/elimination—The complexity of the metabolism of fluoxetine has several consequences that may potentially affect fluoxetine's clinical use.

Variability in metabolism—A subset (about 7%) of the population has reduced activity of the drug metabolizing enzyme cytochrome P450 2D6 (CYP2D6). Such individuals are referred to as "poor metabolizers" of drugs such as debrisoquin, dextromethorphan, and the TCAs. In a study involving labeled and unlabeled enantiomers administered as a racemate, these individuals metabolized *S*-fluoxetine at a slower rate and thus achieved higher concentrations of *S*-fluoxetine. Consequently, concentrations of *S*-norfluoxetine at steady state were lower. The metabolism of *R*-fluoxetine in these poor metabolizers appears normal. When compared with normal metabolizers, the total sum at steady state of the plasma concentrations of the 4 active enantiomers was not significantly greater among poor metabolizers. Thus, the net pharmacodynamic activities were essentially the same. Alternative, nonsaturable pathways (non-2D6) also contribute to the metabolism of fluoxetine. This explains how fluoxetine achieves a steady-state concentration rather than increasing without limit.

Because fluoxetine's metabolism, like that of a number of other compounds including TCAs and other selective serotonin reuptake (SSRIs), involves the CYP2D6 system, concomitant therapy with drugs also metabolized by this enzyme system (such as the TCAs) may lead to drug interactions (*see* Drug Interactions *under* PRECAUTIONS).

Accumulation and slow elimination—The relatively slow elimination of fluoxetine (elimination half-life of 1 to 3 days after acute administration and 4 to 6 days after chronic administration) and its active metabolite, norfluoxetine (elimination half-life of 4 to 16 days after acute and chronic administration), leads to significant accumulation of these active species in chronic use and delayed attainment of steady state, even when a fixed dose is used. After 30 days of dosing at 40 mg/day, plasma concentrations of fluoxetine in the range of 91 to 302 ng/mL and norfluoxetine in the range of 72 to 258 ng/mL have been observed. Plasma concentrations of fluoxetine were higher than those predicted by single-dose studies, because fluoxetine's metabolism is not proportional to dose. Norfluoxetine, however, appears to have linear pharmacokinetics. Its mean terminal half-life after a single dose was 8.6 days and after multiple dosing was 9.3 days. Steady-state levels after prolonged dosing are similar to levels seen at 4 to 5 weeks.

The long elimination half-lives of fluoxetine and norfluoxetine assure that, even when dosing is stopped, active drug substance will persist in the body for weeks (primarily depending on individual patient characteristics, previous dosing regimen, and length of previous therapy at discontinuation). This is of potential consequence when drug discontinuation is required or when drugs are prescribed that might interact with fluoxetine and norfluoxetine following the discontinuation of Prozac.

Weekly dosing—Administration of Prozac Weekly once weekly results in increased fluctuation between peak and trough concentrations of fluoxetine and norfluoxetine compared with once-daily dosing [for fluoxetine: 24% (daily) to 164% (weekly) and for norfluoxetine: 17% (daily) to 43% (weekly)]. Plasma concentrations may not necessarily be predictive of clinical response. Peak concentrations from once-weekly doses of Prozac Weekly capsules of fluoxetine are in the range of the average concentration for 20-mg once-daily dosing. Average trough concentrations are 76% lower for fluoxetine and 47% lower for norfluoxetine than the concentrations maintained by 20-mg once-daily dosing. Average steady-state concentrations of either once-daily or once-weekly dosing are in relative proportion to the total dose administered. Average steady-state fluoxetine concentrations are approximately 50% lower following the once-weekly regimen compared with the once-daily regimen.

C_{max} for fluoxetine following the 90-mg dose was approximately 1.7-fold higher than the C_{max} value for the established 20-mg once-daily regimen following transition the next day to the once-weekly regimen. In contrast, when the first 90-mg once-weekly dose and the last 20-mg once-daily dose were separated by 1 week, C_{max} values were similar. Also, there was a transient increase in the average steady-state concentrations of fluoxetine observed following transition the next day to the once-weekly regimen. From a pharmacokinetic perspective, it may be better to separate the first 90-mg weekly dose and the last 20-mg once-daily dose by 1 week (*see* DOSAGE AND ADMINISTRATION).

Liver disease—As might be predicted from its primary site of metabolism, liver impairment can affect the elimination of fluoxetine. The elimination half-life of fluoxetine was prolonged in a study of cirrhotic patients, with a mean of 7.6 days compared with the range of 2 to 3 days seen in subjects without liver disease; norfluoxetine elimination was also delayed, with a mean duration of 12 days for cirrhotic patients compared with the range of 7 to 9 days in normal subjects. This suggests that the use of fluoxetine in patients with liver disease must be approached with caution. If fluoxetine is administered to patients with liver disease, a lower or less frequent dose should be used (*see* PRECAUTIONS *and* DOSAGE AND ADMINISTRATION).

Renal disease—In depressed patients on dialysis (N=12), fluoxetine administered as 20 mg once daily for 2 months produced steady-state fluoxetine and norfluoxetine plasma concentrations comparable with those seen in patients with normal renal function. While the possibility exists that renally excreted metabolites of fluoxetine may accumulate to

Continued on next page

*** Identi-Code® symbol. This product information was prepared in June 2004. Current information on these and other products of Eli Lilly and Company may be obtained by direct inquiry to Lilly Research Laboratories, Lilly Corporate Center, Indianapolis, Indiana 46285, (800) 545-5979.**

Prozac—Cont.

higher levels in patients with severe renal dysfunction, use of a lower or less frequent dose is not routinely necessary in renally impaired patients (*see* Use in patients with concomitant illness *under* PRECAUTIONS *and* DOSAGE AND ADMINISTRATION).

Age

Geriatric pharmacokinetics—The disposition of single doses of fluoxetine in healthy elderly subjects (>65 years of age) did not differ significantly from that in younger normal subjects. However, given the long half-life and nonlinear disposition of the drug, a single-dose study is not adequate to rule out the possibility of altered pharmacokinetics in the elderly, particularly if they have systemic illness or are receiving multiple drugs for concomitant diseases. The effects of age upon the metabolism of fluoxetine have been investigated in 260 elderly but otherwise healthy depressed patients (≥60 years of age) who received 20 mg fluoxetine for 6 weeks. Combined fluoxetine plus norfluoxetine plasma concentrations were 209.3 ± 85.7 ng/mL at the end of 6 weeks. No unusual age-associated pattern of adverse events was observed in those elderly patients.

Pediatric pharmacokinetics (children and adolescents)—Fluoxetine pharmacokinetics were evaluated in 21 pediatric patients (10 children ages 6 to <13, 11 adolescents ages 13 to <18) diagnosed with major depressive disorder or obsessive-compulsive disorder (OCD). Fluoxetine 20 mg/day was administered for up to 62 days. The average steady-state concentrations of fluoxetine in these children were 2-fold higher than in adolescents (171 and 86 ng/mL, respectively). The average norfluoxetine steady-state concentrations in these children were 1.5-fold higher than in adolescents (195 and 113 ng/mL, respectively). These differences can be almost entirely explained by differences in weight. No gender-associated difference in fluoxetine pharmacokinetics was observed. Similar ranges of fluoxetine and norfluoxetine plasma concentrations were observed in another study in 94 pediatric patients (ages 8 to <18) diagnosed with major depressive disorder.

Higher average steady-state fluoxetine and norfluoxetine concentrations were observed in children relative to adults; however, these concentrations were within the range of concentrations observed in the adult population. As in adults, fluoxetine and norfluoxetine accumulated extensively following multiple oral dosing; steady-state concentrations were achieved within 3 to 4 weeks of daily dosing.

CLINICAL TRIALS

Major Depressive Disorder

Daily Dosing

Adult—The efficacy of Prozac for the treatment of patients with major depressive disorder (≥18 years of age) has been studied in 5- and 6-week placebo-controlled trials. Prozac was shown to be significantly more effective than placebo as measured by the Hamilton Depression Rating Scale (HAM-D). Prozac was also significantly more effective than placebo on the HAM-D subscores for depressed mood, sleep disturbance, and the anxiety subfactor.

Two 6-week controlled studies (N=671, randomized) comparing Prozac 20 mg and placebo have shown Prozac 20 mg daily to be effective in the treatment of elderly patients (≥60 years of age) with major depressive disorder. In these studies, Prozac produced a significantly higher rate of response and remission as defined, respectively, by a 50% decrease in the HAM-D score and a total endpoint HAM-D score of ≤8. Prozac was well tolerated and the rate of treatment discontinuations due to adverse events did not differ between Prozac (12%) and placebo (9%).

A study was conducted involving depressed outpatients who had responded (modified HAMD-17 score of ≤7 during each of the last 3 weeks of open-label treatment and absence of major depressive disorder by DSM-III-R criteria) by the end of an initial 12-week open-treatment phase on Prozac 20 mg/day. These patients (N=298) were randomized to continuation on double-blind Prozac 20 mg/day or placebo. At 38 weeks (50 weeks total), a statistically significantly lower relapse rate (defined as symptoms sufficient to meet a diagnosis of major depressive disorder for 2 weeks or a modified HAMD-17 score of ≥14 for 3 weeks) was observed for patients taking Prozac compared with those on placebo.

Pediatric (children and adolescents)—The efficacy of Prozac 20 mg/day for the treatment of major depressive disorder in pediatric outpatients (N=315 randomized; 170 children ages 8 to <13, 145 adolescents ages 13 to ≤18) has been studied in two 8- to 9-week placebo-controlled clinical trials.

In both studies independently, Prozac produced a statistically significantly greater mean change on the Childhood Depression Rating Scale-Revised (CDRS-R) total score from baseline to endpoint than did placebo.

Subgroup analyses on the CDRS-R total score did not suggest any differential responsiveness on the basis of age or gender.

Weekly dosing for maintenance/continuation treatment

A longer-term study was conducted involving adult outpatients meeting DSM-IV criteria for major depressive disorder who had responded (defined as having a modified HAMD-17 score of ≤9, a CGI-Severity rating of ≤2, and no longer meeting criteria for major depressive disorder) for 3 consecutive weeks at the end of 13 weeks of open-label treatment with Prozac 20 mg once daily. These patients were randomized to double-blind, once-weekly continuation treatment with Prozac Weekly, Prozac 20 mg once daily, or placebo. Prozac Weekly once weekly and Prozac 20 mg once daily demonstrated superior efficacy (having a significantly longer time to relapse of depressive symptoms) compared with placebo for a period of 25 weeks. However, the equivalence of these 2 treatments during continuation therapy has not been established.

Obsessive-Compulsive Disorder

Adult—The effectiveness of Prozac for the treatment of obsessive-compulsive disorder (OCD) was demonstrated in two 13-week, multicenter, parallel group studies (Studies 1 and 2) of adult outpatients who received fixed Prozac doses of 20, 40, or 60 mg/day (on a once-a-day schedule, in the morning) or placebo. Patients in both studies had moderate to severe OCD (DSM-III-R), with mean baseline ratings on the Yale-Brown Obsessive Compulsive Scale (YBOCS, total score) ranging from 22 to 26. In Study 1, patients receiving Prozac experienced mean reductions of approximately 4 to 6 units on the YBOCS total score, compared with a 1-unit reduction for placebo patients. In Study 2, patients receiving Prozac experienced mean reductions of approximately 4 to 9 units on the YBOCS total score, compared with a 1-unit reduction for placebo patients. While there was no indication of a dose-response relationship for effectiveness in Study 1, a dose-response relationship was observed in Study 2, with numerically better responses in the 2 higher dose groups. The following table provides the outcome classification by treatment group on the Clinical Global Impression (CGI) improvement scale for Studies 1 and 2 combined:

Outcome Classification (%) on CGI Improvement Scale for Completers in Pool of Two OCD Studies

		Prozac		
Outcome Classification	Placebo	20 mg	40 mg	60 mg
Worse	8%	0%	0%	0%
No change	64%	41%	33%	29%
Minimally improved	17%	23%	28%	24%
Much improved	8%	28%	27%	28%
Very much improved	3%	8%	12%	19%

Exploratory analyses for age and gender effects on outcome did not suggest any differential responsiveness on the basis of age or sex.

Pediatric (children and adolescents)—In one 13-week clinical trial in pediatric patients (N=103 randomized; 75 children ages 7 to <13, 28 adolescents ages 13 to <18) with OCD, patients received Prozac 10 mg/day for 2 weeks, followed by 20 mg/day for 2 weeks. The dose was then adjusted in the range of 20 to 60 mg/day on the basis of clinical response and tolerability. Prozac produced a statistically significantly greater mean change from baseline to endpoint than did placebo as measured by the Children's Yale-Brown Obsessive Compulsive Scale (CY-BOCS).

Subgroup analyses on outcome did not suggest any differential responsiveness on the basis of age or gender.

Bulimia Nervosa

The effectiveness of Prozac for the treatment of bulimia was demonstrated in two 8-week and one 16-week, multicenter, parallel group studies of adult outpatients meeting DSM-III-R criteria for bulimia. Patients in the 8-week studies received either 20 or 60 mg/day of Prozac or placebo in the morning. Patients in the 16-week study received a fixed Prozac dose of 60 mg/day (once a day) or placebo. Patients in these 3 studies had moderate to severe bulimia with median binge-eating and vomiting frequencies ranging from 7 to 10 per week and 5 to 9 per week, respectively. In these 3 studies, Prozac 60 mg, but not 20 mg, was statistically significantly superior to placebo in reducing the number of binge-eating and vomiting episodes per week. The statistically significantly superior effect of 60 mg versus placebo was present as early as Week 1 and persisted throughout each study. The Prozac-related reduction in bulimic episodes appeared to be independent of baseline depression as assessed by the Hamilton Depression Rating Scale. In each of these 3 studies, the treatment effect, as measured by differences between Prozac 60 mg and placebo on median reduction from baseline in frequency of bulimic behaviors at endpoint, ranged from 1 to 2 episodes per week for binge-eating and 2 to 4 episodes per week for vomiting. The size of the effect was related to baseline frequency, with greater reductions seen in patients with higher baseline frequencies. Although some patients achieved freedom from binge-eating and purging as a result of treatment, for the majority, the benefit was a partial reduction in the frequency of binge-eating and purging.

In a longer-term trial, 150 patients meeting DSM-IV criteria for bulimia nervosa, purging subtype, who had responded during a single-blind, 8-week acute treatment phase with Prozac 60 mg/day, were randomized to continuation of Prozac 60 mg/day or placebo, for up to 52 weeks of observation for relapse. Response during the single-blind phase was defined by having achieved at least a 50% decrease in vomiting frequency compared with baseline. Relapse during the double-blind phase was defined as a persistent return to baseline vomiting frequency or physician judgment that the patient had relapsed. Patients receiving continued Prozac 60 mg/day experienced a significantly longer time to relapse over the subsequent 52 weeks compared with those receiving placebo.

Panic Disorder

The effectiveness of Prozac in the treatment of panic disorder was demonstrated in 2 double-blind, randomized, placebo-controlled, multicenter studies of adult outpatients who had a primary diagnosis of panic disorder (DSM-IV), with or without agoraphobia.

Study 1 (N=180 randomized) was a 12-week flexible-dose study. Prozac was initiated at 10 mg/day for the first week, after which patients were dosed in the range of 20 to 60 mg/day on the basis of clinical response and tolerability. A statistically significantly greater percentage of Prozac-treated patients were free from panic attacks at endpoint than placebo-treated patients, 42% versus 28%, respectively.

Study 2 (N=214 randomized) was a 12-week flexible-dose study. Prozac was initiated at 10 mg/day for the first week, after which patients were dosed in a range of 20 to 60 mg/day on the basis of clinical response and tolerability. A statistically significantly greater percentage of Prozac-treated patients were free from panic attacks at endpoint than placebo-treated patients, 62% versus 44%, respectively.

INDICATIONS AND USAGE

Major Depressive Disorder

Prozac is indicated for the treatment of major depressive disorder.

Adult—The efficacy of Prozac was established in 5- and 6-week trials with depressed adult and geriatric outpatients (≥18 years of age) whose diagnoses corresponded most closely to the DSM-III (currently DSM-IV) category of major depressive disorder (*see* CLINICAL TRIALS).

A major depressive episode (DSM-IV) implies a prominent and relatively persistent (nearly every day for at least 2 weeks) depressed or dysphoric mood that usually interferes with daily functioning, and includes at least 5 of the following 9 symptoms: depressed mood, loss of interest in usual activities, significant change in weight and/or appetite, insomnia or hypersomnia, psychomotor agitation or retardation, increased fatigue, feelings of guilt or worthlessness, slowed thinking or impaired concentration, a suicide attempt or suicidal ideation.

The effects of Prozac in hospitalized depressed patients have not been adequately studied.

The efficacy of Prozac 20 mg once daily in maintaining a response in major depressive disorder for up to 38 weeks following 12 weeks of open-label acute treatment (50 weeks total) was demonstrated in a placebo-controlled trial.

The efficacy of Prozac Weekly once weekly in maintaining a response in major depressive disorder has been demonstrated in a placebo-controlled trial for up to 25 weeks following open-label acute treatment of 13 weeks with Prozac 20 mg daily for a total treatment of 38 weeks. However, it is unknown whether or not Prozac Weekly given on a once-weekly basis provides the same level of protection from relapse as that provided by Prozac 20 mg daily (*see* CLINICAL TRIALS).

Pediatric (children and adolescents)—The efficacy of Prozac in children and adolescents was established in two 8- to 9-week placebo-controlled clinical trials in depressed outpatients whose diagnoses corresponded most closely to the DSM-III-R or DSM-IV category of major depressive disorder (*see* CLINICAL TRIALS).

The usefulness of the drug in adult and pediatric patients receiving fluoxetine for extended periods should be reevaluated periodically.

Obsessive-Compulsive Disorder

Adult—Prozac is indicated for the treatment of obsessions and compulsions in patients with obsessive-compulsive disorder (OCD), as defined in the DSM-III-R; i.e., the obsessions or compulsions cause marked distress, are time-consuming, or significantly interfere with social or occupational functioning.

The efficacy of Prozac was established in 13-week trials with obsessive-compulsive outpatients whose diagnoses corresponded most closely to the DSM-III-R category of OCD (*see* CLINICAL TRIALS).

OCD is characterized by recurrent and persistent ideas, thoughts, impulses, or images (obsessions) that are ego-dystonic and/or repetitive, purposeful, and intentional behaviors (compulsions) that are recognized by the person as excessive or unreasonable.

The effectiveness of Prozac in long-term use, i.e., for more than 13 weeks, has not been systematically evaluated in placebo-controlled trials. Therefore, the physician who elects to use Prozac for extended periods should periodically reevaluate the long-term usefulness of the drug for the individual patient (*see* DOSAGE AND ADMINISTRATION).

Pediatric (children and adolescents)—The efficacy of Prozac in children and adolescents was established in a 13-week, dose titration, clinical trial in patients with OCD, as defined in DSM-IV (*see* CLINICAL TRIALS).

Bulimia Nervosa

Prozac is indicated for the treatment of binge-eating and vomiting behaviors in patients with moderate to severe bulimia nervosa.

The efficacy of Prozac was established in 8- to 16-week trials for adult outpatients with moderate to severe bulimia nervosa, i.e., at least 3 bulimic episodes per week for 6 months (*see* CLINICAL TRIALS).

The efficacy of Prozac 60 mg/day in maintaining a response, in patients with bulimia who responded during an 8-week acute treatment phase while taking Prozac 60 mg/day and were then observed for relapse during a period of up to 52 weeks, was demonstrated in a placebo-controlled trial (*see* CLINICAL TRIALS). Nevertheless, the physician who elects to use Prozac for extended periods should periodically reevaluate the long-term usefulness of the drug for the individual patient (*see* DOSAGE AND ADMINISTRATION).

Panic Disorder

Prozac is indicated for the treatment of panic disorder, with or without agoraphobia, as defined in DSM-IV. Panic disorder is characterized by the occurrence of unexpected panic attacks, and associated concern about having additional attacks, worry about the implications or consequences of the attacks, and/or a significant change in behavior related to the attacks.

The efficacy of Prozac was established in two 12-week clinical trials in patients whose diagnoses corresponded to the DSM-IV category of panic disorder (*see* CLINICAL TRIALS).

Panic disorder (DSM-IV) is characterized by recurrent, unexpected panic attacks, i.e., a discrete period of intense fear or discomfort in which 4 or more of the following symptoms develop abruptly and reach a peak within 10 minutes: 1) palpitations, pounding heart, or accelerated heart rate; 2) sweating; 3) trembling or shaking; 4) sensations of shortness of breath or smothering; 5) feeling of choking; 6) chest pain or discomfort; 7) nausea or abdominal distress; 8) feeling dizzy, unsteady, lightheaded, or faint; 9) fear of losing control; 10) fear of dying; 11) paresthesias (numbness or tingling sensations); 12) chills or hot flashes.

The effectiveness of Prozac in long-term use, i.e., for more than 12 weeks, has not been established in placebo-controlled trials. Therefore, the physician who elects to use Prozac for extended periods should periodically reevaluate the long-term usefulness of the drug for the individual patient (*see* DOSAGE AND ADMINISTRATION).

CONTRAINDICATIONS

Prozac is contraindicated in patients known to be hypersensitive to it.

Monoamine oxidase inhibitors—There have been reports of serious, sometimes fatal, reactions (including hyperthermia, rigidity, myoclonus, autonomic instability with possible rapid fluctuations of vital signs, and mental status changes that include extreme agitation progressing to delirium and coma) in patients receiving fluoxetine in combination with a monoamine oxidase inhibitor (MAOI), and in patients who have recently discontinued fluoxetine and are then started on an MAOI. Some cases presented with features resembling neuroleptic malignant syndrome. Therefore, Prozac should not be used in combination with an MAOI, or within a minimum of 14 days of discontinuing therapy with an MAOI. Since fluoxetine and its major metabolite have very long elimination half-lives, at least 5 weeks [perhaps longer, especially if fluoxetine has been prescribed chronically and/or at higher doses (*see* Accumulation and slow elimination *under* CLINICAL PHARMACOLOGY)] should be allowed after stopping Prozac before starting an MAOI.

Thioridazine—Thioridazine should not be administered with Prozac or within a minimum of 5 weeks after Prozac has been discontinued (*see* WARNINGS).

WARNINGS

Rash and possibly allergic events—In US fluoxetine clinical trials as of May 8, 1995, 7% of 10,782 patients developed various types of rashes and/or urticaria. Among the cases of rash and/or urticaria reported in premarketing clinical trials, almost a third were withdrawn from treatment because of the rash and/or systemic signs or symptoms associated with the rash. Clinical findings reported in association with rash include fever, leukocytosis, arthralgias, edema, carpal tunnel syndrome, respiratory distress, lymphadenopathy, proteinuria, and mild transaminase elevation. Most patients improved promptly with discontinuation of fluoxetine and/or adjunctive treatment with antihistamines or steroids, and all patients experiencing these events were reported to recover completely.

In premarketing clinical trials, 2 patients are known to have developed a serious cutaneous systemic illness. In neither patient was there an unequivocal diagnosis, but one was considered to have a leukocytoclastic vasculitis, and the other, a severe desquamating syndrome that was considered variously to be a vasculitis or erythema multiforme. Other patients have had systemic syndromes suggestive of serum sickness.

Since the introduction of Prozac, systemic events, possibly related to vasculitis and including lupus-like syndrome, have developed in patients with rash. Although these events are rare, they may be serious, involving the lung, kidney, or liver. Death has been reported to occur in association with these systemic events.

Anaphylactoid events, including bronchospasm, angioedema, laryngospasm, and urticaria alone and in combination, have been reported.

Pulmonary events, including inflammatory processes of varying histopathology and/or fibrosis, have been reported rarely. These events have occurred with dyspnea as the only preceding symptom.

Whether these systemic events and rash have a common underlying cause or are due to different etiologies or pathogenic processes is not known. Furthermore, a specific underlying immunologic basis for these events has not been identified. Upon the appearance of rash or of other possibly allergic phenomena for which an alternative etiology cannot be identified, Prozac should be discontinued.

Potential interaction with thioridazine—In a study of 19 healthy male subjects, which included 6 slow and 13 rapid hydroxylators of debrisoquin, a single 25-mg oral dose of thioridazine produced a 2.4-fold higher C_{max} and a 4.5-fold higher AUC for thioridazine in the slow hydroxylators compared with the rapid hydroxylators. The rate of debrisoquin hydroxylation is felt to depend on the level of CYP2D6 isozyme activity. Thus, this study suggests that drugs which inhibit CYP2D6, such as certain SSRIs, including fluoxetine, will produce elevated plasma levels of thioridazine (*see* PRECAUTIONS).

Thioridazine administration produces a dose-related prolongation of the QT_c interval, which is associated with serious ventricular arrhythmias, such as torsades de pointes-type arrhythmias, and sudden death. This risk is expected to increase with fluoxetine-induced inhibition of thioridazine metabolism (*see* CONTRAINDICATIONS).

PRECAUTIONS

General

Abnormal Bleeding—Published case reports have documented the occurrence of bleeding episodes in patients treated with psychotropic drugs that interfere with serotonin reuptake. Subsequent epidemiological studies, both of the case-control and cohort design, have demonstrated an association between use of psychotropic drugs that interfere with serotonin reuptake and the occurrence of upper gastrointestinal bleeding. In two studies, concurrent use of a nonsteroidal anti-inflammatory drug (NSAID) or aspirin potentiated the risk of bleeding (*see* DRUG INTERACTIONS). Although these studies focused on upper gastrointestinal bleeding, there is reason to believe that bleeding at other sites may be similarly potentiated. Patients should be cautioned regarding the risk of bleeding associated with the concomitant use of Prozac with NSAIDs, aspirin, or other drugs that affect coagulation.

Anxiety and insomnia—In US placebo-controlled clinical trials for major depressive disorder, 12% to 16% of patients treated with Prozac and 7% to 9% of patients treated with placebo reported anxiety, nervousness, or insomnia.

In US placebo-controlled clinical trials for OCD, insomnia was reported in 28% of patients treated with Prozac and in 22% of patients treated with placebo. Anxiety was reported in 14% of patients treated with Prozac and in 7% of patients treated with placebo.

In US placebo-controlled clinical trials for bulimia nervosa, insomnia was reported in 33% of patients treated with Prozac 60 mg, and 13% of patients treated with placebo. Anxiety and nervousness were reported, respectively, in 15% and 11% of patients treated with Prozac 60 mg and in 9% and 5% of patients treated with placebo.

Among the most common adverse events associated with discontinuation (incidence at least twice that for placebo and at least 1% for Prozac in clinical trials collecting only a primary event associated with discontinuation) in US placebo-controlled fluoxetine clinical trials were anxiety (2% in OCD), insomnia (1% in combined indications and 2% in bulimia), and nervousness (1% in major depressive disorder) (*see* Table 3).

Altered appetite and weight—Significant weight loss, especially in underweight depressed or bulimic patients may be an undesirable result of treatment with Prozac.

In US placebo-controlled clinical trials for major depressive disorder, 11% of patients treated with Prozac and 2% of patients treated with placebo reported anorexia (decreased appetite). Weight loss was reported in 1.4% of patients treated with Prozac and in 0.5% of patients treated with placebo. However, only rarely have patients discontinued treatment with Prozac because of anorexia or weight loss (*see also* Pediatric Use *under* PRECAUTIONS).

In US placebo-controlled clinical trials for OCD, 17% of patients treated with Prozac and 10% of patients treated with placebo reported anorexia (decreased appetite). One patient discontinued treatment with Prozac because of anorexia (*see also* Pediatric Use *under* PRECAUTIONS).

In US placebo-controlled clinical trials for bulimia nervosa, 8% of patients treated with Prozac 60 mg and 4% of patients treated with placebo reported anorexia (decreased appetite). Patients treated with Prozac 60 mg on average lost 0.45 kg compared with a gain of 0.16 kg by patients treated with placebo in the 16-week double-blind trial. Weight change should be monitored during therapy.

Activation of mania/hypomania—In US placebo-controlled clinical trials for major depressive disorder, mania/hypomania was reported in 0.1% of patients treated with Prozac and 0.1% of patients treated with placebo. Activation of mania/hypomania has also been reported in a small proportion of patients with Major Affective Disorder treated with other marketed drugs effective in the treatment of major depressive disorder (*see also* Pediatric Use *under* PRECAUTIONS).

In US placebo-controlled clinical trials for OCD, mania/hypomania was reported in 0.8% of patients treated with Prozac and no patients treated with placebo. No patients reported mania/hypomania in US placebo-controlled clinical trials for bulimia. In all US Prozac clinical trials as of May 8, 1995, 0.7% of 10,782 patients reported mania/hypomania (*see also* Pediatric Use *under* PRECAUTIONS).

Seizures—In US placebo-controlled clinical trials for major depressive disorder, convulsions (or events described as possibly having been seizures) were reported in 0.1% of patients treated with Prozac and 0.2% of patients treated with placebo. No patients reported convulsions in US placebo-controlled clinical trials for either OCD or bulimia. In all US Prozac clinical trials as of May 8, 1995, 0.2% of 10,782 patients reported convulsions. The percentage appears to be similar to that associated with other marketed drugs effective in the treatment of major depressive disorder. Prozac should be introduced with care in patients with a history of seizures.

Suicide—The possibility of a suicide attempt is inherent in major depressive disorder and may persist until significant remission occurs. Close supervision of high-risk patients should accompany initial drug therapy. Prescriptions for Prozac should be written for the smallest quantity of capsules consistent with good patient management, in order to reduce the risk of overdose.

Because of well-established comorbidity between both OCD and major depressive disorder and bulimia and major depressive disorder, the same precautions observed when treating patients with major depressive disorder should be observed when treating patients with OCD or bulimia.

The long elimination half-lives of fluoxetine and its metabolites—Because of the long elimination half-lives of the parent drug and its major active metabolite, changes in dose will not be fully reflected in plasma for several weeks, affecting both strategies for titration to final dose and withdrawal from treatment (*see* CLINICAL PHARMACOLOGY *and* DOSAGE AND ADMINISTRATION).

Use in patients with concomitant illness—Clinical experience with Prozac in patients with concomitant systemic illness is limited. Caution is advisable in using Prozac in patients with diseases or conditions that could affect metabolism or hemodynamic responses.

Fluoxetine has not been evaluated or used to any appreciable extent in patients with a recent history of myocardial infarction or unstable heart disease. Patients with these diagnoses were systematically excluded from clinical studies during the product's premarket testing. However, the electrocardiograms of 312 patients who received Prozac in double-blind trials were retrospectively evaluated; no conduction abnormalities that resulted in heart block were observed. The mean heart rate was reduced by approximately 3 beats/min.

In subjects with cirrhosis of the liver, the clearances of fluoxetine and its active metabolite, norfluoxetine, were decreased, thus increasing the elimination half-lives of these substances. A lower or less frequent dose should be used in patients with cirrhosis.

Studies in depressed patients on dialysis did not reveal excessive accumulation of fluoxetine or norfluoxetine in plasma (*see* Renal disease *under* CLINICAL PHARMACOLOGY). Use of a lower or less frequent dose for renally impaired patients is not routinely necessary (*see* DOSAGE AND ADMINISTRATION).

In patients with diabetes, Prozac may alter glycemic control. Hypoglycemia has occurred during therapy with Prozac, and hyperglycemia has developed following discontinuation of the drug. As is true with many other types of medication when taken concurrently by patients with diabetes, insulin and/or oral hypoglycemic dosage may need to be adjusted when therapy with Prozac is instituted or discontinued.

Interference with cognitive and motor performance—Any psychoactive drug may impair judgment, thinking, or motor skills, and patients should be cautioned about operating hazardous machinery, including automobiles, until they are reasonably certain that the drug treatment does not affect them adversely.

Information for Patients

Physicians are advised to discuss the following issues with patients for whom they prescribe Prozac:

Because Prozac may impair judgment, thinking, or motor skills, patients should be advised to avoid driving a car or operating hazardous machinery until they are reasonably certain that their performance is not affected.

Patients should be advised to inform their physician if they are taking or plan to take any prescription or over-the-counter drugs, or alcohol.

Patients should be cautioned about the concomitant use of Prozac and nonsteroidal anti-inflammatory drugs (NSAIDs) or aspirin since combined use of these drug products have been associated with an increased risk of bleeding.

Patients should be advised to notify their physician if they become pregnant or intend to become pregnant during therapy.

Patients should be advised to notify their physician if they are breast-feeding an infant.

Patients should be advised to notify their physician if they develop a rash or hives.

Laboratory Tests

There are no specific laboratory tests recommended.

Drug Interactions

As with all drugs, the potential for interaction by a variety of mechanisms (e.g., pharmacodynamic, pharmacokinetic

Continued on next page

*** Identi-Code® symbol. This product information was prepared in June 2004. Current information on these and other products of Eli Lilly and Company may be obtained by direct inquiry to Lilly Research Laboratories, Lilly Corporate Center, Indianapolis, Indiana 46285, (800) 545-5979.**

Prozac—Cont.

drug inhibition or enhancement, etc.) is a possibility (*see* Accumulation and slow elimination *under* CLINICAL PHARMACOLOGY).

Drugs metabolized by CYP2D6—Approximately 7% of the normal population has a genetic defect that leads to reduced levels of activity of the cytochrome P450 isoenzyme 2D6. Such individuals have been referred to as "poor metabolizers" of drugs such as debrisoquin, dextromethorphan, and TCAs. Many drugs, such as most drugs effective in the treatment of major depressive disorder, including fluoxetine and other selective uptake inhibitors of serotonin, are metabolized by this isoenzyme; thus, both the pharmacokinetic properties and relative proportion of metabolites are altered in poor metabolizers. However, for fluoxetine and its metabolite, the sum of the plasma concentrations of the 4 active enantiomers is comparable between poor and extensive metabolizers (*see* Variability in metabolism *under* CLINICAL PHARMACOLOGY).

Fluoxetine, like other agents that are metabolized by CYP2D6, inhibits the activity of this isoenzyme, and thus may make normal metabolizers resemble poor metabolizers. Therapy with medications that are predominantly metabolized by the CYP2D6 system and that have a relatively narrow therapeutic index (see list below) should be initiated at the low end of the dose range if a patient is receiving fluoxetine concurrently or has taken it in the previous 5 weeks. Thus, his/her dosing requirements resemble those of poor metabolizers. If fluoxetine is added to the treatment regimen of a patient already receiving a drug metabolized by CYP2D6, the need for decreased dose of the original medication should be considered. Drugs with a narrow therapeutic index represent the greatest concern (e.g., flecainide, vinblastine, and TCAs). Due to the risk of serious ventricular arrhythmias and sudden death potentially associated with elevated plasma levels of thioridazine, thioridazine should not be administered with fluoxetine or within a minimum of 5 weeks after fluoxetine has been discontinued (*see* CONTRAINDICATIONS *and* WARNINGS).

Drugs metabolized by CYP3A4—In an in vivo interaction study involving coadministration of fluoxetine with single doses of terfenadine (a CYP3A4 substrate), no increase in plasma terfenadine concentrations occurred with concomitant fluoxetine. In addition, in vitro studies have shown ketoconazole, a potent inhibitor of CYP3A4 activity, to be at least 100 times more potent than fluoxetine or norfluoxetine as an inhibitor of the metabolism of several substrates for this enzyme, including astemizole, cisapride, and midazolam. These data indicate that fluoxetine's extent of inhibition of CYP3A4 activity is not likely to be of clinical significance.

CNS active drugs—The risk of using Prozac in combination with other CNS active drugs has not been systematically evaluated. Nonetheless, caution is advised if the concomitant administration of Prozac and such drugs is required. In evaluating individual cases, consideration should be given to using lower initial doses of the concomitantly administered drugs, using conservative titration schedules, and monitoring of clinical status (*see* Accumulation and slow elimination *under* CLINICAL PHARMACOLOGY).

Anticonvulsants—Patients on stable doses of phenytoin and carbamazepine have developed elevated plasma anticonvulsant concentrations and clinical anticonvulsant toxicity following initiation of concomitant fluoxetine treatment.

Antipsychotics—Some clinical data suggests a possible pharmacodynamic and/or pharmacokinetic interaction between SSRIs and antipsychotics. Elevation of blood levels of haloperidol and clozapine has been observed in patients receiving concomitant fluoxetine. A single case report has suggested possible additive effects of pimozide and fluoxetine leading to bradycardia. For thioridazine, see CONTRAINDICATIONS and WARNINGS.

Benzodiazepines—The half-life of concurrently administered diazepam may be prolonged in some patients (*see* Accumulation and slow elimination *under* CLINICAL PHARMACOLOGY). Coadministration of alprazolam and fluoxetine has resulted in increased alprazolam plasma concentrations and in further psychomotor performance decrement due to increased alprazolam levels.

Lithium—There have been reports of both increased and decreased lithium levels when lithium was used concomitantly with fluoxetine. Cases of lithium toxicity and increased serotonergic effects have been reported. Lithium levels should be monitored when these drugs are administered concomitantly.

Tryptophan—Five patients receiving Prozac in combination with tryptophan experienced adverse reactions, including agitation, restlessness, and gastrointestinal distress.

Monoamine oxidase inhibitors—See CONTRAINDICATIONS.

Other drugs effective in the treatment of major depressive disorder—In 2 studies, previously stable plasma levels of imipramine and desipramine have increased greater than 2- to 10-fold when fluoxetine has been administered in combination. This influence may persist for 3 weeks or longer after fluoxetine is discontinued. Thus, the dose of TCA may need to be reduced and plasma TCA concentrations may need to be monitored temporarily when fluoxetine is coadministered or has been recently discontinued (*see* Accumulation and slow elimination *under* CLINICAL PHARMACOLOGY, *and* Drugs metabolized by CYP2D6 *under* Drug Interactions).

Sumatriptan—There have been rare postmarketing reports describing patients with weakness, hyperreflexia, and incoordination following the use of an SSRI and sumatriptan. If concomitant treatment with sumatriptan and an SSRI (e.g., fluoxetine, fluvoxamine, paroxetine, sertraline, or citalopram) is clinically warranted, appropriate observation of the patient is advised.

Potential effects of coadministration of drugs tightly bound to plasma proteins—Because fluoxetine is tightly bound to plasma protein, the administration of fluoxetine to a patient taking another drug that is tightly bound to protein (e.g., Coumadin, digitoxin) may cause a shift in plasma concentrations potentially resulting in an adverse effect. Conversely, adverse effects may result from displacement of protein-bound fluoxetine by other tightly-bound drugs (*see* Accumulation and slow elimination *under* CLINICAL PHARMACOLOGY).

Drugs that interfere with hemostasis (NSAIDs, aspirin, warfarin, etc.)—Serotonin release by platelets plays an important role in hemostasis. Epidemiological studies of the case-control and cohort design that have demonstrated an association between use of psychotropic drugs that interfere with serotonin reuptake and the occurrence of upper gastrointestinal bleeding have also shown that concurrent use of an NSAID or aspirin potentiated the risk of bleeding.

Warfarin—Altered anticoagulant effects, including increased bleeding, have been reported when fluoxetine is coadministered with warfarin. Patients receiving warfarin therapy should receive careful coagulation monitoring when fluoxetine is initiated or stopped.

Electroconvulsive therapy (ECT)—There are no clinical studies establishing the benefit of the combined use of ECT and fluoxetine. There have been rare reports of prolonged seizures in patients on fluoxetine receiving ECT treatment.

Carcinogenesis, Mutagenesis, Impairment of Fertility

There is no evidence of carcinogenicity, mutagenicity, or impairment of fertility with Prozac.

Carcinogenicity—The dietary administration of fluoxetine to rats and mice for 2 years at doses of up to 10 and 12 mg/kg/day, respectively [approximately 1.2 and 0.7 times, respectively, the maximum recommended human dose (MRHD) of 80 mg on a mg/m^2 basis], produced no evidence of carcinogenicity.

Mutagenicity—Fluoxetine and norfluoxetine have been shown to have no genotoxic effects based on the following assays: bacterial mutation assay, DNA repair assay in cultured rat hepatocytes, mouse lymphoma assay, and in vivo sister chromatid exchange assay in Chinese hamster bone marrow cells.

Impairment of fertility—Two fertility studies conducted in rats at doses of up to 7.5 and 12.5 mg/kg/day (approximately 0.9 and 1.5 times the MRHD on a mg/m^2 basis) indicated that fluoxetine had no adverse effects on fertility.

Pregnancy

Pregnancy Category C —In embryo-fetal development studies in rats and rabbits, there was no evidence of teratogenicity following administration of up to 12.5 and 15 mg/kg/day, respectively (1.5 and 3.6 times, respectively, the MRHD of 80 mg on a mg/m^2 basis) throughout organogenesis. However, in rat reproduction studies, an increase in stillborn pups, a decrease in pup weight, and an increase in pup deaths during the first 7 days postpartum occurred following maternal exposure to 12 mg/kg/day (1.5 times the MRHD on a mg/m^2 basis) during gestation or 7.5 mg/kg/day (0.9 times the MRHD on a mg/m^2 basis) during gestation and lactation. There was no evidence of developmental neurotoxicity in the surviving offspring of rats treated with 12 mg/kg/day during gestation. The no-effect dose for rat pup mortality was 5 mg/kg/day (0.6 times the MRHD on a mg/m^2 basis). Prozac should be used during pregnancy only if the potential benefit justifies the potential risk to the fetus.

Labor and Delivery

The effect of Prozac on labor and delivery in humans is unknown. However, because fluoxetine crosses the placenta and because of the possibility that fluoxetine may have adverse effects on the newborn, fluoxetine should be used during labor and delivery only if the potential benefit justifies the potential risk to the fetus.

Nursing Mothers

Because Prozac is excreted in human milk, nursing while on Prozac is not recommended. In one breast-milk sample, the concentration of fluoxetine plus norfluoxetine was 70.4 ng/mL. The concentration in the mother's plasma was 295.0 ng/mL. No adverse effects on the infant were reported. In another case, an infant nursed by a mother on Prozac developed crying, sleep disturbance, vomiting, and watery stools. The infant's plasma drug levels were 340 ng/mL of fluoxetine and 208 ng/mL of norfluoxetine on the second day of feeding.

Pediatric Use

The efficacy of Prozac for the treatment of major depressive disorder was demonstrated in two 8- to 9-week placebo-controlled clinical trials with 315 pediatric outpatients ages 8 to ≤18. (*see* CLINICAL TRIALS).

The efficacy of Prozac for the treatment of OCD was demonstrated in one 13-week placebo-controlled clinical trial with 103 pediatric outpatients ages 7 to <18 (*see* CLINICAL TRIALS).

The safety and effectiveness in pediatric patients <8 years of age in major depressive disorder and <7 years of age in OCD have not been established.

Fluoxetine pharmacokinetics were evaluated in 21 pediatric patients (ages 6 to ≤ 18) with major depressive disorder or OCD (*see* Pharmacokinetics *under* CLINICAL PHARMACOLOGY).

The acute adverse event profiles observed in the 3 studies (N=418 randomized; 228 fluoxetine-treated, 190 placebo-treated) were generally similar to that observed in adult studies with fluoxetine. The longer-term adverse event profile observed in the 19-week major depressive disorder study (N=219 randomized; 109 fluoxetine-treated, 110 placebo-treated) was also similar to that observed in adult trials with fluoxetine (*see* ADVERSE REACTIONS).

Manic reaction, including mania and hypomania, was reported in 6 (1 mania, 5 hypomania) out of 228 (2.6%) fluoxetine-treated patients and in 0 out of 190 (0%) placebo-treated patients. Mania/hypomania led to the discontinuation of 4 (1.8%) fluoxetine-treated patients from the acute phases of the 3 studies combined. Consequently, regular monitoring for the occurrence of mania/hypomania is recommended.

As with other SSRIs, decreased weight gain has been observed in association with the use of fluoxetine in children and adolescent patients. After 19 weeks of treatment in a clinical trial, pediatric subjects treated with fluoxetine gained an average of 1.1 cm less in height (p=0.004) and 1.1 kg less in weight (p=0.008) than subjects treated with placebo. In addition, fluoxetine treatment was associated with a decrease in alkaline phosphatase levels. The safety of fluoxetine treatment for pediatric patients has not been systematically assessed for chronic treatment longer than several months in duration. In particular, there are no studies that directly evaluate the longer-term effects of fluoxetine on the growth, development, and maturation of children and adolescent patients. Therefore, height and weight should be monitored periodically in pediatric patients receiving fluoxetine.

Geriatric Use

US fluoxetine clinical trials as of May 8, 1995 (10,782 patients) included 687 patients ≥65 years of age and 93 patients ≥75 years of age. The efficacy in geriatric patients has been established (*see* CLINICAL TRIALS). For pharmacokinetic information in geriatric patients, see Age under CLINICAL PHARMACOLOGY. No overall differences in safety or effectiveness were observed between these subjects and younger subjects, and other reported clinical experience has not identified differences in responses between the elderly and younger patients, but greater sensitivity of some older individuals cannot be ruled out. As with other SSRIs, fluoxetine has been associated with cases of clinically significant hyponatremia in elderly patients (*see* Hyponatremia *under* PRECAUTIONS).

Hyponatremia

Cases of hyponatremia (some with serum sodium lower than 110 mmol/L) have been reported. The hyponatremia appeared to be reversible when Prozac was discontinued. Although these cases were complex with varying possible etiologies, some were possibly due to the syndrome of inappropriate antidiuretic hormone secretion (SIADH). The majority of these occurrences have been in older patients and in patients taking diuretics or who were otherwise volume depleted. In two 6-week controlled studies in patients ≥60 years of age, 10 of 323 fluoxetine patients and 6 of 327 placebo recipients had a lowering of serum sodium below the reference range; this difference was not statistically significant. The lowest observed concentration was 129 mmol/L. The observed decreases were not clinically significant.

ADVERSE REACTIONS

Multiple doses of Prozac had been administered to 10,782 patients with various diagnoses in US clinical trials as of May 8, 1995. In addition, there have been 425 patients administered Prozac in panic clinical trials. Adverse events were recorded by clinical investigators using descriptive terminology of their own choosing. Consequently, it is not possible to provide a meaningful estimate of the proportion of individuals experiencing adverse events without first grouping similar types of events into a limited (i.e., reduced) number of standardized event categories.

In the tables and tabulations that follow, COSTART Dictionary terminology has been used to classify reported adverse events. The stated frequencies represent the proportion of individuals who experienced, at least once, a treatment-emergent adverse event of the type listed. An event was considered treatment-emergent if it occurred for the first time or worsened while receiving therapy following baseline evaluation. It is important to emphasize that events reported during therapy were not necessarily caused by it.

The prescriber should be aware that the figures in the tables and tabulations cannot be used to predict the incidence of side effects in the course of usual medical practice where patient characteristics and other factors differ from those that prevailed in the clinical trials. Similarly, the cited frequencies cannot be compared with figures obtained from other clinical investigations involving different treatments, uses, and investigators. The cited figures, however, do provide the prescribing physician with some basis for estimating the relative contribution of drug and nondrug factors to the side effect incidence rate in the population studied.

Incidence in major depressive disorder, OCD, bulimia, and panic disorder placebo-controlled clinical trials (excluding data from extensions of trials)—Table 1 enumerates the most common treatment-emergent adverse events associated with the use of Prozac (incidence of at least 5% for

Prozac and at least twice that for placebo within at least 1 of the indications) for the treatment of major depressive disorder, OCD, and bulimia in US controlled clinical trials and panic disorder in US plus non-US controlled trials. Table 2 enumerates treatment-emergent adverse events that occurred in 2% or more patients treated with Prozac and with incidence greater than placebo who participated in US major depressive disorder, OCD, and bulimia controlled clinical trials and US plus non-US panic disorder controlled clinical trials. Table 2 provides combined data for the pool of studies that are provided separately by indication in Table 1.

[See table 1 at right]

Table 2: Treatment-Emergent Adverse Events: Incidence in Major Depressive Disorder, OCD, Bulimia, and Panic Disorder Placebo-Controlled Clinical Trials[1]

	Percentage of Patients Reporting Event	
	Major Depressive Disorder, OCD, Bulimia, and Panic Disorder Combined	
Body System/ Adverse Event[2]	Prozac (N=2869)	Placebo (N=1673)
Body as a Whole		
Headache	21	19
Asthenia	11	6
Flu syndrome	5	4
Fever	2	1
Cardiovascular System		
Vasodilatation	2	1
Digestive System		
Nausea	22	9
Diarrhea	11	7
Anorexia	10	3
Dry mouth	9	6
Dyspepsia	8	4
Constipation	5	4
Flatulence	3	2
Vomiting	3	2
Metabolic and Nutritional Disorders		
Weight loss	2	1
Nervous System		
Insomnia	19	10
Nervousness	13	8
Anxiety	12	6
Somnolence	12	5
Dizziness	9	6
Tremor	9	2
Libido decreased	4	1
Thinking abnormal	2	1
Respiratory System		
Yawn	3	—
Skin and Appendages		
Sweating	7	3
Rash	4	3
Pruritus	3	2
Special Senses		
Abnormal vision	2	1

[1] Includes US data for major depressive disorder, OCD, bulimia, and panic disorder clinical trials, plus non-US data for panic disorder clinical trials.

[2] Included are events reported by at least 2% of patients taking Prozac, except the following events, which had an incidence on placebo ≥ Prozac (major depressive disorder, OCD, bulimia, and panic disorder combined): abdominal pain, abnormal dreams, accidental injury, back pain, cough increased, major depressive disorder (includes suicidal thoughts), dysmenorrhea, infection, myalgia, pain, paresthesia, pharyngitis, rhinitis, sinusitis.

—Incidence less than 1%.

Table 1: Most Common Treatment-Emergent Adverse Events: Incidence in Major Depressive Disorder, OCD, Bulimia, and Panic Disorder Placebo-Controlled Clinical Trials[1]

	Percentage of Patients Reporting Event							
	Major Depressive Disorder		OCD		Bulimia		Panic Disorder	
Body System/ Adverse Event	Prozac (N=1728)	Placebo (N=975)	Prozac (N=266)	Placebo (N=89)	Prozac (N=450)	Placebo (N=267)	Prozac (N=425)	Placebo (N=342)
Body as a Whole								
Asthenia	9	5	15	11	21	9	7	7
Flu syndrome	3	4	10	7	8	3	5	5
Cardiovascular System								
Vasodilatation	3	2	5	—	2	1	1	—
Digestive System								
Nausea	21	9	26	13	29	11	12	7
Diarrhea	12	8	18	13	8	6	9	4
Anorexia	11	2	17	10	8	4	4	1
Dry mouth	10	7	12	3	9	6	4	4
Dyspepsia	7	5	10	4	10	6	6	2
Nervous System								
Insomnia	16	9	28	22	33	13	10	7
Anxiety	12	7	14	7	15	9	6	2
Nervousness	14	9	14	15	11	5	8	6
Somnolence	13	6	17	7	13	5	5	2
Tremor	10	3	9	1	13	1	3	1
Libido decreased	3	—	11	2	5	1	1	2
Abnormal dreams	1	1	5	2	5	3	1	1
Respiratory System								
Pharyngitis	3	3	11	9	10	5	3	3
Sinusitis	1	4	5	2	6	4	2	3
Yawn	—	—	7	—	11	—	1	—
Skin and Appendages								
Sweating	8	3	7	—	8	3	2	2
Rash	4	3	6	3	4	4	2	2
Urogenital System								
Impotence[2]	2	—	—	—	7	—	1	—
Abnormal ejaculation[2]	—	—	7	—	7	—	2	1

[1] Includes US data for major depressive disorder, OCD, bulimia, and panic disorder clinical trials, plus non-US data for panic disorder clinical trials.

[2] Denominator used was for males only (N=690 Prozac major depressive disorder; N=410 placebo major depressive disorder; N=116 Prozac OCD; N=43 placebo OCD; N=14 Prozac bulimia; N=1 placebo bulimia; N=162 Prozac panic; N=121 placebo panic).

—Incidence less than 1%.

Associated with discontinuation in major depressive disorder, OCD, bulimia, and panic disorder placebo-controlled clinical trials (excluding data from extensions of trials)—Table 3 lists the adverse events associated with discontinuation of Prozac treatment (incidence at least twice that for placebo and at least 1% for Prozac in clinical trials collecting only a primary event associated with discontinuation) in major depressive disorder, OCD, bulimia, and panic disorder clinical trials, plus non-US panic disorder clinical trials.

[See table 3 at top of next page]

Other adverse events in pediatric patients (children and adolescents)—Treatment-emergent adverse events were collected in 322 pediatric patients (180 fluoxetine-treated, 142 placebo-treated). The overall profile of adverse events was generally similar to that seen in adult studies, as shown in Tables 1 and 2. However, the following adverse events (excluding those which appear in the body or footnotes of Tables 1 and 2 and those for which the COSTART terms were uninformative or misleading) were reported at an incidence of at least 2% for fluoxetine and greater than placebo: thirst, hyperkinesia, agitation, personality disorder, epistaxis, urinary frequency, and menorrhagia.

The most common adverse event (incidence at least 1% for fluoxetine and greater than placebo) associated with discontinuation in 3 pediatric placebo-controlled trials (N=418 randomized; 228 fluoxetine-treated; 190 placebo-treated) was mania/hypomania (1.8% for fluoxetine-treated, 0% for placebo-treated). In these clinical trials, only a primary event associated with discontinuation was collected.

Events observed in Prozac Weekly clinical trials—Treatment-emergent adverse events in clinical trials with Prozac Weekly were similar to the adverse events reported by patients in clinical trials with Prozac daily. In a placebo-controlled clinical trial, more patients taking Prozac Weekly reported diarrhea than patients taking placebo (10% versus 3%, respectively) or taking Prozac 20 mg daily (10% versus 5%, respectively).

Male and female sexual dysfunction with SSRIs—Although changes in sexual desire, sexual performance, and sexual satisfaction often occur as manifestations of a psychiatric disorder, they may also be a consequence of pharmacologic treatment. In particular, some evidence suggests that SSRIs can cause such untoward sexual experiences. Reliable estimates of the incidence and severity of untoward experiences involving sexual desire, performance, and satisfaction are difficult to obtain, however, in part because patients and physicians may be reluctant to discuss them. Accordingly,

Continued on next page

*** Identi-Code® symbol. This product information was prepared in June 2004. Current information on these and other products of Eli Lilly and Company may be obtained by direct inquiry to Lilly Research Laboratories, Lilly Corporate Center, Indianapolis, Indiana 46285, (800) 545-5979.**

Prozac—Cont.

estimates of the incidence of untoward sexual experience and performance, cited in product labeling, are likely to underestimate their actual incidence. In patients enrolled in US major depressive disorder, OCD, and bulimia placebo-controlled clinical trials, decreased libido was the only sexual side effect reported by at least 2% of patients taking fluoxetine (4% fluoxetine, <1% placebo). There have been spontaneous reports in women taking fluoxetine of orgasmic dysfunction, including anorgasmia.

There are no adequate and well-controlled studies examining sexual dysfunction with fluoxetine treatment.

Priapism has been reported with all SSRIs.

While it is difficult to know the precise risk of sexual dysfunction associated with the use of SSRIs, physicians should routinely inquire about such possible side effects.

Other Events Observed in Clinical Trials

Following is a list of all treatment-emergent adverse events reported at anytime by individuals taking fluoxetine in US clinical trials as of May 8, 1995 (10,782 patients) except (1) those listed in the body or footnotes of Tables 1 or 2 above or elsewhere in labeling; (2) those for which the COSTART terms were uninformative or misleading; (3) those events for which a causal relationship to Prozac use was considered remote; and (4) events occurring in only 1 patient treated with Prozac and which did not have a substantial probability of being acutely life-threatening.

Events are classified within body system categories using the following definitions: frequent adverse events are defined as those occurring on one or more occasions in at least 1/100 patients; infrequent adverse events are those occurring in 1/100 to 1/1000 patients; rare events are those occurring in less than 1/1000 patients.

Body as a Whole—*Frequent:* chest pain, chills; *Infrequent:* chills and fever, face edema, intentional overdose, malaise, pelvic pain, suicide attempt; *Rare:* abdominal syndrome acute, hypothermia, intentional injury, neuroleptic malignant syndrome[1], photosensitivity reaction.

Cardiovascular System—*Frequent:* hemorrhage, hypertension, palpitation; *Infrequent:* angina pectoris, arrhythmia, congestive heart failure, hypotension, migraine, myocardial infarct, postural hypotension, syncope, tachycardia, vascular headache; *Rare:* atrial fibrillation, bradycardia, cerebral embolism, cerebral ischemia, cerebrovascular accident, extrasystoles, heart arrest, heart block, pallor, peripheral vascular disorder, phlebitis, shock, thrombophlebitis, thrombosis, vasospasm, ventricular arrhythmia, ventricular extrasystoles, ventricular fibrillation.

Digestive System—*Frequent:* increased appetite, nausea and vomiting; *Infrequent:* aphthous stomatitis, cholelithiasis, colitis, dysphagia, eructation, esophagitis, gastritis, gastroenteritis, glossitis, gum hemorrhage, hyperchlorhydria, increased salivation, liver function tests abnormal, melena, mouth ulceration, nausea/vomiting/diarrhea, stomach ulcer, stomatitis, thirst; *Rare:* biliary pain, bloody diarrhea, cholecystitis, duodenal ulcer, enteritis, esophageal ulcer, fecal incontinence, gastrointestinal hemorrhage, hematemesis, hemorrhage of colon, hepatitis, intestinal obstruction, liver fatty deposit, pancreatitis, peptic ulcer, rectal hemorrhage, salivary gland enlargement, stomach ulcer hemorrhage, tongue edema.

Endocrine System—*Infrequent:* hypothyroidism; *Rare:* diabetic acidosis, diabetes mellitus.

Hemic and Lymphatic System—*Infrequent:* anemia, ecchymosis; *Rare:* blood dyscrasia, hypochromic anemia, leukopenia, lymphedema, lymphocytosis, petechia, purpura, thrombocythemia, thrombocytopenia.

Metabolic and Nutritional—*Frequent:* weight gain; *Infrequent:* dehydration, generalized edema, gout, hypercholesteremia, hyperlipemia, hypokalemia, peripheral edema; *Rare:* alcohol intolerance, alkaline phosphatase increased, BUN increased, creatine phosphokinase increased, hyperkalemia, hyperuricemia, hypocalcemia, iron deficiency anemia, SGPT increased.

Musculoskeletal System—*Infrequent:* arthritis, bone pain, bursitis, leg cramps, tenosynovitis; *Rare:* arthrosis, chondrodystrophy, myasthenia, myopathy, myositis, osteomyelitis, osteoporosis, rheumatoid arthritis.

Nervous System—*Frequent:* agitation, amnesia, confusion, emotional lability, sleep disorder; *Infrequent:* abnormal gait, acute brain syndrome, akathisia, apathy, ataxia, buccoglossal syndrome, CNS depression, CNS stimulation, depersonalization, euphoria, hallucinations, hostility, hyperkinesia, hypertonia, hypesthesia, incoordination, libido increased, myoclonus, neuralgia, neuropathy, neurosis, paranoid reaction, personality disorder[2], psychosis, vertigo; *Rare:* abnormal electroencephalogram, antisocial reaction, circumoral paresthesia, coma, delusions, dysarthria, dystonia, extrapyramidal syndrome, foot drop, hyperesthesia, neuritis, paralysis, reflexes decreased, reflexes increased, stupor.

Respiratory System—*Infrequent:* asthma, epistaxis, hiccup, hyperventilation; *Rare:* apnea, atelectasis, cough decreased, emphysema, hemoptysis, hypoventilation, hypoxia, larynx edema, lung edema, pneumothorax, stridor.

Skin and Appendages—*Infrequent:* acne, alopecia, contact dermatitis, eczema, maculopapular rash, skin discoloration, skin ulcer, vesiculobullous rash; *Rare:* furunculosis, herpes zoster, hirsutism, petechial rash, psoriasis, purpuric rash, pustular rash, seborrhea.

Special Senses—*Frequent:* ear pain, taste perversion, tinnitus; *Infrequent:* conjunctivitis, dry eyes, mydriasis, photophobia; *Rare:* blepharitis, deafness, diplopia, exophthalmos, eye hemorrhage, glaucoma, hyperacusis, iritis, parosmia, scleritis, strabismus, taste loss, visual field defect.

Urogenital System—*Frequent:* urinary frequency; *Infrequent:* abortion[3], albuminuria, amenorrhea[3], anorgasmia, breast enlargement, breast pain, cystitis, dysuria, female lactation[3], fibrocystic breast[3], hematuria, leukorrhea[3], menorrhagia[3], metrorrhagia[3], nocturia, polyuria, urinary incontinence, urinary retention, urinary urgency, vaginal hemorrhage[3]; *Rare:* breast engorgement, glycosuria, hypomenorrhea[3], kidney pain, oliguria, priapism[3], uterine hemorrhage[3], uterine fibroids enlarged[3].

[1] Neuroleptic malignant syndrome is the COSTART term which best captures serotonin syndrome.

[2] Personality disorder is the COSTART term for designating nonaggressive objectionable behavior.

[3] Adjusted for gender.

Table 3: Most Common Adverse Events Associated with Discontinuation in Major Depressive Disorder, OCD, Bulimia, and Panic Disorder Placebo-Controlled Clinical Trials[1]

Major Depressive Disorder, OCD, Bulimia, and Panic Disorder Combined (N=1533)	Major Depressive Disorder (N=392)	OCD (N=266)	Bulimia (N=450)	Panic Disorder (N=425)
Anxiety (1%)	—	Anxiety (2%)	—	Anxiety (2%)
—	—	—	Insomnia (2%)	—
—	Nervousness (1%)	—	—	Nervousness (1%)
—	—	Rash (1%)	—	—

[1] Includes US major depressive disorder, OCD, bulimia, and panic disorder clinical trials, plus non-US panic disorder clinical trials.

Postintroduction Reports

Voluntary reports of adverse events temporally associated with Prozac that have been received since market introduction and that may have no causal relationship with the drug include the following: aplastic anemia, atrial fibrillation, cataract, cerebral vascular accident, cholestatic jaundice, confusion, dyskinesia (including, for example, a case of buccal-lingual-masticatory syndrome with involuntary tongue protrusion reported to develop in a 77-year-old female after 5 weeks of fluoxetine therapy and which completely resolved over the next few months following drug discontinuation), eosinophilic pneumonia, epidermal necrolysis, erythema nodosum, exfoliative dermatitis, gynecomastia, heart arrest, hepatic failure/necrosis, hyperprolactinemia, hypoglycemia, immune-related hemolytic anemia, kidney failure, misuse/abuse, movement disorders developing in patients with risk factors including drugs associated with such events and worsening of preexisting movement disorders, neuroleptic malignant syndrome-like events, optic neuritis, pancreatitis, pancytopenia, priapism, pulmonary embolism, pulmonary hypertension, QT prolongation, serotonin syndrome (a range of signs and symptoms that can rarely, in its most severe form, resemble neuroleptic malignant syndrome), Stevens-Johnson syndrome, sudden unexpected death, suicidal ideation, thrombocytopenia, thrombocytopenic purpura, vaginal bleeding after drug withdrawal, ventricular tachycardia (including torsades de pointes-type arrhythmias), and violent behaviors.

DRUG ABUSE AND DEPENDENCE

Controlled substance class—Prozac is not a controlled substance.

Physical and psychological dependence—Prozac has not been systematically studied, in animals or humans, for its potential for abuse, tolerance, or physical dependence. While the premarketing clinical experience with Prozac did not reveal any tendency for a withdrawal syndrome or any drug seeking behavior, these observations were not systematic and it is not possible to predict on the basis of this limited experience the extent to which a CNS active drug will be misused, diverted, and/or abused once marketed. Consequently, physicians should carefully evaluate patients for history of drug abuse and follow such patients closely, observing them for signs of misuse or abuse of Prozac (e.g., development of tolerance, incrementation of dose, drug-seeking behavior).

OVERDOSAGE

Human Experience

Worldwide exposure to fluoxetine hydrochloride is estimated to be over 38 million patients (circa 1999). Of the 1578 cases of overdose involving fluoxetine hydrochloride, alone or with other drugs, reported from this population, there were 195 deaths.

Among 633 adult patients who overdosed on fluoxetine hydrochloride alone, 34 resulted in a fatal outcome, 378 completely recovered, and 15 patients experienced sequelae after overdosage, including abnormal accommodation, abnormal gait, confusion, unresponsiveness, nervousness, pulmonary dysfunction, vertigo, tremor, elevated blood pressure, impotence, movement disorder, and hypomania. The remaining 206 patients had an unknown outcome. The most common signs and symptoms associated with non-fatal overdosage were seizures, somnolence, nausea, tachycardia, and vomiting. The largest known ingestion of fluoxetine hydrochloride in adult patients was 8 grams in a patient who took fluoxetine alone and who subsequently recovered. However, in an adult patient who took fluoxetine alone, an ingestion as low as 520 mg has been associated with lethal outcome, but causality has not been established.

Among pediatric patients (ages 3 months to 17 years), there were 156 cases of overdose involving fluoxetine alone or in combination with other drugs. Six patients died, 127 patients completely recovered, 1 patient experienced renal failure, and 22 patients had an unknown outcome. One of the six fatalities was a 9-year-old boy who had a history of OCD, Tourette's syndrome with tics, attention deficit disorder, and fetal alcohol syndrome. He had been receiving 100 mg of fluoxetine daily for 6 months in addition to clonidine, methylphenidate, and promethazine. Mixed-drug ingestion or other methods of suicide complicated all 6 overdoses in children that resulted in fatalities. The largest ingestion in pediatric patients was 3 grams which was nonlethal.

Other important adverse events reported with fluoxetine overdose (single or multiple drugs) include coma, delirium, ECG abnormalities (such as QT interval prolongation and ventricular tachycardia, including torsades de pointes-type arrhythmias), hypotension, mania, neuroleptic malignant syndrome-like events, pyrexia, stupor, and syncope.

Animal Experience

Studies in animals do not provide precise or necessarily valid information about the treatment of human overdose. However, animal experiments can provide useful insights into possible treatment strategies.

The oral median lethal dose in rats and mice was found to be 452 and 248 mg/kg, respectively. Acute high oral doses produced hyperirritability and convulsions in several animal species.

Among 6 dogs purposely overdosed with oral fluoxetine, 5 experienced grand mal seizures. Seizures stopped immediately upon the bolus intravenous administration of a standard veterinary dose of diazepam. In this short-term study, the lowest plasma concentration at which a seizure occurred was only twice the maximum plasma concentration seen in humans taking 80 mg/day, chronically.

In a separate single-dose study, the ECG of dogs given high doses did not reveal prolongation of the PR, QRS, or QT intervals. Tachycardia and an increase in blood pressure were observed. Consequently, the value of the ECG in predicting cardiac toxicity is unknown. Nonetheless, the ECG should ordinarily be monitored in cases of human overdose (*see* Management of Overdose).

Management of Overdose

Treatment should consist of those general measures employed in the management of overdosage with any drug effective in the treatment of major depressive disorder.

Ensure an adequate airway, oxygenation, and ventilation. Monitor cardiac rhythm and vital signs. General supportive and symptomatic measures are also recommended. Induction of emesis is not recommended. Gastric lavage with a large-bore orogastric tube with appropriate airway protection, if needed, may be indicated if performed soon after ingestion, or in symptomatic patients.

Activated charcoal should be administered. Due to the large volume of distribution of this drug, forced diuresis, dialysis, hemoperfusion, and exchange transfusion are unlikely to be of benefit. No specific antidotes for fluoxetine are known.

A specific caution involves patients who are taking or have recently taken fluoxetine and might ingest excessive quantities of a TCA. In such a case, accumulation of the parent tricyclic and/or an active metabolite may increase the possibility of clinically significant sequelae and extend the time needed for close medical observation (*see* Other drugs effective in the treatment of major depressive disorder *under* PRECAUTIONS).

Based on experience in animals, which may not be relevant to humans, fluoxetine-induced seizures that fail to remit spontaneously may respond to diazepam.

In managing overdosage, consider the possibility of multiple drug involvement. The physician should consider contacting a poison control center for additional information on the treatment of any overdose. Telephone numbers for certified poison control centers are listed in the *Physicians' Desk Reference (PDR)*.

DOSAGE AND ADMINISTRATION

Major Depressive Disorder

Initial Treatment

Adult—In controlled trials used to support the efficacy of fluoxetine, patients were administered morning doses ranging from 20 to 80 mg/day. Studies comparing fluoxetine 20, 40, and 60 mg/day to placebo indicate that 20 mg/day is suf-

ficient to obtain a satisfactory response in major depressive disorder in most cases. Consequently, a dose of 20 mg/day, administered in the morning, is recommended as the initial dose.
A dose increase may be considered after several weeks if insufficient clinical improvement is observed. Doses above 20 mg/day may be administered on a once-a-day (morning) or BID schedule (i.e., morning and noon) and should not exceed a maximum dose of 80 mg/day.
Pediatric (children and adolescents)—In the short-term (8 to 9 week) controlled clinical trials of fluoxetine supporting its effectiveness in the treatment of major depressive disorder, patients were administered fluoxetine doses of 10 to 20 mg/day (*see* CLINICAL TRIALS). Treatment should be initiated with a dose of 10 or 20 mg/day. After 1 week at 10 mg/day, the dose should be increased to 20 mg/day.
However, due to higher plasma levels in lower weight children, the starting and target dose in this group may be 10 mg/day. A dose increase to 20 mg/day may be considered after several weeks if insufficient clinical improvement is observed.
All patients—As with other drugs effective in the treatment of major depressive disorder, the full effect may be delayed until 4 weeks of treatment or longer.
As with many other medications, a lower or less frequent dosage should be used in patients with hepatic impairment. A lower or less frequent dosage should also be considered for the elderly (*see* Geriatric Use *under* PRECAUTIONS), and for patients with concurrent disease or on multiple concomitant medications. Dosage adjustments for renal impairment are not routinely necessary (*see* Liver disease *and* Renal disease *under* CLINICAL PHARMACOLOGY, *and* Use in patients with concomitant illness *under* PRECAUTIONS).
Maintenance/Continuation/Extended Treatment
It is generally agreed that acute episodes of major depressive disorder require several months or longer of sustained pharmacologic therapy. Whether the dose needed to induce remission is identical to the dose needed to maintain and/or sustain euthymia is unknown.
Daily Dosing
Systematic evaluation of Prozac in adult patients has shown that its efficacy in major depressive disorder is maintained for periods of up to 38 weeks following 12 weeks of open-label acute treatment (50 weeks total) at a dose of 20 mg/day (*see* CLINICAL TRIALS).
Weekly Dosing
Systematic evaluation of Prozac Weekly in adult patients has shown that its efficacy in major depressive disorder is maintained for periods of up to 25 weeks with once-weekly dosing following 13 weeks of open-label treatment with Prozac 20 mg once daily. However, therapeutic equivalence of Prozac Weekly given on a once-weekly basis with Prozac 20 mg given daily for delaying time to relapse has not been established (*see* CLINICAL TRIALS).
Weekly dosing with Prozac Weekly capsules is recommended to be initiated 7 days after the last daily dose of Prozac 20 mg (*see* Weekly dosing *under* CLINICAL PHARMACOLOGY).
If satisfactory response is not maintained with Prozac Weekly, consider reestablishing a daily dosing regimen (*see* CLINICAL TRIALS).
Switching Patients to a Tricyclic Antidepressant (TCA)
Dosage of a TCA may need to be reduced, and plasma TCA concentrations may need to be monitored temporarily when fluoxetine is coadministered or has been recently discontinued (*see* Other drugs effective in the treatment of major depressive disorder *under* Drug Interactions).
Switching Patients to or from a Monoamine Oxidase Inhibitor (MAOI)
At least 14 days should elapse between discontinuation of an MAOI and initiation of therapy with Prozac. In addition, at least 5 weeks, perhaps longer, should be allowed after stopping Prozac before starting an MAOI (*see* CONTRAINDICATIONS *and* PRECAUTIONS).

Obsessive-Compulsive Disorder
Initial Treatment
Adult—In the controlled clinical trials of fluoxetine supporting its effectiveness in the treatment of OCD, patients were administered fixed daily doses of 20, 40, or 60 mg of fluoxetine or placebo (*see* CLINICAL TRIALS). In 1 of these studies, no dose-response relationship for effectiveness was demonstrated. Consequently, a dose of 20 mg/day, administered in the morning, is recommended as the initial dose. Since there was a suggestion of a possible dose-response relationship for effectiveness in the second study, a dose increase may be considered after several weeks if insufficient clinical improvement is observed. The full therapeutic effect may be delayed until 5 weeks of treatment or longer.
Doses above 20 mg/day may be administered on a once-a-day (i.e., morning) or BID schedule (i.e., morning and noon). A dose range of 20 to 60 mg/day is recommended; however, doses of up to 80 mg/day have been well tolerated in open studies of OCD. The maximum fluoxetine dose should not exceed 80 mg/day.
Pediatric (children and adolescents)—In the controlled clinical trial of fluoxetine supporting its effectiveness in the treatment of OCD, patients were administered fluoxetine doses in the range of 10 to 60 mg/day (*see* CLINICAL TRIALS).
In adolescents and higher weight children, treatment should be initiated with a dose of 10 mg/day. After 2 weeks, the dose should be increased to 20 mg/day. Additional dose increases may be considered after several more weeks if insufficient clinical improvement is observed. A dose range of 20 to 60 mg/day is recommended.
In lower weight children, treatment should be initiated with a dose of 10 mg/day. Additional dose increases may be considered after several more weeks if insufficient clinical improvement is observed. A dose range of 20 to 30 mg/day is recommended. Experience with daily doses greater than 20 mg is very minimal, and there is no experience with doses greater than 60 mg.
All patients—As with the use of Prozac in the treatment of major depressive disorder, a lower or less frequent dosage should be used in patients with hepatic impairment. A lower or less frequent dosage should also be considered for the elderly (*see* Geriatric Use *under* PRECAUTIONS), and for patients with concurrent disease or on multiple concomitant medications. Dosage adjustments for renal impairment are not routinely necessary (*see* Liver disease *and* Renal disease *under* CLINICAL PHARMACOLOGY, *and* Use in patients with concomitant illness *under* PRECAUTIONS).
Maintenance/Continuation Treatment
While there are no systematic studies that answer the question of how long to continue Prozac, OCD is a chronic condition and it is reasonable to consider continuation for a responding patient. Although the efficacy of Prozac after 13 weeks has not been documented in controlled trials, adult patients have been continued in therapy under double-blind conditions for up to an additional 6 months without loss of benefit. However, dosage adjustments should be made to maintain the patient on the lowest effective dosage, and patients should be periodically reassessed to determine the need for treatment.

Bulimia Nervosa
Initial Treatment
In the controlled clinical trials of fluoxetine supporting its effectiveness in the treatment of bulimia nervosa, patients were administered fixed daily fluoxetine doses of 20 or 60 mg, or placebo (*see* CLINICAL TRIALS). Only the 60-mg dose was statistically significantly superior to placebo in reducing the frequency of binge-eating and vomiting. Consequently, the recommended dose is 60 mg/day, administered in the morning. For some patients it may be advisable to titrate up to this target dose over several days. Fluoxetine doses above 60 mg/day have not been systematically studied in patients with bulimia.
As with the use of Prozac in the treatment of major depressive disorder and OCD, a lower or less frequent dosage should be used in patients with hepatic impairment. A lower or less frequent dosage should also be considered for the elderly (*see* Geriatric Use *under* PRECAUTIONS), and for patients with concurrent disease or on multiple concomitant medications. Dosage adjustments for renal impairment are not routinely necessary (*see* Liver disease *and* Renal disease *under* CLINICAL PHARMACOLOGY, *and* Use in patients with concomitant illness *under* PRECAUTIONS).
Maintenance/Continuation Treatment
Systematic evaluation of continuing Prozac 60 mg/day for periods of up to 52 weeks in patients with bulimia who have responded while taking Prozac 60 mg/day during an 8-week acute treatment phase has demonstrated a benefit of such maintenance treatment (*see* CLINICAL TRIALS). Nevertheless, patients should be periodically reassessed to determine the need for maintenance treatment.

Panic Disorder
Initial Treatment
In the controlled clinical trials of fluoxetine supporting its effectiveness in the treatment of panic disorder, patients were administered fluoxetine doses in the range of 10 to 60 mg/day (*see* CLINICAL TRIALS). Treatment should be initiated with a dose of 10 mg/day. After 1 week, the dose should be increased to 20 mg/day. The most frequently administered dose in the 2 flexible-dose clinical trials was 20 mg/day.
A dose increase may be considered after several weeks if no clinical improvement is observed. Fluoxetine doses above 60 mg/day have not been systematically evaluated in patients with panic disorder.
As with the use of Prozac in other indications, a lower or less frequent dosage should be used in patients with hepatic impairment. A lower or less frequent dosage should also be considered for the elderly (*see* Geriatric Use *under* PRECAUTIONS), and for patients with concurrent disease or on multiple concomitant medications. Dosage adjustments for renal impairment are not routinely necessary (*see* Liver disease *and* Renal disease *under* CLINICAL PHARMACOLOGY, *and* Use in patients with concomitant illness *under* PRECAUTIONS).
Maintenance/Continuation Treatment
While there are no systematic studies that answer the question of how long to continue Prozac, panic disorder is a chronic condition and it is reasonable to consider continuation for a responding patient. Nevertheless, patients should be periodically reassessed to determine the need for continued treatment.

HOW SUPPLIED

The following products are manufactured by Eli Lilly and Company for Dista Products Company.
Prozac® Pulvules®, USP, are available in:
The 10-mg[1] Pulvule is opaque green and green, imprinted with DISTA 3104 on the cap and Prozac 10 mg on the body:
NDC 0777-3104-02 (PU3104[2]) – Bottles of 100
NDC 0777-3104-07 (PU3104[2]) – Bottles of 2000
NDC 0777-3104-82 (PU3104[2]) – 20 FlexPak™[3] blister cards of 31
The 20-mg[1] Pulvule is an opaque green cap and off-white body, imprinted with DISTA 3105 on the cap and Prozac 20 mg on the body:
NDC 0777-3105-30 (PU3105[2]) – Bottles of 30
NDC 0777-3105-02 (PU3105[2]) – Bottles of 100
NDC 0777-3105-07 (PU3105[2]) – Bottles of 2000
NDC 0777-3105-33 (PU3105[2]) – (ID[4]100) Blisters
NDC 0777-3105-82 (PU3105[2]) – 20 FlexPak™[3] blister cards of 31
The 40-mg[1] Pulvule is an opaque green cap and opaque orange body, imprinted with DISTA 3107 on the cap and Prozac 40 mg on the body:
NDC 0777-3107-30 (PU3107[2]) – Bottles of 30
The following is manufactured by OSG Norwich Pharmaceuticals, Inc., North Norwich, NY, 13814, for Dista Products Company:
Liquid, Oral Solution is available in:
20 mg[1] per 5 mL with mint flavor:
NDC 0777-5120-58 (MS-5120[5]) – Bottles of 120 mL
The following products are manufactured and distributed by Eli Lilly and Company.
Prozac® Tablets are available in:
The 10-mg[1] tablet is green, elliptical shaped, and scored, with PROZAC 10 debossed on opposite side of score.
NDC 0002-4006-30 (TA4006) – Bottles of 30
NDC 0002-4006-02 (TA4006) – Bottles of 100
Prozac® Weekly™ Capsules are available in:
The 90-mg[1] capsule is an opaque green cap and clear body containing discretely visible white pellets through the clear body of the capsule, imprinted with Lilly on the cap and 3004 and 90 mg on the body.
NDC 0002-3004-75 (PU3004) – Blister package of 4

[1]Fluoxetine base equivalent.
[2]Protect from light.
[3]FlexPak™ (flexible blister card, Lilly).
[4]Identi-Dose® (unit dose medication, Lilly).
[5]Dispense in a tight, light-resistant container.
Store at Controlled Room Temperature, 15° to 30°C (59° to 86°F).

ANIMAL TOXICOLOGY

Phospholipids are increased in some tissues of mice, rats, and dogs given fluoxetine chronically. This effect is reversible after cessation of fluoxetine treatment. Phospholipid accumulation in animals has been observed with many cationic amphiphilic drugs, including fenfluramine, imipramine, and ranitidine. The significance of this effect in humans is unknown.
Literature revised November 17, 2003
www.lilly.com
PV 3455 DPP
Shown in Product Identification Guide, page 320

REOPRO® ℞

[*rē-ō-prō*]
(abciximab)
For intravenous administration

DESCRIPTION

Abciximab, ReoPro®, is the Fab fragment of the chimeric human-murine monoclonal antibody 7E3. Abciximab binds to the glycoprotein (GP) IIb/IIIa receptor of human platelets and inhibits platelet aggregation. Abciximab also binds to the vitronectin ($\alpha_v\beta_3$) receptor found on platelets and vessel wall endothelial and smooth muscle cells.
The chimeric 7E3 antibody is produced by continuous perfusion in mammalian cell culture. The 47,615 dalton Fab fragment is purified from cell culture supernatant by a series of steps involving specific viral inactivation and removal procedures, digestion with papain and column chromatography.
ReoPro® is a clear, colorless, sterile, non-pyrogenic solution for intravenous (IV) use. Each single use vial contains 2 mg/mL of Abciximab in a buffered solution (pH 7.2) of 0.01 M sodium phosphate, 0.15 M sodium chloride and 0.001% polysorbate 80 in Water for Injection. No preservatives are added.

CLINICAL PHARMACOLOGY

General—Abciximab binds to the intact platelet GPIIb/IIIa receptor, which is a member of the integrin family of adhesion receptors and the major platelet surface receptor involved in platelet aggregation. Abciximab inhibits platelet aggregation by preventing the binding of fibrinogen, von Willebrand factor, and other adhesive molecules to GPIIb/IIIa receptor sites on activated platelets. The mechanism of action is thought to involve steric hindrance and/or conformational effects to block access of large molecules to the receptor rather than direct interaction with the RGD (arginine-glycine-aspartic acid) binding site of GPIIb/IIIa.

Continued on next page

*** Identi-Code® symbol. This product information was prepared in June 2004. Current information on these and other products of Eli Lilly and Company may be obtained by direct inquiry to Lilly Research Laboratories, Lilly Corporate Center, Indianapolis, Indiana 46285, (800) 545-5979.**

ReoPro—Cont.

Abciximab binds with similar affinity to the vitronectin receptor, also known as the $\alpha_v\beta_3$ integrin. The vitronectin receptor mediates the procoagulant properties of platelets and the proliferative properties of vascular endothelial and smooth muscle cells. In *in vitro* studies using a model cell line derived from melanoma cells, Abciximab blocked $\alpha_v\beta_3$-mediated effects including cell adhesion (IC_{50} = 0.34 µg/mL). At concentrations which, *in vitro*, provide > 80% GPIIb/IIIa receptor blockade, but above the *in vivo* therapeutic range, Abciximab more effectively blocked the burst of thrombin generation that followed platelet activation than select comparator antibodies which inhibit GPIIb/IIIa alone (1). The relationship of these *in vitro* data to clinical efficacy is unknown.
Abciximab also binds to the activated Mac-1 receptor on monocytes and neutrophils (2). In *in vitro* studies, Abciximab and 7E3 IgG blocked Mac-1 receptor function as evidenced by inhibition of monocyte adhesion (3). In addition, the degree of activated Mac-1 expression on circulating leukocytes and the numbers of circulating leukocyte-platelet complexes has been shown to be reduced in patients treated with Abciximab compared to control patients (4). The relationship of these *in vitro* data to clinical efficacy is uncertain.
Pre-clinical experience—Maximal inhibition of platelet aggregation was observed when ≥ 80% of GPIIb/IIIa receptors were blocked by Abciximab. In non-human primates, Abciximab bolus doses of 0.25 mg/kg generally achieved a blockade of at least 80% of platelet receptors and fully inhibited platelet aggregation. Inhibition of platelet function was temporary following a bolus dose, but receptor blockade could be sustained at ≥ 80% by continuous intravenous infusion. The inhibitory effects of Abciximab were substantially reversed by the transfusion of platelets in monkeys. The antithrombotic efficacy of prototype antibodies [murine 7E3 Fab and $F(ab')_2$] and Abciximab was evaluated in dog, monkey and baboon models of coronary, carotid, and femoral artery thrombosis. Doses of the murine version of 7E3 or Abciximab sufficient to produce high-grade (≥ 80%) GPIIb/IIIa receptor blockade prevented acute thrombosis and yielded lower rates of thrombosis compared with aspirin and/or heparin.
Pharmacokinetics—Following intravenous bolus administration, free plasma concentrations of Abciximab decrease rapidly with an initial half-life of less than 10 minutes and a second phase half-life of about 30 minutes, probably related to rapid binding to the platelet GPIIb/IIIa receptors. Platelet function generally recovers over the course of 48 hours (5,6), although Abciximab remains in the circulation for 15 days or more in a platelet-bound state. Intravenous administration of a 0.25 mg/kg bolus dose of Abciximab followed by continuous infusion of 10 µg/min (or a weight-adjusted infusion of 0.125 µg/kg/min to a maximum of 10 µg/min) produces approximately constant free plasma concentrations throughout the infusion. At the termination of the infusion period, free plasma concentrations fall rapidly for approximately six hours then decline at a slower rate.
Pharmacodynamics—Intravenous administration in humans of single bolus doses of Abciximab from 0.15 mg/kg to 0.30 mg/kg produced rapid dose-dependent inhibition of platelet function as measured by *ex vivo* platelet aggregation in response to adenosine diphosphate (ADP) or by prolongation of bleeding time. At the two highest doses (0.25 and 0.30 mg/kg) at two hours post injection (the first time point evaluated), over 80% of the GPIIb/IIIa receptors were blocked and platelet aggregation in response to 20 µM ADP was almost abolished. The median bleeding time increased to over 30 minutes at both doses compared with a baseline value of approximately five minutes.
Intravenous administration in humans of a single bolus dose of 0.25 mg/kg followed by a continuous infusion of 10 µg/min for periods of 12 to 96 hours produced sustained high-grade GPIIb/IIIa receptor blockade (≥ 80%) and inhibition of platelet function (*ex vivo* platelet aggregation in response to 5 µM or 20 µM ADP less than 20% of baseline and bleeding time greater than 30 minutes) for the duration of the infusion in most patients. Similar results were obtained when a weight-adjusted infusion dose (0.125 µg/kg/min to a maximum of 10 µg/min) was used in patients weighing up to 80 kg. Results in patients who received the 0.25 mg/kg bolus followed by a 5 µg/min infusion for 24 hours showed a similar initial receptor blockade and inhibition of platelet aggregation, but the response was not maintained throughout the infusion period. The onset of Abciximab-mediated platelet inhibition following a 0.25 mg/kg bolus and 0.125 µg/kg/min infusion was rapid and platelet aggregation was reduced to less than 20% of baseline in 8 of 10 patients at 10 minutes after treatment initiation.
Low levels of GPIIb/IIIa receptor blockade are present for more than 10 days following cessation of the infusion. After discontinuation of Abciximab infusion, platelet function returns gradually to normal. Bleeding time returned to ≤ 12 minutes within 12 hours following the end of infusion in 15 of 20 patients (75%), and within 24 hours in 18 of 20 patients (90%). *Ex vivo* platelet aggregation in response to 5 µM ADP returned to ≥ 50% of baseline within 24 hours following the end of infusion in 11 of 32 patients (34%) and within 48 hours in 23 of 32 patients (72%). In response to 20 µM ADP, *ex vivo* platelet aggregation returned to ≥ 50% of baseline within 24 hours in 20 of 32 patients (62%) and within 48 hours in 28 of 32 patients (88%).

Table 1
ENDPOINT EVENT RATES AT 30 DAYS - EPILOG TRIAL

	Placebo + Standard Dose Heparin (n=939)	Abciximab + Standard Dose Heparin (n=918)	Abciximab + Low Dose Heparin (n=935)
		Number of Patients (%)	
Death or MI[a]	85 (9.1)	38 (4.2)	35 (3.8)
p-value vs. placebo		<0.001	<0.001
Death, MI, or urgent intervention[a]	109 (11.7)	49 (5.4)	48 (5.2)
p-value vs. placebo		<0.001	<0.001
Components of Composite Endpoints[b]			
Death	7 (0.8)	4 (0.4)	3 (0.3)
Acute myocardial infarctions in surviving patients	78 (8.4)	34 (3.7)	32 (3.4)
Urgent interventions in surviving patients without an acute myocardial infarction	24 (2.6)	11 (1.2)	13 (1.4)

[a] Patients who experienced more than one event in the first 30 days are counted only once.
[b] Patients are counted only once under the most serious component (death > acute MI > urgent intervention).

Table 2
PRIMARY ENDPOINT EVENT RATE AT 30 DAYS - EPISTENT TRIAL

	Placebo + Stent (n=809)	Abciximab + Stent (n=794)	Abciximab + PTCA (n=796)
		Number of Patients (%)	
Death, MI, or urgent intervention[a]	87 (10.8%)	42 (5.3%)	55 (6.9%)
p-value vs. placebo		<0.001	0.007
Components of Composite Endpoint[b]			
Death	5 (0.6%)	2 (0.3%)	6 (0.8%)
Acute myocardial infarctions in surviving patients	77 (9.6%)	35 (4.4%)	40 (5.0%)
Urgent interventions in surviving patients without an acute myocardial infarction	5 (0.6%)	5 (0.6%)	9 (1.1%)

[a] Patients who experienced more than one event in the first 30 days are counted only once.
[b] Patients are counted only once under the most serious component (death > acute MI > urgent intervention).

CLINICAL STUDIES

Abciximab has been studied in four Phase 3 clinical trials, all of which evaluated the effect of Abciximab in patients undergoing percutaneous coronary intervention (PCI): in patients at high risk for abrupt closure of the treated coronary vessel (EPIC), in a broader group of patients (EPILOG), in unstable angina patients not responding to conventional medical therapy (CAPTURE), and in patients suitable for either conventional angioplasty/atherectomy or primary stent implantation (EPILOG Stent; EPISTENT). Percutaneous intervention included balloon angioplasty, atherectomy, or stent placement. All trials involved the use of various, concomitant heparin dose regimens and, unless contraindicated, aspirin (325 mg) was administered orally two hours prior to the planned procedure and then once daily.
EPIC was a multicenter, double-blind, placebo-controlled trial of Abciximab in patients undergoing percutaneous transluminal coronary angioplasty or atherectomy (PTCA) who were at high risk for abrupt closure of the treated coronary vessel (7). Patients were allocated to treatment with: 1) Abciximab bolus plus infusion for 12 hours; 2) Abciximab bolus plus placebo infusion, or; 3) placebo bolus plus infusion. All patients received concomitant heparin (10,000 to 12,000 U bolus followed by an infusion for 12 hours).
The primary endpoint was the composite of death, myocardial infarction (MI), or urgent intervention for recurrent ischemia within 30 days of randomization. The primary endpoint event rates in the Abciximab bolus plus infusion group were reduced mostly in the first 48 hours and this benefit was sustained through 30 days (7), 6 months (8), and three years (9).
EPILOG was a randomized, double-blind, multicenter, placebo-controlled trial which evaluated Abciximab in a broad population of patients undergoing PCI (excluding patients with myocardial infarction and unstable angina meeting the EPIC high risk criteria) (10). Study procedures emphasized discontinuation of heparin after the procedure with early femoral arterial sheath removal and careful access site management (see PRECAUTIONS). EPILOG was a three-arm trial comparing Abciximab plus standard-dose heparin, Abciximab plus low-dose heparin, and placebo plus standard-dose heparin. Abciximab and heparin infusions were weight-adjusted in all arms. The Abciximab bolus plus infusion regimen was: 0.25 mg/kg bolus followed by a 0.125 µg/kg/min infusion (to a maximum of 10 µg/min) for 12 hours. The heparin regimen was either a standard-dose regimen (initial 100 U/kg bolus, target ACT ≥ 300 seconds) or a low-dose regimen (initial 70 U/kg bolus, target ACT ≥ 200 seconds).
The primary endpoint of the EPILOG trial was the composite of death or MI occurring within 30 days of PCI. The composite of death, MI, or urgent intervention was an important secondary endpoint. The endpoint events in the Abciximab treatment group were reduced mostly in the first 48 hours and this benefit was sustained through 30 days and six months (10) and one year (11). The (Kaplan-Meier) endpoint event rates at 30 days are shown in Table 1.
[See table 1 above]
At the six-month follow up visit, the event rate for death, MI, or repeat (urgent or non-urgent) intervention remained lower in the Abciximab treatment arms (22.3% and 22.8%, respectively, for the standard- and low-dose heparin arms) than in the placebo arm (25.8%) and the event rate for death, MI, or urgent intervention was substantially lower in the Abciximab treatment arms (8.3% and 8.4%, respectively, for the standard- and low-dose heparin arms) than in the placebo arm (14.7%). The treatment associated effects continued to persist at the one-year follow up visit. The proportionate reductions in endpoint event rates were similar irrespective of the type of coronary intervention used (balloon angioplasty, atherectomy, or stent placement). Risk assessment using the American College of Cardiology/American Heart Association clinical/morphological criteria had large inter-observer variability. Consequently, a low risk subgroup could not be reproducibly identified in which to evaluate efficacy.
The EPISTENT trial was a randomized, multicenter trial evaluating three different treatment strategies in patients undergoing PCI: conventional PTCA with Abciximab plus low-dose heparin, primary intracoronary stent implantation with Abciximab plus low-dose heparin, and primary intracoronary stent implantation with placebo plus standard-dose heparin (12). The heparin dose was weight-adjusted in all arms. The JJIS Palmaz-Schatz stent was used in over 90% of the patients receiving stents. The two stent arms were blinded with respect to study agent (Abciximab or placebo) and heparin dose; the PCI arm with Abciximab was open-label. The Abciximab bolus plus infusion regimen was the same as that used in the EPILOG trial. The standard-dose and low-dose heparin regimens were the same as those used in the EPILOG trial. All patients were to receive aspirin; ticlopidine, if given, was to be started prior to study agent. Patient and access site management guidelines were the same as those for EPILOG, including a strong recommendation for early sheath removal.
The results demonstrated benefit in both Abciximab arms (i.e., with and without stents) compared with stenting alone on the composite of death, MI, or urgent intervention (repeat PCI or CABG) within 30 days of PCI (12). The (Kaplan-Meier) endpoint event rates at 30 days are shown in Table 2.
[See table 2 above]
This benefit was maintained at 6 months: 12.1% of patients in the placebo/stent group experienced death, MI, or urgent revascularization compared with 6.4% of patients in the Abciximab/stent group (p<0.001 vs placebo/stent) and 9.2% in the Abciximab/PTCA group (p=0.051 vs placebo/stent). At 6 months, a reduction in the composite of death, MI, or all repeat (urgent or non-urgent) intervention was observed in the Abciximab/stent group compared with the placebo/stent group (15.4% vs 20.4%, p=0.006); the rate of this composite endpoint was similar in the Abciximab/PTCA and placebo/stent groups (22.4% vs 20.4%, p=0.467). (13)
CAPTURE was a randomized, double-blind, multicenter, placebo-controlled trial of the use of Abciximab in unstable angina patients not responding to conventional medical therapy for whom PCI was planned, but not immediately performed (14). The CAPTURE trial involved the administration of placebo or Abciximab starting 18 to 24 hours prior to PCI and continuing until one hour after completion of the intervention.
Patients were assessed as having unstable angina not responding to conventional medical therapy if they had at least one episode of myocardial ischemia despite bed rest

and at least two hours of therapy with intravenous heparin and oral or intravenous nitrates. These patients were enrolled into the CAPTURE trial, if during a screening angiogram, they were determined to have a coronary lesion amenable to PCI. Patients received a bolus dose and intravenous infusion of placebo or Abciximab for 18 to 24 hours. At the end of the infusion period, the intervention was performed. The Abciximab or placebo infusion was discontinued one hour following the intervention. Patients were treated with intravenous heparin and oral or intravenous nitrates throughout the 18- to 24-hour Abciximab infusion period prior to the PCI.

The Abciximab dose was a 0.25 mg/kg bolus followed by a continuous infusion at a rate of 10 μg/min. The CAPTURE trial incorporated weight adjustment of the standard heparin dose only during the performance of the intervention, but did not investigate the effect of a lower heparin dose, and arterial sheaths were left in place for approximately 40 hours. The primary endpoint of the CAPTURE trial was the occurrence of any of the following events within 30 days of PCI: death, MI, or urgent intervention. The 30-day (Kaplan-Meier) primary endpoint event rates are shown in Table 3. [See table 3 at right]

Table 3
PRIMARY ENDPOINT EVENT RATE AT 30 DAYS - CAPTURE TRIAL

	Placebo (n=635)	Abciximab (n=630)
	Number of Patients (%)	
Death, MI, or urgent intervention[a]	101 (15.9)	71 (11.3)
p-value vs. placebo		0.012
Components of Primary Endpoint[b]		
Death	8 (1.3)	6 (1.0)
MI in surviving patients	49 (7.7)	24 (3.8)
Urgent intervention in surviving patients without an acute MI	44 (6.9)	41 (6.6)

[a] Patients who experienced more than one event in the first 30 days are counted only once. Urgent interventions included any unplanned PCI after the planned intervention, as well as any stent placement for immediate patency and any unplanned CABG or use of an intra-aortic balloon pump.

[b] Patients are counted only once under the most serious component (death > acute MI > urgent intervention).

The 30-day results are consistent with the results of the other three trials, with the greatest effects on the myocardial infarction and urgent intervention components of the composite endpoint. As secondary endpoints, the components of the composite endpoint were analyzed separately for the period prior to the PCI and the period from the beginning of the intervention through Day 30. The greatest difference in MI occurred in the post-intervention period: the rates of MI were lower in the Abciximab group compared with placebo (Abciximab 3.6%, placebo 6.1%). There was also a reduction in MI occurring prior to the PCI (Abciximab 0.6%, placebo 2.0%). An Abciximab-associated reduction in the incidence of urgent intervention occurred in the post-intervention period. No effect on mortality was observed in either period. At six months of follow up, the composite endpoint of death, MI, or all repeat intervention (urgent or non-urgent) was not different between the Abciximab and placebo groups (Abciximab 31.0%, placebo 30.8%, p=0.77).

Mortality was uncommon in all four trials. Similar mortality rates were observed in all arms within each trial. Patient follow-up through one year of the EPISTENT trial suggested decreased mortality among patients treated with Abciximab and stent placement compared to patients treated with stent alone (8/794 vs. 19/809, p=0.037). Data from earlier studies with balloon angioplasty were not suggestive of the same benefit. In all four trials, the rates of acute MI were significantly lower in the groups treated with Abciximab. Most of the Abciximab treatment effect was seen in reduction in the rate of acute non-Q-wave MI. Urgent intervention rates were also lower in Abciximab-treated groups in these trials.

Anticoagulation:

EPILOG and EPISTENT: Weight-adjusted low dose heparin, weight-adjusted Abciximab, careful vascular access site management and discontinuation of heparin after the procedure with early femoral arterial sheath removal were used.

The initial heparin bolus was based upon the results of the baseline ACT, according to the following regimen:

ACT < 150 seconds: administer 70 U/kg heparin
ACT 150 - 199 seconds: administer 50 U/kg heparin
ACT ≥ 200 seconds: administer no heparin

Additional 20 U/kg heparin boluses were given to achieve and maintain an ACT of ≥ 200 seconds during the procedure.

Discontinuation of heparin immediately after the procedure and removal of the arterial sheath within six hours were strongly recommended in the trials. If prolonged heparin therapy or delayed sheath removal was clinically indicated, heparin was adjusted to keep the APTT at a target of 60 to 85 seconds (EPILOG) or 55 to 75 seconds (EPISTENT).

CAPTURE trial: Anticoagulation was initiated prior to the administration of Abciximab. Anticoagulation was initiated with an intravenous heparin infusion to achieve a target APTT of 60 to 85 seconds. The heparin infusion was not uniformly weight adjusted in this trial. The heparin infusion was maintained during the Abciximab infusion and was adjusted to achieve an ACT of 300 seconds or an APTT of 70 seconds during the PCI. Following the intervention, heparin management was as outlined above for the EPILOG trial.

INDICATIONS AND USAGE

Abciximab is indicated as an adjunct to percutaneous coronary intervention for the prevention of cardiac ischemic complications.

- in patients undergoing percutaneous coronary intervention
- in patients with unstable angina not responding to conventional medical therapy when percutaneous coronary intervention is planned within 24 hours

Safety and efficacy ofAbciximab use in patients not undergoing percutaneous coronary intervention have not been established.

Abciximab is intended for use with aspirin and heparin and has been studied only in that setting, as described in CLINICAL STUDIES.

CONTRAINDICATIONS

Because Abciximab may increase the risk of bleeding, Abciximab is contraindicated in the following clinical situations:

- Active internal bleeding
- Recent (within six weeks) gastrointestinal (GI) or genitourinary (GU) bleeding of clinical significance.
- History of cerebrovascular accident (CVA) within two years, or CVA with a significant residual neurological deficit
- Bleeding diathesis
- Administration of oral anticoagulants within seven days unless prothrombin time is ≤ 1.2 times control
- Thrombocytopenia (< 100,000 cells/μL)
- Recent (within six weeks) major surgery or trauma
- Intracranial neoplasm, arteriovenous malformation, or aneurysm
- Severe uncontrolled hypertension
- Presumed or documented history of vasculitis
- Use of intravenous dextran before PCI, or intent to use it during an intervention

Abciximab is also contraindicated in patients with known hypersensitivity to any component of this product or to murine proteins.

WARNINGS

Abciximab has the potential to increase the risk of bleeding, particularly in the presence of anticoagulation, e.g., from heparin, other anticoagulants, or thrombolytics (see ADVERSE REACTIONS: Bleeding).

The risk of major bleeds due to Abciximab therapy is increased in patients receiving thrombolytics and should be weighed against the anticipated benefits.

Should serious bleeding occur that is not controllable with pressure, the infusion of Abciximab and any concomitant heparin should be stopped.

PRECAUTIONS

Bleeding Precautions—To minimize the risk of bleeding with Abciximab, it is important to use a low-dose, weight-adjusted heparin regimen, a weight-adjusted Abciximab bolus and infusion, strict anticoagulation guidelines, careful vascular access site management, discontinuation of heparin after the procedure and early femoral arterial sheath removal.

Therapy with Abciximab requires careful attention to all potential bleeding sites including catheter insertion sites, arterial and venous puncture sites, cutdown sites, needle puncture sites, and gastrointestinal, genitourinary, pulmonary (alveolar), and retroperitoneal sites.

Arterial and venous punctures, intramuscular injections, and use of urinary catheters, nasotracheal intubation, nasogastric tubes and automatic blood pressure cuffs should be minimized. When obtaining intravenous access, noncompressible sites (e.g., subclavian or jugular veins) should be avoided. Saline or heparin locks should be considered for blood drawing. Vascular puncture sites should be documented and monitored. Gentle care should be provided when removing dressings.

Femoral artery access site: Arterial access site care is important to prevent bleeding. Care should be taken when attempting vascular access that only the anterior wall of the femoral artery is punctured, avoiding a Seldinger (through and through) technique for obtaining sheath access. Femoral vein sheath placement should be avoided unless needed. While the vascular sheath is in place, patients should be maintained on complete bed rest with the head of the bed ≤ 30° and the affected limb restrained in a straight position. Patients may be medicated for back/groin pain as necessary. Discontinuation of heparin immediately upon completion of the procedure and removal of the arterial sheath within six hours is strongly recommended if APTT ≤ 50 sec or ACT ≤ 175 sec (See PRECAUTIONS: Laboratory Tests). In all circumstances, heparin should be discontinued at least two hours prior to arterial sheath removal.

Following sheath removal, pressure should be applied to the femoral artery for at least 30 minutes using either manual compression or a mechanical device for hemostasis. A pressure dressing should be applied following hemostasis. The patient should be maintained on bed rest for six to eight hours following sheath removal or discontinuation of Abciximab, or four hours following discontinuation of heparin, whichever is later. The pressure dressing should be removed prior to ambulation. The sheath insertion site and distal pulses of affected leg(s) should be frequently checked while the femoral artery sheath is in place and for six hours after femoral artery sheath removal. Any hematoma should be measured and monitored for enlargement.

The following conditions have been associated with an increased risk of bleeding and may be additive with the effect of Abciximab in the angioplasty setting: PCI within 12 hours of the onset of symptoms for acute myocardial infarction, prolonged PCI (lasting more than 70 minutes) and failed PCI.

Use of Thrombolytics, Anticoagulants and Other Antiplatelet Agents—In the EPIC, EPILOG, CAPTURE, and EPISTENT trials, Abciximab was used concomitantly with heparin and aspirin. For details of the anticoagulation algorithms used in these clinical trials, see CLINICAL STUDIES: Anticoagulation. Because Abciximab inhibits platelet aggregation, caution should be employed when it is used with other drugs that affect hemostasis, including thrombolytics, oral anticoagulants, non-steroidal anti-inflammatory drugs, dipyridamole, and ticlopidine.

In the EPIC trial, there was limited experience with the administration of Abciximab with low molecular weight dextran. Low molecular weight dextran was usually given for the deployment of a coronary stent, for which oral anticoagulants were also given. In the 11 patients who received low molecular weight dextran with Abciximab, five had major bleeding events and four had minor bleeding events. None of the five placebo patients treated with low molecular weight dextran had a major or minor bleeding event (see CONTRAINDICATIONS).

Because of observed synergistic effects on bleeding, Abciximab therapy should be used judiciously in patients who have received systemic thrombolytic therapy. The GUSTO V trial randomized patients with acute myocardial infarction to treatment with combined Abciximab and half-dose Reteplase, or full-dose Reteplase alone (15). In this trial, the incidence of moderate or severe nonintracranial bleeding was increased in those patients receiving Abciximab and half-dose Reteplase versus those receiving Reteplase alone (4.6% versus 2.3%, respectively).

Thrombocytopenia—Thrombocytopenia, including severe thrombocytopenia, has been observed with Abciximab administration (See Adverse Reactions: Thrombocytopenia). Platelet counts should be monitored prior to, during, and after treatment with Abciximab. Acute decreases in platelet count should be differentiated between true thrombocytopenia and pseudothrombocytopenia (See Precautions: Laboratory Tests). If true thrombocytopenia is verified, Abciximab should be immediately discontinued and the condition appropriately monitored and treated.

In clinical trials, patients who developed thrombocytopenia were followed with daily platelet counts until their platelet count returned to normal. Heparin and aspirin were discontinued for platelet counts below 60,000 cells/μL and platelets were transfused for a platelet count below 50,000 cells/μL. Most cases of severe thrombocytopenia (< 50,000 cells/μL) occurred within the first 24 hours of Abciximab administration.

In a registry study of Abciximab readministration, a history of thrombocytopenia associated with prior use of Abciximab was predictive of an increased risk of recurrent thrombocytopenia (See Adverse Reactions: Thrombocytopenia). Readministration within 30 days was associated with an increased incidence and severity of thrombocytopenia, as was a positive human anti-chimeric antibody (HACA) test at baseline, compared to the rates seen in studies with first administration.

Restoration of Platelet Function—In the event of serious uncontrolled bleeding or the need for emergency surgery, Abciximab should be discontinued. If platelet function does not return to normal, it may be restored, at least in part, with platelet transfusions.

Laboratory Tests—Before infusion of Abciximab, prothrombin time, ACT, APTT, and platelet count should be measured to identify pre-existing hemostatic abnormalities.

Based on an integrated analysis of data from all studies, the following guidelines may be utilized to minimize the risk for bleeding:

- When Abciximab is initiated 18 to 24 hours before PCI, the APTT should be maintained between 60 and 85 seconds during the Abciximab and heparin infusion period.

Continued on next page

*** Identi-Code® symbol. This product information was prepared in June 2004. Current information on these and other products of Eli Lilly and Company may be obtained by direct inquiry to Lilly Research Laboratories, Lilly Corporate Center, Indianapolis, Indiana 46285, (800) 545-5979.**

ReoPro—Cont.

- During PCI the ACT should be maintained between 200 and 300 seconds.
- If anticoagulation is continued in these patients following PCI, the APTT should be maintained between 55 and 75 seconds.

The APTT or ACT should be checked prior to arterial sheath removal. The sheath should not be removed unless APTT ≤ 50 seconds or ACT ≤ 175 seconds.

Platelet counts should be monitored prior to treatment, two to four hours following the bolus dose of Abciximab and at 24 hours or prior to discharge, whichever is first. If a patient experiences an acute platelet decrease (e.g., a platelet decrease to less than 100,000 cells/µL and a decrease of at least 25% from pre-treatment value), additional platelet counts should be determined. Platelet monitoring should continue until platelet counts return to normal.

To exclude pseudothrombocytopenia, a laboratory artifact due to *in vitro* anticoagulant interaction, blood samples should be drawn in three separate tubes containing ethylenediaminetetraacetic acid (EDTA), citrate and heparin, respectively. A low platelet count in EDTA but not in heparin and/or citrate is supportive of a diagnosis of pseudothrombocytopenia.

Readministration—Administration of Abciximab may result in the formation of HACA that could potentially cause allergic or hypersensitivity reactions (including anaphylaxis), thrombocytopenia or diminished benefit upon readministration of Abciximab (See Adverse Reactions: Immunogenicity).

Readministration of Abciximab to patients undergoing PCI was assessed in a registry that included 1342 treatments in 1286 patients. Most patients were receiving their second Abciximab exposure; 15% were receiving the third or subsequent exposure. The overall rate of HACA positivity prior to the readministration was 6% and increased to 27% post-readministration. There were no reports of serious allergic reactions or anaphylaxis. Thrombocytopenia was observed at higher rates in the readministration study than in the phase 3 studies of first-time administration (See Precautions: Thrombocytopenia and Adverse Reactions: Thrombocytopenia), suggesting that readministration may be associated with an increased incidence and severity of thrombocytopenia.

Allergic Reactions—Anaphylaxis has not been reported for Abciximab-treated patients in any of the Phase 3 clinical trials. However, anaphylaxis may occur. If it does, administration of Abciximab should be immediately stopped and standard appropriate resuscitative measures should be initiated.

Drug Interactions—Formal drug interaction studies with Abciximab have not been conducted. Abciximab has been administered to patients with ischemic heart disease treated concomitantly with a broad range of medications used in the treatment of angina, myocardial infarction and hypertension. These medications have included heparin, warfarin, beta-adrenergic receptor blockers, calcium channel antagonists, angiotensin converting enzyme inhibitors, intravenous and oral nitrates, ticlopidine, and aspirin. Heparin, other anticoagulants, thrombolytics, and antiplatelet agents are associated with an increase in bleeding. Patients with HACA titers may have allergic or hypersensitivity reactions when treated with other diagnostic or therapeutic monoclonal antibodies.

Carcinogenesis, Mutagenesis and Impairment of Fertility—*In vitro* and *in vivo* mutagenicity studies have not demonstrated any mutagenic effect. Long-term studies in animals have not been performed to evaluate the carcinogenic potential or effects on fertility in male or female animals.

Pregnancy Category C—Animal reproduction studies have not been conducted with Abciximab. It is also not known whether Abciximab can cause fetal harm when administered to a pregnant woman or can affect reproduction capacity. Abciximab should be given to a pregnant woman only if clearly needed.

Nursing Mothers—It is not known whether this drug is excreted in human milk or absorbed systemically after ingestion. Because many drugs are excreted in human milk, caution should be exercised when Abciximab is administered to a nursing woman.

Pediatric Use—Safety and effectiveness in pediatric patients have not been studied.

Geriatric Use—Of the total number of 7860 patients in the four Phase 3 trials, 2933 (37%) were 65 and over, while 653 (8%) were 75 and over. No overall differences in safety or efficacy were observed between patients of age 65 to less than 75 as compared to younger patients. The clinical experience is not adequate to determine whether patients of age 75 or greater respond differently than younger patients.

ADVERSE REACTIONS

Bleeding—Abciximab has the potential to increase the risk of bleeding, particularly in the presence of anticoagulation, e.g., from heparin, other anticoagulants or thrombolytics. Bleeding in the Phase 3 trials was classified as major, minor or insignificant by the criteria of the Thrombolysis in Myocardial Infarction study group (16). Major bleeding events were defined as either an intracranial hemorrhage or a decrease in hemoglobin greater than 5 g/dL. Minor bleeding events included spontaneous gross hematuria, spontaneous hematemesis, observed blood loss with a hemoglobin decrease of more than 3 g/dL, or a decrease in hemoglobin of at least 4 g/dL without an identified bleeding site. Insignificant bleeding events were defined as a decrease in hemoglobin of less than 3 g/dL or a decrease in hemoglobin between 3-4 g/dL without observed bleeding. In patients who received transfusions, the number of units of blood lost was estimated through an adaptation of the method of Landefeld, et al. (17).

In the EPIC trial, in which a non-weight-adjusted, longer-duration heparin dose regimen was used, the most common complication during Abciximab therapy was bleeding during the first 36 hours. The incidences of major bleeding, minor bleeding and transfusion of blood products were significantly increased. Major bleeding occurred in 10.6% of patients in the Abciximab bolus plus infusion arm compared with 3.3% of patients in the placebo arm. Minor bleeding was seen in 16.8% of Abciximab bolus plus infusion patients and 9.2% of placebo patients (7). Approximately 70% of Abciximab-treated patients with major bleeding had bleeding at the arterial access site in the groin. Abciximab-treated patients also had a higher incidence of major bleeding events from gastrointestinal, genitourinary, retroperitoneal, and other sites.

Bleeding rates were reduced in the CAPTURE trial, and further reduced in the EPILOG and EPISTENT trials by use of modified dosing regimens and specific patient management techniques. In EPILOG and EPISTENT, using the heparin and Abciximab dosing, sheath removal and arterial access site guidelines described under PRECAUTIONS, the incidence of major bleeding in patients treated with Abciximab and low-dose, weight-adjusted heparin was not significantly different from that in patients receiving placebo.

Subgroup analyses in the EPIC and CAPTURE trials showed that non-CABG major bleeding was more common in Abciximab patients weighing ≤ 75 kg. In the EPILOG and EPISTENT trials, which used weight-adjusted heparin dosing, the non-CABG major bleeding rates for Abciximab-treated patients did not differ substantially by weight subgroup.

Although data are limited, Abciximab treatment was not associated with excess major bleeding in patients who underwent CABG surgery. (The range among all treatment arms was 3-5% in EPIC, and 1-2% in the CAPTURE, EPILOG, and EPISTENT trials.) Some patients with prolonged bleeding times received platelet transfusions to correct the bleeding time prior to surgery. (See PRECAUTIONS: Restoration of Platelet Function.)

The rates of major bleeding, minor bleeding and bleeding events requiring transfusions in the CAPTURE, EPILOG, and EPISTENT trials are shown in Table 4. The rates of insignificant bleeding events are not included in Table 4.

Pulmonary alveolar hemorrhage has been rarely reported during use of Abciximab. This can present with any or all of the following in close association with ReoPro administration: hypoxemia, alveolar infiltrates on chest x-ray, hemoptysis, or an unexplained drop in hemoglobin.

[See table 4 below]

Table 4
NON-CABG BLEEDING IN TRIALS OF PERCUTANEOUS CORONARY INTERVENTION (EPILOG, EPISTENT and CAPTURE)
Number of Patients with Bleeds (%)

	Placebo[c] (n = 1748)	Abciximab + Low-dose Heparin[d] (n=2525)	Abciximab + Standard-dose Heparin[e] (n=918)
EPILOG and EPISTENT:			
Major[a]	18 (1.0)	21 (0.8)	17 (1.9)
Minor	46 (2.6)	82 (3.2)	70 (7.6)
Requiring transfusion[b]	15 (0.9)	13 (0.5)	7 (0.8)
CAPTURE:	Placebo[f] (n=635)		Abciximab[f] (n=630)
Major[a]	12 (1.9)		24 (3.8)
Minor	13 (2.0)		30 (4.8)
Requiring transfusion[b]	9 (1.4)		15 (2.4)

[a] Patients who had bleeding in more than one classification are counted only once according to the most severe classification. Patients with multiple bleeding events of the same classification are also counted once within that classification.
[b] Patients with major non-CABG bleeding who received packed red blood cells or whole blood transfusion.
[c] Standard-dose heparin with or without stent (EPILOG and EPISTENT)
[d] Low-dose heparin with or without stent (EPILOG and EPISTENT)
[e] Standard-dose heparin (EPILOG)
[f] Standard-dose heparin (CAPTURE)

Intracranial Hemorrhage and Stroke—The total incidence of intracranial hemorrhage and non-hemorrhagic stroke across all four trials was not significantly different, 9/3023 for placebo patients and 15/4680 for Abciximab-treated patients. The incidence of intracranial hemorrhage was 3/3023 for placebo patients and 7/4680 for Abciximab patients.

Thrombocytopenia—In the clinical trials, patients treated with Abciximab were more likely than patients treated with placebo to experience decreases in platelet counts.

Among patients in the EPILOG and EPISTENT trials who were treated with Abciximab plus low-dose heparin, the proportion of patients with any thrombocytopenia (platelets less than 100,000 cells/µL) ranged from 2.5 to 3.0%. The incidence of severe thrombocytopenia (platelets less than 50,000 cells/µL) ranged from 0.4 to 1.0% and platelet transfusions were required in 0.9 to 1.1%, respectively. Modestly lower rates were observed among patients treated with placebo plus standard-dose heparin. Overall higher rates were observed among patients in the EPIC and CAPTURE trials treated with Abciximab plus longer duration heparin: 2.6 to 5.2% were found to have any thrombocytopenia, 0.9 to 1.7% had severe thrombocytopenia, and 2.1 to 5.5% required platelet transfusion, respectively.

In a readministration registry study of patients receiving a second or subsequent exposure to Abciximab (See Precautions: Readministration) the incidence of any degree of thrombocytopenia was 5%, with an incidence of profound thrombocytopenia of 2% (<20,000 cell/µL). Factors associated with an increased risk of thrombocytopenia were a history of thrombocytopenia on previous Abciximab exposure, readministration within 30 days, and a positive HACA assay prior to the readministration.

Among 14 patients who had thrombocytopenia associated with a prior exposure to Abciximab, 7 (50%) had recurrent thrombocytopenia. In 130 patients with a readministration interval of 30 days or less, 25 (19%) developed thrombocytopenia. Severe thrombocytopenia occurred in 19 of these patients. Among the 71 patients who had a positive HACA assay at baseline, 11 (15%) developed thrombocytopenia, 7 of which were severe.

Other Adverse Reactions—Table 5 shows adverse events other than bleeding and thrombocytopenia from the combined EPIC, EPILOG and CAPTURE trials which occurred in patients in the bolus plus infusion arm at an incidence of more than 0.5% higher than in those treated with placebo.

Table 5
ADVERSE EVENTS AMONG TREATED PATIENTS IN THE EPIC, EPILOG, AND CAPTURE TRIALS

Event	Placebo (n=2226)	Bolus + Infusion (n=3111)
	Number of Patients (%)	
Cardiovascular system		
Hypotension	230 (10.3)	447 (14.4)
Bradycardia	79 (3.5)	140 (4.5)
Gastrointestinal system		
Nausea	255 (11.5)	423 (13.6)
Vomiting	152 (6.8)	226 (7.3)
Abdominal pain	49 (2.2)	97 (3.1)
Miscellaneous		
Back pain	304 (13.7)	546 (17.6)
Chest pain	208 (9.3)	356 (11.4)
Headache	122 (5.5)	200 (6.4)
Puncture site pain	58 (2.6)	113 (3.6)
Peripheral edema	25 (1.1)	49 (1.6)

The following additional adverse events from the EPIC, EPILOG and CAPTURE trials were reported by investigators for patients treated with a bolus plus infusion of Abciximab at incidences which were less than 0.5% higher than for patients in the placebo arm.

Cardiovascular System: ventricular tachycardia (1.4%), pseudoaneurysm (0.8%), palpitation (0.5%), arteriovenous fistula (0.4%), incomplete AV block (0.3%), nodal arrhythmia (0.2%), complete AV block (0.1%), embolism (limb)(0.1%); thrombophlebitis (0.1%);

Gastrointestinal System: dyspepsia (2.1%), diarrhea (1.1%), ileus (0.1%), gastroesophageal reflux (0.1%);

Hemic and Lymphatic System: anemia (1.3%), leukocytosis (0.5%), petechiae (0.2%);

Nervous System: dizziness (2.9%), anxiety (1.7%), abnormal thinking (1.3%), agitation (0.7%), hypesthesia (0.6%), confusion (0.5%) muscle contractions (0.4%), coma (0.2%), hypertonia (0.2%), diplopia (0.1%);

Respiratory System: pneumonia (0.4%), rales (0.4%), pleural effusion (0.3%), bronchitis (0.3%) bronchospasm (0.3%), pleurisy (0.2%), pulmonary embolism (0.2%), rhonchi (0.1%);

Musculoskeletal System: myalgia (0.2%);

Urogenital System: urinary retention (0.7%), dysuria (0.4%), abnormal renal function (0.4%), frequent micturition (0.1%), cystalgia (0.1%), urinary incontinence (0.1%), prostatitis (0.1%);

Miscellaneous: pain (5.4%), sweating increased (1.0%), asthenia (0.7%), incisional pain (0.6%), pruritus (0.5%), abnormal vision (0.3%), edema (0.3%), wound (0.2%), abscess (0.2%), cellulitis (0.2%), peripheral coldness (0.2%), injection site pain (0.1%), dry mouth (0.1%), pallor (0.1%), diabetes mellitus (0.1%), hyperkalemia (0.1%), enlarged abdomen (0.1%), bullous eruption (0.1%), inflammation (0.1%), drug toxicity (0.1%).

Immunogenicity

As with all therapeutic proteins, there is a potential for immunogenicity. In the EPIC, EPILOG, and CAPTURE trials, positive HACA responses occurred in approximately 5.8% of these patients receiving a first exposure to Abciximab. No increase in hypersensitivity or allergic reactions was observed with Abciximab treatment.

In a study of readministration of Abciximab to patients (See Precautions: Readministration) the overall rate of HACA positivity prior to the readministration was 6% and increased post-readministration to 27%. Among the 36 subjects receiving a fourth or greater Abciximab exposure, HACA positive assays were observed post-readministration in 16 subjects (44%). There were no reports of serious allergic reactions or anaphylaxis. HACA positive status was associated with an increased risk of thrombocytopenia (See Precautions: Thrombocytopenia).

The data reflect the percentage of patients whose test results were considered positive for antibodies to Abciximab using an ELISA assay, and are highly dependent on the sensitivity and specificity of the assay. Additionally, the observed incidence of antibody positivity in an assay may be influenced by several factors including sample handling, timing of sample collection, concomitant medications, and underlying disease. For these reasons, comparison of the incidence of antibodies to Abciximab with the incidence of antibodies to other products may be misleading.

OVERDOSAGE

There has been no experience of overdosage in human clinical trials.

DOSAGE AND ADMINISTRATION

The safety and efficacy of Abciximab have only been investigated with concomitant administration of heparin and aspirin as described in CLINICAL STUDIES.

In patients with failed PCIs, the continuous infusion of Abciximab should be stopped because there is no evidence for Abciximab efficacy in that setting.

In the event of serious bleeding that cannot be controlled by compression, Abciximab and heparin should be discontinued immediately.

The recommended dosage of Abciximab in adults is a 0.25 mg/kg intravenous bolus administered 10-60 minutes before the start of PCI, followed by a continuous intravenous infusion of 0.125 μg/kg/min (to a maximum of 10 μg/min) for 12 hours.

Patients with unstable angina not responding to conventional medical therapy and who are planned to undergo PCI within 24 hours may be treated with an Abciximab 0.25 mg/kg intravenous bolus followed by an 18- to 24-hour intravenous infusion of 10 μg/min, concluding one hour after the PCI.

Instructions for Administration

1. Parenteral drug products should be inspected visually for particulate matter prior to administration. Preparations of Abciximab containing visibly opaque particles should NOT be used.

2. Hypersensitivity reactions should be anticipated whenever protein solutions such as Abciximab are administered. Epinephrine, dopamine, theophylline, antihistamines and corticosteroids should be available for immediate use. If symptoms of an allergic reaction or anaphylaxis appear, the infusion should be stopped and appropriate treatment given.

3. As with all parenteral drug products, aseptic procedures should be used during the administration of Abciximab.

4. Withdraw the necessary amount of Abciximab for bolus injection into a syringe. Filter the bolus injection using a sterile, non-pyrogenic, low protein-binding 0.2 or 5μm syringe filter (Millipore SLGV025LS or SLSV025LS or equivalent).

5. Withdraw the necessary amount of Abciximab for the continuous infusion into a syringe. Inject into an appropriate container of sterile 0.9% saline or 5% dextrose and infuse at the calculated rate via a continuous infusion pump. The continuous infusion should be filtered either upon admixture using a sterile, non-pyrogenic, low protein-binding 0.2 or 5 μm syringe filter (Millipore SLGV025LS or SLSV025LS or equivalent) or upon administration using an in-line, sterile, non-pyrogenic, low protein-binding 0.2 or 0.22 μm filter (Abbott #4524 or equivalent). Discard the unused portion at the end of the infusion.

6. No incompatibilities have been shown with intravenous infusion fluids or commonly used cardiovascular drugs. Nevertheless, Abciximab should be administered in a separate intravenous line whenever possible and not mixed with other medications.

7. No incompatibilities have been observed with glass bottles or polyvinyl chloride bags and administration sets.

HOW SUPPLIED

Abciximab (ReoPro®) 2 mg/mL is supplied in 5 mL vials containing 10 mg (NDC 0002-7140-01).

Vials should be stored at 2 to 8 °C (36 to 46 °F). Do not freeze. Do not shake. Do not use beyond the expiration date. Discard any unused portion left in the vial.

REFERENCES

1. Reverter JC, Beguin S, Kessels H, Kumar R, Hemmer HC, Coller BS. Inhibition of platelet-mediated, tissue-factor-induced thrombin generation by the mouse/human chimeric 7E3 antibody; potential implications for the effect of c7E3 Fab treatment on acute thrombosis and "clinical restenosis". *J Clin Invest.* 1996;**98**:863-874.
2. Alteri D, Edgington T, A monoclonal antibody reacting with distinct adhesion molecules defines a transition in the functional state of the receptor CD11b/CD18 (Mac-1). The Journal of Immunology. 1988;**141**:2656-2660.
3. Simon DI, Xu H, Ortlepp S, Rogers C, Rao NK. 7E3 monoclonal antibody directed against the platelet glycoprotein IIb/IIIa cross-reacts with the leukocyte integrin Mac-1 and blocks adhesion to fibrinogen and ICAM-1. Arterioscler Thromb Vasc Biol. 1997;**17**:528-535.
4. Mickelson JK, Ali MN, Kleiman NS, Lakkis NM, Chow TW, Hughes BJ. Chimeric 7E3 Fab (ReoPro) decreases detectable CD11b on neutrophils from patients undergoing coronary angioplasty. J Am Coll Cardiol. 1999;**33**:97-106.
5. Tcheng J, Ellis SG, George BS. Pharmacodynamics of chimeric glycoprotein IIb/IIIa integrin antiplatelet antibody Fab 7E3 in high risk coronary angioplasty. *Circulation.* 1994;**90**:1757-1764.
6. Simoons ML, de Boer MJ, van der Brand MJBM, et al. Randomized trial of a GPIIb/IIIa platelet receptor blocker in refractory unstable angina. *Circulation.* 1994;**89**:596-603.
7. EPIC Investigators. Use of a monoclonal antibody directed against the platelet glycoprotein IIb/IIIa receptor in high-risk coronary angioplasty. *N Engl J Med.* 1994;**330**:956-961.
8. Topol EJ, Califf RM, Weisman HF, et al. Randomised trial of coronary intervention with antibody against platelet IIb/IIIa integrin for reduction of clinical restenosis: results at six months. *Lancet.* 1994;**343**:881-886.
9. Topol EJ, Ferguson JJ, Weisman HF, et al. for the EPIC Investigators. Long-term protection from myocardial ischemic events in a randomized trial of brief integrin blockade with percutaneous coronary intervention. *JAMA.*1997;**278**:479-484.
10. EPILOG Investigators. Platelet glycoprotein IIb/IIIa receptor blockade and low dose heparin during percutaneous coronary revascularization. *N Eng J Med.* 1997;**336**:1689-1696.
11. Lincoff AM, Tcheng JE, Califf RM, et al. for the EPILOG Investigators. Sustained suppression of ischemic complications of coronary intervention by platelet GP IIb/IIIa blockade with abciximab. *Circ.* 1999;**99**:1951-1958.
12. EPISTENT Investigators. Randomised placebo-controlled and balloon angioplasty-controlled trial to assess safety of coronary stenting with use of platelet glycoprotein-IIb/IIIa blockade. *Lancet.* 1998;**352**:87-92.
13. Lincoff AM, Califf RM, Moliterno DJ, et al. for the EPI STENT Investigator. Complementary clinical benefits of coronary stenting and blockade of platelet glycoprotein IIb/IIIa receptors. *N Engl J Med* 1999;**341**:319-327.
14. CAPTURE Investigators. Randomised placebo-controlled trial of abciximab before, during and after coronary intervention in refractory unstable angina: the CAPTURE study. *Lancet.* 1997;**349**:1429-1435.
15. Data on file.
16. Rao, AK, Pratt C, Berke A, et al. Thrombolysis in Myocardial Infarction (TIMI) Trial - Phase I: Hemorrhagic manifestations and changes in plasma fibrinogen and the fibrinolytic system in patients treated with recombinant tissue plasminogen activator and streptokinase. *J Am Coll Cardiol.* 1988;**11**:1-11.
17. Landefeld, CS, Cook EF, Flatley M, et al. Identification and preliminary validation of predictors of major bleeding in hospitalized patients starting anticoagulant therapy. *Am J Med.* 1987;**82**:703-713.

Manufactured by:
Centocor B.V.
Leiden, The Netherlands
U.S. License Number: 1178

Distributed by:
Eli Lilly and Company
Indianapolis, IN 46285

Revision Date: November 21, 2003

Shown in Product Identification Guide, page 320

SEROMYCIN® ℞

CYCLOSERINE CAPSULES, USP

DESCRIPTION

Seromycin® (Cycloserine Capsules, USP), 3-isoxazolidinone, 4-amino-, (R)- is a broad- spectrum antibiotic that is produced by a strain of *Streptomyces orchidaceus* and has also been synthesized. Cycloserine is a white to off-white powder that is soluble in water and stable in alkaline solution. It is rapidly destroyed at a neutral or acid pH.

Cycloserine has a pH between 5.5 and 6.5 in a solution containing 100 mg/mL. The molecular weight of cycloserine is 102.09, and it has an empirical formula of $C_3H_6N_2O_2$. The structural formula of cycloserine is as follows:

Each capsule contains cycloserine, 250 mg (2.45 mmol); D & C Yellow No. 10, F D & C Blue No. 1, F D & C Red No. 3, F D & C Yellow No. 6, gelatin, iron oxide, talc, titanium dioxide, and other inactive ingredients.

CLINICAL PHARMACOLOGY

After oral administration, cycloserine is readily absorbed from the gastrointestinal tract, with peak blood levels occurring in 4 to 8 hours. Blood levels of 25 to 30 μg/mL can generally be maintained with the usual dosage of 250 mg twice a day, although the relationship of plasma levels to dosage is not always consistent. Concentrations in the cerebrospinal fluid, pleural fluid, fetal blood, and mother's milk approach those found in the serum. Detectable amounts are found in ascitic fluid, bile, sputum, amniotic fluid, and lung and lymph tissues. Approximately 65% of a single dose of cycloserine can be recovered in the urine within 72 hours after oral administration. The remaining 35% is apparently metabolized to unknown substances. The maximum excretion rate occurs 2 to 6 hours after administration, with 50% of the drug eliminated in 12 hours.

Microbiology

Cycloserine inhibits cell-wall synthesis in susceptible strains of gram-positive and gram-negative bacteria and in *Mycobacterium tuberculosis*.

Susceptibility Tests

Cycloserine clinical laboratory standard powder is available for both direct and indirect methods[1] of determining the susceptibility of strains of mycobacteria. Cycloserine MICs for susceptible strains are 25 μg/mL or lower.

INDICATIONS AND USAGE

Seromycin is indicated in the treatment of active pulmonary and extrapulmonary tuberculosis (including renal disease) when the causative organisms are susceptible to this drug and when treatment with the primary medications (streptomycin, isoniazid, rifampin, and ethambutol) has proved inadequate. Like all antituberculosis drugs, Seromycin should be administered in conjunction with other effective chemotherapy and not as the sole therapeutic agent.

Seromycin may be effective in the treatment of acute urinary tract infections caused by susceptible strains of gram-positive and gram-negative bacteria, especially *Enterobacter* spp. and *Escherichia coli*. It is generally no more and is usually less effective than other antimicrobial agents in the treatment of urinary tract infections caused by bacteria other than mycobacteria. Use of Seromycin in these infections should be considered only when more conventional therapy has failed and when the organism has been demonstrated to be susceptible to the drug.

CONTRAINDICATIONS

Administration is contraindicated in patients with any of the following:

- Hypersensitivity to cycloserine
- Epilepsy
- Depression, severe anxiety, or psychosis
- Severe renal insufficiency
- Excessive concurrent use of alcohol

WARNINGS

Administration of Seromycin should be discontinued or the dosage reduced if the patient develops allergic dermatitis or symptoms of CNS toxicity, such as convulsions, psychosis, somnolence, depression, confusion, hyperreflexia, headache, tremor, vertigo, paresis, or dysarthria.

The toxicity of Seromycin is closely related to excessive blood levels (above 30 μg/mL), as determined by high dosage or inadequate renal clearance. The ratio of toxic dose to effective dose in tuberculosis is small.

The risk of convulsions is increased in chronic alcoholics.

Patients should be monitored by hematologic, renal excretion, blood level, and liver function studies.

PRECAUTIONS

General

Before treatment with Seromycin is initiated, cultures should be taken and the organism's susceptibility to the drug should be established. In tuberculous infections, the organism's susceptibility to the other antituberculosis agents in the regimen should also be demonstrated.

Anticonvulsant drugs or sedatives may be effective in controlling symptoms of CNS toxicity, such as convulsions, anxiety, and tremor. Patients receiving more than 500 mg of Seromycin daily should be closely observed for such symptoms. The value of pyridoxine in preventing CNS toxicity from Seromycin has not been proved.

Administration of Seromycin and other antituberculosis drugs has been associated in a few instances with vitamin B_{12} and/or folic-acid deficiency, megaloblastic anemia, and sideroblastic anemia. If evidence of anemia develops during treatment, appropriate studies and therapy should be instituted.

Laboratory Tests

Blood levels should be determined at least weekly for patients with reduced renal function, for individuals receiving a daily dosage of more than 500 mg, and for those showing

Continued on next page

*** Identi-Code® symbol. This product information was prepared in June 2004. Current information on these and other products of Eli Lilly and Company may be obtained by direct inquiry to Lilly Research Laboratories, Lilly Corporate Center, Indianapolis, Indiana 46285, (800) 545-5979.**

Seromycin—Cont.

signs and symptoms suggestive of toxicity. The dosage should be adjusted to keep the blood level below 30 µg/mL.

Drug Interactions

Concurrent administration of ethionamide has been reported to potentiate neurotoxic side effects.

Alcohol and Seromycin are incompatible, especially during a regimen calling for large doses of the latter. Alcohol increases the possibility and risk of epileptic episodes.

Concurrent administration of isoniazid may result in increased incidence of CNS effects, such as dizziness or drowsiness. Dosage adjustments may be necessary and patients should be monitored closely for signs of CNS toxicity.

Carcinogenesis, Mutagenicity, and Impairment of Fertility

Studies have not been performed to determine potential for carcinogenicity. The Ames test and unscheduled DNA repair test were negative. A study in 2 generations of rats showed no impairment of fertility relative to controls for the first mating but somewhat lower fertility in the second mating.

Pregnancy Category C

A study in 2 generations of rats given doses up to 100 mg/kg/day demonstrated no teratogenic effect in offspring. It is not known whether Seromycin can cause fetal harm when administered to a pregnant woman or can affect reproduction capacity. Seromycin should be given to a pregnant woman only if clearly needed.

Nursing Mothers

Because of the potential for serious adverse reactions in nursing infants from Seromycin, a decision should be made whether to discontinue nursing or to discontinue the drug, taking into account the importance of the drug to the mother.

Usage in Pediatric Patients

Safety and effectiveness in pediatric patients have not been established.

ADVERSE REACTIONS

Most adverse reactions occurring during therapy with Seromycin involve the nervous system or are manifestations of drug hypersensitivity. The following side effects have been observed in patients receiving Seromycin:

Nervous system symptoms (which appear to be related to higher dosages of the drug, i.e., more than 500 mg daily)

- Convulsions
- Drowsiness and somnolence
- Headache
- Tremor
- Dysarthria
- Vertigo
- Confusion and disorientation with loss of memory
- Psychoses, possibly with suicidal tendencies
- Character changes
- Hyperirritability
- Aggression
- Paresis
- Hyperreflexia
- Paresthesia
- Major and minor (localized) clonic seizures
- Coma

Cardiovascular

Sudden development of congestive heart failure in patients receiving 1 to 1.5 g of Seromycin daily has been reported

Allergy (apparently not related to dosage)

Skin rash

Miscellaneous

Elevated serum transaminase, especially in patients with preexisting liver disease

OVERDOSAGE

Signs and Symptoms

Acute toxicity from cycloserine can occur if more than 1 g is ingested by an adult. Chronic toxicity from cycloserine is dose related and can occur if more than 500 mg is administered daily. Patients with renal impairment will accumulate cycloserine and may develop toxicity if the dosing regimen is not modified. Patients with severe renal impairment should not receive the drug. The central nervous system is the most common organ system involved with toxicity. Toxic effects may include headache, vertigo, confusion, drowsiness, hyperirritability, paresthesias, dysarthria, and psychosis. Following larger ingestions, paresis, convulsions, and coma often occur. Ethyl alcohol may increase the risk of seizures in patients receiving cycloserine.

The oral median lethal dose in mice is 5290 mg/kg.

Treatment

To obtain up-to-date information about the treatment of overdose, a good resource is your certified Regional Poison Control Center. Telephone numbers of certified poison control centers are listed in the *Physicians' Desk Reference (PDR)*. In managing overdosage, consider the possibility of multiple drug overdoses, interaction among drugs, and unusual drug kinetics in your patient.

Overdoses of cycloserine have been reported rarely. The following is provided to serve as a guide should such an overdose be encountered.

Protect the patient's airway and support ventilation and perfusion. Meticulously monitor and maintain, within acceptable limits, the patient's vital signs, blood gases, serum electrolytes, etc. Absorption of drugs from the gastrointestinal tract may be decreased by giving activated charcoal, which, in many cases, is more effective than emesis or lavage; consider charcoal instead of or in addition to gastric emptying. Repeated doses of charcoal over time may hasten elimination of some drugs that have been absorbed. Safeguard the patient's airway when employing gastric emptying or charcoal.

In adults, many of the neurotoxic effects of cycloserine can be both treated and prevented with the administration of 200 to 300 mg of pyridoxine daily.

The use of hemodialysis has been shown to remove cycloserine from the bloodstream. This procedure should be reserved for patients with life-threatening toxicity that is unresponsive to less invasive therapy.

DOSAGE AND ADMINISTRATION

Seromycin is effective orally and is currently administered only by this route. The usual dosage is 500 mg to 1 g daily in divided doses monitored by blood levels.[2] The initial adult dosage most frequently given is 250 mg twice daily at 12-hour intervals for the first 2 weeks. A daily dosage of 1 g should not be exceeded.

HOW SUPPLIED

Seromycin® is available as a 250 mg capsule with an opaque red cap and opaque gray body imprinted with "PU0012"and "F04" in edible black ink on both the cap and the body.

Bottles of 40 (No.12) NDC 0002-0604-40

Store at controlled room temperature, 20 ° to 25°C (68° to 77°F) [see USP].

REFERENCES

1. Kubica GP, Dye WE: Laboratory methods for clinical and public health — mycobacteriology. US Department of Health, Education and Welfare, Public Health Service, 1967, pp 47–55, 66–70.
2. Jones LR: Colorimetric determination of cycloserine, a new antibiotic. Anal Chem 1956;28:39.

Literature revised December 8, 2003

Eli Lilly and Company
Indianapolis, IN 46285, USA
PV 4810 AMP PRINTED IN USA

STRATTERA® ℞

[*stră-tĕr-ă*]

(atomoxetine HCl)

DESCRIPTION

STRATTERA® (atomoxetine HCl) is a selective norepinephrine reuptake inhibitor. Atomoxetine HCl is the *R*(-) isomer as determined by x-ray diffraction. The chemical designation is (-)-*N*-Methyl-3-phenyl-3-(*o*-tolyloxy)-propylamine hydrochloride. The molecular formula is $C_{17}H_{21}NO{\bullet}HCl$, which corresponds to a molecular weight of 291.82. The chemical structure is:

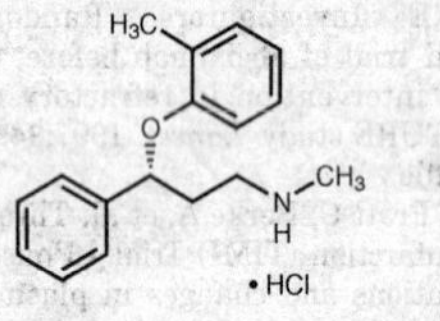

Atomoxetine HCl is a white to practically white solid, which has a solubility of 27.8 mg/mL in water.

STRATTERA capsules are intended for oral administration only.

Each capsule contains atomoxetine HCl equivalent to 10, 18, 25, 40, or 60 mg of atomoxetine. The capsules also contain pregelatinized starch and dimethicone. The capsule shells contain gelatin, sodium lauryl sulfate, and other inactive ingredients. The capsule shells also contain one or more of the following: FD&C Blue No. 2, synthetic yellow iron oxide, titanium dioxide. The capsules are imprinted with edible black ink.

CLINICAL PHARMACOLOGY

Pharmacodynamics and Mechanism of Action

The precise mechanism by which atomoxetine produces its therapeutic effects in Attention-Deficit/Hyperactivity Disorder (ADHD) is unknown, but is thought to be related to selective inhibition of the pre-synaptic norepinephrine transporter, as determined in ex vivo uptake and neurotransmitter depletion studies.

Human Pharmacokinetics

Atomoxetine is well-absorbed after oral administration and is minimally affected by food. It is eliminated primarily by oxidative metabolism through the cytochrome P450 2D6 (CYP2D6) enzymatic pathway and subsequent glucuronidation. Atomoxetine has a half-life of about 5 hours. A fraction of the population (about 7% of Caucasians and 2% of African Americans) are poor metabolizers (PMs) of CYP2D6 metabolized drugs. These individuals have reduced activity in this pathway resulting in 10-fold higher AUCs, 5-fold higher peak plasma concentrations, and slower elimination (plasma half-life of about 24 hours) of atomoxetine compared with people with normal activity [extensive metabolizers (EMs)]. Drugs that inhibit CYP2D6, such as fluoxetine, paroxetine, and quinidine, cause similar increases in exposure.

The pharmacokinetics of atomoxetine have been evaluated in more than 400 children and adolescents in selected clinical trials, primarily using population pharmacokinetic studies. Single-dose and steady-state individual pharmacokinetic data were also obtained in children, adolescents, and adults. When doses were normalized to a mg/kg basis, similar half-life, C_{max}, and AUC values were observed in children, adolescents, and adults. Clearance and volume of distribution after adjustment for body weight were also similar.

<u>Absorption and distribution</u> — Atomoxetine is rapidly absorbed after oral administration, with absolute bioavailability of about 63% in EMs and 94% in PMs. Maximal plasma concentrations (C_{max}) are reached approximately 1 to 2 hours after dosing.

STRATTERA can be administered with or without food. Administration of STRATTERA with a standard high-fat meal in adults did not affect the extent of oral absorption of atomoxetine (AUC), but did decrease the rate of absorption, resulting in a 37% lower C_{max}, and delayed T_{max} by 3 hours. In clinical trials with children and adolescents, administration of STRATTERA with food resulted in a 9% lower C_{max}.

The steady-state volume of distribution after intravenous administration is 0.85 L/kg indicating that atomoxetine distributes primarily into total body water. Volume of distribution is similar across the patient weight range after normalizing for body weight.

At therapeutic concentrations, 98% of atomoxetine in plasma is bound to protein, primarily albumin.

<u>Metabolism and elimination</u> — Atomoxetine is metabolized primarily through the CYP2D6 enzymatic pathway. People with reduced activity in this pathway (PMs) have higher plasma concentrations of atomoxetine compared with people with normal activity (EMs). For PMs, AUC of atomoxetine is approximately 10-fold and $C_{ss,max}$ is about 5-fold greater than EMs. Laboratory tests are available to identify CYP2D6 PMs. Coadministration of STRATTERA with potent inhibitors of CYP2D6, such as fluoxetine, paroxetine, or quinidine, results in a substantial increase in atomoxetine plasma exposure, and dosing adjustment may be necessary (*see* Drug-Drug Interactions). Atomoxetine did not inhibit or induce the CYP2D6 pathway.

The major oxidative metabolite formed, regardless of CYP2D6 status, is 4-hydroxyatomoxetine, which is glucuronidated. 4-Hydroxyatomoxetine is equipotent to atomoxetine as an inhibitor of the norepinephrine transporter but circulates in plasma at much lower concentrations (1% of atomoxetine concentration in EMs and 0.1% of atomoxetine concentration in PMs). 4-Hydroxyatomoxetine is primarily formed by CYP2D6, but in PMs, 4-hydroxyatomoxetine is formed at a slower rate by several other cytochrome P450 enzymes. N-Desmethylatomoxetine is formed by CYP2C19 and other cytochrome P450 enzymes, but has substantially less pharmacological activity compared with atomoxetine and circulates in plasma at lower concentrations (5% of atomoxetine concentration in EMs and 45% of atomoxetine concentration in PMs).

Mean apparent plasma clearance of atomoxetine after oral administration in adult EMs is 0.35 L/hr/kg and the mean half-life is 5.2 hours. Following oral administration of atomoxetine to PMs, mean apparent plasma clearance is 0.03 L/hr/kg and mean half-life is 21.6 hours. For PMs, AUC of atomoxetine is approximately 10-fold and $C_{ss,max}$ is about 5-fold greater than EMs. The elimination half-life of 4-hydroxyatomoxetine is similar to that of N-desmethylatomoxetine (6 to 8 hours) in EM subjects, while the half-life of N-desmethylatomoxetine is much longer in PM subjects (34 to 40 hours).

Atomoxetine is excreted primarily as 4-hydroxyatomoxetine-*O*-glucuronide, mainly in the urine (greater than 80% of the dose) and to a lesser extent in the feces (less than 17% of the dose). Only a small fraction of the STRATTERA dose is excreted as unchanged atomoxetine (less than 3% of the dose), indicating extensive biotransformation.

Special Populations

<u>Hepatic insufficiency</u> — Atomoxetine exposure (AUC) is increased, compared with normal subjects, in EM subjects with moderate (Child-Pugh Class B) (2-fold increase) and severe (Child-Pugh Class C) (4-fold increase) hepatic insufficiency. Dosage adjustment is recommended for patients with moderate or severe hepatic insufficiency (*see* DOSAGE AND ADMINISTRATION).

<u>Renal insufficiency</u> — EM subjects with end stage renal disease had higher systemic exposure to atomoxetine than healthy subjects (about a 65% increase), but there was no difference when exposure was corrected for mg/kg dose. STRATTERA can therefore be administered to ADHD patients with end stage renal disease or lesser degrees of renal insufficiency using the normal dosing regimen.

<u>Geriatric</u> — The pharmacokinetics of atomoxetine have not been evaluated in the geriatric population.

<u>Pediatric</u> — The pharmacokinetics of atomoxetine in children and adolescents are similar to those in adults. The pharmacokinetics of atomoxetine have not been evaluated in children under 6 years of age.

<u>Gender</u> — Gender did not influence atomoxetine disposition.

<u>Ethnic origin</u> — Ethnic origin did not influence atomoxetine disposition (except that PMs are more common in Caucasians).

Drug-Drug Interactions

<u>CYP2D6 activity and atomoxetine plasma concentration</u> — Atomoxetine is primarily metabolized by the CYP2D6 pathway to 4-hydroxyatomoxetine. In EMs, inhibitors of CYP2D6 increase atomoxetine steady-state plasma concentrations to exposures similar to those observed in PMs. Dosage adjustment of STRATTERA in EMs may be necessary when coadministered with CYP2D6 inhibitors, e.g., parox-

etine, fluoxetine, and quinidine (*see* Drug-Drug Interactions *under* PRECAUTIONS). In vitro studies suggest that coadministration of cytochrome P450 inhibitors to PMs will not increase the plasma concentrations of atomoxetine.

Effect of atomoxetine on P450 enzymes — Atomoxetine did not cause clinically important inhibition or induction of cytochrome P450 enzymes, including CYP1A2, CYP3A, CYP2D6, and CYP2C9.

Albuterol — Albuterol (600 mcg iv over 2 hours) induced increases in heart rate and blood pressure. These effects were potentiated by atomoxetine (60 mg BID for 5 days) and were most marked after the initial coadministration of albuterol and atomoxetine (*see* Drug-Drug Interactions *under* PRECAUTIONS).

Alcohol — Consumption of ethanol with STRATTERA did not change the intoxicating effects of ethanol.

Desipramine — Coadministration of STRATTERA (40 or 60 mg BID for 13 days) with desipramine, a model compound for CYP2D6 metabolized drugs (single dose of 50 mg), did not alter the pharmacokinetics of desipramine. No dose adjustment is recommended for drugs metabolized by CYP2D6.

Methylphenidate — Coadministration of methylphenidate with STRATTERA did not increase cardiovascular effects beyond those seen with methylphenidate alone.

Midazolam — Coadministration of STRATTERA (60 mg BID for 12 days) with midazolam, a model compound for CYP3A4 metabolized drugs (single dose of 5 mg), resulted in 15% increase in AUC of midazolam. No dose adjustment is recommended for drugs metabolized by CYP3A.

Drugs highly bound to plasma protein — In vitro drug-displacement studies were conducted with atomoxetine and other highly-bound drugs at therapeutic concentrations. Atomoxetine did not affect the binding of warfarin, acetylsalicylic acid, phenytoin, or diazepam to human albumin. Similarly, these compounds did not affect the binding of atomoxetine to human albumin.

Drugs that affect gastric pH — Drugs that elevate gastric pH (magnesium hydroxide/aluminum hydroxide, omeprazole) had no effect on STRATTERA bioavailability.

CLINICAL STUDIES

The effectiveness of STRATTERA in the treatment of ADHD was established in 6 randomized, double-blind, placebo-controlled studies in children, adolescents, and adults who met Diagnostic and Statistical Manual 4th edition (DSM-IV) criteria for ADHD (*see* INDICATIONS AND USAGE).

Children and Adolescents

The effectiveness of STRATTERA in the treatment of ADHD was established in 4 randomized, double-blind, placebo-controlled studies of pediatric patients (ages 6 to 18). Approximately one-third of the patients met DSM-IV criteria for inattentive subtype and two-thirds met criteria for both inattentive and hyperactive/impulsive subtypes (*see* INDICATIONS AND USAGE).

Signs and symptoms of ADHD were evaluated by a comparison of mean change from baseline to endpoint for STRATTERA- and placebo-treated patients using an intent-to-treat analysis of the primary outcome measure, the investigator administered and scored ADHD Rating Scale-IV-Parent Version (ADHDRS) total score including hyperactive/impulsive and inattentive subscales. Each item on the ADHDRS maps directly to one symptom criterion for ADHD in the DSM-IV.

In Study 1, an 8-week randomized, double-blind, placebo-controlled, dose-response, acute treatment study of children and adolescents aged 8 to 18 (N=297), patients received either a fixed dose of STRATTERA (0.5, 1.2, or 1.8 mg/kg/day) or placebo. STRATTERA was administered as a divided dose in the early morning and late afternoon/early evening. At the 2 higher doses, improvements in ADHD symptoms were statistically significantly superior in STRATTERA-treated patients compared with placebo-treated patients as measured on the ADHDRS scale. The 1.8-mg/kg/day STRATTERA dose did not provide any additional benefit over that observed with the 1.2-mg/kg/day dose. The 0.5-mg/kg/day STRATTERA dose was not superior to placebo.

In Study 2, a 6-week randomized, double-blind, placebo-controlled, acute treatment study of children and adolescents aged 6 to 16 (N=171), patients received either STRATTERA or placebo. STRATTERA was administered as a single dose in the early morning and titrated on a weight-adjusted basis according to clinical response, up to a maximum dose of 1.5 mg/kg/day. The mean final dose of STRATTERA was approximately 1.3 mg/kg/day. ADHD symptoms were statistically significantly improved on STRATTERA compared with placebo, as measured on the ADHDRS scale. This study shows that STRATTERA is effective when administered once daily in the morning.

In 2 identical, 9-week, acute, randomized, double-blind, placebo-controlled studies of children aged 7 to 13 (Study 3, N=147; Study 4, N=144), STRATTERA and methylphenidate were compared with placebo. STRATTERA was administered as a divided dose in the early morning and late afternoon (after school) and titrated on a weight-adjusted basis according to clinical response. The maximum recommended STRATTERA dose was 2.0 mg/kg/day. The mean final dose of STRATTERA for both studies was approximately 1.6 mg/kg/day. In both studies, ADHD symptoms statistically significantly improved more on STRATTERA than on placebo, as measured on the ADHDRS scale.

Examination of population subsets based on gender and age (<12 and 12 to 17) did not reveal any differential responsiveness on the basis of these subgroupings. There was not sufficient exposure of ethnic groups other than Caucasian to allow exploration of differences in these subgroups.

Adults

The effectiveness of STRATTERA in the treatment of ADHD was established in 2 randomized, double-blind, placebo-controlled clinical studies of adult patients, age 18 and older, who met DSM-IV criteria for ADHD.

Signs and symptoms of ADHD were evaluated using the investigator-administered Conners Adult ADHD Rating Scale Screening Version (CAARS), a 30-item scale. The primary effectiveness measure was the 18-item Total ADHD Symptom score (the sum of the inattentive and hyperactivity/impulsivity subscales from the CAARS) evaluated by a comparison of mean change from baseline to endpoint using an intent-to-treat analysis.

In 2 identical, 10-week, randomized, double-blind, placebo-controlled acute treatment studies (Study 5, N=280; Study 6, N=256), patients received either STRATTERA or placebo. STRATTERA was administered as a divided dose in the early morning and late afternoon/early evening and titrated according to clinical response in a range of 60 to 120 mg/day. The mean final dose of STRATTERA for both studies was approximately 95 mg/day. In both studies, ADHD symptoms were statistically significantly improved on STRATTERA, as measured on the ADHD Symptom score from the CAARS scale.

Examination of population subsets based on gender and age (<42 and ≥42) did not reveal any differential responsiveness on the basis of these subgroupings. There was not sufficient exposure of ethnic groups other than Caucasian to allow exploration of differences in these subgroups.

INDICATIONS AND USAGE

STRATTERA is indicated for the treatment of Attention-Deficit/Hyperactivity Disorder (ADHD).

The effectiveness of STRATTERA in the treatment of ADHD was established in 2 placebo-controlled trials in children, 2 placebo-controlled trials in children and adolescents, and 2 placebo-controlled trials in adults who met DSM-IV criteria for ADHD (*see* CLINICAL STUDIES).

A diagnosis of ADHD (DSM-IV) implies the presence of hyperactive-impulsive or inattentive symptoms that cause impairment and that were present before age 7 years. The symptoms must be persistent, must be more severe than is typically observed in individuals at a comparable level of development, must cause clinically significant impairment, e.g., in social, academic, or occupational functioning, and must be present in 2 or more settings, e.g., school (or work) and at home. The symptoms must not be better accounted for by another mental disorder. For the Inattentive Type, at least 6 of the following symptoms must have persisted for at least 6 months: lack of attention to details/careless mistakes, lack of sustained attention, poor listener, failure to follow through on tasks, poor organization, avoids tasks requiring sustained mental effort, loses things, easily distracted, forgetful. For the Hyperactive-Impulsive Type, at least 6 of the following symptoms must have persisted for at least 6 months: fidgeting/squirming, leaving seat, inappropriate running/climbing, difficulty with quiet activities, "on the go," excessive talking, blurting answers, can't wait turn, intrusive. For a Combined Type diagnosis, both inattentive and hyperactive-impulsive criteria must be met.

Special Diagnostic Considerations

The specific etiology of ADHD is unknown, and there is no single diagnostic test. Adequate diagnosis requires the use not only of medical but also of special psychological, educational, and social resources. Learning may or may not be impaired. The diagnosis must be based upon a complete history and evaluation of the patient and not solely on the presence of the required number of DSM-IV characteristics.

Need for Comprehensive Treatment Program

STRATTERA is indicated as an integral part of a total treatment program for ADHD that may include other measures (psychological, educational, social) for patients with this syndrome. Drug treatment may not be indicated for all patients with this syndrome. Drug treatment is not intended for use in the patient who exhibits symptoms secondary to environmental factors and/or other primary psychiatric disorders, including psychosis. Appropriate educational placement is essential in children and adolescents with this diagnosis and psychosocial intervention is often helpful. When remedial measures alone are insufficient, the decision to prescribe drug treatment medication will depend upon the physician's assessment of the chronicity and severity of the patient's symptoms.

Long-Term Use

The effectiveness of STRATTERA for long-term use, ie, for more than 9 weeks in child and adolescent patients and 10 weeks in adult patients, has not been systematically evaluated in controlled trials. Therefore, the physician who elects to use STRATTERA for extended periods should periodically reevaluate the long-term usefulness of the drug for the individual patient (*see* DOSAGE AND ADMINISTRATION).

CONTRAINDICATIONS

Hypersensitivity

STRATTERA is contraindicated in patients known to be hypersensitive to atomoxetine or other constituents of the product (*see* WARNINGS).

Monoamine Oxidase Inhibitors (MAOI)

STRATTERA should not be taken with an MAOI, or within 2 weeks after discontinuing an MAOI. Treatment with an MAOI should not be initiated within 2 weeks after discontinuing STRATTERA. With other drugs that affect brain monoamine concentrations, there have been reports of serious, sometimes fatal reactions (including hyperthermia, rigidity, myoclonus, autonomic instability with possible rapid fluctuations of vital signs, and mental status changes that include extreme agitation progressing to delirium and coma) when taken in combination with an MAOI. Some cases presented with features resembling neuroleptic malignant syndrome. Such reactions may occur when these drugs are given concurrently or in close proximity.

Narrow Angle Glaucoma

In clinical trials, STRATTERA use was associated with an increased risk of mydriasis and therefore its use is not recommended in patients with narrow angle glaucoma.

WARNINGS

Allergic Events

Although uncommon, allergic reactions, including angioneurotic edema, urticaria, and rash, have been reported in patients taking STRATTERA.

Growth

Growth should be monitored during treatment with STRATTERA. During acute treatment studies (up to 9 weeks), STRATTERA-treated patients lost an average of 0.4 kg, while placebo patients gained an average of 1.5 kg. In a controlled trial that randomized patients to placebo or 1 of 3 atomoxetine doses, 1.3%, 7.1%, 19.3%, and 29.1% of patients lost at least 3.5% of their body weight in the placebo, 0.5, 1.2, and 1.8 mg/kg/day STRATTERA dose groups, respectively. During acute treatment studies, STRATTERA-treated patients grew an average of 0.9 cm, while placebo-treated patients grew an average of 1.1 cm. There are no long-term, placebo-controlled data to evaluate the effect of STRATTERA on growth. Weight and height were assessed during open-label studies of 12 and 18 months, and mean rates of growth were compared with normal growth curves. Patients treated with STRATTERA for at least 18 months gained an average of 6.5 kg while mean weight percentile decreased slightly from 68 to 60. For this same group of patients, the average gain in height was 9.3 cm with a slight decrease in mean height percentile from 54 to 50. Among patients treated for at least 6 months, mean weight gain was lower for poor metabolizer (PM) patients compared with extensive metabolizer (EM) patients (+0.7 kg compared with +3.0 kg), while mean growth for PM patients was 4.3 cm and mean growth for EM patients was 4.4 cm. Whether final adult height or weight is affected by treatment with STRATTERA is unknown. Patients requiring long-term therapy should be monitored and consideration should be given to interrupting therapy in patients who are not growing or gaining weight satisfactorily.

PRECAUTIONS

General

Effects on blood pressure and heart rate — STRATTERA should be used with caution in patients with hypertension, tachycardia, or cardiovascular or cerebrovascular disease because it can increase blood pressure and heart rate. Pulse and blood pressure should be measured at baseline, following STRATTERA dose increases, and periodically while on therapy.

In pediatric placebo-controlled trials, STRATTERA-treated subjects experienced a mean increase in heart rate of about 6 beats/minute compared with placebo subjects. At the final study visit before drug discontinuation, 3.6% (12/335) of STRATTERA-treated subjects had heart rate increases of at least 25 beats/minute and a heart rate of at least 110 beats/minute, compared with 0.5% (1/204) of placebo subjects. No pediatric subject had a heart rate increase of at least 25 beats/minute and a heart rate of at least 110 beats/minute on more than one occasion. Tachycardia was identified as an adverse event for 1.5% (5/340) of these pediatric subjects compared with 0.5% (1/207) of placebo subjects. The mean heart rate increase in extensive metabolizer (EM) patients was 6.7 beats/minute, and in poor metabolizer (PM) patients 10.4 beats/minute.

STRATTERA-treated pediatric subjects experienced mean increases of about 1.5 mm Hg in systolic and diastolic blood pressures compared with placebo. At the final study visit before drug discontinuation, 6.8% (22/324) of STRATTERA-treated pediatric subjects had high systolic blood pressure measurements compared with 3.0% (6/197) of placebo subjects. High systolic blood pressures were measured on 2 or more occasions in 8.6% (28/324) of STRATTERA-treated subjects and 3.6% (7/197) of placebo subjects. At the final study visit before drug discontinuation, 2.8% (9/326) of STRATTERA-treated pediatric subjects had high diastolic blood pressure measurements compared with 0.5% (1/200) of placebo subjects. High diastolic blood pressures were measured on 2 or more occasions in 5.2% (17/326) of STRATTERA-treated subjects and 1.5% (3/200) of placebo subjects. (High systolic and diastolic blood pressure measurements were defined as those exceeding the 95th percentile, stratified by age, gender, and height percentile - National High Blood Pressure Education Working Group on Hypertension Control in Children and Adolescents.)

Continued on next page

*** Identi-Code® symbol. This product information was prepared in June 2004. Current information on these and other products of Eli Lilly and Company may be obtained by direct inquiry to Lilly Research Laboratories, Lilly Corporate Center, Indianapolis, Indiana 46285, (800) 545-5979.**

Strattera—Cont.

In adult placebo-controlled trials, STRATTERA-treated subjects experienced a mean increase in heart rate of 5 beats/minute compared with placebo subjects. Tachycardia was identified as an adverse event for 3% (8/269) of these adult atomoxetine subjects compared with 0.8% (2/263) of placebo subjects.

STRATTERA-treated adult subjects experienced mean increases in systolic (about 3 mm Hg) and diastolic (about 1 mm Hg) blood pressures compared with placebo. At the final study visit before drug discontinuation, 1.9% (5/258) of STRATTERA-treated adult subjects had systolic blood pressure measurements ≥150 mm Hg compared with 1.2% (3/256) of placebo subjects. At the final study visit before drug discontinuation, 0.8% (2/257) of STRATTERA-treated adult subjects had diastolic blood pressure measurements ≥100 mm Hg compared with 0.4% (1/257) of placebo subjects. No adult subject had a high systolic or diastolic blood pressure detected on more than one occasion.

Orthostatic hypotension has been reported in subjects taking STRATTERA. In short-term, child- and adolescent-controlled trials, 1.8% (6/340) of STRATTERA-treated subjects experienced symptoms of postural hypotension compared with 0.5% (1/207) of placebo-treated subjects. STRATTERA should be used with caution in any condition that may predispose patients to hypotension.

Effects on urine outflow from the bladder — In adult ADHD controlled trials, the rates of urinary retention (3%, 7/269) and urinary hesitation (3%, 7/269) were increased among atomoxetine subjects compared with placebo subjects (0%, 0/263). Two adult atomoxetine subjects and no placebo subjects discontinued from controlled clinical trials because of urinary retention. A complaint of urinary retention or urinary hesitancy should be considered potentially related to atomoxetine.

Information for Patients

Patients should read *Information for Patients* before starting therapy with STRATTERA and when the prescription is renewed.

Patients should consult a physician if they are taking or plan to take any prescription or over-the-counter medicines, dietary supplements, or herbal remedies.

Patients should consult a physician if they are nursing, pregnant, or thinking of becoming pregnant while taking STRATTERA.

Patients may take STRATTERA with or without food.

If patients miss a dose, they should take it as soon as possible, but should not take more than the prescribed total daily amount of STRATTERA in any 24-hour period.

Patients should use caution when driving a car or operating hazardous machinery until they are reasonably certain that their performance is not affected by atomoxetine.

Laboratory Tests

Routine laboratory tests are not required.

CYP2D6 metabolism — Poor metabolizers (PMs) of CYP2D6 have a 10-fold higher AUC and a 5-fold higher peak concentration to a given dose of STRATTERA compared with extensive metabolizers (EMs). Approximately 7% of a Caucasian population are PMs. Laboratory tests are available to identify CYP2D6 PMs. The blood levels in PMs are similar to those attained by taking strong inhibitors of CYP2D6. The higher blood levels in PMs lead to a higher rate of some adverse effects of STRATTERA (*see* ADVERSE REACTIONS).

Drug-Drug Interactions

Albuterol — STRATTERA should be administered with caution to patients being treated with systemically-administered (oral or intravenous) albuterol (or other $beta_2$ agonists) because the action of albuterol on the cardiovascular system can be potentiated.

CYP2D6 inhibitors — Atomoxetine is primarily metabolized by the CYP2D6 pathway to 4-hydroxyatomoxetine. In EMs, selective inhibitors of CYP2D6 increase atomoxetine steady-state plasma concentrations to exposures similar to those observed in PMs. Dosage adjustment of STRATTERA may be necessary when coadministered with CYP2D6 inhibitors, e.g., paroxetine, fluoxetine, and quinidine (*see* DOSAGE AND ADMINISTRATION). In EM individuals treated with paroxetine or fluoxetine, the AUC of atomoxetine is approximately 6- to 8-fold and $C_{ss,max}$ is about 3- to 4-fold greater than atomoxetine alone.

In vitro studies suggest that coadministration of cytochrome P450 inhibitors to PMs will not increase the plasma concentrations of atomoxetine.

Monoamine oxidase inhibitors — See CONTRAINDICATIONS.

Pressor agents — Because of possible effects on blood pressure, STRATTERA should be used cautiously with pressor agents.

Carcinogenesis, Mutagenesis, Impairment of Fertility

Carcinogenesis — Atomoxetine HCl was not carcinogenic in rats and mice when given in the diet for 2 years at time-weighted average doses up to 47 and 458 mg/kg/day, respectively. The highest dose used in rats is approximately 8 and 5 times the maximum human dose in children and adults, respectively, on a mg/m^2 basis. Plasma levels (AUC) of atomoxetine at this dose in rats are estimated to be 1.8 times (extensive metabolizers) or 0.2 times (poor metabolizers) those in humans receiving the maximum human dose. The highest dose used in mice is approximately 39 and 26 times the maximum human dose in children and adults, respectively, on a mg/m^2 basis.

Mutagenesis — Atomoxetine HCl was negative in a battery of genotoxicity studies that included a reverse point mutation assay (Ames Test), an in vitro mouse lymphoma assay, a chromosomal aberration test in Chinese hamster ovary cells, an unscheduled DNA synthesis test in rat hepatocytes, and an in vivo micronucleus test in mice. However, there was a slight increase in the percentage of Chinese hamster ovary cells with diplochromosomes, suggesting endoreduplication (numerical aberration).

The metabolite N-desmethylatomoxetine HCl was negative in the Ames Test, mouse lymphoma assay, and unscheduled DNA synthesis test.

Impairment of fertility — Atomoxetine HCl did not impair fertility in rats when given in the diet at doses of up to 57 mg/kg/day, which is approximately 6 times the maximum human dose on a mg/m^2 basis.

Pregnancy

Pregnancy Category C — Pregnant rabbits were treated with up to 100 mg/kg/day of atomoxetine by gavage throughout the period of organogenesis. At this dose, in 1 of 3 studies, a decrease in live fetuses and an increase in early resorptions was observed. Slight increases in the incidences of atypical origin of carotid artery and absent subclavian artery were observed. These findings were observed at doses that caused slight maternal toxicity. The no effect dose for these findings was 30 mg/kg/day. The 100-mg/kg dose is approximately 23 times the maximum human dose on a mg/m^2 basis; plasma levels (AUC) of atomoxetine at this dose in rabbits are estimated to be 3.3 times (extensive metabolizers) or 0.4 times (poor metabolizers) those in humans receiving the maximum human dose.

Rats were treated with up to approximately 50 mg/kg/day of atomoxetine (approximately 6 times the maximum human dose on a mg/m^2 basis) in the diet from 2 weeks (females) or 10 weeks (males) prior to mating through the periods of organogenesis and lactation. In 1 of 2 studies, decreases in pup weight and pup survival were observed. The decreased pup survival was also seen at 25 mg/kg (but not at 13 mg/kg). In a study in which rats were treated with atomoxetine in the diet from 2 weeks (females) or 10 weeks (males) prior to mating throughout the period of organogenesis, a decrease in fetal weight (female only) and an increase in the incidence of incomplete ossification of the vertebral arch in fetuses were observed at 40 mg/kg/day (approximately 5 times the maximum human dose on a mg/m^2 basis) but not at 20 mg/kg/day.

No adverse fetal effects were seen when pregnant rats were treated with up to 150 mg/kg/day (approximately 17 times the maximum human dose on a mg/m^2 basis) by gavage throughout the period of organogenesis.

No adequate and well-controlled studies have been conducted in pregnant women. STRATTERA should not be used during pregnancy unless the potential benefit justifies the potential risk to the fetus.

Labor and Delivery

Parturition in rats was not affected by atomoxetine. The effect of STRATTERA on labor and delivery in humans is unknown.

Nursing Mothers

Atomoxetine and/or its metabolites were excreted in the milk of rats. It is not known if atomoxetine is excreted in human milk. Caution should be exercised if STRATTERA is administered to a nursing woman.

Pediatric Use

The safety and efficacy of STRATTERA in pediatric patients less than 6 years of age have not been established. The efficacy of STRATTERA beyond 9 weeks and safety of STRATTERA beyond 1 year of treatment have not been systematically evaluated.

A study was conducted in young rats to evaluate the effects of atomoxetine on growth and neurobehavioral and sexual development. Rats were treated with 1, 10, or 50 mg/kg/day (approximately 0.2, 2, and 8 times, respectively, the maximum human dose on a mg/m^2 basis) of atomoxetine given by gavage from the early postnatal period (Day 10 of age) through adulthood. Slight delays in onset of vaginal patency (all doses) and preputial separation (10 and 50 mg/kg), slight decreases in epididymal weight and sperm number (10 and 50 mg/kg), and a slight decrease in corpora lutea (50 mg/kg) were seen, but there were no effects on fertility or reproductive performance. A slight delay in onset of incisor eruption was seen at 50 mg/kg. A slight increase in motor activity was seen on Day 15 (males at 10 and 50 mg/kg and females at 50 mg/kg) and on Day 30 (females at 50 mg/kg) but not on Day 60 of age. There were no effects on learning and memory tests. The significance of these findings to humans is unknown.

Geriatric Use

The safety and efficacy of STRATTERA in geriatric patients have not been established.

ADVERSE REACTIONS

STRATTERA was administered to 2067 children or adolescent patients with ADHD and 270 adults with ADHD in clinical studies. During the ADHD clinical trials, 169 patients were treated for longer than 1 year and 526 patients were treated for over 6 months.

The data in the following tables and text cannot be used to predict the incidence of side effects in the course of usual medical practice where patient characteristics and other factors differ from those that prevailed in the clinical trials. Similarly, the cited frequencies cannot be compared with data obtained from other clinical investigations involving different treatments, uses, or investigators. The cited data provide the prescribing physician with some basis for estimating the relative contribution of drug and non-drug factors to the adverse event incidence in the population studied.

Child and Adolescent Clinical Trials

Reasons for discontinuation of treatment due to adverse events in child and adolescent clinical trials — In acute child and adolescent placebo-controlled trials, 3.5% (15/427) of atomoxetine subjects and 1.4% (4/294) placebo subjects discontinued for adverse events. For all studies, (including open-label and long-term studies), 5% of extensive metabolizer (EM) patients and 7% of poor metabolizer (PM) patients discontinued because of an adverse event. Among STRATTERA-treated patients, aggression (0.5%, N=2); irritability (0.5%, N=2); somnolence (0.5%, N=2); and vomiting (0.5%, N=2) were the reasons for discontinuation reported by more than 1 patient.

Commonly observed adverse events in acute child and adolescent, placebo-controlled trials — Commonly observed adverse events associated with the use of STRATTERA (incidence of 2% or greater) and not observed at an equivalent incidence among placebo-treated patients (STRATTERA incidence greater than placebo) are listed in Table 1 for the BID trials. Results were similar in the QD trial except as shown in Table 2, which shows both BID and QD results for selected adverse events. The most commonly observed adverse events in patients treated with STRATTERA (incidence of 5% or greater and at least twice the incidence in placebo patients, for either BID or QD dosing) were: dyspepsia, nausea, vomiting, fatigue, appetite decreased, dizziness, and mood swings (*see* Tables 1 *and* 2).

Table 1: Common Treatment-Emergent Adverse Events Associated with the Use of STRATTERA in Acute (up to 9 weeks) Child and Adolescent Trials

Adverse Event[1]	Percentage of Patients Reporting Events from BID Trials	
	STRATTERA (N=340)	Placebo (N=207)
Gastrointestinal Disorders		
Abdominal pain upper	20	16
Constipation	3	1
Dyspepsia	4	2
Vomiting	11	9
Infections		
Ear infection	3	1
Influenza	3	1
Investigations		
Weight decreased	2	0
Metabolism and Nutritional Disorders		
Appetite decreased	14	6
Nervous System Disorders		
Dizziness (exc vertigo)	6	3
Headache	27	25
Somnolence	7	5
Psychiatric Disorders		
Crying	2	1
Irritability	8	5
Mood swings	2	0
Respiratory, Thoracic, and Mediastinal Disorders		
Cough	11	7
Rhinorrhea	4	3
Skin and Subcutaneous Tissue Disorders		
Dermatitis	4	1

[1] Events reported by at least 2% of patients treated with atomoxetine, and greater than placebo. The following events did not meet this criterion but were reported by more atomoxetine-treated patients than placebo-treated patients and are possibly related to atomoxetine treatment: anorexia, blood pressure increased, early morning awakening, flushing, mydriasis, sinus tachycardia, tearfulness. The following events were reported by at least 2% of patients treated with atomoxetine, and equal to or less than placebo: arthralgia, gastroenteritis viral, insomnia,

sore throat, nasal congestion, nasopharyngitis, pruritus, sinus congestion, upper respiratory tract infection.

[See table 2 at right]

The following adverse events occurred in at least 2% of PM patients and were either twice as frequent or statistically significantly more frequent in PM patients compared with EM patients: decreased appetite (23% of PMs, 16% of EMs); insomnia (13% of PMs, 7% of EMs); sedation (4% of PMs, 2% of EMs); depression (6% of PMs, 2% of EMs); tremor (4% of PMs, 1% of EMs); early morning awakening (3% of PMs, 1% of EMs); pruritus (2% of PMs, 1% of EMs); mydriasis (2% of PMs, 1% of EMs).

Adult Clinical Trials

Reasons for discontinuation of treatment due to adverse events in acute adult placebo-controlled trials — In the acute adult placebo-controlled trials, 8.5% (23/270) atomoxetine subjects and 3.4% (9/266) placebo subjects discontinued for adverse events. Among STRATTERA-treated patients, insomnia (1.1%, N=3); chest pain (0.7%, N=2); palpitations (0.7%, N=2); and urinary retention (0.7%, N=2) were the reasons for discontinuation reported by more than 1 patient.

Commonly observed adverse events in acute adult placebo-controlled trials — Commonly observed adverse events associated with the use of STRATTERA (incidence of 2% or greater) and not observed at an equivalent incidence among placebo-treated patients (STRATTERA incidence greater than placebo) are listed in Table 3. The most commonly observed adverse events in patients treated with STRATTERA (incidence of 5% or greater and at least twice the incidence in placebo patients) were: constipation, dry mouth, nausea, appetite decreased, dizziness, insomnia, decreased libido, ejaculatory problems, impotence, urinary hesitation and/or urinary retention and/or difficulty in micturition, and dysmenorrhea (*see* Table 3).

Table 2: Common Treatment-Emergent Adverse Events Associated with the Use of STRATTERA in Acute (up to 9 weeks) Child and Adolescent Trials

Adverse Event	Percentage of Patients Reporting Events from BID Trials		Percentage of Patients Reporting Events from QD Trials	
	STRATTERA (N=340)	Placebo (N=207)	STRATTERA (N=85)	Placebo (N=85)
Gastrointestinal Disorders				
Abdominal pain upper	20	16	16	9
Constipation	3	1	0	0
Diarrhea	3	6	4	1
Dry mouth	1	2	4	1
Dyspepsia	4	2	8	0
Nausea	7	8	12	2
Vomiting	11	9	15	1
General Disorders				
Fatigue	4	5	9	1
Psychiatric Disorders				
Mood swings	2	0	5	2

Table 3: Common Treatment-Emergent Adverse Events Associated with the Use of STRATTERA in Acute (up to 10 weeks) Adult Trials

Adverse Event[1]	Percentage of Patients Reporting Events	
System Organ Class/ Adverse Event	STRATTERA (N=269)	Placebo (N=263)
Cardiac Disorders		
Palpitations	4	1
Gastrointestinal Disorders		
Constipation	10	4
Dry mouth	21	6
Dyspepsia	6	4
Flatulence	2	1
Nausea	12	5
General Disorders and Administration Site Conditions		
Fatigue and/or lethargy	7	4
Pyrexia	3	2
Rigors	3	1
Infections		
Sinusitis	6	4
Investigations		
Weight decreased	2	1
Metabolism and Nutritional Disorders		
Appetite decreased	10	3
Musculoskeletal, Connective Tissue, and Bone Disorders		
Myalgia	3	2
Nervous System Disorders		
Dizziness	6	2
Headache	17	17
Insomnia and/or middle insomnia	16	8
Paraesthesia	4	2
Sinus headache	3	1
Psychiatric Disorders		
Abnormal dreams	4	3
Libido decreased	6	2
Sleep disorder	4	2
Renal and Urinary Disorders		
Urinary hesitation and/or urinary retention and/or difficulty in micturition	8	0
Reproductive System and Breast Disorders		
Dysmenorrhea[3]	7	3
Ejaculation failure[2] and/or ejaculation disorder[2]	5	2
Erectile disturbance[2]	7	1
Impotence[2]	3	0
Menses delayed[3]	2	1
Menstrual disorder[3]	3	2
Menstruation irregular[3]	2	0
Orgasm abnormal	2	1
Prostatitis[2]	3	0
Skin and Subcutaneous Tissue Disorders		
Dermatitis	2	1
Sweating increased	4	1
Vascular Disorders		
Hot flushes	3	1

[1] Events reported by at least 2% of patients treated with atomoxetine, and greater than placebo. The following events did not meet this criterion but were reported by more atomoxetine-treated patients than placebo-treated patients and are possibly related to atomoxetine treatment: early morning awakening, peripheral coldness, tachycardia. The following events were reported by at least 2% of patients treated with atomoxetine, and equal to or less than placebo: abdominal pain upper, arthralgia, back pain, cough, diarrhea, influenza, irritability, nasopharyngitis, sore throat, upper respiratory tract infection, vomiting.

[2] Based on total number of males (STRATTERA, N=174; placebo, N=172).

[3] Based on total number of females (STRATTERA, N=95; placebo, N=91).

Male and female sexual dysfunction — Atomoxetine appears to impair sexual function in some patients. Changes in sexual desire, sexual performance, and sexual satisfaction are not well assessed in most clinical trials because they need special attention and because patients and physicians may be reluctant to discuss them. Accordingly, estimates of the incidence of untoward sexual experience and performance cited in product labeling are likely to underestimate the actual incidence. The table below displays the incidence of sexual side effects reported by at least 2% of adult patients taking STRATTERA in placebo-controlled trials.

Table 4

	STRATTERA	Placebo
Erectile disturbance[1]	7%	1%
Impotence[1]	3%	0%
Orgasm abnormal	2%	1%

[1] Males only.

There are no adequate and well-controlled studies examining sexual dysfunction with STRATTERA treatment. While it is difficult to know the precise risk of sexual dysfunction associated with the use of STRATTERA, physicians should routinely inquire about such possible side effects.

DRUG ABUSE AND DEPENDENCE

Controlled Substance Class

STRATTERA is not a controlled substance.

Physical and Psychological Dependence

In a randomized, double-blind, placebo-controlled, abuse-potential study in adults comparing effects of STRATTERA and placebo, STRATTERA was not associated with a pattern of response that suggested stimulant or euphoriant properties.

Clinical study data in over 2000 children, adolescents, and adults with ADHD and over 1200 adults with depression showed only isolated incidents of drug diversion or inappropriate self-administration associated with STRATTERA. There was no evidence of symptom rebound or adverse events suggesting a drug-discontinuation or withdrawal syndrome.

Animal Experience

Drug discrimination studies in rats and monkeys showed inconsistent stimulus generalization between atomoxetine and cocaine.

OVERDOSAGE

Human Experience

There is limited clinical trial experience with STRATTERA overdose and no fatalities were observed. During post-marketing, there have been reports of acute and chronic overdoses of STRATTERA. No fatal overdoses of STRATTERA alone have been reported. The most commonly reported symptoms accompanying acute and chronic overdoses were somnolence, agitation, hyperactivity, abnormal behavior, and gastrointestinal symptoms. Signs and symptoms consistent with sympathetic nervous system activation (e.g., mydriasis, tachycardia, dry mouth) have also been observed.

Management of Overdose

An airway should be established. Monitoring of cardiac and vital signs is recommended, along with appropriate symptomatic and supportive measures. Gastric lavage may be indicated if performed soon after ingestion. Activated charcoal

Continued on next page

*** Identi-Code® symbol. This product information was prepared in June 2004. Current information on these and other products of Eli Lilly and Company may be obtained by direct inquiry to Lilly Research Laboratories, Lilly Corporate Center, Indianapolis, Indiana 46285, (800) 545-5979.**

Strattera—Cont.

may be useful in limiting absorption. Because atomoxetine is highly protein-bound, dialysis is not likely to be useful in the treatment of overdose.

DOSAGE AND ADMINISTRATION

Initial Treatment

Dosing of children and adolescents up to 70 kg body weight — STRATTERA should be initiated at a total daily dose of approximately 0.5 mg/kg and increased after a minimum of 3 days to a target total daily dose of approximately 1.2 mg/kg administered either as a single daily dose in the morning or as evenly divided doses in the morning and late afternoon/early evening. No additional benefit has been demonstrated for doses higher than 1.2 mg/kg/day (*see* CLINICAL STUDIES).

The total daily dose in children and adolescents should not exceed 1.4 mg/kg or 100 mg, whichever is less.

Dosing of children and adolescents over 70 kg body weight and adults — STRATTERA should be initiated at a total daily dose of 40 mg and increased after a minimum of 3 days to a target total daily dose of approximately 80 mg administered either as a single daily dose in the morning or as evenly divided doses in the morning and late afternoon/early evening. After 2 to 4 additional weeks, the dose may be increased to a maximum of 100 mg in patients who have not achieved an optimal response. There are no data that support increased effectiveness at higher doses (*see* CLINICAL STUDIES).

The maximum recommended total daily dose in children and adolescents over 70 kg and adults is 100 mg.

Maintenance/Extended Treatment

There is no evidence available from controlled trials to indicate how long the patient with ADHD should be treated with STRATTERA. It is generally agreed, however, that pharmacological treatment of ADHD may be needed for extended periods. Nevertheless, the physician who elects to use STRATTERA for extended periods should periodically reevaluate the long-term usefulness of the drug for the individual patient.

General Dosing Information

STRATTERA may be taken with or without food.

The safety of single doses over 120 mg and total daily doses above 150 mg have not been systematically evaluated.

Dosing adjustment for hepatically impaired patients — For those ADHD patients who have hepatic insufficiency (HI), dosage adjustment is recommended as follows: For patients with moderate HI (Child-Pugh Class B), initial and target doses should be reduced to 50% of the normal dose (for patients without HI). For patients with severe HI (Child-Pugh Class C), initial dose and target doses should be reduced to 25% of normal (*see* Special Populations *under* CLINICAL PHARMACOLOGY).

Dosing adjustment for use with a strong CYP2D6 inhibitor — In children and adolescents up to 70 kg body weight administered strong CYP2D6 inhibitors, e.g., paroxetine, fluoxetine, and quinidine, STRATTERA should be initiated at 0.5 mg/kg/day and only increased to the usual target dose of 1.2 mg/kg/day if symptoms fail to improve after 4 weeks and the initial dose is well tolerated.

In children and adolescents over 70 kg body weight and adults administered strong CYP2D6 inhibitors, e.g., paroxetine, fluoxetine, and quinidine, STRATTERA should be initiated at 40 mg/day and only increased to the usual target dose of 80 mg/day if symptoms fail to improve after 4 weeks and the initial dose is well tolerated.

Atomoxetine can be discontinued without being tapered.

HOW SUPPLIED

STRATTERA capsules are supplied in 10-, 18-, 25-, 40-, and 60-mg strengths.

[See table below]

Store at 25°C (77°F); excursions permitted to 15° to 30°C (59° to 86°F) [see USP Controlled Room Temperature].

Literature revised September 3, 2003

www.strattera.com

PV 3753 AMP

INFORMATION FOR PATIENTS OR THEIR PARENTS OR CAREGIVERS

STRATTERA®

(atomoxetine HCl)

Read this information before you start taking STRATTERA (Stra-TAIR-a). Read this information you get each time you get more STRATTERA. There may be new information. This information does not take the place of talking to your doctor about your medical condition or treatment.

What is STRATTERA?

STRATTERA is a non-stimulant medicine used to treat Attention-Deficit/Hyperactivity Disorder (ADHD). STRATTERA contains atomoxetine hydrochloride, a selective norepinephrine reuptake inhibitor. Your doctor has prescribed this medicine as part of an overall treatment plan to control your symptoms of ADHD.

What is ADHD?

ADHD has 3 main types of symptoms: inattention, hyperactivity, and impulsiveness. Symptoms of inattention include not paying attention, making careless mistakes, not listening, not finishing tasks, not following directions, and being easily distracted. Symptoms of hyperactivity and impulsiveness include fidgeting, talking excessively, running around at inappropriate times, and interrupting others. Some patients have more symptoms of hyperactivity and impulsiveness while others have more symptoms of inattentiveness. Some patients have all 3 types of symptoms.

Symptoms of ADHD in adults may include a lack of organization, problems starting tasks, impulsive actions, daydreaming, daytime drowsiness, slow processing of information, difficulty learning new things, irritability, lack of motivation, sensitivity to criticism, forgetfulness, low self-esteem, and excessive effort to maintain some organization. The symptoms shown by adults who primarily have attention problems but not hyperactivity have been commonly described as Attention-Deficit Disorder (ADD).

Many people have symptoms like these from time to time, but patients with ADHD have these symptoms more than others their age. Symptoms must be present for at least 6 months to be certain of the diagnosis.

Who should NOT take STRATTERA?

Do not take STRATTERA if:

- you took a medicine known as a monoamine oxidase inhibitor (MAOI) in the last 2 weeks. An MAOI is a medicine sometimes used for depression and other mental problems. Some names of MAOI medicines are Nardil® (phenelzine sulfate) and Parnate® (tranylcypromine sulfate). Taking STRATTERA with an MAOI could cause serious side effects or be life-threatening.
- you have narrow angle glaucoma, an eye disease.
- you are allergic to STRATTERA or any of its ingredients. The active ingredient is atomoxetine. The inactive ingredients are listed at the end of this leaflet.

What should I tell my doctor before taking STRATTERA?

Talk to your doctor before taking STRATTERA if you:

- have or had liver problems. You may need a lower dose.
- have high blood pressure. STRATTERA can increase blood pressure.
- have problems with your heart or an irregular heartbeat. STRATTERA can increase heart rate (pulse).
- have low blood pressure. STRATTERA can cause dizziness or fainting in people with low blood pressure.

Tell your doctor about all the medicines you take or plan to take, including prescription and non-prescription medicines, dietary supplements, and herbal remedies. Your doctor will decide if you can take STRATTERA with your other medicines.

Certain medicines may change the way your body reacts to STRATTERA. These include medicines used to treat depression [like Paxil® (paroxetine hydrochloride) and Prozac® (fluoxetine hydrochloride)], and certain other medicines (like quinidine). Your doctor may need to change your dose of STRATTERA if you are taking it with these medicines.

STRATTERA may change the way your body reacts to oral or intravenous albuterol (or drugs with similar actions), but the effectiveness of these drugs will not be changed. Talk with your doctor before taking STRATTERA if you are taking albuterol.

How should I take STRATTERA?

- Take STRATTERA according to your doctor's instructions. This is usually taken 1 or 2 times a day (morning and late afternoon/early evening).
- You can take STRATTERA with or without food.
- If you miss a dose, take it as soon as possible, but do not take more than your total daily dose in any 24-hour period.
- Taking STRATTERA at the same time each day may help you remember.
- STRATTERA is available in several dosage strengths: 10, 18, 25, 40, and 60 mg.

Call your doctor right away if you take more than your prescribed dose of STRATTERA.

Other important safety information about STRATTERA

Use caution when driving a car or operating heavy machinery until you know how STRATTERA affects you.

Talk to your doctor if you are:

- pregnant or planning to become pregnant
- breast-feeding. We do not know if STRATTERA can pass into your breast milk.

What are the possible side effects of STRATTERA?

The most common side effects of STRATTERA used in teenagers and children over 6 years old are:

- upset stomach
- decreased appetite
- nausea or vomiting
- dizziness
- tiredness
- mood swings

Weight loss may occur after starting STRATTERA. It is not known if growth will be slowed in children who use STRATTERA for a long period of time. Your doctor will watch your weight and height. If you are not growing or gaining weight as expected, your doctor may change your treatment of STRATTERA.

The most common side effects of STRATTERA used in adults are:

- constipation
- dry mouth
- nausea
- decreased appetite
- dizziness
- problems sleeping
- sexual side effects
- problems urinating
- menstrual cramps

Stop taking STRATTERA and call your doctor right away if you get swelling or hives. STRATTERA can cause a serious allergic reaction in rare cases.

This is not a complete list of side effects. Talk to your doctor if you develop any symptoms that concern you.

General advice about STRATTERA

STRATTERA has not been studied in children under 6 years old.

Medicines are sometimes prescribed for conditions that are not mentioned in patient information leaflets. Do not use STRATTERA for a condition for which it was not prescribed. Do not give STRATTERA to other people, even if they have the same symptoms you have.

This leaflet summarizes the most important information about STRATTERA. If you would like more information, talk with your doctor. You can ask your doctor or pharmacist for information on STRATTERA that is written for health professionals. You can also call 1-800-Lilly-Rx (1-800-545-5979) or visit our website at www.strattera.com.

What are the ingredients in STRATTERA?

Active ingredient: atomoxetine.

Inactive ingredients: pregelatinized starch, dimethicone, gelatin, sodium lauryl sulfate, FD&C Blue No. 2, synthetic yellow iron oxide, titanium dioxide, and edible black ink.

Store STRATTERA at room temperature.

This patient information summary has been approved by the US Food and Drug Administration.

Literature revised January 9, 2004

www.strattera.com

PV 3741 AMP

Shown in Product Identification Guide, page 320

STRATTERA® Capsules	10 mg*	18 mg*	25 mg*	40 mg*	60 mg*
Color	Opaque White, Opaque White	Gold, Opaque White	Opaque Blue, Opaque White	Opaque Blue, Opaque Blue	Opaque Blue, Gold
Identification	LILLY 3227 10 mg	LILLY 3238 18 mg	LILLY 3228 25 mg	LILLY 3229 40 mg	LILLY 3239 60 mg
NDC Codes:					
Bottles of 30	0002-3227-30	0002-3238-30	0002-3228-30	0002-3229-30	0002-3239-30

*Atomoxetine base equivalent.

SYMBYAX™ ℞

[sim-bee-ax]

(olanzapine and fluoxetine HCl capsules)

DESCRIPTION

SYMBYAX™ (olanzapine and fluoxetine HCl capsules) combines 2 psychotropic agents, olanzapine (the active ingredient in Zyprexa®, and Zyprexa Zydis®) and fluoxetine hydrochloride (the active ingredient in Prozac®, Prozac Weekly™, and Sarafem®).

Olanzapine belongs to the thienobenzodiazepine class. The chemical designation is 2-methyl-4-(4-methyl-1-piperazinyl)-10*H*-thieno[2,3-b] [1,5]benzodiazepine. The molecular formula is $C_{17}H_{20}N_4S$, which corresponds to a molecular weight of 312.44.

Fluoxetine hydrochloride is a selective serotonin reuptake inhibitor (SSRI). The chemical designation is (±)-N-methyl-3-phenyl-3-[(α,α,α-trifluoro-*p*-tolyl)oxy]propylamine hydrochloride. The molecular formula is $C_{17}H_{18}F_3NO \cdot HCl$, which corresponds to a molecular weight of 345.79.

The chemical structures are:

olanzapine

[See chemical structure at top of next column]

Olanzapine is a yellow crystalline solid, which is practically insoluble in water.

Fluoxetine hydrochloride is a white to off-white crystalline solid with a solubility of 14 mg/mL in water.

fluoxetine hydrochloride

SYMBYAX capsules are available for oral administration in the following strength combinations:

	6 mg/ 25 mg	6 mg/ 50 mg	12 mg/ 25 mg	12 mg/ 50 mg
olanzapine equivalent	6	6	12	12
fluoxetine base equivalent	25	50	25	50

Each capsule also contains pregelatinized starch, gelatin, dimethicone, titanium dioxide, sodium lauryl sulfate, edible black ink, red iron oxide, yellow iron oxide, and/or black iron oxide.

CLINICAL PHARMACOLOGY

Pharmacodynamics

Although the exact mechanism of SYMBYAX is unknown, it has been proposed that the activation of 3 monoaminergic neural systems (serotonin, norepinephrine, and dopamine) is responsible for its enhanced antidepressant effect. This is supported by animal studies in which the olanzapine/fluoxetine combination has been shown to produce synergistic increases in norepinephrine and dopamine release in the prefrontal cortex compared with either component alone, as well as increases in serotonin.

Olanzapine is a psychotropic agent with high affinity binding to the following receptors: serotonin $5HT_{2A/2C}$ (K_i=4 and 11 nM, respectively), dopamine D_{1-4} (K_i=11 to 31 nM), muscarinic M_{1-5} (K_i=1.9 to 25 nM), histamine H_1 (K_i=7 nM), and adrenergic α_1 receptors (K_i=19 nM). Olanzapine binds weakly to $GABA_A$, BZD, and β-adrenergic receptors (K_i>10 μM). Fluoxetine is an inhibitor of the serotonin transporter and is a weak inhibitor of the norepinephrine and dopamine transporters.

Antagonism at receptors other than dopamine and $5HT_2$ with similar receptor affinities may explain some of the other therapeutic and side effects of olanzapine. Olanzapine's antagonism of muscarinic M_{1-5} receptors may explain its anticholinergic effects. The antagonism of histamine H_1 receptors by olanzapine may explain the somnolence observed with this drug. The antagonism of α_1-adrenergic receptors by olanzapine may explain the orthostatic hypotension observed with this drug. Fluoxetine has relatively low affinity for muscarinic, α_1-adrenergic, and histamine H_1 receptors.

Pharmacokinetics

Fluoxetine (administered as a 60-mg single dose or 60 mg daily for 8 days) caused a small increase in the mean maximum concentration of olanzapine (16%) following a 5-mg dose, an increase in the mean area under the curve (17%) and a small decrease in mean apparent clearance of olanzapine (16%). In another study, a similar decrease in apparent clearance of olanzapine of 14% was observed following olanzapine doses of 6 or 12 mg with concomitant fluoxetine doses of 25 mg or more. The decrease in clearance reflects an increase in bioavailability. The terminal half-life is not affected, and therefore the time to reach steady state should not be altered. The overall steady-state plasma concentrations of olanzapine and fluoxetine when given as the combination in the therapeutic dose ranges were comparable with those typically attained with each of the monotherapies. The small change in olanzapine clearance, observed in both studies, likely reflects the inhibition of a minor metabolic pathway for olanzapine via CYP2D6 by fluoxetine, a potent CYP2D6 inhibitor, and was not deemed clinically significant. Therefore, the pharmacokinetics of the individual components is expected to reasonably characterize the overall pharmacokinetics of the combination.

Absorption and Bioavailability

SYMBYAX — Following a single oral 12-mg/50-mg dose of SYMBYAX, peak plasma concentrations of olanzapine and fluoxetine occur at approximately 4 and 6 hours, respectively. The effect of food on the absorption and bioavailability of SYMBYAX has not been evaluated. The bioavailability of olanzapine given as Zyprexa, and the bioavailability of fluoxetine given as Prozac were not affected by food. It is unlikely that there would be a significant food effect on the bioavailability of SYMBYAX.

Olanzapine — Olanzapine is well absorbed and reaches peak concentration approximately 6 hours following an oral dose. Food does not affect the rate or extent of olanzapine absorption when olanzapine is given as Zyprexa. It is eliminated extensively by first pass metabolism, with approximately 40% of the dose metabolized before reaching the systemic circulation.

Fluoxetine — Following a single oral 40-mg dose, peak plasma concentrations of fluoxetine from 15 to 55 ng/mL are observed after 6 to 8 hours. Food does not appear to affect the systemic bioavailability of fluoxetine given as Prozac, although it may delay its absorption by 1 to 2 hours, which is probably not clinically significant.

Distribution

SYMBYAX — The in vitro binding to human plasma proteins of the olanzapine/fluoxetine combination is similar to the binding of the individual components.

Olanzapine — Olanzapine is extensively distributed throughout the body, with a volume of distribution of approximately 1000 L. It is 93% bound to plasma proteins over the concentration range of 7 to 1100 ng/mL, binding primarily to albumin and α_1-acid glycoprotein.

Fluoxetine — Over the concentration range from 200 to 1000 ng/mL, approximately 94.5% of fluoxetine is bound in vitro to human serum proteins, including albumin and α_1-glycoprotein. The interaction between fluoxetine and other highly protein-bound drugs has not been fully evaluated (*see* PRECAUTIONS, Drugs tightly bound to plasma proteins).

Metabolism and Elimination

SYMBYAX — SYMBYAX therapy yielded steady-state concentrations of norfluoxetine similar to those seen with fluoxetine in the therapeutic dose range.

Olanzapine — Olanzapine displays linear pharmacokinetics over the clinical dosing range. Its half-life ranges from 21 to 54 hours (5th to 95th percentile; mean of 30 hr), and apparent plasma clearance ranges from 12 to 47 L/hr (5th to 95th percentile; mean of 25 L/hr). Administration of olanzapine once daily leads to steady-state concentrations in about 1 week that are approximately twice the concentrations after single doses. Plasma concentrations, half-life, and clearance of olanzapine may vary between individuals on the basis of smoking status, gender, and age (*see* Special Populations).

Following a single oral dose of ^{14}C-labeled olanzapine, 7% of the dose of olanzapine was recovered in the urine as unchanged drug, indicating that olanzapine is highly metabolized. Approximately 57% and 30% of the dose was recovered in the urine and feces, respectively. In the plasma, olanzapine accounted for only 12% of the AUC for total radioactivity, indicating significant exposure to metabolites. After multiple dosing, the major circulating metabolites were the 10-N-glucuronide, present at steady state at 44% of the concentration of olanzapine, and 4′-N-desmethyl olanzapine, present at steady state at 31% of the concentration of olanzapine. Both metabolites lack pharmacological activity at the concentrations observed.

Direct glucuronidation and CYP450-mediated oxidation are the primary metabolic pathways for olanzapine. In vitro studies suggest that CYP1A2, CYP2D6, and the flavin-containing monooxygenase system are involved in olanzapine oxidation. CYP2D6-mediated oxidation appears to be a minor metabolic pathway in vivo, because the clearance of olanzapine is not reduced in subjects who are deficient in this enzyme.

Fluoxetine — Fluoxetine is a racemic mixture (50/50) of *R*-fluoxetine and *S*-fluoxetine enantiomers. In animal models, both enantiomers are specific and potent serotonin uptake inhibitors with essentially equivalent pharmacologic activity. The *S*-fluoxetine enantiomer is eliminated more slowly and is the predominant enantiomer present in plasma at steady state.

Fluoxetine is extensively metabolized in the liver to its only identified active metabolite, norfluoxetine, via the CYP2D6 pathway. A number of unidentified metabolites exist.

In animal models, *S*-norfluoxetine is a potent and selective inhibitor of serotonin uptake and has activity essentially equivalent to *R*- or *S*-fluoxetine. *R*-norfluoxetine is significantly less potent than the parent drug in the inhibition of serotonin uptake. The primary route of elimination appears to be hepatic metabolism to inactive metabolites excreted by the kidney.

Clinical issues related to metabolism and elimination — The complexity of the metabolism of fluoxetine has several consequences that may potentially affect the clinical use of SYMBYAX.

Variability in metabolism — A subset (about 7%) of the population has reduced activity of the drug metabolizing enzyme CYP2D6. Such individuals are referred to as "poor metabolizers" of drugs such as debrisoquin, dextromethorphan, and the tricyclic antidepressants (TCAs). In a study involving labeled and unlabeled enantiomers administered as a racemate, these individuals metabolized *S*-fluoxetine at a slower rate and thus achieved higher concentrations of *S*-fluoxetine. Consequently, concentrations of *S*-norfluoxetine at steady state were lower. The metabolism of *R*-fluoxetine in these poor metabolizers appears normal. When compared with normal metabolizers, the total sum at steady state of the plasma concentrations of the 4 enantiomers was not significantly greater among poor metabolizers. Thus, the net pharmacodynamic activities were essentially the same. Alternative nonsaturable pathways (non-CYP2D6) also contribute to the metabolism of fluoxetine. This explains how fluoxetine achieves a steady-state concentration rather than increasing without limit.

Because the metabolism of fluoxetine, like that of a number of other compounds including TCAs and other selective serotonin antidepressants, involves the CYP2D6 system, concomitant therapy with drugs also metabolized by this enzyme system (such as the TCAs) may lead to drug interactions (*see* PRECAUTIONS, Drug Interactions).

Accumulation and slow elimination — The relatively slow elimination of fluoxetine (elimination half-life of 1 to 3 days after acute administration and 4 to 6 days after chronic administration) and its active metabolite, norfluoxetine (elimination half-life of 4 to 16 days after acute and chronic administration), leads to significant accumulation of these active species in chronic use and delayed attainment of steady state, even when a fixed dose is used. After 30 days of dosing at 40 mg/day, plasma concentrations of fluoxetine in the range of 91 to 302 ng/mL and norfluoxetine in the range of 72 to 258 ng/mL have been observed. Plasma concentrations of fluoxetine were higher than those predicted by single-dose studies, because the metabolism of fluoxetine is not proportional to dose. However, norfluoxetine appears to have linear pharmacokinetics. Its mean terminal half-life after a single dose was 8.6 days and after multiple dosing was 9.3 days. Steady-state levels after prolonged dosing are similar to levels seen at 4 to 5 weeks.

The long elimination half-lives of fluoxetine and norfluoxetine assure that, even when dosing is stopped, active drug substance will persist in the body for weeks (primarily depending on individual patient characteristics, previous dosing regimen, and length of previous therapy at discontinuation). This is of potential consequence when drug discontinuation is required or when drugs are prescribed that might interact with fluoxetine and norfluoxetine following the discontinuation of fluoxetine.

Special Populations

Geriatric — Based on the individual pharmacokinetic profiles of olanzapine and fluoxetine, the pharmacokinetics of SYMBYAX may be altered in geriatric patients. Caution should be used in dosing the elderly, especially if there are other factors that might additively influence drug metabolism and/or pharmacodynamic sensitivity.

In a study involving 24 healthy subjects, the mean elimination half-life of olanzapine was about 1.5 times greater in elderly subjects (>65 years of age) than in non-elderly subjects (≤65 years of age).

The disposition of single doses of fluoxetine in healthy elderly subjects (>65 years of age) did not differ significantly from that in younger normal subjects. However, given the long half-life and nonlinear disposition of the drug, a single-dose study is not adequate to rule out the possibility of altered pharmacokinetics in the elderly, particularly if they have systemic illness or are receiving multiple drugs for concomitant diseases. The effects of age upon the metabolism of fluoxetine have been investigated in 260 elderly but otherwise healthy depressed patients (≥60 years of age) who received 20 mg fluoxetine for 6 weeks. Combined fluoxetine plus norfluoxetine plasma concentrations were 209.3 ± 85.7 ng/mL at the end of 6 weeks. No unusual age-associated pattern of adverse events was observed in those elderly patients.

Renal impairment — The pharmacokinetics of SYMBYAX has not been studied in patients with renal impairment. However, olanzapine and fluoxetine individual pharmacokinetics do not differ significantly in patients with renal impairment. SYMBYAX dosing adjustment based upon renal impairment is not routinely required.

Because olanzapine is highly metabolized before excretion and only 7% of the drug is excreted unchanged, renal dysfunction alone is unlikely to have a major impact on the pharmacokinetics of olanzapine. The pharmacokinetic characteristics of olanzapine were similar in patients with severe renal impairment and normal subjects, indicating that dosage adjustment based upon the degree of renal impairment is not required. In addition, olanzapine is not removed by dialysis. The effect of renal impairment on olanzapine metabolite elimination has not been studied.

In depressed patients on dialysis (N=12), fluoxetine administered as 20 mg once daily for 2 months produced steady-state fluoxetine and norfluoxetine plasma concentrations comparable with those seen in patients with normal renal function. While the possibility exists that renally excreted metabolites of fluoxetine may accumulate to higher levels in patients with severe renal dysfunction, use of a lower or less frequent dose is not routinely necessary in renally impaired patients.

Hepatic impairment — Based on the individual pharmacokinetic profiles of olanzapine and fluoxetine, the pharmacokinetics of SYMBYAX may be altered in patients with hepatic impairment. The lowest starting dose should be considered for patients with hepatic impairment (*see* PRECAUTIONS, Use in patients with concomitant illness *and* DOSAGE AND ADMINISTRATION, Special Populations).

Although the presence of hepatic impairment may be expected to reduce the clearance of olanzapine, a study of the effect of impaired liver function in subjects (N=6) with clinically significant cirrhosis (Childs-Pugh Classification A and B) revealed little effect on the pharmacokinetics of olanzapine.

As might be predicted from its primary site of metabolism, liver impairment can affect the elimination of fluoxetine. The elimination half-life of fluoxetine was prolonged in a study of cirrhotic patients, with a mean of 7.6 days compared with the range of 2 to 3 days seen in subjects without liver disease; norfluoxetine elimination was also delayed, with a mean duration of 12 days for cirrhotic patients compared with the range of 7 to 9 days in normal subjects.

Continued on next page

*** Identi-Code® symbol. This product information was prepared in June 2004. Current information on these and other products of Eli Lilly and Company may be obtained by direct inquiry to Lilly Research Laboratories, Lilly Corporate Center, Indianapolis, Indiana 46285, (800) 545-5979.**

Symbyax—Cont.

Gender — Clearance of olanzapine is approximately 30% lower in women than in men. There were, however, no apparent differences between men and women in effectiveness or adverse effects. Dosage modifications based on gender should not be needed.

Smoking status — Olanzapine clearance is about 40% higher in smokers than in nonsmokers, although dosage modifications are not routinely required.

Race — No SYMBYAX pharmacokinetic study was conducted to investigate the effects of race. Results from an olanzapine cross-study comparison between data obtained in Japan and data obtained in the US suggest that exposure to olanzapine may be about 2-fold greater in the Japanese when equivalent doses are administered. Olanzapine clinical study safety and efficacy data, however, did not suggest clinically significant differences among Caucasian patients, patients of African descent, and a 3rd pooled category including Asian and Hispanic patients. Dosage modifications for race, therefore, are not routinely required.

Combined effects — The combined effects of age, smoking, and gender could lead to substantial pharmacokinetic differences in populations. The clearance of olanzapine in young smoking males, for example, may be 3 times higher than that in elderly nonsmoking females. SYMBYAX dosing modification may be necessary in patients who exhibit a combination of factors that may result in slower metabolism of the olanzapine component (*see* DOSAGE AND ADMINISTRATION, Special Populations).

CLINICAL STUDIES

The efficacy of SYMBYAX for the treatment of depressive episodes associated with bipolar disorder was established in 2 identically designed, 8-week, randomized, double-blind, controlled studies of patients who met Diagnostic and Statistical Manual 4th edition (DSM-IV) criteria for Bipolar I Disorder, Depressed utilizing flexible dosing of SYMBYAX (6/25, 6/50, or 12/50 mg/day), olanzapine (5 to 20 mg/day), and placebo. These studies included patients (≥18 years of age) with or without psychotic symptoms and with or without a rapid cycling course.

The primary rating instrument used to assess depressive symptoms in these studies was the Montgomery-Asberg Depression Rating Scale (MADRS), a 10-item clinician-rated scale with total scores ranging from 0 to 60. The primary outcome measure of these studies was the change from baseline to endpoint in the MADRS total score. In both studies, SYMBYAX was statistically significantly superior to both olanzapine monotherapy and placebo in reduction of the MADRS total score. The results of the studies are summarized below (Table 1).

Table 1: MADRS Total Score Mean Change from Baseline to Endpoint

	Treatment Group	Baseline Mean	Change to Endpoint Mean[1]
Study 1	SYMBYAX (N=40)	30	-16[a]
	Olanzapine (N=182)	32	-12
	Placebo (N=181)	31	-10
Study 2	SYMBYAX (N=42)	32	-18[a]
	Olanzapine (N=169)	33	-14
	Placebo (N=174)	31	-9

[1] Negative number denotes improvement from baseline.
[a] Statistically significant compared to both olanzapine and placebo.

INDICATIONS AND USAGE

SYMBYAX is indicated for the treatment of depressive episodes associated with bipolar disorder. The efficacy of SYMBYAX was established in 2 identically designed, 8-week, randomized, double-blind clinical studies.

Unlike with unipolar depression, there are no established guidelines for the length of time patients with bipolar disorder experiencing a major depressive episode should be treated with agents containing antidepressant drugs.

The effectiveness of SYMBYAX for maintaining antidepressant response in this patient population beyond 8 weeks has not been established in controlled clinical studies. Physicians who elect to use SYMBYAX for extended periods should periodically reevaluate the benefits and long-term risks of the drug for the individual patient.

CONTRAINDICATIONS

Hypersensitivity — SYMBYAX is contraindicated in patients with a known hypersensitivity to the product or any component of the product.

Monoamine oxidase inhibitors (MAOI) — There have been reports of serious, sometimes fatal reactions (including hyperthermia, rigidity, myoclonus, autonomic instability with possible rapid fluctuations of vital signs, and mental status changes that include extreme agitation progressing to delirium and coma) in patients receiving fluoxetine in combination with an MAOI, and in patients who have recently discontinued fluoxetine and are then started on an MAOI. Some cases presented with features resembling neuroleptic malignant syndrome. Therefore, SYMBYAX should not be used in combination with an MAOI, or within a minimum of 14 days of discontinuing therapy with an MAOI. Since fluoxetine and its major metabolite have very long elimination half-lives, at least 5 weeks [perhaps longer, especially if fluoxetine has been prescribed chronically and/or at higher doses (*see* CLINICAL PHARMACOLOGY, Accumulation and slow elimination)] should be allowed after stopping SYMBYAX before starting an MAOI.

Thioridazine — Thioridazine should not be administered with SYMBYAX or administered within a minimum of 5 weeks after discontinuation of SYMBYAX (*see* WARNINGS, Thioridazine).

WARNINGS

Hyperglycemia and Diabetes Mellitus — Hyperglycemia, in some cases extreme and associated with ketoacidosis or hyperosmolar coma or death, has been reported in patients treated with atypical antipsychotics, including olanzapine alone, as well as olanzapine taken concomitantly with fluoxetine. Assessment of the relationship between atypical antipsychotic use and glucose abnormalities is complicated by the possibility of an increased background risk of diabetes mellitus in patients with schizophrenia and the increasing incidence of diabetes mellitus in the general population. Given these confounders, the relationship between atypical antipsychotic use and hyperglycemia-related adverse events is not completely understood. However, epidemiological studies suggest an increased risk of treatment-emergent hyperglycemia-related adverse events in patients treated with the atypical antipsychotics. Precise risk estimates for hyperglycemia-related adverse events in patients treated with atypical antipsychotics are not available.

Patients with an established diagnosis of diabetes mellitus who are started on atypical antipsychotics should be monitored regularly for worsening of glucose control. Patients with risk factors for diabetes mellitus (e.g., obesity, family history of diabetes) who are starting treatment with atypical antipsychotics should undergo fasting blood glucose testing at the beginning of treatment and periodically during treatment. Any patient treated with atypical antipsychotics should be monitored for symptoms of hyperglycemia including polydipsia, polyuria, polyphagia, and weakness. Patients who develop symptoms of hyperglycemia during treatment with atypical antipsychotics should undergo fasting blood glucose testing. In some cases, hyperglycemia has resolved when the atypical antipsychotic was discontinued; however, some patients required continuation of anti-diabetic treatment despite discontinuation of the suspect drug.

Cerebrovascular adverse events (CVAE), including stroke, in elderly patients with dementia — Cerebrovascular adverse events (e.g., stroke, transient ischemic attack), including fatalities, were reported in patients in trials of olanzapine in elderly patients with dementia-related psychosis. In placebo-controlled trials, there was a significantly higher incidence of cerebrovascular adverse events in patients treated with olanzapine compared to patients treated with placebo. Olanzapine is not approved for the treatment of patients with dementia-related psychosis.

Orthostatic hypotension — SYMBYAX may induce orthostatic hypotension associated with dizziness, tachycardia, bradycardia, and in some patients, syncope, especially during the initial dose-titration period.

In the bipolar depression studies, statistically significantly more orthostatic changes occurred with the SYMBYAX group compared to placebo and olanzapine groups. Orthostatic systolic blood pressure decrease of at least 30 mm Hg occurred in 7.3% (6/82), 1.4% (5/346), and 1.4% (5/352) of the SYMBYAX, olanzapine and placebo groups, respectively. Among the group of controlled clinical studies with SYMBYAX, an orthostatic systolic blood pressure decrease of ≥30 mm Hg occurred in 4% (21/512) of SYMBYAX-treated patients, 5% (10/204) of fluoxetine-treated patients, 2% (16/644) of olanzapine-treated patients, and 2% (8/445) of placebo-treated patients. In this group of studies, the incidence of syncope in SYMBYAX-treated patients was 0.4% (2/571) compared to placebo 0.2% (1/477).

In a clinical pharmacology study of SYMBYAX, three healthy subjects were discontinued from the trial after experiencing severe, but self-limited, hypotension and bradycardia that occurred 2 to 9 hours following a single 12-mg/50-mg dose of SYMBYAX. Reactions consisting of this combination of hypotension and bradycardia (and also accompanied by sinus pause) have been observed in at least three other healthy subjects treated with various formulations of olanzapine (one oral, two intramuscular). In controlled clinical studies, the incidence of patients with a ≥20 bpm decrease in orthostatic pulse concomitantly with a ≥20 mm Hg decrease in orthostatic systolic blood pressure was 0.4% (2/549) in the SYMBYAX group, 0.2% (1/455) in the placebo group, 0.8% (5/659) in the olanzapine group, and 0% (0/241) in the fluoxetine group.

SYMBYAX should be used with particular caution in patients with known cardiovascular disease (history of myocardial infarction or ischemia, heart failure, or conduction abnormalities), cerebrovascular disease, or conditions that would predispose patients to hypotension (dehydration, hypovolemia, and treatment with antihypertensive medications).

Allergic events and rash — In SYMBYAX premarketing controlled clinical studies, the overall incidence of rash or allergic events in SYMBYAX-treated patients [4.6% (26/571)] was similar to that of placebo [5.2% (25/477)]. The majority of the cases of rash and/or urticaria were mild; however, three patients discontinued (one due to rash, which was moderate in severity, and two due to allergic events, one of which included face edema).

In fluoxetine US clinical studies, 7% of 10,782 fluoxetine-treated patients developed various types of rashes and/or urticaria. Among the cases of rash and/or urticaria reported in premarketing clinical studies, almost a third were withdrawn from treatment because of the rash and/or systemic signs or symptoms associated with the rash. Clinical findings reported in association with rash include fever, leukocytosis, arthralgias, edema, carpal tunnel syndrome, respiratory distress, lymphadenopathy, proteinuria, and mild transaminase elevation. Most patients improved promptly with discontinuation of fluoxetine and/or adjunctive treatment with antihistamines or steroids, and all patients experiencing these events were reported to recover completely.

In fluoxetine premarketing clinical studies, 2 patients are known to have developed a serious cutaneous systemic illness. In neither patient was there an unequivocal diagnosis, but 1 was considered to have a leukocytoclastic vasculitis, and the other, a severe desquamating syndrome that was considered variously to be a vasculitis or erythema multiforme. Other patients have had systemic syndromes suggestive of serum sickness.

Since the introduction of fluoxetine, systemic events, possibly related to vasculitis, have developed in patients with rash. Although these events are rare, they may be serious, involving the lung, kidney, or liver. Death has been reported to occur in association with these systemic events.

Anaphylactoid events, including bronchospasm, angioedema, and urticaria alone and in combination, have been reported.

Pulmonary events, including inflammatory processes of varying histopathology and/or fibrosis, have been reported rarely. These events have occurred with dyspnea as the only preceding symptom.

Whether these systemic events and rash have a common underlying cause or are due to different etiologies or pathogenic processes is not known. Furthermore, a specific underlying immunologic basis for these events has not been identified. Upon the appearance of rash or of other possible allergic phenomena for which an alternative etiology cannot be identified, SYMBYAX should be discontinued.

Neuroleptic malignant syndrome (NMS) — A potentially fatal symptom complex sometimes referred to as NMS has been reported in association with administration of antipsychotic drugs, including olanzapine. Clinical manifestations of NMS are hyperpyrexia, muscle rigidity, altered mental status, and evidence of autonomic instability (irregular pulse or blood pressure, tachycardia, diaphoresis, and cardiac dysrhythmia). Additional signs may include elevated creatinine phosphokinase, myoglobinuria (rhabdomyolysis), and acute renal failure.

The diagnostic evaluation of patients with this syndrome is complicated. In arriving at a diagnosis, it is important to exclude cases where the clinical presentation includes both serious medical illness (e.g., pneumonia, systemic infection, etc.) and untreated or inadequately treated extrapyramidal signs and symptoms (EPS). Other important considerations in the differential diagnosis include central anticholinergic toxicity, heat stroke, drug fever, and primary central nervous system pathology.

The management of NMS should include: 1) immediate discontinuation of antipsychotic drugs and other drugs not essential to concurrent therapy, 2) intensive symptomatic treatment and medical monitoring, and 3) treatment of any concomitant serious medical problems for which specific treatments are available. There is no general agreement about specific pharmacological treatment regimens for NMS.

If after recovering from NMS, a patient requires treatment with an antipsychotic, the patient should be carefully monitored, since recurrences of NMS have been reported.

Tardive dyskinesia — A syndrome of potentially irreversible, involuntary, dyskinetic movements may develop in patients treated with antipsychotic drugs. Although the prevalence of the syndrome appears to be highest among the elderly, especially elderly women, it is impossible to rely upon prevalence estimates to predict, at the inception of antipsychotic treatment, which patients are likely to develop the syndrome. Whether antipsychotic drug products differ in their potential to cause tardive dyskinesia is unknown.

The risk of developing tardive dyskinesia and the likelihood that it will become irreversible are believed to increase as the duration of treatment and the total cumulative dose of antipsychotic drugs administered to the patient increase. However, the syndrome can develop, although much less commonly, after relatively brief treatment periods at low doses or may even arise after discontinuation of treatment.

There is no known treatment for established cases of tardive dyskinesia, although the syndrome may remit, partially or completely, if antipsychotic treatment is withdrawn. Antipsychotic treatment itself, however, may suppress (or partially suppress) the signs and symptoms of the syndrome and thereby may possibly mask the underlying process. The effect that symptomatic suppression has upon the long-term course of the syndrome is unknown.

The incidence of dyskinetic movement in SYMBYAX-treated patients was infrequent. The mean score on the Abnormal

Involuntary Movement Scale (AIMS) across clinical studies involving SYMBYAX-treated patients decreased from baseline. Nonetheless, SYMBYAX should be prescribed in a manner that is most likely to minimize the risk of tardive dyskinesia. If signs and symptoms of tardive dyskinesia appear in a patient on SYMBYAX, drug discontinuation should be considered. However, some patients may require treatment with SYMBYAX despite the presence of the syndrome. The need for continued treatment should be reassessed periodically.

Thioridazine — In a study of 19 healthy male subjects, which included 6 slow and 13 rapid hydroxylators of debrisoquin, a single 25-mg oral dose of thioridazine produced a 2.4-fold higher C_{max} and a 4.5-fold higher AUC for thioridazine in the slow hydroxylators compared with the rapid hydroxylators. The rate of debrisoquin hydroxylation is felt to depend on the level of CYP2D6 isozyme activity. Thus, this study suggests that drugs that inhibit CYP2D6, such as certain SSRIs, including fluoxetine, will produce elevated plasma levels of thioridazine (*see* PRECAUTIONS).

Thioridazine administration produces a dose-related prolongation of the QT_c interval, which is associated with serious ventricular arrhythmias, such as torsades de pointes-type arrhythmias and sudden death. This risk is expected to increase with fluoxetine-induced inhibition of thioridazine metabolism (*see* CONTRAINDICATIONS, Thioridazine).

PRECAUTIONS

General

Concomitant use of olanzapine and fluoxetine products — SYMBYAX contains the same active ingredients that are in Zyprexa and Zyprexa Zydis (olanzapine) and in Prozac, Prozac Weekly, and Sarafem (fluoxetine HCl). Caution should be exercised when prescribing these medications concomitantly with SYMBYAX.

Abnormal bleeding — Published case reports have documented the occurrence of bleeding episodes in patients treated with psychotropic drugs that interfere with serotonin reuptake. Subsequent epidemiological studies, both of the case-control and cohort design, have demonstrated an association between use of psychotropic drugs that interfere with serotonin reuptake and the occurrence of upper gastrointestinal bleeding. In two studies, concurrent use of a nonsteroidal anti-inflammatory drug (NSAID) or aspirin potentiated the risk of bleeding (*see* DRUG INTERACTIONS). Although these studies focused on upper gastrointestinal bleeding, there is reason to believe that bleeding at other sites may be similarly potentiated. Patients should be cautioned regarding the risk of bleeding associated with the concomitant use of SYMBYAX with NSAIDs, aspirin, or other drugs that affect coagulation.

Mania/Hypomania — In the two controlled bipolar depression studies there was no statistically significant difference in the incidence of manic events (manic reaction or manic depressive reaction) between SYMBYAX- and placebo-treated patients. In one of the studies, the incidence of manic events was (7% [3/43]) in SYMBYAX-treated patients compared to (3% [5/184]) in placebo-treated patients. In the other study, the incidence of manic events was (2% [1/43]) in SYMBYAX-treated patients compared to (8% [15/193]) in placebo-treated patients. This limited controlled trial experience of SYMBYAX in the treatment of bipolar depression makes it difficult to interpret these findings until additional data is obtained. Because of this and the cyclical nature of bipolar disorder, patients should be monitored closely for the development of symptoms of mania/hypomania during treatment with SYMBYAX.

Body temperature regulation — Disruption of the body's ability to reduce core body temperature has been attributed to antipsychotic drugs. Appropriate care is advised when prescribing SYMBYAX for patients who will be experiencing conditions which may contribute to an elevation in core body temperature, e.g., exercising strenuously, exposure to extreme heat, receiving concomitant medication with anticholinergic activity, or being subject to dehydration.

Cognitive and motor impairment — Somnolence was a commonly reported adverse event associated with SYMBYAX treatment, occurring at an incidence of 22% in SYMBYAX patients compared with 11% in placebo patients. Somnolence led to discontinuation in 2% (10/571) of patients in the premarketing controlled clinical studies.

As with any CNS-active drug, SYMBYAX has the potential to impair judgment, thinking, or motor skills. Patients should be cautioned about operating hazardous machinery, including automobiles, until they are reasonably certain that SYMBYAX therapy does not affect them adversely.

Dysphagia — Dysphagia was observed infrequently in SYMBYAX-treated patients in premarketing clinical studies. Nonetheless, like other psychotropic drugs, SYMBYAX should be used cautiously in patients at risk for aspiration pneumonia.

Esophageal dysmotility and aspiration have been associated with antipsychotic drug use. Two olanzapine-treated patients (2/407) in 2 olanzapine studies in patients with Alzheimer's disease died from aspiration pneumonia during or within 30 days of the termination of the double-blind portion of their respective studies; there were no deaths in the placebo-treated patients. One of these patients had experienced dysphagia prior to the development of aspiration pneumonia. Aspiration pneumonia is a common cause of morbidity and mortality in patients with advanced Alzheimer's disease.

Half-life — Because of the long elimination half-lives of fluoxetine and its major active metabolite, changes in dose will not be fully reflected in plasma for several weeks, affecting both strategies for titration to final dose and withdrawal from treatment (*see* CLINICAL PHARMACOLOGY, Accumulation and slow elimination).

Hyperprolactinemia — As with other drugs that antagonize dopamine D_2 receptors, SYMBYAX elevates prolactin levels, and a modest elevation persists during administration; however, possibly associated clinical manifestations (e.g., galactorrhea and breast enlargement) were infrequently observed.

Tissue culture experiments indicate that approximately one-third of human breast cancers are prolactin dependent in vitro, a factor of potential importance if the prescription of these drugs is contemplated in a patient with previously detected breast cancer of this type. Although disturbances such as galactorrhea, amenorrhea, gynecomastia, and impotence have been reported with prolactin-elevating compounds, the clinical significance of elevated serum prolactin levels is unknown for most patients. As is common with compounds that increase prolactin release, an increase in mammary gland neoplasia was observed in the olanzapine carcinogenicity studies conducted in mice and rats (*see* Carcinogenesis). However, neither clinical studies nor epidemiologic studies have shown an association between chronic administration of this class of drugs and tumorigenesis in humans; the available evidence is considered too limited to be conclusive.

Hyponatremia — Hyponatremia has been observed in SYMBYAX premarketing clinical studies. In controlled trials, no SYMBYAX-treated patients had a treatment-emergent serum sodium below 130 mmol/L; however, a lowering of serum sodium below the reference range occurred at an incidence of 2% (10/500) of SYMBYAX patients compared with 0.5% (2/380) of placebo patients. In open label studies, 0.3% (5/1889) of these SYMBYAX-treated patients had a treatment-emergent serum sodium below 130 mmol/L.

Cases of hyponatremia (some with serum sodium lower than 110 mmol/L) have been reported with fluoxetine. The hyponatremia appeared to be reversible when fluoxetine was discontinued. Although these cases were complex with varying possible etiologies, some were possibly due to the syndrome of inappropriate antidiuretic hormone secretion (SIADH). The majority of these occurrences have been in older patients and in patients taking diuretics or who were otherwise volume depleted. In two 6-week controlled studies in patients ≥60 years of age, 10 of 323 fluoxetine patients and 6 of 327 placebo recipients had a lowering of serum sodium below the reference range; this difference was not statistically significant. The lowest observed concentration was 129 mmol/L. The observed decreases were not clinically significant.

Seizures — Seizures occurred in 0.2% (4/2066) of SYMBYAX-treated patients during open-label premarketing clinical studies. No seizures occurred in the premarketing controlled SYMBYAX studies. Seizures have also been reported with both olanzapine and fluoxetine monotherapy. Therefore, SYMBYAX should be used cautiously in patients with a history of seizures or with conditions that potentially lower the seizure threshold. Conditions that lower the seizure threshold may be more prevalent in a population of ≥65 years of age.

Suicide — The possibility of a suicide attempt is inherent in bipolar disorder and may persist until significant remission occurs. Close supervision of high-risk patients should accompany drug therapy. Prescriptions for SYMBYAX should be written for the smallest quantity consistent with good patient management in order to reduce the risk of overdose.

Transaminase elevations — As with olanzapine, asymptomatic elevations of hepatic transaminases [ALT (SGPT), AST (SGOT), and GGT] and alkaline phosphatase have been observed with SYMBYAX. In the SYMBYAX-controlled database, ALT (SGPT) elevations (≥3 times the upper limit of the normal range) were observed in 6.3% (31/495) of patients exposed to SYMBYAX compared with 0.5% (2/384) of the placebo patients and 4.5% (25/560) of olanzapine-treated patients. The difference between SYMBYAX and placebo was statistically significant. None of these 31 SYMBYAX-treated patients experienced jaundice and three had transient elevations >200 IU/L.

In olanzapine placebo-controlled studies, clinically significant ALT (SGPT) elevations (≥3 times the upper limit of the normal range) were observed in 2% (6/243) of patients exposed to olanzapine compared with 0% (0/115) of the placebo patients. None of these patients experienced jaundice. In 2 of these patients, liver enzymes decreased toward normal despite continued treatment, and in 2 others, enzymes decreased upon discontinuation of olanzapine. In the remaining 2 patients, 1, seropositive for hepatitis C, had persistent enzyme elevations for 4 months after discontinuation, and the other had insufficient follow-up to determine if enzymes normalized.

Within the larger olanzapine premarketing database of about 2400 patients with baseline SGPT ≤90 IU/L, the incidence of SGPT elevation to >200 IU/L was 2% (50/2381). Again, none of these patients experienced jaundice or other symptoms attributable to liver impairment and most had transient changes that tended to normalize while olanzapine treatment was continued. Among all 2500 patients in olanzapine clinical studies, approximately 1% (23/2500) discontinued treatment due to transaminase increases.

Caution should be exercised in patients with signs and symptoms of hepatic impairment, in patients with pre-existing conditions associated with limited hepatic functional reserve, and in patients who are being treated with potentially hepatotoxic drugs. Periodic assessment of transaminases is recommended in patients with significant hepatic disease (*see* Laboratory Tests).

Weight gain — In clinical studies, the mean weight increase for SYMBYAX-treated patients was statistically significantly greater than placebo-treated (3.6 kg vs -0.3 kg) and fluoxetine-treated (3.6 kg vs -0.7 kg) patients, but was not statistically significantly different from olanzapine-treated patients (3.6 kg vs 3.0 kg). Fourteen percent of SYMBYAX-treated patients met criterion for having gained >10% of their baseline weight. This was statistically significantly greater than placebo-treated (<1%) and fluoxetine-treated patients (<1%) but was not statistically significantly different than olanzapine-treated patients (11%).

Use in Patients with Concomitant Illness

Clinical experience with SYMBYAX in patients with concomitant systemic illnesses is limited (*see* CLINICAL PHARMACOLOGY, Renal impairment *and* Hepatic impairment). The following precautions for the individual components may be applicable to SYMBYAX.

Olanzapine exhibits in vitro muscarinic receptor affinity. In premarketing clinical studies, SYMBYAX was associated with constipation, dry mouth, and tachycardia, all adverse events possibly related to cholinergic antagonism. Such adverse events were not often the basis for study discontinuations; SYMBYAX should be used with caution in patients with clinically significant prostatic hypertrophy, narrow angle glaucoma, a history of paralytic ileus, or related conditions.

In a fixed-dose study of olanzapine (olanzapine at doses of 5, 10, and 15 mg/day) and placebo in nursing home patients (mean age: 83 years, range: 61 to 97; median Mini-Mental State Examination (MMSE): 5, range: 0 to 22) having various psychiatric symptoms in association with Alzheimer's disease, the following treatment-emergent adverse events were reported in all (each and every) olanzapine-treated groups at an incidence of either (1) 2-fold or more in excess of the placebo-treated group, where at least 1 placebo-treated patient was reported to have experienced the event, or (2) at least 2 cases if no placebo-treated patient was reported to have experienced the event: somnolence, abnormal gait, fever, dehydration, and back pain. The rate of discontinuation in this study for olanzapine was 12% vs 4% with placebo. Discontinuations due to abnormal gait (1% for olanzapine vs 0% for placebo), accidental injury (1% for olanzapine vs 0% for placebo), and somnolence (3% for olanzapine vs 0% for placebo) were considered to be drug related.

As with other CNS-active drugs, SYMBYAX should be used with caution in elderly patients with dementia.

SYMBYAX has not been evaluated or used to any appreciable extent in patients with a recent history of myocardial infarction or unstable heart disease. Patients with these diagnoses were excluded from clinical studies during the premarket testing.

Caution is advised when using SYMBYAX in cardiac patients and in patients with diseases or conditions that could affect hemodynamic responses (*see* WARNINGS, Orthostatic hypotension).

In subjects with cirrhosis of the liver, the clearances of fluoxetine and its active metabolite, norfluoxetine, were decreased, thus increasing the elimination half-lives of these substances. A lower dose of the fluoxetine-component of SYMBYAX should be used in patients with cirrhosis. Caution is advised when using SYMBYAX in patients with diseases or conditions that could affect its metabolism (*see* CLINICAL PHARMACOLOGY, Hepatic impairment *and* DOSING AND ADMINISTRATION, Special Populations).

Olanzapine and fluoxetine individual pharmacokinetics do not differ significantly in patients with renal impairment. SYMBYAX dosing adjustment based upon renal impairment is not routinely required (*see* CLINICAL PHARMACOLOGY, Renal impairment).

Information for Patients

Physicians are advised to discuss the following issues with patients for whom they prescribe SYMBYAX:

Abnormal bleeding — Patients should be cautioned about the concomitant use of SYMBYAX and NSAIDs, aspirin, or other drugs that affect coagulation since the combined use of psychotropic drugs that interfere with serotonin reuptake and these agents has been associated with an increased risk of bleeding (*see* PRECAUTIONS, Abnormal bleeding).

Alcohol — Patients should be advised to avoid alcohol while taking SYMBYAX.

Cognitive and motor impairment — As with any CNS-active drug, SYMBYAX has the potential to impair judgment, thinking, or motor skills. Patients should be cautioned about operating hazardous machinery, including automobiles, until they are reasonably certain that SYMBYAX therapy does not affect them adversely.

Concomitant medication — Patients should be advised to inform their physician if they are taking Prozac®, Prozac Weekly™, Sarafem®, fluoxetine, Zyprexa®, or Zyprexa

Continued on next page

*** Identi-Code® symbol. This product information was prepared in June 2004. Current information on these and other products of Eli Lilly and Company may be obtained by direct inquiry to Lilly Research Laboratories, Lilly Corporate Center, Indianapolis, Indiana 46285, (800) 545-5979.**

Symbyax—Cont.

Zydis®. Patients should also be advised to inform their physicians if they are taking or plan to take any prescription or over-the-counter drugs, including herbal supplements, since there is a potential for interactions.

Heat exposure and dehydration — Patients should be advised regarding appropriate care in avoiding overheating and dehydration.

Nursing — Patients, if taking SYMBYAX, should be advised not to breast-feed.

Orthostatic hypotension — Patients should be advised of the risk of orthostatic hypotension, especially during the period of initial dose titration and in association with the use of concomitant drugs that may potentiate the orthostatic effect of olanzapine, e.g., diazepam or alcohol (*see* WARNINGS *and* Drug Interactions).

Pregnancy — Patients should be advised to notify their physician if they become pregnant or intend to become pregnant during SYMBYAX therapy.

Rash — Patients should be advised to notify their physician if they develop a rash or hives while taking SYMBYAX.

Treatment adherence — Patients should be advised to take SYMBYAX exactly as prescribed, and to continue taking SYMBYAX as prescribed even after their mood symptoms improve. Patients should be advised that they should not alter their dosing regimen, or stop taking SYMBYAX, without consulting their physician.

Patient information is printed at the end of this insert. Physicians should discuss this information with their patients and instruct them to read the patient package insert before starting therapy with SYMBYAX and each time their prescription is refilled.

Laboratory Tests

Periodic assessment of transaminases is recommended in patients with significant hepatic disease (*see* Transaminase elevations).

Drug Interactions

The risks of using SYMBYAX in combination with other drugs have not been extensively evaluated in systematic studies. The drug-drug interactions of the individual components are applicable to SYMBYAX. As with all drugs, the potential for interaction by a variety of mechanisms (e.g., pharmacodynamic, pharmacokinetic drug inhibition or enhancement, etc.) is a possibility. Caution is advised if the concomitant administration of SYMBYAX and other CNS-active drugs is required. In evaluating individual cases, consideration should be given to using lower initial doses of the concomitantly administered drugs, using conservative titration schedules, and monitoring of clinical status (*see* CLINICAL PHARMACOLOGY, Accumulation and slow elimination).

Antihypertensive agents — Because of the potential for olanzapine to induce hypotension, SYMBYAX may enhance the effects of certain antihypertensive agents (*see* WARNINGS, Orthostatic hypotension).

Anti-Parkinsonian — The olanzapine component of SYMBYAX may antagonize the effects of levodopa and dopamine agonists.

Benzodiazepines — Multiple doses of olanzapine did not influence the pharmacokinetics of diazepam and its active metabolite N-desmethyldiazepam. However, the coadministration of diazepam with olanzapine potentiated the orthostatic hypotension observed with olanzapine.

When concurrently administered with fluoxetine, the half-life of diazepam may be prolonged in some patients (*see* CLINICAL PHARMACOLOGY, Accumulation and slow elimination). Coadministration of alprazolam and fluoxetine has resulted in increased alprazolam plasma concentrations and in further psychomotor performance decrement due to increased alprazolam levels.

Biperiden — Multiple doses of olanzapine did not influence the pharmacokinetics of biperiden.

Carbamazepine — Carbamazepine therapy (200 mg BID) causes an approximate 50% increase in the clearance of olanzapine. This increase is likely due to the fact that carbamazepine is a potent inducer of CYP1A2 activity. Higher daily doses of carbamazepine may cause an even greater increase in olanzapine clearance.

Patients on stable doses of carbamazepine have developed elevated plasma anticonvulsant concentrations and clinical anticonvulsant toxicity following initiation of concomitant fluoxetine treatment.

Clozapine — Elevation of blood levels of clozapine has been observed in patients receiving concomitant fluoxetine.

Electroconvulsive therapy (ECT) — There are no clinical studies establishing the benefit of the combined use of ECT and fluoxetine. There have been rare reports of prolonged seizures in patients on fluoxetine receiving ECT treatment (*see* Seizures).

Ethanol — Ethanol (45 mg/70 kg single dose) did not have an effect on olanzapine pharmacokinetics. The coadministration of ethanol with SYMBYAX may potentiate sedation and orthostatic hypotension.

Fluvoxamine — Fluvoxamine, a CYP1A2 inhibitor, decreases the clearance of olanzapine. This results in a mean increase in olanzapine C_{max} following fluvoxamine administration of 54% in female nonsmokers and 77% in male smokers. The mean increase in olanzapine AUC is 52% and 108%, respectively. Lower doses of the olanzapine component of SYMBYAX should be considered in patients receiving concomitant treatment with fluvoxamine.

Haloperidol — Elevation of blood levels of haloperidol has been observed in patients receiving concomitant fluoxetine.

Lithium — Multiple doses of olanzapine did not influence the pharmacokinetics of lithium.

There have been reports of both increased and decreased lithium levels when lithium was used concomitantly with fluoxetine. Cases of lithium toxicity and increased serotonergic effects have been reported. Lithium levels should be monitored in patients taking SYMBYAX concomitantly with lithium.

Monoamine oxidase inhibitors — See CONTRAINDICATIONS.

Phenytoin — Patients on stable doses of phenytoin have developed elevated plasma levels of phenytoin with clinical phenytoin toxicity following initiation of concomitant fluoxetine.

Pimozide — A single case report has suggested possible additive effects of pimozide and fluoxetine leading to bradycardia.

Sumatriptan — There have been rare postmarketing reports describing patients with weakness, hyperreflexia, and incoordination following the use of an SSRI and sumatriptan. If concomitant treatment with sumatriptan and an SSRI (e.g., fluoxetine, fluvoxamine, paroxetine, sertraline, or citalopram) is clinically warranted, appropriate observation of the patient is advised.

Theophylline — Multiple doses of olanzapine did not affect the pharmacokinetics of theophylline or its metabolites.

Thioridazine — See CONTRAINDICATIONS and WARNINGS, Thioridazine.

Tricyclic antidepressants (TCAs) — Single doses of olanzapine did not affect the pharmacokinetics of imipramine or its active metabolite desipramine.

In two fluoxetine studies, previously stable plasma levels of imipramine and desipramine have increased >2- to 10-fold when fluoxetine has been administered in combination. This influence may persist for three weeks or longer after fluoxetine is discontinued. Thus, the dose of TCA may need to be reduced and plasma TCA concentrations may need to be monitored temporarily when SYMBYAX is coadministered or has been recently discontinued (*see* Drugs metabolized by CYP2D6 *and* CLINICAL PHARMACOLOGY, Accumulation and slow elimination).

Tryptophan — Five patients receiving fluoxetine in combination with tryptophan experienced adverse reactions, including agitation, restlessness, and gastrointestinal distress.

Valproate — In vitro studies using human liver microsomes determined that olanzapine has little potential to inhibit the major metabolic pathway, glucuronidation, of valproate. Further, valproate has little effect on the metabolism of olanzapine in vitro. Thus, a clinically significant pharmacokinetic interaction between olanzapine and valproate is unlikely.

Warfarin — Warfarin (20-mg single dose) did not affect olanzapine pharmacokinetics. Single doses of olanzapine did not affect the pharmacokinetics of warfarin.

Altered anticoagulant effects, including increased bleeding, have been reported when fluoxetine is coadministered with warfarin (*see* PRECAUTIONS, Abnormal bleeding). Patients receiving warfarin therapy should receive careful coagulation monitoring when SYMBYAX is initiated or stopped.

Drugs that interfere with hemostasis (NSAIDs, aspirin, warfarin, etc.) — Serotonin release by platelets plays an important role in hemostasis. Epidemiological studies of the case-control and cohort design that have demonstrated an association between use of psychotropic drugs that interfere with serotonin reuptake and the occurrence of upper gastrointestinal bleeding have also shown that concurrent use of an NSAID or aspirin potentiated the risk of bleeding (*see* PRECAUTIONS, Abnormal bleeding). Thus, patients should be cautioned about the use of such drugs concurrently with SYMBYAX.

Drugs metabolized by CYP2D6 — In vitro studies utilizing human liver microsomes suggest that olanzapine has little potential to inhibit CYP2D6. Thus, olanzapine is unlikely to cause clinically important drug interactions mediated by this enzyme.

Approximately 7% of the normal population has a genetic variation that leads to reduced levels of activity of CYP2D6. Such individuals have been referred to as poor metabolizers of drugs such as debrisoquin, dextromethorphan, and TCAs. Many drugs, such as most antidepressants, including fluoxetine and other selective uptake inhibitors of serotonin, are metabolized by this isoenzyme; thus, both the pharmacokinetic properties and relative proportion of metabolites are altered in poor metabolizers. However, for fluoxetine and its metabolite, the sum of the plasma concentrations of the 4 enantiomers is comparable between poor and extensive metabolizers (*see* CLINICAL PHARMACOLOGY, Variability in metabolism).

Fluoxetine, like other agents that are metabolized by CYP2D6, inhibits the activity of this isoenzyme, and thus may make normal metabolizers resemble poor metabolizers. Therapy with medications that are predominantly metabolized by the CYP2D6 system and that have a relatively narrow therapeutic index should be initiated at the low end of the dose range if a patient is receiving fluoxetine concurrently or has taken it in the previous five weeks. If fluoxetine is added to the treatment regimen of a patient already receiving a drug metabolized by CYP2D6, the need for a decreased dose of the original medication should be considered. Drugs with a narrow therapeutic index represent the greatest concern (including but not limited to, flecainide, vinblastine, and TCAs). Due to the risk of serious ventricular arrhythmias and sudden death potentially associated with elevated thioridazine plasma levels, thioridazine should not be administered with fluoxetine or within a minimum of five weeks after fluoxetine has been discontinued (*see* CONTRAINDICATIONS, Monoamine oxidase inhibitors (MAOI) *and* WARNINGS, Thioridazine).

Drugs metabolized by CYP3A — In vitro studies utilizing human liver microsomes suggest that olanzapine has little potential to inhibit CYP3A. Thus, olanzapine is unlikely to cause clinically important drug interactions mediated by these enzymes.

In an in vivo interaction study involving the coadministration of fluoxetine with single doses of terfenadine (a CYP3A substrate), no increase in plasma terfenadine concentrations occurred with concomitant fluoxetine. In addition, in vitro studies have shown ketoconazole, a potent inhibitor of CYP3A activity, to be at least 100 times more potent than fluoxetine or norfluoxetine as an inhibitor of the metabolism of several substrates for this enzyme, including astemizole, cisapride, and midazolam. These data indicate that fluoxetine's extent of inhibition of CYP3A activity is not likely to be of clinical significance.

Effect of olanzapine on drugs metabolized by other CYP enzymes — In vitro studies utilizing human liver microsomes suggest that olanzapine has little potential to inhibit CYP1A2, CYP2C9, and CYP2C19. Thus, olanzapine is unlikely to cause clinically important drug interactions mediated by these enzymes.

The effect of other drugs on olanzapine — Fluoxetine, an inhibitor of CYP2D6, decreases olanzapine clearance a small amount (*see* CLINICAL PHARMACOLOGY, Pharmacokinetics). Agents that induce CYP1A2 or glucuronyl transferase enzymes, such as omeprazole and rifampin, may cause an increase in olanzapine clearance. Fluvoxamine, an inhibitor of CYP1A2, decreases olanzapine clearance (*see* Drug Interactions, Fluvoxamine). The effect of CYP1A2 inhibitors, such as fluvoxamine and some fluoroquinolone antibiotics, on SYMBYAX has not been evaluated. Although olanzapine is metabolized by multiple enzyme systems, induction or inhibition of a single enzyme may appreciably alter olanzapine clearance. Therefore, a dosage increase (for induction) or a dosage decrease (for inhibition) may need to be considered with specific drugs.

Drugs tightly bound to plasma proteins — The in vitro binding of SYMBYAX to human plasma proteins is similar to the individual components. The interaction between SYMBYAX and other highly protein-bound drugs has not been fully evaluated. Because fluoxetine is tightly bound to plasma protein, the administration of fluoxetine to a patient taking another drug that is tightly bound to protein (e.g., Coumadin, digitoxin) may cause a shift in plasma concentrations potentially resulting in an adverse effect. Conversely, adverse effects may result from displacement of protein-bound fluoxetine by other tightly bound drugs (*see* CLINICAL PHARMACOLOGY, Distribution *and* PRECAUTIONS, Drug Interactions).

Carcinogenesis, Mutagenesis, Impairment of Fertility

No carcinogenicity, mutagenicity, or fertility studies were conducted with SYMBYAX. The following data are based on findings in studies performed with the individual components.

Carcinogenesis

Olanzapine — Oral carcinogenicity studies were conducted in mice and rats. Olanzapine was administered to mice in two 78-week studies at doses of 3, 10, and 30/20 mg/kg/day [equivalent to 0.8 to 5 times the maximum recommended human daily dose (MRHD) on a mg/m^2 basis] and 0.25, 2, and 8 mg/kg/day (equivalent to 0.06 to 2 times the MRHD on a mg/m^2 basis). Rats were dosed for 2 years at doses of 0.25, 1, 2.5, and 4 mg/kg/day (males) and 0.25, 1, 4, and 8 mg/kg/day (females) (equivalent to 0.1 to 2 and 0.1 to 4 times the MRHD on a mg/m^2 basis, respectively). The incidence of liver hemangiomas and hemangiosarcomas was significantly increased in one mouse study in females dosed at 8 mg/kg/day (2 times the MRHD on a mg/m^2 basis). These tumors were not increased in another mouse study in females dosed at 10 or 30/20 mg/kg/day (2 to 5 times the MRHD on a mg/m^2 basis); in this study, there was a high incidence of early mortalities in males of the 30/20 mg/kg/day group. The incidence of mammary gland adenomas and adenocarcinomas was significantly increased in female mice dosed at ≥2 mg/kg/day and in female rats dosed at ≥4 mg/kg/day (0.5 and 2 times the MRHD on a mg/m^2 basis, respectively). Antipsychotic drugs have been shown to chronically elevate prolactin levels in rodents. Serum prolactin levels were not measured during the olanzapine carcinogenicity studies; however, measurements during subchronic toxicity studies showed that olanzapine elevated serum prolactin levels up to 4-fold in rats at the same doses used in the carcinogenicity study. An increase in mammary gland neoplasms has been found in rodents after chronic administration of other antipsychotic drugs and is considered to be prolactin-mediated. The relevance for human risk of the finding of prolactin-mediated endocrine tumors in rodents is unknown (*see* PRECAUTIONS, Hyperprolactinemia).

Fluoxetine — The dietary administration of fluoxetine to rats and mice for two years at doses of up to 10 and 12 mg/kg/day, respectively (approximately 1.2 and 0.7 times, respectively, the MRHD on a mg/m^2 basis), produced no evidence of carcinogenicity.

Mutagenesis

Olanzapine — No evidence of mutagenic potential for olanzapine was found in the Ames reverse mutation test, in vivo micronucleus test in mice, the chromosomal aberration test in Chinese hamster ovary cells, unscheduled DNA synthesis test in rat hepatocytes, induction of forward mutation test in mouse lymphoma cells, or in vivo sister chromatid exchange test in bone marrow of Chinese hamsters.

Fluoxetine — Fluoxetine and norfluoxetine have been shown to have no genotoxic effects based on the following assays: bacterial mutation assay, DNA repair assay in cultured rat hepatocytes, mouse lymphoma assay, and in vivo sister chromatid exchange assay in Chinese hamster bone marrow cells.

Impairment of Fertility

SYMBYAX — Fertility studies were not conducted with SYMBYAX. However in a repeat-dose rat toxicology study of three months duration, ovary weight was decreased in females treated with the low-dose [2 and 4 mg/kg/day (1 and 0.5 times the MRHD on a mg/m^2 basis), respectively] and high-dose [4 and 8 mg/kg/day (2 and 1 times the MRHD on a mg/m^2 basis), respectively] combinations of olanzapine and fluoxetine. Decreased ovary weight, and corpora luteal depletion and uterine atrophy were observed to a greater extent in the females receiving the high-dose combination than in females receiving either olanzapine or fluoxetine alone. In a 3-month repeat-dose dog toxicology study, reduced epididymal sperm and reduced testicular and prostate weights were observed with the high-dose combination of olanzapine and fluoxetine (5 and 5 mg/kg/day (9 and 2 times the MRHD on a mg/m^2 basis, respectively) and with olanzapine alone (5 mg/kg/day or 9 times the MRHD on a mg/m^2 basis).

Olanzapine — In a fertility and reproductive performance study in rats, male mating performance, but not fertility, was impaired at a dose of 22.4 mg/kg/day and female fertility was decreased at a dose of 3 mg/kg/day (11 and 1.5 times the MRHD on a mg/m^2 basis, respectively). Discontinuance of olanzapine treatment reversed the effects on male-mating performance. In female rats, the precoital period was increased and the mating index reduced at 5 mg/kg/day (2.5 times the MRHD on a mg/m^2 basis). Diestrous was prolonged and estrous was delayed at 1.1 mg/kg/day (0.6 times the MRHD on a mg/m^2 basis); therefore, olanzapine may produce a delay in ovulation.

Fluoxetine — Two fertility studies conducted in rats at doses of up to 7.5 and 12.5 mg/kg/day (approximately 0.9 and 1.5 times the MRHD on a mg/m^2 basis) indicated that fluoxetine had no adverse effects on fertility.

Pregnancy — Pregnancy Category C

SYMBYAX

Embryo fetal development studies were conducted in rats and rabbits with olanzapine and fluoxetine in low-dose and high-dose combinations. In rats, the doses were: 2 and 4 mg/kg/day (low-dose) [1 and 0.5 times the MRHD on a mg/m^2 basis, respectively], and 4 and 8 mg/kg/day (high-dose) [2 and 1 times the MRHD on a mg/m^2 basis, respectively]. In rabbits, the doses were 4 and 4 mg/kg/day (low-dose) [4 and 1 times the MRHD on a mg/m^2 basis, respectively], and 8 and 8 mg/kg/day (high-dose) [9 and 2 times the MRHD on a mg/m^2 basis, respectively]. In these studies, olanzapine and fluoxetine were also administered alone at the high-doses (4 and 8 mg/kg/day, respectively, in the rat; 8 and 8 mg/kg/day, respectively, in the rabbit). In the rabbit, there was no evidence of teratogenicity; however, the high-dose combination produced decreases in fetal weight and retarded skeletal ossification in conjunction with maternal toxicity. Similarly, in the rat there was no evidence of teratogenicity; however, a decrease in fetal weight was observed with the high-dose combination.

In a pre- and postnatal study conducted in rats, olanzapine and fluoxetine were administered during pregnancy and throughout lactation in combination (low-dose: 2 and 4 mg/kg/day [1 and 0.5 times the MRHD on a mg/m^2 basis], respectively, high-dose: 4 and 8 mg/kg/day [2 and 1 times the MRHD on a mg/m^2 basis], respectively, and alone: 4 and 8 mg/kg/day [2 and 1 times the MRHD on a mg/m^2 basis], respectively). Administration of the high-dose combination resulted in a marked elevation in offspring mortality and growth retardation in comparison to the same doses of olanzapine and fluoxetine administered alone. These effects were not observed with the low-dose combination; however, there were a few cases of testicular degeneration and atrophy, depletion of epididymal sperm and infertility in the male progeny. The effects of the high-dose combination on postnatal endpoints could not be assessed due to high progeny mortality.

There are no adequate and well-controlled studies with SYMBYAX in pregnant women.

SYMBYAX should be used during pregnancy only if the potential benefit justifies the potential risk to the fetus.

Olanzapine

In reproduction studies in rats at doses up to 18 mg/kg/day and in rabbits at doses up to 30 mg/kg/day (9 and 30 times the MRHD on a mg/m^2 basis, respectively), no evidence of teratogenicity was observed. In a rat teratology study, early resorptions and increased numbers of nonviable fetuses were observed at a dose of 18 mg/kg/day (9 times the MRHD on a mg/m^2 basis). Gestation was prolonged at 10 mg/kg/day (5 times the MRHD on a mg/m^2 basis). In a rabbit teratology study, fetal toxicity (manifested as increased resorptions and decreased fetal weight) occurred at a maternally toxic dose of 30 mg/kg/day (30 times the MRHD on a mg/m^2 basis).

Placental transfer of olanzapine occurs in rat pups.

There are no adequate and well-controlled clinical studies with olanzapine in pregnant women. Seven pregnancies were observed during premarketing clinical studies with olanzapine, including two resulting in normal births, one resulting in neonatal death due to a cardiovascular defect, three therapeutic abortions, and one spontaneous abortion.

Fluoxetine

In embryo fetal development studies in rats and rabbits, there was no evidence of teratogenicity following administration of up to 12.5 and 15 mg/kg/day, respectively (1.5 and 3.6 times the MRHD on a mg/m^2 basis, respectively) throughout organogenesis. However, in rat reproduction studies, an increase in stillborn pups, a decrease in pup weight, and an increase in pup deaths during the first 7 days postpartum occurred following maternal exposure to 12 mg/kg/day (1.5 times the MRHD on a mg/m^2 basis) during gestation or 7.5 mg/kg/day (0.9 times the MRHD on a mg/m^2 basis) during gestation and lactation. There was no evidence of developmental neurotoxicity in the surviving offspring of rats treated with 12 mg/kg/day during gestation. The no-effect dose for rat pup mortality was 5 mg/kg/day (0.6 times the MRHD on a mg/m^2 basis).

Labor and Delivery

SYMBYAX

The effect of SYMBYAX on labor and delivery in humans is unknown. Parturition in rats was not affected by SYMBYAX. SYMBYAX should be used during labor and delivery only if the potential benefit justifies the potential risk.

Olanzapine

Parturition in rats was not affected by olanzapine. The effect of olanzapine on labor and delivery in humans is unknown.

Fluoxetine

The effect of fluoxetine on labor and delivery in humans is unknown. Fluoxetine crosses the placenta; therefore, there is a possibility that fluoxetine may have adverse effects on the newborn.

Nursing Mothers

SYMBYAX

There are no adequate and well-controlled studies with SYMBYAX in nursing mothers or infants. No studies have been conducted to examine the excretion of olanzapine or fluoxetine in breast milk following SYMBYAX treatment. It is recommended that women not breast-feed when receiving SYMBYAX.

Olanzapine

Olanzapine was excreted in milk of treated rats during lactation.

Fluoxetine

Fluoxetine is excreted in human breast milk. In one breast milk sample, the concentration of fluoxetine plus norfluoxetine was 70.4 ng/mL. The concentration in the mother's plasma was 295.0 ng/mL. No adverse effects on the infant were reported. In another case, an infant nursed by a mother on fluoxetine developed crying, sleep disturbance, vomiting, and watery stools. The infant's plasma drug levels were 340 ng/mL of fluoxetine and 208 ng/mL of norfluoxetine on the 2nd day of feeding.

Pediatric Use

Safety and effectiveness of SYMBYAX in pediatric patients have not been established.

Geriatric Use

SYMBYAX

Clinical studies of SYMBYAX did not include sufficient numbers of patients ≥65 years of age to determine whether they respond differently from younger patients. Other reported clinical experience has not identified differences in responses between the elderly and younger patients. In general, dose selection for an elderly patient should be cautious, usually starting at the low end of the dosing range, reflecting the greater frequency of decreased hepatic, renal, or cardiac function, and of concomitant disease or other drug therapy (*see* DOSAGE AND ADMINISTRATION).

Olanzapine

Of the 2500 patients in premarketing clinical studies with olanzapine, 11% (263 patients) were ≥65 years of age. In patients with schizophrenia, there was no indication of any different tolerability of olanzapine in the elderly compared with younger patients. Studies in patients with various psychiatric symptoms in association with Alzheimer's disease have suggested that there may be a different tolerability profile in this population compared with younger patients with schizophrenia. In placebo-controlled studies of olanzapine in elderly patients with dementia-related psychosis, there was a significantly higher incidence of cerebrovascular adverse events (e.g., stroke, transient ischemic attack) in patients treated with olanzapine compared to patients treated with placebo. Olanzapine is not approved for the treatment of patients with dementia-related psychosis (*see* WARNINGS, Cerebrovascular adverse events).

As with other CNS-active drugs, olanzapine should be used with caution in elderly patients with dementia. Also, the presence of factors that might decrease pharmacokinetic clearance or increase the pharmacodynamic response to olanzapine should lead to consideration of a lower starting dose for any geriatric patient.

Fluoxetine

US fluoxetine clinical studies (10,782 patients) included 687 patients ≥65 years of age and 93 patients ≥75 years of age. No overall differences in safety or effectiveness were observed between these subjects and younger subjects, and other reported clinical experience has not identified differences in responses between the elderly and younger patients, but greater sensitivity of some older individuals cannot be ruled out. As with other SSRIs, fluoxetine has been associated with cases of clinically significant hyponatremia in elderly patients.

ADVERSE REACTIONS

The information below is derived from a premarketing clinical study database for SYMBYAX consisting of 2066 patients with various diagnoses with approximately 1061 patient-years of exposure. The conditions and duration of treatment with SYMBYAX varied greatly and included (in overlapping categories) open-label and double-blind phases of studies, inpatients and outpatients, fixed-dose and dose-titration studies, and short-term or long-term exposure.

Adverse events were recorded by clinical investigators using descriptive terminology of their own choosing. Consequently, it is not possible to provide a meaningful estimate of the proportion of individuals experiencing adverse events without first grouping similar types of events into a limited (i.e., reduced) number of standardized event categories.

In the tables and tabulations that follow, COSTART Dictionary terminology has been used to classify reported adverse events. The data in the tables represent the proportion of individuals who experienced, at least once, a treatment-emergent adverse event of the type listed. An event was considered treatment-emergent if it occurred for the first time or worsened while receiving therapy following baseline evaluation. It is possible that events reported during therapy were not necessarily related to drug exposure.

The prescriber should be aware that the figures in the tables and tabulations cannot be used to predict the incidence of side effects in the course of usual medical practice where patient characteristics and other factors differ from those that prevailed in the clinical studies. Similarly, the cited frequencies cannot be compared with figures obtained from other clinical investigations involving different treatments, uses, and investigators. The cited figures, however, do provide the prescribing clinician with some basis for estimating the relative contribution of drug and non-drug factors to the side effect incidence rate in the population studied.

Incidence in Controlled Clinical Studies

The following findings are based on the short-term, controlled premarketing studies in various diagnoses including bipolar depression.

Adverse events associated with discontinuation of treatment — Overall, 10% of the patients in the SYMBYAX group discontinued due to adverse events compared with 4.6% for placebo. Table 2 enumerates the adverse events leading to discontinuation associated with the use of SYMBYAX (incidence of at least 1% for SYMBYAX and greater than that for placebo). The bipolar depression column shows the incidence of adverse events with SYMBYAX in the bipolar depression studies and the "SYMBYAX-Controlled" column shows the incidence in the controlled SYMBYAX studies; the placebo column shows the incidence in the pooled controlled studies that included a placebo arm.

Table 2: Adverse Events Associated with Discontinuation*

Adverse Event	Percentage of Patients Reporting Event		
	SYMBYAX		Placebo
	Bipolar Depression (N=86)	SYMBYAX-Controlled (N=571)	(N=477)
Asthenia	0	1	0
Somnolence	0	2	0
Weight gain	0	2	0
Chest pain	1	0	0

* Table includes events associated with discontinuation of at least 1% and greater than placebo

Commonly observed adverse events in controlled clinical studies — The most commonly observed adverse events associated with the use of SYMBYAX (incidence of ≥5% and at least twice that for placebo in the SYMBYAX-controlled database) were: asthenia, edema, increased appetite, peripheral edema, pharyngitis, somnolence, thinking abnormal, tremor, and weight gain.

Adverse events occurring at an incidence of 2% or more in controlled clinical studies — Table 3 enumerates the treatment-emergent adverse events associated with the use of SYMBYAX (incidence of at least 2% for SYMBYAX and twice or more that for placebo).

Continued on next page

*** Identi-Code® symbol. This product information was prepared in June 2004. Current information on these and other products of Eli Lilly and Company may be obtained by direct inquiry to Lilly Research Laboratories, Lilly Corporate Center, Indianapolis, Indiana 46285, (800) 545-5979.**

Symbyax—Cont.

Table 3: Treatment-Emergent Adverse Events: Incidence in Controlled Clinical Studies

Body System/ Adverse Event[1]	Percentage of Patients Reporting Event		
	SYMBYAX		Placebo
	Bipolar Depression (N=86)	SYMBYAX-Controlled (N=571)	(N=477)
Body as a Whole			
Asthena	13	15	3
Accidental injury	5	3	2
Fever	4	3	1
Cardiovascular System			
Hypertension	2	2	1
Tachycardia	2	2	0
Digestive System			
Diarrhea	19	8	7
Dry Mouth	16	11	6
Increased appetite	13	16	4
Tooth disorder	1	2	1
Metabolic and Nutritional Disorders			
Weight gain	17	21	3
Peripheral edema	4	8	1
Edema	0	5	0
Musculoskeletal System			
Joint disorder	1	2	1
Twitching	6	2	1
Arthralgia	5	3	1
Nervous System			
Somnolence	21	22	11
Tremor	9	8	3
Thinking abnormal	6	6	3
Libido decreased	4	2	1
Hyperkinesia	2	1	1
Personality disorder	2	1	1
Sleep disorder	2	1	1
Amnesia	1	3	0
Respiratory System			
Pharyngitis	4	6	3
Dyspnea	1	2	1
Special Senses			
Amblyopia	5	4	2
Ear pain	2	1	1
Otitis media	2	0	0
Speech disorder	0	2	0
Urogenital System			
Abnormal ejaculation[2]	7	2	1
Impotence[2]	4	2	1
Anorgasmia	3	1	0

[1] Included are events reported by at least 2% of patients taking SYMBYAX except the following events, which had an incidence on placebo ≥SYMBYAX: abdominal pain, abnormal dreams, agitation, akathisia, anorexia, anxiety, apathy, back pain, chest pain, constipation, cough increased, depression, dizziness, dysmenorrhea[2], dyspepsia, flatulence, flu syndrome, headache, hypertonia, insomnia, manic reaction, myalgia, nausea, nervousness, pain, palpitation, paresthesia, rash, rhinitis, sinusitis, sweating, vomiting.

[2] Adjusted for gender.

Additional Findings Observed in Clinical Studies

The following findings are based on clinical studies.

Effect on cardiac repolarization — The mean increase in QT_c interval for SYMBYAX-treated patients (4.9 msec) in clinical studies was significantly greater than that for placebo-treated (-0.9 msec) and olanzapine-treated (0.6 msec) patients, but was not significantly different from fluoxetine-treated (3.7 msec) patients. There were no differences between patients treated with SYMBYAX, placebo, olanzapine, or fluoxetine in the incidence of QT_c outliers (>500 msec).

Laboratory changes — In clinical studies, SYMBYAX was associated with asymptomatic mean increases in alkaline phosphatase, cholesterol, GGT, and uric acid compared with placebo (*see* PRECAUTIONS, Transaminase elevations).

SYMBYAX was associated with a slight decrease in hemoglobin that was statistically significantly greater than that seen with placebo, olanzapine, and fluoxetine.

An elevation in serum prolactin was observed with SYMBYAX. This elevation was not statistically different than that seen with olanzapine (*see* PRECAUTIONS, Hyperprolactinemia).

Sexual dysfunction — In the pool of controlled SYMBYAX studies, there were higher rates of the treatment–emergent adverse events decreased libido, anorgasmia, impotence and abnormal ejaculation in the SYMBYAX group than in the placebo group. One case of decreased libido led to discontinuation in the SYMBYAX group. In the controlled studies that contained a fluoxetine arm, the rates of decreased libido and abnormal ejaculation in the SYMBYAX group were less than the rates in the fluoxetine group. None of the differences were statistically significant.

Sexual dysfunction, including priapism, has been reported with all SSRIs. While it is difficult to know the precise risk of sexual dysfunction associated with the use of SSRIs, physicians should routinely inquire about such possible side effects.

Vital signs — Tachycardia, bradycardia, and orthostatic hypotension have occurred in SYMBYAX-treated patients (*see* WARNINGS, Orthostatic hypotension). The mean pulse of SYMBYAX-treated patients was reduced by 1.6 beats/min.

Other Events Observed in Clinical Studies

Following is a list of all treatment-emergent adverse events reported at anytime by individuals taking SYMBYAX in clinical studies except (1) those listed in the body or footnotes of Tables 2 and 3 above or elsewhere in labeling, (2) those for which the COSTART terms were uninformative or misleading, (3) those events for which a causal relationship to SYMBYAX use was considered remote, and (4) events occurring in only 1 patient treated with SYMBYAX and which did not have a substantial probability of being acutely life-threatening.

Events are classified within body system categories using the following definitions: frequent adverse events are defined as those occurring on 1 or more occasions in at least 1/100 patients, infrequent adverse events are those occurring in 1/100 to 1/1000 patients, and rare events are those occurring in <1/1000 patients.

Body as a Whole — *Frequent:* chills, infection, neck pain, neck rigidity, photosensitivity reaction; *Infrequent:* cellulitis, cyst, hernia, intentional injury, intentional overdose, malaise, moniliasis, overdose, pelvic pain, suicide attempt; *Rare:* death, tolerance decreased.

Cardiovascular System — *Frequent:* migraine, vasodilatation; *Infrequent:* arrhythmia, bradycardia, cerebral ischemia, electrocardiogram abnormal, hypotension, QT-interval prolonged; *Rare:* angina pectoris, atrial arrhythmia, atrial fibrillation, bundle branch block, congestive heart failure, myocardial infarct, peripheral vascular disorder, T-wave inverted.

Digestive System — *Frequent:* increased salivation, thirst; *Infrequent:* cholelithiasis, colitis, eructation, esophagitis, gastritis, gastroenteritis, gingivitis, hepatomegaly, nausea and vomiting, peptic ulcer, periodontal abscess, stomatitis, tooth caries; *Rare:* aphthous stomatitis, fecal incontinence, gastrointestinal hemorrhage, gum hemorrhage, intestinal obstruction, liver fatty deposit, pancreatitis.

Endocrine System — *Infrequent:* hypothyroidism.

Hemic and Lymphatic System — *Frequent:* ecchymosis; *Infrequent:* anemia, leukocytosis, lymphadenopathy; *Rare:* coagulation disorder, leukopenia, purpura, thrombocythemia.

Metabolic and Nutritional — *Frequent:* generalized edema, weight loss; *Infrequent:* alcohol intolerance, dehydration, glycosuria, hyperlipemia, hypoglycemia, hypokalemia, obesity; *Rare:* acidosis, bilirubinemia, creatinine increased, gout, hyperkalemia, hypoglycemic reaction.

Musculoskeletal System — *Infrequent:* arthritis, bone disorder, generalized spasm, leg cramps, tendinous contracture, tenosynovitis; *Rare:* arthrosis, bursitis, myasthenia, myopathy, osteoporosis, rheumatoid arthritis.

Nervous System — *Infrequent:* abnormal gait, ataxia, buccoglossal syndrome, cogwheel rigidity, coma, confusion, depersonalization, dysarthria, emotional lability, euphoria, extrapyramidal syndrome, hostility, hypesthesia, hypokinesia, incoordination, movement disorder, myoclonus, neuralgia, neurosis, vertigo; *Rare:* acute brain syndrome, aphasia, dystonia, libido increased, subarachnoid hemorrhage, withdrawal syndrome.

Respiratory System — *Frequent:* bronchitis, lung disorder; *Infrequent:* apnea, asthma, epistaxis, hiccup, hyperventilation, laryngitis, pneumonia, voice alteration, yawn; *Rare:* emphysema, hemoptysis, laryngismus.

Skin and Appendages — *Infrequent:* acne, alopecia, contact dermatitis, dry skin, eczema, pruritis, psoriasis, skin discoloration, vesiculobullous rash; *Rare:* exfoliative dermatitis, maculopapular rash, seborrhea, skin ulcer.

Special Senses — *Frequent:* abnormal vision, taste perversion, tinnitus; *Infrequent:* abnormality of accommodation, conjunctivitis, deafness, diplopia, dry eyes, eye pain, miosis; *Rare:* eye hemorrhage.

Urogenital System — *Frequent:* breast pain, menorrhagia[1], urinary frequency, urinary incontinence, urinary tract infection; *Infrequent:* amenorrhea[1], breast enlargement, breast neoplasm, cystitis, dysuria, female lactation[1], fibrocystic breast[1], hematuria, hypomenorrhea[1], leukorrhea[1], menopause[1], metrorrhagia[1], oliguria, ovarian disorder[1], polyuria, urinary retention, urinary urgency, urination impaired, vaginal hemorrhage[1], vaginal moniliasis[1], vaginitis[1]; *Rare:* breast carcinoma, breast engorgement, endometrial disorder[1], gynecomastia[1], kidney calculus, uterine fibroids enlarged[1].

[1] Adjusted for gender.

Other Events Observed with Olanzapine or Fluoxetine Monotherapy

The following adverse events were not observed in SYMBYAX-treated patients during premarketing clinical studies but have been reported with olanzapine or fluoxetine monotherapy: aplastic anemia, cholestatic jaundice, diabetic coma, dyskinesia, eosinophilic pneumonia, hepatitis, idiosyncratic hepatitis, priapism, pulmonary embolism, serotonin syndrome, serum sickness-like reaction, sudden unexpected death, suicidal ideation, vasculitis, violent behaviors.

DRUG ABUSE AND DEPENDENCE

Controlled substance class — SYMBYAX is not a controlled substance.

Physical and psychological dependence — SYMBYAX, as with fluoxetine and olanzapine, has not been systematically studied in humans for its potential for abuse, tolerance, or physical dependence. While the clinical studies did not reveal any tendency for any drug-seeking behavior, these observations were not systematic, and it is not possible to predict on the basis of this limited experience the extent to which a CNS-active drug will be misused, diverted, and/or abused once marketed. Consequently, physicians should carefully evaluate patients for history of drug abuse and follow such patients closely, observing them for signs of misuse or abuse of SYMBYAX (e.g., development of tolerance, incrementation of dose, drug-seeking behavior).

In studies in rats and Rhesus monkeys designed to assess abuse and dependence potential, olanzapine alone was shown to have acute depressive CNS effects but little or no potential of abuse or physical dependence at oral doses up to 15 (rat) and 8 (monkey) times the MRHD (20 mg) on a mg/m^2 basis.

OVERDOSAGE

SYMBYAX

During premarketing clinical studies of the olanzapine/fluoxetine combination, overdose of both fluoxetine and olanzapine were reported in five study subjects. Four of the five subjects experienced loss of consciousness (3) or coma (1). No fatalities occurred.

Since the market introduction of olanzapine in October 1996, adverse event cases involving combination use of fluoxetine and olanzapine have been reported to Eli Lilly and Company. An overdose of combination therapy is defined as confirmed or suspected ingestion of a dose of olanzapine 20 mg or greater in combination with a dose of fluoxetine 80 mg or greater. As of 1 February 2002, 12 cases of combination therapy overdose were reported, most of which involved additional substances. Adverse events associated with these reports included somnolence; impaired consciousness (coma, lethargy); impaired neurologic function (ataxia, confusion, convulsions, dysarthria); arrhythmias; and fatality. Fatalities have been confounded by exposure to additional substances including alcohol, thioridazine, oxycodone, and propoxyphene.

Olanzapine

In postmarketing reports of overdose with olanzapine alone, symptoms have been reported in the majority of cases. In symptomatic patients, symptoms with ≥10% incidence included agitation/aggressiveness, dysarthria, tachycardia, various extrapyramidal symptoms, and reduced level of consciousness ranging from sedation to coma. Among less commonly reported symptoms were the following potentially medically serious events: aspiration, cardiopulmonary arrest, cardiac arrhythmias (such as supraventricular tachycardia as well as a patient that experienced sinus pause with spontaneous resumption of normal rhythm), delirium, possible neuroleptic malignant syndrome, respiratory depression/arrest, convulsion, hypertension, and hypotension. Eli Lilly and Company has received reports of fatality in association with overdose of olanzapine alone. In 1 case of death, the amount of acutely ingested olanzapine was reported to be possibly as low as 450 mg; however, in another case, a patient was reported to survive an acute olanzapine ingestion of 1500 mg.

Fluoxetine

Worldwide exposure to fluoxetine is estimated to be over 38 million patients (circa 1999). Of the 1578 cases of overdose involving fluoxetine, alone or with other drugs, reported from this population, there were 195 deaths.

Among 633 adult patients who overdosed on fluoxetine alone, 34 resulted in a fatal outcome, 378 completely recovered, and 15 patients experienced sequelae after overdose, including abnormal accommodation, abnormal gait, confusion, unresponsiveness, nervousness, pulmonary dysfunction, vertigo, tremor, elevated blood pressure, impotence, movement disorder, and hypomania. The remaining 206 patients had an unknown outcome. The most common signs and symptoms associated with non-fatal overdose were seizures, somnolence, nausea, tachycardia, and vomiting. The largest known ingestion of fluoxetine in adult patients was 8 grams in a patient who took fluoxetine alone and who subsequently recovered. However, in an adult patient who took fluoxetine alone, an ingestion as low as 520 mg has been associated with lethal outcome, but causality has not been established.

Among pediatric patients (ages 3 months to 17 years), there were 156 cases of overdose involving fluoxetine alone or in combination with other drugs. Six patients died, 127 patients completely recovered, 1 patient experienced renal failure, and 22 patients had an unknown outcome. One of the 6 fatalities was a 9-year-old boy who had a history of OCD, Tourette's Syndrome with tics, attention deficit disorder, and fetal alcohol syndrome. He had been receiving 100 mg of fluoxetine daily for 6 months in addition to clonidine, methylphenidate, and promethazine. Mixed-drug ingestion or other methods of suicide complicated all 6 overdoses in children that resulted in fatalities. The largest ingestion in pediatric patients was 3 grams, which was nonlethal.

Other important adverse events reported with fluoxetine overdose (single or multiple drugs) included coma, delirium, ECG abnormalities (such as QT-interval prolongation and ventricular tachycardia, including torsades de pointes-type arrhythmias), hypotension, mania, neuroleptic malignant syndrome-like events, pyrexia, stupor, and syncope.

Management of overdose — In managing overdose, the possibility of multiple drug involvement should be considered. In case of acute overdose, establish and maintain an airway and ensure adequate ventilation, which may include intubation. Induction of emesis is not recommended as the possibility of obtundation, seizures, or dystonic reactions of the head and neck following overdose may create a risk for aspiration. Gastric lavage (after intubation, if patient is unconscious) and administration of activated charcoal together with a laxative should be considered. Cardiovascular monitoring should commence immediately and should include continuous electrocardiographic monitoring to detect possible arrhythmias.

A specific precaution involves patients who are taking or have recently taken SYMBYAX and may have ingested excessive quantities of a TCA (tricyclic antidepressant). In such cases, accumulation of the parent TCA and/or an active metabolite may increase the possibility of serious sequelae and extend the time needed for close medical observation.

Due to the large volume of distribution of olanzapine and fluoxetine, forced diuresis, dialysis, hemoperfusion, and exchange transfusion are unlikely to be of benefit. No specific antidote for either fluoxetine or olanzapine overdose is known. Hypotension and circulatory collapse should be treated with appropriate measures such as intravenous fluids and/or sympathomimetic agents. Do not use epinephrine, dopamine, or other sympathomimetics with β-agonist activity, since beta stimulation may worsen hypotension in the setting of olanzapine-induced alpha blockade.

The physician should consider contacting a poison control center for additional information on the treatment of any overdose. Telephone numbers for certified poison control centers are listed in the *Physicians' Desk Reference (PDR)*.

DOSAGE AND ADMINISTRATION

SYMBYAX should be administered once daily in the evening, generally beginning with the 6-mg/25-mg capsule. While food has no appreciable effect on the absorption of olanzapine and fluoxetine given individually, the effect of food on the absorption of SYMBYAX has not been studied. Dosage adjustments, if indicated, can be made according to efficacy and tolerability. Antidepressant efficacy was demonstrated with SYMBYAX in a dose range of olanzapine 6 to 12 mg and fluoxetine 25 to 50 mg (*see* CLINICAL STUDIES).

The safety of doses above 18 mg/75 mg has not been evaluated in clinical studies.

Special Populations

The starting dose of SYMBYAX 6 mg/25 mg should be used for patients with a predisposition to hypotensive reactions, patients with hepatic impairment, or patients who exhibit a combination of factors that may slow the metabolism of SYMBYAX (female gender, geriatric age, nonsmoking status). When indicated, dose escalation should be performed with caution in these patients. SYMBYAX has not been systematically studied in patients over 65 years of age or in patients <18 years of age (*see* WARNINGS, Orthostatic Hypotension, PRECAUTIONS, Pediatric Use, *and* Geriatric Use, *and* CLINICAL PHARMACOLOGY, Pharmacokinetics).

HOW SUPPLIED

SYMBYAX capsules are supplied in 6/25-, 6/50-, 12/25-, and 12/50-mg (mg equivalent olanzapine/mg equivalent fluoxetine[a]) strengths.

SYMBYAX	CAPSULE STRENGTH			
	6 mg/25 mg	6 mg/50 mg	12 mg/25 mg	12 mg/50 mg
Color	Mustard Yellow & Light Yellow	Mustard Yellow & Light Grey	Red & Light Yellow	Red & Light Grey
Capsule No.	PU3231	PU3233	PU3232	PU3234
Identification	Lilly 3231 6/25	Lilly 3233 6/50	Lilly 3232 12/25	Lilly 3234 12/50
NDC Codes				
Bottles 30	0002-3231-30	0002-3233-30	0002-3232-30	0002-3234-30
Bottles 100	0002-3231-02	0002-3233-02	0002-3232-02	0002-3234-02
Bottles 1000	0002-3231-04	0002-3233-04	0002-3232-04	0002-3234-04
Blisters ID[b] 100	0002-3231-33	0002-3233-33	0002-3232-33	0002-3234-33

[a] Fluoxetine base equivalent.
[b] IDENTI-DOSE®, Unit Dose Medication, Lilly.

[See table above]

Store at 25°C (77°F); excursions permitted to 15–30°C (59–86°F) [see USP Controlled Room Temperature].

Keep tightly closed and protect from moisture.

Patient Information

SYMBYAX™ (SIM-bee-ax)
(olanzapine and fluoxetine HCl capsules)

Read the Patient Information that comes with SYMBYAX before you start using it and each time you get a refill. There may be new information. This information does not take the place of talking with your doctor about your medical condition or treatment. It is important to stay under a doctor's care while taking SYMBYAX. **Do not change or stop treatment without first talking with your doctor.** Talk to your doctor or pharmacist if you have any questions about SYMBYAX.

What is SYMBYAX?

SYMBYAX is a prescription medicine used to treat adults who have depression with bipolar disorder. SYMBYAX contains two medicines, olanzapine and fluoxetine hydrochloride.

Olanzapine is also the active ingredient in Zyprexa® and Zyprexa Zydis®. Fluoxetine hydrochloride is also the active ingredient in Prozac®, Prozac Weekly™, and Sarafem®.

SYMBYAX has not been studied in children.

What is bipolar disorder?

Bipolar disorder, once called manic-depressive illness, is a brain disorder that causes unusual changes in a person's mood, energy level, and ability to function. Bipolar disorder is a long-term illness that can be treated with medicines, but it usually requires life-long treatment.

Who should not take SYMBYAX?

Do not take SYMBYAX if you are:

- **Taking a medicine known as a monoamine oxidase inhibitor (MAOI) or have stopped taking a MAOI within the last 2 weeks.** An MAOI is a medicine sometimes used for depression and other mental problems. Examples of MAOI medicines are Nardil® (phenylzine sulfate) and Parnate® (tranylcypromine sulfate). Taking SYMBYAX with a MAOI may cause serious side effects that can be life threatening. Do not take a MAOI for at least 5 weeks after you stop taking SYMBYAX.
- **Taking Mellaril® (thioridazine) for mental problems.** Mellaril® (thioridazine) can cause a heart problem (prolongation of the QT_c interval) **that can cause death.** Taking SYMBYAX with Mellaril® (thioridazine) can increase your chances of having this serious and life-threatening heart problem. Do not take Mellaril® (thioridazine) for at least 5 weeks after you stop taking SYMBYAX.
- **Allergic to SYMBYAX or any of its ingredients.** The active ingredients are olanzapine and fluoxetine hydrochloride. See the end of this leaflet for a complete list of ingredients in SYMBYAX.

What should I tell my doctor before taking SYMBYAX?

- **Tell your doctor if you are taking fluoxetine, Prozac, Prozac Weekly, Sarafem, olanzapine, Zyprexa, or Zyprexa Zydis.** These medicines each contain an active ingredient that is also found in SYMBYAX.
- **Tell your doctor about all the medicines you take, including prescription and non-prescription medicines, vitamins and herbal supplements. SYMBYAX can interact with many other medicines, causing serious or life-threatening side effects.** Your doctor will decide if you can take SYMBYAX with your other medicines, or if your dose should be adjusted. Keep a list of your medicines with you and show it to your doctor and pharmacist every time you are prescribed a new medicine or start a new non-prescription medicine, vitamin, or herbal supplement.
- **Tell your doctor if you are taking SYMBYAX and are taking or plan to take nonsteroidal anti-inflammatory drugs or aspirin** since combined use of these drug products has been associated with an increased risk of bleeding.

Before taking SYMBYAX, tell your doctor if you have or had the following medical conditions:

- **Are pregnant or plan to become pregnant.** It is not known if SYMBYAX can harm your unborn baby. You and your doctor should decide if SYMBYAX is right for you during pregnancy.
- **Are breast-feeding or plan to breast-feed.** SYMBYAX may pass into your milk and may harm your baby. You should choose either to breast-feed or take SYMBYAX, but not both.
- **Are older than age 65 and have a mental problem called dementia** (slow loss of mental function)
- **High blood sugar, diabetes or family history of diabetes**
- **Liver problems.** You may need a lower dose of SYMBYAX.
- **Seizures** (convulsions or fits)
- **Low blood pressure.** SYMBYAX may cause dizziness or fainting in people with low blood pressure.
- **Heart problems including heart attacks**
- **Strokes, or mini-strokes called transient ischemic attacks (TIA)**
- **High blood pressure**
- **An enlarged prostate** (men)
- **An eye problem called narrow angle glaucoma**
- **A stomach problem called a paralytic ileus**

Also, tell your doctor if you

- **Currently smoke**
- **Drink alcohol,** especially if you drink a lot
- **Exercise a lot** or are often in **hot places**

How should I take SYMBYAX?

- Take SYMBYAX exactly as instructed by your doctor. Your doctor will usually start you on a low dose of SYMBYAX. Your dose may be adjusted depending on your body's response to SYMBYAX. Your dose will also depend on certain medical problems you have. **Do not stop taking SYMBYAX or change your dose even if you feel better, without talking with your doctor.**
- SYMBYAX is usually taken once a day in the evening. Take SYMBYAX at the same time each day. SYMBYAX may be taken with or without food.
- If you miss a dose, take it as soon as you remember. However, if it is almost time for your next dose, skip the missed dose and take only your regularly scheduled dose. Do not take more than your doctor has prescribed for you.
- Tell your doctor if your depression does not get better while taking SYMBYAX. Your doctor may adjust your dose or give you a different medicine.
- If you take too much SYMBYAX or overdose, call your doctor or poison control center right away, or go to the nearest emergency room.

What should I avoid while taking SYMBYAX?

- Do not drive or operate other dangerous machinery until you know how SYMBYAX affects you. SYMBYAX can impair your judgment, thinking, and motor skills.
- Do not take medicines, including prescription and nonprescription medicines, vitamins and herbal supplements unless you have talked to your doctor about them.
- Do not get pregnant.
- Do not breast-feed.
- Do not drink alcohol.
- Do not get over-heated or dehydrated (loss of body fluids) during hot weather or exercise, or when using a hot tub.
- Do not take a MAOI medicine or Mellaril® (thioridazine) for **at least 5 weeks** after you stop taking SYMBYAX.

Continued on next page

*** Identi-Code® symbol. This product information was prepared in June 2004. Current information on these and other products of Eli Lilly and Company may be obtained by direct inquiry to Lilly Research Laboratories, Lilly Corporate Center, Indianapolis, Indiana 46285, (800) 545-5979.**

Symbyax—Cont.

What are the possible side effects of SYMBYAX?
All medicines may cause side effects in some patients. Serious side effects reported by patients treated with SYMBYAX follow below:

- **Severe allergic reactions** that cause hives, swelling of your face, eyes, mouth, or tongue, trouble breathing or a rash with fever and joint pain. Tell your doctor right away if you get these symptoms. Your doctor may stop SYMBYAX and prescribe medicines to treat your allergic reaction.
- **Strokes and "mini-strokes" called transient ischemic attacks (TIAs).** These are more common in elderly patients with dementia. As with other mental health drugs, SYMBYAX should be used with caution in elderly patients with dementia. SYMBYAX is not approved for the treatment of elderly patients with dementia.
- **High blood sugar or diabetes.** Patients who already have diabetes should have their blood sugar checked regularly during treatment with SYMBYAX. Patients at risk for diabetes (for example, those who are overweight or have a family history of diabetes) who are starting treatment with SYMBYAX should undergo blood sugar testing on an empty stomach at the beginning of treatment and regularly during treatment. Any patient treated with SYMBYAX should be monitored for signs of high blood sugar including being thirsty, going to the bathroom a lot, eating a lot, and feeling weak. Patients who develop signs of high blood sugar during treatment with SYMBYAX should undergo blood sugar testing on an empty stomach. In some cases, high blood sugar has gone away when SYMBYAX was stopped; however, some patients had to keep taking medicine for diabetes even though they stopped taking SYMBYAX.
- **Neuroleptic malignant syndrome (NMS).** NMS is a rare, but life-threatening reaction to certain medicines for mental problems, including SYMBYAX. Stop taking SYMBYAX and call your doctor right away if you get any of the following symptoms of NMS, such as a high fever, sweating, muscle stiffness, trouble thinking clearly, a change in mental functioning, sleepiness, or changes in your breathing, heartbeat, and blood pressure. NMS can cause death and must be treated in a hospital.
- **Tardive dyskinesia.** This is a condition caused by certain medicines for mental problems, including SYMBYAX. It causes body movements, mostly in your face or tongue, that keep happening and that you cannot control. It may start after you stop taking SYMBYAX. Tardive dyskinesia may not go away, even if you stop taking SYMBYAX. Tell your doctor if you get body movements that you can't control.
- **Low blood pressure.** SYMBYAX may cause low blood pressure in some patients. Low blood pressure is more likely in patients who have heart problems, who have brain problems such as strokes, who take certain medicines, or who drink alcohol. Signs of low blood pressure include dizziness, fast heartbeat, and fainting. To lower your chances of fainting while taking SYMBYAX, stand up slowly if you have been sitting or lying down.
- **Seizures.** SYMBYAX should be used cautiously in people who have had seizures in the past or who have conditions that increase their risk for seizures.
- **Impaired judgment, thinking, and motor skills**
- **Trouble swallowing**
- **Abnormal bleeding.** When SYMBYAX is used alone, and especially with certain other medicines that can increase bleeding risk (for example; ibuprofen or aspirin), your risk of bleeding can increase. If you notice increased or unusual bruising or other bleeding, contact your doctor.
- **Low salt levels in the blood.** SYMBYAX can cause a low salt level in the blood. Weakness, confusion, or trouble thinking can be caused by low salt levels in the blood. If you develop any of these symptoms, contact your doctor.
- **Body temperature problems.** SYMBYAX can cause problems in keeping your body temperature regular. Do not become overheated or dehydrated during hot weather or exercise, or when using a hot tub.

Common side effects of SYMBYAX are:

- Weight gain
- Sleepiness
- Diarrhea
- Dry mouth
- Increased appetite
- Feeling weak
- Swelling of your hands and feet
- Tremors (shakes)
- Sore throat
- Trouble concentrating
- SYMBYAX can cause problems in keeping your body temperature regulated.

Tell your doctor about any side effect that bothers you or won't go away. Your doctor may be able to help you manage the side effect.
These are not all the side effects of SYMBYAX. For more information ask your doctor or pharmacist.

Other important safety information about SYMBYAX

- The symptoms of bipolar disorder may include thoughts of harming yourself or others or committing suicide. Tell your doctor immediately or go to an emergency center if you have any of these thoughts.
- Symptoms of bipolar disorder may include mania. If you experience manic symptoms (for example; racing thoughts, poor sleep, irritability, mood swings, extra energy), contact your doctor.
- If your depression becomes worse, contact your doctor.
- Rarely, people taking medicines of this type have started to leak milk from their breasts, and women have missed periods or had irregular periods. If these symptoms occur, contact your doctor.
- If you gain weight while taking SYMBYAX, contact your doctor to discuss changes you can make in your activities or eating habits to help manage your weight.
- Problems with sexual functioning have commonly occurred in patients taking SYMBYAX. If these symptoms occur, contact your doctor.

How do I store SYMBYAX?

- Store SYMBYAX at room temperature, 59° to 86°F (15° to 30°C).
- Keep the container tightly closed and protect from moisture.
- **Keep SYMBYAX and all medicines away from children.**

General information about SYMBYAX
Medicines are sometimes prescribed for conditions that are not mentioned in patient information leaflets. Do not take SYMBYAX for a condition for which it was not prescribed. Do not give SYMBYAX to other people, even if they have the same symptoms that you have. It may harm them.
This leaflet summarizes important information about SYMBYAX. If you would like more information, talk with your doctor. You can ask your doctor or pharmacist for information that is written for health professionals. You can also call 1-800-Lilly-Rx (1-800-545-5979) or visit our website at www.SYMBYAX.com.

What are the ingredients in SYMBYAX?
Active ingredients: olanzapine and fluoxetine hydrochloride
Inactive ingredients: pregelatinized starch, gelatin, dimethicone, titanium dioxide, sodium lauryl sulfate, edible black ink, red iron oxide, yellow iron oxide, and/or black iron oxide.
Rx Only
This patient information has been approved by the US Food and Drug Administration.
Literature revised December 30, 2003
Eli Lilly and Company
Indianapolis, IN 46285
www.SYMBYAX.com
PV 4201 AMP

Shown in Product Identification Guide, page 320

VANCOCIN® HCl ℞

[văn 'kō-sĭn ăch 'sē-ĕl]
Vancomycin Hydrochloride
Capsules, USP
Pulvules®

To reduce the development of drug-resistant bacteria and maintain the effectiveness of Vancocin® HCl and other antibacterial drugs, Vancocin HCl should be used only to treat or prevent infections that are proven or strongly suspected to be caused by bacteria.

This preparation for the treatment of colitis is for oral use only and is not systemically absorbed. Vancocin® HCl must be given orally for treatment of staphylococcal enterocolitis and antibiotic-associated pseudomembranous colitis caused by *Clostridium difficile*. Orally administered Vancocin HCl is not effective for other types of infection. Parenteral administration of Vancocin HCl is *not* effective for treatment of staphylococcal enterocolitis and antibiotic-associated pseudomembranous colitis caused by *C. difficile*. If parenteral vancomycin therapy is desired, use Vancocin® HCl (Sterile Vancomycin Hydrochloride, USP), IntraVenous, and consult package insert accompanying that preparation.

DESCRIPTION

Pulvules® Vancocin® HCl (Vancomycin Hydrochloride Capsules, USP) contain chromatographically purified vancomycin hydrochloride, a tricyclic glycopeptide antibiotic derived from *Amycolatopsis orientalis* (formerly *Nocardia orientalis*), which has the chemical formula $C_{66}H_{75}Cl_2N_9O_{24}$•HCl. The molecular weight of vancomycin hydrochloride is 1485.73; 500 mg of the base is equivalent to 0.34 mmol.
The Pulvules contain vancomycin hydrochloride equivalent to 125 mg (0.08 mmol) or 250 mg (0.17 mmol) vancomycin. The Pulvules also contain F D & C Blue No. 2, gelatin, iron oxide, polyethylene glycol, titanium dioxide, and other inactive ingredients.
Vancomycin hydrochloride has the following structural formula:
[See chemical structure at top of next column]

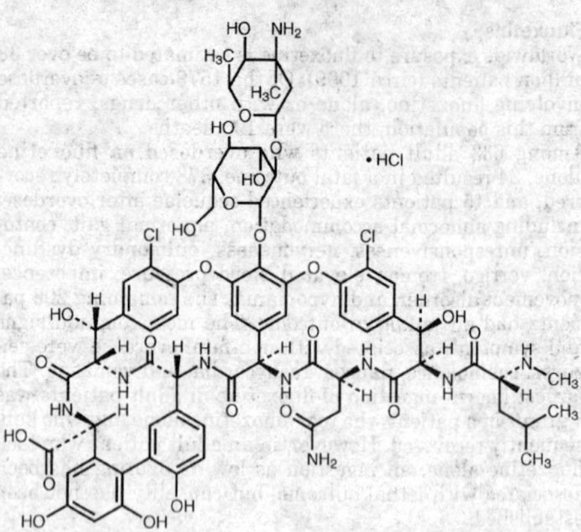

CLINICAL PHARMACOLOGY

Vancomycin is poorly absorbed after oral administration. During multiple dosing of 250 mg every 8 hours for 7 doses, fecal concentrations of vancomycin in volunteers exceeded 100 mg/kg in the majority of samples. No blood concentrations were detected and urinary recovery did not exceed 0.76%. Additional data using an oral solution follow. In anephric patients with no inflammatory bowel disease, blood concentrations of vancomycin were barely measurable (0.66 µg/mL) in 2 of 5 subjects who received 2 g of Vancocin HCl for Oral Solution daily for 16 days. No measurable blood concentrations were attained in the other 3 patients. With doses of 2 g daily, very high concentrations of drug can be found in the feces (>3100 mg/kg) and very low concentrations (<1 µg/mL) can be found in the serum of patients with normal renal function who have pseudomembranous colitis. Orally administered vancomycin does not usually enter the systemic circulation even when inflammatory lesions are present. After multiple-dose oral administration of vancomycin, measurable serum concentrations may infrequently occur in patients with active *C. difficile*-induced pseudomembranous colitis, and, in the presence of renal impairment, the possibility of accumulation exists.

Microbiology
The bactericidal action of vancomycin results primarily from inhibition of cell-wall biosynthesis. In addition, vancomycin alters bacterial-cell-membrane permeability and RNA synthesis. There is no cross-resistance between vancomycin and other antibiotics.
NOTE: The oral form of vancomycin is effective only for the infections noted in the **INDICATIONS AND USAGE** section. The oral form is ***not*** effective for any other type of infection.
Vancomycin has been shown to be active against most strains of the following microorganisms in clinical infections as described in the **INDICATIONS AND USAGE** section.
Aerobic gram-positive microorganisms
Staphylococcus aureus (including methicillin-resistant strains) associated with enterocolitis
Anaerobic gram-positive microorganisms
Clostridium difficile antibiotic-associated pseudomembranous colitis

INDICATIONS AND USAGE

Vancocin HCl Pulvules may be administered orally for treatment of enterocolitis caused by *Staphylococcus aureus* (including methicillin-resistant strains) and antibiotic-associated pseudomembranous colitis caused by *C. difficile*. Parenteral administration of Vancocin HCl is not effective for the above indications; therefore, Vancocin HCl must be given orally for these indications. **Orally administered Vancocin HCl is not effective for other types of infection.**
To reduce the development of drug-resistant bacteria and maintain the effectiveness of Vancocin HCl and other antibacterial drugs, Vancocin HCl should be used only to treat or prevent infections that are proven or strongly suspected to be caused by susceptible bacteria. When culture and susceptibility information are available, they should be considered in selecting or modifying antibacterial therapy. In the absence of such data, local epidemiology and susceptibility patterns may contribute to the empiric selection of therapy.

CONTRAINDICATION

Vancocin HCl is contraindicated in patients with known hypersensitivity to this antibiotic.

PRECAUTIONS

General
Prescribing Vancocin HCl in the absence of a proven or strongly suspected bacterial infection or a prophylactic indication is unlikely to provide benefit to the patient and increases the risk of the development of drug-resistant bacteria.
Clinically significant serum concentrations have been reported in some patients who have taken multiple oral doses of vancomycin for active *C. difficile*-induced pseudomembranous colitis; therefore, monitoring of serum concentrations may be appropriate in some instances, e.g., in patients with renal insufficiency and/or colitis.
Some patients with inflammatory disorders of the intestinal mucosa may have significant systemic absorption of vancomycin and, therefore, may be at risk for the development of adverse reactions associated with the parenteral administration of vancomycin. (See package insert accompanying the intravenous preparation.) The risk is greater if renal impairment is present. It should be noted that the total systemic and renal clearances of vancomycin are reduced in the elderly.
Ototoxicity has occurred in patients receiving Vancocin HCl. It may be transient or permanent. It has been reported mostly in patients who have been given excessive intravenous doses, who have an underlying hearing loss, or who are receiving concomitant therapy with another ototoxic

agent, such as an aminoglycoside. Serial tests of auditory function may be helpful in order to minimize the risk of ototoxicity.

When patients with underlying renal dysfunction or those receiving concomitant therapy with an aminoglycoside are being treated, serial monitoring of renal function should be performed.

Use of vancomycin may result in the overgrowth of nonsusceptible organisms. If superinfection occurs during therapy, appropriate measures should be taken.

Information for Patients

Patients should be counseled that antibacterial drugs including Vancocin HCl should only be used to treat bacterial infections. They do not treat viral infections (e.g., the common cold). When Vancocin HCl is prescribed to treat a bacterial infection, patients should be told that although it is common to feel better early in the course of therapy, the medication should be taken exactly as directed. Skipping doses or not completing the full course of therapy may (1) decrease the effectiveness of the immediate treatment and (2) increase the likelihood that bacteria will develop resistance and will not be treatable by Vancocin HCl or other antibacterial drugs in the future.

Carcinogenesis, Mutagenesis, Impairment of Fertility

No long-term carcinogenesis studies in animals have been conducted.

At concentrations up to 1000 µg/mL, vancomycin had no mutagenic effect *in vitro* in the mouse lymphoma forward mutation assay or the primary rat hepatocyte unscheduled DNA synthesis assay. The concentrations tested *in vitro* were above the peak plasma vancomycin concentrations of 20 to 40 µg/mL usually achieved in humans after slow infusion of the maximum recommended dose of 1 g. Vancomycin had no mutagenic effect *in vivo* in the Chinese hamster sister chromatid exchange assay (400 mg/kg IP) or the mouse micronucleus assay (800 mg/kg IP).

No definitive fertility studies have been conducted.

Pregnancy

Teratogenic Effects—Pregnancy Category B—The highest doses of vancomycin tested were not teratogenic in rats given up to 200 mg/kg/day IV (1180 mg/m^2 or 1 times the recommended maximum human dose based on a mg/m^2 basis) or in rabbits given up to 120 mg/kg/day IV (1320 mg/m^2 or 1.1 times the recommended maximum human dose based on a mg/m^2 basis). No effects on fetal weight or development were seen in rats at the highest dose tested or in rabbits given 80 mg/kg/day (880 mg/m^2 or 0.74 times the recommended maximum human dose based on mg/m^2).

In a controlled clinical study, the potential ototoxic and nephrotoxic effects of Vancocin HCl on infants were evaluated when the drug was administered intravenously to pregnant women for serious staphylococcal infections complicating intravenous drug abuse. Vancocin HCl was found in cord blood. No sensorineural hearing loss or nephrotoxicity attributable to Vancocin HCl was noted. One infant whose mother received Vancocin HCl in the third trimester experienced conductive hearing loss that was not attributed to the administration of Vancocin HCl. Because the number of patients treated in this study was limited and Vancocin HCl was administered only in the second and third trimesters, it is not known whether Vancocin HCl causes fetal harm. Because animal reproduction studies are not always predictive of human response, Vancocin HCl should be given to a pregnant woman only if clearly needed.

Nursing Mothers

Vancomycin is excreted in human milk based on information obtained with the intravenous administration of Vancocin HCl. However, systemic absorption of vancomycin is very low following oral administration of Vancocin HCl Pulvules (*see* **CLINICAL PHARMACOLOGY**). It is not known whether oral vancomycin is excreted in human milk, as no studies of vancomycin concentration in human milk after oral administration have been done. Caution should be exercised when Vancocin HCl is administered to a nursing woman. Because of the potential for adverse events, a decision should be made whether to discontinue nursing or discontinue the drug, taking into account the importance of the drug to the mother.

Pediatric Use

Safety and effectiveness in pediatric patients have not been established.

ADVERSE REACTIONS

Nephrotoxicity—Rarely, renal failure, principally manifested by increased serum creatinine or BUN concentrations, especially in patients given large doses of intravenously administered Vancocin HCl has been reported. Rare cases of interstitial nephritis have been reported. Most of these have occurred in patients who were given aminoglycosides concomitantly or who had preexisting kidney dysfunction. When Vancocin HCl was discontinued, azotemia resolved in most patients.

Ototoxicity—A few dozen cases of hearing loss associated with intravenously administered Vancocin HCl have been reported. Most of these patients had kidney dysfunction or a preexisting hearing loss or were receiving concomitant treatment with an ototoxic drug. Vertigo, dizziness, and tinnitus have been reported rarely.

Hematopoietic—Reversible neutropenia, usually starting 1 week or more after onset of intravenous therapy with Vancocin HCl or after a total dose of more than 25 g, has been reported for several dozen patients. Neutropenia appears to be promptly reversible when Vancocin HCl is discontinued. Thrombocytopenia has rarely been reported.

Miscellaneous—Infrequently, patients have been reported to have had anaphylaxis, drug fever, chills, nausea, eosinophilia, rashes (including exfoliative dermatitis), Stevens-Johnson syndrome, toxic epidermal necrolysis, and rare cases of vasculitis in association with the administration of Vancocin HCl.

A condition has been reported that is similar to the IV-induced syndrome with symptoms consistent with anaphylactoid reactions, including hypotension, wheezing, dyspnea, urticaria, pruritus, flushing of the upper body ("Red Man Syndrome"), pain and muscle spasm of the chest and back. These reactions usually resolve within 20 minutes but may persist for several hours.

OVERDOSAGE

Supportive care is advised, with maintenance of glomerular filtration. Vancomycin is poorly removed by dialysis. Hemofiltration and hemoperfusion with polysulfone resin have been reported to result in increased vancomycin clearance.

Treatment—To obtain up-to-date information about the treatment of overdose, a good resource is your certified Regional Poison Control Center. Telephone numbers of certified poison control centers are listed in the *Physicians' Desk Reference (PDR)*. In managing overdosage, consider the possibility of multiple drug overdoses, interaction among drugs, and unusual drug kinetics in your patient.

DOSAGE AND ADMINISTRATION

Adults—Oral Vancocin HCl is used in treating antibiotic-associated pseudomembranous colitis caused by *C. difficile* and staphylococcal enterocolitis. Vancocin HCl is not effective by the oral route for other types of infections. The usual adult total daily dosage is 500 mg to 2 g administered orally in 3 or 4 divided doses for 7 to 10 days.

Pediatric Patients—The usual daily dosage is 40 mg/kg in 3 or 4 divided doses for 7 to 10 days. The total daily dosage should not exceed 2 g.

HOW SUPPLIED

Vancocin® HCl Pulvules® (or Vancomycin Hydrochloride Capsules, USP) are available in:

The 125 mg* Pulvules have an opaque blue cap and opaque brown body imprinted with "3125" on the cap and "VANCOCIN HCL 125 MG" on the body in white ink. They are available in:

ID†20 NDC 0002-3125-42 (PU3125)

The 250 mg* Pulvules have an opaque blue cap and opaque lavender body imprinted with "3126" on the cap and "VANCOCIN HCL 250 MG" on the body in white ink. They are available in:

ID†20 NDC 0002-3126-42 (PU3126)

Store at controlled room temperature, 59° to 86°F (15° to 30°C).

*Equivalent to vancomycin.

†Identi-Dose® (unit dose medication, Lilly).

Literature revised March 5, 2003

Eli Lilly and Company
Indianapolis, IN 46285, USA
www.lilly.com

PV 1985 AMP PRINTED IN USA

XIGRIS® ℞

[zī′grĭs]

Drotrecogin alfa (activated)

DESCRIPTION

Xigris® (drotrecogin alfa (activated)) is a recombinant form of human Activated Protein C. An established human cell line possessing the complementary DNA for the inactive human Protein C zymogen secretes the protein into the fermentation medium. Fermentation is carried out in a nutrient medium containing the antibiotic geneticin sulfate. Geneticin sulfate is not detectable in the final product. Human Protein C is enzymatically activated by cleavage with thrombin and subsequently purified.

Drotrecogin alfa (activated) is a serine protease with the same amino acid sequence as human plasma-derived Activated Protein C. Drotrecogin alfa (activated) is a glycoprotein of approximately 55 kilodalton molecular weight, consisting of a heavy chain and a light chain linked by a disulfide bond. Drotrecogin alfa (activated) and human plasma-derived Activated Protein C have the same sites of glycosylation, although some differences in the glycosylation structures exist.

Xigris is supplied as a sterile, lyophilized, white to off-white powder for intravenous infusion. The 5 and 20 mg vials of Xigris contain 5.3 mg and 20.8 mg of drotrecogin alfa (activated), respectively. The 5 and 20 mg vials of Xigris also contain 40.3 and 158.1 mg of sodium chloride, 10.9 and 42.9 mg of sodium citrate, and 31.8 and 124.9 mg of sucrose, respectively.

CLINICAL PHARMACOLOGY

General Pharmacology

Activated Protein C exerts an antithrombotic effect by inhibiting Factors Va and VIIIa. *In vitro* data indicate that Activated Protein C has indirect profibrinolytic activity through its ability to inhibit plasminogen activator inhibitor-1 (PAI-1) and limiting generation of activated thrombin-activatable-fibrinolysis-inhibitor. Additionally, *in vitro* data indicate that Activated Protein C may exert an anti-inflammatory effect by inhibiting human tumor necrosis factor production by monocytes, by blocking leukocyte adhesion to selectins, and by limiting the thrombin-induced inflammatory responses within the microvascular endothelium.

Pharmacodynamics

The specific mechanisms by which Xigris exerts its effect on survival in patients with severe sepsis are not completely understood. In patients with severe sepsis, Xigris infusions of 48 or 96 hours produced dose dependent declines in D-dimer and IL-6. Compared to placebo, Xigris-treated patients experienced more rapid declines in D-dimer, PAI-1 levels, thrombin-antithrombin levels, prothrombin F1.2, IL-6, more rapid increases in protein C and antithrombin levels, and normalization of plasminogen. As assessed by infusion duration, the maximum observed pharmacodynamic effect of drotrecogin alfa (activated) on D-dimer levels occurred at the end of 96 hours of infusion for the 24 µg/kg/hr treatment group.

Human Pharmacokinetics

Xigris and endogenous Activated Protein C are inactivated by endogenous plasma protease inhibitors. Plasma concentrations of endogenous Activated Protein C in healthy subjects and patients with severe sepsis are usually below detection limits.

In patients with severe sepsis, Xigris infusions of 12 µg/kg/hr to 30 µg/kg/hr rapidly produce steady state concentrations (C_{ss}) that are proportional to infusion rates. In the Phase 3 trial (*see* **CLINICAL STUDIES**), the median clearance of Xigris was 40 L/hr (interquartile range of 27 to 52 L/hr). The median C_{ss} of 45 ng/mL (interquartile range of 35 to 62 ng/mL) was attained within 2 hours after starting infusion. In the majority of patients, plasma concentrations of Xigris fell below the assay's quantitation limit of 10 ng/mL within 2 hours after stopping infusion. Plasma clearance of Xigris in patients with severe sepsis is approximately 50% higher than that in healthy subjects.

Special Populations

In adult patients with severe sepsis, small differences were detected in the plasma clearance of Xigris with regard to age, gender, hepatic dysfunction or renal dysfunction. Dose adjustment is not required based on these factors alone or in combination (*see* **PRECAUTIONS**).

End stage renal disease—Patients with end stage renal disease requiring chronic renal replacement therapy were excluded from the Phase 3 study. In patients without sepsis undergoing hemodialysis (n=6), plasma clearance (mean ± SD) of Xigris administered on non-dialysis days was 30 ± 8 L/hr. Plasma clearance of Xigris was 23 ± 4 L/hr in patients without sepsis undergoing peritoneal dialysis (n=5). These clearance rates did not meaningfully differ from those in normal healthy subjects (28 ± 9 L/hr) (n=190).

Pediatrics—Safety and efficacy have not been established in pediatric patients with severe sepsis (*see* **INDICATIONS AND USAGE**), therefore no dosage recommendation can be made. The pharmacokinetics of a dose of 24 µg/kg/hr of Xigris appear to be similar in pediatric and adult patients with severe sepsis.

Drug-Drug Interactions—Formal drug interactions studies have not been conducted.

CLINICAL STUDIES

The efficacy of Xigris was studied in an international, multicenter, randomized, double-blind, placebo-controlled trial (PROWESS) of 1690 patients with severe sepsis.[1] Entry criteria included a systemic inflammatory response presumed due to infection and at least one associated acute organ dysfunction. Acute organ dysfunction was defined as one of the following: cardiovascular dysfunction (shock, hypotension, or the need for vasopressor support despite adequate fluid resuscitation); respiratory dysfunction (relative hypoxemia (PaO_2/FiO_2 ratio <250)); renal dysfunction (oliguria despite adequate fluid resuscitation); thrombocytopenia (platelet count <80,000/mm^3 or 50% decrease from the highest value the previous 3 days); or metabolic acidosis with elevated lactic acid concentrations. Patients received a 96 hour infusion of Xigris at 24 µg/kg/hr or placebo starting within 48 hours after the onset of the first sepsis induced organ dysfunction. Exclusion criteria encompassed patients at high risk for bleeding (*see* **CONTRAINDICATIONS** *and* **WARNINGS**), patients who were not expected to survive for 28 days due to a pre-existing, non-sepsis related medical condition, HIV positive patients whose most recent CD_4 count was ≤50/mm^3, patients on chronic dialysis, and patients who had undergone bone marrow, lung, liver, pancreas or small bowel transplantation.

The primary efficacy endpoint was all-cause mortality assessed 28 days after the start of study drug administration. Prospectively defined subsets for mortality analyses included groups defined by APACHE II score[2] (a score designed to assess risk of mortality based on acute physiology and chronic health evaluation, see http://www.sfar.org/scores2/scores2.html), protein C activity, and the number of acute organ dysfunctions at baseline. The APACHE II score

Continued on next page

*** Identi-Code® symbol. This product information was prepared in June 2004. Current information on these and other products of Eli Lilly and Company may be obtained by direct inquiry to Lilly Research Laboratories, Lilly Corporate Center, Indianapolis, Indiana 46285, (800) 545-5979.**

Xigris—Cont.

was calculated from physiologic and laboratory data obtained within the 24-hour period immediately preceding the start of study drug administration irrespective of the preceding length of stay in the Intensive Care Unit.

The study was terminated after a planned interim analysis due to significantly lower mortality in patients on Xigris than in patients on placebo (210/850, 25% vs. 259/840, 31% p=0.005, see Table 1).

Baseline APACHE II score, as measured in PROWESS, was correlated with risk of death; among patients receiving placebo, those with the lowest APACHE II scores had a 12% mortality rate, while those in the 2nd, 3rd, and 4th APACHE quartiles had mortality rates of 26%, 36% and 49%, respectively. The observed mortality difference between Xigris and placebo was limited to the half of patients with higher risk of death, i.e., APACHE II score ≥25, the 3rd and 4th quartile APACHE II scores (Table 1). The efficacy of Xigris has not been established in patients with lower risk of death, e.g., APACHE II score <25.

[See table 1 below]

Of measures used, the APACHE II score was most effective in classifying patients by risk of death within 28 days and by likelihood of benefit from Xigris, but other important indicators of risk or severity also supported an association between likelihood of Xigris benefit and risk of death. Absolute reductions in mortality of 2%, 5%, 8% and 11% with Xigris were observed for patients with 1, 2, 3, and 4 or more organ dysfunctions, respectively. Similarly, each of the three major components of the APACHE II score (acute physiology score, chronic health score, age score) identified a higher risk population with larger mortality differences associated with treatment. That is, the reduction in mortality was greater in patients with more severe physiologic disturbances, in patients with serious underlying disease predating sepsis, and in older patients.

Treatment-associated reductions in mortality were observed in patients with normal protein C levels and those with low protein C levels. No substantial differences in Xigris treatment effects were observed in subgroups defined by gender, ethnic origin, or infectious agent.

Long-Term Follow-Up

The one-year survival status was provided for 93% of the 1690 PROWESS subjects. For patients with APACHE II score ≥25, mortality was lower for the Xigris group compared to the placebo group through 90-days (41% versus 52%; RR: 0.72, 95% CI: 0.59–0.88) and through 1 year (48% versus 59%; RR: 0.73, 95% CI: 0.60–0.88). However, for patients with APACHE II score <25, mortality was higher for the Xigris group compared to the placebo group through 90-days (27% versus 25%; RR: 1.09, 95% CI: 0.84–1.42) and through 1 year (35% versus 28%; RR: 1.24, 95% CI: 0.97–1.58).

INDICATIONS AND USAGE

Xigris is indicated for the reduction of mortality in adult patients with severe sepsis (sepsis associated with acute organ dysfunction) who have a high risk of death (e.g., as determined by APACHE II, *see* **CLINICAL STUDIES**).

Safety and efficacy have not been established in adult patients with severe sepsis and lower risk of death (*see* **CLINICAL STUDIES, Long-Term Follow-Up**). Safety and efficacy have not been established in pediatric patients with severe sepsis.

CONTRAINDICATIONS

Xigris increases the risk of bleeding. Xigris is contraindicated in patients with the following clinical situations in which bleeding could be associated with a high risk of death or significant morbidity:

- Active internal bleeding
- Recent (within 3 months) hemorrhagic stroke
- Recent (within 2 months) intracranial or intraspinal surgery, or severe head trauma
- Trauma with an increased risk of life-threatening bleeding
- Presence of an epidural catheter
- Intracranial neoplasm or mass lesion or evidence of cerebral herniation

Xigris is contraindicated in patients with known hypersensitivity to drotrecogin alfa (activated) or any component of this product.

WARNINGS

Bleeding is the most common serious adverse effect associated with Xigris therapy. Each patient being considered for therapy with Xigris should be carefully evaluated and anticipated benefits weighed against potential risks associated with therapy.

Certain conditions, many of which led to exclusion from the Phase 3 trial, are likely to increase the risk of bleeding with Xigris therapy. For individuals with one or more of the following conditions, the increased risk of bleeding should be carefully considered when deciding whether to use Xigris therapy:

- Concurrent therapeutic dosing of heparin to treat an active thrombotic or embolic event (*see* **PRECAUTIONS, Drug Interactions**)
- Platelet count $<30{,}000 \times 10^6$/L, even if the platelet count is increased after transfusions
- Prothrombin time-INR >3.0
- Recent (within 6 weeks) gastrointestinal bleeding
- Recent administration (within 3 days) of thrombolytic therapy
- Recent administration (within 7 days) of oral anticoagulants or glycoprotein IIb/IIIa inhibitors
- Recent administration (within 7 days) of aspirin >650 mg per day or other platelet inhibitors
- Recent (within 3 months) ischemic stroke (*see* **CONTRAINDICATIONS**)
- Intracranial arteriovenous malformation or aneurysm
- Known bleeding diathesis
- Chronic severe hepatic disease
- Any other condition in which bleeding constitutes a significant hazard or would be particularly difficult to manage because of its location

Should clinically important bleeding occur, immediately stop the infusion of Xigris. Continued use of other agents affecting the coagulation system should be carefully assessed. Once adequate hemostasis has been achieved, continued use of Xigris may be reconsidered.

Xigris should be discontinued 2 hours prior to undergoing an invasive surgical procedure or procedures with an inherent risk of bleeding. Once adequate hemostasis has been achieved, initiation of Xigris may be reconsidered 12 hours after major invasive procedures or surgery or restarted immediately after uncomplicated less invasive procedures.

PRECAUTIONS

Laboratory Tests

Most patients with severe sepsis have a coagulopathy that is commonly associated with prolongation of the activated partial thromboplastin time (APTT) and the prothrombin time (PT). Xigris may variably prolong the APTT. Therefore, the APTT cannot be reliably used to assess the status of the coagulopathy during Xigris infusion. Xigris has minimal effect on the PT and the PT can be used to monitor the status of the coagulopathy in these patients.

Immunogenicity

As with all therapeutic proteins, there is a potential for immunogenicity. The incidence of antibody development in patients receiving Xigris has not been adequately determined, as the assay sensitivity is inadequate to reliably detect all potential antibody responses. One patient in the Phase 2 trial developed antibodies to Xigris without clinical sequelae. One patient in the Phase 3 trial who developed antibodies to Xigris developed superficial and deep vein thrombi during the study, and died of multi-organ failure on day 36 post-treatment but the relationship of this event to antibody is not clear.

Xigris has not been readministered to patients with severe sepsis.

Drug Interactions

Drug interaction studies with Xigris have not been performed in patients with severe sepsis. However, since there is an increased risk of bleeding with Xigris, caution should be employed when Xigris is used with other drugs that affect hemostasis (*see* **CLINICAL PHARMACOLOGY, WARNINGS**). Approximately 2/3 of the patients in the Phase 3 study received either prophylactic low dose heparin (unfractionated heparin up to 15,000 units/day) or prophylactic doses of low molecular weight heparins as indicated in the prescribing information for the specific products. Concomitant use of prophylactic low dose heparin did not appear to affect safety, however, its effects on the efficacy of Xigris have not been evaluated in an adequate and well-controlled clinical trial.

Drug/Laboratory Test Interaction

Because Xigris may affect the APTT assay, Xigris present in plasma samples may interfere with one-stage coagulation assays based on the APTT (such as factor VIII, IX, and XI assays). This interference may result in an apparent factor concentration that is lower than the true concentration. Xigris present in plasma samples does not interfere with one-stage factor assays based on the PT (such as factor II, V, VII, and X assays).

Carcinogenesis, Mutagenesis, Impairment of Fertility

Long-term studies in animals to evaluate potential carcinogenicity of Xigris have not been performed.

Xigris was not mutagenic in an *in vivo* micronucleus study in mice or in an *in vitro* chromosomal aberration study in human peripheral blood lymphocytes with or without rat liver metabolic activation.

The potential of Xigris to impair fertility has not been evaluated in male or female animals.

Pregnancy Category C

Animal reproductive studies have not been conducted with Xigris. It is not known whether Xigris can cause fetal harm when administered to a pregnant woman or can affect reproduction capacity. Xigris should be given to pregnant women only if clearly needed.

Nursing Mothers

It is not known whether Xigris is excreted in human milk or absorbed systemically after ingestion. Because many drugs are excreted in human milk, and because of the potential for adverse effects on the nursing infant, a decision should be made whether to discontinue nursing or discontinue the drug, taking into account the importance of the drug to the mother.

Pediatric Use

The safety and effectiveness of Xigris have not been established in the age group newborn (38 weeks gestational age) to 18 years. The efficacy of Xigris in adult patients with severe sepsis and high risk of death cannot be extrapolated to pediatric patients with severe sepsis.

Geriatric Use

In clinical studies evaluating 1821 patients with severe sepsis, approximately 50% of the patients were 65 years or older. No overall differences in safety or effectiveness were observed between these patients and younger patients.

ADVERSE REACTIONS

Bleeding

Bleeding is the most common adverse reaction associated with Xigris.

In the Phase 3 study, serious bleeding events were observed during the 28-day study period in 3.5% of Xigris-treated and 2.0% of placebo-treated patients, respectively. The difference in serious bleeding between Xigris and placebo occurred primarily during the infusion period and is shown in Table 2.[1] Serious bleeding events were defined as any intracranial hemorrhage, any life-threatening bleed, any bleeding event requiring the administration of ≥3 units of packed red blood cells per day for 2 consecutive days, or any bleeding event assessed as a serious adverse event.

Table 2: Number of Patients Experiencing a Serious Bleeding Event by Site of Hemorrhage During the Study Drug Infusion Period[a] in PROWESS[1]

	Xigris N=850	Placebo N=840
Total	**20 (2.4%)**	**8 (1.0%)**
Site of Hemorrhage		
Gastrointestinal	5	4
Intra-abdominal	2	3
Intra-thoracic	4	0
Retroperitoneal	3	0
Intracranial	2	0
Genitourinary	2	0
Skin/soft tissue	1	0
Other[b]	1	1

[a] Study drug infusion period is defined as the date of initiation of study drug to the date of study drug discontinuation plus the next calendar day.

[b] Patients requiring the administration of ≥3 units of packed red blood cells per day for 2 consecutive days without an identified site of bleeding.

In PROWESS, 2 cases of intracranial hemorrhage (ICH) occurred during the infusion period for Xigris-treated patients and no cases were reported in the placebo patients. The incidence of ICH during the 28-day study period was 0.2% for Xigris-treated patients and 0.1% for placebo-treated patients. ICH has been reported in patients receiving Xigris in non-placebo controlled trials with an incidence of approximately 1% during the infusion period. The risk of ICH may be increased in patients with risk factors for bleeding such as severe coagulopathy and severe thrombocytopenia (*see* **WARNINGS**).

In PROWESS, 25% of the Xigris-treated patients and 18% of the placebo-treated patients experienced at least one bleeding event during the 28-day study period. In both treatment groups, the majority of bleeding events were ecchymoses or gastrointestinal tract bleeding.

Other Adverse Reactions

Patients administered Xigris as treatment for severe sepsis experience many events which are potential sequelae of severe sepsis and may or may not be attributable to Xigris

Table 1: 28-Day All-Cause Mortality for All Patients and for Subgroups Defined by APACHE II Score[a]

	Xigris Total N[b]	N[c] (%)	Placebo Total N	N (%)	Absolute Mortality Difference (%)	Relative Risk (RR)	95% CI for RR
Overall	850	210 (25)	840	259 (31)	-6	0.81	0.70, 0.93
APACHE II quartile (score)							
1st + 2nd (3–24)	436	82 (19)	437	83 (19)	0	0.99	0.75, 1.30
3rd + 4th (25–53)	414	128 (31)	403	176 (44)	-13	0.71	0.59, 0.85

[a] For more information on calculating the APACHE II score, see: http://www.sfar.org/scores2/scores2.html

[b] Total N = Total number of patients in group.

[c] N = Number of deaths in group.

therapy. In clinical trials, there were no types of non-bleeding adverse events suggesting a causal association with Xigris.

OVERDOSAGE

There is no known antidote for Xigris. In case of overdose, immediately stop the infusion and monitor closely for hemorrhagic complications (*see* **Human Pharmacokinetics**).

Post-marketing experience: There have been some reports of accidental overdosing. In the majority of these cases (which included patients receiving up to 60 times the recommended dose administration rate), no reactions have been observed. For the other reports, the observed events were consistent with known effects of the drug and/or sequelae of the underlying condition of sepsis.

DOSAGE AND ADMINISTRATION

Xigris should be administered intravenously at an infusion rate of 24 µg/kg/hr for a total duration of infusion of 96 hours. Dose adjustment based on clinical or laboratory parameters is not recommended (*see* **PRECAUTIONS**).

If the infusion is interrupted, Xigris should be restarted at the 24 µg/kg/hr infusion rate. Dose escalation or bolus doses of Xigris are not recommended.

In the event of clinically important bleeding, immediately stop the infusion (*see* **WARNINGS**).

Preparation and administration instructions:

1. Use appropriate aseptic technique during the preparation of Xigris for intravenous administration.
2. Calculate the dose and the number of Xigris vials needed. Each 5 mg and 20 mg vial of Xigris contains an excess of Xigris to facilitate delivery of the labeled amount.
3. Prior to administration, 5 mg vials must be reconstituted with 2.5 mL of Sterile Water for Injection, USP, and 20 mg vials of Xigris must be reconstituted with 10 mL of Sterile Water for Injection, USP. The resulting concentration of the solution is approximately 2 mg/mL of Xigris. Slowly add the Sterile Water for Injection, USP to the vial and avoid inverting or shaking the vial. Gently swirl each vial until the powder is completely dissolved.
4. Because Xigris contains no antibacterial preservatives, the intravenous solution should be prepared immediately upon reconstitution of the Xigris in the vial(s). If the vial of reconstituted Xigris is not used immediately, it may be held at controlled room temperature 20° to 25°C (68° to 77°F), but must be used within 3 hours.
5. Before further dilution or administration, the product should be inspected visually for particulate matter and discoloration. Do not use vials if particulate matter is visible or solution is discolored.
6. Xigris should be administered via a dedicated intravenous line or a dedicated lumen of a multilumen central venous catheter. The ONLY other solutions that can be administered through the same line are 0.9% Sodium Chloride Injection, USP; Lactated Ringer's Injection, USP; Dextrose Injection, USP; and Dextrose and Sodium Chloride Injection, USP.
7. Avoid exposing Xigris solutions to heat and/or direct sunlight. Studies conducted at the recommended concentrations indicate the Xigris intravenous solution to be compatible with glass infusion bottles, and infusion bags and syringes made of polyvinylchloride, polyethylene, polypropylene, or polyolefin.

Dilution and Administration Instructions for an Intravenous Infusion Pump:

8. The solution of reconstituted Xigris must be further diluted into an infusion bag containing 0.9% Sodium Chloride Injection, USP to a final concentration of between 100 µg/mL and 200 µg/mL. Slowly withdraw the reconstituted Xigris solution from the vial(s) and add the reconstituted Xigris into a prepared infusion bag of 0.9% Sodium Chloride Injection, USP. When injecting the Xigris into the infusion bag, direct the stream to the side of the bag to minimize the agitation of the solution. Gently invert the infusion bag to obtain a homogeneous solution. Do not transport the infusion bag using mechanical transport systems such as pneumatic-tube systems that may cause vigorous agitation of the solution.
9. After preparation, the intravenous solution should be used at controlled room temperature 20° to 25°C (68° to 77°F) within 14 hours. If the intravenous solution is not administered immediately, the solution may be stored refrigerated 2° to 8°C (36° to 46°F) for up to 12 hours. If the prepared solution is refrigerated prior to administration, **the maximum time limit for use of the intravenous solution, including preparation, refrigeration, and administration, is 24 hours.**

Dilution and Administration Instructions for a Syringe Pump:

10. The solution of reconstituted Xigris must be further diluted with 0.9% Sodium Chloride Injection, USP to a final concentration of between 100 µg/mL and 1000 µg/mL. Slowly withdraw the reconstituted Xigris solution from the vial(s) into a syringe that will be used in the syringe pump. Into the same syringe, slowly withdraw 0.9% Sodium Chloride Injection, USP to obtain the desired final concentration of Xigris. Gently invert and/or rotate the syringe to obtain a homogenous solution. When administering Xigris using a syringe pump at low concentrations (less than approximately 200 µg/mL) at low flow rates (less than approximately 5 mL/hr), the infusion set must be primed for approximately 15 minutes at a flow rate of approximately 5 mL/hr.
11. After preparation, the intravenous solution should be used at controlled room temperature 20° to 25°C (68° to 77°F) within 12 hours. **The maximum time limit for use of the intravenous solution, including preparation and administration, is 12 hours.**

HOW SUPPLIED

Xigris is available in 5 mg and 20 mg single-use vials containing sterile, preservative-free, lyophilized drotrecogin alfa (activated).

Vials:

5 mg Vials
NDC 0002-7559-01

20 mg Vials
NDC 0002-7561-01

Xigris should be stored in a refrigerator 2° to 8°C (36° to 46°F). Do not freeze. Protect unreconstituted vials of Xigris from light. Retain in carton until time of use. Do not use beyond the expiration date stamped on the vial.

REFERENCES

1. Bernard GR, et al. Efficacy and Safety of Recombinant Human Activated Protein C for Severe Sepsis. *N Engl J Med.* 2001;344:699–709
2. Knaus WA, et al. APACHE II: a severity of disease classification system. *Crit Care Med.* 1985;13:818–29

Literature revised November 14, 2003

Eli Lilly and Company
Indianapolis, IN 46285, USA
www.lilly.com
PV 3425 AMP PRINTED IN USA

Shown in Product Identification Guide, page 320

ZYPREXA® ℞

[zī-prex-ah]

Olanzapine Tablets

ZYPREXA® ZYDIS®

Olanzapine Orally Disintegrating Tablets

ZYPREXA® IntraMuscular

Olanzapine for Injection

DESCRIPTION

ZYPREXA (olanzapine) is a psychotropic agent that belongs to the thienobenzodiazepine class. The chemical designation is 2-methyl-4-(4-methyl-1-piperazinyl)-10*H*-thieno[2,3-*b*][1,5]benzodiazepine. The molecular formula is $C_{17}H_{20}N_4S$, which corresponds to a molecular weight of 312.44. The chemical structure is:

[chemical structure of olanzapine]

Olanzapine is a yellow crystalline solid, which is practically insoluble in water.

ZYPREXA tablets are intended for oral administration only.

Each tablet contains olanzapine equivalent to 2.5 mg (8 µmol), 5 mg (16 µmol), 7.5 mg (24 µmol), 10 mg (32 µmol), 15 mg (48 µmol), or 20 mg (64 µmol). Inactive ingredients are carnauba wax, crospovidone, hydroxypropyl cellulose, hypromellose, lactose, magnesium stearate, microcrystalline cellulose, and other inactive ingredients. The color coating contains Titanium Dioxide (all strengths), FD&C Blue No. 2 Aluminum Lake (15 mg), or Synthetic Red Iron Oxide (20 mg). The 2.5, 5.0, 7.5, and 10 mg tablets are imprinted with edible ink which contains FD&C Blue No. 2 Aluminum Lake.

ZYPREXA ZYDIS (olanzapine orally disintegrating tablets) is intended for oral administration only.

Each orally disintegrating tablet contains olanzapine equivalent to 5 mg (16 µmol), 10 mg (32 µmol), 15 mg (48 µmol) or 20 mg (64 µmol). It begins disintegrating in the mouth within seconds, allowing its contents to be subsequently swallowed with or without liquid. ZYPREXA ZYDIS (olanzapine orally disintegrating tablets) also contains the following inactive ingredients: gelatin, mannitol, aspartame, sodium methyl paraben and sodium propyl paraben.

ZYPREXA IntraMuscular (olanzapine for injection) is intended for intramuscular use only.

Each vial provides for the administration of 10 mg (32 µmol) olanzapine with inactive ingredients 50 mg lactose monohydrate and 3.5 mg tartaric acid. Hydrochloric acid and/or sodium hydroxide may have been added during manufacturing to adjust pH.

CLINICAL PHARMACOLOGY

Pharmacodynamics

Olanzapine is a selective monoaminergic antagonist with high affinity binding to the following receptors: serotonin $5HT_{2A/2C}$ (K_i=4 and 11 nM, respectively), dopamine D_{1-4} (K_i=11–31 nM), muscarinic M_{1-5} (K_i=1.9–25 nM), histamine H_1 (K_i=7 nM), and adrenergic α_1 receptors (K_i=19 nM). Olanzapine binds weakly to $GABA_A$, BZD, and β adrenergic receptors (K_i>10 µM).

The mechanism of action of olanzapine, as with other drugs having efficacy in schizophrenia, is unknown. However, it has been proposed that this drug's efficacy in schizophrenia is mediated through a combination of dopamine and serotonin type 2 ($5HT_2$) antagonism. The mechanism of action of olanzapine in the treatment of acute manic episodes associated with Bipolar I Disorder is unknown.

Antagonism at receptors other than dopamine and $5HT_2$ with similar receptor affinities may explain some of the other therapeutic and side effects of olanzapine. Olanzapine's antagonism of muscarinic M_{1-5} receptors may explain its anticholinergic effects. Olanzapine's antagonism of histamine H_1 receptors may explain the somnolence observed with this drug. Olanzapine's antagonism of adrenergic α_1 receptors may explain the orthostatic hypotension observed with this drug.

Pharmacokinetics

Oral Administration

Olanzapine is well absorbed and reaches peak concentrations in approximately 6 hours following an oral dose. It is eliminated extensively by first pass metabolism, with approximately 40% of the dose metabolized before reaching the systemic circulation. Food does not affect the rate or extent of olanzapine absorption. Pharmacokinetic studies showed that ZYPREXA tablets and ZYPREXA ZYDIS (olanzapine orally disintegrating tablets) dosage forms of olanzapine are bioequivalent.

Olanzapine displays linear kinetics over the clinical dosing range. Its half-life ranges from 21 to 54 hours (5th to 95th percentile; mean of 30 hr), and apparent plasma clearance ranges from 12 to 47 L/hr (5th to 95th percentile; mean of 25 L/hr).

Administration of olanzapine once daily leads to steady-state concentrations in about one week that are approximately twice the concentrations after single doses. Plasma concentrations, half-life, and clearance of olanzapine may vary between individuals on the basis of smoking status, gender, and age (*see* Special Populations).

Olanzapine is extensively distributed throughout the body, with a volume of distribution of approximately 1000 L. It is 93% bound to plasma proteins over the concentration range of 7 to 1100 ng/mL, binding primarily to albumin and α_1-acid glycoprotein.

Metabolism and Elimination — Following a single oral dose of ^{14}C labeled olanzapine, 7% of the dose of olanzapine was recovered in the urine as unchanged drug, indicating that olanzapine is highly metabolized. Approximately 57% and 30% of the dose was recovered in the urine and feces, respectively. In the plasma, olanzapine accounted for only 12% of the AUC for total radioactivity, indicating significant exposure to metabolites. After multiple dosing, the major circulating metabolites were the 10-N-glucuronide, present at steady state at 44% of the concentration of olanzapine, and 4'-N-desmethyl olanzapine, present at steady state at 31% of the concentration of olanzapine. Both metabolites lack pharmacological activity at the concentrations observed.

Direct glucuronidation and cytochrome P450 (CYP) mediated oxidation are the primary metabolic pathways for olanzapine. In vitro studies suggest that CYPs 1A2 and 2D6, and the flavin-containing monooxygenase system are involved in olanzapine oxidation. CYP2D6 mediated oxidation appears to be a minor metabolic pathway in vivo, because the clearance of olanzapine is not reduced in subjects who are deficient in this enzyme.

Intramuscular Administration

ZYPREXA IntraMuscular results in rapid absorption with peak plasma concentrations occurring within 15 to 45 minutes. Based upon a pharmacokinetic study in healthy volunteers, a 5 mg dose of intramuscular olanzapine for injection produces, on average, a maximum plasma concentration approximately 5 times higher than the maximum plasma concentration produced by a 5 mg dose of oral olanzapine. Area under the curve achieved after an intramuscular dose is similar to that achieved after oral administration of the same dose. The half-life observed after intramuscular administration is similar to that observed after oral dosing. The pharmacokinetics are linear over the clinical dosing range. Metabolic profiles after intramuscular administration are qualitatively similar to metabolic profiles after oral administration.

Special Populations

Renal Impairment — Because olanzapine is highly metabolized before excretion and only 7% of the drug is excreted unchanged, renal dysfunction alone is unlikely to have a major impact on the pharmacokinetics of olanzapine. The pharmacokinetic characteristics of olanzapine were similar in patients with severe renal impairment and normal subjects, indicating that dosage adjustment based upon the degree of renal impairment is not required. In addition, olanzapine is not removed by dialysis. The effect of renal

Continued on next page

*** Identi-Code® symbol. This product information was prepared in June 2004. Current information on these and other products of Eli Lilly and Company may be obtained by direct inquiry to Lilly Research Laboratories, Lilly Corporate Center, Indianapolis, Indiana 46285, (800) 545-5979.**

Zyprexa—Cont.

impairment on metabolite elimination has not been studied.
Hepatic Impairment — Although the presence of hepatic impairment may be expected to reduce the clearance of olanzapine, a study of the effect of impaired liver function in subjects (n=6) with clinically significant (Childs Pugh Classification A and B) cirrhosis revealed little effect on the pharmacokinetics of olanzapine.
Age — In a study involving 24 healthy subjects, the mean elimination half-life of olanzapine was about 1.5 times greater in elderly (>65 years) than in non-elderly subjects (≤65 years). Caution should be used in dosing the elderly, especially if there are other factors that might additively influence drug metabolism and/or pharmacodynamic sensitivity (*see* DOSAGE AND ADMINISTRATION).
Gender — Clearance of olanzapine is approximately 30% lower in women than in men. There were, however, no apparent differences between men and women in effectiveness or adverse effects. Dosage modifications based on gender should not be needed.
Smoking Status — Olanzapine clearance is about 40% higher in smokers than in nonsmokers, although dosage modifications are not routinely recommended.
Race — In vivo studies have shown that exposures are similar among Japanese, Chinese and Caucasians, especially after normalization for body weight differences. Dosage modifications for race are, therefore, not recommended.
Combined Effects — The combined effects of age, smoking, and gender could lead to substantial pharmacokinetic differences in populations. The clearance in young smoking males, for example, may be 3 times higher than that in elderly nonsmoking females. Dosing modification may be necessary in patients who exhibit a combination of factors that may result in slower metabolism of olanzapine (*see* DOSAGE AND ADMINISTRATION).
For specific information about the pharmacology of lithium or valproate, refer to the CLINICAL PHARMACOLOGY section of the package inserts for these other products.

Clinical Efficacy Data

Schizophrenia

The efficacy of oral olanzapine in the treatment of schizophrenia was established in 2 short-term (6-week) controlled trials of inpatients who met DSM III-R criteria for schizophrenia. A single haloperidol arm was included as a comparative treatment in one of the two trials, but this trial did not compare these two drugs on the full range of clinically relevant doses for both.
Several instruments were used for assessing psychiatric signs and symptoms in these studies, among them the Brief Psychiatric Rating Scale (BPRS), a multi-item inventory of general psychopathology traditionally used to evaluate the effects of drug treatment in schizophrenia. The BPRS psychosis cluster (conceptual disorganization, hallucinatory behavior, suspiciousness, and unusual thought content) is considered a particularly useful subset for assessing actively psychotic schizophrenic patients. A second traditional assessment, the Clinical Global Impression (CGI), reflects the impression of a skilled observer, fully familiar with the manifestations of schizophrenia, about the overall clinical state of the patient. In addition, two more recently developed scales were employed; these included the 30-item Positive and Negative Symptoms Scale (PANSS), in which are embedded the 18 items of the BPRS, and the Scale for Assessing Negative Symptoms (SANS). The trial summaries below focus on the following outcomes: PANSS total and/or BPRS total; BPRS psychosis cluster; PANSS negative subscale or SANS; and CGI Severity. The results of the trials follow:
(1) In a 6-week, placebo-controlled trial (n=149) involving two fixed olanzapine doses of 1 and 10 mg/day (once daily schedule), olanzapine, at 10 mg/day (but not at 1 mg/day), was superior to placebo on the PANSS total score (also on the extracted BPRS total), on the BPRS psychosis cluster, on the PANSS Negative subscale, and on CGI Severity.
(2) In a 6-week, placebo-controlled trial (n=253) involving 3 fixed dose ranges of olanzapine (5.0 ± 2.5 mg/day, 10.0 ± 2.5 mg/day, and 15.0 ± 2.5 mg/day) on a once daily schedule, the two highest olanzapine dose groups (actual mean doses of 12 and 16 mg/day, respectively) were superior to placebo on BPRS total score, BPRS psychosis cluster, and CGI severity score; the highest olanzapine dose group was superior to placebo on the SANS. There was no clear advantage for the high dose group over the medium dose group.
Examination of population subsets (race and gender) did not reveal any differential responsiveness on the basis of these subgroupings.
In a longer-term trial, adult outpatients (n=326) who predominantly met DSM-IV criteria for schizophrenia and who remained stable on olanzapine during open label treatment for at least 8 weeks were randomized to continuation on their current olanzapine doses (ranging from 10 to 20 mg/day) or to placebo. The follow-up period to observe patients for relapse, defined in terms of increases in BPRS positive symptoms or hospitalization, was planned for 12 months, however, criteria were met for stopping the trial early due to an excess of placebo relapses compared to olanzapine relapses, and olanzapine was superior to placebo on time to relapse, the primary outcome for this study. Thus, olanzapine was more effective than placebo at maintaining efficacy in patients stabilized for approximately 8 weeks and followed for an observation period of up to 8 months.

Bipolar Disorder

Monotherapy — The efficacy of oral olanzapine in the treatment of acute manic or mixed episodes was established in 2 short-term (one 3-week and one 4-week) placebo-controlled trials in patients who met the DSM-IV criteria for Bipolar I Disorder with manic or mixed episodes. These trials included patients with or without psychotic features and with or without a rapid-cycling course.
The primary rating instrument used for assessing manic symptoms in these trials was the Young Mania Rating Scale (Y-MRS), an 11-item clinician-rated scale traditionally used to assess the degree of manic symptomatology (irritability, disruptive/aggressive behavior, sleep, elevated mood, speech, increased activity, sexual interest, language/thought disorder, thought content, appearance, and insight) in a range from 0 (no manic features) to 60 (maximum score). The primary outcome in these trials was change from baseline in the Y-MRS total score. The results of the trials follow:
(1) In one 3-week placebo-controlled trial (n=67) which involved a dose range of olanzapine (5–20 mg/day, once daily, starting at 10 mg/day), olanzapine was superior to placebo in the reduction of Y-MRS total score. In an identically designed trial conducted simultaneously with the first trial, olanzapine demonstrated a similar treatment difference, but possibly due to sample size and site variability, was not shown to be superior to placebo on this outcome.
(2) In a 4-week placebo-controlled trial (n=115) which involved a dose range of olanzapine (5–20 mg/day, once daily, starting at 15 mg/day), olanzapine was superior to placebo in the reduction of Y-MRS total score.
(3) In another trial, 361 patients meeting DSM-IV criteria for a manic or mixed episode of bipolar disorder who had responded during an initial open-label treatment phase for about two weeks, on average, to olanzapine 5 to 20 mg/day were randomized to either continuation of olanzapine at their same dose (n=225) or to placebo (n=136), for observation of relapse. Approximately 50% of the patients had discontinued from the olanzapine group by day 59 and 50% of the placebo group had discontinued by day 23 of double-blind treatment. Response during the open-label phase was defined by having a decrease of the Y-MRS total score to ≤12 and HAM-D 21 to ≤8. Relapse during the double-blind phase was defined as an increase of the Y-MRS or HAM-D 21 total score to ≥15, or being hospitalized for either mania or depression. In the randomized phase, patients receiving continued olanzapine experienced a significantly longer time to relapse.
Combination Therapy — The efficacy of oral olanzapine with concomitant lithium or valproate in the treatment of acute manic episodes was established in two controlled trials in patients who met the DSM-IV criteria for Bipolar I Disorder with manic or mixed episodes. These trials included patients with or without psychotic features and with or without a rapid-cycling course. The results of the trials follow:
(1) In one 6-week placebo-controlled combination trial, 175 outpatients on lithium or valproate therapy with inadequately controlled manic or mixed symptoms (Y-MRS ≥16) were randomized to receive either olanzapine or placebo, in combination with their original therapy. Olanzapine (in a dose range of 5–20 mg/day, once daily, starting at 10 mg/day) combined with lithium or valproate (in a therapeutic range of 0.6 mEq/L to 1.2 mEq/L or 50 μg/mL to 125 μg/mL, respectively) was superior to lithium or valproate alone in the reduction of Y-MRS total score.
(2) In a second 6-week placebo-controlled combination trial, 169 outpatients on lithium or valproate therapy with inadequately controlled manic or mixed symptoms (Y-MRS ≥16) were randomized to receive either olanzapine or placebo, in combination with their original therapy. Olanzapine (in a dose range of 5–20 mg/day, once daily, starting at 10 mg/day) combined with lithium or valproate (in a therapeutic range of 0.6 mEq/L to 1.2 mEq/L or 50 μg/mL to 125 μg/mL, respectively) was superior to lithium or valproate alone in the reduction of Y-MRS total score.

Agitation Associated with Schizophrenia and Bipolar I Mania

The efficacy of intramuscular olanzapine for injection for the treatment of agitation was established in 3 short-term (24 hours of IM treatment) placebo-controlled trials in agitated inpatients from two diagnostic groups: schizophrenia and Bipolar I Disorder (manic or mixed episodes). Each of the trials included a single active comparator treatment arm of either haloperidol injection (schizophrenia studies) or lorazepam injection (bipolar mania study). Patients enrolled in the trials needed to be: (1) judged by the clinical investigators as clinically agitated and clinically appropriate candidates for treatment with intramuscular medication, and (2) exhibiting a level of agitation that met or exceeded a threshold score of ≥14 on the five items comprising the Positive and Negative Syndrome Scale (PANSS) Excited Component (i.e., poor impulse control, tension, hostility, uncooperativeness and excitement items) with at least one individual item score ≥4 using a 1–7 scoring system (1=absent, 4=moderate, 7=extreme). In the studies, the mean baseline PANSS Excited Component score was 18.4, with scores ranging from 13 to 32 (out of a maximum score of 35), thus suggesting predominantly moderate levels of agitation with some patients experiencing mild or severe levels of agitation. The primary efficacy measure used for assessing agitation signs and symptoms in these trials was the change from baseline in the PANSS Excited Component at 2 hours post-injection. Patients could receive up to three injections during the 24 hour IM treatment periods; however, patients could not receive the second injection until after the initial 2 hour period when the primary efficacy measure was assessed. The results of the trials follow:
(1) In a placebo-controlled trial in agitated inpatients meeting DSM-IV criteria for schizophrenia (n=270), four fixed intramuscular olanzapine for injection doses of 2.5 mg, 5 mg, 7.5 mg and 10 mg were evaluated. All doses were statistically superior to placebo on the PANSS Excited Component at 2 hours post-injection. However, the effect was larger and more consistent for the three highest doses. There were no significant pairwise differences for the 7.5 and 10 mg doses over the 5 mg dose.
(2) In a second placebo-controlled trial in agitated inpatients meeting DSM-IV criteria for schizophrenia (n=311), one fixed intramuscular olanzapine for injection dose of 10 mg was evaluated. Olanzapine for injection was statistically superior to placebo on the PANSS Excited Component at 2 hours post-injection.
(3) In a placebo-controlled trial in agitated inpatients meeting DSM-IV criteria for Bipolar I Disorder (and currently displaying an acute manic or mixed episode with or without psychotic features) (n=201), one fixed intramuscular olanzapine for injection dose of 10 mg was evaluated. Olanzapine for injection was statistically superior to placebo on the PANSS Excited Component at 2 hours post-injection.
Examination of population subsets (age, race, and gender) did not reveal any differential responsiveness on the basis of these subgroupings.

INDICATIONS AND USAGE

Schizophrenia

Oral ZYPREXA is indicated for the treatment of schizophrenia.
The efficacy of ZYPREXA was established in short-term (6-week) controlled trials of schizophrenic inpatients (*see* CLINICAL PHARMACOLOGY).
The effectiveness of oral ZYPREXA at maintaining a treatment response in schizophrenic patients who had been stable on ZYPREXA for approximately 8 weeks and were then followed for a period of up to 8 months has been demonstrated in a placebo-controlled trial (*see* CLINICAL PHARMACOLOGY). Nevertheless, the physician who elects to use ZYPREXA for extended periods should periodically re-evaluate the long-term usefulness of the drug for the individual patient (*see* DOSAGE AND ADMINISTRATION).

Bipolar Disorder

Acute Monotherapy — Oral ZYPREXA is indicated for the treatment of acute mixed or manic episodes associated with Bipolar I Disorder.
The efficacy of ZYPREXA was established in two placebo-controlled trials (one 3-week and one 4-week) with patients meeting DSM-IV criteria for Bipolar I Disorder who currently displayed an acute manic or mixed episode with or without psychotic features (*see* CLINICAL PHARMACOLOGY).
Maintenance Monotherapy — The benefit of maintaining bipolar patients on monotherapy with oral ZYPREXA after achieving a responder status for an average duration of two weeks was demonstrated in a controlled trial (*see* Clinical Efficacy Data *under* CLINICAL PHARMACOLOGY). The physician who elects to use ZYPREXA for extended periods should periodically re-evaluate the long-term usefulness of the drug for the individual patient (*see* DOSAGE AND ADMINISTRATION).
Combination Therapy — The combination of oral ZYPREXA with lithium or valproate is indicated for the short-term treatment of acute manic episodes associated with Bipolar I Disorder.
The efficacy of ZYPREXA in combination with lithium or valproate was established in two placebo-controlled (6-week) trials with patients meeting DSM-IV criteria for Bipolar I Disorder who currently displayed an acute manic or mixed episode with or without psychotic features (*see* CLINICAL PHARMACOLOGY).

Agitation Associated with Schizophrenia and Bipolar I Mania

ZYPREXA IntraMuscular is indicated for the treatment of agitation associated with schizophrenia and bipolar I mania. "Psychomotor agitation" is defined in DSM-IV as "excessive motor activity associated with a feeling of inner tension." Patients experiencing agitation often manifest behaviors that interfere with their diagnosis and care, e.g., threatening behaviors, escalating or urgently distressing behavior, or self-exhausting behavior, leading clinicians to the use of intramuscular antipsychotic medications to achieve immediate control of the agitation.
The efficacy of ZYPREXA IntraMuscular for the treatment of agitation associated with schizophrenia and bipolar I mania was established in 3 short-term (24 hours) placebo-controlled trials in agitated inpatients with schizophrenia or Bipolar I Disorder (manic or mixed episodes) (*see* CLINICAL PHARMACOLOGY).

CONTRAINDICATIONS

ZYPREXA is contraindicated in patients with a known hypersensitivity to the product.
For specific information about the contraindications of lithium or valproate, refer to the CONTRAINDICATIONS section of the package inserts for these other products.

WARNINGS

Hyperglycemia and Diabetes Mellitus — Hyperglycemia, in some cases extreme and associated with ketoacidosis or hyperosmolar coma or death, has been reported in patients treated with atypical antipsychotics including olanzapine.

Assessment of the relationship between atypical antipsychotic use and glucose abnormalities is complicated by the possibility of an increased background risk of diabetes mellitus in patients with schizophrenia and the increasing incidence of diabetes mellitus in the general population. Given these confounders, the relationship between atypical antipsychotic use and hyperglycemia-related adverse events is not completely understood. However, epidemiological studies suggest an increased risk of treatment-emergent hyperglycemia-related adverse events in patients treated with the atypical antipsychotics. Precise risk estimates for hyperglycemia-related adverse events in patients treated with atypical antipsychotics are not available.

Patients with an established diagnosis of diabetes mellitus who are started on atypical antipsychotics should be monitored regularly for worsening of glucose control. Patients with risk factors for diabetes mellitus (e.g., obesity, family history of diabetes) who are starting treatment with atypical antipsychotics should undergo fasting blood glucose testing at the beginning of treatment and periodically during treatment. Any patient treated with atypical antipsychotics should be monitored for symptoms of hyperglycemia including polydipsia, polyuria, polyphagia, and weakness. Patients who develop symptoms of hyperglycemia during treatment with atypical antipsychotics should undergo fasting blood glucose testing. In some cases, hyperglycemia has resolved when the atypical antipsychotic was discontinued; however, some patients required continuation of anti-diabetic treatment despite discontinuation of the suspect drug.

Safety Experience in Elderly Patients with Dementia-Related Psychosis — In placebo-controlled clinical trials of elderly patients with dementia-related psychosis, the incidence of death in olanzapine-treated patients was significantly greater than placebo-treated patients (3.5% vs. 1.5%, respectively). Risk factors that may predispose this patient population to increased mortality when treated with olanzapine include age >80 years, sedation, concomitant use of benzodiazepines or presence of pulmonary conditions (e.g., pneumonia, with or without aspiration). Olanzapine is not approved for the treatment of patients with dementia-related psychosis.

Cerebrovascular Adverse Events, Including Stroke, in Elderly Patients with Dementia — Cerebrovascular adverse events (e.g., stroke, transient ischemic attack), including fatalities, were reported in patients in trials of olanzapine in elderly patients with dementia-related psychosis. In placebo-controlled trials, there was a significantly higher incidence of cerebrovascular adverse events in patients treated with olanzapine compared to patients treated with placebo. Olanzapine is not approved for the treatment of patients with dementia-related psychosis.

Neuroleptic Malignant Syndrome (NMS) — A potentially fatal symptom complex sometimes referred to as Neuroleptic Malignant Syndrome (NMS) has been reported in association with administration of antipsychotic drugs, including olanzapine. Clinical manifestations of NMS are hyperpyrexia, muscle rigidity, altered mental status and evidence of autonomic instability (irregular pulse or blood pressure, tachycardia, diaphoresis and cardiac dysrhythmia). Additional signs may include elevated creatinine phosphokinase, myoglobinuria (rhabdomyolysis), and acute renal failure.

The diagnostic evaluation of patients with this syndrome is complicated. In arriving at a diagnosis, it is important to exclude cases where the clinical presentation includes both serious medical illness (e.g., pneumonia, systemic infection, etc.) and untreated or inadequately treated extrapyramidal signs and symptoms (EPS). Other important considerations in the differential diagnosis include central anticholinergic toxicity, heat stroke, drug fever, and primary central nervous system pathology.

The management of NMS should include: 1) immediate discontinuation of antipsychotic drugs and other drugs not essential to concurrent therapy; 2) intensive symptomatic treatment and medical monitoring; and 3) treatment of any concomitant serious medical problems for which specific treatments are available. There is no general agreement about specific pharmacological treatment regimens for NMS.

If a patient requires antipsychotic drug treatment after recovery from NMS, the potential reintroduction of drug therapy should be carefully considered. The patient should be carefully monitored, since recurrences of NMS have been reported.

Tardive Dyskinesia — A syndrome of potentially irreversible, involuntary, dyskinetic movements may develop in patients treated with antipsychotic drugs. Although the prevalence of the syndrome appears to be highest among the elderly, especially elderly women, it is impossible to rely upon prevalence estimates to predict, at the inception of antipsychotic treatment, which patients are likely to develop the syndrome. Whether antipsychotic drug products differ in their potential to cause tardive dyskinesia is unknown.

The risk of developing tardive dyskinesia and the likelihood that it will become irreversible are believed to increase as the duration of treatment and the total cumulative dose of antipsychotic drugs administered to the patient increase. However, the syndrome can develop, although much less commonly, after relatively brief treatment periods at low doses.

There is no known treatment for established cases of tardive dyskinesia, although the syndrome may remit, partially or completely, if antipsychotic treatment is withdrawn. Antipsychotic treatment, itself, however, may suppress (or partially suppress) the signs and symptoms of the syndrome and thereby may possibly mask the underlying process. The effect that symptomatic suppression has upon the long-term course of the syndrome is unknown.

Given these considerations, olanzapine should be prescribed in a manner that is most likely to minimize the occurrence of tardive dyskinesia. Chronic antipsychotic treatment should generally be reserved for patients (1) who suffer from a chronic illness that is known to respond to antipsychotic drugs, and (2) for whom alternative, equally effective, but potentially less harmful treatments are not available or appropriate. In patients who do require chronic treatment, the smallest dose and the shortest duration of treatment producing a satisfactory clinical response should be sought. The need for continued treatment should be reassessed periodically.

If signs and symptoms of tardive dyskinesia appear in a patient on olanzapine, drug discontinuation should be considered. However, some patients may require treatment with olanzapine despite the presence of the syndrome.

For specific information about the warnings of lithium or valproate, refer to the WARNINGS section of the package inserts for these other products.

PRECAUTIONS

General

Hemodynamic Effects — Olanzapine may induce orthostatic hypotension associated with dizziness, tachycardia, and in some patients, syncope, especially during the initial dose-titration period, probably reflecting its α_1-adrenergic antagonistic properties. Hypotension, bradycardia with or without hypotension, tachycardia, and syncope were also reported during the clinical trials with intramuscular olanzapine for injection. In an open-label clinical pharmacology study in non-agitated patients with schizophrenia in which the safety and tolerability of intramuscular olanzapine were evaluated under a maximal dosing regimen (three 10 mg doses administered 4 hours apart), approximately one-third of these patients experienced a significant orthostatic decrease in systolic blood pressure (i.e., decrease ≥30 mmHg) (*see* DOSAGE AND ADMINISTRATION). Syncope was reported in 0.6% (15/2500) of olanzapine-treated patients in phase 2–3 oral olanzapine studies and in 0.3% (2/722) of olanzapine-treated patients with agitation in the intramuscular olanzapine for injection studies. Three normal volunteers in phase 1 studies with intramuscular olanzapine experienced hypotension, bradycardia, and sinus pauses of up to 6 seconds that spontaneously resolved (in 2 cases the events occurred on intramuscular olanzapine, and in 1 case, on oral olanzapine). The risk for this sequence of hypotension, bradycardia, and sinus pause may be greater in nonpsychiatric patients compared to psychiatric patients who are possibly more adapted to certain effects of psychotropic drugs.

For oral olanzapine therapy, the risk of orthostatic hypotension and syncope may be minimized by initiating therapy with 5 mg QD (*see* DOSAGE AND ADMINISTRATION). A more gradual titration to the target dose should be considered if hypotension occurs.

For intramuscular olanzapine for injection therapy, patients should remain recumbent if drowsy or dizzy after injection until examination has indicated that they are not experiencing postural hypotension and/or bradycardia.

Olanzapine should be used with particular caution in patients with known cardiovascular disease (history of myocardial infarction or ischemia, heart failure, or conduction abnormalities), cerebrovascular disease, and conditions which would predispose patients to hypotension (dehydration, hypovolemia, and treatment with antihypertensive medications) where the occurrence of syncope, or hypotension and/or bradycardia might put the patient at increased medical risk.

Seizures — During premarketing testing, seizures occurred in 0.9% (22/2500) of olanzapine-treated patients. There were confounding factors that may have contributed to the occurrence of seizures in many of these cases. Olanzapine should be used cautiously in patients with a history of seizures or with conditions that potentially lower the seizure threshold, e.g., Alzheimer's dementia. Conditions that lower the seizure threshold may be more prevalent in a population of 65 years or older.

Hyperprolactinemia — As with other drugs that antagonize dopamine D_2 receptors, olanzapine elevates prolactin levels, and a modest elevation persists during chronic administration. Tissue culture experiments indicate that approximately one-third of human breast cancers are prolactin dependent in vitro, a factor of potential importance if the prescription of these drugs is contemplated in a patient with previously detected breast cancer of this type. Although disturbances such as galactorrhea, amenorrhea, gynecomastia, and impotence have been reported with prolactin-elevating compounds, the clinical significance of elevated serum prolactin levels is unknown for most patients. As is common with compounds which increase prolactin release, an increase in mammary gland neoplasia was observed in the olanzapine carcinogenicity studies conducted in mice and rats (*see* Carcinogenesis). However, neither clinical studies nor epidemiologic studies have shown an association between chronic administration of this class of drugs and tumorigenesis in humans; the available evidence is considered too limited to be conclusive.

Transaminase Elevations — In placebo-controlled studies, clinically significant ALT (SGPT) elevations (≥3 times the upper limit of the normal range) were observed in 2% (6/243) of patients exposed to olanzapine compared to none (0/115) of the placebo patients. None of these patients experienced jaundice. In two of these patients, liver enzymes decreased toward normal despite continued treatment and in two others, enzymes decreased upon discontinuation of olanzapine. In the remaining two patients, one, seropositive for hepatitis C, had persistent enzyme elevation for four months after discontinuation, and the other had insufficient follow-up to determine if enzymes normalized.

Within the larger premarketing database of about 2400 patients with baseline SGPT ≤90 IU/L, the incidence of SGPT elevation to >200 IU/L was 2% (50/2381). Again, none of these patients experienced jaundice or other symptoms attributable to liver impairment and most had transient changes that tended to normalize while olanzapine treatment was continued.

Among 2500 patients in oral olanzapine clinical trials, about 1% (23/2500) discontinued treatment due to transaminase increases.

Caution should be exercised in patients with signs and symptoms of hepatic impairment, in patients with pre-existing conditions associated with limited hepatic functional reserve, and in patients who are being treated with potentially hepatotoxic drugs. Periodic assessment of transaminases is recommended in patients with significant hepatic disease (*see* Laboratory Tests).

Potential for Cognitive and Motor Impairment — Somnolence was a commonly reported adverse event associated with olanzapine treatment, occurring at an incidence of 26% in olanzapine patients compared to 15% in placebo patients. This adverse event was also dose related. Somnolence led to discontinuation in 0.4% (9/2500) of patients in the premarketing database.

Since olanzapine has the potential to impair judgment, thinking, or motor skills, patients should be cautioned about operating hazardous machinery, including automobiles, until they are reasonably certain that olanzapine therapy does not affect them adversely.

Body Temperature Regulation — Disruption of the body's ability to reduce core body temperature has been attributed to antipsychotic agents. Appropriate care is advised when prescribing olanzapine for patients who will be experiencing conditions which may contribute to an elevation in core body temperature, e.g., exercising strenuously, exposure to extreme heat, receiving concomitant medication with anticholinergic activity, or being subject to dehydration.

Dysphagia — Esophageal dysmotility and aspiration have been associated with antipsychotic drug use. Aspiration pneumonia is a common cause of morbidity and mortality in patients with advanced Alzheimer's disease. Olanzapine and other antipsychotic drugs should be used cautiously in patients at risk for aspiration pneumonia.

Suicide — The possibility of a suicide attempt is inherent in schizophrenia and in bipolar disorder, and close supervision of high-risk patients should accompany drug therapy. Prescriptions for olanzapine should be written for the smallest quantity of tablets consistent with good patient management, in order to reduce the risk of overdose.

Use in Patients with Concomitant Illness — Clinical experience with olanzapine in patients with certain concomitant systemic illnesses (*see* Renal Impairment and Hepatic Impairment *under* CLINICAL PHARMACOLOGY, Special Populations) is limited.

Olanzapine exhibits in vitro muscarinic receptor affinity. In premarketing clinical trials with olanzapine, olanzapine was associated with constipation, dry mouth, and tachycardia, all adverse events possibly related to cholinergic antagonism. Such adverse events were not often the basis for discontinuations from olanzapine, but olanzapine should be used with caution in patients with clinically significant prostatic hypertrophy, narrow angle glaucoma, or a history of paralytic ileus.

In five placebo-controlled studies of olanzapine in elderly patients with dementia-related psychosis (n=1184), the following treatment-emergent adverse events were reported in olanzapine-treated patients at an incidence of at least 2% and significantly greater than placebo-treated patients: falls, somnolence, peripheral edema, abnormal gait, urinary incontinence, lethargy, increased weight, asthenia, pyrexia, pneumonia, dry mouth and visual hallucinations. The rate of discontinuation due to adverse events was significantly greater with olanzapine than placebo (13% vs 7%). As with other CNS-active drugs, olanzapine should be used with caution in elderly patients with dementia. Olanzapine is not approved for the treatment of patients with dementia-related psychosis. If the prescriber elects to treat elderly patients with dementia-related psychosis, vigilance should be exercised (*see* WARNINGS).

Olanzapine has not been evaluated or used to any appreciable extent in patients with a recent history of myocardial infarction or unstable heart disease. Patients with these diagnoses were excluded from premarketing clinical studies. Because of the risk of orthostatic hypotension with olanzapine, caution should be observed in cardiac patients (*see* Hemodynamic Effects).

Continued on next page

*** Identi-Code® symbol. This product information was prepared in June 2004. Current information on these and other products of Eli Lilly and Company may be obtained by direct inquiry to Lilly Research Laboratories, Lilly Corporate Center, Indianapolis, Indiana 46285, (800) 545-5979.**

Zyprexa—Cont.

For specific information about the precautions of lithium or valproate, refer to the PRECAUTIONS section of the package inserts for these other products.

Information for Patients

Physicians are advised to discuss the following issues with patients for whom they prescribe olanzapine:

Orthostatic Hypotension — Patients should be advised of the risk of orthostatic hypotension, especially during the period of initial dose titration and in association with the use of concomitant drugs that may potentiate the orthostatic effect of olanzapine, e.g., diazepam or alcohol (*see* Drug Interactions).

Interference with Cognitive and Motor Performance — Because olanzapine has the potential to impair judgment, thinking, or motor skills, patients should be cautioned about operating hazardous machinery, including automobiles, until they are reasonably certain that olanzapine therapy does not affect them adversely.

Pregnancy — Patients should be advised to notify their physician if they become pregnant or intend to become pregnant during therapy with olanzapine.

Nursing — Patients should be advised not to breast-feed an infant if they are taking olanzapine.

Concomitant Medication — Patients should be advised to inform their physicians if they are taking, or plan to take, any prescription or over-the-counter drugs, since there is a potential for interactions.

Alcohol — Patients should be advised to avoid alcohol while taking olanzapine.

Heat Exposure and Dehydration — Patients should be advised regarding appropriate care in avoiding overheating and dehydration.

Phenylketonurics — ZYPREXA ZYDIS (olanzapine orally disintegrating tablets) contains phenylalanine (0.34, 0.45, 0.67, or 0.90 mg per 5, 10, 15, or 20 mg tablet, respectively).

Laboratory Tests

Periodic assessment of transaminases is recommended in patients with significant hepatic disease (*see* Transaminase Elevations).

Drug Interactions

The risks of using olanzapine in combination with other drugs have not been extensively evaluated in systematic studies. Given the primary CNS effects of olanzapine, caution should be used when olanzapine is taken in combination with other centrally acting drugs and alcohol.

Because of its potential for inducing hypotension, olanzapine may enhance the effects of certain antihypertensive agents.

Olanzapine may antagonize the effects of levodopa and dopamine agonists.

The Effect of Other Drugs on Olanzapine — Agents that induce CYP1A2 or glucuronyl transferase enzymes, such as omeprazole and rifampin, may cause an increase in olanzapine clearance. Inhibitors of CYP1A2 could potentially inhibit olanzapine clearance. Although olanzapine is metabolized by multiple enzyme systems, induction or inhibition of a single enzyme may appreciably alter olanzapine clearance. Therefore, a dosage increase (for induction) or a dosage decrease (for inhibition) may need to be considered with specific drugs.

Charcoal — The administration of activated charcoal (1 g) reduced the Cmax and AUC of oral olanzapine by about 60%. As peak olanzapine levels are not typically obtained until about 6 hours after dosing, charcoal may be a useful treatment for olanzapine overdose.

Cimetidine and Antacids — Single doses of cimetidine (800 mg) or aluminum- and magnesium-containing antacids did not affect the oral bioavailability of olanzapine.

Carbamazepine — Carbamazepine therapy (200 mg bid) causes an approximately 50% increase in the clearance of olanzapine. This increase is likely due to the fact that carbamazepine is a potent inducer of CYP1A2 activity. Higher daily doses of carbamazepine may cause an even greater increase in olanzapine clearance.

Ethanol — Ethanol (45 mg/70 kg single dose) did not have an effect on olanzapine pharmacokinetics.

Fluoxetine — Fluoxetine (60 mg single dose or 60 mg daily for 8 days) causes a small (mean 16%) increase in the maximum concentration of olanzapine and a small (mean 16%) decrease in olanzapine clearance. The magnitude of the impact of this factor is small in comparison to the overall variability between individuals, and therefore dose modification is not routinely recommended.

Fluvoxamine — Fluvoxamine, a CYP1A2 inhibitor, decreases the clearance of olanzapine. This results in a mean increase in olanzapine Cmax following fluvoxamine of 54% in female nonsmokers and 77% in male smokers. The mean increase in olanzapine AUC is 52% and 108%, respectively. Lower doses of olanzapine should be considered in patients receiving concomitant treatment with fluvoxamine.

Warfarin — Warfarin (20 mg single dose) did not affect olanzapine pharmacokinetics.

Effect of Olanzapine on Other Drugs — In vitro studies utilizing human liver microsomes suggest that olanzapine has little potential to inhibit CYP1A2, CYP2C9, CYP2C19, CYP2D6, and CYP3A. Thus, olanzapine is unlikely to cause clinically important drug interactions mediated by these enzymes.

Lithium — Multiple doses of olanzapine (10 mg for 8 days) did not influence the kinetics of lithium. Therefore, concomitant olanzapine administration does not require dosage adjustment of lithium.

Valproate — Studies in vitro using human liver microsomes determined that olanzapine has little potential to inhibit the major metabolic pathway, glucuronidation, of valproate. Further, valproate has little effect on the metabolism of olanzapine in vitro. In vivo administration of olanzapine (10 mg daily for 2 weeks) did not affect the steady state plasma concentrations of valproate. Therefore, concomitant olanzapine administration does not require dosage adjustment of valproate.

Single doses of olanzapine did not affect the pharmacokinetics of imipramine or its active metabolite desipramine, and warfarin. Multiple doses of olanzapine did not influence the kinetics of diazepam and its active metabolite N-desmethyldiazepam, ethanol, or biperiden. However, the co-administration of either diazepam or ethanol with olanzapine potentiated the orthostatic hypotension observed with olanzapine. Multiple doses of olanzapine did not affect the pharmacokinetics of theophylline or its metabolites.

Lorazepam — Administration of intramuscular lorazepam (2 mg) 1 hour after intramuscular olanzapine for injection (5 mg) did not significantly affect the pharmacokinetics of olanzapine, unconjugated lorazepam, or total lorazepam. However, this co-administration of intramuscular lorazepam and intramuscular olanzapine for injection added to the somnolence observed with either drug alone.

Carcinogenesis, Mutagenesis, Impairment of Fertility

Carcinogenesis — Oral carcinogenicity studies were conducted in mice and rats. Olanzapine was administered to mice in two 78-week studies at doses of 3, 10, 30/20 mg/kg/day (equivalent to 0.8–5 times the maximum recommended human daily oral dose on a mg/m^2 basis) and 0.25, 2, 8 mg/kg/day (equivalent to 0.06–2 times the maximum recommended human daily oral dose on a mg/m^2 basis). Rats were dosed for 2 years at doses of 0.25, 1, 2.5, 4 mg/kg/day (males) and 0.25, 1, 4, 8 mg/kg/day (females) (equivalent to 0.13–2 and 0.13–4 times the maximum recommended human daily oral dose on a mg/m^2 basis, respectively). The incidence of liver hemangiomas and hemangiosarcomas was significantly increased in one mouse study in female mice dosed at 8 mg/kg/day (2 times the maximum recommended human daily oral dose on a mg/m^2 basis). These tumors were not increased in another mouse study in females dosed at 10 or 30/20 mg/kg/day (2–5 times the maximum recommended human daily oral dose on a mg/m^2 basis); in this study, there was a high incidence of early mortalities in males of the 30/20 mg/kg/day group. The incidence of mammary gland adenomas and adenocarcinomas was significantly increased in female mice dosed at ≥2 mg/kg/day and in female rats dosed at ≥4 mg/kg/day (0.5 and 2 times the maximum recommended human daily oral dose on a mg/m^2 basis, respectively). Antipsychotic drugs have been shown to chronically elevate prolactin levels in rodents. Serum prolactin levels were not measured during the olanzapine carcinogenicity studies; however, measurements during subchronic toxicity studies showed that olanzapine elevated serum prolactin levels up to 4-fold in rats at the same doses used in the carcinogenicity study. An increase in mammary gland neoplasms has been found in rodents after chronic administration of other antipsychotic drugs and is considered to be prolactin mediated. The relevance for human risk of the finding of prolactin mediated endocrine tumors in rodents is unknown (*see* Hyperprolactinemia *under* PRECAUTIONS, General).

Mutagenesis — No evidence of mutagenic potential for olanzapine was found in the Ames reverse mutation test, in vivo micronucleus test in mice, the chromosomal aberration test in Chinese hamster ovary cells, unscheduled DNA synthesis test in rat hepatocytes, induction of forward mutation test in mouse lymphoma cells, or in vivo sister chromatid exchange test in bone marrow of Chinese hamsters.

Impairment of Fertility — In an oral fertility and reproductive performance study in rats, male mating performance, but not fertility, was impaired at a dose of 22.4 mg/kg/day and female fertility was decreased at a dose of 3 mg/kg/day (11 and 1.5 times the maximum recommended human daily oral dose on a mg/m^2 basis, respectively). Discontinuance of olanzapine treatment reversed the effects on male mating performance. In female rats, the precoital period was increased and the mating index reduced at 5 mg/kg/day (2.5 times the maximum recommended human daily oral dose on a mg/m^2 basis). Diestrous was prolonged and estrous delayed at 1.1 mg/kg/day (0.6 times the maximum recommended human daily oral dose on a mg/m^2 basis); therefore olanzapine may produce a delay in ovulation.

Pregnancy

Pregnancy Category C — In oral reproduction studies in rats at doses up to 18 mg/kg/day and in rabbits at doses up to 30 mg/kg/day (9 and 30 times the maximum recommended human daily oral dose on a mg/m^2 basis, respectively) no evidence of teratogenicity was observed. In an oral rat teratology study, early resorptions and increased numbers of nonviable fetuses were observed at a dose of 18 mg/kg/day (9 times the maximum recommended human daily oral dose on a mg/m^2 basis). Gestation was prolonged at 10 mg/kg/day (5 times the maximum recommended human daily oral dose on a mg/m^2 basis). In an oral rabbit teratology study, fetal toxicity (manifested as increased resorptions and decreased fetal weight) occurred at a maternally toxic dose of 30 mg/kg/day (30 times the maximum recommended human daily oral dose on a mg/m^2 basis).

Placental transfer of olanzapine occurs in rat pups.

There are no adequate and well-controlled trials with olanzapine in pregnant females. Seven pregnancies were observed during clinical trials with olanzapine, including 2 resulting in normal births, 1 resulting in neonatal death due to a cardiovascular defect, 3 therapeutic abortions, and 1 spontaneous abortion. Because animal reproduction studies are not always predictive of human response, this drug should be used during pregnancy only if the potential benefit justifies the potential risk to the fetus.

Labor and Delivery

Parturition in rats was not affected by olanzapine. The effect of olanzapine on labor and delivery in humans is unknown.

Nursing Mothers

Olanzapine was excreted in milk of treated rats during lactation. It is not known if olanzapine is excreted in human milk. It is recommended that women receiving olanzapine should not breast-feed.

Pediatric Use

Safety and effectiveness in pediatric patients have not been established.

Geriatric Use

Of the 2500 patients in premarketing clinical studies with oral olanzapine, 11% (263) were 65 years of age or over. In patients with schizophrenia, there was no indication of any different tolerability of olanzapine in the elderly compared to younger patients. Studies in elderly patients with dementia-related psychosis have suggested that there may be a different tolerability profile in this population compared to younger patients with schizophrenia. As with other CNS-active drugs, olanzapine should be used with caution in elderly patients with dementia. Olanzapine is not approved for the treatment of patients with dementia-related psychosis. If the prescriber elects to treat elderly patients with dementia-related psychosis, vigilance should be exercised. Also, the presence of factors that might decrease pharmacokinetic clearance or increase the pharmacodynamic response to olanzapine should lead to consideration of a lower starting dose for any geriatric patient (*see* WARNINGS, PRECAUTIONS, *and* DOSAGE AND ADMINISTRATION).

ADVERSE REACTIONS

The information below is derived from a clinical trial database for olanzapine consisting of 8661 patients with approximately 4165 patient-years of exposure to oral olanzapine and 722 patients with exposure to intramuscular olanzapine for injection. This database includes: (1) 2500 patients who participated in multiple-dose oral olanzapine premarketing trials in schizophrenia and Alzheimer's disease representing approximately 1122 patient-years of exposure as of February 14, 1995; (2) 182 patients who participated in oral olanzapine premarketing bipolar mania trials representing approximately 66 patient-years of exposure; (3) 191 patients who participated in an oral olanzapine trial of patients having various psychiatric symptoms in association with Alzheimer's disease representing approximately 29 patient-years of exposure; (4) 5788 patients from 88 additional oral olanzapine clinical trials as of December 31, 2001; and (5) 722 patients who participated in intramuscular olanzapine for injection premarketing trials in agitated patients with schizophrenia, Bipolar I Disorder (manic or mixed episodes), or dementia. In addition, information from the premarketing 6-week clinical study database for olanzapine in combination with lithium or valproate, consisting of 224 patients who participated in bipolar mania trials with approximately 22 patient-years of exposure, is included below.

The conditions and duration of treatment with olanzapine varied greatly and included (in overlapping categories) open-label and double-blind phases of studies, inpatients and outpatients, fixed-dose and dose-titration studies, and short-term or longer-term exposure. Adverse reactions were assessed by collecting adverse events, results of physical examinations, vital signs, weights, laboratory analytes, ECGs, chest x-rays, and results of ophthalmologic examinations.

Certain portions of the discussion below relating to objective or numeric safety parameters, namely, dose-dependent adverse events, vital sign changes, weight gain, laboratory changes, and ECG changes are derived from studies in patients with schizophrenia and have not been duplicated for bipolar mania or agitation. However, this information is also generally applicable to bipolar mania and agitation.

Adverse events during exposure were obtained by spontaneous report and recorded by clinical investigators using terminology of their own choosing. Consequently, it is not possible to provide a meaningful estimate of the proportion of individuals experiencing adverse events without first grouping similar types of events into a smaller number of standardized event categories. In the tables and tabulations that follow, standard COSTART dictionary terminology has been used initially to classify reported adverse events.

The stated frequencies of adverse events represent the proportion of individuals who experienced, at least once, a treatment-emergent adverse event of the type listed. An event was considered treatment emergent if it occurred for the first time or worsened while receiving therapy following baseline evaluation. The reported events do not include those event terms that were so general as to be uninformative. Events listed elsewhere in labeling may not be repeated below. It is important to emphasize that, although the events occurred during treatment with olanzapine, they were not necessarily caused by it. The entire label should be read to gain a complete understanding of the safety profile of olanzapine.

The prescriber should be aware that the figures in the tables and tabulations cannot be used to predict the incidence of side effects in the course of usual medical practice where patient characteristics and other factors differ from those that prevailed in the clinical trials. Similarly, the cited frequencies cannot be compared with figures obtained from other clinical investigations involving different treatments, uses, and investigators. The cited figures, however, do provide the prescribing physician with some basis for estimating the relative contribution of drug and nondrug factors to the adverse event incidence in the population studied.

Incidence of Adverse Events in Short-Term, Placebo-Controlled and Combination Trials

The following findings are based on premarketing trials of (1) oral olanzapine for schizophrenia, bipolar mania, a subsequent trial of patients having various psychiatric symptoms in association with Alzheimer's disease, and premarketing combination trials, and (2) intramuscular olanzapine for injection in agitated patients with schizophrenia or bipolar mania.

Adverse Events Associated with Discontinuation of Treatment in Short-Term, Placebo-Controlled Trials

Schizophrenia — Overall, there was no difference in the incidence of discontinuation due to adverse events (5% for oral olanzapine vs 6% for placebo). However, discontinuations due to increases in SGPT were considered to be drug related (2% for oral olanzapine vs 0% for placebo) (*see* PRECAUTIONS).

Bipolar Mania Monotherapy — Overall, there was no difference in the incidence of discontinuation due to adverse events (2% for oral olanzapine vs 2% for placebo).

Agitation — Overall, there was no difference in the incidence of discontinuation due to adverse events (0.4% for intramuscular olanzapine for injection vs 0% for placebo).

Adverse Events Associated with Discontinuation of Treatment in Short-Term Combination Trials

Bipolar Mania Combination Therapy — In a study of patients who were already tolerating either lithium or valproate as monotherapy, discontinuation rates due to adverse events were 11% for the combination of oral olanzapine with lithium or valproate compared to 2% for patients who remained on lithium or valproate monotherapy. Discontinuations with the combination of oral olanzapine and lithium or valproate that occurred in more than 1 patient were: somnolence (3%), weight gain (1%), and peripheral edema (1%).

Commonly Observed Adverse Events in Short-Term, Placebo-Controlled Trials

The most commonly observed adverse events associated with the use of oral olanzapine (incidence of 5% or greater) and not observed at an equivalent incidence among placebo-treated patients (olanzapine incidence at least twice that for placebo) were:

Common Treatment-Emergent Adverse Events Associated with the Use of Oral Olanzapine in 6-Week Trials — SCHIZOPHRENIA

Adverse Event	Percentage of Patients Reporting Event	
	Olanzapine (N=248)	Placebo (N=118)
Postural hypotension	5	2
Constipation	9	3
Weight gain	6	1
Dizziness	11	4
Personality disorder[1]	8	4
Akathisia	5	1

[1] Personality disorder is the COSTART term for designating non-aggressive objectionable behavior.

Common Treatment-Emergent Adverse Events Associated with the Use of Oral Olanzapine in 3-Week and 4-Week Trials — BIPOLAR MANIA

Adverse Event	Percentage of Patients Reporting Event	
	Olanzapine (N=125)	Placebo (N=129)
Asthenia	15	6
Dry mouth	22	7
Constipation	11	5
Dyspepsia	11	5
Increased appetite	6	3
Somnolence	35	13
Dizziness	18	6
Tremor	6	3

There was one adverse event (somnolence) observed at an incidence of 5% or greater among intramuscular olanzapine for injection-treated patients and not observed at an equivalent incidence among placebo-treated patients (olanzapine incidence at least twice that for placebo) during the placebo-controlled premarketing studies. The incidence of somnolence during the 24 hour IM treatment period in clinical trials in agitated patients with schizophrenia or bipolar mania was 6% for intramuscular olanzapine for injection and 3% for placebo.

Adverse Events Occurring at an Incidence of 2% or More Among Oral Olanzapine-Treated Patients in Short-Term, Placebo-Controlled Trials

Table 1 enumerates the incidence, rounded to the nearest percent, of treatment-emergent adverse events that occurred in 2% or more of patients treated with oral olanzapine (doses ≥2.5 mg/day) and with incidence greater than placebo who participated in the acute phase of placebo-controlled trials.

Table 1
Treatment-Emergent Adverse Events: Incidence in Short-Term, Placebo-Controlled Clinical Trials[1] with Oral Olanzapine

Body System/Adverse Event	Percentage of Patients Reporting Event	
	Olanzapine (N=532)	Placebo (N=294)
Body as a Whole		
Accidental injury	12	8
Asthenia	10	9
Fever	6	2
Back pain	5	2
Chest pain	3	1
Cardiovascular System		
Postural hypotension	3	1
Tachycardia	3	1
Hypertension	2	1
Digestive System		
Dry mouth	9	5
Constipation	9	4
Dyspepsia	7	5
Vomiting	4	3
Increased appetite	3	2
Hemic and Lymphatic System		
Ecchymosis	5	3
Metabolic and Nutritional Disorders		
Weight gain	5	3
Peripheral edema	3	1
Musculoskeletal System		
Extremity pain (other than joint)	5	3
Joint pain	5	3
Nervous System		
Somnolence	29	13
Insomnia	12	11
Dizziness	11	4
Abnormal gait	6	1
Tremor	4	3
Akathisia	3	2
Hypertonia	3	2
Articulation impairment	2	1
Respiratory System		
Rhinitis	7	6
Cough increased	6	3
Pharyngitis	4	3
Special Senses		
Amblyopia	3	2
Urogenital System		
Urinary incontinence	2	1
Urinary tract infection	2	1

[1] Events reported by at least 2% of patients treated with olanzapine, except the following events which had an incidence equal to or less than placebo: abdominal pain, agitation, anorexia, anxiety, apathy, confusion, depression, diarrhea, dysmenorrhea[2], hallucinations, headache, hostility, hyperkinesia, myalgia, nausea, nervousness, paranoid reaction, personality disorder[3], rash, thinking abnormal, weight loss.

[2] Denominator used was for females only (olanzapine, N=201; placebo, N=114).

[3] Personality disorder is the COSTART term for designating non-aggressive objectionable behavior.

Commonly Observed Adverse Events in Short-Term Combination Trials

In the bipolar mania combination placebo-controlled trials, the most commonly observed adverse events associated with the combination of olanzapine and lithium or valproate (incidence of ≥5% and at least twice placebo) were:

Common Treatment-Emergent Adverse Events Associated with the Use of Oral Olanzapine in 6-Week Combination Trials — BIPOLAR MANIA

Adverse Event	Percentage of Patients Reporting Event	
	Olanzapine with lithium or valproate (N=229)	Placebo with lithium or valproate (N=115)
Dry mouth	32	9
Weight gain	26	7
Increased appetite	24	8
Dizziness	14	7
Back pain	8	4
Constipation	8	4
Speech disorder	7	1
Increased salivation	6	2
Amnesia	5	2
Paresthesia	5	2

Adverse Events Occurring at an Incidence of 2% or More Among Oral Olanzapine-Treated Patients in Short-Term Combination Trials

Table 2 enumerates the incidence, rounded to the nearest percent, of treatment-emergent adverse events that occurred in 2% or more of patients treated with the combination of olanzapine (doses ≥5 mg/day) and lithium or valproate and with incidence greater than lithium or valproate alone who participated in the acute phase of placebo-controlled combination trials.

Table 2
Treatment-Emergent Adverse Events: Incidence in Short-Term, Placebo-Controlled Combination Clinical Trials[1] with Oral Olanzapine

Body System/Adverse Event	Percentage of Patients Reporting Event	
	Olanzapine with lithium or valproate (N=229)	Placebo with lithium or valproate (N=115)
Body as a Whole		
Asthenia	18	13
Back pain	8	4
Accidental injury	4	2
Chest pain	3	2
Cardiovascular System		
Hypertension	2	1
Digestive System		
Dry mouth	32	9
Increased appetite	24	8
Thirst	10	6
Constipation	8	4
Increased salivation	6	2
Metabolic and Nutritional Disorders		
Weight gain	26	7
Peripheral edema	6	4
Edema	2	1
Nervous System		
Somnolence	52	27
Tremor	23	13
Depression	18	17
Dizziness	14	7
Speech disorder	7	1
Amnesia	5	2
Paresthesia	5	2
Apathy	4	3
Confusion	4	1
Euphoria	3	2
Incoordination	2	0

Continued on next page

*** Identi-Code® symbol. This product information was prepared in June 2004. Current information on these and other products of Eli Lilly and Company may be obtained by direct inquiry to Lilly Research Laboratories, Lilly Corporate Center, Indianapolis, Indiana 46285, (800) 545-5979.**

Zyprexa—Cont.

Respiratory System		
Pharyngitis	4	1
Dyspnea	3	1
Skin and Appendages		
Sweating	3	1
Acne	2	0
Dry skin	2	0
Special Senses		
Amblyopia	9	5
Abnormal vision	2	0
Urogenital System		
Dysmenorrhea[2]	2	0
Vaginitis[2]	2	0

[1] Events reported by at least 2% of patients treated with olanzapine, except the following events which had an incidence equal to or less than placebo: abdominal pain, abnormal dreams, abnormal ejaculation, agitation, akathisia, anorexia, anxiety, arthralgia, cough increased, diarrhea, dyspepsia, emotional lability, fever, flatulence, flu syndrome, headache, hostility, insomnia, libido decreased, libido increased, menstrual disorder[2], myalgia, nausea, nervousness, pain, paranoid reaction, personality disorder, rash, rhinitis, sleep disorder, thinking abnormal, vomiting.

[2] Denominator used was for females only (olanzapine, N=128; placebo, N=51).

For specific information about the adverse reactions observed with lithium or valproate, refer to the ADVERSE REACTIONS section of the package inserts for these other products.

Adverse Events Occurring at an Incidence of 1% or More Among Intramuscular Olanzapine for Injection-Treated Patients in Short-Term, Placebo-Controlled Trials

Table 3 enumerates the incidence, rounded to the nearest percent, of treatment-emergent adverse events that occurred in 1% or more of patients treated with intramuscular olanzapine for injection (dose range of 2.5–10.0 mg/injection) and with incidence greater than placebo who participated in the short-term, placebo-controlled trials in agitated patients with schizophrenia or bipolar mania.

Table 3

Treatment-Emergent Adverse Events: Incidence in Short-Term (24 Hour), Placebo-Controlled Clinical Trials with Intramuscular Olanzapine for Injection in Agitated Patients with Schizophrenia or Bipolar Mania[1]

	Percentage of Patients Reporting Event	
Body System/Adverse Event	**Olanzapine (N=415)**	**Placebo (N=150)**
Body as a Whole		
Asthenia	2	1
Cardiovascular System		
Hypotension	2	0
Postural hypotension	1	0
Nervous System		
Somnolence	6	3
Dizziness	4	2
Tremor	1	0

[1] Events reported by at least 1% of patients treated with olanzapine for injection, except the following events which had an incidence equal to or less than placebo: agitation, anxiety, dry mouth, headache, hypertension, insomnia, nervousness.

Additional Findings Observed in Clinical Trials

The following findings are based on clinical trials.

Dose Dependency of Adverse Events in Short-Term, Placebo-Controlled Trials

Extrapyramidal Symptoms — The following table enumerates the percentage of patients with treatment-emergent extrapyramidal symptoms as assessed by categorical analyses of formal rating scales during acute therapy in a controlled clinical trial comparing oral olanzapine at 3 fixed doses with placebo in the treatment of schizophrenia.

[See first table above]

The following table enumerates the percentage of patients with treatment-emergent extrapyramidal symptoms as assessed by spontaneously reported adverse events during acute therapy in the same controlled clinical trial comparing olanzapine at 3 fixed doses with placebo in the treatment of schizophrenia.

[See second table above]

The following table enumerates the percentage of patients with treatment-emergent extrapyramidal symptoms as assessed by categorical analyses of formal rating scales during controlled clinical trials comparing fixed doses of intramuscular olanzapine for injection with placebo in agitation. Patients in each dose group could receive up to three injections during the trials (*see* CLINICAL PHARMACOLOGY). Patient assessments were conducted during the 24 hours following the initial dose of intramuscular olanzapine for injection. There were no statistically significant differences from placebo.

[See third table above]

The following table enumerates the percentage of patients with treatment-emergent extrapyramidal symptoms as assessed by spontaneously reported adverse events in the same controlled clinical trial comparing fixed doses of intramuscular olanzapine for injection with placebo in agitated patients with schizophrenia. There were no statistically significant differences from placebo.

[See first table at top of next page]

TREATMENT-EMERGENT EXTRAPYRAMIDAL SYMPTOMS ASSESSED BY RATING SCALES INCIDENCE IN A FIXED DOSAGE RANGE, PLACEBO-CONTROLLED CLINICAL TRIAL OF ORAL OLANZAPINE IN SCHIZOPHRENIA — ACUTE PHASE*

	Percentage of Patients Reporting Event			
	Placebo	Olanzapine 5± 2.5 mg/day	Olanzapine 10 ± 2.5 mg/day	Olanzapine 15 ± 2.5 mg/day
Parkinsonism[1]	15	14	12	14
Akathisia[2]	23	16	19	27

* No statistically significant differences.

[1] Percentage of patients with a Simpson-Angus Scale total score >3.

[2] Percentage of patients with a Barnes Akathisia Scale global score ≥2.

TREATMENT-EMERGENT EXTRAPYRAMIDAL SYMPTOMS ASSESSED BY ADVERSE EVENTS INCIDENCE IN A FIXED DOSAGE RANGE, PLACEBO-CONTROLLED CLINICAL TRIAL OF ORAL OLANZAPINE IN SCHIZOPHRENIA — ACUTE PHASE

	Percentage of Patients Reporting Event			
	Placebo (N=68)	Olanzapine 5 ± 2.5 mg/day (N=65)	Olanzapine 10± 2.5 mg/day (N=64)	Olanzapine 15 ± 2.5 mg/day (N=69)
Dystonic events[1]	1	3	2	3
Parkinsonism events[2]	10	8	14	20
Akathisia events[3]	1	5	11*	10*
Dyskinetic events[4]	4	0	2	1
Residual events[5]	1	2	5	1
Any extrapyramidal event	16	15	25	32*

* Statistically significantly different from placebo.

[1] Patients with the following COSTART terms were counted in this category: dystonia, generalized spasm, neck rigidity, oculogyric crisis, opisthotonos, torticollis.

[2] Patients with the following COSTART terms were counted in this category: akinesia, cogwheel rigidity, extrapyramidal syndrome, hypertonia, hypokinesia, masked facies, tremor.

[3] Patients with the following COSTART terms were counted in this category: akathisia, hyperkinesia.

[4] Patients with the following COSTART terms were counted in this category: buccoglossal syndrome, choreoathetosis, dyskinesia, tardive dyskinesia.

[5] Patients with the following COSTART terms were counted in this category: movement disorder, myoclonus, twitching.

TREATMENT-EMERGENT EXTRAPYRAMIDAL SYMPTOMS ASSESSED BY RATING SCALES INCIDENCE IN A FIXED DOSE, PLACEBO-CONTROLLED CLINICAL TRIAL OF INTRAMUSCULAR OLANZAPINE FOR INJECTION IN AGITATED PATIENTS WITH SCHIZOPHRENIA*

	Percentage of Patients Reporting Event				
	Placebo	Olanzapine IM 2.5 mg	Olanzapine IM 5 mg	Olanzapine IM 7.5 mg	Olanzapine IM 10 mg
Parkinsonism[1]	0	0	0	0	3
Akathisia[2]	0	0	5	0	0

* No statistically significant differences.

[1] Percentage of patients with a Simpson-Angus Scale total score >3.

[2] Percentage of patients with a Barnes Akathisia Scale global score ≥2.

Other Adverse Events — The following table addresses dose relatedness for other adverse events using data from a schizophrenia trial involving fixed dosage ranges of oral olanzapine. It enumerates the percentage of patients with treatment-emergent adverse events for the three fixed-dose range groups and placebo. The data were analyzed using the Cochran-Armitage test, excluding the placebo group, and the table includes only those adverse events for which there was a statistically significant trend.

[See second table at top of next page]

Vital Sign Changes — Oral olanzapine was associated with orthostatic hypotension and tachycardia in clinical trials. Intramuscular olanzapine for injection was associated with bradycardia, hypotension, and tachycardia in clinical trials (*see* PRECAUTIONS).

Weight Gain — In placebo-controlled, 6-week studies, weight gain was reported in 5.6% of olanzapine patients compared to 0.8% of placebo patients. Olanzapine patients gained an average of 2.8 kg, compared to an average 0.4 kg weight loss in placebo patients; 29% of olanzapine patients gained greater than 7% of their baseline weight, compared to 3% of placebo patients. A categorization of patients at baseline on the basis of body mass index (BMI) revealed a significantly greater effect in patients with low BMI compared to normal or overweight patients; nevertheless, weight gain was greater in all 3 olanzapine groups compared to the placebo group. During long-term continuation therapy with olanzapine (238 median days of exposure), 56% of olanzapine patients met the criterion for having gained greater than 7% of their baseline weight. Average weight gain during long-term therapy was 5.4 kg.

Laboratory Changes — An assessment of the premarketing experience for olanzapine revealed an association with asymptomatic increases in SGPT, SGOT, and GGT (*see* PRECAUTIONS). Olanzapine administration was also associated with increases in serum prolactin (*see* PRECAUTIONS), with an asymptomatic elevation of the eosinophil count in 0.3% of patients, and with an increase in CPK.

Given the concern about neutropenia associated with other psychotropic compounds and the finding of leukopenia associated with the administration of olanzapine in several animal models (*see* ANIMAL TOXICOLOGY), careful attention was given to examination of hematologic parameters in premarketing studies with olanzapine. There was no indication of a risk of clinically significant neutropenia associated with olanzapine treatment in the premarketing database for this drug.

ECG Changes — Between-group comparisons for pooled placebo-controlled trials revealed no statistically significant olanzapine/placebo differences in the proportions of patients experiencing potentially important changes in ECG parameters, including QT, QTc, and PR intervals. Olanzapine use was associated with a mean increase in heart rate of 2.4 beats per minute compared to no change among placebo patients. This slight tendency to tachycardia may be related to olanzapine's potential for inducing orthostatic changes (*see* PRECAUTIONS).

Other Adverse Events Observed During the Clinical Trial Evaluation of Olanzapine

Following is a list of terms that reflect treatment-emergent adverse events reported by patients treated with oral olanzapine (at multiple doses ≥1 mg/day) in clinical trials (8661 patients, 4165 patient-years of exposure). This listing may not include those events already listed in previous tables or elsewhere in labeling, those events for which a drug cause was remote, those event terms which were so general as to be uninformative, and those events reported only once or twice which did not have a substantial probability of being acutely life-threatening.

Events are further categorized by body system and listed in order of decreasing frequency according to the following definitions: frequent adverse events are those occurring in at least 1/100 patients (only those not already listed in the tabulated results from placebo-controlled trials appear in this listing); infrequent adverse events are those occurring in 1/100 to 1/1000 patients; rare events are those occurring in fewer than 1/1000 patients.

Body as a Whole — *Frequent:* dental pain and flu syndrome; *Infrequent:* abdomen enlarged, chills, face edema, intentional injury, malaise, moniliasis, neck pain, neck rigidity, pelvic pain, photosensitivity reaction, and suicide attempt; *Rare:* chills and fever, hangover effect, and sudden death.

Cardiovascular System — *Frequent:* hypotension; *Infrequent:* atrial fibrillation, bradycardia, cerebrovascular accident, congestive heart failure, heart arrest, hemorrhage, migraine, pallor, palpitation, vasodilatation, and ventricular extrasystoles; *Rare:* arteritis, heart failure, and pulmonary embolus.

Digestive System — *Frequent:* flatulence, increased salivation, and thirst; *Infrequent:* dysphagia, esophagitis, fecal impaction, fecal incontinence, gastritis, gastroenteritis, gingivitis, hepatitis, melena, mouth ulceration, nausea and vomiting, oral moniliasis, periodontal abscess, rectal hemorrhage, stomatitis, tongue edema, and tooth caries; *Rare:* aphthous stomatitis, enteritis, eructation, esophageal ulcer, glossitis, ileus, intestinal obstruction, liver fatty deposit, and tongue discoloration.

Endocrine System — *Infrequent:* diabetes mellitus; *Rare:* diabetic acidosis and goiter.

Hemic and Lymphatic System — *Infrequent:* anemia, cyanosis, leukocytosis, leukopenia, lymphadenopathy, and thrombocytopenia; *Rare:* normocytic anemia and thrombocythemia.

Metabolic and Nutritional Disorders — *Infrequent:* acidosis, alkaline phosphatase increased, bilirubinemia, dehydration, hypercholesteremia, hyperglycemia, hyperlipemia, hyperuricemia, hypoglycemia, hypokalemia, hyponatremia, lower extremity edema, and upper extremity edema; *Rare:* gout, hyperkalemia, hypernatremia, hypoproteinemia, ketosis, and water intoxication.

Musculoskeletal System — *Frequent:* joint stiffness and twitching; *Infrequent:* arthritis, arthrosis, leg cramps, and myasthenia; *Rare:* bone pain, bursitis, myopathy, osteoporosis, and rheumatoid arthritis.

Nervous System — *Frequent:* abnormal dreams, amnesia, delusions, emotional lability, euphoria, manic reaction, paresthesia, and schizophrenic reaction; *Infrequent:* akinesia, alcohol misuse, antisocial reaction, ataxia, CNS stimulation, cogwheel rigidity, delirium, dementia, depersonalization, dysarthria, facial paralysis, hypesthesia, hypokinesia, hypotonia, incoordination, libido decreased, libido increased, obsessive compulsive symptoms, phobias, somatization, stimulant misuse, stupor, stuttering, tardive dyskinesia, vertigo, and withdrawal syndrome; *Rare:* circumoral paresthesia, coma, encephalopathy, neuralgia, neuropathy, nystagmus, paralysis, subarachnoid hemorrhage, and tobacco misuse.

Respiratory System — *Frequent:* dyspnea; *Infrequent:* apnea, asthma, epistaxis, hemoptysis, hyperventilation, hypoxia, laryngitis, and voice alteration; *Rare:* atelectasis, hiccup, hypoventilation, lung edema, and stridor.

Skin and Appendages — *Frequent:* sweating; *Infrequent:* alopecia, contact dermatitis, dry skin, eczema, maculopapular rash, pruritus, seborrhea, skin discoloration, skin ulcer, urticaria, and vesiculobullous rash; *Rare:* hirsutism and pustular rash.

Special Senses — *Frequent:* conjunctivitis; *Infrequent:* abnormality of accommodation, blepharitis, cataract, deafness, diplopia, dry eyes, ear pain, eye hemorrhage, eye inflammation, eye pain, ocular muscle abnormality, taste perversion, and tinnitus; *Rare:* corneal lesion, glaucoma, keratoconjunctivitis, macular hypopigmentation, miosis, mydriasis, and pigment deposits lens.

Urogenital System — *Frequent:* vaginitis*; *Infrequent:* abnormal ejaculation*, amenorrhea*, breast pain, cystitis, decreased menstruation*, dysuria, female lactation*, glycosuria, gynecomastia, hematuria, impotence*, increased menstruation*, menorrhagia*, metrorrhagia*, polyuria, premenstrual syndrome*, pyuria, urinary frequency, urinary retention, urinary urgency, urination impaired, uterine fibroids enlarged*, and vaginal hemorrhage*; *Rare:* albuminuria, breast enlargement, mastitis, and oliguria.

*Adjusted for gender.

Following is a list of terms that reflect treatment-emergent adverse events reported by patients treated with intramuscular olanzapine for injection (at one or more doses ≥2.5 mg/injection) in clinical trials (722 patients). This listing may not include those events already listed in previous tables or elsewhere in labeling, those events for which a drug cause was remote, those event terms which were so general as to be uninformative, and those events reported only once which did not have a substantial probability of being acutely life-threatening.

Events are further categorized by body system and listed in order of decreasing frequency according to the following definitions: frequent adverse events are those occurring in at least 1/100 patients (only those not already listed in the tabulated results from placebo-controlled trials appear in this listing); infrequent adverse events are those occurring in 1/100 to 1/1000 patients.

TREATMENT-EMERGENT EXTRAPYRAMIDAL SYMPTOMS ASSESSED BY ADVERSE EVENTS INCIDENCE IN A FIXED DOSE, PLACEBO-CONTROLLED CLINICAL TRIAL OF INTRAMUSCULAR OLANZAPINE FOR INJECTION IN AGITATED PATIENTS WITH SCHIZOPHRENIA*

	Percentage of Patients Reporting Event				
	Placebo (N=45)	Olanzapine IM 2.5 mg (N=48)	Olanzapine IM 5 mg (N=45)	Olanzapine IM 7.5 mg (N=46)	Olanzapine IM 10 mg (N=46)
Dystonic events[1]	0	0	0	0	0
Parkinsonism events[2]	0	4	2	0	0
Akathisia events[3]	0	2	0	0	0
Dyskinetic events[4]	0	0	0	0	0
Residual events[5]	0	0	0	0	0
Any extrapyramidal event	0	4	2	0	0

* No statistically significant differences.

[1] Patients with the following COSTART terms were counted in this category: dystonia, generalized spasm, neck rigidity, oculogyric crisis, opisthotonos, torticollis.

[2] Patients with the following COSTART terms were counted in this category: akinesia, cogwheel rigidity, extrapyramidal syndrome, hypertonia, hypokinesia, masked facies, tremor.

[3] Patients with the following COSTART terms were counted in this category: akathisia, hyperkinesia.

[4] Patients with the following COSTART terms were counted in this category: buccoglossal syndrome, choreoathetosis, dyskinesia, tardive dyskinesia.

[5] Patients with the following COSTART terms were counted in this category: movement disorder, myoclonus, twitching.

	Percentage of Patients Reporting Event			
Adverse Event	Placebo (N=68)	Olanzapine 5 ± 2.5 mg/day (N=65)	Olanzapine 10 ± 2.5 mg/day (N=64)	Olanzapine 15 ± 2.5 mg/day (N=69)
Asthenia	15	8	9	20
Dry mouth	4	3	5	13
Nausea	9	0	2	9
Somnolence	16	20	30	39
Tremor	3	0	5	7

at least 1/100 patients (only those not already listed in the tabulated results from placebo-controlled trials appear in this listing); infrequent adverse events are those occurring in 1/100 to 1/1000 patients.

Body as a Whole — *Frequent:* injection site pain; *Infrequent:* abdominal pain and fever.

Cardiovascular System — *Infrequent:* AV block, heart block, and syncope.

Digestive System — *Infrequent:* diarrhea and nausea.

Hemic and Lymphatic System — *Infrequent:* anemia.

Metabolic and Nutritional Disorders — *Infrequent:* creatine phosphokinase increased, dehydration, and hyperkalemia.

Musculoskeletal System — *Infrequent:* twitching.

Nervous System — *Infrequent:* abnormal gait, akathisia, articulation impairment, confusion, and emotional lability.

Skin and Appendages — *Infrequent:* sweating.

Postintroduction Reports

Adverse events reported since market introduction that were temporally (but not necessarily causally) related to ZYPREXA therapy include the following: allergic reaction (e.g., anaphylactoid reaction, angioedema, pruritus or urticaria), diabetic coma, pancreatitis, priapism, rhabdomyolysis, and venous thromboembolic events (including pulmonary embolism and deep venous thrombosis).

DRUG ABUSE AND DEPENDENCE

Controlled Substance Class

Olanzapine is not a controlled substance.

Physical and Psychological Dependence

In studies prospectively designed to assess abuse and dependence potential, olanzapine was shown to have acute depressive CNS effects but little or no potential of abuse or physical dependence in rats administered oral doses up to 15 times the maximum recommended human daily oral dose (20 mg) and rhesus monkeys administered oral doses up to 8 times the maximum recommended human daily oral dose on a mg/m^2 basis.

Olanzapine has not been systematically studied in humans for its potential for abuse, tolerance, or physical dependence. While the clinical trials did not reveal any tendency for any drug-seeking behavior, these observations were not systematic, and it is not possible to predict on the basis of this limited experience the extent to which a CNS-active drug will be misused, diverted, and/or abused once marketed. Consequently, patients should be evaluated carefully for a history of drug abuse, and such patients should be observed closely for signs of misuse or abuse of olanzapine (e.g., development of tolerance, increases in dose, drug-seeking behavior).

OVERDOSAGE

Human Experience

In premarketing trials involving more than 3100 patients and/or normal subjects, accidental or intentional acute overdosage of olanzapine was identified in 67 patients. In the patient taking the largest identified amount, 300 mg, the only symptoms reported were drowsiness and slurred speech. In the limited number of patients who were evaluated in hospitals, including the patient taking 300 mg, there were no observations indicating an adverse change in laboratory analytes or ECG. Vital signs were usually within normal limits following overdoses.

In postmarketing reports of overdose with olanzapine alone, symptoms have been reported in the majority of cases. In symptomatic patients, symptoms with ≥10% incidence included agitation/aggressiveness, dysarthria, tachycardia, various extrapyramidal symptoms, and reduced level of consciousness ranging from sedation to coma. Among less commonly reported symptoms were the following potentially medically serious events: aspiration, cardiopulmonary arrest, cardiac arrhythmias (such as supraventricular tachycardia and one patient experiencing sinus pause with spontaneous resumption of normal rhythm), delirium, possible neuroleptic malignant syndrome, respiratory depression/arrest, convulsion, hypertension, and hypotension. Eli Lilly and Company has received reports of fatality in association with overdose of olanzapine alone. In one case of death, the amount of acutely ingested olanzapine was reported to be possibly as low as 450 mg; however, in another case, a patient was reported to survive an acute olanzapine ingestion of 1500 mg.

Overdosage Management

The possibility of multiple drug involvement should be considered. In case of acute overdosage, establish and maintain an airway and ensure adequate oxygenation and ventilation, which may include intubation. Gastric lavage (after intubation, if patient is unconscious) and administration of activated charcoal together with a laxative should be considered. The possibility of obtundation, seizures, or dystonic reaction of the head and neck following overdose may create a risk of aspiration with induced emesis. Cardiovascular monitoring should commence immediately and should include continuous electrocardiographic monitoring to detect possible arrhythmias.

There is no specific antidote to olanzapine. Therefore, appropriate supportive measures should be initiated. Hypotension and circulatory collapse should be treated with appropriate measures such as intravenous fluids and/or sympathomimetic agents. (Do not use epinephrine, dopamine, or other sympathomimetics with beta-agonist activity, since beta stimulation may worsen hypotension in the setting of olanzapine-induced alpha blockade.) Close medical supervision and monitoring should continue until the patient recovers.

Continued on next page

*** Identi-Code® symbol. This product information was prepared in June 2004. Current information on these and other products of Eli Lilly and Company may be obtained by direct inquiry to Lilly Research Laboratories, Lilly Corporate Center, Indianapolis, Indiana 46285, (800) 545-5979.**

Zyprexa—Cont.

DOSAGE AND ADMINISTRATION

Schizophrenia

Usual Dose — Oral olanzapine should be administered on a once-a-day schedule without regard to meals, generally beginning with 5 to 10 mg initially, with a target dose of 10 mg/day within several days. Further dosage adjustments, if indicated, should generally occur at intervals of not less than 1 week, since steady state for olanzapine would not be achieved for approximately 1 week in the typical patient. When dosage adjustments are necessary, dose increments/decrements of 5 mg QD are recommended.

Efficacy in schizophrenia was demonstrated in a dose range of 10 to 15 mg/day in clinical trials. However, doses above 10 mg/day were not demonstrated to be more efficacious than the 10 mg/day dose. An increase to a dose greater than the target dose of 10 mg/day (i.e., to a dose of 15 mg/day or greater) is recommended only after clinical assessment. The safety of doses above 20 mg/day has not been evaluated in clinical trials.

Dosing in Special Populations — The recommended starting dose is 5 mg in patients who are debilitated, who have a predisposition to hypotensive reactions, who otherwise exhibit a combination of factors that may result in slower metabolism of olanzapine (e.g., nonsmoking female patients ≥65 years of age), or who may be more pharmacodynamically sensitive to olanzapine (*see* CLINICAL PHARMACOLOGY; also *see* Use in Patients with Concomitant Illness and Drug Interactions *under* PRECAUTIONS). When indicated, dose escalation should be performed with caution in these patients.

Maintenance Treatment — While there is no body of evidence available to answer the question of how long the patient treated with olanzapine should remain on it, the effectiveness of oral olanzapine, 10 mg/day to 20 mg/day, in maintaining treatment response in schizophrenic patients who had been stable on ZYPREXA for approximately 8 weeks and were then followed for a period of up to 8 months has been demonstrated in a placebo-controlled trial (*see* CLINICAL PHARMACOLOGY). Patients should be periodically reassessed to determine the need for maintenance treatment with appropriate dose.

Bipolar Disorder

Usual Monotherapy Dose — Oral olanzapine should be administered on a once-a-day schedule without regard to meals, generally beginning with 10 or 15 mg. Dosage adjustments, if indicated, should generally occur at intervals of not less than 24 hours, reflecting the procedures in the placebo-controlled trials. When dosage adjustments are necessary, dose increments/decrements of 5 mg QD are recommended.

Short-term (3–4 weeks) antimanic efficacy was demonstrated in a dose range of 5 mg to 20 mg/day in clinical trials. The safety of doses above 20 mg/day has not been evaluated in clinical trials.

Maintenance Monotherapy — The benefit of maintaining bipolar patients on monotherapy with oral ZYPREXA at a dose of 5 to 20 mg/day, after achieving a responder status for an average duration of two weeks, was demonstrated in a controlled trial (*see* Clinical Efficacy Data *under* CLINICAL PHARMACOLOGY). The physician who elects to use ZYPREXA for extended periods should periodically re-evaluate the long-term usefulness of the drug for the individual patient.

Bipolar Mania Usual Dose in Combination with Lithium or Valproate — When administered in combination with lithium or valproate, oral olanzapine dosing should generally begin with 10 mg once-a-day without regard to meals.

Short-term (6 weeks) antimanic efficacy was demonstrated in a dose range of 5 mg to 20 mg/day in clinical trials. The safety of doses above 20 mg/day has not been evaluated in clinical trials.

Dosing in Special Populations — *See* Dosing in Special Populations *under* DOSAGE AND ADMINISTRATION, Schizophrenia.

Administration of ZYPREXA ZYDIS (olanzapine orally disintegrating tablets)

After opening sachet, peel back foil on blister. Do not push tablet through foil. Immediately upon opening the blister, using dry hands, remove tablet and place entire ZYPREXA ZYDIS in the mouth. Tablet disintegration occurs rapidly in saliva so it can be easily swallowed with or without liquid.

Agitation Associated with Schizophrenia and Bipolar I Mania

Usual Dose for Agitated Patients with Schizophrenia or Bipolar Mania — The efficacy of intramuscular olanzapine for injection in controlling agitation in these disorders was demonstrated in a dose range of 2.5 mg to 10 mg. The recommended dose in these patients is 10 mg. A lower dose of 5 or 7.5 mg may be considered when clinical factors warrant (*see* CLINICAL PHARMACOLOGY). If agitation warranting additional intramuscular doses persists following the initial dose, subsequent doses up to 10 mg may be given. However, the efficacy of repeated doses of intramuscular olanzapine for injection in agitated patients has not been systematically evaluated in controlled clinical trials. Also, the safety of total daily doses greater than 30 mg, or 10 mg injections given more frequently than 2 hours after the initial dose, and 4 hours after the second dose have not been evaluated in clinical trials. Maximal dosing of intramuscular olanzapine (e.g., three doses of 10 mg administered 2–4 hours apart) may be associated with a substantial occurrence of significant orthostatic hypotension (*see* PRECAUTIONS, Hemodynamic Effects). Thus, it is recommended that patients requiring subsequent intramuscular injections be assessed for orthostatic hypotension prior to the administration of any subsequent doses of intramuscular olanzapine for injection. The administration of an additional dose to a patient with a clinically significant postural change in systolic blood pressure is not recommended.

If ongoing olanzapine therapy is clinically indicated, oral olanzapine may be initiated in a range of 5–20 mg/day as soon as clinically appropriate (*see* Schizophrenia or Bipolar Disorder *under* DOSAGE AND ADMINISTRATION).

Intramuscular Dosing in Special Populations — A dose of 5 mg per injection should be considered for geriatric patients or when other clinical factors warrant. A lower dose of 2.5 mg per injection should be considered for patients who otherwise might be debilitated, be predisposed to hypotensive reactions, or be more pharmacodynamically sensitive to olanzapine*see* CLINICAL PHARMACOLOGY; also *see* Use in Patients with Concomitant Illness and Drug Interactions *under* PRECAUTIONS).

Administration of ZYPREXA IntraMuscular

ZYPREXA IntraMuscular is intended for intramuscular use only. Do not administer intravenously or subcutaneously. Inject slowly, deep into the muscle mass.

Parenteral drug products should be inspected visually for particulate matter and discoloration prior to administration, whenever solution and container permit.

Directions for preparation of ZYPREXA IntraMuscular with Sterile Water for Injection

Dissolve the contents of the vial using 2.1 mL of Sterile Water for Injection to provide a solution containing approximately 5 mg/mL of olanzapine. The resulting solution should appear clear and yellow. ZYPREXA IntraMuscular reconstituted with Sterile Water for Injection should be used immediately (within 1 hour) after reconstitution. **Discard any unused portion.**

The following table provides injection volumes for delivering various doses of intramuscular olanzapine for injection reconstituted with Sterile Water for Injection.

Dose, mg Olanzapine	Volume of Injection, mL
10.0	Withdraw total contents of vial
7.5	1.5
5.0	1.0
2.5	0.5

Physical Incompatibility Information

ZYPREXA IntraMuscular should be reconstituted only with Sterile Water for Injection. ZYPREXA IntraMuscular should not be combined in a syringe with diazepam injection because precipitation occurs when these products are mixed. Lorazepam injection should not be used to reconstitute ZYPREXA IntraMuscular as this combination results in a delayed reconstitution time. ZYPREXA IntraMuscular should not be combined in a syringe with haloperidol injection because the resulting low pH has been shown to degrade olanzapine over time.

HOW SUPPLIED

The ZYPREXA 2.5 mg, 5 mg, 7.5 mg, and 10 mg tablets are white, round, and imprinted in blue ink with LILLY and tablet number. The 15 mg tablets are elliptical, blue, and debossed with LILLY and tablet number. The 20 mg tablets are elliptical, pink, and debossed with LILLY and tablet number. The tablets are available as follows:

[See first table above]

	TABLET STRENGTH 2.5 mg	5 mg	7.5 mg	10 mg	15 mg	20 mg
Tablet No.	4112	4115	4116	4117	4415	4420
Identification	LILLY 4112	LILLY 4115	LILLY 4116	LILLY 4117	LILLY 4415	LILLY 4420
NDC Codes:						
Bottles 60	NDC 0002-4112-60	NDC 0002-4115-60	NDC 0002-4116-60	NDC 0002-4117-60	NDC 0002-4415-60	NDC 0002-4420-60
Blisters - ID* 100	NDC 0002-4112-33	NDC 0002-4115-33	NDC 0002-4116-33	NDC 0002-4117-33	NDC 0002-4415-33	NDC 0002-4420-33
Bottles 1000	NDC 0002-4112-04	NDC 0002-4115-04	NDC 0002-4116-04	NDC 0002-4117-04	NDC 0002-4415-04	NDC 0002-4420-04

*Identi-Dose® (unit dose medication, Lilly)

ZYPREXA ZYDIS (olanzapine orally disintegrating tablets) are yellow, round, and debossed with the tablet strength. The tablets are available as follows:

[See second table above]

ZYPREXA ZYDIS Tablets*	TABLET STRENGTH 5 mg	10 mg	15 mg	20 mg
Tablet No.	4453	4454	4455	4456
Debossed	5	10	15	20
NDC Codes:				
Dose Pack 30 (Child-Resistant)	NDC 0002-4453-85	NDC 0002-4454-85	NDC 0002-4455-85	NDC 0002-4456-85

ZYPREXA is a registered trademark of Eli Lilly and Company.
ZYDIS is a registered trademark of R. P. Scherer Corporation.
*ZYPREXA ZYDIS (olanzapine orally disintegrating tablets) is manufactured for Eli Lilly and Company by Scherer DDS Limited, United Kingdom, SN5 8RU.

ZYPREXA IntraMuscular is available in:

NDC 0002-7597-01 (No. VL7597) – 10 mg vial (1s)

Store ZYPREXA tablets, ZYPREXA ZYDIS, and ZYPREXA IntraMuscular vials (before reconstitution) at controlled room temperature, 20° to 25°C (68° to 77°F) [*see* USP]. Reconstituted ZYPREXA IntraMuscular may be stored at controlled room temperature, 20° to 25°C (68° to 77°F) [*see* USP] for up to 1 hour if necessary. **Discard any unused portion of reconstituted ZYPREXA IntraMuscular.** The USP defines controlled room temperature as a temperature maintained thermostatically that encompasses the usual and customary working environment of 20° to 25°C (68° to 77°F); that results in a mean kinetic temperature calculated to be not more than 25°C; and that allows for excursions between 15° and 30°C (59° and 86°F) that are experienced in pharmacies, hospitals, and warehouses.

Protect ZYPREXA tablets and ZYPREXA ZYDIS from light and moisture. Protect ZYPREXA IntraMuscular from light, do not freeze.

ANIMAL TOXICOLOGY

In animal studies with olanzapine, the principal hematologic findings were reversible peripheral cytopenias in individual dogs dosed at 10 mg/kg (17 times the maximum recommended human daily oral dose on a mg/m[2] basis), dose-related decreases in lymphocytes and neutrophils in mice, and lymphopenia in rats. A few dogs treated with 10 mg/kg developed reversible neutropenia and/or reversible hemolytic anemia between 1 and 10 months of treatment. Dose-related decreases in lymphocytes and neutrophils were seen in mice given doses of 10 mg/kg (equal to 2 times the maximum recommended human daily oral dose on a mg/m[2] basis) in studies of 3 months' duration. Nonspecific lymphopenia, consistent with decreased body weight gain, occurred in rats receiving 22.5 mg/kg (11 times the maximum recommended human daily oral dose on a mg/m[2] basis) for 3 months or 16 mg/kg (8 times the maximum recommended human daily oral dose on a mg/m[2] basis) for 6 or 12 months. No evidence of bone marrow cytotoxicity was found in any of the species examined. Bone marrows were normocellular or hypercellular, indicating that the reductions in circulating blood cells were probably due to peripheral (non-marrow) factors.

Literature revised May 13, 2004

Eli Lilly and Company
Indianapolis, IN 46285, USA
www.ZYPREXA.com

PV 3513 AMP PRINTED IN USA

Shown in Product Identification Guide, page 320

Lilly ICOS LLC

c/o ELI LILLY AND COMPANY
LILLY CORPORATE CENTER
INDIANAPOLIS, IN 46285

Direct Inquiries to:
Lilly ICOS LLC
c/o Eli Lilly and Company
Lilly Corporate Center
Indianapolis, IN 46285
(317) 276-2000
www.cialis.com

For Medical Information Contact:
Lilly ICOS LLC
1-877-Cialis-1

CIALIS® ℞
[see-AL-iss]
(tadalafil)
tablets

DESCRIPTION

CIALIS® (tadalafil), an oral treatment for erectile dysfunction, is a selective inhibitor of cyclic guanosine monophosphate (cGMP)-specific phosphodiesterase type 5 (PDE5). Tadalafil has the empirical formula $C_{22}H_{19}N_3O_4$ representing a molecular weight of 389.41. The structural formula is:

The chemical designation is pyrazino[1′,2′:1,6]pyrido[3,4-b]-indole-1,4-dione, 6-(1,3-benzodioxol-5-yl)-2,3,6,7,12,12a-hexahydro-2-methyl-, (6R,12aR)-. It is a crystalline solid that is practically insoluble in water and very slightly soluble in ethanol.

CIALIS is available as film-coated, almond-shaped tablets for oral administration. Each tablet contains 5, 10, or 20 mg of tadalafil and the following inactive ingredients: croscarmellose sodium, hydroxypropyl cellulose, hypromellose, iron oxide, lactose monohydrate, magnesium stearate, microcrystalline cellulose, sodium lauryl sulfate, talc, titanium dioxide, and triacetin.

CLINICAL PHARMACOLOGY

Mechanism of Action

Penile erection during sexual stimulation is caused by increased penile blood flow resulting from the relaxation of penile arteries and corpus cavernosal smooth muscle. This response is mediated by the release of nitric oxide (NO) from nerve terminals and endothelial cells, which stimulates the synthesis of cGMP in smooth muscle cells. Cyclic GMP causes smooth muscle relaxation and increased blood flow into the corpus cavernosum. The inhibition of phosphodiesterase type 5 (PDE5) enhances erectile function by increasing the amount of cGMP. Tadalafil inhibits PDE5. Because sexual stimulation is required to initiate the local release of nitric oxide, the inhibition of PDE5 by tadalafil has no effect in the absence of sexual stimulation.

Studies *in vitro* have demonstrated that tadalafil is a selective inhibitor of PDE5. PDE5 is found in corpus cavernosum smooth muscle, vascular and visceral smooth muscle, skeletal muscle, platelets, kidney, lung, cerebellum, and pancreas.

In vitro studies have shown that the effect of tadalafil is more potent on PDE5 than on other phosphodiesterases. These studies have shown that tadalafil is >10,000-fold more potent for PDE5 than for PDE1, PDE2, PDE4, and PDE7 enzymes, which are found in the heart, brain, blood vessels, liver, leukocytes, skeletal muscle, and other organs. Tadalafil is >10,000-fold more potent for PDE5 than for PDE3, an enzyme found in the heart and blood vessels. Additionally, tadalafil is 700-fold more potent for PDE5 than for PDE6, which is found in the retina and is responsible for phototransduction. Tadalafil is >9,000-fold more potent for PDE5 than for PDE8, PDE9, and PDE10 and 14-fold more potent for PDE5 than for PDE11A1, an enzyme found in human skeletal muscle. Tadalafil inhibits human recombinant PDE11A1 activity at concentrations within the therapeutic range. The physiological role and clinical consequence of PDE11 inhibition in humans have not been defined.

Pharmacokinetics

Over a dose range of 2.5 to 20 mg, tadalafil exposure (AUC) increases proportionally with dose in healthy subjects. Steady-state plasma concentrations are attained within 5 days of once-daily dosing, and exposure is approximately 1.6-fold greater than after a single dose. Tadalafil is eliminated predominantly by hepatic metabolism, mainly by cytochrome P450 3A4 (CYP3A4). The concomitant use of potent CYP3A4 inhibitors such as ritonavir or ketoconazole resulted in significant increases in tadalafil AUC values (*see* **PRECAUTIONS** *and* **DOSAGE AND ADMINISTRATION**). Mean tadalafil concentrations measured after the administration of a single oral dose of 20 mg to healthy male subjects are depicted in Figure 1.

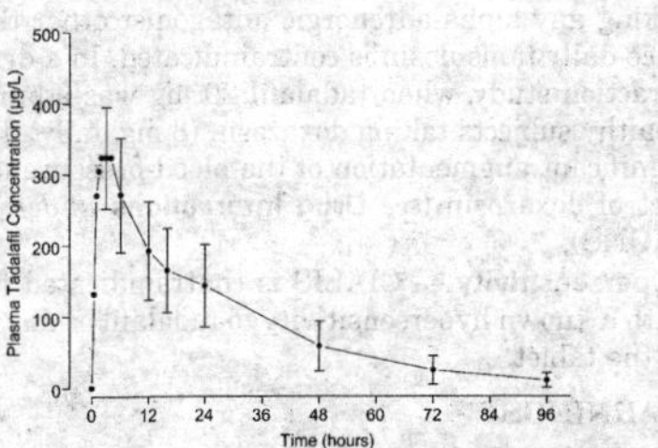

Figure 1: Plasma tadalafil concentrations (mean ± SD) following a single 20-mg tadalafil dose

Absorption — After single oral-dose administration, the maximum observed plasma concentration (C_{max}) of tadalafil is achieved between 30 minutes and 6 hours (median time of 2 hours). Absolute bioavailability of tadalafil following oral dosing has not been determined.

The rate and extent of absorption of tadalafil are not influenced by food; thus CIALIS may be taken with or without food.

Distribution — The mean apparent volume of distribution following oral administration is approximately 63 L, indicating that tadalafil is distributed into tissues. At therapeutic concentrations, 94% of tadalafil in plasma is bound to proteins.

Less than 0.0005% of the administered dose appeared in the semen of healthy subjects.

Metabolism — Tadalafil is predominantly metabolized by CYP3A4 to a catechol metabolite. The catechol metabolite undergoes extensive methylation and glucuronidation to form the methylcatechol and methylcatechol glucuronide conjugate, respectively. The major circulating metabolite is the methylcatechol glucuronide. Methylcatechol concentrations are less than 10% of glucuronide concentrations. *In vitro* data suggests that metabolites are not expected to be pharmacologically active at observed metabolite concentrations.

Elimination — The mean oral clearance for tadalafil is 2.5 L/hr and the mean terminal half-life is 17.5 hours in healthy subjects. Tadalafil is excreted predominantly as metabolites, mainly in the feces (approximately 61% of the dose) and to a lesser extent in the urine (approximately 36% of the dose).

Pharmacokinetics in Special Populations

Geriatric — Healthy male elderly subjects (65 years or over) had a lower oral clearance of tadalafil, resulting in 25% higher exposure (AUC) with no effect on C_{max} relative to that observed in healthy subjects 19 to 45 years of age. No dose adjustment is warranted based on age alone. However, greater sensitivity to medications in some older individuals should be considered (*see* **Geriatric Use** *under* **PRECAUTIONS**).

Pediatric — Tadalafil has not been evaluated in individuals less than 18 years old.

Hepatic Impairment — In clinical pharmacology studies, tadalafil exposure (AUC) in subjects with mild or moderate hepatic impairment (Child-Pugh Class A or B) was comparable to exposure in healthy subjects when a dose of 10 mg was administered. There are no available data for doses higher than 10 mg of tadalafil in patients with hepatic impairment. Insufficient data are available for subjects with severe hepatic impairment (Child-Pugh Class C). Therefore, for patients with mild or moderate hepatic impairment, the maximum dose should not exceed 10 mg, and use in patients with severe hepatic impairment is not recommended (*see* **DOSAGE AND ADMINISTRATION**).

Renal Insufficiency — In clinical pharmacology studies using single-dose tadalafil (5 to 10 mg), tadalafil exposure (AUC) doubled in subjects with mild (creatinine clearance 51 to 80 mL/min) or moderate (creatinine clearance 31 to 50 mL/min) renal insufficiency. In subjects with end-stage renal disease on hemodialysis, there was a two-fold increase in C_{max} and 2.7- to 4.1-fold increase in AUC following single-dose administration of 10 or 20 mg tadalafil. Exposure to total methylcatechol (unconjugated plus glucuronide) was 2- to 4-fold higher in subjects with renal impairment, compared to those with normal renal function. Hemodialysis (performed between 24 and 30 hours post-dose) contributed negligibly to tadalafil or metabolite elimination. In a clinical pharmacology study (N=28) at a dose of 10 mg, back pain was reported as a limiting adverse event in male patients with moderate renal impairment. At a dose of 5 mg, the incidence and severity of back pain was not significantly different than in the general population. In patients on hemodialysis taking 10- or 20-mg tadalafil, there were no reported cases of back pain. The dose of tadalafil should be limited to 5 mg not more than once daily in patients with severe renal insufficiency or end-stage renal disease. A starting dose of 5 mg not more than once daily is recommended for patients with moderate renal insufficiency; the maximum recommended dose is 10 mg not more than once in every 48 hours. No dose adjustment is required in patients with mild renal insufficiency (*see* **DOSAGE AND ADMINISTRATION**).

Patients with Diabetes Mellitus — In male patients with diabetes mellitus after a 10 mg tadalafil dose, exposure (AUC) was reduced approximately 19% and C_{max} was 5% lower than that observed in healthy subjects. No dose adjustment is warranted.

Pharmacodynamics

Effects on Blood Pressure — Tadalafil 20 mg administered to healthy male subjects produced no significant difference compared to placebo in supine systolic and diastolic blood pressure (difference in the mean maximal decrease of 1.6/0.8 mm Hg, respectively) and in standing systolic and diastolic blood pressure (difference in the mean maximal decrease of 0.2/4.6 mm Hg, respectively). In addition, there was no significant effect on heart rate.

Effects on Blood Pressure when CIALIS is Administered with Nitrates — In clinical pharmacology studies, tadalafil (5 to 20 mg) was shown to potentiate the hypotensive effect of nitrates. Therefore, the use of CIALIS in patients taking any form of nitrates is contraindicated (*see* **CONTRAINDICATIONS**).

A study was conducted to assess the degree of interaction between nitroglycerin and tadalafil, should nitroglycerin be required in an emergency situation after tadalafil was taken. This was a double-blind, placebo-controlled, crossover study in 150 male subjects at least 40 years of age (including subjects with diabetes mellitus and/or controlled hypertension) and receiving daily doses of tadalafil 20 mg or matching placebo for 7 days. Subjects were administered a single dose of 0.4 mg sublingual nitroglycerin (NTG) at prespecified timepoints, following their last dose of tadalafil (2, 4, 8, 24, 48, 72, and 96 hours after tadalafil). The objective of the study was to determine when, after tadalafil dosing, no apparent blood pressure interaction was observed. In this study, a significant interaction between tadalafil and NTG was observed at each timepoint up to and including 24 hours. At 48 hours, by most hemodynamic measures, the interaction between tadalafil and NTG was not observed, although a few more tadalafil subjects compared to placebo experienced greater blood-pressure lowering at this timepoint. After 48 hours, the interaction was not detectable (*see* Figure 2).

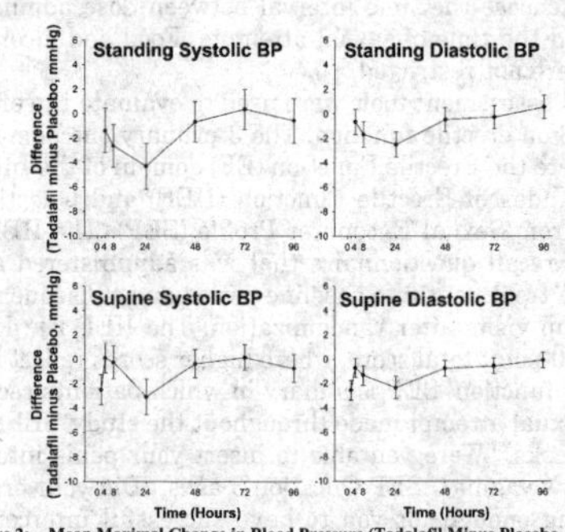

Figure 2: Mean Maximal Change in Blood Pressure (Tadalafil Minus Placebo, Point Estimate with 90% CI) in Response to Sublingual Nitroglycerin at 2 (Supine Only), 4, 8, 24, 48, 72, and 96 Hours after the Last Dose of Tadalafil 20 mg or Placebo

Therefore, CIALIS administration with nitrates is contraindicated. In a patient who has taken CIALIS, where nitrate administration is deemed medically necessary in a life-threatening situation, at least 48 hours should elapse after the last dose of CIALIS before nitrate administration is considered. In such circumstances, nitrates should still only be administered under close medical supervision with appropriate hemodynamic monitoring (*see* **CONTRAINDICATIONS**).

Effects on Exercise Stress Testing — The effects of tadalafil on cardiac function, hemodynamics, and exercise tolerance were investigated in a single clinical pharmacology study. In this blinded crossover trial, 23 subjects with stable coronary artery disease and evidence of exercise-induced cardiac ischemia were enrolled. The primary endpoint was time to cardiac ischemia. The mean difference in total exercise time was 3 seconds (tadalafil 10 mg minus placebo), which represented no clinically meaningful difference. Further statistical analysis demonstrated that tadalafil was non-inferior to placebo with respect to time to ischemia. Of note, in this study, in some subjects who received tadalafil followed by sublingual nitroglycerin in the post-exercise period, clinically significant reductions in blood pressure were observed, consistent with the augmentation by tadalafil of the blood-pressure-lowering effects of nitrates.

Effects on Vision — Single oral doses of phosphodiesterase inhibitors have demonstrated transient dose-related impairment of color discrimination (blue/green), using the Farnsworth-Munsell 100-hue test, with peak effects near the time of peak plasma levels. This finding is consistent with the inhibition of PDE6, which is involved in phototransduction in the retina. In a study to assess the effects of a single dose of tadalafil 40 mg on vision (N=59), no effects were observed on visual acuity, intraocular pressure, or pupillometry. Across all clinical studies with CIALIS, reports of changes in color vision were rare (<0.1% of patients).

Effects on Sperm Characteristics — There were no clinically relevant effects on sperm concentration, sperm count, motility, or morphology in humans in placebo-controlled studies of daily doses of tadalafil 10 mg (N=204) or 20 mg (N=217) for 6 months. In addition, tadalafil had no effect on serum levels of testosterone, luteinizing hormone, or follicle stimulating hormone.

Effects on Cardiac Electrophysiology — The effect of a single 100-mg dose of tadalafil on the QT interval was evaluated at the time of peak tadalafil concentration in a randomized, double-blinded, placebo, and active (intravenous ibutilide)-controlled crossover study in 90 healthy males aged 18 to 53 years. The mean change in QT_c (Fridericia QT correction) for tadalafil, relative to placebo, was 3.5 milliseconds (two-sided 90% CI=1.9, 5.1). The mean change in QT_c (Individual QT correction) for tadalafil, relative to placebo, was 2.8 milliseconds (two-sided 90% CI=1.2, 4.4). A 100-mg dose of tadalafil (5 times the highest recommended dose) was chosen because this dose yields exposures covering those observed upon coadministration of tadalafil with potent CYP3A4 inhibitors or those observed in renal impairment. In this study, the mean increase in heart rate associated with a 100-mg dose of tadalafil compared to placebo was 3.1 beats per minute.

Clinical Studies

The efficacy and safety of tadalafil in the treatment of erectile dysfunction has been evaluated in 22 clinical trials of up to 24-weeks duration, involving over 4000 patients. CIALIS, when taken as needed up to once daily, was shown to be effective in improving erectile function in men with erectile dysfunction (ED).

Study Design — CIALIS was studied in the general ED population in 7 randomized, multicenter, double-blinded, placebo-controlled, parallel-arm design, primary efficacy and safety studies of 12-weeks duration. Two of these studies were conducted in the United States and 5 were conducted in centers outside the US. Additional efficacy and safety

Continued on next page

Cialis—Cont.

studies were performed in ED patients with diabetes mellitus and in patients who developed ED status post bilateral nerve-sparing radical prostatectomy.
In these 7 trials, CIALIS was taken as needed, at doses ranging from 2.5 to 20 mg, up to once daily. Patients were free to choose the time interval between dose administration and the time of sexual attempts. Food and alcohol intake were not restricted.
Several assessment tools were used to evaluate the effect of CIALIS on erectile function. The 3 primary outcome measures were the Erectile Function (EF) domain of the International Index of Erectile Function (IIEF) and Questions 2 and 3 from Sexual Encounter Profile (SEP). The IIEF is a 4-week recall questionnaire that was administered at the end of a treatment-free baseline period and subsequently at follow-up visits after randomization. The IIEF EF domain has a 30-point total score, where higher scores reflect better erectile function. SEP is a diary in which patients recorded each sexual attempt made throughout the study. SEP Question 2 asks, "Were you able to insert your penis into your partner's vagina?" SEP Question 3 asks, "Did your erection last long enough for you to have successful intercourse?" The overall percentage of successful attempts to insert the penis into the vagina (SEP2) and to maintain the erection for successful intercourse (SEP3) is derived for each patient.

Study Results —

ED Population in US Trials — The 2 primary US efficacy and safety trials included a total of 402 men with erectile dysfunction, with a mean age of 59 years (range 27 to 87 years). The population was 78% White, 14% Black, 7% Hispanic, and 1% of other ethnicities, and included patients with ED of various severities, etiologies (organic, psychogenic, mixed), and with multiple co-morbid conditions, including diabetes mellitus, hypertension, and other cardiovascular disease. Most (>90%) patients reported ED of at least 1-year duration. Study A was conducted primarily in academic centers. Study B was conducted primarily in community-based urology practices. In each of these 2 trials, CIALIS 20 mg showed clinically meaningful and statistically significant improvements in all 3 primary efficacy variables (*see* Table 1). The treatment effect of CIALIS did not diminish over time.
[See table 1 above]

Table 1: Mean Endpoint and Change from Baseline for the Primary Efficacy Variables in the Two Primary US Trials

	Study A			Study B		
	Placebo	CIALIS 20 mg		Placebo	CIALIS 20 mg	
	(N=49)	(N=146)	p-value	(N=48)	(N=159)	p-value
EF Domain Score						
Endpoint	13.5	19.5		13.6	22.5	
Change from baseline	-0.2	6.9	<.001	0.3	9.3	<.001
Insertion of Penis (SEP2)						
Endpoint	39%	62%		43%	77%	
Change from baseline	2%	26%	<.001	2%	32%	<.001
Maintenance of Erection (SEP3)						
Endpoint	25%	50%		23%	64%	
Change from baseline	5%	34%	<.001	4%	44%	<.001

General ED Population in Trials Outside the US — The 5 primary efficacy and safety studies conducted in the general ED population outside the US included 1112 patients, with a mean age of 59 years (range 21 to 82 years). The population was 76% White, 1% Black, 3% Hispanic, and 20% of other ethnicities, and included patients with ED of various severities, etiologies (organic, psychogenic, mixed), and with multiple co-morbid conditions, including diabetes mellitus, hypertension, and other cardiovascular disease. Most (90%) patients reported ED of at least 1-year duration. In these 5 trials, CIALIS 5, 10, and 20 mg showed clinically meaningful and statistically significant improvements in all 3 primary efficacy variables (*see* Tables 2, 3, and 4). The treatment effect of CIALIS did not diminish over time.
[See table 2 at right]
[See table 3 at top of next page]
[See table 4 on next page]

Table 2: Mean Endpoint and Change from Baseline for the EF Domain of the IIEF in the General ED Population in Five Primary Trials Outside the US

	Placebo	CIALIS 5 mg	CIALIS 10 mg	CIALIS 20 mg
Study C				
Endpoint [Change from baseline]	15.0 [0.7]	17.9 [4.0]	20.0 [5.6]	
		p=.006	*p<.001*	
Study D				
Endpoint [Change from baseline]	14.4 [1.1]	17.5 [5.1]	20.6 [6.0]	
		p=.002	*p<.001*	
Study E				
Endpoint [Change from baseline]	18.1 [2.6]		22.6 [8.1]	25.0 [8.0]
			p<.001	*p<.001*
Study F*				
Endpoint [Change from baseline]	12.7 [-1.6]			22.8 [6.8]
				p<.001
Study G				
Endpoint [Change from baseline]	14.5 [-0.9]		21.2 [6.6]	23.3 [8.0]
			p<.001	*p<.001*

* Treatment duration in Study F was 6 months

In addition, there were improvements in EF domain scores, success rates based upon SEP Questions 2 and 3, and patient-reported improvement in erections across patients with ED of all degrees of disease severity while taking CIALIS, compared to patients on placebo.
Therefore, in all 7 primary efficacy and safety studies, CIALIS showed statistically significant improvement in patients' ability to achieve an erection sufficient for vaginal penetration and to maintain the erection long enough for successful intercourse, as measured by the IIEF questionnaire and by SEP diaries.

Efficacy in ED Patients with Diabetes Mellitus — CIALIS was shown to be effective in treating ED in patients with diabetes mellitus. Patients with diabetes were included in all 7 primary efficacy studies in the general ED population (N=235) and in 1 study that specifically assessed CIALIS in ED patients with type 1 or type 2 diabetes (N=216). In this randomized, placebo-controlled, double-blinded, parallel-arm design prospective trial, CIALIS demonstrated clinically meaningful and statistically significant improvement in erectile function, as measured by the EF domain of the IIEF questionnaire and Questions 2 and 3 of the SEP diary (*see* Table 5).
[See table 5 at top of page 1910]

Efficacy in ED Patients following Radical Prostatectomy — CIALIS was shown to be effective in treating patients who developed ED following bilateral nerve-sparing radical prostatectomy. In 1 randomized, placebo-controlled, double-blinded, parallel-arm design prospective trial in this population (N=303), CIALIS demonstrated clinically meaningful and statistically significant improvement in erectile function, as measured by the EF domain of the IIEF questionnaire and Questions 2 and 3 of the SEP diary (*see* Table 6).
[See table 6 at top of page 1910]

Studies to Determine the Optimal Use of CIALIS — Several studies were conducted with the objective of determining the optimal use of CIALIS in the treatment of ED. In 1 of these studies, the percentage of patients reporting successful erections within 30 minutes of dosing was determined. In this randomized, placebo-controlled, double-blinded trial, 223 patients were randomized to placebo, CIALIS 10, or 20 mg. Using a stopwatch, patients recorded the time following dosing at which a successful erection was obtained. A successful erection was defined as at least 1 erection in 4 attempts that led to successful intercourse. At or prior to 30 minutes, 35% (26/74), 38% (28/74), and 52% (39/75) of patients in the placebo, 10-, and 20-mg groups, respectively, reported successful erections as defined above.
Two studies were conducted to assess the efficacy of CIALIS at a given timepoint after dosing, specifically at 24 hours and at 36 hours after dosing.
In the first of these studies, 348 patients with ED were randomized to placebo or CIALIS 20 mg. Patients were encouraged to make 4 total attempts at intercourse; 2 attempts were to occur at 24 hours after dosing and 2 completely separate attempts were to occur at 36 hours after dosing. The results demonstrated a difference between the placebo group and the CIALIS group at each of the pre-specified timepoints. At the 24-hour timepoint, (more specifically, 22 to 26 hours), 53/144 (37%) patients reported at least 1 successful intercourse in the placebo group versus 84/138 (61%) in the CIALIS 20-mg group. At the 36-hour timepoint (more specifically, 33 to 39 hours), 49/133 (37%) of patients reported at least 1 successful intercourse in the placebo group versus 88/137 (64%) in the CIALIS 20-mg group.
In the second of these studies, a total of 483 patients were evenly randomized to 1 of 6 groups: 3 different dosing groups (placebo, CIALIS 10, or 20 mg) that were instructed to attempt intercourse at 2 different times (24 and 36 hours post-dosing). Patients were encouraged to make 4 separate attempts at their assigned dose and assigned timepoint. In this study, the results demonstrated a statistically significant difference between the placebo group and the CIALIS groups at each of the pre-specified timepoints. At the 24-hour timepoint, the mean, per-patient percentage of attempts resulting in successful intercourse were 42, 56, and 67% for the placebo, CIALIS 10-, and 20-mg groups, respectively. At the 36-hour timepoint, the mean, per-patient percentage of attempts resulting in successful intercourse were 33, 56, and 62% for placebo, CIALIS 10-, and 20-mg groups, respectively.

INDICATIONS AND USAGE

CIALIS is indicated for the treatment of erectile dysfunction.

CONTRAINDICATIONS

Nitrates — Administration of CIALIS to patients who are using any form of organic nitrate, either regularly and/or intermittently, is contraindicated. In clinical pharmacology studies, tadalafil was shown to potentiate the hypotensive effect of nitrates. This is thought to result from the combined effects of nitrates and tadalafil on the nitric oxide/cGMP pathway (*see* **Pharmacodynamics, Effects on Blood Pressure when CIALIS is Administered with Nitrates** *under* **CLINICAL PHARMACOLOGY**).

Alpha Blockers — Administration of CIALIS to patients taking any alpha-adrenergic antagonist other than 0.4 mg once-daily tamsulosin is contraindicated. In a drug-drug interaction study, when tadalafil 20 mg was administered to healthy subjects taking doxazosin (8 mg daily), there was a significant augmentation of the blood-pressure-lowering effect of doxazosin (*see* **Drug Interactions** *under* **PRECAUTIONS**).

Hypersensitivity — CIALIS is contraindicated for patients with a known hypersensitivity to tadalafil or any component of the tablet.

WARNINGS

Cardiovascular

General — Physicians should consider the cardiovascular status of their patients, since there is a degree of cardiac risk associated with sexual activity. Therefore, treatments for erectile dysfunction, including CIALIS, should not be used in men for whom sexual activity is inadvisable as a result of their underlying cardiovascular status.

Left Ventricular Outflow Obstruction — Patients with left ventricular outflow obstruction, (e.g., aortic stenosis and idiopathic hypertrophic subaortic stenosis) can be sensitive to the action of vasodilators, including PDE5 inhibitors.

Patients Not Studied in Clinical Trials

The following groups of patients with cardiovascular disease were not included in clinical safety and efficacy trials for CIALIS, and, therefore, the use of CIALIS is not recommended in these groups until further information is available:

— patients with a myocardial infarction within the last 90 days
— patients with unstable angina or angina occurring during sexual intercourse
— patients with New York Heart Association Class 2 or greater heart failure in the last 6 months
— patients with uncontrolled arrhythmias, hypotension (<90/50 mm Hg), or uncontrolled hypertension (>170/100 mm Hg)
— patients with a stroke within the last 6 months

In addition, patients with known hereditary degenerative retinal disorders, including retinitis pigmentosa, were not included in the clinical trials, and use in these patients is not recommended.

Prolonged Erection

There have been rare reports of prolonged erections greater than 4 hours and priapism (painful erections greater than 6 hours in duration) for this class of compounds. Priapism, if not treated promptly, can result in irreversible damage to the erectile tissue. Patients who have an erection lasting greater than 4 hours, whether painful or not, should seek emergency medical attention.

PRECAUTIONS

Evaluation of erectile dysfunction should include an appropriate medical assessment to identify potential underlying causes, as well as treatment options.

Before prescribing CIALIS, it is important to note the following:

Renal Insufficiency

CIALIS should be limited to 5 mg not more than once daily in patients with severe renal insufficiency or end-stage renal disease. The starting dose of CIALIS in patients with a moderate degree of renal insufficiency should be 5 mg not more than once daily, and the maximum dose should be limited to 10 mg not more than once in every 48 hours. No dose adjustment is required in patients with mild renal insufficiency (*see* **Pharmacokinetics in Special Populations** *under* **CLINICAL PHARMACOLOGY**).

Hepatic Impairment

In patients with mild or moderate hepatic impairment, the dose of CIALIS should not exceed 10 mg. Because of insufficient information in patients with severe hepatic impairment, use of CIALIS in this group is not recommended (*see* **Pharmacokinetics in Special Populations** *under* **CLINICAL PHARMACOLOGY**).

Concomitant Use of Potent Inhibitors of Cytochrome P450 3A4 (CYP3A4)

CIALIS is metabolized predominantly by CYP3A4 in the liver. The dose of CIALIS should be limited to 10 mg no more than once every 72 hours in patients taking potent inhibitors of CYP3A4 such as ritonavir, ketoconazole, and itraconazole (*see* Effects of Other Drugs on CIALIS *under* **Drug Interactions**).

General

As with other PDE5 inhibitors, tadalafil has mild systemic vasodilatory properties that may result in transient decreases in blood pressure. In a clinical pharmacology study, tadalafil 20 mg resulted in a mean maximal decrease in supine blood pressure, relative to placebo, of 1.6/0.8 mm Hg in healthy subjects (*see* **Clinical Studies** *under* **CLINICAL PHARMACOLOGY**). While this effect should not be of consequence in most patients, prior to prescribing CIALIS, physicians should carefully consider whether their patients with underlying cardiovascular disease could be affected adversely by such vasodilatory effects. Patients with significant left ventricular outflow obstruction or severely impaired autonomic control of blood pressure may be particularly sensitive to the actions of vasodilators.

The safety and efficacy of combinations of CIALIS and other treatments for erectile dysfunction have not been studied. Therefore, the use of such combinations is not recommended.

CIALIS should be used with caution in patients who have conditions that might predispose them to priapism (such as sickle cell anemia, multiple myeloma, or leukemia), or in patients with anatomical deformation of the penis (such as angulation, cavernosal fibrosis, or Peyronie's disease).

When administered in combination with aspirin, tadalafil 20 mg did not prolong bleeding time, relative to aspirin alone. CIALIS has not been administered to patients with bleeding disorders or significant active peptic ulceration. Although CIALIS has not been shown to increase bleeding times in healthy subjects, use in patients with bleeding disorders or significant active peptic ulceration should be based upon a careful risk-benefit assessment and caution.

Information for Patients

Physicians should discuss with patients the contraindication of CIALIS with regular and/or intermittent use of organic nitrates. Patients should be counseled that concomitant use of CIALIS with nitrates could cause blood pressure to suddenly drop to an unsafe level, resulting in dizziness, syncope, or even heart attack or stroke.

Physicians should discuss with patients the appropriate action in the event that they experience anginal chest pain requiring nitroglycerin following intake of CIALIS. In such a patient, who has taken CIALIS, where nitrate administration is deemed medically necessary for a life-threatening situation, at least 48 hours should have elapsed after the last dose of CIALIS before nitrate administration is considered. In such circumstances, nitrates should still only be administered under close medical supervision with appropriate hemodynamic monitoring. Therefore, patients who experience anginal chest pain after taking CIALIS should seek immediate medical attention.

Table 3: Mean Post-Baseline Success Rate and Change from Baseline for SEP Question 2 ("Were you able to insert your penis into the partner's vagina?") in the General ED Population in Five Pivotal Trials Outside the US

	Placebo	CIALIS 5 mg	CIALIS 10 mg	CIALIS 20 mg
Study C				
Endpoint [Change from baseline]	49% [6%]	57% [15%]	73% [29%]	
		p=.063	*p<.001*	
Study D				
Endpoint [Change from baseline]	46% [2%]	56% [18%]	68% [15%]	
		p=.008	*p<.001*	
Study E				
Endpoint [Change from baseline]	55% [10%]		77% [35%]	85% [35%]
			p<.001	*p<.001*
Study F*				
Endpoint [Change from baseline]	42% [-8%]			81% [27%]
				p<.001
Study G				
Endpoint [Change from baseline]	45% [-6%]		73% [21%]	76% [21%]
			p<.001	*p<.001*

* Treatment duration in Study F was 6 months

Table 4: Mean Post-Baseline Success Rate and Change from Baseline for SEP Question 3 ("Did your erection last long enough for you to have successful intercourse?") in the General ED Population in Five Pivotal Trials Outside the US

	Placebo	CIALIS 5 mg	CIALIS 10 mg	CIALIS 20 mg
Study C				
Endpoint [Change from baseline]	26% [4%]	38% [19%]	58% [32%]	
		p=.040	*p<.001*	
Study D				
Endpoint [Change from baseline]	28% [4%]	42% [24%]	51% [26%]	
		p<.001	*p<.001*	
Study E				
Endpoint [Change from baseline]	43% [15%]		70% [48%]	78% [50%]
			p<.001	*p<.001*
Study F*				
Endpoint [Change from baseline]	27% [1%]			74% [40%]
				p<.001
Study G				
Endpoint [Change from baseline]	32% [5%]		57% [33%]	62% [29%]
			p<.001	*p<.001*

* Treatment duration in Study F was 6 months

Physicians should inform their patients that concomitant use of CIALIS with alpha-adrenergic antagonists (other than 0.4 mg once-daily tamsulosin) is contraindicated because coadministration can lead to significant reductions in blood pressure.

Physicians should discuss with patients the potential for CIALIS to augment the blood-pressure-lowering effect of other anti-hypertensive medications.

Patients should be made aware that both alcohol and CIALIS, a PDE5 inhibitor, act as mild vasodilators. When mild vasodilators are taken in combination, blood-pressure-lowering effects of each individual compound may be increased. Therefore, physicians should inform patients that substantial consumption of alcohol (e.g., 5 units or greater) in combination with CIALIS can increase the potential for orthostatic signs and symptoms, including increase in heart rate, decrease in standing blood pressure, dizziness, and headache.

Physicians should consider the potential cardiac risk of sexual activity in patients with preexisting cardiovascular disease. Patients who experience symptoms upon initiation of sexual activity should be advised to refrain from further sexual activity and seek immediate medical attention.

There have been rare reports of prolonged erections greater than 4 hours and priapism (painful erections greater than 6 hours in duration) for this class of compounds. Priapism, if not treated promptly, can result in irreversible damage to the erectile tissue. Patients who have an erection lasting greater than 4 hours, whether painful or not, should seek emergency medical attention.

The use of CIALIS offers no protection against sexually transmitted diseases. Counseling of patients about the protective measures necessary to guard against sexually transmitted diseases, including Human Immunodeficiency Virus (HIV) should be considered.

Patients should read the patient leaflet entitled "INFORMATION FOR THE PATIENT" before starting therapy with CIALIS and each time the prescription is renewed or refilled.

Drug Interactions

Effects of Other Drugs on CIALIS

Cytochrome P450 Inhibitors

CIALIS is a substrate of and predominantly metabolized by CYP3A4. Studies have shown that drugs that inhibit CYP3A4 can increase tadalafil exposure (*see* **PRECAUTIONS** *and* **DOSAGE AND ADMINISTRATION**).

Ketoconazole — Ketoconazole (400 mg daily), a selective and potent inhibitor of CYP3A4, increased tadalafil 20-mg single-dose exposure (AUC) by 312% and C_{max} by 22%, relative to the values for tadalafil 20 mg alone. Ketoconazole (200 mg daily) increased tadalafil 10-mg single-dose exposure (AUC) by 107% and C_{max} by 15%, relative to the values for tadalafil 10 mg alone.

Continued on next page

Cialis—Cont.

HIV Protease inhibitor — Ritonavir (200 mg twice daily), an inhibitor of CYP3A4, CYP2C9, CYP2C19, and CYP2D6, increased tadalafil 20-mg single-dose exposure (AUC) by 124% with no change in C_{max}, relative to the values for tadalafil 20 mg alone. Although specific interactions have not been studied, other HIV protease inhibitors would likely increase tadalafil exposure (*see* **DOSAGE AND ADMINISTRATION**).

Based upon these results, in patients taking concomitant potent CYP3A4 inhibitors, the dose of CIALIS should not exceed 10 mg, and CIALIS should not be taken more frequently than once in every 72 hours (*see* **DOSAGE AND ADMINISTRATION**).

Other cytochrome P450 inhibitors — Although specific interactions have not been studied, other CYP3A4 inhibitors, such as erythromycin, itraconazole, and grapefruit juice, would likely increase tadalafil exposure.

Cytochrome P450 Inducers

Studies have shown that drugs that induce CYP3A4 can decrease tadalafil exposure.

Rifampin — Rifampin (600 mg daily), a CYP3A4 inducer, reduced tadalafil 10-mg single-dose exposure (AUC) by 88% and C_{max} by 46%, relative to the values for tadalafil 10 mg alone. Although specific interactions have not been studied, other CYP3A4 inducers, such as carbamazepine, phenytoin, and phenobarbitol, would likely decrease tadalafil exposure. No dose adjustment is warranted.

Gastrointestinal Drugs

H_2 antagonists — An increase in gastric pH resulting from administration of nizatidine had no significant effect on tadalafil pharmacokinetics.

Antacids — Simultaneous administration of an antacid (magnesium hydroxide/aluminum hydroxide) and tadalafil reduced the apparent rate of absorption of tadalafil without altering exposure (AUC) to tadalafil.

Effects of CIALIS on Other Drugs

Drugs Metabolized by Cytochrome P450

CIALIS is not expected to cause clinically significant inhibition or induction of the clearance of drugs metabolized by cytochrome P450 (CYP) isoforms. Studies have shown that tadalafil does not inhibit or induce P450 isoforms CYP1A2, CYP3A4, CYP2C9, CYP2C19, CYP2D6, and CYP2E1.

CYP1A2 substrate — Tadalafil had no clinically significant effect on the pharmacokinetics of theophylline. When tadalafil was administered to subjects taking theophylline, a small augmentation (3 beats per minute) of the increase in heart rate associated with theophylline was observed.

CYP3A4 substrates — Tadalafil had no clinically significant effect on exposure (AUC) to midazolam or lovastatin.

CYP2C9 substrate — Tadalafil had no clinically significant effect on exposure (AUC) to S-warfarin or R-warfarin, nor did tadalafil affect changes in prothrombin time induced by warfarin.

Alcohol

Alcohol and PDE5 inhibitors, including tadalafil, are mild systemic vasodilators. The interaction of tadalafil with alcohol was evaluated in 3 clinical pharmacology studies. In 2 of these, alcohol was administered at a dose of 0.7 g/kg, which is equivalent to approximately 6 ounces of 80-proof vodka in an 80-kg male, and tadalafil was administered at a dose of 10 mg in 1 study and 20 mg in another. In both these studies, all patients imbibed the entire alcohol dose within 10 minutes of starting. In one of these two studies, blood alcohol levels of 0.08% were confirmed. In these two studies, more patients had clinically significant decreases in blood pressure on the combination of tadalafil and alcohol as compared to alcohol alone. Some subjects reported postural dizziness, and orthostatic hypotension was observed in some subjects. When tadalafil 20 mg was administered with a lower dose of alcohol (0.6 g/kg, which is equivalent to approximately 4 ounces of 80-proof vodka, administered in less than 10 minutes), orthostatic hypotension was not observed, dizziness occurred with similar frequency to alcohol alone, and the hypotensive effects of alcohol were not potentiated.

Tadalafil did not affect alcohol plasma concentrations and alcohol did not affect tadalafil plasma concentrations.

Both alcohol and CIALIS, a PDE5 inhibitor, act as mild vasodilators. When mild vasodilators are taken in combination, blood-pressure-lowering effects of each individual compound may be increased. Substantial consumption of alcohol (e.g., 5 units or greater) in combination with CIALIS can increase the potential for orthostatic signs and symptoms, including increase in heart rate, decrease in standing blood pressure, dizziness, and headache.

Anti-Hypertensives

PDE5 inhibitors, including tadalafil, are mild systemic vasodilators. Clinical pharmacology studies were conducted to assess the effect of tadalafil on the potentiation of the blood-pressure-lowering effects of selected anti-hypertensive medications.

Alpha Blockers

Doxazosin — When tadalafil 20 mg was administered to healthy subjects taking doxazosin (8 mg daily), an alpha[1]-adrenergic blocker, there was significant augmentation of the blood-pressure-lowering effect of doxazosin.

Tamsulosin — In a clinical pharmacology study, when a single dose of tadalafil 20 mg was administered to healthy subjects taking 0.4 mg once-daily tamsulosin, a selective alpha[1A]-adrenergic blocker, no significant decreases in blood pressure were observed.

Table 5: Mean Endpoint and Change from Baseline for the Primary Efficacy Variables in a Study in ED Patients with Diabetes

	Placebo	CIALIS 10 mg	CIALIS 20 mg	
	(N=71)	(N=73)	(N=72)	p-value
EF Domain Score				
Endpoint [Change from baseline]	12.2 [0.1]	19.3 [6.4]	18.7 [7.3]	<.001
Insertion of Penis (SEP2)				
Endpoint [Change from baseline]	30% [-4%]	57% [22%]	54% [23%]	<.001
Maintenance of Erection (SEP3)				
Endpoint [Change from baseline]	20% [2%]	48% [28%]	42% [29%]	<.001

Table 6: Mean Endpoint and Change from Baseline for the Primary Efficacy Variables in a Study in Patients who Developed ED Following Bilateral Nerve-Sparing Radical Prostatectomy

	Placebo	CIALIS 20 mg	
	(N=102)	(N=201)	p-value
EF Domain Score			
Endpoint [Change from baseline]	13.3 [1.1]	17.7 [5.3]	<.001
Insertion of Penis (SEP2)			
Endpoint [Change from baseline]	32% [2%]	54% [22%]	<.001
Maintenance of Erection (SEP3)			
Endpoint [Change from baseline]	19% [4%]	41% [23%]	<.001

Therefore, based upon significant augmentation of the blood-pressure-lowering effect of doxazosin, an alpha[1]-adrenergic blocker, and no significant effect seen with 0.4 mg once-daily tamsulosin, a selective alpha[1A]-adrenergic blocker, administration of CIALIS to patients taking any alpha-adrenergic blocker other than 0.4 mg once-daily tamsulosin is contraindicated.

Other Anti-Hypertensive Agents

Amlodipine — A study was conducted to assess the interaction of amlodipine (5 mg daily) and tadalafil 10 mg. There was no effect of tadalafil on amlodipine blood levels and no effect of amlodipine on tadalafil blood levels. The mean reduction in supine systolic/diastolic blood pressure due to tadalafil 10 mg in subjects taking amlodipine was 3/2 mm Hg, compared to placebo. In a similar study using tadalafil 20 mg, there were no clinically significant differences between tadalafil and placebo in subjects taking amlodipine.

Metoprolol — A study was conducted to assess the interaction of sustained-release metoprolol (25 to 200 mg daily) and tadalafil 10 mg. Following dosing, the mean reduction in supine systolic/diastolic blood pressure due to tadalafil 10 mg in subjects taking metoprolol was 5/3 mm Hg, compared to placebo.

Bendrofluazide — A study was conducted to assess the interaction of bendrofluazide (2.5 mg daily) and tadalafil 10 mg. Following dosing, the mean reduction in supine systolic/diastolic blood pressure due to tadalafil 10 mg in subjects taking bendrofluazide was 6/4 mm Hg, compared to placebo.

Enalapril — A study was conducted to assess the interaction of enalapril (10 to 20 mg daily) and tadalafil 10 mg. Following dosing, the mean reduction in supine systolic/diastolic blood pressure due to tadalafil 10 mg in subjects taking enalapril was 4/1 mm Hg, compared to placebo.

Angiotensin II receptor blocker (and other anti-hypertensives) — A study was conducted to assess the interaction of angiotensin II receptor blockers and tadalafil 20 mg. Subjects in the study were taking any marketed angiotensin II receptor blocker, either alone, as a component of a combination product, or as part of a multiple anti-hypertensive regimen. Following dosing, ambulatory measurements of blood pressure revealed differences between tadalafil and placebo of 8/4 mm Hg in systolic/diastolic blood pressure.

Aspirin

Tadalafil did not potentiate the increase in bleeding time caused by aspirin.

Carcinogenesis, Mutagenesis, Impairment of Fertility

Tadalafil was not carcinogenic to rats or mice when administered daily for 2 years at doses up to 400 mg/kg/day. Systemic drug exposures, as measured by AUC of unbound tadalafil, were approximately 10-fold for mice, and 14- and 26-fold for male and female rats, respectively, the exposures in human males given Maximum Recommended Human Dose (MRHD) of 20 mg.

Tadalafil was not mutagenic in the *in vitro* bacterial Ames assays or the forward mutation test in mouse lymphoma cells. Tadalafil was not clastogenic in the *in vitro* chromosomal aberration test in human lymphocytes or the *in vivo* rat micronucleus assays.

There were no effects on fertility, reproductive performance or reproductive organ morphology in male or female rats given oral doses of tadalafil up to 400 mg/kg/day, a dose producing AUCs for unbound tadalafil of 14-fold for males or 26-fold for females the exposures observed in human males given the MRHD of 20 mg. In beagle dogs given tadalafil daily for 3 to 12 months, there was treatment-related non-reversible degeneration and atrophy of the seminiferous tubular epithelium in the testes in 20-100% of the dogs that resulted in a decrease in spermatogenesis in 40-75% of the dogs at doses of ≥10 mg/kg/day. Systemic exposure (based on AUC) at no-observed-adverse-effect-level (NOAEL) (10 mg/kg/day) for unbound tadalafil was similar to that expected in humans at the MRHD of 20 mg.

There were no treatment-related testicular findings in rats or mice treated with doses up to 400 mg/kg/day for 2 years. In men, there were no clinically relevant effects on sperm concentration, sperm count, motility, or morphology in placebo-controlled studies of daily doses of tadalafil 10 mg (N=204) or 20 mg (N=217) for 6 months. In addition, tadalafil had no effect on serum levels of testosterone, luteinizing hormone, or follicle stimulating hormone in males.

Animal Toxicology

Animal studies showed vascular inflammation in tadalafil-treated mice, rats, and dogs. In mice and rats, lymphoid necrosis and hemorrhage were seen in the spleen, thymus, and mesenteric lymph nodes at unbound tadalafil exposure of 2- to 33-fold above the human exposure (AUCs) at the MRHD of 20 mg. In dogs, an increased incidence of disseminated arteritis was observed in 1- and 6-month studies at unbound tadalafil exposure of 1- to 54-fold above the human exposure (AUC) at the MRHD of 20 mg. In a 12-month dog study, no disseminated arteritis was observed, but 2 dogs exhibited marked decreases in white blood cells (neutrophils) and moderate decreases in platelets with inflammatory signs at unbound tadalafil exposures of approximately 14- to 18-fold the human exposure at the MRHD of 20 mg. The abnormal blood-cell findings were reversible within 2 weeks upon removal of the drug.

Pregnancy, Nursing Mothers, and Pediatric Use

CIALIS is not indicated for use in newborns, children, or women.

Tadalafil and/or its metabolites cross the placenta, resulting in fetal exposure in rats. Tadalafil and/or its metabolites were secreted into the milk in lactating rats at concentrations approximately 2.4-fold greater than found in the plasma. Following a single-oral dose of 10 mg/kg, approximately 0.1% of the total radioactive dose was excreted into the milk within 3 hours. It is not known if tadalafil and/or its metabolites is excreted in human breast milk. Use of tadalafil in nursing mothers is not recommended.

Pregnancy Category B — There was no evidence of teratogenicity, embryotoxicity, or fetotoxicity in rat or mouse fetuses that received up to 1000 mg/kg/day during the major organ development. Plasma exposure at this dose is approximately 11-fold greater than the AUC values for unbound tadalafil in humans given the MRHD of 20 mg. In a rat prenatal and postnatal development study at doses of 60, 200, and 1000 mg/kg, there was a reduction in postnatal survival of pups. The no-observed-effect-level (NOEL) for maternal toxicity was 200 mg/kg/day and for developmental toxicity was 30 mg/kg/day, which gives approximately 16- and 10-fold exposure multiples, respectively, of the human AUC for the MRHD dose of 20 mg. There are no adequate and well-controlled studies of tadalafil in pregnant women.

Table 7: **Treatment-Emergent Adverse Events Reported by ≥2% of Patients Treated with Tadalafil (10 or 20 mg) and More Frequent on Drug than Placebo in the Eight Primary Placebo-Controlled Phase 3 Studies (Including a Study in Patients with Diabetes)**

	Placebo	Tadalafil 5 mg	Tadalafil 10 mg	Tadalafil 20 mg
Adverse Event	**(N=476)**	**(N=151)**	**(N=394)**	**(N=635)**
Headache	5%	11%	11%	15%
Dyspepsia	1%	4%	8%	10%
Back pain	3%	3%	5%	6%
Myalgia	1%	1%	4%	3%
Nasal congestion	1%	2%	3%	3%
Flushing*	1%	2%	3%	3%
Pain in limb	1%	1%	3%	3%

* The term flushing includes: facial flushing and flushing

Geriatric Use
Approximately 25% of patients in the primary efficacy and safety studies of tadalafil were greater than 65 years of age. No overall differences in efficacy and safety were observed between older and younger patients. No dose adjustment is warranted based on age alone. However, greater sensitivity to medications in some older individuals should be considered (*see* **Special Populations** *under* **CLINICAL PHARMACOLOGY**).

ADVERSE REACTIONS

Tadalafil was administered to over 5700 men (mean age 59, range 19 to 87 years) during clinical trials worldwide. Over 1000 patients were treated for 1 year or longer and over 1300 patients were treated for 6 months or more.

In placebo-controlled Phase 3 clinical trials, the discontinuation rate due to adverse events in patients treated with tadalafil 10 or 20 mg was 3.1%, compared to 1.4% in placebo-treated patients.

When tadalafil was taken as recommended in the placebo-controlled clinical trials, the following adverse events were reported (*see* Table 7):

[See table 7 above]

Back pain or myalgia was reported at incidence rates described in Table 7. In tadalafil clinical pharmacology trials, back pain or myalgia generally occurred 12 to 24 hours after dosing and typically resolved within 48 hours. The back pain/myalgia associated with tadalafil treatment was characterized by diffuse bilateral lower lumbar, gluteal, thigh, or thoracolumbar muscular discomfort and was exacerbated by recumbancy. In general, pain was reported as mild or moderate in severity and resolved without medical treatment, but severe back pain was reported infrequently (<5% of all reports). When medical treatment was necessary, acetaminophen or non-steroidal anti-inflammatory drugs were generally effective; however, in a small percentage of subjects who required treatment, a mild narcotic (e.g. codeine) was used. Overall, approximately 0.5% of all tadalafil-treated subjects discontinued treatment as a consequence of back pain/myalgia. Diagnostic testing, including measures for inflammation, muscle injury, or renal damage revealed no evidence of medically significant underlying pathology.

Across all studies with any tadalafil dose, reports of changes in color vision were rare (<0.1% of patients).

The following section identifies additional, less frequent events (<2%) reported in controlled clinical trials; a causal relationship of these events to CIALIS is uncertain. Excluded from this list are those events that were minor, those with no plausible relation to drug use, and reports too imprecise to be meaningful:

Body as a whole: asthenia, face edema, fatigue, pain
Cardiovascular: angina pectoris, chest pain, hypotension, hypertension, myocardial infarction, postural hypotension, palpitations, syncope, tachycardia
Digestive: abnormal liver function tests, diarrhea, dry mouth, dysphagia, esophagitis, gastroesophageal reflux, gastritis, GGTP increased, loose stools, nausea, upper abdominal pain, vomiting
Musculoskeletal: arthralgia, neck pain
Nervous: dizziness, hypesthesia, insomnia, paresthesia, somnolence, vertigo
Respiratory: dyspnea, epistaxis, pharyngitis
Skin and Appendages: pruritus, rash, sweating
Ophthalmologic: blurred vision, changes in color vision, conjunctivitis (including conjunctival hyperemia), eye pain, lacrimation increase, swelling of eyelids
Urogenital: erection increased, spontaneous penile erection

OVERDOSAGE

Single doses up to 500 mg have been given to healthy subjects, and multiple daily doses up to 100 mg have been given to patients. Adverse events were similar to those seen at lower doses. In cases of overdose, standard supportive measures should be adopted as required. Hemodialysis contributes negligibly to tadalafil elimination.

DOSAGE AND ADMINISTRATION

The recommended starting dose of CIALIS in most patients is 10 mg, taken prior to anticipated sexual activity. The dose may be increased to 20 mg or decreased to 5 mg, based on individual efficacy and tolerability. The maximum recommended dosing frequency is once per day in most patients. CIALIS was shown to improve erectile function compared to placebo up to 36 hours following dosing. Therefore, when advising patients on optimal use of CIALIS, this should be taken into consideration.

CIALIS may be taken without regard to food.

Renal Insufficiency — No dose adjustment is required in patients with mild renal insufficiency. For patients with moderate (creatinine clearance 31 to 50 mL/min) renal insufficiency, a starting dose of 5 mg not more than once daily is recommended, and the maximum dose should be limited to 10 mg not more than once in every 48 hours. For patients with severe (creatinine clearance <30 mL/min) renal insufficiency on hemodialysis, the maximum recommended dose is 5 mg (*see* **General** *and* **Patients with Renal Insufficiency** *under* **PRECAUTIONS** *and* **Pharmacokinetics in Special Populations** *under* **CLINICAL PHARMACOLOGY**).

Hepatic Impairment — For patients with mild or moderate degrees of hepatic impairment (Child-Pugh Class A or B), the dose of CIALIS should not exceed 10 mg once daily. In patients with severe hepatic impairment (Child-Pugh Class C), the use of CIALIS is not recommended (*see* **Patients with Hepatic Impairment** *under* **PRECAUTIONS** *and* **Pharmacokinetics in Special Populations** *under* **CLINICAL PHARMACOLOGY**).

Concomitant Medications — For patients taking concomitant potent inhibitors of CYP3A4, such as ketoconazole or ritonavir, the maximum recommended dose of CIALIS is 10 mg, not to exceed once every 72 hours (*see* **General** *and* **Drug Interactions** *under* **PRECAUTIONS**).

Concomitant use of nitrates in any form and alpha-adrenergic blockers (other than 0.4 mg once-daily tamsulosin) is contraindicated (*see* **CONTRAINDICATIONS** *and* **Drug Interactions** *under* **PRECAUTIONS**).

Geriatrics — No dose adjustment is required in patients >65 years of age.

HOW SUPPLIED

CIALIS® (tadalafil) is supplied as follows:

Three strengths of film-coated, almond-shaped tablets are available in different sizes and different shades of yellow, and supplied in the following package sizes:

5-mg tablets debossed with "C 5"
Bottles of 30 NDC 0002-4462-30
10-mg tablets debossed with "C 10"
Bottles of 30 NDC 0002-4463-30
20-mg tablets debossed with "C 20"
Bottles of 30 NDC 0002-4464-30

Store at 25°C (77°F); excursions permitted to 15-30°C (59-86°F) [see USP Controlled Room Temperature].

Keep out of reach of children.

Literature issued November, 2003
Manufactured for Lilly ICOS LLC
by Eli Lilly and Company
Indianapolis, IN 46285, USA
PV 3530 AMP

Shown in Product Identification Guide, page 320

NOTICE
Before prescribing or administering any product described in PHYSICIANS' DESK REFERENCE check the **PDR Supplements** for revised information.

3M Pharmaceuticals

3M CENTER, BLDG. 275-6W-13
P.O. BOX 33275
ST. PAUL, MN 55144

Commercial Customers:
Orders, Returns, Accounting
(800) 447-4537

Trade and Government:
(800) 328-6523

For Medical Information Contact:
Drug Surveillance & Information
3M Pharmaceuticals
3M Center, Bldg. 275-6W-13
P.O. Box 33275
St. Paul, MN 55144
(800) 328-0255
For Aldara™:
(800) 814-1795

In Emergencies:
(800) 328-0255 (all hours)

Website:
www.3M.com/pharma

ALDARA™ ℞

[al dar' a]
(imiquimod)
Cream, 5%
For Dermatologic Use Only
Not for Ophthalmic Use.

DESCRIPTION

Aldara ™ is the brand name for imiquimod which is an immune response modifier. Each gram of the 5% cream contains 50 mg of imiquimod in an off-white oil-in-water vanishing cream base consisting of isostearic acid, cetyl alcohol, stearyl alcohol, white petrolatum, polysorbate 60, sorbitan monostearate, glycerin, xanthan gum, purified water, benzyl alcohol, methylparaben, and propylparaben.

Chemically, imiquimod is 1-(2-methylpropyl)-1*H*-imidazo [4,5-c]quinolin-4-amine. Imiquimod has a molecular formula of $C_{14}H_{16}N_4$ and a molecular weight of 240.3. Its structural formula is:

CLINICAL PHARMACOLOGY

Pharmacodynamics

Actinic Keratosis

The mechanism of action of Aldara Cream in treating actinic keratosis (AK) lesions is unknown. In a study of 18 patients with AK comparing Aldara Cream to vehicle, increases from baseline in week 2 biomarker levels were reported for CD3, CD4, CD8, CD11c, and CD68 for Aldara Cream treated patients; however, the clinical relevance of these findings is unknown.

Superficial Basal Cell Carcinoma

The mechanism of action of Aldara Cream in treating superficial basal cell carcinoma (sBCC) lesions is unknown. An open label study in six subjects with sBCC suggests that treatment with Aldara Cream may increase the infiltration of lymphocytes, dendritic cells, and macrophages into the tumor lesion; however, the clinical significance of these findings is unknown.

External Genital Warts

Imiquimod has no direct antiviral activity in cell culture. A study in 22 patients with genital/perianal warts comparing Aldara Cream and vehicle shows that Aldara Cream induces mRNA encoding cytokines including interferon-α at the treatment site. In addition HPVL1 mRNA and HPV DNA are significantly decreased following treatment. However, the clinical relevance of these findings is unknown.

PHARMACOKINETICS

Systemic absorption of imiquimod was observed across the affected skin of 12 patients with genital/perianal warts, with an average dose of 4.6 mg. Mean peak drug concentration of approximately 0.4 ng/mL was seen during the study. Mean urinary recoveries of imiquimod and metabolites combined over the whole course of treatment, expressed as percent of the estimated applied dose, were 0.11 and 2.41% in the males and females, respectively.

Systemic absorption of imiquimod across the affected skin of 58 patients with AK was observed with a dosing frequency of 3 applications per week for 16 weeks. Mean peak serum drug concentrations at the end of week 16 were approximately 0.1, 0.2, and 3.5 ng/mL for the applications to face (12.5 mg imiquimod, 1 single-use packet), scalp (25 mg, 2 packets) and hands/arms (75 mg, 6 packets), respectively.

Continued on next page

Aldara—Cont.

Mean Serum Imiquimod Concentration Following Administration of the Last Topical Dose During Week 16	
Amount of Aldara Cream applied	**Mean peak serum imiquimod concentration [Cmax]**
12.5 mg (1 packet)	0.1 ng/mL
25 mg (2 packets)	0.2 ng/mL
75 mg (6 packets)	3.5 ng/mL

The application surface area was not controlled when more than one packet was used. Dose proportionality was not observed. However it appears that systemic exposure may be more dependent on surface area of application than amount of applied dose. The apparent half-life was approximately 10 times greater with topical dosing than the 2 hour apparent half-life seen following subcutaneous dosing, suggesting prolonged retention of drug in the skin. Mean urinary recoveries of imiquimod and metabolites combined were 0.08 and 0.15% of the applied dose in the group using 75 mg (6 packets) for males and females, respectively following 3 applications per week for 16 weeks.

CLINICAL STUDIES

Actinic Keratosis

In two double-blind, vehicle-controlled clinical studies, 436 patients with actinic keratosis (AK) were treated with Aldara Cream or vehicle cream 2 times per week for 16 weeks. Patients with 4 to 8 clinically typical, visible, discrete, nonhyperkeratotic, nonhypertrophic AK lesions within a 25 cm^2 contiguous treatment area on either the face or scalp were enrolled and randomized to active or vehicle treatment. The population studied ranged from 37-88 years of age (median 66 years) and 55% had Fitzpatrick skin type I or II. All imiquimod-treated patients were Caucasians. The 25 cm^2 contiguous treatment area could be of any dimensions e.g., 5 cm × 5 cm, 3 cm by 8.3 cm, 2 cm by 12.5 cm, etc. On a scheduled dosing day, the study cream was applied to the entire treatment area prior to normal sleeping hours and left on for approximately 8 hours. Twice weekly dosing was continued for a total of 16 weeks. Eight weeks after the patient's last scheduled application of study cream, the clinical response of each patient was evaluated. The primary efficacy variable was the complete clearance rate. Complete clearance (designated below as "clear") was defined as the proportion of subjects at the 8-week post-treatment visit with no (zero) clinically visible AK lesions in the treatment area. Complete clearance included clearance of all baseline lesions, as well as any new or subclinical AK lesions which appeared during therapy. Patient outcomes are shown in the figure below.

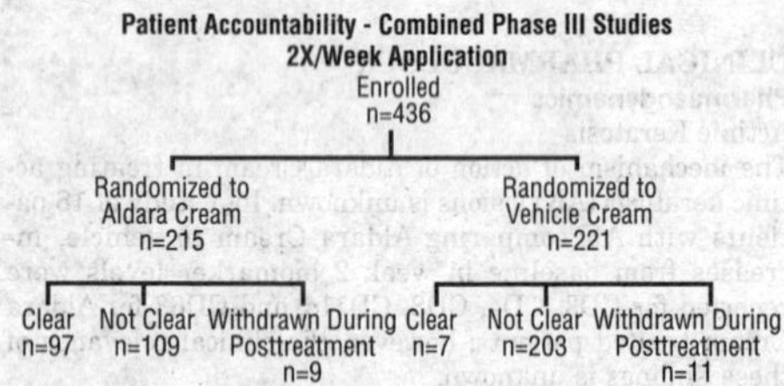

Complete and partial clearance rates are shown in the table below. The partial clearance rate was defined as the percentage of patients in whom 75% or more baseline AK lesions were cleared.

Complete Clearance Rates (100% Lesions Cleared)

Study	Aldara Cream	Vehicle
Study A	46% (49/107)	3% (3/110)
Study B	44% (48/108)	4% (4/111)

Partial Clearance Rates (75% or More Baseline Lesions Cleared)

Study	Aldara Cream	Vehicle
Study A	60% (64/107)	10% (11/110)
Study B	58% (63/108)	14% (15/111)

Sub-clinical AK lesions may become apparent in the treatment area during treatment with Aldara Cream. During the course of treatment, 48% (103/215) of patients experienced an increase in AK lesions relative to the number present at baseline within the treatment area. Patients with an increase in AK lesions had a similar response to those with no increase in AK lesions.

Of the 206 imiquimod subjects with both baseline and 8-week post-treatment scarring assessments, only 6 (2.9%) had a greater degree of scarring scores at 8-weeks post-treatment than at baseline.

Superficial Basal Cell Carcinoma

In two double-blind, vehicle-controlled clinical studies, 364 patients with primary superficial basal cell carcinoma (sBCC) were treated with Aldara Cream or vehicle cream 5×/week for 6 weeks. Patients with one biopsy-confirmed sBCC tumor were enrolled and randomized in a 1:1 ratio to active or vehicle treatment. Target tumors were to have a minimum area of 0.5 cm^2 and a maximum diameter of 2.0 cm (4.0 cm^2). Target tumors were not to be located within 1.0 cm of the hairline, eyes, nose, mouth, ears, on the anogenital area or on the hands or feet, or have any atypical features. On a scheduled dosing day, the study cream was applied to the target tumor and approximately 1 cm (about 1/3 inch) beyond the target tumor prior to normal sleeping hours; 5×/week dosing was continued for a total of 6 weeks. Twelve weeks after the last scheduled application of study cream, the target tumor area was clinically assessed. The entire target tumor was then excised and examined histologically for the presence of tumor.

The primary efficacy variable was the complete response rate defined as the proportion of patients with clinical (visual) and histological clearance of the sBCC lesion at 12 weeks post-treatment. The population ranged from 31-89 years of age (median 60 years) and 65% had Fitzpatrick skin type I or II. Patient outcomes are shown in the figure below.

[See first graphic above]

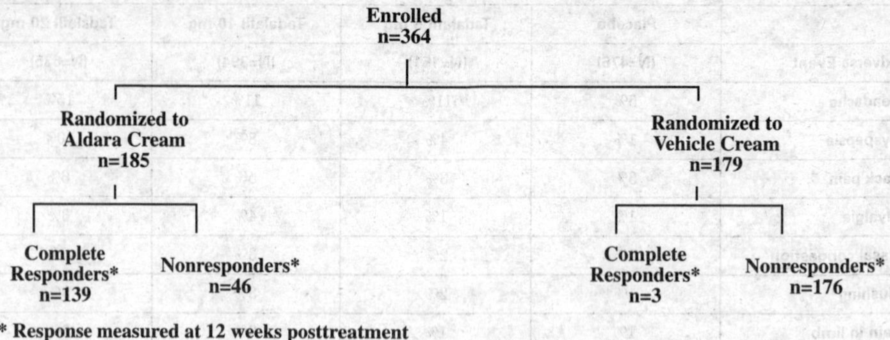

Of Aldara-treated patients 6% (11/178) who had both clinical and histological assessments post-treatment, and appeared to be clinically clear in Studies C and D had evidence of tumor on excision of the clinically clear treatment area. Data on composite clearance (defined as both clinical and histological clearance) are shown in the table below.

Composite Clearance Rates at 12 Weeks Post-treatment for Superficial Basal Cell Carcinoma 5×/Week Application

Study	Aldara Cream	Vehicle Cream
Study C	70% (66/94)	2% (2/89)
Study D	80% (73/91)	1% (1/90)
Total	75% (139/185)	2% (3/179)

An open-label 5-year study (Study E) is ongoing to assess the recurrence of sBCC treated with Aldara Cream applied once daily 5 days per week for 6 weeks. Target tumor inclusion criteria were the same as for Studies C and D as described above. At 12-weeks post-treatment, patients were clinically (no histological assessment) evaluated for evidence of persistent sBCC. Subjects with no clinical evidence of BCC entered the long-term follow-up period. At the 12 week post-treatment assessment 163/182 (90%) of the subjects enrolled had no clinical evidence of sBCC at their target site and 162 subjects entered the long-term follow-up period for up to 5 years. Two year (24 month) follow-up data are available from this study and are presented in the table below:

[See table above]

Estimated Clinical Clearance Rates for Superficial Basal Cell Carcinoma

	Follow-up Period			
Follow-up visit after 12-week post-treatment assessment	No. of Subjects who remained clinically clear	No. of Subjects with sBCC recurrence	No. of Subjects who discontinued at this visit with no sBCC[a]	Estimated Rate of Patients who Clinically Cleared and remained Clear[b]
Month 3	153	4	5	87%
Month 6	149	4	0	85%
Month 12	143	2	4	84%
Month 24	139	4	0	79%

[a]Reasons for discontinuation included death, non-compliance, entry criteria violations, personal reasons, and treatment of nearby sBCC tumor

[b]Estimated rate of patients who clinically cleared and remained clear are estimated based on the time to event analysis employing the life table method beginning with the rate of clinical clearance at 12 weeks post-treatment.

External Genital Warts

In a double-blind, placebo-controlled clinical study, 209 otherwise healthy patients 18 years of age and older with genital/perianal warts were treated with Aldara Cream or vehicle control 3×/week for a maximum of 16 weeks. The median baseline wart area was 69 mm^2 (range 8 to 5525 mm^2). Patient accountability is shown in the figure below.

[See graphic above]

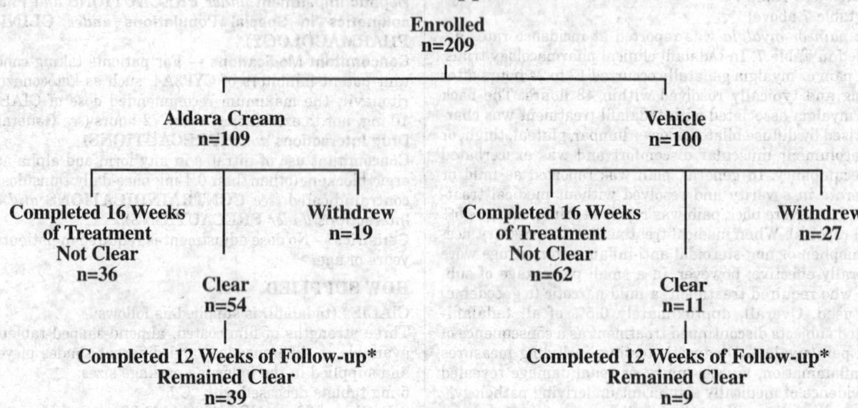

Data on complete clearance are listed in the table below. The median time to complete wart clearance was 10 weeks.

[See table at top of next page]

INDICATIONS AND USAGE

Aldara Cream is indicated for the topical treatment of clinically typical, nonhyperkeratotic, nonhypertrophic actinic keratoses on the face or scalp in immunocompetent adults.

Aldara Cream is indicated for the topical treatment of biopsy-confirmed, primary superficial basal cell carcinoma (sBCC) in immunocompetent adults, with a maximum tumor diameter of 2.0 cm, located on the trunk (excluding anogenital skin), neck, or extremities (excluding hands and feet), only when surgical methods are medically less appropriate and patient follow-up can be reasonably assured. The histological diagnosis of superficial basal cell carcinoma should be established prior to treatment, since safety and effectiveness of Aldara Cream have not been established for other types of basal cell carcinomas, including nodular, morpheaform (fibrosing or sclerosing) types.

Aldara Cream is indicated for the treatment of external genital and perianal warts/condyloma acuminata in individuals 12 years old and above.

CONTRAINDICATIONS

This drug is contraindicated in individuals with a history of sensitivity reactions to any of its components. It should be discontinued if hypersensitivity to any of its ingredients is noted.

WARNINGS

The diagnosis of sBCC should be confirmed prior to treatment, since safety and effectiveness of Aldara Cream have not been established for other types of basal cell carcinomas, including nodular, morpheaform (fibrosing or sclerosing) types and is not recommended for treatment of BCC subtypes other than the superficial variant (i.e., sBCC). Patients with sBCC treated with Aldara Cream are recommended to have regular follow-up of the treatment site. See table of Estimated Clinical Clearance Rates for Superficial Basal Cell Carcinoma in the CLINICAL STUDIES section.

Aldara Cream has not been evaluated for the treatment of urethral, intra-vaginal, cervical, rectal, or intra-anal human papilloma viral disease and is not recommended for these conditions.

PRECAUTIONS

General

The safety and efficacy of Aldara Cream in immunosuppressed patients have not been established.

Aldara Cream administration is not recommended until the skin is completely healed from any previous drug or surgical treatment.

Aldara Cream has the potential to exacerbate inflammatory conditions of the skin.

Exposure to sunlight (including sunlamps) should be avoided or minimized during use of Aldara Cream because of concern for heightened sunburn susceptibility. Patients should be warned to use protective clothing (hat) when using Aldara Cream. Patients with sunburn should be advised not to use Aldara Cream until fully recovered. Patients who may have considerable sun exposure, e.g., due to their occupation, and those patients with inherent sensitivity to sunlight should exercise caution when using Aldara Cream.

Phototoxicity has not been adequately assessed for Aldara Cream. The enhancement of ultraviolet carcinogenicity is not necessarily dependent on phototoxic mechanisms. Despite the absence of observed phototoxicity in humans *(see ADVERSE REACTIONS),* Aldara Cream shortened the time to skin tumor formation in an animal photoco-carcinogenicity study *(see Carcinogenesis, Mutagenesis, Impairment of Fertility).* Therefore, it is prudent for patients to minimize or avoid natural or artificial sunlight exposure.

Actinic Keratosis

Safety and efficacy have not been established for Aldara Cream in the treatment of actinic keratosis with repeated use, i.e. more than one treatment course, in the same 25 cm^2 area.

The safety of Aldara Cream applied to areas of skin greater than 25 cm^2 (e.g. 5 cm × 5 cm) for the treatment of actinic keratosis has not been established *(see CLINICAL PHARMACOLOGY; Pharmacokinetics section* regarding systemic absorption).

Superficial Basal Cell Carcinoma

The safety and efficacy of treating superficial basal cell carcinoma (sBCC) lesions on the face, head and anogenital area have not been established.

The efficacy and safety of Aldara Cream have not been established for patients with Basal Cell Nevus Syndrome or Xeroderma Pigmentosum.

Information for Patients

General Information

Patients using Aldara Cream should receive the following information and instructions:

1. This medication is to be used as directed by a physician. It is for external use only. Eye contact should be avoided.
2. The treatment area should not be bandaged or otherwise covered or wrapped as to be occlusive.
3. Some reports have been received of localized hypopigmentation and hyperpigmentation following Aldara Cream use. Follow-up information suggests that these skin color changes may be permanent in some patients.

Patients Being Treated for Actinic Keratosis (AK)

1. It is recommended that the treatment area be washed with mild soap and water 8 hours following Aldara Cream application.
2. It is common for patients to experience local skin reactions (can range from mild to severe in intensity) during treatment with Aldara Cream, and these reactions may extend beyond the application site onto the surrounding skin. Skin reactions generally decrease in intensity or resolve after cessation of Aldara Cream therapy. Potential local skin reactions include erythema, edema, vesicles, erosion/ulceration, weeping/exudate, flaking/scaling/dryness, and scabbing/crusting. Most patients using Aldara Cream for the treatment of AK experience erythema, flaking/scaling/dryness and scabbing/crusting at the application site with normal dosing. Patients may also experience application site reactions such as itching and/or burning. Local skin reactions may be of such an intensity that patients may require rest periods from treatment. Treatment with Aldara Cream can be resumed after the skin reaction has subsided, as determined by the physician. Patients should contact their physician promptly if they experience any sign or symptom at the application site that restricts or prohibits their daily activity or makes continued application of the cream difficult.
3. Because of local skin reactions, during treatment and until healed, the treatment area is likely to appear noticeably different from normal skin. The skin surrounding the treatment area may also be affected, but less intensely so.
4. Contact with the eyes, lips and nostrils should be avoided.
5. Use of sunscreen is encouraged, and patients should minimize or avoid exposure to natural or artificial sunlight (tanning beds or UVA/B treatment) while using Aldara Cream.
6. During treatment, sub-clinical AK lesions may become apparent in the treatment area and may subsequently resolve.
7. Partially-used packets should be discarded and not reused.
8. Dosing is twice weekly for the full 16 weeks, unless otherwise directed by the physician. However, the treatment period should not be extended beyond 16 weeks due to missed doses or rest periods.

Patients Being Treated for Superficial Basal Cell Carcinoma (sBCC)

1. It is recommended that the treatment area be washed with mild soap and water 8 hours following Aldara Cream application.
2. Most patients using Aldara Cream for the treatment of sBCC experience erythema, edema, induration, erosion, scabbing/crusting and flaking/scaling at the application site with normal dosing. These local skin reactions generally decrease in intensity or resolve after cessation of Aldara Cream therapy. Patients may also experience application site reactions such as itching and/or burning. Local skin reactions may be of such an intensity that patients may require rest periods from treatment. Treatment with Aldara Cream can be resumed after the skin reaction has subsided, as determined by the physician.
3. During treatment and until healed, affected skin is likely to appear noticeably different from normal skin.
4. It is prudent for patients to minimize or avoid exposure to natural or artificial sunlight.
5. The clinical outcome of therapy can be determined after regeneration of the treated skin, approximately 12 weeks after the end of treatment.
6. Patients should contact their physician if they experience any sign or symptom at the application site that restricts or prohibits their daily activity or makes continued application of the cream difficult.
7. Patients with sBCC treated with Aldara Cream are recommended to have regular follow-up to re-evaluate the treatment site.

Patients Being Treated for External Genital Warts

1. It is recommended that the treatment area be washed with mild soap and water 6-10 hours following Aldara Cream application.
2. It is common for patients to experience local skin reactions such as erythema, erosion, excoriation/flaking, and edema at the site of application or surrounding areas. Most skin reactions are mild to moderate. Severe skin reactions can occur and should be promptly reported to the prescribing physician. Should severe local skin reaction occur, the cream should be removed by washing the treatment area with mild soap and water. Treatment with Aldara Cream can be resumed after the skin reaction has subsided.
3. Sexual (genital, anal, oral) contact should be avoided while the cream is on the skin.
4. Application of Aldara Cream in the vagina is considered internal and should be avoided. Female patients should take special care if applying the cream at the opening of the vagina because local skin reactions on the delicate moist surfaces can result in pain or swelling, and may cause difficulty in passing urine.
5. Uncircumcised males treating warts under the foreskin should retract the foreskin and clean the area daily.
6. Patients should be aware that new warts may develop during therapy, as Aldara Cream is not a cure.
7. The effect of Aldara Cream on the transmission of genital/perianal warts is unknown.
8. Aldara Cream may weaken condoms and vaginal diaphragms, therefore concurrent use is not recommended.

Complete Clearance Rates — Study 1004-IMIQ

Treatment	Patients with Complete Clearance of Warts	Patients Without Follow-up	Patients with Warts Remaining at Week 16
Overall			
Aldara Cream (n=109)	50%	17%	33%
Vehicle (n=100)	11%	27%	62%
Females			
Aldara Cream (n=46)	72%	11%	17%
Vehicle (n=40)	20%	33%	48%
Males			
Aldara Cream (n=63)	33%	22%	44%
Vehicle (n=60)	5%	23%	72%

Carcinogenesis, Mutagenesis, and Impairment of Fertility

Note: The Maximum Recommended Human Dose (MRHD) was set at 2 packets per treatment of Aldara Cream (25 mg imiquimod) for the animal multiple of human exposure ratios presented in this label. If higher doses than 2 packets of Aldara Cream are used clinically, then the animal multiple of human exposure would be reduced for that dose. A nonproportional increase in systemic exposure with increased dose of Aldara Cream was noted in the clinical pharmacokinetic study conducted in actinic keratosis subjects (*see Pharmacokinetics*). The AUC after topical application of 6 packets of Aldara Cream was 8 fold greater than the AUC after topical application of 2 packets of Aldara Cream in actinic keratosis subjects. Therefore, if a dose of 6 packets per treatment of Aldara Cream was topically administered to an individual, then the animal multiple of human exposure would be either 1/3 of the value provided in the label (based on body surface area comparisons) or 1/8 of the value provided in the label (based on AUC comparisons). The animal multiples of human exposure calculations were based on weekly dose comparisons for the carcinogenicity studies described in this label. The animal multiples of human exposure calculations were based on daily dose comparisons for the reproductive toxicology studies described in this label.

In an oral (gavage) rat carcinogenicity study, imiquimod was administered to Wistar rats on a 2×/week (up to 6 mg/kg/day) or daily (3 mg/kg/day) dosing schedule for 24 months. No treatment related tumors were noted in the oral rat carcinogenicity study up to the highest doses tested in this study of 6 mg/kg administered 2×/week in female rats (87× MRHD based on weekly AUC comparisons), 4 mg/kg administered 2×/week in male rats (75× MRHD based on weekly AUC comparisons) or 3 mg/kg administered 7×/week to male and female rats (153× MRHD based on weekly AUC comparisons).

In a dermal mouse carcinogenicity study, imiquimod cream (up to 5 mg/kg/application imiquimod or 0.3% imiquimod cream) was applied to the backs of mice 3×/week for 24 months. A statistically significant increase in the incidence of liver adenomas and carcinomas was noted in high dose male mice compared to control male mice (251× MRHD based on weekly AUC comparisons). An increased number of skin papillomas was observed in vehicle cream control group animals at the treated site only. The quantitative composition of the vehicle cream used in the dermal mouse carcinogenicity study is the same as the vehicle cream used for Aldara Cream, minus the active moiety (imiquimod).

In a 52-week dermal photoco-carcinogenicity study, the median time to onset of skin tumor formation was decreased in hairless mice following chronic topical dosing (3×/week; 40 weeks of treatment followed by 12 weeks of observation) with concurrent exposure to UV radiation (5 days per week) with the Aldara Cream vehicle alone. No additional effect on tumor development beyond the vehicle effect was noted with the addition of the active ingredient, imiquimod, to the vehicle cream.

Imiquimod revealed no evidence of mutagenic or clastogenic potential based on the results of five in vitro genotoxicity tests (Ames assay, mouse lymphoma L5178Y assay, Chinese hamster ovary cell chromosome aberration assay, human lymphocyte chromosome aberration assay and SHE cell transformation assay) and three in vivo genotoxicity tests (rat and hamster bone marrow cytogenetics assay and a mouse dominant lethal test).

Daily oral administration of imiquimod to rats, throughout mating, gestation, parturition and lactation, demonstrated no effects on growth, fertility or reproduction, at doses up to 87× MRHD based on AUC comparisons.

Pregnancy

Pregnancy Category C:

Systemic embryofetal development studies were conducted in rats and rabbits. Oral doses of 1, 5 and 20 mg/kg/day imiquimod were administered during the period of organogenesis (gestational days 6 – 15) to pregnant female rats. In the

Continued on next page

Aldara—Cont.

presence of maternal toxicity, fetal effects noted at 20 mg/kg/day [8× MRHD based on body surface area (BSA) comparisons] included increased resorptions, decreased fetal body weights, delays in skeletal ossification, bent limb bones, and two fetuses in one litter (2 of 1567 fetuses) demonstrated exencephaly, protruding tongues and low-set ears. No treatment related effects on embryofetal toxicity or teratogenicity were noted at 5 mg/kg/day (55× MRHD based on AUC comparisons).

Intravenous doses of 0.5, 1 and 2 mg/kg/day imiquimod were administered during the period of organogenesis (gestational days 6 – 18) to pregnant female rabbits. No treatment related effects on embryofetal toxicity or teratogenicity were noted at 2 mg/kg/day (1.5× MRHD based on BSA comparisons), the highest dose evaluated in this study, or 1 mg/kg/day (407× MRHD based on AUC comparisons).

A combined fertility and peri- and post-natal development study was conducted in rats. Oral doses of 1, 1.5, 3 and 6 mg/kg/day imiquimod were administered to male rats from 70 days prior to mating through the mating period and to female rats from 14 days prior to mating through parturition and lactation. No effects on growth, fertility, reproduction or post-natal development were noted at doses up to 6 mg/kg/day (87× MRHD based on AUC comparisons), the highest dose evaluated in this study. In the absence of maternal toxicity, bent limb bones were noted in the F1 fetuses at a dose of 6 mg/kg/day (87× MRHD based on AUC comparisons). This fetal effect was also noted in the oral rat embryofetal development study conducted with imiquimod. No treatment related effects on teratogenicity were noted at 3 mg/kg/day (41× MRHD based on AUC comparisons).

There are no adequate and well-controlled studies in pregnant women. Aldara Cream should be used during pregnancy only if the potential benefit justifies the potential risk to the fetus.

Nursing Mothers

It is not known whether topically applied imiquimod is excreted in breast milk.

Pediatric Use

Safety and efficacy in patients with external genital/perianal warts below the age of 12 years have not been established.

AK and sBCC are not conditions generally seen within the pediatric population. The safety and efficacy of Aldara Cream for AK or sBCC in patients less than 18 years of age have not been established.

Geriatric Use

Of the 215 patients in the 2X/week clinical studies evaluating the treatment of AK lesions with Aldara Cream, 127 patients (59%) were 65 years and older, while 60 patients (28%) were 75 years and older. Of the 185 patients in the 5×/week treatment groups of clinical studies evaluating the treatment of sBCC with Aldara Cream, 65 patients (35%) were 65 years and older, while 25 patients (14%) were 75 years and older. No overall differences in safety or effectiveness were observed between these patients and younger patients. No other clinical experience has identified differences in responses between the elderly and younger patients, but greater sensitivity of some older individuals cannot be ruled out.

ADVERSE REACTIONS

Healthcare providers and patients may contact 3M or FDA's Medwatch to report adverse reactions by calling 1-800-814-1795 or 1-800-FDA-1088, or on the internet at http://www.fda.gov/medwatch.

Dermal safety studies involving induction and challenge phases produced no evidence that Aldara Cream causes photoallergenicity or contact sensitization in healthy skin; however, cumulative irritancy testing revealed the potential for Aldara Cream to cause irritation, and in the clinical studies application site reactions were reported in a significant percentage of study patients. Phototoxicity testing was incomplete as wavelengths in the UVB range were not included and Aldara Cream has peak absorption in the UVB range (320 nm) of the light spectrum.

Actinic Keratosis

The data described below reflect exposure to Aldara Cream or vehicle in 436 patients enrolled in two double-blind, vehicle-controlled, 2×/week studies. Patients applied Aldara Cream or vehicle to a 25 cm² contiguous treatment area on the face or scalp 2×/week for 16 weeks.

Summary of All Adverse Events Reported by > 1% of Patients in the Combined 2×/Week Studies

Body System Preferred Term	Imiq 2×/Week (n= 215)	Vehicle 2×/Week (n= 221)
APPLICATION SITE DISORDERS		
APPLICATION SITE REACTION	71 (33.0%)	32 (14.5%)
BODY AS A WHOLE - GENERAL DISORDERS		
BACK PAIN	3 (1.4%)	2 (0.9%)
FATIGUE	3 (1.4%)	2 (0.9%)
FEVER	3 (1.4%)	0 (0.0%)
HEADACHE	11 (5.1%)	7 (3.2%)
HERNIA NOS	4 (1.9%)	1 (0.5%)
INFLUENZA-LIKE SYMPTOMS	4 (1.9%)	4 (1.8%)
PAIN	3 (1.4%)	3 (1.4%)
RIGORS	3 (1.4%)	0 (0.0%)
CARDIOVASCULAR DISORDERS, GENERAL		
CHEST PAIN	1 (0.5%)	4 (1.8%)
HYPERTENSION	3 (1.4%)	5 (2.3%)
CENTR & PERIPH NERVOUS SYSTEM DISORDERS		
DIZZINESS	3 (1.4%)	1 (0.5%)
GASTRO-INTESTINAL SYSTEM DISORDERS		
DIARRHOEA	6 (2.8%)	2 (0.9%)
DYSPEPSIA	6 (2.8%)	4 (1.8%)
GASTROESOPHAGEAL REFLUX	3 (1.4%)	3 (1.4%)
NAUSEA	3 (1.4%)	3 (1.4%)
VOMITING	3 (1.4%)	1 (0.5%)
HEART RATE AND RHYTHM DISORDERS		
FIBRILLATION ATRIAL	3 (1.4%)	2 (0.9%)
METABOLIC AND NUTRITIONAL DISORDERS		
HYPERCHOLESTEROLAEMIA	4 (1.9%)	0 (0.0%)
MUSCULO-SKELETAL SYSTEM DISORDERS		
ARTHRALGIA	2 (0.9%)	4 (1.8%)
ARTHRITIS	2 (0.9%)	3 (1.4%)
MYALGIA	3 (1.4%)	3 (1.4%)
SKELETAL PAIN	1 (0.5%)	3 (1.4%)
NEOPLASM		
BASAL CELL CARCINOMA	5 (2.3%)	5 (2.3%)
CARCINOMA SQUAMOUS	8 (3.7%)	5 (2.3%)
RESISTANCE MECHANISM DISORDERS	9 (4.2%)	11 (5.0%)
HERPES SIMPLEX	4 (1.9%)	4 (1.8%)
INFECTION VIRAL	3 (1.4%)	2 (0.9%)
RESPIRATORY SYSTEM DISORDERS		
BRONCHITIS	2 (0.9%)	3 (1.4%)
COUGHING	6 (2.8%)	10 (4.5%)
PHARYNGITIS	4 (1.9%)	4 (1.8%)
PULMONARY CONGESTION	1 (0.5%)	3 (1.4%)
RHINITIS	7 (3.3%)	8 (3.6%)
SINUSITIS	16 (7.4%)	14 (6.3%)
UPPER RESP TRACT INFECTION	33 (15.3%)	27 (12.2%)
SECONDARY TERMS		
ABRASION NOS	7 (3.3%)	5 (2.3%)
CYST NOS	0 (0.0%)	4 (1.8%)
INFLICTED INJURY	19 (8.8%)	21 (9.5%)
POST-OPERATIVE PAIN	3 (1.4%)	4 (1.8%)
SKIN AND APPENDAGES DISORDERS	47 (21.9%)	42 (19.0%)
ALOPECIA	3 (1.4%)	0 (0.0%)
DERMATITIS	3 (1.4%)	7 (3.2%)
ECZEMA	4 (1.9%)	3 (1.4%)
HYPERKERATOSIS	19 (8.8%)	12 (5.4%)
PHOTOSENSITIVITY REACTION	2 (0.9%)	4 (1.8%)
PRURITUS	2 (0.9%)	3 (1.4%)
RASH	5 (2.3%)	5 (2.3%)
SKIN DISORDER	6 (2.8%)	7 (3.2%)
VERRUCA	1 (0.5%)	3 (1.4%)
URINARY SYSTEM DISORDERS	8 (3.7%)	10 (4.5%)
URINARY TRACT INFECTION	3 (1.4%)	1 (0.5%)
VISION DISORDERS		
CONJUNCTIVITIS	1 (0.5%)	3 (1.4%)
EYE ABNORMALITY	4 (1.9%)	1 (0.5%)
EYE INFECTION	0 (0.0%)	3 (1.4%)

Local Skin Reactions in the Treatment Area as Assessed by the Investigator (Percentage of Patients) 2×/Week Application

	Mild/Moderate/Severe		Severe	
	Aldara Cream n=215	Vehicle n=220	Aldara Cream n=215	Vehicle n=220
Erythema	209 (97%)	206 (93%)	38 (18%)	5 (2%)
Edema	106 (49%)	22 (10%)	0 (0%)	0 (0%)
Weeping/Exudate	45 (22%)	3 (1%)	0 (0%)	0 (0%)
Vesicles	19 (9%)	2 (1%)	0 (0%)	0 (0%)
Erosion/Ulceration	103 (48%)	20 (9%)	5 (2%)	0 (0%)
Flaking/Scaling/Dryness	199 (93%)	199 (91%)	16 (7%)	7 (3%)
Scabbing/Crusting	169 (79%)	92 (42%)	18 (8%)	4 (2%)

Summary of All Application Site Reactions Reported by > 1% of Patients in the Combined 2×/Week Studies

Included Term	Imiq 2×/Week (n= 215)	Vehicle 2×/Week (n= 221)
BLEEDING AT TARGET SITE	7 (3.3%)	1 (0.5%)
BURNING AT REMOTE SITE	4 (1.9%)	0 (0.0%)
BURNING AT TARGET SITE	12 (5.6%)	4 (1.8%)
INDURATION AT REMOTE SITE	3 (1.4%)	0 (0.0%)
INDURATION AT TARGET SITE	5 (2.3%)	3 (1.4%)
IRRITATION AT REMOTE SITE	3 (1.4%)	0 (0.0%)
ITCHING AT REMOTE SITE	7 (3.3%)	3 (1.4%)
ITCHING AT TARGET SITE	44 (20.5%)	15 (6.8%)
PAIN AT TARGET SITE	5 (2.3%)	2 (0.9%)
STINGING AT TARGET SITE	6 (2.8%)	2 (0.9%)
TENDERNESS AT TARGET SITE	4 (1.9%)	3 (1.4%)

Local skin reactions were collected independently of the adverse event "application site reaction" in an effort to provide a better picture of the specific types of local reactions that might be seen. The most frequently reported local skin reactions were erythema, flaking/scaling/dryness, and scabbing/crusting. The prevalence and severity of local skin reactions that occurred during controlled studies are shown in the following table.

[See table below]

The adverse reactions that most frequently resulted in clinical intervention (e.g., rest periods, withdrawal from study) were local skin and application site reactions. Overall, in the clinical studies, 2% (5/215) of patients discontinued for local skin/application site reactions. Of the 215 patients treated, 35 patients (16%) on Aldara Cream and 3 of 220 patients (1%) on vehicle cream had at least one rest period. Of these Aldara Cream patients, 32 (91%) resumed therapy after a rest period.

In the AK studies, 22 of 678 imiquimod treated patients developed treatment site infections that required a rest period off Aldara Cream and were treated with antibiotics (19 with oral and 3 with topical).

Superficial Basal Cell Carcinoma

The data described below reflect exposure to Aldara Cream or vehicle in 364 patients enrolled in two double-blind, vehicle-controlled, 5×/week studies. Patients applied Aldara Cream or vehicle 5×/week for 6 weeks. The incidence of adverse events reported by > 1% of subjects during the 6 week treatment period is summarized below.

Summary of All Adverse Events Reported by > 1% of Patients in the Combined 5×/Week Studies

Body System Preferred Term	Imiquimod 5×/Week (n= 185) N %	Vehicle 5×/Week (n= 179) N %
APPLICATION SITE DISORDERS		
APPLICATION SITE REACTION	52 (28.1%)	5 (2.8%)
BODY AS A WHOLE - GENERAL DISORDERS		
ALLERGY AGGRAVATED	2 (1.1%)	1 (0.6%)
BACK PAIN	7 (3.8%)	1 (0.6%)
CHEST PAIN	2 (1.1%)	0 (0.0%)
FATIGUE	4 (2.2%)	2 (1.1%)
FEVER	3 (1.6%)	0 (0.0%)
PAIN	3 (1.6%)	2 (1.1%)
CARDIOVASCULAR DISORDERS, GENERAL		
HYPERTENSION	5 (2.7%)	1 (0.6%)
CENTR & PERIPH NERVOUS SYSTEM DISORDERS		
DIZZINESS	2 (1.1%)	1 (0.6%)
HEADACHE	14 (7.6%)	4 (2.2%)
GASTRO-INTESTINAL SYSTEM DISORDERS		
ABDOMINAL PAIN	1 (0.5%)	2 (1.1%)
DIARRHOEA	1 (0.5%)	2 (1.1%)
DYSPEPSIA	3 (1.6%)	2 (1.1%)
GASTRO-INTESTINAL DISORDER NOS	1 (0.5%)	2 (1.1%)
NAUSEA	2 (1.1%)	0 (0.0%)
TOOTH DISORDER	0 (0.0%)	2 (1.1%)
METABOLIC AND NUTRITIONAL DISORDERS		
GOUT	2 (1.1%)	0 (0.0%)
MUSCULO-SKELETAL SYSTEM DISORDERS		
SKELETAL PAIN	3 (1.6%)	2 (1.1%)
PSYCHIATRIC DISORDERS		
ANXIETY	2 (1.1%)	1 (0.6%)
RESISTANCE MECHANISM DISORDERS		
INFECTION	1 (0.5%)	3 (1.7%)
INFECTION FUNGAL	2 (1.1%)	2 (1.1%)
RESPIRATORY SYSTEM DISORDERS		
COUGHING	3 (1.6%)	1 (0.6%)
PHARYNGITIS	2 (1.1%)	1 (0.6%)
RHINITIS	5 (2.7%)	1 (0.6%)
SINUSITIS	4 (2.2%)	1 (0.6%)
UPPER RESP TRACT INFECTION	6 (3.2%)	2 (1.1%)
SECONDARY TERMS		
INFLICTED INJURY	3 (1.6%)	3 (1.7%)
PROCEDURAL SITE REACTION	2 (1.1%)	3 (1.7%)

Wart Site Reaction as Assessed by Investigator (Percentage of Patients)
3×/Week Application

	Mild/Moderate/Severe				Severe			
	Females		Males		Females		Males	
	Aldara Cream n=114	Vehicle n=99	Aldara Cream n=156	Vehicle n=157	Aldara Cream n=114	Vehicle n=99	Aldara Cream n=156	Vehicle n=157
Erythema	74 (65%)	21 (21%)	90 (58%)	34 (22%)	4 (4%)	0 (0%)	6 (4%)	0 (0%)
Erosion	35 (31%)	8 (8%)	47 (30%)	10 (6%)	1 (1%)	0 (0%)	2 (1%)	0 (0%)
Excoriation/Flaking	21 (18%)	8 (8%)	40 (26%)	12 (8%)	0 (0%)	0 (0%)	1 (1%)	0 (0%)
Edema	20 (18%)	5 (5%)	19 (12%)	1 (1%)	1 (1%)	0 (0%)	0 (0%)	0 (0%)
Induration	6 (5%)	2 (2%)	11 (7%)	3 (2%)	0 (0%)	0 (0%)	0 (0%)	0 (0%)
Ulceration	9 (8%)	1 (1%)	7 (4%)	1 (1%)	3 (3%)	0 (0%)	0 (0%)	0 (0%)
Scabbing	4 (4%)	0 (0%)	20 (13%)	4 (3%)	0 (0%)	0 (0%)	0 (0%)	0 (0%)
Vesicles	3 (3%)	0 (0%)	3 (2%)	0 (0%)	0 (0%)	0 (0%)	0 (0%)	0 (0%)

SKIN AND APPENDAGES DISORDERS		
HYPERKERATOSIS	3 (1.6%)	2 (1.1%)
RASH	3 (1.6%)	1 (0.6%)
SKIN DISORDER	1 (0.5%)	3 (1.7%)
WHITE CELL AND RES DISORDERS		
LYMPHADENOPATHY	5 (2.7%)	1 (0.6%)

In controlled clinical studies, the most frequently reported adverse reactions were local skin and application site reactions including erythema, edema, induration, erosion, flaking/scaling, scabbing/crusting, itching and burning at the application site. The incidence of the application site reactions reported by > 1% of the subjects during the 6 week treatment period is summarized in the table below.

Summary of All Application Site Reactions Reported by > 1% of Patients in the Combined 5×/Week Studies

Included Term	Imiquimod 5×/Week (n= 185) N %	Vehicle 5×/Week (n= 179) N %
ITCHING AT TARGET SITE	30 (16.2%)	1 (0.6%)
BURNING AT TARGET SITE	11 (5.9%)	2 (1.1%)
PAIN AT TARGET SITE	6 (3.2%)	0 (0.0%)
TENDERNESS AT TARGET SITE	2 (1.1%)	0 (0.0%)
ERYTHEMA AT REMOTE SITE	3 (1.6%)	0 (0.0%)
PAPULE(S) AT TARGET SITE	3 (1.6%)	0 (0.0%)
BLEEDING AT TARGET SITE	4 (2.2%)	0 (0.0%)
TINGLING AT TARGET SITE	1 (0.5%)	2 (1.1%)
INFECTION AT TARGET SITE	2 (1.1%)	0 (0.0%)

Local skin reactions were collected independently of the adverse event "application site reaction" in an effort to provide a better picture of the specific types of local reactions that might be seen. The prevalence and severity of local skin reactions that occurred during controlled studies are shown in the following table.

Most Intense Local Skin Reactions in the Treatment Area as Assessed by the Investigator (Percentage of Patients)
5X/Week Application

	Mild/Moderate		Severe	
	Aldara Cream n=184	Vehicle n=178	Aldara Cream n=184	Vehicle n=178
Edema	71%	36%	7%	0%
Erosion	54%	14%	13%	0%
Erythema	69%	95%	31%	2%
Flaking/Scaling	87%	76%	4%	0%
Induration	78%	53%	6%	0%
Scabbing/Crusting	64%	34%	19%	0%
Ulceration	34%	3%	6%	0%
Vesicles	29%	2%	2%	0%

The adverse reactions that most frequently resulted in clinical intervention (e.g., rest periods, withdrawal from study) were local skin and application site reactions; 10% (19/185) of patients received rest periods. The average number of doses not received per patient due to rest periods was 7 doses with a range of 2 to 22 doses; 79% of patients (15/19) resumed therapy after a rest period. Overall, in the clinical studies, 2% (4/185) of patients discontinued for local skin/application site reactions.

In the sBCC studies, 17 of 1266 (1.3%) imiquimod-treated patients developed treatment site infections that required a rest period off Aldara Cream and were treated with antibiotics.

External Genital Warts

In controlled clinical trials for genital warts, the most frequently reported adverse reactions were local skin and application site reactions.

These reactions were usually mild to moderate in intensity; however, severe reactions were reported with 3×/week application. **These reactions were more frequent and more intense with daily application than with 3×/week application.** Some patients also reported systemic reactions. Overall, in the 3×/week application clinical studies, 1.2% (4/327) of the patients discontinued due to local skin/application site reactions. The incidence and severity of local skin reactions during controlled clinical trials are shown in the following table.

[See table above]

Remote site skin reactions were also reported in female and male patients treated 3X/week with Aldara Cream. The severe remote site skin reactions reported for females were erythema (3%), ulceration (2%), and edema (1%); and for males, erosion (2%), and erythema, edema, induration, and excoriation/flaking (each 1%).

Adverse events judged to be probably or possibly related to Aldara Cream reported by more than 5% of patients are listed below; also included are soreness, influenza-like symptoms and myalgia.

3×/Week Application

	Females		Males	
	Aldara Cream N=117	Vehicle n=103	Aldara Cream n=156	Vehicle n=158
Application Site Disorders:				
Application Site Reactions				
Wart Site:				
Itching	32%	20%	22%	10%
Burning	26%	12%	9%	5%
Pain	8%	2%	2%	1%
Soreness	3%	0%	0%	1%
Fungal Infection*	11%	3%	2%	1%
Systemic Reactions:				
Headache	4%	3%	5%	2%
Influenza-like symptoms	3%	2%	1%	0%
Myalgia	1%	0%	1%	1%

*Incidences reported without regard to causality with Aldara Cream.

Adverse events judged to be possibly or probably related to Aldara Cream and reported by more than 1% of patients included: **Application Site Disorders: Wart Site Reactions** (burning, hypopigmentation, irritation, itching, pain, rash, sensitivity, soreness, stinging, tenderness); **Remote Site Reactions** (bleeding, burning, itching, pain, tenderness, tinea cruris); **Body as a Whole:** fatigue, fever, influenza-like symptoms; **Central and Peripheral Nervous System Disorders:** headache; **Gastro-Intestinal System Disorders:** diarrhea; **Musculo-Skeletal System Disorders:** myalgia.

OVERDOSAGE

Persistent topical overdosing of Aldara Cream could result in an increased incidence of severe local skin reactions and may increase the risk for systemic reactions. The most clinically serious adverse event reported following multiple oral imiquimod doses of >200 mg (equivalent to imiquimod content of >16 packets) was hypotension, which resolved following oral or intravenous fluid administration.

DOSAGE AND ADMINISTRATION

The application frequency for Aldara Cream is different for each indication.

Actinic Keratosis

Aldara Cream is to be applied 2 times per week for 16 weeks to a defined treatment area on the face or scalp (but not both concurrently). The treatment area should be one contiguous area of approximately 25 cm² (e.g., 5 cm × 5 cm). Imiquimod cream should be applied to the entire treatment area (e.g., the forehead, scalp, or one cheek).

Aldara Cream is packaged in single-use packets, with 12 packets supplied per box. Patients should be prescribed no more than 3 boxes (36 packets) for the 16 week treatment period. Unused packets should be discarded. Partially-used packets should be discarded and not reused. Before applying the cream, the patient should wash the treatment area with mild soap and water and allow the area to dry thoroughly (at least 10 minutes). The patient should apply no more than one packet of Aldara Cream to the contiguous treatment area at each application. **Aldara Cream is applied prior to normal sleeping hours, and left on the skin for approximately 8 hours, after which time the cream should be removed by washing the area with mild soap and water.** The cream should be rubbed into the treatment area until the cream is no longer visible. Contact with the eyes, lips and nostrils should be avoided. Examples of two times per week application schedules are Monday and Thursday, or Tuesday and Friday prior to sleeping hours. **Aldara Cream treatment should continue for the full 16 weeks. However, the treatment period should not be extended beyond 16 weeks due to missed doses or rest periods.** Local skin reactions in the treatment area are common. Patients should contact their physician if they experience any sign or symptom in the treatment area that restricts or prohibits their daily activity or makes continued application of the cream difficult. A rest period of several days may be taken if required by the patient's discomfort or severity of the local skin reaction. The technique for proper dose administration should be demonstrated by the prescriber to maximize the benefit of Aldara Cream therapy. Handwashing before and after cream application is recommended.

Lesions that do not respond to therapy should be carefully re-evaluated and management reconsidered.

Superficial Basal Cell Carcinoma

Aldara Cream is to be applied 5 times per week for 6 weeks to a biopsy-confirmed superficial basal cell carcinoma. The target tumor should have a maximum diameter of no more than 2 cm and be located on the trunk (excluding anogenital skin), neck, or extremities (excluding hands and feet). The treatment area should include a 1 cm margin of skin around the tumor.

Target Tumor Diameter	Size of Cream Droplet to be Used (diameter)	Approximate Amount of Cream to be Used
0.5 to < 1.0 cm	4 mm	10 mg
≥1.0 to < 1.5 cm	5 mm	25 mg
≥ 1.5 to 2.0 cm	7 mm	40 mg

Aldara Cream is packaged in single-use packets, with 12 packets supplied per box. Patients should be prescribed no more than 3 boxes (36 packets) for the 6 week treatment period. Unused packets should be discarded. Partially-used packets should be discarded and not reused.

Aldara Cream is to be applied 5 times per week, prior to normal sleeping hours, and left on the skin for approximately 8 hours. Before applying the cream, the patient should wash the treatment area with mild soap and water and allow the area to dry thoroughly. Sufficient cream should be applied to cover the treatment area, including one centimeter of skin surrounding the tumor. The cream should be rubbed into the treatment area until the cream is no longer visible. Eye contact should be avoided. Following the treatment period, cream should be removed by washing the area with mild soap and water. An example of a 5 times per week application schedule is to apply Aldara Cream, once per day, Monday through Friday, prior to sleeping hours. **Aldara Cream treatment should continue for 6 weeks.** Local skin reactions in the treatment area are common. Patients should contact their physician if they experience any sign or symptom in the treatment area that restricts or prohibits their daily activity or makes continued application of the cream difficult. A rest period of several days may be taken if required by the patient's discomfort or severity of the local skin reaction. The technique for proper dose administration should be demonstrated by the prescriber to maximize the benefit of Aldara Cream therapy. Handwashing before and after cream application is recommended.

Early clinical clearance cannot be adequately assessed until resolution of local skin reactions. It is appropriate to have the first follow-up visit at approximately 12 weeks post-treatment to assess the treatment site for clinical clearance. Local skin reactions or other findings (e.g. infection) may require that a patient be seen sooner than the 12 week post-treatment visit. If there is clinical evidence of persistent tumor at the 12 week post-treatment assessment, a biopsy or other alternative intervention should be considered; the safety and efficacy of a repeat course of Aldara Cream treatment have not been established. If any suspicious lesion arises in the treatment area at any time after 12 weeks, the patient should seek a medical evaluation. See table of Estimated Clinical Clearance Rates for Superficial Basal Cell Carcinoma in the CLINICAL STUDIES section.

External Genital Warts

Aldara Cream is to be applied 3 times per week, prior to normal sleeping hours, and left on the skin for 6-10 hours. Patients should be instructed to apply Aldara Cream to external genital/perianal warts. A thin layer is applied to the wart area and rubbed in until the cream is no longer visible. The application site is not to be occluded. Following the treatment period cream should be removed by washing the treated area with mild soap and water. Examples of 3 times per week application schedules are: Monday, Wednesday, Friday; or Tuesday, Thursday, Saturday application prior to sleeping hours. Aldara Cream treatment should continue until there is total clearance of the genital/perianal warts or for a maximum of 16 weeks. Local skin reactions (erythema) at the treatment site are common. A rest period of several days may be taken if required by the patient's discomfort or severity of the local skin reaction. Treatment may resume once the reaction subsides. Non-occlusive dressings such as cotton gauze or cotton underwear may be used in the management of skin reactions. The technique for proper dose administration should be demonstrated by the prescriber to maximize the benefit of Aldara Cream therapy. Handwashing before and after cream application is recommended.

Aldara Cream is packaged in single-use packets which contain sufficient cream to cover a wart area of up to 20 cm²; use of excessive amounts of cream should be avoided.

HOW SUPPLIED

Aldara (imiquimod) Cream, 5%, is supplied in single-use packets which contain 250 mg of the cream. Available as: box of 12 packets NDC 0089-0610-12.

Continued on next page

Aldara—Cont.

Store below 25°C (77°F).
Avoid freezing.
Keep out of reach of children.
Rx only
Manufactured by
3M Health Care Limited
Loughborough LE11 1EP England
Distributed by
3M Pharmaceuticals
Northridge, CA 91324
July 2004
662600
3M and Aldara are trademarks
of the 3M Company
Shown in Product Identification Guide, page 320

ALU-CAP™ Capsules OTC
(aluminum hydroxide)

For indications, actions, warnings, dosage, and precautions see container label or call 800-328-0255 for a copy.

HOW SUPPLIED

Bottles of 100 red and green Alu-Cap capsules (NDC **0089-0105-10**).

CALCIUM DISODIUM VERSENATE ℞
(edetate calcium disodium injection, USP)

> **WARNINGS:**
> Calcium Disodium Versenate is capable of producing toxic effects which can be fatal. Lead encephalopathy is relatively rare in adults, but occurs more often in pediatric patients in whom it may be incipient and thus overlooked. The mortality rate in pediatric patients has been high. Patients with lead encephalopathy and cerebral edema may experience a lethal increase in intracranial pressure following intravenous infusion; the intramuscular route is preferred for these patients. In cases where the intravenous route is necessary, avoid rapid infusion. The dosage schedule should be followed and at no time should the recommended daily dose be exceeded.

DESCRIPTION

Calcium Disodium Versenate (edetate calcium disodium injection, USP) is a sterile, injectable, chelating agent in concentrated solution for intravenous infusion or intramuscular injection. Each 5 ml ampul contains 1000 mg of edetate calcium disodium (equivalent to 200 mg/ml) in water for injection. Chemically, this product is called [[N,N′-1,2-ethanediyl-bis[N-(carboxymethyl)-glycinato]](4-)-N,N′,O,O′,O^N,O^N′]-,disodium,hydrate, (OC-6-21)-Calciate (2-).
Structural Formula:

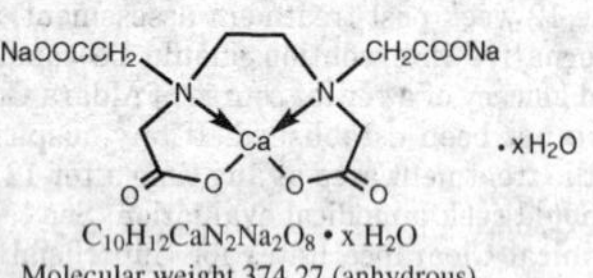

$C_{10}H_{12}CaN_2Na_2O_8 \cdot x\ H_2O$
Molecular weight 374.27 (anhydrous)

CLINICAL PHARMACOLOGY

The pharmacologic effects of edetate calcium disodium are due to the formation of chelates with divalent and trivalent metals. A stable chelate will form with any metal that has the ability to displace calcium from the molecule, a feature shared by lead, zinc, cadmium, manganese, iron and mercury. The amounts of manganese and iron mobilized are not significant. Copper[1] is not mobilized and mercury is unavailable for chelation because it is too tightly bound to body ligands or it is stored in inaccessible body compartments. The excretion of calcium by the body is not increased following intravenous administration of edetate calcium disodium, but the excretion of zinc is considerably increased.[1]
Edetate calcium disodium is poorly absorbed from the gastrointestinal tract. In blood, all the drug is found in the plasma. Edetate calcium disodium does not appear to penetrate cells; it is distributed primarily in the extracellular fluid with only about 5% of the plasma concentration found in the spinal fluid.
The half life of edetate calcium disodium is 20 to 60 minutes. It is excreted primarily by the kidney, with about 50% excreted in one hour and over 95% within 24 hours.[2] Almost none of the compound is metabolized.
The primary source of lead chelated by Calcium Disodium Versenate is from bone; subsequently, soft-tissue lead is redistributed to bone when chelation is stopped.[3,4] There is also some reduction in kidney lead levels following chelation therapy.
It has been shown in animals that following a single dose of Calcium Disodium Versenate urinary lead output increases, blood lead concentration decreases, but brain lead is significantly increased due to internal redistribution of lead.[5] (See **WARNINGS**.) These data are in agreement with the recent results of others in experimental animals showing that after a five day course of treatment there is no net reduction in brain lead.[6]

INDICATIONS AND USAGE

Edetate calcium disodium is indicated for the reduction of blood levels and depot stores of lead in lead poisoning (acute and chronic) and lead encephalopathy, in both pediatric populations and adults.
Chelation therapy should not replace effective measures to eliminate or reduce further exposure to lead.

CONTRAINDICATIONS

Edetate calcium disodium should not be given during periods of anuria, nor to patients with active renal disease or hepatitis.

WARNINGS

See boxed warning.

PRECAUTIONS

General Precautions: Edetate calcium disodium may produce the same renal damage as lead poisoning, such as proteinuria and microscopic hematuria. Treatment-induced nephrotoxicity is dose-dependent and may be reduced by assuring adequate diuresis before therapy begins. Urine flow must be monitored throughout therapy which must be stopped if anuria or severe oliguria develop. The proximal tubule hydropic degeneration usually recovers upon cessation of therapy. Edetate calcium disodium must be used in reduced doses in patients with pre-existing mild renal disease.
Patients should be monitored for cardiac rhythm irregularities and other ECG changes during intravenous therapy.
Information for patients: Patients should be instructed to immediately inform their physician if urine output stops for a period of 12 hours.
Laboratory tests: Urinalysis and urine sediment, renal and hepatic function and serum electrolyte levels should be checked before each course of therapy and then be monitored daily during therapy in severe cases, and in less serious cases after the second and fifth day of therapy. Therapy must be discontinued at the first sign of renal toxicity. The presence of large renal epithelial cells or increasing number of red blood cells in urinary sediment or greater proteinuria call for immediate stopping of edetate calcium disodium administration. Alkaline phosphatase values are frequently depressed (possibly due to decreased serum zinc levels), but return to normal within 48 hours after cessation of therapy. Elevated erythrocyte protoporphyrin levels (>35 mcg/dl of whole blood) indicate the need to perform a venous blood lead determination. If the whole blood lead concentration is between 25–55 mcg/dl a mobilization test can be considered.[7,8] (See **Diagnostic Test.**) An elevation of urinary coproporphyrin (adults: >250 mcg/day; pediatric patients under 80 lbs: >75 mcg/day) and elevation of urinary delta aminolevulinic acid (ALA) (adults: >4 mg/day; pediatric patients: >3 mg/m²/day) are associated with blood lead levels >40 mcg/dl. Urinary coproporphyrin may be falsely negative in terminal patients and in severely iron-depleted pediatric patients who are not regenerating heme.[9] In growing pediatric patients long bone x-rays showing lead lines and abdominal x-rays showing radio-opaque material in the abdomen may be of help in estimating the level of exposure to lead.
Drug Interactions: There is no known drug interference with standard clinical laboratory tests. Steroids enhance the renal toxicity of edetate calcium disodium in animals.[7] Edetate calcium disodium interferes with the action of zinc insulin preparations by chelating the zinc.[7]
Carcinogenesis, Mutagenesis, Impairment of Fertility: Long term animal studies have not been conducted with edetate calcium disodium to evaluate its carcinogenic potential, mutagenic potential or its effect on fertility.
Pregnancy: Category B: One reproduction study was performed in rats at doses up to 13 times the human dose and revealed no evidence of impaired fertility or harm to the fetus due to Calcium Disodium Versenate.[10] Another reproduction study performed in rats at doses up to about 25 to 40 times the human dose revealed evidence of fetal malformations due to Calcium Disodium Versenate, which were prevented by simultaneous supplementation of dietary zinc.[11] There are, however, no adequate and well-controlled studies in pregnant women. Because animal reproduction studies are not always predictive of human response, this drug should be used during pregnancy only if clearly needed.
Labor and Delivery: Calcium Disodium Versenate has no recognized use during labor and delivery, and its effects during these processes are unknown.
Nursing Mothers: It is not known whether this drug is excreted in human milk. Because many drugs are excreted in human milk, caution should be exercised when Calcium Disodium Versenate is administered to a nursing woman.
Pediatric Use: Since lead poisoning occurs in pediatric populations and adults but is frequently more severe in pediatric patients, Calcium Disodium Versenate is used in patients of all ages. The intramuscular route is preferred by some for young pediatric patients. In cases where the intravenous route is necessary, avoid rapid infusion. (See **WARNINGS.**) Urine flow must be monitored throughout therapy; Calcium Disodium Versenate therapy must be stopped if anuria or severe oliguria develops. (See **General Precautions.**) At no time should the recommended daily dosage be exceeded. (See **DOSAGE AND ADMINISTRATION.**)

ADVERSE REACTIONS

The following adverse effects have been associated with the use of edetate calcium disodium:
Body as a Whole: pain at intramuscular injection site, fever, chills, malaise, fatigue, myalgia, arthralgia.
Cardiovascular: hypotension, cardiac rhythm irregularities.
Renal: acute necrosis of proximal tubules (which may result in fatal nephrosis), infrequent changes in distal tubules and glomeruli.
Urinary: glycosuria, proteinuria, microscopic hematuria and large epithelial cells in urinary sediment.
Nervous System: tremors, headache, numbness, tingling.
Gastrointestinal: cheilosis, nausea, vomiting, anorexia, excessive thirst.
Hepatic: mild increases in SGOT and SGPT are common, and return to normal within 48 hours after cessation of therapy.
Immunogenic: histamine-like reactions (sneezing, nasal congestion, lacrimation), rash.
Hematopoietic: transient bone marrow depression, anemia.
Metabolic: zinc deficiency, hypercalcemia.

OVERDOSAGE

Symptoms: Inadvertent administration of 5 times the recommended dose, infused intravenously over a 24 hour period, to an asymptomatic 16 month old patient with a blood lead content of 56 mcg/dl did not cause any ill effects. Edetate calcium disodium can aggravate the symptoms of severe lead poisoning, therefore, most toxic effects (cerebral edema, renal tubular necrosis) appear to be associated with lead poisoning.
Because of cerebral edema, a therapeutic dose may be lethal to an adult or a pediatric patient with lead encephalopathy. Higher dosage of edetate calcium disodium may produce a more severe zinc deficiency.
Treatment: Cerebral edema should be treated with repeated doses of mannitol. Steroids enhance the renal toxicity of edetate calcium disodium in animals and, therefore, are no longer recommended.[7] Zinc levels must be monitored. Good urinary output must be maintained because diuresis will enhance drug elimination. It is not known if edetate calcium disodium is dialyzable.

DOSAGE AND ADMINISTRATION

When a source for the lead intoxication has been identified, the patient should be removed from the source, if possible. The recommended dose of Calcium Disodium Versenate for asymptomatic adults and pediatric patients whose blood lead level is <70 mcg/dl but >20 mcg/dl (World Health Organization recommended upper allowable level) is 1000 mg/m²/day whether given intravenously or intramuscularly. (See Surface Area Nomogram.)

SURFACE AREA NOMOGRAM

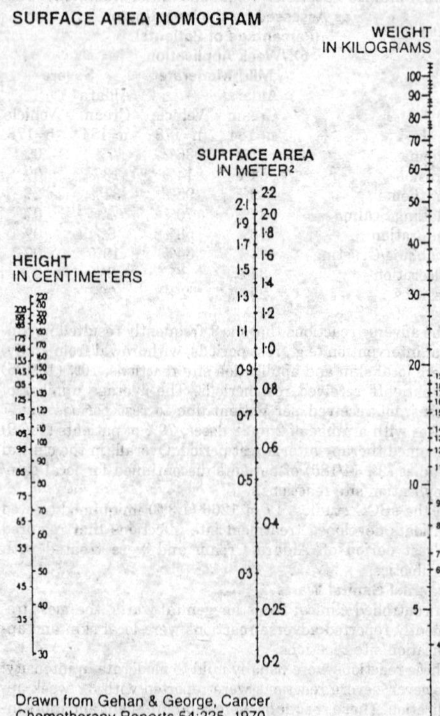

Drawn from Gehan & George, Cancer Chemotherapy Reports 54:225, 1970.

For adults with lead nephropathy, the following dosing regimen has been suggested: 500 mg/m² every 24 hours for 5 days for patients with serum creatinine levels of 2–3 mg/dl, every 48 hours for 3 doses for patients with creatinine levels of 3–4 mg/dl, and once weekly for patients with creatinine levels above 4 mg/dl. These regimens may be repeated at one month intervals.[12]
Calcium Disodium Versenate, used alone, may aggravate symptoms in patients with very high blood lead levels.

When the blood lead level is >70 mcg/dl or clinical symptoms consistent with lead poisoning are present, it is recommended that Calcium Disodium Versenate be used in conjunction with BAL (dimercaprol). Please consult published protocols and specialized references for dosage recommendations of combination therapy.[14–18]
Therapy of lead poisoning in adults and pediatric patients with Calcium Disodium Versenate is continued over a period of five days. Therapy is then interrupted for 2 to 4 days to allow redistribution of the lead and to prevent severe depletion of zinc and other essential metals. Two courses of treatment are usually employed; however, it depends on severity of the lead toxicity and the patient's tolerance of the drug.
Calcium Disodium Versenate is equally effective whether administered intravenously or intramuscularly. The intramuscular route is used for all patients with overt lead encephalopathy and this route is preferred by some for young pediatric patients.
Acutely ill individuals may be dehydrated from vomiting. Since edetate calcium disodium is excreted almost exclusively in the urine, it is very important to establish urine flow with intravenous fluid administration before the first dose of the chelating agent is given; however, excessive fluid must be avoided in patients with encephalopathy. Once urine flow is established, further intravenous fluid is restricted to basal water and electrolyte requirements. Administration of Calcium Disodium Versenate should be stopped whenever there is cessation of urine flow in order to avoid unduly high tissue levels of the drug. Edetate calcium disodium must be used in reduced doses in patients with pre-existing mild renal disease.
Intravenous Administration: Add the total daily dose of Calcium Disodium Versenate (1000 mg/m^2/day) to 250–500 ml of 5% dextrose or 0.9% sodium chloride injection. The total daily dose should be infused over a period of 8–12 hours. Calcium Disodium Versenate injection is incompatible with 10% dextrose, 10% invert sugar in 0.9% sodium chloride, lactate Ringer's, Ringer's, one-sixth molar sodium lactate injections, and with injectable amphotericin B and hydralazine hydrochloride.
Intramuscular Administration: The total daily dosage (1000 mg/m^2/day) should be divided into equal doses spaced 8–12 hours apart. Lidocaine or procaine should be added to the Calcium Disodium Versenate injection to minimize pain at the injection site. The final lidocaine or procaine concentration of 5 mg/ml (0.5%) can be obtained as follows: 0.25 ml of 10% lidocaine solution per 5 ml (entire content of ampul) concentrated Calcium Disodium Versenate; 1 ml of 1% lidocaine or procaine solution per ml of concentrated Calcium Disodium Versenate. When used alone, regardless of method of administration, Calcium Disodium Versenate should not be given at doses larger than those recommended.
Diagnostic Test: Several methods have been described for lead mobilization tests using edetate calcium disodium to assess body stores.[7,9,12,13,18]
These procedures have advantages and disadvantages that should be reviewed in current references. Edetate calcium disodium mobilization tests should not be performed in symptomatic patients and in patients with blood lead levels above 55 mcg/dl for whom appropriate therapy is indicated.
Parenteral drugs should be inspected visually for particulate matter and discoloration prior to administration, whenever solution and container permit.

HOW SUPPLIED

Calcium Disodium Versenate injection, 5 ml ampul containing 200 mg of edetate calcium disodium per ml (1 g per ampul), in boxes containing 6 ampuls (NDC **0089-0510-06**).
Store at controlled room temperature 15°–30°C (59°–86°F).
Rx only

REFERENCES

1. Thomas DJ, Chisolm JJ. Lead, zinc and copper decorporation during calcium disodium ethylenediamine tetraacetate treatment of lead-poisoned children. J Pharmacol Exp Therapeu 1986; 239: 829–835.
2. The Pharmacological Basis of Therapeutics, 7th edition, Goodman and Gilman, editors. MacMillan Publishing Company, New York, 1985, pp. 1619–1622.
3. Hammond PB, Aronson AL, Olson WC. The mechanism of mobilization of lead by ethylenediaminetetraacetate. J Pharmacol Exp Therapeu 1967; 157: 196–206.
4. Van deVyver FL, D'Haese PC, Visser WJ, et al. Bone lead in dialysis patients. Kidney Intl 1988; 33:601–607.
5. Cory-Slecta DA, Weiss B, Cox C. Mobilization and redistribution of lead over the course of calcium disodium ethylenediamine tetraacetate chelation therapy. J Pharmacol Exp Therapeu 1987; 243:804–813.
6. Chisolm JJ. Mobilization of lead by calcium disodium edetate. Am J Dis Child 1987; 141:1256–1257.
7. Drug Evaluations, 6th Edition, American Medical Association, Saunders, Philadelphia, 1986, pp. 1637–1639.
8. Centers for Disease Control: Preventing lead poisoning in young children. Atlanta, GA, Department of Health and Human Services, 1985 Jan.
9. Finberg L, Rajagopal V. Diagnosis and treatment of lead poisoning in children. J Family Med 1985 April: 3–12.
10. Schardein JL, Sakowski R, Petrere J, et al. Teratogenesis studies with EDTA and its salts in rats. Toxicol Appl Pharmacol 1981; 61:423–428.
11. Swenerton H, Hurley LS. Teratogenic effects of a chelating agent and their prevention by zinc. Science 1971; 173:62–64.
12. American Hospital Formulary Service, Drug Information, 1988, pp. 1695–1698.
13. Markowitz ME, Rosen JF. Assessment of lead stores in chidren: Validation of an 8-hour $CaNa_2EDTA$ (Calcium Disodium Versenate) provocative test. J Pediatrics 1984; 104:337–341.
14. Piomelli S, Rosen JF, Chisolm JJ, et al. Management of childhood lead poisoning. J Pediatrics 1984; 105:523–532.
15. Sachs HK, Blanksma LA, Murray EF, et al. Ambulatory treatment of lead poisoning: Report of 1,155 cases. Pediatrics 1970; 46:389.
16. Chisolm JJ. The use of chelating agents in the treatment of acute and chronic lead intoxication in childhood. J Pediatrics 1968; 73:1.
17. Coffin R, Phillips JL, Staples WI, et al. Treatment of lead encephalopathy in children. J Pediatrics 1966;69: 198–206.
18. Chisolm JJ. Increased lead absorption and acute lead poisoning. Current Pediatric Therapy 12, Gillis and Kagan, editors, WB Saunders, Philadelphia, 1986, pp. 667–671.

Manufactured for
3M Pharmaceuticals
Northridge, CA 91324
By Abbott Laboratories
North Chicago, IL 60064
994004 January 2000

MAXAIR™ AUTOHALER™ ℞

(pirbuterol acetate inhalation aerosol)
For Oral Inhalation Only

DESCRIPTION

The active component of MAXAIR AUTOHALER (pirbuterol acetate) is (R,S)α^6-{[(1,1-dimethylethyl)amino]methyl}-3-hydroxy-2,6-pyridinedimethanol monoacetate salt, a beta-2 adrenergic bronchodilator, having the following chemical structure:

HO–CH₂–(3-hydroxypyridin-2-yl)–CH(OH)–CH₂–NH–C(CH₃)₂–CH₃•CH₃COOH

Pirbuterol acetate is a white, crystalline racemic mixture of two optically active isomers. It is a powder, freely soluble in water, with a molecular weight of 300.3 and empirical formula of $C_{12}H_{20}N_2O_3 \cdot C_2H_4O_2$.
MAXAIR AUTOHALER is a pressurized metered-dose aerosol unit for oral inhalation. It provides a fine-particle suspension of pirbuterol acetate in the propellant mixture of trichloromonofluoromethane and dichlorodifluoromethane, with sorbitan trioleate. Each actuation delivers 253 mcg of pirbuterol (as pirbuterol acetate) from the valve and 200 mcg of pirbuterol (as pirbuterol acetate) from the mouthpiece. The unit is breath-actuated such that the medication is delivered automatically during inspiration without the need for the patient to coordinate actuation with inspiration. Each 14.0 g canister provides 400 inhalations.
As with all aerosol medications, it is recommended to prime (test) MAXAIR AUTOHALER before using for the first time. MAXAIR AUTOHALER should also be primed if it has not been used in 48 hours. As described in the priming procedure, use the test fire slide to release two priming sprays into the air away from yourself and other people. (See "Patient's Instructions For Use" portion of this package insert.)

CLINICAL PHARMACOLOGY

In vitro studies and *in vivo* pharmacologic studies have demonstrated that pirbuterol has a preferential effect on beta-2 adrenergic receptors compared with isoproterenol. While it is recognized that beta-2 adrenergic receptors are the predominant receptors in bronchial smooth muscle, data indicate that there is a population of beta-2 receptors in the human heart, existing in a concentration between 10–50%. The precise function of these receptors has not been established (see WARNINGS section).
The pharmacologic effects of beta adrenergic agonist drugs, including pirbuterol, are at least in part attributable to stimulation through beta adrenergic receptors of intracellular adenyl cyclase, the enzyme which catalyzes the conversion of adenosine triphosphate (ATP) to cyclic-3′,5′-adenosine monophosphate (c-AMP). Increased c-AMP levels are associated with relaxation of bronchial smooth muscle and inhibition of release of mediators of immediate hypersensitivity from cells, especially from mast cells.
Bronchodilator activity of pirbuterol was manifested clinically by an improvement in various pulmonary function parameters (FEV_1, MMF, PEFR, airway resistance [RAW] and conductance [GA/V_{tg}]).
Clinical Trials: In controlled double-blind single-dose clinical trials, the onset of improvement in pulmonary function occurred within 5 minutes in most patients as determined by forced expiratory volume in one second (FEV_1). FEV_1 and MMF measurements also showed that maximum improvement in pulmonary function generally occurred 30–60 minutes following one (1) or two (2) inhalations of pirbuterol (200–400 mcg). The duration of action of pirbuterol is maintained for 5 hours (the time at which the last observations were made) in a substantial number of patients, based on a 15% or greater increase in FEV_1. In controlled repetitive-dose studies of 12 weeks' duration, 74% of 156 patients on pirbuterol and 62% of 141 patients on metaproterenol showed a clinically significant improvement based on a 15% or greater increase in FEV_1 on at least half of the days. Onset and duration were equivalent to that seen in single-dose studies. Continued effectiveness was demonstrated over the 12-week period in the majority (94%) of responding patients; however, chronic dosing was associated with the development of tachyphylaxis (tolerance) to the bronchodilator effect in some patients in both treatment groups.
A placebo-controlled, double-blind, single-dose study (24 patients per treatment group), utilizing continuous Holter monitoring for 5 hours after drug administration, showed no significant difference in ectopic activity between the placebo control group and pirbuterol at the recommended dose (200-400 mcg), and twice the recommended dose (800 mcg). As with other inhaled beta adrenergic agonists, supraventricular and ventricular ectopic beats have been seen with pirbuterol (see WARNINGS).
Two randomized, double-blind, cross-over studies in a total of 97 patients, have compared the clinical effects of either one inhalation or two inhalations of the pirbuterol formulations in the AUTOHALER actuator and the conventional inhaler and demonstrated no significant difference between the formulations for the means of peak changes in FEV_1, time to peak FEV_1, onset, duration, or area under the FEV_1 curve.
Preclinical: Studies in laboratory animals (minipigs, rodents, and dogs) have demonstrated the occurrence of cardiac arrhythmias and sudden death (with histologic evidence of myocardial necrosis) when beta-agonists and methylxanthines were administered concurrently. The clinical significance of these findings when applied to humans is unknown.
Pharmacokinetics: As expected by extrapolation from oral data, systemic blood levels of pirbuterol are below the limit of assay sensitivity (2–5 ng/ml) following inhalation of doses up to 800 mcg (twice the maximum recommended dose).
A mean of 51% of the dose is recovered in urine as pirbuterol plus its sulfate conjugate following administration by aerosol. Pirbuterol is not metabolized by catechol-O-methyltransferase.
The percent of administered dose recovered as pirbuterol plus its sulfate conjugate does not change significantly over the dose range of 400 mcg to 800 mcg and is not significantly different from that after oral administration of pirbuterol. The plasma half-life measured after oral administration is about two hours.

INDICATIONS AND USAGE

MAXAIR AUTOHALER is indicated for the prevention and reversal of bronchospasm in patients 12 years of age and older with reversible bronchospasm including asthma. It may be used with or without concurrent theophylline and/or corticosteroid therapy.

CONTRAINDICATIONS

MAXAIR AUTOHALER is contraindicated in patients with a history of hypersensitivity to pirbuterol or any of its ingredients.

WARNINGS

Cardiovascular: MAXAIR AUTOHALER, like other inhaled beta adrenergic agonists, can produce a clinically significant cardiovascular effect in some patients, as measured by pulse rate, blood pressure and/or symptoms. Although such effects are uncommon after administration of MAXAIR AUTOHALER at recommended doses, if they occur, the drug may need to be discontinued. In addition, beta-agonists have been reported to produce ECG changes, such as flattening of the T wave, prolongation of the QTc interval, and ST segment depression. The clinical significance of these findings is unknown. Therefore, MAXAIR AUTOHALER, like all sympathomimetic amines, should be used with caution in patients with cardiovascular disorders, especially coronary insufficiency, cardiac arrhythmias, and hypertension.
Paradoxical Bronchospasm: MAXAIR AUTOHALER can produce paradoxical bronchospasm, which can be life threatening. If paradoxical bronchospasm occurs, MAXAIR AUTOHALER should be discontinued immediately and alternative therapy instituted. It should be recognized that paradoxical bronchospasm, when associated with inhaled formulations, frequently occurs with the first use of a new canister or vial.
Use of Anti-Inflammatory Agents: The use of beta adrenergic agonist bronchodilators alone may not be adequate to control asthma in many patients. Early consideration should be given to adding anti-inflammatory agents, e.g., corticosteroids.
Deterioration of Asthma: Asthma may deteriorate acutely over a period of hours or chronically over several days or longer. If the patient needs more doses of MAXAIR AUTOHALER than usual, this may be a marker of destabilization of asthma and requires reevaluation of the patient and the treatment regimen, giving special consideration to the possible need for anti-inflammatory treatment, e.g., corticosteroids.

PRECAUTIONS

General: Since pirbuterol is a sympathomimetic amine, it should be used with caution in patients with cardiovascular disorders, including ischemic heart disease, hypertension,

Continued on next page

Maxair Autohaler—Cont.

or cardiac arrhythmias, in patients with hyperthyroidism or diabetes mellitus, and in patients who are unusually responsive to sympathomimetic amines or who have convulsive disorders. Significant changes in systolic and diastolic blood pressure could be expected to occur in some patients after use of any beta adrenergic aerosol bronchodilator.

Beta adrenergic agonist medications may produce significant hypokalemia in some patients, possibly through intracellular shunting, which has the potential to produce adverse cardiovascular effects. The decrease is usually transient, not requiring supplementation.

Information for Patients: The action of MAXAIR AUTOHALER should last up to five hours or longer. MAXAIR AUTOHALER should not be used more frequently than recommended. Do not increase the dose or frequency of MAXAIR AUTOHALER without consulting your physician. If you find that treatment with MAXAIR AUTOHALER becomes less effective for symptomatic relief, or your symptoms become worse, and/or you need to use the product more frequently than usual, you should seek medical attention immediately. While you are using MAXAIR AUTOHALER, other inhaled drugs and asthma medications should be taken only as directed by your physician. Common adverse effects include palpitations, chest pain, rapid heart rate, tremor or nervousness. If you are pregnant or nursing, contact your physician about use of MAXAIR AUTOHALER. Effective and safe use includes an understanding of the way the medication should be administered.

As with all aerosol medications, it is recommended to prime (test) MAXAIR AUTOHALER before using for the first time. MAXAIR AUTOHALER should also be primed if it has not been used in 48 hours. As described in the priming procedure, use the test fire slide to release two priming sprays into the air away from yourself and other people (See "Patient's Instructions For Use" portion of this package insert.) The MAXAIR AUTOHALER actuator should not be used with any other inhalation aerosol canister. In addition, canisters for use with MAXAIR AUTOHALER should not be utilized with any other actuator.

Drug Interactions: Other short-acting beta adrenergic aerosol bronchodilators should not be used concomitantly with MAXAIR AUTOHALER because they may have additive effects.

Monoamine Oxidase Inhibitors or Tricyclic Antidepressants: Pirbuterol should be administered with extreme caution to patients being treated with monoamine oxidase inhibitors or tricyclic antidepressants, or within 2 weeks of discontinuation of such agents, because the action of pirbuterol on the vascular system may be potentiated.

Beta Blockers: Beta adrenergic receptor blocking agents not only block the pulmonary effect of beta-agonists, such as MAXAIR AUTOHALER, but may produce severe bronchospasm in asthmatic patients. Therefore, patients with asthma should not normally be treated with beta blockers. However, under certain circumstances, e.g., as prophylaxis after myocardial infarction, there may be no acceptable alternatives to the use of beta adrenergic blocking agents in patients with asthma. In this setting, cardioselective beta blockers could be considered, although they should be administered with caution.

Diuretics: The ECG changes and/or hypokalemia that may result from the administration of non-potassium sparing diuretics (such as loop or thiazide diuretics) can be acutely worsened by beta-agonists, especially when the recommended dose of the beta-agonist is exceeded. Although the clinical significance of these effects is not known, caution is advised in the coadministration of beta-agonists with non-potassium sparing diuretics.

Carcinogenesis, Mutagenesis and Impairment of Fertility: In a 2-year study in Sprague-Dawley rats, pirbuterol hydrochloride administered at dietary doses of 1.0, 3.0, and 10 mg/kg (approximately 3, 10, and 35 times the maximum recommended daily inhalation dose for adults and children on a mg/m^2 basis) showed no evidence of carcinogenicity. In an 18-month study in mice at dietary doses of 1.0, 3.0, and 10 mg/kg (approximately 2, 5, and 15 times the maximum recommended daily inhalation dose for adults and children on a mg/m^2 basis) no evidence of tumorigenicity was seen. Reproduction studies in rats administered pirbuterol hydrochloride at oral doses of 1, 3, and 10 mg/kg (approximately 3, 10, and 35 times the maximum recommended daily inhalation dose for adults on a mg/m^2 basis) revealed no evidence of impaired fertility.

Pirbuterol dihydrochloride showed no evidence of mutagenicity in *in vitro* assays and host-mediated microbial (Ames) assays for point mutations and *in vivo* tests for somatic or germ cell effects following acute and subchronic treatment in mice (cytogenicity assays).

Teratogenic Effects—Pregnancy Category C: Pirbuterol was not teratogenic in rats administered oral doses of 30, 100, and 300 mg/kg (approximately 100, 340, and 1000 times the maximum recommended daily inhalation dose for adults on a mg/m^2 basis). Pirbuterol was not teratogenic in rabbits administered oral doses of 30 and 100 mg/kg (approximately 200 and 680 times the maximum recommended inhalation dose for adults on a mg/m^2 basis). However, pirbuterol at an oral dose of 300 mg/kg (approximately 2000 times the maximum recommended daily inhalation dose in adults on a mg/m^2 basis) caused abortions and fetal death. There are no adequate and well-controlled studies in pregnant women. Pirbuterol should be used during pregnancy only if the potential benefit justifies the potential risk to the fetus.

Labor and Delivery: Because of the potential for beta-agonist interference with uterine contractility, use of MAXAIR AUTOHALER for relief of bronchospasm during labor should be restricted to those patients in whom the benefits clearly outweigh the risk.

Nursing Mothers: It is not known whether pirbuterol is excreted in human milk. Therefore, MAXAIR AUTOHALER should be used during nursing only if the potential benefit justifies the possible risk to the newborn.

Pediatric Use: MAXAIR AUTOHALER is not recommended for patients under the age of 12 years because of insufficient clinical data to establish safety and effectiveness.

ADVERSE REACTIONS

The following rates of adverse reactions to pirbuterol are based on single- and multiple-dose clinical trials involving 761 patients, 400 of whom received multiple doses (mean duration of treatment was 2.5 months and maximum was 19 months).

The following were the adverse reactions reported more frequently than 1 in 100 patients:

CNS: nervousness (6.9%), tremor (6.0%), headache (2.0%), dizziness (1.2%).

Cardiovascular: palpitations (1.7%), tachycardia (1.2%).

Respiratory: cough (1.2%).

Gastrointestinal: nausea (1.7%).

The following adverse reactions occurred less frequently than 1 in 100 patients and there may be a causal relationship with pirbuterol:

CNS: depression, anxiety, confusion, insomnia, weakness, hyperkinesia, syncope.

Cardiovascular: hypotension, skipped beats, chest pain.

Gastrointestinal: dry mouth, glossitis, abdominal pain/cramps, anorexia, diarrhea, stomatitis, nausea and vomiting.

Ear, Nose and Throat: smell/taste changes, sore throat.

Dermatological: rash, pruritus.

Other: numbness in extremities, alopecia, bruising, fatigue, edema, weight gain, flushing.

Other adverse reactions were reported with a frequency of less than 1 in 100 patients but a causal relationship between pirbuterol and the reaction could not be determined: migraine, productive cough, wheezing, and dermatitis.

The following rates of adverse reactions during three-month controlled clinical trials involving 310 patients are noted. The table does not include mild reactions.

PERCENT OF PATIENTS WITH MODERATE TO SEVERE ADVERSE REACTIONS

Reaction	Pirbuterol N=157	Metaproterenol N=153
Central Nervous System		
tremors	1.3%	3.3%
nervousness	4.5%	2.6%
headache	1.3%	2.0%
weakness	.0%	1.3%
drowsiness	.0%	0.7%
dizziness	0.6%	.0%
Cardiovascular		
palpitations	1.3%	1.3%
tachycardia	1.3%	2.0%
Respiratory		
chest pain/tightness	1.3%	.0%
cough	.0%	0.7%
Gastrointestinal		
nausea	1.3%	2.0%
diarrhea	1.3%	0.7%
dry mouth	1.3%	1.3%
vomiting	.0%	0.7%
Dermatological		
skin reaction	.0%	0.7%
rash	.0%	1.3%
Other		
bruising	0.6%	.0%
smell/taste change	0.6%	.0%
backache	.0%	0.7%
fatigue	.0%	0.7%
hoarseness	.0%	0.7%
nasal congestion	.0%	0.7%

Electrocardiograms: Electrocardiograms, obtained during a randomized, double-blind, cross-over study in 57 patients, showed no observations or findings considered clinically significant, or related to drug administration. Most electrocardiographic observations, obtained during a randomized, double-blind, cross-over study in 40 patients, were judged not clinically significant or related to drug administration. One patient was noted to have some changes on the one hour postdose electrocardiogram consisting of ST and T wave abnormality suggesting possible inferior ischemia. This abnormality was not observed on the predose or the six hours postdose ECG. A treadmill was subsequently performed and all the findings were normal.

OVERDOSAGE

The expected symptoms with overdosage are those of excessive beta-stimulation and/or any of the symptoms listed under ADVERSE REACTIONS, e.g., seizures, angina, hypertension or hypotension, tachycardia with rates up to 200 beats per minute, arrhythmias, nervousness, headache, tremor, dry mouth, palpitation, nausea, dizziness, fatigue, malaise, and insomnia. Hypokalemia may also occur. As with all sympathomimetic aerosol medication, cardiac arrest and even death may be associated with abuse of MAXAIR AUTOHALER.

Treatment consists of discontinuation of pirbuterol together with appropriate symptomatic therapy. The judicious use of a cardioselective beta-receptor blocker may be considered, bearing in mind that such medication can produce bronchospasm. There is insufficient evidence to determine if dialysis is beneficial for overdosage.

The oral median lethal dose of pirbuterol dihydrochloride in mice and rats is greater than 2000 mg/kg (approximately 3400 and 6800 times the maximum recommended daily inhalation dose for adults on a mg/m^2 basis).

DOSAGE AND ADMINISTRATION

The usual dose for adults and children 12 years and older is two inhalations (400 mcg) repeated every 4–6 hours. One inhalation (200 mcg) repeated every 4–6 hours may be sufficient for some patients.

A total daily dose of 12 inhalations should not be exceeded.

If a previously effective dosage regimen fails to provide the usual relief, medical advice should be sought immediately as this is often a sign of seriously worsening asthma which would require reassessment of therapy.

HOW SUPPLIED

MAXAIR AUTOHALER, box of one, is supplied in a pressurized aluminum canister with a light blue plastic breath-activated actuator and a light blue mouthpiece cover. DO NOT USE WITH OTHER CANISTERS OR MOUTHPIECES. Each actuation delivers 253 mcg of pirbuterol (as pirbuterol acetate) from the valve and 200 mcg of pirbuterol (as pirbuterol acetate) from the mouthpiece.

Canister net content weight 14.0 g, 400 inhalations (NDC **0089-0815-21**).

The correct amount of medication in each canister cannot be assured after 400 actuations from the 14.0 g canister, even though the canister is not completely empty. The canister should be discarded when the labeled numbers of actuations have been used.

Note: The indented statement below is required by the Federal government's Clean Air Act for all products containing or manufactured with chlorofluorocarbons (CFC's).

> **WARNING:** Contains trichloromonofluoromethane and dichlorodifluoromethane, substances which harm public health and environment by destroying ozone in the upper atmosphere.

A notice similar to the above WARNING has been placed in the "Patient's Instructions For Use" portion of this package insert under the Environmental Protection Agency's (EPA's) regulations. The patient's warning states that the patient should consult his or her physician if there are questions about alternatives.

Rx only

Store between 15° and 30°C (59° to 86°F). Failure to use this product within this temperature range may result in improper dosing. For optimal results, the canister should be at room temperature before use. Shake well before using.

The contents of MAXAIR AUTOHALER are under pressure. Do not puncture. Do not use or store near heat or open flame. Exposure to temperature above 120°F may cause bursting. Never throw container into fire or incinerator. Keep out of reach of children. Avoid spraying in eyes.

The light blue plastic actuator supplied with MAXAIR AUTOHALER should not be used with any other product canisters, and actuators from other product should not be used with MAXAIR AUTOHALER canister.

3M Pharmaceuticals
Northridge, CA 91324
654600 SEPTEMBER 2000

MAXAIR™ AUTOHALER™ (pirbuterol acetate inhalation aerosol)

Patient's Instructions For Use

Questions? Call our Patient Assistance Line at 1-(800)-841-3885 24 hours a day. To talk to an operator call between 8:30 AM and 5PM EST (Weekdays).

Priming Procedure for MAXAIR™ AUTOHALER™

As with all aerosol medications, it is recommended to prime (test) MAXAIR AUTOHALER before using for the first time. MAXAIR AUTOHALER should also be primed if it has not been used in 48 hours. As described in the priming procedure, use the test fire slide to release two priming sprays into the air away from yourself and other people.

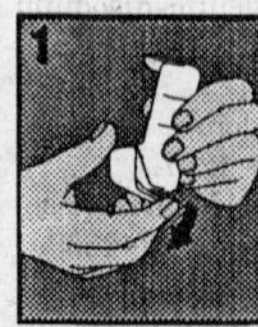

Remove mouthpiece cover by pulling down lip on **back** of cover.

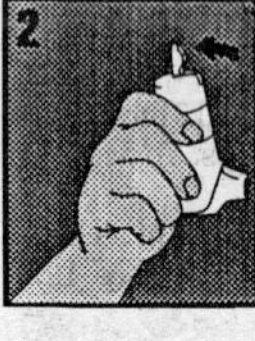

Point the mouthpiece away from yourself and other people so that the priming sprays will go into the air. Push the lever up so that it stays up.

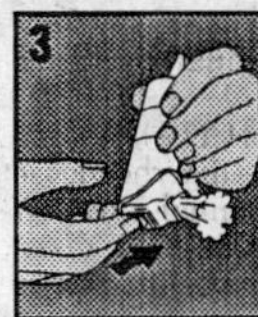

To release a priming spray, push the white test fire slide on the bottom of the mouthpiece in the direction indicated by the arrow on the test fire slide.

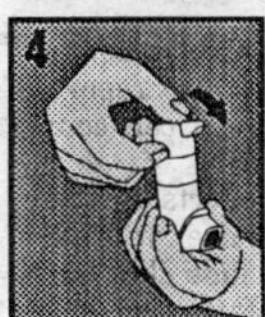

To release the second priming spray, return the lever to its down position and repeat steps 2 and 3. After releasing the second priming spray, return the lever to its down position.

Using Your MAXAIR™ AUTOHALER™

IMPORTANT NOTE: Use MAXAIR AUTOHALER according to the instructions given to you by your physician, who will advise you on the number of inhalations to take. If you have previously been using MAXAIR Inhaler, you should take the same number of inhalations through your MAXAIR AUTOHALER as you did through the MAXAIR Inhaler.

Before using your MAXAIR AUTOHALER, read complete instructions carefully.

The light blue plastic actuator supplied with MAXAIR AUTOHALER should not be used with any other product canisters, and actuators from other products should not be used with a MAXAIR AUTOHALER canister.

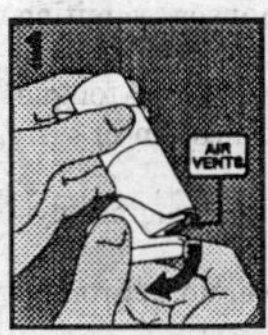

Remove mouthpiece cover by pulling down lip on **back** of cover.

Inspect mouthpiece for foreign objects.

Locate "Up" arrows on MAXAIR AUTOHALER.

Locate air vents at bottom of MAXAIR AUTOHALER.

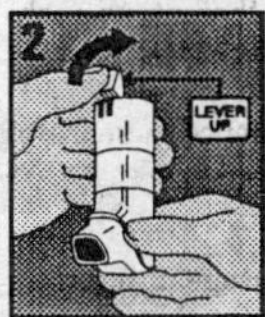

Hold MAXAIR AUTOHALER **upright** as shown in figure 2. The arrows should point up.

MAXAIR AUTOHALER must be held upright while raising lever.

Raise lever so that is stays up. It will "snap" into place.

Do not lower lever until step 6.

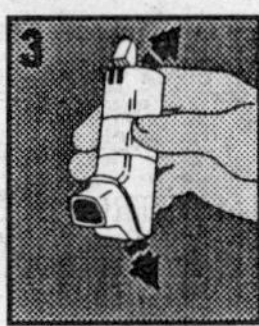

Hold MAXAIR AUTOHALER around the middle as shown in figure 3.

Shake MAXAIR AUTOHALER gently several times.

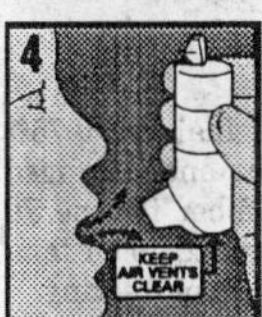

Continue to hold MAXAIR AUTOHALER upright as shown in figure 4.

Do not block air vents at bottom of MAXAIR AUTOHALER.

Exhale normally before use.

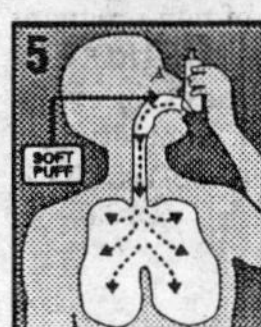

Seal your lips tightly around mouthpiece as shown in figure 5.

Inhale deeply through mouthpiece with **steady, moderate force.** You will hear a "click" and feel a **soft** puff when your inhaling triggers the release of medicine. **Do not stop when you hear and feel the puff.** Continue to take a **full, deep breath.**

Take MAXAIR AUTOHALER away from your mouth when done inhaling. Hold your breath for 10 seconds, then exhale slowly.

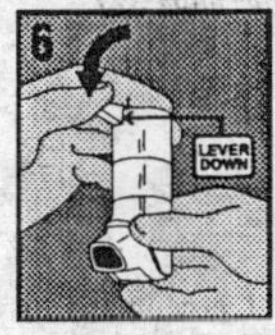

Continue to hold MAXAIR AUTOHALER upright while lowering the lever as shown in figure 6. Lower lever after each inhalation.

If your physician has prescribed additional inhalations, wait one minute then repeat steps 2 through 6. Following use, make sure lever is down and replace mouthpiece cover.

How to Clean and Care for MAXAIR™ AUTOHALER™

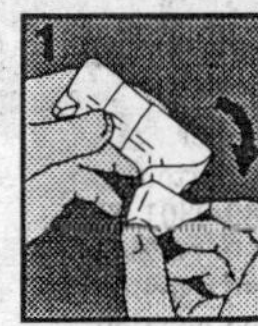

Remove mouthpiece cover by pulling down lip on **back** of cover.

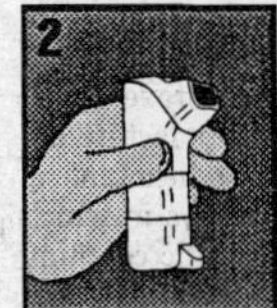

Turn MAXAIR AUTOHALER upside down. Wipe mouthpiece with a clean dry cloth.

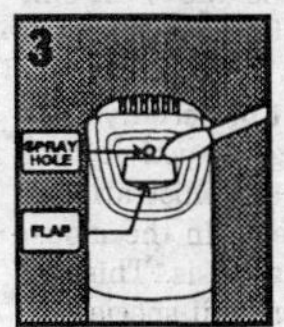

Gently tap back of MAXAIR AUTOHALER so flap comes down and spray hole can be seen. With white flap down as shown in the picture, clean the surface of the flap with a dry cotton swab.

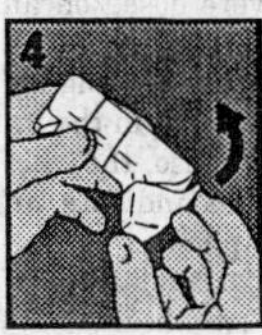

Replace mouthpiece cover. When you are not using MAXAIR AUTOHALER, make sure lever is down and mouthpiece cover is in place.

Repeat cleaning instructions weekly or as often as required.

Note: The indented statement below is required by the Federal Government's Clean Air Act for all products containing or manufactured with chlorofluorocarbons (CFC's).

> This product contains trichloromonofluromethane and dichlorodifluoromethane, substances which harm the environment by destroying ozone in the upper atmosphere.

Your physician has determined that this product is likely to help your personal health. USE THIS PRODUCT AS DIRECTED, UNLESS INSTRUCTED TO DO OTHERWISE BY YOUR PHYSICIAN. If you have any questions about alternatives, consult with your physician.

The correct amount of medication in each canister cannot be assured after 400 actuations from the 14.0 g canister, even though the canister is not completely empty. You should keep track of the number of actuations used from each MAXAIR AUTOHALER and discard the MAXAIR AUTOHALER after 400 actuations from the 14.0 g canister. MAXAIR AUTOHALER should be discarded when the labeled numbers of actuations have been used. Before you reach the specified number of actuations, you should consult your physician to determine whether a refill is needed. Just as you should not take extra doses without consulting your physician, you also should not stop using MAXAIR AUTOHALER without consulting your physician.

Dosage: Use only as directed by your physician.

WARNINGS: The effects of MAXAIR AUTOHALER may last up to five hours or longer. Therefore, it should not be used more frequently than recommended. Do not increase the number or frequency of doses without speaking with the prescribing physician. If the recommended dosage does not provide relief of symptoms, or your symptoms get worse, speak with your physician. While taking MAXAIR AUTOHALER, other inhaled medicines should not be used unless prescribed.

Important Information:

Store between 15° and 30° C (59° to 86° F). Failure to use this product within this temperature range may result in improper dosing. For optimal results, the canister should be at room temperature before use. Shake well before using.

Caution: Contents of canister under pressure. Do not puncture. Do not use near heat or open flame. Exposure to temperatures above 120°F may cause bursting. Never throw container into fire or incinerator. Avoid spraying in eyes. Keep out of reach of children.

Rx only

Use MAXAIR AUTOHALER only as prescribed by your physician.

Handle with care.

DO NOT USE WITH OTHER CANISTERS OR MOUTHPIECES.

For information on the drug, refer to your doctor or pharmacist.

General Information about MAXAIR™ AUTOHALER™ (pirbuterol acetate inhalation aerosol)

Your MAXAIR AUTOHALER is a new type of inhaler designed to be very easy to use. MAXAIR AUTOHALER automatically releases an inhalation of medicine when you inhale.

What will I feel when I use MAXAIR AUTOHALER?

MAXAIR AUTOHALER provides a soft spray of medicine. It is designed to automatically deliver a precisely measured dose of your medicine with each inhalation, so you can be assured of a consistent dose of medicine.

When medicine is delivered, you will hear a "click" and feel a **soft** inhalation.

How will I know when there's no more medicine in MAXAIR AUTOHALER?

The MAXAIR AUTOHALER you receive from the pharmacy contains 400 inhalations (the MAXAIR AUTOHALER sample contains 80 inhalations and says "SAMPLE" on the back). You can estimate how many days it will last by dividing 80 or 400 (total inhalations in a unit) by the number of inhalations you normally use in a day. The chart below can help you calculate about how long your 400 inhalation MAXAIR AUTOHALER will last. Actual usage may vary depending on how many inhalations you use each day. A total daily dose of 12 inhalations should not be exceeded.

Average Number of Inhalations Per Day	Approximate Days of Therapy Available
2 inhalations/day	200 days
4 inhalations/day	100 days
6 inhalations/day	65 days
8 inhalations/day	50 days

3M Pharmaceuticals
Northridge, CA 91324 SEPTEMBER 2000

Shown in Product Identification Guide, page 321

METROGEL-VAGINAL® ℞

(metronidazole vaginal gel)
0.75% Vaginal Gel
FOR INTRAVAGINAL USE ONLY
NOT FOR OPHTHALMIC, DERMAL, OR ORAL USE

DESCRIPTION

METROGEL-VAGINAL is the intravaginal dosage form of the synthetic antibacterial agent, metronidazole, USP at a concentration of 0.75%. Metronidazole is a member of the imidazole class of antibacterial agents and is classified therapeutically as an antiprotozoal and antibacterial agent. Chemically, metronidazole is a 2-methyl-5-nitroimidazole-1-ethanol. It has a chemical formula of $C_6H_9N_3O_3$, a molecular weight of 171.16, and has the following structure:

CH_2CH_2OH ; O_2N ; CH_3 ; N

METROGEL-VAGINAL is a gelled, purified water solution, containing metronidazole at a concentration of 7.5 mg/g (0.75%). The gel is formulated at pH 4.0. The gel also contains carbomer 934P, edetate disodium, methyl paraben, propyl paraben, propylene glycol, and sodium hydroxide. Each applicator full of 5 grams of vaginal gel contains approximately 37.5 mg of metronidazole.

CLINICAL PHARMACOLOGY

Normal Subjects:

Following a single, intravaginal 5 gram dose of metronidazole vaginal gel (equivalent to 37.5 mg of metronidazole) to 12 normal subjects, a mean maximum serum metronidazole concentration of 237 ng/mL was reported (range: 152 to 368 ng/mL). This is approximately 2% of the mean maximum serum metronidazole concentration reported in the same subjects administered a single, oral 500 mg dose of metronidazole (mean C_{max} = 12,785 ng/mL, range: 10,013 to 17,400 ng/mL). These peak concentrations were obtained in 6 to 12 hours after dosing with metronidazole vaginal gel and 1 to 3 hours after dosing with oral metronidazole.

The extent of exposure [area under the curve (AUC)] of metronidazole, when administered as a single intravaginal 5 gram dose of metronidazole vaginal gel (equivalent to 37.5 mg of metronidazole), was approximately 4% of the AUC of a single oral 500 mg dose of metronidazole (4977 ng-hr/mL and approximately 125,000 ng-hr/mL, respectively).

Dose-adjusted comparisons of AUCs demonstrated that, on a mg to mg comparison basis, the absorption of metronidazole, when administered vaginally, was approximately half that of an equivalent oral dosage.

Patients with Bacterial Vaginosis:

Following single and multiple 5 gram doses of metronidazole vaginal gel to 4 patients with bacterial vaginosis, a mean maximum serum metronidazole concentration of 214 ng/mL on day 1 and 294 ng/mL (range: 228 to 349 ng/mL) on day five were reported. Steady-state metronidazole serum concentrations following oral dosages of 400 to 500 mg BID have been reported to range from 6,000 to 20,000 ng/mL.

Microbiology:

The intracellular targets of action of metronidazole on anaerobes are largely unknown. The 5-nitro group of metronidazole is reduced by metabolically active anaerobes, and studies have demonstrated that the reduced form of the drug interacts with bacterial DNA. However, it is not clear whether interaction with DNA alone is an important component in the bactericidal action of metronidazole on anaerobic organisms.

Culture and sensitivity testing of bacteria are not routinely performed to establish the diagnosis of bacterial vaginosis. (See **INDICATIONS AND USAGE.**)

Standard methodology for the susceptibility testing of the potential bacterial vaginosis pathogens, *Gardnerella vagi-*

Continued on next page

Metrogel-Vaginal—Cont.

nalis, Mobiluncus spp., and *Mycoplasma hominis*, has not been defined. Nonetheless, metronidazole is an antimicrobial agent active *in vitro* against most strains of the following organisms that have been reported to be associated with bacterial vaginosis:
Bacteroides spp.
Gardnerella vaginalis
Mobiluncus spp.
Peptostreptococcus spp.

INDICATIONS AND USAGE

METROGEL-VAGINAL is indicated in the treatment of bacterial vaginosis (formerly referred to as *Haemophilus* vaginitis, *Gardnerella* vaginitis, nonspecific vaginitis, *Corynebacterium* vaginitis, or anaerobic vaginosis).

NOTE: For purposes of this indication, a clinical diagnosis of bacterial vaginosis is usually defined by the presence of a homogeneous vaginal discharge that (a) has a pH of greater than 4.5, (b) emits a "fishy" amine odor when mixed with a 10% KOH solution, and (c) contains clue cells on microscopic examination. Gram's stain results consistent with a diagnosis of bacterial vaginosis include (a) markedly reduced or absent *Lactobacillus* morphology, (b) predominance of *Gardnerella* morphotype, and (c) absent or few white blood cells. Other pathogens commonly associated with vulvovaginitis, e.g., *Trichomonas vaginalis, Chlamydia trachomatis, N. gonorrhoeae, Candida albicans*, and *Herpes simplex* virus should be ruled out.

CONTRAINDICATIONS

METROGEL-VAGINAL is contraindicated in patients with a prior history of hypersensitivity to metronidazole, parabens, other ingredients of the formulation, or other nitroimidazole derivatives.

WARNINGS

Convulsive Seizures and Peripheral Neuropathy:
Convulsive seizures and peripheral neuropathy, the latter characterized mainly by numbness or paresthesia of an extremity, have been reported in patients treated with oral or intravenous metronidazole. The appearance of abnormal neurologic signs demands the prompt discontinuation of metronidazole vaginal gel therapy. Metronidazole vaginal gel should be administered with caution to patients with central nervous system diseases.

Psychotic Reactions:
Psychotic reactions have been reported in alcoholic patients who were using oral metronidazole and disulfiram concurrently. Metronidazole vaginal gel should not be administered to patients who have taken disulfiram within the last two weeks.

PRECAUTIONS

METROGEL-VAGINAL affords minimal peak serum levels and systemic exposure (AUCs) of metronidazole compared to 500 mg oral metronidazole dosing. Although these lower levels of exposure are less likely to produce the common reactions seen with oral metronidazole, the possibility of these and other reactions cannot be excluded presently. Data from well-controlled trials directly comparing metronidazole administered orally to metronidazole administered vaginally are not available.

General: Patients with severe hepatic disease metabolize metronidazole slowly. This results in the accumulation of metronidazole and its metabolites in the plasma. Accordingly, for such patients, metronidazole vaginal gel should be administered cautiously.

Known or previously unrecognized vaginal candidiasis may present more prominent symptoms during therapy with metronidazole vaginal gel. Approximately 6–10% of patients treated with METROGEL-VAGINAL developed symptomatic *Candida* vaginitis during or immediately after therapy.

Disulfiram-like reaction to alcohol has been reported with oral metronidazole, thus the possibility of such a reaction occurring while on metronidazole vaginal gel therapy cannot be excluded.

METROGEL-VAGINAL contains ingredients that may cause burning and irritation of the eye. In the event of accidental contact with the eye, rinse the eye with copious amounts of cool tap water.

Information for the Patient: The patient should be cautioned about drinking alcohol while being treated with metronidazole vaginal gel. While blood levels are significantly lower with METROGEL-VAGINAL than with usual doses of oral metronidazole, a possible interaction with alcohol cannot be excluded.

The patient should be instructed not to engage in vaginal intercourse during treatment with this product.

Drug Interactions: Oral metronidazole has been reported to potentiate the anticoagulant effect of warfarin and other coumarin anticoagulants, resulting in a prolongation of prothrombin time. This possible drug interaction should be considered when metronidazole vaginal gel is prescribed for patients on this type of anticoagulant therapy.

In patients stabilized on relatively high doses of lithium, short-term oral metronidazole therapy has been associated with elevation of serum lithium levels and, in a few cases, signs of lithium toxicity.

Use of cimetidine with oral metronidazole may prolong the half-life and decrease plasma clearance of metronidazole.

Drug/Laboratory Test Interactions: Metronidazole may interfere with certain types of determinations of serum chemistry values, such as aspartate aminotransferase (AST, SGOT), alanine aminotransferase (ALT, SGPT), lactate dehydrogenase (LDH), triglycerides, and glucose hexokinase. Values of zero may be observed. All of the assays in which interference has been reported involve enzymatic coupling of the assay to oxidation-reduction of nicotinamide-adenine dinucleotides (NAD+NADH). Interference is due to the similarity in absorbance peaks of NADH (340 nm) and metronidazole (322 nm) at pH 7.

Carcinogenesis, Mutagenesis, Impairment of Fertility: Metronidazole has shown evidence of carcinogenic activity in a number of studies involving chronic oral administration in mice and rats. Prominent among the effects in the mouse was the promotion of pulmonary tumorigenesis. This has been observed in all six reported studies in that species, including one study in which the animals were dosed on an intermittent schedule (administration during every fourth week only). At very high dose levels (approx. 500 mg/kg/day), there was a statistically significant increase in the incidence of malignant liver tumors in males. Also, the published results of one of the mouse studies indicate an increase in the incidence of malignant lymphomas as well as pulmonary neoplasms associated with lifetime feeding of the drug. All these effects are statistically significant. Several long-term oral dosing studies in the rat have been completed. There were statistically significant increases in the incidence of various neoplasms, particularly in mammary and hepatic tumors, among female rats administered metronidazole over those noted in the concurrent female control groups. Two lifetime tumorigenicity studies in hamsters have been performed and reported to be negative.

These studies have not been conducted with 0.75% metronidazole vaginal gel, which would result in significantly lower systemic blood levels than those obtained with oral formulations.

Although metronidazole has shown mutagenic activity in a number of *in vitro* assay systems, studies in mammals (*in vivo*) have failed to demonstrate a potential for genetic damage.

Fertility studies have been performed in mice up to six times the recommended human oral dose (based on mg/m^2) and have revealed no evidence of impaired fertility.

Pregnancy: Teratogenic Effects: Pregnancy Category B
There has been no experience to date with the use of METROGEL-VAGINAL in pregnant patients. Metronidazole crosses the placental barrier and enters the fetal circulation rapidly. No fetotoxicity or teratogenicity was observed when metronidazole was administered orally to pregnant mice at six times the recommended human dose (based on mg/m^2); however, in a single small study where the drug was administered intraperitoneally, some intrauterine deaths were observed. The relationship of these findings to the drug is unknown.

There are, however, no adequate and well-controlled studies in pregnant women. Because animal reproduction studies are not always predictive of human response, and because metronidazole is a carcinogen in rodents, this drug should be used during pregnancy only if clearly needed.

Nursing Mothers: Specific studies of metronidazole levels in human milk following intravaginally administered metronidazole have not been performed. However, metronidazole is secreted in human milk in concentrations similar to those found in plasma following oral administration of metronidazole.

Because of the potential for tumorigenicity shown for metronidazole in mouse and rat studies, a decision should be made whether to discontinue nursing or to discontinue the drug, taking into account the importance of the drug to the mother.

Pediatric Use: Safety and effectiveness in children have not been established.

ADVERSE EVENTS

Clinical Trials:
There were no deaths or serious adverse events related to drug therapy in clinical trials involving 800 non-pregnant women who received METROGEL-VAGINAL.

In a randomized, single-blind clinical trial of 505 non-pregnant women who received METROGEL-VAGINAL once or twice a day, 2 patients (one from each regimen) discontinued therapy early due to drug-related adverse events. One patient discontinued drug because of moderate abdominal cramping and loose stools, while the other patient discontinued drug because of mild vaginal burning. These symptoms resolved after discontinuation of drug.

Medical events judged to be related, probably related, or possibly related to administration of METROGEL-VAGINAL once or twice a day were reported for 195/505 (39%) patients. The incidence of individual adverse reactions were not significantly different between the two regimens. Unless percentages are otherwise stipulated, the incidence of individual adverse reactions listed below was less than 1%:

Reproductive: Vaginal discharge (12%), symptomatic *Candida* cervicitis/vaginitis (10%), vulva/vaginal irritative symptoms (9%), pelvic discomfort (3%).
Gastrointestinal: Gastrointestinal discomfort (7%), nausea and/or vomiting (4%), unusual taste (2%), diarrhea/loose stools (1%), decreased appetite (1%), abdominal bloating/gas; thirsty, dry mouth. *Neurologic:* Headache (5%), dizziness (2%), depression. *Dermatologic:* Generalized itching or rash. *Other:* Unspecified cramping (1%), fatigue, darkened urine.

In previous clinical trials submitted for approved labeling of METROGEL-VAGINAL the following was also reported: *Laboratory:* Increased/decreased white blood cell counts (1.7%).

Other Metronidazole Formulations: Other effects that have been reported in association with the use of **topical (dermal)** formulations of metronidazole include skin irritation, transient skin erythema, and mild skin dryness and burning. None of these adverse events exceeded an incidence of 2% of patients.

METROGEL-VAGINAL affords minimal peak serum levels and systemic exposure (AUC) of metronidazole compared to 500 mg oral metronidazole dosing. Although these lower levels of exposure are less likely to produce the common reactions seen with oral metronidazole, the possibility of these and other reactions cannot be excluded presently.

The following adverse reactions and altered laboratory tests have been reported with the **oral or parenteral** use of metronidazole:

Cardiovascular: Flattening of the T-wave may be seen in electrocardiographic tracings.
Central Nervous System: (See **WARNINGS.**) Headache, dizziness, syncope, ataxia, confusion, convulsive seizures, peripheral neuropathy, vertigo, incoordination, irritability, depression, weakness, insomnia.
Gastrointestinal: Abdominal discomfort, nausea, vomiting, diarrhea, an unpleasant metallic taste, anorexia, epigastric distress, abdominal cramping, constipation, "furry" tongue, glossitis, stomatitis, pancreatitis, and modification of taste of alcoholic beverages.
Genitourinary: Overgrowth of *Candida* in the vagina, dyspareunia, decreased libido, proctitis.
Hematopoietic: Reversible neutropenia, reversible thrombocytopenia.
Hypersensitivity Reactions: Urticaria; erythematous rash; flushing; nasal congestion; dryness of the mouth, vagina, or vulva; fever; pruritus; fleeting joint pains.
Renal: Dysuria, cystitis, polyuria, incontinence, a sense of pelvic pressure, darkened urine.

OVERDOSAGE

There is no human experience with overdosage of metronidazole vaginal gel. Vaginally applied metronidazole gel, 0.75% could be absorbed in sufficient amounts to produce systemic effects.
(See **WARNINGS.**)

DOSAGE AND ADMINISTRATION

The recommended dose is one applicator full of METROGEL-VAGINAL (approximately 5 grams containing approximately 37.5 mg of metronidazole) intravaginally once or twice a day for 5 days. For once a day dosing, METROGEL-VAGINAL should be administered at bedtime.

HOW SUPPLIED

METROGEL-VAGINAL (metronidazole vaginal gel) 0.75% Vaginal Gel is supplied in a 70 gram tube and packaged with 5 vaginal applicators. The NDC number for the 70 gram tube is 0089-0200-25. Store at controlled room temperature 15° to 30°C (59° to 86°F). Protect from freezing.

Clinical Studies
In a randomized, single-blind clinical trial of non-pregnant women with bacterial vaginosis who received METROGEL-VAGINAL daily for 5 days, the clinical cure rates for evaluable patients determined at 4 weeks after completion of therapy for the QD and BID regimens were 98/185 (53%) and 109/190 (57%), respectively.

Rx only
January 2003

Manufactured for
3M Pharmaceuticals
Northridge, CA 91324
Manufactured by
DPT Laboratories, Inc.
San Antonio, TX, 78215

Shown in Product Identification Guide, page 321

MINITRAN™ ℞
(nitroglycerin)
Transdermal Delivery System

For full prescribing information see leaflet accompanying product or call 800-328-0255 for a copy.

HOW SUPPLIED

[See table below]

MINITRAN System Rated Release In Vivo	System Size	Total Nitroglycerin in System	NDC Number (30 per carton)
0.1 mg/hr	3.3 cm^2	9 mg	NDC-0089-0301-02
0.2 mg/hr	6.7 cm^2	18 mg	NDC-0089-0302-02
0.4 mg/hr	13.3 cm^2	36 mg	NDC-0089-0303-02
0.6 mg/hr	20.0 cm^2	54 mg	NDC-0089-0304-02

NORFLEX™ ℞
(orphenadrine citrate)
Extended-release
Tablets and Injection

DESCRIPTION
Orphenadrine citrate is the citrate salt of orphenadrine (2-dimethylaminoethyl 2-methylbenzhydryl ether citrate). It occurs as a white, crystalline powder having a bitter taste. It is practically odorless; sparingly soluble in water, slightly soluble in alcohol.
Each Norflex Extended-release tablet contains 100 mg orphenadrine citrate. Norflex Extended-release tablets also contain: calcium stearate, ethylcellulose, and lactose. Norflex Injection contains 60 mg of orphenadrine citrate in aqueous solution in each ampul. Norflex Injection also contains: sodium bisulfite NF, 2.0 mg; sodium chloride USP, 5.8 mg; sodium hydroxide, to adjust pH; and water for injection USP, q.s. to 2 mL.

ACTIONS
The mode of therapeutic action has not been clearly identified, but may be related to its analgesic properties. Orphenadrine citrate also possesses anticholinergic actions.

INDICATIONS
Orphenadrine citrate is indicated as an adjunct to rest, physical therapy, and other measures for the relief of discomfort associated with acute painful musculoskeletal conditions. The mode of action of the drug has not been clearly identified, but may be related to its analgesic properties. Orphenadrine citrate does not directly relax tense skeletal muscles in man.

CONTRAINDICATIONS
Contraindicated in patients with glaucoma, pyloric or duodenal obstruction, stenosing peptic ulcers, prostatic hypertrophy or obstruction of the bladder neck, cardio-spasm (megaesophagus) and myasthenia gravis. Contraindicated in patients who have demonstrated a previous hypersensitivity to the drug.

WARNINGS
Some patients may experience transient episodes of light-headedness, dizziness or syncope. Norflex may impair the ability of the patient to engage in potentially hazardous activities such as operating machinery or driving a motor vehicle; ambulatory patients should therefore be cautioned accordingly.
Norflex Injection contains sodium bisulfite, a sulfite that may cause allergic-type reactions including anaphylactic symptoms and life-threatening or less severe asthmatic episodes in certain susceptible people. The overall prevalence of sulfite sensitivity in the general population is unknown and probably low. Sulfite sensitivity is seen more frequently in asthmatic than nonasthmatic people.

PREGNANCY
Pregnancy Category C. Animal reproduction studies have not been conducted with Norflex. It is also not known whether Norflex can cause fetal harm when administered to a pregnant woman or can affect reproduction capacity. Norflex should be given to a pregnant woman only if clearly needed.

PEDIATRIC USE
Safety and effectiveness in pediatric patients have not been established.

PRECAUTIONS
Confusion, anxiety and tremors have been reported in few patients receiving propoxyphene and orphenadrine concomitantly. As these symptoms may be simply due to an additive effect, reduction of dosage and/or discontinuation of one or both agents is recommended in such cases.
Orphenadrine citrate should be used with caution in patients with tachycardia, cardiac decompensation, coronary insufficiency, cardiac arrhythmias.
Safety of continuous long-term therapy with orphenadrine has not been established. Therefore, if orphenadrine is prescribed for prolonged use, periodic monitoring of blood, urine and liver function values is recommended.

ADVERSE REACTIONS
Adverse reactions of orphenadrine are mainly due to the mild anticholinergic action of orphenadrine, and are usually associated with higher dosage. Dryness of the mouth is usually the first adverse effect to appear. When the daily dose is increased, possible adverse effects include: tachycardia, palpitation, urinary hesitancy or retention, blurred vision, dilatation of pupils, increased ocular tension, weakness, nausea, vomiting, headache, dizziness, constipation, drowsiness, hypersensitivity reactions, pruritus, hallucinations, agitation, tremor, gastric irritation, and rarely urticaria and other dermatoses. Infrequently, an elderly patient may experience some degree of mental confusion. These adverse reactions can usually be eliminated by reduction in dosage. Very rare cases of aplastic anemia associated with the use of orphenadrine tablets have been reported. No causal relationship has been established.
Rare instances of anaphylactic reaction have been reported associated with the intramuscular injection of Norflex Injection.

DOSAGE AND ADMINISTRATION
TABLETS: Adults—Two tablets per day; one in the morning and one in the evening.
INJECTION: Adults—One 2 mL ampul (60 mg) intravenously or intramuscularly; may be repeated every 12 hours. Relief may be maintained by 1 Norflex Extended-release tablet twice daily.

HOW SUPPLIED
TABLETS: Each round, white tablet imprinted with "3M" on one side and "221" on the other. Bottles of 100 (NDC **0089-0221-10**). Each tablet contains 100 mg of orphenadrine citrate.
INJECTION: Boxes of 6 (NDC **0089-0540-06**) 2 mL ampuls, each ampul containing 60 mg of orphenadrine citrate in aqueous solution.
Store at controlled room temperature 15°–30°C (59°–86°F).
Rx only
994103 July 2000

Tablets Manufactured by
3M Pharmaceuticals
Northridge, CA 91324

Injection Manufactured for
3M Pharmaceuticals
Northridge, CA 91324
By Abbott Laboratories
North Chicago, IL 60064

NORGESIC™ ℞

NORGESIC™ FORTE ℞
Tablets

For full prescribing information see leaflet accompanying product or call 800-328-0255 for a copy.

ACTIONS
Orphenadrine citrate is a centrally acting (brain stem) compound which in animals selectively blocks facilitatory functions of the reticular formation. Orphenadrine does not produce myoneural block, nor does it affect crossed extensor reflexes. Orphenadrine prevents nicotine-induced convulsions but not those produced by strychnine.
Chronic administration of Norgesic to dogs and rats has revealed no drug-related toxicity. No blood or urine changes were observed, nor were there any macroscopic or microscopic pathological changes detected. Extensive experience with combinations containing aspirin and caffeine has established them as safe agents. The addition of orphenadrine citrate does not alter the toxicity of aspirin and caffeine.
The mode of therapeutic action of orphenadrine has not been clearly identified, but may be related to its analgesic properties. Orphenadrine citrate also possesses anticholinergic actions.

HOW SUPPLIED
Norgesic tablets can be identified by their two layers colored white and yellow. Each round tablet is embossed "NORGESIC" on one side and "3M" on the other and contains orphenadrine citrate (2-dimethylaminoethyl 2-methylbenzhydryl ether citrate) 25 mg, aspirin 385 mg, and caffeine 30 mg.
Norgesic Forte tablets are exactly twice the strength of Norgesic. They are identified by their scored capsule shape and by their two layers colored white and yellow. Each capsule shaped tablet is embossed "NORGESIC FORTE" on one side and "3M" on the other and contains orphenadrine citrate 50 mg, aspirin 770 mg, and caffeine 60 mg.
Norgesic and Norgesic Forte also contain: lactose, polyethylene glycol, povidone, starch, sucrose, zinc stearate, and D&C yellow #10.
Norgesic: Bottles of 100 tablets (NDC **0089-0231-10**).
Norgesic Forte: Bottles of 100 tablets (NDC **0089-0233-10**).
Store below 30°C (86°F).
Rx only.

TAMBOCOR™ ℞
[tăm-ba-kōr]
(flecainide acetate)
Tablets

DESCRIPTION
TAMBOCOR™ (flecainide acetate) is an antiarrhythmic drug available in tablets of 50, 100, or 150 mg for oral administration.
Flecainide acetate is benzamide, N-(2-piperidinylmethyl)-2,5-bis(2,2,2-trifluoroethoxy)-monoacetate. The structural formula is given below.

Flecainide acetate is a white crystalline substance with a pK_a of 9.3. It has an aqueous solubility of 48.4 mg/mL at 37°C.
TAMBOCOR tablets also contain: croscarmellose sodium, hydrogenated vegetable oil, magnesium stearate, microcrystalline cellulose and starch.

CLINICAL PHARMACOLOGY
TAMBOCOR has local anesthetic activity and belongs to the membrane stabilizing (Class 1) group of antiarrhythmic agents; it has electrophysiologic effects characteristic of the 1C class of antiarrhythmics.
Electrophysiology. In man, TAMBOCOR produces a dose-related decrease in intracardiac conduction in all parts of the heart with the greatest effect on the His-Purkinje system (H-V conduction). Effects upon atrioventricular (AV) nodal conduction time and intra-atrial conduction times, although present, are less pronounced than those on ventricular conduction velocity. Significant effects on refractory periods were observed only in the ventricle. Sinus node recovery times (corrected) following pacing and spontaneous cycle lengths are somewhat increased. This latter effect may become significant in patients with sinus node dysfunction. (See Warnings.)
TAMBOCOR causes a dose-related and plasma-level related decrease in single and multiple PVCs and can suppress recurrence of ventricular tachycardia. In limited studies of patients with a history of ventricular tachycardia, TAMBOCOR has been successful 30–40% of the time in fully suppressing the inducibility of arrhythmias by programmed electrical stimulation. Based on PVC suppression, it appears that plasma levels of 0.2 to 1.0 μg/mL may be needed to obtain the maximal therapeutic effect. It is more difficult to assess the dose needed to suppress serious arrhythmias, but trough plasma levels in patients successfully treated for recurrent ventricular tachycardia were between 0.2 and 1.0 μg/mL. Plasma levels above 0.7–1.0 μg/mL are associated with a higher rate of cardiac adverse experiences such as conduction defects or bradycardia. The relation of plasma levels to proarrhythmic events is not established, but dose reduction in clinical trials of patients with ventricular tachycardia appears to have led to a reduced frequency and severity of such events.
Hemodynamics. TAMBOCOR does not usually alter heart rate, although bradycardia and tachycardia have been reported occasionally.
In animals and isolated myocardium, a negative inotropic effect of flecainide has been demonstrated. Decreases in ejection fraction, consistent with a negative inotropic effect, have been observed after single administration of 200 to 250 mg of the drug in man; both increases and decreases in ejection fraction have been encountered during multidose therapy in patients at usual therapeutic doses. (See Warnings.)
Metabolism in Humans. Following oral administration, the absorption of TAMBOCOR is nearly complete. Peak plasma levels are attained at about three hours in most individuals (range, 1 to 6 hours). Flecainide does not undergo any consequential presystemic biotransformation (first-pass effect). Food or antacid do not affect absorption. Milk, however, may inhibit absorption in infants. A reduction in TAMBOCOR dosage should be considered when milk is removed from the diet of infants.
The apparent plasma half-life averages about 20 hours and is quite variable (range, 12 to 27 hours) after multiple oral doses in patients with premature ventricular contractions (PVCs). With multiple dosing, plasma levels increase because of its long half-life with steady-state levels approached in 3 to 5 days; once at steady-state, no additional (or unexpected) accumulation of drug in plasma occurs during chronic therapy. Over the usual therapeutic range, data suggest that plasma levels in an individual are approximately proportional to dose, deviating upwards from linearity only slightly (about 10 to 15% per 100 mg on average).
In healthy subjects, about 30% of a single oral dose (range, 10 to 50%) is excreted in urine as unchanged drug. The two major urinary metabolites are meta-O-dealkylated flecainide (active, but about one-fifth as potent) and the meta-O-dealkylated lactam of flecainide (non-active metabolite). These two metabolites (primarily conjugated) account for most of the remaining portion of the dose. Several minor metabolites (3% of the dose or less) are also found in urine; only 5% of an oral dose is excreted in feces. In patients, free (unconjugated) plasma levels of the two major metabolites are very low (less than 0.05 μg/mL).
In vitro metabolic studies have confirmed that cytochrome P450IID6 is involved in the metabolism of flecainide.
When urinary pH is very alkaline (8 or higher), as may occur in rare conditions (e.g., renal tubular acidosis, strict vegetarian diet), flecainide elimination from plasma is much slower.
The elimination of flecainide from the body depends on renal function (i.e., 10 to 50% appears in urine as unchanged drug). With increasing renal impairment, the extent of unchanged drug excretion in urine is reduced and the plasma half-life of flecainide is prolonged. Since flecainide is also extensively metabolized, there is no simple relationship between creatinine clearance and the rate of flecainide elimination from plasma. (See Dosage and Administration.)
In patients with NYHA class III congestive heart failure (CHF), the rate of flecainide elimination from plasma (mean half-life, 19 hours) is moderately slower than for healthy subjects (mean half-life, 14 hours), but similar to the rate for patients with PVCs without CHF. The extent of excretion of unchanged drug in urine is also similar. (See Dosage and Administration.)
Under one year of age, currently available data are limited but suggest that the half-life at birth may be as long as 29

Continued on next page

Tambocor—Cont.

hours, decreasing to 11–12 hours by three months of age and 6 hours by one year of age. The pharmacokinetics in hydropic infants have not been studied, but case reports suggest prolonged elimination. In children aged 1 year to 12 years the half-life is approximately 8 hours. In adolescents (age 12 to 15) the plasma elimination half-life is approximately 11–12 hours. Since milk may inhibit absorption in infants, a reduction in TAMBOCOR dosage should be considered when milk is removed from the diet (e.g., gastroenteritis, weaning). Plasma trough flecainide levels should be monitored during major changes in dietary milk intake.

From age 20 to 80, plasma levels are only slightly higher with advancing age; flecainide elimination from plasma is somewhat slower in elderly subjects than in younger subjects. Patients up to age 80+ have been safely treated with usual dosages.

The extent of flecainide binding to human plasma proteins is about 40% and is independent of plasma drug level over the range of 0.015 to about 3.4 μg/mL. Thus, clinically significant drug interactions based on protein binding effects would not be expected.

Hemodialysis removes only about 1% of an oral dose as unchanged flecainide.

Small increases in plasma digoxin levels are seen during coadministration of TAMBOCOR with digoxin. Small increases in both flecainide and propranolol plasma levels are seen during coadministration of these two drugs. (See Precautions, Drug Interactions.)

Clinical Trials. In two randomized, crossover, placebo-controlled clinical trials of 16 weeks double-blind duration, 79% of patients with paroxysmal supraventricular tachycardia (PSVT) receiving flecainide were attack free, whereas 15% of patients receiving placebo remained attack free. The median time-before-recurrence of PSVT in patients receiving placebo was 11 to 12 days, whereas over 85% of patients receiving flecainide had no recurrence at 60 days.

In two randomized, crossover, placebo-controlled clinical trials of 16 weeks double-blind duration, 31% of patients with paroxysmal atrial fibrillation/flutter (PAF) receiving flecainide were attack free, whereas 8% receiving placebo remained attack free. The median time-before-recurrence of PAF in patients receiving placebo was about 2 to 3 days, whereas for those receiving flecainide the median time-before-recurrence was 15 days.

INDICATIONS AND USAGE

In patients without structural heart disease, TAMBOCOR is indicated for the prevention of

- paroxysmal supraventricular tachycardias (PSVT), including atrioventricular nodal reentrant tachycardia, atrioventricular reentrant tachycardia and other supraventricular tachycardias of unspecified mechanism associated with disabling symptoms
- paroxysmal atrial fibrillation/flutter (PAF) associated with disabling symptoms

TAMBOCOR is also indicated for the prevention of

- documented ventricular arrhythmias, such as sustained ventricular tachycardia (sustained VT), that in the judgment of the physician are life-threatening.

Use of TAMBOCOR for the treatment of sustained VT, like other antiarrhythmics, should be initiated in the hospital. The use of TAMBOCOR is not recommended in patients with less severe ventricular arrhythmias even if the patients are symptomatic.

Because of the proarrhythmic effects of TAMBOCOR, its use should be reserved for patients in whom, in the opinion of the physician, the benefits of treatment outweigh the risks.

TAMBOCOR should not be used in patients with recent myocardial infarction. (See Boxed Warnings.)

Use of TAMBOCOR in chronic atrial fibrillation has not been adequately studied and is not recommended. (See Boxed Warnings.)

As is the case for other antiarrhythmic agents, there is no evidence from controlled trials that the use of TAMBOCOR favorably affects survival or the incidence of sudden death.

CONTRAINDICATIONS

TAMBOCOR is contraindicated in patients with pre-existing second- or third-degree AV block, or with right bundle branch block when associated with a left hemiblock (bifascicular block), unless a pacemaker is present to sustain the cardiac rhythm should complete heart block occur. TAMBOCOR is also contraindicated in the presence of cardiogenic shock or known hypersensitivity to the drug.

WARNINGS

Mortality. TAMBOCOR was included in the National Heart Lung and Blood Institute's Cardiac Arrhythmia Suppression Trial (CAST), a long-term, multicenter, randomized, double-blind study in patients with asymptomatic non-life-threatening ventricular arrhythmias who had a myocardial infarction more than six days but less than two years previously. An excessive mortality or non-fatal cardiac arrest rate was seen in patients treated with TAMBOCOR compared with that seen in patients assigned to a carefully matched placebo-treated group. This rate was 16/315 (5.1%) for TAMBOCOR and 7/309 (2.3%) for the matched placebo. The average duration of treatment with TAMBOCOR in this study was ten months.

The applicability of the CAST results to other populations (e.g., those without recent myocardial infarction) is uncertain, but at present, it is prudent to consider the risks of Class IC agents (including TAMBOCOR), coupled with the lack of any evidence of improved survival, generally unacceptable in patients without life-threatening ventricular arrhythmias, even if the patients are experiencing unpleasant, but not life-threatening, symptoms or signs.

Ventricular Pro-arrhythmic Effects in Patients with Atrial Fibrillation/Flutter. A review of the world literature revealed reports of 568 patients treated with oral TAMBOCOR for paroxysmal atrial fibrillation/flutter (PAF). Ventricular tachycardia was experienced in 0.4% (2/568) of these patients. Of 19 patients in the literature with chronic atrial fibrillation (CAF), 10.5% (2) experienced VT or VF. FLECAINIDE IS NOT RECOMMENDED FOR USE IN PATIENTS WITH CHRONIC ATRIAL FIBRILLATION. Case reports of ventricular proarrhythmic effects in patients treated with TAMBOCOR for atrial fibrillation/flutter have included increased PVCs, VT, ventricular fibrillation (VF), and death.

As with other Class I agents, patients treated with TAMBOCOR for atrial flutter have been reported with 1:1 atrioventricular conduction due to slowing the atrial rate. A paradoxical increase in the ventricular rate also may occur in patients with atrial fibrillation who receive TAMBOCOR. Concomitant negative chronotropic therapy such as digoxin or beta-blockers may lower the risk of this complication.

PROARRHYTHMIC EFFECTS

TAMBOCOR, like other antiarrhythmic agents, can cause new or worsened supraventricular or ventricular arrhythmias. Ventricular proarrhythmic effects range from an increase in frequency of PVCs to the development of more severe ventricular tachycardia, e.g., tachycardia that is more sustained or more resistant to conversion to sinus rhythm, with potentially fatal consequences. In studies of ventricular arrhythmia patients treated with TAMBOCOR, three-fourths of proarrhythmic events were new or worsened ventricular tachyarrhythmias, the remainder being increased frequency of PVCs or new supraventricular arrhythmias. In patients treated with flecainide for sustained ventricular tachycardia, 80% (51/64) of proarrhythmic events occurred within 14 days of the onset of therapy. In studies of 225 patients with supraventricular arrhythmia (108 with paroxysmal supraventricular tachycardia and 117 with paroxysmal atrial fibrillation), there were 9 (4%) proarrhythmic events, 8 of them in patients with paroxysmal atrial fibrillation. Of the 9, 7 (including the one in a PSVT patient) were exacerbations of supraventricular arrhythmias (longer duration, more rapid rate, harder to reverse) while 2 were ventricular arrhythmias, including one fatal case of VT/VF and one wide complex VT (the patient showed inducible VT, however, after withdrawal of flecainide), both in patients with paroxysmal atrial fibrillation and known coronary artery disease.

It is uncertain if TAMBOCOR's risk of proarrhythmia is exaggerated in patients with chronic atrial fibrillation (CAF), high ventricular rate, and/or exercise. Wide complex tachycardia and ventricular fibrillation have been reported in two of 12 CAF patients undergoing maximal exercise tolerance testing.

In patients with complex ventricular arrhythmias, it is often difficult to distinguish a spontaneous variation in the patient's underlying rhythm disorder from drug-induced worsening, so that the following occurrence rates must be considered approximations. Their frequency appears to be related to dose and to the underlying cardiac disease.

Among patients treated for sustained VT (who frequently also had CHF, a low ejection fraction, a history of myocardial infarction and/or an episode of cardiac arrest), the incidence of proarrhythmic events was 13% when dosage was initiated at 200 mg/day with slow upward titration, and did not exceed 300 mg/day in most patients. In early studies in patients with sustained VT utilizing a higher initial dose (400 mg/day) the incidence of proarrhythmic events was 26%; moreover, in about 10% of the patients treated proarrhythmic events resulted in death, despite prompt medical attention. With lower initial doses, the incidence of proarrhythmic events resulting in death decreased to 0.5% of these patients. Accordingly, it is extremely important to follow the recommended dosage schedule. (See Dosage and Administration.)

The relatively high frequency of proarrhythmic events in patients with sustained VT and serious underlying heart disease, and the need for careful titration and monitoring, requires that therapy of patients with sustained VT be started in the hospital. (See Dosage and Administration.)

HEART FAILURE

TAMBOCOR has a negative inotropic effect and may cause or worsen CHF, particularly in patients with cardiomyopathy, preexisting severe heart failure (NYHA functional class III or IV) or low ejection fractions (less than 30%). In patients with supraventricular arrhythmias new or worsened CHF developed in 0.4% (1/225) of patients. In patients with sustained ventricular tachycardia during a mean duration of 7.9 months of TAMBOCOR therapy, 6.3% (20/317) developed new CHF. In patients with sustained ventricular tachycardia and a history of CHF, during a mean duration of 5.4 months of TAMBOCOR therapy, 25.7% (78/304) developed worsened CHF. Exacerbation of preexisting CHF occurred more commonly in studies which included patients with class III or IV failure than in studies which excluded such patients. TAMBOCOR should be used cautiously in patients who are known to have a history of CHF or myocardial dysfunction. The initial dosage in such patients should be no more than 100 mg bid (see Dosage and Administration) and patients should be monitored carefully. Close attention must be given to maintenance of cardiac function, including optimization of digitalis, diuretic, or other therapy. In cases where CHF has developed or worsened during treatment with TAMBOCOR, the time of onset has ranged from a few hours to several months after starting therapy. Some patients who develop evidence of reduced myocardial function while on TAMBOCOR can continue on TAMBOCOR with adjustment of digitalis or diuretics, others may require dosage reduction or discontinuation of TAMBOCOR. When feasible, it is recommended that plasma flecainide levels be monitored. Attempts should be made to keep trough plasma levels below 0.7 to 1.0 μg/mL.

Effects on Cardiac Conduction. TAMBOCOR slows cardiac conduction in most patients to produce dose-related increases in PR, QRS, and QT intervals.

PR interval increases on average about 25% (0.04 seconds) and as much as 118% in some patients. Approximately one-third of patients may develop new first-degree AV heart block (PR interval ≥ 0.20 seconds). The QRS complex increases on average about 25% (0.02 seconds) and as much as 150% in some patients. Many patients develop QRS complexes with a duration of 0.12 seconds or more. In one study, 4% of patients developed new bundle branch block while on TAMBOCOR. The degree of lengthening of PR and QRS intervals does not predict either efficacy or the development of cardiac adverse effects. In clinical trials, it was unusual for PR intervals to increase to 0.30 seconds or more, or for QRS intervals to increase to 0.18 seconds or more. Thus, caution should be used when such intervals occur, and dose reductions may be considered. The QT interval widens about 8%, but most of this widening (about 60% to 90%) is due to widening of the QRS duration. The JT interval (QT minus QRS) only widens about 4% on the average. Significant JT prolongation occurs in less than 2% of patients. There have been rare cases of Torsade de Pointes-type arrhythmia associated with TAMBOCOR therapy.

Clinically significant conduction changes have been observed at these rates: sinus node dysfunction such as sinus pause, sinus arrest and symptomatic bradycardia (1.2%), second-degree AV block (0.5%) and third-degree AV block (0.4%). An attempt should be made to manage the patient on the lowest effective dose in an effort to minimize these effects. (See Dosage and Administration.) If second- or third-degree AV block, or right bundle branch block associated with a left hemiblock occur, TAMBOCOR therapy should be discontinued unless a temporary or implanted ventricular pacemaker is in place to ensure an adequate ventricular rate.

Sick Sinus Syndrome (Bradycardia-Tachycardia Syndrome). TAMBOCOR should be used only with extreme caution in patients with sick sinus syndrome because it may cause sinus bradycardia, sinus pause, or sinus arrest.

Effects on Pacemaker Thresholds. TAMBOCOR is known to increase endocardial pacing thresholds and may suppress ventricular escape rhythms. These effects are reversible if flecainide is discontinued. It should be used with caution in patients with permanent pacemakers or temporary pacing electrodes and should not be administered to patients with existing poor thresholds or nonprogrammable pacemakers unless suitable pacing rescue is available.

The pacing threshold in patients with pacemakers should be determined prior to instituting therapy with TAMBOCOR, again after one week of administration and at regular intervals thereafter. Generally threshold changes are within the range of multiprogrammable pacemakers and, when these occur, a doubling of either voltage or pulse width is usually sufficient to regain capture.

Electrolyte Disturbances. Hypokalemia or hyperkalemia may alter the effects of Class I antiarrhythmic drugs. Preexisting hypokalemia or hyperkalemia should be corrected before administration of TAMBOCOR.

Pediatric Use. The safety and efficacy of TAMBOCOR in the fetus, infant, or child have not been established in double-blind, randomized, placebo-controlled trials. The proarrhythmic effects of TAMBOCOR, as described previously, apply also to children. In pediatric patients with structural heart disease, TAMBOCOR has been associated with cardiac arrest and sudden death. TAMBOCOR should be started in the hospital with rhythm monitoring. Any use of TAMBOCOR in children should be directly supervised by a cardiologist skilled in the treatment of arrhythmias in children.

PRECAUTIONS

Drug Interactions. TAMBOCOR has been administered to patients receiving **digitalis** preparations or **beta-adrenergic blocking agents** without adverse effects. During administration of multiple oral doses of TAMBOCOR to healthy subjects stabilized on a maintenance dose of **digoxin**, a 13%–19% increase in plasma **digoxin** levels occurred at six hours postdose.

In a study involving healthy subjects receiving TAMBOCOR and **propranolol** concurrently, plasma flecainide levels were increased about 20% and **propranolol** levels were increased about 30% compared to control values. In this formal interaction study, TAMBOCOR and **propranolol** were each found to have negative inotropic effects; when the drugs were administered together, the effects were additive. The effects of concomitant administration of TAMBOCOR and **propranolol** on the PR interval were less than additive. In TAMBOCOR clinical trials, patients who were receiving **beta blockers** concurrently did not experience an increased incidence of side effects. Nevertheless, the possibility of additive negative inotropic effects of **beta blockers** and flecainide should be recognized.

Flecainide is not extensively bound to plasma proteins. In vitro studies with several drugs which may be administered concomitantly showed that the extent of flecainide binding to human plasma proteins is either unchanged or only slightly less. Consequently, interactions with other drugs which are highly protein bound (e.g., **anticoagulants**) would not be expected. TAMBOCOR has been used in a large number of patients receiving **diuretics** without apparent interaction. Limited data in patients receiving known enzyme inducers (**phenytoin, phenobarbital, carbamazepine**) indicate only a 30% increase in the rate of flecainide elimination. In healthy subjects receiving **cimetidine** (1 gm daily) for one week, plasma flecainide levels increased by about 30% and half-life increased by about 10%.

When **amiodarone** is added to flecainide therapy, plasma flecainide levels may increase two-fold or more in some patients, if flecainide dosage is not reduced. (See Dosage and Administration.)

Drugs that inhibit cytochrome P450IID6, such as **quinidine**, might increase the plasma concentrations of flecainide in patients that are on chronic flecainide therapy, especially if these patients are extensive metabolizers.

There has been little experience with the coadministration of TAMBOCOR and either **disopyramide** or **verapamil**. Because both of these drugs have negative inotropic properties and the effects of coadministration with TAMBOCOR are unknown, neither **disopyramide** nor **verapamil** should be administered concurrently with TAMBOCOR unless, in the judgment of the physician, the benefits of this combination outweigh the risks. There has been too little experience with the coadministration of TAMBOCOR with **nifedipine** or **diltiazem** to recommend concomitant use.

Carcinogenesis, Mutagenesis, Impairment of Fertility. Long-term studies with flecainide in rats and mice at doses up to 60 mg/kg/day have not revealed any compound-related carcinogenic effects. Mutagenicity studies (Ames test, mouse lymphoma and in vivo cytogenetics) did not reveal any mutagenic effects. A rat reproduction study at doses up to 50 mg/kg/day (seven times the usual human dose) did not reveal any adverse effect on male or female fertility.

Pregnancy. Pregnancy Category C. Flecainide has been shown to have teratogenic effects (club paws, sternebrae and vertebrae abnormalities, pale hearts with contracted ventricular septum) and an embryotoxic effect (increased resorptions) in one breed of rabbit (New Zealand White) when given doses of 30 and 35 mg/kg/day, but not in another breed of rabbit (Dutch Belted) when given doses up to 30 mg/kg/day. No teratogenic effects were observed in rats and mice given doses up to 50 and 80 mg/kg/day, respectively; however, delayed sternebral and vertebral ossification was observed at the high dose in rats. Because there are no adequate and well-controlled studies in pregnant women, TAMBOCOR should be used during pregnancy only if the potential benefit justifies the potential risk to the fetus.

Labor and Delivery. It is not known whether the use of TAMBOCOR during labor or delivery has immediate or delayed adverse effects on the mother or fetus, affects the duration of labor or delivery, or increases the possibility of forceps delivery or other obstetrical intervention.

Nursing Mothers. Results from a multiple dose study conducted in mothers soon after delivery indicates that flecainide is excreted in human breast milk in concentrations as high as 4 times (with average levels about 2.5 times) corresponding plasma levels; assuming a maternal plasma level at the top of the therapeutic range (1 μg/mL), the calculated daily dose to a nursing infant (assuming about 700 mL breast milk over 24 hours) would be less than 3 mg.

Pediatric Use. The safety and efficacy of TAMBOCOR in the fetus, infant, or child have not been established in double-blind, randomized, placebo-controlled trials (see CLINICAL PHARMACOLOGY, WARNINGS, and DOSAGE AND ADMINISTRATION).

Hepatic Impairment. Since flecainide elimination from plasma can be markedly slower in patients with significant hepatic impairment, TAMBOCOR should not be used in such patients unless the potential benefits clearly outweigh the risks. If used, frequent and early plasma level monitoring is required to guide dosage (see Plasma Level Monitoring); dosage increases should be made very cautiously when plasma levels have plateaued (after more than four days).

ADVERSE REACTIONS

In post-myocardial infarction patients with asymptomatic PVCs and non-sustained ventricular tachycardia, TAMBOCOR therapy was found to be associated with a 5.1% rate of death and non-fatal cardiac arrest, compared with a 2.3% rate in a matched placebo group. (See Warnings.)

Adverse effects reported for TAMBOCOR, described in detail in the Warnings section, were new or worsened arrhythmias which occurred in 1% of 108 patients with PSVT and in 7% of 117 patients with PAF; and new or exacerbated ventricular arrhythmias which occurred in 7% of 1330 patients with PVCs, non-sustained or sustained VT. In patients treated with flecainide for sustained VT, 80% (51/64) of proarrhythmic events occurred within 14 days of the onset of therapy. 198 patients with sustained VT experienced a 13% incidence of new or exacerbated ventricular arrhythmias when dosage was initiated at 200 mg/day with slow upward titration, and did not exceed 300 mg/day in most patients. In some patients, TAMBOCOR treatment has been associated with episodes of unresuscitatable VT or ventricular fibrillation (cardiac arrest). (See Warnings.)

New or worsened CHF occurred in 6.3% of 1046 patients with PVCs, non-sustained or sustained VT. Of 297 patients with sustained VT, 9.1% experienced new or worsened CHF. New or worsened CHF was reported in 0.4% of 225 patients with supraventricular arrhythmias. There have also been instances of second- (0.5%) or third-degree (0.4%) AV block. Patients have developed sinus bradycardia, sinus pause, or sinus arrest, about 1.2% altogether (see Warnings). The frequency of most of these serious adverse events probably increases with higher trough plasma levels, especially when these trough levels exceed 1.0 μg/mL.

There have been rare reports of isolated elevations of serum alkaline phosphatase and isolated elevations of serum transaminase levels. These elevations have been asymptomatic and no cause and effect relationship with TAMBOCOR has been established. In foreign postmarketing surveillance studies, there have been rare reports of hepatic dysfunction including reports of cholestasis and hepatic failure, and extremely rare reports of blood dyscrasias. Although no cause and effect relationship has been established, it is advisable to discontinue TAMBOCOR in patients who develop unexplained jaundice or signs of hepatic dysfunction or blood dyscrasias in order to eliminate TAMBOCOR as the possible causative agent.

Incidence figures for other adverse effects in patients with ventricular arrhythmias are based on a multicenter efficacy study, utilizing starting doses of 200 mg/day with gradual upward titration to 400 mg/day. Patients were treated for an average of 4.7 months, with some receiving up to 22 months of therapy. In this trial, 5.4% of patients discontinued due to non-cardiac adverse effects.

[See table 1 above]

Table 1
Most Common Non-Cardiac Adverse Effects in Ventricular Arrhythmia Patients Treated with TAMBOCOR in the Multicenter Study

Adverse Effect	Incidence All 429 Patients at Any Dose	Incidence By Dose During Upward Titration 200 mg/Day (N=426)	300 mg/Day (N=293)	400 mg/Day (N=100)
Dizziness*	18.9%	11.0%	10.6%	13.0%
Visual Disturbances†	15.9%	5.4%	12.3%	18.0%
Dyspnea	10.3%	5.2%	7.5%	4.0%
Headache	9.6%	4.5%	6.1%	9.0%
Nausea	8.9%	4.9%	4.8%	6.0%
Fatigue	7.7%	4.5%	4.4%	3.0%
Palpitation	6.1%	3.5%	2.4%	7.0%
Chest Pain	5.4%	3.1%	3.8%	1.0%
Asthenia	4.9%	2.6%	2.0%	4.0%
Tremor	4.7%	2.4%	3.4%	2.0%
Constipation	4.4%	2.8%	2.1%	1.0%
Edema	3.5%	1.9%	1.4%	2.0%
Abdominal pain	3.3%	1.9%	2.4%	1.0%

* Dizziness includes reports of dizziness, lightheadedness, faintness, unsteadiness, near syncope, etc.
† Visual disturbance includes reports of blurred vision, difficulty in focusing, spots before eyes, etc.

The following additional adverse experiences, possibly related to TAMBOCOR therapy and occurring in 1% to less than 3% of patients, have been reported in acute and chronic studies: *Body as a Whole* —malaise, fever; *Cardiovascular*—tachycardia, sinus pause or arrest; *Gastrointestinal* —vomiting, diarrhea, dyspepsia, anorexia; *Skin* —rash; *Visual*—diplopia; *Nervous System* —hypoesthesia, paresthesia, paresis, ataxia, flushing, increased sweating, vertigo, syncope, somnolence, tinnitus; *Psychiatric* —anxiety, insomnia, depression.

The following additional adverse experiences, possibly related to TAMBOCOR, have been reported in less than 1% of patients: *Body as a Whole* —swollen lips, tongue and mouth; arthralgia, bronchospasm, myalgia; *Cardiovascular* —angina pectoris, second-degree and third-degree AV block, bradycardia, hypertension, hypotension; *Gastrointestinal* —flatulence; *Urinary System* —polyuria, urinary retention; *Hematologic* —leukopenia, granulocytopenia, thrombocytopenia; *Skin* —urticaria, exfoliative dermatitis, pruritus, alopecia; *Visual* —eye pain or irritation, photophobia, nystagmus; *Nervous System* —twitching, weakness, change in taste, dry mouth, convulsions, impotence, speech disorder, stupor, neuropathy; *Respiratory* —pneumonitis/pulmonary infiltration possibly due to chronic flecainide treatment: *Psychiatric*—amnesia, confusion, decreased libido, depersonalization, euphoria, morbid dreams, apathy.

For patients with supraventricular arrhythmias, the most commonly reported noncardiac adverse experiences remain consistent with those known for patients treated with TAMBOCOR for ventricular arrhythmias. Dizziness is possibly more frequent in PAF patients.

OVERDOSAGE

No specific antidote has been identified for the treatment of TAMBOCOR overdosage. Overdoses ranging up to 8000 mg have been survived, with peak plasma flecainide concentrations as high as 5.3 μg/mL. Untoward effects in these cases included nausea and vomiting, convulsions, hypotension, bradycardia, syncope, extreme widening of the QRS complex, widening of the QT interval, widening of the PR interval, ventricular tachycardia, AV nodal block, asystole, bundle branch block, cardiac failure, and cardiac arrest. The spectrum of events observed in fatal cases was much the same as that seen in the non-fatal cases. Death has resulted following ingestion of as little as 1000 mg; concomitant overdose of other drugs and/or alcohol in many instances undoubtedly contributed to the fatal outcome. Treatment of overdosage should be supportive and may include the following: removal of unabsorbed drug from the gastrointestinal tract, administration of inotropic agents or cardiac stimulants such as dopamine, dobutamine or isoproterenol; mechanically assisted respiration; circulatory assists such as intra-aortic balloon pumping; and transvenous pacing in the event of conduction block. Because of the long plasma half-life of flecainide (12 to 27 hours in patients receiving usual doses), and the possibility of markedly non-linear elimination kinetics at very high doses, these supportive treatments may need to be continued for extended periods of time.

Hemodialysis is not an effective means of removing flecainide from the body. Since flecainide elimination is much slower when urine is very alkaline (pH 8 or higher), theoretically, acidification of urine to promote drug excretion may be beneficial in overdose cases with very alkaline urine. There is no evidence that acidification from normal urinary pH increases excretion.

DOSAGE AND ADMINISTRATION

For patients with sustained VT, no matter what their cardiac status, TAMBOCOR, like other antiarrhythmics, should be initiated in-hospital with rhythm monitoring.

Flecainide has a long half-life (12 to 27 hours in patients). Steady-state plasma levels, in patients with normal renal and hepatic function, may not be achieved until the patient has received 3 to 5 days of therapy at a given dose. Therefore, **increases in dosage should be made no more frequently than once every four days,** since during the first 2 to 3 days of therapy the optimal effect of a given dose may not be achieved.

For patients with PSVT and patients with PAF the recommended starting dose is 50 mg every 12 hours. TAMBOCOR doses may be increased in increments of 50 mg bid every four days until efficacy is achieved. For PAF patients, a substantial increase in efficacy without a substantial increase in discontinuations for adverse experiences may be achieved by increasing the TAMBOCOR dose from 50 to 100 mg bid. The maximum recommended dose for patients with paroxysmal supraventricular arrhythmias is 300 mg/day.

For sustained VT the recommended starting dose is 100 mg every 12 hours. This dose may be increased in increments of 50 mg bid every four days until efficacy is achieved. Most patients with sustained VT do not require more than 150 mg every 12 hours (300 mg/day), and the maximum dose recommended is 400 mg/day.

In patients with sustained VT, use of higher initial doses and more rapid dosage adjustments have resulted in an increased incidence of proarrhythmic events and CHF, particularly during the first few days of dosing (see Warnings). Therefore, a loading dose is not recommended.

Intravenous lidocaine has been used occasionally with TAMBOCOR while awaiting the therapeutic effect of TAMBOCOR. No adverse drug interactions were apparent. However, no formal studies have been performed to demonstrate the usefulness of this regimen.

An occasional patient not adequately controlled by (or intolerant to) a dose given at 12-hour intervals may be dosed at eight-hour intervals.

Once adequate control of the arrhythmia has been achieved, it may be possible in some patients to reduce the dose as necessary to minimize side effects or effects on conduction. In such patients, efficacy at the lower dose should be evaluated.

TAMBOCOR should be used cautiously in patients with a history of CHF or myocardial dysfunction (see Warnings).

Any use of TAMBOCOR in children should be directly supervised by a cardiologist skilled in the treatment of arrhythmias in children. Because of the evolving nature of information in this area, specialized literature should be

Continued on next page

Tambocor—Cont.

consulted. Under six months of age, the initial starting dose of TAMBOCOR in children is approximately 50 mg/M^2 body surface area daily, divided into two or three equally spaced doses. Over six months of age, the initial starting dose may be increased to 100 mg/M^2 per day. The maximum recommended dose is 200 mg/M^2 per day. This dose should not be exceeded. In some children on higher doses, despite previously low plasma levels, the level has increased rapidly to far above therapeutic values while taking the same dose. Small changes in dose may also lead to disproportionate increases in plasma levels. Plasma trough (less than one hour pre-dose) flecainide levels and electrocardiograms should be obtained at presumed steady state (after at least five doses) either after initiation or change in TAMBOCOR dose, whether the dose was increased for lack of effectiveness, or increased growth of the patient. For the first year on therapy, whenever the patient is seen for reasons of clinical follow-up, it is suggested that a 12-lead electrocardiogram and plasma trough flecainide level are obtained. The usual therapeutic level of flecainide in children is 200–500 ng/mL. In some cases, levels as high as 800 ng/mL may be required for control.

In patients with severe renal impairment (creatinine clearance of 35 mL/min/1.73 square meters or less), the initial dosage should be 100 mg once daily (or 50 mg bid); when used in such patients, frequent plasma level monitoring is required to guide dosage adjustments (see Plasma Level Monitoring). In patients with less severe renal disease, the initial dosage should be 100 mg every 12 hours; plasma level monitoring may also be useful in these patients during dosage adjustment. In both groups of patients, dosage increases should be made very cautiously when plasma levels have plateaued (after more than four days), observing the patient closely for signs of adverse cardiac effects or other toxicity. It should be borne in mind that in these patients it may take longer than four days before a new steady-state plasma level is reached following a dosage change.

Based on theoretical considerations, rather than experimental data, the following suggestion is made: when transferring patients from another antiarrhythmic drug to TAMBOCOR allow at least two to four plasma half-lives to elapse for the drug being discontinued before starting TAMBOCOR at the usual dosage. In patients where withdrawal of a previous antiarrhythmic agent is likely to produce life-threatening arrhythmias, the physician should consider hospitalizing the patient.

When flecainide is given in the presence of amiodarone, reduce the usual flecainide dose by 50% and monitor the patient closely for adverse effects. Plasma level monitoring is strongly recommended to guide dosage with such combination therapy (see below).

Plasma Level Monitoring. The large majority of patients successfully treated with TAMBOCOR were found to have trough plasma levels between 0.2 and 1.0 µg/mL. The probability of adverse experiences, especially cardiac, may increase with higher trough plasma levels, especially when these exceed 1.0 µg/mL. Periodic monitoring of trough plasma levels may be useful in patient management. Plasma level monitoring is required in patients with severe renal failure or severe hepatic disease, since elimination of flecainide from plasma may be markedly slower. Monitoring of plasma levels is strongly recommended in patients on concurrent amiodarone therapy and may also be helpful in patients with CHF and in patients with moderate renal disease.

HOW SUPPLIED

All tablets are embossed with 3M on one side and TR 50, TR 100 or TR 150 on the other side.

Tambocor, 50 mg per white, round tablet, is available in
Bottles of 100—NDC #0089-0305-10.

Tambocor, 100 mg per white, round, scored tablet, is available in
Bottles of 100—NDC #0089-0307-10.

Tambocor, 150 mg per white, oval, scored tablet, is available in
Bottles of 100—NDC #0089-0314-10.

Store at controlled room temperature 15°–30°C (59°–86°F) in a tight, light-resistant container.

Rx only

600900 June 1998

Manufactured by
3M Pharmaceuticals
Northridge, CA 91324

Shown in Product Identification Guide, page 321

MAGNA Pharmaceuticals, Inc.

11802 BRINLEY AVENUE, SUITE 201
LOUISVILLE, KY 40243

DIRECT INQUIRIES TO:
Customer Service Department
Toll free (888) 206-5525
FAX: (502) 254-9279
www.magnaweb.com

The following is a listing of MAGNA Pharmaceuticals, Inc. products:

STAHIST™ Tablets
STA-D™ Tablets
STAMOIST™ E Tablets
STAFLEX Caplets
STAGESIC™ Capsules CIII
ZTUSS™ ZT Caplets CIII
ZTUSS™ Tablets CIII
ZTUSS™ Expectorant Syrup CIII
STATUSS™ DM Syrup
STATUSS™ Green Syrup CIII
Z-Xtra™ Medicated Lotion
www.Z-Xtra.com

Mallinckrodt Inc.

675 McDONNELL BLVD
ST. LOUIS, MO 63134

Direct Inquiries to:
Medical Information
888-744-1414, option 2, then 1
Customer Service (Sales and Ordering)
800-325-8888
www.mallinckrodt.com

The following list of Mallinckrodt Generic products is provided to facilitate identification.

PRODUCT Description Color(s) Shape	IDENTIFICATION CODE
ACETAMINOPHEN AND CODEINE PHOSPHATE TABLETS, USP Tablets 300/15mg CIII white to off-white round tab	Debossed "2" on one side and an "M" in a box on other side
ACETAMINOPHEN AND CODEINE PHOSPHATE TABLETS, USP Tablets 300/30mg CIII white to off-white round tab	Debossed "3" on one side and an "M" in a box on other side
ACETAMINOPHEN AND CODEINE PHOSPHATE TABLETS, USP Tablets 300/60mg CIII white to off-white round tab	Debossed "4" on one side and an "M" in a box on other side
BUTALBITAL, ACETAMINOPHEN AND CAFFEINE TABLETS, USP Tablets 50/325/40mg White/Round Tab	Debossed "970" on one side and an "M" in a box on reverse side, unscored
DEXTROAMPHETAMINE SACCHARATE, AMPHETAMINE ASPARTATE, DEXTROAMPHETAMINE SULFATE AND AMPHETAMINE SULFATE TABLETS (Mixed Salts of a Single Entity Amphetamine Product) Tablets 5 mg CII White to cream colored pillow shaped tablet	Debossed with a "5" and a partial quadrisect on one side and a "M" in a box on other side
DEXTROAMPHETAMINE SACCHARATE, AMPHETAMINE ASPARTATE, DEXTROAMPHETAMINE SULFATE AND AMPHETAMINE SULFATE TABLETS (Mixed Salts of a Single Entity Amphetamine Product) Tablets 7.5 mg CII White to cream colored pillow shaped tablet	Debossed with a "7.5" and a partial quadrisect on one side and a "M" in a box on other side
DEXTROAMPHETAMINE SACCHARATE, AMPHETAMINE ASPARTATE, DEXTROAMPHETAMINE SULFATE AND AMPHETAMINE SULFATE TABLETS (Mixed Salts of a Single Entity Amphetamine Product) Tablets 10 mg CII White to cream colored pillow shaped tablet	Debossed with a "10" and a partial quadrisect on one side and a "M" in a box on other side
DEXTROAMPHETAMINE SACCHARATE, AMPHETAMINE ASPARTATE, DEXTROAMPHETAMINE SULFATE AND AMPHETAMINE SULFATE TABLETS (Mixed Salts of a Single Entity Amphetamine Product) Tablets 12.5 mg CII White to cream colored octagon shaped tablet	Debossed with a "12.5" and a partial quadrisect on one side and a "M" in a box on other side
DEXTROAMPHETAMINE SACCHARATE, AMPHETAMINE ASPARTATE, DEXTROAMPHETAMINE SULFATE AND AMPHETAMINE SULFATE TABLETS (Mixed Salts of a Single Entity Amphetamine Product) Tablets 15 mg CII White to cream colored octagon shaped tablet	Debossed with a "15" and a partial quadrisect on one side and a "M" in a box on other side
DEXTROAMPHETAMINE SACCHARATE, AMPHETAMINE ASPARTATE, DEXTROAMPHETAMINE SULFATE AND AMPHETAMINE SULFATE TABLETS (Mixed Salts of a Single Entity Amphetamine Product) Tablets 20 mg CII White to cream colored octagon shaped tablet	Debossed with a "20" and a partial quadrisect on one side and a "M" in a box on other side
DEXTROAMPHETAMINE SACCHARATE, AMPHETAMINE ASPARTATE, DEXTROAMPHETAMINE SULFATE AND AMPHETAMINE SULFATE TABLETS (Mixed Salts of a Single Entity Amphetamine Product) Tablets 30 mg CII White to cream colored octagon shaped tablet	Debossed with a "30" and a partial quadrisect on one side and a "M" in a box on other side
DEXTROAMPHETAMINE SULFATE ER CAPSULES hard gel capsule 5mg CII white	Boxed "M"® on the cap and is imprinted "8960 5mg" on the body in black
DEXTROAMPHETAMINE SULFATE ER CAPSULES hard gel capsule 10mg CII white	Boxed "M"® on the cap and is imprinted "8961 10mg" on the body in blue
DEXTROAMPHETAMINE SULFATE ER CAPSULES hard gel capsule 15mg CII white	Boxed "M"® on the cap and is imprinted "8962 15mg" on the body in pink
DEXTROAMPHETAMINE SULFATE TABLETS, USP Tablets 5mg CII white, triangle tab	"5" and a bisect on one side and an "M" within a box on the other side
DEXTROAMPHETAMINE SULFATE TABLETS, USP Tablets 10mg CII white, diamond tab	"10" and a partial quadrisect on one side and an "M" within a box on the other side
FLUOXETINE CAPSULES, USP Capsules 10mg opaque lt green body and cap/ hard gel capsule	Boxed "M" over 0661 in black print
FLUOXETINE CAPSULES, USP Capsules 20mg opaq white body/ opaq lt green cap, hard gel capsule	Boxed "M" over 0663 in black print
FLUOXETINE ORAL SOLUTION, USP 20 mg per 5 mL liquid, mint flavor	
HYDROCODONE BITARTRATE AND ACETAMINOPHEN TABLETS, USP Tablets 5mg/325mg CIII White capsule shaped tablet	Debossed with M365 bisect on other side
HYDROCODONE BITARTRATE AND ACETAMINOPHEN CAPSULES Capsules 5mg/500mg CIII opaque maroon capsule	Boxed M 4357 imprinted in white

HYDROCODONE BITARTRATE AND ACETAMINOPHEN TABLETS, USP
Tablets 7.5mg/325mg CIII
White oval shaped tablet
Debossed with M366 on other side, unscored

HYDROCODONE BITARTRATE AND ACETAMINOPHEN ORAL SOLUTION
7.5/500mg per 15mL CIII
yellow liquid, tropical fruit punch flavor

HYDROCODONE BITARTRATE AND ACETAMINOPHEN TABLETS, USP
Tablets 5mg/500mg CIII
white capsule shaped tablet
Debossed M357; bisect on other side

HYDROCODONE BITARTRATE AND ACETAMINOPHEN TABLETS, USP
Tablets 7.5mg/500mg CIII
white capsule shaped tablet
Debossed with M358; bisect on other side

HYDROCODONE BITARTRATE AND ACETAMINOPHEN TABLETS, USP
Tablets 7.5mg/650mg CIII
white capsule shaped tablet
Debossed with M359; bisect on other side

HYDROCODONE BITARTRATE AND ACETAMINOPHEN TABLETS, USP
Tablets 7.5mg/750mg CIII
white capsule shaped tablet
Debossed with M360; bisect on other side

HYDROCODONE BITARTRATE AND ACETAMINOPHEN TABLETS, USP
Tablets 10mg/650mg CIII
blue capsule shaped tablet
Debossed with M361; bisect on other side

HYDROCODONE BITARTRATE AND ACETAMINOPHEN TABLETS, USP
Tablets 10mg/660mg CIII
white capsule shaped tablet
Debossed with M362; bisect on other side

HYDROCODONE BITARTRATE AND ACETAMINOPHEN TABLETS, USP
Tablets 10mg/500mg CIII
white capsule shaped tablet
Debossed with M363; bisect on other side

HYDROCODONE BITARTRATE AND ACETAMINOPHEN TABLETS, USP
Tablets 10mg/325mg CIII
white oval shaped tablet
Debossed with M367; bisect on other side

HYDROCODONE BITARTRATE AND ACETAMINOPHEN TABLETS, USP
Tablets 10mg/750mg CIII
White Oval Shaped Tablet
Debossed M364 one side and a bisect on the side

HYDROMORPHONE HYDROCHLORIDE TABLETS, USP
Tablets 2mg CII
white/round tab
Debossed with "M" one side; 2 on the reverse side

HYDROMORPHONE HYDROCHLORIDE TABLETS, USP
Tablets 4mg CII
white/round tab
Debossed with "M" one side; 4 on the reverse side

MEPERIDINE HYDROCHLORIDE TABLETS, USP
Tablets 50mg CII
white to off-white scored/round tab
Debossed Boxed "M" on one side; Semicircle arc "7113" on reverse side

MEPERIDINE HYDROCHLORIDE TABLETS, USP
Tablets 100mg CII
white to off-white scored/round tab
Debossed Boxed "M" on one side; Semicircle arc "7115" on reverse side

METHADOSE® ORAL TABLETS (methadone hydrochloride tablets, USP)
5 mg CII
white tab
Scored, (identified METHADOSE 5)

METHADOSE® ORAL TABLETS (methadone hydrochloride tablets, USP)
10 mg CII
white tab
Scored, (identified METHADOSE 10)

METHYLIN® (methylphenidate hydrochloride tablets, USP)
5 mg CII
white/round tab
Unscored/boxed M; 5 on reverse side

METHYLIN® (methylphenidate hydrochloride tablet, USP)
10 mg CII
white/round tab
Scored M; 10 on reverse side

METHYLIN® (methylphenidate hydrochloride tablet, USP)
20 mg CII
white/round tab
Scored/boxed M; 20 on reverse side

METHYLIN® ER (methylphenidate hydrochloride extended-release tablets, USP)
10 mg CII
white to off white round tab
Boxed "M"; 1423 on reverse side

METHYLIN® ER (methylphenidate hydrochloride extended-release tablets, USP)
20 mg CII
white to off-white round tab
Boxed "M"; 1451 on reverse side

MORPHINE SULFATE EXTENDED-RELEASE TABLETS
Tablets 15mg CII
Blue, round convex tablet
Debossed with 15 on one side, boxed "M" on reverse side

MORPHINE SULFATE EXTENDED-RELEASE TABLETS
Tablets 30mg CII
Purple, round convex tablet
Debossed with 30 on one side, boxed "M" on reverse side

MORPHINE SULFATE EXTENDED-RELEASE TABLETS
Tablets 60mg CII
Orange, round convex tablet
Debossed with 60 on one side, boxed "M" on reverse side

MORPHINE SULFATE EXTENDED-RELEASE TABLETS
Tablets 100mg CII
Gray, round convex tablet
Debossed with 100 on one side, boxed "M" on reverse side

MORPHINE SULFATE EXTENDED-RELEASE TABLETS
Tablets 200mg CII
Green, capsule shaped convex tablet
Debossed with 200 on one side, boxed "M" on reverse side

NALTREXONE HYDROCHLORIDE TABLETS, USP
Tablets 50mg
yellow, film coated capsule-shaped tablet
Debossed A 105 on bisected side

OXYCODONE HYDROCHLORIDE TABLETS, USP
Tablets 5mg CII
white/round convex, tab
Debossed with a boxed "M" on one side, "0552" with a vertical bisect between the fives on reverse side

OXYCODONE HYDROCHLORIDE TABLETS, USP
Tablets 15mg CII
Light Green/Round Convex Tablet
Debossed with a "15" above a bisect on one side and a "M" in a box on the other side

OXYCODONE HYDROCHLORIDE TABLETS, USP
Tablets 30mg CII
Light Blue/Round Convex Tablet
Debossed with a "30" above a bisect on one side and a "M" in a box on the other side

OXYCODONE HYDROCHLORIDE CAPSULES
Capsules 5mg CII
opaque brown/ opaque lt. brown
Printed with "0554"/ "M" in a box over "5mg" in black ink

OXYCODONE HYDROCHLORIDE ORAL SOLUTION, USP
5mg/5mL CII
red raspberry flavored liquid

OXYCODONE HYDROCHLORIDE ORAL CONCENTRATE SOLUTION
20mg/mL CII
yellow unflavored liquid

OXYCODONE AND ACETAMINOPHEN CAPSULES, USP
Capsules 5mg/500mg CII
red&beige hard gel capsule
Boxed "M" 532

OXYCODONE AND ACETAMINOPHEN TABLETS, USP
Tablets 5mg/325mg CII
white/round tab
Scored, debossed 512

OXYCODONE AND ACETAMINOPHEN TABLETS, USP
Tablets 7.5/325mg CII
White to off-white/Caplet Shaped Tablet
Debossed with a "M522" on one side and "7.5/325" on the other side

OXYCODONE AND ACETAMINOPHEN TABLETS, USP
Tablets 7.5/500mg CII
White to off-white/Oval Shaped Tablet
Debossed with a "M582" on one side and plain on the other side

OXYCODONE AND ACETAMINOPHEN TABLETS, USP
Tablets 10/325mg CII
White to off-white/Caplet Shaped Tablet
Debossed with a "M523" on one side and "10/325" on the other side

OXYCODONE AND ACETAMINOPHEN TABLETS, USP
Tablets 10/650mg CII
White to off-white/Capsule Shaped Tablet
Debossed with a "M562" on one side and plain on the other

PEMOLINE TABLETS
Tablets 18.75 mg CIV
white, round bisected tablet
Debossed A197 on bisected side

PEMOLINE TABLETS
Tablets 37.5 mg CIV
peach, round bisected tablet
Debossed A161 on bisected side

PEMOLINE TABLETS
Tablets 75 mg CIV
peach, round bisected tablet
Debossed A162 on bisected side

PEMOLINE (CHEWABLE) TABLETS
Tablets 37.5 mg CIV
peach, square bisected tablet
A186 on bisected side

PROPOXYPHENE NAPSYLATE AND ACETAMINOPHEN TABLETS, USP
White Tablets 100/650 mg CIV
white capsule-shaped coated tablet
Debossed "1721" on one side, boxed "M" on the other side

PROPOXYPHENE NAPSYLATE AND ACETAMINOPHEN TABLETS, USP
Pink Tablets 100/650 mg CIV
pink capsule-shaped coated tablet
Debossed "1772" on one side, boxed "M" on the other side

TRAMADOL HYDROCHLORIDE TABLETS,
Tablets 50 mg
white to off-white capsule coated tablet
Debossed "7171" on one side, debossed "M" on the other side

TUSSIZONE-12 RF™ TABLETS
carbetapentane tannate 60 mg, chlorpheniramine tannate 5 mg
Tablets 60mg/5mg
mauve capsule-shaped tablet
Scored one side, imprinted with 0037 0681 on reverse side

TUSSIZONE-12 RF™ SUSPENSION
carbetapentane tannate 30 mg, chlorpheniramine tannate 4 mg (per 5 mL)
30mg/4mg per 5 mL
pink suspension strawberry-currant flavor

The following list of Mallinckrodt Brand Products is provided to facilitate identification.

PRODUCT
Description
Color(s) Shape
IDENTIFICATION CODE

ANAFRANIL® (clomipramine hydrochloride capsules)
Capsules 25 mg
ivory/melon yellow capsule
ANAFRANIL 25 mg

ANAFRANIL® (clomipramine hydrochloride capsules)
Capsules 50 mg
ivory/aqua-blue capsule
ANAFRANIL 50 mg

ANAFRANIL® (clomipramine hydrochloride capsules)
Capsules 75 mg
ivory/yellow capsule
ANAFRANIL 75 mg

ANEXSIA® (hydrocodone bitartrate and acetaminophen tablets, USP)
Tablets 5mg/500mg CIII
white capsule shaped tablet
Bisected with 5361; Anexsia on reverse side

ANEXSIA® (hydrocodone bitartrate and acetaminophen tablets, USP)
Tablets 7.5/650mg CIII
white capsule shaped tablet
Bisected with 5362; Anexsia on reverse side

DEPADE® (naltrexone hydrochloride tablets, USP)
Tablets 25 mg
pink, film coated capsule-shaped tablet
Debossed "25" on one side, "DEPADE" on the reverse side

DEPADE® (naltrexone hydrochloride tablets, USP)
Tablets 50 mg
yellow, film coated capsule-shaped tablet
Debossed "50" on bisected side and "DEPADE" on the reverse side.

Continued on next page

Mallinckrodt brands—Cont.

DEPADE® (naltrexone hydrochloride tablets, USP) Tablets 100 mg beige, film coated capsule-shaped tablet	Debossed "100" and a partial score on one side, "DEPADE" and partial score on the reverse side
METHADOSE® DISPERSIBLE TABLETS (methadone hydrochloride tablets, USP) Dispersible Tablets 40mg CII white tab	Quadrisected (identified Methadose 40)
METHADOSE® ORAL CONCENTRATE (methadone hydrochloride oral concentrate, USP) CII Oral Concentrate 10mg/mL CII a cherry flavored liquid concentrate	
METHADOSE® SUGAR FREE ORAL CONCENTRATE (methadone hydrochloride oral concentrate, USP) Oral Concentrate 10mg/mL CII dye-free, sugar-free, unflavored	
PAMELOR® (nortriptyline hydrochloride capsules, USP) Capsules 10 mg white/orange capsule	SANDOZ - on one half PAMELOR 10 mg - on other half
PAMELOR® (nortriptyline hydrochloride capsules, USP) Capsules 25 mg white/orange capsule	SANDOZ - on one half PAMELOR 25 mg - on other half
PAMELOR® (nortriptyline hydrochloride capsules, USP) Capsules 50 mg white/white capsule	SANDOZ - on one half PAMELOR 50 mg - on other half
PAMELOR® (nortriptyline hydrochloride capsules, USP) Capsules 75 mg orange/orange capsule	SANDOZ - on one half PAMELOR 75 mg - on other half
PAMELOR® (nortriptyline hydrochloride oral solution, USP) Oral Solution 10 mg/5 mL liquid-cherry flavor clear, colorless	
RESTORIL® (temazepam capsules, USP) Capsules 7.5 mg CIV pink/blue capsule	Pink body imprinted "FOR SLEEP" on one side and [M] ® on the other side in red, and a blue cap imprinted "RESTORIL 7.5 mg" twice in red.
RESTORIL® (temazepam capsules, USP) Capsules 15 mg CIV pink/maroon capsule	Pink body imprinted "FOR SLEEP" on one side and [M] ® on the other side in red, and a maroon cap imprinted "RESTORIL 15 mg" twice in white.
RESTORIL® (temazepam capsules, USP) Capsules 30 mg CIV blue/maroon capsule	Blue body imprinted "FOR SLEEP" on one side and [M] ® on the other side in red, and a maroon cap imprinted "RESTORIL 30 mg" twice in white.
TOFRANIL® (imipramine hydrochloride tablets, USP) Tablets 10 mg tablet, triangular sugar-coated, coral	Geigy 32 (in black)
TOFRANIL® (imipramine hydrochloride tablets, USP) Tablets 25 mg tablet, round, biconvex sugar-coated, coral	Geigy 140 (in black)
TOFRANIL® (imipramine hydrochloride tablets, USP) Tablets 50 mg tablet, round, biconvex sugar-coated, coral	Geigy 136 (in black)
TOFRANIL-PM® (imipramine pamoate capsules) Capsules 75 mg coral capsule	Geigy 20 (in black)
TOFRANIL-PM® (imipramine pamoate capsules) Capsules 100 mg dark yellow/coral capsule	Geigy 40 (in black)
TOFRANIL-PM® (imipramine pamoate capsules) Capsules 125 mg ivory/coral capsule	Geigy 45 (in black)
TOFRANIL-PM® (imipramine pamoate capsules) Capsules 150 mg coral capsule	Geigy 22 (in black)

RESTORIL® ℂ ℞
(temazepam)
capsules, USP
Rx only

DESCRIPTION

Restoril® (temazepam) is a benzodiazepine hypnotic agent. The chemical name is 7-chloro-1,3-dihydro-3-hydroxy-1-methyl-5-phenyl-2*H*-1,4-benzodiazepin-2-one, and the structural formula is:

$C_{16}H_{13}ClN_2O_2$ Mol. wt. 300.74

Temazepam is a white, crystalline substance, very slightly soluble in water and sparingly soluble in alcohol, USP.

Restoril® (temazepam) capsules, 7.5 mg, 15 mg, and 30 mg, are for oral administration.

7.5 mg, 15 mg, and 30 mg Capsules

Active Ingredient: temazepam, USP

7.5 mg Capsules

Inactive Ingredients: FD&C Blue #1, FD&C Red #3, gelatin, lactose, magnesium stearate, sodium lauryl sulfate, synthetic red ferric oxide, titanium dioxide, and other ingredients.

May also include: benzyl alcohol, butylparaben, carboxymethylcellulose sodium, edetate calcium disodium, methylparaben, propylparaben, silicon dioxide, and sodium propionate.

15 mg Capsules

Inactive Ingredients: FD&C Blue #1, FD&C Red #3, gelatin, lactose, magnesium stearate, sodium lauryl sulfate, synthetic red ferric oxide, titanium dioxide, and other ingredients.

May also include: benzyl alcohol, butylparaben, carboxymethylcellulose sodium, edetate calcium disodium, methylparaben, propylparaben, silicon dioxide, and sodium propionate.

30 mg Capsules

Inactive Ingredients: FD&C Blue #1, FD&C Red #3, gelatin, lactose, magnesium stearate, sodium lauryl sulfate, titanium dioxide, and other ingredients.

May also include: benzyl alcohol, butylparaben, carboxymethylcellulose sodium, edetate calcium disodium, methylparaben, propylparaben, silicon dioxide, and sodium propionate.

HOW SUPPLIED

Restoril® (temazepam capsules, USP)

7.5 mg

Blue and pink capsules, with the pink body imprinted "FOR SLEEP" on one side and [M] ® on the other side in red, and a blue cap imprinted "RESTORIL 7.5 mg" twice in red.

Bottle of 30 .... NDC 0406-9915-03
Bottle of 100 .... NDC 0406-9915-01

15 mg

Maroon and pink capsules, with the pink body imprinted "FOR SLEEP" on one side and [M] ® on the other side in red, and a maroon cap imprinted "RESTORIL 15 mg" twice in white.

Bottle 100 .... NDC 0406-9916-01
Bottle of 500 .... NDC 0406-9916-05

30 mg

Maroon and blue capsules, with the blue body imprinted "FOR SLEEP" on one side and [M] ® on the other side in red, and a maroon cap imprinted "RESTORIL 30 mg" twice in white.

Bottle 100 .... NDC 0406-9917-01
Bottle of 500 .... NDC 0406-9917-05

Dispense in a well-closed, light resistant container with a child-resistant closure.

Storage: Store at 20° to 25°C (68° to 77°F) [**see** USP Controlled Room Temperature].

[M] and Restoril are registered trademarks of Mallinckrodt Inc.

Rev 040204

Shown in Product Identification Guide, page 321

TOFRANIL-PM® ℞
imipramine pamoate
Capsules of 75 mg
Capsules of 100 mg
Capsules of 125 mg
Capsules of 150 mg
For oral administration
℞ only

Prescribing Information

DESCRIPTION

Tofranil-PM®, imipramine pamoate, is a tricyclic antidepressant, available as capsules for oral administration. The 75-, 100-, 125-, and 150-mg capsules contain imipramine pamoate equivalent to 75, 100, 125, and 150 mg of imipramine hydrochloride. Imipramine pamoate is 5-[3-(dimethylamino) propyl]-10,11-dihydro-5*H*-dibenz[b,f]azepine 4, 4'-methylenebis-(3-hydroxy-2-naphthoate) (2:1), and its structural formula is

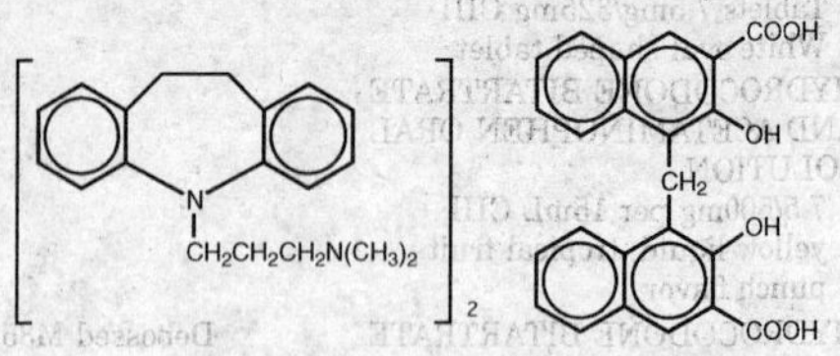

Imipramine pamoate is a fine, yellow, tasteless, odorless powder. It is soluble in ethanol, in acetone, in ether, in chloroform, and in carbon tetrachloride, and is insoluble in water. Its molecular weight is 949.21.

Inactive Ingredients. D&C Red No. 28, FD&C Blue No. 1, FD&C Yellow No. 6, D&C Yellow No. 10 (100 mg and 125 mg capsules only), gelatin, magnesium stearate, parabens, silicon dioxide, sodium lauryl sulfate, starch, talc, and titanium dioxide.

HOW SUPPLIED

Capsules 75 mg—coral (imprinted black Geigy 20) equivalent to 75 mg imipramine hydrochloride

Bottles of 30 .... NDC 0406-9923-03
Bottles of 100 .... NDC 0406-9923-01

Capsules 100 mg—dark yellow/coral (imprinted black Geigy 40) equivalent to 100 mg imipramine hydrochloride

Bottles of 30 .... NDC 0406-9924-03
Bottles of 100 .... NDC 0406-9924-01

Capsules 125 mg—ivory/coral (imprinted black Geigy 45) equivalent to 125 mg imipramine hydrochloride

Bottles of 30 .... NDC 0406-9925-03
Bottles of 100 .... NDC 0406-9925-01

Capsules 150 mg—coral (imprinted black Geigy 22) equivalent to 150 mg imipramine hydrochloride

Bottles of 30 .... NDC 0406-9926-03
Bottles of 100 .... NDC 0406-9926-01

Do not store above 30°C (86°F).

Dispense in a tight container (USP).

Manufactured by
Novartis Pharmaceuticals Corporation
East Hanover, New Jersey 07936
Manufactured for
Mallinckrodt Inc.
St. Louis, MO 63134
tyco
Healthcare
Mallinckrodt

Rev 041701

Shown in Product Identification Guide, page 321

Marlyn Nutraceuticals, Inc.
4404 E. ELWOOD ST.
PHOENIX, AZ 85040

Direct Inquiries to:
Joe Lehmann
4404 E. Elwood St.
Phoenix, AZ 85040
(800) 899-4499
480 991-0200
EMAIL info@naturallyvitamins.com

HEP-FORTE® OTC
[*hep-for 'tay*]

DESCRIPTION

Hep-Forte is a comprehensive formulation of protein, B factors and other nutritional factors which can be important as a dietary supplement for maintenance and support of normal hepatic function.

COMPOSITION

Each capsule contains:

Vitamin A (Palmitate)	1,200I.U.
Vitamin E (d-Alpha Tocopherol)	10I.U.
Vitamin C (Ascorbic Acid)	10mg.
Folic Acid	0.06mg.
Vitamin B1 (Thiamine Mononitrate)	1mg.
Vitamin B2 (Riboflavin)	1mg.
Niacinamide	10mg.
Vitamin B6 (Pyridoxine HCl)	0.5mg.
Vitamin B12 (Cobalamin)	1mcg.
Biotin	3.3mcg.
Pantothenic Acid	2mg.
Choline Bitartrate	21mg.
Zinc (Zinc Sulfate)	2mg.
Desiccated Liver	194.4mg.
Liver Concentrate	64.8mg.
Liver Fraction Number 2	64.8mg.
Yeast (Dried)	64.8mg.
dl-Methionine	10mg.
Inositol	10mg.

INDICATIONS

Hep-Forte is a balanced formulation of vitamins, minerals, lipotropic factors, and vitamin-protein supplements. It is of value as a nutritional supplement for persons who are receiving professional treatment for alcoholism, hepatic dysfunction due to hepatotoxic drugs and liver poisons, male and female infertility due to hormonal imbalance caused by hepatic dysfunction, and for nutritional supplementation after treatment.

CONTRAINDICATIONS

There are no known contraindications to Hep-Forte.

DOSAGE

Three to six capsules daily.

HOW SUPPLIED

Bottles of 100, 200 or 500 capsules.
Literature Available.

MARLYN FORMULA 50® OTC

PRODUCT OVERVIEW

KEY FACTS

Marlyn Formula 50 is a dietary supplement providing a combination of amino acids and B6 in a gelatin capsule which provides protein "building blocks" important to growth and development of all protein containing tissue including nails, hair, and skin.

MAJOR USES

Dermatologists recommend Formula 50 for splitting, peeling nails. Since splitting and peeling nails are often associated with nail fungus, Formula 50 may be recommended in conjunction with drug therapy for nail fungus in order to provide protein necessary for growth and development of nails. OB-Gyn's recommend it for help in controlling excessive hair fall-out after child birth.

SAFETY INFORMATION

There are no known contraindications or adverse reactions.

PRESCRIBING INFORMATION

MARLYN FORMULA 50®

COMPOSITION

Each capsule contains:
Amino Acids .... 0.3 Gm*
Vitamin B6 (pyridoxine HCl) .... 1.0 mg.

*Approximate analysis of the amino acids: indispensable amino acids (lysine, tryptophan, phenylalanine, methionine, threonine, leucine, isoleucine, valine), 35.30%; semi-dispensable amino acids (arginine, histidine, tyrosine, cystine, glycine), 19.18%; dispensable amino acids (glutamic acid, alanine, aspartic acid, serine, proline), 45.56%.

Amino acids: Protein "building blocks" important to growth and development of all protein containing tissue including nails, hair, and skin.

DOSAGE AND ADMINISTRATION

The recommended daily dose is 6 capsules daily.

SUPPLY

Bottles of 100, 250 capsules.
Literature Available.

WOBENZYM®N OTC

[*wō-bĕn-zīm*]

KEY FACTS

Wobenzym, a combination of proteolytic enzymes and the antioxidant rutin, works systemically by targeting various tissues and organs in the body. Wobenzym modulates the immune response by restoring a healthy balance between anti-inflammatory and pro-inflammatory cytokines.

MAJOR USES

Orally administered enzymes work as biocatalysts, which accelerate and control the bodily metabolism without themselves being altered. They support enzymatic catabolism—for example in inflammatory diseases. They have great significance for optimal functioning of the immune system and the body's own defense forces against pathogens, harmful substances and foreign bodies. Inflammation plays a role as a defense of the body against damaged tissue for almost every disease. Enzymes are responsible for the physiological discharge of inflammation and re-establishment of the affected tissue's function.

SAFETY INFORMATION

The use of Wobenzym should be graduated when taken in conjunction with blood thinners.

DOSAGE AND ADMINISTRATION

As a preventive measure, three tablets on a relatively empty stomach two to three times a day (3 b.i.d./t.i.d.).

HOW SUPPLIED

Bottles of 100, 200, 400 and 800 tablets. Literature available upon request.

McNeil Consumer & Specialty Pharmaceuticals

Division of McNeil-PPC, Inc.
FORT WASHINGTON, PA 19034

Direct Inquiries to:
Consumer Relationship Center
Fort Washington, PA 19034
800-962-5357
For Concerta, Direct Inquiries to:
888-440-7903

CONCERTA® ℂ ℞

(methylphenidate HCl)
Extended-release Tablets

DESCRIPTION

CONCERTA® is a central nervous system (CNS) stimulant. CONCERTA® is available in four tablet strengths. Each extended-release tablet for once-a-day oral administration contains 18, 27, 36, or 54 mg of methylphenidate HCl USP and is designed to have a 12-hour duration of effect. Chemically, methylphenidate HCl is d,l (racemic) methyl α-phenyl-2-piperidineacetate hydrochloride. Its empirical formula is $C_{14}H_{19}NO_2$•HCl. Its structural formula is:

Methylphenidate HCl USP is a white, odorless crystalline powder. Its solutions are acid to litmus. It is freely soluble in water and in methanol, soluble in alcohol, and slightly soluble in chloroform and in acetone. Its molecular weight is 269.77.

CONCERTA® also contains the following inert ingredients: butylated hydroxytoluene, carnauba wax, cellulose acetate, hypromellose, lactose, phosphoric acid, poloxamer, polyethylene glycol, polyethylene oxides, povidone, propylene glycol, sodium chloride, stearic acid, succinic acid, synthetic iron oxides, titanium dioxide, and triacetin.

System Components and Performance

CONCERTA® uses osmotic pressure to deliver methylphenidate HCl at a controlled rate. The system, which resembles a conventional tablet in appearance, comprises an osmotically active trilayer core surrounded by a semipermeable membrane with an immediate-release drug overcoat. The trilayer core is composed of two drug layers containing the drug and excipients, and a push layer containing osmotically active components. There is a precision-laser drilled orifice on the drug-layer end of the tablet. In an aqueous environment, such as the gastrointestinal tract, the drug overcoat dissolves within one hour, providing an initial dose of methylphenidate. Water permeates through the membrane into the tablet core. As the osmotically active polymer excipients expand, methylphenidate is released through the orifice. The membrane controls the rate at which water enters the tablet core, which in turn controls drug delivery. The biologically inert components of the tablet remain intact during gastrointestinal transit and are eliminated in the stool as a tablet shell along with insoluble core components.

CLINICAL PHARMACOLOGY

Pharmacodynamics

Methylphenidate HCl is a central nervous system (CNS) stimulant. The mode of therapeutic action in Attention Deficit Hyperactivity Disorder (ADHD) is not known. Methylphenidate is thought to block the reuptake of norepinephrine and dopamine into the presynaptic neuron and increase the release of these monoamines into the extraneuronal space. Methylphenidate is a racemic mixture comprised of the d- and l-isomers. The d-isomer is more pharmacologically active than the l-isomer.

Pharmacokinetics

Absorption

Methylphenidate is readily absorbed. Following oral administration of CONCERTA® to adults, plasma methylphenidate concentrations increase rapidly reaching an initial maximum at about 1 to 2 hours, then increase gradually over the next several hours. Peak plasma concentrations are achieved at about 6 to 8 hours after which a gradual decrease in plasma levels of methylphenidate begins. CONCERTA® qd minimizes the fluctuations between peak and trough concentrations associated with immediate-release methylphenidate tid (see Figure 1). The relative bioavailability of CONCERTA® qd and methylphenidate tid in adults is comparable.

[See figure at top of next column]

Figure 1. Mean methylphenidate plasma concentrations in 36 adults, following a single dose of CONCERTA® 18 mg qd and immediate-release methylphenidate 5 mg tid administered every 4 hours.

The mean pharmacokinetic parameters in 36 adults following the administration of CONCERTA® 18 mg qd and methylphenidate 5 mg tid are summarized in Table 1.

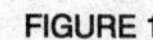

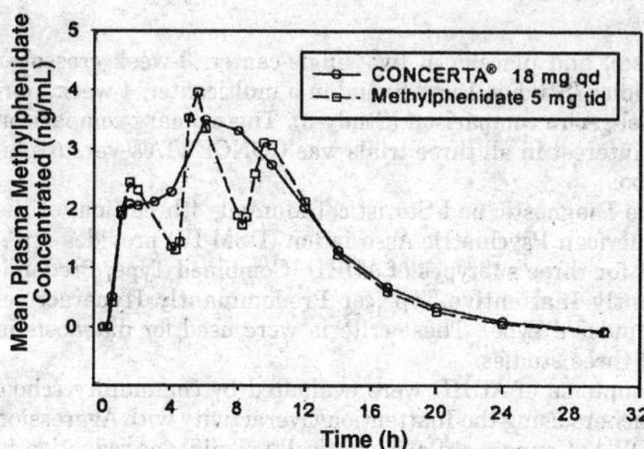

TABLE 1
Mean ± SD Pharmacokinetic Parameters

Parameters	CONCERTA® (18 mg qd) (n=36)	Methylphenidate (5 mg tid) (n=35)
C_{max} (ng/mL)	3.7 ± 1.0	4.2 ± 1.0
T_{max} (h)	6.8 ± 1.8	6.5 ± 1.8
AUC_{inf} (ng•h/mL)	41.8 ± 13.9	38.0 ± 11.0
$t_{1/2}$ (h)	3.5 ± 0.4	3.0 ± 0.5

No differences in the pharmacokinetics of CONCERTA® were noted following single and repeated qd dosing indicating no significant drug accumulation. The AUC and $t_{1/2}$ following repeated qd dosing are similar to those following the first dose of CONCERTA® 18 mg.

Dose Proportionality

Following administration of CONCERTA® in single doses of 18, 36, and 54 mg/day to adults, C_{max} and $AUC_{(0-inf)}$ of d-methylphenidate were proportional to dose, whereas l-methylphenidate C_{max} and $AUC_{(0-inf)}$ increased disproportionately with respect to dose. Following administration of CONCERTA®, plasma concentrations of the l-isomer were approximately 1/40th the plasma concentrations of the d-isomer.

Distribution

Plasma methylphenidate concentrations in adults decline biexponentially following oral administration. The half-life of methylphenidate in adults following oral administration of CONCERTA® was approximately 3.5 h.

Metabolism and Excretion

In humans, methylphenidate is metabolized primarily by de-esterification to α-phenyl-piperidine acetic acid (PPA) which has little or no pharmacologic activity. In adults the metabolism of CONCERTA® qd as evaluated by metabolism to PPA is similar to that of methylphenidate tid. The metabolism of single and repeated qd doses of CONCERTA® is similar.

After oral dosing of radiolabeled methylphenidate in humans, about 90% of the radioactivity was recovered in urine. The main urinary metabolite was PPA, accounting for approximately 80% of the dose.

Food Effects

In patients, there were no differences in either the pharmacokinetics or the pharmacodynamic performance of CONCERTA® when administered after a high fat breakfast. There is no evidence of dose dumping in the presence or absence of food.

Special Populations

Gender

In healthy adults, the mean dose-adjusted $AUC_{(0-inf)}$ values for CONCERTA® were 36.7 ng•h/mL in men and 37.1 ng•h/mL in women, with no differences noted between the two groups.

Race

In adults receiving CONCERTA®, dose-adjusted $AUC_{(0-inf)}$ was consistent across ethnic groups; however, the sample size may have been insufficient to detect ethnic variations in pharmacokinetics.

Age

The pharmacokinetics of CONCERTA® has not been studied in children less than 6 years of age.

Renal Insufficiency

There is no experience with the use of CONCERTA® in patients with renal insufficiency. After oral administration of radiolabeled methylphenidate in humans, methylphenidate was extensively metabolized and approximately 80% of the radioactivity was excreted in the urine in the form of PPA. Since renal clearance is not an important route of methylphenidate clearance, renal insufficiency is expected to have little effect on the pharmacokinetics of CONCERTA®.

Hepatic Insufficiency

There is no experience with the use of CONCERTA® in patients with hepatic insufficiency.

Clinical Studies

CONCERTA® was demonstrated to be effective in the treatment of Attention Deficit Hyperactivity Disorder (ADHD) in three double-blind, active- and placebo-controlled studies in 416 children 6 to 12 years old. The controlled studies compared CONCERTA® given qd (18, 36, or 54 mg), methylphenidate given tid over 12 hours (15, 30, or 45 mg total daily

Continued on next page

Concerta—Cont.

dose), and placebo in two single-center, 3-week crossover studies (Studies 1 and 2) and in a multicenter, 4-week, parallel-group comparison (Study 3). The primary comparison of interest in all three trials was CONCERTA® versus placebo.

The Diagnostic and Statistical Manual, 4th edition, of the American Psychiatric Association (DSM-IV) provides criteria for three subtypes of ADHD (Combined Type, Predominantly Inattentive Type, or Predominantly Hyperactive-Impulsive Type). These criteria were used for diagnosis in all three studies.

Symptoms of ADHD were evaluated by community school teachers using the Inattention/Overactivity with Aggression (IOWA) Conners scale. Statistically significant reduction in the Inattention/Overactivity subscale versus placebo was shown consistently across all three controlled studies for CONCERTA® qd. The scores for CONCERTA® and placebo for the three studies are presented in Figure 2.

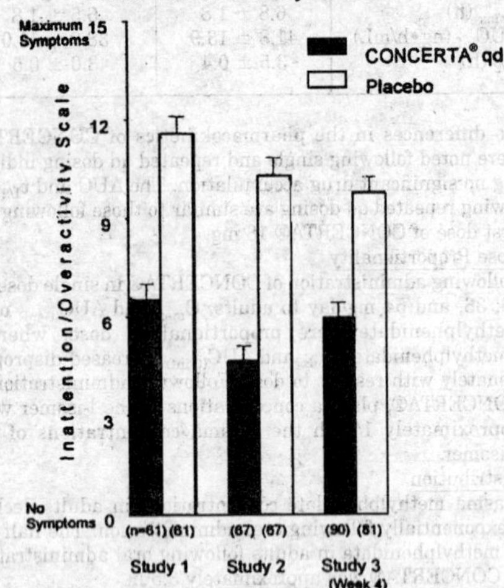

Figure 2: Mean Community School Teacher IOWA Conners Inattention/Overactivity Scores with CONCERTA® qd (18, 36, or 54 mg) and placebo. Studies 1 and 2 involved a 3-way crossover of 1 week per treatment arm. Study 3 involved 4 weeks of parallel group treatments with a Last Observation Carried Forward analysis at week 4. Error bars represent the mean plus standard error of the mean.

In two controlled studies (Studies 1 and 2), symptoms of ADHD were evaluated by laboratory school teachers using the SKAMP* laboratory school rating scale. The combined results from these two studies demonstrated significant improvements in attention and behavior in patients treated with CONCERTA® versus placebo that were maintained through 12 hours after dosing. Figure 3 presents the laboratory school teacher SKAMP ratings for CONCERTA® and placebo.

*Swanson, Kotkin, Agler, M-Fynn and Pelham

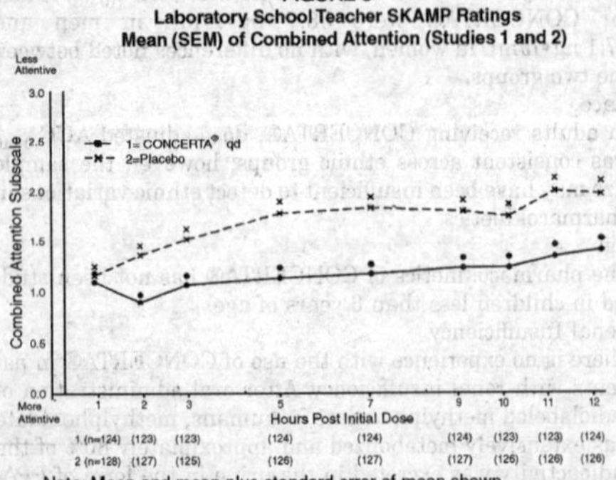

Note: Mean and mean plus standard error of mean shown

INDICATION AND USAGE

Attention Deficit Hyperactivity Disorder (ADHD)

CONCERTA® is indicated for the treatment of Attention Deficit Hyperactivity Disorder (ADHD).

The efficacy of CONCERTA® in the treatment of ADHD was established in three controlled trials of children aged 6 to 12 who met DSM-IV criteria for ADHD (see CLINICAL PHARMACOLOGY).

A diagnosis of Attention Deficit Hyperactivity Disorder (ADHD; DSM-IV) implies the presence of hyperactive-impulsive or inattentive symptoms that caused impairment and were present before age 7 years. The symptoms must cause clinically significant impairment, eg, in social, academic, or occupational functioning, and be present in two or more settings, eg, school (or work) and at home. The symptoms must not be better accounted for by another mental disorder. For the Inattentive Type, at least six of the following symptoms must have persisted for at least 6 months: lack of attention to details/careless mistakes; lack of sustained attention; poor listener; failure to follow through on tasks; poor organization; avoids tasks requiring sustained mental effort; loses things; easily distracted; forgetful. For the Hyperactive-Impulsive Type, at least six of the following symptoms must have persisted for at least 6 months: fidgeting/squirming; leaving seat; inappropriate running/climbing; difficulty with quiet activities; "on the go;" excessive talking; blurting answers; can't wait turn; intrusive. The Combined Type requires both inattentive and hyperactive-impulsive criteria to be met.

Special Diagnostic Considerations

Specific etiology of this syndrome is unknown, and there is no single diagnostic test. Adequate diagnosis requires the use of medical and special psychological, educational, and social resources. Learning may or may not be impaired. The diagnosis must be based upon a complete history and evaluation of the child and not solely on the presence of the required number of DSM-IV characteristics.

Need for Comprehensive Treatment Program

CONCERTA® is indicated as an integral part of a total treatment program for ADHD that may include other measures (psychological, educational, social) for patients with this syndrome. Drug treatment may not be indicated for all children with this syndrome. Stimulants are not intended for use in the child who exhibits symptoms secondary to environmental factors and/or other primary psychiatric disorders, including psychosis. Appropriate educational placement is essential and psychosocial intervention is often helpful. When remedial measures alone are insufficient, the decision to prescribe stimulant medication will depend upon the physician's assessment of the chronicity and severity of the child's symptoms.

Long-Term Use

The effectiveness of CONCERTA® for long-term use, ie, for more than 4 weeks, has not been systematically evaluated in controlled trials. Therefore, the physician who elects to use CONCERTA® for extended periods should periodically re-evaluate the long-term usefulness of the drug for the individual patient (see DOSAGE AND ADMINISTRATION).

CONTRAINDICATIONS

Agitation

CONCERTA® is contraindicated in patients with marked anxiety, tension, and agitation, since the drug may aggravate these symptoms.

Hypersensitivity to Methylphenidate

CONCERTA® is contraindicated in patients known to be hypersensitive to methylphenidate or other components of the product.

Glaucoma

CONCERTA® is contraindicated in patients with glaucoma.

Tics

CONCERTA® is contraindicated in patients with motor tics or with a family history or diagnosis of Tourette's syndrome (see ADVERSE REACTIONS).

Monoamine Oxidase Inhibitors

CONCERTA® is contraindicated during treatment with monoamine oxidase (MAO) inhibitors, and also within a minimum of 14 days following discontinuation of a MAO-inhibitor (hypertensive crises may result) (see PRECAUTIONS, Drug Interactions).

WARNINGS

Depression

CONCERTA® should not be used to treat severe depression.

Fatigue

CONCERTA® should not be used for the prevention or treatment of normal fatigue states.

Long-Term Suppression of Growth

Sufficient data on the safety of long-term use of methylphenidate in children are not yet available. Although a causal relationship has not been established, suppression of growth (ie, weight gain, and/or height) has been reported with the long-term use of stimulants in children. Therefore, patients requiring long-term therapy should be carefully monitored. Patients who are not growing or gaining weight as expected should have their treatment interrupted.

Psychosis

Clinical experience suggests that in psychotic patients, administration of methylphenidate may exacerbate symptoms of behavior disturbance and thought disorder.

Seizures

There is some clinical evidence that methylphenidate may lower the convulsive threshold in patients with prior history of seizures, in patients with prior EEG abnormalities in absence of seizures, and, very rarely, in absence of history of seizures and no prior EEG evidence of seizures. In the presence of seizures, the drug should be discontinued.

Potential for Gastrointestinal Obstruction

Because the CONCERTA® tablet is nondeformable and does not appreciably change in shape in the GI tract, CONCERTA® should not ordinarily be administered to patients with preexisting severe gastrointestinal narrowing (pathologic or iatrogenic, for example: esophageal motility disorders small bowel inflammatory disease, "short gut" syndrome due to adhesions or decreased transit time, past history of peritonitis, cystic fibrosis, chronic intestinal pseudoobstruction, or Meckel's diverticulum). There have been rare reports of obstructive symptoms in patients with known strictures in association with the ingestion of drugs in nondeformable controlled-release formulations. Due to the controlled-release design of the tablet, CONCERTA® should only be used in patients who are able to swallow the tablet whole (see PRECAUTIONS: Information for Patients).

Hypertension and other Cardiovascular Conditions

Use cautiously in patients with hypertension. Blood pressure should be monitored at appropriate intervals in patients taking CONCERTA®, especially patients with hypertension. In the laboratory classroom clinical trials (Studies 1 and 2), both CONCERTA® and methylphenidate tid increased resting pulse by an average of 2–6 bpm and produced average increases of systolic and diastolic blood pressure of roughly 1–4 mm Hg during the day, relative to placebo. Therefore, caution is indicated in treating patients whose underlying medical conditions might be compromised by increases in blood pressure or heart rate, eg, those with preexisting hypertension, heart failure, recent myocardial infarction, or hyperthyroidism.

Visual Disturbance

Symptoms of visual disturbances have been encountered in rare cases. Difficulties with accommodation and blurring of vision have been reported.

Use in Children Under Six Years of Age

CONCERTA® should not be used in children under six years, since safety and efficacy in this age group have not been established.

DRUG DEPENDENCE

CONCERTA® should be given cautiously to patients with a history of drug dependence or alcoholism. Chronic abusive use can lead to marked tolerance and psychological dependence with varying degrees of abnormal behavior. Frank psychotic episodes can occur, especially with parenteral abuse. Careful supervision is required during withdrawal from abusive use since severe depression may occur. Withdrawal following chronic therapeutic use may unmask symptoms of the underlying disorder that may require follow-up.

PRECAUTIONS

Hematologic Monitoring

Periodic CBC, differential, and platelet counts are advised during prolonged therapy.

Information for Patients

Patients should be informed that CONCERTA® should be swallowed whole with the aid of liquids. Tablets should not be chewed, divided, or crushed. The medication is contained within a nonabsorbable shell designed to release the drug at a controlled rate. The tablet shell, along with insoluble core components, is eliminated from the body; patients should not be concerned if they occasionally notice in their stool something that looks like a tablet.

Patient information is printed at the end of this insert. To assure safe and effective use of CONCERTA®, the information and instructions provided in the patient information section should be discussed with patients.

Drug Interactions

CONCERTA® should not be used in patients being treated (currently or within the proceeding 2 weeks) with MAO inhibitors (see CONTRAINDICATIONS, Monoamine Oxidase Inhibitors).

Because of possible effects on blood pressure, CONCERTA® should be used cautiously with vasopressor agents.

Human pharmacologic studies have shown that methylphenidate may inhibit the metabolism of coumarin anticoagulants, anticonvulsants (eg, phenobarbital, phenytoin, primidone), and some antidepressants (tricyclics and selective serotonin reuptake inhibitors). Downward dose adjustment of these drugs may be required when given concomitantly with methylphenidate. It may be necessary to adjust the dosage and monitor plasma drug concentrations (or, in the case of coumarin, coagulation times), when initiating or discontinuing concomitant methylphenidate.

Serious adverse events have been reported in concomitant use with clonidine, although no causality for the combination has been established. The safety of using methylphenidate in combination with clonidine or other centrally acting alpha-2 agonists has not been systematically evaluated.

Carcinogenesis, Mutagenesis, and Impairment of Fertility

In a lifetime carcinogenicity study carried out in B6C3F1 mice, methylphenidate caused an increase in hepatocellular adenomas and, in males only, an increase in hepatoblastomas at a daily dose of approximately 60 mg/kg/day. This dose is approximately 30 times and 4 times the maximum recommended human dose of CONCERTA® on a mg/kg and mg/m^2 basis, respectively. Hepatoblastoma is a relatively rare rodent malignant tumor type. There was no increase in total malignant hepatic tumors. The mouse strain used is sensitive to the development of hepatic tumors, and the significance of these results to humans is unknown.

Methylphenidate did not cause any increases in tumors in a lifetime carcinogenicity study carried out in F344 rats; the highest dose used was approximately 45 mg/kg/day, which is approximately 22 times and 5 times the maximum recommended human dose of CONCERTA® on a mg/kg and mg/m^2 basis, respectively.

In a 24-week carcinogenicity study in the transgenic mouse strain p53+/−, which is sensitive to genotoxic carcinogens, there was no evidence of carcinogenicity. Male and female mice were fed diets containing the same concentration of methylphenidate as in the lifetime carcinogenicity study; the high-dose groups were exposed to 60 to 74 mg/kg/day of methylphenidate.

Methylphenidate was not mutagenic in the in vitro Ames reverse mutation assay or the in vitro mouse lymphoma cell forward mutation assay. Sister chromatid exchanges and chromosome aberrations were increased, indicative of a weak clastogenic response, in an in vitro assay in cultured Chinese Hamster Ovary cells. Methylphenidate was negative in vivo in males and females in the mouse bone marrow micronucleus assay.

Methylphenidate did not impair fertility in male or female mice that were fed diets containing the drug in an 18-week Continuous Breeding study. The study was conducted at doses up to 160 mg/kg/day, approximately 80-fold and 8-fold the highest recommended human dose of CONCERTA® on a mg/kg and mg/m^2 basis, respectively.

Pregnancy: Teratogenic Effects

Pregnancy Category C: Methylphenidate has been shown to have teratogenic effects in rabbits when given in doses of 200 mg/kg/day, which is approximately 100 times and 40 times the maximum recommended human dose on a mg/kg and mg/m^2 basis, respectively.

A reproduction study in rats revealed no evidence of harm to the fetus at oral doses up to 30 mg/kg/day, approximately 15-fold and 3-fold the maximum recommended human dose of CONCERTA® on a mg/kg and mg/m^2 basis, respectively. The approximate plasma exposure to methylphenidate plus its main metabolite PPA in pregnant rats was 2 times that seen in trials in volunteers and patients with the maximum recommended dose of CONCERTA® based on the AUC.

The safety of methylphenidate for use during human pregnancy has not been established. There are no adequate and well-controlled studies in pregnant women. CONCERTA® should be used during pregnancy only if the potential benefit justifies the potential risk to the fetus.

Nursing Mothers

It is not known whether methylphenidate is excreted in human milk. Because many drugs are excreted in human milk, caution should be exercised if CONCERTA® is administered to a nursing woman.

Pediatric Use

The safety and efficacy of CONCERTA® in children under 6 years old have not been established. Long-term effects of methylphenidate in children have not been well established (see WARNINGS).

ADVERSE REACTIONS

The premarketing development program for CONCERTA® included exposures in a total of 755 participants in clinical trials (469 patients, 286 healthy adult subjects). These participants received CONCERTA® 18, 36, and/or 54 mg/day. The 469 patients (ages 6 to 13) were evaluated in three controlled clinical studies (Studies 1, 2, and 3), two uncontrolled clinical studies (including a long-term safety study), and one clinical pharmacology study in children with ADHD. Of the 469 patients in this program, 68 CONCERTA®-treated patients in one uncontrolled dose-initiation study were näive to any pharmacologic therapy for their ADHD. Safety data on all patients are included in the discussion that follows. Adverse reactions were assessed by collecting adverse events, results of physical examinations, vital signs, weights, laboratory analyses, and ECGs.

Adverse events during exposure were obtained primarily by general inquiry and recorded by clinical investigators using terminology of their own choosing. Consequently, it is not possible to provide a meaningful estimate of the proportion of individuals experiencing adverse events without first grouping similar types of events into a smaller number of standardized event categories. In the tables and listings that follow, COSTART terminology has been used to classify reported adverse events.

The stated frequencies of adverse events represent the proportion of individuals who experienced, at least once, a treatment-emergent adverse event of the type listed. An event was considered treatment emergent if it occurred for the first time or worsened while receiving therapy following baseline evaluation.

Adverse Findings in Clinical Trials with CONCERTA®

Adverse Events Associated with Discontinuation of Treatment

In the 4-week placebo-controlled, parallel-group trial one CONCERTA®-treated patient (0.9%; 1/106) and one placebo-treated patient (1.0%; 1/99) discontinued due to an adverse event (sadness and increase in tics, respectively).

In uncontrolled studies up to 12 months with CONCERTA®, 6.6% (29/441) patients discontinued for adverse events. Those events associated with discontinuation of CONCERTA® in more than one patient included the following: twitching (tics, 1.8%); anorexia (loss of appetite, 0.9%); aggravation reaction (0.7%); hostility (0.7%); insomnia (0.7%); and somnolence (0.5%).

Adverse Events Occurring at an Incidence of 1% or more Among CONCERTA®-Treated Patients

Table 2 enumerates, for a 4-week placebo-controlled, parallel-group trial in children with ADHD at CONCERTA® doses of 18, 36, or 54 mg/day, the incidence of treatment-emergent adverse events. The table includes only those events that occurred in 1% or more of patients treated with CONCERTA® where the incidence in patients treated with CONCERTA® was greater than the incidence in placebo-treated patients.

The prescriber should be aware that these figures cannot be used to predict the incidence of adverse events in the course of usual medical practice where patient characteristics and other factors differ from those which prevailed in the clinical trials. Similarly, the cited frequencies cannot be compared with figures obtained from other clinical investigations involving different treatments, uses, and investigators. The cited figures, however, do provide the prescribing physician with some basis for estimating the relative contribution of drug and non-drug factors to the adverse event incidence rate in the population studied.

[See table 2 above]

TABLE 2
Incidence of Treatment-Emergent Events[1] in a 4-Week Placebo-Controlled Clinical Trial of CONCERTA®

Body System	Preferred Term	CONCERTA® (n=106)	Placebo (n=99)
General	Headache	14%	10%
	Abdominal pain (stomachache)	7%	1%
Digestive	Vomiting	4%	3%
	Anorexia (loss of appetite)	4%	0%
Nervous	Dizziness	2%	0%
	Insomnia	4%	1%
Respiratory	Upper Respiratory Tract Infection	8%	5%
	Cough Increased	4%	2%
	Pharyngitis	4%	3%
	Sinusitis	3%	0%

[1]: Events, regardless of causality, for which the incidence for patients treated with CONCERTA® was at least 1% and greater than the incidence among placebo-treated patients. Incidence greater than 1% has been rounded to the nearest whole number.

Tics

In a long-term uncontrolled study (n=407 children), the cumulative incidence of new onset of tics was 8% after 10 months of treatment with CONCERTA®.

Post-Marketing Experience with CONCERTA®:

Additional very rare undesirable effects were reported during the marketing experience: difficulties in visual accomodation, blurred vision, abnormal liver function tests (eg, transaminase elevation), palpitations, arrhythmia, leukopenia, and thrombocytopenia.

Adverse Events with Other Methylphenidate HCl Products

Nervousness and insomnia are the most common adverse reactions reported with other methylphenidate products. Other reactions include hypersensitivity (including skin rash, urticaria, fever, arthralgia, exfoliative dermatitis, erythema multiforme with histopathological findings of necrotizing vasculitis, and thrombocytopenic purpura); anorexia; nausea; dizziness; headache; dyskinesia; drowsiness; blood pressure and pulse changes, both up and down; tachycardia; angina; abdominal pain; weight loss during prolonged therapy. There have been rare reports of Tourette's syndrome. Toxic psychosis has been reported. Although a definite causal relationship has not been established, the following have been reported in patients taking this drug: hepatic coma; isolated cases of cerebral arteritis and/or occlusion; anemia; transient depressed mood; a few instances of scalp hair loss. Very rare reports of neuroleptic malignant syndrome (NMS) have been received, and, in most of these, patients were concurrently receiving therapies associated with NMS. In a single report, a ten year old boy who had been taking methylphenidate for approximately 18 months experienced an NMS-like event within 45 minutes of ingesting his first dose of venlafaxine. It is uncertain whether this case represented a drug-drug interaction, a response to either drug alone, or some other cause.

In children, loss of appetite, abdominal pain, weight loss during prolonged therapy, insomnia, and tachycardia may occur more frequently; however, any of the other adverse reactions listed above may also occur.

DRUG ABUSE AND DEPENDENCE

Controlled Substance Class

CONCERTA®, like other methylphenidate products, is classified as a Schedule II controlled substance by federal regulation.

Abuse, Dependence, and Tolerance

See WARNINGS for boxed warning containing drug abuse and dependence information.

OVERDOSAGE

Signs and Symptoms

Signs and symptoms of acute methylphenidate overdosage, resulting principally from overstimulation of the CNS and from excessive sympathomimetic effects, may include the following: vomiting, agitation, tremors, hyperreflexia, muscle twitching, convulsions (may be followed by coma), euphoria, confusion, hallucinations, delirium, sweating, flushing, headache, hyperpyrexia, tachycardia, palpitations, cardiac arrhythmias, hypertension, mydriasis, and dryness of mucous membranes.

Recommended Treatment

Treatment consists of appropriate supportive measures. The patient must be protected against self-injury and against external stimuli that would aggravate overstimulation already present. Gastric contents may be evacuated by gastric lavage as indicated. Before performing gastric lavage, control agitation and seizures if present and protect the airway. Other measures to detoxify the gut include administration of activated charcoal and a cathartic. Intensive care must be provided to maintain adequate circulation and respiratory exchange; external cooling procedures may be required for hyperpyrexia.

Efficacy of peritoneal dialysis or extracorporeal hemodialysis for CONCERTA® overdosage has not been established.

The prolonged release of methylphenidate from CONCERTA® should be considered when treating patients with overdose.

Poison Control Center

As with the management of all overdosage, the possibility of multiple drug ingestion should be considered. The physician may wish to consider contacting a poison control center for up-to-date information on the management of overdosage with methylphenidate.

DOSAGE AND ADMINISTRATION

CONCERTA® is administered orally once daily in the morning.

CONCERTA® must be swallowed whole with the aid of liquids, and must not be chewed, divided, or crushed (see PRECAUTIONS: Information for Patients).

CONCERTA® may be administered with or without food and should be administered once daily in the morning as it has been shown to improve attention and behavior through 12 hours after dosing.

Dosage should be individualized according to the needs and responses of the patient.

Patients New to Methylphenidate

The recommended starting dose of CONCERTA® for patients who are not currently taking methylphenidate, or for patients who are on stimulants other than methylphenidate, is 18 mg once daily.

Dosage may be adjusted to a maximum of 54 mg/day taken once daily in the morning. In general, dosage adjustment may proceed at approximately weekly intervals.

Patients Currently Using Methylphenidate

The recommended dose of CONCERTA® for patients who are currently taking methylphenidate bid, tid, or sustained-release (SR) at doses of 10 to 60 mg/day is provided in Table 3. Dosing recommendations are based on current dose regimen and clinical judgement.

Dosage may be adjusted to a maximum of 54 mg/day taken once daily in the morning. In general, dosage adjustment may proceed at approximately weekly intervals.

TABLE 3
Recommended Dose Conversion from Methylphenidate Regimens to CONCERTA®

Previous Methylphenidate Daily Dose	Recommended CONCERTA® Dose
5 mg Methylphenidate bid or 5 mg Methylphenidate tid or 20 mg Methylphenidate-SR	18 mg q am
10 mg Methylphenidate bid or 10 mg Methylphenidate tid or 40 mg Methylphenidate-SR	36 mg q am
15 mg Methylphenidate bid or 15 mg Methylphenidate tid or 60 mg Methylphenidate-SR	54 mg q am

Other methylphenidate regimens: Clinical judgement should be used when selecting the starting dose.

A 27 mg dosage strength is available for physicians who wish to prescribe between the 18 mg and 36 mg dosages. Daily dosage above 54 mg is not recommended.

Maintenance/Extended Treatment

There is no body of evidence available from controlled trials to indicate how long the patient with ADHD should be treated with CONCERTA®. It is generally agreed, however, that pharmacological treatment of ADHD may be needed for extended periods. Nevertheless, the physician who elects to use CONCERTA® for extended periods in patients with ADHD should periodically re-evaluate the long-term useful-

Continued on next page

Concerta—Cont.

ness of the drug for the individual patient with trials off medication to assess the patient's functioning without pharmacotherapy. Improvement may be sustained when the drug is either temporarily or permanently discontinued.

Dose Reduction and Discontinuation

If paradoxical aggravation of symptoms or other adverse events occur, the dosage should be reduced, or, if necessary, the drug should be discontinued.

If improvement is not observed after appropriate dosage adjustment over a one-month period, the drug should be discontinued.

HOW SUPPLIED

CONCERTA® (methylphenidate HCl) Extended-release Tablets are available in 18 mg, 27 mg, 36 mg, and 54 mg dosage strengths. The 18 mg tablets are yellow and imprinted with "alza 18". The 27 mg tablets are gray and imprinted with "alza 27". The 36 mg tablets are white and imprinted with "alza 36". The 54 mg tablets are brownish-red and imprinted with "alza 54". All four dosage strengths are supplied in bottles containing 100 tablets.

18 mg	100 count bottle	NDC 17314-5850-2
27 mg	100 count bottle	NDC 17314-5853-2
36 mg	100 count bottle	NDC 17314-5851-2
54 mg	100 count bottle	NDC 17314-5852-2

Storage

Store at 25°C (77°F); excursions permitted to 15–30°C (59–86°F) [see USP Controlled Room Temperature]. Protect from humidity.

REFERENCE

American Psychiatric Association. Diagnosis and Statistical Manual of Mental Disorders. 4th ed. Washington DC: American Psychiatric Association 1994.

Rx Only.

For more information call 1-888-440-7903 or visit www.concerta.net

Manufactured by
ALZA Corporation, Mountain View, CA 94043.
Distributed and Marketed by
McNeil Consumer & Specialty Pharmaceuticals, Fort Washington, PA 19034.
10025000 Edition: March 2004
An ALZA OROS® Technology Product
Concerta® and OROS® are Registered Trademarks of ALZA Corporation

INFORMATION FOR PATIENTS TAKING CONCERTA® OR THEIR PARENTS OR CAREGIVERS

CONCERTA® ℞
(methylphenidate HCl)
Extended-release Tablets CII

This information is for patients taking CONCERTA® Extended-release Tablets CII for the treatment of Attention Deficit Hyperactivity Disorder, or their parents or caregivers.

Please read this before you start taking CONCERTA®. Remember, this information does not take the place of your doctor's instructions. If you have any questions about this information or about CONCERTA®, talk to your doctor or pharmacist.

What is CONCERTA®?

CONCERTA® is a once-a-day treatment for Attention Deficit Hyperactivity Disorder, or ADHD. CONCERTA® contains the drug methylphenidate, a central nervous system stimulant that has been used to treat ADHD for more than 30 years. CONCERTA® is taken by mouth, once each day in the morning.

What is Attention Deficit Hyperactivity Disorder?

ADHD has three main types of symptoms: inattention, hyperactivity, and impulsiveness. Symptoms of inattention include not paying attention, making careless mistakes, not listening, not finishing tasks, not following directions, and being easily distracted. Symptoms of hyperactivity and impulsiveness include fidgeting, talking excessively, running around at inappropriate times, and interrupting others. Some patients have more symptoms of hyperactivity and impulsiveness while others have more symptoms of inattentiveness. Some patients have all three types of symptoms.

Many people have symptoms like these from time to time, but patients with ADHD have these symptoms more than others their age. Symptoms must be present for at least 6 months to be certain of the diagnosis.

How does CONCERTA® work?

Part of the CONCERTA® tablet dissolves right after you swallow it in the morning, giving you an initial dose of methylphenidate. The remaining drug is slowly released during the day to continue to help lessen the symptoms of ADHD. Methylphenidate, the active ingredient in CONCERTA®, helps increase attention and decrease impulsiveness and hyperactivity in patients with ADHD.

Who should NOT take CONCERTA®?

You should NOT take CONCERTA® if:

- You have significant anxiety, tension, or agitation since CONCERTA® may make these conditions worse.
- You are allergic to methylphenidate or any of the other ingredients in CONCERTA®.
- You have glaucoma, an eye disease.
- You have tics or Tourette's syndrome, or a family history of Tourette's syndrome.

Talk to your doctor if you believe any of these conditions apply to you.

How should I take CONCERTA®?

Do not chew, crush, or divide the tablets. Swallow CONCERTA® tablets whole with the help of water or other liquids, such as milk or juice.

Take CONCERTA® once each day in the morning.

You may take CONCERTA® before or after you eat.

Take the dose prescribed by your doctor. Your doctor may adjust the amount of drug you take until it is right for you. From time to time, your doctor may interrupt your treatment to check your symptoms while you are not taking the drug.

What are the possible side effects of CONCERTA®?

In the clinical studies with patients using CONCERTA®, the most common side effects were headache, stomach pain, sleeplessness, and decreased appetite. Other side effects seen with methylphenidate, the active ingredient in CONCERTA®, include nausea, vomiting, dizziness, nervousness, tics, allergic reactions, increased blood pressure and psychosis (abnormal thinking or hallucinations).

This is not a complete list of possible side effects. Ask your doctor about other side effects. If you develop any side effect, talk to your doctor.

What must I discuss with my doctor before taking CONCERTA®?

Talk to your doctor ***before*** taking CONCERTA® if you:

- Are being treated for depression or have symptoms of depression such as feelings of sadness, worthlessness, and hopelessness.
- Have motion tics (hard-to-control, repeated twitching of any parts of your body) or verbal tics (hard-to-control repeating of sounds or words).
- Have someone in your family with motion tics, verbal tics, or Tourette's syndrome.
- Have abnormal thoughts or visions, hear abnormal sounds, or have been diagnosed with psychosis.
- Have had seizures (convulsions, epilepsy) or abnormal EEGs (electroencephalograms).
- Have high blood pressure.
- Have a narrowing or blockage of your gastrointestinal tract (your esophagus, stomach, or small or large intestine).

Tell your doctor ***immediately*** if you develop any of the above conditions or symptoms while taking CONCERTA®.

Can I take CONCERTA® with other medicines?

Tell your doctor about ***all*** medicines that you are taking. Your doctor should decide whether you can take CONCERTA® with other medicines. These include:

Other medicines that a doctor has prescribed.

Medicines that you buy yourself without a prescription.

Any herbal remedies that you may be taking.

You should not take CONCERTA® with monoamine oxidase (MAO) inhibitors.

While on CONCERTA®, do not start taking a new medicine or herbal remedy before checking with your doctor.

CONCERTA® may change the way your body reacts to certain medicines. These include medicines used to treat depression, prevent seizures, or prevent blood clots (commonly called "blood thinners"). Your doctor may need to change your dose of these medicines if you are taking them with CONCERTA®.

Other Important Safety Information

Abuse of methylphenidate can lead to dependence.

Tell your doctor if you have ever abused or been dependent on alcohol or drugs, or if you are now abusing or dependent on alcohol or drugs.

Before taking CONCERTA®, tell your doctor if you are pregnant or plan on becoming pregnant. If you take methylphenidate, it may be in your breast milk. Tell your doctor if you are nursing a baby.

Tell your doctor if you have blurred vision when taking CONCERTA®.

Slower growth (weight gain and/or height) has been reported with long-term use of methylphenidate in children. Your doctor will be carefully watching your height and weight. If you are not growing or gaining weight as your doctor expects, your doctor may stop your CONCERTA® treatment.

Call your doctor ***immediately*** if you take more than the amount of CONCERTA® prescribed by your doctor.

What else should I know about CONCERTA®?

CONCERTA® has not been studied in children under 6 years of age.

The CONCERTA® tablet does not dissolve completely after all the drug has been released, and you may sometimes notice it in your stool. This is normal.

CONCERTA® may be a part of your overall treatment for ADHD. Your doctor may also recommend that you have counseling or other therapy.

As with all medicines, never share CONCERTA® with anyone else and take only the number of CONCERTA® tablets prescribed by your doctor.

CONCERTA® should be stored in a safe place at room temperature (between 59°–86° F). Do not store this medicine in hot, damp, or humid places.

Keep out of the reach of children.

For more information call 1-888-440-7903 or visit www.concerta.net

Manufactured by
ALZA Corporation, Mountain View, CA 94043.
Distributed and Marketed by
McNeil Consumer & Specialty Pharmaceuticals, Fort Washington, PA 19034.
An ALZA OROS® Technology Product
Concerta® and OROS® are Registered Trademarks of ALZA Corporation
10025000 PPI Edition: March 2004

Shown in Product Identification Guide, page 321

FLEXERIL® ℞
(CYCLOBENZAPRINE HCl) TABLETS

DESCRIPTION

Cyclobenzaprine hydrochloride is a white, crystalline tricyclic amine salt with the empirical formula $C_{20}H_{21}N \cdot HCl$ and a molecular weight of 311.9. It has a melting point of 217°C, and a pK_a of 8.47 at 25°C. It is freely soluble in water and alcohol, sparingly soluble in isopropanol, and insoluble in hydrocarbon solvents. If aqueous solutions are made alkaline, the free base separates. Cyclobenzaprine HCl is designated chemically as 3-(5*H*-dibenzo[*a,d*] cyclohepten-5-ylidene)-*N*, *N*-dimethyl-1-propanamine hydrochloride, and has the following structural formula:

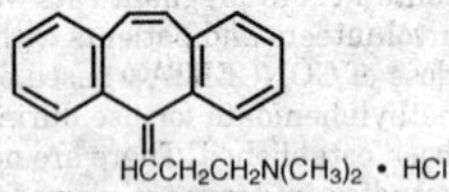

FLEXERIL 5 mg (Cyclobenzaprine HCl) is supplied as a 5 mg tablet for oral administration. FLEXERIL 10 mg (Cyclobenzaprine HCl) is supplied as a 10 mg tablet for oral administration.

FLEXERIL tablets contain the following inactive ingredients: hydroxypropyl cellulose, hypromellose, iron oxide, lactose, magnesium stearate, starch, and titanium dioxide. FLEXERIL 5 mg tablets also contain Yellow D&C #10 Aluminum Lake HT, and Yellow FD&C #6 Aluminum Lake.

CLINICAL PHARMACOLOGY

Cyclobenzaprine HCl relieves skeletal muscle spasm of local origin without interfering with muscle function. It is ineffective in muscle spasm due to central nervous system disease.

Cyclobenzaprine reduced or abolished skeletal muscle hyperactivity in several animal models. Animal studies indicate that cyclobenzaprine does not act at the neuromuscular junction or directly on skeletal muscle. Such studies show that cyclobenzaprine acts primarily within the central nervous system at brain stem as opposed to spinal cord levels, although its action on the latter may contribute to its overall skeletal muscle relaxant activity. Evidence suggests that the net effect of cyclobenzaprine is a reduction of tonic somatic motor activity, influencing both gamma (γ) and alpha (α) motor systems.

Pharmacological studies in animals showed a similarity between the effects of cyclobenzaprine and the structurally related tricyclic antidepressants, including reserpine antagonism, norepinephrine potentiation, potent peripheral and central anticholinergic effects, and sedation. Cyclobenzaprine caused slight to moderate increase in heart rate in animals.

Pharmacokinetics

Estimates of mean oral bioavailability of cyclobenzaprine range from 33% to 55%. Cyclobenzaprine exhibits linear pharmacokinetics over the dose range 2.5 mg to 10 mg, and is subject to enterohepatic circulation. It is highly bound to plasma proteins. Drug accumulates when dosed three times a day, reaching steady-state within 3–4 days at plasma concentrations about four-fold higher than after a single dose. At steady state in healthy subjects receiving 10 mg t.i.d. (n=18), peak plasma concentration was 25.9 ng/mL (range, 12.8–46.1 ng/mL), and area under the concentration-time (AUC) curve over an 8-hour dosing interval was 177 ng.hr/mL (range, 80–319 ng.hr/mL).

Cyclobenzaprine is extensively metabolized, and is excreted primarily as glucuronides via the kidney. Cytochromes P-450 3A4, 1A2, and, to a lesser extent, 2D6, mediate N-demethylation, one of the oxidative pathways for cyclobenzaprine. Cyclobenzaprine is eliminated quite slowly, with an effective half-life of 18 hours (range 8–37 hours; n=18); plasma clearance is 0.7 L/min.

The plasma concentration of cyclobenzaprine is generally higher in the elderly and in patients with hepatic impairment. (See PRECAUTIONS, *Use in the Elderly* and PRECAUTIONS, *Impaired Hepatic Function.*)

Elderly

In a pharmacokinetic study in elderly individuals (≥65yrs old), mean (n=10) steady-state cyclobenzaprine AUC values were approximately 1.7 fold (171.0 ng.hr/mL, range 96.1–255.3) higher than those seen in a group of eighteen younger adults (101.4 ng.hr/mL, range 36.1–182.9) from another study. Elderly male subjects had the highest observed mean increase, approximately 2.4 fold (198.3 ng.hr/mL, range 155.6–255.3 versus 83.2 ng.hr/mL, range 41.1–142.5 for younger males) while levels in elderly females were increased to a much lesser extent, approximately 1.2 fold (143.8 ng.hr/mL, range 96.1–196.3 versus 115.9 ng.hr/mL, range 36.1–182.9 for younger females).

In light of these findings, therapy with FLEXERIL in the elderly should be initiated with a 5 mg dose and titrated slowly upward.

Hepatic Impairment

In a pharmacokinetic study of sixteen subjects with hepatic impairment (15 mild, 1 moderate per Child-Pugh score), both AUC and C_{max} were approximately double the values seen in the healthy control group. Based on the findings, FLEXERIL should be used with caution in subjects with mild hepatic impairment starting with the 5 mg dose and titrating slowly upward. Due to the lack of data in subjects with more severe hepatic insufficiency, the use of FLEXERIL in subjects with moderate to severe impairment is not recommended.

No significant effect on plasma levels or bioavailability of FLEXERIL or aspirin was noted when single or multiple doses of the two drugs were administered concomitantly. Concomitant administration of FLEXERIL and naproxen or diflunisal was well tolerated with no reported unexpected adverse effects. However combination therapy of FLEXERIL with naproxen was associated with more side effects than therapy with naproxen alone, primarily in the form of drowsiness. No well-controlled studies have been performed to indicate whether FLEXERIL enhances the clinical effect of aspirin or other analgesics, or whether analgesics enhance the clinical effect of FLEXERIL in acute musculoskeletal conditions.

Clinical Studies

Eight double-blind controlled clinical studies were performed in 642 patients comparing FLEXERIL 10 mg, diazepam**, and placebo. Muscle spasm, local pain and tenderness, limitation of motion, and restriction in activities of daily living were evaluated. In three of these studies there was a significantly greater improvement with FLEXERIL than with diazepam, while in the other studies the improvement following both treatments was comparable.

Although the frequency and severity of adverse reactions observed in patients treated with FLEXERIL were comparable to those observed in patients treated with diazepam, dry mouth was observed more frequently in patients treated with FLEXERIL and dizziness more frequently in those treated with diazepam. The incidence of drowsiness, the most frequent adverse reaction, was similar with both drugs.

The efficacy of FLEXERIL 5 mg was demonstrated in two seven-day, double-blind, controlled clinical trials enrolling 1405 patients. One study compared FLEXERIL 5 mg and 10 mg t.i.d. to placebo; and a second study compared FLEXERIL 5 mg and 2.5 mg t.i.d. to placebo. Primary endpoints for both trials were determined by patient-generated data and included global impression of change, medication helpfulness, and relief from starting backache. Each endpoint consisted of a score on a 5-point rating scale (from 0 or worst outcome to 4 or best outcome). Secondary endpoints included a physician's evaluation of the presence and extent of palpable muscle spasm.

Comparisons of FLEXERIL 5 mg and placebo groups in both trials established the statistically significant superiority of the 5 mg dose for all three primary endpoints at day 8 and, in the study comparing 5 and 10 mg, at day 3 or 4 as well. A similar effect was observed with FLEXERIL 10 mg (all endpoints). Physician-assessed secondary endpoints also showed that FLEXERIL 5 mg was associated with a greater reduction in palpable muscle spasm than placebo.

Analysis of the data from controlled studies shows that FLEXERIL produces clinical improvement whether or not sedation occurs.

Surveillance Program

A post-marketing surveillance program was carried out in 7607 patients with acute musculoskeletal disorders, and included 297 patients treated with FLEXERIL 10 mg for 30 days or longer. The overall effectiveness of FLEXERIL was similar to that observed in the double-blind controlled studies; the overall incidence of adverse effects was less (see ADVERSE REACTIONS).

INDICATIONS AND USAGE

FLEXERIL is indicated as an adjunct to rest and physical therapy for relief of muscle spasm associated with acute, painful musculoskeletal conditions.

Improvement is manifested by relief of muscle spasm and its associated signs and symptoms, namely, pain, tenderness, limitation of motion, and restriction in activities of daily living.

FLEXERIL should be used only for short periods (up to two or three weeks) because adequate evidence of effectiveness for more prolonged use is not available and because muscle spasm associated with acute, painful musculoskeletal conditions is generally of short duration and specific therapy for longer periods is seldom warranted.

FLEXERIL has not been found effective in the treatment of spasticity associated with cerebral or spinal cord disease, or in children with cerebral palsy.

CONTRAINDICATIONS

Hypersensitivity to any component of this product.

Concomitant use of monoamine oxidase (MAO) inhibitors or within 14 days after their discontinuation. Hyperpyretic crisis seizures, and deaths have occurred in patients receiving cyclobenzaprine (or structurally similar tricyclic antidepressants) concomitantly with MAO inhibitor drugs.

Acute recovery phase of myocardial infarction, and patients with arrhythmias, heart block or conduction disturbances, or congestive heart failure.

Hyperthyroidism.

WARNINGS

Cyclobenzaprine is closely related to the tricyclic antidepressants, e.g., amitriptyline and imipramine. In short term studies for indications other than muscle spasm associated with acute musculoskeletal conditions, and usually at doses somewhat greater than those recommended for skeletal muscle spasm, some of the more serious central nervous system reactions noted with the tricyclic antidepressants have occurred (see WARNINGS, below, and ADVERSE REACTIONS).

Tricyclic antidepressants have been reported to produce arrhythmias, sinus tachycardia, prolongation of the conduction time leading to myocardial infarction and stroke.

FLEXERIL may enhance the effects of alcohol, barbiturates, and other CNS depressants.

PRECAUTIONS

General

Because of its atropine-like action, FLEXERIL should be used with caution in patients with a history of urinary retention, angle-closure glaucoma, increased intraocular pressure, and in patients taking anticholinergic medication.

Impaired Hepatic Function

The plasma concentration of cyclobenzaprine is increased in patients with hepatic impairment (see CLINICAL PHARMACOLOGY, *Pharmacokinetics, Hepatic Impairment*). These patients are generally more susceptible to drugs with potentially sedating effects, including cyclobenzaprine. FLEXERIL should be used with caution in subjects with mild hepatic impairment starting with a 5 mg dose and titrating slowly upward. Due to the lack of data in subjects with more severe hepatic insufficiency, the use of FLEXERIL in subjects with moderate to severe impairment is not recommended.

Information for Patients

FLEXERIL, especially when used with alcohol or other CNS depressants, may impair mental and/or physical abilities required for performance of hazardous tasks, such as operating machinery or driving a motor vehicle. In the elderly, the frequency and severity of adverse events associated with the use of cyclobenzaprine, with or without concomitant medications, is increased. In elderly patients, FLEXERIL should be initiated with a 5 mg dose and titrated slowly upward.

Drug Interactions

FLEXERIL may have life-threatening interactions with MAO inhibitors. (See CONTRAINDICATIONS.)

FLEXERIL may enhance the effects of alcohol, barbiturates, and other CNS depressants.

Tricyclic antidepressants may block the antihypertensive action of guanethidine and similarly acting compounds.

Tricyclic antidepressants may enhance the seizure risk in patients taking tramadol.[†]

Carcinogenesis, Mutagenesis, Impairment of Fertility

In rats treated with FLEXERIL for up to 67 weeks at doses of approximately 5 to 40 times the maximum recommended human dose, pale, sometimes enlarged, livers were noted and there was a dose-related hepatocyte vacuolation with lipidosis. In the higher dose groups this microscopic change was seen after 26 weeks and even earlier in rats which died prior to 26 weeks; at lower doses, the change was not seen until after 26 weeks.

Cyclobenzaprine did not affect the onset, incidence or distribution of neoplasia in an 81-week study in the mouse or in a 105-week study in the rat.

At oral doses of up to 10 times the human dose, cyclobenzaprine did not adversely affect the reproductive performance or fertility of male or female rats. Cyclobenzaprine did not demonstrate mutagenic activity in the male mouse at dose levels of up to 20 times the human dose.

Pregnancy

Pregnancy Category B: Reproduction studies have been performed in rats, mice and rabbits at doses up to 20 times the human dose, and have revealed no evidence of impaired fertility or harm to the fetus due to FLEXERIL. There are, however, no adequate and well-controlled studies in pregnant women. Because animal reproduction studies are not always predictive of human response, this drug should be used during pregnancy only if clearly needed.

Nursing Mothers

It is not known whether this drug is excreted in human milk. Because cyclobenzapine is closely related to the tricyclic antidepressants, some of which are known to be excreted in human milk, caution should be exercised when FLEXERIL is administered to a nursing woman.

Pediatric Use

Safety and effectiveness of FLEXERIL in pediatric patients below 15 years of age have not been established.

Use in the Elderly

The plasma concentration of cyclobenzaprine is increased in the elderly (see CLINICAL PHARMACOLOGY, *Pharmacokinetics, Elderly*). The elderly may also be more at risk for CNS adverse events such as hallucinations and confusion, cardiac events resulting in falls or other sequelae, drug-drug and drug-disease interactions. For these reasons, in the elderly, cyclobenzaprine should be used only if clearly needed. In such patients FLEXERIL should be initiated with a 5 mg dose and titrated slowly upward.

ADVERSE REACTIONS

Incidence of most common adverse reactions in the 2 double-blind[‡], placebo-controlled 5 mg studies (incidence of > 3% on FLEXERIL 5 mg):

	FLEXERIL 5 mg N=464	FLEXERIL 10 mg N=249	Placebo N=469
Drowsiness	29%	38%	10%
Dry Mouth	21%	32%	7%
Fatigue	6%	6%	3%
Headache	5%	5%	8%

Adverse reactions which were reported in 1% to 3% of the patients were: abdominal pain, acid regurgitation, constipation, diarrhea, dizziness, nausea, irritability, mental acuity decreased, nervousness, upper respiratory infection, and pharyngitis.

The following list of adverse reactions is based on the experience in 473 patients treated with FLEXERIL 10 mg in additional controlled clinical studies, 7607 patients in the post-marketing surveillance program, and reports received since the drug was marketed. The overall incidence of adverse reactions among patients in the surveillance program was less than the incidence in the controlled clinical studies.

The adverse reactions reported most frequently with FLEXERIL were drowsiness, dry mouth and dizziness. The incidence of these common adverse reactions was lower in the surveillance program than in the controlled clinical studies.

[‡]Note: FLEXERIL 10 mg data are from one clinical trial. FLEXERIL 5 mg and placebo data are from two studies.

	Clinical Studies With FLEXERIL 10 mg	*Surveillance Program With FLEXERIL 10 mg*
Drowsiness	39%	16%
Dry Mouth	27%	7%
Dizziness	11%	3%

Among the less frequent adverse reactions, there was no appreciable difference in incidence in controlled clinical studies or in the surveillance program. Adverse reactions which were reported in 1% to 3% of the patients were: fatigue/tiredness, asthenia, nausea, constipation, dyspepsia, unpleasant taste, blurred vision, headache, nervousness, and confusion.

The following adverse reactions have been reported in post-marketing experience or with an incidence of less than 1% of patients in clinical trials with the 10 mg tablet:

Body as a Whole: Syncope; malaise.

Cardiovascular: Tachycardia; arrhythmia; vasodilatation; palpitation; hypotension.

Digestive: Vomiting; anorexia; diarrhea; gastrointestinal pain; gastritis; thirst; flatulence; edema of the tongue; abnormal liver function and rare reports of hepatitis, jaundice and cholestasis.

Hypersensitivity: Anaphylaxis; angioedema; pruritus; facial edema; urticaria; rash.

Musculoskeletal: Local weakness.

Nervous System and Psychiatric: Seizures; ataxia; vertigo; dysarthria; tremors; hypertonia; convulsions; muscle twitching; disorientation; insomnia; depressed mood; abnormal sensations; anxiety; agitation; psychosis, abnormal thinking and dreaming; hallucinations; excitement; paresthesia; diplopia.

Skin: Sweating.

Special Senses: Ageusia; tinnitus.

Urogenital: Urinary frequency and/or retention.

Causal Relationship Unknown

Other reactions, reported rarely for FLEXERIL under circumstances where a causal relationship could not be established or reported for other tricyclic drugs, are listed to serve as alerting information to physicians:

Body as a Whole: Chest pain; edema.

Cardiovascular: Hypertension; myocardial infarction; heart block; stroke.

Digestive: Paralytic ileus; tongue discoloration; stomatitis; parotid swelling.

Endocrine: Inappropriate ADH syndrome.

Hematic and Lymphatic: Purpura; bone marrow depression; leukopenia; eosinophilia; thrombocytopenia.

Metabolic, Nutritional and Immune: Elevation and lowering of blood sugar levels; weight gain or loss.

Musculoskeletal: Myalgia.

Nervous System and Psychiatric: Decreased or increased libido; abnormal gait; delusions; aggressive behavior; paranoia; peripheral neuropathy; Bell's palsy; alteration in EEG patterns; extrapyramidal symptoms.

Respiratory: Dyspnea.

Skin: Photosensitization; alopecia.

Urogenital: Impaired urination; dilatation of urinary tract; impotence; testicular swelling; gynecomastia; breast enlargement; galactorrhea.

DRUG ABUSE AND DEPENDENCE

Pharmacologic similarities among the tricyclic drugs require that certain withdrawal symptoms be considered when FLEXERIL is administered even though they have not been reported to occur with this drug. Abrupt cessation of treatment after prolonged administration rarely may produce nausea, headache, and malaise. These are not indicative of addiction.

Continued on next page

Flexeril—Cont.

OVERDOSAGE

Although rare, deaths may occur from overdosage with FLEXERIL. Multiple drug ingestion (including alcohol) is common in deliberate cyclobenzaprine overdose. **As management of overdose is complex and changing, it is recommended that the physician contact a poison control center for current information on treatment.** Signs and symptoms of toxicity may develop rapidly after cyclobenzaprine overdose; therefore, hospital monitoring is required as soon as possible. The acute oral LD_{50} of FLEXERIL is approximately 338 and 425 mg/kg in mice and rats, respectively.

MANIFESTATIONS

The most common effects associated with cyclobenzaprine overdose are drowsiness and tachycardia. Less frequent manifestations include tremor, agitation, coma, ataxia, hypertension, slurred speech, confusion, dizziness, nausea, vomiting, and hallucinations. Rare but potentially critical manifestations of overdose are cardiac arrest, chest pain, cardiac dysrhythmias, severe hypotension, seizures, and neuroleptic malignant syndrome.

Changes in the electrocardiogram, particularly in QRS axis or width, are clinically significant indicators of cyclobenzaprine toxicity.

Other potential effects of overdosage include any of the symptoms listed under ADVERSE REACTIONS.

MANAGEMENT

General

As management of overdose is complex and changing, it is recommended that the physician contact a poison control center for current information on treatment.

In order to protect against the rare but potentially critical manifestations described above, obtain an ECG and immediately initiate cardiac monitoring. Protect the patient's airway, establish an intravenous line and initiate gastric decontamination. Observation with cardiac monitoring and observation for signs of CNS or respiratory depression, hypotension, cardiac dysrhythmias and/or conduction blocks, and seizures is necessary. If signs of toxicity occur at any time during this period, extended monitoring is required. Monitoring of plasma drug levels should not guide management of the patient. Dialysis is probably of no value because of low plasma concentrations of the drug.

Gastrointestinal Decontamination

All patients suspected of an overdose with FLEXERIL should receive gastrointestinal decontamination. This should include large volume gastric lavage followed by activated charcoal. If consciousness is impaired, the airway should be secured prior to lavage and emesis is contraindicated.

Cardiovascular

A maximal limb-lead QRS duration of ≥0.10 seconds may be the best indication of the severity of the overdose. Serum alkalinization, to a pH of 7.45 to 7.55, using intravenous sodium bicarbonate and hyperventilation (as needed), should be instituted for patients with dysrhythmias and/or QRS widening. A pH >7.60 or a pCO_2 <20 mmHg is undesirable. Dysrhythmias unresponsive to sodium bicarbonate therapy/hyperventilation may respond to lidocaine, bretylium or phenytoin. Type 1A and 1C antiarrhythmics are generally contraindicated (e.g., quinidine, disopyramide, and procainamide).

CNS

In patients with CNS depression, early intubation is advised because of the potential for abrupt deterioration. Seizures should be controlled with benzodiazepines or, if these are ineffective, other anticonvulsants (e.g. phenobarbital, phenytoin). Physostigmine is not recommended except to treat life-threatening symptoms that have been unresponsive to other therapies, and then only in close consultation with a poison control center.

PSYCHIATRIC FOLLOW-UP

Since overdosage is often deliberate, patients may attempt suicide by other means during the recovery phase. Psychiatric referral may be appropriate.

PEDIATRIC MANAGEMENT

The principles of management of child and adult overdosages are similar. It is strongly recommended that the physician contact the local poison control center for specific pediatric treatment.

DOSAGE AND ADMINISTRATION

For most patients, the recommended dose of FLEXERIL is 5 mg three times a day. Based on individual patient response, the dose may be increased to 10 mg three times a day. Use of FLEXERIL for periods longer than two or three weeks is not recommended. (See INDICATIONS AND USAGE).

Less frequent dosing should be considered for hepatically impaired or elderly patients (see PRECAUTIONS, *Impaired Hepatic Function*, and *Use in the Elderly*).

HOW SUPPLIED

FLEXERIL tablets are available in 5 mg and 10 mg dosage strengths. The 5 mg tablets are yellow-orange, 5-sided D-shaped, film coated tablets, coded FLEXERIL on one side and without coding on the other. The 10 mg tablets are butterscotch yellow, 5-sided D-shaped, film coated tablets, coded FLEXERIL on one side and without coding on the other. The two dosage strengths are supplied as follows:

5 mg	100 count bottle	NDC 50580-280-10
10 mg	100 count bottle	NDC 50580-874-11

STORAGE

Store at 25°C (77°F); excursions permitted to 15–30°C (59–86°F). [See USP Controlled Room Temperature].

Rx only

For more information call 1-888-440-7903 or visit www.flexeril.info

Distributed by
McNeil Consumer & Specialty Pharmaceuticals
Fort Washington, PA 19034.

FLEXERIL is a registered trademark of ALZA Corporation

Revised March 2004

†ULTRAM® (tramadol HCl, Ortho-McNeil Pharmaceutical) ULTRACET® (tramadol HCl and acetaminophen tablets, Ortho-McNeil Pharmaceutical)

Shown in Product Identification Guide, page 321

MAXIMUM STRENGTH GAS AID SOFTGELS OTC

DESCRIPTION

Each softgel of Maximum Strength GasAid contains simethicone 125 mg.

ACTIONS

Simethicone acts in the stomach and intestines by altering the surface tension of gas bubbles enabling them to coalesce, thereby freeing and eliminating the gas more easily by belching or passing flatus.

USES

Relieves bloating, pressure, fullness or stuffed feeling commonly referred to as gas.

DIRECTIONS

Adults and children 12 years and over: take 1–2 softgels as needed after meals and at bedtime. Do not take more than 4 softgels in 24 hours unless directed by a doctor.

WARNINGS

Keep out of reach of children.

OTHER INFORMATION

- **do not use if carton or any blister unit is open or broken**
- store at room temperature. Avoid high humidity and excessive heat (40°C).

INACTIVE INGREDIENTS

FD&C blue #1, FD&C red #40, gelatin, glycerin, peppermint oil, titanium dioxide.

HOW SUPPLIED

Softgels in 12s, 24s blister packaging. Each Maximum Strength GasAid softgel is oval, green in color, and imprinted with "I-G" on one side.

Shown in Product Identification Guide, page 321

IMODIUM® ℞
(loperamide HCl) Capsules

DESCRIPTION

IMODIUM® (loperamide hydrochloride), 4-(p-chlorophenyl)-4-hydroxy-N, N-dimethyl-α,α-diphenyl-1-piperidinebutyramide monohydrochloride, is a synthetic antidiarrheal for oral use.

IMODIUM® is available in 2 mg capsules.

The inactive ingredients are: Lactose, cornstarch, talc, and magnesium stearate. IMODIUM® capsules contain FD&C Yellow No. 6.

CLINICAL PHARMACOLOGY

In vitro and animal studies show that IMODIUM® (loperamide hydrochloride) acts by slowing intestinal motility and by affecting water and electrolyte movement through the bowel. IMODIUM® inhibits peristaltic activity by a direct effect on the circular and longitudinal muscles of the intestinal wall.

In man, IMODIUM® prolongs the transit time of the intestinal contents. It reduces the daily fecal volume, increases the viscosity and bulk density, and diminishes the loss of fluid and electrolytes. Tolerance to the antidiarrheal effect has not been observed.

Clinical studies have indicated that the apparent elimination half-life of loperamide in man is 10.8 hours with a range of 9.1–14.4 hours. Plasma levels of unchanged drug remain below 2 nanograms per ml after the intake of a 2 mg capsule of IMODIUM®. Plasma levels are highest approximately five hours after administration of the capsule and 2.5 hours after the liquid. The peak plasma levels of loperamide were similar for both formulations. Of the total excreted in urine and feces, most of the administered drug was excreted in feces.

In those patients in whom biochemical and hematological parameters were monitored during clinical trials, no trends toward abnormality during IMODIUM® therapy were noted. Similarly, urinalyses, EKG and clinical ophthalmological examinations did not show trends toward abnormality.

INDICATIONS AND USAGE

IMODIUM® (loperamide hydrochloride) is indicated for the control and symptomatic relief of acute nonspecific diarrhea and of chronic diarrhea associated with inflammatory bowel disease. IMODIUM® is also indicated for reducing the volume of discharge from ileostomies.

CONTRAINDICATIONS

IMODIUM® (loperamide hydrochloride) is contraindicated in patients with known hypersensitivity to the drug and in those in whom constipation must be avoided.

WARNINGS

IMODIUM® (loperamide hydrochloride) should not be used in the case of acute dysentery, which is characterized by blood in stools and high fever.

Fluid and electrolyte depletion often occur in patients who have diarrhea. In such cases, administration of appropriate fluid and electrolytes is very important. The use of IMODIUM® does not preclude the need for appropriate fluid and electrolyte therapy.

In some patients with acute ulcerative colitis, and in pseudomembranous colitis associated with broad-spectrum antibiotics, agents which inhibit intestinal motility or delay intestinal transit time have been reported to induce toxic megacolon.

IMODIUM® therapy should be discontinued promptly if abdominal distention, constipation, or ileus occurs.

IMODIUM® should be used with special caution in young children because of the greater variability of response in this age group. Dehydration, particularly in younger children, may further influence the variability of response to IMODIUM®.

PRECAUTIONS

General

Extremely rare allergic reactions including anaphylaxis and anaphylactic shock have been reported.

In acute diarrhea, if clinical improvement is not observed in 48 hours, the administration of IMODIUM® (loperamide hydrochloride) should be discontinued. Patients with hepatic dysfunction should be monitored closely for signs of CNS toxicity because of the apparent large first pass biotransformation.

Information for Patients

Patients should be advised to check with their physician if their diarrhea does not improve after a couple of days or if they note blood in their stools or develop a fever.

Drug Interactions

There was no evidence in clinical trials of drug interactions with concurrent medications.

Carcinogenesis, mutagenesis, impairment of fertility

In an 18-month rat study with doses up to 133 times the maximum human dose (on a mg/kg basis), there was no evidence of carcinogenesis. Mutagenicity studies were not conducted. Reproduction studies in rats indicated that high doses (150–200 times the human dose) could cause marked female infertility and reduced male fertility.

Pregnancy

Teratogenic Effects

Pregnancy Category B

Reproduction studies in rats and rabbits have revealed no evidence of impaired fertility or harm to the fetus at doses up to 30 times the human dose. Higher doses impaired the survival of mothers and nursing young. The studies offered no evidence of teratogenic activity. There are, however, no adequate and well controlled studies in pregnant women. Because animal reproduction studies are not always predictive of human response, this drug should be used during pregnancy only if clearly needed.

Nursing Mothers

It is not known whether this drug is excreted in human milk. Because many drugs are excreted in human milk, caution should be exercised when IMODIUM® is administered to a nursing woman.

Pediatric Use

See the "Warnings" Section for information on the greater variability of response in this age group.

In case of accidental overdosage of IMODIUM® by children, see "Overdosage" Section for suggested treatment.

ADVERSE REACTIONS

The adverse effects reported during clinical investigations of IMODIUM® (loperamide hydrochloride) are difficult to distinguish from symptoms associated with the diarrheal syndrome. Adverse experiences recorded during clinical studies with IMODIUM® were generally of a minor and self-limiting nature. They were more commonly observed during the treatment of chronic diarrhea.

The following adverse events have been reported: hypersensitivity reactions such as skin rash and urticaria, and extremely rare cases of anaphylactic shock and bullous erup-

tion including Toxic Epidermal Necrolysis. In the majority of these cases, the patients were on other medications which may have caused or contributed to the events.
The following patient complaints have also been reported: abdominal pain, distention or discomfort, nausea, vomiting, constipation, tiredness, drowsiness or dizziness and dry mouth.
There have been rare reports of paralytic ileus associated with abdominal distention. Most of these reports occurred in the setting of acute dysentery, overdose, and with very young children of less than two years of age.

DRUG ABUSE AND DEPENDENCE

Abuse

A specific clinical study designed to assess the abuse potential of loperamide at high doses resulted in a finding of extremely low abuse potential.

Dependence

Studies in morphine-dependent monkeys demonstrated that loperamide hydrochloride at doses above those recommended for humans prevented signs of morphine withdrawal. However, in humans, the naloxone challenge pupil test, which when positive indicates opiate-like effects, performed after a single high dose, or after more than two years of therapeutic use of IMODIUM® (loperamide hydrochloride), was negative. Orally administered IMODIUM® (loperamide formulated with magnesium stearate) is both highly insoluble and penetrates the CNS poorly.

OVERDOSAGE

In cases of overdosage, paralytic ileus and CNS depression may occur. Children may be more sensitive to CNS effects than adults. Clinical trials have demonstrated that a slurry of activated charcoal administered promptly after ingestion of loperamide hydrochloride can reduce the amount of drug which is absorbed into the systemic circulation by as much as ninefold. If vomiting occurs spontaneously upon ingestion, a slurry of 100 gms of activated charcoal should be administered orally as soon as fluids can be retained.
If vomiting has not occurred, gastric lavage should be performed followed by administration of 100 gms of the activated charcoal slurry through the gastric tube. In the event of overdosage, patients should be monitored for signs of CNS depression for at least 24 hours. Children may be more sensitive to central nervous system effects than adults. If CNS depression is observed, naloxone may be administered. If responsive to naloxone, vital signs must be monitored carefully for recurrence of symptoms of drug overdose for at least 24 hours after the last dose of naloxone.
In view of the prolonged action of loperamide and the short duration (one to three hours) of naloxone, the patient must be monitored closely and treated repeatedly with naloxone as indicated. Since relatively little drug is excreted in the urine, forced diuresis is not expected to be effective for IMODIUM® (loperamide hydrochloride) overdosage.
In clinical trials an adult who took three 20 mg doses within a 24 hour period was nauseated after the second dose and vomited after the third dose. In studies designed to examine the potential for side effects, intentional ingestion of up to 60 mg of loperamide hydrochloride in a single dose to healthy subjects resulted in no significant adverse effects.

DOSAGE AND ADMINISTRATION

(1 capsule = 2 mg)
Patients should receive appropriate fluid and electrolyte replacement as needed.

Acute Diarrhea

Adults: The recommended initial dose is 4 mg (two capsules) followed by 2 mg (one capsule) after each unformed stool. Daily dosage should not exceed 16 mg (eight capsules). Clinical improvement is usually observed within 48 hours.
Children: IMODIUM® (loperamide hydrochloride) use is not recommended for children under 2 years of age. In children 2 to 5 years of age (20 kg or less), the non-prescription liquid formulation (IMODIUM A-D 1 mg/5 ml) should be used; for ages 6 to 12, either IMODIUM® Capsules of IMODIUM® A-D liquid may be used. For children 2 to 12 years of age, the following schedule for capsules or liquid will usually fulfill initial dosage requirements:

Recommended First Day Dosage Schedule •

Two to five years: 1 mg t.i.d. (3 mg daily dose) (13 to 20 kg)
Six to eight years: 2 mg b.i.d. (4 mg daily dose) (20 to 30 kg)
Eight to twelve years: 2 mg t.i.d. (6 mg daily dose) (greater than 30 kg)

Recommended Subsequent Daily Dosage

Following the first treatment day, it is recommended that subsequent IMODIUM® doses (1 mg/10 kg body weight) be administered only after a loose stool. Total daily dosage should not exceed recommended dosages for the first day.

Chronic Diarrhea

Children: Although IMODIUM® has been studied in a limited number of children with chronic diarrhea, the therapeutic dose for the treatment of chronic diarrhea in a pediatric population has not been established.
Adults: The recommended initial dose is 4 mg (two capsules) followed by 2 mg (one capsule) after each unformed stool until diarrhea is controlled, after which the dosage of IMODIUM® should be reduced to meet individual requirements. When the optimal daily dosage has been established, this amount may then be administered as a single dose or in divided doses.
The average daily maintenance dosage in clinical trials was 4 to 8 mg (two to four capsules). A dosage of 16 mg (eight capsules) was rarely exceeded. If clinical improvement is not observed after treatment with 16 mg per day for at least 10 days, symptoms are unlikely to be controlled by further administration. IMODIUM® administration may be continued if diarrhea cannot be adequately controlled with diet or specific treatment.

HOW SUPPLIED

Capsules—each capsule contains 2 mg of loperamide hydrochloride. The capsules have a light green body and a dark green cap with "JANSSEN" imprinted on one segment and "IMODIUM" on the other segment. IMODIUM® capsules are supplied in bottles of 100.
NDC 50458-400-10
(100 capsules)
Store at 15°–25°C (59°–77°F).
Revised September 1996, July 1998
©Janssen Pharmaceutica Inc. 1998
CAUTION: FEDERAL LAW PROHIBITS DISPENSING WITHOUT A PRESCRIPTION
U.S. Patent 3,714,159 7502205
Distributed by
McNeil Consumer Specialty Pharmaceuticals

IMODIUM® A–D LIQUID AND CAPLETS OTC
(loperamide hydrochloride)

DESCRIPTION

Each 5 mL (teaspoonful) of *IMODIUM® A-D* liquid contains loperamide hydrochloride 1 mg. *IMODIUM® A-D* liquid is stable, cherry-mint flavored, and clear in color.
Each caplet of *IMODIUM® A-D* contains 2 mg of loperamide hydrochloride and is scored and colored green.

ACTIONS

IMODIUM® A-D contains a clinically proven antidiarrheal medication. Loperamide HCl acts by slowing intestinal motility and by affecting water and electrolyte movement through the bowel.

USES

controls symptoms of diarrhea, including Travelers' Diarrhea.

DIRECTIONS

- **drink plenty of clear fluids to help prevent dehydration caused by diarrhea**
- find right dose on chart. If possible, use weight to dose; otherwise, use age

adults and children 12 years and over	4 teaspoonfuls (1 dosage cup) or 2 caplets after the first loose stool; 2 teaspoonfuls or 1 caplet after each subsequent loose stool; but no more than 8 teaspoonfuls or 4 caplets in 24 hours
children 9–11 years (60–95 lbs)	2 teaspoonfuls (½ dosage cup) or 1 caplet after first loose stool; 1 teaspoonful or ½ caplet after each subsequent loose stool; but no more than 6 teaspoonfuls or 3 caplets in 24 hours
children 6–8 years (48–59 lbs)	2 teaspoonfuls (½ dosage cup) or 1 caplet after first loose stool; 1 teaspoonful or ½ caplet after each subsequent loose stool; but no more than 4 teaspoonfuls or 2 caplets in 24 hours
children under 6 years (up to 47 lbs)	ask a doctor

Imodium A-D Liquid Professional Dosage Schedule for children 2–5 years old (24–47 lbs): 1 teaspoonful after first loose bowel movement, followed by 1 after each subsequent loose bowel movement. Do not exceed 3 teaspoonfuls a day.

WARNINGS

Allergy alert: Do not use if you have ever had a rash or other allergic reaction to loperamide HCl
Do not use if you have bloody or black stool
Ask a doctor before use if you have
• fever • mucus in the stool • a history of liver disease
Stop use and ask a doctor if
• symptoms get worse • diarrhea lasts for more than 2 days
If pregnant or breast feeding, ask a health professional before use. **Keep out of reach of children.** In case of overdose, get medical help or contact a Poison Control Center right away.

OTHER INFORMATION

Liquid:
- **do not use if carton is opened or if printed plastic neck wrap is broken or missing**
- store between 20–25°C (68–77°F)

Caplets:
- store between 20–25°C (68–77°F)
- **do not use if carton or blister unit is open or torn**

Professional Information:

Overdosage Information

Overdosage of loperamide HCl in man may result in constipation, CNS depression and nausea. A slurry of activated charcoal administered promptly after ingestion of loperamide hydrochloride can reduce the amount of drug which is absorbed. If vomiting occurs spontaneously upon ingestion, a slurry of 100 grams of activated charcoal should be administered orally as soon as fluids can be retained. If vomiting has not occurred, and CNS depression is evident, gastric lavage should be performed followed by administration of 100 gms of the activated charcoal slurry through the gastric tube. In the event of overdosage, patients should be monitored for signs of CNS depression for at least 24 hours. Children may be more sensitive to central nervous system effects than adults. If CNS depression is observed, naloxone may be administered. If responsive to naloxone, vital signs must be monitored carefully for recurrence of symptoms of drug overdose for at least 24 hours after the last dose of naloxone.

INACTIVE INGREDIENTS

Liquid: alcohol 0.5%, benzoic acid, citric acid, flavors, glycerin, propylene glycol, purified water, sodium benzoate, sorbitol, sucrose.
Caplets: colloidal silicon dioxide, D&C yellow no. 10, dibasic calcium phosphate, FD&C blue no. 1, magnesium stearate, microcrystalline cellulose.

HOW SUPPLIED

Liquid: Cherry-mint flavored liquid (clear) 2 fl. oz. and 4 fl. oz. tamper evident bottles with child resistant safety caps and special dosage cups.
Caplets: Green scored caplets in 6s, 12s, 18s, 24s, 48s and 72s blister packaging which is tamper evident and child resistant.

Shown in Product Identification Guide, page 321

IMODIUM® ADVANCED OTC
(loperamide HCl/simethicone)
Caplets & Chewable Tablets

DESCRIPTION

Each easy to swallow caplet and mint-flavored chewable tablet of *Imodium® Advanced* contains loperamide HCl 2 mg/simethicone 125 mg.

ACTIONS

Imodium® Advanced combines original prescription strength Imodium® to control the symptoms of diarrhea plus simethicone to relieve bloating, pressure and cramps commonly referred to as gas. Loperamide HCl acts by slowing intestinal motility and by affecting water and electrolyte movement through the bowel. Simethicone acts in the stomach and intestines by altering the surface tension of gas bubbles enabling them to coalesce, thereby freeing and eliminating the gas more easily by belching or passing flatus.

USE

Controls symptoms of diarrhea plus bloating, pressure, and cramps commonly referred to as gas.

DIRECTIONS

- **drink plenty of clear fluids to help prevent dehydration caused by diarrhea**
- find right dose on chart. If possible, use weight to dose; otherwise use age

adults and children 12 years and over	swallow 2 caplets or chew 2 tablets and take with water (for chewables) after the first loose stool; 1 caplet/tablet and take with water (for chewables) after each subsequent loose stool; but no more than 4 caplets/tablets in 24 hours
children 9–11 years (60–95 lbs)	swallow 1 caplet or chew 1 tablet and take with water (for chewables) after the first loose stool; ½ caplet/tablet and take with water (for chewables) after each subsequent loose stool; but no more than 3 caplets/tablets in 24 hours
children 6–8 years (48–59 lbs)	swallow 1 caplet or chew 1 tablet and take with water (for chewables) after the first loose stool; ½ caplet/tablet and take with water (for chewables) after each subsequent loose stool; but no more than 2 caplets/tablets in 24 hours
children under 6 years (up to 47 lbs)	ask a doctor

Continued on next page

Imodium Advanced—Cont.

WARNINGS

Allergy alert: Do not use if you have ever had a rash or other allergic reaction to loperamide HCl

Do not use if you have bloody or black stool

Ask a doctor before use if you have • fever • mucus in the stool • a history of liver disease

Ask a doctor or pharmacist before use if you are taking antibiotics

Stop use and ask a doctor if • symptoms get worse • diarrhea lasts for more than 2 days

If pregnant or breast-feeding, ask a health professional before use.

Keep out of reach of children. In case of overdose, get medical help or contact a Poison Control Center right away.

OTHER INFORMATION

Caplets:
- store between 20–25°C (68–77°F)
- protect from light

Blister statement:
- do not use if carton is open or if blister unit is open or torn

Bottle statement:
- do not use if carton if open or if printed foil seal under bottle cap is open or torn

Chewable Tablets:
- do not use if carton is opened or if blister unit is broken
- store between 20–25°C (68–77°F)

Professional Information:

Overdosage Information:

Overdosage of loperamide HCl in man may result in constipation, CNS depression and nausea. A slurry of activated charcoal administered promptly after ingestion of loperamide hydrochloride can reduce the amount of drug which is absorbed. If vomiting occurs spontaneously upon ingestion, a slurry of 100 grams of activated charcoal should be administered orally as soon as fluids can be retained. If vomiting has not occurred, and CNS depression is evident, gastric lavage should be performed followed by administration of 100 gms of the activated charcoal slurry through the gastric tube. In the event of overdosage, patients should be monitored for signs of CNS depression for at least 24 hours. Children may be more sensitive to central nervous system effects than adults. If CNS depression is observed, naloxone may be administered. If responsive to naloxone, vital signs must be monitored carefully for recurrence of symptoms of drug overdose for at least 24 hours after the last dose of naloxone. No treatment is necessary for the simethicone ingestion in this circumstance.

INACTIVE INGREDIENTS

Caplets: acesulfame K, cellulose, dibasic calcium phosphate, flavor, sodium starch glycolate, stearic acid **Chewable Tablets:** cellulose acetate, corn starch, D&C Yellow No. 10, dextrates, FD&C Blue No. 1, flavors, microcrystalline cellulose, polymethacrylates, saccharin sodium, sorbitol, stearic acid, sucrose, tribasic calcium phosphate.

HOW SUPPLIED

Mint Chewable Tablets in 6's, 12's, 18's, 30's, and blister packaging which is tamper evident and child resistant. Each Imodium® Advanced tablet is round, light green in color and has "IMODIUM" embossed on one side and "2/125" on the other side. Imodium Advanced Caplets are available in blister packs of 12's and 18's and bottles of 30's and 42's. Each Imodium® Advanced Caplet is oval, white color and has "IMO" embossed on one side and "2/125" on the other side.

Shown in Product Identification Guide, page 321

LACTAID® ORIGINAL STRENGTH CAPLETS OTC
(lactase enzyme)

LACTAID® EXTRA STRENGTH CAPLETS
(lactase enzyme)

LACTAID® ULTRA CAPLETS AND CHEWABLE TABLETS
(lactase enzyme)

DESCRIPTION

Each serving size (3 caplets) of *LACTAID® Original Strength* contains 9000 FCC (Food Chemical Codex) units of lactase enzyme (derived from *Aspergillus oryzae*).

Each serving size (2 caplets) of *LACTAID® Extra Strength* contains 9000 FCC units of lactase enzyme (derived from *Aspergillus oryzae*).

Each serving size (1 caplet) of *LACTAID® Ultra Caplet* contains 9000 FCC units of lactase enzyme (derived from *Aspergillus oryzae*).

Each serving size (1 tablet) of *LACTAID® Ultra Chewable Tablet* contains 9000 FCC units of lactase enzyme (derived from *Aspergillus oryzae*).

LACTAID® is the original lactase dietary supplement that makes milk and dairy foods more digestible for individuals with lactose intolerance. *LACTAID®* lactase enzyme hydrolyzes lactose into two digestible simple sugars: glucose and galactose. *LACTAID® Caplets/Chewable Tablets* are taken orally for *in vivo* hydrolysis of lactose.

ACTIONS

LACTAID® Caplets/Chewable Tablets work by providing the enzyme that hydrolyzes the milk sugar lactose (disaccharide) into the two monosaccharides, glucose and galactose.

USES

LACTAID contains a natural enzyme that helps your body break down lactose, the complex sugar found in dairy foods. If not properly digested, lactose can cause flatulence, bloating, cramps or diarrhea.*

*This statement has not been evaluated by the Food and Drug Administration. This product is not intended to diagnose, treat, cure, or prevent any disease.

DIRECTIONS

Original Strength: Swallow 3 caplets with your first bite of dairy foods to help prevent symptoms. **Extra Strength:** Swallow 2 caplets with your first bite of dairy foods to help prevent synptoms. **Ultra Caplets:** Take 1 caplet with your first bite of dairy foods to help prevent symptoms. You may have to take more than 1 caplet, but no more than 2 at a time. **Ultra Chewables:** Chew 1 chewable tablet with your first bite of dairy foods to help prevent symptoms. You may have to take more than 1 chewable tablet but no more than 2 at a time.

WARNINGS

Consult your doctor if your symptoms continue after using the product or if your symptoms are unusual and seem unrelated to eating dairy. Keep out of reach of children. **Do not use if carton is open or if printed plastic neckwrap is broken or if single serve packet is open.**

LACTAID® Ultra Chewable Tablets: **Phenylketonurics Contains: Phenylalanine.**

INGREDIENTS

LACTAID® Original Strength Caplets: Lactase Enzyme (9000 FCC Lactase units/3 caplets), Mannitol, Cellulose, Sodium Citrate, Magnesium Stearate.

LACTAID® Extra Strength Caplets: Lactase Enzyme (9000 FCC Lactase units/2 caplets), Mannitol, Cellulose, Sodium Citrate, Magnesium Stearate.

LACTAID® Ultra Caplets: Lactase Enzyme (9000 FCC Lactase units/Caplet), Cellulose, Sodium Citrate, Magnesium Stearate, Colloidal Silicon Dioxide.

LACTAID® Ultra Chewable Tablets: Lactase Enzyme (9000 FCC Lactase units/tablet), Mannitol, Cellulose, Sodium Citrate, Magnesium Stearate, Natural and Artificial Flavor, Citric Acid, Acesulfame K, Aspartame.

HOW SUPPLIED

LACTAID® Original Strength Caplets are available in bottles of 120 count. Store at or below room temperature (below 77°F) but do not refrigerate. Keep away from heat.

LACTAID® Extra Strength Caplets are available in bottles of 50 count. Store at or below room temperature (below 77°F) but do not refrigerate. Keep away from heat.

LACTAID® Ultra Caplets are available in single serve packets in 12, 32, 60 and 90 count packages. Store at or below 86°F. Keep away from heat. *LACTAID® Ultra Chewable Tablets* are available in single serve packets of 32 and 60 counts. Store at or below room temperature (below 77°F), but do not refrigerate. Keep away from heat and moisture.

LACTAID® Caplets and *LACTAID® Ultra Chewable Tablets* are certified kosher from the Orthodox Union.

Also available: 100% lactose-free Lactaid Milk.

Shown in Product Identification Guide, page 321

MOTRIN® IB Ibuprofen Pain Reliever/Fever Reducer OTC
Tablets, Caplets and Gelcaps

DESCRIPTION

Each *MOTRIN® IB Tablet, Caplet and Gelcap* contains ibuprofen 200 mg.

USES

Temporarily relieves minor aches and pains due to:
• headache • muscular aches • minor pain of arthritis • toothache • backache • the common cold • menstrual cramps

Temporarily reduces fever

DIRECTIONS
- **do not take more than directed**

adults and children 12 years and older	• take 1 tablet, caplet, or gelcap every 4 to 6 hours while symptoms persist • if pain or fever does not respond to 1 tablet, caplet or gelcap, 2 tablets, caplets or gelcaps may be used, • do not exceed 6 tablets, caplets or gelcaps in 24 hours, unless directed by a doctor • the smallest effective dose should be used
children under 12 years	• ask a doctor

WARNINGS

Allergy alert: Ibuprofen may cause a severe allergic reaction which may include:
- hives • facial swelling
- asthma (wheezing) • shock

Stomach bleeding warning: Taking more than recommended may cause stomach bleeding.

Alcohol Warning: If you consume 3 or more alcoholic drinks every day, ask your doctor whether you should take ibuprofen or other pain relievers/fever reducers. Ibuprofen may cause stomach bleeding.

Do not use if you have ever had an allergic reaction to any other pain reliever/fever reducer.

Ask a doctor before use if you have
- problems or serious side effects from taking pain relievers or fever reducers
- stomach problems that last or come back, such as heartburn, upset stomach, or pain
- ulcers
- bleeding problems
- high blood pressure, heart or kidney disease, are taking a diuretic, or are over 65 years of age.

Ask a doctor or pharmacist before use if you are
- under a doctor's care for any serious condition
- taking any other product that contains ibuprofen, or any other pain reliever/fever reducer
- taking a prescription drug for anticoagulation (blood thinning)
- taking any other drug

When using this product take with food or milk if stomach upset occurs.

Stop use and ask a doctor if
- an allergic reaction occurs. Seek medical help right away.
- pain gets worse or lasts more than 10 days
- fever gets worse or lasts more than 3 days
- stomach pain or upset gets worse or lasts
- redness or swelling is present in the painful area
- any new symptoms appear.

If pregnant or breast-feeding, ask a health professional before use. It is especially important not to use ibuprofen during the last 3 months of pregnancy unless definitely directed to do so by a doctor because it may cause problems in the unborn child or complications during delivery.

Keep out of reach of children. In case of overdose, get medical help or contact a Poison Control Center right away.

Other Information
- **Do not use if neck wrap or foil inner seal imprinted "Safety Seal®" is broken or missing.**
- Store at 20°–25°C (68°–77°F) (applies to gelcaps only)
- avoid high humidity and excessive heat above 40°C (104°F) (applies to gelcaps only)

Professional Information:

Overdosage Information for Adult Motrin®

IBUPROFEN

The *toxicity of ibuprofen* overdose is dependent upon the amount of drug ingested and the time elapsed since ingestion, though individual response may vary, which makes it necessary to evaluate each case individually. Although uncommon, serious toxicity and death have been reported in the medical literature with ibuprofen overdosage. The most frequently reported symptoms of ibuprofen overdose include abdominal pain, nausea, vomiting, lethargy and drowsiness. Other central nervous system symptoms include headache, tinnitus, CNS depression and seizures. Metabolic acidosis, coma, acute renal failure and apnea (primarily in very young children) may rarely occur. Cardiovascular toxicity, including hypotension, bradycardia, tachycardia and atrial fibrillation, also have been reported. The *treatment of acute ibuprofen overdose* is primarily supportive. Management of hypotension, acidosis and gastrointestinal bleeding may be necessary. In cases of acute overdose, the stomach should be emptied through ipecac-induced emesis or lavage. Emesis is most effective if initiated within 30 minutes of ingestion. Orally administered activated charcoal may help in reducing the absorption and reabsorption of ibuprofen. In children, the estimated amount of ibuprofen ingested per body weight may be helpful to predict the potential for development of toxicity although each case must be evaluated. Ingestion of less than 100 mg/kg is unlikely to produce toxicity. Children ingesting 100 to 200 mg/kg may be managed with induced emesis and a minimal observation time of four hours. Children ingesting 200 to 400 mg/kg of ibuprofen should have immediate gastric emptying and at least four hours observation in a health care facility. Children ingesting greater than 400 mg/kg require immediate medical referral, careful observation and appropriate supportive therapy. Ipecac-induced emesis is not recommended in overdoses greater than 400 mg/kg because of the risk of convulsions and the potential for aspiration of gastric contents. In adult patients the history of the dose reportedly ingested does not appear to be predictive of toxicity. The need for referral and follow-up must be judged by the circumstances at the time of the overdose ingestion. Symptomatic adults should be admitted to a health care facility for observation.

Our Adult MOTRIN® combination products contain pseudoephedrine in addition to ibuprofen. For basic overdose information regarding pseudoephedrine, please see below. For additional emergency information, please contact your local poison control center.

PSEUDOEPHEDRINE

Symptoms from pseudoephedrine overdose consist most often of mild anxiety, tachycardia and/or mild hypertension. Symptoms usually appear within 4 to 8 hours and are transient, usually requiring no treatment.

INACTIVE INGREDIENTS

Tablets and Caplets: carnauba wax, corn starch, FD&C Yellow #6, hypromellose, iron oxide, polydextrose, polyethylene glycol, silicon dioxide, stearic acid, titanium dioxide.

Gelcaps: benzyl alcohol, butylparaben, castor oil, cellulose, corn starch, edetate calcium disodium, FD&C Yellow No. 6, gelatin, hypromellose, iron oxide, methylparaben, povidone, propylparaben, silicon dioxide, sodium lauryl sulfate, sodium propionate, sodium starch glycolate, titanium dioxide.

HOW SUPPLIED

Tablets: (orange, printed "MOTRIN IB" in black) in tamper evident packaging of 24, 50, 100, and 165.

Caplets: (orange, printed "MOTRIN IB" in black) in tamper evident packaging of 24, 50, 100, 165, 250, 300 and

Gelcaps: (colored orange and white, printed "MOTRIN IB" in black) in tamper evident packaging of 24, 50 and 100.

Shown in Product Identification Guide, page 321

MOTRIN® Ibuprofen Suspension ℞
100 mg/5 mL

DESCRIPTION

The active ingredient in MOTRIN is ibuprofen, which is a member of the propionic acid group of nonsteroidal anti-inflammatory drugs (NSAIDs). Ibuprofen is a racemic mixture of [+]S- and [−]R-enantiomers. It is a white to off-white crystalline powder, with a melting point of 74° to 77°C. It is practically insoluble in water (<0.1 mg/mL), but readily soluble in organic solvents such as ethanol and acetone. Ibuprofen has a pKa of 4.43±0.03 and an n-octanol/water partition coefficient of 11.7 at pH 7.4. The chemical name for ibuprofen is (±)-2-(p-isobutylphenyl) propionic acid. The molecular weight of ibuprofen is 206.28. Its molecular formula is $C_{13}H_{18}O_2$ and it has the following structural formula:

MOTRIN Suspension is a sucrose-sweetened, orange-colored, berry-flavored liquid suspension containing 100 mg of ibuprofen in 5 mL (20 mg/mL). Inactive ingredients include citric acid, glycerin, polysorbate 80, pregelatinized starch, purified water, sodium benzoate, sucrose, xanthan gum, D&C Yellow #10 and FD&C Red #40, and artificial flavors.

MOTRIN Oral Drops (intended for pediatric use only) is a sucrose-sweetened, pink-colored, berry-flavored liquid suspension containing 40 mg of ibuprofen per mL. Inactive ingredients include citric acid, glycerin, polysorbate 80, pregelatinized starch, purified water, sodium benzoate, sorbitol, sucrose, xanthan gum, FD&C Red #40, and artificial flavors.

MOTRIN Chewable Tablets are aspartame-sweetened, citrus-tasting, orange-colored tablets, that contain 50 mg or 100 mg of ibuprofen per tablet. Inactive ingredients include aspartame, citric acid, hydroxyethyl cellulose, hydroxypropyl methylcellulose, magnesium stearate, mannitol, microcrystalline cellulose, povidone, sodium lauryl sulfate, sodium starch glycolate, FD&C Yellow #6, and artificial flavors.

MOTRIN Caplets are unsweetened, white-colored, unflavored, film-coated, capsule-shaped tablets, containing 100 mg of ibuprofen per tablet. Inactive ingredients include carnauba wax, colloidal silicone dioxide, cornstarch, hydroxypropyl methylcellulose, microcrystalline cellulose, polydextrose, polyethylene glycol, pregelatinized starch, propylene glycol, sodium starch glycolate, titanium dioxide, triacetin, D&C Yellow #10, and FD&C Yellow #6.

CLINICAL PHARMACOLOGY

Pharmacodynamics—Ibuprofen is a nonsteroidal anti-inflammatory drug (NSAID) that possesses anti-inflammatory, analgesic and antipyretic activity. Its mode of action, like that of other NSAIDs, is not completely understood, but may be related to prostaglandin synthetase inhibition. After absorption of the racemic ibuprofen, the [−]R-enantiomer undergoes interconversion to the [+]S-form. The biological activities of ibuprofen are associated with the [+]S-enantiomer.

In clinical studies in adult patients with rheumatoid arthritis and osteoarthritis, ibuprofen has been shown to be comparable to aspirin in controlling pain and inflammation, though causing fewer of the mild gastrointestinal side effects (see ADVERSE REACTIONS). MOTRIN may be well tolerated in some patients who have had gastrointestinal side effects with aspirin, but these patients, when treated with MOTRIN, should be carefully followed for signs and symptoms of gastrointestinal ulceration and bleeding. Although it is not definitely known whether ibuprofen causes

Table 1
Pharmacokinetic Parameters of Ibuprofen Formulations [Mean Values (% coefficient of variation)]

Dose	200mg (= 2.8 mg/kg) in Adults				10 mg/kg in Febrile Children	
Formulation	Suspension	Drops	Caplet	Chewable Tablet	Suspension	Chewable Tablet
Number of Patients	24	24	25	24	18	18
AUCinf (μg·h/mL)	64 (27%)	74 (19%)	60 (19%)	66 (22%)	155 (24%)	176 (25%)
Cmax (μg/mL)	19 (22%)	24 (21%)	20 (18%)	15 (24%)	55 (23%)	43 (39%)
Tmax (h)	0.79 (69%)	1.0 (60%)	1.04 (50%)	2.0 (56%)	0.97 (57%)	1.43 (69%)
Cl/F (mL/h/kg)	45.6 (22%)	43.4 (18%)	45.0 (19%)	42.8 (18%)	68.6 (22%)	60.9 (27%)

Legend: AUCinf = Area-under-the-curve to infinity
Tmax = Time-to-peak plasma concentration
Cmax = Peak plasma concentration
Cl/F = Clearance divided by fraction at drug absorbed

less peptic ulceration than aspirin, in one study involving 885 adult patients with rheumatoid arthritis treated for up to one year (438 patients on ibuprofen and 447 patients on aspirin), there were no reports of gastric ulceration with ibuprofen whereas frank ulceration was reported in 13 patients in the aspirin group (statistically significant p<.001). Gastroscopic studies at varying doses of ibuprofen showed an increased tendency toward endoscopic lesions at higher doses. However, at clinically comparable doses (2,400 mg of ibuprofen vs. 3,600 mg of aspirin), endoscopic lesions were approximately half that seen with aspirin. Studies using ^{51}Cr-tagged red cells indicate that fecal blood loss associated with ibuprofen in doses up to 2400 mg daily did not exceed the range of normal, and was significantly less than that seen in aspirin-treated patients. The clinical significance of these findings is unknown.

Pharmacokinetics—As noted in the DESCRIPTION section, ibuprofen is a racemic mixture of [−]R-and [+]S-isomers. *In vivo* and *in vitro* studies indicate that the [+]S-isomer is responsible for clinial activity. The [−]R-form, while thought to be pharmacologically inactive, is slowly and incompletely (~60%) interconverted into the active [+]S species in adults. The degree of interconversion in children is unknown, but is thought to be similar. The [−]R-isomer serves as a circulating reservoir to maintain levels of active drug. Ibuprofen is well absorbed orally, with less than 1% being excreted in the urine unchanged. It has a biphasic elimination time curve with a plasma half-life of approximately 2 hours. Studies in febrile children have established the dose-proportionality of 5 and 10 mg/kg doses of ibuprofen. Studies in adults have established the dose-proportionality of ibuprofen as a single oral dose from 50 to 600 mg for total drug and up to 1200 mg for free drug.

Absorption—*In vivo* studies indicate that ibuprofen is well absorbed orally from the suspension, drops, caplet and chewable tablet formulations, with peak plasma levels usually occurring within 1 to 2 hours. The pharmacokinetic differences between the products in adults (see Table 1) are due to differences in the rate of absorption of ibuprofen from the various dosage forms. The observed differences in the table between adults and children, in terms of AUC and C_{max}, are due to both differences in dose per body weight and age-or fever-related change in volume of distribution (Vd/F). All of the formulations are equally bioavailable in terms of peak plasma levels (C_{max}) and extent of absorption (AUC), however, the time-to-peak (T_{max}) is different between the products. Clinically, this has been shown to have no effect on either onset or peak fever reduction in children. [See table 1 above]

Antacid—A bioavailability study in adults has shown that there was no interference with the absorption of ibuprofen when given in conjunction with an antacid containing both aluminum hydroxide and magnesium hydroxide.

Food Effects—Absorption is most rapid when MOTRIN is given under fasting conditions. Administration of MOTRIN Suspension, MOTRIN Oral Drops, MOTRIN Chewable Tablets and MOTRIN Caplets with food affects the rate but not the extent of absorption. When taken with food, T_{max} is delayed by approximately 30 to 60 minutes, and peak levels are reduced by approximately 30 to 50%.

Distribution—Ibuprofen, like most other drugs of its class, is highly protein bound (>99% bound at 20 μg/mL). Protein binding is saturable and at concentrations >20 μg/mL binding is non-linear. Based on oral dosing data there is an age-or fever-related change in volume of distribution for ibuprofen. Febrile children <11 years old have a volume of approximately 0.2 L/kg while adults have a volume of approximately 0.12 L/kg. The clinical significance of these findings is unknown.

Metabolism—Following oral administration, the majority of the dose was recovered in the urine within 24 hours as the hydroxy-(25%) and carboxypropyl-(37%) phenylpropionic acid metabolites. The percentages of free and conjugated ibuprofen found in the urine were approximately 1% and 14%, respectively. The remainder of the drug was found in the stool as both metabolites and unabsorbed drug.

Elimination—Ibuprofen is rapidly metabolized and eliminated in the urine. The excretion of ibuprofen is virtually complete 24 hours after the last dose. It has a biphasic plasma elimination time curve with a half-life of approximately 2.0 hours. There is no difference in the observed terminal elimination rate or half-life between children and adults, however, there is an age-or fever-related change in total clearance. This suggests that the observed change in clearance is due to changes in the volume of distribution of ibuprofen (see Table 1 for Cl/F values).

Clinical Studies—Controlled clinical trials comparing doses of 5 and 10 mg/kg ibuprofen suspension and 10-15 mg/kg of acetaminophen elixir have been conducted in children 6 months to 12 years of age with fever primarily do to viral illnesses. In these studies there were no differences between treatments in fever reduction for the first hour and maximum fever reduction occurred between 2 and 4 hours. Response after 1 hour was dependent on both the level of temperature elevation as well as the treatment. In children with baseline temperatures at or below 102.5°F both ibuprofen doses and acetaminophen were equally effective in their maximum effect. In children with temperatures above 102.5°F, the ibuprofen 10 mg/kg dose was more effective. By 6 hours, children treated with ibuprofen 5mg/kg tended to have recurrence of fever, whereas children treated with ibuprofen 10 mg/kg still had significant fever reduction at 8 hours. In control groups treated with 10 mg/kg acetaminophen, fever reduction resembled that seen in children treated with 5 mg/kg of ibuprofen, with the exception that temperature elevation tended to return 1-2 hours earlier.

A comparison of MOTRIN Chewable Tablets and MOTRIN Suspension in febrile children showed similar antipyretic effects of the two formulations, lasting between 6 and 8 hours. No clinical studies of fever reduction in children have been performed with MOTRIN Caplets or MOTRIN Oral Drops.

Controlled single-dose clinical analgesia trials comparing doses of 5 and 10 mg/kg ibuprofen suspension with acetaminophen suspension 12.5 mg/kg and placebo, have been conducted in children 5 to 12 years of age, with sore throat pain due to an infectious agent, or ear pain due to acute otitis media. Onset of pain relief provided by ibuprofen was similar to that of acetaminophen, occurring within the first hour, usually around the half-hour mark. All active treatments showed significant pain relief versus placebo, and the 10 mg/kg dose of ibuprofen had a duration of analgesic effect of 6 to 8 hours. Ibuprofen 10 mg/kg provided more overall pain relief than the 5 mg/kg dose.

Controlled studies have demonstrated that ibuprofen is a more effective analgesic than propoxyphene for the relief of episiotomy pain, pain following dental extraction procedures, and for the relief of the symptoms of primary dysmenorrhea.

In patients with primary dysmenorrhea, ibuprofen has been shown to reduce elevated levels of prostaglandin activity in the menstrual fluid and to reduce resting and active intrauterine pressure, as well as the frequency of uterine contractions. The probable mechanism of action is to inhibit prostaglandin synthesis rather than simply to provide analgesia.

In clinical studies in adult patients with rheumatoid arthritis, ibuprofen has been shown to be comparable to indomethacin in controlling the signs and symptoms of disease activity, with a lower incidence of milder gastrointestinal and CNS side effects than indomethacin.

MOTRIN may be used in combination with gold salts and/or corticosteroids.

INDICATIONS AND USAGE

In Children MOTRIN is indicated:

- For reduction of fever in patients aged 6 months and older.
- For relief of mild to moderate pain in patients aged 6 months and older.
- For relief of signs and symptoms of juvenile arthritis.

In Adults MOTRIN is indicated:

- For relief of mild to moderate pain.

Continued on next page

Motrin—Cont.

- For treatment of primary dysmenorrhea.
- For relief of the signs and symptoms of rheumatoid arthritis and osteoarthritis.

Since there have been no controlled trials to demonstrate whether there is any beneficial effect or harmful interaction with the use of ibuprofen in conjuction with aspirin, the combination cannot be recommended (see PRECAUTIONS—Drug Interactions).

CONTRAINDICATIONS

MOTRIN should not be used in patients with previously demonstrated hypersensitivity to ibuprofen, or in individuals with a history of allergic manifestations to aspirin or other NSAIDs. Severe anaphylactic-like reactions to ibuprofen have been reported in such patients, some with fatal outcome.

WARNINGS

Risk of GI Ulceration, Bleeding and Perforation with NSAID Therapy. Serious gastrointestinal toxicity such as bleeding, ulceration, and perforation, can occur at any time, with or without warning symptoms, in patients treated chronically with NSAID therapy. Although minor upper gastrointestinal problems, such as dyspepsia, are common, usually developing early in therapy, physicians should remain alert for ulceration and bleeding in patients treated chronically with NSAIDs even in the absence of previous GI tract symptoms. In patients observed in clinical trials of several months to two years duration, symptomatic upper GI ulcers, gross bleeding or perforation appear to occur in approximately 1% of patients treated for 3–6 months, and in about 2–4% of patients treated for one year. Physicians should inform patients about the signs and/or symptoms of serious GI toxicity and what steps to take if they occur.

Studies to date have not identified any subset of patients not at risk of developing peptic ulceration and bleeding. Except for a prior history of serious GI events and other risk factors known to be associated with peptic ulcer disease, such as alcoholism, smoking, etc., no risk factors (e.g., age, sex) have been associated with increased risk. Elderly or debilitated patients seem to tolerate ulceration or bleeding less well than other individuals and most spontaneous reports of fatal GI events are in this population. Studies to date are inconclusive concerning the relative risk of various NSAIDs in causing such reactions. High doses of any NSAID probably carry a greater risk of these reactions, although controlled clinical trials showing this do not exist in most cases. In considering the use of relatively large doses (within the recommended dosage range), sufficient benefit should be anticipated to offset the potential increased risk of GI toxicity.

Anaphylactoid Reactions: Anaphylactoid reactions may occur even in patients without prior exposure to ibuprofen. Extreme caution should be exercised when giving MOTRIN to patients with bronchospastic reactivity (e.g., asthma), nasal polyps, or those with a history of angiodema. Emergency help should be sought in case such anaphylactoid reaction occurs.

Advanced Renal Disease: In cases with advanced kidney disease, treatment with MOTRIN should not be initiated; if MOTRIN is used in such cases, close monitoring of the patient's kidney functions is advisable (see PRECAUTIONS—Renal Effects).

PRECAUTIONS

Renal Effects: Caution should be used when initiating treatment with MOTRIN in patients with considerable dehydration. It is advisable to rehydrate patients first and then start therapy with MOTRIN. Caution is also recommended in patients with pre-existing kidney disease (see WARNINGS—Advanced Renal Disease).

As with other NSAIDs, long-term administration of ibuprofen to animals has resulted in renal papillary necrosis and other abnormal renal pathology. In humans, there have been reports of acute interstitial nephritis with hematuria, proteinuria, and occasionally nephrotic syndrome.

A second form of renal toxicity has been seen in patients with prerenal conditions leading to a reduction in renal blood flow or blood volume, where the renal prostaglandins have a supportive role in the maintenance of renal perfusion. In these patients, administration of an NSAID may cause a dose-dependent reduction in prostaglandin formation and may precipitate overt renal decompensation. Patients at greatest risk of this reaction are those with impaired renal function, heart failure, liver dysfunction, those taking diuretics and the elderly. Discontinuation of NSAID therapy is typically followed by recovery to the pre-treatment state.

Those patients at high risk, who chronically take ibuprofen, should have renal function monitored if they have signs or symptoms which may be consistent with mild azotemia, such as malaise, fatigue, loss of appetite, etc. Occasional patients may develop some elevation of serum creatinine and BUN levels without signs or symptoms.

Since ibuprofen is eliminated primarily by the kidneys, patients with significantly impaired renal function should be closely monitored and a reduction in dosage should be anticipated to avoid drug accumulation. Prospective studies on the safety of ibuprofen in patients with chronic renal failure have not been conducted.

Fluid Retention: Fluid retention and edema have been reported in association with ibuprofen, therefore, the drug should be used with caution in patients with a history of cardiac decompensation or hypertension.

Hematologic Effects: MOTRIN can inhibit platelet aggregation but, unlike aspirin, its effect on platelet function is reversible, quantitatively less, and of shorter duration. Because this prolonged bleeding effect may be exaggerated in patients with underlying hemostatic defects, MOTRIN should be used with caution in persons with intrinsic coagulation defects and those on anticoagulant therapy.

Hepatic Effects: As with other nonsteroidal anti-inflammatory drugs, borderline elevations of one or more liver laboratory tests may occur in up to 15% of patients. These abnormalities may progress, may remain essentially unchanged, or may be transient with continued therapy. The ALT (SGPT) test is probably the most sensitive indicator of liver dysfunction. Meaningful (3 times the upper limit of normal) elevations of ALT and AST (SGOT) occurred in controlled clinical trials in less than 1% of patients. A patient with symptoms and/or signs suggesting liver dysfunction, or in whom an abnormal liver test has occurred, should be evaluated for evidence of the development of more severe hepatic reactions while on therapy with MOTRIN. Severe hepatic reactions, including jaundice and cases of fatal hepatitis, have been reported with ibuprofen as with other nonsteroidal anti-inflammatory drugs. Although such reactions are rare, if abnormal liver tests persist or worsen, if clinical signs and symptoms consistent with liver disease develop, or if systemic manifestations occur (e.g., eosinophilia, rash, etc.), treatment with MOTRIN should be discontinued.

Aseptic Meningitis: Aseptic meningitis, with fever and coma, has been observed on rare occasions in patients on ibuprofen therapy. Although it is probably more likely to occur in patients with systemic lupus erythematosus and related connective tissue diseases, it has been reported in patients who do not have an underlying chronic disease. If signs or symptoms of meningitis develop in a patient receiving MOTRIN, the possibility of its being related to ibuprofen should be considered.

Other Precautions—The pharmacological activity of MOTRIN may induce reduction of fever and inflammation, thus diminishing their utility as diagnostic signs in detecting underlying conditions.

In order to avoid exacerbation of manifestations of adrenal insufficiency, patients who have been on prolonged corticosteroid therapy should have their therapy tapered slowly rather than discontinued abruptly when ibuprofen is added to the treatment program.

Blurred and/or diminished vision, scotomata, and/or changes in color vision have been reported. If a patient develops such complaints while receiving MOTRIN Chewable Tablets, the drug should be discontinued and the patient should have an ophthalmologic examination which includes central visual fields and color vision testing.

Phenylketonurics: MOTRIN Chewable Tablets 50 mg contain phenylalanine 3 mg per tablet, and the 100 mg tablets contain phenylalanine 6 mg per tablet.

Diabetics: MOTRIN Suspension and MOTRIN Oral Drops contain 0.3 g sucrose and 1.6 calories per mL, or 1.5 g sucrose and 8 calories per teaspoon, which should be taken into consideration when treating diabetic patients with this product.

Information for Patients—MOTRIN, like other drugs of its class, is not free of side effects. The side effects of these drugs can cause discomfort and, rarely, there are more serious side effects, such as gastrointestinal bleeding, which may result in hospitalization and even fatal outcomes.

NSAIDs are often essential agents in the management of arthritis, pain and fever, but they also may be commonly employed for conditions which are less serious.

Physicians may wish to discuss with their patients the potential risks (see WARNINGS, PRECAUTIONS, and ADVERSE REACTIONS) and likely benefits of NSAID treatment, particularly when the drugs are used for less serious conditions where treatment without NSAIDs may represent an acceptable alternative to both the patient and physician.

Patients on MOTRIN should report to their physicians signs or symptoms of gastrointestinal ulceration or bleeding, blurred vision or other eye symptoms, skin rash, weight gain, or edema.

Because serious GI tract ulceration and bleeding can occur without warning symptoms, physicians should follow chronically treated patients for the signs and symptoms of ulceration and bleeding and should inform them of the importance of this follow-up (see WARNINGS).

Patients should also be instructed to seek medical emergency help in case of an occurrence of an anaphylactoid reaction (see WARNINGS).

LABORATORY TESTS

Hemoglobin Levels: In cross-study comparisons, in adults, with doses ranging from 1200 mg to 3200 mg daily for several weeks, a slight dose-response decrease in hemoglobin/hematocrit was noted. This has been observed with other nonsteroidal anti-inflammatory drugs; the mechanism is unknown. However, even with daily doses of 3200 mg, the total decrease in hemoglobin usually does not exceed 1 g/dL; if there are no signs of bleeding, it is probably not clinically important.

In two postmarketing clinical studies with ibuprofen, the incidence of a decreased hemoglobin level was greater than previously reported. Decrease in hemoglobin of 1 g/dL or more was observed in 17.1% of 193 patients on 1600 mg ibuprofen daily (osteoarthritis), and 22.8% of 189 patients taking 2400mg of ibuprofen daily (rheumatoid arthritis). Positive stool occult blood tests and elevated serum creatinine levels were also observed in these studies.

DRUG INTERACTIONS

Coumarin-type anticoagulants: Several short-term controlled studies failed to show that iburprofen significantly affected prothrombin times or a variety of other clotting factors administered to individuals on coumarin-type anticoagulants. Because bleeding has been reported when ibuprofen and other nonsteroidal anti-inflammatory agents have been administered to patients on coumarin-type anticoagulants, the physician should be cautious when administering MOTRIN to patients on anticoagulants.

Aspirin: Animal studies show that aspirin given with NSAIDs, including ibuprofen, yields a net decrease in anti-inflammatory activity with lowered blood levels of the non-aspirin drug. Single-dose bioavailability studies in normal volunteers have failed to show an effect of aspirin on ibuprofen blood levels. Correlative clinical studies have not been done.

Methotrexate: Ibuprofen, as well as other NSAIDs, has been reported to competitively inhibit methotrexate accumulation in rabbit kidney slices. This may indicate that ibuprofen could enhance the toxicity of methotrexate. Caution should be used, therefore, if MOTRIN is administered concomitantly with methotrexate.

H-2 Antagonists: In studies with human volunteers, coadministration of cimetidine or ranitidine with ibuprofen had no substantive effect on ibuprofen serum concentrations.

ACE-inhibitors: Reports suggest that NSAIDs, including ibuprofen, may diminish the antihypertensive effect of ACE-inhibitors. This interaction should be given consideration in patients taking MOTRIN concomitantly with ACE-inhibitors.

Furosemide: Clinical studies, as well as random observations, have shown that ibuprofen can reduce the natriuretic effect of furosemide and thiazides in some patients. This response has been attributed to inhibition of renal prostaglandin synthesis. During concomitant therapy with MOTRIN, the patient should be observed closely for signs of renal failure (see PRECAUTIONS, Renal Effects), as well as to assure diuretic efficacy.

Lithium: Ibuprofen produced an elevation of plasma lithium levels and a reduction in renal lithium clearance in a study of eleven normal volunteers. The mean minimum lithium concentration increased 15% and the renal clearance of lithium was decreased by 19% during this period of concomitant drug administration. This effect has been attributed to inhibition of renal prostaglandin synthesis by ibuprofen. Thus, when MOTRIN and lithium are administered concurrently, subjects should be observed carefully for signs of lithium toxicity. (Read circulars for lithium preparation before use of such concurrent therapy.)

Teratogenic Effects—Pregnancy Category B: Reproductive studies conducted in rats and rabbits at doses somewhat less than the maximal clinical dose did not demonstrate evidence of developmental abnormalities. However, animal reproduction studies are not always predictive of human response. As there are no adequate and well-controlled studies in pregnant women, this drug should be used during pregnancy only if clearly needed. Because of the known effects of nonsteroidal anti-inflammatory drugs on the fetal cardiovascular system (closure of ductus arteriosus), use during late pregnancy should be avoided. Administration of MOTRIN is not recommended during pregnancy.

Labor and Delivery: As with other drugs known to inhibit prostaglandin synthesis, an increased incidence of dystocia and delayed parturition occurred in rats. Administration of MOTRIN is not recommended during labor and delivery.

Nursing Mothers: In limited studies, an assay capable of detecting 1 μg/mL did not demonstrate ibuprofen in the milk of lactating mothers. Because of the limited nature of these studies, however, and the possible adverse effects of prostaglandin inhibiting drugs on neonates, MOTRIN is not recommended for use in nursing mothers.

Pediatric Use: Safety and efficacy of MOTRIN in children below the age of 6 months has not been established (see CLINICAL PHARMACOLOGY-Clinical Studies). There is no evidence of age-dependent kinetics in patients 2 to 11 years old (see CLINICAL PHARMACOLOGY-Pharmacokinetics). Dosing of MOTRIN in children 6 months or older should be guided by their body weight (see DOSAGE AND ADMINISTRATION).

ADVERSE REACTIONS

The most frequent type of adverse reaction occurring with ibuprofen is gastrointestinal. In controlled clinical trials, the percentage of adult patients reporting one or more gastrointestinal complaints ranged from 4% to 16%.

In controlled studies in adults, when ibuprofen was compared to aspirin and indomethacin in equally effective doses, the overall incidence of gastrointestinal complaints was about half that seen in either the aspirin- or indomethacin-treated patients.

Adverse reactions observed during controlled clinical trials in adults at an incidence greater than 1% are listed in the chart. Those reactions listed under the heading "Incidence Greater than 1% (but less than 3%) Probable Causal Relationship," encompass observations in approximately 3,000 patients. More than 500 of these patients were treated for periods of at least 54 weeks.

Still other reactions, occurring less frequently than 1 in 100, were reported in controlled clinical trials and from marketing experience. These reactions have been divided into two categories: "Incidence less than 1%—Probable Causal Relationships," lists reactions with Ibuprofen therapy for which the probability of a causal relationship exists; this category was completed over time with postmarketing serious adverse reactions. "Incidence less than 1% —Causal Relationship Unknown," lists reactions with ibuprofen therapy for which a causal relationship has not been established, but are presented as alerting information for physicians.

INCIDENCE OF 1% OR GREATER

Probable Causal Relationship

*Incidence between 3 and 9%=ADR marked with**

Incidence between 1 and <3%=unmarked ADR

Cardiovascular system: Edema, fluid retention (generally responds promptly to drug discontinuation) (See PRECAUTIONS).

Digestive system: Nausea*, epigastric pain*, heartburn*, diarrhea, abdominal distress, nausea and vomiting, indigestion, constipation, abdominal cramps or pain, fullness of GI tract (bloating and flatulence).

Nervous system: Dizziness*, headache, nervousness.

Skin and appendages: Rash* (including maculopapular type), pruritus

Specal senses: Tinnitus.

INCIDENCE LESS THAN 1%

Probable Causal Relationship: The following adverse reactions were reported in clincial trials at an incidence of less than 1%, or were reported from postmarketing or foreign experience. The probability exists between the drug and these adverse reactions.

Body as a whole: Anaphylaxis and anaphylactoid reactions (see WARNINGS).

Cardiovascular system: Cerebrovascular accident, hypotension, congestive heart failure in patients with marginal cardiac function, elevated blood pressure, palpitations.

Digestive system: Gastric or duodenal ulcer with bleeding and/or perforation, gastrointestinal hemorrhage, pancreatitis, melena, gastritis, duodenitis, esophagitis, hematemesis, hepatorenal syndrome, liver necrosis, liver failure, hepatitis, jaundice, abnormal liver tests.

Hematologic system: Neutropenia, agranulocytosis, aplastic anemia, hemolytic anemia (sometimes Coombs positive), thrombocytopenia with or without purpura, eosinophilia, decrease in hemoglobin and hematocrit (see PRECAUTIONS), pancytopenia.

Nervous system: Depression, insomnia, confusion, emotional lability, somnolence, convulsions, aseptic meningitis with fever and coma (see PRECAUTIONS).

Respiratory: Bronchospasm, dyspnea, apnea.

Skin and appendages: Vesiculobullous eruptions, urticaria, erythema multiforme, Stevens-Johnson syndrome, alopecia, exfoliative dermatitis, Lyell's syndrome (toxic epidermal necrolysis), photosensitivity reactions.

Special senses: Hearing loss, amblyopia (blurred and/or diminished vision, scotomata and/or changes in color vision) (see PRECAUTIONS—Other Precautions).

Urogenital system: Acute renal failure in patients with pre-existing significantly impaired renal function (see PRECAUTIONS), renal papillary necrosis, tubular necrosis, glomerulitis, decreased creatinine clearance, polyuria, azotemia, cystitis, hematuria.

Miscellaneous: Dry eyes and mouth, gingival ulcer, rhinitis.

INCIDENCE LESS THAN 1%

Causal Relationship Unknown: The following adverse reactions occurred at an incidence of less than 1% in clinical trials, or were suggested by marketing experience under circumstances where a causal relationship could not be definitely established. They are listed as alerting information for the physician.

Allergic: Serum sickness, lupus erythematosus syndrome, Henoch-Schonlein vasculitis, angioedema.

Cardivascular system: Arrhythmias (sinus tachycardia, sinus bradycardia).

Hematologic system: Bleeding episodes (e.g., epistaxis, menorrhagia).

Metabolic/endocrine: Gynecomastia, hypoglycemic reaction, acidosis.

Nervous system: Paresthesias, hallucinations, dream abnormalities, pseudo-tumor cerebri.

Special senses: Conjunctivitis, diplopia, optic neuritis, cataracts.

OVERDOSAGE

The *toxicity of ibuprofen overdose* is dependent upon the amount of drug ingested and the time elapsed since ingestion, though individual response may vary, which makes it necessary to evaluate each case individually. Although uncommon, serious toxicity and death have been reported in the medical literature with ibuprofen overdosage. The most frequently reported symptoms of ibuprofen overdose include abdominal pain, nausea, vomiting, lethargy and drowsiness. Other central nervous system symptoms include headache, tinnitus, CNS depression and seizures. Metabolic acidosis, coma, acute renal failure and apnea (primarily in very young children) may rarely occur. Cardiovascular toxicity, including hypotension, bradycardia, tachycardia and atrial fibrillation, also have been reported.

The *treatment of acute ibuprofen overdose* is primarily supportive. Management of hypotension, acidosis and gastrointestinal bleeding may be necessary. In cases of acute overdose, the stomach should be emptied through ipecac-induced emesis or lavage. Emesis is most effective if initiated within 30 mintues of ingestion. Orally administered activated charcoal may help in reducing the absorption and reabsorption of ibuprofen.

In children, the estimated amount of ibuprofen ingested per body weight may be helpful to predict the potential for development of toxicity although each case must be evaluated. Ingestion of less than 100 mg/kg is unlikely to produce toxicity. Children ingesting 100 to 200 mg/kg may be managed with induced emesis and a minimal observation time of four hours. Children ingesting 200 to 400 mg/kg of ibuprofen should have immediate gastric emptying and at least four hours observation in a health care facility. Children ingesting greater than 400 mg/kg require immediate medical referral, careful observation and appropriate supportive therapy. Ipecac-induced emesis is not recommended in overdoses greater than 400 mg/kg because of the risk for convulsions and the potential for aspiration of gastric contents.

In adult patients the history of the dose reportedly ingested does not appear to be predictive of toxicity. The need for referral and follow-up must be judged by the circumstances at the time of the overdose ingestion. Symptomatic adults should be admitted to a health care facility for observation.

DOSAGE AND ADMINISTRATION

CHILDREN

Fever reduction: For reduction of fever in children, 6 months to 12 years of age, the dosage should be adjusted on the basis of the initial temperature level (see CLINICAL PHARMACOLOGY). The recommended dose is 5 mg/kg if the baseline temperature is less than 102.5°F, or 10 mg/kg if the baseline temperature is 102.5°F or greater. The duration of fever reduction is generally 6 to 8 hours. The recommended maximum daily dose is 40 mg/kg.

Analgesia: For relief of mild to moderate pain in children, 6 months to 12 years of age, the recommended dosage is 10 mg/kg, every 6 to 8 hours. The recommended maximum daily dose is 40 mg/kg. Doses should be given so as not to disturb the child's sleep pattern. Taking fluids after chewing MOTRIN Chewable Tablets may help to promote absorption of the drug (see CLINICAL PHARMACOLOGY—Pharmacokinetics, and "Individualization of Dosage" in this section).

Juvenile Arthritis: The recommended dose is 30 to 40 mg/kg/day divided into three to four doses (see Individualization of Dosage). Patients with milder disease may be adequately treated with 20 mg/kg/day.

ADULTS

Analgesia: 400 mg every 4 to 6 hours as necessary for the relief of mild to moderate pain in adults. In controlled analgesic clincial trials, doses of MOTRIN greater than 400 mg were no more effective than the 400 mg dose.

Primary Dysmenorrhea: For the treatment of primary dysmenorrhea, beginning with the earliest onset of such pain, MOTRIN should be given in a dose of 400 mg every 4 hours, as necessary, for the relief of pain.

Rheumatoid arthritis and osteoarthritis, including flare-ups of chronic disease: Suggested dosage: 1200-3200 mg daily (300 mg q.i.d or 400 mg, 600 mg or 800 mg t.i.d. or q.i.d). Individual patients may show a better response to 3200 mg daily, as compared with 2400 mg, although in well-controlled clinical trials patients on 3200 mg did not show a better mean response in terms of efficacy. Therefore, when treating patients with 3200 mg/day, the physician should observe sufficient increased clincial benefits to offset potential increased risk.

Individualization of Dosage The dose of MOTRIN should be tailored to each patient, and may be lowered or raised from the suggested doses depending on the severity of symptoms either at time of initiating drug therapy or as the patient responds or fails to respond.

One fever study showed that, after the initial dose of MOTRIN, subsequent doses may be lowered and still provide adequate fever control.

In a situation when low fever would require the MOTRIN 5 mg/kg dose in a child with pain, the dose that will effectively treat the predominant symptom should be chosen.

In chronic conditions, a therapeutic response to MOTRIN therapy is sometimes seen in a few days to a week, but most often is observed by two weeks. After a satisfactory response has been achieved, the patient's dose should be reviewed and adjusted as required.

In patients with juvenile arthritis, doses above 50 mg/kg/day are not recommended because they have not been studied and doses exceeding the upper recommended dose of 40 mg/kg/day may increase the risk of causing serious adverse events. The therapeutic response may require from a few days to several weeks to be achieved. Once a clincial effect is obtained, the dosage should be lowered to the smallest dose of MOTRIN needed to maintain adequate control of symptoms.

In general, patients with rheumatoid arthritis seem to require higher doses than do patients with osteoarthritis. The smallest dose of MOTRIN that yields acceptable control should be employed.

HOW SUPPLIED

MOTRIN® (ibuprofen) Suspension 100 mg/5 mL

Orange-colored, berry-flavored suspension

–Bottles of 120 mL—NDC 0045-0448-04

–Bottles of 480 mL—NDC 0045-0448-16

Shake well before using. Store at controlled room temperature [15° to 30°C (59° to 86°F)]

MOTRIN® (ibuprofen) Oral Drops, 40mg/mL

(intended for pediatric use only)

Pink-colored, berry flavored suspension

–Bottles of 15 ml—NDC 0045-0446-15

Shake well before using. Store at controlled room temperature [15° to 30°C (59° to 86°F)].

MOTRIN® (ibuprofen) Chewable Tablets, 50 mg

Round, orange-colored, citrus-tasting, scored tablet, debossed "MOTRIN 50"

–Bottles of 100 Chewable Tablets—NDC 0045-0361-10

Store at controlled room temperature [15° to 30°C (59° to 86°F)]

MOTRIN® (ibuprofen) Chewable Tablets, 100 mg

Round, orange-colored, citrus-tasting, scored tablet, debossed "MOTRIN 100"

–Bottles of 100 Chewable Tablets—NDC 0045-0431-10

Store at controlled room temperature [15° to 30°C (59° to 86°F)]

MOTRIN® (ibuprofen) Caplets, 100 mg

White-colored, scored capsule-shaped tablet, imprinted "M 100"

–Bottles of 100 Caplets—NDC 0045-0445-10

Store at controlled room temperature [15° to 30°C (59° to 86°F)]

Caution: Federal Law prohibits dispensing without prescription.

McNeil Consumer & Specialty Pharmaceuticals

DIVISION OF McNEIL-PPC, INC.

FORT WASHINGTON, PA 19034-USA

JUNE 1995

Shown in Product Identification Guide, page 321

MOTRIN® COLD & SINUS CAPLETS OTC

DESCRIPTION

Each MOTRIN® Cold & Sinus Caplet contains ibuprofen 200 mg and pseudoephedrine HCl 30 mg.

USES

temporarily relieves these symptoms associated with the common cold, sinusitis, and flu:

• headache • nasal congestion

• fever • minor body aches and pains

DIRECTIONS

Adults and children 12 years of age and older	• take 1 caplet every 4 to 6 hours while symptoms persist • If symptoms do not respond to 1 caplet, 2 caplets may be used. • do not use more than 6 caplets in any 24-hour period unless directed by a doctor • the smallest effective dose should be used
Children under 12 years of age	Consult a doctor

WARNINGS

Allergy alert: Ibuprofen may cause a severe allergic reaction which may include:

• hives • facial swelling

• asthma (wheezing) • shock

Alcohol warning: If you consume 3 or more alcoholic drinks every day, ask your doctor whether you should take ibuprofen or other pain relievers/fever reducers. Ibuprofen may cause stomach bleeding.

Do not use if you

• have ever had an allergic reaction to any other pain reliever/fever reducer

• are now taking a prescription monoamine oxidase inhibitor (MAOI) (certain drugs for depression, psychiatric or emotional conditions, or Parkinson's disease), or for 2 weeks after stopping the MAOI drug. If you do not know if your prescription drug contains an MAOI, ask a doctor or pharmacist before taking this product.

Ask a doctor before use if you have

• heart disease • high blood pressure

• thyroid disease • diabetes

• trouble urinating due to an enlarged prostate gland

• had serious side effects from taking any pain reliever/fever reducers.

Ask a doctor or pharmacist before use if you are

• taking any other product that contains ibuprofen or pseudoephedrine.

• taking any other pain reliever/fever reducer or nasal decongestant

• under a doctor's care for any continuing medical condition

• taking other drugs on a regular basis

When using this product

• **do not use more than directed**

• give with food or milk if stomach upset occurs

Stop use and ask a doctor if

• an allergic reaction occurs. Seek medical help right away

• you get nervous, dizzy, or sleepless

Continued on next page

Motrin Cold & Sinus—Cont.

- nasal congestion lasts for more than 7 days
- fever lasts for more than 3 days
- symptoms continue or get worse
- new or unexpected symptoms occur
- stomach pain occurs with use of this product or even if mild symptoms persist

If pregnant or breast-feeding, ask a health professional before use. It is especially important not to use this product during the last 3 months of pregnancy unless definitely directed to do so by a doctor because it may cause problems in the unborn child or complications during delivery.
Keep out of reach of children. In case of overdose, get medical help or contact a Poison Control Center right away.

OTHER INFORMATION
- **do not use if blister unit is broken or open**
- store between 20–25°C (68–77°F).
- avoid excessive heat above 40°C (104°F)
- read all warnings and directions before use. Keep carton.

Professional Information:
Overdosage Information:

For overdosage information, please refer to pgs. 1934–1935

INACTIVE INGREDIENTS
Caplets: carnauba wax, cellulose, corn starch, FD&C Red #40, hypromellose, silicon dioxide, sodium lauryl sulfate, sodium starch glycolate, stearic acid, titanium dioxide, triacetin.

HOW SUPPLIED
Caplets: (white, printed "Cold & Sinus" in red) in blister packs of 20 and 40.
Shown in Product Identification Guide, page 321

Infants' MOTRIN® ibuprofen OTC
Concentrated Drops
Children's MOTRIN® ibuprofen Oral Suspension and Chewable Tablets
Junior Strength MOTRIN® ibuprofen Caplets and Chewable Tablets

Product information for all dosages of Children's MOTRIN have been combined under this heading

DESCRIPTION
Infants' MOTRIN® Concentrated Drops are available in an alcohol-free, berry-flavored suspension and a non-staining, dye-free, berry-flavored suspension. Each 1.25 mL contains ibuprofen 50 mg. *Children's MOTRIN® Oral Suspension* is available as an alcohol-free, berry, dye-free berry, bubblegum or grape-flavored suspension. Each 5 mL (teaspoon) of *Children's MOTRIN® Oral Suspension* contains ibuprofen 100 mg. Each *Children's MOTRIN® Chewable Tablet* contains 50 mg of ibuprofen and is available as orange or grape-flavored chewable tablets. *Junior Strength MOTRIN® Chewable Tablets* and *Junior Strength MOTRIN® Caplets* contain ibuprofen 100 mg. *Junior Strength MOTRIN® Chewable Tablets* are available in orange or grape flavors. *Junior Strength MOTRIN® Caplets* are available as easy-to-swallow caplets (capsule-shaped tablet).

USES
temporarily:
- reduces fever
- relieves minor aches and pains due to the common cold, flu, sore throat, headaches and toothaches

DIRECTIONS
See Table 2: Children's Motrin Dosing Chart on pg. 1939

WARNINGS
Allergy alert: Ibuprofen may cause a severe allergic reaction which may include:
- hives • facial swelling
- asthma (wheezing) • shock

Sore throat warning: Severe or persistent sore throat or sore throat accompanied by high fever, headache, nausea, and vomiting may be serious. Consult doctor promptly. Do not use more than 2 days or administer to children under 3 years of age unless directed by doctor.
Do not use if the child has ever had an allergic reaction to any other fever reducer/pain reliever
Ask a doctor before use if the child has
- not been drinking fluids
- lost a lot of fluid due to continued vomiting or diarrhea
- stomach pain
- problems or serious side effects from taking fever reducers or pain relievers

Ask a doctor or pharmacist before use if the child
- under a doctor's care for any serious condition
- taking any other drug
- taking any other product that contains ibuprofen, or any other fever reducer/pain reliever

When using this product
- mouth or throat burning may occur; give with food or water (*Children's MOTRIN® Chewable Tablets and Junior Strength MOTRIN® Chewable Tablets* only)
- give with food or milk if stomach upset occurs

Stop use and ask a doctor if
- an allergic reaction occurs. Seek medical help right away.
- fever or pain gets worse or lasts more than 3 days
- the child does not get any relief within first day (24 hours) of treatment
- stomach pain or upset gets worse or lasts
- redness or swelling is present in the painful area
- any new symptoms appear

Keep out of reach of children. In case of overdose, get medical help or contact a Poison Control Center right away.

Other Information: *Infants', Children's and Junior Strength MOTRIN® products:*
- Store at 20–25°C *(68–77°F)*

Infants' MOTRIN® Concentrated Drops:
- **do not use if plastic carton wrap or bottle wrap imprinted "Safety Seal®" and "Use with Enclosed Dosage Device" is broken or missing.**

Children's MOTRIN® Suspension Liquid:
- **do not use if plastic carton wrap or bottle wrap imprinted "Safety Seal®" is broken or missing**

Children's MOTRIN® Chewable Tablets:
- Phenylketonurics: Contains phenylalanine 1.4 mg per tablet
- **do not use if neck wrap or foil inner seal imprinted "Safety Seal®" is broken or missing**

Junior Strength MOTRIN® Caplets and Chewable Tablets:
- **do not use if neck wrap or foil inner seal imprinted "Safety Seal®" is broken or missing**

Junior Strength MOTRIN® Chewable Tablets:
- phenylketonurics: contains phenylalanine 2.8 mg per tablet (tablet only)

Professional Information:
Overdosage Information for all Infants', Children's & Junior Strength Motrin® Products

IBUPROFEN: The *toxicity of ibuprofen* overdose is dependent upon the amount of drug ingested and the time elapsed since ingestion, though individual response may vary, which makes it necessary to evaluate each case individually. Although uncommon, serious toxicity and death have been reported in the medical literature with ibuprofen overdosage. The most frequently reported symptoms of ibuprofen overdose include abdominal pain, nausea, vomiting, lethargy and drowsiness. Other central nervous system symptoms include headache, tinnitus, CNS depression and seizures. Metabolic acidosis, coma, acute renal failure and apnea (primarily in very young children) may rarely occur. Cardiovascular toxicity, including hypotension, bradycardia, tachycardia and atrial fibrillation, also have been reported.
The *treatment of acute ibuprofen overdose* is primarily supportive. Management of hypotension, acidosis and gastrointestinal bleeding may be necessary. In cases of acute overdose, the stomach should be emptied through ipecac-induced emesis or lavage. Emesis is most effective if initiated within 30 minutes of ingestion. Orally administered activated charcoal may help in reducing the absorption and reabsorption of ibuprofen. In children, the estimated amount of ibuprofen ingested per body weight may be helpful to predict the potential for development of toxicity although each case must be evaluated. Ingestion of less than 100 mg/kg is unlikely to produce toxicity. Children ingesting 100 to 200 mg/kg may be managed with induced emesis and a minimal observation time of four hours. Children ingesting 200 to 400 mg/kg of ibuprofen should have immediate gastric emptying and at least four hours observation in a health care facility. Children ingesting greater than 400 mg/kg require immediate medical referral, careful observation and appropriate supportive therapy. Ipecac-induced emesis is not recommended in overdoses greater than 400 mg/kg because of the risk of convulsions and the potential for aspiration of gastric contents.
In adult patients the history of the dose reportedly ingested does not appear to be predictive of toxicity. The need for referral and follow-up must be judged by the circumstances at the time of the overdose ingestion. Symptomatic adults should be admitted to a health care facility for observation.
Our Children's MOTRIN® Cold products contain pseudoephedrine in addition to ibuprofen. The following is basic overdose information regarding pseudoephedrine.
PSEUDOEPHEDRINE: Symptoms from pseudoephedrine overdose consist most often of mild anxiety, tachycardia and/or mild hypertension. Symptoms usually appear within 4 to 8 hours of ingestion and are transient, usually requiring no treatment.
For additional emergency information, please contact your local poison control center.

INACTIVE INGREDIENTS
Infants' MOTRIN® Concentrated Drops:
Berry-Flavored: citric acid, corn starch, FD&C Red #40, flavors, glycerin, polysorbate 80, purified water, sodium benzoate, sorbitol, sucrose, xanthan gum. **Dye-Free Berry-Flavored:** artificial flavors, citric acid, corn starch, glycerin, polysorbate 80, purified water, sodium benzoate, sorbitol, sucrose, xanthan gum.
Children's MOTRIN® Oral Suspension: **Berry-Flavored:** acesulfame potassium, citric acid, corn starch, D&C Yellow #10, FD&C Red #40, glycerin, natural and artificial flavors, polysorbate 80, purified water, sodium benzoate, sucrose, xanthan gum. **Dye-Free Berry-Flavored:** acesulfame potassium, citric acid, corn starch, glycerin, natural and artificial flavors, polysorbate 80, purified water, sodium benzoate, sucrose, xanthan gum. **Bubble Gum-Flavored:** acesulfame potassium, citric acid, corn starch, FD&C Red #40, glycerin, natural and artificial flavors, polysorbate 80, purified water, sodium benzoate, sucrose, xanthan gum. **Grape-Flavored:** acesulfame potassium, citric acid, corn starch, D&C Red #33, FD&C Blue #1, FD&C Red #40 flavors, glycerin, natural and artificial flavors, polysorbate 80, purified water, sodium benzoate, sucrose, xanthan gum.
Children's MOTRIN® Chewable Tablets: **Orange-Flavored:** acesulfame K, aspartame, cellulose, citric acid, FD&C Yellow #6, flavor, fumaric acid, hydroxymethyl cellulose, hypromellose, magnesium stearate, mannitol, povidone, sodium lauryl sulfate, sodium starch glycolate. **Grape-Flavored:** acesulfame K, aspartame, cellulose, citric acid, D&C Red #7, D&C Red #30, FD&C Blue #1, flavor, fumaric acid, hydroxyethyl cellulose, hypromellose, magnesium stearate, mannitol, povidone, sodium lauryl sulfate, sodium starch glycolate.
Junior Strength MOTRIN® Chewable Tablets: **Orange-Flavored:** acesulfame K, aspartame, cellulose, citric acid, FD&C yellow #6, flavor, fumaric acid, hydroxyethyl cellulose, hypromellose, magnesium stearate, mannitol, povidone, sodium lauryl sulfate, sodium starch glycolate. **Grape-Flavored:** acesulfame K, aspartame, cellulose, citric acid, D&C Red #7, D&C Red #30, FD&C Blue #1, flavor, fumaric acid, hydroxyethyl cellulose, hypromellose, magnesium stearate, mannitol, povidone, sodium lauryl sulfate, sodium starch glycolate. **Easy-To-Swallow Caplets:** carnauba wax, cellulose, corn starch, D&C Yellow #10, FD&C Yellow #6, hypromellose, polydextrose, polyethylene glycol, propylene glycol, silicon dioxide, sodium starch glycolate, titanium dioxide, triacetin.

HOW SUPPLIED
Infants' MOTRIN® Concentrated Drops: Berry-flavored, pink-colored liquid and Berry-Flavored, Dye-Free, white-colored liquid in ½ fl. oz. bottles w/calibrated plastic syringe.
Children's MOTRIN® Oral Suspension: Berry-flavored, pink-colored; (2 and 4 fl. oz) Berry-Flavored, Dye-Free white-colored, Bubble Gum-flavored, pink-colored and Grape-flavored, purple-colored liquid in tamper evident bottles (4 fl. oz.)
Children's MOTRIN® Chewable Tablets: Orange-flavored, orange-colored and Grape-flavored, purple-colored chewable tablets in 24 count bottles.
Junior Strength MOTRIN® Chewable Tablets: Orange-flavored, orange-colored chewable tablets or Grape-flavored, purple-colored chewable tablets in 24 count bottles.
Junior Strength MOTRIN® Caplets: Easy-to-swallow caplets (capsule shaped tablets) in 24 count bottles.
Shown in Product Identification Guide, page 321

Children's MOTRIN® Cold ibuprofen/pseudoephedrine HCl Oral Suspension OTC

DESCRIPTION
Children's MOTRIN® Cold Oral Suspension is an alcohol-free berry, dye-free berry, or grape-flavored suspension. Each 5 mL (teaspoonful) contains the pain reliever/fever reducer ibuprofen 100 mg and the nasal decongestant pseudoephedrine HCl 15 mg.

USES
temporarily relieves these cold, sinus and flu symptoms:
- nasal and sinus congestion
- stuffy nose • headache • sore throat
- minor body aches and pains • fever

DIRECTIONS
See Table 2: Children's Motrin Dosing Chart on pg. 1939

WARNINGS
Allergy alert: Ibuprofen may cause a severe allergic reaction which may include:
- hives • facial swelling
- asthma (wheezing) • shock

Sore throat warning: Severe or persistent sore throat or sore throat accompanied by high fever, headache, nausea, and vomiting may be serious. Consult a doctor promptly. Do not use more than 2 days or administer to children under 3 years of age unless directed by doctor.
Do not use
- if the child has ever had an allergic reaction to any other pain reliever/fever reducer and/or nasal decongestant
- in a child who is taking a prescription monoamine oxidase inhibitor [MAOI] (certain drugs for depression, psychiatric or emotional conditions, or Parkinson's disease), or for 2 weeks after stopping the MAOI drug. If you do not know if your child's prescription drug contains an MAOI, ask a doctor or pharmacist before giving this product.

Ask a doctor before use if the child has
- not been drinking fluids
- lost a lot of fluid due to continued vomiting or diarrhea
- problems or serious side effects from taking pain relievers, fever reducers or nasal decongestants
- stomach pain
- heart disease
- high blood pressure
- thyroid disease
- diabetes

Ask a doctor or pharmacist before use if the child is
- under a doctor's care for any continuing medical condition
- taking any other drug
- taking any other product that contains ibuprofen or pseudoephedrine

Table 2. Children's Motrin Dosing Chart

AGE GROUP*		0-5 mos*	6-11 mos	12-23 mos	2-3 yrs	4-5 yrs	6-8 yrs	9-10 yrs	11 yrs	
WEIGHT	(if possible use weight to dose; otherwise use age)	6-11 lbs	12-17 lbs	18-23 lbs	24-35 lbs	36-47 lbs	48-59 lbs	60-71 lbs	72-95 lbs	
PRODUCT FORM	**INGREDIENTS Dose to be administered based on weight or age†**									**Maximum doses/ 24 hrs**
Infants' Drops	**Per 1.25 mL**									
Infants' Motrin Concentrated Drops	Ibuprofen 50 mg	—	1.25 mL	1.875 mL	—	—	—	—	—	4 times in 24 hrs
Children's Liquid	**Per 5 mL teaspoonful (TSP)**									
Children's Motrin Suspension	Ibuprofen 100 mg	—	—	—	1 TSP	1 ½ TSP	2 TSP	2 ½ TSP	3 TSP	4 times in 24 hrs
Children's Motrin Cold Suspension Liquid†	Ibuprofen 100 mg Pseudoephedrine HCl 15 mg	—	—	—	1 TSP	1 TSP	2 TSP	2 TSP	2 TSP	4 times in 24 hrs
Children's Tablets & Caplets	**Per tablet/ caplet**									
Children's Motrin Chewable Tablets	Ibuprofen 50 mg	—	—	—	2 tablets	3 tablets	4 tablets	5 tablets	6 tablets	4 times in 24 hrs
Junior Strength Motrin Chewable Tablets	Ibuprofen 100 mg	—	—	—	—	—	2 tablets	2 ½ tablets	3 tablets	4 times in 24 hrs
Junior Strength Motrin Caplets	Ibuprofen 100 mg	—	—	—	—	—	2 caplets	2 ½ caplets	3 caplets	4 times in 24 hrs

†Do not give, take or chew more than directed. If needed, repeat dose every 6-8 hours; except for Children's Motrin Cold which is every 6 hours, shake well before using.
* Under 6 mos, call a doctor.

- Infant drops: dispense liquid slowly into the child's mouth, toward the inner cheek.
- Infants' Motrin Drops are more concentrated than Children's Motrin Liquids. The Infants' Concentrated Drops have been specifically designed for use only with enclosed dosing device. Do not use any other dosing device with this product.
- Children's Motrin Liquids are less concentrated than Infants' Motrin Drops. The Children's Motrin Liquids have been specifically designed for use with the enclosed measuring cup. Use only enclosed measuring cup to dose this product.
- Children's Motrin Suspensions (including cold)—replace original bottle cap to maintain child resistance
- Children's Motrin Chewable Tablets are not the same concentration as Junior Strength Motrin Chewable Tablets.
- Junior Strength Motrin Chewable Tablets contain twice as much medicine as Children's Motrin Chewable Tablets.

- taking any other pain reliever/fever reducer and/or nasal decongestant

When using this product
- **do not exceed recommended dosage**
- give with food or milk if stomach upset occurs

Stop use and ask a doctor if
- an allergic reaction occurs. Seek medical help right away.
- the child does not get any relief within first day (24 hours) of treatment
- fever, pain or nasal congestion gets worse, or lasts for more than 3 days
- stomach pain or upset gets worse or lasts
- symptoms continue or get worse
- redness or swelling is present in the painful area
- the child gets nervous, dizzy, sleepless or sleepy
- any new symptoms appear

Keep out of reach of children. In case of overdose, get medical help or contact a Poison Control Center right away.

OTHER INFORMATION
- **do not use if plastic carton wrap or bottle wrap imprinted "Safety Seal®" is broken or missing.**
- Store at 20–25°C (68–77°F)

Professional Information:
Overdosage Information

For overdosage information, please refer to pg. 1938

INACTIVE INGREDIENTS
Berry Flavor: acesulfame potassium, citric acid, corn starch, D&C Yellow #10, FD&C Red #40, flavors, glycerin, polysorbate 80, purified water, sodium benzoate, sucrose, xanthan gum. **Dye-Free Berry Flavor:** acesulfame potassium, citric acid, corn starch, flavors, glycerin, polysorbate 80, purified water, sodium benzoate, sucrose, xanthan gum. **Grape Flavor:** acesulfame potassium, citric acid, corn starch, D&C Red #33, FD&C Blue #1, FD&C Red #40, flavors, glycerin, polysorbate 80, purified water, sodium benzoate, sucrose, xanthan gum.

HOW SUPPLIED
Berry-flavored, pink-colored; Grape-flavored, purple-colored, and Dye-Free Berry-flavored, white-colored liquid in child resistant tamper-evident bottles of 4 fl. oz.

Shown in Product Identification Guide, page 321

Children's Motrin® Dosing Chart

[See table 2 above]

NIZORAL® ℞
[*nī 'zōr-ăl*]
(ketoconazole) 2% Shampoo

DESCRIPTION
NIZORAL® (ketoconazole) 2% Shampoo is a red-orange liquid for topical application, containing the broad-spectrum synthetic antifungal agent ketoconazole in a concentration of 2% in an aqueous suspension. It also contains: coconut fatty acid diethanolamide, disodium monolauryl ether sulfosuccinate, F.D. & C. Red No. 40, hydrochloric acid, imidurea, laurdimonium hydrolyzed animal collagen, macrogol 120 methyl-glucose dioleate, perfume bouquet, sodium chloride, sodium hydroxide, sodium lauryl ether sulfate, and purified water.

Ketoconazole is cis-1-acetyl-4-[4-[[2-(2,4-di-chlorophenyl)-2-(1H-imidazol-1-ylmethyl)-1,3-dioxolan-4-yl]methoxy]phenyl]piperazine and has the following structural formula:

CLINICAL PHARMACOLOGY
Tinea (pityriasis) versicolor is a non-contagious infection of the skin caused by *Pityrosporum orbiculare (Malassezia furfur)*. This commensal organism is part of the normal skin flora. In susceptible individuals the condition is often recurrent and may give rise to hyperpigmented or hypopigmented patches on the trunk which may extend to the neck, arms and upper thighs. Treatment of the infection may not immediately result in restoration of pigment to the affected sites. Normalization of pigment following successful therapy is variable and may take months, depending on individual skin type and incidental skin exposure. The rate of recurrence of infection is variable.

When ketoconazole 2% shampoo was applied dermally to intact or abraded skin of rabbits for 28 days at doses up to 50 mg/kg and allowed to remain one hour before being washed away, there were no detectable plasma ketoconazole levels using an assay method having a lower detection limit of 5 ng/mL. NIZORAL® (ketoconazole) was not detected in plasma in 39 patients who shampooed 4–10 times per week for 6 months or in 33 patients who shampooed 2–3 times per week for 3–26 months (mean: 16 months).

An exaggerated use washing test on the sensitive antecubital skin of 10 subjects twice daily for five consecutive days showed that the irritancy potential of ketoconazole 2% shampoo was significantly less than that of 2.5% selenium sulfide shampoo.

A human sensitization test, a phototoxicity study, and a photoallergy study conducted in 38 male and 22 female volunteers showed no contact sensitization of the delayed hypersensitivity type, no phototoxicity and no photoallergenic potential due to NIZORAL® (ketoconazole) 2% Shampoo.

Mode of Action: Interpretations of *in vivo* studies suggest that ketoconazole impairs the synthesis of ergosterol, which is a vital component of fungal cell membranes. It is postulated, but not proven, that the therapeutic effect of ketoconazole in tinea (pityriasis) versicolor is due to the reduction of *Pityrosporum orbiculare (Malassezia furfur)* and that the therapeutic effect in dandruff is due to the reduction of *Pityrosporum ovale*. Support for the therapeutic effect in tinea versicolor comes from a three-arm, parallel, double-blind, placebo-controlled study in patients who had moderately severe tinea (pityriasis) versicolor. Successful response rates in the primary efficacy population for each of both three-day and single-day regimens of ketoconazole 2% shampoo were statistically significantly greater (73% and 69%, respectively) than a placebo regimen (5%). There had been mycological confirmation of fungal disease in all cases at baseline. Mycological clearing rates were 84% and 78%, respectively, for the three-day and one-day regimens of the 2% shampoo and 11% in the placebo regimen. While the differences in the rates of successful response between either of the two active treatments and placebo were statistically significant, the difference between the two active regimens was not.

Microbiology: NIZORAL® (ketoconazole) is a broad-spectrum synthetic antifungal agent which inhibits the growth of the following common dermatophytes and yeasts by altering the permeability of the cell membrane: dermatophytes: *Trichophyton rubrum, T. mentagrophytes, T. tonsurans, Microsporum canis, M. audouini, M. gypseum* and *Epidermophyton floccosum*; yeasts: *Candida albicans, C. tropicalis, Pityrosporum ovale (Malassezia ovale)* and *Pityrosporum orbiculare (M. furfur)*. Development of resistance by these microorganisms to ketoconazole has not been reported.

INDICATIONS AND USAGE
NIZORAL® (ketoconazole) 2% Shampoo is indicated for the treatment of tinea (pityriasis) versicolor caused by or presumed to be caused by *Pityrosporum orbiculare* (also known as *Malassezia furfur* or *M. orbiculare*).

Note: Tinea (pityriasis) versicolor may give rise to hyperpigmented or hypopigmented patches on the trunk which may extend to the neck, arms and upper thighs. Treatment of the

Continued on next page

Nizoral Shampoo—Cont.

infection may not immediately result in normalization of pigment to the affected sites. Normalization of pigment following successful therapy is variable and may take months, depending on individual skin type and incidental sun exposure. Although tinea versicolor is not contagious, it may recur because the organism that causes the disease is part of the normal skin flora.

CONTRAINDICATIONS

NIZORAL® (ketoconazole) 2% Shampoo is contraindicated in persons who have shown hypersensitivity to the active ingredient or excipients of this formulation.

PRECAUTIONS

General: If a reaction suggesting sensitivity or chemical irritation should occur, use of the medication should be discontinued.

Information for Patients: May be irritating to mucous membranes of the eyes and contact with this area should be avoided.

There have been reports that use of the shampoo resulted in removal of the curl from permanently waved hair.

Carcinogenesis, Mutagenesis, Impairment of Fertility: The dominant lethal mutation test in male and female mice revealed that single oral doses of ketoconazole as high as 80 mg/kg produced no mutation in any stage of germ cell development. The Ames Salmonella microsomal activator assay was also negative. A long-term feeding study of ketoconazole in Swiss Albino mice and in Wistar rats showed no evidence of oncogenic activity.

Pregnancy: Teratogenic effects: Pregnancy Category C: Ketoconazole is not detected in plasma after chronic shampooing. Ketoconazole has been shown to be teratogenic (syndactylia and oligodactylia) in the rat when given orally in the diet at 80 mg/kg/day (10 times the maximum recommended human oral dose). However, these effects may be related to maternal toxicity, which was seen at this and higher dose levels.

There are no adequate and well-controlled studies in pregnant women. Ketoconazole should be used during pregnancy only if the potential benefit justifies the potential risk to the fetus.

Nursing mothers: Ketoconazole is not detected in plasma after chronic shampooing. Nevertheless, caution should be exercised when NIZORAL® (ketoconazole) 2% Shampoo is administered to a nursing woman.

Pediatric Use: Safety and effectiveness in children have not been established.

ADVERSE REACTIONS

In 11 double-blind trials in 264 patients using ketoconazole 2% shampoo for the treatment of dandruff or seborrheic dermatitis, an increase in normal hair loss and irritation occurred in less than 1% of patients. In three open-label safety trials in which 41 patients shampooed 4–10 times weekly for six months, the following adverse experiences each occurred once: abnormal hair texture, scalp pustules, mild dryness of the skin, and itching. As with other shampoos, oiliness and dryness of hair and scalp have been reported. In a double-blind, placebo-controlled trial in which patients with tinea versicolor were treated with either a single application of NIZORAL® (ketoconazole) 2% Shampoo (n=106), a daily application for three consecutive days (n=107), or placebo (n=105), drug-related adverse events occurred in 5 (5%), 7 (7%) and 4 (4%) of patients, respectively. The only events that occurred in more than one patient in any one of the three treatment groups were pruritus, application site reaction, and dry skin; none of these events occurred in more than 3% of the patients in any one of the three groups.

In worldwide experience with NIZORAL® Shampoo there have been rare reports of hair discoloration.

OVERDOSAGE

NIZORAL® (ketoconazole) 2% Shampoo is intended for external use only. In the event of accidental ingestion, supportive measures should be employed. Induced emesis and gastric lavage should usually be avoided.

DOSAGE AND ADMINISTRATION

Apply the shampoo to the damp skin of the affected area and a wide margin surrounding this area. Lather, leave in place for 5 minutes, and then rinse off with water.

One application of the shampoo should be sufficient.

HOW SUPPLIED

NIZORAL® (ketoconazole) 2% Shampoo is a red-orange liquid supplied in a 4-fluid ounce nonbreakable plastic bottle (NDC 50580-380-08).

Storage conditions: Store at a temperature not above 25°C (77°F). Protect from light.

Rx only

Distributed by:
McNeil Consumer & Specialty Pharmaceuticals
DIVISION OF McNeil-PPC, INC.
FORT WASHINGTON, PA 19034 USA
MCN-PPC, INC. 04
Revised August 1997, May 1999, October 2003.
U.S. Patent No. 4,335,125

Shown in Product Identification Guide, page 321

NIZORAL® A-D OTC
KETOCONAZOLE SHAMPOO 1%

DESCRIPTION

Nizoral® A-D (Ketoconazole Shampoo 1%) Anti-Dandruff Shampoo is a light-blue liquid for topical application, containing the broad spectrum synthetic antifungal agent Ketoconazole in a concentration of 1%.

USE

Controls flaking, scaling and itching associated with dandruff.

DIRECTIONS

Adults and children 12 years and over:	• wet hair thoroughly • apply shampoo, generously lather, rinse thoroughly. Repeat. • use every 3–4 days for up to 8 weeks or as directed by a doctor. Then use only as needed to control dandruff.
children under 12 years	• ask a doctor

WARNINGS

• **For external use only**

Do Not Use
• on scalp that is broken or inflamed
• if you are allergic to ingredients in this product

When Using This Product
• avoid contact with eyes
• if product gets into eyes, rinse thoroughly with water

Stop use and ask a doctor if
• rash appears
• condition worsens or does not improve in 2–4 weeks

If pregnant or breast-feeding, ask a doctor before use.

Keep out of the reach of children.
If swallowed get medical help or contact a Poison Control Center right away.

Other Information
• store between 35° and 86°F (2° and 30°C)
• protect from light • protect from freezing

Professional Information:

Overdosage Information ***Nizoral® A-D (Ketoconazole) 1% Shampoo*** is intended for external use only. In the event of accidental ingestion, supportive measures should be employed. Induced emesis and gastric lavage should usually be avoided.

INACTIVE INGREDIENTS

acrylic acid polymer (carbomer 1342), butylated hydroxytoluene, cocamide MEA, FD&C Blue #1, fragrance, glycol distearate, polyquaternium-7, quaternium-15, sodium chloride, sodium cocoyl sarcosinate, sodium hydroxide and/or hydrochloric acid, sodium laureth sulfate, tetrasodium EDTA, water.

HOW SUPPLIED

Available in 4 and 7 fl oz bottles

Shown in Product Identification Guide, page 321

SIMPLY COUGH™ LIQUID OTC

DESCRIPTION

Simply Cough™ Liquid is Cherry Berry-flavored and contains no alcohol or aspirin. Each teaspoonful (5 mL) contains dextromethorphan HBr 5 mg.

ACTIONS

Simply Cough™ Liquid is a single ingredient product that contains the cough suppressant dextromethorphan hydrobromide to provide fast, effective, temporary relief of your child's cough.

USES

temporarily relieves cough occurring with a cold

DIRECTIONS

• find right dose on chart below. If possible, use weight to dose; otherwise use age.
• only use with enclosed measuring cup
• if needed, repeat dose every 4 hours
• do not use more than 4 times in 24 hours

AccuDose™ Chart

Weight (lb)	Age (yr)	Dose (teaspoon)
under 24	under 2	call a doctor
24–47	2–5	1 tsp
48–95	6–11	2 tsp

Professional Dosage Schedule: 4–11 mos (12–17 lbs): ½ teaspoonful; 12–23 mos (18–23 lbs): ¾ teaspoonful; 2–3 years (24–35 lbs) 1 teaspoonful; 4–5 yrs (36–47 lbs): 1½ teaspoonsful; 6–8 yrs (48–59 lbs): 2 teaspoonsful; 9–10 yrs (60–71 lbs): 2½ teaspoonsful; 11 yrs (72–95 lbs): 3 teaspoonsful.

If needed, repeat dose every 4 hours. Do not use more than 4 times in 24 hours.

WARNINGS

Do not use in a child who is taking a prescription monoamine oxidase inhibitor (MAOI) (certain drugs for depression, psychiatric or emotional conditions, or Parkinson's disease), or for 2 weeks after stopping the MAOI drug. If you do not know if your child's prescription drug contains an MAOI, ask a doctor or pharmacist before giving this product.

Ask a doctor before use if this child has
• cough that occurs with too much phlegm (mucus)
• chronic cough that lasts or occurs with asthma

Stop use and ask a doctor if
• cough gets worse or lasts for more than 5 days, comes back or occurs with fever, rash or headache that lasts. These could be signs of a serious condition.

Keep out of reach of children. In case of overdose, get medical help or contact a Poison Control Center right away.

OTHER INFORMATION
• **do not use if carton is opened, or if neck wrap or foil inner seal imprinted with "Safety Seal®" is broken or missing**
• store at room temperature

Professional Information:

Overdosage Information:

Acute dextromethorphan overdose usually does not result in serious signs and symptoms unless massive amounts have been ingested. Signs and symptoms of a substantial overdose may include nausea and vomiting, visual disturbances, CNS disturbances and urinary retention.

INACTIVE INGREDIENTS

citric acid, corn syrup, FD&C Red #40, flavor, glycerin, purified water, sodium benzoate, sucralose

HOW SUPPLIED

Cherry Berry flavored liquid in child resistant tamper-evident bottles of 4 fl. oz.

Shown in Product Identification Guide, page 321

SIMPLY SLEEP™ OTC

Nighttime Sleep Aid

DESCRIPTION

SIMPLY SLEEP™ is a non habit-forming nighttime sleep aid. Each *SIMPLY SLEEP™* Caplet contains diphenhydramine HCl 25 mg.

ACTIONS

SIMPLY SLEEP™ contains an antihistamine (diphenhydramine HCl) which has sedative properties.

USE

relief of occasional sleeplessness

DIRECTIONS

adults and children 12 years and over	take 2 caplets at bedtime if needed or as directed by a doctor
children under 12 years	do not use

WARNINGS

Do not use
• with any other product containing diphenhydramine, even one used on skin
• in children under 12 years of age

Ask a doctor before use if you have
• a breathing problem such as emphysema or chronic bronchitis
• trouble urinating due to an enlarged prostate gland
• glaucoma

Ask a doctor or pharmacist before use if you are taking sedatives or tranquilizers

When using this product
• drowsiness may occur
• avoid alcoholic drinks
• do not drive a motor vehicle or operate machinery

Stop use and ask a doctor if
• sleeplessness persists continuously for more than 2 weeks. Insomnia may be a symptom of serious underlying medical illness.

If pregnant or breast-feeding, ask a health professional before use.

Keep out of reach of children. In case of overdose, get medical help or contact a Poison Control Center right away.

Other Information:
• **Do not use if blister carton is opened or if blister unit is broken.**
• Store at room temperature

INACTIVE INGREDIENTS

carnauba wax, cellulose, croscarmellose sodium, dibasic calcium phosphate, FD&C Blue #1, hypromellose, magnesium stearate, polyethylene glycol, polysorbate 80, titanium dioxide.

HOW SUPPLIED

Light blue mini-caplets embossed with "SL" on one side in blister packs of 24 and 48.

Shown in Product Identification Guide, page 321

SIMPLY STUFFY™ LIQUID OTC

DESCRIPTION

Simply Stuffy™ Liquid is Cherry Berry-flavored and contains no alcohol or aspirin. Each teaspoonful (5 mL) contains pseudoephedrine HCL 15 mg.

ACTIONS

Simply Stuffy™ Liquid is a single ingredient product that contains the decongestant pseudoephedrine hydrochloride to provide fast, effective, temporary relief of your child's nasal congestion.

USES

temporarily relieves nasal congestion due to:
• the common cold • hay fever • upper respiratory allergies
• sinusitis

DIRECTIONS

- find right dose on chart below. If possible, use weight to dose; otherwise use age.
- only use with enclosed measuring cup
- if needed, repeat dose every 4 to 6 hours
- do not use more than 4 times in 24 hours

AccuDose™ Chart

Weight (lb)	Age (yr)	Dose (teaspoon)
under 24	under 2	call a doctor
24–47	2–5	1 tsp
48–95	6–11	2 tsp

Professional Dosage Schedule: 4–11 mos (12–17 lbs): ½ teaspoonful; 12–23 mos (18–23 lbs): ¾ teaspoonful; 2–3 yrs (24–35 lbs) 1 teaspoonful; 4–5 yrs (36–47 lbs): 1½ teaspoonsful; 6–8 yrs (48–59 lbs): 2 teaspoonsful; 9–10 yrs (60–71 lbs): 2½ teaspoonsful; 11 yrs (72–95 lbs): 3 teaspoonsful

If needed, repeat dose every 4 hours. Do not use more than 4 times in 24 hours.

WARNINGS

Do not use in a child who is taking a prescription monoamine oxidase inhibitor (MAOI) (certain drugs for depression, psychiatric or emotional conditions, or Parkinson's disease), or for 2 weeks after stopping the MAOI drug. If you do not know if your child's prescription drug contains an MAOI, ask a doctor or pharmacist before giving this product.

Ask a doctor before use if this child has
• heart disease • high blood pressure • thyroid disease
• diabetes

When using this product
- **do not exceed recommended dosage**

Stop use and ask a doctor if
- nervousness, dizziness, or sleeplessness occur
- symptoms do not get better within 7 days or occur with a fever

Keep out of reach of children. In case of overdose, get medical help or contact a Poison Control Center right away.

Other Information:
- **do not use if carton is opened, of if neck wrap or foil inner seal imprinted with "Safety Seal®" is broken or missing**
- store at room temperature

Professional Information:
Overdosage Information:

Symptoms from pseudoephedrine overdose consist most often of mild anxiety, tachycardia and/or mild hypertension. Symptoms usually appear within 4 to 8 hours of ingestion and are transient, usually requiring no treatment.

INACTIVE INGREDIENTS

citric acid, corn syrup, FD&C Red #40, flavor, glycerin, purified water, sodium benzoate, sucralose

HOW SUPPLIED

Cherry Berry flavored liquid in child resistant tamper-evident bottles of 4 fl. oz.

Shown in Product Identification Guide, page 321

ST. JOSEPH 81 mg Aspirin OTC
ST. JOSEPH 81 mg Adult Low Strength Aspirin Chewable & Enteric Coated Tablets

DESCRIPTION

Each St. Joseph Adult Low Strength Aspirin tablet contains 81 mg of aspirin.

USES

- temporarily relieves minor aches and pains or as recommended by your doctor
- ask your doctor about other uses for St. Joseph Adult 81 mg Aspirin

DIRECTIONS

- drink a full glass of water with each dose
- **adults and children 12 years and over:**
  - take 4 to 8 tablets every 4 hours while symptoms persist
  - do not exceed 48 tablets in 24 hours or as directed by a doctor
- **children under 12:**
  - do not use unless directed by a doctor

WARNINGS

Reye's syndrome: Children and teenagers should not use this drug for chicken pox or flu symptoms before a doctor is consulted about Reye's syndrome, a rare but serious illness reported to be associated with aspirin.

Allergy alert: Aspirin may cause a severe allergic reaction which may include:
- hives
- facial swelling
- asthma (wheezing)
- shock

Alcohol warning: If you consume 3 or more alcoholic drinks every day, ask your doctor whether you should take aspirin or other pain relievers/fever reducers. Aspirin may cause stomach bleeding.

Do not use
- if you have ever had an allergic reaction to any other pain reliever/fever reducer
- for at least 7 days after tonsillectomy or oral surgery unless directed by a doctor *(chewable tablet formulation only)*

Ask a doctor before use if you have
- asthma
- ulcers
- bleeding problems
- stomach problems that last or come back such as heartburn, upset stomach or pain

Ask a doctor or pharmacist before use if you are taking a prescription for:
- anticoagulation (blood thinning)
- gout
- diabetes
- arthritis

Stop use and ask a doctor if
- allergic reaction occurs. Seek medical help right away.
- ringing in the ears or loss of hearing occurs
- pain gets worse or lasts more than 10 days
- new symptoms occur
- redness or swelling is present

If pregnant or breast-feeding, ask a health professional before use. It is especially important not to use aspirin during the last three months of pregnancy unless definitely directed to do so by a doctor because it may cause problems in the unborn child or complications during delivery.

Keep out of reach of children. In case of overdose, get medical help or contact a Poison Control Center right away.

OTHER INFORMATION
- **do not use if carton is opened or neck wrap or foil inner seal imprinted with "Safety Seal®" is broken**
- store at room temperature. Avoid high humidity and excessive heat (40° C).

INACTIVE INGREDIENTS

St. Joseph 81 mg Adult Low Strength Aspirin Chewable Tablets: corn starch, FD&C yellow #6 aluminum lake, flavor, mannitol, saccharin, silicon dioxide, stearic acid. *Enteric Coated Tablets:* cellulose, corn starch, FD&C Red #40, FD&C Yellow #6, glyceryl monostearate, iron oxide, methacrylic acid, silicon dioxide, simethicone, stearic acid, triethyl citrate.

HOW SUPPLIED

St. Joseph 81 mg Adult Low Strength Chewable Aspirin Tablets: tamper evident bottles of 36 108 (Tri-Pack). *Enteric Coated Tablets:* tamper evident bottles of 36 100, 180, 300 and 395.

Comprehensive Prescribing Information
DESCRIPTION

St. Joseph Adult Low Strength Aspirin Chewable & Enteric Coated Tablets (acetylsalicylic acid) are available in 81 mg for oral administration. *St. Joseph 81 mg Adult Low Strength Aspirin Chewable Tablets* contain the following inactive ingredients: corn starch, FD&C yellow #6 aluminum lake, flavor, mannitol, saccharin, silicon dioxide, stearic acid. *St. Joseph 81 mg Adult Low Strength Aspirin Enteric Coated Tablets* contain the following inactive ingredients: cellulose, corn starch, FD&C Red #40, FD&C Yellow #6, glyceryl monostearate, iron oxide, methacrylic acid, silicon dioxide, simethicone, stearic acid, triethyl citrate. Aspirin is an odorless white, needle-like crystalline or powdery substance. When exposed to moisture, aspirin hydrolyzes into salicylic and acetic acids, and gives off a vinegary-odor. It is highly lipid soluble and slightly soluble in water.

CLINICAL PHARMACOLOGY

Mechanism of Action: Aspirin is a more potent inhibitor of both prostaglandin synthesis and platelet aggregation than other salicylic acid derivatives. The differences in activity between aspirin and salicylic acid are thought to be due to the acetyl group on the aspirin molecule. This acetyl group is responsible for the inactivation of cyclo-oxygenase via acetylation.

PHARMACOKINETICS

Absorption: In general, immediate release aspirin is well and completely absorbed from the gastrointestinal (GI) tract. Following absorption, aspirin is hydrolyzed to salicylic acid with peak plasma levels of salicylic acid occurring within 1–2 hours of dosing (see Pharmacokinetics—Metabolism). The rate of absorption from the GI tract is dependent upon the dosage form, the presence or absence of food, gastric pH (the presence or absence of GI antacids or buffering agents), and other physiologic factors. Enteric coated aspirin products are erratically absorbed from the GI tract.

Distribution: Salicylic acid is widely distributed to all tissues and fluids in the body including the central nervous system (CNS), breast milk, and fetal tissues. The highest concentrations are found in the plasma, liver, renal cortex, heart, and lungs. The protein binding of salicylate is concentration-dependent, i.e., nonlinear. At low concentrations (<100 micrograms/milliliter µg/mL), approximately 90 percent of plasma salicylate is bound to albumin while at higher concentrations (400 µg/mL), only about 75 percent is bound. The early signs of salicylic overdose (salicylism), including tinnitus (ringing in the ears), occur at plasma concentrations approximating 200 µg/mL. Severe toxic effects are associated with levels 400 µg/mL. (See Adverse Reactions and Overdosage.)

Metabolism: Aspirin is rapidly hydrolyzed in the plasma to salicylic acid such that plasma levels of aspirin are essentially undetectable 1–2 hours after dosing. Salicylic acid is primarily conjugated in the liver to form salicyluric acid, a phenolic glucuronide, an acyl glucuronide, and a number of minor metabolites. Salicylic acid has a plasma half-life of approximately 6 hours. Salicylate metabolism is saturable and total body clearance decreases at higher serum concentrations due to the limited ability of the liver to form both salicyluric acid and phenolic glucuronide. Following toxic doses (10–20 grams (g)), the plasma half-life may be increased to over 20 hours.

Elimination: The elimination of salicylic acid follows zero order pharmacokinetics; (i.e., the rate of drug elimination is constant in relation to plasma concentration). Renal excretion of unchanged drug depends upon urine pH. As urinary pH rises above 6.5, the renal clearance of free salicylate increases from <5 percent to 80 percent. Alkalinization of the urine is a key concept in the management of salicylate overdose. (See Overdosage.) Following therapeutic doses, approximately 10 percent is found excreted in the urine as salicylic acid, 75 percent as salicyluric acid, and 10 percent phenolic and 5 percent acyl glucuronides of salicylic acid.

Pharmacodynamics: Aspirin affects platelet aggregation by irreversibly inhibiting prostaglandin cyclo-oxygenase. The effect lasts for the life of the platelet and prevents the formation of the platelet aggregating factor thromboxane A2. Nonacetylated salicylates do not inhibit this enzyme and have no effect on platelet aggregation. At somewhat higher doses, aspirin reversibly inhibits the formation of prostaglandin I2 (prostacyclin), which is an arterial vasodilator and inhibits platelet aggregation.

At higher doses, aspirin is an effective anti-inflammatory agent, partially due to inhibition of inflammatory mediators via cyclo-oxygenase inhibition in peripheral tissues. In vitro studies suggest that other mediators of inflammation may also be suppressed by aspirin administration, although the precise mechanism of action has not been elucidated. It is this nonspecific suppression of cyclo-oxygenase activity in peripheral tissues following large doses that leads to its primary side effect of gastric irritation. (See Adverse Reactions.)

CLINICAL STUDIES

Ischemic Stroke and Transient Ischemic Attack (TIA): In clinical trials of subjects with TIA's due to fibrin platelet emboli or ischemic stroke, aspirin has been shown to significantly reduce the risk of the combined endpoint of stroke or death and the combined endpoint of TIA, stroke, or death by about 13–18 percent.

Suspected Acute Myocardial Infarction (MI): In a large, multi-center study of aspirin, streptokinase, and the combination of aspirin and streptokinase in 17,187 patients with suspected acute MI, aspirin treatment produced a 23-percent reduction in the risk of vascular mortality. Aspirin was also shown to have an additional benefit in patients given a thrombolytic agent.

Prevention of Recurrent MI and Unstable Angina Pectoris: These indications are supported by the results of six large, randomized, multi-center, placebo-controlled trials of predominantly male post-MI subjects and one randomized placebo-controlled study of men with unstable angina pectoris. Aspirin therapy in MI subjects was associated with a significant reduction (about 20 percent) in the risk of the combined endpoint of subsequent death and/or nonfatal reinfarction in these patients. In aspirin-treated unstable angina patients, the event rate was reduced to 5 percent from the 10 percent rate in the placebo group.

Chronic Stable Angina Pectoris: In a randomized, multicenter, double-blind trial designed to assess the role of aspirin for prevention of MI in patients with chronic stable angina pectoris, aspirin significantly reduced the primary combined endpoint of nonfatal MI, fatal MI, and sudden death by 34 percent. The secondary endpoint for vascular events (first occurrence of MI, stroke, or vascular death) was also significantly reduced (32 percent).

Revascularization Procedures: Most patients who undergo coronary artery revascularization procedures have already had symptomatic coronary artery disease for which aspirin is indicated. Similarly, patients with lesions of the carotid bifurcation sufficient to require carotid endarterectomy are likely to have had a precedent event. Aspirin is recom-

Continued on next page

St. Joseph Aspirin—Cont.

mended for patients who undergo revascularization procedures if there is a preexisting condition for which aspirin is already indicated.
Rheumatologic Diseases: In clinical studies in patients with rheumatoid arthritis, juvenile rheumatoid arthritis, ankylosing spondylitis and osteoarthritis, aspirin has been shown to be effective in controlling various indices of clinical disease activity.

ANIMAL TOXICOLOGY

The acute oral 50 percent lethal dose in rats is about 1.5 g/kilogram (kg) and in mice 1.1 g/kg. Renal papillary necrosis and decreased urinary concentrating ability occur in rodents chronically administered high doses. Dose-dependent gastric mucosal injury occurs in rats and humans. Mammals may develop aspirin toxicosis associated with GI symptoms, circulatory effects, and central nervous system depression. (See Overdosage.)

INDICATIONS AND USAGE

Vascular Indications (Ischemic Stroke, TIA, Acute MI, Prevention of Recurrent MI, Unstable Angina Pectoris, and Chronic Stable Angina Pectoris): Aspirin is indicated to: (1) Reduce the combined risk of death and nonfatal stroke in patients who have had ischemic stroke or transient ischemia of the brain due to fibrin platelet emboli, (2) reduce the risk of vascular mortality in patients with a suspected acute MI, (3) reduce the combined risk of death and nonfatal MI in patients with a previous MI or unstable angina pectoris, and (4) reduce the combined risk of MI and sudden death in patients with chronic stable angina pectoris.
Revascularization Procedures (Coronary Artery Bypass Graft (CABG), Percutaneous Transminase Coronary Angioplasty (PTCA), and Carotid Endarterectomy): Aspirin is indicated in patients who have undergone revascularization procedures (i.e., CABG, PTCA, or carotid endarterectomy) when there is a preexisting condition for which aspirin is already indicated.
Rheumatologic Disease Indications (Rheumatoid Arthritis, Juvenile Rheumatoid Arthritis, Spondyloarthropathies, Osteoarthritis, and the Arthritis and Pleurisy of Systemic Lupus Erythematosus (SLE)): Aspirin is indicated for the relief of the signs and symptoms of rheumatoid arthritis, juvenile rheumatoid arthritis, osteoarthritis, spondyloarthopathies, and arthritis and pleurisy associated with SLE.

CONTRAINDICATIONS

Allergy: Aspirin is contraindicated in patients with known allergy to nonsteroidal anti-inflammatory drug products and in patients with the syndrome of asthma, rhinitis, and nasal polyps. Aspirin may cause severe urticaria, angioedema, or bronchospasm (asthma).
Reye's Syndrome: Aspirin should not be used in children or teenagers for viral infections, with or without fever, because of the risk of Reye's syndrome with concomitant use of aspirin in certain viral illnesses.

WARNINGS

Alcohol Warning: Patients who consume three or more alcoholic drinks every day should be counseled about the bleeding risks involved with chronic, heavy alcohol use while taking aspirin.
Coagulation Abnormalities: Even low doses of aspirin can inhibit platelet function leading to an increase in bleeding time. This can adversely affect patients with inherited (hemophilia) or acquired (liver disease or vitamin K deficiency) bleeding disorders.
GI Side Effects: GI side effects include stomach pain, heartburn, nausea, vomiting, and gross GI bleeding. Although minor upper GI symptoms, such as dyspepsia, are common and can occur anytime during therapy, physicians should remain alert for signs of ulceration and bleeding, even in the absence of previous GI symptoms. Physicians should inform patients about the signs and symptoms of GI side effects and what steps to take if they occur.
Peptic Ulcer Disease: Patients with a history of active peptic ulcer disease should avoid using aspirin, which can cause gastric mucosal irritation and bleeding.

PRECAUTIONS

General: Renal Failure: Avoid aspirin in patients with severe renal failure (glomerular filtration rate less than 10 mL/minute)
Hepatic Insufficiency: Avoid aspirin in patients with severe hepatic insufficiency.
Sodium Restricted Diets: Patients with sodium-retaining states, such as congestive heart failure or renal failure, should avoid sodium-containing buffered aspirin preparations because of their high sodium content.
Laboratory Tests: Aspirin has been associated with elevated hepatic enzymes, blood urea nitrogen and serum creatinine, hyperkalemia, proteinuria, and prolonged bleeding time.
DRUG INTERACTIONS
Angiotensin Converting Enzyme (ACE) Inhibitors: The hyponatremic and hypotensive effects of ACE inhibitors may be diminished by the concomitant administration of aspirin due to its indirect effect on the renin-angiotensin conversion pathway.
Acetazolamide: Concurrent use of aspirin and acetazolamide can lead to high serum concentrations of acetazolamide (and toxicity) due to competition at the renal tubule for secretion.
Anticoagulant Therapy (Heparin and Warfarin): Patients on anticoagulation therapy are at increased risk for bleeding because of drug-drug interactions and the effect on platelets. Aspirin can displace warfarin from protein binding sites, leading to prolongation of both the prothrombin time and the bleeding time. Aspirin can increase the anticoagulant activity of heparin, increasing bleeding risk.
Anticonvulsants: Salicylate can displace protein-bound phenytoin and valproic acid, leading to a decrease in the total concentration of phenytoin and an increase in serum valproic acid levels.
Beta Blockers: The hypotensive effects of beta blockers may be diminished by the concomitant administration of aspirin due to inhibition of renal prostaglandins, leading to decreased renal blood flow, and salt and fluid retention.
Diuretics: The effectiveness of diuretics in patients with underlying renal or cadiovascular disease may be diminished by the concomitant administration of aspirin due to inhibition of renal prostaglandins, leading to decreased renal blood flow and salt and fluid retention.
Methotrexate: Salicylate can inhibit renal clearance of methotrexate, leading to bone marrow toxicity, especially in the elderly or renal impaired.
Nonsteroidal Anti-Inflammatory Drugs (NSAID's): The concurrent use of aspirin with other NSAID's should be avoided because this may increase bleeding or lead to decreased renal function.
Oral Hypoglycemics: Moderate doses of aspirin may increase the effectiveness of oral hypoglycemic drugs, leading to hypoglycemia.
Uricosuric Agents (Probenecid and Sulfinpyrazone): Salicylates antagonize the uricosuric action of uricosuric agents.
Carcinogenesis, Mutagenesis, Impairment of Fertility: Administration of aspirin for 68 weeks at 0.5 percent in the feed of rats was not carcinogenic. In the Ames Salmonella assay, aspirin was not mutagenic; however, aspirin did induce chromosome aberrations in cultured human fibroblasts. Aspirin inhibits ovulation in rats. (See Pregnancy.)
Pregnancy: Pregnant women should only take aspirin if clearly needed. Because of the known effects of NSAID's on the fetal cardiovascular system (closure of the ductus arteriosus), use during the third trimester of pregnancy should be avoided. Salicylate products have also been associated with alterations in maternal and neonatal hemostasis mechanisms, decreased birth weight, and with perinatal mortality.
Labor and Delivery: Aspirin should be avoided 1 week prior to and during labor and delivery because it can result in excessive blood loss at delivery. Prolonged gestation and prolonged labor due to prostaglandin inhibition have been reported.
Nursing Mothers: Nursing mothers should avoid using aspirin because salicylate is excreted in breast milk. Use of high doses may lead to rashes, platelet abnormalities, and bleeding in nursing infants.
Pediatric Use: Pediatric dosing recommendations for juvenile rheumatoid arthritis are based on well-controlled clinical studies. An initial dose of 90–130 mg/kg/day in divided doses, with an increase as needed for anti-inflammatory efficacy (target plasma salicylate levels of 150–300 μg/mL) are effective. At high doses (i.e., plasma levels of greater than 200 μg/mL), the incidence of toxicity increases.

ADVERSE REACTIONS

Many adverse reactions due to aspirin ingestion are dose-related. The following is a list of adverse reactions that have been reported in the literature. (See Warnings.)
Body as a Whole: Fever, hypothermia, thirst.
Cardiovascular: Dysrhythmias, hypotension, tachycardia.
Central Nervous System: Agitation, cerebral edema, coma, confusion, dizziness, headache, subdural or intracranial hemorrhage, lethargy, seizures.
Fluid and Electrolyte: Dehydration, hyperkalemia, metabolic acidosis, respiratory alkalosis.
Gastrointestinal: Dyspepsia, GI bleeding, ulceration and perforation, nausea, vomiting, transient elevations of hepatic enzymes, hepatitis, Reye's Syndrome, pancreatitis.
Hematologic: Prolongation of the prothrombin time, disseminated intravascular coagulation, coagulopathy, thrombocytopenia.
Hypersensitivity: Acute anaphylaxis, angioedema, asthma, bronchospasm, laryngeal edema, urticaria.
Musculoskeletal: Rhabdomyolysis.
Metabolism: Hypoglycemia (in children), hyperglycemia.
Reproductive: Prolonged pregnancy and labor, stillbirths, lower birth weight infants, antepartum and postpartum bleeding.
Special Senses: Hearing loss, tinnitus. Patients with high frequency hearing loss may have difficulty perceiving tinnitus. In these patients, tinnitus cannot be used as a clinical indicator of salicylism.
Urogenital: Interstitial nephritis, papillary necrosis, proteinuria, renal insufficiency and failure.

DRUG ABUSE AND DEPENDENCE

Aspirin is nonnarcotic. There is no known potential for addiction associated with the use of aspirin.

OVERDOSAGE

Salicylate toxicity may result from acute ingestion (overdose) or chronic intoxication. The early signs of salicylic overdose (salicylism), including tinnitus (ringing in the ears), occur at plasma concentrations approaching 200 μg/mL. Plasma concentrations of aspirin above 300 μg/mL are clearly toxic. Severe toxic effects are associated with levels above 400 μg/mL (See Clinical Pharmacology.) A single lethal dose of aspirin in adults is not known with certainty but death may be expected at 30 g. For real or suspected overdose, a Poison Control Center should be contacted immediately. Careful medical management is essential.
Signs and Symptoms: In acute overdose, severe acid-base and electrolyte disturbances may occur and are complicated by hyperthermia and dehydration. Respiratory alkalosis occurs early while hyperventilation is present, but is quickly followed by metabolic acidosis.
Treatment: Treatment consists primarily of supporting vital functions, increasing salicylate elimination, and correcting the acid-base disturbance. Gastric emptying and/or lavage is recommended as soon as possible after ingestion, even if the patient has vomited spontaneously. After lavage and/or emesis, administration of activated charcoal, as a slurry, is beneficial, if less than 3 hours have passed since ingestion. Charcoal adsorption should not be employed prior to emesis and lavage. Severity of aspirin intoxication is determined by measuring the blood salicylate level. Acid-base status should be closely followed with serial blood gas and serum pH measurements. Fluid and electrolyte balance should also be maintained. In severe cases, hyperthermia and hypovolemia are the major immediate threats to life. Children should be sponged with tepid water. Replacement fluids should be administered intravenously and augmented with correction of acidosis. Plasma electrolytes and pH should be monitored to promote alkaline diuresis of salicylate if renal function is normal. Infusion of glucose may be required to control hypoglycemia. Hemodialysis and peritoneal dialysis can be performed to reduce the body drug content. In patients with renal insufficiency or in cases of life-threatening intoxication, dialysis is usually required. Exchange transfusion may be indicated in infants and young children.

DOSAGE AND ADMINISTRATION

Each dose of aspirin should be taken with a full glass of water unless the patient is fluid restricted. Anti-inflammatory and analgesic dosages should be individualized. When aspirin is used in high doses, the development of tinnitus may be used as a clinical sign of elevated plasma salicylate levels except in patients with high frequency hearing loss.
Ischemic Stroke and TIA: 50–325 mg once a day. Continue therapy indefinitely
Suspected Acute MI: The initial dose of 160–162.5 mg is administered as soon as an MI is suspected. The maintenance dose of 160–162.5 mg a day is continued for 30 days post-infarction. After 30 days, consider further therapy based on dosage and administration for prevention of recurrent MI.
Prevention of Recurrent MI: 75–325 mg once a day. Continue therapy indefinitely.
Unstable Angina Pectoris: 75–325 mg once a day. Continue therapy indefinitely.
Chronic Stable Angina Pectoris: 75–325 mg once a day. Continue therapy indefinitely.
CABG: 325 mg daily starting 6 hours post-procedure. Continue therapy for 1 year post-procedure.
PTCA: The initial dose of 325 mg daily should be given 2 hours pre-surgery. Maintenance dose is 160–325 mg daily. Continue therapy indefinitely.
Carotid Endarterectomy: Doses of 80 mg once daily to 650 mg twice daily, started presurgery, are recommended. Continue therapy indefinitely.
Rheumatoid Arthritis: The initial dose is 3 g a day in divided doses. Increase as needed for anti-inflammatory efficacy with target plasma salicylate levels of 150–300 μg/mL. At high doses (i.e., plasma levels of greater than 200 μg/mL), the incidence of toxicity increases.
Juvenile Rheumatoid Arthritis: Initial dose is 90–130 mg/kg/day in divided doses. Increase as needed for anti-inflammatory efficacy with target plasma salicylate levels of 150–300 μg/mL. At high doses (i.e., plasma levels of greater than 200 μg/mL), the incidence of toxicity increases.
Spondyloarthropathies: Up to 4 g per day in divided doses.
Osteoarthritis: Up to 3 g per day in divided doses.
Arthritis and Pleurisy of SLE: The initial dose is 3 g a day in divided doses. Increase as needed for anti-inflammatory efficacy with target plasma salicylate levels of 150–300 μg/mL. At high doses (i.e., plasma levels of greater than 200 μg/mL), the incidence of toxicity increases.

HOW SUPPLIED

St. Joseph Adult Low Strength Aspirin Chewable Tablets are round, concave, orange-flavored, orange-colored tablets that are debossed with the "SJ" logo. Available as follows:
NDC 50580-173-36 Bottle of 36 tablets
NDC Coated Tablets 50580-173-08 Tri-Pack
St Joseph Adult Low Strength Enteric Coated Tablets are round, concave, pink-coated tablets that are printed with the "St J" logo. Available as follows:
NDC 50580-126-36 Bottle of 36 tablets
NDC 50580-126-10 Bottle of 100 tablets
NDC 50580-126-18 Bottle of 180 tablets
Store in tight container at 25 deg.C (77 deg.F); excursions permitted to 15–30 deg.C (59–86 deg.F).

Shown in Product Identification Guide, page 321

Regular Strength TYLENOL® acetaminophen Tablets OTC

Extra Strength TYLENOL® acetaminophen Gelcaps, Geltabs, Caplets, Tablets

Extra Strength TYLENOL® acetaminophen Rapid Release Gels

Extra Strength TYLENOL® acetaminophen Adult Liquid Pain Reliever

TYLENOL® Arthritis Pain Acetaminophen Extended Release Geltabs/Caplets

TYLENOL® 8 Hour Acetaminophen Extended Release Geltabs/Caplets

Product information for all dosage forms of Adult TYLENOL actaminophen have been combined under this heading.

DESCRIPTION

Each Regular Strength TYLENOL® Tablet contains acetaminophen 325 mg. *Each Extra Strength TYLENOL® Gelcap, Geltab, Caplet, Tablet or Rapid Release Gel* contains acetaminophen 500 mg. *Extra Strength TYLENOL® Adult Liquid* is alcohol-free and each 15 mL (1/2 fl oz or one tablespoonful) contains 500 mg acetaminophen. *Each TYLENOL® Arthritis Pain Extended Relief Caplet* and each *TYLENOL® 8 Hour Extended Release Geltab/caplet* contains acetaminophen 650 mg.

ACTIONS

Acetaminophen is a clinically proven analgesic/antipyretic. Acetaminophen produces analgesia by elevation of the pain threshold and antipyresis through action on the hypothalamic heat-regulating center. Acetaminophen is equal to aspirin in analgesic and antipyretic effectiveness and it is unlikely to produce many of the side effects associated with aspirin and aspirin-containing products. *Tylenol Arthritis Pain Extended Relief* and *TYLENOL 8 Hour Extended Release* use a unique, patented, bilayer caplet. The first layer dissolves quickly to provide prompt relief while the second layer is time released to provide up to 8 hours of relief.

USES

Regular Strength TYLENOL® Tablets, Extra Strength TYLENOL® Gelcaps, Geltabs, Caplets, Tablets, or Rapid Release Gels: temporarily relieves minor aches and pains due to:
• headache • muscular aches • backache • arthritis
• the common cold • toothache • menstrual cramps
• temporarily reduces fever

Extra Strength TYLENOL® Adult Liquid: temporarily relieves minor aches and pains due to:
• headache • muscular aches • backache • arthritis
• the common cold • toothache • menstrual cramps
• reduces fever

TYLENOL® Arthritis Pain Extended Release Geltabs/Caplets: temporarily relieves minor aches and pains due to:
• arthritis • the common cold • headache • toothache
• muscular aches • backache • menstrual cramps

TYLENOL® 8 Hour Extended Release Geltabs/Caplets: temporarily relieves minor aches and pains due to:
• muscular aches • backache • headache • toothache • the common cold
• menstrual cramps • minor pain of arthritis
• temporarily reduces fever

DIRECTIONS

Regular Strength TYLENOL® Tablets:
• **do not take more than directed (see overdose warning)**

adults and children 12 years and over	• take 2 tablets every 4 to 6 hours as needed • do not take more than 12 tablets in 24 hours
children 6–11 years	• take 1 tablet every 4 to 6 hours as needed • do not take more than 5 in 24 hours
children under 6 years	do not use this adult Regular Strength product in children under 6 years of age; this will provide more than the recommended dose (overdose) of TYLENOL® and may cause liver damage

Extra Strength TYLENOL® Gelcaps, Geltabs, Caplets, Tablets, or Rapid Release Gels:
• **do not take more than directed (see overdose warning)**

adults and children 12 years and over	• take 2 gelcaps, geltabs, caplets, or tablets every 4 to 6 hours as needed • do not take more than 8 gelcaps, geltabs, caplets, or tablets in 24 hours
children under 12 years	do not use this adult Extra Strength product in children under 12 years of age; this will provide more than the recommended dose (overdose) of TYLENOL® and may cause liver damage

Extra Strength TYLENOL® Adult Liquid:
• **do not take more than directed (see overdose warning)**

adults and children 12 years and over	• take 2 tablespoons (tbsp.) in dose cup provided every 4 to 6 hours as needed • do not take more than 8 tablespoons in 24 hours
children under 12 years	do not use this adult Extra Strength product in children under 12 years of age; this will provide more than the recommended dose (overdose) of TYLENOL® and may cause liver damage

TYLENOL® 8 Hour Extended Release Geltabs/Caplets
• **do not take more than directed (see overdose warning)**

adults and children 12 years and over	• take 2 geltabs/caplets every 8 hours with water • swallow whole – do not crush, chew or dissolve • do not take more than 6 geltabs/caplets in 24 hours • do not use for more than 10 days unless directed by a doctor
children under 12 years	• do not use

TYLENOL® Arthritis Pain Extended Release Geltabs/Caplets
• **do not take more than directed (see overdose warning)**

adults	• take 2 geltabs or caplets every 8 hours with water • swallow whole – do not crush, chew or dissolve • do not take more than 6 geltabs or caplets in 24 hours • do not use for more than 10 days unless directed by a doctor
under 18 years of age	• ask a doctor

WARNINGS

Regular Strength TYLENOL® Tablets, Extra Strength TYLENOL® Gelcaps, Geltabs, Caplets, Tablets or Rapid Release Gels, Extra Strength TYLENOL® Liquid

Alcohol warning: If you consume 3 or more alcoholic drinks every day, ask your doctor whether you should take acetaminophen or other pain relievers/fever reducers. Acetaminophen may cause liver damage.

Do not use:
• with any other product containing acetaminophen.

Stop using and ask a doctor if:
• new symptoms occur
• redness or swelling is present
• pain gets worse or lasts for more than 10 days
• fever gets worse or lasts for more than 3 days

If pregnant or breast-feeding, ask a health professional before use.

Keep out of reach of children.

Overdose warning: Taking more than the recommended dose (overdose) may cause liver damage. In case of overdose, get medical help or contact a Poison Control Center right away. Quick medical attention is critical for adults as well as for children even if you do not notice any signs or symptoms.

TYLENOL® Arthritis Pain Extended Release Geltabs/Caplets:

Alcohol warning: If you consume 3 or more alcoholic drinks every day, ask your doctor whether you should take acetaminophen or other pain relievers/fever reducers. Acetaminophen may cause liver damage.

Do not use
• with any other product containing acetaminophen.

Stop use and ask a doctor if
• new symptoms occur
• redness or swelling is present
• pain gets worse or lasts for more than 10 days

If pregnant or breast-feeding, ask a health professional before use.

Keep out of reach of children.

Overdose warning: Taking more than the recommended dose (overdose) may cause liver damage. In case of overdose, get medical help or contact a Poison Control Center right away. Quick medical attention is critical for adults as well as for children even if you do not notice any signs or symptoms.

TYLENOL® 8 Hour Extended Release Geltab/Caplets:

Alcohol warning: If you consume 3 or more alcoholic drinks every day, ask your doctor whether you should take acetaminophen or other pain relievers/fever reducers. Acetaminophen may cause liver damage.

Do not use
• with any other product containing acetaminophen.

Stop use and ask a doctor if
• new symptoms occur
• redness or swelling is present
• pain gets worse or lasts for more than 10 days
• fever gets worse or lasts for more than 3 days.

If pregnant or breast-feeding, ask a health professional before use.

Keep out of reach of children.

Overdose warning: Taking more than the recommended dose (overdose) may cause liver damage. In case of overdose, get medical help or contact a Poison Control Center right away. Quick medical attention is critical for adults as well as for children even if you do not notice any signs or symptoms.

OTHER INFORMATION

Regular Strength TYLENOL® Tablets
• **do not use if carton is opened or red neck wrap or foil inner seal imprinted with "Safety Seal®" is broken**
• store between 20–25°C (68–77°F)

Extra Strength TYLENOL® Gelcaps, Geltabs, Caplets, Tablets, or Rapid Release Gels:
• **do not use if carton is opened or red neck wrap or foil inner seal imprinted with "Safety Seal®" is broken**
• store between 20–25°C (68–77°F) (*tablet and caplet*)
• store between 20–25°C (68–77°F); avoid high humidity (*Gelcap, Geltab, and Rapid Release Gel*)

Extra Strength TYLENOL® Adult Liquid
• **do not use if carton is opened, or if bottle wrap or foil inner seal imprinted "Safety Seal®" is broken or missing.**
• store between 20–25°C (68–77°F)

TYLENOL® Arthritis Pain Extended Release Geltabs/Caplets and *TYLENOL® 8 Hour Extended Release Geltabs/Caplets*
• **do not use if carton is opened or neck wrap or foil inner seal with "Safety Seal®" is broken**
• store at 20–25°C (68–77°F)
• avoid excessive heat at 40°C (104°F)

Professional Information:

Overdosage Information for all Adult Tylenol products

ACETAMINOPHEN: Acetaminophen in massive overdosage may cause hepatic toxicity in some patients. In adults and adolescents (≧ 12 years of age), hepatic toxicity may occur following ingestion of greater than 7.5 to 10 grams over a period of 8 hours or less. Fatalities are infrequent (less than 3–4% of untreated cases) and have rarely been reported with overdoses of less than 15 grams. In children (<12 years of age), an acute overdosage of less than 150 mg/kg has not been associated with hepatic toxicity. Early symptoms following a potentially hepatotoxic overdose may include: nausea, vomiting, diaphoresis and general malaise. Clinical and laboratory evidence of hepatic toxicity may not be apparent until 48 to 72 hours postingestion. In adults and adolescents, any individual presenting with an unknown amount of acetaminophen ingested or with a questionable or unreliable history about the time of ingestion should have a plasma acetaminophen level drawn and be treated with *N*-acetylcysteine. For full prescribing information, refer to the *N*-acetylcysteine package insert. Do not await results of assays for plasma acetaminophen levels before initiating treatment with *N*-acetylcysteine. The following additional procedures are recommended: Promptly initiate gastric decontamination of the stomach. A plasma acetaminophen assay should be obtained as early as possible, but no sooner than four hours following ingestion. If an acetaminophen *extended release* product is involved, it may be appropriate to obtain an additional plasma acetaminophen level 4–6 hours following the initial acetaminophen level. If either acetaminophen level plots above the treatment line on the acetaminophen overdose nomogram, *N*-acetylcysteine treatment should be continued for a full course of therapy. Liver function studies should be obtained initially and repeated at 24-hour intervals. Serious toxicity or fatalities have been extremely infrequent following an acute acetaminophen overdose in young children, possibly because of differences in the way they metabolize acetaminophen. In children, the maximum potential amount ingested can be more easily estimated. If more than 150 mg/kg or an unknown amount was ingested, obtain a plasma acetaminophen level as soon as possible, but no sooner than 4 hours following ingestion. If an acetaminophen *extended release* product is involved, it may be appropriate to obtain an additional plasma acetaminophen level 4–6 hours following the initial acetaminophen level. If either acetaminophen level plots above the treatment line on the acetaminophen overdose nomogram, *N*-acetylcysteine treatment should be initiated and continued for a full course of therapy. If an assay cannot be obtained and the estimated acetaminophen ingestion exceeds 150 mg/kg, dosing with *N*-acetylcysteine should be initiated and continued for a full course of therapy. For additional emergency information, call your regional poison

Continued on next page

Tylenol—Cont.

center or call the Rocky Mountain Poison Center toll-free, (1-800-525-6115).

Our adult Tylenol® combination products contain active ingredients in addition to acetaminophen. The following is basic overdose information regarding those ingredients.

CHLORPHENIRAMINE: Chlorpheniramine toxicity should be treated as you would an anthihistamine/anticholinergic overdose and is likely to be present within a few hours after acute ingestion.

DEXTROMETHORHPHAN: Acute dextromethorphan overdose usually does not result in serious signs and symptoms unless massive amounts have been ingested. Signs and symptoms of a substantial overdose may include nausea and vomiting, visual disturbances, CNS disturbances and urinary retention.

DIPHENHYDRAMINE: Diphenhydramine toxicity should be treated as you would an antihistamine/anticholinergic overdose and is likely to be present within a few hours after acute ingestion.

DOXYLAMINE: Doxylamine toxicity should be treated as you would an antihistamine/anticholinergic overdose and is likely to be present within a few hours after acute ingestion.

GUAIFENESIN: Guaifenesin should be treated as a nontoxic ingestion.

PAMABROM: Acute overexposure of diuretics is primarily associated with fluid and electrolyte loss. Fluid loss should be treated with the appropriate intravenous and/or oral fluids.

PSEUDOEPHEDRINE: Symptoms from pseudoephedrine overdose consist most often of mild anxiety, tachycardia and/or mild hypertension. Symptoms usually appear within 4 to 8 hours of ingestion and are transient, usually requiring no treatment.

For additional emergency information, please contact your local poison control center.

Alcohol Information: Chronic heavy alcohol abusers may be at increased risk of liver toxicity from excessive acetaminophen use, although reports of this event are rare. Reports usually involve cases of severe chronic alcoholics and the dosages of acetaminophen most often exceed recommended doses and often involve substantial overdose. Healthcare professionals should alert their patients who regularly consume large amounts of alcohol not to exceed recommended doses of acetaminophen.

INACTIVE INGREDIENTS

Regular Strength TYLENOL® Tablets: cellulose, corn starch, magnesium stearate, sodium starch glycolate.

Extra Strength TYLENOL® **Tablets**: cellulose, corn starch, magnesium stearate, sodium starch glycolate. **Caplets**: cellulose, corn starch, FD&C Red #40, hypromellose, magnesium stearate, polyethylene glycol, sodium starch glycolate, titanium dioxide. **Gelcaps**: benzyl alcohol, butylparaben, castor oil, cellulose, corn starch, D&C Yellow #10, edetate calcium disodium, FD&C Blue #1, FD&C Blue #2, FD&C Red #40, gelatin, hypromellose, magnesium stearate, methylparaben, propylparaben, sodium lauryl sulfate, sodium propionate, sodium starch glycolate, titanium dioxide. **Geltabs**: benzyl alcohol, butylparaben, castor oil, cellulose, corn starch, D&C Yellow #10, edetate calcium disodium, FD&C Blue #1, FD&C Blue #2, FD&C Red #40, gelatin, hypromellose, magnesium stearate, methylparaben, propylparaben, sodium lauryl sulfate, sodium propionate, sodium starch glycolate, titanium dioxide. **Rapid Release Gels**: benzyl alcohol, black iron oxide, butylparaben, cellulose, corn starch, D&C yellow #10, edetate calcium disodium, FD&C blue #2, FD&C red #40 gelatin, hypromellose, magnesium stearate, methylparaben, polyethylene glycol, polysorbate 80, propylparaben, red iron oxide, sodium lauryl sulfate, sodium propionate, sodium starch glycolate, titanium dioxide, yellow iron oxide.

Extra Strength TYLENOL® Adult Liquid: citric acid, corn syrup, D&C Red #33, FD&C Red #40, flavor, polyethylene glycol, purified water, saccharin sodium, sodium benzoate, sorbitol

TYLENOL® Arthritis Pain Extended Relief Caplets: corn starch, hydroxyethyl cellulose, hypromellose, magnesium stearate, microcrystalline cellulose, povidone, powdered cellulose, pregelatinized starch, sodium starch glycolate, titanium dioxide, triacetin. **Geltabs**: benzyl alcohol, butylparaben, castor oil, cellulose, corn starch, edetate calcium disodium, FD&C Blue #1, FD&C Blue #2, gelatin, hydroxyethyl cellulose, hypromellose, magnesium stearate, methylparaben, povidone, propylparaben, sodium lauryl sulfate, sodium propionate, sodium starch glycolate, titanium dioxide.

Tylenol 8 Hour Extended Release **Caplets**: corn starch, D&C Yellow #10, FD&C Red #40, FD&C Yellow #6, hydroxyethyl cellulose, magnesium stearate, microcrystalline cellulose, polyethylene glycol, polyvinyl alcohol, povidone, powdered cellulose, pregelatinized starch, sodium starch glycolate, sucralose, talc, titanium dioxide. **Geltabs**: benzyl alcohol, butylparaben, castor oil, cellulose, corn starch, edetate calcium disodium, FD & C Blue #1, FD & C Blue #2, FD & C Red #40, gelatin, hydroxyethyl cellulose, hypromellose, magnesium stearate, methylparaben, povidone, propylparaben, sodium lauryl sulfate, sodium propionate, sodium starch glycolate, titanium dioxide

HOW SUPPLIED

Regular Strength TYLENOL® Tablets: (colored white, scored, imprinted "TYLENOL" and "325")—tamper-evident bottles of 100.

Extra Strength TYLENOL® Tablets: (colored white, imprinted "TYLENOL" and "500")—tamper-evident bottles of 30, 60, 100, and 200. *Caplets* (colored white, imprinted "TYLENOL 500 mg")—vials of 10, and tamper-evident bottles of 8, 16, 40, 325, 24, 50, 100, 150, and 250. *Gelcaps* (colored yellow and red, imprinted "Tylenol 500") tamper-evident bottles of 40, 24, 50, 100, 150 and 225. *Geltabs* (colored yellow and red, imprinted "Tylenol 500") tamper-evident bottles of 24, 50, 40, 100, and 150. *Rapid Release Gels* (colored red and light blue with an exposed grey band; gelcaps are imprinted with "TY 500") tamper-evident bottles of 8, 24, 50, 100, 150, and 290.

Extra Strength TYLENOL® Adult Liquid: Cherry-flavored liquid (colored red) 8 fl. oz. tamper-evident bottle with child resistant safety cap and special dosage cup.

TYLENOL® Arthritis Pain Extended Relief Caplets: (colored white, engraved "TYLENOL ER") tamper-evident bottles of 24, 50, and 100, 150, 250 and 290

TYLENOL® 8 Hour Extended Release Geltabs: (colored white and red, imprinted "8 HOUR") tamper-evident bottles of 20, 40 and 80. *Caplets:* (colored red, imprinted "8 hour") available in 24's, 50's, 100's, 150's and 200's.

Shown in Product Identification Guide, page 321

TYLENOL® Severe Allergy — OTC
Caplets
Maximum Strength

TYLENOL® Allergy Sinus
Night Time Caplets
Maximum Strength

TYLENOL® Allergy Sinus
Day Time Caplets, Gelcaps and Geltabs

Product information for all dosage forms of TYLENOL Allergy have been combined under this heading.

DESCRIPTION

Each *TYLENOL® Severe Allergy Caplet* contains acetaminophen 500 mg and diphenhydramine HCl 12.5 mg. Each *Maximum Strength TYLENOL® Allergy Sinus Night Time Caplet* contains acetaminophen 500 mg, diphenhydramine HCl 25 mg, and pseudoephedrine HCl 30 mg. Each *Maximum Strength TYLENOL® Allergy Sinus Day Time Caplet Gelcap and Geltab* contains acetaminophen 500 mg, chlorpheniramine maleate 2 mg, and pseudoephedrine HCl 30 mg.

ACTIONS

TYLENOL® Severe Allergy Caplets contain a clinically proven analgesic-antipyretic and antihistamine. Acetaminophen produces analgesia by elevation of the pain threshold and antipyresis through action on the hypothalamic heat regulating center. Acetaminophen is equal to aspirin in analgesic and antipyretic effectiveness, and it is unlikely to produce many of the side effects associated with aspirin and aspirin-containing products.

Diphenhydramine HCl is an antihistamine which helps provide temporary relief of itchy, watery eyes, runny nose, sneezing, itching of the nose or throat due to hay fever or other respiratory allergies.

Maximum Strength TYLENOL® Allergy Sinus Night Time Caplets contain, in addition to the above ingredients, a decongestant, pseudoephedrine HCl. Pseudoephedrine is a sympathomimetic amine which provides temporary relief of nasal and sinus congestion.

Maximum Strength TYLENOL® Allergy Sinus Day Time Caplets, Gelcaps and Geltabs contain acetaminophen, pseudoephedrine HCl and the antihistamine, chlorpheniramine maleate. Chlorpheniramine is an antihistamine which helps provide temporary relief of runny nose, sneezing and watery and itchy eyes.

USES

TYLENOL® Severe Allergy: temporarily relieves these symptoms due to hay fever or other upper respiratory allergies:
- itchy, watery eyes • runny nose
- sneezing • sore throat
- itching of nose or throat

Maximum Strength TYLENOL® Allergy Sinus Night Time and TYLENOL® Allergy Sinus Day Time: temporarily relieves these symptoms due to hay fever or other upper respiratory allergies:
- nasal congestion • sinus pressure
- sinus pain • headache
- runny nose • sneezing
- itchy, watery eyes • itchy throat

DIRECTIONS

TYLENOL® Severe Allergy:
- **do not take more than directed (see overdose warning)**

adults and children 12 years and over	• take 2 caplets every 4 to 6 hours as needed • do not take more than 8 caplets in 24 hours
children under 12 years	• do not use this adult product in children under 12 years of age; this will provide more than the recommended dose (overdose) and may cause liver damage.

Maximum Strength TYLENOL® Allergy Sinus Night Time:
- **do not take more than directed (see overdose warning)**

adults and children 12 years and over	• take 2 caplets every 4 to 6 hours as needed • do not take more than 8 caplets in 24 hours
children under 12 years	• do not use this adult product in children under 12 years of age; this will provide more than the recommended dose (overdose) and may cause liver damage.

Maximum Strength TYLENOL® Allergy Sinus Day Time:
- **do not take more than directed (see overdose warning)**

adults and children 12 years and over	• take two caplets, gelcaps, or geltabs every 4 to 6 hours as needed • do not take more than 8 caplets, gelcaps, or geltabs in 24 hours
children under 12 years	• do not use this adult product in children under 12 years of age; this will provide more than the recommended dose (overdose) and may cause liver damage.

WARNINGS

Alcohol warning: If you consume 3 or more alcoholic drinks every day, ask your doctor whether your should take acetaminophen or other pain relievers/fever reducers. Acetaminophen may cause liver damage.

Sore throat warning: If sore throat is severe, persists for more than 2 days, is accompanied or followed by fever, headache, rash, nausea or vomiting, consult a doctor promptly. *(applies to TYLENOL® Severe Allergy only)*

Do not use
- if you are now taking a prescription monoamine oxidase inhibitor (MAOI) (certain drugs for depression, psychiatric or emotional conditions, or Parkinson's disease) or for 2 weeks after stopping the MAOI drug. If you do not know if your prescription drug contains an MAOI, ask a doctor or pharmacist before taking this product (does not apply to *TYLENOL® Severe Allergy)*
- with any other product containing acetaminophen
- with any other product containing diphenhydramine, even one used on skin. (does not apply to TYLENOL® Allergy Sinus Day Time)

Ask a doctor or pharmacist before use if you are taking sedatives or tranquilizers

Stop use and ask a doctor if
- new symptoms occur
- redness or swelling is present
- pain gets worse or lasts for more than 7 days
- fever gets worse or lasts for more than 3 days
- you get nervous, dizzy or sleepless (does not apply to TYLENOL® Severe Allergy)

If pregnant or breast feeding, ask a health professional before use.

Keep out of reach of children.

Overdose warning: Taking more than the recommended dose (overdose) may cause liver damage. In case of overdose, get medical help or contact a Poison Control Center right away. Quick medical attention is critical for adults as well as for children even if you do not notice any signs or symptoms.

When using this product
- **do not exceed recommended dosage**
- marked drowsiness may occur (does not apply to TYLENOL® Allergy Sinus Day Time)
- drowsiness may occur (applies to TYLENOL® Allergy Sinus Day Time only)
- avoid alcoholic drinks
- alcohol, sedatives and tranquilizers may increase drowsiness
- be careful when driving a motor vehicle or operating machinery
- excitability may occur, especially in children

TYLENOL® Severe Allergy

Ask a doctor before use if you have
- glaucoma
- trouble urinating due to an enlarged prostate gland
- a breathing problem such as emphysema or chronic bronchitis

Maximum Strength TYLENOL® Allergy Sinus Night Time and Maximum Strength TYLENOL® Allergy Sinus Day Time

Ask a doctor before use if you have
• heart disease • glaucoma • diabetes
• thyroid disease • high blood pressure
• trouble urinating due to an enlarged prostate gland
• a breathing problem such as emphysema or chronic bronchitis

Other Information:
• do not use if carton is opened or if blister unit is broken
Tylenol Severe Allergy Caplets:
• store between 20–25°C (68–77°F)
TYLENOL® Allergy Sinus Day Time Caplet and TYLENOL® Allergy Sinus Night Time Caplet:
• store at room temperature
TYLENOL® Allergy Sinus Day Time Gelcap & Geltabs
• store at room temperature. Avoid high humidity and excessive heat 40°C (104°F)

Professional Information:
Overdosage Information:
For overdosage information, please refer to pgs. 1934–1935

INACTIVE INGREDIENTS
TYLENOL® Severe Allergy: **Caplets:** carnauba wax, cellulose, corn starch, D&C Yellow #10, FD&C Yellow #6, hydroxpropyl cellulose, hypromellose, iron oxide, magnesium stearate, polyethylene glycol, sodium citrate, sodium starch glycolate, titanium dioxide.
Maximum Strength TYLENOL® Allergy Sinus Night Time: **Caplets:** carnauba wax, cellulose, corn starch, D&C Yellow #10, FD&C Blue #1, hypromellose, iron oxide, magnesium stearate, polyethylene glycol, polysorbate 80, sodium citrate, sodium starch glycolate, titanium dioxide.
Maximum Strength TYLENOL® Allergy Sinus Day Time: **Caplets:** carnauba wax, cellulose, corn starch, D&C Yellow #10, FD&C Blue #1, FD&C Yellow #6, hydroxypropyl cellulose, hypromellose, iron oxide, magnesium stearate, polyethylene glycol, sodium starch glycolate, titanium dioxide.
Gelcaps and Geltabs: benzyl alcohol, butylparaben, castor oil, cellulose, corn starch, D&C Yellow #10, edetate calcium disodium, FD&C Blue #1, FD&C Blue #2, gelatin, hypromellose, magnesium stearate, methylparaben, propylparaben, sodium lauryl sulfate, sodium propionate, sodium starch glycolate, titanium dioxide.

HOW SUPPLIED
TYLENOL® Severe Allergy: **Caplets:** Yellow film-coated, imprinted with "TYLENOL Severe Allergy" on one side—blister packs of 24.
Maximum Strength TYLENOL® Allergy Sinus Night Time: **Caplets:** Light blue film-coated, imprinted with "TYLENOL A/S Night Time" on one side—blister packs of 24.
Maximum Strength TYLENOL® Allergy Sinus Day Time: **Caplets:** Yellow film-coated, imprinted with "TYLENOL Allergy Sinus" on one side—blister packs of 24.
Gelcaps and Geltabs: Green and yellow-colored, imprinted with "TYLENOL A/S"—blister packs of 24 and 48.
These products are also available in a convenience pack containing Maximum Strength Tylenol Allergy Sinus Day (pack of 12) and Maximum Strength Tylenol Allergy Sinus Night (pack of 12).
Shown in Product Identification Guide, page 322

Multi-Symptom TYLENOL® Cold Day Non-Drowsy Caplets and Gelcaps — OTC

Multi-Symptom TYLENOL® Cold Night Caplets

Product information for all dosage forms of TYLENOL Cold have been combined under this heading.

DESCRIPTION
Each *Multi-Symptom TYLENOL® Cold Day Non-Drowsy Caplet and Gelcap* contains acetaminophen 325 mg, dextromethorphan HBr 15 mg, and pseudoephedrine HCl 30 mg. Each *Multi-Symptom TYLENOL® Cold Night Time Complete Formula Caplet* contains acetaminophen 325 mg, chlorpheniramine maleate 2 mg, dextromethorphan HBr 15 mg, and pseudoephedrine HCl 30 mg.

ACTIONS
Multi-Symptom TYLENOL® Cold Day Non-Drowsy contains a clinically proven analgesic-antipyretic, a decongestant and a cough suppressant. Acetaminophen produces analgesia by elevation of the pain threshold and antipyresis through action on the hypothalamic heat regulating center. Acetaminophen is equal to aspirin in analgesic and antipyretic effectiveness and it is unlikely to produce many of the side effects associated with aspirin and aspirin-containing products. Pseudoephedrine is a sympathomimetic amine which provides temporary relief of nasal congestion. Dextromethorphan is a cough suppressant which provides temporary relief of coughs due to minor throat irritations that may occur with the common cold.
Multi-Symptom TYLENOL® Cold Night Time Complete Formula Caplets contain, in addition to the above ingredients, an antihistamine. Chlorpheniramine is an antihistamine which helps provide temporary relief of runny nose, sneezing and watery and itchy eyes.

USES
Multi-Symptom TYLENOL® Cold Day Non-Drowsy: temporarily relieves these cold symptoms:
• cough • sore throat • minor aches and pains • headaches
• nasal congestion
• temporarily reduces fever
Multi-Symptom TYLENOL® Cold Night Time Complete Formula: temporarily relieves these cold symptoms:
• cough • sore throat • minor aches and pains • headache
• nasal congestion • runny nose • sneezing • watery and itchy eyes
• temporarily reduces fever

DIRECTIONS
Multi-Symptom TYLENOL® Cold Day Non-Drowsy and Multi-Symptom TYLENOL® Cold Night Time Complete Formula:
• do not take more than directed (see overdose warning)

adults and children 12 years and over	• take 2 gelcaps or caplets every 6 hours as needed • do not take more than 8 gelcaps or caplets in 24 hours.
children under 12 years	• not intended for use in children under 12. Ask your doctor.

WARNINGS
Alcohol Warning: If you consume 3 or more alcoholic drinks every day, ask your doctor whether you should take acetaminophen or other pain relievers/fever reducers. Acetaminophen may cause liver damage.
Sore throat warning: If sore throat is severe, persists for more than 2 days, is accompanied or followed by fever, headache, rash, nausea or vomiting, consult a doctor promptly.
Do not use
• if you are now taking a prescription monoamine oxidase inhibitor (MAOI) (certain drugs for depression, psychiatric or emotional conditions or Parkinson's disease), or for 2 weeks after stopping the MAOI drug. If you do not know if your prescription drug contains an MAOI, ask a doctor or pharmacist before taking this product.
• with any other product containing acetaminophen
Stop use and ask a doctor if
• new symptoms occur
• redness or swelling is present
• pain gets worse or lasts for more than 7 days
• fever gets worse or lasts for more than 3 days
• you get nervous, dizzy or sleepless
• cough lasts more than 7 days, comes back or occurs with fever, rash or headache that lasts. These could be signs of a serious condition.
If pregnant or breast-feeding, ask a health professional before use.
Keep out of reach of children.
Overdose warning: Taking more than the recommended dose (overdose) may cause liver damage. In case of overdose, get medical help or contact a Poison Control Center right away. Quick medical attention is critical for adults as well as for children even if you do not notice any signs or symptoms.
Multi-Symptom TYLENOL® Cold Day Non-Drowsy
Ask a doctor before use if you have
• heart disease • diabetes • thyroid disease • cough that occurs with too much phlegm (mucus) • high blood pressure
• trouble urinating due to an enlarged prostate gland
• chronic cough that lasts as occurs with smoking, asthma, chronic bronchitis or emphysema
When using this product
• do not exceed recommended dosage
Multi-Symptom TYLENOL® Cold Night Time Complete Formula:
Ask a doctor before use if you have
• heart disease • glaucoma • diabetes • thyroid disease
• cough that occurs with too much phlegm (mucus) • high blood pressure • a breathing problem or chronic cough that lasts as occurs with smoking, asthma, chronic bronchitis or emphysema • trouble urinating due to an enlarged prostate gland
Ask a doctor or pharmacist before use if you are taking sedatives or tranquilizers
When using this product
• do not exceed recommended dosage
• drowsiness may occur • avoid alcoholic drinks • alcohol, sedatives and tranquilizers may increase drowsiness • be careful when driving a motor vehicle or operating machinery • excitability may occur, especially in children
OTHER INFORMATION
• do not use if carton is opened or if blister unit is broken
• store at room temperature
Avoid high humidity and excessive heat 40°C (104°F)
Applies to TYLENOL® Cold Non-Drowsy Gelcap only

Professional Information:
Overdosage Information
For overdosage information, please refer to pgs. 1934–1935

INACTIVE INGREDIENTS
Multi-Symptom TYLENOL® Cold Day Non Drowsy Formula: **Caplets:** carnauba wax, cellulose, corn starch, D&C Yellow #10, FD&C Blue #1, hypromellose, iron oxide, magnesium stearate, sodium starch glycolate, titanium dioxide, triacetin.
Gelcaps: benzyl alcohol, butylparaben, castor oil, cellulose, corn starch, D&C Yellow #10, edetate calcium disodium, FD&C Red #40, gelatin, hypromellose, iron oxide, magnesium stearate, methylparaben, propylparaben, sodium lauryl sulfate, sodium propionate, sodium starch glycolate, titanium dioxide.
Multi-Symptom TYLENOL® Cold Night Time Complete Formula: **Caplets:** carnauba wax, cellulose, corn starch, D&C Yellow #10, D&C Blue #1, FD&C Yellow #6, hypromellose, iron oxide, magnesium stearate, sodium starch glycolate, titanium dioxide, triacetin.

HOW SUPPLIED
Multi-Symptom TYLENOL® Cold Day Non Drowsy Caplets: White-colored, imprinted with "TYLENOL Cold"—blister packs of 12 & 24. **Gelcaps:** Red- and tan-colored, imprinted with "TYLENOL COLD"—blister packs of 24.
Multi-Symptom TYLENOL® Cold Night Time Complete Formula Caplets: Yellow-colored, imprinted with "TYLENOL Cold"—blister packs of 12 & 24.
These products are also available in a convenience pack containing Multi-Symptom TYLENOL® Cold Day Non-Drowsy (pack of 12) and Multi-Symptom TYLENOL® Cold Night Time Complete Formula (pack of 12).
Shown in Product Identification Guide, page 322

TYLENOL® COLD — OTC
Severe Congestion Non-Drowsy

DESCRIPTION
Each *TYLENOL® Cold Severe Congestion Non-Drowsy Caplet* contains acetaminophen 325 mg, dextromethorphan HBr 15 mg, guaifenesin 200 mg and pseudoephedrine HCl 30 mg.

ACTIONS
TYLENOL® Cold Severe Congestion Non-Drowsy Caplets contain a clinically proven analgesic-antipyretic, decongestant, expectorant and cough suppressant. Acetaminophen produces analgesia by elevation of the pain threshold and antipyresis through action on the hypothalamic heat regulating center. Acetaminophen is equal to aspirin in analgesic and antipyretic effectiveness and is unlikely to produce many of the side effects associated with aspirin and aspirin-containing products. Pseudoephedrine is a sympathomimetic amine which provides temporary relief of nasal congestion. Guaifenesin is an expectorant which helps loosen phlegm (mucus) and thin bronchial secretions to make coughs more productive. Dextromethorphan is a cough suppressant which provides temporary relief of coughs due to minor throat irritations that may occur with the common cold.

USES
temporarily relieves these cold symptoms:
• cough • sore throat • minor aches and pains • headaches
• nasal congestion
• helps loosen phlegm (mucus) and thin bronchial secretions to make coughs more productive
• temporarily reduces fever

DIRECTIONS
• do not take more than directed (see overdose warning)

adults and children 12 years and over	• take 2 caplets every 6–8 hours as needed • do not take more than 8 caplets in 24 hours
children under 12 years	• not intended for use in children under 12. Ask your doctor.

WARNINGS
Alcohol warning: If you consume 3 or more alcoholic drinks every day, ask your doctor whether you should take acetaminophen or other pain relievers/fever reducers. Acetaminophen may cause liver damage.
Sore throat warning: If sore throat is severe, persists for more than 2 days, is accompanied or followed by fever, headache, rash, nausea or vomiting, consult a doctor promptly.
Do not use
• if you are now taking a prescription monoamine oxidase inhibitor (MAOI) (certain drugs for depression, psychiatric or emotional conditions, or Parkinson's disease), or for 2 weeks after stopping the MAOI drug. If you do not know if your prescription drug contains an MAOI, ask a doctor or pharmacist before taking this product.
• with any other product containing acetaminophen
Ask a doctor before use if you have
• heart disease • diabetes • thyroid disease • cough that occurs with too much phlegm (mucus) • high blood pressure • trouble urinating due to an enlarged prostate gland • chronic cough that lasts as occurs with smoking, asthma, chronic bronchitis or emphysema

Continued on next page

Tylenol Cold Severe—Cont.

When using this product
- **do not exceed recommended dosage**

Stop use and ask a doctor if
- new symptoms occur
- redness or swelling is present
- pain gets worse or lasts for more than 7 days
- fever gets worse or lasts for more than 3 days
- you get nervous, dizzy or sleepless
- cough lasts more than 7 days, comes back or occurs with fever, rash or headache that lasts. These could be signs of a serious condition.

If pregnant or breast-feeding, ask a health professional before use.

Keep out of reach of children.

Overdose warning: Taking more than the recommended dose (overdose) may cause liver damage. In case of overdose, get medical help or contact a Poison Control Center right away. Quick medical attention is critical for adults as well as for children even if you do not notice any signs or symptoms.

OTHER INFORMATION
- **do not use if carton is opened or if blister unit is broken**
- Store at room temperature. Avoid high humidity and excessive heat (40°C)

Professional Information:
Overdosage Information: For overdosage information, please refer to pgs. 1934–1935

INACTIVE INGREDIENTS

carnauba wax, cellulose, corn starch, D&C Yellow #10, FD&C Blue #1, FD&C Yellow #6, hypromellose, iron oxide, povidone, silicon dioxide, sodium starch glycolate, stearic acid, titanium dioxide, triacetin.

HOW SUPPLIED

Caplets: Buttery-tan-colored, imprinted with *"TYLENOL COLD SC"* in green ink—blister packs of 24 & 48 ct.

Shown in Product Identification Guide, page 322

TYLENOL® OTC
Flu Day Non-Drowsy Gelcaps
TYLENOL® Flu NightTime Gelcaps
TYLENOL® Cold & Flu Severe Nighttime Liquid
TYLENOL® Cold & Flu Severe Daytime Liquid

Product information for all dosage forms of TYLENOL Flu have been combined under this heading.

DESCRIPTION

Each *TYLENOL® Flu Day Non-Drowsy Gelcap* contains acetaminophen 500 mg, dextromethorphan HBr 15 mg and pseudoephedrine HCl 30 mg. Each *TYLENOL® Flu NightTime Gelcap* contains acetaminophen 500 mg, diphenhydramine HCl 25 mg and pseudoephedrine HCl 30 mg. *TYLENOL® Cold & Flu Severe NightTime Liquid:* Each 30 mL (2 tablespoonsful) contains acetaminophen 1000 mg, dextromethorphan HBr 30 mg, doxylamine succinate 12.5 mg, and pseudoephedrine HCl 60 mg. *TYLENOL Cold & Flu Severe Daytime Liquid:* Each 30mL (2 tablespoonful) contains acetaminophen 1000 mg, dextromethorphan HBr 30 mg, pseudoephedrine HCl 60 mg.

ACTIONS

TYLENOL® Flu Day Non-Drowsy Gelcaps contain a clinically proven analgesic-antipyretic, a decongestant and a cough suppressant. Acetaminophen produces analgesia by elevation of the pain threshold and antipyresis through action on the hypothalamic heat regulating center. Acetaminophen is equal to aspirin in analgesic and antipyretic effectiveness and it is unlikely to produce many of the side effects associated with aspirin and aspirin-containing products. Pseudoephedrine hydrochloride is a sympathomimetic amine which provides temporary relief of nasal congestion. Dextromethorphan is a cough suppressant which provides temporary relief of coughs due to minor throat irritations that may occur with the common cold.

TYLENOL® Flu NightTime Gelcaps contains the same clinically proven analgesic-antipyretic and decongestant as *TYLENOL Flu Day Non-Drowsy Gelcaps* along with an antihistamine. Diphenhydramine is an antihistamine which helps provide temporary relief of runny nose and sneezing. *TYLENOL Cold & Flu Severe Daytime* contains the same clinically proven analgesic antipyretic decongestant and cough suppressant as *TYLENOL Flu Day Non-Drowsy Gelcaps. TYLENOL® Cold & Flu Severe NightTime Liquid* contains the same clinically proven analgesic-antipyretic, decongestant and cough suppressant as *TYLENOL Flu Day Non-Drowsy Gelcaps* along with an antihistamine. Doxylamine succinate is an antihistamine which helps provide temporary relief of runny nose and sneezing.

USES

TYLENOL® Flu Day Non-Drowsy Gelcaps:
temporarily relieves these cold and flu symptoms:
- minor aches and pains • headaches
- sore throat • nasal congestion
- coughs
- temporarily reduces fever

TYLENOL® Flu NightTime Gelcaps:
temporarily relieves these cold and flu symptoms:
- minor aches and pains • headaches
- sore throat • nasal congestion • runny nose • sneezing
- temporarily reduces fever

TYLENOL® Cold & Flu Severe Daytime and TYLENOL Cold & Flu Severe NightTime Liquid:
temporarily relieves these cold and flu symptoms:
- body aches and headaches • coughs
- nasal congestion • sore throat • runny nose • sneezing
- temporarily reduces fever

DIRECTIONS

- **do not take more than directed (see overdose warning)**

TYLENOL® Flu Day Non-Drowsy Gelcaps:

adults and children 12 years and over	• take 2 gelcaps every 6 hours as needed • do not take more than 8 gelcaps in 24 hours
children under 12 years	• do not use this adult product in children under 12 years of age; this will provide more than the recommended dose (overdose) and may cause liver damage.

TYLENOL® Flu NightTime Gelcaps:
- **do not take more than directed (see overdose warnings)**

adults and children 12 years and over	• take 2 gelcaps at bedtime may repeat every 6 hours • do not take more than 8 gelcaps in 24 hours
children under 12 years	• do not use this adult product in children under 12 years of age; this will provide more than the recommended dose (overdose) and may cause liver damage.

TYLENOL® Cold & Flu Severe Daytime and TYLENOL Cold & Flu Severe NightTime Liquid:
- **do not take more than directed (see overdose warnings)**

adults and children 12 years and over	• take 2 tablespoons (tbsp) in dose cup provided every 6 hours as needed • do not take more than 8 tablespoons in 24 hours
children under 12 years	• do not use this adult product in children under 12 years of age; this will provide more than the recommended dose (overdose) and may cause serious liver damage.

WARNINGS

Alcohol Warning: If you consume 3 or more alcoholic drinks every day, ask your doctor whether you should take acetaminophen or other pain relievers/fever reducers. Acetaminophen may cause liver damage.

Sore throat warning: If sore throat is severe, persists for more than 2 days, is accompanied or followed by fever, headache, rash, nausea or vomiting, consult a doctor promptly.

Do not use
- if you are now taking a prescription monoamine-oxidase inhibitor (MAOI) (certain drugs for depression, psychiatric or emotional conditions, or Parkinson's disease), or for 2 weeks after stopping the MAOI drug. If you do not know if your prescription drug contains an MAOI, ask a doctor or pharmacist before taking this product.
- with any other product containing acetaminophen
- with any other product containing diphenhydramine, even one used on skin (applies to *TYLENOL Flu Nighttime Gelcaps*)

If pregnant or breast-feeding, ask a health professional before use.

Keep out of reach of children.

OVERDOSE WARNING Taking more than the recommended dose (overdose) may cause liver damage. In case of overdose, get medical help or contact a Poison Control Center right away. Quick medical attention is critical for adults as well as for children even if you do not notice any signs or symptoms.

TYLENOL® Flu Day Non-Drowsy Gelcaps
Ask a doctor before use if you have
- heart disease • diabetes • thyroid disease • cough that occurs with too much phlegm (mucus) • high blood pressure • trouble urinating due to an enlarged prostate gland • chronic cough that lasts as occurs with smoking, asthma, chronic bronchitis or emphysema

When using this product
- **do not exceed recommended dosage**

Stop use and ask a doctor if
- new symptoms occur
- redness or swelling is present
- pain gets worse or lasts for more than 7 days
- fever gets worse or lasts for more than 3 days
- you get nervous, dizzy or sleepless
- cough lasts more than 7 days, comes back or occurs with fever, rash or headache that lasts. These could be signs of a serious condition.

TYLENOL® Flu NightTime Gelcaps
Ask a doctor before use if you have
- heart disease • glaucoma • diabetes
- thyroid disease • high blood pressure
- trouble urinating due to an enlarged prostate gland • a breathing problem such as emphysema or chronic bronchitis

Ask a doctor or pharmacist before use if you are taking sedatives or tranquilizers

When using this product
- **do not exceed recommended dosage**
- marked drowsiness may occur
- avoid alcoholic drinks
- alcohol, sedatives and tranquilizers may increase drowsiness
- be careful when driving a motor vehicle or operating machinery
- excitability may occur, especially in children

Stop use and ask a doctor if
- new symptoms occur
- redness or swelling is present
- pain gets worse or lasts for more than 7 days
- fever gets worse or lasts for more than 3 days
- you get nervous, dizzy or sleepless

TYLENOL® Cold & Flu Severe Daytime and TYLENOL Cold & Flu Severe Nighttime Liquid
Ask a doctor before use if you have
- heart disease • glaucoma • diabetes
- thyroid disease • cough that occurs with too much phlegm (mucus)
- high blood pressure • a breathing problem such as emphysema or chronic bronchitis • trouble urinating due to an enlarged prostate gland

Ask a doctor or pharmacist before use if you are taking sedatives or tranquilizers (applies to *TYLENOL Cold & Flu Severe Nighttime* only)

When using this product
- **do not exceed recommended dosage**
- The following apply to *TYLENOL Cold & Flu Severe Nighttime* only
  - marked drowsiness may occur
  - avoid alcoholic drinks
  - alcohol, sedatives and tranquilizers may increase drowsiness
  - be careful when driving a motor vehicle or operating machinery
  - excitability may occur, especially in children

Stop use and ask a doctor if
- pain, cough or nasal congestion gets worse or lasts for more than 7 days
- redness or swelling is present
- new symptoms occur
- fever gets worse or lasts for more than 3 days
- you get nervous, dizzy or sleepless (applies to *TYLENOL Cold & Flu Severe NightTime* only)
- cough with rash or headache that lasts. These could be signs of a serious condition.

OTHER INFORMATION
TYLENOL® Flu Day Non-Drowsy Gelcaps and TYLENOL® Flu NightTime Gelcaps:
- **do not use if carton is opened or if blister unit is broken**
- Store at room temperature; Avoid high humidity and excessive heat 40°C (104°F)

TYLENOL® NightTime Severe Cold & Flu Liquid
- **do not use if carton is opened or if bottle wrap or foil inner seal imprinted "Safety Seal®" is broken or missing**
- Store at room temperature

Professional Information:
Overdosage Information
For overdosage information, please refer to pgs. 1934–1935

INACTIVE INGREDIENTS

TYLENOL® Flu Day Non-Drowsy Gelcaps: benzyl alcohol, butylparaben, castor oil, cellulose, corn starch, edetate calcium disodium, FD&C Blue #1, FD&C Red #40, gelatin, hypromellose, iron oxide, magnesium stearate, methylparaben, propylparaben, sodium lauryl sulfate, sodium propionate, sodium starch glycolate, titanium dioxide.

TYLENOL® Flu NightTime Gelcaps: benzyl alcohol, butylparaben, castor oil, cellulose, corn starch, D&C Red #28, edetate calcium disodium, FD&C Blue #1, gelatin, hypromellose, iron oxide, magnesium stearate, methylparaben, propylparaben, sodium citrate, sodium lauryl sulfate, sodium propionate, sodium starch glycolate, titanium dioxide.

TYLENOL® NightTime Severe Cold & Flu Liquid: citric acid, corn syrup, D&C Red #33, FD&C Red #40, flavors, polyethylene glycol, propylene glycol, purified water, saccharin sodium, sodium benzoate, sorbitol.

HOW SUPPLIED

TYLENOL® Flu Day Non-Drowsy Gelcaps: Burgundy- and white-colored gelcap, imprinted with "TYLENOL FLU" in gray ink—blister packs of 12 & 24. Liquid: Blue-colored—bottles of 8 fl oz with child resistant safety cap and tamper evident packaging.

TYLENOL® Flu NightTime: **Gelcaps**: Blue and white-colored gelcap, imprinted with "TYLENOL FLU NT" gray ink—blister packs of 12 and 24. **Liquid**: Blue-colored—bottles of 8 fl. oz with child resistant safety cap and tamper evident packaging.

These products are also available in a convenience pack containing *TYLENOL Flu Day* (pack of 12) and *TYLENOL Flu Night* (pack of 12).

Shown in Product Identification Guide, page 322

Extra Strength **OTC**
TYLENOL® PM
Pain Reliever/Sleep Aid Caplets, Geltabs and Gelcaps

DESCRIPTION

Each *Extra Strength TYLENOL® PM Caplet, Geltab* or *Gelcap* contains acetaminophen 500 mg and diphenhydramine HCl 25 mg.

ACTIONS

Extra Strength TYLENOL® PM Caplets, Geltabs and *Gelcaps* contain a clinically proven analgesic-antipyretic and an antihistamine. Maximum allowable non-prescription levels of acetaminophen and diphenhydramine provide temporary relief of occasional headaches and minor aches and pains accompanying sleeplessness. Acetaminophen is equal to aspirin in analgesic and antipyretic effectiveness and it is unlikely to produce many of the side effects associated with aspirin-containing products. Acetaminophen produces analgesia by elevation of the pain threshold. Diphenhydramine HCl is an antihistamine with sedative properties.

USES

temporary relief of occasional headaches and minor aches and pains with accompanying sleeplessness.

DIRECTIONS

- **do not take more than directed (see overdose warning)**

adults and children 12 years and over: Take 2 caplets, geltabs or gelcaps at bedtime or as directed by a doctor. Children under 12 years: do not use this adult product in children under 12 years of age; this will provide more than the recommended dose (overdose) and may cause liver damage.

WARNINGS

Alcohol Warning: If you consume 3 or more alcoholic drinks every day, ask your doctor whether you should take acetaminophen or other pain relievers/fever reducers. Acetaminophen may cause liver damage.

Do not use
- with any other product containing acetaminophen
- with any other product containing diphenhydramine, even one used on skin.
- in children under 12 years of age

Ask a doctor before use if you have
- a breathing problem such as emphysema or chronic bronchitis
- trouble urinating due to an enlarged prostate gland
- glaucoma

Ask a doctor or pharmacist before use if you are
- taking sedatives or tranquilizers.

When using this product
- drowsiness will occur
- avoid alcoholic drinks
- do not drive a motor vehicle or operate machinery

Stop use and ask a doctor if
- sleeplessness persists continuously for more than 2 weeks. Insomnia may be a symptom of serious underlying medical illness.
- new symptoms occur
- redness or swelling is present
- pain gets worse or lasts for more than 10 days
- fever gets worse or lasts for more than 3 days

If pregnant or breast-feeding, ask a health professional before use.

Keep out of reach of children.

Overdose warning: Taking more than the recommended dose (overdose) may cause liver damage. In case of overdose, get medical help or contact a Poison Control Center right away. Quick medical attention is critical for adults as well as for children even if you do not notice any signs or symptoms.

OTHER INFORMATION
- **do not use if carton is opened or neck wrap or foil inner seal imprinted with "Safety Seal®" is broken**
- Store between 20–25°C (68–77°F). Avoid high humidity. (Applies only to Tylenol® PM Geltabs/Gelcaps)

Professional Information:
Overdosage Information:

For overdosage information, please refer to pgs. 1934–1935

INACTIVE INGREDIENTS

Caplets: carnauba wax, cellulose, corn starch, FD&C Blue #1, FD&C Blue #2, hypromellose, magnesium stearate, polyethylene glycol, polysorbate 80, sodium citrate, sodium starch glycolate, titanium dioxide.

Geltabs/Gelcaps: benzyl alcohol, butylparaben, castor oil, cellulose, corn starch, D&C Red #28, edetate calcium disodium, FD&C Blue #1, gelatin, hypromellose, iron oxide magnesium stearate, methylparaben, propylparaben, sodium citrate, sodium lauryl sulfate, sodium propionate, sodium starch glycolate, titanium dioxide,

HOW SUPPLIED

Caplets (colored light blue imprinted "Tylenol PM") tamper evident bottles of 24, 50, 100, and 150 and 225.

Gelcaps (colored blue and white imprinted "TYLENOL PM") tamper-evident bottles of 24 and 50.

Geltabs (colored blue and white imprinted "TYLENOL PM") tamper-evident bottles of 24, 50, and 100 and 150.

Shown in Product Identification Guide, page 322

Maximum Strength **OTC**
TYLENOL® Sinus Day Non-Drowsy
Geltabs, Gelcaps and Caplets

Maximum Strength
TYLENOL® Sinus
Night Time Caplets

TYLENOL® Sinus Severe Congestion
Caplets

Product information for all dosage forms of TYLENOL Sinus have been combined under this heading.

DESCRIPTION

Each *Maximum Strength TYLENOL® Sinus Day Non-Drowsy Geltab, Gelcap, or Caplet* contains acetaminophen 500 mg and pseudoephedrine HCl 30 mg. Each *Maximum Strength TYLENOL® Sinus Night Time Caplet* contains acetaminophen 500 mg, doxylamine succinate 6.25 mg and pseudoephedrine HCl 30 mg. Each *Tylenol Sinus Severe Congestion Caplet* contains acetaminophen 325 mg, guaifenesin 200 mg, and pseudoephedrine HCl 30 mg.

ACTIONS

Maximum Strength TYLENOL® Sinus Day Non-Drowsy contains a clinically proven analgesic-antipyretic and a decongestant. Maximum allowable non-prescription levels of acetaminophen and pseudoephedrine provide temporary relief of sinus pain and headache and congestion. Acetaminophen is equal to aspirin in analgesic and antipyretic effectiveness and it is unlikely to produce many of the side effects associated with aspirin and aspirin-containing products. Acetaminophen produces analgesia by elevation of the pain threshold and antipyresis through action on the hypothalamic heat regulating center. Pseudoephedrine hydrochloride is a sympathomimetic amine which promotes sinus cavity drainage by reducing nasopharyngeal mucosal congestion.

Maximum Strength TYLENOL® Sinus Night Time Caplets contain, in addition to the above ingredients, an antihistamine which provides temporary relief of runny nose and itching of the nose or throat.

Tylenol Sinus Severe Congestion contains a clinically proven analgesic-antipyretic, an expectorant, and a decongestant. Maximum allowable non-prescription levels of acetaminophen, guaifenesin, and pseudoephedrine HCl provide temporary relief of sinus pain, headache, and congestion. Acetaminophen is equal to aspirin in analgesic and antipyretic effectiveness and its unlikely to produce many of the side effects associated with aspirin and aspirin-containing products. Acetaminophen produces analgesia by elevation of the pain threshold and antipyresis through action on the hypothalamic heat regulating center. Guaifenesin is an expectorant which helps loosen phlegm (mucus) and thin bronchial secretions to make coughs more productive. Pseudoephedrine hydrochloride is a sympathomimetic amine which promotes sinus cavity drainage by reducing nasopharyngeal mucosal congestion.

USES

Maximum Strength TYLENOL® Sinus Day Non-Drowsy: temporarily relieves:
- sinus pain • headache • nasal and sinus congestion

Maximum Strength TYLENOL® Sinus Night Time: temporarily relieves:
- nasal congestion • sinus pressure • sinus pain • headache • runny nose • sneezing • itchy, watery eyes • itching of the nose or throat

Tylenol Sinus Severe Congestion temporarily relieves:
- minor aches and pains
- sinus headache
- temporarily relieves nasal congestion associated with sinusitis
- promotes nasal and/or sinus drainage
- helps loosen phlegm (mucus) and thin bronchial secretions to make coughs more productive

DIRECTIONS

Maximum Strength TYLENOL® Sinus Day Non-Drowsy:
- **do not take more than directed (see overdose warning)**

adults and children 12 years and over	• take 2 Geltabs, Gelcaps or Caplets every 4–6 hours as needed • do not take more than 8 Geltabs, Gelcaps or Caplets in 24 hours
children under 12 years	• do not use this adult product in children under 12 years of age; this will provide more than the recommended dose (overdose) and may cause liver damage.

Maximum Strength TYLENOL® Sinus Night Time;
- **do not take more than directed (see overdose warning)**

adults and children 12 years and over	• take 2 caplets every 4–6 hours as needed • do not take more than 8 caplets in 24 hours
children under 12 years	• do not use this adult product in children under 12 years of age; this will provide more than the recommended dose (overdose) and may cause liver damage.

Tylenol Sinus Severe Congestion
- **Do not take more than directed (see overdose warning)**

adults and children 12 years and over	• take 2 caplets every 4–6 hours as needed • swallow whole—do not crush, chew or dissolve • do not take more than 8 caplets in 24 hours
children under 12 years	• not intended for use in children under 12. Ask your doctor.

WARNINGS

Alcohol warning: If you consume 3 or more alcoholic drinks every day, ask your doctor whether you should take acetaminophen or other pain relievers/fever reducers. Acetaminophen may cause liver damage.

Do not use
- if you are now taking a prescription monamine oxidase inhibitor (MAOI) (certain drugs for depression, psychiatric or emotional conditions or Parkinson's disease), or for 2 weeks after stopping the MAOI drug. If you do not know if your prescription drug contains an MAOI, ask a doctor or pharmacist before taking this product
- with any other product containing acetaminophen

Maximum Strength TYLENOL® Sinus Day Non-Drowsy Geltabs, Gelcaps and Caplets

Ask a doctor before use if you have
- heart disease • high blood pressure
- thyroid disease • diabetes
- trouble urinating due to an enlarged prostate gland

When using this product
- **do not exceed recommend dosage**

Maximum Strength TYLENOL® Sinus Night Time Caplets

Ask a doctor before use if you have
- heart disease • glaucoma • diabetes
- thyroid disease • high blood pressure
- trouble urinating due to an enlarged prostate gland • a breathing problem such as emphysema or chronic bronchitis

Ask a doctor or pharmacist before use if you are taking sedatives or tranquilizers

When using this product
- **do not exceed recommended dosage**
- marked drowsiness may occur
- avoid alcoholic drinks
- alcohol, sedatives and tranquilizers may increase drowsiness
- be careful when driving a motor vehicle or operating machinery
- excitability may occur, especially in children

Tylenol Sinus Severe Congestion Caplets

Ask a doctor before use if you have
- heart disease • diabetes • thyroid disease • cough that occurs with too much phlegm (mucus) • high blood pressure • trouble urinating due to an enlarged prostate gland • chronic cough that lasts as occurs with smoking, asthma, chronic bronchitis or emphysema

Continued on next page

Tylenol Sinus—Cont.

When using this product
- **do not exceed recommended dosage**

Stop use and ask a doctor if
- new symptoms occur
- redness or swelling is present
- pains gets worse or last for more than 7 days
- fever gets worse or lasts for more than 3 days
- you get nervous, dizzy or sleepless

Tylenol Sinus Severe Congestion
Stop use and ask a doctor if
- new symptoms occur
- redness or swelling is present
- pain, nasal congestion, or cough gets worse or lasts for more than 7 days
- you get nervous, dizzy or sleepless
- cough comes back or occurs with rash or headache that lasts. These could be signs of a serious condition.

If pregnant or breast feeding, ask a health professional before use.
Keep out of reach of children.

OVERDOSE WARNING Taking more than the recommended dose (overdose) may cause liver damage. In case of overdose get medical help or contact a Poison Control Center right away. Quick medical attention is critical for adults as well as for children even if you do not notice any signs or symptoms.

OTHER INFORMATION
- **do not use if carton is opened or if blister unit is broken**

Maximum Strength TYLENOL® Sinus Geltabs and Gelcaps
- store at room temperature; avoid high humidity and excessive heat 40°C (104°F)

Maximum Strength TYLENOL® Sinus Caplets and Maximum Strength TYLENOL® Sinus Night Time Caplets
- store at room temperature

Tylenol Sinus Severe Congestion
- Store at 20–25° C (68–77° F)

Professional Information:
Overdosage Information
For overdosage information, please refer to pgs. 1934–1935

INACTIVE INGREDIENTS
Maximum Strength TYLENOL® Sinus Day Non-Drowsy Formula: **Caplets:** carnauba wax, cellulose, corn starch, D&C Yellow #10, FD&C Blue #1, FD&C Red #40, hypromellose, iron oxide, magnesium stearate, polyethylene glycol, polysorbate 80, sodium starch glycolate, titanium dioxide.
Gelcaps and Geltabs: benzyl alcohol, butylparaben, castor oil, cellulose, corn starch, D&C Yellow #10, edetate calcium disodium, FD&C Blue #1, gelatin, hypromellose, iron oxide, magnesium stearate, methylparaben, propylparaben, sodium lauryl sulfate, sodium propionate, sodium starch glycolate, titanium dioxide.
Maximum Strength TYLENOL® Sinus Night Time Caplets: black iron oxide, carnauba wax, cellulose, corn starch, FD&C Blue #1, FD&C Blue #2, hypromellose, propylene glycol, silicon dioxide, sodium starch glycolate, stearic acid, titanium dioxide, triacetin, yellow iron oxide.
Tylenol Sinus Severe Congestion: cellulose, corn starch, croscarmellose sodium, D&C Yellow #10, FD&C Blue #1, FD&C Red #40, flavor, iron oxide, mannitol, polyethylene glycol, polyvinyl alcohol, povidone, silicon dioxide, stearic acid, sucralose, talc, titanium dioxide

HOW SUPPLIED
Maximum Strength TYLENOL® Sinus Day Non-Drowsy Formula:
Caplets: Light green-colored, imprinted with "TYLENOL Sinus" in green ink—blister packs of 24 and 48.
Gelcaps: Green- and white-colored, imprinted with "TYLENOL Sinus" in dark green ink—blister packs of 24 and 48.
Geltabs: Green-colored on one side and white-colored on opposite side, imprinted with "TYLENOL Sinus" in gray ink—blister packs of 24 and 48.
Maximum Strength TYLENOL® Sinus Night Time Caplets: Green-colored, imprinted with "Tylenol Sinus NT"—blister packs of 24.
These products are also available in a convenience pack containing Maximum Strength TYLENOL® Sinus Day Non-Drowsy (pack of 12) and Maximum Strength TYLENOL® Sinus Night Time (pack of 12).
Tylenol Sinus Severe Congestion are light green-colored caplets printed with "Tylenol Sinus SC" in black ink and are available in blister packs of 12, 24, and 48.
Shown in Product Identification Guide, page 322

Maximum Strength TYLENOL® Sore Throat Adult Liquid — OTC

DESCRIPTION
Maximum Strength TYLENOL® Sore Throat Liquid is available in Honey Lemon Flavor or Wild Cherry Flavor and contains acetaminophen 1000 mg in each 30 mL (2 Tablespoonsful).

ACTIONS
Acetaminophen is a clinically proven analgesic/antipyretic. Acetaminophen produces analgesia by elevation of the pain threshold and antipyresis through action on the hypothalamic heat regulating center. Acetaminophen is equal to aspirin in analgesic and antipyretic effectiveness and it is unlikely to produce many of the side effects associated with aspirin and aspirin-containing products.

USES
temporarily relieves minor aches and pains due to:
- sore throat • headache • muscular aches • the common cold
- temporarily reduces fever

DIRECTIONS
- **do not take more than directed (see overdose warning)**

adults and children 12 years and over	• take 2 tablespoons (tbsp) in dose cup provided every 4 to 6 hours as needed • do not take more than 8 tablespoons in 24 hours
children under 12 years	do not use this adult product in children under 12 years of age; this will provide more than the recommended dose (overdose) of TYLENOL® and may cause liver damage.

WARNINGS
Alcohol warning: If you consume 3 or more alcoholic drinks every day, ask your doctor whether you should take acetaminophen or other pain relievers/fever reducers. Acetaminophen may cause liver damage.
Sore throat warning: If sore throat is severe, persists for more than 2 days, is accompanied or followed by fever, headache, rash, nausea or vomiting, consult a doctor promptly.
Do not use
- with any other product containing acetaminophen

Stop use and ask a doctor if
- new symptoms occur
- redness or swelling is present
- pain gets worse or lasts for more than 10 days
- fever gets worse or lasts for more than 3 days

If pregnant or breast-feeding, ask a health professional before use.
Keep out of the reach of children.
Overdose warning: Taking more than the recommended dose (overdose) may cause liver damage. In case of overdose, get medical help or contact a Poison Control Center right away. Quick medical attention is critical for adults as well as for children even if you do not notice any signs or symptoms.
OTHER INFORMATION
- **Do not use if carton is opened or if bottle wrap or foil inner seal imprinted "Safety Seal®" is broken or missing**
- store at room temperature

Professional Information:
Overdosage Information
For overdosage information, please refer to pgs. 1934–1935

INACTIVE INGREDIENTS
Maximum Strength TYLENOL® Sore Throat Honey-Lemon-Flavored Adult Liquid: caramel color, citric acid, flavor, high fructose corn syrup, polyethylene glycol, propylene glycol, purified water, saccharin sodium, sodium benzoate, sorbitol
Maximum Strength TYLENOL® Sore Throat Wild Cherry-Flavored Adult Liquid: citric acid, D&C Red # 33, FD&C Red # 40, flavor, high fructose corn syrup, polyethylene glycol, propylene glycol, purified water, saccharin sodium, sodium benzoate, sorbitol

HOW SUPPLIED
Honey lemon-flavored or wild cherry-flavored liquid in child-resistant tamper-evident bottles of 8 fl. oz.
Shown in Product Identification Guide, page 322

WOMEN'S TYLENOL® — OTC
Menstrual Relief Pain Reliever/ Diuretic Caplets

DESCRIPTION
Each *Women's Tylenol® Menstrual Relief Caplet* contains acetaminophen 500 mg and pamabrom 25 mg.

ACTIONS
Women's TYLENOL® Menstrual Relief Caplets contain a clinically proven analgesic-antipyretic and a diuretic. Maximum allowable non-prescription levels of acetaminophen and pamabrom provide temporary relief of minor aches and pains due to cramps, headache, and backache and water retention, weight gain, bloating, swelling and full feeling associated with the premenstrual and menstrual periods. Acetaminophen is equal to aspirin in analgesic and antipyretic effectiveness and it is unlikely to produce many of the side effects associated with aspirin containing products. Acetaminophen produces analgesia by elevation of the pain threshold. Pamabrom is a diuretic which relieves water retention.

USES
- temporarily relieves minor aches and pains due to:
  - cramps • headache • backache
- temporarily relieves water-weight gain, bloating, swelling and full feeling associated with the premenstrual and menstrual periods

DIRECTIONS
- **do not take more than directed (see overdose warning)**

adults and children 12 years and over: take 2 caplets every 4 to 6 hours; do not take more than 8 caplets in 24 hours
children under 12 years: do not use this adult product in children under 12 years of age; this will provide more than the recommended dose (overdose) and may cause liver damage

WARNINGS
Alcohol warning: If you consume 3 or more alcoholic drinks every day, ask your doctor whether you should take acetaminophen or other pain relievers/fever reducers. Acetaminophen may cause liver damage.
Do not use
- with any other product containing acetaminophen

Stop use and ask a doctor if
- new symptoms occur
- redness or swelling is present
- pain gets worse or lasts for more than 10 days

If pregnant or breast-feeding, ask a health professional before use.
Keep out of reach of children.
Overdose Warning: Taking more than the recommended dose (overdose) may cause liver damage. In case of overdose, get medical help or contact a Poison Control Center right away. Quick medical attention is critical for adults as well as for children even if you do not notice any signs or symptoms.
OTHER INFORMATION
- **do not use if carton is opened, or if neck wrap or foil inner seal imprinted "Safety Seal®" is broken or missing**
- store below 20–25°C (68–77°F)

Professional Information:
Overdosage Information
For overdosage information, please refer to pgs. 1934–1935

INACTIVE INGREDIENTS
cellulose, corn starch, hypromellose, magnesium stearate, polydextrose, polyethylene glycol, sodium starch glycolate, titanium dioxide, triacetin.

HOW SUPPLIED
White capsule shaped caplets with TYME printed on one side in tamper-evident bottles of 24.
Shown in Product Identification Guide, page 321

Concentrated TYLENOL® — OTC
acetaminophen Infants' Drops
Children's TYLENOL®
acetaminophen Suspension Liquid and Meltaways
Jr. TYLENOL®
acetaminophen Meltaways
Product information for all dosages of Children's TYLENOL have been combined under this heading

DESCRIPTION
Concentrated TYLENOL® Infants' Drops are stable, alcohol-free, grape-flavored and purple in color or cherry-flavored and red in color. Each 1.6 mL contains 160 mg acetaminophen. *Concentrated TYLENOL® Infants' Drops* features the SAFE-TY-LOCK™ Bottle. The SAFE-TY-LOCK™ Bottle has a unique safety barrier inside the bottle which helps make administration easier. The integrated dropper promotes proper administration. The innovative design eliminates excess product on dropper. The star-shaped barrier inside the bottle minimizes spills and discourages pouring into a spoon. *Children's TYLENOL® Suspension Liquid* is stable, alcohol-free, cherry blast-flavored and red in color, or bubblegum yum-flavored and pink in color, grape splash-flavored and purple in color, or very berry strawberry-flavored and red in color. Each 5 mL (one teaspoonful) contains 160 mg acetaminophen. Each *Children's TYLENOL® Meltaways* contains 80 mg acetaminophen in a grape punch, bubblegum burst or wacky watermelon flavor. *Each Jr. TYLENOL® Meltaways* contains 160 mg acetaminophen in grape punch or bubblegum burst flavor.

ACTIONS
Acetaminophen is a clinically proven analgesic/antipyretic. Acetaminophen produces analgesia by elevation of the pain threshold and antipyresis through action on the hypothalamic heat-regulating center. Acetaminophen is equal to aspirin in analgesic and antipyretic effectiveness and it is unlikely to produce many of the side effects associated with aspirin and aspirin-containing products.

USES
Concentrated TYLENOL® Infants' Drops: temporarily:
- reduces fever
- relieves minor aches and pains due to: • the common cold • flu • headaches • sore throat • immunizations • toothaches

Children's TYLENOL® Suspension Liquid and Children's TYLENOL® Meltaways: temporarily relieves minor aches and pains due to: • the common cold • flu • headaches • sore throat • immunizations • toothache
• temporarily reduces fever
Jr. TYLENOL® Meltaways: temporarily relieves minor aches and pains due to: • the common cold • flu • headache • muscle aches • sprains • overexertion
• temporarily reduces fever

DIRECTIONS

See Table 1: Children's Tylenol Dosing Chart on pg. 1951

WARNINGS

Sore throat warning: if sore throat is severe, persists for more than 2 days, is accompanied or followed by fever, headache, rash, nausea, or vomiting, consult a doctor promptly (excluding *Jr. TYLENOL® Meltaways*).
Do not use
• with any other product containing acetaminophen
When using this product
• **do not exceed recommended dose (see overdose warning)**
Stop use and ask a doctor if
• new symptoms occur
• redness or swelling is present
• pain gets worse or lasts for more than 5 days
• fever gets worse or lasts for more than 3 days
Keep out of the reach of children.
OVERDOSE WARNING: Taking more than the recommended dose (overdose) may cause liver damage. In case of overdose, get medical help or contact a Poison Control Center right away. Quick medical attention is critical even if you do not notice any signs or symptoms.
OTHER INFORMATION
Concentrated TYLENOL® Infants' Drops:
• **Do not use if plastic carton wrap or bottle wrap imprinted "Safety Seal®" is broken or missing.**
• Store at room temperature
Children's TYLENOL® Suspension Liquid:
•**Do not use if bottle wrap, or foil inner seal imprinted "Safety Seal®" is broken or missing**
• Store between 20–25°C (68–77°F)
Children's TYLENOL® Meltaways:
• **Do not use if carton is opened or if neck wrap or foil inner seal imprinted "Safety Seal®" is broken or missing.** Store between 20–25°C (68–77°F). (Grape Punch: Protect from light). Avoid high humidity. *Jr. TYLENOL® Meltaways:*
• **Do not use if carton is opened or if blister unit is broken**
• Store between 20–25°C (68–77°F). (Grape Punch: Protect from light). Avoid high humidity.

Professional Information:
Overdosage Information for all Infants', Children's & Jr. Tylenol® Products

ACETAMINOPHEN: Acetaminophen in massive overdosage may cause hepatic toxicity in some patients. In adults and adolescents (≥ 12 years of age), hepatic toxicity may occur following ingestion of greater than 7.5 to 10 grams over a period of 8 hours or less. Fatalities are infrequent (less than 3–4% of untreated cases) and have rarely been reported with overdoses of less than 15 grams. In children (<12 years of age), an acute overdosage of less than 150 mg/kg has not been associated with hepatic toxicity. Early symptoms following a potentially hepatotoxic overdose may include: nausea, vomiting, diaphoresis and general malaise. Clinical and laboratory evidence of hepatic toxicity may not be apparent until 48 to 72 hours postingestion. In adults and adolescents, any individual presenting with an unknown amount of acetaminophen ingested or with a questionable or unreliable history about the time of ingestion should have a plasma acetaminophen level drawn and be treated with *N*-acetylcysteine. For full prescribing information, refer to the *N*-acetylcysteine package insert. Do not await results of assays for plasma acetaminophen levels before initiating treatment with *N*-acetylcysteine. The following additional procedures are recommended: Promptly initiate gastric decontamination of the stomach. A plasma acetaminophen assay should be obtained as early as possible, but no sooner than four hours following ingestion. If an acetaminophen *extended release* product is involved, it may be appropriate to obtain an additional plasma acetaminophen level 4–6 hours following the initial acetaminophen level. If either acetaminophen level plots above the treatment line on the acetaminophen overdose nomogram, *N*-acetylcysteine treatment should be continued for a full course of therapy. Liver function studies should be obtained initially and repeated at 24-hour intervals. Serious toxicity or fatalities have been extremely infrequent following an acute acetaminophen overdose in young children, possibly because of differences in the way they metabolize acetaminophen. In children, the maximum potential amount ingested can be more easily estimated. If more than 150 mg/kg or an unknown amount was ingested, obtain a plasma acetaminophen level as soon as possible, but no sooner than 4 hours following ingestion. If an acetaminophen *extended release* product is involved, it may be appropriate to obtain an additional plasma acetaminophen level 4–6 hours following the initial acetaminophen level. If either acetaminophen level plots above the treatment line on the acetaminophen overdose nomogram, *N*-acetylcysteine treatment should be initiated and continued for a full course of therapy. If an assay cannot be obtained and the estimated acetaminophen ingestion exceeds 150 mg/kg, dosing with *N*-acetylcysteine should be initiated and continued for a full course of therapy. For additional emergency information, call your regional poison center or call the Rocky Mountain Poison Center toll-free, (1-800-525-6115).

Our pediatric Tylenol® combination products contain active ingredients in addition to acetaminophen. The following is basic overdose information regarding those ingredients.

CHLORPHENIRAMINE: Chlorphenir amine toxicity should be treated as you would an anthihistamine/anticholinergic overdose and is likely to be present within a few hours after acute ingestion.

DEXTROMETHORPHAN: Acute dextromethorphan overdose usually does not result in serious signs and symptoms unless massive amounts have been ingested. Signs and symptoms of a substantial overdose may include nausea and vomiting, visual disturbances, CNS disturbances and urinary retention.

DIPHENHYDRAMINE: Diphenhydramine toxicity should be treated as you would an antihistamine/anticholinergic overdose and is likely to be present within a few hours after acute ingestion.

PSEUDOEPHEDRINE: Symptoms from pseudoephedrine overdose consist most often of mild anxiety, tachycardia and/or mild hypertension. Symptoms usually appear within 4 to 8 hours of ingestion and are transient, usually requiring no treatment.

For additional emergency information, please contact your local poison control center.

INACTIVE INGREDIENTS

***Concentrated TYLENOL® Infants' Drops:* Cherry-Flavored:** cellulose, citric acid, corn syrup, FD&C Red #40, flavors, glycerin, purified water, sodium benzoate, sorbitol, xanthan gum. **Grape-Flavored:** cellulose, citric acid, corn syrup, D&C Red #33, FD&C Blue #1, flavors, glycerin, purified water, sodium benzoate, sorbitol, xanthan gum.
Children's TYLENOL® Suspension Liquid: butylparaben, carboxymethyl cellulose sodium, cellulose, citric acid, corn syrup, flavors, glycerin, propylene glycol, purified water, sodium benzoate, sorbitol sucralose, xanthan gum. In addition to the above ingredients cherry blast-flavored suspension contains FD&C Red #40, bubblegum-yum suspension contains D&C Red #33 and FD&C Red #40, grape splash-flavored suspension contains D&C Red #33 and FD&C Blue #1 and very berry strawberry-flavored suspension contains FD&C Red #40.
***Children's TYLENOL® Meltaways:* Wacky Watermelon-Flavored:** cellulose acetate, citric acid, crospovidone, D&C Red #30, dextrose, flavors, magnesium stearate, povidone, sucralose. **Grape-Punch-Flavored:** cellulose acetate, citric acid, crospovidone, dextrose, D&C Red #7, D&C Red #30, FD&C Blue #1, flavors, magnesium stearate, povidone, sucralose. **Bubblegum Burst-Flavored:** cellulose acetate citric acid, crospovidone, D&C Red #7, dextrose, flavors, magnesium stearate, povidone, sucralose.
***Jr. TYLENOL® Meltaways* Bubblegum Burst Flavored:** cellulose acetate, citric acid, crospovidone, D&C red #7, dextrose, flavors, magnesium stearate, povidone, sucralose. **Grape Punch Flavored:** cellulose acetate, citric acid, crospovidone, D&C Red #7, D&C Red #30, dextrose, FD&C Blue #1, flavors, magnesium stearate, povidone, sucralose.

HOW SUPPLIED

Concentrated TYLENOL® Infants' Drops: (purple-colored grape): bottles of ½ oz (15 mL) and 1 oz (30 mL); (red-colored cherry): bottles of ½ oz and 1 oz, each with calibrated plastic dropper.
Children's TYLENOL® Suspension Liquid: (red-colored cherry blast): bottles of 2 and 4 fl oz. (pink-colored bubblegum yum, purple-colored grape splash and red-colored very berry strawberry): bottles of 4 fl. oz.
Children's TYLENOL® Meltaways: (red-colored wacky watermelon, purple-colored grape punch, pink-colored bubblegum burst, scored, imprinted "TY80"). Bottles of 30 and also blister packaged 48's and 64's.
Jr. TYLENOL® Meltaways: (purple-colored grape punch or pink-colored bubblegum burst, imprinted "TY 160"). Blister packaged 24's and 48's. All packages listed above are safety sealed and use child-resistant safety caps or blisters.

Shown in Product Identification Guide, page 321

CHILDREN'S TYLENOL Plus Cold & Allergy OTC

DESCRIPTION

Children's TYLENOL® Plus Cold & Allergy is Bubble Gum flavored and contains no alcohol or aspirin. Each teaspoon (5 mL) contains acetaminophen 160 mg, diphenhydramine HCl 12.5 mg and pseudoephedrine HCl 15 mg.

ACTIONS

Children's TYLENOL® Plus Cold & Allergy combines the analgesic-antipyretic acetaminophen with the antihistamine diphenhydramine hydrochloride and the decongestant pseudoephedrine hydrochloride to provide fast, effective, temporary relief of all your child's symptoms associated with hay fever and other respiratory allergies including sneezing, sore throat, itchy throat, itchy/watery eyes, runny nose, stuffy nose and nasal congestion. Acetaminophen is equal to aspirin in analgesic and antipyretic effectiveness and it is unlikely to produce the side effects often associated with aspirin or aspirin-containing products.

USES

temporarily relieves these cold and upper respiratory allergy symptoms:
• sore throat • headache
• runny nose • sneezing
• stuffy nose • minor aches and pains
• itchy, watery eyes
• temporarily reduces fever

DIRECTIONS

See Table 1: Children's Tylenol Dosing Chart on pg. 1951

WARNINGS

Sore throat warning: If sore throat is severe, persists for more than 2 days, is accompanied or followed by fever, headache, rash, nausea or vomiting, consult a doctor promptly.
Do not use
• in a child who is taking a prescription monoamine oxidase inhibitor (MAOI) (certain drugs for depression, psychiatric, or emotional conditions, or Parkinson's disease) or for 2 weeks after stopping the MAOI drug. If you do not know if your child's prescription drug contains an MAOI, ask a doctor or pharmacist before giving this product.
• with any other product containing acetaminophen.
• with any other product containing diphenhydramine, even one used on skin
Ask a doctor before use if the child has
• heart disease • high blood pressure
• thyroid disease • diabetes
• glaucoma • a breathing problem such as chronic bronchitis
When using this product
• **do not exceed recommended dosage (see overdose warning)**
• marked drowsiness may occur
• excitability may occur, especially in children
Stop use and ask a doctor if
• pain or nasal congestion gets worse or lasts for more than 5 days
• fever gets worse or lasts for more than 3 days
• redness or swelling is present
• new symptoms occur
• nervousness, dizziness or sleeplessness occurs
Keep out of reach of children.
OVERDOSE WARNING
Taking more than the recommended dose (overdose) may cause liver damage. In case of overdose, get medical help or contact a Poison Control Center right away. Quick medical attention is critical even if you do not notice any signs or symptoms
OTHER INFORMATION
• **do not use if plastic carton wrap or bottle wrap imprinted "Safety Seal®" is broken or missing.**
• store between 20–25° C (68–77° F)

Professional Information:
Overdosage Information:

For overdosage information, please refer to pg. 1949

INACTIVE INGREDIENTS

carboxymethylcellulose sodium, cellulose, citric acid, corn syrup, D&C Red #33, FD&C Red #40, flavors, glycerin, purified water, sodium benzoate, sorbitol, sucralose, xanthan gum

HOW SUPPLIED

Pink-colored, Bubble Gum flavored liquid in child resistant tamper-evident bottles of 4 fl. oz.

Shown in Product Identification Guide, page 322

Concentrated TYLENOL® Infants' Drops Plus Cold Nasal Decongestant, Fever Reducer & Pain Reliever OTC

Concentrated TYLENOL® Infants' Drops Plus Cold & Cough Nasal Decongestant, Fever Reducer & Pain Reliever

Children's TYLENOL® Plus Cold Nighttime Suspension Liquid

Children's TYLENOL® Plus Cold Chewable Tablets

Children's TYLENOL® Plus Cold & Cough Suspension Liquid and Chewable Tablets

DESCRIPTION

Concentrated TYLENOL® Infants' Drops Plus Cold are alcohol-free, aspirin-free, BubbleGum-flavored and red in color. Each 1.6 mL contains acetaminophen 160 mg and pseudoephedrine HCl 15 mg. *Concentrated TYLENOL® Infants' Drops Plus Cold & Cough* are alcohol-free, aspirin-free, Cherry-flavored and red in color. Each 1.6 mL contains acetaminophen 160 mg, dextromethorphan HBr 5 mg, and pseudoephedrine HCl 15 mg. *Children's TYLENOL® Plus Cold Nighttime Suspension Liquid* is Grape-flavored and contains no alcohol or aspirin. Each teaspoon (5 mL) contains acetaminophen 160 mg, chlorpheniramine maleate 1 mg and pseudoephedrine HCl 15 mg. *Children's TYLENOL® Plus Cold Chewable Tablets* are Grape-flavored and each tablet contains acetaminophen 80 mg, chlorpheniramine maleate 0.5 mg and pseudoephedrine HCl 7.5 mg.

Continued on next page

Tylenol Infants'/Children's Cold—Cont.

Children's
TYLENOL® Plus Cold & Cough Suspension Liquid is Cherry-flavored and contains no alcohol or aspirin. Each teaspoonful (5 mL) contains acetaminophen 160 mg, chlorpheniramine maleate 1 mg, dextromethorphan HBr 5 mg and pseudoephedrine HCl 15 mg. *Children's TYLENOL® Plus Cold & Cough Chewable Tablets* are Cherry-flavored and each tablet contains acetaminophen 80 mg, chlorpheniramine maleate 0.5 mg, dextromethorphan HBr 2.5 mg, and pseudoephedrine HCl 7.5 mg.

ACTIONS

Acetaminophen is a clinically proven analgesic/antipyretic. Acetaminophen produces analgesia by elevation of the pain threshold and antipyresis through action on the hypothalamic heat-regulating center. Acetaminophen is equal to aspirin in analgesic and antipyretic effectiveness and it is unlikely to produce many of the side effects associated with aspirin and aspirin-containing products.
Pseudoephedrine hydrochloride is a sympathomimetic amine which provides temporary relief of nasal congestion. Chlorpheniramine maleate is an antihistamine that provides temporary relief of runny nose, sneezing and watery and itchy eyes.
Dextromethorphan hydrobromide is a cough suppressant which helps relieve coughs.

USES

Concentrated TYLENOL® Infants' Drops Plus Cold, temporarily relieves these cold symptoms:
- minor aches and pains
- nasal congestion • headaches
- temporarily reduces fever

Concentrated TYLENOL® Infants' Drops Plus Cold & Cough, temporarily relieves these cold symptoms:
- coughs • nasal congestion
- minor aches and pains
- sore throat • headaches
- temporarily reduces fever

Children's TYLENOL® Plus Cold Nighttime Suspension Liquid: temporarily relieves these cold symptoms:
- nasal congestion • sore throat • runny nose • sneezing
- headache • minor aches and pains
- temporarily reduces fever

Children's TYLENOL® Plus Cold Chewable Tablets: temporarily relieves these cold symptoms:
- nasal congestion • sore throat • runny nose • sneezing
- headache • minor aches and pains
- temporarily reduces fever

Children's TYLENOL® Plus Cold & Cough Suspension Liquid and *Chewable Tablets:* temporarily relieves these cold symptoms:
- nasal congestion • sore throat • runny nose • sneezing
- headache • minor aches and pains • coughs

temporarily reduces fever

DIRECTIONS

See Table 1: Children's Tylenol Dosing Chart on pg. 1951

WARNINGS

Sore throat warning: If sore throat is severe, persists for more than 2 days, is accompanied by or followed by fever, headache, rash, nausea or vomiting, consult a doctor promptly (does not apply to *Concentrated TYLENOL® Infants' Drops Plus Cold)*

Do not use
- in a child who is taking a prescription monoamine oxidase inhibitor (MAOI) (certain drugs for depression, psychiatric or emotional conditions, or Parkinson's disease), or for 2 weeks after stopping the MAOI drug. If you do not know if your child's prescription drug contains an MAOI, ask a doctor or pharmacist before giving this product.
- with any other products containing acetaminophen

Keep out of reach of children.

Overdose Warning: Taking more than the recommended dose (overdose) may cause liver damage. In case of overdose, get medical help or contact a Poison Control Center right away. Quick medical attention is critical even if you do not notice any signs or symptoms.

Stop use and ask a doctor if
- new symptoms occur
- redness or swelling is present
- pain gets worse or lasts for more than 5 days *for Children's Tyl. Plus Cold N.T. liquid: pain or nasal congestion gets worse or lasts more than 5 days *for Children's TYLENOL® cold plus cough suspension liquid:—pain, cough, or nasal congestion gets worse or lasts more than 5 days. comes back or occurs with rash or headache that lasts. These could be signs of a serious condition
- fever gets worse or lasts for more than 3 days
- nervousness, dizziness or sleeplessness occurs
- cough lasts for more than 7 days, comes back or occurs with fever, rash or headache that lasts. These could be signs of a serious condition. (*Concentrated TYLENOL® Infants' Drops Plus Cold & Cough and Children's TYLENOL® Plus Cold & Cough Products* only)

Concentrated TYLENOL® Infants' Drops Plus Cold,
Ask a doctor before use if the child has
- heart disease • high blood pressure • thyroid disease
- diabetes

When using this product
- **do not exceed recommended dosage (see overdose warning)**

Concentrated TYLENOL® Infants' Drops Plus Cold & Cough
Ask a doctor before use if the child has
- heart disease • high blood pressure
- cough that occurs with too much phlegm (mucus) • thyroid disease • diabetes • chronic cough that lasts as occurs with asthma

When using this product
- **do not exceed recommended dosage (see Overdose warning)**

Children's TYLENOL® Plus Cold Nighttime Suspension Liquid and Plus Cold Chewable Tablets
Ask a doctor before use if the child has
- heart disease • thyroid disease • glaucoma • high blood pressure • diabetes
- a breathing problem such as chronic bronchitis

When using this product
- **do not exceed recommended dosage (see overdose warning)**
- drowsiness may occur
- excitability may occur, especially in children

Children's TYLENOL® Plus Cold & Cough Nighttime Suspension Liquid and Chewable Tablets
Ask a doctor before use if the child has
- heart disease • thyroid disease • glaucoma • high blood pressure • diabetes
- cough that occurs with too much phlegm (mucus)
- chronic cough that lasts as occurs with asthma

When using this product
- **do not exceed recommended dosage (see overdose warning)**
- drowsiness may occur
- excitability may occur, especially in children

OTHER INFORMATION

Concentrated TYLENOL® Infants' Drops Plus Cold, Concentrated TYLENOL® Infants' Drops Plus Cold & Cough
- **do not use if plastic carton wrap or bottle wrap imprinted "Safety Seal®" is broken or missing**
- store at room temperature

Children's TYLENOL® Plus Cold & Cough Suspension Liquid, Children's TYLENOL® Plus Cold Nighttime Suspension Liquid
- **do not use if bottle wrap or foil inner seal imprinted "Safety Seal®" is broken or missing**
- store between 20°–25°C (68°–77°F)

Children's TYLENOL® Plus Cold Chewable Tablets
- phenylketonurics: contains phenylalanine 6 mg per tablet
- **do not use if carton is opened or if blister unit is broken**
- store at room temperature

Children's TYLENOL® Plus Cold & Cough Chewable Tablets
- phenylketonurics: contains phenylalanine 4 mg per tablet
- **do not use if carton is opened or if blister unit is broken**
- store at room temperature

Professional Information:
Overdosage Information: For overdosage information, please refer to pg. 1941

INACTIVE INGREDIENTS

Concentrated TYLENOL® Infants' Drops Plus Cold: citric acid, corn syrup, FD&C Red #40, flavors, polyethylene glycol, propylene glycol, sodium benzoate, sodium saccharin.
Concentrated TYLENOL® Infants' Drops Plus Cold & Cough: acesulfame potassium, citric acid, corn syrup, FD&C Red #40, flavors, polyethylene glycol, propylene glycol, sodium benzoate.
***Children's TYLENOL® Plus Cold:* Nighttime Suspension Liquid:** acesulfame potassium, carboxymethylcellulose sodium, cellulose, citric acid, corn syrup, D&C Red #33, FD&C Blue #1, FD&C Red #40, flavors, glycerin, propylene glycol, purified water, sodium benzoate, sorbitol, xanthan gum. **Chewable Tablets:** aspartame, basic polymethacrylate, cellulose, cellulose acetate, citric acid, D&C Red #7, FD&C Blue #1, flavors, hypromellose, magnesium stearate, mannitol.
***Children's TYLENOL® Plus Cold & Cough:* Suspension Liquid:** acesulfame potassium, carboxymethylcellulose sodium, cellulose, citric acid, corn syrup, D&C Red #33, FD&C Red #40, flavors, glycerin, purified water, sodium benzoate, sorbitol, xanthan gum. **Chewable Tablets:** aspartame, basic polymethacrylate, cellulose, cellulose acetate, D&C Red #7, flavors, hypromellose, magnesium stearate, mannitol.

HOW SUPPLIED

Concentrated TYLENOL® Infants' Drops Plus Cold: Red colored, Bubble Gum flavored drops in child resistant tamper-evident bottles of $^1/_2$ fl. oz.
Concentrated TYLENOL® Infants' Drops Plus Cold & Cough: Red colored, Cherry Flavored drops in Child resistant tamper evident bottles of $^1/_2$ fl. oz.
***Children's TYLENOL® Plus Cold:* Nighttime Suspension Liquid:** Purple-colored-bottles of 4 fl. oz. Store between 20°–25°C (68°–77°F). **Chewable Tablets:** Purple-colored, imprinted "TYLENOL COLD" on one side and "TC" on opposite side- blisters of 24.
***Children's TYLENOL® Plus Cold & Cough:* Suspension Liquid:** Red colored, Cherry flavored liquid in child resistant tamper-evident bottles of 4 fl. oz.
Chewable Tablets: Red-colored, imprinted TYLENOL C/C" on one side and "TC/C" on the opposite side- blisters of 24. Check cold bottle color – clear or white (opaque)
Shown in Product Identification Guide, pages 321 & 322

Children's TYLENOL® Plus Flu OTC

DESCRIPTION

Children's TYLENOL® Plus Flu Suspension Liquid is Bubble Gum flavored and contains no alcohol or aspirin. Each teaspoon (5 mL) contains acetaminophen 160 mg, chlorpheniramine maleate 1 mg, dextromethorphan HBr 7.5 mg and pseudoephedrine HCl 15 mg.

ACTIONS

Children's TYLENOL® Plus Flu Suspension Liquid combines the analgesic-antipyretic acetaminophen with the decongestant pseudoephedrine hydrochloride, the cough suppressant dextromethorphan hydrobromide and the antihistamine chlorpheniramine maleate to provide fast, effective, temporary relief of all your child's symptoms associated with flu including fever, body aches, headache, stuffy nose, runny nose, sore throat and coughs. Acetaminophen is equal to aspirin in analgesic and antipyretic effectiveness and it is unlikely to produce the side effects often associated with aspirin and aspirin-containing products.

USES

temporarily relieves these cold and flu symptoms:
- nasal congestion • sore throat
- runny nose • sneezing
- headache • minor aches and pains
- coughs
- temporarily reduces fever

DIRECTIONS

See Table 1: Children's Tylenol Dosing Chart on pg. 1951

WARNINGS

Sore throat warning:
If sore throat is severe, persists for more than 2 days, is accompanied or followed by fever, headache, rash, nausea or vomiting, consult a doctor promptly.

Do not use
- in a child who is taking a prescription monoamine oxidase inhibitor (MAOI) (certain drugs for depression, psychiatric or emotional conditions, or Parkinson's disease), or for 2 weeks after stopping the MAOI drug. If you do not know if your child's prescription drug contains an MAOI, ask a doctor or pharmacist before giving this product.
- with any other product containing acetaminophen.

Ask a doctor before use if the child has
- heart disease • thyroid disease
- glaucoma • high blood pressure
- diabetes • cough that occurs with too much phlegm (mucus)
- chronic cough that lasts as occurs with asthma

When using this product
- **do not exceed recommended dosage (see overdose warning)**
- drowsiness may occur
- excitability may occur, especially in children

Stop use and ask a doctor if
- new symptoms occur
- fever gets worse or lasts for more than 3 days
- redness or swelling is present
- nervousness, dizziness or sleeplessness occurs
- pain, cough or nasal congestion gets worse or lasts for more than 5 days
- cough comes back or occurs with rash or headache that lasts. These could be signs of a serious condition.

Keep out of reach of children.

Overdose Warning: Taking more than the recommended dose (overdose) may cause liver damage. In case of overdose, get medical help or contact a Poison Control Center right away. Quick medical attention is critical even if you do not notice any signs or symptoms.

OTHER INFORMATION
- **do not use if bottle wrap or foil inner seal imprinted "Safety Seal®" is broken or missing.**
- store between 20–25°C (68–77°F).

Professional Information:
Overdosage Information: For overdosage information, please refer to pg. 1941

INACTIVE INGREDIENTS

acesulfame potassium, carboxymethylcellulose sodium, cellulose, citric acid, corn syrup, D&C Red #33, FD&C Red #40, flavors, glycerin, purified water, sodium benzoate, sorbitol, xanthan gum.

HOW SUPPLIED

Pink colored, Bubble Gum flavored liquid in child resistant tamper-evident bottle of 4 fl. oz.
Shown in Product Identification Guide, page 322

CHILDREN'S TYLENOL® Plus Cold Daytime Non-Drowsy OTC

DESCRIPTION

Children's TYLENOL® Plus Cold Daytime Non-Drowsy Suspension Liquid is Fruit Burst-flavored and contains no alcohol or aspirin. Each teaspoon (5 mL) contains acetaminophen 160 mg and pseudoephedrine HCl 15 mg.

TABLE 1
Children's Tylenol® Dosing Chart

AGE GROUP		0–3 mos	4–11 mos	12–23 mos	2–3 yrs	4–5 yrs	6–8 yrs	9–10 yrs	11 yrs	12 yrs	
WEIGHT	(if possible use weight to dose; otherwise use age)	6–11 lbs	12–17 lbs	18–23 lbs	24–35 lbs	36–47 lbs	48–59 lbs	60–71 lbs	72–95 lbs	96 lbs and over	
PRODUCT FORM	**INGREDIENTS Dose to be administered based on weight or age†**										**Maximum doses/24 hrs**
Infants' Drops	**in each (0.8 mL)**										
Concentrated Tylenol Infants' Drops	Acetaminophen 80 mg	(0.4 mL)*	(0.8 mL)*	1.2 mL (0.8 + 0.4 mL)*	1.6 mL (0.8 + 0.8 mL)	—	—	—	—	—	5 times in 24 hrs
Concentrated Tylenol Infants' Drops Plus Cold	Acetaminophen 80 mg Pseudoephedrine HCl 7.5 mg	(0.4 mL)*	(0.8 mL)*	1.2 mL (0.8 + 0.4 mL)*	1.6 mL (0.8 + 0.8 mL)	—	—	—	—	—	4 times in 24 hrs
Concentrated Tylenol Infants' Drops Plus Cold & Cough	Acetaminophen 80 mg Dextromethorphan HBr 2.5 mg Pseudoephedrine HCl 7.5 mg	(0.4 mL)*	(0.8 mL)*	1.2 mL (0.8 + 0.4 mL)*	1.6 mL (0.8 + 0.8 mL)	—	—	—	—		4 times in 24 hrs
Children's Liquids	**Per 5 mL teaspoonful (TSP)**										
Children's Tylenol Suspension Liquid	Acetaminophen 160 mg	—	1/2 TSP*	3/4 TSP*	1 TSP	1 1/2 TSP	2 TSP	2 1/2 TSP	3 TSP	—	5 times in 24 hrs
Children's Tylenol Plus Cold Nighttime Suspension Liquid	Acetaminophen 160 mg Chlorpheniramine Maleate 1 mg Pseudoephedrine HCl 15 mg	—	1/2 TSP**	3/4 TSP**	1 TSP**	1 1/2 TSP**	2 TSP	2 1/2 TSP	3 TSP	—	4 times in 24 hrs
Children's Tylenol Plus Cold & Cough Suspension Liquid	Acetaminophen 160 mg Chlorpheniramine Maleate 1 mg Dextromethorphan HBr 5 mg Pseudoephedrine HCl 15 mg	—	1/2 TSP**	3/4 TSP**	1 TSP**	1 1/2 TSP**	2 TSP	2 1/2 TSP	3 TSP	—	4 times in 24 hrs
Children's Tylenol Plus Flu Suspension Liquid†	Acetaminophen 160 mg Chlorpheniramine Maleate 1 mg Dextromethorphan HBr 7.5 mg Pseudoephedrine HCl 15 mg	—	1/2 TSP**	3/4 TSP**	1 TSP**	1 1/2 TSP**	2 TSP	2 1/2 TSP	3 TSP	—	4 times in 24 hrs
Children's Tylenol Plus Cold Daytime Suspension Liquid	Acetaminophen 160 mg Pseudoephedrine HCl 15 mg	—	1/2 TSP*	3/4 TSP*	1 TSP	1 1/2 TSP	2 TSP	2 1/2 TSP	3 TSP	—	4 times in 24 hrs
Children's Tylenol Plus Cold & Allergy Liquid	Acetaminophen 160 mg Diphenhydramine HCl 12.5 mg Pseudoephedrine HCl 15 mg	—	1/2 TSP**	3/4 TSP**	1 TSP**	1 1/2 TSP**	2 TSP	2 1/2 TSP	3 TSP	—	4 times in 24 hrs
Children's Tablets	**Per tablet**										
Children's Tylenol Meltaways	Acetaminophen 80 mg	—	—	—	2 tablets	3 tablets	4 tablets	5 tablets	6 tablets	—	5 times in 24 hrs
Children's Tylenol Plus Cold Chewable Tablets	Acetaminophen 80 mg Chlorpheniramine Maleate 0.5 mg Pseudoephedrine HCl 7.5 mg	—	—	—	2 tablets**	3 tablets**	4 tablets	5 tablets	6 tablets	—	4 times in 24 hrs
Children's Tylenol Plus Cold & Cough Chewable Tablets	Acetaminophen 80 mg Chlorpheniramine Maleate 0.5 mg Dextromethorphan HBr 2.5 mg Pseudoephedrine HCl 7.5 mg	—	—	—	2 tablets**	3 tablets**	4 tablets	5 tablets	6 tablets	—	4 times in 24 hrs
JR Tylenol Meltaways	Acetaminophen 160 mg	—	—	—	—	—	2 tablets	2 1/2 tablets	3 tablets	4 tablets	5 times in 24 hrs
Simply Stuffy Liquid	pseudoephedrine HCl 15 mg	—	1/2 tsp.*	3/4 tsp.*	1 tsp	1 1/2 tsp	2 tsp	2 1/2 tsp	3 tsp	—	4 times in 24 hours
Simply Cough Liquid	dextromethorphan HBr 5 mg	—	1/2 tsp*	3/4 tsp*	1 tsp	1 1/2 tsp	2 tsp	2 1/2 tsp	3 tsp	—	4 times in 24 hrs

†All products may be dosed every 4 hours, if needed; except for Children's Tylenol Flu which is dosed every 6–8 hrs, if needed.
*Under 2 years (under 24 lbs), consult a doctor. **Under 6 years (under 48 lbs), consult a doctor.

- Infants' Tylenol Drops are more concentrated than Children's Tylenol Liquids. The Infants' Concentrated Drops have been specifically designed for use only with enclosed dropper. Do not use any other dosing device with this product. Shake well before using; fill to prescribed level and dispense liquid slowly into child's mouth, toward inner cheek. Use original bottle cap or dropper to maintain child resistance.
- Children's Tylenol Liquids are less concentrated than Infants' Tylenol Concentrated Drops. The Children's Tylenol Liquids have been specifically designed for use with the enclosed measuring cup. Use only enclosed measuring cup to dose this product. Shake well before using.
- Children's Tylenol Meltaways Tablets are not the same concentration as Junior Strength Tylenol Meltaways Tablets; dissolve in mouth or chew before swallowing.
- Junior Strength Tylenol Meltaways Tablets and Caplets contain twice as much medicine as Children's Tylenol Meltaways Tablets; dissolve in mouth or chew before swallowing.

ACTIONS

Children's TYLENOL® Plus Cold Daytime Non-Drowsy Suspension Liquid combines the analgesic-antipyretic acetaminophen with the decongestant pseudoephedrine hydrochloride to provide fast, effective, temporary relief of all your child's sinus symptoms including stuffy nose, sinus headache, sinus pressure, sinus pain, and nasal congestion. Acetaminophen is equal to aspirin in analgesic and antipyretic effectiveness and is unlikely to produce the side effects often associated with aspirin or aspirin-containing products.

USES

temporarily relieves:
• sinus congestion • stuffy nose • sinus pressure • minor aches, pains and headache • temporarily reduces fever

Continued on next page

Tylenol Children's Plus Cold—Cont.

DIRECTIONS

See Table 1: Children's Tylenol Dosing Chart on pg. 1951

WARNINGS

Do not use

- in a child who is taking a prescription monoamine oxidase inhibitor (MAOI) (certain drugs for depression, psychiatric, or emotional conditions, or Parkinson's disease), or for 2 weeks after stopping the MAOI drug. If you do not know if your child's prescription drug contains an MAOI, ask a doctor or pharmacist before giving this product.
- with any other product containing acetaminophen

Ask a doctor before use if the child has

- heart disease • high blood pressure • thyroid disease
- diabetes

When using this product

- **do not exceed recommended dosage (see overdose warning)**

Stop use and ask a doctor if

- new symptoms occur
- redness or swelling is present
- pain or nasal congestion gets worse or lasts for more than 5 days
- fever gets worse or lasts for more than 3 days
- nervousness, dizziness or sleeplessness occurs

Keep out of reach of children.

OVERDOSE WARNING Taking more than the recommended dose (overdose) may cause liver damage. In case of overdose, get medical help or contact a Poison Control Center right away. Quick medical attention is critical even if you do not notice any signs or symptoms.

OTHER INFORMATION

- **do not use if plastic carton wrap or bottle wrap imprinted "Safety Seal®" is broken or missing**
- store between 20–25°C (68–77°F)

Professional Information:
Overdosage Information:

For overdosage information, please refer to pg. 1941

INACTIVE INGREDIENTS

acesulfame potassium, carboxymethylcellulose sodium, cellulose, citric acid, corn syrup, D&C Red #33, FD&C Red #40, flavors, glycerin, purified water, sodium benzoate, sorbitol, xanthan gum.

HOW SUPPLIED

Red-colored, Fruit flavored liquid in child resistant tamper-evident bottles of 4 fl. oz.

Shown in Product Identification Guide, page 322

Children's TYLENOL® Dosing Chart

[See table 1 at top of previous page]

VERMOX® ℞

[vĕr - 'mŏx]
(mebendazole)
Chewable Tablets

DESCRIPTION

VERMOX® (mebendazole) is a (synthetic) broad-spectrum anthelmintic available as chewable tablets, each containing 100 mg of mebendazole. Inactive ingredients are: colloidal silicon dioxide, corn starch, hydrogenated vegetable oil, magnesium stearate, microcrystalline cellulose, sodium lauryl sulfate, sodium saccharin, sodium starch glycolate, talc, tetrarome orange, and FD&C yellow No. 6.

Mebendazole is methyl 5-benzoylbenzimidazole-2-carbamate and has the following structural formula:

[structural formula: H, N, HN—C(=O)—O—CH₃, C(=O), N]

Mebendazole is a white to slightly yellow powder with a molecular weight of 295.29. It is less than 0.05% soluble in water, dilute mineral acid solutions, alcohol, ether and chloroform, but is soluble in formic acid.

CLINICAL PHARMACOLOGY

Following administration of 100 mg twice daily for three consecutive days, plasma levels of VERMOX® (mebendazole) and its primary metabolite, the 2-amine, do not exceed 0.03 µg/ml and 0.09 µg/ml, respectively. All metabolites are devoid of anthelmintic activity. In man, approximately 2% of administered VERMOX® is excreted in urine and the remainder in the feces as unchanged drug or a primary metabolite.

Mode of Action: VERMOX® inhibits the formation of the worms' microtubules and causes the worms' glucose depletion.

INDICATIONS AND USAGE

VERMOX® (mebendazole) is indicated for the treatment of *Enterobius vermicularis* (pinworm), *Trichuris trichiura* (whipworm), *Ascaris lumbricoides* (common roundworm), *Ancylostoma duodenale* (common hookworm), *Necator americanus* (American hookworm) in single or mixed infections.

Efficacy varies as a function of such factors as pre-existing diarrhea and gastrointestinal transit time, degree of infection, and helminth strains. Efficacy rates derived from various studies are shown in the table below:

[See first table above]

	Pinworm (enterobiasis)	Whipworm (trichuriasis)	Common Roundworm (ascariasis)	Hookworm
Cure rates mean	95%	68%	98%	96%
Egg reduction mean	—	93%	99%	99%

CONTRAINDICATIONS

VERMOX® (mebendazole) is contraindicated in persons who have shown hypersensitivity to the drug.

WARNINGS

There is no evidence that VERMOX® (mebendazole), even at high doses, is effective for hydatid disease. There have been rare reports of neutropenia and agranulocytosis when VERMOX® was taken for prolonged periods and at dosages substantially above those recommended.

PRECAUTIONS

General: Periodic assessment of organ system functions, including hematopoietic and hepatic, is advisable during prolonged therapy.

Information for Patients: Patients should be informed of the potential risk to the fetus in women taking VERMOX® (mebendazole) during pregnancy, especially during the first trimester (see **Pregnancy**).

Patients should also be informed that cleanliness is important to prevent reinfection and transmission of the infection.

Drug Interactions: Preliminary evidence suggests that cimetidine inhibits mebendazole metabolism and may result in an increase in plasma concentrations of mebendazole.

Carcinogenesis, Mutagenesis, Impairment of Fertility: In carcinogenicity tests of mebendazole in mice and rats, no carcinogenic effects were seen at doses as high as 40 mg/kg (one to two times the human dose, based on mg/m^2) given daily over two years. Dominant lethal mutation tests in mice showed no mutagenicity at single doses as high as 640 mg/kg (18 times the human dose, based on mg/m^2). Neither the spermatocyte test, the F_1 translocation test, nor the Ames test indicated mutagenic properties. Doses up to 40 mg/kg in mice (equal to the human dose, based on mg/m^2), given to males for 60 days and to females for 14 days prior to gestation, had no effect upon fetuses and offspring, though there was slight maternal toxicity.

Pregnancy: Teratogenic effects. Pregnancy Category C. Mebendazole has shown embryotoxic and teratogenic activity in pregnant rats at single oral doses as low as 10 mg/kg (approximately equal to the human dose, based on mg/m^2). In view of these findings the use of VERMOX® is not recommended in pregnant women. Although there are no adequate and well-controlled studies in pregnant women, a post-marketing survey has been done of a limited number of women who inadvertently had consumed VERMOX® during the first trimester of pregnancy. The incidence of spontaneous abortion and malformation did not exceed that in the general population. In 170 deliveries on term, no teratogenic risk of VERMOX® was identified.

Nursing Mothers: It is not known whether VERMOX® is excreted in human milk. Because many drugs are excreted in human milk, caution should be exercised when VERMOX® is administered to a nursing woman.

Pediatric Use: The drug has not been extensively studied in children under two years; therefore, in the treatment of children under two years the relative benefit/risk should be considered.

ADVERSE REACTIONS

Gastrointestinal: Transient symptoms of abdominal pain and diarrhea in cases of massive infection and expulsion of worms.

Hypersensitivity: Rash, urticaria and angioedema have been observed on rare occasions.

Central Nervous System: Very rare cases of convulsions have been reported.

Liver: There have been liver function test elevations [AST (SGOT), ALT (SGPT), and GGT] and rare reports of hepatitis when VERMOX® was taken for prolonged periods and at dosages substantially above those recommended.

Hematologic: Neutropenia and agranulocytosis. (See **WARNINGS**).

OVERDOSAGE

In the event of accidental overdosage gastrointestinal complaints lasting up to a few hours may occur. Vomiting and purging should be induced.

DOSAGE AND ADMINISTRATION

The same dosage schedule applies to children and adults. The tablet may be chewed, swallowed, or crushed and mixed with food.

[See second table above]

Vermox®

	Pinworm (enterobiasis)	Whipworm (trichuriasis)	Common Roundworm (ascariasis)	Hookworm
Dose	1 tablet, once	1 tablet morning and evening for 3 consecutive days.	1 tablet morning and evening for 3 consecutive days.	1 tablet morning and evening for 3 consecutive days.

If the patient is not cured three weeks after treatment, a second course of treatment is advised. No special procedures, such as fasting or purging, are required.

HOW SUPPLIED

VERMOX® (mebendazole) is available as chewable tablets, each containing 100 mg of mebendazole, and is supplied in boxes of twelve tablets and boxes of sixty tablets.

Store at controlled room temperature 59°–77°F (15°–25°C).

McNeil Consumer & Specialty Pharmaceuticals
Fort Washington, PA 19034
Rev. October 1999
NDC 50580-070-12 (blister package of 12)
NDC 50580-070-60 (blister package of 60)
Distributed by:
McNeil Consumer Healthcare
DIVISION OF McNEIL-PPC, INC.
FORT WASHINGTON, PA 19034 USA

Revised October 1999
U.S. Patent 3,657,267

Shown in Product Identification Guide, page 322

MDR Fitness Corp.

MEDICAL DOCTORS' RESEARCH
14101 NW 4th STREET
SUNRISE, FL 33325

Direct Inquiries to:
1-800-637-8227 ext 5111 or 5445
www.mdri.com

MDR FITNESS TABS FOR MEN OTC
MDR FITNESS TABS FOR WOMEN

DESCRIPTION

The original AM/PM Fitness Tabs® from Medical Doctors' Research are patented because of their ability to increase blood levels of nutrients that can increase immune defenses and support a healthy cardiovascular system within weeks of taking the formula. MDR Fitness Tabs. The A.M. and P.M. dosage allows more absorption of the water soluble vitamins (B-complex and C) which are not readily stored by the body. The AM tablet provides more micronutrients required for energy producing reactions when physical activity is greater. The MDR Fitness Tabs formulas are free of dyes, yeast, preservatives, fillers, soy, wheat gluten, lactose and other sugars.

INDICATIONS AND USAGE

MDR Fitness Tabs are designed for the maintenance of good health and nutrition for men and women, 11 years of age or older, whenever a multi-vitamin, mineral supplement is indicated to help provide nutrients missing from the diet or to replace nutrient loss from oral contraceptives, antacids, excessive alcohol, smoking, physical or emotional stress, exercise, weight loss diets, or illness. Daily use of MDR Fitness Tabs may also play a protective role for good health by assuring adequate intake of essential nutrients, including antioxidant nutrients shown in recent research to enhance the body's natural defenses.

Directions: After the first meal of the day, take one "AM" Fitness Tab (and one Stress Defense Performance Tab, or

one MDR CardioTone if needed.) After lunch or dinner, take one "PM" Fitness Tab. Swallow Fitness Tab with a full glass of water.

PRECAUTIONS

Not recommended for persons with severe kidney disease or those undergoing renal dialysis, unless under a physician's supervision. Diabetics may need to adjust insulin dosage and should be monitored. Not recommended for those suffering from pernicious anemia, or Parkinson patients on levodopa therapy, due to the presence of vitamin B-6 which may decrease levodopa's efficacy. Pregnant and lactating women may need additional supplementation.

Note: MDR also provides a Stress Defense supplement to be taken with MDR Fitness Tabs when higher dosages are indicated. MDR has formulated Vital Factors for persons over 40 years of age to supply secretagogues that help enhance the body's natural release of Human Growth Hormone, and to supply other vital factors which decline with age. A majority of users report increased vitality, energy, better sleep, reduced depression, improved flexibility and greater mental function after using Vital Factors.

Also available: Nite-Cal Calcium, Vitamin B-12 Liquid B Complex, Chondro-Pro Arthritis Formula, Cholesterol Defense, CardioTone Cardiovascular Nutritional Support, Longevity Antioxidants, Prostate Health Tabs, Cranberry Capsules, Triple Bioflavenoids, Healthy Tract Digestive Enzymes, AM/PM Slimming Factors.

For Samples, Product or Order Information Call
1-800-MDR-TABS ext. 5111 or 5445 or fax (954) 845-9505
att: L. Giordano
www.mdri.com
or write: (MDR) Medical Doctors' Research
14101 NW 4th Street
SUNRISE, FL 33325

Mead Johnson & Company

2400 WEST LLOYD EXPRESSWAY
EVANSVILLE, IN 47721-0001

For Medical Information Contact:
Generally:
FAX: (609) 897-6859
EMAIL: drug.information@bms.com
In Emergencies:
(800) 321-1335
Adverse Event Experiences and Product Defects Reporting:
(866) 232-2557
Sales and Ordering:
(800) 457-3550

CAFCIT® ℞
[kaf-sit]
(caffeine citrate) Injection
CAFCIT®
(caffeine citrate) Oral Solution
Rx only

DESCRIPTION

Both CAFCIT® (caffeine citrate) Injection for intravenous administration and CAFCIT® (caffeine citrate) Oral Solution are clear, colorless, sterile, non-pyrogenic, preservative-free, aqueous solutions adjusted to pH 4.7. Each mL contains 20 mg caffeine citrate (equivalent to 10 mg of caffeine base) prepared in solution by the addition of 10 mg caffeine anhydrous to 5.0 mg citric acid monohydrate, 8.3 mg sodium citrate dihydrate and Water for Injection.

Caffeine, a central nervous system stimulant, is an odorless white crystalline powder or granule, with a bitter taste. It is sparingly soluble in water and ethanol at room temperature. The chemical name of caffeine is 3,7-dihydro-1,3,7-trimethyl-*1H*-purine-2,6-dione. In the presence of citric acid it forms caffeine citrate salt in solution. The structural formula and molecular weight of caffeine citrate follows.

Caffeine citrate
$C_{14}H_{18}N_4O_9$ Mol. Wt. 386.31

CLINICAL PHARMACOLOGY

Mechanism of Action

Caffeine is structurally related to other methylxanthines, theophylline and theobromine. It is a bronchial smooth muscle relaxant, a CNS stimulant, a cardiac muscle stimulant and a diuretic.

Although the mechanism of action of caffeine in apnea of prematurity is not known, several mechanisms have been hypothesized. These include: (1) stimulation of the respiratory center, (2) increased minute ventilation, (3) decreased threshold to hypercapnia, (4) increased response to hypercapnia, (5) increased skeletal muscle tone, (6) decreased diaphragmatic fatigue, (7) increased metabolic rate, and (8) increased oxygen consumption.

Most of these effects have been attributed to antagonism of adenosine receptors, both A_1 and A_2 subtypes, by caffeine, which has been demonstrated in receptor binding assays and observed at concentrations approximating those achieved therapeutically.

Pharmacokinetics

Absorption: After oral administration of 10 mg caffeine base/kg to preterm neonates, the peak plasma level (C_{max}) for caffeine ranged from 6–10 mg/L and the mean time to reach peak concentration (T_{max}) ranged from 30 minutes to 2 hours. The T_{max} was not affected by formula feeding. The absolute bioavailability, however, was not fully examined in preterm neonates.

Distribution: Caffeine is rapidly distributed into the brain. Caffeine levels in the cerebrospinal fluid of preterm neonates approximate their plasma levels. The mean volume of distribution of caffeine in infants (0.8-0.9 L/kg) is slightly higher than that in adults (0.6 L/kg). Plasma protein binding data are not available for neonates or infants. In adults, the mean plasma protein binding *in vitro* is reported to be approximately 36%.

Metabolism: Hepatic cytochrome P450 1A2 (CYP1A2) is involved in caffeine biotransformation. Caffeine metabolism in preterm neonates is limited due to their immature hepatic enzyme systems.

Interconversion between caffeine and theophylline has been reported in preterm neonates; caffeine levels are approximately 25% of theophylline levels after theophylline administration and approximately 3-8% of caffeine administered would be expected to convert to theophylline.

Elimination: In young infants, the elimination of caffeine is much slower than that in adults due to immature hepatic and/or renal function. Mean half-life ($T_{1/2}$) and fraction excreted unchanged in urine (A_e) of caffeine in infants have been shown to be inversely related to gestational/postconceptual age. In neonates, the $T_{1/2}$ is approximately 3-4 days and the A_e is approximately 86% (within 6 days). By 9 months of age, the metabolism of caffeine approximates that seen in adults ($T_{1/2}$ = 5 hours and A_e = 1%).

Special Populations: Studies examining the pharmacokinetics of caffeine in neonates with hepatic or renal insufficiency have not been conducted. CAFCIT (caffeine citrate) should be administered with caution in preterm neonates with impaired renal or hepatic function. Serum concentrations of caffeine should be monitored and dose administration of CAFCIT should be adjusted to avoid toxicity in this population.

Clinical Studies

One multicenter, randomized, double-blind trial compared CAFCIT (caffeine citrate) to placebo in eighty-five (85) preterm infants (gestational age 28 to <33 weeks) with apnea of prematurity. Apnea of prematurity was defined as having at least 6 apnea episodes of greater than 20 seconds duration in a 24-hour period with no other identifiable cause of apnea. A 1 mL/kg (20 mg/kg caffeine citrate providing 10 mg/kg as caffeine base) loading dose of CAFCIT was administered intravenously, followed by a 0.25 mL/kg (5 mg/kg caffeine citrate providing 2.5 mg/kg of caffeine base) daily maintenance dose administered either intravenously or orally (generally through a feeding tube). The duration of treatment in this study was limited to 10 to 12 days. The protocol allowed infants to be "rescued" with open-label caffeine citrate treatment if their apnea remained uncontrolled during the double-blind phase of the trial.

The percentage of patients without apnea on day 2 of treatment (24–48 hours after the loading dose) was significantly greater with CAFCIT than placebo. The following table summarizes the clinically relevant endpoints evaluated in this study:

	CAFCIT	Placebo	p-value
Number of patients evaluated[1]	45	37	
% of patients with zero apnea events on day 2	26.7	8.1	0.03
Apnea rate on day 2 (per 24 hrs.)	4.9	7.2	0.134
% of patients with 50% reduction in apnea events from baseline on day 2	76	57	0.07

[1] Of 85 patients who received drug, 3 were not included in the efficacy analysis because they had <6 apnea episodes/24 hours at baseline.

In this 10-12 day trial, the mean number of days with zero apnea events was 3.0 in the CAFCIT group and 1.2 in the placebo group. The mean number of days with a 50% reduction from baseline in apnea events was 6.8 in the CAFCIT group and 4.6 in the placebo group.

INDICATIONS AND USAGE

CAFCIT (caffeine citrate) is indicated for the short term treatment of apnea of prematurity in infants between 28 and <33 weeks gestational age.

CONTRAINDICATIONS

CAFCIT is contraindicated in patients who have demonstrated hypersensitivity to any of its components.

WARNINGS

During the double-blind, placebo-controlled clinical trial, six cases of necrotizing enterocolitis developed among the 85 infants studied (caffeine=46, placebo=39), with three cases resulting in death. Five of the six patients with necrotizing enterocolitis were randomized to or had been exposed to CAFCIT.

Reports in the published literature have raised a question regarding the possible association between the use of methylxanthines and development of necrotizing enterocolitis, although a causal relationship between methylxanthine use and necrotizing enterocolitis has not been established. Therefore, as with all preterm infants, patients being treated with CAFCIT should be carefully monitored for the development of necrotizing enterocolitis.

PRECAUTIONS

General

Apnea of prematurity is a diagnosis of exclusion. Other causes of apnea (e.g., central nervous system disorders, primary lung disease, anemia, sepsis, metabolic disturbances, cardiovascular abnormalities, or obstructive apnea) should be ruled out or properly treated prior to initiation of CAFCIT.

Caffeine is a central nervous system stimulant and in cases of caffeine overdose, seizures have been reported. CAFCIT should be used with caution in infants with seizure disorders.

The duration of treatment of apnea of prematurity in the placebo-controlled trial was limited to 10 to 12 days. The safety and efficacy of CAFCIT for longer periods of treatment have not been established. Safety and efficacy of CAFCIT for use in the prophylactic treatment of sudden infant death syndrome (SIDS) or prior to extubation in mechanically ventilated infants have also not been established.

Cardiovascular

Although no cases of cardiac toxicity were reported in the placebo-controlled trial, caffeine has been shown to increase heart rate, left ventricular output, and stroke volume in published studies. Therefore, CAFCIT (caffeine citrate) should be used with caution in infants with cardiovascular disease.

Renal and Hepatic Systems

CAFCIT should be administered with caution in infants with impaired renal or hepatic function. Serum concentrations of caffeine should be monitored and dose administration of CAFCIT should be adjusted to avoid toxicity in this population. (See **CLINICAL PHARMACOLOGY**, *Elimination, Special Populations*).

Information for Patients

Parents/caregivers of patients receiving CAFCIT Oral Solution should receive the following instructions:

1. CAFCIT does not contain any preservatives and each vial is for single use only. Any unused portion of the medication should be discarded.
2. It is important that the dose of CAFCIT be measured accurately, i.e., with a 1cc or other appropriate syringe.
3. Consult your physician if the baby continues to have apnea events; do not increase the dose of CAFCIT without medical consultation.
4. Consult your physician if the baby begins to demonstrate signs of gastrointestinal intolerance, such as abdominal distention, vomiting, or bloody stools, or seems lethargic.
5. CAFCIT should be inspected visually for particulate matter and discoloration prior to its administration. Vials containing discolored solution or visible particulate matter should be discarded.

Laboratory Tests

Prior to initiation of CAFCIT, baseline serum levels of caffeine should be measured in infants previously treated with theophylline, since preterm infants metabolize theophylline to caffeine. Likewise, baseline serum levels of caffeine should be measured in infants born to mothers who consumed caffeine prior to delivery, since caffeine readily crosses the placenta.

In the placebo-controlled clinical trial, caffeine levels ranged from 8 to 40 mg/L. A therapeutic plasma concentration range of caffeine could not be determined from the placebo-controlled clinical trial. Serious toxicity has been reported in the literature when serum caffeine levels exceed 50 mg/L. Serum concentrations of caffeine may need to be monitored periodically throughout treatment to avoid toxicity.

In clinical studies reported in the literature, cases of hypoglycemia and hyperglycemia have been observed. Therefore, serum glucose may need to be periodically monitored in infants receiving CAFCIT.

Drug Interactions

Cytochrome P450 1A2 (CYP1A2) is known to be the major enzyme involved in the metabolism of caffeine. Therefore, caffeine has the potential to interact with drugs that are substrates for CYP1A2, inhibit CYP1A2, or induce CYP1A2. Few data exist on drug interactions with caffeine in preterm neonates. Based on adult data, lower doses of caffeine may be needed following coadministration of drugs which are reported to decrease caffeine elimination (e.g., cimetidine and ketoconazole) and higher caffeine doses may be needed following coadministration of drugs that increase caffeine elimination (e.g., phenobarbital and phenytoin).

Caffeine administered concurrently with ketoprofen reduced the urine volume in 4 healthy volunteers. The clinical significance of this interaction in preterm neonates is not known.

Interconversion between caffeine and theophylline has been reported in preterm neonates. The concurrent use of these drugs is not recommended.

Continued on next page

Cafcit—Cont.

Carcinogenesis, Mutagenesis, Impairment of Fertility
In a 2-year study in Sprague-Dawley rats, caffeine (as caffeine base) administered in drinking water was not carcinogenic in male rats at doses up to 102 mg/kg or in female rats at doses up to 170 mg/kg (approximately 2 and 4 times, respectively, the maximum recommended intravenous loading dose for infants on a mg/m^2 basis). In an 18-month study in C57BL/6 mice, no evidence of tumorigenicity was seen at dietary doses up to 55 mg/kg (less than the maximum recommended intravenous loading dose for infants on a mg/m^2 basis).
Caffeine (as caffeine base) increased the sister chromatid exchange (SCE) SCE/cell metaphase (exposure time dependent) in an *in vivo* mouse metaphase analysis. Caffeine also potentiated the genotoxicity of known mutagens and enhanced the micronuclei formation (5-fold) in folate-deficient mice. However, caffeine did not increase chromosomal aberrations in *in vitro* Chinese hamster ovary cell (CHO) and human lymphocyte assays and was not mutagenic in an *in vitro* CHO/hypoxanthine guanine phosphoribosyltransferase (HGPRT) gene mutation assay, except at cytotoxic concentrations. In addition, caffeine was not clastogenic in an *in vivo* mouse micronucleus assay.
Caffeine (as caffeine base) administered to male rats at 50 mg/kg/day subcutaneously (approximately equal to the maximum recommended intravenous loading dose for infants on a mg/m^2 basis) for four days prior to mating with untreated females, caused decreased male reproductive performance in addition to causing embryotoxicity. In addition, long-term exposure to high oral doses of caffeine (3.0 g over 7 weeks) was toxic to rat testes as manifested by spermatogenic cell degeneration.
Pregnancy: ***Pregnancy Category C***
Concern for the teratogenicity of caffeine is not relevant when administered to infants. In studies performed in adult animals, caffeine (as caffeine base) administered to pregnant mice as sustained release pellets at 50 mg/kg (less than the maximum recommended intravenous loading dose for infants on a mg/m^2 basis), during the period of organogenesis, caused a low incidence of cleft palate and exencephaly in the fetuses. There are no adequate and well-controlled studies in pregnant women.

ADVERSE REACTIONS

Overall, the reported number of adverse events in the double-blind period of the controlled trial was similar for the CAFCIT (caffeine citrate) and placebo groups. The following table shows adverse events that occurred in the double-blind period of the controlled trial and that were more frequent in CAFCIT treated patients than placebo.

ADVERSE EVENTS THAT OCCURRED MORE FREQUENTLY IN CAFCIT TREATED PATIENTS THAN PLACEBO DURING DOUBLE-BLIND THERAPY

Adverse Event (AE)	CAFCIT N=46 n (%)	Placebo N=39 n (%)
BODY AS A WHOLE		
Accidental Injury	1 (2.2)	0 (0.0)
Feeding Intolerance	4 (8.7)	2 (5.1)
Sepsis	2 (4.3)	0 (0.0)
CARDIOVASCULAR SYSTEM		
Hemorrhage	1 (2.2)	0 (0.0)
DIGESTIVE SYSTEM		
Necrotizing Enterocolitis	2 (4.3)	1 (2.6)
Gastritis	1 (2.2)	0 (0.0)
Gastrointestinal Hemorrhage	1 (2.2)	0 (0.0)
HEMIC AND LYMPHATIC SYSTEM		
Disseminated Intravascular Coagulation	1 (2.2)	0 (0.0)
METABOLIC AND NUTRITIVE DISORDERS		
Acidosis	1 (2.2)	0 (0.0)
Healing Abnormal	1 (2.2)	0 (0.0)
NERVOUS SYSTEM		
Cerebral Hemorrhage	1 (2.2)	0 (0.0)
RESPIRATORY SYSTEM		
Dyspnea	1 (2.2)	0 (0.0)
Lung Edema	1 (2.2)	0 (0.0)
SKIN AND APPENDAGES		
Dry Skin	1 (2.2)	0 (0.0)
Rash	4 (8.7)	3 (7.7)
Skin Breakdown	1 (2.2)	0 (0.0)
SPECIAL SENSES		
Retinopathy of Prematurity	1 (2.2)	0 (0.0)
UROGENITAL SYSTEM		
Kidney Failure	1 (2.2)	0 (0.0)

In addition to the cases above, three cases of necrotizing enterocolitis were diagnosed in patients receiving CAFCIT during the open-label phase of the study.

	Dose of CAFCIT Volume	Dose of CAFCIT mg/kg	Route	Frequency
Loading Dose	1 mL/kg	20 mg/kg	Intravenous* (over 30 minutes)	One Time
Maintenance Dose	0.25 mL/kg	5 mg/kg	Intravenous* (over 10 minutes) or Orally	Every 24 hours**

* using a syringe infusion pump
** beginning 24 hours after the loading dose

Three of the infants who developed necrotizing enterocolitis during the trial died. All had been exposed to caffeine. Two were randomized to caffeine, and one placebo patient was "rescued" with open-label caffeine for uncontrolled apnea.
Adverse events described in the published literature include: central nervous system stimulation (i.e., irritability, restlessness, jitteriness), cardiovascular effects (i.e., tachycardia, increased left ventricular output, and increased stroke volume), gastrointestinal effects (i.e., increased gastric aspirate, gastrointestinal intolerance), alterations in serum glucose (hypoglycemia and hyperglycemia) and renal effects (increased urine flow rate, increased creatinine clearance, and increased sodium and calcium excretion). Published long-term follow-up studies have not shown caffeine to adversely affect neurological development or growth parameters.

OVERDOSAGE

Following overdose, serum caffeine levels have ranged from approximately 24 mg/L (a post marketing spontaneous case report in which an infant exhibited irritability, poor feeding and insomnia) to 350 mg/L. Serious toxicity has been associated with serum levels greater than 50 mg/L (see **PRECAUTIONS—Laboratory Tests** and **DOSAGE AND ADMINISTRATION**). Signs and symptoms reported in the literature after caffeine overdose in preterm infants include fever, tachypnea, jitteriness, insomnia, fine tremor of the extremities, hypertonia, opisthotonos, tonic-clonic movements, nonpurposeful jaw and lip movements, vomiting, hyperglycemia, elevated blood urea nitrogen, and elevated total leukocyte concentration. Seizures have also been reported in cases of overdose. One case of caffeine overdose complicated by development of intraventricular hemorrhage and long-term neurological sequelae has been reported. Another case of caffeine citrate overdose (from New Zealand; not CAFCIT) of an estimated 600 mg caffeine citrate (approximately 322 mg/kg) administered over 40 minutes was complicated by tachycardia, ST depression, respiratory distress, heart failure, gastric distention, acidosis and a severe extravasation burn with tissue necrosis at the peripheral intravenous injection site. No deaths associated with caffeine overdose have been reported in preterm infants.
Treatment of caffeine overdose is primarily symptomatic and supportive. Caffeine levels have been shown to decrease after exchange transfusions. Convulsions may be treated with intravenous administration of diazepam or a barbiturate such as pentobarbital sodium.

DOSAGE AND ADMINISTRATION

Prior to initiation of CAFCIT (caffeine citrate), baseline serum levels of caffeine should be measured in infants previously treated with theophylline, since preterm infants metabolize theophylline to caffeine. Likewise, baseline serum levels of caffeine should be measured in infants born to mothers who consumed caffeine prior to delivery, since caffeine readily crosses the placenta.
The recommended loading dose and maintenance doses of CAFCIT follow.
[See table above]
NOTE THAT THE DOSE OF CAFFEINE BASE IS ONE-HALF THE DOSE WHEN EXPRESSED AS CAFFEINE CITRATE (e.g., 20 mg of caffeine citrate is equivalent to 10 mg of caffeine base).
Serum concentrations of caffeine may need to be monitored periodically throughout treatment to avoid toxicity. Serious toxicity has been associated with serum levels greater than 50 mg/L.
CAFCIT should be inspected visually for particulate matter and discoloration prior to administration. Vials containing discolored solution or visible particulate matter should be discarded.
Drug Compatibility
To test for drug compatibility with common intravenous solutions or medications, 20 mL of CAFCIT (caffeine citrate) Injection were combined with 20 mL of a solution or medication, with the exception of an Intralipid® admixture, which was combined as 80 mL/80 mL. The physical appearance of the combined solutions was evaluated for precipitation. The admixtures were mixed for 10 minutes and then assayed for caffeine. The admixtures were then continually mixed for 24 hours, with further sampling for caffeine assays at 2, 4, 8, and 24 hours.
Based on this testing, CAFCIT Injection, 60 mg/3 mL is chemically stable for 24 hours at room temperature when combined with the following test products.
- Dextrose Injection, USP 5%
- 50% Dextrose Injection USP
- Intralipid® 20% IV Fat Emulsion
- Aminosyn® 8.5% Crystalline Amino Acid Solution
- Dopamine HCI Injection, USP 40 mg/mL diluted to 0.6 mg/mL with Dextrose Injection, USP 5%
- Calcium Gluconate Injection, USP 10% (0.465 mEq/Ca^{+2}/mL)
- Heparin Sodium Injection, USP 1000 units/mL diluted to 1 unit/mL with Dextrose Injection, USP 5%
- Fentanyl Citrate Injection, USP 50 µg/mL diluted to 10 µg/mL with Dextrose Injection, USP 5%

HOW SUPPLIED

Both CAFCIT Injection and CAFCIT Oral Solution are available as clear, colorless, sterile, non-pyrogenic, preservative-free, aqueous solutions in 3 mL colorless glass vials. The vials of CAFCIT Injection are sealed with a teflon-faced gray rubber stopper and an aluminum overseal with a white flip-off polypropylene disk inset. The vials of CAFCIT Oral Solution are sealed with a teflon-faced gray rubber stopper and a peel-off aluminum overseal with a blue flip-off polypropylene disk inset.
Both the injection and oral solution vials contain 3 mL solution at a concentration of 20 mg/mL caffeine citrate (60 mg/vial) equivalent to 10 mg/mL caffeine base (30 mg/vial).
CAFCIT® (caffeine citrate) Injection
NDC 0087-6011-42: 3 mL vial, individually packaged in a carton.
CAFCIT® (caffeine citrate) Oral Solution
NDC 0087-6111-42: 3 mL vial (NOT CHILD-RESISTANT), 10 vials per white polypropylene child resistant container.
Store at 15°-30°C (59°-86°F).
Preservative Free. For single use only. Discard unused portion.
ATTENTION PHARMACIST: Detach "Instructions for Use" from the package insert and dispense with CAFCIT Oral Solution prescription.

CAFCIT®
(caffeine citrate) Oral Solution
Rx only
Each bottle (vial) of CAFCIT contains a total of 60 mg of caffeine citrate in 3 mL (20 mg/mL).

Information and Instructions for Use

This leaflet tells you about CAFCIT (KAF-sit) and how to give it to your baby. Read the following information before giving this medicine to your baby. Completely discuss CAFCIT with your baby's doctor. Continue to discuss any questions you have about this medicine at your baby's checkups.
After you remove your baby's dose, throw away the open bottle (vial) and all medicine left in it. Use each vial of CAFCIT for only one dose. There will be extra medicine left in the vial after one dose is removed. Leftover medicine should not be used because CAFCIT does not contain preservatives. Once the vial is open, any medicine that is not used right away must be discarded.

What is CAFCIT?
The main ingredient of CAFCIT is caffeine citrate. CAFCIT is a clear, colorless, medicine to treat apnea of prematurity - short periods when premature babies stop breathing. Apnea of prematurity is due to the baby's breathing centers not being fully developed.

How do I give CAFCIT to my baby?
Give CAFCIT to your baby once a day, at about the same time each day. Your baby's doctor will prescribe the right amount of CAFCIT based on your baby's weight and age. Carefully follow the doctor's dosing instructions.
Measure the dose of CAFCIT carefully. Your baby's doctor, nurse, or pharmacist will give you a suitable syringe or supply of syringes to measure small but accurate doses of CAFCIT.
Never change (increase or decrease) your baby's dose without speaking to your baby's doctor.
If your baby continues to have periods of apnea, call your baby's doctor right away.
CAFCIT can be swallowed by mouth or given through a feeding tube. Based on your baby's own situation, your baby's doctor or other healthcare professional should teach you how to give CAFCIT correctly.
CAFCIT should be clear and colorless. Before giving CAFCIT, look for small particles, cloudiness, or discoloration in the medicine. **Do not use vials that contain cloudy or discolored medicine, or any visible particles.**
CAFCIT does NOT contain any preservatives. Do not open the vial until it is time for your baby to receive the dose of medicine. Use each vial only once. After you remove your baby's dose, throw away the vial and all medicine left in the opened vial.
Ten (10) vials of CAFCIT are packaged in a child-resistant container. CAFCIT vials are **NOT CHILD-RESISTANT.** Always store vials of CAFCIT in the child-resistant container. Follow the instructions below to open the child-resistant container, to open a vial of CAFCIT, and to remove a dose of medicine from the vial.

To open the child-resistant container that holds the vials of CAFCIT:

(Instructions with pictures are also printed on the top of the container)

1. Hold the bottom-half of the child-resistant container with one hand and push the lower semicircular section on the front of the container with your thumb.
2. With your other hand, pull the cover up until you hear it click.
3. While holding the ends of the bottom-half of the container with both hands, place both index fingers on the two semicircular locking tabs on the sides of the container.
4. Press the two tabs and raise the cover up.

To open a vial of CAFCIT (caffeine citrate):

1. Hold the blue plastic top between the thumb and index finger. Use your thumb to flip the blue plastic top completely off the vial.
2. Carefully lift up the metal ring.
3. Pull the metal ring away from the vial and then pull it down towards the bottom of the vial without twisting the ring.
4. After you pull the ring down and the metal band around the top of the vial is completely broken through, carefully remove the rest of the metal band by pulling it out and away from the vial.
5. Being careful not to spill any medicine, remove the rubber stopper from the top of the vial.

To remove the prescribed dose from the vial:

You will need a small syringe to measure the exact amount of medicine that your baby's doctor prescribed. Your baby's doctor, nurse or pharmacist will give you this small syringe.

Note that a milliliter (mL) is the same as a cubic centimeter (cc).

1. Insert the tip of the syringe in the medicine and pull up on the plunger to draw the medicine into the syringe. Remove slightly more of the medicine than the exact amount to be given to your baby.
2. Turn the syringe tip up so that any air in it rises to the top. Remove the air by gently pushing up on the syringe plunger. Continue to push the syringe plunger up to remove any extra medicine in the syringe, until only the exact number of milliliters (or cubic centimeters) that your baby's doctor prescribed remains in the syringe.
3. Give the CAFCIT to your baby as your baby's doctor instructed.
4. Throw away the sharp metal pieces, the rubber stopper, the open vial, and any medicine that remains in it after your baby receives the dose.

What are possible side effects of CAFCIT (caffeine citrate)?

Your baby may or may not develop side effects from taking CAFCIT. Each baby is different. If your baby develops one or more of the following symptoms, speak with your baby's doctor right away:

- restlessness, jitteriness or shakiness
- faster heart beat
- increased urination (increased diaper wetting)

The following symptoms may be caused by serious bowel or stomach problems. Call your baby's doctor right away if your baby develops:

- bloated abdomen (stomach area)
- vomiting
- bloody stools (bloody bowel movements)
- loss of energy, lethargy (acting sluggish)

This is not a complete list of side effects reported with CAFCIT. If you have a concern about your baby, speak with your baby's doctor. If you want more information about CAFCIT, speak with your baby's doctor or pharmacist.

Manufactured by:
Ben Venue Laboratories, Inc., Bedford, Ohio 44146.
Distributed by:
Mead Johnson & Company, Evansville, IN 47721 U.S.A.
Mead Johnson™ Nutritionals

 Revised (2) May 2003
LB1976P

Shown in Product Identification Guide, page 322

The Medicines Company

8 CAMPUS DRIVE
PARSIPPANY, NJ 07054

Direct Inquiries to:
(800) 264-4662

ANGIOMAX® ℞

[*ăn-jē-ō-măks*]
(bivalirudin)
FOR INJECTION

DESCRIPTION

ANGIOMAX® (bivalirudin) is a specific and reversible direct thrombin inhibitor. The active substance is a synthetic, 20 amino acid peptide. The chemical name is D-phenylalanyl-L-prolyl-L-arginyl-L-prolyl-glycyl-glycyl-glycyl-glycyl-L-asparagyl-glycyl-L-aspartyl-L-phenylalanyl-L-glutamyl-L-glutamyl-L-isoleucyl-L-prolyl-L-glutamyl-L-glutamyl-L-tyrosyl-L-leucine trifluoroacetate (salt) hydrate (Figure 1). The molecular weight of Angiomax is 2180 daltons (anhydrous free base peptide). Angiomax is supplied in single-use vials as a white lyophilized cake, which is sterile. Each vial contains 250 mg bivalirudin, 125 mg mannitol, and sodium hydroxide to adjust the pH to 5–6 (equivalent of approximately 12.5 mg sodium). When reconstituted with Sterile Water for Injection the product yields a clear to opalescent, colorless to slightly yellow solution, pH 5–6.

[See chemical structure above]

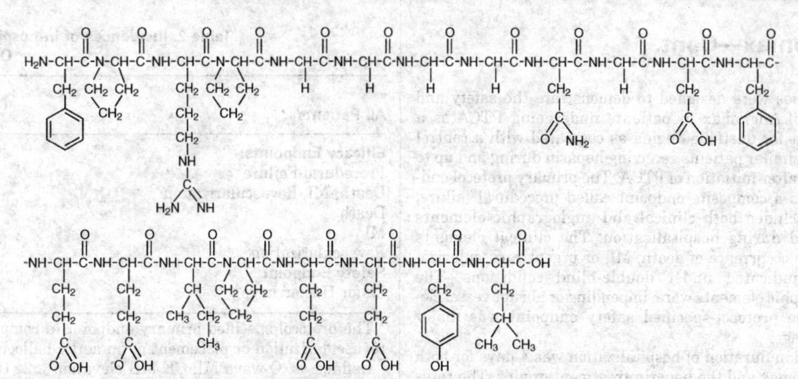

Table 1. PK Parameters and Dose Adjustments in Renal Impairment*

Renal Function (GFR, mL/min)	Clearance (mL/min/kg)	Half-life (minutes)	% Reduction in Infusion Dose
Normal renal function (≥90 mL/min)	3.4	25	0
Mild renal impairment (60-89 mL/min)	3.4	22	0
Moderate renal impairment (30-59 mL/min)	2.7	34	20
Severe renal impairment (10-29 mL/min)	2.8	57	60
Dialysis-dependent patients (off dialysis)	1.0	3.5 hours	90

* The ACT should be monitored in renally-impaired patients.

CLINICAL PHARMACOLOGY

General:

Angiomax directly inhibits thrombin by specifically binding both to the catalytic site and to the anion-binding exosite of circulating and clot-bound thrombin. Thrombin is a serine proteinase that plays a central role in the thrombotic process, acting to cleave fibrinogen into fibrin monomers and to activate Factor XIII to Factor XIIIa, allowing fibrin to develop a covalently cross-linked framework which stabilizes the thrombus; thrombin also activates Factors V and VIII, promoting further thrombin generation, and activates platelets, stimulating aggregation and granule release. The binding of Angiomax to thrombin is reversible as thrombin slowly cleaves the Angiomax-Arg_3-Pro_4 bond, resulting in recovery of thrombin active site functions.

In *in vitro* studies, bivalirudin inhibited both soluble (free) and clot-bound thrombin, was not neutralized by products of the platelet release reaction, and prolonged the activated partial thromboplastin time (aPTT), thrombin time (TT), and prothrombin time (PT) of normal human plasma in a concentration-dependent manner. The clinical relevance of these findings is unknown.

Pharmacokinetics:

Bivalirudin exhibits linear pharmacokinetics following intravenous (IV) administration to patients undergoing percutaneous transluminal coronary angioplasty (PTCA). In these patients, a mean steady state bivalirudin concentration of 12.3 ± 1.7 mcg/mL is achieved following an IV bolus of 1 mg/kg and a 4-hour 2.5 mg/kg/h IV infusion. Bivalirudin is cleared from plasma by a combination of renal mechanisms and proteolytic cleavage, with a half-life in patients with normal renal function of 25 min. The disposition of bivalirudin was studied in PTCA patients with mild and moderate renal impairment and in patients with severe renal impairment. Drug elimination was related to glomerular filtration rate (GFR). Total body clearance was similar for patients with normal renal function and with mild renal impairment (60-89 mL/min). Clearance was reduced approximately 20% in patients with moderate and severe renal impairment and was reduced approximately 80% in dialysis-dependent patients. See Table 1 for pharmacokinetic parameters and dose reduction recommendations. For patients with renal impairment the activated clotting time (ACT) should be monitored. Bivalirudin is hemodialyzable. Approximately 25% is cleared by hemodialysis.

Bivalirudin does not bind to plasma proteins (other than thrombin) or to red blood cells.

[See table 1 above]

Pharmacodynamics:

In healthy volunteers and patients (with ≥70%) vessel occlusion undergoing routine angioplasty), bivalirudin exhibits linear dose- and concentration-dependent anticoagulant activity as evidenced by prolongation of the ACT, aPTT, PT, and TT. Intravenous administration of Angiomax produces an immediate anticoagulant effect. Coagulation times return to baseline approximately 1 hour following cessation of Angiomax administration.

In 291 patients with ≥70% vessel occlusion undergoing routine angioplasty, a positive correlation was observed between the dose of Angiomax and the proportion of patients achieving ACT values of 300 sec or 350 sec. At an Angiomax dose of 1.0 mg/kg IV bolus plus 2.5 mg/kg/h IV infusion for 4 hours, followed by 0.2 mg/kg/h, all patients reached maximal ACT values >300 sec.

Clinical Trials:

Angiomax was evaluated in patients with unstable angina undergoing PTCA in two randomized, double-blind, multicenter studies with identical protocols. Patients must have had unstable angina defined as: (1) a new onset of severe or accelerated angina or rest pain within the month prior to study entry or (2) angina or ischemic rest pain which developed between four hours and two weeks after an acute myocardial infarction (MI). Overall, 4312 patients with unstable angina, including 741 (17%) patients with post-MI angina, were treated in a 1:1 randomized fashion with Angiomax or heparin. Patients ranged in age from 29-90 (median 63) years, their weight was a median of 80 kg (39-120 kg), 68% were male, and 91% were Caucasian. Twenty-three percent of patients were treated with heparin within one hour prior to randomization. All patients were administered aspirin 300-325 mg prior to PTCA and daily thereafter. Patients randomized to Angiomax were started on an intravenous infusion of Angiomax (2.5 mg/kg/h). Within 5 min after starting the infusion, and prior to PTCA, a 1 mg/kg loading dose was administered as an intravenous bolus. The infusion was continued for 4 hours, then the infusion was changed under double-blinded conditions to Angiomax (0.2 mg/kg/h) for up to an additional 20 hours (patients received this infusion for an average of 14 hours). The ACT was checked at 5 min and at 45 min following commencement. If on either occasion the ACT was <350 sec, an additional double-blinded bolus of placebo was administered. The Angiomax dose was not titrated to ACT. Median ACT values were: ACT in sec (5th percentile-95th percentile): 345 sec (240–595 sec) at 5 min and 346 sec (range 269-583 sec) at 45 min after initiation of dosing. Patients randomized to heparin were given a loading dose (175 IU/kg) as an intravenous bolus 5 min before the planned procedure, with immediate commencement of an infusion of heparin (15 IU/kg/h). The infusion was continued for 4 hours. After 4 hours of infusion, the heparin infusion was changed under double-blinded conditions to heparin (15 IU/kg/h) for up to 20 additional hours. The ACT was checked at 5 min and at 45 min following commencement. If on either occasion the ACT was <350 sec, an additional double-blind bolus of heparin (60 IU/kg) was administered. Once the target ACT was achieved for heparin patients, no further ACT measurements were performed. All ACTs were determined with the Hemochron® device. The protocol allowed use of open-label heparin at the discretion of the investigator after discontinuation of blinded study medication, whether or not an endpoint event (procedural failure) had occurred. The use of open-label heparin was similar between Angiomax® (bivalirudin) and heparin treatment groups (about 20% in both groups).

Continued on next page

Angiomax—Cont.

The studies were designed to demonstrate the safety and efficacy of Angiomax in patients undergoing PTCA as a treatment for unstable angina as compared with a control group of similar patients receiving heparin during and up to 24 hours after initiation of PTCA. The primary protocol endpoint was a composite endpoint called procedural failure, which included both clinical and angiographic elements measured during hospitalization. The clinical elements were: the occurrence of death, MI, or urgent revascularization, adjudicated under double-blind conditions. The angiographic elements were: impending or abrupt vessel closure. The protocol-specified safety endpoint was major hemorrhage.

The median duration of hospitalization was 4 days for both the Angiomax and the heparin treatment groups. The rates of procedural failure were similar in the Angiomax and heparin treatment groups. Study outcomes are shown in Table 2.

[See table 2 at right]

Table 2. Incidences of In-hospital Clinical Endpoints In Randomized Clinical Trials Occurring within 7 Days

All Patients	ANGIOMAX® n=2161	HEPARIN n=2151
Efficacy Endpoints:		
Procedural Failure[1]	7.9%	9.3%
Death, MI, Revascularization	6.2%	7.9%
Death	0.2%	0.2%
MI[2]	3.3%	4.2%
Revascularization[3]	4.2%	5.6%
Safety Endpoint:		
Major Hemorrhage[4]	3.5%	9.3%

[1] The protocol specified primary endpoint (a composite of death or MI or clinical deterioration of cardiac origin requiring revascularization or placement of an aortic balloon pump or angiographic evidence of abrupt vessel closure).

[2] Defined as: Q-wave MI; CK-MB elevation ≥2×ULN, new ST- or T-wave abnormality, and chest pain ≥30 min; OR new LBBB with chest pain ≥30 min and/or elevated CK-MB enzymes; OR elevated CK-MB and new ST- or T-wave abnormality without chest pain; OR elevated CK-MB.

[3] Defined as: any revascularization procedure, including angioplasty, CABG, stenting, or placement of an intra-aortic balloon pump.

[4] Defined as the occurrence of any of the following: intracranial bleeding, retroperitoneal bleeding, clinically overt bleeding with a decrease in hemoglobin ≥3 g/dL or leading to a transfusion of ≥2 units of blood.

INDICATIONS AND USAGE

Angiomax is indicated for use as an anticoagulant in patients with unstable angina undergoing percutaneous transluminal coronary angioplasty (PTCA). Angiomax is intended for use with aspirin and has been studied only in patients receiving concomitant aspirin (see Clinical Trials and DOSAGE AND ADMINISTRATION).

The safety and effectiveness of Angiomax have not been established when used in conjunction with platelet inhibitors other than aspirin, such as glycoprotein IIb/IIIa inhibitors (see PRECAUTIONS, Drug Interactions).

The safety and effectiveness of Angiomax have not been established in patients with unstable angina who are not undergoing PTCA or in patients with other acute coronary syndromes.

CONTRAINDICATIONS

Angiomax is contraindicated in patients with:

— active major bleeding;

— hypersensitivity to Angiomax or its components.

WARNINGS

Angiomax is not intended for intramuscular administration. Although most bleeding associated with the use of Angiomax in PTCA occurs at the site of arterial puncture, hemorrhage can occur at any site. An unexplained fall in blood pressure or hematocrit, or any unexplained symptom, should lead to serious consideration of a hemorrhagic event and cessation of Angiomax administration.

An increased risk of thrombus formation has been associated with the use of Angiomax in gamma brachytherapy, including fatal outcomes.

There is no known antidote to Angiomax. Angiomax is hemodialyzable (see CLINICAL PHARMACOLOGY, Pharmacokinetics).

PRECAUTIONS

General:

Clinical trials have provided limited information for use of Angiomax in patients with heparin-induced thrombocytopenia/heparin-induced thrombocytopenia-thrombosis syndrome (HIT/HITTS) undergoing PTCA. The number of HIT/HITTS patients treated is inadequate to reliably assess efficacy and safety in these patients undergoing PTCA. Angiomax was administered to a small number of patients with a history of HIT/HITTS or active HIT/HITTS and undergoing PTCA in an uncontrolled, open-label study and in an emergency treatment program and appeared to provide adequate anticoagulation in these patients. In *in vitro* studies, bivalirudin exhibited no platelet aggregation response against sera from patients with a history of HIT/HITTS.

Caution should be used when Angiomax is used as the antithrombin brachytherapy procedures. Operators are advised to maintain meticulous catheter technique, with frequent aspiration and flushing, paying special attention to minimizing conditions of stasis within the catheter or vessels.

Drug Interactions:

Bivalirudin does not exhibit binding to plasma proteins (other than thrombin) or red blood cells.

Drug-drug interaction studies have been conducted with the adenosine diphosphate (ADP) antagonist, ticlopidine, and the glycoprotein IIb/IIIa inhibitor, abciximab, and with low molecular weight heparin. Although data are limited, precluding conclusions regarding efficacy and safety in combination with these agents, the results do not suggest pharmacodynamic interactions. In patients treated with low molecular weight heparin, low molecular weight heparin was discontinued at least 8 hours prior to the procedure and administration of Angiomax.

The safety and effectiveness of Angiomax have not been established when used in conjunction with platelet inhibitors other than aspirin, such as glycoprotein IIb/IIIa inhibitors. In clinical trials in patients undergoing PTCA, co-administration of Angiomax with heparin, warfarin or thrombolytics was associated with increased risks of major bleeding events compared to patients not receiving these concomitant medications. There is no experience with co-administration of Angiomax and plasma expanders such as dextran. Angiomax should be used with caution in patients with disease states associated with an increased risk of bleeding.

Pediatric Use:

The safety and effectiveness of Angiomax in pediatric patients have not been established.

Table 3. Major Bleeding and Transfusions: All Patients[1]

	ANGIOMAX® n=2161	HEPARIN n=2151
No. (%) Patients with Major Hemorrhage[2]	79 (3.7)	199 (9.3)
- with ≥3g/dL fall in Hgb	41 (1.9)	124 (5.8)
- with ≥5g/dL fall in Hgb	14 (<1)	47 (2.2)
- Retroperitoneal Bleeding	5 (<1)	15 (<1)
- Intracranial Bleeding	1 (<1)	2 (<1)
- Required Transfusion	43 (2.0)	123 (5.7)

[1] No monitoring of ACT (or PTT) was done after a target ACT was achieved.

[2] Major hemorrhage was defined as the occurrence of any of the following: intracranial bleeding, retroperitoneal bleeding, clinically overt bleeding with a decrease in hemoglobin ≥3 g/dL or leading to a transfusion of ≥2 units of blood. This table includes data from the entire hospitalization period.

Table 4. Adverse Events Other Than Bleeding Occurring in ≥5% Of Patients In Either Treatment Group In Randomized Clinical Trials

EVENT	Treatment Group ANGIOMAX® n=2161	HEPARIN n=2151
	Number of Patients (%)	
Cardiovascular		
Hypotension	262 (12)	371 (17)
Hypertension	135 (6)	115 (5)
Bradycardia	118 (5)	164 (8)
Gastrointestinal		
Nausea	318 (15)	347 (16)
Vomiting	138 (6)	169 (8)
Dyspepsia	100 (5)	111 (5)
Genitourinary		
Urinary retention	89 (4)	98 (5)
Miscellaneous		
Back pain	916 (42)	944 (44)
Pain	330 (15)	358 (17)
Headache	264 (12)	225 (10)
Injection site pain	174 (8)	274 (13)
Insomnia	142 (7)	139 (6)
Pelvic pain	130 (6)	169 (8)
Anxiety	127 (6)	140 (7)
Abdominal pain	103 (5)	104 (5)
Fever	103 (5)	108 (5)
Nervousness	102 (5)	87 (4)

Immunogenicity/Re-exposure:

Among 494 subjects who received Angiomax in clinical trials and were tested for antibodies, 2 subjects had treatment-emergent positive bivalirudin antibody tests. Neither subject demonstrated clinical evidence of allergic or anaphylactic reactions and repeat testing was not performed. Nine additional patients who had initial positive tests were negative on repeat testing.

Carcinogenesis, Mutagenesis, and Impairment of Fertility:

No long-term studies in animals have been performed to evaluate the carcinogenic potential of Angiomax. Bivalirudin displayed no genotoxic potential in the *in vitro* bacterial cell reverse mutation assay (Ames test), the *in vitro* Chinese hamster ovary cell forward gene mutation test (CHO/HGPRT), the *in vitro* human lymphocyte chromosomal aberration assay, the *in vitro* rat hepatocyte unscheduled DNA synthesis (UDS) assay, and the *in vivo* rat micronucleus assay. Fertility and general reproductive performance in rats were unaffected by subcutaneous doses of bivalirudin up to 150 mg/kg/day, about 1.6 times the dose on a body surface area basis (mg/m^2) of a 50 kg person given the maximum recommended dose of 15 mg/kg/day.

Pregnancy:

Angiomax® (bivalirudin) is intended for use with aspirin (see INDICATIONS AND USAGE). Because of possible adverse effects on the neonate and the potential for increased maternal bleeding, particularly during the third trimester, Angiomax and aspirin should be used together during pregnancy only if clearly needed.

Pregnancy Category B:

Teratogenicity studies have been performed in rats at subcutaneous doses up to 150 mg/kg/day, (1.6 times the maximum recommended human dose based on body surface area) and rabbits at subcutaneous doses up to 150 mg/kg/day (3.2 times the maximum recommended human dose based on body surface area). These studies revealed no evidence of impaired fertility or harm to the fetus attributable to bivalirudin. There are, however, no adequate and well-controlled studies in pregnant women. Because animal reproduction studies are not always predictive of human response, this drug should be used during pregnancy only if clearly needed.

Nursing Mothers:

It is not known whether bivalirudin is excreted in human milk. Because many drugs are excreted in human milk, caution should be exercised when Angiomax is administered to a nursing woman.

Geriatric Patients:

Of the total number of patients in clinical studies of Angiomax undergoing PTCA, 41% were ≥65 years of age, while 11% were >75 years old. A difference of ≥5% between age groups was observed for heparin-treated but not Angiomax-treated patients with regard to the percentage of patients with major bleeding events. There were no individual bleeding events which were observed with a difference of ≥5% between treatment groups, although puncture site hemorrhage and catheterization site hematoma were each observed in a higher percentage of patients ≥65 years than

Table 5. Dosing Table

	Using 5 mg/mL Concentration		Using 0.5 mg/mL Concentration
Weight (kg)	Bolus (1 mg/kg) (mL)	Initial 4-hour Infusion (2.5 mg/kg/h) (mL/h)	Subsequent Low-rate Infusion (0.2mg/kg/h) (mL/h)
43-47	9	22.5	18
48-52	10	25	20
53-57	11	27.5	22
58-62	12	30	24
63-67	13	32.5	26
68-72	14	35	28
73-77	15	37.5	30
78-82	16	40	32
83-87	17	42.5	34
88-92	18	45	36
93-97	19	47.5	38
98-102	20	50	40
103-107	21	52.5	42
108-112	22	55	44
113-117	23	57.5	46
118-122	24	60	48
123-127	25	62.5	50
128-132	26	65	52
133-137	27	67.5	54
138-142	28	70	56
143-147	29	72.5	58
148-152	30	75	60

in patients <65 years. This difference between age groups was more pronounced for heparin-treated than Angiomax-treated patients.

ADVERSE REACTIONS

Bleeding:

In 4312 patients undergoing PTCA for treatment of unstable angina in 2 randomized, double-blind studies comparing Angiomax to heparin, Angiomax patients exhibited lower rates of major bleeding and lower requirements for blood transfusions. The incidence of major bleeding is presented in Table 3. The incidence of major bleeding was lower in the Angiomax group than in the heparin group.

[See table 3 at top of previous page]

Other Adverse Events:

In the 2 randomized double-blind clinical trials of Angiomax in patients undergoing PTCA, 82% of 2161 Angiomax-treated patients and 83% of 2151 heparin-treated patients experienced at least one treatment-emergent adverse event. The most frequent treatment-emergent events were back pain (42%), pain (15%), nausea (15%), headache (12%), and hypotension (12%) in the Angiomax-treated group. Treatment-emergent adverse events other than bleeding reported for ≥5% of patients in either treatment group are shown in Table 4.

[See table 4 on previous page]

Serious, non-bleeding adverse events were experienced in 2% of 2161 Angiomax-treated patients and 2% of 2151 heparin-treated patients. The following individual serious non-bleeding adverse events were rare (>0.1% to <1%) and similar in incidence between Angiomax- and heparin-treated patients. These events are listed by body system: *Body as a Whole:* fever, infection, sepsis: *Cardiovascular:* hypotension, syncope, vascular anomaly, ventricular fibrillation; *Nervous:* cerebral ischemia, confusion, facial paralysis; *Respiratory:* lung edema; *Urogenital:* kidney failure, oliguria.

Postmarketing events:

There have been reports of thrombus formation with the use of Angiomax during percutaneous coronary intervention (PCI), including intracoronary brachytherapy. Fatal outcomes have been reported.

OVERDOSAGE

Discontinuation of Angiomax leads to a gradual reduction in anticoagulant effects due to metabolism of the drug. There has been no experience of overdosage in human clinical trials. In case of overdosage, Angiomax should be discontinued and the patient should be closely monitored for signs of bleeding. There is no known antidote to Angiomax. Angiomax is hemodialyzable (see CLINICAL PHARMACOLOGY, Pharmacokinetics).

DOSAGE AND ADMINISTRATION

The recommended dosage of Angiomax is an intravenous (IV) bolus dose of 1.0 mg/kg followed by a 4-hour IV infusion at a rate of 2.5 mg/kg/h. After completion of the initial 4-hour infusion, an additional IV infusion of Angiomax may be initiated at a rate of 0.2 mg/kg/h for up to 20 hours, if needed. Angiomax is intended for use with aspirin (300-325 mg daily) and has been studied only in patients receiving concomitant aspirin. Treatment with Angiomax should be initiated just prior to PTCA. The dose of Angiomax may need to be reduced, and anticoagulation status monitored, in patients with renal impairment (see CLINICAL PHARMACOLOGY, Pharmacokinetics).

Instructions for Administration:

Angiomax® (bivalirudin) is intended for intravenous injection and infusion. To each 250 mg vial add 5 mL of Sterile Water for Injection, USP. Gently swirl until all material is dissolved. Each reconstituted vial should be further diluted in 50 mL of 5% Dextrose in Water or 0.9% Sodium Chloride for Injection to yield a final concentration of 5 mg/mL (e.g., 1 vial in 50 mL; 2 vials in 100 mL; 5 vials in 250 mL). The dose to be administered is adjusted according to the patient's weight, see Table 5.

If the low-rate infusion is used after the initial infusion, a lower concentration bag should be prepared. In order to prepare this bag, reconstitute the 250 mg vial with 5 mL of Sterile Water for Injection, USP. Gently swirl until all material is dissolved. Each reconstituted vial should be further diluted in 500 mL of 5% Dextrose in Water or 0.9% Sodium Chloride for Injection to yield a final concentration of 0.5 mg/mL. The infusion rate to be administered should be selected from the right-hand column in Table 5.

[See table 5 above]

Angiomax should be administered via an intravenous line. No incompatibilities have been observed with glass bottles or polyvinyl chloride bags and administration sets. The following nine drugs should not be administered in the same intravenous line with Angiomax, since they resulted in haze formation, microparticulate formation, or gross precipitation when mixed with Angiomax: alteplase, amiodarone HCl, amphotericin B, chlorpromazine HCl, diazepam, prochlorperazine edisylate, reteplase, streptokinase, and vancomycin HCl.

Parenteral drug products should be inspected visually for particulate matter and discoloration prior to administration. Preparations of Angiomax containing particulate matter should not be used. Reconstituted material will be a clear to slightly opalescent, colorless to slightly yellow solution.

Storage after Reconstitution:

Do not freeze reconstituted or diluted Angiomax. Reconstituted material may be stored at 2–8°C for up to 24 hours. Diluted Angiomax with a concentration of between 0.5 mg/mL and 5 mg/mL is stable at room temperature for up to 24 hours. Discard any unused portion of reconstituted solution remaining in the vial.

HOW SUPPLIED

Angiomax® (bivalirudin) is supplied as a sterile, lyophilized product in single-use, glass vials. After reconstitution, each vial delivers 250 mg of Angiomax.

Store Angiomax dosage units at 20-25°C (68-77°F). Excursions to 15-30°C permitted. [See USP Controlled Room Temperature.]

NDC 65293-001-01

Manufactured by:
Ben Venue Laboratories
Bedford, OH

Distributed by:
ICS
Louisville, KY

Marketed by:
THE **MEDICINES** COMPANY
Parsippany, NJ 07054
For information call: (800) 264-4662

U.S. Patent 5,196,404

Rx only

Hemochron® is a registered trademark of International Technidyne Corporation, Edison, NJ.

TMC PN 1002-6 (February 10, 2004)

Shown in Product Identification Guide, page 322

MEDICIS, The Dermatology Company®

**8125 NORTH HAYDEN ROAD
SCOTTSDALE, AZ 85258**

For Medical Information Contact:
Generally:
Medical Affairs Department
(602) 808-8800
FAX: (602) 808-0822

In Emergencies:
(602) 808-8800

DYNACIN® ℞

[*dī 'nă-sən*]
(minocycline hcl tablets, usp)
℞ Only

To reduce the development of drug-resistant bacteria and maintain the effectiveness of the antibacterial drug product and other antibacterial drugs, the drug product should be used only to treat or prevent infections that are proven or strongly suspected to be caused by bacteria.

DESCRIPTION

Minocycline hydrochloride, a semisynthetic derivative of tetracycline, is 4,7-Bis(dimethylamino)-1,4,4a,5,5a,6,11,12a-octahydro-3,10,12,12a-tetrahydroxy-1,11-dioxo-2-naphthacenecarboxamide monohydrochloride. Its structural formula is:

$C_{23}H_{27}N_3O_7{\bullet}HCL$ M.W. 493.94

Minocycline hydrochloride tablets for oral administration contain minocycline HCl equivalent to 50 mg, 75 mg or 100 mg of minocycline. In addition, 50 mg, 75 mg and 100 mg tablets contain the following inactive ingredients: Colloidal Silicon Dioxide, Lactose Anhydrous, Magnesium Stearate, Microcrystalline Cellulose, Povidone and Sodium Starch Glycolate. The 50 mg tablets also contain Opadry White which contains: Titanium Dioxide, Hydroxypropyl Methylcellulose, Polyethylene Glycol and Polysorbate 80. The 75 mg and 100 mg tablets contain Opadry Gray which contains: Titanium Dioxide, Hydroxypropyl Methylcellulose, Polyethylene Glycol and Iron Oxide Black.

CLINICAL PHARMACOLOGY

Minocycline hydrochloride tablets are rapidly absorbed from the gastrointestinal tract following oral administration. Following a single dose of one 100 mg tablet of minocycline hydrochloride administered to 30 normal fasting adult volunteers, maximum serum concentrations were attained in 1 to 3 hours (average 1.71 hours) and ranged from 491.71 to 1292.70 ng/mL (average 758.29 ng/mL). The serum half-life in the normal volunteers ranged from 11.38 to 24.31 hours (average 17.03 hours).

When minocycline hydrochloride tablets were given concomitantly with a meal, which included dairy products, the extent of absorption of minocycline hydrochloride tablets was not noticeably influenced. The peak plasma concentrations were slightly decreased (12%) and delayed by 1.09 hours when administered with food, compared to dosing under fasting conditions.

In previous studies with other minocycline dosage forms, the minocycline serum half-life ranged from 11 to 16 hours in 7 patients with hepatic dysfunction, and from 18 to 69 hours in 5 patients with renal dysfunction. The urinary and fecal recovery of minocycline when administered to 12 normal volunteers is one-half to one-third that of other tetracyclines.

Microbiology

The tetracyclines are primarily bacteriostatic and are thought to exert their antimicrobial effect by the inhibition of protein synthesis. The tetracyclines, including minocycline, have similar antimicrobial spectra of activity against a wide range of gram-positive and gram-negative organisms. Cross-resistance of these organisms to tetracyclines is common.

Minocycline has been shown to be active against most strains of the following microorganisms, both *in vitro* and in clinical infections as described in the **INDICATIONS AND USAGE** section:

AEROBIC GRAM-POSITIVE MICROORGANISMS

Because many strains of the following gram-positive microorganisms have been shown to be resistant to tetracyclines, culture and susceptibility testing are especially recommended. Tetracycline antibiotics should not be used for streptococcal diseases unless the organism has been demonstrated to be susceptible. Tetracyclines are not the drug of choice in the treatment of any type of staphylococcal infection.

Continued on next page

Dynacin—Cont.

Bacillus anthracis†
Listeria monocytogenes†
Staphylococcus aureus
Streptococcus pneumoniae
AEROBIC GRAM-NEGATIVE MICROORGANISMS
Bartonella bacilliformis
Brucella species
Calymmatobacterium granulomatis
Campylobacter fetus
Francisella tularensis
Haemophilus ducreyi
Vibrio cholerae
Yersinia pestis
Because many strains of the following groups of gram-negative microorganisms have been shown to be resistant to tetracyclines, culture and susceptibility tests are especially recommended.
Acinetobacter species
Enterobacter aerogenes
Escherichia coli
Haemophilus influenzae
Klebsiella species
Neisseria gonorrhoeae†
Neisseria meningitidis†
Shigella species
"OTHER" MICROORGANISMS
Actinomyces species†
Borrelia recurrentis
Chlamydia psittaci
Chlamydia trachomatis
Clostridium species†
Entamoeba species
Fusobacterium nucleatum ssp. *fusiforme*†
Mycobacterium marinum
Mycoplasma pneumoniae
Propionibacterium acnes
Rickettsiae
Treponema pallidum subspecies *pallidum*†
Treponema pallidum subspecies *pertenue*†
Ureaplasma urealyticum

†When penicillin is contraindicated, tetracyclines are alternative drugs in the treatment of infections caused by the cited microorganisms.

Susceptibility Tests

Susceptibility testing should be performed with tetracycline since it predicts susceptibility to minocycline. However, certain organisms (e.g., some staphylococci, and *Acinetobacter* ssp.) may be more susceptible to minocycline and doxycycline than tetracycline.

Dilution techniques:

Quantitative methods are used to determine antimicrobial minimal inhibitory concentrations (MICs). These MICs provide estimates of the susceptibility of bacteria to antimicrobial compounds. The MICs should be determined using a standardized procedure. Standardized procedures are based on a dilution method[1,3] (broth or agar) or equivalent with standardized inoculum concentrations and standardized concentrations of tetracycline powder. The MIC values should be interpreted according to the following criteria:

For testing aerobic gram-negative microorganisms (Enterobacteriaceae), *Acinetobacter* ssp. and *Staphylococcus aureus.*

MIC (mcg/mL)	Interpretation
≤ 4	Susceptible (S)
8	Intermediate (I)
≥ 16	Resistant (R)

For testing *Haemophilus influenzae*[a] and *Streptococcus pneumoniae*[b]:

MIC (mcg/mL)	Interpretation
≤ 2	Susceptible (S)
4	Intermediate (I)
≥ 8	Resistant (R)

[a] These interpretative standards are applicable only to broth microdilution susceptibility testing with *Haemophilus influenzae* using *Haemophilus* Test Medium.[1]

[b] These interpretative standards are applicable only to broth microdilution susceptibility testing using cation-adjusted Muller-Hinton broth with 2 – 5% lysed horse blood.[1]

For testing Neisseria gonorrhoeae[c]:

MIC (mcg/mL)	Interpretation
≤ 0.25	Susceptible (S)
0.5-1	Intermediate (I)
≥ 2	Resistant (R)

[c] These interpretative standards are applicable only to agar dilution susceptibility testing using GC agar base and 1% defined growth supplements.[1]

A report of "Susceptible" indicates that the pathogen is likely to be inhibited if the antimicrobial compound in the blood reaches the concentrations usually achievable. A report of "Intermediate" indicates that the result should be considered equivocal, and, if the microorganism is not fully susceptible to alternative, clinically feasible drugs, the test should be repeated. This category implies possible clinical applicability in body sites where the drug is physiologically concentrated or in situations where high dosage of drug can be used. This category also provides a buffer zone which prevents small uncontrolled technical factors from causing major discrepancies in interpretation. A report of "Resistant" indicates that the pathogen is not likely to be inhibited if the antimicrobial compound in the blood reaches the concentrations usually achievable; other therapy should be selected.

Standardized susceptibility test procedures require the use of laboratory control microorganisms to control the technical aspects of the laboratory procedures. Standard tetracycline powder should provide the following MIC values:

Microorganism		MIC Range (mcg/mL)
Escherichia coli	ATCC 25922	0.5-2
Enterococcus faecalis	ATCC 29212	8-32
Staphylococcus aureus	ATCC 29213	0.25-1
Haemophilus influenzae	ATCC 49247	4-32
Streptococcus pneumoniae	ATCC 49619	0.12-0.5
Neisseria gonorrhoeae	ATCC 49226	0.25-1

Diffusion techniques:

Quantitative methods that require measurement of zone diameters also provide reproducible estimates of the susceptibility of bacteria to antimicrobial compounds. One such standardized procedure[2,3] requires the use of standardized inoculum concentrations. This procedure uses paper disks impregnated with 30 mcg tetracycline (class disk) or 30 mcg minocycline to test the susceptibility of microorganisms to minocycline. Reports from the laboratory providing results of the standard single-disk susceptibility test with a 30 mcg tetracycline or minocycline disk should be interpreted according to the following criteria:

For testing aerobic gram-negative microorganisms (Enterobacteriaceae). *Acinetobacter* spp. and *Staphylococcus aureus:*

Zone Diameter (mm)	Interpretation
≥ 19	Susceptible (S)
15-18	Intermediate (I)
≤ 14	Resistant (R)

For testing *Haemophilus influenzae*[d]:

Zone Diameter (mm)	Interpretation
≥ 29	Susceptible (S)
26-28	Intermediate (I)
≤ 25	Resistant (R)

[d] These zone diameter standards are applicable only to susceptibility testing with *Haemophilus influenzae* using Haemophilus Test Medium and a 30 mcg tetracycline disk.[2]

For testing *Neisseria gonorrhoeae*[e]:

Zone Diameter (mm)	Interpretation
≥ 38	Susceptible (S)
31-37	Intermediate (I)
≤ 30	Resistant (R)

[e] These interpretative standards are applicable only to disk diffusion testing using GC agar and 1% growth supplements, and a 30 mcg tetracycline disk.[2]

For testing *Streptococcus pneumoniae*[f]:

Zone Diameter (mm)	Interpretation
≥ 23	Susceptible (S)
19-22	Intermediate (I)
≤ 18	Resistant (R)

[f] These interpretative standards are applicable only to disk diffusion testing using Muller-Hinton agar adjusted with 5% sheep blood and a 30 mcg tetracycline-class disk.[2]

For testing *Vibrio cholerae*[g]:

Zone Diameter (mm)	Interpretation
≥ 19	Susceptible (S)
15-18	Intermediate (I)
≤ 14	Resistant (R)

[g] These interpretative standards are applicable only to disk diffusion testing performed with a 30 mcg tetracycline-class disk.[2]

Interpretation should be as stated above for results using dilution techniques. Interpretation involves correlation of the diameter obtained in the disk test with the MIC for tetracycline.

As with standardized dilution techniques, diffusion methods require the use of laboratory control microorganisms that are used to control the technical aspects of the laboratory procedures. For the diffusion technique, the 30 mcg tetracycline or minocycline disk should provide the following zone diameters in these laboratory test quality control strains:

[See table below]

Microorganism		Zone Diameter Range (mm) Tetracycline	Minocycline
Escherichia coli	ATCC 25922	18-25	19-25
Staphylococcus aureus	ATCC 25923	24-30	25-30
Haemophilus influenzae	ATCC 49247	14-22	
Neisseria gonorrhoeae	ATCC 49226	30-42	
Streptococcus pneumoniae	ATCC 49619	27-31	

INDICATIONS AND USAGE

Minocycline hydrochloride tablets are indicated in the treatment of the following infections due to susceptible strains of the designated microorganisms:

Rocky Mountain spotted fever, typhus fever and the typhus group, Q fever, rickettsialpox and tick fevers caused by *Rickettsiae.*
Respiratory tract infections caused by *Mycoplasma pneumoniae.*
Lymphogranuloma venereum caused by *Chlamydia trachomatis.*
Psittacosis (Ornithosis) due to *Chlamydia psittaci.*
Trachoma caused by *Chlamydia trachomatis,* although the infectious agent is not always eliminated, as judged by immunoflourescence.
Inclusion conjunctivitis caused by *Chlamydia trachomatis.*
Nongonococcal urethritis, endocervical, or rectal infections in adults caused by *Ureaplasma urealyticum* or *Chlamydia trachomatis.*
Relapsing fever due to *Borrelia recurrentis.*
Chancroid caused by *Haemophilus ducreyi.*
Plague due to *Yersinia pestis.*
Tularemia due to *Francisella tularensis.*
Cholera caused by *Vibrio cholerae.*
Campylobacter fetus infections caused by *Campylobacter fetus.*
Brucellosis due to *Brucella* species (in conjunction with streptomycin).
Bartonellosis due to *Bartonella bacilliforms.*
Granuloma inguinale caused by *Calymmatobacterium granulomatis.*

Minocycline is indicated for treatment of infections caused by the following gram-negative microorganisms, when bacteriologic testing indicates appropriate susceptibility to the drug:

Escherichia coli.
Enterobacter aerogenes.
Shigella species.
Acinetobacter species.
Respiratory tract infections caused by *Haemophilus influenzae.*
Respiratory tract and urinary tract infections caused by *Klebsiella* species.

Minocycline hydrochloride tablets are indicated for the treatment of infections caused by the following gram-positive microorganisms when bacteriologic testing indicates appropriate susceptibility to the drug:

Upper respiratory tract infections caused by *Streptococcus pneumoniae.*
Skin and skin structure infections caused by *Staphylococcus aureus.*
(Note: Minocycline is not the drug of choice in the treatment of any type of staphylococcal infection.)

Minocycline is an alternative drug in the treatment of the following gonococcal infections:

Uncomplicated urethritis in men due to *Neisseria gonorrhoeae* and for the treatment of other gonococcal infections when penicillin is contraindicated.
Infections in women caused by *Neisseria gonorrhoeae.*
Syphilis caused by *Treponema pallidum* subspecies *pallidum.*
Yaws caused by *Treponema pallidum* subspecies *pertenue.*
Listeriosis due to *Listeria monocytogenes.*
Anthrax due to *Bacillus anthracis.*
Vincent's infection caused by *Fusobacterium fusiforme.*
Actinomycosis caused by *Actinomyces israelii.*
Infections caused by *Clostridium* species.

In *acute intestinal amebiasis,* minocycline may be useful adjunct to amebicides.

In severe acne, minocycline may be useful adjunctive therapy.

Oral minocycline is indicated in the treatment of asymptomatic carriers of *Neisseria meningitidis* to eliminate the meningococci from the nasopharynx. In order to preserve the usefulness of minocycline in the treatment of asymptomatic meningococcal carrier, diagnostic laboratory procedures, including serotyping and susceptibility testing, should be performed to establish the carrier state and the correct treatment. It is recommended that the prophylactic use of minocycline be reserved for situations in which the risk of meningococcal meningitis is high.

Oral minocycline is not indicated for the treatment of meningococcal infection.

Although no controlled clinical efficacy studies have been conducted, limited clinical data show that oral minocycline hydrochloride has been used successfully in the treatment of infections caused by *Mycobacterium marinum.*

To reduce the development of drug-resistant bacteria and maintain the effectiveness of the antibacterial drug product and other antibacterial drugs, the drug product should be used only to treat or prevent infections that are proven or strongly suspected to be caused by susceptible bacteria. When culture and susceptibility information are available, they should be considered in selecting or modifying antimicrobial therapy. In the absence of such data, local and susceptibility patterns may contribute to the empiric selection of therapy.

CONTRAINDICATIONS

This drug is contraindicated in persons who have shown hypersensitivity to any of the tetracyclines.

WARNINGS

MINOCYCLINE HYDROCHLORIDE TABLETS, LIKE OTHER TETRACYCLINES-CLASS ANTIBIOTICS, CAN CAUSE FETAL HARM WHEN ADMINISTERED TO A PREGNANT WOMAN. IF ANY TETRACYCLINE IS USED DURING PREGNANCY OR IF THE PATIENT BECOMES PREGNANT WHILE TAKING THESE DRUGS, THE PATIENT SHOULD BE APPRISED OF THE POTENTIAL HAZARD TO THE FETUS. THE USE OF DRUGS OF THE TETRACYCLINE CLASS DURING TOOTH DEVELOPMENT (LAST HALF OF PREGNANCY, INFANCY, AND CHILDHOOD TO THE AGE OF 8 YEARS) MAY CAUSE PERMANENT DISCOLORATION OF THE TEETH (YELLOW-GRAY-BROWN).

This adverse reaction is more common during long-term use of the drug but has been observed following repeated short-term courses. Enamel hypoplasia has also been reported. TETRACYCLINE DRUGS, THEREFORE, SHOULD NOT BE USED DURING TOOTH DEVELOPMENT UNLESS OTHER DRUGS ARE NOT LIKELY TO BE EFFECTIVE OR ARE CONTRAINDICATED.

All tetracyclines form a stable calcium complex in any bone-forming tissue. A decrease in fibula growth rate has been observed in premature human infants given oral tetracycline in doses of 25 mg/kg every six hours. This reaction was shown to be reversible when the drug was discontinued.

Results of animal studies indicate that tetracyclines cross the placenta, are found in fetal tissues, and can have toxic effects on the developing fetus (often related to retardation of skeletal development). Evidence of embryotoxicity has been noted in animals treated early in pregnancy.

The anti-anabolic action of the tetracyclines may cause an increase in BUN. While this is not a problem in those with normal renal function, in patients with significantly impaired function, higher serum levels of tetracycline may lead to azotemia, hyperphosphatemia, and acidosis. If renal impairment exists, even usual oral or parenteral doses may lead to excessive systemic accumulations of the drug and possible liver toxicity. Under such conditions, lower than usual total doses are indicated, and if therapy is prolonged, serum level determinations of the drug may be advisable.

Photosensitivity manifested by an exaggerated sunburn reaction has been observed in some individuals taking tetracyclines. This has been reported rarely with minocycline.

Central nervous system side effects including light headedness, dizziness, or vertigo have been reported with minocycline therapy. Patients who experience these symptoms should be cautioned about driving vehicles or using hazardous machinery while on minocycline therapy. These symptoms may disappear during therapy and usually disappear rapidly when the drug is discontinued.

PRECAUTIONS

General

As with other antibiotic preparations, use of this drug may result in overgrowth of non-susceptible organisms, including fungi. If superinfection occurs, the antibiotic should be discontinued and appropriate therapy instituted.

Pseudotumor cerebri (benign intracranial hypertension) in adults has been associated with the use of tetracyclines. The usual clinical manifestations are headaches and blurred vision. Bulging fontanels have been associated with the use of tetracyclines in infants. While both of these conditions and related symptoms usually resolve after discontinuation of the tetracycline, the possibility for permanent sequelae exists.

Incision and drainage or other surgical procedures should be performed in conjunction with antibiotic therapy when indicated.

Prescribing the antibacterial drug product in the absence of a proven or strongly suspected bacterial infection of a prophylactic indication is unlikely to provide benefit to the patient and increases the risk of the development of drug resistant bacteria.

Information For Patients

Photosensitivity manifested by an exaggerated sunburn reaction has been observed in some individuals taking tetracyclines. Patients apt to be exposed to direct sunlight or ultraviolet light should be advised that this reaction can occur with tetracycline drugs, and treatment should be discontinued at the first evidence of skin erythema. This reaction has been reported rarely with use of minocycline.

Patients who experience central nervous system symptoms (see **WARNINGS**) should be cautioned about driving vehicles or using hazardous machinery while on minocycline therapy.

Concurrent use of tetracycline may render oral contraceptives less effective (see **Drug Interactions**).

Patients should be counseled that antibacterial drugs, including the antibacterial drug prescribed, should only be used to treat bacterial infections and that they do not treat viral infections (e.g., the common cold). When an antibacterial drug product is prescribed to treat a bacterial infection, patients should be told that, although it is common to feel better early in the course of therapy, the medication should be taken exactly as directed. Physicians should counsel patients that skipping doses or not completing the full course of therapy may: (1) decrease the effectiveness of the immediate treatment, and (2) increase the likelihood that bacteria will develop resistance and will not be treatable by the antibacterial drug product or other antibacterial drugs in the future.

Laboratory Tests

In long-term therapy, periodic laboratory evaluations of organ systems, including hematopoietic, renal, and hepatic studies should be performed.

All patients with gonorrhea should have a serologic test for syphilis at the time of diagnosis. Patients treated with minocycline should have a follow-up serologic test for syphilis after 3 months.

Drug Interactions

Because tetracyclines have been shown to depress plasma prothrombin activity, patients who are on anticoagulant therapy may require downward adjustment of their anticoagulant dosage.

Since bacteriostatic drugs may interfere with the bactericidal action of penicillin, it is advisable to avoid giving tetracycline-class drugs in conjunction with penicillin.

Absorption of tetracyclines is impaired by antacids containing aluminum, calcium or magnesium, and iron-containing preparations.

The concurrent use of tetracycline and methoxyflurane has been reported to result in fatal renal toxicity.

Concurrent use of tetracyclines with oral contraceptives may render oral contraceptives less effective.

Drug Laboratory Interactions

False elevations of urinary catecholamine levels may occur due to interference with the fluorescence test.

Carcinogenesis, Mutagenesis, Impairment of Fertility

Dietary administration of minocycline in long term tumorigenicity studies in rats resulted in evidence of thyroid tumor production. Minocycline has also been found to produce thyroid hyperplasia in rats and dogs. In addition, there has been evidence of oncogenic activity in rats in studies with a related antibiotic, oxytetracycline (i.e., adrenal and pituitary tumors). Likewise, although mutagenicity studies of minocycline have not been conducted, positive results in *in vitro* mammalian cell assays (i.e., mouse lymphoma and Chinese hamster lung cells) have been reported for related antibiotics (tetracycline hydrochloride and oxytetracycline). Segment I (fertility and general reproduction) studies have provided evidence that minocycline impairs fertility in male rats.

Pregnancy

Teratogenic Effects

Pregnancy Category D.

(See **WARNINGS**)

Nonteratogenic Effects

(See **WARNINGS**).

Labor and Delivery

The effect of tetracyclines on labor and delivery is unknown.

Nursing Mothers

Tetracyclines are excreted in human milk. Because of the potential for serious adverse reactions in nursing infants from the tetracyclines, a decision should be made whether to discontinue nursing or discontinue the drug, taking into account the importance of the drug to the mother (see **WARNINGS**).

Pediatric Use

See **WARNINGS**.

ADVERSE REACTIONS

Due to oral minocycline's virtually complete absorption, side effects to the lower bowel, particularly diarrhea, have been infrequent. The following adverse reactions have been observed in patients receiving tetracyclines.

Gastrointestinal: Anorexia, nausea, vomiting, diarrhea, glossitis, dysphagia, enterocolitis, pancreatitis, inflammatory lesions (with monilial overgrowth) in the anogenital region, and increases in liver enzymes have been reported. Rare instances of esophagitis and esophageal ulcerations have been reported in patients taking the tetracycline-class antibiotics in capsule and tablet form. Most of these patients took the medication immediately before going to bed (see **DOSAGE AND ADMINISTRATION**).

Skin: Maculopapular and erythematous rashes. Exfoliative dermatitis has been reported but is uncommon. Fixed drug eruptions have been rarely reported. Lesions occurring on the glans penis have caused balanitis. Erythema multiforme and rarely Stevens-Johnson syndrome have been reported. Photosensitivity is discussed above (see **WARNINGS**). Pigmentation of the skin and mucous membranes has been reported.

Renal toxicity: Elevations in BUN have been reported and are apparently dose related (see **WARNINGS**). Acute renal failure has been rarely reported and, in most cases is reversible.

Hypersensitivity reactions: Urticaria, angioneurotic edema, polyarthralgia, anaphylaxis, anaphylactoid purpura, pericarditis, exacerbation of systemic lupus erythematosus and rarely pulmonary infiltrates with eosinophilia have been reported. A transient lupus-like syndrome and serum sickness-like reaction have also been reported.

Blood: Hemolytic anemia, thrombocytopenia, neutropenia, and eosinophilia have been reported.

Central nervous system: Bulging fontanels in infants and benign intracranial hypertension (pseudotumor cerebri) in adults (see **PRECAUTIONS-General**) have been reported. Headache has also been reported.

Other: When given over prolonged periods, tetracyclines have been reported to produce brown-black microscopic discoloration of the thyroid glands. Very rare cases of abnormal thyroid function have been reported.

Tooth discoloration in pediatric patients less than 8 years of age (see **WARNINGS**) and also, rarely, in adults have been reported.

Tinnitus and decreased hearing has been rarely reported in patients on minocycline hydrochloride.

OVERDOSAGE

In case of overdosage, discontinue medication, treat symptomatically and institute supportive measures. Minocycline is not removed in significant quantities by hemodialysis or peritoneal dialysis.

DOSAGE AND ADMINISTRATION

THE USUAL DOSAGE AND FREQUENCY OF ADMINISTRATION OF MINOCYCLINE DIFFERS FROM THAT OF THE OTHER TETRACYCLINES. EXCEEDING THE RECOMMENDED DOSAGE MAY RESULT IN AN INCREASED INCIDENCE OF SIDE EFFECTS.

Minocycline hydrochloride tablets should be taken at least one hour before meals or 2 hours after meals (see **CLINICAL PHARMACOLOGY**).

For Pediatric Patients Above 8 Years of Age:

Usual pediatric dose: 4 mg/kg initially followed by 2 mg/kg every 12 hours.

Adults:

The usual dosage of minocycline hydrochloride tablets is 200 mg initially followed by 100 mg every 12 hours. Alternatively, if more frequent doses are preferred, two or four 50 mg tablets may be given initially followed by one 50 mg tablets four times daily.

Uncomplicated gonococcal infections other than urethritis and anorectal infections in men: 200 mg initially, followed by 100 mg every 12 hours for a minimum of four days, with post-therapy cultures within 2 to 3 days.

In the treatment of uncomplicated gonococcal urethritis in men, 100 mg every 12 hours for 5 days is recommended.

For the treatment of syphilis, the usual dosage of minocycline hydrochloride should be administered over a period of 10 to 15 days. Close follow-up, including laboratory tests, is recommended.

In the treatment of meningococcal carrier state, the recommended dosage is 100 mg every 12 hours for five days.

Mycobacterium marinum infections: Although optimal doses have not been established, 100 mg every 12 hours for 6 to 8 weeks have been used successfully in a limited number of cases.

Uncomplicated urethra, endocervical, or rectal infection in adults caused by *Chlamydia trachomatis* or *Ureaplasma urealyticum:* 100 mg orally, every 12 hours for at least seven days.

Ingestion of adequate amounts of fluids along with tablet form of drugs in the tetracycline-class is recommended to reduce the risk of esophageal irritation and ulceration.

In patients with renal impairment (see **WARNINGS**), the total dosage should be decreased by either reducing the recommended individual doses and/or by extending the time intervals between doses.

HOW SUPPLIED

Minocycline hydrochloride tablets are supplied as aqueous film coated tablets containing minocycline hydrochloride equivalent to 100 mg, 75 mg and 50 mg minocycline.

The 100 mg tablets are dark gray, unscored, modified capsule shaped, coated tablet debossed "DYN-100" on one side and "749" on the other. Each tablet contains minocycline hydrochloride equivalent to 100 mg minocycline, supplied as follows:

NDC 99207-492-50 Bottle of 50
NDC 99207-492-11 Bottle of 1000

The 75 mg tablets are gray, unscored, modified capsule shaped, coated tablet debossed "DYN 75" on one side and "748" on the other. Each tablet contains minocycline hydrochloride equivalent to 75 mg minocycline, supplied as follows:

NDC 99207-491-10 Bottle of 100
NDC 99207-491-11 Bottle of 1000

The 50 mg tablets are white, unscored, modified capsule shaped, coated tablet debossed "DYN-50" on one side and "747" on the other. Each tablet contains minocycline hydrochloride equivalent to 50 mg minocycline, supplied as follows:

NDC 99207-490-10 Bottle of 100
NDC 99207-490-11 Bottle of 1000

Continued on next page

Dynacin—Cont.

Store at 20°-25°C (68°-77°F) [See USP Controlled Room Temperature].
Protect from light, moisture and excessive heat.

ANIMAL PHARMACOLOGY AND TOXICOLOGY

Minocycline hydrochloride has been observed to cause a dark discoloration of the thyroid in experimental animals (rats, minipigs, dogs and monkeys). In the rat, chronic treatment with minocycline hydrochloride has resulted in goiter accompanied by elevated radioactive iodine uptake and evidence of thyroid tumor production. Minocycline hydrochloride has also been found to produce thyroid hyperplasia in rats and dogs.

REFERENCES

1. National Committee for Clinical Laboratory Standards, Methods for Dilution Antimicrobial Susceptibility Tests for Bacteria that Grow Aerobically – Fourth Edition; Approved Standard. NCCLS Document M7-A4, Vol. 17, No. 2, NCCLS, 940 West Valley Road, Suite 1400, Wayne, PA. January 1997.
2. National Committee for Clinical Laboratory Standards, Performance Standards for Antimicrobial Disks Susceptibility Tests – Sixth Edition; Approved Standard. NCCLS Document M2-A6, Vol. 17, No. 1, NCCLS, 940 West Valley Road, Suite 1400, Wayne, PA. January 1997.
3. National Committee for Clinical Laboratory Standards, Performance Standards for Antimicrobial Disk Susceptibility Tests – Eighth Edition; Approved Standard. NCCLS Document M100-S8, Vol. 18, No. 1, NCCLS, 940 West Valley Road, Suite 1400, Wayne, PA. January 1998.

Manufactured for:
MEDICIS, The Dermatology Company®
Scottsdale, AZ 85258
by:
PAR PHARMACEUTICAL, INC.
Spring Valley, NY 10977
Issued: 04/03 49010-08A

LOPROX® GEL ℞

[lō' prŏx]
(ciclopirox) 0.77%
FOR DERMATOLOGIC USE ONLY
NOT FOR USE IN EYES
℞ Only

DESCRIPTION

Loprox® (ciclopirox) Gel 0.77% contains a synthetic antifungal agent, ciclopirox. It is intended for topical dermatologic use only.
Each gram of LOPROX Gel contains 7.70 mg of Ciclopirox in a gel consisting of Purified Water USP, Isopropyl Alcohol USP, Octyldodecanol NF, Dimethicone Copolyol 190, Carbomer 980, Sodium Hydroxide NF, and Docusate Sodium USP.
LOPROX Gel is a white, slightly fluid gel.
The chemical name for ciclopirox is 6-cyclohexyl-1-hydroxy-4-methyl-2(1*H*)-pyridinone, with the empirical formula $C_{12}H_{17}NO_2$ and a molecular weight of 207.27. The CAS Registry Number is [29342-05-0]. The chemical structure is:

OH N O CH₃

CLINICAL PHARMACOLOGY

Mechanism of Action

Ciclopirox acts by chelation of polyvalent cations (Fe^{3+} or Al^{3+}) resulting in the inhibition of the metal-dependent enzymes that are responsible for the degradation of peroxides within the fungal cell.
In vitro studies showed that ciclopirox inhibited the formation of 5-lipoxygenase inflammatory mediators (5-HETE and LTB_4) and also inhibited PGE_2 release in a cell culture model. *In vivo*, ciclopirox inhibited inflammation in an arachidonic acid-induced murine ear edema model. The clinical significance of these findings is unknown.

Pharmacokinetics

A comparative study of the pharmacokinetics of LOPROX Gel and Loprox® (ciclopirox) Cream 0.77% in 18 healthy males indicated that systemic absorption of ciclopirox from LOPROX Gel was higher than that of LOPROX Cream. A 5 gm dose of LOPROX Gel produced a mean (±SD) peak serum concentration of 25.02 (±20.6) ng/mL total ciclopirox and 5 gm of LOPROX Cream produced 18.62 (±13.56) ng/mL total ciclopirox. Approximately 3% of the applied ciclopirox was excreted in the urine within 48 hours after application, with a renal elimination half-life of about 5.5 hours.
In a study of LOPROX Gel, 16 men with moderate to severe tinea cruris applied approximately 15 grams/day of the gel for 14.5 days. The mean (±SD) dose-normalized values of C_{max} for total ciclopirox in serum were 100 (±42) ng/mL on Day 1 and 238 (±144) ng/mL on Day 15. During the 10 hours after dosing on Day 1, approximately 10% of the administered dose was excreted in the urine.

Microbiology

Ciclopirox is a hydroxypyridinone antifungal agent that inhibits the growth of pathogenic dermatophytes. Ciclopirox has been shown to be active against most strains of the following microorganisms both *in vitro* and in clinical infections as described in the INDICATIONS AND USAGE section:
Trichophyton rubrum, Trichophyton mentagrophytes, and Epidermophyton floccosum.

INDICATIONS AND USAGE

Superficial Dermatophyte Infections
LOPROX Gel is indicated for the topical treatment of interdigital tinea pedis and tinea corporis due to *Trichophyton rubrum, Trichophyton mentagrophytes,* or *Epidermophyton floccosum.*
Seborrheic Dermatitis
LOPROX Gel is indicated for the topical treatment of seborrheic dermatitis of the scalp.

CONTRAINDICATIONS

LOPROX Gel is contraindicated in individuals who have shown hypersensitivity to any of its components.

WARNINGS

LOPROX Gel is not for ophthalmic, oral, or intravaginal use.
Keep out of reach of children.

PRECAUTIONS

If a reaction suggesting sensitivity or chemical irritation should occur with the use of LOPROX Gel, treatment should be discontinued and appropriate therapy instituted.
A transient burning sensation may occur, especially after application to sensitive areas. Avoid contact with eyes. Efficacy of LOPROX Gel in immunosuppressed individuals has not been studied. Seborrheic dermatitis in association with acne, atopic dermatitis, Parkinsonism, psoriasis and rosacea has not been studied with LOPROX Gel. Efficacy in the treatment of plantar and vesicular types of tinea pedis has not been established.

Information for Patients

The patient should be told the following:
1. Use LOPROX Gel as directed by the physician. Avoid contact with the eyes and mucous membranes. LOPROX Gel is for external use only.
2. Use the medication for fungal infections for the full treatment time even though symptoms may have improved, and notify the physician if there is no improvement after 4 weeks.
3. A transient burning/stinging sensation may be felt. This may occur in approximately 15% to 20% of cases, when LOPROX Gel is used to treat seborrheic dermatitis of the scalp.
4. Inform the physician if the area of application shows signs of increased irritation or possible sensitization (redness with itching, burning, blistering, swelling, and/or oozing).
5. Avoid the use of occlusive dressings.
6. Do not use this medication for any disorder other than that for which it is prescribed.

Carcinogenesis, Mutagenesis, Impairment of Fertility

A carcinogenicity study of ciclopirox (1% and 5% solutions in polyethylene glycol 400) in female mice dosed cutaneously twice per week for 50 weeks followed by a 6-month drug-free observation period prior to necropsy revealed no evidence of tumors at the application site.
The following battery of *in vitro* genotoxicity tests was conducted with ciclopirox: evaluation of gene mutation in the Ames *Salmonella* and *E. coli* assays (negative); chromosome aberration assays in V79 Chinese hamster cells, with and without metabolic activation (positive); gene mutation assays in the HGPRT-test with V79 Chinese hamster cells (negative); and a primary DNA damage assay (i.e., unscheduled DNA synthesis assay in A549 human cells) (negative). An *in vitro* cell transformation assay in BALB/c 3T3 cells was negative for cell transformation. In an *in vivo* Chinese hamster bone marrow cytogenetic assay, ciclopirox was negative for chromosome aberrations at 5000 mg/kg.

Pregnancy

Teratogenic effects: Pregnancy Category B

Reproduction studies of ciclopirox revealed no significant evidence of impaired fertility in rats exposed orally up to 5 mg/kg body weight (approximately 5 times the maximum recommended topical human dose based on surface area). No fetotoxicity was shown due to ciclopirox in the mouse, rat, rabbit, and monkey at oral doses up to 100, 30, 30, and 50 mg/kg body weight, respectively (approximately 37.5, 30, 44, and 77 times the maximum recommended topical human dose based on surface area). By the dermal route of administration, no fetotoxicity was shown due to ciclopirox in the rat and rabbit at doses up to 120 and 100 mg/kg body weight, respectively (approximately 121 and 147 times, respectively, the maximum recommended topical human dose based on surface area).
There are no adequate or well-controlled studies of topically applied ciclopirox in pregnant women. LOPROX Gel Should be used during pregnancy only if the potential benefit justifies the potential risk to the fetus.

Nursing Mothers

It is not known whether this drug is excreted in human milk. Since many drugs are excreted in human milk, caution should be exercised when LOPROX Gel is administered to a nursing woman.

Pediatric Use

The efficacy and safety of LOPROX Gel in pediatric patients below the age of 16 years have not been established.

ADVERSE REACTIONS

In clinical trials, 140 (39%) of 359 subjects treated with LOPROX Gel reported adverse experiences, irrespective of relationship to test materials, which resulted in 8 subjects discontinuing treatment. The most frequent experience reported was skin burning sensation upon application, which occurred in approximately 34% of seborrheic dermatitis patients and 7% of tinea pedis patients. Adverse experiences occurring between 1% to 5% were contact dermatitis and pruritus. Other reactions that occurred in less than 1% included dry skin, acne, rash, alopecia, pain upon application, eye pain, and facial edema.

DOSAGE AND ADMINISTRATION

Superficial Dermatophyte Infections
Gently massage LOPROX Gel into the affected areas and surrounding skin twice daily, in the morning and evening immediately after cleaning or washing the areas to be treated. Interdigital tinea pedis and tinea corporis should be treated for 4 weeks. If a patient shows no clinical improvement after 4 weeks of treatment, the diagnosis should be reviewed.
Seborrheic Dermatitis of the Scalp
Apply LOPROX Gel to affected scalp areas twice daily, in the morning and evening for 4 weeks. Clinical improvement usually occurs within the first week with continuing resolution of signs and symptoms through the fourth week of treatment. If a patient shows no clinical improvement after 4 weeks of treatment, the diagnosis should be reviewed.

HOW SUPPLIED

Loprox® (ciclopirox) Gel 0.77% is supplied in 30 g tubes (NDC 99207-013-30), 45 g tubes (NDC 99207-013-45), and 100 g tubes (NDC 99207-013-01).
Store between 15° and 30°C (59° and 86°F).
Prescribing Information as of March 2002.
Manufactured for:
MEDICIS, The Dermatology Company®
Scottsdale, AZ 85258
By: Aventis Pharma Deutschland GmbH
D-65926 Frankfurt am Main
GERMANY
Made in Germany
REG TM MEDICIS
148286 A

LOPROX® TOPICAL SUSPENSION ℞

[lō' prŏx]
(ciclopirox) 0.77% (w/w)
FOR DERMATOLOGIC USE ONLY.
NOT FOR USE IN EYES.
℞ Only

DESCRIPTION

LOPROX® Topical Suspension (ciclopirox) 0.77% is for topical use.
Each gram of LOPROX® Topical Suspension contains 7.70 mg of ciclopirox (as ciclopirox olamine) in a water miscible suspension base consisting of Purified Water USP, Cocamide DEA, Octyldodecanol NF, Mineral Oil USP, Stearyl Alcohol NF, Cetyl Alcohol NF, Polysorbate 60 NF, Myristyl Alcohol NF, Lactic Acid USP, Sorbitan Monostearate NF, and Benzyl Alcohol NF (1%) as preservative.
LOPROX® Topical Suspension contains a synthetic, broad-spectrum, antifungal agent ciclopirox (as ciclopirox olamine). The chemical name is 6-cyclohexyl-1-hydroxy-4-methyl-2(1*H*)-pyridone, 2-aminoethanol salt.
The CAS Registry Number is 41621-49-2.
LOPROX® Topical Suspension has a pH of 7.
The chemical structure is:

OH N O • $H_2NCH_2CH_2OH$ CH₃

CLINICAL PHARMACOLOGY

Ciclopirox is a broad-spectrum, antifungal agent that inhibits the growth of pathogenic dermatophytes, yeasts, and *Malassezia furfur.* Ciclopirox exhibits fungicidal activity *in vitro* against isolates of *Trichophyton rubrum, Trichophyton mentagrophytes, Epidermophyton floccosum, Microsporum canis,* and *Candida albicans.* Pharmacokinetic studies in men with radiolabeled ciclopirox solution in polyethylene glycol 400 showed an average of 1.3% absorption of the dose when it was applied topically to 750 cm^2 on the back followed by occlusion for 6 hours. The biological half-life was 1.7 hours and excretion occurred via the kidney. Two days after application only 0.01% of the dose applied could be found in the urine. Fecal excretion was negligible. Autoradiographic studies with human cadaver skin showed that ciclopirox penetrates into the hair and through the epidermis and hair follicles into the sebaceous glands and dermis, while a portion of the drug remains in the stratum corneum. *In vitro* penetration studies in frozen or fresh excised human cadaver and pig skin indicated that the penetration of

LOPROX® Topical Suspension is equivalent to that of LOPROX® Cream (ciclopirox olamine) 0.77%. Therapeutic equivalence of cream and suspension formulations also was indicated by studies of experimentally induced guinea pig and human trichophytosis.

INDICATIONS AND USAGE

LOPROX® Topical Suspension is indicated for the topical treatment of the following dermal infections: tinea pedis, tinea cruris and tinea corporis due to *Trichophyton rubrum, Trichophyton mentagrophytes, Epidermophyton floccosum,* and *Microsporum canis;* cutaneous candidiasis (moniliasis) due to *Candida albicans;* and tinea (pityriasis) versicolor due to *Malassezia furfur.*

CONTRAINDICATIONS

LOPROX® Topical Suspension is contraindicated in individuals who have shown hypersensitivity to any of its components.

WARNINGS

General

LOPROX® Topical Suspension is not for ophthalmic use.

Keep out of reach of children.

PRECAUTIONS

If a reaction suggesting sensitivity or chemical irritation should occur with the use of LOPROX® Topical Suspension, treatment should be discontinued and appropriate therapy instituted.

Information for Patients

The patient should be told to:

1. Use the medication for the full treatment time even though signs/symptoms may have improved and notify the physician if there is no improvement after four weeks.
2. Inform the physician if the area of application shows signs of increased irritation (redness, itching, burning, blistering, swelling, oozing) indicative of possible sensitization.
3. Avoid the use of occlusive wrappings or dressings.

Carcinogenesis, Mutagenesis, Impairment of Fertility

A carcinogenicity study in female mice dosed cutaneously twice per week for 50 weeks followed by a 6-month drug-free observation period prior to necropsy revealed no evidence of tumors at the application site. The following *in vitro* and *in vivo* genotoxicity tests have been conducted with ciclopirox olamine: studies to evaluate gene mutation in the Ames *Salmonella*/Mammalian Microsome Assay (negative) and Yeast Saccharomyces Cerevisiae Assay (negative) and studies to evaluate chromosome aberrations *in vivo* in the Mouse Dominant Lethal Assay and in the Mouse Micronucleus Assay at 500 mg/kg (negative). The following battery of *in vitro* genotoxicity tests were conducted with ciclopirox: a chromosome aberration assay in V79 Chinese Hamster Cells, with and without metabolic activation (positive); a gene mutation assay in the HGPRT - test with V79 Chinese Hamster Cells (negative); and a primary DNA damage assay (i.e., unscheduled DNA Synthesis Assay in A549 Human Cells (negative)). An *in vitro* Cell Transformation Assay in BALB/C3T3 Cells was negative for cell transformation. In an *in vivo* Chinese Hamster Bone Marrow Cytogenetic Assay, ciclopirox was negative for chromosome aberrations at 5000 mg/kg.

Pregnancy Category B

Reproduction studies have been performed in the mouse, rat, rabbit, and monkey, via various routes of administration, at doses 10 times or more the topical human dose and have revealed no significant evidence of impaired fertility or harm to the fetus due to ciclopirox. There are, however, no adequate or well-controlled studies in pregnant women. Because animal reproduction studies are not always predictive of human response, this drug should be used during pregnancy only if clearly needed.

Nursing Mothers

It is not known whether this drug is excreted in human milk. Caution should be exercised when LOPROX® Topical Suspension is administered to a nursing woman.

Pediatric Use

Safety and effectiveness in pediatric patients below the age of 10 years have not been established.

ADVERSE REACTIONS

In the controlled clinical trial with 89 patients using LOPROX® Topical Suspension and 89 patients using the vehicle, the incidence of adverse reactions was low. Those considered possibly related to treatment or occurring in more than one patient were pruritus, which occurred in two patients using ciclopirox topical suspension and one patient using the suspension vehicle, and burning, which occurred in one patient using ciclopirox topical suspension.

DOSAGE AND ADMINISTRATION

Gently massage LOPROX® Topical Suspension into the affected and surrounding skin areas twice daily, in the morning and evening. Clinical improvement with relief of pruritus and other symptoms usually occurs within the first week of treatment. If a patient shows no clinical improvement after four weeks of treatment with LOPROX® Topical Suspension the diagnosis should be redetermined. Patients with tinea versicolor usually exhibit clinical and mycological clearing after two weeks of treatment.

HOW SUPPLIED

LOPROX® Topical Suspension (ciclopirox) 0.77% is supplied in 30 mL bottles (NDC 99207-022-30), and 60 mL bottles (NDC 99207-022-60).

Bottle space provided to allow for vigorous shaking before each use.

Store between 5°-25°C (41°-77°F).

US Patent Pending

Prescribing Information as of May 2003

Manufactured for:

MEDICIS, The Dermatology Company

Scottsdale, AZ 85258

by: Patheon, Inc.

Missisauga, Ontario L5N 7K9 CANADA

Made in Canada

REG TM MEDICIS

MEDICIS®

The Dermatology Company

LOPROX® SHAMPOO ℞

[*lō'prŏks*]

(ciclopirox) 1%

℞ Only

FOR TOPICAL USE ONLY

NOT FOR OPHTHALMIC, ORAL OR INTRAVAGINAL USE

KEEP OUT OF REACH OF CHILDREN

DESCRIPTION

LOPROX® (ciclopirox) Shampoo 1% contains the synthetic antifungal agent, ciclopirox.

Each gram (equivalent to 0.96 mL) of LOPROX Shampoo contains 10 mg ciclopirox in a shampoo base consisting of Purified Water USP, Sodium Laureth Sulfate, Disodium Laureth Sulfosuccinate, Sodium Chloride USP, and Laureth-2.

LOPROX Shampoo is a colorless, translucent solution. The chemical name for ciclopirox is 6-cyclohexyl-1-hydroxy-4-methyl-2(1*H*)-pyridone, with the empirical formula $C_{12}H_{17}NO_2$ and a molecular weight of 207.27. The CAS Registry Number is [29342-05-0]. The chemical structure is:

OH N O CH3

CLINICAL PHARMACOLOGY

Mechanism of Action

Ciclopirox is a hydroxypyridone antifungal agent although the relevance of this property for the indication of seborrheic dermatitis is not known. Ciclopirox acts by chelation of polyvalent cations (Fe^{3+} or Al^{3+}), resulting in the inhibition of the metal-dependent enzymes that are responsible for the degradation of peroxides within the fungal cell.

Pharmacokinetics and Pharmacodynamics

In a study in patients with seborrheic dermatitis of the scalp, application of 5 mL ciclopirox shampoo 1% twice weekly for 4 weeks, with an exposure time of 3 minutes per application, resulted in detectable serum concentrations of ciclopirox in 6 out of 18 patients. The serum concentrations measured throughout the dosing interval on Days 1 and 29 ranged from 10.3 ng/mL to 13.2 ng/mL. Total urinary excretion of ciclopirox was less than 0.5% of the administered dose.

CLINICAL STUDIES

In two randomized, double-blind clinical trials, patients 16 years and older with seborrheic dermatitis of the scalp applied LOPROX Shampoo or its vehicle two times per week for 4 weeks. Patients who were immunocompromised, those with psoriasis or atopic dermatitis, women of childbearing potential not using adequate contraception, and pregnant or lactating women were excluded from the clinical studies. An evaluation of the overall status of the seborrheic dermatitis, and the presence and severity of erythema or inflammation, and scaling, was made at week 4, using a scale of 0 = none, 1 = slight, 2 = mild, 3 = moderate, 4 = pronounced, and 5 = severe. Effective treatment was defined as achieving a score of 0 (or a score of 1 if the baseline score was ≥ 3) simultaneously for status of the seborrheic dermatitis, erythema or inflammation, and scaling at Week 4. Ciclopirox shampoo was shown to be statistically significantly more effective than vehicle in both studies. Efficacy results for the two studies are presented in the following table.

Effective Treatment Rates at Week 4 in Studies 1 and 2

	Ciclopirox Shampoo	Vehicle
Study 1	220/380 (58%)	60/192 (31%)
Study 2	65/250 (26%)	32/249 (13%)

Efficacy for black patients was not demonstrated, although only 53 black patients were enrolled in the two pivotal studies.

Microbiology

Ciclopirox is fungicidal *in vitro* against *Malassezia furfur* (*Pityrosporum* spp.), *P. ovale*, and *P. orbiculare*. Ciclopirox acts by chelation of polyvalent cations (Fe^{3+} or Al^{3+}), resulting in the inhibition of the metal-dependent enzymes that are responsible for the degradation of peroxides within the fungal cell.

The clinical significance of antifungal activity in the treatment of seborrheic dermatitis is not known.

INDICATIONS AND USAGE

LOPROX Shampoo is indicated for the topical treatment of seborrheic dermatitis of the scalp in adults.

CONTRAINDICATIONS

LOPROX Shampoo is contraindicated in individuals who have shown hypersensitivity to any of its components.

WARNINGS

LOPROX Shampoo is not for ophthalmic, oral, or intravaginal use.

Keep out of reach of children.

PRECAUTIONS

General

If a reaction suggesting sensitivity or irritation should occur with the use of LOPROX Shampoo, treatment should be discontinued and appropriate therapy instituted.

Contact of LOPROX Shampoo with the eyes should be avoided. If contact occurs, rinse thoroughly with water.

Seborrheic dermatitis may appear at puberty, however, no clinical studies have been done in patients younger than 16 years.

There is no relevant clinical experience with patients who have a history of immunosuppression (e.g., extensive, persistent, or unusual distribution of dermatomycoses, recent or recurring herpes zoster, or persistent herpes simplex), who are immunocompromised (e.g., HIV-infected patients and transplant patients), or who have a diabetic neuropathy.

Information for Patients

The patient should be instructed to:

1. Use LOPROX Shampoo as directed by the physician. Avoid contact with the eyes and mucous membranes. If contact occurs, rinse thoroughly with water. LOPROX Shampoo is for external use on the scalp only. Do not swallow.
2. Use the medication for seborrheic dermatitis for the full treatment time even though symptoms may have improved. Notify the physician if there is no improvement after 4 weeks.
3. Inform the physician if the area of application shows signs of increased irritation (redness, itching, burning, blistering, swelling, or oozing) indicative of possible allergic reaction.
4. Not use the medication for any disorder other than that for which it is prescribed.

Carcinogenesis, Mutagenesis, and Impairment of Fertility:

Long-term animal studies have not been performed to evaluate the carcinogenic potential of LOPROX Shampoo or ciclopirox.

The following *in vitro* genotoxicity tests have been conducted with ciclopirox: evaluation of gene mutation in the Ames *Salmonella* and *E. coli* assays (negative); chromosome aberration assays in V79 Chinese hamster lung fibroblast cells, with and without metabolic activation (positive); chromosome aberration assays in V79 Chinese hamster lung fibroblast cells in the presence of supplemental Fe^{3+}, with and without metabolic activation (negative); gene mutation assays in the HGPRT-test with V79 Chinese hamster lung fibroblast cells (negative); and a primary DNA damage assay (i.e., unscheduled DNA synthesis assay in A549 human cells) (negative). An *in vitro* cell transformation assay in BALB/c 3T3 cells was negative for cell transformation. In an *in vivo* Chinese hamster bone marrow cytogenetic assay, ciclopirox was negative for chromosome aberrations at a dosage of 5000 mg/kg body weight.

A combined oral fertility and embryofetal developmental study was conducted in rats with ciclopirox olamine. No effect on fertility or reproductive performance was noted at the highest dose tested of 3.85 mg/kg/day ciclopirox (approximately 1.3 times the maximum recommended human dose based on body surface area comparisons).

Pregnancy:

Teratogenic effects: Pregnancy Category B

Oral embryofetal developmental studies were conducted in mice, rats, rabbits and monkeys. Ciclopirox or ciclopirox olamine was orally administered during the period of organogenesis. No maternal toxicity, embryotoxicity or teratogenicity were noted at the highest doses of 77, 125, 80 and 38.5 mg/kg/day ciclopirox in mice, rats, rabbits and monkeys, respectively (approximately 13, 42, 54 and 26 times the maximum recommended human dose based on body surface area comparisons, respectively).

Dermal embryofetal developmental studies were conducted in rats and rabbits with ciclopirox olamine dissolved in PEG 400. Ciclopirox olamine was topically administered during the period of organogenesis. No maternal toxicity, embryotoxicity or teratogenicity were noted at the highest doses of 92 mg/kg/day and 77 mg/kg/day ciclopirox in rats and rabbits, respectively (approximately 31 and 54 times the maximum recommended human dose based on body surface area comparisons, respectively).

There are no adequate or well-controlled studies of topically applied ciclopirox in pregnant women. Because animal reproduction studies are not always predictive of human response, LOPROX Shampoo should be used during pregnancy only if clearly needed.

Nursing Mothers:

It is not known whether this drug is excreted in human milk. Because many drugs are excreted in human milk, caution should be exercised when LOPROX Shampoo is administered to a nursing woman.

Continued on next page

Loprox Shampoo—Cont.

Pediatric Use:
Seborrheic dermatitis may appear at puberty, however, no clinical studies have been done in patients younger than 16 years.

Geriatric Use:
In clinical studies, the safety and tolerability of LOPROX Shampoo in the population 65 years and older was comparable to that of younger subjects. Results of the efficacy analysis in those patients 65 years and older showed effectiveness in 25 of 85 (29%) patients treated with LOPROX Shampoo, and in 15 of 61 (25%) patients treated with the vehicle; due to the small sample size, a statistically significant difference was not demonstrated. Other reported clinical experience has not identified differences in responses between the elderly and younger subjects, but greater sensitivity to adverse effects in some older individuals cannot be ruled out.

ADVERSE REACTIONS

In 626 patients treated with LOPROX Shampoo twice weekly in the two pivotal clinical studies, the most frequent adverse events were increased itching in 1% of patients, and application site reactions, such as burning, erythema, and itching, also in 1% of patients. Other adverse events occurred in individual patients only.
Adverse events that led to early study medication termination in clinical trials occurred in 1.5% (26/1738) of patients treated with LOPROX Shampoo and 2.0% (12/661) of patients treated with shampoo vehicle. The most common adverse events leading to termination of study medication in either group was seborrhea. In the LOPROX Shampoo group, other adverse events included rash, pruritus, headache, ventricular tachycardia, and skin disorder. In the shampoo vehicle group, other adverse events included skin disorder and rash.

DOSAGE AND ADMINISTRATION

Wet hair and apply approximately 1 teaspoon (5 mL) of LOPROX Shampoo to the scalp. Up to 2 teaspoons (10 mL) may be used for long hair. Lather and leave on hair and scalp for 3 minutes. A timer may be used. Avoid contact with eyes. Rinse off. Treatment should be repeated twice per week for 4 weeks, with a minimum of 3 days between applications.
If a patient with seborrheic dermatitis shows no clinical improvement after 4 weeks of treatment with LOPROX Shampoo, the diagnosis should be reviewed.

HOW SUPPLIED

LOPROX ® (ciclopirox) Shampoo 1% is supplied in 120 mL plastic bottles (NDC 99207-010-10). Discard unused product after initial treatment duration. Store between 15°C and 30°C (59°F and 86°F).

Manufactured for:
MEDICIS® Pharmaceutical Corp.
Scottsdale, AZ 85258
by: Patheon, Inc.
Mississauga, Ontario L5N 7K9
CANADA
PRESCRIBING INFORMATION AS OF FEBRUARY 2003

PLEXION™ ℞

[plĕx' ēōn]
(sodium sulfacetamide 10% and sulfur 5%)
Cleanser

PLEXION™ TS ℞

(sodium sulfacetamide 10% and sulfur 5%)
Topical Suspension

Rx Only

DESCRIPTION

Sodium sulfacetamide is a sulfonamide with antibacterial activity while sulfur acts as a keratolytic agent. Chemically sodium sulfacetamide is N-[(4-aminophenyl) sulfonyl]-acetamide, monosodium salt, monohydrate. The structural formula is:

NH_2–(benzene ring)–$SO_2N(Na)COCH_3 \cdot H_2O$

Each gram of Plexion™ (sodium sulfacetamide 10% and sulfur 5%) Cleanser contains 100 mg of Sodium Sulfacetamide USP and 50 mg of Sulfur USP in a cleanser base containing Purified Water USP, Sodium Methyl Oleyltaurate, Sodium Cocoyl Isethionate, Disodium Oleamido MEA Sulfosuccinate, Cetyl Alcohol NF, Glyceryl Stearate (and) PEG-100 Stearate, Stearyl Alcohol NF, PEG-55 Propylene Glycol Oleate, Magnesium Aluminum Silicate NF, Methylparaben NF, Disodium EDTA USP, Butylated Hydroxytoluene NF, Sodium Thiosulfate USP, Fragrance, Xanthan Gum NF, and Propylparaben NF.
Each gram of Plexion™ (sodium sulfacetamide 10% and sulfur 5%) Topical Suspension contains 100 mg of Sodium Sulfacetamide USP and 50 mg of Sulfur USP in a suspension containing Purified Water USP, Propylene Glycol USP, Isopropyl Myristate NF, Light Mineral Oil NF, Polysorbate 60 NF, Sorbitan Monostearate NF, Cetyl Alcohol NF, Hydrogenated Coco-Glycerides USP, Stearyl Alcohol NF, Fragrances, Benzyl Alcohol NF, Glyceryl Stearate (and) PEG-100 Stearate, Dimethicone NF, Zinc Ricinoleate, Xanthan Gum NF, Disodium EDTA USP, and Sodium Thiosulfate USP.

CLINICAL PHARMACOLOGY

The most widely accepted mechanism of action of sulfonamides is the Woods-Fildes theory which is based on the fact that sulfonamides act as competitive antagonists to para-aminobenzoic acid (PABA), an essential component for bacterial growth. While absorption through intact skin has not been determined, sodium sulfacetamide is readily absorbed from the gastrointestinal tract when taken orally and
excreted in the urine, largely unchanged. The biological half-life has variously been reported as 7 to 12.8 hours. The exact mode of action of sulfur in the treatment of acne is unknown, but it has been reported that it inhibits the growth of Propionibacterium acnes and the formation of free fatty acids.

INDICATIONS

PLEXION Cleanser and PLEXION TS are indicated in the topical control of acne vulgaris, acne rosacea and seborrheic dermatitis.

CONTRAINDICATIONS

PLEXION Cleanser and PLEXION TS are contraindicated for use by patients having known hypersensitivity to sulfonamides, sulfur or any other component of this preparation. PLEXION Cleanser and PLEXION TS are not to be used by patients with kidney disease.

WARNINGS

Although rare, sensitivity to sodium sulfacetamide may occur. Therefore, caution and careful supervision should be observed when prescribing this drug for patients who may be prone to hypersensitivity to topical sulfonamides. Systemic toxic reactions such as agranulocytosis, acute hemolytic anemia, purpura hemorrhagica, drug fever, jaundice, and contact dermatitis indicate hypersensitivity to sulfonamides. Particular caution should be employed if areas of denuded or abraded skin are involved.
FOR EXTERNAL USE ONLY. Keep away from eyes. Keep out of reach of children. Keep tube tightly closed.

PRECAUTIONS

General—If irritation develops, use of the product should be discontinued and appropriate therapy instituted. Patients should be carefully observed for possible local irritation or sensitization during long-term therapy. The object of this therapy is to achieve desquamation without irritation, but sodium sulfacetamide and sulfur can cause reddening and scaling of the epidermis. These side effects are not unusual in the treatment of acne vulgaris, but patients should be cautioned about the possibility.
Information for Patients: Avoid contact with eyes, eyelids, lips and mucous membranes. If accidental contact occurs, rinse with water. If excessive irritation develops, discontinue use and consult your physician.
Carcinogenesis, Mutagenesis and Impairment of Fertility—Long-term studies in animals have not been performed to evaluate carcinogenic potential.
Pregnancy—Category C. Animal reproduction studies have not been conducted with PLEXION Cleanser or PLEXION TS. It is also not known whether PLEXION Cleanser and PLEXION TS can cause fetal harm when administered to a pregnant woman or can affect reproduction capacity. PLEXION Cleanser and PLEXION TS should be given to a pregnant woman only if clearly needed.
Nursing Mothers—It is not known whether sodium sulfacetamide is excreted in the human milk following topical use of PLEXION Cleanser or PLEXION TS. However, small amounts of orally administered sulfonamides have been reported to be eliminated in human milk. In view of this and because many drugs are excreted in human milk, caution should be exercised when PLEXION Cleanser or PLEXION TS are administered to a nursing woman.
Pediatric Use—Safety and effectiveness in children under the age of 12 have not been established.

ADVERSE REACTIONS

Although rare, sodium sulfacetamide may cause local irritation.

DOSAGE AND ADMINISTRATION

PLEXION Cleanser: Wash affected areas once or twice daily, or as directed by your physician. Avoid contact with eyes or mucous membranes. Wet skin and liberally apply to areas to be cleansed, massage gently into skin for 10–20 seconds working into a full lather, rinse thoroughly and pat dry. If drying occurs, it may be controlled by rinsing cleanser off sooner or using less often.
PLEXION TS: Cleanse affected areas. Apply a thin film of PLEXION TS to affected areas 1 to 3 times daily, or as directed by a physician.

HOW SUPPLIED

Plexion™ (sodium sulfacetamide 10% and sulfur 5%) Cleanser is available in 6 oz. (170.3 g) tube, NDC 99207-741-06 and 12 oz. (340.2 g) bottle, NDC 99207-741-12. Plexion™ (sodium sulfacetamide 10% and sulfur 5%) Topical Suspension is available in 30 g tube (NDC 99207-743-30).
Store at 15°–25°C (59°–77°F).

Manufactured for:
MEDICIS, The Dermatology Company®
Scottsdale, AZ 85258
by: Contract Pharmaceuticals Limited
Mississauga, Ontario CANADA
Prescribing information as of November 2000
U.S. Patent Pending
74330-08A

PLEXION SCT™ ℞

[plĕxēŏn]
(sodium sulfacetamide 10% and sulfur 5%)
Rx Only

DESCRIPTION

Each gram of Plexion SCT™ (sodium sulfacetamide 10% and sulfur 5%) contains 100 mg of Sodium Sulfacetamide USP and 50 mg of Sulfur USP in a cream containing Purified Water USP, Kaolin USP, Glyceryl Stearate (and) PEG-100 Stearate, Witch Hazel USP, Silicon Dioxide NF, Magnesium Aluminum Silicate NF, Benzyl Alcohol NF, Water (and) Propylene Glycol (and) Quillaja Saponaria Extract, Xanthan Gum NF, Sodium Thiosulfate USP, Fragrance.
Sodium sulfacetamide is a sulfonamide with antibacterial activity while sulfur acts as a keratolytic agent. Chemically sodium sulfacetamide is N-[(4-aminophenyl) sulfonyl]-acetamide, monosodium salt, monohydrate. The structural formula is:

NH_2–(benzene ring)–$SO_2N(Na)COCH_3 \cdot H_2O$

CLINICAL PHARMACOLOGY

The most widely accepted mechanism of action of sulfonamides is the Woods-Fildes theory which is based on the fact that sulfonamides act as competitive antagonists to para-aminobenzoic acid (PABA), an essential component for bacterial growth. While absorption through intact skin has not been determined, sodium sulfacetamide is readily absorbed from the gastrointestinal tract when taken orally and excreted in the urine, largely unchanged. The biological half-life has variously been reported as 7 to 12.8 hours. The exact mode of action of sulfur in the treatment of acne is unknown, but it has been reported that it inhibits the growth of Propionibacterium acnes and the formation of free fatty acids.

INDICATIONS

PLEXION SCT is indicated in the topical control of acne vulgaris, acne rosacea and seborrheic dermatitis.

CONTRAINDICATIONS

PLEXION SCT is contraindicated for use by patients having known hypersensitivity to sulfonamides, sulfur or any other component of this preparation. PLEXION SCT is not to be used by patients with kidney disease.

WARNINGS

Although rare, sensitivity to sodium sulfacetamide may occur. Therefore, caution and careful supervision should be observed when prescribing this drug for patients who may be prone to hypersensitivity to topical sulfonamides. Systemic toxic reactions such as agranulocytosis, acute hemolytic anemia, purpura hemorrhagica, drug fever, jaundice, and contact dermatitis indicate hypersensitivity to sulfonamides. Particular caution should be employed if areas of denuded or abraded skin are involved.
FOR EXTERNAL USE ONLY. Keep away from eyes. **Keep out of reach of children.** Keep tube tightly closed.

PRECAUTIONS

General—If irritation develops, use of the product should be discontinued and appropriate therapy instituted. Patients should be carefully observed for possible local irritation or sensitization during long-term therapy. The object of this therapy is to achieve desquamation without irritation, but sodium sulfacetamide and sulfur can cause reddening and scaling of the epidermis. These side effects are not unusual in the treatment of acne vulgaris, but patients should be cautioned about the possibility.
Carcinogenesis, Mutagenesis and Impairment of Fertility—Long-term studies in animals have not been performed to evaluate carcinogenic potential.
Pregnancy—Category C. Animal reproduction studies have not been conducted with PLEXION SCT. It is also not known whether PLEXION SCT can cause fetal harm when administered to a pregnant woman or can affect reproduction capacity. PLEXION SCT should be given to a pregnant woman only if clearly needed.
Nursing Mothers—It is not known whether sodium sulfacetamide is excreted in the human milk following topical use of PLEXION SCT. However, small amounts of orally administered sulfonamides have been reported to be eliminated in human milk. In view of this and because many drugs are excreted in human milk, caution should be exercised when PLEXION SCT is administered to a nursing woman.
Pediatric Use—Safety and effectiveness in children under the age of 12 have not been established.

ADVERSE REACTIONS

Although rare, sodium sulfacetamide may cause local irritation.

DOSAGE AND ADMINISTRATION

Use once daily or as directed by physician.
Wet skin. Apply in a film to entire face, avoiding contact with eyes or mucous membranes. Wait 10 minutes or until dry. Rinse thoroughly with water and pat dry.

HOW SUPPLIED

Plexion SCT™ (sodium sulfacetamide 10% and sulfur 5%) is available in a 4 oz tube (NDC 99207-744-04).
Store at 15°–25°C (59°–77°F).
Manufactured for:
MEDICIS, The Dermatology Company
Scottsdale, AZ 85258
by: Contract Pharmaceuticals Limited
Mississauga, Ontario
CANADA L5N 6L6
Prescribing Information as of November 2001
U.S. Patent Pending
74404-08A

TRIAZ® ℞

[trē' ăz]
(benzoyl peroxide)
℞ Only

DESCRIPTION

TRIAZ® (benzoyl peroxide) 3%, 6%, and 9% Gels, TRIAZ® (benzoyl peroxide) 3%, 6%, and 9% Cleansers and TRIAZ® (benzoyl peroxide) 3%, 6%, and 9% Pads are topical, gel-based, benzoyl peroxide containing preparations for use in the treatment of acne vulgaris. Benzoyl peroxide is an oxidizing agent that possesses antibacterial properties and is classified as a keratolytic. Benzoyl peroxide ($C_{14}H_{10}O_4$) is represented by the following chemical structure:

O=C—O—O—C=O

TRIAZ 3% Gel contains Hydrous Benzoyl Peroxide USP 3% as the active ingredient in a gel-based formulation consisting of: Purified Water USP, C12-15 Alkyl Benzoate, Glycerin USP, Cetyl Stearyl Alcohol, Polyacrylamide (and) C13-14 Isoparaffin (and) Laureth-7, Glyceryl Stearate (and) PEG-100 Stearate, Steareth S-2, Steareth S-20, Dimethicone 200, Glycolic Acid, Zinc Lactate, Lactic Acid USP, Disodium EDTA USP, Sodium Hydroxide NF.
TRIAZ 6% and 9% Gels contain, respectively, Hydrous Benzoyl Peroxide USP 6% and 9% as the active ingredient in a gel-based formulation consisting of: Purified Water USP, C12-15 Alkyl Benzoate, Glycerin USP, Cetyl Stearyl Alcohol, Glycolic Acid, Polyacrylamide (and) C13-14 Isoparaffin (and) Laureth-7, Glyceryl Stearate (and) PEG-100 Stearate, Steareth S-2, Sodium Hydroxide NF, Steareth S-20, Dimethicone 200, Zinc Lactate, Disodium EDTA USP.
TRIAZ 3% Cleanser contains Hydrous Benzoyl Peroxide USP 3% as the active ingredient in a vehicle consisting of: Glycerin USP, Petrolatum USP, C12-15 Alkyl Benzoate, Sodium Cocoyl Isethionate, Sodium C14-16 Olefin Sulfonate, Special Petrolatum Fraction, Zinc Lactate, Carbomer, Potassium Polymetaphosphate NF, Titanium Dioxide USP, Triethanolamine NF, Glycolic Acid, Lavender Extract, Menthol Crystals USP.
TRIAZ 6% and 9% Cleansers contain, respectively, Hydrous Benzoyl Peroxide USP 6% and 9% as the active ingredient in a vehicle consisting of: Glycerin USP, White Petrolatum USP, C12-15 Alkyl Benzoate, Sodium Cocoyl Isethionate, Special Petrolatum Fraction, Sodium C14-16 Olefin Sulfonate, Zinc Lactate, Carbomer, Potassium Polymetaphosphate NF, Titanium Dioxide USP, Triethanolamine NF, Glycolic Acid, Lavender Extract, Menthol Crystals USP.
TRIAZ 3%, 6% and 9% Pads contain, respectively, Hydrous Benzoyl Peroxide 3%, 6% and 9% as the active ingredient in a gel-based formulation consisting of: Purified Water USP, C12-15 Alkyl Benzoate NF, Glycerin 99% USP, Cetyl Stearyl Alcohol NF, Steareth S-2, Polysorbate 20 NF, Corn Starch Modified, Dimethicone NF, PEG 100 Stearate, Steareth S-20, Disodium EDTA USP, Glycolic Acid, Carbopol, Sodium Hydroxide NF, Zinc Lactate.

CLINICAL PHARMACOLOGY

The mechanism of action of benzoyl peroxide is not totally understood but its antibacterial activity against *Propionibacterium acnes* is thought to be a major mode of action. In addition, patients treated with benzoyl peroxide show a reduction in lipids and free fatty acids, and mild desquamation (drying and peeling activity) with simultaneous reduction in comedones and acne lesions. Little is known about the percutaneous penetration, metabolism, and excretion of benzoyl peroxide, although it has been shown that benzoyl peroxide absorbed by the skin is metabolized to benzoic acid and then excreted as benzoate in the urine. There is no evidence of systemic toxicity caused by benzoyl peroxide in humans.

INDICATIONS AND USAGE

TRIAZ 3%, 6%, and 9% Gels, TRIAZ 3%, 6%, and 9% Cleansers and TRIAZ 3%, 6%, and 9% Pads are indicated for the topical treatment of acne vulgaris.

CONTRAINDICATIONS

These preparations are contraindicated in patients with a history of hypersensitivity to any of their components.

WARNINGS

When using this product, avoid unnecessary sun exposure and use a sunscreen.

PRECAUTIONS

General: For external use only. If severe irritation develops, discontinue use and institute appropriate therapy. After reaction clears, treatment may often be resumed with less frequent application. These preparations should not be used in or near the eyes or on mucous membranes.
Information for Patients: Avoid contact with eyes, eyelids, lips and mucous membranes. If accidental contact occurs, rinse with water. Contact with any colored material (including hair and fabric) may result in bleaching or discoloration. If excessive irritation develops, discontinue use and consult your physician.
Carcinogenesis, Mutagenesis, Impairment of Fertility: Data from several studies employing a strain of mice that are highly susceptible to developing cancer suggest that benzoyl peroxide acts as a tumor promoter. The clinical significance of these findings to humans is unknown. Benzoyl peroxide has not been found to be mutagenic (Ames Test) and there are no published data indicating it impairs fertility.
Pregnancy: Teratogenic Effects: *Pregnancy Category C:* Animal reproduction studies have not been conducted with benzoyl peroxide. It is not known whether benzoyl peroxide can cause fetal harm when administered to a pregnant woman or can effect reproduction capacity. Benzoyl peroxide should be used by a pregnant woman only if clearly needed. There are no available data on the effect of benzoyl peroxide on the later growth, development and functional maturation of the unborn child.
Nursing Mothers: It is not known whether this drug is excreted in human milk. Because many drugs are excreted in human milk, caution should be exercised when benzoyl peroxide is administered to a nursing woman.
Pediatric Use: Safety and effectiveness in children have not been established.

ADVERSE REACTIONS

Allergic contact dermatitis and dryness have been reported with topical benzoyl peroxide therapy.

OVERDOSAGE

If excessive scaling, erythema or edema occurs, the use of these preparations should be discontinued. To hasten resolution of the adverse effects, cool compresses may be used. After symptoms and signs subside, a reduced dosage schedule may be cautiously tried if the reaction is judged to be due to excessive use and not allergenicity.

DOSAGE AND ADMINISTRATION

TRIAZ Gels: Apply once or twice daily to cover affected areas, or as directed by your dermatologist. Use after washing with a mild cleanser, such as one of the TRIAZ Cleansers, and water. **TRIAZ Cleansers:** Wash affected areas once or twice daily, or as directed by your dermatologist. Avoid contact with eyes or mucous membranes. Wet skin and liberally apply to areas to be cleansed, massage gently into skin for 10–20 seconds working into a full lather, rinse thoroughly and pat dry. If drying occurs, it may be controlled by rinsing cleanser off sooner or using less often. **TRIAZ Pads:** Apply once or twice daily to cover affected areas, or as directed by your dermatologist. Use after washing with a mild cleanser, such as one of the TRIAZ Cleansers, and water.

HOW SUPPLIED

TRIAZ 3% Gel – 1.5 oz. (42.5 g) tube, NDC 99207-209-01.
TRIAZ 6% Gel – 1.5 oz. (42.5 g) tube, NDC 99207-051-01.
TRIAZ 9% Gel – 1.5 oz (42.5 g) tube, NDC 99207-207-01.
TRIAZ 3% Cleanser – 6 oz. (170.3 g) tube, NDC 99207-206-12. **TRIAZ 3% Cleanser** – 12 oz. (340.2 g) bottle, NDC 99207-206-09. **TRIAZ 6% Cleanser** – 6 oz. (170.3 g) tube, NDC 99207-116-12. **TRIAZ 6% Cleanser** – 12 oz. (340.2 g) bottle, NDC 99207-116-09. **TRIAZ 9% Cleanser** – 6 oz. (170.3 g) tube, NDC 99207-208-12.**TRIAZ 9% Cleanser** – 12 oz. (340.2 g) bottle, NDC 99207-208-09.
TRIAZ 3% Pads – 1.0 g. Individual foil-wrapped pads, 30 per box, NDC 99207-221-30.
TRIAZ 6% Pads – 1.0 g. Individual foil-wrapped pads, 30 per box, NDC 99207-222-30.
TRIAZ 9% Pads – 1.0 g. Individual foil-wrapped pads, 30 per box, NDC 99207-223-30.
Store at 15° – 25°C (59° – 77°F).
TRIAZ Gels and TRIAZ Cleansers covered by US Patents: 5,648,389; 5,254,334; 5,409,706; and 5,632,996.
TRIAZ Gels and TRIAZ Cleansers manufactured for:
MEDICIS, The Dermatology Company®, Scottsdale, AZ 85258
by: Contract Pharmaceuticals Limited, Mississauga, Ontario L5N 6L6 CANADA
Made in Canada
TRIAZ Pads manufactured for:
MEDICIS, The Dermatology Company®, Scottsdale, AZ 85258
by: Tapemark, West St. Paul, MN 55118
Made in U.S.
Prescribing information as of November 2002
22130-08C

MedImmune, Inc.

ONE MEDIMMUNE WAY
GAITHERSBURG, MD 20878

For Medical Information Contact:
(800) 949-3789 or (877) 633-4411
Adverse Drug Experience:
(800) 949-3789 or (877) 633-4411
In Emergencies:
24-hour emergency
(800) 949-3789 or (877) 633-4411
Sales and Ordering/Customer Service:
(800) 527-7130 or (877) 633-4411
Customer Support Network
(877) 633-4411

CYTOGAM® ℞

[sī-tō-găm]
CYTOMEGALOVIRUS IMMUNE GLOBULIN INTRAVENOUS (HUMAN)
Liquid Formulation
Solvent Detergent Treated

DESCRIPTION

CytoGam®, Cytomegalovirus Immune Globulin Intravenous (Human) (CMV-IGIV), is an immunoglobulin G (IgG) containing a standardized amount of antibody to Cytomegalovirus (CMV). CMV-IGIV is formulated in final vial as a sterile liquid. The globulin is stabilized with 5% sucrose and 1% Albumin (Human). CytoGam® contains no preservative. The purified immunoglobulin is derived from pooled adult human plasma selected for high titers of antibody for Cytomegalovirus (CMV) (1). Source material for fractionation may be obtained from another U.S. licensed manufacturer. Pooled plasma was fractionated by ethanol precipitation of the proteins according to Cohn Methods 6 and 9, modified to yield a product suitable for intravenous administration. A widely utilized solvent-detergent viral inactivation process is also used (2). Certain manufacturing operations may be performed by other firms. Each milliliter contains: 50 ± 10 mg of immunoglobulin, primarily IgG, and trace amounts of IgA and IgM; 50 mg of sucrose; 10 mg of Albumin (Human). The sodium content is 20-30 mEq per liter, i.e., 0.4–0.6 mEq per 20 mL or 1.0-1.5 mEq per 50 mL. The solution should appear colorless and translucent.

CLINICAL PHARMACOLOGY

CytoGam® contains IgG antibodies representative of the large number of normal persons who contributed to the plasma pools from which the product was derived. The globulin contains a relatively high concentration of antibodies directed against Cytomegalovirus (CMV). In the case of persons who may be exposed to CMV, CytoGam® can raise the relevant antibodies to levels sufficient to attenuate or reduce the incidence of serious CMV disease.

INDICATIONS AND USAGE

Cytomegalovirus Immune Globulin Intravenous (Human) is indicated for the prophylaxis of cytomegalovirus disease associated with transplantation of kidney, lung, liver, pancreas and heart. In transplants of these organs other than kidney from CMV seropositive donors into seronegative recipients, prophylactic CMV-IGIV should be considered in combination with ganciclovir.

CLINICAL STUDIES

Clinical studies have shown a 50% reduction in primary CMV disease in renal transplant patients given CMV-IGIV (3) and a 56% reduction in serious CMV disease (4) in liver transplant patients given CMV-IGIV. CMV-IGIV prophylaxis was associated with increased survival in liver transplant recipients (5).
In two separate clinical trials, CytoGam® was shown to provide effective prophylaxis in renal transplant recipients at risk for primary CMV disease. In the first randomized trial, (3) the incidence of virologically confirmed CMV-associated syndromes was reduced from 60% in controls (n=35) to 21% in recipients of CMV immune globulin (n=24) ($P < 0.01$); marked leukopenia was reduced from 37% in controls to 4% in globulin recipients ($P < 0.01$); and fungal or parasitic superinfections were not seen in globulin recipients but occurred in 20% of controls ($P = 0.05$). Serious CMV disease was reduced from 46% to 13%. There was a concomitant but not statistically significant reduction in the incidence of CMV pneumonia (17% of controls as compared with 4% of globulin recipients). There was no effect on rates of viral isolation or seroconversion although the rate of viremia was less in CytoGam® recipients. In a subsequent non-randomized trial in renal transplant recipients (n=36), (6) the incidence of virologically confirmed CMV-associated syndrome was reduced to 36% in the globulin recipients in comparison to a 60% incidence in control patients (n=35) in the randomized trial. The rates of serious CMV disease, and concomitant fungal and parasitic superinfection were similar to patients receiving CMV-IGIV in the first trial.
In a randomized, double-blind, placebo-controlled trial in liver transplant recipients (4), the incidence of serious CMV-

Continued on next page

CytoGam—Cont.

associated disease was reduced from 26% in the 72 control patients to 12% in the 69 CMV-IGIV recipients (p=0.02); serious CMV-associated disease included CMV disease in 2 or more organs, CMV pneumonia, or CMV-associated invasive fungal infection, the incidence of which was 18% in controls and 7% in CMV-IGIV recipients (p=0.04). In follow-up (5) of the liver transplant patients studied in this randomized controlled trial and a subsequent open-label trial (7), the one year survival of the 72 control patients was 72% versus 86% in the 90 recipients of CMV-IGIV (p=0.03). In the randomized control trial, the reduction in serious CMV-associated disease in CMV seronegative recipients of livers from a CMV seropositive donor (7/19 in the CMV-IGIV group vs. 9/19 in control) was less than in transplants with other donor and recipient serologic status (1/50 in the CMV-IGIV group vs. 10/53 in the control group). This finding was similar to that of Merigan et al. (8) in a study of ganciclovir prophylaxis after heart transplantation. In this study, patients received ganciclovir IV at 5 mg/kg bid for the initial 14 days post-transplant, then at 6 mg/kg each day for 5 days per week through day 28.

Recent studies of combined prophylaxis with CMV-IGIV and ganciclovir have shown reductions in the incidence of serious CMV associated disease in CMV seronegative recipients of CMV seropositive organs below that expected from one drug alone (9-12).

Ham et al. (9) used CMV-IGIV with a dosage schedule of 150 mg/kg CMV-IGIV within 72 hours of transplant; 100 mg/kg at two, four, six and eight weeks following liver transplant and then 50 mg/kg at 12 and 16 weeks post-transplant in combination with ganciclovir (10 mg/kg/day for 14 days). The incidence of CMV disease was reduced from an expected 60-80% rate to 7% in 15 seronegative recipients of a seropositive organ.

Snydman (10) using the CMV-IGIV dosage schedule listed under DOSAGE AND ADMINISTRATION section in combination with ganciclovir (10 mg/kg/day for 14 days) reduced the incidence of serious CMV disease in D+R− liver transplant recipients receiving placebo or one drug from 16/47 (34%) to 3/41 (7%) in patients receiving both drugs for prophylaxis.

Martin (11) using CMV-IGIV 100 mg/kg every two weeks for six weeks followed by 50 mg/kg every two weeks with a final dose at week 16, in combination with ganciclovir 10 mg/kg/day for 14 days after transplantation, observed severe CMV disease in 1/74 (1%) of CMV seronegative recipients of a kidney from a CMV seropositive donor, in 0/14 (0%) of CMV seronegative recipients of a kidney-pancreas transplant from a CMV seropositive donor and in 1/12 (8%) of CMV seronegative recipients of a liver from a CMV seropositive donor. The incidence of serious CMV disease with combined CMV-IGIV and ganciclovir prophylaxis was lower than previous experience with single drug prophylaxis.

Valantine and Luikart (12) compared prophylaxis with CMV-IGIV (biweekly for three months) in combination with ganciclovir prophylaxis (IV at 5 mg/kg bid for the initial 14 days post-transplant, then at 6 mg/kg through day 28) in 16 CMV seronegative recipients of hearts from CMV seropositive donors with 16 matched controls receiving ganciclovir alone. The actuarial incidence of CMV disease was reduced from 55% in the ganciclovir group to 46% in the combined group ($p \leq 0.06$) and survival was increased from 61% to 94% ($p \leq 0.001$). In heart-lung or lung transplant patients in whom either the donor or recipient was CMV seropositive, the actuarial incidence of CMV disease in patients receiving ganciclovir alone (n=25) was 85% as compared to 36% of the 33 patients receiving both CMV-IGIV and ganciclovir ($p \leq 0.05$). Survival was 60% in the ganciclovir group and 80% in patients receiving CMV-IGIV and ganciclovir ($p \leq 0.01$).

CONTRAINDICATIONS

CytoGam® should not be used in individuals with a history of a prior severe reaction associated with the administration of this or other human immunoglobulin preparations. Persons with selective immunoglobulin A deficiency have the potential for developing antibodies to immunoglobulin A and could have anaphylactic reactions to subsequent administration of blood products that contain immunoglobulin A, including CytoGam®.

WARNINGS

CMV-IGIV is made from human plasma and, like other plasma products, carries the possibility for transmission of blood-borne viral agents and theoretically, the Creutzfeldt-Jakob disease (CJD) agent. The risk of transmission of recognized blood-borne viruses is considered to be low because of the viral inactivation and removal properties in the Cohn-Oncley cold ethanol precipitation procedure used for purification of immune globulin products (13-15). Until 1993, cold ethanol manufactured immune globulins licensed in the United States had not been documented to transmit any viral agent. However, during a brief period in late 1993 to early 1994, intravenous immune globulin made by one U.S. manufacturer was associated with transmission of Hepatitis C virus (16). To further guard against possible transmission of blood-borne viruses, including Hepatitis C, CMV-IGIV is treated with a solvent detergent viral inactivation procedure (2) known to inactivate a wide spectrum of lipid enveloped viruses, including HIV-1, HIV-2, Hepatitis B, and Hepatitis C (17). However, because new blood-borne viruses may yet emerge, some of which may not be inactivated by the manufacturing process or by solvent detergent treatment, CMV-IGIV, like any other blood product, should be given only if a benefit is expected.

Immune Globulin Intravenous (Human) products have been reported to be associated with renal dysfunction, acute renal failure, osmotic nephrosis and death (18-25). Patients predisposed to acute renal failure include patients with any degree of pre-existing renal insufficiency, diabetes mellitus, age greater than 65, volume depletion, sepsis, paraproteinemia or patients receiving known nephrotoxic drugs. Especially in such patients, IGIV products should be administered at the minimum concentrations available and the minimum rate of infusion practicable. While these reports of renal dysfunction and acute renal failure have been associated with the use of many IGIV products, those containing sucrose as a stabilizer (and given at daily doses of 350 mg/kg or greater) account for a disproportionate share of the total number (18). CytoGam® contains sucrose as a stabilizer. See PRECAUTIONS and DOSAGE AND ADMINISTRATION sections for important information intended to reduce the risk of acute renal failure.

During administration, the patient's vital signs should be monitored continuously and careful observation made for any symptoms throughout the infusion. Epinephrine should be available for the treatment of an acute anaphylactic reaction (see PRECAUTIONS section).

PRECAUTIONS

General:

CytoGam® does not contain a preservative. The vial should be entered only once for administration purposes and the infusion should begin within 6 hours. The infusion schedule should be adhered to closely (see INFUSION section). Do not use if the solution is turbid.

Although systemic allergic reactions are rare (see ADVERSE REACTIONS section), epinephrine and diphenhydramine should be available for treatment of acute allergic symptoms. If hypotension or anaphylaxis occur, the administration of the immunoglobulin should be discontinued immediately and an antidote should be given as noted above.

Renal Function:

Assure that patients are not volume depleted prior to the initiation of IGIV. Periodic monitoring of renal function tests and urine output is particularly important in patients judged to have a potential increased risk for developing acute renal failure. Renal function, including the measurement of blood urea nitrogen (BUN) and serum creatinine should be assessed prior to the initial infusion of CytoGam® and again at appropriate intervals thereafter. If renal function deteriorates, discontinuation of the product should be considered. The recommended rate of CytoGam® infusion for prophylaxis of CMV disease in solid organ transplant patients is 60 mg Ig/kg/hr (see DOSAGE AND ADMINISTRATION).

Aseptic Meningitis Syndrome:

An aseptic meningitis syndrome (AMS) has been reported to occur infrequently in association with Immune Globulin Intravenous (Human) (IGIV) treatment (26–29). The syndrome usually begins within several hours to two days following IGIV treatment. It is characterized by symptoms and signs including severe headache, nuchal rigidity, drowsiness, fever, photophobia, painful eye movements, and nausea and vomiting. Cerebrospinal fluid (CSF) studies are frequently positive with pleocytosis up to several thousand cells per cu.mm., predominantly from the granulocytic series, and elevated protein levels up to several hundred mg/dl. Patients exhibiting such symptoms and signs should receive a thorough neurological examination, including CSF studies, to rule out other causes of meningitis. AMS may occur more frequently in association with high dose (2 g/kg) IGIV treatment. Discontinuation of IGIV treatment has resulted in remission of AMS within several days without sequelae.

Hemolysis:

Immune Globulin Intravenous (Human) (IGIV) products can contain blood group antibodies which may act as hemolysins and induce in vivo coating of red blood cells with immunoglobulin, causing a positive direct antiglobulin reaction and, rarely, hemolysis (30–32). Hemolytic anemia can develop subsequent to IGIV therapy due to enhanced RBC sequestration (33) [See ADVERSE REACTIONS]. IGIV recipients should be monitored for clinical signs and symptoms of hemolysis [See PRECAUTIONS: Laboratory Tests].

Transfusion-Related Acute Lung Injury (TRALI):

There have been reports of noncardiogenic pulmonary edema [Transfusion-Related Acute Lung Injury (TRALI)] in patients administered IGIV (34). TRALI is characterized by severe respiratory distress, pulmonary edema, hypoxemia, normal left ventricular function, and fever and typically occurs within 1–6 hours after transfusion. Patients with TRALI may be managed using oxygen therapy with adequate ventilatory support.

IGIV recipents should be monitored for pulmonary adverse reactions. If TRALI is suspected, appropriate tests should be performed for the presence of anti-neutrophil antibodies in both the product and patient serum [See PRECAUTIONS: Laboratory Tests].

Thrombotic Events:

Thrombotic events have been reported in association with IGIV (35–37) (See ADVERSE REACTIONS). Patients at risk may include those with a history of atherosclerosis, multiple cardiovascular risk factors, advanced age, impaired cardiac output, and/or known or suspected hyperviscosity. The potential risks and benefits of IGIV should be weighed against those of alternative therapies for all patients for whom IGIV administration is being considered. Baseline assessment of blood viscosity should be considered in patients at risk for hyperviscosity, including those with cryoglobulins, fasting chylomicronemia/markedly high triacylglycerols (triglycerides), or monoclonal gammopathies [See PRECAUTIONS: Laboratory Tests].

Laboratory Tests:

If signs and/or symptoms of hemolysis are present after IGIV infusion, appropriate confirmatory laboratory testing should be done [See PRECAUTIONS].

If TRALI is suspected, appropriate tests should be performed for the presence of anti-neutrophil antibodies in both the product and the patient serum [See PRECAUTIONS].

Because of the potentially increased risk of thrombosis, baseline assessment of blood viscosity should be considered in patients at risk for hyperviscosity, including those with cryoglobulins, fasting chylomicronemia/markedly high triacylglycerols (triglycerides), or monoclonal gammopathies [See PRECAUTIONS].

Drug Interactions:

Antibodies present in immune globulin preparations may interfere with the immune response to live virus vaccines such as measles, mumps, and rubella; therefore, vaccination with live virus vaccines should be deferred until approximately three months after administration of CytoGam®. If such vaccinations were given shortly after CytoGam®, a revaccination may be necessary. Admixtures of CytoGam® with other drugs have not been evaluated. It is recommended that CytoGam® be administered separately from other drugs or medications which the patient may be receiving (see DOSAGE AND ADMINISTRATION section).

Pregnancy Category C:

Animal reproduction studies have not been conducted with Cytomegalovirus Immune Globulin Intravenous (Human). It is also not known whether Cytomegalovirus Immune Globulin Intravenous (Human) can cause fetal harm when administered to a pregnant woman or can affect reproduction capacity. Cytomegalovirus Immune Globulin Intravenous (Human) should be given to a pregnant woman only if clearly needed.

Information for Patients:

Patients should be instructed to report all infections directly to their physician and to the Massachusetts Public Health Biologic Laboratories at (617)983-6400. The risks and benefits of this product should be discussed with the patient. In addition, patients should be instructed to immediately report symptoms of decreased urine output, sudden weight gain, and/or shortness of breath (which may suggest kidney damage) to their physician.

ADVERSE REACTIONS

Minor reactions such as flushing, chills, muscle cramps, back pain, fever, nausea, vomiting, arthralgia, and wheezing were the most frequent adverse reactions observed during the clinical trials of CytoGam®, Cytomegalovirus Immune Globulin Intravenous (Human). The incidence of these reactions during the clinical trials was less than 6.0% of all infusions and such reactions were most often related to infusion rates. A decrease in blood pressure was observed in 1 of 1039 infusions in clinical trials of CytoGam®. If a patient develops a minor side effect, *slow the rate* immediately or temporarily interrupt the infusion.

Increases in serum creatinine and blood urea nitrogen (BUN) have been observed as soon as one to two days following IGIV infusion. Progression to oliguria or anuria requiring dialysis has been observed. Types of severe renal adverse events that have been seen following IGIV therapy include acute renal failure, acute tubular necrosis, proximal tubular nephropathy and osmotic nephrosis (18–25).

Severe reactions such as angioneurotic edema and anaphylactic shock, although not observed during clinical trials, are a possibility. Clinical anaphylaxis may occur even when the patient is not known to be sensitized to immune globulin products. A reaction may be related to the rate of infusion; therefore, carefully adhere to the infusion rates as outlined under "DOSAGE AND ADMINISTRATION." If anaphylaxis or drop in blood pressure occurs, *discontinue infusion* and use antidote such as diphenhydramine and adrenalin.

Postmarketing:

The following adverse reactions have been identified and reported during the post-approval use of IVIG products (38):

Respiratory: Apnea, Acute Respiratory Distress Syndrome (ARDS), Transfusion Associated Lung Injury (TRALI), cyanosis, hypoxemia, pulmonary edema, dyspnea, bronchospasm

Cardiovascular: Cardiac arrest, thromboembolism, vascular collapse, hypotension

Neurological: Coma, loss of consciousness, seizures, tremor

Integumentary: Stevens-Johnson syndrome, epidermolysis, erythema multiforme, bullous dermatitis

Hematologic: Pancytopenia, leukopenia, hemolysis, positive direct antiglobulin (Coombs) test

General/Body as a Whole: Pyrexia, Rigors

Musculoskeletal: Back pain

Gastrointestinal: Hepatic dysfunction, abdominal pain

Because postmarketing reporting of these reactions is voluntary and the at-risk populations are of uncertain size, it is not always possible to reliably estimate the frequency of the reaction or establish a causal relationship to exposure to the product. Such is also the case with literature reports authored independently.

OVERDOSAGE

Although few data are available, clinical experience with other immunoglobulin preparations suggests that the major manifestations would be those related to volume overload.

DOSAGE AND ADMINISTRATION

The maximum recommended total dosage per infusion is 150 mg Ig/kg, administered according to the following schedule:

[See first table at right]

	Type of Transplant	
	Kidney	Liver, Pancreas Lung, Heart
Within 72 hours of transplant:	150 mg/kg	150 mg/kg
2 weeks post transplant:	100 mg/kg	150 mg/kg
4 weeks post transplant:	100 mg/kg	150 mg/kg
6 weeks post transplant:	100 mg/kg	150 mg/kg
8 weeks post transplant:	100 mg/kg	150 mg/kg
12 weeks post transplant:	50 mg/kg	100 mg/kg
16 weeks post transplant:	50 mg/kg	100 mg/kg

Preparation for Administration. Remove the tab portion of the vial cap and clean the rubber stopper with 70% alcohol or equivalent. DO NOT SHAKE VIAL; AVOID FOAMING. Parenteral drug products should be inspected visually for particulate matter and discoloration prior to administration whenever solution and container permit. Infuse the solution only if it is colorless, free of particulate matter and not turbid.

Infusion. Infusion should begin within 6 hours after entering the vial and should be complete within 12 hours of entering the vial. Vital signs should be taken preinfusion, midway and post-infusion as well as before any rate increase. CytoGam® should be administered through an intravenous line using an administration set that contains an in-line filter (pore size 15μ) and a constant infusion pump (i.e., IVAC pump or equivalent). A smaller in-line filter (0.2μ) is also acceptable. Pre-dilution of CytoGam® before infusion is not recommended. CytoGam® should be administered through a separate intravenous line. If this is not possible, CytoGam® may be "piggybacked" into a pre-existing line if that line contains either Sodium Chloride, Injection, USP, or one of the following dextrose solutions (with or without NaCl added): 2.5% dextrose in water, 5% dextrose in water, 10% dextrose in water, 20% dextrose in water. If a pre-existing line must be used, the CytoGam® should not be diluted more than 1:2 with any of the above-named solutions. Admixtures of CytoGam® with any other solutions have not been evaluated.

Initial Dose. Administer intravenously at 15 mg Ig per kg body weight per hour. If no adverse reactions occur after 30 minutes, the rate may be increased to 30 mg Ig/kg/hr; if no adverse reactions occur after a subsequent 30 minutes, then the infusion may be increased to 60 mg Ig/kg/hr (volume not to exceed 75 ml/hour). DO NOT EXCEED THIS RATE OF ADMINISTRATION. The patient should be monitored closely during and after each rate change.

Subsequent Doses. Administer at 15 mg Ig/kg/hr for 15 minutes. If no adverse reactions occur, increase to 30 mg Ig/kg/hr for 15 minutes and then increase to a maximum rate of 60 mg Ig/kg/hr (volume not to exceed 75 ml/hour). DO NOT EXCEED THIS RATE OF ADMINISTRATION. The patient should be monitored closely during each rate change.

CytoGam® should be used with caution in patients with pre-existing renal insufficiency and in patients judged to be at increased risk of developing renal insufficiency (including, but not limited to those with diabetes mellitus, age greater than 65, volume depletion, paraproteinemia, sepsis and patients receiving known nephrotoxic drugs). In these cases especially, it is important to assure that patients are not volume depleted prior to CytoGam® infusion. While most cases of renal insufficiency have occurred in patients receiving total doses of 350 mg Ig/kg or greater, no prospective data are presently available to identify a maximum safe dose, concentration or rate of infusion in patients determined to be at increased risk of acute renal failure. In the absence of prospective data, recommended doses should not be exceeded and the concentration and infusion rate selected should be the minimum practicable.

Potential adverse reactions are: flushing, chills, muscle cramps, back pain, fever, nausea, vomiting, wheezing, drop in blood pressure. Minor adverse reactions have been infusion rate related – if the patient develops a minor side effect (i.e., nausea, back pain, flushing), slow the rate or temporarily interrupt the infusion. If anaphylaxis or drop in blood pressure occurs, discontinue infusion and use antidote such as diphenhydramine and adrenalin.

To prevent the transmission of hepatitis viruses or other infectious agents from one person to another, sterile disposable syringes and needles should be used. The syringes and needles should not be reused.

HOW SUPPLIED

CytoGam®, Cytomegalovirus Immune Globulin Intravenous (Human), is supplied in two single-dose vial forms:

[See second table above]

NDC No.	Total Quantity of Immunoglobulin	Volume	Concentration
60574-3102-1	1000 mg ± 200 mg	20 ml	50 ± 10 mg/ml
60574-3101-1	2500 mg ± 500 mg	50 ml	50 ± 10 mg/ml

STORAGE

CytoGam® should be stored between 2° C and 8° C (35.6°F and 46.4°F), and used within 6 hours after entering the vial.

REFERENCES

1. Snydman DR, Mclver J, Leszczynski J, et al. A pilot trial of a novel cytomegalovirus immune globulin in renal transplant recipients. Transplantation 38:553-557, 1984.
2. Horowitz B, Wiebe ME, Lippin A, et al. Inactivation of viruses in labile blood derivatives. Transfusion; 25: 516-522, 1985.
3. Snydman DR, Werner BG, Heinze-Lacey BH, et al. Use of cytomegalovirus immune globulin to prevent cytomegalovirus disease in renal transplant recipients. NEJM 317:1049-1054, 1987.
4. Snydman DR, Werner BG, Dougherty NN, et al. Cytomegalovirus Immune Globulin prophylaxis in liver transplantation. A randomized, double-blind, placebo-controlled trial. Ann Int Med 119:984-991, 1993.
5. Falagas ME, Snydman DR, Ruthazer R, et al. Cytomegalovirus Immune Globulin (CMVIG) prophylaxis is associated with increased survival after orthotopic liver transplantation. Clin Transplantation, 11:432-437, 1997.
6. Snydman DR, Werner BG, Tilney NL, et al. A final analysis of primary cytomegalovirus disease prevention in renal transplant recipients with a cytomegalovirus immune globulin: Comparison of randomized and open-label trials. Transplant Proceed 23:1357-1360, 1991.
7. Snydman DR, Werner BG, Dougherty NN, et al. A further analysis of the use of Cytomegalovirus Immune Globulin in orthotopic liver transplant patients at risk for primary infection. Transplant Proceed 26, suppl 1:23-27, 1994.
8. Merigan TC, Renlund DG, Keay S, et al. A controlled trial of ganciclovir to prevent cytomegalovirus disease after heart transplantation. NEJM 326:1182-1186, 1992.
9. Ham JM, Shelden SR, Godkin RR, et al. Cytomegalovirus prophylaxis with ganciclovir, acyclovir and CMV hyperimmune globulin in liver transplant patients receiving OKT3 induction. Transplant Proc; 27 (5 suppl 1):31-33, 1995.
10. Snydman DR. Combined CMV-IGIV and ganciclovir prophylaxis in CMV seronegative transplant recipients from CMV seropositive donors. Report on file, MedImmune, Inc.
11. Martin M. CMV prophylaxis with combination ganciclovir and CMV hyperimmune globulin followed by high-dose acyclovir in solid organ transplant recipients. Report on file, MedImmune, Inc.
12. Valantine H and Luikart H. Impact of CMV hyperimmune globulin on outcome after cardiothoracic transplantation: A comparative study of combined prophylaxis with CMVIG plus ganciclovir vs. ganciclovir alone. Report on file, MedImmune, Inc.
13. Bossell, et al. Safety of therapeutic immune globulin preparations with respect to transmission of human T-lymphotropic virus type III/lymphadenopathy-associated virus infection. MMWR vol. 35:231-233, April 11, 1996.
14. Wells MA, Wittek AE, Epstein JS, et al. Inactivation and partition of human T-cell lymphotropic virus, type III, during ethanol fractionation of plasma. Transfusion 26:210-213, 1986.
15. McIver J, Grady G. Immunoglobulin preparations. In: Churchill WH and Kurtz SR, (ed): Transfusion Medicine. Boston: Blackwell; 1988.
16. Schneider L, Geha R. Outbreak of Hepatitis C associated with intravenous immunoglobulin administration – United States, October 1993–June 1994. MMWR vol. 43:505-509, 43:505-509, July 22, 1994.
17. Edwards CA, Piet MPJ, Chin S, et al. Tri(nButyl) phosphate detergent treatment of licensed therapeutic and experimental blood derivatives. Vox Sang 52: 53-59, 1987.
18. Cayco AV, Perazella MA, Hayslett JP. Renal insufficiency after intravenous immune globulin therapy: A report of two cases and an analysis of the literature. J Am Soc Nephrology; 8: 1788-1793, 1997.
19. Cantu TG, Hoehn-Saric EW, Burgess KM, et al. Acute renal failure associated with immunoglobulin therapy. Am J Kidney Dis; 25: 228-234, 1995.
20. Hansen-Schmidt S, Silomon J, Keller F. Osmotic nephrosis due to high-dose intravenous immunoglobulin therapy containing sucrose (but not with glycine) in a patient with immunoglobulin A nephritis. Am J Kidney Dis; 28: 451-453, 1996.
21. Tan E, Hajinazarian M, Bay W, Neff J, Mendell JR. Acute renal failure resulting from intravenous immunoglobulin therapy. Arch Neurol.; 50:137-139, 1993.
22. Winward D and Brophy MT. Acute renal failure after administration of intravenous immunoglobulin: Review of the literature and case report. Pharmacotherapy; 15(6): 765-772, 1995.
23. Phillips AO. Renal failure and intravenous immunoglobulin. Clin Nephrol; 37:217, 1992.
24. Lindberg HA, Wald MH, Barker MH. Renal changes following administration of hypertonic solutions. Arch Int. Med; 63:907-918, 1939.
25. Rigdon RH, and Cardwell ES. Renal lesions following the intravenous injection of a hypertonic solution of sucrose. Arch Int Med; 69:670-690, 1942.
26. Sekul E, Culper E, Dalaks M. Aseptic meningitis associated with high-dose intravenous immunoglobulin therapy; Frequency and risk factors. Ann Int Med; 121:259-262, 1994.
27. Kato E, Shindo S, Eto Y, et al. Administration of immune globulin associated with aseptic meningitis. JAMA; 259:3269-3270, 1988.
28. Casteels Van Daele M, Wijndaele L, Hunnick, et al. Intravenous immunoglobulin and acute aseptic meningitis. NEJM; 323:614-615, 1990.
29. Scribner C, Kapit R, Philips E, et al. Aseptic meningitis and intravenous immunoglobulin therapy. Ann Intern Med; 121:305-306, 1994.
30. Copelan EA, Strohm PL, Kennedy MS, Tutschka PJ. Hemolysis following intravenous immune globulin therapy. Transfusion; 26:410-412, 1986.
31. Thomas MJ, Misbah SA, Chapel HM, Jones M, Elrington G. Newsom-Davis J. Hemolysis after high-dose intravenous Ig. Blood; 15:3789, 1993.
32. Reinhart WH, Berchtold PE. Effect of high dose intravenous immunoglobulin therapy on blood rheology. Lancet; 339:662-664, 1992.
33. Kessary-Shoham H, Levy Y, Shoenfeld Y, Lorber M, Gershon H. In vivo administration of intravenous immunoglobulin (IVIg) can lead to enhanced erythrocyte sequestration. J. Autoimmune; 13:129-135, 1999.
34. Rizk A, Gorson KC, Kenney L, Weinstein R. Transfusion-related acute lung injury after the infusion of IVIG. Transfusion; 41:264-268, 2001.
35. Dalakas MC. High-dose intravenous Immunoglobulin and serum viscosity: risk of precipitating thromboembolic events. Neurology, 44: 223-226, 1994.
36. Woodruff RK, Grigg AP, Firkin FC, Smith IL. Fatal thrombotic events during treatment of autoimmune thrombocytopenia with intravenous immunoglobulin in elderly patients. Lancet; 2:217-218, 1986.
37. Wolberg AS, Kon RH, Monroe DM, Hoffman M. Coagulation factor XI is a contaminant in intravenous immunoglobulin preparations. Am J. Hematol; 65:30-34, 2000.
38. Pierce LR, Jain N. Risks associated with the use of intravenous immunoglobulin. Trans Med Rev; 17:241-251, 2003.

For additional information concerning Cytomegalovirus Immune Globulin Intravenous (Human) contact:
Professional Services
MedImmune, Inc.
Gaithersburg, MD 20878, USA
1-800-949-3789
Manufactured by:
MASSACHUSETTS PUBLIC HEALTH BIOLOGIC LABORATORIES
Boston, Massachusetts 02130, USA
US Govt. License No. 64
Revised January 2004
Marketed by:
MedImmune, Inc.
Gaithersburg, MD 20878, USA

Shown in Product Identification Guide, page 322

SYNAGIS® ℞

[*sĭ-nă-jĭs*]
(palivizumab)
for Intramuscular Administration

DESCRIPTION

Synagis® (palivizumab) is a humanized monoclonal antibody (IgG1κ) produced by recombinant DNA technology, directed to an epitope in the A antigenic site of the F protein of respiratory syncytial virus (RSV). Synagis® is a composite of human (95%) and murine (5%) antibody sequences. The human heavy chain sequence was derived from the constant domains of human IgG1 and the variable framework regions of the V_H genes Cor (1) and Cess (2). The human light chain sequence was derived from the constant domain of Cκ and the variable framework regions of the V_L gene K104 with Jκ-4 (3). The murine sequences were derived from a murine monoclonal antibody, Mab 1129 (4), in a process that involved the grafting of the murine complementarity deter-

Continued on next page

Synagis—Cont.

mining regions into the human antibody frameworks. Synagis® is composed of two heavy chains and two light chains and has a molecular weight of approximately 148,000 Daltons.

Synagis® is available in two formulations: a lyophilized powder and a liquid solution.

Lyophilized Powder: Synagis® is supplied as a sterile lyophilized product for reconstitution with sterile water for injection. Reconstituted Synagis® (100 mg/mL) is to be administered by intramuscular injection (IM) only. The reconstituted solution should appear clear or slightly opalescent with pH of 6.0.

Each 100 mg single-use vial of Synagis® lyophilized powder is formulated in 67.5 mg of mannitol, 8.7 mg histidine and 0.3 mg of glycine and is designed to deliver 100 mg of Synagis® in 1.0 mL when reconstituted with 1.0 mL of sterile water for injection.

Each 50 mg single-use vial of Synagis® lyophilized powder is formulated in 40.5 mg mannitol, 5.2 mg of histidine and 0.2 mg of glycine and is designed to deliver 50 mg of Synagis® in 0.5 mL when reconstituted with 0.6 mL of sterile water for injection.

Liquid Solution: Synagis® (100 mg/mL) is supplied as a sterile, preservative-free solution to be administered by intramuscular injection (IM) only. The solution should appear clear or slightly opalescent with pH of 6.0.

Each 100 mg single-use vial of Synagis® liquid solution is formulated in 4.7 mg of histidine and 0.1 mg of glycine in a volume of 1.2 mL to and is designed to deliver 100 mg of Synagis® in 1.0 mL.

Each 50 mg single-use vial of Synagis® liquid solution is formulated in 2.7 mg of histidine and 0.08 mg of glycine in a volume of 0.7 mL to and is designed to deliver 50 mg of Synagis® in 0.5 mL.

CLINICAL PHARMACOLOGY:

Mechanism of Action: Synagis® exhibits neutralizing and fusion-inhibitory activity against RSV. These activities inhibit RSV replication in laboratory experiments. Although resistant RSV strains may be isolated in laboratory studies, a panel of 57 clinical RSV isolates were all neutralized by Synagis® (5). Synagis® serum concentrations of ≥ 40 µg/mL have been shown to reduce pulmonary RSV replication in the cotton rat model of RSV infection by 100-fold (5). The *in vivo* neutralizing activity of the active ingredient in Synagis® was assessed in a randomized, placebo-controlled study of 35 pediatric patients tracheally intubated because of RSV disease. In these patients, Synagis® significantly reduced the quantity of RSV in the lower respiratory tract compared to control patients (6).

Pharmacokinetics: In pediatric patients less than 24 months of age without congenital heart disease, the mean half-life of Synagis® was 20 days and monthly intramuscular doses of 15 mg/kg achieved mean ± SD 30 day trough serum drug concentrations of 37 ± 21 µg/mL after the first injection, 57 ± 41 µg/mL after the second injection, 68 ± 51 µg/mL after the third injection and 72 ± 50 µg/mL after the fourth injection (7). Trough concentrations following the first and fourth Synagis® dose were similar in children with congenital heart disease and in non-cardiac patients. In pediatric patients given Synagis® for a second season, the mean ±SD serum concentrations following the first and fourth injections were 61 ± 17 µg/mL and 86 ± 31 µg/mL, respectively.

In 139 pediatric patients ≤ 24 months of age with hemodynamically significant congenital heart disease (CHD) who received Synagis® and underwent cardio-pulmonary bypass for open-heart surgery, the mean ± SD serum Synagis® concentration was 98 ± 52 µg/mL before bypass and declined to 41 ± 33 µg/mL after bypass, a reduction of 58% (see *DOSAGE AND ADMINISTRATION*). The clinical significance of this reduction is unknown.

Specific studies were not conducted to evaluate the effects of demographic parameters on Synagis® systemic exposure. However, no effects of gender, age, body weight or race on Synagis® serum trough concentrations were observed in a clinical study with 639 pediatric patients with congenital heart disease (≤24 months of age) receiving five monthly intramuscular injections of 15 mg/kg of Synagis®.

Trough serum Synagis® concentrations were comparable between the Synagis® liquid and Synagis® lyophilized formulations administered IM at 15 mg/kg in a cross-over trial in 153 pediatric patients ≤6 months of age with a history of prematurity.

CLINICAL STUDIES

The safety and efficacy of Synagis® (palivizumab) were assessed in two randomized, double-blind, placebo-controlled trials of prophylaxis against RSV infection in pediatric patients at high risk of an RSV-related hospitalization. Trial 1 was conducted during a single RSV season and studied a total of 1,502 patients ≤ 24 months of age with bronchopulmonary dysplasia (BPD) or infants with premature birth (≤ 35 weeks gestation) who were ≤ 6 months of age at study entry (7). Trial 2 was conducted over four consecutive seasons among a total of 1287 patients ≤ 24 months of age with hemodynamically significant congenital heart disease. In both trials participants received 15 mg/kg Synagis® or an equivalent volume of placebo IM monthly for five injections and were followed for 150 days from randomization. In Trial 1, 99% of all subjects completed the study and 93% completed all five injections. In Trial 2, 96% of all subjects completed the study and 92% completed all five injections. The incidence of RSV hospitalization is shown in Table 1.

[See table 1 above]

Table 1: Incidence of RSV Hospitalization by Treatment Group

Trial		Placebo	Synagis	Difference between groups	Relative Reduction	p-Value
Tiral 1 Impact-RSV	n	500	1002			
	Hospitalization	53 (10.6%)	48 (4.8%)	5.8%	55%	<0.001
Trial 2 CHD	n	648	639			
	Hospitalization	63 (9.7%)	34 (5.3%)	4.4%	45%	0.003

In Trial 1, the reduction of RSV hospitalization was observed both in patients with BPD (34/266 [12.8%] placebo vs. 39/496 [7.9%] Synagis®), and in premature infants without BPD (19/234 [8.1%] placebo vs. 9/506 [1.8%] Synagis®). In Trial 2, reductions were observed in acyanotic (36/305 [11.8%] placebo versus 15/300 [5.0%] Synagis® and cyanotic children (27/343 [7.9%]) placebo versus 19/339 [5.6%] Synagis®).

The clinical studies do not suggest that RSV infection was less severe among RSV hospitalized patients who received Synagis® compared to those who received placebo.

INDICATIONS AND USAGE

Synagis® is indicated for the prevention of serious lower respiratory tract disease caused by respiratory syncytial virus (RSV) in pediatric patients at high risk of RSV disease. Safety and efficacy were established in infants with bronchopulmonary dysplasia (BPD), infants with a history of premature birth (≤ 35 weeks gestational age), and children with hemodynamically significant CHD. (See *CLINICAL STUDIES*)

CONTRAINDICATIONS

Synagis® should not be used in pediatric patients with a history of a severe prior reaction to Synagis® or other components of this product.

WARNINGS

Very rare cases of anaphylaxis (<1 case per 100,000 patients) have been reported following re-exposure to Synagis® (see *ADVERSE REACTIONS, POST-MARKETING EXPERIENCE*). Rare severe acute hypersensitivity reactions have also been reported on initial exposure or re-exposure to Synagis®. If a severe hypersensitivity reaction occurs, therapy with Synagis® should be permanently discontinued. If milder hypersensitivity reactions occur, caution should be used on readministration of Synagis®. **If anaphylaxis or severe allergic reactions occur, administer appropriate medications (e.g., epinephrine) and provide supportive care as required.**

PRECAUTIONS

General: Synagis® is for intramuscular use only. As with any intramuscular injection, Synagis® should be given with caution to patients with thrombocytopenia or any coagulation disorder.

The safety and efficacy of Synagis® have not been demonstrated for treatment of established RSV disease.

The single-use vial of Synagis® (palivizumab) does not contain a preservative. Lyophilized Synagis® must be used within 6 hours of reconstitution. Administration of either reconstituted Synagis® or liquid Synagis® should occur immediately after withdrawal from vial. The vial should not be re-entered. Discard any unused portion.

Drug Interactions: No formal drug-drug interaction studies were conducted. In Trial 1, the proportions of patients in the placebo and Synagis® groups who received routine childhood vaccines, influenza vaccine, bronchodilators or corticosteroids were similar and no incremental increase in adverse reactions was observed among patients receiving these agents.

Carcinogenesis, Mutagenesis, Impairment of Fertility: Carcinogenesis, mutagenesis and reproductive toxicity studies have not performed.

Pregnancy: Pregnancy Category C: Synagis® is not indicated for adult usage and animal reproduction studies have not been conducted. It is also not known whether Synagis® can cause fetal harm when administered to a pregnant woman or could affect reproductive capacity.

ADVERSE REACTIONS

The most serious adverse reactions occurring with Synagis® treatment are anaphylaxis and other acute hypersensitivity reactions (see *WARNINGS*). The adverse reactions most commonly observed in Synagis®-treated patients were upper respiratory tract infection, otitis media, fever, rhinitis, rash, diarrhea, cough, vomiting, gastroenteritis, and wheezing. Upper respiratory tract infection, otitis media, fever, and rhinitis occurred at a rate of 1% or greater in the Synagis® group compared to placebo (Table 2).

Because clinical trials are conducted under widely varying conditions, adverse event rates observed in the clinical trials of a drug cannot be directly compared to rates in the clinical trials of another drug and may not reflect the rates observed in practice. The adverse reaction information does, however, provide a basis for identifying the adverse events that appear to be related to drug use and a basis for approximating rates.

The data described reflect Synagis® exposure for 1641 pediatric patients of age 3 days to 24.1 months in Trials 1 and 2. Among these patients, 496 had bronchopulmonary dysplasia, 506 were premature birth infants less than 6 months of age, and 639 had congenital heart disease. Adverse events observed in the 153 patient crossover study comparing the liquid and lyophilized formulations were similar between the two formulations, and similar to the adverse events observed with Synagis® in Trials 1 and 2.

[See table 2 above]

Table 2 - adverse events occurring at a rate of 1% or greater more frequently in patients† receiving Synagis®

Event	Synagis® (n=1641) n (%)	Placebo (n=1148) n (%)
Upper respiratory infection	830 (50.6)	544 (47.4)
Otitis media	597 (36.4)	397 (34.6)
Fever	446 (27.1)	289 (25.2)
Rhinitis	439 (26.8)	282 (24.6)
Hernia	68 (4.1)	30 (2.6)
SGOT Increase	49 (3.0)	20 (1.7)

†Cyanosis (Synagis® [9.1%]/placebo [6.9%]) and arrhythmia (Synagis® [3.1%]/placebo [1.7%]) were reported during Trial 2 in congenital heart disease patients.

Immunogenicity

In Trial 1, the incidence of anti-Synagis® antibody following the fourth injection was 1.1% in the placebo group and 0.7% in the Synagis® group. In pediatric patients receiving Synagis® for a second season, one of the fifty-six patients had transient, low titer reactivity. This reactivity was not associated with adverse events or alteration in serum concentrations. Immunogenicity was not assessed in Trial 2.

These data reflect the percentage of patients whose test results were considered positive for antibodies to Synagis® (palivizumab) in an ELISA assay, and are highly dependent on the sensitivity and specificity of the assay. Additionally, the observed incidence of antibody positivity in an assay may be influenced by several factors including sample handling, concomitant medications, and underlying disease. For these reasons, comparison of the incidence of antibodies to Synagis® with the incidence of antibodies to other products may be misleading.

Post-Marketing Experience

The following adverse reactions have been identified and reported during post-approval use of Synagis®. Because the reports of these reactions are voluntary and the population is of uncertain size, it is not always possible to reliably estimate the frequency of the reaction or establish a causal relationship to drug exposure.

Based on experience in over 400,000 patients who have received Synagis® (>2 million doses), rare severe acute hypersensitivity reactions have been reported on initial or subsequent exposure. Very rare cases of anaphylaxis (<1 case per 100,000 patients) have also been reported following re-exposure (See *WARNINGS*). None of the reported hypersensitivity reactions were fatal. Hypersensitivity reactions may include dyspnea, cyanosis, respiratory failure, urticaria, pruritus, angioedema, hypotonia and unresponsiveness. The relationship between these reactions and the development of antibodies to Synagis® is unknown.

Limited information from post-marketing reports suggests that, within a single RSV season, adverse events after a sixth or greater dose of Synagis® are similar in character and frequency to those after the initial five doses.

OVER DOSAGE

No data from clinical studies are available on over dosage. No toxicity was observed in rabbits administered a single intramuscular or subcutaneous injection of Synagis® at a dose of 50 mg/kg.

DOSAGE AND ADMINISTRATION

The recommended dose of Synagis® is 15 mg/kg of body weight. Patients, including those who develop an RSV infection, should continue to receive monthly doses throughout the RSV season. The first dose should be administered prior to commencement of the RSV season. In the northern hemisphere, the RSV season typically commences in November and lasts through April, but it may begin earlier or persist later in certain communities.

Synagis® serum levels are decreased after cardio-pulmonary bypass (See *CLINICAL PHARMACOLOGY*). Patients undergoing cardio-pulmonary bypass should receive a dose of Synagis® as soon as possible after the cardio-pulmonary bypass procedure (even if sooner than a month from the previous dose). Thereafter, doses should be administered monthly.

Synagis® should be administered in a dose of 15 mg/kg intramuscularly using aseptic technique, preferably in the anterolateral aspect of the thigh. The gluteal muscle should not be used routinely as an injection site because of the risk of damage to the sciatic nerve. The dose per month = patient weight (kg) × 15 mg/kg ÷ 100 mg/mL of Synagis®. Injection volumes over 1 mL should be given as a divided dose.

Preparation of Lyophilized Product for Administration:

- To reconstitute, remove the tab portion of the vial cap and clean the rubber stopper with 70% ethanol or equivalent.
- Both the 50 mg and 100 mg vials contain an overfill to allow the withdrawal of 50 milligrams or 100 milligrams respectively when reconstituted following the directions described below.
- SLOWLY add 0.6 mL of sterile water for injection to the 50 mg vial or add 1.0 mL of sterile water for injection to the 100 mg vial. The vial should be tilted slightly and gently rotated for 30 seconds to avoid foaming. DO NOT SHAKE or VIGOROUSLY AGITATE the VIAL. This is a critical step to avoid prolonged foaming.
- Reconstituted Synagis® should stand undisturbed at room temperature for a minimum of 20 minutes until the solution clarifies.
- Reconstituted Synagis® (palivizumab) should be inspected visually for particulate matter or discoloration prior to administration. The reconstituted solution should appear clear or slightly opalescent (a thin layer of microbubbles on the surface is normal and will not affect dosage). Do not use if there is particulate matter or if the solution is discolored.
- Reconstituted Synagis® does not contain a preservative and should be administered within 6 hours of reconstitution. Administer immediately after withdrawal from vial. Synagis® is supplied in single-use vials DO NOT re-enter the vial. Discard any unused portion.

Preparation of Liquid Product for Administration:

- Remove the tab portion of the vial cap and clean the rubber stopper with 70% ethanol or equivalent.
- Both the 50 mg and 100 mg vials contain an overfill to allow the withdrawal of 50 milligrams or 100 milligrams.
- Synagis® does not contain a preservative and should be administered immediately after withdrawal from vial. Synagis® is supplied in single-use vials. DO NOT re-enter the vial. Discard any unused portion.

To prevent the transmission of hepatitis viruses or other infectious agents from one person to another, sterile disposable syringes and needles should be used. Do not reuse syringes and needles.

HOW SUPPLIED

Synagis® is available in two formulations: a lyophilized powder and liquid solution.

Lyophilized Powder: Synagis® is supplied in single-use vials as lyophilized powder to deliver either 50 milligrams or 100 milligrams when reconstituted with sterile water for injection.

50 mg vial NDC 60574-4112-1

Upon reconstitution the 50 mg vial contains 50 milligrams Synagis® in 0.5 mL.

100 mg vial NDC 60574-4111-1

Liquid Solution: Synagis® is supplied in single-use vials as a preservative free, sterile solution at 100 mg/mL in 0.5 mL and 1.0 mL to deliver either 50 milligrams or 100 milligrams, respectively for IM injection.

50 mg vial NDC 60574-4114-1

The 50 mg vial contains 50 milligrams Synagis® in 0.5 mL.

100 mg vial NDC 60574-4113-1

The 100 mg vial contains 100 milligrams Synagis® in 1.0 mL.

Upon receipt and until use, Synagis® should be stored between 2 and 8°C (35.6° and 46.4°F) in its original container. Do not freeze. Do not use beyond the expiration date.

REFERENCES

1. Press E, and Hogg N. The amino acid sequences of the Fd Fragments of Two Human gamma-1 heavy chains. Biochem. J. 1970;117:641–660.
2. Takahashi N, Noma T, and Honjo T. Rearranged immunoglobulin heavy chain variable region (V_H) pseudogene that deletes the second complementary-determining region. Proc. Nat. Acad. Sci. USA 1984;81:5194–5198.
3. Bentley D, and Rabbitts T. Human immunoglobulin variable region genes - DNA sequences of two Vκ genes and a pseudogene. Nature 1980;288:730–733.
4. Beeler JA, and Van Wyke Coelingh K. Neutralization epitopes of the F Protein of Respiratory Syncytial Virus: Effect of mutation upon fusion function. J. Virology 1989;63:2941–2950.
5. Johnson S, Oliver C, Prince GA, et al. Development of a humanized monoclonal antibody (MEDI-493) with potent in vitro and in vivo activity against respiratory syncytial virus. J. Infect. Dis. 1997; 176:1215–1224.
6. Malley R, DeVincenzo J, Ramilo O, et al. Reduction of Respiratory Syncytial Virus (RSV) in Tracheal Aspirates in Intubated Infants by Use of Humanized Monoclonal Antibody to RSV F Protein. J. Infect. Dis. 1998;178:1555–1561.
7. The IMpact RSV Study Group. Palivizumab, a Humanized Respiratory Syncytial Virus Monoclonal Antibody, Reduces Hospitalization From Respiratory Syncytial Virus Infection in High-risk Infants. Pediatrics 1998;102:531–537.

Manufactured by:
MedImmune, Inc.
Gaithersburg, MD 20878
U.S. Gov't. License No. 1252
(1-877-633-4411)
Date: July 23, 2004
Co-Marketed by:
Ross Products Division
Abbott Laboratories, Inc.
Columbus, OH 43215-1724

Shown in Product Identification Guide, page 322

MedImmune Oncology, Inc.

ONE MEDIMMUNE WAY
GAITHERSBURG, MD 20878

Direct Inquiries to:
MedImmune Oncology, Inc.
1-(877)-633-4411
For Medical Information, adverse drug experiences, product sales, and ordering, and other inquiries please contact:
1-(877)-633-4411
internet—www.medimmune.com
For Emergencies, 24 hours.
1-(877)-633-4411

Ethyol® (amifostine), see Listing under MedImmune Oncology, Inc.

ETHYOL® ℞

[a-thī-ol]
AMIFOSTINE for Injection
℞ only

DESCRIPTION

ETHYOL® (amifostine) is an organic thiophosphate cytoprotective agent known chemically as 2-[(3-aminopropyl)amino]ethanethiol dihydrogen phosphate (ester) and has the following structural formula:

$$H_2N(CH_2)_3NH(CH_2)_2S\text{-}PO_3H_2$$

Amifostine is a white crystalline powder which is freely soluble in water. Its empirical formula is $C_5H_{15}N_2O_3PS$ and it has a molecular weight of 214.22.

ETHYOL® is the trihydrate form of amifostine and is supplied as a sterile lyophilized powder requiring reconstitution for intravenous infusion. Each single-use 10 mL vial contains 500 mg of amifostine on the anhydrous basis.

CLINICAL PHARMACOLOGY

ETHYOL® is a prodrug that is dephosphorylated by alkaline phosphatase in tissues to a pharmacologically active free thiol metabolite. This metabolite is believed to be responsible for the reduction of the cumulative renal toxicity of cisplatin and for the reduction of the toxic effects of radiation on normal oral tissues. The ability of ETHYOL® to differentially protect normal tissues is attributed to the higher capillary alkaline phosphatase activity, higher pH and better vascularity of normal tissues relative to tumor tissue, which results in a more rapid generation of the active thiol metabolite as well as a higher rate constant for uptake into cells. The higher concentration of the thiol metabolite in normal tissues is available to bind to, and thereby detoxify, reactive metabolites of cisplatin. This thiol metabolite can also scavenge reactive oxygen species generated by exposure to either cisplatin or radiation.

Pharmacokinetics: Clinical pharmacokinetic studies show that ETHYOL® is rapidly cleared from the plasma with a distribution half-life of <1 minute and an elimination half-life of approximately 8 minutes. Less than 10% of ETHYOL® remains in the plasma 6 minutes after drug administration. ETHYOL® is rapidly metabolized to an active free thiol metabolite. A disulfide metabolite is produced subsequently and is less active than the free thiol. After a 10-second bolus dose of 150 mg/m² of ETHYOL®, renal excretion of the parent drug and its two metabolites was low during the hour following drug administration, averaging 0.69%, 2.64% and 2.22% of the administered dose for the parent, thiol and disulfide, respectively. Measurable levels of the free thiol metabolite have been found in bone marrow cells 5–8 minutes after intravenous infusion of ETHYOL®. Pretreatment with dexamethasone or metoclopramide has no effect on ETHYOL® pharmacokinetics.

Clinical Studies

Chemotherapy for Ovarian Cancer and Non-Small Cell Lung Cancer. A randomized controlled trial compared six cycles of cyclophosphamide 1000 mg/m², and cisplatin 100 mg/m² with or without ETHYOL® pretreatment at 910 mg/m², in two successive cohorts of 121 patients with advanced ovarian cancer. In both cohorts, after multiple cycles of chemotherapy, pretreatment with ETHYOL® significantly reduced the cumulative renal toxicity associated with cisplatin as assessed by the proportion of patients who had ≥40% decrease in creatinine clearance from pretreatment values, protracted elevations in serum creatinine (>1.5 mg/dL), or severe hypomagnesemia. Subgroup analyses suggested that the effect of ETHYOL® was present in patients who had received nephrotoxic antibiotics, or who had preexisting diabetes or hypertension (and thus may have been at increased risk for significant nephrotoxicity), as well as in patients who lacked these risks. Selected analyses of the effects of ETHYOL® in reducing the cumulative renal toxicity of cisplatin in the randomized ovarian cancer study are provided in TABLES 1 and 2, below.

TABLE 1
Proportion of Patients with ≥40% Reduction in Calculated Creatinine Clearance*

	ETHYOL® + CP	CP	p-value (2-sided)
All Patients	16/122 (13%)	36/120 (30%)	0.001
First Cohort	10/63	20/58	0.018
Second Cohort	6/59	16/62	0.026

*Creatinine clearance values were calculated using the Cockcroft-Gault formula, *Nephron* 1976;16:31–41.

[See table 2 below]

In the randomized ovarian cancer study, ETHYOL® had no detectable effect on the antitumor efficacy of cisplatin-cyclophosphamide chemotherapy. Objective response rates (including pathologically confirmed complete remission rates), time to progression, and survival duration were all similar in the ETHYOL® and control study groups. The table below summarizes the principal efficacy findings of the randomized ovarian cancer study.

[See table 3 at top of next page]

A Phase II trial of ETHYOL®, 740–910 mg/m², and cisplatin, 120 mg/m², administered on day 1 and vinblastine,

Continued on next page

TABLE 2
NCI Toxicity Grades of Serum Magnesium Levels for Each Patient's Last Cycle of Therapy

NCI-CTC Grade: (mEq/L)	0 >1.4	1 ≤1.4–>1.1	2 ≤1.1–>0.8	3 ≤0.8–>0.5	4 ≤0.5	p-value*
All Patients						0.001
ETHYOL® + CP	92	13	3	0	0	
CP	73	18	7	5	1	
First Cohort						0.017
ETHYOL® + CP	49	10	3	0	0	
CP	35	8	6	3	1	
Second Cohort						0.012
ETHYOL® + CP	43	3	0	0	0	
CP	38	10	1	2	0	

*Based on 2-sided Mantel-Haenszel Chi-Square statistic.

Ethyol—Cont.

5 mg/m^2, administered on days 1, 8, 15 and 22 of each monthly cycle was conducted in 25 patients with Stage IV non-small cell lung cancer. This regimen was repeated until disease progression or unacceptable toxicity occurred, or a maximum of six cycles had been administered. Among 13 patients who received 4 or more cycles of this intensive cisplatin regimen, 1 had a ≥40% reduction in creatinine clearance. These results are consistent with the randomized ovarian cancer trial.

Sixteen of the 25 patients treated demonstrated a partial response to chemotherapy. With a median follow-up of 19 months, the median survival was 17 months. At one year, 64% of the patients were alive. These results indicate that ETHYOL® may not adversely affect the efficacy of this chemotherapy for non-small cell lung cancer.

Radiotherapy for Head and Neck Cancer. A randomized controlled trial of standard fractionated radiation (1.8 Gy–2.0 Gy/day for 5 days/week for 5–7 weeks) with or without ETHYOL®, administered at 200 mg/m^2 as a 3 minute i.v. infusion 15–30 minutes prior to each fraction of radiation, was conducted in 315 patients with head and neck cancer. Patients were required to have at least 75% of both parotid glands in the radiation field. The incidence of Grade 2 or higher acute (90 days or less from start of radiation) and late xerostomia (9–12 months following radiation) as assessed by RTOG Acute and Late Morbidity Scoring Criteria, was significantly reduced in patients receiving ETHYOL® (TABLE 4).

[See table 4 at right]

At one year following radiation, whole saliva collection following radiation showed that more patients given ETHYOL® produced >0.1 gm of saliva (72% vs. 49%). In addition, the median saliva production at one year was higher in those patients who received ETHYOL® (0.26 gm vs. 0.1 gm). Stimulated saliva collections did not show a difference between treatment arms. These improvements in saliva production were supported by the patients' subjective responses to a questionnaire regarding oral dryness.

In the randomized head and neck cancer study, locoregional control, disease-free survival and overall survival were all comparable in the two treatment groups after one year of follow-up (see TABLE 5).

[See table 5 at right]

INDICATIONS AND USAGE

ETHYOL® (amifostine) is indicated to reduce the cumulative renal toxicity associated with repeated administration of cisplatin in patients with advanced ovarian cancer or non-small cell lung cancer.

ETHYOL® is indicated to reduce the incidence of moderate to severe xerostomia in patients undergoing post-operative radiation treatment for head and neck cancer, where the radiation port includes a substantial portion of the parotid glands (see Clinical Studies).

For the approved indications, the clinical data do not suggest that the effectiveness of cisplatin based chemotherapy regimens or radiation therapy is altered by ETHYOL®. There are at present only limited data on the effects of ETHYOL® on the efficacy of chemotherapy or radiotherapy in other settings. ETHYOL® should not be administered to patients in other settings where chemotherapy can produce a significant survival benefit or cure, or in patients receiving definitive radiotherapy, except in the context of a clinical study (see WARNINGS).

CONTRAINDICATIONS

ETHYOL® is contraindicated in patients with known sensitivity to aminothiol compounds.

WARNINGS

1. Effectiveness of the Cytotoxic Regimen

Limited data are currently available regarding the preservation of antitumor efficacy when ETHYOL® is administered prior to cisplatin therapy in settings other than advanced ovarian cancer or non-small cell lung cancer. Although some animal data suggest interference is possible, in most tumor models the antitumor effects of chemotherapy are not altered by amifostine. ETHYOL® should not be used in patients receiving chemotherapy for other malignancies in which chemotherapy can produce a significant survival benefit or cure (e.g., certain malignancies of germ cell origin), except in the context of a clinical study.

2. Effectiveness of Radiotherapy

ETHYOL® should not be administered in patients receiving definitive radiotherapy, except in the context of a clinical trial, since there are at present insufficient data to exclude a tumor-protective effect in this setting. ETHYOL® was studied only with standard fractionated radiotherapy and only when ≥75% of both parotid glands were exposed to radiation. The effects of ETHYOL® on the incidence of xerostomia and on toxicity in the setting of combined chemotherapy and radiotherapy and in the setting of accelerated and hyperfractionated therapy have not been systematically studied.

3. Hypotension

Patients who are hypotensive or in a state of dehydration should not receive ETHYOL®. Patients receiving ETHYOL® at doses recommended for chemotherapy should have antihypertensive therapy interrupted 24 hours preceding administration of ETHYOL®. Patients receiving ETHYOL® at doses recommended for chemotherapy who are taking anti-

TABLE 3
Comparison of Principal Efficacy Findings

	ETHYOL® + CP	CP
Complete pathologic tumor response rate	21.3%	15.8%
Time to progression (months)		
Median (± 95% CI)	15.8 (13.2, 25.1)	18.1 (12.5, 20.4)
Mean (± Std error)	19.8 (±1.04)	19.1 (±1.58)
Hazard ratio (95% Confidence Interval)	.98 (.64, 1.4)	
Survival (months)		
Median (± 95% CI)	31.3 (28.3, 38.2)	31.8 (26.3, 39.8)
Mean (± Std error)	33.7 (±2.03)	34.3 (±2.04)
Hazard ratio (95% Confidence Interval)	.97 (.69, 1.32)	

TABLE 4
Incidence of Grade 2 or Higher Xerostomia
(RTOG criteria)

	ETHYOL® + RT	RT	p-value
Acute (≤90 days from start of radiation)	51% (75/148)	78% (120/153)	p<0.0001
Late[a] (9–12 months post radiation)	35% (36/103)	57% (63/111)	p=0.0016

[a]Based on the number of patients for whom actual data were available.

TABLE 5
Comparison of Principal Efficacy Findings at 1 Year

	ETHYOL® + RT	RT
Locoregional Control Rate[a]	76.1%	75.0%
Hazard Ratio[b] 95% Confidence Interval	1.013 (0.671, 1.530)	
Disease-Free Survival Rate[a]	74.6%	70.4%
Hazard Ratio[b] 95% Confidence Interval	1.035 (0.702, 1.528)	
Overall Survival Rate[a]	89.4%	82.4%
Hazard Ratio[b] 95% Confidence Interval	1.585 (0.961, 2.613)	

[a]1 year rates estimated using Kaplan-Meier method
[b]Hazard ratio >1.0 is in favor of the ETHYOL® + RT arm

hypertensive therapy that cannot be stopped for 24 hours preceding ETHYOL® treatment, should not receive ETHYOL®.

Prior to ETHYOL® infusion patients should be adequately hydrated. During ETHYOL® infusion patients should be kept in a supine position. Blood pressure should be monitored every 5 minutes during the infusion, and thereafter as clinically indicated. It is important that the duration of the 910 mg/m^2 infusion not exceed 15 minutes, as administration of ETHYOL® as a longer infusion is associated with a higher incidence of side effects. For infusion durations less than 5 minutes, blood pressure should be monitored at least before and immediately after the infusion, and thereafter as clinically indicated. If hypotension occurs, patients should be placed in the Trendelenburg position and be given an infusion of normal saline using a separate i.v. line. During and after ETHYOL® infusion, care should be taken to monitor the blood pressure of patients whose antihypertensive medication has been interrupted since hypertension may be exacerbated by discontinuation of antihypertensive medication and other causes such as i.v. hydration.

Guidelines for interrupting and restarting ETHYOL® infusion if a decrease in systolic blood pressure should occur are provided in the DOSAGE AND ADMINISTRATION section.

Hypotension may occur during or shortly after ETHYOL® infusion, despite adequate hydration and positioning of the patient (see ADVERSE REACTIONS and PRECAUTIONS). Hypotension has been reported to be associated with dyspnea, apnea, hypoxia, and in rare cases seizures, unconsciousness, respiratory arrest and renal failure.

4. Hypersensitivity

Allergic manifestations including anaphylaxis and severe cutaneous reactions have been associated rarely with ETHYOL® administration. Serious cutaneous hypersensitivity reactions have included erythema multiforme, Stevens-Johnson syndrome, toxic epidermal necrolysis, toxoderma and exfoliative dermatitis, which have been reported more frequently when ETHYOL® is used as a radioprotectant (see ADVERSE REACTIONS). Some of these reactions have been fatal or have required hospitalization and/or discontinuance of therapy. Patients should be carefully monitored prior to, during and after ETHYOL® administration (see PRECAUTIONS).

5. Nausea and Vomiting

Antiemetic medication should be administered prior to and in conjunction with ETHYOL® (see DOSAGE AND ADMINISTRATION). When ETHYOL® is administered with highly emetogenic chemotherapy, the fluid balance of the patient should be carefully monitored.

6. Hypocalcemia

Serum calcium levels should be monitored in patients at risk of hypocalcemia, such as those with nephrotic syndrome or patients receiving multiple doses of ETHYOL® (see ADVERSE REACTIONS). If necessary, calcium supplements can be administered.

PRECAUTIONS

General

Patients should be adequately hydrated prior to the ETHYOL® infusion and blood pressure should be monitored (see DOSAGE AND ADMINISTRATION).

The safety of ETHYOL® administration has not been established in elderly patients, or in patients with preexisting cardiovascular or cerebrovascular conditions such as ischemic heart disease, arrhythmias, congestive heart failure, or history of stroke or transient ischemic attacks. ETHYOL® should be used with particular care in these and other patients in whom the common ETHYOL® adverse effects of nausea/vomiting and hypotension may be more likely to have serious consequences.

Prior to chemotherapy, ETHYOL® should be administered as a 15-minute infusion (see DOSAGE AND ADMINISTRATION). Blood pressure should be monitored every 5 minutes during the infusion, and thereafter as clinically indicated.

Prior to radiation therapy, ETHYOL® should be administered as a 3-minute infusion (see DOSAGE AND ADMINISTRATION). Blood pressure should be monitored at least before and immediately after the infusion, and thereafter as clinically indicated.

Allergic Reactions

In case of severe acute allergic reaction ETHYOL® should be immediately and permanently discontinued. Epinephrine and other appropriate measures should be available for treatment of serious allergic events such as anaphylaxis. ETHYOL® should also be permanently discontinued for serious or severe cutaneous reactions (see WARNINGS and ADVERSE REACTIONS) or for cutaneous reactions associated with fever or other constitutional symptoms not known to be due to another etiology. ETHYOL® should be withheld and dermatologic consultation and biopsy considered for cutaneous reactions or mucosal lesions of unknown etiology appearing outside of the injection site or radiation port and for erythematous, edematous or bullous lesions on the palms of the hand or soles of the feet. Reinitiation of

ETHYOL® should be at the physician's discretion based on medical judgment and appropriate dermatologic evaluation.

Drug Interactions

Special consideration should be given to the administration of ETHYOL® in patients receiving antihypertensive medications or other drugs that could cause or potentiate hypotension.

Carcinogenesis, Mutagenesis, Impairment of Fertility

No long term animal studies have been performed to evaluate the carcinogenic potential of ETHYOL®. ETHYOL® was negative in the Ames test and in the mouse micronucleus test. The free thiol metabolite was positive in the Ames test with S9 microsomal fraction in the TA1535 *Salmonella typhimurium* strain and at the TK locus in the mouse L5178Y cell assay. The metabolite was negative in the mouse micronucleus test and negative for clastogenicity in human lymphocytes.

Pregnancy

Pregnancy Category C. ETHYOL® has been shown to be embryotoxic in rabbits at doses of 50 mg/kg, approximately sixty percent of the recommended dose in humans on a body surface area basis. There are no adequate and well-controlled studies in pregnant women. ETHYOL® should be used during pregnancy only if the potential benefit justifies the potential risk to the fetus.

Nursing Mothers

No information is available on the excretion of ETHYOL® or its metabolites into human milk. Because many drugs are excreted in human milk and because of the potential for adverse reactions in nursing infants, it is recommended that breast feeding be discontinued if the mother is treated with ETHYOL®.

Pediatric Use

The safety and effectiveness in pediatric patients have not been established.

Geriatric Use

The clinical studies did not include sufficient number of subjects aged 65 and over to determine whether they respond differently from younger subjects. Other reported clinical experience has not identified differences in responses between elderly and younger patients. In general, dose selection for an elderly patient should be cautious, reflecting the greater frequency of decreased hepatic, renal, or cardiac function and of concomitant disease of other drug therapy in elderly patients.

ADVERSE REACTIONS

Controlled Trials

In the randomized study of patients with ovarian cancer given ETHYOL® at a dose of 910 mg/m^2 prior to chemotherapy, transient hypotension was observed in 62% of patients treated. The mean time of onset was 14 minutes into the 15-minute period of ETHYOL® infusion, and the mean duration was 6 minutes. In some cases, the infusion had to be prematurely terminated due to a more pronounced drop in systolic blood pressure. In general, the blood pressure returned to normal within 5–15 minutes. Fewer than 3% of patients discontinued ETHYOL® due to blood pressure reductions. In the randomized study of patients with head and neck cancer given ETHYOL® at a dose of 200 mg/m^2 prior to radiotherapy, hypotension was observed in 15% of patients treated (see TABLE 6).

[See table 6 above]

TABLE 6
Incidence of Common Adverse Events in Patients Receiving ETHYOL®

	Phase III Ovarian Cancer Trial (WR-1) 910 mg/m^2		Phase III Head and Neck Cancer Trial (WR-38) 200 mg/m^2	
	Per Patient	**Per Infusion**	**Per Patient**	**Per Infusion**
Nausea/Vomiting				
≥Grade 3	36/122 (30%)	53/592 (9%)	12/150 (8%)	13/4314 (<1%)
All Grades	117/122 (96%)	520/592 (88%)	80/150 (53%)	233/4314 (5%)
Hypotension				
≥Grade 3[a]	10/122 (8%)		4/150 (3%)	
All Grades	75/122 (61%)	159/592 (27%)	22/150 (15%)	46/4314 (1%)

[a]According to protocol-defined criteria. WR-1: requiring interruption of infusion; WR-38: drop of >20mm Hg.

In the randomized study of patients with head and neck cancer, 17% (26/150) discontinued ETHYOL® due to adverse events. All but one of these patients continued to receive radiation treatment until completion.

Hypotension that requires interruption of the ETHYOL® infusion should be treated with fluid infusion and postural management of the patient (supine or Trendelenburg position). If the blood pressure returns to normal within 5 minutes and the patient is asymptomatic, the infusion may be restarted, so that the full dose of ETHYOL® can be administered.

Short term, reversible loss of consciousness has been reported rarely.

Nausea and/or vomiting occur frequently after ETHYOL® infusion and may be severe. In the ovarian cancer randomized study, the incidence of severe nausea/vomiting on day 1 of cyclophosphamide-cisplatin chemotherapy was 10% in patients who did not receive ETHYOL®, and 19% in patients who did receive ETHYOL®. In the randomized study of patients with head and neck cancer, the incidence of severe nausea/vomiting was 8% in patients who received ETHYOL® and 1% in patients who did not receive ETHYOL®.

Decrease in serum calcium concentrations is a known pharmacological effect of ETHYOL®. At the recommended doses, clinically significant hypocalcemia has occurred rarely (<1%) (see WARNINGS).

Other effects which have been described during or following ETHYOL® infusion are flushing/feeling of warmth, chills/feeling of coldness, fever, dizziness, somnolence, hiccups and sneezing. These effects have not generally precluded the completion of therapy.

Clinical Trials and Pharmacovigilance Reports

Allergic reactions characterized by one or more of the following manifestations have been observed during or after ETHYOL® administration: hypotension, fever, chills/rigors, dyspnea, hypoxia, chest tightness, cutaneous eruptions, urticaria and laryngeal edema. Serious, sometimes fatal skin reactions including erythema multiforme, and in rare cases, exfoliative dermatitis, Stevens-Johnson syndrome and toxic epidermal necrolysis have occurred. The reported incidence of serious skin reactions associated with ETHYOL® is higher in patients receiving ETHYOL® as a radioprotectant than in patients receiving ETHYOL® as a chemoprotectant. Rare anaphylactoid reactions and cardiac arrest have also been reported.

Hypotension, usually brief systolic and diastolic, has been associated with one or more of the following adverse events: apnea, dyspnea, hypoxia, tachycardia, bradycardia, extrasystoles, chest pain, myocardial ischemia and convulsion. Rare cases of renal failure, myocardial infarction, respiratory and cardiac arrest have been observed during or after hypotension. (See WARNINGS and PRECAUTIONS)

Rare cases of arrythmias such as atrial fibrillation/flutter and supraventricular tachycardia have been reported. These are sometimes associated with hypotension or allergic reactions.

Transient hypertension and exacerbations of preexisting hypertension have been observed rarely after ETHYOL® administration.

Seizures and syncope have been reported rarely. (See WARNINGS and PRECAUTIONS)

OVERDOSAGE

In clinical trials, the maximum single dose of ETHYOL® was 1300 mg/m^2. No information is available on single doses higher than this in adults. In the setting of a clinical trial, pediatric patients have received single ETHYOL® doses of up to 2700 mg/m^2. At the higher doses, anxiety and reversible urinary retention occurred.

Administration of ETHYOL® at 2 and 4 hours after the initial dose has not led to increased nausea and vomiting or hypotension. The most likely symptom of overdosage is hypotension, which should be managed by infusion of normal saline and other supportive measures, as clinically indicated.

DOSAGE AND ADMINISTRATION

For Reduction of Cumulative Renal Toxicity with Chemotherapy: The recommended starting dose of ETHYOL® is 910 mg/m^2 administered once daily as a 15-minute i.v. infusion, starting 30 minutes prior to chemotherapy.

The 15-minute infusion is better tolerated than more extended infusions. Further reductions in infusion times for chemotherapy regimens have not been systematically investigated.

Patients should be adequately hydrated prior to ETHYOL® infusion and kept in a supine position during the infusion. Blood pressure should be monitored every 5 minutes during the infusion, and thereafter as clinically indicated.

The infusion of ETHYOL® should be interrupted if the systolic blood pressure decreases significantly from the baseline value as listed in the guideline below:

[See second table above]

Guideline for Interrupting ETHYOL® Infusion Due to Decrease in Systolic Blood Pressure

	Baseline Systolic Blood Pressure (mm Hg)				
	<100	100–119	120–139	140–179	≥180
Decrease in systolic blood pressure during infusion of ETHYOL® (mm Hg)	20	25	30	40	50

If the blood pressure returns to normal within 5 minutes and the patient is asymptomatic, the infusion may be restarted so that the full dose of ETHYOL® may be administered. If the full dose of ETHYOL® cannot be administered, the dose of ETHYOL® for subsequent chemotherapy cycles should be 740 mg/m^2.

It is recommended that antiemetic medication, including dexamethasone 20 mg i.v. and a serotonin 5HT$_3$ receptor antagonist, be administered prior to and in conjunction with ETHYOL®. Additional antiemetics may be required based on the chemotherapy drugs administered.

For Reduction of Moderate to Severe Xerostomia from Radiation of the Head and Neck: The recommended dose of ETHYOL® is 200 mg/m^2 administered once daily as a 3-minute i.v. infusion, starting 15–30 minutes prior to standard fraction radiation therapy (1.8–2.0 Gy).

Patients should be adequately hydrated prior to ETHYOL® infusion. Blood pressure should be monitored at least before and immediately after the infusion, and thereafter as clinically indicated.

It is recommended that antiemetic medication be administered prior to and in conjunction with ETHYOL®. Oral 5HT$_3$ receptor antagonists, alone or in combination with other antiemetics, have been used effectively in the radiotherapy setting.

Reconstitution

ETHYOL® (amifostine) for Injection is supplied as a sterile lyophilized powder requiring reconstitution for intravenous infusion. Each single-use vial contains 500 mg of amifostine on the anhydrous basis.

Prior to intravenous injection, ETHYOL® is reconstituted with 9.7 mL of sterile 0.9% Sodium Chloride Injection, USP. This reconstituted solution (500 mg amifostine/10 mL) is chemically stable for up to 5 hours at room temperature (approximately 25°C) or up to 24 hours under refrigeration (2°C to 8°C).

ETHYOL® prepared in polyvinylchloride (PVC) bags at concentrations ranging from 5 mg/mL to 40 mg/mL is chemically stable for up to 5 hours when stored at room temperature (approximately 25°C) or up to 24 hours when stored under refrigeration (2°C to 8°C). CAUTION: Parenteral products should be inspected visually for particulate matter and discoloration prior to administration whenever solution and container permit. Do not use if cloudiness or precipitate is observed.

Incompatibilities

The compatibility of ETHYOL® with solutions other than 0.9% Sodium Chloride for Injection, or Sodium Chloride solutions with other additives, has not been examined. The use of other solutions is not recommended.

HOW SUPPLIED

ETHYOL® (amifostine) for injection is supplied as a sterile lyophilized powder in 10 mL single-use vials (NDC 58178-017-01). Each single-use vial contains 500 mg of amifostine on the anhydrous basis. The vials are available packaged as follows:

3 pack - 3 vials per carton (NDC 58178-017-03)

Store the lyophilized dosage form at Controlled Room Temperature 20°–25°C (68°–77°F) [See USP].

U.S. Patents 5,424,471; 5,591,731; 5,994,409

Manufactured by:
MedImmune Pharma B.V.
6545 CG Nijmegan
The Netherlands
Or:
Ben Venue, Inc.
Bedford, Ohio 44146
Marketed by:
MedImmune Oncology, Inc.
a subsidiary of MedImmune, Inc.
Gaithersburg, MD 20878
MedImmune
Oncology, Inc.
For product information, please call 1-877-633-4411

Revision Date 3/2003 **N-LB2022 PI**

MedImmune Vaccines, Inc.
ONE MEDIMMUNE WAY
GAITHERSBURG, MD 20878

For Medical Information, please contact:
(800) 949-3789 or
(877) 633-4411
Adverse Drug Experience:
(800) 949-3789 or
(877) 633-4411
In Emergencies:
24-hour emergency
(800) 949-3789 or
(877) 633-4411
Sales and Ordering/Customer Services:
(877) FLUMIST
Customer Support Network:
(877) 633-4411

FLUMIST™ ℞
[flew' mĭst]
Influenza Virus Vaccine Live, Intranasal
2004-2005 Formula
FOR NASAL ADMINISTRATION ONLY
℞ *only*

DESCRIPTION

Influenza Virus Vaccine Live, Intranasal (FluMist™) is a live trivalent nasally administered vaccine intended for active immunization for the prevention of influenza.

Each 0.5 mL dose is formulated to contain $10^{6.5\text{-}7.5}$ $TCID_{50}$ (median tissue culture infectious dose) of live attenuated influenza virus reassortants of the strains recommended by the U.S. Public Health Service (USPHS) for the 2004-2005 season: A/New Caledonia/20/99 (H1N1), A/Wyoming/3/2003 (H3N2) (A/Fujian/411/2002-like), and B/Jilin/20/2003 (B/Shanghai/361/2002-like) [1]. These strains are (a) *antigenically representative* of influenza viruses that may circulate in humans during the 2004-2005 influenza season; (b) *cold-adapted (ca)* (i.e., they replicate efficiently at 25°C, a temperature that is restrictive for replication of many wild-type viruses); (c) *temperature-sensitive (ts)* (i.e., they are restricted in replication at 37°C (Type B strains) or 39°C (Type A strains), temperatures at which many wild-type influenza viruses grow efficiently); and (d) *attenuated (att)* so as not to produce classic influenza-like illness in the ferret model of human influenza infection. The cumulative effect of the antigenic properties and the *ca, ts,* and *att* phenotype is that the attenuated vaccine viruses replicate in the nasopharynx to induce protective immunity.

Each of the three influenza virus strains contained in FluMist is a genetic reassortant of a Master Donor Virus (MDV) and a wild-type influenza virus. The MDVs (A/Ann Arbor/6/60 and B/Ann Arbor/1/66) were developed by serial passage at sequentially lower temperatures in specific pathogen-free (SPF) primary chick kidney cells [2]. During this process, the MDVs acquired the *ca, ts,* and *att* phenotype and multiple mutations in the gene segments that encode viral proteins other than the surface glycoproteins. The individual contribution of the genetic sequences of the six non-glycoprotein MDV genes ("internal gene segments") to the *ca, ts,* and *att* phenotype is not completely understood. However, for the Type A MDV, at least five genetic loci in three different internal gene segments contribute to the *ts* and *att* phenotype. For the Type B MDV, at least three genetic loci in two different internal gene segments contribute to both the *ts* and *att* properties; two additional genetic loci in a third gene segment also contribute to the *att* property. No evidence of reversion has been observed in the recovered vaccine strains that have been tested (135 of possible 250 recovered isolates) (see TRANSMISSION) [3, 4]. For each of the three strains in FluMist, the six internal gene segments responsible for *ca, ts,* and *att* phenotypes are derived from the MDV, and the two segments that encode the two surface glycoproteins, hemagglutinin (HA) and neuraminidase (NA), are derived from the corresponding antigenically relevant wild-type influenza viruses that have been recommended by the USPHS for inclusion in the annual vaccine formulation. Thus, the three viruses contained in FluMist maintain the replication characteristics and phenotypic properties of the MDV and express the HA and NA of wild-type viruses that are related to strains expected to circulate during the 2004-2005 influenza season.

Viral harvests used in the production of FluMist are produced by inoculating each of the three reassortant viruses into specific pathogen-free (SPF) eggs that are incubated to allow for vaccine virus replication. The allantoic fluid of these eggs is harvested, clarified by centrifugation, and stabilized with buffer containing sucrose, potassium phosphate, and monosodium glutamate (0.47 mg/dose). Viral harvests from the three strains (H1N1, H3N2, and B) are subsequently blended and diluted to desired potency with allantoic fluid derived from uninfected SPF eggs to produce trivalent bulk vaccine. Each lot of viral harvest is tested for *ca, ts,* and *att* and is also tested extensively by *in vitro* and *in vivo* methods to detect adventitious agents. The bulk vaccine is then filled directly into individual sprayers for nasal administration. These sprayers are labeled and stored at ≤−15°C.

Gentamicin sulfate is added early in the manufacturing process during preparation of reassortant viruses at a calculated concentration of approximately 1 μg/mL. Later steps of the manufacturing process do not use gentamicin, resulting in a diluted residual concentration in the final product of <0.015 μg/mL (limit of detection of the assay). FluMist does not contain any preservatives.

Each pre-filled FluMist sprayer contains a single 0.5 mL dose. The teflon tip attached to the sprayer is equipped with a one-way valve that produces a fine mist that is primarily deposited in the nose and nasopharynx. When thawed for administration, FluMist is a colorless to pale yellow liquid and is clear to slightly cloudy (see DOSAGE AND ADMINISTRATION).

CLINICAL PHARMACOLOGY

Influenza is a highly infectious respiratory viral infection that causes recurrent winter epidemics of acute disease in persons of all ages. Highest rates of illness are generally reported among 5-14 year-olds [5, 6]. Influenza-associated deaths have been reported in previously healthy children and young adults. Among healthy individuals 15-44 years of age, the average rate of excess hospitalizations attributable to influenza is 23-25 per 100,000 per year [7], with an annual influenza-associated mortality rate of 0.2-1.5 per 100,000 person-years [8].

Types A and B influenza viruses are the principal causes of influenza in humans. Type A influenza viruses are divided into subtypes on the basis of the two surface antigens, hemagglutinin (HA) and neuraminidase (NA), while influenza virus B is classified as a single subtype. Continuous mutation of the influenza virus genome leads to an accumulation of genetic and accompanying antigenic changes that result in the evolution of viruses into recognizable antigenic lineages or strains within a subtype. Protective immune responses following natural infection result in population-based immunity to circulating strains. However, this immune barrier eventually results in the emergence of strains that have undergone antigenic change, or "drift." Because these "drifted" strains can escape immunity to HA and NA antigens of previously circulating strains, vaccines may require annual updating to match the contemporary strains.

Vaccination is the principal means of prevention of influenza and influenza-associated complications [1].

Mechanism of Action

Immune mechanisms conferring protection against influenza following receipt of FluMist vaccine are not fully understood. Likewise, naturally acquired immunity to wild-type influenza has not been completely elucidated. Serum antibodies, mucosal antibodies and influenza-specific T cells may play a role in prevention and recovery from infection [9, 10]. Vaccination with FluMist has been demonstrated to induce influenza strain-specific serum antibodies [11, 12].

Clinical Studies

FluMist was administered to 20,228 subjects in clinical studies. The population evaluated included 10,297 healthy children 5-17 years of age (14,058 doses of FluMist received) and 3297 healthy adults 18-49 years of age (3335 doses of FluMist received) who received at least one dose of vaccine. Second and third annual doses have been given to 1766 and 128 children 5-17 years of age, respectively. In randomized, placebo-controlled trials, 4719 healthy children 5-17 years of age and 2864 healthy adults 18-49 years of age received FluMist.

The efficacy of FluMist against culture-confirmed influenza disease for Types A/H3N2 and B was assessed in a field trial in children. The effectiveness of FluMist against Types A/H3N2 and B, defined as a reduction in influenza-like illness and illness-associated health care utilization, was assessed in a field trial in adults. Type A/H1N1 did not circulate during either trial, and no field efficacy data against this strain are available.

Pediatric Study

The Pediatric Efficacy Study was a multi-center, randomized, double-blind, placebo-controlled trial performed in healthy U.S. children to evaluate the efficacy of FluMist against culture-confirmed influenza over two successive seasons [13, 14]. The primary endpoint for the first year of the trial was the prevention of culture-confirmed influenza illness due to antigenically matched wild-type influenza in healthy children who received two doses of vaccine. During the first year of the study a subset of 312 children 60-71 months of age were randomized 2:1 (vaccine:placebo). All children with culture-confirmed influenza experienced respiratory symptoms (cough, runny nose, or sore throat) and most experienced fever (68%), health care provider visits (68%), and missed school days (74%).

As shown in Table 1, when compared with placebo recipients, FluMist recipients 60-71 months of age who received two doses of vaccine (n=238) experienced a significant reduction in the incidence of culture-confirmed influenza (efficacy 87.4%, 95% CI: 59.4, 97.9). In the 60-71 month old age group, children who received one dose of FluMist when compared to one dose of placebo experienced a significant reduction in the incidence of culture-confirmed influenza (0 of 54 FluMist recipients vs 3 of 20 placebo recipients; efficacy 100%, 95% CI: 47.0, 100).

Approximately 85% of the participants in the first year returned for the second year of the Pediatric Efficacy Study, including a subset of 544 children 60-84 months of age [15]. During the second year of the trial, the H3N2 strain included in the vaccine was A/Wuhan/359/95, which was antigenically distinct from the A/Sydney/05/97 H3N2 strain that was the primary circulating strain. Type A/Wuhan/359/95 (H3N2) also circulated as did Type B strains. Children remained in the same treatment group as in year one and received a single dose of FluMist or placebo. The primary endpoint of the trial was the prevention of culture-confirmed influenza illness due to antigenically matched wild-type influenza after a single annual revaccination dose of FluMist. In the subset of 544 children 60-84 months of age, illness associated with culture-confirmed illness in the second year was similar in scope and severity to that in the first year.

The overall efficacy of FluMist against culture-confirmed wild-type influenza, regardless of antigenic match, was 86.9% (95% CI: 70.8, 94.1).

[See table 1 below]

Table 1
Efficacy of FluMist Against Culture-Confirmed Influenza in Children ≥60 Months of Age

Endpoint	Cases FluMist	Cases Placebo	Efficacy (%)	(95% CI)
	N=163	N=75		
Year One (60-71 mo of age)	n (%)	n (%)		
Culture-confirmed influenza[a]	3 (1.8)	11 (14.7)	**87.4**	(59.4, 97.9)*
	N=375	N=169		
Year Two (60-84 mo of age)	n (%)	n (%)		
Culture-confirmed influenza[a,b]	7 (1.9)	24 (14.2)	**86.9**	(70.8, 94.1)*

*Denotes statistically significant, p≤0.05.
[a] Overall efficacy against Type A (H3N2) and Type B wild-type viruses. Field efficacy against wild Type A (H1N1) viruses could not be determined because those strains did not circulate during the study period.
[b] Includes illness caused by A/Sydney/05/97 (H3N2), an antigenic variant not included in the vaccine.

Studies in Adults

The Adult Effectiveness Study was a multi-center, randomized, double-blind, placebo-controlled trial in which healthy adults were enrolled, including 3920 adults 18-49 years of age (2150 women and 1770 men). Participants were randomized 2:1, vaccine:placebo. The trial was designed to evaluate the effectiveness of FluMist in the reduction of influenza-like illness during the peak influenza outbreak period at each site, based on community surveillance [16]. Cultures for influenza virus were not obtained from subjects in the trial, so that the efficacy against culture-confirmed influenza was not assessed. The A/Wuhan/359/95 (H3N2) strain, which was contained in FluMist, was antigenically distinct from the predominant circulating strain of influenza virus during the trial period, A/Sydney/05/97 (H3N2). Type A/Wuhan (H3N2) and Type B strains also circulated in the U.S. during the study period. The primary endpoint of the trial was the reduction in the proportion of participants with one or more episodes of any febrile illness (AFI). Two other, more specific febrile influenza-like illness definitions were also prospectively assessed: severe febrile illness (SFI), and febrile upper respiratory illness (FURI). Adults were characterized as having AFI if they had symptoms for at least two consecutive days with fever on at least one day and if they had two or more symptoms (fever, chills, headache, runny nose, sore throat, cough, muscle aches, tiredness/weakness) on at least one day. SFI was defined as having at least three consecutive days of symptoms, at least one day of fever, and two or more symptoms on at least three days. FURI was defined as at least two consecutive days of upper respiratory infection (URI) symptoms (runny nose, sore throat, or cough), fever on at least one day, and at least two URI symptoms on at least one day. Adults meeting the three illness definitions often had associated health care provider visits (25-31%), used antibiotics (28-32%), and missed at least one day of work (51-58%).

During the seven-week site-specific outbreak period, in the subset of subjects age 18-49 years, FluMist recipients did not experience a significant reduction in AFI; significant reductions were observed for SFI and FURI (Table 2). An additional measure of the severity of disease was illness-associated days of health care provider visits; FluMist recipients experienced significant reductions in days of health care provider visits associated with SFI (17.8%, 95% CI: 2.0, 31.0), and FURI (36.9%, 95% CI: 24.4, 47.3) when compared to placebo recipients. However, no significant reduction in days of health care provider visits associated with AFI was observed among FluMist recipients when compared to placebo recipients.

[See table 2 at top of next page]

Challenge Study
The ability of FluMist to protect adults from influenza illness after challenge with wild-type influenza was assessed in a multi-center, randomized, double-blind, placebo-controlled trial in healthy adults 18-41 years of age who were serosusceptible to at least one strain included in the vaccine [12]. Adults were randomized to receive FluMist (n=29) or placebo (n=31). Each subject was challenged intranasally with only a single strain of wild-type virus (Type A/H3N2, Type A/H1N1 or Type B) to which he/she was serosusceptible, and the results were pooled for all three strains combined within each treatment group. Laboratory-documented influenza illness due to all three strains combined was reduced compared to placebo by 85% (95% CI: 28, 100) in FluMist recipients.

Transmission
FluMist contains live attenuated influenza viruses that must infect and replicate in cells lining the nasopharynx of the recipient to induce immunity. Vaccine viruses capable of infection and replication can be cultured from nasal secretions obtained from vaccine recipients. The relationship of viral replication in a vaccine recipient and transmission of vaccine viruses to other individuals has not been established.

A prospective, randomized, double-blind, placebo-controlled trial in a daycare setting in children less than three years of age was performed with the primary objective of assessing the probability that vaccine viruses will be transmitted from a vaccinated individual to a non-vaccinated individual [17]. Children enrolled in the study attended daycare at least three days per week for four hours per day, and were in a playroom with at least four children, at least one of whom was vaccinated with FluMist. A total of 197 children 8-36 months of age were randomized to receive one dose of FluMist (n=98) or placebo (n=99). Virus shedding was evaluated for 21 days by culture of nasal swab specimens obtained from each subject approximately three times per week. Wild-type A (H3N2) influenza virus was documented to have circulated in the community and in the study population during the trial, whereas Type A (H1N1) and Type B strains did not.

At least one vaccine strain was isolated from 80% of FluMist recipients. Viruses were recovered from specimens obtained over a range of 1-21 days (mean duration of 7.6 days ± 3.4 days). The cold-adapted *(ca)* and temperature-sensitive *(ts)* phenotypes were preserved in all recovered viruses tested (n=135 tested of 250 strains isolated at the local laboratory). Ten influenza isolates were cultured from a total of seven placebo subjects. One placebo subject became infected with a Type B virus confirmed as a transmitted vaccine virus by a FluMist recipient in the same playgroup. Of the 11 nasal swabs obtained from the subject on Days 0-21, vaccine virus was cultured only from the Day 15 specimen. This Type B isolate retained the *ca*, *ts*, and *att* phenotypes of the vaccine strain, and had the same genetic sequence when compared to a Type B virus cultured from a vaccine recipient within the same playgroup. This placebo recipient experienced cough, coryza, and irritability similar to the symptoms observed among some FluMist vaccinees in the trial. No viruses were cultured from any of the other placebo recipients in this playgroup. Nine isolates identified as Type A were cultured from six placebo subjects; two of these subjects had two cultures that grew Type A strains (four isolates) confirmed as wild-type A/Panama (H3N2). Type A isolates that could not be further characterized were cultured from the four remaining placebo subjects; because the isolates could not be further characterized, the possibility that they were vaccine strains could not be excluded.

Assuming that a single transmission event occurred (isolation of the Type B vaccine strain), the probability of a young child acquiring vaccine virus following close contact with a single FluMist vaccinee in this daycare setting was 0.58% (95% CI: 0, 1.7) based on the Reed Frost model [18]. With documented transmission of one Type B in one placebo subject and possible transmission of Type A viruses in four placebo subjects, the probability of acquiring a transmitted vaccine virus was estimated to be 2.4% (95% CI: 0.13, 4.6), using the Reed Frost model.

The duration of FluMist vaccine virus replication and the potential for transmission of vaccine viruses by recipients 5-49 years of age have not been established.

INDICATIONS AND USAGE

FOR NASAL ADMINISTRATION ONLY
FluMist is indicated for active immunization for the prevention of disease caused by influenza A and B viruses in healthy children and adolescents, 5-17 years of age, and healthy adults, 18-49 years of age.

FluMist is not indicated for immunization of individuals less than 5 years of age, or 50 years of age and older, or for therapy of influenza, nor will it protect against infections and illness caused by infectious agents other than influenza A or B viruses.

CONTRAINDICATIONS

Under no circumstances should FluMist™ be administered parenterally.
Individuals with a history of hypersensitivity, especially anaphylactic reactions, to any component of FluMist, including eggs or egg products, should not receive FluMist (see DESCRIPTION).

Table 2
Effectiveness of FluMist in Adults 18-49 Years of Age During the 7-week Site-Specific Outbreak Period

Endpoint	FluMist N=2411[a] n (%)	Placebo N=1226[a] n (%)	Percent Reduction	(95% CI)
Participants with one or more events of:[b]				
Any febrile illness	331 (13.73)	189 (15.42)	**10.9**	(-5.1, 24.4)
Severe febrile illness	250 (10.37)	158 (12.89)	**19.5**	(3.0, 33.2)*
Febrile upper respiratory illness	213 (8.83)	142 (11.58)	**23.7**	(6.7, 37.5)*

*Denotes p-value ≤0.05.
Note: The proportion of participants with any febrile illness (AFI) was the primary study endpoint; effectiveness was not demonstrated for this endpoint (p-value >0.05).
[a] Number of evaluable subjects (92.7% and 93.0% of FluMist and placebo recipients, respectively).
[b] The predominantly circulating virus during the trial period was A/Syndey/05/97 (H3N2), an antigenic variant not included in the vaccine.

FluMist is contraindicated in children and adolescents (5-17 years of age) receiving aspirin therapy or aspirin-containing therapy, because of the association of Reye syndrome with aspirin and wild-type influenza infection.

FluMist should not be administered to individuals who have a history of Guillain-Barré syndrome.

As with other live virus vaccines, FluMist should not be administered to individuals with known or suspected immune deficiency diseases such as combined immunodeficiency, agammaglobulinemia, and thymic abnormalities and conditions such as human immunodeficiency virus infection, malignancy, leukemia, or lymphoma. FluMist is also contraindicated in patients who may be immunosuppressed or have altered or compromised immune status as a consequence of treatment with systemic corticosteroids, alkylating drugs, antimetabolites, radiation, or other immunosuppressive therapies.

WARNINGS

The safety of FluMist in individuals with asthma or reactive airways disease has not been established. In a large safety study in children 1-17 years of age, children <5 years of age who received FluMist were found to have an increased rate of asthma within 42 days of vaccination when compared to placebo recipients (see ADVERSE REACTIONS). FluMist should not be administered to individuals with a history of asthma or reactive airways disease.

The safety of FluMist in individuals with underlying medical conditions that may predispose them to severe disease following wild-type influenza infection has not been established. FluMist is not indicated for these individuals. High-risk individuals include, but are not limited to, adults and children with chronic disorders of the cardiovascular and pulmonary systems, including asthma; pregnant women; adults and children who required regular medical follow-up or hospitalization during the preceding year because of chronic metabolic diseases (including diabetes), renal dysfunction, or hemoglobinopathies; and adults and children with congenital or acquired immunosuppression caused by underlying disease or immunosuppressive therapy (see CONTRAINDICATIONS). Intramuscularly administered inactivated influenza vaccines are available to immunize high-risk individuals [1].

As with any vaccine, FluMist may not protect 100% of individuals receiving the vaccine.

PRECAUTIONS

General
CARE IS TO BE TAKEN BY THE HEALTH CARE PROVIDER FOR THE SAFE AND EFFECTIVE USE OF THIS PRODUCT.

Prior to administration of FluMist, individuals or their parent/guardian should be asked about their current health status and their personal medical history, including immune status, to determine the existence of any contraindications to immunization with FluMist (see CONTRAINDICATIONS and WARNINGS) FluMist recipients should avoid close contact (e.g., within the same household) with immunocompromised individuals for at least 21 days.

EPINEPHRINE INJECTION (1:1000) OR COMPARABLE TREATMENT MUST BE READILY AVAILABLE IN THE EVENT OF AN ACUTE ANAPHYLACTIC REACTION FOLLOWING VACCINATION. The health care provider should ensure prevention of any allergic or other adverse reactions by reviewing the individual's history for possible sensitivity to influenza vaccine components, including eggs and egg products.

Administration of FluMist should be postponed until after the acute phase (at least 72 hours) of febrile and/or respiratory illnesses.

Information for Vaccine Recipients or Parents/Guardians
Vaccine recipients or their parents/guardians should be informed by the health care provider of the potential benefits and risks of FluMist, and the need for two doses for the first use of FluMist in 5-8 year olds. Due to the possible transmission of vaccine virus, vaccine recipients or their parents/guardians should be advised that vaccine recipients should avoid close contact (e.g., within the same household) with immunocompromised individuals for at least 21 days.

The vaccine recipient or the parent/guardian accompanying the vaccine recipient should be told to report any suspected adverse events to the physician or clinic where the vaccine was administered (see ADVERSE EVENT REPORTING).

Drug Interactions
Children or adolescents who are receiving aspirin therapy or aspirin-containing therapy should not receive FluMist (see CONTRAINDICATIONS). FluMist should not be administered to persons on immunosuppressive therapy.

The concurrent use of FluMist with antiviral compounds that are active against influenza A and/or B viruses has not been evaluated. However, based upon the potential for interference between such compounds and FluMist, it is advisable not to administer FluMist until 48 hours after the cessation of antiviral therapy and that antiviral agents not be administered until two weeks after administration of FluMist unless medically indicated.

There are no data regarding co-administration of FluMist with other intranasal preparations, including steroids.

Concurrent Administration with Other Vaccines
The safety and immunogenicity of FluMist when administered concurrently with other vaccines have not been determined. Therefore, FluMist should not be administered concurrently with other vaccines. Studies of FluMist in healthy individuals excluded subjects who received any live virus vaccine within one month of enrollment and any inactivated or subunit vaccine within two weeks of enrollment; therefore, health care providers should adhere to these intervals when administering FluMist.

Laboratory Interactions
Data related to the length of time that FluMist can be recovered from nasal specimens of children and adults are limited. Nasopharyngeal secretions or swabs collected from vaccinees may test positive for influenza virus for up to three weeks.

Carcinogenesis, Mutagenesis, Impairment of Fertility
FluMist has not been evaluated for its carcinogenic or mutagenic potential or its potential to impair fertility.

Pregnancy (Category C)
Animal reproduction studies have not been conducted with FluMist. It is also not known whether FluMist can cause fetal harm when administered to a pregnant woman or affect reproduction capacity. Therefore, FluMist should not be administered to pregnant women.

Nursing Mothers
It is not known whether FluMist is excreted in human milk. Therefore, as some viruses are excreted in human milk and additionally, because of the possibility of shedding of vaccine virus and the close proximity of a nursing infant and mother, caution should be exercised if FluMist is administered to nursing mothers.

Pediatric Use
The safety of FluMist in infants and children <60 months of age has not been established (see CLINICAL STUDIES, INDICATIONS AND USAGE, and ADVERSE REACTIONS).

Geriatric Use
Clinical studies with FluMist did not include sufficient numbers of adults age 65 years and older to determine if they respond differently from younger individuals. The safe use of FluMist in persons 65 years and older has not been established (see CLINICAL PHARMACOLOGY and DOSAGE AND ADMINISTRATION).

ADVERSE REACTIONS

See CLINICAL STUDIES for a description of the number of participants in clinical trials.

Serious Adverse Events
Across all clinical trials, serious adverse events (SAEs) were monitored after vaccination for 42 days in children and for 28 days in adults. SAEs occurred at a similar rate (<1%) in FluMist and placebo recipients for both healthy children and healthy adults.

Overall, across the placebo-controlled trials in adults and children, the incidence of selected adverse reactions that may be complications of wild-type influenza (such as pneumonia, bronchitis, bronchiolitis, or central nervous system events) was similar in FluMist and placebo groups.

Adverse Events in Placebo-Controlled Trials
In all placebo-controlled studies, allantoic fluid from uninfected eggs was used as the placebo. In randomized, placebo-controlled trials, 4719 healthy children 5-17 years of age and 2864 healthy adults 18-49 years of age received FluMist and 2327 healthy children and 1454 healthy adults received the placebo. In placebo-controlled clinical trials

Continued on next page

FluMist—Cont.

conducted in healthy populations, solicited adverse events and daily temperatures were collected on diary cards. These solicited events included runny nose/nasal congestion, sore throat, cough, irritability, headache, chills, vomiting, muscle aches, and decreased activity and a feeling of tiredness/weakness.

Solicited Adverse Events in Children

Table 3 shows an analysis of solicited events for the Pediatric Efficacy Study in the subset of healthy children 60-71 months of age. The largest absolute differences between FluMist and placebo after Dose One were observed in the incidences of headache and runny nose/nasal congestion. No differences were observed for fever (>100°F oral). Following Dose Two, the largest absolute differences between FluMist and placebo were runny nose/nasal congestion and cough. There was no significant increase in influenza-like illness (ILI) as defined by the CDC in the FluMist group compared to the placebo group. CDC has defined CDC-ILI as having fever (temperature ≥100°F oral) plus either cough or sore throat on the same day or on consecutive days.

[See table 3 below]

For the cohort of 128 children who received FluMist across three consecutive years, rates of solicited adverse events were not significantly increased when compared to placebo recipients [15].

Medically Attended Events in Children and Adolescents

A large randomized, double-blind, placebo-controlled trial in healthy children 1 through 17 years of age was conducted at 31 clinics in the Northern California Kaiser-Permanente Health Maintenance Organization (HMO) to assess the rate of medically attended events (MAEs) within 42 days of vaccination. Participants were randomized 2:1 (vaccine:placebo). A total of 6657 evaluable children 5-17 years of age were enrolled, including 3244 boys and 3413 girls. Of these 6657 children, 2606 were 5-8 years of age and 4051 were 9-17 years of age. Dose Two for children less than nine years of age was to be administered 28 to 42 days after Dose One. Data regarding MAEs were obtained from the Kaiser-Permanente computerized health care utilization databases for hospitalizations, emergency department visits and clinical visits. MAEs were analyzed individually and within four pre-specified grouped diagnoses: acute respiratory tract events, systemic bacterial infections, acute gastrointestinal tract events, and rare events potentially related to influenza. For these four pre-specified grouped diagnoses, no significant increase in risk for FluMist recipients was seen in the combined analyses across all utilization settings, doses, and age groups. Selected respiratory tract illnesses of special interest (pneumonia, bronchitis, bronchiolitis, and croup) were included in acute respiratory tract events and were not associated with increased risk for FluMist recipients in any protocol-specified analysis. No systemic bacterial infection occurred. In FluMist recipients, an increased risk was not observed for rare events that have been reported with naturally occurring influenza virus infection, including seizures, febrile seizures, and epilepsy. No cases of encephalitis, acute idiopathic polyneuritis (Guillain-Barré syndrome), Reye syndrome, or myocarditis (influenza-associated rare disorders) were reported in this study.

In this study, in individuals 5-17 years of age, four individual MAEs were significantly increased and 11 were significantly decreased. Of the four individual MAEs associated with increased risk, a biological association with FluMist is plausible for one: abdominal pain. Of the 11 individual MAEs associated with decreased risk, a biologically plausible association with FluMist exists for seven: asthma, bronchitis, conjunctivitis, cough, viral syndrome, otitis media, and wheezing/shortness of breath. However, in the same study, a statistically significant increase in asthma or reactive airways disease was observed for children 12-59 months of age following Dose One (Relative Risk 3.53, 90% CI: 1.1,15.7). As a result of this finding, FluMist is not indicated for children <60 months of age.

Solicited Adverse Events in Adults

In the placebo-controlled Adult Effectiveness Study, the rates of solicited adverse events in the subset of healthy adults 18-49 years of age are shown in Table 4. Statistically significant differences were observed for any event, cough, runny nose, sore throat, chills, and tiredness/weakness. Fever >100°F was similar in FluMist and placebo recipients after a single dose. There was no significant increase in influenza-like illness (ILI) as defined by the CDC in the FluMist group compared to the placebo group.

Table 4
Summary of Solicited Events Observed within 7 Days after Each Dose for Vaccine and Placebo Recipients; Healthy Adults 18-49 Years of Age

	FluMist N=2548[a]	Placebo N=1290[a]
Event	%	%
Any event	71.9*	62.6
Cough	13.9*	10.8
Runny Nose	44.5*	27.1
Sore Throat	27.8*	17.1
Headache	40.4	38.4
Chills	8.6*	6.0
Muscle Aches	16.7	14.6
Tiredness/Weakness	25.7*	21.6
Fever		
Oral Temp >100°F	1.5	1.3
Oral Temp >101°F	0.5	0.7
Oral Temp >102°F	0.1	0.2
Oral Temp >103°F	0.0	0.0

*Denotes statistically significant p-value ≤0.05; no adjustments for multiple comparisons; Fisher's exact method.
[a] Number of evaluable subjects (those who returned diary cards). [97.9% of FluMist recipients and 97.9% of placebo recipients.]

Other Adverse Events in Children and Adults

In addition to the solicited events, parents of subjects in the Pediatric Efficacy Trial also reported other adverse events that occurred during the course of the trial. Among healthy children age 60-71 months, the events that occurred in at least 1% of FluMist recipients and at a higher rate compared to placebo were: abdominal pain (3.7% FluMist vs 0% placebo), otitis media (1.4% FluMist vs 0% placebo), accidental injury (2.3% FluMist vs 2.1% placebo), diarrhea (3.7% FluMist vs 1.1% placebo), following Dose One and otitis media (3.1% FluMist vs 1.3% placebo) following Dose Two. None of these differences were statistically significant.

In addition to the solicited events, adults who participated in the Adult Effectiveness Study also reported other adverse events that occurred during the course of the clinical trial. For adults 18-49 years of age in the Adult Effectiveness Study, nasal congestion (9.2% FluMist vs 2.2% placebo), rhinitis (6.3% FluMist vs 3.1% placebo), and sinusitis (4.1% FluMist vs 2.2% placebo) were reported significantly more often by FluMist recipients compared to placebo recipients.

Adverse events reported post-licensure have included nausea, rash, hypersensitivity reactions (including anaphylaxis, facial edema, and urticaria). These events occurred at similar rates in FluMist versus placebo recipients in prelicensure studies.

Table 3
Summary of Solicited Events Observed within 10 Days after Each Dose for Vaccine and Placebo Recipients; Healthy Children 60-71 Months of Age

	Post-Dose One		Post-Dose Two	
	FluMist 214[a]	Placebo 95[a]	FluMist 161[a]	Placebo 75[a]
Event	%	%	%	%
Any event	65.4	61.4	66.5	53.3
Cough	26.8	32.7	38.5	30.7
Runny Nose/Nasal Congestion	48.1	44.2	46.0	32.0
Sore Throat	12.6	19.8	9.3	16.0
Irritability	19.5	16.8	9.9	9.3
Headache	17.8	11.6	6.8	16.0
Chills	6.1	5.3	2.5	4.0
Vomiting	4.7	3.2	5.6	12.0
Muscle Aches	6.1	4.2	5.0	4.0
Decreased Activity	14.0	12.6	10.6	13.3
Fever[b]				
Temp 1	9.5	9.9	4.3	4.0
Temp 2	2.2	2.0	0.6	1.3
Temp 3	0.0	0.0	0.0	0.0

Note: There were no statistically significant differences in any of these events (p-value >0.05); Fisher's exact method.
[a] Number of evaluable subjects (those who returned diary cards) for each event.
[b] Fever
Temp 1: Oral >100°F, rectal or aural >100.6°F, or axillary >99.6°F.
Temp 2: Oral >102°F, rectal or aural >102.6°F, or axillary >101.6°F.
Temp 3: Oral >104°F, rectal or aural >104.6°F, or axillary >103.6°F.

Annually, 20-40 cases of Guillain-Barré syndrome (GBS) that occur within 42 days of administration of inactivated influenza vaccine are reported to VAERS. In 2003-2004, one case of GBS with temporal association with FluMist was reported. Evidence of a causal relationship between influenza vaccines, including FluMist, has not been established.

Guillain-Barré Syndrome and Influenza Vaccines

The 1976 swine influenza vaccine was associated with an increased frequency of Guillain-Barré syndrome (GBS). Among persons who received the swine influenza vaccine in 1976, the rate of GBS that exceeded the background rate was <10 cases/1 million persons vaccinated with the risk for influenza vaccine-associated GBS higher among persons aged >25 years than persons <25 years. Evidence for a causal relation of GBS with subsequent vaccines prepared from other influenza viruses is unclear. Obtaining strong epidemiologic evidence for a possible limited increase in risk is difficult for such a rare condition as GBS, which has an annual incidence of 10-20 cases/1 million adults. Thus, investigations to date indicate no substantial increase GBS associated with influenza vaccines (other than the swine influenza vaccine in 1976), and that, if influenza vaccine does pose a risk, it is probably slightly more than one additional case/1 million persons vaccinated. Cases of GBS after influenza infection have been reported, but no epidemiologic studies have documented such an association [1].

The incidence of GBS among the general population is low, but persons with a history of GBS have a substantially greater likelihood of subsequently experiencing GBS than persons without such a history. Thus, the likelihood of coincidentally experiencing GBS after influenza vaccination is expected to be greater among persons with a history of GBS than among persons with no history of this syndrome [1].

ADVERSE EVENT REPORTING

Reporting by vaccine recipients or the parents/guardians of vaccinees and health care providers of all adverse events occurring after vaccine administration is encouraged. The U.S. Department of Health and Human Services (DHHS) has established a Vaccine Adverse Event Reporting System (VAERS) to accept all reports of suspected adverse events after the administration of any vaccine. The VAERS toll-free number is 1-800-822-7967. Reporting forms may also be obtained at the FDA Web site at: http://www.vaers.org.

DOSAGE AND ADMINISTRATION

FOR NASAL USE ONLY. DO NOT ADMINISTER PARENTERALLY.

FluMist™ should be administered according to the following schedule:

Age Group	Vaccination Status	Dosage Schedule
Children age 5 years through 8 years	Not previously vaccinated with FluMist	2 doses (0.5 mL each, 60 days apart ± 14 days) for initial season
Children age 5 years through 8 years	Previously vaccinated with FluMist	1 dose (0.5 mL) per season
Children and Adults age 9 through 49 years	Not applicable	1 dose (0.5 mL) per season

For healthy children age 5 years through 8 years who have not previously received FluMist vaccine, the recommended dosage schedule for nasal administration is one 0.5 mL dose followed by a second 0.5 mL dose given at least 6 weeks later. Only limited data are available on the degree of protection in children who receive one dose (see CLINICAL PHARMACOLOGY).

For all other healthy individuals, including children age 5-8 years who have previously received at least one dose of FluMist, the recommended schedule is one dose.

FluMist should be administered prior to exposure to influenza. The peak of influenza activity is variable from year to year, but generally occurs in the U.S. between late December and early March. Because the duration of protection induced by FluMist over multiple seasons is not known and yearly antigenic variation in the influenza strains is possible, annual revaccination may increase the likelihood of protection.

FluMist must be thawed prior to administration. FluMist may be thawed by holding the sprayer in the palm of the hand and supporting the plunger rod with the thumb (see ADMINISTRATION INSTRUCTIONS); the vaccine should be administered immediately thereafter. Alternatively, FluMist may be thawed in a refrigerator and stored at 2-8°C (36-46°F) for no more than 60 hours prior to use. When thawed for administration, FluMist is a colorless to pale yellow liquid and is clear to slightly cloudy; some proteinaceous particulates may be present but do not affect the use of the product.

Approximately 0.25 mL (i.e., half of the dose from a single FluMist sprayer) is administered into each nostril while the recipient is in an upright position. Insert the tip of the sprayer just inside the nose and depress the plunger to spray. The dose-divider clip is removed from the sprayer to administer the second half of the dose (approximately 0.25 mL) into the other nostril. Once FluMist has been ad-

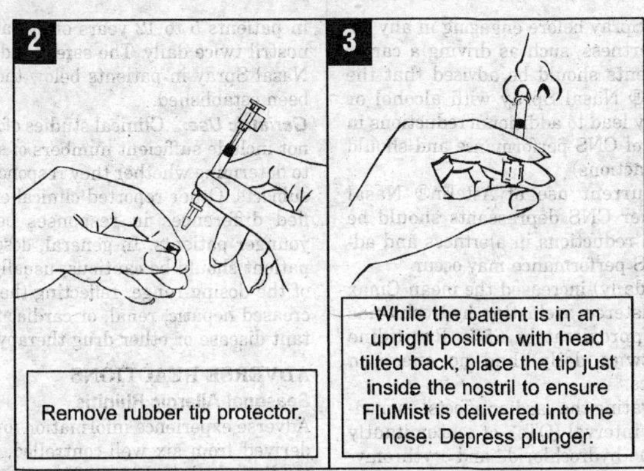

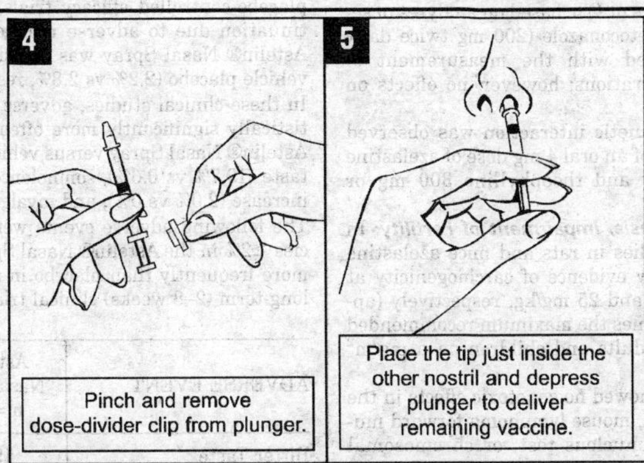

ministered, the used sprayer should be disposed of according to the standard procedures for biohazardous waste products.

ADMINISTRATION INSTRUCTIONS

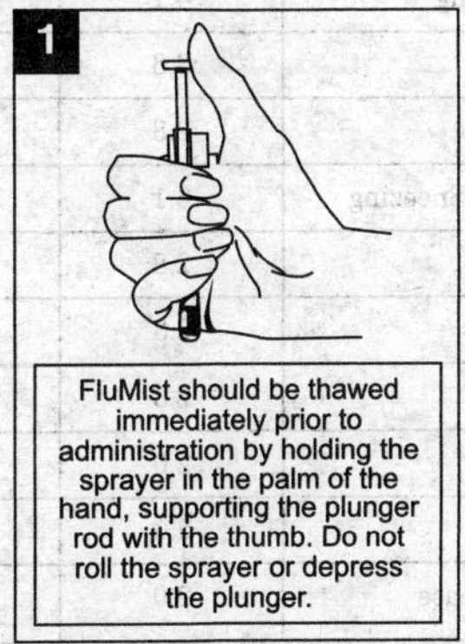

1
FluMist should be thawed immediately prior to administration by holding the sprayer in the palm of the hand, supporting the plunger rod with the thumb. Do not roll the sprayer or depress the plunger.

[See figures 2 and 3 above]
[See figures 4 and 5 above]

HOW SUPPLIED

FluMist is supplied for intranasal delivery in a package of 10 pre-filled, single-use sprayers (NDC 66019-101-01).

STORAGE

STORE AT OR BELOW −15°C (5°F).

DO NOT REFREEZE AFTER THAWING.

UPON RECEIPT, FluMist SHOULD BE IMMEDIATELY STORED AT −15°C (5°F) OR BELOW.

FluMist may be stored in a non-frost-free freezer to be maintained continuously at −15°C (5°F) or below.

Storage of FluMist in a frost-free freezer should be avoided because the temperature could cycle above −15°C (5°F) and can therefore negatively impact the stability of the product.

FluMist may be thawed in a refrigerator and stored at 2-8°C (36-46°F) for no more than 60 hours prior to use.

The cold chain must be maintained when transporting FluMist prior to use.

For information regarding product storage and stability under conditions other than those recommended, call 1-877-FLUMIST.

REFERENCES

1. Centers for Disease Control and Prevention. Prevention and control of Influenza: recommendations of the Advisory Committee on Immunization Practices (ACIP). *MMWR*. 2004;53 (Early release) (No. RR-6):1-40.
2. Murphy BR, Coelingh KC. Principles underlying the development and use of live attenuated cold-adapted influenza A and influenza B virus vaccines. *Viral Immunol*. 2002;15:295-323.
3. Jin H, et al. Multiple amino acid residues confer temperature sensitivity to human influenza virus vaccine strains (FluMist) derived from cold-adapted A/Ann Arbor/6/60. *Virology*. 2003;306:18-24.
4. Hoffmann, et al. Molecular basis for temperature sensitivity and attenuation of the human vaccine strain B/Ann Arbor/1/66. Presented at the International Conference on Options for the Control of Influenza V, (Okinawa, Japan). 2003.
5. Monto AS, Sullivan KM. Acute respiratory illness in the community. Frequency of illness and the agents involved. *Epidemiol Infect*. 1993;110:145-160.
6. Sullivan KM. Health impact of influenza in the United States. *Pharmacoeconomics*. 1996;9 Suppl. 3:26-33.
7. Barker WH, Mullooly JP. Impact of epidemic Type A influenza in a defined adult population. *Am J Epi*. 1980;112:798-811.
8. Thompson WW, et al. Mortality associated with influenza and respiratory syncytial virus in the United States. *JAMA*. 2003;289:179-186.
9. Murphy BR, Clements ML. The systemic and mucosal immune response of humans to influenza A virus. *Curr Topics in Micro Immun*. 1989;146:107-116.
10. McMichael AJ, et al. Cytotoxic T-cell immunity to influenza. *N Engl J Med*. 1983;309:13-17.
11. Belshe RB, et al. Correlates of immune protection induced by live, attenuated, cold-adapted, trivalent, intranasal influenza virus vaccine. *J Infect Dis*. 2000a;181:1133-1137.
12. Treanor JJ, et al. Evaluation of trivalent, live, cold-adapted (CAIV-T) and inactivated (TIV) influenza vaccines in prevention of virus infection and illness following challenge of adults with wild-type influenza A (H1N1), A (H3N2), and B viruses. *Vaccine*. 2000;18:899-906.
13. Belshe RB, et al. The efficacy of live attenuated, cold-adapted, trivalent, intranasal influenza virus vaccine in children. *N Engl J Med*. 1998;338:1405-1412.
14. Belshe RB, et al. Efficacy of vaccination with live attenuated, cold-adapted, trivalent, intranasal influenza virus vaccine against a variant (A/Sydney) not contained in the vaccine. *J Peds*. 2000b;136:168-175.
15. MedImmune data on file.
16. Nichol KL, et al. Effectiveness of live, attenuated intranasal influenza virus vaccine in healthy, working adults. *JAMA*. 1999;282:137-144.
17. Vesikari T, et al. A randomized, double-blind, placebo-controlled trial of the safety, transmissibility and phenotypic stability of a live, attenuated, cold-adapted influenza virus vaccine (CAIV-T) in children attending day care. Presented at the 41st Annual Interscience Conference on Antimicrobial Agents and Chemotherapy (Chicago, IL). 2001.
18. Longini IM, et al. Estimating household and community transmission parameters for influenza. *Am J Epidemiol*. 1982;115:736-751.

Manufactured and Marketed by:
MedImmune Vaccines, Inc.
Gaithersburg, MD 20878
MedImmune
Vaccines, Inc.
Component No. FLU04-072
Issue Date: September 2004
U.S. Govt. License No. 1652

Shown in Product Identification Guide, page 322

MedPointe Pharmaceuticals
MedPointe Healthcare Inc.
SOMERSET, NJ 08873

For Medical Information, Contact:
Generally:
Medical Information
800-526-3840
After Hours and Weekend Emergencies:
800-526-3840

MedPointe Pharmaceuticals
MedPointe Healthcare Inc.
Sales and Ordering
Somerset, NJ 08873

ASTELIN®
(azelastine hydrochloride)
Nasal Spray, 137 mcg
IN-023S6-02
For Intranasal Use Only

DESCRIPTION

Astelin® (azelastine hydrochloride) Nasal Spray, 137 micrograms (mcg), is an antihistamine formulated as a metered-spray solution for intranasal administration. Azelastine hydrochloride occurs as a white, almost odorless, crystalline powder with a bitter taste. It has a molecular weight of 418.37. It is sparingly soluble in water, methanol, and propylene glycol and slightly soluble in ethanol, octanol, and glycerine. It has a melting point of about 225°C and the pH of a saturated solution is between 5.0 and 5.4. Its chemical name is (±)-1-(2H)-phthalazinone,4-[(4-chlorophenyl) methyl]-2-(hexahydro-1-methyl-1H-azepin-4-yl)-, monohydrochloride. Its molecular formula is $C_{22}H_{24}ClN_3O \cdot HCl$ with the following chemical structure:

Astelin® Nasal Spray contains 0.1% azelastine hydrochloride in an aqueous solution at pH 6.8 ± 0.3. It also contains benzalkonium chloride (125 mcg/mL), edetate disodium, hypromellose, citric acid, dibasic sodium phosphate, sodium chloride, and purified water.

After priming, each metered spray delivers a 0.137 mL mean volume containing 137 mcg of azelastine hydrochloride (equivalent to 125 mcg of azelastine base). The bottle can deliver 200 metered sprays.

CLINICAL PHARMACOLOGY

Azelastine hydrochloride, a phthalazinone derivative, exhibits histamine H_1-receptor antagonist activity in isolated tissues, animal models, and humans. Astelin® Nasal Spray is administered as a racemic mixture with no difference in pharmacologic activity noted between the enantiomers in *in vitro* studies. The major metabolite, desmethylazelastine, also possesses H_1-receptor antagonist activity.

Pharmacokinetics and Metabolism

After intranasal administration, the systemic bioavailability of azelastine hydrochloride is approximately 40%. Maximum plasma concentrations (Cmax) are achieved in 2–3 hours. Based on intravenous and oral administration, the elimination half-life, steady-state volume of distribution, and plasma clearance are 22 hours, 14.5 L/kg, and 0.5 L/h/kg, respectively. Approximately 75% of an oral dose of radiolabeled azelastine hydrochloride was excreted in the feces with less than 10% as unchanged azelastine. Azelastine is oxidatively metabolized to the principal active metabolite, desmethylazelastine, by the cytochrome P450 enzyme system. The specific P450 isoforms responsible for the biotransformation of azelastine have not been identified; however, clinical interaction studies with the known CYP3A4 inhibitor erythromycin failed to demonstrate a pharmacokinetic interaction. In a multiple-dose, steady-state drug interaction study in normal volunteers, cimetidine (400 mg twice daily), a nonspecific P450 inhibitor, raised orally administered mean azelastine (4 mg twice daily) concentrations by approximately 65%.

The major active metabolite, desmethylazelastine, was not measurable (below assay limits) after single-dose intranasal administration of azelastine hydrochloride. After intranasal dosing of azelastine hydrochloride to steady-state, plasma concentrations of desmethylazelastine range from 20–50% of azelastine concentrations. When azelastine hydrochloride is administered orally, desmethylazelastine has an elimination half-life of 54 hours. Limited data indicate that the metabolite profile is similar when azelastine hydrochloride is administered via the intranasal or oral route.

In vitro studies with human plasma indicate that the plasma protein binding of azelastine and desmethylazelastine are approximately 88% and 97%, respectively.

Continued on next page

Astelin—Cont.

Azelastine hydrochloride administered intranasally at doses above two sprays per nostril twice daily for 29 days resulted in greater than proportional increases in Cmax and area under the curve (AUC) for azelastine.
Studies in healthy subjects administered oral doses of azelastine hydrochloride demonstrated linear responses in Cmax and AUC.

Special Populations
Following oral administration, pharmacokinetic parameters were not influenced by age, gender, or hepatic impairment. Based on oral, single-dose studies, renal insufficiency (creatinine clearance <50 mL/min) resulted in a 70–75% higher Cmax and AUC compared to normal subjects. Time to maximum concentration was unchanged.
Oral azelastine has been safely administered to over 1400 asthmatic subjects, supporting the safety of administering Astelin® Nasal Spray to allergic rhinitis patients with asthma.

Pharmacodynamics
In a placebo-controlled study (95 subjects with allergic rhinitis), there was no evidence of an effect of Astelin® Nasal Spray (2 sprays per nostril twice daily for 56 days) on cardiac repolarization as represented by the corrected QT interval (QTc) of the electrocardiogram. At higher oral exposures (≥4 mg twice daily), a nonclinically significant mean change on the QTc (3–7 millisecond increase) was observed.
Interaction studies investigating the cardiac repolarization effects of concomitantly administered oral azelastine hydrochloride and erythromycin or ketoconazole were conducted. Oral erythromycin had no effect on azelastine pharmacokinetics or QTc based on analysis of serial electrocardiograms. Ketoconazole interfered with the measurement of azelastine plasma levels; however, no effects on QTc were observed (see PRECAUTIONS, Drug Interactions).

Clinical Trials
U.S. placebo-controlled clinical trials of Astelin® Nasal Spray included 322 patients with seasonal allergic rhinitis who received two sprays per nostril twice a day for up to 4 weeks. These trials included 55 pediatric patients ages 12 to 16 years. Astelin® Nasal Spray significantly improved a complex of symptoms, which included rhinorrhea, sneezing, and nasal pruritus.
In dose-ranging trials, Astelin® Nasal Spray administration resulted in a decrease in symptoms, which reached statistical significance from saline placebo within 3 hours after initial dosing and persisted over the 12-hour dosing interval.
There were no findings on nasal examination in an 8-week study that suggested any adverse effect of azelastine on the nasal mucosa.
Two hundred sixteen patients with vasomotor rhinitis received Astelin® Nasal Spray two sprays per nostril twice a day in two U.S. placebo controlled trials. These patients had vasomotor rhinitis for at least one year, negative skin tests to indoor and outdoor aeroallergens, negative nasal smears for eosinophils, and negative sinus X-rays, Astelin® Nasal Spray significantly improved a symptom complex comprised of rhinorrhea, post nasal drip, nasal congestion, and sneezing.

INDICATIONS AND USAGE
Astelin® Nasal Spray is indicated for the treatment of the symptoms of seasonal allergic rhinitis such as rhinorrhea, sneezing, and nasal pruritus in adults and children 5 years and older, and for the treatment of the symptoms of vasomotor rhinitis, such as rhinorrhea, nasal congestion and postnasal drip in adults and children 12 years and older.

CONTRAINDICATIONS
Astelin® Nasal Spray is contraindicated in patients with a known hypersensitivity to azelastine hydrochloride or any of its components.

PRECAUTIONS
Activities Requiring Mental Alertness: In clinical trials, the occurrence of somnolence has been reported in some patients taking Astelin® Nasal Spray; due caution should therefore be exercised when driving a car or operating potentially dangerous machinery. Concurrent use of Astelin® Nasal Spray with alcohol or other CNS depressants should be avoided because additional reductions in alertness and additional impairment of CNS performance may occur.
Information for Patients: Patients should be instructed to use Astelin® Nasal Spray only as prescribed. For the proper use of the nasal spray and to attain maximum improvement, the patient should read and follow carefully the accompanying patient instructions. Patients should be instructed to prime the delivery system before initial use and after storage for 3 or more days (see PATIENT INSTRUCTIONS FOR USE). Patients should also be instructed to store the bottle upright at room temperature with the pump tightly closed and out of the reach of children. In case of accidental ingestion by a young child, seek professional assistance or contact a poison control center immediately.
Patients should be advised against the concurrent use of Astelin® Nasal Spray with other antihistamines without consulting a physician. Patients who are, or may become, pregnant should be told that this product should be used in pregnancy or during lactation only if the potential benefit justifies the potential risks to the fetus or nursing infant. Patients should be advised to assess their individual responses to Astelin® Nasal Spray before engaging in any activity requiring mental alertness, such as driving a car or operating machinery. Patients should be advised that the concurrent use of Astelin® Nasal Spray with alcohol or other CNS depressants may lead to additional reductions in alertness and impairment of CNS performance and should be avoided (see Drug Interactions).
Drug Interactions: Concurrent use of Astelin® Nasal Spray with alcohol or other CNS depressants should be avoided because additional reductions in alertness and additional impairment of CNS performance may occur.
Cimetidine (400 mg twice daily) increased the mean Cmax and AUC of orally administered azelastine hydrochloride (4 mg twice daily) by approximately 65%. Ranitidine hydrochloride (150 mg twice daily) had no effect on azelastine pharmacokinetics.
Interaction studies investigating the cardiac effects, as measured by the corrected QT interval (QTc), of concomitantly administered oral azelastine hydrochloride and erythromycin or ketoconazole were conducted. Oral erythromycin (500 mg three times daily for seven days) had no effect on azelastine pharmacokinetics or QTc based on analyses of serial electrocardiograms. Ketoconazole (200 mg twice daily for seven days) interfered with the measurement of azelastine plasma concentrations; however, no effects on QTc were observed.
No significant pharmacokinetic interaction was observed with the coadministration of an oral 4 mg dose of azelastine hydrochloride twice daily and theophylline 300 mg or 400 mg twice daily.
Carcinogenesis, Mutagenesis, Impairment of Fertility: In 2 year carcinogenicity studies in rats and mice azelastine hydrochloride did not show evidence of carcinogenicity at oral doses up to 30 mg/kg and 25 mg/kg, respectively (approximately 240 and 100 times the maximum recommended daily intranasal dose in adults and children on a mg/m^2 basis).
Azelastine hydrochloride showed no genotoxic effects in the Ames test, DNA repair test, mouse lymphoma forward mutation assay, mouse micronucleus test, or chromosomal aberration test in rat bone marrow.
Reproduction and fertility studies in rats showed no effects on male or female fertility at oral doses up to 30 mg/kg (approximately 240 times the maximum recommended daily intranasal dose in adults on a mg/m^2 basis). At 68.6 mg/kg (approximately 560 times the maximum recommended daily intranasal dose in adults on a mg/m^2 basis), the duration of estrous cycles was prolonged and copulatory activity and the number of pregnancies were decreased. The numbers of corpora lutea and implantations were decreased; however, pre-implantation loss was not increased.
Pregnancy Category C: Azelastine hydrochloride has been shown to cause developmental toxicity. Treatment of mice with an oral dose of 68.6 mg/kg (approximately 280 times the maximum recommended daily intranasal dose in adults on a mg/m^2 basis) caused embryo-fetal death, malformations (cleft palate; short or absent tail; fused, absent or branched ribs), delayed ossification and decreased fetal weight. This dose also caused maternal toxicity as evidenced by decreased body weight. Neither fetal nor maternal effects occurred at a dose of 3 mg/kg (approximately 10 times the maximum recommended daily intranasal dose in adults on a mg/m^2 basis).
In rats, an oral dose of 30 mg/kg (approximately 240 times the maximum recommended daily intranasal dose in adults on a mg/m^2 basis) caused malformations (oligo-and brachydactylia), delayed ossification and skeletal variations, in the absence of maternal toxicity. At 68.6 mg/kg (approximately 560 times the maximum recommended daily intranasal dose in adults on a mg/m^2 basis) azelastine hydrochloride also caused embryo-fetal death and decreased fetal weight; however, the 68.6 mg/kg dose caused severe maternal toxicity. Neither fetal nor maternal effects occurred at a dose of 3 mg/kg (approximately 25 times the maximum recommended daily intranasal dose in adults on a mg/m^2 basis).
In rabbits, oral doses of 30 mg/kg and greater (approximately 500 times the maximum recommended daily intranasal dose in adults on a mg/m^2 basis) caused abortion, delayed ossification and decreased fetal weight; however, these doses also resulted in severe maternal toxicity. Neither fetal nor maternal effects occurred at a dose of 0.3 mg/kg (approximately 5 times the maximum recommended daily intranasal dose in adults on a mg/m^2 basis).
There are no adequate and well-controlled clinical studies in pregnant women. Astelin® Nasal Spray should be used during pregnancy only if the potential benefit justifies the potential risk to the fetus.
Nursing Mothers: It is not known whether azelastine hydrochloride is excreted in human milk. Because many drugs are excreted in human milk, caution should be exercised when Astelin® Nasal Spray is administered to a nursing woman.
Pediatric Use: The safety and effectiveness of Astelin® Nasal Spray at a dose of 1 spray per nostril twice daily has been established for patients 5 through 11 years of age for the treatment of symptoms of seasonal allergic rhinitis. The safety of this dosage of Astelin® Nasal Spray was established in well-controlled studies of this dose in 176 patients 5 to 12 years of age treated for up to 6 weeks. The efficacy of Astelin® Nasal Spray at this dose is based on an extrapolation of the finding of efficacy in adults, on the likelihood that the disease course, pathophysiology and response to treatment are substantially similar in children compared to adults, and on supportive data from controlled clinical trials in patients 5 to 12 years of age at the dose of 1 spray per nostril twice daily. The safety and effectiveness of Astelin® Nasal Spray in patients below the age of 5 years have not been established.
Geriatric Use: Clinical studies of Astelin® Nasal Spray did not include sufficient numbers of subjects aged 65 and over to determine whether they respond differently from younger subjects. Other reported clinical experience has not identified differences in responses between the elderly and younger patients. In general, dose selection for an elderly patient should be cautious, usually starting at the low end of the dosing range, reflecting the greater frequency of decreased hepatic, renal, or cardiac function, and of concomitant disease or other drug therapy.

ADVERSE REACTIONS
Seasonal Allergic Rhinitis
Adverse experience information for Astelin® Nasal Spray is derived from six well-controlled, 2-day to 8-week clinical studies which included 391 patients who received Astelin® Nasal Spray at a dose of 2 sprays per nostril twice daily. In placebo-controlled efficacy trials, the incidence of discontinuation due to adverse reactions in patients receiving Astelin® Nasal Spray was not significantly different from vehicle placebo (2.2% vs 2.8%, respectively).
In these clinical studies, adverse events that occurred statistically significantly more often in patients treated with Astelin® Nasal Spray versus vehicle placebo included bitter taste (19.7% vs 0.6%), somnolence (11.5% vs 5.4%), weight increase (2.0% vs 0%), and myalgia (1.5% vs 0%).
The following adverse events were reported with frequencies ≥2% in the Astelin® Nasal Spray treatment group and more frequently than placebo in short-term (≤2 days) and long-term (2–8 weeks) clinical trials.

ADVERSE EVENT	Astelin® Nasal Spray n = 391	Vehicle Placebo n = 353
Bitter Taste	19.7	0.6
Headache	14.8	12.7
Somnolence	11.5	5.4
Nasal Burning	4.1	1.7
Pharyngitis	3.8	2.8
Dry Mouth	2.8	1.7
Paroxysmal Sneezing	3.1	1.1
Nausea	2.8	1.1
Rhinitis	2.3	1.4
Fatigue	2.3	1.4
Dizziness	2.0	1.4
Epistaxis	2.0	1.4
Weight Increase	2.0	0.0

A total of 176 patients 5 to 12 years of age were exposed to Astelin® Nasal Spray at a dose of 1 spray each nostril twice daily in 3 placebo-controlled studies. In these studies, adverse events that occurred more frequently in patients treated with Astelin® Nasal Spray than with placebo, and that were not represented in the adult adverse event table above include rhinitis/cold symptoms (17.0% vs 9.5%), cough (11.4% vs 8.3%), conjunctivitis (5.1% vs 1.8%), and asthma (4.5% vs 4.1%).
The following events were observed infrequently (<2% and exceeding placebo incidence) in patients who received Astelin® Nasal Spray (2 sprays/nostril twice daily) in U.S. clinical trials.
Cardiovascular: flushing, hypertension, tachycardia.
Dermatological: contact dermatitis, eczema, hair and follicle infection, furunculosis.
Digestive: constipation, gastroenteritis, glossitis, ulcerative stomatitis, vomiting, increased SGPT, aphthous stomatitis.
Metabolic and Nutritional: increased appetite.
Musculoskeletal: myalgia, temporomandibular dislocation.
Neurological: hyperkinesia, hypoesthesia, vertigo.
Psychological: anxiety, depersonalization, depression, nervousness, sleep disorder, thinking abnormal.
Respiratory: bronchospasm, coughing, throat burning, laryngitis.
Special Senses: conjunctivitis, eye abnormality, eye pain, watery eyes, taste loss.
Urogenital: albuminuria, amenorrhea, breast pain, hematuria, increased urinary frequency.
Whole Body: allergic reaction, back pain, herpes simplex, viral infection, malaise, pain in extremities, abdominal pain.

ADVERSE REACTIONS
Vasomotor Rhinitis
Adverse experience information for Astelin® Nasal Spray is derived from two placebo-controlled clinical studies which included 216 patients who received Astelin® Nasal Spray at a dose of 2 sprays per nostril twice daily for up to 28 days.

The incidence of discontinuation due to adverse reactions in patients receiving Astelin® Nasal Spray was not different from vehicle placebo (2.8% vs 2.9%, respectively).
The following adverse events were reported with frequencies ≥2% in the Astelin® Nasal Spray treatment group and more frequently than placebo.

ADVERSE EVENT	Astelin® Nasal Spray n = 216	Vehicle Placebo n = 210
Bitter Taste	19.4	2.4
Headache	7.9	7.6
Dysesthesia	7.9	3.3
Rhinitis	5.6	2.4
Epistaxis	3.2	2.4
Sinusitis	3.2	1.9
Somnolence	3.2	1.0

Events observed infrequently (<2% and exceeding placebo incidence) in patients who received Astelin® Nasal Spray (2 sprays/nostril twice daily) in U.S. clinical trials in vasomotor rhinitis were similar to those observed in U.S. clinical trials in seasonal allergic rhinitis.
In controlled trials involving nasal and oral azelastine hydrochloride formulations, there were infrequent occurrences of hepatic transaminase elevations. The clinical relevance of these reports has not been established.
In addition, the following spontaneous adverse events have been reported during the marketing of Astelin® Nasal Spray and causal relationship with the drug is unknown: anaphylactoid reaction, application site irritation, chest pain, nasal congestion, confusion, diarrhea, dyspnea, facial edema, involuntary muscle contractions, paresthesia, parosmia, pruritus, rash, tolerance, urinary retention, vision abnormal and xerophthalmia.

OVERDOSAGE

There have been no reported overdosages with Astelin® Nasal Spray. Acute overdosage by adults with this dosage form is unlikely to result in clinically significant adverse events, other than increased somnolence, since one bottle of Astelin® Nasal Spray contains 30 mg of azelastine hydrochloride. Clinical studies in adults with single doses of the oral formulation of azelastine hydrochloride (up to 16 mg) have not resulted in increased incidence of serious adverse events. General supportive measures should be employed if overdosage occurs. There is no known antidote to Astelin® Nasal Spray. Oral ingestion of antihistamines has the potential to cause serious adverse effects in young children. Accordingly, Astelin® Nasal Spray should be kept out of the reach of children. Oral doses of 120 mg/kg and greater (approximately 460 times the maximum recommended daily intranasal dose in adults and children on a mg/m^2 basis) were lethal in mice. Responses seen prior to death were tremor, convulsions, decreased muscle tone, and salivation. In dogs, single oral doses as high as 10 mg/kg (approximately 260 times the maximum recommended daily intranasal dose in adults and children on a mg/m^2 basis) were well tolerated, but single oral doses of 20 mg/kg were lethal.

DOSAGE AND ADMINISTRATION

Seasonal Allergic Rhinitis
The recommended dose of Astelin® Nasal Spray in adults and children 12 years and older with seasonal allergic rhinitis is two sprays per nostril twice daily. The recommended dose of Astelin® Nasal Spray in children 5 years to 11 years of age is one spray per nostril twice daily.
Vasomotor Rhinitis
The recommended dose of Astelin® Nasal Spray in adults and children 12 years and older with vasomotor rhinitis is two sprays per nostril twice daily.
Before initial use, the screw cap on the bottle should be replaced with the pump unit and the delivery system should be primed with 4 sprays or until a fine mist appears. When 3 or more days have elapsed since the last use, the pump should be reprimed with 2 sprays or until a fine mist appears.
CAUTION: Avoid spraying in the eyes.
Directions for Use: Illustrated patient instructions for proper use accompany each package of Astelin® Nasal Spray.

HOW SUPPLIED

Astelin® (azelastine hydrochloride) Nasal Spray, 137 mcg, (NDC 0037-0241-30) is supplied as a package containing 200 metered sprays in a high-density polyethylene (HDPE) bottle fitted with a metered-dose spray pump unit. A leaflet of patient instructions is also provided. The spray pump unit consists of a nasal spray pump fitted with a blue safety clip and a blue plastic dust cover.
The Astelin® (azelastine hydrochloride) Nasal Spray, 137 mcg, bottle contains 30 mg (1 mg/mL) of azelastine hydrochloride. The bottle can deliver 200 metered sprays. Each spray delivers a mean of 0.137 mL solution containing 137 mcg of azelastine hydrochloride.
Storage: Store at controlled room temperature 20°–25°C (68°–77°F). Protect from freezing.

U.S. Patents 5,164,194; D447,419.
Manufactured by
MedPointe Pharmaceuticals
MedPointe Healthcare Inc.
Somerset, NJ 08873

IN-023S6-02 Rev. 5/03
Shown in Product Identification Guide, page 322

OPTIVAR® ℞

[ŏp-tĭ-vər]
(azelastine hydrochloride ophthalmic solution), 0.05%

DESCRIPTION

OPTIVAR® (azelastine hydrochloride ophthalmic solution), 0.05% is a sterile ophthalmic solution containing azelastine hydrochloride, a relatively selective H_1-receptor antagonist for topical administration to the eyes. Azelastine hydrochloride is a white crystalline powder with a molecular weight of 418.37. Azelastine hydrochloride is sparingly soluble in water, methanol and propylene glycol, and slightly soluble in ethanol, octanol, and glycerine. Azelastine hydrochloride is a racemic mixture with a melting point of 225°C. The chemical name for azelastine hydrochloride is (±)-1-(2H)-phthalazinone,4-[(4-chlorophenyl) methyl]-2-(hexahydro-1-methyl-1H-azepin-4-yl)-, monohydrochloride and is represented by the following chemical structure:

Empirical chemical structure: $C_{22}H_{24}ClN_3O \bullet HCl$

Each mL of OPTIVAR® contains: **Active:** 0.5 mg azelastine hydrochloride, equivalent to 0.457 mg of azelastine base; **Preservative:** 0.125 mg benzalkonium chloride; **Inactives:** disodium edetate dihydrate, hydroxypropylmethylcellulose, sorbitol solution, sodium hydroxide and water for injection. It has a pH of approximately 5.0 to 6.5 and an osmolality of approximately 271 to 312 mOsmol/L.

CLINICAL PHARMACOLOGY

Azelastine hydrochloride is a relatively selective histamine H_1 antagonist and an inhibitor of the release of histamine and other mediators from cells (e.g. mast cells) involved in the allergic response. Based on *in-vitro* studies using human cell lines, inhibition of other mediators involved in allergic reactions (e.g. leukotrienes and PAF) has been demonstrated with azelastine hydrochloride. Decreased chemotaxis and activation of eosinophils has also been demonstrated.
Pharmacokinetics and Metabolism
Absorption of azelastine following ocular administration was relatively low. A study in symptomatic patients receiving one drop of OPTIVAR® in each eye two to four times a day (0.06 to 0.12 mg azelastine hydrochloride) demonstrated plasma concentrations of azelastine hydrochloride to generally be between 0.02 and 0.25 ng/mL after 56 days of treatment. Three of nineteen patients had quantifiable amounts of N-desmethylazelastine that ranged from 0.25–0.87 ng/mL at Day 56.
Based on intravenous and oral administration, the elimination half-life, steady-state volume of distribution and plasma clearance were 22 hours, 14.5 L/kg and 0.5 L/h/kg, respectively. Approximately 75% of an oral dose of radiolabeled azelastine hydrochloride was excreted in the feces with less than 10% as unchanged azelastine. Azelastine hydrochloride is oxidatively metabolized to the principal metabolite, N-desmethylazelastine, by the cytochrome P450 enzyme system. *In-vitro* studies in human plasma indicate that the plasma protein binding of azelastine and N-desmethylazelastine are approximately 88% and 97% respectively.
Clinical Trials
In a conjunctival antigen challenge study, OPTIVAR® was more effective than its vehicle in preventing itching associated with allergic conjunctivitis. OPTIVAR® had a rapid (within 3 minutes) onset of effect and a duration of effect of approximately 8 hours for the prevention of itching.
In environmental studies, adult and pediatric, patients with seasonal allergic conjunctivitis were treated with OPTIVAR® for two to eight weeks. In these studies, OPTIVAR® was more effective than its vehicle in relieving itching associated with allergic conjunctivitis.

INDICATIONS AND USAGE

OPTIVAR® is indicated for the treatment of itching of the eye associated with allergic conjunctivitis.

CONTRAINDICATIONS

OPTIVAR® is contraindicated in persons with known or suspected hypersensitivity to any of its components.

WARNINGS

OPTIVAR® is for ocular use only and not for injection or oral use.

PRECAUTIONS

Information for Patients:
To prevent contaminating the dropper tip and solution, care should be taken not to touch any surface, the eyelids, or surrounding areas with the dropper tip of the bottle. Keep bottle tightly closed when not in use. This product is sterile when packaged.
Patients should be advised not to wear a contact lens if their eye is red. OPTIVAR® should not be used to treat contact lens related irritation. The preservative in OPTIVAR®, benzalkonium chloride, may be absorbed by soft contact lenses. Patients who wear soft contact lenses and **whose eyes are not red**, should be instructed to wait at least ten minutes after instilling OPTIVAR® before they insert their contact lenses.
Carcinogenesis, Mutagenesis, Impairment of Fertility:
Azelastine hydrochloride administered orally for 24 months was not carcinogenic in rats and mice at doses up to 30 mg/kg/day and 25 mg/kg/day, respectively. Based on a 30 µL drop size, these doses were approximately 25,000 and 21,000 times higher than the maximum recommended ocular human use level of 0.001 mg/kg/day for a 50 kg adult.
Azelastine hydrochloride showed no genotoxic effects in the Ames test, DNA repair test, mouse lymphoma forward mutation assay, mouse micronucleus test, or chromosomal aberration test in rat bone marrow. Reproduction and fertility studies in rats showed no effects on male or female fertility at oral doses of up to 25,000 times the maximum recommended ocular human use level. At 68.6 mg/kg/day (57,000 times the maximum recommended ocular human use level), the duration of the estrous cycle was prolonged and copulatory activity and the number of pregnancies were decreased. The numbers of corpora lutea and implantations were decreased; however, the implantation ratio was not affected.
Pregnancy:
Teratogenic Effects: Pregnancy Category C. Azelastine hydrochloride has been shown to be embryotoxic, fetotoxic, and teratogenic (external and skeletal abnormalities) in mice at an oral dose of 68.6 mg/kg/day (57,000 times the recommended ocular human use level). At an oral dose of 30 mg/kg/day (25,000 times the recommended ocular human use level), delayed ossification (undeveloped metacarpus), and the incidence of 14th rib were increased in rats. At 68.6 mg/kg/day (57,000 times the maximum recommended ocular human use level) azelastine hydrochloride caused resorption and fetotoxic effects in rats. The relevance to humans of these skeletal findings noted at only high drug exposure levels in unknown.
There are no adequate and well-controlled studies in pregnant women. OPTIVAR® should be used during pregnancy only if the potential benefit justifies the potential risk to the fetus.
Nursing Mothers:
It is not known whether azelastine hydrochloride is excreted in human milk. Because many drugs are excreted in human milk, caution should be exercised when OPTIVAR® is administered to a nursing woman.
Pediatric Use:
Safety and effectiveness in pediatric patients below the age of 3 have not been established.
Geriatric Use:
No overall differences in safety or effectiveness have been observed between elderly and younger adult patients.

ADVERSE REACTIONS

In controlled multiple-dose studies where patients were treated for up to 56 days, the most frequently reported adverse reactions were transient eye burning/stinging (approximately 30%), headaches (approximately 15%) and bitter taste (approximately 10%). The occurrence of these events was generally mild.
The following events were reported in 1–10% of patients: asthma, conjunctivitis, dyspnea, eye pain, fatigue, influenza-like symptoms, pharyngitis, pruritus, rhinitis and temporary blurring. Some of these events were similar to the underlying disease being studied.

DOSAGE AND ADMINISTRATION

The recommended dose is one drop instilled into each affected eye twice a day.

HOW SUPPLIED

OPTIVAR® (azelastine hydrochloride ophthalmic solution), 0.05% is supplied as follows: 6 mL (NDC# 0037-7025-06) solution in a translucent 10 mL HDPE container with a LDPE dropper tip, and a white HDPE screw cap.
Storage
Store UPRIGHT between 2° and 25°C (36° and 77°F)
℞ only
U.S. Patent No 5,164,194

Manufactured by: Vetter Pharma Fertigung GmbH & Co. KG, Germany

Distributed by:
MedPointe Pharmaceuticals
MedPointe Healthcare Inc.
Somerset, New Jersey 08873

Made in Germany
Issued July 2003
Shown in Product Identification Guide, page 323
Continued on next page

SOMA® ℞
(carisoprodol)
Tablets, USP

DESCRIPTION

'SOMA' (carisoprodol) Tablets, USP is available as 350 mg round, white tablets. Chemically, carisoprodol is N-isopropyl-2-methyl-2-propyl-1,3-propanediol dicarbamate. Carisoprodol is a white, crystalline powder, having a mild, characteristic odor and a bitter taste. It is very slightly soluble in water; freely soluble in alcohol, in chloroform, and in acetone; its solubility is practically independent of pH. Carisoprodol is present as a racemic mixture. The molecular formula is $C_{12}H_{24}N_2O_4$, with a molecular weight of 260.33. The structural formula is:

$CH_2CH_2CH_3$
$H_2NCOOCH_2CCH_2OOCNHCH(CH_3)_2$
CH_3

Other ingredients: alginic acid, magnesium stearate, potassium sorbate, starch, tribasic calcium phosphate.

ACTIONS

Carisoprodol produces muscle relaxation in animals by blocking interneuronal activity in the descending reticular formation and spinal cord. The onset of action is rapid and effects last four to six hours.

INDICATIONS

Carisoprodol is indicated as an adjunct to rest, physical therapy, and other measures for the relief of discomfort associated with acute, painful musculoskeletal conditions. The mode of action of this drug has not been clearly identified, but may be related to its sedative properties. Carisoprodol does not directly relax tense skeletal muscles in man.

CONTRAINDICATIONS

Acute intermittent porphyria as well as allergic or idiosyncratic reactions to carisoprodol or related compounds.

WARNINGS

Idiosyncratic Reactions—On very rare occasions, the first dose of carisoprodol has been followed by idiosyncratic symptoms appearing within minutes or hours. Symptoms reported include: extreme weakness, transient quadriplegia, dizziness, ataxia, temporary loss of vision, diplopia, mydriasis, dysarthria, agitation, euphoria, confusion, and disorientation. Symptoms usually subside over the course of the next several hours. Supportive and symptomatic therapy, including hospitalization, may be necessary.

Usage in Pregnancy and Lactation—Safe usage of this drug in pregnancy or lactation has not been established. Therefore, use of this drug in pregnancy, in nursing mothers, or in women of childbearing potential requires that the potential benefits of the drug be weighed against the potential hazards to mother and child. Carisoprodol is present in breast milk of lactating mothers at concentrations two to four times that of maternal plasma. This factor should be taken into account when use of the drug is contemplated in breast-feeding patients.

Usage in Children—Because of limited clinical experience, 'SOMA' is not recommended for use in patients under 12 years of age.

Potentially Hazardous Tasks—Patients should be warned that this drug may impair the mental and/or physical abilities required for the performance of potentially hazardous tasks such as driving a motor vehicle or operating machinery.

Additive Effects—Since the effects of carisoprodol and alcohol or carisoprodol and other CNS depressants or psychotropic drugs may be additive, appropriate caution should be exercised with patients who take more than one of these agents simultaneously.

Drug Dependence—In dogs, no withdrawal symptoms occurred after abrupt cessation of carisoprodol from dosages as high as 1 gm/kg/day. In a study in man, abrupt cessation of 100 mg/kg/day (about five times the recommended daily adult dosage) was followed in some subjects by mild withdrawal symptoms such as abdominal cramps, insomnia, chilliness, headache, and nausea. Delirium and convulsions did not occur. In clinical use, psychological dependence and abuse have been rare, and there have been no reports of significant abstinence signs. Nevertheless, the drug should be used with caution in addiction prone individuals.

PRECAUTIONS

Carisoprodol is metabolized in the liver and excreted by the kidney; to avoid its excess accumulation, caution should be exercised in administration to patients with compromised liver or kidney function.

ADVERSE REACTIONS

Central Nervous System —Drowsiness and other CNS effects may require dosage reduction. Also observed: dizziness, vertigo, ataxia, tremor, agitation, irritability, headache, depressive reactions, syncope, and insomnia. (See also Idiosyncratic Reactions under "Warnings.")

Allergic or Idiosyncratic —Allergic or idiosyncratic reactions occasionally develop. They are usually seen within the period of the first to fourth dose in patients having had no previous contact with the drug. Skin rash, erythema multiforme, pruritus, eosinophilia, and fixed drug eruption with cross reaction to meprobamate have been reported with carisoprodol. Severe reactions have been manifested by asthmatic episodes, fever, weakness, dizziness, angioneurotic edema, smarting eyes, hypotension, and anaphylactoid shock. (See also Idiosyncratic Reactions under "Warnings.") In case of allergic or idiosyncratic reactions to carisoprodol, discontinue the drug and initiate appropriate symptomatic therapy, which may include epinephrine, antihistamines, and in severe cases corticosteroids. In evaluating possible allergic reactions, also consider allergy to excipients (information on excipients is available to physicians on request).

Cardiovascular —Tachycardia, postural hypotension, and facial flushing.

Gastrointestinal —Nausea, vomiting, hiccup, and epigastric distress.

Hematologic —Leukopenia, in which other drugs or viral infection may have been responsible, and pancytopenia, attributed to phenylbutazone, have been reported. No serious blood dyscrasias have been attributed to carisoprodol.

DOSAGE AND ADMINISTRATION

The usual adult dosage of 'SOMA' (carisoprodol) Tablets, USP is one 350 mg tablet, three times daily and at bedtime. Usage in patients under age 12 is not recommended.

OVERDOSAGE

Overdosage of carisoprodol has produced stupor, coma, shock, respiratory depression, and, very rarely, death. The effects of an overdosage of carisoprodol and alcohol or other CNS depressants or psychotropic agents can be additive even when one of the drugs has been taken in the usual recommended dosage. Any drug remaining in the stomach should be removed and symptomatic therapy given. Should respiration or blood pressure become compromised, respiratory assistance, central nervous system stimulants, and pressor agents should be administered cautiously as indicated. Carisoprodol is metabolized in the liver and excreted by the kidney. Although carisoprodol overdosage experience is limited, the following types of treatment have been used successfully with the related drug meprobamate: diuresis, osmotic (mannitol) diuresis, peritoneal dialysis, and hemodialysis (carisoprodol is dialyzable). Careful monitoring of urinary output is necessary and caution should be taken to avoid overhydration. Observe for possible relapse due to incomplete gastric emptying and delayed absorption. Carisoprodol can be measured in biological fluids by gas chromatography (Douglas, J. F. et al.: *J Pharm Sci 58:* 145, 1969).

HOW SUPPLIED

'SOMA' (carisoprodol) Tablets, USP 350 mg: Round, convex, white tablets, inscribed with 'SOMA' on one side and 37-WALLACE 2001 on the other side, are available in bottles of 100 (NDC 0037-2001-01) and 500 (NDC 0037-2001-03), and unit-dose packages of 100 (NDC 0037-2001-85).

Storage: Store at controlled room temperature 15°–30°C (59°–86°F).

Dispense in a tight container.

MedPointe Pharmaceuticals
MedPointe Healthcare Inc.
Somerset, NJ 08873

IN-090H2-12 Rev. 10/01

Shown in Product Identification Guide, page 323

ZOMIG® ℞
[zō'mig]
(zolmitriptan)
TABLETS

ZOMIG-ZMT®
(zolmitriptan)
Orally Disintegrating Tablets

DESCRIPTION

ZOMIG® (zolmitriptan) Tablets and ZOMIG-ZMT® (zolmitriptan) Orally Disintegrating Tablets contain zolmitriptan, which is a selective 5 hydroxytryptamine 1B/1D ($5\text{-}HT_{1B/1D}$) receptor agonist. Zolmitriptan is chemically designated as (S)-4-[[3-[2-(dimethylamino)ethyl]-1H-indol-5-yl]methyl]-2-oxazolidinone and has the following chemical structure:

The empirical formula is $C_{16}H_{21}N_3O_2$, representing a molecular weight of 287.36. Zolmitriptan is a white to almost white powder that is readily soluble in water. ZOMIG Tablets are available as 2.5 mg (yellow) and 5 mg (pink) film coated tablets for oral administration. The film coated tablets contain anhydrous lactose NF, microcrystalline cellulose NF, sodium starch glycolate NF, magnesium stearate NF, hydroxypropyl methylcellulose USP, titanium dioxide USP, polyethylene glycol 400 NF, yellow iron oxide NF (2.5 mg tablet), red iron oxide NF (5 mg tablet), and polyethylene glycol 8000 NF.

ZOMIG-ZMT® Orally Disintegrating Tablets are available as 2.5 mg and 5.0 mg white uncoated tablets for oral administration. The orally disintegrating tablets contain mannitol USP, microcrystalline cellulose NF, crospovidone NF, aspartame NF, sodium bicarbonate USP, citric acid anhydrous USP, colloidal silicon dioxide NF, magnesium stearate NF and orange flavor SN 027512.

CLINICAL PHARMACOLOGY

Mechanism of Action

Zolmitriptan binds with high affinity to human recombinant $5\text{-}HT_{1D}$ and $5\text{-}HT_{1B}$ receptors. Zolmitriptan exhibits modest affinity for $5\text{-}HT_{1A}$ receptors, but has no significant affinity (as measured by radioligand binding assays) or pharmacological activity at $5\text{-}HT_2$, $5\text{-}HT_3$, $5\text{-}HT_4$, $alpha_1$-, $alpha_2$- or $beta_1$-adrenergic; H_1, H_2, histaminic; muscarinic; $dopamine_1$, or $dopamine_2$ receptors. The N-desmethyl metabolite also has high affinity for $5\text{-}HT_{1B/1D}$ and modest affinity for $5\text{-}HT_{1A}$ receptors.

Current theories proposed to explain the etiology of migraine headache suggest that symptoms are due to local cranial vasodilatation and/or to the release of sensory neuropeptides (vasoactive intestinal peptide, substance P and calcitonin gene-related peptide) through nerve endings in the trigeminal system. The therapeutic activity of zolmitriptan for the treatment of migraine headache can most likely be attributed to the agonist effects at the $5\text{-}HT_{1B/1D}$ receptors on intracranial blood vessels (including the arterio-venous anastomoses) and sensory nerves of the trigeminal system which result in cranial vessel constriction and inhibition of pro-inflammatory neuropeptide release.

Clinical Pharmacokinetics and Bioavailability

Absorption

Zolmitriptan is well absorbed after oral administration for both the conventional tablets and the orally disintegrating tablets. Zolmitriptan displays linear kinetics over the dose range of 2.5 to 50 mg.

The AUC and C_{max} of zolmitriptan are similar following administration of ZOMIG Tablets and ZOMIG-ZMT Orally Disintegrating Tablets, but the T_{max} is somewhat later with ZOMIG-ZMT, with a median T_{max} of 3 hours for the orally disintegrating tablet compared with 1.5 hours for the conventional tablet. The AUC, C_{max}, and T_{max} for the active N-desmethyl metabolite are similar for the two formulations.

During a moderate to severe migraine attack, mean $AUC_{0\text{-}4}$ and C_{max} for zolmitriptan, dosed as a conventional tablet, were decreased by 40% and 25%, respectively, and mean T_{max} was delayed by one-half hour compared to the same patients during a migraine free period.

Food has no significant effect on the bioavailability of zolmitriptan. No accumulation occurred on multiple dosing.

Distribution:

Mean absolute bioavailability is approximately 40%. The mean apparent volume of distribution is 7.0 L/kg. Plasma protein binding of zolmitriptan is 25% over the concentration range of 10–1000ng/mL.

Metabolism:

Zolmitriptan is converted to an active N-desmethyl metabolite such that the metabolite concentrations are about two-thirds that of zolmitriptan. Because the $5HT_{1B/1D}$ potency of the metabolite is 2 to 6 times that of the parent, the metabolite may contribute a substantial portion of the overall effect after zolmitriptan administration.

Elimination:

Total radioactivity recovered in urine and feces was 65% and 30% of the administered dose, respectively. About 8% of the dose was recovered in the urine as unchanged zolmitriptan. Indole acetic acid metabolite accounted for 31% of the dose, followed by N-oxide (7%) and N-desmethyl (4%) metabolites. The indole acetic acid and N-oxide metabolites are inactive.

Mean total plasma clearance is 31.5mL/min/kg, of which one-sixth is renal clearance. The renal clearance is greater than the glomerular filtration rate suggesting renal tubular secretion.

Special Populations:

Age: Zolmitriptan pharmacokinetics in healthy elderly non-migraineur volunteers (age 65–76 yrs) were similar to those in younger non-migraineur volunteers (age 18–39 yrs).

Gender: Mean plasma concentrations of zolmitriptan were up to 1.5-fold higher in females than males.

Renal Impairment: Clearance of zolmitriptan was reduced by 25% in patients with severe renal impairment (Clcr ≥ 5 ≤ 25 mL/min) compared to the normal group (Clcr > = 70 mL/min); no significant change in clearance was observed in the moderately renally impaired group (Clcr ≥ 26 ≤ 50 mL/min).

Hepatic Impairment: In severely hepatically impaired patients, the mean C_{max}, T_{max}, and $AUC_{0\text{-}\infty}$ of zolmitriptan were increased 1.5, 2 (2 vs 4 hr), and 3-fold, respectively, compared to normals. Seven out of 27 patients experienced 20 to 80 mm Hg elevations in systolic and/or diastolic blood pressure after a 10 mg dose. Zolmitriptan should be administered with caution in subjects with liver disease, generally using doses less than 2.5 mg (see WARNINGS and PRECAUTIONS).

Hypertensive Patients: No differences in the pharmacokinetics of zolmitriptan or its effects on blood pressure were seen in mild to moderate hypertensive volunteers compared to normotensive controls.

Race: Retrospective analysis of pharmacokinetic data between Japanese and Caucasians revealed no significant differences.

Drug Interactions

All drug interaction studies were performed in healthy volunteers using a single 10 mg dose of zolmitriptan and a single dose of the other drug except where otherwise noted.

Fluoxetine: The pharmacokinetics of zolmitriptan, as well as its effect on blood pressure, were unaffected by 4 weeks of pretreatment with oral fluoxetine (20 mg/day).

MAO Inhibitors: Following one week of administration of 150 mg bid moclobemide, a specific MAO-A inhibitor, there was an increase of about 25% in both C_{max} and AUC for zolmitriptan and a 3-fold increase in the C_{max} and AUC of the active N-desmethyl metabolite of zolmitriptan (see CONTRAINDICATIONS and PRECAUTIONS).

Selegiline, a selective MAO-B inhibitor, at a dose of 10 mg/day for 1 week, had no effect on the pharmacokinetics of zolmitriptan and its metabolite.

Propranolol: C_{max} and AUC of zolmitriptan increased 1.5-fold after one week of dosing with propranolol (160 mg/day). C_{max} and AUC of the N-desmethyl metabolite were reduced by 30% and 15%, respectively. There were no interactive effects on blood pressure or pulse rate following administration of propranolol with zolmitriptan.

Acetaminophen: A single 1 g dose of acetaminophen does not alter the pharmacokinetics of zolmitriptan and its N-desmethyl metabolite. However, zolmitriptan delayed the T_{max} of acetaminophen by one hour.

Metoclopramide: A single 10 mg dose of metoclopramide had no effect on the pharmacokinetics of zolmitriptan or its metabolites.

Oral Contraceptives: Retrospective analysis of pharmacokinetic data across studies indicated that mean plasma concentrations of zolmitriptan were generally higher in females taking oral contraceptives compared to those not taking oral contraceptives. Mean C_{max} and AUC of zolmitriptan were found to be higher by 30% and 50%, respectively, and T_{max} was delayed by one-half hour in females taking oral contraceptives. The effect of zolmitriptan on the pharmacokinetics of oral contraceptives has not been studied.

Cimetidine: Following the administration of cimetidine, the half-life and AUC of a 5 mg dose of zolmitriptan and its active metabolite were approximately doubled (see PRECAUTIONS).

Clinical Studies

The efficacy of ZOMIG Tablets in the acute treatment of migraine headaches was demonstrated in five randomized, double-blind, placebo controlled studies, of which 2 utilized the 1 mg dose, 2 utilized the 2.5 mg dose and 4 utilized the 5 mg dose; all studies used the marketed formulation. In study 1, patients treated their headaches in a clinic setting. In the other studies, patients treated their headaches as outpatients. In study 4, patients who had previously used sumatriptan were excluded, whereas in the other studies no such exclusion was applied. Patients enrolled in these five studies were predominantly female (82%) and Caucasian (97%) with a mean age of 40 years (range 12–65). Patients were instructed to treat a moderate to severe headache. Headache response, defined as a reduction in headache severity from moderate or severe pain to mild or no pain, was assessed at 1, 2, and, in most studies, 4 hours after dosing. Associated symptoms such as nausea, photophobia, and phonophobia were also assessed. Maintenance of response was assessed for up to 24 hours postdose. A second dose of ZOMIG Tablets or other medication was allowed 2 to 24 hours after the initial treatment for persistent and recurrent headache. The frequency and time to use of these additional treatments were also recorded. In all studies, the effect of zolmitriptan was compared to placebo in the treatment of a single migraine attack.

In all five studies, the percentage of patients achieving headache response 2 hours after treatment was significantly greater among patients receiving ZOMIG Tablets at all doses (except for the 1 mg dose in the smallest study) compared to those who received placebo. In the two studies that evaluated the 1 mg dose, there was a statistically significant greater percentage of patients with headache response at 2 hours in the higher dose groups (2.5 and/or 5 mg) compared to the 1 mg dose group. There were no statistically significant differences between the 2.5 and 5 mg dose groups (or of doses up to 20 mg) for the primary end point of headache response at 2 hours in any study. The results of these controlled clinical studies are summarized in Table 1.

Comparisons of drug performance based upon results obtained in different clinical trials are never reliable. Because studies are conducted at different times, with different samples of patients, by different investigators, employing different criteria and/or different interpretations of the same criteria, under different conditions (dose, dosing regimen, etc.), quantitative estimates of treatment response and the timing of response may be expected to vary considerably from study to study.

Table 1: Percentage of Patients with Headache Response (Mild or no Headache) 2 Hours Following Treatment (n=number of patients randomized)

	Placebo	ZOMIG 1.0 mg	ZOMIG 2.5 mg	ZOMIG 5 mg
Study 1[a]	16% (n=19)	27% (n=22)	NA	60%*# (n=20)
Study 2	19% (n=88)	NA	NA	66%* (n=179)
Study 3	34% (n=121)	50%* (n=140)	65%*# (n=260)	67%*# (n=245)
Study 4[b]	44% (n=55)	NA	NA	59%* (n=491)
Study 5	36% (n=92)	NA NA	62%* (n=178)	NA

* $p<0.05$ in comparison with placebo.
\# $p<0.05$ in comparison with 1 mg.
a This was the only study in which patients treated the headache in a clinic setting.
b This was the only study where patients were excluded who had previously used sumatriptan.
NA - not applicable

The estimated probability of achieving an initial headache response by 4 hours following treatment is depicted in Figure 1.

Figure 1: Estimated Probability of achieving initial headache response within 4 hours*

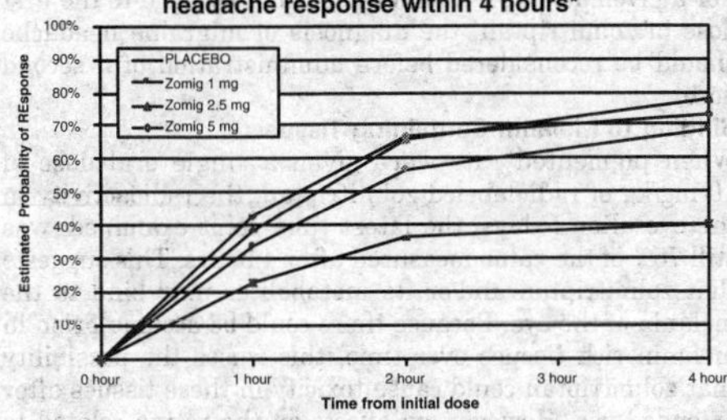

*Figure 1 shows the Kaplan-Meier plot of the probability over time of obtaining headache response (no or mild pain) following treatment with zolmitriptan. The averages displayed are based on pooled data from 3 placebo-controlled, outpatient trials providing evidence of efficacy (Trials 2, 3 and 5). Patients not achieving headache response or taking additional treatment prior to 4 hours were censored to 4 hours.

For patients with migraine associated photophobia, phonophobia, and nausea at baseline, there was a decreased incidence of these symptoms following administration of ZOMIG as compared to placebo.

Two to 24 hours following the initial dose of study treatment, patients were allowed to use additional treatment for pain relief in the form of a second dose of study treatment or other medication. The estimated probability of patients taking a second dose or other medication for migraine over the 24 hours following the initial dose of study treatment is summarized in Figure 2.

Figure 2: The Estimated Probability Of Patients Taking A Second Dose Or Other Medication For Migraines Over The 24 Hours Following The Initial Dose Of Study Treatment*

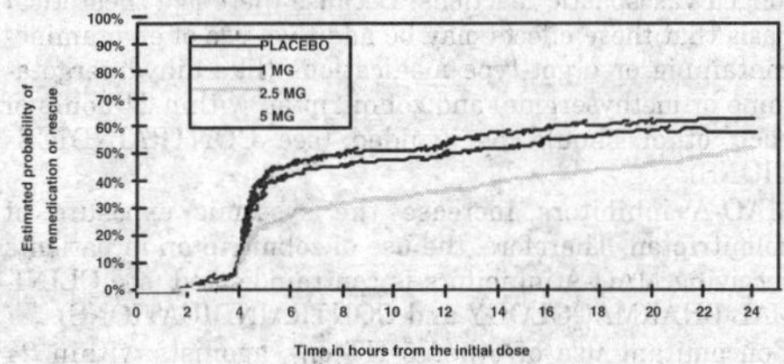

*This Kaplan-Meier plot is based on data obtained in 3 placebo controlled clinical trials (Study 2, 3 and 5). Patients not using additional treatments were censored at 24 hours. The plot includes both patients who had headache response at 2 hours and those who had no response to the initial dose. It should be noted that the protocols did not allow remedication within 2 hours postdose.

The efficacy of ZOMIG was unaffected by presence of aura; duration of headache prior to treatment; relationship to menses; gender, age, or weight of the patient; pretreatment nausea, or concomitant use of common migraine prophylactic drugs.

ZOMIG-ZMT Orally Disintegrating Tablets

The efficacy of ZOMIG-ZMT 2.5 mg was demonstrated in a randomized, placebo-controlled trial that was similar in design to the trials of ZOMIG Tablets. Patients were instructed to treat a moderate to severe headache. Of the 471 patients treated in the study, 87% were female and 97% were Caucasian, with a mean age of 41 years (range 18–62).

At 2 hours post-dosing response rates in patients treated with ZOMIG-ZMT 2.5 mg were 63% compared to 22% in the placebo group. The difference was statistically significant. The estimated probability of achieving an initial headache response by 2 hours following treatment with ZOMIG-ZMT Tablets is depicted in Figure 3.

Figure 3: Estimated Probability of Achieving Initial Headache Response by 2 Hours

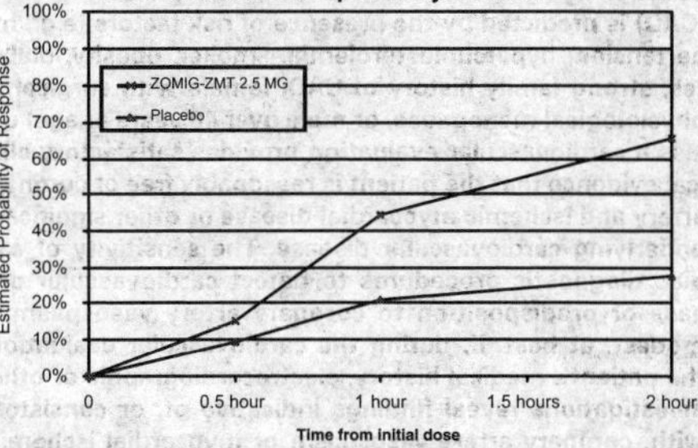

Figure 3 shows the Kaplan-Meier plot of the probability over time of obtaining headache response (no or mild pain) following treatment with ZOMIG-ZMT Tablets or placebo. Patients taking additional treatment or not achieving headache response prior to 2 hours were censored at 2 hours.

For patients with migraine-associated photophobia, phonophobia and nausea at baseline, there was a decreased incidence of these symptoms following administration of ZOMIG-ZMT as compared to placebo.

Two to 24 hours following the initial dose of study treatment, patients were allowed to use additional treatment in the form of a second dose of study treatment or other medication. The estimated probability of patients taking a second dose or other medication for migraine over the 24 hours following the initial dose of study treatment is summarized in Figure 4.

Figure 4: The Estimated Probability of Patients Taking a Second Dose or Other Medication for Migraines Over the 24 Hours Following The Initial Dose of Study Treatment

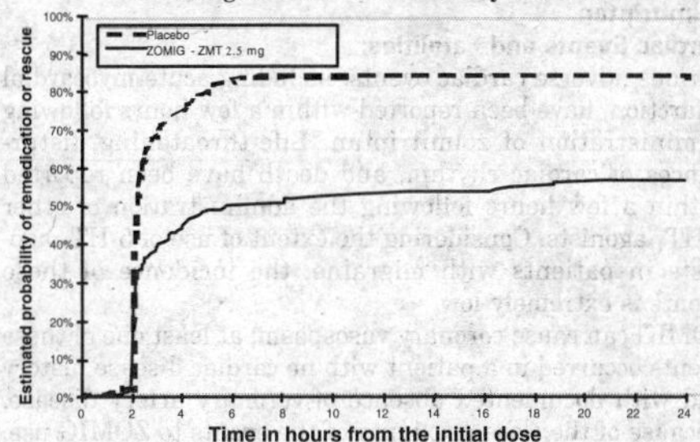

In this Kaplan-Meier plot, patients not using additional treatments were censored at 24 hours. The plot includes both patients who had headache response at 2 hours and those who had no response to the initial dose. Remedication was allowed 2 hours post-dose, and unlike the conventional tablet, remedication prior to 4 hours was not discouraged.

INDICATIONS AND USAGE

ZOMIG is indicated for the acute treatment of migraine with or without aura in adults.

ZOMIG is not intended for the prophylactic therapy of migraine or for use in the management of hemiplegic or basilar migraine (see CONTRAINDICATIONS). Safety and effectiveness of ZOMIG have not been established for cluster headache, which is present in an older, predominantly male population.

CONTRAINDICATIONS

ZOMIG should not be given to patients with ischemic heart disease (angina pectoris, history of myocardial infarction, or documented silent ischemia) or to patients who have symptoms or findings consistent with ischemic heart disease, coronary artery vasospasm, including Prinzmetal's variant angina, or other significant underlying cardiovascular disease (see WARNINGS).

Because ZOMIG may increase blood pressure, it should not be given to patients with uncontrolled hypertension (see WARNINGS).

ZOMIG should not be used within 24 hours of treatment with another 5-HT1 agonist, or an ergotamine-containing or ergot-type medication like dihydroergotamine or methysergide.

ZOMIG should not be administered to patients with hemiplegic or basilar migraine.

Concurrent administration of MAO-A inhibitors or use of zolmitriptan within 2 weeks of discontinuation of MAO-A inhibitor therapy is contraindicated (see CLINICAL PHARMACOLOGY: Drug Interactions and PRECAUTIONS: Drug Interactions).

ZOMIG is contraindicated in patients who are hypersensitive to zolmitriptan or any of its inactive ingredients.

WARNINGS

ZOMIG should only be used where a clear diagnosis of migraine has been established.

Continued on next page

Zomig/Zomig ZMT—Cont.

Risk of Myocardial Ischemia and/or Infarction and Other Adverse Cardiac Events: ZOMIG should not be given to patients with documented ischemic or vasospastic coronary artery disease (see CONTRAINDICATIONS). It is strongly recommended that zolmitriptan not be given to patients in whom unrecognized coronary artery disease (CAD) is predicted by the presence of risk factors (e.g., hypertension, hypercholesterolemia, smoker, obesity, diabetes, strong family history of CAD, female with surgical or physiological menopause, or male over 40 years of age) unless a cardiovascular evaluation provides satisfactory clinical evidence that the patient is reasonably free of coronary artery and ischemic myocardial disease or other significant underlying cardiovascular disease. The sensitivity of cardiac diagnostic procedures to detect cardiovascular disease or predisposition to coronary artery vasospasm is modest, at best. If, during the cardiovascular evaluation, the patient's medical history, electrocardiographic or other investigations reveal findings indicative of, or consistent with, coronary artery vasospasm or myocardial ischemia, zolmitriptan should not be administered (see CONTRAINDICATIONS). For patients with risk factors predictive of CAD, who are determined to have a satisfactory cardiovascular evaluation, it is strongly recommended that administration of the first dose of zolmitriptan take place in the setting of a physician's office or similar medically staffed and equipped facility unless the patient has previously received zolmitriptan. Because cardiac ischemia can occur in the absence of clinical symptoms, consideration should be given to obtaining on the first occasion of use an electrocardiogram (ECG) during the interval immediately following ZOMIG, in these patients with risk factors.

It is recommended that patients who are intermittent long-term users of ZOMIG and who have or acquire risk factors predictive of CAD, as described above, undergo periodic interval cardiovascular evaluation as they continue to use ZOMIG.

The systematic approach described above is intended to reduce the likelihood that patients with unrecognized cardiovascular disease will be inadvertently exposed to zolmitriptan.

Cardiac Events and Fatalities:
Serious adverse cardiac events, including acute myocardial infarction, have been reported within a few hours following administration of zolmitriptan. Life-threatening disturbances of cardiac rhythm, and death have been reported within a few hours following the administration of other 5-HT_1 agonists. Considering the extent of use of 5-HT_1 agonists in patients with migraine, the incidence of these events is extremely low.

ZOMIG can cause coronary vasospasm; at least one of these events occurred in a patient with no cardiac disease history and with documented absence of coronary artery disease. Because of the close proximity of the events to ZOMIG use, a causal relationship cannot be excluded. In the cases where there has been known underlying coronary artery disease, the relationship is uncertain.

Patients with symptomatic Wolff-Parkinson-White syndrome or arrhythmias associated with other cardiac accessory conduction pathway disorders should not receive ZOMIG.

Premarketing experience with zolmitriptan:
Among the more than 2,500 patients with migraine who participated in premarketing controlled clinical trials of ZOMIG Tablets, no deaths or serious cardiac events were reported.

Postmarketing experience with zolmitriptan:
Serious cardiovascular events have been reported in association with the use of ZOMIG Tablets, and in very rare cases, these events have occurred in the absence of known cardiovascular disease. The uncontrolled nature of postmarketing surveillance, however, makes it impossible to determine definitively the proportion of the reported cases that were actually caused by zolmitriptan or to reliably assess causation in individual cases.

Cerebrovascular Events and Fatalities with 5-HT_1 agonists:
Cerebral hemorrhage, subarachnoid hemorrhage, stroke, and other cerebrovascular events have been reported in patients treated with 5-HT_1 agonists; and some have resulted in fatalities. In a number of cases, it appears possible that the cerebrovascular events were primary, the agonist having been administered in the incorrect belief that the symptoms experienced were a consequence of migraine, when they were not. It should be noted that patients with migraine may be at increased risk of certain cerebrovascular events (eg, stroke, hemorrhage, transient ischemic attack).

Other Vasospasm-Related Events:
5-HT_1 agonists may cause vasospastic reactions other than coronary artery vasospasm such as peripheral and gastrointestinal vascular ischemia. As with other serotonin 5HT_1 agonists, very rare gastrointestinal ischemic events including ischemic colitis and gastrointestinal infarction or necrosis have been reported with ZOMIG Tablets; these may present as bloody diarrhea or abdominal pain.

Increase in Blood Pressure:
As with other 5-HT_1 agonists, significant elevations in systemic blood pressure have been reported on rare occasions with ZOMIG Tablet use, in patients with and without a history of hypertension; very rarely these increases in blood pressure have been associated with significant clinical events. Zolmitriptan is contraindicated in patients with uncontrolled hypertension. In volunteers, an increase of 1 and 5 mm Hg in the systolic and diastolic blood pressure, respectively, was seen at 5 mg. In the headache trials, vital signs were measured only in the small inpatient study and no effect on blood pressure was seen. In a study of patients with moderate to severe liver disease, 7 of 27 experienced 20 to 80 mm Hg elevations in systolic and/or diastolic blood pressure after a dose of 10 mg of zolmitriptan (see CONTRAINDICATIONS).

An 18% increase in mean pulmonary artery pressure was seen following dosing with another 5-HT_1 agonist in a study evaluating subjects undergoing cardiac catheterization.

PRECAUTIONS

General
As with other 5-$HT_{1B/1D}$ agonists, sensations of tightness, pain, pressure, and heaviness have been reported after treatment with ZOMIG Tablets in the precordium, throat, neck, and jaw. Because zolmitriptan may cause coronary artery vasospasm, patients who experience signs or symptoms suggestive of angina following dosing should be evaluated for the presence of CAD or a predisposition to Prinzmetal's variant angina before receiving additional doses of medication, and should be monitored electrocardiographically if dosing is resumed and similar symptoms recur. Similarly, patients who experience other symptoms or signs suggestive of decreased arterial flow, such as ischemic bowel syndrome or Raynaud's syndrome following the use of any 5-HT_1 agonist are candidates for further evaluation. (see WARNINGS).

Zolmitriptan should also be administered with caution to patients with diseases that may alter the absorption, metabolism, or excretion of drugs, such as impaired hepatic function (see CLINICAL PHARMACOLOGY).

For a given attack, if a patient does not respond to the first dose of zolmitriptan, the diagnosis of migraine headache should be reconsidered before administration of a second dose.

Binding to Melanin-Containing Tissues:
When pigmented rats were given a single oral dose of 10 mg/kg of radiolabeled zolmitriptan, the radioactivity in the eye after 7 days, the latest time point examined, was still 75% of the value measured after 4 hours. This suggests that zolmitriptan and/or its metabolites may bind to the melanin of the eye. Because there could be accumulation in melanin rich tissues over time, this raises the possibility that zolmitriptan could cause toxicity in these tissues after extended use. However, no effects on the retina related to treatment with zolmitriptan were noted in any of the toxicity studies. Although no systematic monitoring of ophthalmologic function was undertaken in clinical trials, and no specific recommendations for ophthalmologic monitoring are offered, prescribers should be aware of the possibility of long-term ophthalmologic effects.

Phenylketonurics:
Phenylketonuric patients should be informed that ZOMIG-ZMT contain phenylalanine (a component of aspartame). Each 2.5 mg orally disintegrating tablet contains 2.81 mg phenylalanine. Each 5 mg orally disintegrating tablet contains 5.62 mg phenylalanine.

Information for Patients:
See PATIENT INFORMATION at the end of this labeling for the text of the separate leaflet provided for patients.

ZOMIG-ZMT Orally Disintegrating Tablets:
The orally disintegrating tablet is packaged in a blister. Patients should be instructed not to remove the tablet from the blister until just prior to dosing. The blister pack should then be peeled open, and the orally disintegrating tablet placed on the tongue, where it will dissolve and be swallowed with the saliva.

Laboratory Tests:
No monitoring of specific laboratory tests is recommended.

Drug Interactions:
Ergot-containing drugs have been reported to cause prolonged vasospastic reactions. Because there is a theoretical basis that these effects may be additive, use of ergotamine-containing or ergot-type medications (like dihydroergotamine or methysergide) and zolmitriptan within 24 hours of each other should be avoided (see CONTRAINDICATIONS).

MAO-A inhibitors increase the systemic exposure of zolmitriptan. Therefore, the use of zolmitriptan in patients receiving MAO-A inhibitors is contraindicated (see CLINICAL PHARMACOLOGY and CONTRAINDICATIONS).

Concomitant use of other 5-$HT_{1B/1D}$ agonists within 24 hours of ZOMIG treatment is not recommended. (see CONTRAINDICATIONS).

Following administration of cimetidine, the half-life and AUC of zolmitriptan and its active metabolites were approximately doubled (see CLINICAL PHARMACOLOGY).

Selective serotonin reuptake inhibitors (SSRIs) (eg, fluoxetine, fluvoxamine, paroxetine, sertraline) have been reported, rarely, to cause weakness, hyperreflexia, and incoordination when coadministered with 5-HT_1 agonists. If concomitant treatment with zolmitriptan and an SSRI is clinically warranted, appropriate observation of the patient is advised.

Drug/Laboratory Test Interactions:
Zolmitriptan is not known to interfere with commonly employed clinical laboratory tests.

Carcinogenesis, Mutagenesis, Impairment of Fertility:
Carcinogenicity studies by oral gavage were carried out in mice and rats at doses up to 400 mg/kg/day. Mice were dosed for 85 weeks (males) and 92 weeks (females). The exposure (plasma AUC of parent drug) at the highest dose level was approximately 800 times that seen in humans after a single 10 mg dose (the maximum recommended total daily dose). There was no effect of zolmitriptan on tumor incidence. Control, low dose, and middle dose rats were dosed for 104–105 weeks; the high dose group was sacrificed after 101 weeks (males) and 86 weeks (females) due to excess mortality. Aside from an increase in the incidence of thyroid follicular cell hyperplasia and thyroid follicular cell adenomas seen in male rats receiving 400 mg/kg/day, an exposure approximately 3000 times that seen in humans after dosing with 10 mg, no tumors were noted.

Mutagenesis:
Zolmitriptan was mutagenic in an Ames test, in 2 of 5 strains of *S. typhimurium* tested, in the presence of, but not in the absence of, metabolic activation. It was not mutagenic in an *in vitro* mammalian gene cell mutation (CHO/HGPRT) assay. Zolmitriptan was clastogenic in an *in vitro* human lymphocyte assay both in the absence of and the presence of metabolic activation; it was not clastogenic in an *in vivo* mouse micronucleus assay. It was also not genotoxic in an unscheduled DNA synthesis study.

Impairment of Fertility:
Studies of male and female rats administered zolmitriptan prior to and during mating and up to implantation have shown no impairment of fertility at doses up to 400 mg/kg/day. Exposure at this dose was approximately 3000 times exposure at the maximum recommended human dose of 10 mg/day.

Pregnancy

Pregnancy Category C
There are no adequate and well controlled studies in pregnant women; therefore, zolmitriptan should be used during pregnancy only if the potential benefit justifies the potential risk to the fetus.

In reproductive toxicity studies in rats and rabbits, oral administration of zolmitriptan to pregnant animals was associated with embryolethality and fetal abnormalities. When pregnant rats were administered oral zolmitriptan during the period of organogenesis at doses of 100, 400, and 1200 mg/kg/day, there was a dose-related increase in embryolethality which became statistically significant at the high dose. The maternal plasma exposures at these doses were approximately 280, 1100, and 5000 times the exposure in humans receiving the maximum recommended total daily dose of 10 mg. The high dose was maternally toxic, as evidenced by a decreased maternal body weight gain during gestation. In a similar study in rabbits, embryolethality was increased at the maternally toxic doses of 10 and 30 mg/kg/day (maternal plasma exposures equivalent to 11 and 42 times exposure in humans receiving the maximum recommended total daily dose of 10 mg), and increased incidences of fetal malformations (fused sternebrae, rib anomalies) and variations (major blood vessel variations, irregular ossification pattern of ribs) were observed at 30 mg/kg/day. Three mg/kg/day was a no effect dose (equivalent to human exposure at a dose of 10 mg). When female rats were given zolmitriptan during gestation, parturition, and lactation, an increased incidence of hydronephrosis was found in the offspring at the maternally toxic dose of 400 mg/kg/day (1100 times human exposure).

Nursing Mothers
It is not known whether zolmitriptan is excreted in human milk. Because many drugs are excreted in human milk, caution should be exercised when zolmitriptan is administered to a nursing woman. Lactating rats dosed with zolmitriptan had milk levels equivalent to maternal plasma levels at 1 hour and 4 times higher than plasma levels at 4 hours

Pediatric Use
Safety and effectiveness of ZOMIG in pediatric patients have not been established therefore, ZOMIG is not recommended for use in patients under 18 years of age.

Postmarketing experience with other triptans includes a limited number of reports that describe pediatric patients who have experienced clinically serious adverse events that are similar in nature to those reported rarely in adults.

Geriatric Use
Although the pharmacokinetic disposition of the drug in the elderly is similar to that seen in younger adults, there is no information about the safety and effectiveness of zolmitriptan in this population because patients over age 65 were excluded from the controlled clinical trials. (see CLINICAL PHARMACOLOGY: Special Populations)

ADVERSE REACTIONS

Serious cardiac events, including myocardial infarction, have occurred following the use of ZOMIG Tablets. These events are extremely rare and most have been reported in patients with risk factors predictive of CAD. Events reported, in association with drugs of this class, have included coronary artery vasospasm, transient myocardial ischemia, myocardial infarction, ventricular tachycardia, and ventricular fibrillation (see CONTRAINDICATIONS, WARNINGS, and PRECAUTIONS).

Incidence in Controlled Clinical Trials:
Among 2,633 patients treated with ZOMIG Tablets in the active and placebo controlled trials, no patients withdrew for reasons related to adverse events, but as patients treated a single headache in these trials, the opportunity for discontinuation was limited. In a long-term, open label study where patients were allowed to treat multiple migraine attacks for up to 1 year, 8% (167 out of 2,058) withdrew from the trial because of adverse experience. The most

common events were paresthesia, asthenia, nausea, dizziness, pain, chest or neck tightness or heaviness, somnolence, and warm sensation.

Table 2 lists the adverse events that occurred in ≥ 2% of the 2,074 patients in any one of the ZOMIG 1 mg, ZOMIG 2.5 mg or ZOMIG 5 mg Tablets dose groups of the controlled clinical trials. Only events that were more frequent in a ZOMIG Tablets group compared to the placebo groups are included. The events cited reflect experience gained under closely monitored conditions of clinical trials in a highly selected patient population. In actual clinical practice or in other clinical trials, these frequency estimates may not apply, as the conditions of use, reporting behavior, and the kinds of patients treated may differ.

Several of the adverse events appear dose related, notably paresthesia, sensation of heaviness or tightness in chest, neck, jaw, and throat, dizziness, somnolence, and possibly asthenia and nausea.

[See table 2 at right]

ZOMIG is generally well tolerated. Across all doses, most adverse reactions were mild and transient and did not lead to long-lasting effects. The incidence of adverse events in controlled clinical trials was not affected by gender, weight, or age of the patients; use of prophylactic medications; or presence of aura. There were insufficient data to assess the impact of race on the incidence of adverse events.

Other Events:

In the paragraphs that follow, the frequencies of less commonly reported adverse clinical events are presented. Because the reports include events observed in open and uncontrolled studies, the role of ZOMIG in their causation cannot be reliably determined. Furthermore, variability associated with adverse event reporting, the terminology used to describe adverse events, etc., limit the value of the quantitative frequency estimates provided. Event frequencies are calculated as the number of patients who used ZOMIG Tablets (n=4,027) and reported an event divided by the total number of patients exposed to ZOMIG Tablets. All reported events are included except those already listed in the previous table, those too general to be informative, and those not reasonably associated with the use of the drug. Events are further classified within body system categories and enumerated in order of decreasing frequency using the following definitions: infrequent adverse events are those occurring in 1/100 to 1/1,000 patients and rare adverse events are those occurring in fewer than 1/1,000 patients.

Atypical sensation: Infrequent was hyperesthesia.

General: Infrequent were allergy reaction, chills, facial edema, fever, malaise, and photosensitivity.

Cardiovascular: Infrequent were arrhythmias, hypertension, and syncope. Rare were bradycardia, extrasystoles, postural hypotension, QT prolongation, tachycardia, and thrombophlebitis.

Digestive: Infrequent were increased appetite, tongue edema, esophagitis, gastroenteritis, liver function abnormality, and thirst. Rare were anorexia, constipation, gastritis, hematemesis, pancreatitis, melena, and ulcer.

Hemic: Infrequent was ecchymosis. Rare were cyanosis, thrombocytopenia, eosinophilia, and leukopenia.

Metabolic: Infrequent was edema. Rare were hyperglycemia and alkaline phosphatase increased.

Musculoskeletal: Infrequent were back pain, leg cramps, and tenosynovitis. Rare were arthritis, asthenia, tetany, and twitching.

Neurological: Infrequent were agitation, anxiety, depression, emotional lability, and insomnia; Rare were akathisia, amnesia, apathy, ataxia, dystonia, euphoria, hallucinations, cerebral ischemia, hyperkinesia, hypotonia, hypertonia, and irritability.

Respiratory: Infrequent were bronchitis, bronchospasm, epistaxis, hiccup, laryngitis, and yawn. Rare were apnea and voice alteration.

Skin: Infrequent were pruritus, rash, and urticaria.

Special Senses: Infrequent were dry eye, eye pain, hyperacusis, ear pain, parosmia, and tinnitus. Rare were diplopia and lacrimation.

Urogenital: Infrequent were hematuria, cystitis, polyuria, urinary frequency, urinary urgency. Rare were miscarriage and dysmenorrhea.

The adverse experiences profile seen with ZOMIG-ZMT Tablets was similar to that seen with ZOMIG Tablets.

Postmarketing Experience with ZOMIG Tablets:

The following section enumerates potentially important adverse events that have occurred in clinical practice and which have been reported spontaneously to various surveillance systems. The events enumerated represent reports arising from both domestic and non-domestic use of oral zolmitriptan. The events enumerated include all except those already listed in the ADVERSE REACTIONS section above or those too general to be informative. Because the reports cite events reported spontaneously from worldwide postmarketing experience, frequency of events and the role of zolmitriptan in their causation cannot be reliably determined.

Cardiovascular

Coronary artery vasospasm; transient myocardial ischemia, angina pectoris, and myocardial infarction.

Digestive

Very rare gastrointestinal ischemic events including splenic infarction, ischemic colitis and gastrointestinal infarction or necrosis have been reported; these may present as bloody diarrhea or abdominal pain. (See WARNINGS.)

Table 2:
Adverse Experience Incidence in Five Placebo-Controlled Migraine Clinical Trials:
Events Reported By ≥ 2% Patients Treated With ZOMIG Tablets

Adverse Event Type	Placebo (n=401)	ZOMIG 1 mg (n=163)	ZOMIG 2.5 mg (n=498)	ZOMIG 5 mg (n=1012)
ATYPICAL SENSATIONS	**6%**	**12%**	**12%**	**18%**
Hypesthesia	1%	1%	1%	2%
Paresthesia (all types)	2%	5%	7%	9%
Sensation warm/cold	4%	6%	5%	7%
PAIN AND PRESSURE SENSATIONS	**7%**	**13%**	**14%**	**22%**
Chest - pain/tightness/pressure and/or heaviness	1%	2%	3%	4%
Neck/throat/jaw - pain/tightness/pressure	3%	4%	7%	10%
Heaviness other than chest or neck	1%	1%	2%	5%
Pain – location specified	1%	2%	2%	3%
Other – Pressure/tightness/heaviness	0%	2%	2%	2%
DIGESTIVE	**8%**	**11%**	**16%**	**14%**
Dry mouth	2%	5%	3%	3%
Dyspepsia	1%	3%	2%	1%
Dysphagia	0%	0%	0%	2%
Nausea	4%	4%	9%	6%
NEUROLOGICAL	**10%**	**11%**	**17%**	**21%**
Dizziness	4%	6%	8%	10%
Somnolence	3%	5%	6%	8%
Vertigo	0%	0%	0%	2%
OTHER				
Asthenia	3%	5%	3%	9%
Palpitations	1%	0%	<1%	2%
Myalgia	<1%	1%	1%	2%
Myasthenia	<1%	0%	1%	2%
Sweating	1%	0%	2%	3%

Neurological: As with other acute migraine treatments including other $5HT_1$ agonists, there have been rare reports of headache.

General

As with other $5\text{-}HT_{1B/1D}$ agonists, there have been very rare reports of anaphylaxis or anaphylactoid reactions in patients receiving ZOMIG. There have been rare reports of hypersensitivity reactions, including angioedema.

DRUG ABUSE AND DEPENDENCE

The abuse potential of ZOMIG has not been assessed in clinical trials.

OVERDOSAGE

There is no experience with clinical overdose. Volunteers receiving single 50 mg oral doses of zolmitriptan commonly experienced sedation.

The elimination half-life of ZOMIG is 3 hours (see CLINICAL PHARMACOLOGY), and therefore monitoring of patients after overdose with ZOMIG should continue for at least 15 hours or while symptoms or signs persist.

There is no specific antidote to zolmitriptan. In cases of severe intoxication, intensive care procedures are recommended, including establishing and maintaining a patent airway, ensuring adequate oxygenation and ventilation, and monitoring and support of the cardiovascular system.

It is unknown what effect hemodialysis or peritoneal dialysis has on the plasma concentrations of zolmitriptan.

DOSAGE AND ADMINISTRATION

ZOMIG Tablets

In controlled clinical trials, single doses of 1, 2.5 and 5 mg of ZOMIG Tablets were effective for the acute treatment of migraines in adults. A greater proportion of patients had headache response following a 2.5 or 5 mg dose than following a 1 mg dose (see Table 1). In the only direct comparison of 2.5 and 5 mg, there was little added benefit from the larger dose but side effects are generally increased at 5 mg (see Table 2). Patients should, therefore, be started on 2.5 mg or lower. A dose lower than 2.5 mg can be achieved by manually breaking the scored 2.5 mg tablet in half.

If the headache returns, the dose may be repeated after 2 hours, not to exceed 10 mg within a 24 hour period. Controlled trials have not adequately established the effectiveness of a second dose if the initial dose is ineffective.

The safety of treating an average of more than three headaches in a 30-day period has not been established.

ZOMIG-ZMT Orally Disintegrating Tablets

In a controlled clinical trial, a single dose of 2.5 mg of ZOMIG-ZMT Tablets was effective for the acute treatment of migraines in adults.

If the headache returns, the dose may be repeated after 2 hours, not to exceed 10 mg within a 24 hour period. Controlled trials have not adequately established the effectiveness of a second dose if the initial dose is ineffective.

The safety of treating an average of more than three headaches in a 30-day period has not been established.

Administration with liquid is not necessary. The orally disintegrating tablet is packaged in a blister. Patients should be instructed not to remove the tablet from the blister until just prior to dosing. The blister pack should then be peeled open, and the orally disintegrating tablet placed on the tongue, where it will dissolve and be swallowed with the saliva. It is not recommended to break the orally disintegrating tablet.

Hepatic Impairment

Patients with moderate to severe hepatic impairment have decreased clearance of zolmitriptan and significant elevation in blood pressure was observed in some patients. Use of a low dose with blood pressure monitoring is recommended (see CLINICAL PHARMACOLOGY AND WARNINGS).

HOW SUPPLIED

2.5 mg Tablets - Yellow, biconvex, round film-coated, scored tablets containing 2.5 mg of zolmitriptan identified with "ZOMIG" and "2.5" debossed on one side are supplied in cartons containing a blister pack of 6 tablets (NDC 0037-7210-20).

2.5 mg Orally Disintegrating Tablets - White, flat faced, uncoated, bevelled tablet containing 2.5 mg of zolmitriptan identified with a debossed "Z" on one side are supplied in cartons containing a blister pack of 6 tablets (NDC 0037-7209-20).

5 mg Tablets - Pink, biconvex, film-coated tablets containing 5 mg of zolmitriptan identified with "ZOMIG" and "5" debossed on one side are supplied in cartons containing a blister pack of 3 tablets (NDC 0037-7211-25).

5 mg Orally Disintegrating Tablets - White, flat faced, round, uncoated, bevelled tablet containing 5.0 mg of zolmitriptan identified with a debossed "Z" and "5" on one side and plain on the other are supplied in cartons containing a blister pack of 3 tablets (NDC 0037-7213-21).

Storage:

Store both ZOMIG Tablets and ZOMIG-ZMT Tablets at controlled room temperature, 20–25°C (68–77°F) [see USP]. Protect from light and moisture.

ZOMIG®
(zolmitriptan)
TABLETS
ZOMIG-ZMT®
(zolmitriptan)
ORALLY DISINTEGRATING TABLETS
PATIENT INFORMATION

The following wording is contained in a separate leaflet provided for patients.

ZOMIG® (zolmitriptan) Tablets

ZOMIG-ZMT® (zolmitriptan) Orally Disintegrating Tablets

Patient Information about ZOMIG (Zo-mig) for Migraines

Generic Name: zolmitriptan (zol-mi-trip-tan)

Information for the Consumer on ZOMIG (zolmitriptan) Tablets

Please read this leaflet carefully before you administer ZOMIG Tablets. This provides a summary of the information available on your medicine. Please do not throw away this leaflet until you have finished your medicine. You may need to read this leaflet again. This leaflet does not contain all the information on ZOMIG Tablets. For further information or advice, ask your doctor or pharmacist.

Information About Your Medicine

The name of your medicine is ZOMIG Tablets. It can be obtained only by prescription from your doctor. The decision to use ZOMIG Tablets is one that you and your doctor should make jointly, taking into account your individual preferences and medical circumstances. If you have risk factors for heart disease (such as high blood pressure, high cholesterol, obesity, diabetes, smoking, strong family history of heart disease, or you are postmenopausal or a male over the age of 40), you should tell your doctor, who should evaluate you for heart disease in order to determine if ZOMIG Tablets are appropriate for you.

1. The Purpose of Your Medicine: ZOMIG Tablets are intended to relieve your migraine, but not to prevent or reduce the number of attacks you experience. Use ZOMIG Tablets only to treat an actual migraine attack.

2. Important Questions to Consider Before Using ZOMIG Tablets: If the answer to any of the following questions is **YES** or if you do not know the answer, then you must discuss it with your doctor before you use ZOMIG Tablets.

Continued on next page

Zomig/Zomig ZMT—Cont.

- Do you have any chest pain, heart disease, shortness of breath, or irregular heartbeats? Have you had a heart attack?
- Do you have risk factors for heart disease (such as high blood pressure, high cholesterol, obesity, diabetes, smoking, strong family history of heart disease, or you are postmenopausal or a male over the age of 40)?
- Do you have high blood pressure?
- Are you pregnant? Do you think you might be pregnant? Are you trying to become pregnant? Are you not using adequate contraception? Are you breast feeding an infant?
- If you are taking ZOMIG-ZMT®, are you sensitive to phenylalanine (a component of the artificial sweetener aspartame)?
- Have you ever had to stop taking this or any other medication because of an allergy or other problems?
- Are you taking any other migraine medications, including 5-HT_1 agonists (triptans) or migraine medications containing ergotamine, dihydroergotamine, or methysergide?
- Are you taking any medication for depression (monoamine oxidase inhibitors or selective serotonin reuptake inhibitors [SSRIs])?
- Are you taking cimetidine for gastrointestinal symptoms?
- Have you had, or do you have, any disease of the liver or kidney?
- Have you had, or do you have, epilepsy or seizures?
- Is this headache different from your usual migraine attacks?

Remember, if you answered **YES** to any of the above questions, then you must discuss it with your doctor.

3. The Use of ZOMIG Tablets During Pregnancy: Do not use ZOMIG Tablets if you are pregnant, think you might be pregnant, are trying to become pregnant, or are not using adequate contraception unless you have discussed this with your doctor.

4. How to Use ZOMIG Tablets and ZOMIG-ZMT Orally Disintegrating Tablets: Adults should be started on a 2.5 mg dose or lower administered by mouth. A dose lower than 2.5 mg can be achieved by manually breaking the conventional film-coated, scored 2.5 mg tablet in half. It is not recommended to break the ZOMIG-ZMT Tablet. If your headache comes back after your initial dose, a second dose may be administered anytime after 2 hours of administering the dose. For any attack where you have no response to the first dose, do not take a second dose without first consulting with your doctor. Do not administer more than a total of 10 mg of ZOMIG in any 24-hour period. Discard any unused tablets or its portion that have been removed from the blister packaging. Do not take ZOMIG with any other drug in the same class (triptans) within 24 hours or within 24 hours of taking ergotamine-type medications such as ergotamine, dihydroergotamine or methysergide to treat your migraine.

Additionally for ZOMIG-ZMT Tablets, the blister pack should be peeled open and the orally disintegrating tablet placed on the tongue, where it will dissolve and be swallowed with the saliva.

5. Side Effects to Watch for: Some patients experience pain or tightness in the chest or throat, including muscle aches and pains, when using ZOMIG. If this happens to you, then discuss it with your doctor before using any more ZOMIG. If the chest pain is severe or does not go away, call your doctor immediately. As with other drugs in this class (triptans), there have been very rare reports of heart attack occurring in patients with and without risk factors for heart and blood vessel disease.

- Some people experience; alterations of heart rate; temporary increase in blood pressure; sudden and severe stomach pain.
- Shortness of breath; wheeziness; heart throbbing; swelling of eyelids, face, or lips; or a skin rash, skin lumps, or hives happens rarely. If it happens to you, then tell your doctor immediately. Do not take any more ZOMIG unless your doctor tells you to do so.
- Some people may have feelings of dry mouth, tingling, heat, heaviness, or pressure after treatment with ZOMIG. A few people may feel drowsy, dizzy, tired, or sick. Tell your doctor immediately if you have symptoms that you do not understand.

6. What to Do if an Overdose Is Taken: If you have taken more medication than you have been told, contact either your doctor, hospital emergency department, or nearest poison control center immediately. This medicine was prescribed for your particular condition and should not be used by others or for any other condition.

7. Storing Your Medicine: Keep your medicine in a safe place where children cannot reach it. It may be harmful to children. Store your medication away from light and moisture, and at a controlled room temperature. If your medication has expired (the expiration date is printed on the treatment pack), throw it away as instructed. If your doctor decides to stop your treatment, do not keep any leftover medicine unless your doctor tells you to. Throw away your medicine as instructed. Be sure that discarded tablets are out of the reach of children.

ZOMIG® (zolmitriptan) Tablets
Manufactured for:
AstraZeneca Pharmaceuticals LP
Wilmington, Delaware 19850
By: IPR Pharmaceuticals, Inc.
Carolina, Puerto Rico 00984-1967

ZOMIG-ZMT® (zolmitriptan) Orally Disintegrating Tablets
Manufactured for:
AstraZeneca Pharmaceuticals LP
Wilmington, Delaware 19850
By: CIMA Labs, Inc.
Eden Prairie, Minnesota 55344

Distributed by:
MedPointe Pharmaceuticals
MedPointe Healthcare Inc.
Somerset, New Jersey 08873

Rev 10/03

Shown in Product Identification Guide, page 323

ZOMIG® NASAL SPRAY ℞

[*zō-mĭg*]
(zolmitriptan)
FOR NASAL USE ONLY

DESCRIPTION

ZOMIG® (zolmitriptan) Nasal Spray contains zolmitriptan, which is a selective 5-hydroxytryptamine $_{1B/1D}$ (5-$HT_{1B/1D}$) receptor agonist. Zolmitriptan is chemically designated as (S)-4-[[3-[2-(dimethylamino)ethyl]-1H-indol-5-yl]methyl]-2-oxazolidinone and has the following chemical structure:

The empirical formula is $C_{16}H_{21}N_3O_2$, representing a molecular weight of 287.36. Zolmitriptan is a white to almost white powder that is readily soluble in water. ZOMIG Nasal Spray is supplied as a clear to pale yellow solution of zolmitriptan, buffered to a pH 5.0. Each ZOMIG Nasal Spray contains 5 mg of zolmitriptan in a 100-µL unit dose aqueous buffered solution containing citric acid, anhydrous, USP, disodium phosphate dodecahydrate USP and purified water USP.

ZOMIG Nasal Spray is hypertonic. The osmolarity of ZOMIG Nasal Spray 5 mg is 420 to 470 mOsmol.

CLINICAL PHARMACOLOGY

Mechanism of Action: Zolmitriptan binds with high affinity to human recombinant 5-HT_{1D} and 5-HT_{1B} receptors. Zolmitriptan exhibits modest affinity for 5-HT_{1A} receptors, but has no significant affinity (as measured by radioligand binding assays) or pharmacological activity at 5-HT_2, 5-HT_3, 5-HT_4, alpha$_1$-, alpha$_2$, or beta$_1$-adrenergic; H_1, H_2, histaminic; muscarinic; dopamine$_1$, or dopamine$_2$ receptors. The N-desmethyl metabolite also has high affinity for 5-$HT_{1B/1D}$ and modest affinity for 5-HT_{1A} receptors.

Current theories proposed to explain the etiology of migraine headache suggest that symptoms are due to local cranial vasodilatation and/or to the release of sensory neuropeptides (vasoactive intestinal peptide, substance P and calcitonin gene-related peptide) through nerve endings in the trigeminal system. The therapeutic activity of zolmitriptan for the treatment of migraine headache can most likely be attributed to the agonist effects at the 5-$HT_{1B/1D}$ receptors on intracranial blood vessels (including the arterio-venous anastomoses) and sensory nerves of the trigeminal system which result in cranial vessel constriction and inhibition of pro-inflammatory neuropeptide release.

Clinical Pharmacokinetics and Bioavailability:

Absorption: Zolmitriptan nasal spray is rapidly absorbed via the nasopharynx as detected in a Photon Emission Tomography (PET) study using ^{11}C zolmitriptan. Zolmitriptan was detected in plasma by 5 minutes and peak plasma concentration generally was achieved by 3 hours. The time at which maximum plasma concentrations were observed was similar after single (1 day) or multiple (4 day) nasal dosing. Plasma concentrations of zolmitriptan are sustained for 4 to 6 hours after dosing. Zolmitriptan displays linear kinetics after multiple doses of 2.5 mg, 5 mg, or 10 mg. The mean relative bioavailability of the nasal spray formulation is 102%, compared to the oral tablet.

Zolmitriptan and its active metabolite display dose proportionality after single or multiple dosing. Dose proportional increases in zolmitriptan and N-desmethyl metabolite C_{max} and AUC were observed for 2.5 and 5 mg nasal spray doses. The pharmacokinetics for elimination of zolmitriptan and its active N-desmethyl metabolite are similar for all nasal spray dosages. The N-desmethyl metabolite is detected in plasma by 15 minutes and peak plasma concentration is generally achieved by 3 hours after administration.

Food has no significant effect on the bioavailability of zolmitriptan.

Distribution: Plasma protein binding of zolmitriptan is 25% over the concentration range of 10 - 1000 ng/mL. The mean (±SD) apparent volume of distribution for zolmitriptan nasal spray formulation is 8.6±3.3 L/kg.

Metabolism: Zolmitriptan is converted to an active N-desmethyl metabolite such that the metabolite concentrations are about two- thirds that of zolmitriptan. Because the 5-$HT_{1B/1D}$ potency of the metabolite is 2 to 6 times that of the parent compound, the metabolite may contribute a substantial portion of the overall effect after zolmitriptan administration.

Excretion: The mean elimination half-life for zolmitriptan and its active N-desmethyl metabolite following nasal spray administration are approximately 3 hours, which is similar to the half-life values seen after oral tablet administration. The half-life values were similar for zolmitriptan and the N-desmethyl metabolite after single (1 day) and multiple (4 day) nasal dosing.

Mean total plasma clearance is 25.9 mL/min/kg, of which one-sixth is renal clearance. The renal clearance is greater than the glomerular filtration rate suggesting renal tubular secretion.

Special Populations

Age: The pharmacokinetics of oral zolmitriptan in healthy elderly non-migraineur volunteers (age 65 - 76 yrs) was similar to those in younger non-migraineur volunteers (age 18-39 yrs).

Gender: Mean plasma concentrations of orally administered zolmitriptan were up to 1.5-fold higher in females than males.

Renal Impairment: The effect of renal impairment on the pharmacokinetics of zolmitriptan nasal spray has not been evaluated. After orally dosing zolmitriptan, renal clearance was reduced by 25% in patients with severe renal impairment (Clcr ≥ 5 ≤ 25 mL/min) compared to the normal group (Clcr ≥ 70 mL/min); no significant change in renal clearance was observed in the moderately renally impaired group (Clcr ≥ 26 ≤ 50 mL/min).

Hepatic Impairment: The effect of hepatic disease on the pharmacokinetics of zolmitriptan nasal spray has not been evaluated. In severely hepatically impaired patients, the mean C_{max}, T_{max}, and $AUC_{0-\infty}$ of zolmitriptan dosed orally were increased 1.5, 2, and 3-fold, respectively, compared to normals. Seven out of 27 patients experienced 20 to 80 mm Hg elevations in systolic and/or diastolic blood pressure after a 10 mg dose. Because of the similarity in exposure, zolmitriptan tablets and nasal spray should have similar dosage adjustments and should be administered with caution in subjects with liver disease, generally using doses less than 2.5 mg. Doses lower than 5 mg can only be achieved through the use of an oral formulation. (see WARNINGS and PRECAUTIONS).

Hypertensive Patients: No differences in the pharmacokinetics of oral zolmitriptan or its effects on blood pressure were seen in mild to moderate hypertensive volunteers compared to normotensive controls.

Race: Retrospective analysis of pharmacokinetic data between Japanese and Caucasians revealed no significant differences for orally dosed zolmitriptan.

Drug Interactions: All drug interaction studies were performed in healthy volunteers using a single 10 mg dose of zolmitriptan and a single dose of the other drug except where otherwise noted. Eight drug interaction studies have been performed with zolmitriptan tablets and one study (xylometazoline) was performed with nasal spray.

Xylometazoline: An in vivo drug interaction study with ZOMIG Nasal Spray indicated that 1 spray (100µL dose) of xylometazoline (0.1% w/v), a decongestant, administered 30 minutes prior to a 5 mg nasal dose of zolmitriptan did not alter the pharmacokinetics of zolmitriptan.

Fluoxetine: The pharmacokinetics of zolmitriptan, as well as its effect on blood pressure, were unaffected by 4 weeks of pretreatment with oral fluoxetine (20 mg/day).

MAO Inhibitors: Following one week of administration of 150 mg bid moclobemide, a specific MAO-A inhibitor, there was an increase of about 25% in both C_{max} and AUC for zolmitriptan and a 3-fold increase in the C_{max} and AUC of the active N-desmethyl metabolite of zolmitriptan (see CONTRAINDICATIONS and PRECAUTIONS).

Selegiline, a selective MAO-B inhibitor, at a dose of 10 mg/day for 1 week, had no effect on the pharmacokinetics of zolmitriptan and its metabolite.

Propranolol: C_{max} and AUC of zolmitriptan increased 1.5-fold after one week of dosing with propranolol (160 mg/day). C_{max} and AUC of the N-desmethyl metabolite were reduced by 30% and 15%, respectively. There were no interactive effects on blood pressure or pulse rate following administration of propranolol with zolmitriptan.

Acetaminophen: A single 1 g dose of acetaminophen does not alter the pharmacokinetics of zolmitriptan and its N-desmethyl metabolite. However, zolmitriptan delayed the T_{max} of acetaminophen by one hour.

Metoclopramide: A single 10 mg dose of metoclopramide had no effect on the pharmacokinetics of zolmitriptan or its metabolites.

Oral Contraceptives: Retrospective analysis of pharmacokinetic data across studies indicated that mean plasma concentrations of zolmitriptan were generally higher in females taking oral contraceptives compared to those not taking oral contraceptives. Mean C_{max} and AUC of zolmitriptan were found to be higher by 30% and 50%, respectively, and T_{max} was delayed by one-half hour in females taking oral contraceptives. The effect of zolmitriptan on the pharmacokinetics of oral contraceptives has not been studied.

Cimetidine: Following the administration of cimetidine, the half-life and AUC of a 5 mg dose of zolmitriptan and its active metabolite were approximately doubled (see PRECAUTIONS).

Clinical Studies: The efficacy of ZOMIG Nasal Spray 5 mg in the acute treatment of migraine headache with or without aura was demonstrated in a randomized, outpatient, double-blind, placebo-controlled trial.

Patients were instructed to treat a moderate to severe headache. Headache response, defined as a reduction in headache severity from moderate or severe pain to mild or no pain, was assessed 15, 30, 45 minutes and 1, 2, and 4 hours after dosing. Pain free response rates and associated symptoms such as nausea, photophobia, and phonophobia were also assessed. A dose of escape medication was allowed 4 to 24 hours after the initial treatment for persistent and recurrent headache.

Of the 1372 patients treated in the study, 83% were female and 99% were Caucasian, with a mean age of 40.6 years (range 18 to 65 years).

The two hour headache response rates in patients treated with ZOMIG Nasal Spray were statistically significant among patients receiving ZOMIG Nasal Spray compared to placebo. There was a greater percentage of patients with a headache response at 2 hours in the higher dose groups. The headache response efficacy endpoints of the controlled clinical study, analyzed from the first attack data, are shown in Table 1.

Table 1
First Attack Data: Percentage of Patients with Headache Response to ZOMIG Nasal Spray (Mild or No Headache) 2 Hours Following Treatment (N = number of randomized patients treating a migraine attack)
The 2 hour headache response was the primary end-point

N	PLACEBO (226)	ZOMIG 5 mg (235)
2 hours	31%	69%†

†p <0.0001 in comparison with placebo

The estimated probability of achieving an initial headache response by 4 hours following treatment with ZOMIG Nasal Spray is depicted in Figure 1.

Figure 1
Estimated probability of achieving an initial headache response within 4 hours of initial treatment

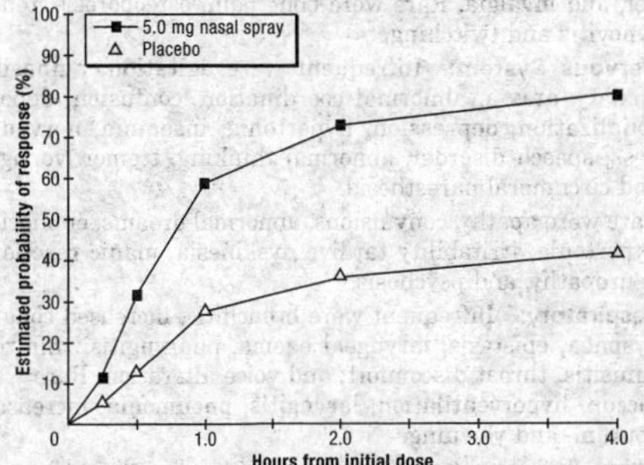

Note: Figure 1 shows the Kaplan-Meier plot of the probability over time of obtaining headache response (moderate or severe headache improving to mild or no pain) following treatment with zolmitriptan nasal spray. The averages displayed are based on a placebo controlled, outpatient trial providing evidence of efficacy. Patients not achieving headache response or taking additional treatment prior to 4 hours were censored to 4 hours.

For patients with migraine associated photophobia, phonophobia, and nausea at baseline, there was a decreased incidence of these symptoms following administration of ZOMIG Nasal Spray as compared to placebo.

Four to 24 hours following the initial dose of study treatment, patients were allowed to use additional treatment for pain relief in the form of a second dose of study treatment or other medication. The estimated probability of patients taking a second dose or other medication for migraine over the 24 hours following the initial dose of study treatment is summarized in Figure 2.

Figure 2: Estimated probability of patients taking an escape medication within the 24 hours following the initial dose of study treatment

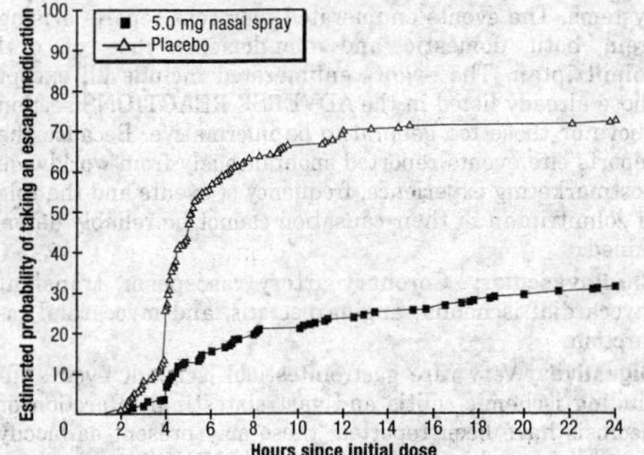

*This Kaplan-Meier plot is based on data obtained from the placebo controlled clinical trial. Patients not using additional treatments were censored at 24 hours. The plot includes both patients who had headache response at 2 hours and those who had no response to the initial dose. It should be noted that the protocol did not allow remedication within 4 hours post dose.

The efficacy of ZOMIG was unaffected by presence of aura; presence of headache upon awakening, relationship to menses; gender, age or weight of the patient; or presence of pretreatment nausea.

The efficacy of ZOMIG Nasal Spray 5 mg was further supported by an interim analysis of another similarly designed trial. The 2 hour headache response rates for the first 210 subjects in that study for ZOMIG 5 mg and placebo were 70% and 47%, respectively (N=108 and 102, respectively, p=0.0006).

INDICATIONS AND USAGE

ZOMIG Nasal Spray is indicated for the acute treatment of migraine with or without aura in adults.

ZOMIG is not intended for the prophylactic therapy of migraine or for use in the management of hemiplegic or basilar migraine (see CONTRAINDICATIONS). Safety and effectiveness of ZOMIG have not been established for cluster headache, which is present in an older, predominantly male population.

CONTRAINDICATIONS

ZOMIG should not be given to patients with ischemic heart disease (angina pectoris, history of myocardial infarction, or documented silent ischemia) or to patients who have symptoms or findings consistent with ischemic heart disease, coronary artery vasospasm, including Prinzmetal's variant angina, or other significant underlying cardiovascular disease (see WARNINGS).

ZOMIG should not be given to patients with cerebrovascular syndromes including (but not limited to) stroke of any type as well as transient ischemic attacks.

Because ZOMIG may increase blood pressure, it should not be given to patients with uncontrolled hypertension (see WARNINGS).

ZOMIG should not be used within 24 hours of treatment with another 5-HT$_1$ agonist, or an ergotamine-containing or ergot-type medication like dihydroergotamine or methysergide.

ZOMIG should not be administered to patients with hemiplegic or basilar migraine.

Concurrent administration of MAO-A inhibitors or use of zolmitriptan within 2 weeks of discontinuation of MAO-A inhibitor therapy is contraindicated (see CLINICAL PHARMACOLOGY: Drug Interactions and PRECAUTIONS: Drug Interactions).

ZOMIG is contraindicated in patients who are hypersensitive to zolmitriptan or any of its inactive ingredients.

WARNINGS

ZOMIG should only be used where a clear diagnosis of migraine has been established.

Risk of Myocardial Ischemia and/or Infarction and Other Adverse Cardiac Events:

ZOMIG should not be given to patients with documented ischemic or vasospastic coronary artery disease (see CONTRAINDICATIONS). It is strongly recommended that zolmitriptan not be given to patients in whom unrecognized coronary artery disease (CAD) is predicted by the presence of risk factors (eg, hypertension, hypercholesterolemia, smoker, obesity, diabetes, strong family history of CAD, female with surgical or physiological menopause, or male over 40 years of age) unless a cardiovascular evaluation provides satisfactory clinical evidence that the patient is reasonably free of coronary artery and ischemic myocardial disease or other significant underlying cardiovascular disease. The sensitivity of cardiac diagnostic procedures to detect cardiovascular disease or predisposition to coronary artery vasospasm is modest, at best. If, during the cardiovascular evaluation, the patient's medical history, electrocardiographic or other investigations reveal findings indicative of, or consistent with, coronary artery vasospasm or myocardial ischemia, zolmitriptan should not be administered (see CONTRAINDICATIONS). For patients with risk factors predictive of CAD, who are determined to have a satisfactory cardiovascular evaluation, it is strongly recommended that administration of the first dose of zolmitriptan take place in the setting of a physician's office or similar medically staffed and equipped facility unless the patient has previously received zolmitriptan.

Because cardiac ischemia can occur in the absence of clinical symptoms, consideration should be given to obtaining on the first occasion of use an electrocardiogram (ECG) during the interval immediately following ZOMIG, in these patients with risk factors.

It is recommended that patients who are intermittent long-term users of ZOMIG and who have or acquire risk factors predictive of CAD, as described above, undergo periodic interval cardiovascular evaluation as they continue to use ZOMIG.

The systematic approach described above is intended to reduce the likelihood that patients with unrecognized cardiovascular disease will be inadvertently exposed to zolmitriptan.

Cardiac Events and Fatalities: Serious adverse cardiac events, including acute myocardial infarction, have been reported within a few hours following administration of zolmitriptan. Life-threatening disturbances of cardiac rhythm, and death have been reported within a few hours following the administration of other 5-HT$_1$ agonists. Considering the extent of use of 5-HT$_1$ agonists in patients with migraine, the incidence of these events is extremely low.

ZOMIG can cause coronary vasospasm; at least one of these events occurred in a patient with no cardiac disease history and with documented absence of coronary artery disease. Because of the close proximity of the events to ZOMIG use, a causal relationship cannot be excluded. In the cases where there has been known underlying coronary artery disease, the relationship is uncertain.

Patients with symptomatic Wolff-Parkinson-White syndrome or arrhythmias associated with other cardiac accessory conduction pathway disorders should not receive ZOMIG.

Premarketing experience with zolmitriptan: Among the more than 2500 patients with migraine who participated in premarketing controlled clinical trials of ZOMIG Tablets, no deaths or serious cardiac events were reported. In premarketing controlled clinical trial of ZOMIG Nasal Spray, more than 1300 patients participated and there were no deaths or serious cardiac events to report.

Postmarketing experience with zolmitriptan: Serious cardiovascular events have been reported in association with the use of ZOMIG Tablets, and in very rare cases, these events have occurred in the absence of known cardiovascular disease. The uncontrolled nature of postmarketing surveillance, however, makes it impossible to determine definitively the proportion of the reported cases that were actually caused by zolmitriptan or to reliably assess causation in individual cases.

Cerebrovascular Events and Fatalities with 5-HT$_1$ agonists: Cerebral hemorrhage, subarachnoid hemorrhage, stroke, and other cerebrovascular events have been reported in patients treated with 5-HT$_1$ agonists; and some have resulted in fatalities. In a number of cases, it appears possible that the cerebrovascular events were primary, the agonist having been administered in the incorrect belief that the symptoms experienced were a consequence of migraine, when they were not. It should be noted that patients with migraine may be at increased risk of certain cerebrovascular events (eg, stroke, hemorrhage, transient ischemic attack).

Other Vasospasm-Related Events: 5-HT$_1$ agonists may cause vasospastic reactions other than coronary artery vasospasm such as peripheral and gastrointestinal vascular ischemia. As with other serotonin 5HT$_1$ agonists, very rare gastrointestinal ischemic events including ischemic colitis and gastrointestinal infarction or necrosis have been reported with ZOMIG Tablets; these may present as bloody diarrhea or abdominal pain.

Increase in Blood Pressure: As with other 5-HT$_1$ agonists, significant elevations in systemic blood pressure have been reported on rare occasions with ZOMIG Tablet use, in patients with and without a history of hypertension; very rarely these increases in blood pressure have been associated with significant clinical events. Zolmitriptan is contraindicated in patients with uncontrolled hypertension. In volunteers, an increase of 1 and 5 mm Hg in the systolic and diastolic blood pressure, respectively, was seen at 5 mg. In the headache trials, vital signs were measured only in the small inpatient study and no effect on blood pressure was seen. In a study of patients with moderate to severe liver disease, 7 of 27 experienced 20 to 80 mm Hg elevations in systolic and/or diastolic blood pressure after a dose of 10 mg of zolmitriptan (see CONTRAINDICATIONS).

An 18% increase in mean pulmonary artery pressure was seen following dosing with another 5-HT$_1$ agonist in a study evaluating subjects undergoing cardiac catheterization.

Local Adverse Reactions: Among 922 patients using the zolmitriptan nasal spray to treat 2311 attacks in the controlled clinical study who were exposed, across all doses (0.5 to 5 mg), approximately 3% noted local irritation or soreness at the site of administration. Adverse events of any kind, perceived in the nasopharynx (which may include systemic effects of triptans) were severe in about 1% of patients and approximately 60% resolved in 1 hour. Nasopharyngeal examinations, in a subset of patients participating in two long term trials of up to one year duration, failed to demonstrate any clinically significant changes with repeated use of ZOMIG Nasal Spray.

All nasopharyngeal adverse events with an incidence of ≥ 2% of patients in any zolmitriptan nasal spray dose groups are included in ADVERSE REACTIONS Table 2.

PRECAUTIONS

General: As with other 5-HT$_{1B/1D}$ agonists, sensations of tightness, pain, pressure, and heaviness have been reported after treatment with ZOMIG Tablets in the precordium, throat, neck, and jaw. Because zolmitriptan may cause coronary artery vasospasm, patients who experience signs or symptoms suggestive of angina following dosing should be evaluated for the presence of CAD or a predisposition to Prinzmetal's variant angina before receiving additional doses of medication, and should be monitored electrocardiographically if dosing is resumed and similar symptoms recur. Similarly, patients who experience other symptoms or signs suggestive of decreased arterial flow following the use of any 5-HT agonist, such as ischemic bowel syndrome or Raynaud's syndrome, are candidates for further evaluation. (see WARNINGS).

Zolmitriptan should also be administered with caution to patients with diseases that may alter the absorption, metabolism, or excretion of drugs, such as impaired hepatic function (see CLINICAL PHARMACOLOGY).

Continued on next page

Zomig Nasal Spray—Cont.

For a given attack, if a patient does not respond to the first dose of zolmitriptan, the diagnosis of migraine headache should be reconsidered before administration of a second dose.

Binding to Melanin-Containing Tissues: When pigmented rats were given a single oral dose of 10 mg/kg of radiolabeled zolmitriptan, the radioactivity in the eye after 7 days, the latest time point examined, was still 75% of the value measured after 4 hours. This suggests that zolmitriptan and/or its metabolites may bind to the melanin of the eye. Because there could be accumulation in melanin rich tissues over time, this raises the possibility that zolmitriptan could cause toxicity in these tissues after extended use. However, no effects on the retina related to treatment with zolmitriptan were noted in any of the toxicity studies including those conducted by the nasal route. Although no systematic monitoring of ophthalmologic function was undertaken in clinical trials, and no specific recommendations for ophthalmologic monitoring are offered, prescribers should be aware of the possibility of long-term ophthalmologic effects.

Information for Patients: See PATIENT INFORMATION at the end of this labeling for the figures and text of the separate leaflet provided for patients.

The ZOMIG Nasal Spray device is packaged in a carton and is a blue colored plastic device with a gray protection cap, labeled to indicate the nominal dose. Patients should be cautioned to not remove the gray protection cap until prior to dosing. The ZOMIG Nasal Spray device is placed in a nostril and actuated to deliver a single dose. **Patients should be cautioned to avoid spraying the contents of the device in their eyes.**

Laboratory Tests: No monitoring of specific laboratory tests is recommended.

Drug Interactions: Ergot-containing drugs have been reported to cause prolonged vasospastic reactions. Because there is a theoretical basis that these effects may be additive, use of ergotamine-containing or ergot-type medications (like dihydroergotamine or methysergide) and zolmitriptan within 24 hours of each other should be avoided (see CONTRAINDICATIONS).

MAO-A inhibitors increase the systemic exposure of zolmitriptan.

Therefore, the use of zolmitriptan in patients receiving MAO-A inhibitors is contraindicated (see CLINICAL PHARMACOLOGY and CONTRAINDICATIONS).

Concomitant use of other $5\text{-HT}_{1B/1D}$ agonists within 24 hours of ZOMIG treatment is not recommended. (see CONTRAINDICATIONS).

Following administration of cimetidine, the half-life and AUC of zolmitriptan and its active metabolites were approximately doubled (see CLINICAL PHARMACOLOGY).

Selective serotonin reuptake inhibitors (SSRIs) (eg, fluoxetine, fluvoxamine, paroxetine, sertraline) have been reported, rarely, to cause weakness, hyperreflexia, and incoordination when coadministered with 5-HT_1 agonists. If concomitant treatment with zolmitriptan and an SSRI is clinically warranted, appropriate observation of the patient is advised.

Drug/Laboratory Test Interactions: Zolmitriptan is not known to interfere with commonly employed clinical laboratory tests.

Carcinogenesis, Mutagenesis, Impairment of Fertility:

Carcinogenesis: Carcinogenicity studies by oral gavage were carried out in mice and rats at doses up to 400 mg/kg/day. Mice were dosed for 85 weeks (males) and 92 weeks (females). The exposure (plasma AUC of parent drug) at the highest dose level was approximately 800 times that seen in humans after a single 10 mg dose (the maximum recommended total daily dose). There was no effect of zolmitriptan on tumor incidence. Control, low dose, and middle dose rats were dosed for 104-105 weeks; the high dose group was sacrificed after 101 weeks (males) and 86 weeks (females) due to excess mortality. Aside from an increase in the incidence of thyroid follicular cell hyperplasia and thyroid follicular cell adenomas seen in male rats receiving 400 mg/kg/day, an exposure approximately 3000 times that seen in humans after dosing with 10 mg, no tumors were noted.

Mutagenesis: Zolmitriptan was mutagenic in an Ames test, in 2 of 5 strains of S. typhimurium tested, in the presence of, but not in the absence of, metabolic activation. It was not mutagenic in an *in vitro* mammalian gene cell mutation (CHO/HGPRT) assay. Zolmitriptan was clastogenic in an *in vitro* human lymphocyte assay both in the absence of and the presence of metabolic activation. Zolmitriptan was not clastogenic in *in vivo* mouse and rat micronucleus assays. Zolmitriptan was not genotoxic in an unscheduled DNA synthesis study.

Impairment of Fertility: Studies of male and female rats administered zolmitriptan prior to and during mating and up to implantation have shown no impairment of fertility at doses up to 400 mg/kg/day. Exposure at this dose was approximately 3000 times exposure at the maximum recommended human dose of 10 mg/day.

Pregnancy: Pregnancy Category C: There are no adequate and well controlled studies in pregnant women; therefore, zolmitriptan should be used during pregnancy only if the potential benefit justifies the potential risk to the fetus.

In reproductive toxicity studies in rats and rabbits, oral administration of zolmitriptan to pregnant animals was associated with embryolethality and fetal abnormalities. When pregnant rats were administered oral zolmitriptan during the period of organogenesis at doses of 100, 400, and 1200 mg/kg/day, there was a dose-related increase in embryolethality which became statistically significant at the high dose. The maternal plasma exposures at these doses were approximately 280, 1100, and 5000 times the exposure in humans receiving the maximum recommended total daily dose of 10 mg. The high dose was maternally toxic, as evidenced by a decreased maternal body weight gain during gestation. In a similar study in rabbits, embryolethality was increased at the maternally toxic doses of 10 and 30 mg/kg/day (maternal plasma exposures equivalent to 11 and 42 times exposure in humans receiving the maximum recommended total daily dose of 10 mg), and increased incidences of fetal malformations (fused sternebrae, rib anomalies) and variations (major blood vessel variations, irregular ossification pattern of ribs) were observed at 30 mg/kg/day. Three mg/kg/day was a no effect dose (equivalent to human exposure at a dose of 10 mg). When female rats were given zolmitriptan during gestation, parturition, and lactation, an increased incidence of hydronephrosis was found in the offspring at the maternally toxic dose of 400 mg/kg/day (1100 times human exposure).

Nursing Mothers: It is not known whether zolmitriptan is excreted in human milk. Because many drugs are excreted in human milk, caution should be exercised when zolmitriptan is administered to a nursing woman. Lactating rats dosed with zolmitriptan had levels in milk equivalent to maternal plasma levels at 1 hour and 4 times higher than plasma levels at 4 hours.

Pediatric Use: Safety and effectiveness of ZOMIG in pediatric patients have not been established therefore ZOMIG is not recommended for use in patients under 18 years of age. Postmarketing experience with other triptans includes a limited number of reports that describe pediatric patients who have experienced clinically serious adverse events that are similar in nature to those reported rarely in adults.

Geriatric Use: Although the pharmacokinetic disposition of the drug in the elderly is similar to that seen in younger adults, there is no information about the safety and effectiveness of zolmitriptan in this population because patients over age 65 were excluded from the controlled clinical trials. (see CLINICAL PHARMACOLOGY: Special Populations).

ADVERSE REACTIONS

Serious cardiac events, including myocardial infarction, have occurred following the use of ZOMIG Tablets. These events are extremely rare and most have been reported in patients with risk factors predictive of CAD. Events reported, in association with drugs of this class, have included coronary artery vasospasm, transient myocardial ischemia, myocardial infarction, ventricular tachycardia, and ventricular fibrillation (see CONTRAINDICATIONS, WARNINGS, and PRECAUTIONS).

Incidence in Controlled Clinical Trials: Among 464 patients treating single attacks with zolmitriptan nasal spray in a blinded placebo controlled trial, there was a low withdrawal rate related to adverse events: 5 mg (1.3%), and placebo (0.4%). None of the withdrawals were due to a serious event. One patient was withdrawn due to abnormal ECG changes from baseline that were incidentally found 23 days after the last dose of ZOMIG Nasal Spray. The most common adverse events in clinical trials for ZOMIG Nasal Spray were: unusual taste, paresthesia, hyperesthesia, and dizziness. Table 2 lists the adverse events that occurred in ≥ 2% of the 236 patients in the 5 mg dose group of the controlled clinical trial.

Table 2
Adverse events with an incidence of ≥ 2% of patients in the zolmitriptan 5 mg nasal spray treatment group by body system and greater than placebo.

Body System and Adverse event	Zolmitriptan nasal spray Placebo (N=228)	5.0 mg (N=236)
ATYPICAL SENSATIONS		
Hyperesthesia	0%	5%
Paraesthesia	6%	10%
EAR/NOSE/THROAT		
Disorder/Discomfort of nasal cavity	2%	3%
PAIN AND PRESSURE SENSATIONS		
Pain Location Specified	1%	4%
Pain Throat	1%	4%
Tightness Throat	1%	2%
DIGESTIVE		
Dry Mouth	0%	2%
Nausea	1%	4%
NEUROLOGICAL		
Dizziness	4%	3%
Somnolence	2%	4%
Unusual Taste	3%	21%
OTHER		
Asthenia	1%	3%

Adverse clinical events occurring in ≥ 1% and < 2% of patients in all attacks of the controlled clinical trial were pain abdominal, pressure throat, vomiting, headache, tightness chest, dysphagia, insomnia, palpitation and reaction aggravation.

ZOMIG is generally well tolerated. Across all doses, most adverse reactions were mild and transient and did not lead to long-lasting effects. The incidence of adverse events in controlled clinical trials was not affected by gender, weight, or age of the patients (18-39 vs. 40-65 years of age), or presence of aura. There were insufficient data to assess the impact of race on the incidence of adverse events.

Other Events: In the paragraphs that follow, the frequencies of less commonly reported adverse clinical events are presented. Because the reports include events observed in open and uncontrolled studies, the role of ZOMIG in their causation cannot be reliably determined. Furthermore, variability associated with adverse event reporting, the terminology used to describe adverse events, etc., limit the value of the quantitative frequency estimates provided. Event frequencies are calculated as the number of patients who used ZOMIG Nasal Spray and reported an event divided by the total number of patients exposed to ZOMIG Nasal Spray (n=3059). All reported events are included except those already listed in the previous table, those too general to be informative, and those not reasonably associated with the use of the drug. Events are further classified within body system categories and enumerated in order of decreasing frequency using the following definitions: infrequent adverse events are those occurring in 1/100 to 1/1000 patients and rare adverse events are those occurring in fewer than 1/1000 patients.

Body: Infrequent was allergic reaction, back pain, chills, cyst, flu syndrome, infection, jaw pain, pressure other, jaw tightening, edema of the face, abnormal laboratory test, neck pain, neoplasm, and neck tightness, chest heaviness, chest pain, and chest pressure. Rare were cellulitis, fever, jaw pressure, and neck heaviness.

Cardiovascular: Infrequent were arrhythmias, hypertension, syncope, thrombophlebitis, and tachycardia. Rare were angina pectoris, bradycardia, atrial fibrillation, myocardial infarct, vasodilation, and vascular disorder.

Digestive: Infrequent were diarrhea, dyspepsia, tongue edema, gastrointestinal disorder, increased saliva, and thirst. Rare were increased appetite, colitis, constipation, eructation, gastritis, gastrointestinal carcinoma, gingivitis, hepatic neoplasia, intestinal obstruction, jaundice, sialadenitis, and stomatitis.

Endocrine System: Rare were hyperthyroidism and thyroid edema.

Hemic: Infrequent was cyanosis. Rare were ecchymosis, lymphadenopathy and leukopenia.

Metabolic Nutritional: Rare were increased weight, dehydration, and peripheral edema.

Musculoskeletal: Infrequent were arthralgia, joint disorder, and myalgia. Rare were bone pain, osteoporosis, tenosynovitis and twitching.

Nervous System: Infrequent were agitation, amnesia, anxiety, ataxia, abnormal coordination, confusion, depersonalization, depression, hypertonia, insomnia, nervousness, speech disorder, abnormal thinking, tremor, vertigo, and circumoral paresthesia.

Rare were apathy, convulsions, abnormal dreams, euphoria, hypertonia, irritability tardive dyskinesia, manic reaction, neuropathy, and psychosis.

Respiratory: Infrequent were bronchitis, increased cough, dyspnea, epistasis, laryngeal edema, pharyngitis, rhinitis, sinusitis, throat discomfort, and voice alteration. Rare was hiccup, hyperventilation, laryngitis, pneumonia, increased sputum, and yawning.

Skin: Infrequent was pruritus, rash, skin disorder, and sweating. Rare were eczema, erythema, erythema multiform, hair disorder, and neoplasm.

Special Senses: Infrequent were amblyopia, disorder of lacrimation, ear pain, eye pain, parosmia and tinnitus. Rare were conjunctivitis, dry eye, photophobia, and visual field defect.

Urogenital: Infrequent was polyuria and menorrhagia. Rare were breast carcinoma, dysmenorrhea, metrorrhagia, breast neoplasm, unintended pregnancy, suspicious PAP smear, uterine disorder, enlarged uterine fibroids, fibrocytic breast, vaginitis, urogenital neoplasm, cystitis, urinary tract infection, kidney pain, pyelonephritis, urinary frequency, urine impaired, and urinary tract disorder.

The adverse experience profile seen with ZOMIG Nasal Spray is similar to that seen with ZOMIG tablets and Zomig-ZMT tablets except for the occurrence of local adverse effects from the nasal spray (see ZOMIG Tablet Prescribing information).

Postmarketing Experience with ZOMIG Tablets: The following section enumerates potentially important adverse events that have occurred in clinical practice and which have been reported spontaneously to various surveillance systems. The events enumerated represent reports arising from both domestic and non-domestic use of oral zolmitriptan. The events enumerated include all except those already listed in the ADVERSE REACTIONS section above or those too general to be informative. Because the reports cite events reported spontaneously from worldwide postmarketing experience, frequency of events and the role of zolmitriptan in their causation cannot be reliably determined.

Cardiovascular: Coronary artery vasospasm, transient myocardial ischemia, angina pectoris, and myocardial infarction.

Digestive: Very rare gastrointestinal ischemic events including ischemic colitis and gastrointestinal infarction or necrosis have been reported; these may present as bloody diarrhea or abdominal pain. (See WARNINGS.)

Neurological: As with other acute migraine treatments including other $5HT_1$ agonists, there have been rare reports of headache.

General: As with other $5\text{-}HT_{1B/1D}$ agonists, there have been very rare reports of anaphylaxis or anaphylactoid reactions in patients receiving ZOMIG. There have been rare reports of hypersensitivity reactions, including angioedema.

DRUG ABUSE AND DEPENDENCE

The abuse potential of ZOMIG has not been assessed in clinical trials.

OVERDOSAGE

There is no experience with clinical overdose. Volunteers receiving single 50 mg oral doses of zolmitriptan commonly experienced sedation.

The elimination half-life of ZOMIG is 3 hours (see CLINICAL PHARMACOLOGY) and therefore monitoring of patients after overdose with ZOMIG should continue for at least 15 hours or while symptoms or signs persist.

There is no specific antidote to zolmitriptan. In cases of severe intoxication, intensive care procedures are recommended, including establishing and maintaining a patent airway, ensuring adequate oxygenation and ventilation, and monitoring and support of the cardiovascular system.

It is unknown what effect hemodialysis or peritoneal dialysis has on the plasma concentrations of zolmitriptan.

DOSAGE AND ADMINISTRATION

Administer one dose of ZOMIG Nasal Spray 5 mg for the treatment of acute migraine. If the headache returns the dose may be repeated after 2 hours. The maximum daily dose should not exceed 10 mg in any 24-hour period.

In controlled clinical trials, single doses of 5 mg zolmitriptan nasal spray were administered into one nostril and were effective for the treatment of acute migraines in adults.

Individuals may vary in response to ZOMIG Nasal Spray. The pharmacokinetics of a 5 mg nasal spray dose is similar to the 5 mg oral formulations. Doses lower than 5 mg can only be achieved through the use of an oral formulation. The choice of dose, and route of administration should therefore be made on an individual basis. The effectiveness of a second dose has not been established in placebo-controlled trials.

The safety of treating an average of more than four headaches in a 30 day period has not been established.

Hepatic Impairment: Patients with moderate to severe hepatic impairment have decreased clearance of zolmitriptan and significant elevation in blood pressure was observed in some patients. Use of a lower dose of an alternate formulation with blood pressure monitoring is recommended (see CLINICAL PHARMACOLOGY AND WARNINGS).

HOW SUPPLIED

The ZOMIG Nasal Spray device is a blue colored plastic device with a gray protection cap, labeled to indicate the nominal dose. Each ZOMIG Nasal Spray device administers a single dose of ZOMIG.

ZOMIG Nasal Spray is supplied as a clear to pale yellow solution of zolmitriptan, buffered to a pH 5.0. Each ZOMIG Nasal Spray device contains 5 mg of zolmitriptan in a 100-µL unit dose aqueous buffered solution containing citric acid, anhydrous, USP, disodium phosphate dodecahydrate USP and purified water USP.

5 mg ZOMIG® Nasal Spray is supplied in boxes of 6 single use nasal spray units. (NDC 0037-7208-60).

Each ZOMIG® Nasal Spray single dose unit spray supplies 5 mg of zolmitriptan. The ZOMIG® Nasal Spray unit must be discarded after use.

Store at controlled room temperature, 20-25°C (68-77°F) [see USP].

ZOMIG is a trademark of the AstraZeneca group of companies.

Manufactured for:
AstraZeneca Pharmaceuticals LP
Wilmington, Delaware 19850
By: AstraZeneca UK Limited
Macclesfield, Cheshire, UK

Distributed by:
MedPointe Pharmaceuticals
MedPointe Healthcare Inc.
Somerset, New Jersey, 08873

Made in the United Kingdom

PATIENT SUMMARY OF INFORMATION

Zomig® Nasal Spray
ZOLMITRIPTAN

Please read this information before you start taking ZOMIG® Nasal Spray and each time you renew your prescription just in case anything has changed. Remember, this summary does not take the place of discussions with your doctor. You and your doctor should discuss ZOMIG Nasal Spray when you start taking your medication and at regular checkups.

What is ZOMIG Nasal Spray?

ZOMIG Nasal Spray is a prescription medication used to treat migraine headaches in adults. ZOMIG Nasal Spray is not for other types of headaches. The safety and efficacy of ZOMIG in patients under 18 have not been established.

What is a Migraine Headache?

Migraine is an intense, throbbing headache. You may have pain on one or both sides of your head. You may have nausea and vomiting, and be sensitive to light and noise. The pain and symptoms of a migraine headache can be worse than a common headache. Some women get migraines around the time of their menstrual period. Some people have visual symptoms before the headache, such as flashing lights or wavy lines, called an aura.

How does ZOMIG Nasal Spray work?

Treatment with ZOMIG Nasal Spray reduces swelling of blood vessels surrounding the brain. This swelling is associated with the headache pain of a migraine attack. ZOMIG Nasal Spray blocks the release of substances from nerve endings that cause more pain and other symptoms like nausea, and sensitivity to light and sound.

It is thought that these actions contribute to relief of your symptoms by ZOMIG Nasal Spray.

Who should not take ZOMIG Nasal Spray?

Do not take ZOMIG Nasal Spray if you:

- Have heart disease or a history of heart disease
- Have uncontrolled high blood pressure
- Have hemiplegic or basilar migraine (if you are not sure about this, ask your doctor)
- Have or had a stroke or problems with your blood circulation
- Have serious liver problems
- Have taken any of the following medicines in the last 24 hours: other "triptans" like almotriptan (Axert®), eletriptan (Relpax®), frovatriptan (Frova™), naratriptan (Amerge®), rizatriptan (Maxalt®), sumatriptan (Imitrex®); ergotamines like Bellergal-S®, Cafergot®, Ergomar®, Wigraine®; dihydroergotamine like D.H.E. 45® or Migranal®; or methysergide (Sansert®). These medications have side effects similar to ZOMIG Nasal Spray.
- Have taken monoamine oxidase (MAO) inhibitors such as phenelzine sulfate (Nardil®) or tranylcypromaine sulfate (Parnate®) for depression or other conditions, or if it has been less than 2 weeks since you stopped taking a MAO inhibitor.
- Are allergic to ZOMIG Nasal Spray or any of its ingredients. The active ingredient is zolmitriptan. The inactive ingredients are listed at the end of this leaflet.

Tell your doctor about all the medicines you take or plan to take, including prescription and nonprescription medicines, supplements, and herbal remedies. Your doctor will decide if you can take ZOMIG Nasal Spray with your other medicines.

Tell your doctor if you know that you have any of the following: risk factors for heart disease like high cholesterol, diabetes, smoking, obesity (overweight), menopause, or a family history of heart disease or stroke.

Tell your doctor if you are pregnant, planning to become pregnant, breast feeding, planning to breast feed, or not using effective birth control.

How should I take ZOMIG Nasal Spray?

The ZOMIG Nasal Spray device is a blue colored plastic sprayer device with a gray protection cap, labeled to indicate the dose. For adults, the usual dose is a single nasal spray taken into one nostril. If your headache comes back after your first dose, you may take a second dose anytime after 2 hours of taking the first dose. For any attack where the first dose didn't work, do not take a second dose without talking with your doctor. Do not take more than a total of 10 mg of ZOMIG (tablets or spray combined) in any 24-hour period. If you take too much medicine, contact your doctor, hospital emergency department, or poison control center right away.

The ZOMIG Nasal Spray device consists of the following parts:

A) The Tip: This is the part that you put into your nostril. The medicine comes out of a tiny hole in the top.

B) The Protective Cap: This covers the tip to protect it. Do not remove the protective cap until just before you are ready to take your ZOMIG Nasal Spray.

C) The Finger-grip: This is the part that you hold when you use the sprayer.

D) The Plunger: This is the part that you press when you put the tip into your nostril. This sprayer works only once.

Steps for using ZOMIG Nasal Spray
(Please read all steps before using for the first time):

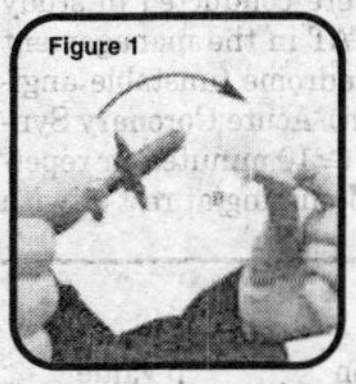

1. Blow your nose gently before use. Remove the protective cap (B) (Figure 1).

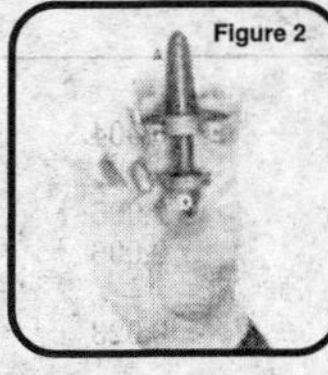

Hold the nasal sprayer device gently with your fingers and thumb as shown in the picture to the right (Figure 2). Do not press the plunger until you have put the tip into your nostril or you will lose the dose.

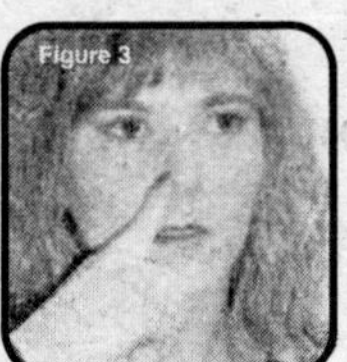

2. Block one nostril by pressing firmly on the side of your nose (Figure 3). Either nostril can be used.

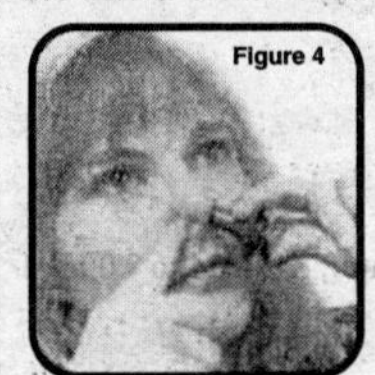

Put the tip (A) of the sprayer device into the other nostril as far as feels comfortable and tilt your head slightly as shown in the picture to the right (Figure 4).

Do not press the plunger yet.

Do not spray the contents of the device in your eyes.

3. Breathe in gently through your nose and at the same time press the plunger (D) firmly with your thumb. The plunger may feel stiff and you may hear a click. Keep your head slightly tilted back and remove the tip from your nose. Breathe gently through your mouth for 5-10 seconds. You may feel liquid in your nose or the back of your throat. This is normal and will soon pass.

What are the possible side effects of ZOMIG Nasal Spray?

ZOMIG Nasal Spray is generally well tolerated. As with any medicine, people taking ZOMIG Nasal Spray may have side effects. The side effects are usually mild and do not last long.

The most common side effects of ZOMIG Nasal Spray are:

- unusual taste, dry mouth
- tingling sensation, skin sensitivity, especially around the nose
- pain, pressure, and tightness sensations (eg, in the nose, throat, or chest)
- drowsiness, weakness, dizziness
- nausea

In very rare cases, patients taking triptans may experience serious side effects, such as heart attacks, high blood pressure, stroke, or serious allergic reactions. Extremely rarely, patients have died. **Call your doctor right away if you have any of the following problems after taking ZOMIG Nasal Spray:**

- **severe tightness, pain, pressure or heaviness in your chest, throat, neck, or jaw**
- **shortness of breath or wheezing**
- **sudden or severe stomach pain**
- **hives; tongue, mouth, or throat swelling**
- **problems seeing**
- **unusual weakness or numbness**

This is not a complete list of side effects. Talk to your doctor if you develop any symptoms that concern you.

What to do in case of an overdose?

Call your doctor or poison control center or go to the ER.

General advice about ZOMIG Nasal Spray

Medicines are sometimes prescribed for conditions that are not mentioned in patient information leaflets. Do not use ZOMIG Nasal Spray for a condition for which it was not prescribed. Do not give ZOMIG Nasal Spray to other people, even if they have the same symptoms as you. People may be harmed if they take medicines that have not been prescribed for them.

This leaflet summarizes the most important information about ZOMIG Nasal Spray. If you would like more information about ZOMIG Nasal Spray, talk to your doctor. You can ask your doctor or pharmacist for information on ZOMIG Nasal Spray that is written for health professionals. You can also call **1-800-236-9933** or visit our web site at **www.ZOMIG.com.**

What are the Ingredients in ZOMIG Nasal Spray?

Active ingredient: zolmitriptan

Inactive ingredients: anhydrous citric acid, dibasic sodium phosphate, and purified water

Store your medication at controlled room temperature, 20–25°C (68–77°F), and away from children. Discard after use or when it expires.

ZOMIG is a trademark of the AstraZeneca group of companies.

Manufactured for:
AstraZeneca Pharmaceuticals LP,
Wilmington, Delaware 19850
By: AstraZeneca UK Limited,
Macclesfield, Cheshire, UK

Distributed by:
MedPointe Pharmaceuticals
MedPointe Healthcare, Inc.
Somerset, New Jersey 08873

Made in the United Kingdom
Rev. 11/03

Shown in Product Identification Guide, page 323

Merck & Co., Inc.
PO BOX 4 WP39-206
WEST POINT, PA 19486-0004

For Medical Information Contact:
Generally:
Product and service information:
Call the Merck National Service Center, 8:00 AM to 7:00 PM (ET), Monday through Friday:
(800) NSC-MERCK
(800) 672-6372
FAX: (800) MERCK-68
FAX: (800) 637-2568
Adverse Drug Experiences:
Call the Merck National Service Center, 8:00 AM to 7:00 PM (ET), Monday through Friday:
(800) NSC-MERCK
(800) 672-6372
Pregnancy Registries
(800) 986-8999
In Emergencies:
24-hour emergency information for healthcare professionals:
(800) NSC-MERCK
(800) 672-6372
Sales and Ordering:
For product orders and direct account inquiries only, call the Order Management Center,
8:00 AM to 7:00 PM (ET), Monday through Friday:
(800) MERCK RX
(800) 637-2579

AGGRASTAT® ℞
(tirofiban hydrochloride injection premixed)
AGGRASTAT®
(tirofiban hydrochloride injection)

DESCRIPTION

AGGRASTAT* (tirofiban hydrochloride), a non-peptide antagonist of the platelet glycoprotein (GP) IIb/IIIa receptor, inhibits platelet aggregation.
Tirofiban hydrochloride monohydrate, a non-peptide molecule, is chemically described as *N*-(butylsulfonyl)-*O*-[4-(4-piperidinyl)butyl]-L-tyrosine monohydrochloride monohydrate.
Its molecular formula is $C_{22}H_{36}N_2O_5S \cdot HCl \cdot H_2O$ and its structural formula is:

Tirofiban hydrochloride monohydrate is a white to off-white, non-hygroscopic, free-flowing powder, with a molecular weight of 495.08. It is very slightly soluble in water.
AGGRASTAT Injection Premixed is supplied as a sterile solution in water for injection, for intravenous use only, in plastic containers of 100 mL or 250 mL. Each 100 mL of the premixed, iso-osmotic intravenous injection contains 5.618 mg tirofiban hydrochloride monohydrate equivalent to 5 mg tirofiban (50 mcg/mL) and the following inactive ingredients: 0.9 mg sodium chloride, 54 mg sodium citrate dihydrate, and 3.2 mg citric acid anhydrous. Each 250 mL of the premixed, iso-osmotic intravenous injection contains 14.045 mg tirofiban hydrochloride monohydrate equivalent to 12.5 mg tirofiban (50 mcg/mL) and the following inactive ingredients: 2.25 g sodium chloride, 135 mg sodium citrate dihydrate, and 8 mg citric acid anhydrous.
The pH of the solution ranges from 5.5 to 6.5 and may have been adjusted with hydrochloric acid and/or sodium hydroxide. The flexible container is manufactured from a specially designed multilayer plastic (PL2408). Solutions in contact with the plastic container leach out certain chemical components from the plastic in very small amounts; however, biological testing was supportive of the safety of the plastic container materials.
AGGRASTAT Injection is a sterile concentrated solution for intravenous infusion after dilution and is supplied in a 25 mL or a 50 mL vial. Each mL of the solution contains 0.281 mg of tirofiban hydrochloride monohydrate equivalent to 0.25 mg of tirofiban and the following inactive ingredients: 0.16 mg citric acid anhydrous, 2.7 mg sodium citrate dihydrate, 8 mg sodium chloride, and water for injection. The pH ranges from 5.5 to 6.5 and may have been adjusted with hydrochloric acid and/or sodium hydroxide.

*Registered trademark of MERCK & CO., Inc.

CLINICAL PHARMACOLOGY

Mechanism of Action
AGGRASTAT is a reversible antagonist of fibrinogen binding to the GP IIb/IIIa receptor, the major platelet surface receptor involved in platelet aggregation. When administered intravenously, AGGRASTAT inhibits *ex vivo* platelet aggregation in a dose- and concentration-dependent manner. When given according to the recommended regimen, >90% inhibition is attained by the end of the 30-minute infusion. Platelet aggregation inhibition is reversible following cessation of the infusion of AGGRASTAT.
Pharmacokinetics
Tirofiban has a half-life of approximately 2 hours. It is cleared from the plasma largely by renal excretion, with about 65% of an administered dose appearing in urine and about 25% in feces, both largely as unchanged tirofiban. Metabolism appears to be limited.
Tirofiban is not highly bound to plasma proteins and protein binding is concentration independent over the range of 0.01 to 25 mcg/mL. Unbound fraction in human plasma is 35%. The steady state volume of distribution of tirofiban ranges from 22 to 42 liters.
In healthy subjects, the plasma clearance of tirofiban ranges from 213 to 314 mL/min. Renal clearance accounts for 39 to 69% of plasma clearance. The recommended regimen of a loading infusion followed by a maintenance infusion produces a peak tirofiban plasma concentration that is similar to the steady state concentration during the infusion. In patients with coronary artery disease, the plasma clearance of tirofiban ranges from 152 to 267 mL/min; renal clearance accounts for 39% of plasma clearance.
Special Populations
Gender
Plasma clearance of tirofiban in patients with coronary artery disease is similar in males and females.
Elderly
Plasma clearance of tirofiban is about 19 to 26% lower in elderly (>65 years) patients with coronary artery disease than in younger (≤65 years) patients.
Race
No difference in plasma clearance was detected in patients of different races.
Hepatic Insufficiency
In patients with mild to moderate hepatic insufficiency, plasma clearance of tirofiban is not significantly different from clearance in healthy subjects.
Renal Insufficiency
Plasma clearance of tirofiban is significantly decreased (>50%) in patients with creatinine clearance <30 mL/min, including patients requiring hemodialysis (see DOSAGE AND ADMINISTRATION, *Recommended Dosage*). Tirofiban is removed by hemodialysis.
Pharmacodynamics
AGGRASTAT inhibits platelet function, as demonstrated by its ability to inhibit *ex vivo* adenosine phosphate (ADP)-induced platelet aggregation and prolong bleeding time in healthy subjects and patients with coronary artery disease. The time course of inhibition parallels the plasma concentration profile of the drug. Following discontinuation of an infusion of AGGRASTAT, 0.10 mcg/kg/min, *ex vivo* platelet aggregation returns to near baseline in approximately 90% of patients with coronary artery disease in 4 to 8 hours. The addition of heparin to this regimen does not significantly alter the percentage of subjects with >70% inhibition of platelet aggregation (IPA), but does increase the average bleeding time, as well as the number of patients with bleeding times prolonged to >30 minutes.
In patients with unstable angina, a two-staged intravenous infusion regimen of AGGRASTAT (loading infusion of 0.4 mcg/kg/min for 30 minutes followed by 0.1 mcg/kg/min for up to 48 hours in the presence of heparin and aspirin), produces approximately 90% inhibition of *ex vivo* ADP-induced platelet aggregation with a 2.9-fold prolongation of bleeding time during the loading infusion. Inhibition persists over the duration of the maintenance infusion.
Clinical Trials
Three large-scale clinical studies were conducted to study the efficacy and safety of AGGRASTAT in the management of patients with Acute Coronary Syndrome (unstable angina/non-Q-wave myocardial infarction). Acute Coronary Syndrome is characterized by prolonged (≥10 minutes) or repetitive symptoms of cardiac ischemia occurring at rest or with minimal exertion, associated with either ischemic ST-T wave changes on electrocardiogram (ECG) or elevated cardiac enzymes. The definition includes "unstable angina" and "non-Q-wave myocardial infarction" but excludes myocardial infarction that is associated with Q-waves or non-transient ST-segment elevation. The three studies examined AGGRASTAT alone and as an addition to heparin, prior to and after angioplasty (if indicated) (PRISM-PLUS), in comparison to heparin in a similar population (PRISM), and in addition to heparin in patients undergoing percutaneous transluminal coronary angioplasty (PTCA) or atherectomy (RESTORE). These trials are discussed in detail below.
PRISM-PLUS (Platelet Receptor Inhibition for Ischemic Syndrome Management–Patients Limited by Unstable Signs and Symptoms)
In the multi-center, randomized, parallel, double-blind PRISM-PLUS trial, the use of AGGRASTAT in combination with heparin (n=773) was compared to heparin alone (n=797) in patients with documented unstable angina/non-Q-wave myocardial infarction within 12 hours of entry into the study and initiation of treatment. All patients with unstable angina/non-Q-wave myocardial infarction had cardiac ischemia documented by ECG or had elevated cardiac enzymes. Patients who were medically managed or who subsequently underwent revascularization procedures were studied. The mean age of the population was 63 years; 32% of patients were female and approximately half of the population presented with non-Q-wave myocardial infarction. Exclusions included contraindications to anticoagulation (see CONTRAINDICATIONS), decompensated heart failure, platelet count <150,000/mm^3, and creatinine >2.5 mg/dL. In this study, patients were randomized to either AGGRASTAT (30 minute loading infusion of 0.4 mcg/kg/min followed by a maintenance infusion of 0.10 mcg/kg/min) and heparin (bolus of 5,000 units (U) followed by an infusion of 1,000 U/hr titrated to maintain an activated partial thromboplastin time (APTT) of approximately 2 times control), or heparin alone (bolus of 5,000 U followed by an infusion of 1,000 U/hr titrated to maintain an APTT of approximately 2 times control). All patients received concomitant aspirin unless contraindicated. Patients underwent 48 hours of medical stabilization on study drug therapy, and they were to undergo angiography before 96 hours (and, if indicated, angioplasty/atherectomy, while continuing on AGGRASTAT and heparin for 12–24 hours after the procedure). Some patients went on to coronary artery bypass grafting (CABG) after cessation of drug therapy. AGGRASTAT and heparin could be continued for up to 108 hours. On average, patients received AGGRASTAT for 71.3 hours. A third group of patients was initially randomized to AGGRASTAT alone (no heparin). This arm was stopped when the group was found, at an interim look, to have greater mortality than the other two groups. Note, however, that a direct comparison of heparin and tirofiban alone in the PRISM study (see below) did not show excess mortality
The primary endpoint of the study was a composite of refractory ischemia, new myocardial infarction and death at 7 days after initiation of AGGRASTAT and heparin. At the primary endpoint, there was a 32% risk reduction in the overall composite. The components of the composite were examined separately (they total more than the composite because a patient could have more than one, e.g., by dying after having a new infarction). There was a 47% risk reduction in myocardial infarction and a 30% risk reduction in refractory ischemia. The results are shown in Table 1.
[See table 1 below]
The benefit seen at 7 days was maintained over time. At 30 days, the risk of the composite endpoint was reduced by 22% (p=0.029) and there was a 30% reduction in the composite of myocardial infarction and death (p=0.027). At 6 months, the risk of the composite endpoint was reduced by 19% (p=0.024). The risk reduction in the composite endpoint at 30 days and 6 months is shown in the Kaplan-Meier curve below.

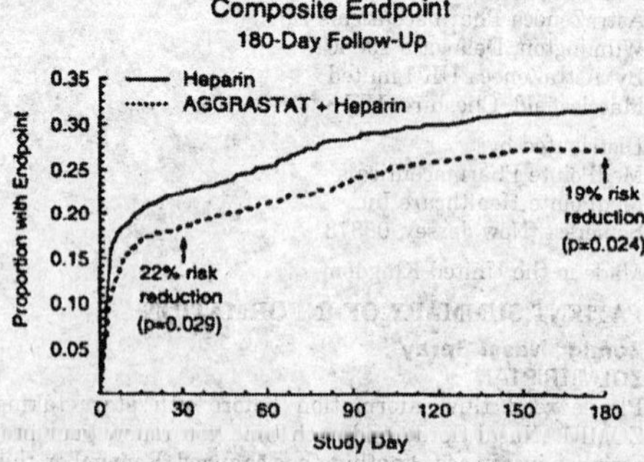

PRISM-PLUS was not designed to provide definitive results in subsets of the overall population. Nonetheless, results were examined for demographic (age, gender, race) subsets and for people who did and did not receive PTCA, atherectomy, or CABG.
In PRISM-PLUS, there was a consistent treatment effect in patients either greater or less than 65 years old, and in men and women. Too few non-Caucasians were enrolled to make a definite statement about racial differences in treatment effect.
Approximately 90% of patients in the PRISM-PLUS study underwent coronary angiography and 30% underwent angi-

Table 1
Cardiac Ischemic Events (7 Days)

Endpoint	AGGRASTAT+ Heparin (n=773)	Heparin (n=797)	Risk Reduction	p-value
Composite Endpoint	12.9%	17.9%	32%	0.004
Components				
Myocardial Infarction and Death	4.9%	8.3%	43%	0.006
Myocardial Infarction	3.9%	7.0%	47%	0.006
Death	1.9%	1.9%	—	—
Refractory Ischemia	9.3%	12.7%	30%	0.023

oplasty/atherectomy during the first 30 days of the study. The majority of these patients continued on study drug throughout these procedures. AGGRASTAT was continued for 12-24 hours (average 15 hours) after angioplasty/atherectomy. The effects of AGGRASTAT at Day 30 did not appear to differ among the sub-populations that did or did not receive PTCA or CABG, both prior to and after the procedure.

A sub-study in PRISM-PLUS of angiograms after 48 to 96 hours found that there was a significant decrease in the extent of angiographically apparent thrombus in patients treated with AGGRASTAT in combination with heparin compared to heparin alone. In addition, flow in the affected coronary artery was significantly improved.

PRISM (Platelet Receptor Inhibition for Ischemic Syndrome Management)

In the PRISM study, a randomized, parallel, double-blind, active control study, AGGRASTAT alone (n=1616) was compared to heparin (n=1616) alone as medical management in patients with unstable angina/non-Q-wave myocardial infarction. In this study, the drug was started within 24 hours of the time the patient experienced chest pain. The mean age of the population was 62 years; 32% of the population was female and 25% had non-Q-wave myocardial infraction on presentation. Thirty percent had no ECG evidence of cardiac ischemia. Exclusion criteria were similar to PRISM-PLUS. The primary, prospectively identified endpoint was the composite endpoint of refractory ischemia, myocardial infarction or death after a 48-hour drug infusion with AGGRASTAT. The results are shown in Table 2.

[See table 2 above]

In the PRISM study, no adverse effect of AGGRASTAT on mortality at either 7 or 30 days was detected. This result is in conflict with the PRISM-PLUS study, where the arm that included AGGRASTAT without heparin (n=345) was dropped at an interim analysis by the Data Safety Monitoring Committee due to increased mortality at 7 days. A pooled analysis of the data from these two trials (PRISM and PRISM-PLUS) demonstrated that the effect of AGGRASTAT alone on mortality (at 7 and 30 days) was comparable to that of heparin alone.

RESTORE (Randomized Efficacy Study of Tirofiban for Outcomes and Restenosis)

The RESTORE study (n=2141) was a randomized, controlled comparison of AGGRASTAT and placebo, each added to heparin, in patients undergoing PTCA or atherectomy within 72 hours of presentation with unstable angina or acute myocardial infarction. The mean age of the population was 59 years; 27% were female. Two-thirds of patients underwent angioplasty for unstable angina and the remainder in association with acute myocardial infarction. Exclusions included anatomy not amenable to angioplasty, contraindications to anticoagulation (see CONTRAINDICATIONS), platelet count <150,000/mm^3, and creatinine >2.0 mg/dL. AGGRASTAT (with heparin) was initiated immediately prior to the angioplasty/atherectomy at a dose of 10 mcg/kg bolus (over 3 minutes) followed by an infusion of 0.15 mcg/kg/min along with a heparin bolus (bolus of 10,000 U, or 150 U/kg for patients <70 kg). The infusion dose of AGGRASTAT is 50% higher than the dose used in the PRISM-PLUS trial. AGGRASTAT was administered for a total of 36 hours. In general, heparin was to be discontinued at the conclusion of the angioplasty/atherectomy. Reasons for continued heparin included: imperfect outcome (e.g., large tear, intraluminal filling defect, or residual stenosis >40%), large thrombus load, continuing rest angina through the procedure, abrupt closure or very active artery during the procedure, or side branch occlusion. The primary endpoint was the composite of all deaths, non-fatal myocardial infarctions, and all repeat revascularization procedures at 30 days. For results see Table 3. A sub-study in RESTORE of angiograms after approximately 6 months found that AGGRASTAT had no significant effect on the extent of coronary artery restenosis following angioplasty.

[See table 3 above]

The risk reduction in the composite endpoint at 180 days is shown in the Kaplan-Meier curve below.

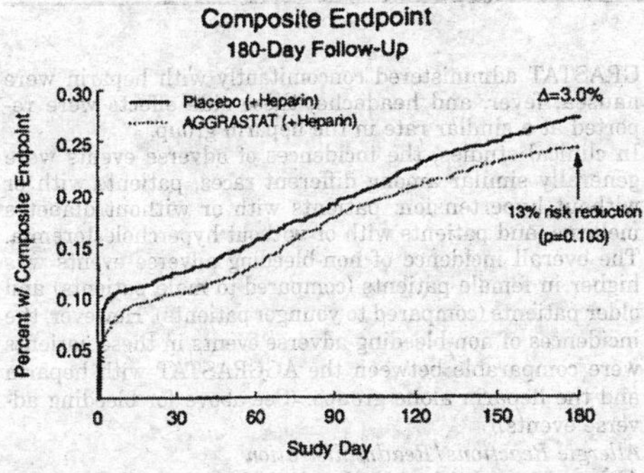

INDICATIONS AND USAGE

AGGRASTAT, in combination with heparin, is indicated for the treatment of acute coronary syndrome, including patients who are to be managed medically and those undergoing PTCA or atherectomy. In this setting, AGGRASTAT has been shown to decrease the rate of a combined endpoint of death, new myocardial infarction or refractory ischemia/repeat cardiac procedure (for discussion of trial results and for definition of acute coronary syndrome see CLINICAL PHARMACOLOGY, *Clinical Trials*).

AGGRASTAT has been studied in a setting, as described in *Clinical Trials*, that included aspirin and heparin.

Table 2
Cardiac Ischemic Events

Composite Endpoint	AGGRASTAT (n=1616)	Heparin (n=1616)	Risk Reduction	p-value
2 Days	3.8%	5.6%	33%	0.015
7 Days	10.3%	11.3%	10%	0.33
30 Days	15.9%	17.1%	8%	0.34

Table 3
Cardiac Ischemic Events

Composite Endpoint	AGGRASTAT (n=1071)	Placebo (n=1070)	Risk Reduction	p-value
2 Days	5.4%	8.7%	38%	0.004
7 Days	7.6%	10.4%	28%	0.023
30 Days	10.3%	12.2%	17%	0.17

CONTRAINDICATIONS

AGGRASTAT is contraindicated in patients with:

- known hypersensitivity to any component of the product
- active internal bleeding or a history of bleeding diathesis within the previous 30 days
- a history of intracranial hemorrhage, intracranial neoplasm, arteriovenous malformation, or aneurysm
- a history of thrombocytopenia following prior exposure to AGGRASTAT
- history of stroke within 30 days or any history of hemorrhagic stroke
- major surgical procedure or severe physical trauma within the previous month
- history, symptoms, or findings suggestive of aortic dissection
- severe hypertension (systolic blood pressure >180 mmHg and/or diastolic blood pressure >110 mmHg)
- concomitant use of another parenteral GP IIb/IIIa inhibitor
- acute pericarditis

WARNINGS

Bleeding is the most common complication encountered during therapy with AGGRASTAT. Administration of AGGRASTAT is associated with an increase in bleeding events classified as both major and minor bleeding events by criteria developed by the Thrombolysis in Myocardial Infarction Study group (TIMI).** Most major bleeding associated with AGGRASTAT occurs at the arterial access site for cardiac catheterization. Fatal bleedings have been reported (see ADVERSE REACTIONS).

AGGRASTAT should be used with caution in patients with platelet count <150,000/mm^3, in patients with hemorrhagic retinopathy, and in chronic hemodialysis patients.

Because AGGRASTAT inhibits platelet aggregation, caution should be employed when it is used with other drugs that affect hemostasis. The safety of AGGRASTAT when used in combination with thrombolytic agents has not been established.

During therapy with AGGRASTAT, patients should be monitored for potential bleeding. When bleeding cannot be controlled with pressure, infusion of AGGRASTAT and heparin should be discontinued.

** Bovill, E.G.; et al.: Hemorrhagic Events during Therapy with Recombinant Tissue-Type Plasminogen Activator, Heparin, and Aspirin for Acute Myocardial Infarction, Results of the Thrombolysis in Myocardial Infarction (TIMI) Phase II Trial, Annals of Internal Medicine,*115*(4):256-265, 1991.

PRECAUTIONS

Bleeding Precautions

Percutaneous Coronary Intervention—Care of the femoral artery access site: Therapy with AGGRASTAT is associated with increases in bleeding rates particularly at the site of arterial access for femoral sheath placement. Care should be taken when attempting vascular access that only the anterior wall of the femoral artery is punctured. Prior to pulling the sheath, heparin should be discontinued for 3-4 hours and activated clotting time (ACT) <180 seconds or APTT <45 seconds should be documented. Care should be taken to obtain proper hemostasis after removal of the sheaths using standard compressive techniques followed by close observation. While the vascular sheath is in place, patients should be maintained on complete bed rest with the head of the bed elevated 30° and the affected limb restrained in a straight position. Sheath hemostasis should be achieved at least 4 hours before hospital discharge.

Minimize Vascular and Other Trauma: Other arterial and venous punctures, epidural procedures, intramuscular injections, and the use of urinary catheters, nasotracheal intubation and nasogastric tubes should be minimized. When obtaining intravenous access, non-compressible sites (e.g., subclavian or jugular veins) should be avoided.

Laboratory Monitoring: Platelet counts, and hemoglobin and hematocrit should be monitored prior to treatment, within 6 hours following the loading infusion, and at least daily thereafter during therapy with AGGRASTAT (or more frequently if there is evidence of significant decline). In patients who have previously received GP IIb/IIIa receptor antagonists, consideration should be given to earlier monitoring of platelet count. If the patient experiences a platelet decrease to <90,000/mm^3, additional platelet counts should be performed to exclude pseudothrombocytopenia. If thrombocytopenia is confirmed, AGGRASTAT and heparin should be discontinued and the condition appropriately monitored and treated.

In addition, the activated partial thromboplastin time (APTT) should be determined before treatment and the anticoagulant effects of heparin should be carefully monitored by repeated determinations of APTT and the dose should be adjusted accordingly (see also DOSAGE AND ADMINISTRATION). Potentially life-threatening bleeding may occur especially when heparin is administered with other products affecting hemostasis, such as GP IIb/IIIa receptor antagonists. To monitor unfractionated heparin, APTT should be monitored 6 hours after the start of the heparin infusion; heparin should be adjusted to maintain APTT at approximately 2 times control.

Severe Renal Insufficiency

In clinical studies, patients with severe renal insufficiency (creatinine clearance <30 mL/min) showed decreased plasma clearance of AGGRASTAT. The dosage of AGGRASTAT should be reduced in these patients (see DOSAGE AND ADMINISTRATION and CLINICAL PHARMACOLOGY, *Clinical Trials*).

Drug Interactions

AGGRASTAT has been studied on a background of aspirin and heparin.

The use of AGGRASTAT, in combination with heparin and aspirin, has been associated with an increase in bleeding compared to heparin and aspirin alone (see ADVERSE REACTIONS). Caution should be employed when AGGRASTAT is used with other drugs that affect hemostasis (e.g., warfarin). No information is available about the concomitant use of AGGRASTAT with thrombolytic agents (see PRECAUTIONS, *Bleeding Precautions*).

In a sub-set of patients (n=762) in the PRISM study, the plasma clearance of tirofiban in patients receiving one of the following drugs was compared to that in patients not receiving that drug. There were no clinically significant effects of co-administration of these drugs on the plasma clearance of tirofiban: acebutolol, acetaminophen, alprazolam, amlodipine, aspirin preparations, atenolol, bromazepam, captopril, diazepam, digoxin, diltiazem, docusate sodium, enalapril, furosemide, glyburide, heparin, insulin, isosorbide, lorazepam, lovastatin, metoclopramide, metoprolol, morphine, nifedipine, nitrate preparations, oxazepam, potassium chloride, propranolol, ranitidine, simvastatin, sucralfate and temazepam. Patients who received levothyroxine or omeprazole along with AGGRASTAT had a higher rate of clearance of AGGRASTAT. The clinical significance of this is unknown.

Carcinogenesis, Mutagenesis, Impairment of Fertility

The carcinogenic potential of AGGRASTAT has not been evaluated.

Tirofiban HCl was negative in the *in vitro* microbial mutagenesis and V-79 mammalian cell mutagenesis assays. In addition, there was no evidence of direct genotoxicity in the *in vitro* alkaline elution and *in vitro* chromosomal aberration assays. There was no induction of chromosomal aberrations in bone marrow cells of male mice after the administration of intravenous doses up to 5 mg tirofiban/kg (about 3 times the maximum recommended daily human dose when compared on a body surface area basis).

Fertility and reproductive performance were not affected in studies with male and female rats given intravenous doses of tirofiban hydrochloride up to 5 mg/kg/day (about 5 times the maximum recommended daily human dose when compared on a body surface area basis).

Pregnancy

Pregnancy Category B

Tirofiban has been shown to cross the placenta in pregnant rats and rabbits. Studies with tirofiban HCl at intravenous

Continued on next page

Information on the Merck & Co., Inc., products listed on these pages is from the prescribing information in use October 1, 2004. For information, please call 1-800-NSC-MERCK [1-800-672-6372].

Aggrastat—Cont.

doses up to 5 mg/kg/day (about 5 and 13 times the maximum recommended daily human dose for rat and rabbit, respectively, when compared on a body surface area basis) have revealed no harm to the fetus. There are, however, no adequate and well-controlled studies in pregnant women. Because animal reproduction studies are not always predictive of human response, this drug should be used during pregnancy only if clearly needed.

Nursing Mothers

It is not known whether tirofiban is excreted in human milk. However, significant levels of tirofiban were shown to be present in rat milk. Because many drugs are excreted in human milk, and because of the potential for adverse effects on the nursing infant, a decision should be made whether to discontinue nursing or discontinue the drug, taking into account the importance of the drug to the mother.

Pediatric Use

Safety and effectiveness of AGGRASTAT in pediatric patients (<18 years old) have not been established.

Geriatric Use

Of the total number of patients in controlled clinical studies of AGGRASTAT, 42.8% were 65 years and over, while 11.7% were 75 and over. With respect to efficacy, the effect of AGGRASTAT in the elderly (≥65 years) appeared similar to that seen in younger patients (<65 years). Elderly patients receiving AGGRASTAT with heparin or heparin alone had a higher incidence of bleeding complications than younger patients, but the incremental risk of bleeding in patients treated with AGGRASTAT in combination with heparin compared to the risk in patients treated with heparin alone was similar regardless of age. The overall incidence of non-bleeding adverse events was higher in older patients (compared to younger patients) but this was true both for AGGRASTAT with heparin and heparin alone. No dose adjustment is recommended for the elderly population (see DOSAGE AND ADMINISTRATION, *Recommended Dosage*).

ADVERSE REACTIONS

In clinical trials, 1946 patients received AGGRASTAT in combination with heparin and 2002 patients received AGGRASTAT alone. Duration of exposure was up to 116 hours. 43% of the population was >65 years of age and approximately 30% of patients were female.

BLEEDING

The most common drug-related adverse event reported during therapy with AGGRASTAT when used concomitantly with heparin and aspirin, was bleeding (usually reported by the investigators as oozing or mild). The incidences of major and minor bleeding using the TIMI criteria in the PRISM-PLUS and RESTORE studies are shown below.

[See first table above]

There were no reports of intracranial bleeding in the PRISM-PLUS study for AGGRASTAT in combination with heparin or in the heparin control group. The incidence of intracranial bleeding in the RESTORE study was 0.1% for AGGRASTAT in combination with heparin and 0.3% for the control group (which received heparin). In the PRISM-PLUS study, the incidences of retroperitoneal bleeding reported for AGGRASTAT in combination with heparin, and for the heparin control group were 0.0% and 0.1%, respectively. In the RESTORE study, the incidences of retroperitoneal bleeding reported for AGGRASTAT in combination with heparin, and the control group were 0.6% and 0.3%, respectively. The incidences of TIMI major gastrointestinal and genitourinary bleeding for AGGRASTAT in combination with heparin in the PRISM-PLUS study were 0.1% and 0.1%, respectively; the incidences in the RESTORE study for AGGRASTAT in combination with heparin were 0.2% and 0.0%, respectively.

The incidence rates of TIMI major bleeding in patients undergoing percutaneous procedures in PRISM-PLUS are shown below.

[See second table above]

The incidence rates of TIMI major bleeding (in some cases possibly reflecting hemodilution rather than actual bleeding) in patients undergoing CABG in the PRISM-PLUS and RESTORE studies within one day of discontinuation of AGGRASTAT are shown below.

[See third table above]

Female patients and elderly patients receiving AGGRASTAT with heparin or heparin alone had a higher incidence of bleeding complications than male patients or younger patients. The incremental risk of bleeding in patients treated with AGGRASTAT in combination with heparin over the risk in patients treated with heparin alone was comparable regardless of age or gender. No dose adjustment is recommended for these populations (see DOSAGE AND ADMINISTRATION, *Recommended Dosage*).

NON-BLEEDING

The incidences of non-bleeding adverse events that occurred at an incidence of >1% and numerically higher than control, regardless of drug relationship, are shown below:

	PRISM-PLUS* (UAP/Non-Q-Wave MI Study)		RESTORE* (Angioplasty/Atherectomy Study)	
Bleeding	AGGRASTAT** + Heparin*** (n=773) % (n)	Heparin*** (n=797) % (n)	AGGRASTAT† + Heparin†† (n=1071) % (n)	Heparin†† (n=1070) % (n)
Major Bleeding (TIMI Criteria)‡	1.4 (11)	0.8 (6)	2.2 (24)	1.6 (17)
Minor Bleeding (TIMI Criteria)§	10.5 (81)	8.0 (64)	12.0 (129)	6.3 (67)
Transfusions	4.0 (31)	2.8 (22)	4.3 (46)	2.5 (27)

* Patients received aspirin unless contraindicated.
** 0.4 mcg/kg/min loading infusion; 0.10 mcg/kg/min maintenance infusion.
*** 5,000 U bolus followed by 1,000 U/hr titrated to maintain an APTT of approximately 2 times control.
† 10 mcg/kg bolus followed by infusion of 0.15 mcg/kg/min.
†† Bolus of 10,000 U or 150 U/kg for patients <70 kg followed by administration as necessary to maintain ACT in approximate range of 300 to 400 seconds during procedure.
‡ Hemoglobin drop of >50 g/L with or without an identified site, intracranial hemorrhage, or cardiac tamponade.
§ Hemoglobin drop of >30 g/L with bleeding from a known site, spontaneous gross hematuria, hematemesis or hemoptysis.

	AGGRASTAT + Heparin		Heparin	
	n	%	n	%
Prior to Procedures	2/773	0.3	1/797	0.1
Following Angiography	9/697	1.3	5/708	0.7
Following PTCA	6/239	2.5	5/236	2.2

	AGGRASTAT + Heparin		Heparin	
	n	%	n	%
PRISM-PLUS	5/29	17.2	11/31	35.4
RESTORE	3/12	25.0	6/16	37.5

	Most Patients		Severe Renal Impairment	
Patient Weight (kg)	30 Min Loading Infusion Rate (mL/hr)	Maintenance Infusion Rate (mL/hr)	30 Min Loading Infusion Rate (mL/hr)	Maintenance Infusion Rate (mL/hr)
30–37	16	4	8	2
38–45	20	5	10	3
46–54	24	6	12	3
55–62	28	7	14	4
63–70	32	8	16	4
71–79	36	9	18	5
80–87	40	10	20	5
88–95	44	11	22	6
96–104	48	12	24	6
105–112	52	13	26	7
113–120	56	14	28	7
121–128	60	15	30	8
129–137	64	16	32	8
138–145	68	17	34	9
146–153	72	18	36	9

	AGGRASTAT+ Heparin (n=1953) %	Heparin (n=1887) %
Body as a Whole		
Edema/swelling	2	1
Pain, pelvic	6	5
Reaction, vasovagal	2	1
Cardiovascular System		
Bradycardia	4	3
Dissection, coronary artery	5	4
Musculoskeletal System		
Pain, leg	3	2
Nervous System/Psychiatric		
Dizziness	3	2
Skin and Skin Appendage		
Sweating	2	1

Other non-bleeding side effects (considered at least possibly related to treatment) reported at a >1% rate with AGGRASTAT administered concomitantly with heparin were nausea, fever, and headache; these side effects were reported at a similar rate in the heparin group.

In clinical studies, the incidences of adverse events were generally similar among different races, patients with or without hypertension, patients with or without diabetes mellitus, and patients with or without hypercholesteremia. The overall incidence of non-bleeding adverse events was higher in female patients (compared to male patients) and older patients (compared to younger patients). However, the incidences of non-bleeding adverse events in these patients were comparable between the AGGRASTAT with heparin and the heparin alone groups. (See above for bleeding adverse events.)

Allergic Reactions/Readministration

Although no patients in the clinical trial database developed anaphylaxis and/or hives requiring discontinuation of the infusion of tirofiban, anaphylaxis has been reported in post-marketing experience (see also *Post-Marketing Experience, Hypersensitivity*). No information is available regarding the development of antibodies to tirofiban.

Laboratory Findings

The most frequently observed laboratory adverse events in patients receiving AGGRASTAT concomitantly with heparin were related to bleeding. Decreases in hemoglobin (2.1%) and hematocrit (2.2%) were observed in the group receiving AGGRASTAT compared to 3.1% and 2.6%, respectively, in the heparin group. Increases in the presence of urine and fecal occult blood were also observed (10.7% and 18.3%, respectively) in the group receiving AGGRASTAT compared to 7.8% and 12.2%, respectively, in the heparin group.

Patients treated with AGGRASTAT, with heparin, were more likely to experience decreases in platelet counts than the control group. These decreases were reversible upon discontinuation of AGGRASTAT. The percentage of patients with a decrease of platelets to <90,000/mm^3 was 1.5%, compared with 0.6% in the patients who received heparin alone. The percentage of patients with a decrease of platelets to <50,000/mm^3 was 0.3%, compared with 0.1% of the patients who received heparin alone. Platelet decreases have been observed in patients with no prior history of thrombocytopenia upon readministration of GP IIb/IIIa receptor antagonists.

Post-Marketing Experience

The following additional adverse reactions have been reported in post-marketing experience: *Bleeding:* Intracranial bleeding, retroperitoneal bleeding, hemopericardium, pulmonary (alveolar) hemorrhage, and spinal-epidural hematoma. Fatal bleeding events have been reported; *Body as a Whole:* Acute and/or severe decreases in platelet counts which may be associated with chills, low-grade fever, or bleeding complications (see *Laboratory Findings* above); *Hypersensitivity:* Severe allergic reactions including anaphylactic reactions. The reported cases have occurred during the first day of tirofiban infusion, during initial treatment, and during readministration of tirofiban. Some cases have been associated with severe thrombocytopenia (platelet counts <10,000/mm^3).

OVERDOSAGE

In clinical trials, inadvertent overdosage with AGGRASTAT occurred in doses up to 5 times and 2 times the recommended dose for bolus administration and loading infusion, respectively. Inadvertent overdosage occurred in doses up to 9.8 times the 0.15 µg/kg/min maintenance infusion rate.

The most frequently reported manifestation of overdosage was bleeding, primarily minor mucocutaneous bleeding events and minor bleeding at the sites of cardiac catheterization (see PRECAUTIONS, *Bleeding Precautions*).

Overdosage of AGGRASTAT should be treated by assessment of the patient's clinical condition and cessation or adjustment of the drug infusion as appropriate.

AGGRASTAT can be removed by hemodialysis.

DOSAGE AND ADMINISTRATION

AGGRASTAT Injection must first be diluted to the same strength as AGGRASTAT Injection Premixed, as noted under *Directions for Use.*

Use with Aspirin and Heparin

In the clinical studies, patients received aspirin, unless it was contraindicated, and heparin. AGGRASTAT and heparin can be administered through the same intravenous catheter.

Precautions

AGGRASTAT is intended for intravenous delivery using sterile equipment and technique. Do not add other drugs or remove solution directly from the bag with a syringe. Do not use plastic containers in series connections; such use can result in air embolism by drawing air from the first container if it is empty of solution. Any unused solution should be discarded.

Directions for Use

Prior to use, AGGRASTAT Injection (250 mcg/mL) must be diluted to the same strength as AGGRASTAT Injection Premixed (50 mcg/mL). This may be achieved, for example, using one of the following three methods:

1. If using a 500 mL bag of sterile 0.9% sodium chloride or 5% dextrose in water, withdraw and discard 100 mL from the bag and replace this volume with 100 mL of AGGRASTAT Injection (from four 25 mL vials or two 50 mL vials), **OR**
2. If using a 250 mL bag of sterile 0.9% sodium chloride or 5% dextrose in water, withdraw and discard 50 mL from the bag and replace this volume with 50 mL of AGGRASTAT Injection (from two 25 mL vials or one 50 mL vial), **OR**
3. If using a 100 mL bag of sterile 0.9% sodium chloride or 5% dextrose in water, add the contents of a 25 mL vial to the bag.

Mix well prior to administration.

AGGRASTAT Injection Premixed is supplied as 100 mL or 250 mL of 0.9% sodium chloride containing 50 mcg/mL tirofiban. It is supplied in IntraVia*** containers (PL 2408 plastic). To open the IntraVia® container, first tear off its foil overpouch. The plastic may be somewhat opaque because of moisture absorption during sterilization; the opacity will diminish gradually. Check for leaks by squeezing the inner bag firmly; if any leaks are found, the sterility is suspect and the solution should be discarded. Do not use unless the solution is clear and the seal is intact. Suspend the container from its eyelet support, remove the plastic protector from the outlet port, and attach a conventional administration set.

***Registered trademark of Baxter International, Inc.

AGGRASTAT may be administered in the same intravenous line as dopamine, lidocaine, potassium chloride, and PEPCID* (famotidine) Injection. AGGRASTAT should not be administered in the same intravenous line as diazepam.

Recommended Dosage

In most patients, AGGRASTAT should be administered intravenously, at an initial rate of 0.4 mcg/kg/min for 30 minutes and then continued at 0.1 mcg/kg/min. Patients with severe renal insufficiency (creatinine clearance <30 mL/min) should receive half the usual rate of infusion (see PRECAUTIONS, *Severe Renal Insufficiency* and CLINICAL PHARMACOLOGY, *Pharmacokinetics, Special Populations, Renal Insufficiency*). The table below is provided as a guide to dosage adjustment by weight.

AGGRASTAT Injection must first be diluted to the same strength as AGGRASTAT Injection Premixed, as noted under *Directions for Use.*

[See fourth table on previous page]

No dosage adjustment is recommended for elderly or female patients (see PRECAUTIONS, *Geriatric Use*). In PRISM-PLUS, AGGRASTAT was administered in combination with heparin for 48 to 108 hours. The infusion should be continued through angiography and for 12 to 24 hours after angioplasty or atherectomy.

*Registered trademark of MERCK & CO., Inc.

HOW SUPPLIED

FOR INTRAVENOUS USE ONLY

No. 3713—AGGRASTAT Injection 6.25 mg per 25 mL (250 mcg per mL) and 12.5 mg per 50 mL (250 mcg per mL) are non-preserved, clear, colorless concentrated sterile solutions for intravenous infusion after dilution and are supplied as follows:

NDC 0006-3713-25, 25 mL vials.

NDC 0006-3713-50, 50 mL vials.

No. 3739—AGGRASTAT Injection Premixed 5 mg tirofiban per 100 mL (50 mcg per mL) and 12.5 mg tirofiban per 250 mL (50 mcg per mL) are clear, non-preserved, sterile solutions premixed in a vehicle made iso-osmotic with sodium chloride, and is supplied as follows:

NDC 0006-3739-55, 100 mL single-dose IntraVia® containers (PL 2408 Plastic).

NDC 0006-3739-96, 250 mL single-dose IntraVia® containers (PL 2408 Plastic).

Storage

AGGRASTAT Injection

Store at 25°C (77°F) with excursions permitted between 15–30°C (59–86°F) (see USP Controlled Room Temperature). Do not freeze. Protect from light during storage.

AGGRASTAT Injection Premixed

Store at 25°C (77°F) with excursions permitted between 15–30°C (59–86°F) (see USP Controlled Room Temperature). Do not freeze. Protect from light during storage.

AGGRASTAT (Tirofiban Hydrochloride Injection Premixed) is manufactured for:

MERCK & CO., INC., Whitehouse Station, NJ 08889, USA

by:

BAXTER HEALTHCARE CORPORATION

Deerfield, Illinois 60015 USA

AGGRASTAT (Tirofiban Hydrochloride Injection) is manufactured for:

MERCK & CO., INC., Whitehouse Station, NJ 08889, USA

by:

BEN VENUE LABORATORIES

Bedford, Ohio 44146 USA

9123311 Issued May 2002

ALDOCLOR® Tablets ℞
(Methyldopa-Chlorothiazide)

WARNING

This fixed combination drug is not indicated for initial therapy of hypertension. Hypertension requires therapy titrated to the individual patient. If the fixed combination represents the dosage so determined, its use may be more convenient in patient management. The treatment of hypertension is not static, but must be re-evaluated as conditions in each patient warrant.

DESCRIPTION

ALDOCLOR* (Methyldopa-Chlorothiazide) combines two antihypertensives: methyldopa and chlorothiazide.

Methyldopa

Methyldopa is an antihypertensive and is the *L* - isomer of alpha-methyldopa. It is levo-3-(3,4-dihydroxyphenyl)-2- methylalanine. Its empirical formula is $C_{10}H_{13}NO_4$, with a molecular weight of 211.22, and its structural formula is:

[See chemical structure at top of next column]

Methyldopa is a white to yellowish white, odorless fine powder, and is soluble in water.

Chlorothiazide

Chlorothiazide is a diuretic and antihypertensive. It is 6-chloro-2*H* -1, 2, 4-benzothiadiazine-7-sulfonamide 1, 1-dioxide. Its empirical formula is $C_7H_6ClN_3O_4S_2$ and its structural formula is:

*Registered trademark of MERCK & CO., INC.

It is a white, or practically white crystalline powder with a molecular weight of 295.73, which is very slightly soluble in water, but readily soluble in dilute aqueous sodium hydroxide. It is soluble in urine to the extent of about 150 mg per 100 mL at pH 7.

ALDOCLOR is supplied as tablets for oral use, each containing 250 mg of methyldopa and 250 mg of chlorothiazide. Each tablet contains the following inactive ingredients: calcium disodium edetate, cellulose, citric acid, D&C Yellow 10 aluminum lake, ethylcellulose, FD&C Yellow 6 aluminum lake, gelatin, glycerin, guar gum, hydroxypropyl methylcellulose, magnesium stearate, starch, talc, titanium dioxide, and FD&C Blue 2 aluminum lake.

CLINICAL PHARMACOLOGY

Methyldopa

Methyldopa is an aromatic-amino-acid decarboxylase inhibitor in animals and in man. Although the mechanism of action has yet to be conclusively demonstrated, the antihypertensive effect of methyldopa probably is due to its metabolism to alpha-methylnorepinephrine, which then lowers arterial pressure by stimulation of central inhibitory alpha-adrenergic receptors, false neurotransmission, and/or reduction of plasma renin activity. Methyldopa has been shown to cause a net reduction in the tissue concentration of serotonin, dopamine, norepinephrine, and epinephrine.

Only methyldopa, the *L* -isomer of alpha-methyldopa, has the ability to inhibit dopa decarboxylase and to deplete animal tissues of norepinephrine. In man, the antihypertensive activity appears to be due solely to the *L* -isomer. About twice the dose of the racemate (*DL* -alpha-methyldopa) is required for equal antihypertensive effect.

Methyldopa has no direct effect on cardiac function and usually does not reduce glomerular filtration rate, renal blood flow, or filtration fraction. Cardiac output usually is maintained without cardiac acceleration. In some patients the heart rate is slowed.

Normal or elevated plasma renin activity may decrease in the course of methyldopa therapy.

Methyldopa reduces both supine and standing blood pressure. It usually produces highly effective lowering of the supine pressure with infrequent symptomatic postural hypotension. Exercise hypotension and diurnal blood pressure variations rarely occur.

Chlorothiazide

The mechanism of the antihypertensive effect of thiazides is unknown. Chlorothiazide does not usually affect normal blood pressure.

Chlorothiazide affects the distal renal tubular mechanism of electrolyte reabsorption. At maximal therapeutic dosage all thiazides are approximately equal in their diuretic efficacy.

Chlorothiazide increases excretion of sodium and chloride in approximately equivalent amounts. Natriuresis may be accompanied by some loss of potassium and bicarbonate.

After oral use diuresis begins within 2 hours, peaks in about 4 hours and lasts about 6 to 12 hours.

Pharmacokinetics and Metabolism

Methyldopa

The maximum decrease in blood pressure occurs four to six hours after oral dosage. After withdrawal, blood pressure usually returns to pretreatment levels within 24–48 hours.

Methyldopa is extensively metabolized. The known urinary metabolites are: α-methyldopa mono-0-sulfate; 3-0 methyl-α- methyldopa; 3,4,-dihydroxyphenylacetone; α-methyldopamine; 3-0-methyl-α-methyldopamine and their conjugates.

Approximately 70 percent of the drug which is absorbed is excreted in the urine as methyldopa and its mono-0-sulfate conjugate. The renal clearance is about 130 mL/min in normal subjects and is diminished in renal insufficiency. The plasma half-life of methyldopa is 105 minutes. After oral doses, excretion is essentially complete in 36 hours.

Methyldopa crosses the placental barrier, appears in cord blood, and appears in breast milk.

Continued on next page

Information on the Merck & Co., Inc., products listed on these pages is from the prescribing information in use October 1, 2004. For information, please call 1-800-NSC-MERCK [1-800-672-6372].

Aldoclor—Cont.

Chlorothiazide
Chlorothiazide is not metabolized but is eliminated rapidly by the kidney. The plasma half-life is 45–120 minutes. After oral doses, 20–24 percent of the dose is excreted unchanged in the urine. Chlorothiazide crosses the placental but not the blood-brain barrier and is excreted in breast milk.

INDICATION AND USAGE

Hypertension (see box warning).

CONTRAINDICATIONS

ALDOCLOR is contraindicated in patients:
— with active hepatic disease, such as acute hepatitis and active cirrhosis
— with liver disorders previously associated with methyldopa therapy (see WARNINGS)
— with anuria
— with hypersensitivity to methyldopa, or to chlorothiazide or other sulfonamide-derived drugs
— on therapy with monoamine oxidase (MAO) inhibitors.

WARNINGS

Methyldopa
It is important to recognize that a positive Coombs test, hemolytic anemia, and liver disorders may occur with methyldopa therapy. The rare occurrences of hemolytic anemia or liver disorders could lead to potentially fatal complications unless properly recognized and managed. Read this section carefully to understand these reactions.
With prolonged methyldopa therapy, 10 to 20 percent of patients develop a positive direct Coombs test which usually occurs between 6 and 12 months of methyldopa therapy. Lowest incidence is at daily dosage of 1 g or less. This on rare occasions may be associated with hemolytic anemia, which could lead to potentially fatal complications. One cannot predict which patients with a positive direct Coombs test may develop hemolytic anemia.
Prior existence or development of a positive direct Coombs test is not in itself a contraindication to use of methyldopa. If a positive Coombs test develops during methyldopa therapy, the physician should determine whether hemolytic anemia exists and whether the positive Coombs test may be a problem. For example, in addition to a positive direct Coombs test there is less often a positive indirect Coombs test which may interfere with cross matching of blood.
Before treatment is started, it is desirable to do a blood count (hematocrit, hemoglobin, or red cell count) for a baseline or to establish whether there is anemia. Periodic blood counts should be done during therapy to detect hemolytic anemia. It may be useful to do a direct Coombs test before therapy and at 6 and 12 months after the start of therapy.
If Coombs-positive hemolytic anemia occurs, the cause may be methyldopa and the drug should be discontinued. Usually the anemia remits promptly. If not, corticosteroids may be given and other causes of anemia should be considered. If the hemolytic anemia is related to methyldopa, the drug should not be reinstituted.
When methyldopa causes Coombs positivity alone or with hemolytic anemia, the red cell is usually coated with gamma globulin of the IgG (gamma G) class only. The positive Coombs test may not revert to normal until weeks to months after methyldopa is stopped.
Should the need for transfusion arise in a patient receiving methyldopa, both a direct and an indirect Coombs test should be performed. In the absence of hemolytic anemia, usually only the direct Coombs test will be positive. A positive direct Coombs test alone will not interfere with typing or cross matching. If the indirect Coombs test is also positive, problems may arise in the major cross match and the assistance of a hematologist or transfusion expert will be needed.
Occasionally, fever has occurred within the first three weeks of methyldopa therapy, associated in some cases with eosinophilia or abnormalities in one or more liver function tests, such as serum alkaline phosphatase, serum transaminases (SGOT, SGPT), bilirubin, and prothrombin time. Jaundice, with or without fever, may occur with onset usually within the first two to three months of therapy. In some patients the findings are consistent with those of cholestasis. In others the findings are consistent with hepatitis and hepatocellular injury.
Rarely, fatal hepatic necrosis has been reported after use of methyldopa. These hepatic changes may represent hypersensitivity reactions. Periodic determination of hepatic function should be done particularly during the first 6 to 12 weeks of therapy or whenever an unexplained fever occurs. If fever, abnormalities in liver function tests, or jaundice appear, stop therapy with methyldopa. If caused by methyldopa, the temperature and abnormalities in liver function characteristically have reverted to normal when the drug was discontinued. Methyldopa should not be reinstituted in such patients.
Rarely, a reversible reduction of the white blood cell count with a primary effect on the granulocytes has been seen. The granulocyte count returned promptly to normal on discontinuance of the drug. Rare cases of granulocytopenia have been reported. In each instance, upon stopping the drug, the white cell count returned to normal. Reversible thrombocytopenia has occurred rarely.

Chlorothiazide
Use with caution in severe renal disease. In patients with renal disease, thiazides may precipitate azotemia. Cumulative effects of the drug may develop in patients with impaired renal function.
Thiazides should be used with caution in patients with impaired hepatic function or progressive liver disease, since minor alterations of fluid and electrolyte balance may precipitate hepatic coma.
Thiazides may add to or potentiate the action of other antihypertensive drugs.
Sensitivity reactions may occur in patients with or without a history of allergy or bronchial asthma.
The possibility of exacerbation or activation of systemic lupus erythematosus has been reported.
Lithium generally should not be given with diuretics (see PRECAUTIONS, *Drug Interactions*).

PRECAUTIONS

General
Methyldopa
Methyldopa should be used with caution in patients with a history of previous liver disease or dysfunction (see WARNINGS).
Some patients taking methyldopa experience clinical edema or weight gain which may be controlled by use of a diuretic. Methyldopa should not be continued if edema progresses or signs of heart failure appear.
Hypertension has recurred occasionally after dialysis in patients given methyldopa because the drug is removed by this procedure.
Rarely, involuntary choreoathetotic movements have been observed during therapy with methyldopa in patients with severe bilateral cerebrovascular disease. Should these movements occur, stop therapy.
Chlorothiazide
All patients receiving diuretic therapy should be observed for evidence of fluid or electrolyte imbalance: namely, hyponatremia, hypochloremic alkalosis, and hypokalemia.
Serum and urine electrolyte determinations are particularly important when the patient is vomiting excessively or receiving parenteral fluids. Warning signs or symptoms of fluid and electrolyte imbalance, irrespective of cause include dryness of mouth, thirst, weakness, lethargy, drowsiness, restlessness, confusion, seizures, muscle pains or cramps, muscular fatigue, hypotension, oliguria, tachycardia, and gastrointestinal disturbances such as nausea and vomiting.
Hypokalemia may develop, especially after prolonged therapy or when severe cirrhosis is present (see CONTRAINDICATIONS and WARNINGS).
Interference with adequate oral electrolyte intake will also contribute to hypokalemia. Hypokalemia may cause cardiac arrhythmia and may also sensitize or exaggerate the response of the heart to the toxic effects of digitalis (e.g., increased ventricular irritability). Hypokalemia may be avoided or treated by use of potassium sparing diuretics or potassium supplements such as foods with a high potassium content.
Although any chloride deficit is generally mild and usually does not require specific treatment except under extraordinary circumstances (as in liver disease or renal disease), chloride replacement may be required in the treatment of metabolic alkalosis.
Dilutional hyponatremia may occur in edematous patients in hot weather; appropriate therapy is water restriction, rather than administration of salt, except in rare instances when the hyponatremia is life threatening. In actual salt depletion, appropriate replacement is the therapy of choice.
Hyperuricemia may occur or acute gout may be precipitated in certain patients receiving thiazides.
In diabetic patients dosage adjustments of insulin or oral hypoglycemic agents may be required. Hyperglycemia may occur with thiazide diuretics. Thus latent diabetes mellitus may become manifest during thiazide therapy.
The antihypertensive effects of the drug may be enhanced in the postsympathectomy patient.
If progressive renal impairment becomes evident, consider withholding or discontinuing diuretic therapy.
Thiazides have been shown to increase the urinary excretion of magnesium; this may result in hypomagnesemia.
Thiazides may decrease urinary calcium excretion. Thiazides may cause intermittent and slight elevation of serum calcium in the absence of known disorders of calcium metabolism. Marked hypercalcemia may be evidence of hidden hyperparathyroidism. Thiazides should be discontinued before carrying out tests for parathyroid function.
Increases in cholesterol and triglyceride levels may be associated with thiazide diuretic therapy.
Laboratory Tests
Methyldopa
Blood count, Coombs test and liver function tests are recommended before initiating therapy and at periodic intervals (see WARNINGS).
Chlorothiazide
Periodic determination of serum electrolytes to detect possible electrolyte imbalance should be done at appropriate intervals.
Drug Interactions
Methyldopa
When methyldopa is used with other antihypertensive drugs, potentiation of antihypertensive effect may occur. Patients should be followed carefully to detect side reactions or unusual manifestations of drug idiosyncrasy.
Patients may require reduced doses of anesthetics when on methyldopa. If hypotension does occur during anesthesia, it usually can be controlled by vasopressors. The adrenergic receptors remain sensitive during treatment with methyldopa.
When methyldopa and lithium are given concomitantly the patient should be carefully monitored for symptoms of lithium toxicity. Read the prescribing information for lithium preparations.
Several studies demonstrate a decrease in the bioavailability of methyldopa when it is ingested with ferrous sulfate or ferrous gluconate. This may adversely affect blood pressure control in patients treated with methyldopa. Coadministration of methyldopa with ferrous sulfate or ferrous gluconate is not recommended.
Monoamine oxidase (MAO) inhibitors: See CONTRAINDICATIONS.
Chlorothiazide
When given concurrently the following drugs may interact with thiazide diuretics.
Alcohol, barbiturates, or narcotics —potentiation of orthostatic hypotension may occur.
Antidiabetic drugs (oral agents and insulin)—dosage adjustment of the antidiabetic drug may be required.
Other antihypertensive drugs —additive effect or potentiation.
Cholestyramine and colestipol resins —Both cholestyramine and colestipol resins have the potential of binding thiazide diuretics and reducing diuretic absorption from the gastrointestinal tract.
Corticosteroids, ACTH —intensified electrolyte depletion, particularly hypokalemia.
Pressor amines (e.g., norepinephrine) —possible decreased response to pressor amines but not sufficient to preclude their use.
Skeletal muscle relaxants, nondepolarizing (e.g., tubocurarine) —possible increased responsiveness to the muscle relaxant.
Lithium —generally should not be given with diuretics. Diuretic agents reduce the renal clearance of lithium and add a high risk of lithium toxicity. Refer to the package insert for lithium preparations before use of such preparations with ALDOCLOR.
Non-steroidal Anti-inflammatory Drugs —In some patients, the administration of a non-steroidal anti-inflammatory agent can reduce the diuretic, natriuretic, and antihypertensive effects of loop, potassium-sparing and thiazide diuretics. Therefore, when ALDOCLOR and non-steroidal anti-inflammatory agents are used concomitantly, the patient should be observed closely to determine if the desired effect of the diuretic is obtained.
Drug/Laboratory Test Interactions
Methyldopa
Methyldopa may interfere with measurement of: urinary uric acid by the phosphotungstate method, serum creatinine by the alkaline picrate method, and SGOT by colorimetric methods. Interference with spectrophotometric methods for SGOT analysis has not been reported.
Since methyldopa causes fluorescence in urine samples at the same wave lengths as catecholamines, falsely high levels of urinary catecholamines may be reported. This will interfere with the diagnosis of pheochromocytoma. It is important to recognize this phenomenon before a patient with a possible pheochromocytoma is subjected to surgery. Methyldopa does not interfere with measurement of VMA (vanillylmandelic acid), a test for pheochromocytoma, by those methods which convert VMA to vanillin. Methyldopa is not recommended for the treatment of patients with pheochromocytoma. Rarely, when urine is exposed to air after voiding, it may darken because of breakdown of methyldopa or its metabolites.
Chlorothiazide
Thiazides should be discontinued before carrying out tests for parathyroid function (see PRECAUTIONS, *General*).
Carcinogenesis, Mutagenesis, Impairment of Fertility
Studies to evaluate the carcinogenic or mutagenic potential of the methyldopa-chlorothiazide combination, or the effects of this combination on fertility have not been performed.
Methyldopa
No evidence of a tumorigenic effect was seen when methyldopa was given for two years to mice at doses up to 1800 mg/kg/day or to rats at doses up to 240 mg/kg/day (30 and 4 times the maximum recommended human dose in mice and rats, respectively, when compared on the basis of body weight; 2.5 and 0.6 times the maximum recommended human dose in mice and rats, respectively, when compared on the basis of body surface area; calculations assume a patient weight of 50 kg).
Methyldopa was not mutagenic in the Ames Test and did not increase chromosomal aberration or sister chromatid exchanges in Chinese hamster ovary cells. These *in vitro* studies were carried out both with and without exogenous metabolic activation.
Fertility was unaffected when methyldopa was given to male and female rats at 100 mg/kg/day (1.7 times the maximum daily human dose when compared on the basis of body weight; 0.2 times the maximum daily human dose when compared on the basis of body surface area). Methyldopa decreased sperm count, sperm motility, the number of late spermatids and the male fertility index when given to male rats of 200 and 400 mg/kg/day (3.3 and 6 times the maximum daily human dose when compared on the basis of body weight; 0.5 and 1 times the maximum daily human dose when compared on the basis of body surface area).

Chlorothiazide
Carcinogenicity studies have not been done with chlorothiazide.
Chlorothiazide was not mutagenic *in vitro* in the Ames microbial mutagen test (using a maximum concentration of 5 mg/plate and *Salmonella typhimurium* strains TA 98 and TA 100) and was not mutagenic and did not induce miotic nondis junction to diploid-strains of *Aspergillus nidulans.*
Chlorothiazide had no adverse effects on fertility in female rats at doses up to 60/mg/kg/day and no adverse effects on fertility in male rats at doses up to 40 mg/kg/day. These doses are 1.5 and 1.0 times* the recommended maximum human dose, respectively, when compared on a body weight basis.

*Calculations based on a human body weight of 50 kg.

Pregnancy
Use of diuretics during normal pregnancy is inappropriate and exposes mother and fetus to unnecessary hazard. Diuretics do not prevent development of toxemia of pregnancy and there is no satisfactory evidence that they are useful in treatment of toxemia.
Teratogenic Effects —Pregnancy Category C: Reproduction studies in the rat, at doses up to 40 mg/kg/day (3–4 times the maximum recommended human dose), did not impair fertility or cause abnormalities of the fetus due to ALDOCLOR.
There are no adequate and well-controlled studies with ALDOCLOR in pregnant women. Because animal reproduction studies are not always predictive of human response, this drug should be used during pregnancy only if clearly needed.
Chlorothiazide: Thiazides cross the placental barrier and appear in cord blood.
Although reproduction studies performed with chlorothiazide doses of 50 mg/kg/day in rabbits, 60 mg/kg/day in rats and 500 mg/kg/day in mice revealed no external abnormalities or impairment of neonatal growth and survival due to chlorothiazide, such studies did not include complete visceral and skeletal examinations.
Methyldopa: Reproduction studies performed with methyldopa at oral doses up to 1000 mg/kg in mice, 200 mg/kg in rabbits, and 100 mg/kg in rats revealed no evidence of harm to the fetus. These doses are 16.6 times, 3.3 times and 1.7 times, respectively, the maximum daily human dose when compared on the basis of body weight: 1.4 times, 1.1 times and 0.2 times, respectively, when compared on the basis of body surface area: calculations assume a patient weight of 50 kg. There are, however, no adequate and well-controlled studies in pregnant women in the first trimester of pregnancy. Because animal reproduction studies are not always predictive of human response, methyldopa should be used during pregnancy only if clearly needed.
Published reports of the use of methyldopa during all trimesters indicate that if this drug is used during pregnancy the possibility of fetal harm appears remote. In five studies, three of which were controlled, involving 332 pregnant hypertensive women, treatment with methyldopa was associated with an improved fetal outcome. The majority of these women were in the third trimester when methyldopa therapy was begun.
In one study, women who had begun methyldopa treatment between weeks 16 and 20 of pregnancy gave birth to infants whose average head circumference was reduced by a small amount (34.2 ± 1.7 cm vs. 34.6 ± 1.3 cm [mean ± 1 S.D.]). Long-term follow up of 195 (97.5%) of the children born to methyldopa-treated pregnant women (including those who began treatment between weeks 16 and 20) failed to uncover any significant adverse effect on the children. At four years of age, the developmental delay commonly seen in children born to hypertensive mothers was less evident in those whose mothers were treated with methyldopa during pregnancy than those whose mothers were untreated. The children of the treated group scored consistently higher than the children of the untreated group on five major indices of intellectual and motor development. At age seven and one-half developmental scores and intelligence indices showed no significant differences in children of treated or untreated hypertensive women.
Nonteratogenic Effects: These may include fetal or neonatal jaundice, thrombocytopenia, and possibly other adverse reactions which have occurred in the adult.
Nursing Mothers
Methyldopa and thiazides appear in breast milk. Therefore, because of the potential for serious adverse reactions in nursing infants from chlorothiazide, a decision should be made whether to discontinue nursing or to discontinue the drug, taking into account the importance of the drug to the mother.
Pediatric Use
Safety and effectiveness of ALDOCLOR in pediatric patients have not been established.

ADVERSE REACTIONS

The following adverse reactions have been reported and, within each category, are listed in order of decreasing severity.
Methyldopa
Sedation, usually transient, may occur during the initial period of therapy or whenever the dose is increased. Headache, asthenia, or weakness may be noted as early and transient symptoms. However, significant adverse effects due to methyldopa have been infrequent and this agent usually is well tolerated.
Cardiovascular: Aggravation of angina pectoris, congestive heart failure, prolonged carotid sinus hypersensitivity, orthostatic hypotension (decrease daily dosage), edema or weight gain, bradycardia.
Digestive: Pancreatitis, colitis, vomiting, diarrhea, sialadenitis, sore or "black" tongue, nausea, constipation, distension, flatus, dryness of mouth.
Endocrine: Hyperprolactinemia.
Hematologic: Bone marrow depression, leukopenia, granulocytopenia, thrombocytopenia, hemolytic anemia; positive tests for antinuclear antibody, LE cells, and rheumatoid factor, positive Coombs test.
Hepatic: Liver disorders including hepatitis, jaundice, abnormal liver function tests (see WARNINGS).
Hypersensitivity: Myocarditis, pericarditis, vasculitis, lupus-like syndrome, drug-related fever, eosinophilia.
Nervous System / Psychiatric: Parkinsonism, Bell's palsy, decreased mental acuity, involuntary choreoathetotic movements, symptoms of cerebrovascular insufficiency, psychic disturbances including nightmares and reversible mild psychoses or depression, headache, sedation, asthenia or weakness, dizziness, lightheadedness, paresthesias.
Metabolic: Rise in BUN.
Musculoskeletal: Arthralgia, with or without joint swelling; myalgia.
Respiratory: Nasal stuffiness.
Skin: Toxic epidermal necrolysis, rash.
Urogenital: Amenorrhea, breast enlargement, gynecomastia, lactation, impotence, decreased libido.
Chlorothiazide
Body as a Whole: Weakness.
Cardiovascular: Hypotension including orthostatic hypotension (may be aggravated by alcohol, barbiturates, narcotics or antihypertensive drugs).
Digestive: Pancreatitis, jaundice (intrahepatic cholestatic jaundice), diarrhea, vomiting, sialadenitis, cramping, constipation, gastric irritation, nausea, anorexia.
Hematologic: Aplastic anemia, agranulocytosis, leukopenia, hemolytic anemia, thrombocytopenia.
Hypersensitivity: Anaphylactic reactions, necrotizing angiitis (vasculitis and cutaneous vasculitis), respiratory distress including pneumonitis and pulmonary edema, photosensitivity, fever, urticaria, rash, purpura.
Metabolic: Electrolyte imbalance (see PRECAUTIONS), hyperglycemia, glycosuria, hyperuricemia.
Musculoskeletal: Muscle spasm.
Nervous System / Psychiatric: Vertigo, paresthesias, dizziness, headache, restlessness.
Renal: Renal failure, renal dysfunction, interstitial nephritis. (See WARNINGS.)
Skin: Erythema multiforme including Stevens-Johnson syndrome, exfoliative dermatitis including toxic epidermal necrolysis, alopecia.
Special Senses: Transient blurred vision, xanthopsia.
Urogenital: Impotence.

OVERDOSAGE

Acute overdosage may produce acute hypotension with other responses attributable to brain and gastrointestinal malfunction (excessive sedation, weakness, bradycardia, dizziness, lightheadedness, constipation, distention, flatus, diarrhea, nausea, vomiting).
In the event of overdosage, symptomatic and supportive measures should be employed. When ingestion is recent, gastric lavage or emesis may reduce absorption. Otherwise, management includes special attention to cardiac rate and output, blood volume, electrolyte imbalance, paralytic ileus, urinary function and cerebral activity.
Sympathomimetic drugs [e.g., levarterenol, epinephrine, ARAMINE* (Metaraminol Bitartrate)] may be indicated. Methyldopa is dialyzable. The degree to which chlorothiazide is removed by hemodialysis has not been established.
The oral LD_{50} of methyldopa is greater than 1.5 g/kg in both the mouse and the rat. The oral LD_{50} of chlorothiazide is 8.5 g/kg, greater than 10 g/kg, and greater than 1 g/kg in the mouse, rat, and dog respectively.

*Registered trademark of MERCK & CO., INC.

DOSAGE AND ADMINISTRATION

DOSAGE MUST BE INDIVIDUALIZED, AS DETERMINED BY TITRATION OF THE INDIVIDUAL COMPONENTS (see box warning). Once the patient has been successfully titrated, ALDOCLOR may be substituted if the previously determined titrated doses are the same as in the combination. The usual starting dosage is one tablet of ALDOCLOR 250 two or three times a day.
When administered individually, the usual daily dosage of chlorothiazide is 0.5 g to 1.0 g in single or divided doses and that of methyldopa is 500 mg to 2 g. To minimize the sedation associated with methyldopa, start dosage increases in the evening.
Occasionally tolerance to methyldopa may occur, usually between the second and third month of therapy. Additional separate doses of methyldopa or replacement of ALDOCLOR with single entity agents is necessary until the new effective dose ratio is re-established by titration. The maximum recommended daily dose of methyldopa is 3 g. When ALDOCLOR 250 is used to provide 1 g of methyldopa, 1 g of chlorothiazide is delivered. It is prudent, if greater than 1 g of methyldopa per day is required, to provide the additional methyldopa as methyldopa alone.
If ALDOCLOR does not adequately control blood pressure, additional doses of other agents may be given. When ALDOCLOR is given with antihypertensives other than thiazides, the initial dosage of methyldopa should be limited to 500 mg daily in divided doses and the dose of these other agents may need to be adjusted to effect a smooth transition.
Since both components of ALDOCLOR have a relatively short duration of action, withdrawal is followed by return of hypertension usually within 48 hours. This is not complicated by an overshoot of blood pressure.
Since methyldopa is largely excreted by the kidney, patients with impaired renal function may respond to smaller doses. Syncope in older patients may be related to an increased sensitivity and advanced arteriosclerotic vascular disease. This may be avoided by lower doses.

HOW SUPPLIED

No. 3319—Tablets ALDOCLOR 250 are green, oval, film coated tablets coded MSD 634 on one side and ALDOCLOR on the other. Each tablet contains 250 mg of methyldopa and 250 mg of chlorothiazide. They are supplied as follows:
NDC 0006-0634-68 bottles of 100.
Storage
Keep container tightly closed. Protect from moisture, light, and freezing, −20°C (−4°F) and store at room temperature, 15–30°C (59–86°F).
7899646 Issued February 1999

Shown in Product Identification Guide, page 323

ALDORIL® Tablets ℞
(Methyldopa-Hydrochlorothiazide)

WARNING
This fixed combination drug is not indicated for initial therapy of hypertension. Hypertension requires therapy titrated to the individual patient. If the fixed combination represents the dosage so determined, its use may be more convenient in patient management. The treatment of hypertension is not static, but must be re-evaluated as conditions in each patient warrant.

DESCRIPTION

ALDORIL* (Methyldopa-Hydrochlorothiazide) combines two antihypertensives: methyldopa and hydrochlorothiazide.
Methyldopa
Methyldopa is an antihypertensive and is the *L* -isomer of alphamethyldopa. It is levo-3-(3,4-dihydroxyphenyl)-2-methylalanine. Its empirical formula is $C_{10}H_{13}NO_4$, with a molecular weight of 211.22, and its structural formula is:

Methyldopa is a white to yellowish white, odorless fine powder, and is soluble in water.
Hydrochlorothiazide
Hydrochlorothiazide is a diuretic and antihypertensive. It is the 3,4-dihydro derivative of chlorothiazide. Its chemical name is 6-chloro-3,4-dihydro-2*H* -1,2,4-benzothiadiazine-7-sulfonamide 1,1-dioxide. Its empirical formula is $C_7H_8ClN_3O_4S_2$ and its structural formula is:

Hydrochlorothiazide is a white, or practically white, crystalline powder with a molecular weight of 297.74, which is slightly soluble in water, but freely soluble in sodium hydroxide solution.
ALDORIL is supplied as tablets in four strengths for oral use:
ALDORIL 15, contains 250 mg of methyldopa and 15 mg of hydrochlorothiazide.

*Registered trademark of MERCK & CO., Inc.

Continued on next page

Information on the Merck & Co., Inc., products listed on these pages is from the prescribing information in use October 1, 2004. For information, please call 1-800-NSC-MERCK [1-800-672-6372].

Aldoril—Cont.

ALDORIL 25, contains 250 mg of methyldopa and 25 mg of hydrochlorothiazide.
ALDORIL D30, contains 500 mg of methyldopa and 30 mg of hydrochlorothiazide.
ALDORIL D50, contains 500 mg of methyldopa and 50 mg of hydrochlorothiazide.
Each tablet contains the following inactive ingredients: calcium disodium edetate, calcium phosphate, cellulose, citric acid, colloidal silicon dioxide, ethylcellulose, guar gum, hydroxypropyl methylcellulose, magnesium stearate, propylene glycol, talc, and titanium dioxide. ALDORIL 15 and ALDORIL D30 also contain iron oxide.

CLINICAL PHARMACOLOGY

Methyldopa
Methyldopa is an aromatic-amino-acid decarboxylase inhibitor in animals and in man. Although the mechanism of action has yet to be conclusively demonstrated, the antihypertensive effect of methyldopa probably is due to its metabolism to alpha-methylnorepinephrine, which then lowers arterial pressure by stimulation of central inhibitory alpha-adrenergic receptors, false neurotransmission, and/or reduction of plasma renin activity. Methyldopa has been shown to cause a net reduction in the tissue concentration of serotonin, dopamine, norepinephrine, and epinephrine.
Only methyldopa, the *L* -isomer of alpha-methyldopa, has the ability to inhibit dopa decarboxylase and to deplete animal tissues of norepinephrine. In man, the antihypertensive activity appears to be due solely to the *L*-isomer. About twice the dose of the racemate (*DL* -alpha-methyldopa) is required for equal antihypertensive effect.
Methyldopa has no direct effect on cardiac function and usually does not reduce glomerular filtration rate, renal blood flow, or filtration fraction. Cardiac output usually is maintained without cardiac acceleration. In some patients the heart rate is slowed.
Normal or elevated plasma renin activity may decrease in the course of methyldopa therapy.
Methyldopa reduces both supine and standing blood pressure. It usually produces highly effective lowering of the supine pressure with infrequent symptomatic postural hypotension. Exercise hypotension and diurnal blood pressure variations rarely occur.
Hydrochlorothiazide
The mechanism of the antihypertensive effect of thiazides is unknown. Hydrochlorothiazide does not usually affect normal blood pressure.
Hydrochlorothiazide affects the distal renal tubular mechanism of electrolyte reabsorption. At maximal therapeutic dosage all thiazides are approximately equal in their diuretic efficacy.
Hydrochlorothiazide increases excretion of sodium and chloride in approximately equivalent amounts. Natriuresis may be accompanied by some loss of potassium and bicarbonate.
After oral use diuresis begins within 2 hours, peaks in about 4 hours and lasts about 6 to 12 hours.
Pharmacokinetics and Metabolism
Methyldopa
The maximum decrease in blood pressure occurs four to six hours after oral dosage. Once an effective dosage level is attained, a smooth blood pressure response occurs in most patients in 12 to 24 hours. After withdrawal, blood pressure usually returns to pretreatment levels within 24–48 hours.
Methyldopa is extensively metabolized. The known urinary metabolites are: α-methyldopa mono-0-sulfate; 3-0-methyl-α-methyldopa; 3,4-dihydroxyphenylacetone; α-methyldopamine; 3-0-methyl-α-methyldopamine and their conjugates.
Approximately 70 percent of the drug which is absorbed is excreted in the urine as methyldopa and its mono-0-sulfate conjugate. The renal clearance is about 130 mL/min in normal subjects and is diminished in renal insufficiency. The plasma half-life of methyldopa is 105 minutes. After oral doses, excretion is essentially complete in 36 hours.
Methyldopa crosses the placental barrier, appears in cord blood, and appears in breast milk.
Hydrochlorothiazide
Hydrochlorothiazide is not metabolized but is eliminated rapidly by the kidney. When plasma levels have been followed for at least 24 hours, the plasma half-life has been observed to vary between 5.6 and 14.8 hours. At least 61 percent of the oral dose is eliminated unchanged within 24 hours. Hydrochlorothiazide crosses the placental but not the blood-brain barrier and is excreted in breast milk.

INDICATION AND USAGE

Hypertension (see box warning).

CONTRAINDICATIONS

ALDORIL is contraindicated in patients:
— with active hepatic disease, such as acute hepatitis and active cirrhosis
— with liver disorders previously associated with methyldopa therapy (see WARNINGS)
— with anuria
— with hypersensitivity to methyldopa, or to hydrochlorothiazide or other sulfonamide-derived drugs
— on therapy with monoamine oxidase (MAO) inhibitors.

WARNINGS

Methyldopa
It is important to recognize that a positive Coombs test, hemolytic anemia, and liver disorders may occur with methyldopa therapy. The rare occurrences of hemolytic anemia or liver disorders could lead to potentially fatal complications unless properly recognized and managed. Read this section carefully to understand these reactions.
With prolonged methyldopa therapy, 10 to 20 percent of patients develop a positive direct Coombs test which usually occurs between 6 and 12 months of methyldopa therapy. Lowest incidence is at daily dosage of 1 g or less. This on rare occasions may be associated with hemolytic anemia, which could lead to potentially fatal complications. One cannot predict which patients with a positive direct Coombs test may develop hemolytic anemia.
Prior existence or development of a positive direct Coombs test is not in itself a contraindication to use of methyldopa. If a positive Coombs test develops during methyldopa therapy, the physician should determine whether hemolytic anemia exists and whether the positive Coombs test may be a problem. For example, in addition to a positive direct Coombs test there is less often a positive indirect Coombs test which may interfere with cross matching of blood.
Before treatment is started it is desirable to do a blood count (hematocrit, hemoglobin, or red cell count) for a baseline or to establish whether there is anemia. Periodic blood counts should be done during therapy to detect hemolytic anemia. It may be useful to do a direct Coombs test before therapy and at 6 and 12 months after the start of therapy.
If Coombs-positive hemolytic anemia occurs, the cause may be methyldopa and the drug should be discontinued. Usually the anemia remits promptly. If not, corticosteroids may be given and other causes of anemia should be considered. If the hemolytic anemia is related to methyldopa, the drug should not be reinstituted.
When methyldopa causes Coombs positivity alone or with hemolytic anemia, the red cell is usually coated with gamma globulin of the IgG (gamma G) class only. The positive Coombs test may not revert to normal until weeks to months after methyldopa is stopped.
Should the need for transfusion arise in a patient receiving methyldopa, both a direct and an indirect Coombs test should be performed. In the absence of hemolytic anemia, usually only the direct Coombs test will be positive. A positive direct Coombs test alone will not interfere with typing or cross matching. If the indirect Coombs test is also positive, problems may arise in the major cross match and the assistance of a hematologist or transfusion expert will be needed.
Occasionally, fever has occurred within the first three weeks of methyldopa therapy, associated in some cases with eosinophilia or abnormalities in one or more liver function tests, such as serum alkaline phosphatase, serum transaminases (SGOT, SGPT), bilirubin, and prothrombin time. Jaundice, with or without fever, may occur with onset usually within the first two to three months of therapy. In some patients the findings are consistent with those of cholestasis. In others the findings are consistent with hepatitis and hepatocellular injury.
Rarely, fatal hepatic necrosis has been reported after use of methyldopa. These hepatic changes may represent hypersensitivity reactions. Periodic determination of hepatic function should be done particularly during the first 6 to 12 weeks of therapy or whenever an unexplained fever occurs. If fever, abnormalities in liver function tests, or jaundice appear, stop therapy with methyldopa. If caused by methyldopa, the temperature and abnormalities in liver function characteristically have reverted to normal when the drug was discontinued. Methyldopa should not be reinstituted in such patients.
Rarely, a reversible reduction of the white blood cell count with a primary effect on the granulocytes has been seen. The granulocyte count returned promptly to normal on discontinuance of the drug. Rare cases of granulocytopenia have been reported. In each instance, upon stopping the drug, the white cell count returned to normal. Reversible thrombocytopenia has occurred rarely.
Hydrochlorothiazide
Use with caution in severe renal disease. In patients with renal disease, thiazides may precipitate azotemia. Cumulative effects of the drug may develop in patients with impaired renal function.
Thiazides should be used with caution in patients with impaired hepatic function or progressive liver disease, since minor alterations of fluid and electrolyte balance may precipitate hepatic coma.
Thiazides may add to or potentiate the action of other antihypertensive drugs.
Sensitivity reactions may occur in patients with or without a history of allergy or bronchial asthma.
The possibility of exacerbation or activation of systemic lupus erythematosus has been reported.
Lithium generally should not be given with diuretics (see PRECAUTIONS, *Drug Interactions*).

PRECAUTIONS

General
Methyldopa
Methyldopa should be used with caution in patients with a history of previous liver disease or dysfunction (see WARNINGS).
Some patients taking methyldopa experience clinical edema or weight gain which may be controlled by use of a diuretic. Methyldopa should not be continued if edema progresses or signs of heart failure appear.
Hypertension has recurred occasionally after dialysis in patients given methyldopa because the drug is removed by this procedure.
Rarely, involuntary choreoathetotic movements have been observed during therapy with methyldopa in patients with severe bilateral cerebrovascular disease. Should these movements occur, stop therapy.
Hydrochlorothiazide
All patients receiving diuretic therapy should be observed for evidence of fluid or electrolyte imbalance: namely; hyponatremia, hypochloremic alkalosis, and hypokalemia. Serum and urine electrolyte determinations are particularly important when the patient is vomiting excessively or receiving parenteral fluids. Warning signs or symptoms of fluid and electrolyte imbalance, irrespective of cause, include dryness of mouth, thirst, weakness, lethargy, drowsiness, restlessness, confusion, seizures, muscle pains or cramps, muscular fatigue, hypotension, oliguria, tachycardia, and gastrointestinal disturbances such as nausea and vomiting.
Hypokalemia may develop especially after prolonged therapy or when severe cirrhosis is present (see CONTRAINDICATIONS and WARNINGS).
Interference with adequate oral electrolyte intake will also contribute to hypokalemia. Hypokalemia may cause cardiac arrhythmia and may also sensitize or exaggerate the response of the heart to the toxic effects of digitalis (e.g., increased ventricular irritability). Hypokalemia may be avoided or treated by use of potassium sparing diuretics or potassium supplements such as foods with a high potassium content.
Although any chloride deficit is generally mild and usually does not require specific treatment except under extraordinary circumstances (as in liver disease or renal disease), chloride replacement may be required in the treatment of metabolic alkalosis.
Dilutional hyponatremia may occur in edematous patients in hot weather; appropriate therapy is water restriction, rather than administration of salt, except in rare instances when the hyponatremia is life threatening. In actual salt depletion, appropriate replacement is the therapy of choice.
Hyperuricemia may occur or acute gout may be precipitated in certain patients receiving thiazides.
In diabetic patients dosage adjustment of insulin or oral hypoglycemic agents may be required. Hyperglycemia may occur with thiazide diuretics. Thus latent diabetes mellitus may become manifest during thiazide therapy.
The antihypertensive effects of the drug may be enhanced in the postsympathectomy patient.
If progressive renal impairment becomes evident, consider withholding or discontinuing diuretic therapy.
Thiazides have been shown to increase the urinary excretion of magnesium; this may result in hypomagnesemia.
Thiazides may decrease urinary calcium excretion. Thiazides may cause intermittent and slight elevation of serum calcium in the absence of known disorders of calcium metabolism. Marked hypercalcemia may be evidence of hidden hyperparathyroidism. Thiazides should be discontinued before carrying out tests for parathyroid function.
Increases in cholesterol and triglyceride levels may be associated with thiazide diuretic therapy.
Laboratory Tests
Methyldopa
Blood count, Coombs test and liver function test, are recommended before initiating therapy and at periodic intervals (see WARNINGS).
Hydrochlorothiazide
Periodic determination of serum electrolytes to detect possible electrolyte imbalance should be done at appropriate intervals.
Drug Interactions
Methyldopa
When methyldopa is used with other antihypertensive drugs, potentiation of antihypertensive effect may occur. Patients should be followed carefully to detect side reactions or unusual manifestations of drug idiosyncrasy.
Patients may require reduced doses of anesthetics when on methyldopa. If hypotension does occur during anesthesia, it usually can be controlled by vasopressors. The adrenergic receptors remain sensitive during treatment with methyldopa.
When methyldopa and lithium are given concomitantly the patient should be carefully monitored for symptoms of lithium toxicity. Read the prescribing information for lithium preparations.
Several studies demonstrate a decrease in the bioavailability of methyldopa when it is ingested with ferrous sulfate or ferrous gluconate. This may adversely affect blood pressure control in patients treated with methyldopa. Coadministration of methyldopa with ferrous sulfate or ferrous gluconate is not recommended.
Monoamine oxidase (MAO) inhibitors: see CONTRAINDICATIONS.
Hydrochlorothiazide
When given concurrently the following drugs may interact with thiazide diuretics.
Alcohol, barbiturates, or narcotics —potentiation of orthostatic hypotension may occur.
Antidiabetic drugs (oral agents and insulin) —dosage adjustment of the antidiabetic drug may be required.

Other antihypertensive drugs —additive effect or potentiation.
Cholestyramine and colestipol resins—Absorption of hydrochlorothiazide is impaired in the presence of anionic exchange resins. Single doses of either cholestyramine or colestipol resins bind the hydrochlorothiazide and reduce its absorption from the gastrointestinal tract by up to 85 and 43 percent, respectively.
Corticosteroids, ACTH —intensified electrolyte depletion, particularly hypokalemia.
Pressor amines (e.g., norepinephrine) —possible decreased response to pressor amines but not sufficient to preclude their use.
Skeletal muscle relaxants, nondepolarizing (e.g., tubocurarine) —possible increased responsiveness to the muscle relaxant.
Lithium —generally should not be given with diuretics. Diuretic agents reduce the renal clearance of lithium and add a high risk of lithium toxicity. Refer to the package insert for lithium preparations before use of such preparations with ALDORIL.
Non-steroidal Anti-inflammatory Drugs —In some patients, the administration of a non-steroidal anti-inflammatory agent can reduce the diuretic, natriuretic, and antihypertensive effects of loop, potassium-sparing and thiazide diuretics. Therefore, when ALDORIL and non-steroidal anti-inflammatory agents are used concomitantly, the patient should be observed closely to determine if the desired effect of the diuretic is obtained.
Drug/Laboratory Test Interactions
Methyldopa
Methyldopa may interfere with measurement of: urinary uric acid by the phosphotungstate method, serum creatinine by the alkaline picrate method, and SGOT by colorimetric methods. Interference with spectrophotometric methods for SGOT analysis has not been reported.
Since methyldopa causes fluorescence in urine samples at the same wave lengths as catecholamines, falsely high levels of urinary catecholamines may be reported. This will interfere with the diagnosis of pheochromocytoma. It is important to recognize this phenomenon before a patient with a possible pheochromocytoma is subjected to surgery. Methyldopa does not interfere with measurement of VMA (vanillylmandelic acid), a test for pheochromocytoma, by those methods which convert VMA to vanillin. Methyldopa is not recommended for the treatment of patients with pheochromocytoma. Rarely, when urine is exposed to air after voiding, it may darken because of breakdown of methyldopa or its metabolites.
Hydrochlorothiazide
Thiazides should be discontinued before carrying out tests for parathyroid function (see PRECAUTIONS, *General*).
Carcinogenesis, Mutagenesis, Impairment of Fertility
Long-term studies in animals have not been performed to evaluate the effects upon fertility, mutagenic or carcinogenic potential of the combination.
Methyldopa
No evidence of a tumorigenic effect was seen when methyldopa was given for two years to mice at doses up to 1800 mg/kg/day or to rats at doses up to 240 mg/kg/day (30 and 4 times the maximum recommended human dose in mice and rats, respectively, when compared on the basis of body weight; 2.5 and 0.6 times the maximum recommended human dose in mice and rats, respectively, when compared on the basis of body surface area; calculations assume a patient weight of 50 kg).
Methyldopa was not mutagenic in the Ames Test and did not increase chromosomal aberration or sister chromatid exchanges in Chinese hamster ovary cells. These *in vitro* studies were carried out both with and without exogenous metabolic activation.
Fertility was unaffected when methyldopa was given to male and female rats at 100 mg/kg/day (1.7 times the maximum daily human dose when compared on the basis of body weight; 0.2 times the maximum daily human dose when compared on the basis of body surface area). Methyldopa decreased sperm count, sperm motility, the number of late spermatids and the male fertility index when given to male rats at 200 and 400 mg/kg/day (3.3 and 6.7 times the maximum daily human dose when compared on the basis of body weight; 0.5 and 1 times the maximum daily human dose when compared on the basis of body surface area).
Hydrochlorothiazide
Two-year feeding studies in mice and rats conducted under the auspices of the National Toxicology Program (NTP) uncovered no evidence of a carcinogenic potential of hydrochlorothiazide in female mice (at doses of up to approximately 600 mg/kg/day) or in male and female rats (at doses of up to approximately 100 mg/kg/day). The NTP, however, found equivocal evidence for hepatocarcinogenicity in male mice.
Hydrochlorothiazide was not genotoxic *in vitro* in the Ames mutagenicity assay of *Salmonella typhimurium* strains TA 98, TA 100, TA 1535, TA 1537, and TA 1538 and in the Chinese Hamster Ovary (CHO) test for chromosomal aberrations, or *in vivo* in assays using mouse germinal cell chromosomes, Chinese hamster bone marrow chromosomes, and the *Drosophila* sex-linked recessive lethal trait gene. Positive test results were obtained only in the *in vitro* CHO Sister Chromatid Exchange (clastogenicity) and in the Mouse Lymphoma Cell (mutagenicity) assays, using concentrations of hydrochlorothiazide from 43 to 1300 µg/mL, and in the *Aspergillus nidulans* non-disjunction assay at an unspecified concentration.
Hydrochlorothiazide had no adverse effects on the fertility of mice and rats of either sex in studies wherein these species were exposed, via their diet, to doses of up to 100 and 4 mg/kg, respectively, prior to conception and throughout gestation.
Pregnancy
Use of diuretics during normal pregnancy is inappropriate and exposes mother and fetus to unnecessary hazard. Diuretics do not prevent development of toxemia of pregnancy and there is no satisfactory evidence that they are useful in the treatment of toxemia.
Teratogenic Effects—Pregnancy Category C: Animal reproduction studies have not been conducted with ALDORIL. It is also not known whether ALDORIL can affect reproduction capacity or can cause fetal harm when given to a pregnant woman. ALDORIL should be given to a pregnant woman only if clearly needed.
Hydrochlorothiazide: Studies in which hydrochlorothiazide was orally administered to pregnant mice and rats during their respective periods of major organogenesis at doses up to 3000 and 1000 mg hydrochlorothiazide/kg, respectively, provided no evidence of harm to the fetus. There are, however, no adequate and well-controlled studies in pregnant women.
Methyldopa: Reproduction studies performed with methyldopa at oral doses up to 1000 mg/kg in mice, 200 mg/kg in rabbits and 100 mg/kg in rats revealed no evidence of harm to the fetus. These doses are 16.6 times, 3.3 times and 1.7 times, respectively, the maximum daily human dose when compared on the basis of body weight; 1.4 times, 1.1 times and 0.2 times, respectively, when compared on the basis of body surface area; calculations assume a patient weight of 50 kg. There are, however, no adequate and well-controlled studies in pregnant women in the first trimester of pregnancy. Because animal reproduction studies are not always predictive of human response, methyldopa should be used during pregnancy only if clearly needed.
Published reports of the use of methyldopa during all trimesters indicate that if this drug is used during pregnancy the possibility of fetal harm appears remote. In five studies, three of which were controlled, involving 332 pregnant hypertensive women, treatment with methyldopa was associated with an improved fetal outcome. The majority of these women were in the third trimester when methyldopa therapy was begun.
In one study, women who had begun methyldopa treatment between weeks 16 and 20 of pregnancy gave birth to infants whose average head circumference was reduced by a small amount (34.2 ± 1.7 cm vs. 34.6 ± 1.3 cm [mean ± 1 S.D.]). Long term follow-up of 195 (97.5%) of the children born to methyldopa-treated pregnant women (including those who began treatment between weeks 16 and 20) failed to uncover any significant adverse effect on the children. At four years of age, the developmental delay commonly seen in children born to hypertensive mothers was less evident in those whose mothers were treated with methyldopa during pregnancy than those whose mothers were untreated. The children of the treated group scored consistently higher than the children of the untreated group on five major indices of intellectual and motor development. At age 7 and one-half developmental scores and intelligence indices showed no significant differences in children of treated or untreated hypertensive women.
Nonteratogenic Effects: Thiazides cross the placental barrier and appear in cord blood. There is a risk of fetal or neonatal jaundice, thrombocytopenia, and possibly other adverse reactions that have occurred in adults.
Nursing Mothers
Methyldopa and thiazides appear in breast milk. Therefore, because of the potential for serious adverse reactions in nursing infants from hydrochlorothiazide, a decision should be made whether to discontinue nursing or to discontinue the drug, taking into account the importance of the drug to the mother.
Pediatric Use
Safety and effectiveness of ALDORIL in pediatric patients have not been established.

ADVERSE REACTIONS

The following adverse reactions have been reported and, within each category, are listed in order of decreasing severity.
Methyldopa
Sedation, usually transient, may occur during the initial period of therapy or whenever the dose is increased. Headache, asthenia, or weakness may be noted as early and transient symptoms. However, significant adverse effects due to methyldopa have been infrequent and this agent usually is well tolerated.
Cardiovascular: Aggravation of angina pectoris, congestive heart failure, prolonged carotid sinus hypersensitivity, orthostatic hypotension (decrease daily dosage), edema or weight gain, bradycardia.
Digestive: Pancreatitis, colitis, vomiting, diarrhea, sialadenitis, sore or "black" tongue, nausea, constipation, distention, flatus, dryness of mouth.
Endocrine: Hyperprolactinemia.
Hematologic: Bone marrow depression, leukopenia, granulocytopenia, thrombocytopenia, hemolytic anemia; positive tests for antinuclear antibody, LE cells, and rheumatoid factor, positive Coombs test.
Hepatic: Liver disorders including hepatitis, jaundice, abnormal liver function tests (see WARNINGS).
Hypersensitivity: Myocarditis, pericarditis, vasculitis, lupus-like syndrome, drug-related fever, eosinophilia.
Nervous System/Psychiatric: Parkinsonism, Bell's palsy, decreased mental acuity, involuntary choreoathetotic movements, symptoms of cerebrovascular insufficiency, psychic disturbances including nightmares and reversible mild psychoses or depression, headache, sedation, asthenia or weakness, dizziness, lightheadedness, paresthesias.
Metabolic: Rise in BUN.
Musculoskeletal: Arthralgia, with or without joint swelling; myalgia.
Respiratory: Nasal stuffiness.
Skin: Toxic epidermal necrolysis, rash.
Urogenital: Amenorrhea, breast enlargement, gynecomastia, lactation, impotence, decreased libido.
Hydrochlorothiazide
Body as a Whole: Weakness.
Cardiovascular: Hypotension including orthostatic hypotension (may be aggravated by alcohol, barbiturates, narcotics or antihypertensive drugs).
Digestive: Pancreatitis, jaundice (intrahepatic cholestatic jaundice), diarrhea, vomiting, sialadenitis, cramping, constipation, gastric irritation, nausea, anorexia.
Hematologic: Aplastic anemia, agranulocytosis, leukopenia, hemolytic anemia, thrombocytopenia.
Hypersensitivity: Anaphylactic reactions, necrotizing angiitis (vasculitis and cutaneous vasculitis), respiratory distress including pneumonitis and pulmonary edema, photosensitivity, fever, urticaria, rash, purpura.
Metabolic: Electrolyte imbalance (see PRECAUTIONS), hyperglycemia, glycosuria, hyperuricemia.
Musculoskeletal: Muscle spasm.
Nervous System/Psychiatric: Vertigo, paresthesias, dizziness, headache, restlessness.
Renal: Renal failure, renal dysfunction, interstitial nephritis. (See WARNINGS.)
Skin: Erythema multiforme including Stevens-Johnson syndrome, exfoliative dermatitis including toxic epidermal necrolysis, alopecia.
Special Senses: Transient blurred vision, xanthopsia.
Urogenital: Impotence.

OVERDOSAGE

Acute overdosage may produce acute hypotension with other responses attributable to brain and gastrointestinal malfunction (excessive sedation, weakness, bradycardia, dizziness, lightheadedness, constipation, distention, flatus, diarrhea, nausea, vomiting).
In the event of overdosage, symptomatic and supportive measures should be employed. When ingestion is recent, gastric lavage or emesis may reduce absorption. When ingestion has been earlier, infusions may be helpful to promote urinary excretion. Otherwise, management includes special attention to cardiac rate and output, blood volume, electrolyte balance, paralytic ileus, urinary function and cerebral activity.
Sympathomimetic drugs [e.g., levarterenol, epinephrine, ARAMINE* (Metaraminol Bitartrate)] may be indicated.
Methyldopa is dialyzable. The degree to which hydrochlorothiazide is removed by hemodialysis has not been established.
The oral LD_{50} of methyldopa is greater than 1.5 g/kg in both the mouse and the rat. The oral LD_{50} of hydrochlorothiazide is greater than 10 g/kg in the mouse and rat.

*Registered trademark of MERCK & CO., Inc.

DOSAGE AND ADMINISTRATION

DOSAGE MUST BE INDIVIDUALIZED, AS DETERMINED BY TITRATION OF THE INDIVIDUAL COMPONENTS (see box warning). Once the patient has been successfully titrated, ALDORIL may be substituted if the previously determined titrated doses are the same as in the combination. The usual starting dosage is one tablet of ALDORIL 15 two or three times a day or one tablet of ALDORIL 25 two times a day. Alternatively, one tablet of ALDORIL D30 or ALDORIL D50 once daily may be used. Hydrochlorothiazide doses greater than 50 mg daily should be avoided.
Hydrochlorothiazide can be given at doses of 12.5 to 50 mg per day when used alone. The usual daily dosage of methyldopa is 500 mg to 2 g. To minimize the sedation associated with methyldopa, start dosage increases in the evening. The maximum recommended daily dose of methyldopa is 3 g.
Occasionally tolerance to methyldopa may occur, usually between the second and third month of therapy. Additional separate doses of methyldopa or replacement of ALDORIL with single entity agents is necessary until the new effective dose ratio is re-established by titration. If ALDORIL does not adequately control blood pressure, additional doses of other agents may be given. When ALDORIL is given with antihypertensives other than thiazides, the initial dosage of

Continued on next page

Information on the Merck & Co., Inc., products listed on these pages is from the prescribing information in use October 1, 2004. For information, please call 1-800-NSC-MERCK [1-800-672-6372].

Aldoril—Cont.

methyldopa should be limited to 500 mg daily in divided doses and the dose of these other agents may need to be adjusted to effect a smooth transition.
Since both components of ALDORIL have a relatively short duration of action, withdrawal is followed by return of hypertension usually within 48 hours. This is not complicated by an overshoot of blood pressure.
Since methyldopa is largely excreted by the kidney, patients with impaired renal function may respond to smaller doses. Syncope in older patients may be related to an increased sensitivity and advanced arteriosclerotic vascular disease. This may be avoided by lower doses.

HOW SUPPLIED

No. 3294—Tablets ALDORIL 15 are salmon, round, film coated tablets, coded MSD 423 on one side and ALDORIL on the other. Each tablet contains 250 mg of methyldopa and 15 mg of hydrochlorothiazide. They are supplied as follows:
NDC 0006-0423-68 bottles of 100
No. 3295—Tablets ALDORIL 25 are white, round, film coated tablets, coded MSD 456 on one side and ALDORIL on the other. Each tablet contains 250 mg of methyldopa and 25 mg of hydrochlorothiazide. They are supplied as follows:
NDC 0006-0456-68 bottles of 100
NDC 0006-0456-82 bottles of 1000.
No. 3362—Tablets ALDORIL D30 are salmon, oval, film coated tablets, coded MSD 694 on one side and ALDORIL on the other. Each tablet contains 500 mg of methyldopa and 30 mg of hydrochlorothiazide. They are supplied as follows:
NDC 0006-0694-68 bottles of 100.
No. 3363—Tablets ALDORIL D50 are white, oval, film coated tablets, coded MSD 935 on one side and ALDORIL on the other. Each tablet contains 500 mg of methyldopa and 50 mg of hydrochlorothiazide. They are supplied as follows:
NDC 0006-0935-68 bottles of 100.
Storage
Keep container tightly closed. Protect from light, moisture, freezing, −20°C (−4°F) and store at controlled room temperature, 15–30°C (59–86°F).
7843554 Issued March 1999

Shown in Product Identification Guide, page 323

AMINOHIPPURATE SODIUM "PAH" ℞
Injection

DESCRIPTION

Aminohippurate sodium* is an agent to measure effective renal plasma flow (ERPF). It is the sodium salt of para-aminohippuric acid, commonly abbreviated "PAH."It is water soluble, lipid-insoluble, and has a pKa of 3.83. The empirical formula of the anhydrous salt is $C_9H_9N_2NaO_3$ and its structural formula is:

H_2N— —$CONHCH_2COONa$

It is provided as a sterile, non-preserved 20 percent aqueous solution for injection, with a pH of 6.7 to 7.6. Each 10 mL contains: Aminohippurate sodium 2 g. Inactive ingredients: Sodium hydroxide to adjust pH, water for injection, q.s.

*Formerly referred to as Sodium para-Aminohippurate.

CLINICAL PHARMACOLOGY

PAH is filtered by the glomeruli and is actively secreted by the proximal tubules. At low plasma concentrations (1.0 to 2.0 mg/100 mL), an average of 90 percent of PAH is cleared by the kidneys from the renal blood stream in a single circulation. It is ideally suited for measurement of ERPF since it has a high clearance, is essentially nontoxic at the plasma concentrations reached with recommended doses and its analytical determination is relatively simple and accurate.
PAH is also used to measure the functional capacity of the renal tubular secretory mechanism or transport maximum (Tm_{PAH}). This is accomplished by elevating the plasma concentration to levels (40–60 mg/100 mL) sufficient to saturate the maximal capacity of the tubular cells to secrete PAH.
Inulin clearance is generally measured during Tm_{PAH} determinations since glomerular filtration rate (GFR) must be known before calculations of secretory Tm measurements can be done (see DOSAGE AND ADMINISTRATION, *Calculations*).

INDICATIONS AND USAGE

Estimation of effective renal plasma flow.
Measurement of the functional capacity of the renal tubular secretory mechanism.

CONTRAINDICATIONS

Hypersensitivity to this product or to its components.

PRECAUTIONS

General
Intravenous solutions must be given with caution to patients with low cardiac reserve, since a rapid increase in plasma volume can precipitate congestive heart failure.
For measurement of ERPF, small doses of PAH are used. However, in research procedures to measure Tm_{PAH}, high plasma levels are required to saturate the capacity of the tubular cells. During these procedures, the intravenous administration of PAH solutions should be carried out slowly and with caution. The patient should be continuously observed for any adverse reactions.
Drug Interactions
Renal clearance measurements of PAH cannot be made with any significant accuracy in patients receiving sulfonamides, procaine, or thiazolesulfone. These compounds interfere with chemical color development essential to the analytical procedures.
Probenecid depresses tubular secretion of certain weak acids such as PAH. Therefore, patients receiving probenecid will have erroneously low ERPF and Tm_{PAH} values.
Carcinogenesis, Mutagenesis, Impairment of Fertility
Long-term studies in animals have not been done to evaluate any effects upon fertility or carcinogenic potential of PAH.
Pregnancy
Pregnancy Category C. Animal reproduction studies have not been done with PAH. It is also not known whether PAH can cause fetal harm when given to a pregnant woman or can affect reproduction capacity. PAH should be given to a pregnant woman only if clearly needed.
Nursing Mothers
It is not known whether this drug is excreted in human milk. Because many drugs are excreted in human milk, caution should be exercised when PAH is administered to a nursing woman.
Pediatric Use
Safety and effectiveness in pediatric patients have not been established.
Geriatric Use
Clinical studies of PAH did not include sufficient numbers of subjects aged 65 and over to determine whether they respond differently from younger subjects. Other reported clinical experience has not identified differences in responses between the elderly and younger patients.

ADVERSE REACTIONS

Hypersensitivity reactions (including angioedema and urticaria), vasomotor disturbances, flushing, tingling, nausea, vomiting, and cramps may occur.
Patients may have a sensation of warmth or the desire to defecate or urinate during or shortly following initiation of infusion.

OVERDOSAGE

The intravenous LD_{50} in female mice is 7.22 g/kg.

DOSAGE AND ADMINISTRATION

For intravenous use only
Clearance measurements using single injection techniques are generally inaccurate, particularly in the measurement of ERPF. For this reason, intravenous infusions at fixed rates are used to sustain the plasma PAH concentration at the desired level.
To measure ERPF, the concentration of PAH in the plasma should be maintained at 2 mg per 100 mL, which can be achieved with a priming dose of 6 to 10 mg/kg and an infusion dose of 10 to 24 mg/min.
As a research procedure for the measurement of Tm_{PAH}, the plasma level of PAH must be sufficient to saturate the capacity of the tubular secretory cells. Concentrations from 40 to 60 mg per 100 mL are usually necessary.
Technical details of these tests may be found in Smith[1]; Wesson[2]; Bauer[3]; Pitts[4]; and Schnurr.[5]
Parenteral drug products should be inspected visually for particulate matter and discoloration prior to use, whenever solution and container permit. NOTE: The normal color range for this product is a colorless to yellow/brown solution. The efficacy is not affected by color changes within this range.
Calculations
Effective Renal Plasma Flow (ERPF)
The clearance of PAH, which is extracted almost completely from the plasma during its passage through the renal circulation, constitutes a measure of ERPF. Hence:

$$ERPF = \frac{U_{PAH}V}{P_{PAH}}$$

Where U_{PAH} = concentration of PAH (mg/mL) in the urine
V = rate of urine excretion (mL/min), and
P_{PAH} = plasma concentration of PAH (mg/mL).

Example: U_{PAH} = 8.0 mg/mL
V = 1.5 mL/min
P_{PAH} = 0.02 mg/mL

$$ERPF = \frac{8.0 \times 1.5}{0.02} = 600 \text{ mL/min}$$

Based on PAH clearance studies, the normal values for ERPF are:

men 675 ± 150 mL/min
women 595 ± 125 mL/min.

Maximum Tubular Secretory Mechanism (Tm_{PAH})
The quantity of PAH, secreted by the tubules (Tm_{PAH}) is given by the difference between the total rate of excretion ($U_{PAH}V$) and the quantity filtered by the glomeruli (GFR × P_{PAH}). Hence:

$$Tm_{PAH} = U_{PAH}V - (GFR \times P_{PAH} \times 0.83)$$

The factor, 0.83, corrects for that portion of PAH which is bound to plasma protein and hence is unfilterable.

Example: U_{PAH} = 9.55 mg/mL
V = 16.68 mL/min
GFR = 120 mL/min
P_{PAH} = 0.60 mg/mL

Then $Tm_{PAH} = 9.55 \times 16.68 - (120 \times 0.60 \times 0.83) =$ 100 mg/min.
Average normal values of Tm_{PAH} are 80–90 mg/min.
The value of the expression $U_{PAH}V$, used in calculations of ERPF and Tm_{PAH}, may be found by determining the amount of PAH in a measured volume of urine excreted within a specific period of time.
These calculations are based on a body surface area of 1.73 m^2. Corrections for variations in surface area are made by multiplying the values obtained for ERPF and Tm_{PAH} by 1.73/A, where A is the subject surface area.

HOW SUPPLIED

No. 95—Aminohippurate Sodium, 20 percent sterile solution for intravenous injection, is supplied as follows:
NDC 0006-3395-11 in 10 mL vials.
Storage
Store at 25°C (77°F); excursions permitted to 15–30°C (59–86°F) [see USP Controlled Room Temperature].

REFERENCES

1. Smith, H. W.: Lectures on the kidney, University Extension Division, University of Kansas, Lawrence, Kansas, 1943.
2. Wesson, L. G., Jr.: "Physiology of the Human Kidney," New York, Grune & Stratton, 1969, pp. 632–655.
3. Bauer, J. D.; Ackermann, P. G.; Toro, G.: "Brays Clinical Laboratory Methods," ed. 7, St. Louis, Mosby, 1968.
4. Pitts, R. F.: "Physiology of the Kidney and Body Fluids," ed. 2, Chicago, Year Book Medical Publishers, 1968.
5. Schnurr, E., Lahme, W., Kuppers, H.: Measurement of renal clearance of inulin and PAH in the steady state without urine collection; Clinical Nephrology, *13* (1): (26–29), 1980.
9051023 Issued January 2002

ANTIVENIN ℞
(Latrodectus mactans)
(Black Widow Spider Antivenin)
Equine Origin

DESCRIPTION

Antivenin (Latrodectus mactans) is a sterile, non-pyrogenic preparation derived by drying a frozen solution of specific venom-neutralizing globulins obtained from the blood serum of healthy horses immunized against venom of black widow spiders (Latrodectus mactans). It is standardized by biological assay on mice, in terms of one dose of antivenin neutralizing the venom in not less than 6000 mouse LD_{50} of Latrodectus mactans. Thimerosal (mercury derivative) 1:10,000 is added as a preservative. When constituted as specified, it is opalescent, ranging in color from light (straw) to very dark (iced tea), and contains not more than 20.0 percent of solids.
Each vial contains not less than 6000 Antivenin units. One unit of Antivenin will neutralize one average mouse lethal dose of black widow spider venom when the Antivenin and the venom are injected simultaneously in mice under suitable conditions.

CLINICAL PHARMACOLOGY

The pharmacological mode of action is unknown and metabolic and pharmacokinetic data in humans are unavailable.

INDICATIONS AND USAGE

Antivenin (Latrodectus mactans) is used to treat patients with symptoms due to bites by the black widow spider (Latrodectus mactans). Early use of the Antivenin is emphasized for prompt relief.
Local muscular cramps begin from 15 minutes to several hours after the bite which usually produces a sharp pain

similar to that caused by puncture with a needle. The exact sequence of symptoms depends somewhat on the location of the bite. The venom acts on the myoneural junctions or on the nerve endings, causing an ascending motor paralysis or destruction of the peripheral nerve endings. The groups of muscles most frequently affected at first are those of the thigh, shoulder, and back. After a varying length of time, the pain becomes more severe, spreading to the abdomen, and weakness and tremor usually develop. The abdominal muscles assume a boardlike rigidity, but tenderness is slight. Respiration is thoracic. The patient is restless and anxious. Feeble pulse, cold, clammy skin, labored breathing and speech, light stupor, and delirium may occur. Convulsions also may occur, particularly in small children. The temperature may be normal or slightly elevated. Urinary retention, shock, cyanosis, nausea and vomiting, insomnia, and cold sweats also have been reported. The syndrome following the bite of the black widow spider may be confused easily with any medical or surgical condition with acute abdominal symptoms.

The symptoms of black widow spider bite increase in severity for several hours, perhaps a day, and then very slowly become less severe, gradually passing off in the course of two or three days except in fatal cases. Residual symptoms such as general weakness, tingling, nervousness, and transient muscle spasm may persist for weeks or months after recovery from the acute stage.

If possible, the patient should be hospitalized. Other additional measures giving greatest relief are prolonged warm baths and intravenous injection of 10 mL of 10 percent solution of calcium gluconate repeated as necessary to control muscle pain. Morphine also may be required to control pain. Barbiturates may be used for extreme restlessness. However, as the venom is a neurotoxin, it can cause respiratory paralysis. This must be borne in mind when considering use of morphine or a barbiturate. Adrenocorticosteroids have been used with varying degrees of success. Supportive therapy is indicated by the condition of the patient. Local treatment of the site of the bite is of no value. Nothing is gained by applying a tourniquet or by attempting to remove venom from the site of the bite by incision and suction.

In otherwise healthy individuals between the ages of 16 and 60, the use of Antivenin may be deferred and treatment with muscle relaxants may be considered.

WARNINGS

Prior to treatment with any product prepared from horse serum, a careful review of the patient's history should be taken emphasizing prior exposure to horse serum or any allergies. Serious sickness and even death could result from the use of horse serum in a sensitive patient. A skin or conjunctival test should be performed prior to administration of Antivenin.

Skin test: Inject into (not under) the skin not more than 0.02 mL of the test material (1:10 dilution of normal horse serum in physiologic saline). Evaluate result in 10 minutes. A positive reaction is an urticarial wheal surrounded by a zone of erythema. A control test using Sodium Chloride Injection facilitates interpretation of the results.

Conjunctival test: For adults instill into the conjunctival sac one drop of a 1:10 dilution of horse serum and for children one drop of 1:100 dilution. Itching of the eye and reddening of the conjunctiva indicate a positive reaction, usually within 10 minutes.

Patients should be observed for serum sickness for an average of 8 to 12 days following administration of Antivenin.

Desensitization should be attempted only when the administration of Antivenin is considered necessary to save life. Epinephrine must be available in case of untoward reaction.

Desensitization: If the history is positive or the results of the sensitivity tests are mildly or quetionably positive, Antivenin should be administered as follows to reduce the risk of an immediate severe allergic reaction:

1. In separate sterile vials or syringes prepare 1:10 or 1:100 dilutions of Antivenin in Sodium Chloride for Injection.
2. Allow at least 15 but preferably 30 minutes between injections and only proceed with the next dose if no reactions occurred following the previous dose.
3. Using a tuberculin syringe, inject subcutaneously 0.1, 0.2 and 0.5 mL of the 1:100 dilution at 15 or 30 minute intervals; repeat with the 1:10 dilution, and finally the undiluted Antivenin.
4. If there is a reaction after any of the injections, place a tourniquet proximal to the sites of injection and administer epinephrine, 1:1000 (0.3 to 1.0 mL subcutaneously, 0.05 to 0.1 mL intravenously), proximal to the tourniquet or into another extremity. Wait at least 30 minutes before giving another injection of Antivenin, the amount of which should be the same as the last one not evoking a reaction.
5. If no reaction has occurred after 0.5 mL of undiluted Antivenin has been given, it is probably safe to continue the dose at 15 minute intervals until the entire dose has been injected.

PRECAUTIONS

Carcinogenesis, Mutagenesis, Impairment of Fertility

No long term studies in animals have been performed to evaluate the potential for carcinogenesis, mutagenesis, or impairment of fertility.

Pregnancy

Pregnancy Category C. Animal reproduction studies have not been conducted with Black Widow Spider Antivenin. It is also not known whether Black Widow Spider Antivenin can cause fetal harm when administered to a pregnant woman or can affect reproduction capacity. Black Widow Spider Antivenin should be given to a pregnant woman only if clearly needed.

Nursing Mothers

It is not known whether this drug is excreted in human milk. Because many drugs are excreted in human milk, caution should be exercised when Black Widow Spider Antivenin is administered to a nursing woman.

Pediatric Use

Controlled clinical studies for safety and effectiveness in children have not been conducted; however, there have been virtually no adverse effects reported in those children who have received the product.

Geriatric Use

Reported clinical experience has not identified differences in responses between the elderly and younger patients. Because of the increased risk of complications from envenomation in elderly patients, the standard of care described in the literature suggests that patients older than 60 years of age should be given Antivenin as a preferred initial therapy (see INDICATIONS AND USAGE).

ADVERSE REACTIONS

Anaphylaxis and serum sickness have been reported following use of Antivenin.

DOSAGE AND ADMINISTRATION

Using a sterile syringe, remove from the accompanying vial 2.5 mL of Sterile Diluent for Antivenin and inject into the vial of Antivenin. With the needle still in the rubber stopper, shake the vial to dissolve the contents completely.

Parenteral drug products should be inspected visually for particulate matter prior to administration, whenever solution and container permit (see DESCRIPTION).

The dose for adults and children is the entire contents of a restored vial (2.5 mL) of Antivenin. It may be given intramuscularly, preferably in the region of the anterolateral thigh so that a tourniquet may be applied in the event of a systemic reaction. Symptoms usually subside in 1 to 3 hours. Although one dose of Antivenin usually is adequate, a second dose may be necessary in some cases.

Antivenin also may be given intravenously in 10 to 50 mL of saline solution over a 15 minute period. It is the preferred route in severe cases, or when the patient is under 12, or in shock. One restored vial usually is enough.

HOW SUPPLIED

No. 4084—Antivenin (Latrodectus mactans) equine origin is a white to grey crystalline powder, each vial containing not less than 6000 Antivenin units. Thimerosal (mercury derivative) 1:10,000 is added as preservative, **NDC** 0006-4084-00. A 2.5 mL vial of Sterile Diluent for Antivenin is included. Also supplied is a 1 mL vial of normal horse serum (1:10 dilution) for sensitivity testing. Thimerosal (mercury derivative) 1:10,000 is added as preservative.

Storage

Antivenin must be stored and shipped at 2–8°C (36–46°F). When reconstituted as directed, the color of Antivenin ranges from light (straw) to very dark (iced tea), but the color has no effect on potency. *Do not freeze.*

A.H.F.S. Category: 80:04

7972115 October 2003

AquaMEPHYTON® Injection ℞
(Phytonadione)
Aqueous Colloidal Solution of Vitamin K_1

> **WARNING—INTRAVENOUS AND INTRAMUSCULAR USE**
>
> Severe reactions, including fatalities, have occurred during and immediately after INTRAVENOUS injection of AquaMEPHYTON* (Phytonadione), even when precautions have been taken to dilute the AquaMEPHYTON and to avoid rapid infusion. Severe reactions, including fatalities, have also been reported following INTRAMUSCULAR administration. Typically these severe reactions have resembled hypersensitivity or anaphylaxis, including shock and cardiac and/or respiratory arrest. Some patients have exhibited these severe reactions on receiving AquaMEPHYTON for the first time. Therefore the INTRAVENOUS and INTRAMUSCULAR routes should be restricted to those situations where the subcutaneous route is not feasible and the serious risk involved is considered justified.

*Registered trademark of MERCK & CO., INC.

DESCRIPTION

Phytonadione is a vitamin, which is a clear, yellow to amber, viscous, odorless or nearly odorless liquid. It is insoluble in water, soluble in chloroform and slightly soluble in ethanol. It has a molecular weight of 450.70.

Phytonadione is 2-methyl-3-phytyl-1,4-naphthoquinone. Its empirical formula is $C_{31}H_{46}O_2$ and its structural formula is:

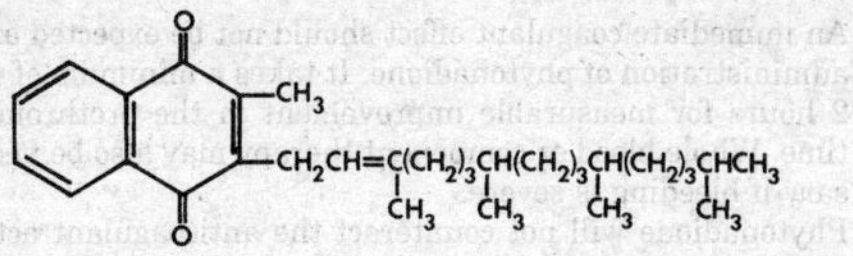

AquaMEPHYTON injection is a yellow, sterile, aqueous colloidal solution of vitamin K_1, with a pH of 5.0 to 7.0, available for injection by the intravenous, intramuscular, and subcutaneous routes. Each milliliter contains:

Phytonadione	2 mg or 10 mg
Inactive ingredients:	
Polyoxyethylated fatty acid derivative	70 mg
Dextrose	37.5 mg
Water for Injection, q.s.	1 mL
Added as preservative:	
Benzyl alcohol	0.9%

CLINICAL PHARMACOLOGY

AquaMEPHYTON aqueous colloidal solution of vitamin K_1 for parenteral injection, possesses the same type and degree of activity as does naturally-occurring vitamin K, which is necessary for the production via the liver of active prothrombin (factor II), proconvertin (factor VII), plasma thromboplastin component (factor IX), and Stuart factor (factor X). The prothrombin test is sensitive to the levels of three of these four factors—II, VII, and X. Vitamin K is an essential cofactor for a microsomal enzyme that catalyzes the post-translational carboxylation of multiple, specific, peptide-bound glutamic acid residues in inactive hepatic precursors of factors II, VII, IX, and X. The resulting gamma-carboxyglutamic acid residues convert the precursors into active coagulation factors that are subsequently secreted by liver cells into the blood.

Phytonadione is readily absorbed following intramuscular administration. After absorption, phytonadione is initially concentrated in the liver, but the concentration declines rapidly. Very little vitamin K accumulates in tissues. Little is known about the metabolic fate of vitamin K. Almost no free unmetabolized vitamin K appears in bile or urine.

In normal animals and humans, phytonadione is virtually devoid of pharmacodynamic activity. However, in animals and humans deficient in vitamin K, the pharmacological action of vitamin K is related to its normal physiological function, that is, to promote the hepatic biosynthesis of vitamin K dependent clotting factors.

The action of the aqueous colloidal solution, when administered intravenously, is generally detectable within an hour or two and hemorrhage is usually controlled within 3 to 6 hours. A normal prothrombin level may often be obtained in 12 to 14 hours.

In the prophylaxis and treatment of hemorrhagic disease of the newborn, phytonadione has demonstrated a greater margin of safety than that of the water-soluble vitamin K analogues.

INDICATIONS AND USAGE

AquaMEPHYTON is indicated in the following coagulation disorders which are due to faulty formation of factors II, VII, IX and X when caused by vitamin K deficiency or interference with vitamin K activity.

AquaMEPHYTON injection is indicated in:

- anticoagulant-induced prothrombin deficiency caused by coumarin or indanedione derivatives;
- prophylaxis and therapy of hemorrhagic disease of the newborn;
- hypoprothrombinemia due to antibacterial therapy;
- hypoprothrombinemia secondary to factors limiting absorption or synthesis of vitamin K, e.g., obstructive jaundice, biliary fistula, sprue, ulcerative colitis, celiac disease, intestinal resection, cystic fibrosis of the pancreas, and regional enteritis;
- other drug-induced hypoprothrombinemia where it is definitely shown that the result is due to interference with vitamin K metabolism, e.g., salicylates.

CONTRAINDICATION

Hypersensitivity to any component of this medication.

WARNINGS

Benzyl alcohol as a preservative in Bacteriostatic Sodium Chloride Injection has been associated with toxicity in newborns. Data are unavailable on the toxicity of other preservatives in this age group. There is no evidence to suggest that the small amount of benzyl alcohol contained in AquaMEPHYTON, when used as recommended, is associated with toxicity.

Continued on next page

Information on the Merck & Co., Inc., products listed on these pages is from the prescribing information in use October 1, 2004. For information, please call 1-800-NSC-MERCK [1-800-672-6372].

AquaMephyton—Cont.

An immediate coagulant effect should not be expected after administration of phytonadione. It takes a minimum of 1 to 2 hours for measurable improvement in the prothrombin time. Whole blood or component therapy may also be necessary if bleeding is severe.

Phytonadione will not counteract the anticoagulant action of heparin.

When vitamin K_1 is used to correct excessive anticoagulant-induced hypoprothrombinemia, anticoagulant therapy still being indicated, the patient is again faced with the clotting hazards existing prior to starting the anticoagulant therapy. Phytonadione is not a clotting agent, but overzealous therapy with vitamin K_1 may restore conditions which originally permitted thromboembolic phenomena. Dosage should be kept as low as possible, and prothrombin time should be checked regularly as clinical conditions indicate.

Repeated large doses of vitamin K are not warranted in liver disease if the response to initial use of the vitamin is unsatisfactory. Failure to respond to vitamin K may indicate that the condition being treated is inherently unresponsive to vitamin K.

PRECAUTIONS

General

Vitamin K_1 is fairly rapidly degraded by light; therefore, always protect AquaMEPHYTON from light. Store AquaMEPHYTON in closed original carton until contents have been used. (See also HOW SUPPLIED, *Storage*.)

Drug Interactions

Temporary resistance to prothrombin-depressing anticoagulants may result, especially when larger doses of phytonadione are used. If relatively large doses have been employed, it may be necessary when reinstituting anticoagulant therapy to use somewhat larger doses of the prothrombin-depressing anticoagulant, or to use one which acts on a different principle, such as heparin sodium.

Laboratory Tests

Prothrombin time should be checked regularly as clinical conditions indicate.

Carcinogenesis, Mutagenesis, Impairment of Fertility

Studies of carcinogenicity, mutagenesis or impairment of fertility have not been conducted with AquaMEPHYTON.

Pregnancy

Pregnancy Category C: Animal reproduction studies have not been conducted with AquaMEPHYTON. It is also not known whether AquaMEPHYTON can cause fetal harm when administered to a pregnant woman or can affect reproduction capacity. AquaMEPHYTON should be given to a pregnant woman only if clearly needed.

Nursing Mothers

It is not known whether this drug is excreted in human milk. Because many drugs are excreted in human milk, caution should be exercised when AquaMEPHYTON is administered to a nursing woman.

Pediatric Use

Hemolysis, jaundice, and hyperbilirubinemia in newborns, particularly in premature infants, may be related to the dose of AquaMEPHYTON. Therefore, the recommended dose should not be exceeded (see ADVERSE REACTIONS and DOSAGE AND ADMINISTRATION).

ADVERSE REACTIONS

Deaths have occurred after intravenous and intramuscular administration. (See Box Warning.)

Transient "flushing sensations" and "peculiar" sensations of taste have been observed, as well as rare instances of dizziness, rapid and weak pulse, profuse sweating, brief hypotension, dyspnea, and cyanosis.

Pain, swelling, and tenderness at the injection site may occur.

The possibility of allergic sensitivity, including an anaphylactoid reaction, should be kept in mind.

Infrequently, usually after repeated injection, erythematous, indurated, pruritic plaques have occurred; rarely, these have progressed to sclerodermalike lesions that have persisted for long periods. In other cases, these lesions have resembled erythema perstans.

Hyperbilirubinemia has been observed in the newborn following administration of phytonadione. This has occurred rarely and primarily with doses above those recommended. (See PRECAUTIONS, *Pediatric Use.*)

OVERDOSAGE

The intravenous LD_{50} of AquaMEPHYTON in the mouse is 41.5 and 52 mL/kg for the 0.2% and 1% concentrations respectively.

DOSAGE AND ADMINISTRATION

Whenever possible, AquaMEPHYTON should be given by the subcutaneous route (see Box Warning). When intravenous administration is considered unavoidable, the drug should be injected very slowly, not exceeding 1 mg per minute.

Protect from light at all times.

Parenteral drug products should be inspected visually for particulate matter and discoloration prior to administration, whenever solution and container permit.

Directions for Dilution

AquaMEPHYTON may be diluted with 0.9% Sodium Chloride Injection, 5% Dextrose Injection, or 5% Dextrose and Sodium Chloride Injection. Benzyl alcohol as a preservative has been associated with toxicity in newborns. *Therefore, all of the above diluents should be preservative-free* (see WARNINGS). *Other diluents should not be used.* When dilutions are indicated, administration should be started immediately after mixture with the diluent, and unused portions of the dilution should be discarded, as well as unused contents of the ampul.

Prophylaxis of Hemorrhagic Disease of the Newborn

The American Academy of Pediatrics recommends that vitamin K_1 be given to the newborn. A single intramuscular dose of AquaMEPHYTON 0.5 to 1 mg within one hour of birth is recommended.

Treatment of Hemorrhagic Disease of the Newborn

Empiric administration of vitamin K_1 should not replace proper laboratory evaluation of the coagulation mechanism. A prompt response (shortening of the prothrombin time in 2 to 4 hours) following administration of vitamin K_1 is usually diagnostic of hemorrhagic disease of the newborn, and failure to respond indicates another diagnosis or coagulation disorder.

AquaMEPHYTON 1 mg should be given either subcutaneously or intramuscularly. Higher doses may be necessary if the mother has been receiving oral anticoagulants.

[See table below]

Whole blood or component therapy may be indicated if bleeding is excessive. This therapy, however, does not correct the underlying disorder and AquaMEPHYTON should be given concurrently.

Anticoagulant-Induced Prothrombin Deficiency in Adults

To correct excessively prolonged prothrombin time caused by oral anticoagulant therapy—2.5 to 10 mg or up to 25 mg initially is recommended. In rare instances 50 mg may be required. Frequency and amount of subsequent doses should be determined by prothrombin time response or clinical condition (see WARNINGS). If in 6 to 8 hours after parenteral administration the prothrombin time has not been shortened satisfactorily, the dose should be repeated.

In the event of shock or excessive blood loss, the use of whole blood or component therapy is indicated.

Hypoprothrombinemia Due to Other Causes in Adults

A dosage of 2.5 to 25 mg or more (rarely up to 50 mg) is recommended, the amount and route of administration depending upon the severity of the condition and response obtained.

If possible, discontinuation or reduction of the dosage of drugs interfering with coagulation mechanisms (such as salicylates, antibiotics) is suggested as an alternative to administering concurrent AquaMEPHYTON. The severity of the coagulation disorder should determine whether the immediate administration of AquaMEPHYTON is required in addition to discontinuation or reduction of interfering drugs.

AquaMEPHYTON
Summary of Dosage Guidelines
(See circular text for details)

Newborns	Dosage
Hemorrhagic Disease of the Newborn	
Prophylaxis	0.5–1 mg IM within 1 hour of birth
Treatment	1 mg SC or IM (Higher doses may be necessary if the mother has been receiving oral anticoagulants)
Adults	**Initial Dosage**
Anticoagulant-Induced Prothrombin Deficiency (caused by coumarin or indanedione derivatives)	2.5 mg–10 mg or up to 25 mg (rarely 50 mg)
Hypoprothrombinemia due to other causes (Antibiotics; Salicylates or other drugs; Factors limiting absorption or synthesis)	2.5 mg–25 mg or more (rarely up to 50 mg)

HOW SUPPLIED

Injection AquaMEPHYTON is a yellow, sterile, aqueous colloidal solution and is supplied in the following concentrations:

No. 7780—10 mg of vitamin K_1 per mL

NDC 0006-7780-38 boxes of 5 × 1 mL ampuls

NDC 0006-7780-66 five boxes of 5 × 1 mL ampuls.

No. 7784—1 mg of vitamin K_1 per 0.5 mL

NDC 0006-7784-33 five boxes of 5 × 0.5 mL ampuls.

Storage

Store container in original carton. Always protect AquaMEPHYTON from light. Store container in closed original carton until contents have been used. (See PRECAUTIONS, *General*.)

9073025 Issued February 2002

ARAMINE® Injection ℞
(Metaraminol Bitartrate)

DESCRIPTION

Metaraminol bitartrate is a potent sympathomimetic amine that increases both systolic and diastolic blood pressure.

Metaraminol bitartrate is [*R*-(*R**,*S**)]-α-(1-aminoethyl)-3-hydroxybenzenemethanol [*R*-(*R**,*R**)]-2,3-dihydroxybutanedioate (1:1) (salt), which is levorotatory. Its empirical formula is $C_9H_{13}NO_2 \cdot C_4H_6O_6$ and its structural formula is:

Metaraminol bitartrate is a white, crystalline powder with a molecular weight of 317.29, is freely soluble in water, slightly soluble in alcohol, and practically insoluble in chloroform and in ether.

Injection ARAMINE* (Metaraminol Bitartrate) is a sterile solution. Each mL contains:

Metaraminol bitartrate equivalent to
metaraminol .... 10 mg

Inactive ingredients:
Sodium chloride .... 4.4 mg
Water for Injection q.s. ad .... 1 mL
Methylparaben 0.15%, propylparaben 0.02%, and sodium bisulfite 0.2% added as preservatives.

*Registered trademark of MERCK & CO., INC.

CLINICAL PHARMACOLOGY

The pressor effect of ARAMINE begins in 1 to 2 minutes after intravenous infusion, in about 10 minutes after intramuscular injection, and in 5 to 20 minutes after subcutaneous injection. The effect lasts from about 20 minutes to one hour. ARAMINE has a positive inotropic effect on the heart and a peripheral vasoconstrictor action.

Renal, coronary, and cerebral blood flow are a function of perfusion pressure and regional resistance. In patients with insufficient or failing vasoconstriction, there is additional advantage to the peripheral action of ARAMINE, but in most patients with shock, vasoconstriction is adequate and any further increase is unnecessary. Blood flow to vital organs may decrease with ARAMINE if regional resistance increases excessively.

The pressor effect of ARAMINE is decreased but not reversed by alpha-adrenergic blocking agents. Primary or secondary fall in blood pressure and tachyphylactic response to repeated use are uncommon.

INDICATIONS AND USAGE

ARAMINE is indicated for prevention and treatment of the acute hypotensive state occurring with spinal anesthesia. It is also indicated as adjunctive treatment of hypotension due to hemorrhage, reactions to medications, surgical complications, and shock associated with brain damage due to trauma or tumor.

CONTRAINDICATIONS

Use of ARAMINE with cyclopropane or halothane anesthesia should be avoided, unless clinical circumstances demand such use.

Hypersensitivity to any component of this product, including sulfites (see WARNINGS).

WARNINGS

Use of sympathomimetic amines with monoamine oxidase inhibitors or tricyclic antidepressants may result in potentiation of the pressor effect. (See PRECAUTIONS, *Drug Interactions.*)

ARAMINE contains sodium bisulfite, a sulfite that may cause allergic-type reactions including anaphylactic symptoms and life-threatening or less severe asthmatic episodes in certain susceptible people. The overall prevalence of sulfite sensitivity in the general population is unknown and probably low. Sulfite sensitivity is seen more frequently in asthmatic than in nonasthmatic people.

PRECAUTIONS

General

Caution should be used to avoid excessive blood pressure response. Rapidly induced hypertensive responses have been reported to cause acute pulmonary edema, arrhythmias, cerebral hemorrhage, or cardiac arrest.

Patients with cirrhosis should be treated with caution, with adequate restoration of electrolytes if diuresis ensues. Fatal ventricular arrhythmia was reported in one patient with Laennec's cirrhosis while receiving metaraminol bitartrate. In several instances, ventricular extrasystoles that appeared during infusion of this vasopressor subsided promptly when the rate of infusion was reduced.

With the prolonged action of ARAMINE, a cumulative effect is possible. If there is an excessive vasopressor response there may be a prolonged elevation of blood pressure even after discontinuation of therapy.

When vasopressor amines are used for long periods, the resulting vasoconstriction may prevent adequate expansion of circulating volume and may cause perpetuation of shock. There is evidence that plasma volume may be reduced in all types of shock, and that the measurement of central venous pressure is useful in assessing the adequacy of the circulating blood volume. Therefore, blood or plasma volume expanders should be used when the principal reason for hypotension or shock is decreased circulating volume.

Because of its vasoconstrictor effect, ARAMINE should be given with caution in heart or thyroid disease, hypertension, or diabetes. Sympathomimetic amines may provoke a relapse in patients with a history of malaria.

Drug Interactions

ARAMINE should be used with caution in digitalized patients, since the combination of digitalis and sympathomimetic amines may cause ectopic arrhythmias.

Monoamine oxidase inhibitors or tricyclic antidepressants may potentiate the action of sympathomimetic amines. Therefore, when initiating pressor therapy in patients receiving these drugs, the initial dose should be small and given with caution. (See WARNINGS.)

Carcinogenesis, Mutagenesis, Impairment of Fertility

Studies in animals have not been performed to evaluate the mutagenic or carcinogenic potential of ARAMINE or its potential to affect fertility.

Pregnancy

Pregnancy Category C. Animal reproduction studies have not been conducted with ARAMINE. It is not known whether ARAMINE can cause fetal harm when given to a pregnant woman or can affect reproduction capacity. ARAMINE should be given to a pregnant woman only if clearly needed.

Nursing Mothers

It is not known whether this drug is secreted in human milk. Because many drugs are secreted in human milk, caution should be exercised when ARAMINE is given to a nursing woman.

Pediatric Use

Safety and effectiveness in pediatric patients have not been established.

ADVERSE REACTIONS

Sympathomimetic amines, including ARAMINE, may cause sinus or ventricular tachycardia, or other arrhythmias, especially in patients with myocardial infarction. (See PRECAUTIONS.)

In patients with a history of malaria, these compounds may provoke a relapse.

Abscess formation, tissue necrosis, or sloughing rarely may follow the use of ARAMINE. In choosing the site of injection, it is important to avoid those areas recognized as *not* suitable for use of any pressor agent and to discontinue the infusion immediately if infiltration or thrombosis occurs. Although the physician may be forced by the urgent nature of the patient's condition to choose injection sites that are not recognized as suitable, he should, when possible, use the preferred areas of injection. The larger veins of the antecubital fossa or the thigh are preferred to veins in the dorsum of the hand or ankle veins, particularly in patients with peripheral vascular disease, diabetes mellitus, Buerger's disease, or conditions with coexistent hypercoagulability.

OVERDOSAGE

Overdosage may result in severe hypertension accompanied by headache, constricting sensation in the chest, nausea, vomiting, euphoria, diaphoresis, pulmonary edema, tachycardia, bradycardia, sinus arrhythmia, atrial or ventricular arrhythmias, cerebral hemorrhage, myocardial infarction, cardiac arrest or convulsions.

Should an excessive elevation of blood pressure occur, it may be immediately relieved by a sympatholytic agent, e.g., phentolamine. An appropriate antiarrhythmic agent may also be required.

The oral LD_{50} in the rat and mouse is 240 mg/kg and 99 mg/kg, respectively.

DOSAGE AND ADMINISTRATION

ARAMINE may be given intramuscularly, subcutaneously, or intravenously, the route depending on the nature and severity of the indication.

Parenteral drug products should be inspected visually for particulate matter and discoloration prior to use, whenever solution and container permit.

Allow at least 10 minutes to elapse before increasing the dose because the maximum effect is not immediately apparent. When the vasopressor is discontinued, observe the patient carefully as the effect of the drug tapers off, so that therapy can be reinitiated promptly if the blood pressure falls too rapidly. The response to vasopressors may be poor in patients with coexistent shock and acidosis. When indicated, established methods of shock management should be used, such as blood or fluid replacement.

Intramuscular or Subcutaneous Injection (for prevention of hypotension—see INDICATIONS): The recommended dose is 2 to 10 mg (0.2 to 1 mL). As with other agents given subcutaneously, only the preferred sites of injection, as set forth in standard texts, should be used.

Intravenous Infusion (for adjunctive treatment of hypotension—see INDICATIONS): The recommended dose is 15 to 100 mg (1.5 to 10 mL) in 500 mL of Sodium Chloride Injection or 5% Dextrose Injection, adjusting the rate of infusion to maintain the blood pressure at the desired level. Higher concentrations of ARAMINE, 150 to 500 mg per 500 mL of infusion fluid, have been used.

If the patient needs more saline or dextrose solution at a rate of flow that would provide an excessive dose of the vasopressor, the recommended volume of infusion fluid (500 mL) should be increased accordingly. ARAMINE may also be added to *less* than 500 mL of infusion fluid if a smaller volume is desired.

Compatibility Information

In addition to Sodium Chloride Injection and Dextrose Injection 5%, the following infusion solutions were found physically and chemically compatible with Injection ARAMINE when 5 mL of Injection ARAMINE, 10 mg/mL (metaraminol equivalent), was added to 500 mL of infusion solution: Ringer's Injection, Lactated Ringer's Injection, Dextran 6% in Saline**, Normosol®-R pH 7.4**, and Normosol®-M in D5-W**.

When Injection ARAMINE is mixed with an infusion solution, sterile precautions should be observed. Since infusion solutions generally do not contain preservatives, mixtures should be used within 24 hours.

Direct Intravenous Injection: In severe shock, when time is of great importance, this agent should be given by direct intravenous injection. The suggested dose is 0.5 to 5 mg (0.05 to 0.5 mL), followed by an infusion of 15 to 100 mg (1.5 to 10 mL) in 500 mL of infusion fluid as described previously. Vials may be sterilized by autoclaving or by immersion in a sterilizing solution.

**Product of Abbott Laboratories

HOW SUPPLIED

No. 3222X—Injection ARAMINE 1%, containing metaraminol bitartrate equivalent to 10 mg of metaraminol per mL, is a clear, colorless solution and is supplied as follows:
NDC 0006-3222-10 in 10 mL vials.

Storage

Store at 25°C (77°F); excursions permitted to 15–30°C (59–86°F) [see USP Controlled Room Temperature]. Store container in carton until contents have been used. Protect from light. Protect from freezing.

9050625 Issued August 1999

ATTENUVAX® ℞
(Measles Virus Vaccine Live)

DESCRIPTION

ATTENUVAX* (Measles Virus Vaccine Live) is a live virus vaccine for vaccination against measles (rubeola).

ATTENUVAX is a sterile lyophilized preparation of a more attenuated line of measles virus derived from Enders' attenuated Edmonston strain and propagated in chick embryo cell culture.

The growth medium for measles is Medium 199 (a buffered salt solution containing vitamins and amino acids and supplemented with fetal bovine serum) containing SPGA (sucrose, phosphate, glutamate, and human albumin) as stabilizer and neomycin.

The cells, virus pools, fetal bovine serum, and human albumin are all screened for the absence of adventitious agents. Human albumin is processed using the Cohn cold ethanol fractionation procedure.

The reconstituted vaccine is for subcutaneous administration. Each 0.5 mL dose contains not less than 1,000 $TCID_{50}$ (tissue culture infectious doses) of measles virus. Each dose of the vaccine is calculated to contain sorbitol (14.5 mg), sodium phosphate, sucrose (1.9 mg), sodium chloride, hydrolyzed gelatin (14.5 mg), human albumin (0.3 mg), fetal bovine serum (<1 ppm), other buffer and media ingredients and approximately 25 mcg of neomycin. The product contains no preservative.

Before reconstitution, the lyophilized vaccine is a light yellow compact crystalline plug. ATTENUVAX, when reconstituted as directed, is clear yellow.

*Registered trademark of MERCK & CO., Inc.

CLINICAL PHARMACOLOGY

Measles is a common childhood disease, caused by measles virus (paramyxovirus), that may be associated with serious complications and/or death. For example, pneumonia and encephalitis are caused by measles.

The impact of measles vaccination on the natural history of each disease in the United States can be quantified by comparing the maximum number of measles cases reported in a given year prior to vaccine use to the number of cases of each disease reported in 1995. A total of 894,134 cases reported in 1941 compared to 288 cases reported in 1995 resulted in a 99.97% decrease in reported cases of measles.

Extensive clinical trials have demonstrated that ATTENUVAX is highly immunogenic and generally well tolerated. A single injection of the vaccine has been shown to induce measles hemagglutination-inhibition (HI) antibodies in 97% or more of susceptible persons. However, a small percentage (1–5%) of vaccinees may fail to seroconvert after the primary dose (see also INDICATIONS AND USAGE, *Recommended Vaccination Schedule*).

A study of 6 month old and 15 month old infants born to vaccine-immunized mothers demonstrated that, following vaccination with ATTENUVAX, 74% of the 6 month old infants developed detectable neutralizing antibody (NT) titers while 100% of the 15 month old infants developed NT. This rate of seroconversion is higher than that previously reported for 6 month old infants born to naturally immune mothers tested by HI assay. When the 6 month old infants of immunized mothers were revaccinated at 15 months, they developed antibody titers equivalent to the 15 month old vaccinees. The lower seroconversion rate in 6 month olds has two possible explanations: 1) Due to the limit of the detection level of the assays (NT and enzyme immunoassay [EIA]), the presence of trace amounts of undetectable maternal antibody might interfere with the seroconversion of infants; or 2) the immune system of 6 month olds is not always capable of mounting a response to measles vaccine as measured by the two antibody assays.

There is some evidence to suggest that infants who are born to mothers who had natural measles and who are vaccinated at less than one year of age may not develop sustained antibody levels when later revaccinated. The advantage of early protection must be weighed against the chance for failure to respond adequately on reimmunization.

Efficacy of measles vaccine was established in a series of double-blind controlled field trials which demonstrated a high degree of protective efficacy. These studies also established that seroconversion in response to measles vaccination paralleled protection from these diseases.

Following vaccination, antibodies associated with protection can be measured by neutralization assays, HI, or ELISA (enzyme linked immunosorbent assay) tests. Neutralizing and ELISA antibodies to measles virus are still detectable in most individuals 11–13 years after primary vaccination.

INDICATIONS AND USAGE

Recommended Vaccination Schedule

ATTENUVAX is indicated for vaccination against measles in persons 12 months of age or older.

Individuals first vaccinated with ATTENUVAX at 12 months of age or older should be revaccinated with M-M-R* II (Measles, Mumps, and Rubella Virus Vaccine Live) prior to elementary school entry. Revaccination is intended to seroconvert those who do not respond to the first dose. The Advisory Committee on Immunization Practices (ACIP) recommends administration of the first dose of M-M-R II at 12–15 months of age and administration of the second dose of M-M-R II at 4–6 years of age. In addition, some public health jurisdictions mandate the age for revaccination. Consult the complete text of applicable guidelines regarding routine revaccination including that of high-risk adult populations.

Measles Outbreak Schedule

Infants Between 6–12 Months of Age

Local health authorities may recommend measles vaccination of infants between 6–12 months of age in outbreak situations. This population may fail to respond to the measles component of the vaccine. The younger the infant, the lower the likelihood of seroconversion (see CLINICAL PHARMACOLOGY). Such infants should receive a second dose of M-M-R II between 12 to 15 months of age followed by revaccination prior to elementary school entry.

Unnecessary doses of a vaccine are best avoided by ensuring that written documentation of vaccination is preserved and a copy given to each vaccinee's parent or guardian.

Other Vaccination Considerations

Other Populations

Individuals planning travel outside the United States, if not immune, can acquire measles, mumps or rubella and import

Continued on next page

Information on the Merck & Co., Inc., products listed on these pages is from the prescribing information in use October 1, 2004. For information, please call 1-800-NSC-MERCK [1-800-672-6372].

Attenuvax—Cont.

these diseases into the United States. Therefore, prior to international travel, individuals known to be susceptible to one or more of these diseases can receive either a monovalent vaccine (measles, mumps or rubella), or a combination vaccine as appropriate. However, M-M-R II is preferred for persons likely to be susceptible to mumps and rubella; and if monovalent measles vaccine is not readily available, travelers should receive M-M-R II regardless of their immune status to mumps or rubella.

Vaccination is recommended for susceptible individuals in high-risk groups such as college students, health-care workers, and military personnel.

According to ACIP recommendations, most persons born in 1956 or earlier are likely to have been infected with measles naturally and generally need not be considered susceptible. All children, adolescents, and adults born after 1956 are considered susceptible and should be vaccinated, if there are no contraindications. This includes persons who may be immune to measles but who lack adequate documentation of immunity such as: (1) physician-diagnosed measles, (2) laboratory evidence of measles immunity, or (3) adequate immunization with live measles vaccine on or after the first birthday.

The ACIP recommends that "Persons vaccinated with inactivated vaccine followed within 3 months by live vaccine should be revaccinated with two doses of live vaccine. Revaccination is particularly important when the risk of exposure to natural measles virus is increased, as may occur during international travel."

Post-Exposure Vaccination

ATTENUVAX given immediately after exposure to natural measles may provide some protection if the vaccine can be administered within 72 hours of exposure. If, however, the vaccine is given a few days before exposure, substantial protection may be provided.

Use With Other Vaccines

See DOSAGE AND ADMINISTRATION, *Use With Other Vaccines.*

CONTRAINDICATIONS

Hypersensitivity to any component of the vaccine, including gelatin.

Do not give ATTENUVAX to pregnant females; the possible effects of the vaccine on fetal development are unknown at this time. If vaccination of postpubertal females is undertaken, pregnancy should be avoided for 3 months following vaccination (see PRECAUTIONS, *Pregnancy*).

Anaphylactic or anaphylactoid reactions to neomycin (each dose of reconstituted vaccine contains approximately 25 mcg of neomycin).

Febrile respiratory illness or other active febrile infection. However, the ACIP has recommended that all vaccines can be administered to persons with minor illnesses such as diarrhea, mild upper respiratory infection with or without low-grade fever, or other low-grade febrile illness.

Patients receiving immunosuppressive therapy. This contraindication does not apply to patients who are receiving corticosteroids as replacement therapy, e.g., for Addison's disease.

Individuals with blood dyscrasias, leukemia, lymphomas of any type, or other malignant neoplasms affecting the bone marrow or lymphatic systems.

Primary and acquired immunodeficiency states, including patients who are immunosuppressed in association with AIDS or other clinical manifestations of infection with human immunodeficiency viruses; cellular immune deficiencies; and hypogammaglobulinemic and dysgammaglobulinemic states. Measles inclusion body encephalitis (MIBE), pneumonitis and death as a direct consequence of disseminated measles vaccine virus infection has been reported in immunocompromised individuals inadvertently vaccinated with measles-containing vaccine.

Individuals with a family history of congenital or hereditary immunodeficiency, until the immune competence of the potential vaccine recipient is demonstrated.

WARNINGS

Due caution should be employed in administration of ATTENUVAX to persons with a history of cerebral injury, individual or family histories of convulsions, or any other condition in which stress due to fever should be avoided. The physician should be alert to the temperature elevation which may occur following vaccination (see ADVERSE REACTIONS).

This product contains albumin, a derivative of human blood. Based on effective donor screening and product manufacturing processes, it carries an extremely remote risk for transmission of viral diseases. Although there is a theoretical risk for transmission of Creutzfeldt-Jacob disease (CJD), no cases of transmission of CJD or viral disease have ever been identified that were associated with the use of albumin.

Hypersensitivity To Eggs

Live measles vaccine is produced in chick embryo cell culture. Persons with a history of anaphylactic, anaphylactoid or other immediate reactions (e.g., hives, swelling of the mouth and throat, difficulty breathing, hypotension and shock) subsequent to egg ingestion may be at an enhanced risk of immediate-type hypersensitivity reactions after receiving vaccines containing traces of chick embryo antigen. The potential risk to benefit ratio should be carefully evaluated before considering vaccination in such cases. Such individuals may be vaccinated with extreme caution, having adequate treatment on hand should a reaction occur (see PRECAUTIONS).

However, the AAP has stated, "Most children with a history of anaphylactic reactions to eggs have no untoward reactions to measles or MMR vaccine. Persons are not at increased risk if they have egg allergies that are not anaphylactic, and they should be vaccinated in the usual manner. In addition, skin testing of egg-allergic children with vaccine has not been predictive of which children will have an immediate hypersensitivity reaction. Persons with allergies to chickens or chicken feathers are not at increased risk of reaction to the vaccine."

Hypersensitivity to Neomycin

The AAP states, "Persons who have experienced anaphylactic reactions to topically or systemically administered neomycin should not receive measles vaccine. Most often, however, neomycin allergy manifests as a contact dermatitis, which is a delayed-type (cell-mediated) immune response rather than anaphylaxis. In such persons, an adverse reaction to neomycin in the vaccine would be an erythematous, pruritic nodule or papule, 48 to 96 hours after vaccination. A history of contact dermatitis to neomycin is not a contraindication to receiving measles vaccine."

Thrombocytopenia

Individuals with current thrombocytopenia may develop more severe thrombocytopenia following vaccination. In addition, individuals who experienced thrombocytopenia with the first dose of M-M-R II (or its component vaccines) may develop thrombocytopenia with repeat doses. Serologic status may be evaluated to determine whether or not additional doses of vaccine are needed. The potential risk to benefit ratio should be carefully evaluated before considering vaccination in such cases (see ADVERSE REACTIONS).

PRECAUTIONS

General

Adequate treatment provisions including epinephrine injection (1:1000), should be available for immediate use should an anaphylactic or anaphylactoid reaction occur.

Special care should be taken to ensure that the injection does not enter a blood vessel.

Children and young adults who are known to be infected with human immunodeficiency viruses and are not immunosuppressed may be vaccinated. However, vaccinees who are infected with HIV should be monitored closely for vaccine-preventable diseases because immunization may be less effective than for uninfected persons (see CONTRAINDICATIONS).

Vaccination should be deferred for 3 months or longer following blood or plasma transfusions, or administration of immune globulin (human).

There are no reports of transmission of live attenuated measles virus from vaccinees to susceptible contacts.

It has been reported that attenuated measles virus vaccine live may result in a temporary depression of tuberculin skin sensitivity. Therefore, if a tuberculin test is to be done, it should be administered either before or simultaneously with ATTENUVAX.

Children under treatment for tuberculosis have not experienced exacerbation of the disease when immunized with live measels virus vaccine; no studies have been reported to date of the effect of measles virus vaccines on untreated tuberculosis children. However, individuals with active untreated tuberculosis should not be vaccinated.

As for any vaccine, vaccination with ATTENUVAX may not result in protection in 100% of vaccinees.

The health-care provider should determine the current health status and previous vaccination history of the vaccinee.

The health-care provider should question the patient, parent, or guardian about reactions to a previous dose of ATTENUVAX or other measles-containing vaccines.

Drug Interactions

See DOSAGE AND ADMINISTRATION, *Use With Other Vaccines.*

Information For Patients

The health-care provider should provide the vaccine information required to be given with each vaccination to the patient, parent or guardian.

The health-care provider should inform the patient, parent or guardian of the benefits and risks associated with vaccination. For risks associated with vaccination see WARNINGS, PRECAUTIONS, ADVERSE REACTIONS.

Patients, parents or guardians should be instructed to report any serious adverse reactions to their health-care provider who in turn should report such events to the U.S. Department of Health and Human Services through the Vaccine Adverse Event Reporting System (VAERS), 1-800-822-7967.

Pregnancy should be avoided for 3 months following vaccination, and patients should be informed of the reasons for this precaution (see CONTRAINDICATIONS and PRECAUTIONS, *Pregnancy*).

Immunosuppressive Therapy

The immune status of patients about to undergo immunosuppressive therapy should be evaluated so that the physician can consider whether vaccination prior to the initiation of treatment is indicated (see CONTRAINDICATIONS and PRECAUTIONS).

The ACIP has stated that "patients with leukemia in remission who have not received chemotherapy for at least 3 months may receive live-virus vaccines. Short-term (<2 weeks), low- to moderate-dose systemic corticosteroid therapy, topical steroid therapy (e.g., nasal, skin), long-term alternate-day treatment with low to moderate doses of short-acting systemic steroid, and intra-articular, bursal, or tendon injection of corticosteroids are not immunosuppressive in their usual doses and do not contraindicate the administration of measles vaccine."

Immune Globulin

Administration of immune globulins concurrently with ATTENUVAX may interfere with the expected immune response.

See also PRECAUTIONS, *General.*

Carcinogenesis, Mutagenesis, Impairment of Fertility

ATTENUVAX has not been evaluated for carcinogenic or mutagenic potential, or potential to impair fertility.

Pregnancy

Pregnancy Category C

Animal reproduction studies have not been conducted with ATTENUVAX. It is also not known whether ATTENUVAX can cause fetal harm when administered to a pregnant woman or can affect reproduction capacity. Therefore, the vaccine should not be administered to pregnant females; furthermore, pregnancy should be avoided for 3 months following vaccination (see CONTRAINDICATIONS).

In counseling women who are inadvertently vaccinated when pregnant or who become pregnant within 3 months of vaccination, the physician should be aware that reports have indicated that contracting natural measles during pregnancy enhances fetal risk. Increased rates of spontaneous abortion, stillbirth, congenital defects and prematurity have been observed subsequent to natural measles during pregnancy. There are no adequate studies of the attenuated (vaccine) strain of measles virus in pregnancy. However, it would be prudent to assume that the vaccine strain of virus is also capable of inducing adverse fetal effects.

Nursing Mothers

It is not known whether measles vaccine virus is secreted in human milk. Therefore, because many drugs are excreted in human milk, caution should be exercised when ATTENUVAX is administered to a nursing woman.

Pediatric Use

Safety and effectiveness in infants below the age of 6 months have not been established (see also CLINICAL PHARMACOLOGY).

Geriatric Use

Clinical studies of ATTENUVAX did not include sufficient numbers of seronegative subjects aged 65 and over to determine whether they respond differently from younger subjects. Other reported clinical experience has not identified differences in responses between the elderly and younger subjects.

ADVERSE REACTIONS

The following adverse reactions are listed in decreasing order of severity, without regard to causality, within each body system category and have been reported during clinical trials, with use of the marketed vaccine, or with use of polyvalent vaccine containing measles:

Body as a Whole

Panniculitis; atypical measles; fever; syncope; headache; dizziness; malaise; irritability.

Cardiovascular System

Vasculitis.

Digestive System

Diarrhea.

Hemic and Lymphatic System

Thrombocytopenia (see WARNINGS, *Thrombocytopenia*); purpura; lymphadenopathy; leukocytosis.

Immune System

Anaphylaxis and anaphylactoid reactions have been reported as well as related phenomena such as angioneurotic edema (including peripheral or facial edema) and bronchial spasm in individuals with or without an allergic history.

Nervous System

Encephalitis; encephalopathy; measles inclusion body encephalitis (MIBE) (see CONTRAINDICATIONS); subacute sclerosing panencephalitis (SSPE); Guillain-Barré Syndrome (GBS); febrile convulsions; afebrile convulsions or seizures; ataxia; ocular palsies.

Experience from more than 80 million doses of all live measles vaccines given in the U.S. through 1975 indicates that significant central nervous system reactions such as encephalitis and encephalopathy, occurring within 30 days after vaccination, have been temporally associated with measles vaccine very rarely. In no case has it been shown that reactions were actually caused by vaccine. The Centers for Disease Control and Prevention has pointed out that "a certain number of cases of encephalitis may be expected to occur in a large childhood population in a defined period of time even when no vaccines are administered". However, the data suggest the possibility that some of these cases may have been caused by measles vaccines. The risk of such serious neurological disorders following live measles virus vaccine administration remains far less than that for encephalitis and encephalopathy with natural measles (one per two thousand reported cases).

Post-marketing surveillance of the more than 200 million doses of M-M-R and M-M-R II that have been distributed

worldwide over 25 years (1971–1996) indicates that serious adverse events such as encephalitis and encephalopathy continue to be rarely reported.
There have been reports of subacute sclerosing panencephalitis (SSPE) in children who did not have a history of natural measles but did receive measles vaccine. Some of these cases may have resulted from unrecognized measles in the first year of life or possibly from the measles vaccination. Based on estimated nationwide measles vaccine distribution, the association of SSPE cases to measles vaccination is about one case per million vaccine doses distributed. This is far less than the association with natural measles, 6–22 cases of SSPE per million cases of measles. The results of a retrospective case-controlled study conducted by the Centers for Disease Control and Prevention suggest that the overall effect of measles vaccine has been to protect against SSPE by preventing measles with its inherent higher risk of SSPE.
Respiratory System
Pneumonitis (see CONTRAINDICATIONS); cough; rhinitis.
Skin
Stevens-Johnson Syndrome; erythema multiforme; urticaria; rash.
Local reactions including burning/stinging at injection site; wheal and flare; redness (erythema); swelling; vesiculation at injection site.
Special Senses—Ear
Nerve deafness; otitis media.
Special Senses—Eye
Retinitis; optic neuritis; papillitis; retrobulbar neuritis; conjunctivitis.
Other
Death from various, and in some cases unknown, causes has been reported rarely following vaccination with measles, mumps, and rubella vaccines; however, a causal relationship has not been established. No deaths or permanent sequelae were reported in a published post-marketing surveillance study in Finland involving 1.5 million children and adults who were vaccinated with M-M-R II during 1982–1993.
Under the National Childhood Vaccine Injury Act of 1986, health-care providers and manufacturers are required to record and report certain suspected adverse events occurring within specific time periods after vaccination. However, the U.S. Department of Health and Human Services (DHHS) has established a Vaccine Adverse Event Reporting System (VAERS) which will accept all reports of suspected events. A VAERS report form as well as information regarding reporting requirements can be obtained by calling VAERS 1-800-822-7967.

DOSAGE AND ADMINISTRATION

FOR SUBCUTANEOUS ADMINISTRATION
Do not inject intravenously.
The dose for any age is 0.5 mL administered subcutaneously, preferably into the outer aspect of the upper arm.
The recommended age for primary vaccination is 12 to 15 months.
Revaccination with M-M-R II is recommended prior to elementary school entry. See also INDICATIONS AND USAGE, *Recommended Vaccination Schedule.*
Children first vaccinated when younger than 12 months of age should receive another dose between 12 to 15 months of age followed by revaccination prior to elementary school entry. See also INDICATIONS AND USAGE, *Measles Outbreak Schedule.*
Immune Globulin (IG) is not to be given concurrently with ATTENUVAX.
CAUTION: A sterile syringe free of preservatives, antiseptics, and detergents should be used for each injection and/or reconstitution of the vaccine because these substances may inactivate the live virus vaccine. A 25 gauge, 5/8″ needle is recommended.
To reconstitute, use only the diluent supplied, since it is free of preservatives or other antiviral substances which might inactivate the vaccine.
Single Dose Vial—First withdraw the entire volume of diluent into the syringe to be used for reconstitution. Inject all the diluent in the syringe into the vial of lyophilized vaccine, and agitate to mix thoroughly. If the lyophilized vaccine cannot be dissolved, discard. Withdraw the entire contents into a syringe and inject the total volume of restored vaccine subcutaneously.
It is important to use a separate sterile syringe and needle for each individual patient to prevent transmission of hepatitis B and other infectious agents from one person to another.
Parenteral drug products should be inspected visually for particulate matter and discoloration prior to administration whenever solution and container permit. ATTENUVAX, when reconstituted, is clear yellow.
Use With Other Vaccines
ATTENUVAX should not be given less than one month before or after administration of other live viral vaccines.
M-M-R II has been administered concurrently with VARIVAX* [Varicella Virus Vaccine Live (Oka/Merck)], and PedvaxHIB* [Haemophilus b Conjugate Vaccine (Meningococcal Protein Conjugate)] using separate sites and syringes. No impairment of immune response to individual tested vaccine antigens was demonstrated. The type, frequency, and severity of adverse experiences observed with M-M-R II were similar to those seen when each vaccine was given alone.
Routine administration of DTP (diphtheria, tetanus, pertussis) and/or OPV (oral poliovirus vaccine) concurrently with measles, mumps and rubella vaccines is not recommended because there are limited data relating to the simultaneous administration of these antigens.
However, other schedules have been used. The ACIP has stated "Although data are limited concerning the simultaneous administration of the entire recommended vaccine series (i.e., DTP, OPV, MMR, and Hib vaccines, with or without hepatitis B vaccine), data from numerous studies have indicated no interference between routinely recommended childhood vaccines (either live, attenuated, or killed). These findings support the simultaneous use of all vaccines as recommended."

HOW SUPPLIED

No. 4709—ATTENUVAX is supplied as a single-dose vial of lyophilized vaccine, **NDC** 0006-4709-00, and a vial of diluent.
No. 4589X/4309—ATTENUVAX is supplied as follows: (1) a box of 10 single-dose vials of lyophilized vaccine (package A), **NDC** 0006-4589-00; and (2) a box of 10 vials of diluent (package B). To conserve refrigerator space, the diluent may be stored separately at room temperature.
Storage
During shipment, to ensure that there is no loss of potency, the vaccine must be maintained at a temperature of 10°C (50°F) or colder. Freezing during shipment will not affect potency.
Protect the vaccine from light at all times, since such exposure may inactivate the virus.
Before reconstitution, store the vial of lyophilized vaccine at 2–8°C (36–46°F) or colder. The diluent may be stored in the refrigerator with the lyophilized vaccine or separately at room temperature.
It is recommended that the vaccine be used as soon as possible after reconstitution. Store reconstituted vaccine in the vaccine vial in a dark place at 2–8°C (36–46°F) and discard if not used within 8 hours.
9243205 Issued September 2002

BLOCADREN® Tablets ℞
(Timolol Maleate)

DESCRIPTION

BLOCADREN* (Timolol Maleate) is a non-selective beta-adrenergic receptor blocking agent. The chemical name for timolol maleate is (*S*)-1-[(1,1-dimethylethyl)amino] -3-[[4-(4-morpholinyl)-1,2,5-thiadiazol-3-yl]oxy]-2-propanol (*Z*)-2-butenedioate (1:1) salt. It possesses an asymmetric carbon atom in its structure and is provided as the levo isomer. Its empirical formula is $C_{13}H_{24}N_4O_3S{\cdot}C_4H_4O_4$ and its structural formula is:

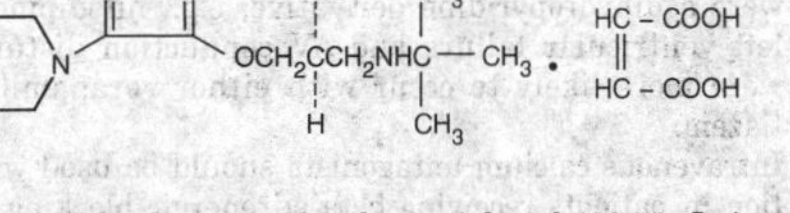

Timolol maleate has a molecular weight of 432.50. It is a white, odorless, crystalline powder which is soluble in water, methanol, and alcohol.
BLOCADREN is supplied as tablets in three strengths containing 5 mg, 10 mg or 20 mg timolol maleate for oral administration. Inactive ingredients are cellulose, FD&C Blue 2, magnesium stearate, and starch.

*Registered trademark of MERCK & CO., INC.

CLINICAL PHARMACOLOGY

BLOCADREN is a $beta_1$ and $beta_2$ (non-selective) adrenergic receptor blocking agent that does not have significant intrinsic sympathomimetic, direct myocardial depressant, or local anesthetic activity.
Pharmacodynamics
Clinical pharmacology studies have confirmed the beta-adrenergic blocking activity as shown by (1) changes in resting heart rate and response of heart rate to changes in posture; (2) inhibition of isoproterenol-induced tachycardia; (3) alteration of the response to the Valsalva maneuver and amyl nitrite administration; and (4) reduction of heart rate and blood pressure changes on exercise.
BLOCADREN decreases the positive chronotropic, positive inotropic, bronchodilator, and vasodilator responses caused by beta-adrenergic receptor agonists. The magnitude of this decreased response is proportional to the existing sympathetic tone and the concentration of BLOCADREN at receptor sites.
In normal volunteers, the reduction in heart rate response to a standard exercise was dose dependent over the test range of 0.5 to 20 mg, with a peak reduction at 2 hours of approximately 30% at higher doses.
Beta-adrenergic receptor blockade reduces cardiac output in both healthy subjects and patients with heart disease. In patients with severe impairment of myocardial function beta-adrenergic receptor blockade may inhibit the stimulatory effect of the sympathetic nervous system necessary to maintain adequate cardiac function.
Beta-adrenergic receptor blockade in the bronchi and bronchioles results in increased airway resistance from unopposed parasympathetic activity. Such an effect in patients with asthma or other bronchospastic conditions is potentially dangerous.
Clinical studies indicate that BLOCADREN at a dosage of 20–60 mg/day reduces blood pressure without causing postural hypotension in most patients with essential hypertension. Administration of BLOCADREN to patients with hypertension results initially in a decrease in cardiac output, little immediate change in blood pressure, and an increase in calculated peripheral resistance. With continued administration of BLOCADREN, blood pressure decreases within a few days, cardiac output usually remains reduced, and peripheral resistance falls toward pretreatment levels. Plasma volume may decrease or remain unchanged during therapy with BLOCADREN. In the majority of patients with hypertension BLOCADREN also decreases plasma renin activity. Dosage adjustment to achieve optimal antihypertensive effect may require a few weeks. When therapy with BLOCADREN is discontinued, the blood pressure tends to return to pretreatment levels gradually. In most patients the antihypertensive activity of BLOCADREN is maintained with long-term therapy and is well tolerated.
The mechanism of the antihypertensive effects of beta-adrenergic receptor blocking agents is not established at this time. Possible mechanisms of action include reduction in cardiac output, reduction in plasma renin activity, and a central nervous system sympatholytic action.
A Norwegian multi-center, double-blind study, which included patients 20 to 75 years of age, compared the effects of timolol maleate with placebo in 1,884 patients who had survived the acute phase of a myocardial infarction. Patients with systolic blood pressure below 100 mm Hg, sick sinus syndrome and contraindications to beta blockers, including uncontrolled heart failure, second or third degree AV block and bradycardia (<50 beats per minute), were excluded from the multi-center trial. Therapy with BLOCADREN, begun 7 to 28 days following infarction, was shown to reduce overall mortality; this was primarily attributable to a reduction in cardiovascular mortality. BLOCADREN significantly reduced the incidence of sudden deaths (deaths occurring without symptoms or within 24 hours of the onset of symptoms), including those occurring within one hour, and particularly instantaneous deaths (those occurring without preceding symptoms). The protective effect of BLOCADREN was consistent regardless of age, sex or site of infarction. The effect was clearest in patients with a first infarction who were considered at a high risk of dying, defined as those with one or more of the following characteristics during the acute phase: transient left ventricular failure, cardiomegaly, newly appearing atrial fibrillation or flutter, systolic hypotension, or SGOT (ASAT) levels greater than four times the upper limit of normal. Therapy with BLOCADREN also reduced the incidence of non-fatal reinfarction. The mechanism of the protective effect of BLOCADREN is unknown.
BLOCADREN was studied for the prophylactic treatment of migraine headache in placebo-controlled clinical trials involving 400 patients, mostly women between the ages of 18 and 66 years. Common migraine was the most frequent diagnosis. All patients had at least two headaches per month at baseline. Approximately 50 percent of patients who received BLOCADREN had a reduction in the frequency of migraine headache of at least 50 percent, compared to a similar decrease in frequency in 30 percent of patients receiving placebo. The most common cardiovascular adverse effect was bradycardia (5%).
Pharmacokinetics and Metabolism
BLOCADREN is rapidly and nearly completely absorbed (about 90%) following oral ingestion. Detectable plasma levels of timolol occur within one-half hour and peak plasma levels occur in about one to two hours. The drug half-life in plasma is approximately 4 hours and this is essentially unchanged in patients with moderate renal insufficiency. Timolol is partially metabolized by the liver and timolol and its metabolites are excreted by the kidney. Timolol is not extensively bound to plasma proteins; i.e., <10% by equilibrium dialysis and approximately 60% by ultrafiltration. An *in vitro* hemodialysis study, using ^{14}C timolol added to human plasma or whole blood, showed that timolol was readily dialyzed from these fluids; however, a study of patients with renal failure showed that timolol did not dialyze readily. Plasma levels following oral administration are about half those following intravenous administration indicating approximately 50% first pass metabolism. The level of beta sympathetic activity varies widely among individuals, and no simple correlation exists between the dose or plasma level of timolol maleate and its therapeutic activity. Therefore, objective clinical measurements such as reduction of heart rate and/or blood pressure should be used as guides in determining the optimal dosage for each patient.

Continued on next page

Information on the Merck & Co., Inc., products listed on these pages is from the prescribing information in use October 1, 2004. For information, please call 1-800-NSC-MERCK [1-800-672-6372].

Blocadren—Cont.

INDICATIONS AND USAGE

Hypertension
BLOCADREN is indicated for the treatment of hypertension. It may be used alone or in combination with other antihypertensive agents, especially thiazide-type diuretics.
Myocardial Infarction
BLOCADREN is indicated in patients who have survived the acute phase of a myocardial infarction, and are clinically stable, to reduce cardiovascular mortality and the risk of reinfarction.
Migraine
BLOCADREN is indicated for the prophylaxis of migraine headache.

CONTRAINDICATIONS

BLOCADREN is contraindicated in patients with bronchial asthma or with a history of bronchial asthma, or severe chronic obstructive pulmonary disease (see WARNINGS); sinus bradycardia; second and third degree atrioventricular block; overt cardiac failure (see WARNINGS); cardiogenic shock; hypersensitivity to this product.

WARNINGS

Cardiac Failure
Sympathetic stimulation may be essential for support of the circulation in individuals with diminished myocardial contractility, and its inhibition by beta-adrenergic receptor blockade may precipitate more severe failure. Although beta blockers should be avoided in overt congestive heart failure, they can be used, if necessary, with caution in patients with a history of failure who are well-compensated, usually with digitalis and diuretics. Both digitalis and timolol maleate slow AV conduction. If cardiac failure persists, therapy with BLOCADREN should be withdrawn.
In Patients Without a History of Cardiac Failure continued depression of the myocardium with beta-blocking agents over a period of time can, in some cases, lead to cardiac failure. At the first sign or symptom of cardiac failure, patients receiving BLOCADREN should be digitalized and/or be given a diuretic, and the response observed closely. If cardiac failure continues, despite adequate digitalization and diuretic therapy, BLOCADREN should be withdrawn.

Exacerbation of Ischemic Heart Disease Following Abrupt Withdrawal—Hypersensitivity to catecholamines has been observed in patients withdrawn from beta blocker therapy; exacerbation of angina and, in some cases, myocardial infarction have occurred after *abrupt* discontinuation of such therapy. When discontinuing chronically administered timolol maleate, particularly in patients with ischemic heart disease, the dosage should be gradually reduced over a period of one to two weeks and the patient should be carefully monitored. If angina markedly worsens or acute coronary insufficiency develops, timolol maleate administration should be reinstituted promptly, at least temporarily, and other measures appropriate for the management of unstable angina should be taken. Patients should be warned against interruption or discontinuation of therapy without the physician's advice. Because coronary artery disease is common and may be unrecognized, it may be prudent not to discontinue timolol maleate therapy abruptly even in patients treated only for hypertension.

Obstructive Pulmonary Disease
PATIENTS WITH CHRONIC OBSTRUCTIVE PULMONARY DISEASE (e.g., CHRONIC BRONCHITIS, EMPHYSEMA) OF MILD OR MODERATE SEVERITY, BRONCHOSPASTIC DISEASE OR A HISTORY OF BRONCHOSPASTIC DISEASE (OTHER THAN BRONCHIAL ASTHMA OR A HISTORY OF BRONCHIAL ASTHMA, IN WHICH 'BLOCADREN' IS CONTRAINDICATED, see CONTRAINDICATIONS), SHOULD IN GENERAL NOT RECEIVE BETA BLOCKERS, INCLUDING 'BLOCADREN'. However, if BLOCADREN is necessary in such patients, then the drug should be administered with caution since it may block bronchodilation produced by endogenous and exogenous catecholamine stimulation of $beta_2$ receptors.
Major Surgery
The necessity or desirability of withdrawal of beta-blocking therapy prior to major surgery is controversial. Beta-adrenergic receptor blockade impairs the ability of the heart to respond to beta-adrenergically mediated reflex stimuli. This may augment the risk of general anesthesia in surgical procedures. Some patients receiving beta-adrenergic receptor blocking agents have been subject to protracted severe hypotension during anesthesia. Difficulty in restarting and maintaining the heartbeat has also been reported. For these reasons, in patients undergoing elective surgery, some authorities recommend gradual withdrawal of beta-adrenergic receptor blocking agents.
If necessary during surgery, the effects of beta-adrenergic blocking agents may be reversed by sufficient doses of such agonists as isoproterenol, dopamine, dobutamine or levarterenol (see OVERDOSAGE).
Diabetes Mellitus
BLOCADREN should be administered with caution in patients subject to spontaneous hypoglycemia or to diabetic patients (especially those with labile diabetes) who are receiving insulin or oral hypoglycemic agents. Beta-adrenergic receptor blocking agents may mask the signs and symptoms of acute hypoglycemia.
Thyrotoxicosis
Beta-adrenergic blockade may mask certain clinical signs (e.g., tachycardia) of hyperthyroidism. Patients suspected of developing thyrotoxicosis should be managed carefully to avoid abrupt withdrawal of beta blockade which might precipitate a thyroid storm.

PRECAUTIONS

General
Impaired Hepatic or Renal Function: Since BLOCADREN is partially metabolized in the liver and excreted mainly by the kidneys, dosage reductions may be necessary when hepatic and/or renal insufficiency is present.
Dosing in the Presence of Marked Renal Failure: Although the pharmacokinetics of BLOCADREN are not greatly altered by renal impairment, marked hypotensive responses have been seen in patients with marked renal impairment undergoing dialysis after 20 mg doses. Dosing in such patients should therefore be especially cautious.
Muscle Weakness: Beta-adrenergic blockade has been reported to potentiate muscle weakness consistent with certain myasthenic symptoms (e.g., diplopia, ptosis, and generalized weakness). Timolol has been reported rarely to increase muscle weakness in some patients with myasthenia gravis or myasthenic symptoms.
Cerebrovascular Insufficiency: Because of potential effects of beta-adrenergic blocking agents relative to blood pressure and pulse, these agents should be used with caution in patients with cerebrovascular insufficiency. If signs or symptoms suggesting reduced cerebral blood flow are observed, consideration should be given to discontinuing these agents.
Drug Interactions
Catecholamine-depleting drugs: Close observation of the patient is recommended when BLOCADREN is administered to patients receiving catecholamine-depleting drugs such as reserpine, because of possible additive effects and the production of hypotension and/or marked bradycardia, which may produce vertigo, syncope, or postural hypotension.
Non-steroidal anti-inflammatory drugs: Blunting of the antihypertensive effect of beta-adrenoceptor blocking agents by non-steroidal anti-inflammatory drugs has been reported. When using these agents concomitantly, patients should be observed carefully to confirm that the desired therapeutic effect has been obtained.
Calcium antagonists: Literature reports suggest that oral calcium antagonists may be used in combination with beta-adrenergic blocking agents when heart function is normal, but should be avoided in patients with impaired cardiac function. Hypotension, AV conduction disturbances, and left ventricular failure have been reported in some patients receiving beta-adrenergic blocking agents when an oral calcium antagonist was added to the treatment regimen. Hypotension was more likely to occur if the calcium antagonist were a dihydropyridine derivative, e.g., nifedipine, while left ventricular failure and AV conduction disturbances were more likely to occur with either verapamil or diltiazem.
Intravenous calcium antagonists should be used with caution in patients receiving beta-adrenergic blocking agents.
Digitalis and either diltiazem or verapamil: The concomitant use of beta-adrenergic blocking agents with digitalis and either diltiazem or verapamil may have additive effects in prolonging AV conduction time.
Quinidine: Potentiated systemic beta-blockade (e.g., decreased heart rate) has been reported during combined treatment with quinidine and timolol, possibly because quinidine inhibits the metabolism of timolol via the P-450 enzyme, CYP2D6.
Clonidine: Beta adrenergic blocking agents may exacerbate the rebound hypertension which can follow the withdrawal of clonidine. If the two drugs are coadministered, the beta adrenergic blocking agent should be withdrawn several days before the gradual withdrawal of clonidine. If replacing clonidine by beta-blocker therapy, the introduction of beta adrenergic blocking agents should be delayed for several days after clonidine administration has stopped.
Risk from Anaphylactic Reaction: While taking beta-blockers, patients with a history of atopy or a history of severe anaphylactic reaction to a variety of allergens may be more reactive to repeated accidental, diagnostic, or therapeutic challenge with such allergens. Such patients may be unresponsive to the usual doses of epinephrine used to treat anaphylactic reactions.
Carcinogenesis, Mutagenesis, Impairment of Fertility
In a two-year study of timolol maleate in rats, there was a statistically significant increase in the incidence of adrenal pheochromocytomas in male rats administered 300 mg/kg/day (250 times** the maximum recommended human dose). Similar differences were not observed in rats administered doses equivalent to approximately 20 or 80 times** the maximum recommended human dose.
In a lifetime study in mice, there were statistically significant increases in the incidence of benign and malignant pulmonary tumors, benign uterine polyps and mammary adenocarcinoma in female mice at 500 mg/kg/day (approximately 400 times** the maximum recommended human dose), but not at 5 or 50 mg/kg/day. In a subsequent study in female mice, in which post-mortem examinations were limited to uterus and lungs, a statistically significant increase in the incidence of pulmonary tumors was again observed at 500 mg/kg/day.
The increased occurrence of mammary adenocarcinoma was associated with elevations in serum prolactin that occurred in female mice administered timolol at 500 mg/kg/day, but not at doses of 5 or 50 mg/kg/day. An increased incidence of mammary adenocarcinomas in rodents has been associated with administration of several other therapeutic agents which elevate serum prolactin, but no correlation between serum prolactin levels and mammary tumors has been established in man. Furthermore, in adult human female subjects who received oral dosages of up to 60 mg of timolol maleate, the maximum recommended human oral dosage, there were no clinically meaningful changes in serum prolactin.
Timolol maleate was devoid of mutagenic potential when evaluated *in vivo* (mouse) in the micronucleus test and cytogenetic assay (doses up to 800 mg/kg) and *in vitro* in a neoplastic cell transformation assay (up to 100 μg/mL). In Ames tests the highest concentrations of timolol employed, 5000 or 10,000 μg/plate, were associated with statistically significant elevations of revertants observed with tester strain TA100 (in seven replicate assays), but not in three additional strains. In the assays with tester strain TA100, no consistent dose response relationship was observed, nor did the ratio of test to control revertants reach 2. A ratio of 2 is usually considered the criterion for a positive Ames test.
Reproduction and fertility studies in rats showed no adverse effect on male or female fertility at doses up to 125 times** the maximum recommended human dose.

**Based on patient weight of 50 kg

Pregnancy
Pregnancy Category C. Teratogenicity studies with timolol in mice, rats and rabbits at doses up to 50 mg/kg/day (approximately 40 times** the maximum recommended daily human dose) showed no evidence of fetal malformations. Although delayed fetal ossification was observed at this dose in rats, there were no adverse effects on postnatal development of offspring. Doses of 1000 mg/kg/day (approximately 830 times** the maximum recommended daily human dose) were maternotoxic in mice and resulted in an increased number of fetal resorptions. Increased fetal resorptions were also seen in rabbits at doses of approximately 40 times** the maximum recommended daily human dose, in this case without apparent maternotoxicity. There are no adequate and well-controlled studies in pregnant women. BLOCADREN should be used during pregnancy only if the potential benefit justifies the potential risk to the fetus.

**Based on patient weight of 50 kg

Nursing Mothers
Timolol maleate has been detected in human milk.
Because of the potential for serious adverse reactions from timolol in nursing infants, a decision should be made whether to discontinue nursing or to discontinue the drug, taking into account the importance of the drug to the mother.
Pediatric Use
Safety and effectiveness in pediatric patients have not been established.
Geriatric Use
Clinical studies of BLOCADREN for the treatment of hypertension or migraine did not include sufficient numbers of subjects aged 65 and over to determine whether they respond differently from younger subjects.
In a clinical study of BLOCADREN in patients who had survived the acute phase of a myocardial infarction, approximately 350 patients (37%) were 65–75 years of age. Safety and efficacy were not different between these patients and younger patients (see CLINICAL PHARMACOLOGY, *Pharmacodynamics*).
Other reported clinical experience has not identified differences in responses between the elderly and younger patients. In general, dose selection for an elderly patient should be cautious, usually starting at the low end of the dosing range, reflecting the greater frequency of decreased hepatic, renal or cardiac function, and of concomitant disease or other drug therapy.
This drug is known to be substantially excreted by the kidney, and the risk of toxic reactions to this drug may be greater in patients with impaired renal function. Because elderly patients are more likely to have decreased renal function, care should be taken in dose selection, and it may be useful to monitor renal function. (See PRECAUTIONS, *Impaired Hepatic or Renal Function* and *Dosing in the Presence of Marked Renal Failure*.)

ADVERSE REACTIONS

BLOCADREN is usually well tolerated in properly selected patients. Most adverse effects have been mild and transient.
In a multicenter (12-week) clinical trial comparing timolol maleate and placebo in hypertensive patients, the following adverse reactions were reported spontaneously and considered to be causally related to timolol maleate:

	Timolol Maleate (n = 176) %	Placebo (n = 168) %
BODY AS A WHOLE		
fatigue/tiredness	3.4	0.6
headache	1.7	1.8
chest pain	0.6	0
asthenia	0.6	0
CARDIOVASCULAR		
bradycardia	9.1	0
arrhythmia	1.1	0.6
syncope	0.6	0
edema	0.6	1.2
DIGESTIVE		
dyspepsia	0.6	0.6
nausea	0.6	0
SKIN		
pruritus	1.1	0
NERVOUS SYSTEM		
dizziness	2.3	1.2
vertigo	0.6	0
paresthesia	0.6	0
PSYCHIATRIC		
decreased libido	0.6	0
RESPIRATORY		
dyspnea	1.7	0.6
bronchial spasm	0.6	0
rales	0.6	0
SPECIAL SENSES		
eye irritation	1.1	0.6
tinnitus	0.6	0

These data are representative of the incidence of adverse effects that may be observed in properly selected patients treated with BLOCADREN, i.e., excluding patients with bronchospastic disease, congestive heart failure or other contraindications to beta blocker therapy.

In patients with migraine the incidence of bradycardia was 5 percent.

In a coronary artery disease population studied in the Norwegian multi-center trial (see CLINICAL PHARMACOLOGY), the frequency of the principal adverse reactions and the frequency with which these resulted in discontinuation of therapy in the timolol and placebo groups were:

[See table above]

BLOCADREN	Adverse Reaction***		Withdrawal†	
	Timolol (n = 945) %	Placebo (n = 939) %	Timolol (n = 945) %	Placebo (n = 939) %
Asthenia or Fatigue	5	1	<1	<1
Heart Rate <40 beats/minute	5	<1	4	<1
Cardiac Failure—Nonfatal	8	7	3	2
Hypotension	3	2	3	1
Pulmonary Edema—Nonfatal	2	<1	<1	<1
Claudication	3	3	1	<1
AV Block 2nd or 3rd degree	<1	<1	<1	<1
Sinoatrial Block	<1	<1	<1	<1
Cold Hands and Feet	8	<1	<1	0
Nausea or Digestive Disorders	8	6	1	<1
Dizziness	6	4	1	0
Bronchial Obstruction	2	<1	1	<1

***When an adverse reaction recurred in a patient, it is listed only once.
†Only principal reason for withdrawal in each patient is listed.
These adverse reactions can also occur in patients treated for hypertension.

The following additional adverse effects have been reported in clinical experience with the drug: *Body as a Whole:* anaphylaxis, extremity pain, decreased exercise tolerance, weight loss, fever; *Cardiovascular:* cardiac arrest, cardiac failure, cerebral vascular accident, worsening of angina pectoris, worsening of arterial insufficiency, Raynaud's phenomenon, palpitations, vasodilatation; *Digestive:* gastrointestinal pain, hepatomegaly, vomiting, diarrhea, dyspepsia; *Hematologic:* nonthrombocytopenic purpura; *Endocrine:* hyperglycemia, hypoglycemia; *Skin:* rash, skin irritation, increased pigmentation, sweating, alopecia; *Musculoskeletal:* arthralgia; *Nervous System:* local weakness, increase in signs and symptoms of myasthenia gravis; *Psychiatric:* depression, nightmares, somnolence, insomnia, nervousness, diminished concentration, hallucinations; *Respiratory:* cough; *Special Senses:* visual disturbances, diplopia, ptosis, dry eyes; *Urogenital:* impotence, urination difficulties.

There have been reports of retroperitoneal fibrosis in patients receiving timolol maleate and in patients receiving other beta-adrenergic blocking agents. A causal relationship between this condition and therapy with beta-adrenergic blocking agents has not been established.

Potential Adverse Effects: In addition, a variety of adverse effects not observed in clinical trials with BLOCADREN, but reported with other beta-adrenergic blocking agents, should be considered potential adverse effects of BLOCADREN: *Nervous System:* Reversible mental depression progressing to catatonia; an acute reversible syndrome characterized by disorientation for time and place, short-term memory loss, emotional lability, slightly clouded sensorium, and decreased performance on neuropsychometrics; *Cardiovascular:* Intensification of AV block (see CONTRAINDICATIONS); *Digestive:* Mesenteric arterial thrombosis, ischemic colitis; *Hematologic:* Agranulocytosis, thrombocytopenic purpura; *Allergic:* Erythematous rash, fever combined with aching and sore throat, laryngospasm with respiratory distress; *Miscellaneous:* Peyronie's disease.

There have been reports of a syndrome comprising psoriasiform skin rash, conjunctivitis sicca, otitis, and sclerosing serositis attributed to the beta-adrenergic receptor blocking agent, practolol. This syndrome has not been reported with BLOCADREN.

Clinical Laboratory Test Findings: Clinically important changes in standard laboratory parameters were rarely associated with the administration of BLOCADREN. Slight increases in blood urea nitrogen, serum potassium, uric acid, and triglycerides, and slight decreases in hemoglobin, hematocrit and HDL cholesterol occurred, but were not progressive or associated with clinical manifestations. Increases in liver function tests have been reported.

OVERDOSAGE

Overdosage has been reported with Tablets BLOCADREN. A 30-year-old female ingested 650 mg of BLOCADREN (maximum recommended daily dose—60 mg) and experienced second and third degree heart block. She recovered without treatment but approximately two months later developed irregular heartbeat, hypertension, dizziness, tinnitus, faintness, increased pulse rate and borderline first degree heart block.

The oral LD_{50} of the drug is 1190 and 900 mg/kg in female mice and female rats, respectively.

An *in vitro* hemodialysis study, using ^{14}C timolol added to human plasma or whole blood, showed that timolol was readily dialyzed from these fluids; however, a study of patients with renal failure showed that timolol did not dialyze readily.

The most common signs and symptoms to be expected with overdosage with a beta-adrenergic receptor blocking agent are symptomatic bradycardia, hypotension, bronchospasm, and acute cardiac failure. Therapy with BLOCADREN should be discontinued and the patient observed closely. The following additional therapeutic measures should be considered:

(1) *Gastric lavage*

(2) *Symptomatic bradycardia:* Use atropine sulfate intravenously in a dosage of 0.25 mg to 2 mg to induce vagal blockade. If bradycardia persists, intravenous isoproterenol hydrochloride should be administered cautiously. In refractory cases the use of a transvenous cardiac pacemaker may be considered.

(3) *Hypotension:* Use sympathomimetic pressor drug therapy, such as dopamine, dobutamine or levarterenol. In refractory cases the use of glucagon hydrochloride has been reported to be useful.

(4) *Bronchospasm:* Use isoproterenol hydrochloride. Additional therapy with aminophylline may be considered.

(5) *Acute cardiac failure:* Conventional therapy with digitalis, diuretics, and oxygen should be instituted immediately. In refractory cases the use of intravenous aminophylline is suggested. This may be followed if necessary by glucagon hydrochloride which has been reported to be useful.

(6) *Heart block (second or third degree):* Use isoproterenol hydrochloride or a transvenous cardiac pacemaker.

DOSAGE AND ADMINISTRATION

Hypertension

The usual initial dosage of BLOCADREN is 10 mg twice a day, whether used alone or added to diuretic therapy. Dosage may be increased or decreased depending on heart rate and blood pressure response. The usual total maintenance dosage is 20–40 mg per day. Increases in dosage to a maximum of 60 mg per day divided into two doses may be necessary. There should be an interval of at least seven days between increases in dosages.

BLOCADREN may be used with a thiazide diuretic or with other antihypertensive agents. Patients should be observed carefully during initiation of such concomitant therapy.

Myocardial Infarction

The recommended dosage for long-term prophylactic use in patients who have survived the acute phase of a myocardial infarction is 10 mg given twice daily (see CLINICAL PHARMACOLOGY).

Migraine

The usual initial dosage of BLOCADREN is 10 mg twice a day. During maintenance therapy the 20 mg daily dosage may be administered as a single dose. Total daily dosage may be increased to a maximum of 30 mg, given in divided doses, or decreased to 10 mg once per day, depending on clinical response and tolerability. If a satisfactory response is not obtained after 6-8 weeks use of the maximum daily dosage, therapy with BLOCADREN should be discontinued.

HOW SUPPLIED

No. 3343—Tablets BLOCADREN, 5 mg, are light blue, round, compressed tablets, with code MSD 59 on one side and BLOCADREN on the other. They are supplied as follows:

NDC 0006-0059-68 bottles of 100.

No. 3344—Tablets BLOCADREN, 10 mg, are light blue, round, scored, compressed tablets, with code MSD 136 on one side and BLOCADREN on the other. They are supplied as follows:

NDC 0006-0136-68 bottles of 100.

No. 3371—Tablets BLOCADREN, 20 mg, are light blue, capsule shaped, scored, compressed tablets, with code MSD 437 on one side and BLOCADREN on the other. They are supplied as follows:

NDC 0006-0437-68 bottles of 100.

Storage

Store at controlled room temperature. 15–30°C (59–86°F). Keep container tightly closed. Protect from light.

7901233 Issued March 2002

Shown in Product Identification Guide, page 323

INTRAVENOUS INFUSION (not for IV Bolus Injection)

CANCIDAS® ℞
(caspofungin acetate) FOR INJECTION

DESCRIPTION

CANCIDAS* is a sterile, lyophilized product for intravenous (IV) infusion that contains a semisynthetic lipopeptide (echinocandin) compound synthesized from a fermentation product of *Glarea lozoyensis*. CANCIDAS is the first of a new class of antifungal drugs (glucan synthesis inhibitors) that inhibit the synthesis of β (1,3)-D-glucan, an integral component of the fungal cell wall.

CANCIDAS (caspofungin acetate) is 1-[(4*R*,5*S*)-5-[(2-amino-ethyl)amino]-N^2-(10,12-dimethyl-1-oxotetradecyl)-4-hydroxy-L-ornithine]-5-[(3*R*)-3-hydroxy-L-ornithine] pneumocandin B_0 diacetate (salt). In addition to the active ingredient caspofungin acetate, CANCIDAS contains the following inactive ingredients: sucrose, mannitol, acetic acid, and sodium hydroxide. Caspofungin acetate is a hygroscopic, white to off-white powder. It is freely soluble in water and methanol, and slightly soluble in ethanol. The pH of a saturated aqueous solution of caspofungin acetate is approximately 6.6. The empirical formula is $C_{52}H_{88}N_{10}O_{15} \bullet 2C_2H_4O_2$ and the formula weight is 1213.42. The structural formula is:

*Registered trademark of MERCK & CO., Inc.

CLINICAL PHARMACOLOGY

Pharmacokinetics

Distribution

Plasma concentrations of caspofungin decline in a polyphasic manner following single 1-hour IV infusions. A short α-phase occurs immediately postinfusion, followed by a

Continued on next page

Information on the Merck & Co., Inc., products listed on these pages is from the prescribing information in use October 1, 2004. For information, please call 1-800-NSC-MERCK [1-800-672-6372].

Cancidas—Cont.

β-phase (half-life of 9 to 11 hours) that characterizes much of the profile and exhibits clear log-linear behavior from 6 to 48 hours postdose during which the plasma concentration decreases 10-fold. An additional, longer half-life phase, γ-phase, (half-life of 40-50 hours), also occurs. Distribution, rather than excretion or biotransformation, is the dominant mechanism influencing plasma clearance. Caspofungin is extensively bound to albumin (~97%), and distribution into red blood cells is minimal. Mass balance results showed that approximately 92% of the administered radioactivity was distributed to tissues by 36 to 48 hours after a single 70-mg dose of [^{3}H] caspofungin acetate. There is little excretion or biotransformation of caspofungin during the first 30 hours after administration.

Metabolism

Caspofungin is slowly metabolized by hydrolysis and N-acetylation. Caspofungin also undergoes spontaneous chemical degradation to an open-ring peptide compound, L-747969. At later time points (≥5 days postdose), there is a low level (≤7 picomoles/mg protein, or ≤ 1.3% of administered dose) of covalent binding of radiolabel in plasma following single-dose administration of [^{3}H] caspofungin acetate, which may be due to two reactive intermediates formed during the chemical degradation of caspofungin to L-747969. Additional metabolism involves hydrolysis into constitutive amino acids and their degradates, including dihydroxyhomotyrosine and N-acetyl-dihydroxyhomotyrosine. These two tyrosine derivatives are found only in urine, suggesting rapid clearance of these derivatives by the kidneys.

Excretion

Two single-dose radiolabeled pharmacokinetic studies were conducted. In one study, plasma, urine, and feces were collected over 27 days, and in the second study plasma was collected over 6 months. Plasma concentrations of radioactivity and of caspofungin were similar during the first 24 to 48 hours postdose; thereafter drug levels fell more rapidly. In plasma, caspofungin concentrations fell below the limit of quantitation after 6 to 8 days postdose, while radiolabel fell below the limit of quantitation at 22.3 weeks postdose. After single intravenous administration of [^{3}H] caspofungin acetate, excretion of caspofungin and its metabolites in humans were 35% of dose in feces and 41% of dose in urine. A small amount of caspofungin is excreted unchanged in urine (~1.4% of dose). Renal clearance of parent drug is low (~0.15 mL/min) and total clearance of caspofungin is 12 mL/min.

Special Populations

Gender

Plasma concentrations of caspofungin in healthy men and women were similar following a single 70-mg dose. After 13 daily 50-mg doses, caspofungin plasma concentrations in women were elevated slightly (approximately 22% in area under the curve [AUC]) relative to men. No dosage adjustment is necessary based on gender.

Geriatric

Plasma concentrations of caspofungin in healthy older men and women (≥65 years of age) were increased slightly (approximately 28% AUC) compared to young healthy men after a single 70-mg dose of caspofungin. In patients with candidemia or other *Candida* infections (intra-abdominal abscesses, peritonitis, or pleural space infections), a similar modest effect of age was seen in older patients relative to younger patients. No dosage adjustment is necessary for the elderly (see PRECAUTIONS, *Geriatric Use*).

Race

Regression analyses of patient pharmacokinetic data indicated that no clinically significant differences in the pharmacokinetics of caspofungin were seen among Caucasians, Blacks, and Hispanics. No dosage adjustment is necessary on the basis of race.

Renal Insufficiency

In a clinical study of single 70-mg doses, caspofungin pharmacokinetics were similar in volunteers with mild renal insufficiency (creatinine clearance 50 to 80 mL/min) and control subjects. Moderate (creatinine clearance 31 to 49 mL/min), advanced (creatinine clearance 5 to 30 mL/min), and end-stage (creatinine clearance <10 mL/min and dialysis dependent) renal insufficiency moderately increased caspofungin plasma concentrations after single-dose administration (range: 30 to 49% for AUC). However, in patients with invasive aspergillosis, candidemia, or other *Candida* infections (intra-abdominal abscesses, peritonitis, or pleural space infections) who received multiple daily doses of CANCIDAS 50 mg, there was no significant effect of mild to end-stage renal impairment on caspofungin concentrations. No dosage adjustment is necessary for patients with renal insufficiency. Caspofungin is not dialyzable, thus supplementary dosing is not required following hemodialysis.

Hepatic Insufficiency

Plasma concentrations of caspofungin after a single 70-mg dose in patients with mild hepatic insufficiency (Child-Pugh score 5 to 6) were increased by approximately 55% in AUC compared to healthy control subjects. In a 14-day multiple-dose study (70 mg on Day 1 followed by 50 mg daily thereafter), plasma concentrations in patients with mild hepatic insufficiency were increased modestly (19 to 25% in AUC) on Days 7 and 14 relative to healthy control subjects. No dosage adjustment is recommended for patients with mild hepatic insufficiency. Patients with moderate hepatic insufficiency (Child-Pugh score 7 to 9) who received a single 70-mg dose of CANCIDAS had an average plasma caspofungin increase of 76% in AUC compared to control subjects. A dosage reduction is recommended for patients with moderate hepatic insufficiency (see DOSAGE AND ADMINISTRATION). There is no clinical experience in patients with severe hepatic insufficiency (Child-Pugh score >9).

Pediatric Patients

CANCIDAS has not been adequately studied in patients under 18 years of age.

MICROBIOLOGY

Mechanism of Action

Caspofungin acetate, the active ingredient of CANCIDAS, inhibits the synthesis of β (1,3)-D-glucan, an essential component of the cell wall of susceptible *Aspergillus* species and *Candida* species. β (1,3)-D-glucan is not present in mammalian cells. Caspofungin has shown activity against *Candida* species and in regions of active cell growth of the hyphae of *Aspergillus fumigatus*.

Activity in vitro

Caspofungin exhibits *in vitro* activity against *Aspergillus* species (*Aspergillus fumigatus, Aspergillus flavus,* and *Aspergillus terreus*) and *Candida* species (*Candida albicans, Candida glabrata, Candida guilliermondii, Candida krusei, Candida parapsilosis,* and *Candida tropicalis*). Susceptibility testing was performed according to the National Committee for Clinical Laboratory Standards (NCCLS) method M38-A (for *Aspergillus* species) and M27-A (for *Candida* species). Standardized susceptibility testing methods for β (1,3)-D-glucan synthesis inhibitors have not been established for yeasts and filamentous fungi, and results of susceptibility studies do not correlate with clinical outcome.

Activity in vivo

Caspofungin was active when parenterally administered to immunocompetent and immunosuppressed mice as long as 24 hours after disseminated infections with *C. albicans*, in which the endpoints were prolonged survival of infected mice and reduction of *C. albicans* from target organs. Caspofungin, administered parenterally to immunocompetent and immunosuppressed rodents, as long as 24 hours after disseminated or pulmonary infection with *Aspergillus fumigatus*, has shown prolonged survival, which has not been consistently associated with a reduction in mycological burden.

Drug Resistance

Mutants of *Candida* with reduced susceptibility to caspofungin have been identified in some patients during treatment. Similar observations were made in a study in mice infected with *C. albicans* and treated with orally administered doses of caspofungin. MIC values for caspofungin should not be used to predict clinical outcome, since a correlation between MIC values and clinical outcome has not been established.

Drug Interactions

Studies *in vitro* and *in vivo* of caspofungin, in combination with amphotericin B, suggest no antagonism of antifungal activity against either *A. fumigatus* or *C. albicans*. The clinical significance of these results is unknown.

CLINICAL STUDIES

Candidemia and the following other Candida infections: intra-abdominal abscesses, peritonitis and pleural space infections

In a Phase III randomized, double-blind study, patients with a proven diagnosis of invasive candidiasis received daily doses of CANCIDAS (50 mg/day following a 70-mg loading dose on Day 1) or amphotericin B deoxycholate (0.6 to 0.7 mg/kg/day for non-neutropenic patients and 0.7 to 1.0 mg/kg/day for neutropenic patients). Patients were stratified by both neutropenic status and APACHE II score. Patients with *Candida* endocarditis, meningitis, or osteomyelitis were excluded from this study.

Patients who met the entry criteria and received one or more doses of IV study therapy were included in the primary (modified intention-to-treat [MITT]) analysis of response at the end of IV study therapy. A favorable response at this time point required both symptom/sign resolution/improvement and microbiological clearance of the *Candida* infection.

Two hundred thirty-nine patients were enrolled. Patient disposition is shown in Table 1.

[See table 1 below]

Of the 239 patients enrolled, 224 met the criteria for inclusion in the MITT population (109 treated with CANCIDAS and 115 treated with amphotericin B). Of these 224 patients, 186 patients had candidemia (92 treated with CANCIDAS and 94 treated with amphotericin B). The majority of the patients with candidemia were non-neutropenic (87%) and had an APACHE II score less than or equal to 20 (77%) in both arms. Most candidemia infections were caused by *C. albicans* (39%), followed by *C. parapsilosis* (20%), *C. tropicalis* (17%), *C. glabrata* (8%), and *C. krusei* (3%).

At the end of the IV study therapy, CANCIDAS was comparable to amphotericin B in the treatment of candidemia in the MITT population. For the other efficacy time points (Day 10 of IV study therapy, end of all antifungal therapy, 2-week post-therapy follow-up, and 6- to 8-week post-therapy follow-up), CANCIDAS was as effective as amphotericin B.

Outcome, relapse and mortality data are shown in Table 2.

[See table 2 at top of next page]

In this study, the efficacy of CANCIDAS in patients with intra-abdominal abscesses, peritonitis and pleural space *Candida* infections was evaluated in 19 non-neutropenic patients. Two of these patients had concurrent candidemia. *Candida* was part of a polymicrobial infection that required adjunctive surgical drainage in 11 of these 19 patients. A favorable response was seen in 9 of 9 patients with peritonitis, 3 of 4 with abscesses (liver, parasplenic, and urinary bladder abscesses), 2 of 2 with pleural space infections, 1 of 2 with mixed peritoneal and pleural infection, 1 of 1 with mixed abdominal abscess and peritonitis, and 0 of 1 with *Candida* pneumonia.

Overall, across all sites of infection included in the study, the efficacy of CANCIDAS was comparable to that of amphotericin B for the primary endpoint.

In this study, the efficacy data for CANCIDAS in neutropenic patients with candidemia were limited. In a separate compassionate use study, 4 patients with hepatosplenic candidiasis received prolonged therapy with CANCIDAS following other long-term antifungal therapy; three of these patients had a favorable response.

Esophageal Candidiasis (and information on oropharyngeal candidiasis)

The safety and efficacy of CANCIDAS in the treatment of esophageal candidiasis was evaluated in one large, controlled, noninferiority, clinical trial and two smaller dose-response studies.

In all 3 studies, patients were required to have symptoms and microbiological documentation of esophageal candidiasis; most patients had advanced AIDS (with CD4 counts <50/mm^3).

Of the 166 patients in the large study who had culture-confirmed esophageal candidiasis at baseline, 120 had *Candida albicans* and 2 had *Candida tropicalis* as the sole baseline pathogen whereas 44 had mixed baseline cultures containing *C. albicans* and one or more additional *Candida* species.

In the large, randomized, double-blind study comparing CANCIDAS 50 mg/day versus intravenous fluconazole 200 mg/day for the treatment of esophageal candidiasis, patients were treated for an average of 9 days (range 7-21 days). The primary endpoint was favorable overall response at 5 to 7 days following discontinuation of study therapy, which required both complete resolution of symptoms and significant endoscopic improvement. The definition of endoscopic response was based on severity of disease at baseline using a 4-grade scale and required at least a two-grade reduction from baseline endoscopic score or reduction to grade 0 for patients with a baseline score of 2 or less.

The proportion of patients with a favorable overall response for the primary endpoint was comparable for CANCIDAS and fluconazole as shown in Table 3.

TABLE 1
Disposition in Candidemia and Other *Candida* Infections
(Intra-abdominal abscesses, peritonitis, and pleural space infections)

	CANCIDAS*	Amphotericin B
Randomized patients	114	125
Patients completing study**	63 (55.3%)	69 (55.2%)
DISCONTINUATIONS OF STUDY**		
All Study Discontinuations	51 (44.7%)	56 (44.8%)
Study Discontinuations due to clinical adverse events	39 (34.2%)	43 (34.4%)
Study Discontinuations due to laboratory adverse events	0 (0%)	1 (0.8%)
DISCONTINUATIONS OF STUDY THERAPY		
All Study Therapy Discontinuations	48 (42.1%)	58 (46.4%)
Study Therapy Discontinuations due to clinical adverse events	30 (26.3%)	37 (29.6%)
Study Therapy Discontinuations due to laboratory adverse events	1 (0.9%)	7 (5.6%)
Study Therapy Discontinuations due to all drug-related*** adverse events	3 (2.6%)	29 (23.2%)

*Patients received CANCIDAS 70 mg on Day 1, then 50 mg daily for the remainder of their treatment.
**Study defined as study treatment period and 6-8 week follow-up period.
***Determined by the investigator to be possibly, probably, or definitely drug-related.

[See table 3 at right]

The proportion of patients with a favorable symptom response was also comparable (90.1% and 89.4% for CANCIDAS and fluconazole, respectively). In addition, the proportion of patients with a favorable endoscopic response was comparable (85.2% and 86.2% for CANCIDAS and fluconazole, respectively).

As shown in Table 4, the esophageal candidiasis relapse rates at the Day 14 post-treatment visit were similar for the two groups. At the Day 28 post-treatment visit, the group treated with CANCIDAS had a numerically higher incidence of relapse, however, the difference was not statistically significant.

[See table 4 at top of next page]

In this trial, which was designed to establish noninferiority of CANCIDAS to fluconazole for the treatment of esophageal candidiasis, 122 (70%) patients also had oropharyngeal candidiasis. A favorable response was defined as complete resolution of all symptoms of oropharyngeal disease and all visible oropharyngeal lesions. The proportion of patients with a favorable oropharyngeal response at the 5- to 7-day post-treatment visit was numerically lower for CANCIDAS, however, the difference was not statistically significant. The results are shown in Table 5.

[See table 5 at top of next page]

As shown in Table 6, the oropharyngeal candidiasis relapse rates at the Day 14 and the Day 28 post-treatment visits were statistically significantly higher for CANCIDAS than for fluconazole.

[See table 6 at top of next page]

The results from the two smaller dose-ranging studies corroborate the efficacy of CANCIDAS for esophageal candidiasis that was demonstrated in the larger study.

CANCIDAS was associated with favorable outcomes in 7 of 10 esophageal *C. albicans* infections refractory to at least 200 mg of fluconazole given for 7 days, although the *in vitro* susceptibility of the infecting isolates to fluconazole was not known.

Invasive Aspergillosis

Sixty-nine patients between the ages of 18 and 80 with invasive aspergillosis (IA) were enrolled in an open-label, noncomparative study to evaluate the safety, tolerability, and efficacy of CANCIDAS. Enrolled patients had previously been refractory to or intolerant of other antifungal therapy(ies). Refractory patients were classified as those who had disease progression or failed to improve despite therapy for at least 7 days with amphotericin B, lipid formulations of amphotericin B, itraconazole, or an investigational azole with reported activity against *Aspergillus*. Intolerance to previous therapy was defined as a doubling of creatinine (or creatinine ≥2.5 mg/dL while on therapy), other acute reactions, or infusion-related toxicity. To be included in the study, patients with pulmonary disease must have had definite (positive tissue histopathology or positive culture from tissue obtained by an invasive procedure) or probable (positive radiographic or computed tomography evidence with supporting culture from bronchoalveolar lavage or sputum, galactomannan enzyme-linked immunosorbent assay, and/or polymerase chain reaction) invasive aspergillosis. Patients with extrapulmonary disease had to have definite invasive aspergillosis. The definitions were modeled after the Mycoses Study Group Criteria.[1] Patients were administered a single 70-mg loading dose of CANCIDAS and subsequently dosed with 50 mg daily. The mean duration of therapy was 33.7 days, with a range of 1 to 162 days.

[1] Denning DW, Lee JY, Hostetler JS, et al. NIAID Mycoses Study Group multicenter trial of oral itraconazole therapy for invasive aspergillosis. *Am J Med* 1994; 97:135-144.

An independent expert panel evaluated patient data, including diagnosis of invasive aspergillosis, response and tolerability to previous antifungal therapy, treatment course on CANCIDAS, and clinical outcome.

A favorable response was defined as either complete resolution (complete response) or clinically meaningful improvement (partial response) of all signs and symptoms and attributable radiographic findings. Stable, nonprogressive disease was considered to be an unfavorable response.

Among the 69 patients enrolled in the study, 63 met entry diagnostic criteria and had outcome data; and of these, 52 patients received treatment for >7 days. Fifty-three (84%) were refractory to previous antifungal therapy and 10 (16%) were intolerant. Forty-five patients had pulmonary disease and 18 had extrapulmonary disease. Underlying conditions were hematologic malignancy (N=24), allogeneic bone marrow transplant or stem cell transplant (N=18), organ transplant (N=8), solid tumor (N=3), or other conditions (N=10). All patients in the study received concomitant therapies for their other underlying conditions. Eighteen patients received tacrolimus and CANCIDAS concomitantly, of whom 8 also received mycophenolate mofetil.

Overall, the expert panel determined that 41% (26/63) of patients receiving at least one dose of CANCIDAS had a favorable response. For those patients who received >7 days of therapy with CANCIDAS, 50% (26/52) had a favorable response. The favorable response rates for patients who were either refractory to or intolerant of previous therapies were 36% (19/53) and 70% (7/10), respectively. The response rates among patients with pulmonary disease and extrapulmonary disease were 47% (21/45) and 28% (5/18), respectively. Among patients with extrapulmonary disease, 2 of 8 patients who also had definite, probable, or possible CNS involvement had a favorable response. Two of these 8 patients had progression of disease and manifested CNS involvement while on therapy.

There is substantial evidence that CANCIDAS is well tolerated and effective for the treatment of invasive aspergillosis in patients who are refractory to or intolerant of itraconazole, amphotericin B, and/or lipid formulations of amphotericin B. However, the efficacy of CANCIDAS has not been evaluated in concurrently controlled clinical studies, with other antifungal therapies.

TABLE 2
Outcomes, Relapse, & Mortality in Candidemia and Other *Candida* Infections (Intra-abdominal abscesses, peritonitis, and pleural space infections)

	CANCIDAS*	Amphotericin B	% Difference** after adjusting for strata (Confidence Interval)***
Number of MITT[†] patients	109	115	
FAVORABLE OUTCOMES (MITT) AT THE END OF IV STUDY THERAPY			
All MITT patients	81/109 (74.3%)	78/115 (67.8%)	7.5 (-5.4, 20.3)
Candidemia	67/92 (72.8%)	63/94 (67%)	7.0 (-7.0, 21.1)
Neutropenic	6/14 (43%)	5/10 (50%)	
Non-neutropenic	61/78 (78%)	58/84 (69%)	
Endophthalmitis	0/1	2/3	
Multiple Sites	4/5	4/4	
Blood / Pleural	1/1	1/1	
Blood / Peritoneal	1/1	1/1	
Blood / Urine	–	1/1	
Peritoneal / Pleural	½	–	
Abdominal / Peritoneal	–	1/1	
Subphrenic / Peritoneal	1/1		
DISSEMINATED INFECTIONS, RELAPSES AND MORTALITY			
Disseminated Infections in neutropenic patients	4/14 (28.6%)	3/10 (30%)	
All relapses[††]	7/81 (8.6%)	8/78 (10.3%)	
Culture-confirmed relapse	5/81 (6%)	2/78 (3%)	
Overall study[†††] mortality in MITT	36/109 (33.0%)	35/115 (30.4%)	
Mortality during study therapy	18/109 (17%)	13/115 (11%)	
Mortality attributed to *Candida*	4/109 (4%)	7/115 (6%)	

*Patients received CANCIDAS 70 mg on Day 1, then 50 mg daily for the remainder of their treatment.
**Calculated as CANCIDAS – amphotericin B
***95% CI for candidemia, 95.6% for all patients
[†]Modified intention-to-treat
[††]Includes all patients who either developed a culture-confirmed recurrence of *Candida* infection or required antifungal therapy for the treatment of a proven or suspected *Candida* infection in the follow-up period.
[†††]Study defined as study treatment period and 6-8 week follow-up period.

TABLE 3
Favorable Response Rates for Patients with Esophageal Candidiasis

	CANCIDAS	Fluconazole	% Difference* (95% CI)
Day 5-7 post-treatment	66/81 (81.5%)	80/94 (85.1%)	-3.6 (-14.7, 7.5)

*calculated as CANCIDAS – fluconazole

INDICATIONS AND USAGE

CANCIDAS is indicated for the treatment of:

- Candidemia and the following *Candida* infections: intra-abdominal abscesses, peritonitis and pleural space infections. CANCIDAS has not been studied in endocarditis, osteomyelitis, and meningitis due to *Candida*.
- Esophageal Candidiasis (see CLINICAL STUDIES).
- Invasive Aspergillosis in patients who are refractory to or intolerant of other therapies (i.e., amphotericin B, lipid formulations of amphotericin B, and/or itraconazole). CANCIDAS has not been studied as initial therapy for invasive aspergillosis.

CONTRAINDICATIONS

CANCIDAS is contraindicated in patients with hypersensitivity to any component of this product.

WARNINGS

Concomitant use of CANCIDAS with cyclosporine is not recommended unless the potential benefit outweighs the potential risk to the patient. In one clinical study, 3 of 4 healthy subjects who received CANCIDAS 70 mg on Days 1 through 10, and also received two 3 mg/kg doses of cyclosporine 12 hours apart on Day 10, developed transient elevations of alanine transaminase (ALT) on Day 11 that were 2 to 3 times the upper limit of normal (ULN). In a separate panel of subjects in the same study, 2 of 8 who received CANCIDAS 35 mg daily for 3 days and cyclosporine (two 3 mg/kg doses administered 12 hours apart) on Day 1 had small increases in ALT (slightly above the ULN) on Day 2. In both groups, elevations in aspartate transaminase (AST) paralleled ALT elevations, but were of lesser magnitude (see ADVERSE REACTIONS). Hence, concomitant use of CANCIDAS with cyclosporine is not recommended until multiple-dose use in patients is studied.

PRECAUTIONS

General

The efficacy of a 70-mg dose regimen in patients with invasive aspergillosis who are not clinically responding to the 50 mg daily dose is not known. Limited safety data suggest that an increase in dose to 70 mg daily is well tolerated. For candidiasis, see CLINICAL STUDIES. The safety and efficacy of doses above 70 mg have not been adequately studied in patients. However, CANCIDAS was generally well tolerated at a dose of 100 mg once daily for 21 days when administered to 15 healthy subjects.

The safety information on treatment durations longer than 2 weeks is limited, however, available data suggest that CANCIDAS continues to be well tolerated with longer courses of therapy (112 patients received from 15 to 60 days of therapy; 14 patients received from 61 to 162 days of therapy).

Drug Interactions

Studies *in vitro* show that caspofungin acetate is not an inhibitor of any enzyme in the cytochrome P450 (CYP) system. In clinical studies, caspofungin did not induce the CYP3A4 metabolism of other drugs. Caspofungin is not a substrate for P-glycoprotein and is a poor substrate for cytochrome P450 enzymes.

Clinical studies in healthy volunteers show that the pharmacokinetics of CANCIDAS are not altered by itraconazole, amphotericin B, mycophenolate, nelfinavir, or tacrolimus. CANCIDAS has no effect on the pharmacokinetics of itraconazole, amphotericin B, or the active metabolite of mycophenolate.

CANCIDAS reduced the blood AUC_{0-12} of tacrolimus (FK-506, Prograf®[2]) by approximately 20%, peak blood concentration (C_{max}) by 16%, and 12-hour blood concentration (C_{12hr}) by 26% in healthy subjects when tacrolimus (2 doses of 0.1 mg/kg 12 hours apart) was administered on the 10th day of CANCIDAS 70 mg daily, as compared to results from a control period in which tacrolimus was administered

Continued on next page

Information on the Merck & Co., Inc., products listed on these pages is from the prescribing information in use October 1, 2004. For information, please call 1-800-NSC-MERCK [1-800-672-6372].

Cancidas—Cont.

alone. For patients receiving both therapies, standard monitoring of tacrolimus blood concentrations and appropriate tacrolimus dosage adjustments are recommended.

[2] Registered trademark of Fujisawa Healthcare, Inc.

In two clinical studies, cyclosporine (one 4 mg/kg dose or two 3 mg/kg doses) increased the AUC of caspofungin by approximately 35%. CANCIDAS did not increase the plasma levels of cyclosporine. There were transient increases in liver ALT and AST when CANCIDAS and cyclosporine were coadministered (see WARNINGS and ADVERSE REACTIONS).

A drug-drug interaction study with rifampin in healthy volunteers has shown a 30% decrease in caspofungin trough concentrations. Patients on rifampin should receive 70 mg of CANCIDAS daily. In addition, results from regression analyses of patient pharmacokinetic data suggest that coadministration of other inducers of drug clearance (efavirenz, nevirapine, phenytoin, dexamethasone, or carbamazepine) with CANCIDAS may result in clinically meaningful reductions in caspofungin concentrations. It is not known which drug clearance mechanism involved in caspofungin disposition may be inducible. When CANCIDAS is co-administered with inducers of drug clearance, such as efavirenz, nevirapine, phenytoin, dexamethasone, or carbamazepine, use of a daily dose of 70 mg of CANCIDAS should be considered.

Carcinogenesis, Mutagenesis, and Impairment of Fertility

No long-term studies in animals have been performed to evaluate the carcinogenic potential of caspofungin.

Caspofungin did not show evidence of mutagenic or genotoxic potential when evaluated in the following *in vitro* assays: bacterial (Ames) and mammalian cell (V79 Chinese hamster lung fibroblasts) mutagenesis assays, the alkaline elution/rat hepatocyte DNA strand break test, and the chromosome aberration assay in Chinese hamster ovary cells. Caspofungin was not genotoxic when assessed in the mouse bone marrow chromosomal test at doses up to 12.5 mg/kg (equivalent to a human dose of 1 mg/kg based on body surface area comparisons), administered intravenously.

Fertility and reproductive performance were not affected by the intravenous administration of caspofungin to rats at doses up to 5 mg/kg. At 5 mg/kg exposures were similar to those seen in patients treated with the 70-mg dose.

Pregnancy

Pregnancy Category C. CANCIDAS was shown to be embryotoxic in rats and rabbits. Findings included incomplete ossification of the skull and torso and an increased incidence of cervical rib in rats. An increased incidence of incomplete ossifications of the talus/calcaneus was seen in rabbits. Caspofungin also produced increases in resorptions in rats and rabbits and periimplantation losses in rats. These findings were observed at doses which produced exposures similar to those seen in patients treated with a 70-mg dose. Caspofungin crossed the placental barrier in rats and rabbits and was detected in the plasma of fetuses of pregnant animals dosed with CANCIDAS. There are no adequate and well-controlled studies in pregnant women. CANCIDAS should be used during pregnancy only if the potential benefit justifies the potential risk to the fetus.

Nursing Mothers

Caspofungin was found in the milk of lactating, drug-treated rats. It is not known whether caspofungin is excreted in human milk. Because many drugs are excreted in human milk, caution should be exercised when caspofungin is administered to a nursing woman.

Patients with Hepatic Insufficiency

Patients with mild hepatic insufficiency (Child-Pugh score 5 to 6) do not need a dosage adjustment. For patients with moderate hepatic insufficiency (Child-Pugh score 7 to 9), CANCIDAS 35 mg daily is recommended. However, where recommended, a 70-mg loading dose should still be administered on Day 1 (see DOSAGE AND ADMINISTRATION). There is no clinical experience in patients with severe hepatic insufficiency (Child-Pugh score >9).

Pediatric Use

Safety and effectiveness in pediatric patients have not been established.

Geriatric Use

Clinical studies of CANCIDAS did not include sufficient numbers of patients aged 65 and over to determine whether they respond differently from younger patients. Although the number of elderly patients was not large enough for a statistical analysis, no overall differences in safety or efficacy were observed between these and younger patients. Plasma concentrations of caspofungin in healthy older men and women (≥65 years of age) were increased slightly (approximately 28% in AUC) compared to young healthy men. A similar effect of age on pharmacokinetics was seen in patients with candidemia or other *Candida* infections (intra-abdominal abscesses, peritonitis, or pleural space infections). No dose adjustment is recommended for the elderly; however, greater sensitivity of some older individuals cannot be ruled out.

ADVERSE REACTIONS

General

Possible histamine-mediated symptoms have been reported including reports of rash, facial swelling, pruritus, sensation of warmth, or bronchospasm. Anaphylaxis has been reported during administration of CANCIDAS.

TABLE 4
Relapse Rates at 14 and 28 Days Post-Therapy in Patients with Esophageal Candidiasis at Baseline

	CANCIDAS	Fluconazole	% Difference* (95% CI)
Day 14 post-treatment	7/66 (10.6%)	6/76 (7.9%)	2.7 (-6.9, 12.3)
Day 28 post-treatment	18/64 (28.1%)	12/72 (16.7%)	11.5 (-2.5, 25.4)

*calculated as CANCIDAS – fluconazole

TABLE 5
Oropharyngeal Candidiasis Response Rates at 5 to 7 Days Post-Therapy in Patients with Oropharyngeal and Esophageal Candidiasis at Baseline

	CANCIDAS	Fluconazole	% Difference* (95% CI)
Day 5-7 post-treatment	40/56 (71.4%)	55/66 (83.3%)	-11.9 (-26.8, 3.0)

*calculated as CANCIDAS – fluconazole

TABLE 6
Oropharyngeal Candidiasis Relapse Rates at 14 and 28 Days Post-Therapy in Patients with Oropharyngeal and Esophageal Candidiasis at Baseline

	CANCIDAS	Fluconazole	% Difference* (95% CI)
Day 14 post-treatment	17/40 (42.5%)	7/53 (13.2%)	29.3 (11.5, 47.1)
Day 28 post-treatment	23/39 (59.0%)	18/51 (35.3%)	23.7 (3.4, 43.9)

*calculated as CANCIDAS – fluconazole

Clinical Adverse Experiences

The overall safety of caspofungin was assessed in 876 individuals who received single or multiple doses of caspofungin acetate. There were 125 patients with candidemia and/or intra-abdominal abscesses, peritonitis, or pleural space infections, including 4 patients with chronic disseminated candidiasis; 285 patients with esophageal and/or oropharyngeal candidiasis; and 72 patients with invasive aspergillosis enrolled in phase II and phase III clinical studies. The remaining 394 individuals were enrolled in phase I studies. The majority of the patients with *Candida* infections had serious underlying medical conditions (e.g., hematologic or other malignancy, recent major surgery, HIV) requiring multiple concomitant medications. Patients in the noncomparative *Aspergillus* study often had serious predisposing medical conditions (e.g., bone marrow or peripheral stem cell transplants, hematologic malignancy, solid tumors or organ transplants) requiring multiple concomitant medications.

In the randomized, double-blinded invasive candidiasis study, patients received either CANCIDAS 50 mg/day (following a 70-mg loading dose) or amphotericin B 0.6 to 1.0 mg/kg/day. Drug-related clinical adverse experiences occurring in ≥2% of the patients in either treatment group are presented in Table 7.

TABLE 7
Drug-Related* Clinical Adverse Experiences Among Patients with Candidemia or other *Candida* Infections**
Incidence ≥2% for at least one treatment group by Body System

	CANCIDAS 50 mg*** N=114 (percent)	Amphotericin B N=125 (percent)
Body as a Whole		
Chills	5.3	26.4
Fever	7.0	23.2
Cardiovascular System		
Hypertension	1.8	6.4
Hypotension	0.9	2.4
Tachycardia	1.8	10.4
Peripheral Vascular System		
Phlebitis/thrombophlebitis	3.5	4.8
Digestive System		
Diarrhea	2.6	0.8
Jaundice	0.9	3.2
Nausea	1.8	5.6
Vomiting	3.5	8.0
Metabolic/Nutritional/Immune		
Hypokalemia	0.9	5.6
Nervous System & Psychiatric		
Tremor	1.8	2.4
Respiratory System		
Tachypnea	0.0	10.4
Skin & Skin Appendage		
Erythema	0.0	2.4
Rash	0.9	3.2
Sweating	0.9	3.2
Urogenital System		
Renal insufficiency	0.9	5.6
Renal insufficiency, acute	0.0	5.6

*Determined by the investigator to be possibly, probably, or definitely drug-related.
**Intra-abdominal abscesses, peritonitis and pleural space infections
***Patients received CANCIDAS 70 mg on Day 1, then 50 mg daily for the remainder of their treatment.

The incidence of drug-related clinical adverse experiences was significantly lower among patients treated with CANCIDAS (28.9%) than among patients treated with amphotericin B (58.4%). Also, the proportion of patients who experienced an infusion-related adverse event was significantly lower in the group treated with CANCIDAS (20.2%) than in the group treated with amphotericin B (48.8%).

Drug-related laboratory adverse experiences occurring in ≥2% of the patients in either treatment group are presented in Table 8.

TABLE 8
Drug-Related* Laboratory Adverse Experiences Among Patients with Candidemia or other *Candida* Infections**
Incidence ≥2% for at least one treatment group by Laboratory Test Category

	CANCIDAS 50 mg*** N=114 (percent)	Amphotericin B N=125 (percent)
Blood Chemistry		
ALT increased	3.7	8.1
AST increased	1.9	9.0
Blood urea increased	1.9	15.8
Direct serum bilirubin increased	3.8	8.4
Serum alkaline phosphatase increased	8.3	15.6
Serum bicarbonate decreased	0.0	3.6
Serum creatinine increased	3.7	22.6
Serum phosphate increased	0.0	2.7
Serum potassium decreased	9.9	23.4
Serum potassium increased	0.9	2.4
Total serum bilirubin increased	2.8	8.9
Hematology		
Hematocrit decreased	0.9	7.3
Hemoglobin decreased	0.9	10.5
Urinalysis		
Urine protein increased	0.0	3.7

*Determined by the investigator to be possibly, probably, or definitely drug-related.
**Intra-abdominal abscesses, peritonitis and pleural space infections
***Patients received CANCIDAS 70 mg on Day 1, then 50 mg daily for the remainder of their treatment.

The incidence of drug-related laboratory adverse experiences was signficantly lower among patients receiving CANCIDAS (24.3%) than among patients receiving amphotericin B (54.0%).

The percentage of patients with either a drug-related clinical adverse experience or a drug-related laboratory adverse experience was significantly lower among patients receiving CANCIDAS (42.1%) than among patients receiving amphotericin B (75.2%). Furthermore, a significant difference between the two treatment groups was observed with regard to incidence of discontinuation due to drug-related clinical or laboratory adverse experience; incidences were 3/114 (2.6%) in the group treated with CANCIDAS and 29/125 (23.2%) in the group treated with amphotericin B.

To evaluate the effect of CANCIDAS and amphotericin B on renal function, nephrotoxicity was defined as doubling of serum creatinine relative to baseline or an increase of

TABLE 9
Drug-Related Clinical Adverse Experiences Among Patients with Esophageal and/or Oropharyngeal Candidiasis*
Incidence ≥2% for at least one treatment dose (per comparison) by Body System

	CANCIDAS 50 mg** N=83 (percent)	Fluconazole IV 200 mg** N=94 (percent)	CANCIDAS 50 mg*** N=80 (percent)	CANCIDAS 70 mg*** N=65 (percent)	Amphotericin B 0.5 mg/kg*** N=89 (percent)
Body as a Whole					
Asthenia/fatigue	0.0	0.0	0.0	0.0	6.7
Chills	0.0	0.0	2.5	1.5	75.3
Edema/swelling	0.0	0.0	0.0	0.0	5.6
Edema, facial	0.0	0.0	0.0	3.1	0.0
Fever	3.6	1.1	21.3	26.2	69.7
Flu-like illness	0.0	0.0	0.0	3.1	0.0
Malaise	0.0	0.0	0.0	0.0	5.6
Pain	0.0	0.0	1.3	4.6	5.6
Pain, abdominal	3.6	2.1	2.5	0.0	9.0
Warm sensation	0.0	0.0	0.0	1.5	4.5
Peripheral Vascular System					
Infused vein complication	12.0	8.5	2.5	1.5	0.0
Phlebitis/thrombophlebitis	15.7	8.5	11.3	13.8	22.5
Cardiovascular System					
Tachycardia	0.0	0.0	1.3	0.0	4.5
Vasculitis	0.0	0.0	0.0	0.0	3.4
Digestive System					
Anorexia	0.0	0.0	1.3	0.0	3.4
Diarrhea	3.6	2.1	1.3	3.1	11.2
Gastritis	0.0	2.1	0.0	0.0	0.0
Nausea	6.0	6.4	2.5	3.1	21.3
Vomiting	1.2	3.2	1.3	3.1	13.5
Hemic & Lymphatic System					
Anemia	0.0	0.0	3.8	0.0	9.0
Metabolic/Nutritional/ Immune					
Anaphylaxis	0.0	0.0	0.0	0.0	2.2
Musculoskeletal System					
Myalgia	1.2	0.0	0.0	3.1	2.2
Pain, back	0.0	0.0	0.0	0.0	2.2
Pain, musculoskeletal	0.0	0.0	1.3	0.0	4.5
Nervous System & Psychiatric					
Dizziness	0.0	2.1	0.0	1.5	1.1
Headache	6.0	1.1	11.3	7.7	19.1
Insomnia	1.2	0.0	0.0	0.0	2.2
Paresthesia	0.0	0.0	1.3	3.1	1.1
Tremor	0.0	0.0	0.0	0.0	7.9
Respiratory System					
Tachypnea	0.0	0.0	1.3	0.0	4.5
Skin & Skin Appendage					
Erythema	1.2	0.0	1.3	1.5	7.9
Induration	0.0	0.0	0.0	3.1	6.7
Pruritus	1.2	0.0	2.5	1.5	0.0
Rash	0.0	0.0	1.3	4.6	3.4
Sweating	0.0	0.0	1.3	0.0	3.4

*Relationship to drug was determined by the investigator to be possibly, probably or definitely drug-related.
**Derived from a Phase III comparator-controlled clinical study.
***Derived from Phase II comparator-controlled clinical studies.

TABLE 10
Drug-Related Laboratory Abnormalities Reported Among Patients with Esophageal and/or Oropharyngeal Candidiasis*
Incidence ≥2% (for at least one treatment dose) by Laboratory Test Category

	CANCIDAS 50 mg** N=163 (percent)	CANCIDAS 70 mg*** N=65 (percent)	Fluconazole IV 200 mg** N=94 (percent)	Amphotericin B 0.5 mg/kg*** N=89 (percent)
Blood Chemistry				
ALT increased	10.6	10.8	11.8	22.7
AST increased	13.0	10.8	12.9	22.7
Blood urea increased	0.0	0.0	1.2	10.3
Direct serum bilirubin increased	0.6	0.0	3.3	2.5
Serum albumin decreased	8.6	4.6	5.4	14.9
Serum alkaline phosphatase increased	10.5	7.7	11.8	19.3
Serum bicarbonate decreased	0.9	0.0	0.0	6.6
Serum calcium decreased	1.9	0.0	3.2	1.1
Serum creatinine increased	0.0	1.5	2.2	28.1
Serum potassium decreased	3.7	10.8	4.3	31.5
Serum potassium increased	0.6	0.0	2.2	1.1
Serum sodium decreased	1.9	1.5	3.2	1.1
Serum uric acid increased	0.6	0.0	0.0	3.4
Total serum bilirubin increased	0.0	0.0	3.2	4.5
Total serum protein decreased	3.1	0.0	3.2	3.4

(Table continued on next page)

≥1 mg/dL in serum creatinine if baseline serum creatinine was above the upper limit of the normal range. In a subgroup of patients whose baseline creatinine clearance was >30 mL/min, the incidence of nephrotoxicity was significantly lower in the group treated with CANCIDAS than in the group treated with amphotericin B.

Drug-related clinical adverse experiences occurring in ≥2% of patients with esophageal and/or oropharyngeal candidiasis are presented in Table 9.

[See table 9 above]

Laboratory abnormalities occurring in ≥2% of patients with esophageal and/or oropharyngeal candidiasis are presented in Table 10.

[See table 10 above and on next page]

In the open-label, noncomparative aspergillosis study, in which 69 patients received CANCIDAS (70-mg loading dose on Day 1 followed by 50 mg daily), the following drug-related clinical adverse experiences were observed with an incidence of ≥2%; fever (2.9%), infused-vein complications (2.9%), nausea (2.9%), vomiting (2.9%) and flushing (2.9%). Also reported infrequently in this patient population were pulmonary edema, ARDS, and radiographic infiltrates.

Drug-related laboratory abnormalities reported with an incidence ≥2% in patients treated with CANCIDAS in the noncomparative aspergillosis study were: serum alkaline phosphatase increased (2.9%), serum potassium decreased (2.9%), eosinophils increased (3.2%), urine protein increased (4.9%), and urine RBCs increased (2.2%).

Post Marketing Experience:

The following postmarketing adverse events have been reported:

Hepatobiliary: Rare cases of clinically significant hepatic dysfunction

Cardiovascular: swelling and peripheral edema

Metabolic: hypercalcemia

Concomitant Therapy

OVERDOSAGE

In clinical studies the highest dose was 210 mg, administered as a single dose to 6 healthy subjects. This dose was generally well tolerated. In addition, 100 mg once daily for 21 days has been administered to 15 healthy subjects and was generally well tolerated. Caspofungin is not dialyzable. The minimum lethal dose of caspofungin in rats was 50 mg/kg, a dose which is equivalent to 10 times the recommended daily dose based on relative body surface area comparison.

ANIMAL PHARMACOLOGY AND TOXICOLOGY

In one 5-week study in monkeys at doses which produced exposures approximately 4 to 6 times those seen in patients treated with a 70-mg dose, scattered small foci of subcapsular necrosis were observed microscopically in the livers of some animals (2/8 monkeys at 5 mg/kg and 4/8 monkeys at 8 mg/kg); however, this histopathological finding was not seen in another study of 27 weeks duration at similar doses.

DOSAGE AND ADMINISTRATION

Do not mix or co-infuse CANCIDAS with other medications, as there are no data available on the compatibility of CANCIDAS with other intravenous substances, additives, or medications. DO NOT USE DILUENTS CONTAINING DEXTROSE (α-D-GLUCOSE), as CANCIDAS is not stable in diluents containing dextrose.

Candidemia and other Candida infections (see CLINICAL STUDIES)

A single 70-mg loading dose should be administered on Day 1, followed by 50 mg daily thereafter. CANCIDAS should be administered by slow IV infusion over approximately 1 hour. Duration of treatment should be dictated by the patient's clinical and microbiological response. In general, antifungal therapy should continue for at least 14 days after the last positive culture. Patients who remain persistently neutropenic may warrant a longer course of therapy pending resolution of the neutropenia.

Esophageal Candidiasis

50 mg daily should be administered by slow IV infusion over approximately 1 hour. Because of the risk of relapse of oropharyngeal candidiasis in patients with HIV infections, suppressive oral therapy could be considered (see CLINICAL STUDIES). A 70-mg loading dose has not been studied with this indication.

Invasive Aspergillosis

A single 70-mg loading dose should be administered on Day 1, followed by 50 mg daily thereafter. CANCIDAS should be administered by slow IV infusion over approximately 1 hour. Duration of treatment should be based upon the severity of the patient's underlying disease, recovery from immunosuppression, and clinical response. The efficacy of a 70-mg dose regimen in patients who are not clinically responding to the 50-mg daily dose is not known. Limited safety data suggests that an increase in dose to 70 mg daily is well tolerated. The safety and efficacy of doses above 70 mg have not been adequately studied.

Hepatic Insufficiency

Patients with mild hepatic insufficiency (Child-Pugh score 5 to 6) do not need a dosage adjustment. For patients with moderate hepatic insufficiency (Child-Pugh score 7 to 9), CANCIDAS 35 mg daily is recommended. However, where recommended, a 70-mg loading dose should still be administered on Day 1. There is no clinical experience in patients with severe hepatic insufficiency (Child-Pugh score >9).

Concomitant Medication with Inducers of Drug Clearance

Patients on rifampin should receive 70 mg of CANCIDAS daily. Patients on nevirapine, efavirenz, carbamazepine, dexamethasone, or phenytoin may require an increase in dose to 70 mg of CANCIDAS daily (see PRECAUTIONS, *Drug Interactions*).

Preparation of CANCIDAS for use:

Do not mix or co-infuse CANCIDAS with other medications, as there are no data available on the compatibility of CANCIDAS with other intravenous substances, additives, or medications. DO NOT USE DILUENTS CONTAINING DEXTROSE (α-D-GLUCOSE), as CANCIDAS is not stable in diluents containing dextrose.

Preparation of the 70-mg infusion

1. Equilibrate the refrigerated vial of CANCIDAS to room temperature.
2. Aseptically add 10.5 mL of 0.9% Sodium Chloride Injection, Sterile Water for Injection, Bacteriostatic Water for In-

Continued on next page

Information on the Merck & Co., Inc., products listed on these pages is from the prescribing information in use October 1, 2004. For information, please call 1-800-NSC-MERCK [1-800-672-6372].

TABLE 10 *(cont.)*
Drug-Related Laboratory Abnormalities Reported Among Patients with Esophageal and/or Oropharyngeal Candidiasis*
Incidence ≥2% (for at least one treatment dose) by Laboratory Test Category

	CANCIDAS 50 mg** N=163 (percent)	CANCIDAS 70 mg*** N=65 (percent)	Fluconazole IV 200 mg** N=94 (percent)	Amphotericin B 0.5 mg/kg*** N=89 (percent)
Hematology				
Eosinophils increased	3.1	3.1	1.1	1.1
Hematocrit decreased	11.1	1.5	5.4	32.6
Hemoglobin decreased	12.3	3.1	5.4	37.1
Lymphocytes increased	0.0	1.6	2.2	0.0
Neutrophils decreased	1.9	3.1	3.2	1.1
Platelet count decreased	3.1	1.5	2.2	3.4
Prothrombin time increased	1.3	1.5	0.0	2.3
WBC count decreased	6.2	4.6	8.6	7.9
Urinalysis				
Urine blood increased	0.0	0.0	0.0	4.0
Urine casts increased	0.0	0.0	0.0	8.0
Urine pH increased	0.8	0.0	0.0	3.6
Urine protein increased	1.2	0.0	3.3	4.5
Urine RBCs increased	1.1	3.8	5.1	12.0
Urine WBCs increased	0.0	7.7	0.0	24.0

*Relationship to drug was determined by the investigator to be possibly, probably or definitely drug-related.
**Derived from Phase II and Phase III comparator-controlled clinical studies.
***Derived from Phase II comparator-controlled clinical studies.

TABLE 11
CANCIDAS Concentrations

Dose	Reconstituted Solution Concentration	Infusion Volume	Infusion Solution Concentration
70-mg initial dose	7.2 mg/mL	260 mL	0.28 mg/mL
50-mg daily dose	5.2 mg/mL	260 mL	0.20 mg/mL
70-mg initial dose* (from two 50 mg vials)	5.2 mg/mL	264 mL	0.28 mg/mL
50-mg daily dose* (reduced volume)	5.2 mg/mL	110 mL	0.47 mg/mL
35-mg daily dose* (from one 50 mg vial) for Moderate Hepatic Insufficiency	5.2 mg/mL or 5.2 mg/mL	257 mL or 107 mL	0.14 mg/mL or 0.34 mg/mL

*See preceding text for these special situations.

Cancidas—Cont.

jection with methylparaben and propylparaben, or Bacteriostatic Water for Injection with 0.9% benzyl alcohol to the vial.[a] This reconstituted solution may be stored for up to one hour at ≤25°C (≤77°F).[b]

3. Aseptically transfer 10 mL[c] of reconstituted CANCIDAS to an IV bag (or bottle) containing 250 mL 0.9%, 0.45%, or 0.225% Sodium Chloride Injection, or Lactated Ringer's Injection. This infusion solution must be used within 24 hours if stored at ≤25°C (≤77°F) or within 48 hours if stored refrigerated at 2 to 8°C (36 to 46°F). (If a 70-mg vial is unavailable, see below: *Alternative Infusion Preparation Methods, Preparation of 70-mg Day 1 loading dose from two 50-mg vials.*)

Preparation of the daily 50-mg infusion

1. Equilibrate the refrigerated vial of CANCIDAS to room temperature.
2. Aseptically add 10.5 mL of 0.9% Sodium Chloride Injection, Sterile Water for Injection, Bacteriostatic Water for Injection with methylparaben and propylparaben, or Bacteriostatic Water for Injection with 0.9% benzyl alcohol to the vial.[a] This reconstituted solution may be stored for up to one hour at ≤25°C (≤77°F).[b]
3. Aseptically transfer 10 mL[c] of reconstituted CANCIDAS to an IV bag (or bottle) containing 250 mL 0.9%, 0.45%, or 0.225% Sodium Chloride Injection, or Lactated Ringer's Injection. This infusion solution must be used within 24 hours if stored at ≤25°C (≤77°F) or within 48 hours if stored refrigerated at 2 to 8°C (36 to 46°F). (If a reduced infusion volume is medically necessary, see below: *Alternative Infusion Preparation Methods, Preparation of 50-mg daily doses at reduced volume.*)

Alternative Infusion Preparation Methods

Preparation of 70-mg dose from two 50-mg vials

Reconstitute two 50-mg vials with 10.5 mL of diluent each (see *Preparation of the daily 50-mg infusion*). Aseptically transfer a total of 14 mL of the reconstituted CANCIDAS from the two vials to 250 mL of 0.9%, 0.45%, or 0.225% Sodium Chloride Injection, or Lactated Ringer's Injection.

Preparation of 50-mg daily doses at reduced volume

When medically necessary, the 50-mg daily doses can be prepared by adding 10 mL of reconstituted CANCIDAS to 100 mL of 0.9%, 0.45%, or 0.225% Sodium Chloride Injection, or Lactated Ringer's Injection (see *Preparation of the daily 50-mg infusion*).

Preparation of a 35-mg daily dose for patients with moderate Hepatic Insufficiency

Reconstitute one 50-mg vial (see above: *Preparation of the daily 50-mg infusion*). Aseptically transfer 7 mL of the reconstituted CANCIDAS from the vial to 250 mL or, if medically necessary, to 100 mL of 0.9%, 0.45%, or 0.225% Sodium Chloride Injection or Lactated Ringer's Injection.

Preparation notes:
[a]The white to off-white cake will dissolve completely. Mix gently until a clear solution is obtained.
[b]Visually inspect the reconstituted solution for particulate matter or discoloration during reconstitution and prior to infusion. Do not use if the solution is cloudy or has precipitated.
[c]CANCIDAS is formulated to provide the full labeled vial dose (70 mg or 50 mg) when 10 mL is withdrawn from the vial.

[See table 11 above]

HOW SUPPLIED

No. 3822 — CANCIDAS 50 mg is a white to off-white powder/cake for infusion in a vial labeled with a red aluminum band and a plastic cap.
NDC 0006-3822-10 one single-use vial.
No. 3823 — CANCIDAS 70 mg is a white to off-white powder/cake for infusion in a vial with a yellow/orange aluminum band and a plastic cap.
NDC 0006-3823-10 one single-use vial.

Storage

Vials

The lyophilized vials should be stored refrigerated at 2° to 8°C (36° to 46°F).

Reconstituted Concentrate

Reconstituted CANCIDAS may be stored at ≤25°C(≤77°F) for one hour prior to the preparation of the patient infusion solution.

Diluted Product

The final patient infusion solution in the IV bag or bottle can be stored at ≤25°C(≤77°F) for 24 hours or at 2 to 8°C (36 to 46°F) for 48 hours.

9344304 Issued March 2004

CLINORIL® Tablets ℞
(Sulindac)

DESCRIPTION

Sulindac is a non-steroidal, anti-inflammatory indene derivative designated chemically as (Z)- 5-fluoro-2-methyl - 1 - [[*p* - (methylsulfinyl) phenyl]methylene]-1*H*-indene-3-acetic acid. It is not a salicylate, pyrazolone or propionic acid derivative. Its empirical formula is $C_{20}H_{17}FO_3S$, with a molecular weight of 356.42. Sulindac, a yellow crystalline compound, is a weak organic acid practically insoluble in water below pH 4.5, but very soluble as the sodium salt or in buffers of pH 6 or higher.

CLINORIL* (Sulindac) is available in 150 and 200 mg tablets for oral administration. Each tablet contains the following inactive ingredients: cellulose, magnesium stearate, starch.

Following absorption, sulindac undergoes two major biotransformations—reversible reduction to the sulfide metabolite, and irreversible oxidation to the sulfone metabolite. Available evidence indicates that the biological activity resides with the sulfide metabolite.

The structural formulas of sulindac and its metabolites are:

(sulfide)

SULINDAC (sulfoxide)

(sulfone)

*Registered trademark of MERCK & CO., INC.

CLINICAL PHARMACOLOGY

CLINORIL is a non-steroidal anti-inflammatory drug, also possessing analgesic and antipyretic activities. Its mode of action, like that of other non-steroidal anti-inflammatory agents, is not known; however, its therapeutic action is not due to pituitary-adrenal stimulation. Inhibition of prostaglandin synthesis by the sulfide metabolite may be involved in the anti-inflammatory action of CLINORIL.

Sulindac is approximately 90% absorbed in man after oral administration. The peak plasma concentrations of the biologically active sulfide metabolite are achieved in about two hours when sulindac is administered in the fasting state, and in about three to four hours when sulindac is administered with food. The mean half-life of sulindac is 7.8 hours while the mean half-life of the sulfide metabolite is 16.4 hours. Sustained plasma levels of the sulfide metabolite are consistent with a prolonged anti-inflammatory action which is the rationale for a twice per day dosage schedule.

Sulindac and its sulfone metabolite undergo extensive enterohepatic circulation relative to the sulfide metabolite in animals. Studies in man have also demonstrated that recirculation of the parent drug, sulindac, and its sulfone metabolite, is more extensive than that of the active sulfide metabolite. The active sulfide metabolite accounts for less than six percent of the total intestinal exposure to sulindac and its metabolites.

The primary route of excretion in man is via the urine as both sulindac and its sulfone metabolite (free and glucuronide conjugates). Approximately 50% of the administered dose is excreted in the urine, with the conjugated sulfone metabolite accounting for the major portion. Less than 1% of the administered dose of sulindac appears in the urine as the sulfide metabolite. Approximately 25% is found in the feces, primarily as the sulfone and sulfide metabolites.

The bioavailability of sulindac, as assessed by urinary excretion, was not changed by concomitant administration of an antacid containing magnesium hydroxide 200 mg and aluminum hydroxide 225 mg per 5 mL.

Because CLINORIL is excreted in the urine primarily as biologically inactive forms, it may possibly affect renal function to a lesser extent than other non-steroidal anti-inflammatory drugs, however, renal adverse experiences have been reported with CLINORIL (see ADVERSE REACTIONS). In a study of patients with chronic glomerular disease treated with therapeutic doses of CLINORIL, no effect was demonstrated on renal blood flow, glomerular filtration rate, or urinary excretion of prostaglandin E_2 and the primary metabolite of prostacyclin, 6-keto-PGF$_{1}\alpha$. However, in other studies in healthy volunteers and patients with liver disease, CLINORIL was found to blunt the renal responses to intravenous furosemide, i.e., the diuresis, natriuresis, increments in plasma renin activity and urinary excretion of prostaglandins. These observations may represent a differentiation of the effects of CLINORIL on renal functions based on differences in pathogenesis of the renal prostaglandin dependence associated with differing dose-response relationships of different NSAIDs to the various renal functions influenced by prostaglandins. These observations need further clarification and in the interim, sulindac should be used with caution in patients whose renal function may be impaired (see PRECAUTIONS).

In healthy men, the average fecal blood loss, measured over a two-week period during administration of 400 mg per day of CLINORIL, was similar to that for placebo, and was statistically significantly less than that resulting from 4800 mg per day of aspirin.

In controlled clinical studies CLINORIL was evaluated in the following five conditions:

1. *Osteoarthritis*

In patients with osteoarthritis of the hip and knee, the anti-inflammatory and analgesic activity of CLINORIL was demonstrated by clinical measurements that included: assessments by both patient and investigator of overall response; decrease in disease activity as assessed by both patient and investigator; improvement in ARA Functional Class; relief of night pain; improvement in overall evaluation of pain, including pain on weight bearing and pain on active and passive motion; improvement in joint mobility, range of motion, and functional activities; decreased swelling and tenderness; and decreased duration of stiffness following prolonged inactivity.

In clinical studies in which dosages were adjusted according to patient needs, CLINORIL 200 to 400 mg daily was shown to be comparable in effectiveness to aspirin 2400 to 4800 mg daily. CLINORIL was generally well tolerated, and patients on it had a lower overall incidence of total adverse effects, of milder gastrointestinal reactions, and of tinnitus than did patients on aspirin. (See ADVERSE REACTIONS.)

2. *Rheumatoid Arthritis*

In patients with rheumatoid arthritis, the anti-inflammatory and analgesic activity of CLINORIL was demonstrated by clinical measurements that included: assessments by both patient and investigator of overall response; decrease in disease activity as assessed by both patient and investigator; reduction in overall joint pain; reduction in duration and severity of morning stiffness; reduction in day and night pain; decrease in time required to walk 50 feet; decrease in general pain as measured on a visual analog scale; improvement in the Ritchie articular index; decrease in proximal interphalangeal joint size; improvement in ARA Functional Class; increase in grip strength; reduction in painful joint count and score; reduction in swollen joint count and score; and increased flexion and extension of the wrist.

In clinical studies in which dosages were adjusted according to patient needs, CLINORIL 300 to 400 mg daily was shown to be comparable in effectiveness to aspirin 3600 to 4800 mg daily. CLINORIL was generally well tolerated, and patients on it had a lower overall incidence of total adverse effects, of milder gastrointestinal reactions, and of tinnitus than did patients on aspirin. (See ADVERSE REACTIONS.)

In patients with rheumatoid arthritis, CLINORIL may be used in combination with gold salts at usual dosage levels. In clinical studies, CLINORIL added to the regimen of gold salts usually resulted in additional symptomatic relief but did not alter the course of the underlying disease.

3. *Ankylosing spondylitis*

In patients with ankylosing spondylitis, the anti-inflammatory and analgesic activity of CLINORIL was demonstrated by clinical measurements that included: assessments by both patient and investigator of overall response; decrease in disease activity as assessed by both patient and investigator; improvement in ARA Functional Class; improvement in patient and investigator evaluation of spinal pain, tenderness and/or spasm; reduction in the duration of morning stiffness; increase in the time to onset of fatigue; relief of night pain; increase in chest expansion; and increase in spinal mobility evaluated by fingers-to-floor distance, occiput to wall distance, the Schober Test, and the Wright Modification of the Schober Test. In a clinical study in which dosages were adjusted according to patient need, CLINORIL 200 to 400 mg daily was as effective as indomethacin 75 to 150 mg daily. In a second study, CLINORIL 300 to 400 mg daily was comparable in effectiveness to phenylbutazone 400 to 600 mg daily. CLINORIL was better tolerated than phenylbutazone. (See ADVERSE REACTIONS.)

4. *Acute painful shoulder (Acute subacromial bursitis/supraspinatus tendinitis)*

In patients with acute painful shoulder (acute subacromial bursitis/supraspinatus tendinitis), the anti-inflammatory and analgesic activity of CLINORIL was demonstrated by clinical measurements that included: assessments by both patient and investigator of overall response; relief of night pain, spontaneous pain, and pain on active motion; decrease in local tenderness; and improvement in range of motion measured by abduction, and internal and external rotation. In clinical studies in acute painful shoulder, CLINORIL 300 to 400 mg daily and oxyphenbutazone 400 to 600 mg daily were shown to be equally effective and well tolerated.

5. *Acute gouty arthritis*

In patients with acute gouty arthritis, the anti-inflammatory and analgesic activity of CLINORIL was demonstrated by clinical measurements that included: assessments by both the patient and investigator of overall response; relief of weight-bearing pain; relief of pain at rest and on active and passive motion; decrease in tenderness; reduction in warmth and swelling; increase in range of motion; and improvement in ability to function. In clinical studies, CLINORIL at 400 mg daily and phenylbutazone at 600 mg daily were shown to be equally effective. In these short-term studies in which reduction of dosage was permitted according to response, both drugs were equally well tolerated.

INDICATIONS AND USAGE

CLINORIL is indicated for acute or long-term use in the relief of signs and symptoms of the following:

1. Osteoarthritis
2. Rheumatoid arthritis**
3. Ankylosing spondylitis
4. Acute painful shoulder (Acute subacromial bursitis/supraspinatus tendinitis)
5. Acute gouty arthritis

**The safety and effectiveness of CLINORIL have not been established in rheumatoid arthritis patients who are designated in the American Rheumatism Association classification as Functional Class IV (incapacitated, largely or wholly bedridden, or confined to wheelchair; little or no self-care).

CONTRAINDICATIONS

CLINORIL should not be used in:

Patients who are hypersensitive to this product.

Patients in whom acute asthmatic attacks, urticaria, or rhinitis are precipitated by aspirin or other non-steroidal anti-inflammatory agents.

WARNINGS

Gastrointestinal Effects

Peptic ulceration and gastrointestinal bleeding have been reported in patients receiving CLINORIL. Fatalities have occurred. Gastrointestinal bleeding is associated with higher morbidity and mortality in patients acutely ill with other conditions, the elderly and patients with hemorrhagic disorders. In patients with active gastrointestinal bleeding or an active peptic ulcer, an appropriate ulcer regimen should be instituted, and the physician must weigh the benefits of therapy with CLINORIL against possible hazards, and carefully monitor the patient's progress. When CLINORIL is given to patients with a history of either upper or lower gastrointestinal tract disease, it should be given under close supervision and only after consulting the ADVERSE REACTIONS section.

Risk of GI Ulcerations, Bleeding and Perforation with NSAID Therapy

Serious gastrointestinal toxicity such as bleeding, ulceration, and perforation can occur at any time, with or without warning symptoms, in patients treated chronically with NSAID therapy. Although minor upper gastrointestinal problems, such as dyspepsia, are common, usually developing early in therapy, physicians should remain alert for ulceration and bleeding in patients treated chronically with NSAIDs even in the absence of previous GI tract symptoms. In patients observed in clinical trials of several months to two years duration, symptomatic upper GI ulcers, gross bleeding or perforation appear to occur in approximately 1% of patients treated for 3-6 months, and in about 2-4% of patients treated for one year. Physicians should inform patients about the signs and/or symptoms of serious GI toxicity and what steps to take if they occur.

Studies to date have not identified any subset of patients not at risk of developing peptic ulceration and bleeding. Except for a prior history of serious GI events and other risk factors known to be associated with peptic ulcer disease, such as alcoholism, smoking, etc., no risk factors (e.g., age, sex) have been associated with increased risk. Elderly or debilitated patients seem to tolerate ulceration or bleeding less well than other individuals and most spontaneous reports of fatal GI events are in this population. Studies to date are inconclusive concerning the relative risk of various NSAIDs in causing such reactions. High doses of any NSAID probably carry a greater risk of these reactions, although controlled clinical trials showing this do not exist in most cases. In considering the use of relatively large doses (within the recommended dosage range), sufficient benefit should be anticipated to offset the potential increased risk of GI toxicity.

Hypersensitivity

Rarely, fever and other evidence of hypersensitivity (see ADVERSE REACTIONS) including abnormalities in one or more liver function tests and severe skin reactions have occurred during therapy with CLINORIL. Fatalities have occurred in these patients. Hepatitis, jaundice, or both, with or without fever, may occur usually within the first one to three months of therapy. Determinations of liver function should be considered whenever a patient on therapy with CLINORIL develops unexplained fever, rash or other dermatologic reactions or constitutional symptoms. If unexplained fever or other evidence of hypersensitivity occurs, therapy with CLINORIL should be discontinued. The elevated temperature and abnormalities in liver function caused by CLINORIL characteristically have reverted to normal after discontinuation of therapy. Administration of CLINORIL should not be reinstituted in such patients.

Hepatic Effects

In addition to hypersensitivity reactions involving the liver, in some patients the findings are consistent with those of cholestatic hepatitis. As with other non-steroidal anti-inflammatory drugs, borderline elevations of one or more liver tests without any other signs and symptoms may occur in up to 15% of patients. These abnormalities may progress, may remain essentially unchanged, or may be transient with continued therapy. The SGPT (ALT) test is probably the most sensitive indicator of liver dysfunction. Meaningful (3 times the upper limit of normal) elevations of SGPT or SGOT (AST) occurred in controlled clinical trials in less than 1% of patients. A patient with symptoms and/or signs suggesting liver dysfunction, or in whom an abnormal liver test has occurred, should be evaluated for evidence of the development of more severe hepatic reaction while on therapy with CLINORIL. Although such reactions as described above are rare, if abnormal liver tests persist or worsen, if clinical signs and symptoms consistent with liver disease develop, or if systemic manifestations occur (e.g. eosinophilia, rash, etc.), CLINORIL should be discontinued.

In clinical trials with CLINORIL, the use of doses of 600 mg/ day has been associated with an increased incidence of mild liver test abnormalities (see DOSAGE AND ADMINISTRATION for maximum dosage recommendation).

PRECAUTIONS

General

Non-steroidal anti-inflammatory drugs, including CLINORIL, may mask the usual signs and symptoms of infection. Therefore, the physician must be continually on the alert for this and should use the drug with extra care in the presence of existing infection.

Although CLINORIL has less effect on platelet function and bleeding time than aspirin, it is an inhibitor of platelet function; therefore, patients who may be adversely affected should be carefully observed when CLINORIL is administered.

Pancreatitis has been reported in patients receiving CLINORIL (see ADVERSE REACTIONS). Should pancreatitis be suspected, the drug should be discontinued and not restarted, supportive medical therapy instituted, and the patient monitored closely with appropriate laboratory studies (e.g., serum and urine amylase, amylase/creatinine clearance ratio, electrolytes, serum calcium, glucose, lipase, etc.). A search for other causes of pancreatitis as well as those conditions which mimic pancreatitis should be conducted.

Because of reports of adverse eye findings with non-steroidal anti-inflammatory agents, it is recommended that patients who develop eye complaints during treatment with CLINORIL have ophthalmologic studies.

In patients with poor liver function, delayed, elevated and prolonged circulating levels of the sulfide and sulfone metabolites may occur. Such patients should be monitored closely; a reduction of daily dosage may be required.

Edema has been observed in some patients taking CLINORIL. Therefore, as with other non-steroidal anti-inflammatory drugs, CLINORIL should be used with caution in patients with compromised cardiac function, hypertension, or other conditions predisposing to fluid retention.

CLINORIL may allow a reduction in dosage or the elimination of chronic corticosteroid therapy in some patients with rheumatoid arthritis. However, it is generally necessary to reduce corticosteroids gradually over several months in order to avoid an exacerbation of disease or signs and symptoms of adrenal insufficiency. Abrupt withdrawal of chronic corticosteroid treatment is generally not recommended even when patients have had a serious complication of chronic corticosteroid therapy.

Renal Effects

As with other non-steroidal anti-inflammatory drugs, long-term administration of sulindac to animals has resulted in renal papillary necrosis and other abnormal renal pathology. In humans, there have been reports of acute interstitial nephritis with hematuria, proteinuria, and occasionally nephrotic syndrome.

A second form of renal toxicity has been seen in patients with prerenal and renal conditions leading to a reduction in renal blood flow or blood volume, where the renal prostaglandins have a supportive role in the maintenance of renal perfusion. In these patients, administration of an NSAID may cause a dose dependent reduction in prostaglandin formation and may precipitate overt renal decompensation. CLINORIL may affect renal function less than other NSAIDs in patients with chronic glomerular renal disease (see CLINICAL PHARMACOLOGY). Until these observations are better understood and clarified, however, and because renal adverse experiences have been reported with CLINORIL (see ADVERSE REACTIONS), caution should be exercised when administering the drug to patients with conditions associated with increased risk of the effects of non-steroidal anti-inflammatory drugs on renal function, such as those with renal or hepatic dysfunction, diabetes mellitus, advanced age, extracellular volume depletion from any cause, congestive heart failure, septicemia, pyelonephritis, or concomitant use of any nephrotoxic drug. Discontinuation of NSAID therapy is typically followed by recovery to the pretreatment state.

Since CLINORIL is eliminated primarily by the kidneys, patients with significantly impaired renal function should be closely monitored; a lower daily dosage should be anticipated to avoid excessive drug accumulation.

Sulindac metabolites have been reported rarely as the major or a minor component in renal stones in association with other calculus components. CLINORIL should be used with caution in patients with a history of renal lithiasis, and they should be kept well hydrated while receiving CLINORIL.

Continued on next page

Information on the Merck & Co., Inc., products listed on these pages is from the prescribing information in use October 1, 2004. For information, please call 1-800-NSC-MERCK [1-800-672-6372].

Clinoril—Cont.

Information for Patients

CLINORIL, like other drugs of its class, is not free of side effects. The side effects of these drugs can cause discomfort and, rarely, there are more serious side effects such as gastrointestinal bleeding, which may result in hospitalization and even fatal outcomes.

NSAIDs (Non-steroidal Anti-inflammatory Drugs) are often essential agents in the management of arthritis, but they also may be commonly employed for conditions which are less serious.

Physicians may wish to discuss with their patients the potential risks (see WARNINGS, PRECAUTIONS and ADVERSE REACTIONS) and likely benefits of NSAID treatment, particularly when the drugs are used for less serious conditions where treatment without NSAIDs may represent an acceptable alternative to both the patient and physician.

Laboratory Tests

Because serious GI tract ulceration and bleeding can occur without warning symptoms, physicians should follow chronically treated patients for the signs and symptoms of ulceration and bleeding and should inform them of the importance of this follow-up (see WARNINGS, *Risk of GI Ulcerations, Bleeding and Perforation with NSAID Therapy).*

Use in Pregnancy

CLINORIL is not recommended for use in pregnant women, since safety for use has not been established. The known effects of drugs of this class on the human fetus during the third trimester of pregnancy include: constriction of the ductus arteriosus prenatally, tricuspid incompetence, and pulmonary hypertension; non-closure of the ductus arteriosus postnatally which may be resistant to medical management; myocardial degenerative changes, platelet dysfunction with resultant bleeding, intracranial bleeding, renal dysfunction or failure, renal injury/dysgenesis which may result in prolonged or permanent renal failure, oligohydramnios, gastrointestinal bleeding or perforation, and increased risk of necrotizing enterocolitis.

In reproduction studies in the rat, a decrease in average fetal weight and an increase in numbers of dead pups were observed on the first day of the postpartum period at dosage levels of 20 and 40 mg/kg/day ($2^1/_2$ and 5 times the usual maximum daily dose in humans), although there was no adverse effect on the survival and growth during the remainder of the postpartum period. CLINORIL prolongs the duration of gestation in rats, as do other compounds of this class which also may cause dystocia and delayed parturition in pregnant animals. Visceral and skeletal malformations observed in low incidence among rabbits in some teratology studies did not occur at the same dosage levels in repeat studies, nor at a higher dosage level in the same species.

Nursing Mothers

Nursing should not be undertaken while a patient is on CLINORIL. It is not known whether sulindac is secreted in human milk; however, it is secreted in the milk of lactating rats.

Pediatric Use

Safety and effectiveness in pediatric patients have not been established.

Geriatric Use

As with any NSAID, caution should be exercised in treating the elderly (65 years and older) since advancing age appears to increase the possibility of adverse reactions. Elderly patients seem to tolerate ulceration or bleeding less well than other individuals and many spontaneous reports of fatal GI events are in this population (see WARNINGS, *Gastrointestinal Effects* and *Risk of GI Ulcerations, Bleeding and Perforation with NSAID Therapy*).

This drug is known to be substantially excreted by the kidney and the risk of toxic reactions to this drug may be greater in patients with impaired renal function. Because elderly patients are more likely to have decreased renal function, care should be taken in dose selection and it may be useful to monitor renal function (see PRECAUTIONS, *Renal Effects*).

Drug Interactions

DMSO should not be used with sulindac. Concomitant administration has been reported to reduce the plasma levels of the active sulfide metabolite and potentially reduce efficacy. In addition, this combination has been reported to cause peripheral neuropathy.

Although sulindac and its sulfide metabolite are highly bound to protein, studies, in which CLINORIL was given at a dose of 400 mg daily, have shown no clinically significant interaction with oral anticoagulants or oral hypoglycemic agents. However, patients should be monitored carefully until it is certain that no change in their anticoagulant or hypoglycemic dosage is required. Special attention should be paid to patients taking higher doses than those recommended and to patients with renal impairment or other metabolic defects that might increase sulindac blood levels.

The concomitant administration of aspirin with sulindac significantly depressed the plasma levels of the active sulfide metabolite. A double-blind study compared the safety and efficacy of CLINORIL 300 or 400 mg daily given alone or with aspirin 2.4 g/day for the treatment of osteoarthritis. The addition of aspirin did not alter the types of clinical or laboratory adverse experiences for CLINORIL; however, the combination showed an increase in the incidence of gastrointestinal adverse experiences. Since the addition of aspirin did not have a favorable effect on the therapeutic response to CLINORIL, the combination is not recommended.

The concomitant use of CLINORIL with other NSAIDs is not recommended due to the increased possibility of gastrointestinal toxicity, with little or no increase in efficacy.

Caution should be used if CLINORIL is administered concomitantly with methotrexate. Nonsteroidal anti-inflammatory drugs have been reported to decrease the tubular secretion of methotrexate and to potentiate its toxicity.

Administration of non-steroidal anti-inflammatory drugs concomitantly with cyclosporine has been associated with an increase in cyclosporine-induced toxicity, possibly due to decreased synthesis of renal prostacyclin. NSAIDs should be used with caution in patients taking cyclosporine, and renal function should be carefully monitored.

The concomitant administration of CLINORIL and diflunisal in normal volunteers resulted in lowering of the plasma levels of the active sulindac sulfide metabolite by approximately one-third.

Probenecid given concomitantly with sulindac had only a slight effect on plasma sulfide levels, while plasma levels of sulindac and sulfone were increased. Sulindac was shown to produce a modest reduction in the uricosuric action of probenecid, which probably is not significant under most circumstances.

Neither propoxyphene hydrochloride nor acetaminophen had any effect on the plasma levels of sulindac or its sulfide metabolite.

ADVERSE REACTIONS

The following adverse reactions were reported in clinical trials or have been reported since the drug was marketed. The probability exists of a causal relationship between CLINORIL and these adverse reactions. The adverse reactions which have been observed in clinical trials encompass observations in 1,865 patients, including 232 observed for at least 48 weeks.

Incidence Greater Than 1%

Gastrointestinal

The most frequent types of adverse reactions occurring with CLINORIL are gastrointestinal; these include gastrointestinal pain (10%), dyspepsia***, nausea*** with or without vomiting, diarrhea***, constipation***, flatulence, anorexia and gastrointestinal cramps.

Dermatologic

Rash***, pruritus.

Central Nervous System

Dizziness***, headache***, nervousness.

Special Senses

Tinnitus.

Miscellaneous

Edema (see PRECAUTIONS).

***Incidence between 3% and 9%. Those reactions occurring in 1% to 3% of patients are not marked with an asterisk.

Incidence Less Than 1 in 100

Gastrointestinal

Gastritis, gastroenteritis or colitis. Peptic ulcer and gastrointestinal bleeding have been reported. GI perforation and intestinal strictures (diaphragms) have been reported rarely.

Liver function abnormalities; jaundice, sometimes with fever; cholestasis; hepatitis; hepatic failure.

There have been rare reports of sulindac metabolites in common bile duct "sludge" and in biliary calculi in patients with symptoms of cholecystitis who underwent a cholecystectomy.

Pancreatitis (see PRECAUTIONS).

Ageusia; glossitis.

Dermatologic

Stomatitis, sore or dry mucous membranes, alopecia, photosensitivity.

Erythema multiforme, toxic epidermal necrolysis, Stevens-Johnson syndrome, and exfoliative dermatitis have been reported.

Cardiovascular

Congestive heart failure, especially in patients with marginal cardiac function; palpitation; hypertension.

Hematologic

Thrombocytopenia; ecchymosis; purpura; leukopenia; agranulocytosis; neutropenia; bone marrow depression, including aplastic anemia; hemolytic anemia; increased prothrombin time in patients on oral anticoagulants (see PRECAUTIONS).

Genitourinary

Urine discoloration; dysuria; vaginal bleeding; hematuria; proteinuria; crystalluria; renal impairment, including renal failure; interstitial nephritis; nephrotic syndrome.

Renal calculi containing sulindac metabolites have been observed rarely.

Metabolic

Hyperkalemia.

Musculoskeletal

Muscle weakness.

Psychiatric

Depression; psychic disturbances including acute psychosis.

Nervous System

Vertigo; insomnia; somnolence; paresthesia; convulsions; syncope; aseptic meningitis.

Special Senses

Blurred vision; visual disturbances; decreased hearing; metallic or bitter taste.

Respiratory

Epistaxis.

Hypersensitivity Reactions

Anaphylaxis; angioneurotic edema; bronchial spasm; dyspnea.

Hypersensitivity vasculitis.

A potentially fatal apparent hypersensitivity syndrome has been reported. This syndrome may include constitutional symptoms (fever, chills, diaphoresis, flushing), cutaneous findings (rash or other dermatologic reactions—see above), conjunctivitis, involvement of major organs (changes in liver function including hepatic failure, jaundice, pancreatitis, pneumonitis with or without pleural effusion, leukopenia, leukocytosis, eosinophilia, disseminated intravascular coagulation, anemia, renal impairment, including renal failure), and other less specific findings (adenitis, arthralgia, arthritis, myalgia, fatigue, malaise, hypotension, chest pain, tachycardia).

Causal Relationship Unknown

A rare occurrence of fulminant necrotizing fasciitis, particularly in association with Group A β-hemolytic streptococcus, has been described in persons treated with non-steroidal anti-inflammatory agents, sometimes with fatal outcome (see also PRECAUTIONS, *General*).

Other reactions have been reported in clinical trials or since the drug was marketed, but occurred under circumstances where a causal relationship could not be established. However, in these rarely reported events, that possibility cannot be excluded. Therefore, these observations are listed to serve as alerting information to physicians.

Cardiovascular

Arrhythmia.

Metabolic

Hyperglycemia.

Nervous System

Neuritis.

Special Senses

Disturbances of the retina and its vasculature.

Miscellaneous

Gynecomastia.

MANAGEMENT OF OVERDOSAGE

Cases of overdosage have been reported and rarely, deaths have occurred. The following signs and symptoms may be observed following overdosage: stupor, coma, diminished urine output and hypotension.

In the event of overdosage, the stomach should be emptied by inducing vomiting or by gastric lavage, and the patient carefully observed and given symptomatic and supportive treatment.

Animal studies show that absorption is decreased by the prompt administration of activated charcoal and excretion is enhanced by alkalinization of the urine.

DOSAGE AND ADMINISTRATION

CLINORIL should be administered orally twice a day with food. The maximum dosage is 400 mg per day. Dosages above 400 mg per day are not recommended.

In osteoarthritis, rheumatoid arthritis, and ankylosing spondylitis, the recommended starting dosage is 150 mg twice a day. The dosage may be lowered or raised depending on the response.

A prompt response (within one week) can be expected in about one-half of patients with osteoarthritis, ankylosing spondylitis, and rheumatoid arthritis. Others may require longer to respond.

In acute painful shoulder (acute subacromial bursitis/supraspinatus tendinitis) and acute gouty arthritis, the recommended dosage is 200 mg twice a day. After a satisfactory response has been achieved, the dosage may be reduced according to the response. In acute painful shoulder, therapy for 7–14 days is usually adequate. In acute gouty arthritis, therapy for 7 days is usually adequate.

HOW SUPPLIED

No. 3360—Tablets CLINORIL 150 mg are bright yellow, hexagon-shaped, compressed tablets, coded MSD 941 on one side and CLINORIL on the other. They are supplied as follows:

NDC 0006-0941-68 in bottles of 100
(6505-01-071-5559, 150 mg 100's).

No. 3353—Tablets CLINORIL 200 mg are bright yellow, hexagon-shaped, scored, compressed tablets, coded MSD 942 on one side and CLINORIL on the other. They are supplied as follows:

NDC 0006-0942-68 in bottles of 100
(6505-01-072-3426, 200 mg 100's).

7858637 Issued July 1998

Shown in Product Identification Guide, page 323

COGENTIN® Injection ℞
(Benztropine Mesylate)

DESCRIPTION

Benztropine mesylate is a synthetic compound containing structural features found in atropine and diphenhydramine.

It is designated chemically as 8-azabicyclo[3.2.1] octane, 3-(diphenylmethoxy)-,*endo*, methanesulfonate. Its empirical formula is $C_{21}H_{25}NO \cdot CH_4O_3S$, and its structural formula is:

Benztropine mesylate is a crystalline white powder, very soluble in water, and has a molecular weight of 403.54.
COGENTIN* (Benztropine Mesylate) is supplied as a sterile injection for intravenous and intramuscular use.
Each milliliter of the injection contains:

Benztropine mesylate .... 1 mg
Sodium chloride .... 9 mg
Water for Injection q.s. .... 1 mL

*Registered trademark of MERCK & CO., INC.

ACTIONS

COGENTIN possesses both anticholinergic and antihistaminic effects, although only the former have been established as therapeutically significant in the management of parkinsonism.
In the isolated guinea pig ileum, the anticholinergic activity of this drug is about equal to that of atropine; however, when administered orally to unanesthetized cats, it is only about half as active as atropine.
In laboratory animals, its antihistaminic activity and duration of action approach those of pyrilamine maleate.

INDICATIONS

For use as an adjunct in the therapy of all forms of parkinsonism.
Useful also in the control of extrapyramidal disorders (except tardive dyskinesia—see PRECAUTIONS) due to neuroleptic drugs (e.g., phenothiazines).

CONTRAINDICATIONS

Hypersensitivity to any component of COGENTIN injection.
Because of its atropine-like side effects, this drug is contraindicated in pediatric patients under three years of age, and should be used with caution in older pediatric patients.

WARNINGS

Safe use in pregnancy has not been established.
COGENTIN may impair mental and/or physical abilities required for performance of hazardous tasks, such as operating machinery or driving a motor vehicle.
When COGENTIN is given concomitantly with phenothiazines, haloperidol, or other drugs with anticholinergic or antidopaminergic activity, patients should be advised to report gastrointestinal complaints, fever or heat intolerance promptly. Paralytic ileus, hyperthermia and heat stroke, all of which have sometimes been fatal, have occurred in patients taking anticholinergic-type antiparkinsonism drugs, including COGENTIN, in combination with phenothiazines and/or tricyclic antidepressants.
Since COGENTIN contains structural features of atropine, it may produce anhidrosis. For this reason, it should be administered with caution during hot weather, especially when given concomitantly with other atropine-like drugs to the chronically ill, the alcoholic, those who have central nervous system disease, and those who do manual labor in a hot environment. Anhidrosis may occur more readily when some disturbance of sweating already exists. If there is evidence of anhidrosis, the possibility of hyperthermia should be considered. Dosage should be decreased at the discretion of the physician so that the ability to maintain body heat equilibrium by perspiration is not impaired. Severe anhidrosis and fatal hyperthermia have occurred.

PRECAUTIONS

General
Since COGENTIN has cumulative action, continued supervision is advisable. Patients with a tendency to tachycardia and patients with prostatic hypertrophy should be observed closely during treatment.
Dysuria may occur, but rarely becomes a problem. Urinary retention has been reported with COGENTIN.
The drug may cause complaints of weakness and inability to move particular muscle groups, especially in large doses. For example, if the neck has been rigid and suddenly relaxes, it may feel weak, causing some concern. In this event, dosage adjustment is required.
Mental confusion and excitement may occur with large doses, or in susceptible patients. Visual hallucinations have been reported occasionally. Furthermore, in the treatment of extrapyramidal disorders due to neuroleptic drugs (e.g., phenothiazines), in patients with mental disorders, occasionally there may be intensification of mental symptoms. In such cases, antiparkinsonian drugs can precipitate a toxic psychosis. Patients with mental disorders should be kept under careful observation, especially at the beginning of treatment or if dosage is increased.
Tardive dyskinesia may appear in some patients on long-term therapy with phenothiazines and related agents, or may occur after therapy with these drugs has been discontinued. Antiparkinsonism agents do not alleviate the symptoms of tardive dyskinesia, and in some instances may aggravate them. COGENTIN is not recommended for use in patients with tardive dyskinesia.
The physician should be aware of the possible occurrence of glaucoma. Although the drug does not appear to have any adverse effect on simple glaucoma, it probably should not be used in angle-closure glaucoma.
Drug Interactions
Antipsychotic drugs such as phenothiazines or haloperidol; tricyclic antidepressants (see WARNINGS).
Pediatric use
Because of the atropine-like side effects, COGENTIN should be used with caution in pediatric patients over three years of age (see CONTRAINDICATIONS).

ADVERSE REACTIONS

The adverse reactions below, most of which are anticholinergic in nature, have been reported and within each category are listed in order of decreasing severity.
Cardiovascular
Tachycardia.
Digestive
Paralytic ileus, constipation, vomiting, nausea, dry mouth. If dry mouth is so severe that there is difficulty in swallowing or speaking, or loss of appetite and weight, reduce dosage, or discontinue the drug temporarily.
Slight reduction in dosage may control nausea and still give sufficient relief of symptoms. Vomiting may be controlled by temporary discontinuation, followed by resumption at a lower dosage.
Nervous System
Toxic psychosis, including confusion, disorientation, memory impairment, visual hallucinations; exacerbation of preexisting psychotic symptoms; nervousness; depression; listlessness; numbness of fingers.
Special Senses
Blurred vision, dilated pupils.
Urogenital
Urinary retention, dysuria.
Metabolic/Immune or Skin
Occasionally, an allergic reaction, e.g., skin rash, develops. If this can not be controlled by dosage reduction, the medication should be discontinued.
Other
Heat stroke, hyperthermia, fever.

DOSAGE AND ADMINISTRATION

Since there is no significant difference in onset of effect after intravenous or intramuscular injection, usually there is no need to use the intravenous route. The drug is quickly effective after either route, with improvement sometimes noticeable a few minutes after injection. In emergency situations, when the condition of the patient is alarming, 1 to 2 mL of the injection normally will provide quick relief. If the parkinsonism effect begins to return, the dose can be repeated.
Because of cumulative action, therapy should be initiated with a low dose which is increased gradually at five or six-day intervals to the smallest amount necessary for optimal relief. Increases should be made in increments of 0.5 mg, to a maximum of 6 mg, or until optimal results are obtained without excessive adverse reactions.
Postencephalitic and Idiopathic Parkinsonism—
The usual daily dose is 1 to 2 mg, with a range of 0.5 to 6 mg parenterally.
As with any agent used in parkinsonism, dosage must be individualized according to age and weight, and the type of parkinsonism being treated. Generally, older patients and thin patients cannot tolerate large doses. Most patients with postencephalitic parkinsonism need fairly large doses and tolerate them well. Patients with a poor mental outlook are usually poor candidates for therapy.
In idiopathic parkinsonism, therapy may be initiated with a single daily dose of 0.5 to 1 mg at bedtime. In some patients, this will be adequate; in others 4 to 6 mg a day may be required.
In postencephalitic parkinsonism, therapy may be initiated in most patients with 2 mg a day in one or more doses. In highly sensitive patients, therapy may be initiated with 0.5 mg at bedtime, and increased as necessary.
Some patients experience greatest relief when given the entire dose at bedtime; others react more favorably to divided doses, two to four times a day. Frequently, one dose a day is sufficient, and divided doses may be unnecessary or undesirable.
The long duration of action of this drug makes it particularly suitable for bedtime medication when its effects may last throughout the night, enabling patients to turn in bed during the night more easily, and to rise in the morning.
When COGENTIN is started, do not terminate therapy with other antiparkinsonian agents abruptly. If the other agents are to be reduced or discontinued, it must be done gradually. Many patients obtain greatest relief with combination therapy.
COGENTIN may be used concomitantly with SINEMET* (Carbidopa-Levodopa), or with levodopa, in which case periodic dosage adjustment may be required in order to maintain optimum response.
Drug-Induced Extrapyramidal Disorders—In treating extrapyramidal disorders due to neuroleptic drugs (e.g., phenothiazines), the recommended dosage is 1 to 4 mg once or twice a day parenterally. Dosage must be individualized according to the need of the patient. Some patients require more than recommended; others do not need as much.
In acute dystonic reactions, 1 to 2 mL of the injection usually relieves the condition quickly.
When extrapyramidal disorders develop soon after initiation of treatment with neuroleptic drugs (e.g., phenothiazines), they are likely to be transient. One to 2 mg of COGENTIN two or three times a day usually provides relief within one or two days. After one or two weeks, the drug should be withdrawn to determine the continued need for it. If such disorders recur, COGENTIN can be reinstituted.
Certain drug-induced extrapyramidal disorders that develop slowly may not respond to COGENTIN.

*Registered trademark of MERCK & CO., INC.

OVERDOSAGE

Manifestations—May be any of those seen in atropine poisoning or antihistamine overdosage: CNS depression, preceded or followed by stimulation; confusion; nervousness; listlessness; intensification of mental symptoms or toxic psychosis in patients with mental illness being treated with neuroleptic drugs (e.g., phenothiazines); hallucinations (especially visual); dizziness; muscle weakness; ataxia; dry mouth; mydriasis; blurred vision; palpitations; tachycardia; elevated blood pressure; nausea; vomiting; dysuria; numbness of fingers; dysphagia; allergic reactions, e.g., skin rash; headache; hot, dry, flushed skin; delirium; coma; shock; convulsions; respiratory arrest; anhidrosis; hyperthermia; glaucoma; constipation.
Treatment—Physostigmine salicylate, 1 to 2 mg, SC or IV, reportedly will reverse symptoms of anticholinergic intoxication.** A second injection may be given after 2 hours if required. Otherwise treatment is symptomatic and supportive. Induce emesis or perform gastric lavage (contraindicated in precomatose, convulsive, or psychotic states). Maintain respiration. A short-acting barbiturate may be used for CNS excitement, but with caution to avoid subsequent depression; supportive care for depression (avoid convulsant stimulants such as picrotoxin, pentylenetetrazol, or bemegride); artificial respiration for severe respiratory depression; a local miotic for mydriasis and cycloplegia; ice bags or other cold applications and alcohol sponges for hyperpyrexia, a vasopressor and fluids for circulatory collapse. Darken room for photophobia.

**Duvoisin, R.C.; Katz, R.J.; Amer. Med. Ass. *206*:1963–1965, Nov. 25, 1968.

HOW SUPPLIED

No. 3275—Injection COGENTIN, 1 mg per mL, is a clear, colorless solution and is supplied as follows:
NDC 0006-3275-38 in boxes of 5×2 mL ampuls.
7924125 Issued October 2001

COMVAX® ℞

[Haemophilus b conjugate (meningococcal protein conjugate) and hepatitis B (recombinant) vaccine]

DESCRIPTION

COMVAX* [Haemophilus b Conjugate (Meningococcal Protein Conjugate) and Hepatitis B (Recombinant) Vaccine] is a sterile bivalent vaccine made of the antigenic components used in producing PedvaxHIB* [Haemophilus b Conjugate Vaccine (Meningococcal Protein Conjugate)] and RECOMBIVAX HB* [Hepatitis B Vaccine (Recombinant)]. These components are the *Haemophilus influenzae* type b capsular polysaccharide [polyribosylribitol phosphate (PRP)] that is covalently bound to an outer membrane protein complex (OMPC) of *Neisseria meningitidis* and hepatitis B surface antigen (HBsAg) from recombinant yeast cultures.
Haemophilus influenzae type b and *Neisseria meningitidis* serogroup B are grown in complex fermentation media. The primary ingredients of the phenol-inactivated fermentation medium for *Haemophilus influenzae* include an extract of yeast, nicotinamide adenine dinucleotide, hemin chloride, soy peptone, dextrose, and mineral salts and for *Neisseria meningitidis* include an extract of yeast, amino acids and

Continued on next page

Information on the Merck & Co., Inc., products listed on these pages is from the prescribing information in use October 1, 2004. For information, please call 1-800-NSC-MERCK [1-800-672-6372].

Comvax—Cont.

mineral salts. The PRP is purified from the culture broth by purification procedures which include ethanol fractionation, enzyme digestion, phenol extraction and diafiltration. The OMPC from *Neisseria meningitidis* is purified by detergent extraction, ultracentrifugation, diafiltration and sterile filtration.

The PRP-OMPC conjugate is prepared by the chemical coupling of the highly purified PRP (polyribosylribitol phosphate) of *Haemophilus influenzae* type b (Haemophilus b, Ross strain) to an OMPC of the B11 strain of *Neisseria meningitidis* serogroup B. The coupling of the PRP to the OMPC is necessary for enhanced immunogenicity of the PRP. This coupling is confirmed by analysis of the components of the conjugate following chemical treatment which yields a unique amino acid. After conjugation, the aqueous bulk is then adsorbed onto an amorphous aluminum hydroxyphosphate sulfate adjuvant (previously referred to as aluminum hydroxide).

HBsAg is produced in recombinant yeast cells. A portion of the hepatitis B virus gene, coding for HBsAg, is cloned into yeast, and the vaccine for hepatitis B is produced from cultures of this recombinant yeast strain according to methods developed in the Merck Research Laboratories. The antigen is harvested and purified from fermentation cultures of a recombinant strain of the yeast *Saccharomyces cerevisiae* containing the gene for the *adw* subtype of HBsAg. The fermentation process involves growth of *Saccharomyces cerevisiae* on a complex fermentation medium which consists of an extract of yeast, soy peptone, dextrose, amino acids and mineral salts.

The HBsAg protein is released from the yeast cells by mechanical cell disruption and detergent extraction, and purified by a series of physical and chemical methods, which includes ion and hydrophobic chromatography, and diafiltration. The purified protein is treated in phosphate buffer with formaldehyde and then coprecipitated with alum (potassium aluminum sulfate) to form bulk vaccine adjuvanted with amorphous aluminum hydroxyphosphate sulfate. The vaccine contains no detectable yeast DNA, and 1% or less of the protein is of yeast origin.

The individual PRP-OMPC and HBsAg adjuvanted bulks are combined to produce COMVAX. Each 0.5 mL dose of COMVAX is formulated to contain 7.5 mcg PRP conjugated to approximately 125 mcg OMPC, 5 mcg HBsAg, approximately 225 mcg aluminum as amorphous aluminum hydroxyphosphate sulfate, and 35 mcg sodium borate (decahydrate) as a pH stabilizer, in 0.9% sodium chloride. The vaccine contains not more than 0.0004% (w/v) residual formaldehyde.

The potency of the PRP-OMPC component is measured by quantitating the polysaccharide concentration by an HPLC method. The potency of the HBsAg component is measured relative to a standard by an *in vitro* immunoassay.

The product contains no preservative.

COMVAX is a sterile suspension for intramuscular injection.

*Registered trademark of MERCK & CO., Inc.

CLINICAL PHARMACOLOGY

Haemophilus influenzae type b Disease

Prior to the introduction of *Haemophilus b* conjugate vaccines, *Haemophilus influenzae* type b (Hib) was the most frequent cause of bacterial meningitis and a leading cause of serious, systemic bacterial disease in young children worldwide.

Hib disease occurred primarily in children under 5 years of age, and in the United States prior to the initiation of a vaccine program was estimated to account for nearly 20,000 cases of invasive infections annually, approximately 12,000 of which were meningitis. The mortality rate from Hib meningitis is about 5%. In addition, up to 35% of survivors develop neurologic sequelae including seizures, deafness, and mental retardation. Other invasive diseases caused by this bacterium include cellulitis, epiglottitis, sepsis, pneumonia, septic arthritis, osteomyelitis, and pericarditis.

Prior to the introduction of the vaccine, it was estimated that 17% of all cases of Hib disease occurred in infants less than 6 months of age. The peak incidence of Hib meningitis occurred between 6 to 11 months of age. Forty-seven percent of all cases occurred by one year of age with the remaining 53% of cases occurring over the next four years.

Among children under 5 years of age, the risk of invasive Hib disease is increased in certain populations including the following:

- Daycare attendees
- Lower socio-economic groups
- Blacks (especially those who lack the Km(1) immunoglobulin allotype)
- Caucasians who lack the G2m(23) immunoglobulin allotype
- Native Americans
- Household contacts of cases
- Individuals with asplenia, sickle cell disease, or antibody deficiency syndromes.

Prevention of Hib Disease with Vaccine

An important virulence factor of the Hib bacterium is its polysaccharide capsule (PRP). Antibody to PRP (anti-PRP) has been shown to correlate with protection against Hib disease. While the anti-PRP level associated with protection using conjugated vaccines has not yet been determined, the level of anti-PRP associated with protection in studies using bacterial polysaccharide immune globulin or nonconjugated PRP vaccines ranged from ≥0.15 to ≥1.0 mcg/mL.

Nonconjugated PRP vaccines are capable of stimulating B-lymphocytes to produce antibody without the help of T-lymphocytes (T-independent). The responses to many other antigens are augmented by helper T-lymphocytes (T-dependent). PedvaxHIB is a PRP-conjugate vaccine in which the PRP is covalently bound to the OMPC carrier producing an antigen which is postulated to convert the T-independent antigen (PRP alone) into a T-dependent antigen resulting in both an enhanced antibody response and immunologic memory.

Clinical Trials with PedvaxHIB

The protective efficacy of the PRP-OMPC component of COMVAX was demonstrated in a randomized, double-blind, placebo-controlled study involving 3486 Native American (Navajo) infants (The Protective Efficacy Study) who completed the primary two-dose regimen for lyophilized PedvaxHIB. This population has a much higher incidence of Hib disease than the United States population as a whole and also has a lower antibody response to Haemophilus b conjugate vaccines, including PedvaxHIB.

Each infant in this study received two doses of either placebo or lyophilized PedvaxHIB (15 mcg Haemophilus b PRP) with the first dose administered at a mean of 8 weeks of age and the second administered approximately two months later; DTP (Diphtheria and Tetanus Toxoids and Pertussis Vaccine, Adsorbed) and OPV (Poliovirus Vaccine Live Oral Trivalent) were administered concomitantly. In a subset of 416 subjects, lyophilized PedvaxHIB (15 mcg Haemophilus b PRP) induced anti-PRP levels >0.15 mcg/mL in 88% and >1.0 mcg/mL in 52% with a geometric mean titer (GMT) of 0.95 mcg/mL one to three months after the first dose; the corresponding anti-PRP levels one to three months following the second dose were 91% and 60%, respectively, with a GMT of 1.43 mcg/mL. These antibody responses were associated with a high level of protection.

Most subjects were initially followed until 15 to 18 months of age. During this time, 22 cases of invasive Hib disease occurred in the placebo group (8 cases after the first dose and 14 cases after the second dose) and only 1 case in the vaccine group (none after the first dose and 1 after the second dose). Following the primary two-dose regimen, the protective efficacy of lyophilized PedvaxHIB was calculated to be 93% with a 95% confidence interval (C.I.) of 57–98%. In the two months between the first and second doses, the difference in number of cases of disease between placebo and vaccine recipients (8 vs 0 cases, respectively) was statistically significant (p=0.008). At termination of the study, placebo recipients were offered vaccine. All original participants were then followed two years and nine months from termination of the study. During this extended follow-up, invasive Hib disease occurred in an additional 7 of the original placebo recipients prior to receiving vaccine and in 1 of the original vaccine recipients (who had received only 1 dose of vaccine). No cases of invasive Hib disease were observed in placebo recipients after they received at least one dose of vaccine. Efficacy for this follow-up period, estimated from person-days at risk, was 96.6% (95 C.I., 72.2–99.9%) in children under 18 months of age and 100% (95 C.I., 23.5–100%) in children over 18 months of age. Thus, in this study, a protective efficacy of 93% was achieved with an anti-PRP level of >1.0 mcg/mL in 60% of vaccinees and a GMT of 1.43 mcg/mL one to three months after the second dose.

Hepatitis B Disease

Hepatitis B virus is an important cause of viral hepatitis. According to the Centers for Disease Control (CDC), there are an estimated 200,000–300,000 new cases of Hepatitis B infection annually in the United States. There is no specific treatment for this disease. The incubation period for hepatitis B is relatively long; six weeks to six months may elapse between exposure and the onset of clinical symptoms. The prognosis following infection with hepatitis B virus is variable and dependent on at least three factors: (1) Age—infants and younger children usually experience milder initial disease than older persons but are much more likely to remain persistently infected and become at risk of developing serious chronic liver disease; (2) Dose of virus—the higher the dose, the more likely acute icteric hepatitis B will result; and, (3) Severity of associated underlying disease—underlying malignancy or pre-existing hepatic disease predisposes to increased mortality and morbidity.

Hepatitis B infection fails to resolve and progresses to a chronic carrier state in 5 to 10% of older children and adults and in up to 90% of infants; chronic infection also occurs more frequently after initial anicteric hepatitis B than after initial icteric disease. Consequently, carriers of HBsAg frequently give no history of having had recognized acute hepatitis. It has been estimated that more than 285 million people in the world today are persistently infected with hepatitis B virus. The CDC estimates that there are approximately 1 million–1.25 million chronic carriers of hepatitis B virus in the USA. Chronic carriers represent the largest human reservoir of hepatitis B virus.

A serious complication of acute hepatitis B virus infection is massive hepatic necrosis while sequelae of chronic hepatitis B include cirrhosis of the liver, chronic active hepatitis, and hepatocellular carcinoma. Chronic carriers of HBsAg appear to be at increased risk of developing hepatocellular carcinoma. Although a number of etiologic factors are associated with development of hepatocellular carcinoma, the single most important etiologic factor appears to be chronic infection with hepatitis B virus. According to the CDC, hepatitis B vaccine is recognized as the first anti-cancer vaccine because it can prevent primary liver cancer.

The vehicles for transmission of the virus are most often blood and blood products but the viral antigen has also been found in tears, saliva, breast milk, urine, semen, and vaginal secretions. Hepatitis B virus is capable of surviving for days on environmental surfaces exposed to body fluids containing hepatitis B virus. Infection may occur when hepatitis B virus, transmitted by infected body fluids, is implanted via mucous surfaces or percutaneously introduced through accidental or deliberate breaks in the skin. Transmission of hepatitis B virus infection is often associated with close interpersonal contact with an infected individual and with crowded living conditions.

Prevention of Hepatitis B Disease with Vaccine

Hepatitis B infection and disease can be prevented through immunization with vaccines that contain viral surface antigen (HBsAg) and induce formation of protective antibody (anti-HBs).

Multiple clinical studies have defined a protective level of anti-HBs as 1) 10 or more sample ratio units (SRU or S/N) as determined by radioimmunoassay or 2) a positive result as determined by enzyme immunoassay. Note: 10 SRU is comparable to 10 mIU/mL of antibody. The ACIP and an international group of hepatitis B experts consider an anti-HBs titer ≥10 mIU/mL an adequate response to a complete course of hepatitis B vaccine and protective against clinically significant infection (antigenemia with or without clinical disease).

Clinical Trials with RECOMBIVAX HB

In clinical studies, 100% of 92 infants under 1 year of age born of non-carrier mothers developed a protective level of antibody (anti-HBs ≥10 mIU/mL) after receiving three 5—mcg doses of RECOMBIVAX HB at intervals of 0, 1, and 6 months.

In one clinical study of RECOMBIVAX HB (2.5 mcg), which examined a different regimen of RECOMBIVAX HB, protective levels of antibody were achieved in 98% of 52 healthy infants vaccinated at 2, 4, and 12 months of age. Protective anti-HBs levels were achieved in 100% of 50 infants vaccinated at 2, 4, and 15 months of age.

The protective efficacy of three 5—mcg doses of RECOMBIVAX HB, given at birth (with Hepatitis B Immune Globulin), 1, and 6 months of age, has been demonstrated in neonates born of mothers positive for both HBsAg and HBeAg (a core-associated antigenic complex which correlates with high infectivity). In this trial, after nine months of follow-up, chronic infection had not occurred in 96% of 130 infants. The estimated efficacy in prevention of chronic hepatitis B infection was 95% as compared to the infection rate in untreated historical controls.

Immunogenicity of COMVAX

The immunogenicity of COMVAX (7.5 mcg Haemophilus b PRP, 5 mcg HBsAg) was assessed in 1602 infants and children 6 weeks to 15 months of age in 5 clinical studies. In 2 controlled clinical trials (n=684, the immune response of COMVAX was compared with that obtained using the monovalent vaccines, PedvaxHIB (7.5 mcg Haemophilus b PRP) and RECOMBIVAX HB (5 mcg HBsAg) given at separate sites, either concurrently or one month apart. The immunogenicity of COMVAX was further assessed in 2 uncontrolled studies (n=852). In the first, a complete three—dose series of COMVAX was administered concurrently with other routine pediatric vaccines. In the second, COMVAX was administered as the third dose of Haemophilus b PRP and HBsAg concurrently with routine pediatric vaccines. COMVAX was also administered as the control arm in the evaluation of an investigational vaccine (n=66).

These studies demonstrate COMVAX to be highly immunogenic. The antibody responses are summarized below.

Antibody Responses to COMVAX in Infants Not Previously Vaccinated with Hib or Hepatitis B Vaccine

In the pivotal, controlled, multicenter, randomized, open-label study 882 infants approximately 2 months of age, who had not previously received any Hib or hepatitis B vaccine, were assigned to receive a three-dose regimen of either COMVAX or PedvaxHIB plus RECOMBIVAX HB at approximately 2, 4, and 12–15 months of age. The proportions of evaluable vaccinees developing clinically important levels of anti-PRP (percent with >1.0 mcg/mL after the second dose, n=762) and anti-HBs (percent with ≥10 mIU/mL after the third dose, n=750) were similar in children given COMVAX or concurrent PedvaxHIB and RECOMBIVAX HB (Table 1). The anti-PRP response after the second dose among infants given COMVAX in this study was 72.4% (C.I. 68.7, 76.0) >1.0 mcg/mL with a GMT=2.5 mcg/mL (C.I. 2.2, 2.8) and was comparable to that of infants given the Pedvax HIB and RECOMBIVAX HB controls which was 76.3% (C.I. 70.2, 82.5) with a GMT=2.8 mcg/mL (C.I. 2.2, 3.5). These responses exceed the response of Native American (Navajo) infants in a previous study of lyophilized PedvaxHIB (60% >1.0 mcg/mL; GMT=1.43 mcg/mL) that was associated with a 93% reduction in the incidence of invasive Hib disease. The efficacy of COMVAX in the prevention of invasive Hib disease is expected to be similar to that obtained with monovalent lyophilized PedvaxHIB in the Protective Efficacy Trial (see CLINICAL PHARMACOLOGY, *Clinical Trials with PedvaxHIB*).

The anti-HBs response after the third dose among infants given COMVAX in this study was 98.4% ≥10 mIU/mL (C.I. 97.0, 99.3) with a GMT of 4467.5 (C.I. 3786.3, 5271.3) compared to 100.0% (C.I. 97.9, 100.0) with a GMT of 6943.9 (C.I. 5555.9, 8678.7) among infants given COMVAX or concurrent PedvaxHIB and RECOMBIVAX HB.

Although the difference in anti-HBs GMT is statistically significant (p=0.011), both values are much greater than the level of 10 mIU/mL previously established as marking a protective response to hepatitis B. These GMTs are higher than those observed in young infants who received the currently licensed regimen of RECOMBIVAX HB consisting of 5-mcg doses administered on the standard 0, 1, and 6-month schedule (GMT ~ 1359.9 mIU/mL). In addition, two studies have shown that infants given 2.5-mcg doses of RECOMBIVAX HB according to the schedule used for COMVAX (2, 4, and 12–15 months of age) developed GMTs of 1245–3424 mIU/mL. While a difference in GMT may result in differential retention of ≥10 mIU/mL of anti-HBs after a number of years, this is of no apparent clinical significance because of immunologic memory.

Because the HBsAg component of COMVAX induces a comparable anti-HBs response to that obtained with RECOMBIVAX HB, the efficacy of COMVAX is expected to be similar (Table 1).

[See table 1 at right]

Antibody Responses to COMVAX in Infants Previously Vaccinated with Hepatitis B Vaccine at Birth

Two clinical studies assessed antibody responses to a three—dose series of COMVAX in 128 evaluable infants who were previously given a birth dose of hepatitis B vaccine. Table 2 summarizes the anti-PRP and anti-HBs responses of these infants. The antibody responses were clinically comparable to those observed in the pivotal trial of COMVAX (Table 1).

[See table 2 at right]

Interchangeability of COMVAX and Licensed Haemophilus b Conjugate Vaccines or Recombinant Hepatitis B Vaccines

Among 58 children previously given a primary course of PedvaxHIB, 90% (95% C.I. 78.8%, 96.1%) developed an anti-PRP response >1 mcg/mL with a GMT of 9.6 mcg/mL (95% C.I. 6.6, 14.1) in response to a dose of COMVAX at 12–15 months of age. Among 683 children previously given a primary course of another HIB or HIB-containing vaccine, 99% (95% C.I. 97.9%, 99.6%) developed an anti-PRP response >1 mcg/mL with a GMT of 14.9 mcg/mL (95% C.I. 13.7, 16.3) in response to a dose of COMVAX at 12–15 months of age. In another study, COMVAX was administered either concomitantly or six weeks after vaccination with M-M-R II and VARIVAX* (Varicella Virus Vaccine Live, Oka/Merck). Among 149 children who previously received 2 doses of monovalent Hepatitis B vaccine, 100% (95% C.I. 97.6%, 100.0%) developed an anti-HBs response ≥10 mIU/mL with a GMT of 2194.6 mIU/mL (95% C.I. 1667.8, 2887.8) in response to a dose of COMVAX at 12–15 months of age.

Antibody Responses to COMVAX and Concurrently Administered Vaccines

Immunogenicity results from open-labeled studies indicate that COMVAX can be administered concomitantly with DTP, DTaP, OPV, IPV (inactivated poliomyelitis vaccine), M-M-R II, and VARIVAX using separate sites and syringes for injectable vaccines.

DTP and DTaP

After a primary series of DTP (2, 4, 6 months of age (given concomitantly with COMVAX (2 and 4 months of age), 98.2% of 57 infants developed a 4-fold rise in antibody to diphtheria, 100% of 57 infants developed a 4-fold rise in antibody to tetanus, and 89.5% to 96.5% of 57 infants developed a 4-fold rise in antibody to pertussis antigens, depending on the assay used and adjusted for maternal antibody. In this trial, after 2 doses of COMVAX, 79.0% of 62 infants developed anti-PRP >1.0 mcg/mL and after 3 doses (2, 4, and 15 months of age), 100% of 59 infants developed ≥10 mIU/mL of anti-HBs.

After a primary series of DTaP and COMVAX given concomitantly at 2, 4, and 6 months of age, 100% of 18 infants had ≥0.01 antitoxin units/mL to diphtheria and tetanus and 94.4% to 100% of 18 infants developed a ≥4-fold rise in antibody to pertussis antigens, depending on the assay used and adjusted for maternal antibody. In this trial, after 2 doses of COMVAX, 85.7% of 63 infants developed anti-PRP >1.0 mcg/mL and after 3 doses administered on the compressed schedule of 2, 4, and 6 months of age, 92.9% of 56 infants developed ≥10 mIU/mL of anti-HBs.

OPV and IPV

After a primary series of OPV (2, 4, 6 months of age) given concomitantly with COMVAX (2 and 4 months of age), 98.3% of 60 infants had neutralizing antibody ≥1:4 to poliovirus type 1, 100% of 57 infants had neutralizing antibody ≥1:4 to poliovirus type 2 and 98.1% of 53 infants had neutralizing antibody ≥1:4 to poliovirus type 3. In this trial, after 2 doses of COMVAX, 79.0% of 62 infants developed anti-PRP >1.0 mcg/mL and after 3 doses, 100% of 59 infants developed ≥10 mIU/mL of anti-HBs.

After a primary series of IPV and COMVAX given concomitantly at 2, 4, and 6 months of age, 100% of 38 infants had neutralizing antibody ≥1:4 to poliovirus types 1, 2, and 3. In this trial, after 2 doses of COMVAX, 85.7% of 63 infants developed anti-PRP >1.0 mcg/mL and after 3 doses administered on the compressed schedule of 2, 4, and 6 months of age, 92.9% of 56 infants developed ≥10 mIU/mL of anti-HBs.

M-M-R II and VARIVAX

After concomitant vaccination of M-M-R II and VARIVAX with COMVAX (12 to 15 months of age), 99.4% of 313 children developed antibody to measles, 99.2% of 354 children developed antibody to mumps, 100% of 358 children developed antibody to rubella and 100% of 276 children developed antibody to varicella. In this trial, infants received the primary series of Hib vaccine and the first two doses of Hepatitis B vaccine in the first year of life. After the dose of COMVAX, 97.8% of 368 infants developed >1.0 mcg/mL of anti-PRP and 99.2% developed ≥10 mIU/mL of anti-HBs.

Table 1
Antibody Responses to COMVAX, PedvaxHIB, and RECOMBIVAX HB in Infants Not Previously Vaccinated with Hib or Hepatitis B Vaccine

Vaccine	Age (months)	Time	n	Anti-PRP % Subjects with >0.15 mcg/mL	Anti-PRP % Subjects with >1.0 mcg/mL	Anti-PRP GMT (mcg/mL)	n	Anti-HBs % Subjects ≥10 mIU/mL	Anti-HBs GMT (mIU/mL)
COMVAX		Prevaccination	633	34.4	4.7	0.1	603	10.6	0.6
(7.5 mcg PRP,	2	Dose 1*	620	88.9	51.5	1.0	595	34.3	4.2
5 mcg HBsAg)	4	Dose 2*	576	94.8	72.4***	2.5***	571	92.1	113.9
[N=661]	12/15	Dose 3**	570	99.3	92.6	9.5	571	98.4	4467.5***
PedvaxHIB		Prevaccination	208	33.7	5.8	0.1	196	7.1	0.5
(7.5 mcg PRP)	2	Dose 1*	202	90.1	53.5	1.1	198	41.9	5.3
+	4	Dose 2*	186	95.2	76.3***	2.8***	185	98.4***	255.7
RECOMBIVAX HB	12/15	Dose 3**	181	98.9	92.3	10.2	179	100.0***	6943.9***
(5 mcg HBsAg) [N=221]									

* Postvaccination responses were determined approximately two months after doses 1 and 2.

** Postvaccination responses were determined approximately one month after administration of dose 3.

More than three-quarters of the infants in the study received DTP and OPV concomitantly with the first two doses of COMVAX or PedvaxHIB plus RECOMBIVAX HB, and approximately one-third received M-M-R II* (Measles, Mumps, and Rubella Virus Vaccine Live) with the third dose of these vaccines at 12 or 15 months of age.

*** C.I.'s of comparisons:

Dose 2 Anti-PRP: 95% C.I. on difference in % >1.0 mcg/ml (−11.2, 3.1); 95% C.I. on ratio of GMT (0.69, 1.17)

Dose 3 Anti-HBs: 95% C.I. on difference in % ≥10 mIU/mL (−2.9, −0.6); 95% C.I. on ratio of GMT (0.49, 0.91)

Table 2
Antibody Responses to COMVAX in Infants Previously Vaccinated with Hepatitis B Vaccine at Birth

Study	Age (months) at Vaccination	Time	n	Anti-PRP % Subjects with >0.15 mcg/mL	Anti-PRP % Subjects with >1.0 mcg/mL	Anti-PRP GMT (mcg/mL)	n	Anti-HBs % Subjects ≥10mIU/mL	Anti-HBs GMT (mIU/mL)
		Prevaccination	119	24.4	5.9	0.1	71	25.4	2.9
Study 1	2	Dose 1	— Not Measured —						
[N=126]	4	Dose 2*	111	94.6	81.1	3.3	111	98.2	417.2
	14/15	Dose 3*	88	100	93.2	11.0	87	98.9	3500.7
		Prevaccination	17	58.8	0	0.2	15	6.7	0.7
Study 2	2	Dose 1**	17	88.2	47.1	0.9	16	81.3	35.2
[N=19]	4	Dose 2**	17	100	76.5	2.8	16	100	281.8
	15	Dose 3**	15	100	100	8.5	16	100	3913.4

*Postvaccination responses were determined approximately 2 months after dose 2 and 1 month after dose 3.

**Postvaccination responses were determined approximately 2 months after doses 1, 2, and 3.

Infants in these studies received DTP and OPV or eIPV (enhanced inactivated poliovirus vaccine) concomitantly with the first two doses of COMVAX, while the third dose of COMVAX was given concomitantly with DTaP (diphtheria and tetanus and acellular pertussis), OPV, and M-M-R II at 14–15 months of age (Study 1) or with just M-M-R II at 15 months of age (Study 2).

INDICATIONS AND USAGE

COMVAX is indicated for vaccination against invasive disease caused by *Haemophilus influenzae* type b and against infection caused by all known subtypes of hepatitis B virus in infants 6 weeks to 15 months of age born of HBsAg negative mothers.

Infants born to HBsAg positive mothers should receive Hepatitis B Immune Globulin and Hepatitis B Vaccine (Recombinant) at birth and should complete the hepatitis B vaccination series given according to a particular schedule (see manufacturer's circular for Hepatitis B Vaccine [Recombinant]).

Infants born to mothers of unknown HBsAg status should receive Hepatitis B Vaccine (Recombinant) at birth and should complete the hepatitis B vaccination series given according to a particular schedule (see manufacturer's circular for Hepatitis B Vaccine [Recombinant]).

Vaccination with COMVAX should ideally begin at approximately 2 months of age or as soon thereafter as possible. In order to complete the three-dose regimen of COMVAX, vaccination should be initiated no later than 10 months of age. Infants in whom vaccination with a PRP-OMPC-containing product (i.e., PedvaxHIB, COMVAX) is not initiated until 11 months of age do not require three doses of PRP-OMPC; however, three doses of an HBsAg-containing product are required for complete vaccination against hepatitis B, regardless of age. For infants and children not vaccinated according to the recommended schedule see DOSAGE AND ADMINISTRATION.

COMVAX will not protect against invasive disease caused by *Haemophilus influenzae* other than type b or against invasive disease (such as meningitis or sepsis) caused by other microorganisms. COMVAX will not prevent hepatitis caused by other viruses known to infect the liver. Because of the long incubation period for hepatitis B, it is possible for unrecognized infection to be present at the time the vaccine is given. The vaccine may not prevent hepatitis B in such patients.

As with other vaccines, COMVAX may not induce protective antibody levels immediately following vaccination and may not result in a protective antibody response in all individuals given the vaccine.

Use With Other Vaccines

Immunogenicity results from open-labeled studies indicate that COMVAX can be administered concomitantly with DTP, DTaP, OPV, IPV, M-M-R II, and VARIVAX using separate sites and syringes for injectable vaccines (see CLINICAL PHARMACOLOGY).

CONTRAINDICATIONS

Hypersensitivity to yeast or any component of the vaccine. The decision to administer or delay vaccination because of current or recent febrile illness depends on the severity of symptoms and on the etiology of the disease. The ACIP has recommended that immunization should be delayed during the course of an acute febrile illness. All vaccines can be administered to persons with minor illnesses such as diarrhea, mild upper-respiratory infection with or without low-grade fever, or other low-grade febrile illness. Persons with moderate or severe febrile illness should be vaccinated as soon as they have recovered from the acute phase of the illness.

WARNINGS

Patients who develop symptoms suggestive of hypersensitivity after an injection should not receive further injections of the vaccine (see CONTRAINDICATIONS).

PRECAUTIONS

General

General care is to be taken by the Health Care Provider for the safe and effective use of this product.

As for any vaccine, adequate treatment provisions, including epinephrine, should be available for immediate use should an anaphylactic or anaphylactoid reaction occur.

As reported with Haemophilus b Polysaccharide Vaccine and another Haemophilus b Conjugate Vaccine, cases of Haemophilus b disease may occur in the week after vaccination, prior to the onset of the protective effects of the vaccines.

Continued on next page

Information on the Merck & Co., Inc., products listed on these pages is from the prescribing information in use October 1, 2004. For information, please call 1-800-NSC-MERCK [1-800-672-6372].

Comvax—Cont.

The packaging stopper of this product contains natural rubber latex which may cause allergic reactions.
Instructions to Health-care Provider
The health-care provider should determine the current health status and previous vaccination history of the vaccinee.
The health-care provider should question the patient, parent, or guardian about reactions to a previous dose of COMVAX, PedvaxHIB or other Haemophilus b conjugate vaccines or RECOMBIVAX HB or other hepatitis B vaccines.
Injection of a blood vessel should be avoided.
COMVAX should be given with caution in infants with bleeding disorders such as hemophilia or thrombocytopenia, with steps taken to avoid the risk of hematoma following the injection.
If COMVAX is used in persons with malignancies or those receiving immunosuppressive therapy or who are otherwise immunocompromised, the expected immune response may not be obtained.
COMVAX is not contraindicated in the presence of HIV infection.
Information for Vaccine Recipients and Parents / Guardians
The health-care provider should provide the vaccine information required to be given with each vaccination to the patient, parent or guardian.
The health-care provider should inform the patient, parent or guardian of the benefits and risks associated with vaccination. For risks associated with vaccination, see WARNINGS, PRECAUTIONS, and ADVERSE REACTIONS.
Laboratory Test Interactions
Sensitive tests (e.g., Latex Agglutination Kits) may detect PRP derived from the vaccine in the urine of some vaccinees for at least 30 days following vaccination with lyophilized PedvaxHIB; in clinical studies with lyophilized PedvaxHIB, such children demonstrated a normal immune response to the vaccine. It is not known whether antigenuria will occur after vaccination with COMVAX.
Drug Interaction
Deferral of immunization may be considered in individuals receiving immunosuppressive therapy.
Carcinogenesis, Mutagenesis, Impairment of Fertility
COMVAX has not been evaluated for its carcinogenic or mutagenic potential, or its potential to impair fertility.
Pregnancy
Pregnancy Category C: Animal reproduction studies have not been conducted with COMVAX. It is also not known whether COMVAX can cause fetal harm when administered to a pregnant woman or can affect reproduction capacity. COMVAX is not recommended for use in women of child-bearing age.
Pediatric Use
Safety and effectiveness of COMVAX in infants below the age of 6 weeks and above the age of 15 months have not been established. However, studies have demonstrated that PedvaxHIB is safe and immunogenic when administered to infants and children up to the age of 71 months and RECOMBIVAX HB is safe and immunogenic in persons of all ages.
COMVAX should not be used in infants younger than 6 weeks of age because this will lead to a reduced anti-PRP response and may lead to immune tolerance (impaired ability to respond to subsequent exposure to the PRP antigen).
Infants born to HBsAg-positive mothers should not receive COMVAX but instead should receive Hepatitis B Immune Globulin and Hepatitis B Vaccine (Recombinant) at birth and should complete the hepatitis B vaccination series given according to a particular schedule (see manufacturer's circular for Hepatitis B Vaccine [Recombinant]). (See DOSAGE AND ADMINISTRATION.)
Geriatric Use
This vaccine is NOT recommended for use in adult populations.

ADVERSE REACTIONS

In clinical trials involving the administration of 7918 doses of COMVAX to 3561 healthy infants 6 weeks to 15 months of age, COMVAX was generally well tolerated. In these studies, infants received COMVAX with licensed pediatric vaccines (n=1745) or investigational vaccines (n=1816). Serious adverse experience data were available for all 3561 infants and non-serious adverse experience data were available for a subset of 1678 infants.
Pivotal Immunogenicity and Safety Study
In the pivotal, randomized, multicenter study, 882 infants were assigned in a 3:1 ratio to receive either COMVAX or PedvaxHIB plus RECOMBIVAX HB at separate injection sites at 2, 4, and 12–15 months of age. Children may have also received routine pediatric immunizations. The children were monitored daily for five days after each injection for injection-site and systemic adverse experiences. During this time, adverse experiences in infants who received COMVAX were generally similar in type and frequency to those observed in infants who received PedvaxHIB plus RECOMBIVAX HB.
The most frequently cited events were mild, transient signs and symptoms of inflammation at the injection site (i.e., pain/soreness, erythema, and swelling/induration), somnolence, and irritability, all of which were prompted for on report cards filled out by parents of vaccinated children. Table 3 summarizes the frequencies of injection-site and systemic adverse experiences within five days of vaccination that were reported among ≥1.0% of children in this pivotal trial.
[See table 3 above]

Table 3
Local Reactions and Systemic Complaints Within 5 Days After Injection Reported to Occur in ≥1.0%† of Children Given a 3-Dose Course of COMVAX Compared to These Events in Children Given Concomitant Injections of PedvaxHIB and RECOMBIVAX HB

	Injection 1‡		Injection 2‡		Injection 3	
Event	COMVAX® (N=660) %	PedvaxHIB and RECOMBIVAX HB*** (N=221) %	COMVAX® (N=645) %	PedvaxHIB and RECOMBIVAX HB*** (N=213) %	COMVAX® (N=593) %	PedvaxHIB and RECOMBIVAX HB*** (N=193) %
Injection Site Reactions						
Pain/Soreness*	34.5	37.6	24.3	25.8	23.9	21.2
Erythema (>1 in.)*	22.4 (2.7)	25.8 (2.7)	25.7 (1.4)	23.5 (3.3)	27.2 (3.0)	24.4 (1.6)
Swelling/Induration (>1 in.)*	27.6 (3.0)	33.5 (4.1)	30.4 (2.9)	31.0 (3.8)	27.2 (3.2)	29.5 (4.1)
Systemic Complaints						
Irritability*	57.0	46.6	50.7	44.1	32.2	29.0
Somnolence*	49.5	47.1	37.4	31.9	21.1	22.3
Crying—						
unusual, high pitched*	10.6	8.6	6.7	2.3	2.9	3.6
not otherwise specified	2.3	2.3	1.4	2.3	0.7	1.6
prolonged (>4 hrs.)*	2.4	2.3	0.8	1.4	0.2	0
Anorexia	3.9	2.3	2.0	0.9	0.8	0.5
Vomiting	2.1	1.8	2.5	0.9	1.0	1.6
Otitis media	0.5	0	2.0	1.4	2.7	1.6
Fever (°F, rectal equiv.)**						
101.0–102.9	14.2	11.9	13.8	12.2	10.5	6.4
≥103.0	0.8	0	1.6	1.4	2.7	4.3
Diarrhea	1.7	1.8	0.8	0.9	2.2	0.5
Upper respiratory infection	0.5	0.5	1.1	0.9	1.3	0.5
Rash	0.8	0	0.9	0	0.8	0.5
Rhinorrhea	0.2	0	1.1	0.9	1.3	2.1
Respiratory congestion	0.6	0.5	1.2	0.9	0.3	0.5
Cough	0.2	0	0.9	0.5	0.2	1.0
Candidiasis, oral	0.3	0.5	0.8	0	0.2	0
Rash, diaper	0.5	0.5	0.5	0.9	0.2	0

† Overall frequency of each event listed above is ≥1% even though the frequency after a given dose may be <1%.
‡ Most children received DTP and OPV concomitantly with the first two doses of COMVAX or PedvaxHIB and RECOMBIVAX HB.
* Events prompted for on Vaccination Report Card given to parents/guardians of vaccinees.
** N for injections 1, 2, and 3 equals 655, 639, and 588, respectively, for COMVAX; N for injections 1, 2, and 3 equals 218, 213, and 187, respectively, for PedvaxHIB and RECOMBIVAX HB.
*** Injection site reactions for PedvaxHIB and RECOMBIVAX HB based on occurrence with either of the monovalent components.

Infants Previously Vaccinated with Hepatitis B Vaccine
In a group of infants (N=126) given a three-dose course of COMVAX after previously receiving a dose of Hepatitis B Vaccine (Recombinant) at or shortly after birth, the type, frequency, and severity of adverse experiences did not appear to be greater than those observed in infants in the pivotal study who did not receive hepatitis B vaccine at birth.
Infants 6 Weeks to 15 Months of Age
In clinical trials, 3285 doses of COMVAX were administered to 1678 infants who were monitored for injection-site and systemic adverse experiences from Days 0 to 5 after each injection of vaccine. Of these, 855 infants had safety data following vaccination at approximately 2 months of age, 836 infants at approximately 4 months of age and 1573 infants at 12 to 15 months of age. The most frequently reported adverse experiences (≥1% of subjects for at least one injection), without regard to causality are listed in decreasing order of frequency within each body system:
Injection Site Reactions: Pain/tenderness/soreness, swelling/induration, erythema; *Body as a Whole:* Fever; *Digestive System:* Anorexia, diarrhea, vomiting; *Nervous System / Psychiatric:* Irritability, somnolence, crying; *Respiratory System:* Upper respiratory infection, rhinorrhea, cough, rhinitis; *Skin:* Rash; *Special Senses:* Otitis media.
Post-Marketing Experience
As with any vaccine, there is the possibility that broad use of COMVAX could reveal adverse experiences not observed in clinical trials. The following additional adverse reactions have been reported with the use of the marketed vaccine.
Hypersensitivity
Anaphylaxis, angioedema, urticaria, erythema multiforme
Hematologic
Thrombocytopenia
Nervous System
Seizure, febrile seizures
Potential Adverse Effects
In addition, a variety of adverse effects have been reported with marketed use of either PedvaxHIB or RECOMBIVAX HB in infants and children through 71 months of age. These adverse effects are listed below.
PedvaxHIB
Hematologic / Lymphatic
Lymphadenopathy
Skin
Sterile injection-site abscess; pain at the injection site
RECOMBIVAX HB
Hypersensitivity
Symptoms of hypersensitivity including reports of rash, pruritus, edema, arthralgia, dyspnea, hypotension, and ecchymoses
Cardiovascular System
Tachycardia; syncope
Digestive System
Elevation of liver enzymes
Hematologic
Increased erythrocyte sedimentation rate
Musculoskeletal System
Arthritis
Nervous System
Bell's Palsy; Guillain-Barré Syndrome
Psychiatric / Behavioral
Agitation; somnolence; irritability
Skin
Stevens-Johnson Syndrome; alopecia
Special Senses
Conjunctivitis; visual disturbances
Adverse Event Reporting
Patients, parents and guardians should be instructed to report any serious adverse reactions to their health-care provider who in turn should report such events to the U.S. Department of Health and Human Services through the Vaccine Adverse Event Reporting System (VAERS), 1-800-822-7967. The health-care provider should inform the parent or guardian of the National Vaccine Injury Compensation Program (NVICP), 1-888-338-2382 or http://www.hrsa.dhhs.gov/bhpr/vicp.

DOSAGE AND ADMINISTRATION

FOR INTRAMUSCULAR ADMINISTRATION
Do not inject intravenously, intradermally, or subcutaneously.
Recommended Schedule
Infants born to HBsAg negative mothers should be vaccinated with three 0.5 mL doses of COMVAX, ideally at 2, 4, and 12–15 months of age. If the recommended schedule cannot be followed, the interval between the first two doses should be at least six weeks and the interval between the second and third dose should be as close as possible to eight to eleven months.
Infants born to HBsAg-positive mothers should receive Hepatitis B Immune Globulin and Hepatitis B Vaccine (Recombinant) at birth and should complete the hepatitis B vaccination series given according to a particular schedule (see manufacturer's circular for Hepatitis B Vaccine [Recombinant]).
Infants born to mothers of unknown HBsAg status should receive Hepatitis B Vaccine (Recombinant) at birth and should complete the hepatitis B vaccination series given according to a particular schedule (see manufacturer's circular for Hepatitis B Vaccine [Recombinant]).
The subsequent administration of COMVAX for completion of the hepatitis B vaccination series in infants who were

born to HBsAg positive mothers and received HBIG or infants born to mothers of unknown status has not been studied.
COMVAX should not be administered to any infant before the age of 6 weeks.
Modified Schedules
Children previously vaccinated with one or more doses of either hepatitis B vaccine or Haemophilus b conjugate vaccine
Children who receive one dose of hepatitis B vaccine at or shortly after birth may be administered COMVAX on the schedule of 2, 4, and 12–15 months of age. There are no data to support the use of a three-dose series of COMVAX in infants who have previously received more than one dose of hepatitis B vaccine. However, COMVAX may be administered to children otherwise scheduled to receive concurrent RECOMBIVAX HB and PedvaxHIB.
Children not vaccinated according to recommended schedule for COMVAX
Vaccination schedules for children not vaccinated according to the recommended schedule should be considered on an individual basis. The number of doses of a PRP-OMPC-containing product (i.e., COMVAX, PedvaxHIB) depends on the age that vaccination is begun. An infant 2 to 10 months of age should receive three doses of a product containing PRP-OMPC. An infant 11 to 14 months of age should receive two doses of a product containing PRP-OMPC. A child 15 to 71 months of age should receive one dose of a product containing PRP-OMPC. Infants and children, regardless of age, should receive three doses of an HBsAg-containing product.
COMVAX is for intramuscular injection. The *anterolateral thigh* is the recommended site for intramuscular injection in infants. Data suggests that injections given in the buttocks frequently are given into fatty tissue instead of into muscle. Such injections have resulted in a lower seroconversion rate (for hepatitis B vaccine) than was expected.
Injection must be accomplished with a needle long enough to ensure intramuscular deposition of the vaccine. The ACIP has recommended that for intramuscular injections, the needle should be of sufficient length to reach the muscle mass itself. In a clinical trial with COMVAX (see CLINICAL PHARMACOLOGY, *Antibody Responses to COMVAX in Infants Not Previously Vaccinated with Hib or Hepatitis B Vaccine*, Table 1) vaccination was accomplished with a needle length of 5/8 inches in accordance with ACIP recommendations in effect at that time. ACIP currently recommends that needles of longer length (7/8 to 1 inch) be used.
The vaccine should be used as supplied; no reconstitution is necessary.
Shake well before withdrawal and use. Thorough agitation is necessary to maintain suspension of the vaccine.
Parenteral drug products should be inspected visually for extraneous particulate matter and discoloration prior to administration whenever solution and container permit. After thorough agitation, COMVAX is a slightly opaque, white suspension.
It is important to use a separate sterile syringe and needle for each patient to prevent transmission of infectious agents from one person to another.
Interchangeability of COMVAX and Licensed Haemophilus b Conjugate Vaccines or Recombinant Hepatitis B Vaccines
Since 1990, the Advisory Committee on Immunization Practices (ACIP) and the Committee on Infectious Diseases of the American Academy of Pediatrics (AAP) have recommended routine immunization of infants starting at 2 months of age with a polysaccharide – protein conjugate vaccine to prevent invasive Hib disease.
Three Hib vaccines are licensed for infant vaccination: 1) oligosaccharide conjugate Hib vaccine (HbOC) (HibTITER®**), 2) polyribosylribitol phosphate-tetanus toxoid conjugate (PRP-T) (ActHIB®** and OmniHIB®**), and 3) Haemophilus b conjugate vaccine (meningococcal protein conjugate) (PRP-OMP) (PedvaxHIB®). According to the ACIP, these products are now considered interchangeable for primary as well as booster vaccination.
Because vaccination recommendations limited to high-risk individuals have failed to substantially lower the overall incidence of hepatitis B infection, both the Advisory Committee on Immunization Practices (ACIP) and the Committee on Infectious Diseases of the American Academy of Pediatrics (AAP) have endorsed universal infant immunization as part of a comprehensive strategy for the control of hepatitis B infection.

**HibTITER is a registered trademark of Lederle Laboratories, ActHIB is a registered trademark of Aventis Pasteur Inc. and OmniHIB is a registered trademark of GlaxoSmithKline.

HOW SUPPLIED

No. 4898 — COMVAX is supplied as 7.5 mcg PRP polysaccharide conjugated to approximately 125 mcg OMPC and 5 mcg HBsAg in a box of 10 single dose vials.
NDC 0006-4898-00.
Storage
Store vaccine at 2–8°C (36–46°F). Storage above or below the recommended temperature may reduce potency.
DO NOT FREEZE since freezing destroys potency.
9376601 Issued March 2002

COSMEGEN® for Injection ℞
(Dactinomycin for Injection)
(Actinomycin D)

> **WARNING**
> COSMEGEN* (Dactinomycin for Injection) should be administered only under the supervision of a physician who is experienced in the use of cancer chemotherapeutic agents.
> This drug is **HIGHLY TOXIC** and both powder and solution must be handled and administered with care. Inhalation of dust or vapors and contact with skin or mucous membranes, especially those of the eyes, must be avoided. Avoid exposure during pregnancy. Due to the toxic properties of dactinomycin (e.g., corrosivity, carcinogenicity, mutagenicity, teratogenicity), special handling procedures should be reviewed prior to handling and followed diligently. Dactinomycin is extremely corrosive to soft tissue. If extravasation occurs during intravenous use, severe damage to soft tissues will occur. In at least one instance, this has led to contracture of the arms.

*Registered trademark of MERCK & CO., Inc.

DESCRIPTION

Dactinomycin is one of the actinomycins, a group of antibiotics produced by various species of *Streptomyces*. Dactinomycin is the principal component of the mixture of actinomycins produced by *Streptomyces parvullus*. Unlike other species of *Streptomyces*, this organism yields an essentially pure substance that contains only traces of similar compounds differing in the amino acid content of the peptide side chains. The empirical formula is $C_{62}H_{86}N_{12}O_{16}$ and the structural formula is:

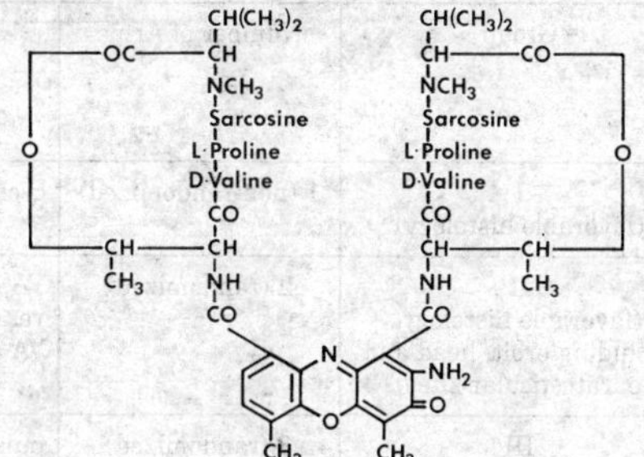

COSMEGEN is a sterile, yellow lyophilized powder for injection by the intravenous route or by regional perfusion after reconstitution. Each vial contains 0.5 mg (500 mcg) of dactinomycin and 20.0 mg of mannitol.

CLINICAL PHARMACOLOGY

Action
Generally, the actinomycins exert an inhibitory effect on gram-positive and gram-negative bacteria and on some fungi. However, the toxic properties of the actinomycins (including dactinomycin) in relation to antibacterial activity are such as to preclude their use as antibiotics in the treatment of infectious diseases.
Because the actinomycins are cytotoxic, they have an antineoplastic effect which has been demonstrated in experimental animals with various types of tumor implant. This cytotoxic action is the basis for their use in the treatment of certain types of cancer. Dactinomycin is believed to produce its cytotoxic effects by binding DNA and inhibiting RNA synthesis.
Pharmacokinetics and Metabolism
Results of a study in patients with malignant melanoma indicate that dactinomycin (^3H actinomycin D) is minimally metabolized, is concentrated in nucleated cells, and does not penetrate the blood-brain barrier. Approximately 30% of the dose was recovered in urine and feces in one week. The terminal plasma half-life for radioactivity was approximately 36 hours.

CLINICAL STUDIES

A wide variety of single agent and combination chemotherapy regimens with COSMEGEN have been studied. Because chemotherapeutic regimens are constantly changing, the decision to employ COSMEGEN should be directly supervised by physicians familiar with current oncologic practices and new advances in therapy.
Wilms' Tumor
The neoplasm responding most frequently to COSMEGEN is Wilms' tumor. Data from the National Wilms' Tumor Studies (NWTS-1, NWTS-2, NWTS-3 and NWTS-4) support the use of COSMEGEN in Wilms' tumor. The NWTS-3 evaluated results in 1,439 patients randomized to various regimens incorporating COSMEGEN (see table below).
[See first table at top of next page]
It should be noted that the complete results from NWTS-4 have not yet been published. Changes in NWTS-4 and NWTS-5 have consisted of alterations in duration as well as dose intensity of COSMEGEN. As a consequence, appropriate consultation with physicians experienced in the management of Wilms' tumor should be sought.
Childhood Rhabdomyosarcoma
The Third Intergroup Rhabdomyosarcoma Study (IRS-III) studied 1,062 previously untreated pediatric patients and young adults (≤21 years of age) and compared outcomes amongst a number of treatment regimens. COSMEGEN was included in all arms as a standard component of the treatment regimen; thus, comparative data are not available from this study. Nevertheless, it does provide information on treatment outcomes in a large group of closely studied patients. For treatment purposes, patients were stratified according to clinical group, histologic subtype, and site of disease. Patients in most strata were randomized, but clinical group I patients with favorable histology were not randomized and treated according to a single regimen.
[See second table on next page]
Metastatic Nonseminomatous Testicular Cancer
Combinations of vinblastine, cyclophosphamide, COSMEGEN, bleomycin and cisplatin (VAB-6 regimen) have been employed in the treatment of metastatic nonseminomatous testicular cancer. In a retrospective analysis of 142 evaluable patients with primary advanced stage II or clinical stage III testicular cancer 112 (79%) achieved a complete response (CR) after treatment with VAB-6 alone or in combination with surgery. Relapses were uncommon (12%) and 117 of 166 patients (71%) were categorized as alive without evidence of disease during the four years covered by the study.
Ewing's Sarcoma
COSMEGEN in conjunction with vincristine, doxorubicin, cyclophosphamide and radiotherapy has been used in the management of both metastatic and non-metastatic Ewing's sarcoma. Of 120 previously untreated patients with non-metastatic disease treated with COSMEGEN as part of maintenance therapy in the United Kingdom Children's Cancer Study Group Ewing's Tumor Study (ET-1), 49 (41%) were free of disease at 5 years and 53 (44%) were alive at 5 years. Outcomes in regional and metastatic disease for previously untreated patients administered COSMEGEN resulted in 31 of 44 patients (70%) achieving a CR after a median time on study of 83 weeks. Eight of 44 (18%) patients achieved a partial response (PR) and the remaining 5 (11%) demonstrated no response to the regimen.
Gestational Trophoblastic Neoplasia
Single agent COSMEGEN has been used in the management of nonmetastatic gestational trophoblastic neoplasia. In a series of 31 patients with nonmetastatic disease, complete and sustained remissions were achieved with COSMEGEN alone in 94% of treated patients. Alternating combination regimens incorporating COSMEGEN in conjunction with etoposide, methotrexate, vincristine and cyclophosphamide (EMA-CO regimen) have also been used in the treatment of poor prognosis gestational trophoblastic neoplasia. Administration of EMA-CO to 148 women with poor prognosis gestational trophoblastic neoplasia resulted in 110 (80%) complete and 25 (18%) partial responses after a mean follow-up of 50.4 months. Overall survival during the study period was 85% and relapses were uncommon (5.4%). Meticulous monitoring of beta-hCG (human chorionic gonadotropin) must be incorporated into the treatment regimen.
Regional Perfusion in Locally Recurrent and Locoregional Solid Malignancies
COSMEGEN, as a component of regional perfusion, has been administered as palliative treatment and as an adjunct to tumor resection in the management of locally recurrent and locoregional sarcomas, carcinomas and adenocarcinomas.

INDICATIONS AND USAGE

COSMEGEN, as part of a combination chemotherapy and/or multi-modality treatment regimen, is indicated for the treatment of Wilms' tumor, childhood rhabdomyosarcoma, Ewing's sarcoma and metastatic, nonseminomatous testicular cancer.
COSMEGEN is indicated as a single agent, or as part of a combination chemotherapy regimen, for the treatment of gestational trophoblastic neoplasia.
COSMEGEN, as a component of regional perfusion, is indicated for the palliative and/or adjunctive treatment of locally recurrent or locoregional solid malignancies.

CONTRAINDICATIONS

COSMEGEN should not be given at or about the time of infection with chickenpox or herpes zoster because of the risk of severe generalized disease which may result in death.

WARNINGS

Reports indicate an increased incidence of second primary tumors (including leukemia) following treatment with radi-

Continued on next page

Information on the Merck & Co., Inc., products listed on these pages is from the prescribing information in use October 1, 2004. For information, please call 1-800-NSC-MERCK [1-800-672-6372].

Cosmegen—Cont.

ation and antineoplastic agents, such as COSMEGEN. Multi-modal therapy creates the need for careful, long-term observation of cancer survivors.

Pregnancy Category D

COSMEGEN may cause fetal harm when administered to a pregnant woman. COSMEGEN has been shown to cause malformations and embryotoxicity in rat, rabbit, and hamster when given in doses of 50–100 mcg/kg (approximately 0.5–2 times the maximum recommended daily human dose on a body surface area basis). If this drug is used during pregnancy, or if the patient becomes pregnant while receiving this drug, the patient should be apprised of the potential hazard to the fetus. Women of childbearing potential must be warned to avoid becoming pregnant.

PRECAUTIONS

General

This drug is **HIGHLY TOXIC** and both powder and solution must be handled and administered with care (see boxed warning and HOW SUPPLIED, *Special Handling*). Since COSMEGEN is extremely corrosive to soft tissues, it is intended for intravenous use. Inhalation of dust or vapors and contact with skin or mucous membranes, especially those of the eyes, must be avoided. Appropriate protective equipment should be worn when handling COSMEGEN. Should accidental eye contact occur, copious irrigation for at least 15 minutes with water, normal saline or a balanced salt ophthalmic irrigating solution should be instituted immediately, followed by prompt ophthalmologic consultation. Should accidental skin contact occur, the affected part must be irrigated immediately with copious amounts of water for at least 15 minutes while removing contaminated clothing and shoes. Medical attention should be sought immediately. Contaminated clothing should be destroyed and shoes cleaned thoroughly before reuse (see HOW SUPPLIED, *Special Handling*).

As with all antineoplastic agents, COSMEGEN is a toxic drug and very careful and frequent observation of the patient for adverse reactions is necessary. These reactions may involve any tissue of the body, most commonly the hematopoietic system resulting in myelosuppression. The possibility of an anaphylactoid reaction should be borne in mind. It is extremely important to observe the patient daily for toxic side effects when combination chemotherapy is employed, since a full course of therapy occasionally is not tolerated. If stomatitis, diarrhea, or severe hematopoietic depression appear during therapy, these drugs should be discontinued until the patient has recovered.

COSMEGEN (Dactinomycin for Injection) and Radiation Therapy

An increased incidence of gastrointestinal toxicity and marrow suppression has been reported with combined therapy incorporating COSMEGEN and radiation. Moreover, the normal skin, as well as the buccal and pharyngeal mucosa, may show early erythema. A smaller than usual radiation dose administered in combination with COSMEGEN causes erythema and vesiculation, which progress more rapidly through the stages of tanning and desquamation. Healing may occur in four to six weeks rather than two to three months. Erythema from previous radiation therapy may be reactivated by COSMEGEN alone, even when radiotherapy was administered many months earlier, and especially when the interval between the two forms of therapy is brief. This potentiation of radiation effect represents a special problem when the radiotherapy involves the mucous membrane. When irradiation is directed toward the nasopharynx, the combination may produce severe oropharyngeal mucositis. *Severe reactions may ensue if high doses of both COSMEGEN and radiation therapy are used or if the patient is particularly sensitive to such combined therapy.*

Particular caution is necessary when administering COSMEGEN within two months of irradiation for the treatment of right-sided Wilms' tumor, since hepatomegaly and elevated AST levels have been noted. In general, COSMEGEN should not be concomitantly administered with radiotherapy in the treatment of Wilms' tumor unless the benefit outweighs the risk.

COSMEGEN (Dactinomycin for Injection) and Regional Perfusion Therapy

Complications of the perfusion technique are related mainly to the amount of drug that escapes into the systemic circulation and may consist of hematopoietic depression, absorption of toxic products from massive destruction of neoplastic tissue, increased susceptibility to infection, impaired wound healing, and superficial ulceration of the gastric mucosa. Other side effects may include edema of the extremity involved, damage to soft tissues of the perfused area, and (potentially) venous thrombosis.

Laboratory Tests

Many abnormalities of renal, hepatic, and bone marrow function have been reported in patients with neoplastic diseases receiving COSMEGEN. Renal, hepatic, and bone marrow functions should be assessed frequently.

Drug/Laboratory Test Interactions

Dactinomycin may interfere with bioassay procedures for the determination of antibacterial drug levels.

Carcinogenesis, Mutagenesis, Impairment of Fertility

Reports indicate an increased incidence of second primary tumors (including leukemia) following treatment with radi-

The Third National Wilms' Tumor Study

Stage	Regimen	4-Year Relapse Free Survival (%)	4-Year Overall Survival (%)
I (favorable histology)	L	89.0	95.6
	EE	91.8	97.4
II (favorable histology)	DD	87.9	93.6
	DD2	86.9	89.6
	K	87.4	91.1
	K2	90.1	94.9
III (favorable histology)	DD1	82.0	90.9
	DD2	85.9	86.7
	K1	71.4	85.2
	K2	76.8	85.1
IV (favorable histology)	DD-RT	71.9	78.4
	J	77.9	86.6
I-III (unfavorable histology)	DD-RT	67.1	68.3
	J	62.4	68.4
IV (unfavorable histology)	DD-RT	58.3	58.3
	J	52.9	52.3

L = COSMEGEN and vincristine (10 weeks)
EE = COSMEGEN and vincristine (26 weeks)
DD = COSMEGEN, doxorubicin, and vincristine (65 weeks)
DD1 = COSMEGEN, doxorubicin, and vincristine (65 weeks) preceded by radiation therapy (1000 rads)
DD2 = COSMEGEN, doxorubicin, and vincristine (65 weeks) preceded by radiation therapy (2000 rads)
DD-RT = COSMEGEN, doxorubicin, and vincristine (65 weeks) preceded by radiation therapy (dose according to age)
K = COSMEGEN and vincristine (65 weeks)
K1 = COSMEGEN and vincristine (65 weeks) preceded by radiation therapy (1000 rads)
K2 = COSMEGEN and vincristine (65 weeks) preceded by radiation therapy (2000 rads)
J = COSMEGEN, doxorubicin, cyclophosphamide, and vincristine (65 weeks)

The Third Intergroup Rhabdomyosarcoma Study

Group	Number of Arms	Chemotherapy Regimen	5-Year Progression Free Survival (%) (mean±SEM)	5-Year Overall Survival (%) (mean±SEM)
I (favorable histology)	1 (non-randomized)	cyclic sequential VA (1 year)	83±3	93±2
II (favorable histology, excluding orbit, head and paratesticular sites)	2 (randomized)	VA, doxorubicin and RT (1 year)	77±6	89±5
		VA and RT (1 year)	56±10	54±13
III (excluding special pelvic, orbit, scalp, parotid, oral cavity, larynx, oropharynx and cheek)	3 (randomized)	pulsed VAC and RT (2 years)	70±6	70±6
		pulsed VADRC-VAC, CDDP and RT (2 years)	62±5	63±5
		pulsed VADRC-VAC, CDDP, VP-16 and RT (2 years)	56±4	64±5
IV (all)	3 (randomized)	pulsed VAC and RT (2 years)	27±8	27±6
		pulsed VADRC-VAC, CDDP and RT (2 years)	27±8	31±6
		pulsed VADRC-VAC, CDDP, VP-16 and RT (2 years)	30±6	29±7

VA = vincristine/COSMEGEN
VADRC = vincristine/doxorubicin/cyclophosphamide
VAC = vincristine/COSMEGEN/cyclophosphamide
CDDP = cisplatin
VP-16 = etoposide
RT = radiation therapy

ation and antineoplastic agents, such as COSMEGEN. Multi-modal therapy creates the need for careful, long-term observation of cancer survivors.

The International Agency on Research on Cancer has judged that dactinomycin is a positive carcinogen in animals. Local sarcomas were produced in mice and rats after repeated subcutaneous or intraperitoneal injection. Mesenchymal tumors occurred in male F344 rats given intraperitoneal injections of 50 mcg/kg, 2 to 5 times per week for 18 weeks. The first tumor appeared at 23 weeks.

Dactinomycin has been shown to be mutagenic in a number of test systems *in vitro* and *in vivo* including human fibroblasts and leukocytes, and HeLa cells. DNA damage and cytogenetic effects have been demonstrated in the mouse and the rat.

Adequate fertility studies have not been reported, although, reports suggest an increased incidence of infertility following treatment with other antineoplastic agents.

Pregnancy

Pregnancy Category D

(See WARNINGS.)

Nursing Mothers

It is not known whether this drug is excreted in human milk. Because many drugs are excreted in human milk and because of the potential for serious adverse reactions in nursing infants from COSMEGEN, a decision should be made as to discontinuation of nursing and/or drug, taking into account the importance of the drug to the mother.

Pediatric Use

The greater frequency of toxic effects of COSMEGEN in infants suggest that this drug should be administered to infants only over the age of 6 to 12 months.

Geriatric Use

Clinical studies of COSMEGEN did not include sufficient numbers of subjects aged 65 and over to determine whether they respond differently from younger subjects. Other reported clinical experience has not identified differences in responses between the elderly and younger patients. However, a published meta-analysis of all studies performed by the Eastern Cooperative Oncology Group (ECOG) over a 13-year period suggests that administration of COSMEGEN to elderly patients may be associated with an increased risk of myelosuppression compared to younger patients. In general, dose selection for an elderly patient should be cautious, usually starting at the low end of the dosing range, reflecting the greater frequency of decreased hepatic, renal, or cardiac function, and of concomitant disease or other drug therapy.

ADVERSE REACTIONS

Toxic effects (excepting nausea and vomiting) usually do not become apparent until two to four days after a course of therapy is stopped, and may not peak until one to two weeks have elapsed. Deaths have been reported. However, adverse reactions are usually reversible on discontinuance of therapy. They include the following.

Miscellaneous: malaise, fatigue, lethargy, fever, myalgia, proctitis, hypocalcemia, growth retardation, infection.

Oral: cheilitis, dysphagia, esophagitis, ulcerative stomatitis, pharyngitis.

Lung: pneumonitis.

Gastrointestinal: anorexia, nausea, vomiting, abdominal pain, diarrhea, gastrointestinal ulceration, liver toxicity in-

cluding ascites, hepatomegaly, hepatic veno-occlusive disease, hepatitis, and liver function test abnormalities. Nausea and vomiting, which occur early during the first few hours of administration, may be alleviated by the administration of anti-emetics.
Hematologic: anemia, even to the point of aplastic anemia, agranulocytosis, leukopenia, thrombocytopenia, pancytopenia, reticulocytopenia. Platelet and white cell counts should be performed *frequently* to detect severe hematopoietic depression. If either count markedly decreases, the drug should be withheld to allow marrow recovery. This often takes up to three weeks.
Dermatologic: alopecia, skin eruptions, acne, flare-up of erythema or increased pigmentation of previously irradiated skin.
Soft tissues: Dactinomycin is extremely corrosive. If extravasation occurs during intravenous use, severe damage to soft tissues will occur. In at least one instance, this has led to contracture of the arms. Epidermolysis, erythema, and edema, at times severe, have been reported with regional limb perfusion.
Laboratory Tests
Many abnormalities of renal, hepatic, and bone marrow function have been reported in patients with neoplastic diseases receiving COSMEGEN. Renal, hepatic, and bone marrow functions should be assessed frequently.

OVERDOSAGE

Dactinomycin was lethal to mice and rats at intravenous doses of 700 and 500 mcg/kg, respectively (approximately 3.8 and 5.4 times the maximum recommended daily human dose on a body surface area basis, respectively). The oral LD_{50} of dactinomycin is 7.8 mg/kg and 7.2 mg/kg in the mouse and rat, respectively.

DOSAGE AND ADMINISTRATION

Not for oral administration
Toxic reactions due to COSMEGEN are frequent and may be severe (see ADVERSE REACTIONS), thus limiting in many instances the amount that may be administered. However, the severity of toxicity varies markedly and is only partly dependent on the dose employed.
Intravenous Use
The dosage of COSMEGEN varies depending on the tolerance of the patient, the size and location of the neoplasm, and the use of other forms of therapy. It may be necessary to decrease the usual dosages suggested below when additional chemotherapy or radiation therapy is used concomitantly or has been used previously.
The dosage for COSMEGEN is calculated in micrograms (mcg). The dose intensity per 2-week cycle for adults or children should not exceed 15 mcg/kg/day or 400–600 mcg/m^2/day intravenously for five days. Calculation of the dosage for obese or edematous patients should be performed on the basis of surface area in an effort to more closely relate dosage to lean body mass.
A wide variety of single agent and combination chemotherapy regimens with COSMEGEN may be employed. Because chemotherapeutic regimens are constantly changing, dosing and administration should be performed under the direct supervision of physicians familiar with current oncologic practices and new advances in therapy. The following suggested regimens are based upon a review of current literature concerning therapy with COSMEGEN and are on a per cycle basis.
Wilms' Tumor, Childhood Rhabdomyosarcoma and Ewing's Sarcoma
Regimens of 15 mcg/kg intravenously daily for five days administered in various combinations and schedules with other chemotherapeutic agents have been utilized in the treatment of Wilms' tumor, rhabdomyosarcoma and Ewing's sarcoma.
Metastatic Nonseminomatous Testicular Cancer
1000 mcg/m^2 intravenously on Day 1 as part of a combination regimen with cyclophosphamide, bleomycin, vinblastine, and cisplatin.
Gestational Trophoblastic Neoplasia
12 mcg/kg intravenously daily for five days as a single agent.
500 mcg intravenously on Days 1 and 2 as part of a combination regimen with etoposide, methotrexate, folinic acid, vincristine, cyclophosphamide and cisplatin.
Regional Perfusion in Locally Recurrent and Locoregional Solid Malignancies
The dosage schedules and the technique itself vary from one investigator to another; the published literature, therefore, should be consulted for details. In general, the following doses are suggested.
50 mcg (0.05 mg) per kilogram of body weight for lower extremity or pelvis.
35 mcg (0.035 mg) per kilogram of body weight for upper extremity.
It may be advisable to use lower doses in obese patients, or when previous chemotherapy or radiation therapy has been employed.
Preparation of Solution for Intravenous Administration
This drug is **HIGHLY TOXIC** and both powder and solution must be handled and administered with care (see boxed warning and HOW SUPPLIED, *Special Handling*). Since COSMEGEN is extremely corrosive to soft tissues, it is intended for intravenous use. Inhalation of dust or vapors and contact with skin or mucous membranes, especially those of the eyes, must be avoided. Appropriate protective equipment should be worn when handling COSMEGEN. Should accidental eye contact occur, copious irrigation for at least 15 minutes with water, normal saline or a balanced salt ophthalmic irrigating solution should be instituted immediately, followed by prompt ophthalmologic consultation. Should accidental skin contact occur, the affected part must be irrigated immediately with copious amounts of water for at least 15 minutes while removing contaminated clothing and shoes. Medical attention should be sought immediately. Contaminated clothing should be destroyed and shoes cleaned thoroughly before reuse. (See HOW SUPPLIED, *Special Handling*.)
Reconstitute COSMEGEN by adding 1.1 mL of **Sterile Water for Injection (without preservative)** using aseptic precautions. The resulting solution of COSMEGEN will contain approximately 500 mcg (0.5 mg) per mL.
Parenteral drug products should be inspected visually for particulate matter and discoloration prior to administration, whenever solution and container permit. When reconstituted, COSMEGEN is a clear, gold-colored solution.
Once reconstituted, the solution of COSMEGEN can be added to infusion solutions of Dextrose Injection 5 percent or Sodium Chloride Injection either directly or to the tubing of a running intravenous infusion.
Although reconstituted COSMEGEN is chemically stable, the product does not contain a preservative and accidental microbial contamination might result. Any unused portion should be discarded. Use of water containing preservatives (benzyl alcohol or parabens) to reconstitute COSMEGEN for Injection, results in the formation of a precipitate.
Partial removal of COSMEGEN from intravenous solutions by cellulose ester membrane filters used in some intravenous in-line filters has been reported.
Since dactinomycin is extremely corrosive to soft tissue, precautions for materials of this nature should be observed.
If the drug is given directly into the vein without the use of an infusion, the "two-needle technique" should be used. Reconstitute and withdraw the calculated dose from the vial with one sterile needle. Use another sterile needle for direct injection into the vein.
Discard any unused portion of the COSMEGEN solution.
Management of Extravasation
Care in the administration of COSMEGEN will reduce the chance of perivenous infiltration (see boxed warning and ADVERSE REACTIONS). It may also decrease the chance of local reactions such as urticaria and erythematous streaking. On intravenous administration of COSMEGEN, extravasation may occur with or without an accompanying burning or stinging sensation, even if blood returns well on aspiration of the infusion needle. If any signs or symptoms of extravasation have occurred, the injection or infusion should be immediately terminated and restarted in another vein. If extravasation is suspected, intermittent application of ice to the site for 15 minutes q.i.d. for 3 days may be useful. The benefit of local administration of drugs has not been clearly established. Because of the progressive nature of extravasation reactions, close observation and plastic surgery consultation is recommended. Blistering, ulceration and/or persistent pain are indications for wide excision surgery, followed by split-thickness skin grafting.

HOW SUPPLIED

No. 3298—COSMEGEN for Injection is a lyophilized powder. In the dry form the compound is an amorphous yellow to orange powder. The solution is clear and gold-colored.
COSMEGEN for Injection is supplied as follows:
NDC 0006-3298-22 in vials containing 0.5 mg (500 micrograms) of dactinomycin and 20.0 mg of mannitol.
Storage
Store at 25°C (77°F); excursions permitted to 15–30°C (59–86°F) [see USP Controlled Room Temperature]. Protect from light and humidity.
Special Handling
Animal studies have shown dactinomycin to be corrosive to skin, irritating to the eyes and mucous membranes of the respiratory tract and highly toxic by the oral route. It has also been shown to be carcinogenic, mutagenic, embryotoxic and teratogenic. Due to the drug's toxic properties, appropriate precautions including the use of appropriate safety equipment are recommended for the preparation of COSMEGEN for parenteral administration. Inhalation of dust or vapors and contact with skin or mucous membranes, especially those of the eyes, must be avoided. Avoid exposure during pregnancy. The National Institutes of Health presently recommends that the preparation of injectable antineoplastic drugs should be performed in a Class II laminar flow biological safety cabinet. Personnel preparing drugs of this class should wear chemical resistant, impervious gloves, safety goggles, outer garments and shoe covers. Additional body garments should be used based upon the task being performed (e.g., sleevelets, apron, gauntlets, disposable suits) to avoid exposed skin surfaces and inhalation of vapors and dust. Appropriate techniques should be used to remove potentially contaminated clothing.
Several other guidelines for proper handling and disposal of antineoplastic drugs have been published and should be considered.
Accidental Contact Measures
Should accidental eye contact occur, copious irrigation for at least 15 minutes with water, normal saline or a balanced salt ophthalmic irrigating solution should be instituted immediately, followed by prompt ophthalmologic consultation. Should accidental skin contact occur, the affected part must be irrigated immediately with copious amounts of water for at least 15 minutes while removing contaminated clothing and shoes. Medical attention should be sought immediately. Contaminated clothing should be destroyed and shoes cleaned thoroughly before reuse (see PRECAUTIONS, *General* and DOSAGE AND ADMINISTRATION, *Preparation of Solution for Intravenous Administration*).

9000833 Issued December 2002

COSOPT® ℞

(dorzolamide hydrochloride-timolol maleate ophthalmic solution)
Sterile Ophthalmic Solution

DESCRIPTION

COSOPT* (dorzolamide hydrochloride-timolol maleate ophthalmic solution) is the combination of a topical carbonic anhydrase inhibitor and a topical beta-adrenergic receptor blocking agent.
Dorzolamide hydrochloride is described chemically as: (4*S-trans*)-4-(ethylamino)-5,6-dihydro-6-methyl-4*H*-thieno[2,3-*b*]thiopyran-2-sulfonamide 7,7-dioxide monohydrochloride. Dorzolamide hydrochloride is optically active. The specific rotation is:

$$[\alpha]^{25^\circ C}_{405\ nm} \ (C=1, \text{water}) = \sim -17^\circ.$$

Its empirical formula is $C_{10}H_{16}N_2O_4S_3 \bullet HCl$ and its structural formula is:

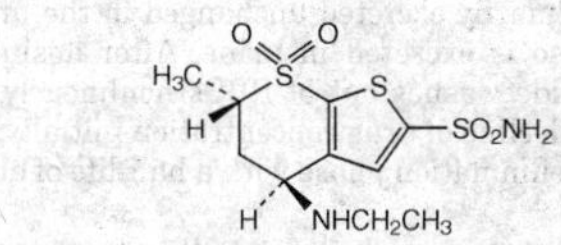

H_3C, H, O, O, S, S, $SO_2NH_2 \bullet HCl$, H, $NHCH_2CH_3$

Dorzolamide hydrochloride has a molecular weight of 360.91. It is a white to off-white, crystalline powder, which is soluble in water and slightly soluble in methanol and ethanol.
Timolol maleate is described chemically as: (-)-1-(*tert*-butylamino)-3-[(4-morpholino-1,2,5-thiadiazol-3-yl)oxy]-2-propanol maleate (1:1) (salt). Timolol maleate possesses an asymmetric carbon atom in its structure and is provided as the levo-isomer. The nominal optical rotation of timolol maleate is:

$$[\alpha]^{25^\circ C}_{405\ nm} \ \text{in 1N HCl } (C=5) = -12.2^\circ \ (-11.7^\circ \text{ to } -12.5^\circ).$$

Its molecular formula is $C_{13}H_{24}N_4O_3S \bullet C_4H_4O_4$ and its structural formula is:

N, S, N, O, N, OH, CH_3, $OCH_2CCH_2NHC—CH_3 \bullet$, H, CH_3, HC–COOH, HC–COOH

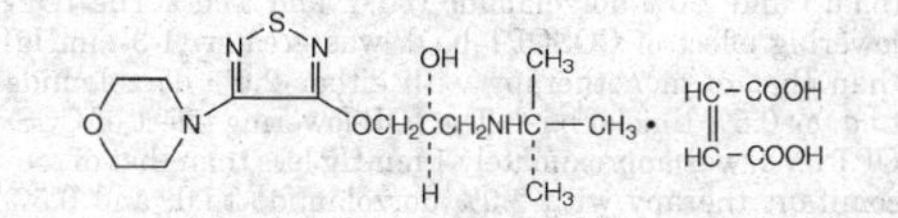

Timolol maleate has a molecular weight of 432.50. It is a white, odorless, crystalline powder which is soluble in water, methanol, and alcohol. Timolol maleate is stable at room temperature.
COSOPT is supplied as a sterile, isotonic, buffered, slightly viscous, aqueous solution. The pH of the solution is approximately 5.65, and the osmolarity is 242-323 mOsM. Each mL of COSOPT contains 20 mg dorzolamide (22.26 mg of dorzolamide hydrochloride) and 5 mg timolol (6.83 mg timolol maleate). Inactive ingredients are sodium citrate, hydroxyethyl cellulose, sodium hydroxide, mannitol, and water for injection. Benzalkonium chloride 0.0075% is added as a preservative.

*Registered trademark of MERCK & CO., Inc.

CLINICAL PHARMACOLOGY

Mechanism of Action
COSOPT is comprised of two components: dorzolamide hydrochloride and timolol maleate. Each of these two components decreases elevated intraocular pressure, whether or not associated with glaucoma, by reducing aqueous humor secretion. Elevated intraocular pressure is a major risk factor in the pathogenesis of optic nerve damage and glauco-

Continued on next page

Information on the Merck & Co., Inc., products listed on these pages is from the prescribing information in use October 1, 2004. For information, please call 1-800-NSC-MERCK [1-800-672-6372].

Cosopt—Cont.

matous visual field loss. The higher the level of intraocular pressure, the greater the likelihood of glaucomatous field loss and optic nerve damage.
Dorzolamide hydrochloride is an inhibitor of human carbonic anhydrase II. Inhibition of carbonic anhydrase in the ciliary processes of the eye decreases aqueous humor secretion, presumably by slowing the formation of bicarbonate ions with subsequent reduction in sodium and fluid transport. Timolol maleate is a $beta_1$ and $beta_2$ (non-selective) adrenergic receptor blocking agent that does not have significant intrinsic sympathomimetic, direct myocardial depressant, or local anesthetic (membrane-stabilizing) activity. The combined effect of these two agents administered as COSOPT b.i.d. results in additional intraocular pressure reduction compared to either component administered alone, but the reduction is not as much as when dorzolamide t.i.d. and timolol b.i.d. are administered concomitantly (see *Clinical Studies*).
Pharmacokinetics/Pharmacodynamics
Dorzolamide Hydrochloride
When topically applied, dorzolamide reaches the systemic circulation. To assess the potential for systemic carbonic anhydrase inhibition following topical administration, drug and metabolite concentrations in RBCs and plasma and carbonic anhydrase inhibition in RBCs were measured. Dorzolamide accumulates in RBCs during chronic dosing as a result of binding to CA-II. The parent drug forms a single N-desethyl metabolite, which inhibits CA-II less potently than the parent drug but also inhibits CA-I. The metabolite also accumulates in RBCs where it binds primarily to CA-I. Plasma concentrations of dorzolamide and metabolite are generally below the assay limit of quantitation (15nM). Dorzolamide binds moderately to plasma proteins (approximately 33%).
Dorzolamide is primarily excreted unchanged in the urine; the metabolite also is excreted in urine. After dosing is stopped, dorzolamide washes out of RBCs nonlinearly, resulting in a rapid decline of drug concentration initially, followed by a slower elimination phase with a half-life of about four months.
To simulate the systemic exposure after long-term topical ocular administration, dorzolamide was given orally to eight healthy subjects for up to 20 weeks. The oral dose of 2 mg b.i.d. closely approximates the amount of drug delivered by topical ocular administration of dorzolamide 2% t.i.d. Steady state was reached within 8 weeks. The inhibition of CA-II and total carbonic anhydrase activities was below the degree of inhibition anticipated to be necessary for a pharmacological effect on renal function and respiration in healthy individuals.
Timolol Maleate
In a study of plasma drug concentrations in six subjects, the systemic exposure to timolol was determined following twice daily topical administration of timolol maleate ophthalmic solution 0.5%. The mean peak plasma concentration following morning dosing was 0.46 ng/mL.
Clinical Studies
Clinical studies of 3 to 15 months duration were conducted to compare the IOP-lowering effect over the course of the day of COSOPT b.i.d. (dosed morning and bedtime) to individually- and concomitantly-administered 0.5% timolol (b.i.d.) and 2.0% dorzolamide (b.i.d. and t.i.d.). The IOP-lowering effect of COSOPT b.i.d. was greater (1-3 mmHg) than that of monotherapy with either 2.0% dorzolamide t.i.d. or 0.5% timolol b.i.d. The IOP-lowering effect of COSOPT b.i.d. was approximately 1 mmHg less than that of concomitant therapy with 2.0% dorzolamide t.i.d. and 0.5% timolol b.i.d.
Open-label extensions of two studies were conducted for up to 12 months. During this period, the IOP-lowering effect of COSOPT b.i.d. was consistent during the 12 month follow-up period.

INDICATIONS AND USAGE

COSOPT is indicated for the reduction of elevated intraocular pressure in patients with open-angle glaucoma or ocular hypertension who are insufficiently responsive to beta-blockers (failed to achieve target IOP determined after multiple measurements over time). The IOP-lowering of COSOPT b.i.d. was slightly less than that seen with the concomitant administration of 0.5% timolol b.i.d. and 2.0% dorzolamide t.i.d. (see CLINICAL PHARMACOLOGY, *Clinical Studies*).

CONTRAINDICATIONS

COSOPT is contraindicated in patients with (1) bronchial asthma; (2) a history of bronchial asthma; (3) severe chronic obstructive pulmonary disease (see WARNINGS); (4) sinus bradycardia; (5) second or third degree atrioventricular block; (6) overt cardiac failure (see WARNINGS); (7) cardiogenic shock; or (8) hypersensitivity to any component of this product.

WARNINGS

Systemic Exposure
COSOPT contains dorzolamide, a sulfonamide, and timolol maleate, a beta-adrenergic blocking agent; and although administered topically, is absorbed systemically. Therefore, the same types of adverse reactions that are attributable to sulfonamides and/or systemic administration of beta-adrenergic blocking agents may occur with topical administration. For example, severe respiratory reactions and cardiac reactions, including death due to bronchospasm in patients with asthma, and rarely death in association with cardiac failure, have been reported following systemic or ophthalmic administration of timolol maleate (see CONTRAINDICATIONS). Fatalities have occurred, although rarely, due to severe reactions to sulfonamides including Stevens-Johnson syndrome, toxic epidermal necrolysis, fulminant hepatic necrosis, agranulocytosis, aplastic anemia, and other blood dyscrasias. Sensitization may recur when a sulfonamide is readministered irrespective of the route of administration. If signs of serious reactions or hypersensitivity occur, discontinue the use of this preparation.
Cardiac Failure
Sympathetic stimulation may be essential for support of the circulation in individuals with diminished myocardial contractility, and its inhibition by beta-adrenergic receptor blockade may precipitate more severe failure.
In Patients Without a History of Cardiac Failure continued depression of the myocardium with beta-blocking agents over a period of time can, in some cases, lead to cardiac failure. At the first sign or symptom of cardiac failure, COSOPT should be discontinued.
Obstructive Pulmonary Disease
Patients with chronic obstructive pulmonary disease (e.g., chronic bronchitis, emphysema) of mild or moderate severity, bronchospastic disease, or a history of bronchospastic disease (other than bronchial asthma or a history of bronchial asthma, in which COSOPT is contraindicated [see CONTRAINDICATIONS]) should, in general, not receive beta-blocking agents, including COSOPT.
Major Surgery
The necessity or desirability of withdrawal of beta-adrenergic blocking agents prior to major surgery is controversial. Beta-adrenergic receptor blockade impairs the ability of the heart to respond to beta-adrenergically mediated reflex stimuli. This may augment the risk of general anesthesia in surgical procedures. Some patients receiving beta-adrenergic receptor blocking agents have experienced protracted severe hypotension during anesthesia. Difficulty in restarting and maintaining the heartbeat has also been reported. For these reasons, in patients undergoing elective surgery, some authorities recommend gradual withdrawal of beta-adrenergic receptor blocking agents.
If necessary during surgery, the effects of beta-adrenergic blocking agents may be reversed by sufficient doses of adrenergic agonists.
Diabetes Mellitus
Beta-adrenergic blocking agents should be administered with caution in patients subject to spontaneous hypoglycemia or to diabetic patients (especially those with labile diabetes) who are receiving insulin or oral hypoglycemic agents. Beta-adrenergic receptor blocking agents may mask the signs and symptoms of acute hypoglycemia.
Thyrotoxicosis
Beta-adrenergic blocking agents may mask certain clinical signs (e.g., tachycardia) of hyperthyroidism. Patients suspected of developing thyrotoxicosis should be managed carefully to avoid abrupt withdrawal of beta-adrenergic blocking agents that might precipitate a thyroid storm.

PRECAUTIONS

General
Dorzolamide has not been studied in patients with severe renal impairment (CrCl <30 mL/min). Because dorzolamide and its metabolite are excreted predominantly by the kidney, COSOPT is not recommended in such patients.
Dorzolamide has not been studied in patients with hepatic impairment and should therefore be used with caution in such patients.
While taking beta-blockers, patients with a history of atopy or a history of severe anaphylactic reactions to a variety of allergens may be more reactive to repeated accidental, diagnostic, or therapeutic challenge with such allergens. Such patients may be unresponsive to the usual doses of epinephrine used to treat anaphylactic reactions.
In clinical studies, local ocular adverse effects, primarily conjunctivitis and lid reactions, were reported with chronic administration of COSOPT. Many of these reactions had the clinical appearance and course of an allergic-type reaction that resolved upon discontinuation of drug therapy. If such reactions are observed, COSOPT should be discontinued and the patient evaluated before considering restarting the drug. (See ADVERSE REACTIONS.)
The management of patients with acute angle-closure glaucoma requires therapeutic interventions in addition to ocular hypotensive agents. COSOPT has not been studied in patients with acute angle-closure glaucoma.
Choroidal detachment after filtration procedures has been reported with the administration of aqueous suppressant therapy (e.g., timolol).
Beta-adrenergic blockade has been reported to potentiate muscle weakness consistent with certain myasthenic symptoms (e.g., diplopia, ptosis, and generalized weakness). Timolol has been reported rarely to increase muscle weakness in some patients with myasthenia gravis or myasthenic symptoms.
There have been reports of bacterial keratitis associated with the use of multiple dose containers of topical ophthalmic products. These containers had been inadvertently contaminated by patients who, in most cases, had a concurrent corneal disease or a disruption of the ocular epithelial surface. (See PRECAUTIONS, *Information for Patients*.)
Information for Patients
Patients with bronchial asthma, a history of bronchial asthma, severe chronic obstructive pulmonary disease, sinus bradycardia, second or third degree atrioventricular block, or cardiac failure should be advised not to take this product. (See CONTRAINDICATIONS.)
COSOPT contains dorzolamide (which is a sulfonamide) and although administered topically is absorbed systemically. Therefore the same types of adverse reactions that are attributable to sulfonamides may occur with topical administration. Patients should be advised that if serious or unusual reactions or signs of hypersensitivity occur, they should discontinue the use of the product (see WARNINGS).
Patients should be advised that if they develop any ocular reactions, particularly conjunctivitis and lid reactions, they should discontinue use and seek their physician's advice.
Patients should be instructed to avoid allowing the tip of the dispensing container to contact the eye or surrounding structures.
Patients should also be instructed that ocular solutions, if handled improperly or if the tip of the dispensing container contacts the eye or surrounding structures, can become contaminated by common bacteria known to cause ocular infections. Serious damage to the eye and subsequent loss of vision may result from using contaminated solutions. (See PRECAUTIONS, *General*.)
Patients also should be advised that if they have ocular surgery or develop an intercurrent ocular condition (e.g., trauma or infection), they should immediately seek their physician's advice concerning the continued use of the present multidose container.
If more than one topical ophthalmic drug is being used, the drugs should be administered at least ten minutes apart.
Patients should be advised that COSOPT contains benzalkonium chloride which may be absorbed by soft contact lenses. Contact lenses should be removed prior to administration of the solution. Lenses may be reinserted 15 minutes following administration of COSOPT.
Drug Interactions
Carbonic anhydrase inhibitors: There is a potential for an additive effect on the known systemic effects of carbonic anhydrase inhibition in patients receiving an oral carbonic anhydrase inhibitor and COSOPT. The concomitant administration of COSOPT and oral carbonic anhydrase inhibitors is not recommended.
Acid-base disturbances: Although acid-base and electrolyte disturbances were not reported in the clinical trials with dorzolamide hydrochloride ophthalmic solution, these disturbances have been reported with oral carbonic anhydrase inhibitors and have, in some instances, resulted in drug interactions (e.g., toxicity associated with high-dose salicylate therapy). Therefore, the potential for such drug interactions should be considered in patients receiving COSOPT.
Beta-adrenergic blocking agents: Patients who are receiving a beta-adrenergic blocking agent orally and COSOPT should be observed for potential additive effects of beta-blockade, both systemic and on intraocular pressure. The concomitant use of two topical beta-adrenergic blocking agents is not recommended.
Calcium antagonists: Caution should be used in the coadministration of beta-adrenergic blocking agents, such as COSOPT, and oral or intravenous calcium antagonists because of possible atrioventricular conduction disturbances, left ventricular failure, and hypotension. In patients with impaired cardiac function, coadministration should be avoided.
Catecholamine-depleting drugs: Close observation of the patient is recommended when a beta-blocker is administered to patients receiving catecholamine-depleting drugs such as reserpine, because of possible additive effects and the production of hypotension and/or marked bradycardia, which may result in vertigo, syncope, or postural hypotension.
Digitalis and calcium antagonists: The concomitant use of beta-adrenergic blocking agents with digitalis and calcium antagonists may have additive effects in prolonging atrioventricular conduction time.
Quinidine: Potentiated systemic beta-blockade (e.g., decreased heart rate) has been reported during combined treatment with quinidine and timolol, possibly because quinidine inhibits the metabolism of timolol via the P-450 enzyme, CYP2D6.
Clonidine: Oral beta-adrenergic blocking agents may exacerbate the rebound hypertension which can follow the withdrawal of clonidine. There have been no reports of exacerbation of rebound hypertension with ophthalmic timolol maleate.
Injectable Epinephrine: (See PRECAUTIONS, *General, Anaphylaxis*.)
Carcinogenesis, Mutagenesis, Impairment of Fertility
In a two-year study of dorzolamide hydrochloride administered orally to male and female Sprague-Dawley rats, urinary bladder papillomas were seen in male rats in the highest dosage group of 20 mg/kg/day (250 times the recommended human ophthalmic dose). Papillomas were not seen in rats given oral doses equivalent to approximately 12 times the recommended human ophthalmic dose. No treatment-related tumors were seen in a 21-month study in female and male mice given oral doses up to 75 mg/kg/day (~900 times the recommended human ophthalmic dose).
The increased incidence of urinary bladder papillomas seen in the high-dose male rats is a class-effect of carbonic anhy-

drase inhibitors in rats. Rats are particularly prone to developing papillomas in response to foreign bodies, compounds causing crystalluria, and diverse sodium salts.

No changes in bladder urothelium were seen in dogs given oral dorzolamide hydrochloride for one year at 2 mg/kg/day (25 times the recommended human ophthalmic dose) or monkeys dosed topically to the eye at 0.4 mg/kg/day (~5 times the recommended human ophthalmic dose) for one year.

In a two-year study of timolol maleate administered orally to rats, there was a statistically significant increase in the incidence of adrenal pheochromocytomas in male rats administered 300 mg/kg/day (approximately 42,000 times the systemic exposure following the maximum recommended human ophthalmic dose). Similar differences were not observed in rats administered oral doses equivalent to approximately 14,000 times the maximum recommended human ophthalmic dose.

In a lifetime oral study of timolol maleate in mice, there were statistically significant increases in the incidence of benign and malignant pulmonary tumors, benign uterine polyps and mammary adenocarcinomas in female mice at 500 mg/kg/day, (approximately 71,000 times the systemic exposure following the maximum recommended human ophthalmic dose), but not at 5 or 50 mg/kg/day (approximately 700 or 7,000, respectively, times the systemic exposure following the maximum recommended human ophthalmic dose). In a subsequent study in female mice, in which post-mortem examinations were limited to the uterus and the lungs, a statistically significant increase in the incidence of pulmonary tumors was again observed at 500 mg/kg/day.

The increased occurrence of mammary adenocarcinomas was associated with elevations in serum prolactin which occurred in female mice administered oral timolol at 500 mg/kg/day, but not at doses of 5 or 50 mg/kg/day. An increased incidence of mammary adenocarcinomas in rodents has been associated with administration of several other therapeutic agents that elevate serum prolactin, but no correlation between serum prolactin levels and mammary tumors has been established in humans. Furthermore, in adult human female subjects who received oral dosages of up to 60 mg of timolol maleate (the maximum recommended human oral dosage), there were no clinically meaningful changes in serum prolactin.

The following tests for mutagenic potential were negative for dorzolamide: (1) *in vivo* (mouse) cytogenetic assay; (2) *in vitro* chromosomal aberration assay; (3) alkaline elution assay; (4) V-79 assay; and (5) Ames test.

Timolol maleate was devoid of mutagenic potential when tested *in vivo* (mouse) in the micronucleus test and cytogenetic assay (doses up to 800 mg/kg) and *in vitro* in a neoplastic cell transformation assay (up to 100 µg/mL). In Ames tests the highest concentrations of timolol employed, 5,000 or 10,000 µg/plate, were associated with statistically significant elevations of revertants observed with tester strain TA100 (in seven replicate assays), but not in the remaining three strains. In the assays with tester strain TA100, no consistent dose response relationship was observed, and the ratio of test to control revertants did not reach 2. A ratio of 2 is usually considered the criterion for a positive Ames test.

Reproduction and fertility studies in rats with either timolol maleate or dorzolamide hydrochloride demonstrated no adverse effect on male or female fertility at doses up to approximately 100 times the systemic exposure following the maximum recommended human ophthalmic dose.

Pregnancy

Teratogenic Effects. Pregnancy Category C. Developmental toxicity studies with dorzolamide hydrochloride in rabbits at oral doses of ≥2.5 mg/kg/day (31 times the recommended human ophthalmic dose) revealed malformations of the vertebral bodies. These malformations occurred at doses that caused metabolic acidosis with decreased body weight gain in dams and decreased fetal weights. No treatment-related malformations were seen at 1.0 mg/kg/day (13 times the recommended human ophthalmic dose).

Teratogenicity studies with timolol in mice, rats, and rabbits at oral doses up to 50 mg/kg/day (7,000 times the systemic exposure following the maximum recommended human ophthalmic dose) demonstrated no evidence of fetal malformations. Although delayed fetal ossification was observed at this dose in rats, there were no adverse effects on postnatal development of offspring. Doses of 1000 mg/kg/day (142,000 times the systemic exposure following the maximum recommended human ophthalmic dose) were maternotoxic in mice and resulted in an increased number of fetal resorptions. Increased fetal resorptions were also seen in rabbits at doses of 14,000 times the systemic exposure following the maximum recommended human ophthalmic dose, in this case without apparent maternotoxicity.

There are no adequate and well-controlled studies in pregnant women. COSOPT should be used during pregnancy only if the potential benefit justifies the potential risk to the fetus.

Nursing Mothers

It is not known whether dorzolamide is excreted in human milk. Timolol maleate has been detected in human milk following oral and ophthalmic drug administration. Because of the potential for serious adverse reactions from COSOPT in nursing infants, a decision should be made whether to discontinue nursing or to discontinue the drug, taking into account the importance of the drug to the mother.

Pediatric Use

Safety and effectiveness in pediatric patients have not been established.

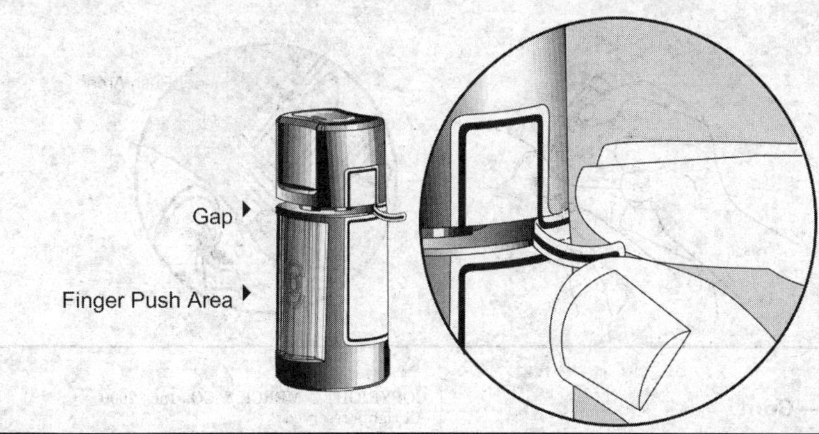

Geriatric Use

No overall differences in safety or effectiveness have been observed between elderly and younger patients.

ADVERSE REACTIONS

COSOPT was evaluated for safety in 1035 patients with elevated intraocular pressure treated for open-angle-glaucoma or ocular hypertension. Approximately 5% of all patients discontinued therapy with COSOPT because of adverse reactions. The most frequently reported adverse events were taste perversion (bitter, sour, or unusual taste) or ocular burning and/or stinging in up to 30% of patients. Conjunctival hyperemia, blurred vision, superficial punctate keratitis or eye itching were reported between 5-15% of patients. The following adverse events were reported in 1-5% of patients: abdominal pain, back pain, blepharitis, bronchitis, cloudy vision, conjunctival discharge, conjunctival edema, conjunctival follicles, conjunctival injection, conjunctivitis, corneal erosion, corneal staining, cortical lens opacity, cough, dizziness, dryness of eyes, dyspepsia, eye debris, eye discharge, eye pain, eye tearing, eyelid edema, eyelid erythema, eyelid exudate/scales, eyelid pain or discomfort, foreign body sensation, glaucomatous cupping, headache, hypertension, influenza, lens nucleus coloration, lens opacity, nausea, nuclear lens opacity, pharyngitis, post-subcapsular cataract, sinusitis, upper respiratory infection, urinary tract infection, visual field defect, vitreous detachment.

The following adverse events have occurred either at low incidence (<1%) during clinical trials or have been reported during the use of COSOPT in clinical practice where these events were reported voluntarily from a population of unknown size and frequency of occurrence cannot be determined precisely. They have been chosen for inclusion based on factors such as seriousness, frequency of reporting, possible causal connection to COSOPT, or a combination of these factors: bradycardia, cardiac failure, cerebral vascular accident, chest pain, choroidal detachment following filtration surgery (see PRECAUTIONS, *General*), depression, diarrhea, dry mouth, dyspnea, heart block, hypotension, iridocyclitis, myocardial infarction, nasal congestion, paresthesia, photophobia, respiratory failure, skin rashes, urolithiasis, and vomiting.

Other adverse reactions that have been reported with the individual components are listed below:

Dorzolamide — Allergic/Hypersensitivity: Signs and symptoms of local reactions including palpebral reactions and systemic allergic reactions including angioedema, bronchospasm, pruritus, urticaria; *Body as a Whole:* Asthenia/fatigue; *Skin/Mucous Membranes:* Contact dermatitis, epistaxis, throat irritation; *Special Senses:* Eyelid crusting, signs and symptoms of ocular allergic reaction, and transient myopia.

Timolol (ocular administration) — Body as a Whole: Asthenia/fatigue; *Cardiovascular:* Arrhythmia, syncope, cerebral ischemia, worsening of angina pectoris, palpitation, cardiac arrest, pulmonary edema, edema, claudication, Raynaud's phenomenon, and cold hands and feet; *Digestive:* Anorexia; *Immunologic:* Systemic lupus erythematosus; *Nervous System/Psychiatric:* Increase in signs and symptoms of myasthenia gravis, somnolence, insomnia, nightmares, behavioral changes and psychic disturbances including confusion, hallucinations, anxiety, disorientation, nervousness, and memory loss; *Skin:* Alopecia, psoriasiform rash or exacerbation of psoriasis; *Hypersensitivity:* Signs and symptoms of systemic allergic reactions, including anaphylaxis, angioedema, urticaria, and localized and generalized rash; *Respiratory:* Bronchospasm (predominantly in patients with preexisting bronchospastic disease); *Endocrine:* Masked symptoms of hypoglycemia in diabetic patients (see WARNINGS); *Special Senses:* Ptosis; decreased corneal sensitivity; cystoid macular edema; visual disturbances including refractive changes and diplopia; pseudopemphigoid; and tinnitus; *Urogenital:* Retroperitoneal fibrosis, decreased libido, impotence, and Peyronie's disease.

The following additional adverse effects have been reported in clinical experience with ORAL timolol maleate or other ORAL beta-blocking agents and may be considered potential effects of ophthalmic timolol maleate: *Allergic:* Erythematous rash, fever combined with aching and sore throat, laryngospasm with respiratory distress; *Body as a Whole:* Extremity pain, decreased exercise tolerance, weight loss; *Cardiovascular:* Worsening of arterial insufficiency, vasodilatation; *Digestive:* Gastrointestinal pain, hepatomegaly, mesenteric arterial thrombosis, ischemic colitis; *Hematologic:* Nonthrombocytopenic purpura; thrombocytopenic purpura, agranulocytosis; *Endocrine:* Hyperglycemia, hypoglycemia; *Skin:* Pruritus, skin irritation, increased pigmentation, sweating; *Musculoskeletal:* Arthralgia; *Nervous System/Psychiatric:* Vertigo, local weakness, diminished concentration, reversible mental depression progressing to catatonia, an acute reversible syndrome characterized by disorientation for time and place, emotional lability, slightly clouded sensorium, and decreased performance on neuropsychometrics; *Respiratory:* Rales, bronchial obstruction; *Urogenital:* Urination difficulties.

OVERDOSAGE

There are no human data available on overdosage with COSOPT.

Symptoms consistent with systemic administration of beta-blockers or carbonic anhydrase inhibitors may occur, including electrolyte imbalance, development of an acidotic state, dizziness, headache, shortness of breath, bradycardia, bronchospasm, cardiac arrest and possible central nervous system effects. Serum electrolyte levels (particularly potassium) and blood pH levels should be monitored (see also ADVERSE REACTIONS).

A study of patients with renal failure showed that timolol did not dialyze readily.

DOSAGE AND ADMINISTRATION

The dose is one drop of COSOPT in the affected eye(s) two times daily.

If more than one topical ophthalmic drug is being used, the drugs should be administered at least ten minutes apart (see also PRECAUTIONS, *Drug Interactions*).

HOW SUPPLIED

COSOPT Ophthalmic Solution is a clear, colorless to nearly colorless, slightly viscous solution.

No. 3628 — COSOPT Ophthalmic Solution is supplied in an OCUMETER®* PLUS container, a white, translucent, HDPE plastic ophthalmic dispenser with a controlled drop tip and a white polystyrene cap with dark blue label as follows:

NDC 0006-3628-35, 5 mL in a 7.5 mL bottle

NDC 0006-3628-36, 10 mL in an 18 mL bottle.

Storage

Store COSOPT at 25°C (77°F), excursions permitted to 15–30°C (59–86°F) [see USP Controlled Room Temperature]. Protect from light.

INSTRUCTIONS FOR USE

Please follow these instructions carefully when using COSOPT*. Use COSOPT as prescribed by your doctor.

1. If you use other topically applied ophthalmic medications, they should be administered at least 10 minutes before or after COSOPT.
2. Wash hands before each use.
3. Before using the medication for the first time, be sure the Safety Strip on the front of the bottle is unbroken. A gap between the bottle and the cap is normal for an unopened bottle.

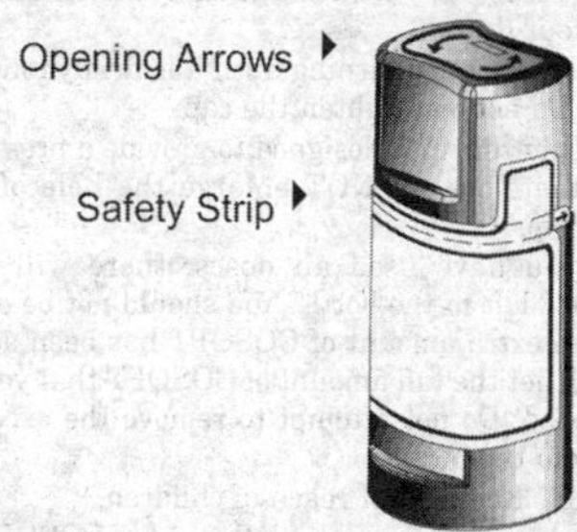

Continued on next page

Information on the Merck & Co., Inc., products listed on these pages is from the prescribing information in use October 1, 2004. For information, please call 1-800-NSC-MERCK [1-800-672-6372].

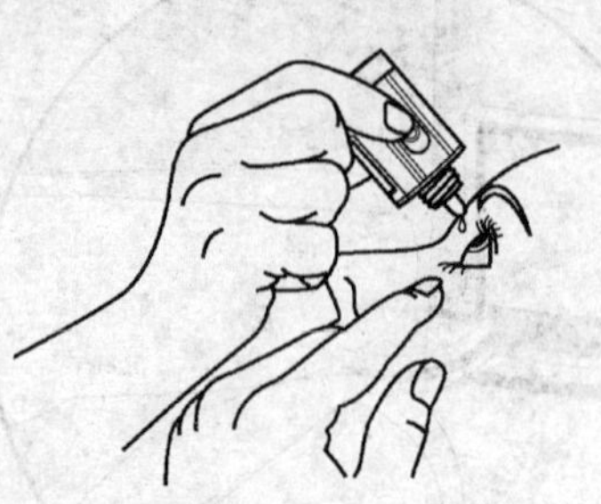

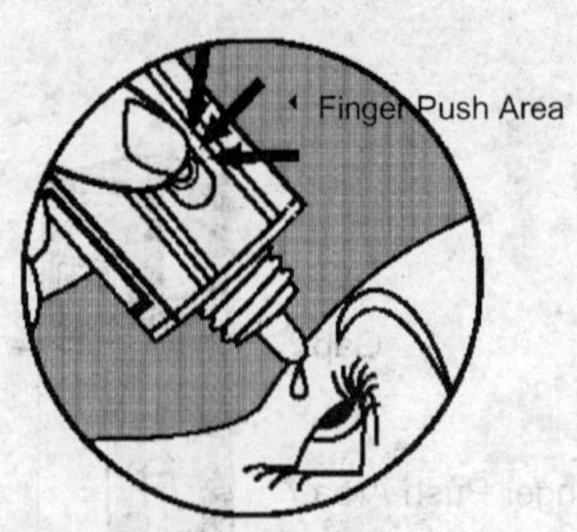

Cosopt—Cont.

4. Tear off the Safety Strip to break the seal.
[See figure at top of previous page]
5. To open the bottle, unscrew the cap by turning as indicated by the arrows.

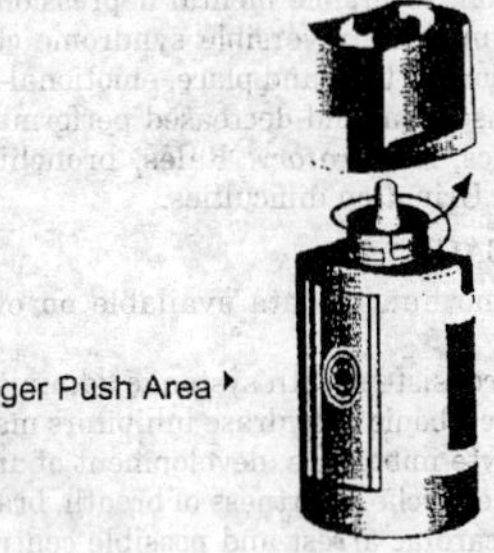

6. Tilt your head back and pull your lower eyelid down slightly to form a pocket between your eyelid and your eye.

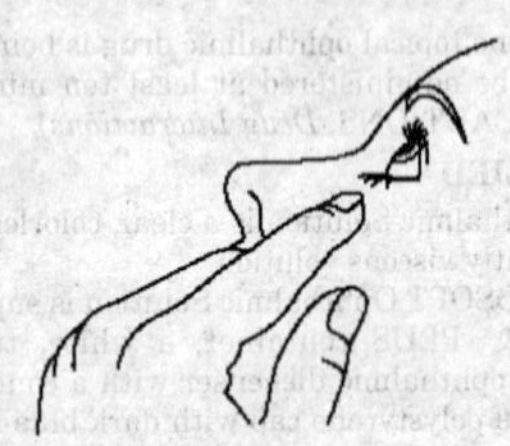

7. Invert the bottle, and press lightly with the thumb or index finger over the "Finger Push Area" (as shown) until a single drop is dispensed into the eye as directed by your doctor.
[See figure above]
DO NOT TOUCH YOUR EYE OR EYELID WITH THE DROPPER TIP.
Ophthalmic medications, if handled improperly, can become contaminated by common bacteria known to cause eye infections. Serious damage to the eye and subsequent loss of vision may result from using contaminated ophthalmic medications. If you think your medication may be contaminated, or if you develop an eye infection, contact your doctor immediately concerning continued use of this bottle.
8. Repeat steps 6 & 7 with the other eye if instructed to do so by your doctor.
9. Replace the cap by turning until it is firmly touching the bottle. Do not overtighten the cap.
10. The dispenser tip is designed to provide a pre-measured drop; therefore, do NOT enlarge the hole of the dispenser tip.
11. After you have used all doses, there will be some COSOPT left in the bottle. You should not be concerned since an extra amount of COSOPT has been added and you will get the full amount of COSOPT that your doctor prescribed. Do not attempt to remove the excess medicine from the bottle.

WARNING: Keep out of reach of children.
If you have any questions about the use of COSOPT, please consult your doctor.

* Registered trademark of MERCK & CO., Inc.
Manuf. for:
Merck & Co., Inc., Whitehouse Station, NJ 08889, USA
By: Laboratories Merck Sharp & Dohme-Chibret
63963 Clermont-Ferrand Cedex 9, France
9359302 Issued January 2004

Shown in Product Identification Guide, page 104

COZAAR®
[*cō'zâr*]
(losartan potassium tablets)

USE IN PREGNANCY
When used in pregnancy during the second and third trimesters, drugs that act directly on the renin-angiotensin system can cause injury and even death to the developing fetus. When pregnancy is detected, COZAAR should be discontinued as soon as possible. See WARNINGS: *Fetal/Neonatal Morbidity and Mortality*.

DESCRIPTION

COZAAR* (losartan potassium) is an angiotensin II receptor (type AT_1) antagonist. Losartan potassium, a non-peptide molecule, is chemically described as 2-butyl-4-chloro-1-[*p*-(*o*-1*H*-tetrazol-5-ylphenyl)benzyl]imidazole-5-methanol monopotassium salt.
Its empirical formula is $C_{22}H_{22}ClKN_6O$, and its structural formula is:

Losartan potassium is a white to off-white free-flowing crystalline powder with a molecular weight of 461.01. It is freely soluble in water, soluble in alcohols, and slightly soluble in common organic solvents, such as acetonitrile and methyl ethyl ketone. Oxidation of the 5-hydroxymethyl group on the imidazole ring results in the active metabolite of losartan.
COZAAR is available as tablets for oral administration containing either 25 mg, 50 mg or 100 mg of losartan potassium and the following inactive ingredients: microcrystalline cellulose, lactose hydrous, pregelatinized starch, magnesium stearate, hydroxypropyl cellulose, hypromellose, titanium dioxide, D&C yellow No. 10 aluminum lake and FD&C blue No. 2 aluminum lake.
COZAAR 25 mg, 50 mg and 100 mg tablets contain potassium in the following amounts: 2.12 mg (0.054 mEq), 4.24 mg (0.108 mEq) and 8.48 mg (0.216 mEq), respectively.

*Registered trademark of E.I. du Pont de Nemours and Company, Wilmington, Delaware, USA

CLINICAL PHARMACOLOGY

Mechanism of Action
Angiotensin II [formed from angiotensin I in a reaction catalyzed by angiotensin converting enzyme (ACE, kininase II)], is a potent vasoconstrictor, the primary vasoactive hormone of the renin-angiotensin system and an important component in the pathophysiology of hypertension. It also stimulates aldosterone secretion by the adrenal cortex. Losartan and its principal active metabolite block the vasoconstrictor and aldosterone-secreting effects of angiotensin II by selectively blocking the binding of angiotensin II to the AT_1 receptor found in many tissues, (e.g., vascular smooth muscle, adrenal gland). There is also an AT_2 receptor found in many tissues but it is not known to be associated with cardiovascular homeostasis. Both losartan and its principal active metabolite do not exhibit any partial agonist activity at the AT_1 receptor and have much greater affinity (about 1000-fold) for the AT_1 receptor than for the AT_2 receptor. *In vitro* binding studies indicate that losartan is a reversible, competitive inhibitor of the AT_1 receptor. The active metabolite is 10 to 40 times more potent by weight than losartan and appears to be a reversible, non-competitive inhibitor of the AT_1 receptor.
Neither losartan nor its active metabolite inhibits ACE (kininase II, the enzyme that converts angiotensin I to angiotensin II and degrades bradykinin); nor do they bind to or block other hormone receptors or ion channels known to be important in cardiovascular regulation.
Pharmacokinetics
General
Losartan is an orally active agent that undergoes substantial first-pass metabolism by cytochrome P450 enzymes. It is converted, in part, to an active carboxylic acid metabolite that is responsible for most of the angiotensin II receptor antagonism that follows losartan treatment. Losartan metabolites have been identified in human plasma and urine. In addition to the active carboxylic acid metabolite, several inactive metabolites are formed. Following oral and intravenous administration of ^{14}C-labeled losartan potassium, circulating plasma radioactivity is primarily attributed to losartan and its active metabolite. *In vitro* studies indicate that cytochrome P450 2C9 and 3A4 are involved in the biotransformation of losartan to its metabolites. Minimal conversion of losartan to the active metabolite (less than 1% of the dose compared to 14% of the dose in normal subjects) was seen in about one percent of individuals studied.
The terminal half-life of losartan is about 2 hours and of the metabolite is about 6-9 hours.
The pharmacokinetics of losartan and its active metabolite are linear with oral losartan doses up to 200 mg and do not change over time. Neither losartan nor its metabolite accumulate in plasma upon repeated once-daily dosing.
Following oral administration, losartan is well absorbed (based on absorption of radiolabeled losartan) and undergoes substantial first-pass metabolism; the systemic bioavailability of losartan is approximately 33%. About 14% of an orally-administered dose of losartan is converted to the active metabolite. Mean peak concentrations of losartan and its active metabolite are reached in 1 hour and in 3-4 hours, respectively. While maximum plasma concentrations of losartan and its active metabolite are approximately equal, the AUC of the metabolite is about 4 times as great as that of losartan. A meal slows absorption of losartan and decreases its C_{max} but has only minor effects on losartan AUC or on the AUC of the metabolite (about 10% decreased).
The pharmacokinetics of losartan and its active metabolite were also determined after IV doses of each component separately in healthy volunteers. The volume of distribution of losartan and the active metabolite is about 34 liters and 12 liters, respectively. Total plasma clearance of losartan and the active metabolite is about 600 mL/min and 50 mL/min, respectively, with renal clearance of about 75 mL/min and 25 mL/min, respectively. After single doses of losartan administered orally, about 4% of the dose is excreted unchanged in the urine and about 6% is excreted in urine as active metabolite. Biliary excretion contributes to the elimination of losartan and its metabolites. Following oral ^{14}C-labeled losartan, about 35% of radioactivity is recovered in the urine and about 60% in the feces. Following an intravenous dose of ^{14}C-labeled losartan, about 45% of radioactivity is recovered in the urine and 50% in the feces.
Both losartan and its active metabolite are highly bound to plasma proteins, primarily albumin, with plasma free fractions of 1.3% and 0.2%, respectively. Plasma protein binding is constant over the concentration range achieved with recommended doses. Studies in rats indicate that losartan crosses the blood-brain barrier poorly, if at all.
Special Populations
Pediatric: Pharmacokinetic parameters after multiple doses of losartan (average dose 0.7 mg/kg, range 0.36 to 0.97 mg/kg) as a tablet to 25 hypertensive patients aged 6 to 16 years are shown in Table 1 below. Pharmacokinetics of losartan and its active metabolite were generally similar across the studied age groups and similar to historical pharmacokinetic data in adults. The principal pharmacokinetic parameters in adults and children are shown in the table below.
[See table 1 at top of next page]
The bioavailability of the suspension formulation was compared with losartan tablets in healthy adults. The suspension and tablet are similar in their bioavailability with respect to both losartan and the active metabolite (see DOSAGE AND ADMINISTRATION, *Preparation of Suspension*).
Geriatric and Gender: Losartan pharmacokinetics have been investigated in the elderly (65-75 years) and in both genders. Plasma concentrations of losartan and its active metabolite are similar in elderly and young hypertensives. Plasma concentrations of losartan were about twice as high in female hypertensives as male hypertensives, but concentrations of the active metabolite were similar in males and females. No dosage adjustment is necessary (see DOSAGE AND ADMINISTRATION).
Race: Pharmacokinetic differences due to race have not been studied. (see also PRECAUTIONS, *Race* and CLINICAL PHARMACOLOGY, *Pharmacodynamics and Clinical Effects, Reduction in the Risk of Stroke, Race*).
Renal Insufficiency: Following oral administration, plasma concentrations and AUCs of losartan and its active metabolite are increased by 50-90% in patients with mild (creatinine clearance of 50 to 74 mL/min) or moderate (creatinine clearance 30 to 49 mL/min) renal insufficiency. In this study, renal clearance was reduced by 55-85% for both losartan and its active metabolite in patients with mild or moderate renal insufficiency. Neither losartan nor its active metabolite can be removed by hemodialysis. No dosage adjustment

is necessary for patients with renal impairment unless they are volume-depleted (see WARNINGS, *Hypotension — Volume-Depleted Patients* and DOSAGE AND ADMINISTRATION).

Hepatic Insufficiency: Following oral administration in patients with mild to moderate alcoholic cirrhosis of the liver, plasma concentrations of losartan and its active metabolite were, respectively, 5-times and about 1.7-times those in young male volunteers. Compared to normal subjects the total plasma clearance of losartan in patients with hepatic insufficiency was about 50% lower and the oral bioavailability was about 2-times higher. A lower starting dose is recommended for patients with a history of hepatic impairment (see DOSAGE AND ADMINISTRATION).

Drug Interactions

Losartan, administered for 12 days, did not affect the pharmacokinetics or pharmacodynamics of a single dose of warfarin. Losartan did not affect the pharmacokinetics of oral or intravenous digoxin. There is no pharmacokinetic interaction between losartan and hydrochlorothiazide. Coadministration of losartan and cimetidine led to an increase of about 18% in AUC of losartan but did not affect the pharmacokinetics of its active metabolite. Coadministration of losartan and phenobarbital led to a reduction of about 20% in the AUC of losartan and that of its active metabolite. A somewhat greater interaction (approximately 40% reduction in the AUC of active metabolite and approximately 30% reduction in the AUC of losartan) has been reported with rifampin. Fluconazole, an inhibitor of cytochrome P450 2C9, decreased the AUC of the active metabolite by approximately 40%, but increased the AUC of losartan by approximately 70% following multiple doses. Conversion of losartan to its active metabolite after intravenous administration is not affected by ketoconazole, an inhibitor of P450 3A4. The AUC of active metabolite following oral losartan was not affected by erythromycin, another inhibitor of P450 3A4, but the AUC of losartan was increased by 30%.

Pharmacodynamics and Clinical Effects

Adult Hypertension

Losartan inhibits the pressor effect of angiotensin II (as well as angiotensin I) infusions. A dose of 100 mg inhibits the pressor effect by about 85% at peak with 25-40% inhibition persisting for 24 hours. Removal of the negative feedback of angiotensin II causes a 2- to 3-fold rise in plasma renin activity and consequent rise in angiotensin II plasma concentration in hypertensive patients. Losartan does not affect the response to bradykinin, whereas ACE inhibitors increase the response to bradykinin. Aldosterone plasma concentrations fall following losartan administration. In spite of the effect of losartan on aldosterone secretion, very little effect on serum potassium was observed.

In a single-dose study in normal volunteers, losartan had no effects on glomerular filtration rate, renal plasma flow or filtration fraction. In multiple-dose studies in hypertensive patients, there were no notable effects on systemic or renal prostaglandin concentrations, fasting triglycerides, total cholesterol or HDL-cholesterol or fasting glucose concentrations. There was a small uricosuric effect leading to a minimal decrease in serum uric acid (mean decrease <0.4 mg/dL) during chronic oral administration.

The antihypertensive effects of COZAAR were demonstrated principally in 4 placebo-controlled, 6- to 12-week trials of dosages from 10 to 150 mg per day in patients with baseline diastolic blood pressures of 95-115. The studies allowed comparisons of two doses (50-100 mg/day) as once-daily or twice-daily regimens, comparisons of peak and trough effects, and comparisons of response by gender, age, and race. Three additional studies examined the antihypertensive effects of losartan and hydrochlorothiazide in combination.

The 4 studies of losartan monotherapy included a total of 1075 patients randomized to several doses of losartan and 334 to placebo. The 10- and 25-mg doses produced some effect at peak (6 hours after dosing) but small and inconsistent trough (24 hour) responses. Doses of 50, 100 and 150 mg once daily gave statistically significant systolic/diastolic mean decreases in blood pressure, compared to placebo in the range of 5.5-10.5/3.5-7.5 mmHg, with the 150-mg dose giving no greater effect than 50-100 mg. Twice-daily dosing at 50-100 mg/day gave consistently larger trough responses than once-daily dosing at the same total dose. Peak (6 hour) effects were uniformly, but moderately, larger than trough effects, with the trough-to-peak ratio for systolic and diastolic responses 50-95% and 60-90%, respectively.

Addition of a low dose of hydrochlorothiazide (12.5 mg) to losartan 50 mg once daily resulted in placebo-adjusted blood pressure reductions of 15.5/9.2 mmHg.

Analysis of age, gender, and race subgroups of patients showed that men and women, and patients over and under 65, had generally similar responses. COZAAR was effective in reducing blood pressure regardless of race, although the effect was somewhat less in Black patients (usually a low-renin population).

The effect of losartan is substantially present within one week but in some studies the maximal effect occurred in 3-6 weeks. In long-term follow-up studies (without placebo control) the effect of losartan appeared to be maintained for up to a year. There is no apparent rebound effect after abrupt withdrawal of losartan. There was essentially no change in average heart rate in losartan-treated patients in controlled trials.

Pediatric Hypertension

The antihypertensive effect of losartan was studied in one trial enrolling 177 hypertensive pediatric patients aged 6 to 16 years old. Children who weighed <50 kg received 2.5, 25 or 50 mg of losartan daily and patients who weighed ≥50 kg received 5, 50 or 100 mg of losartan daily. Children in the lowest dose group were given losartan in a suspension formulation (see DOSAGE AND ADMINISTRATION, *Preparation of Suspension*). The majority of the children had hypertension associated with renal and urogenital disease. The sitting diastolic blood pressure (SiDBP) on entry into the study was higher than the 95th percentile level for the patient's age, gender, and height. At the end of three weeks, losartan reduced systolic and diastolic blood pressure, measured at trough, in a dose-dependent manner. Overall, the two higher doses (25 to 50 mg in patients <50 kg; 50 to 100 mg in patients ≥50 kg) reduced diastolic blood pressure by 5 to 6 mmHg more than the lowest dose used (2.5 mg in patients <50 kg; 5 mg in patients ≥50 kg). The lowest dose, corresponding to an average daily dose of 0.07 mg/kg, did not appear to offer consistent antihypertensive efficacy. When patients were randomized to continue losartan at the two higher doses or to placebo after 3 weeks of therapy, trough diastolic blood pressure rose in patients on placebo between 5 and 7 mmHg more than patients randomized to continuing losartan. When the low dose of losartan was randomly withdrawn, the rise in trough diastolic blood pressure was the same in patients receiving placebo and in those continuing losartan, again suggesting that the lowest dose did not have significant antihypertensive efficacy. Overall, no significant differences in the overall antihypertensive effect of losartan were detected when the patients were analyzed according to age (<, ≥12 years old) or gender. While blood pressure was reduced in all racial subgroups examined, too few non-White patients were enrolled to compare the dose-response of losartan in the non-White subgroup.

Table 1 Pharmacokinetic Parameters in Hypertensive Adults and Children Age 6-16 Following Multiple Dosing

	Adults given 50 mg once daily for 7 days N=12		Age 6-16 given 0.7 mg/kg once daily for 7 days N=25	
	Parent	Active Metabolite	Parent	Active Metabolite
AUC_{0-24}[a] (ng•h/mL)	442 ± 173	1685 ± 452	368 ± 169	1866 ± 1076
C_{MAX} (ng/mL)[a]	224 ± 82	212 ± 73	141 ± 88	222 ± 127
$T_{1/2}$ (h) [b]	2.1 ± 0.70	7.4 ± 2.4	2.3 ± 0.8	5.6 ± 1.2
T_{PEAK} (h) [c]	0.9	3.5	2.0	4.1
CL_{REN} (mL/min)[a]	56 ± 23	20 ± 3	53 ± 33	17 ± 8

[a] Mean ± standard deviation
[b] Harmonic mean and standard deviation
[c] Median

Reduction in the Risk of Stroke: The Losartan Intervention For Endpoint reduction in hypertension (LIFE) study was a multinational, double-blind study comparing COZAAR and atenolol in 9193 hypertensive patients with ECG-documented left ventricular hypertrophy. Patients with myocardial infarction or stroke within six months prior to randomization were excluded. Patients were randomized to receive once daily COZAAR 50 mg or atenolol 50 mg. If goal blood pressure (<140/90 mmHg) was not reached, hydrochlorothiazide (12.5 mg) was added first and, if needed, the dose of COZAAR or atenolol was then increased to 100 mg once daily. If necessary, other antihypertensive treatments (e.g., increase in dose of hydrochlorothiazide therapy to 25 mg or addition of other diuretic therapy, calcium-channel blockers, alpha-blockers, or centrally acting agents, but not ACE inhibitors, angiotensin II antagonists, or beta-blockers) were added to the treatment regimen to reach the goal blood pressure.

Of the randomized patients, 4963 (54%) were female and 533 (6%) were Black. The mean age was 67 with 5704 (62%) age ≥65. At baseline, 1195 (13%) had diabetes, 1326 (14%) had isolated systolic hypertension, 1469 (16%) had coronary heart disease, and 728 (8%) had cerebrovascular disease. Baseline mean blood pressure was 174/98 mmHg in both treatment groups. The mean length of follow-up was 4.8 years. At the end of study or at the last visit before a primary endpoint, 77% of the group treated with COZAAR and 73% of the group treated with atenolol were still taking study medication. Of the patients still taking study medication, the mean doses of COZAAR and atenolol were both about 80 mg/day, and 15% were taking atenolol or losartan as monotherapy, while 77% were also receiving hydrochlorothiazide (at a mean dose of 20 mg/day in each group). Blood pressure reduction measured at trough was similar for both treatment groups but blood pressure was not measured at any other time of the day. At the end of study or at the last visit before a primary endpoint, the mean blood pressures were 144.1/81.3 mmHg for the group treated with COZAAR and 145.4/80.9 mmHg for the group treated with atenolol [the difference in systolic blood pressure (SBP) of 1.3 mmHg was significant (p<0.001), while the difference of 0.4 mmHg in diastolic blood pressure (DBP) was not significant (p=0.098)].

The primary endpoint was the first occurrence of cardiovascular death, nonfatal stroke, or nonfatal myocardial infarction. Patients with non-fatal events remained in the trial, so that there was also an examination of the first event of each type even if it was not the first event (e.g., a stroke following an initial myocardial infarction would be counted in the analysis of stroke). Treatment with COZAAR resulted in a 13% reduction (p=0.021) in risk of the primary endpoint compared to the atenolol group (see Figure 1 and Table 2); this difference was primarily the result of an effect on fatal and nonfatal stroke. Treatment with COZAAR reduced the risk of stroke by 25% relative to atenolol (p=0.001) (see Figure 2 and Table 2).

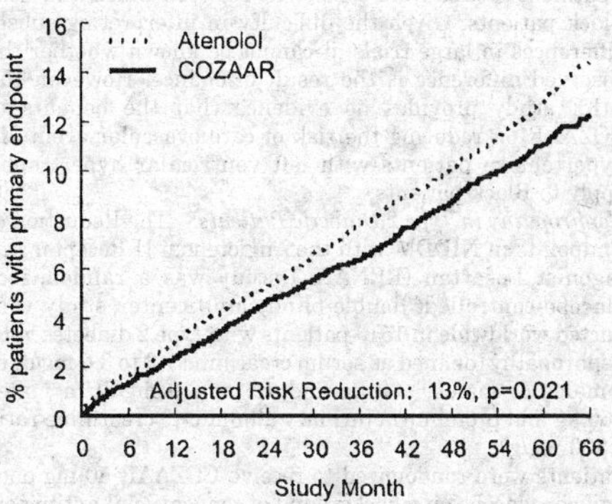

Figure 1. Kaplan-Meier estimates of the primary endpoint of time to cardiovascular death, nonfatal stroke, or nonfatal myocardial infarction in the groups treated with COZAAR and atenolol. The Risk Reduction is adjusted for baseline Framingham risk score and level of electrocardiographic left ventricular hypertrophy.

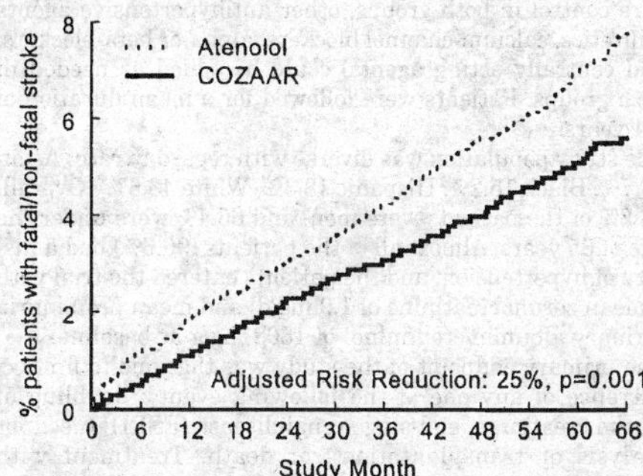

Figure 2. Kaplan-Meier estimates of the time to fatal/nonfatal stroke in the groups treated with COZAAR and atenolol. The Risk Reduction is adjusted for baseline Framingham risk score and level of electrocardiographic left ventricular hypertrophy.

Table 2 shows the results for the primary composite endpoint and the individual endpoints. The primary endpoint was the first occurrence of stroke, myocardial infarction or cardiovascular death, analyzed using an intention-to-treat (ITT) approach. The table shows the number of events for each component in two different ways. The Components of Primary Endpoint (as a first event) counts only the events that define the primary endpoint, while the Secondary Endpoints count all first events of a particular type, whether or not they were preceded by a different type of event.

[See table 2 at top of next page]

Although the LIFE study favored COZAAR over atenolol with respect to the primary endpoint (p=0.021), this result is from a single study and, therefore, is less compelling than the difference between COZAAR and placebo. Although not measured directly, the difference between COZAAR and placebo is compelling because there is evidence that atenolol is itself effective (vs. placebo) in reducing cardiovascular events, including stroke, in hypertensive patients.

Other clinical endpoints of the LIFE study were: total mortality, hospitalization for heart failure or angina pectoris,

Continued on next page

Information on the Merck & Co., Inc., products listed on these pages is from the prescribing information in use October 1, 2004. For information, please call 1-800-NSC-MERCK [1-800-672-6372].

Cozaar—Cont.

coronary or peripheral revascularization procedures, and resuscitated cardiac arrest. There were no significant differences in the rates of these endpoints between the COZAAR and atenolol groups.

For the primary endpoint and stroke, the effects of COZAAR in patient subgroups defined by age, gender, race and presence or absence of isolated systolic hypertension (ISH), diabetes, and history of cardiovascular disease (CVD) are shown in Figure 3 below. Subgroup analyses can be difficult to interpret and it is not known whether these represent true differences or chance effects.

[See figure 3 at right]

Race: In the LIFE study, Black patients treated with atenolol were at lower risk of experiencing the primary composite endpoint compared with Black patients treated with COZAAR. In the subgroup of Black patients (n=533; 6% of the LIFE study patients), there were 29 primary endpoints among 263 patients on atenolol (11%, 26 per 1000 patient-years) and 46 primary endpoints among 270 patients (17%, 42 per 1000 patient-years) on COZAAR. This finding could not be explained on the basis of differences in the populations other than race or on any imbalances between treatment groups. In addition, blood pressure reductions in both treatment groups were consistent between Black and non-Black patients. Given the difficulty in interpreting subset differences in large trials, it cannot be known whether the observed difference is the result of chance. However, the LIFE study provides no evidence that the benefits of COZAAR on reducing the risk of cardiovascular events in hypertensive patients with left ventricular hypertrophy apply to Black patients.

Nephropathy in Type 2 Diabetic Patients: The Reduction of Endpoints in NIDDM with the Angiotensin II Receptor Antagonist Losartan (RENAAL) study was a randomized, placebo-controlled, double-blind, multicenter study conducted worldwide in 1513 patients with type 2 diabetes with nephropathy (defined as serum creatinine 1.3 to 3.0 mg/dl in females or males ≤60 kg and 1.5 to 3.0 mg/dl in males >60 kg and proteinuria [urinary albumin to creatinine ratio ≥300 mg/g]).

Patients were randomized to receive COZAAR 50 mg once daily or placebo on a background of conventional antihypertensive therapy excluding ACE inhibitors and angiotensin II antagonists. After one month, investigators were instructed to titrate study drug to 100 mg once daily if the trough blood pressure goal (140/90 mmHg) was not achieved. Overall, 72% of patients received the 100-mg daily dose more than 50% of the time they were on study drug. Because the study was designed to achieve equal blood pressure control in both groups, other antihypertensive agents (diuretics, calcium-channel blockers, alpha-or beta-blockers, and centrally acting agents) could be added as needed in both groups. Patients were followed for a mean duration of 3.4 years.

The study population was diverse with regard to race (Asian 16.7%, Black 15.2%, Hispanic 18.3%, White 48.6%). Overall, 63.2% of the patients were men, and 66.4% were under the age of 65 years. Almost all of the patients (96.6%) had a history of hypertension, and the patients entered the trial with a mean serum creatinine of 1.9 mg/dl and mean proteinuria (urinary albumin/creatinine) of 1808 mg/g at baseline.

The primary endpoint of the study was the time to first occurrence of any one of the following events: doubling of serum creatinine, end-stage renal disease (ESRD) (need for dialysis or transplantation), or death. Treatment with COZAAR resulted in a 16% risk reduction in this endpoint (see Figure 4 and Table 3). Treatment with COZAAR also reduced the occurrence of sustained doubling of serum creatinine by 25% and ESRD by 29% as separate endpoints, but had no effect on overall mortality (see Table 3).

The mean baseline blood pressures were 152/82 mmHg for COZAAR plus conventional antihypertensive therapy and 153/82 mmHg for placebo plus conventional antihypertensive therapy. At the end of the study, the mean blood pressures were 143/76 mmHg for the group treated with COZAAR and 146/77 mmHg for the group treated with placebo.

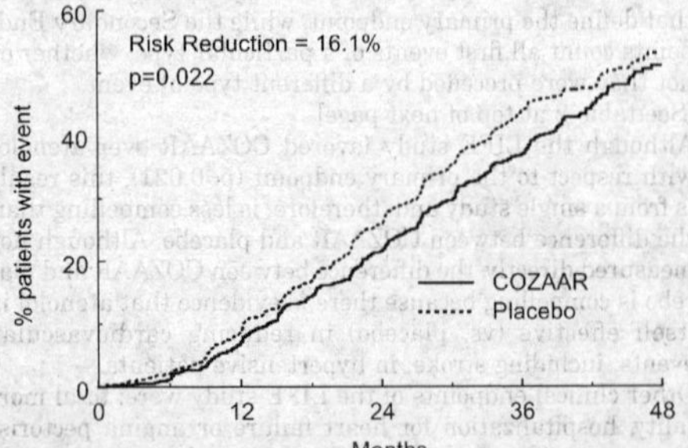

Figure 4. Kaplan-Meier curve for the primary composite endpoint of doubling of serum creatinine, end stage renal disease (need for dialysis or transplantation) or death.

[See table 3 at top of next page]

The secondary endpoints of the study were change in proteinuria, change in the rate of progression of renal disease, and the composite of morbidity and mortality from cardio-

Table 2 Incidence of Primary Endpoint Events

	COZAAR		Atenolol		Risk Reduction†	95% CI	p-Value
	N (%)	Rate*	N (%)	Rate*			
Primary Composite Endpoint	508 (11)	23.8	588 (13)	27.9	13%	2% to 23%	0.021
Components of Primary Composite Endpoint (as a first event)							
Stroke (nonfatal‡)	209 (5)		286 (6)				
Myocardial infarction (nonfatal‡)	174 (4)		168 (4)				
Cardiovascular mortality	125 (3)		134 (3)				
Secondary Endpoints (any time in study)							
Stroke (fatal/nonfatal)	232 (5)	10.8	309 (7)	14.5	25%	11% to 37%	0.001
Myocardial infarction (fatal/nonfatal)	198 (4)	9.2	188 (4)	8.7	-7%	-13% to 12%	0.491
Cardiovascular mortality	204 (4)	9.2	234 (5)	10.6	11%	-7% to 27%	0.206
Due to CHD	125 (3)	5.6	124 (3)	5.6	-3%	-32% to 20%	0.839
Due to Stroke	40 (1)	1.8	62 (1)	2.8	35%	4% to 67%	0.032
Other§	39 (1)	1.8	48 (1)	2.2	16%	-28% to 45%	0.411

*Rate per 1000 patient-years of follow-up

†Adjusted for baseline Framingham risk score and level of electrocardiographic left ventricular hypertrophy

‡First report of an event, in some cases the patient died subsequently to the event reported

§Death due to heart failure, non-coronary vascular disease, pulmonary embolism, or a cardiovascular cause other than stroke or coronary heart disease

Figure 3 Primary Endpoint Events† within Demographic Subgroups

	No. of Patients	Primary Composite: COZAAR Event Rate (%)	Primary Composite: Atenolol Event Rate (%)	Stroke (Fatal/Non-fatal): COZAAR Event Rate (%)	Stroke (Fatal/Non-fatal): Atenolol Event Rate (%)
Overall Results	9193	11	13	5	7
Age					
<65 years	3489	7	7	3	3
≥65 years	5704	13	16	6	9
Gender					
Female	4963	9	11	4	6
Male	4230	14	15	6	7
Race					
Black	533	17	11	9	5
White	8503	11	13	5	7
Other#	157	9	14	5	5
ISH					
Yes	1326	11	16	5	8
No	7867	11	12	5	6
Diabetes					
Yes	1195	18	23	9	11
No	7998	10	11	5	6
History of CVD					
Yes	2307	19	21	9	11
No	6886	8	10	4	6

Hazard Ratio (95% CI): 0.3 0.5 1 2 3 ← Favors COZAAR Favors Atenolol →

Symbols are proportional to sample size.

#Other includes Asian, Hispanic, Asiatic, Multi-race, Indian, Native American, European.

†Adjusted for baseline Framingham risk score and level of electrocardiographic left ventricular hypertrophy.

vascular causes (hospitalization for heart failure, myocardial infarction, revascularization, stroke, hospitalization for unstable angina, or cardiovascular death). Compared with placebo, COZAAR significantly reduced proteinuria by an average of 34%, an effect that was evident within 3 months of starting therapy, and significantly reduced the rate of decline in glomerular filtration rate during the study by 13%, as measured by the reciprocal of the serum creatinine concentration. There was no significant difference in the incidence of the composite endpoint of cardiovascular morbidity and mortality.

The favorable effects of COZAAR were seen in patients also taking other anti-hypertensive medications (angiotensin II receptor antagonists and angiotensin converting enzyme inhibitors were not allowed), oral hypoglycemic agents and lipid-lowering agents.

For the primary endpoint and ESRD, the effects of COZAAR in patient subgroups defined by age, gender and race are shown in Table 4 below. Subgroup analyses can be difficult to interpret and it is not known whether these represent true differences or chance effects.

[See table 4 on next page]

INDICATIONS AND USAGE

Hypertension
COZAAR is indicated for the treatment of hypertension. It may be used alone or in combination with other antihypertensive agents, including diuretics.

Hypertensive Patients with Left Ventricular Hypertrophy
COZAAR is indicated to reduce the risk of stroke in patients with hypertension and left ventricular hypertrophy, but there is evidence that this benefit does not apply to Black patients. (See PRECAUTIONS, *Race* and CLINICAL PHARMACOLOGY, *Pharmacodynamics and Clinical Effects, Reduction in the Risk of Stroke, Race.*)

Nephropathy in Type 2 Diabetic Patients
COZAAR is indicated for the treatment of diabetic nephropathy with an elevated serum creatinine and proteinuria (urinary albumin to creatinine ratio ≥300 mg/g) in patients with type 2 diabetes and a history of hypertension. In this population, COZAAR reduces the rate of progression of nephropathy as measured by the occurrence of doubling of serum creatinine or end stage renal disease (need for dialysis or renal transplantation) (see CLINICAL PHARMACOLOGY, *Pharmacodynamics and Clinical Effects*).

CONTRAINDICATIONS

COZAAR is contraindicated in patients who are hypersensitive to any component of this product.

WARNINGS

Fetal/Neonatal Morbidity and Mortality
Drugs that act directly on the renin-angiotensin system can cause fetal and neonatal morbidity and death when administered to pregnant women. Several dozen cases have been reported in the world literature in patients who were taking angiotensin converting enzyme inhibitors. When pregnancy is detected, COZAAR should be discontinued as soon as possible.

The use of drugs that act directly on the renin-angiotensin system during the second and third trimesters of pregnancy has been associated with fetal and neonatal injury, including hypotension, neonatal skull hypoplasia, anuria, reversible or irreversible renal failure, and death. Oligohydramnios has also been reported, presumably resulting from decreased fetal renal function; oligohydramnios in this setting has been associated with fetal limb contractures, craniofacial deformation, and hypoplastic lung development.

Prematurity, intrauterine growth retardation, and patent ductus arteriosus have also been reported, although it is not clear whether these occurrences were due to exposure to the drug.
These adverse effects do not appear to have resulted from intrauterine drug exposure that has been limited to the first trimester.
Mothers whose embryos and fetuses are exposed to an angiotensin II receptor antagonist only during the first trimester should be so informed. Nonetheless, when patients become pregnant, physicians should have the patient discontinue the use of COZAAR as soon as possible.
Rarely (probably less often than once in every thousand pregnancies), no alternative to an angiotensin II receptor antagonist will be found. In these rare cases, the mothers should be apprised of the potential hazards to their fetuses, and serial ultrasound examinations should be performed to assess the intra-amniotic environment.
If oligohydramnios is observed, COZAAR should be discontinued unless it is considered life-saving for the mother. Contraction stress testing (CST), a non-stress test (NST), or biophysical profiling (BPP) may be appropriate, depending upon the week of pregnancy. Patients and physicians should be aware, however, that oligohydramnios may not appear until after the fetus has sustained irreversible injury.
Infants with histories of *in utero* exposure to an angiotensin II receptor antagonist should be closely observed for hypotension, oliguria, and hyperkalemia. If oliguria occurs, attention should be directed toward support of blood pressure and renal perfusion. Exchange transfusion or dialysis may be required as means of reversing hypotension and/or substituting for disordered renal function.
Losartan potassium has been shown to produce adverse effects in rat fetuses and neonates, including decreased body weight, delayed physical and behavioral development, mortality and renal toxicity. With the exception of neonatal weight gain (which was affected at doses as low as 10 mg/kg/day), doses associated with these effects exceeded 25 mg/kg/day (approximately three times the maximum recommended human dose of 100 mg on a mg/m^2 basis). These findings are attributed to drug exposure in late gestation and during lactation. Significant levels of losartan and its active metabolite were shown to be present in rat fetal plasma during late gestation and in rat milk.
Hypotension — Volume-Depleted Patients
In patients who are intravascularly volume-depleted (e.g., those treated with diuretics), symptomatic hypotension may occur after initiation of therapy with COZAAR. These conditions should be corrected prior to administration of COZAAR, or a lower starting dose should be used (see DOSAGE AND ADMINISTRATION).

PRECAUTIONS

General
Hypersensitivity: Angioedema. See ADVERSE REACTIONS, *Post-Marketing Experience.*
Impaired Hepatic Function
Based on pharmacokinetic data which demonstrate significantly increased plasma concentrations of losartan in cirrhotic patients, a lower dose should be considered for patients with impaired liver function (see DOSAGE AND ADMINISTRATION and CLINICAL PHARMACOLOGY, *Pharmacokinetics*).
Impaired Renal Function
As a consequence of inhibiting the renin-angiotensin-aldosterone system, changes in renal function have been reported in susceptible individuals treated with COZAAR; in some patients, these changes in renal function were reversible upon discontinuation of therapy.
In patients whose renal function may depend on the activity of the renin-angiotensin-aldosterone system (e.g., patients with severe congestive heart failure), treatment with angiotensin converting enzyme inhibitors has been associated with oliguria and/or progressive azotemia and (rarely) with acute renal failure and/or death. Similar outcomes have been reported with COZAAR.
In studies of ACE inhibitors in patients with unilateral or bilateral renal artery stenosis, increases in serum creatinine or blood urea nitrogen (BUN) have been reported. Similar effects have been reported with COZAAR; in some patients, these effects were reversible upon discontinuation of therapy.
Electrolyte Imbalance
Electrolyte imbalances are common in patients with renal impairment, with or without diabetes, and should be addressed. In a clinical study conducted in type 2 diabetic patients with proteinuria, the incidence of hyperkalemia was higher in the group treated with COZAAR as compared to the placebo group; however, few patients discontinued therapy due to hyperkalemia (see ADVERSE REACTIONS).
Information for Patients
Pregnancy: Female patients of childbearing age should be told about the consequences of second-and third-trimester exposure to drugs that act on the renin-angiotensin system, and they should also be told that these consequences do not appear to have resulted from intrauterine drug exposure that has been limited to the first trimester. These patients should be asked to report pregnancies to their physicians as soon as possible.
Potassium Supplements: A patient receiving COZAAR should be told not to use potassium supplements or salt substitutes containing potassium without consulting the prescribing physician (see PRECAUTIONS, *Drug Interactions*).

Table 3 Incidence of Primary Endpoint Events

	Incidence		Risk Reduction	95% C.I.	p-Value
	Losartan	Placebo			
Primary Composite Endpoint	43.5%	47.1%	16.1%	2.3% to 27.9%	0.022
Doubling of Serum Creatinine, ESRD and Death Occurring as a First Event					
Doubling of Serum Creatinine	21.6%	26.0%			
ESRD	8.5%	8.5%			
Death	13.4%	12.6%			
Overall Incidence of Doubling of Serum Creatinine, ESRD and Death					
Doubling of Serum Creatinine	21.6%	26.0%	25.3%	7.8% to 39.4%	0.006
ESRD	19.6%	25.5%	28.6%	11.5% to 42.4%	0.002
Death	21.0%	20.3%	-1.7%	-26.9% to 18.6%	0.884

Table 4 Efficacy Outcomes within Demographic Subgroups

		Primary Composite Endpoint			ESRD		
	No. of Patients	COZAAR Event Rate %	Placebo Event Rate %	Hazard Ratio (95% CI)	COZAAR Event Rate %	Placebo Event Rate %	Hazard Ratio (95% CI)
Overall Results	1513	43.5	47.1	0.839 (0.721, 0.977)	19.6	25.5	0.714 (0.576, 0.885)
Age							
<65 years	1005	44.1	49.0	0.784 (0.653, 0.941)	21.1	28.5	0.670 (0.521, 0.863)
≥65 years	508	42.3	43.5	0.978 (0.749, 1.277)	16.5	19.6	0.847 (0.560, 1.281)
Gender							
Female	557	47.8	54.1	0.762 (0.603, 0.962)	22.8	32.8	0.601 (0.436, 0.828)
Male	956	40.9	43.3	0.892 (0.733, 1.085)	17.5	21.5	0.809 (0.605, 1.081)
Race							
Asian	252	41.9	54.8	0.655 (0.453, 0.947)	18.8	27.4	0.625 (0.367, 1.066)
Black	230	40.0	39.0	0.983 (0.647, 1.495)	17.6	21.0	0.831 (0.456, 1.516)
Hispanic	277	55.0	54.0	1.003 (0.728, 1.380)	30.0	28.5	1.024 (0.661, 1.586)
White	735	40.5	43.2	0.809 (0.645, 1.013)	16.2	23.9	0.596 (0.427, 0.831)

Drug Interactions
No significant drug-drug pharmacokinetic interactions have been found in interaction studies with hydrochlorothiazide, digoxin, warfarin, cimetidine and phenobarbital. Rifampin, an inducer of drug metabolism, decreased the concentrations of losartan and its active metabolite. (See CLINICAL PHARMACOLOGY, *Drug Interactions.*) In humans, two inhibitors of P450 3A4 have been studied. Ketoconazole did not affect the conversion of losartan to the active metabolite after intravenous administration of losartan, and erythromycin had no clinically significant effect after oral administration. Fluconazole, an inhibitor of P450 2C9, decreased active metabolite concentration and increased losartan concentration. The pharmacodynamic consequences of concomitant use of losartan and inhibitors of P450 2C9 have not been examined. Subjects who do not metabolize losartan to active metabolite have been shown to have a specific, rare defect in cytochrome P450 2C9. These data suggest that the conversion of losartan to its active metabolite is mediated primarily by P450 2C9 and not P450 3A4.
As with other drugs that block angiotensin II or its effects, concomitant use of potassium-sparing diuretics (e.g., spironolactone, triamterene, amiloride), potassium supplements, or salt substitutes containing potassium may lead to increases in serum potassium.
As with other antihypertensive agents, the antihypertensive effect of losartan may be blunted by the non-steroidal anti-inflammatory drug indomethacin.
Carcinogenesis, Mutagenesis, Impairment of Fertility
Losartan potassium was not carcinogenic when administered at maximally tolerated dosages to rats and mice for 105 and 92 weeks, respectively. Female rats given the highest dose (270 mg/kg/day) had a slightly higher incidence of pancreatic acinar adenoma. The maximally tolerated dosages (270 mg/kg/day in rats, 200 mg/kg/day in mice) provided systemic exposures for losartan and its pharmacologically active metabolite that were approximately 160- and 90-times (rats) and 30- and 15-times (mice) the exposure of a 50 kg human given 100 mg per day.
Losartan potassium was negative in the microbial mutagenesis and V-79 mammalian cell mutagenesis assays and in the *in vitro* alkaline elution and *in vitro* and *in vivo* chromosomal aberration assays. In addition, the active metabolite showed no evidence of genotoxicity in the microbial mutagenesis, *in vitro* alkaline elution, and *in vitro* chromosomal aberration assays.
Fertility and reproductive performance were not affected in studies with male rats given oral doses of losartan potassium up to approximately 150 mg/kg/day. The administration of toxic dosage levels in females (300/200 mg/kg/day) was associated with a significant ($p<0.05$) decrease in the number of corpora lutea/female, implants/female, and live fetuses/female at C-section. At 100 mg/kg/day only a decrease in the number of corpora lutea/female was observed. The relationship of these findings to drug-treatment is uncertain since there was no effect at these dosage levels on implants/pregnant female, percent post-implantation loss, or live animals/litter at parturition. In nonpregnant rats dosed at 135 mg/kg/day for 7 days, systemic exposure (AUCs) for losartan and its active metabolite were approximately 66 and 26 times the exposure achieved in man at the maximum recommended human daily dosage (100 mg).
Pregnancy
Pregnancy Categories C (first trimester) and D (second and third trimesters). See WARNINGS, *Fetal / Neonatal Morbidity and Mortality.*
Nursing Mothers
It is not known whether losartan is excreted in human milk, but significant levels of losartan and its active metabolite were shown to be present in rat milk. Because of the potential for adverse effects on the nursing infant, a decision should be made whether to discontinue nursing or discontinue the drug, taking into account the importance of the drug to the mother.
Pediatric Use
Antihypertensive effects of COZAAR have been established in hypertensive pediatric patients aged 6 to 16 years. There are no data on the effect of COZAAR on blood pressure in pediatric patients under the age of 6 or in pediatric patients with glomerular filtration rate <30 mL/min/1.73 m^2 (see CLINICAL PHARMACOLOGY, *Pharmacokinetics, Special Populations* and *Pharmacodynamics and Clinical Effects,* and DOSAGE AND ADMINISTRATION).
Geriatric Use
Of the total number of patients receiving COZAAR in controlled clinical studies for hypertension, 391 patients (19%) were 65 years and over, while 37 patients (2%) were 75

Continued on next page

Information on the Merck & Co., Inc., products listed on these pages is from the prescribing information in use October 1, 2004. For information, please call 1-800-NSC-MERCK [1-800-672-6372].

Cozaar—Cont.

years and over. In a controlled clinical study for renal protection in type 2 diabetic patients with proteinuria, 248 patients (33%) were 65 years and over. In a controlled clinical study for the reduction in the combined risk of cardiovascular death, stroke and myocardial infarction in hypertensive patients with left ventricular hypertrophy, 2857 patients (62%) were 65 years and over, while 808 patients (18%) were 75 years and over. No overall differences in effectiveness or safety were observed between these patients and younger patients, but greater sensitivity of some older individuals cannot be ruled out.

Race

In the LIFE study, Black patients with hypertension and left ventricular hypertrophy had a lower risk of stroke on atenolol than on COZAAR. Given the difficulty in interpreting subset differences in large trials, it cannot be known whether the observed difference is the result of chance. However, the LIFE study does not provide evidence that the benefits of COZAAR on reducing the risk of cardiovascular events in hypertensive patients with left ventricular hypertrophy apply to Black patients. (See CLINICAL PHARMACOLOGY, *Pharmacodynamics and Clinical Effects*; *Reduction in the Risk of Stroke*.)

ADVERSE REACTIONS

Hypertension

COZAAR has been evaluated for safety in more than 3300 adult patients treated for essential hypertension and 4058 patients/subjects overall. Over 1200 patients were treated for over 6 months and more than 800 for over one year. In general, treatment with COZAAR was well-tolerated. The overall incidence of adverse experiences reported with COZAAR was similar to placebo.

In controlled clinical trials, discontinuation of therapy due to clinical adverse experiences was required in 2.3 percent of patients treated with COZAAR and 3.7 percent of patients given placebo.

The following table of adverse events is based on four 6- to 12-week, placebo-controlled trials involving over 1000 patients on various doses (10-150 mg) of losartan and over 300 patients given placebo. All doses of losartan are grouped because none of the adverse events appeared to have a dose-related frequency. The adverse experiences reported in ≥1% of patients treated with COZAAR and more commonly than placebo are shown in the table below.

	Losartan (n=1075) Incidence %	Placebo (n=334) Incidence %
Musculoskeletal		
Cramp, muscle	1	0
Pain, back	2	1
Pain, leg	1	0
Nervous System/Psychiatric		
Dizziness	3	2
Respiratory		
Congestion, nasal	2	1
Infection, upper respiratory	8	7
Sinusitis	1	0

The following adverse events were also reported at a rate of 1% or greater in patients treated with losartan, but were as, or more frequent, in the placebo group: asthenia/fatigue, edema/swelling, abdominal pain, chest pain, nausea, headache, pharyngitis, diarrhea, dyspepsia, myalgia, insomnia, cough, sinus disorder.

Adverse events occurred at about the same rates in men and women, older and younger patients, and Black and non-Black patients.

A patient with known hypersensitivity to aspirin and penicillin, when treated with COZAAR, was withdrawn from study due to swelling of the lips and eyelids and facial rash, reported as angioedema, which returned to normal 5 days after therapy was discontinued.

Superficial peeling of palms and hemolysis were reported in one subject.

In addition to the adverse events above, potentially important events that occurred in at least two patients/subjects exposed to losartan or other adverse events that occurred in <1% of patients in clinical studies are listed below. It cannot be determined whether these events were causally related to losartan: *Body as a Whole:* facial edema, fever, orthostatic effects, syncope; *Cardiovascular:* angina pectoris, second degree AV block, CVA, hypotension, myocardial infarction, arrhythmias including atrial fibrillation, palpitation, sinus bradycardia, tachycardia, ventricular tachycardia, ventricular fibrillation; *Digestive:* anorexia, constipation, dental pain, dry mouth, flatulence, gastritis, vomiting; *Hematologic:* anemia; *Metabolic:* gout; *Musculoskeletal:* arm pain, hip pain, joint swelling, knee pain, musculoskeletal pain, shoulder pain, stiffness, arthralgia, arthritis, fibromyalgia, muscle weakness; *Nervous System/Psychiatric:* anxiety, anxiety disorder, ataxia, confusion, depression, dream abnormality, hypesthesia, decreased libido, memory impairment, migraine, nervousness, paresthesia, peripheral neuropathy, panic disorder, sleep disorder, somnolence, tremor, vertigo; *Respiratory:* dyspnea, bronchitis, pharyngeal discomfort, epistaxis, rhinitis, respiratory congestion; *Skin:* alopecia, dermatitis, dry skin, ecchymosis, erythema, flushing, photosensitivity, pruritus, rash, sweating, urticaria; *Special Senses:* blurred vision, burning/stinging in the eye, conjunctivitis, taste perversion, tinnitus, decrease in visual acuity; *Urogenital:* impotence, nocturia, urinary frequency, urinary tract infection.

Persistent dry cough (with an incidence of a few percent) has been associated with ACE-inhibitor use and in practice can be a cause of discontinuation of ACE-inhibitor therapy. Two prospective, parallel-group, double-blind, randomized, controlled trials were conducted to assess the effects of losartan on the incidence of cough in hypertensive patients who had experienced cough while receiving ACE-inhibitor therapy. Patients who had typical ACE-inhibitor cough when challenged with lisinopril, whose cough disappeared on placebo, were randomized to losartan 50 mg, lisinopril 20 mg, or either placebo (one study, n=97) or 25 mg hydrochlorothiazide (n=135). The double-blind treatment period lasted up to 8 weeks. The incidence of cough is shown below.

Study 1[†]	HCTZ	Losartan	Lisinopril
Cough	25%	17%	69%
Study 2[††]	**Placebo**	**Losartan**	**Lisinopril**
Cough	35%	29%	62%

[†]Demographics = (89% caucasian, 64% female)
[††]Demographics = (90% caucasian, 51% female)

These studies demonstrate that the incidence of cough associated with losartan therapy, in a population that all had cough associated with ACE-inhibitor therapy, is similar to that associated with hydrochlorothiazide or placebo therapy.

Cases of cough, including positive re-challenges, have been reported with the use of losartan in post-marketing experience.

Pediatric Patients: No relevant differences between the adverse experience profile for pediatric patients and that previously reported for adult patients were identified.

Hypertensive Patients with Left Ventricular Hypertrophy

In the LIFE study, adverse events with COZAAR were similar to those reported previously for patients with hypertension.

Nephropathy in Type 2 Diabetic Patients

In the RENAAL study involving 1513 patients treated with COZAAR or placebo, the overall incidences of reported adverse experiences were similar for the two groups. COZAAR was generally well tolerated as evidenced by a similar incidence of discontinuations due to side effects compared to placebo (19% for COZAAR, 24% for placebo). The adverse experiences, regardless of drug relationship, reported with an incidence of ≥4% of patients treated with COZAAR and occurring more commonly than placebo, on a background of conventional antihypertensive therapy, are shown in the table below.

[See table below]

	Losartan and Conventional Antihypertensive Therapy Incidence % (n=751)	Placebo and Conventional Antihypertensive Therapy Incidence % (n=762)
Body as a Whole		
Asthenia/Fatigue	14	10
Chest Pain	12	8
Fever	4	3
Infection	5	4
Influenza-like disease	10	9
Trauma	4	3
Cardiovascular		
Hypotension	7	3
Orthostatic hypotension	4	1
Digestive		
Diarrhea	15	10
Dyspepsia	4	3
Gastritis	5	4
Endocrine		
Diabetic neuropathy	4	3
Diabetic vascular disease	10	9
Eyes, Ears, Nose and Throat		
Cataract	7	5
Sinusitis	6	5
Hemic		
Anemia	14	11
Metabolic and Nutrition		
Hyperkalemia	7	3
Hypoglycemia	14	10
Weight gain	4	3
Musculoskeletal		
Back pain	12	10
Leg pain	5	4
Knee pain	5	4
Muscular weakness	7	4
Nervous System		
Hypesthesia	5	4
Respiratory		
Bronchitis	10	9
Cough	11	10
Skin		
Cellulitis	7	6
Urogenital		
Urinary tract infection	16	13

Post-Marketing Experience

The following additional adverse reactions have been reported in post-marketing experience:

Hypersensitivity: Angioedema, including swelling of the larynx and glottis, causing airway obstruction and/or swelling of the face, lips, pharynx, and/or tongue has been reported rarely in patients treated with losartan; some of these patients previously experienced angioedema with other drugs including ACE inhibitors. Vasculitis, including Henoch-Schönlein purpura, has been reported. Anaphylactic reactions have been reported.

Digestive: Hepatitis (reported rarely).

Respiratory: Dry cough (see above).

Hyperkalemia and hyponatremia have been reported.

Laboratory Test Findings

In controlled clinical trials, clinically important changes in standard laboratory parameters were rarely associated with administration of COZAAR.

Creatinine, Blood Urea Nitrogen: Minor increases in blood urea nitrogen (BUN) or serum creatinine were observed in less than 0.1 percent of patients with essential hypertension treated with COZAAR alone (see PRECAUTIONS, *Impaired Renal Function*).

Hemoglobin and Hematocrit: Small decreases in hemoglobin and hematocrit (mean decreases of approximately 0.11 grams percent and 0.09 volume percent, respectively) occurred frequently in patients treated with COZAAR alone, but were rarely of clinical importance. No patients were discontinued due to anemia.

Liver Function Tests: Occasional elevations of liver enzymes and/or serum bilirubin have occurred. In patients with essential hypertension treated with COZAAR alone, one patient (<0.1%) was discontinued due to these laboratory adverse experiences.

OVERDOSAGE

Significant lethality was observed in mice and rats after oral administration of 1000 mg/kg and 2000 mg/kg, respectively, about 44 and 170 times the maximum recommended human dose on a mg/m[2] basis.

Limited data are available in regard to overdosage in humans. The most likely manifestation of overdosage would be

hypotension and tachycardia; bradycardia could occur from parasympathetic (vagal) stimulation. If symptomatic hypotension should occur, supportive treatment should be instituted.
Neither losartan nor its active metabolite can be removed by hemodialysis.

DOSAGE AND ADMINISTRATION

Adult Hypertensive Patients
COZAAR may be administered with other antihypertensive agents, and with or without food.
Dosing must be individualized. The usual starting dose of COZAAR is 50 mg once daily, with 25 mg used in patients with possible depletion of intravascular volume (e.g., patients treated with diuretics) (see WARNINGS, *Hypotension — Volume-Depleted Patients*) and patients with a history of hepatic impairment (see PRECAUTIONS, *General*). COZAAR can be administered once or twice daily with total daily doses ranging from 25 mg to 100 mg.
If the antihypertensive effect measured at trough using once-a-day dosing is inadequate, a twice-a-day regimen at the same total daily dose or an increase in dose may give a more satisfactory response. The effect of losartan is substantially present within one week but in some studies the maximal effect occurred in 3-6 weeks (see CLINICAL PHARMACOLOGY, *Pharmacodynamics and Clinical Effects, Hypertension*).
If blood pressure is not controlled by COZAAR alone, a low dose of a diuretic may be added. Hydrochlorothiazide has been shown to have an additive effect (see CLINICAL PHARMACOLOGY, *Pharmacodynamics and Clinical Effects, Hypertension*).
No initial dosage adjustment is necessary for elderly patients or for patients with renal impairment, including patients on dialysis.
Pediatric Hypertensive Patients ≥6 years of age
The usual recommended starting dose is 0.7 mg/kg once daily (up to 50 mg total) administered as a tablet or a suspension (see *Preparation of Suspension*). Dosage should be adjusted according to blood pressure response. Doses above 1.4 mg/kg (or in excess of 100 mg) daily have not been studied in pediatric patients. See CLINICAL PHARMACOLOGY, *Pharmacokinetics, Special Populations* and *Pharmacodynamics and Clinical Effects*.
COZAAR is not recommended in pediatric patients <6 years of age or in pediatric patients with glomerular filtration rate <30 mL/min/1.73 m^2 (see CLINICAL PHARMACOLOGY, *Pharmacokinetics, Special Populations, Pharmacodynamics and Clinical Effects*, and PRECAUTIONS).
Preparation of Suspension (for 200 mL of a 2.5 mg/mL suspension)
Add 10 mL of Purified Water USP to an 8 ounce (240 mL) amber polyethylene terephthalate (PET) bottle containing ten 50 mg COZAAR tablets. Immediately shake for at least 2 minutes. Let the concentrate stand for 1 hour and then shake for 1 minute to disperse the tablet contents. Separately prepare a 50/50 volumetric mixture of Ora-Plus™*** and Ora-Sweet SF™***. Add 190 mL of the 50/50 Ora-Plus™/Ora-Sweet SF™ mixture to the tablet and water slurry in the PET bottle and shake for 1 minute to disperse the ingredients. The suspension should be refrigerated at 2-8°C (36-46°F) and can be stored for up to 4 weeks. Shake the suspension prior to each use and return promptly to the refrigerator.

***Trademark of Paddock Laboratories, Inc.

Hypertensive Patients with Left Ventricular Hypertrophy
The usual starting dose is 50 mg of COZAAR once daily. Hydrochlorothiazide 12.5 mg daily should be added and/or the dose of COZAAR should be increased to 100 mg once daily followed by an increase in hydrochlorothiazide to 25 mg once daily based on blood pressure response (see CLINICAL PHARMACOLOGY, *Pharmacodynamics and Clinical Effects, Reduction in the Risk of Stroke*).
Nephropathy in Type 2 Diabetic Patients
The usual starting dose is 50 mg once daily. The dose should be increased to 100 mg once daily based on blood pressure response (see CLINICAL PHARMACOLOGY, *Pharmacodynamics and Clinical Effects, Nephropathy in Type 2 Diabetic Patients*). COZAAR may be administered with insulin and other commonly used hypoglycemic agents (e.g., sulfonylureas, glitazones and glucosidase inhibitors).

HOW SUPPLIED

No. 3612 — Tablets COZAAR, 25 mg, are light green, teardrop-shaped, film-coated tablets with code MRK on one side and 951 on the other. They are supplied as follows:
NDC 0006-0951-54 unit of use bottles of 90
NDC 0006-0951-58 unit of use bottles of 100
NDC 0006-0951-28 unit dose packages of 100
NDC 0006-0951-82 bottles of 1,000.
No. 3613 — Tablets COZAAR, 50 mg, are green, teardrop-shaped, film-coated tablets with code MRK 952 on one side and COZAAR on the other. They are supplied as follows:
NDC 0006-0952-31 unit of use bottles of 30
NDC 0006-0952-54 unit of use bottles of 90
NDC 0006-0952-58 unit of use bottles of 100
NDC 0006-0952-28 unit dose packages of 100
NDC 0006-0952-82 bottles of 1,000.
No. 6536 — Tablets COZAAR, 100 mg, are dark green, teardrop-shaped, film-coated tablets with code 960 on one side and MRK on the other. They are supplied as follows:
NDC 0006-0960-31 unit of use bottles of 30
NDC 0006-0960-54 unit of use bottles of 90
NDC 0006-0960-58 unit of use bottles of 100
NDC 0006-0960-28 unit dose packages of 100
NDC 0006-0960-82 bottles of 1,000.
Storage
Store at 25°C (77°F); excursions permitted to 15-30°C (59-86°F) [see USP Controlled Room Temperature]. Keep container tightly closed. Protect from light.
MERCK & CO., INC., Whitehouse Station, NJ 08889, USA
9573525 Issued February 2004

Shown in Product Identification Guide, page 323

CRIXIVAN® ℞
(INDINAVIR SULFATE)
CAPSULES

DESCRIPTION

CRIXIVAN* (indinavir sulfate) is an inhibitor of the human immunodeficiency virus (HIV) protease. CRIXIVAN Capsules are formulated as a sulfate salt and are available for oral administration in strengths of 100, 200, 333, and 400 mg of indinavir (corresponding to 125, 250, 416.3, and 500 mg indinavir sulfate, respectively). Each capsule also contains the inactive ingredients anhydrous lactose and magnesium stearate. The capsule shell has the following inactive ingredients and dyes: gelatin, titanium dioxide, silicon dioxide and sodium lauryl sulfate.
The chemical name for indinavir sulfate is [1(1*S*,2*R*),5(*S*)]-2,3,5-trideoxy-*N*-(2,3-dihydro-2-hydroxy-1*H*-inden-1-yl)-5-[2-[[(1,1-dimethylethyl)amino]carbonyl]-4-(3-pyridinylmethyl)-1-piperazinyl]-2-(phenylmethyl)-D-*erythro*-pentonamide sulfate (1:1) salt. Indinavir sulfate has the following structural formula:

Indinavir sulfate is a white to off-white, hygroscopic, crystalline powder with the molecular formula $C_{36}H_{47}N_5O_4 \cdot H_2SO_4$ and a molecular weight of 711.88. It is very soluble in water and in methanol.

*Registered trademark of MERCK & CO., Inc.

MICROBIOLOGY

Mechanism of Action: HIV-1 protease is an enzyme required for the proteolytic cleavage of the viral polyprotein precursors into the individual functional proteins found in infectious HIV-1. Indinavir binds to the protease active site and inhibits the activity of the enzyme. This inhibition prevents cleavage of the viral polyproteins resulting in the formation of immature non-infectious viral particles.
Antiretroviral Activity In Vitro: The *in vitro* activity of indinavir was assessed in cell lines of lymphoblastic and monocytic origin and in peripheral blood lymphocytes. HIV-1 variants used to infect the different cell types include laboratory-adapted variants, primary clinical isolates and clinical isolates resistant to nucleoside analogue and nonnucleoside inhibitors of the HIV-1 reverse transcriptase. The IC_{95} (95% inhibitory concentration) of indinavir in these test systems was in the range of 25 to 100 nM. In drug combination studies with the nucleoside analogues zidovudine and didanosine, indinavir showed synergistic activity in cell culture. The relationship between *in vitro* susceptibility of HIV-1 to indinavir and inhibition of HIV-1 replication in humans has not been established.
Drug Resistance: Isolates of HIV-1 with reduced susceptibility to the drug have been recovered from some patients treated with indinavir. Viral resistance was correlated with the accumulation of mutations that resulted in the expression of amino acid substitutions in the viral protease. Eleven amino acid residue positions, (L10I/V/R, K20I/M/R, L24I, M46I/L, I54A/V, L63P, I64V, A71T/V, V82A/F/T, I84V, and L90M), at which substitutions are associated with resistance, have been identified. Resistance was mediated by the co-expression of multiple and variable substitutions at these positions. No single substitution was either necessary or sufficient for measurable resistance (≥4-fold increase in IC_{95}). In general, higher levels of resistance were associated with the co-expression of greater numbers of substitutions, although their individual effects varied and were not additive. At least 3 amino acid substitutions must be present for phenotypic resistance to indinavir to reach measurable levels. In addition, mutations in the p7/ p1 and p1/ p6 gag cleavage sites were observed in some indinavir resistant HIV-1 isolates.
In vitro phenotypic susceptibilities to indinavir were determined for 38 viral isolates from 13 patients who experienced virologic rebounds during indinavir monotherapy. Pre-treatment isolates from five patients exhibited indinavir IC_{95} values of 50-100 nM. At or following viral RNA rebound (after 12-76 weeks of therapy), IC_{95} values ranged from 25 to >3000 nM, and the viruses carried 2 to 10 mutations in the protease gene relative to baseline.
Cross-Resistance to Other Antiviral Agents: Varying degrees of HIV-1 cross-resistance have been observed between indinavir and other HIV-1 protease inhibitors. In studies with ritonavir, saquinavir, and amprenavir, the extent and spectrum of cross-resistance varied with the specific mutational patterns observed. In general, the degree of cross-resistance increased with the accumulation of resistance-associated amino acid substitutions. Within a panel of 29 viral isolates from indinavir-treated patients that exhibited measurable (≥4-fold) phenotypic resistance to indinavir, all were resistant to ritonavir. Of the indinavir resistant HIV-1 isolates, 63% showed resistance to saquinavir and 81% to amprenavir.

CLINICAL PHARMACOLOGY

Pharmacokinetics
Absorption: Indinavir was rapidly absorbed in the fasted state with a time to peak plasma concentration (T_{max}) of 0.8 ± 0.3 hours (mean ± S.D.) (n=11). A greater than dose-proportional increase in indinavir plasma concentrations was observed over the 200-1000 mg dose range. At a dosing regimen of 800 mg every 8 hours, steady-state area under the plasma concentration time curve (AUC) was 30,691 ± 11,407 nM•hour (n=16), peak plasma concentration (C_{max}) was 12,617 ± 4037 nM (n=16), and plasma concentration eight hours post dose (trough) was 251 ± 178 nM (n=16).
Effect of Food on Oral Absorption: Administration of indinavir with a meal high in calories, fat, and protein (784 kcal, 48.6 g fat, 31.3 g protein) resulted in a 77% ± 8% reduction in AUC and an 84% ± 7% reduction in C_{max} (n=10). Administration with lighter meals (e.g., a meal of dry toast with jelly, apple juice, and coffee with skim milk and sugar or a meal of corn flakes, skim milk and sugar) resulted in little or no change in AUC, C_{max} or trough concentration.
Distribution: Indinavir was approximately 60% bound to human plasma proteins over a concentration range of 81 nM to 16,300 nM.
Metabolism: Following a 400-mg dose of ^{14}C-indinavir, 83 ± 1% (n=4) and 19 ± 3% (n=6) of the total radioactivity was recovered in feces and urine, respectively; radioactivity due to parent drug in feces and urine was 19.1% and 9.4%, respectively. Seven metabolites have been identified, one glucuronide conjugate and six oxidative metabolites. *In vitro* studies indicate that cytochrome P-450 3A4 (CYP3A4) is the major enzyme responsible for formation of the oxidative metabolites.
Elimination: Less than 20% of indinavir is excreted unchanged in the urine. Mean urinary excretion of unchanged drug was 10.4 ± 4.9% (n=10) and 12.0 ± 4.9% (n=10) following a single 700-mg and 1000-mg dose, respectively. Indinavir was rapidly eliminated with a half-life of 1.8 ± 0.4 hours (n=10). Significant accumulation was not observed after multiple dosing at 800 mg every 8 hours.
Special Populations
Hepatic Insufficiency: Patients with mild to moderate hepatic insufficiency and clinical evidence of cirrhosis had evidence of decreased metabolism of indinavir resulting in approximately 60% higher mean AUC following a single 400-mg dose (n=12). The half-life of indinavir increased to 2.8 ± 0.5 hours. Indinavir pharmacokinetics have not been studied in patients with severe hepatic insufficiency (see DOSAGE AND ADMINISTRATION, *Hepatic Insufficiency*).
Renal Insufficiency: The pharmacokinetics of indinavir have not been studied in patients with renal insufficiency.
Gender: The effect of gender on the pharmacokinetics of indinavir was evaluated in 10 HIV seropositive women who received CRIXIVAN 800 mg every 8 hours with zidovudine 200 mg every 8 hours and lamivudine 150 mg twice a day for one week. Indinavir pharmacokinetic parameters in these women were compared to those in HIV seropositive men (pooled historical control data). Differences in indinavir exposure, peak concentrations, and trough concentrations between males and females are shown in Table 1 below:
[See table 1 at bottom of next page]
The clinical significance of these gender differences in the pharmacokinetics of indinavir is not known.
Race: Pharmacokinetics of indinavir appear to be comparable in Caucasians and Blacks based on pharmacokinetic studies including 42 Caucasians (26 HIV-positive) and 16 Blacks (4 HIV-positive).
Pediatric: The optimal dosing regimen for use of indinavir in pediatric patients has not been established. In HIV-infected pediatric patients (age 4-15 years), a dosage regimen of indinavir capsules, 500 mg/m^2 every 8 hours, produced AUC_{0-8hr} of 38,742 ± 24,098 nM•hour (n=34), C_{max} of 17,181 ± 9809 nM (n=34), and trough concentrations of 134 ± 91 nM (n=28). The pharmacokinetic profiles of indinavir in pediatric patients were not comparable to profiles

Continued on next page

Information on the Merck & Co., Inc., products listed on these pages is from the prescribing information in use October 1, 2004. For information, please call 1-800-NSC-MERCK [1-800-672-6372].

Crixivan—Cont.

previously observed in HIV-infected adults receiving the recommended dose of 800 mg every 8 hours. The AUC and C_{max} values were slightly higher and the trough concentrations were considerably lower in pediatric patients. Approximately 50% of the pediatric patients had trough values below 100 nM; whereas, approximately 10% of adult patients had trough levels below 100 nM. The relationship between specific trough values and inhibition of HIV replication has not been established.

Drug Interactions (also see CONTRAINDICATIONS, WARNINGS, PRECAUTIONS, *Drug Interactions*)
Indinavir is an inhibitor of the cytochrome P450 isoform CYP3A4. Coadministration of CRIXIVAN and drugs primarily metabolized by CYP3A4 may result in increased plasma concentrations of the other drug, which could increase or prolong its therapeutic and adverse effects (see CONTRAINDICATIONS and WARNINGS). Based on *in vitro* data in human liver microsomes, indinavir does not inhibit CYP1A2, CYP2C9, CYP2E1 and CYP2B6. However, indinavir may be a weak inhibitor of CYP2D6.
Indinavir is metabolized by CYP3A4. Drugs that induce CYP3A4 activity would be expected to increase the clearance of indinavir, resulting in lowered plasma concentrations of indinavir. Coadministration of CRIXIVAN and other drugs that inhibit CYP3A4 may decrease the clearance of indinavir and may result in increased plasma concentrations of indinavir.
Drug interaction studies were performed with CRIXIVAN and other drugs likely to be coadministered and some drugs commonly used as probes for pharmacokinetic interactions. The effects of coadministration of CRIXIVAN on the AUC, C_{max} and C_{min} are summarized in Table 2 (effect of other drugs on indinavir) and Table 3 (effect of indinavir on other drugs). For information regarding clinical recommendations, see Table 9 in PRECAUTIONS.

[See table 2 below and on next page]
[See table 3 on pages 2023 and 2024]

Delavirdine: Delavirdine inhibits the metabolism of indinavir such that coadministration of 400-mg or 600-mg indinavir three times daily with 400-mg delavirdine three times daily alters indinavir AUC, C_{max} and C_{min} (see Table 2). Indinavir had no effect on delavirdine pharmacokinetics (see DOSAGE AND ADMINISTRATION, *Concomitant Therapy, Delavirdine*), based on a comparison to historical delavirdine pharmacokinetic data.
Methadone: Administration of indinavir (800 mg every 8 hours) with methadone (20 mg to 60 mg daily) for one week in subjects on methadone maintenance resulted in no change in methadone AUC. Based on a comparison to historical data, there was little or no change in indinavir AUC.
Ritonavir: Compared to historical data in patients who received indinavir 800 mg every 8 hours alone, twice-daily coadministration to volunteers of indinavir 800 mg and ritonavir with food for two weeks resulted in an 2.7-fold of indinavir AUC_{24h}, a 1.6-fold increase in indinavir C_{max}, and an 11-fold increase in indinavir C_{min} for a 100-mg ritonavir dose and a 3.6-fold increase of indinavir AUC_{24h}, a 1.8-fold increase in indinavir C_{max}, and a 24-fold increase in indinavir C_{min} for a 200-mg ritonavir dose. In the same study, twice-daily coadministration of indinavir (800 mg) and ritonavir (100 or 200 mg) resulted in ritonavir AUC_{24h} increases versus the same doses of ritonavir alone (see Table 3).
Sildenafil: The results of one published study in HIV-infected men (n=6) indicated that coadministration of indinavir (800 mg every 8 hours chronically) with a single 25-mg dose of sildenafil resulted in an 11% increase in average $AUC_{0\text{-}8hr}$ of indinavir and a 48% increase in average indinavir peak concentration (C_{max}) compared to 800 mg every 8 hours alone. Average sildenafil AUC was increased by 340% following coadministration of sildenafil and indinavir compared to historical data following administration of sildenafil alone (see WARNINGS, *Drug Interactions* and PRECAUTIONS, *Drug Interactions*).
Vardenafil: Indinavir (800 mg every 8 hours) coadministered with a single 10-mg dose of vardenafil resulted in a 16-fold increase in vardenafil AUC, a 7-fold increase in vardenafil C_{max}, and a 2-fold increase in vardenafil half-life (see WARNINGS, *Drug Interactions* and PRECAUTIONS, *Drug Interactions*).

Table 1

PK Parameter	% change in PK parameter for females relative to males	90% Confidence Interval
$AUC_{0\text{-}8h}$ (nM•hr)	↓13%	(↓32%, ↑12%)
C_{max} (nM)	↓13%	(↓32%, ↑10%)
C_{8h} (nM)	↓22%	(↓47%, ↑15%)

↓ Indicates a decrease in the PK parameter;
↑ indicates an increase in the PK parameter.

Table 2
Drug Interactions: Pharmacokinetic Parameters for Indinavir in the Presence of the Coadministered Drug
(See PRECAUTIONS, Table 9 for Recommended Alterations in Dose or Regimen)

Coadministered drug	Dose of Coadministered drug (mg)	Dose of CRIXIVAN (mg)	n	Ratio (with/without coadministered drug) of Indinavir Pharmacokinetic Parameters (90% CI); No Effect =1.00		
				C_{max}	AUC	C_{min}
Cimetidine	600 twice daily, 6 days	400 single dose	12	1.07 (0.77, 1.49)	0.98 (0.81, 1.19)	0.82 (0.69, 0.99)
Clarithromycin	500 q12h, 7 days	800 three times daily, 7 days	10	1.08 (0.85, 1.38)	1.19 (1.00, 1.42)	1.57 (1.16, 2.12)
Delavirdine	400 three times daily	400 three times daily, 7 days	28	0.64[1] (0.48, 0.86)	No significant change[1]	2.18[1] (1.16, 4.12)
Delavirdine	400 three times daily	600 three times daily, 7 days	28	No significant change	1.53[1] (1.07, 2.20)	3.98[1] (2.04, 7.78)
Efavirenz[2]	600 once daily, 10 days	1000 three times daily, 10 days	20			
		After morning dose		No significant change[1]	0.67[1] (0.61, 0.74)	0.61[1] (0.49, 0.76)
		After afternoon dose		No significant change[1]	0.63[1] (0.54, 0.74)	0.48[1] (0.43, 0.53)
		After evening dose		0.71[1] (0.57, 0.89)	0.54[1] (0.46, 0.63)	0.43[1] (0.37, 0.50)
Fluconazole[2]	400 once daily, 8 days	1000 three times daily, 7 days	11	0.87 (0.72, 1.05)	0.76 (0.59, 0.98)	0.90 (0.72, 1.12)
Grapefruit Juice	8 oz.	400 single dose	10	0.65 (0.53, 0.79)	0.73 (0.60, 0.87)	0.90 (0.71, 1.15)
Isoniazid	300 once daily in the morning, 8 days	800 three times daily, 7 days	11	0.95 (0.88, 1.03)	0.99 (0.87, 1.13)	0.89 (0.75, 1.06)
Itraconazole	200 twice daily, 7 days	600 three times daily, 7 days	12	0.78[3] (0.69, 0.88)	0.99[3] (0.91, 1.06)	1.49[3] (1.28, 1.74)
Ketoconazole	400 once daily, 7 days	600 three times daily, 7 days	10	1.14[3] (0.93, 1.40)	1.62[3] (1.38, 1.92)	2.80[3] (2.20, 3.57)
Methadone	20-60 once daily in the morning, 8 days	800 three times daily, 8 days	10	See text below for discussion of interaction.		
Quinidine	200 single dose	400 single dose	10	0.96 (0.79, 1.18)	1.07 (0.89, 1.28)	0.93 (0.73, 1.19)
Rifabutin	150 once daily in the morning, 10 days	800 three times daily, 10 days	14	0.80 (0.72, 0.89)	0.68 (0.60, 0.76)	0.60 (0.51, 0.72)
Rifabutin	300 once daily in the morning, 10 days	800 three times daily, 10 days	10	0.75 (0.61, 0.91)	0.66 (0.56, 0.77)	0.61 (0.50, 0.75)
Rifampin	600 once daily in the morning, 8 days	800 three times daily, 7 days	12	0.13 (0.08, 0.22)	0.08 (0.06, 0.11)	Not Done
Ritonavir	100 twice daily, 14 days	800 twice daily, 14 days	10, 16[3]	See text below for discussion of interaction.		
Ritonavir	200 twice daily, 14 days	800 twice daily, 14 days	9, 16[3]	See text below for discussion of interaction.		
Sildenafil	25 single dose	800 three times daily	6	See text below for discussion of interaction.		

(Table continued on next page)

INDICATIONS AND USAGE

CRIXIVAN in combination with antiretroviral agents is indicated for the treatment of HIV infection.
This indication is based on two clinical trials of approximately 1 year duration that demonstrated: 1) a reduction in the risk of AIDS-defining illnesses or death; 2) a prolonged suppression of HIV RNA.

Description of Studies
In all clinical studies, with the exception of ACTG 320, the AMPLICOR HIV MONITOR assay was used to determine the level of circulating HIV RNA in serum. This is an experimental use of the assay. HIV RNA results should not be directly compared to results from other trials using different HIV RNA assays or using other sample sources.
Study ACTG 320 was a multicenter, randomized, double-blind clinical endpoint trial to compare the effect of CRIXIVAN in combination with zidovudine and lamivudine with that of zidovudine plus lamivudine on the progression to an AIDS-defining illness (ADI) or death. Patients were protease inhibitor and lamivudine naive and zidovudine experienced, with CD4 cell counts of ≤200 cells/mm³. The study enrolled 1156 HIV-infected patients (17% female, 28% Black, 18% Hispanic, mean age 39 years). The mean baseline CD4 cell count was 87 cells/mm³. The mean baseline HIV RNA was 4.95 $\log_{10}$ copies/mL (89,035 copies/mL). The study was terminated after a planned interim analysis, resulting in a median follow-up of 38 weeks and a maximum follow-up of 52 weeks. Results are shown in Table 4 and Figures 1 & 2.

Table 4
ACTG 320

Endpoint	Number (%) of Patients with AIDS-defining Illness or Death: IDV+ZDV+L (n=577)	ZDV+L (n=579)
HIV Progression or Death	35 (6.1)	63 (10.9)
Death*	10 (1.7)	19 (3.3)

*The number of deaths is inadequate to assess the impact of indinavir on survival.
IDV = Indinavir, ZDV = Zidovudine, L = Lamivudine

[See figure 1 at top of next column]
[See figure 2 at top of next column]

Study 028, a double-blind, multicenter, randomized, clinical endpoint trial conducted in Brazil, compared the effects of CRIXIVAN plus zidovudine with those of CRIXIVAN alone or zidovudine alone on the progression to an ADI or death, and on surrogate marker responses. All patients were antiretroviral naive with CD4 cell counts of 50 to 250 cells/mm³. The study enrolled 996 HIV-1 seropositive patients [28% female, 11% Black, 1% Asian/Other, median age 33 years,

Study ACTG 320: Figure 1

Indinavir Protocol ACTG 320 Zidovudine Experienced
Plasma Viral RNA - Proportions Below 400 copies/mL

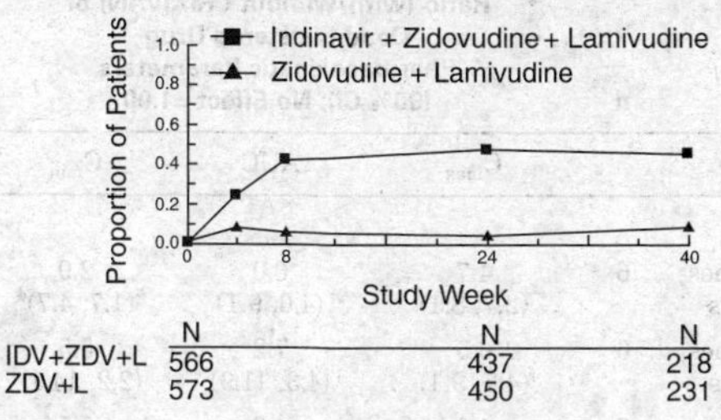

Study ACTG 320: Figure 2

ACTG 320 Zidovudine Experienced
CD4 Cell Counts - Mean Change from Baseline

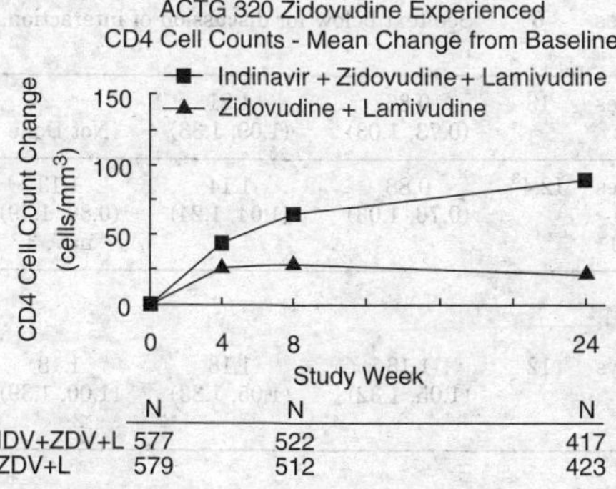

mean baseline CD4 cell count of 152 cells/mm^3, mean serum viral RNA of 4.44 $\log_{10}$ copies/mL (27,824 copies/mL)]. Treatment regimens containing zidovudine were modified in a blinded manner with the optional addition of lamivudine (median time: week 40). The median length of follow-up was 56 weeks with a maximum of 97 weeks. The study was terminated after a planned interim analysis, resulting in a median follow-up of 56 weeks and a maximum follow-up of 97 weeks. Results are shown in Table 5 and Figures 3 and 4.

Table 5
Protocol 028

Endpoint	Number (%) of Patients with AIDS-defining Illness or Death IDV+ZDV (n=332)	IDV (n=332)	ZDV (n=332)
HIV Progression or Death	21 (6.3)	27 (8.1)	62 (18.7)
Death*	8 (2.4)	5 (1.5)	11 (3.3)

*The number of deaths is inadequate to assess the impact of Indinavir on survival.

Study 028: Figure 3

Indinavir Protocol 028 Zidovudine Naive
Viral RNA - Proportions Below 500 Copies/mL in Serum

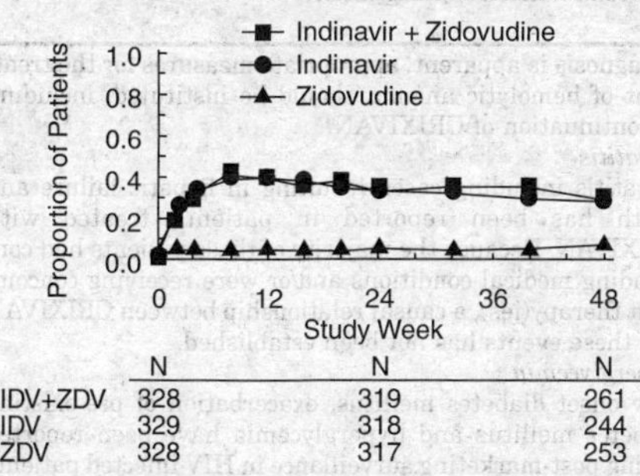

Study 028: Figure 4

Indinavir Protocol 028 Zidovudine Naive
CD4 Cell Counts - Mean Change from Baseline

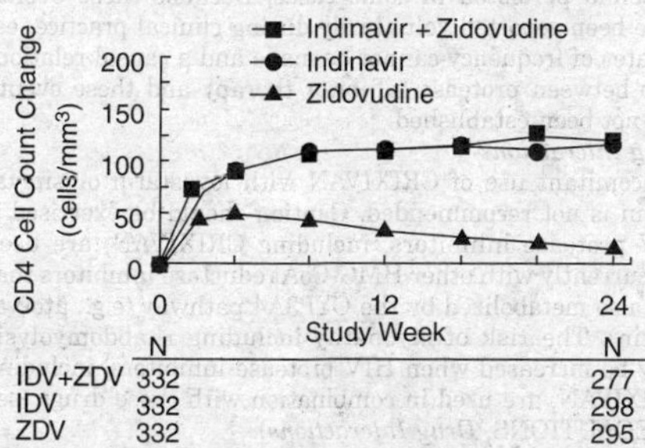

Study 035 was a multicenter, randomized trial in 97 HIV-1 seropositive patients who were zidovudine-experienced (median exposure 30 months), protease-inhibitor- and lamivu-

Table 2 *(cont.)*
Drug Interactions: Pharmacokinetic Parameters for Indinavir in the Presence of the Coadministered Drug
(See PRECAUTIONS, Table 9 for Recommended Alterations in Dose or Regimen)

Coadministered drug	Dose of Coadministered drug (mg)	Dose of CRIXIVAN (mg)	n	Ratio (with/without coadministered drug) of Indinavir Pharmacokinetic Parameters (90% CI); No Effect =1.00 C_{max}	AUC	C_{min}
St. John's wort (*Hypericum perforatum*, standardized to 0.3% hypericin)	300 three times daily with meals, 14 days	800 three times daily	8	Not Available	0.46 (0.34, 0.58)[4]	0.19 (0.06, 0.33)[4]
Stavudine (d4T)[2]	40 twice daily, 7 days	800 three times daily, 7 days	11	0.95 (0.80, 1.11)	0.95 (0.80, 1.12)	1.13 (0.83, 1.53)
Trimethoprim/ Sulfamethoxazole	800 Trimethoprim/ 160 Sulfamethoxazole q12h, 7 days	400 four times daily, 7 days	12	1.12 (0.87, 1.46)	0.98 (0.81, 1.18)	0.83 (0.72, 0.95)
Zidovudine[2]	200 three times daily, 7 days	1000 three times daily, 7 days	12	1.06 (0.91, 1.25)	1.05 (0.86, 1.28)	1.02 (0.77, 1.35)
Zidovudine/ Lamivudine (3TC)[2]	200/150 three times daily, 7 days	800 three times daily, 7 days	6, 9[5]	1.05 (0.83, 1.33)	1.04 (0.67, 1.61)	0.98 (0.56, 1.73)

All interaction studies conducted in healthy, HIV-negative adult subjects, unless otherwise indicated.
[1]Relative to indinavir 800 mg three times daily alone.
[2]Study conducted in HIV-positive subjects.
[3]Comparison to historical data on 16 subjects receiving indinavir alone.
[4]95% CI.
[5]Parallel group design; n for indinavir + coadministered drug, n for indinavir alone.

Table 3
Drug Interactions: Pharmacokinetic Parameters for Coadministered Drug in the Presence of Indinavir
(See PRECAUTIONS, Table 9 for Recommended Alterations in Dose or Regimen)

Coadministered drug	Dose of Coadministered drug (mg)	Dose of CRIXIVAN (mg)	n	Ratio (with/without CRIXIVAN) of Coadministered Drug Pharmacokinetic Parameters (90% CI); No Effect =1.00 C_{max}	AUC	C_{min}
Clarithromycin	500 twice daily, 7 days	800 three times daily, 7 days	12	1.19 (1.02, 1.39)	1.47 (1.30, 1.65)	1.97 (1.58, 2.46) n=11
Efavirenz	200 once daily, 14 days	800 three times daily, 14 days	20	No significant change	No significant change	—
Ethinyl Estradiol (ORTHO-NOVUM 1/35)	35 mcg, 8 days	800 three times daily, 8 days	18	1.02 (0.96, 1.09)	1.22 (1.15, 1.30)	1.37 (1.24, 1.51)
Isoniazid	300 once daily in the morning, 8 days	800 three times daily, 8 days	11	1.34 (1.12, 1.60)	1.12 (1.03, 1.22)	1.00 (0.92, 1.08)
Methadone[2]	20-60 once daily in the morning, 8 days	800 three times daily, 8 days	12	0.93 (0.84, 1.03)	0.96 (0.86, 1.06)	1.06 (0.96, 1.19)
Norethindrone (ORTHO-NOVUM 1/35)	1 mcg, 8 days	800 three times daily, 8 days	18	1.05 (0.95, 1.16)	1.26 (1.20, 1.31)	1.44 (1.32, 1.57)
Rifabutin *150 mg once daily in the morning, 11 days + indinavir compared to 300 mg once daily in the morning, 11 days alone	150 once daily in the morning, 10 days	800 three times daily, 10 days	14	1.29 (1.05, 1.59)	1.54 (1.33, 1.79)	1.99 (1.71, 2.31) n=13
	300 once daily in the morning, 10 days	800 three times daily, 10 days	10	2.34 (1.64, 3.35)	2.73 (1.99, 3.77)	3.44 (2.65, 4.46) n=9
Ritonavir	100 twice daily, 14 days	800 twice daily, 14 days	10,4[3]	1.61 (1.13, 2.29)	1.72 (1.20, 2.48)	1.62 (0.93, 2.85)
	200 twice daily, 14 days	800 twice daily, 14 days	9,5[3]	1.19 (0.85, 1.66)	1.96 (1.39, 2.76)	4.71 (2.66, 8.33) n=9, 4

(Table continued on next page)

dine-naive, with mean baseline CD4 count 175 cells/mm^3 and mean baseline serum viral RNA 4.62 $\log_{10}$ copies/mL (41,230 copies/mL). Comparisons included CRIXIVAN plus zidovudine plus lamivudine vs. CRIXIVAN alone vs. zidovudine plus lamivudine. After at least 24 weeks of randomized, double-blind therapy, patients were switched to open-label CRIXIVAN plus lamivudine plus zidovudine. Mean changes in $\log_{10}$ viral RNA in serum, the proportions of patients with viral RNA below 500 copies/mL in serum, and mean changes in CD4 cell counts, during 24 weeks of randomized, double-blinded therapy are summarized in Figures 5, 6, and 7, respectively. A limited number of patients remained on randomized, double-blind treatment for longer periods; based on this extended treatment experience, it appears that a greater number of subjects randomized to CRIXIVAN plus zidovudine plus lamivudine demonstrated HIV RNA levels below 500 copies/mL during one year of therapy as compared to those in other treatment groups.

Continued on next page

Information on the Merck & Co., Inc., products listed on these pages is from the prescribing information in use October 1, 2004. For information, please call 1-800-NSC-MERCK [1-800-672-6372].

Crixivan—Cont.

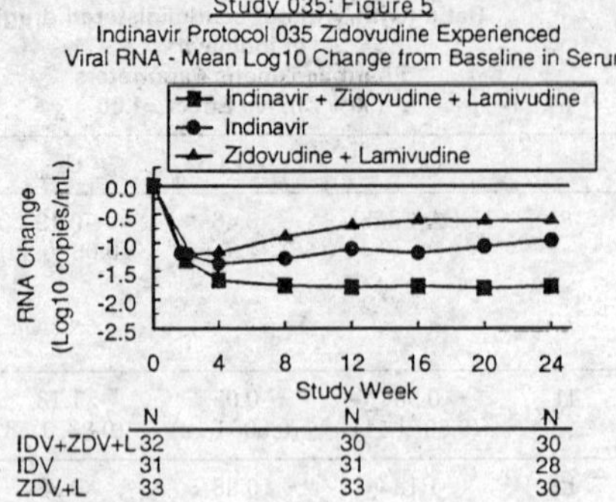

Study 035: Figure 6
Indinavir Protocol 035 Zidovudine Experienced
Viral RNA - Proportions Below 500 Copies/mL in Serum

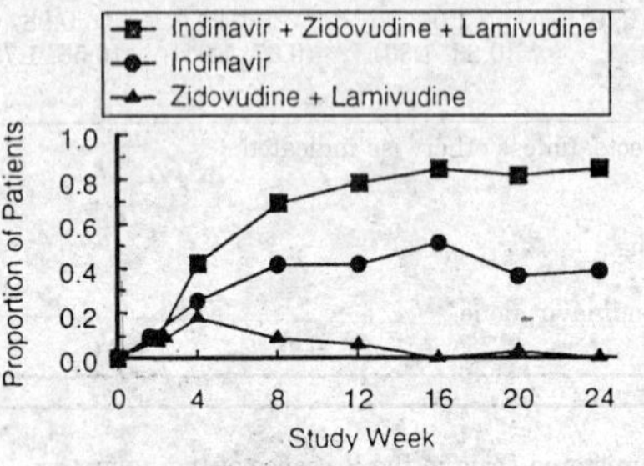

Study 035: Figure 7
Indinavir Protocol 035 Zidovudine Experienced
CD4 Cell Counts - Mean Change from Baseline

Indinavir + Zidovudine + Lamivudine
Indinavir
Zidovudine + Lamivudine
CD4 Cell Count Change (cells/mm³)
150
100
50
0
0 4 8 12 16 20 24
Study Week

	N	N	N
IDV+ZDV+L	33	31	31
IDV	31	31	27
ZDV+L	33	33	29

Genotypic Resistance in Clinical Studies

Study 006 (10/15/93-10/12/94) was a dose-ranging study in which patients were initially treated with CRIXIVAN at a dose of <2.4 g/day followed by 2.4 g/day. Study 019 (6/23/94-4/10/95) was a randomized comparison of CRIXIVAN 600 mg every 6 hours, CRIXIVAN plus zidovudine, and zidovudine alone. Table 6 shows the incidence of genotypic resistance at 24 weeks in these studies.

Table 6
Genotypic Resistance at 24 Weeks

Treatment Group	Resistance to IDV n/N*	Resistance to ZDV n/N*
IDV	—	—
<2.4 g/day	31/37 (84%)	—
2.4 g/day	9/21 (43%)	1/17 (6%)
IDV/ZDV	4/22 (18%)	1/22 (5%)
ZDV	1/18 (6%)	11/17 (65%)

*N – includes patients with non-amplifiable virus at 24 weeks who had amplifiable virus at week 0.

CONTRAINDICATIONS

CRIXIVAN is contraindicated in patients with clinically significant hypersensitivity to any of its components.

Inhibition of CYP3A4 by CRIXIVAN can result in elevated plasma concentrations of the following drugs, potentially causing serious or life-threatening reactions:

Table 7
Drug Interactions With Crixivan: Contraindicated Drugs

Drug Class	Drugs Within Class That Are Contraindicated With CRIXIVAN
Antiarrhythmics	amiodarone
Ergot derivatives	dihydroergotamine, ergonovine, ergotamine, methylergonovine
Sedative/ hypnotics	midazolam, triazolam
GI motility agents	cisapride
Neuroleptics	pimozide

Table 3 *(cont.)*
Drug Interactions: Pharmacokinetic Parameters for Coadministered Drug in the Presence of Indinavir
(See PRECAUTIONS, Table 9 for Recommended Alterations in Dose or Regimen)

Coadministered drug	Dose of Coadministered drug (mg)	Dose of CRIXIVAN (mg)	n	Ratio (with/without CRIXIVAN) of Coadministered Drug Pharmacokinetic Parameters (90% CI); No Effect =1.00		
				C_{max}	AUC	C_{min}
Saquinavir						
Hard gel formulation	600 single dose	800 three times daily, 2 days	6	4.7 (2.7, 8.1)	6.0 (4.0, 9.1)	2.9 (1.7, 4.7)[4]
Soft gel formulation	800 single dose	800 three times daily, 2 days	6	6.5 (4.7, 9.1)	7.2 (4.3, 11.9)	5.5 (2.2, 14.1)[4]
Soft gel formulation	1200 single dose	800 three times daily, 2 days	6	4.0 (2.7, 5.9)	4.6 (3.2, 6.7)	5.5 (3.7, 8.3)[4]
Sildenafil	25 single dose	800 three times daily	6	See text below for discussion of interaction.		
Stavudine[1]	40 twice daily, 7 days	800 three times daily, 7 days	13	0.86 (0.73, 1.03)	1.21 (1.09, 1.33)	Not Done
Theophylline	250 single dose (on Days 1 and 7)	800 three times daily, 6 days (Days 2 to 7)	12,4[3]	0.88 (0.76, 1.03)	1.14 (1.04, 1.24)	1.13 (0.86, 1,49) n=7, 3
Trimethoprim/ Sulfamethoxazole						
Trimethoprim	800 Trimethoprim/ 160 Sulfamethoxazole q12h, 7 days	400 q6h, 7 days	12	1.18 (1.05, 1.32)	1.18 (1.05, 1.33)	1.18 (1.00, 1.39)
Trimethoprim/ Sulfamethoxazole						
Sulfamethoxazole	800 Trimethoprim/ 160 Sulfamethoxazole q12h, 7 days	400 q6h, 7 days	12	1.01 (0.95, 1.08)	1.05 (1.01, 1.09)	1.05 (0.97, 1.14)
Vardenafil	2.5 single dose	800 three times daily	18	See text below for discussion of interaction.		
Zidovudine[1]	200 three times daily, 7 days	1000 three times daily, 7 days	12	0.89 (0.73, 1.09)	1.17 (1.07, 1.29)	1.51 (0.71, 3.20) n=4
Zidovudine/ Lamivudine[1]						
Zidovudine	200/150 three times daily, 7 days	800 three times daily, 7 days	6, 7[3]	1.23 (0.74, 2.03)	1.39 (1.02, 1.89)	1.08 (0.77, 1.50) n=5, 5
Zidovudine/ Lamivudine[1]						
Lamivudine	200/150 three times daily, 7 days	800 three times daily, 7 days	6, 7[3]	0.73 (0.52, 1.02)	0.91 (0.66, 1.26)	0.88 (0.59, 1.33)

All interaction studies conducted in healthy, HIV-negative adult subjects, unless otherwise indicated.
[1]Study conducted in HIV-positive subjects.
[2]Study conducted in subjects on methadone maintenance.
[3]Parallel group design; n for coadministered drug + indinavir, n for coadministered drug alone.
[4]C_{6hr}

WARNINGS

ALERT: Find out about medicines that should not be taken with CRIXIVAN. This statement is included on the product's bottle label.

Nephrolithiasis/Urolithiasis

Nephrolithiasis/urolithiasis has occurred with CRIXIVAN therapy. The cumulative frequency of nephrolithiasis is substantially higher in pediatric patients (29%) than in adult patients (12.4%; range across individual trials: 4.7% to 34.4%). The cumulative frequency of nephrolithiasis events increases with increasing exposure to CRIXIVAN; however, the risk over time remains relatively constant. In some cases, nephrolithiasis/urolithiasis has been associated with renal insufficiency or acute renal failure, pyelonephritis with or without bacteremia. If signs or symptoms of nephrolithiasis/urolithiasis occur, (including flank pain, with or without hematuria or microscopic hematuria), temporary interruption (e.g., 1-3 days) or discontinuation of therapy may be considered. **Adequate hydration is recommended in all patients treated with CRIXIVAN. (See ADVERSE REACTIONS and DOSAGE AND ADMINISTRATION, *Nephrolithiasis/Urolithiasis*.)**

Hemolytic Anemia

Acute hemolytic anemia, including cases resulting in death, has been reported in patients treated with CRIXIVAN. Once a diagnosis is apparent, appropriate measures for the treatment of hemolytic anemia should be instituted, including discontinuation of CRIXIVAN.

Hepatitis

Hepatitis including cases resulting in hepatic failure and death has been reported in patients treated with CRIXIVAN. Because the majority of these patients had confounding medical conditions and/or were receiving concomitant therapy(ies), a causal relationship between CRIXIVAN and these events has not been established.

Hyperglycemia

New onset diabetes mellitus, exacerbation of pre-existing diabetes mellitus and hyperglycemia have been reported during post-marketing surveillance in HIV-infected patients receiving protease inhibitor therapy. Some patients required either initiation or dose adjustments of insulin or oral hypoglycemic agents for treatment of these events. In some cases, diabetic ketoacidosis has occurred. In those patients who discontinued protease inhibitor therapy, hyperglycemia persisted in some cases. Because these events have been reported voluntarily during clinical practice, estimates of frequency cannot be made and a causal relationship between protease inhibitor therapy and these events has not been established.

Drug Interactions

Concomitant use of CRIXIVAN with lovastatin or simvastatin is not recommended. Caution should be exercised if HIV protease inhibitors, including CRIXIVAN, are used concurrently with other HMG-CoA reductase inhibitors that are also metabolized by the CYP3A4 pathway (e.g., atorvastatin). The risk of myopathy including rhabdomyolysis may be increased when HIV protease inhibitors, including CRIXIVAN, are used in combination with these drugs (see PRECAUTIONS, *Drug Interactions*).

Particular caution should be used when prescribing sildenafil, tadalafil, or vardenafil in patients receiving indinavir. Coadministration of CRIXIVAN with these medications is expected to substantially increase plasma concentrations of sildenafil, tadalafil, and vardenafil and may result in an increase in adverse events, including hypotension, visual changes, and priapism, which have been associated with sildenafil, tadalafil, and vardenafil (see PRECAUTIONS, *Drug Interactions* and *Information for Patients*, and the manufacturer's complete prescribing information for sildenafil, tadalafil, or vardenafil).

Concomitant use of CRIXIVAN and St. John's wort (*Hypericum perforatum*) or products containing St. John's wort is not recommended. Coadministration of CRIXIVAN and St. John's wort has been shown to substantially decrease indinavir concentrations (see CLINICAL PHARMACOLOGY, *Drug Interactions*) and may lead to loss of virologic response and possible resistance to CRIXIVAN or to the class of protease inhibitors.

PRECAUTIONS

General

Indirect hyperbilirubinemia has occurred frequently during treatment with CRIXIVAN and has infrequently been associated with increases in serum transaminases (see also ADVERSE REACTIONS, *Clinical Trials* and *Post-Marketing Experience*). It is not known whether CRIXIVAN will exacerbate the physiologic hyperbilirubinemia seen in neonates. (See *Pregnancy*.)

Tubulointerstitial Nephritis

Reports of tubulointerstitial nephritis with medullary calcification and cortical atrophy have been observed in patients with asymptomatic severe leukocyturia (>100 cells/high power field). Patients with asymptomatic severe leukocyturia should be followed closely and monitored frequently with urinalyses. Further diagnostic evaluation may be warranted, and discontinuation of CRIXIVAN should be considered in all patients with severe leukocyturia.

Immune reconstitution syndrome has been reported in patients treated with combination antiretroviral therapy (CART), including CRIXIVAN. During the initial phase of treatment, patients responding to antiretroviral therapy whose immune system responds to CART may develop an inflammatory response to indolent or residual opportunistic infections (such as MAI, CMV, PCP, or TB), which may necessitate further evaluation and treatment.

Coexisting Conditions

Patients with hemophilia: There have been reports of spontaneous bleeding in patients with hemophilia A and B treated with protease inhibitors. In some patients, additional factor VIII was required. In many of the reported cases, treatment with protease inhibitors was continued or restarted. A causal relationship between protease inhibitor therapy and these episodes has not been established. (See ADVERSE REACTIONS, *Post-Marketing Experience*).

Patients with hepatic insufficiency due to cirrhosis: In these patients, the dosage of CRIXIVAN should be lowered because of decreased metabolism of CRIXIVAN (see DOSAGE AND ADMINISTRATION).

Patients with renal insufficiency: Patients with renal insufficiency have not been studied.

Fat Redistribution

Redistribution/accumulation of body fat including central obesity, dorsocervical fat enlargement (buffalo hump), peripheral wasting, facial wasting, breast enlargement, and "cushingoid appearance" have been observed in patients receiving antiretroviral therapy. The mechanism and long-term consequences of these events are currently unknown. A causal relationship has not been established.

Information for Patients

A statement to patients and health care providers is included on the product's bottle label. **ALERT: Find out about medicines that should NOT be taken with CRIXIVAN.** A Patient Package Insert (PPI) for CRIXIVAN is available for patient information.

CRIXIVAN is not a cure for HIV infection and patients may continue to develop opportunistic infections and other complications associated with HIV disease. The long-term effects of CRIXIVAN are unknown at this time. CRIXIVAN has not been shown to reduce the risk of transmission of HIV to others through sexual contact or blood contamination.

Patients should be advised to remain under the care of a physician when using CRIXIVAN and should not modify or discontinue treatment without first consulting the physician. Therefore, if a dose is missed, patients should take the next dose at the regularly scheduled time and should not double this dose. Therapy with CRIXIVAN should be initiated and maintained at the recommended dosage.

CRIXIVAN may interact with some drugs; therefore, patients should be advised to report to their doctor the use of any other prescription, non-prescription medication or herbal products, particularly St. John's wort.

For optimal absorption, CRIXIVAN should be administered without food but with water 1 hour before or 2 hours after a meal. Alternatively, CRIXIVAN may be administered with other liquids such as skim milk, juice, coffee, or tea, or with a light meal, e.g., dry toast with jelly, juice, and coffee with skim milk and sugar; or corn flakes, skim milk and sugar (see CLINICAL PHARMACOLOGY, *Effect of Food on Oral Absorption* and DOSAGE AND ADMINISTRATION). Ingestion of CRIXIVAN with a meal high in calories, fat, and protein reduces the absorption of indinavir.

Patients receiving a phosphodiesterase type 5 (PDE5) inhibitor (sildenafil, tadalafil, or vardenafil) should be advised that they may be at an increased risk of PDE5 inhibitor-associated adverse events including hypotension, visual changes, and priapism, and should promptly report any symptoms to their doctors.

Table 8
Drugs That Should Not Be Coadministered with CRIXIVAN

Drug Class: Drug Name	Clinical Comment
Antiarrhythmics: amiodarone	CONTRAINDICATED due to potential for serious and/or life-threatening reactions such as cardiac arrhythmias.
Ergot derivatives: dihydroergotamine, ergonovine, ergotamine, methylergonovine	CONTRAINDICATED due to potential for serious and/or life-threatening reactions such as acute ergot toxicity characterized by peripheral vasospasm and ischemia of the extremitites and other tissues.
Sedative/hypnotics: midazolam, triazolam	CONTRAINDICATED due to potential for serious and/or life-threatening reactions such as prolonged or increased sedation or respiratory depression.
GI motility agents: cisapride	CONTRAINDICATED due to potential for serious and/or life-threatening reactions such as cardiac arrhythmias.
Neuroleptic: pimozide	CONTRAINDICATED due to potential for serious and/or life-threatening reactions such as cardiac arrhythmias.
Herbal products: St. John's wort (*Hypericum perforatum*)	May lead to loss of virologic response and possible resistance to CRIXIVAN or to the class of protease inhibitors.
Antimycobacterial: rifampin	May lead to loss of virologic response and possible resistance to CRIXIVAN or to the class of protease inhibitors or other coadministered antiretroviral agents.
HMG-CoA Reductase inhibitors: lovastatin, simvastatin	Potential for serious reactions such as risk of myopathy including rhabdomyolysis.
Protease inhibitor: atazanavir	Both CRIXIVAN and atazanavir are associated with indirect (unconjugated) hyperbilirubinemia. Combinations of these drugs have not been studied and coadministration of CRIXIVAN and atazanavir is not recommended.

Patients should be informed that redistribution or accumulation of body fat may occur in patients receiving antiretroviral therapy and that the cause and long-term health effects of these conditions are not known at this time.

CRIXIVAN Capsules are sensitive to moisture. Patients should be informed that CRIXIVAN should be stored and used in the original container and the desiccant should remain in the bottle.

Drug Interactions

Indinavir is an inhibitor of the cytochrome P450 isoform CYP3A4. Coadministration of CRIXIVAN and drugs primarily metabolized by CYP3A4 may result in increased plasma concentrations of the other drug, which could increase or prolong its therapeutic and adverse effects (see CONTRAINDICATIONS and WARNINGS).

Indinavir is metabolized by CYP3A4. Drugs that induce CYP3A4 activity would be expected to increase the clearance of indinavir, resulting in lowered plasma concentrations of indinavir. Coadministration of CRIXIVAN and other drugs that inhibit CYP3A4 may decrease the clearance of indinavir and may result in increased plasma concentrations of indinavir.

[See table 8 above]
[See table 9 at top of next page]

Carcinogenesis, Mutagenesis, Impairment of Fertility

Carcinogenicity studies were conducted in mice and rats. In mice, no increased incidence of any tumor type was observed. The highest dose tested in rats was 640 mg/kg/day; at this dose a statistically significant increased incidence of thyroid adenomas was seen only in male rats. At that dose, daily systemic exposure in rats was approximately 1.3 times higher than daily systemic exposure in humans. No evidence of mutagenicity or genotoxicity was observed in *in vitro* microbial mutagenesis (Ames) tests, *in vitro* alkaline elution assays for DNA breakage, *in vitro* and *in vivo* chromosomal aberration studies, and *in vitro* mammalian cell mutagenesis assays. No treatment-related effects on mating, fertility, or embryo survival were seen in female rats and no treatment-related effects on mating performance were seen in male rats at doses providing systemic exposure comparable to or slightly higher than that with the clinical dose. In addition, no treatment-related effects were observed in fecundity or fertility of untreated females mated to treated males.

Pregnancy

Pregnancy Category C: Developmental toxicity studies were performed in rabbits (at doses up to 240 mg/kg/day), dogs (at doses up to 80 mg/kg/day), and rats (at doses up to 640 mg/kg/day). The highest doses in these studies produced systemic exposures in these species comparable to or slightly greater than human exposure. No treatment-related external, visceral, or skeletal changes were observed in rabbits or dogs. No treatment-related external or visceral changes were observed in rats. Treatment-related increases over controls in the incidence of supernumerary ribs (at exposures at or below those in humans) and of cervical ribs (at exposures comparable to or slightly greater than those in humans) were seen in rats. In all three species, no treatment-related effects on embryonic/fetal survival or fetal weights were observed.

In rabbits, at a maternal dose of 240 mg/kg/day, no drug was detected in fetal plasma 1 hour after dosing. Fetal plasma drug levels 2 hours after dosing were approximately 3% of maternal plasma drug levels. In dogs, at a maternal dose of 80 mg/kg/day, fetal plasma drug levels were approximately 50% of maternal plasma drug levels both 1 and 2 hours after dosing. In rats, at maternal doses of 40 and 640 mg/kg/day, fetal plasma drug levels were approximately 10 to 15% and 10 to 20% of maternal plasma drug levels 1 and 2 hours after dosing, respectively.

Indinavir was administered to Rhesus monkeys during the third trimester of pregnancy (at doses up to 160 mg/kg twice daily) and to neonatal Rhesus monkeys (at doses up to 160 mg/kg twice daily). When administered to neonates, indinavir caused an exacerbation of the transient physiologic hyperbilirubinemia seen in this species after birth; serum bilirubin values were approximately fourfold above controls at 160 mg/kg twice daily. A similar exacerbation did not occur in neonates after *in utero* exposure to indinavir during the third trimester of pregnancy. In Rhesus monkeys, fetal plasma drug levels were approximately 1 to 2% of maternal plasma drug levels approximately 1 hour after maternal dosing at 40, 80, or 160 mg/kg twice daily.

Hyperbilirubinemia has occurred during treatment with CRIXIVAN (see PRECAUTIONS and ADVERSE REACTIONS). It is unknown whether CRIXIVAN administered to the mother in the perinatal period will exacerbate physiologic hyperbilirubinemia in neonates.

There are no adequate and well-controlled studies in pregnant women. CRIXIVAN should be used during pregnancy only if the potential benefit justifies the potential risk to the fetus.

Antiviral Pregnancy Registry

To monitor maternal-fetal outcomes of pregnant women exposed to CRIXIVAN, an Antiretroviral Pregnancy Registry has been established. Physicians are encouraged to register patients by calling 1-800-258-4263.

Nursing Mothers

Studies in lactating rats have demonstrated that indinavir is excreted in milk. Although it is not known whether CRIXIVAN is excreted in human milk, there exists the potential for adverse effects from indinavir in nursing infants. Mothers should be instructed to discontinue nursing if they are receiving CRIXIVAN. This is consistent with the recommendation by the U.S. Public Health Service Centers for Disease Control and Prevention that HIV-infected mothers not breast-feed their infants to avoid risking postnatal transmission of HIV.

Pediatric Use

The optimal dosing regimen for use of indinavir in pediatric patients has not been established. A dose of 500 mg/m^2 every eight hours has been studied in uncontrolled studies of 70 children, 3 to 18 years of age. The pharmacokinetic profiles of indinavir at this dose were not comparable to profiles previously observed in adults receiving the recommended dose (see CLINICAL PHARMACOLOGY, *Pediatric*). Although viral suppression was observed in some of the 32 children who were followed on this regimen through 24 weeks, a substantially higher rate of nephrolithiasis was reported when compared to adult historical data (see WARNINGS, *Nephrolithiasis/Urolithiasis*). Physicians considering the use of indinavir in pediatric patients without other protease inhibitor options should be aware of the limited data available in this population and the increased risk of nephrolithiasis.

Geriatric Use

Clinical studies of CRIXIVAN did not include sufficient numbers of subjects aged 65 and over to determine whether

Continued on next page

Information on the Merck & Co., Inc., products listed on these pages is from the prescribing information in use October 1, 2004. For information, please call 1-800-NSC-MERCK [1-800-672-6372].

Crixivan—Cont.

they respond differently from younger subjects. In general, dose selection for an elderly patient should be cautious, reflecting the greater frequency of decreased hepatic, renal or cardiac function and of concomitant disease or other drug therapy.

ADVERSE REACTIONS

Clinical Trials in Adults

Nephrolithiasis/urolithiasis, including flank pain with or without hematuria (including microscopic hematuria), has been reported in approximately 12.4% (301/2429; range across individual trials: 4.7% to 34.4%) of patients receiving CRIXIVAN at the recommended dose in clinical trials with a median follow-up of 47 weeks (range: 1 day to 242 weeks; 2238 patient-years follow-up). The cumulative frequency of nephrolithiasis events increases with duration of exposure to CRIXIVAN; however, the risk over time remains relatively constant. Of the patients treated with CRIXIVAN who developed nephrolithiasis/urolithiasis in clinical trials during the double-blind phase, 2.8% (7/246) were reported to develop hydronephrosis and 4.5% (11/246) underwent stent placement. Following the acute episode, 4.9% (12/246) of patients discontinued therapy. (See WARNINGS and DOSAGE AND ADMINISTRATION, *Nephrolithiasis/Urolithiasis.*)

Asymptomatic hyperbilirubinemia (total bilirubin ≥2.5 mg/dL), reported predominantly as elevated indirect bilirubin, has occurred in approximately 14% of patients treated with CRIXIVAN. In <1% this was associated with elevations in ALT or AST.

Hyperbilirubinemia and nephrolithiasis/urolithiasis occurred more frequently at doses exceeding 2.4 g/day compared to doses ≤2.4 g/day.

Clinical adverse experiences reported in ≥2% of patients treated with CRIXIVAN alone, CRIXIVAN in combination with zidovudine or zidovudine plus lamivudine, zidovudine alone, or zidovudine plus lamivudine are presented in Table 10.

[See table 10 at top of next page]

In Phase I and II controlled trials, the following adverse events were reported significantly more frequently by those randomized to the arms containing CRIXIVAN than by those randomized to nucleoside analogues: rash, upper respiratory infection, dry skin, pharyngitis, taste perversion.

Selected laboratory abnormalities of severe or life-threatening intensity reported in patients treated with CRIXIVAN alone, CRIXIVAN in combination with zidovudine or zidovudine plus lamivudine, zidovudine alone, or zidovudine plus lamivudine are presented in Table 11.

[See table 11 on next page]

Post-Marketing Experience

Body As A Whole: redistribution/accumulation of body fat (see PRECAUTIONS, *Fat Redistribution*).

Cardiovascular System: cardiovascular disorders including myocardial infarction and angina pectoris; cerebrovascular disorder.

Digestive System: liver function abnormalities; hepatitis including reports of hepatic failure (see WARNINGS); pancreatitis; jaundice; abdominal distention; dyspepsia.

Hematologic: increased spontaneous bleeding in patients with hemophilia (see PRECAUTIONS); acute hemolytic anemia (see WARNINGS).

Endocrine/Metabolic: new onset diabetes mellitus, exacerbation of pre-existing diabetes mellitus, hyperglycemia (see WARNINGS).

Hypersensitivity: anaphylactoid reactions; urticaria; vasculitis.

Musculoskeletal System: arthralgia.

Nervous System/Psychiatric: oral paresthesia; depression.

Skin and Skin Appendage: rash including erythema multiforme and Stevens-Johnson syndrome; hyperpigmentation; alopecia; ingrown toenails and/or paronychia; pruritus.

Urogenital System: nephrolithiasis/urolithiasis; in some cases resulting in renal insufficiency or acute renal failure; pyelonephritis with or without bacteremia (see WARNINGS); interstitial nephritis sometimes with indinavir crystal deposits; in some patients, the interstitial nephritis did not resolve following discontinuation of CRIXIVAN; leukocyturia; (see PRECAUTIONS), crystalluria; dysuria.

Laboratory Abnormalities

Increased serum triglycerides; increased serum cholesterol.

OVERDOSAGE

There have been more than 60 reports of acute or chronic human overdosage (up to 23 times the recommended total daily dose of 2400 mg) with CRIXIVAN. The most commonly reported symptoms were renal (e.g., nephrolithiasis/urolithiasis, flank pain, hematuria) and gastrointestinal (e.g., nausea, vomiting, diarrhea).

It is not known whether CRIXIVAN is dialyzable by peritoneal or hemodialysis.

DOSAGE AND ADMINISTRATION

The recommended dosage of CRIXIVAN is 800 mg (usually **two** 400-mg capsules) orally every 8 hours.

CRIXIVAN must be taken at intervals of 8 hours. For optimal absorption, CRIXIVAN should be administered without food but with water 1 hour before or 2 hours after a meal. Alternatively, CRIXIVAN may be administered with other liquids such as skim milk, juice, coffee, or tea, or with a light meal, e.g., dry toast with jelly, juice, and coffee with skim milk and sugar; or corn flakes, skim milk and sugar. (See CLINICAL PHARMACOLOGY, *Effect of Food on Oral Absorption.*)

To ensure adequate hydration, it is recommended that adults drink at least 1.5 liters (approximately 48 ounces) of liquids during the course of 24 hours.

Concomitant Therapy (See CLINICAL PHARMACOLOGY, *Drug Interactions*, and/or PRECAUTIONS, *Drug Interactions*.)

Delavirdine

Dose reduction of CRIXIVAN to 600 mg every 8 hours should be considered when administering delavirdine 400 mg three times a day.

Didanosine

If indinavir and didanosine are administered concomitantly, they should be administered at least one hour apart on an empty stomach (consult the manufacturer's product circular for didanosine).

Itraconazole

Dose reduction of CRIXIVAN to 600 mg every 8 hours is recommended when administering itraconazole 200 mg twice daily concurrently.

Table 9
Established and Other Potentially Significant Drug Interactions: Alteration in Dose or Regimen May Be Recommended Based on Drug Interaction Studies or Predicted Interaction
(See also CLINICAL PHARMACOLOGY for magnitude of interaction, WARNINGS and DOSAGE AND ADMINISTRATION.)

Drug Name	Effect	Clinical Comment
HIV Antiviral Agents		
Delavirdine	↑ indinavir concentration	Dose reduction of CRIXIVAN to 600 mg every 8 hours should be considered when taking delavirdine 400 mg three times a day.
Didanosine		Indinavir and didanosine formulations containing buffer should be administered at least one hour apart on an empty stomach.
Efavirenz	↓ indinavir concentration	The optimal dose of indinavir, when given in combination with efavirenz, is not known. Increasing the indinavir dose to 1000 mg every 8 hours does not compensate for the increased indinavir metabolism due to efavirenz.
Nelfinavir	↑ indinavir concentration	The appropriate doses for this combination, with respect to efficacy and safety, have not been established.
Nevirapine	↓ indinavir concentration	Indinavir concentrations may be decreased in the presence of nevirapine. The appropriate doses for this combination, with respect to efficacy and safety, have not been established.
Ritonavir	↑ indinavir concentration ↑ ritonavir concentration	The appropriate doses for this combination, with respect to efficacy and safety, have not been established. Preliminary clinical data suggest that the incidence of nephrolithiasis is higher in patients receiving indinavir in combination with ritonavir than those receiving CRIXIVAN 800 mg q8h.
Saquinavir	↑ saquinavir concentration	The appropriate doses for this combination, with respect to efficacy and safety, have not been established.
Other Agents		
Antiarrhythmics: bepridil, lidocaine (systemic) and quinidine	↑ antiarrhythmic agents concentration	Caution is warranted and therapeutic concentration monitoring is recommended for antiarrhythmics when coadministered with CRIXIVAN.
Anticonvulsants: carbamazepine, phenobarbital phenytoin	↓ indinavir concentration	Use with caution. CRIXIVAN may not be effective due to decreased indinavir concentrations in patients taking these agents concomitantly.
Calcium Channel Blockers, Dihydropyridine: e.g., felodipine, nifedipine, nicardipine	↑ dihydropyridine calcium channel blockers concentration	Caution is warranted and clinical monitoring of patients is recommended.
Clarithromycin	↑ clarithromycin concentration ↑ indinavir concentration	The appropriate doses for this combination, with respect to efficacy and safety, have not been established.
HMG-CoA Reductase Inhibitor: atorvastatin	↑ atorvastatin concentration	Use lowest possible dose of atorvastatin with careful monitoring, or consider HMG-CoA reductase inhibitors that are not primarily metabolized by CYP3A4, such as pravastatin, fluvastatin, or rosuvastatin in combination with CRIXIVAN.
Immunosuppressants: cyclosporine, tacrolimus, sirolimus	↑ immunosuppressant agents concentration	Plasma concentrations may be increased by CRIXIVAN.
Itraconazole	↑ indinavir concentration	Dose reduction of CRIXIVAN to 600 mg every 8 hours is recommended when administering itraconazole concurrently.
Ketoconazole	↑ indinavir concentration	Dose reduction of CRIXIVAN to 600 mg every 8 hours should be considered.
Rifabutin	↓ indinavir concentration ↑ rifabutin concentration	Dose reduction of rifabutin to half the standard dose and a dose increase of CRIXIVAN to 1000 mg (three 333-mg capsules) every 8 hours are recommended when rifabutin and CRIXIVAN are coadministered.
Sildenafil	↑ sildenafil concentration	Sildenafil dose should not exceed a maximum of 25 mg in a 48-hour period in patients receiving concomitant indinavir therapy.
Tadalafil	↑ tadalafil concentration	Tadalafil dose should not exceed a maximum of 10 mg in a 72-hour period in patients receiving concomitant indinavir therapy.
Vardenafil	↑ vardenafil concentration	Vardenafil dose should not exceed a maximum of 2.5 mg in a 24-hour period in patients receiving concomitant indinavir therapy.

Note: ↑ = increase; ↓ = decrease

Ketoconazole
Dose reduction of CRIXIVAN to 600 mg every 8 hours is recommended when administering ketoconazole concurrently.
Rifabutin
Dose reduction of rifabutin to half the standard dose (consult the manufacturer's product circular for rifabutin) and a dose increase of CRIXIVAN to 1000 mg (**three** 333-mg capsules) every 8 hours are recommended when rifabutin and CRIXIVAN are coadministered.
Hepatic Insufficiency
The dosage of CRIXIVAN should be reduced to 600 mg every 8 hours in patients with mild-to-moderate hepatic insufficiency due to cirrhosis.
Nephrolithiasis/Urolithiasis
In addition to adequate hydration, medical management in patients who experience nephrolithiasis/urolithiasis may include temporary interruption (e.g., 1 to 3 days) or discontinuation of therapy.

HOW SUPPLIED

CRIXIVAN Capsules are supplied as follows:
No. 3755 — 100 mg capsules: semi-translucent white capsules coded **"CRIXIVAN™ 100 mg"** in green. Available as:
NDC 0006-0570-62 unit-of-use bottles of 180 (with desiccant).
No. 3756 — 200 mg capsules: semi-translucent white capsules coded **"CRIXIVAN™ 200 mg"** in blue. Available as:
NDC 0006-0571-43 unit-of-use bottles of 360 (with desiccant).
No. 3802 — 333 mg capsules: semi-translucent white capsules coded **"CRIXIVAN™ 333 mg"** in red and a radial red band on the body. Available as:
NDC 0006-0574-65 unit-of-use bottles of 135 (with desiccant).
No. 3758 — 400 mg capsules: semi-translucent white capsules coded **"CRIXIVAN™ 400 mg"** in green. Available as:
NDC 0006-0573-42 unit-dose packages of 42
NDC 0006-0573-40 unit-of-use bottles of 120 (with desiccant)
NDC 0006-0573-62 unit-of-use bottles of 180 (with desiccant)
NDC 0006-0573-54 unit-of-use bottles of 90 (with desiccant)
NDC 0006-0573-18 unit-of-use bottles of 18 (with desiccant).
Storage
Bottles: Store in a tightly-closed container at room temperature, 15-30°C (59-86°F). Protect from moisture.
CRIXIVAN Capsules are sensitive to moisture. CRIXIVAN should be dispensed and stored in the original container. The desiccant should remain in the original bottle.
Unit-Dose Packages: Store at room temperature, 15-30°C (59-86°F). Protect from moisture.
MERCK & CO., INC., Whitehouse Station, NJ 08889, USA
7979827 Issued May 2004

CRIXIVAN®* (indinavir sulfate) Capsules
Patient Information about
CRIXIVAN (KRIK-sih-van)
for HIV (Human Immunodeficiency Virus) Infection
Generic name: indinavir (in-DIH-nuh-veer) sulfate
ALERT: Find out about medicines that should NOT be taken with CRIXIVAN. Please also read the section "MEDICINES YOU SHOULD NOT TAKE WITH CRIXIVAN".
Please read this information before you start taking CRIXIVAN. Also, read the leaflet each time you renew your prescription, just in case anything has changed. Remember, this leaflet does not take the place of careful discussions with your doctor. You and your doctor should discuss CRIXIVAN when you start taking your medication and at regular checkups. You should remain under a doctor's care when using CRIXIVAN and should not change or stop treatment without first talking with your doctor.

*Registered trademark of MERCK & CO., Inc.

What is CRIXIVAN?
CRIXIVAN is an oral capsule used for the treatment of HIV (Human Immunodeficiency Virus). HIV is the virus that causes AIDS (acquired immune deficiency syndrome).
CRIXIVAN is a type of HIV drug called a protease (PRO-tee-ase) inhibitor.
How does CRIXIVAN work?
CRIXIVAN is a protease inhibitor that fights HIV. CRIXIVAN can help reduce your chances of getting illnesses associated with HIV. CRIXIVAN can also help lower the amount of HIV in your body (called "viral load") and raise your CD4 (T) cell count. CRIXIVAN may not have these effects in all patients.
CRIXIVAN is usually prescribed with other anti-HIV drugs such as ZDV (also called AZT), 3TC, ddI, ddC, or d4T. CRIXIVAN works differently from these other anti-HIV drugs. Talk with your doctor about how you should take CRIXIVAN.
How should I take CRIXIVAN?
There are six important things you must do to help you benefit from CRIXIVAN:

1. **Take CRIXIVAN capsules every day as prescribed by your doctor.** Continue taking CRIXIVAN unless your doctor tells you to stop. Take the exact amount of CRIXIVAN that your doctor tells you to take, right from the very

Table 10
Clinical Adverse Experiences Reported in ≥2% of Patients

	Study 028 Considered Drug-Related and of Moderate or Severe Intensity		Study ACTG 320 of Unknown Drug Relationship and of Severe or Life-threatening Intensity		
Adverse Experience	CRIXIVAN Percent (n=332)	CRIXIVAN plus Zidovudine Percent (n=332)	Zidovudine Percent (n=332)	CRIXIVAN plus Zidovudine plus Lamivudine Percent (n=571)	Zidovudine plus Lamivudine Percent (n=575)
Body as a Whole					
Abdominal pain	16.6	16.0	12.0	1.9	0.7
Asthenia/fatigue	2.1	4.2	3.6	2.4	4.5
Fever	1.5	1.5	2.1	3.8	3.0
Malaise	2.1	2.7	1.8	0	0
Digestive System					
Nausea	11.7	31.9	19.6	2.8	1.4
Diarrhea	3.3	3.0	2.4	0.9	1.2
Vomiting	8.4	17.8	9.0	1.4	1.4
Acid regurgitation	2.7	5.4	1.8	0.4	0
Anorexia	2.7	5.4	3.0	0.5	0.2
Appetite increase	2.1	1.5	1.2	0	0
Dyspepsia	1.5	2.7	0.9	0	0
Jaundice	1.5	2.1	0.3	0	0
Hemic and Lymphatic System					
Anemia	0.6	1.2	2.1	2.4	3.5
Musculoskeletal System					
Back pain	8.4	4.5	1.5	0.9	0.7
Nervous System/Psychiatric					
Headache	5.4	9.6	6.0	2.4	2.8
Dizziness	3.0	3.9	0.9	0.5	0.7
Somnolence	2.4	3.3	3.3	0	0
Skin and Skin Appendage					
Pruritus	4.2	2.4	1.8	0.5	0
Rash	1.2	0.6	2.4	1.1	0.5
Respiratory System					
Cough	1.5	0.3	0.6	1.6	1.0
Difficulty breathing/ dyspnea/shortness of breath	0	0.6	0.3	1.8	1.0
Urogenital System					
Nephrolithiasis/urolithiasis*	8.7	7.8	2.1	2.6	0.3
Dysuria	1.5	2.4	0.3	0.4	0.2
Special Senses					
Taste perversion	2.7	8.4	1.2	0.2	0

*Including renal colic, and flank pain with and without hematuria

Table 11
Selected Laboratory Abnormalities of Severe or Life-threatening Intensity Reported in Studies 028 and ACTG 320

	Study 028		Study ACTG 320		
	CRIXIVAN Percent (n=329)	CRIXIVAN plus Zidovudine Percent (n=320)	Zidovudine Percent (n=330)	CRIXIVAN plus Zidovudine plus Lamivudine Percent (n=571)	Zidovudine plus Lamivudine Percent (n=575)
Hematology					
Decreased hemoglobin <7.0 g/dL	0.6	0.9	3.3	2.4	3.5
Decreased platelet count <50 THS/mm^3	0.9	0.9	1.8	0.2	0.9
Decreased neutrophils <0.75 THS/mm^3	2.4	2.2	6.7	5.1	14.6
Blood chemistry					
Increased ALT >500% ULN*	4.9	4.1	3.0	2.6	2.6
Increased AST >500% ULN	3.7	2.8	2.7	3.3	2.8
Total serum bilirubin >250% ULN	11.9	9.7	0.6	6.1	1.4
Increased serum amylase >200% ULN	2.1	1.9	1.8	0.9	0.3
Increased glucose >250 mg/dL	0.9	0.9	0.6	1.6	1.9
Increased creatinine >300% ULN	0	0	0.6	0.2	0

*Upper limit of the normal range.

start. To help make sure you will benefit from CRIXIVAN, you must not skip doses or take "drug holidays". If you don't take CRIXIVAN as prescribed, the activity of CRIXIVAN may be reduced (due to resistance).

2. **Take CRIXIVAN capsules every 8 hours around the clock, *every day*.** It may be easier to remember to take CRIXIVAN if you take it at the same time every day. If you have questions about when to take CRIXIVAN, your doctor or health care provider can help you decide what schedule works for you.
3. **If you miss a dose by more than 2 hours, wait and then take the next dose at the regularly scheduled time.** However, if you miss a dose by less than 2 hours, take your missed dose immediately. Then take your next dose at the regularly scheduled time. Do not take more or less than your prescribed dose of CRIXIVAN at any one time.

Continued on next page

Information on the Merck & Co., Inc., products listed on these pages is from the prescribing information in use October 1, 2004. For information, please call 1-800-NSC-MERCK [1-800-672-6372].

Crixivan—Cont.

4. **Take CRIXIVAN with water.** You can also take CRIXIVAN with other beverages such as skim or non-fat milk, juice, coffee, or tea.
5. **Ideally, take each dose of CRIXIVAN without food but with water at least one hour before or two hours after a meal.** Or you can take CRIXIVAN with a light meal. Examples of light meals include:
   dry toast with jelly, juice, and coffee (with skim or non-fat milk and sugar if you want)
   cornflakes with skim or non-fat milk and sugar

   Do not take CRIXIVAN at the same time as any meals that are high in calories, fat, and protein (for example—a bacon and egg breakfast). When taken at the same time as CRIXIVAN, these foods can interfere with CRIXIVAN being absorbed into your bloodstream and may lessen its effect.
6. **It is critical to drink plenty of fluids while taking CRIXIVAN.** Adults should drink at least six 8-ounce glasses of liquids (preferably water) throughout the day, every day. Your health care provider will give you further instructions on the amount of fluid that you should drink. **CRIXIVAN can cause kidney stones.** Having enough fluids in your body should help reduce the chances of forming a kidney stone. Call your doctor or other health care provider if you develop kidney pains (middle to lower stomach or back pain) or blood in the urine.

Does CRIXIVAN cure HIV or AIDS?

CRIXIVAN is not a cure for HIV or AIDS. People taking CRIXIVAN may still develop infections or other conditions associated with HIV. Because of this, it is very important for you to remain under the care of a doctor. Although CRIXIVAN is not a cure for HIV or AIDS, CRIXIVAN can help reduce your chances of getting illnesses, including death, associated with HIV. CRIXIVAN may not have these effects in all patients.

Does CRIXIVAN reduce the risk of passing HIV to others?

CRIXIVAN has not been shown to reduce the risk of passing HIV to others through sexual contact or blood contamination.

Who should not take CRIXIVAN?

Do not take CRIXIVAN if you have had a serious allergic reaction to CRIXIVAN or any of its components.

What other medical problems or conditions should I discuss with my doctor?

Talk to your doctor if:

- You are pregnant or if you become pregnant while you are taking CRIXIVAN. We do not yet know how CRIXIVAN affects pregnant women or their developing babies.
- You are breast-feeding. You should stop breast-feeding if you are taking CRIXIVAN

Also talk to your doctor if you have:

- Problems with your liver, especially if you have mild or moderate liver disease caused by cirrhosis
- Problems with your kidneys
- Diabetes
- Hemophilia
- High cholesterol and you are taking cholesterol-lowering medicines called "statins".

Tell you doctor about any medicines you are taking or plan to take, including non-prescription medicines, herbal products including St. John's wort (*Hypericum perforatum*), or dietary supplements.

Can CRIXIVAN be taken with other medications?**

MEDICINES YOU SHOULD NOT TAKE WITH CRIXIVAN

VERSED®
(midazolam)
ORAP®
(pimozide)
PROPULSID®
(cisapride)
CORDARONE®
(amiodarone)
HISMANAL®
(astemizole)
HALCION®
(triazolam)
Ergot medications
(e.g., Wigraine®, Cafergot®,
D.H.E. 45®, Migranal®,
Ergotrate®, and Methergine®)

Taking CRIXIVAN with the above medications could result in serious or life-threatening problems (such as irregular heartbeat or excessive sleepiness).

In addition, you should not take CRIXIVAN with the following:

Rifampin, known as RIFADIN®, RIFAMATE®, RIFATER®, or RIMACTANE®.

It is not recommended to take CRIXIVAN with the cholesterol-lowering drugs MEVACOR* (lovastatin) or ZOCOR* (simvastatin) because of possible drug interactions. There is also an increased risk of drug interactions between CRIXIVAN and LIPITOR® (atorvastatin); talk to your doctor before you take any of these cholesterol-reducing drugs with CRIXIVAN.

Taking CRIXIVAN with REYATAZ® (atazanavir) is not recommended because they can both sometimes cause increased levels of bilirubin in the blood.

Taking CRIXIVAN with St. John's wort (*Hypericum perforatum*), an herbal product sold as a dietary supplement, or products containing St. John's wort is not recommended. Taking St. John's wort has been shown to decrease CRIXIVAN levels and may lead to increased viral load and possible resistance to CRIXIVAN or cross resistance to other antiretroviral drugs.

Before you take VIAGRA® (sildenafil), CIALIS® (tadalafil), or LEVITRA® (vardenafil) with CRIXIVAN, talk to your doctor about possible drug interactions and side effects. If you take any of these medicines together with CRIXIVAN, you may be at increased risk of side effects such as low blood pressure, visual changes, and penile erection lasting more than 4 hours, which have been associated with sildenafil, tadalafil, and vardenafil. If an erection lasts longer than 4 hours, you should seek immediate medical assistance to avoid permanent damage to your penis. Your doctor can explain these symptoms to you.

MEDICINES YOU CAN TAKE WITH CRIXIVAN

RETROVIR®
(zidovudine, ZDV
also called AZT)
ZERIT®
(stavudine, d4T)
BACTRIM®/SEPTRA®
(trimethopim/
sulfamethoxazole)
BIAXIN®
(clarithromycin)
TAGAMET®
(cimetidine)
CRESTOR®
(rosuvastatin)
EPIVIR™
(lamivudine, 3TC)
isonaizid
(INH)
DIFLUCAN®
(fluconazole)
ORTHO-NOVUM 1/35®
(oral contraceptive)
Methadone

VIDEX® (didanosine, ddl)—If you take CRIXIVAN with VIDEX, take them at least one hour apart.

MYCOBUTIN® (rifabutin)—If you take CRIXIVAN with MYCOBUTIN, your doctor may adjust both the dose of MYCOBUTIN and the dose of CRIXIVAN.

NIZORAL® (ketoconazole)—If you take CRIXIVAN with NIZORAL, your doctor may adjust the dose of CRIXIVAN.

RESCRIPTOR® (delaviridine)—If you take CRIXIVAN with RESCRIPTOR, your doctor may adjust the dose of CRIXIVAN.

SPORANOX® (itraconazole)—If you take CRIXIVAN with SPORANOX, your doctor may adjust the dose of CRIXIVAN.

SISTIVA™ (efavirenz)—If you take CRIXIVAN with SUSTIVA, your doctor may adjust the dose of CRIXIVAN.

Talk to your doctor about any medications you are taking.

Calcium Channel Blockers: Tell your doctor if you are taking calcium channel blockers (e.g., amlodipine, felodipine).

Antiarrhythmics: Tell your doctor if you are taking antiarrhythmics (e.g., quinidine).

Anticonvulsants: Tell your doctor if you are taking anticonvulsants (e.g., phenobarbital, phenytoin, or carbamazepine).

Steroids: Tell your doctor if you are taking steroids (e.g., dexamethasone).

**The brands listed are the registered trademarks of their respective owners and are not trademarks of Merck & Co., Inc.

What are the possible side effects of CRIXIVAN?

Like all prescription drugs, CRIXIVAN can cause side effects. The following is **not** a complete list of side effects reported with CRIXIVAN when taken either alone or with other anti-HIV drugs. Do not rely on this leaflet alone for information about side effects. Your doctor can discuss with you a more complete list of side effects.

Some patients treated with CRIXIVAN developed kidney stones. In some of these patients this led to more severe kidney problems, including kidney failure or inflammation of the kidneys or kidney infection which sometimes spread to the blood. Drinking at least six 8-ounce glasses of liquids (preferably water) each day should help reduce the chances of forming a kidney stone (see How should I take CRIXIVAN?). Call your doctor or other health care provider if you develop kidney pains (middle to lower stomach or back pain) or blood in the urine.

Some patients treated with CRIXIVAN have had rapid breakdown of red blood cells (hemolytic anemia) which in some cases was severe or resulted in death.

Some patients treated with CRIXIVAN have had liver problems including liver failure and death. Some patients had other illnesses or were taking other drugs. It is uncertain if CRIXIVAN caused these liver problems.

Diabetes and high blood sugar (hyperglycemia) have occurred in patients taking protease inhibitors. In some of these patients, this led to ketoacidosis, a serious condition caused by poorly controlled blood sugar. Some patients had diabetes before starting protease inhibitors, others did not. Some patients required adjustments to their diabetes medication. Others needed new diabetes medication.

In some patients with hemophilia, increased bleeding has been reported.

Severe muscle pain and weakness have occurred in patients taking protease inhibitors, including CRIXIVAN, together with some of the cholesterol-lowering medicines called "statins". Call your doctor if you develop severe muscle pain or weakness.

Changes in body fat have been seen in some patients taking antiretroviral therapy. These changes may include increased amount of fat in the upper back and neck ("buffalo hump"), breast, and around the trunk. Loss of fat from the legs, arms and face may also happen. The cause and long term health effects of these conditions are not known at this time.

In some patients with advanced HIV infection (AIDS), signs and symptoms of inflammation from opportunistic infections may occur when combination antiretroviral treatment is started.

Clinical Studies

Increases in bilirubin (one laboratory test of liver function) have been reported in approximately 14% of patients. Usually, this finding has not been associated with liver problems. However, on rare occasions, a person may develop yellowing of the skin and/or eyes.

Side effects occurring in 2% or more of patients included: abdominal pain, fatigue or weakness, low red blood cell count, flank pain, painful urination, feeling unwell, nausea, upset stomach, diarrhea, vomiting, acid regurgitation, increased or decreased appetite, back pain, headache, dizziness, taste changes, rash, itchy skin, yellowing of the skin and/or eyes, upper respiratory infection, dry skin, and sore throat.

Swollen kidneys due to blocked urine flow occurred rarely.

Marketing Experience

Other side effects reported since CRIXIVAN has been marketed include: allergic reactions; severe skin reactions; yellowing of the skin and/or eyes; heart problems including heart attack; stroke; abdominal swelling; indigestion; inflammation of the kidneys; inflammation of the pancreas; joint pain; depression; itching; hives; change in skin color; hair loss; ingrown toenails with or without infection; crystals in the urine; painful urination; numbness of the mouth and increased cholesterol.

Tell your doctor promptly about these or any other unusual symptoms. If the condition persists or worsens, seek medical attention.

How should I store CRIXIVAN capsules?

- Keep CRIXIVAN capsules in the bottle they came in and at room temperature (59°–86°F).
- Keep CRIXIVAN capsules dry by leaving the small dessicant in the bottle. Keep the bottle closed.

This medication was prescribed for your particular condition. Do not use it for any other condition or give it to anybody else. Keep CRIXIVAN and all medicines out of the reach of children. If you suspect that more than the prescribed dose of this medicine has been taken, contact your local poison control center or emergency room immediately.

This leaflet provides a summary of information about CRIXIVAN. If you have any questions or concerns about either CRIXIVAN or HIV, talk to your doctor.

MERCK & CO., INC.

9024519 Issued May 2004

Whitehouse Station, NJ 08889, USA

Shown in Product Identification Guide, page 323

CUPRIMINE® Capsules ℞
(Penicillamine)

> Physicians planning to use penicillamine should thoroughly familiarize themselves with its toxicity, special dosage considerations, and therapeutic benefits. Penicillamine should never be used casually. Each patient should remain constantly under the close supervision of the physician. Patients should be warned to report promptly any symptoms suggesting toxicity.

DESCRIPTION

Penicillamine is a chelating agent used in the treatment of Wilson's disease. It is also used to reduce cystine excretion in cystinuria and to treat patients with severe, active rheumatoid arthritis unresponsive to conventional therapy (see INDICATIONS). It is 3-mercapto-D-valine. It is a white or practically white, crystalline powder, freely soluble in water, slightly soluble in alcohol, and insoluble in ether, acetone, benzene, and carbon tetrachloride. Although its configuration is D, it is levorotatory as usually measured:

$[\alpha]^{25°}_{D} = -62.5° \pm 2°$ (c = 1, 1N NaOH),

calculated on a dried basis.

The empirical formula is $C_5H_{11}NO_2S$, giving it a molecular weight of 149.21. The structural formula is:

$$(CH_3)_2C(SH)—CH(NH_2)COOH$$

It reacts readily with formaldehyde or acetone to form a thiazolidine-carboxylic acid.

Capsules CUPRIMINE* (Penicillamine) for oral administration contain either 125 mg or 250 mg of penicillamine. Each capsule contains the following inactive ingredients: D

& C Yellow 10, gelatin, lactose, magnesium stearate, and titanium dioxide. The 125 mg capsule also contains iron oxide.

*Registered trademark of MERCK & CO., Inc.

CLINICAL PHARMACOLOGY

Penicillamine is a chelating agent recommended for the removal of excess copper in patients with Wilson's disease. From *in vitro* studies which indicate that one atom of copper combines with two molecules of penicillamine, it would appear that one gram of penicillamine should be followed by the excretion of about 200 milligrams of copper; however, the actual amount excreted is about one percent of this.

Penicillamine also reduces excess cystine excretion in cystinuria. This is done, at least in part, by disulfide interchange between penicillamine and cystine, resulting in formation of penicillamine-cysteine disulfide, a substance that is much more soluble than cystine and is excreted readily.

Penicillamine interferes with the formation of cross-links between tropocollagen molecules and cleaves them when newly formed.

The mechanism of action of penicillamine in rheumatoid arthritis is unknown although it appears to suppress disease activity. Unlike cytotoxic immunosuppressants, penicillamine markedly lowers IgM rheumatoid factor but produces no significant depression in absolute levels of serum immunoglobulins. Also unlike cytotoxic immunosuppressants which act on both, penicillamine *in vitro* depresses T-cell activity but not B-cell activity.

In vitro, penicillamine dissociates macroglobulins (rheumatoid factor) although the relationship of the activity to its effect in rheumatoid arthritis is not known.

In rheumatoid arthritis, the onset of therapeutic response to CUPRIMINE may not be seen for two or three months. In those patients who respond, however, the first evidence of suppression of symptoms such as pain, tenderness, and swelling is generally apparent within three months. The optimum duration of therapy has not been determined. If remissions occur, they may last from months to years, but usually require continued treatment (see DOSAGE AND ADMINISTRATION).

In all patients receiving penicillamine, it is important that CUPRIMINE be given on an empty stomach, at least one hour before meals or two hours after meals, and at least one hour apart from any other drug, food, or milk. This permits maximum absorption and reduces the likelihood of inactivation by metal binding in the gastrointestinal tract.

Pharmacokinetics

Penicillamine is absorbed rapidly but incompletely (40–70%) from the gastrointestinal tract, with wide inter-individual variations. Food, antacids, and iron reduce absorption of the drug. The peak plasma concentration of penicillamine occurs 1–3 hours after ingestion. It is approximately 1–2 mg/L after an oral dose of 250 mg. The drug appears in the plasma as free penicillamine, penicillamine disulfide, and cysteine-penicillamine disulfide. When prolonged treatment is stopped, there is a slow elimination phase lasting 4–6 days.

More than 80% of plasma penicillamine is bound to proteins. The drug also binds to erythrocytes and macrophages. A small fraction of the dose is metabolized in the liver to s-methyl-D-penicillamine. Drug excretion is primarily renal, mainly as disulfides.

INDICATIONS

CUPRIMINE is indicated in the treatment of Wilson's disease, cystinuria, and in patients with severe, active rheumatoid arthritis who have failed to respond to an adequate trial of conventional therapy. Available evidence suggests that CUPRIMINE is not of value in ankylosing spondylitis.

Wilson's Disease—Wilson's disease (hepatolenticular degeneration) occurs in individuals who have inherited an autosomal recessive defect that leads to an accumulation of copper far in excess of metabolic requirements. The excess copper is deposited in several organs and tissues, and eventually produces pathological effects primarily in the liver, where damage progresses to postnecrotic cirrhosis, and in the brain, where degeneration is widespread. Copper is also deposited as characteristic, asymptomatic, golden-brown Kayser-Fleisher rings in the corneas of all patients with cerebral symptomatology and some patients who are either asymptomatic or manifest only hepatic symptomatology.

Two types of patients require treatment for Wilson's disease: (1) the symptomatic, and (2) the asymptomatic in whom it can be assumed the disease will develop in the future if the patient is not treated.

The diagnosis, if suspected on the basis of family or individual history or physical examination, can be confirmed if the plasma copper-protein ceruloplasmin** is <20 mg/dL and either a quantitative determination in a liver biopsy specimen shows an abnormally high concentration of copper (>250 mcg/g dry weight) or Kayser-Fleischer rings are present.

Treatment has two objectives:

(1) to minimize dietary intake of copper;

(2) to promote excretion and complex formation (i.e., detoxification) of excess tissue copper.

The first objective is attained by a daily diet that contains no more than one or two milligrams of copper. Such a diet should exclude, most importantly, chocolate, nuts, shellfish, mushrooms, liver, molasses, broccoli, and cereals and dietary supplements enriched with copper, and be composed to as great an extent as possible of foods with a low copper content. Distilled or demineralized water should be used if the patient's drinking water contains more than 0.1 mg of copper per liter.

For the second objective, a copper chelating agent is used. In symptomatic patients this treatment usually produces marked neurologic improvement, fading of Kayser-Fleischer rings, and gradual amelioration of hepatic dysfunction and psychic disturbances.

Clinical experience to date suggests that life is prolonged with the above regimen.

Noticeable improvement may not occur for one to three months. Occasionally, neurologic symptoms become worse during initiation of therapy with CUPRIMINE. Despite this, the drug should not be withdrawn. Temporary interruption carries an increased risk of developing a sensitivity reaction upon resumption of therapy, although it may result in clinical improvement of neurological symptoms (see WARNINGS). If the neurological symptoms and signs continue to worsen for a month after the initiation of CUPRIMINE therapy, several short courses of treatment with 2,3-dimercaprol (BAL) while continuing CUPRIMINE may be considered.

Treatment of asymptomatic patients has been carried out for over thirty years. Symptoms and signs of the disease appear to be prevented indefinitely if daily treatment with CUPRIMINE is continued.

Cystinuria—Cystinuria is characterized by excessive urinary excretion of the dibasic amino acids, arginine, lysine, ornithine, and cystine, and the mixed disulfide of cysteine and homocysteine. The metabolic defect that leads to cystinuria is inherited as an autosomal, recessive trait. Metabolism of the affected amino acids is influenced by at least two abnormal factors: (1) defective gastrointestinal absorption and (2) renal tubular dysfunction.

Arginine, lysine, ornithine, and cysteine are soluble substances, readily excreted. There is no apparent pathology connected with their excretion in excessive quantities.

Cystine, however, is so slightly soluble at the usual range of urinary pH that it is not excreted readily, and so crystallizes and forms stones in the urinary tract. Stone formation is the only known pathology in cystinuria.

Normal daily output of cystine is 40 to 80 mg. In cystinuria, output is greatly increased and may exceed 1 g/day. At 500 to 600 mg/day, stone formation is almost certain. When it is more than 300 mg/day, treatment is indicated.

Conventional treatment is directed at keeping urinary cystine diluted enough to prevent stone formation, keeping the urine alkaline enough to dissolve as much cystine as possible, and minimizing cystine production by a diet low in methionine (the major dietary precursor of cystine). Patients must drink enough fluid to keep urine specific gravity below 1.010, take enough alkali to keep urinary pH at 7.5 to 8, and maintain a diet low in methionine. This diet is not recommended in growing children and probably is contraindicated in pregnancy because of its low protein content (see PRECAUTIONS).

When these measures are inadequate to control recurrent stone formation, CUPRIMINE may be used as additional therapy, and when patients refuse to adhere to conventional treatment, CUPRIMINE may be a useful substitute. It is capable of keeping cystine excretion to near normal values, thereby hindering stone formation and the serious consequences of pyelonephritis and impaired renal function that develop in some patients.

Bartter and colleagues depict the process by which penicillamine interacts with cystine to form penicillamine-cysteine mixed disulfide as:

$$\text{CSSC} + \text{PS}' \rightleftarrows \text{CS}' + \text{CSSP}$$
$$\text{PSSP} + \text{CS}' \rightleftarrows \text{PS}' + \text{CSSP}$$
$$\text{CSSC} + \text{PSSP} \rightleftarrows 2\ \text{CSSP}$$

CSSC = cystine
CS′ = deprotonated cysteine
PSSP = penicillamine disulfide
PS′ = deprotonated penicillamine sulfhydryl
CSSP = penicillamine-cysteine mixed disulfide

In this process, it is assumed that the deprotonated form of penicillamine, PS′, is the active factor in bringing about the disulfide interchange.

Rheumatoid Arthritis —Because CUPRIMINE can cause severe adverse reactions, its use in rheumatoid arthritis should be restricted to patients who have severe, active disease and who have failed to respond to an adequate trial of conventional therapy. Even then, benefit-to-risk ratio should be carefully considered. Other measures, such as rest, physiotherapy, salicylates, and corticosteroids should be used, when indicated, in conjunction with CUPRIMINE (see PRECAUTIONS).

**For quantitative test for serum ceruloplasmin see: Morell, A.G.; Windsor, J.; Sternlieb, I.; Scheinberg, I.H.: Measurement of the concentration of ceruloplasmin in serum by determination of its oxidase activity, in "Laboratory Diagnosis of Liver Disease", F.W. Sunderman; F.W. Sunderman, Jr. (eds.), St. Louis, Warren H. Green, Inc., 1968, pp. 193-195.

CONTRAINDICATIONS

Except for the treatment of Wilson's disease or certain patients with cystinuria, use of penicillamine during pregnancy is contraindicated (see WARNINGS).

Although breast milk studies have not been reported in animals or humans, mothers on therapy with penicillamine should not nurse their infants.

Patients with a history of penicillamine-related aplastic anemia or agranulocytosis should not be restarted on penicillamine (see WARNINGS and ADVERSE REACTIONS).

Because of its potential for causing renal damage, penicillamine should not be administered to rheumatoid arthritis patients with a history or other evidence of renal insufficiency.

WARNINGS

The use of penicillamine has been associated with fatalities due to certain diseases such as aplastic anemia, agranulocytosis, thrombocytopenia, Goodpasture's syndrome, and myasthenia gravis.

Because of the potential for serious hematological and renal adverse reactions to occur at any time, routine urinalysis, white and differential blood cell count, hemoglobin determination, and direct platelet count must be done twice weekly, together with monitoring of the patient's skin, lymph nodes and body temperature, during the first month of therapy, every two weeks for the next five months, and monthly thereafter. Patients should be instructed to report promptly the development of signs and symptoms of granulocytopenia and/or thrombocytopenia such as fever, sore throat, chills, bruising or bleeding. The above laboratory studies should then be promptly repeated.

Leukopenia and thrombocytopenia have been reported to occur in up to five percent of patients during penicillamine therapy. Leukopenia is of the granulocytic series and may or may not be associated with an increase in eosinophils. A confirmed reduction in WBC below 3500/mm^3 mandates discontinuance of penicillamine therapy. Thrombocytopenia may be on an idiosyncratic basis, with decreased or absent megakaryocytes in the marrow, when it is part of an aplastic anemia. In other cases the thrombocytopenia is presumably on an immune basis since the number of megakaryocytes in the marrow has been reported to be normal or sometimes increased. The development of a platelet count below 100,000/mm^3, even in the absence of clinical bleeding, requires at least temporary cessation of penicillamine therapy. A progressive fall in either platelet count or WBC in three successive determinations, even though values are still within the normal range, likewise requires at least temporary cessation.

Proteinuria and/or hematuria may develop during therapy and may be warning signs of membranous glomerulopathy which can progress to a nephrotic syndrome. Close observation of these patients is essential. In some patients the proteinuria disappears with continued therapy; in others, penicillamine must be discontinued. When a patient develops proteinuria or hematuria the physician must ascertain whether it is a sign of drug-induced glomerulopathy or is unrelated to penicillamine.

Rheumatoid arthritis patients who develop moderate degrees of proteinuria may be continued cautiously on penicillamine therapy, provided that quantitative 24-hour urinary protein determinations are obtained at intervals of one to two weeks. Penicillamine dosage should not be increased under these circumstances. Proteinuria which exceeds 1 g/24 hours, or proteinuria which is progressively increasing, requires either discontinuance of the drug or a reduction in the dosage. In some patients, proteinuria has been reported to clear following reduction in dosage.

In rheumatoid arthritis patients, penicillamine should be discontinued if unexplained gross hematuria or persistent microscopic hematuria develops.

In patients with Wilson's disease or cystinuria the risks of continued penicillamine therapy in patients manifesting potentially serious urinary abnormalities must be weighed against the expected therapeutic benefits.

When penicillamine is used in cystinuria, an annual x-ray for renal stones is advised. Cystine stones form rapidly, sometimes in six months.

Up to one year or more may be required for any urinary abnormalities to disappear after penicillamine has been discontinued.

Because of rare reports of intrahepatic cholestasis and toxic hepatitis, liver function tests are recommended every six months for the duration of therapy. In Wilson's disease, these are recommended every three months, at least during the first year of treatment.

Goodpasture's syndrome has occurred rarely. The development of abnormal urinary findings associated with hemoptysis and pulmonary infiltrates on x-ray requires immediate cessation of penicillamine.

Obliterative bronchiolitis has been reported rarely. The patient should be cautioned to report immediately pulmonary symptoms such as exertional dyspnea, unexplained cough or wheezing. Pulmonary function studies should be considered at that time.

Onset of new neurological symptoms has been reported with CUPRIMINE (see ADVERSE REACTIONS). Occasionally, neurological symptoms become worse during initiation of

Continued on next page

Cuprimine—Cont.

therapy with CUPRIMINE (see INDICATIONS). Myasthenic syndrome sometimes progressing to myasthenia gravis has been reported. Ptosis and diplopia, with weakness of the extraocular muscles, are often early signs of myasthenia. In the majority of cases, symptoms of myasthenia have receded after withdrawal of penicillamine.

Most of the various forms of pemphigus have occurred during treatment with penicillamine. Pemphigus vulgaris and pemphigus foliaceus are reported most frequently, usually as a late complication of therapy. The seborrhea-like characteristics of pemphigus foliaceus may obscure an early diagnosis. When pemphigus is suspected, CUPRIMINE should be discontinued. Treatment has consisted of high doses of corticosteroids alone or, in some cases, concomitantly with an immunosuppressant. Treatment may be required for only a few weeks or months, but may need to be continued for more than a year.

Once instituted for Wilson's disease or cystinuria, treatment with penicillamine should, as a rule, be continued on a daily basis. Interruptions for even a few days have been followed by sensitivity reactions after reinstitution of therapy.

Pregnancy

Penicillamine has been shown to be teratogenic in rats when given in doses 6 times higher than the highest dose recommended for human use. Skeletal defects, cleft palates and fetal toxicity (resorptions) have been reported.

There are no controlled studies on the use of penicillamine in pregnant women. Although normal outcomes have been reported, characteristic congenital cutis laxa and associated birth defects have been reported in infants born of mothers who received therapy with penicillamine during pregnancy. Penicillamine should be used in women of childbearing potential only when the expected benefits outweigh the possible hazards. Women on therapy with penicillamine who are of childbearing potential should be apprised of this risk, advised to report promptly any missed menstrual periods or other indications of possible pregnancy, and followed closely for early recognition of pregnancy.

Wilson's Disease—Reported experience*** shows that continued treatment with penicillamine throughout pregnancy protects the mother against relapse of the Wilson's disease, and that discontinuation of penicillamine has deleterious effects on the mother, which may be fatal.

If penicillamine is administered during pregnancy to patients with Wilson's disease, it is recommended that the daily dosage be limited to 750 mg. If cesarean section is planned the daily dose should be reduced to 250 mg, but not lower, for the last six weeks of pregnancy and postoperatively until wound healing is complete.

Cystinuria —If possible, penicillamine should not be given during pregnancy to women with cystinuria (see CONTRAINDICATIONS). There are reports of women with cystinuria on therapy with penicillamine who gave birth to infants with generalized connective tissue defects who died following abdominal surgery. If stones continue to form in these patients, the benefits of therapy to the mother must be evaluated against the risk to the fetus.

Rheumatoid Arthritis—Penicillamine should not be administered to rheumatoid arthritis patients who are pregnant (see CONTRAINDICATIONS) and should be discontinued promptly in patients in whom pregnancy is suspected or diagnosed.

There is a report that a woman with rheumatoid arthritis treated with less than one gram a day of penicillamine during pregnancy gave birth (cesarean delivery) to an infant with growth retardation, flattened face with broad nasal bridge, low set ears, short neck with loose skin folds, and unusually lax body skin.

***Scheinberg, I.H., Sternlieb, I.: N. Engl. J. Med. *293*: 1300-1302, Dec. 18, 1975.

PRECAUTIONS

Some patients may experience drug fever, a marked febrile response to penicillamine, usually in the second to third week following initiation of therapy. Drug fever may sometimes be accompanied by a macular cutaneous eruption.

In the case of drug fever in patients with Wilson's disease or cystinuria, penicillamine should be temporarily discontinued until the reaction subsides. Then penicillamine should be reinstituted with a small dose that is gradually increased until the desired dosage is attained. Systemic steroid therapy may be necessary, and is usually helpful, in such patients in whom drug fever and rash develop several times.

In the case of drug fever in rheumatoid arthritis patients, because other treatments are available, penicillamine should be discontinued and another therapeutic alternative tried since experience indicates that the febrile reaction will recur in a very high percentage of patients upon readministration of penicillamine.

The skin and mucous membranes should be observed for allergic reactions. Early and late rashes have occurred. Early rash occurs during the first few months of treatment and is more common. It is usually a generalized pruritic, erythematous, maculopapular or morbilliform rash and resembles the allergic rash seen with other drugs. Early rash usually disappears within days after stopping penicillamine and seldom recurs when the drug is restarted at a lower dosage. Pruritus and early rash may often be controlled by the concomitant administration of antihistamines. Less commonly, a late rash may be seen, usually after six months or more of treatment, and requires discontinuation of penicillamine. It is usually on the trunk, is accompanied by intense pruritus, and is usually unresponsive to topical corticosteroid therapy. Late rash may take weeks to disappear after penicillamine is stopped and usually recurs if the drug is restarted.

The appearance of a drug eruption accompanied by fever, arthralgia, lymphadenopathy or other allergic manifestations usually requires discontinuation of penicillamine.

Certain patients will develop a positive antinuclear antibody (ANA) test and some of these may show a lupus erythematosus-like syndrome similar to drug-induced lupus associated with other drugs. The lupus erythematosus-like syndrome is not associated with hypocomplementemia and may be present without nephropathy. The development of a positive ANA test does not mandate discontinuance of the drug; however, the physician should be alerted to the possibility that a lupus erythematosus-like syndrome may develop in the future.

Some patients may develop oral ulcerations which in some cases have the appearance of aphthous stomatitis. The stomatitis usually recurs on rechallenge but often clears on a lower dosage. Although rare, cheilosis, glossitis and gingivostomatitis have also been reported. These oral lesions are frequently dose-related and may preclude further increase in penicillamine dosage or require discontinuation of the drug.

Hypogeusia (a blunting or diminution in taste perception) has occurred in some patients. This may last two to three months or more and may develop into a total loss of taste; however, it is usually self-limited despite continued penicillamine treatment. Such taste impairment is rare in patients with Wilson's disease.

Penicillamine should not be used in patients who are receiving concurrently gold therapy, antimalarial or cytotoxic drugs, oxyphenbutazone or phenylbutazone because these drugs are also associated with similar serious hematologic and renal adverse reactions. Patients who have had gold salt therapy discontinued due to a major toxic reaction may be at greater risk of serious adverse reactions with penicillamine but not necessarily of the same type.

Patients who are allergic to penicillin may theoretically have cross-sensitivity to penicillamine. The possibility of reactions from contamination of penicillamine by trace amounts of penicillin has been eliminated now that penicillamine is being produced synthetically rather than as a degradation product of penicillin.

Patients with Wilson's disease or cystinuria should be given 25 mg/day of pyridoxine during therapy, since penicillamine increases the requirement for this vitamin. Patients also may receive benefit from a multivitamin preparation, although there is no evidence that deficiency of any vitamin other than pyridoxine is associated with penicillamine. In Wilson's disease, multivitamin preparations must be copper-free.

Rheumatoid arthritis patients whose nutrition is impaired should also be given a daily supplement of pyridoxine. Mineral supplements should not be given, since they may block the response to penicillamine.

Iron deficiency may develop, especially in pediatric patients and in menstruating women. In Wilson's disease, this may be a result of adding the effects of the low copper diet, which is probably also low in iron, and the penicillamine to the effects of blood loss or growth. In cystinuria, a low methionine diet may contribute to iron deficiency, since it is necessarily low in protein. If necessary, iron may be given in short courses, but a period of two hours should elapse between administration of penicillamine and iron, since orally administered iron has been shown to reduce the effects of penicillamine.

Penicillamine causes an increase in the amount of soluble collagen. In the rat this results in inhibition of normal healing and also a decrease in tensile strength of intact skin. In man this may be the cause of increased skin friability at sites especially subject to pressure or trauma, such as shoulders, elbows, knees, toes, and buttocks. Extravasations of blood may occur and may appear as purpuric areas, with external bleeding if the skin is broken, or as vesicles containing dark blood. Neither type is progressive. There is no apparent association with bleeding elsewhere in the body and no associated coagulation defect has been found. Therapy with penicillamine may be continued in the presence of these lesions. They may not recur if dosage is reduced. Other reported effects probably due to the action of penicillamine on collagen are excessive wrinkling of the skin and development of small, white papules at venipuncture and surgical sites.

The effects of penicillamine on collagen and elastin make it advisable to consider a reduction in dosage to 250 mg/day, when surgery is contemplated. Reinstitution of full therapy should be delayed until wound healing is complete.

Carcinogenesis

Long-term animal carcinogenicity studies have not been done with penicillamine. There is a report that five of ten autoimmune disease-prone NZB hybrid mice developed lymphocytic leukemia after 6 months' intraperitoneal treatment with a dose of 400 mg/kg penicillamine 5 days per week.

Nursing Mothers

See CONTRAINDICATIONS.

Pediatric Use

The efficacy of CUPRIMINE in juvenile rheumatoid arthritis has not been established.

ADVERSE REACTIONS

Penicillamine is a drug with a high incidence of untoward reactions, some of which are potentially fatal. Therefore, it is mandatory that patients receiving penicillamine therapy remain under close medical supervision throughout the period of drug administration (see WARNINGS and PRECAUTIONS).

Reported incidences (%) for the most commonly occurring adverse reactions in rheumatoid arthritis patients are noted, based on 17 representative clinical trials reported in the literature (1270 patients).

Allergic—Generalized pruritus, early and late rashes (5%), pemphigus (see WARNINGS), and drug eruptions which may be accompanied by fever, arthralgia, or lymphadenopathy have occurred (see WARNINGS and PRECAUTIONS). Some patients may show a lupus erythematosus-like syndrome similar to drug-induced lupus produced by other pharmacological agents (see PRECAUTIONS).

Urticaria and exfoliative dermatitis have occurred.

Thyroiditis has been reported; hypoglycemia in association with anti-insulin antibodies has been reported. These reactions are extremely rare.

Some patients may develop a migratory polyarthralgia, often with objective synovitis (see DOSAGE AND ADMINISTRATION).

Gastrointestinal—Anorexia, epigastric pain, nausea, vomiting, or occasional diarrhea may occur (17%).

Isolated cases of reactivated peptic ulcer have occurred, as have hepatic dysfunction including hepatic failure, and pancreatitis. Intrahepatic cholestasis and toxic hepatitis have been reported rarely. There have been a few reports of increased serum alkaline phosphatase, lactic dehydrogenase, and positive cephalin flocculation and thymol turbidity tests.

Some patients may report a blunting, diminution, or total loss of taste perception (12%); or may develop oral ulcerations. Although rare, cheilosis, glossitis, and gingivostomatitis have been reported (see PRECAUTIONS).

Gastrointestinal side effects are usually reversible following cessation of therapy.

Hematological—Penicillamine can cause bone marrow depression (see WARNINGS). Leukopenia (2%) and thrombocytopenia (4%) have occurred. Fatalities have been reported as a result of thrombocytopenia, agranulocytosis, aplastic anemia, and sideroblastic anemia.

Thrombotic thrombocytopenic purpura, hemolytic anemia, red cell aplasia, monocytosis, leukocytosis, eosinophilia, and thrombocytosis have also been reported.

Renal—Patients on penicillamine therapy may develop proteinuria (6%) and/or hematuria which, in some, may progress to the development of the nephrotic syndrome as a result of an immune complex membranous glomerulopathy (see WARNINGS). Renal failure has been reported.

Central Nervous System—Tinnitus, optic neuritis and peripheral sensory and motor neuropathies (including polyradiculoneuropathy, i.e., Guillain-Barre syndrome) have been reported. Muscular weakness may or may not occur with the peripheral neuropathies. Visual and psychic disturbances; mental disorders; and agitation and anxiety have been reported.

Neuromuscular—Myasthenia gravis (see WARNINGS); dystonia.

Other—Adverse reactions that have been reported rarely include thrombophlebitis; hyperpyrexia (see PRECAUTIONS); falling hair or alopecia; lichen planus; polymyositis; dermatomyositis; mammary hyperplasia; elastosis perforans serpiginosa; toxic epidermal necrolysis; anetoderma (cutaneous macular atrophy); and Goodpasture's syndrome, a severe and ultimately fatal glomerulonephritis associated with intra-alveolar hemorrhage (see WARNINGS). Vasculitis, including fatal renal vasculitis, has also been reported. Allergic alveolitis, obliterative bronchiolitis, interstitial pneumonitis and pulmonary fibrosis have been reported in patients with severe rheumatoid arthritis, some of whom were receiving penicillamine. Bronchial asthma also has been reported.

Increased skin friability, excessive wrinkling of skin, and development of small white papules at venipuncture and surgical sites have been reported (see PRECAUTIONS); yellow nail syndrome.

The chelating action of the drug may cause increased excretion of other heavy metals such as zinc, mercury and lead. There have been reports associating penicillamine with leukemia. However, circumstances involved in these reports are such that a cause and effect relationship to the drug has not been established.

DOSAGE AND ADMINISTRATION

In all patients receiving penicillamine, it is important that CUPRIMINE be given on an empty stomach, at least one hour before meals or two hours after meals, and at least one hour apart from any other drug, food, or milk. Because penicillamine increases the requirement for pyridoxine, patients may require a daily supplement of pyridoxine (see PRECAUTIONS).

Wilson's Disease— Optimal dosage can be determined by measurement of urinary copper excretion and the determination of free copper in the serum. The urine must be collected in copper-free glassware, and should be quantitatively analyzed for copper before and soon after initiation of therapy with CUPRIMINE.

Determination of 24-hour urinary copper excretion is of greatest value in the first week of therapy with penicillamine. In the absence of any drug reaction, a dose between 0.75 and 1.5 g that results in an initial 24-hour cupriuresis of over 2 mg should be continued for about three months, by which time the most reliable method of monitoring maintenance treatment is the determination of free copper in the serum. This equals the difference between quantitatively determined total copper and ceruloplasmin-copper. Adequately treated patients will usually have less than 10 mcg free copper/dL of serum. It is seldom necessary to exceed a dosage of 2 g/day. If the patient is intolerant to therapy with CUPRIMINE, alternative treatment is trientine hydrochloride.

In patients who cannot tolerate as much as 1 g/day initially, initiating dosage with 250 mg/day, and increasing gradually to the requisite amount, gives closer control of the effects of the drug and may help to reduce the incidence of adverse reactions.

Cystinuria—It is recommended that CUPRIMINE be used along with conventional therapy. By reducing urinary cystine, it decreases crystalluria and stone formation. In some instances, it has been reported to decrease the size of, and even to dissolve, stones already formed.

The usual dosage of CUPRIMINE in the treatment of cystinuria is 2 g/day for adults, with a range of 1 to 4 g/day. For pediatric patients, dosage can be based on 30 mg/kg/day. The total daily amount should be divided into four doses. If four equal doses are not feasible, give the larger portion at bedtime. If adverse reactions necessitate a reduction in dosage, it is important to retain the bedtime dose.

Initiating dosage with 250 mg/day, and increasing gradually to the requisite amount, gives closer control of the effects of the drug and may help to reduce the incidence of adverse reactions.

In addition to taking CUPRIMINE, patients should drink copiously. It is especially important to drink about a pint of fluid at bedtime and another pint once during the night when urine is more concentrated and more acid than during the day. The greater the fluid intake, the lower the required dosage of CUPRIMINE.

Dosage must be individualized to an amount that limits cystine excretion to 100-200 mg/day in those with no history of stones, and below 100 mg/day in those who have had stone formation and/or pain. Thus, in determining dosage, the inherent tubular defect, the patient's size, age, and rate of growth, and his diet and water intake all must be taken into consideration.

The standard nitroprusside cyanide test has been reported useful as a qualitative measure of the effective dose:† Add 2 mL of freshly prepared 5 percent sodium cyanide to 5 mL of a 24-hour aliquot of protein-free urine and let stand ten minutes. Add 5 drops of freshly prepared 5 percent sodium nitroprusside and mix. Cystine will turn the mixture magenta. If the result is negative, it can be assumed that cystine excretion is less than 100 mg/g creatinine.

Although penicillamine is rarely excreted unchanged, it also will turn the mixture magenta. If there is any question as to which substance is causing the reaction, a ferric chloride test can be done to eliminate doubt: Add 3 percent ferric chloride dropwise to the urine. Penicillamine will turn the urine an immediate and quickly fading blue. Cystine will not produce any change in appearance.

† Lotz, M., Potts, J.T. and Bartter, F.C.: Brit. Med. J. *2* :521, Aug. 28, 1965 (in Medical Memoranda).

Rheumatoid Arthritis—The principal rule of treatment with CUPRIMINE in rheumatoid arthritis is patience. The onset of therapeutic response is typically delayed. Two or three months may be required before the first evidence of a clinical response is noted (see CLINICAL PHARMACOLOGY).

When treatment with CUPRIMINE has been interrupted because of adverse reactions or other reasons, the drug should be reintroduced cautiously by starting with a lower dosage and increasing slowly.

Initial Therapy—The currently recommended dosage regimen in rheumatoid arthritis begins with a single daily dose of 125 mg or 250 mg which is thereafter increased at one to three month intervals, by 125 mg or 250 mg/day, as patient response and tolerance indicate. If a satisfactory remission of symptoms is achieved, the dose associated with the remission should be continued (see *Maintenance Therapy*). If there is no improvement and there are no signs of potentially serious toxicity after two to three months of treatment with doses of 500-750 mg/day, increases of 250 mg/day at two to three month intervals may be continued until a satisfactory remission occurs (see *Maintenance Therapy*) or signs of toxicity develop (see WARNINGS and PRECAUTIONS). If there is no discernible improvement after three to four months of treatment with 1000 to 1500 mg of penicillamine/day, it may be assumed the patient will not respond and CUPRIMINE should be discontinued.

Maintenance Therapy—The maintenance dosage of CUPRIMINE must be individualized, and may require adjustment during the course of treatment. Many patients respond satisfactorily to a dosage within the 500-750 mg/day range. Some need less.

Changes in maintenance dosage levels may not be reflected clinically or in the erythrocyte sedimentation rate for two to three months after each dosage adjustment.

Some patients will subsequently require an increase in the maintenance dosage to achieve maximal disease suppression. In those patients who do respond, but who evidence incomplete suppression of their disease after the first six to nine months of treatment, the daily dosage of CUPRIMINE may be increased by 125 mg or 250 mg/day at three-month intervals. It is unusual in current practice to employ a dosage in excess of 1 g/day, but up to 1.5 g/day has sometimes been required.

Management of Exacerbations—During the course of treatment some patients may experience an exacerbation of disease activity following an initial good response. These may be self-limited and can subside within twelve weeks. They are usually controlled by the addition of non-steroidal anti-inflammatory drugs, and only if the patient has demonstrated a true "escape" phenomenon (as evidenced by failure of the flare to subside within this time period) should an increase in the maintenance dose ordinarily be considered.

In the rheumatoid patient, migratory polyarthralgia due to penicillamine is extremely difficult to differentiate from an exacerbation of the rheumatoid arthritis. Discontinuance or a substantial reduction in dosage of CUPRIMINE for up to several weeks will usually determine which of these processes is responsible for the arthralgia.

Duration of Therapy—The optimum duration of therapy with CUPRIMINE in rheumatoid arthritis has not been determined. If the patient has been in remission for six months or more, a gradual, stepwise dosage reduction in decrements of 125 mg or 250 mg/day at approximately three month intervals may be attempted.

Concomitant Drug Therapy—CUPRIMINE should not be used in patients who are receiving gold therapy, antimalarial or cytotoxic drugs, oxyphenbutazone, or phenylbutazone (see PRECAUTIONS). Other measures, such as salicylates, other non-steroidal anti-inflammatory drugs, or systemic corticosteroids, may be continued when penicillamine is initiated. After improvement commences, analgesic and anti-inflammatory drugs may be slowly discontinued as symptoms permit. Steroid withdrawal must be done gradually, and many months of treatment with CUPRIMINE may be required before steroids can be completely eliminated.

Dosage Frequency—Based on clinical experience dosages up to 500 mg/day can be given as a single daily dose. Dosages in excess of 500 mg/day should be administered in divided doses.

HOW SUPPLIED

No. 3299—Capsules CUPRIMINE, 250 mg, are ivory-colored capsules containing a white or nearly white powder, and are coded CUPRIMINE and MSD 602. They are supplied as follows:

NDC 0006-0602-68 in bottles of 100.

No. 3350—Capsules CUPRIMINE, 125 mg, are opaque ivory and gray capsules containing a white or nearly white powder, and are coded CUPRIMINE and MSD 672. They are supplied as follows:

NDC 0006-0672-68 in bottles of 100.

Storage

Keep container tightly closed.

7873243 Issued November 2003

Shown in Product Identification Guide, page 323

DARANIDE® Tablets ℞
(Dichlorphenamide)

DESCRIPTION

DARANIDE* (Dichlorphenamide) is an oral carbonic anhydrase inhibitor. Dichlorphenamide, a dichlorinated benzenedisulfonamide, is known chemically as 4,5-dichloro-1,3-benzenedisulfonamide. Its empirical formula is $C_6H_6Cl_2N_2O_4S_2$ and its structural formula is:

Dichlorphenamide is a white or practically white, crystalline compound with a molecular weight of 305.16. It is very slightly soluble in water but soluble in dilute solutions of sodium carbonate and sodium hydroxide. Dilute alkaline solutions of dichlorphenamide are stable at room temperature.

DARANIDE is supplied as tablets, for oral administration, each containing 50 mg dichlorphenamide. Inactive ingredients are D&C Yellow 10, lactose, magnesium stearate, and starch.

*Registered trademark of MERCK & CO., Inc.

CLINICAL PHARMACOLOGY

Carbonic anhydrase inhibitors reduce intraocular pressure by partially suppressing the secretion of aqueous humor (inflow), although the mechanism by which they do this is not fully understood. Evidence suggests that HCO_3^- ions are produced in the ciliary body by hydration of carbon dioxide under the influence of carbonic anhydrase and diffuse into the posterior chamber with Na^+ ions. The aqueous fluid contains more Na^+ and HCO_3^- ions than does plasma and consequently is hypertonic. Water is attracted to the posterior chamber by osmosis. Systemic administration of a carbonic anhydrase inhibitor has been shown to inactivate carbonic anhydrase in the ciliary body of the rabbit's eye and to reduce the high concentration of HCO_3^- ions in ocular fluids. As is the case with all carbonic anhydrase inhibitors, DARANIDE in high doses causes some decrease in renal blood flow and glomerular filtration rate.

In man, DARANIDE begins to act within an hour and maximal effect is observed in two to four hours. The lowered intraocular tension may be maintained for approximately 6 to 12 hours.

INDICATIONS AND USAGE

For adjunctive treatment of: chronic simple (open-angle) glaucoma, secondary glaucoma, and preoperatively in acute angle-closure glaucoma where delay of surgery is desired in order to lower intraocular pressure.

CONTRAINDICATIONS

DARANIDE is contraindicated in hepatic insufficiency, renal failure, adrenocortical insufficiency, hyperchloremic acidosis, or in conditions in which serum levels of sodium or potassium are depressed. DARANIDE should not be used in patients with severe pulmonary obstruction who are unable to increase their alveolar ventilation since their acidosis may be increased.

DARANIDE is contraindicated in patients who are hypersensitive to this product.

PRECAUTIONS

General

Potassium excretion is increased by DARANIDE and hypokalemia may develop with brisk diuresis, when severe cirrhosis is present, or during concomitant use of steroids or ACTH.

Interference with adequate oral electrolyte intake will also contribute to hypokalemia. Hypokalemia can sensitize or exaggerate the response of the heart to the toxic effects of digitalis (e.g., increased ventricular irritability). Hypokalemia may be avoided or treated by use of potassium supplements such as foods with a high potassium content. DARANIDE should be used with caution in patients with respiratory acidosis.

Drug Interactions

Caution is advised in patients receiving concomitant high-dose aspirin and carbonic anhydrase inhibitors, as anorexia, tachypnea, lethargy and coma have been rarely reported due to a possible drug interaction.

Carcinogenesis, Mutagenesis, Impairment of Fertility

Long-term studies in animals have not been performed to evaluate the effects upon fertility or carcinogenic potential of DARANIDE.

Pregnancy

Pregnancy Category C. Diclorphenamide has been shown to be teratogenic in the rat (skeletal anomalies) when given in doses 100 times the human dose. There are no adequate and well-controlled studies in pregnant women. DARANIDE should not be used in women of childbearing age or in pregnancy, especially during the first trimester, unless the potential benefits outweigh the potential risks.

Nursing Mothers

It is not known whether diclorphenamide is excreted in human milk. Because many drugs are excreted in human milk, caution should be exercised when diclorphenamide is administered to a nursing woman.

Pediatric Use

Safety and effectiveness in pediatric patients have not been established.

ADVERSE REACTIONS

Certain side effects characteristic of carbonic anhydrase inhibitors may occur with DARANIDE, particularly with increasing doses.

The most common effects include gastrointestinal disturbances (anorexia, nausea, and vomiting), drowsiness and paresthesias.

Included in the listing which follows are some adverse reactions which have not been reported with DARANIDE. However, pharmacological similarities among the carbonic anhydrase inhibitors make it advisable to consider the following reactions when diclorphenamide is administered.

Central Nervous System / Psychiatric: ataxia, tremor, tinnitus, headache, weakness, nervousness, globus hystericus, lassitude, depression, confusion, disorientation, dizziness;

Gastrointestinal: constipation, hepatic insufficiency;

Metabolic: loss of weight, metabolic acidosis, electrolyte imbalance (hypokalemia, hyperchloremia), hyperuricemia;

Continued on next page

Information on the Merck & Co., Inc., products listed on these pages is from the prescribing information in use October 1, 2004. For information, please call 1-800-NSC-MERCK [1-800-672-6372].

Daranide—Cont.

Hypersensitivity: skin eruptions, pruritus, fever;
Hematologic: leukopenia, agranulocytosis, thrombocytopenia;
Genitourinary: urinary frequency, renal colic, renal calculi, phosphaturia.

OVERDOSAGE

The oral LD_{50} of DARANIDE is 1710 and 2600 mg/kg in the mouse and rat respectively.
Symptoms of overdosage or toxicity may include drowsiness, anorexia, nausea, vomiting, dizziness, paresthesias, ataxia, tremor and tinnitus.
In the event of overdosage, induce emesis or perform gastric lavage. The electrolyte disturbance most likely to be encountered from overdosage is hyperchloremic acidosis that may respond to bicarbonate administration. Potassium supplementation may be required. The patient should be carefully observed and given supportive treatment.

DOSAGE AND ADMINISTRATION

DARANIDE is usually given in conjunction with topical ocular hypotensive agents. In acute angle-closure glaucoma, it may be used together with miotics and osmotic agents in an attempt to reduce intraocular tension rapidly. If this is not quickly relieved, surgery may be mandatory.
Dosage must be adjusted carefully to meet the requirements of the individual patient. A priming dose of 100 to 200 mg of DARANIDE (2 to 4 tablets) is suggested for adults, followed by 100 mg (2 tablets) every 12 hours until the desired response has been obtained. The recommended maintenance dosage for adults is 25 to 50 mg (1/2 to 1 tablet) once to three times daily.

HOW SUPPLIED

No. 3256—Tablets DARANIDE, 50 mg each, are yellow, round, scored, compressed tablets, coded MSD 49 on one side and DARANIDE on the other. They are supplied as follows:
NDC 0006-0049-68 bottles of 100.
7870319 Issued October 1996

DECADRON® Tablets ℞
(Dexamethasone)

DESCRIPTION

Glucocorticoids are adrenocortical steroids, both naturally occurring and synthetic, which are readily absorbed from the gastrointestinal tract.
Dexamethasone, a synthetic adrenocortical steroid, is a white to practically white, odorless, crystalline powder. It is stable in air. It is practically insoluble in water. The molecular weight is 392.47. It is designated chemically as 9-fluoro-11β, 17, 21-trihydroxy-16α-methylpregna-1, 4-diene-3,20-dione. The empirical formula is $C_{22}H_{29}FO_5$ and the structural formula is:

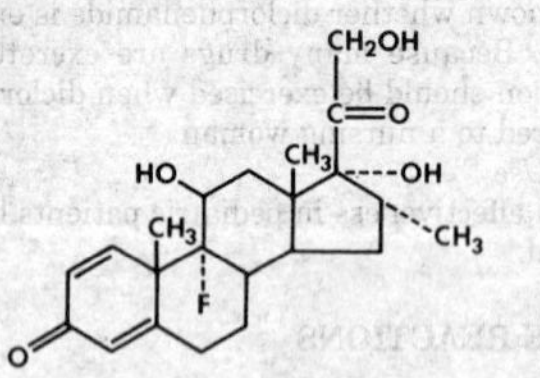

DECADRON* (Dexamethasone) tablets are supplied in three potencies, 0.5 mg, 0.75 mg, and 4 mg. Inactive ingredients are calcium phosphate, lactose, magnesium stearate, and starch. Tablets DECADRON 0.5 mg also contain D&C Yellow 10 and FD&C Yellow 6. Tablets DECADRON 0.75 mg also contain FD&C Blue 1.

*Registered trademark of MERCK & CO., INC.

ACTIONS

Naturally occurring glucocorticoids (hydrocortisone and cortisone), which also have salt-retaining properties, are used as replacement therapy in adrenocortical deficiency states. Their synthetic analogs including dexamethasone are primarily used for their potent anti-inflammatory effects in disorders of many organ systems.
Glucocorticoids cause profound and varied metabolic effects. In addition, they modify the body's immune responses to diverse stimuli.
At equipotent anti-inflammatory doses, dexamethasone almost completely lacks the sodium-retaining property of hydrocortisone and closely related derivatives of hydrocortisone.

INDICATIONS

1. *Endocrine Disorders*
Primary or secondary adrenocortical insufficiency (hydrocortisone or cortisone is the first choice; synthetic analogs may be used in conjunction with mineralocorticoids where applicable; in infancy mineralocorticoid supplementation is of particular importance)
Congenital adrenal hyperplasia
Nonsuppurative thyroiditis
Hypercalcemia associated with cancer
2. *Rheumatic Disorders*
As adjunctive therapy for short-term administration (to tide the patient over an acute episode or exacerbation) in:
Psoriatic arthritis
Rheumatoid arthritis, including juvenile rheumatoid arthritis (selected cases may require low-dose maintenance therapy)
Ankylosing spondylitis
Acute and subacute bursitis
Acute nonspecific tenosynovitis
Acute gouty arthritis
Post-traumatic osteoarthritis
Synovitis of osteoarthritis
Epicondylitis
3. *Collagen Diseases*
During an exacerbation or as maintenance therapy in selected cases of—
Systemic lupus erythematosus
Acute rheumatic carditis
4. *Dermatologic Diseases*
Pemphigus
Bullous dermatitis herpetiformis
Severe erythema multiforme (Stevens-Johnson syndrome)
Exfoliative dermatitis
Mycosis fungoides
Severe psoriasis
Severe seborrheic dermatitis
5. *Allergic States*
Control of severe or incapacitating allergic conditions intractable to adequate trials of conventional treatment:
Seasonal or perennial allergic rhinitis
Bronchial asthma
Contact dermatitis
Atopic dermatitis
Serum sickness
Drug hypersensitivity reactions
6. *Ophthalmic Diseases*
Severe acute and chronic allergic and inflammatory processes involving the eye and its adnexa, such as—
Allergic conjunctivitis
Keratitis
Allergic corneal marginal ulcers
Herpes zoster ophthalmicus
Iritis and iridocyclitis
Chorioretinitis
Anterior segment inflammation
Diffuse posterior uveitis and choroiditis
Optic neuritis
Sympathetic ophthalmia
7. *Respiratory Diseases*
Symptomatic sarcoidosis
Loeffler's syndrome not manageable by other means
Berylliosis
Fulminating or disseminated pulmonary tuberculosis when used concurrently with appropriate antituberculous chemotherapy
Aspiration pneumonitis
8. *Hematologic Disorders*
Idiopathic thrombocytopenic purpura in adults
Secondary thrombocytopenia in adults
Acquired (autoimmune) hemolytic anemia
Erythroblastopenia (RBC anemia)
Congenital (erythroid) hypoplastic anemia
9. *Neoplastic Diseases*
For palliative management of:
Leukemias and lymphomas in adults
Acute leukemia of childhood
10. *Edematous States*
To induce a diuresis or remission of proteinuria in the nephrotic syndrome, without uremia, of the idiopathic type or that due to lupus erythematosus
11. *Gastrointestinal Diseases*
To tide the patient over a critical period of the disease in:
Ulcerative colitis
Regional enteritis
12. *Cerebral Edema* associated with primary or metastatic brain tumor, craniotomy, or head injury. Use in cerebral edema is not a substitute for careful neurosurgical evaluation and definitive management such as neurosurgery or other specific therapy
13. *Miscellaneous*
Tuberculous meningitis with subarachnoid block or impending block when used concurrently with appropriate antituberculous chemotherapy
Trichinosis with neurologic or myocardial involvement
14. *Diagnostic testing of adrenocortical hyperfunction*

CONTRAINDICATIONS

Systemic fungal infections
Hypersensitivity to this drug

WARNINGS

In patients on corticosteroid therapy subjected to unusual stress, increased dosage of rapidly acting corticosteroids before, during, and after the stressful situation is indicated.
Drug-induced secondary adrenocortical insufficiency may result from too rapid withdrawal of corticosteroids and may be minimized by gradual reduction of dosage. This type of relative insufficiency may persist for months after discontinuation of therapy; therefore, in any situation of stress occurring during that period, hormone therapy should be reinstituted. If the patient is receiving steroids already, dosage may have to be increased. Since mineralocorticoid secretion may be impaired, salt and/or a mineralocorticoid should be administered concurrently. (See PRECAUTIONS.)
Corticosteroids may mask some signs of infection, and new infections may appear during their use. There may be decreased resistance and inability to localize infection when corticosteroids are used. Moreover, corticosteroids may affect the nitroblue-tetrazolium test for bacterial infection and produce false negative results.
In cerebral malaria, a double-blind trial has shown that the use of corticosteroids is associated with prolongation of coma and a higher incidence of pneumonia and gastrointestinal bleeding.
Corticosteroids may activate latent amebiasis. Therefore, it is recommended that latent or active amebiasis be ruled out before initiating corticosteroid therapy in any patient who has spent time in the tropics or any patient with unexplained diarrhea.
Prolonged use of corticosteroids may produce posterior subcapsular cataracts, glaucoma with possible damage to the optic nerves, and may enhance the establishment of secondary ocular infections due to fungi or viruses.
Usage in pregnancy: Since adequate human reproduction studies have not been done with corticosteroids, use of these drugs in pregnancy or in women of childbearing potential requires that the anticipated benefits be weighed against the possible hazards to the mother and embryo or fetus. Infants born of mothers who have received substantial doses of corticosteroids during pregnancy should be carefully observed for signs of hypoadrenalism.
Corticosteroids appear in breast milk and could suppress growth, interfere with endogenous corticosteroid production, or cause other unwanted effects. Mothers taking pharmacologic doses of corticosteroids should be advised not to nurse.
Average and large doses of hydrocortisone or cortisone can cause elevation of blood pressure, salt and water retention, and increased excretion of potassium. These effects are less likely to occur with the synthetic derivatives except when used in large doses. Dietary salt restriction and potassium supplementation may be necessary. All corticosteroids increase calcium excretion.
Administration of live virus vaccines, including smallpox, is contraindicated in individuals receiving immunosuppressive doses of corticosteroids. If inactivated viral or bacterial vaccines are administered to individuals receiving immunosuppressive doses of corticosteroid the expected serum antibody response may not be obtained. However, immunization procedures may be undertaken in patients who are receiving corticosteroids as replacement therapy, e.g., for Addison's disease.
Patients who are on drugs which suppress the immune system are more susceptible to infections than healthy individuals. Chickenpox and measles, for example, can have a more serious or even fatal course in non-immune patients on corticosteroids. In such patients who have not had these diseases, particular care should be taken to avoid exposure. The risk of developing a disseminated infection varies among individuals and can be related to the dose, route and duration of corticosteroid administration as well as to the underlying disease. If exposed to chickenpox, prophylaxis with varicella zoster immune globulin (VZIG) may be indicated. If chickenpox develops, treatment with antiviral agents may be considered. If exposed to measles, prophylaxis with immune globulin (IG) may be indicated. (See the respective package inserts for VZIG and IG for complete prescribing information.)
Similarly, corticosteroids should be used with great care in patients with known or suspected Strongyloides (threadworm) infestation. In such patients, corticosteroid-induced immunosuppression may lead to Strongyloides hyperinfection and dissemination with widespread larval migration, often accompanied by severe enterocolitis and potentially fatal gram-negative septicemia.
The use of DECADRON tablets in active tuberculosis should be restricted to those cases of fulminating or disseminated tuberculosis in which the corticosteroid is used for the management of the disease in conjunction with an appropriate antituberculous regimen.
If corticosteroids are indicated in patients with latent tuberculosis or tuberculin reactivity, close observation is necessary as reactivation of the disease may occur. During prolonged corticosteroid therapy, these patients should receive chemoprophylaxis.
Literature reports suggest an apparent association between use of corticosteroids and left ventricular free wall rupture after a recent myocardial infarction; therefore, therapy with corticosteroids should be used with great caution in these patients.

PRECAUTIONS

Following prolonged therapy, withdrawal of corticosteroids may result in symptoms of the corticosteroid withdrawal syndrome including fever, myalgia, arthralgia, and malaise. This may occur in patients even without evidence of adrenal insufficiency.

There is an enhanced effect of corticosteroids in patients with hypothyroidism and in those with cirrhosis.

Corticosteroids should be used cautiously in patients with ocular herpes simplex because of possible corneal perforation.

The lowest possible dose of corticosteroids should be used to control the condition under treatment, and when reduction in dosage is possible, the reduction should be gradual.

Psychic derangements may appear when corticosteroids are used, ranging from euphoria, insomnia, mood swings, personality changes, and severe depression, to frank psychotic manifestations. Also, existing emotional instability or psychotic tendencies may be aggravated by corticosteroids.

Co-administration of thalidomide with DECADRON tablets should be employed cautiously, as toxic epidermal necrolysis has been reported with concomitant use.

Aspirin should be used cautiously in conjunction with corticosteroids in hypoprothrombinemia.

Steroids should be used with caution in nonspecific ulcerative colitis, if there is a probability of impending perforation, abscess, or other pyogenic infection, diverticulitis, fresh intestinal anastomoses, active or latent peptic ulcer, renal insufficiency, hypertension, osteoporosis, and myasthenia gravis. Signs of peritoneal irritation following gastrointestinal perforation in patients receiving large doses of corticosteroids may be minimal or absent. Fat embolism has been reported as a possible complication of hypercortisonism.

When large doses are given, some authorities advise that corticosteroids be taken with meals and antacids taken between meals to help to prevent peptic ulcer.

Steroids may increase or decrease motility and number of spermatozoa in some patients.

Cytochrome P450 3A4 (CYP 3A4) enzyme inducers, such as phenytoin, barbiturates (e.g., phenobarbital), carbamazepine, and rifampin may enhance the metabolic clearance of corticosteroids, resulting in decreased blood levels and lessened physiologic activity, thus requiring an increase in corticosteroid dosage.

Dexamethasone is metabolized by CYP 3A4. Concomitant administration of dexamethasone with inducers of CYP 3A4 (as listed above) has the potential to result in decreased plasma concentrations of dexamethasone. In addition, concomitant administration of dexamethasone with known inhibitors of CYP 3A4 (e.g., ketoconazole, macrolide antibiotics such as erythromycin) has the potential to result in increased plasma concentrations of dexamethasone. Effects of other drugs on the metabolism of dexamethasone may interfere with dexamethasone suppression tests, which should be interpreted with caution during administration of such drugs.

Dexamethasone is a moderate inducer of CYP 3A4. Co-administration of dexamethasone with other drugs that are metabolized by CYP 3A4 (e.g., indinavir, erythromycin) may increase their clearance, resulting in decreased plasma concentrations.

In post-marketing experience, there have been reports of both increases and decreases in phenytoin levels with dexamethasone co-administration, leading to alterations in seizure control.

Although ketoconazole may increase dexamethasone plasma concentrations through inhibition of CYP 3A4, ketoconazole alone can inhibit adrenal corticosteroid synthesis and may cause adrenal insufficiency during corticosteroid withdrawal (see WARNINGS).

Ephedrine may enhance the metabolic clearance of corticosteroids, resulting in decreased blood levels and lessened physiologic activity, thus requiring an increase in corticosteroid dosage.

False-negative results in the dexamethasone suppression test (DST) in patients being treated with indomethacin have been reported. Thus, results of the DST should be interpreted with caution in these patients.

The prothrombin time should be checked frequently in patients who are receiving corticosteroids and coumarin anticoagulants at the same time because of reports that corticosteroids have altered the response to these anticoagulants. Studies have shown that the usual effect produced by adding corticosteroids is inhibition of response to coumarins, although there have been some conflicting reports of potentiation not substantiated by studies.

When corticosteroids are administered concomitantly with potassium-depleting diuretics, patients should be observed closely for development of hypokalemia.

Information for Patients

Susceptible patients who are on immunosuppressant doses of corticosteroids should be warned to avoid exposure to chickenpox or measles. Patients should also be advised that if they are exposed, medical advice should be sought without delay.

Pediatric Use

Growth and development of pediatric patients on prolonged corticosteroid therapy should be carefully followed.

ADVERSE REACTIONS

Fluid and Electrolyte Disturbances
- Sodium retention
- Fluid retention
- Congestive heart failure in susceptible patients
- Potassium loss
- Hypokalemic alkalosis
- Hypertension

Musculoskeletal
- Muscle weakness
- Steroid myopathy
- Loss of muscle mass
- Osteoporosis
- Vertebral compression fractures
- Aseptic necrosis of femoral and humeral heads
- Pathologic fracture of long bones
- Tendon rupture

Gastrointestinal
- Peptic ulcer with possible perforation and hemorrhage
- Perforation of the small and large bowel, particularly in patients with inflammatory bowel disease
- Pancreatitis
- Abdominal distention
- Ulcerative esophagitis

Dermatologic
- Impaired wound healing
- Thin fragile skin
- Petechiae and ecchymoses
- Erythema
- Increased sweating
- May suppress reactions to skin tests
- Other cutaneous reactions, such as allergic dermatitis, urticaria, angioneurotic edema

Neurologic
- Convulsions
- Increased intracranial pressure with papilledema (pseudotumor cerebri) usually after treatment
- Vertigo
- Headache
- Psychic disturbances

Endocrine
- Menstrual irregularities
- Development of cushingoid state
- Suppression of growth in children
- Secondary adrenocortical and pituitary unresponsiveness, particularly in times of stress, as in trauma, surgery, or illness
- Decreased carbohydrate tolerance
- Manifestations of latent diabetes mellitus
- Hyperglycemia
- Increased requirements for insulin or oral hypoglycemic agents in diabetics
- Hirsutism

Ophthalmic
- Posterior subcapsular cataracts
- Increased intraocular pressure
- Glaucoma
- Exophthalmos

Metabolic
- Negative nitrogen balance due to protein catabolism

Cardiovascular
- Myocardial rupture following recent myocardial infarction (see WARNINGS)

Other
- Hypersensitivity
- Thromboembolism
- Weight gain
- Increased appetite
- Nausea
- Malaise
- Hiccups

OVERDOSAGE

Reports of acute toxicity and/or death following overdosage of glucocorticoids are rare. In the event of overdosage, no specific antidote is available; treatment is supportive and symptomatic.

The oral LD_{50} of dexamethasone in female mice was 6.5 g/kg.

DOSAGE AND ADMINISTRATION

For oral administration

DOSAGE REQUIREMENTS ARE VARIABLE AND MUST BE INDIVIDUALIZED ON THE BASIS OF THE DISEASE AND THE RESPONSE OF THE PATIENT.

The initial dosage varies from 0.75 to 9 mg a day depending on the disease being treated. In less severe diseases doses lower than 0.75 mg may suffice, while in severe diseases doses higher than 9 mg may be required. The initial dosage should be maintained or adjusted until the patient's response is satisfactory. If satisfactory clinical response does not occur after a reasonable period of time, discontinue DECADRON tablets and transfer the patient to other therapy.

After a favorable initial response, the proper maintenance dosage should be determined by decreasing the initial dosage in small amounts to the lowest dosage that maintains an adequate clinical response.

Patients should be observed closely for signs that might require dosage adjustment, including changes in clinical status resulting from remissions or exacerbations of the disease, individual drug responsiveness, and the effect of stress (e.g., surgery, infection, trauma). During stress it may be necessary to increase dosage temporarily.

If the drug is to be stopped after more than a few days of treatment, it usually should be withdrawn gradually.

The following milligram equivalents facilitate changing to DECADRON from other glucocorticoids:

DECADRON	Methylprednisolone and Triamcinolone	Prednisolone and Prednisone	Hydrocortisone	Cortisone
0.75 mg =	4 mg =	5 mg =	20 mg =	25 mg

[See table above]

In *acute, self-limited allergic disorders or acute exacerbations of chronic allergic disorders,* the following dosage schedule combining parenteral and oral therapy is suggested:

DECADRON Phosphate (Dexamethasone Sodium Phosphate) injection, 4 mg per mL:

First Day
- 1 or 2 mL, intramuscularly

DECADRON tablets, 0.75 mg:

Second Day
- 4 tablets in two divided doses

Third Day
- 4 tablets in two divided doses

Fourth Day
- 2 tablets in two divided doses

Fifth Day
- 1 tablet

Sixth Day
- 1 tablet

Seventh Day
- No treatment

Eighth Day
- Follow-up visit

This schedule is designed to ensure adequate therapy during acute episodes, while minimizing the risk of overdosage in chronic cases.

In *cerebral edema,* DECADRON Phosphate (Dexamethasone Sodium Phosphate) injection is generally administered initially in a dosage of 10 mg intravenously followed by 4 mg every six hours intramuscularly until the symptoms of cerebral edema subside. Response is usually noted within 12 to 24 hours and dosage may be reduced after two to four days and gradually discontinued over a period of five to seven days. For palliative management of patients with recurrent or inoperable brain tumors, maintenance therapy with either DECADRON Phosphate (Dexamethasone Sodium Phosphate) injection or DECADRON tablets in a dosage of two mg two or three times daily may be effective.

Dexamethasone suppression tests.

1. Tests for Cushing's syndrome
   Give 1.0 mg of DECADRON orally at 11:00 p.m. Blood is drawn for plasma cortisol determination at 8:00 a.m. the following morning.
   For greater accuracy, give 0.5 mg of DECADRON orally every 6 hours for 48 hours. Twenty-four hour urine collections are made for determination of 17-hydroxycorticosteroid excretion.
2. Test to distinguish Cushing's syndrome due to pituitary ACTH excess from Cushing's syndrome due to other causes
   Give 2.0 mg of DECADRON orally every 6 hours for 48 hours. Twenty-four hour urine collections are made for determination of 17-hydroxycorticosteroid excretion.

HOW SUPPLIED

Tablets DECADRON are compressed, pentagonal-shaped tablets, colored to distinguish potency. They are scored and coded on one side and embossed with DECADRON on the other. They are available as follows:

No. 7645—4 mg, white in color and coded MSD 97.
NDC 0006-0097-50 bottles of 50

No. 7601—0.75 mg, bluish-green in color and coded MSD 63.
NDC 0006-0063-12 5-12 PAK* (package of 12)
NDC 0006-0063-68 bottles of 100.

No. 7598—0.5 mg, yellow in color and coded MSD 41.
NDC 0006-0041-68 bottles of 100.

*Registered trademark of MERCK & CO., INC.

7921150 Issued November 2001

Shown in Product Identification Guide, page 323

Continued on next page

Information on the Merck & Co., Inc., products listed on these pages is from the prescribing information in use October 1, 2004. For information, please call 1-800-NSC-MERCK [1-800-672-6372].

DECADRON® Phosphate Injection ℞
(Dexamethasone Sodium Phosphate)

DESCRIPTION

Dexamethasone sodium phosphate, a synthetic adrenocortical steroid, is a white or slightly yellow, crystalline powder. It is freely soluble in water and is exceedingly hygroscopic. The molecular weight is 516.41. It is designated chemically as 9-fluoro-11β, 17-dihydroxy-16α-methyl-21-(phosphonooxy)pregna-1, 4-diene-3, 20-dione disodium salt. The empirical formula is $C_{22}H_{28}FNa_2O_8P$ and the structural formula is:

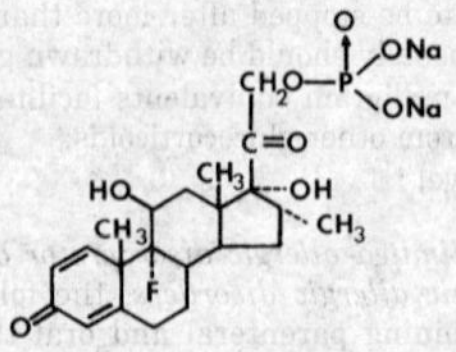

DECADRON* Phosphate (Dexamethasone Sodium Phosphate) injection is a sterile solution (pH 7.0 to 8.5) of dexamethasone sodium phosphate, sealed under nitrogen, and is supplied in two concentrations: 4 mg/mL and 24 mg/mL. The 24 mg/mL concentration offers the advantage of less volume in indications where high doses of corticosteroids by the intravenous route are needed.

Each milliliter of DECADRON Phosphate injection, 4 mg/mL, contains dexamethasone sodium phosphate equivalent to 4 mg dexamethasone phosphate or 3.33 mg dexamethasone. Inactive ingredients per mL: 8 mg creatinine, 10 mg sodium citrate, sodium hydroxide to adjust pH, and Water for Injection q.s., with 1 mg sodium bisulfite, 1.5 mg methylparaben, and 0.2 mg propylparaben added as preservatives.

Each milliliter of DECADRON Phosphate injection, 24 mg/mL, contains dexamethasone sodium phosphate equivalent to 24 mg dexamethasone phosphate or 20 mg dexamethasone. Inactive ingredients per mL: 8 mg creatinine, 10 mg sodium citrate, 0.5 mg disodium edetate, sodium hydroxide to adjust pH, and Water for Injection q.s., with 1 mg sodium bisulfite, 1.5 mg methylparaben, and 0.2 mg propylparaben added as preservatives.

*Registered trademark of MERCK & CO., INC.

ACTIONS

DECADRON Phosphate injection has a rapid onset but short duration of action when compared with less soluble preparations. Because of this, it is suitable for the treatment of acute disorders responsive to adrenocortical steroid therapy.

Naturally occurring glucocorticoids (hydrocortisone and cortisone), which also have salt-retaining properties, are used as replacement therapy in adrenocortical deficiency states. Their synthetic analogs, including dexamethasone, are primarily used for their potent anti-inflammatory effects in disorders of many organ systems.

Glucocorticoids cause profound and varied metabolic effects. In addition, they modify the body's immune responses to diverse stimuli.

At equipotent anti-inflammatory doses, dexamethasone almost completely lacks the sodium-retaining property of hydrocortisone and closely related derivatives of hydrocortisone.

INDICATIONS

A. By intravenous or intramuscular injection when oral therapy is not feasible:

1. *Endocrine disorders*

Primary or secondary adrenocortical insufficiency (hydrocortisone or cortisone is the drug of choice; synthetic analogs may be used in conjunction with mineralocorticoids where applicable; in infancy, mineralocorticoid supplementation is of particular importance)

Acute adrenocortical insufficiency (hydrocortisone or cortisone is the drug of choice; mineralocorticoid supplementation may be necessary, particularly when synthetic analogs are used)

Preoperatively, and in the event of serious trauma or illness, in patients with known adrenal insufficiency or when adrenocortical reserve is doubtful

Shock unresponsive to conventional therapy if adrenocortical insufficiency exists or is suspected

Congenital adrenal hyperplasia

Nonsuppurative thyroiditis

Hypercalcemia associated with cancer

2. *Rheumatic disorders*

As adjunctive therapy for short-term administration (to tide the patient over an acute episode or exacerbation) in:

Post-traumatic osteoarthritis

Synovitis of osteoarthritis

Rheumatoid arthritis, including juvenile rheumatoid arthritis (selected cases may require low-dose maintenance therapy)

Acute and subacute bursitis

Epicondylitis

Acute nonspecific tenosynovitis

Acute gouty arthritis

Psoriatic arthritis

Ankylosing spondylitis

3. *Collagen diseases*

During an exacerbation or as maintenance therapy in selected cases of:

Systemic lupus erythematosus

Acute rheumatic carditis

4. *Dermatologic diseases*

Pemphigus

Severe erythema multiforme (Stevens-Johnson syndrome)

Exfoliative dermatitis

Bullous dermatitis herpetiformis

Severe seborrheic dermatitis

Severe psoriasis

Mycosis fungoides

5. *Allergic states*

Control of severe or incapacitating allergic conditions intractable to adequate trials of conventional treatment in:

Bronchial asthma

Contact dermatitis

Atopic dermatitis

Serum sickness

Seasonal or perennial allergic rhinitis

Drug hypersensitivity reactions

Urticarial transfusion reactions

Acute noninfectious laryngeal edema (epinephrine is the drug of first choice)

6. *Ophthalmic diseases*

Severe acute and chronic allergic and inflammatory processes involving the eye, such as:

Herpes zoster ophthalmicus

Iritis, iridocyclitis

Chorioretinitis

Diffuse posterior uveitis and choroiditis

Optic neuritis

Sympathetic ophthalmia

Anterior segment inflammation

Allergic conjunctivitis

Keratitis

Allergic corneal marginal ulcers

7. *Gastrointestinal diseases*

To tide the patient over a critical period of the disease in:

Ulcerative colitis (Systemic therapy)

Regional enteritis (Systemic therapy)

8. *Respiratory diseases*

Symptomatic sarcoidosis

Berylliosis

Fulminating or disseminated pulmonary tuberculosis when used concurrently with appropriate antituberculous chemotherapy

Loeffler's syndrome not manageable by other means

Aspiration pneumonitis

9. *Hematologic disorders*

Acquired (autoimmune) hemolytic anemia

Idiopathic thrombocytopenic purpura in adults (I.V. only; I.M. administration is contraindicated)

Secondary thrombocytopenia in adults

Erythroblastopenia (RBC anemia)

Congenital (erythroid) hypoplastic anemia

10. *Neoplastic diseases*

For palliative management of:

Leukemias and lymphomas in adults

Acute leukemia of childhood

11. *Edematous states*

To induce diuresis or remission of proteinuria in the nephrotic syndrome, without uremia, of the idiopathic type, or that due to lupus erythematosus

12. *Miscellaneous*

Tuberculous meningitis with subarachnoid block or impending block when used concurrently with appropriate antituberculous chemotherapy

Trichinosis with neurologic or myocardial involvement

13. *Diagnostic testing of adrenocortical hyperfunction*

14. *Cerebral Edema* associated with primary or metastatic brain tumor, craniotomy, or head injury. Use in cerebral edema is not a substitute for careful neurosurgical evaluation and definitive management such as neurosurgery or other specific therapy.

B. By intra-articular or soft tissue injection:

As adjunctive therapy for short-term administration (to tide the patient over an acute episode or exacerbation) in:

Synovitis of osteoarthritis

Rheumatoid arthritis

Acute and subacute bursitis

Acute gouty arthritis

Epicondylitis

Acute nonspecific tenosynovitis

Post-traumatic osteoarthritis.

C. By intralesional injection:

Keloids

Localized hypertrophic, infiltrated, inflammatory lesions of: lichen planus, psoriatic plaques, granuloma annulare, and lichen simplex chronicus (neurodermatitis)

Discoid lupus erythematosus

Necrobiosis lipoidica diabeticorum

Alopecia areata

May also be useful in cystic tumors of an aponeurosis or tendon (ganglia).

CONTRAINDICATIONS

Systemic fungal infections. (See WARNINGS regarding amphotericin B.)

Hypersensitivity to any component of this product, including sulfites (see WARNINGS).

WARNINGS

Because rare instances of anaphylactoid reactions have occurred in patients receiving parenteral corticosteroid therapy, appropriate precautionary measures should be taken prior to administration, especially when the patient has a history of allergy to any drug. Anaphylactoid and hypersensitivity reactions have been reported for Injection DECADRON Phosphate (see ADVERSE REACTIONS).

Injection DECADRON Phosphate contains sodium bisulfite, a sulfite that may cause allergic-type reactions including anaphylactic symptoms and life-threatening or less severe asthmatic episodes in certain susceptible people. The overall prevalence of sulfite sensitivity in the general population is unknown and probably low. Sulfite sensitivity is seen more frequently in asthmatic than in nonasthmatic people.

Corticosteroids may exacerbate systemic fungal infections and therefore should not be used in the presence of such infections unless they are needed to control drug reactions due to amphotericin B. Moreover, there have been cases reported in which concomitant use of amphotericin B and hydrocortisone was followed by cardiac enlargement and congestive failure.

In patients on corticosteroid therapy subjected to any unusual stress, increased dosage of rapidly acting corticosteroids before, during, and after the stressful situation is indicated.

Drug-induced secondary adrenocortical insufficiency may result from too rapid withdrawal of corticosteroids and may be minimized by gradual reduction of dosage. This type of relative insufficiency may persist for months after discontinuation of therapy; therefore, in any situation of stress occurring during that period, hormone therapy should be reinstituted. If the patient is receiving steroids already, dosage may have to be increased. Since mineralocorticoid secretion may be impaired, salt and/or a mineralocorticoid should be administered concurrently. (See PRECAUTIONS.)

Corticosteroids may mask some signs of infection, and new infections may appear during their use. There may be decreased resistance and inability to localize infection when corticosteroids are used. Moreover, corticosteroids may affect the nitroblue-tetrazolium test for bacterial infection and produce false negative results.

In cerebral malaria, a double-blind trial has shown that the use of corticosteroids is associated with prolongation of coma and a higher incidence of pneumonia and gastrointestinal bleeding.

Corticosteroids may activate latent amebiasis. Therefore, it is recommended that latent or active amebiasis be ruled out before initiating corticosteroid therapy in any patient who has spent time in the tropics or any patient with unexplained diarrhea.

Prolonged use of corticosteroids may produce posterior subcapsular cataracts, glaucoma with possible damage to the optic nerves, and may enhance the establishment of secondary ocular infections due to fungi or viruses.

Usage in pregnancy. Since adequate human reproduction studies have not been done with corticosteroids, use of these drugs in pregnancy or in women of childbearing potential requires that the anticipated benefits be weighed against the possible hazards to the mother and embryo or fetus. Infants born of mothers who have received substantial doses of corticosteroids during pregnancy should be carefully observed for signs of hypoadrenalism.

Corticosteroids appear in breast milk and could suppress growth, interfere with endogenous corticosteroid production, or cause other unwanted effects. Mothers taking pharmacologic doses of corticosteroids should be advised not to nurse.

Average and large doses of cortisone or hydrocortisone can cause elevation of blood pressure, salt and water retention, and increased excretion of potassium. These effects are less likely to occur with the synthetic derivatives except when used in large doses. Dietary salt restriction and potassium supplementation may be necessary. All corticosteroids increase calcium excretion.

Administration of live virus vaccines, including smallpox, is contraindicated in individuals receiving immunosuppressive doses of corticosteroids. If inactivated viral or bacterial vaccines are administered to individuals receiving immunosuppressive doses of corticosteroids, the expected serum antibody response may not be obtained. However, immunization procedures may be undertaken in patients who are receiving corticosteroids as replacement therapy, e.g., for Addison's disease.

Patients who are on drugs which suppress the immune system are more susceptible to infections than healthy individuals. Chickenpox and measles, for example, can have a more serious or even fatal course in non-immune patients on corticosteroids. In such patients who have not had these diseases, particular care should be taken to avoid exposure. The risk of developing a disseminated infection varies among individuals and can be related to the dose, route and duration of corticosteroid administration as well as to the underlying disease. If exposed to chickenpox, prophylaxis with varicella zoster immune globulin (VZIG) may be indicated. If chickenpox develops, treatment with antiviral agents may be considered. If exposed to measles, prophy-

laxis with immune globulin (IG) may be indicated. (See the respective package inserts for VZIG and IG for complete prescribing information.)
Similarly, corticosteroids should be used with great care in patients with known or suspected Strongyloides (threadworm) infestation. In such patients, corticosteroid-induced immunosuppression may lead to Strongyloides hyperinfection and dissemination with widespread larval migration, often accompanied by severe enterocolitis and potentially fatal gram-negative septicemia.
The use of DECADRON Phosphate injection in active tuberculosis should be restricted to those cases of fulminating or disseminated tuberculosis in which the corticosteroid is used for the management of the disease in conjunction with an appropriate antituberculous regimen.
If corticosteroids are indicated in patients with latent tuberculosis or tuberculin reactivity, close observation is necessary as reactivation of the disease may occur. During prolonged corticosteroid therapy, these patients should receive chemoprophylaxis.
Literature reports suggest an apparent association between use of corticosteroids and left ventricular free wall rupture after a recent myocardial infarction; therefore, therapy with corticosteroids should be used with great caution in these patients.

PRECAUTIONS

This product, like many other steroid formulations, is sensitive to heat. Therefore, it should not be autoclaved when it is desirable to sterilize the exterior of the vial.
Following prolonged therapy, withdrawal of corticosteroids may result in symptoms of the corticosteroid withdrawal syndrome including fever, myalgia, arthralgia, and malaise. This may occur in patients even without evidence of adrenal insufficiency.
There is an enhanced effect of corticosteroids in patients with hypothyroidism and in those with cirrhosis.
Corticosteroids should be used cautiously in patients with ocular herpes simplex for fear of corneal perforation.
The lowest possible dose of corticosteroid should be used to control the condition under treatment, and when reduction in dosage is possible, the reduction must be gradual.
Psychic derangements may appear when corticosteroids are used, ranging from euphoria, insomnia, mood swings, personality changes, and severe depression to frank psychotic manifestations. Also, existing emotional instability or psychotic tendencies may be aggravated by corticosteroids.
Co-administration of thalidomide with DECADRON Phosphate injection should be employed cautiously, as toxic epidermal necrolysis has been reported with concomitant use.
Aspirin should be used cautiously in conjunction with corticosteroids in hypoprothrombinemia.
Steroids should be used with caution in nonspecific ulcerative colitis, if there is a probability of impending perforation, abscess, or other pyogenic infection, also in diverticulitis, fresh intestinal anastomoses, active or latent peptic ulcer, renal insufficiency, hypertension, osteoporosis, and myasthenia gravis. Signs of peritoneal irritation following gastrointestinal perforation in patients receiving large doses of corticosteroids may be minimal or absent. Fat embolism has been reported as a possible complication of hypercortisonism.
When large doses are given, some authorities advise that antacids be administered between meals to help to prevent peptic ulcer.
Steroids may increase or decrease motility and number of spermatozoa in some patients.
Cytochrome P450 3A4 (CYP 3A4) enzyme inducers, such as phenytoin, barbiturates (e.g., phenobarbital), carbamazepine, and rifampin may enhance the metabolic clearance of corticosteroids resulting in decreased blood levels and lessened physiologic activity, thus requiring an increase in corticosteroid dosage.
Dexamethasone is metabolized by CYP 3A4. Concomitant administration of dexamethasone with inducers of CYP 3A4 (as listed above) has the potential to result in decreased plasma concentrations of dexamethasone. In addition, concomitant administration of dexamethasone with known inhibitors of CYP 3A4 (e.g., ketoconazole, macrolide antibiotics such as erythromycin) has the potential to result in increased plasma concentrations of dexamethasone. Effects of other drugs on the metabolism of dexamethasone may interfere with dexamethasone suppression tests, which should be interpreted with caution during administration of such drugs.
Dexamethasone is a moderate inducer of CYP 3A4. Co-administration of dexamethasone with other drugs that are metabolized by CYP 3A4 (e.g., indinavir, erythromycin) may increase their clearance, resulting in decreased plasma concentrations.
In post-marketing experience, there have been reports of both increases and decreases in phenytoin levels with dexamethasone co-administration, leading to alterations in seizure control.
Although ketoconazole may increase dexamethasone plasma concentrations through inhibition of CYP 3A4, ketoconazole alone can inhibit adrenal corticosteroid synthesis and may cause adrenal insufficiency during corticosteroid withdrawal (see WARNINGS).
Ephedrine may enhance the metabolic clearance of corticosteroids, resulting in decreased blood levels and lessened physiologic activity, thus requiring an increase in corticosteroid dosage.
False negative results in the dexamethasone suppression test (DST) in patients being treated with indomethacin have been reported. Thus, results of the DST should be interpreted with caution in these patients.
The prothrombin time should be checked frequently in patients who are receiving corticosteroids and coumarin anticoagulants at the same time because of reports that corticosteroids have altered the response to these anticoagulants. Studies have shown that the usual effect produced by adding corticosteroids is inhibition of response to coumarins, although there have been some conflicting reports of potentiation not substantiated by studies.
When corticosteroids are administered concomitantly with potassium-depleting diuretics, patients should be observed closely for development of hypokalemia.
Intra-articular injection of a corticosteroid may produce systemic as well as local effects.
Appropriate examination of any joint fluid present is necessary to exclude a septic process.
A marked increase in pain accompanied by local swelling, further restriction of joint motion, fever, and malaise is suggestive of septic arthritis. If this complication occurs and the diagnosis of sepsis is confirmed, appropriate antimicrobial therapy should be instituted.
Injection of a steroid into an infected site is to be avoided.
Corticosteroids should not be injected into unstable joints.
Patients should be impressed strongly with the importance of not overusing joints in which symptomatic benefit has been obtained as long as the inflammatory process remains active.
Frequent intra-articular injection may result in damage to joint tissues.
The slower rate of absorption by intramuscular administration should be recognized.
Information for Patients
Susceptible patients who are on immunosuppressant doses of corticosteroids should be warned to avoid exposure to chickenpox or measles. Patients should also be advised that if they are exposed, medical advice should be sought without delay.
Pediatric Use
Growth and development of pediatric patients on prolonged corticosteroid therapy should be carefully followed.

ADVERSE REACTIONS

Fluid and electrolyte disturbances
Sodium retention
Fluid retention
Congestive heart failure in susceptible patients
Potassium loss
Hypokalemic alkalosis
Hypertension
Musculoskeletal
Muscle weakness
Steroid myopathy
Loss of muscle mass
Osteoporosis
Vertebral compression fractures
Aseptic necrosis of femoral and humeral heads
Pathologic fracture of long bones
Tendon rupture
Gastrointestinal
Peptic ulcer with possible subsequent perforation and hemorrhage
Perforation of the small and large bowel, particularly in patients with inflammatory bowel disease
Pancreatitis
Abdominal distention
Ulcerative esophagitis
Dermatologic
Impaired wound healing
Thin fragile skin
Petechiae and ecchymoses
Erythema
Increased sweating
May suppress reactions to skin tests
Burning or tingling, especially in the perineal area (after I.V. injection)
Other cutaneous reactions, such as allergic dermatitis, urticaria, angioneurotic edema
Neurologic
Convulsions
Increased intracranial pressure with papilledema (pseudotumor cerebri) usually after treatment
Vertigo
Headache
Psychic disturbances
Cerebral palsy in preterm infants
Endocrine
Menstrual irregularities
Development of cushingoid state
Suppression of growth in pediatric patients
Secondary adrenocortical and pituitary unresponsiveness, particularly in times of stress, as in trauma, surgery, or illness
Decreased carbohydrate tolerance
Manifestations of latent diabetes mellitus
Hyperglycemia
Increased requirements for insulin or oral hypoglycemic agents in diabetics
Hirsutism
Ophthalmic
Posterior subcapsular cataracts
Increased intraocular pressure
Glaucoma
Exophthalmos
Retinopathy of prematurity
Metabolic
Negative nitrogen balance due to protein catabolism
Cardiovascular
Myocardial rupture following recent myocardial infarction (see WARNINGS)
Hypertrophic cardiomyopathy in low birth weight infants
Other
Anaphylactoid or hypersensitivity reactions
Thromboembolism
Weight gain
Increased appetite
Nausea
Malaise
Hiccups
The following *additional* adverse reactions are related to parenteral corticosteroid therapy:
Rare instances of blindness associated with intralesional therapy around the face and head
Hyperpigmentation or hypopigmentation
Subcutaneous and cutaneous atrophy
Sterile abscess
Postinjection flare (following intra-articular use)
Charcot-like arthropathy

OVERDOSAGE

Reports of acute toxicity and/or death following overdosage of glucocorticoids are rare. In the event of overdosage, no specific antidote is available; treatment is supportive and symptomatic.
Significant lethality was observed in female mice at single oral doses of 3630 mg/m^2 (1210 mg/kg) and single intravenous doses of 2382 mg/m^2 (794 mg/kg).

DOSAGE AND ADMINISTRATION

DECADRON Phosphate injection, 4 mg/mL—*For intravenous, intramuscular, intra-articular, intralesional, and soft tissue injection.*
DECADRON Phosphate injection, 24 mg/mL—*For intravenous injection only.*
DECADRON Phosphate injection can be given directly from the vial, or it can be added to Sodium Chloride Injection or Dextrose Injection and administered by intravenous drip.
Solutions used for intravenous administration or further dilution of this product should be preservative-free when used in the neonate, especially the premature infant.
When it is mixed with an infusion solution, sterile precautions should be observed. Since infusion solutions generally do not contain preservatives, mixtures should be used within 24 hours.
Parenteral drug products should be inspected visually for particulate matter and discoloration prior to administration, whenever solution and container permit.
DOSAGE REQUIREMENTS ARE VARIABLE AND MUST BE INDIVIDUALIZED ON THE BASIS OF THE DISEASE AND THE RESPONSE OF THE PATIENT.

Intravenous and Intramuscular Injection

The initial dosage of DECADRON Phosphate injection varies from 0.5 to 9 mg a day depending on the disease being treated. In less severe diseases doses lower than 0.5 mg may suffice, while in severe diseases doses higher than 9 mg may be required.
The initial dosage should be maintained or adjusted until the patient's response is satisfactory. If a satisfactory clinical response does not occur after a reasonable period of time, discontinue DECADRON Phosphate injection and transfer the patient to other therapy.
After a favorable initial response, the proper maintenance dosage should be determined by decreasing the initial dosage in small amounts to the lowest dosage that maintains an adequate clinical response.
Patients should be observed closely for signs that might require dosage adjustment, including changes in clinical status resulting from remissions or exacerbations of the disease, individual drug responsiveness, and the effect of stress (e.g., surgery, infection, trauma). During stress it may be necessary to increase dosage temporarily.
If the drug is to be stopped after more than a few days of treatment, it usually should be withdrawn gradually.
When the intravenous route of administration is used, dosage usually should be the same as the oral dosage. In certain overwhelming, acute, life-threatening situations, however, administration in dosages exceeding the usual dosages may be justified and may be in multiples of the oral dosages.
The slower rate of absorption by intramuscular administration should be recognized.
Shock
There is a tendency in current medical practice to use high (pharmacologic) doses of corticosteroids for the treatment of

Continued on next page

Information on the Merck & Co., Inc., products listed on these pages is from the prescribing information in use October 1, 2004. For information, please call 1-800-NSC-MERCK [1-800-672-6372].

Decadron Phosphate Inj.—Cont.

unresponsive shock. The following dosages of DECADRON phosphate injection have been suggested by various authors:

*Author***	*Dosage*
Cavanagh[1]	3 mg/kg of body weight per 24 hours by constant intravenous infusion after an initial intravenous injection of 20 mg
Dietzman[2]	2 to 6 mg/kg of body weight as a single intravenous injection
Frank[3]	40 mg initially followed by repeat intravenous injection every 4 to 6 hours while shock persists
Oaks[4]	40 mg initially followed by repeat intravenous injection every 2 to 6 hours while shock persists
Schumer[5]	1 mg/kg of body weight as a single intravenous injection

Administration of high dose corticosteroid therapy should be continued only until the patient's condition has stabilized and usually not longer than 48 to 72 hours.
Although adverse reactions associated with high dose, short term corticosteroid therapy are uncommon, peptic ulceration may occur.

**1. Cavanagh, D.; Singh, K. B.: Endotoxin shock in pregnancy and abortion, in "Corticosteroids in the Treatment of Shock", Schumer, W.; Nyhus, L. M., Editors, Urbana, University of Illinois Press, 1970, pp. 86-96.
2. Dietzman, R. H.; Ersek, R. A.; Bloch, J. M.; Lillehei, R. C.: High-output, low-resistance gram-negative septic shock in man, Angiology *20:* 691-700, Dec. 1969.
3. Frank, E.: Clinical observations in shock and management (In: Shields, T. F., ed.: Symposium on current concepts and management of shock), J. Maine Med. Ass. *59:* 195-200, Oct. 1968.
4. Oaks, W. W.; Cohen, H. E.: Endotoxin shock in the geriatric patient, Geriat. *22:* 120-130, Mar. 1967.
5. Schumer, W.; Nyhus, L. M.: Corticosteroid effect on biochemical parameters of human oligemic shock, Arch. Surg. *100:* 405-408, Apr. 1970.

Cerebral Edema
DECADRON Phosphate injection is generally administered initially in a dosage of 10 mg intravenously followed by 4 mg every six hours intramuscularly until the symptoms of cerebral edema subside. Response is usually noted within 12 to 24 hours and dosage may be reduced after two to four days and gradually discontinued over a period of five to seven days. For palliative management of patients with recurrent or inoperable brain tumors, maintenance therapy with two mg two or three times a day may be effective.
Acute Allergic Disorders
In acute, self-limited allergic disorders or acute exacerbations of chronic allergic disorders, the following dosage schedule combining parenteral and oral therapy is suggested:
DECADRON Phosphate injection, 4 mg/mL: *first day,* 1 or 2 mL (4 or 8 mg), intramuscularly.
DECADRON (Dexamethasone) tablets, 0.75 mg: *second and third days,* 4 tablets in two divided doses each day; *fourth day,* 2 tablets in two divided doses; *fifth and sixth days,* 1 tablet each day; *seventh day,* no treatment; *eighth day,* follow-up visit.
This schedule is designed to ensure adequate therapy during acute episodes, while minimizing the risk of overdosage in chronic cases.

Intra-articular, Intralesional, and Soft Tissue Injection
Intra-articular, intralesional, and soft tissue injections are generally employed when the affected joints or areas are limited to one or two sites. Dosage and frequency of injection varies depending on the condition and the site of injection. The usual dose is from 0.2 to 6 mg. The frequency usually ranges from once every three to five days to once every two to three weeks. Frequent intra-articular injection may result in damage to joint tissues.
Some of the usual single doses are:

Site of Injection	Amount of Dexamethasone Phosphate (mg)
Large Joints (e.g., Knee)	2 to 4
Small Joints (e.g., Interphalangeal, Temporomandibular)	0.8 to 1
Bursae	2 to 3
Tendon Sheaths	0.4 to 1
Soft Tissue Infiltration	2 to 6
Ganglia	1 to 2

DECADRON Phosphate injection is particularly recommended for use in conjunction with one of the less soluble, longer-acting steroids for intra-articular and soft tissue injection.

HOW SUPPLIED

No 7628X—Injection DECADRON Phosphate, 4 mg per mL, is a clear, colorless solution, and is available in 5 mL and 25 mL vials as follows:
NDC 0006-7628-03, 5 mL vial
NDC 0006-7628-25, 25 mL vial.
FOR INTRAVENOUS USE ONLY:
No. 7646—Injection DECADRON Phosphate, 24 mg per mL, is a clear, colorless to light yellow solution and is available in 5 mL vials as follows:
NDC 0006-7646-03, 5 mL vial.
Storage
Store at 25°C (77°F), excursions permitted to 15–30°C (59–86°F) [See USP Controlled Room Temperature].
Sensitive to heat. Do not autoclave.
Protect from freezing.
Protect from light. Store container in carton until contents have been used.
9051534 Issued November 2001

DEMSER® Capsules (Metyrosine) ℞

DESCRIPTION

DEMSER* (Metyrosine) is (−)-α-methyl-*L* -tyrosine or (α-MPT). It has the following structural formula:

HO–C₆H₄–CH₂–C(CH₃)(NH₂)–COOH

Metyrosine is a white, crystalline compound of molecular weight 195. It is very slightly soluble in water, acetone, and methanol, and insoluble in chloroform and benzene. It is soluble in acidic aqueous solutions. It is also soluble in alkaline aqueous solutions, but is subject to oxidative degradation under these conditions.
DEMSER is supplied as capsules, for oral administration. Each capsule contains 250 mg metyrosine. Inactive ingredients are colloidal silicon dioxide, gelatin, hydroxypropyl cellulose, magnesium stearate, titanium dioxide, and FD&C Blue 2.

*Registered trademark of MERCK & CO., INC.

CLINICAL PHARMACOLOGY

DEMSER inhibits tyrosine hydroxylase, which catalyzes the first transformation in catecholamine biosynthesis, i.e., the conversion of tyrosine to dihydroxyphenylalanine (DOPA). Because the first step is also the rate-limiting step, blockade of tyrosine hydroxylase activity results in decreased endogenous levels of catecholamines, usually measured as decreased urinary excretion of catecholamines and their metabolites.
In patients with pheochromocytoma, who produce excessive amounts of norepinephrine and epinephrine, administration of one to four grams of DEMSER per day has reduced catecholamine biosynthesis from about 35 to 80 percent as measured by the total excretion of catecholamines and their metabolites (metanephrine and vanillylmandelic acid). The maximum biochemical effect usually occurs within two to three days, and the urinary concentration of catecholamines and their metabolites usually returns to pretreatment levels within three to four days after DEMSER is discontinued. In some patients the total excretion of catecholamines and catecholamine metabolites may be lowered to normal or near normal levels (less than 10 mg/24 hours). In most patients the duration of treatment has been two to eight weeks, but several patients have received DEMSER for periods of one to 10 years.
Most patients with pheochromocytoma treated with DEMSER experience decreased frequency and severity of hypertensive attacks with their associated headache, nausea, sweating, and tachycardia. In patients who respond, blood pressure decreases progressively during the first two days of therapy with DEMSER; after withdrawal, blood pressure usually increases gradually to pretreatment values within two to three days.
Metyrosine is well absorbed from the gastrointestinal tract. From 53 to 88 percent (mean 69 percent) was recovered in the urine as unchanged drug following maintenance oral doses of 600 to 4000 mg/24 hours in patients with pheochromocytoma or essential hypertension. Less than 1% of the dose was recovered as catechol metabolites. These metabolites are probably not present in sufficient amounts to contribute to the biochemical effects of metyrosine. The quantities excreted, however, are sufficient to interfere with accurate determination of urinary catecholamines determined by routine techniques.
Plasma half-life of metyrosine determined over an 8-hour period after single oral doses was 3.4–3.7 hours in three patients.
For further information, refer to: Sjoerdsma, A.; Engelman, K.; Waldman, T. A.; Cooperman, L. H.; Hammond, W. G.: Pheochromocytoma: Current concepts of diagnosis and treatment, Ann. Intern. Med. *65:* 1302–1326, Dec. 1966.

INDICATIONS AND USAGE

DEMSER is indicated in the treatment of patients with pheochromocytoma for:
1. Preoperative preparation of patients for surgery
2. Management of patients when surgery is contraindicated
3. Chronic treatment of patients with malignant pheochromocytoma.

DEMSER is not recommended for the control of essential hypertension.

CONTRAINDICATIONS

DEMSER is contraindicated in persons known to be hypersensitive to this compound.

WARNINGS

Maintain Fluid Volume During and After Surgery
When DEMSER is used preoperatively, alone or especially in combination with alpha-adrenergic blocking drugs, adequate intravascular volume must be maintained intraoperatively (especially after tumor removal) and postoperatively to avoid hypotension and decreased perfusion of vital organs resulting from vasodilatation and expanded volume capacity. Following tumor removal, large volumes of plasma may be needed to maintain blood pressure and central venous pressure within the normal range.
In addition, life-threatening arrhythmias may occur during anesthesia and surgery, and may require treatment with a beta blocker or lidocaine. During surgery, patients should have continuous monitoring of blood pressure and electrocardiogram.
Intraoperative Effects
While the preoperative use of DEMSER in patients with pheochromocytoma is thought to decrease intraoperative problems with blood pressure control, DEMSER does not eliminate the danger of hypertensive crises or arrhythmias during manipulation of the tumor, and the alpha-adrenergic blocking drug, phentolamine, may be needed.
Interaction with Alcohol
DEMSER may add to the sedative effects of alcohol and other CNS depressants, e.g., hypnotics, sedatives, and tranquilizers. (See PRECAUTIONS, *Information for Patients and Drug Interactions.*)

PRECAUTIONS

General
Metyrosine Crystalluria: **Crystalluria and urolithiasis have been found in dogs treated with DEMSER (Metyrosine) at doses similar to those used in humans, and crystalluria has also been observed in a few patients. To minimize the risk of crystalluria, patients should be urged to maintain water intake sufficient to achieve a daily urine volume of 2000 mL or more, particularly when doses greater than 2 g per day are given. Routine examination of the urine should be carried out. Metyrosine will crystallize as needles or rods. If metyrosine crystalluria occurs, fluid intake should be increased further. If crystalluria persists, the dosage should be reduced or the drug discontinued.**
Relatively Little Data Regarding Long-term Use: The total human experience with the drug is quite limited and few patients have been studied long-term. Chronic animal studies have not been carried out. Therefore, suitable laboratory tests should be carried out periodically in patients requiring prolonged use of DEMSER and caution should be observed in patients with impaired hepatic or renal function.
Information for Patients
When receiving DEMSER, patients should be warned about engaging in activities requiring mental alertness and motor coordination, such as driving a motor vehicle or operating machinery. DEMSER may have additive sedative effects with alcohol and other CNS depressants, e.g., hypnotics, sedatives, and tranquilizers.
Patients should be advised to maintain a liberal fluid intake. (See PRECAUTIONS, *General.*)
Drug Interactions
Caution should be observed in administering DEMSER to patients receiving phenothiazines or haloperidol because the extrapyramidal effects of these drugs can be expected to be potentiated by inhibition of catecholamine synthesis.
Concurrent use of DEMSER with alcohol or other CNS depressants can increase their sedative effects. (See WARNINGS and PRECAUTIONS, *Information for Patients.*)
Laboratory Test Interference
Spurious increases in urinary catecholamines may be observed in patients receiving DEMSER due to the presence of metabolites of the drug.
Carcinogenesis, Mutagenesis, Impairment of Fertility
Long-term carcinogenic studies in animals and studies on mutagenesis and impairment of fertility have not been performed with metyrosine.
Pregnancy
Pregnancy Category C. Animal reproduction studies have not been conducted with DEMSER. It is also not known whether DEMSER can cause fetal harm when administered to a pregnant woman or can affect reproduction capacity. DEMSER should be given to a pregnant woman only if clearly needed.

Nursing Mothers
It is not known whether DEMSER is excreted in human milk. Because many drugs are excreted in human milk, caution should be exercised when DEMSER is administered to a nursing woman.
Pediatric Use
Safety and effectiveness in pediatric patients below the age of 12 years have not been established.
Geriatric Use
Clinical studies of DEMSER did not include sufficient numbers of subjects aged 65 and over to determine whether they respond differently from younger subjects. Other reported clinical experience has not identified differences in responses between the elderly and younger patients. In general, dose selection for an elderly patient should be cautious, usually starting at the low end of the dosing range, reflecting the greater frequency of decreased hepatic, renal, or cardiac function, and of concomitant disease or other drug therapy.

ADVERSE REACTIONS

Central Nervous System
Sedation: The most common adverse reaction to DEMSER is moderate to severe sedation, which has been observed in almost all patients. It occurs at both low and high dosages. Sedative effects begin within the first 24 hours of therapy, are maximal after two to three days, and tend to wane during the next few days. Sedation usually is not obvious after one week unless the dosage is increased, but at dosages greater than 2000 mg/day some degree of sedation or fatigue may persist.
In most patients who experience sedation, temporary changes in sleep pattern occur following withdrawal of the drug. Changes consist of insomnia that may last for two or three days and feelings of increased alertness and ambition. Even patients who do not experience sedation while on DEMSER may report symptoms of psychic stimulation when the drug is discontinued.
Extrapyramidal Signs: Extrapyramidal signs such as drooling, speech difficulty, and tremor have been reported in approximately 10 percent of patients. These occasionally have been accompanied by trismus and frank parkinsonism.
Anxiety and Psychic Disturbances: Anxiety and psychic disturbances such as depression, hallucinations, disorientation, and confusion may occur. These effects seem to be dose-dependent and may disappear with reduction of dosage.
Diarrhea
Diarrhea occurs in about 10 percent of patients and may be severe. Anti-diarrheal agents may be required if continuation of DEMSER is necessary.
Miscellaneous
Infrequently, slight swelling of the breast, galactorrhea, nasal stuffiness, decreased salivation, dry mouth, headache, nausea, vomiting, abdominal pain, and impotence or failure of ejaculation may occur. Crystalluria (see PRECAUTIONS) and transient dysuria and hematuria have been observed in a few patients. Hematologic disorders (including eosinophilia, anemia, thrombocytopenia, and thrombocytosis), increased SGOT levels, peripheral edema, and hypersensitivity reactions such as urticaria and pharyngeal edema have been reported rarely.

OVERDOSAGE

Signs of metyrosine overdosage include those central nervous system effects observed in some patients even at low dosages.
At doses exceeding 2000 mg/day, some degree of sedation or feeling of fatigue may persist. Doses of 2000–4000 mg/day can result in anxiety or agitated depression, neuromuscular effects (including fine tremor of the hands, gross tremor of the trunk, tightening of the jaw with trismus), diarrhea, and decreased salivation with dry mouth.
Reduction of drug dose or cessation of treatment results in the disappearance of these symptoms.
The acute toxicity of metyrosine was 442 mg/kg and 752 mg/kg in the female mouse and rat respectively.

DOSAGE AND ADMINISTRATION

The recommended initial dosage of DEMSER for adults and children 12 years of age and older is 250 mg orally four times daily. This may be increased by 250 mg to 500 mg every day to a maximum of 4.0 g/day in divided doses. When used for preoperative preparation, the optimally effective dosage of DEMSER should be given for at least five to seven days.
Optimally effective dosages of DEMSER usually are between 2.0 and 3.0 g/day, and the dose should be titrated by monitoring clinical symptoms and catecholamine excretion. In patients who are hypertensive, dosage should be titrated to achieve normalization of blood pressure and control of clinical symptoms. In patients who are usually normotensive, dosage should be titrated to the amount that will reduce urinary metanephrines and/or vanillylmandelic acid by 50 percent or more.
If patients are not adequately controlled by the use of DEMSER, an alpha-adrenergic blocking agent (phenoxybenzamine) should be added.
Use of DEMSER in children under 12 years of age has been limited and a dosage schedule for this age group cannot be given.

HOW SUPPLIED

No. 3355—Capsules DEMSER, 250 mg, are opaque, two-toned blue capsules coded MSD 690 on one side and DEMSER on the other. They are supplied as follows:
NDC 0006-0690-68 bottles of 100.
7900809 Issued April 2002

Shown in Product Identification Guide, page 323

DIURIL® Sodium Intravenous (Chlorothiazide Sodium) ℞

DESCRIPTION
Intravenous Sodium DIURIL* (Chlorothiazide Sodium) is a diuretic and antihypertensive. It is 6-chloro-2*H* -1,2,4-benzothiadiazine-7-sulfonamide 1,1-dioxide monosodium salt and its molecular weight is 317.71. Its empirical formula is $C_7H_5ClN_3NaO_4S_2$ and its structural formula is:

Intravenous Sodium DIURIL is a sterile lyophilized white powder and is supplied in a vial containing:

Chlorothiazide sodium equivalent
to chlorothiazide .... 0.5 g
Inactive ingredients:
Mannitol .... 0.25 g
Sodium hydroxide to adjust pH.

DIURIL* (Chlorothiazide) is a diuretic and antihypertensive. It is 6-chloro-2*H* -1,2,4-benzothiadiazine-7-sulfonamide 1,1-dioxide. Its empirical formula is $C_7H_6ClN_3O_4S_2$ and its structural formula is:

It is a white, or practically white, crystalline powder with a molecular weight of 295.72, which is very slightly soluble in water, but readily soluble in dilute aqueous sodium hydroxide. It is soluble in urine to the extent of about 150 mg per 100 mL at pH 7.

*Registered trademark of MERCK & CO., INC.

CLINICAL PHARMACOLOGY

The mechanism of the antihypertensive effect of thiazides is unknown. DIURIL (Chlorothiazide) does not usually affect normal blood pressure.
DIURIL (Chlorothiazide) affects the distal renal tubular mechanism of electrolyte reabsorption. At maximal therapeutic dosage all thiazides are approximately equal in their diuretic efficacy.
DIURIL (Chlorothiazide) increases excretion of sodium and chloride in approximately equivalent amounts. Natriuresis may be accompanied by some loss of potassium and bicarbonate.
After oral use diuresis begins within 2 hours, peaks in about 4 hours and lasts about 6 to 12 hours. Following intravenous use of Sodium DIURIL, onset of the diuretic action occurs in 15 minutes and the maximal action in 30 minutes.
Pharmacokinetics and Metabolism
DIURIL is not metabolized but is eliminated rapidly by the kidney; 96 percent of an intravenous dose is excreted unchanged in the urine within 23 hours. The plasma half-life of chlorothiazide is 45–120 minutes. Chlorothiazide crosses the placental but not the blood-brain barrier and is excreted in breast milk.

INDICATIONS AND USAGE

Intravenous Sodium DIURIL is indicated as adjunctive therapy in edema associated with congestive heart failure, hepatic cirrhosis, and corticosteroid and estrogen therapy.
Intravenous Sodium DIURIL has also been found useful in edema due to various forms of renal dysfunction such as nephrotic syndrome, acute glomerulonephritis, and chronic renal failure.
Use in Pregnancy. Routine use of diuretics during normal pregnancy is inappropriate and exposes mother and fetus to unnecessary hazard. Diuretics do not prevent development of toxemia of pregnancy and there is no satisfactory evidence that they are useful in the treatment of toxemia.
Edema during pregnancy may arise from pathologic causes or from the physiologic and mechanical consequences of pregnancy. Thiazides are indicated in pregnancy when edema is due to pathologic causes, just as they are in the absence of pregnancy (see PRECAUTIONS, *Pregnancy*). Dependent edema in pregnancy, resulting from restriction of venous return by the gravid uterus, is properly treated through elevation of the lower extremities and use of support stockings. Use of diuretics to lower intravascular volume in this instance is illogical and unnecessary. During normal pregnancy there is hypervolemia which is not harmful to the fetus or the mother in the absence of cardiovascular disease. However, it may be associated with edema, rarely generalized edema. If such edema causes discomfort, increased recumbency will often provide relief. Rarely this edema may cause extreme discomfort which is not relieved by rest. In these instances, a short course of diuretic therapy may provide relief and be appropriate.

CONTRAINDICATIONS

Anuria.
Hypersensitivity to any component of this product or to other sulfonamide-derived drugs.

WARNINGS

Intravenous use in infants and children has been limited and is not generally recommended.
Use with caution in severe renal disease. In patients with renal disease, thiazides may precipitate azotemia. Cumulative effects of the drug may develop in patients with impaired renal function.
Thiazides should be used with caution in patients with impaired hepatic function or progressive liver disease, since minor alterations of fluid and electrolyte balance may precipitate hepatic coma.
Thiazides may add to or potentiate the action of other antihypertensive drugs.
Sensitivity reactions may occur in patients with or without a history of allergy or bronchial asthma.
The possibility of exacerbation or activation of systemic lupus erythematosus has been reported.
Lithium generally should not be given with diuretics (see PRECAUTIONS, *Drug Interactions*).

PRECAUTIONS

General
All patients receiving diuretic therapy should be observed for evidence of fluid or electrolyte imbalance: namely, hyponatremia, hypochloremic alkalosis, and hypokalemia. Serum and urine electrolyte determinations are particularly important when the patient is vomiting excessively or receiving parenteral fluids. Warning signs or symptoms of fluid and electrolyte imbalance, irrespective of cause, include dryness of mouth, thirst, weakness, lethargy, drowsiness, restlessness, confusion, seizures, muscle pains or cramps, muscular fatigue, hypotension, oliguria, tachycardia, and gastrointestinal disturbances such as nausea and vomiting.
Hypokalemia may develop especially with brisk diuresis, when severe cirrhosis is present or after prolonged therapy. Interference with adequate oral electrolyte intake will also contribute to hypokalemia. Hypokalemia may cause cardiac arrhythmias and may also sensitize or exaggerate the response of the heart to the toxic effects of digitalis (e.g., increased ventricular irritability). Hypokalemia may be avoided or treated by use of potassium-sparing diuretics or potassium supplements such as foods with a high potassium content.
Although any chloride deficit is generally mild and usually does not require specific treatment except under extraordinary circumstances (as in liver disease or renal disease), chloride replacement may be required in the treatment of metabolic alkalosis.
Dilutional hyponatremia may occur in edematous patients in hot weather; appropriate therapy is water restriction, rather than administration of salt, except in rare instances when the hyponatremia is life threatening. In actual salt depletion, appropriate replacement is the therapy of choice.
Hyperuricemia may occur or acute gout may be precipitated in certain patients receiving thiazides.
In diabetic patients dosage adjustments of insulin or oral hypoglycemic agents may be required. Hyperglycemia may occur with thiazide diuretics. Thus latent diabetes mellitus may become manifest during thiazide therapy.
The antihypertensive effects of the drug may be enhanced in the postsympathectomy patient.
If progressive renal impairment becomes evident, consider withholding or discontinuing diuretic therapy.
Thiazides have been shown to increase the urinary excretion of magnesium; this may result in hypomagnesemia.
Thiazides may decrease urinary calcium excretion. Thiazides may cause intermittent and slight elevation of serum calcium in the absence of known disorders of calcium metabolism. Marked hypercalcemia may be evidence of hidden hyperparathyroidism. Thiazides should be discontinued before carrying out tests for parathyroid function.
Increases in cholesterol and triglyceride levels may be associated with thiazide diuretic therapy.

Continued on next page

Information on the Merck & Co., Inc., products listed on these pages is from the prescribing information in use October 1, 2004. For information, please call 1-800-NSC-MERCK [1-800-672-6372].

Diuril I.V.—Cont.

Laboratory Tests
Periodic determination of serum electrolytes to detect possible electrolyte imbalance should be done at appropriate intervals.
Drug Interactions
When given concurrently the following drugs may interact with thiazide diuretics.
Alcohol, barbiturates, or narcotics —potentiation of orthostatic hypotension may occur.
Antidiabetic drugs —(oral agents and insulin)—dosage adjustment of the antidiabetic drug may be required.
Other antihypertensive drugs —additive effect or potentiation.
Corticosteroids, ACTH —intensified electrolyte depletion, particularly hypokalemia.
Pressor amines (e.g., norepinephrine) —possible decreased response to pressor amines but not sufficient to preclude their use.
Skeletal muscle relaxants, nondepolarizing (e.g., tubocurarine) —possible increased responsiveness to the muscle relaxant.
Lithium —generally should not be given with diuretics. Diuretic agents reduce the renal clearance of lithium and add a high risk of lithium toxicity. Refer to the package insert for lithium preparations before use of such preparations with Sodium DIURIL.
Non-steroidal Anti-inflammatory Drugs —In some patients, the administration of a non-steroidal anti-inflammatory agent can reduce the diuretic, natriuretic, and antihypertensive effects of loop, potassium-sparing and thiazide diuretics. Therefore, when Sodium DIURIL and non-steroidal anti-inflammatory agents are used concomitantly, the patient should be observed closely to determine if the desired effect of the diuretic is obtained.
Drug/Laboratory Test Interactions
Thiazides should be discontinued before carrying out tests for parathyroid function (see PRECAUTIONS, *General*).
Carcinogenesis, Mutagenesis, Impairment of Fertility
Carcinogenicity studies have not been conducted with chlorothiazide.
Chlorothiazide was not mutagenic *in vitro* in the Ames microbial mutagen test (using a maximum concentration of 5 mg/plate and *Salmonella typhimurium* strains TA98 and TA100) and was not mutagenic and did not induce mitotic nondisjunction in diploid-strains of *Aspergillus nidulans*.
Chlorothiazide had no adverse effects on fertility in female rats at doses up to 60 mg/kg/day and no adverse effects on fertility in male rats at doses up to 40 mg/kg/day. These doses are 1.5 and 1.0 times** the recommended maximum human dose, respectively, when compared on a body weight basis.

**Calculations based on a human body weight of 50 kg

Pregnancy
Teratogenic Effects —Pregnancy Category C: Although reproduction studies performed with chlorothiazide doses of 50 mg/kg/day in rabbits, 60 mg/kg/day in rats and 500 mg/kg/day in mice revealed no external abnormalities of the fetus or impairment of growth and survival of the fetus due to chlorothiazide, such studies did not include complete examinations for visceral and skeletal abnormalities. It is not known whether chlorothiazide can cause fetal harm when administered to a pregnant woman; however, thiazides cross the placental barrier and appear in cord blood. DIURIL should be used during pregnancy only if clearly needed (see INDICATIONS AND USAGE).
Nonteratogenic Effects: Chlorothiazide may cause fetal or neonatal jaundice, thrombocytopenia, and possibly other adverse reactions which have occurred in the adult.
Nursing Mothers
Because of the potential for serious adverse reactions in nursing infants from Intravenous Sodium DIURIL, a decision should be made whether to discontinue nursing or to discontinue the drug, taking into account the importance of the drug to the mother.
Pediatric Use
Safety and effectiveness of Intravenous Sodium DIURIL in pediatric patients have not been established.

ADVERSE REACTIONS

The following adverse reactions have been reported and, within each category, are listed in order of decreasing severity.
Body as a Whole: Weakness.
Cardiovascular: Hypotension including orthostatic hypotension (may be aggravated by alcohol, barbiturates, narcotics or antihypertensive drugs).
Digestive: Pancreatitis, jaundice (intrahepatic cholestatic jaundice), diarrhea, vomiting, sialadenitis, cramping, constipation, gastric irritation, nausea, anorexia.
Hematologic: Aplastic anemia, agranulocytosis, leukopenia, hemolytic anemia, thrombocytopenia.
Hypersensitivity: Anaphylactic reactions, necrotizing angiitis (vasculitis and cutaneous vasculitis), respiratory distress including pneumonitis and pulmonary edema, photosensitivity, fever, urticaria, rash, purpura.
Metabolic: Electrolyte imbalance (see PRECAUTIONS), hyperglycemia, glycosuria, hyperuricemia.
Musculoskeletal: Muscle spasm.
Nervous System/Psychiatric: Vertigo, paresthesias, dizziness, headache, restlessness.
Skin: Erythema multiforme including Stevens-Johnson syndrome, exfoliative dermatitis including toxic epidermal necrolysis, alopecia.
Special Senses: Transient blurred vision, xanthopsia.
Renal: Renal failure, renal dysfunction, interstitial nephritis (see WARNINGS); hematuria (following intravenous use).
Urogenital: Impotence.
Whenever adverse reactions are moderate or severe, thiazide dosage should be reduced or therapy withdrawn.

OVERDOSAGE

The most common signs and symptoms observed are those caused by electrolyte depletion (hypokalemia, hypochloremia, hyponatremia) and dehydration resulting from excessive diuresis. If digitalis has also been administered, hypokalemia may accentuate cardiac arrhythmias.
In the event of overdosage, symptomatic and supportive measures should be employed. Correct dehydration, electrolyte imbalance, hepatic coma and hypotension by established procedures. If required, give oxygen or artificial respiration for respiratory impairment.
The degree to which chlorothiazide sodium is removed by hemodialysis has not been established.
The intravenous LD_{50} of chlorothiazide in the mouse is 1.1 g/kg.

DOSAGE AND ADMINISTRATION

Intravenous Sodium DIURIL should be reserved for patients unable to take oral medication or for emergency situations.
Therapy should be individualized according to patient response. Use the smallest dosage necessary to achieve the required response.
Intravenous use in infants and children has been limited and is not generally recommended.
When medication can be taken orally, therapy with DIURIL tablets or oral suspension may be substituted for intravenous therapy, using the same dosage schedule as for the parenteral route.
Intravenous Sodium DIURIL may be given slowly by direct intravenous injection or by intravenous infusion.
Extravasation must be rigidly avoided. Do not give subcutaneously or intramuscularly.
The usual adult dosage is 0.5 to 1.0 g once or twice a day. Many patients with edema respond to intermittent therapy, i.e., administration on alternate days or on three to five days each week. With an intermittent schedule, excessive response and the resulting undesirable electrolyte imbalance are less likely to occur.
Directions for Reconstitution
Use aseptic technique. Because Intravenous Sodium DIURIL contains no preservative, a fresh solution should be prepared immediately prior to each administration, and the unused portion should be discarded.
Add 18 mL of Sterile Water for Injection to the vial to form an isotonic solution for intravenous injection. Never add less than 18 mL. When reconstituted with 18 mL of Sterile Water, the final concentration of Intravenous Sodium DIURIL is 28 mg/mL. Parenteral drug products should be inspected visually for particulate matter and discoloration prior to use whenever solution and container permit. The solution is compatible with dextrose or sodium chloride solutions for intravenous infusion. Avoid simultaneous administration of solutions of chlorothiazide with whole blood or its derivatives.

HOW SUPPLIED

No. 3619—Intravenous Sodium DIURIL is a dry, sterile lyophilized white powder usually in plug form, supplied in vials containing chlorothiazide sodium equivalent to 0.5 g of chlorothiazide.
NDC 0006-3619-32.
Storage
Store lyophilized powder between 2–25°C (36–77°F).
For single dose only. Use solution immediately after reconstitution. (See DOSAGE AND ADMINISTRATION, *Directions for Reconstitution*.) Discard unused portion of the reconstituted solution.

9273238 Issued April 2004

DIURIL® Tablets ℞
(Chlorothiazide)
DIURIL® Oral Suspension ℞
(Chlorothiazide)

DESCRIPTION

DIURIL* (Chlorothiazide) is a diuretic and antihypertensive. It is 6-chloro-*2H* -1,2,4 -benzothiadiazine-7-sulfonamide 1,1-dioxide. Its empirical formula is $C_7H_6ClN_3O_4S_2$ and its structural formula is:
[See chemical structure at top of next column]
It is a white, or practically white, crystalline powder with a molecular weight of 295.73, which is very slightly soluble in water, but readily soluble in dilute aqueous sodium hydroxide. It is soluble in urine to the extent of about 150 mg per 100 mL at pH 7.
DIURIL is supplied as 250 mg and 500 mg tablets, for oral use. Each tablet contains the following inactive ingredients: gelatin, magnesium stearate, starch and talc. The 250 mg tablet also contains lactose.
Oral Suspension DIURIL contains 250 mg of chlorothiazide per 5 mL, alcohol 0.5 percent, with methylparaben 0.12 percent, propylparaben 0.02 percent, and benzoic acid 0.1 percent added as preservatives. The inactive ingredients are D&C Yellow 10, flavors, glycerin, purified water, sodium saccharin, sucrose and tragacanth.

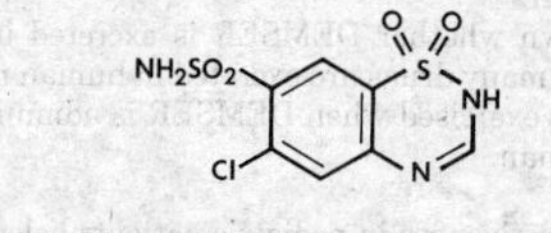

*Registered trademark of MERCK & CO., INC.

CLINICAL PHARMACOLOGY

The mechanism of the antihypertensive effect of thiazides is unknown. DIURIL does not usually affect normal blood pressure.
DIURIL affects the distal renal tubular mechanism of electrolyte reabsorption. At maximal therapeutic dosage all thiazides are approximately equal in their diuretic efficacy.
DIURIL increases excretion of sodium and chloride in approximately equivalent amounts. Natriuresis may be accompanied by some loss of potassium and bicarbonate.
After oral use diuresis begins within 2 hours, peaks in about 4 hours and lasts about 6 to 12 hours.
Pharmacokinetics and Metabolism
DIURIL is not metabolized but is eliminated rapidly by the kidney. The plasma half-life of chlorothiazide is 45–120 minutes. After oral doses, 10–15 percent of the dose is excreted unchanged in the urine. Chlorothiazide crosses the placental but not the blood-brain barrier and is excreted in breast milk.

INDICATIONS AND USAGE

DIURIL is indicated as adjunctive therapy in edema associated with congestive heart failure, hepatic cirrhosis, and corticosteroid and estrogen therapy.
DIURIL has also been found useful in edema due to various forms of renal dysfunction such as nephrotic syndrome, acute glomerulonephritis, and chronic renal failure.
DIURIL is indicated in the management of hypertension either as the sole therapeutic agent or to enhance the effectiveness of other antihypertensive drugs in the more severe forms of hypertension.
Use in Pregnancy. Routine use of diuretics during normal pregnancy is inappropriate and exposes mother and fetus to unnecessary hazard. Diuretics do not prevent development of toxemia of pregnancy and there is no satisfactory evidence that they are useful in the treatment of toxemia.
Edema during pregnancy may arise from pathologic causes or from the physiologic and mechanical consequences of pregnancy. Thiazides are indicated in pregnancy when edema is due to pathologic causes, just as they are in the absence of pregnancy (see PRECAUTIONS, *Pregnancy*). Dependent edema in pregnancy, resulting from restriction of venous return by the gravid uterus, is properly treated through elevation of the lower extremities and use of support stockings. Use of diuretics to lower intravascular volume in this instance is illogical and unnecessary. During normal pregnancy there is hypervolemia which is not harmful to the fetus or the mother in the absence of cardiovascular disease. However, it may be associated with edema, rarely generalized edema. If such edema causes discomfort, increased recumbency will often provide relief. Rarely this edema may cause extreme discomfort which is not relieved by rest. In these instances, a short course of diuretic therapy may provide relief and be appropriate.

CONTRAINDICATIONS

Anuria.
Hypersensitivity to this product or to other sulfonamide-derived drugs.

WARNINGS

Use with caution in severe renal disease. In patients with renal disease, thiazides may precipitate azotemia. Cumulative effects of the drug may develop in patients with impaired renal function.
Thiazides should be used with caution in patients with impaired hepatic function or progressive liver disease, since minor alterations of fluid and electrolyte balance may precipitate hepatic coma.
Thiazides may add to or potentiate the action of other antihypertensive drugs.
Sensitivity reactions may occur in patients with or without a history of allergy or bronchial asthma.
The possibility of exacerbation or activation of systemic lupus erythematosus has been reported.
Lithium generally should not be given with diuretics (see PRECAUTIONS, *Drug Interactions*).

PRECAUTIONS

General
All patients receiving diuretic therapy should be observed for evidence of fluid or electrolyte imbalance: namely, hyponatremia, hypochloremic alkalosis, and hypokalemia. Serum and urine electrolyte determinations are particularly important when the patient is vomiting excessively or receiving parenteral fluids. Warning signs or symptoms of fluid and electrolyte imbalance, irrespective of cause, include dryness of mouth, thirst, weakness, lethargy, drowsiness, restlessness, confusion, seizures, muscle pains or cramps, muscular fatigue, hypotension, oliguria, tachycardia, and gastrointestinal disturbances such as nausea and vomiting.
Hypokalemia may develop, especially with brisk diuresis, when severe cirrhosis is present or after prolonged therapy. Interference with adequate oral electrolyte intake will also contribute to hypokalemia. Hypokalemia may cause cardiac arrhythmias and may also sensitize or exaggerate the response of the heart to the toxic effects of digitalis (e.g., increased ventricular irritability). Hypokalemia may be avoided or treated by use of potassium sparing diuretics or potassium supplements such as foods with a high potassium content.
Although any chloride deficit is generally mild and usually does not require specific treatment except under extraordinary circumstances (as in liver disease or renal disease), chloride replacement may be required in the treatment of metabolic alkalosis.
Dilutional hyponatremia may occur in edematous patients in hot weather; appropriate therapy is water restriction, rather than administration of salt, except in rare instances when the hyponatremia is life-threatening. In actual salt depletion, appropriate replacement is the therapy of choice.
Hyperuricemia may occur or acute gout may be precipitated in certain patients receiving thiazides.
In diabetic patients dosage adjustments of insulin or oral hypoglycemic agents may be required. Hyperglycemia may occur with thiazide diuretics. Thus latent diabetes mellitus may become manifest during thiazide therapy.
The antihypertensive effects of the drug may be enhanced in the post-sympathectomy patient.
If progressive renal impairment becomes evident, consider withholding or discontinuing diuretic therapy.
Thiazides have been shown to increase the urinary excretion of magnesium; this may result in hypomagnesemia.
Thiazides may decrease urinary calcium excretion. Thiazides may cause intermittent and slight elevation of serum calcium in the absence of known disorders of calcium metabolism. Marked hypercalcemia may be evidence of hidden hyperparathyroidism. Thiazides should be discontinued before carrying out tests for parathyroid function.
Increases in cholesterol and triglyceride levels may be associated with thiazide diuretic therapy.
Laboratory Tests
Periodic determination of serum electrolytes to detect possible electrolyte imbalance should be done at appropriate intervals.
Drug Interactions
When given concurrently the following drugs may interact with thiazide diuretics.
Alcohol, barbiturates, or narcotics —potentiation of orthostatic hypotension may occur.
Antidiabetic drugs (oral agents and insulin)—dosage adjustment of the antidiabetic drug may be required.
Other antihypertensive drugs —additive effect or potentiation.
Cholestyramine and colestipol resins—Both cholestyramine and colestipol resins have the potential of binding thiazide diuretics and reducing diuretic absorption from the gastrointestinal tract.
Corticosteroids, ACTH —intensified electrolyte depletion, particularly hypokalemia.
Pressor amines (e.g., norepinephrine) —possible decreased response to pressor amines but not sufficient to preclude their use.
Skeletal muscle relaxants, nondepolarizing (e.g., tubocurarine) —possible increased responsiveness to the muscle relaxant.
Lithium —generally should not be given with diuretics. Diuretic agents reduce the renal clearance of lithium and add a high risk of lithium toxicity. Refer to the package insert for lithium preparations before use of such preparations with DIURIL.
Non-steroidal Anti-inflammatory Drugs —In some patients, the administration of a non-steroidal anti-inflammatory agent can reduce the diuretic, natriuretic, and antihypertensive effects of loop, potassium-sparing and thiazide diuretics. Therefore, when DIURIL and non-steroidal anti-inflammatory agents are used concomitantly, the patient should be observed closely to determine if the desired effect of the diuretic is obtained.
Drug/Laboratory Test Interactions
Thiazides should be discontinued before carrying out tests for parathyroid function (see PRECAUTIONS, *General*).
Carcinogenesis, Mutagenesis, Impairment of Fertility
Carcinogenicity studies have not been conducted with chlorothiazide.
Chlorothiazide was not mutagenic *in vitro* in the Ames microbial mutagen test (using a maximum concentration of 5 mg/plate and *Salmonella typhimurium* strains TA98 and TA100) and was not mutagenic and did not induce mitotic nondisjunction in diploid-strains of *Aspergillus nidulans.*
Chlorothiazide had no adverse effects on fertility in female rats at doses up to 60 mg/kg/day and no adverse effects on fertility in male rats at doses up to 40 mg/kg/day. These doses are 1.5 and 1.0 times** the recommended maximum human dose, respectively, when compared on a body weight basis.

**Calculations based on a human body weight of 50 kg

Pregnancy
Teratogenic Effects —Pregnancy Category C: Although reproduction studies performed with chlorothiazide doses of 50 mg/kg/day in rabbits, 60 mg/kg/day in rats and 500 mg/kg/day in mice revealed no external abnormalities of the fetus or impairment of growth and survival of the fetus due to chlorothiazide, such studies did not include complete examinations for visceral and skeletal abnormalities. It is not known whether chlorothiazide can cause fetal harm when administered to a pregnant woman; however, thiazides cross the placental barrier and appear in cord blood. DIURIL should be used during pregnancy only if clearly needed (see INDICATIONS AND USAGE).
Nonteratogenic Effects: Chlorothiazide may cause fetal or neonatal jaundice, thrombocytopenia, and possibly other adverse reactions which have occurred in the adult.
Nursing Mothers
Because of the potential for serious adverse reactions in nursing infants from DIURIL, a decision should be made whether to discontinue nursing or to discontinue the drug, taking into account the importance of the drug to the mother.
Pediatric Use
There are no well-controlled clinical trials in pediatric patients. Information on dosing in this age group is supported by evidence from empiric use in pediatric patients and published literature regarding the treatment of hypertension in such patients. (See DOSAGE AND ADMINISTRATION, *Infants and Children.*)

ADVERSE REACTIONS

The following adverse reactions have been reported and, within each category, are listed in order of decreasing severity.
Body as a Whole: Weakness.
Cardiovascular: Hypotension including orthostatic hypotension (may be aggravated by alcohol, barbiturates, narcotics or antihypertensive drugs).
Digestive: Pancreatitis, jaundice (intrahepatic cholestatic jaundice), diarrhea, vomiting, sialadenitis, cramping, constipation, gastric irritation, nausea, anorexia.
Hematologic: Aplastic anemia, agranulocytosis, leukopenia, hemolytic anemia, thrombocytopenia.
Hypersensitivity: Anaphylactic reactions, necrotizing angiitis (vasculitis and cutaneous vasculitis), respiratory distress including pneumonitis and pulmonary edema, photosensitivity, fever, urticaria, rash, purpura.
Metabolic: Electrolyte imbalance (see PRECAUTIONS), hyperglycemia, glycosuria, hyperuricemia.
Musculoskeletal: Muscle spasm.
Nervous System/Psychiatric: Vertigo, paresthesias, dizziness, headache, restlessness.
Renal: Renal failure, renal dysfunction, interstitial nephritis. (See WARNINGS.)
Skin: Erythema multiforme including Stevens-Johnson syndrome, exfoliative dermatitis including toxic epidermal necrolysis, alopecia.
Special Senses: Transient blurred vision, xanthopsia.
Urogenital: Impotence.
Whenever adverse reactions are moderate or severe, thiazide dosage should be reduced or therapy withdrawn.

OVERDOSAGE

The most common signs and symptoms observed are those caused by electrolyte depletion (hypokalemia, hypochloremia, hyponatremia) and dehydration resulting from excessive diuresis. If digitalis has also been administered, hypokalemia may accentuate cardiac arrhythmias.
In the event of overdosage, symptomatic and supportive measures should be employed. Emesis should be induced or gastric lavage performed. Correct dehydration, electrolyte imbalance, hepatic coma and hypotension by established procedures. If required, give oxygen or artificial respiration for respiratory impairment.
The degree to which chlorothiazide sodium is removed by hemodialysis has not been established.
The oral LD_{50} of chlorothiazide is 8.5 g/kg, greater than 10 g/kg, and greater than 1 g/kg, in the mouse, rat and dog respectively.

DOSAGE AND ADMINISTRATION

Therapy should be individualized according to patient response. Use the smallest dosage necessary to achieve the required response.

Adults

For Edema
The usual adult dosage is 0.5 to 1.0 g once or twice a day. Many patients with edema respond to intermittent therapy, i.e., administration on alternate days or on three to five days each week. With an intermittent schedule, excessive response and the resulting undesirable electrolyte imbalance are less likely to occur.
For Control of Hypertension
The usual adult starting dosage is 0.5 or 1.0 g a day as a single or divided dose. Dosage is increased or decreased according to blood pressure response. Rarely some patients may require up to 2.0 g a day in divided doses.

Infants and Children

For Diuresis and For Control of Hypertension
The usual pediatric dosage is 5 to 10 mg per pound (10 to 20 mg/kg) per day in single or two divided doses, not to exceed 375 mg per day (2.5 to 7.5 mL or $^1/_2$ to $1^1/_2$ teaspoonfuls of the oral suspension daily) in infants up to 2 years of age or 1 g per day in children 2 to 12 years of age. In infants less than 6 months of age, doses up to 15 mg per pound (30 mg/kg) per day in two divided doses may be required. (See PRECAUTIONS, *Pediatric Use.*)

HOW SUPPLIED

No. 3244—Tablets DIURIL, 250 mg, are white, round, scored, compressed tablets, coded MSD 214 on one side and DIURIL on the other. They are supplied as follows:
NDC 0006-0214-68 bottles of 100.
No. 3245—Tablets DIURIL, 500 mg, are white, round, scored, compressed tablets, coded MSD 432 on one side and DIURIL on the other. They are supplied as follows:
NDC 0006-0432-68 bottles of 100.
No. 3239—Oral Suspension DIURIL, 250 mg of chlorothiazide per 5 mL, is a yellow, creamy suspension, and is supplied as follows:
NDC 0006-3239-66 bottles of 237 mL
(6505-01-156-1600, 250 mg/5 mL, 237 mL).
Storage
Tablets DIURIL: Keep container tightly closed. Protect from moisture, freezing, -20°C (-4°F) and store at room temperature, 15–30°C (59–86°F).
Oral Suspension DIURIL: Keep container tightly closed. Protect from freezing, -20°C (-4°F) and store at room temperature, 15–30°C (59–86°F).
7897959 Issued June 1998

Shown in Product Identification Guide, page 323

DOLOBID® Tablets ℞
(Diflunisal)

DESCRIPTION

Diflunisal is 2′, 4′-difluoro-4-hydroxy-3-biphenylcarboxylic acid. Its empirical formula is $C_{13}H_8F_2O_3$ and its structural formula is:

Diflunisal has a molecular weight of 250.20. It is a stable, white, crystalline compound with a melting point of 211–213°C. It is practically insoluble in water at neutral or acidic pH. Because it is an organic acid, it dissolves readily in dilute alkali to give a moderately stable solution at room temperature. It is soluble in most organic solvents including ethanol, methanol, and acetone.
DOLOBID* (Diflunisal) is available in 250 and 500 mg tablets for oral administration. Tablets DOLOBID contain the following inactive ingredients: cellulose, FD&C Yellow 6 hydroxypropyl cellulose, hydroxypropyl methylcellulose, magnesium stearate, starch, talc, and titanium dioxide.

*Registered trademark of MERCK & CO., INC.

CLINICAL PHARMACOLOGY

Action
DOLOBID is a non-steroidal drug with analgesic, anti-inflammatory and antipyretic properties. It is a peripherally-acting non-narcotic analgesic drug. Habituation, tolerance and addiction have not been reported.
Diflunisal is a difluorophenyl derivative of salicylic acid. Chemically, diflunisal differs from aspirin (acetylsalicylic acid) in two respects. The first of these two is the presence of a difluorophenyl substituent at carbon 1. The second difference is the removal of the 0-acetyl group from the carbon 4 position. Diflunisal is not metabolized to salicylic acid, and the fluorine atoms are not displaced from the difluorophenyl ring structure.
The precise mechanism of the analgesic and anti-inflammatory actions of diflunisal is not known. Diflunisal is a prostaglandin synthetase inhibitor. In animals, prostaglandins

Continued on next page

Information on the Merck & Co., Inc., products listed on these pages is from the prescribing information in use October 1, 2004. For information, please call 1-800-NSC-MERCK [1-800-672-6372].

Dolobid—Cont.

sensitize afferent nerves and potentiate the action of bradykinin in inducing pain. Since prostaglandins are known to be among the mediators of pain and inflammation, the mode of action of diflunisal may be due to a decrease of prostaglandins in peripheral tissues.

Pharmacokinetics and Metabolism

DOLOBID is rapidly and completely absorbed following oral administration with peak plasma concentrations occurring between 2 to 3 hours. The drug is excreted in the urine as two soluble glucuronide conjugates accounting for about 90% of the administered dose. Little or no diflunisal is excreted in the feces. Diflunisal appears in human milk in concentrations of 2–7% of those in plasma. More than 99% of diflunisal in plasma is bound to proteins.

As is the case with salicylic acid, concentration-dependent pharmacokinetics prevail when DOLOBID is administered; a doubling of dosage produces a greater than doubling of drug accumulation. The effect becomes more apparent with repetitive doses. Following single doses, peak plasma concentrations of 41 ± 11 μg/mL (mean ± S.D.) were observed following 250 mg doses, 87 ± 17 μg/mL were observed following 500 mg and 124 ± 11 μg/mL following single 1000 mg doses. However, following administration of 250 mg b.i.d., a mean peak level of 56 ± 14 μg/mL was observed on day 8, while the mean peak level after 500 mg b.i.d. for 11 days was 190 ± 33 μg/mL. In contrast to salicylic acid which has a plasma half-life of $2^1/_2$ hours, the plasma half-life of diflunisal is 3 to 4 times longer (8 to 12 hours), because of a difluorophenyl substituent at carbon 1. Because of its long half-life and nonlinear pharmacokinetics, several days are required for diflunisal plasma levels to reach steady state following multiple doses. For this reason, an initial loading dose is necessary to shorten the time to reach steady state levels, and 2 to 3 days of observation are necessary for evaluating changes in treatment regimens if a loading dose is not used.

Studies in baboons to determine passage across the blood-brain barrier have shown that only small quantities of diflunisal, under normal or acidotic conditions are transported into the cerebrospinal fluid (CSF). The ratio of blood/CSF concentrations after intravenous doses of 50 mg/kg or oral doses of 100 mg/kg of diflunisal was 100:1. In contrast, oral doses of 500 mg/kg of aspirin resulted in a blood/CSF ratio of 5:1.

Mild to Moderate Pain

DOLOBID is a peripherally-acting analgesic agent with a long duration of action. DOLOBID produces significant analgesia within 1 hour and maximum analgesia within 2 to 3 hours.

Consistent with its long half-life, clinical effects of DOLOBID mirror its pharmacokinetic behavior, which is the basis for recommending a loading dose when instituting therapy. Patients treated with DOLOBID, on the first dose, tend to have a slower onset of pain relief when compared with drugs achieving comparable peak effects. However, DOLOBID produces longer-lasting responses than the comparative agents.

Comparative single dose clinical studies have established the analgesic efficacy of DOLOBID at various dose levels relative to other analgesics. Analgesic effect measurements were derived from hourly evaluations by patients during eight and twelve-hour postdosing observation periods. The following information may serve as a guide for prescribing DOLOBID.

DOLOBID 500 mg was comparable in analgesic efficacy to aspirin 650 mg, acetaminophen 600 mg or 650 mg, and acetaminophen 650 mg with propoxyphene napsylate 100 mg. Patients treated with DOLOBID had longer lasting responses than the patients treated with the comparative analgesics.

DOLOBID 1000 mg was comparable in analgesic efficacy to acetaminophen 600 mg with codeine 60 mg. Patients treated with DOLOBID had longer lasting responses than the patients who received acetaminophen with codeine.

A loading dose of 1000 mg provides faster onset of pain relief, shorter time to peak analgesic effect, and greater peak analgesic effect than an initial 500 mg dose.

In contrast to the comparative analgesics, a significantly greater proportion of patients treated with DOLOBID did not remedicate and continued to have a good analgesic effect eight to twelve hours after dosing. Seventy-five percent (75%) of patients treated with DOLOBID continued to have a good analgesic response at four hours. When patients having a good analgesic response at four hours were followed, 78% of these patients continued to have a good analgesic response at eight hours and 64% at twelve hours.

Chronic Anti-inflammatory Therapy in Osteoarthritis and Rheumatoid Arthritis

In the controlled, double-blind clinical trials in which DOLOBID (500 mg to 1000 mg a day) was compared with anti-inflammatory doses of aspirin (2–4 grams a day), patients treated with DOLOBID had a significantly lower incidence of tinnitus and of adverse effects involving the gastrointestinal system than patients treated with aspirin. (See also *Effect on Fecal Blood Loss*).

Osteoarthritis

The effectiveness of DOLOBID for the treatment of osteoarthritis was studied in patients with osteoarthritis of the hip and/or knee. The activity of DOLOBID was demonstrated by clinical improvement in the signs and symptoms of disease activity.

In a double-blind multicenter study of 12 weeks' duration in which dosages were adjusted according to patient response, DOLOBID, 500 or 750 mg daily, was shown to be comparable in effectiveness to aspirin, 2000 or 3000 mg daily. In open-label extensions of this study to 24 or 48 weeks, DOLOBID continued to show similar effectiveness and generally was well tolerated.

Rheumatoid Arthritis

In controlled clinical trials, the effectiveness of DOLOBID was established for both acute exacerbations and long-term management of rheumatoid arthritis. The activity of DOLOBID was demonstrated by clinical improvement in the signs and symptoms of disease activity.

In a double-blind multicenter study of 12 weeks' duration in which dosages were adjusted according to patient response, DOLOBID 500 or 750 mg daily was comparable in effectiveness to aspirin 2,600 or 3,900 mg daily. In open-label extensions of this study to 52 weeks, DOLOBID continued to be effective and was generally well tolerated.

DOLOBID 500, 750, or 1000 mg daily was compared with aspirin 2000, 3000, or 4000 mg daily in a multicenter study of 8 weeks' duration in which dosages were adjusted according to patient response. In this study, DOLOBID was comparable in efficacy to aspirin.

In a double-blind multicenter study of 12 weeks' duration in which dosages were adjusted according to patient needs, DOLOBID 500 or 750 mg daily and ibuprofen 1600 or 2400 mg daily were comparable in effectiveness and tolerability.

In a double-blind multicenter study of 12 weeks' duration, DOLOBID 750 mg daily was comparable in efficacy to naproxen 750 mg daily. The incidence of gastrointestinal adverse effects and tinnitus was comparable for both drugs. This study was extended to 48 weeks on an open-label basis. DOLOBID continued to be effective and generally well tolerated.

In patients with rheumatoid arthritis, DOLOBID and gold salts may be used in combination at their usual dosage levels. In clinical studies, DOLOBID added to the regimen of gold salts usually resulted in additional symptomatic relief but did not alter the course of the underlying disease.

Antipyretic Activity

DOLOBID is not recommended for use as an antipyretic agent. In single 250 mg, 500 mg, or 750 mg doses, DOLOBID produced measurable but not clinically useful decreases in temperature in patients with fever; however, the possibility that it may mask fever in some patients, particularly with chronic or high doses, should be considered.

Uricosuric Effect

In normal volunteers, an increase in the renal clearance of uric acid and a decrease in serum uric acid was observed when DOLOBID was administered at 500 mg or 750 mg daily in divided doses. Patients on long-term therapy taking DOLOBID at 500 mg to 1000 mg daily in divided doses showed a prompt and consistent reduction across studies in mean serum uric acid levels, which were lowered as much as 1.4 mg%. It is not known whether DOLOBID interferes with the activity of other uricosuric agents.

Effect on Platelet Function

As an inhibitor of prostaglandin synthetase, DOLOBID has a dose-related effect on platelet function and bleeding time. In normal volunteers, 250 mg b.i.d. for 8 days had no effect on platelet function, and 500 mg b.i.d., the usual recommended dose, had a slight effect. At 1000 mg b.i.d., which exceeds the maximum recommended dosage, however, DOLOBID inhibited platelet function. In contrast to aspirin, these effects of DOLOBID were reversible, because of the absence of the chemically labile and biologically reactive 0-acetyl group at the carbon 4 position. Bleeding time was not altered by a dose of 250 mg b.i.d., and was only slightly increased at 500 mg b.i.d. At 1000 mg b.i.d., a greater increase occurred, but was not statistically significantly different from the change in the placebo group.

Effect on Fecal Blood Loss

When DOLOBID was given to normal volunteers at the usual recommended dose of 500 mg twice daily, fecal blood loss was not significantly different from placebo. Aspirin at 1000 mg four times daily produced the expected increase in fecal blood loss. DOLOBID at 1000 mg twice daily (NOTE: exceeds the recommended dosage) caused a statistically significant increase in fecal blood loss, but this increase was only one-half as large as that associated with aspirin 1300 mg twice daily.

Effect on Blood Glucose

DOLOBID did not affect fasting blood sugar in diabetic patients who were receiving tolbutamide or placebo.

INDICATIONS AND USAGE

DOLOBID is indicated for acute or long-term use for symptomatic treatment of the following:

1. Mild to moderate pain
2. Osteoarthritis
3. Rheumatoid arthritis

CONTRAINDICATIONS

Patients who are hypersensitive to this product.

Patients in whom acute asthmatic attacks, urticaria, or rhinitis are precipitated by aspirin or other non-steroidal anti-inflammatory drugs.

WARNINGS

Peptic ulceration and gastrointestinal bleeding have been reported in patients receiving DOLOBID. Fatalities have occurred rarely. Gastrointestinal bleeding is associated with higher morbidity and mortality in patients acutely ill with other conditions, the elderly and patients with hemorrhagic disorders. In patients with active gastrointestinal bleeding or an active peptic ulcer, the physician must weigh the benefits of therapy with DOLOBID against possible hazards, institute an appropriate ulcer regimen, and carefully monitor the patient's progress. When DOLOBID is given to patients with a history of either upper or lower gastrointestinal tract disease, it should be given only after consulting the ADVERSE REACTIONS section and under close supervision.

Risk of GI Ulcerations, Bleeding and Perforation with NSAID Therapy

Serious gastrointestinal toxicity such as bleeding, ulceration, and perforation, can occur at any time, with or without warning symptoms, in patients treated chronically with NSAID therapy. Although minor upper gastrointestinal problems, such as dyspepsia, are common, usually developing early in therapy, physicians should remain alert for ulceration and bleeding in patients treated chronically with NSAIDs even in the absence of previous GI tract symptoms. In patients observed in clinical trials of several months to two years duration, symptomatic upper GI ulcers, gross bleeding or perforation appear to occur in approximately 1% of patients treated for 3–6 months, and in about 2–4% of patients treated for one year. Physicians should inform patients about the signs and/or symptoms of serious GI toxicity and what steps to take if they occur.

Studies to date have not identified any subset of patients not at risk of developing peptic ulceration and bleeding. Except for a prior history of serious GI events and other risk factors known to be associated with peptic ulcer disease, such as alcoholism, smoking, etc., no risk factors (e.g., age, sex) have been associated with increased risk. Elderly or debilitated patients seem to tolerate ulceration or bleeding less well than other individuals and most spontaneous reports of fatal GI events are in this population. Studies to date are inconclusive concerning the relative risk of various NSAIDs in causing such reactions. High doses of any NSAID probably carry a greater risk of these reactions, although controlled clinical trials showing this do not exist in most cases. In considering the use of relatively large doses (within the recommended dosage range), sufficient benefit should be anticipated to offset the potential increased risk of GI toxicity.

PRECAUTIONS

General

Non-steroidal anti-inflammatory drugs, including DOLOBID, may mask the usual signs and symptoms of infection. Therefore, the physician must be continually on the alert for this and should use the drug with extra care in the presence of existing infection.

Although DOLOBID has less effect on platelet function and bleeding time than aspirin, at higher doses it is an inhibitor of platelet function; therefore, patients who may be adversely affected should be carefully observed when DOLOBID is administered (see CLINICAL PHARMACOLOGY).

Because of reports of adverse eye findings with agents of this class, it is recommended that patients who develop eye complaints during treatment with DOLOBID have ophthalmologic studies.

Peripheral edema has been observed in some patients taking DOLOBID. Therefore, as with other drugs in this class, DOLOBID should be used with caution in patients with compromised cardiac function, hypertension, or other conditions predisposing to fluid retention.

Acetylsalicylic acid has been associated with Reye syndrome. Because diflunisal is a derivative of salicylic acid, the possibility of its association with Reye syndrome cannot be excluded.

Hypersensitivity Syndrome

A potentially life-threatening, apparent hypersensitivity syndrome has been reported. This multisystem syndrome includes constitutional symptoms (fever, chills), and cutaneous findings (see ADVERSE REACTIONS, *Dermatologic*). It may also include involvement of major organs (changes in liver function, jaundice, leukopenia, thrombocytopenia, eosinophilia, disseminated intravascular coagulation, renal impairment, including renal failure), and less specific findings (adenitis, arthralgia, myalgia, arthritis, malaise, anorexia, disorientation). If evidence of hypersensitivity occurs, therapy with DOLOBID should be discontinued.

Renal Effects

As with other non-steroidal anti-inflammatory drugs, long term administration of diflunisal to animals has resulted in renal papillary necrosis and other abnormal renal pathology. In humans, there have been reports of acute interstitial nephritis with hematuria and proteinuria and occasionally nephrotic syndrome.

A second form of renal toxicity has been seen in patients with prerenal and renal conditions leading to a reduction in renal blood flow or blood volume, where the renal prostaglandins have a supportive role in the maintenance of renal perfusion. In these patients administration of an NSAID may cause a dose dependent reduction in prostaglandin formation and may precipitate overt renal decompensation. Patients at greatest risk of this reaction are those with conditions such as renal or hepatic dysfunction, diabetes mellitus, advanced age, extracellular volume depletion from any cause, congestive heart failure, septicemia, pyelonephritis, or concomitant use of any nephrotoxic drug. DOLOBID or other NSAIDs should be given with caution and renal function should be monitored in any patient who may have reduced renal reserve. Discontinuation of NSAID therapy is typically followed by recovery to the pretreatment state.

Since DOLOBID is eliminated primarily by the kidneys, patients with significantly impaired renal function should be closely monitored; a lower daily dosage should be anticipated to avoid excessive drug accumulation.

Information for Patients

DOLOBID, like other drugs of its class, is not free of side effects. The side effects of these drugs can cause discomfort and, rarely, there are more serious side effects such as gastrointestinal bleeding, which may result in hospitalization and even fatal outcomes.

NSAIDs (Non-steroidal Anti-inflammatory Drugs) are often essential agents in the management of arthritis and have a major role in the treatment of pain, but they also may be commonly employed for conditions which are less serious.

Physicians may wish to discuss with their patients the potential risks (see WARNINGS, PRECAUTIONS and ADVERSE REACTIONS) and likely benefits of NSAID treatment, particularly when the drugs are used for less serious conditions where treatment without NSAIDs may represent an acceptable alternative to both the patient and physician.

Laboratory Tests

Liver Function Tests: As with other non-steroidal anti-inflammatory drugs, borderline elevations of one or more liver tests may occur in up to 15% of patients. These abnormalities may progress, may remain essentially unchanged, or may be transient with continued therapy. The SGPT (ALT) test is probably the most sensitive indicator of liver dysfunction. Meaningful (3 times the upper limit of normal) elevations of SGPT or SGOT (AST) occurred in controlled clinical trials in less than 1% of patients. A patient with symptoms and/or signs suggesting liver dysfunction, or in whom an abnormal liver test has occurred, should be evaluated for evidence of the development of more severe hepatic reactions while on therapy with DOLOBID. Severe hepatic reactions, including jaundice, have been reported with DOLOBID as well as with other non-steroidal anti-inflammatory drugs. Although such reactions are rare, if abnormal liver tests persist or worsen, if clinical signs and symptoms consistent with liver disease develop, or if systemic manifestations occur (e.g., eosinophilia, rash, etc.), DOLOBID should be discontinued, since liver reactions can be fatal.

Gastrointestinal: Because serious GI tract ulceration and bleeding can occur without warning symptoms, physicians should follow chronically treated patients for the signs and symptoms of ulceration and bleeding and should inform them of the importance of this follow-up (see WARNINGS, *Risk of GI Ulcerations, Bleeding and Perforation with NSAID Therapy*).

Drug Interactions

Oral Anticoagulants: In some normal volunteers, the concomitant administration of DOLOBID and warfarin, acenocoumarol, or phenprocoumon resulted in prolongation of prothrombin time. This may occur because diflunisal competitively displaces coumarins from protein binding sites. Accordingly, when DOLOBID is administered with oral anticoagulants, the prothrombin time should be closely monitored during and for several days after concomitant drug administration. Adjustment of dosage of oral anticoagulants may be required.

Tolbutamide: In diabetic patients receiving DOLOBID and tolbutamide, no significant effects were seen on tolbutamide plasma levels or fasting blood glucose.

Hydrochlorothiazide: In normal volunteers, concomitant administration of DOLOBID and hydrochlorothiazide resulted in significantly increased plasma levels of hydrochlorothiazide. DOLOBID decreased the hyperuricemic effect of hydrochlorothiazide.

Furosemide: In normal volunteers, the concomitant administration of DOLOBID and furosemide had no effect on the diuretic activity of furosemide. DOLOBID decreased the hyperuricemic effect of furosemide.

Antacids: Concomitant administration of antacids may reduce plasma levels of DOLOBID. This effect is small with occasional doses of antacids, but may be clinically significant when antacids are used on a continuous schedule.

Acetaminophen: In normal volunteers, concomitant administration of DOLOBID and acetaminophen resulted in an approximate 50% increase in plasma levels of acetaminophen. Acetaminophen had no effect on plasma levels of DOLOBID. Since acetaminophen in high doses has been associated with hepatotoxicity, concomitant administration of DOLOBID and acetaminophen should be used cautiously, with careful monitoring of patients.

Concomitant administration of DOLOBID and acetaminophen in dogs, but not in rats, at approximately 2 times the recommended maximum human therapeutic dose of each (40-52 mg/kg/day of DOLOBID/acetaminophen), resulted in greater gastrointestinal toxicity than when either drug was administered alone. The clinical significance of these findings has not been established.

Methotrexate: Caution should be used if DOLOBID is administered concomitantly with methotrexate. Non-steroidal anti-inflammatory drugs have been reported to decrease the tubular secretion of methotrexate and to potentiate its toxicity.

Cyclosporine: Administration of non-steroidal anti-inflammatory drugs concomitantly with cyclosporine has been associated with an increase in cyclosporine-induced toxicity, possibly due to decreased synthesis of renal prostacyclin. NSAIDs should be used with caution in patients taking cyclosporine, and renal function should be carefully monitored.

Drug Interactions: Non-steroidal Anti-inflammatory Drugs

The administration of diflunisal to normal volunteers receiving indomethacin decreased the renal clearance and significantly increased the plasma levels of indomethacin. In some patients the combined use of indomethacin and DOLOBID has been associated with fatal gastrointestinal hemorrhage. Therefore, indomethacin and DOLOBID should not be used concomitantly.

The concomitant use of DOLOBID and other NSAIDs is not recommended due to the increased possibility of gastrointestinal toxicity, with little or no increase in efficacy. The following information was obtained from studies in normal volunteers.

Aspirin: In normal volunteers, a small decrease in diflunisal levels was observed when multiple doses of DOLOBID and aspirin were administered concomitantly.

Sulindac: The concomitant administration of DOLOBID and sulindac in normal volunteers resulted in lowering of the plasma levels of the active sulindac sulfide metabolite by approximately one-third.

Naproxen: The concomitant administration of DOLOBID and naproxen in normal volunteers had no effect on the plasma levels of naproxen, but significantly decreased the urinary excretion of naproxen and its glucuronide metabolite. Naproxen had no effect on plasma levels of DOLOBID.

Drug/Laboratory Test Interactions

Serum Salicylate Assays: Caution should be used in interpreting the results of serum salicylate assays when diflunisal is present. Salicylate levels have been found to be falsely elevated with some assay methods.

Carcinogenesis, Mutagenesis, Impairment of Fertility

Diflunisal did not affect the type or incidence of neoplasia in a 105-week study in the rat given doses up to 40 mg/kg/day (equivalent to approximately 1.3 times the maximum recommended human dose), or in long-term carcinogenic studies in mice given diflunisal at doses up to 80 mg/kg/day (equivalent to approximately 2.7 times the maximum recommended human dose). It was concluded that there was no carcinogenic potential for DOLOBID.

Diflunisal passes the placental barrier to a minor degree in the rat. Diflunisal had no mutagenic activity after oral administration in the dominant lethal assay, in the Ames microbial mutagen test or in the V-79 Chinese hamster lung cell assay.

No evidence of impaired fertility was found in reproduction studies in rats at doses up to 50 mg/kg/day.

Pregnancy

Pregnancy Category C. A dose of 60 mg/kg/day of diflunisal (equivalent to two times the maximum human dose) was maternotoxic, embryotoxic, and teratogenic in rabbits. In three of six studies in rabbits, evidence of teratogenicity was observed at doses ranging from 40 to 50 mg/kg/day. Teratology studies in mice, at doses up to 45 mg/kg/day, and in rats at doses up to 100 mg/kg/day, revealed no harm to the fetus due to diflunisal. Aspirin and other salicylates have been shown to be teratogenic in a wide variety of species, including the rat and rabbit, at doses ranging from 50 to 400 mg/kg/day (approximately one to eight times the human dose). There are no adequate and well controlled studies with diflunisal in pregnant women. DOLOBID should be used during the first two trimesters of pregnancy only if the potential benefit justifies the potential risk to the fetus. The known effects of drugs of this class on the human fetus during the third trimester of pregnancy include: constriction of the ductus arteriosus prenatally, tricuspid incompetence, and pulmonary hypertension; non-closure of the ductus arteriosus postnatally which may be resistant to medical management; myocardial degenerative changes, platelet dysfunction with resultant bleeding, intracranial bleeding, renal dysfunction or failure, renal injury/dysgenesis which may result in prolonged or permanent renal failure, oligohydramnios, gastrointestinal bleeding or perforation, and increased risk of necrotizing enterocolitis. Use during the third trimester of pregnancy is not recommended.

In rats at a dose of one and one-half times the maximum human dose, there was an increase in the average length of gestation. Similar increases in the length of gestation have been observed with aspirin, indomethacin, and phenylbutazone, and may be related to inhibition of prostaglandin synthetase. Drugs of this class may cause dystocia and delayed parturition in pregnant animals.

Nursing Mothers

Diflunisal is excreted in human milk in concentrations of 2–7% of those in plasma. Because of the potential for serious adverse reactions in nursing infants from DOLOBID, a decision should be made whether to discontinue nursing or to discontinue the drug, taking into account the importance of the drug to the mother.

Pediatric Use

Safety and effectiveness of DOLOBID in pediatric patients have not been established. Use of DOLOBID in pediatric patients below the age of 12 years is not recommended.

The adverse effects observed following diflunisal administration to neonatal animals appear to be species, age, and dose-dependent. At dose levels approximately 3 times the usual human therapeutic dose, both aspirin (200 to 400 mg/kg/day) and diflunisal (80 mg/kg/day) resulted in death, leukocytosis, weight loss, and bilateral cataracts in neonatal (4 to 5-day-old) beagle puppies after 2 to 10 doses. Administration of an 80 mg/kg/day dose of diflunisal to 25-day-old puppies resulted in lower mortality, and did not produce cataracts. In newborn rats, a 400 mg/kg/day dose of aspirin resulted in increased mortality and some cataracts, whereas the effects of diflunisal administration at doses up to 140 mg/kg/day were limited to a decrease in average body weight gain.

Geriatric Use

As with any NSAID, caution should be exercised in treating the elderly (65 years and older) since advancing age appears to increase the possibility of adverse reactions. Elderly patients seem to tolerate ulceration or bleeding less well than other individuals and many spontaneous reports of fatal GI events are in this population (see WARNINGS, *Risk of GI Ulcerations, Bleeding and Perforation with NSAID Therapy*).

This drug is known to be substantially excreted by the kidney and the risk of toxic reactions to this drug may be greater in patients with impaired renal function. Because elderly patients are more likely to have decreased renal function, care should be taken in dose selection and it may be useful to monitor renal function (see PRECAUTIONS, *Renal Effects*).

ADVERSE REACTIONS

The adverse reactions observed in controlled clinical trials encompass observations in 2,427 patients.

Listed below are the adverse reactions reported in the 1,314 of these patients who received treatment in studies of two weeks or longer. Five hundred thirteen patients were treated for at least 24 weeks, 255 patients were treated for at least 48 weeks, and 46 patients were treated for 96 weeks. In general, the adverse reactions listed below were 2 to 14 times less frequent in the 1,113 patients who received short-term treatment for mild to moderate pain.

Incidence Greater Than 1%

Gastrointestinal

The most frequent types of adverse reactions occurring with DOLOBID are gastrointestinal: these include nausea**, vomiting, dyspepsia**, gastrointestinal pain**, diarrhea**, constipation, and flatulence.

Psychiatric

Somnolence, insomnia.

Central Nervous System

Dizziness.

Special Senses

Tinnitus.

Dermatologic

Rash**.

Miscellaneous

Headache**, fatigue/tiredness.

Incidence Less Than 1 in 100

The following adverse reactions, occurring less frequently than 1 in 100, were reported in clinical trials or since the drug was marketed. The probability exists of a causal relationship between DOLOBID and these adverse reactions.

Dermatologic

Erythema multiforme, exfoliative dermatitis, Stevens-Johnson syndrome, toxic epidermal necrolysis, urticaria, pruritus, sweating, dry mucous membranes, stomatitis, photosensitivity.

Gastrointestinal

Peptic ulcer, gastrointestinal bleeding, anorexia, eructation, gastrointestinal perforation, gastritis.

Liver function abnormalities; jaundice, sometimes with fever; cholestasis; hepatitis.

Hematologic

Thrombocytopenia; agranulocytosis; hemolytic anemia.

Genitourinary

Dysuria; renal impairment, including renal failure; interstitial nephritis; hematuria; proteinuria.

Psychiatric

Nervousness, depression, hallucinations, confusion, disorientation.

Central Nervous System

Vertigo; light-headedness; paresthesias.

Special Senses

Transient visual disturbances including blurred vision.

Hypersensitivity Reactions

Acute anaphylactic reaction with bronchospasm; angioedema; flushing.

Hypersensitivity vasculitis.

Hypersensitivity syndrome (see PRECAUTIONS).

Miscellaneous

Asthenia, edema.

Causal Relationship Unknown

Other reactions have been reported in clinical trials or since the drug was marketed, but occurred under circumstances where a causal relationship could not be established. However, in these rarely reported events, that possibility cannot be excluded. Therefore, these observations are listed to serve as alerting information to physicians.

Continued on next page

Information on the Merck & Co., Inc., products listed on these pages is from the prescribing information in use October 1, 2004. For information, please call 1-800-NSC-MERCK [1-800-672-6372].

Dolobid—Cont.

Respiratory
Dyspnea.
Cardiovascular
Palpitation, syncope.
Musculoskeletal
Muscle cramps.
Genitourinary
Nephrotic syndrome.
Special Senses
Hearing loss.
Miscellaneous
Chest pain.

A rare occurrence of fulminant necrotizing fasciitis, particularly in association with Group A β-hemolytic streptococcus, has been described in persons treated with non-steroidal anti-inflammatory agents, including diflunisal, sometimes with fatal outcome (see also PRECAUTIONS, *General*).

Potential Adverse Effects

In addition, a variety of adverse effects not observed with DOLOBID in clinical trials or in marketing experience, but reported with other non-steroidal analgesic/anti-inflammatory agents, should be considered potential adverse effects of DOLOBID.

**Incidence between 3% and 9%. Those reactions occurring in 1% to 3% are not marked with an asterisk.

OVERDOSAGE

Cases of overdosage have occurred and deaths have been reported. Most patients recovered without evidence of permanent sequelae. The most common signs and symptoms observed with overdosage were drowsiness, vomiting, nausea, diarrhea, hyperventilation, tachycardia, sweating, tinnitus, disorientation, stupor and coma. Diminished urine output and cardiorespiratory arrest have also been reported. The lowest dosage of DOLOBID at which a death has been reported was 15 grams without the presence of other drugs. In a mixed drug overdose, ingestion of 7.5 grams of DOLOBID resulted in death.

In the event of overdosage, the stomach should be emptied by inducing vomiting or by gastric lavage, and the patient carefully observed and given symptomatic and supportive treatment. Because of the high degree of protein binding, hemodialysis may not be effective.

The oral LD_{50} of the drug is 500 mg/kg and 826 mg/kg in female mice and female rats respectively.

DOSAGE AND ADMINISTRATION

Concentration-dependent pharmacokinetics prevail when DOLOBID is administered; a doubling of dosage produces a greater than doubling of drug accumulation. The effect becomes more apparent with repetitive doses.

For mild to moderate pain, an initial dose of 1000 mg followed by 500 mg every 12 hours is recommended for most patients. Following the initial dose, some patients may require 500 mg every 8 hours.

A lower dosage may be appropriate depending on such factors as pain severity, patient response, weight, or advanced age; for example, 500 mg initially, followed by 250 mg every 8–12 hours.

For osteoarthritis and rheumatoid arthritis, the suggested dosage range is 500 mg to 1000 mg daily in two divided doses. The dosage of DOLOBID may be increased or decreased according to patient response.

Maintenance doses higher than 1500 mg a day are not recommended.

DOLOBID may be administered with water, milk or meals. Tablets should be swallowed whole, not crushed or chewed.

HOW SUPPLIED

Tablets DOLOBID are capsule-shaped, film-coated tablets supplied as follows:

No. 3390—250 mg peach colored, coded DOLOBID on one side and MSD 675 on the other.
NDC 0006-0675-61 unit of use bottles of 60
(6505-01-164-0501, 250 mg 60's).

No. 3392—500 mg orange colored, coded DOLOBID on one side and MSD 697 on the other.
NDC 0006-0697-61 unit of use bottles of 60
(6505-01-144-9724, 500 mg 60's).

7928833 Issued July 1998

Shown in Product Identification Guide, page 323

EDECRIN® Tablets ℞
(Ethacrynic Acid)

Intravenous
SODIUM EDECRIN® ℞
(Ethacrynate Sodium)

EDECRIN* (Ethacrynic Acid) is a potent diuretic which, if given in excessive amounts, may lead to profound diuresis with water and electrolyte depletion. Therefore, careful medical supervision is required, and dose and dose schedule must be adjusted to the individual patient's needs (see DOSAGE AND ADMINISTRATION).

DESCRIPTION

Ethacrynic acid is an unsaturated ketone derivative of an aryloxyacetic acid. It is designated chemically as [2,3-dichloro-4-(2-methylene-1-oxobutyl)phenoxy] acetic acid, and has a molecular weight of 303.14. Ethacrynic acid is a white, or practically white, crystalline powder, very slightly soluble in water, but soluble in most organic solvents such as alcohols, chloroform, and benzene. Its empirical formula is $C_{13}H_{12}Cl_2O_4$ and its structural formula is:

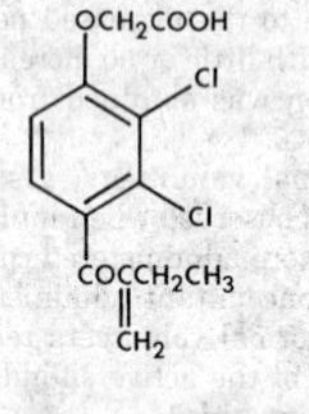

Ethacrynate sodium, the sodium salt of ethacrynic acid, is soluble in water at 25°C to the extent of about 7 percent. Solutions of the sodium salt are relatively stable at about pH 7 at room temperature for short periods, but as the pH or temperature increases the solutions are less stable. The molecular weight of ethacrynate sodium is 325.12. Its empirical formula is $C_{13}H_{11}Cl_2NaO_4$ and its structural formula is:

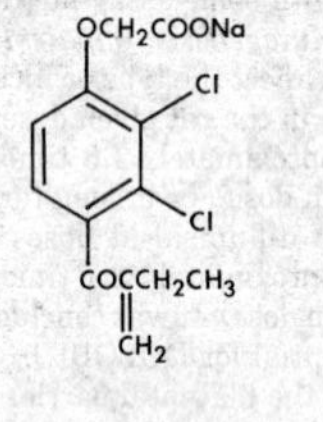

EDECRIN is supplied as 25 mg and 50 mg tablets for oral use. Each tablet contains the following inactive ingredients: colloidal silicon dioxide, lactose, magnesium stearate, starch and talc. The 50 mg tablet also contains D&C Yellow 10, FD&C Blue 1 and FD&C Yellow 6. Intravenous SODIUM EDECRIN* (Ethacrynate Sodium) is a sterile freeze-dried powder and is supplied in a vial containing:

Ethacrynate sodium equivalent to ethacrynic acid	50.0 mg
Inactive ingredients:	
Mannitol	62.5 mg

*Registered trademark of MERCK & CO., INC.

CLINICAL PHARMACOLOGY

Pharmacokinetics and Metabolism

EDECRIN acts on the ascending limb of the loop of Henle and on the proximal and distal tubules. Urinary output is usually dose dependent and related to the magnitude of fluid accumulation. Water and electrolyte excretion may be increased several times over that observed with thiazide diuretics, since EDECRIN inhibits reabsorption of a much greater proportion of filtered sodium than most other diuretic agents. Therefore, EDECRIN is effective in many patients who have significant degrees of renal insufficiency (see WARNINGS concerning deafness). EDECRIN has little or no effect on glomerular filtration or on renal blood flow, except following pronounced reductions in plasma volume when associated with rapid diuresis.

The electrolyte excretion pattern of ethacrynic acid varies from that of the thiazides and mercurial diuretics. Initial sodium and chloride excretion is usually substantial and chloride loss exceeds that of sodium. With prolonged administration, chloride excretion declines, and potassium and hydrogen ion excretion may increase. EDECRIN is effective whether or not there is clinical acidosis or alkalosis.

Although EDECRIN, in carefully controlled studies in animals and experimental subjects, produces a more favorable sodium/potassium excretion ratio than the thiazides, in patients with increased diuresis excessive amounts of potassium may be excreted.

Onset of action is rapid, usually within 30 minutes after an oral dose of EDECRIN or within 5 minutes after an intravenous injection of SODIUM EDECRIN. After oral use, diuresis peaks in about 2 hours and lasts about 6 to 8 hours. The sulfhydryl binding propensity of ethacrynic acid differs somewhat from that of the organomercurials. Its mode of action is not by carbonic anhydrase inhibition.

Ethacrynic acid does not cross the blood-brain barrier.

INDICATIONS AND USAGE

EDECRIN is indicated for treatment of edema when an agent with greater diuretic potential than those commonly employed is required.

1. Treatment of the edema associated with congestive heart failure, cirrhosis of the liver, and renal disease, including the nephrotic syndrome.
2. Short-term management of ascites due to malignancy, idiopathic edema, and lymphedema.
3. Short-term management of hospitalized pediatric patients, other than infants, with congenital heart disease or the nephrotic syndrome.
4. Intravenous SODIUM EDECRIN is indicated when a rapid onset of diuresis is desired, e.g., in acute pulmonary edema, or when gastrointestinal absorption is impaired or oral medication is not practicable.

CONTRAINDICATIONS

All diuretics, including ethacrynic acid, are contraindicated in anuria. If increasing electrolyte imbalance, azotemia, and/or oliguria occur during treatment of severe, progressive renal disease, the diuretic should be discontinued.

In a few patients this diuretic has produced severe, watery diarrhea. If this occurs, it should be discontinued and not used again.

Until further experience in infants is accumulated, therapy with oral and parenteral EDECRIN is contraindicated.

Hypersensitivity to any component of this product.

WARNINGS

The effects of EDECRIN on electrolytes are related to its renal pharmacologic activity and are dose dependent. The possibility of profound electrolyte and water loss may be avoided by weighing the patient throughout the treatment period, by careful adjustment of dosage, by initiating treatment with small doses, and by using the drug on an intermittent schedule when possible. When excessive diuresis occurs, the drug should be withdrawn until homeostasis is restored. When excessive electrolyte loss occurs, the dosage should be reduced or the drug temporarily withdrawn.

Initiation of diuretic therapy with EDECRIN in the cirrhotic patient with ascites is best carried out in the hospital. When maintenance therapy has been established, the individual can be satisfactorily followed as an outpatient.

EDECRIN should be given with caution to patients with advanced cirrhosis of the liver, particularly those with a history of previous episodes of electrolyte imbalance or hepatic encephalopathy. Like other diuretics it may precipitate hepatic coma and death.

Too vigorous a diuresis, as evidenced by rapid and excessive weight loss, may induce an acute hypotensive episode. In elderly cardiac patients, rapid contraction of plasma volume and the resultant hemoconcentration should be avoided to prevent the development of thromboembolic episodes, such as cerebral vascular thromboses and pulmonary emboli which may be fatal. Excessive loss of potassium in patients receiving digitalis glycosides may precipitate digitalis toxicity. Care should also be exercised in patients receiving potassium-depleting steroids.

A number of possibly drug-related deaths have occurred in critically ill patients refractory to other diuretics. These generally have fallen into two categories: (1) patients with severe myocardial disease who have been receiving digitalis and presumably developed acute hypokalemia with fatal arrhythmia; (2) patients with severely decompensated hepatic cirrhosis with ascites, with or without accompanying encephalopathy, who were in electrolyte imbalance and died because of intensification of the electrolyte defect.

Deafness, tinnitus, and vertigo with a sense of fullness in the ears have occurred, most frequently in patients with severe impairment of renal function. These symptoms have been associated most often with intravenous administration and with doses in excess of those recommended. The deafness has usually been reversible and of short duration (one to 24 hours). However, in some patients the hearing loss has been permanent. A number of these patients were also receiving drugs known to be ototoxic. EDECRIN may increase the ototoxic potential of other drugs (see PRECAUTIONS, *Drug Interactions*).

Lithium generally should not be given with diuretics (see PRECAUTIONS, *Drug Interactions*).

PRECAUTIONS

General

Weakness, muscle cramps, paresthesias, thirst, anorexia, and signs of hyponatremia, hypokalemia, and/or hypochloremic alkalosis may occur following vigorous or excessive diuresis and these may be accentuated by rigid salt restriction. Rarely tetany has been reported following vigorous diuresis. *During therapy with ethacrynic acid, liberalization of salt intake and supplementary potassium chloride are often necessary.*

When a metabolic alkalosis may be anticipated, e.g., in cirrhosis with ascites, the use of potassium chloride or a potassium-sparing agent before and during therapy with EDECRIN may mitigate or prevent the hypokalemia.

Loop diuretics have been shown to increase the urinary excretion of magnesium; this may result in hypomagnesemia.

The safety and efficacy of ethacrynic acid in hypertension have not been established. However, the dosage of coadministered antihypertensive agents may require adjustment.

Orthostatic hypotension may occur in patients receiving other antihypertensive agents when given ethacrynic acid.

EDECRIN has little or no effect on glomerular filtration or on renal blood flow, except following pronounced reductions in plasma volume when associated with rapid diuresis. A transient increase in serum urea nitrogen may occur. Usually, this is readily reversible when the drug is discontinued. As with other diuretics used in the treatment of renal edema, hypoproteinemia may reduce responsiveness to ethacrynic acid and the use of salt-poor albumin should be considered.

A number of drugs, including ethacrynic acid, have been shown to displace warfarin from plasma protein; a reduction in the usual anticoagulant dosage may be required in patients receiving both drugs.

EDECRIN may increase the risk of gastric hemorrhage associated with corticosteroid treatment.

Laboratory Tests

Frequent serum electrolyte, CO_2 and BUN determinations should be performed early in therapy and periodically thereafter during active diuresis. Any electrolyte abnormalities should be corrected or the drug temporarily withdrawn.

Increases in blood glucose and alterations in glucose tolerance tests have been observed in patients receiving EDECRIN.

Drug Interactions

Lithium generally should not be given with diuretics because they reduce its renal clearance and add a high risk of lithium toxicity. Read circulars for lithium preparations before use of such concomitant therapy.

EDECRIN may increase the ototoxic potential of other drugs such as aminoglycoside and some cephalosporin antibiotics. Their concurrent use should be avoided.

A number of drugs, including ethacrynic acid, have been shown to displace warfarin from plasma protein; a reduction in the usual anticoagulant dosage may be required in patients receiving both drugs.

In some patients, the administration of a non-steroidal anti-inflammatory agent can reduce the diuretic, natriuretic, and antihypertensive effects of loop, potassium-sparing and thiazide diuretics. Therefore, when EDECRIN and non-steroidal anti-inflammatory agents are used concomitantly, the patient should be observed closely to determine if the desired effect of the diuretic is obtained.

Carcinogenesis, Mutagenesis, Impairment of Fertility

There was no evidence of a tumorigenic effect in a 79-week oral chronic toxicity study in rats at doses up to 45 times the human dose.

Ethacrynic acid had no effect on fertility in a two-litter study in rats or a two-generation study in mice at 10 times the human dose.

Pregnancy

Pregnancy Category B: Reproduction studies in the mouse and rabbit at doses up to 50 times the human dose showed no evidence of external abnormalities of the fetus due to EDECRIN.

In a two-litter study in the dog and rat, oral doses of 5 or 20 mg/kg/day ($2^1/_2$ or 10 times the human dose), respectively, did not interfere with pregnancy or with growth and development of the pups. Although there was reduction in the mean body weights of the fetuses in a teratogenic study in the rat at a dose level of 100 mg/kg (50 times the human dose), there was no effect on mortality or postnatal development. Functional and morphologic abnormalities were not observed.

There are, however, no adequate and well-controlled studies in pregnant women. Since animal reproduction studies are not always predictive of human response, EDECRIN should be used during pregnancy only if clearly needed.

Nursing Mothers

It is not known whether this drug is excreted in human milk. Because many drugs are excreted in human milk and because of the potential for serious adverse reactions in nursing infants from EDECRIN, a decision should be made whether to discontinue nursing or to discontinue the drug, taking into account the importance of the drug to the mother.

Pediatric Use

There are no well-controlled clinical trials in pediatric patients. The information on oral dosing in pediatric patients, other than infants, is supported by evidence from empiric use in this age group.

For information on oral use in pediatric patients, other than infants, see INDICATIONS AND USAGE and DOSAGE AND ADMINISTRATION.

Safety and effectiveness of oral and parenteral use in infants have not been established (see CONTRAINDICATIONS).

Safety and effectiveness of intravenous use in pediatric patients have not been established (see DOSAGE AND ADMINISTRATION, *Intravenous Use).*

Geriatric Use

Of the total number of subjects in clinical studies of EDECRIN/SODIUM EDECRIN, approximately 224 patients (21%) were 65 to 74 years of age, while approximately 100 patients (9%) were 75 years of age and over. No overall differences in safety or effectiveness were observed between these subjects and younger subjects, and other reported clinical experience has not identified differences in responses between the elderly and younger patients, but greater sensitivity of some older individuals cannot be ruled out. (See WARNINGS.)

This drug is known to be substantially excreted by the kidney, and the risk of toxic reactions to this drug may be greater in patients with impaired renal function. Because elderly patients are more likely to have decreased renal function, care should be taken in dose selection, and it may be useful to monitor renal function. (See CONTRAINDICATIONS.)

ADVERSE REACTIONS

Gastrointestinal

Anorexia, malaise, abdominal discomfort or pain, dysphagia, nausea, vomiting, and diarrhea have occurred. These are more frequent with large doses or after one to three months of continuous therapy. A few patients have had sudden onset of profuse, watery diarrhea. Discontinue EDECRIN if diarrhea is severe and do not give it again. Gastrointestinal bleeding has occurred in some patients. Rarely, acute pancreatitis has been reported.

Metabolic

Reversible hyperuricemia and acute gout have been reported. Acute symptomatic hypoglycemia with convulsions occurred in two uremic patients who received doses above those recommended. Hyperglycemia has been reported. Rarely, jaundice and abnormal liver function tests have been reported in seriously ill patients receiving multiple drug therapy, including EDECRIN.

Hematologic

Agranulocytosis or severe neutropenia has been reported in a few critically ill patients also receiving agents known to produce this effect. Thrombocytopenia has been reported rarely. Henoch-Schönlein purpura has been reported rarely in patients with rheumatic heart disease receiving multiple drug therapy, including EDECRIN.

Special Senses (See WARNINGS)

Deafness, tinnitus and vertigo with a sense of fullness in the ears, and blurred vision have occurred.

Central Nervous System

Headache, fatigue, apprehension, confusion.

Miscellaneous

Skin rash, fever, chills, hematuria.

SODIUM EDECRIN occasionally has caused local irritation and pain after intravenous use.

OVERDOSAGE

Overdosage may lead to excessive diuresis with electrolyte depletion and dehydration.

In the event of overdosage, symptomatic and supportive measures should be employed. Emesis should be induced or gastric lavage performed. Correct dehydration, electrolyte imbalance, hepatic coma, and hypotension by established procedures. If required, give oxygen or artificial respiration for respiratory impairment.

In the mouse, the oral LD_{50} of ethacrynic acid is 627 mg/kg and the intravenous LD_{50} of ethacrynate sodium is 175 mg/kg.

DOSAGE AND ADMINISTRATION

Dosage must be regulated carefully to prevent a more rapid or substantial loss of fluid or electrolyte than is indicated or necessary. The magnitude of diuresis and natriuresis is largely dependent on the degree of fluid accumulation present in the patient. Similarly, the extent of potassium excretion is determined in large measure by the presence and magnitude of aldosteronism.

Oral Use

EDECRIN is available for oral use as 25 mg and 50 mg tablets.

Dosage: To Initiate Diuresis

In Adults: The smallest dose required to produce gradual weight loss (about 1 to 2 pounds per day) is recommended. Onset of diuresis usually occurs at 50 to 100 mg for adults. After diuresis has been achieved, the minimally effective dose (usually from 50 to 200 mg daily) may be given on a continuous or intermittent dosage schedule. Dosage adjustments are usually in 25 to 50 mg increments to avoid derangement of water and electrolyte excretion.

The patient should be weighed under standard conditions before and during the institution of diuretic therapy with this compound. Small alterations in dose should effectively prevent a massive diuretic response. The following schedule may be helpful in determining the smallest effective dose.

Day 1—50 mg (single dose) after a meal
Day 2—50 mg twice daily after meals, if necessary
Day 3—100 mg in the morning and 50 to 100 mg following the afternoon or evening meal, depending upon response to the morning dose.

A few patients may require initial and maintenance doses as high as 200 mg twice daily. These higher doses, which should be achieved gradually, are most often required in patients with severe, refractory edema.

In Pediatric Patients (excluding infants, see CONTRAINDICATIONS): The initial dose should be 25 mg. Careful stepwise increments in dosage of 25 mg should be made to achieve effective maintenance.

Maintenance Therapy

It is usually possible to reduce the dosage and frequency of administration once dry weight has been achieved.

EDECRIN (Ethacrynic Acid) may be given intermittently after an effective diuresis is obtained with the regimen outlined above. Dosage may be on an alternate daily schedule or more prolonged periods of diuretic therapy may be interspersed with rest periods. Such an intermittent dosage schedule allows time for correction of any electrolyte imbalance and may provide a more efficient diuretic response.

The chloruretic effect of this agent may give rise to retention of bicarbonate and a metabolic alkalosis. This may be corrected by giving chloride (ammonium chloride or arginine chloride). Ammonium chloride should not be given to cirrhotic patients.

EDECRIN has additive effects when used with other diuretics. For example, a patient who is on maintenance dosage of an oral diuretic may require additional intermittent diuretic therapy, such as an organomercurial, for the maintenance of basal weight. The intermittent use of EDECRIN orally may eliminate the need for injections of organomercurials. Small doses of EDECRIN may be added to existing diuretic regimens to maintain basal weight. This drug may potentiate the action of carbonic anhydrase inhibitors, with augmentation of natriuresis and kaliuresis. Therefore, when adding EDECRIN the initial dose and changes of dose should be in 25 mg increments, to avoid electrolyte depletion. Rarely, patients who failed to respond to ethacrynic acid have responded to older established agents.

While many patients do not require supplemental potassium, the use of potassium chloride or potassium-sparing agents, or both, during treatment with EDECRIN is advisable, especially in cirrhotic or nephrotic patients and in patients receiving digitalis.

Salt liberalization usually prevents the development of hyponatremia and hypochloremia. During treatment with EDECRIN, salt may be liberalized to a greater extent than with other diuretics. Cirrhotic patients, however, usually require at least moderate salt restriction concomitant with diuretic therapy.

Intravenous Use

Intravenous SODIUM EDECRIN is for intravenous use when oral intake is impractical or in urgent conditions, such as acute pulmonary edema.

The usual intravenous dose for the average sized adult is 50 mg, or 0.5 to 1.0 mg per kg of body weight. Usually only one dose has been necessary; occasionally a second dose at a new injection site, to avoid possible thrombophlebitis, may be required. A single intravenous dose not exceeding 100 mg has been used in critical situations.

Insufficient pediatric experience precludes recommendation for this age group.

To reconstitute the dry material, add 50 mL of 5 percent Dextrose Injection, or Sodium Chloride Injection to the vial. Occasionally, some 5 percent Dextrose Injection solutions may have a low pH (below 5). The resulting solution with such a diluent may be hazy or opalescent. Intravenous use of such a solution is not recommended. Inspect the vial containing Intravenous SODIUM EDECRIN for particulate matter and discoloration before use.

The solution may be given slowly through the tubing of a running infusion or by direct intravenous injection over a period of several minutes. Do not mix this solution with whole blood or its derivatives. Discard unused reconstituted solution after 24 hours.

SODIUM EDECRIN should not be given subcutaneously or intramuscularly because of local pain and irritation.

HOW SUPPLIED

No. 3321—Tablets EDECRIN, 25 mg, are white, capsule shaped, scored tablets, coded MSD 65 on one side and EDECRIN on the other. They are supplied as follows:
NDC 0006-0065-68 in bottles of 100.

No. 3322—Tablets EDECRIN, 50 mg, are green, capsule shaped, scored tablets, coded MSD 90 on one side and EDECRIN on the other. They are supplied as follows:
NDC 0006-0090-68 in bottles of 100

No. 3620—Intravenous SODIUM EDECRIN is a dry white material either in a plug form or as a powder. It is supplied in vials containing ethacrynate sodium equivalent to 50 mg of ethacrynic acid, **NDC** 0006-3620-50.

Storage:

Store in a tightly closed container at 25°C (77°F); excursions permitted to 15–30°C (59–86°F) [see USP Controlled Room Temperature].

9350229 Issued April 2003

Shown in Product Identification Guide, page 323

ELSPAR® ℞
(Asparaginase)

WARNINGS

It is recommended that asparaginase be administered to patients only in a hospital setting under the supervision of a physician who is qualified by training and experience to administer cancer chemotherapeutic agents, because of the possibility of severe reactions, including anaphylaxis and sudden death. The physician must be prepared to treat anaphylaxis at each administration of the drug. In the treatment of each patient the physician

Continued on next page

Information on the Merck & Co., Inc., products listed on these pages is from the prescribing information in use October 1, 2004. For information, please call 1-800-NSC-MERCK [1-800-672-6372].

Elspar—Cont.

must weigh carefully the possibility of achieving therapeutic benefit versus the risk of toxicity.
Special handling procedures should be followed (see DOSAGE AND ADMINISTRATION, *Special Handling*).

DESCRIPTION

ELSPAR* (Asparaginase) contains the enzyme L-asparagine amidohydrolase, type EC-2, derived from *Escherichia coli*. It is a white crystalline powder that is freely soluble in water and practically insoluble in methanol, acetone and chloroform. Its activity is expressed in terms of International Units (I.U.) according to the recommendation of the International Union of Biochemistry. The specific activity of ELSPAR is at least 225 I.U. per milligram of protein and each vial contains 10,000 I.U. of asparaginase and 80 mg of mannitol, an inactive ingredient, as a sterile, white lyophilized plug or powder for intravenous or intramuscular injection after reconstitution.

*Registered trademark of MERCK & CO., INC.

CLINICAL PHARMACOLOGY

Action
In a significant number of patients with acute leukemia, particularly lymphocytic, the malignant cells are dependent on an exogenous source of asparagine for survival. Normal cells, however, are able to synthesize asparagine and thus are affected less by the rapid depletion produced by treatment with the enzyme asparaginase. This is a unique approach to therapy based on a metabolic defect in asparagine synthesis of some malignant cells. ELSPAR, derived from *Escherichia coli*, is effective in inducing remissions in some patients with acute lymphocytic leukemia.

Asparagine Dependence Test
An asparagine dependence test has been utilized during the investigational studies. In this test leukemic cells obtained from some marrow cultures could be shown to require asparagine in *vitro*, suggesting sensitivity to asparaginase therapy in *vivo*. However, present data indicate that the correlation between asparagine dependence in such tests and the final response to therapy is sufficiently poor that the test is not recommended as a basis for selection of patients for treatment.

Pharmacokinetics and Metabolism
In a study in patients with metastatic cancer and leukemia, initial plasma levels of L-asparaginase following intravenous administration were correlated to dose. Daily administration resulted in a cumulative increase in plasma levels. Plasma half-life varied from 8 to 30 hours; it did not appear to be influenced by dosage, either single or repetitive, and could not be correlated with age, sex, surface area, renal or hepatic function, diagnosis or extent of disease. Apparent volume of distribution was approximately 70–80% of estimated plasma volume. There was some slow movement of asparaginase from vascular to extravascular, extracellular space. L-asparaginase was detected in the lymph. Cerebrospinal fluid levels were less than 1% of concurrent plasma levels. Only trace amounts appeared in the urine.
In a study in which patients with leukemia and metastatic cancer received intramuscular L-asparaginase, peak plasma levels of asparaginase were reached 14 to 24 hours after dosing. Plasma half-life was 39 to 49 hours. No asparaginase was detected in the urine.

INDICATIONS AND USAGE

ELSPAR is indicated in the therapy of patients with acute lymphocytic leukemia. This agent is useful primarily in combination with other chemotherapeutic agents in the induction of remissions of the disease in pediatric patients. ELSPAR should not be used as the sole induction agent unless combination therapy is deemed inappropriate. ELSPAR is not recommended for maintenance therapy.

CONTRAINDICATIONS

ELSPAR is contraindicated in patients with pancreatitis or a history of pancreatitis. Acute hemorrhagic pancreatitis, in some instances fatal, has been reported following asparaginase administration. Asparaginase is also contraindicated in patients who have had previous anaphylactic reactions to it.

WARNINGS

Allergic reactions to asparaginase are frequent and may occur during the primary course of therapy. They are not completely predictable on the basis of the intradermal skin test. Anaphylaxis and death have occurred even in a hospital setting with experienced observers.
Once a patient has received ELSPAR as part of a treatment regimen, retreatment with this agent at a later time is associated with increased risk of hypersensitivity reactions. In patients found by skin testing to be hypersensitive to asparaginase, and in any patient who has received a previous course of therapy with asparaginase, therapy with this agent should be instituted or reinstituted only after successful desensitization, and then only if in the judgement of the physician the possible benefit is greater than the increased risk. Desensitization itself may be hazardous. (See DOSAGE AND ADMINISTRATION, *Intradermal Skin Test.*)
In view of the unpredictability of the adverse reactions to asparaginase, it is recommended that this product be used in a hospital setting. Asparaginase has an adverse effect on liver function in the majority of patients. Therapy with asparaginase may increase pre-existing liver impairment caused by prior therapy or the underlying disease. Because of this there is a possibility that asparaginase may increase the toxicity of other medications.
The administration of ELSPAR *intravenously concurrently with or immediately before* a course of vincristine and prednisone may be associated with increased toxicity. (See DOSAGE AND ADMINISTRATION, *Recommended Induction Regimens.*)

PRECAUTIONS

General
This drug may have toxic properties and must be handled and administered with care. ELSPAR may be irritating to eyes, skin, and the upper respiratory tract. Inhalation of dust or aerosols and contact with skin or mucous membranes, especially those of the eyes, must be avoided. (See DOSAGE AND ADMINISTRATION, *Special Handling.*)
Asparaginase has been reported to have immunosuppressive activity in animal experiments. Accordingly, the possibility that use of the drug in man may predispose to infection should be considered.
Asparaginase toxicity is reported to be greater in adults than in pediatric patients.

Laboratory Tests
The fall in circulating lymphoblasts often is quite marked; normal or below normal leukocyte counts are noted frequently within the first several days after initiating therapy. This may be accompanied by a marked rise in serum uric acid. The possible development of uric acid nephropathy should be borne in mind. Appropriate preventive measures should be taken, e.g., allopurinol, increased fluid intake, alkalization of urine. As a guide to the effects of therapy, the patient's peripheral blood count and bone marrow should be monitored frequently.
Frequent serum amylase determinations should be obtained to detect early evidence of pancreatitis. If pancreatitis occurs, therapy should be stopped and not reinstituted. Blood sugar should be monitored during therapy with ELSPAR because hyperglycemia may occur.

Drug Interactions
Tissue culture and animal studies indicate that ELSPAR can diminish or abolish the effect of methotrexate on malignant cells. This effect on methotrexate activity persists as long as plasma asparagine levels are suppressed. These results would seem to dictate against the clinical use of methotrexate with ELSPAR, or during the period following ELSPAR therapy when plasma asparagine levels are below normal.

Drug/Laboratory Test Interactions
L-asparaginase has been reported to interfere with the interpretation of thyroid function tests by producing a rapid and marked reduction in serum concentrations of thyroxine-binding globulin within two days after the first dose. Serum concentrations of thyroxine-binding globulin returned to pretreatment values within four weeks of the last dose of L-asparaginase.

Animal Toxicology
A one-month intravenous toxicity study of ELSPAR in dogs at doses of 250, 1000, and 2000 I.U./kg/day revealed reduced serum total protein and albumin with loss of body weight at the highest dose level and anorexia, emesis, and diarrhea at all dosage levels. A similar study in monkeys at doses of 100, 300, and 1000 I.U./kg/day also revealed reduction of serum total protein and albumin and body weight loss at all dosage levels. Bromsulfalein retention and fatty changes in the liver were noted in monkeys that were given 300 and 1000 I.U./kg/day. The rabbit was unusually sensitive to ELSPAR since a single intravenous dose of 1000 I.U./kg caused hypocalcemia associated with necrosis of the parathyroid cells, convulsions, and death in about one third of the animals. Some rabbits that died showed small thymic and lymph node hemorrhages and necrosis of the germinal centers in the lymph nodes and spleen. The intravenous administration of calcium gluconate alleviated or prevented the adverse effects.
Changes in the pancreatic islets (not pancreatitis) ranging from edema to necrosis were observed in the rabbits in the acute intravenous toxicity studies (doses of 12,500 to 50,000 I.U./kg) but not in rabbits that received 1000 I.U./kg. The anatomical changes and the hypocalcemia found in the rabbits were not observed in the subacute intravenous studies in the dogs and monkeys.

Carcinogenesis, Mutagenesis, Impairment of Fertility
The intraperitoneal injection of 2500 I.U./kg/ day for 4 days in newborn Swiss mice resulted in a small increase in pulmonary adenomas; lymphatic leukemia was not increased. L-asparaginase at concentrations of 152-909 I.U./plate was not mutagenic in the Ames microbial mutagen test with or without metabolic activation.
There are no adequate studies on the effects of asparaginase on fertility.

Pregnancy
Pregnancy Category C. In mice and rats ELSPAR has been shown to retard the weight gain of mothers and fetuses when given in doses of more than 1000 I.U./kg (the recommended human dose). Resorptions, gross abnormalities and skeletal abnormalities were observed. The intravenous administration of 50 or 100 I.U./kg (one-twentieth or one-tenth of the human dose) to pregnant rabbits on Day 8 and 9 of gestation resulted in dose dependent embryotoxicity and gross abnormalities. There are no adequate and well-controlled studies in pregnant women. ELSPAR should be used during pregnancy only if the potential benefit justifies the potential risk to the fetus.

Nursing Mothers
It is not known whether this drug is secreted in human milk. Because many drugs are secreted in human milk and because of the potential for serious adverse reactions in nursing infants from ELSPAR, a decision should be made whether to discontinue nursing or to discontinue the drug, taking into account the importance of the drug to the mother.

Pediatric Use
Asparaginase toxicity is reported to be greater in adults than in pediatric patients.

Geriatric Use
Clinical studies of ELSPAR did not include sufficient numbers of subjects aged 65 and over to determine whether they respond differently from younger subjects. Other reported clinical experience has not identified differences in responses between the elderly and younger patients. In general, dose selection for an elderly patient should be cautious, usually starting at the low end of the dosing range, reflecting the greater frequency of decreased hepatic, renal, or cardiac function, and of concomitant disease or other drug therapy.

ADVERSE REACTIONS

Allergic reactions, including skin rashes, urticaria, arthralgia, respiratory distress, and acute anaphylaxis have been reported. (See WARNINGS.) Acute reactions have occurred in the absence of a positive skin test and during continued maintenance of therapeutic serum levels of ELSPAR.
In pediatric patients with advanced leukemia, a lower incidence of anaphylaxis has been reported with intramuscular administration, although there was a higher incidence of milder hypersensitivity reactions than with intravenous administration.
Fatal hyperthermia has been reported.
Pancreatitis, sometimes fulminant and fatal, has occurred during or following therapy with ELSPAR.
Hyperglycemia with glucosuria and polyuria has been reported in low incidence. Serum and urine acetone usually have been absent or negligible in these patients; this syndrome thus resembles hyperosmolar, nonketotic, hyperglycemia induced by a variety of other agents. This complication usually responds to discontinuance of ELSPAR, judicious use of intravenous fluid, and insulin, but may be fatal on occasion.
In addition to hypofibrinogenemia, depression of various other clotting factors has been reported. Most marked has been a decrease in plasma levels of factors V and VIII with a variable decrease in factors VII and IX. A decrease in circulating platelets has occurred in low incidence which, together with the increased levels of fibrin degradation products in the serum, may indicate development of a consumption coagulopathy. Bleeding has been a problem in only a minority of patients with demonstrable coagulopathy. However, intracranial hemorrhage and fatal bleeding associated with low fibrinogen levels have been reported. Increased fibrinolytic activity, apparently compensatory in nature, also has occurred.
Some patients have shown central nervous system effects consisting of depression, somnolence, fatigue, coma, confusion, agitation, and hallucinations varying from mild to severe. Rarely, a Parkinson-like syndrome has occurred, with tremor and a progressive increase in muscular tone. These side effects usually have reversed spontaneously after treatment was stopped. Therapy with ELSPAR is associated with an increase in blood ammonia during the conversion of asparagine to aspartic acid by the enzyme. No clear correlation exists between the degree of elevation of blood ammonia levels and the appearance of CNS changes. Chills, fever, nausea, vomiting, anorexia, abdominal cramps, weight loss, headache, and irritability may occur and usually are mild. Azotemia, usually pre-renal, occurs frequently. Acute renal shut down and fatal renal insufficiency have been reported during treatment. Proteinuria has occurred infrequently.
A variety of liver function abnormalities have been reported, including elevations of AST (SGOT), ALT (SGPT), alkaline phosphatase, bilirubin (direct and indirect), and depression of serum albumin, cholesterol (total and esters), and plasma fibrinogen. Increases and decreases of total lipids have occurred. Marked hypoalbuminemia associated with peripheral edema has been reported. However, these abnormalities usually are reversible on discontinuance of therapy and some reversal may occur during the course of therapy. Fatty changes in the liver have been documented by biopsy. Malabsorption syndrome has been reported.
Rarely, transient bone marrow depression has been observed, as evidenced by a delay in return of hemoglobin or hematocrit levels to normal in patients undergoing hematologic remission of leukemia. Marked leukopenia has been reported.

OVERDOSAGE

The acute intravenous LD_{50} of ELSPAR for mice was about 500,000 I.U./kg and for rabbits about 22,000 I.U./kg.

DOSAGE AND ADMINISTRATION

This drug may have toxic properties and must be handled and administered with care. Special handling procedures should be reviewed prior to handling and followed diligently during reconstitution and administration. Inhalation of dust or aerosols and contact with skin or mucous membranes, especially those of the eyes, must be avoided. (See DOSAGE AND ADMINISTRATION, *Special Handling*.)

As a component of selected multiple agent induction regimens, ELSPAR may be administered by either the intravenous or the intramuscular route. When administered intravenously this enzyme should be given over a period of not less than thirty minutes through the side arm of an already running infusion of Sodium Chloride Injection or Dextrose Injection 5% (D_5W). ELSPAR has little tendency to cause phlebitis when given intravenously. Anaphylactic reactions require the immediate use of epinephrine, oxygen, and intravenous steroids.

When administering ELSPAR intramuscularly, the volume at a single injection site should be limited to 2 ml. If a volume greater than 2 ml is to be administered, two injection sites should be used.

Unfavorable interactions of ELSPAR with some antitumor agents have been demonstrated. It is recommended therefore, that ELSPAR be used in combination regimens only by physicians familiar with the benefits and risks of a given regimen. During the period of its inhibition of protein synthesis and cell replication ELSPAR may interfere with the action of drugs such as methotrexate which require cell replication for their lethal effect. ELSPAR may interfere with the enzymatic detoxification of other drugs, particularly in the liver.

Recommended Induction Regimens:

When using chemotherapeutic agents in combination for the induction of remissions in patients with acute lymphocytic leukemia, regimens are sought which provide maximum chance of success while avoiding excessive cumulative toxicity or negative drug interactions.

One of the following combination regimens incorporating ELSPAR is recommended for acute lymphocytic leukemia in pediatric patients:

In the regimens below, Day 1 is considered to be the first day of therapy.

Regimen I

Prednisone 40 mg/square meter of body surface area per day orally in three divided doses for 15 days, followed by tapering of the dosage as follows:

20 mg/square meter for 2 days, 10 mg/square meter for 2 days, 5 mg/square meter for 2 days, 2.5 mg/square meter for 2 days and then discontinue.

Vincristine sulfate 2 mg/square meter of body surface area intravenously once weekly on Days 1, 8, and 15 of the treatment period. The maximum single dose should not exceed 2.0 mg.

Asparaginase 1,000 I.U./kg/day intravenously for ten successive days beginning on Day 22 of the treatment period.

Regimen II

Prednisone 40 mg/square meter of body surface area per day orally in three divided doses for 28 days (the total daily dose should be to the nearest 2.5 mg), following which the dosage of prednisone should be discontinued gradually over a 14 day period.

Vincristine sulfate 1.5 mg/square meter of body surface area intravenously weekly for four doses, on Days 1, 8, 15, and 22 of the treatment period. The maximum single dose should not exceed 2.0 mg.

Asparaginase 6,000 I.U./square meter of body surface area intramuscularly on Days 4, 7, 10, 13, 16, 19, 22, 25, and 28 of the treatment period. When a remission is obtained with either of the above regimens, appropriate maintenance therapy must be instituted. ELSPAR should not be used as part of a maintenance regimen. The above regimens do not preclude a need for special therapy directed toward the prevention of central nervous system leukemia.

It should be noted that ELSPAR has been used in combination regimens other than those recommended above. It is important to keep in mind that ELSPAR administered intravenously concurrently with or immediately before a course of vincristine and prednisone may be associated with increased toxicity. Physicians using a given regimen should be thoroughly familiar with its benefits and risks. Clinical data are insufficient for a recommendation concerning the use of combination regimens in adults. Asparaginase toxicity is reported to be greater in adults than in pediatric patients.

Use of ELSPAR as the sole induction agent should be undertaken only in an unusual situation when a combined regimen is inappropriate because of toxicity or other specific patient-related factors, or in cases refractory to other therapy. When ELSPAR is to be used as the sole induction agent for pediatric patients or adults the recommended dosage regimen is 200 I.U./kg/ day intravenously for 28 days. When complete remissions were obtained with this regimen, they were of short duration, 1 to 3 months. ELSPAR has been used as the sole induction agent in other regimens. Physicians using a given regimen should be thoroughly familiar with its benefits and risks.

Patients undergoing induction therapy must be carefully monitored and the therapeutic regimen adjusted according to response and toxicity.

Such adjustments should always involve decreasing dosages of one or more agents or discontinuation depending on the degree of toxicity. Patients who have received a course of ELSPAR, if retreated, have an increased risk of hypersensitivity reactions. Therefore, retreatment should be undertaken only when the benefit of such therapy is weighed against the increased risk.

Intradermal Skin Test:

Because of the occurrence of allergic reactions, an intradermal skin test should be performed prior to the initial administration of ELSPAR and when ELSPAR is given after an interval of a week or more has elapsed between doses. The skin test solution may be prepared as follows: Reconstitute the contents of a 10,000 I.U. vial with 5.0 ml of diluent. From this solution (2,000 I.U./ml) withdraw 0.1 ml and inject it into another vial containing 9.9 ml of diluent, yielding a skin test solution of approximately 20.0 I.U./ml. Use 0.1 ml of this solution (about 2.0 I.U.) for the intradermal skin test. The skin test site should be observed for at least one hour for the appearance of a wheal or erythema either of which indicates a positive reaction. An allergic reaction even to the skin test dose in certain sensitized individuals may rarely occur. A negative skin test reaction does not preclude the possibility of the development of an allergic reaction.

Desensitization:

Desensitization should be performed before administering the first dose of ELSPAR on initiation of therapy in positive reactors, and on retreatment of any patient in whom such therapy is deemed necessary after carefully weighing the increased risk of hypersensitivity reactions. Rapid desensitization of the patient may be attempted with progressively increasing amounts of intravenously administered ELSPAR provided adequate precautions are taken to treat an acute allergic reaction should it occur. One reported schedule begins with a total of 1 I.U. given intravenously and doubles the dose every 10 minutes, provided no reaction has occurred, until the accumulated total amount given equals the planned doses for that day.

For convenience the following table is included to calculate the number of doses necessary to reach the patient's total dose for that day:

Injection Number	ELSPAR Dose in I.U.	Accumulated Total Dose
1	1	1
2	2	3
3	4	7
4	8	15
5	16	31
6	32	63
7	64	127
8	128	255
9	256	511
10	512	1023
11	1024	2047
12	2048	4095
13	4096	8191
14	8192	16383
15	16384	32767
16	32768	65535
17	65536	131071
18	131072	262143

For example: A patient weighing 20 kg who is to receive 200 I.U./kg (total dose 4000 I.U.) would receive injections 1 through 12 during desensitization.

Directions for Reconstitution

This drug may have toxic properties and must be handled and administered with care. Inhalation of dust or aerosols and contact with skin or mucous membranes, especially those of the eyes, must be avoided. Appropriate protective equipment should be worn when handling ELSPAR. (See *Special Handling*.)

Parenteral drug products should be inspected visually for particulate matter and discoloration prior to administration whenever solution and container permit. When reconstituted, ELSPAR should be a clear, colorless solution. If the solution becomes cloudy, discard.

For Intravenous Use

Reconstitute with Sterile Water for Injection or with Sodium Chloride Injection. The volume recommended for reconstitution is 5 ml for the 10,000 unit vials. Ordinary shaking during reconstitution does not inactivate the enzyme. This solution may be used for direct intravenous administration within an eight hour period following restoration. For administration by infusion, solutions should be diluted with the isotonic solutions, Sodium Chloride Injection or Dextrose Injection 5%. These solutions should be infused within eight hours and only if clear.

Occasionally, a very small number of gelatinous fiber-like particles may develop on standing. Filtration through a 5.0 micron filter during administration will remove the particles with no resultant loss in potency. Some loss of potency has been observed with the use of a 0.2 micron filter.

For Intramuscular Use

When ELSPAR is administered intramuscularly according to the schedule cited in the induction regimen, reconstitution is carried out by adding 2 ml Sodium Chloride Injection to the 10,000 unit vial. The resulting solution should be used within eight hours and only if clear.

Special Handling

L-asparaginase may be irritating to eyes, skin and the upper respiratory tract. It has also been shown to be embryotoxic and teratogenic by the intravenous route in animal studies. Due to the drug's potential toxic properties, appropriate precautions including the use of appropriate safety equipment are recommended for the preparation of ELSPAR for administration. Inhalation of dust or aerosols and contact with skin or mucous membranes, especially those of the eyes, must be avoided. The National Institutes of Health presently recommends that the preparation of injectable anti-neoplastic drugs should be performed in a Class II laminar flow biological safety cabinet. Personnel preparing drugs of this class should wear chemical resistant, impervious gloves, safety goggles, outer garments and shoe covers. Additional body garments should be used based upon the task being performed (e.g., sleevelets, apron, gauntlets, disposable suits) to avoid exposed skin surfaces and inhalation of vapors and dust. Appropriate techniques should be used to remove potentially contaminated clothing. Several other guidelines for proper handling and disposal of antineoplastic drugs have been published and should be considered.

Accidental Contact Measures

Should accidental eye contact occur, copious irrigation for at least 15 minutes with water, normal saline or a balanced salt ophthalmic irrigating solution should be instituted immediately, followed by prompt ophthalmologic consultation. Should accidental skin contact occur, the affected part should be washed immediately with soap and water. Medical attention should be sought. If inhaled, remove from exposure and seek medical attention. (See PRECAUTIONS, *General* and DOSAGE AND ADMINISTRATION.)

HOW SUPPLIED

No. 4612 — ELSPAR is a white lyophilized plug or powder supplied as follows:

NDC 0006-4612-00 in a sterile 10 ml vial containing 10,000 I.U. of asparaginase and 80 mg mannitol, an inactive ingredient

(6505-01-153-9650 10 mL vial).

Storage

Store at 2–8°C (36–46°F). ELSPAR does not contain a preservative. Unused, reconstituted solution should be stored at 2–8°C (36–46°F) and discarded after eight hours, or sooner if it becomes cloudy.

9463116 Issued August 2002.

EMEND® Capsules ℞

[ē′mĕnd]
(aprepitant)

DESCRIPTION

EMEND* (aprepitant) is a substance P/neurokinin 1 (NK_1) receptor antagonist, chemically described as 5-[[(2*R*,3*S*)-2-[(1*R*)-1-[3,5-bis(trifluoromethyl)phenyl]ethoxy]-3-(4-fluorophenyl)-4-morpholinyl]methyl]-1,2-dihydro-3*H*-1,2,4-triazol-3-one.

Its empirical formula is $C_{23}H_{21}F_7N_4O_3$, and its structural formula is:

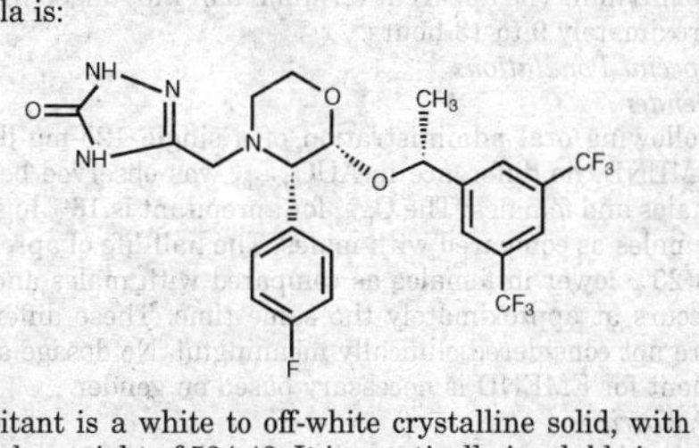

Aprepitant is a white to off-white crystalline solid, with a molecular weight of 534.43. It is practically insoluble in water. Aprepitant is sparingly soluble in ethanol and isopropyl acetate and slightly soluble in acetonitrile.

Each capsule of EMEND for oral administration contains either 80 mg or 125 mg of aprepitant and the following inactive ingredients: sucrose, microcrystalline cellulose, hydroxypropyl cellulose and sodium lauryl sulfate. The capsule shell excipients are gelatin and titanium dioxide. The 125-mg capsule also contains red ferric oxide and yellow ferric oxide.

*Registered trademark of MERCK & CO., Inc., Whitehouse Station, New Jersey, 08889 USA

CLINICAL PHARMACOLOGY

Mechanism of Action

Aprepitant is a selective high-affinity antagonist of human substance P/neurokinin 1 (NK_1) receptors. Aprepitant has

Continued on next page

Information on the Merck & Co., Inc., products listed on these pages is from the prescribing information in use October 1, 2004. For information, please call 1-800-NSC-MERCK [1-800-672-6372].

Emend—Cont.

little or no affinity for serotonin (5-HT_3), dopamine, and corticosteroid receptors, the targets of existing therapies for chemotherapy-induced nausea and vomiting (CINV).
Aprepitant has been shown in animal models to inhibit emesis induced by cytotoxic chemotherapeutic agents, such as cisplatin, via central actions. Animal and human Positron Emission Tomography (PET) studies with aprepitant have shown that it crosses the blood brain barrier and occupies brain NK_1 receptors. Animal and human studies show that aprepitant augments the antiemetic activity of the 5-HT_3-receptor antagonist ondansetron and the corticosteroid dexamethasone and inhibits both the acute and delayed phases of cisplatin-induced emesis.

Pharmacokinetics

Absorption

The mean absolute oral bioavailability of aprepitant is approximately 60 to 65% and the mean peak plasma concentration (C_{max}) of aprepitant occurred at approximately 4 hours (T_{max}). Oral administration of the capsule with a standard breakfast had no clinically meaningful effect on the bioavailability of aprepitant.
The pharmacokinetics of aprepitant are non-linear across the clinical dose range. In healthy young adults, the increase in $AUC_{0\text{-}\infty}$ was 26% greater than dose proportional between 80-mg and 125-mg single doses administered in the fed state.
Following oral administration of a single 125-mg dose of EMEND on Day 1 and 80 mg once daily on Days 2 and 3, the $AUC_{0\text{-}24hr}$ was approximately 19.6 mcg•hr/mL and 21.2 mcg•hr/mL on Day 1 and Day 3, respectively. The C_{max} of 1.6 mcg/mL and 1.4 mcg/mL were reached in approximately 4 hours (T_{max}) on Day 1 and Day 3, respectively.

Distribution

Aprepitant is greater than 95% bound to plasma proteins. The mean apparent volume of distribution at steady state (Vd_{ss}) is approximately 70 L in humans.
Aprepitant crosses the placenta in rats and rabbits and crosses the blood brain barrier in humans (see CLINICAL PHARMACOLOGY, *Mechanism of Action*).

Metabolism

Aprepitant undergoes extensive metabolism. *In vitro* studies using human liver microsomes indicate that aprepitant is metabolized primarily by CYP3A4 with minor metabolism by CYP1A2 and CYP2C19. Metabolism is largely via oxidation at the morpholine ring and its side chains. No metabolism by CYP2D6, CYP2C9, or CYP2E1 was detected. In healthy young adults, aprepitant accounts for approximately 24% of the radioactivity in plasma over 72 hours following a single oral 300-mg dose of [^{14}C]-aprepitant, indicating a substantial presence of metabolites in the plasma. Seven metabolites of aprepitant, which are only weakly active, have been identified in human plasma.

Excretion

Following administration of a single IV 100-mg dose of [^{14}C]-aprepitant prodrug to healthy subjects, 57% of the radioactivity was recovered in urine and 45% in feces. A study was not conducted with radiolabeled capsule formulation. The results after oral administration may differ.
Aprepitant is eliminated primarily by metabolism; aprepitant is not renally excreted. The apparent plasma clearance of aprepitant ranged from approximately 62 to 90 mL/min. The apparent terminal half-life ranged from approximately 9 to 13 hours.

Special Populations

Gender

Following oral administration of a single 125-mg dose of EMEND, no difference in $AUC_{0\text{-}24hr}$ was observed between males and females. The C_{max} for aprepitant is 16% higher in females as compared with males. The half-life of aprepitant is 25% lower in females as compared with males and T_{max} occurs at approximately the same time. These differences are not considered clinically meaningful. No dosage adjustment for EMEND is necessary based on gender.

Geriatric

Following oral administration of a single 125-mg dose of EMEND on Day 1 and 80 mg once daily on Days 2 through 5, the $AUC_{0\text{-}24hr}$ of aprepitant was 21% higher on Day 1 and 36% higher on Day 5 in elderly (≥65 years) relative to younger adults. The C_{max} was 10% higher on Day 1 and 24% higher on Day 5 in elderly relative to younger adults. These differences are not considered clinically meaningful. No dosage adjustment for EMEND is necessary in elderly patients.

Pediatric

The pharmacokinetics of EMEND have not been evaluated in patients below 18 years of age.

Race

Following oral administration of a single 125-mg dose of EMEND, the $AUC_{0\text{-}24hr}$ is approximately 25% and 29% higher in Hispanics as compared with Whites and Blacks, respectively. The C_{max} is 22% and 31% higher in Hispanics as compared with Whites and Blacks, respectively. These differences are not considered clinically meaningful. There was no difference in $AUC_{0\text{-}24hr}$ or C_{max} between Whites and Blacks. No dosage adjustment for EMEND is necessary based on race.

Hepatic Insufficiency

EMEND was well tolerated in patients with mild to moderate hepatic insufficiency. Following administration of a single 125-mg dose of EMEND on Day 1 and 80 mg once daily on Days 2 and 3 to patients with mild hepatic insufficiency (Child-Pugh score 5 to 6), the $AUC_{0\text{-}24hr}$ of aprepitant was 11% lower on Day 1 and 36% lower on Day 3, as compared with healthy subjects given the same regimen. In patients with moderate hepatic insufficiency (Child-Pugh score 7 to 9), the $AUC_{0\text{-}24hr}$ of aprepitant was 10% higher on Day 1 and 18% higher on Day 3, as compared with healthy subjects given the same regimen. These differences in $AUC_{0\text{-}24hr}$ are not considered clinically meaningful; therefore, no dosage adjustment for EMEND is necessary in patients with mild to moderate hepatic insufficiency.
There are no clinical or pharmacokinetic data in patients with severe hepatic insufficiency (Child-Pugh score >9) (see PRECAUTIONS).

Renal Insufficiency

A single 240-mg dose of EMEND was administered to patients with severe renal insufficiency (CrCl<30 mL/min) and to patients with end stage renal disease (ESRD) requiring hemodialysis.
In patients with severe renal insufficiency, the $AUC_{0\text{-}\infty}$ of total aprepitant (unbound and protein bound) decreased by 21% and C_{max} decreased by 32%, relative to healthy subjects. In patients with ESRD undergoing hemodialysis, the $AUC_{0\text{-}\infty}$ of total aprepitant decreased by 42% and C_{max} decreased by 32%. Due to modest decreases in protein binding of aprepitant in patients with renal disease, the AUC of pharmacologically active unbound drug was not significantly affected in patients with renal insufficiency compared with healthy subjects. Hemodialysis conducted 4 or 48 hours after dosing had no significant effect on the pharmacokinetics of aprepitant; less than 0.2% of the dose was recovered in the dialysate.
No dosage adjustment for EMEND is necessary for patients with renal insufficiency or for patients with ESRD undergoing hemodialysis.

Clinical Studies

Oral administration of EMEND in combination with ondansetron and dexamethasone (aprepitant regimen) has been shown to prevent acute and delayed nausea and vomiting associated with highly emetogenic chemotherapy including high-dose cisplatin.
In 2 multicenter, randomized, parallel, double-blind, controlled clinical studies, the aprepitant regimen (see table below) was compared with standard therapy in patients receiving a chemotherapy regimen that included cisplatin >50 mg/m^2 (mean cisplatin dose = 80.2 mg/m^2). Of the 550 patients who were randomized to receive the aprepitant regimen, 42% were women, 58% men, 59% White, 3% Asian, 5% Black, 12% Hispanic American, and 21% Multi-Racial. The aprepitant-treated patients in these clinical studies ranged from 14 to 84 years of age, with a mean age of 56 years. 170 patients were 65 years or older, with 29 patients being 75 years or older.
Patients (N = 1105) were randomized to either the aprepitant regimen (N = 550) or standard therapy (N = 555). The treatment regimens are defined in the table below.

[See first table above]

Treatment Regimens

Treatment Regimen	Day 1	Days 2 to 4
Aprepitant	Aprepitant 125 mg PO Dexamethasone 12 mg PO Ondansetron 32 mg IV	Aprepitant 80 mg PO Daily (Days 2 and 3 only) Dexamethasone 8 mg PO Daily (morning)
Standard Therapy	Dexamethasone 20 mg PO Ondansetron 32 mg IV	Dexamethasone 8 mg PO Daily (morning) Dexamethasone 8 mg PO Daily (evening)

Aprepitant placebo and dexamethasone placebo were used to maintain blinding.

During these studies 95% of the patients in the aprepitant group received a concomitant chemotherapeutic agent in addition to protocol-mandated cisplatin. The most common chemotherapeutic agents and the number of aprepitant patients exposed follows: etoposide (106), fluorouracil (100), gemcitabine (89), vinorelbine (82), paclitaxel (52), cyclophosphamide (50), doxorubicin (38), docetaxel (11).
The antiemetic activity of EMEND was evaluated during the acute phase (0 to 24 hours post-cisplatin treatment), the delayed phase (25 to 120 hours post-cisplatin treatment) and overall (0 to 120 hours post-cisplatin treatment) in Cycle 1. Efficacy was based on evaluation of the following endpoints:
Primary endpoint:
- complete response (defined as no emetic episodes and no use of rescue therapy)

Other prespecified (secondary and exploratory) endpoints:
- complete protection (defined as no emetic episodes, no use of rescue therapy, and a maximum nausea visual analogue scale [VAS] score <25 mm on a 0 to 100 mm scale)
- no emesis (defined as no emetic episodes regardless of use of rescue therapy)
- no nausea (maximum VAS <5 mm on a 0 to 100 mm scale)

Table 1
Percent of Patients Responding by Treatment Group and Phase for Study 1 — Cycle 1

ENDPOINTS	Aprepitant Regimen (N= 260)† %	Standard Therapy (N= 261)† %	p-Value
PRIMARY ENDPOINT			
Complete Response			
Overall‡	73	52	<0.001
OTHER PRESPECIFIED (SECONDARY AND EXPLORATORY) ENDPOINTS			
Complete Response			
Acute phase§	89	78	<0.001
Delayed phase‖	75	56	<0.001
Complete Protection			
Overall	63	49	0.001
Acute phase	85	75	0.005
Delayed phase	66	52	<0.001
No Emesis			
Overall	78	55	<0.001
Acute phase	90	79	0.001
Delayed phase	81	59	<0.001
No Nausea			
Overall	48	44	>0.050
Delayed phase	51	48	>0.050
No Significant Nausea			
Overall	73	66	>0.050
Delayed phase	75	69	>0.050

†N: Number of patients (older than 18 years of age) who received cisplatin, study drug, and had at least one post-treatment efficacy evaluation.
‡Overall: 0 to 120 hours post-cisplatin treatment.
§Acute phase: 0 to 24 hours post-cisplatin treatment.
‖Delayed phase: 25 to 120 hours post-cisplatin treatment.
Visual analogue scale (VAS) score range: 0 mm = no nausea; 100 mm = nausea as bad as it could be.
Table 1 includes nominal p-values not adjusted for multiplicity.

- no significant nausea (maximum VAS <25 mm on a 0 to 100 mm scale)

A summary of the key study results from each individual study analysis is shown in Table 1 and in Table 2.

[See table 1 at top of previous page]

[See table 2 at right]

In both studies, a statistically significantly higher proportion of patients receiving the aprepitant regimen in Cycle 1 had a complete response (primary endpoint), compared with patients receiving standard therapy. A statistically significant difference in complete response in favor of the aprepitant regimen was also observed when the acute phase and the delayed phase were analyzed separately.

In both studies, the estimated time to first emesis after initiation of cisplatin treatment was longer with the aprepitant regimen, and the incidence of first emesis was reduced in the aprepitant regimen group compared with standard therapy group as depicted in the Kaplan-Meier curves in Figure 1.

[See figure 1 at right]

Patient-Reported Outcomes: The impact of nausea and vomiting on patients' daily lives was assessed in Cycle 1 of both Phase III studies using the Functional Living Index–Emesis (FLIE), a validated nausea- and vomiting-specific patient-reported outcome measure. Minimal or no impact of nausea and vomiting on patients' daily lives is defined as a FLIE total score >108. In each of the 2 studies, a higher proportion of patients receiving the aprepitant regimen reported minimal or no impact of nausea and vomiting on daily life (Study 1: 74% versus 64%; Study 2: 75% versus 64%).

Multiple-Cycle Extension: In the same 2 clinical studies, patients continued into the Multiple-Cycle extension for up to 5 additional cycles of chemotherapy. The proportion of patients with no emesis and no significant nausea by treatment group at each cycle is depicted in Figure 2. Antiemetic effectiveness for the patients receiving the aprepitant regimen is maintained throughout repeat cycles for those patients continuing in each of the multiple cycles.

[See figure 2 at top of next page]

INDICATIONS AND USAGE

EMEND, in combination with other antiemetic agents, is indicated for the prevention of acute and delayed nausea and vomiting associated with initial and repeat courses of highly emetogenic cancer chemotherapy, including high-dose cisplatin (see DOSAGE AND ADMINISTRATION).

CONTRAINDICATIONS

EMEND is a moderate CYP3A4 inhibitor. EMEND should not be used concurrently with pimozide, terfenadine, astemizole, or cisapride. Inhibition of cytochrome P450 isoenzyme 3A4 (CYP3A4) by aprepitant could result in elevated plasma concentrations of these drugs, potentially causing serious or life-threatening reactions (see PRECAUTIONS, *Drug Interactions*).

EMEND is contraindicated in patients who are hypersensitive to any component of the product.

PRECAUTIONS

General

EMEND should be used with caution in patients receiving concomitant medicinal products, including chemotherapy agents that are primarily metabolized through CYP3A4. Inhibition of CYP3A4 by aprepitant could result in elevated plasma concentrations of these concomitant medicinal products. The effect of EMEND on the pharmacokinetics of orally administered CYP3A4 substrates is expected to be greater than the effect of EMEND on the pharmacokinetics of intravenously administered CYP3A4 substrates (see PRECAUTIONS, *Drug Interactions*).

Chemotherapy agents that are known to be metabolized by CYP3A4 include docetaxel, paclitaxel, etoposide, irinotecan, ifosfamide, imatinib, vinorelbine, vinblastine and vincristine. In clinical studies, EMEND was administered commonly with etoposide, vinorelbine, or paclitaxel. The doses of these agents were not adjusted to account for potential drug interactions.

Due to the small number of patients in clinical studies who received the CYP3A4 substrates docetaxel, vinblastine, vincristine, or ifosfamide, particular caution and careful monitoring are advised in patients receiving these agents or other chemotherapy agents metabolized primarily by CYP3A4 that were not studied (see PRECAUTIONS, *Drug Interactions*).

Chronic continuous use of EMEND for prevention of nausea and vomiting is not recommended because it has not been studied and because the drug interaction profile may change during chronic continuous use.

Coadministration of EMEND with warfarin may result in a clinically significant decrease in International Normalized Ratio (INR) of prothrombin time. In patients on chronic warfarin therapy, the INR should be closely monitored in the 2-week period, particularly at 7 to 10 days, following initiation of the 3-day regimen of EMEND with each chemotherapy cycle (see PRECAUTIONS, *Drug Interactions*).

The efficacy of oral contraceptives during administration of EMEND may be reduced. Although effects on contraception with a 3-day regimen of EMEND given concomitantly with oral contraceptives has not been studied, alternative or back-up methods of contraception should be used (see PRECAUTIONS, *Drug Interactions*).

Table 2
Percent of Patients Responding by Treatment Group and Phase for Study 2 — Cycle 1

ENDPOINTS	Aprepitant Regimen (N= 261)[†] %	Standard Therapy (N= 263)[†] %	p-Value
PRIMARY ENDPOINT			
Complete Response			
Overall[‡]	63	43	<0.001
OTHER PRESPECIFIED (SECONDARY AND EXPLORATORY) ENDPOINTS			
Complete Response			
Acute phase[§]	83	68	<0.001
Delayed phase[‖]	68	47	<0.001
Complete Protection			
Overall	56	41	<0.001
Acute phase	80	65	<0.001
Delayed phase	61	44	<0.001
No Emesis			
Overall	66	44	<0.001
Acute phase	84	69	<0.001
Delayed phase	72	48	<0.001
No Nausea			
Overall	49	39	0.021
Delayed phase	53	40	0.004
No Significant Nausea			
Overall	71	64	>0.050
Delayed phase	73	65	>0.050

[†]N: Number of patients (older than 18 years of age) who received cisplatin, study drug, and had at least one post-treatment efficacy evaluation.
[‡]Overall: 0 to 120 hours post-cisplatin treatment.
[§]Acute phase: 0 to 24 hours post-cisplatin treatment.
[‖]Delayed phase: 25 to 120 hours post-cisplatin treatment.
Visual analogue scale (VAS) score range: 0 mm = no nausea; 100 mm = nausea as bad as it could be.
Table 2 includes nominal p-values not adjusted for multiplicity.

Figure 1: Percent of Patients Who Remain Emesis Free Over Time – Cycle 1

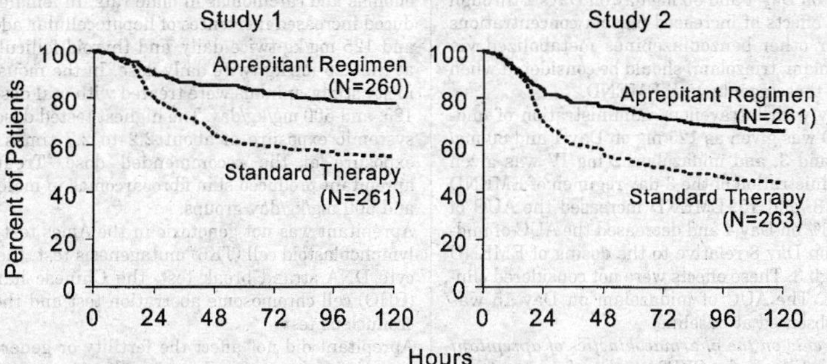

p-Value <0.001 based on a log rank test for Study 1 and Study 2; nominal p-values not adjusted for multiplicity.

There are no clinical or pharmacokinetic data in patients with severe hepatic insufficiency (Child-Pugh score > 9). Therefore, caution should be exercised when EMEND is administered in these patients (see CLINICAL PHARMACOLOGY, *Special Populations, Hepatic Insufficiency* and DOSAGE AND ADMINISTRATION).

Information for Patients

Physicians should instruct their patients to read the patient package insert before starting therapy with EMEND and to reread it each time the prescription is renewed.

Patients should be instructed to take EMEND only as prescribed. Patients should be advised to take their first dose (125 mg) of EMEND 1 hour prior to chemotherapy treatment.

EMEND may interact with some drugs including chemotherapy; therefore, patients should be advised to report to their doctor the use of any other prescription, nonprescription medication or herbal products.

Patients on chronic warfarin therapy should be instructed to have their clotting status closely monitored in the 2-week period, particularly at 7 to 10 days, following initiation of the 3-day regimen of EMEND with each chemotherapy cycle.

Administration of EMEND may reduce the efficacy of oral contraceptives. Patients should be advised to use alternative or back-up methods of contraception.

Drug Interactions

Aprepitant is a substrate, a moderate inhibitor, and an inducer of CYP3A4. Aprepitant is also an inducer of CYP2C9.

Effect of aprepitant on the pharmacokinetics of other agents

As a moderate inhibitor of CYP3A4, aprepitant can increase plasma concentrations of coadministered medicinal products that are metabolized through CYP3A4 (see CONTRAINDICATIONS).

Aprepitant has been shown to induce the metabolism of S(-) warfarin and tolbutamide, which are metabolized through CYP2C9. Coadministration of EMEND with these drugs or other drugs that are known to be metabolized by CYP2C9, such as phenytoin, may result in lower plasma concentrations of these drugs.

EMEND is unlikely to interact with drugs that are substrates for the P-glycoprotein transporter, as demonstrated by the lack of interaction of EMEND with digoxin in a clinical drug interaction study.

5-HT_3 antagonists: In clinical drug interaction studies, aprepitant did not have clinically important effects on the pharmacokinetics of ondansetron or granisetron. No clinical or drug interaction study was conducted with dolasetron.

Corticosteroids:

Dexamethasone: EMEND, when given as a regimen of 125 mg with dexamethasone coadministered orally as 20 mg on Day 1, and EMEND when given as 80 mg/day with dexamethasone coadministered orally as 8 mg on Days 2 through 5, increased the AUC of dexamethasone, a CYP3A4 substrate by 2.2-fold, on Days 1 and 5. The oral dexamethasone doses should be reduced by approximately 50% when coadministered with EMEND, to achieve exposures of dexamethasone similar to those obtained when it is given with-

Continued on next page

Information on the Merck & Co., Inc., products listed on these pages is from the prescribing information in use October 1, 2004. For information, please call 1-800-NSC-MERCK [1-800-672-6372].

Emend—Cont.

out EMEND. The daily dose of dexamethasone administered in clinical studies with EMEND reflects an approximate 50% reduction of the dose of dexamethasone (see DOSAGE AND ADMINISTRATION).

Methylprednisolone: EMEND, when given as a regimen of 125 mg on Day 1 and 80 mg/day on Days 2 and 3, increased the AUC of methylprednisolone, a CYP3A4 substrate, by 1.34-fold on Day 1 and by 2.5-fold on Day 3, when methylprednisolone was coadministered intravenously as 125 mg on Day 1 and orally as 40 mg on Days 2 and 3. The IV methylprednisolone dose should be reduced by approximately 25%, and the oral methylprednisolone dose should be reduced by approximately 50% when coadministered with EMEND to achieve exposures of methylprednisolone similar to those obtained when it is given without EMEND.

Chemotherapeutic agents: See PRECAUTIONS, *General.*

Warfarin: A single 125-mg dose of EMEND was administered on Day 1 and 80 mg/day on Days 2 and 3 to healthy subjects who were stabilized on chronic warfarin therapy. Although there was no effect of EMEND on the plasma AUC of R(+) or S(-) warfarin determined on Day 3, there was a 34% decrease in S(-) warfarin (a CYP2C9 substrate) trough concentration accompanied by a 14% decrease in the prothrombin time (reported as International Normalized Ratio or INR) 5 days after completion of dosing with EMEND. In patients on chronic warfarin therapy, the prothrombin time (INR) should be closely monitored in the 2-week period, particularly at 7 to 10 days, following initiation of the 3-day regimen of EMEND with each chemotherapy cycle.

Tolbutamide: EMEND, when given as 125 mg on Day 1 and 80 mg/day on Days 2 and 3, decreased the AUC of tolbutamide (a CYP2C9 substrate) by 23% on Day 4, 28% on Day 8, and 15% on Day 15, when a single dose of tolbutamide 500 mg was administered orally prior to the administration of the 3-day regimen of EMEND and on Days 4, 8, and 15.

Oral contraceptives: Aprepitant, when given once daily for 14 days as a 100-mg capsule with an oral contraceptive containing 35 mcg of ethinyl estradiol and 1 mg of norethindrone, decreased the AUC of ethinyl estradiol by 43%, and decreased the AUC of norethindrone by 8%; therefore, the efficacy of oral contraceptives during administration of EMEND may be reduced. Although a 3-day regimen of EMEND given concomitantly with oral contraceptives has not been studied, alternative or back-up methods of contraception should be used.

Midazolam: EMEND increased the AUC of midazolam, a sensitive CYP3A4 substrate, by 2.3-fold on Day 1 and 3.3-fold on Day 5, when a single oral dose of midazolam 2 mg was coadministered on Day 1 and Day 5 of a regimen of EMEND 125 mg on Day 1 and 80 mg/day on Days 2 through 5. The potential effects of increased plasma concentrations of midazolam or other benzodiazepines metabolized via CYP3A4 (alprazolam, triazolam) should be considered when coadministering these agents with EMEND.

In another study with intravenous administration of midazolam, EMEND was given as 125 mg on Day 1 and 80 mg/day on Days 2 and 3, and midazolam 2 mg IV was given prior to the administration of the 3-day regimen of EMEND and on Days 4, 8, and 15. EMEND increased the AUC of midazolam by 25% on Day 4 and decreased the AUC of midazolam by 19% on Day 8 relative to the dosing of EMEND on Days 1 through 3. These effects were not considered clinically important. The AUC of midazolam on Day 15 was similar to that observed at baseline.

Effect of other agents on the pharmacokinetics of aprepitant

Aprepitant is a substrate for CYP3A4; therefore, coadministration of EMEND with drugs that inhibit CYP3A4 activity may result in increased plasma concentrations of aprepitant. Consequently, concomitant administration of EMEND with strong CYP3A4 inhibitors (e.g., ketoconazole, itraconazole, nefazodone, troleandomycin, clarithromycin, ritonavir, nelfinavir) should be approached with caution. Because moderate CYP3A4 inhibitors (e.g., diltiazem) result in 2-fold increase in plasma concentrations of aprepitant, concomitant administration should also be approached with caution.

Aprepitant is a substrate for CYP3A4; therefore, coadministration of EMEND with drugs that strongly induce CYP3A4 activity (e.g., rifampin, carbamazepine, phenytoin) may result in reduced plasma concentrations of aprepitant that may result in decreased efficacy of EMEND.

Ketoconazole: When a single 125-mg dose of EMEND was administered on Day 5 of a 10-day regimen of 400 mg/day of ketoconazole, a strong CYP3A4 inhibitor, the AUC of aprepitant increased approximately 5-fold and the mean terminal half-life of aprepitant increased approximately 3-fold. Concomitant administration of EMEND with strong CYP3A4 inhibitors should be approached cautiously.

Rifampin: When a single 375-mg dose of EMEND was administered on Day 9 of a 14-day regimen of 600 mg/day of rifampin, a strong CYP3A4 inducer, the AUC of aprepitant decreased approximately 11-fold and the mean terminal half-life decreased approximately 3-fold.

Coadministration of EMEND with drugs that induce CYP3A4 activity may result in reduced plasma concentrations and decreased efficacy of EMEND.

Additional interactions

Diltiazem: In patients with mild to moderate hypertension, administration of aprepitant once daily, as a tablet formulation comparable to 230 mg of the capsule formulation,

Figure 2: Proportion of Patients With No Emesis and No Significant Nausea by Treatment Group and Cycle

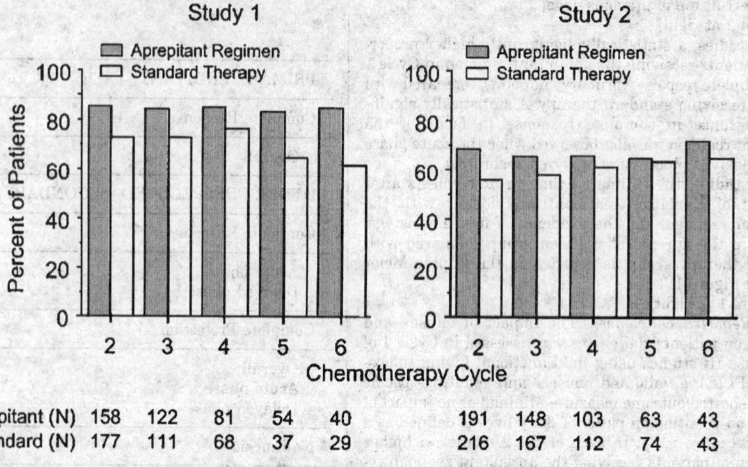

with diltiazem 120 mg 3 times daily for 5 days, resulted in a 2-fold increase of aprepitant AUC and a simultaneous 1.7-fold increase of diltiazem AUC. These pharmacokinetic effects did not result in clinically meaningful changes in ECG, heart rate or blood pressure beyond those changes induced by diltiazem alone.

Paroxetine: Coadministration of once daily doses of aprepitant, as a tablet formulation comparable to 85 mg or 170 mg of the capsule formulation, with paroxetine 20 mg once daily, resulted in a decrease in AUC by approximately 25% and C_{max} by approximately 20% of both aprepitant and paroxetine.

Carcinogenesis, Mutagenesis, Impairment of Fertility

Three 2-year carcinogenicity studies of aprepitant (two in Sprague-Dawley rats and one in CD-1 mice) were conducted with aprepitant. Dose selection for the studies was based on saturation of absorption in both species. In the rat carcinogenicity studies, animals were treated with oral doses of 0.05, 0.25, 1, 5, 25, 125 mg/kg twice daily. The highest dose tested produced a systemic exposure to aprepitant (plasma $AUC_{0\text{-}24hr}$) of 0.4 to 1.4 times the human exposure ($AUC_{0\text{-}24hr}$ = 19.6 mcg•hr/mL) at the recommended dose of 125 mg/day. Treatment with aprepitant at doses of 5 to 125 mg/kg twice per day produced thyroid follicular cell adenomas and carcinomas in male rats. In female rats, it produced increased incidences of hepatocellular adenoma at 25 and 125 mg/kg twice daily, and thyroid follicular adenoma at the 125 mg/kg twice daily dose. In the mouse carcinogenicity study, animals were treated with oral doses of 2.5, 25, 125, and 500 mg/kg/day. The highest tested dose produced a systemic exposure of about 2.2 to 2.7 times the human exposure at the recommended dose. Treatment with aprepitant produced skin fibrosarcomas in male mice of 125 and 500 mg/kg/day groups.

Aprepitant was not genotoxic in the Ames test, the human lymphoblastoid cell (TK6) mutagenesis test, the rat hepatocyte DNA strand break test, the Chinese hamster ovary (CHO) cell chromosome aberration test and the mouse micronucleus test.

Aprepitant did not affect the fertility or general reproductive performance of male or female rats at doses up to the maximum feasible dose of 1000 mg/kg twice daily (providing exposure in male rats lower than the exposure at the recommended human dose and exposure in female rats at about 1.6 times the human exposure).

Pregnancy. Teratogenic Effects: Category B. Teratology studies have been performed in rats at oral doses up to 1000 mg/kg twice daily (plasma $AUC_{0\text{-}24hr}$ of 31.3 mcg•hr/mL, about 1.6 times the human exposure at the recommended dose) and in rabbits at oral doses up to 25 mg/kg/day (plasma $AUC_{0\text{-}24hr}$ of 26.9 mcg•hr/mL, about 1.4 times the human exposure at the recommended dose) and have revealed no evidence of impaired fertility or harm to the fetus due to aprepitant. There are, however, no adequate and well-controlled studies in pregnant women. Because animal reproduction studies are not always predictive of human response, this drug should be used during pregnancy only if clearly needed.

Nursing Mothers

Aprepitant is excreted in the milk of rats. It is not known whether this drug is excreted in human milk. Because many drugs are excreted in human milk and because of the potential for possible serious adverse reactions in nursing infants from aprepitant and because of the potential for tumorigenicity shown for aprepitant in rodent carcinogenicity studies, a decision should be made whether to discontinue nursing or to discontinue the drug, taking into account the importance of the drug to the mother.

Pediatric Use

Safety and effectiveness of EMEND in pediatric patients have not been established.

Geriatric Use

In 2 well-controlled clinical studies, of the total number of patients (N=544) treated with EMEND, 31% were 65 and over, while 5% were 75 and over. No overall differences in safety or effectiveness were observed between these subjects and younger subjects. Greater sensitivity of some older individuals cannot be ruled out. Dosage adjustment in the elderly is not necessary.

ADVERSE REACTIONS

The overall safety of aprepitant was evaluated in approximately 3300 individuals.

In 2 well-controlled clinical trials in patients receiving highly emetogenic cancer chemotherapy, 544 patients were treated with aprepitant during Cycle 1 of chemotherapy and 413 of these patients continued into the Multiple-Cycle extension for up to 6 cycles of chemotherapy. EMEND was given in combination with ondansetron and dexamethasone and was generally well tolerated. Most adverse experiences reported in these clinical studies were described as mild to moderate in intensity.

In Cycle 1, clinical adverse experiences were reported in approximately 69% of patients treated with the aprepitant regimen compared with approximately 68% of patients treated with standard therapy. Table 3 shows the percent of patients with clinical adverse experiences reported at an incidence ≥3% during Cycle 1 of the 2 combined Phase III studies.

Table 3
Percent of Patients With Clinical Adverse Experiences (Incidence ≥3%) in CINV Phase III Studies (Cycle 1)

	Aprepitant Regimen (N = 544)	Standard Therapy (N = 550)
Body as a Whole/Site Unspecified		
Abdominal Pain	4.6	3.3
Asthenia/Fatigue	17.8	11.8
Dehydration	5.9	5.1
Dizziness	6.6	4.4
Fever	2.9	3.5
Mucous Membrane Disorder	2.6	3.1
Digestive System		
Constipation	10.3	12.2
Diarrhea	10.3	7.5
Epigastric Discomfort	4.0	3.1
Gastritis	4.2	3.1
Heartburn	5.3	4.9
Nausea	12.7	11.8
Vomiting	7.5	7.6
Eyes, Ears, Nose, and Throat		
Tinnitus	3.7	3.8
Hemic and Lymphatic System		
Neutropenia	3.1	2.9
Metabolism and Nutrition		
Anorexia	10.1	9.5
Nervous System		
Headache	8.5	8.7
Insomnia	2.9	3.1
Respiratory System		
Hiccups	10.8	5.6

The following additional clinical adverse experiences (incidence >0.5% and greater than standard therapy), regardless of causality, were reported in patients treated with aprepitant regimen:

Body as a whole: diaphoresis, edema, flushing, malaise, malignant neoplasm, pelvic pain, septic shock, upper respiratory infection.

Cardiovascular system: deep venous thrombosis, hypertension, hypotension, myocardial infarction, pulmonary embolism, tachycardia.
Digestive system: acid reflux, deglutition disorder, dysgeusia, dyspepsia, dysphagia, flatulence, obstipation, salivation increased, taste disturbance.
Endocrine system: diabetes mellitus.
Eyes, ears, nose, and throat: nasal secretion, pharyngitis, vocal disturbance.
Hemic and lymphatic system: anemia, febrile neutropenia, thrombocytopenia.
Metabolism and nutrition: appetite decreased, hypokalemia, weight loss.
Musculoskeletal system: muscular weakness, musculoskeletal pain, myalgia.
Nervous system: peripheral neuropathy, sensory neuropathy.
Psychiatric disorder: anxiety disorder, confusion, depression.
Respiratory system: cough, dyspnea, lower respiratory infection, non-small cell lung carcinoma, pneumonitis, respiratory insufficiency.
Skin and skin appendages: alopecia, rash.
Urogenital system: dysuria, renal insufficiency.
Laboratory Adverse Experiences
Table 4 shows the percent of patients with laboratory adverse experiences reported at an incidence ≥3% during Cycle 1 of the 2 combined Phase III studies.

Table 4
Percent of Patients With Laboratory Adverse Experiences (Incidence ≥3%) in CINV Phase III Studies (Cycle 1)

	Aprepitant Regimen (N = 544)	Standard Therapy (N = 550)
ALT Increased	6.0	4.3
AST Increased	3.0	1.3
Blood Urea Nitrogen Increased	4.7	3.5
Serum Creatinine Increased	3.7	4.3
Proteinuria	6.8	5.3

The following additional laboratory adverse experiences (incidence >0.5% and greater than standard therapy), regardless of causality, were reported in patients treated with aprepitant regimen: alkaline phosphatase increased, hyperglycemia, hyponatremia, leukocytes increased, erythrocyturia, leukocyturia.
The adverse experiences of increased AST and ALT were generally mild and transient.
The adverse experience profile in the Multiple-Cycle extension for up to 6 cycles of chemotherapy was generally similar to that observed in Cycle 1.
In addition, isolated cases of serious adverse experiences, regardless of causality, of bradycardia, disorientation, and perforating duodenal ulcer were reported in CINV clinical studies.
Stevens-Johnson syndrome was reported in a patient receiving aprepitant with cancer chemotherapy in another CINV study. Angioedema and urticaria were reported in a patient receiving aprepitant in a non-CINV study.

OVERDOSAGE

No specific information is available on the treatment of overdosage with EMEND. Single doses up to 600 mg of aprepitant were generally well tolerated in healthy subjects. Aprepitant was generally well tolerated when administered as 375 mg once daily for up to 42 days to patients in non-CINV studies. In 33 cancer patients, administration of a single 375-mg dose of aprepitant on Day 1 and 250 mg once daily on Days 2 to 5 was generally well tolerated.
Drowsiness and headache were reported in one patient who ingested 1440 mg of aprepitant.
In the event of overdose, EMEND should be discontinued and general supportive treatment and monitoring should be provided. Because of the antiemetic activity of aprepitant, drug-induced emesis may not be effective.
Aprepitant cannot be removed by hemodialysis.

DOSAGE AND ADMINISTRATION

EMEND is given for 3 days as part of a regimen that includes a corticosteroid and a 5-HT_3 antagonist. The recommended dose of EMEND is 125 mg orally 1 hour prior to chemotherapy treatment (Day 1) and 80 mg once daily in the morning on Days 2 and 3. EMEND has not been studied for the treatment of established nausea and vomiting.
In clinical studies, the following regimen was used:
[See table above]

	Day 1	Day 2	Day 3	Day 4
EMEND*	125 mg	80 mg	80 mg	none
Dexamethasone**	12 mg orally	8 mg orally	8 mg orally	8 mg orally
Ondansetron[†]	32 mg IV	none	none	none

*EMEND was administered orally 1 hour prior to chemotherapy treatment on Day 1 and in the morning on Days 2 and 3.
**Dexamethasone was administered 30 minutes prior to chemotherapy treatment on Day 1 and in the morning on Days 2 through 4. The dose of dexamethasone was chosen to account for drug interactions.
[†]Ondansetron was administered 30 minutes prior to chemotherapy treatment on Day 1.

Chronic continuous administration is not recommended (see PRECAUTIONS).
See PRECAUTIONS, *Drug Interactions* for additional information on dose adjustment for corticosteroids when coadministered with EMEND.
Refer to the full prescribing information for coadministered antiemetic agents.
EMEND may be taken with or without food.
No dosage adjustment is necessary for the elderly.
No dosage adjustment is necessary for patients with renal insufficiency or for patients with end stage renal disease undergoing hemodialysis.
No dosage adjustment is necessary for patients with mild to moderate hepatic insufficiency (Child-Pugh score 5 to 9). There are no clinical data in patients with severe hepatic insufficiency (Child-Pugh score >9).

HOW SUPPLIED

No. 3854 — 80 mg capsules: White, opaque, hard gelatin capsule with "461" and "80 mg" printed radially in black ink on the body. They are supplied as follows:
NDC 0006-0461-30 bottles of 30 (with desiccant)
NDC 0006-0461-05 unit-dose packages of 5.
No. 3855 — 125 mg capsules: Opaque, hard gelatin capsule with white body and pink cap with "462" and "125 mg" printed radially in black ink on the body. They are supplied as follows:
NDC 0006-0462-30 bottles of 30 (with desiccant)
NDC 0006-0462-05 unit-dose packages of 5.
No. 3862 — Unit-of-use tri-fold pack containing one 125 mg capsule and two 80 mg capsules.
NDC 0006-3862-03.
Storage
Bottles: Store at 20-25°C (68-77°F) [see USP Controlled Room Temperature]. The desiccant should remain in the original bottle.
Blisters: Store at 20-25°C (68-77°F) [see USP Controlled Room Temperature].
Rx only

9565001 Issued May 2003

Patient Information

EMEND® (EE mend)
(aprepitant) Capsules
You should read this information before you start taking EMEND*. Also, read the leaflet each time you refill your prescription, in case any information has changed. This leaflet provides only a summary of certain information about EMEND. Your doctor or pharmacist can give you an additional leaflet that is written for health professionals that contains more complete information. This leaflet does not take the place of careful discussions with your doctor. You and your doctor should discuss EMEND when you start taking your medicine.

*Registered trademark of MERCK & CO., Inc.

What is EMEND?
EMEND is an antiemetic medicine for use in adult patients. An antiemetic is a medicine used to prevent and control nausea and vomiting. EMEND is always used WITH OTHER MEDICINES to prevent and control nausea and vomiting caused by your chemotherapy treatment. EMEND is not used to treat nausea and vomiting that you already have.
Who should not take EMEND?**
Do not take EMEND if you:
- are taking any of the following medicines:
  - ORAP® (pimozide)
  - SELDANE® (terfenadine)
  - HISMANAL® (astemizole)
  - PROPULSID® (cisapride)

Taking EMEND with these medicines could cause serious or life-threatening problems.
- are allergic to any of the ingredients in EMEND. The active ingredient is aprepitant. See the end of this leaflet for a list of all the ingredients in EMEND.

**The brands listed are the registered trademarks of their respective owners and are not trademarks of Merck & Co., Inc.

What should I tell my doctor before and during treatment with EMEND?
Tell your doctor:
- if you are pregnant or plan to become pregnant. It is not known if EMEND can harm your unborn baby.
- if you are breast-feeding. It is not known if EMEND passes into your milk and if it can harm your baby.
- if you have liver problems.
- about all your medical problems.
- about all the medicines that you are taking or plan to take, prescription and nonprescription medicines, vitamins, and herbal supplements. EMEND may cause **serious life-threatening reactions** if used with certain medicines (see the section **Who should not take EMEND?**). Some medicines can affect EMEND. EMEND may also affect some medicines, including chemotherapy, causing them to work differently in your body.

Your doctor may check to make sure your other medicines are working, while you are taking EMEND. Patients who take COUMADIN® (warfarin) may need to have blood tests after each 3-day treatment with EMEND to check their blood clotting.
Women who use birth control pills while taking EMEND should also use a back-up method of contraception to avoid pregnancy.
How should I take EMEND?
- Take EMEND exactly as prescribed.
- EMEND is a capsule that you swallow with a drink.

The recommended dose of EMEND is:
- Take one 125-mg capsule (white/pink) by mouth 1 hour before you start your chemotherapy treatment;

AND
- Take one 80-mg capsule (white) each morning for the 2 days following your chemotherapy treatment.
- EMEND may be taken with or without food.
- Do not start taking EMEND if you already have nausea and vomiting. Ask your doctor what to do.
- If you take too much EMEND, call your doctor, local emergency room or poison control center right away.

What are the possible side effects of EMEND?
The most common side effects with EMEND are:
- tiredness
- nausea
- hiccups
- constipation
- diarrhea
- loss of appetite

These are not all of the possible side effects of EMEND. For further information ask your doctor or pharmacist. Talk to your doctor about any side effect that bothers you.
General information about the use of EMEND
Medicines are sometimes prescribed for conditions that are not mentioned in patient information leaflets. Do not use EMEND for a condition for which it was not prescribed. Do not give EMEND to other people, even if they have the same symptoms you have. It may harm them. Keep EMEND and all medicines out of the reach of children.
This leaflet summarizes the most important information about EMEND. If you would like to know more information, talk with your doctor. You can ask your doctor or pharmacist for information about EMEND that is written for health professionals.
What are the ingredients in EMEND?
Active ingredient: aprepitant
Inactive Ingredients: Sucrose, microcrystalline cellulose, hydroxypropyl cellulose and sodium lauryl sulfate. The capsule shell excipients are gelatin and titanium dioxide. The 125-mg capsule shell also contains red ferric oxide and yellow ferric oxide.

9565100 Issued March 2003

Shown in Product Identification Guide, page 323

FOSAMAX® ℞

(alendronate sodium)
Tablets and Oral Solution

DESCRIPTION

FOSAMAX* (alendronate sodium) is a bisphosphonate that acts as a specific inhibitor of osteoclast-mediated bone resorption. Bisphosphonates are synthetic analogs of pyrophosphate that bind to the hydroxyapatite found in bone.
Alendronate sodium is chemically described as (4-amino-1-hydroxybutylidene) bisphosphonic acid monosodium salt trihydrate.
The empirical formula of alendronate sodium is $C_4H_{12}NNaO_7P_2 \cdot 3H_2O$ and its formula weight is 325.12. The structural formula is:

Continued on next page

Information on the Merck & Co., Inc., products listed on these pages is from the prescribing information in use October 1, 2004. For information, please call 1-800-NSC-MERCK [1-800-672-6372].

Fosamax—Cont.

```
                NH2
                |
                CH2
                |
                CH2
        O       CH2 O
        ||      |   ||
   HO — P — C — P — ONa • 3H2O
        |   |   |
        OH  OH  OH
```

Alendronate sodium is a white, crystalline, nonhygroscopic powder. It is soluble in water, very slightly soluble in alcohol, and practically insoluble in chloroform.

Tablets FOSAMAX for oral administration contain 6.53, 13.05, 45.68, 52.21 or 91.37 mg of alendronate monosodium salt trihydrate, which is the molar equivalent of 5, 10, 35, 40 and 70 mg, respectively, of free acid, and the following inactive ingredients: microcrystalline cellulose, anhydrous lactose, croscarmellose sodium, and magnesium stearate. Tablets FOSAMAX 10 mg also contain carnauba wax.

Each bottle of the oral solution contains 91.35 mg of alendronate monosodium salt trihydrate, which is the molar equivalent to 70 mg of free acid. Each bottle also contains the following inactive ingredients: sodium citrate dihydrate and citric acid anhydrous as buffering agents, sodium saccharin, artificial raspberry flavor, and purified water. Added as preservatives are sodium propylparaben 0.0225% and sodium butylparaben 0.0075%.

*Registered trademark of MERCK & CO., Inc.

CLINICAL PHARMACOLOGY

Mechanism of Action

Animal studies have indicated the following mode of action. At the cellular level, alendronate shows preferential localization to sites of bone resorption, specifically under osteoclasts. The osteoclasts adhere normally to the bone surface but lack the ruffled border that is indicative of active resorption. Alendronate does not interfere with osteoclast recruitment or attachment, but it does inhibit osteoclast activity. Studies in mice on the localization of radioactive [^{3}H]alendronate in bone showed about 10-fold higher uptake on osteoclast surfaces than on osteoblast surfaces. Bones examined 6 and 49 days after [^{3}H]alendronate administration in rats and mice, respectively, showed that normal bone was formed on top of the alendronate, which was incorporated inside the matrix. While incorporated in bone matrix, alendronate is not pharmacologically active. Thus, alendronate must be continuously administered to suppress osteoclasts on newly formed resorption surfaces. Histomorphometry in baboons and rats showed that alendronate treatment reduces bone turnover (i.e., the number of sites at which bone is remodeled). In addition, bone formation exceeds bone resorption at these remodeling sites, leading to progressive gains in bone mass.

Pharmacokinetics

Absorption

Relative to an intravenous (IV) reference dose, the mean oral bioavailability of alendronate in women was 0.64% for doses ranging from 5 to 70 mg when administered after an overnight fast and two hours before a standardized breakfast. Oral bioavailability of the 10 mg tablet in men (0.59%) was similar to that in women when administered after an overnight fast and 2 hours before breakfast.

FOSAMAX 70 mg oral solution and FOSAMAX 70 mg tablet are equally bioavailable.

A study examining the effect of timing of a meal on the bioavailability of alendronate was performed in 49 postmenopausal women. Bioavailability was decreased (by approximately 40%) when 10 mg alendronate was administered either 0.5 or 1 hour before a standardized breakfast, when compared to dosing 2 hours before eating. In studies of treatment and prevention of osteoporosis, alendronate was effective when administered at least 30 minutes before breakfast.

Bioavailability was negligible whether alendronate was administered with or up to two hours after a standardized breakfast. Concomitant administration of alendronate with coffee or orange juice reduced bioavailability by approximately 60%.

Distribution

Preclinical studies (in male rats) show that alendronate transiently distributes to soft tissues following 1 mg/kg IV administration but is then rapidly redistributed to bone or excreted in the urine. The mean steady-state volume of distribution, exclusive of bone, is at least 28 L in humans. Concentrations of drug in plasma following therapeutic oral doses are too low (less than 5 ng/mL) for analytical detection. Protein binding in human plasma is approximately 78%.

Metabolism

There is no evidence that alendronate is metabolized in animals or humans.

Excretion

Following a single IV dose of [^{14}C]alendronate, approximately 50% of the radioactivity was excreted in the urine within 72 hours and little or no radioactivity was recovered in the feces. Following a single 10 mg IV dose, the renal clearance of alendronate was 71 mL/min (64, 78; 90% confidence interval [CI]), and systemic clearance did not exceed 200 mL/min. Plasma concentrations fell by more than 95% within 6 hours following IV administration. The terminal half-life in humans is estimated to exceed 10 years, probably reflecting release of alendronate from the skeleton. Based on the above, it is estimated that after 10 years of oral treatment with FOSAMAX (10 mg daily) the amount of alendronate released daily from the skeleton is approximately 25% of that absorbed from the gastrointestinal tract.

Special Populations

Pediatric: Alendronate pharmacokinetics have not been investigated in patients <18 years of age.

Gender: Bioavailability and the fraction of an IV dose excreted in urine were similar in men and women.

Geriatric: Bioavailability and disposition (urinary excretion) were similar in elderly and younger patients. No dosage adjustment is necessary (see DOSAGE AND ADMINISTRATION).

Race: Pharmacokinetic differences due to race have not been studied.

Renal Insufficiency: Preclinical studies show that, in rats with kidney failure, increasing amounts of drug are present in plasma, kidney, spleen, and tibia. In healthy controls, drug that is not deposited in bone is rapidly excreted in the urine. No evidence of saturation of bone uptake was found after 3 weeks dosing with cumulative IV doses of 35 mg/kg in young male rats. Although no clinical information is available, it is likely that, as in animals, elimination of alendronate via the kidney will be reduced in patients with impaired renal function. Therefore, somewhat greater accumulation of alendronate in bone might be expected in patients with impaired renal function.

No dosage adjustment is necessary for patients with mild-to-moderate renal insufficiency (creatinine clearance 35 to 60 mL/min). **FOSAMAX is not recommended for patients with more severe renal insufficiency (creatinine clearance <35 mL/min) due to lack of experience with alendronate in renal failure.**

Hepatic Insufficiency: As there is evidence that alendronate is not metabolized or excreted in the bile, no studies were conducted in patients with hepatic insufficiency. No dosage adjustment is necessary.

Drug Interactions (also see PRECAUTIONS, *Drug Interactions*)

Intravenous ranitidine was shown to double the bioavailability of oral alendronate. The clinical significance of this increased bioavailability and whether similar increases will occur in patients given oral H_2-antagonists is unknown.

In healthy subjects, oral prednisone (20 mg three times daily for five days) did not produce a clinically meaningful change in the oral bioavailability of alendronate (a mean increase ranging from 20 to 44%).

Products containing calcium and other multivalent cations are likely to interfere with absorption of alendronate.

Pharmacodynamics

Alendronate is a bisphosphonate that binds to bone hydroxyapatite and specifically inhibits the activity of osteoclasts, the bone-resorbing cells. Alendronate reduces bone resorption with no direct effect on bone formation, although the latter process is ultimately reduced because bone resorption and formation are coupled during bone turnover.

Osteoporosis in postmenopausal women

Osteoporosis is characterized by low bone mass that leads to an increased risk of fracture. The diagnosis can be confirmed by the finding of low bone mass, evidence of fracture on x-ray, a history of osteoporotic fracture, or height loss or kyphosis, indicative of vertebral (spinal) fracture. Osteoporosis occurs in both males and females but is most common among women following the menopause, when bone turnover increases and the rate of bone resorption exceeds that of bone formation. These changes result in progressive bone loss and lead to osteoporosis in a significant proportion of women over age 50. Fractures, usually of the spine, hip, and wrist, are the common consequences. From age 50 to age 90, the risk of hip fracture in white women increases 50-fold and the risk of vertebral fracture 15- to 30-fold. It is estimated that approximately 40% of 50-year-old women will sustain one or more osteoporosis-related fractures of the spine, hip, or wrist during their remaining lifetimes. Hip fractures, in particular, are associated with substantial morbidity, disability, and mortality.

Daily oral doses of alendronate (5, 20, and 40 mg for six weeks) in postmenopausal women produced biochemical changes indicative of dose-dependent inhibition of bone resorption, including decreases in urinary calcium and urinary markers of bone collagen degradation (such as deoxypyridinoline and cross-linked N-telopeptides of type I collagen). These biochemical changes tended to return toward baseline values as early as 3 weeks following the discontinuation of therapy with alendronate and did not differ from placebo after 7 months.

Long-term treatment of osteoporosis with FOSAMAX 10 mg/day (for up to five years) reduced urinary excretion of markers of bone resorption, deoxypyridinoline and cross-linked N-telopeptides of type I collagen, by approximately 50% and 70%, respectively, to reach levels similar to those seen in healthy premenopausal women. Similar decreases were seen in patients in osteoporosis prevention studies who received FOSAMAX 5 mg/day. The decrease in the rate of bone resorption indicated by these markers was evident as early as one month and at three to six months reached a plateau that was maintained for the entire duration of treatment with FOSAMAX. In osteoporosis treatment studies FOSAMAX 10 mg/day decreased the markers of bone formation, osteocalcin and bone specific alkaline phosphatase by approximately 50%, and total serum alkaline phosphatase by approximately 25 to 30% to reach a plateau after 6 to 12 months. In osteoporosis prevention studies FOSAMAX 5 mg/day decreased osteocalcin and total serum alkaline phosphatase by approximately 40% and 15%, respectively. Similar reductions in the rate of bone turnover were observed in postmenopausal women during one-year studies with once weekly FOSAMAX 70 mg for the treatment of osteoporosis and once weekly FOSAMAX 35 mg for the prevention of osteoporosis. These data indicate that the rate of bone turnover reached a new steady-state, despite the progressive increase in the total amount of alendronate deposited within bone.

As a result of inhibition of bone resorption, asymptomatic reductions in serum calcium and phosphate concentrations were also observed following treatment with FOSAMAX. In the long-term studies, reductions from baseline in serum calcium (approximately 2%) and phosphate (approximately 4 to 6%) were evident the first month after the initiation of FOSAMAX 10 mg. No further decreases in serum calcium were observed for the five-year duration of treatment; however, serum phosphate returned toward prestudy levels during years three through five. Similar reductions were observed with FOSAMAX 5 mg/day. In one-year studies with once weekly FOSAMAX 35 and 70 mg, similar reductions were observed at 6 and 12 months. The reduction in serum phosphate may reflect not only the positive bone mineral balance due to FOSAMAX but also a decrease in renal phosphate reabsorption.

Osteoporosis in men

Treatment of men with osteoporosis with FOSAMAX 10 mg/day for two years reduced urinary excretion of cross-linked N-telopeptides of type I collagen by approximately 60% and bone-specific alkaline phosphatase by approximately 40%. Similar reductions were observed in a one-year study in men with osteoporosis receiving once weekly FOSAMAX 70 mg.

Glucocorticoid-induced Osteoporosis

Sustained use of glucocorticoids is commonly associated with development of osteoporosis and resulting fractures (especially vertebral, hip, and rib). It occurs both in males and females of all ages. Osteoporosis occurs as a result of inhibited bone formation and increased bone resorption resulting in net bone loss. Alendronate decreases bone resorption without directly inhibiting bone formation.

In clinical studies of up to two years' duration, FOSAMAX 5 and 10 mg/day reduced cross-linked N-telopeptides of type I collagen (a marker of bone resorption) by approximately 60% and reduced bone-specific alkaline phosphatase and total serum alkaline phosphatase (markers of bone formation) by approximately 15 to 30% and 8 to 18%, respectively. As a result of inhibition of bone resorption, FOSAMAX 5 and 10 mg/day induced asymptomatic decreases in serum calcium (approximately 1 to 2%) and serum phosphate (approximately 1 to 8%).

Paget's disease of bone

Paget's disease of bone is a chronic, focal skeletal disorder characterized by greatly increased and disorderly bone remodeling. Excessive osteoclastic bone resorption is followed by osteoblastic new bone formation, leading to the replacement of the normal bone architecture by disorganized, enlarged, and weakened bone structure.

Clinical manifestations of Paget's disease range from no symptoms to severe morbidity due to bone pain, bone deformity, pathological fractures, and neurological and other complications. Serum alkaline phosphatase, the most frequently used biochemical index of disease activity, provides an objective measure of disease severity and response to therapy.

FOSAMAX decreases the rate of bone resorption directly, which leads to an indirect decrease in bone formation. In clinical trials, FOSAMAX 40 mg once daily for six months produced significant decreases in serum alkaline phosphatase as well as in urinary markers of bone collagen degradation. As a result of the inhibition of bone resorption, FOSAMAX induced generally mild, transient, and asymptomatic decreases in serum calcium and phosphate.

Clinical Studies

Treatment of osteoporosis

Postmenopausal women

Effect on bone mineral density

The efficacy of FOSAMAX 10 mg once daily in postmenopausal women, 44 to 84 years of age, with osteoporosis (lumbar spine bone mineral density [BMD] of at least 2 standard deviations below the premenopausal mean) was demonstrated in four double-blind, placebo-controlled clinical studies of two or three years' duration. These included two three-year, multicenter studies of virtually identical design, one performed in the United States (U.S.) and the other in 15 different countries (Multinational), which enrolled 478 and 516 patients, respectively. The following graph shows the mean increases in BMD of the lumbar spine, femoral neck, and trochanter in patients receiving FOSAMAX 10 mg/day relative to placebo-treated patients at three years for each of these studies.

[See figure at top of next column]

At three years significant increases in BMD, relative both to baseline and placebo, were seen at each measurement site in each study in patients who received FOSAMAX 10 mg/day. Total body BMD also increased significantly in each study, suggesting that the increases in bone mass of the spine and hip did not occur at the expense of other skeletal sites. Increases in BMD were evident as early as three months and continued throughout the three years of treat-

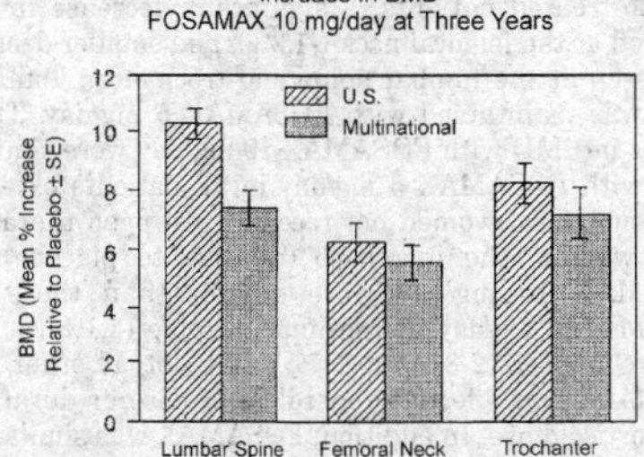

ment. (See figures below for lumbar spine results.) In the two-year extension of these studies, treatment of 147 patients with FOSAMAX 10 mg/day resulted in continued increases in BMD at the lumbar spine and trochanter (absolute additional increases between years 3 and 5: lumbar spine, 0.94%; trochanter, 0.88%). BMD at the femoral neck, forearm and total body were maintained. FOSAMAX was similarly effective regardless of age, race, baseline rate of bone turnover, and baseline BMD in the range studied (at least 2 standard deviations below the premenopausal mean). Thus, overall FOSAMAX reverses the loss of bone mineral density, a central factor in the progression of osteoporosis.

[See figure above]

In patients with postmenopausal osteoporosis treated with FOSAMAX 10 mg/day for one or two years, the effects of treatment withdrawal were assessed. Following discontinuation, there were no further increases in bone mass and the rates of bone loss were similar to those of the placebo groups. These data indicate that continued treatment with FOSAMAX is required to maintain the effect of the drug.

The therapeutic equivalence of once weekly FOSAMAX 70 mg (n=519) and FOSAMAX 10 mg daily (n=370) was demonstrated in a one-year, double-blind, multicenter study of postmenopausal women with osteoporosis. In the primary analysis of completers, the mean increases from baseline in lumbar spine BMD at one year were 5.1% (4.8, 5.4%; 95% CI) in the 70-mg once-weekly group (n=440) and 5.4% (5.0, 5.8%; 95% CI) in the 10-mg daily group (n=330). The two treatment groups were also similar with regard to BMD increases at other skeletal sites. The results of the intention-to-treat analysis were consistent with the primary analysis of completers.

Effect on fracture incidence

Data on the effects of FOSAMAX on fracture incidence are derived from three clinical studies: 1) U.S. and Multinational combined: a study of patients with a BMD T-score at or below minus 2.5 with or without a prior vertebral fracture, 2) Three-Year Study of the Fracture Intervention Trial (FIT): a study of patients with at least one baseline vertebral fracture, and 3) Four-Year Study of FIT: a study of patients with low bone mass but without a baseline vertebral fracture.

To assess the effects of FOSAMAX on the incidence of vertebral fractures (detected by digitized radiography; approximately one third of these were clinically symptomatic), the U.S. and Multinational studies were combined in an analysis that compared placebo to the pooled dosage groups of FOSAMAX (5 or 10 mg for three years or 20 mg for two years followed by 5 mg for one year). There was a statistically significant reduction in the proportion of patients treated with FOSAMAX experiencing one or more new vertebral fractures relative to those treated with placebo (3.2% vs. 6.2%; a 48% relative risk reduction). A reduction in the total number of new vertebral fractures (4.2 vs. 11.3 per 100 patients) was also observed. In the pooled analysis, patients who received FOSAMAX had a loss in stature that was statistically significantly less than was observed in those who received placebo (-3.0 mm vs. -4.6 mm).

The Fracture Intervention Trial (FIT) consisted of two studies in postmenopausal women: the Three-Year Study of patients who had at least one baseline radiographic vertebral fracture and the Four-Year Study of patients with low bone mass but without a baseline vertebral fracture. In both studies of FIT, 96% of randomized patients completed the studies (i.e., had a closeout visit at the scheduled end of the study); approximately 80% of patients were still taking study medication upon completion.

Fracture Intervention Trial: Three-Year Study (patients with at least one baseline radiographic vertebral fracture)

This randomized, double-blind, placebo-controlled, 2027-patient study (FOSAMAX, n=1022; placebo, n=1005) demonstrated that treatment with FOSAMAX resulted in statistically significant reductions in fracture incidence at three years as shown in the table below.

[See first table above]

Furthermore, in this population of patients with baseline vertebral fracture, treatment with FOSAMAX significantly reduced the incidence of hospitalizations (25.0% vs. 30.7%).

In the Three-Year Study of FIT, fractures of the hip occurred in 22 (2.2%) of 1005 patients on placebo and 11 (1.1%) of 1022 patients on FOSAMAX, p=0.047. The figure below displays the cumulative incidence of hip fractures in this study.

Osteoporosis Treatment Studies in Postmenopausal Women

Time Course of Effect of FOSAMAX 10 mg/day Versus Placebo: Lumbar Spine BMD Percent Change From Baseline

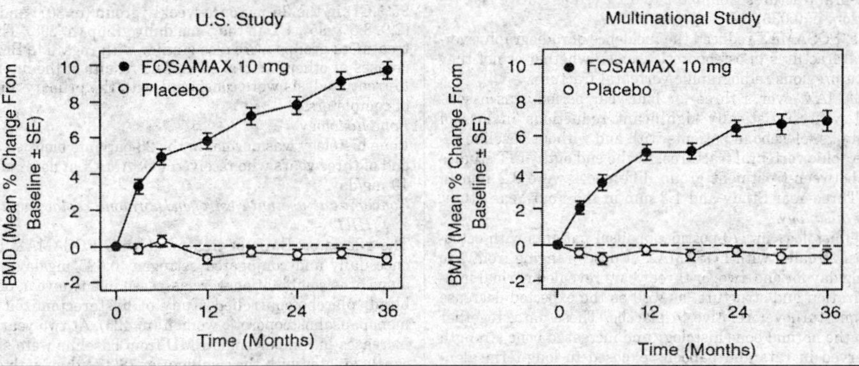

Effect of FOSAMAX on Fracture Incidence in the Three-Year Study of FIT
(patients with vertebral fracture at baseline)

	Percent of Patients		Absolute Reduction in Fracture Incidence	Relative Reduction in Fracture Risk %
	FOSAMAX (n=1022)	Placebo (n=1005)		
Patients with:				
Vertebral fractures (diagnosed by X-ray)†				
≥1 new vertebral fracture	7.9	15.0	7.1	47***
≥2 new vertebral fractures	0.5	4.9	4.4	90***
Clinical (symptomatic) fractures				
Any clinical (symptomatic) fracture	13.8	18.1	4.3	26‡
≥1 clinical (symptomatic) vertebral fracture	2.3	5.0	2.7	54**
Hip fracture	1.1	2.2	1.1	51*
Wrist (forearm) fracture	2.2	4.1	1.9	48*

†Number evaluable for vertebral fractures: FOSAMAX, n=984; placebo, n=966
*p<0.05, **p<0.01, ***p<0.001, ‡p=0.007

Effect of FOSAMAX on Fracture Incidence in Osteoporotic† Patients in the Four-Year Study of FIT
(patients without vertebral fracture at baseline)

	Percent of Patients		Absolute Reduction in Fracture Incidence	Relative Reduction in Fracture Risk (%)
	FOSAMAX (n=1545)	Placebo (n=1521)		
Patients with:				
Vertebral fractures (diagnosed by X-ray)††				
≥1 new vertebral fracture	2.5	4.8	2.3	48***
≥2 new vertebral fractures	0.1	0.6	0.5	78*
Clinical (symptomatic) fractures				
Any clinical (symptomatic) fracture	12.9	16.2	3.3	22**
≥1 clinical (symptomatic) vertebral fracture	1.0	1.6	0.6	41 (NS)†††
Hip fracture	1.0	1.4	0.4	29 (NS)†††
Wrist (forearm) fracture	3.9	3.8	-0.1	NS†††

†Baseline femoral neck BMD at least 2 SD below the mean for young adult women
††Number evaluable for vertebral fractures: FOSAMAX, n=1426; placebo, n=1428
†††Not significant. This study was not powered to detect differences at these sites.
*p=0.035, **p=0.01, ***p<0.001

Cumulative Incidence of Hip Fractures in the Three-Year Study of FIT
(patients with radiographic vertebral fracture at baseline)

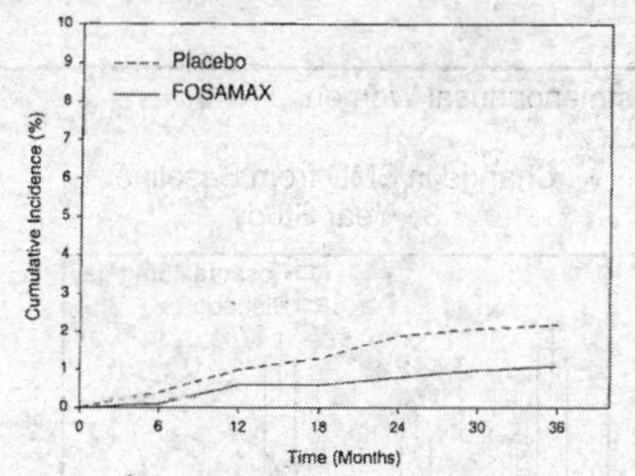

Fracture Intervention Trial: Four-Year Study (patients with low bone mass but without a baseline radiographic vertebral fracture)

This randomized, double-blind, placebo-controlled, 4432-patient study (FOSAMAX, n=2214; placebo, n=2218) further investigated the reduction in fracture incidence due to FOSAMAX. The intent of the study was to recruit women with osteoporosis, defined as a baseline femoral neck BMD at least two standard deviations below the mean for young adult women. However, due to subsequent revisions to the normative values for femoral neck BMD, 31% of patients were found not to meet this entry criterion and thus this study included both osteoporotic and non-osteoporotic women. The results are shown in the table below for the patients with osteoporosis.

[See second table above]

Fracture results across studies

In the Three-Year Study of FIT, FOSAMAX reduced the percentage of women experiencing at least one new radiographic vertebral fracture from 15.0% to 7.9% (47% relative risk reduction, p<0.001); in the Four-Year Study of FIT, the percentage was reduced from 3.8% to 2.1% (44% relative risk reduction, p=0.001); and in the combined U.S./Multinational studies, from 6.2% to 3.2% (48% relative risk reduction, p=0.034).

FOSAMAX reduced the percentage of women experiencing multiple (two or more) new vertebral fractures from 4.2% to 0.6% (87% relative risk reduction, p<0.001) in the combined U.S./Multinational studies and from 4.9% to 0.5% (90% relative risk reduction, p<0.001) in the Three-Year Study of

Continued on next page

Fosamax—Cont.

FIT. In the Four-Year Study of FIT, FOSAMAX reduced the percentage of osteoporotic women experiencing multiple vertebral fractures from 0.6% to 0.1% (78% relative risk reduction, p=0.035).

Thus, FOSAMAX reduced the incidence of radiographic vertebral fractures in osteoporotic women whether or not they had a previous radiographic vertebral fracture.

FOSAMAX, over a three- or four-year period, was associated with statistically significant reductions in loss of height vs. placebo in patients with and without baseline radiographic vertebral fractures. At the end of the FIT studies the between-treatment group differences were 3.2 mm in the Three-Year Study and 1.3 mm in the Four-Year Study.

Bone histology

Bone histology in 270 postmenopausal patients with osteoporosis treated with FOSAMAX at doses ranging from 1 to 20 mg/day for one, two, or three years revealed normal mineralization and structure, as well as the expected decrease in bone turnover relative to placebo. These data, together with the normal bone histology and increased bone strength observed in rats and baboons exposed to long-term alendronate treatment, support the conclusion that bone formed during therapy with FOSAMAX is of normal quality.

Men

The efficacy of FOSAMAX in men with hypogonadal or idiopathic osteoporosis was demonstrated in two clinical studies.

A two-year, double-blind, placebo-controlled, multicenter study of FOSAMAX 10 mg once daily enrolled a total of 241 men between the ages of 31 and 87 (mean, 63). All patients in the trial had either: 1) a BMD T-score ≤-2 at the femoral neck and ≤-1 at the lumbar spine, or 2) a baseline osteoporotic fracture and a BMD T-score ≤-1 at the femoral neck. At two years, the mean increases relative to placebo in BMD in men receiving FOSAMAX 10 mg/day were significant at the following sites: lumbar spine, 5.3%; femoral neck, 2.6%; trochanter, 3.1%; and total body, 1.6%. Treatment with FOSAMAX also reduced height loss (FOSAMAX, -0.6 mm vs. placebo, -2.4 mm).

A one-year, double-blind, placebo-controlled, multicenter study of once weekly FOSAMAX 70 mg enrolled a total of 167 men between the ages of 38 and 91 (mean, 66). Patients in the study had either: 1) a BMD T-score ≤-2 at the femoral neck and ≤-1 at the lumbar spine, 2) a BMD T-score ≤-2 at the lumbar spine and ≤-1 at the femoral neck, or 3) a baseline osteoporotic fracture and a BMD T-score ≤-1 at the femoral neck. At one year, the mean increases relative to placebo in BMD in men receiving FOSAMAX 70 mg once weekly were significant at the following sites: lumbar spine, 2.8%; femoral neck, 1.9%; trochanter, 2.0%; and total body, 1.2%. These increases in BMD were similar to those seen at one year in the 10 mg once-daily study.

In both studies, BMD responses were similar regardless of age (≥65 years vs. <65 years), gonadal function (baseline testosterone <9 ng/dL vs. ≥9 ng/dL), or baseline BMD (femoral neck and lumbar spine T-score ≤-2.5 vs. >-2.5).

Prevention of osteoporosis in postmenopausal women

Prevention of bone loss was demonstrated in two double-blind, placebo-controlled studies of postmenopausal women 40-60 years of age. One thousand six hundred nine patients (FOSAMAX 5 mg/day; n=498) who were at least six months postmenopausal were entered into a two-year study without regard to their baseline BMD. In the other study, 447 patients (FOSAMAX 5 mg/day; n=88), who were between six months and three years postmenopause, were treated for up to three years. In the placebo-treated patients BMD losses of approximately 1% per year were seen at the spine, hip (femoral neck and trochanter) and total body. In contrast, FOSAMAX 5 mg/day prevented bone loss in the majority of patients and induced significant increases in mean bone mass at each of these sites (see figures below). In addition, FOSAMAX 5 mg/day reduced the rate of bone loss at the forearm by approximately half relative to placebo. FOSAMAX 5 mg/day was similarly effective in this population regardless of age, time since menopause, race and baseline rate of bone turnover.

[See figure below]

The therapeutic equivalence of once weekly FOSAMAX 35 mg (n=362) and FOSAMAX 5 mg daily (n=361) was demonstrated in a one-year, double-blind, multicenter study of postmenopausal women without osteoporosis. In the primary analysis of completers, the mean increases from baseline in lumbar spine BMD at one year were 2.9% (2.6, 3.2%; 95% CI) in the 35-mg once-weekly group (n=307) and 3.2% (2.9, 3.5%; 95% CI) in the 5-mg daily group (n=298). The two treatment groups were also similar with regard to BMD increases at other skeletal sites. The results of the intention-to-treat analysis were consistent with the primary analysis of completers.

Bone histology

Bone histology was normal in the 28 patients biopsied at the end of three years who received FOSAMAX at doses of up to 10 mg/day.

Concomitant use with estrogen/hormone replacement therapy (HRT)

The effects on BMD of treatment with FOSAMAX 10 mg once daily and conjugated estrogen (0.625 mg/day) either alone or in combination were assessed in a two-year, double-blind, placebo-controlled study of hysterectomized postmenopausal osteoporotic women (n=425). At two years, the increases in lumbar spine BMD from baseline were significantly greater with the combination (8.3%) than with either estrogen or FOSAMAX alone (both 6.0%).

The effects on BMD when FOSAMAX was added to stable doses (for at least one year) of HRT (estrogen ± progestin) were assessed in a one-year, double-blind, placebo-controlled study in postmenopausal osteoporotic women (n=428). The addition of FOSAMAX 10 mg once daily to HRT produced, at one year, significantly greater increases in lumbar spine BMD (3.7%) vs. HRT alone (1.1%).

In these studies, significant increases or favorable trends in BMD for combined therapy compared with HRT alone were seen at the total hip, femoral neck, and trochanter. No significant effect was seen for total body BMD.

Histomorphometric studies of transiliac biopsies in 92 subjects showed normal bone architecture. Compared to placebo there was a 98% suppression of bone turnover (as assessed by mineralizing surface) after 18 months of combined treatment with FOSAMAX and HRT, 94% on FOSAMAX alone, and 78% on HRT alone. The long-term effects of combined FOSAMAX and HRT on fracture occurrence and fracture healing have not been studied.

Glucocorticoid-induced osteoporosis

The efficacy of FOSAMAX 5 and 10 mg once daily in men and women receiving glucocorticoids (at least 7.5 mg/day of prednisone or equivalent) was demonstrated in two, one-year, double-blind, randomized, placebo-controlled, multicenter studies of virtually identical design, one performed in the United States and the other in 15 different countries (Multinational [which also included FOSAMAX 2.5 mg/day]). These studies enrolled 232 and 328 patients, respectively, between the ages of 17 and 83 with a variety of glucocorticoid-requiring diseases. Patients received supplemental calcium and vitamin D. The following figure shows the mean increases relative to placebo in BMD of the lumbar spine, femoral neck, and trochanter in patients receiving FOSAMAX 5 mg/day for each study.

Studies in Glucocorticoid - Treated Patients
Increase in BMD
FOSAMAX 5 mg/day at One Year

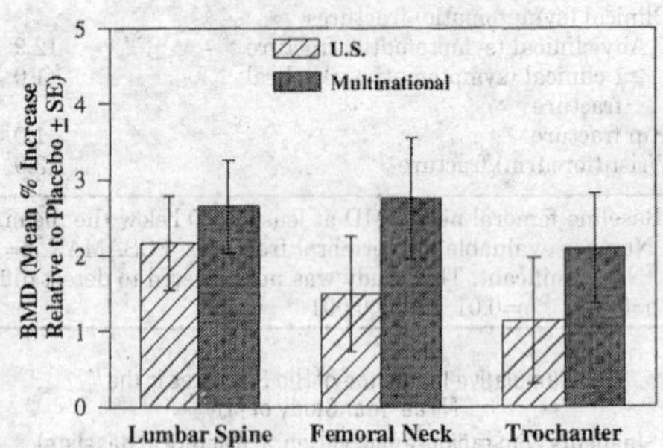

After one year, significant increases relative to placebo in BMD were seen in the combined studies at each of these sites in patients who received FOSAMAX 5 mg/day. In the placebo-treated patients, a significant decrease in BMD occurred at the femoral neck (-1.2%), and smaller decreases were seen at the lumbar spine and trochanter. Total body BMD was maintained with FOSAMAX 5 mg/day. The increases in BMD with FOSAMAX 10 mg/day were similar to those with FOSAMAX 5 mg/day in all patients except for postmenopausal women not receiving estrogen therapy. In these women, the increases (relative to placebo) with FOSAMAX 10 mg/day were greater than those with FOSAMAX 5 mg/day at the lumbar spine (4.1% vs. 1.6%) and trochanter (2.8% vs. 1.7%), but not at other sites. FOSAMAX was effective regardless of dose or duration of glucocorticoid use. In addition, FOSAMAX was similarly effective regardless of age (<65 vs. ≥65 years), race (Caucasian vs. other races), gender, underlying disease, baseline BMD, baseline bone turnover, and use with a variety of common medications.

Bone histology was normal in the 49 patients biopsied at the end of one year who received FOSAMAX at doses of up to 10 mg/day.

Of the original 560 patients in these studies, 208 patients who remained on at least 7.5 mg/day of prednisone or equivalent continued into a one-year double-blind extension. After two years of treatment, spine BMD increased by 3.7% and 5.0% relative to placebo with FOSAMAX 5 and 10 mg/day, respectively. Significant increases in BMD (relative to placebo) were also observed at the femoral neck, trochanter, and total body.

After one year, 2.3% of patients treated with FOSAMAX 5 or 10 mg/day (pooled) vs. 3.7% of those treated with placebo experienced a new vertebral fracture (not significant). However, in the population studied for two years, treatment with FOSAMAX (pooled dosage groups: 5 or 10 mg for two years or 2.5 mg for one year followed by 10 mg for one year) significantly reduced the incidence of patients with a new vertebral fracture (FOSAMAX 0.7% vs. placebo 6.8%).

Paget's disease of bone

The efficacy of FOSAMAX 40 mg once daily for six months was demonstrated in two double-blind clinical studies of male and female patients with moderate to severe Paget's disease (alkaline phosphatase at least twice the upper limit of normal): a placebo-controlled, multinational study and a U.S. comparative study with etidronate disodium 400 mg/day. The following figure shows the mean percent changes from baseline in serum alkaline phosphatase for up to six months of randomized treatment.

Studies in Paget's Disease of Bone

Effect on Serum Alkaline Phospatase of FOSAMAX 40 mg/day Versus Placebo or Etidronate 400 mg/day

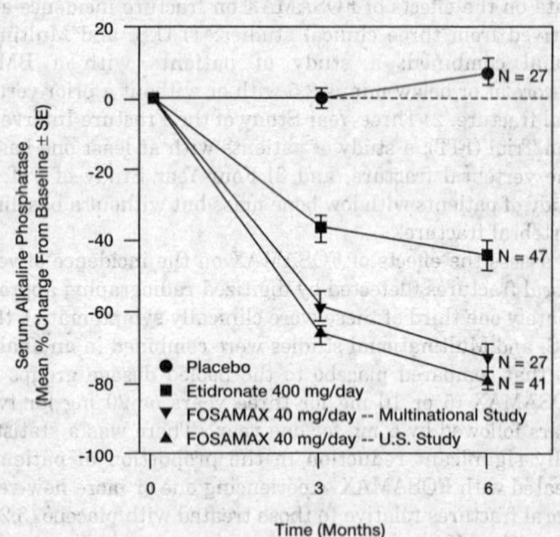

At six months the suppression in alkaline phosphatase in patients treated with FOSAMAX was significantly greater than that achieved with etidronate and contrasted with the complete lack of response in placebo-treated patients. Response (defined as either normalization of serum alkaline phosphatase or decrease from baseline ≥60%) occurred in approximately 85% of patients treated with FOSAMAX in the combined studies vs. 30% in the etidronate group and 0% in the placebo group. FOSAMAX was similarly effective regardless of age, gender, race, prior use of other bisphosphonates, or baseline alkaline phosphatase within the range studied (at least twice the upper limit of normal).

Bone histology was evaluated in 33 patients with Paget's disease treated with FOSAMAX 40 mg/day for 6 months. As in patients treated for osteoporosis (see *Clinical Studies, Treatment of osteoporosis in postmenopausal women, Bone histology*), FOSAMAX did not impair mineralization, and the expected decrease in the rate of bone turnover was observed. Normal lamellar bone was produced during treatment with FOSAMAX, even where preexisting bone was woven and disorganized. Overall, bone histology data support the conclusion that bone formed during treatment with FOSAMAX is of normal quality.

ANIMAL PHARMACOLOGY

The relative inhibitory activities on bone resorption and mineralization of alendronate and etidronate were compared in the Schenk assay, which is based on histological examination of the epiphyses of growing rats. In this assay, the lowest dose of alendronate that interfered with bone

Osteoporosis Prevention Studies in Postmenopausal Women

Change in BMD from Baseline
2 - Year Study

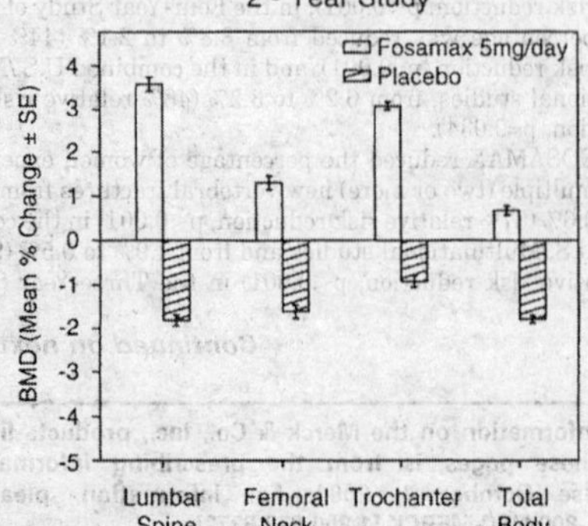

Change in BMD from Baseline
3 - Year Study

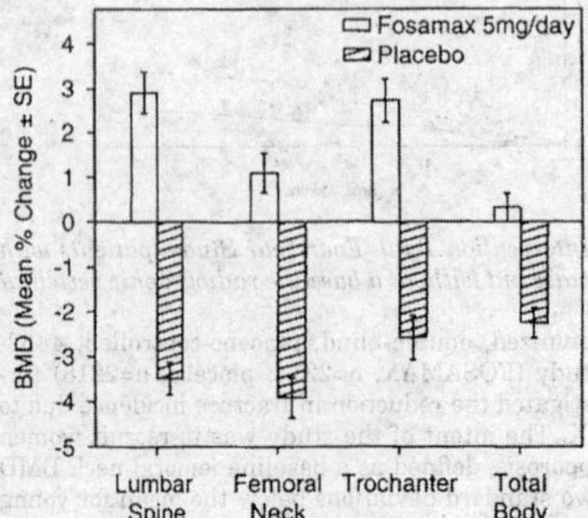

mineralization (leading to osteomalacia) was 6000-fold the antiresorptive dose. The corresponding ratio for etidronate was one to one. These data suggest that alendronate administered in therapeutic doses is highly unlikely to induce osteomalacia.

INDICATIONS AND USAGE

FOSAMAX is indicated for:

- Treatment and prevention of osteoporosis in postmenopausal women
  - For the treatment of osteoporosis, FOSAMAX increases bone mass and reduces the incidence of fractures, including those of the hip and spine (vertebral compression fractures). Osteoporosis may be confirmed by the finding of low bone mass (for example, at least 2 standard deviations below the premenopausal mean) or by the presence or history of osteoporotic fracture. (See CLINICAL PHARMACOLOGY, *Pharmacodynamics*.)
  - For the prevention of osteoporosis, FOSAMAX may be considered in postmenopausal women who are at risk of developing osteoporosis and for whom the desired clinical outcome is to maintain bone mass and to reduce the risk of future fracture.

    Bone loss is particularly rapid in postmenopausal women younger than age 60. Risk factors often associated with the development of postmenopausal osteoporosis include early menopause; moderately low bone mass (for example, at least 1 standard deviation below the mean for healthy young adult women); thin body build; Caucasian or Asian race; and family history of osteoporosis. The presence of such risk factors may be important when considering the use of FOSAMAX for prevention of osteoporosis.
- Treatment to increase bone mass in men with osteoporosis
- Treatment of glucocorticoid-induced osteoporosis in men and women receiving glucocorticoids in a daily dosage equivalent to 7.5 mg or greater of prednisone and who have low bone mineral density (see PRECAUTIONS, *Glucocorticoid-induced osteoporosis*). Patients treated with glucocorticoids should receive adequate amounts of calcium and vitamin D.
- Treatment of Paget's disease of bone in men and women
  - Treatment is indicated in patients with Paget's disease of bone having alkaline phosphatase at least two times the upper limit of normal, or those who are symptomatic, or those at risk for future complications from their disease.

CONTRAINDICATIONS

- Abnormalities of the esophagus which delay esophageal emptying such as stricture or achalasia
- Inability to stand or sit upright for at least 30 minutes
- Patients at increased risk of aspiration should not receive FOSAMAX oral solution.
- Hypersensitivity to any component of this product
- Hypocalcemia (see PRECAUTIONS, *General*)

WARNINGS

FOSAMAX, like other bisphosphonates, may cause local irritation of the upper gastrointestinal mucosa.

Esophageal adverse experiences, such as esophagitis, esophageal ulcers and esophageal erosions, occasionally with bleeding and rarely followed by esophageal stricture or perforation, have been reported in patients receiving treatment with FOSAMAX. In some cases these have been severe and required hospitalization. Physicians should therefore be alert to any signs or symptoms signaling a possible esophageal reaction and patients should be instructed to discontinue FOSAMAX and seek medical attention if they develop dysphagia, odynophagia, retrosternal pain or new or worsening heartburn.

The risk of severe esophageal adverse experiences appears to be greater in patients who lie down after taking FOSAMAX and/or who fail to swallow it with the recommended amount of water, and/or who continue to take FOSAMAX after developing symptoms suggestive of esophageal irritation. Therefore, it is very important that the full dosing instructions are provided to, and understood by, the patient (see DOSAGE AND ADMINISTRATION). In patients who cannot comply with dosing instructions due to mental disability, therapy with FOSAMAX should be used under appropriate supervision.

Because of possible irritant effects of FOSAMAX on the upper gastrointestinal mucosa and a potential for worsening of the underlying disease, caution should be used when FOSAMAX is given to patients with active upper gastrointestinal problems (such as dysphagia, esophageal diseases, gastritis, duodenitis, or ulcers).

There have been post-marketing reports of gastric and duodenal ulcers, some severe and with complications, although no increased risk was observed in controlled clinical trials.

PRECAUTIONS

General

Causes of osteoporosis other than estrogen deficiency, aging, and glucocorticoid use should be considered.

Hypocalcemia must be corrected before initiating therapy with FOSAMAX (see CONTRAINDICATIONS). Other disorders affecting mineral metabolism (such as vitamin D deficiency) should also be effectively treated. In patients with these conditions, serum calcium and symptoms of hypocalcemia should be monitored during therapy with FOSAMAX.

Presumably due to the effects of FOSAMAX on increasing bone mineral, small, asymptomatic decreases in serum calcium and phosphate may occur, especially in patients with Paget's disease, in whom the pretreatment rate of bone turnover may be greatly elevated and in patients receiving glucocorticoids, in whom calcium absorption may be decreased.

Ensuring adequate calcium and vitamin D intake is especially important in patients with Paget's disease of bone and in patients receiving glucocorticoids.

Renal insufficiency

FOSAMAX is not recommended for patients with renal insufficiency (creatinine clearance <35 mL/min). (See DOSAGE AND ADMINISTRATION.)

Glucocorticoid-induced osteoporosis

The risk versus benefit of FOSAMAX for treatment at daily dosages of glucocorticoids less than 7.5 mg of prednisone or equivalent has not been established (see INDICATIONS AND USAGE). Before initiating treatment, the hormonal status of both men and women should be ascertained and appropriate replacement considered.

A bone mineral density measurement should be made at the initiation of therapy and repeated after 6 to 12 months of combined FOSAMAX and glucocorticoid treatment.

The efficacy of FOSAMAX for the treatment of glucocorticoid-induced osteoporosis has been shown in patients with a median bone mineral density which was 1.2 standard deviations below the mean for healthy young adults.

The efficacy of FOSAMAX has been established in studies of two years' duration. The greatest increase in bone mineral density occurred in the first year with maintenance or smaller gains during the second year. Efficacy of FOSAMAX beyond two years has not been studied.

The efficacy of FOSAMAX in respect to fracture prevention has been demonstrated for vertebral fractures. However, this finding was based on very few fractures that occurred primarily in postmenopausal women. The efficacy for prevention of non-vertebral fractures has not been demonstrated.

Information for Patients

General

Physicians should instruct their patients to read the patient package insert before starting therapy with FOSAMAX and to reread it each time the prescription is renewed.

Patients should be instructed to take supplemental calcium and vitamin D, if daily dietary intake is inadequate. Weight-bearing exercise should be considered along with the modification of certain behavioral factors, such as cigarette smoking and/or excessive alcohol consumption, if these factors exist.

Dosing Instructions

Patients should be instructed that the expected benefits of FOSAMAX may only be obtained when it is taken with plain water the first thing upon arising for the day at least 30 minutes before the first food, beverage, or medication of the day. Even dosing with orange juice or coffee has been shown to markedly reduce the absorption of FOSAMAX (see CLINICAL PHARMACOLOGY, *Pharmacokinetics Absorption*).

To facilitate delivery to the stomach and thus reduce the potential for esophageal irritation patients should be instructed to swallow each tablet of FOSAMAX with a full glass of water (6-8 oz). To facilitate gastric emptying patients should drink at least 2 oz (a quarter of a cup) of water after taking FOSAMAX oral solution. Patients should be instructed not to lie down for at least 30 minutes and until after their first food of the day. Patients should not chew or suck on the tablet because of a potential for oropharyngeal ulceration. Patients should be specifically instructed not to take FOSAMAX at bedtime or before arising for the day. Patients should be informed that failure to follow these instructions may increase their risk of esophageal problems. Patients should be instructed that if they develop symptoms of esophageal disease (such as difficulty or pain upon swallowing, retrosternal pain or new or worsening heartburn) they should stop taking FOSAMAX and consult their physician.

Patients should be instructed that if they miss a dose of once weekly FOSAMAX, they should take one dose on the morning after they remember. They should not take two doses on the same day but should return to taking one dose once a week, as originally scheduled on their chosen day.

Drug Interactions (also see CLINICAL PHARMACOLOGY, *Pharmacokinetics, Drug Interactions*)

Estrogen/hormone replacement therapy (HRT)

Concomitant use of HRT (estrogen $\pm$ progestin) and FOSAMAX was assessed in two clinical studies of one or two years' duration in postmenopausal osteoporotic women. In these studies, the safety and tolerability profile of the combination was consistent with those of the individual treatments; however, the degree of suppression of bone turnover (as assessed by mineralizing surface) was significantly greater with the combination than with either component alone. The long-term effects of combined FOSAMAX and HRT on fracture occurrence have not been studied (see CLINICAL PHARMACOLOGY, *Clinical Studies, Concomitant use with estrogen/hormone replacement therapy (HRT)* and ADVERSE REACTIONS, *Clinical Studies, Concomitant use with estrogen/hormone replacement therapy*).

Calcium Supplements/Antacids

It is likely that calcium supplements, antacids, and some oral medications will interfere with absorption of FOSAMAX. Therefore, patients must wait at least one-half hour after taking FOSAMAX before taking any other oral medications.

Aspirin

In clinical studies, the incidence of upper gastrointestinal adverse events was increased in patients receiving concomitant therapy with daily doses of FOSAMAX greater than 10 mg and aspirin-containing products.

Nonsteroidal Anti-inflammatory Drugs (NSAIDs)

FOSAMAX may be administered to patients taking NSAIDs. In a 3-year, controlled, clinical study (n=2027) during which a majority of patients received concomitant NSAIDs, the incidence of upper gastrointestinal adverse events was similar in patients taking FOSAMAX 5 or 10 mg/day compared to those taking placebo. However, since NSAID use is associated with gastrointestinal irritation, caution should be used during concomitant use with FOSAMAX.

Carcinogenesis, Mutagenesis, Impairment of Fertility

Harderian gland (a retro-orbital gland not present in humans) adenomas were increased in high-dose female mice (p=0.003) in a 92-week oral carcinogenicity study at doses of alendronate of 1, 3, and 10 mg/kg/day (males) or 1, 2, and 5 mg/kg/day (females). These doses are equivalent to 0.12 to 1.2 times a maximum recommended daily dose of 40 mg (Paget's disease) based on surface area, mg/m^2. The relevance of this finding to humans is unknown.

Parafollicular cell (thyroid) adenomas were increased in high-dose male rats (p=0.003) in a 2-year oral carcinogenicity study at doses of 1 and 3.75 mg/kg body weight. These doses are equivalent to 0.26 and 1 times a 40 mg human daily dose based on surface area, mg/m^2. The relevance of this finding to humans is unknown.

Alendronate was not genotoxic in the *in vitro* microbial mutagenesis assay with and without metabolic activation, in an *in vitro* mammalian cell mutagenesis assay, in an *in vitro* alkaline elution assay in rat hepatocytes, and in an *in vivo* chromosomal aberration assay in mice. In an *in vitro* chromosomal aberration assay in Chinese hamster ovary cells, however, alendronate gave equivocal results.

Alendronate had no effect on fertility (male or female) in rats at oral doses up to 5 mg/kg/day (1.3 times a 40 mg human daily dose based on surface area, mg/m^2).

Pregnancy

Pregnancy Category C:

Reproduction studies in rats showed decreased postimplantation survival at 2 mg/kg/day and decreased body weight gain in normal pups at 1 mg/kg/day. Sites of incomplete fetal ossification were statistically significantly increased in rats beginning at 10 mg/kg/day in vertebral (cervical, thoracic, and lumbar), skull, and sternebral bones. The above doses ranged from 0.26 times (1 mg/kg) to 2.6 times (10 mg/kg) a maximum recommended daily dose of 40 mg (Paget's disease) based on surface area, mg/m^2. No similar fetal effects were seen when pregnant rabbits were treated at doses up to 35 mg/kg/day (10.3 times a 40 mg human daily dose based on surface area, mg/m^2).

Both total and ionized calcium decreased in pregnant rats at 15 mg/kg/day (3.9 times a 40 mg human daily dose based on surface area, mg/m^2) resulting in delays and failures of delivery. Protracted parturition due to maternal hypocalcemia occurred in rats at doses as low as 0.5 mg/kg/day (0.13 times a 40 mg human daily dose based on surface area, mg/m^2) when rats were treated from before mating through gestation. Maternotoxicity (late pregnancy deaths) occurred in the female rats treated with 15 mg/kg/day for varying periods of time ranging from treatment only during pre-mating to treatment only during early, middle, or late gestation; these deaths were lessened but not eliminated by cessation of treatment. Calcium supplementation either in the drinking water or by minipump could not ameliorate the hypocalcemia or prevent maternal and neonatal deaths due to delays in delivery; calcium supplementation IV prevented maternal, but not fetal deaths.

Bisphosphonates are incorporated into the bone matrix, from which they are gradually released over a period of years. The amount of bisphosphonate incorporated into adult bone, and hence, the amount available for release back into the systemic circulation, is directly related to the dose and duration of bisphosphonate use. There are no data on fetal risk in humans. However, there is a theoretical risk of fetal harm, predominantly skeletal, if a woman becomes pregnant after completing a course of bisphosphonate therapy. The impact of variables such as time between cessation of bisphosphonate therapy to conception, the particular bisphosphonate used, and the route of administration (intravenous versus oral) on the risk has not been studied.

There are no studies in pregnant women. FOSAMAX should be used during pregnancy only if the potential benefit justifies the potential risk to the mother and fetus.

Nursing Mothers

It is not known whether alendronate is excreted in human milk. Because many drugs are excreted in human milk, caution should be exercised when FOSAMAX is administered to nursing women.

Pediatric Use

Safety and effectiveness in pediatric patients have not been established.

Continued on next page

Information on the Merck & Co., Inc., products listed on these pages is from the prescribing information in use October 1, 2004. For information, please call 1-800-NSC-MERCK [1-800-672-6372].

Fosamax—Cont.

Geriatric Use
Of the patients receiving FOSAMAX in the Fracture Intervention Trial (FIT), 71% (n=2302) were ≥65 years of age and 17% (n=550) were ≥75 years of age. Of the patients receiving FOSAMAX in the United States and Multinational osteoporosis treatment studies in women, osteoporosis studies in men, glucocorticoid-induced osteoporosis studies, and Paget's disease studies (see CLINICAL PHARMACOLOGY, *Clinical Studies*), 45%, 54%, 37%, and 70%, respectively, were 65 years of age or over. No overall differences in efficacy or safety were observed between these patients and younger patients, but greater sensitivity of some older individuals cannot be ruled out.

ADVERSE REACTIONS
Clinical Studies
In clinical studies of up to five years in duration adverse experiences associated with FOSAMAX usually were mild, and generally did not require discontinuation of therapy.
FOSAMAX has been evaluated for safety in approximately 8000 postmenopausal women in clinical studies.
Treatment of osteoporosis
Postmenopausal women
In two identically designed, three-year, placebo-controlled, double-blind, multicenter studies (United States and Multinational; n=994), discontinuation of therapy due to any clinical adverse experience occurred in 4.1% of 196 patients treated with FOSAMAX 10 mg/day and 6.0% of 397 patients treated with placebo. In the Fracture Intervention Trial (n=6459), discontinuation of therapy due to any clinical adverse experience occurred in 9.1% of 3236 patients treated with FOSAMAX 5 mg/day for 2 years and 10 mg/day for either one or two additional years and 10.1% of 3223 patients treated with placebo. Discontinuations due to upper gastrointestinal adverse experiences were: FOSAMAX, 3.2%; placebo, 2.7%. In these study populations, 49-54% had a history of gastrointestinal disorders at baseline and 54-89% used nonsteroidal anti-inflammatory drugs or aspirin at some time during the studies. Adverse experiences from these studies considered by the investigators as possibly, probably, or definitely drug related in ≥1% of patients treated with either FOSAMAX or placebo are presented in the following table.
[See first table above]
Rarely, rash and erythema have occurred.
One patient treated with FOSAMAX (10 mg/day), who had a history of peptic ulcer disease and gastrectomy and who was taking concomitant aspirin developed an anastomotic ulcer with mild hemorrhage, which was considered drug related. Aspirin and FOSAMAX were discontinued and the patient recovered.
The adverse experience profile was similar for the 401 patients treated with either 5 or 20 mg doses of FOSAMAX in the United States and Multinational studies. The adverse experience profile for the 296 patients who received continued treatment with either 5 or 10 mg doses of FOSAMAX in the two-year extension of these studies (treatment years 4 and 5) was similar to that observed during the three-year placebo-controlled period. During the extension period, of the 151 patients treated with FOSAMAX 10 mg/day, the proportion of patients who discontinued therapy due to any clinical adverse experience was similar to that during the first three years of the study.
In a one-year, double-blind, multicenter study, the overall safety and tolerability profiles of once weekly FOSAMAX 70 mg and FOSAMAX 10 mg daily were similar. The adverse experiences considered by the investigators as possibly, probably, or definitely drug related in ≥1% of patients in either treatment group are presented in the following table.

Osteoporosis Treatment Studies in Postmenopausal Women Adverse Experiences Considered Possibly, Probably, or Definitely Drug Related by the Investigators and Reported in ≥1% of Patients

	Once Weekly FOSAMAX 70 mg % (n=519)	FOSAMAX 10 mg/day % (n=370)
Gastrointestinal		
abdominal pain	3.7	3.0
dyspepsia	2.7	2.2
acid regurgitation	1.9	2.4
nausea	1.9	2.4
abdominal distention	1.0	1.4
constipation	0.8	1.6
flatulence	0.4	1.6
gastritis	0.2	1.1
gastric ulcer	0.0	1.1
Musculoskeletal		
musculoskeletal (bone, muscle, joint) pain	2.9	3.2
muscle cramp	0.2	1.1

Men
In two placebo-controlled, double-blind, multicenter studies in men (a two-year study of FOSAMAX 10 mg/day and a one-year study of once weekly FOSAMAX 70 mg) the rates of discontinuation of therapy due to any clinical adverse experience were 2.7% for FOSAMAX 10 mg/day vs. 10.5% for placebo, and 6.4% for once weekly FOSAMAX 70 mg vs. 8.6% for placebo. The adverse experiences considered by the investigators as possibly, probably, or definitely drug related in ≥2% of patients treated with either FOSAMAX or placebo are presented in the following table.
[See second table above]

Osteoporosis Treatment Studies in Postmenopausal Women Adverse Experiences Considered Possibly, Probably, or Definitely Drug Related by the Investigators and Reported in ≥1% of Patients

	United States/Multinational Studies		Fracture Intervention Trial	
	FOSAMAX* % (n=196)	Placebo % (n=397)	FOSAMAX** % (n=3236)	Placebo % (n=3223)
Gastrointestinal				
abdominal pain	6.6	4.8	1.5	1.5
nausea	3.6	4.0	1.1	1.5
dyspepsia	3.6	3.5	1.1	1.2
constipation	3.1	1.8	0.0	0.2
diarrhea	3.1	1.8	0.6	0.3
flatulence	2.6	0.5	0.2	0.3
acid regurgitation	2.0	4.3	1.1	0.9
esophageal ulcer	1.5	0.0	0.1	0.1
vomiting	1.0	1.5	0.2	0.3
dysphagia	1.0	0.0	0.1	0.1
abdominal distention	1.0	0.8	0.0	0.0
gastritis	0.5	1.3	0.6	0.7
Musculoskeletal				
musculoskeletal (bone, muscle or joint) pain	4.1	2.5	0.4	0.3
muscle cramp	0.0	1.0	0.2	0.1
Nervous System/Psychiatric				
headache	2.6	1.5	0.2	0.2
dizziness	0.0	1.0	0.0	0.1
Special Senses				
taste perversion	0.5	1.0	0.1	0.0

*10 mg/day for three years
**5 mg/day for 2 years and 10 mg/day for either 1 or 2 additional years

Osteoporosis Studies in Men Adverse Experiences Considered Possibly, Probably, or Definitely Drug Related by the Investigators and Reported in ≥2% of Patients

	Two-year Study		One-year Study	
	FOSAMAX 10 mg/day % (n=146)	Placebo % (n=95)	Once Weekly FOSAMAX 70 mg/day % (n=109)	Placebo % (n=58)
Gastrointestinal				
acid regurgitation	4.1	3.2	0.0	0.0
flatulence	4.1	1.1	0.0	0.0
gastroesophageal reflux disease	0.7	3.2	2.8	0.0
dyspepsia	3.4	0.0	2.8	1.7
diarrhea	1.4	1.1	2.8	0.0
abdominal pain	2.1	1.1	0.9	3.4
nausea	2.1	0.0	0.0	0.0

Osteoporosis Prevention Studies in Postmenopausal Women Adverse Experiences Considered Possibly, Probably, or Definitely Drug Related by the Investigators and Reported in ≥1% of Patients

	Two/Three-Year Studies		One-Year Study	
	FOSAMAX 5 mg/day % (n=642)	Placebo % (n=648)	FOSAMAX 5 mg/day % (n=361)	Once Weekly FOSAMAX 35 mg % (n=362)
Gastrointestinal				
dyspepsia	1.9	1.4	2.2	1.7
abdominal pain	1.9	3.4	4.2	2.2
acid regurgitation	1.7	2.5	4.2	4.7
nausea	1.4	1.4	2.5	1.4
diarrhea	1.1	1.7	1.1	0.6
constipation	0.9	0.5	1.7	0.3
abdominal distention	0.2	0.3	1.4	1.1
Musculoskeletal				
musculoskeletal (bone, muscle or joint) pain	0.8	0.9	1.9	2.2

Prevention of osteoporosis in postmenopausal women
The safety of FOSAMAX 5 mg/day in postmenopausal women 40-60 years of age has been evaluated in three double-blind, placebo-controlled studies involving over 1,400 patients randomized to receive FOSAMAX for either two or three years. In these studies the overall safety profiles of FOSAMAX 5 mg/day and placebo were similar. Discontinuation of therapy due to any clinical adverse experience occurred in 7.5% of 642 patients treated with FOSAMAX 5 mg/day and 5.7% of 648 patients treated with placebo.
In a one-year, double-blind multicenter study, the overall safety and tolerability profiles of once weekly FOSAMAX 35 mg and FOSAMAX 5 mg daily were similar.
The adverse experiences from these studies considered by the investigators as possibly, probably, or definitely drug related in ≥1% of patients treated with either once weekly FOSAMAX 35 mg, FOSAMAX 5 mg/day or placebo are presented in the following table.
[See third table above]
Concomitant use with estrogen/hormone replacement therapy
In two studies (of one and two years' duration) of postmenopausal osteoporotic women (total: n=853), the safety and tolerability profile of combined treatment with FOSAMAX 10 mg once daily and estrogen ± progestin (n=354) was consistent with those of the individual treatments.
Treatment of glucocorticoid-induced osteoporosis
In two, one-year, placebo-controlled, double-blind, multicenter studies in patients receiving glucocorticoid treat-

ment, the overall safety and tolerability profiles of FOSAMAX 5 and 10 mg/day were generally similar to that of placebo. The adverse experiences considered by the investigators as possibly, probably, or definitely drug related in ≥1% of patients treated with either FOSAMAX 5 or 10 mg/day or placebo are presented in the following table. [See table above]

The overall safety and tolerability profile in the glucocorticoid-induced osteoporosis population that continued therapy for the second year of the studies (FOSAMAX: n=147) was consistent with that observed in the first year.

Paget's disease of bone

In clinical studies (osteoporosis and Paget's disease), adverse experiences reported in 175 patients taking FOSAMAX 40 mg/day for 3-12 months were similar to those in postmenopausal women treated with FOSAMAX 10 mg/day. However, there was an apparent increased incidence of upper gastrointestinal adverse experiences in patients taking FOSAMAX 40 mg/day (17.7% FOSAMAX vs. 10.2% placebo). One case of esophagitis and two cases of gastritis resulted in discontinuation of treatment.

Additionally, musculoskeletal (bone, muscle or joint) pain, which has been described in patients with Paget's disease treated with other bisphosphonates, was considered by the investigators as possibly, probably, or definitely drug related in approximately 6% of patients treated with FOSAMAX 40 mg/day versus approximately 1% of patients treated with placebo, but rarely resulted in discontinuation of therapy. Discontinuation of therapy due to any clinical adverse experience occurred in 6.4% of patients with Paget's disease treated with FOSAMAX 40 mg/day and 2.4% of patients treated with placebo.

Laboratory Test Findings

In double-blind, multicenter, controlled studies, asymptomatic, mild, and transient decreases in serum calcium and phosphate were observed in approximately 18% and 10%, respectively, of patients taking FOSAMAX versus approximately 12% and 3% of those taking placebo. However, the incidences of decreases in serum calcium to <8.0 mg/dL (2.0 mM) and serum phosphate to ≤2.0 mg/dL (0.65 mM) were similar in both treatment groups.

Post-Marketing Experience

The following adverse reactions have been reported in post-marketing use:

Body as a Whole: hypersensitivity reactions including urticaria and rarely angioedema. Transient symptoms of myalgia, malaise and rarely, fever have been reported with FOSAMAX, typically in association with initiation of treatment. Rarely, symptomatic hypocalcemia has occurred, generally in association with predisposing conditions.

Gastrointestinal: esophagitis, esophageal erosions, esophageal ulcers, rarely esophageal stricture or perforation, and oropharyngeal ulceration. Gastric or duodenal ulcers, some severe and with complications have also been reported (see WARNINGS, PRECAUTIONS, *Information for Patients*, and DOSAGE AND ADMINISTRATION).

Skin: rash (occasionally with photosensitivity), pruritus, rarely severe skin reactions, including Stevens-Johnson syndrome and toxic epidermal necrolysis.

Special Senses: rarely uveitis, rarely scleritis.

OVERDOSAGE

Significant lethality after single oral doses was seen in female rats and mice at 552 mg/kg (3256 mg/m^2) and 966 mg/kg (2898 mg/m^2), respectively. In males, these values were slightly higher, 626 and 1280 mg/kg, respectively. There was no lethality in dogs at oral doses up to 200 mg/kg (4000 mg/m^2).

No specific information is available on the treatment of overdosage with FOSAMAX. Hypocalcemia, hypophosphatemia, and upper gastrointestinal adverse events, such as upset stomach, heartburn, esophagitis, gastritis, or ulcer, may result from oral overdosage. Milk or antacids should be given to bind alendronate. Due to the risk of esophageal irritation, vomiting should not be induced and the patient should remain fully upright.

Dialysis would not be beneficial.

DOSAGE AND ADMINISTRATION

FOSAMAX must be taken *at least* one-half hour before the first food, beverage, or medication of the day with plain water only (see PRECAUTIONS, *Information for Patients*). Other beverages (including mineral water), food, and some medications are likely to reduce the absorption of FOSAMAX (see PRECAUTIONS, *Drug Interactions*). Waiting less than 30 minutes, or taking FOSAMAX with food, beverages (other than plain water) or other medications will lessen the effect of FOSAMAX by decreasing its absorption into the body.

FOSAMAX should only be taken upon arising for the day. To facilitate delivery to the stomach and thus reduce the potential for esophageal irritation, a FOSAMAX tablet should be swallowed with a full glass of water (6-8 oz). To facilitate gastric emptying FOSAMAX oral solution should be followed by at least 2 oz (a quarter of a cup) of water. Patients should not lie down for at least 30 minutes and until after their first food of the day. FOSAMAX should not be taken at bedtime or before arising for the day. Failure to follow these instructions may increase the risk of esophageal adverse experiences (see WARNINGS, PRECAUTIONS, *Information for Patients*).

Patients should receive supplemental calcium and vitamin D, if dietary intake is inadequate (see PRECAUTIONS, *General*).

One-Year Studies in Glucocorticoid-Treated Patients Adverse Experiences Considered Possibly, Probably, or Definitely Drug Related by the Investigators and Reported in ≥1% of Patients

	FOSAMAX 10 mg/day % (n=157)	FOSAMAX 5 mg/day % (n=161)	Placebo % (n=159)
Gastrointestinal			
abdominal pain	3.2	1.9	0.0
acid regurgitation	2.5	1.9	1.3
constipation	1.3	0.6	0.0
melena	1.3	0.0	0.0
nausea	0.6	1.2	0.6
diarrhea	0.0	0.0	1.3
Nervous System / Psychiatric			
headache	0.6	0.0	1.3

No dosage adjustment is necessary for the elderly or for patients with mild-to-moderate renal insufficiency (creatinine clearance 35 to 60 mL/min). FOSAMAX is not recommended for patients with more severe renal insufficiency (creatinine clearance <35 mL/min) due to lack of experience.

Treatment of osteoporosis in postmenopausal women (see INDICATIONS AND USAGE)

The recommended dosage is:

- one 70 mg tablet once weekly

  or

- one bottle of 70 mg oral solution once weekly

  or

- one 10 mg tablet once daily

Treatment to increase bone mass in men with osteoporosis

The recommended dosage is:

- one 70 mg tablet once weekly

  or

- one bottle of 70 mg oral solution once weekly

  or

- one 10 mg tablet once daily

Prevention of osteoporosis in postmenopausal women (see INDICATIONS AND USAGE)

The recommended dosage is:

- one 35 mg tablet once weekly

  or

- one 5 mg tablet once daily

The safety of treatment and prevention of osteoporosis with FOSAMAX has been studied for up to 7 years.

Treatment of glucocorticoid-induced osteoporosis in men and women

The recommended dosage is one 5 mg tablet once daily, except for postmenopausal women not receiving estrogen, for whom the recommended dosage is one 10 mg tablet once daily.

Paget's disease of bone in men and women

The recommended treatment regimen is 40 mg once a day for six months.

Retreatment of Paget's disease

In clinical studies in which patients were followed every six months, relapses during the 12 months following therapy occurred in 9% (3 out of 32) of patients who responded to treatment with FOSAMAX. Specific retreatment data are not available, although responses to FOSAMAX were similar in patients who had received prior bisphosphonate therapy and those who had not. Retreatment with FOSAMAX may be considered, following a six-month post-treatment evaluation period in patients who have relapsed, based on increases in serum alkaline phosphatase, which should be measured periodically. Retreatment may also be considered in those who failed to normalize their serum alkaline phosphatase.

HOW SUPPLIED

No. 3759—Tablets FOSAMAX, 5 mg, are white, round, uncoated tablets with an outline of a bone image on one side and code MRK 925 on the other. They are supplied as follows:

NDC 0006-0925-31 unit-of-use bottles of 30
NDC 0006-0925-58 unit-of-use bottles of 100.

No. 3797—Tablets FOSAMAX, 10 mg, are white, oval, wax-polished tablets with code MRK on one side and 936 on the other. They are supplied as follows:

NDC 0006-0936-31 unit-of-use bottles of 30
NDC 0006-0936-58 unit-of-use bottles of 100
NDC 0006-0936-28 unit dose packages of 100
NDC 0006-0936-82 bottles of 1,000.

No. 3813—Tablets FOSAMAX, 35 mg, are white, oval, uncoated tablets with code 77 on one side and a bone image on the other. They are supplied as follows:

NDC 0006-0077-44 unit-of-use blister package of 4
NDC 0006-0077-21 unit dose packages of 20.

No. 3592—Tablets FOSAMAX, 40 mg, are white, triangular-shaped, uncoated tablets with code MRK 212 on one side and FOSAMAX on the other. They are supplied as follows:

NDC 0006-0212-31 unit-of-use bottles of 30.

No. 3814—Tablets FOSAMAX, 70 mg, are white, oval, uncoated tablets with code 31 on one side and an outline of a bone image on the other. They are supplied as follows:

NDC 0006-0031-44 unit-of-use blister package of 4
NDC 0006-0031-21 unit dose packages of 20.

No. 3833—Oral Solution FOSAMAX, 70 mg, is a clear, colorless solution with a raspberry flavor and is supplied as follows:

NDC 0006-0033-34 unit-of-use cartons of 4 single-dose bottles containing 75 mL each.

Storage

FOSAMAX Tablets:

Store in a well-closed container at room temperature, 15-30°C (59-86°F).

FOSAMAX Oral Solution:

Store at 25°C (77°F), excursions permitted to 15-30°C (59-86°F). [See USP Controlled Room Temperature.] Do not freeze.

7957025 Issued April 2004

Patient Information about
FOSAMAX® (FOSS-ah-max) for Osteoporosis

Generic name: alendronate sodium (a-LEN-dro-nate)

Please read this information before you start taking FOSAMAX*. Also, read the leaflet each time you renew your prescription, just in case anything has changed. Remember, this leaflet does not take the place of careful discussions with your doctor. You and your doctor should discuss FOSAMAX when you start taking your medication and at regular checkups.

*Registered trademark of MERCK & CO., Inc.

How should I take FOSAMAX?

These are the important things you must do to help make sure you will benefit from FOSAMAX:

1. **After getting up for the day and before taking your first food, beverage, or other medication, swallow your FOSAMAX tablet with a full glass (6–8 oz) of plain water only.**
   Not mineral water
   Not coffee or tea
   Not juice
   Do not chew or suck on a tablet of FOSAMAX.
2. **After swallowing your FOSAMAX tablet do not lie down—stay fully upright (sitting, standing or walking) for at least 30 minutes and do not lie down until after your first food of the day.** This will help the FOSAMAX tablet reach your stomach quickly and help reduce the potential for irritation of your esophagus (the tube that connects your mouth with your stomach).
3. **After swallowing your FOSAMAX tablet, wait at least 30 minutes before taking your first food, beverage, or other medication of the day,** including antacids, calcium supplements and vitamins. FOSAMAX is effective only if taken when your stomach is empty.
4. **Do not take FOSAMAX at bedtime or before getting up for the day.**
5. **If you have difficulty or pain upon swallowing, chest pain, or new or worsening heartburn, stop taking FOSAMAX and call your doctor.**
6. Take one FOSAMAX tablet once a day, every day.
7. It is important that you continue taking FOSAMAX for as long as your doctor prescribes it. FOSAMAX can treat your osteoporosis or help you from getting osteoporosis only if you continue to take it.
8. If you miss a dose do not take it later in the day. Continue your usual schedule of 1 tablet once a day the next morning.

What is FOSAMAX?

FOSAMAX is for:

- **The treatment or prevention of osteoporosis (thinning of bone) in women after menopause. It reduces the chance of having a hip or spinal fracture.**
- **Treatment to increase bone mass in men with osteoporosis.**
- **The treatment of osteoporosis in both men and women receiving corticosteroid medications (for example, prednisone).**

You will find more information about osteoporosis at the end of this leaflet.

How does FOSAMAX work?

FOSAMAX works by:

- Reducing the activity of the cells that cause bone loss
- Decreasing the faster rate of bone loss that occurs after menopause or with use of corticosteroid medications

Continued on next page

Information on the Merck & Co., Inc., products listed on these pages is from the prescribing information in use October 1, 2004. For information, please call 1-800-NSC-MERCK [1-800-672-6372].

Fosamax—Cont.

- Increasing the amount of bone in most patients

These effects are seen as soon as three months after therapy with FOSAMAX has begun. These effects continue as long as you keep taking FOSAMAX. The density of bone is maintained or increased and the bone is less likely to fracture.

Who should not take FOSAMAX?

Patients with:
- Certain disorders of the esophagus (the tube that connects your mouth with your stomach)
- Inability to stand or sit upright for at least 30 minutes
- Low levels of calcium in their blood
- Severe kidney disease
- Allergy to FOSAMAX

Patients who are:
- Pregnant or Nursing
  If you are pregnant or nursing, you should not be taking FOSAMAX. Talk to your doctor.

What other medical problems should I discuss with my doctor?

Talk to your doctor about any:
- Problems with swallowing
- Stomach or digestive problems
- Other medical problems you have or have had in the past

What are the possible side effects of FOSAMAX?

Some patients may develop severe digestive reactions including irritation, inflammation or ulceration (occasionally severe and/or with bleeding) of the esophagus (the tube that connects your mouth with your stomach). These reactions can cause chest pain, heartburn or difficulty or pain upon swallowing. This may occur especially if patients do not drink a full glass of water with FOSAMAX and/or if they lie down in less than 30 minutes or before their first food of the day. Esophageal reactions may worsen if patients continue to take FOSAMAX after developing symptoms suggesting irritation of the esophagus.

Like all prescription drugs, FOSAMAX may cause side effects. Side effects usually have been mild. They generally have not caused patients to stop taking FOSAMAX. Some patients treated with FOSAMAX experienced abdominal (stomach) pain. This is the most commonly reported side effect. Less frequently reported side effects are:

Nausea, heartburn, irritation or pain of the esophagus (the tube that connects your mouth with your stomach), vomiting, difficulty swallowing, a full or bloated feeling in the stomach, constipation, diarrhea, black and/or bloody stools, stomach or other peptic ulcers (some severe), and gas.

Bone, muscle or joint pain (rarely, with flu-like symptoms or fever), headache, or an altered sense of taste were also experienced by some patients. Rarely, a rash (occasionally made worse by sunlight), itching, or eye pain have occurred. Rarely, severe skin reactions have occurred. Allergic reactions such as hives or, rarely, swelling of the face, lips, tongue and/or throat which may cause difficulty in breathing or swallowing have also been reported. Mouth ulcers have occurred when the tablet was chewed or dissolved in the mouth.

Anytime you have a medical problem you think may be related to FOSAMAX, talk to your doctor.

What should I know about osteoporosis?

Normally your bones are being rebuilt all the time. First, old bone is removed (resorbed). Then a similar amount of new bone is formed. This balanced process keeps your skeleton healthy and strong.

Osteoporosis is a thinning and weakening of the bones. It is common in women after menopause and may also occur in men. It may also be caused by certain medications called corticosteroids in both men and women. At the start osteoporosis usually has no symptoms, but it can result in fractures (broken bones). Fractures usually cause pain. Fractures of the bones of the spine may not be painful, but over time they cause height loss. Eventually the spine becomes curved and the body becomes bent over. Fractures may happen during normal, everyday activity, such as lifting, or from minor injury that would normally not cause bone to break. Fractures most often occur at the hip, spine, or wrist. This can lead to pain, severe disability, or loss of mobility.

Osteoporosis in men and in postmenopausal women

Osteoporosis often occurs in women several years after the menopause, which happens when the ovaries stop producing the female hormone, estrogen, or are removed (which may occur, for example, at the time of a hysterectomy). Osteoporosis can also occur in men due to several causes, including aging and/or a low level of the male hormone, testosterone. In all instances, bone is removed faster than it is formed, so bone loss occurs and bones become weaker. Therefore, maintaining bone mass is important to keep your bones healthy.

Osteoporosis in men and women caused by corticosteroids

Corticosteroids can cause bone to be removed faster than it is formed, so bone loss occurs and bones become weaker. Therefore, maintaining bone mass is important to keep your bones healthy. It is important to take your corticosteroid medication as recommended by your doctor.

How can osteoporosis be treated or prevented?

- **Medication.**
  Your doctor has prescribed FOSAMAX. FOSAMAX acts specifically on your bones. FOSAMAX is not a hormone and does not have the benefits and risks of estrogen (hormone replacement therapy used in postmenopausal women) elsewhere in your body.
- **Lifestyle changes.**
  In addition to FOSAMAX, your doctor may recommend one or more of the following lifestyle changes:
  - **Stop smoking.** Smoking appears to increase the risk of osteoporosis.
  - **Reduce the use of alcohol.** Too much alcohol appears to increase the risk of osteoporosis and injuries that may cause fractures.
  - **Exercise regularly.** Like muscles, bones need exercise to stay strong and healthy. Exercise must be safe to prevent injuries including fractures. You should consult your doctor before you begin any exercise program.
  - **Eat a balanced diet.** Adequate dietary calcium is important. Your doctor can advise you whether you need to change your diet or take any dietary supplements such as calcium or vitamin D.

This medication was prescribed for your particular condition. Do not use it for another condition or give the drug to others. Keep FOSAMAX and all medicines out of the reach of children. If you suspect that more than the prescribed dose of this medicine has been taken, drink a full glass of milk and contact your local poison control center or emergency room immediately. Do not induce vomiting. Do not lie down.

This leaflet provides a summary of information about FOSAMAX. If you have any questions or concerns about either FOSAMAX or osteoporosis, talk to your doctor. In addition, talk to your pharmacist or other health care provider.

7969413 Issued April 2003

Patient Information about
Once Weekly FOSAMAX® (FOSS-ah-max) for Osteoporosis

Generic name: alendronate sodium (a-LEN-dro-nate)

Please read this information before you start taking once weekly FOSAMAX*. Also, read the leaflet each time you renew your prescription, just in case anything has changed. Remember, this leaflet does not take the place of careful discussions with your doctor. You and your doctor should discuss FOSAMAX when you start taking your medication and at regular checkups.

*Registered trademark of MERCK & CO., Inc.

How should I take once weekly FOSAMAX?

These are the important things you must do to help make sure you will benefit from FOSAMAX:

1. **Choose the day of the week that best fits your schedule. Every week, take one dose of FOSAMAX (one tablet or one entire bottle of solution) on your chosen day.**
2. **After getting up for the day and before taking your first food, beverage, or other medication, take your FOSAMAX with plain water only as follows:**
   - **TABLETS: Swallow one tablet with a full glass (6–8 oz) of plain water.**
   - **ORAL SOLUTION: Drink one entire bottle of solution followed by at least 2 ounces (a quarter of a cup) of plain water.**

   Do not take FOSAMAX with:
   Mineral water
   Coffee or tea
   Juice
   Do not chew or suck on a tablet of FOSAMAX.
3. **After taking your FOSAMAX do not lie down—stay fully upright (sitting, standing or walking) for at least 30 minutes and do not lie down until after your first food of the day.** This will help FOSAMAX reach your stomach quickly and help reduce the potential for irritation of your esophagus (the tube that connects your mouth with your stomach).
4. **After taking your FOSAMAX, wait at least 30 minutes before taking your first food, beverage, or other medication of the day,** including antacids, calcium supplements and vitamins. FOSAMAX is effective only if taken when your stomach is empty.
5. **Do not take FOSAMAX at bedtime or before getting up for the day.**
6. **If you have difficulty or pain upon swallowing, chest pain, or new or worsening heartburn, stop taking FOSAMAX and call your doctor.**
7. If you miss a dose, take only one dose of FOSAMAX on the morning after you remember. *Do not take two doses on the same day.* Return to taking one dose once a week, as originally scheduled on your chosen day.
8. It is important that you continue taking FOSAMAX for as long as your doctor prescribes it. FOSAMAX can treat your osteoporosis or help you from getting osteoporosis only if you continue to take it.

What is FOSAMAX?

FOSAMAX is for:
- **The treatment or prevention of osteoporosis (thinning of bone) in women after menopause. It reduces the chance of having a hip or spinal fracture.**
- **Treatment to increase bone mass in men with osteoporosis.**

FOSAMAX tablets are for treatment and prevention, and FOSAMAX oral solution is for treatment of osteoporosis.

You will find more information about osteoporosis at the end of this leaflet.

How does FOSAMAX work?

FOSAMAX works by:
- Reducing the activity of the cells that cause bone loss
- Decreasing the faster rate of bone loss that occurs after menopause
- Increasing the amount of bone in most patients

These effects are seen as soon as three months after therapy with FOSAMAX has begun. These effects continue as long as you keep taking FOSAMAX. The density of bone is maintained or increased and the bone is less likely to fracture.

Who should not take FOSAMAX?

Patients with:
- Certain disorders of the esophagus (the tube that connects your mouth with your stomach)
- Inability to stand or sit upright for at least 30 minutes
- Difficulty swallowing liquids should not take FOSAMAX oral solution
- Low levels of calcium in their blood
- Severe kidney disease
- Allergy to FOSAMAX

Patients who are:
- Pregnant or Nursing
  If you are pregnant or nursing, you should not be taking FOSAMAX. Talk to your doctor.

What other medical problems should I discuss with my doctor?

Talk to your doctor about any:
- Problems with swallowing
- Stomach or digestive problems
- Other medical problems you have or have had in the past

What are the possible side effects of FOSAMAX?

Some patients may develop severe digestive reactions including irritation, inflammation or ulceration (occasionally severe and/or with bleeding) of the esophagus (the tube that connects your mouth with your stomach). These reactions can cause chest pain, heartburn or difficulty or pain upon swallowing. This may occur especially if patients do not drink the recommended amount of water with FOSAMAX and/or if they lie down in less than 30 minutes or before their first food of the day. Esophageal reactions may worsen if patients continue to take FOSAMAX after developing symptoms suggesting irritation of the esophagus.

Like all prescription drugs, FOSAMAX may cause side effects. Side effects usually have been mild. They generally have not caused patients to stop taking FOSAMAX. Some patients treated with FOSAMAX experienced abdominal (stomach) pain. This is the most commonly reported side effect. Less frequently reported side effects are:

Nausea, heartburn, irritation or pain of the esophagus (the tube that connects your mouth with your stomach), vomiting, difficulty swallowing, a full or bloated feeling in the stomach, constipation, diarrhea, black and/or bloody stools, stomach or other peptic ulcers (some severe), and gas.

Bone, muscle or joint pain (rarely, with flu-like symptoms or fever), headache, or an altered sense of taste were also experienced by some patients. Rarely, a rash (occasionally made worse by sunlight), itching, or eye pain have occurred. Rarely, severe skin reactions have occurred. Allergic reactions such as hives or, rarely, swelling of the face, lips, tongue and/or throat which may cause difficulty in breathing or swallowing have also been reported. Mouth ulcers have occurred when the tablet was chewed or dissolved in the mouth.

Anytime you have a medical problem you think may be related to FOSAMAX, talk to your doctor.

What should I know about osteoporosis?

Normally your bones are being rebuilt all the time. First, old bone is removed (resorbed). Then a similar amount of new bone is formed. This balanced process keeps your skeleton healthy and strong.

Osteoporosis is a thinning and weakening of the bones. It is common in women after menopause and may also occur in men. Osteoporosis often occurs in women several years after the menopause, which happens when the ovaries stop producing the female hormone, estrogen, or are removed (which may occur, for example, at the time of a hysterectomy). Osteoporosis can also occur in men due to several causes, including aging and/or a low level of the male hormone, testosterone. In all instances of osteoporosis bone is removed faster than it is formed, so bone loss occurs and bones become weaker. Therefore, maintaining bone mass is important to keep your bones healthy. At the start osteoporosis usually has no symptoms, but it can result in fractures (broken bones). Fractures usually cause pain. Fractures of the bones of the spine may not be painful, but over time they cause height loss. Eventually the spine becomes curved and the body becomes bent over. Fractures may happen during normal, everyday activity, such as lifting, or from minor injury that would normally not cause bone to break. Fractures most often occur at the hip, spine, or wrist. This can lead to pain, severe disability, or loss of mobility.

How can osteoporosis be treated or prevented?

- **Medication.**
  Your doctor has prescribed FOSAMAX. FOSAMAX acts specifically on your bones. FOSAMAX is not a hormone and does not have the benefits and risks of estrogen (hormone replacement therapy used in postmenopausal women) elsewhere in your body.
- **Lifestyle changes.**
  In addition to FOSAMAX, your doctor may recommend one or more of the following lifestyle changes:
  - **Stop smoking.** Smoking appears to increase the risk of osteoporosis.
  - **Reduce the use of alcohol.** Too much alcohol appears to increase the risk of osteoporosis and injuries that may cause fractures.
  - **Exercise regularly.** Like muscles, bones need exercise to stay strong and healthy. Exercise must be safe to pre-

vent injuries including fractures. You should consult your doctor before you begin any exercise program

- **Eat a balanced diet.** Adequate dietary calcium is important. Your doctor can advise you whether you need to change your diet or take any dietary supplements such as calcium or vitamin D.

This medication was prescribed for your particular condition. Do not use it for another condition or give the drug to others. Keep FOSAMAX and all medicines out of the reach of children. If you suspect that more than the prescribed dose of this medicine has been taken, drink a full glass of milk and contact your local poison control center or emergency room immediately. Do not induce vomiting. Do not lie down.

This leaflet provides a summary of information about FOSAMAX. If you have any questions or concerns about either FOSAMAX or osteoporosis, talk to your doctor. In addition, talk to your pharmacist or other health care provider.

9364105 Issued September 2003

Shown in Product Identification Guide, page 323

HYDROCORTONE® Phosphate Injection, Sterile ℞
(Hydrocortisone Sodium Phosphate)

FOR USE AS A SINGLE DOSE VIAL ONLY

DESCRIPTION

Hydrocortisone sodium phosphate, a synthetic adrenocortical steroid, is a white to light yellow, odorless or practically odorless powder. It is freely soluble in water and is exceedingly hygroscopic. The molecular weight is 486.41. It is designated chemically as 11β,17-dihydroxy-21-(phosphonooxy)-pregn-4-ene-3,20-dione disodium salt. The empirical formula is $C_{21}H_{29}Na_2O_8P$ and the structural formula is:

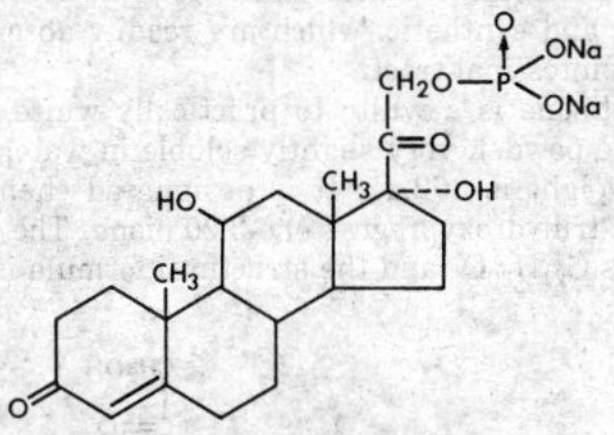

HYDROCORTONE* Phosphate (Hydrocortisone Sodium Phosphate) injection is a sterile solution (pH 7.5 to 8.5), sealed under nitrogen, for intravenous, intramuscular, and subcutaneous administration.

Each milliliter contains hydrocortisone sodium phosphate equivalent to 50 mg hydrocortisone. Inactive ingredients per mL: 8 mg creatinine, 10 mg sodium citrate, sodium hydroxide to adjust pH, and Water for Injection, q.s. 1 mL, with 3.2 mg sodium bisulfite, 1.5 mg methylparaben, and 0.2 mg propylparaben added as preservatives.

*Registered trademark of MERCK & CO., INC.

ACTIONS

HYDROCORTONE Phosphate injection has a rapid onset but short duration of action when compared with less soluble preparations. Because of this, it is suitable for the treatment of acute disorders responsive to adrenocortical steroid therapy.

Naturally occurring glucocorticoids (hydrocortisone and cortisone), which also have salt-retaining properties, are used as replacement therapy in adrenocortical deficiency states. They are also used for their potent anti-inflammatory effects in disorders of many organ systems.

Glucocorticoids cause profound and varied metabolic effects. In addition, they modify the body's immune responses to diverse stimuli.

INDICATIONS

When oral therapy is not feasible:

1. *Endocrine disorders*

Primary or secondary adrenocortical insufficiency (hydrocortisone or cortisone is the drug of choice; synthetic analogs may be used in conjunction with mineralocorticoids where applicable; in infancy, mineralocorticoid supplementation is of particular importance)

Acute adrenocortical insufficiency (hydrocortisone or cortisone is the drug of choice; mineralocorticoid supplementation may be necessary, particularly when synthetic analogs are used)

Preoperatively, and in the event of serious trauma or illness, in patients with known adrenal insufficiency or when adrenocortical reserve is doubtful

Shock unresponsive to conventional therapy if adrenocortical insufficiency exists or is suspected

Congenital adrenal hyperplasia
Nonsuppurative thyroiditis
Hypercalcemia associated with cancer

2. *Rheumatic disorders*

As adjunctive therapy for short-term administration (to tide the patient over an acute episode or exacerbation) in:

Post-traumatic osteoarthritis
Synovitis of osteoarthritis
Rheumatoid arthritis, including juvenile rheumatoid arthritis (selected cases may require low-dose maintenance therapy)
Acute and subacute bursitis
Epicondylitis
Acute nonspecific tenosynovitis
Acute gouty arthritis
Psoriatic arthritis
Ankylosing spondylitis

3. *Collagen diseases*

During an exacerbation or as maintenance therapy in selected cases of:

Systemic lupus erythematosus
Acute rheumatic carditis
Systemic dermatomyositis (polymyositis)

4. *Dermatologic diseases*

Pemphigus
Severe erythema multiforme (Stevens-Johnson syndrome)
Exfoliative dermatitis
Bullous dermatitis herpetiformis
Severe seborrheic dermatitis
Severe psoriasis
Mycosis fungoides

5. *Allergic states*

Control of severe or incapacitating allergic conditions intractable to adequate trials of conventional treatment in:

Bronchial asthma
Contact dermatitis
Atopic dermatitis
Serum sickness
Seasonal or perennial allergic rhinitis
Drug hypersensitivity reactions
Urticarial transfusion reactions
Acute noninfectious laryngeal edema (epinephrine is the drug of first choice)

6. *Ophthalmic diseases*

Severe acute and chronic allergic and inflammatory processes involving the eye, such as:

Herpes zoster ophthalmicus
Iritis, iridocyclitis
Chorioretinitis
Diffuse posterior uveitis and choroiditis
Optic neuritis
Sympathetic ophthalmia
Anterior segment inflammation
Allergic conjunctivitis
Keratitis
Allergic corneal marginal ulcers

7. *Gastrointestinal diseases*

To tide the patient over a critical period of the disease in:

Ulcerative colitis (Systemic therapy)
Regional enteritis (Systemic therapy)

8. *Respiratory diseases*

Symptomatic sarcoidosis
Berylliosis
Fulminating or disseminated pulmonary tuberculosis when used concurrently with appropriate antituberculous chemotherapy
Loeffler's syndrome not manageable by other means
Aspiration pneumonitis

9. *Hematologic disorders*

Acquired (autoimmune) hemolytic anemia
Idiopathic thrombocytopenic purpura in adults (I.V. only; I.M. administration is contraindicated)
Secondary thrombocytopenia in adults
Erythroblastopenia (RBC anemia)
Congenital (erythroid) hypoplastic anemia

10. *Neoplastic diseases*

For palliative management of:

Leukemias and lymphomas in adults
Acute leukemia of childhood

11. *Edematous states*

To induce diuresis or remission of proteinuria in the nephrotic syndrome, without uremia, of the idiopathic type, or that due to lupus erythematosus

12. *Miscellaneous*

Tuberculous meningitis with subarachnoid block or impending block when used concurrently with appropriate antituberculous chemotherapy
Trichinosis with neurologic or myocardial involvement

CONTRAINDICATIONS

Systemic fungal infections (see WARNINGS regarding amphotericin B)

Hypersensitivity to any component of this product, including sulfites (see WARNINGS)

WARNINGS

Because rare instances of anaphylactoid reactions have occurred in patients receiving parenteral corticosteroid therapy, appropriate precautionary measures should be taken prior to administration, especially when the patient has a history of allergy to any drug. Anaphylactoid and hypersensitivity reactions have been reported for Injection HYDROCORTONE Phosphate (see ADVERSE REACTIONS).

Injection HYDROCORTONE Phosphate contains sodium bisulfite, a sulfite that may cause allergic-type reactions including anaphylactic symptoms and life-threatening or less severe asthmatic episodes in certain susceptible people. The overall prevalence of sulfite sensitivity in the general population is unknown and probably low. Sulfite sensitivity is seen more frequently in asthmatic than in nonasthmatic people.

Corticosteroids may exacerbate systemic fungal infections and therefore should not be used in the presence of such infections unless they are needed to control life-threatening drug reactions due to amphotericin B. Moreover, there have been cases reported in which concomitant use of amphotericin B and hydrocortisone was followed by cardiac enlargement and congestive failure.

In patients on corticosteroid therapy subjected to any unusual stress, increased dosage of rapidly acting corticosteroids before, during, and after the stressful situation is indicated.

Drug-induced secondary adrenocortical insufficiency may result from too rapid withdrawal of corticosteroids and may be minimized by gradual reduction of dosage. This type of relative insufficiency may persist for months after discontinuation of therapy; therefore, in any situation of stress occurring during that period, hormone therapy should be reinstituted. If the patient is receiving steroids already, dosage may have to be increased. Since mineralocorticoid secretion may be impaired, salt and/or a mineralocorticoid should be administered concurrently. (See PRECAUTIONS.)

Corticosteroids may mask some signs of infection, and new infections may appear during their use. There may be decreased resistance and inability to localize infection when corticosteroids are used. Moreover, corticosteroids may affect the nitroblue-tetrazolium test for bacterial infection and produce false negative results.

In cerebral malaria, a double-blind trial has shown that the use of corticosteroids is associated with prolongation of coma and a higher incidence of pneumonia and gastrointestinal bleeding.

Corticosteroids may activate latent amebiasis. Therefore, it is recommended that latent or active amebiasis be ruled out before initiating corticosteroid therapy in any patient who has spent time in the tropics or any patient with unexplained diarrhea.

Prolonged use of corticosteroids may produce posterior subcapsular cataracts, glaucoma with possible damage to the optic nerves, and may enhance the establishment of secondary ocular infections due to fungi or viruses.

Usage in pregnancy. Since adequate human reproduction studies have not been done with corticosteroids, use of these drugs in pregnancy or in women of childbearing potential requires that the anticipated benefits be weighed against the possible hazards to the mother and embryo or fetus. Infants born of mothers who have received substantial doses of corticosteroids during pregnancy should be carefully observed for signs of hypoadrenalism.

Corticosteroids appear in breast milk and could suppress growth, interfere with endogenous corticosteroid production, or cause other unwanted effects. Mothers taking pharmacologic doses of corticosteroids should be advised not to nurse.

Average and large doses of cortisone or hydrocortisone can cause elevation of blood pressure, salt and water retention, and increased excretion of potassium. These effects are less likely to occur with the synthetic derivatives except when used in large doses. Dietary salt restriction and potassium supplementation may be necessary. All corticosteroids increase calcium excretion.

Administration of live virus vaccines, including smallpox, is contraindicated in individuals receiving immunosuppressive doses of corticosteroids. If inactivated viral or bacterial vaccines are administered to individuals receiving immunosuppressive doses of corticosteroids, the expected serum antibody response may not be obtained. However, immunization procedures may be undertaken in patients who are receiving corticosteroids as replacement therapy, e.g., for Addison's disease.

Patients who are on drugs which suppress the immune system are more susceptible to infections than healthy individuals. Chickenpox and measles, for example, can have a more serious or even fatal course in non-immune patients on corticosteroids. In such patients who have not had these diseases, particular care should be taken to avoid exposure. The risk of developing a disseminated infection varies among individuals and can be related to the dose, route and duration of corticosteroid administration as well as to the underlying disease. If exposed to chickenpox, prophylaxis with varicella zoster immune globulin (VZIG) may be indicated. If chickenpox develops, treatment with antiviral agents may be considered. If exposed to measles, prophylaxis with immune globulin (IG) may be indicated. (See the respective package inserts for VZIG and IG for complete prescribing information.)

Similarly, corticosteroids should be used with great care in patients with known or suspected Strongyloides (threadworm) infestation. In such patients, corticosteroid-induced immunosuppression may lead to Strongyloides hyperinfec-

Continued on next page

Information on the Merck & Co., Inc., products listed on these pages is from the prescribing information in use October 1, 2004. For information, please call 1-800-NSC-MERCK [1-800-672-6372].

Hydrocortone Phosphate Inj.—Cont.

tion and dissemination with widespread larval migration, often accompanied by severe enterocolitis and potentially fatal gram-negative septicemia.
The use of HYDROCORTONE Phosphate injection in active tuberculosis should be restricted to those cases of fulminating or disseminated tuberculosis in which the corticosteroid is used for the management of the disease in conjunction with an appropriate antituberculous regimen.
If corticosteroids are indicated in patients with latent tuberculosis or tuberculin reactivity, close observation is necessary as reactivation of the disease may occur. During prolonged corticosteroid therapy, these patients should receive chemoprophylaxis.
Literature reports suggest an apparent association between use of corticosteroids and left ventricular free wall rupture after a recent myocardial infarction; therefore, therapy with corticosteroids should be used with great caution in these patients.

PRECAUTIONS

This product, like many other steroid formulations, is sensitive to heat. Therefore, it should not be autoclaved when it is desirable to sterilize the exterior of the vial.
Following prolonged therapy, withdrawal of corticosteroids may result in symptoms of the corticosteroid withdrawal syndrome including fever, myalgia, arthralgia, and malaise. This may occur in patients even without evidence of adrenal insufficiency.
There is an enhanced effect of corticosteroids in patients with hypothyroidism and in those with cirrhosis.
Corticosteroids should be used cautiously in patients with ocular herpes simplex for fear of corneal perforation.
The lowest possible dose of corticosteroid should be used to control the condition under treatment, and when reduction in dosage is possible, the reduction must be gradual.
Psychic derangements may appear when corticosteroids are used, ranging from euphoria, insomnia, mood swings, personality changes, and severe depression to frank psychotic manifestations. Also, existing emotional instability or psychotic tendencies may be aggravated by corticosteroids.
Aspirin should be used cautiously in conjunction with corticosteroids in hypoprothrombinemia.
Steroids should be used with caution in nonspecific ulcerative colitis, if there is a probability of impending perforation, abscess, or other pyogenic infection, also in diverticulitis, fresh intestinal anastomoses, active or latent peptic ulcer, renal insufficiency, hypertension, osteoporosis, and myasthenia gravis. Signs of peritoneal irritation following gastrointestinal perforation in patients receiving large doses of corticosteroids may be minimal or absent. Fat embolism has been reported as a possible complication of hypercortisonism.
When large doses are given, some authorities advise that antacids be administered between meals to help to prevent peptic ulcer.
Steroids may increase or decrease motility and number of spermatozoa in some patients.
Phenytoin, phenobarbital, ephedrine, and rifampin may enhance the metabolic clearance of corticosteroids, resulting in decreased blood levels and lessened physiologic activity, thus requiring adjustment in corticosteroid dosage.
Ketoconazole alone can inhibit adrenal corticosteroid synthesis and may cause adrenal insufficiency during corticosteroid withdrawal (see WARNINGS).
The prothrombin time should be checked frequently in patients who are receiving corticosteroids and coumarin anticoagulants at the same time because of reports that corticosteroids have altered the response to these anticoagulants. Studies have shown that the usual effect produced by adding corticosteroids is inhibition of response to coumarins, although there have been some conflicting reports of potentiation not substantiated by studies.
When corticosteroids are administered concomitantly with potassium-depleting diuretics, patients should be observed closely for development of hypokalemia.
Injection of a steroid into an infected site is to be avoided.
The slower rate of absorption by intramuscular administration should be recognized.
Information for Patients
Susceptible patients who are on immunosuppressant doses of corticosteroids should be warned to avoid exposure to chickenpox or measles. Patients should also be advised that if they are exposed, medical advice should be sought without delay.
Pediatric Use
Growth and development of pediatric patients on prolonged corticosteroid therapy should be carefully followed.

ADVERSE REACTIONS

Fluid and electrolyte disturbances
Sodium retention
Fluid retention
Congestive heart failure in susceptible patients
Potassium loss
Hypokalemic alkalosis
Hypertension
Musculoskeletal
Muscle weakness
Steroid myopathy
Loss of muscle mass
Osteoporosis
Vertebral compression fractures
Aseptic necrosis of femoral and humeral heads
Pathologic fracture of long bones
Tendon rupture
Gastrointestinal
Peptic ulcer with possible subsequent perforation and hemorrhage
Perforation of the small and large bowel, particularly in patients with inflammatory bowel disease
Pancreatitis
Abdominal distention
Ulcerative esophagitis
Dermatologic
Impaired wound healing
Thin fragile skin
Petechiae and ecchymoses
Erythema
Increased sweating
May suppress reactions to skin tests
Burning or tingling, especially in the perineal area (after I.V. injection)
Other cutaneous reactions, such as allergic dermatitis, urticaria, angioneurotic edema
Neurologic
Convulsions
Increased intracranial pressure with papilledema (pseudotumor cerebri) usually after treatment
Vertigo
Headache
Psychic disturbances
Endocrine
Menstrual irregularities
Development of cushingoid state
Suppression of growth in children
Secondary adrenocortical and pituitary unresponsiveness, particularly in times of stress, as in trauma, surgery, or illness
Decreased carbohydrate tolerance
Manifestations of latent diabetes mellitus
Hyperglycemia
Increased requirements for insulin or oral hypoglycemic agents in diabetics
Hirsutism
Ophthalmic
Posterior subcapsular cataracts
Increased intraocular pressure
Glaucoma
Exophthalmos
Metabolic
Negative nitrogen balance due to protein catabolism
Cardiovascular
Myocardial rupture following recent myocardial infarction (see WARNINGS)
Other
Anaphylactoid or hypersensitivity reactions
Thromboembolism
Weight gain
Increased appetite
Nausea
Malaise
The following *additional* adverse reactions are related to parenteral corticosteroid therapy:
Rare instances of blindness associated with intralesional therapy around the face and head
Hyperpigmentation or hypopigmentation
Subcutaneous and cutaneous atrophy
Sterile abscess

OVERDOSAGE

Reports of acute toxicity and/or death following overdosage of glucocorticoids are rare. In the event of overdosage, no specific antidote is available; treatment is supportive and symptomatic.
The intraperitoneal LD_{50} of hydrocortisone in female mice was 1740 mg/kg.

DOSAGE AND ADMINISTRATION

For intravenous, intramuscular, and subcutaneous injection. For single dose use only. Maintenance of sterility cannot be assured when used as a multiple dose vial.
HYDROCORTONE Phosphate injection can be given directly from the vial, or it can be added to Sodium Chloride Injection or Dextrose Injection and administered by intravenous drip.
Benzyl alcohol as a preservative has been associated with toxicity in premature infants. Solutions used for intravenous administration or further dilution of this product should be preservative-free when used in the neonate, especially the premature infant.
When it is mixed with an infusion solution, sterile precautions should be observed. Since infusion solutions generally do not contain preservatives, mixtures should be used within 24 hours.
DOSAGE REQUIREMENTS ARE VARIABLE AND MUST BE INDIVIDUALIZED ON THE BASIS OF THE DISEASE AND THE RESPONSE OF THE PATIENT.
The initial dosage varies from 15 to 240 mg a day depending on the disease being treated. In less severe diseases doses lower than 15 mg may suffice, while in severe diseases doses higher than 240 mg may be required. Usually the parenteral dosage ranges are one-third to one-half the oral dose given every 12 hours. However, in certain overwhelming, acute, life-threatening situations, administration in dosages exceeding the usual dosages may be justified and may be in multiples of the oral dosages.
The initial dosage should be maintained or adjusted until the patient's response is satisfactory. If a satisfactory clinical response does not occur after a reasonable period of time, discontinue HYDROCORTONE Phosphate injection and transfer the patient to other therapy.
After a favorable initial response, the proper maintenance dosage should be determined by decreasing the initial dosage in small amounts to the lowest dosage that maintains an adequate clinical response.
Patients should be observed closely for signs that might require dosage adjustment, including changes in clinical status resulting from remissions or exacerbations of the disease, individual drug responsiveness, and the effect of stress (e.g., surgery, infection, trauma). During stress it may be necessary to increase dosage temporarily.
If the drug is to be stopped after more than a few days of treatment, it usually should be withdrawn gradually.

HOW SUPPLIED

No. 7633—Injection HYDROCORTONE Phosphate, 50 mg hydrocortisone equivalent per mL, is a clear, light yellow solution, and is supplied as follows:
NDC 0006-7633-04 in 2 mL single dose vials.
Storage
Sensitive to heat. Do not autoclave.
9024030 Issued November 2001

HYDROCORTONE® Tablets ℞
(Hydrocortisone)

DESCRIPTION

Glucocorticoids are adrenocortical steroids, both naturally occurring and synthetic, which are readily absorbed from the gastrointestinal tract.
Hydrocortisone is a white to practically white, odorless, crystalline powder, very slightly soluble in water. The molecular weight is 362.47. It is designated chemically as 11β,17,21-trihydroxypregn-4-ene-3,20-dione. The empirical formula is $C_{21}H_{30}O_5$ and the structural formula is:

Hydrocortisone is believed to be the principal hormone secreted by the adrenal cortex.
HYDROCORTONE* (Hydrocortisone) tablets contain 10 mg of hydrocortisone in each tablet.
Inactive ingredients are lactose, magnesium stearate, and starch.

*Registered trademark of MERCK & CO., INC.

ACTIONS

Naturally occurring glucocorticoids (hydrocortisone and cortisone), which also have salt-retaining properties, are used as replacement therapy in adrenocortical deficiency states. They are also used for their potent anti-inflammatory effects in disorders of many organ systems.
Glucocorticoids cause profound and varied metabolic effects. In addition, they modify the body's immune responses to diverse stimuli.

INDICATIONS

1. *Endocrine Disorders*
Primary or secondary adrenocortical insufficiency (hydrocortisone or cortisone is the first choice; synthetic analogs may be used in conjunction with mineralocorticoids where applicable; in infancy mineralocorticoid supplementation is of particular importance)
Congenital adrenal hyperplasia
Nonsuppurative thyroiditis
Hypercalcemia associated with cancer
2. *Rheumatic Disorders*
As adjunctive therapy for short-term administration (to tide the patient over an acute episode or exacerbation) in:
Psoriatic arthritis
Rheumatoid arthritis, including juvenile rheumatoid arthritis (selected cases may require low-dose maintenance therapy)
Ankylosing spondylitis
Acute and subacute bursitis
Acute nonspecific tenosynovitis
Acute gouty arthritis
Post-traumatic osteoarthritis

Synovitis of osteoarthritis
Epicondylitis
3. *Collagen Diseases*
During an exacerbation or as maintenance therapy in selected cases of—
Systemic lupus erythematosus
Acute rheumatic carditis
Systemic dermatomyositis (polymyositis)
4. *Dermatologic Diseases*
Pemphigus
Bullous dermatitis herpetiformis
Severe erythema multiforme (Stevens-Johnson syndrome)
Exfoliative dermatitis
Mycosis fungoides
Severe psoriasis
Severe seborrheic dermatitis
5. *Allergic States*
Control of severe or incapacitating allergic conditions intractable to adequate trials of conventional treatment:
Seasonal or perennial allergic rhinitis
Bronchial asthma
Contact dermatitis
Atopic dermatitis
Serum sickness
Drug hypersensitivity reactions
6. *Ophthalmic Diseases*
Severe acute and chronic allergic and inflammatory processes involving the eye and its adnexa, such as—
Allergic conjunctivitis
Keratitis
Allergic corneal marginal ulcers
Herpes zoster ophthalmicus
Iritis and iridocyclitis
Chorioretinitis
Anterior segment inflammation
Diffuse posterior uveitis and choroiditis
Optic neuritis
Sympathetic ophthalmia
7. *Respiratory Diseases*
Symptomatic sarcoidosis
Loeffler's syndrome not manageable by other means
Berylliosis
Fulminating or disseminated pulmonary tuberculosis when used concurrently with appropriate antituberculous chemotherapy
Aspiration pneumonitis
8. *Hematologic Disorders*
Idiopathic thrombocytopenic purpura in adults
Secondary thrombocytopenia in adults
Acquired (autoimmune) hemolytic anemia
Erythroblastopenia (RBC anemia)
Congenital (erythroid) hypoplastic anemia
9. *Neoplastic Diseases*
For palliative management of:
Leukemias and lymphomas in adults
Acute leukemia of childhood
10. *Edematous States*
To induce a diuresis or remission of proteinuria in the nephrotic syndrome, without uremia, of the idiopathic type or that due to lupus erythematosus
11. *Gastrointestinal Diseases*
To tide the patient over a critical period of the disease in:
Ulcerative colitis
Regional enteritis
12. *Miscellaneous*
Tuberculous meningitis with subarachnoid block or impending block when used concurrently with appropriate antituberculous chemotherapy
Trichinosis with neurologic or myocardial involvement

CONTRAINDICATIONS

Systemic fungal infections
Hypersensitivity to this product

WARNINGS

In patients on corticosteroid therapy subjected to unusual stress, increased dosage of rapidly acting corticosteroids before, during, and after the stressful situation is indicated.
Drug-induced secondary adrenocortical insufficiency may result from too rapid wthdrawal of corticosteroids and may be minimized by gradual reduction of dosage. This type of relative insufficiency may persist for months after discontinuation of therapy; therefore, in any situation of stress occurring during that period, hormone therapy should be reinstituted. If the patient is receiving steroids already, dosage may have to be increased. Since mineralocorticoid secretion may be impaired, salt and/or a mineralocorticoid should be administered concurrently. (See PRECAUTIONS.)
Corticosteroids may mask some signs of infection, and new infections may appear during their use. There may be decreased resistance and inability to localize infection when corticosteroids are used. Moreover, corticosteroids may affect the nitroblue-tetrazolium test for bacterial infection and produce false negative results.
In cerebral malaria, a double-blind trial has shown that the use of corticosteroids is associated with prolongation of coma and a higher incidence of pneumonia and gastrointestinal bleeding.
Corticosteroids may activate latent amebiasis. Therefore, it is recommended that latent or active amebiasis be ruled out before initiating corticosteroid therapy in any patient who has spent time in the tropics or any patient with unexplained diarrhea.
Prolonged use of corticosteroids may produce posterior subcapsular cataracts, glaucoma with possible damage to the optic nerves, and may enhance the establishment of secondary ocular infections due to fungi or viruses.
Usage in pregnancy: Since adequate human reproduction studies have not been done with corticosteroids, use of these drugs in pregnancy or in women of childbearing potential requires that the anticipated benefits be weighed against the possible hazards to the mother and embryo or fetus. Infants born of mothers who have received substantial doses of corticosteroids during pregnancy should be carefully observed for signs of hypoadrenalism.
Corticosteroids appear in breast milk and could suppress growth, interfere with endogenous corticosteroid production, or cause other unwanted effects. Mothers taking pharmacologic doses of corticosteroids should be advised not to nurse.
Average and large doses of hydrocortisone or cortisone can cause elevation of blood pressure, salt and water retention, and increased excretion of potassium. These effects are less likely to occur with the synthetic derivatives except when used in large doses. Dietary salt restriction and potassium supplementation may be necessary. All corticosteroids increase calcium excretion.
Administration of live virus vaccines, including smallpox, is contraindicated in individuals receiving immunosuppressive doses of corticosteroids. If inactivated viral or bacterial vaccines are administered to individuals receiving immunosuppressive doses of corticosteroids, the expected serum antibody response may not be obtained. However, immunization procedures may be undertaken in patients who are receiving corticosteroids as replacement therapy, e.g., for Addison's disease.
Patients who are on drugs which suppress the immune system are more susceptible to infections than healthy individuals. Chickenpox and measles, for example, can have a more serious or even fatal course in non-immune patients on corticosteroids. In such patients who have not had these diseases, particular care should be taken to avoid exposure. The risk of developing a disseminated infection varies among individuals and can be related to the dose, route and duration of corticosteroid administration as well as to the underlying disease. If exposed to chickenpox, prophylaxis with varicella zoster immune globulin (VZIG) may be indicated. If chickenpox develops, treatment with antiviral agents may be considered. If exposed to measles, prophylaxis with immune globulin (IG) may be indicated. (See the respective package inserts for VZIG and IG for complete prescribing information.)
Similarly, corticosteroids should be used with great care in patients with known or suspected Strongyloides (threadworm) infestation. In such patients, corticosteroid-induced immunosuppression may lead to Strongyloides hyperinfection and dissemination with widespread larval migration, often accompanied by severe enterocolitis and potentially fatal gram-negative septicemia.
The use of HYDROCORTONE tablets in active tuberculosis should be restricted to those cases of fulminating or disseminated tuberculosis in which the corticosteroid is used for the management of the disease in conjunction with an appropriate antituberculous regimen.
If corticosteroids are indicated in patients with latent tuberculosis or tuberculin reactivity, close observation is necessary as reactivation of the disease may occur. During prolonged corticosteroid therapy, these patients should receive chemoprophylaxis.
Literature reports suggest an apparent association between use of corticosteroids and left ventricular free wall rupture after a recent myocardial infarction; therefore, therapy with corticosteroids should be used with great caution in these patients.

PRECAUTIONS

Following prolonged therapy, withdrawal of corticosteroids may result in symptoms of the corticosteroid withdrawal syndrome including fever, myalgia, arthralgia, and malaise. This may occur in patients even without evidence of adrenal insufficiency.
There is an enhanced effect of corticosteroids in patients with hypothyroidism and in those with cirrhosis.
Corticosteroids should be used cautiously in patients with ocular herpes simplex because of possible corneal perforation.
The lowest possible dose of corticosteroid should be used to control the condition under treatment, and when reduction in dosage is possible, the reduction should be gradual.
Psychic derangements may appear when corticosteroids are used, ranging from euphoria, insomnia, mood swings, personality changes, and severe depression, to frank psychotic manifestations. Also, existing emotional instability or psychotic tendencies may be aggravated by corticosteroids.
Aspirin should be used cautiously in conjunction with corticosteroids in hypoprothrombinemia.
Steroids should be used with caution in nonspecific ulcerative colitis, if there is a probability of impending perforation, abscess, or other pyogenic infection, diverticulitis, fresh intestinal anastomoses, active or latent peptic ulcer, renal insufficiency, hypertension, osteoporosis, and myasthenia gravis. Signs of peritoneal irritation following gastrointestinal perforation in patients receiving large doses of corticosteroids may be minimal or absent. Fat embolism has been reported as a possible complication of hypercortisonism.
When large doses are given, some authorities advise that corticosteroids be taken with meals and antacids taken between meals to help to prevent peptic ulcer.
Steroids may increase or decrease motility and number of spermatozoa in some patients.
Phenytoin, phenobarbital, ephedrine, and rifampin may enhance the metabolic clearance of corticosteroids, resulting in decreased blood levels and lessened physiologic activity, thus requiring adjustment in corticosteroid dosage.
Ketoconazole alone can inhibit adrenal corticosteroid synthesis and may cause adrenal insufficiency during corticosteroid withdrawal (see WARNINGS).
The prothrombin time should be checked frequently in patients who are receiving corticosteroids and coumarin anticoagulants at the same time because of reports that corticosteroids have altered the response to these anticoagulants. Studies have shown that the usual effect produced by adding corticosteroids is inhibition of response to coumarins, although there have been some conflicting reports of potentiation not substantiated by studies.
When corticosteroids are administered concomitantly with potassium-depleting diuretics, patients should be observed closely for development of hypokalemia.
Information for Patients
Susceptible patients who are on immunosuppressant doses of corticosteroids should be warned to avoid exposure to chickenpox or measles. Patients should also be advised that if they are exposed, medical advice should be sought without delay.
Pediatric Use
Growth and development of pediatric patients on prolonged corticosteroid therapy should be carefully followed.

ADVERSE REACTIONS

Fluid and Electrolyte Disturbances
Sodium retention
Fluid retention
Congestive heart failure in susceptible patients
Potassium loss
Hypokalemic alkalosis
Hypertension
Musculoskeletal
Muscle weakness
Steroid myopathy
Loss of muscle mass
Osteoporosis
Vertebral compression fractures
Aseptic necrosis of femoral and humeral heads
Pathologic fracture of long bones
Tendon rupture
Gastrointestinal
Peptic ulcer with possible perforation and hemorrhage
Perforation of the small and large bowel, particularly in patients with inflammatory bowel disease
Pancreatitis
Abdominal distention
Ulcerative esophagitis
Dermatologic
Impaired wound healing
Thin fragile skin
Petechiae and ecchymoses
Erythema
Increased sweating
May suppress reactions to skin tests
Other cutaneous reactions, such as allergic dermatitis, urticaria, angioneurotic edema
Neurologic
Convulsions
Increased intracranial pressure with papilledema (pseudotumor cerebri) usually after treatment
Vertigo
Headache
Psychic disturbances
Endocrine
Menstrual irregularities
Development of cushingoid state
Suppression of growth in children
Secondary adrenocortical and pituitary unresponsiveness, particularly in times of stress, as in trauma, surgery, or illness
Decreased carbohydrate tolerance
Manifestations of latent diabetes mellitus
Hyperglycemia
Increased requirements for insulin or oral hypoglycemic agents in diabetics
Hirsutism
Ophthalmic
Posterior subcapsular cataracts
Increased intraocular pressure
Glaucoma
Exophthalmos

Continued on next page

Information on the Merck & Co., Inc., products listed on these pages is from the prescribing information in use October 1, 2004. For information, please call 1-800-NSC-MERCK [1-800-672-6372].

Hydrocortone Tablets—Cont.

Metabolic
Negative nitrogen balance due to protein catabolism
Cardiovascular
Myocardial rupture following recent myocardial infarction (see WARNINGS)
Other
Hypersensitivity
Thromboembolism
Weight gain
Increased appetite
Nausea
Malaise

OVERDOSAGE

Reports of acute toxicity and/or death following overdosage of glucocorticoids are rare. In the event of overdosage, no specific antidote is available; treatment is supportive and symptomatic.

The intraperitoneal LD_{50} of hydrocortisone in female mice was 1740 mg/kg.

DOSAGE AND ADMINISTRATION

For oral administration
DOSAGE REQUIREMENTS ARE VARIABLE AND MUST BE INDIVIDUALIZED ON THE BASIS OF THE DISEASE AND THE RESPONSE OF THE PATIENT.

The initial dosage varies from 20 to 240 mg a day depending on the disease being treated. In less severe diseases doses lower than 20 mg may suffice, while in severe diseases doses higher than 240 mg may be required. The initial dosage should be maintained or adjusted until the patient's response is satisfactory. If satisfactory clinical response does not occur after a reasonable period of time, discontinue HYDROCORTONE tablets and transfer the patient to other therapy.

After a favorable initial response, the proper maintenance dosage should be determined by decreasing the initial dosage in small amounts to the lowest dosage that maintains an adequate clinical response.

Patients should be observed closely for signs that might require dosage adjustment, including changes in clinical status resulting from remissions or exacerbations of the disease, individual drug responsiveness, and the effect of stress (e.g, surgery, infection, trauma). During stress it may be necessary to increase dosage temporarily.

If the drug is to be stopped after more than a few days of treatment, it usually should be withdrawn gradually.

HOW SUPPLIED

No. 7604—Tablets HYDROCORTONE, 10 mg each, are white, oval shaped compressed tablets, scored and imprinted MSD 619 on one side and HYDROCORTONE on the other, and are supplied as follows:
NDC 0006-0619-68 in bottles of 100.

7920529 Issued November 2001

Shown in Product Identification Guide, page 323

HYDRODIURIL® Tablets ℞
(Hydrochlorothiazide)

DESCRIPTION

HydroDIURIL* (Hydrochlorothiazide) is a diuretic and antihypertensive. It is the 3,4-dihydro derivative of chlorothiazide. Its chemical name is 6-chloro-3,4-dihydro-2*H* -1,2,4-benzothiadiazine-7-sulfonamide 1,1-dioxide. Its empirical formula is $C_7H_8ClN_3O_4S_2$ and its structural formula is:

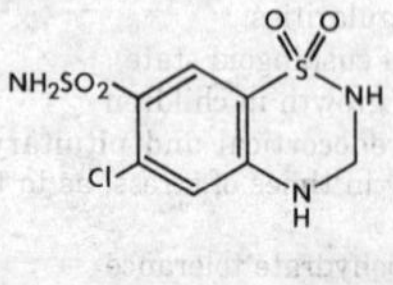

It is a white, or practically white, crystalline powder with a molecular weight of 297.74, which is slightly soluble in water, but freely soluble in sodium hydroxide solution.

HydroDIURIL is supplied as 25 mg and 50 mg tablets for oral use. Each tablet contains the following inactive ingredients: calcium phosphate, FD&C Yellow 6, gelatin, lactose, magnesium stearate, starch and talc.

*Registered trademark of MERCK & CO., INC.

CLINICAL PHARMACOLOGY

The mechanism of the antihypertensive effect of thiazides is unknown. HydroDIURIL does not usually affect normal blood pressure.

HydroDIURIL affects the distal renal tubular mechanism of electrolyte reabsorption. At maximal therapeutic dosage all thiazides are approximately equal in their diuretic efficacy.

HydroDIURIL increases excretion of sodium and chloride in approximately equivalent amounts. Natriuresis may be accompanied by some loss of potassium and bicarbonate.

After oral use diuresis begins within 2 hours, peaks in about 4 hours and lasts about 6 to 12 hours.

Pharmacokinetics and Metabolism
HydroDIURIL is not metabolized but is eliminated rapidly by the kidney. When plasma levels have been followed for at least 24 hours, the plasma half-life has been observed to vary between 5.6 and 14.8 hours. At least 61 percent of the oral dose is eliminated unchanged within 24 hours. Hydrochlorothiazide crosses the placental but not the blood-brain barrier and is excreted in breast milk.

INDICATIONS AND USAGE

HydroDIURIL is indicated as adjunctive therapy in edema associated with congestive heart failure, hepatic cirrhosis, and corticosteroid and estrogen therapy.

HydroDIURIL has also been found useful in edema due to various forms of renal dysfunction such as nephrotic syndrome, acute glomerulonephritis, and chronic renal failure.

HydroDIURIL is indicated in the management of hypertension either as the sole therapeutic agent or to enhance the effectiveness of other antihypertensive drugs in the more severe forms of hypertension.

Use in Pregnancy. Routine use of diuretics during normal pregnancy is inappropriate and exposes mother and fetus to unnecessary hazard. Diuretics do not prevent development of toxemia of pregnancy and there is no satisfactory evidence that they are useful in the treatment of toxemia.

Edema during pregnancy may arise from pathologic causes or from the physiologic and mechanical consequences of pregnancy. Thiazides are indicated in pregnancy when edema is due to pathologic causes, just as they are in the absence of pregnancy (see PRECAUTIONS, *Pregnancy*). Dependent edema in pregnancy, resulting from restriction of venous return by the gravid uterus, is properly treated through elevation of the lower extremities and use of support stockings. Use of diuretics to lower intravascular volume in this instance is illogical and unnecessary. During normal pregnancy there is hypervolemia which is not harmful to the fetus or the mother in the absence of cardiovascular disease. However, it may be associated with edema, rarely generalized edema. If such edema causes discomfort, increased recumbency will often provide relief. Rarely this edema may cause extreme discomfort which is not relieved by rest. In these instances, a short course of diuretic therapy may provide relief and be appropriate.

CONTRAINDICATIONS

Anuria.
Hypersensitivity to this product or to other sulfonamide-derived drugs.

WARNINGS

Use with caution in severe renal disease. In patients with renal disease, thiazides may precipitate azotemia. Cumulative effects of the drug may develop in patients with impaired renal function.

Thiazides should be used with caution in patients with impaired hepatic function or progressive liver disease, since minor alterations of fluid and electrolyte balance may precipitate hepatic coma.

Thiazides may add to or potentiate the action of other antihypertensive drugs.

Sensitivity reactions may occur in patients with or without a history of allergy or bronchial asthma.

The possibility of exacerbation or activation of systemic lupus erythematosus has been reported.

Lithium generally should not be given with diuretics (see PRECAUTIONS, *Drug Interactions*).

PRECAUTIONS

General
All patients receiving diuretic therapy should be observed for evidence of fluid or electrolyte imbalance: namely, hyponatremia, hypochloremic alkalosis, and hypokalemia. Serum and urine electrolyte determinations are particularly important when the patient is vomiting excessively or receiving parenteral fluids. Warning signs or symptoms of fluid and electrolyte imbalance, irrespective of cause, include dryness of mouth, thirst, weakness, lethargy, drowsiness, restlessness, confusion, seizures, muscle pains or cramps, muscular fatigue, hypotension, oliguria, tachycardia, and gastrointestinal disturbances such as nausea and vomiting.

Hypokalemia may develop, especially with brisk diuresis, when severe cirrhosis is present or after prolonged therapy. Interference with adequate oral electrolyte intake will also contribute to hypokalemia. Hypokalemia may cause cardiac arrhythmia and may also sensitize or exaggerate the response of the heart to the toxic effects of digitalis (e.g., increased ventricular irritability). Hypokalemia may be avoided or treated by use of potassium sparing diuretics or potassium supplements such as foods with a high potassium content.

Although any chloride deficit is generally mild and usually does not require specific treatment except under extraordinary circumstances (as in liver disease or renal disease), chloride replacement may be required in the treatment of metabolic alkalosis.

Dilutional hyponatremia may occur in edematous patients in hot weather; appropriate therapy is water restriction, rather than administration of salt, except in rare instances when the hyponatremia is life threatening. In actual salt depletion, appropriate replacement is the therapy of choice.

Hyperuricemia may occur or acute gout may be precipitated in certain patients receiving thiazides.

In diabetic patients dosage adjustments of insulin or oral hypoglycemic agents may be required. Hyperglycemia may occur with thiazide diuretics. Thus latent diabetes mellitus may become manifest during thiazide therapy.

The antihypertensive effects of the drug may be enhanced in the post-sympathectomy patient.

If progressive renal impairment becomes evident, consider withholding or discontinuing diuretic therapy.

Thiazides have been shown to increase the urinary excretion of magnesium; this may result in hypomagnesemia.

Thiazides may decrease urinary calcium excretion. Thiazides may cause intermittent and slight elevation of serum calcium in the absence of known disorders of calcium metabolism. Marked hypercalcemia may be evidence of hidden hyperparathyroidism. Thiazides should be discontinued before carrying out tests for parathyroid function.

Increases in cholesterol and triglyceride levels may be associated with thiazide diuretic therapy.

Laboratory Tests
Periodic determination of serum electrolytes to detect possible electrolyte imbalance should be done at appropriate intervals.

Drug Interactions
When given concurrently the following drugs may interact with thiazide diuretics.

Alcohol, barbiturates, or narcotics —potentiation of orthostatic hypotension may occur.

Antidiabetic drugs —(oral agents and insulin)—dosage adjustment of the antidiabetic drug may be required.

Other antihypertensive drugs —additive effect or potentiation.

Cholestyramine and colestipol resins—Absorption of hydrochlorothiazide is impaired in the presence of anionic exchange resins. Single doses of either cholestyramine or colestipol resins bind the hydrochlorothiazide and reduce its absorption from the gastrointestinal tract by up to 85 and 43 percent, respectively.

Corticosteroids, ACTH —intensified electrolyte depletion, particularly hypokalemia.

Pressor amines (e.g., norepinephrine) —possible decreased response to pressor amines but not sufficient to preclude their use.

Skeletal muscle relaxants, nondepolarizing (e.g., tubocurarine) —possible increased responsiveness to the muscle relaxant.

Lithium —generally should not be given with diuretics. Diuretic agents reduce the renal clearance of lithium and add a high risk of lithium toxicity. Refer to the package insert for lithium preparations before use of such preparations with HydroDIURIL.

Non-steroidal Anti-inflammatory Drugs —In some patients, the administration of a non-steroidal anti-inflammatory agent can reduce the diuretic, natriuretic, and antihypertensive effects of loop, potassium-sparing and thiazide diuretics. Therefore, when HydroDIURIL and non-steroidal anti-inflammatory agents are used concomitantly, the patient should be observed closely to determine if the desired effect of the diuretic is obtained.

Drug/Laboratory Test Interactions
Thiazides should be discontinued before carrying out tests for parathyroid function (see PRECAUTIONS, *General*).

Carcinogenesis, Mutagenesis, Impairment of Fertility
Two-year feeding studies in mice and rats conducted under the auspices of the National Toxicology Program (NTP) uncovered no evidence of a carcinogenic potential of hydrochlorothiazide in female mice (at doses of up to approximately 600 mg/kg/day) or in male and female rats (at doses of up to approximately 100 mg/kg/day). The NTP, however, found equivocal evidence for hepatocarcinogenicity in male mice.

Hydrochlorothiazide was not genotoxic *in vitro* in the Ames mutagenicity assay of *Salmonella typhimurium* strains TA 98, TA 100, TA 1535, TA 1537, and TA 1538 and in the Chinese Hamster Ovary (CHO) test for chromosomal aberrations, or *in vivo* in assays using mouse germinal cell chromosomes, Chinese hamster bone marrow chromosomes, and the *Drosophila* sex-linked recessive lethal trait gene. Positive test results were obtained only in the *in vitro* CHO Sister Chromatid Exchange (clastogenicity) and in the Mouse Lymphoma Cell (mutagenicity) assays, using concentrations of hydrochlorothiazide from 43 to 1300 µg/mL, and in the *Aspergillus nidulans* non-disjunction assay at an unspecified concentration.

Hydrochlorothiazide had no adverse effects on the fertility of mice and rats of either sex in studies wherein these species were exposed, via their diet, to doses of up to 100 and 4 mg/kg, respectively, prior to conception and throughout gestation.

Pregnancy
Teratogenic Effects—Pregnancy Category B: Studies in which hydrochlorothiazide was orally administered to pregnant mice and rats during their respective periods of major organogenesis at doses up to 3000 and 1000 mg hydrochlorothiazide/kg, respectively, provided no evidence of harm to the fetus.

There are, however, no adequate and well-controlled studies in pregnant women. Because animal reproduction studies are not always predictice of human response, this drug should be used during pregnancy only if clearly needed.
Nonteratogenic Effects: Thiazides cross the placental barrier and appear in cord blood. There is a risk of fetal or neonatal jaundice, thrombocytopenia, and possibly other adverse reactions that have occurred in adults.
Nursing Mothers
Thiazides are excreted in breast milk. Because of the potential for serious adverse reactions in nursing infants, a decision should be made whether to discontinue nursing or to discontinue hydrochlorothiazide, taking into account the importance of the drug to the mother.
Pediatric Use
There are no well-controlled clinical trials in pediatric patients. Information on dosing in this age group is supported by evidence from empiric use in pediatric patients and published literature regarding the treatment of hypertension in such patients. (See DOSAGE AND ADMINISTRATION, *Infants and Children.*)

ADVERSE REACTIONS

The following adverse reactions have been reported and, within each category, are listed in order of decreasing severity.
Body as a Whole: Weakness.
Cardiovascular: Hypotension including orthostatic hypotension (may be aggravated by alcohol, barbiturates, narcotics or antihypertensive drugs).
Digestive: Pancreatitis, jaundice (intrahepatic cholestatic jaundice), diarrhea, vomiting, sialadenitis, cramping, constipation, gastric irritation, nausea, anorexia.
Hematologic: Aplastic anemia, agranulocytosis, leukopenia, hemolytic anemia, thrombocytopenia.
Hypersensitivity: Anaphylactic reactions, necrotizing angiitis (vasculitis and cutaneous vasculitis), respiratory distress including pneumonitis and pulmonary edema, photosensitivity, fever, urticaria, rash, purpura.
Metabolic: Electrolyte imbalance (see PRECAUTIONS), hyperglycemia, glycosuria, hyperuricemia.
Musculoskeletal: Muscle spasm.
Nervous System/Psychiatric: Vertigo, paresthesias, dizziness, headache, restlessness.
Renal: Renal failure, renal dysfunction, interstitial nephritis. (See WARNINGS.)
Skin: Erythema multiforme including Stevens-Johnson syndrome, exfoliative dermatitis including toxic epidermal necrolysis, alopecia.
Special Senses: Transient blurred vision, xanthopsia.
Urogenital: Impotence.
Whenever adverse reactions are moderate or severe, thiazide dosage should be reduced or therapy withdrawn.

OVERDOSAGE

The most common signs and symptoms observed are those caused by electrolyte depletion (hypokalemia, hypochloremia, hyponatremia) and dehydration resulting from excessive diuresis. If digitalis has also been administered, hypokalemia may accentuate cardiac arrhythmias.
In the event of overdosage, symptomatic and supportive measures should be employed. Emesis should be induced or gastric lavage performed. Correct dehydration, electrolyte imbalance, hepatic coma and hypotension by established procedures. If required, give oxygen or artificial respiration for respiratory impairment. The degree to which hydrochlorothiazide is removed by hemodialysis has not been established.
The oral LD_{50} of hydrochlorothiazide is greater than 10 g/kg in the mouse and rat.

DOSAGE AND ADMINISTRATION

Therapy should be individualized according to patient response. Use the smallest dosage necessary to achieve the required response.

Adults
For Edema
The usual adult dosage is 25 to 100 mg daily as a single or divided dose. Many patients with edema respond to intermittent therapy, i.e., administration on alternate days or on three to five days each week. With an intermittent schedule, excessive response and the resulting undesirable electrolyte imbalance are less likely to occur.
For Control of Hypertension
The usual initial dose in adults is 25 mg daily given as a single dose. The dose may be increased to 50 mg daily, given as a single or two divided doses. Doses above 50 mg are often associated with marked reductions in serum potassium (see also PRECAUTIONS).
Patients usually do not require doses in excess of 50 mg of hydrochlorothiazide daily when used concomitantly with other antihypertensive agents.

Infants and Children
For Diuresis and For Control of Hypertension
The usual pediatric dosage is 0.5 to 1 mg per pound (1 to 2 mg/kg) per day in single or two divided doses, not to exceed 37.5 mg per day in infants up to 2 years of age or 100 mg per day in children 2 to 12 years of age. In infants less than 6 months of age, doses up to 1.5 mg per pound (3 mg/kg) per day in two divided doses may be required. (See PRECAUTIONS, *Pediatric Use.*)

HOW SUPPLIED
No. 3263—Tablets HydroDIURIL, 25 mg, are peach-colored, round, scored, compressed tablets, coded MSD 42 on one side and HydroDIURIL on the other. They are supplied as follows:
NDC 0006-0042-68 bottles of 100
NDC 0006-0042-82 bottles of 1000.
No. 3264—Tablets HydroDIURIL, 50 mg, are peach-colored, round, scored, compressed tablets, coded MSD 105 on one side and HydroDIURIL on the other. They are supplied as follows:
NDC 0006-0105-68 bottles of 100
NDC 0006-0105-86 bottles of 5000.
Storage
Keep container tightly closed. Protect from light, moisture, freezing, −20°C (−4°F) and store at room temperature, 15–30°C (59–86°F).
7897450 Issued June 1998

HYZAAR® 50-12.5 ℞
(losartan potassium-hydrochlorothiazide tablets)
HYZAAR® 100-25 ℞
(losartan potassium-hydrochlorothiazide tablets)

USE IN PREGNANCY
When used in pregnancy during the second and third trimesters, drugs that act directly on the renin-angiotensin system can cause injury and even death to the developing fetus. When pregnancy is detected, HYZAAR should be discontinued as soon as possible. See WARNINGS: *Fetal/Neonatal Morbidity and Mortality.*

DESCRIPTION

HYZAAR* 50-12.5 (losartan potassium-hydrochlorothiazide) and HYZAAR* 100-25 (losartan potassium-hydrochlorothiazide), combines an angiotensin II receptor (type AT_1) antagonist and a diuretic, hydrochlorothiazide.
Losartan potassium, a non-peptide molecule, is chemically described as 2-butyl-4-chloro-1-[*p*-(*o*-1*H*-tetrazol-5-ylphenyl)benzyl]imidazole-5-methanol monopotassium salt. Its empirical formula is $C_{22}H_{22}ClKN_6O$, and its structural formula is:

N Cl
$CH_3CH_2CH_2CH_2$ N CH_2OH
CH_2 N N N N K+

Losartan potassium is a white to off-white free-flowing crystalline powder with a molecular weight of 461.01. It is freely soluble in water, soluble in alcohols, and slightly soluble in common organic solvents, such as acetonitrile and methyl ethyl ketone.
Oxidation of the 5-hydroxymethyl group on the imidazole ring results in the active metabolite of losartan.
Hydrochlorothiazide is 6-chloro-3,4-dihydro-2*H*-1,2,4-benzothiadiazine-7-sulfonamide 1,1-dioxide. Its empirical formula is $C_7H_8ClN_3O_4S_2$ and its structural formula is:

O O
NH_2SO_2 S NH
Cl N H

Hydrochlorothiazide is a white, or practically white, crystalline powder with a molecular weight of 297.74, which is slightly soluble in water, but freely soluble in sodium hydroxide solution.
HYZAAR is available for oral administration in two tablet combinations of losartan and hydrochlorothiazide. HYZAAR 50-12.5 contains 50 mg of losartan potassium and 12.5 mg of hydrochlorothiazide. HYZAAR 100-25 contains 100 mg of losartan potassium and 25 mg of hydrochlorothiazide. Inactive ingredients are microcrystalline cellulose, lactose hydrous, pregelatinized starch, magnesium stearate, hydroxypropyl cellulose, hypromellose, titanium dioxide and D&C yellow No. 10 aluminum lake.
HYZAAR 50-12.5 contains 4.24 mg (0.108 mEq) of potassium and HYZAAR 100-25 contains 8.48 mg (0.216 mEq) of potassium.

*Registered trademark of E.I. du Pont de Nemours and Company, Wilmington, Delaware, USA

CLINICAL PHARMACOLOGY

Mechanism of Action
Angiotensin II [formed from angiotensin I in a reaction catalyzed by angiotensin converting enzyme (ACE, kininase II)], is a potent vasoconstrictor, the primary vasoactive hormone of the renin-angiotensin system and an important component in the pathophysiology of hypertension. It also stimulates aldosterone secretion by the adrenal cortex. Losartan and its principal active metabolite block the vasoconstrictor and aldosterone-secreting effects of angiotensin II by selectively blocking the binding of angiotensin II to the AT_1 receptor found in many tissues, (e.g., vascular smooth muscle, adrenal gland). There is also an AT_2 receptor found in many tissues but it is not known to be associated with cardiovascular homeostasis. Both losartan and its principal active metabolite do not exhibit any partial agonist activity at the AT_1 receptor and have much greater affinity (about 1000-fold) for the AT_1 receptor than for the AT_2 receptor. *In vitro* binding studies indicate that losartan is a reversible, competitive inhibitor of the AT_1 receptor. The active metabolite is 10 to 40 times more potent by weight than losartan and appears to be a reversible, non-competitive inhibitor of the AT_1 receptor.
Neither losartan nor its active metabolite inhibits ACE (kininase II, the enzyme that converts angiotensin I to angiotensin II and degrades bradykinin); nor do they bind to or block other hormone receptors or ion channels known to be important in cardiovascular regulation.
Hydrochlorothiazide is a thiazide diuretic. Thiazides affect the renal tubular mechanisms of electrolyte reabsorption, directly increasing excretion of sodium and chloride in approximately equivalent amounts. Indirectly, the diuretic action of hydrochlorothiazide reduces plasma volume, with consequent increases in plasma renin activity, increases in aldosterone secretion, increases in urinary potassium loss, and decreases in serum potassium. The renin-aldosterone link is mediated by angiotensin II, so coadministration of an angiotensin II receptor antagonist tends to reverse the potassium loss associated with these diuretics.
The mechanism of the antihypertensive effect of thiazides is unknown.
Pharmacokinetics
General
Losartan Potassium
Losartan is an orally active agent that undergoes substantial first-pass metabolism by cytochrome P450 enzymes. It is converted, in part, to an active carboxylic acid metabolite that is responsible for most of the angiotensin II receptor antagonism that follows losartan treatment. The terminal half-life of losartan is about 2 hours and of the metabolite is about 6–9 hours. The pharmacokinetics of losartan and its active metabolite are linear with oral losartan doses up to 200 mg and do not change over time. Neither losartan nor its metabolite accumulate in plasma upon repeated once-daily dosing.
Following oral administration, losartan is well absorbed (based on absorption of radiolabeled losartan) and undergoes substantial first-pass metabolism; the systemic bioavailability of losartan is approximately 33%. About 14% of an orally-administered dose of losartan is converted to the active metabolite. Mean peak concentrations of losartan and its active metabolite are reached in 1 hour and in 3–4 hours, respectively. While maximum plasma concentrations of losartan and its active metabolite are approximately equal, the AUC of the metabolite is about 4 times as great as that of losartan. A meal slows absorption of losartan and decreases its C_{max} but has only minor effects on losartan AUC or on the AUC of the metabolite (about 10% decreased).
Both losartan and its active metabolite are highly bound to plasma proteins, primarily albumin, with plasma free fractions of 1.3% and 0.2% respectively. Plasma protein binding is constant over the concentration range achieved with recommended doses. Studies in rats indicate that losartan crosses the blood-brain barrier poorly, if at all.
Losartan metabolites have been identified in human plasma and urine. In addition to the active carboxylic acid metabolite, several inactive metabolites are formed. Following oral and intravenous administration of ^{14}C-labeled losartan potassium, circulating plasma radioactivity is primarily attributed to losartan and its active metabolite. *In vitro* studies indicate that cytochrome P450 2C9 and 3A4 are involved in the biotransformation of losartan to its metabolites. Minimal conversion of losartan to the active metabolite (less than 1% of the dose compared to 14% of the dose in normal subjects) was seen in about one percent of individuals studied.
The volume of distribution of losartan is about 34 liters and of the active metabolite is about 12 liters. Total plasma clearance of losartan and the active metabolite is about 600 mL/min and 50 mL/min, respectively, with renal clearance of about 75 mL/min and 25 mL/min, respectively. When losartan is administered orally, about 4% of the dose is excreted unchanged in the urine and about 6% is excreted in urine as active metabolite. Biliary excretion contributes to the elimination of losartan and its metabolites. Following oral ^{14}C-labeled losartan, about 35% of radioactivity is recovered in the urine and about 60% in the feces. Following

Continued on next page

Information on the Merck & Co., Inc., products listed on these pages is from the prescribing information in use October 1, 2004. For information, please call 1-800-NSC-MERCK [1-800-672-6372].

Hyzaar—Cont.

an intravenous dose of ^{14}C-labeled losartan, about 45% of radioactivity is recovered in the urine and 50% in the feces.

Special Populations

Pediatric: Losartan pharmacokinetics have not been investigated in patients <18 years of age.

Geriatric and Gender: Losartan pharmacokinetics have been investigated in the elderly (65–75 years) and in both genders. Plasma concentrations of losartan and its active metabolite are similar in elderly and young hypertensives. Plasma concentrations of losartan were about twice as high in female hypertensives as male hypertensives, but concentrations of the active metabolite were similar in males and females.

Race: Pharmacokinetic differences due to race have not been studied.

Renal Insufficiency:

Losartan: Following oral administration, plasma concentrations and AUCs of losartan and its active metabolite are increased by 50–90% in patients with mild (creatinine clearance of 50 to 74 mL/min) or moderate (creatinine clearance 30 to 49 mL/min) renal insufficiency. In this study, renal clearance was reduced by 55–85% for both losartan and its active metabolite in patients with mild or moderate renal insufficiency. Neither losartan nor its active metabolite can be removed by hemodialysis.

Hydrochlorothiazide: Following oral administration, the AUC for hydrochlorothiazide is increased by 70 and 700% for patients with mild and moderate renal insufficiency, respectively. In this study, renal clearance of hydrochlorothiazide decreased by 45 and 85% in patients with mild and moderate renal impairment, respectively.

The usual regimens of therapy with HYZAAR may be followed as long as the patient's creatinine clearance is >30 mL/min. In patients with more severe renal impairment, loop diuretics are preferred to thiazides, so HYZAAR is not recommended. (See DOSAGE AND ADMINISTRATION.)

Hepatic Insufficiency: Following oral administration in patients with mild to moderate alcoholic cirrhosis of the liver, plasma concentrations of losartan and its active metabolite were, respectively, 5 times and about 1.7 times those in young male volunteers. Compared to normal subjects the total plasma clearance of losartan in patients with hepatic insufficiency was about 50% lower and the oral bioavailability was about 2-times higher. The lower starting dose of losartan recommended for use in patients with hepatic impairment cannot be given using HYZAAR. Its use in such patients as a means of losartan titration is, therefore, not recommended (see DOSAGE AND ADMINISTRATION).

Drug Interactions

Losartan Potassium

Losartan, administered for 12 days, did not affect the pharmacokinetics or pharmacodynamics of a single dose of warfarin. Losartan did not affect the pharmacokinetics of oral or intravenous digoxin. There is no pharmacokinetic interaction between losartan and hydrochlorothiazide. Coadministration of losartan and cimetidine led to an increase of about 18% in AUC of losartan but did not affect the pharmacokinetics of its active metabolite. Coadministration of losartan and phenobarbital led to a reduction of about 20% in the AUC of losartan and that of its active metabolite. A somewhat greater interaction (approximately 40% reduction in the AUC of active metabolite and approximately 30% reduction in the AUC of losartan) has been reported with rifampin. Fluconazole, an inhibitor of cytochrome P450 2C9, decreased the AUC of the active metabolite by approximately 40%, but increased the AUC of losartan by approximately 70% following multiple doses. Conversion of losartan to its active metabolite after intravenous administration is not affected by ketoconazole, an inhibitor of P450 3A4. The AUC of active metabolite following oral losartan was not affected by erythromycin, another inhibitor of P450 3A4, but the AUC of losartan was increased by 30%.

Hydrochlorothiazide

After oral administration of hydrochlorothiazide, diuresis begins within 2 hours, peaks in about 4 hours and lasts about 6 to 12 hours.

Hydrochlorothiazide is not metabolized but is eliminated rapidly by the kidney. When plasma levels have been followed for at least 24 hours, the plasma half-life has been observed to vary between 5.6 and 14.8 hours. At least 61 percent of the oral dose is eliminated unchanged within 24 hours. Hydrochlorothiazide crosses the placental but not the blood-brain barrier and is excreted in breast milk.

Pharmacodynamics and Clinical Effects

Losartan Potassium

Losartan inhibits the pressor effect of angiotensin II (as well as angiotensin I) infusions. A dose of 100 mg inhibits the pressor effect by about 85% at peak with 25–40% inhibition persisting for 24 hours. Removal of the negative feedback of angiotensin II causes a 2- to 3-fold rise in plasma renin activity and consequent rise in angiotensin II plasma concentration in hypertensive patients. Losartan does not affect the response to bradykinin, whereas ACE inhibitors increase the response to bradykinin. Aldosterone plasma concentrations fall following losartan administration. In spite of the effect of losartan on aldosterone secretion, very little effect on serum potassium was observed.

In a single-dose study in normal volunteers, losartan had no effects on glomerular filtration rate, renal plasma flow or filtration fraction. In multiple dose studies in hypertensive patients, there were no notable effects on systemic or renal prostaglandin concentrations, fasting triglycerides, total cholesterol or HDL-cholesterol or fasting glucose concentrations. There was a small uricosuric effect leading to a minimal decrease in serum uric acid (mean decrease <0.4 mg/dL) during chronic oral administration.

The antihypertensive effects of losartan were demonstrated principally in 4 placebo-controlled, 6- to 12-week trials of dosages from 10 to 150 mg per day in patients with baseline diastolic blood pressures of 95–115. The studies allowed comparisons of two doses (50–100 mg/day) as once-daily or twice-daily regimens, comparisons of peak and trough effects, and comparisons of response by gender, age, and race. Three additional studies examined the antihypertensive effects of losartan and hydrochlorothiazide in combination.

The 4 studies of losartan monotherapy included a total of 1075 patients randomized to several doses of losartan and 334 to placebo. The 10 and 25 mg doses produced some effect at peak (6 hours after dosing) but small and inconsistent trough (24 hour) responses. Doses of 50, 100, and 150 mg once daily gave statistically significant systolic/diastolic mean decreases in blood pressure, compared to placebo in the range of 5.5–10.5/3.5–7.5 mmHg, with the 150 mg dose giving no greater effect than 50–100 mg. Twice-daily dosing at 50–100 mg/day gave consistently larger trough responses than once-daily dosing at the same total dose. Peak (6 hour) effects were uniformly, but moderately larger than trough effects, with the trough to peak ratio for systolic and diastolic responses 50–95% and 60–90% respectively.

Analysis of age, gender, and race subgroups of patients showed that men and women, and patients over and under 65, had generally similar responses. Losartan was effective in reducing blood pressure regardless of race, although the effect was somewhat less in Black patients (usually a low-renin population).

The effect of losartan is substantially present within one week but in some studies the maximal effect occurred in 3–6 weeks. In long-term follow-up studies (without placebo control) the effect of losartan appeared to be maintained for up to a year. There is no apparent rebound effect after abrupt withdrawal of losartan. There was essentially no change in average heart rate in losartan-treated patients in controlled trials.

Losartan Potassium-Hydrochlorothiazide

The 3 controlled studies of losartan and hydrochlorothiazide included over 1300 patients assessing the antihypertensive efficacy of various doses of losartan (25, 50 and 100 mg) and concomitant hydrochlorothiazide (6.25, 12.5 and 25 mg). A factorial study compared the combination of losartan/hydrochlorothiazide 50/12.5 mg with its components and placebo. The combination of losartan/hydrochlorothiazide 50/12.5 mg resulted in an approximately additive placebo-adjusted systolic/diastolic response (15.5/9.0 mmHg for the combination compared to 8.5/5.0 mmHg for losartan alone and 7.0/3.0 mmHg for hydrochlorothiazide alone). Another study investigated the dose-response relationship of various doses of hydrochlorothiazide (6.25, 12.5 and 25 mg) or placebo on a background of losartan (50 mg) in patients not adequately controlled (SiDBP 93–120 mmHg) on losartan (50 mg) alone. The third study investigated the dose-response relationship of various doses of losartan (25, 50 and 100 mg) or placebo on a background of hydrochlorothiazide (25 mg) in patients not adequately controlled (SiDBP 93–120 mmHg) on hydrochlorothiazide (25 mg) alone. These studies showed an added antihypertensive response at trough (24 hours post-dosing) of hydrochlorothiazide 12.5 or 25 mg added to losartan 50 mg of 5.5/3.5 and 10.0/6.0 mmHg, respectively. Similarly, there was an added antihypertensive response at trough when losartan 50 or 100 mg was added to hydrochlorothiazide 25 mg of 9.0/5.5 and 12.5/6.5 mmHg, respectively. There was no significant effect on heart rate.

There was no difference in response for men and women or in patients over or under 65 years of age.

Black patients had a larger response to hydrochlorothiazide than non-Black patients and a smaller response to losartan. The overall response to the combination was similar for Black and non-Black patients.

Severe Hypertension (Sitting Diastolic Blood Pressure [SiDBP] ≥110 mmHg)

The safety and efficacy of HYZAAR as initial therapy for severe hypertension (defined as a mean SiDBP ≥110 mmHg confirmed on 2 separate occasions off all antihypertensive therapy) was studied in a 6-week double-blind, randomized, multicenter study. Patients were randomized to either losartan and hydrochlorothiazide (50–12.5 mg, once daily) or to losartan (50 mg, once daily) and followed for blood pressure response. Patients were titrated at 2-week intervals if their SiDBP did not reach goal (<90 mmHg). Patients on combination therapy were titrated from losartan 50 mg/hydrochlorothiazide 12.5 mg to losartan 50 mg/hydrochlorothiazide 12.5 mg (sham titration to maintain the blind) to losartan 100 mg/hydrochlorothiazide 25 mg. Patients on monotherapy were titrated from losartan 50 mg to losartan 100 mg to losartan 150 mg, as needed. The primary endpoint was a comparison at 4 weeks of patients who achieved goal diastolic blood pressure (trough SiDBP <90 mmHg).

The study enrolled 585 patients, including 264 (45%) females, 124 (21%) blacks, and 21 (4%) ≥65 years of age. The mean blood pressure at baseline for the total population was 171/113 mmHg. The mean age was 53 years. After 4 weeks of therapy, the mean SiDBP was 3.1 mmHg lower and the mean SiSBP was 5.6 mmHg lower in the group treated with HYZAAR. As a result, a greater proportion of the patients on HYZAAR reached the target diastolic blood pressure (17.6% for HYZAAR, 9.4% for losartan; p=0.006). Similar trends were seen when the patients were grouped according to gender, race or age (<≥65).

After 6 weeks of therapy, more patients who received the combination regimen reached target diastolic blood pressure than those who received the monotherapy regimen (29.8% versus 12.5%).

During the study period, there were no reported cases of syncope in either treatment group. There were 2 (0.6%) and 0 (0.0%) cases of hypotension reported in the group treated with HYZAAR and the group treated with losartan, respectively. The overall pattern of adverse events reported for patients treated with HYZAAR as initial therapy was similar to the adverse event profile for patients treated with losartan as initial therapy. For information on the specific adverse events observed during the study period, see ADVERSE REACTIONS, *Severe Hypertension*.

INDICATIONS AND USAGE

HYZAAR is indicated for the treatment of hypertension. This fixed dose combination is not indicated for initial therapy of hypertension, except when the hypertension is severe enough that the value of achieving prompt blood pressure control exceeds the risk of initiating combination therapy in these patients (see CLINICAL PHARMACOLOGY, *Pharmacodynamics and Clinical Effects,* and DOSAGE AND ADMINISTRATION).

CONTRAINDICATIONS

HYZAAR is contraindicated in patients who are hypersensitive to any component of this product.

Because of the hydrochlorothiazide component, this product is contraindicated in patients with anuria or hypersensitivity to other sulfonamide-derived drugs.

WARNINGS

Fetal/Neonatal Morbidity and Mortality

Drugs that act directly on the renin-angiotensin system can cause fetal and neonatal morbidity and death when administered to pregnant women. Several dozen cases have been reported in the world literature in patients who were taking angiotensin converting enzyme inhibitors. When pregnancy is detected, HYZAAR should be discontinued as soon as possible.

The use of drugs that act directly on the renin-angiotensin system during the second and third trimesters of pregnancy has been associated with fetal and neonatal injury, including hypotension, neonatal skull hypoplasia, anuria, reversible or irreversible renal failure, and death. Oligohydramnios has also been reported, presumably resulting from decreased fetal renal function; oligohydramnios in this setting has been associated with fetal limb contractures, craniofacial deformation, and hypoplastic lung development. Prematurity, intrauterine growth retardation, and patent ductus arteriosus have also been reported, although it is not clear whether these occurrences were due to exposure to the drug.

These adverse effects do not appear to have resulted from intrauterine drug exposure that has been limited to the first trimester.

Mothers whose embryos and fetuses are exposed to an angiotensin II receptor antagonist only during the first trimester should be so informed. Nonetheless, when patients become pregnant, physicians should have the patient discontinue the use of HYZAAR as soon as possible.

Rarely (probably less often than once in every thousand pregnancies), no alternative to an angiotensin II receptor antagonist will be found. In these rare cases, the mothers should be apprised of the potential hazards to their fetuses, and serial ultrasound examinations should be performed to assess the intra-amniotic environment.

If oligohydramnios is observed, HYZAAR should be discontinued unless it is considered life-saving for the mother. Contraction stress testing (CST), a non-stress test (NST), or biophysical profiling (BPP) may be appropriate, depending upon the week of pregnancy. Patients and physicians should be aware, however, that oligohydramnios may not appear until after the fetus has sustained irreversible injury.

Infants with histories of *in utero* exposure to an angiotensin II receptor antagonist should be closely observed for hypotension, oliguria, and hyperkalemia. If oliguria occurs, attention should be directed toward support of blood pressure and renal perfusion. Exchange transfusion or dialysis may be required as means of reversing hypotension and/or substituting for disordered renal function.

There was no evidence of teratogenicity in rats or rabbits treated with a maximum losartan potassium dose of 10 mg/kg/day in combination with 2.5 mg/kg/day of hydrochlorothiazide. At these dosages, respective exposures (AUCs) of losartan, its active metabolite, and hydrochlorothiazide in rabbits were approximately 5-, 1.5-, and 1.0-times those achieved in humans with 100 mg losartan in combination with 25 mg hydrochlorothiazide. AUC values for losartan, its active metabolite and hydrochlorothiazide, extrapolated from data obtained with losartan administered to rats at a dose of 50 mg/kg/day in combination with 12.5 mg/kg/day of hydrochlorothiazide, were approximately 6, 2, and 2 times greater than those achieved in humans with 100 mg of losartan in combination with 25 mg of hydrochlorothiazide.

Fetal toxicity in rats, as evidenced by a slight increase in supernumerary ribs, was observed when females were treated prior to and throughout gestation with 10 mg/kg/day losartan in combination with 2.5 mg/kg/day hydrochlorothiazide. As also observed in studies with losartan alone, adverse fetal and neonatal effects, including decreased body weight, renal toxicity, and mortality, occurred when pregnant rats were treated during late gestation and/or lactation with 50 mg/kg/day losartan in combination with 12.5 mg/kg/day hydrochlorothiazide. Respective AUCs for losartan, its active metabolite and hydrochlorothiazide at these dosages in rats were approximately 35, 10 and 10 times greater than those achieved in humans with the administration of 100 mg of losartan in combination with 25 mg hydrochlorothiazide. When hydrochlorothiazide was administered without losartan to pregnant mice and rats during their respective periods of major organogenesis, at doses up to 3000 and 1000 mg/kg/day, respectively, there was no evidence of harm to the fetus.

Thiazides cross the placental barrier and appear in cord blood. There is a risk of fetal or neonatal jaundice, thrombocytopenia, and possibly other adverse reactions that have occurred in adults.

Hypotension—Volume-Depleted Patients

In patients who are intravascularly volume-depleted (e.g., those treated with diuretics), symptomatic hypotension may occur after initiation of therapy with HYZAAR. This condition should be corrected prior to administration of HYZAAR (see DOSAGE AND ADMINISTRATION).

Impaired Hepatic Function

Losartan Potassium-Hydrochlorothiazide

HYZAAR is not recommended for patients with hepatic impairment who require titration with losartan. The lower starting dose of losartan recommended for use in patients with hepatic impairment cannot be given using HYZAAR.

Hydrochlorothiazide

Thiazides should be used with caution in patients with impaired hepatic function or progressive liver disease, since minor alterations of fluid and electrolyte balance may precipitate hepatic coma.

Hypersensitivity Reaction

Hypersensitivity reactions to hydrochlorothiazide may occur in patients with or without a history of allergy or bronchial asthma, but are more likely in patients with such a history.

Systemic Lupus Erythematosus

Thiazide diuretics have been reported to cause exacerbation or activation of systemic lupus erythematosus.

Lithium Interaction

Lithium generally should not be given with thiazides (see PRECAUTIONS, *Drug Interactions, Hydrocholorothiazide, Lithium*).

PRECAUTIONS

General

Hypersensitivity. Angioedema. See ADVERSE REACTIONS, *Post-Marketing Experience.*

Losartan Potassium-Hydrochlorothiazide

In double-blind clinical trials of various doses of losartan potassium and hydrochlorothiazide, the incidence of hypertensive patients who developed hypokalemia (serum potassium <3.5 mEq/L) was 6.7% versus 3.5% for placebo; the incidence of hyperkalemia (serum potassium >5.7 mEq/L) was 0.4%. No patient discontinued due to increases or decreases in serum potassium. The mean decrease in serum potassium in patients treated with various doses of losartan and hydrochlorothiazide was 0.123 mEq/L. In patients treated with various doses of losartan and hydrochlorothiazide, there was also a dose-related decrease in the hypokalemic response to hydrochlorothiazide as the dose of losartan was increased, as well as a dose-related decrease in serum uric acid with increasing doses of losartan.

Hydrochlorothiazide

Periodic determination of serum electrolytes to detect possible electrolyte imbalance should be performed at appropriate intervals.

All patients receiving thiazide therapy should be observed for clinical signs of fluid or electrolyte imbalance: hyponatremia, hypochloremic alkalosis, and hypokalemia. Serum and urine electrolyte determinations are particularly important when the patient is vomiting excessively or receiving parenteral fluids. Warning signs or symptoms of fluid and electrolyte imbalance, irrespective of cause, include dryness of mouth, thirst, weakness, lethargy, drowsiness, restlessness, confusion, seizures, muscle pains or cramps, muscular fatigue, hypotension, oliguria, tachycardia, and gastrointestinal disturbances such as nausea and vomiting.

Hypokalemia may develop, especially with brisk diuresis, when severe cirrhosis is present, or after prolonged therapy. Interference with adequate oral electrolyte intake will also contribute to hypokalemia. Hypokalemia may cause cardiac arrhythmia and may also sensitize or exaggerate the response of the heart to the toxic effects of digitalis (e.g., increased ventricular irritability).

Although any chloride deficit is generally mild and usually does not require specific treatment except under extraordinary circumstances (as in liver disease or renal disease), chloride replacement may be required in the treatment of metabolic alkalosis.

Dilutional hyponatremia may occur in edematous patients in hot weather; appropriate therapy is water restriction, rather than administration of salt except in rare instances when the hyponatremia is life-threatening. In actual salt depletion, appropriate replacement is the therapy of choice.

Hyperuricemia may occur or frank gout may be precipitated in certain patients receiving thiazide therapy. Because losartan decreases uric acid, losartan in combination with hydrochlorothiazide attenuates the diuretic-induced hyperuricemia.

In diabetic patients, dosage adjustments of insulin or oral hypoglycemic agents may be required. Hyperglycemia may occur with thiazide diuretics. Thus latent diabetes mellitus may become manifest during thiazide therapy.

The antihypertensive effects of the drug may be enhanced in the postsympathectomy patient.

If progressive renal impairment becomes evident consider withholding or discontinuing diuretic therapy.

Thiazides have been shown to increase the urinary excretion of magnesium; this may result in hypomagnesemia.

Thiazides may decrease urinary calcium excretion. Thiazides may cause intermittent and slight elevation of serum calcium in the absence of known disorders of calcium metabolism. Marked hypercalcemia may be evidence of hidden hyperparathyroidism. Thiazides should be discontinued before carrying out tests for parathyroid function.

Increases in cholesterol and triglyceride levels may be associated with thiazide diuretic therapy.

Impaired Renal Function

As a consequence of inhibiting the renin-angiotensin-aldosterone system, changes in renal function have been reported in susceptible individuals treated with losartan; in some patients, these changes in renal function were reversible upon discontinuation of therapy.

In patients whose renal function may depend on the activity of the renin-angiotensin-aldosterone system (e.g., patients with severe congestive heart failure), treatment with angiotensin converting enzyme inhibitors has been associated with oliguria and/or progressive azotemia and (rarely) with acute renal failure and/or death. Similar outcomes have been reported with losartan.

In studies of ACE inhibitors in patients with unilateral or bilateral renal artery stenosis, increases in serum creatinine or BUN have been reported. Similar effects have been reported with losartan; in some patients, these effects were reversible upon discontinuation of therapy.

Thiazides should be used with caution in severe renal disease. In patients with renal disease, thiazides may precipitate azotemia. Cumulative effects of the drug may develop in patients with impaired renal function.

Information for Patients

Pregnancy: Female patients of childbearing age should be told about the consequences of second- and third-trimester exposure to drugs that act on the renin-angiotensin system, and they should also be told that these consequences do not appear to have resulted from intrauterine drug exposure that has been limited to the first trimester. These patients should be asked to report pregnancies to their physicians as soon as possible.

Symptomatic Hypotension: A patient receiving HYZAAR should be cautioned that lightheadedness can occur, especially during the first days of therapy, and that it should be reported to the prescribing physician. The patients should be told that if syncope occurs, HYZAAR should be discontinued until the physician has been consulted.

All patients should be cautioned that inadequate fluid intake, excessive perspiration, diarrhea, or vomiting can lead to an excessive fall in blood pressure, with the same consequences of lightheadedness and possible syncope.

Potassium Supplements: A patient receiving HYZAAR should be told not to use potassium supplements or salt substitutes containing potassium without consulting the prescribing physician (see PRECAUTIONS, *Drug Interactions, Losartan Potassium*).

Drug Interactions

Losartan Potassium

No significant drug-drug pharmacokinetic interactions have been found in interaction studies with hydrochlorothiazide, digoxin, warfarin, cimetidine and phenobarbital.

Rifampin, an inducer of drug metabolism, decreased the concentrations of losartan and its active metabolite. (See CLINICAL PHARMACOLOGY, *Drug Interactions.*) In humans, two inhibitors of P450 3A4 have been studied. Ketoconazole did not affect the conversion of losartan to the active metabolite after intravenous administration of losartan, and erythromycin had no clinically significant effect after oral administration. Fluconazole, an inhibitor of P450 2C9, decreased active metabolite concentration and increased losartan concentration. The pharmacodynamic consequences of concomitant use of losartan and inhibitors of P450 2C9 have not been examined. Subjects who do not metabolize losartan to active metabolite have been shown to have a specific, rare defect in cytochrome P450 2C9. These data suggest that the conversion of losartan to its active metabolite is mediated primarily by P450 2C9 and not P450 3A4.

As with other drugs that block angiotensin II or its effects, concomitant use of potassium-sparing diuretics (e.g., spironolactone, triamterene, amiloride), potassium supplements, or salt substitutes containing potassium may lead to increases in serum potassium (see PRECAUTIONS, *Information for Patients, Potassium Supplements*).

As with other antihypertensive agents, the antihypertensive effect of losartan may be blunted by the non-steroidal anti-inflammatory drug indomethacin.

Hydrochlorothiazide

When administered concurrently the following drugs may interact with thiazide diuretics:

Alcohol, barbiturates, or narcotics—potentiation of orthostatic hypotension may occur.

Antidiabetic drugs (oral agents and insulin)—dosage adjustment of the antidiabetic drug may be required.

Other antihypertensive drugs—additive effect or potentiation.

Cholestyramine and colestipol resins—Absorption of hydrochlorothiazide is impaired in the presence of anionic exchange resins. Single doses of either cholestyramine or colestipol resins bind the hydrochlorothiazide and reduce its absorption from the gastrointestinal tract by up to 85 and 43 percent, respectively.

Corticosteroids, ACTH—intensified electrolyte depletion, particularly hypokalemia.

Pressor amines (e.g., norepinephrine)—possible decreased response to pressor amines but not sufficient to preclude their use.

Skeletal muscle relaxants, nondepolarizing (e.g., tubocurarine)—possible increased responsiveness to the muscle relaxant.

Lithium—should not generally be given with diuretics. Diuretic agents reduce the renal clearance of lithium and add a high risk of lithium toxicity. Refer to the package insert for lithium preparations before use of such preparations with HYZAAR.

Non-steroidal Anti-inflammatory Drugs—In some patients, the administration of a non-steroidal anti-inflammatory agent can reduce the diuretic, natriuretic, and antihypertensive effects of loop, potassium-sparing and thiazide diuretics. Therefore, when HYZAAR and non-steroidal anti-inflammatory agents are used concomitantly, the patient should be observed closely to determine if the desired effect of the diuretic is obtained.

Carcinogenesis, Mutagenesis, Impairment of Fertility

Losartan Potassium-Hydrochlorothiazide

No carcinogenicity studies have been conducted with the losartan potassium-hydrochlorothiazide combination.

Losartan potassium-hydrochlorothiazide when tested at a weight ratio of 4:1, was negative in the Ames microbial mutagenesis assay and the V-79 Chinese hamster lung cell mutagenesis assay. In addition, there was no evidence of direct genotoxicity in the *in vitro* alkaline elution assay in rat hepatocytes and *in vitro* chromosomal aberration assay in Chinese hamster ovary cells at noncytotoxic concentrations.

Losartan potassium, coadministered with hydrochlorothiazide, had no effect on the fertility or mating behavior of male rats of dosages up to 135 mg/kg/day of losartan and 33.75 mg/kg/day of hydrochlorothiazide. These dosages have been shown to provide respective systemic exposures (AUCs) for losartan, its active metabolite and hydrochlorothiazide that are approximately 60, 60 and 30 times greater than those achieved in humans with 100 mg of losartan potassium in combination with 25 mg of hydrochlorothiazide. In female rats, however, the coadministration of doses as low as 10 mg/kg/day of losartan and 2.5 mg/kg/day of hydrochlorothiazide was associated with slight but statistically significant decreases in fecundity and fertility indices. AUC values for losartan, its active metabolite and hydrochlorothiazide, extrapolated from data obtained with losartan administered to rats at a dose of 50 mg/kg/day in combination with 12.5 mg/kg/day of hydrochlorothiazide, were approximately 6, 2, and 2 times greater than those achieved in humans with 100 mg of losartan in combination with 25 mg of hydrochlorothiazide.

Losartan Potassium

Losartan potassium was not carcinogenic when administered at maximally tolerated dosages to rats and mice for 105 and 92 weeks, respectively. Female rats given the highest dose (270 mg/kg/day) had a slightly higher incidence of pancreatic acinar adenoma. The maximally tolerated dosages (270 mg/kg/day in rats, 200 mg/kg/day in mice) provided systemic exposures for losartan and its pharmacologically active metabolite that were approximately 160 and 90 times (rats) and 30 and 15 times (mice) the exposure of a 50 kg human given 100 mg per day.

Losartan potassium was negative in the microbial mutagenesis and V-79 mammalian cell mutagenesis assays and in the *in vitro* alkaline elution and *in vitro* and *in vivo* chromosomal aberration assays. In addition, the active metabolite showed no evidence of genotoxicity in the microbial mutagenesis, *in vitro* alkaline elution, and *in vitro* chromosomal aberration assays.

Fertility and reproductive performance were not affected in studies with male rats given oral doses of losartan potassium up to approximately 150 mg/kg/day. The administration of toxic dosage levels in females (300/200 mg/kg/day) was associated with a significant ($p<0.05$) decrease in the number of corpora lutea/female, implants/female, and live fetuses/female at C-section. At 100 mg/kg/day only a decrease in the number of corpora lutea/female was observed. The relationship of these findings to drug-treatment is uncertain since there was no effect at these dosage levels on implants/pregnant female, percent post-implantation loss, or live animals/litter at parturition. In nonpregnant rats

Continued on next page

Information on the Merck & Co., Inc., products listed on these pages is from the prescribing information in use October 1, 2004. For information, please call 1-800-NSC-MERCK [1-800-672-6372].

Hyzaar—Cont.

dosed at 135 mg/kg/day for 7 days, systemic exposure (AUCs) for losartan and its active metabolite were approximately 66 and 26 times the exposure achieved in man at the maximum recommended human daily dosage (100 mg).

Hydrochlorothiazide

Two-year feeding studies in mice and rats conducted under the auspices of the National Toxicology Program (NTP) uncovered no evidence of a carcinogenic potential of hydrochlorothiazide in female mice (at doses of up to approximately 600 mg/kg/day) or in male and female rats (at doses of up to approximately 100 mg/kg/day). The NTP, however, found equivocal evidence for hepatocarcinogenicity in male mice.

Hydrochlorothiazide was not genotoxic *in vitro* in the Ames mutagenicity assay of *Salmonella typhimurium* strains TA 98, TA 100, TA 1535, TA 1537, and TA 1538 and in the Chinese Hamster Ovary (CHO) test for chromosomal aberrations, or *in vivo* in assays using mouse germinal cell chromosomes, Chinese hamster bone marrow chromosomes, and the *Drosophila* sex-linked recessive lethal trait gene. Positive test results were obtained only in the *in vitro* CHO Sister Chromatid Exchange (clastogenicity) and in the Mouse Lymphoma Cell (mutagenicity) assays, using concentrations of hydrochlorothiazide from 43 to 1300 μg/mL, and in the *Aspergillus nidulans* non-disjunction assay at an unspecified concentration.

Hydrochlorothiazide had no adverse effects on the fertility of mice and rats of either sex in studies wherein these species were exposed, via their diet, to doses of up to 100 and 4 mg/kg, respectively, prior to mating and throughout gestation.

Pregnancy

Pregnancy Categories C (first trimester) and D (second and third trimesters). See WARNINGS, *Fetal/Neonatal Morbidity and Mortality.*

Nursing Mothers

It is not known whether losartan is excreted in human milk, but significant levels of losartan and its active metabolite were shown to be present in rat milk. Thiazides appear in human milk. Because of the potential for adverse effects on the nursing infant, a decision should be made whether to discontinue nursing or discontinue the drug, taking into account the importance of the drug to the mother.

Pediatric Use

Safety and effectiveness in pediatric patients have not been established.

Geriatric Use

Clinical studies of HYZAAR did not include sufficient numbers of subjects aged 65 and over to determine whether they respond differently from younger subjects. Other reported clinical experience has not identified differences in responses between the elderly and younger patients. In general, dose selection for an elderly patient should be cautious, usually starting at the low end of the dosing range, reflecting the greater frequency of decreased hepatic, renal, or cardiac function, and of concomitant disease or other drug therapy.

Hydrochlorothiazide is known to be substantially excreted by the kidney, and the risk of toxic reactions to this drug may be greater in patients with impaired renal function (see CLINICAL PHARMACOLOGY, *Special Populations*).

ADVERSE REACTIONS

Losartan potassium-hydrochlorothiazide has been evaluated for safety in 858 patients treated for essential hypertension. In clinical trials with losartan potassium-hydrochlorothiazide, no adverse experiences peculiar to this combination have been observed. Adverse experiences have been limited to those that were reported previously with losartan potassium and/or hydrochlorothiazide. The overall incidence of adverse experiences reported with the combination was comparable to placebo.

In general, treatment with losartan potassium-hydrochlorothiazide was well tolerated. For the most part, adverse experiences have been mild and transient in nature and have not required discontinuation of therapy. In controlled clinical trials, discontinuation of therapy due to clinical adverse experiences was required in only 2.8% and 2.3% of patients treated with the combination and placebo, respectively.

In these double-blind controlled clinical trials, the following adverse experiences reported with losartan-hydrochlorothiazide occurred in ≥1 percent of patients, and more often on drug than placebo, regardless of drug relationship:

	Losartan Potassium-Hydrochlorothiazide (n=858)	Placebo (n=173)
Body as a Whole		
Abdominal pain	1.2	0.6
Edema/swelling	1.3	1.2
Cardiovascular		
Palpitation	1.4	0.0
Musculoskeletal		
Back pain	2.1	0.6
Nervous/Psychiatric		
Dizziness	5.7	2.9
Respiratory		
Cough	2.6	2.3
Sinusitis	1.2	0.6
Upper respiratory infection	6.1	4.6
Skin		
Rash	1.4	0.0

The following adverse events were also reported at a rate of 1% or greater, but were as, or more, common in the placebo group: asthenia/fatigue, diarrhea, nausea, headache, bronchitis, pharyngitis.

Adverse events occurred at about the same rates in men and women, older and younger patients, and Black and non-Black patients.

A patient with known hypersensitivity to aspirin and penicillin, when treated with losartan potassium, was withdrawn from study due to swelling of the lips and eyelids and facial rash, reported as angioedema, which returned to normal 5 days after therapy was discontinued.

Superficial peeling of palms and hemolysis were reported in one subject treated with losartan potassium.

Losartan Potassium

Other adverse experiences that have been reported with losartan, without regard to causality, are listed below:

Body as a Whole: chest pain, facial edema, fever, orthostatic effects, syncope; *Cardiovascular:* angina pectoris, arrhythmias including atrial fibrillation, sinus bradycardia, tachycardia, ventricular tachycardia and ventricular fibrillation, CVA, hypotension, myocardial infarction, second degree AV block; *Digestive:* anorexia, constipation, dental pain, dry mouth, dyspepsia, flatulence, gastritis, vomiting; *Hematologic:* anemia; *Metabolic:* gout; *Musculoskeletal:* arm pain, arthralgia, arthritis, fibromyalgia, hip pain, joint swelling, knee pain, leg pain, muscle cramps, muscle weakness, musculoskeletal pain, myalgia, shoulder pain, stiffness; *Nervous System/Psychiatric:* anxiety, anxiety disorder, ataxia, confusion, depression, dream abnormality, hypesthesia, insomnia, libido decreased, memory impairment, migraine, nervousness, panic disorder, paresthesia, peripheral neuropathy, sleep disorder, somnolence, tremor, vertigo; *Respiratory:* dyspnea, epistaxis, nasal congestion, pharyngeal discomfort, respiratory congestion, rhinitis, sinus disorder; *Skin:* alopecia, dermatitis, dry skin, ecchymosis, erythema, flushing, photosensitivity, pruritus, sweating, urticaria; *Special Senses:* blurred vision, burning/stinging in the eye, conjunctivitis, decrease in visual acuity, taste perversion, tinnitus; *Urogenital:* impotence, nocturia, urinary frequency, urinary tract infection.

Hydrochlorothiazide

Other adverse experiences that have been reported with hydrochlorothiazide, without regard to causality, are listed below:

Body as a Whole: weakness; *Digestive:* pancreatitis, jaundice (intrahepatic cholestatic jaundice), sialadenitis, cramping, gastric irritation; *Hematologic:* aplastic anemia, agranulocytosis, leukopenia, hemolytic anemia, thrombocytopenia; *Hypersensitivity:* purpura, photosensitivity, urticaria, necrotizing angiitis (vasculitis and cutaneous vasculitis), fever, respiratory distress including pneumonitis and pulmonary edema, anaphylactic reactions; *Metabolic:* hyperglycemia, glycosuria, hyperuricemia; *Musculoskeletal:* muscle spasm; *Nervous System/Psychiatric:* restlessness; *Renal:* renal failure, renal dysfunction, interstitial nephritis; *Skin:* erythema multiforme including Stevens-Johnson syndrome, exfoliative dermatitis including toxic epidermal necrolysis; *Special Senses:* transient blurred vision, xanthopsia.

Persistent dry cough (with an incidence of a few percent) has been associated with ACE inhibitor use and in practice can be a cause of discontinuation of ACE inhibitor therapy. Two prospective, parallel-group, double-blind, randomized, controlled trials were conducted to assess the effects of losartan on the incidence of cough in hypertensive patients who had experienced cough while receiving ACE inhibitor therapy. Patients who had typical ACE inhibitor cough when challenged with lisinopril, whose cough disappeared on placebo, were randomized to losartan 50 mg, lisinopril 20 mg, or either placebo (one study, n=97) or 25 mg hydrochlorothiazide (n=135). The double-blind treatment period lasted up to 8 weeks. The incidence of cough is shown below.

Study 1†	HCTZ	Losartan	Lisinopril
Cough	25%	17%	69%
Study 2††	**Placebo**	**Losartan**	**Lisinopril**
Cough	35%	29%	62%

†Demographics = (89% caucasian, 64% female)
††Demographics = (90% caucasian, 51% female)

These studies demonstrate that the incidence of cough associated with losartan therapy, in a population that all had cough associated with ACE inhibitor therapy, is similar to that associated with hydrochlorothiazide or placebo therapy.

Cases of cough, including positive re-challenges, have been reported with the use of losartan in post-marketing experience.

Severe Hypertension: In a clinical study in patients with severe hypertension (SiDBP ≥110 mmHg), the overall pattern of adverse events reported through six weeks of follow-up was similar in patients treated with HYZAAR as initial therapy and in patients treated with losartan as initial therapy. There were no reported cases of syncope in either treatment group. There were 2 (0.6%) and 0 (0.0%) cases of hypotension reported in the group treated with HYZAAR and the group treated with losartan, respectively. There were 3 (0.8%) and 2 (1.2%) cases of increased serum creatinine (>0.5 mg/dL) in the group treated with HYZAAR and the group treated with losartan, respectively, during the same time period. (See CLINICAL PHARMACOLOGY, *Pharmacodynamics and Clinical Effects, Severe Hypertension.)*

Post-Marketing Experience

The following additional adverse reactions have been reported in post-marketing experience:

Hypersensitivity: Angioedema, including swelling of the larynx and glottis, causing airway obstruction and/or swelling of the face, lips, pharynx, and/or tongue has been reported rarely in patients treated with losartan; some of these patients previously experienced angioedema with other drugs including ACE inhibitors. Vasculitis, including Henoch-Schönlein purpura, has been reported with losartan. Anaphylactic reactions have been reported.

Digestive: Hepatitis has been reported rarely in patients treated with losartan.

Respiratory: Dry cough (see above) has been reported with losartan.

Hyperkalemia and hyponatremia have been reported with losartan.

Laboratory Test Findings

In controlled clinical trials, clinically important changes in standard laboratory parameters were rarely associated with administration of HYZAAR.

Creatinine, Blood Urea Nitrogen: Minor increases in blood urea nitrogen (BUN) or serum creatinine were observed in 0.6 and 0.8 percent, respectively, of patients with essential hypertension treated with HYZAAR alone. No patient discontinued taking HYZAAR due to increased BUN. One patient discontinued taking HYZAAR due to a minor increase in serum creatinine.

Hemoglobin and Hematocrit: Small decreases in hemoglobin and hematocrit (mean decreases of approximately 0.14 grams percent and 0.72 volume percent, respectively) occurred frequently in patients treated with HYZAAR alone, but were rarely of clinical importance. No patients were discontinued due to anemia.

Liver Function Tests: Occasional elevations of liver enzymes and/or serum bilirubin have occurred. In patients with essential hypertension treated with HYZAAR alone, no patients were discontinued due to these laboratory adverse experiences.

Serum Electrolytes: See PRECAUTIONS.

OVERDOSAGE

Losartan Potassium

Significant lethality was observed in mice and rats after oral administration of 1000 mg/kg and 2000 mg/kg, respectively, about 44 and 170 times the maximum recommended human dose on a mg/m^2 basis.

Limited data are available in regard to overdosage in humans. The most likely manifestation of overdosage would be hypotension and tachycardia; bradycardia could occur from parasympathetic (vagal) stimulation. If symptomatic hypotension should occur, supportive treatment should be instituted.

Neither losartan nor its active metabolite can be removed by hemodialysis.

Hydrochlorothiazide

The oral LD_{50} of hydrochlorothiazide is greater than 10 g/kg in both mice and rats. The most common signs and symptoms observed are those caused by electrolyte depletion (hypokalemia, hypochloremia, hyponatremia) and dehydration resulting from excessive diuresis. If digitalis has also been administered, hypokalemia may accentuate cardiac arrhythmias. The degree to which hydrochlorothiazide is removed by hemodialysis has not been established.

DOSAGE AND ADMINISTRATION

Hypertension

Dosing must be individualized. The usual starting dose of losartan is 50 mg once daily, with 25 mg recommended for patients with intravascular volume depletion (e.g., patients treated with diuretics) (see WARNINGS, *Hypotension—Volume-Depleted Patients*) and patients with a history of hepatic impairment (see WARNINGS, *Impaired Hepatic Function*). Losartan can be administered once or twice daily at total daily doses of 25 to 100 mg. If the antihypertensive effect measured at trough using once-a-day dosing is inadequate, a twice-a-day regimen at the same total daily dose or an increase in dose may give a more satisfactory response.

Hydrochlorothiazide is effective in doses of 12.5 to 50 mg once daily and can be given at doses of 12.5 to 25 mg as HYZAAR.

To minimize dose-independent side effects, it is usually appropriate to begin combination therapy only after a patient has failed to achieve the desired effect with monotherapy.

The side effects (see WARNINGS) of losartan are generally rare and apparently independent of dose; those of hydrochlorothiazide are a mixture of dose-dependent (primarily hypokalemia) and dose-independent phenomena (e.g., pancreatitis), the former much more common than the latter. Therapy with any combination of losartan and hydrochlorothiazide will be associated with both sets of dose-independent side effects.

Replacement Therapy: The combination may be substituted for the titrated components.

Dose Titration by Clinical Effect: A patient whose blood pressure is not adequately controlled with losartan monotherapy (see above) or hydrochlorothiazide alone, may be switched to HYZAAR 50-12.5 (losartan 50 mg/hydrochlorothiazide 12.5 mg) once daily. If blood pressure remains uncontrolled after about 3 weeks of therapy, the dose may be increased to two tablets of HYZAAR 50-12.5 once daily or one tablet of HYZAAR 100-25 (losartan 100 mg/hydrochlorothiazide 25 mg) once daily.

A patient whose blood pressure is inadequately controlled by 25 mg once daily of hydrochlorothiazide, or is controlled but who experiences hypokalemia with this regimen, may be switched to HYZAAR 50-12.5 (losartan 50 mg/hydrochlorothiazide 12.5 mg) once daily, reducing the dose of hydrochlorothiazide without reducing the overall expected antihypertensive response. The clinical response to HYZAAR 50-12.5 should be subsequently evaluated and if blood pressure remains uncontrolled after about 3 weeks of therapy, the dose may be increased to two tablets of HYZAAR 50-12.5 once daily or one tablet of HYZAAR 100-25 (losartan 100 mg/hydrochlorothiazide 25 mg) once daily.

The usual dose of HYZAAR is one tablet of HYZAAR 50-12.5 once daily. More than two tablets of HYZAAR 50-12.5 once daily or more than one tablet of HYZAAR 100-25 once daily is not recommended. The maximal antihypertensive effect is attained about 3 weeks after initiation of therapy.

Use in Patients with Renal Impairment: The usual regimens of therapy with HYZAAR may be followed as long as the patient's creatinine clearance is >30 mL/min. In patients with more severe renal impairment, loop diuretics are preferred to thiazides, so HYZAAR is not recommended.

Patients with Hepatic Impairment: HYZAAR is not recommended for titration in patients with hepatic impairment (see WARNINGS, *Impaired Hepatic Function*) because the appropriate 25 mg starting dose of losartan cannot be given.

Severe Hypertension

The starting dose of HYZAAR for initial treatment of severe hypertension is one tablet of HYZAAR 50-12.5 once daily (see CLINICAL PHARMACOLOGY, *Pharmacodynamics and Clinical Effects*). For patients who do not respond adequately to HYZAAR 50-12.5 after 2 to 4 weeks of therapy, the dosage may be increased to one tablet of HYZAAR 100-25 once daily. The maximum dose is one tablet of HYZAAR 100-25 once daily. HYZAAR is not recommended as initial therapy in patients with hepatic impairment (see WARNINGS, *Impaired Hepatic Function*) because the appropriate 25 mg starting dose of losartan cannot be given. It is also not recommended for use as initial therapy in patients with intravenous volume depletion (e.g., patients treated with diuretics, see WARNINGS, *Hypotension—Volume-Depleted Patients*).

HYZAAR may be administered with other antihypertensive agents.

HYZAAR may be administered with or without food.

HOW SUPPLIED

No. 3502—Tablets HYZAAR, 50-12.5 are yellow, teardrop shaped, film-coated tablets, coded MRK 717 on one side and HYZAAR on the other. Each tablet contains 50 mg of losartan potassium and 12.5 mg of hydrochlorothiazide. They are supplied as follows:

NDC 0006-0717-31 unit of use bottles of 30
NDC 0006-0717-54 unit of use bottles of 90
NDC 0006-0717-58 unit of use bottles of 100
NDC 0006-0717-28 unit dose packages of 100
NDC 0006-0717-82 bottles of 1,000.

No. 3793—Tablets HYZAAR 100-25 are light yellow, teardrop shaped, film-coated tablets, coded MRK 747 on one side and HYZAAR on the other. Each tablet contains 100 mg of losartan potassium and 25 mg of hydrochlorothiazide. They are supplied as follows:

NDC 0006-0747-31 unit of use bottles of 30
NDC 0006-0747-54 unit of use bottles of 90
NDC 0006-0747-58 unit of use bottles of 100
NDC 0006-0747-28 unit dose packages of 100
NDC 0006-0747-82 bottles of 1,000.

Storage

Store at 25°C (77°F); excursions permitted to 15–30°C (59–86°F) [see USP Controlled Room Temperature]. Keep container tightly closed. Protect from light.

Dist. by:
MERCK & CO., INC., Whitehouse Station, NJ 08889, USA
9573622 Issued September 2003

Shown in Product Identification Guide, page 323

INDOCIN® Capsules, Oral Suspension and Suppositories (Indomethacin) ℞

DESCRIPTION

INDOCIN* (Indomethacin) cannot be considered a simple analgesic and should not be used in conditions other than those recommended under INDICATIONS.

INDOCIN is supplied in three dosage forms. Capsules INDOCIN for oral administration contain either 25 mg or 50 mg of indomethacin and the following inactive ingredients: colloidal silicon dioxide, FD & C Blue 1, FD & C Red 3, gelatin, lactose, lecithin, magnesium stearate, and titanium dioxide. Suspension INDOCIN for oral use contains 25 mg of indomethacin per 5 mL, alcohol 1%, and sorbic acid 0.1% added as a preservative and the following inactive ingredients: antifoam AF emulsion, flavors, purified water, sodium hydroxide or hydrochloric acid to adjust pH, sorbitol solution, tragacanth. Suppositories INDOCIN for rectal use contain 50 mg of indomethacin and the following inactive ingredients: butylated hydroxyanisole, butylated hydroxytoluene, edetic acid, glycerin, polyethylene glycol 3350, polyethylene glycol 8000 and sodium chloride. Indomethacin is a non-steroidal anti-inflammatory indole derivative designated chemically as 1-(4-chlorobenzoyl)-5-methoxy-2-methyl-1*H*-indole-3-acetic acid. Indomethacin is practically insoluble in water and sparingly soluble in alcohol. It has a pKa of 4.5 and is stable in neutral or slightly acidic media and decomposes in strong alkali. The suspension has a pH of 4.0–5.0. The structural formula is:

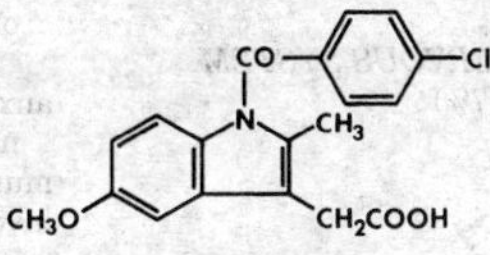

*Registered trademark of MERCK & CO., INC.

CLINICAL PHARMACOLOGY

INDOCIN is a non-steroidal drug with anti-inflammatory, antipyretic and analgesic properties. Its mode of action, like that of other anti-inflammatory drugs, is not known. However, its therapeutic action is not due to pituitary-adrenal stimulation.

INDOCIN is a potent inhibitor of prostaglandin synthesis *in vitro*. Concentrations are reached during therapy which have been demonstrated to have an effect *in vivo* as well. Prostaglandins sensitize afferent nerves and potentiate the action of bradykinin in inducing pain in animal models. Moreover, prostaglandins are known to be among the mediators of inflammation. Since indomethacin is an inhibitor of prostaglandin synthesis, its mode of action may be due to a decrease of prostaglandins in peripheral tissues.

INDOCIN has been shown to be an effective anti-inflammatory agent, appropriate for long-term use in rheumatoid arthritis, ankylosing spondylitis, and osteoarthritis.

INDOCIN affords relief of symptoms; it does not alter the progressive course of the underlying disease.

INDOCIN suppresses inflammation in rheumatoid arthritis as demonstrated by relief of pain, and reduction of fever, swelling and tenderness. Improvement in patients treated with INDOCIN for rheumatoid arthritis has been demonstrated by a reduction in joint swelling, average number of joints involved, and morning stiffness; by increased mobility as demonstrated by a decrease in walking time; and by improved functional capability as demonstrated by an increase in grip strength.

Indomethacin has been reported to diminish basal and CO_2 stimulated cerebral blood flow in healthy volunteers following acute oral and intravenous administration. In one study after one week of treatment with orally administered indomethacin, this effect on basal cerebral blood flow had disappeared. The clinical significance of this effect has not been established.

Capsules INDOCIN have been found effective in relieving the pain, reducing the fever, swelling, redness, and tenderness of acute gouty arthritis—see INDICATIONS.

Following single oral doses of Capsules INDOCIN 25 mg or 50 mg, indomethacin is readily absorbed, attaining peak plasma concentrations of about 1 and 2 mcg/mL, respectively, at about 2 hours. Orally administered Capsules INDOCIN are virtually 100% bioavailable, with 90% of the dose absorbed within 4 hours. A single 50 mg dose of Oral Suspension INDOCIN was found to be bioequivalent to a 50 mg INDOCIN capsule when each was administered with food.

Indomethacin is eliminated via renal excretion, metabolism, and biliary excretion. Indomethacin undergoes appreciable enterohepatic circulation. The mean half-life of indomethacin is estimated to be about 4.5 hours. With a typical therapeutic regimen of 25 or 50 mg t.i.d., the steady-state plasma concentrations of indomethacin are an average 1.4 times those following the first dose.

The rate of absorption is more rapid from the rectal suppository than from Capsules INDOCIN. Ordinarily, therefore, the total amount absorbed from the suppository would be expected to be at least equivalent to the capsule. In controlled clinical trials, however, the amount of indomethacin absorbed was found to be somewhat less (80–90%) than that absorbed from Capsules INDOCIN. This is probably because some subjects did not retain the material from the suppository for the one hour necessary to assure complete absorption. Since the suppository dissolves rather quickly rather than melting slowly, it is seldom recovered in recognizable form if the patient retains the suppository for more than a few minutes.

Indomethacin exists in the plasma as the parent drug and its desmethyl, desbenzoyl, and desmethyl-desbenzoyl metabolites, all in the unconjugated form. About 60 percent of an oral dosage is recovered in urine as drug and metabolites (26 percent as indomethacin and its glucuronide), and 33 percent is recovered in feces (1.5 percent as indomethacin).

About 99% of indomethacin is bound to protein in plasma over the expected range of therapeutic plasma concentrations. Indomethacin has been found to cross the blood-brain barrier and the placenta.

In a gastroscopic study in 45 healthy subjects, the number of gastric mucosal abnormalities was significantly higher in the group receiving Capsules INDOCIN than in the group taking Suppositories INDOCIN or placebo.

In a double-blind comparative clinical study involving 175 patients with rheumatoid arthritis, however, the incidence of upper gastrointestinal adverse effects with Suppositories or Capsules INDOCIN was comparable. The incidence of lower gastrointestinal adverse effects was greater in the suppository group.

INDICATIONS

Indomethacin has been found effective in active stages of the following:

1. Moderate to severe rheumatoid arthritis including acute flares of chronic disease.
2. Moderate to severe ankylosing spondylitis.
3. Moderate to severe osteoarthritis.
4. Acute painful shoulder (bursitis and/or tendinitis).
5. Acute gouty arthritis.

INDOCIN may enable the reduction of steroid dosage in patients receiving steroids for the more severe forms of rheumatoid arthritis. In such instances the steroid dosage should be reduced slowly and the patients followed very closely for any possible adverse effects.

The use of INDOCIN in conjunction with aspirin or other salicylates is not recommended. Controlled clinical studies have shown that the combined use of INDOCIN and aspirin does not produce any greater therapeutic effect than the use of INDOCIN alone. Furthermore, in one of these clinical studies, the incidence of gastrointestinal side effects was significantly increased with combined therapy (see DRUG INTERACTIONS).

CONTRAINDICATIONS

INDOCIN should not be used in:

Patients who are hypersensitive to this product.

Patients in whom acute asthmatic attacks, urticaria, or rhinitis are precipitated by aspirin or other non-steroidal anti-inflammatory agents.

Suppositories INDOCIN are contraindicated in patients with a history of proctitis or recent rectal bleeding.

WARNINGS

General:

Because of the variability of the potential of INDOCIN to cause adverse reactions in the individual patient, the following are strongly recommended:

1. The lowest possible effective dose for the individual patient should be prescribed. Increased dosage tends to increase adverse effects, particularly in doses over 150–200 mg/day, without corresponding increase in clinical benefits.
2. Careful instructions to, and observations of, the individual patient are essential to the prevention of serious adverse reactions. As advancing years appear to increase the possibility of adverse reactions, INDOCIN should be used with greater care in the elderly.
3. Effectiveness of INDOCIN in pediatric patients has not been established. INDOCIN should not be prescribed for pediatric patients 14 years of age and younger unless toxicity or lack of efficacy associated with other drugs warrants the risk.

   In experience with more than 900 pediatric patients reported in the literature or to the manufacturer who were treated with Capsules INDOCIN, side effects in pediatric patients were comparable to those reported in adults. Experience in pediatric patients has been confined to the use of Capsules INDOCIN.

   If a decision is made to use indomethacin for pediatric patients two years of age or older, such patients should be monitored closely and periodic assessment of liver function is recommended. There have been cases of hepatotoxicity reported in pediatric patients with juvenile rheumatoid arthritis, including fatalities. If indomethacin treatment is instituted, a suggested starting dose is 2 mg/kg/day given in divided doses. Maximum daily dosage should not exceed 4 mg/kg/day or 150–200 mg/day, whichever is less. As symptoms subside, the total daily dosage should be reduced to the lowest level required to control symptoms, or the drug should be discontinued.

Gastrointestinal Effects:

Single or multiple ulcerations, including perforation and hemorrhage of the esophagus, stomach, duodenum or small

Continued on next page

Information on the Merck & Co., Inc., products listed on these pages is from the prescribing information in use October 1, 2004. For information, please call 1-800-NSC-MERCK [1-800-672-6372].

Indocin/Caps/O.S./Supp.—Cont.

and large intestine, have been reported to occur with INDOCIN. Fatalities have been reported in some instances. Rarely, intestinal ulceration has been associated with stenosis and obstruction.

Gastrointestinal bleeding without obvious ulcer formation and perforation of pre-existing sigmoid lesions (diverticulum, carcinoma, etc.) have occurred. Increased abdominal pain in ulcerative colitis patients or the development of ulcerative colitis and regional ileitis have been reported to occur rarely.

Because of the occurrence, and at times severity, of gastrointestinal reactions to INDOCIN, the prescribing physician must be continuously alert for any sign or symptom signaling a possible gastrointestinal reaction. The risks of continuing therapy with INDOCIN in the face of such symptoms must be weighed against the possible benefits to the individual patient.

INDOCIN should not be given to patients with active gastrointestinal lesions or with a history of recurrent gastrointestinal lesions except under circumstances which warrant the very high risk and where patients can be monitored very closely.

The gastrointestinal effects may be reduced by giving Capsules INDOCIN immediately after meals, with food, or with antacids.

Risk of GI Ulcerations, Bleeding and Perforation with NSAID Therapy

Serious gastrointestinal toxicity such as bleeding, ulceration, and perforation, can occur at any time, with or without warning symptoms, in patients treated chronically with NSAID therapy. Although minor upper gastrointestinal problems, such as dyspepsia, are common, usually developing early in therapy, physicians should remain alert for ulceration and bleeding in patients treated chronically with NSAIDs even in the absence of previous GI tract symptoms. In patients observed in clinical trials of several months to two years duration, symptomatic upper GI ulcers, gross bleeding or perforation appear to occur in approximately 1% of patients treated for 3–6 months, and in about 2–4% of patients treated for one year. Physicians should inform patients about the signs and/or symptoms of serious GI toxicity and what steps to take if they occur.

Studies to date have not identified any subset of patients not at risk of developing peptic ulceration and bleeding. Except for a prior history of serious GI events and other risk factors known to be associated with peptic ulcer disease, such as alcoholism, smoking, etc., no risk factors (e.g., age, sex) have been associated with increased risk. Elderly or debilitated patients seem to tolerate ulceration or bleeding less well than other individuals and most spontaneous reports of fatal GI events are in this population. Studies to date are inconclusive concerning the relative risk of various NSAIDs in causing such reactions. High doses of any NSAID probably carry a greater risk of these reactions, although controlled clinical trials showing this do not exist in most cases. In considering the use of relatively large doses (within the recommended dosage range), sufficient benefit should be anticipated to offset the potential increased risk of GI toxicity.

Renal Effects:

As with other non-steroidal anti-inflammatory drugs, long term administration of indomethacin to animals has resulted in renal papillary necrosis and other abnormal renal pathology. In humans, there have been reports of acute interstitial nephritis with hematuria, proteinuria, and occasionally nephrotic syndrome.

A second form of renal toxicity has been seen in patients with prerenal and renal conditions leading to a reduction in renal blood flow or blood volume, where the renal prostaglandins have a supportive role in the maintenance of renal perfusion. In these patients administration of an NSAID may cause a dose dependent reduction in prostaglandin formation and may precipitate overt renal decompensation. Patients at greatest risk of this reaction are those with conditions such as renal or hepatic dysfunction, diabetes mellitus, advanced age, extracellular volume depletion from any cause, congestive heart failure, septicemia, pyelonephritis, or concomitant use of any nephrotoxic drug. INDOCIN or other NSAIDs should be given with caution and renal function should be monitored in any patient who may have reduced renal reserve. Discontinuation of NSAID therapy is typically followed by recovery to the pretreatment state.

Increases in serum potassium concentration, including hyperkalemia, have been reported, even in some patients without renal impairment. In patients with normal renal function, these effects have been attributed to a hyporeninemic-hypoaldosteronism state (see PRECAUTIONS, *Drug Interactions*).

Since INDOCIN is eliminated primarily by the kidneys, patients with significantly impaired renal function should be closely monitored; a lower daily dosage should be anticipated to avoid excessive drug accumulation.

Ocular Effects:

Corneal deposits and retinal disturbances, including those of the macula, have been observed in some patients who had received prolonged therapy with INDOCIN. The prescribing physician should be alert to the possible association between the changes noted and INDOCIN. It is advisable to discontinue therapy if such changes are observed. Blurred vision may be a significant symptom and warrants a thorough ophthalmological examination. Since these changes may be asymptomatic, ophthalmologic examination at periodic intervals is desirable in patients where therapy is prolonged.

Incidence greater than 1%	*Incidence less than 1%*	
GASTROINTESTINAL		
nausea* with or without vomiting dyspepsia* (including indigestion, heartburn and epigastric pain) diarrhea abdominal distress or pain constipation	anorexia bloating (includes distention) flatulence peptic ulcer gastroenteritis rectal bleeding proctitis single or multiple ulcerations, including perforation and hemorrhage of the esophagus, stomach, duodenum or small and large intestines intestinal ulceration associated with stenosis and obstruction	gastrointestinal bleeding without obvious ulcer formation and perforation of pre-existing sigmoid lesions (diverticulum, carcinoma, etc.) development of ulcerative colitis and regional ileitis ulcerative stomatitis toxic hepatitis and jaundice (some fatal cases have been reported) intestinal strictures (diaphragms)
CENTRAL NERVOUS SYSTEM		
headache (11.7%) dizziness* vertigo somnolence depression and fatigue (including malaise and listlessness)	anxiety (includes nervousness) muscle weakness involuntary muscle movements insomnia muzziness psychic disturbances including psychotic episodes mental confusion drowsiness	light-headedness syncope paresthesia aggravation of epilepsy and parkinsonism depersonalization coma peripheral neuropathy convulsions dysarthria
SPECIAL SENSES		
tinnitus	ocular—corneal deposits and retinal disturbances, including those of the macula, have been reported in some patients on prolonged therapy with INDOCIN	blurred vision diplopia hearing disturbances, deafness

Central Nervous System Effects:

INDOCIN may aggravate depression or other psychiatric disturbances, epilepsy, and parkinsonism, and should be used with considerable caution in patients with these conditions. If severe CNS adverse reactions develop, INDOCIN should be discontinued.

INDOCIN may cause drowsiness; therefore, patients should be cautioned about engaging in activities requiring mental alertness and motor coordination, such as driving a car. INDOCIN may also cause headache. Headache which persists despite dosage reduction requires cessation of therapy with INDOCIN.

Use in Pregnancy and the Neonatal Period

INDOCIN is not recommended for use in pregnant women, since safety for use has not been established. The known effects of indomethacin and other drugs of this class on the human fetus during the third trimester of pregnancy include: constriction of the ductus arteriosus prenatally, tricuspid incompetence, and pulmonary hypertension; nonclosure of the ductus arteriosus postnatally which may be resistant to medical management; myocardial degenerative changes, platelet dysfunction with resultant bleeding, intracranial bleeding, renal dysfunction or failure, renal injury/dysgenesis which may result in prolonged or permanent renal failure, oligohydramnios, gastrointestinal bleeding or perforation, and increased risk of necrotizing enterocolitis.

Teratogenic studies were conducted in mice and rats at dosages of 0.5, 1.0, 2.0, and 4.0 mg/kg/day. Except for retarded fetal ossification at 4 mg/kg/day considered secondary to the decreased average fetal weights, no increase in fetal malformations was observed as compared with control groups. Other studies in mice reported in the literature using higher doses (5 to 15 mg/kg/day) have described maternal toxicity and death, increased fetal resorptions, and fetal malformations. Comparable studies in rodents using high doses of aspirin have shown similar maternal and fetal effects.

As with other non-steroidal anti-inflammatory agents which inhibit prostaglandin synthesis, indomethacin has been found to delay parturition in rats.

In rats and mice, 4.0 mg/kg/day given during the last three days of gestation caused a decrease in maternal weight gain and some maternal and fetal deaths. An increased incidence of neuronal necrosis in the diencephalon in the live-born fetuses was observed. At 2.0 mg/kg/day, no increase in neuronal necrosis was observed as compared to the control groups. Administration of 0.5 or 4.0 mg/kg/day during the first three days of life did not cause an increase in neuronal necrosis at either dose level.

Use in Nursing Mothers

INDOCIN is excreted in the milk of lactating mothers. INDOCIN is not recommended for use in nursing mothers.

PRECAUTIONS

General

Non-steroidal anti-inflammatory drugs, including INDOCIN, may mask the usual signs and symptoms of infection. Therefore, the physician must be continually on the alert for this and should use the drug with extra care in the presence of existing infection.

Fluid retention and peripheral edema have been observed in some patients taking INDOCIN. Therefore, as with other non-steroidal anti-inflammatory drugs, INDOCIN should be used with caution in patients with cardiac dysfunction, hypertension, or other conditions predisposing to fluid retention.

In a study of patients with severe heart failure and hyponatremia, INDOCIN was associated with significant deterioration of circulatory hemodynamics, presumably due to inhibition of prostaglandin dependent compensatory mechanisms.

INDOCIN, like other non-steroidal anti-inflammatory agents, can inhibit platelet aggregation. This effect is of shorter duration than that seen with aspirin and usually disappears within 24 hours after discontinuation of INDOCIN. INDOCIN has been shown to prolong bleeding time (but within the normal range) in normal subjects. Because this effect may be exaggerated in patients with underlying hemostatic defects, INDOCIN should be used with caution in persons with coagulation defects.

As with other non-steroidal anti-inflammatory drugs, borderline elevations of one or more liver tests may occur in up to 15% of patients. These abnormalities may progress, may remain essentially unchanged, or may be transient with continued therapy. The SGPT (ALT) test is probably the most sensitive indicator of liver dysfunction. Meaningful (3 times the upper limit of normal) elevations of SGPT or SGOT (AST) occurred in controlled clinical trials in less than 1% of patients. A patient with symptoms and/or signs suggesting liver dysfunction, or in whom an abnormal liver test has occurred, should be evaluated for evidence of the development of more severe hepatic reaction while on therapy with INDOCIN. Severe hepatic reactions, including jaundice and cases of fatal hepatitis, have been reported with INDOCIN as with other non-steroidal anti-inflammatory drugs. Although such reactions are rare, if abnormal liver tests persist or worsen, if clinical signs and symptoms consistent with liver disease develop, or if systemic manifestations occur (e.g., eosinophilia, rash, etc.), INDOCIN should be discontinued.

Information for Patients
INDOCIN, like other drugs of its class, is not free of side effects. The side effects of these drugs can cause discomfort and, rarely, there are more serious side effects such as gastrointestinal bleeding, which may result in hospitalization and even fatal outcomes.
NSAIDs (Non-steroidal Anti-inflammatory Drugs) are often essential agents in the management of arthritis; but they also may be commonly employed for conditions which are less serious.
Physicians may wish to discuss with their patients the potential risks (see WARNINGS, PRECAUTIONS and ADVERSE REACTIONS) and likely benefits of NSAID treatment, particularly when the drugs are used for less serious conditions where treatment without NSAIDs may represent an acceptable alternative to both the patient and physician.
Laboratory Tests
Because serious GI tract ulceration and bleeding can occur without warning symptoms, physicians should follow chronically treated patients for the signs and symptoms of ulceration and bleeding and should inform them of the importance of this follow-up (see WARNINGS, *Risk of GI Ulcerations, Bleeding and Perforation with NSAID Therapy*).
Carcinogenesis, Mutagenesis, Impairment of Fertility
In an 81-week chronic oral toxicity study in the rat at doses up to 1 mg/kg/day, indomethacin had no tumorigenic effect. Indomethacin produced no neoplastic or hyperplastic changes related to treatment in carcinogenic studies in the rat (dosing period 73–110 weeks) and the mouse (dosing period 62–88 weeks) at doses up to 1.5 mg/kg/day.
Indomethacin did not have any mutagenic effect in *in vitro* bacterial tests (Ames test and *E. coli* with or without metabolic activation) and a series of *in vivo* tests including the host-mediated assay, sex-linked recessive lethals in *Drosophila,* and the micronucleus test in mice.
Indomethacin at dosage levels up to 0.5 mg/kg/day had no effect on fertility in mice in a two generation reproduction study or a two litter reproduction study in rats.
Drug Interactions
In normal volunteers receiving indomethacin, the administration of diflunisal decreased the renal clearance and significantly increased the plasma levels of indomethacin. In some patients, combined use of INDOCIN and diflunisal has been associated with fatal gastrointestinal hemorrhage. Therefore, diflunisal and INDOCIN should not be used concomitantly.
In a study in normal volunteers, it was found that chronic concurrent administration of 3.6 g of aspirin per day decreases indomethacin blood levels approximately 20%.
The concomitant use of INDOCIN with other NSAIDs is not recommended due to the increased possibility of gastrointestinal toxicity, with little or no increase in efficacy.
Clinical studies have shown that INDOCIN does not influence the hypoprothrombinemia produced by anticoagulants. However, when any additional drug, including INDOCIN, is added to the treatment of patients on anticoagulant therapy, the patients should be observed for alterations of the prothrombin time.
When INDOCIN is given to patients receiving probenecid, the plasma levels of indomethacin are likely to be increased. Therefore, a lower total daily dosage of INDOCIN may produce a satisfactory therapeutic effect. When increases in the dose of INDOCIN are made, they should be made carefully and in small increments.
Caution should be used if INDOCIN is administered simultaneously with methotrexate. INDOCIN has been reported to decrease the tubular secretion of methotrexate and to potentiate its toxicity.
Administration of non-steroidal anti-inflammatory drugs concomitantly with cyclosporine has been associated with an increase in cyclosporine-induced toxicity, possibly due to decreased synthesis of renal prostacyclin. NSAIDs should be used with caution in patients taking cyclosporine, and renal function should be monitored.
Capsules INDOCIN 50 mg t.i.d. produced a clinically relevant elevation of plasma lithium and reduction in renal lithium clearance in psychiatric patients and normal subjects with steady state plasma lithium concentrations. This effect has been attributed to inhibition of prostaglandin synthesis. As a consequence, when INDOCIN and lithium are given concomitantly, the patient should be carefully observed for signs of lithium toxicity. (Read circulars for lithium preparations before use of such concomitant therapy.) In addition, the frequency of monitoring serum lithium concentration should be increased at the outset of such combination drug treatment.
INDOCIN given concomitantly with digoxin has been reported to increase the serum concentration and prolong the half-life of digoxin. Therefore, when INDOCIN and digoxin are used concomitantly, serum digoxin levels should be closely monitored.
In some patients, the administration of INDOCIN can reduce the diuretic, natriuretic, and, antihypertensive effects of loop, potassium-sparing, and thiazide diuretics. Therefore, when INDOCIN and diuretics are used concomitantly, the patient should be observed closely to determine if the desired effect of the diuretic is obtained.
INDOCIN reduces basal plasma renin activity (PRA), as well as those elevations of PRA induced by furosemide administration, or salt or volume depletion. These facts should be considered when evaluating plasma renin activity in hypertensive patients.

Incidence greater than 1%	Incidence less than 1%	
CARDIOVASCULAR		
none	hypertension hypotension tachycardia chest pain	congestive heart failure arrhythmia; palpitations
METABOLIC		
none	edema weight gain fluid retention flushing or sweating	hyperglycemia glycosuria hyperkalemia
INTEGUMENTARY		
none	pruritus rash; urticaria petechiae or ecchymosis	exfoliative dermatitis erythema nodosum loss of hair Stevens-Johnson syndrome erythema multiforme toxic epidermal necrolysis
HEMATOLOGIC		
none	leukopenia bone marrow depression anemia secondary to obvious or occult gastrointestinal bleeding	aplastic anemia hemolytic anemia agranulocytosis thrombocytopenic purpura disseminated intravascular coagulation
HYPERSENSITIVITY		
none	acute anaphylaxis acute respiratory distress rapid fall in blood pressure resembling a shock-like state angioedema	dyspnea asthma purpura angiitis pulmonary edema fever
GENITOURINARY		
none	hematuria vaginal bleeding proteinuria nephrotic syndrome interstitial nephritis	BUN elevation renal insufficiency, including renal failure
MISCELLANEOUS		
none	epistaxis breast changes, including enlargement and tenderness, or gynecomastia	

* Reactions occurring in 3% to 9% of patients treated with INDOCIN. (Those reactions occurring in less than 3% of the patients are unmarked.)

It has been reported that the addition of triamterene to a maintenance schedule of INDOCIN resulted in reversible acute renal failure in two of four healthy volunteers. INDOCIN and triamterene should not be administered together.
INDOCIN and potassium-sparing diuretics each may be associated with increased serum potassium levels. The potential effects of INDOCIN and potassium-sparing diuretics on potassium kinetics and renal function should be considered when these agents are administered concurrently.
Most of the above effects concerning diuretics have been attributed, at least in part, to mechanisms involving inhibition of prostaglandin synthesis by INDOCIN.
Blunting of the antihypertensive effect of beta-adrenoceptor blocking agents by non-steroidal anti-inflammatory drugs including INDOCIN has been reported. Therefore, when using these blocking agents to treat hypertension, patients should be observed carefully in order to confirm that the desired therapeutic effect has been obtained. INDOCIN can reduce the antihypertensive effects of captopril and losartan.
False-negative results in the dexamethasone suppression test (DST) in patients being treated with INDOCIN have been reported. Thus, results of the DST should be interpreted with caution in these patients.
Pediatric Use
Effectiveness in pediatric patients 14 years of age and younger has not been established (see WARNINGS).
Geriatric Use
As with any NSAID, caution should be exercised in treating the elderly (65 years and older) since advancing age appears to increase the possibility of adverse reactions (see WARNINGS, *General*; and DOSAGE AND ADMINISTRATION). Elderly patients seem to tolerate ulceration or bleeding less well than other individuals and many spontaneous reports of fatal GI events are in this population (see WARNINGS, *Risk of GI Ulcerations, Bleeding and Perforation with NSAID Therapy*).
Indomethacin may cause confusion or, rarely, psychosis (see ADVERSE REACTIONS); physicians should remain alert to the possibility of such adverse effects in the elderly.
This drug is known to be substantially excreted by the kidney and the risk of toxic reactions to this drug may be greater in patients with impaired renal function. Because elderly patients are more likely to have decreased renal function, care should be taken in dose selection and it may be useful to monitor renal function (see WARNINGS, *Renal Effects*).

ADVERSE REACTIONS

The adverse reactions for Capsules INDOCIN listed in the following table have been arranged into two groups: (1) incidence greater than 1%; and (2) incidence less than 1%. The incidence for group (1) was obtained from 33 double-blind controlled clinical trials reported in the literature (1,092 patients). The incidence for group (2) was based on reports in clinical trials, in the literature, and on voluntary reports since marketing. The probability of a causal relationship exists between INDOCIN and these adverse reactions, some of which have been reported only rarely.
The adverse reactions reported with Capsules INDOCIN may occur with use of the suppositories. In addition, rectal irritation and tenesmus have been reported in patients who have received the suppositories.
The adverse reactions reported with Capsules INDOCIN may also occur with use of the suspension.
[See table at top of previous page]
[See table above]
Causal relationship unknown: Other reactions have been reported but occurred under circumstances where a causal relationship could not be established. However, in these rarely reported events, the possibility cannot be excluded. Therefore, these observations are being listed to serve as alerting information to physicians:
Cardiovascular: Thrombophlebitis
Hematologic: Although there have been several reports of leukemia, the supporting information is weak.
Genitourinary: Urinary frequency.
A rare occurrence of fulminant necrotizing fasciitis, particularly in association with Group A β-hemolytic streptococcus, has been described in persons treated with non-steroidal anti-inflammatory agents, including indomethacin, sometimes with fatal outcome (see also PRECAUTIONS, *General*).

Continued on next page

Information on the Merck & Co., Inc., products listed on these pages is from the prescribing information in use October 1, 2004. For information, please call 1-800-NSC-MERCK [1-800-672-6372].

Indocin/Caps/O.S./Supp.—Cont.

OVERDOSAGE

The following symptoms may be observed following overdosage: nausea, vomiting, intense headache, dizziness, mental confusion, disorientation, or lethargy. There have been reports of paresthesias, numbness, and convulsions.
Treatment is symptomatic and supportive. The stomach should be emptied as quickly as possible if the ingestion is recent. If vomiting has not occurred spontaneously, the patient should be induced to vomit with syrup of ipecac. If the patient is unable to vomit, gastric lavage should be performed. Once the stomach has been emptied, 25 or 50 g of activated charcoal may be given. Depending on the condition of the patient, close medical observation and nursing care may be required. The patient should be followed for several days because gastrointestinal ulceration and hemorrhage have been reported as adverse reactions of indomethacin. Use of antacids may be helpful.
The oral LD_{50} of indomethacin in mice and rats (based on 14 day mortality response) was 50 and 12 mg/kg, respectively.

DOSAGE AND ADMINISTRATION

INDOCIN is available as 25 and 50 mg Capsules INDOCIN, Oral Suspension INDOCIN, containing 25 mg of indomethacin per 5 mL, and 50 mg Suppositories INDOCIN for rectal use.
Adverse reactions appear to correlate with the size of the dose of INDOCIN in most patients but not all. Therefore, every effort should be made to determine the smallest effective dosage for the individual patient.
Always give Capsules INDOCIN or Oral Suspension INDOCIN with food, immediately after meals, or with antacids to reduce gastric irritation.
Pediatric Use
INDOCIN ordinarily should not be prescribed for pediatric patients 14 years of age and under (see WARNINGS).
Adult Use
Dosage Recommendations for Active Stages of the Following:

1. Moderate to severe rheumatoid arthritis including acute flares of chronic disease; moderate to severe ankylosing spondylitis; and moderate to severe osteoarthritis.
   Suggested Dosage:
   Capsules INDOCIN 25 mg b.i.d. or t.i.d. If this is well tolerated, increase the daily dosage by 25 or by 50 mg, if required by continuing symptoms, at weekly intervals until a satisfactory response is obtained or until a total daily dose of 150–200 mg is reached. DOSES ABOVE THIS AMOUNT GENERALLY DO NOT INCREASE THE EFFECTIVENESS OF THE DRUG.

In patients who have persistent night pain and/or morning stiffness, the giving of a large portion, up to a maximum of 100 mg, of the total daily dose at bedtime, either orally or by rectal suppositories, may be helpful in affording relief. The total daily dose should not exceed 200 mg. In acute flares of chronic rheumatoid arthritis, it may be necessary to increase the dosage by 25 mg or, if required, by 50 mg daily.
If minor adverse effects develop as the dosage is increased, reduce the dosage rapidly to a tolerated dose and OBSERVE THE PATIENT CLOSELY.
If severe adverse reactions occur, STOP THE DRUG. After the acute phase of the disease is under control, an attempt to reduce the daily dose should be made repeatedly until the patient is receiving the smallest effective dose or the drug is discontinued.
Careful instructions to, and observations of, the individual patient are essential to the prevention of serious, irreversible, including fatal, adverse reactions.
As advancing years appear to increase the possibility of adverse reactions, INDOCIN should be used with greater care in the elderly (see PRECAUTIONS, *Geriatric Use*).

2. Acute painful shoulder (bursitis and/or tendinitis).
   Initial Dose:
   75–150 mg daily in 3 or 4 divided doses.
   The drug should be discontinued after the signs and symptoms of inflammation have been controlled for several days. The usual course of therapy is 7–14 days.
3. Acute gouty arthritis.
   Suggested Dosage:
   Capsules INDOCIN 50 mg t.i.d. until pain is tolerable. The dose should then be rapidly reduced to complete cessation of the drug. Definite relief of pain has been reported within 2 to 4 hours. Tenderness and heat usually subside in 24 to 36 hours, and swelling gradually disappears in 3 to 5 days.

HOW SUPPLIED

No. 3316—Capsules INDOCIN, 25 mg are opaque blue and white capsules, coded INDOCIN and MSD 25. They are supplied as follows:
NDC 0006-0025-68 bottles of 100
NDC 0006-0025-82 bottles of 1000
No. 3317—Capsules INDOCIN, 50 mg are opaque blue and white capsules, coded INDOCIN and MSD 50. They are supplied as follows:
NDC 0006-0050-68 bottles of 100
No. 3376—Oral Suspension INDOCIN, 25 mg per 5 mL, is an off-white suspension with a pineapple coconut mint flavor. It is supplied as follows:
NDC 0006-3376-66 in bottles of 237 mL.
No. 3354—Suppositories INDOCIN, 50 mg each, are white, opaque, rectal suppositories and are supplied as follows:
NDC 0006-0150-30, boxes of 30
Storage
Store Oral Suspension INDOCIN below 30°C (86°F). Avoid temperatures above 50°C (122°F). Protect from freezing.
Store Suppositories INDOCIN below 30°C (86°F). Avoid transient temperatures above 40°C (104°F).

Suppositories INDOCIN are distributed by:
MERCK & CO., INC., Whitehouse Station, NJ 08889, USA
Manufactured by:
MERCK SHARP & DOHME
(Italia) S.p.A.
27100—Pavia, Italy
Capsules and Oral Suspension INDOCIN® are distributed and manufactured by:
MERCK & CO., INC., Whitehouse Station, NJ 08889, USA
7873328 Issued February 2002

Shown in Product Identification Guide, page 323

STERILE INDOCIN® I.V. ℞
(Indomethacin for Injection)

DESCRIPTION

Sterile INDOCIN* I.V. (Indomethacin for Injection) for intravenous administration is lyophilized indomethacin for injection. Each vial contains indomethacin for injection equivalent to 1 mg indomethacin as a white to yellow lyophilized powder or plug. Variations in the size of the lyophilized plug and the intensity of color have no relationship to the quality or amount of indomethacin present in the vial.
Indomethacin for injection is designated chemically as 1-(4-chlorobenzoyl) -5- methoxy-2-methyl-1*H* -indole-3-acetic acid, sodium salt, trihydrate. Its molecular weight is 433.82. Its empirical formula is $C_{19}H_{15}ClNNaO_4 \cdot 3H_2O$ and its structural formula is:

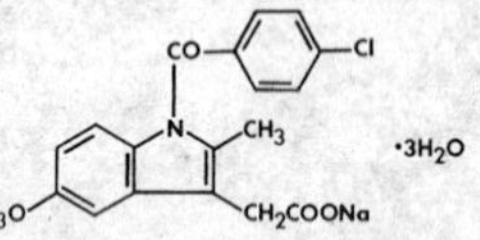

*Registered trademark of MERCK & CO., INC.

CLINICAL PHARMACOLOGY

Although the exact mechanism of action through which indomethacin causes closure of a patent ductus arteriosus is not known, it is believed to be through inhibition of prostaglandin synthesis. Indomethacin has been shown to be a potent inhibitor of prostaglandin synthesis, both *in vitro* and *in vivo*. In human newborns with certain congenital heart malformations, PGE 1 dilates the ductus arteriosus. In fetal and newborn lambs, E type prostaglandins have also been shown to maintain the patency of the ductus, and as in human newborns, indomethacin causes its constriction.
Studies in healthy young animals and in premature infants with patent ductus arteriosus indicated that, after the first dose of intravenous indomethacin, there was a transient reduction in cerebral blood flow velocity and cerebral blood flow. Similar decreases in mesenteric blood flow and velocity have been observed. The clinical significance of these effects has not been established.
In double-blind placebo-controlled studies of INDOCIN I.V. in 460 small pre-term infants, weighing 1750 g or less, the neonates treated with placebo had a ductus closure rate after 48 hours of 25 to 30 percent, whereas those treated with INDOCIN I.V. had a 75 to 80 percent closure rate. In one of these studies, a multicenter study, involving 405 pre-term infants, later re-opening of the ductus arteriosus occurred in 26 percent of neonates treated with INDOCIN I.V., however, 70 percent of these closed subsequently without the need for surgery or additional indomethacin.
Pharmacokinetics and Metabolism
The disposition of indomethacin following intravenous administration (0.2 mg/kg) in pre-term neonates with patent ductus arteriosus has not been extensively evaluated. Even though the plasma half-life of indomethacin was variable among premature infants, it was shown to vary inversely with postnatal age and weight. In one study, of 28 neonates who could be evaluated, the plasma half-life in those less than 7 days old averaged 20 hours (range: 3–60 hours, n = 18). In neonates older than 7 days, the mean plasma half-life of indomethacin was 12 hours (range: 4–38 hours, n = 10). Grouping the neonates by weight, mean plasma half-life in those weighing less than 1000 g was 21 hours (range: 9–60 hours, n = 10); in those neonates weighing more than 1000 g, the mean plasma half-life was 15 hours (range: 3–52 hours, n = 18).
Following intravenous administration in adults, indomethacin is eliminated via renal excretion, metabolism, and biliary excretion. Indomethacin undergoes appreciable enterohepatic circulation. The mean plasma half-life of indomethacin is 4.5 hours. In the absence of enterohepatic circulation, it is 90 minutes. Indomethacin has been found to cross the blood-brain barrier and the placenta.
In adults, about 99 percent of indomethacin is bound to protein in plasma over the expected range of therapeutic plasma concentrations. The percent bound in neonates has not been studied. In controlled trials in premature infants, however, no evidence of bilirubin displacement has been observed as evidenced by increased incidence of bilirubin encephalopathy (kernicterus).

INDICATIONS AND USAGE

INDOCIN I.V. is indicated to close a hemodynamically significant patent ductus arteriosus in premature infants weighing between 500 and 1750 g when after 48 hours usual medical management (e.g., fluid restriction, diuretics, digitalis, respiratory support, etc.) is ineffective. Clear-cut clinical evidence of a hemodynamically significant patent ductus arteriosus should be present, such as respiratory distress, a continuous murmur, a hyperactive precordium, cardiomegaly and pulmonary plethora on chest x-ray.

CONTRAINDICATIONS

INDOCIN I.V. is contraindicated in: neonates with proven or suspected infection that is untreated; neonates who are bleeding, especially those with active intracranial hemorrhage or gastrointestinal bleeding; neonates with thrombocytopenia; neonates with coagulation defects; neonates with or who are suspected of having necrotizing enterocolitis; neonates with significant impairment of renal function; neonates with congenital heart disease in whom patency of the ductus arteriosus is necessary for satisfactory pulmonary or systemic blood flow (e.g., pulmonary atresia, severe tetralogy of Fallot, severe coarctation of the aorta).

WARNINGS

Gastrointestinal Effects:
In the collaborative study, major gastrointestinal bleeding was no more common in those neonates receiving indomethacin than in those neonates on placebo. However, minor gastrointestinal bleeding (i.e., chemical detection of blood in the stool) was more commonly noted in those neonates treated with indomethacin. Severe gastrointestinal effects have been reported in adults with various arthritic disorders treated chronically with oral indomethacin. [For further information, see package circular for Capsules INDOCIN* (Indomethacin)].
Central Nervous System Effects:
Prematurity per se, is associated with an increased incidence of spontaneous intraventricular hemorrhage. Because indomethacin may inhibit platelet aggregation, the potential for intraventricular bleeding may be increased. However, in the large multi-center study of INDOCIN I.V. (see CLINICAL PHARMACOLOGY), the incidence of intraventricular hemorrhage in neonates treated with INDOCIN I.V. was not significantly higher than in the control neonates.
Renal Effects:
INDOCIN I.V. may cause significant reduction in urine output (50 percent or more) with concomitant elevations of blood urea nitrogen and creatinine, and reductions in glomerular filtration rate and creatinine clearance. These effects in most neonates are transient, disappearing with cessation of therapy with INDOCIN I.V. However, because adequate renal function can depend upon renal prostaglandin synthesis, INDOCIN I.V. may precipitate renal insufficiency, including acute renal failure, especially in neonates with other conditions that may adversely affect renal function (e.g., extracellular volume depletion from any cause, congestive heart failure, sepsis, concomitant use of any nephrotoxic drug, hepatic dysfunction). When significant suppression of urine volume occurs after a dose of INDOCIN I.V., no additional dose should be given until the urine output returns to normal levels.
INDOCIN I.V. in pre-term infants may suppress water excretion to a greater extent than sodium excretion. When this occurs, a significant reduction in serum sodium values (i.e., hyponatremia) may result. Neonates should have serum electrolyte determinations done during therapy with INDOCIN I.V. Renal function and serum electrolytes should be monitored (see PRECAUTIONS, *Drug Interactions* and DOSAGE AND ADMINISTRATION).

* Registered trademark of MERCK & CO., INC.

PRECAUTIONS

General
INDOCIN (Indomethacin) may mask the usual signs and symptoms of infection. Therefore, the physician must be continually on the alert for this and should use the drug with extra care in the presence of existing controlled infection.
Severe hepatic reactions have been reported in adults treated chronically with oral indomethacin for arthritic disorders. [For further information, see package circular for Capsules INDOCIN (Indomethacin)]. If clinical signs and symptoms consistent with liver disease develop in the neonate, or if systemic manifestations occur, INDOCIN I.V. should be discontinued.

INDOCIN I.V. may inhibit platelet aggregation. In one small study, platelet aggregation was grossly abnormal after indomethacin therapy (given orally to premature infants to close the ductus arteriosus). Platelet aggregation returned to normal by the tenth day. Premature infants should be observed for signs of bleeding.

The drug should be administered carefully to avoid extravascular injection or leakage as the solution may be irritating to tissue.

Drug Interactions

Since renal function may be reduced by INDOCIN I.V., consideration should be given to reduction in dosage of those medications that rely on adequate renal function for their elimination. Because the half-life of digitalis (given frequently to pre-term infants with patent ductus arteriosus and associated cardiac failure) may be prolonged when given concomitantly with indomethacin, the neonate should be observed closely; frequent ECGs and serum digitalis levels may be required to prevent or detect digitalis toxicity early. Furthermore, in one study of premature infants treated with INDOCIN I.V. and also receiving either gentamicin or amikacin, both peak and trough levels of these aminoglycosides were significantly elevated.

Therapy with indomethacin may blunt the natriuretic effect of furosemide. This response has been attributed to inhibition of prostaglandin synthesis by non-steroidal anti-inflammatory drugs. In a study of 19 premature infants with patent ductus arteriosus treated with either INDOCIN I.V. alone or a combination of INDOCIN I.V. and furosemide, results showed that neonates receiving both INDOCIN I.V. and furosemide had significantly higher urinary output, higher levels of sodium and chloride excretion, and higher glomerular filtration rates than did those receiving INDOCIN I.V. alone. In this study, the data suggested that therapy with furosemide helped to maintain renal function in the premature infant when INDOCIN I.V. was added to the treatment of patent ductus arteriosus.

Neonatal Effects

In rats and mice, oral indomethacin 4.0 mg/kg/day given during the last three days of gestation caused a decrease in maternal weight gain and some maternal and fetal deaths. An increased incidence of neuronal necrosis in the diencephalon in the live-born fetuses was observed. At 2.0 mg/kg/day, no increase in neuronal necrosis was observed as compared to the control groups. Administration of 0.5 or 4.0 mg/kg/day during the first three days of life did not cause an increase in neuronal necrosis at either dose level.

Pregnant rats, given 2.0 mg/kg/day and 4.0 mg/kg/day during the last trimester of gestation, delivered offspring whose pulmonary blood vessels were both reduced in number and excessively muscularized. These findings are similar to those observed in the syndrome of persistent pulmonary hypertension of the neonate.

ADVERSE REACTIONS

In a double-blind placebo-controlled trial of 405 premature infants weighing less than or equal to 1750 g with evidence of large ductal shunting, in those neonates treated with indomethacin (n = 206), there was a statistically significantly greater incidence of bleeding problems, including gross or microscopic bleeding into the gastrointestinal tract, oozing from the skin after needle stick, pulmonary hemorrhage, and disseminated intravascular coagulopathy. There was no statistically significant difference between treatment groups with reference to intracranial hemorrhage.

The neonates treated with indomethacin for injection also had a significantly higher incidence of transient oliguria and elevations of serum creatinine (greater than or equal to 1.8 mg/dL) than did the neonates treated with placebo.

The incidences of retrolental fibroplasia (grades III and IV) and pneumothorax in neonates treated with INDOCIN I.V. were no greater than in placebo controls and were statistically significantly lower than in surgically-treated neonates.

The following additional adverse reactions in neonates have been reported from the collaborative study, anecdotal case reports, from other studies using rectal, oral, or intravenous indomethacin for treatment of patent ductus arteriosus or in marketed use. The rates are calculated from a database which contains experience of 849 indomethacin-treated neonates reported in the medical literature, regardless of the route of administration. One year follow-up is available on 175 neonates and shows no long-term sequelae which could be attributed to indomethacin. In controlled clinical studies, only electrolyte imbalance and renal dysfunction (of the reactions listed below) occurred statistically significantly more frequently after INDOCIN I.V. than after placebo. Reactions marked with a single asterick (*) occurred in 3–9 percent of indomethacin-treated neonates: those marked with a double asterisk (**) occurred in 3–9 percent of both indomethacin- and placebo-treated neonates. Unmarked reactions occurred in less than 3 percent of neonates.

Renal: renal dysfunction in 41 percent of neonates, including one or more of the following: reduced urinary output; reduced urine sodium, chloride, or potassium urine osmolality, free water clearance, or glomerular filtration, rate; elevated serum creatinine or BUN; uremia.

Cardiovascular: intracranial bleeding**, pulmonary hypertension.

Gastrointestinal: gastrointestinal bleeding*, vomiting, abdominal distention, transient ileus, localized perforation(s) of the small and/or large intestine, necrotizing enterocolitis.

Metabolic: hyponatremia*, elevated serum potassium*, reduction in blood sugar, including hypoglycemia, increased weight gain (fluid retention).

Coagulation: decreased platelet aggregation (see PRECAUTIONS).

The following adverse reactions have also been reported in neonates treated with indomethacin, however, a causal relationship to therapy with INDOCIN I.V. has not been established:

Cardiovascular: bradycardia.

Respiratory: apnea, exacerbation of pre-existing pulmonary infection.

Metabolic: acidosis/alkalosis.

Hematologic: disseminated intravascular coagulation.

Ophthalmic: retrolental fibroplasia.**

A variety of additional adverse experiences have been reported in adults treated with oral indomethacin for moderate to severe rheumatoid arthritis, osteoarthritis, ankylosing spondylitis, acute painful shoulder and acute gouty arthritis (see package circular for Capsules INDOCIN (Indomethacin) for additional information concerning adverse reactions and other cautionary statements). Their relevance to the pre-term infant receiving indomethacin for patent ductus arteriosus is unknown, however, the possibility exists that these experiences may be associated with the use of INDOCIN I.V. in pre-term infants.

DOSAGE AND ADMINISTRATION

FOR INTRAVENOUS ADMINISTRATION ONLY.

Dosage recommendations for closure of the ductus arteriosus depend on the age of the infant at the time of therapy. A course of therapy is defined as three intravenous doses of INDOCIN I.V. given at 12–24 hour intervals, with careful attention to urinary output. If anuria or marked oliguria (urinary output < 0.6 mL/kg/hr) is evident at the scheduled time of the second or third dose of INDOCIN I.V., no additional doses should be given until laboratory studies indicate that renal function has returned to normal (see WARNINGS, *Renal Effects*).

Dosage according to age is as follows:

AGE at 1st dose	DOSAGE (mg/kg)		
	1st	2nd	3rd
Less than 48 hours	0.2	0.1	0.1
2–7 days	0.2	0.2	0.2
over 7 days	0.2	0.25	0.25

If the ductus arteriosus closes or is significantly reduced in size after an interval of 48 hours or more from completion of the first course of INDOCIN I.V., no further doses are necessary. If the ductus arteriosus re-opens, a second course of 1–3 doses may be given, each dose separated by a 12–24 hour interval as described above.

If the neonate remains unresponsive to therapy with INDOCIN I.V. after 2 courses, surgery may be necessary for closure of the ductus arteriosus. If severe adverse reactions occur, STOP THE DRUG.

Directions for Use

Parenteral drug products should be inspected visually for particulate matter and discoloration prior to administration whenever solution and container permit.

The solution should be prepared only with 1 to 2 mL of preservative-free sterile Sodium Chloride Injection, 0.9 percent or preservative-free Sterile Water for Injection. Benzyl alcohol as a preservative has been associated with toxicity in neonates. Therefore, all diluents should be preservative-free. If 1 mL of diluent is used, the concentration of indomethacin in the solution will equal approximately 0.1 mg/0.1 mL; if 2 mL of diluent are used, the concentration of the solution will equal approximately 0.05 mg/0.1 mL. Any unused portion of the solution should be discarded because there is no preservative contained in the vial. A fresh solution should be prepared just prior to each administration. Once reconstituted, the indomethacin solution may be injected intravenously. While the optimal rate of injection has not been established, published literature suggests an infusion rate over 20–30 minutes.

INDOCIN I.V. is not buffered. Further dilution with intravenous infusion solutions is not recommended.

HOW SUPPLIED

No. 3406—Sterile INDOCIN I.V. is a lyophilized white to yellow powder or plug supplied as single dose vials containing indomethacin sodium trihydrate, equivalent to 1 mg indomethacin.

NDC 0006-3406-17.

Storage

Store below 30°C (86°F). *Protect from light.* Store container in carton until contents have been used.

9408719 Issued January 2003

INVANZ®
(ertapenem for injection) ℞

To reduce the development of drug-resistant bacteria and maintain the effectiveness of INVANZ and other antibacterial drugs, INVANZ should be used only to treat or prevent infections that are proven or strongly suspected to be caused by bacteria.

For Intravenous or Intramuscular Use

DESCRIPTION

INVANZ* (Ertapenem for Injection) is a sterile, synthetic, parenteral, 1-β methyl-carbapenem that is structurally related to beta-lactam antibiotics.

Chemically, INVANZ is described as [4*R*-[3(3*S**,5*S**),4α,5β,6β(*R**)]]-3-[[5-[[(3-carboxyphenyl)amino]carbonyl-3-pyrrolidinyl]thio]-6-(1-hydroxyethyl)-4-methyl-7-oxo-1-azabicyclo[3.2.0]hept-2-ene-2-carboxylic acid monosodium salt. Its molecular weight is 497.50. The empirical formula is $C_{22}H_{24}N_3O_7SNa$, and its structural formula is:

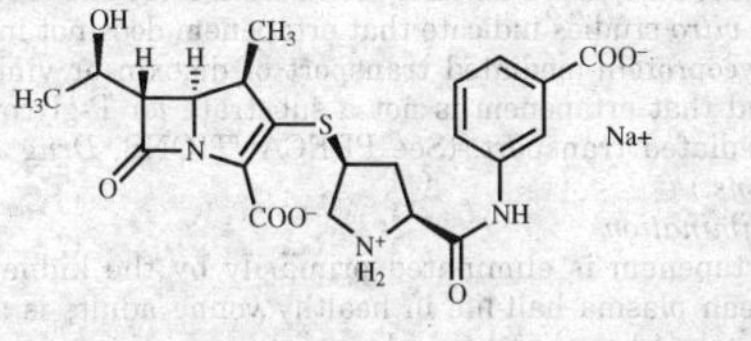

Ertapenem sodium is a white to off-white hygroscopic, weakly crystalline powder. It is soluble in water and 0.9% sodium chloride solution, practically insoluble in ethanol, and insoluble in isopropyl acetate and tetrahydrofuran.

INVANZ is supplied as sterile lyophilized powder for intravenous infusion after reconstitution with appropriate diluent (see DOSAGE AND ADMINISTRATION, PREPARATION OF SOLUTION) and transfer to 50 mL 0.9% Sodium Chloride Injection or for intramuscular injection following reconstitution with 1% lidocaine hydrochloride. Each vial contains 1.046 grams ertapenem sodium, equivalent to 1 gram ertapenem. The sodium content is approximately 137 mg (approximately 6.0 mEq).

Each vial of INVANZ contains the following inactive ingredients: 175 mg sodium bicarbonate and sodium hydroxide to adjust pH to 7.5.

* Trademark of MERCK & CO., Inc.

CLINICAL PHARMACOLOGY

Pharmacokinetics

Average plasma concentrations (mcg/mL) of ertapenem following a single 30-minute infusion of a 1 g intravenous (IV) dose and administration of a single 1 g intramuscular (IM) dose in healthy young adults are presented in Table 1.

[See table 1 at top of next page]

The area under the plasma concentration-time curve (AUC) of ertapenem increased less-than dose-proportional based on total ertapenem concentrations over the 0.5 to 2 g dose range, whereas the AUC increased greater-than dose proportional based on unbound ertapenem concentrations. Ertapenem exhibits non-linear pharmacokinetics due to concentration-dependent plasma protein binding at the proposed therapeutic dose. (See CLINICAL PHARMACOLOGY, *Distribution.*)

There is no accumulation of ertapenem following multiple IV or IM 1g daily doses in healthy adults.

Absorption

Ertapenem, reconstituted with 1% lidocaine HCl injection, USP (in saline without epinephrine), is almost completely absorbed following intramuscular (IM) administration at the recommended dose of 1 g. The mean bioavailability is approximately 90%. Following 1 g daily IM administration, mean peak plasma concentrations (C_{max}) are achieved in approximately 2.3 hours (T_{max}).

Distribution

Ertapenem is highly bound to human plasma proteins, primarily albumin. In healthy young adults, the protein binding of ertapenem decreases as plasma concentrations increase, from approximately 95% bound at an approximate plasma concentration of <100 micrograms (mcg)/mL to approximately 85% bound at an approximate plasma concentration of 300 mcg/mL.

The apparent volume of distribution at steady state (V_{ss}) of ertapenem is approximately 8.2 liters.

The concentrations of ertapenem achieved in suction-induced skin blister fluid at each sampling point on the third day of 1 g once daily IV doses are presented in Table 2. The ratio of AUC_{0-24} in skin blister fluid/AUC_{0-24} in plasma is 0.61.

[See table 2 at top of next page]

The concentration of ertapenem in breast milk from 5 lactating women with pelvic infections (5 to 14 days postpartum) was measured at random time points daily for 5 consecutive days following the last 1 g dose of intravenous therapy (3–10 days of therapy). The concentration of ertapenem in breast milk within 24 hours of the last dose of therapy in all 5 women ranged from <0.13 (lower limit of

Continued on next page

Information on the Merck & Co., Inc., products listed on these pages is from the prescribing information in use October 1, 2004. For information, please call 1-800-NSC-MERCK [1-800-672-6372].

Invanz—Cont.

quantitation) to 0.38 mcg/mL; peak concentrations were not assessed. By day 5 after discontinuation of therapy, the level of ertapenem was undetectable in the breast milk of 4 women and below the lower limit of quantitation (<0.13 mcg/mL) in 1 woman.

Metabolism

In healthy young adults, after infusion of 1 g IV radiolabeled ertapenem, the plasma radioactivity consists predominantly (94%) of ertapenem. The major metabolite of ertapenem is the inactive ring-opened derivative formed by hydrolysis of the beta-lactam ring.

In vitro studies in human liver microsomes indicate that ertapenem does not inhibit metabolism mediated by any of the following cytochrome p450 (CYP) isoforms: 1A2, 2C9, 2C19, 2D6, 2E1 and 3A4. (See DRUG INTERACTIONS.)

In vitro studies indicate that ertapenem does not inhibit P-glycoprotein-mediated transport of digoxin or vinblastine and that ertapenem is not a substrate for P-glycoprotein-mediated transport. (See PRECAUTIONS, *Drug Interactions.*)

Elimination

Ertapenem is eliminated primarily by the kidneys. The mean plasma half-life in healthy young adults is approximately 4 hours and the plasma clearance is approximately 1.8 L/hour.

Following the administration of 1 g IV radiolabeled ertapenem to healthy young adults, approximately 80% is recovered in urine and 10% in feces. Of the 80% recovered in urine, approximately 38% is excreted as unchanged drug and approximately 37% as the ring-opened metabolite.

In healthy young adults given a 1 g IV dose, the mean percentage of the administered dose excreted in urine was 17.4% during 0–2 hours postdose, 5.4% during 4–6 hours postdose, and 2.4% during 12–24 hours postdose.

Special Populations

Renal Insufficiency

Total and unbound fractions of ertapenem pharmacokinetics were investigated in 26 adult subjects (31 to 80 years of age) with varying degrees of renal impairment. Following a single 1 g IV dose of ertapenem, the unbound AUC increased 1.5-fold and 2.3-fold in subjects with mild renal insufficiency (CL_{CR} 60–90 mL/min/1.73 m^2) and moderate renal insufficiency (CL_{CR} 31–59 mL/min/1.73 m^2), respectively, compared with healthy young subjects (25 to 45 years of age). No dosage adjustment is necessary in patients with CL_{CR} ≥31 mL/min/1.73 m^2. The unbound AUC increased 4.4-fold and 7.6-fold in subjects with advanced renal insufficiency (CL_{CR} 5–30 mL/min/1.73 m^2) and end-stage renal insufficiency (CL_{CR} <10 mL/min/1.73 m^2), respectively, compared with healthy young subjects. The effects of renal insufficiency on AUC of total drug were of smaller magnitude. The recommended dose of ertapenem in patients with CL_{CR} ≤30 mL/min/1.73 m^2 is 0.5 grams every 24 hours. Following a single 1 g IV dose given immediately prior to a 4 hour hemodialysis session in 5 patients with end-stage renal insufficiency, approximately 30% of the dose was recovered in the dialysate. A supplementary dose of 150 mg is recommended if ertapenem is administered within 6 hours prior to hemodialysis. (See DOSAGE AND ADMINISTRATION.)

Hepatic Insufficiency

The pharmacokinetics of ertapenem in patients with hepatic insufficiency have not been established. However, ertapenem does not appear to undergo hepatic metabolism based on *in vitro* studies and approximately 10% of an administered dose is recovered in the feces. (See PRECAUTIONS and DOSAGE AND ADMINISTRATION.)

Gender

The effect of gender on the pharmacokinetics of ertapenem was evaluated in healthy male (n=8) and healthy female (n=8) subjects. The differences observed could be attributed to body size when body weight was taken into consideration. No dose adjustment is recommended based on gender.

Geriatric Patients

The impact of age on the pharmacokinetics of ertapenem was evaluated in healthy male (n=7) and healthy female (n=7) subjects ≥65 years of age. The total and unbound AUC increased 37% and 67%, respectively, in elderly adults relative to young adults. These changes were attributed to age-related changes in creatinine clearance. No dosage adjustment is necessary for elderly patients with normal (for their age) renal function.

Pediatric Patients

The pharmacokinetics of ertapenem in pediatric patients have not been established.

Microbiology

Ertapenem has *in vitro* activity against gram-positive and gram-negative aerobic and anaerobic bacteria. The bactericidal activity of ertapenem results from the inhibition of cell wall synthesis and is mediated through ertapenem binding to penicillin binding proteins (PBPs). In *Escherichia coli*, it has strong affinity toward PBPs 1a, 1b, 2, 3, 4 and 5 with preference for PBPs 2 and 3. Ertapenem is stable against hydrolysis by a variety of beta-lactamases, including penicillinases, and cephalosporinases and extended spectrum beta-lactamases. Ertapenem is hydrolyzed by metallo-beta-lactamases.

Ertapenem has been shown to be active against most strains of the following microorganisms *in vitro* and in clinical infections. (See INDICATIONS AND USAGE):

Table 1
Plasma Concentrations of Ertapenem After Single Dose Administration

Dose/Route	Average Plasma Concentrations (mcg/mL) 0.5 hr	1 hr	2 hr	4 hr	6 hr	8 hr	12 hr	18 hr	24 hr
1 g IV*	155	115	83	48	31	20	9	3	1
I g IM	33	53	67	57	40	27	13	4	2

*Infused at a constant rate over 30 minutes

Table 2
Concentrations (mcg/mL) of Ertapenem in Skin Blister Fluid at each Sampling Point on the Third Day of 1-g Once Daily IV Doses

0.5 hr	1 hr	2 hr	4 hr	8 hr	12 hr	24 hr
7	12	17	24	24	21	8

Aerobic gram-positive microorganisms:
Staphylococcus aureus (methicillin susceptible strains only)
Streptococcus agalactiae
Streptococcus pneumoniae (penicillin susceptible strains only)
Streptococcus pyogenes
Note: Methicillin-resistant staphylococci and *Enterococcus* spp. are resistant to ertapenem.

Aerobic gram-negative microorganisms:
Escherichia coli
Haemophilus influenzae (Beta-lactamase negative strains only)
Klebsiella pneumoniae
Moraxella catarrhalis

Anaerobic microorganisms:
Bacteroides fragilis
Bacteroides distasonis
Bacteroides ovatus
Bacteroides thetaiotaomicron
Bacteroides uniformis
Clostridium clostridioforme
Eubacterium lentum
Peptostreptococcus species
Porphyromonas asaccharolytica
Prevotella bivia

The following *in vitro* data are available, **but their clinical significance is unknown.**

At least 90% of the following microorganisms exhibit an *in vitro* minimum inhibitory concentration (MIC) less than or equal to the susceptible breakpoint for ertapenem; however, the safety and effectiveness of ertapenem in treating clinical infections due to these microorganisms have not been established in adequate and well-controlled clinical studies:

Aerobic gram-positive microorganisms:
Streptococcus pneumoniae (penicillin-intermediate strains only)

Aerobic gram-negative microorganisms:
Citrobacter freundii
Citrobacter koseri
Enterobacter aerogenes
Enterobacter cloacae
Haemophilus influenzae (Beta-lactamase positive strains)
Haemophilus parainfluenzae
Klebsiella oxytoca (excluding ESBL producing strains)
Morganella morganii
Proteus mirabilis
Proteus vulgaris
Serratia marcescens

Anaerobic microorganisms:
Clostridium perfringens
Fusobacterium spp.

Susceptibility Tests:

When available, the results of *in vitro* susceptibility tests should be provided to the physician as periodic reports which describe the susceptibility profile of nosocomial and community-acquired pathogens. These reports should aid the physician in selecting the most effective antimicrobial.

Dilution Techniques:

Quantitative methods are used to determine antimicrobial minimum inhibitory concentrations (MICs). These MICs provide estimates of the susceptibility of bacteria to antimicrobial compounds. The MICs should be determined using a standardized procedure. Standardized procedures are based on a broth dilution method[1,4] or equivalent with standardized inoculum concentrations and standardized concentrations of ertapenem powder. The MIC values should be interpreted according to the following criteria:

For testing Enterobacteriaceae and *Staphylococcus* spp.:

MIC (µg/mL)	Interpretation
≤2.0	Susceptible (S)
4.0	Intermediate (I)
≥8.0	Resistant (R)

Note: *Staphylococcus* spp. can be considered susceptible to ertapenem if the penicillin MIC is ≤ 0.12 µg/mL. If the penicillin MIC is >0.12 µg/mL, then test oxacillin. *Staphylococcus aureus* can be considered susceptible to ertapenem if the oxacillin MIC is ≤2.0 µg/mL and resistant to ertapenem if the oxacillin MIC is ≥4.0 µg/mL. Coagulase negative staphylococci can be considered susceptible to ertapenem if the oxacillin MIC is ≤0.25 µg/mL and resistant to ertapenem if the oxacillin MIC ≥0.5 µg/mL.

For testing *Haemophilus* spp.[a]:

MIC (µg/mL)	Interpretation[b]
≤0.5	Susceptible (S)

[a]This interpretive standard is applicable only to broth microdilution susceptibility tests with *Haemophilus* spp. using *Haemophilus* Test Medium (HTM)[1] inoculated with a direct colony suspension and incubated in ambient air at 35°C for 20–24 hrs.

[b]The current absence of data in resistant strains precludes defining any results other than "Susceptible". Strains yielding MIC results suggestive of a "nonsusceptible" category should be submitted to a reference laboratory for further testing.

For testing *Streptococcus pneumoniae*[c,d]:

MIC (µg/mL)	Interpretation[b]
≤1.0	Susceptible (S)

[c]This interpretive standard is applicable only to broth microdilution susceptibility tests using cation-adjusted Mueller-Hinton broth with 2–5% lysed horse blood inoculated with direct colony suspension and incubated in ambient air at 35°C for 20–24 hrs.

[d]*Streptococcus pneumoniae* that are susceptible to penicillin (penicillin MIC ≤0.06 µg/mL) can be considered susceptible to ertapenum. Testing of ertapenem against penicillin-intermediate or penicillin-resistant isolates is not recommended since reliable interpretive criteria for ertapenem are not available.

For testing *Streptococcus* spp. other than *Streptococcus pneumoniae*[c,e]:

MIC (µg/mL)	Interpretation[b]
≤1.0	Susceptible (S)

[e]*Streptococcus* spp. that are susceptible to penicillin (MIC ≤0.12 µg/mL) can be considered susceptible to ertapenem. Testing of ertapenem against penicillin-intermediate or penicillin-resistant isolates is not recommended since reliable interpretive criteria for ertapenum are not available.

A report of "Susceptible" indicates that the pathogen is likely to be inhibited if the antimicrobial compound in blood reaches the concentrations usually achievable. A report of "Intermediate" indicates that the result should be considered equivocal, and, if the microorganism is not fully susceptible to alternative, clinically feasible drugs, the test should be repeated. This category implies possible clinical applicability in body sites where the drug is physiologically concentrated or in situations where high dosage of drug can be used. This category also provides a buffer zone which prevents small uncontrolled technical factors from causing major discrepancies in interpretation. A report of "Resistant" indicates that the pathogen is not likely to be inhibited if the antimicrobial compound in the blood reaches the concentrations usually achievable; other therapy should be selected.

Standardized susceptibility test procedures require the use of laboratory control microorganisms to control the technical aspects of the laboratory procedures. Quality control microorganisms are specific strains of organisms with intrinsic biological properties. QC strains are very stable strains which will give a standard and repeatable susceptibility pattern. The specific strains used for microbiological quality control are not clinically significant. Standard ertapenem powder should provide the following MIC values.

Microorganism	MIC Range (µg/mL)
Enterococcus faecalis ATCC 29212	4.0–16.0
Escherichia coli ATCC 25922	0.004–0.016
Haemophilus influenzae[f] ATCC 49766	0.016–0.06
Pseudomonas aeruginosa ATCC 27853	2.0–8.0
Staphylococcus aureus ATCC 29213	0.06–0.25

Streptococcus pneumoniae[g] ATCC 49619	0.03–0.25

[f]This quality control range is applicable to only *H. influenzae* ATCC 49766 tested by the broth microdilution procedure using HTM[1] inoculated with a direct colony suspension and incubated in ambient air at 35°C for 20–24 hrs.
[g]This quality control range is applicable to only *S. pneumonaie* ATCC 49619 tested by a broth microdilution procedure using cation-adjusted Mueller-Hinton broth with 2–5% lysed horse blood inoculated with a direct colony suspension and incubated in ambient air at 35°C for 20–24 hrs.

Diffusion Techniques:
Quantitative methods that require measurement of zone diameters also provide reproducible estimates of the susceptibility of bacteria to antimicrobial compounds. One such standardized procedure[2,4] requires the use of standardized inoculum concentrations. This procedure uses paper disks impregnated with 10-µg ertapenem to test the suspectibility of microorganisms to ertapenem.
Reports from the laboratory providing results of the standard single-disk susceptibility test with a 10-µg ertapenem disk should be interpreted according to the following criteria:
For testing Enterobacteriaceae and *Staphylococcus* spp.:

Zone Diameter (mm)	Interpretation
≥19	Susceptible (S)
16–18	Intermediate (I)
≤15	Resistant (R)

Note: *Staphylococcus* spp. can be considered susceptible to ertapenem if the penicillin (10 U disk) zone is ≥29 mm. If the penicillin zone is ≤28 mm, then test oxacillin by disk diffusion (1 µg disk). *Staphylococcus aureus* can be considered susceptible to ertapenem if the oxacillin (1 µg disk) zone is ≥13 mm and resistant to ertapenem if the oxacillin zone is ≤10 mm. Coagulase negative staphylococci can be considered susceptible to ertapenem if the oxacillin zone is ≥18 mm and resistant to ertapenem if the oxacillin (1 µg disk) zone is ≤17 mm.

For testing *Haemophilus* spp.[h]:

Zone Diameter (mm)	Interpretation[b]
≥19	Susceptible (S)

[h]This zone diameter standard is applicable only to tests performed by disk diffusion with *Haemophilus* spp. using HTM[2] inoculated with a direct colony suspension and incubated in 5% CO_2 at 35°C for 16–18 hrs.

For testing *Streptococcus pneumoniae*[i,j]:

Zone Diameter (mm)	Interpretation[b]
≥19	Susceptible (S)

[i]These zone diameter standards apply only to tests performed using Mueller-Hinton agar supplemented with 5% sheep blood inoculated with a direct colony suspension and incubated in 5% CO_2 at 35°C for 20–24 hrs.
[j]*Streptococcus pneumoniae* that is susceptible to penicillin (1-µg oxacillin disk zone diameter ≥20 mm), can be considered susceptible to ertapenum. Isolates with 1-µg oxacillin zone diameter ≤19 mm should be tested against ertapenem using an MIC method.

For testing *Streptococcus* spp. other than *Streptococcus pneumoniae*[k,l]:

Zone Diameter (mm)	Interpretation[b]
≥19	Susceptible (S)

[k]These zone diameter standards apply only to tests performed using Mueller-Hinton agar supplemented with 5% sheep blood inoculated with a direct colony suspension and in ambient air at 35°C for 20–24 hrs.
[l]Beta-hemolytic *Streptococcus* spp. that are susceptible to penicillin (10-units penicillin disk zone diameter ≥24 mm), can be considered susceptible to ertapenum. Isolates with 10-units penicillin disk zone diameter <24 mm should be tested against ertapenem using an MIC method. Penicillin disk diffusion interpretive criteria are not available for viridans group streptococci and they should not be tested against ertapenem.

Interpretation should be as stated above for results using dilution techniques. Interpretation involves correlation of the diameter obtained in the disk test with the MIC for ertapenem.
As with standardized dilution techniques, diffusion methods require the use of laboratory control microorganisms that are used to control the technical aspects of the laboratory procedures. Quality control microorganisms are specific strains of organisms with intrinsic biological properties. QC strains are very stable strains that will give a standard and repeatable susceptibility pattern. The specific strains used for microbiological quality control are not clinically significant. For the diffusion technique, the 10-µg ertapenem disk should provide the following zone diameters in these laboratory quality control strains:

Microorganism	Zone Diameter Range (mm)
Escherichia coli ATCC 25922	29–36
Haemophilus influenzae[m] ATCC 49766	27–33
Pseudomonas aeruginosa ATCC 27853	13–21
Staphylococcus aureus ATCC 25923	24–31
Streptococcus pneumoniae[n] ATCC 49619	28–35

[m]This quality control range is applicable to *Haemophilus influenzae* ATCC 49766 tested by disk diffusion using HTM[2] agar inoculated with a direct colony suspension and incubated in 5% CO_2 at 35°C for 16–18 hrs.
[n]This quality control range is applicable to *Streptococcus pneumoniae* ATCC 49619 tested by disk diffusion using Mueller-Hinton agar supplemented with 5% sheep blood inoculated with a direct colony suspension and incubated in 5% CO_2 at 35°C for 20–24 hrs.

Anaerobic Techniques:
For anaerobic bacteria, the susceptibility to ertapenem as MICs can be determined by standardized test methods[3]. The MIC values obtained should be interpreted according to the following criteria:

MIC (µg/mL)	Interpretation
≤4.0	Susceptible (S)
8.0	Intermediate (I)
≥16.0	Resistant (R)

Interpretation is identical to that stated above for results using dilution techniques.
As with other susceptibility techniques, the use of laboratory control microorganisms is required to control the technical aspects of the laboratory standardized procedures. Standardized ertapenem powder should provide the following MIC values:

Microorganism	MIC[o] (µg/mL)
Bacteroides fragilis ATCC 25285	0.06–0.25
Bacteroides thetaiotaomicron ATCC 29741	0.25–1.0
Eubacterium lentum ATCC 43055	0.5–2.0

[o]These quality control ranges are applicable only to agar dilution using *Brucella* agar supplemented with hemin, vitamin K1 and 5% defibrinated or laked sheep blood inoculated with a direct colony suspension or a 6- to 24-hour fresh culture in enriched thioglycollate medium and incubated in an anaerobic jar or chamber at 35–37°C for 42–48 hrs.

INDICATIONS AND USAGE

INVANZ is indicated for the treatment of adult patients with the following moderate to severe infections caused by susceptible strains of the designated microorganisms. (See DOSAGE AND ADMINISTRATION):
Complicated Intra-abdominal Infections due to *Escherichia coli, Clostridium clostridioforme, Eubacterium lentum, Peptostreptococcus* species, *Bacteroides fragilis, Bacteroides distasonis, Bacteroides ovatus, Bacteroides thetaiotaomicron,* or *Bacteroides uniformis*..
Complicated Skin and Skin Structure Infections due to *Staphylococcus aureus* (methicillin susceptible strains only), *Streptococcus pyogenes, Escherichia coli,* or *Peptostreptococcus* species.
Community Acquired Pneumonia due to *Streptococcus pneumoniae* (penicillin susceptible strains only) including cases with concurrent bacteremia, *Haemophilus influenzae* (beta-lactamase negative strains only), or *Moraxella catarrhalis*.
Complicated Urinary Tract Infections including pyelonephritis due to *Escherichia coli,* including cases with concurrent bacteremia, or *Klebsiella pneumoniae*.
Acute Pelvic Infections including postpartum endomyometritis, septic abortion and post surgical gynecologic infections due to *Streptococcus agalactiae, Escherichia coli, Bacteroides fragilis, Porphyromonas asaccharolytica, Peptostreptococcus* species, or *Prevotella bivia*.
Appropriate specimens for bacteriological examination should be obtained in order to isolate and identify the causative organisms and to determine their susceptibility to ertapenem. Therapy with INVANZ (ertapenem) may be initiated empirically before results of these tests are known; once results become available, antimicrobial therapy should be adjusted accordingly.
To reduce the development of drug-resistant bacteria and maintain the effectiveness of INVANZ and other antibacterial drugs, INVANZ should be used only to treat or prevent infections that are proven or strongly suspected to be caused by susceptible bacteria. When culture and susceptibility information are available, they should be considered in selecting or modifying antibacterial therapy. In the absence of such data, local epidemiology and susceptibility patterns may contribute to the empiric selection of therapy.

CONTRAINDICATIONS

INVANZ is contraindicated in patients with known hypersensitivity to any component of this product or to other drugs in the same class or in patients who have demonstrated anaphylactic reactions to beta-lactams.
Due to the use of lidocaine HCl as a diluent, INVANZ administered intramuscularly is contraindicated in patients with a known hypersensitivity to local anesthetics of the amide type. (Refer to the prescribing information for lidocaine HCl.)

WARNINGS

SERIOUS AND OCCASIONALLY FATAL HYPERSENSITIVITY (ANAPHYLACTIC) REACTIONS HAVE BEEN REPORTED IN PATIENTS RECEIVING THERAPY WITH BETA-LACTAMS. THESE REACTIONS ARE MORE LIKELY TO OCCUR IN INDIVIDUALS WITH A HISTORY OF SENSITIVITY TO MULTIPLE ALLERGENS. THERE HAVE BEEN REPORTS OF INDIVIDUALS WITH A HISTORY OF PENICILLIN HYPERSENSITIVITY WHO HAVE EXPERIENCED SEVERE HYPERSENSITIVITY REACTIONS WHEN TREATED WITH ANOTHER BETA-LACTAM. BEFORE INITIATING THERAPY WITH INVANZ, CAREFUL INQUIRY SHOULD BE MADE CONCERNING PREVIOUS HYPERSENSITIVITY REACTIONS TO PENICILLINS, CEPHALOSPORINS, OTHER BETA-LACTAMS AND OTHER ALLERGENS. IF AN ALLERGIC REACTION TO INVANZ OCCURS, DISCONTINUE THE DRUG IMMEDIATELY. **SERIOUS ANAPHYLACTIC REACTIONS REQUIRE IMMEDIATE EMERGENCY TREATMENT WITH EPINEPHRINE, OXYGEN, INTRAVENOUS STEROIDS, AND AIRWAY MANAGEMENT, INCLUDING INTUBATION. OTHER THERAPY MAY ALSO BE ADMINISTERED AS INDICATED.**
Seizures and other CNS adverse experiences have been reported during treatment with INVANZ. (See PRECAUTIONS and ADVERSE REACTIONS.)
Pseudomembranous colitis has been reported with nearly all antibacterial agents, including ertapenem, and may range in severity from mild to life-threatening. Therefore, it is important to consider this diagnosis in patients who present with diarrhea subsequent to the administration of antibacterial agents.
Treatment with antibacterial agents alters the normal flora of the colon and may permit overgrowth of clostridia. Studies indicate that a toxin produced by *Clostridium difficile* is a primary cause of "antibiotic-associated colitis".
After the diagnosis of pseudomembranous colitis has been established, therapeutic measures should be initiated. Mild cases of pseudomembranous colitis usually respond to drug discontinuation alone. In moderate to severe cases, consideration should be given to management with fluids and electrolytes, protein supplementation and treatment with an antibacterial drug clinically effective against *Clostridium difficile* colitis.
Lidocaine HCl is the diluent for intramuscular administration of INVANZ. Refer to the prescribing information for lidocaine HCl.

PRECAUTIONS

General
During clinical investigations in adult patients treated with INVANZ (1 g once a day), seizures, irrespective of drug relationship, occurred in 0.5% of patients during study therapy plus 14-day follow-up period. (See ADVERSE REACTIONS.) These experiences have occurred most commonly in patients with CNS disorders (e.g., brain lesions or history of seizures) and/or comprised renal function. Close adherence to the recommended dosage regimen is urged, especially in patients with known factors that predispose to convulsive activity. Anticonvulsant therapy should be continued in patients with known seizure disorders. If focal tremors, myoclonus, or seizures occur, patients should be evaluated neurologically, placed on anticonvulsant therapy if not already instituted, and the dosage of INVANZ reexamined to determine whether it should be decreased or the antibiotic discontinued. Dosage adjustment of INVANZ is recommended in patients with reduced renal function. (See DOSAGE AND ADMINISTRATION.)
As with other antibiotics, prolonged use of INVANZ may result in overgrowth of non-suspectible organisms. Repeated evaluation of the patient's condition is essential. If superinfection occurs during therapy, appropriate measures should be taken.
Prescribing INVANZ in the absence of a proven or strongly suspected bacterial infection or a prophylactic indication is unlikely to provide benefit to the patient and increases the risk of the development of drug-resistant bacteria.
Caution should be taken when administering INVANZ intramuscularly to avoid inadvertent injection into a blood vessel. (See DOSAGE AND ADMINISTRATION.)
Lidocaine HCl is the diluent for intramuscular administration of INVANZ. Refer to the prescribing information for lidocaine HCl for additional precautions.
Information for patients
Patients should be counseled that antibacterial drugs including INVANZ should only be used to treat bacterial infections. They do not treat viral infections (e.g., the common cold). When INVANZ is prescribed to treat a bacterial infection, patients should be told that although it is common to

Continued on next page

Information on the Merck & Co., Inc., products listed on these pages is from the prescribing information in use October 1, 2004. For information, please call 1-800-NSC-MERCK [1-800-672-6372].

Invanz—Cont.

feel better early in the course of therapy, the medication should be taken exactly as directed. Skipping doses or not completing the full course of therapy may (1) decrease the effectiveness of the immediate treatment and (2) increase the likelihood that bacteria will develop resistance and will not be treatable by INVANZ or other antibacterial drugs in the future.

Laboratory Tests

While INVANZ possesses toxicity similar to the beta-lactam group of antibiotics, periodic assessment of organ system function, including renal, hepatic, and hematopoietic, is advisable during prolonged therapy.

Drug Interactions

When ertapenem is co-administered with probenecid (500 mg p.o. every 6 hours), probenecid competes for active tubular secretion and reduces the renal clearance of ertapenem. Based on total ertapenem concentrations, probenecid increased the AUC by 25% and reduced the plasma and renal clearances by 20% and 35%, respectively. The half-life increased from 4.0 to 4.8 hours. Because of the small effect on half-life, the coadministration with probenecid to extend the half-life of ertapenem is not recommended.

In vitro studies indicate that ertapenem does not inhibit P-glycoprotein-mediated transport of digoxin or vinblastine and that ertapenem is not a substrate for P-glycoprotein-mediated transport. *In vitro* studies in human liver microsomes indicate that ertapenem does not inhibit metabolism mediated by any of the following six cytochrome p450 (CYP) isoforms: 1A2, 2C9, 2C19, 2D6, 2E1 and 3A4. Drug interactions caused by inhibition of P-glycoprotein-mediated drug clearance or CYP-mediated drug clearance with the listed isoforms are unlikely. (See CLINICAL PHARMACOLOGY, *Distribution* and *Metabolism*.)

Other than with probenecid, no specific clinical drug interaction studies have been conducted.

Carcinogenesis, Mutagenesis, Impairment of Fertility

No long-term studies in animals have been performed to evaluate the carcinogenic potential of ertapenem.

Ertapenem was neither mutagenic nor genotoxic in the following *in vitro* assays: alkaline elution/rat hepatocyte assay, chromosomal aberration assay in Chinese hamster ovary cells, and TK6 human lymphoblastoid cell mutagenesis assay; and in the *in vivo* mouse micronucleus assay.

In mice and rats, IV doses of up to 700 mg/kg/day (for mice, approximately 3 times the recommended human dose of 1 g based on body surface area and for rats, approximately 1.2 times the human exposure at the recommended dose of 1 g based on plasma AUCs) resulted in no effects on mating performance, fecundity, fertility, or embryonic survival.

Pregnancy: Teratogenic Effects

Pregnancy Category B: In mice and rats given IV doses of up to 700 mg/kg/day (for mice, approximately 3 times the recommended human dose of 1 g based on body surface area and for rats, approximately 1.2 times the human exposure at the recommended dose of 1 g based on plasma AUCs), there was no evidence of developmental toxicity as assessed by external, visceral, and skeletal examination of the fetuses. However, in mice given 700 mg/kg/day, slight decreases in average fetal weights and an associated decrease in the average number of ossified sacrocaudal vertebrae were observed. Ertapenem crosses the placental barrier in rats.

There are, however, no adequate and well-controlled studies in pregnant women. Because animal reproduction studies are not always predictive of human response, this drug should be used during pregnancy only if clearly needed.

Nursing Mothers

Ertapenem is excreted in human breast milk. (See CLINICAL PHARMACOLOGY, *Distribution*.) Caution should be exercised when INVANZ is administered to a nursing woman. INVANZ should be administered to nursing mothers only when the expected benefit outweighs the risk.

Labor and delivery

INVANZ has not been studied for use during labor and delivery.

Pediatric Use

Safety and effectiveness in pediatric patients have not been established. Therefore, use in patients under 18 years of age is not recommended.

Geriatric Use

Of the 1,835 patients in Phase llb/lll studies treated with INVANZ, approximately 26 percent were 65 and over, while approximately 12 percent were 75 and over. No overall differences in safety or effectiveness were observed between these patients and younger patients. Other reported clinical experience has not identified differences in responses between the elderly and younger patients, but greater sensitivity of some older individuals cannot be ruled out.

This drug is known to be substantially excreted by the kidney, and the risk of toxic reactions to this drug may be greater in patients with impaired renal function. Because elderly patients are more likely to have decreased renal function, care should be taken in dose selection, and it may be useful to monitor renal function. (See DOSAGE AND ADMINISTRATION.)

Hepatic Insufficiency

The pharmacokinetics of ertapenem in patients with hepatic insufficiency have not been established. Of the total number of patients in clinical studies, 37 patients receiving ertapenem 1 g daily and 36 patients receiving comparator drugs were considered to have Child-Pugh Class A, B, or C liver impairment. The incidence of adverse experiences in patients with hepatic impairment was similar between the ertapenem group and the comparator groups.

ANIMAL PHARMACOLOGY

In repeat-dose studies in rats, treatment-related neutropenia occurred at every dose-level tested, including the lowest dose (2 mg/kg, 12 mg/m^2).

Studies in rabbits and Rhesus monkeys were inconclusive with regard to the effect on neutrophil counts.

ADVERSE REACTIONS

Clinical studies enrolled 1954 patients treated with ertapenem; in some of the clinical studies, parenteral therapy was followed by a switch to an appropriate oral antimicrobial. (See CLINICAL STUDIES.) Most adverse experiences reported in these clinical studies were described as mild to moderate in severity. Ertapenem was discontinued due to adverse experiences in 4.7% of patients. Table 3 shows the incidence of adverse experiences reported in ≥1.0% of patients in these studies. The most common drug-related adverse experiences in patients treated with INVANZ, including those who were switched to therapy with an oral antimicrobial, were diarrhea (5.5%), infused vein complication (3.7%), nausea (3.1%), headache (2.2%), vaginitis in females (2.1%), phlebitis/thrombophlebitis (1.3%), and vomiting (1.1%).

[See table 3 below]

Table 3
Incidence (%) of Adverse Experiences Reported
During Study Therapy Plus 14-Day Follow-Up in ≥1.0% of Patients
Treated With INVANZ in Clinical Studies

Adverse Events	INVANZ* 1 g daily (N=802)	Piperacillin/ Tazobactam* 3.375 g q6h (N=774)	INVANZ† 1 g daily (N=1152)	Ceftriaxone† 1 or 2 g daily (N=942)
Local:				
Extravasation	1.9	1.7	0.7	1.1
Infused vein complication	7.1	7.9	5.4	6.7
Phlebitis/thrombophlebitis	1.9	2.7	1.6	2.0
Systemic:				
Asthenia/fatigue	1.2	0.9	1.2	1.1
Death	2.5	1.6	1.3	1.6
Edema/swelling	3.4	2.5	2.9	3.3
Fever	5.0	6.6	2.3	3.4
Abdominal pain	3.6	4.8	4.3	3.9
Chest pain	1.5	1.4	1.0	2.5
Hypertension	1.6	1.4	0.7	1.0
Hypotension	2.0	1.4	1.0	1.2
Tachycardia	1.6	1.3	1.3	0.7
Acid regurgitation	1.6	0.9	1.1	0.6
Oral candidiasis	0.1	1.3	1.4	1.9
Constipation	4.0	5.4	3.3	3.1
Diarrhea	10.3	12.1	9.2	9.8
Dyspepsia	1.1	0.6	1.0	1.6
Nausea	8.5	8.7	6.4	7.4
Vomiting	3.7	5.3	4.0	4.0
Leg pain	1.1	0.5	0.4	0.3
Anxiety	1.4	1.3	0.8	1.2
Altered mental status‡	5.1	3.4	3.3	2.5
Dizziness	2.1	3.0	1.5	2.1
Headache	5.6	5.4	6.8	6.9
Insomnia	3.2	5.2	3.0	4.1
Cough	1.6	1.7	1.3	0.5
Dyspnea	2.6	1.8	1.0	2.4
Pharyngitis	0.7	1.4	1.1	0.6
Rales/rhonchi	1.1	1.0	0.5	1.0
Respiratory distress	1.0	0.4	0.2	0.2
Erythema	1.6	1.7	1.2	1.2
Pruritus	2.0	2.6	1.0	1.9
Rash	2.5	3.1	2.3	1.5
Vaginitis	1.4	1.0	3.3	3.7

* Includes Phase IIb/III Complicated intra-abdominal infections, Complicated skin and skin structure infections and Acute pelvic infections studies

† Includes Phase IIb/III Community acquired pneumonia and Complicated urinary tract infections, and Phase IIa studies

‡ Includes agitation, confusion, disorientation, decreased mental acuity, changed mental status, somnolence, stupor

In patients treated for complicated intra-abdominal infections, death occurred in 4.7% (15/316) of patients receiving ertapenem and 2.6% (8/307) of patients receiving comparator drug. These deaths occurred in patients with significant co-morbidity and/or severe baseline infections. Deaths were considered unrelated to study drugs by investigators.

In clinical studies, seizure was reported during study therapy plus 14-day follow-up period in 0.5% of patients treated with ertapenem, 0.3% of patients treated with piperacillin/tazobactam and 0% of patients treated with ceftriaxone. (See PRECAUTIONS.)

Additional adverse experiences that were reported with INVANZ with an incidence >0.1% within each body system are listed below:

Body as a whole: abdominal distention, pain, chills, septicemia, septic shock, dehydration, gout, malaise, necrosis, candidiasis, weight loss, facial edema, injection site induration, injection site pain, flank pain, and syncope;

Cardiovascular System: heart failure, hematoma, cardiac arrest, bradycardia, arrhythmia, atrial fibrillation, heart murmur, ventricular tachycardia, asystole, and subdural hemorrhage;

Digestive System: gastrointestinal hemorrhage, anorexia, flatulence, *C. difficile* associated diarrhea, stomatitis, dysphagia, hemorrhoids, ileus, cholelithiasis, duodenitis, esophagitis, gastritis, jaundice, mouth ulcer, pancreatitis, and pyloric stenosis;

Nervous System & Psychiatric: nervousness, seizure (see WARNINGS and PRECAUTIONS), tremor, depression, hypesthesia, spasm, paresthesia, aggressive behavior, and vertigo;

Respiratory System: pleural effusion, hypoxemia, bronchoconstriction, pharyngeal discomfort, epistaxis, pleuritic pain, asthma, hemoptysis, hiccups, and voice disturbance;

Skin & Skin Appendage: sweating, dermatitis, desquamation, flushing, and urticaria;

Special Senses: taste perversion;

Urogenital System: renal insufficiency, oliguria/anuria, vaginal pruritus, hematuria, urinary retention, bladder dysfunction, vaginal candidiasis, and vulvovaginitis.

Post-Marketing Experience:

The following post-marketing adverse experiences have been reported:

Immune System: anaphylaxis including anaphylactoid reactions

Nervous System & Psychiatric: hallucinations

Adverse Laboratory Changes

Laboratory adverse experiences that were reported during therapy in ≥1.0% of patients treated with INVANZ in clinical studies are presented in Table 4. Drug-related laboratory adverse experiences that were reported during therapy in ≥1.0% of patients treated with INVANZ, including those who were switched to therapy with an oral antimicrobial, in clinical studies were ALT increased (6.0%), AST increased (5.2%), serum alkaline phosphatase increased (3.4%), platelet count increased (2.8%), and eosinophils increased (1.1%). Ertapenem was discontinued due to laboratory adverse experiences in 0.3% of patients.

[See table 4 at top of next page]

Additional laboratory adverse experiences that were reported during therapy in >0.1% but <1.0% of patients treated with INVANZ in clinical studies include: increases in BUN, direct and indirect serum bilirubin, serum sodium, monocytes, PTT, urine epithelial cells; decreases in serum bicarbonate.

OVERDOSAGE

No specific information is available on the treatment of overdosage with INVANZ. Intentional overdosing of

INVANZ is unlikely. Intravenous administration of INVANZ at a dose of 2 g over 30 min or 3 g over 1–2h in healthy volunteers resulted in an increased incidence of nausea. In clinical studies, inadvertent administration of three 1 g doses of INVANZ in a 24 hour period resulted in diarrhea and transient dizziness in one patient.
In the event of an overdose, INVANZ should be discontinued and general supportive treatment given until renal elimination takes place.
INVANZ can be removed by hemodialysis; the plasma clearance of the total fraction of ertapenem was increased 30% in subjects with end-stage renal insufficiency when hemodialysis (4 hour session) was performed immediately following administration. However, no information is available on the use of hemodialysis to treat overdosage.

DOSAGE AND ADMINISTRATION

The dose of INVANZ in adults is 1 gram (g) given once a day. INVANZ may be administered by intravenous infusion for up to 14 days or intramuscular injection for up to 7 days. When administered intravenously, INVANZ should be infused over a period of 30 minutes.
Intramuscular administration of INVANZ may be used as an alternative to intravenous administration in the treatment of those infections for which intramuscular therapy is appropriate.
DO NOT MIX OR CO-INFUSE INVANZ WITH OTHER MEDICATIONS. DO NOT USE DILUENTS CONTAINING DEXTROSE (α-D-GLUCOSE).
Table 5 presents dosage guidelines for INVANZ.
[See table 5 at right]
Patients with Renal Insufficiency: INVANZ may be used for the treatment of infections in patients with renal insufficiency. In patients whose creatinine clearance is >30 mL/min/1.73 m^2, no dosage adjustment is necessary. Patients with advanced renal insufficiency (creatinine clearance ≤30 mL/min/1.73 m^2) and end-stage renal insufficiency (creatinine clearance ≤10 mL/min/1.73 m^2) should receive 500 mg daily.
Patients on Hemodialysis: When patients on hemodialysis are given the recommended daily dose of 500 mg of INVANZ within 6 hours prior to hemodialysis, a supplementary dose of 150 mg is recommended following the hemodialysis session. If INVANZ is given at least 6 hours prior to hemodialysis, no supplementary dose is needed. There are no data in patients undergoing peritoneal dialysis or hemofiltration.
When only the serum creatinine is available, the following formula** may be used to estimate creatinine clearance. The serum creatinine should represent a steady state of renal function.

$$\text{Males: } \frac{(\text{weight in kg}) \times (140\text{-age in years})}{(72) \times \text{serum creatinine (mg/100 mL)}}$$

Females: (0.85) × (value calculated for males)

Patients with Hepatic Insufficiency: No dose adjustment recommendations can be made in patients with impaired hepatic function. (See CLINICAL PHARMACOLOGY, *Special Populations, Hepatic Insufficiency* and PRECAUTIONS.)
No dosage adjustment is recommended based on age or gender. (See CLINICAL PHARMACOLOGY, *Special Populations.*)

** Cockcroft and Gault equation: Cockcroft DW, Gault MH. Prediction of creatinine clearance from serum creatinine. Nephron. 1976

PREPARATION OF SOLUTION
Preparation for intravenous administration:
DO NOT MIX OR CO-INFUSE INVANZ WITH OTHER MEDICATIONS. DO NOT USE DILUENTS CONTAINING DEXTROSE (α-D-GLUCOSE).
INVANZ MUST BE RECONSTITUTED AND THEN DILUTED PRIOR TO ADMINISTRATION.

1. Reconstitute the contents of a 1 g vial of INVANZ with 10 mL of one of the following: Water for Injection, 0.9% Sodium Chloride Injection or Bacteriostatic Water for Injection.
2. Shake well to dissolve and immediately transfer contents of the reconstituted vial to 50 mL of 0.9% Sodium Chloride Injection.
3. Complete the infusion within 6 hours of reconstitution.

Preparation for intramuscular administration:
INVANZ MUST BE RECONSTITUTED PRIOR TO ADMINISTRATION.

1. Reconstitute the contents of a 1 g vial of INVANZ with 3.2 mL of 1.0% lidocaine HCl injection*** **(without epinephrine)**. Shake vial thoroughly to form solution.
2. Immediately withdraw the contents of the vial and administer by deep intramuscular injection into a large muscle mass (such as the gluteal muscles or lateral part of the thigh).
3. The reconstituted IM solution should be used within 1 hour after preparation. **NOTE: THE RECONSTITUTED SOLUTION SHOULD NOT BE ADMINISTERED INTRAVENOUSLY.**

Parenteral drug products should be inspected visually for particulate matter and discoloration prior to use, whenever solution and container permit. Solutions of INVANZ range from colorless to pale yellow. Variations of color within this range do not affect the potency of the product.

Table 4
Incidence* (%) of Specific Laboratory Adverse Experiences Reported During Study Therapy Plus 14-Day Follow-Up in ≥1.0% of Patients Treated With INVANZ in Clinical Studies

Adverse laboratory experiences	INVANZ‡ 1 g daily (n†=766)	Piperacillin/ Tazobactam‡ 3.375 g q6h (n†=755)	INVANZ§ 1 g daily (n†=1122)	Ceftriaxone§ 1 or 2 g daily (n†=920)
ALT increased	8.8	7.3	8.3	6.9
AST increased	8.4	8.3	7.1	6.5
Serum albumin decreased	1.7	1.5	0.9	1.6
Serum alkaline phosphatase increased	6.6	7.2	4.3	2.8
Serum creatinine increased	1.1	2.7	0.9	1.2
Serum glucose increased	1.2	2.3	1.7	2.0
Serum potassium decreased	1.7	2.8	1.8	2.4
Serum potassium increased	1.3	0.5	0.5	0.7
Total serum bilirubin increased	1.7	1.4	0.6	1.1
Eosinophils increased	1.1	1.1	2.1	1.8
Hematocrit decreased	3.0	2.9	3.4	2.4
Hemoglobin decreased	4.9	4.7	4.5	3.5
Platelet count decreased	1.1	1.2	1.1	1.0
Platelet count increased	6.5	6.3	4.3	3.5
Segmented neutrophils decreased	1.0	0.3	1.5	0.8
Prothrombin time increased	1.2	2.0	0.3	0.9
WBC decreased	0.8	0.7	1.5	1.4
Urine RBCs increased	2.5	2.9	1.1	1.0
Urine WBCs increased	2.5	3.2	1.6	1.1

* Number of patients with laboratory adverse experiences/Number of patients with the laboratory test
† Number of patients with one or more laboratory tests
‡ Includes Phase IIb/III Complicated intra-abdominal infections, Complicated skin and skin structure infections and Acute pelvic infections studies
§ Includes Phase IIb/III Community acquired pneumonia and Complicated urinary tract infections, and Phase IIa studies

Table 5
Dosage Guidelines for Adults With Normal Renal Function* and Body Weight

Infection†	Daily Dose (IV or IM)	Recommended Duration of Total Antimcirobial Treatment
Complicated intra-abdominal infections	1 g	5 to 14 days
Complicated skin and skin structure infections	1 g	7 to 14 days
Community acquired pneumonia	1 g	10 to 14 days‡
Complicated urinary tract infections, including pyelonephritis	1 g	10 to 14 days‡
Acute pelvic infections including postpartum endomyometritis, septic abortion and post surgical gynecologic infections	1 g	3 to 10 days

* defined as creatinine clearance >90 mL/min/1.73 m^2
† due to the designated pathogens (see INDICATIONS AND USAGE)
‡ duration includes a possible switch to an appropraite oral therapy, after at least 3 days of parenteral therapy, once clinical improvement has been demonstrated.

***Refer to the prescribing information for lidocaine HCl.

STORAGE AND STABILITY
Before reconstitution
Do not store lyophilized powder above 25°C (77°F).
Reconstituted and infusion solutions
The reconstituted solution, immediately diluted in 0.9% Sodium Chloride Injection (see DOSAGE AND ADMINISTRATION, PREPARATION OF SOLUTION), **may be stored at room temperature (25°C) and used within 6 hours or stored for 24 hours under refrigeration (5°C) and used within 4 hours after removal from refrigeration. Solutions of INVANZ should not be frozen.**

HOW SUPPLIED

INVANZ is supplied as a sterile lyophilized powder in single dose vials containing ertapenem for intravenous infusion or for intramuscular injection as follows:
No. 3843—1 g ertapenem equivalent
NDC 0006-3843-71 in trays of 10 vials
No. 3843—1 g ertapenem equivalent
NDC 0006-3843-45 in trays of 25 vials.

CLINICAL STUDIES

Complicated Intra-Abdominal Infections
Ertapenem was evaluated in adults for the treatment of complicated intra-abdominal infections in a clinical trial. This study compared ertapenem (1 g intravenously once a day) with piperacillin/tazobactam (3.375 g intravenously every 6 hours) for 5 to 14 days and enrolled 665 patients with localized complicated appendicitis, and any other complicated intra-abdominal infection including colonic, small intestinal, and biliary infections and generalized peritonitis. The combined clinical and microbiologic success rates in the microbiologically evaluable population at 4 to 6 weeks posttherapy (test of cure) were 83.6% (163/195) for ertapenem and 80.4% (152/189) for piperacillin/tazobactam.
Complicated Skin and Skin Structure Infections
Ertapenem was evaluated in adults for the treatment of complicated skin and skin structure infections in a clinical trial. This study compared ertapenem (1 g intravenously once a day) with piperacillin/tazobactam (3.375 g intravenously every 6 hours) for 7 to 14 days and enrolled 540 patients including patients with deep soft tissue abscess, posttraumatic wound infection and cellulitis with purulent drainage. The clinical success rates at 10 to 21 days posttherapy (test of cure) were 83.9% (141/168) for ertapenem and 85.3% (145/170) for piperacillin/tazobactam.
Community Acquired Pneumonia
Ertapenem was evaluated in adults for the treatment of community acquired pneumonia in two clinical trials. Both studies compared ertapenem (1 g parenterally once a day) with ceftriaxone (1 g parenterally once a day) and enrolled a total of 866 patients. Both regimens allowed the option to switch to oral amoxicillin/clavulanate for a total of 10 to 14 days of treatment (parenteral and oral). In the first study the primary efficacy parameter was the clinical success rate in the clinically evaluable population and success rates were 92.3% (168/182) for ertapenem and 91.0% (183/201) for ceftriaxone at 7 to 14 days posttherapy (test of cure). In the second study the primary efficacy parameter was the clinical success rates in the microbiologically evaluable population and success rates were 91% (91/100) for ertapenem and 91.8% (45/49) for ceftriaxone at 7 to 14 days posttherapy (test of cure).
Complicated Urinary Tract Infections Including Pyelonephritis
Ertapenem was evaluated in adults for the treatment of complicated urinary tract infections including pyelonephritis in two clinical trials. Both studies compared ertapenem (1 g parenterally once a day) with ceftriaxone (1 g parenterally once a day) and enrolled a total of 850 patients. Both regimens allowed the option to switch to oral ciprofloxacin (500 mg twice daily) for a total of 10 to 14 days of treatment (parenteral and oral). The microbiological success rates (combined studies) at 5 to 9 days posttherapy (test of cure) were 89.5% (229/256) for ertapenem and 91.1% (204/224) for ceftriaxone.
Acute Pelvic Infections Including Endomyometritis, Septic Abortion And Post-Surgical Gynecological Infections
Ertapenem was evaluated in adults for the treatment of acute pelvic infections in a clinical trial. This study com-

Continued on next page

Information on the Merck & Co., Inc., products listed on these pages is from the prescribing information in use October 1, 2004. For information, please call 1-800-NSC-MERCK [1-800-672-6372].

Invanz—Cont.

pared ertapenem (1 g intravenously once a day) with piperacillin/tazobactam (3.375 g intravenously every 6 hours) for 3 to 10 days and enrolled 412 patients including 350 patients with obstetric/postpartum infections and 45 patients with septic abortion. The clinical success rates in the clinically evaluable population at 2 to 4 weeks posttherapy (test of cure) were 93.9% (153/163) for ertapenem and 91.5% (140/153) for piperacillin/tazobactam.

REFERENCES

1. National Committee for Clinical Laboratory Standards. Methods for Dilution Antimicrobial Susceptibility Tests for Bacteria that Grow Aerobically. Fifth Edition; Approved Standard, NCCLS Document M7-A5, Vol. 17, No. 2 NCCLS, Wayne, PA, December 2000.
2. National Committee for Clinical Laboratory Standards. Performance Standards for Antimicrobial Disk Susceptibility Tests. Seventh Edition; Approved Standard, NCCLS Document M2-A7, Vol. 17, No. 1 NCCLS, Wayne, PA, January 2000.
3. National Committee for Clinical Laboratory Standards. *Methods for Antimicrobial Susceptibility Testing of Anaerobic Bacteria* - Fourth Edition; Approved Standard, NCCLS Document M11-A4, Vol. 17, No. 22. NCCLS, Wayne, PA, December 1997.
4. National Committee for Clinical Laboratory Standards. Performance Standards for Antimicrobial Susceptibility Testing - Eleventh Informational Supplement. Approved Standard, NCCLS Document M100-S11, Vol. 21, No. 1. NCCLS, Wayne, PA, January 2001.

MERCK & CO., INC., Whitehouse Station, NJ 08889, USA
9500003 Issued April 2004

LACRISERT® Sterile Ophthalmic Insert ℞
(hydroxypropyl cellulose ophthalmic insert)

DESCRIPTION

LACRISERT* (hydroxypropyl cellulose ophthalmic insert) is a sterile, translucent, rod-shaped, water soluble, ophthalmic insert made of hydroxypropyl cellulose, for administration into the inferior cul-de-sac of the eye.

The chemical name for hydroxypropyl cellulose is cellulose, 2-hydroxypropyl ether. It is an ether of cellulose in which hydroxypropyl groups ($-CH_2CHOHCH_3$) are attached to the hydroxyls present in the anhydroglucose rings of cellulose by ether linkages. A representative structure of the monomer is:

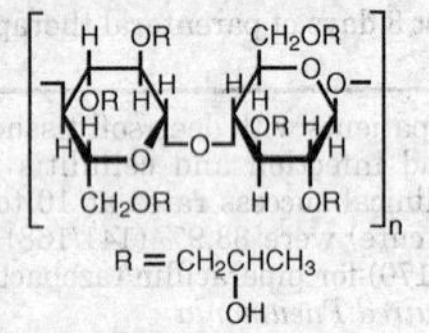

$R = CH_2CHCH_3$ (with OH on the CH)

The molecular weight is typically 1×10^6.

Hydroxypropyl cellulose is an off-white, odorless, tasteless powder. It is soluble in water below 38°C, and in many polar organic solvents such as ethanol, propylene glycol, dioxane, methanol, isopropyl alcohol (95%), dimethyl sulfoxide, and dimethyl formamide.

Each LACRISERT is 5 mg of hydroxypropyl cellulose. LACRISERT contains no preservatives or other ingredients. It is about 1.27 mm in diameter by about 3.5 mm long.

LACRISERT is supplied in packages of 60 units, together with illustrated instructions and a special applicator for removing LACRISERT from the unit dose blister and inserting it into the eye. A spare applicator is included in each package.

*Registered trademark of MERCK & CO., Inc.

CLINICAL PHARMACOLOGY

Pharmacodynamics

LACRISERT acts to stabilize and thicken the precorneal tear film and prolong the tear film breakup time which is usually accelerated in patients with dry eye states. LACRISERT also acts to lubricate and protect the eye.

LACRISERT usually reduces the signs and symptoms resulting from moderate to severe dry eye syndromes, such as conjunctival hyperemia, corneal and conjunctival staining with rose bengal, exudation, itching, burning, foreign body sensation, smarting, photophobia, dryness and blurred or cloudy vision. Progressive visual deterioration which occurs in some patients may be retarded, halted, or sometimes reversed.

In a multicenter crossover study the 5 mg LACRISERT administered once a day during the waking hours was compared to artificial tears used four or more times daily. There was a prolongation of tear film breakup time and a decrease in foreign body sensation associated with dry eye syndrome in patients during treatment with inserts as compared to artificial tears; these findings were statistically significantly different between the treatment groups. Improvement, as measured by amelioration of symptoms, by slit-lamp examination and by rose bengal staining of the cornea and conjunctiva, was greater in most patients with moderate to severe symptoms during treatment with LACRISERT. Patient comfort was usually better with LACRISERT than with artificial tears solution, and most patients preferred LACRISERT.

In most patients treated with LACRISERT for over one year, improvement was observed as evidenced by amelioration of symptoms generally associated with keratoconjunctivitis sicca such as burning, tearing, foreign body sensation, itching, photophobia and blurred or cloudy vision.

During studies in healthy volunteers, a thickened precorneal tear film was usually observed through the slit-lamp while LACRISERT was present in the conjunctival sac.

Pharmacokinetics and Metabolism

Hydroxypropyl cellulose is a physiologically inert substance. In a study of rats fed hydroxypropyl cellulose or unmodified cellulose at levels up to 5% of their diet, it was found that the two were biologically equivalent in that neither was metabolized.

Studies conducted in rats fed ^{14}C-labeled hydroxypropyl cellulose demonstrated that when orally administered, hydroxypropyl cellulose is not absorbed from the gastrointestinal tract and is quantitatively excreted in the feces.

Dissolution studies in rabbits showed that hydroxypropyl cellulose inserts became softer within 1 hour after they were placed in the conjunctival sac. Most of the inserts dissolved completely in 14 to 18 hours; with a single exception, all had disappeared by 24 hours after insertion. Similar dissolution of the inserts was observed during prolonged administration (up to 54 weeks).

INDICATIONS AND USAGE

LACRISERT is indicated in patients with moderate to severe dry eye syndromes, including keratoconjunctivitis sicca. LACRISERT is indicated especially in patients who remain symptomatic after an adequate trial of therapy with artificial tear solutions.

LACRISERT is also indicated for patients with:
- Exposure keratitis
- Decreased corneal sensitivity
- Recurrent corneal erosions

CONTRAINDICATIONS

LACRISERT is contraindicated in patients who are hypersensitive to hydroxypropyl cellulose.

WARNINGS

Instructions for inserting and removing LACRISERT should be carefully followed.

PRECAUTIONS

General

If improperly placed, LACRISERT may result in corneal abrasion (see DOSAGE AND ADMINISTRATION).

Information for Patients

Patients should be advised to follow the instructions for using LACRISERT which accompany the package.

Because this product may produce transient blurring of vision, patients should be instructed to exercise caution when operating hazardous machinery or driving a motor vehicle.

Drug Interactions

Application of hydroxypropyl cellulose ophthalmic inserts to the eyes of unanesthetized rabbits immediately prior to or two hours before instilling pilocarpine, proparacaine HCl (0.5%), or phenylephrine (5%) did not markedly alter the magnitude and/or duration of the miotic, local corneal anesthetic, or mydriatic activity, respectively, of these agents.

Under various treatment schedules, the anti-inflammatory effect of ocularly instilled dexamethasone (0.1%) in unanesthetized rabbits with primary uveitis was not affected by the presence of hydroxypropyl cellulose inserts.

Carcinogenesis, Mutagenesis, Impairment of Fertility

Feeding of hydroxypropyl cellulose to rats at levels up to 5% of their diet produced no gross or histopathologic changes or other deleterious effects.

Pediatric Use

Safety and effectiveness in pediatric patients have not been established.

Geriatric Use

No overall differences in safety or effectiveness have been observed between elderly and younger patients.

ADVERSE REACTIONS

The following adverse reactions have been reported in patients treated with LACRISERT, but were in most instances mild and transient:
- Transient blurring of vision (See PRECAUTIONS)
- Ocular discomfort or irritation
- Matting or stickiness of eyelashes
- Photophobia
- Hypersensitivity
- Edema of the eyelids
- Hyperemia

DOSAGE AND ADMINISTRATION

One LACRISERT ophthalmic insert in each eye once daily is usually sufficient to relieve the symptoms associated with moderate to severe dry eye syndromes. Individual patients may require more flexibility in the use of LACRISERT; some patients may require twice daily use for optimal results.

Clinical experience with LACRISERT indicates that in some patients several weeks may be required before satisfactory improvement of symptoms is achieved.

LACRISERT is inserted into the inferior cul-de-sac of the eye beneath the base of the tarsus, not in apposition to the cornea, nor beneath the eyelid at the level of the tarsal plate. If not properly positioned, it will be expelled into the interpalpebral fissure, and may cause symptoms of a foreign body. Illustrated instructions are included in each package. While in the licensed practitioner's office, the patient should read the instructions, then practice insertion and removal of LACRISERT until proficiency is achieved.

NOTE: Occasionally LACRISERT is inadvertently expelled from the eye, especially in patients with shallow conjunctival fornices. The patient should be cautioned against rubbing the eye(s) containing LACRISERT, especially upon awakening, so as not to dislodge or expel the insert. If required, another LACRISERT ophthalmic insert may be inserted. If experience indicates that transient blurred vision develops in an individual patient, the patient may want to remove LACRISERT a few hours after insertion to avoid this. Another LACRISERT ophthalmic insert may be inserted if needed.

If LACRISERT causes worsening of symptoms, the patient should be instructed to inspect the conjunctival sac to make certain LACRISERT is in the proper location, deep in the inferior cul-de-sac of the eye beneath the base of the tarsus. If these symptoms persist, LACRISERT should be removed and the patient should contact the practitioner.

HOW SUPPLIED

No. 3380—LACRISERT, a sterile, translucent, rod-shaped, water soluble, ophthalmic insert made of hydroxypropyl cellulose, 5 mg, is supplied as follows:

NDC 0006-3380-60 in packages containing 60 unit doses (each wrapped in an aluminum blister), two reusable applicators, and a plastic storage container to store the applicators after use.

Storage

Store below 30°C (86°F).

9246112 Issued June 2002

M-M-R®$_{II}$ ℞
(Measles, Mumps, and Rubella Virus Vaccine Live)

DESCRIPTION

M-M-R* II (Measles, Mumps, and Rubella Virus Vaccine Live) is a live virus vaccine for vaccination against measles (rubeola), mumps and rubella (German measles).

M-M-R II is a sterile lyophilized preparation of (1) ATTENUVAX* (Measles Virus Vaccine Live), a more attenuated line of measles virus, derived from Enders' attenuated Edmonston strain and propagated in chick embryo cell culture; (2) MUMPSVAX* (Mumps Virus Vaccine Live), the Jeryl Lynn** (B level) strain of mumps virus propagated in chick embryo cell culture; and (3) MERUVAX* II (Rubella Virus Vaccine Live), the Wistar RA 27/3 strain of live attenuated rubella virus propagated in WI-38 human diploid lung fibroblasts.

The growth medium for measles and mumps is Medium 199 (a buffered salt solution containing vitamins and amino acids and supplemented with fetal bovine serum) containing SPGA (sucrose, phosphate, glutamate, and human albumin) as stabilizer and neomycin.

The growth medium for rubella is Minimum Essential Medium (MEM) [a buffered salt solution containing vitamins and amino acids and supplemented with fetal bovine serum] containing human serum albumin and neomycin. Sorbitol and hydrolyzed gelatin stabilizer are added to the individual virus harvests.

The cells, virus pools, fetal bovine serum, and human albumin are all screened for the absence of adventitious agents. Human albumin is processed using the Cohn cold ethanol fractionation procedure.

The reconstituted vaccine is for subcutaneous administration. Each 0.5 mL dose contains not less than 1,000 $TCID_{50}$ (tissue culture infectious doses) of measles virus; 20,000 $TCID_{50}$ of mumps virus; and 1,000 $TCID_{50}$ of rubella virus. Each dose of the vaccine is calculated to contain sorbitol (14.5 mg), sodium phosphate, sucrose (1.9 mg), sodium chloride, hydrolyzed gelatin (14.5 mg), human albumin (0.3 mg), fetal bovine serum (<1 ppm), other buffer and media ingredients and approximately 25 mcg of neomycin. The product contains no preservative.

Before reconstitution, the lyophilized vaccine is a light yellow compact crystalline plug. M-M-R II, when reconstituted as directed, is clear yellow.

*Registered trademark of MERCK & CO., Inc.
**Trademark of MERCK & CO., Inc.

CLINICAL PHARMACOLOGY

Measles, mumps, and rubella are three common childhood diseases, caused by measles virus, mumps virus (paramyxoviruses), and rubella virus (togavirus), respectively, that may be associated with serious complications and/or death. For example, pneumonia and encephalitis are caused by measles. Mumps is associated with aseptic meningitis, deafness and orchitis; and rubella during pregnancy may cause congenital rubella syndrome in the infants of infected mothers.

The impact of measles, mumps, and rubella vaccination on the natural history of each disease in the United States can be quantified by comparing the maximum number of measles, mumps, and rubella cases reported in a given year prior to vaccine use to the number of cases of each disease reported in 1995. For measles, 894,134 cases reported in 1941 compared to 288 cases reported in 1995 resulted in a 99.97% decrease in reported cases; for mumps, 152,209 cases reported in 1968 compared to 840 cases reported in 1995 resulted in a 99.45% decrease in reported cases; and for rubella, 57,686 cases reported in 1969 compared to 200 cases reported in 1995 resulted in a 99.65% decrease.

Clinical studies of 279 triple seronegative children, 11 months to 7 years of age, demonstrated that M-M-R II is highly immunogenic and generally well tolerated. In these studies, a single injection of the vaccine induced measles hemagglutination-inhibition (HI) antibodies in 95%, mumps neutralizing antibodies in 96%, and rubella HI antibodies in 99% of susceptible persons. However, a small percentage (1–5%) of vaccines may fail to seroconvert after the primary dose (see also INDICATIONS AND USAGE, *Recommended Vaccination Schedule*).

A study of 6 month old and 15 month old infants born to vaccine-immunized mothers demonstrated that, following vaccination with ATTENUVAX, 74% of the 6 month old infants developed detectable neutralizing antibody (NT) titers while 100% of the 15 month old infants developed NT. This rate of seroconversion is higher than that previously reported for 6 month old infants born to naturally immune mothers tested by HI assay. When the 6 month old infants of immunized mothers were revaccinated at 15 months, they developed antibody titers equivalent to the 15 month old vaccinees. The lower seroconversion rate in 6 month olds has two possible explanations: 1) Due to the limit of the detection level of the assays (NT and enzyme immunoassay [EIA]), the presence of trace amounts of undetectable maternal antibody might interfere with the seroconversion of infants; or 2) The immune system of 6 month olds is not always capable of mounting a response to measles vaccine as measured by the two antibody assays.

There is some evidence to suggest that infants who are born to mothers who had natural measles and who are vaccinated at less than one year of age may not develop sustained antibody levels when later revaccinated. The advantage of early protection must be weighed against the chance for failure to respond adequately on reimmunization.

Efficacy of measles, mumps, and rubella vaccine was established in a series of double-blind controlled field trials which demonstrated a high degree of protective efficacy afforded by the individual vaccine components. These studies also established that seroconversion in response to vaccination against measles, mumps, and rubella paralleled protection from these diseases.

Following vaccination, antibodies associated with protection can be measured by neutralization assays, HI, or ELISA (enzyme linked immunosorbent assay) tests. Neutralizing and ELISA antibodies to measles, mumps, and rubella viruses are still detectable in most individuals 11–13 years after primary vaccination. See INDICATIONS AND USAGE, *Non-Pregnant Adolescents and Adult Females*, for Rubella Susceptibility Testing.

The RA 27/3 rubella strain in M-M-R II elicits higher immediate post-vaccination HI, complement-fixing and neutralizing antibody levels than other strains of rubella vaccine and has been shown to induce a broader profile of circulating antibodies including anti-theta and anti-iota precipitating antibodies. The RA 27/3 rubella strain immunologically simulates natural infection more closely than other rubella vaccine viruses. The increased levels and broader profile of antibodies produced by RA 27/3 strain rubella virus vaccine appear to correlate with greater resistance to subclinical reinfection with the wild virus, and provide greater confidence for lasting immunity.

INDICATIONS AND USAGE

Recommended Vaccination Schedule

M-M-R II is indicated for simultaneous vaccination against measles, mumps, and rubella in individuals 12 months of age or older.

Individuals first vaccinated at 12 months of age or older should be revaccinated prior to elementary school entry. Revaccination is intended to seroconvert those who do not respond to the first dose. The Advisory Committee on Immunization Practices (ACIP) recommends administration of the first dose of M-M-R II at 12–15 months of age and administration of the second dose of M-M-R II at 4–6 years of age. In addition, some public health jurisdictions mandate the age for revaccination. Consult the complete text of applicable guidelines regarding routine revaccination including that of high-risk adult populations.

Measles Outbreak Schedule

Infants Between 6–12 Months of Age

Local health authorities may recommend measles vaccination of infants between 6–12 months of age in outbreak situations. This population may fail to respond to the components of the vaccine. Safety and effectiveness of mumps and rubella vaccine in infants less than 12 months of age have not been established. The younger the infant, the lower the likelihood of seroconversion (see CLINICAL PHARMACOLOGY). Such infants should receive a second dose of M-M-R II between 12 to 15 months of age followed by revaccination at elementary school entry.

Unnecessary doses of a vaccine are best avoided by ensuring that written documentation of vaccination is preserved and a copy given to each vaccinee's parent or guardian.

Other Vaccination Considerations

Non-Pregnant Adolescent and Adult Females

Immunization of susceptible non-pregnant adolescent and adult females of childbearing age with live attenuated rubella virus vaccine is indicated if certain precautions are observed (see below and PRECAUTIONS). Vaccinating susceptible postpubertal females confers individual protection against subsequently acquiring rubella infection during pregnancy, which in turn prevents infection of the fetus and consequent congenital rubella injury.

Women of childbearing age should be advised not to become pregnant for 3 months after vaccination and should be informed of the reasons for this precaution.

The ACIP has stated "If it is practical and if reliable laboratory services are available, women of childbearing age who are potential candidates for vaccination can have serologic tests to determine susceptibility to rubella. However, with the exception of premarital and prenatal screening, routinely performing serologic tests for all women of childbearing age to determine susceptibility (so that vaccine is given only to proven susceptible women) can be effective but is expensive. Also, 2 visits to the health-care provider would be necessary—one for screening and one for vaccination. Accordingly, rubella vaccination of a woman who is not known to be pregnant and has no history of vaccination is justifiable without serologic testing—and may be preferable, particularly when costs of serology are high and follow-up of identified susceptible women for vaccination is not assured."

Postpubertal females should be informed of the frequent occurrence of generally self-limited arthralgia and/or arthritis beginning 2 to 4 weeks after vaccination (see ADVERSE REACTIONS).

Postpartum Women

It has been found convenient in many instances to vaccinate rubella-susceptible women in the immediate postpartum period (see PRECAUTIONS, *Nursing Mothers*).

Other Populations

Previously unvaccinated children older than 12 months who are in contact with susceptible pregnant women should receive live attenuated rubella vaccine (such as that contained in monovalent rubella vaccine or in M-M-R II) to reduce the risk of exposure of the pregnant woman.

Individuals planning travel outside the United States, if not immune, can acquire measles, mumps or rubella and import these diseases into the United States. Therefore, prior to international travel, individuals known to be susceptible to one or more of these diseases can receive either a monovalent vaccine (measles, mumps or rubella), or a combination vaccine as appropriate. However, M-M-R II is preferred for persons likely to be susceptible to mumps and rubella; and if monovalent measles vaccine is not readily available, travelers should receive M-M-R II regardless of their immune status to mumps or rubella.

Vaccination is recommended for susceptible individuals in high-risk groups such as college students, health-care workers, and military personnel.

According to ACIP recommendations, most persons born in 1956 or earlier are likely to have been infected with measles naturally and generally need not be considered susceptible. All children, adolescents, and adults born after 1956 are considered susceptible and should be vaccinated, if there are no contraindications. This includes persons who may be immune to measles but who lack adequate documentation of immunity such as: (1) physician-diagnosed measles, (2) laboratory evidence of measles immunity, or (3) adequate immunization with live measles vaccine on or after the first birthday.

The ACIP recommends that "Persons vaccinated with inactivated vaccine followed within 3 months by live vaccine should be revaccinated with two doses of live vaccine. Revaccination is particularly important when the risk of exposure to natural measles virus is increased, as may occur during international travel."

Post-Exposure Vaccination

Vaccination of individuals exposed to natural measles may provide some protection if the vaccine can be administered within 72 hours of exposure. If, however, vaccine is given a few days before exposure, substantial protection may be afforded. There is no conclusive evidence that vaccination of individuals recently exposed to natural mumps or natural rubella will provide protection.

Use With Other Vaccines

See DOSAGE AND ADMINISTRATION, *Use With Other Vaccines.*

CONTRAINDICATIONS

Hypersensitivity to any component of the vaccine, including gelatin.

Do not give M-M-R II to pregnant females; the possible effects of the vaccine on fetal development are unknown at this time. If vaccination of postpubertal females is undertaken, pregnancy should be avoided for three months following vaccination (see INDICATIONS AND USAGE, *Non-Pregnant Adolescent and Adult Females* and PRECAUTIONS, *Pregnancy*).

Anaphylactic or anaphylactoid reactions to neomycin (each dose of reconstituted vaccine contains approximately 25 mcg of neomycin).

Febrile respiratory illness or other active febrile infection. However, the ACIP has recommended that all vaccines can be administered to persons with minor illnesses such as diarrhea, mild upper respiratory infection with or without low-grade fever, or other low-grade febrile illness.

Patients receiving immunosuppressive therapy. This contraindication does not apply to patients who are receiving corticosteroids as replacement therapy, e.g., for Addison's disease.

Individuals with blood dyscrasias, leukemia, lymphomas of any type, or other malignant neoplasms affecting the bone marrow or lymphatic systems.

Primary and acquired immunodeficiency states, including patients who are immunosuppressed in association with AIDS or other clinical manifestations of infection with human immunodeficiency viruses; cellular immune deficiencies; and hypogammaglobulinemic and dysgammaglobulinemic states. Measles inclusion body encephalitis (MIBE), pneumonitis and death as a direct consequence of disseminated measles vaccine virus infection has been reported in immunocompromised individuals inadvertently vaccinated with measles-containing vaccine.

Individuals with a family history of congenital or hereditary immunodeficiency, until the immune competence of the potential vaccine recipient is demonstrated.

WARNINGS

Due caution should be employed in administration of M-M-R II to persons with a history of cerebral injury, individual or family histories of convulsions, or any other condition in which stress due to fever should be avoided. The physician should be alert to the temperature elevation which may occur following vaccination (see ADVERSE REACTIONS).

This product contains albumin, a derivative of human blood. Based on effective donor screening and product manufacturing processes, it carries an extremely remote risk for transmission of viral diseases. Although there is a theoretical risk for transmission of Creutzfeldt-Jacob disease (CJD), no cases of transmission of CJD or viral disease have ever been identified that were associated with the use of albumin.

Hypersensitivity To Eggs

Live measles vaccine and live mumps vaccine are produced in chick embryo cell culture. Persons with a history of anaphylactic, anaphylactoid, or other immediate reactions (e.g., hives, swelling of the mouth and throat, difficulty breathing, hypotension, or shock) subsequent to egg ingestion may be at an enhanced risk of immediate-type hypersensitivity reactions after receiving vaccines containing traces of chick embryo antigen. The potential risk to benefit ratio should be carefully evaluated before considering vaccination in such cases. Such individuals may be vaccinated with extreme caution, having adequate treatment on hand should a reaction occur (see PRECAUTIONS).

However, the AAP has stated, "Most children with a history of anaphylactic reactions to eggs have no untoward reactions to measles or MMR vaccine. Persons are not at increased risk if they have egg allergies that are not anaphylactic, and they should be vaccinated in the usual manner. In addition, skin testing of egg-allergic children with vaccine has not been predictive of which children will have an immediate hypersensitivity reaction...Persons with allergies to chickens or chicken feathers are not at increased risk of reaction to the vaccine."

Hypersensitivity to Neomycin

The AAP states, "Persons who have experienced anaphylactic reactions to topically or systemically administered neomycin should not receive measles vaccine. Most often, however, neomycin allergy manifests as a contact dermatitis, which is a delayed-type (cell-mediated) immune response rather than anaphylaxis. In such persons, an adverse reaction to neomycin in the vaccine would be an erythematous, pruritic nodule or papule, 48 to 96 hours after vaccination. A history of contact dermatitis to neomycin is not a contraindication to receiving measles vaccine."

Thrombocytopenia

Individuals with current thrombocytopenia may develop more severe thrombocytopenia following vaccination. In addition, individuals who experienced thrombocytopenia with the first dose of M-M-R II (or its component vaccines) may develop thrombocytopenia with repeat doses. Serologic status may be evaluated to determine whether or not additional doses of vaccine are needed. The potential risk to benefit ratio should be carefully evaluated before considering vaccination in such cases (see ADVERSE REACTIONS).

PRECAUTIONS

General

Adequate treatment provisions including epinephrine injection (1:1000), should be available for immediate use should an anaphylactic or anaphylactoid reaction occur.

Continued on next page

Information on the Merck & Co., Inc., products listed on these pages is from the prescribing information in use October 1, 2004. For information, please call 1-800-NSC-MERCK [1-800-672-6372].

M-M-R II—Cont.

Special care should be taken to ensure that the injection does not enter a blood vessel.
Children and young adults who are known to be infected with human immunodeficiency viruses and are not immunosuppressed may be vaccinated. However, vaccinees who are infected with HIV should be monitored closely for vaccine-preventable diseases because immunization may be less effective than for uninfected persons (see CONTRAINDICATIONS).
Vaccination should be deferred for 3 months or longer following blood or plasma transfusions, or administration of immune globulin (human).
Excretion of small amounts of the live attenuated rubella virus from the nose or throat has occurred in the majority of susceptible individuals 7–28 days after vaccination. There is no confirmed evidence to indicate that such virus is transmitted to susceptible persons who are in contact with the vaccinated individuals. Consequently, transmission through close personal contact, while accepted as a theoretical possibility, is not regarded as a significant risk. However, transmission of the rubella vaccine virus to infants via breast milk has been documented (see *Nursing Mothers*).
There are no reports of transmission of live attenuated measles or mumps viruses from vaccinees to susceptible contacts.
It has been reported that live attenuated measles, mumps and rubella virus vaccines given individually may result in a temporary depression of tuberculin skin sensitivity. Therefore, if a tuberculin test is to be done, it should be administered either before or simultaneously with M-M-R II.
Children under treatment for tuberculosis have not experienced exacerbation of the disease when immunized with live measles virus vaccine; no studies have been reported to date of the effect of measles virus vaccines on untreated tuberculous children. However, individuals with active untreated tuberculosis should not be vaccinated.
As for any vaccine, vaccination with M-M-R II may not result in protection in 100% of vaccinees.
The health-care provider should determine the current health status and previous vaccination history of the vaccinee.
The health-care provider should question the patient, parent, or guardian about reactions to a previous dose of M-M-R II or other measles-, mumps-, or rubella-containing vaccines.

Information for Patients

The health-care provider should provide the vaccine information required to be given with each vaccination to the patient, parent or guardian.
The health-care provider should inform the patient, parent or guardian of the benefits and risks associated with vaccination. For risks associated with vaccination see WARNINGS, PRECAUTIONS, ADVERSE REACTIONS.
Patients, parents or guardians should be instructed to report any serious adverse reactions to their health-care provider who in turn should report such events to the U.S. Department of Health and Human Services through the Vaccine Adverse Event Reporting System (VAERS), 1-800-822-7967.
Pregnancy should be avoided for 3 months following vaccination, and patients should be informed of the reasons for this precaution (see INDICATIONS AND USAGE, *Non-Pregnant Adolescent and Adult Females*, CONTRAINDICATIONS, and PRECAUTIONS, *Pregnancy*).

Laboratory Tests

See INDICATIONS AND USAGE, *Non-Pregnant Adolescents and Adult Females*, for Rubella Susceptibility Testing, and CLINICAL PHARMACOLOGY.

Drug Interactions

See DOSAGE AND ADMINISTRATION, *Use With Other Vaccines.*

Immunosuppressive Therapy

The immune status of patients about to undergo immunosuppressive therapy should be evaluated so that the physician can consider whether vaccination prior to the initiation of treatment is indicated. (see CONTRAINDICATIONS and PRECAUTIONS)
The ACIP has stated that "patients with leukemia in remission who have not received chemotherapy for at least 3 months may receive live-virus vaccines. Short-term (<2 weeks), low- to moderate-dose systemic corticosteroid therapy, topical steroid therapy (e.g. nasal, skin), long-term alternate-day treatment with low to moderate doses of short-acting systemic steroid, and intra-articular, bursal, or tendon injection of corticosteroids are not immunosuppressive in their usual doses and do not contraindicate the administration of [measles, mumps or rubella vaccine]."

Immune Globulin

Administration of immune globulins concurrently with M-M-R II may interfere with the expected immune response.
See also PRECAUTIONS, *General.*

Carcinogenesis, Mutagenesis, Impairment of Fertility

M-M-R II has not been evaluated for carcinogenic or mutagenic potential, or potential to impair fertility.

Pregnancy

Pregnancy Category C

Animal reproduction studies have not been conducted with M-M-R II. It is also not known whether M-M-R II can cause fetal harm when administered to a pregnant woman or can affect reproduction capacity. Therefore, the vaccine should not be administered to pregnant females; furthermore, pregnancy should be avoided for 3 months following vaccination (see INDICATIONS AND USAGE, *Non-Pregnant Adolescent and Adult Females* and CONTRAINDICATIONS).
In counseling women who are inadvertently vaccinated when pregnant or who become pregnant within 3 months of vaccination, the physician should be aware of the following: (1) In a 10 year survey involving over 700 pregnant women who received rubella vaccine within 3 months before or after conception (of whom 189 received the Wistar RA 27/3 strain), none of the newborns had abnormalities compatible with congenital rubella syndrome; (2) Mumps infection during the first trimester of pregnancy may increase the rate of spontaneous abortion. Although mumps vaccine virus has been shown to infect the placenta and fetus, there is no evidence that it causes congenital malformations in humans; and (3) Reports have indicated that contracting natural measles during pregnancy enhances fetal risk. Increased rates of spontaneous abortion, stillbirth, congenital defects and prematurity have been observed subsequent to natural measles during pregnancy. There are no adequate studies of the attenuated (vaccine) strain of measles virus in pregnancy. However, it would be prudent to assume that the vaccine strain of virus is also capable of inducing adverse fetal effects.

Nursing Mothers

It is not known whether measles or mumps vaccine virus is secreted in human milk. Recent studies have shown that lactating postpartum women immunized with live attenuated rubella vaccine may secrete the virus in breast milk and transmit it to breast-fed infants. In the infants with serological evidence of rubella infection, none exhibited severe disease; however, one exhibited mild clinical illness typical of acquired rubella. Caution should be exercised when M-M-R II is administered to a nursing woman.

Pediatric Use

Safety and effectiveness of measles vaccine in infants below the age of 6 months have not been established (see also CLINICAL PHARMACOLOGY). Safety and effectiveness of mumps and rubella vaccine in infants less than 12 months of age have not been established.

Geriatric Use

Clinical studies of M-M-R II did not include sufficient numbers of seronegative subjects aged 65 and over to determine whether they respond differently from younger subjects. Other reported clinical experience has not identified differences in responses between the elderly and younger subjects.

ADVERSE REACTIONS

The following adverse reactions are listed in decreasing order of severity, without regard to causality, within each body system category and have been reported during clinical trials, with use of the marketed vaccine, or with use of monovalent or bivalent vaccine containing measles, mumps, or rubella:

Body as a Whole

Panniculitis; atypical measles; fever; syncope, headache; dizziness; malaise; irritability.

Cardiovascular System

Vasculitis.

Digestive System

Pancreatitis; diarrhea; vomiting; parotitis; nausea.

Endocrine System

Diabetes mellitus.

Hemic and Lymphatic System

Thrombocytopenia (see WARNINGS, *Thrombocytopenia*); purpura; regional lymphadenopathy; leukocytosis.

Immune System

Anaphylaxis and anaphylactoid reactions have been reported as well as related phenomena such as angioneurotic edema (including peripheral or facial edema) and bronchial spasm in individuals with or without an allergic history.

Musculoskeletal System

Arthritis; arthralgia; myalgia.
Arthralgia and/or arthritis (usually transient and rarely chronic), and polyneuritis are features of natural rubella and vary in frequency and severity with age and sex, being greatest in adult females and least in prepubertal children. This type of involvement as well as myalgia and paresthesia, have also been reported following administration of MERUVAX II.
Chronic arthritis has been associated with natural rubella infection and has been related to persistent virus and/or viral antigen isolated from body tissues. Only rarely have vaccine recipients developed chronic joint symptoms.
Following vaccination in children, reactions in joints are uncommon and generally of brief duration. In women, incidence rates for arthritis and arthralgia are generally higher than those seen in children (children: 0–3%; women: 12–26%), and the reactions tend to be more marked and of longer duration. Symptoms may persist for a matter of months or on rare occasions for years. In adolescent girls, the reactions appear to be intermediate in incidence between those seen in children and in adult women. Even in women older than 35 years, these reactions are generally well tolerated and rarely interfere with normal activities.

Nervous System

Encephalitis; encephalopathy; measles inclusion body encephalitis (MIBE) (see CONTRAINDICATIONS); subacute sclerosing panencephalitis (SSPE); Guillain-Barré Syndrome (GBS); febrile convulsions; afebrile convulsions or seizures; ataxia; polyneuritis; polyneuropathy; ocular palsies; paresthesia.
Experience from more than 80 million doses of all live measles vaccines given in the U.S. through 1975 indicates that significant central nervous system reactions such as encephalitis and encephalopathy, occurring within 30 days after vaccination, have been temporally associated with measles vaccine very rarely. In no case has it been shown that reactions were actually caused by vaccine. The Centers for Disease Control and Prevention has pointed out that "a certain number of cases of encephalitis may be expected to occur in a large childhood population in a defined period of time even when no vaccines are administered". However, the data suggest the possibility that some of these cases may have been caused by measles vaccines. The risk of such serious neurological disorders following live measles virus vaccine administration remains far less than that for encephalitis and encephalopathy with natural measles (one per two thousand reported cases).
Post-marketing surveillance of the more than 200 million doses of M-M-R and M-M-R II that have been distributed worldwide over 25 years (1971–1996) indicates that serious adverse events such as encephalitis and encephalopathy continue to be rarely reported.
There have been reports of subacute sclerosing panencephalitis (SSPE) in children who did not have a history of natural measles but did receive measles vaccine. Some of these cases may have resulted from unrecognized measles in the first year of life or possibly from the measles vaccination. Based on estimated nationwide measles vaccine distribution, the association of SSPE cases to measles vaccination is about one case per million vaccine doses distributed. This is far less than the association with natural measles, 6–22 cases of SSPE per million cases of measles. The results of a retrospective case-controlled study conducted by the Centers for Disease Control and Prevention suggest that the overall effect of measles vaccine has been to protect against SSPE by preventing measles with its inherent higher risk of SSPE.
Cases of aseptic meningitis have been reported to VAERS following measles, mumps, and rubella vaccination. Although a causal relationship between the Urabe strain of mumps vaccine and aseptic meningitis has been shown, there are no data to link Jeryl Lynn mumps vaccine to aseptic meningitis.

Respiratory System

Pneumonitis (see CONTRAINDICATIONS); sore throat; cough; rhinitis.

Skin

Stevens-Johnson Syndrome; erythema multiforme; urticaria; rash.
Local reactions including burning/stinging at injection site; wheal and flare; redness (erythema); swelling; induration; tenderness; vesiculation at injection site.

Special Senses—Ear

Nerve deafness; otitis media.

Special Senses—Eye

Retinitis; optic neuritis; papillitis; retrobulbar neuritis; conjunctivitis.

Urogenital System

Orchitis.

Other

Death from various, and in some cases unknown, causes has been reported rarely following vaccination with measles, mumps, and rubella vaccines; however, a causal relationship has not been established. No deaths or permanent sequelae were reported in a published post-marketing surveillance study in Finland involving 1.5 million children and adults who were vaccinated with M-M-R II during 1982–1993.
Under the National Childhood Vaccine Injury Act of 1986, health-care providers and manufacturers are required to record and report certain suspected adverse events occurring within specific time periods after vaccination. However, the U.S. Department of Health and Human Services (DHHS) has established a Vaccine Adverse Event Reporting System (VAERS) which will accept all reports of suspected events. A VAERS report form as well as information regarding reporting requirements can be obtained by calling VAERS 1-800-822-7967.

DOSAGE AND ADMINISTRATION

FOR SUBCUTANEOUS ADMINISTRATION

Do not inject intravenously

The dose for any age is 0.5 mL administered subcutaneously, preferably into the outer aspect of the upper arm.
The recommended age for primary vaccination is 12 to 15 months.
Revaccination with M-M-R II is recommended prior to elementary school entry. See also INDICATIONS AND USAGE, *Recommended Vaccination Schedule.*
Children first vaccinated when younger than 12 months of age should receive another dose between 12 to 15 months of age followed by revaccination prior to elementary school entry. See also INDICATIONS AND USAGE, *Measles Outbreak Schedule.*

Immune Globulin (IG) is not to be given concurrently with M-M-R II.

CAUTION: A sterile syringe free of preservatives, antiseptics, and detergents should be used for each injection and/or reconstitution of the vaccine because these substances may inactivate the live virus vaccine. A 25 gauge, 5/8" needle is recommended.

To reconstitute, use only the diluent supplied, since it is free of preservatives or other antiviral substances which might inactivate the vaccine.

Single Dose Vial—First withdraw the entire volume of diluent into the syringe to be used for reconstitution. Inject all the diluent in the syringe into the vial of lyophilized vaccine, and agitate to mix thoroughly. If the lyophilized vaccine cannot be dissolved, discard. Withdraw the entire contents into a syringe and inject the total volume of restored vaccine subcutaneously.

It is important to use a separate sterile syringe and needle for each individual patient to prevent transmission of hepatitis B and other infectious agents from one person to another.

10 Dose Vial (available only to government agencies/institutions)—Withdraw the entire contents (7 mL) of the diluent vial into the sterile syringe to be used for reconstitution, and introduce into the 10 dose vial of lyophilized vaccine. Agitate to ensure thorough mixing. If the lyophilized vaccine cannot be dissolved, discard. The outer labeling suggests "For Jet Injector or Syringe Use." Use with separate sterile syringes is permitted for containers of 10 doses or less. The vaccine and diluent do not contain preservatives; therefore, the user must recognize the potential contamination hazards and exercise special precautions to protect the sterility and potency of the product. The use of aseptic techniques and proper storage prior to and after restoration of the vaccine and subsequent withdrawal of the individual doses is essential. Use 0.5 mL of the reconstituted vaccine for subcutaneous injection.

It is important to use a separate sterile syringe and needle for each individual patient to prevent transmission of hepatitis B and other infectious agents from one person to another.

Parenteral drug products should be inspected visually for particulate matter and discoloration prior to administration whenever solution and container permit. M-M-R II, when reconstituted, is clear yellow.

Use With Other Vaccines

M-M-R II should be given one month before or after administration of other live viral vaccines.

M-M-R II has been administered concurrently with VARIVAX* [Varicella Virus Vaccine Live (Oka/Merck)], and PedvaxHIB* [Haemophilus b Conjugate Vaccine (Meningococcal Protein Conjugate)] using separate sites and syringes. No impairment of immune response to individual tested vaccine antigens was demonstrated. The type, frequency, and severity of adverse experiences observed with M-M-R II were similar to those seen when each vaccine was given alone.

Routine administration of DTP (diphtheria, tetanus, pertussis) and/or OPV (oral poliovirus vaccine) concurrently with measles, mumps and rubella vaccines is not recommended because there are limited data relating to the simultaneous administration of these antigens.

However, other schedules have been used. The ACIP has stated "Although data are limited concerning the simultaneous administration of the entire recommended vaccine series (i.e., DTP, OPV, MMR, and Hib vaccines, with or without hepatitis B vaccine), data from numerous studies have indicated no interference between routinely recommended childhood vaccines (either live, attenuated, or killed). These findings support the simultaneous use of all vaccines as recommended."

HOW SUPPLIED

No. 4749—M-M-R II is supplied as a single-dose vial of lyophilized vaccine, **NDC** 0006-4749-00, and a vial of diluent.

No. 4681/4309—M-M-R II is supplied as follows: (1) a box of 10 single-dose vials of lyophilized vaccine (package A), **NDC** 0006-4681-00; and (2) a box of 10 vials of diluent (package B). To conserve refrigerator space, the diluent may be stored separately at room temperature.

Available only to government agencies/institutions:

No. 4682X—M-M-R II is supplied as one 10 dose vial of lyophilized vaccine.

NDC 0006-4682-00, and one 7 mL vial of diluent.

Storage

During shipment, to ensure that there is no loss of potency, the vaccine must be maintained at a temperature of 10°C (50°F) or colder. Freezing during shipment will not affect potency.

Protect the vaccine from light at all times, since such exposure may inactivate the virus.

Before reconstitution, store the vial of lyophilized vaccine at 2–8°C (36–46°F) or colder. The diluent may be stored in the refrigerator with the lyophilized vaccine or separately at room temperature.

It is recommended that the vaccine be used as soon as possible after reconstitution. Store reconstituted vaccine in the vaccine vial in a dark place at 2–8°C (36–46°F) and discard if not used within 8 hours.

9265208 Issued October 2003

MAXALT® ℞
(rizatriptan benzoate)
TABLETS
MAXALT-MLT® ℞
(rizatriptan benzoate)
ORALLY DISINTEGRATING TABLETS

DESCRIPTION

MAXALT* contains rizatriptan benzoate, a selective 5-hydroxytryptamine$_{1B/1D}$ (5-HT$_{1B/1D}$) receptor agonist.

Rizatriptan benzoate is described chemically as: *N,N*-dimethyl-5-(1*H*-1,2,4-triazol-1-ylmethyl)-1*H*-indole-3-ethanamine monobenzoate and its structural formula is:

Its empirical formula is $C_{15}H_{19}N_5 \bullet C_7H_6O_2$, representing a molecular weight of the free base of 269.4. Rizatriptan benzoate is a white to off-white, crystalline solid that is soluble in water at about 42 mg per mL (expressed as free base) at 25°C.

MAXALT Tablets and MAXALT-MLT* Orally Disintegrating Tablets are available for oral administration in strengths of 5 and 10 mg (corresponding to 7.265 mg or 14.53 mg of the benzoate salt, respectively). Each compressed tablet contains the following inactive ingredients: lactose monohydrate, microcrystalline cellulose, pregelatinized starch, ferric oxide (red), and magnesium stearate.

Each lyophilized orally disintegrating tablet contains the following inactive ingredients: gelatin, mannitol, glycine, aspartame, and peppermint flavor.

* Registered trademark of MERCK & CO., Inc.

CLINICAL PHARMACOLOGY

Mechanism of Action

Rizatriptan binds with high affinity to human cloned 5-HT$_{1B}$ and 5-HT$_{1D}$ receptors. Rizatriptan has weak affinity for other 5-HT$_1$ receptor subtypes (5-HT$_{1A}$, 5-HT$_{1E}$, 5-HT$_{1F}$) and the 5-HT$_7$ receptor, but has no significant activity at 5-HT$_2$, 5-HT$_3$, alpha- and beta-adrenergic, dopaminergic, histaminergic, muscarinic or benzodiazepine receptors.

Current theories on the etiology of migraine headache suggest that symptoms are due to local cranial vasodilatation and/or to the release of vasoactive and pro-inflammatory peptides from sensory nerve endings in an activated trigeminal system. The therapeutic activity of rizatriptan in migraine can most likely be attributed to agonist effects at 5-HT$_{1B/1D}$ receptors on the extracerebral, intracranial blood vessels that become dilated during a migraine attack and on nerve terminals in the trigeminal system. Activation of these receptors results in cranial vessel constriction, inhibition of neuropeptide release and reduced transmission in trigeminal pain pathways.

Pharmacokinetics

Rizatriptan is completely absorbed following oral administration. The mean oral absolute bioavailability of the MAXALT Tablet is about 45%, and mean peak plasma concentrations (C_{max}) are reached in approximately 1–1.5 hours (T_{max}). The presence of a migraine headache did not appear to affect the absorption or pharmacokinetics of rizatriptan. Food has no significant effect on the bioavailability of rizatriptan but delays the time to reach peak concentration by an hour. In clinical trials, MAXALT was administered without regard to food. The plasma half-life of rizatriptan in males and females averages 2–3 hours.

The bioavailability and C_{max} of rizatriptan were similar following administration of MAXALT Tablets and MAXALT-MLT Orally Disintegrating Tablets, but the rate of absorption is somewhat slower with MAXALT-MLT, with T_{max} averaging 1.6–2.5 hours. AUC of rizatriptan is approximately 30% higher in females than in males. No accumulation occurred on multiple dosing.

The mean volume of distribution is approximately 140 liters in male subjects and 110 liters in female subjects. Rizatriptan is minimally bound (14%) to plasma proteins.

The primary route of rizatriptan metabolism is via oxidative deamination by monoamine oxidase-A (MAO-A) to the indole acetic acid metabolite, which is not active at the 5-HT$_{1B/1D}$ receptor. N-monodesmethyl-rizatriptan, a metabolite with activity similar to that of parent compound at the 5-HT$_{1B/1D}$ receptor, is formed to a minor degree. Plasma concentrations of N-monodesmethyl-rizatriptan are approximately 14% of those of parent compound, and it is eliminated at a similar rate. Other minor metabolites the N-oxide, the 6-hydroxy compound, and the sulfate conjugate of the 6-hydroxy metabolite are not active at the 5-HT$_{1B/1D}$ receptor.

The total radioactivity of the administered dose recovered over 120 hours in urine and feces was 82% and 12%, respectively, following a single 10 mg oral administration of ^{14}C-rizatriptan. Following oral administration of ^{14}C-rizatriptan, rizatriptan accounted for about 17% of circulating plasma radioactivity. Approximately 14% of an oral dose is excreted in urine as unchanged rizatriptan while 51% is excreted as indole acetic acid metabolite, indicating substantial first pass metabolism.

Cytochrome P450 Isoforms: Rizatriptan is not an inhibitor of the activities of human liver cytochrome P450 isoforms 3A4/5, 1A2, 2C9, 2C19, or 2E1; rizatriptan is a competitive inhibitor (Ki=1400 nM) of cytochrome P450 2D6, but only at high, clinically irrelevant concentrations.

Special Populations

Age: Rizatriptan pharmacokinetics in healthy elderly non-migraineur volunteers (age 65–77 years) were similar to those in younger non-migraineur volunteers (age 18–45 years).

Gender: The mean $AUC_{0-\infty}$ and C_{max} of rizatriptan (10 mg orally) were about 30% and 11% higher in females as compared to males, respectively, while T_{max} occurred at approximately the same time.

Hepatic impairment: Following oral administration in patients with hepatic impairment caused by mild to moderate alcoholic cirrhosis of the liver, plasma concentrations of rizatriptan were similar in patients with mild hepatic insufficiency compared to a control group of healthy subjects; plasma concentrations of rizatriptan were approximately 30% greater in patients with moderate hepatic insufficiency. (See PRECAUTIONS.)

Renal impairment: In patients with renal impairment (creatinine clearance 10–60 mL/min/1.73 m^2), the $AUC_{0-\infty}$ of rizatriptan was not significantly different from that in healthy subjects. In hemodialysis patients, (creatinine clearance < 2 mL/min/1.73 m^2), however, the AUC for rizatriptan was approximately 44% greater than that in patients with normal renal function. (See PRECAUTIONS.)

Race: Pharmacokinetic data revealed no significant differences between African American and Caucasian subjects.

Drug Interactions (See also PRECAUTIONS, *Drug Interactions.*)

Monoamine oxidase inhibitors: Rizatriptan is principally metabolized via monoamine oxidase, 'A' subtype (MAO-A). Plasma concentrations of rizatriptan may be increased by drugs that are selective MAO-A inhibitors (e.g., moclobemide) or nonselective MAO inhibitors [type A and B] (e.g., isocarboxazid, phenelzine, tranylcypromine, and pargyline). In a drug interaction study, when MAXALT 10 mg was administered to subjects (n=12) receiving concomitant therapy with the selective, reversible MAO-A inhibitor, moclobemide 150 mg t.i.d., there were mean increases in rizatriptan AUC and C_{max} of 119% and 41% respectively; and the AUC of the active N-monodesmethyl metabolite of rizatriptan was increased more than 400%. The interaction would be expected to be greater with irreversible MAO inhibitors. No pharmacokinetic interaction is anticipated in patients receiving selective MAO-B inhibitors. (See CONTRAINDICATIONS; PRECAUTIONS, *Drug Interactions.*)

Propranolol: In a study of concurrent administration of propranolol 240 mg/day and a single dose of rizatriptan 10 mg in healthy subjects (n=11), mean plasma AUC for rizatriptan was increased by 70% during propranolol administration, and a fourfold increase was observed in one subject. The AUC of the active N-monodesmethyl metabolite of rizatriptan was not affected by propranolol. (See PRECAUTIONS; DOSAGE AND ADMINISTRATION.)

Nadolol/Metoprolol: In a drug interactions study, effects of multiple doses of nadolol 80 mg or metoprolol 100 mg every 12 hours on the pharmacokinetics of a single dose of 10 mg rizatriptan were evaluated in healthy subjects (n=12). No pharmacokinetic interactions were observed.

Paroxetine: In a study of the interaction between the selective serotonin reuptake inhibitor (SSRI) paroxetine 20 mg/day for two weeks and a single dose of MAXALT 10 mg in healthy subjects (n=12), neither the plasma concentrations of rizatriptan nor its safety profile were affected by paroxetine.

Oral contraceptives: In a study of concurrent administration of an oral contraceptive during 6 days of administration of MAXALT (10–30 mg/day) in healthy female volunteers (n=18), rizatriptan did not affect plasma concentrations of ethinyl estradiol or norethindrone.

Clinical Studies

The efficacy of MAXALT Tablets was established in four multicenter, randomized, placebo-controlled trials. Patients enrolled in these studies were primarily female (84%) and Caucasian (88%), with a mean age of 40 years (range of 18 to 71). Patients were instructed to treat a moderate to severe headache. Headache response, defined as a reduction of moderate or severe headache pain to no or mild headache pain, was assessed for up to 2 hours (Study 1) or up to 4 hours after dosing (Studies 2, 3 and 4). Associated symptoms of nausea, photophobia, and phonophobia and maintenance of response up to 24 hours postdose were evaluated. A second dose of MAXALT Tablets was allowed 2 to 24 hours after dosing for treatment of recurrent headache in Studies 1 and 2. Additional analgesics and/or antiemetics were allowed 2 hours after initial treatment for rescue in all four studies.

In all studies, the percentage of patients achieving headache response 2 hours after treatment was significantly greater in patients who received either MAXALT 5 or 10 mg compared to those who received placebo. In a separate study, doses of 2.5 mg were not different from placebo. Doses greater than 10 mg were associated with an increased incidence of adverse effects. The results from the 4 controlled studies using the marketed formulation are summarized in Table 1.

Continued on next page

Information on the Merck & Co., Inc., products listed on these pages is from the prescribing information in use October 1, 2004. For information, please call 1-800-NSC-MERCK [1-800-672-6372].

Maxalt—Cont.

Table 1
Response Rates 2 Hours Following Treatment of Initial Headache

Study	Placebo	MAXALT Tablets 5 mg	MAXALT Tablets 10 mg
1	35% (n=304)	62%* (n=458)	71%*,** (n=456)
2†	37% (n=82)	—	77%* (n=320)
3	23% (n=80)	63%* (n=352)	
4	40% (n=159)	60%* (n=164)	67%* (n=385)

*p value <0.05 in comparison with placebo
**p value <0.05 in comparison with 5 mg
†Results for initial headache only.

Comparisons of drug performance based upon results obtained in different clinical trials are never reliable. Because studies are conducted at different times, with different samples of patients, by different investigators, employing different criteria and/or different interpretations of the same criteria, under different conditions (dose, dosing regimen, etc.), quantitative estimates of treatment response and the timing of response may be expected to vary considerably from study to study.

The estimated probability of achieving an initial headache response within 2 hours following treatment is depicted in Figure 1.

Figure 1: Estimated Probability of Achieving an Initial Headache Response by 2 Hours††

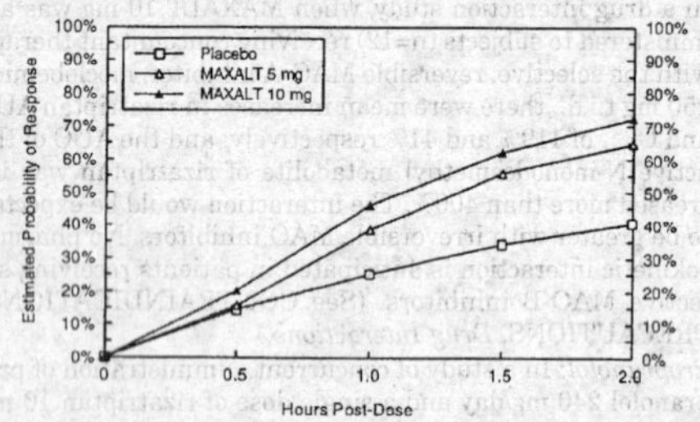

†† Figure 1 shows the Kaplan-Meier plot of the probability over time of obtaining headache response (no or mild pain) following treatment with rizatriptan or placebo. The averages displayed are based on pooled data from 4 placebo-controlled, outpatient trials providing evidence of efficacy (Studies 1, 2, 3, and 4). Patients taking additional treatment or not achieving headache response prior to 2 hours were censored at 2 hours.

For patients with migraine-associated photophobia, phonophobia, and nausea at baseline, there was a decreased incidence of these symptoms following administration of MAXALT compared to placebo.

Two to 24 hours following the initial dose of study treatment, patients were allowed to use additional treatment for pain response in the form of a second dose of study treatment or other medication. The estimated probability of patients taking a second dose or other medication for migraine over the 24 hours following the initial dose of study treatment is summarized in Figure 2.

Figure 2: Estimated Probability of Patients Taking a Second Dose of MAXALT Tablets or Other Medication for Migraines Over the 24 Hours Following the Initial Dose of Study Treatment†††

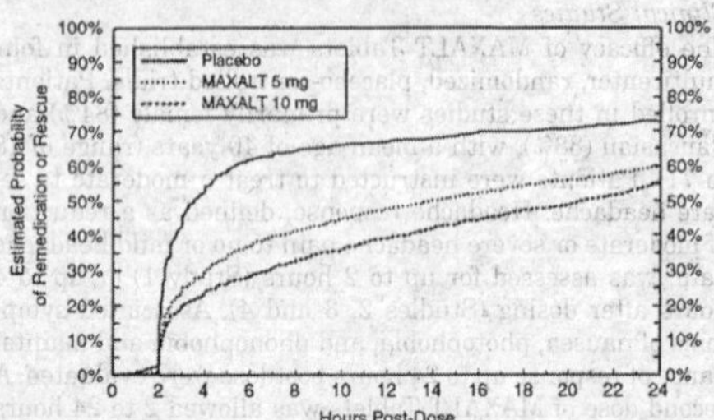

††† This Kaplan-Meier plot is based on data obtained in 4 placebo-controlled outpatient clinical trials (Studies 1, 2, 3, and 4). Patients not using additional treatments were censored at 24 hours. The plot includes both patients who had headache response at 2 hours and those who had no response to the initial dose. Remedication was not allowed within 2 hours post-dose.

Efficacy was unaffected by the presence of aura; by the gender, or age of the patient; or by concomitant use of common migraine prophylactic drugs (e.g., beta-blockers, calcium channel blockers, tricyclic antidepressants) or oral contraceptives. In two additional similar studies, efficacy was unaffected by relationship to menses. There were insufficient data to assess the impact of race on efficacy.

In a single study in adolescents (n=291), there were no statistically significant differences between treatment groups. The headache response rates at 2 hours were 66% and 56% for MAXALT 5 mg Tablets and placebo, respectively.

MAXALT-MLT Orally Disintegrating Tablets

The efficacy of MAXALT-MLT was established in two multicenter, randomized, placebo-controlled trials that were similar in design to the trials of MAXALT Tablets. Patients were instructed to treat a moderate to severe headache. Patients treated in these studies were primarily female (88%) and Caucasian (95%), with a mean age of 42 years (range 18–72).

In both studies, the percentage of patients achieving headache response 2 hours after treatment was significantly greater in patients who received either MAXALT-MLT 5 or 10 mg compared to those who received placebo. The results from the 2 controlled studies using the marketed formulation are summarized in Table 2.

Table 2
Response Rates 2 Hours Following Treatment of Initial Headache

Study	Placebo	MAXALT-MLT 5 mg	MAXALT-MLT 10 mg
1	47% (n=98)	66%* (n=100)	66%* (n=113)
2	28% (n=180)	59%* (n=181)	74%*,** (n=186)

*p value <0.01 in comparison with placebo
**p value <0.01 in comparison with 5 mg

The estimated probability of achieving an initial headache response by 2 hours following treatment with MAXALT-MLT is depicted in Figure 3.

Figure 3: Estimated Probability of Achieving an Initial Headache Response with MAXALT-MLT by 2 Hours‡

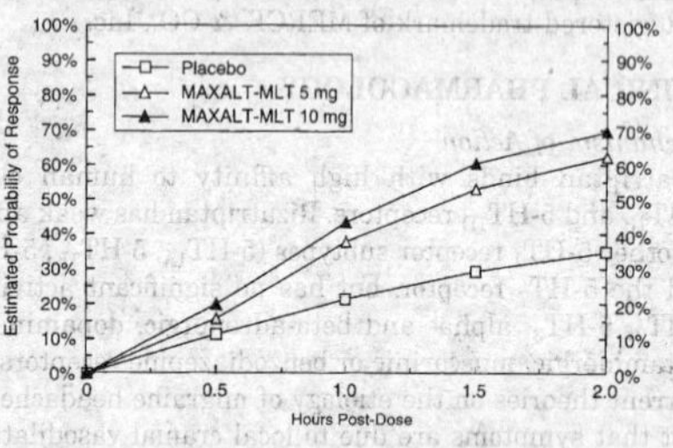

‡Figure 3 shows the Kaplan-Meier plot of the probability over time of obtaining headache responses (no or mild pain) following treatment with MAXALT-MLT or placebo. The averages displayed are based on pooled data from 2 placebo-controlled, outpatient trials providing evidence of efficacy (Studies 1 and 2). Patients taking additional treatment or not achieving headache response prior to 2 hours were censored at 2 hours.

For patients with migraine-associated photophobia and phonophobia at baseline, there was a decreased incidence of these symptoms following administration of MAXALT-MLT as compared to placebo.

Two to 24 hours following the initial dose of study treatment, patients were allowed to use additional treatment for pain response in the form of a second dose of study treatment or other medication. The estimated probability of patients taking a second dose or other medication for migraine over the 24 hours following the initial dose of study treatment is summarized in Figure 4.

Figure 4: Estimated Probability of Patients Taking a Second Dose of MAXALT-MLT or Other Medication for Migraines Over the 24 Hours Following the Initial Dose of Study Treatment‡‡

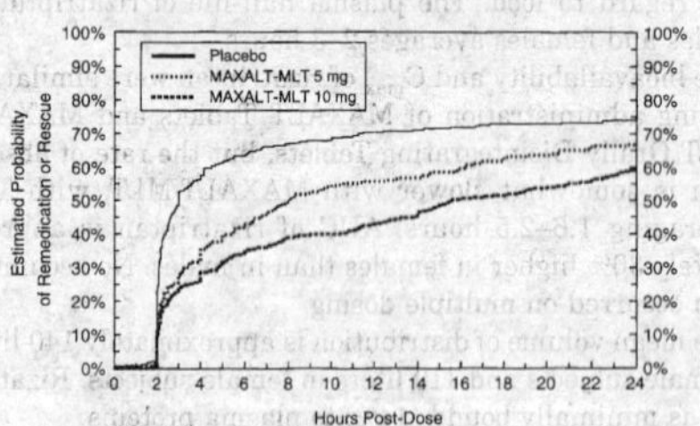

The Kaplan-Meier plot is based on data obtained in 2 placebo-controlled outpatient clinical trials (Studies 1 and 2). Patients not using additional treatments were censored at 24 hours. The plot includes both patients who had headache response at 2 hours and those who had no response to the initial dose. Remedication was not allowed within 2 hours post-dose.

INDICATIONS AND USAGE

MAXALT is indicated for the acute treatment of migraine attacks with or without aura in adults.

MAXALT is not intended for the prophylactic therapy of migraine or for use in the management of hemiplegic or basilar migraine (see CONTRAINDICATIONS). Safety and effectiveness of MAXALT have not been established for cluster headache, which is present in an older, predominantly male population.

CONTRAINDICATIONS

MAXALT should not be given to patients with ischemic heart disease (e.g., angina pectoris, history of myocardial infarction, or documented silent ischemia) or to patients who have symptoms or findings consistent with ischemic heart disease, coronary artery vasospasm, including Prinzmetal's variant angina, or other significant underlying cardiovascular disease (see WARNINGS).

Because MAXALT may increase blood pressure, it should not be given to patients with uncontrolled hypertension (see WARNINGS).

MAXALT should not be used within 24 hours of treatment with another 5-HT$_1$ agonist, or an ergotamine-containing or ergot-type medication like dihydroergotamine or methysergide.

MAXALT should not be administered to patients with hemiplegic or basilar migraine.

Concurrent administration of MAO inhibitors or use of rizatriptan within 2 weeks of discontinuation of MAO inhibitor therapy is contraindicated (see CLINICAL PHARMACOLOGY, *Drug Interactions* and PRECAUTIONS, *Drug Interactions*).

MAXALT is contraindicated in patients who are hypersensitive to rizatriptan or any of its inactive ingredients.

WARNINGS

MAXALT should only be used where a clear diagnosis of migraine has been established.

***Risk of Myocardial Ischemia and/or Infarction and Other Adverse Cardiac Events:* Because of the potential of this class of compounds (5-HT$_{1B/1D}$ agonists) to cause coronary vasospasm, MAXALT should not be given to patients with documented ischemic or vasospastic coronary artery disease (see CONTRAINDICATIONS). It is strongly recommended that rizatriptan not be given to patients in whom unrecognized coronary artery disease (CAD) is predicted by the presence of risk factors (e.g., hypertension, hypercholesterolemia, smoker, obesity, diabetes, strong family history of CAD, female with surgical or physiological menopause, or male over 40 years of age) unless a cardiovascular evaluation provides satisfactory clinical evidence that the patient is reasonably free of coronary artery and ischemic myocardial disease or other significant underlying cardiovascular disease. The sensitivity of cardiac diagnostic procedures to detect cardiovascular disease or predisposition to coronary artery vasospasm is modest, at best. If, during the cardiovascular evaluation, the patient's medical history, electrocardiographic or other investigations reveal findings indicative of, or consistent with, coronary artery vasospasm or myocardial ischemia, rizatriptan should not be administered (see CONTRAINDICATIONS).**

For patients with risk factors predictive of CAD, who are determined to have a satisfactory cardiovascular evaluation, it is strongly recommended that administration of the first dose of rizatriptan take place in the setting of a physician's office or similar medically staffed and equipped facility unless the patient has previously received rizatriptan. Because cardiac ischemia can occur in the absence of clinical symptoms, consideration should be given to obtaining on the first occasion of use an electrocardiogram (ECG) during the interval immediately following MAXALT, in these patients with risk factors.

It is recommended that patients who are intermittent long-term users of MAXALT and who have or acquire risk factors predictive of CAD, as described above, undergo periodic interval cardiovascular evaluation as they continue to use MAXALT.

The systematic approach described above is intended to reduce the likelihood that patients with unrecognized cardiovascular disease will be inadvertently exposed to rizatriptan.

Cardiac Events and Fatalities Associated with 5-HT$_1$ Agonists: Serious adverse cardiac events, including acute myocardial infarction, have been reported within a few hours following the administration of rizatriptan. Life-threatening disturbances of cardiac rhythm and death have been reported within a few hours following the administration of other 5-HT$_1$ agonists. Considering the extent of use of 5-HT$_1$ agonists in patients with migraine, the incidence of these events is extremely low. MAXALT can cause coronary vasospasm. Because of the close proximity of the events to MAXALT use, a causal relationship cannot be excluded. In the cases where there has been known underlying coronary artery disease, the relationship is uncertain.

Premarketing experience with rizatriptan: Among the 3700 patients with migraine who participated in premarketing clinical trials of MAXALT, one patient was reported to have chest pain with possible ischemic ECG changes following a single dose of 10 mg.

Postmarketing experience with rizatriptan: Serious cardiovascular events have been reported in association with the use of MAXALT. The uncontrolled nature of postmarketing surveillance, however, makes it impossible to determine definitively the proportion of the reported cases that were actually caused by rizatriptan or to reliably assess causation in individual cases.

Cerebrovascular Events and Fatalities Associated with 5-HT$_1$ Agonists: Cerebral hemorrhage, subarachnoid hemorrhage, stroke, and other cerebrovascular events have been reported in patients treated with 5-HT$_1$ agonists; and some have resulted in fatalities. In a number of cases, it appears possible that the cerebrovascular events were primary, the agonist having been administered in the incorrect belief that the symptoms experienced were a consequence of migraine, when they were not. It should be noted that patients with migraine may be at increased risk of certain cerebrovascular events (e.g., stroke, hemorrhage, transient ischemic attack).

Other Vasospasm-Related Events: 5-HT$_1$ agonists may cause vasospastic reactions other than coronary artery vasospasm. Both peripheral vascular ischemia and colonic ischemia with abdominal pain and bloody diarrhea have been reported with 5-HT$_1$ agonists.

Increase in Blood Pressure: Significant elevation in blood pressure, including hypertensive crisis, has been reported on rare occasions in patients receiving 5-HT_1 agonists with and without a history of hypertension. In healthy young male and female subjects who received maximal doses of MAXALT (10 mg every 2 hours for 3 doses), slight increases in blood pressure (approximately 2–3 mmHg) were observed. Rizatriptan is contraindicated in patients with uncontrolled hypertension (see CONTRAINDICATIONS).

An 18% increase in mean pulmonary artery pressure was seen following dosing with another 5-HT_1 agonist in a study evaluating subjects undergoing cardiac catheterization.

PRECAUTIONS

General

As with other 5-$HT_{1B/1D}$ agonists, sensations of tightness, pain, pressure, and heaviness have been reported after treatment with MAXALT in the precordium, throat, neck and jaw. These events have not been associated with arrhythmias or definite ischemic ECG changes in clinical trials (one patient experienced chest pain with possible ischemic ECG changes). Because drugs in this class may cause coronary artery vasospasm, patients who experience signs or symptoms suggestive of angina following dosing should be evaluated for the presence of CAD or a predisposition to Prinzmetal's variant angina before receiving additional doses of medication, and should be monitored electrocardiographically if dosing is resumed and similar symptoms recur. Similarly, patients who experience other symptoms or signs suggestive of decreased arterial flow, such as ischemic bowel syndrome or Raynaud's syndrome following the use of any 5-HT_1 agonist are candidates for further evaluation (see WARNINGS).

Rizatriptan should also be administered with caution to patients with diseases that may alter the absorption, metabolism, or excretion of drugs (see CLINICAL PHARMACOLOGY, *Special Populations*).

Renally Impaired Patients: Rizatriptan should be used with caution in dialysis patients due to a decrease in the clearance of rizatriptan (see CLINICAL PHARMACOLOGY, *Special Populations*).

Hepatically Impaired Patients: Rizatriptan should be used with caution in patients with moderate hepatic insufficiency due to an increase in plasma concentrations of approximately 30% (see CLINICAL PHARMACOLOGY, *Special Populations*).

For a given attack, if a patient has no response to the first dose of rizatriptan, the diagnosis of migraine should be reconsidered before administration of a second dose.

Binding to Melanin-Containing Tissues

The propensity for rizatriptan to bind melanin has not been investigated. Based on its chemical properties, rizatriptan may bind to melanin and accumulate in melanin rich tissue (e.g., eye) over time. This raises the possibility that rizatriptan could cause toxicity in these tissues after extended use. There were, however, no adverse ophthalmologic changes related to treatment with rizatriptan in the one year dog toxicity study. Although no systematic monitoring of ophthalmologic function was undertaken in clinical trials, and no specific recommendations for ophthalmologic monitoring are offered, prescribers should be aware of the possibility of long-term ophthalmologic effects.

Phenylketonurics

Phenylketonuric patients should be informed that MAXALT-MLT Orally Disintegrating Tablets contain phenylalanine (a component of aspartame). Each 5-mg orally disintegrating tablet contains 1.05 mg phenylalanine, and each 10-mg orally disintegrating tablet contains 2.10 mg phenylalanine.

Information for Patients

Migraine or treatment with MAXALT may cause somnolence in some patients. Dizziness has also been reported in some patients receiving MAXALT. Patients should, therefore, evaluate their ability to perform complex tasks during migraine attacks and after administration of MAXALT.

Physicians should instruct their patients to read the patient package insert before taking MAXALT. See the accompanying PATIENT INFORMATION leaflet.

MAXALT-MLT Orally Disintegrating Tablets

Patients should be instructed not to remove the blister from the outer pouch until just prior to dosing. The blister pack should then be peeled open with dry hands and the orally disintegrating tablet placed on the tongue, where it will dissolve and be swallowed with the saliva.

Laboratory Tests

No specific laboratory tests are recommended for monitoring patients prior to and/or after treatment with MAXALT.

Drug Interactions (See also CLINICAL PHARMACOLOGY, *Drug Interactions.*)

Propranolol: Rizatriptan 5 mg should be used in patients taking propranolol, as propranolol has been shown to increase the plasma concentrations of rizatriptan by 70% (see CLINICAL PHARMACOLOGY, *Drug Interactions*; DOSAGE AND ADMINISTRATION).

Ergot-containing drugs: Ergot-containing drugs have been reported to cause prolonged vasospastic reactions. Because there is a theoretical basis that these effects may be additive, use of ergotamine-containing or ergot-type medications (like dihydroergotamine or methysergide) and rizatriptan within 24 hours is contraindicated (see CONTRAINDICATIONS).

Other 5-HT_1 agonists: The administration of rizatriptan with other 5-HT_1 agonists has not been evaluated in migraine patients. Because their vasospastic effects may be additive, coadministration of rizatriptan and other 5-HT_1 agonists within 24 hours of each other is not recommended (see CONTRAINDICATIONS).

Selective serotonin reuptake inhibitors (SSRIs): SSRIs (e.g., fluoxetine, fluvoxamine, paroxetine, sertraline) have been reported, rarely, to cause weakness, hyperreflexia, and incoordination when coadministered with 5-HT_1 agonists. If concomitant treatment with rizatriptan and an SSRI is clinically warranted, appropriate observation of the patient is advised. No clinical or pharmacokinetic interactions were observed when MAXALT 10 mg was administered with paroxetine.

Monoamine oxidase inhibitors: Rizatriptan should not be administered to patients taking MAO-A inhibitors and nonselective MAO inhibitors; it has been shown that moclobemide (a specific MAO-A inhibitor) increased the systemic exposure of rizatriptan and its metabolite (see CLINICAL PHARMACOLOGY, *Drug Interactions*; CONTRAINDICATIONS).

Drug/Laboratory Test Interactions

MAXALT is not known to interfere with commonly employed clinical laboratory tests.

Carcinogenesis, Mutagenesis, Impairment of Fertility

Carcinogenesis: The lifetime carcinogenic potential of rizatriptan was evaluated in a 100-week study in mice and a 106-week study in rats at oral gavage doses of up to 125 mg/kg/day. Exposure data were not obtained in those studies, but plasma AUC's of parent drug measured in other studies after 5 and 21 weeks of oral dosing in mice and rats, respectively, indicate that the exposures to parent drug at the highest dose level in the carcinogenicity studies would have been approximately 150 times (mice) and 240 times (rats) average AUC's measured in humans after three 10 mg doses, the maximum recommended total daily dose. There was no evidence of an increase in tumor incidence related to rizatriptan in either species.

Mutagenesis: Rizatriptan, with and without metabolic activation, was neither mutagenic, nor clastogenic in a battery of *in vitro* and *in vivo* genetic toxicity studies, including: the microbial mutagenesis (Ames) assay, the *in vitro* mammalian cell mutagenesis assay in V-79 Chinese hamster lung cells, the *in vitro* alkaline elution assay in rat hepatocytes, the *in vitro* chromosomal aberration assay in Chinese hamster ovary cells and the *in vivo* chromosomal aberration assay in mouse bone marrow.

Impairment of Fertility: In a fertility study in rats, altered estrus cyclicity and delays in time to mating were observed in females treated orally with 100 mg/kg/day rizatriptan. Plasma drug exposure (AUC) at this dose was approximately 225 times the exposure in humans receiving the maximum recommended daily dose (MRDD) of 30 mg. The no-effect dose was 10 mg/kg/day (approximately 15 times the human exposure at the MRDD). There were no other fertility-related effects in the female rats. There was no impairment of fertility or reproductive performance in male rats treated with up to 250 mg/kg/day (approximately 550 times the human exposure at the MRDD).

Pregnancy: Pregnancy Category C

In a general reproductive study in rats, birth weights and pre- and post-weaning weight gain were reduced in the offspring of females treated prior to and during mating and throughout gestation and lactation with doses of 10 and 100 mg/kg/day. Maternal drug exposures (AUC) at these doses were approximately 15 and 225 times, respectively, the exposure in humans receiving the maximum recommended daily dose (MRDD) of 30 mg. In a pre- and postnatal developmental toxicity study in rats, an increase in mortality of the offspring at birth and for the first three days after birth, a decrease in pre- and post-weaning weight gain, and decreased performance in a passive avoidance test (which indicates a decrease in learning capacity of the offspring) were observed at doses of 100 and 250 mg/kg/day. The no-effect dose for all of these effects was 5 mg/kg/day, approximately 7.5 times the exposure in humans receiving the MRDD. With doses of 100 and 250 mg/kg/day, the decreases in average weight of both the male and female offspring persisted into adulthood. All of these effects on the offspring in both reproductive toxicity studies occurred in the absence of any apparent maternal toxicity.

In embryofetal development studies, no teratogenic effects were observed when pregnant rats and rabbits were administered doses of 100 and 50 mg/kg/day, respectively, during organogenesis. Fetal weights were decreased in conjunction with decreased maternal weight gain at the highest doses (maternal exposures approximately 225 and 115 times the human exposure at the MRDD in rats and rabbits, respectively). The developmental no-effect dose in these studies was 10 mg/kg/day in both rats and rabbits (maternal exposures approximately 15 times human exposure at the MRDD). Toxicokinetic studies demonstrated placental transfer of drug in both species.

There are no adequate and well-controlled studies in pregnant women; therefore, rizatriptan should be used during pregnancy only if the potential benefit justifies the potential risk to the fetus.

Merck & Co., Inc. maintains a registry to monitor the pregnancy outcomes of women exposed to MAXALT while pregnant. Healthcare providers are encouraged to report any prenatal exposure to MAXALT by calling the Pregnancy Registry at (800) 986-8999.

Nursing Mothers

It is not known whether this drug is excreted in human milk. Because many drugs are excreted in human milk, caution should be exercised when MAXALT is administered to women who are breast-feeding. Rizatriptan is extensively excreted in rat milk, at a level of 5-fold or greater than maternal plasma levels.

Pediatric Use

Safety and effectiveness of rizatriptan in pediatric patients have not been established; therefore, MAXALT is not recommended for use in patients under 18 years of age.

The efficacy of MAXALT Tablets (5 mg) in patients aged 12 to 17 years was not established in a randomized placebo-controlled trial of 291 adolescent migraineurs (see *Clinical Studies*). Adverse events observed were similar in nature to those reported in clinical trials in adults. Postmarketing experience with other triptans includes a limited number of reports that describe pediatric patients who have experienced clinically serious adverse events that are similar in nature to those reported rarely in adults. The long-term safety of rizatriptan in pediatric patients has not been studied.

Geriatric Use

The pharmacokinetics of rizatriptan were similar in elderly (aged ≥ 65 years) and in younger adults. Because migraine occurs infrequently in the elderly, clinical experience with MAXALT is limited in such patients. In clinical trials, there were no apparent differences in efficacy or in overall adverse experience rates between patients under 65 years of age and those 65 and above (n=17).

ADVERSE REACTIONS

Serious cardiac events, including some that have been fatal, have occurred following use of 5-HT_1 agonists. These events are extremely rare and most have been reported in patients with risk factors predictive of CAD. Events reported have included coronary artery vasospasm, transient myocardial ischemia, myocardial infarction, ventricular tachycardia, and ventricular fibrillation (see CONTRAINDICATIONS, WARNINGS, and PRECAUTIONS).

Incidence in Controlled Clinical Trials: Adverse experiences to rizatriptan were assessed in controlled clinical trials that included over 3700 patients who received single or multiple doses of MAXALT Tablets. The most common adverse events during treatment with MAXALT were asthenia/fatigue, somnolence, pain/pressure sensation and dizziness. These events appeared to be dose related. In long term extension studies where patients were allowed to treat multiple attacks for up to 1 year, 4% (59 out of 1525 patients) withdrew because of adverse experiences.

Table 3 lists the adverse events regardless of drug relationship (incidence ≥2% and greater than placebo) after a single dose of MAXALT. The events cited reflect experience gained under closely monitored conditions of clinical trials in a highly selected patient population. In actual clinical practice or in other clinical trials, these frequency estimates may not apply, as the conditions of use, reporting behavior, and the kinds of patients treated may differ.

Table 3
Incidence (≥ 2% and Greater than Placebo) of Adverse Experiences After a Single Dose of MAXALT Tablets or Placebo

Adverse Experiences	% of Patients		
	MAXALT 5 mg (N=977)	MAXALT 10 mg (N=1167)	Placebo (N=627)
Atypical Sensations	4	5	4
Paresthesia	3	4	<2
Pain and other Pressure Sensations	6	9	3
Chest Pain: tightness/pressure and/or heaviness	<2	3	1
Neck/throat/jaw: pain/tightness/pressure	<2	2	1
Regional Pain: tightness/pressure/ heaviness	<1	2	0
Pain, location unspecified	3	3	<2
Digestive	9	13	8
Dry Mouth	3	3	1
Nausea	4	6	4
Neurological	14	20	11
Dizziness	4	9	5
Headache	<2	2	<1
Somnolence	4	8	4
Other			
Asthenia/fatigue	4	7	2

MAXALT was generally well-tolerated. Adverse experiences were typically mild in intensity and were transient. The frequencies of adverse experiences in clinical trials did not increase when up to three doses were taken within 24 hours. Adverse event frequencies were also unchanged by concomitant use of drugs commonly taken for migraine prophylaxis

Continued on next page

Information on the Merck & Co., Inc., products listed on these pages is from the prescribing information in use October 1, 2004. For information, please call 1-800-NSC-MERCK [1-800-672-6372].

Maxalt—Cont.

(including propranolol), oral contraceptives, or analgesics. The incidences of adverse experiences were not affected by age or gender. There were insufficient data to assess the impact of race on the incidence of adverse events.

Other Events Observed in Association with the Administration of MAXALT: In the section that follows, the frequencies of less commonly reported adverse clinical events are presented. Because the reports include events observed in open studies, the role of MAXALT in their causation cannot be reliably determined. Furthermore, variability associated with adverse event reporting, the terminology used to describe adverse events, etc., limit the value of the quantitative frequency estimates provided. Event frequencies are calculated as the number of patients who used MAXALT (N=3716) and reported an event divided by the total number of patients exposed to MAXALT. All reported events are included, except those already listed in the previous table, those too general to be informative, and those not reasonably associated with the use of the drug. Events are further classified within body system categories and enumerated in order of decreasing frequency using the following definitions: frequent adverse events are those defined as those occurring in at least (>)1/100 patients; infrequent adverse experiences are those occurring in 1/100 to 1/1000 patients; and rare adverse experiences are those occurring in fewer than 1/1000 patients.

General: Infrequent were chills, heat sensitivity, facial edema, hangover effect, and abdominal distention. Rare were fever, orthostatic effects, syncope and edema/swelling.

Atypical Sensations: Frequent were warm/cold sensations.

Cardiovascular: Frequent was palpitation. Infrequent were tachycardia, cold extremities, hypertension, arrhythmia, and bradycardia. Rare was angina pectoris.

Digestive: Frequent were diarrhea and vomiting. Infrequent were dyspepsia, thirst, acid regurgitation, dysphagia, constipation, flatulence, and tongue edema. Rare were anorexia, appetite increase, gastritis, paralysis (tongue), and eructation.

Metabolic: Infrequent was dehydration.

Musculoskeletal: Infrequent were muscle weakness, stiffness, myalgia, muscle cramp, musculoskeletal pain, arthralgia, and muscle spasm.

Neurological/Psychiatric: Frequent were hypesthesia, mental acuity decreased, euphoria and tremor. Infrequent were nervousness, vertigo, insomnia, anxiety, depression, disorientation, ataxia, dysarthria, confusion, dream abnormality, gait abnormality, irritability, memory impairment, agitation and hyperesthesia. Rare were: dysesthesia, depersonalization, akinesia/bradykinesia, apprehension, hyperkinesia, hypersomnia, and hyporeflexia.

Respiratory: Frequent was dyspnea. Infrequent were pharyngitis, irritation (nasal), congestion (nasal), dry throat, upper respiratory infection, yawning, respiratory congestion (nasal), dry nose, epistaxis, and sinus disorder. Rare were cough, hiccups, hoarseness, rhinorrhea, sneezing, tachypnea, and pharyngeal edema.

Special Senses: Infrequent were blurred vision, tinnitus, dry eyes, burning eye, eye pain, eye irritation, ear pain, and tearing. Rare were hyperacusis, smell perversion, photophobia, photopsia, itching eye, and eye swelling.

Skin and Skin Appendage: Frequent was flushing. Infrequent were sweating, pruritus, rash, and urticaria. Rare were erythema, acne, and photosensitivity.

Urogenital System: Frequent was hot flashes. Infrequent were urinary frequency, polyuria, and menstruation disorder. Rare was dysuria.

The adverse experience profile seen with MAXALT-MLT Orally Disintegrating Tablets was similar to that seen with MAXALT Tablets.

Postmarketing Experience

The following section enumerates potentially important adverse events that have occurred in clinical practice and which have been reported spontaneously to various surveillance systems. The events enumerated represent reports arising from both domestic and non-domestic use of rizatriptan. The events enumerated include all except those already listed in the ADVERSE REACTIONS section above or those too general to be informative. Because the reports cite events reported spontaneously from worldwide postmarketing experience, frequency of events and the role of rizatriptan in their causation cannot be reliably determined.

Cardiovascular: Myocardial ischemia, Myocardial infarction (See WARNINGS).

Cerebrovascular: Stroke.

Special Senses: Dysgeusia.

General: *Hypersensitivity:* angioedema (e.g., facial edema, tongue swelling, pharyngeal edema), wheezing, toxic epidermal necrolysis.

DRUG ABUSE AND DEPENDENCE

Although the abuse potential of MAXALT has not been specifically assessed, no abuse of, tolerance to, withdrawal from, or drug-seeking behavior was observed in patients who received MAXALT in clinical trials or their extensions. The 5-$HT_{1B/1D}$ agonists, as a class, have not been associated with drug abuse.

OVERDOSAGE

No overdoses of MAXALT were reported during clinical trials.

Rizatriptan 40 mg (administered as either a single dose or as two doses with a 2-hour interdose interval) was generally well tolerated in over 300 patients; dizziness and somnolence were the most common drug-related adverse effects.

In a clinical pharmacology study in which 12 subjects received rizatriptan, at total cumulative doses of 80 mg (given within four hours), two subjects experienced syncope and/or bradycardia. One subject, a female aged 29 years, developed vomiting, bradycardia, and dizziness beginning three hours after receiving a total of 80 mg rizatriptan (administered over two hours); a third degree AV block, responsive to atropine, was observed an hour after the onset of the other symptoms. The second subject, a 25 year old male, experienced transient dizziness, syncope, incontinence, and a 5-second systolic pause (on ECG monitor) immediately after a painful venipuncture. The venipuncture occurred two hours after the subject had received a total of 80 mg rizatriptan (administered over four hours).

In addition, based on the pharmacology of rizatriptan, hypertension or other more serious cardiovascular symptoms could occur after overdosage. Gastrointestinal decontamination, (i.e., gastric lavage followed by activated charcoal) should be considered in patients suspected of an overdose with MAXALT. Clinical and electrocardiographic monitoring should be continued for at least 12 hours, even if clinical symptoms are not observed.

The effects of hemo- or peritoneal dialysis on serum concentrations of rizatriptan are unknown.

DOSAGE AND ADMINISTRATION

In controlled clinical trials, single doses of 5 and 10 mg of MAXALT Tablets or MAXALT-MLT were effective for the acute treatment of migraines in adults. There is evidence that the 10-mg dose may provide a greater effect than the 5-mg dose (see CLINICAL PHARMACOLOGY, *Clinical Studies*). Individuals may vary in response to doses of MAXALT Tablets. The choice of dose should therefore be made on an individual basis, weighing the possible benefit of the 10-mg dose with the potential risk for increased adverse events.

Redosing: Doses should be separated by at least 2 hours; no more than 30 mg should be taken in any 24-hour period.

The safety of treating, on average, more than four headaches in a 30-day period has not been established.

Patients receiving propranolol: In patients receiving propranolol, the 5-mg dose of MAXALT should be used, up to a maximum of 3 doses in any 24-hour period. (See CLINICAL PHARMACOLOGY, *Drug Interactions.*)

For MAXALT-MLT Orally Disintegrating Tablets, administration with liquid is not necessary. The orally disintegrating tablet is packaged in a blister within an outer aluminum pouch. Patients should be instructed not to remove the blister from the outer pouch until just prior to dosing. The blister pack should then be peeled open with dry hands and the orally disintegrating tablet placed on the tongue, where it will dissolve and be swallowed with the saliva.

HOW SUPPLIED

No. 3732—MAXALT Tablets, 5 mg, are pale pink, capsule-shaped, compressed tablets coded MRK on one side and 266 on the other. They are supplied as follows:

NDC 0006-0266-09, carton of 9 tablets.

No. 3733—MAXALT Tablets, 10 mg, are pale pink, capsule-shaped, compressed tablets coded MAXALT on one side and MRK 267 on the other. They are supplied as follows:

NDC 0006-0267-09, carton of 9 tablets.

No. 3800—MAXALT-MLT Orally Disintegrating Tablets, 5 mg, are white to off-white, round lyophilized orally disintegrating tablets debossed with a modified triangle on one side, and measuring 10.0–11.5 mm (side-to-side) with a peppermint flavor. Each orally disintegrating tablet is individually packaged in a blister inside an aluminum pouch (sachet). They are supplied as follows:

NDC 0006-3800-09, 3 × unit of use carrying case of 3 orally disintegrating tablets (9 tablets total).

No. 3801—MAXALT-MLT Orally Disintegrating Tablets, 10 mg, are white to off-white, round lyophilized orally disintegrating tablets debossed with a modified square on one side, and measuring 12.0–13.8 mm (side-to-side) with a peppermint flavor. Each orally disintegrating tablet is individually packaged in a blister inside an aluminum pouch (sachet). They are supplied as follows:

NDC 0006-3801-09, 3 × unit of use carrying case of 3 orally disintegrating tablets (9 tablets total).

Storage

Store MAXALT Tablets at room temperature, 15–30°C (59–86°F). Dispense in a tight container, if product is subdivided.

Store MAXALT-MLT Orally Disintegrating Tablets at room temperature, 15–30°C (59–86°F). The patient should be instructed not to remove the blister from the outer aluminum pouch until the patient is ready to consume the orally disintegrating tablet inside.

MAXALT Tablets are manufactured for:
MERCK & CO., INC., Whitehouse Station, NJ 08889, USA
By:
MSD, Ltd. Cramlington
Northumberland, NE23 9JU, UK

MAXALT-MLT Orally Disintegrating Tablets are manufactured for:
MERCK & CO., INC., Whitehouse Station, NJ 08889, USA
By:
Cardinal Health UK 416 Ltd.
Swindon, Wiltshire, SN5 8RU, UK

9122111 Issued September 2003

Patient Information about MAXALT® (max-awlt) and MAXALT-MLT® for Migraine

Generic name: rizatriptan benzoate

Please read this information before you start taking MAXALT*. Also, read the leaflet each time you renew your prescription, just in case anything has changed. Remember, this leaflet does not take the place of careful discussions with your doctor. You and your doctor should discuss MAXALT when you start taking your medication and at regular checkups.

What is MAXALT and what is it used for?

MAXALT is a medication used for the treatment of migraine attacks in adults. MAXALT is a member of a class of drugs called selective 5-$HT_{1B/1D}$ receptor agonists.

It is available as a traditional tablet (MAXALT) and as an orally disintegrating tablet (MAXALT-MLT*). Unless otherwise stated, the information contained in this leaflet applies both to MAXALT Tablets and to MAXALT-MLT Orally Disintegrating Tablets.

Tell your doctor about your symptoms. Your doctor will decide if you have migraine. Use MAXALT only for a migraine attack. MAXALT should not be used to treat headaches that might be caused by other, more serious conditions.

You will find more information about migraine at the end of this leaflet.

* Registered trademark of MERCK & CO., Inc.

How should I take MAXALT?

Your doctor has prescribed either a 5 mg or 10 mg dosage of MAXALT or MAXALT-MLT for your migraine attack. When you have a migraine headache, take your medication as directed by your doctor.

MAXALT Tablets

If you are using MAXALT Tablets, swallow the tablet whole with liquid.

MAXALT-MLT Orally Disintegrating Tablets

If you are using MAXALT-MLT, leave the orally disintegrating tablet in its package until you are ready to take it. Remove the blister from the foil pouch. Do not push the tablet through the blister; rather, peel open the blister pack with dry hands and place the tablet on your tongue. The tablet will dissolve rapidly and be swallowed with your saliva. No liquid is needed to take the orally disintegrating tablet.

If your headache comes back after your initial dose, a second dose may be taken anytime after 2 hours of administering the first dose. For any attack where you have no response to the first dose, do not take a second dose without first consulting with your doctor. Do not take more than 30 mg of MAXALT in a 24-hour period (for example, do not take more than three 10-mg tablets in a 24-hour period).

If you are receiving propranolol, you should use the 5-mg dose of MAXALT or MAXALT-MLT, up to a maximum of 3 doses (15 mg total) in a 24-hour period.

If your condition worsens, seek medical attention.

Who should not take MAXALT?

Do not take MAXALT if you:

- have had a serious allergic reaction to MAXALT or any of its ingredients
- have uncontrolled high blood pressure
- have heart disease or history of heart disease
- are currently taking monoamine oxidase (MAO) inhibitors** such as phenelzine sulfate (NARDIL®) or tranylcypromine sulfate (PARNATE®) for mental depression, or have taken MAO inhibitors within the last two weeks.

MAXALT should not be used within 24 hours of treatment with another 5-HT_1 agonist** such as sumatriptan (IMITREX®), naratriptan (AMERGE™) or zolmitriptan (ZOMIG™); or ergotamine-type medications such as ergotamine (BELLERGAL-S®, CAFERGOT®, ERGOMAR®, WIGRAINE®), dihydro-ergotamine (D.H.E. 45®), or methysergide (SANSERT®).

** The brands listed are the trademarks of their respective owners and are not trademarks of Merck & Co., Inc.

What should I tell my doctor before and during treatment with MAXALT?

Tell your doctor:

- about any past or present medical problems
- about any history of high blood pressure, chest pain, shortness of breath, heart disease, or stroke
- about any risk factors for heart disease or blood vessel disease
  - high blood pressure or diabetes
  - high cholesterol
  - obesity
  - smoking
  - family history of heart disease or blood vessel disease
  - post menopausal
  - male over 40
- about any allergies you have or have had
- if you are pregnant or plan to become pregnant
- if you are breast-feeding or plan to breast-feed
- about all drugs you are taking or plan to take, including those obtained without a prescription, and those you normally take for a migraine.

MAXALT-MLT orally disintegrating tablets contain aspartame, a source of phenylalanine.
Phenylketonurics: MAXALT-MLT 5-mg and 10-mg orally disintegrating tablets contain 1.05 and 2.10 mg phenylalanine, respectively.

What if I am pregnant?
Do not use MAXALT if you are pregnant, think you might be pregnant, are trying to become pregnant, or are not using adequate contraception, unless you have discussed this with your doctor.

Can I take MAXALT with other medications?**
Do not take MAXALT with any other drug in the same class within 24 hours, such as sumatriptan (IMITREX®), naratriptan (AMERGE™) or zolmitriptan (ZOMIG™).
Do not take MAXALT within 24 hours of taking ergotamine-type medications such as ergotamine (BELLERGAL-S®, CAFERGOT®, ERGOMAR®, WIGRAINE®), dihydro-ergotamine (D.H.E. 45®) or methysergide (SANSERT®) to treat your migraine.
Do not take MAXALT when you are taking monoamine oxidase (MAO) inhibitors, such as phenelzine sulfate (NARDIL®) or tranylcypromine sulfate (PARNATE®) for mental depression, or if it has been less than two weeks since you stopped taking an MAO inhibitor.
Ask your doctor for instructions about taking MAXALT if you are now taking propranolol (INDERAL®). (See **How should I take MAXALT?** section.)

What are the possible side effects of MAXALT?
Like all prescription drugs, MAXALT can cause side effects. In studies, MAXALT was generally well-tolerated. The side effects were usually mild and temporary. The following is **not** a complete list of side effects reported with MAXALT. Do not rely on this leaflet alone for information about side effects. Ask your doctor to discuss with you the more complete list of side effects.
In studies, the **most common** side effects reported were:
- **dizziness**
- **sleepiness, tiredness, fatigue**
- **pain or pressure sensation (e.g., in the chest or throat)**

If you experience dizziness, sleepiness, tiredness or fatigue, you should evaluate your ability to perform complex tasks such as driving or operating heavy machinery.
Other, **less common** side effects reported in studies or general use were related to the:
Heart and blood vessels – Alterations in heartbeat, increased blood pressure and cold extremities.
Muscles – Muscle weakness, stiffness, and spasm; and muscle and bone pain.
Nervous system – Nervousness, decreased mental sharpness, tremor, headache, abnormal sensation, vertigo, sleep disturbance, mood and personality changes, alterations in speech and movement, memory impairment, confusion and dream abnormality.
Digestive system – Stomach upset, diarrhea, dry mouth, constipation, gas, thirst, acid reflux, difficulty swallowing, changes in appetite, burping and inability of the tongue to move.
Skin – Flushing (redness of the face lasting a short time), hot flashes, sweating, itching, rash, acne and skin reaction to sunlight.
Respiratory – Difficult or rapid breathing, dryness or discomfort of the throat or nose, nose bleed, yawning and sinus disorder, cold-like symptoms, cough, and hiccups.
Special Senses – Visual disturbances, ringing in the ears, ear pain, eye discomfort, swelling or tearing, alterations in hearing and smelling, visual intolerance to light, and bad taste.
Miscellaneous – Allergic reactions including swelling of face, lips, tongue and/or throat which may cause difficulty in breathing and/or swallowing, wheezing, hives, rash, and severe sloughing of the skin. Also chills, heat sensitivity, swelling, bloating, hangover effect, fever, fainting, dizziness on standing up, warm/cold sensations, dehydration and changes in urination and menstruation.
As with other drugs in this class, there have been very rare reports of heart attack and stroke generally occurring in patients with risk factors for heart and blood vessel disease (see **What should I tell my doctor before and during treatment with MAXALT?**).
Tell your doctor about these or any other symptoms. If the symptoms persist or worsen, seek medical attention promptly. In addition, tell your doctor if you experience any symptoms that suggest an allergic reaction (see **Miscellaneous** above) after taking MAXALT.

What should I do if I take an overdose?
If you take more medication than you have been told to take, you should contact your doctor, hospital emergency department, or nearest poison control center immediately.

What is migraine and how does it differ from other headaches?
Migraine is an intense, throbbing, typically one-sided headache that often includes nausea, vomiting, sensitivity to light, and sensitivity to sound. According to many migraine sufferers, the pain and symptoms from a migraine headache are more intense than the pain and symptoms of a common headache.
Some people may have visual symptoms before the headache, such as flashing lights or wavy lines, called an aura. Migraine attacks typically last for hours or, rarely, for more than a day, and they can return frequently. The severity and frequency of migraine attacks may vary.
Based on your symptoms, your doctor will decide whether you have migraine.

Who gets migraine?
Migraine headaches tend to occur in members of the same family. Both men and women get migraine, but it is more common in women.

What may trigger a migraine attack?
Certain things are thought to trigger migraine attacks in some people. Some of these triggers are:
- certain foods or beverages (e.g., cheese, chocolate, citrus fruit, caffeine, alcohol)
- stress
- change in a behavior (e.g., under/oversleeping; missing a meal; change in diet)
- hormonal changes in women (e.g., menstruation)

You may be able to prevent migraine attacks or diminish their frequency if you understand what specifically triggers your attacks. Keeping a headache diary may help you identify and monitor the possible migraine triggers you encounter. Once the triggers are identified, you and your doctor can modify your treatment and lifestyle appropriately.

How does MAXALT work during a migraine attack?
Treatment with MAXALT:
1. Reduces swelling of blood vessels surrounding the brain. This swelling results in the headache pain of a migraine attack.
2. Blocks the release of substances from nerve endings that cause more pain and other symptoms of migraine.
3. Interrupts the sending of specific pain signals to your brain.

It is thought that each of these actions contributes to relief of your symptoms by MAXALT.

How should I store MAXALT?
Keep your medicine in a safe place where children cannot reach it. It may be harmful to children. Store your medication away from heat, light, moisture, and at a controlled room temperature 59°–86°F (15°–30°C). If your medication has expired, throw it away as instructed. If your doctor decides to stop your treatment, do not keep any leftover medicine unless your doctor tells you to do so. Throw away your medicine as instructed. Be sure that the discarded tablets are out of the reach of children.
If you are storing MAXALT-MLT, do not remove the blister from the outer aluminum pouch until you are ready to take the medication inside.
This leaflet provides a summary of information about MAXALT. If you have any questions or concerns about either MAXALT or migraine, talk to your doctor. In addition, talk to your pharmacist or other health care provider.

9601304 Issued January 2004

Shown in Product Identification Guide, page 323

MEFOXIN® ℞
(Cefoxitin for Injection)

To reduce the development of drug-resistant bacteria and maintain the effectiveness of MEFOXIN* and other antibacterial drugs, MEFOXIN should be used only to treat or prevent infections that are proven or strongly suspected to be caused by bacteria.

DESCRIPTION

MEFOXIN* (Cefoxitin for Injection) is a semi-synthetic, broad-spectrum cepha antibiotic sealed under nitrogen for intravenous administration. It is derived from cephamycin C, which is produced by *Streptomyces lactamdurans*. Its chemical name is sodium (6*R*, 7*S*)-3-(hydroxymethyl)-7-methoxy-8-oxo-7-[2-(2-thienyl)acetamido]-5-thia-1-azabicyclo[4.2.0]oct-2-ene-2-carboxylate carbamate (ester). The empirical formula is $C_{16}H_{16}N_3NaO_7S_2$, and the structural formula is:

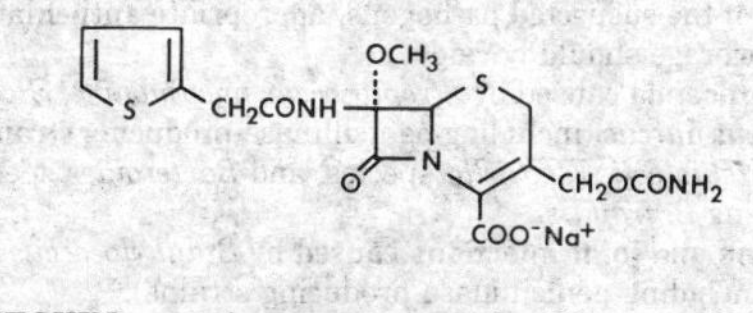

MEFOXIN contains approximately 53.8 mg (2.3 milliequivalents) of sodium per gram of cefoxitin activity. Solutions of MEFOXIN range from colorless to light amber in color. The pH of freshly constituted solutions usually ranges from 4.2 to 7.0.

*Registered trademark of MERCK & CO., Inc.

CLINICAL PHARMACOLOGY

Clinical Pharmacology
Following an intravenous dose of 1 gram, serum concentrations were 110 mcg/mL at 5 minutes, declining to less than 1 mcg/mL at 4 hours. The half-life after an intravenous dose is 41 to 59 minutes. Approximately 85 percent of cefoxitin is excreted unchanged by the kidneys over a 6-hour period, resulting in high urinary concentrations. Probenecid slows tubular excretion and produces higher serum levels and increases the duration of measurable serum concentrations.
Cefoxitin passes into pleural and joint fluids and is detectable in antibacterial concentrations in bile.

Microbiology
The bactericidal action of cefoxitin results from inhibition of cell wall synthesis. Cefoxitin has *in vitro* activity against a wide range of gram-positive and gram-negative organisms. The methoxy group in the 7α position provides cefoxitin with a high degree of stability in the presence of beta-lactamases, both penicillinases and cephalosporinases, of gram-negative bacteria.
Cefoxitin has been shown to be active against most strains of the following microorganisms, both *in vitro* and in clinical infections as described in the INDICATIONS AND USAGE section.

Aerobic gram-positive microorganisms
Staphylococcus aureus[a] (including penicillinase-producing strains)
Staphylococcus epidermidis[a]
Streptococcus agalactiae
Streptococcus pneumoniae
Streptococcus pyogenes

[a] Staphylococci resistant to methicillin/oxacillin should be considered resistant to cefoxitin.

Most strains of enterococci, e.g., *Enterococcus faecalis*, are resistant.

Aerobic gram-negative microorganisms
Escherichia coli
Haemophilus influenzae
Klebsiella spp. (including *K. pneumoniae*)
Morganella morganii
Neisseria gonorrhoeae (including penicillinase-producing strains)
Proteus mirabilis
Proteus vulgaris
Providencia spp. (including *Providencia rettgeri*)

Anaerobic gram-positive microorganisms
Clostridium spp.
Peptococcus niger
Peptostreptococcus spp.

Anaerobic gram-negative microorganisms
Bacteroides distasonis
Bacteroides fragilis
Bacteroides ovatus
Bacteroides thetaiotaomicron
Bacteroides spp.

The following *in vitro* data are available, **but their clinical significance is unknown.**
Cefoxitin exhibits *in vitro* minimum inhibitory concentrations (MIC's) of 8 µg/mL or less for aerobic microorganisms and 16 µg/mL or less for anaerobic microorganisms against most (≥90%) strains of the following microorganisms; however, the safety and effectiveness of cefoxitin in treating clinical infections due to these microorganisms have not been established in adequate and well-controlled clinical trials.

Aerobic gram-negative microorganisms
Eikenella corrodens [non-β-lactamase producers]
Klebsiella oxytoca

Anaerobic gram-positive microorganisms
Clostridium perfringens

Anaerobic gram-negative microorganisms
Prevotella bivia (formerly *Bacteroides bivius*)

Cefoxitin is inactive *in vitro* against most strains of *Pseudomonas aeruginosa* and enterococci and many strains of *Enterobacter cloacae*.

Susceptibility Tests
Dilution Techniques:
Quantitative methods are used to determine antimicrobial minimum inhibitory concentrations (MIC's). These MIC's provide estimates of the susceptibility of bacteria to antimicrobial compounds. The MIC's should be determined using a standardized procedure. Standardized procedures are based on a dilution method[1] (broth or agar) or equivalent with standardized inoculum concentrations and standardized concentrations of cefoxitin powder. The MIC values should be interpreted according to the following criteria:
For testing aerobic microorganisms[a,b,c] other than *Neisseria gonorrhoeae*:

MIC (µg/mL)	Interpretation
≤ 8	Susceptible (S)
16	Intermediate (I)
≥ 32	Resistant (R)

[a] Staphylococci exhibiting resistance to methicillin/oxacillin should be reported as also resistant to cefoxitin despite apparent *in vitro* susceptibility.
[b] For testing *Haemophilus influenzae* these interpretative criteria applicable only to tests performed by broth microdilution method using Haemophilus Test Medium (HTM)[1].
[c] For testing streptococci these interpretative criteria applicable only to tests performed by broth microdilution method using cation-adjusted Mueller-Hinton broth with 2 to 5% lysed horse blood[1].

Continued on next page

Information on the Merck & Co., Inc., products listed on these pages is from the prescribing information in use October 1, 2004. For information, please call 1-800-NSC-MERCK [1-800-672-6372].

Mefoxin—Cont.

For testing *Neisseria gonorrhoeae*[d]:

MIC (μg/mL)	Interpretation
≤ 2	Susceptible (S)
4	Intermediate (I)
≥ 8	Resistant (R)

[d] Interpretative criteria applicable only to tests performed by agar dilution method using GC agar base with 1% defined growth supplement and incubated in 5% CO_2[1]. A report of "Susceptible" indicates that the pathogen is likely to be inhibited if the antimicrobial compound in the blood reaches the concentrations usually achievable. A report of "Intermediate" indicates that the result should be considered equivocal, and, if the microorganism is not fully susceptible to alternative, clinically feasible drugs, the test should be repeated. This category implies possible clinical applicability in body sites where the drug is physiologically concentrated or in situations where high dosage of drug can be used. This category also provides a buffer zone which prevents small uncontrolled technical factors from causing major discrepancies in interpretation. A report of "Resistant" indicates that the pathogen is not likely to be inhibited if the antimicrobial compound in the blood reaches the concentrations usually achievable; other therapy should be selected.

Standardized susceptibility test procedures require the use of laboratory control microorganisms to control the technical aspects of the laboratory procedures. Standard cefoxitin powder should provide the following MIC values:

Microorganism		MIC (μg/mL)
Escherichia coli	ATCC 25922	1-4
Neisseria gonorrhoeae[a]	ATCC 49226	0.5-2
Staphylococcus aureus	ATCC 29213	1-4

[a] Interpretative criteria applicable only to tests performed by agar dilution method using GC agar base with 1% defined growth supplement and incubated in 5% CO_2[1].

Diffusion Techniques:

Quantitative methods that require measurement of zone diameters also provide reproducible estimates of the susceptibility of bacteria to antimicrobial compounds. One such standardized procedure[2] requires the use of standardized inoculum concentrations. This procedure uses paper disks impregnated with 30-μg cefoxitin to test the susceptibility of microorganisms to cefoxitin.

Reports from the laboratory providing results of the standard single-disk susceptibility test with a 30-μg cefoxitin disk should be interpreted according to the following criteria:

For testing aerobic microorganisms[a,b,c] other than *Neisseria gonorrhoeae*:

Zone Diameter (mm)	Interpretation
≥ 18	Susceptible (S)
15-17	Intermediate (I)
≤ 14	Resistant (R)

[a] Staphylococci exhibiting resistance to methicillin/oxacillin should be reported as also resistant to cefoxitin despite apparent *in vitro* susceptibility.

[b] For testing *Haemophilus influenzae* these interpretative criteria applicable only to tests performed by disk diffusion method using Haemophilus Test Medium (HTM)[1].

[c] For testing streptococci these interpretative criteria applicable only to tests performed by disk diffusion method using Mueller-Hinton agar with 5% defibrinated sheep blood and incubated in 5% CO_2[2].

For testing *Neisseria gonorrhoeae*[d]:

Zone Diameter (mm)	Interpretation
≥ 28	Susceptible (S)
24-27	Intermediate (I)
≤ 23	Resistant (R)

[d] Interpretative criteria applicable only to tests performed by disk diffusion method using GC agar base with 1% defined growth supplement and incubated in 5% CO_2[2].

Interpretation should be as stated above for results using dilution techniques.

Interpretation involves correlation of the diameter obtained in the disk test with the MIC for cefoxitin.

As with standardized dilution techniques, diffusion methods require the use of laboratory control microorganisms that are used to control the technical aspects of the laboratory procedures. For the diffusion technique, the 30-μg cefoxitin disk should provide the following zone diameters in these laboratory test quality control strains:

Microorganism		Zone Diameter (mm)
Escherichia coli	ATCC 25922	23-29
Neisseria gonorrhoeae[a]	ATCC 49226	33-41
Staphylococcus aureus	ATCC 25923	23-29

[a] Interpretative criteria applicable only to tests performed by disk diffusion method using GC agar base with 1% defined growth supplement and incubated in 5% CO_2[2].

Anaerobic Techniques:

For anaerobic bacteria, the susceptibility to cefoxitin as MIC's can be determined by standardized test methods[3]. The MIC values obtained should be interpreted according to the following criteria:

MIC (μg/mL)	Interpretation
≤ 16	Susceptible (S)
32	Intermediate (I)
≥ 64	Resistant (R)

Interpretation is identical to that stated above for results using dilution techniques.

As with other susceptibility techniques, the use of laboratory control microorganisms is required to control the technical aspects of the laboratory standardized procedures. Standard cefoxitin powder should provide the following MIC values:

Using either an Agar Dilution Method[a] or Using a Broth[b] Microdilution Method:

Microorganism		MIC (μg/mL)
Bacteroides fragilis	ATCC 25285	4-16
Bacteroides thetaiotaomicron	ATCC 29741	8-32

[a] Range applicable only to tests performed using either Brucella blood or Wilkins-Chalgren agar.

[b] Range applicable only to tests performed in the broth formulation of Wilkins-Chalgren agar[3].

INDICATIONS AND USAGE

Treatment

MEFOXIN is indicated for the treatment of serious infections caused by susceptible strains of the designated microorganisms in the diseases listed below.

(1) **Lower respiratory tract infections**, including pneumonia and lung abscess, caused by *Streptococcus pneumoniae*, other streptococci (excluding enterococci, e.g., *Enterococcus faecalis* [formerly *Streptococcus faecalis*]), *Staphylococcus aureus* (including penicillinase-producing strains), *Escherichia coli, Klebsiella* species, *Haemophilus influenzae*, and *Bacteroides* species.

(2) **Urinary tract infections** caused by *Escherichia coli, Klebsiella* species, *Proteus mirabilis, Morganella morganii, Proteus vulgaris* and *Providencia* species (including *P. rettgeri*).

(3) **Intra-abdominal infections**, including peritonitis and intra-abdominal abscess, caused by *Escherichia coli, Klebsiella* species, *Bacteroides* species including *Bacteroides fragilis*, and *Clostridium* species.

(4) **Gynecological infections**, including endometritis, pelvic cellulitis, and pelvic inflammatory disease caused by *Escherichia coli, Neisseria gonorrhoeae* (including penicillinase-producing strains), *Bacteroides* species including *B. fragilis, Clostridium* species, *Peptococcus niger, Peptostreptococcus* species, and *Streptococcus agalactiae*. MEFOXIN, like cephalosporins, has no activity against *Chlamydia trachomatis*. Therefore, when MEFOXIN is used in the treatment of patients with pelvic inflammatory disease and *C. trachomatis* is one of the suspected pathogens, appropriate anti-chlamydial coverage should be added.

(5) **Septicemia** caused by *Streptococcus pneumoniae, Staphylococcus aureus* (including penicillinase-producing strains), *Escherichia coli, Klebsiella* species, and *Bacteroides* species including *B. fragilis*.

(6) **Bone and joint infections** caused by *Staphylococcus aureus* (including penicillinase-producing strains).

(7) **Skin and skin structure infections** caused by *Staphylococcus aureus* (including penicillinase-producing strains), *Staphylococcus epidermidis, Streptococcus pyogenes* and other streptococci (excluding enterococci e.g., *Enterococcus faecalis* [formerly *Streptococcus faecalis*]), *Escherichia coli, Proteus mirabilis, Klebsiella* species, *Bacteroides* species including *B. fragilis, Clostridium* species, *Peptococcus niger*, and *Peptostreptococcus* species.

Appropriate culture and susceptibility studies should be performed to determine the susceptibility of the causative organisms to MEFOXIN. Therapy may be started while awaiting the results of these studies.

In randomized comparative studies, MEFOXIN and cephalothin were comparably safe and effective in the management of infections caused by gram-positive cocci and gram-negative rods susceptible to the cephalosporins. MEFOXIN has a high degree of stability in the presence of bacterial beta-lactamases, both penicillinases and cephalosporinases.

Many infections caused by aerobic and anaerobic gram-negative bacteria resistant to some cephalosporins respond to MEFOXIN. Similarly, many infections caused by aerobic and anaerobic bacteria resistant to some penicillin antibiotics (ampicillin, carbenicillin, penicillin G) respond to treatment with MEFOXIN. Many infections caused by mixtures of susceptible aerobic and anaerobic bacteria respond to treatment with MEFOXIN.

Prevention

MEFOXIN is indicated for the prophylaxis of infection in patients undergoing uncontaminated gastrointestinal surgery, vaginal hysterectomy, abdominal hysterectomy, or cesarean section.

If there are signs of infection, specimens for culture should be obtained for identification of the causative organism so that appropriate treatment may be instituted.

To reduce the development of drug-resistant bacteria and maintain the effectiveness of MEFOXIN and other antibacterial drugs, MEFOXIN should be used only to treat or prevent infections that are proven or strongly suspected to be caused by susceptible bacteria. When culture and susceptibility information are available, they should be considered in selecting or modifying antibacterial therapy. In the absence of such data, local epidemiology and susceptibility patterns may contribute to the empiric selection of therapy.

CONTRAINDICATIONS

MEFOXIN is contraindicated in patients who have shown hypersensitivity to cefoxitin and the cephalosporin group of antibiotics.

WARNINGS

BEFORE THERAPY WITH 'MEFOXIN' IS INSTITUTED, CAREFUL INQUIRY SHOULD BE MADE TO DETERMINE WHETHER THE PATIENT HAS HAD PREVIOUS HYPERSENSITIVITY REACTIONS TO CEFOXITIN, CEPHALOSPORINS, PENICILLINS, OR OTHER DRUGS. THIS PRODUCT SHOULD BE GIVEN WITH CAUTION TO PENICILLIN-SENSITIVE PATIENTS. ANTIBIOTICS SHOULD BE ADMINISTERED WITH CAUTION TO ANY PATIENT WHO HAS DEMONSTRATED SOME FORM OF ALLERGY, PARTICULARLY TO DRUGS. IF AN ALLERGIC REACTION TO 'MEFOXIN' OCCURS, DISCONTINUE THE DRUG. SERIOUS HYPERSENSITIVITY REACTIONS MAY REQUIRE EPINEPHRINE AND OTHER EMERGENCY MEASURES.

Pseudomembranous colitis has been reported with nearly all antibacterial agents, including cefoxitin, and may range in severity from mild to life threatening. Therefore, it is important to consider this diagnosis in patients who present with diarrhea subsequent to the administration of antibacterial agents.

Treatment with antibacterial agents alters the normal flora of the colon and my permit overgrowth of clostridia. Studies indicate that a toxin produced by *Clostridium difficile* is one primary cause of "antibiotic-associated colitis."

After the diagnosis of pseudomembranous colitis has been established, appropriate therapeutic measures should be initiated. Mild cases of pseudomembranous colitis usually respond to drug discontinuation alone. In moderate to severe cases, consideration should be given to management with fluids and electrolytes, protein supplementation, and treatment with an antibacterial drug clinically effective against *Clostridium difficile* colitis.

PRECAUTIONS

General

The total daily dose should be reduced when MEFOXIN is administered to patients with transient or persistent reduction of urinary output due to renal insufficiency (see DOSAGE AND ADMINISTRATION), because high and prolonged serum antibiotic concentrations can occur in such individuals from usual doses.

Antibiotics (including cephalosporins) should be prescribed with caution in individuals with a history of gastrointestinal disease, particularly colitis.

As with other antibiotics, prolonged use of MEFOXIN may result in overgrowth of nonsusceptible organisms. Repeated evaluation of the patient's condition is essential. If superinfection occurs during therapy, appropriate measures should be taken.

Prescribing MEFOXIN in the absence of a proven or strongly suspected bacterial infection or a prophylactic indication is unlikely to provide benefit to the patient and increases the risk of the development of drug-resistant bacteria.

Information for Patients

Patients should be counseled that antibacterial drugs including MEFOXIN should only be used to treat bacterial infections. They do not treat viral infections (e.g., the common cold). When MEFOXIN is prescribed to treat a bacterial infection, patients should be told that although it is common to feel better early in the course of therapy, the medication should be taken exactly as directed. Skipping doses or not completing the full course of therapy may (1) decrease the effectiveness of the immediate treatment and (2) increase the likelihood that bacteria will develop resistance and will not be treatable by MEFOXIN or other antibacterial drugs in the future.

Laboratory Tests

As with any potent antibacterial agent, periodic assessment of organ system functions, including renal, hepatic, and hematopoietic, is advisable during prolonged therapy.

Drug Interactions
Increased nephrotoxicity has been reported following concomitant administration of cephalosporins and aminoglycoside antibiotics.
Drug/Laboratory Test Interactions
As with cephalothin, high concentrations of cefoxitin (>100 micrograms/mL) may interfere with measurement of serum and urine creatinine levels by the Jaffé reaction, and produce false increases of modest degree in the levels of creatinine reported. Serum samples from patients treated with cefoxitin should not be analyzed for creatinine if withdrawn within 2 hours of drug administration.
High concentrations of cefoxitin in the urine may interfere with measurement of urinary 17-hydroxy-corticosteroids by the Porter-Silber reaction, and produce false increases of modest degree in the levels reported.
A false-positive reaction for glucose in the urine may occur. This has been observed with CLINITEST† reagent tablets.
Carcinogenesis, Mutagenesis, Impairment of Fertility
Long-term studies in animals have not been performed with cefoxitin to evaluate carcinogenic or mutagenic potential. Studies in rats treated intravenously with 400 mg/kg of cefoxitin (approximately three times the maximum recommended human dose) revealed no effects on fertility or mating ability.
Pregnancy
Pregnancy Category B. Reproduction studies performed in rats and mice at parenteral doses of approximately one to seven and one-half times the maximum recommended human dose did not reveal teratogenic or fetal toxic effects, although a slight decrease in fetal weight was observed.
There are, however, no adequate and well-controlled studies in pregnant women. Because animal reproduction studies are not always predictive of human response, this drug should be used during pregnancy only if clearly needed.
In the rabbit, cefoxitin was associated with a high incidence of abortion and maternal death. This was not considered to be a teratogenic effect but an expected consequence of the rabbit's unusual sensitivity to antibiotic-induced changes in the population of the microflora of the intestine.
Nursing Mothers
MEFOXIN is excreted in human milk in low concentrations. Caution should be exercised when MEFOXIN is administered to a nursing woman.
Pediatric Use
Safety and efficacy in pediatric patients from birth to three months of age have not yet been established. In pediatric patients three months of age and older, higher doses of MEFOXIN have been associated with an increased incidence of eosinophilia and elevated SGOT.

† Registered trademark of Ames Company, Division of Miles Laboratories, Inc.

ADVERSE REACTIONS

MEFOXIN is generally well tolerated. The most common adverse reactions have been local reactions following intravenous injection. Other adverse reactions have been encountered infrequently.
Local Reactions
Thrombophlebitis has occurred with intravenous administration.
Allergic Reactions
Rash (including exfoliative dermatitis and toxic epidermal necrolysis), urticaria, flushing, pruritus, eosinophilia, fever, dyspnea, and other allergic reactions including anaphylaxis, interstitial nephritis and angioedema have been noted.
Cardiovascular
Hypotension.
Gastrointestinal
Diarrhea, including documented pseudomembranous colitis which can appear during or after antibiotic treatment. Nausea and vomiting have been reported rarely.
Neuromuscular
Possible exacerbation of myasthenia gravis.
Blood
Eosinophilia, leukopenia, including granulocytopenia, neutropenia, anemia, including hemolytic anemia, thrombocytopenia, and bone marrow depression. A positive direct Coombs test may develop in some individuals, especially those with azotemia.
Liver Function
Transient elevations in SGOT, SGPT, serum LDH, serum alkaline phosphatase; and jaundice have been reported.
Renal Function
Elevations in serum creatinine and/or blood urea nitrogen levels have been observed. As with the cephalosporins, acute renal failure has been reported rarely. The role of MEFOXIN in changes in renal function tests is difficult to assess, since factors predisposing to prerenal azotemia or to impaired renal function usually have been present.
In addition to the adverse reactions listed above which have been observed in patients treated with MEFOXIN, the following adverse reactions and altered laboratory test results have been reported for cephalosporin class antibiotics:
Urticaria, erythema multiforme, Stevens-Johnson syndrome, serum sickness-like reactions, abdominal pain, colitis, renal dysfunction, toxic nephropathy, false-positive test for urinary glucose, hepatic dysfunction including cholestasis, elevated bilirubin, aplastic anemia, hemorrhage, prolonged prothrombin time, pancytopenia, agranulocytosis, superinfection, vaginitis including vaginal candidiasis.

Table 1—Guidelines for Dosage of MEFOXIN

Type of Infection	Daily Dosage	Frequency and Route
Uncomplicated forms+ of infections such as pneumonia, urinary tract infection, cutaneous infection	3-4 grams	1 gram every 6-8 hours IV
Moderately severe or severe infections	6-8 grams	1 gram every 4 hours *or* 2 grams every 6-8 hours IV
Infections commonly needing antibiotics in higher dosage (e.g., gas gangrene)	12 grams	2 grams every 4 hours *or* 3 grams every 6 hours IV

+Including patients in whom bacteremia is absent or unlikely

Table 2—Maintenance Dosage of MEFOXIN in Adults with Reduced Renal Function

Renal Function	Creatinine Clearance (mL/min)	Dose (grams)	Frequency
Mild impairment	50–30	1–2	every 8–12 hours
Moderate impairment	29–10	1–2	every 12–24 hours
Severe impairment	9–5	0.5–1	every 12–24 hours
Essentially no function	<5	0.5–1	every 24–48 hours

Several cephalosporins have been implicated in triggering seizures, particularly in patients with renal impairment when the dosage was not reduced. (See DOSAGE AND ADMINISTRATION.) If seizures associated with drug therapy occur, the drug should be discontinued. Anticonvulsant therapy can be given if clinically indicated.

OVERDOSAGE

The acute intravenous LD_{50} in the adult female mouse and rabbit was about 8.0 g/kg and greater than 1.0 g/kg respectively. The acute intraperitoneal LD_{50} in the adult rat was greater than 10.0 g/kg.

DOSAGE AND ADMINISTRATION

TREATMENT
Adults
The usual adult dosage range is 1 gram to 2 grams every six to eight hours. Dosage should be determined by susceptibility of the causative organisms, severity of infection, and the condition of the patient (see Table 1 for dosage guidelines).
If *C. trachomatis* is a suspected pathogen, appropriate antichlamydial coverage should be added, because cefoxitin sodium has no activity against this organism.
[See table 1 above]
MEFOXIN may be used in patients with reduced renal function with the following dosage adjustments:
In adults with renal insufficiency, an initial loading dose of 1 gram to 2 grams may be given. After a loading dose, the recommendations for *maintenance dosage* (Table 2) may be used as a guide.
[See table 2 above]
When only the serum creatinine level is available, the following formula (based on sex, weight, and age of the patient) may be used to convert this value into creatinine clearance. The serum creatinine should represent a steady state of renal function.

Males: $\dfrac{\text{Weight (kg)} \times (140 - \text{age})}{72 \times \text{serum creatinine (mg/100 mL)}}$

Females: $0.85 \times$ above value

In patients undergoing hemodialysis, the loading dose of 1 to 2 grams should be given after each hemodialysis, and the maintenance dose should be given as indicated in Table 2.
Antibiotic therapy for group A beta-hemolytic streptococcal infections should be maintained for at least 10 days to guard against the risk of rheumatic fever or glomerulonephritis. In staphylococcal and other infections involving a collection of pus, surgical drainage should be carried out where indicated.
Pediatric Patients
The recommended dosage in pediatric patients three months of age and older is 80 to 160 mg/kg of body weight per day divided into four to six equal doses. The higher dosages should be used for more severe or serious infections. The total daily dosage should not exceed 12 grams.
At this time no recommendation is made for pediatric patients from birth to three months of age (see PRECAUTIONS).
In pediatric patients with renal insufficiency, the dosage and frequency of dosage should be modified consistent with the recommendations for adults (see Table 2).
PREVENTION
Effective prophylactic use depends on the time of administration. MEFOXIN usually should be given one-half to one hour before the operation, which is sufficient time to achieve effective levels in the wound during the procedure. Prophylactic administration should usually be stopped within 24 hours since continuing administration of any antibiotic increases the possibility of adverse reactions but, in the majority of surgical procedures, does not reduce the incidence of subsequent infection.
For prophylactic use in uncontaminated gastrointestinal surgery, vaginal hysterectomy, or abdominal hysterectomy, the following doses are recommended:

Adults:
2 grams administered intravenously just prior to surgery (approximately one-half to one hour before the initial incision) followed by 2 grams every 6 hours after the first dose for no more than 24 hours.
Pediatric Patients (3 months and older):
30 to 40 mg/kg doses may be given at the times designated above.
Cesarean section patients:
For patients undergoing cesarean section, either a single 2 gram dose administered intravenously as soon as the umbilical cord is clamped OR a 3-dose regimen consisting of 2 grams given intravenously as soon as the umbilical cord is clamped followed by 2 grams 4 and 8 hours after the initial dose is recommended. (See CLINICAL STUDIES.)
PREPARATION OF SOLUTION
Table 3 is provided for convenience in constituting MEFOXIN for intravenous administration.
For Vials
One gram should be constituted with at least 10 mL, and 2 grams with 10 or 20 mL, of Sterile Water for Injection, Bacteriostatic Water for Injection, 0.9 percent Sodium Chloride Injection, or 5 percent Dextrose Injection. These primary solutions may be further diluted in 50 to 1000 mL of the diluents listed under the *Vials and Bulk Packages* portion of the *COMPATIBILITY AND STABILITY* section.
For Bulk Packages
The 10 gram bulk packages should be constituted with 43 or 93 mL of Sterile Water for Injection, Bacteriostatic Water for Injection, 0.9 percent Sodium Chloride Injection, or 5 percent Dextrose Injection. CAUTION: THE 10 GRAM BULK STOCK SOLUTION IS NOT FOR DIRECT INFUSION. These primary solutions may be further diluted in 50 to 1000 mL of the diluents listed under the *Vials and Bulk Packages* portion of the *COMPATIBILITY AND STABILITY* section.
Benzyl alcohol as a preservative has been associated with toxicity in neonates. While toxicity has not been demonstrated in pediatric patients greater than three months of age, in whom use of MEFOXIN may be indicated, small pediatric patients in this age range may also be at risk for benzyl alcohol toxicity. Therefore, diluent containing benzyl alcohol should not be used when MEFOXIN is constituted for administration to pediatric patients in this age range.
For Infusion Bottles
One or 2 grams of MEFOXIN for infusion may be constituted with 50 or 100 mL of 0.9 percent Sodium Chloride Injection, or 5 percent or 10 percent Dextrose Injection.
For ADD-Vantage®†† Vials
See separate INSTRUCTIONS FOR USE OF MEFOXIN IN ADD-Vantage® VIALS. MEFOXIN in ADD-Vantage® vials should be constituted with ADD-Vantage® diluent containers containing 50 mL or 100 mL of either 0.9 percent Sodium Chloride Injection or 5 percent Dextrose Injection. MEFOXIN in ADD-Vantage® vials is for IV use only.
[See table 3 at top of next page]

†† Registered trademark of Abbott Laboratories.

ADMINISTRATION
MEFOXIN may be administered intravenously after constitution.
Parenteral drug products should be inspected visually for particulate matter and discoloration prior to administration whenever solution and container permit.
Intravenous Administration
The intravenous route is preferable for patients with bacteremia, bacterial septicemia, or other severe or life-threat-

Continued on next page

Information on the Merck & Co., Inc., products listed on these pages is from the prescribing information in use October 1, 2004. For information, please call 1-800-NSC-MERCK [1-800-672-6372].

Table 3—Preparation of Solution

MEFOXIN

Strength	Amount of Diluent to be Added (mL)[++]	Approximate Withdrawable Volume (mL)	Approximate Average Concentration (mg/mL)
1 gram Vial	10	10.5	95
2 gram Vial	10 or 20	11.1 or 21.0	180 or 95
1 gram Infusion Bottle	50 or 100	50 or 100	20 or 10
2 gram Infusion Bottle	50 or 100	50 or 100	40 or 20
10 gram Bulk	43 or 93	49 or 98.5	200 or 100

[++]Shake to dissolve and let stand until clear.

Mefoxin—Cont.

ening infections, or for patients who may be poor risks because of lowered resistance resulting from such debilitating conditions as malnutrition, trauma, surgery, diabetes, heart failure, or malignancy, particularly if shock is present or impending.

For intermittent intravenous administration, a solution containing 1 gram or 2 grams in 10 mL of Sterile Water for Injection can be injected over a period of three to five minutes. Using an infusion system, it may also be given over a longer period of time through the tubing system by which the patient may be receiving other intravenous solutions. However, during infusion of the solution containing MEFOXIN, it is advisable to temporarily discontinue administration of any other solutions at the same site.

For the administration of higher doses by continuous intravenous infusion, a solution of MEFOXIN may be added to an intravenous bottle containing 5 percent Dextrose Injection, 0.9 percent Sodium Chloride Injection, or 5 percent Dextrose and 0.9 percent Sodium Chloride Injection. BUTTERFLY®[††] or scalp vein-type needles are preferred for this type of infusion.

Solutions of MEFOXIN, like those of most beta-lactam antibiotics, should not be added to aminoglycoside solutions (e.g., gentamicin sulfate, tobramycin sulfate, amikacin sulfate) because of potential interaction. However, MEFOXIN and aminoglycosides may be administered separately to the same patient.

[††] Registered trademark of Abbott Laboratories.

COMPATIBILITY AND STABILITY

Vials and Bulk Packages

MEFOXIN, as supplied in vials or the bulk package and constituted to 1 gram/10 mL with Sterile Water for Injection, Bacteriostatic Water for Injection (see *PREPARATION OF SOLUTION*), 0.9 percent Sodium Chloride Injection, or 5 percent Dextrose Injection, maintains satisfactory potency for 6 hours at room temperature or for one week under refrigeration (below 5°C).

These primary solutions may be further diluted in 50 to 1000 mL of the following diluents and maintain potency for an additional 18 hours at room temperature or an additional 48 hours under refrigeration:

- 0.9 percent Sodium Chloride Injection
- 5 percent or 10 percent Dextrose Injection
- 5 percent Dextrose and 0.9 percent Sodium Chloride Injection
- 5 percent Dextrose Injection with 0.2 percent or 0.45 percent saline solution
- Lactated Ringer's Injection
- 5 percent Dextrose in Lactated Ringer's Injection
- 5 percent Sodium Bicarbonate Injection
- M/6 sodium lactate solution
- Mannitol 5% and 10%

Infusion Bottles

MEFOXIN, as supplied in infusion bottles and constituted with 50 to 100 mL of 0.9 percent Sodium Chloride Injection, or 5 percent or 10 percent Dextrose Injection, maintains satisfactory potency for 24 hours at room temperature or for 1 week under refrigeration (below 5°C).

ADD-Vantage® Vials

MEFOXIN is supplied in single dose ADD-Vantage® vials and should be prepared as directed in the accompanying INSTRUCTIONS FOR USE OF MEFOXIN IN ADD-Vantage® VIALS using ADD-Vantage® diluent containers containing 50 mL or 100 mL of either 0.9 percent Sodium Chloride Injection or 5 percent Dextrose Injection. When prepared with either of these diluents, MEFOXIN maintains satisfactory potency for 24 hours at room temperature.

After the periods mentioned above, any unused solutions should be discarded.

HOW SUPPLIED

Sterile MEFOXIN is a dry white to off-white powder supplied in vials and infusion bottles containing cefoxitin sodium as follows:

No. 3356 — 1 gram cefoxitin equivalent
NDC 0006-3356-45 in trays of 25 vials.
No. 3357 — 2 gram cefoxitin equivalent
NDC 0006-3357-53 in trays of 25 vials.
No. 3388 — 10 gram cefoxitin equivalent
NDC 0006-3388-67 in trays of 6 bulk bottles.
No. 3548 — 1 gram cefoxitin equivalent
NDC 0006-3548-45 in trays of 25 ADD-Vantage® vials.
No. 3549 — 2 gram cefoxitin equivalent
NDC 0006-3549-53 in trays of 25 ADD-Vantage® vials.

Special storage instructions

MEFOXIN in the dry state should be stored between 2–25°C (36–77°F). Avoid exposure to temperatures above 50°C. The dry material as well as solutions tend to darken, depending on storage conditions; product potency, however, is not adversely affected.

CLINICAL STUDIES

A prospective, randomized, double-blind, placebo-controlled clinical trial was conducted to determine the efficacy of short-term prophylaxis with MEFOXIN in patients undergoing cesarean section who were at high risk for subsequent endometritis because of ruptured membranes. Patients were randomized to receive either three doses of placebo (n=58), a single dose of MEFOXIN (2 g) followed by two doses of placebo (n=64), or a three-dose regimen of MEFOXIN (each dose consisting of 2 g) (n=60), given intravenously, usually beginning at the time of clamping of the umbilical cord, with the second and third doses given 4 and 8 hours post-operatively. Endometritis occurred in 16/58 (27.6%) patients given placebo, 5/63 (7.9%) patients given a single dose of MEFOXIN, and 3/58 (5.2%) patients given three doses of MEFOXIN. The differences between the two groups treated with MEFOXIN and placebo with respect to endometritis were statistically significant ($p<0.01$) in favor of MEFOXIN. The differences between the one-dose and three-dose regimens of MEFOXIN were not statistically significant.

Two double-blind, randomized studies compared the efficacy of a single 2 gram intravenous dose of MEFOXIN to a single 2 gram dose of cefotetan in the prevention of surgical site-related infection (major morbidity) and non-site-related infections (minor morbidity) in patients following cesarean section. In the first study, 82/98 (83.7%) patients treated with MEFOXIN and 71/95 (74.7%) patients treated with cefotetan experienced no major or minor morbidity. The difference in the outcomes in this study (95% CI: −0.03, +0.21) was not statistically significant. In the second study, 65/75 (86.7%) patients treated with MEFOXIN and 62/76 (81.6%) patients treated with cefotetan experienced no major or minor morbidity. The difference in the outcomes in this study (95% CI: −0.08, +0.18) was not statistically significant.

In clinical trials of patients with intra-abdominal infections due to *Bacteroides fragilis* group microorganisms, eradication rates at 1 to 2 weeks posttreatment for isolates were in the range of 70% to 80%. Eradication rates for individual species are listed below:

Bacteroides distasonis	7/10	(70%)
Bacteroides fragilis	26/33	(79%)
Bacteroides ovatus	10/13	(77%)
B. thetaiotaomicron	13/18	(72%)

REFERENCES

1. National Committee for Clinical Laboratory Standards. Methods for Dilution Antimicrobial Susceptibility Tests for Bacteria that Grow Aerobically - Fourth Edition. Approved Standard NCCLS Document M7-A4, Vol.17, No. 2, NCCLS, Wayne, PA, January 1997.
2. National Committee for Clinical Laboratory Standards. Performance Standards for Antimicrobial Disk Susceptibility Tests - Sixth Edition. Approved Standard NCCLS Document M2-A6, Vol. 17, No. 1, NCCLS, Wayne, PA, January 1997.
3. National Committee for Clinical Laboratory Standards. Methods for Antimicrobial Susceptibility Testing of Anaerobic Bacteria - Fourth Edition. Approved Standard NCCLS Document M11-A4, Vol. 17, No. 22, NCCLS, Villanova, PA, December 1997.

7882341 Issued August 2003

MEFOXIN®
Premixed Intravenous Solution ℞
(Cefoxitin Injection)

To reduce the development of drug-resistant bacteria and maintain the effectiveness of MEFOXIN* and other antibacterial drugs, MEFOXIN should be used only to treat or prevent infections that are proven or strongly suspected to be caused by bacteria.

DESCRIPTION

Cefoxitin sodium is a semi-synthetic, broad-spectrum cepha antibiotic for intravenous administration. It is derived from cephamycin C, which is produced by *Streptomyces lactamdurans*. Its chemical name is sodium (6*R*,7*S*)-3-(hydroxymethyl)-7-methoxy-8-oxo-7-[2- (2-thienyl)acetamido]-5-thia-1-azabicyclo [4.2.0]oct-2-ene-2-carboxylate carbamate (ester). The empirical formula is $C_{16}H_{16}N_3NaO_7S_2$, and the molecular weight is 449.44. The structural formula is:

Cefoxitin sodium contains approximately 53.8 mg (2.3 milliequivalents) of sodium per gram of cefoxitin activity.

Premixed Intravenous Solution MEFOXIN* (Cefoxitin Sodium Injection) is supplied as a sterile, nonpyrogenic, frozen, iso-osmotic solution of cefoxitin sodium. Each 50 mL contains cefoxitin sodium equivalent to either 1 gram or 2 grams cefoxitin. Dextrose hydrous USP has been added to the above dosages to adjust osmolality (approximately 2 grams and 1.1 grams to 1 gram and 2 gram dosages, respectively). The pH is adjusted with sodium bicarbonate and may have been adjusted with hydrochloric acid. The pH is approximately 6.5. After thawing, the solution is intended for intravenous use only. Solutions of MEFOXIN range from colorless to light amber.

The plastic container is fabricated from a specially designed multilayer plastic (PL 2040). Solutions are in contact with the polyethylene layer of this container and can leach out certain chemical components of the plastic in very small amounts within the expiration period. The suitability and safety of the plastic have been confirmed in tests in animals according to the USP biological tests for plastic containers, as well as by tissue culture toxicity studies.

*Registered trademark of MERCK & CO., Inc.

CLINICAL PHARMACOLOGY

Clinical Pharmacology

Following an intravenous dose of 1 gram of cefoxitin, serum concentrations were 110 mcg/mL at 5 minutes, declining to less than 1 mcg/mL at 4 hours. The half-life after an intravenous dose is 41 to 59 minutes. Approximately 85 percent of cefoxitin is excreted unchanged by the kidneys over a 6-hour period, resulting in high urinary concentrations. Probenecid slows tubular excretion and produces higher serum levels and increases the duration of measurable serum concentrations.

Cefoxitin passes into pleural and joint fluids and is detectable in antibacterial concentrations in bile.

Microbiology

The bactericidal action of cefoxitin results from inhibition of cell wall synthesis. Cefoxitin has *in vitro* activity against a wide range of gram-positive and gram-negative organisms. The methoxy group in the 7α position provides cefoxitin with a high degree of stability in the presence of beta-lactamases, both penicillinases and cephalosporinases, of gram-negative bacteria.

Cefoxitin has been shown to be active against most strains of the following microorganisms, both in vitro and in clinical infections as described in the INDICATIONS AND USAGE section.

Aerobic gram-positive microorganisms
- *Staphylococcus aureus*[a] (including penicillinase-producing strains)
- *Staphylococcus epidermidis*[a]
- *Streptococcus agalactiae*
- *Streptococcus pneumoniae*
- *Streptococcus pyogenes*

[a]Staphylococci resistant to methicillin/oxacillin should be considered resistant to cefoxitin.

Most strains of enterococci, e.g., *Enterococcus faecalis,* are resistant.

Aerobic gram-negative microorganisms
- *Escherichia coli*
- *Haemophilus influenzae*
- *Klebsiella* spp. (including *K. pneumoniae)*
- *Morganella morganii*
- *Neisseria gonorrhoeae* (including penicillinase-producing strains)
- *Proteus mirabilis*
- *Proteus vulgaris*
- *Providencia* spp. (including *Providencia rettgeri)*

Anaerobic gram-positive microorganisms
- *Clostridium* spp.
- *Peptococcus niger*
- *Peptostreptococcus* spp.

Anaerobic gram-negative microorganisms
- *Bacteroides distasonis*
- *Bacteroides fragilis*
- *Bacteroides ovatus*
- *Bacteroides thetaiotaomicron*
- *Bacteroides* spp.

The following *in vitro* data are available, **but their clinical significance is unknown.**

Cefoxitin exhibits *in vitro* minimum inhibitory concentrations (MIC's) of 8 µg/mL or less for aerobic microorganisms and 16 µg/mL or less for anaerobic microorganisms against most (≥90%) strains of the following microorganisms; however, the safety and effectiveness of cefoxitin in treating clinical infections due to these microorganisms have not been established in adequate and well-controlled clinical trials.

Aerobic gram-negative microorganisms

Eikenella corrodens [non-β-lactamase producers]

Klebsiella oxytoca

Anaerobic gram-positive microorganisms

Clostridium perfringens

Anaerobic gram-negative microorganisms

Prevotella bivia (formerly *Bacteroides bivius*)

Cefoxitin is inactive *in vitro* against most strains of *Pseudomonas aeruginosa* and eterococci and many strains of *Enterobacter cloacae*.

Susceptibility Tests

Dilution Techniques:

Quantitative methods are used to determine antimicrobial minimum inhibitory concentrations (MIC's). These MIC's provide estimates of the susceptibility of bacteria to antimicrobial compounds. The MIC's should be determined using a standardized procedure. Standardized procedures are based on a dilution method[1] (broth or agar) or equivalent with standardized inoculum concentrations and standardized concentrations of cefoxitin powder. The MIC values should be interpreted according to the following criteria:

For testing aerobic microorganisms[a,b,c] other than *Neisseria gonorrhoeae*:

MIC (μg/mL)	Interpretation
≤ 8	Susceptible (S)
16	Intermediate (I)
≥ 32	Resistant (R)

[a]Staphylococci exhibiting resistance to methicillin/oxacillin should be reported as also resistant to cefoxitin despite apparent *in vitro* susceptibility.

[b]For testing *Haemophilus influenzae* these interpretative criteria applicable only to tests performed by broth microdilution method using Haemophilus Test Medium (HTM)[1].

[c]For testing streptococci these interpretative criteria applicable only to tests performed by broth microdilution method using cation-adjusted Mueller-Hinton broth with 2 to 5% lysed horse blood[1].

For testing *Neisseria gonorrhoeae*[d]:

MIC (μg/mL)	Interpretation
≤ 2	Susceptible (S)
4	Intermediate (I)
≥ 8	Resistant (R)

[d]Interpretative criteria applicable only to tests performed by agar dilution method using GC agar base with 1% defined growth supplement and incubated in 5% CO_2[1]. A report of "Susceptible" indicates that the pathogen is likely to be inhibited if the antimicrobial compound in the blood reaches the concentrations usually achievable. A report of "Intermediate" indicates that the result should be considered equivocal, and, if the microorganism is not fully susceptible to alternative, clinically feasible drugs, the test should be repeated. This category implies possible clinical applicability in body sites where the drug is physiologically concentrated or in situations where high dosage of drug can be used. This category also provides a buffer zone which prevents small uncontrolled technical factors from causing major discrepancies in interpretation. A report of "Resistant" indicates that the pathogen is not likely to be inhibited if the antimicrobial compound in the blood reaches the concentrations usually achievable; other therapy should be selected.

Standardized susceptibility test procedures require the use of laboratory control microorganisms to control the technical aspects of the laboratory procedures. Standard cefoxitin powder should provide the following MIC values:

Microorganism		MIC (μg/mL)
Escherichia coli	ATCC 25922	1-4
Neisseria gonorrhoeae[a]	ATCC 49226	0.5-2
Staphylococcus aureus	ATCC 29213	1-4

[a]Interpretative criteria applicable only to tests performed by agar dilution method using GC agar base with 1% defined growth supplement and incubated in 5% CO_2[1].

Diffusion Techniques:

Quantitative methods that require measurement of zone diameters also provide reproducible estimates of the susceptibility of bacteria to antimicrobial compounds. One such standardized procedure[2] requires the use of standardized inoculum concentrations. This procedure uses paper disks impregnated with 30-μg cefoxitin to test the susceptibility of microorganisms to cefoxitin.

Reports from the laboratory providing results of the standard single-disk susceptibility test with a 30-μg cefoxitin disk should be interpreted according to the following criteria:

For testing aerobic microorganisms[a,b,c] other than *Neisseria gonorrhoeae*:

Zone Diameter (mm)	Interpretation
≥ 18	Susceptible (S)
15-17	Intermediate (I)
≤ 14	Resistant (R)

[a]Staphylococci exhibiting resistance to methicillin/oxacillin should be reported as also resistant to cefoxitin despite apparent *in vitro* susceptibility.

[b]For testing *Haemophilus influenzae* these interpretative criteria applicable only to tests performed by disk diffusion method using Haemophilus Test Medium (HTM)[1].

[c]For testing streptococci these interpretative criteria applicable only to tests performed by disk diffusion method using Mueller-Hinton agar with 5% defibrinated sheep blood and incubated in 5% CO_2[2].

For testing *Neisseria gonorrhoeae*[d]:

Zone Diameter (mm)	Interpretation
≥ 28	Susceptible (S)
24-27	Intermediate (I)
≤ 23	Resistant (R)

[d]Interpretative criteria applicable only to tests performed by disk diffusion method using GC agar base with 1% defined growth supplement and incubated in 5% CO_2[2].

Interpretation should be as stated above for results using dilution techniques.

Interpretation involves correlation of the diameter obtained in the disk test with the MIC for cefoxitin.

As with standardized dilution techniques, diffusion methods require the use of laboratory control microorganisms that are used to control the technical aspects of the laboratory procedures. For the diffusion technique, the 30-μg cefoxitin disk should provide the following zone diameters in these laboratory test quality control strains:

Microorganism		Zone Diameter (mm)
Escherichia coli	ATCC 25922	23-29
Neisseria gonorrhoeae[a]	ATCC 49226	33-41
Staphylococcus aureus	ATCC 25923	23-29

[a]Interpretative criteria applicable only to tests performed by disk diffusion method using GC agar base with 1% defined growth supplement and incubated in 5% CO_2[2].

Anaerobic Techniques:

For anaerobic bacteria, the susceptibility to cefoxitin as MIC's can be determined by standardized test methods[3]. The MIC values obtained should be interpreted according to the following criteria:

MIC (μg/mL)	Interpretation
≤ 16	Susceptible (S)
32	Intermediate (I)
≥ 64	Resistant (R)

Interpretation is identical to that stated above for results using dilution techniques.

As with other susceptibility techniques, the use of laboratory control microorganisms is required to control the technical aspects of the laboratory standardized procedures. Standard cefoxitin powder should provide the following MIC values:

Using either an Agar Dilution Method[a] or Using a Broth[b] Microdilution Method:

Microorganism		MIC (μg/mL)
Bacteroides fragilis	ATCC 25285	4-16
Bacteroides thetaiotaomicron	ATCC 29741	8-32

[a]Range applicable only to tests performed using either Brucella blood or Wilkins-Chalgren agar.

[b]Range applicable only to tests performed in the broth formulation of Wilkins-Chalgren agar[3].

INDICATIONS AND USAGE

MEFOXIN, supplied as a premixed solution in plastic containers, is intended for intravenous use only.

Treatment

MEFOXIN is indicated for the treatment of serious infections caused by susceptible strains of the designated microorganisms in the diseases listed below.

(1) **Lower respiratory tract infections,** including pneumonia and lung abscess, caused by *Streptococcus pneumoniae*, other streptococci (excluding enterococci, e.g., *Enterococcus faecalis* [formerly *Streptococcus faecalis*]), *Staphylococcus aureus* (including penicillinase-producing strains), *Escherichia coli, Klebsiella* species, *Haemophilus influenzae*, and *Bacteroides* species.

(2) **Urinary tract infections** caused by *Escherichia coli, Klebsiella* species, *Proteus mirabilis, Morganella morganii, Proteus vulgaris* and *Providencia* species (including *P. rettgeri*).

(3) **Intra-abdominal infections,** including peritonitis and intra-abdominal abscess, caused by *Escherichia coli, Klebsiella* species, *Bacteroides* species including *Bacteroides fragilis*, and *Clostridium* species.

(4) **Gynecological infections,** including endometritis, pelvic cellulitis, and pelvic inflammatory disease caused by *Escherichia coli, Neisseria gonorrhoeae* (including penicillinase-producing strains), *Bacteroides* species including *B. fragilis*, *Clostridium* species, *Peptococcus niger, Peptostreptococcus* species, and *Streptococcus agalactiae*. MEFOXIN, like cephalosporins, has no activity against *Chlamydia trachomatis*. Therefore, when MEFOXIN is used in the treatment of patients with pelvic inflammatory disease and *C. trachomatis* is one of the suspected pathogens, appropriate anti-chlamydial coverage should be added.

(5) **Septicemia** caused by *Streptococcus pneumoniae, Staphylococcus aureus* (including penicillinase-producing strains), *Escherichia coli, Klebsiella* species, and *Bacteroides* species including *B. fragilis*.

(6) **Bone and joint infections** caused by *Staphylococcus aureus* (including penicillinase-producing strains).

(7) **Skin and skin structure infections** caused by *Staphylococcus aureus* (including penicillinase-producing strains), *Staphylococcus epidermidis, Streptococcus pyogenes* and other streptococci (excluding enterococci, e.g., *Enterococcus faecalis* [formerly *Streptococcus faecalis*]), *Escherichia coli, Proteus mirabilis, Klebsiella* species, *Bacteroides* species including *B. fragilis, Clostridium* species, *Peptococcus niger*, and *Peptostreptococcus* species.

Appropriate culture and susceptibility studies should be performed to determine the susceptibility of the causative organisms to MEFOXIN. Therapy may be started while awaiting the results of these studies.

In randomized comparative studies, cefoxitin and cephalothin were comparably safe and effective in the management of infections caused by gram-positive cocci and gram-negative rods susceptible to the cephalosporins. MEFOXIN has a high degree of stability in the presence of bacterial beta-lactamases, both penicillinases and cephalosporinases.

Many infections caused by aerobic and anaerobic gram-negative bacteria resistant to some cephalosporins respond to MEFOXIN. Similarly, many infections caused by aerobic and anaerobic bacteria resistant to some penicillin antibiotics (ampicillin, carbenicillin, penicillin G) respond to treatment with MEFOXIN. Many infections caused by mixtures of susceptible aerobic and anaerobic bacteria respond to treatment with MEFOXIN.

Prevention

MEFOXIN is indicated for the prophylaxis of infection in patients undergoing uncontaminated gastrointestinal surgery, vaginal hysterectomy, abdominal hysterectomy, or cesarean section.

If there are signs of infection, specimens for culture should be obtained for identification of the causative organism so that appropriate treatment may be instituted.

To reduce the development of drug-resistant bacteria and maintain the effectiveness of MEFOXIN and other antibacterial drugs, MEFOXIN should be used only to treat or prevent infections that are proven or strongly suspected to be caused by susceptible bacteria. When culture and susceptibility information are available, they should be considered in selecting or modifying antibacterial therapy. In the absence of such data, local epidemiology and susceptibility patterns may contribute to the empiric selection of therapy.

CONTRAINDICATIONS

MEFOXIN is contraindicated in patients who have shown hypersensitivity to cefoxitin and the cephalosporin group of antibiotics.

WARNINGS

BEFORE THERAPY WITH 'MEFOXIN' IS INSTITUTED, CAREFUL INQUIRY SHOULD BE MADE TO DETERMINE WHETHER THE PATIENT HAS HAD PREVIOUS HYPERSENSITIVITY REACTIONS TO CEFOXITIN, CEPHALOSPORINS, PENICILLINS, OR OTHER DRUGS. THIS PRODUCT SHOULD BE GIVEN WITH CAUTION TO PENICILLIN-SENSITIVE PATIENTS. ANTIBIOTICS SHOULD BE ADMINISTERED WITH CAUTION TO ANY PATIENT WHO HAS DEMONSTRATED SOME FORM OF ALLERGY, PARTICULARLY TO DRUGS. IF AN ALLERGIC REACTION TO 'MEFOXIN' OCCURS, DISCONTINUE THE DRUG. SERIOUS HYPERSENSITIVITY REACTIONS MAY REQUIRE EPINEPHRINE AND OTHER EMERGENCY MEASURES.

Pseudomembranous colitis has been reported with nearly all antibacterial agents, including cefoxitin, and may range in severity from mild to life threatening. Therefore, it is important to consider this diagnosis in patients who present with diarrhea subsequent to the administration of antibacterial agents.

Treatment with antibacterial agents alters the normal flora of the colon and may permit overgrowth of clostridia. Studies indicate that a toxin produced by *Clostridium difficile* is one primary cause of "antibiotic-associated colitis."

After the diagnosis of pseudomembranous colitis has been established, appropriate therapeutic measures should be initiated. Mild cases of pseudomembranous colitis usually respond to drug discontinuation alone. In moderate to severe cases, consideration should be given to management

Continued on next page

Information on the Merck & Co., Inc., products listed on these pages is from the prescribing information in use October 1, 2004. For information, please call 1-800-NSC-MERCK [1-800-672-6372].

Mefoxin Premixed—Cont.

with fluids and electrolytes, protein supplementation, and treatment with an antibacterial drug clinically effective against *Clostridium difficile* colitis.

PRECAUTIONS

General

The total daily dose should be reduced when MEFOXIN is administered to patients with transient or persistent reduction of urinary output due to renal insufficiency (see DOSAGE AND ADMINISTRATION, *TREATMENT*), because high and prolonged serum antibiotic concentrations can occur in such individuals from usual doses.

Antibiotics (including cephalosporins) should be prescribed with caution in individuals with a history of gastrointestinal disease, particularly colitis.

As with other antibiotics, prolonged use of MEFOXIN may result in overgrowth of nonsusceptible organisms. Repeated evaluation of the patient's condition is essential. If superinfection occurs during therapy, appropriate measures should be taken.

Do not use unless solution is clear and seal is intact.

Prescribing MEFOXIN in the absence of a proven or strongly suspected bacterial infection or a prophylactic indication is unlikely to provide benefit to the patient and increases the risk of the development of drug-resistant bacteria.

Information for Patients

Patients should be counseled that antibacterial drugs including MEFOXIN should only be used to treat bacterial infections. They do not treat viral infections (e.g., the common cold). When MEFOXIN is prescribed to treat a bacterial infection, patients should be told that although it is common to feel better early in the course of therapy, the medication should be taken exactly as directed. Skipping doses or not completing the full course of therapy may (1) decrease the effectiveness of the immediate treatment and (2) increase the likelihood that bacteria will develop resistance and will not be treatable by MEFOXIN or other antibacterial drugs in the future.

Laboratory Tests

As with any potent antibacterial agent, periodic assessment of organ system functions, including renal, hepatic, and hematopoietic, is advisable during prolonged therapy.

Drug Interactions

Increased nephrotoxicity has been reported following concomitant administration of cephalosporins and aminoglycoside antibiotics.

Drug/Laboratory Test Interactions

As with cephalothin, high concentrations of cefoxitin (>100 micrograms/mL) may interfere with measurement of serum and urine creatinine levels by the Jaffé reaction, and produce false increases of modest degree in the levels of creatinine reported. Serum samples from patients treated with cefoxitin should not be analyzed for creatinine if withdrawn within 2 hours of drug administration.

High concentrations of cefoxitin in the urine may interfere with measurement of urinary 17-hydroxy-corticosteroids by the Porter-Silber reaction, and produce false increases of modest degree in the levels reported.

A false-positive reaction for glucose in the urine may occur. This has been observed with CLINITEST[†] reagent tablets.

[†] Registered trademark of Ames Company, Division of Miles Laboratories, Inc.

Carcinogenesis, Mutagenesis, Impairment of Fertility

Long term studies in animals have not been performed with cefoxitin to evaluate carcinogenic or mutagenic potential. Studies in rats treated intravenously with 400 mg/kg of cefoxitin (approximately three times the maximum recommended human dose) revealed no effects on fertility or mating ability.

Pregnancy

Pregnancy Category B. Reproduction studies performed in rats and mice at parenteral doses of approximately one to seven and one-half times the maximum recommended human dose did not reveal teratogenic or fetal toxic effects, although a slight decrease in fetal weight was observed.

There are, however, no adequate and well-controlled studies in pregnant women. Because animal reproduction studies are not always predictive of human response, this drug should be used during pregnancy only if clearly needed.

In the rabbit, cefoxitin was associated with a high incidence of abortion and maternal death. This was not considered to be a teratogenic effect but an expected consequence of the rabbit's unusual sensitivity to antibiotic-induced changes in the population of the microflora of the intestine.

Nursing Mothers

Cefoxitin is excreted in human milk in low concentrations. Caution should be exercised when MEFOXIN is administered to a nursing woman.

Pediatric Use

Safety and efficacy in pediatric patients from birth to three months of age have not yet been established. In pediatric patients three months of age and older, higher doses of cefoxitin have been associated with an increased incidence of eosinophilia and elevated SGOT.

The potential for toxic effects in pediatric patients from chemicals that may leach from the single-dose I.V. preparation in plastic has not been determined.

ADVERSE REACTIONS

Cefoxitin is generally well tolerated. The most common adverse reactions have been local reactions following intravenous injection. Other adverse reactions have been encountered infrequently.

Local Reactions

Thrombophlebitis has occurred with intravenous administration.

Allergic Reactions

Rash (including exfoliative dermatitis and toxic epidermal necrolysis), urticaria, flushing, pruritus, eosinophilia, fever, dyspnea, and other allergic reactions including anaphylaxis, interstitial nephritis and angioedema have been noted.

Cardiovascular

Hypotension

Gastrointestinal

Diarrhea, including documented pseudomembranous colitis which can appear during or after antibiotic treatment. Nausea and vomiting have been reported rarely.

Neuromuscular

Possible exacerbation of myasthenia gravis.

Blood

Eosinophilia, leukopenia including granulocytopenia, neutropenia, anemia, including hemolytic anemia, thrombocytopenia, and bone marrow depression. A positive direct Coombs test may develop in some individuals, especially those with azotemia.

Liver Function

Transient elevations in SGOT, SGPT, serum LDH, and serum alkaline phosphatase; and jaundice have been reported.

Renal Function

Elevations in serum creatinine and/or blood urea nitrogen levels have been observed. As with the cephalosporins, acute renal failure has been reported rarely. The role of MEFOXIN in changes in renal function tests is difficult to assess, since factors predisposing to prerenal azotemia or to impaired renal function usually have been present.

In addition to the adverse reactions listed above which have been observed in patients treated with MEFOXIN, the following adverse reactions and altered laboratory test results have been reported for cephalosporin class antibiotics:

Urticaria, erythema multiforme, Stevens-Johnson syndrome, serum sickness-like reactions, abdominal pain, colitis, renal dysfunction, toxic nephropathy, false-positive test for urinary glucose, hepatic dysfunction including cholestasis, elevated bilirubin, aplastic anemia, hemorrhage, prolonged prothrombin time, pancytopenia, agranulocytosis, superinfection, vaginitis including vaginal candidiasis.

Several cephalosporins have been implicated in triggering seizures, particularly in patients with renal impairment when the dosage was not reduced. (See DOSAGE AND ADMINISTRATION.) If seizures associated with drug therapy occur, the drug should be discontinued. Anticonvulsant therapy can be given if clinically indicated.

OVERDOSAGE

The acute intravenous LD_{50} in the adult female mouse and rabbit was about 8.0 g/kg and greater than 1.0 g/kg respectively. The acute intraperitoneal LD_{50} in the adult rat was greater than 10.0 g/kg.

DOSAGE AND ADMINISTRATION

NOTE: MEFOXIN® in Galaxy[††] container is for intravenous infusion only.

TREATMENT

Adults

The usual adult dosage range is 1 gram to 2 grams every six to eight hours. Dosage should be determined by susceptibility of the causative organisms, severity of infection, and the condition of the patient (see Table 1 for dosage guidelines).

If *C. trachomatis* is a suspected pathogen, appropriate antichlamydial coverage should be added, because cefoxitin sodium has no activity against this organism.

MEFOXIN may be used in patients with reduced renal function with the following dosage adjustments:

In adults with renal insufficiency, an initial loading dose of 1 gram to 2 grams may be given. After a loading dose, the recommendations for *maintenance dosage* (Table 2) may be used as a guide.

When only the serum creatinine level is available, the following formula (based on sex, weight, and age of the patient) may be used to convert this value into creatinine clearance. The serum creatinine should represent a steady state of renal function.

$$\text{Males: } \frac{\text{Weight (kg)} \times (140 - \text{age})}{72 \times \text{serum creatinine (mg/100 mL)}}$$

$$\text{Females: } 0.85 \times \text{male value}$$

In patients undergoing hemodialysis, the loading dose of 1 to 2 grams should be given after each hemodialysis, and the maintenance dose should be given as indicated in Table 2.

Antibiotic therapy for group A beta-hemolytic streptococcal infections should be maintained for at least 10 days to guard against the risk of rheumatic fever or glomerulonephritis. In staphylococcal and other infections involving a collection of pus, surgical drainage should be carried out where indicated.

Pediatric Patients

The recommended dosage in pediatric patients three months of age and older is 80 to 160 mg/kg of body weight per day divided into four to six equal doses. The higher dosages should be used for more severe or serious infections. The total daily dosage should not exceed 12 grams.

At this time no recommendation is made for pediatric patients from birth to three months of age (see PRECAUTIONS).

In pediatric patients with renal insufficiency, the dosage and frequency of dosage should be modified consistent with the recommendations for adults (see Table 2).

PREVENTION

Effective prophylatic use depends on the time of administration. MEFOXIN usually should be given one-half to one hour before the operation, which is sufficient time to achieve effective levels in the wound during the procedure. Prophylactic administration should usually be stopped within 24 hours since continuing administration of any antibiotic increases the possibility of adverse reactions but, in the majority of surgical procedures, does not reduce the incidence of subsequent infection.

For prophylactic use in uncontaminated gastrointestinal surgery, vaginal hysterectomy, or abdominal hysterectomy, the following doses are recommended:

Adults:

2 grams administered intravenously just prior to surgery (approximately one-half to one hour before the initial incision) followed by 2 grams every 6 hours after the first dose for no more than 24 hours.

Pediatric Patients (3 months and older):

30 to 40 mg/kg doses may be given at the times designated above.

Cesarean section patients:

For patients undergoing cesarean section, either a single 2 gram dose administered intravenously as soon as the umbilical cord is clamped OR a 3-dose regimen consisting of 2 grams given intravenously as soon as the umbilical cord is clamped followed by 2 grams 4 and 8 hours after the initial dose is recommended. (See CLINICAL STUDIES.)

[See table 1 below]

[See table 2 at top of next page]

ADMINISTRATION

This premixed solution is for intravenous use only. Premixed Intravenous Solution MEFOXIN in Galaxy® containers (PL 2040 Plastic) is to be administered either as a continuous or intermittent infusion using sterile equipment. Scalp vein-type needles are preferred for this type of infusion. It is recommended that the intravenous administration apparatus be replaced at least once every 48 hours.

The intravenous route is preferred for patients with bacteremia, bacterial septicemia, or other severe or life-threatening infections, or for patients who may be poor risks because of lowered resistance resulting from such debilitating conditions as malnutrition, trauma, surgery, diabetes, heart failure, or malignancy, particularly if shock is present or impending.

Directions for Use of Galaxy® Containers (PL 2040 Plastic)

Thaw frozen container at room temperature, 25°C (77°F), or under refrigeration, 2–8°C (36–46°F). DO NOT FORCE THAW BY IMMERSION IN WATER BATHS OR BY MICROWAVE IRRADIATION.

After thawing, check for minute leaks by squeezing container firmly. If leaks are detected, discard solution as sterility may be impaired.

The container should be visually inspected for particulate matter and discoloration prior to administration. Components of the solution may precipitate in the frozen state and will dissolve upon reaching room temperature with little or no agitation. Agitate after solution has reached room temperature.

Do not use if the solution is cloudy or a precipitate has formed. If any seals or outlet ports are not intact, the con-

Table 1—Guidelines for Dosage of MEFOXIN

Type of Infection	Daily Dosage	Frequency and Route
Uncomplicated forms[‡] of infections such as pneumonia, urinary tract infection, cutaneous infection	3-4 grams	1 gram every 6-8 hours IV
Moderately severe or severe infections	6-8 grams	1 gram every 4 hours *or* 2 grams every 6-8 hours IV
Infections commonly needing antibiotics in higher dosage (e.g., gas gangrene)	12 grams	2 grams every 4 hours *or* 3 grams every 6 hours IV

[‡] Including patients in whom bacteremia is absent or unlikely.

Table 2—Maintenance Dosage of MEFOXIN in Adults with Reduced Renal Function

Renal Function	Creatinine Clearance (mL/min)	Dose (grams)	Frequency
Mild impairment	50-30	1-2	every 8-12 hours
Moderate impairment	29-10	1-2	every 12-24 hours
Severe impairment	9-5	0.5-1	every 12-24 hours
Essentially no function	<5	0.5-1	every 24-48 hours

tainer should be discarded. Solutions of MEFOXIN tend to darken depending on storage conditions; product potency, however, is not adversely affected.
Additives should not be introduced into this solution.
CAUTION: Do not use plastic containers in series connections. Such use would result in air embolism due to residual air being drawn from the primary container before administration of the fluid from the secondary container is complete.

Preparation for Intravenous Administration:

1. Suspend container from eyelet support.
2. Remove plastic protector from outlet port at bottom of container.
3. Attach administration set. Refer to complete directions accompanying set.

MEFOXIN may be administered through the tubing system by which the patient may be receiving other intravenous solutions. However, during infusion of the solution containing MEFOXIN, it is advisable to temporarily discontinue administration of any other solutions at the same site.
Solutions of MEFOXIN, like those of most beta-lactam antibiotics, should not be added to aminoglycoside solutions (e.g., gentamicin sulfate, tobramycin sulfate, amikacin sulfate) because of potential interaction. However, MEFOXIN and aminoglycosides may be administered separately to the same patient.

STABILITY

MEFOXIN, supplied as frozen, premixed, iso-osmotic solution in Galaxy® containers (PL 2040 Plastic), maintains satisfactory potency after thawing for 24 hours at a room temperature of 25°C (77°F) or 21 days under refrigeration, 2-8°C (36-46°F). After these periods, any unused solutions should be discarded.
DO NOT REFREEZE.

††Galaxy® is a registered trademark of Baxter International Inc.

HOW SUPPLIED

Premixed Intravenous Solution MEFOXIN is supplied in single dose Galaxy® containers (PL 2040 Plastic) containing cefoxitin sodium as follows:
No. 2G3506—1 gram cefoxitin equivalent, iso-osmotic in 50 mL diluent containing approximately 2 grams dextrose hydrous USP
NDC 0006-3545-24 in boxes of 24.
No. 2G3507—2 gram cefoxitin equivalent, iso-osmotic in 50 mL diluent containing approximately 1.1 grams dextrose hydrous USP
NDC 0006-3547-25 in boxes of 24.

Special storage instructions

Store at or below −20°C (−4°F). [See Directions for Use of Galaxy® container (PL 2040 Plastic).]
MEFOXIN is also available in dry powder form in vials and infusion bottles containing sterile cefoxitin sodium equivalent to either 1 gram or 2 grams of cefoxitin, and in vials for pharmacy bulk use containing sterile cefoxitin sodium equivalent to 10 grams of cefoxitin, for constitution and intravenous administration (see appropriate product circular).

CLINICAL STUDIES

A prospective, randomized, double-blind, placebo-controlled clinical trial was conducted to determine the efficacy of short-term prophylaxis with MEFOXIN in patients undergoing cesarean section who were at high risk for subsequent endometritis because of ruptured membranes. Patients were randomized to receive either three doses of placebo (n=58), a single dose of MEFOXIN (2 g) followed by two doses of placebo (n=64), or a three-dose regimen of MEFOXIN (each dose consisting of 2 g) (n=60), given intravenously, usually beginning at the time of clamping of the umbilical cord, with the second and third doses given 4 and 8 hours post-operatively. Endometritis occurred in 16/58 (27.6%) patients given placebo, 5/63 (7.9%) patients given a single dose of MEFOXIN, and 3/58 (5.2%) patients given three doses of MEFOXIN. The differences between the two groups treated with MEFOXIN and placebo with respect to endometritis were statistically significant ($p<0.01$) in favor of MEFOXIN. The differences between the one-dose and three-dose regimens of MEFOXIN were not statistically significant.
Two double-blind, randomized studies compared the efficacy of a single 2 gram intravenous dose of MEFOXIN to a single 2 gram dose of cefotetan in the prevention of surgical site-related infection (major morbidity) and non-site-related infections (minor morbidity) in patients following cesarean section. In the first study, 82/98 (83.7%) patients treated with MEFOXIN and 71/95 (74.7%) patients treated with cefotetan experienced no major or minor morbidity. The difference in the outcomes in this study (95% CI: −0.03, +0.21) was not statistically significant. In the second study, 65/75 (86.7%) patients treated with MEFOXIN and 62/76 (81.6%) patients treated with cefotetan experienced no major or minor morbidity. The difference in the outcomes in this study (95% CI: −0.08, +0.18) was not statistically significant.
In clinical trials of patients with intra-abdominal infections due to *Bacteroides fragilis* group microorganisms, eradication rates at 1 to 2 weeks posttreatment for isolates were in the range of 70% to 80%. Eradication rates for individual species are listed below:

Bacteroides distasonis	7/10	(70%)
Bacteroides fragilis	26/33	(79%)
Bacteroides ovatus	10/13	(77%)
B. thetaiotaomicron	13/18	(72%)

REFERENCES

1. National Committee for Clinical Laboratory Standards. Methods for Dilution Antimicrobial Susceptibility Tests for Bacteria that Grow Aerobically - Fourth Edition. Approved Standard NCCLS Document M7-A4, Vol. 17, No. 2, NCCLS, Wayne, PA, January 1997.
2. National Committee for Clinical Laboratory Standards. Performance Standards for Antimicrobial Disk Susceptibility Tests - Sixth Edition. Approved Standard NCCLS Document M2-A6, Vol. 17, No. 1, NCCLS, Wayne, PA, January 1997.
3. National Committee for Clinical Laboratory Standards. Methods for Antimicrobial Susceptibility Testing of Anaerobic Bacteria - Fourth Edition. Approved Standard NCCLS Document M11-A4, Vol. 17, No. 22, NCCLS, Villanova, PA, December 1997.

Manufactured for:
MERCK & CO., INC., Whitehouse Station, NJ 08889, USA
By:
BAXTER HEALTHCARE CORPORATION
Deerfield, Illinois 60015, USA
7948525 Issued August 2003

MEPHYTON® Tablets ℞
(Phytonadione)
Vitamin K_1

DESCRIPTION

Phytonadione is a vitamin which is a clear, yellow to amber, viscous, and nearly odorless liquid. It is insoluble in water, soluble in chloroform and slightly soluble in ethanol. It has a molecular weight of 450.70.
Phytonadione is 2-methyl-3-phytyl-1, 4-naphthoquinone. Its empirical formula is $C_{31}H_{46}O_2$ and its structural formula is:

$$-CH_2CH{=}C(CH_3)(CH_2)_3CH(CH_3)(CH_2)_3CH(CH_3)(CH_2)_3CH(CH_3)CH_3$$

MEPHYTON* (Phytonadione) tablets containing 5 mg of phytonadione are yellow, compressed tablets, scored on one side. Inactive ingredients are acacia, calcium phosphate, colloidal silicon dioxide, lactose, magnesium stearate, starch, and talc.

*Registered trademark of MERCK & CO., INC.

CLINICAL PHARMACOLOGY

MEPHYTON tablets possess the same type and degree of activity as does naturally-occurring vitamin K, which is necessary for the production via the liver of active prothrombin (factor II), proconvertin (factor VII), plasma thromboplastin component (factor IX), and Stuart factor (factor X). The prothrombin test is sensitive to the levels of three of these four factors—II, VII, and X. Vitamin K is an essential cofactor for a microsomal enzyme that catalyzes the post-translational carboxylation of multiple, specific, peptide-bound glutamic acid residues in inactive hepatic precursors of factors II, VII, IX, and X. The resulting gamma-carboxyglutamic acid residues convert the precursors into active coagulation factors that are subsequently secreted by liver cells into the blood.
Oral phytonadione is adequately absorbed from the gastrointestinal tract only if bile salts are present. After absorption, phytonadione is initially concentrated in the liver, but the concentration declines rapidly. Very little vitamin K accumulates in tissues. Little is known about the metabolic fate of vitamin K. Almost no free unmetabolized vitamin K appears in bile or urine.
In normal animals and humans, phytonadione is virtually devoid of pharmacodynamic activity. However, in animals and humans deficient in vitamin K, the pharmacological action of vitamin K is related to its normal physiological function; that is, to promote the hepatic biosynthesis of vitamin K-dependent clotting factors.
MEPHYTON tablets generally exert their effect within 6 to 10 hours.

INDICATIONS AND USAGE

MEPHYTON is indicated in the following coagulation disorders which are due to faulty formation of factors II, VII, IX and X when caused by vitamin K deficiency or interference with vitamin K activity.
MEPHYTON tablets are indicated in:

- — anticoagulant-induced prothrombin deficiency caused by coumarin or indanedione derivatives;
- — hypoprothrombinemia secondary to antibacterial therapy;
- — hypoprothrombinemia secondary to administration of salicylates;
- — hypoprothrombinemia secondary to obstructive jaundice or biliary fistulas but only if bile salts are administered concurrently, since otherwise the oral vitamin K will not be absorbed.

CONTRAINDICATION

Hypersensitivity to any component of this medication.

WARNINGS

An immediate coagulant effect should not be expected after administration of phytonadione.
Phytonadione will not counteract the anticoagulant action of heparin.
When vitamin K_1 is used to correct excessive anticoagulant-induced hypoprothrombinemia, anticoagulant therapy still being indicated, the patient is again faced with the clotting hazards existing prior to starting the anticoagulant therapy. Phytonadione is not a clotting agent, but overzealous therapy with vitamin K_1 may restore conditions which originally permitted thromboembolic phenomena. Dosage should be kept as low as possible, and prothrombin time should be checked regularly as clinical conditions indicate.
Repeated large doses of vitamin K are not warranted in liver disease if the response to initial use of the vitamin is unsatisfactory. Failure to respond to vitamin K may indicate a congenital coagulation defect or that the condition being treated is unresponsive to vitamin K.

PRECAUTIONS

General

Vitamin K_1 is fairly rapidly degraded by light; therefore, always protect MEPHYTON from light. Store MEPHYTON in closed original carton until contents have been used. (See also HOW SUPPLIED, *Storage*).

Drug Interactions

Temporary resistance to prothrombin-depressing anticoagulants may result, especially when larger doses of phytonadione are used. If relatively large doses have been employed, it may be necessary when reinstituting anticoagulant therapy to use somewhat larger doses of the prothrombin-depressing anticoagulant, or to use one which acts on a different principle, such as heparin sodium.

Laboratory Tests

Prothrombin time should be checked regularly as clinical conditions indicate.

Carcinogenesis, Mutagenesis, Impairment of Fertility

Studies of carcinogenicity or impairment of fertility have not been performed with MEPHYTON. MEPHYTON at concentrations up to 2000 mcg/plate with or without metabolic activation, was negative in the Ames microbial mutagen test.

Pregnancy

Pregnancy Category C: Animal reproduction studies have not been conducted with MEPHYTON. It is also not known whether MEPHYTON can cause fetal harm when administered to a pregnant woman or can affect reproduction capacity. MEPHYTON should be given to a pregnant woman only if clearly needed.

Pediatric Use

Safety and effectiveness in pediatric patients have not been established with MEPHYTON. Hemolysis, jaundice, and hyperbilirubinemia in newborns, particularly in premature infants, have been reported with vitamin K.

Nursing Mothers

It is not known whether this drug is excreted in human milk. Because many drugs are excreted in human milk, caution should be exercised when MEPHYTON is administered to a nursing woman.

Continued on next page

Information on the Merck & Co., Inc., products listed on these pages is from the prescribing information in use October 1, 2004. For information, please call 1-800-NSC-MERCK [1-800-672-6372].

Mephyton—Cont.

Geriatric Use
Clinical studies of MEPHYTON did not include sufficient numbers of subjects aged 65 and over to determine whether they respond differently from younger subjects. Other reported clinical experience has not identified differences in responses between the elderly and younger patients. In general, dose selection for an elderly patient should be cautious, usually starting at the low end of the dosing range, reflecting the greater frequency of decreased hepatic, renal, or cardiac function, and of concomitant disease or other drug therapy.

ADVERSE REACTIONS

Transient "flushing sensations" and "peculiar" sensations of taste have been observed with parenteral phytonadione, as well as rare instances of dizziness, rapid and weak pulse, profuse sweating, brief hypotension, dyspnea, and cyanosis. Hyperbilirubinemia has been observed in the newborn following administration of parenteral phytonadione. This has occurred rarely and primarily with doses above those recommended.

OVERDOSAGE

The intravenous and oral LD_{50}s in the mouse are approximately 1.17 g/kg and greater than 24.18 g/kg, respectively.

DOSAGE AND ADMINISTRATION

MEPHYTON
Summary of Dosage Guidelines
(See circular text for details)

Adults	Initial Dosage
Anticoagulant-Induced Prothrombin Deficiency (caused by coumarin or indanedione derivatives)	2.5 mg-10 mg or up to 25 mg (rarely 50 mg)
Hypoprothrombinemia due to other causes (Antibiotics; Salicylates or other drugs; Factors limiting absorption or synthesis)	2.5 mg-25 mg or more (rarely up to 50 mg)

Anticoagulant-Induced Prothrombin Deficiency in Adults
To correct excessively prolonged prothrombin times caused by oral anticoagulant therapy—2.5 to 10 mg or up to 25 mg initially is recommended. In rare instances 50 mg may be required. Frequency and amount of subsequent doses should be determined by prothrombin time response or clinical condition. (See WARNINGS.) If, in 12 to 48 hours after oral administration, the prothrombin time has not been shortened satisfactorily, the dose should be repeated.
Hypoprothrombinemia Due to Other Causes in Adults
If possible, discontinuation or reduction of the dosage of drugs interfering with coagulation mechanisms (such as salicylates, antibiotics) is suggested as an alternative to administering concurrent MEPHYTON. The severity of the coagulation disorder should determine whether the immediate administration of MEPHYTON is required in addition to discontinuation or reduction of interfering drugs.
A dosage of 2.5 to 25 mg or more (rarely up to 50 mg) is recommended, the amount and route of administration depending upon the severity of the condition and response obtained.
The oral route should be avoided when the clinical disorder would prevent proper absorption. Bile salts must be given with the tablets when the endogenous supply of bile to the gastrointestinal tract is deficient.

HOW SUPPLIED

No. 7776—Tablets MEPHYTON, 5 mg vitamin K_1, are yellow, round, scored, compressed tablets, coded MSD 43 on one side and MEPHYTON on the other. They are supplied as follows:
NDC 0006-0043-68 bottles of 100
(6505-00-660-0460, 5 mg 100's).
Storage:
Store in tightly closed original container at 25°C (77°F); excursions permitted to 15-30°C (59-86°F) [See USP Controlled Room Temperature]. Always protect MEPHYTON from light. Store in tightly closed original container and carton until contents have been used. (See PRECAUTIONS, *General.*)

7918718 Issued February 2004

Shown in Product Identification Guide, page 323

MERUVAX®$_{II}$ ℞
(Rubella Virus Vaccine Live)
Wistar RA 27/3 Strain

DESCRIPTION

MERUVAX* II (Rubella Virus Vaccine Live) is a live virus vaccine for vaccination against rubella (German measles). MERUVAX II is a sterile lyophilized preparation of the Wistar Institute RA 27/3 strain of live attenuated rubella virus. The virus was adapted to and propagated in WI-38 human diploid lung fibroblasts.
The growth medium is Minimum Essential Medium (MEM) [a buffered salt solution containing vitamins and amino acids and supplemented with fetal bovine serum] containing human serum albumin and neomycin. Sorbitol and hydrolyzed gelatin stabilizer is added to the individual virus harvests.
The cells, virus pools, fetal bovine serum, and human albumin are all screened for the absence of adventitious agents. Human albumin is processed using the Cohn cold ethanol fractionation procedure.
The reconstituted vaccine is for subcutaneous administration. Each 0.5 mL dose contains not less than 1,000 $TCID_{50}$ (tissue culture infectious doses) of rubella virus. Each dose of the vaccine is calculated to contain sorbitol (14.5 mg), sodium phosphate, sucrose (1.9 mg), sodium chloride, hydrolyzed gelatin (14.5 mg), human albumin (0.3 mg), fetal bovine serum (<1 ppm), other buffer and media ingredients and approximately 25 mcg of neomycin. The product contains no preservative.
Before reconstitution, the lyophilized vaccine is a light yellow compact crystalline plug. MERUVAX II, when reconstituted as directed, is clear yellow.

* Registered trademark of MERCK & CO., Inc.

CLINICAL PHARMACOLOGY

Rubella is a common childhood disease, caused by rubella virus (togavirus), that may be associated with serious complications and/or death. For example, rubella during pregnancy may cause congenital rubella syndrome in the infants of infected mothers.
The impact of measles, mumps, and rubella vaccination on the natural history of each disease in the United States can be quantified by comparing the maximum number of rubella cases reported in a given year prior to vaccine use to the number of cases of each disease reported in 1995. For rubella, 57,686 cases reported in 1969 compared to 200 cases reported in 1995 resulted in a 99.65% decrease.
Extensive clinical trials of rubella virus vaccines, prepared using RA 27/3 strain rubella virus, have been carried out in more than 28,000 human subjects (approximately 11,000 with MERUVAX II) in the U.S.A. and more than 20 additional countries. A single injection of the vaccine has been shown to induce rubella hemagglutination-inhibition (HI) antibodies in 97% or more of susceptible persons. However, a small percentage (1–5%) of vaccinees may fail to seroconvert after the primary dose (see also INDICATIONS AND USAGE, *Recommended Vaccination Schedule*).
Efficacy of rubella vaccine was established in a series of double-blind controlled field trials which demonstrated a high degree of protective efficacy. These studies also established that seroconversion in response to rubella vaccination paralleled protection from this disease.
Following vaccination, antibodies associated with protection can be measured by neutralization assays, HI, or ELISA (enzyme linked immunosorbent assay) tests. Neutralizing and ELISA antibodies to rubella virus are still detectable in most individuals 11–13 years after primary vaccination. See INDICATIONS AND USAGE, *Non-Pregnant Adolescents and Adult Females*, for Rubella Susceptibility Testing.
The RA 27/3 rubella strain elicits higher immediate post-vaccination HI, complement-fixing and neutralizing antibody levels than other strains of rubella vaccine and has been shown to induce a broader profile of circulating antibodies including anti-theta and anti-iota precipitating antibodies. The RA 27/3 rubella strain immunologically simulates natural infection more closely than other rubella vaccine viruses. The increased levels and broader profile of antibodies produced by RA 27/3 strain rubella virus vaccine appear to correlate with greater resistance to subclinical reinfection with the wild virus, and provide greater confidence for lasting immunity.

INDICATIONS AND USAGE

Recommended Vaccination Schedule
MERUVAX II is indicated for vaccination against rubella in persons 12 months of age or older.
It is not recommended for infants younger than 12 months because they may retain maternal rubella neutralizing antibodies that may interfere with the immune response.
Children in kindergarten and the first grades of elementary school deserve priority for vaccination because often they are epidemiologically the major source of virus dissemination in the community. A history of rubella illness is usually not reliable enough to exclude children from immunization.
Previously unimmunized children of susceptible pregnant women should receive live attenuated rubella vaccine, because an immunized child will be less likely to acquire natural rubella and introduce the virus into the household.
Individuals first vaccinated with MERUVAX II at 12 months of age or older should be revaccinated with M-M-R* II (Measles, Mumps, and Rubella Virus Vaccine Live) prior to elementary school entry. Revaccination is intended to seroconvert those who do not respond to the first dose. The Advisory Committee on Immunization Practices (ACIP) recommends administration of the first dose of M-M-R II at 12–15 months of age and administration of the second dose of M-M-R II at 4–6 years of age. In addition, some public health jurisdictions mandate the age for revaccination. Consult the complete text of applicable guidelines regarding routine revaccination including that of high-risk adult populations.
Unnecessary doses of a vaccine are best avoided by ensuring that written documentation of vaccination is preserved and a copy given to each vaccinee's parent or guardian.
Other Vaccination Considerations
Adolescent and Adult Males
Vaccination of adolescent or adult males may be a useful procedure in preventing or controlling outbreaks of rubella in circumscribed population groups (e.g., military bases and schools).
Non-Pregnant Adolescent and Adult Females
Immunization of susceptible non-pregnant adolescent and adult females of childbearing age with live attenuated rubella virus vaccine is indicated if certain precautions are observed (see below and PRECAUTIONS). Vaccinating susceptible postpubertal females confers individual protection against subsequently acquiring rubella infection during pregnancy, which in turn prevents infection of the fetus and consequent congenital rubella injury.
Women of childbearing age should be advised not to become pregnant for 3 months after vaccination and should be informed of the reason for this precaution.**
The ACIP has stated "If it is practical and if reliable laboratory services are available, women of childbearing age who are potential candidates for vaccination can have serologic tests to determine susceptibility to rubella. However, with the exception of premarital and prenatal screening, routinely performing serologic tests for all women of childbearing age to determine susceptibility (so that vaccine is given only to proven susceptible women) can be effective but is expensive. Also, 2 visits to the health-care provider would be necessary—one for screening and one for vaccination. Accordingly, rubella vaccination of a woman who is not known to be pregnant and has no history of vaccination is justifiable without serologic testing—and may be preferable, particularly when costs of serology are high and follow-up of identified susceptible women for vaccination is not assured."
Postpubertal females should be informed of the frequent occurrence of generally self-limited arthralgia and/or arthritis beginning 2 to 4 weeks after vaccination (see ADVERSE REACTIONS).
Other Populations
Previously unvaccinated children in contact with susceptible pregnant women should receive live attenuated rubella vaccine (such as that contained in MERUVAX II) to reduce the risk of exposure of the pregnant woman.
Individuals planning travel outside the United States, if not immune, can acquire measles, mumps or rubella and import these diseases into the United States. Therefore, prior to international travel, individuals known to be susceptible to one or more of these diseases can receive either a monovalent vaccine (measles, mumps or rubella), or a combination vaccine as appropriate. However, M-M-R II is preferred for persons likely to be susceptible to mumps and rubella; and if monovalent measles vaccine is not readily available, travelers should receive M-M-R II regardless or their immune status to mumps or rubella.
Vaccination is recommended for susceptible individuals in high-risk groups such as college students, health-care workers, and military personnel.
Postpartum Women
It has been found convenient in many instances to vaccinate rubella-susceptible women in the immediate postpartum period (see PRECAUTIONS, *Nursing Mothers*).
Post-Exposure Vaccination
There is no conclusive evidence that vaccination of individuals recently exposed to natural rubella will provide protection. There is, however, no contraindication to vaccinating children already exposed to natural rubella.
Use With Other Vaccines
See DOSAGE AND ADMINISTRATION, *Use With Other Vaccines*.

** NOTE: The ACIP has recommended "In view of the importance of protecting this age group against rubella, reasonable practices in a rubella immunization program include a) asking women if they are pregnant, b) excluding those who say they are, c) explaining the concern about risk for the fetus to the others..."

CONTRAINDICATIONS

Hypersensitivity to any component of the vaccine, including gelatin.
Do not give MERUVAX II to pregnant females; the possible effects of the vaccine on fetal development are unknown at this time. If vaccination of postpubertal females is undertaken, pregnancy should be avoided for three months following vaccination (see INDICATIONS AND USAGE, *Non-Pregnant Adolescents and Adult Females* and PRECAUTIONS, *Pregnancy*).
Anaphylactic or anaphylactoid reactions to neomycin (each dose of reconstituted vaccine contains approximately 25 mcg of neomycin).
Febrile respiratory illness or other active febrile infection. However, the ACIP has recommended that all vaccines can be administered to persons with minor illnesses such as diarrhea, mild upper respiratory infection with or without low-grade fever, or other low-grade febrile illness.

Patients receiving immunosuppressive therapy. This contraindication does not apply to patients who are receiving corticosteroids as replacement therapy, e.g., for Addison's disease.
Individuals with blood dyscrasias, leukemia, lymphomas of any type, or other malignant neoplasms affecting the bone marrow or lymphatic systems.
Primary and acquired immunodeficiency states, including patients who are immunosuppressed in association with AIDS or other clinical manifestations of infection with human immunodeficiency viruses; cellular immune deficiencies; and hypogammaglobulinemic and dysgammaglobulinemic states.
Individuals with a family history of congenital or hereditary immunodeficiency, until the immune competence of the potential vaccine recipient is demonstrated.

WARNINGS

The physician should be alert to the temperature elevation which may occur following vaccination (see ADVERSE REACTIONS).
This product contains albumin, a derivative of human blood. Based on effective donor screening and product manufacturing processes, it carries an extremely remote risk for transmission of viral diseases. Although there is a theoretical risk for transmission of Creutzfeldt-Jacob disease (CJD), no cases of transmission of CJD or viral disease have ever been identified that were associated with the use of albumin.
Hypersensitivity to Neomycin
The AAP states, "Persons who have experienced anaphylactic reactions to topically or systemically administered neomycin should not receive measles vaccine. Most often, however, neomycin allergy manifests as a contact dermatitis, which is a delayed-type (cell-mediated) immune response rather than anaphylaxis. In such persons, an adverse reaction to neomycin in the vaccine would be an erythematous, pruritic nodule or papule, 48 to 96 hours after vaccination. A history of contact dermatitis to neomycin is not a contraindication to receiving measles vaccine."
Thrombocytopenia
Individuals with current thrombocytopenia may develop more severe thrombocytopenia following vaccination. In addition, individuals who experienced thrombocytopenia with the first dose of M-M-R II (or its component vaccines) may develop thrombocytopenia with repeat doses. Serologic status may be evaluated to determine whether or not additional doses of vaccine are needed. The potential risk to benefit ratio should be carefully evaluated before considering vaccination in such cases (see ADVERSE REACTIONS).

PRECAUTIONS

General
Adequate treatment provisions including epinephrine injection (1:1000), should be available for immediate use should an anaphylactic or anaphylactoid reaction occur.
Special care should be taken to ensure that the injection does not enter a blood vessel.
Excretion of small amounts of the live attenuated rubella virus from the nose or throat has occurred in the majority of susceptible individuals 7-28 days after vaccination. There is no confirmed evidence to indicate that such virus is transmitted to susceptible persons who are in contact with the vaccinated individuals. Consequently, transmission through close personal contact, while accepted as a theoretical possibility, is not regarded as a significant risk. However, transmission of the vaccine virus to infants via breast milk has been documented (see *Nursing Mothers*).
Children and young adults who are known to be infected with human immunodeficiency viruses and are not immunosuppressed may be vaccinated. However, vaccinees who are infected with HIV should be monitored closely for vaccine-preventable diseases because immunization may be less effective than for uninfected persons (see CONTRAINDICATIONS).
Vaccination should be deferred for 3 months or longer following blood or plasma transfusions, or administration of immune globulin (human). However, susceptible postpartum patients who received blood products may receive MERUVAX II prior to discharge provided that a repeat HI titer is drawn 6-8 weeks after vaccination to insure seroconversion. Similarly, although studies with other live rubella virus vaccines suggest that MERUVAX II may be given in the immediate postpartum period to those non-immune women who have received anti-Rho (D) globulin (human) without interfering with vaccine effectiveness, a follow-up post-vaccination HI titer should also be determined.
It has been reported that attenuated rubella virus vaccine, live, may result in a temporary depression of tuberculin skin sensitivity. Therefore, if a tuberculin test is to be done, it should be administered either before or simultaneously with MERUVAX II.
Individuals with active untreated tuberculosis should not be vaccinated.
As for any vaccine, vaccination with MERUVAX II may not result in protection in 100% of vaccinees.
The health-care provider should determine the current health status and previous vaccination history of the vaccinee.
The health-care provider should question the patient, parent, or guardian about reactions to a previous dose of MERUVAX II or other measles-, mumps-, or rubella-containing vaccines.
Information For Patients
The health-care provider should provide the vaccine information required to be given with each vaccination to the patient, parent or guardian.
The health-care provider should inform the patient, parent or guardian of the benefits and risks associated with vaccination. For risks associated with vaccination see WARNINGS, PRECAUTIONS, ADVERSE REACTIONS.
Patients, parents or guardians should be instructed to report any serious adverse reactions to their health-care provider who in turn should report such events to the U.S. Department of Health and Human Services through the Vaccine Adverse Event Reporting System (VAERS), 1-800-822-7967.
Pregnancy should be avoided for three months following vaccination, and patients should be informed of the reasons for this precaution (see INDICATIONS AND USAGE, *Non-Pregnant Adolescent and Adult Females*, CONTRAINDICATIONS, and PRECAUTIONS, *Pregnancy*).
Laboratory Tests
See INDICATIONS AND USAGE, *Non-Pregnant Adolescents and Adult Females*, for Rubella Susceptibility Testing, and CLINICAL PHARMACOLOGY.
Immunosuppressive Therapy
The immune status of patients about to undergo immunosuppressive therapy should be evaluated so that the physician can consider whether vaccination prior to the initiation of treatment is indicated. (see CONTRAINDICATIONS and PRECAUTIONS).
The ACIP has stated that "patients with leukemia in remission who have not received chemotherapy for at least 3 months may receive live-virus vaccines. Short-term (<2 weeks), low- to moderate-dose systemic corticosteroid therapy, topical steroid therapy (e.g., nasal, skin), long-term alternate-day treatment with low to moderate doses of short-acting systemic steroid, and intra-articular, bursal, or tendon injection of corticosteroids are not immunosuppressive in their usual doses and do not contraindicate the administration of rubella vaccine."
Immune Globulin
Administration of immune globulins concurrently with MERUVAX II may interfere with the expected immune response.
See also PRECAUTIONS, *General*.
Carcinogenesis, Mutagenesis, Impairment of Fertility
MERUVAX II has not been evaluated for carcinogenic or mutagenic potential, or potential to impair fertility.
Pregnancy
Pregnancy Category C
Animal reproduction studies have not been conducted with MERUVAX II. It is also not known whether MERUVAX II can cause fetal harm when administered to a pregnant woman or can affect reproduction capacity. There is evidence suggesting transmission of rubella vaccine viruses to products of conception. Therefore, rubella vaccine should not be administered to pregnant females (see INDICATIONS AND USAGE, *Non-Pregnant Adolescent and Adult Females* and CONTRAINDICATIONS).
In counseling women who are inadvertently vaccinated when pregnant or who become pregnant within 3 months of vaccination, the physician should be aware of the following: In a 10 year survey involving over 700 pregnant women who received rubella vaccine within 3 months before or after conception, (of whom 189 received the Wistar RA 27/3 strain) none of the newborns had abnormalities compatible with congenital rubella syndrome.
Nursing Mothers
Recent studies have shown that lactating postpartum women immunized with live attenuated rubella vaccine may secrete the virus in breast milk and transmit it to breast-fed infants. In the infants with serological evidence of rubella infection, none exhibited severe disease; however, one exhibited mild clinical illness typical of acquired rubella. Caution should be exercised when MERUVAX II is administered to a nursing woman.
Pediatric Use
Safety and effectiveness in infants below the age of 12 months have not been established (see INDICATIONS AND USAGE, *Recommended Vaccination Schedule*).
Geriatric Use
Clinical studies of MERUVAX II did not include sufficient numbers of seronegative subjects aged 65 and over to determine whether they respond differently from younger subjects. Other reported clinical experience has not identified differences in responses between the elderly and younger subjects.

ADVERSE REACTIONS

The following adverse reactions are listed in decreasing order of severity, without regard to causality, within each body system category and have been reported during clinical trials, with use of the marketed vaccine, or with use of polyvalent vaccine containing rubella:
Body as a Whole
Fever; syncope; headache; dizziness; malaise; irritability.
Cardiovascular System
Vasculitis.
Digestive System
Diarrhea; vomiting; nausea.
Hemic and Lymphatic System
Thrombocytopenia (see WARNINGS, *Thrombocytopenia*); purpura; regional lymphadenopathy; leukocytosis.
Immune System
Anaphylaxis and anaphylactoid reactions have been reported as well as related phenomena such as angioneurotic edema (including peripheral or facial edema) and bronchial spasm in individuals with or without an allergic history.
Musculoskeletal System
Arthritis; arthralgia; myalgia.
Chronic arthritis has been associated with natural rubella infection and has been related to persistent virus and/or viral antigen isolated from body tissues. Only rarely have vaccine recipients developed chronic joint symptoms.
Following vaccination in children, reactions in joints are uncommon and generally of brief duration. In women, incidence rates for arthritis and arthralgia are generally higher than those seen in children (children: 0-3%; women: 12-26%) and the reactions tend to be more marked and of longer duration. Symptoms may persist for a matter of months or on rare occasions for years. In adolescent girls, the reactions appear to be intermediate in incidence between those seen in children and in adult women. Even in women older than 35 years, these reactions are generally well tolerated and rarely interfere with normal activities.
Myalgia and paresthesia have been reported rarely after administration of MERUVAX II.
Nervous System
Encephalitis; Guillain-Barré Syndrome (GBS); polyneuritis; polyneuropathy; paresthesia.
Respiratory System
Sore throat; cough; rhinitis.
Skin
Stevens-Johnson Syndrome; erythema multiforme; urticaria; rash.
Local reactions including burning/stinging at injection site; wheal and flare; redness (erythema); pain; induration.
Special Senses — Ear
Nerve deafness; otitis media.
Special Senses — Eye
Optic neuritis; papillitis; retrobulbar neuritis; conjunctivitis.
Other
Death from various, and in some cases unknown, causes has been reported rarely following vaccination with measles, mumps, and rubella vaccines; however, a causal relationship has not been established. No deaths or permanent sequelae were reported in a published post-marketing surveillance study in Finland involving 1.5 million children and adults who were vaccinated with M-M-R II during 1982-1993.
Under the National Childhood Vaccine Injury Act of 1986, health-care providers and manufacturers are required to record and report certain suspected adverse events occurring within specific time periods after vaccination. However, the U.S. Department of Health and Human Services (DHHS) has established a Vaccine Adverse Event Reporting System (VAERS) which will accept all reports of suspected events. A VAERS report form as well as information regarding reporting requirements can be obtained by calling VAERS 1-800-822-7967.

DOSAGE AND ADMINISTRATION

FOR SUBCUTANEOUS ADMINISTRATION
Do not inject intravenously
The dose for any age is 0.5 mL administered subcutaneously, preferably into the outer aspect of the upper arm.
The recommended age for primary vaccination is 12 to 15 months.
Revaccination with M-M-R II is recommended prior to elementary school entry. See also INDICATIONS AND USAGE, *Recommended Vaccination Schedule*.
Immune Globulin (IG) is not to be given concurrently with MERUVAX II.
CAUTION: A sterile syringe free of perservatives, antiseptics, and detergents should be used for each injection and/or reconstitution of the vaccine because these substances may inactivate the live virus vaccine. A 25 gauge, 5/8" needle is recommended.
To reconstitute, use only the diluent supplied, since it is free of preservatives or other antiviral substances which might inactivate the vaccine.
Single Dose Vial — First withdraw the entire volume of diluent into the syringe to be used for reconstitution. Inject all the diluent in the syringe into the vial of lyophilized vaccine, and agitate to mix thoroughly. If the lyophilized vaccine cannot be dissolved, discard. Withdraw the entire contents into a syringe and inject the total volume of restored vaccine subcutaneously.
It is important to use a separate sterile syringe and needle for each individual patient to prevent transmission of hepatitis B and other infectious agents from one person to another.
Parenteral drug products should be inspected visually for particulate matter and discoloration prior to administration whenever solution and container permit. MERUVAX II, when reconstituted, is clear yellow.

Continued on next page

Information on the Merck & Co., Inc., products listed on these pages is from the prescribing information in use October 1, 2004. For information, please call 1-800-NSC-MERCK [1-800-672-6372].

Meruvax II—Cont.

Use With Other Vaccines
MERUVAX II should not be given less than one month before or after administration of other live viral vaccines.
M-M-R II has been administered concurrently with VARIVAX* [Varicella Virus Vaccine Live (Oka/Merck)], and PedvaxHIB* [Haemophilus b Conjugate Vaccine (Meningococcal Protein Conjugate)] using separate sites and syringes. No impairment of immune response to individual tested vaccine antigens was demonstrated. The type, frequency, and severity of adverse experiences observed in these studies with M-M-R II were similar to those seen when each vaccine was given alone.
Routine administration of DTP (diphtheria, tetanus, pertussis) and/or OPV (oral poliovirus vaccine) concurrently with measles, mumps and rubella vaccines is not recommended because there are limited data relating to the simultaneous administration of these antigens.
However, other schedules have been used. The ACIP has stated "Although data are limited concerning the simultaneous administration of the entire recommended vaccine series (i.e., DTP, OPV, MMR, and Hib vaccines, with or without hepatitis B vaccine), data from numerous studies have indicated no interference between routinely recommended childhood vaccines (either live, attenuated, or killed). These findings support the simultaneous use of all vaccines as recommended."

HOW SUPPLIED

No. 4747 — MERUVAX II is supplied as a single-dose vial of lyophilized vaccine **NDC** 0006-4747-00, and a vial of diluent.
No. 4673/4309 — MERUVAX II is supplied as follows: (1) a box of 10 single-dose vials of lyophilized vaccine (package A) **NDC** 0006-4673-00; and (2) a box of 10 vials of diluent (package B). To conserve refrigerator space, the diluent may be stored separately at room temperature.
Storage
During shipment, to ensure that there is no loss of potency, the vaccine must be maintained at a temperature of 10°C (50°F) or colder. Freezing during shipment will not affect potency.
Protect the vaccine from light at all times, since such exposure may inactivate the virus.
Before reconstitution, store the vial of lyophilized vaccine at 2-8°C (36-46°F) or colder. The diluent may be stored in the refrigerator with the lyophilized vaccine or separately at room temperature.
It is recommended that the vaccine be used as soon as possible after reconstitution. Store reconstituted vaccine in the vaccine vial in a dark place at 2-8°C (36-46°F) and discard if not used within 8 hours.
9243404 Issued September 2002

MEVACOR® Tablets ℞
(Lovastatin)

DESCRIPTION

MEVACOR* (Lovastatin), is a cholesterol lowering agent isolated from a strain of *Aspergillus terreus*. After oral ingestion, lovastatin, which is an inactive lactone, is hydrolyzed to the corresponding β-hydroxyacid form. This is a principal metabolite and an inhibitor of 3-hydroxy-3-methylglutaryl-coenzyme A (HMG-CoA) reductase. This enzyme catalyzes the conversion of HMG-CoA to mevalonate, which is an early and rate limiting step in the biosynthesis of cholesterol.
Lovastatin is [1*S* -[1α(*R* *),3α,7β,8β(2*S* *,4*S* *),8aβ]]-1,2,3,7,8,8a-hexahydro-3,7-dimethyl-8-[2-(tetrahydro-4-hydroxy-6-oxo-2*H*-pyran-2-yl)ethyl]-1-naphthalenyl 2-methylbutanoate. The empirical formula of lovastatin is $C_{24}H_{36}O_5$ and its molecular weight is 404.55. Its structural formula is:

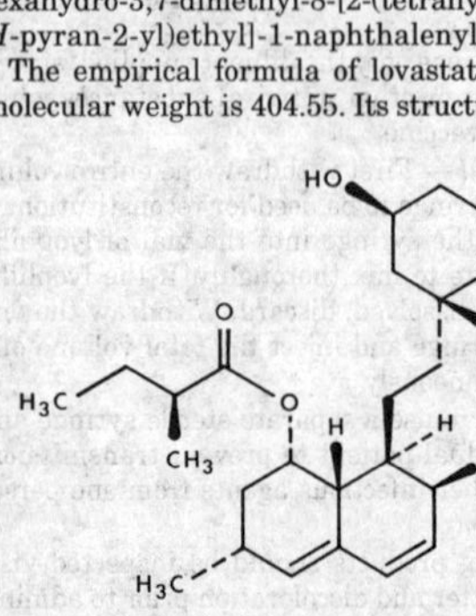

Lovastatin is a white, nonhygroscopic crystalline powder that is insoluble in water and sparingly soluble in ethanol, methanol, and acetonitrile.
Tablets MEVACOR are supplied as 10 mg, 20 mg and 40 mg tablets for oral administration. In addition to the active ingredient lovastatin, each tablet contains the following inactive ingredients: cellulose, lactose, magnesium stearate, and starch. Butylated hydroxyanisole (BHA) is added as a preservative. Tablets MEVACOR 10 mg also contain red ferric oxide and yellow ferric oxide. Tablets MEVACOR 20 mg also contain FD&C Blue 2. Tablets MEVACOR 40 mg also contain D&C Yellow 10 and FD&C Blue 2.

---

* Registered trademark of MERCK & CO., INC.

CLINICAL PHARMACOLOGY

The involvement of low-density lipoprotein cholesterol (LDL-C) in atherogenesis has been well-documented in clinical and pathological studies, as well as in many animal experiments. Epidemiological and clinical studies have established that high LDL-C and low high-density lipoprotein cholesterol (HDL-C) are both associated with coronary heart disease. However, the risk of developing coronary heart disease is continuous and graded over the range of cholesterol levels and many coronary events do occur in patients with total cholesterol (total-C) and LDL-C in the lower end of this range.
MEVACOR has been shown to reduce both normal and elevated LDL-C concentrations. LDL is formed from very low-density lipoprotein (VLDL) and is catabolized predominantly by the high affinity LDL receptor. The mechanism of the LDL-lowering effect of MEVACOR may involve both reduction of VLDL-C concentration, and induction of the LDL receptor, leading to reduced production and/or increased catabolism of LDL-C. Apolipoprotein B also falls substantially during treatment with MEVACOR. Since each LDL particle contains one molecule of apolipoprotein B, and since little apolipoprotein B is found in other lipoproteins, this strongly suggests that MEVACOR does not merely cause cholesterol to be lost from LDL, but also reduces the concentration of circulating LDL particles. In addition, MEVACOR can produce increases of variable magnitude in HDL-C, and modestly reduces VLDL-C and plasma triglycerides (TG) (see Tables I-III under *Clinical Studies*). The effects of MEVACOR on Lp(a), fibrinogen, and certain other independent biochemical risk markers for coronary heart disease are unknown.
MEVACOR is a specific inhibitor of HMG-CoA reductase, the enzyme which catalyzes the conversion of HMG-CoA to mevalonate. The conversion of HMG-CoA to mevalonate is an early step in the biosynthetic pathway for cholesterol.
Pharmacokinetics
Lovastatin is a lactone which is readily hydrolyzed *in vivo* to the corresponding β-hydroxyacid, a potent inhibitor of HMG-CoA reductase. Inhibition of HMG-CoA reductase is the basis for an assay in pharmacokinetic studies of the β-hydroxyacid metabolites (active inhibitors) and, following base hydrolysis, active plus latent inhibitors (total inhibitors) in plasma following administration of lovastatin.
Following an oral dose of ^{14}C-labeled lovastatin in man, 10% of the dose was excreted in urine and 83% in feces. The latter represents absorbed drug equivalents excreted in bile, as well as any unabsorbed drug. Plasma concentrations of total radioactivity (lovastatin plus ^{14}C-metabolites) peaked at 2 hours and declined rapidly to about 10% of peak by 24 hours postdose. Absorption of lovastatin, estimated relative to an intravenous reference dose, in each of four animal species tested, averaged about 30% of an oral dose. In animal studies, after oral dosing, lovastatin had high selectivity for the liver, where it achieved substantially higher concentrations than in non-target tissues. Lovastatin undergoes extensive first-pass extraction in the liver, its primary site of action, with subsequent excretion of drug equivalents in the bile. As a consequence of extensive hepatic extraction of lovastatin, the availability of drug to the general circulation is low and variable. In a single dose study in four hypercholesterolemic patients, it was estimated that less than 5% of an oral dose of lovastatin reaches the general circulation as active inhibitors. Following administration of lovastatin tablets the coefficient of variation, based on between-subject variability, was approximately 40% for the area under the curve (AUC) of total inhibitory activity in the general circulation.
Both lovastatin and its β-hydroxyacid metabolite are highly bound (>95%) to human plasma proteins. Animal studies demonstrated that lovastatin crosses the blood-brain and placental barriers.
The major active metabolites present in human plasma are the β-hydroxyacid of lovastatin, its 6′-hydroxy derivative, and two additional metabolites. Peak plasma concentrations of both active and total inhibitors were attained within 2 to 4 hours of dose administration. While the recommended therapeutic dose range is 10 to 80 mg/day, linearity of inhibitory activity in the general circulation was established by a single dose study employing lovastatin tablet dosages from 60 to as high as 120 mg. With a once-a-day dosing regimen, plasma concentrations of total inhibitors over a dosing interval achieved a steady state between the second and third days of therapy and were about 1.5 times those following a single dose. When lovastatin was given under fasting conditions, plasma concentrations of total inhibitors were on average about two-thirds those found when lovastatin was administered immediately after a standard test meal.
In a study of patients with severe renal insufficiency (creatinine clearance 10–30 mL/min), the plasma concentrations of total inhibitors after a single dose of lovastatin were approximately two-fold higher than those in healthy volunteers.
In a study including 16 elderly patients between 70–78 years of age who received MEVACOR 80 mg/day, the mean plasma level of HMG-CoA reductase inhibitory activity was increased approximately 45% compared with 18 patients between 18-30 years of age (see PRECAUTIONS, *Geriatric Use*).
The risk of myopathy is increased by high levels of HMG-CoA reductase inhibitory activity in plasma. Potent inhibitors of CYP3A4 can raise the plasma levels of HMG-CoA reductase inhibitory activity and increase the risk of myopathy (see WARNINGS, *Myopathy/Rhabdomyolysis* and PRECAUTIONS, *Drug Interactions*).
Lovastatin is a substrate for cytochrome P450 isoform 3A4 (CYP3A4) (see PRECAUTIONS, *Drug Interactions*.) Grapefruit juice contains one or more components that inhibit CYP3A4 and can increase the plasma concentrations of drugs metabolized by CYP3A4. In one study**, 10 subjects consumed 200 mL of double-strength grapefruit juice (one can of frozen concentrate diluted with one rather than 3 cans of water) three times daily for 2 days and an additional 200 mL double-strength grapefruit juice together with and 30 and 90 minutes following a single dose of 80 mg lovastatin on the third day. This regimen of grapefruit juice resulted in a mean increase in the serum concentration of lovastatin and its β-hydroxyacid metabolite (as measured by the area under the concentration-time curve) of 15-fold and 5-fold, respectively [as measured using a chemical assay—high performance liquid chromatography.] In a second study, 15 subjects consumed one 8 oz glass of single-strength grapefruit juice (one can of frozen concentrate diluted with 3 cans of water) with breakfast for 3 consecutive days and a single dose of 40 mg lovastatin in the evening of the third day. This regimen of grapefruit juice resulted in a mean increase in the plasma concentration (as measured by the area under the concentration-time curve) of active and total HMG-CoA reductase inhibitory activity [using an enzyme inhibition assay both before (for active inhibitors) and after (for total inhibitors) base hydrolysis] of 1.34-fold and 1.36-fold, respectively, and of lovastatin and its β-hydroxyacid metabolite [measured using a chemical assay—liquid chromatography/tandem mass spectrometry—different from that used in the first** study] of 1.94-fold and 1.57-fold, respectively. The effect of amounts of grapefruit juice between those used in these two studies of lovastatin pharmacokinetics has not been studied.

**Kantola, T, et al., Clin Pharmacol Ther 1998; 63(4):397–402.

Clinical Studies in Adults
MEVACOR has been shown to be highly effective in reducing total-C and LDL-C in heterozygous familial and non-familial forms of primary hypercholesterolemia and in mixed hyperlipidemia. A marked response was seen within 2 weeks, and the maximum therapeutic response occurred within 4-6 weeks. The response was maintained during continuation of therapy. Single daily doses given in the evening were more effective than the same dose given in the morning, perhaps because cholesterol is synthesized mainly at night.
In multicenter, double-blind studies in patients with familial or non-familial hypercholesterolemia, MEVACOR, administered in doses ranging from 10 mg q.p.m. to 40 mg b.i.d., was compared to placebo. MEVACOR consistently and significantly decreased plasma total-C, LDL-C, total-C/HDL-C ratio and LDL-C/HDL-C ratio. In addition, MEVACOR produced increases of variable magnitude in HDL-C, and modestly decreased VLDL-C and plasma TG (see Tables I through III for dose response results).
The results of a study in patients with primary hypercholesterolemia are presented in Table I.
[See table I at top of next page]
MEVACOR was compared to cholestyramine in a randomized open parallel study. The study was performed with patients with hypercholesterolemia who were at high risk of myocardial infarction. Summary results are presented in Table II.
[See table II at top of next page]
MEVACOR was studied in controlled trials in hypercholesterolemic patients with well-controlled non-insulin dependent diabetes mellitus with normal renal function. The effect of MEVACOR on lipids and lipoproteins and the safety profile of MEVACOR were similar to that demonstrated in studies in nondiabetics. MEVACOR had no clinically important effect on glycemic control or on the dose requirement of oral hypoglycemic agents.
Expanded Clinical Evaluation of Lovastatin (EXCEL) Study
MEVACOR was compared to placebo in 8,245 patients with hypercholesterolemia (total-C 240-300 mg/dL [6.2 mmol/L-7.6 mmol/L], LDL-C >160 mg/dL [4.1 mmol/L]) in the randomized, double-blind, parallel, 48-week EXCEL study. All changes in the lipid measurements (Table III) in MEVACOR treated patients were dose-related and significantly different from placebo (p≤0.001). These results were sustained throughout the study.
[See table III on next page]
Air Force/Texas Coronary Atherosclerosis Prevention Study (AFCAPS/TexCAPS)
The Air Force/Texas Coronary Atherosclerosis Prevention Study (AFCAPS/TexCAPS), a double-blind, randomized, placebo-controlled, primary prevention study, demonstrated that treatment with MEVACOR decreased the rate of acute major coronary events (composite endpoint of myocardial infarction, unstable angina, and sudden cardiac death) compared with placebo during a median of 5.1 years of follow-up. Participants were middle-aged and elderly men (ages 45-73) and women (ages 55-73) without symptomatic cardio-

vascular disease with average to moderately elevated total-C and LDL-C, below average HDL-C, and who were at high risk based on elevated total-C/HDL-C. In addition to age, 63% of the participants had at least one other risk factor (baseline HDL-C <35 mg/dL, hypertension, family history, smoking and diabetes).

AFCAPS/TexCaps enrolled 6,605 participants (5,608 men, 997 women) based on the following lipid entry criteria: total-C range of 180-264 mg/dL, LDL-C range of 130-190 mg/dL, HDL-C of ≤45 mg/dL for men and ≤47 mg/dL for women, and TG of ≤400 mg/dL. Participants were treated with standard care, including diet, and either MEVACOR 20-40 mg daily (n= 3,304) or placebo (n= 3,301). Approximately 50% of the participants treated with MEVACOR were titrated to 40 mg daily when their LDL-C remained >110 mg/dL at the 20-mg starting dose.

MEVACOR reduced the risk of a first acute major coronary event, the primary efficacy endpoint, by 37% (MEVACOR 3.5%, placebo 5.5%; p<0.001; Figure 1). A first acute major coronary event was defined as myocardial infarction (54 participants on MEVACOR, 94 on placebo) or unstable angina (54 vs. 80) or sudden cardiac death (8 vs. 9). Furthermore, among the secondary endpoints, MEVACOR reduced the risk of unstable angina by 32% (1.8 vs. 2.6%; p=0.023), of myocardial infarction by 40% (1.7 vs. 2.9%; p=0.002), and of undergoing coronary revascularization procedures (e.g., coronary artery bypass grafting or percutaneous transluminal coronary angioplasty) by 33% (3.2 vs. 4.8%; p=0.001). Trends in risk reduction associated with treatment with MEVACOR were consistent across men and women, smokers and non-smokers, hypertensives and non-hypertensives, and older and younger participants. Participants with ≥2 risk factors had risk reductions (RR) in both acute major coronary events (RR 43%) and coronary revascularization procedures (RR 37%). Because there were too few events among those participants with age as their only risk factor in this study, the effect of MEVACOR on outcomes could not be adequately assessed in this subgroup.

Figure 1
Acute Major Coronary Events (Primary Endpoint)

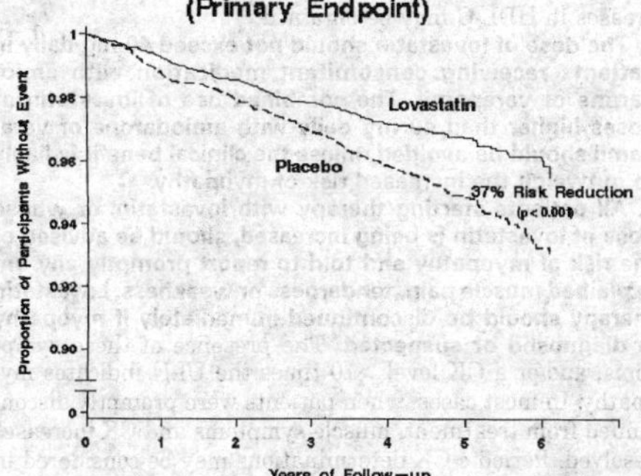

TABLE I
MEVACOR vs Placebo
(Mean Percent Change from Baseline After 6 Weeks)

DOSAGE	N	TOTAL-C	LDL-C	HDL-C	LDL-C/ HDL-C	TOTAL-C/ HDL/C	TRIG.
Placebo	33	−2	−1	−1	0	+1	+9
MEVACOR							
10 mg q.p.m.	33	−16	−21	+5	−24	−19	−10
20 mg q.p.m.	33	−19	−27	+6	−30	−23	+9
10 mg b.i.d.	32	−19	−28	+8	−33	−25	−7
40 mg q.p.m.	33	−22	−31	+5	−33	−25	−8
20 mg b.i.d.	36	−24	−32	+2	−32	−24	−6

TABLE II
MEVACOR vs. Cholestyramine
(Percent Change from Baseline After 12 Weeks)

TREATMENT	N	TOTAL-C (mean)	LDL-C (mean)	HDL-C (mean)	LDL-C/ HDL-C (mean)	TOTAL-C/ HDL-C (mean)	VLDL-C (median)	TRIG. (median)
MEVACOR								
20 mg b.i.d.	85	−27	−32	+9	−36	−31	−34	−21
40 mg b.i.d.	88	−34	−42	+8	−44	−37	−31	−27
Cholestyramine								
12 g b.i.d.	88	−17	−23	+8	−27	−21	+2	+11

TABLE III
MEVACOR vs. Placebo
(Percent Change from Baseline—
Average Values Between Weeks 12 and 48)

DOSAGE	N**	TOTAL-C (mean)	LDL-C (mean)	HDL-C (mean)	LDL-C/ HDL-C (mean)	TOTAL-C/ HDL-C (mean)	TRIG. (median)
Placebo	1663	+0.7	+0.4	+2.0	+0.2	+0.6	+4
MEVACOR							
20 mg q.p.m.	1642	−17	−24	+6.6	−27	−21	−10
40 mg q.p.m.	1645	−22	−30	+7.2	−34	−26	−14
20 mg b.i.d.	1646	−24	−34	+8.6	−38	−29	−16
40 mg b.i.d.	1649	−29	−40	+9.5	−44	−34	−19

**Patients enrolled

TABLE IV
Lipid-lowering Effects of Lovastatin in Adolescent Boys with Heterozygous Familial Hypercholesterolemia
(Mean Percent Change from Baseline at week 48 in Intention-to-Treat Population)

DOSAGE	N	TOTAL-C	LDL-C	HDL-C	TG.*	Apolipoprotein B
Placebo	61	−1.1	−1.4	−2.2	−1.4	−4.4
MEVACOR	64	−19.3	−24.2	+1.1	−1.9	−21

*data presented as median percent changes

Atherosclerosis

In the Canadian Coronary Atherosclerosis Intervention Trial (CCAIT), the effect of therapy with lovastatin on coronary atherosclerosis was assessed by coronary angiography in hyperlipidemic patients. In this randomized, double-blind, controlled clinical trial, patients were treated with conventional measures (usually diet and 325 mg of aspirin every other day) and either lovastatin 20–80 mg daily or placebo. Angiograms were evaluated at baseline and at two years by computerized quantitative coronary angiography (QCA). Lovastatin significantly slowed the progression of lesions as measured by the mean change per-patient in minimum lumen diameter (the primary endpoint) and percent diameter stenosis, and decreased the proportions of patients categorized with disease progression (33% vs. 50%) and with new lesions (16% vs. 32%).

In a similarly designed trial, the Monitored Atherosclerosis Regression Study (MARS), patients were treated with diet and either lovastatin 80 mg daily or placebo. No statistically significant difference between lovastatin and placebo was seen for the primary endpoint (mean change per patient in percent diameter stenosis of all lesions), or for most secondary QCA endpoints. Visual assessment by angiographers who formed a consensus opinion of overall angiographic change (Global Change Score) was also a secondary endpoint. By this endpoint, significant slowing of disease was seen, with regression in 23% of patients treated with lovastatin compared to 11% of placebo patients.

In the Familial Atherosclerosis Treatment Study (FATS), either lovastatin or niacin in combination with a bile acid sequestrant for 2.5 years in hyperlipidemic subjects significantly reduced the frequency of progression and increased the frequency of regression of coronary atherosclerotic lesions by QCA compared to diet and, in some cases, low-dose resin.

The effect of lovastatin on the progression of atherosclerosis in the coronary arteries has been corroborated by similar findings in another vasculature. In the Asymptomatic Carotid Artery Progression Study (ACAPS), the effect of therapy with lovastatin on carotid atherosclerosis was assessed by B-mode ultrasonography in hyperlipidemic patients with early carotid lesions and without known coronary heart disease at baseline. In this double-blind, controlled clinical trial, 919 patients were randomized in a 2 x 2 factorial design to placebo, lovastatin 10-40 mg daily and/or warfarin. Ultrasonograms of the carotid walls were used to determine the change per patient from baseline to three years in mean maximum intimal-medial thickness (IMT) of 12 measured segments. There was a significant regression of carotid lesions in patients receiving lovastatin alone compared to those receiving placebo alone (p=0.001). The predictive value of changes in IMT for stroke has not yet been established. In the lovastatin group there was a significant reduction in the number of patients with major cardiovascular events relative to the placebo group (5 vs. 14) and a significant reduction in all-cause mortality (1 vs. 8).

Eye

There was a high prevalence of baseline lenticular opacities in the patient population included in the early clinical trials with lovastatin. During these trials the appearance of new opacities was noted in both the lovastatin and placebo groups. There was no clinically significant change in visual acuity in the patients who had new opacities reported nor was any patient, including those with opacities noted at baseline, discontinued from therapy because of a decrease in visual acuity.

A three-year, double-blind, placebo-controlled study in hypercholesterolemic patients to assess the effect of lovastatin on the human lens demonstrated that there were no clinically or statistically significant differences between the lovastatin and placebo groups in the incidence, type or progression of lenticular opacities. There are no controlled clinical data assessing the lens available for treatment beyond three years.

Clinical Studies in Adolescent Patients

Efficacy of Lovastatin in Adolescent Boys with Heterozygous Familial Hypercholesterolemia

In a double-blind, placebo-controlled study, 132 boys 10-17 years of age (mean age 12.7 yrs) with heterozygous familial hypercholesterolemia (heFH) were randomized to lovastatin (n=67) or placebo (n=65) for 48 weeks. Inclusion in the study required a baseline LDL-C level between 189 and 500 mg/dL and at least one parent with an LDL-C level >189 mg/dL. The mean baseline LDL-C value was 253.1 mg/dL (range: 171-379 mg/dL) in the MEVACOR group compared to 248.2 mg/dL (range 158.5-413.5 mg/dL) in the placebo group. The dosage of lovastatin (once daily in the evening) was 10 mg for the first 8 weeks, 20 mg for the second 8 weeks, and 40 mg thereafter.

MEVACOR significantly decreased plasma levels of total-C, LDL-C and apolipoprotein B (see Table IV).

[See table IV above]

The mean achieved LDL-C value was 190.9 mg/dL (range: 108-336 mg/dL) in the MEVACOR group compared to 244.8 mg/dL (range: 135-404 mg/dL) in the placebo group.

Efficacy of Lovastatin in Post-menarchal Girls with Heterozygous Familial Hypercholesterolemia

In a double-blind, placebo-controlled study, 54 girls 10-17 years of age who were at least 1 year post-menarche with heFH were randomized to lovastatin (n=35) or placebo (n=19) for 24 weeks. Inclusion in the study required a baseline LDL-C level of 160-400 mg/dL and a parental history of familial hypercholesterolemia. The mean baseline LDL-C value was 218.3 mg/dL (range: 136.3–363.7 mg/dL) in the MEVACOR group compared to 198.8 mg/dL (range: 151.5-283.1 mg/dL) in the placebo group. The dosage of lovastatin (once daily in the evening) was 20 mg for the first 4 weeks, and 40 mg thereafter.

MEVACOR significantly decreased plasma levels of total-C, LDL-C, and apolipoprotein B (see Table V).

[See table V at top of next page]

The mean achieved LDL-C value was 154.5 mg/dL (range: 82-286 mg/dL) in the MEVACOR group compared to 203.5 mg/dL (range: 135-304 mg/dL) in the placebo group.

The safety and efficacy of doses above 40 mg daily have not been studied in children. The long-term efficacy of lovastatin therapy in childhood to reduce morbidity and mortality in adulthood has not been established.

INDICATIONS AND USAGE

Therapy with MEVACOR should be a component of multiple risk factor intervention in those individuals with dyslipidemia at risk for atherosclerotic vascular disease. MEVACOR should be used in addition to a diet restricted in saturated fat and cholesterol as part of a treatment strategy to lower total-C and LDL-C to target levels when the response to diet and other nonpharmacological measures alone has been inadequate to reduce risk.

Primary Prevention of Coronary Heart Disease

In individuals without symptomatic cardiovascular disease, average to moderately elevated total-C and LDL-C, and be-

Continued on next page

Information on the Merck & Co., Inc., products listed on these pages is from the prescribing information in use October 1, 2004. For information, please call 1-800-NSC-MERCK [1-800-672-6372].

Mevacor—Cont.

low average HDL-C, MEVACOR is indicated to reduce the risk of:
— Myocardial infarction
— Unstable angina
— Coronary revascularization procedures
(See CLINICAL PHARMACOLOGY, *Clinical Studies.*)

Coronary Heart Disease
MEVACOR is indicated to slow the progression of coronary atherosclerosis in patients with coronary heart disease as part of a treatment strategy to lower total-C and LDL-C to target levels.

Hypercholesterolemia
Therapy with lipid-altering agents should be a component of multiple risk factor intervention in those individuals at significantly increased risk for artherosclerotic vascular disease due to hypercholesterolemia. MEVACOR is indicated as an adjunct to diet for the reduction of elevated total-C and LDL-C levels in patients with primary hypercholesterolemia (Types IIa and IIb***), when the response to diet restricted in saturated fat and cholesterol and to other nonpharmacological measures alone has been inadequate.

Adolescent Patients with Heterozygous Familial Hypercholesterolemia
MEVACOR is indicated as an adjunct to diet to reduce total-C, LDL-C and apolipoprotein B levels in adolescent boys and girls who are at least one year post-menarche, 10-17 years of age, with heFH if after an adequate trial of diet therapy the following findings are present:
1. LDL-C remains >189 mg/dL or
2. LDL-C remains >160 mg/dL and:
- there is a positive family history of premature cardiovascular disease or
- two or more other CVD risk factors are present in the adolescent patient

General Recommendations
Prior to initiating therapy with lovastatin, secondary causes for hypercholesterolemia (e.g., poorly controlled diabetes mellitus, hypothyroidism, nephrotic syndrome, dysproteinemias, obstructive liver disease, other drug therapy, alcoholism) should be excluded, and a lipid profile performed to measure total-C, HDL-C, and TG. For patients with TG less than 400 mg/dL (<4.5 mmol/L), LDL-C can be estimated using the following equation:
LDL-C = total-C − [0.2 × (TG) + HDL-C]
For TG levels >400 mg/dL (>4.5 mmol/L), this equation is less accurate and LDL-C concentrations should be determined by ultracentrifugation. In hypertriglyceridemic patients, LDL-C may be low or normal despite elevated total-C. In such cases, MEVACOR is not indicated.
The National Cholesterol Education Program (NCEP) Treatment Guidelines are summarized below:
[See second table above]
After the LDL-C goal has been achieved, if the TG is still ≥200 mg/dL, non-HDL-C (total-C minus HDL-C) becomes a secondary target of therapy. Non-HDL-C goals are set 30 mg/dL higher than LDL-C goals for each risk category.
At the time of hospitalization for an acute coronary event, consideration can be given to initiating drug therapy at discharge if the LDL-C is ≥130 mg/dL (see NCEP Guidelines above).
Since the goal of treatment is to lower LDL-C, the NCEP recommends that LDL-C levels be used to initiate and assess treatment response. Only if LDL-C levels are not available, should the total-C be used to monitor therapy.
Although MEVACOR may be useful to reduce elevated LDL-C levels in patients with combined hypercholesterolemia and hypertriglyceridemia where hypercholesterolemia is the major abnormality (Type IIb hyperlipoproteinemia), it has not been studied in conditions where the major abnormality is elevation of chylomicrons, VLDL or IDL (i.e., hyperlipoproteinemia types I, III, IV, or V).***

***Classification of Hyperlipoproteinemias

Type		Lipoproteins elevated	Lipid Elevations major	minor
I	(rare)	chylomicrons	TG	→C
IIa		LDL	C	—
IIb		LDL, VLDL	C	TG
III	(rare)	IDL	C/TG	—
IV		VLDL	TG	→C
V	(rare)	chylomicrons, VLDL	TG	→C

IDL = intermediate-density lipoprotein.

The NCEP classification of cholesterol levels in pediatric patients with a familial history of hypercholesterolemia or premature cardiovascular disease is summarized below:

Category	Total-C (mg/dL)	LDL-C (mg/dL)
Acceptable	<170	<110
Borderline	170-199	110-129
High	≥200	≥130

Children treated with lovastatin in adolescence should be re-evaluated in adulthood and appropriate changes made to their cholesterol-lowering regimen to achieve adult goals for LDL-C.

TABLE V
Lipid-lowering Effects of Lovastatin in Post-menarchal Girls with Heterozygous Familial Hypercholesterolemia
(Mean Percent Change from Baseline at Week 24 in Intention-to-Treat Population)

DOSAGE	N	TOTAL-C	LDL-C	HDL-C	TG.*	Apolipoprotein B
Placebo	18	+3.6	+2.5	+4.8	−3.0	+6.4
MEVACOR	35	−22.4	−29.2	+2.4	−22.7	−24.4

*data presented as median percent changes

NCEP Treatment Guidelines:
LDL-C Goals and Cutpoints for Therapeutic Lifestyle Changes and Drug Therapy in Different Risk Categories

Risk Category	LDL Goal (mg/dL)	LDL Level at Which to Initiate Therapeutic Lifestyle Changes (mg/dL)	LDL Level at Which to Consider Drug Therapy (mg/dL)
CHD[†]or CHD risk equivalents (10-year risk >20%)	<100	≥100	≥130 (100-129: drug optional)[††]
2+ Risk factors (10 year risk ≤20%)	<130	≥130	10-year risk 10-20%: ≥130 10-year risk <10%: ≥160
0-1 Risk factor[†††]	<160	≥160	≥190 (160-189: LDL-lowering drug optional)

[†] CHD, coronary heart disease
[††] Some authorities recommend use of LDL-lowering drugs in this category if an LDL-C level of <100 mg/dL cannot be achieved by therapeutic lifestyle changes. Others prefer use of drugs that primarily modify triglycerides and HDL-C, e.g., nicotinic acid or fibrate. Clinical judgment also may call for deferring drug therapy in this subcategory.
[†††] Almost all people with 0-1 risk factor have a 10-year risk <10%; thus, 10-year risk assessment in people with 0-1 risk factor is not necessary.

CONTRAINDICATIONS

Hypersensitivity to any component of this medication.
Active liver disease or unexplained persistent elevations of serum transaminases (see WARNINGS).
Pregnancy and lactation. Atherosclerosis is a chronic process and the discontinuation of lipid-lowering drugs during pregnancy should have little impact on the outcome of long-term therapy of primary hypercholesterolemia. Moreoever, cholesterol and other products of the cholesterol biosynthesis pathway are essential components for fetal development, including synthesis of steroids and cell membranes. Because of the ability of inhibitors of HMG-CoA reductase such as MEVACOR to decrease the synthesis of cholesterol and possibly other products of the cholesterol biosynthesis pathway, MEVACOR is contraindicated during pregnancy and in nursing mothers. **MEVACOR should be administered to women of childbearing age only when such patients are highly unlikely to conceive.** If the patient becomes pregnant while taking this drug, MEVACOR should be discontinued immediately and the patient should be apprised of the potential hazard to the fetus (see PRECAUTIONS, *Pregnancy*).

WARNINGS

Myopathy/Rhabdomyolysis
Lovastatin, like other inhibitors of HMG-CoA reductase, occasionally causes myopathy manifested as muscle pain, tenderness or weakness with creatine kinase (CK) above 10× the upper limit of normal (ULN). Myopathy sometimes takes the form of rhabdomyolysis with or without acute renal failure secondary to myoglobinuria, and rare fatalities have occurred. The risk of myopathy is increased by high levels of HMG-CoA reductase inhibitory activity in plasma.
- **The risk of myopathy/rhabdomyolysis is increased by concomitant use of lovastatin with the following:**
Potent inhibitors of CYP3A4: Cyclosporine, itraconazole, ketoconazole, erythromycin, clarithromycin, HIV protease inhibitors, nefazodone, or large quantities of grapefruit juice (>1 quart daily), particularly with higher doses of lovastatin (see below; CLINICAL PHARMACOLOGY, *Pharmacokinetics*; PRECAUTIONS, *Drug Interactions, CYP3A4 Interactions*).
Lipid-lowering drugs that can cause myopathy when given alone: Gemfibrozil, other fibrates, or lipid-lowering doses (≥1 g/day) of niacin, particularly with higher doses of lovastatin (see below; CLINICAL PHARMACOLOGY, *Pharmacokinetics*; PRECAUTIONS, *Drug Interactions, Interactions with lipid-lowering drugs that can cause myopathy when given alone*).
Other drugs: The risk of myopathy/rhabdomyolysis is increased when either amiodarone or verapamil is used concomitantly with higher doses of a closely related member of the HMG-CoA reductase inhibitor class (see PRECAUTIONS, *Drug Interactions, Other drug interactions*).
- **The risk of myopathy/rhabdomyolysis is dose related.** In a clinical study (EXCEL) in which patients were carefully monitored and some interacting drugs were excluded, there was one case of myopathy among 4933 patients randomized to lovastatin 20-40 mg daily for 48 weeks, and 4 among 1649 patients randomized to 80 mg daily.

CONSEQUENTLY:
1. Use of lovastatin concomitantly with itraconazole, ketoconazole, erythromycin, clarithromycin, HIV protease inhibitors, nefazodone, or large quantities of grapefruit juice (>1 quart daily) should be avoided. If treatment with itraconazole, ketoconazole, erythromycin, or clarithromycin is unavoidable, therapy with lovastatin should be suspended during the course of treatment. Concomitant use with other medicines labeled as having a potent inhibitory effect on CYP3A4 at therapeutic doses should be avoided unless the benefits of combined therapy outweigh the increased risk.
2. The dose of lovastatin should not exceed 20 mg daily in patients receiving concomitant medication with cyclosporine, gemfibrozil, other fibrates or lipid-lowering doses (≥1 g/day) of niacin. The combined use of lovastatin with fibrates or niacin should be avoided unless the benefit of further alteration in lipid levels is likely to outweigh the increased risk of this drug combination. Addition of these drugs to lovastatin typically provides little additional reduction in LDL-C, but further reductions of TG and further increases in HDL-C may be obtained.
3. The dose of lovastatin should not exceed 40 mg daily in patients receiving concomitant medication with amiodarone or verapamil. The combined use of lovastatin at doses higher than 40 mg daily with amiodarone or verapamil should be avoided unless the clinical benefit is likely to outweigh the increased risk of myopathy.
4. All patients starting therapy with lovastatin, or whose dose of lovastatin is being increased, should be advised of the risk of myopathy and told to report promptly any unexplained muscle pain, tenderness or weakness. Lovastatin therapy should be discontinued immediately if myopathy is diagnosed or suspected. The presence of these symptoms, and/or a CK level >10 times the ULN indicates myopathy. In most cases, when patients were promptly discontinued from treatment, muscle symptoms and CK increases resolved. Periodic CK determinations may be considered in patients starting therapy with lovastatin or whose dose is being increased, but there is no assurance that such monitoring will prevent myopathy.
5. Many of the patients who have developed rhabdomyolysis on therapy with lovastatin have had complicated medical histories, including renal insufficiency usually as a consequence of long-standing diabetes mellitus. Such patients merit closer monitoring. Therapy with lovastatin should be temporarily stopped a few days prior to elective major surgery and when any major medical or surgical condition supervenes.

Liver Dysfunction
Persistent increases (to more than 3 times the upper limit of normal) in serum transaminases occurred in 1.9% of adult patients who received lovastatin for at least one year in early clinical trials (see ADVERSE REACTIONS). When the drug was interrupted or discontinued in these patients, the transaminase levels usually fell slowly to pretreatment levels. The increases usually appeared 3 to 12 months after the start of therapy with lovastatin, and were not associated with jaundice or other clinical signs or symptoms. There was no evidence of hypersensitivity. In the EXCEL study (see CLINICAL PHARMACOLOGY, *Clinical Studies*), the incidence of persistent increases in serum transaminases over 48 weeks was 0.1% for placebo, 0.1% at 20 mg/day, 0.9% at 40 mg/day, and 1.5% at 80 mg/day in patients on lovastatin. However, in post-marketing experience with MEVACOR, symptomatic liver disease has been reported rarely at all dosages (see ADVERSE REACTIONS).
In AFCAPS/TexCAPS, the number of participants with consecutive elevations of either alanine aminotransferase (ALT) or aspartate aminotransferase (AST) (> 3 times the upper limit of normal), over a median of 5.1 years of follow-up, was not significantly different between the MEVACOR and placebo groups (18 [0.6%] vs. 11 [0.3%]). The starting dose of MEVACOR was 20 mg/day; 50% of the MEVACOR treated participants were titrated to 40 mg/day at Week 18. Of the 18 participants on MEVACOR with consecutive elevations of either ALT or AST, 11 (0.7%) elevations occurred in participants taking 20 mg/day, while 7 (0.4%) elevations occurred in participants titrated to 40 mg/day. Elevated transaminases resulted in discontinuation of 6 (0.2%) participants from therapy in the MEVACOR group (n=3,304) and 4 (0.1%) in the placebo group (n=3,301).

It is recommended that liver function tests be performed before the initiation of treatment, at 6 and 12 weeks after initiation of therapy or elevation of dose, and periodically thereafter (e.g., semiannually). Patients who develop increased transaminase levels should be monitored with a second liver function evaluation to confirm the finding and be followed thereafter with frequent liver function tests until the abnormality(ies) return to normal. Should an increase in AST or ALT of three times the upper limit of normal or greater persist, withdrawal of therapy with MEVACOR is recommended.

The drug should be used with caution in patients who consume substantial quantities of alcohol and/or have a past history of liver disease. Active liver disease or unexplained transaminase elevations are contraindications to the use of lovastatin.

As with other lipid-lowering agents, moderate (less than three times the upper limit of normal) elevations of serum transaminases have been reported following therapy with MEVACOR (see ADVERSE REACTIONS). These changes appeared soon after initiation of therapy with MEVACOR, were often transient, were not accompanied by any symptoms and interruption of treatment was not required.

PRECAUTIONS

General

Lovastatin may elevate creatine phosphokinase and transaminase levels (see WARNINGS and ADVERSE REACTIONS). This should be considered in the differential diagnosis of chest pain in a patient on therapy with lovastatin.

Homozygous Familial Hypercholesterolemia

MEVACOR is less effective in patients with the rare homozygous familial hypercholesterolemia, possibly because these patients have no functional LDL receptors. MEVACOR appears to be more likely to raise serum transaminases (see ADVERSE REACTIONS) in these homozygous patients.

Information for Patients

Patients should be advised about substances they should not take concomitantly with lovastatin and be advised to report promptly unexplained muscle pain, tenderness, or weakness (see list below and WARNINGS, *Myopathy/Rhabdomyolysis*). Patients should also be advised to inform other physicians prescribing a new medication that they are taking MEVACOR.

Drug Interactions

CYP3A4 Interactions

Lovastatin is metabolized by CYP3A4 but has no CYP3A4 inhibitory activity; therefore it is not expected to affect the plasma concentrations of other drugs metabolized by CYP3A4. Potent inhibitors of CYP3A4 (below) increase the risk of myopathy by reducing the elimination of lovastatin. **See WARNINGS, *Myopathy/Rhabdomyolysis*, and CLINICAL PHARMACOLOGY, *Pharmacokinetics*.**

- **Itraconazole**
- **Ketoconazole**
- **Erythromycin**
- **Clarithromycin**
- **HIV protease inhibitors**
- **Nefazodone**
- **Cyclosporine**
- **Large quantities of grapefruit juice (>1 quart daily)**

Interactions with lipid-lowering drugs that can cause myopathy when given alone

The risk of myopathy is also increased by the following lipid-lowering drugs that are not potent CYP3A4 inhibitors, but which can cause myopathy when given alone.

See WARNINGS, *Myopathy/Rhabdomyolysis.*

- **Gemfibrozil**
- **Other fibrates**
- **Niacin (nicotinic acid) (≥1 g/day)**

Other drug interactions

Amiodarone or Verapamil: The risk of myopathy/rhabdomyolysis is increased when either amiodarone or verapamil is used concomitantly with a closely related member of the HMG-CoA reductase inhibitor class (see WARNINGS, *Myopathy/Rhabdomyolysis*).

Coumarin Anticoagulants: In a small clinical trial in which lovastatin was administered to warfarin treated patients, no effect on prothrombin time was detected. However, another HMG-CoA reductase inhibitor has been found to produce a less than two seconds increase in prothrombin time in healthy volunteers receiving low doses of warfarin. Also, bleeding and/or increased prothrombin time have been reported in a few patients taking coumarin anticoagulants concomitantly with lovastatin. It is recommended that in patients taking anticoagulants, prothrombin time be determined before starting lovastatin and frequently enough during early therapy to insure that no significant alteration of prothrombin time occurs. Once a stable prothrombin time has been documented, prothrombin times can be monitored at the intervals usually recommended for patients on coumarin anticoagulants. If the dose of lovastatin is changed, the same procedure should be repeated. Lovastatin therapy has not been associated with bleeding or with changes in prothrombin time in patients not taking anticoagulants.

Propranolol: In normal volunteers, there was no clinically significant pharmacokinetic or pharmacodynamic interaction with concomitant administration of single doses of lovastatin and propranolol.

Digoxin: In patients with hypercholesterolemia, concomitant administration of lovastatin and digoxin resulted in no effect on digoxin plasma concentrations.

Oral Hypoglycemic Agents: In pharmacokinetic studies of MEVACOR in hypercholesterolemic non-insulin dependent diabetic patients, there was no drug interaction with glipizide or with chlorpropamide (see CLINICAL PHARMACOLOGY, *Clinical Studies*).

Endocrine Function

HMG-CoA reductase inhibitors interfere with cholesterol synthesis and as such might theoretically blunt adrenal and/or gonadal steroid production. Results of clinical trials with drugs in this class have been inconsistent with regard to drug effects on basal and reserve steroid levels. However, clinical studies have shown that lovastatin does not reduce basal plasma cortisol concentration or impair adrenal reserve, and does not reduce basal plasma testosterone concentration. Another HMG-CoA reductase inhibitor has been shown to reduce the plasma testosterone response to HCG. In the same study, the mean testosterone response to HCG was slightly but not significantly reduced after treatment with lovastatin 40 mg daily for 16 weeks in 21 men. The effects of HMG-CoA reductase inhibitors on male fertility have not been studied in adequate numbers of male patients. The effects, if any, on the pituitary-gonadal axis in premenopausal women are unknown. Patients treated with lovastatin who develop clinical evidence of endocrine dysfunction should be evaluated appropriately. Caution should also be exercised if an HMG-CoA reductase inhibitor or other agent used to lower cholesterol levels is administered to patients also receiving other drugs (e.g., ketoconazole, spironolactone, cimetidine) that may decrease the levels or activity of endogenous steroid hormones.

CNS Toxicity

Lovastatin produced optic nerve degeneration (Wallerian degeneration of retinogeniculate fibers) in clinically normal dogs in a dose-dependent fashion starting at 60 mg/kg/day, a dose that produced mean plasma drug levels about 30 times higher than the mean drug level in humans taking the highest recommended dose (as measured by total enzyme inhibitory activity). Vestibulocochlear Wallerian-like degeneration and retinal ganglion cell chromatolysis were also seen in dogs treated for 14 weeks at 180 mg/kg/day, a dose which resulted in a mean plasma drug level (C_{max}) similar to that seen with the 60 mg/kg/day dose.

CNS vascular lesions, characterized by perivascular hemorrhage and edema, mononuclear cell infiltration of perivascular spaces, perivascular fibrin deposits and necrosis of small vessels, were seen in dogs treated with lovastatin at a dose of 180 mg/kg/day, a dose which produced plasma drug levels (C_{max}) which were about 30 times higher than the mean values in humans taking 80 mg/day.

Similar optic nerve and CNS vascular lesions have been observed with other drugs of this class.

Cataracts were seen in dogs treated for 11 and 28 weeks at 180 mg/kg/day and 1 year at 60 mg/kg/day.

Carcinogenesis, Mutagenesis, Impairment of Fertility

In a 21-month carcinogenic study in mice, there was a statistically significant increase in the incidence of hepatocellular carcinomas and adenomas in both males and females at 500 mg/kg/day. This dose produced a total plasma drug exposure 3 to 4 times that of humans given the highest recommended dose of lovastatin (drug exposure was measured as total HMG-CoA reductase inhibitory activity in extracted plasma). Tumor increases were not seen at 20 and 100 mg/kg/day, doses that produced drug exposures of 0.3 to 2 times that of humans at the 80 mg/day dose. A statistically significant increase in pulmonary adenomas was seen in female mice at approximately 4 times the human drug exposure. (Although mice were given 300 times the human dose [HD] on a mg/kg body weight basis, plasma levels of total inhibitory activity were only 4 times higher in mice than in humans given 80 mg of MEVACOR.)

There was an increase in incidence of papilloma in the non-glandular mucosa of the stomach of mice beginning at exposures of 1 to 2 times that of humans. The glandular mucosa was not affected. The human stomach contains only glandular mucosa.

In a 24-month carcinogenicity study in rats, there was a positive dose response relationship for hepatocellular carcinogenicity in males at drug exposures between 2-7 times that of human exposure at 80 mg/day (doses in rats were 5, 30 and 180 mg/kg/day).

An increased incidence of thyroid neoplasms in rats appears to be a response that has been seen with other HMG-CoA reductase inhibitors.

A chemically similar drug in this class was administered to mice for 72 weeks at 25, 100, and 400 mg/kg body weight, which resulted in mean serum drug levels approximately 3, 15, and 33 times higher than the mean human serum drug concentration (as total inhibitory activity) after a 40 mg oral dose. Liver carcinomas were significantly increased in high dose females and mid- and high dose males, with a maximum incidence of 90 percent in males. The incidence of adenomas of the liver was significantly increased in mid- and high dose females. Drug treatment also significantly increased the incidence of lung adenomas in mid- and high dose males and females. Adenomas of the Harderian gland (a gland of the eye of rodents) were significantly higher in high dose mice than in controls.

No evidence of mutagenicity was observed in a microbial mutagen test using mutant strains of *Salmonella typhimurium* with or without rat or mouse liver metabolic activation. In addition, no evidence of damage to genetic material was noted in an *in vitro* alkaline elution assay using rat or mouse hepatocytes, a V-79 mammalian cell forward mutation study, an *in vitro* chromosome aberration study in CHO cells, or an *in vivo* chromosomal aberration assay in mouse bone marrow.

Drug-related testicular atrophy, decreased spermatogenesis, spermatocytic degeneration and giant cell formation were seen in dogs starting at 20 mg/kg/day. Similar findings were seen with another drug in this class. No drug-related effects on fertility were found in studies with lovastatin in rats. However, in studies with a similar drug in this class, there was decreased fertility in male rats treated for 34 weeks at 25 mg/kg body weight, although this effect was not observed in a subsequent fertility study when this same dose was administered for 11 weeks (the entire cycle of spermatogenesis, including epididymal maturation). In rats treated with this same reductase inhibitor at 180 mg/kg/day, seminiferous tubule degeneration (necrosis and loss of spermatogenic epithelium) was observed. No microscopic changes were observed in the testes from rats of either study. The clinical significance of these findings is unclear.

Pregnancy

Pregnancy Category X

See CONTRAINDICATIONS.

Safety in pregnant women has not been established.

Lovastatin has been shown to produce skeletal malformations at plasma levels 40 times the human exposure (for mouse fetus) and 80 times the human exposure (for rat fetus) based on mg/m^2 surface area (doses were 800 mg/kg/day). No drug-induced changes were seen in either species at multiples of 8 times (rat) or 4 times (mouse) based on surface area. No evidence of malformations was noted in rabbits at exposures up to 3 times the human exposure (dose of 15 mg/kg/day, highest tolerated dose).

Rare reports of congenital anomalies have been received following intrauterine exposure to HMG-CoA reductase inhibitors. In a review[†] of approximately 100 prospectively followed pregnancies in women exposed to MEVACOR or another structurally related HMG-CoA reductase inhibitor, the incidences of congenital anomalies, spontaneous abortions and fetal deaths/stillbirths did not exceed what would be expected in the general population. The number of cases is adequate only to exclude a 3 to 4-fold increase in congenital anomalies over the background incidence. In 89% of the prospectively followed pregnancies, drug treatment was initiated prior to pregnancy and was discontinued at some point in the first trimester when pregnancy was identified.

As safety in pregnant women has not been established and there is no apparent benefit to therapy with MEVACOR during pregnancy (see CONTRAINDICATIONS), treatment should be immediately discontinued as soon as pregnancy is recognized. MEVACOR should be administered to women of child-bearing potential only when such patients are highly unlikely to conceive and have been informed of the potential hazards.

Nursing Mothers

It is not known whether lovastatin is excreted in human milk. Because a small amount of another drug in this class is excreted in human breast milk and because of the potential for serious adverse reactions in nursing infants, women taking MEVACOR should not nurse their infants (see CONTRAINDICATIONS).

Pediatric Use

Safety and effectiveness in patients 10-17 years of age with heFH have been evaluated in controlled clinical trials of 48 weeks duration in adolescent boys and controlled clinical trials of 24 weeks duration in girls who were at least 1 year post-menarche. Patients treated with lovastatin had an adverse experience profile generally similar to that of patients treated with placebo. **Doses greater than 40 mg have not been studied in this population.** In these limited controlled studies, there was no detectable effect on growth or sexual maturation in the adolescent boys or on menstrual cycle length in girls. See CLINICAL PHARMACOLOGY, *Clinical Studies in Adolescent Patients;* ADVERSE REACTIONS, *Adolescent Patients;* and DOSAGE AND ADMINISTRATION, *Adolescent Patients (10-17 years of age) with Heterozygous Familial Hypercholesterolemia*. Adolescent females should be counseled on appropriate contraceptive methods while on lovastatin therapy (see CONTRAINDICATIONS and PRECAUTIONS, *Pregnancy*). **Lovastatin has not been studied in pre-pubertal patients or patients younger than 10 years of age.**

Geriatric Use

A pharmacokinetic study with lovastatin showed the mean plasma level of HMG-CoA reductase inhibitory activity to be approximately 45% higher in elderly patients between 70-78 years of age compared with patients between 18-30 years of age; however, clinical study experience in the elderly indicates that dosage adjustment based on this age-related pharmacokinetic difference is not needed. In the two large clinical studies conducted with lovastatin (EXCEL and AFCAPS/TexCAPS), 21% (3094/14850) of patients were ≥65 years of age. Lipid-lowering efficacy with lovastatin was at least as great in elderly patients compared with younger patients, and there were no overall differences in

Continued on next page

Information on the Merck & Co., Inc., products listed on these pages is from the prescribing information in use October 1, 2004. For information, please call 1-800-NSC-MERCK [1-800-672-6372].

Mevacor—Cont.

safety over the 20 to 80 mg/day dosage range (see CLINICAL PHARMACOLOGY).

[†]Manson, J.M., Freyssinges, C., Ducrocq, M.B., Stephenson, W.P., Postmarketing Surveillance of Lovastatin and Simvastatin Exposure During Pregnancy. *Reproductive Toxicology.* 10(6):439-446. 1996.

ADVERSE REACTIONS

MEVACOR is generally well tolerated; adverse reactions usually have been mild and transient.

Phase III Clinical Studies

In Phase III controlled clinical studies involving 613 patients treated with MEVACOR, the adverse experience profile was similar to that shown below for the 8,245-patient EXCEL study (see *Expanded Clinical Evaluation of Lovastatin [EXCEL] Study*).

Persistent increases of serum transaminases have been noted (see WARNINGS, *Liver Dysfunction*). About 11% of patients had elevations of CK levels of at least twice the normal value on one or more occasions. The corresponding values for the control agent cholestyramine was 9 percent. This was attributable to the noncardiac fraction of CK. Large increases in CK have sometimes been reported (see WARNINGS, *Myopathy/Rhabdomyolysis*).

Expanded Clinical Evaluation of Lovastatin (EXCEL) Study

MEVACOR was compared to placebo in 8,245 patients with hypercholesterolemia (total-C 240-300 mg/dL [6.2-7.8 mmol/L]) in the randomized, double-blind, parallel, 48-week EXCEL study. Clinical adverse experiences reported as possibly, probably or definitely drug-related in ≥1% in any treatment group are shown in the table below. For no event was the incidence on drug and placebo statistically different.

[See table below]

Other clinical adverse experiences reported as possibly, probably or definitely drug-related in 0.5 to 1.0 percent of patients in any drug-treated group are listed below. In all these cases the incidence on drug and placebo was not statistically different. *Body as a Whole:* chest pain; *Gastrointestinal:* acid regurgitation, dry mouth, vomiting; *Musculoskeletal:* leg pain, shoulder pain, arthralgia; *Nervous System/Psychiatric:* insomnia, paresthesia; *Skin:* alopecia, pruritus; *Special Senses:* eye irritation.

In the EXCEL study (see CLINICAL PHARMACOLOGY, *Clinical Studies*), 4.6% of the patients treated up to 48 weeks were discontinued due to clinical or laboratory adverse experiences which were rated by the investigator as possibly, probably or definitely related to therapy with MEVACOR. The value for the placebo group was 2.5%.

Air Force/Texas Coronary Atherosclerosis Prevention Study (AFCAPS/TexCAPS)

In AFCAPS/TexCAPS (see CLINICAL PHARMACOLOGY, *Clinical Studies*) involving 6,605 participants treated with 20-40 mg/day of MEVACOR (n=3,304) or placebo (n=3,301), the safety and tolerability profile of the group treated with MEVACOR was comparable to that of the group treated with placebo during a median of 5.1 years of follow-up. The adverse experiences reported in AFCAPS/TexCAPS were similar to those reported in EXCEL (see ADVERSE REACTIONS, *Expanded Clinical Evaluation of Lovastatin (EXCEL) Study*).

Concomitant Therapy

In controlled clinical studies in which lovastatin was administered concomitantly with cholestyramine, no adverse reactions peculiar to this concomitant treatment were observed. The adverse reactions that occurred were limited to those reported previously with lovastatin or cholestyramine. Other lipid-lowering agents were not administered concomitantly with lovastatin during controlled clinical studies. Preliminary data suggests that the addition of gemfibrozil to therapy with lovastatin is not associated with greater reduction in LDL-C than that achieved with lovastatin alone. In uncontrolled clinical studies, most of the patients who have developed myopathy were receiving concomitant therapy with cyclosporine, gemfibrozil or niacin (nicotinic acid). The combined use of lovastatin at doses exceeding 20 mg/day with cyclosporine, gemfibrozil, other fibrates or lipid-lowering doses (≥1 g/day) of niacin should be avoided (see WARNINGS, *Myopathy/Rhabdomyolysis*).

The following effects have been reported with drugs in this class. Not all the effects listed below have necessarily been associated with lovastatin therapy.

Skeletal: muscle cramps, myalgia, myopathy, rhabdomyolysis, arthralgias.

Neurological: dysfunction of certain cranial nerves (including alteration of taste, impairment of extra-ocular movement, facial paresis), tremor, dizziness, vertigo, memory loss, paresthesia, peripheral neuropathy, peripheral nerve palsy, psychic disturbances, anxiety, insomnia, depression.

Hypersensitivity Reactions: An apparent hypersensitivity syndrome has been reported rarely which has included one or more of the following features: anaphylaxis, angioedema, lupus erythematous-like syndrome, polymyalgia rheumatica, dermatomyositis, vasculitis, purpura, thrombocytopenia, leukopenia, hemolytic anemia, positive ANA, ESR increase, eosinophilia, arthritis, arthralgia, urticaria, asthenia, photosensitivity, fever, chills, flushing, malaise, dyspnea, toxic epidermal necrolysis, erythema multiforme, including Stevens-Johnson syndrome.

Gastrointestinal: pancreatitis, hepatitis, including chronic active hepatitis, cholestatic jaundice, fatty change in liver; and rarely, cirrhosis, fulminant hepatic necrosis, and hepatoma; anorexia, vomiting.

Skin: alopecia, pruritus. A variety of skin changes (e.g., nodules, discoloration, dryness of skin/mucous membranes, changes to hair/nails) have been reported.

Reproductive: gynecomastia, loss of libido, erectile dysfunction.

Eye: progression of cataracts (lens opacities), ophthalmoplegia.

Laboratory Abnormalities: elevated transaminases, alkaline phosphatase, γ-glutamyl transpeptidase, and bilirubin; thyroid function abnormalities.

Adolescent Patients (ages 10-17 years)

In a 48-week controlled study in adolescent boys with heFH (n=132) and a 24-week controlled study in girls who were at least 1 year post-menarche with heFH (n=54), the safety and tolerability profile of the groups treated with MEVACOR (10 to 40 mg daily) was generally similar to that of the groups treated with placebo (see CLINICAL PHARMACOLOGY, *Clinical Studies in Adolescent Patients* and PRECAUTIONS, *Pediatric Use*).

OVERDOSAGE

After oral administration of MEVACOR to mice the median lethal dose observed was >15 g/m².

Five healthy human volunteers have received up to 200 mg of lovastatin as a single dose without clinically significant adverse experiences. A few cases of accidental overdosage have been reported; no patients had any specific symptoms, and all patients recovered without sequelae. The maximum dose taken was 5-6 g.

Until further experience is obtained, no specific treatment of overdosage with MEVACOR can be recommended.

The dialyzability of lovastatin and its metabolites in man is not known at present.

	Placebo (N=1663) %	MEVACOR 20 mg q.p.m. (N=1642) %	MEVACOR 40 mg q.p.m. (N=1645) %	MEVACOR 20 mg b.i.d. (N=1646) %	MEVACOR 40 mg b.i.d. (N=1649) %
Body As a Whole					
Asthenia	1.4	1.7	1.4	1.5	1.2
Gastrointestinal					
Abdominal pain	1.6	2.0	2.0	2.2	2.5
Constipation	1.9	2.0	3.2	3.2	3.5
Diarrhea	2.3	2.6	2.4	2.2	2.6
Dyspepsia	1.9	1.3	1.3	1.0	1.6
Flatulence	4.2	3.7	4.3	3.9	4.5
Nausea	2.5	1.9	2.5	2.2	2.2
Musculoskeletal					
Muscle cramps	0.5	0.0	0.0	1.1	1.0
Myalgia	1.7	2.6	1.8	2.2	3.0
Nervous System/ Psychiatric					
Dizziness	0.7	0.7	1.2	0.5	0.5
Headache	2.7	2.6	2.8	2.1	3.2
Skin					
Rash	0.7	0.8	1.0	1.2	1.3
Special Senses					
Blurred vision	0.8	1.1	0.9	0.9	1.2

DOSAGE AND ADMINISTRATION

The patient should be placed on a standard cholesterol-lowering diet before receiving MEVACOR and should continue on this diet during treatment with MEVACOR (see NCEP Treatment Guidelines for details on dietary therapy). MEVACOR should be given with meals.

Adult Patients

The usual recommended starting dose is 20 mg once a day given with the evening meal. The recommended dosing range is 10-80 mg/day in single or two divided doses; the maximum recommended dose is 80 mg/day. Doses should be individualized according to the recommended goal of therapy (see NCEP Guidelines and CLINICAL PHARMACOLOGY). Patients requiring reductions in LDL-C of 20% or more to achieve their goal (see INDICATIONS AND USAGE) should be started on 20 mg/day of MEVACOR. A starting dose of 10 mg may be considered for patients requiring smaller reductions. Adjustments should be made at intervals of 4 weeks or more.

Cholesterol levels should be monitored periodically and consideration should be given to reducing the dosage of MEVACOR if cholesterol levels fall significantly below the targeted range.

Dosage in Patients taking Cyclosporine

In patients taking cyclosporine concomitantly with lovastatin (see WARNINGS, *Myopathy/Rhabdomyolysis*), therapy should begin with 10 mg of MEVACOR and should not exceed 20 mg/day.

Dosage in Patients taking Amiodarone or Verapamil

In patients taking amiodarone or verapamil concomitantly with MEVACOR, the dose should not exceed 40 mg/day (see WARNINGS, *Myopathy/Rhabdomyolysis* and PRECAUTIONS, *Drug Interactions, Other drug interactions*).

Adolescent Patients (10-17 years of age) with Heterozygous Familial Hypercholesterolemia

The recommended dosing range is 10-40 mg/day; the maximum recommended dose is 40 mg/day. Doses should be individualized according to the recommended goal of therapy (see NCEP Pediatric Panel Guidelines[††], CLINICAL PHARMACOLOGY, and INDICATIONS AND USAGE). Patients requiring reductions in LDL-C of 20% or more to achieve their goal should be started on 20 mg/day of MEVACOR. A starting dose of 10 mg may be considered for patients requiring smaller reductions. Adjustments should be made at intervals of 4 weeks or more.

[††]National Cholesterol Education Program (NCEP): Highlights of the Report of the Expert Panel on Blood Cholesterol Levels in Children and Adolescents. *Pediatrics.* 89(3): 495–501, 1992.

Concomitant Lipid-Lowering Therapy

MEVCOR is effective alone or when used concomitantly with bile-acid sequestrants. If MEVACOR is used in combination with gemfibrozil, other fibrates or lipid-lowering doses (≥1g/day) of niacin, the dose of MEVACOR should not exceed 20 mg/day (see WARNINGS, *Myopathy/Rhabdomyolysis* and PRECAUTIONS, *Drug Interactions*).

Dosage in Patients with Renal Insufficiency

In patients with severe renal insufficiency (creatinine clearance <30 mL/min), dosage increases above 20 mg/day should be carefully considered and, if deemed necessary, implemented cautiously (see CLINICAL PHARMACOLOGY and WARNINGS, *Myopathy/Rhabdomyolysis*).

HOW SUPPLIED

No. 3560—Tablets MEVACOR 10 mg are peach, octagonal tablets, coded MSD 730 on one side and MEVACOR on the other. They are supplied as follows:

NDC 0006-0730-61 unit of use bottles of 60.

No. 3561—Tablets MEVACOR 20 mg are light blue, octagonal tablets, coded MSD 731 on one side and MEVACOR on the other. They are supplied as follows:

NDC 0006-0731-61 unit of use bottles of 60
NDC 0006-0731-94 unit of use bottles of 90
NDC 0006-0731-28 unit dose packages of 100
NDC 0006-0731-82 bottles of 1,000
NDC 0006-0731-87 bottles of 10,000.

No. 3562—Tablets MEVACOR 40 mg are green, octagonal tablets, coded MSD 732 on one side and MEVACOR on the other. They are supplied as follows:

NDC 0006-0732-61 unit of use bottles of 60
NDC 0006-0732-94 unit of use bottles of 90
NDC 0006-0732-82 bottles of 1,000
NDC 0006-0732-87 bottles of 10,000.

Storage

Store between 5-30°C (41-86°F). Tablets MEVACOR must be protected from light and stored in a well-closed, light-resistant container.

7825351 Issued June 2002

Shown in Product Identification Guide, page 323

MIDAMOR® Tablets ℞
(Amiloride HCl)

DESCRIPTION

Amiloride HCl, an antikaliuretic-diuretic agent, is a pyrazine-carbonyl-guanidine that is unrelated chemically to other known antikaliuretic or diuretic agents. It is the salt of a moderately strong base (pKa 8.7). It is designated chemically as 3,5-diamino-6-chloro-*N* -(diaminomethylene) pyrazinecarboxamide monohydrochloride, dihydrate and has a molecular weight of 302.12. Its empirical formula is $C_6H_8ClN_7O{\cdot}HCl{\cdot}2H_2O$ and its structural formula is:

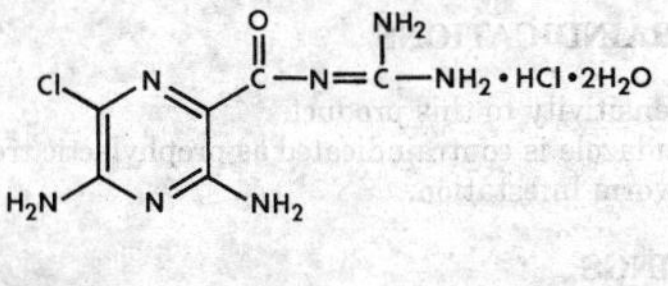

MIDAMOR* (Amiloride HCl) is available for oral use as tablets containing 5 mg of anhydrous amiloride HCl. Each tablet contains the following inactive ingredients: calcium phosphate, D&C Yellow 10, iron oxide, lactose, magnesium stearate and starch.

*Registered trademark of MERCK & CO., Inc.

CLINICAL PHARMACOLOGY

MIDAMOR is a potassium-conserving (antikaliuretic) drug that possesses weak (compared with thiazide diuretics) natriuretic, diuretic, and antihypertensive activity. These effects have been partially additive to the effects of thiazide diuretics in some clinical studies. When administered with a thiazide or loop diuretic, MIDAMOR has been shown to decrease the enhanced urinary excretion of magnesium which occurs when a thiazide or loop diuretic is used alone. MIDAMOR has potassium-conserving activity in patients receiving kaliuretic-diuretic agents.
MIDAMOR is not an aldosterone antagonist and its effects are seen even in the absence of aldosterone.
MIDAMOR exerts its potassium sparing effect through the inhibition of sodium reabsorption at the distal convoluted tubule, cortical collecting tubule and collecting duct; this decreases the net negative potential of the tubular lumen and reduces both potassium and hydrogen secretion and their subsequent excretion. This mechanism accounts in large part for the potassium sparing action of amiloride.
MIDAMOR usually begins to act within 2 hours after an oral dose. Its effect on electrolyte excretion reaches a peak between 6 and 10 hours and lasts about 24 hours. Peak plasma levels are obtained in 3 to 4 hours and the plasma half-life varies from 6 to 9 hours. Effects on electrolytes increase with single doses of amiloride HCl up to approximately 15 mg.
Amiloride HCl is not metabolized by the liver but is excreted unchanged by the kidneys. About 50 percent of a 20 mg dose of MIDAMOR is excreted in the urine and 40 percent in the stool within 72 hours. MIDAMOR has little effect on glomerular filtration rate or renal blood flow. Because amiloride HCl is not metabolized by the liver, drug accumulation is not anticipated in patients with hepatic dysfunction, but accumulation can occur if the hepatorenal syndrome develops.

INDICATIONS AND USAGE

MIDAMOR is indicated as adjunctive treatment with thiazide diuretics or other kaliuretic-diuretic agents in congestive heart failure or hypertension to:

a. help restore normal serum potassium levels in patients who develop hypokalemia on the kaliuretic diuretic
b. prevent development of hypokalemia in patients who would be exposed to particular risk if hypokalemia were to develop, e.g., digitalized patients or patients with significant cardiac arrhythmias.

The use of potassium-conserving agents is often unnecessary in patients receiving diuretics for uncomplicated essential hypertension when such patients have a normal diet. MIDAMOR has little additive diuretic or antihypertensive effect when added to a thiazide diuretic.
MIDAMOR should rarely be used alone. It has weak (compared with thiazides) diuretic and antihypertensive effects. Used as single agents, potassium sparing diuretics, including MIDAMOR, result in an increased risk of hyperkalemia (approximately 10% with amiloride). MIDAMOR should be used alone only when persistent hypokalemia has been documented and only with careful titration of the dose and close monitoring of serum electrolytes.

CONTRAINDICATIONS

Hyperkalemia
MIDAMOR should not be used in the presence of elevated serum potassium levels (greater than 5.5 mEq per liter).
Antikaliuretic Therapy or Potassium Supplementation
MIDAMOR should not be given to patients receiving other potassium conserving agents, such as spironolactone or triamterene. Potassium supplementation in the form of medication, potassium-containing salt substitutes or a potassium-rich diet should not be used with MIDAMOR except in severe and/or refractory cases of hypokalemia. Such concomitant therapy can be associated with rapid increases in serum potassium levels. If potassium supplementation is used, careful monitoring of the serum potassium level is necessary.
Impaired Renal Function
Anuria, acute or chronic renal insufficiency, and evidence of diabetic nephropathy are contraindications to the use of MIDAMOR. Patients with evidence of renal functional impairment (blood urea nitrogen [BUN] levels over 30 mg per 100 mL or serum creatinine levels over 1.5 mg per 100 mL) or diabetes mellitus should not receive the drug without careful, frequent and continuing monitoring of serum electrolytes, creatinine, and BUN levels. Potassium retention associated with the use of an antikaliuretic agent is accentuated in the presence of renal impairment and may result in the rapid development of hyperkalemia.
Hypersensitivity
MIDAMOR is contraindicated in patients who are hypersensitive to this product.

WARNINGS

Hyperkalemia

Like other potassium-conserving agents, amiloride may cause hyperkalemia (serum potassium levels greater than 5.5 mEq per liter) which, if uncorrected, is potentially fatal. Hyperkalemia occurs commonly (about 10%) when amiloride is used without a kaliuretic diuretic. This incidence is greater in patients with renal impairment, diabetes mellitus (with or without recognized renal insufficiency), and in the elderly. When MIDAMOR is used concomitantly with a thiazide diuretic in patients without these complications, the risk of hyperkalemia is reduced to about 1-2 percent. It is thus essential to monitor serum potassium levels carefully in any patient receiving amiloride, particularly when it is first introduced, at the time of diuretic dosage adjustments, and during any illness that could affect renal function.

The risk of hyperkalemia may be increased when potassium-conserving agents, including MIDAMOR, are administered concomitantly with an angiotensin-converting enzyme inhibitor, an angiotensin II receptor antagonist, cyclosporine or tacrolimus. (See PRECAUTIONS, *Drug Interactions.*)
Warning signs or symptoms of hyperkalemia include paresthesias, muscular weakness, fatigue, flaccid paralysis of the extremities, bradycardia, shock, and ECG abnormalities. Monitoring of the serum potassium level is essential because mild hyperkalemia is not usually associated with an abnormal ECG.
When abnormal, the ECG in hyperkalemia is characterized primarily by tall, peaked T waves or elevations from previous tracings. There may also be lowering of the R wave and increased depth of the S wave, widening and even disappearance of the P wave, progressive widening of the QRS complex, prolongation of the PR interval, and ST depression.
Treatment of hyperkalemia: If hyperkalemia occurs in patients taking MIDAMOR, the drug should be discontinued immediately. If the serum potassium level exceeds 6.5 mEq per liter, active measures should be taken to reduce it. Such measures include the intravenous administration of sodium bicarbonate solution or oral or parenteral glucose with a rapid-acting insulin preparation. If needed, a cation exchange resin such as sodium polystyrene sulfonate may be given orally or by enema. Patients with persistent hyperkalemia may require dialysis.

Diabetes Mellitus
In diabetic patients, hyperkalemia has been reported with the use of all potassium-conserving diuretics, including MIDAMOR, even in patients without evidence of diabetic nephropathy. Therefore, MIDAMOR should be avoided, if possible, in diabetic patients and, if it is used, serum electrolytes and renal function must be monitored frequently.
MIDAMOR should be discontinued at least three days before glucose tolerance testing.
Metabolic or Respiratory Acidosis
Antikaliuretic therapy should be instituted only with caution in severely ill patients in whom respiratory or metabolic acidosis may occur, such as patients with cardiopulmonary disease or poorly controlled diabetes. If MIDAMOR is given to these patients, frequent monitoring of acid-base balance is necessary. Shifts in acid-base balance alter the ratio of extracellular/intracellular potassium, and the development of acidosis may be associated with rapid increases in serum potassium levels.

PRECAUTIONS

General
Electrolyte Imbalance and BUN Increases
Hyponatremia and hypochloremia may occur when MIDAMOR is used with other diuretics and increases in BUN levels have been reported. These increases usually have accompanied vigorous fluid elimination, especially when diuretic therapy was used in seriously ill patients, such as those who had hepatic cirrhosis with ascites and metabolic alkalosis, or those with resistant edema. Therefore, when MIDAMOR is given with other diuretics to such patients, careful monitoring of serum electrolytes and BUN levels is important. In patients with pre-existing severe liver disease, hepatic encephalopathy, manifested by tremors, confusion, and coma, and increased jaundice, have been reported in association with diuretics, including amiloride HCl.
Drug Interactions
When amiloride HCl is administered concomitantly with an angiotensin-converting enzyme inhibitor, an angiotensin II receptor antagonist, cyclosporine or tacrolimus, the risk of hyperkalemia may be increased. Therefore, if concomitant use of these agents is indicated because of demonstrated hypokalemia, they should be used with caution and with frequent monitoring of serum potassium. (See WARNINGS.)
Lithium generally should not be given with diuretics because they reduce its renal clearance and add a high risk of lithium toxicity. Read circulars for lithium preparations before use of such concomitant therapy.
In some patients, the administration of a non-steroidal anti-inflammatory agent can reduce the diuretic, natriuretic, and antihypertensive effects of loop, potassium-sparing and thiazide diuretics. Therefore, when MIDAMOR and non-steroidal anti-inflammatory agents are used concomitantly, the patient should be observed closely to determine if the desired effect of the diuretic is obtained. Since indomethacin and potassium-sparing diuretics, including MIDAMOR, may each be associated with increased serum potassium levels, the potential effects on potassium kinetics and renal function should be considered when these agents are administered concurrently.
Carcinogenicity, Mutagenicity, Impairment of Fertility
There was no evidence of a tumorigenic effect when amiloride HCl was administered for 92 weeks to mice at doses up to 10 mg/kg/day (25 times the maximum daily human dose). Amiloride HCl has also been administered for 104 weeks to male and female rats at doses up to 6 and 8 mg/kg/day (15 and 20 times the maximum daily dose for humans, respectively) and showed no evidence of carcinogenicity.
Amiloride HCl was devoid of mutagenic activity in various strains of *Salmonella typhimurium* with or without a mammalian liver microsomal activation system (Ames test).
Pregnancy
Pregnancy Category B. Teratogenicity studies with amiloride HCl in rabbits and mice given 20 and 25 times the maximum human dose, respectively, revealed no evidence of harm to the fetus, although studies showed that the drug crossed the placenta in modest amounts. Reproduction studies in rats at 20 times the expected maximum daily dose for humans showed no evidence of impaired fertility. At approximately 5 or more times the expected maximum daily dose for humans, some toxicity was seen in adult rats and rabbits and a decrease in rat pup growth and survival occurred.
There are, however, no adequate and well-controlled studies in pregnant women. Because animal reproduction studies are not always predictive of human response, this drug should be used during pregnancy only if clearly needed.
Nursing Mothers
Studies in rats have shown that amiloride is excreted in milk in concentrations higher than those found in blood, but it is not known whether MIDAMOR is excreted in human milk. Because many drugs are excreted in human milk and because of the potential for serious adverse reactions in nursing infants from MIDAMOR, a decision should be made whether to discontinue nursing or to discontinue the drug, taking into account the importance of the drug to the mother.
Pediatric Use
Safety and effectiveness in pediatric patients have not been established.
Geriatric Use
Clinical studies of MIDAMOR did not include sufficient numbers of subjects aged 65 and over to determine whether they respond differently from younger subjects. Other reported clinical experience has not identified differences in responses between the elderly and younger patients. In general, dose selection for an elderly patient should be cautious, usually starting at the low end of the dosing range, reflecting the greater frequency of decreased hepatic, renal or cardiac function, and of concomitant disease or other drug therapy.
This drug is known to be substantially excreted by the kidney, and the risk of toxic reactions to this drug may be greater in patients with impaired renal function. Because elderly patients are more likely to have decreased renal function, care should be taken in dose selection, and it may be useful to monitor renal function. (See CONTRAINDICATIONS, *Impaired Renal Function.*)

ADVERSE REACTIONS

MIDAMOR is usually well tolerated and, except for hyperkalemia (serum potassium levels greater than 5.5 mEq per liter—see WARNINGS), significant adverse effects have been reported infrequently. Minor adverse reactions were reported relatively frequently (about 20%) but the relationship of many of the reports to amiloride HCl is uncertain and the overall frequency was similar in hydrochlorothiazide treated groups. Nausea/anorexia, abdominal pain, flatulence, and mild skin rash have been reported and probably are related to amiloride. Other adverse experiences that have been reported with amiloride are generally those known to be associated with diuresis, or with the underlying disease being treated.
The adverse reactions for MIDAMOR listed in the following table have been arranged into two groups: (1) incidence greater than one percent; and (2) incidence one percent or less. The incidence for group (1) was determined from clinical studies conducted in the United States (837 patients treated with MIDAMOR). The adverse effects listed in group (2) include reports from the same clinical studies and voluntary reports since marketing. The probability of a causal relationship exists between MIDAMOR and these adverse reactions, some of which have been reported only rarely.

Continued on next page

Information on the Merck & Co., Inc., products listed on these pages is from the prescribing information in use October 1, 2004. For information, please call 1-800-NSC-MERCK [1-800-672-6372].

Midamor—Cont.

Incidence > 1%	*Incidence ≤ 1%*
Body as a Whole	
Headache**	Back pain
Weakness	Chest pain
Fatigability	Neck/shoulder ache
	Pain, extremeties
Cardiovascular	
None	Angina pectoris
	Orthostatic hypotension
	Arrhythmia
	Palpitation
Digestive	
Nausea/anorexia**	Jaundice
Diarrhea**	GI bleeding
Vomiting**	Abdominal fullness
Abdominal pain	GI disturbance
Gas pain	Thirst
Appetite changes	Heartburn
Constipation	Flatulence
	Dyspepsia
Metabolic	
Elevated serum potassium levels (> 5.5 mEq per liter)***	None
Skin	
None	Skin rash
	Itching
	Dryness of mouth
	Pruritus
	Alopecia
Musculoskeletal	
Muscle cramps	Joint pain
	Leg ache
Nervous	
Dizziness	Paresthesia
Encephalopathy	Tremors
	Vertigo
Psychiatric	
None	Nervousness
	Mental confusion
	Insomnia
	Decreased libido
	Depression
	Somnolence
Respiratory	
Cough	Shortness of breath
Dyspnea	
Special Senses	
None	Visual disturbances
	Nasal congestion
	Tinnitus
	Increased intraocular pressure
Urogenital	
Impotence	Polyuria
	Dysuria
	Urinary frequency
	Bladder spasms
	Gynecomastia

** Reactions occurring in 3% to 8% of patients treated with MIDAMOR. (Those reactions occurring in less than 3% of the patients are unmarked.)
*** See WARNINGS.

Causal Relationship Unknown
Other reactions have been reported but occurred under circumstances where a causal relationship could not be established. However, in these rarely reported events, that possibility cannot be excluded. Therefore, these observations are listed to serve as alerting information to physicians.

- Activation of probable pre-existing peptic ulcer
- Aplastic anemia
- Neutropenia
- Abnormal liver function

OVERDOSAGE

No data are available in regard to overdosage in humans.
The oral LD_{50} of amiloride hydrochloride (calculated as the base) is 56 mg/kg in mice and 36 to 85 mg/kg in rats, depending on the strain.
It is not known whether the drug is dialyzable.
The most likely signs and symptoms to be expected with overdosage are dehydration and electrolyte imbalance. These can be treated by established procedures. Therapy with MIDAMOR should be discontinued and the patient observed closely. There is no specific antidote. Emesis should be induced or gastric lavage performed. Treatment is symptomatic and supportive. If hyperkalemia occurs, active measures should be taken to reduce the serum potassium levels.

DOSAGE AND ADMINISTRATION

MIDAMOR should be administered with food.
MIDAMOR, one 5 mg tablet daily, should be added to the usual antihypertensive or diuretic dosage of a kaliuretic diuretic. The dosage may be increased to 10 mg per day, if necessary. More than two 5 mg tablets of MIDAMOR daily usually are not needed, and there is little controlled experience with such doses. If persistent hypokalemia is documented with 10 mg, the dose can be increased to 15 mg, then 20 mg, with careful monitoring of electrolytes.
In treating patients with congestive heart failure after an initial diuresis has been achieved, potassium loss may also decrease and the need for MIDAMOR should be reevaluated. Dosage adjustment may be necessary. Maintenance therapy may be on an intermittent basis.
If it is necessary to use MIDAMOR alone (see INDICATIONS), the starting dosage should be one 5 mg tablet daily. This dosage may be increased to 10 mg per day, if necessary. More than two 5 mg tablets usually are not needed, and there is little controlled experience with such doses. If persistent hypokalemia is documented with 10 mg, the dose can be increased to 15 mg, then 20 mg, with careful monitoring of electrolytes.

HOW SUPPLIED

No. 3381—Tablets MIDAMOR, 5 mg, are yellow, diamond-shaped, compressed tablets, coded MSD 92 on one side and MIDAMOR on the other. They are supplied as follows:
NDC 0006-0092-68 bottles of 100.
Storage
Protect from moisture, freezing and excessive heat.
7905119 Issued November 2002

Shown in Product Identification Guide, page 323

MINTEZOL® Chewable Tablets ℞
(Thiabendazole)
MINTEZOL® Suspension ℞
(Thiabendazole)

DESCRIPTION

MINTEZOL* (Thiabendazole) is an anthelmintic provided as 500 mg chewable tablets, and as a suspension, containing 500 mg thiabendazole per 5 mL. The suspension also contains sorbic acid 0.1% added as a preservative. Inactive ingredients in the tablets are acacia, calcium phosphate, flavors, lactose, magnesium stearate, mannitol, methylcellulose, and sodium saccharin. Inactive ingredients in the suspension are an antifoam agent, flavors, polysorbate, purified water, sorbitol solution, and tragacanth.
Thiabendazole is a white to off-white odorless powder with a molecular weight of 201.26, which is practically insoluble in water but readily soluble in dilute acid and alkali. Its chemical name is 2-(4-thiazolyl)-1*H*-benzimidazole. The empirical formula is $C_{10}H_7N_3S$ and the structural formula is:

*Registered trademark of MERCK & CO., Inc.

CLINICAL PHARMACOLOGY

In man, thiabendazole is rapidly absorbed and peak plasma concentration is reached within 1 to 2 hours after the oral administration of a suspension. It is metabolized almost completely to the 5-hydroxy form which appears in the urine as glucuronide or sulfate conjugates. In 48 hours, about 5% of the administered dose is recovered from the feces and about 90% from the urine. Most is excreted in the first 24 hours.
Mechanism of Action
The precise mode of action of thiabendazole on the parasite is unknown, but it may inhibit the helminth-specific enzyme fumarate reductase.
Thiabendazole is vermicidal and/or vermifugal against *Ascaris lumbricoides* ("common roundworm"), *Strongyloides stercoralis* (threadworm), *Necator americanus,* and *Ancylostoma duodenale* (hookworm), *Trichuris trichiura* (whipworm), *Ancylostoma braziliense* (dog and cat hookworm), *Toxocara canis* and *Toxocara cati* (ascarids), and *Enterobius vermicularis* (pinworm).
Its effect on larvae of *Trichinella spiralis* that have migrated to muscle is questionable.
Thiabendazole also suppresses egg and/or larval production and may inhibit the subsequent development of those eggs or larvae which are passed in the feces.

INDICATIONS AND USAGE

MINTEZOL is indicated for the treatment of:
- Strongyloidiasis (threadworm)
- Cutaneous larva migrans (creeping eruption)
- Visceral larva migrans
- Trichinosis: Relief of symptoms and fever and a reduction of eosinophilia have followed the use of MINTEZOL during the invasion stage of the disease.

Thiabendazole is usually inappropriate as first line therapy for enterobiasis (pinworm). However, when enterobiasis occurs with any of the conditions listed above, additional therapy is not required for most patients.
MINTEZOL should be used only in the following infestations when more specific therapy is not available or cannot be used or when further therapy with a second agent is desirable: Uncinariasis (hookworm: *Necator americanus* and *Ancylostoma duodenale*); Trichuriasis (whipworm); Ascariasis (large roundworm).

CONTRAINDICATIONS

Hypersensitivity to this product.
Thiabendazole is contraindicated as prophylactic treatment for pinworm infestation.

WARNINGS

If hypersensitivity reactions occur, the drug should be discontinued immediately and not be resumed. Erythema multiforme has been associated with thiabendazole therapy; in severe cases (Stevens-Johnson syndrome), fatalities have occurred.
Because CNS side effects may occur quite frequently, activities requiring mental alertness should be avoided.
Jaundice, cholestasis, and parenchymal liver damage have been reported in patients treated with MINTEZOL. In rare cases, liver damage has been severe and has led to irreversible hepatic failure. (See **ADVERSE REACTIONS**.)
Abnormal sensation in eyes, xanthopsia, blurred vision, drying of mucous membranes, and SICCA syndrome have been reported in patients treated with MINTEZOL. These adverse effects of the eye were in some cases persistent for prolonged intervals which have exceeded one year. (See **ADVERSE REACTIONS**.)
Thiabendazole should not usually be used as first line therapy for the treatment of enterobiasis. It should be reserved for use in patients who have experienced allergic reactions, or resistance to other treatments.

PRECAUTIONS

General
MINTEZOL is not suitable for the treatment of mixed infections with ascaris because it may cause these worms to migrate.
Ideally, supportive therapy is indicated for anemic, dehydrated or malnourished patients prior to initiation of the anthelmintic therapy.
In the presence of hepatic or renal dysfunction, patients should be carefully monitored.
MINTEZOL should be used only in patients in whom susceptible worm infestation has been diagnosed and should not be used prophylactically.
Information for Patients
Because CNS side effects may occur quite frequently, activities requiring mental alertness should be avoided.
Laboratory Tests
Rarely, a transient rise in liver function tests has occurred in patients receiving MINTEZOL.
Drug Interactions
Thiabendazole may compete with other drugs, such as theophylline, for sites of metabolism in the liver, thus elevating the serum levels of such compounds to potentially toxic levels. Therefore, when concomitant use of thiabendazole and xanthine derivatives is anticipated, it may be necessary to monitor blood levels and/or reduce the dosage of such compounds. Such concomitant use should be administered under careful medical supervision.
Carcinogenesis, Mutagenesis, Impairment of Fertility
Thiabendazole has been used in numerous short- and long-term studies in animals at doses up to 15 times the usual human dose and was without carcinogenic effects. It did not adversely affect fertility in the mouse at $2^1/_2$ times the usual human dose or in the rat at a dose equivalent to the usual human dose. Thiabendazole had no mutagenic activity in *in vitro* microbial mutagen test, the micronucleus test and the host mediated assay *in vivo*.
Pregnancy
Pregnancy Category C: Reproduction and teratogenic studies done in the rabbit at a dose up to 15 times the usual human dose, in the rat at a dose equivalent to the human dose, and in the mouse at a dose up to $2^1/_2$ times the usual human dose, revealed no evidence of harm to the fetus. In an additional study in the mouse, no defects were observed when thiabendazole was given in an aqueous suspension, at a dose 10 times the usual human dose; however, cleft palate and axial skeletal defects were observed when thiabendazole was suspended in olive oil and given at the same dose. There are no adequate and well controlled studies in pregnant women. MINTEZOL should be used during pregnancy only if the potential benefit justifies the potential risk to the fetus.
Nursing Mothers
It is not known whether this drug is excreted in human milk. Because of the potential for serious adverse reactions in nursing infants from MINTEZOL, a decision should be made whether to discontinue nursing or to discontinue the drug, taking into account the importance of the drug to the mother.
Pediatric Use
The safety and effectiveness of thiabendazole for the treatment of Strongyloidiasis, Ascariasis, Uncinariasis, Trichuriasis and Trichinosis in pediatric patients weighing less than 30 lbs has been limited.
Geriatric Use
Clinical studies of MINTEZOL did not include sufficient numbers of subjects aged 65 and over to determine whether

Therapeutic Regimens

Indication	*Regimen*	*Comments*
**STRONGYLOIDIASIS	2 doses per day for 2 successive days.	A single dose of 20 mg/lb or 50 mg/kg may be employed as an alternative schedule, but a higher incidence of side effects should be expected.
CUTANEOUS LARVA MIGRANS (Creeping Eruption)	2 doses per day for 2 successive days.	If active lesions are still present 2 days after completion of therapy, a second course is recommended.
VISCERAL LARVA MIGRANS	2 doses per day for 7 successive days.	Safety and efficacy data on the seven-day treatment course are limited.
**TRICHINOSIS	2 doses per day for 2–4 successive days according to the response of the patient.	The optimal dosage for the treatment of trichinosis has not been established.
Other Indications		
**Intestinal roundworms (including Ascariasis, Uncinariasis and Trichuriasis)	2 doses per day for 2 successive days.	A single dose of 20 mg/lb or 50 mg/kg may be employed as an alternative schedule, but a higher incidence of side effects should be expected.

** Clinical experience with thiabendazole for treatment of each of these conditions in pediatric patients weighing less than 30 lbs has been limited.

they respond differently from younger subjects. Other reported clinical experience has not identified differences in responses between the elderly and younger patients. In general, dose selection for an elderly patient should be cautious, usually starting at the low end of the dosing range, reflecting the greater frequency of decreased hepatic, renal, or cardiac function, and of concomitant disease or other drug therapy.

This drug is metabolized almost completely by the liver, and the metabolites are known to be substantially excreted by the kidney, therefore the risk of toxicity may be greater in patients with impaired renal function. Because elderly patients are more likely to have decreased renal function, care should be taken in dose selection, and it may be useful to monitor renal function.

ADVERSE REACTIONS

Gastrointestinal: anorexia, nausea, vomiting, diarrhea, epigastric distress, abdominal pain, jaundice, cholestasis, parenchymal liver damage and hepatic failure. (See **WARNINGS**.)

Central Nervous System: dizziness, weariness, drowsiness, giddiness, headache, numbness, hyperirritability, convulsions, collapse, confusion, depression, floating sensation, weakness and lack of coordination.

Special Senses: tinnitus, abnormal sensation in eyes, xanthopsia, blurred vision, reduced vision, drying of mucous membranes (mouth, eyes, etc.), SICCA syndrome. (See **WARNINGS**.)

Cardiovascular: hypotension.

Metabolic: hyperglycemia.

Hematologic: transient leukopenia.

Genitourinary: hematuria, enuresis, malodor of the urine, crystalluria.

Hypersensitivity: pruritus, fever, facial flush, chills, conjunctival injection, angioedema, anaphylaxis, skin rashes (including perianal), erythema multiforme (including Stevens-Johnson syndrome), and lymphadenopathy.

Miscellaneous: appearance of live Ascaris in the mouth and nose.

OVERDOSAGE

Overdosage may be associated with transient disturbances of vision and psychic alterations.

There is no specific antidote in the event of overdosage. Therefore, symptomatic and supportive measures should be employed. Emesis should be induced or gastric lavage performed carefully.

The oral LD_{50} of MINTEZOL is 3.6 g/kg, 3.1 g/kg and 3.8 g/kg in the mouse, rat, and rabbit respectively.

DOSAGE AND ADMINISTRATION

The recommended maximum daily dose of MINTEZOL *is 3 grams.*

MINTEZOL should be given after meals if possible. Tablets MINTEZOL should be chewed before swallowing. Dietary restriction, complementary medications and cleansing enemas are not needed.

The usual dosage schedule for all conditions is two doses per day. The dosage is determined by the patient's weight.

A weight-dose chart follows:

Weight	Each Dose g	mL
30 lb	0.25 (½ tablet)	2.5 (½ teaspoon)
50 lb	0.5 (1 tablet)	5.0 (1 teaspoon)
75 lb	0.75 (1½ tablets)	7.5 (1½ teaspoons)
100 lb	1.0 (2 tablets)	10.0 (2 teaspoons)
125 lb	1.25 (2½ tablets)	12.5 (2½ teaspoons)
150 lb & over	1.5 (3 tablets)	15.0 (3 teaspoons)

The regimen for each indication follows:
[See table above]

HOW SUPPLIED

No. 3331 — MINTEZOL Suspension, 500 mg per 5 mL, is white to off-white and is supplied as follows:
NDC 0006-3331-60 in bottles of 120 mL
(6505-00-935-5835, 0.5 g/5 mL, 120 mL).

Storage

Store in a well-closed container at controlled room temperature [15–30°C (59–86°F)]. Protect from freezing.

No. 3332 — MINTEZOL Chewable Tablets, 500 mg, are white to off-white, orange-flavored, round, scored, compressed tablets, coded MSD 907 on one side and MINTEZOL on the other.

They are supplied as follows:
NDC 0006-0907-36 unit dose packages of 36
(6505-01-226-9909, 500 mg chewable, individually sealed 36's).

Storage

Store in a well-closed container at controlled room temperature [15–30°C (59–86°F)].

7930815 Issued June 2003

Shown in Product Identification Guide, page 323

MODURETIC® Tablets
(Amiloride HCl-Hydrochlorothiazide)

℞

DESCRIPTION

MODURETIC* (Amiloride HCl-Hydrochlorothiazide) combines the potassium-conserving action of amiloride HCl with the natriuretic action of hydrochlorothiazide.

Amiloride HCl is designated chemically as 3,5-diamino-6-chloro-*N*-(diaminomethylene) pyrazinecarboxamide monohydrochloride, dihydrate and has a molecular weight of 302.12. Its empirical formula is $C_6H_8ClN_7O \cdot HCl \cdot 2H_2O$ and its structural formula is:

Hydrochlorothiazide is designated chemically as 6-chloro-3,4-dihydro-*2H*-1,2,4-benzothiadiazine-7-sulfonamide 1,1-dioxide. Its empirical formula is $C_7H_8ClN_3O_4S_2$ and its structural formula is:

It is a white, or practically white, crystalline powder with a molecular weight of 297.74, which is slightly soluble in water, but freely soluble in sodium hydroxide solution.

MODURETIC is available for oral use as tablets containing 5 mg of anhydrous amiloride HCl and 50 mg of hydrochlorothiazide. Each tablet contains the following inactive ingredients: calcium phosphate, FD&C Yellow 6, guar gum, lactose, magnesium stearate and starch.

*Registered trademark of MERCK & CO., Inc.

CLINICAL PHARMACOLOGY

MODURETIC provides diuretic and antihypertensive activity (principally due to the hydrochlorothiazide component), while acting through the amiloride component to prevent the excessive potassium loss that may occur in patients receiving a thiazide diuretic. Due to its amiloride component, the urinary excretion of magnesium is less with MODURETIC than with a thiazide or loop diuretic used alone (see PRECAUTIONS). The onset of the diuretic action of MODURETIC is within 1 to 2 hours and this action appears to be sustained for approximately 24 hours.

Amiloride HCl

Amiloride HCl is a potassium-conserving (antikaliuretic) drug that possesses weak (compared with thiazide diuretics) natriuretic, diuretic, and antihypertensive activity. These effects have been partially additive to the effects of thiazide diuretics in some clinical studies. Amiloride HCl has potassium-conserving activity in patients receiving kaliuretic-diuretic agents.

Amiloride HCl is not an aldosterone antagonist and its effects are seen even in the absence of aldosterone.

Amiloride HCl exerts its postassium sparing effect through the inhibition of sodium reabsorption at the distal convoluted tubule, cortical collecting tubule and collecting duct; this decreases the net negative potential of the tubular lumen and reduces both potassium and hydrogen secretion and their subsequent excretion. This mechanism accounts in large part for the potassium sparing action of amiloride.

Amiloride HCl usually begins to act within 2 hours after an oral dose. Its effect on electrolyte excretion reaches a peak between 6 and 10 hours and lasts about 24 hours. Peak plasma levels are obtained in 3 to 4 hours and the plasma half-life varies from 6 to 9 hours. Effects on electrolytes increase with single doses of amiloride HCl up to approximately 15 mg.

Amiloride HCl is not metabolized by the liver but is excreted unchanged by the kidneys. About 50 percent of a 20 mg dose of amiloride HCl is excreted in the urine and 40 percent in the stool within 72 hours. Amiloride HCl has little effect on glomerular filtration rate or renal blood flow. Because amiloride HCl is not metabolized by the liver, drug accumulation is not anticipated in patients with hepatic dysfunction, but accumulation can occur if the hepatorenal syndrome develops.

Hydrochlorothiazide

The mechanism of the antihypertensive effect of thiazides is unknown. Thiazides do not usually affect normal blood pressure.

Hydrochlorothiazide is a diuretic and antihypertensive. It affects the distal renal tubular mechanism of electrolyte reabsorption. Hydrochlorothiazide increases excretion of sodium and chloride in approximately equivalent amounts. Natriuresis may be accompanied by some loss of potassium and bicarbonate.

After oral use diuresis begins within two hours, peaks in about four hours and lasts about 6 to 12 hours.

Hydrochlorothiazide is not metabolized but is eliminated rapidly by the kidney. When plasma levels have been followed for at least 24 hours, the plasma half-life has been observed to vary between 5.6 and 14.8 hours. At least 61 percent of the oral dose is eliminated unchanged within 24 hours. Hydrochlorothiazide crosses the placental but not the blood-brain barrier and is excreted in breast milk.

INDICATIONS AND USAGE

MODURETIC is indicated in those patients with hypertension or with congestive heart failure who develop hypokalemia when thiazides or other kaliuretic diuretics are used alone, or in whom maintenance of normal serum potassium levels is considered to be clinically important, e.g., digitalized patients, or patients with significant cardiac arrhythmias.

The use of potassium-conserving agents is often unnecessary in patients receiving diuretics for uncomplicated essential hypertension when such patients have a normal diet.

MODURETIC may be used alone or as an adjunct to other antihypertensive drugs, such as methyldopa or beta blockers. Since MODURETIC enhances the action of these agents, dosage adjustments may be necessary to avoid an excessive fall in blood pressure and other unwanted side effects.

This fixed combination drug is not indicated for the initial therapy of edema or hypertension except in individuals in whom the development of hypokalemia cannot be risked.

Continued on next page

Information on the Merck & Co., Inc., products listed on these pages is from the prescribing information in use October 1, 2004. For information, please call 1-800-NSC-MERCK [1-800-672-6372].

Moduretic—Cont.

CONTRAINDICATIONS

Hyperkalemia
MODURETIC should not be used in the presence of elevated serum potassium levels (greater than 5.5 mEq per liter).
Antikaliuretic Therapy or Potassium Supplementation
MODURETIC should not be given to patients receiving other potassium-conserving agents, such as spironolactone or triamterene. Potassium supplementation in the form of medication, potassium-containing salt substitutes or a potassium-rich diet should not be used with MODURETIC except in severe and/or refractory cases of hypokalemia. Such concomitant therapy can be associated with rapid increases in serum potassium levels. If potassium supplementation is used, careful monitoring of the serum potassium level is necessary.
Impaired Renal Function
Anuria, acute or chronic renal insufficiency, and evidence of diabetic nephropathy are contraindications to the use of MODURETIC. Patients with evidence of renal functional impairment (blood urea nitrogen [BUN] levels over 30 mg per 100 mL or serum creatinine levels over 1.5 mg per 100 mL) or diabetes mellitus should not receive the drug without careful, frequent and continuing monitoring of serum electrolytes, creatinine, and BUN levels. Potassium retention associated with the use of an antikaliuretic agent is accentuated in the presence of renal impairment and may result in the rapid development of hyperkalemia.
Hypersensitivity
MODURETIC is contraindicated in patients who are hypersensitive to this product, or to other sulfonamide-derived drugs.

WARNINGS

Hyperkalemia

Like other potassium-conserving diuretic combinations, MODURETIC may cause hyperkalemia (serum potassium levels greater than 5.5 mEq per liter). In patients without renal impairment or diabetes mellitus, the risk of hyperkalemia with MODURETIC is about 1-2 percent. This risk is higher in patients with renal impairment or diabetes mellitus (even without recognized diabetic nephropathy). Since hyperkalemia, if uncorrected, is potentially fatal, it is essential to monitor serum potassium levels carefully in any patient receiving MODURETIC, particularly when it is first introduced, at the time of dosage adjustments, and during any illness that could affect renal function.

The risk of hyperkalemia may be increased when potassium-conserving agents, including MODURETIC, are administered concomitantly with an angiotensin-converting enzyme inhibitor, an angiotensin II receptor antagonist, cyclosporine or tacrolimus. (See PRECAUTIONS, *Drug Interactions.*) Warning signs or symptoms of hyperkalemia include paresthesias, muscular weakness, fatigue, flaccid paralysis of the extremities, bradycardia, shock, and ECG abnormalities. Monitoring of the serum potassium level is essential because mild hyperkalemia is not usually associated with an abnormal ECG.
When abnormal, the ECG in hyperkalemia is characterized primarily by tall, peaked T waves or elevations from previous tracings. There may also be lowering of the R wave and increased depth of the S wave, widening and even disappearance of the P wave, progressive widening of the QRS complex, prolongation of the PR interval, and ST depression.
Treatment of hyperkalemia: If hyperkalemia occurs in patients taking MODURETIC, the drug should be discontinued immediately. If the serum potassium level exceeds 6.5 mEq per liter, active measures should be taken to reduce it. Such measures include the intravenous administration of sodium bicarbonate solution or oral or parenteral glucose with a rapid-acting insulin preparation. If needed, a cation exchange resin such as sodium polystyrene sulfonate may be given orally or by enema. Patients with persistent hyperkalemia may require dialysis.

Diabetes Mellitus
In diabetic patients, hyperkalemia has been reported with the use of all potassium-conserving diuretics, including amiloride HCl, even in patients without evidence of diabetic nephropathy. Therefore, MODURETIC should be avoided, if possible, in diabetic patients and, if it is used, serum electrolytes and renal function must be monitored frequently.
MODURETIC should be discontinued at least three days before glucose tolerance testing.
Metabolic or Respiratory Acidosis
Antikaliuretic therapy should be instituted only with caution in severely ill patients in whom respiratory or metabolic acidosis may occur, such as patients with cardiopulmonary disease or poorly controlled diabetes. If MODURETIC is given to these patients, frequent monitoring of acid-base balance is necessary. Shifts in acid-base balance alter the ratio of extracellular/intracellular potassium, and the development of acidosis may be associated with rapid increases in serum potassium levels.

PRECAUTIONS

General
Electrolyte Imbalance and BUN Increases
Determination of serum electrolytes to detect possible electrolyte imbalance should be performed at appropriate intervals.
Patients should be observed for clinical signs of fluid or electrolyte imbalance: i.e., hyponatremia, hypochloremic alkalosis, and hypokalemia. Serum and urine electrolyte determinations are particularly important when the patient is vomiting excessively or receiving parenteral fluids. Warning signs or symptoms of fluid and electrolyte imbalance, irrespective of cause, include dryness of mouth, thirst, weakness, lethargy, drowsiness, restlessness, confusion, seizures, muscle pains or cramps, muscular fatigue, hypotension, oliguria, tachycardia, and gastrointestinal disturbances such as nausea and vomiting.
Hyponatremia and hypochloremia may occur during the use of thiazides and other diuretics. Any chloride deficit during thiazide therapy is generally mild and may be lessened by the amiloride HCl component of MODURETIC. Hypochloremia usually does not require specific treatment except under extraordinary circumstances (as in liver disease or renal disease). Dilutional hyponatremia may occur in edematous patients in hot weather; appropriate therapy is water restriction, rather than administration of salt, except in rare instances when the hyponatremia is life-threatening. In actual salt depletion, appropriate replacement is the therapy of choice.
Hypokalemia may develop during thiazide therapy, especially with brisk diuresis, when severe cirrhosis is present, during concomitant use of corticosteroids or ACTH, or after prolonged therapy. However, this usually is prevented by the amiloride HCl component of MODURETIC.
Interference with adequate oral electrolyte intake will also contribute to hypokalemia. Hypokalemia may cause cardiac arrhythmia and may also sensitize or exaggerate the response of the heart to the toxic effects of digitalis (e.g., increased ventricular irritability).
Thiazides have been shown to increase the urinary excretion of magnesium; this may result in hypomagnesemia. Amiloride HCl, a component of MODURETIC, has been shown to decrease the enhanced urinary excretion of magnesium which occurs when a thiazide or loop diuretic is used alone.
Increases in BUN levels have been reported with amiloride HCl and with hydrochlorothiazide. These increases usually have accompanied vigorous fluid elimination, especially when diuretic therapy was used in seriously ill patients, such as those who had hepatic cirrhosis with ascites and metabolic alkalosis, or those with resistant edema. Therefore, when MODURETIC is given to such patients, careful monitoring of serum electrolyte and BUN levels is important. In patients with pre-existing severe liver disease, hepatic encephalopathy, manifested by tremors, confusion, and coma, and increased jaundice, have been reported in association with diuretic therapy including amiloride HCl and hydrochlorothiazide.
In patients with renal disease, diuretics may precipitate azotemia. Cumulative effects of the components of MODURETIC may develop in patients with impaired renal function. If renal impairment becomes evident, MODURETIC should be discontinued (see CONTRAINDICATIONS and WARNINGS).
Drug Interactions
In some patients, the administration of a non-steroidal anti-inflammatory agent can reduce the diuretic, natriuretic, and antihypertensive effects of loop, potassium-sparing and thiazide diuretics. Therefore, when MODURETIC and non-steroidal anti-inflammatory agents are used concomitantly, the patient should be observed closely to determine if the desired effect of the diuretic is obtained. Since indomethacin and potassium-sparing diuretics, including MODURETIC, may each be associated with increased serum potassium levels, the potential effects on potassium kinetics and renal function should be considered when these agents are administered concurrently.
Amiloride HCl
When amiloride HCl is administered concomitantly with an angiotensin-converting enzyme inhibitor, an angiotensin II receptor antagonist, cyclosporine or tacrolimus, the risk of hyperkalemia may be increased. Therefore, if concomitant use of these agents is indicated because of demonstrated hypokalemia, they should be used with caution and with frequent monitoring of serum potassium. (See WARNINGS.)
Hydrochlorothiazide
When given concurrently the following drugs may interact with thiazide diuretics.
Alcohol, barbiturates, or narcotics —potentiation of orthostatic hypotension may occur.
Antidiabetic drugs (oral agents and insulin)—dosage adjustment of the antidiabetic drug may be required.
Other antihypertensive drugs —additive effect or potentiation.
Cholestyramine and colestipol resins—Absorption of hydrochlorothiazide is impaired in the presence of anionic exchange resins. Single doses of either cholestyramine or colestipol resins bind the hydrochlorothiazide and reduce its absorption from the gastrointestinal tract by up to 85 and 43 percent, respectively.
Corticosteroids, ACTH—intensified electrolyte depletion, particularly hypokalemia.
Pressor amines (e.g., norepinephrine) —possible decreased response to pressor amines but not sufficient to preclude their use.
Skeletal muscle relaxants, nondepolarizing (e.g., tubocurarine) —possible increased responsiveness to the muscle relaxant.
Lithium —generally should not be given with diuretics. Diuretic agents reduce the renal clearance of lithium and add a high risk of lithium toxicity. Refer to the package insert for lithium preparations before use of such preparations with MODURETIC.
Metabolic and Endocrine Effects
In diabetic patients, insulin requirements may be increased, decreased, or unchanged due to the hydrochlorothiazide component. Diabetes mellitus that has been latent may become manifest during administration of thiazide diuretics.
Because calcium excretion is decreased by thiazides, MODURETIC should be discontinued before carrying out tests for parathyroid function. Pathologic changes in the parathyroid glands, with hypercalcemia and hypophosphatemia have been observed in a few patients on prolonged thiazide therapy; however, the common complications of hyperparathyroidism such as renal lithiasis, bone resorption, and peptic ulceration have not been seen.
Hyperuricemia may occur or acute gout may be precipitated in certain patients receiving thiazide therapy.
Other Precautions
In patients receiving thiazides, sensitivity reactions may occur with or without a history of allergy or bronchial asthma. The possibility of exacerbation or activation of systemic lupus erythematosus has been reported with the use of thiazides.
Increases in cholesterol and triglyceride levels may be associated with thiazide diuretic therapy.
Carcinogenicity, Mutagenicity, Impairment of Fertility
Long-term studies in animals have not been performed to evaluate the effects upon fertility, mutagenicity or carcinogenic potential of MODURETIC.
Amiloride HCl
There was no evidence of a tumorigenic effect when amiloride HCl was administered for 92 weeks to mice at doses up to 10 mg/kg/day (25 times the maximum daily human dose). Amiloride HCl has also been administered for 104 weeks to male and female rats at doses up to 6 and 8 mg/kg/day (15 and 20 times the maximum daily dose for humans, respectively) and showed no evidence of carcinogenicity.
Amiloride HCl was devoid of mutagenic activity in various strains of *Salmonella typhimurium* with or without a mammalian liver microsomal activation system (Ames test).
Hydrochlorothiazide
Two-year feeding studies in mice and rats conducted under the auspices of the National Toxicology Program (NTP) uncovered no evidence of a carcinogenic potential of hydrochlorothiazide in female mice (at doses of up to approximately 600 mg/kg/day) or in male and female rats (at doses of up to approximately 100 mg/kg/day). The NTP, however, found equivocal evidence for hepatocarcinogenicity in male mice.
Hydrochlorothiazide was not genotoxic *in vitro* in the Ames mutagenicity assay of *Salmonella typhimurium* strains TA 98, TA 100, TA 1535, TA 1537, and TA 1538 and in the Chinese Hamster Ovary (CHO) test for chromosomal aberrations, or *in vivo* in assays using mouse germinal cell chromosomes, Chinese hamster bone marrow chromosomes, and the *Drosophila* sex-linked recessive lethal trait gene. Positive test results were obtained only in the *in vitro* CHO Sister Chromatid Exchange (clastogenicity) and in the Mouse Lymphoma Cell (mutagenicity) assays, using concentrations of hydrochlorothiazide from 43 to 1300 μg/mL, and in the *Asperigillus nidulans* non-disjunction assay at an unspecified concentration.
Hydrochlorothiazide had no adverse effects on the fertility of mice and rats of either sex in studies wherein these species were exposed, via their diet, to doses of up to 100 and 4 mg/kg, respectively, prior to conception and throughout gestation.
Pregnancy
Pregnancy Category B. Teratogenicity studies have been performed with combinations of amiloride HCl and hydrochlorothiazide in rabbits and mice at doses up to 25 times the expected maximum daily dose for humans and have revealed no evidence of harm to the fetus. No evidence of impaired fertility in rats was apparent at dosage levels up to 25 times the expected maximum human daily dose. A perinatal and postnatal study in rats showed a reduction in maternal body weight gain during and after gestation at a daily dose of 25 times the expected maximum daily dose for humans. The body weights of alive pups at birth and at weaning were also reduced at this dose level. There are no adequate and well-controlled studies in pregnant women. Because animal reproduction studies are not always predictive of human responses, and because of the data listed below with the individual components, this drug should be used during pregnancy only if clearly needed.
Amiloride HCl
Teratogenicity studies with amiloride HCl in rabbits and mice given 20 and 25 times the maximum human dose, respectively, revealed no evidence of harm to the fetus, although studies showed that the drug crossed the placenta in modest amounts. Reproduction studies in rats at 20 times the expected maximum daily dose for humans showed no evidence of impaired fertility. At approximately 5 or more

times the expected maximum daily dose for humans, some toxicity was seen in adult rats and rabbits and a decrease in rat pup growth and survival occurred.

Hydrochlorothiazide

Teratogenic Effects: Studies in which hydrochlorothiazide was orally administered to pregnant mice and rats during their respective periods of major organogenesis at doses up to 3000 and 1000 mg hydrochlorothiazide/kg, respectively, provided no evidence of harm to the fetus. There are, however, no adequate and well-controlled studies in pregnant women.

Nonteratogenic Effects: Thiazides cross the placental barrier and appear in cord blood. There is a risk of fetal or neonatal jaundice, thrombocytopenia, and possibly other adverse reactions that have occurred in adults.

Nursing Mothers

Studies in rats have shown that amiloride is excreted in milk in concentrations higher than those found in blood, but it is not known whether amiloride HCl is excreted in human milk. However, thiazides appear in breast milk. Because of the potential for serious adverse reactions in nursing infants, a decision should be made whether to discontinue nursing or to discontinue the drug, taking into account the importance of the drug to the mother.

Pediatric Use

Safety and effectiveness in pediatric patients have not been established.

Geriatric Use

Clinical studies of MODURETIC did not include sufficient numbers of subjects aged 65 and over to determine whether they respond differently from younger subjects. Other reported clinical experience has not identified differences in responses between the elderly and younger patients. In general, dose selection for an elderly patient should be cautious, usually starting at the low end of the dosing range, reflecting the greater frequency of decreased hepatic, renal or cardiac function, and of concomitant disease or other drug therapy.

This drug is known to be substantially excreted by the kidney, and the risk of toxic reactions to this drug may be greater in patients with impaired renal function. Because elderly patients are more likely to have decreased renal function, care should be taken in dose selection, and it may be useful to monitor renal function. (See CONTRAINDICATIONS, *Impaired Renal Function.*)

ADVERSE REACTIONS

MODURETIC is usually well tolerated and significant clinical adverse effects have been reported infrequently. The risk of hyperkalemia (serum potassium levels greater than 5.5 mEq per liter) with MODURETIC is about 1–2 percent in patients without renal impairment or diabetes mellitus (see WARNINGS). Minor adverse reactions to amiloride HCl have been reported relatively frequently (about 20%) but the relationship of many of the reports to amiloride HCl is uncertain and the overall frequency was similar in hydrochlorothiazide treated groups. Nausea/anorexia, abdominal pain, flatulence, and mild skin rash have been reported and probably are related to amiloride. Other adverse experiences that have been reported with MODURETIC are generally those known to be associated with diuresis, thiazide therapy, or with the underlying disease being treated. Clinical trials have not demonstrated that combining amiloride and hydrochlorothiazide increases the risk of adverse reactions over those seen with the individual components.

The adverse reactions for MODURETIC listed in the following table have been arranged into two groups: (1) incidence greater than one percent; and (2) incidence one percent or less. The incidence for group (1) was determined from clinical studies conducted in the United States (607 patients treated with MODURETIC). The adverse effects listed in group (2) include reports from the same clinical studies and voluntary reports since marketing. The probability of a causal relationship exists between MODURETIC and these adverse reactions, some of which have been reported only rarely.

Incidence > 1%	*Incidence ≤ 1%*
Body as a Whole	
Headache**	Malaise
Weakness**	Chest pain
Fatigue/tiredness	Back pain
	Syncope
Cardiovascular	
Arrhythmia	Tachycardia
	Digitalis toxicity
	Orthostatic hypotension
	Angina pectoris
Digestive	
Nausea/anorexia**	Constipation
Diarrhea	GI bleeding
Gastrointestinal pain	GI disturbance
	Appetite changes
Abdominal pain	Abdominal fullness
	Hiccups
	Thirst
	Vomiting
	Anorexia
	Flatulence
Metabolic	
Elevated serum potassium levels (>5.5 mEq per liter)***	Gout
	Dehydration
	Symptomatic hyponatremia†
Musculoskeletal	
Leg ache	Muscle cramps/spasm
	Joint pain
Nervous	
Dizziness**	Paraesthesia/numbness
	Stupor
	Vertigo
Psychiatric	
None	Insomnia
	Nervousness
	Depression
	Sleepiness
	Mental confusion
Respiratory	
Dyspnea	None
Skin	
Rash**	Flushing
Pruritus	Diaphoresis
	Erythema multiforme including Stevens-Johnson syndrome
	Exfoliative dermatits including toxic epidermal necrolysis
	Alopecia
Special Senses	
None	Bad taste
	Visual disturbance
	Nasal congestion
Urogenital	
None	Impotence
	Nocturia
	Dysuria
	Incontinence
	Renal dysfunction including renal failure
	Gynecomastia

** Reactions occurring in 3% to 8% of patients treated with MODURETIC. (Those reactions occurring in less than 3% of the patients are unmarked.)
*** See WARNINGS.
† See PRECAUTIONS.

Other adverse reactions that have been reported with the individual components and within each category are listed in order of decreasing severity:

Amiloride —Body as a Whole: Painful extremities, neck/shoulder ache, fatigability; *Cardiovascular:* Palpitation; *Digestive:* Activation of probable pre-existing peptic ulcer, abnormal liver function, jaundice, dyspepsia, heartburn; *Hematologic:* Aplastic anemia, neutropenia; *Integumentary:* Alopecia, itching, dry mouth; *Nervous System/Psychiatric:* Encephalopathy, tremors, decreased libido; *Respiratory:* Shortness of breath, cough; *Special Senses:* Increased intraocular pressure, tinnitus; *Urogenital:* Bladder spasms, polyuria, urinary frequency.

Hydrochlorothiazide —Digestive: Pancreatitis, jaundice (intrahepatic cholestatic jaundice), sialadenitis, cramping, gastric irritation; *Hematologic:* Aplastic anemia, agranulocytosis, leukopenia, hemolytic anemia, thrombocytopenia; *Hypersensitivity:* Anaphylactic reactions, necrotizing angiitis (vasculitis, cutaneous vasculitis), respiratory distress including pneumonitis and pulmonary edema, photosensitivity, fever, urticaria, purpura; *Metabolic:* Electrolyte imbalance (see PRECAUTIONS), hyperglycemia, glycosuria, hyperuricemia; *Nervous System/Psychiatric:* Restlessness; *Special Senses:* Transient blurred vision, xanthopsia; *Urogenital:* Interstitial nephritis (see WARNINGS).

OVERDOSAGE

No data are available in regard to overdosage in humans. The oral LD_{50} of the combination drug is 189 and 422 mg/kg for female mice and female rats, respectively.

It is not known whether the drug is dialyzable.

No specific information is available on the treatment of overdosage with MODURETIC, and no specific antidote is available. Treatment is symptomatic and supportive. Therapy with MODURETIC should be discontinued and the patient observed closely. Suggested measures include induction of emesis and/or gastric lavage.

Amiloride HCl: No data are available in regard to overdosage in humans.

The oral LD_{50} of amiloride HCl (calculated as the base) is 56 mg/kg in mice and 36 to 85 mg/kg in rats, depending on the strain.

The most common signs and symptoms to be expected with overdosage are dehydration and electrolyte imbalance. If hyperkalemia occurs, active measures should be taken to reduce the serum potassium levels.

Hydrochlorothiazide: The oral LD_{50} of hydrochlorothiazide is greater than 10.0 g/kg in both mice and rats.

The most common signs and symptoms observed are those caused by electrolyte depletion (hypokalemia, hypochloremia, hyponatremia) and dehydration resulting from excessive diuresis. If digitalis has also been administered, hypokalemia may accentuate cardiac arrhythmias.

DOSAGE AND ADMINISTRATION

MODURETIC should be administered with food.

The usual starting dosage is 1 tablet a day. The dosage may be increased to 2 tablets a day, if necessary. More than 2 tablets of MODURETIC daily usually are not needed and there is no controlled experience with such doses. Hydrochlorothiazide can be given at doses of 12.5 to 50 mg per day when used alone. Patients usually do not require doses of hydrochlorothiazide in excess of 50 mg daily when combined with other antihypertensive agents.

The daily dose is usually given as a single dose but may be given in divided doses. Once an initial diuresis has been achieved, dosage adjustment may be necessary. Maintenance therapy may be on an intermittent basis.

HOW SUPPLIED

No. 3385—Tablets MODURETIC are peach-colored, diamond-shaped, scored, compressed tablets, coded MSD 917 on one side and M on the other. Each tablet contains 5 mg of anhydrous amiloride HCl and 50 mg of hydrochlorothiazide. They are supplied as follows:

NDC 0006-0917-68 in bottles of 100.

Storage

Keep container tightly closed. Protect from light, moisture, freezing, -20°C (-4°F) and store at room temperature, 15–30°C (59–86°F).

7887329 Issued November 2002

Shown in Product Identification Guide, page 323

MUMPSVAX® ℞

(Mumps Virus Vaccine Live)
Jeryl Lynn™ Strain

DESCRIPTION

MUMPSVAX* (Mumps Virus Vaccine Live) is a live virus vaccine for vaccination against mumps.

MUMPSVAX is a sterile lyophilized preparation of the Jeryl Lynn** (B level) strain of mumps virus. The virus was adapted to and propagated in chick embryo cell culture.

The growth medium for mumps is Medium 199 (a buffered salt solution containing vitamins and amino acids and supplemented with fetal bovine serum) containing SPGA (sucrose, phosphate, glutamate, and human albumin) as stabilizer and neomycin.

The cells, virus pools, fetal bovine serum, and human albumin are all screened for the absence of adventitious agents. Human albumin is processed using the Cohn cold ethanol fractionation procedure.

The reconstituted vaccine is for subcutaneous administration. Each 0.5 mL dose contains not less than 20,000 $TCID_{50}$ (tissue culture infectious doses) of mumps virus. Each dose of the vaccine is calculated to contain sorbitol (14.5 mg), sodium phosphate, sucrose (1.9 mg), sodium chloride, hydrolyzed gelatin (14.5 mg), human albumin (0.3 mg), fetal bovine serum (<1 ppm), other buffer and media ingredients and approximately 25 mcg of neomycin. The product contains no preservative.

Before reconstitution, the lyophilized vaccine is a light yellow compact crystalline plug. MUMPSVAX, when reconstituted as directed, is clear yellow.

*Registered trademark of MERCK & CO., Inc.
**Trademark of MERCK & CO., Inc.

CLINICAL PHARMACOLOGY

Mumps is a common childhood disease, caused by mumps virus (paramyxovirus), that may be associated with serious complications and/or death. For example, mumps is associated with aseptic meningitis, deafness and orchitis.

The impact of mumps vaccination on the natural history of each disease in the United States can be quantified by comparing the maximum number of mumps cases reported in a given year prior to vaccine use to the number of cases of each disease reported in 1995. For mumps, 152,209 cases reported in 1968 compared to 840 cases reported in 1995 resulted in a 99.45% decrease in reported cases.

Extensive clinical trials have demonstrated that MUMPSVAX is highly immunogenic and well tolerated. A single injection of the vaccine has been shown to induce mumps neutralizing antibodies in approximately 97% of susceptible children and approximately 93% of susceptible adults. The pattern of antibody response closely resembles that observed for natural mumps. Although the antibody level is significantly lower than that following natural infection; it is protective and long lasting. However, a small percentage (1-5%) of vaccinees may fail to seroconvert after the primary dose (see also INDICATIONS AND USAGE, *Recommended Vaccination Schedule*).

Continued on next page

Information on the Merck & Co., Inc., products listed on these pages is from the prescribing information in use October 1, 2004. For information, please call 1-800-NSC-MERCK [1-800-672-6372].

Mumpsvax—Cont.

Efficacy of mumps vaccine was established in a series of double-blind controlled field trials which demonstrated a high degree of protective efficacy. These studies also established that seroconversion in response to mumps vaccination paralleled protection from these diseases.
Following vaccination, antibodies associated with protection can be measured by neutralization assays, hemagglutination-inhibition (HI), or ELISA (enzyme linked immunosorbent assay) tests. Neutralizing and ELISA antibodies to mumps virus are still detectable in most individuals 11-13 years after primary vaccination.

INDICATIONS AND USAGE

Recommended Vaccination Schedule
MUMPSVAX is indicated for vaccination against mumps in persons 12 months of age or older.
It is not recommended for infants younger than 12 months because they may retain maternal mumps neutralizing antibodies which may interfere with the immune response.
Individuals first vaccinated with MUMPSVAX at 12 months of age or older should be revaccinated with M-M-R* II (Measles, Mumps, and Rubella Virus Vaccine Live) prior to elementary school entry. Revaccination is intended to seroconvert those who do not respond to the first dose. The Advisory Committee on Immunization Practices (ACIP) recommends administration of the first dose of M-M-R II at 12-15 months of age and administration of the second dose of M-M-R II at 4-6 years of age. In addition, some public health jurisdictions mandate the age for revaccination. Consult the complete text of applicable guidelines regarding routine revaccination including that of high-risk adult populations.
Unnecessary doses of a vaccine are best avoided by ensuring that written documentation of vaccination is preserved and a copy given to each vaccinee's parent or guardian.
Other Vaccination Considerations
Other Populations
Individuals planning travel outside the United States, if not immune, can acquire measles, mumps or rubella and import these diseases into the United States. Therefore, prior to international travel, individuals known to be susceptible to one or more of these diseases can receive either a monovalent vaccine (measles, mumps or rubella), or a combination vaccine as appropriate. However, M-M-R II is preferred for persons likely to be susceptible to mumps and rebella; and if monovalent measles vaccine is not readily available, travelers should receive M-M-R II regardless of their immune status to mumps or rubella.
Vaccination is recommended for susceptible individuals in high-risk groups such as college students, health-care workers, and military personnel.
Post Exposure Vaccination
There is no conclusive evidence that vaccination of individuals recently exposed to natural mumps will provide protection.
Use With Other Vaccines
See DOSAGE AND ADMINISTRATION, *Use With Other Vaccines*

CONTRAINDICATIONS

Hypersensitivity to any component of the vaccine, including gelatin.
Do not give MUMPSVAX to pregnant females; the possible effects of the vaccine on fetal development are unknown at this time. If vaccination of postpubertal females is undertaken, pregnancy should be avoided for 3 months following vaccination (see PRECAUTIONS, *Pregnancy*).
Anaphylactic or anaphylactoid reactions to neomycin (each dose of reconstituted vaccine contains approximately 25 mcg of neomycin).
Any febrile respiratory illness or other active febrile infection. However, the ACIP has recommended that all vaccines can be administered to persons with minor illnesses such as diarrhea, mild upper respiratory infection with or without low-grade fever, or other low-grade febrile illness.
Patients receiving immunosuppressive therapy. This contraindication does not apply to patients who are receiving corticosteroids as replacement therapy, e.g., for Addison's disease.
Individuals with blood dyscrasias, leukemia, lymphomas of any type, or other malignant neoplasms affecting the bone marrow or lymphatic systems.
Primary and acquired immunodeficiency states, including patients who are immunosuppressed in association with AIDS or other clinical manifestations of infection with human immunodeficiency viruses; cellular immune deficiencies; and hypogammaglobulinemic and dysgammaglobulinemic states.
Individuals with a family history of congenital or hereditary immunodeficiency, until the immune competence of the potential vaccine recipient is demonstrated.

WARNINGS

The physician should be alert to the temperature elevation which may occur following vaccination (see ADVERSE REACTIONS).
This product contains albumin, a derivative of human blood. Based on effective donor screening and product manufacturing processes, it carries an extremely remote risk for transmission of viral diseases. Although there is a theoretical risk for transmission of Creutzfeldt-Jacob disease (CJD), no cases of transmission of CJD or viral disease have ever been identified that were associated with the use of albumin.
Hypersensitivity to Eggs
Live mumps vaccine is produced in chick embryo cell culture. Persons with a history of anaphylactic, anaphylactoid, or other immediate reactions (e.g., hives, swelling of the mouth and throat, difficulty breathing, hypotension, or shock) subsequent to egg ingestion may be at an enhanced risk of immediate-type hypersensitivity reactions after receiving vaccines containing traces of chick embryo antigen. The potential risk to benefit ratio should be carefully evaluated before considering vaccination in such cases. Such individuals may be vaccinated with extreme caution, having adequate treatment on hand should a reaction occur (see PRECAUTIONS).
However, the AAP has stated, "Most children with a history of anaphylactic reactions to eggs have no untoward reactions to measles or MMR vaccine. Persons are not at increased risk if they have egg allergies that are not anaphylactic, and they should be vaccinated in the usual manner. In addition, skin testing of egg-allergic children with vaccine has not been predictive of which children will have an immediate hypersensitivity reaction. Persons with allergies to chickens or chicken feathers are not at increased risk of reaction to the vaccine."
Hypersensitivity to Neomycin
The AAP states, "Persons who have experienced anaphylactic reactions to topically or systemically administered neomycin should not receive measles vaccine. Most often, however, neomycin allergy manifests as a contact dermatitis, which is a delayed-type (cell-mediated) immune response rather than anaphylaxis. In such persons, an adverse reaction to neomycin in the vaccine would be an erythematous, pruritic nodule or papule, 48 to 96 hours after vaccination. A history of contact dermatitis to neomycin is not a contraindication to receiving measles vaccine."
Thrombocytopenia
Individuals with current thrombocytopenia may develop more severe thrombocytopenia following vaccination. In addition, individuals who experienced thrombocytopenia with the first dose of M-M-R II (or its component vaccines) may develop thrombocytopenia with repeat doses. Serologic status may be evaluated to determine whether or not additional doses of vaccine are needed. The potential risk to benefit ratio should be carefully evaluated before considering vaccination in such cases.

PRECAUTIONS

General
Adequate treatment provisions including epinephrine injection (1:1000), should be available for immediate use should an anaphylactic or anaphylactoid reaction occur.
Special care should be taken to ensure that the injection does not enter a blood vessel.
Children and young adults who are known to be infected with human immunodeficiency viruses and are not immunosuppressed may be vaccinated. However, vaccinees who are infected with HIV should be monitored closely for vaccine-preventable diseases because immunization may be less effective than for uninfected persons (see CONTRAINDICATIONS).
Vaccination should be deferred for 3 months or longer following blood or plasma transfusions, or administration of immune globulin (human).
There are no reports of transmission of live mumps virus from vaccinees to susceptible contacts.
It has been reported that mumps virus vaccine live may result in a temporary depression of tuberculin skin sensitivity. Therefore, if a tuberculin test is to be done, it should be administered either before or simultaneously with MUMPSVAX.
Individuals with active untreated tuberculosis should not be vaccinated.
As for any vaccine, vaccination with MUMPSVAX may not result in protection in 100% of vaccinees.
The health-care provider should determine the current health status and previous vaccination history of the vaccinee.
The health-care provider should question the patient, parent, or guardian about reactions to a previous dose of MUMPSVAX or other mumps-containing vaccines.
Drug Interactions
See DOSAGE AND ADMINISTRATION, *Use With Other Vaccines.*
Information for Patients
The health-care provider should provide the vaccine information required to be given with each vaccination to the patient, parent or guardian.
The health-care provider should inform the patient, parent or guardian of the benefits and risks associated with vaccination. For risks associated with vaccination see WARNINGS, PRECAUTIONS, ADVERSE REACTIONS.
Patients, parents or guardians should be instructed to report any serious adverse reactions to their health-care provider who in turn should report such events to the U.S. Department of Health and Human Services through the Vaccine Adverse Event Reporting System (VAERS), 1-800-822-7967.
Pregnancy should be avoided for 3 months following vaccination, and patients should be informed of the reasons for this precaution (see CONTRAINDICATIONS and PRECAUTIONS, *Pregnancy*).
Immunosuppressive Therapy
The immune status of patients about to undergo immunosuppressive therapy should be evaluated so that the physician can consider whether vaccination prior to the initiation of treatment is indicated (see CONTRAINDICATIONS and PRECAUTIONS).
The ACIP has indicated that patients with leukemia in remission who have not received chemotherapy for at least 3 months may receive live virus vaccines. Short-term (<2 weeks), low- to moderate-dose systemic corticosteroid therapy, topical steroid therapy (e.g., nasal, skin), long-term alternate-day treatment with low to moderate doses of short-acting systemic steroid, and intra-articular, bursal, or tendon injection of corticosteroids are not immunosuppressive in their usual doses and do not contraindicate the administration of mumps vaccine.
Immune Globulin
Administration of immune globulins concurrently with MUMPSVAX may interfere with the expected immune response.
See also PRECAUTIONS, *General*.
Carcinogenesis, Mutagenesis, Impairment of Fertility
MUMPSVAX has not been evaluated for carcinogenic or mutagenic potential, or potential to impair fertility.
Pregnancy
Pregnancy Category C
Animal reproduction studies have not been conducted with MUMPSVAX. It is also not known whether MUMPSVAX can cause fetal harm when administered to a pregnant woman or can affect reproduction capacity. Therefore, mumps virus vaccine should not be given to persons known to be pregnant; furthermore, pregnancy should be avoided for 3 months following vaccination (see CONTRAINDICATIONS).
In counseling women who are inadvertently vaccinated when pregnant or who become pregnant within 3 months of vaccination, the physician should be aware that mumps infection during the first trimester of pregnancy may increase the rate of spontaneous abortion. Although mumps vaccine virus has been shown to infect the placenta and fetus, there is no evidence that it causes congenital malformations in humans.
Nursing Mothers
It is not known whether mumps vaccine virus is secreted in human milk. Therefore, because many drugs are excreted in human milk, caution should be exercised when MUMPSVAX is administered to a nursing woman.
Pediatric Use
Safety and effectiveness in infants below the age of 12 months have not been established (see INDICATIONS AND USAGE, *Recommended Vaccination Schedule*).
Geriatric Use
Clinical studies of MUMPSVAX did not include sufficient numbers of seronegative subjects aged 65 and over to determine whether they respond differently from younger subjects. Other reported clinical experience has not identified differences in responses between the elderly and younger subjects.

ADVERSE REACTIONS

The following adverse reactions are listed in decreasing order of severity, without regard to causality, within each body system category and have been reported during clinical trials, with use of the marketed vaccine, or with use of polyvalent vaccine containing mumps:
Body as a Whole
Fever; syncope; irritability.
Cardiovascular System
Vasculitis.
Digestive System
Pancreatitis; diarrhea; parotitis.
Endocrine System
Diabetes mellitus.
Hemic and Lymphatic System
Thrombocytopenia; purpura; lymphadenopathy; leukocytosis.
Immune System
Anaphylaxis and anaphylactoid reactions have been reported as well as related phenomena such as angioneurotic edema (including peripheral or facial edema) and bronchial spasm in individuals with or without an allergic history.
Nervous System
Encephalitis; Guillain-Barré Syndrome (GBS); febrile seizures; ocular palsies.
Cases of aseptic meningitis have been reported to VAERS following measles, mumps, and rubella vaccination. Although a causal relationship between the Urabe strain of mumps vaccine and aseptic meningitis has been shown, there are no data to link Jeryl Lynn mumps vaccine to aseptic meningitis.
Respiratory System
Cough; rhinitis.
Skin
Stevens-Johnson Syndrome; erythema multiforme; urticaria.
Local reactions including burning/stinging at injection site; wheal and flare.
Special Senses—Ear
Nerve deafness; otitis media.

Special Senses—Eye
Optic neuritis; papillitis; retrobulbar neuritis; conjunctivitis.
Urogenital System
Orchitis.
Other
Death from various, and in some cases unknown, causes has been reported rarely following vaccination with measles, mumps, and rubella vaccines; however, a causal relationship has not been established. No deaths or permanent sequelae were reported in a published post-marketing surveillance study in Finland involving 1.5 million children and adults who were vaccinated with M-M-R II during 1982-1993.
Under the National Childhood Vaccine Injury Act of 1986, health-care providers and manufacturers are required to record and report certain suspected adverse events occurring within specific time periods after vaccination. However, the U.S. Department of Health and Human Services (DHHS) has established a Vaccine Adverse Event Reporting System (VAERS) which will accept all reports of suspected events. A VAERS report form as well as information regarding reporting requirements can be obtained by calling VAERS 1-800-822-7967.

DOSAGE AND ADMINISTRATION

FOR SUBCUTANEOUS ADMINISTRATION
Do not inject intravenously
The dose for any age is 0.5 mL administered subcutaneously, preferably into the outer aspect of the upper arm.
The recommended age for primary vaccination is 12 to 15 months.
Revaccination with M-M-R II is recommended prior to elementary school entry. See also INDICATIONS AND USAGE, *Recommended Vaccination Schedule.*
Immune Globulin (IG) is not to be given concurrently with MUMPSVAX.
CAUTION: A sterile syringe free of preservatives, antiseptics, and detergents should be used for each injection and/or reconstitution of the vaccine because these substances may inactivate the live virus vaccine. A 25 gauge, 5/8″ needle is recommended.
To reconstitute, use only the diluent supplied, since it is free of preservatives or other antiviral substances which might inactivate the vaccine.
Single Dose Vial—First withdraw the entire volume of diluent into the syringe to be used for reconstitution. Inject all the diluent in the syringe into the vial of lyophilized vaccine, and agitate to mix thoroughly. If the lyophilized vaccine cannot be dissolved, discard. Withdraw the entire contents into a syringe and inject the total volume of restored vaccine subcutaneously.
It is important to use a separate sterile syringe and needle for each individual patient to prevent transmission of hepatitis B and other infectious agents from one person to another.
Parenteral drug products should be inspected visually for particulate matter and discoloration prior to administration whenever solution and container permit. MUMPSVAX, when reconstituted, is clear yellow.
Use With Other Vaccines
MUMPSVAX should not be given less than one month before or after administration of other live viral vaccines.
M-M-R II has been administered concurrently with VARIVAX* [Varicella Virus Vaccine Live (Oka/Merck)], and PedvaxHIB* [Haemophilus b Conjugate Vaccine (Meningococcal Protein Conjugate)] using separate sites and syringes. No impairment of immune response to individual tested vaccine antigens was demonstrated. The type, frequency, and severity of adverse experiences observed with M-M-R II were similar to those seen when each vaccine was given alone.
Routine administration of DTP (diphtheria, tetanus, pertussis) and/or OPV (oral poliovirus vaccine) concurrently with measles, mumps and rubella vaccines is not recommended because there are limited data relating to the simultaneous administration of these antigens.
However, other schedules have been used. The ACIP has stated "Although data are limited concerning the simultaneous administration of the entire recommended vaccine series (i.e., DTP, OPV, MMR, and Hib vaccines, with or without hepatitis B vaccine), data from numerous studies have indicated no interference between routinely recommended childhood vaccines (either live, attenuated, or killed). These findings support the simultaneous use of all vaccines as recommended."

HOW SUPPLIED

No. 4753—MUMPSVAX is supplied as a single-dose vial of lyophilized vaccine, **NDC** 0006-4753-00, and a vial of diluent.
No. 4584X/4309—MUMPSVAX is supplied as follows: (1) a box of 10 single-dose vials of lyophilized vaccine (package A), **NDC** 0006-4584-00; and (2) a box of 10 vials of diluent (package B). To conserve refrigerator space, the diluent may be stored separately at room temperature.
Storage
During shipment, to ensure that there is not loss of potency, the vaccine must be maintained at a temperature of 10°C (50°F) or colder. Freezing during shipment will not affect potency.
Protect the vaccine from light at all times, since such exposure may inactivate the virus.
Before reconstitution, store the vial of lyophilized vaccine at 2-8°C (36-46°F) or colder. The diluent may be stored in the refrigerator with the lyophilized vaccine or separately at room temperature.
It is recommended that the vaccine be used as soon as possible after reconstitution. Store reconstituted vaccine in the vaccine vial in a dark place at 2-8°C (36-46°F) and discard if not used within 8 hours.

9243504 Issued September 2002

MUSTARGEN®, Trituration of (Mechlorethamine HCl for Injection) ℞

WARNINGS
MUSTARGEN* (Mechlorethamine HCl) should be administered only under the supervision of a physician who is experienced in the use of cancer chemotherapeutic agents.
This drug is **HIGHLY TOXIC** and both powder and solution must be handled and administered with care. Inhalation of dust or vapors and contact with skin or mucous membranes, especially those of the eyes, must be avoided. Avoid exposure during pregnancy. Due to the toxic properties of mechlorethamine (e.g., corrosivity, carcinogenicity, mutagenicity, teratogenicity), special handling procedures should be reviewed prior to handling and followed diligently.
Extravasation of the drug into subcutaneous tissues results in a painful inflammation. The area usually becomes indurated and sloughing may occur. If leakage of drug is obvious, prompt infiltration of the area with sterile isotonic sodium thiosulfate (1/6 molar) and application of an ice compress for 6 to 12 hours may minimize the local reaction. For 1/6 molar solution of sodium thiosulfate, use 4.14 g of sodium thiosulfate per 100 mL of Sterile Water for Injection or 2.64 g of anhydrous sodium thiosulfate per 100 mL or dilute 4 mL of Sodium Thiosulfate Injection (10%) with 6 mL of Sterile Water for Injection.

DESCRIPTION

MUSTARGEN, an antineoplastic nitrogen mustard also known as HN2 hydrochloride, is a nitrogen analog of sulfur mustard. It is a light yellow brown, crystalline, hygroscopic powder that is very soluble in water and also soluble in alcohol.
Mechlorethamine hydrochloride is designated chemically as 2-chloro-*N* -(2-chloroethyl)-*N* -methylethanamine hydrochloride. The molecular weight is 192.52 and the melting point is 108–111°C. The empirical formula is $C_5H_{11}Cl_2N \bullet HCl$, and the structural formula is: $CH_3N(CH_2CH_2Cl)_2 \bullet HCl$.
Trituration of MUSTARGEN is a sterile, light yellow brown crystalline powder for injection by the intravenous or intracavitary routes after dissolution. Each vial of MUSTARGEN contains 10 mg of mechlorethamine hydrochloride triturated with sodium chloride q.s. 100 mg. When dissolved with 10 mL Sterile Water for Injection or 0.9% Sodium Chloride Injection, the resulting solution has a pH of 3–5 at a concentration of 1 mg mechlorethamine HCl per mL.

*Registered trademark of MERCK & CO., INC.

CLINICAL PHARMACOLOGY

Mechlorethamine, a biologic alkylating agent, has a cytotoxic action which inhibits rapidly proliferating cells.
Pharmacokinetics and Metabolism
In water or body fluids, mechlorethamine undergoes rapid chemical transformation and combines with water or reactive compounds of cells, so that the drug is no longer present in active form a few minutes after administration.

INDICATIONS AND USAGE

Before using MUSTARGEN *see CONTRAINDICATIONS, WARNINGS, PRECAUTIONS, ADVERSE REACTIONS, DOSAGE AND ADMINISTRATION, and HOW SUPPLIED, Special Handling.*
MUSTARGEN, administered intravenously, is indicated for the palliative treatment of Hodgkin's disease (Stages III and IV), lymphosarcoma, chronic myelocytic or chronic lymphocytic leukemia, polycythemia vera, mycosis fungoides, and bronchogenic carcinoma.
MUSTARGEN, administered intrapleurally, intraperitoneally, or intrapericardially, is indicated for the palliative treatment of metastatic carcinoma resulting in effusion.

CONTRAINDICATIONS

The use of MUSTARGEN is contraindicated in the presence of known infectious diseases and in patients who have had previous anaphylactic reactions to MUSTARGEN.

WARNINGS

Before using MUSTARGEN, *an accurate histologic diagnosis of the disease, a knowledge of its natural course, and an adequate clinical history are important. The hematologic status of the patient must first be determined. It is essential to understand the hazards and therapeutic effects to be expected. Careful clinical judgment must be exercised in selecting patients. If the indication for its use is not clear, the drug should not be used.*
As nitrogen mustard therapy may contribute to extensive and rapid development of amyloidosis, it should be used only if foci of acute and chronic suppurative inflammation are absent.
Usage in Pregnancy
Mechlorethamine hydrochloride can cause fetal harm when administered to a pregnant woman. MUSTARGEN has been shown to produce fetal malformations in the rat and ferret when given as single subcutaneous injections of 1 mg/kg (2–3 times the maximum recommended human dose). There are no adequate and well controlled studies in pregnant women. If this drug is used during pregnancy, or if the patient becomes pregnant while taking this drug, the patient should be apprised of the potential hazard to the fetus. Women of childbearing potential should be advised to avoid becoming pregnant.

PRECAUTIONS

General
This drug is **HIGHLY TOXIC** and both powder and solution must be handled and administered with care. (See boxed warning and DOSAGE AND ADMINISTRATION, *Special Handling.*) Since MUSTARGEN is a powerful vesicant, it is intended primarily for intravenous use, and in most cases is given by this route. Inhalation of dust or vapors and contact with skin or mucous membranes, especially those of the eyes, must be avoided. Appropriate protective equipment should be worn when handling MUSTARGEN. Should accidental eye contact occur, copious irrigation for at least 15 minutes with water, normal saline or a balanced salt ophthalmic irrigating solution should be instituted immediately, followed by prompt ophthalmologic consultation. Should accidental skin contact occur, the affected part must be irrigated immediately with copious amounts of water, for at least 15 minutes while removing contaminated clothing and shoes, followed by 2% sodium thiosulfate solution. Medical attention should be sought immediately. Contaminated clothing should be destroyed. (See DOSAGE AND ADMINISTRATION, *Special Handling.*)
Because of the toxicity of MUSTARGEN, and the unpleasant side effects following its use, the potential risk and discomfort from the use of this drug in patients with inoperable neoplasms or in the terminal stage of the disease must be balanced against the limited gain obtainable. These gains will vary with the nature and the status of the disease under treatment. The routine use of MUSTARGEN in all cases of widely disseminated neoplasms is to be discouraged.
The use of MUSTARGEN in patients with leukopenia, thrombocytopenia, and anemia, due to invasion of the bone marrow by tumor carries a greater risk. In such patients a good response to treatment with disappearance of the tumor from the bone marrow may be associated with improvement of bone marrow function. However, in the absence of a good response or in patients who have been previously treated with chemotherapeutic agents, hematopoiesis may be further compromised, and leukopenia, thrombocytopenia and anemia may become more severe and lead to the demise of the patient.
Tumors of bone and nervous tissue have responded poorly to therapy. Results are unpredictable in disseminated and malignant tumors of different types.
Precautions must be observed with the use of MUSTARGEN and x-ray therapy or other chemotherapy in alternating courses. Hematopoietic function is characteristically depressed by either form of therapy, and neither MUSTARGEN following x-ray therapy nor x-ray therapy subsequent to the drug should be given until bone marrow function has recovered. In particular, irradiation of such areas as sternum, ribs, and vertebrae shortly after a course of nitrogen mustard may lead to hematologic complications.
MUSTARGEN has been reported to have immunosuppressive activity. Therefore, it should be borne in mind that use of the drug may predispose the patient to bacterial, viral or fungal infection.
Hyperuricemia may develop during therapy with MUSTARGEN. The problem of urate precipitation should be anticipated, particularly in the treatment of the lymphomas, and adequate methods for control of hyperuricemia should be instituted and careful attention directed toward adequate fluid intake before treatment.
Since drug toxicity, especially sensitivity to bone marrow failure, seems to be more common in chronic lymphatic leukemia than in other conditions, the drug should be given in this condition with great caution, if at all.
Extreme caution must be used in exceeding the average recommended dose. (See OVERDOSAGE.)

Continued on next page

Information on the Merck & Co., Inc., products listed on these pages is from the prescribing information in use October 1, 2004. For information, please call 1-800-NSC-MERCK [1-800-672-6372].

Mustargen—Cont.

Laboratory Tests
Many abnormalities of renal, hepatic, and bone marrow function have been reported in patients with neoplastic disease and receiving mechlorethamine. It is advisable to check renal, hepatic, and bone marrow functions frequently.
Carcinogenesis, Mutagenesis, Impairment of Fertility
Therapy with alkylating agents such as MUSTARGEN may be associated with an increased incidence of a second malignant tumor, especially when such therapy is combined with other antineoplastic agents or radiation therapy.
The International Agency on Research on Cancer has judged that mechlorethamine is a probable carcinogen in humans. This is supported by limited evidence of carcinogenicity in humans and sufficient evidence of carcinogenicity in animals. Young-adult female RF mice were injected intravenously with four doses of 2.4 mg/kg of mechlorethamine (0.1% solution) at 2-week intervals with observations for up to 2 years. An increased incidence of thymic lymphomas and pulmonary adenomas was observed. Painting mechlorethamine on the skin of mice for periods up to 33 weeks resulted in squamous cell tumors in 9 of 33 mice.
Mechlorethamine induced mutations in the Ames test, in *E. coli*, and *Neurospora crassa*. Mechlorethamine caused chromosome aberrations in a variety of plant and mammalian cells. Dominant lethal mutations were produced in ICR/Ha Swiss mice.
Mechlorethamine impaired fertility in the rat at a daily dose of 500 mg/kg intravenously for two weeks.
Pregnancy
Pregnancy Category D. See WARNINGS.
Nursing Mothers
It is not known whether this drug is excreted in human milk. Because many drugs are excreted in human milk and because of the potential for serious adverse reactions in nursing infants from MUSTARGEN, a decision should be made whether to discontinue nursing or to discontinue the drug, taking into account the importance of the drug to the mother.
Pediatric Use
Safety and effectiveness in pediatric patients have not been established by well-controlled studies. Use of MUSTARGEN in pediatric patients has been quite limited. MUSTARGEN has been used in Hodgkin's disease, stages III and IV, in combination with other oncolytic agents (MOPP schedule). The MOPP chemotherapy combination includes mechlorethamine, vincristine, procarbazine, and prednisone or prednisolone.
Geriatric Use
Clinical studies of MUSTARGEN did not include sufficient numbers of subjects aged 65 and over to determine whether they respond differently from younger subjects. In general, dose selection for an elderly patient should be cautious, usually starting at the low end of the dosing range, reflecting the greater frequency of decreased hepatic, renal, or cardiac function, and of concomitant disease or other drug therapy.

ADVERSE REACTIONS

Clinical use of MUSTARGEN *usually is accompanied by toxic manifestations.*
Local Toxicity
Thrombosis and thrombophlebitis may result from direct contact of the drug with the intima of the injected vein. Avoid high concentration and prolonged contact with the drug, especially in cases of elevated pressure in the antebrachial vein (e.g., in mediastinal tumor compression from severe vena cava syndrome).
Systemic Toxicity
General: Hypersensitivity reactions, including anaphylaxis, have been reported. Nausea, vomiting and depression of formed elements in the circulating blood are dose-limiting side effects and usually occur with the use of full doses of MUSTARGEN. Jaundice, alopecia, vertigo, tinnitus and diminished hearing may occur infrequently. Rarely, hemolytic anemia associated with such diseases as the lymphomas and chronic lymphocytic leukemia may be precipitated by treatment with alkylating agents including MUSTARGEN. Also, various chromosomal abnormalities have been reported in association with nitrogen mustard therapy.
MUSTARGEN is given preferably at night in case sedation for side effects is required. Nausea and vomiting usually occur 1 to 3 hours after use of the drug. Emesis may disappear in the first 8 hours, but nausea may persist for 24 hours. Nausea and vomiting may be so severe as to precipitate vascular accidents in patients with a hemorrhagic tendency. Premedication with antiemetics, in addition to sedatives, may help control severe nausea and vomiting. Anorexia, weakness and diarrhea may also occur.
Hematologic: The usual course of MUSTARGEN (total dose of 0.4 mg/kg either given as a single intravenous dose or divided into two or four daily doses of 0.2 or 0.1 mg/kg respectively) generally produces a lymphocytopenia within 24 hours after the first injection; significant granulocytopenia occurs within 6 to 8 days and lasts for 10 days to 3 weeks. Agranulocytosis appears to be relatively infrequent and recovery from leukopenia in most cases is complete within two weeks of the maximum reduction. Thrombocytopenia is variable but the time course of the appearance and recovery from reduced platelet counts generally parallels the sequence of granulocyte levels. In some cases severe thrombocytopenia may lead to bleeding from the gums and gastrointestinal tract, petechiae, and small subcutaneous hemorrhages; these symptoms appear to be transient and in most cases disappear with return to a normal platelet count. However, a severe and even uncontrollable depression of the hematopoietic system occasionally may follow the usual dose of MUSTARGEN, particularly in patients with widespread disease and debility and in patients previously treated with other antineoplastic agents or x-ray. Persistent pancytopenia has been reported. In rare instances, hemorrhagic complications may be due to hyperheparinemia. Erythrocyte and hemoglobin levels may decline during the first 2 weeks after therapy but rarely significantly. Depression of the hematopoietic system may be found up to 50 days or more after starting therapy.
Integumentary: Occasionally, a maculopapular skin eruption occurs, but this may be idiosyncratic and does not necessarily recur with subsequent courses of the drug. Erythema multiforme has been observed. Herpes zoster, a common complicating infection in patients with lymphomas, may first appear after therapy is instituted and on occasion may be precipitated by treatment. Further treatment should be discontinued during the acute phase of this illness to avoid progression to generalized herpes zoster.
Reproductive: Since the gonads are susceptible to MUSTARGEN, treatment may be followed by delayed catamenia, oligomenorrhea, or temporary or permanent amenorrhea. Impaired spermatogenesis, azoospermia, and total germinal aplasia have been reported in male patients treated with alkylating agents, especially in combination with other drugs. In some instances spermatogenesis may return in patients in remission, but this may occur only several years after intensive chemotherapy has been discontinued. Patients should be warned of the potential risk to their reproductive capacity.

OVERDOSAGE

With total doses exceeding 0.4 mg/kg of body weight for a single course, severe leukopenia, anemia, thrombocytopenia and a hemorrhagic diathesis with subsequent delayed bleeding may develop. Death may follow. The only treatment in instances of excessive dosage appears to be repeated blood product transfusions, antibiotic treatment of complicating infections and general supportive measures.
The intravenous LD_{50} of MUSTARGEN is 2 mg/kg and 1.6 mg/kg in the mouse and rat, respectively. The oral LD_{50} for mechlorethamine hydrochloride is 20 mg/kg and 10 mg/kg in the mouse and rat, respectively.

DOSAGE AND ADMINISTRATION

Not for oral administration
Intravenous Administration
The dosage of MUSTARGEN varies with the clinical situation, the therapeutic response and the magnitude of hematologic depression. A total dose of 0.4 mg/kg of body weight for each course usually is given either as a single dose or in divided doses of 0.1 to 0.2 mg/kg per day. Dosage should be based on ideal dry body weight. The presence of edema or ascites must be considered so that dosage will be based on actual weight unaugmented by these conditions.
The margin of safety in therapy with MUSTARGEN *is narrow and considerable care must be exercised in the matter of dosage.* Repeated examinations of blood are *mandatory* as a guide to subsequent therapy. (See OVERDOSAGE.)
Within a few minutes after intravenous injection, MUSTARGEN undergoes chemical transformation, combines with reactive compounds, and is no longer present in its active form in the blood stream. Subsequent courses should not be given until the patient has recovered hematologically from the previous course; this is best determined by repeated studies of the peripheral blood elements awaiting their return to normal levels. It is often possible to give repeated courses of MUSTARGEN as early as three weeks after treatment.
Preparation of Solution for Intravenous Administration
This drug is **HIGHLY TOXIC** and both powder and solution must be handled and administered with care. (See boxed warning and DOSAGE AND ADMINISTRATION, *Special Handling*.) Since MUSTARGEN is a powerful vesicant, it is intended primarily for intravenous use, and in most cases is given by this route. Inhalation of dust or vapors and contact with skin or mucous membranes, especially those of the eyes, must be avoided. Appropriate protective equipment should be worn when handling MUSTARGEN. Should accidental eye contact occur, copious irrigation for at least 15 minutes with water, normal saline or a balanced salt ophthalmic irrigating solution should be instituted immediately, followed by prompt ophthalmologic consultation. Should accidental skin contact occur, the affected part must be irrigated immediately with copious amounts of water, for at least 15 minutes while removing contaminated clothing and shoes, followed by 2% sodium thiosulfate solution. Medical attention should be sought immediately. Contaminated clothing should be destroyed. (See DOSAGE AND ADMINISTRATION, *Special Handling*).
Each vial of MUSTARGEN contains 10 mg of mechlorethamine hydrochloride triturated with sodium chloride q.s. 100 mg. In neutral or alkaline aqueous solution it undergoes rapid chemical transformation and is highly unstable. Although solutions prepared according to instructions are acidic and do not decompose as rapidly, they should be prepared immediately before each injection since they will decompose on standing. When reconstituted, MUSTARGEN is a clear colorless solution. *Do not use if the solution is discolored or if droplets of water are visible within the vial prior to reconstitution.*
Using a sterile 10 mL syringe, inject 10 mL of Sterile Water for Injection or 10 mL Sodium Chloride Injection into a vial of MUSTARGEN. With the needle (syringe attached) still in the rubber stopper, shake the vial several times to dissolve the drug completely. The resultant solution contains 1 mg of mechlorethamine hydrochloride per mL.
Parenteral drug products should be inspected visually for particulate matter and discoloration prior to administration whenever solution and container permit.
Special Handling
Animal studies have shown mechlorethamine to be corrosive to skin and eyes, a powerful vesicant, irritating to the mucous membranes of the respiratory tract and highly toxic by the oral route. It has also been shown to be carcinogenic, mutagenic and teratogenic. Due to the drug's toxic properties, appropriate precautions including the use of appropriate safety equipment are recommended for the preparation of MUSTARGEN for parenteral administration. Inhalation of dust or vapors and contact with skin or mucous membranes, especially those of the eyes, must be avoided. Avoid exposure during pregnancy. The National Institutes of Health presently recommends that the preparation of injectable anti-neoplastic drugs should be performed in a Class II laminar flow biological safety cabinet. Personnel preparing drugs of this class should wear chemical resistant, impervious gloves, safety goggles, outer garments and shoe covers. Additional body garments should be used based upon the task being performed (e.g., sleevelets, apron, gauntlets, disposable suits) to avoid exposed skin surfaces and inhalation of vapors and dust. Appropriate techniques should be used to remove potentially contaminated clothing. Several other guidelines for proper handling and disposal of antineoplastic drugs have been published and should be considered.
Accidental Contact Measures
Should accidental eye contact occur, copious irrigation for at least 15 minutes with water, normal saline or a balanced salt ophthalmic irrigating solution should be instituted immediately, followed by prompt ophthalmologic consultation. Should accidental skin contact occur, the affected part must be irrigated immediately with copious amounts of water, for at least 15 minutes while removing contaminated clothing and shoes, followed by 2% sodium thiosulfate solution. Medical attention should be sought immediately. Contaminated clothing should be destroyed. (See PRECAUTIONS, *General* and DOSAGE AND ADMINISTRATION, *Preparation of Solution for Intravenous Administration*.)
Technique for Intravenous Administration
Withdraw into the syringe the calculated volume of solution required for a single injection. *Dispose of any remaining solution after neutralization* (see below). Although the drug may be injected directly into any suitable vein, it is injected preferably into the rubber or plastic tubing of a flowing intravenous infusion set. This reduces the possibility of severe local reactions due to extravasation or high concentration of the drug. Injecting the drug into the tubing rather than adding it to the entire volume of the infusion fluid minimizes a chemical reaction between the drug and the solution. The rate of injection apparently is not critical provided it is completed within a few minutes.
Intracavitary Administration
Nitrogen mustard has been used by intracavitary administration with varying success in certain malignant conditions for the control of pleural, peritoneal, and pericardial effusions caused by malignant cells.
The technique and the dose used by any of these routes varies. Therefore, if MUSTARGEN is given by the intracavitary route, the published articles concerning such use should be consulted. *Because of the inherent risks involved, the physician should be experienced in the appropriate injection techniques, and be thoroughly aware of the indications, dosages, hazards, and precautions as set forth in the published literature. When using* MUSTARGEN *by the intracavitary route, the general precautions concerning this agent should be borne in mind.*
As a general guide, reference is made especially to the techniques of Weisberger et al. Intracavitary use is indicated in the presence of pleural, peritoneal, or pericardial effusion due to metastatic tumors. Local therapy with nitrogen mustard is used only when malignant cells are demonstrated in the effusion. Intracavitary injection is not recommended when the accumulated fluid is chylous in nature, since results are likely to be poor.
Paracentesis is first performed with most of the fluid being removed from the pleural or peritoneal cavity. The intracavitary use of MUSTARGEN may exert at least some of its effect through production of a chemical poudrage. Therefore, the removal of excess fluid allows the drug to more easily contact the peritoneal and pleural linings. For intrapleural or intrapericardial injection nitrogen mustard is introduced directly through the thoracentesis needle. For intraperitoneal injection it is given through a rubber catheter inserted into the trocar used for paracentesis or through a No. 18 gauge needle inserted at another site. This drug should be injected slowly, with frequent aspiration to ensure that a free flow of fluid is present. If fluid cannot be aspirated, pain and necrosis due to injection of solution outside the cavity may occur. Free flow of fluid also is necessary to prevent injection into a loculated pocket and to ensure adequate dissemination of nitrogen mustard.

The usual dose of nitrogen mustard for intracavitary injection is 0.4 mg/kg of body weight, though 0.2 mg/kg (or 10 to 20 mg) has been used by the intrapericardial route. The solution is prepared, as previously described for intravenous injection, by adding 10 mL of Sterile Water for Injection or 10 mL of Sodium Chloride Injection to the vial containing 10 mg of mechlorethamine hydrochloride. (Amounts of diluent of 50 to 100 mL of normal saline have also been used.) The position of the patient should be changed every 5 to 10 minutes for an hour after injection to obtain more uniform distribution of the drug throughout the serous cavity. The remaining fluid may be removed from the pleural or peritoneal cavity by paracentesis 24 to 36 hours later. The patient should be followed carefully by clinical and x-ray examination to detect reaccumulation of fluid.

Pain occurs rarely with intrapleural use; it is common with intraperitoneal injection and is often associated with nausea, vomiting, and diarrhea of 2 to 3 days duration. Transient cardiac irregularities may occur with intrapericardial injection. Death, possibly accelerated by nitrogen mustard, has been reported following the use of this agent by the intracavitary route. Although absorption of MUSTARGEN when given by the intracavitary route is probably not complete because of its rapid deactivation by body fluids, the systemic effect is unpredictable. The acute side effects such as nausea and vomiting are usually mild. Bone marrow depression is generally milder than when the drug is given intravenously. Care should be taken to avoid use by the intracavitary route when other agents which may suppress bone marrow function are being used systemically.

Neutralization of Equipment and Unused Solution

To clean rubber gloves, tubing, glassware, etc., after giving MUSTARGEN, soak them in an aqueous solution containing equal volumes of sodium thiosulfate (5%) and sodium bicarbonate (5%) for 45 minutes. Excess reagents and reaction products are washed away easily with water. Any unused injection solution should be neutralized by mixing with an equal volume of sodium thiosulfate/sodium bicarbonate solution. Allow the mixture to stand for 45 minutes. Vials that have contained MUSTARGEN should be treated in the same way with thiosulfate/bicarbonate solution before disposal.

HOW SUPPLIED

No. 7753—Trituration of MUSTARGEN is a light yellow brown crystalline powder, each vial containing 10 mg mechlorethamine hydrochloride with sodium chloride q.s. 100 mg, and is supplied as follows:

NDC 0006-7753-31 in treatment sets of 4 vials.

Storage

Store at controlled room temperature 15–30°C (59–86°F). Protect from light and humidity. Solutions of mechlorethamine HCl decompose on standing; therefore, solutions of the drug should be prepared immediately before use.

7417934 Issued February 2004

NOROXIN® Tablets ℞
(Norfloxacin)

To reduce the development of drug-resistant bacteria and maintain the effectiveness of NOROXIN† and other antibacterial drugs, NOROXIN should be used only to treat or prevent infections that are proven or strongly suspected to be caused by bacteria.

DESCRIPTION

NOROXIN (Norfloxacin) is a synthetic, broad-spectrum antibacterial agent for oral administration. Norfloxacin, a fluoroquinolone, is 1-ethyl-6-fluoro-1,4-dihydro-4-oxo-7-(1-piperazinyl)-3-quinolinecarboxylic acid. Its empirical formula is $C_{16}H_{18}FN_3O_3$ and the structural formula is:

Norfloxacin is a white to pale yellow crystalline powder with a molecular weight of 319.34 and a melting point of about 221°C. It is freely soluble in glacial acetic acid, and very slightly soluble in ethanol, methanol and water.

NOROXIN is available in 400-mg tablets. Each tablet contains the following inactive ingredients: cellulose, croscarmellose sodium, hydroxypropyl cellulose, hydroxypropyl methylcellulose, iron oxide, magnesium stearate, and titanium dioxide.

Norfloxacin, a fluoroquinolone, differs from non-fluorinated quinolones by having a fluorine atom at the 6 position and a piperazine moiety at the 7 position.

†Registered trademark of MERCK & CO., Inc.

CLINICAL PHARMACOLOGY

In fasting healthy volunteers, at least 30–40% of an oral dose of NOROXIN is absorbed. Absorption is rapid following single doses of 200 mg, 400 mg and 800 mg. At the respective doses, mean peak serum and plasma concentrations of 0.8, 1.5 and 2.4 μg/mL are attained approximately one hour after dosing. The presence of food and/or dairy products may decrease absorption. The effective half-life of norfloxacin in serum and plasma is 3–4 hours. Steady-state concentrations of norfloxacin will be attained within two days of dosing.

In healthy elderly volunteers (65–75 years of age with normal renal function for their age), norfloxacin is eliminated more slowly because of their slightly decreased renal function. Following a single 400-mg dose of norfloxacin, the mean (± SD) AUC and C_{max} of 9.8 (2.83) μg•hr/mL and 2.02 (0.77) μg/mL, respectively, were observed in healthy elderly volunteers. The extent of systemic exposure was slightly higher than that seen in younger adults (AUC 6.4 μg•hr/mL and C_{max} 1.5 μg/mL). Drug absorption appears unaffected. However, the effective half-life of norfloxacin in these elderly subjects is 4 hours.

There is no information on accumulation of norfloxacin with repeated administration in elderly patients. However, no dosage adjustment is required based on age alone. In elderly patients with reduced renal function, the dosage should be adjusted as for other patients with renal impairment (see DOSAGE AND ADMINISTRATION, *Renal Impairment*).

The disposition of norfloxacin in patients with creatinine clearance rates greater than 30 mL/min/1.73m^2 is similar to that in healthy volunteers. In patients with creatinine clearance rates equal to or less than 30 mL/min/1.73m^2, the renal elimination of norfloxacin decreases so that the effective serum half-life is 6.5 hours. In these patients, alteration of dosage is necessary (see DOSAGE AND ADMINISTRATION). Drug absorption appears unaffected by decreasing renal function.

Norfloxacin is eliminated through metabolism, biliary excretion, and renal excretion. After a single 400-mg dose of NOROXIN, mean antimicrobial activities equivalent to 278, 773, and 82 μg of norfloxacin/g of feces were obtained at 12, 24, and 48 hours, respectively. Renal excretion occurs by both glomerular filtration and tubular secretion as evidenced by the high rate of renal clearance (approximately 275 mL/min). Within 24 hours of drug administration, 26 to 32% of the administered dose is recovered in the urine as norfloxacin with an additional 5–8% being recovered in the urine as six active metabolites of lesser antimicrobial potency. Only a small percentage (less than 1%) of the dose is recovered thereafter. Fecal recovery accounts for another 30% of the administered dose. In elderly subjects (average creatinine clearance was 91 mL/min/1.73m^2) approximately 22% of the administered dose was recovered in urine and renal clearance averaged 154 mL/min.

Two to three hours after a single 400-mg dose, urinary concentrations of 200 μg/mL or more are attained in the urine. In healthy volunteers, mean urinary concentrations of norfloxacin remain above 30 μg/mL for at least 12 hours following a 400-mg dose. The urinary pH may affect the solubility of norfloxacin. Norfloxacin is least soluble at urinary pH of 7.5 with greater solubility occurring at pHs above and below this value. The serum protein binding of norfloxacin is between 10 and 15%.

The following are mean concentrations of norfloxacin in various fluids and tissues measured 1 to 4 hours post-dose after two 400-mg doses, unless otherwise indicated:

Renal Parenchyma	7.3 μg/g
Prostate	2.5 μg/g
Seminal Fluid	2.7 μg/mL
Testicle	1.6 μg/g
Uterus/Cervix	3.0 μg/g
Vagina	4.3 μg/g
Fallopian Tube	1.9 μg/g
Bile	6.9 μg/mL (after two 200-mg doses)

Microbiology

Norfloxacin has *in vitro* activity against a broad range of gram-positive and gram-negative aerobic bacteria. The fluorine atom at the 6 position provides increased potency against gram-negative organisms, and the piperazine moiety at the 7 position is responsible for antipseudomonal activity.

Norfloxacin inhibits bacterial deoxyribonucleic acid synthesis and is bactericidal. At the molecular level, three specific events are attributed to norfloxacin in *E. coli* cells:

1) inhibition of the ATP-dependent DNA supercoiling reaction catalyzed by DNA gyrase,
2) inhibition of the relaxation of supercoiled DNA,
3) promotion of double-stranded DNA breakage.

Resistance to norfloxacin due to spontaneous mutation *in vitro* is a rare occurrence (range: 10^{-9} to 10^{-12} cells). Resistant organisms have emerged during therapy with norfloxacin in less than 1% of patients treated. Organisms in which development of resistance is greatest are the following:

Pseudomonas aeruginosa
Klebsiella pneumoniae
Acinetobacter spp.
Enterococcus spp.

For this reason, when there is a lack of satisfactory clinical response, repeat culture and susceptibility testing should be done. Nalidixic acid-resistant organisms are generally susceptible to norfloxacin *in vitro;* however, these organisms may have higher minimum inhibitory concentrations (MIC's) to norfloxacin than nalidixic acid-susceptible strains. There is generally no cross-resistance between norfloxacin and other classes of antibacterial agents. Therefore, norfloxacin may demonstrate activity against indicated organisms resistant to some other antimicrobial agents including the aminoglycosides, penicillins, cephalosporins, tetracyclines, macrolides, and sulfonamides, including combinations of sulfamethoxazole and trimethoprim. Antagonism has been demonstrated *in vitro* between norfloxacin and nitrofurantoin.

Norfloxacin has been shown to be active against most strains of the following microorganisms both *in vitro* and in clinical infections as described in the **INDICATIONS AND USAGE** section.

Gram-positive aerobes:
Enterococcus faecalis
Staphylococcus aureus
Staphylococcus epidermidis
Staphylococcus saprophyticus
Streptococcus agalactiae

Gram-negative aerobes:
Citrobacter freundii
Enterobacter aerogenes
Enterobacter cloacae
Escherichia coli
Klebsiella pneumoniae
Neisseria gonorrhoeae
Proteus mirabilis
Proteus vulgaris
Pseudomonas aeruginosa
Serratia marcescens

The following *in vitro* data are available, **but their clinical significance is unknown.**

Norfloxacin exhibits *in vitro* minimal inhibitory concentrations (MIC's) of ≤4 μg/mL against most (≥90%) strains of the following microorganisms; however, the safety and effectiveness of norfloxacin in treating clinical infections due to these microorganisms have not been established in adequate and well-controlled clinical trials.

Gram-negative aerobes:
Citrobacter diversus
Edwardsiella tarda
Enterobacter agglomerans
Haemophilus ducreyi
Klebsiella oxytoca
Morganella morganii
Providencia alcalifaciens
Providencia rettgeri
Providencia stuartii
Pseudomonas fluorescens
Pseudomonas stutzeri

Other:
Ureaplasma urealyticum

NOROXIN is not generally active against obligate anaerobes.

Norfloxacin has not been shown to be active against *Treponema pallidum.* (See WARNINGS.)

Susceptibility Tests

Dilution Techniques:

Quantitative methods are used to determine antimicrobial minimal inhibitory concentrations (MIC's). These MIC's provide estimates of the susceptibility of bacteria to antimicrobial compounds. The MIC's should be determined using a standardized procedure. Standardized procedures are based on a dilution method[1] (broth, agar, or microdilution) or equivalent with standardized inoculum concentrations and standardized concentrations of norfloxacin powder. The MIC values should be interpreted according to the following criteria*:

MIC (μg/mL)	Interpretation
≤4	Susceptible (S)
8	Intermediate (I)
≥16	Resistant (R)

A report of "Susceptible" indicates that the pathogen is likely to be inhibited if the antimicrobial compound in the blood reaches the concentrations usually achievable. A report of "Intermediate" indicates that the result should be considered equivocal, and, if the microorganism is not fully susceptible to alternative, clinically feasible drugs, the test should be repeated. This category implies possible clinical applicability in body sites where the drug is physiologically concentrated or in situations where high dosage of drug can be used. This category also provides a buffer zone which prevents small uncontrolled technical factors from causing major discrepancies in interpretation. A report of "Resistant"

Continued on next page

Information on the Merck & Co., Inc., products listed on these pages is from the prescribing information in use October 1, 2004. For information, please call 1-800-NSC-MERCK [1-800-672-6372].

Noroxin—Cont.

indicates that the pathogen is not likely to be inhibited if the antimicrobial compound in the blood reaches the concentrations usually achievable; other therapy should be selected.

* These interpretative criteria apply only to isolates from urinary tract infections. There are no established norfloxacin interpretive criteria for *Neisseria gonorrhoeae* or organisms isolated from other infection sites.

Standardized susceptibility test procedures require the use of laboratory control microorganisms to control the technical aspects of the laboratory procedures. Standard norfloxacin powder should provide the following MIC values:

Organism	MIC range (μg/mL)
E. coli ATCC 25922	0.03–0.12
E. faecalis ATCC 29212	2–8
P. aeruginosa ATCC 27853	1–4
S. aureus ATCC 29213	0.5–2

Diffusion Techniques:
Quantitative methods that require measurement of zone diameters also provide reproducible estimates of the susceptibility of bacteria to antimicrobial compounds. One such standardized procedure[2] requires the use of standardized inoculum concentrations. This procedure uses paper disks impregnated with 10-μg norfloxacin to test the susceptibility of microorganisms to norfloxacin. Reports from the laboratory providing results of the standard single-disk susceptibility test with a 10-μg norfloxacin disk should be interpreted according to the following criteria*:

Zone diameter (mm)	Interpretation
≥17	Susceptible (S)
13–16	Intermediate (I)
≤12	Resistant (R)

Interpretation should be as stated above for results using dilution techniques. Interpretation involves correlation of the diameter obtained in the disk test with the MIC for norfloxacin.
As with standard dilution techniques, diffusion methods require the use of laboratory control microorganisms that are used to control the technical aspects of the laboratory procedures. For the diffusion techniques, the 10-μg norfloxacin disk should provide the following zone diameters in these laboratory test quality control strains:

Organism	Zone Diameter (mm)
E. coli ATCC 25922	28–35
P. aeruginosa ATCC 27853	22–29
S. aureus ATCC 25923	17–28

INDICATIONS AND USAGE

NOROXIN is indicated for the treatment of adults with the following infections caused by susceptible strains of the designated microorganisms:
Urinary tract infections:
Uncomplicated urinary tract infections (including cystitis) due to *Enterococcus faecalis, Escherichia coli, Klebsiella pneumoniae, Proteus mirabilis, Pseudomonas aeruginosa, Staphylococcus epidermidis, Staphylococcus saprophyticus, Citrobacter freundii***, *Enterobacter aerogenes***, *Enterobacter cloacae***, *Proteus vulgaris***, *Staphylococcus aureus***, or *Streptococcus agalactiae***.
Complicated urinary tract infections due to *Enterococcus faecalis, Escherichia coli, Klebsiella pneumoniae, Proteus mirabilis, Pseudomonas aeruginosa,* or *Serratia marcescens***.
Sexually transmitted diseases (see WARNINGS):
Uncomplicated urethral and cervical gonorrhea due to *Neisseria gonorrhoeae.*
Prostatitis:
Prostatitis due to *Escherichia coli.*
(See DOSAGE AND ADMINISTRATION for appropriate dosing instructions.)
Penicillinase production should have no effect on norfloxacin activity.
Appropriate culture and susceptibility tests should be performed before treatment in order to isolate and identify organisms causing the infection and to determine their susceptibility to norfloxacin. Therapy with norfloxacin may be initiated before results of these tests are known; once results become available, appropriate therapy should be given. Repeat culture and susceptibility testing performed periodically during therapy will provide information not only on the therapeutic effect of the antimicrobial agents but also on the possible emergence of bacterial resistance.
To reduce the development of drug-resistant bacteria and maintain the effectiveness of NOROXIN and other antibacterial drugs, NOROXIN should be used only to treat or prevent infections that are proven or strongly suspected to be caused by susceptible bacteria. When culture and susceptibility information are available, they should be considered in selecting or modifying antibacterial therapy. In the absence of such data, local epidemiology and susceptibility patterns may contribute to the empiric selection of therapy.

**Efficacy for this organism in this organ system was studied in fewer than 10 infections.

CONTRAINDICATIONS

NOROXIN (norfloxacin) is contraindicated in persons with a history of hypersensitivity, tendinitis, or tendon rupture associated with the use of norfloxacin or any member of the quinolone group of antimicrobial agents.

WARNINGS

Safety in Children, Adolescents, Nursing mothers, and during Pregnancy: THE SAFETY AND EFFICACY OF ORAL NORFLOXACIN IN PEDIATRIC PATIENTS, ADOLESCENTS (UNDER THE AGE OF 18), PREGNANT WOMEN, AND NURSING MOTHERS HAVE NOT BEEN ESTABLISHED. (See PRECAUTIONS, *Pediatric Use, Pregnancy,* and *Nursing Mothers* subsections.) The oral administration of single doses of norfloxacin, 6 times*** the recommended human clinical dose (on a mg/kg basis), caused lameness in immature dogs. Histologic examination of the weight-bearing joints of these dogs revealed permanent lesions of the cartilage. Other quinolones also produced erosions of the cartilage in weight-bearing joints and other signs of arthropathy in immature animals of various species. (See ANIMAL PHARMACOLOGY.)
QT interval prolongation/torsades de pointes: Rare cases of torsades de pointes have been spontaneously reported during post-marketing surveillance in patients receiving quinolones, including norfloxacin. These rare cases were associated with one or more of the following factors: age over 60, female gender, underlying cardiac disease, and/or use of multiple medications. Norfloxacin should be avoided in patients with known prolongation of the QT interval, patients with uncorrected hypokalemia, and patients receiving class IA (quinidine, procainamide), or class III (amiodarone, sotalol) antiarrhythmic agents.
Seizures: Convulsions have been reported in patients receiving norfloxacin. Convulsions, increased intracranial pressure, and toxic psychoses have been reported in patients receiving drugs in this class. Quinolones may also cause central nervous system (CNS) stimulation which may lead to tremors, restlessness, lightheadedness, confusion, and hallucinations. If these reactions occur in patients receiving norfloxacin, the drug should be discontinued and appropriate measures instituted.
The effects of norfloxacin on brain function or on the electrical activity of the brain have not been tested. Therefore, until more information becomes available, norfloxacin, like all other quinolones, should be used with caution in patients with known or suspected CNS disorders, such as severe cerebral arteriosclerosis, epilepsy, and other factors which predispose to seizures. (See ADVERSE REACTIONS.)
Hypersensitivity/anaphylaxis: Serious and occasionally fatal hypersensitivity (anaphylactoid or anaphylactic) reactions, some following the first dose, have been reported in patients receiving quinolone therapy. Some reactions were accompanied by cardiovascular collapse, loss of consciousness, tingling, pharyngeal or facial edema, dyspnea, urticaria and itching. Only a few patients had a history of hypersensitivity reactions. If an allergic reaction to norfloxacin occurs, discontinue the drug. Serious acute hypersensitivity reactions may require immediate emergency treatment with epinephrine. Oxygen, intravenous fluids, antihistamines, corticosteroids, pressor amines, and airway management, including intubation, should be administered as indicated.
***Pseudomembranous colitis:* Pseudomembranous colitis has been reported with nearly all antibacterial agents, including norfloxacin, and may range in severity from mild to life-threatening. Therefore, it is important to consider this diagnosis in patients who present with diarrhea subsequent to the administration of antibacterial agents.**
Treatment with antibacterial agents alters the normal flora of the colon and may permit overgrowth of clostridia. Studies indicate that a toxin produced by *Clostridium difficile* is one primary cause of "antibiotic-associated colitis".
After the diagnosis of pseudomembranous colitis has been established, therapeutic measures should be initiated. Mild cases of pseudomembranous colitis usually respond to drug discontinuation alone. In moderate to severe cases, consideration should be given to management with fluids and electrolytes, protein supplementation, and treatment with an antibacterial drug clinically effective against *C. difficile* colitis.

***Based on a patient weight of 50 kg.

Peripheral neuropathy: Rare cases of sensory or sensorimotor axonal polyneuropathy affecting small and/or large axons resulting in paresthesias, hypoesthesias, dysesthesias and weakness have been reported in patients receiving quinolones, including norfloxacin. Norfloxacin should be discontinued if the patient experiences symptoms of neuropathy including pain, burning, tingling, numbness, and/or weakness, or is found to have deficits in light touch, pain, temperature, position sense, vibratory sensation, and/or motor strength in order to prevent the development of an irreversible condition.
Tendon effects: Ruptures of the shoulder, hand, Achilles tendons or other tendons that required surgical repair or resulted in prolonged disability have been reported in patients receiving quinolones, including norfloxacin. Postmarketing surveillance reports indicate that this risk may be increased in patients receiving concomitant corticosteroids, especially in the elderly. Norfloxacin should be discontinued if the patient experiences pain, inflammation, or rupture of a tendon. Patients should rest and refrain from exercise until the diagnosis of tendinitis or tendon rupture has been excluded. Tendon rupture can occur during or after therapy with quinolones, including norfloxacin.
*Syphilis treatment: Norfloxacin has **not** been shown to be effective in the treatment of syphilis.* Antimicrobial agents used in high doses for short periods of time to treat gonorrhea may mask or delay the symptoms of incubating syphilis. All patients with gonorrhea should have a serologic test for syphilis at the time of diagnosis. Patients treated with norfloxacin should have a follow-up serologic test for syphilis after three months.

PRECAUTIONS

General
Needle-shaped crystals were found in the urine of some volunteers who received either placebo, 800 mg norfloxacin, or 1600 mg norfloxacin (at or twice the recommended daily dose, respectively) while participating in a double-blind, crossover study comparing single doses of norfloxacin with placebo. While crystalluria is not expected to occur under usual conditions with a dosage regimen of 400 mg b.i.d., as a precaution, the daily recommended dosage should not be exceeded and the patient should drink sufficient fluids to ensure a proper state of hydration and adequate urinary output.
Alteration in dosage regimen is necessary for patients with impaired renal function (see DOSAGE AND ADMINISTRATION).
Moderate to severe phototoxicity reactions have been observed in patients who are exposed to excessive sunlight while receiving some members of this drug class. Excessive sunlight should be avoided. Therapy should be discontinued if phototoxicity occurs.
Rarely, hemolytic reactions have been reported in patients with latent or actual defects in glucose-6-phosphate dehydrogenase activity who take quinolone antibacterial agents, including norfloxacin. (See ADVERSE REACTIONS.)
Quinolones, including norfloxacin, may exacerbate the signs of myasthenia gravis and lead to life-threatening weakness of the respiratory muscles. Caution should be exercised when using quinolones, including NOROXIN, in patients with myasthenia gravis (see ADVERSE REACTIONS).
Prescribing NOROXIN in the absence of a proven or strongly suspected bacterial infection or a prophylactic indication is unlikely to provide benefit to the patient and increases the risk of the development of drug-resistant bacteria.
Information for Patients
Patients should be advised:
— that norfloxacin may cause changes in the electrocardiogram (QTc interval prolongation).
— that norfloxacin should be avoided in patients receiving class IA (e.g., quinidine, procainamide) or class III (e.g., amiodarone, sotalol) antiarrhythmic agents.
— that norfloxacin should be used with caution in subjects receiving drugs that affect the QTc interval such as cisapride, erythromycin, antipsychotics, and tricyclic antidepressants.
— to inform their physicians of any personal or family history of QTc prolongation or proarrhythmic conditions such as hypokalemia, bradycardia or recent myocardial ischemia.
— that peripheral neuropathies have been associated with norfloxacin use. If symptoms of peripheral neuropathy including pain, burning, tingling, numbness, and/or weakness develop, they should discontinue treatment and contact their physicians.
— to drink fluids liberally.
— that norfloxacin should be taken at least one hour before or at least two hours after a meal or ingestion of milk and/or other dairy products.
— that multivitamins or other products containing iron or zinc, antacids or Videx®‡ (Didanosine), chewable/buffered tablets or the pediatric powder for oral solution, should not be taken within the two-hour period before or within the two-hour period after taking norfloxacin. (See PRECAUTIONS, *Drug Interactions.*)
— that norfloxacin can cause dizziness and lightheadedness and, therefore, patients should know how they react to norfloxacin before they operate an automobile or machinery or engage in activities requiring mental alertness and coordination.
— to discontinue treatment and inform their physician if they experience pain, inflammation, or rupture of a tendon, and to rest and refrain from exercise until the diagnosis of tendinitis or tendon rupture has been confidently excluded.
— that norfloxacin may be associated with hypersensitivity reactions, even following the first dose, and to discontinue the drug at the first sign of a skin rash or other allergic reaction.
— to avoid undue exposure to excessive sunlight while receiving norfloxacin and to discontinue therapy if phototoxicity occurs.
— that some quinolones may increase the effects of theophylline and/or caffeine. (See PRECAUTIONS, *Drug Interactions.*)

— that convulsions have been reported in patients taking quinolones, including norfloxacin, and to notify their physician before taking this drug if there is a history of this condition.

‡ Registered trademark of Bristol-Myers Squibb Company

Patients should be counseled that antibacterial drugs including NOROXIN should only be used to treat bacterial infections. They do not treat viral infections (e.g., the common cold). When NOROXIN is prescribed to treat a bacterial infection, patients should be told that although it is common to feel better early in the course of therapy, the medication should be taken exactly as directed. Skipping doses or not completing the full course of therapy may (1) decrease the effectiveness of the immediate treatment and (2) increase the likelihood that bacteria will develop resistance and will not be treatable by NOROXIN or other antibacterial drugs in the future.

Laboratory Tests

As with any potent antibacterial agent, periodic assessment of organ system functions, including renal, hepatic, and hematopoietic, is advisable during prolonged therapy.

Drug Interactions

Elevated plasma levels of theophylline have been reported with concomitant quinolone use. There have been reports of theophylline-related side effects in patients on concomitant therapy with norfloxacin and theophylline. Therefore, monitoring of theophylline plasma levels should be considered and dosage of theophylline adjusted as required.

Elevated serum levels of cyclosporine have been reported with concomitant use of cyclosporine with norfloxacin. Therefore, cyclosporine serum levels should be monitored and appropriate cyclosporine dosage adjustments made when these drugs are used concomitantly.

Quinolones, including norfloxacin, may enhance the effects of oral anticoagulants, including warfarin or its derivatives or similar agents. When these products are administered concomitantly, prothrombin time or other suitable coagulation tests should be closely monitored.

The concomitant administration of quinolones including norfloxacin with glyburide (a sulfonylurea agent) has, on rare occasions, resulted in severe hypoglycemia. Therefore, monitoring of blood glucose is recommended when these agents are co-administered.

Diminished urinary excretion of norfloxacin has been reported during the concomitant administration of probenecid and norfloxacin.

The concomitant use of nitrofurantoin is not recommended since nitrofurantoin may antagonize the antibacterial effect of NOROXIN in the urinary tract.

Multivitamins, or other products containing iron or zinc, antacids or sucralfate should not be administered concomitantly with, or within 2 hours of, the administration of norfloxacin, because they may interfere with absorption resulting in lower serum and urine levels of norfloxacin.

Videx® (Didanosine) chewable/buffered tablets or the pediatric powder for oral solution should not be administered concomitantly with, or within 2 hours of, the administration of norfloxacin, because these products may interfere with absorption resulting in lower serum and urine levels of norfloxacin.

Some quinolones have also been shown to interfere with the metabolism of caffeine. This may lead to reduced clearance of caffeine and a prolongation of its plasma half-life.

Carcinogenesis, Mutagenesis, Impairment of Fertility

No increase in neoplastic changes was observed with norfloxacin as compared to controls in a study in rats, lasting up to 96 weeks at doses 8–9 times*** the usual human dose (on a mg/kg basis).

Norfloxacin was tested for mutagenic activity in a number of *in vivo* and *in vitro* tests. Norfloxacin had no mutagenic effect in the dominant lethal test in mice and did not cause chromosomal aberrations in hamsters or rats at doses 30–60 times*** the usual human dose (on a mg/kg basis). Norfloxacin had no mutagenic activity *in vitro* in the Ames microbial mutagen test, Chinese hamster fibroblasts and V-79 mammalian cell assay. Although norfloxacin was weakly positive in the Rec-assay for DNA repair, all other mutagenic assays were negative including a more sensitive test (V-79).

Norfloxacin did not adversely affect the fertility of male and female mice at oral doses up to 30 times*** the usual human dose (on a mg/kg basis).

Pregnancy

Teratogenic Effects. Pregnancy Category C. Norfloxacin has been shown to produce embryonic loss in monkeys when given in doses 10 times*** the maximum daily total human dose (on a mg/kg basis). At this dose, peak plasma levels obtained in monkeys were approximately 2 times those obtained in humans. There has been no evidence of a teratogenic effect in any of the animal species tested (rat, rabbit, mouse, monkey) at 6–50 times*** the maximum daily human dose (on a mg/kg basis). There are, however, no adequate and well-controlled studies in pregnant women. Norfloxacin should be used during pregnancy only if the potential benefit justifies the potential risk to the fetus.

Nursing Mothers

It is not known whether norfloxacin is excreted in human milk.

When a 200-mg dose of NOROXIN was administered to nursing mothers, norfloxacin was not detected in human milk. However, because the dose studied was low, because other drugs in this class are secreted in human milk, and because of the potential for serious adverse reactions from norfloxacin in nursing infants, a decision should be made to discontinue nursing or to discontinue the drug, taking into account the importance of the drug to the mother.

Infection	Description	Unit Dose	Frequency	Duration	Daily Dose
Urinary Tract	Uncomplicated UTI's (crystitis) due to *E. coli, K. pneumoniae,* or *P. mirabilis*	400 mg	q12h	3 days	800 mg
	Uncomplicated UTI's due to other indicated organisms	400 mg	q12h	7–10 days	800 mg
	Complicated UTI's	400 mg	q12h	10–21 days	800 mg
Sexually Transmitted Diseases	Uncomplicated Gonorrhea	800 mg	single dose	1 day	800 mg
Prostatitis	Acute or Chronic	400 mg	q12h	28 days	800 mg

Pediatric Use

The safety and effectiveness of oral norfloxacin in pediatric patients and adolescents below the age of 18 years have not been established. Norfloxacin causes arthropathy in juvenile animals of several animal species. (See WARNINGS and ANIMAL PHARMACOLOGY.)

Geriatric Use

Of the 340 subjects in one large clinical study of NOROXIN for treatment of urinary tract infections, 103 patients were 65 and older, 77 of whom were 70 and older; no overall differences in safety and effectiveness were evident between these subjects and younger subjects. In clinical practice, no difference in the type of reported adverse experiences have been observed between the elderly and younger patients except for a possible increased risk of tendon rupture in elderly patients receiving concomitant corticosteroids (see WARNINGS). In addition, increased risk for other adverse experiences in some older individuals cannot be ruled out (see ADVERSE REACTIONS).

This drug is known to be substantially excreted by the kidney, and the risk of toxic reactions to this drug may be greater in patients with impaired renal function. Because elderly patients are more likely to have decreased renal function, care should be taken in dose selection, and it may be useful to monitor renal function (see DOSAGE AND ADMINISTRATION).

A pharmacokinetic study of NOROXIN in elderly volunteers (65 to 75 years of age with normal renal function for their age) was carried out (see CLINICAL PHARMACOLOGY).

ADVERSE REACTIONS

Single-Dose Studies

In clinical trials involving 82 healthy subjects and 228 patients with gonorrhea, treated with a single dose of norfloxacin, 6.5% reported drug-related adverse experiences. However, the following incidence figures were calculated without reference to drug relationship.

The most common adverse experiences (>1.0%) were: dizziness (2.6%), nausea (2.6%), headache (2.0%), and abdominal cramping (1.6%).

Additional reactions (0.3%–1.0%) were: anorexia, diarrhea, hyperhidrosis, asthenia, anal/rectal pain, constipation, dyspepsia, flatulence, tingling of the fingers, and vomiting.

Laboratory adverse changes considered drug-related were reported in 4.5% of patients/subjects. These laboratory changes were: increased AST (SGOT) (1.6%), decreased WBC (1.3%), decreased platelet count (1.0%), increased urine protein (1.0%), decreased hematocrit and hemoglobin (0.6%), and increased eosinophils (0.6%).

Multiple-Dose Studies

In clinical trials involving 52 healthy subjects and 1980 patients with urinary tract infections or prostatitis treated with multiple doses of norfloxacin, 3.6% reported drug-related adverse experiences. However, the incidence figures below were calculated without reference to drug relationship.

The most common adverse experiences (>1.0%) were: nausea (4.2%), headache (2.8%), dizziness (1.7%), and asthenia (1.3%).

Additional reactions (0.3%–1.0%) were: abdominal pain, back pain, constipation, diarrhea, dry mouth, dyspepsia/heartburn, fever, flatulence, hyperhidrosis, loose stools, pruritus, rash, somnolence, and vomiting.

Less frequent reactions (0.1%–0.2%) included: abdominal swelling, allergies, anorexia, anxiety, bitter taste, blurred vision, bursitis, chest pain, chills, depression, dysmenorrhea, edema, erythema, foot or hand swelling, insomnia, mouth ulcer, myocardial infarction, palpitation, pruritus ani, renal colic, sleep disturbances, and urticaria.

Abnormal laboratory values observed in these patients/subjects were: eosinophilia (1.5%), elevation of ALT (SGPT) (1.4%), decreased WBC and/or neutrophil count (1.4%), elevation of AST (SGOT) (1.4%), and increased alkaline phosphatase (1.1%). Those occurring less frequently included increased BUN, increased LDH, increased serum creatinine, decreased hematocrit, and glycosuria.

Post Marketing

The most frequently reported adverse reaction in postmarketing experience is rash.

CNS effects characterized as generalized seizures, myoclonus and tremors have been reported with NOROXIN (see WARNINGS). Visual disturbances have been reported with drugs in this class.

The following additional adverse reactions have been reported since the drug was marketed:

Hypersensitivity Reactions

Hypersensitivity reactions have been reported including anaphylactoid reactions, angioedema, dyspnea, vasculitis, urticaria, arthritis, arthralgia and myalgia (see WARNINGS).

Skin

Toxic epidermal necrolysis, Stevens-Johnson syndrome and erythema multiforme, exfoliative dermatitis, photosensitivity.

Gastrointestinal

Pseudomembranous colitis, hepatitis, jaundice including cholestatic jaundice and elevated liver function tests, pancreatitis (rare), stomatitis. The onset of pseudomembranous colitis symptoms may occur during or after antibacterial treatment (see WARNINGS).

Cardiovascular

On rare occasions, prolonged QTc interval and ventricular arrhythmia (including torsades de pointes).

Renal

Interstitial nephritis, renal failure.

Nervous System/Psychiatric

Peripheral neuropathy, Guillain-Barré syndrome, ataxia, paresthesia; psychic disturbances including psychotic reactions and confusion.

Musculoskeletal

Tendinitis, tendon rupture; exacerbation of myasthenia gravis (see PRECAUTIONS); elevated creatine kinase (CK).

Hematologic

Neutropenia; leukopenia; agranulocytosis; hemolytic anemia, sometimes associated with glucose-6-phosphate dehydrogenase deficiency; thrombocytopenia.

Special Senses

Hearing loss, tinnitus, diplopia, dysgeusia.

Other adverse events reported with quinolones include: agranulocytosis, albuminuria, candiduria, crystalluria, cylindruria, dysphagia, elevation of blood glucose, elevation of serum cholesterol, elevation of serum potassium, elevation of serum triglycerides, hematuria, hepatic necrosis, symptomatic hypoglycemia, nystagmus, postural hypotension, prolongation of prothrombin time, and vaginal candidiasis.

OVERDOSAGE

No significant lethality was observed in male and female mice and rats at single oral doses up to 4 g/kg.

In the event of acute overdosage, the stomach should be emptied by inducing vomiting or by gastric lavage, and the patient carefully observed and given symptomatic and supportive treatment. Adequate hydration must be maintained.

DOSAGE AND ADMINISTRATION

Tablets NOROXIN should be taken at least one hour before or at least two hours after a meal or ingestion of milk and/or other dairy products. Multivitamins, other products containing iron or zinc, antacids containing magnesium and aluminum, sucralfate, or Videx® (Didanosine), chewable/buffered tablets or the pediatric powder for oral solution, should not be taken within 2 hours of administration of norfloxacin. Tablets NOROXIN should be taken with a glass of water. Patients receiving NOROXIN should be well hydrated (see PRECAUTIONS).

Normal Renal Function

The recommended daily dose of NOROXIN is as described in the following chart:

[See table above]

Renal Impairment

NOROXIN may be used for the treatment of urinary tract infections in patients with renal insufficiency. In patients with a creatinine clearance rate of 30 mL/min/1.73m^2 or less, the recommended dosage is one 400-mg tablet once daily for the duration given above. At this dosage, the urinary concentration exceeds the MICs for most urinary pathogens susceptible to norfloxacin, even when the creatinine clearance is less than 10 mL/min/1.73m^2.

When only the serum creatinine level is available, the following formula (based on sex, weight, and age of the pa-

Continued on next page

Information on the Merck & Co., Inc., products listed on these pages is from the prescribing information in use October 1, 2004. For information, please call 1-800-NSC-MERCK [1-800-672-6372].

Noroxin—Cont.

tient) may be used to convert this value into creatinine clearance. The serum creatinine should represent a steady state of renal function.

Males: $\frac{(\text{weight in kg}) \times (140 - \text{age})}{(72) \times \text{serum creatinine (mg/100 mL)}}$

Females: (0.85) × (above value)

Elderly

Elderly patients being treated for urinary tract infections who have a creatinine clearance of greater than 30 mL/min/1.73m^2 should receive the dosages recommended under *Normal Renal Function*.

Elderly patients being treated for urinary tract infections who have a creatinine clearance of 30 mL/min/1.73m^2 or less should receive 400 mg once daily as recommended under *Renal Impairment*.

HOW SUPPLIED

No. 3522—Tablets NOROXIN 400 mg are dark pink, oval shaped, film-coated tablets, coded MSD 705 on one side and NOROXIN on the other. They are supplied as follows:

NDC 0006-0705-68 bottles of 100

NDC 0006-0705-20 unit of use bottles of 20.

Storage

Store at 25°C (77°F); excursions permitted to 15–30°C (59–86°F) [see USP Controlled Room Temperature]. Keep container tightly closed.

ANIMAL PHARMACOLOGY

Norfloxacin and related drugs have been shown to cause arthropathy in immature animals of most species tested (see WARNINGS).

Crystalluria has occurred in laboratory animals tested with norfloxacin. In dogs, needle-shaped drug crystals were seen in the urine at doses of 50 mg/kg/day. In rats, crystals were reported following doses of 200 mg/kg/day.

Embryo lethality and slight maternotoxicity (vomiting and anorexia) were observed in cynomolgus monkeys at doses of 150 mg/kg/day or higher.

Ocular toxicity, seen with some related drugs, was not observed in any norfloxacin-treated animals.

REFERENCES

1. National Committee for Clinical Laboratory Standards, Methods for dilution antimicrobial susceptibility tests for bacteria that grow aerobically–3rd ed., Approved Standard NCCLS Document M7-A3, Vol. 13, No. 25, NCCLS, Villanova, PA, 1993.
2. National Committee for Clinical Laboratory Standards, Performance standards for antimicrobial disk susceptibility tests–5th ed., Approved Standard NCCLS Document M2-A5, Vol. 13, No. 24, NCCLS, Villanova, PA, 1993.

MERCK & CO., INC., Whitehouse Station, NJ 08889, USA
7898534
Issued March 2004
Printed in USA

Shown in Product Identification Guide, page 323

LIQUID PEDVAXHIB® ℞

[Haemophilus b Conjugate Vaccine (Meningococcal Protein Conjugate)]

DESCRIPTION

PedvaxHIB* [Haemophilus b Conjugate Vaccine (Meningococcal Protein Conjugate)] is a highly purified capsular polysaccharide (polyribosylribitol phosphate or PRP) of *Haemophilus influenzae* type b (Haemophilus b, Ross strain) that is covalently bound to an outer membrane protein complex (OMPC) of the B11 strain of *Neisseria meningitidis* serogroup B. The covalent bonding of the PRP to the OMPC which is necessary for enhanced immunogenicity of the PRP is confirmed by quantitative analysis of the conjugate's components following chemical treatment which yields a unique amino acid. The potency of PedvaxHIB is determined by assay of PRP.

Haemophilus influenzae type b and *Neisseria meningitidis* serogroup B are grown in complex fermentation media. The PRP is purified from the culture broth by purification procedures which include ethanol fractionation, enzyme digestion, phenol extraction and diafiltration. The OMPC from *Neisseria meningitidis* is purified by detergent extraction, ultracentrifugation, diafiltration and sterile filtration.

Liquid PedvaxHIB is ready to use and does not require a diluent. Each 0.5 mL dose of Liquid PedvaxHIB is a sterile product formulated to contain: 7.5 mcg of Haemophilus b PRP, 125 mcg of *Neisseria meningitidis* OMPC and 225 mcg of aluminum as amorphous aluminum hydroxyphosphate sulfate (previously referred to as aluminum hydroxide), in 0.9% sodium chloride, but does not contain lactose or thimerosal. Liquid PedvaxHIB is a slightly opaque white suspension.

This vaccine is for intramuscular administration and not for intravenous injection. (See DOSAGE AND ADMINISTRATION.)

* Registered trademark of MERCK & CO., Inc.

TABLE 1
Antibody Responses in Navajo Infants

Vaccine	No. of Subjects	Time	% Subjects with >0.15 mcg/mL	% Subjects with >1.0 mcg/mL	Anti-PRP GMT (mcg/mL)
Lyophilized PedvaxHIB*	416**	Pre-Vaccination	44	10	0.16
	416	Post-Dose 1	88	52	0.95
	416	Post-Dose 2	91	60	1.43
Placebo*	461**	Pre-Vaccination	44	9	0.16
	461	Post-Dose 1	21	2	0.09
	461	Post-Dose 2	14	1	0.08
Lyophilized PedvaxHIB	27†	Prebooster	70	33	0.51
	27	Postbooster††	100	89	8.39

*Post-Vaccination values obtained approximately 1–3 months after each dose.
**The Protective Efficacy Study
†Immunogenicity Trial
††Booster given at 12 months of age; Post-Vaccination values obtained 1 month after administration of booster dose.

TABLE 2
Antibody Responses to Liquid and Lyophilized PedvaxHIB in Infants From the General U.S. Population

Formulation	Age (Months)	Time	No. of Subjects	% Subjects with anti-PRP >0.15 mcg/mL	% Subjects with anti-PRP >1.0 mcg/mL	Anti-PRP GMT (mcg/mL)
Liquid PedvaxHIB (7.5 mcg PRP)	2–3	Pre-Vaccination	487	32	7	0.12
		Post-Dose 1*	480	94	64	1.55
		Post-Dose 2**	393	97	80	3.22
	12–15	Prebooster	284	80	30	0.49
		Postbooster**	284	99	95	10.23
	24†	Persistence	94	97	55	1.29
Lyophilized PedvaxHIB (15 mcg PRP)	2–3	Pre-Vaccination	171	37	6	0.13
		Post-Dose 1*	169	97	72	1.88
		Post-Dose 2**	133	99	81	2.69
	12–15	Prebooster	87	71	28	0.39
		Postbooster**	87	99	91	7.64
	24†	Persistence	37	97	54	1.10

*Approximately two months Post-Vaccination
**Approximately one month Post-Vaccination
†Approximately

CLINICAL PHARMACOLOGY

Prior to the introduction of Haemophilus b Conjugate Vaccines, *Haemophilus influenzae* type b (Hib) was the most frequent cause of bacterial meningitis and a leading cause of serious, systemic bacterial disease in young children worldwide.

Hib disease occurred primarily in children under 5 years of age in the United States prior to the initiation of a vaccine program and was estimated to account for nearly 20,000 cases of invasive infections annually, approximately 12,000 of which were meningitis. The mortality rate from Hib meningitis is about 5%. In addition, up to 35% of survivors develop neurologic sequelae including seizures, deafness, and mental retardation. Other invasive diseases caused by this bacterium include cellulitis, epiglottitis, sepsis, pneumonia, septic arthritis, osteomyelitis and pericarditis.

Prior to the introduction of the vaccine, it was estimated that 17% of all cases of Hib disease occurred in infants less than 6 months of age. The peak incidence of Hib meningitis occurs between 6 to 11 months of age. Forty-seven percent of all cases occur by one year of age with the remaining 53% of cases occurring over the next four years.

Among children under 5 years of age, the risk of invasive Hib disease is increased in certain populations including the following:

- Daycare attendees
- Lower socio-economic groups
- Blacks (especially those who lack the Km(1) immunoglobulin allotype)
- Caucasians who lack the G2m (n or 23) immunoglobulin allotype
- Native Americans
- Household contacts of cases
- Individuals with asplenia, sickle cell disease, or antibody deficiency syndromes

An important virulence factor of the Hib bacterium is its polysaccharide capsule (PRP). Antibody to PRP (anti-PRP) has been shown to correlate with protection against Hib disease. While the anti-PRP level associated with protection using conjugated vaccines has not yet been determined, the level of anti-PRP associated with protection in studies using bacterial polysaccharide immune globulin or nonconjugated PRP vaccines ranged from >0.15 to >1.0 mcg/mL.

Nonconjugated PRP vaccines are capable of stimulating B-lymphocytes to produce antibody without the help of T-lymphocytes (T-independent). The responses to many other antigens are augmented by helper T-lymphocytes (T-dependent). PedvaxHIB is a PRP-conjugate vaccine in which the PRP is covalently bound to the OMPC carrier producing an antigen which is postulated to convert the T-independent antigen (PRP alone) into a T-dependent antigen resulting in both an enhanced antibody response and immunologic memory.

Clinical Evaluation of PedvaxHIB

PedvaxHIB, in a lyophilized formulation (lyophilized PedvaxHIB), was initially evaluated in 3,486 Native American (Navajo) infants, who completed the primary two-dose regimen in a randomized, double-blind, placebo-controlled study (The Protective Efficacy Study). At the time of the study, this population had a much higher incidence of Hib disease than the United States population as a whole and also had a lower antibody response to Haemophilus b Conjugate Vaccines, including PedvaxHIB.

Each infant in this study received two doses of either placebo or lyophilized PedvaxHIB with the first dose administered at a mean of 8 weeks of age and the second administered approximately two months later; DTP and OPV were administered concomitantly. Antibody levels were measured in a subset of each group (TABLE 1).

[See table 1 above]

Most subjects were initially followed until 15 to 18 months of age. During this time, 22 cases of invasive Hib disease occurred in the placebo group (8 cases after the first dose and 14 cases after the second dose) and only 1 case in the vaccine group (none after the first dose and 1 after the second dose). Following the primary two-dose regimen, the protective efficacy of lyophilized PedvaxHIB was calculated to be 93% with a 95% confidence interval of 57%–98% (p=0.001, two-tailed). In the two months between the first and second doses, the difference in number of cases of disease between placebo and vaccine recipients (8 vs. 0 cases, respectively) was statistically significant (p=0.008, two-tailed); however, a primary two-dose regimen is required for infants 2–14 months of age.

At termination of the study, placebo recipients were offered vaccine. All original participants were then followed two years and nine months from termination of the study. During this extended follow-up, invasive Hib disease occurred in an additional seven of the original placebo recipients prior to receiving vaccine and in one of the original vaccine recipients (who had received only one dose of vaccine). No cases of invasive Hib disease were observed in placebo recipients after they received at least one dose of vaccine. Efficacy for this follow-up period, estimated from person-days at risk, was 96.6% (95 C.I., 72.2–99.9%) in children under 18 months of age and 100% (95 C.I., 23.5–100%) in children over 18 months of age.

Since protective efficacy with lyophilized PedvaxHIB was demonstrated in such a high risk population, it would be expected to be predictive of efficacy in other populations.

The safety and immunogenicity of lyophilized PedvaxHIB were evaluated in infants and children in other clinical studies that were conducted in various locations throughout the United States. PedvaxHIB was highly immunogenic in all age groups studied.

Lyophilized PedvaxHIB induced antibody levels greater than 1.0 mcg/mL in children who were poor responders to nonconjugated PRP vaccines. In a study involving such a subpopulation, 34 children ranging in age from 27 to 61 months who developed invasive Hib disease despite previous vaccination with nonconjugated PRP vaccines were randomly assigned to 2 groups. One group (n=14) was vaccinated with lyophilized PedvaxHIB and the other group (n=20) with a nonconjugated PRP vaccine at a mean interval of approximately 12 months after recovery from disease. All 14 children vaccinated with lyophilized PedvaxHIB but only 6 of 20 children re-vaccinated with a nonconjugated PRP vaccine achieved an antibody level of >1.0 mcg/mL. The 14 children who had not responded to revaccination with the nonconjugated PRP vaccine were then vaccinated with a single dose of lyophilized PedvaxHIB; following this vaccination, all achieved antibody levels of >1.0 mcg/mL.

In addition, lyophilized PedvaxHIB has been studied in children at high risk of Hib disease because of genetically-related deficiencies [Blacks who were Km(1) allotype negative and Caucasians who were G2m(23) allotype negative] and are considered hyporesponsive to nonconjugated PRP vaccines on this basis. The hyporesponsive children had anti-PRP responses comparable to those of allotype positive children of similar age range when vaccinated with lyophilized PedvaxHIB. All children achieved anti-PRP levels of >1.0 mcg/mL.

The safety and immunogenicity of Liquid PedvaxHIB were compared with those of lyophilized PedvaxHIB is a randomized clinical study involving 903 infants 2 to 6 months of age from the general U.S. population. DTP and OPV were administered concomitantly to most subjects. The antibody responses induced by each formulation of PedvaxHIB were similar. TABLE 2 shows antibody responses from this clinical study in subjects who received their first dose at 2 to 3 months of age.

[See table 2 at top of previous page]

A booster dose of PedvaxHIB is required in infants who complete the primary two-dose regimen before 12 months of age. This booster dose will help maintain antibody levels during the first two years of life when children are at highest risk for invasive Hib disease. (See TABLE 2 and DOSAGE AND ADMINISTRATION.)

In four United States studies, antibody responses to lyophilized PedvaxHIB were evaluated in several subpopulations of infants initially vaccinated between 2 to 3 months of age. (See TABLE 3.)

[See table 3 at right]

In two United States studies, antibody responses to Liquid PedvaxHIB were evaluated in several subpopulations of infants initially vaccinated between 2 to 3 months of age. (See TABLE 4.)

[See table 4 at right]

Antibodies to the OMPC of *N. meningitidis* have been demonstrated in vaccinee sera, but the clinical relevance of these antibodies has not been established.

Interchangeability of Licensed Haemophilus b Conjugate Vaccines and PedvaxHIB

Published studies have examined the interchangeability of other licensed Haemophilus b Conjugate Vaccines and PedvaxHIB. According to the American Academy of Pediatrics, excellent immune responses have been achieved when different vaccines have been interchanged in the primary series. If PedvaxHIB is given in a series with one of the other products licensed for infants, the recommended number of doses to complete the series is determined by the other product and not by PedvaxHIB. PedvaxHIB may be interchanged with other licensed Haemophilus b Conjugate Vaccines for the booster dose.

Use with Other Vaccines

Results from clinical studies indicate that Liquid PedvaxHIB can be administered concomitantly with DTP, OPV, eIPV (enhanced inactivated poliovirus vaccine), VARIVAX* [Varicella Virus Vaccine Live (Oka/Merck)], M-M-R* II (Measles, Mumps, and Rubella Virus Vaccine Live) or RECOMBIVAX HB* [Hepatitis B Vaccine (Recombinant)]. No impairment of immune response to individual tested vaccine antigens was demonstrated.

The type, frequency and severity of adverse experiences observed in these studies with PedvaxHIB were similar to those seen when the other vaccines were given alone.

In addition, a PRP-OMPC-containing product, COMVAX* [Haemophilus b Conjugate (Meningococcal Protein Conjugate) and Hepatitis B (Recombinant) Vaccine], was given concomitantly with a booster dose of DTaP [diphtheria, tetanus, acellular pertussis] at approximately 15 months of age, using separate sites and syringes for injectable vaccines. No impairment of immune response to these individually tested vaccine antigens was demonstrated. COMVAX has also been administered concomitantly with the primary series of DTaP to a limited number of infants. PRP antibody responses are satisfactory for COMVAX, but immune responses are currently unavailable for DTaP (see Manufacturer's Product Circular for COMVAX). No serious vaccine-related adverse events were reported.

INDICATIONS AND USAGE

Liquid PedvaxHIB is indicated for routine vaccination against invasive disease caused by *Haemophilus influenzae* type b in infants and children 2 to 71 months of age.

Liquid PedvaxHIB will not protect against disease caused by *Haemophilus influenzae* other than type b or against other microorganisms that cause invasive disease such as meningitis or sepsis. As with any vaccine, vaccination with Liquid PedvaxHIB may not result in a protective antibody response in all individuals given the vaccine.

BECAUSE OF THE POTENTIAL FOR IMMUNE TOLERANCE, Liquid PedvaxHIB IS NOT RECOMMENDED FOR USE IN INFANTS YOUNGER THAN 6 WEEKS OF AGE. (See PRECAUTIONS.)

Revaccination

Infants completing the primary two-dose regimen before 12 months of age should receive a booster dose (see DOSAGE AND ADMINISTRATION).

TABLE 3
Antibody Responses*
After Two Doses of Lyophilized PedvaxHIB Among Infants Initially Vaccinated at 2–3 Months of Age By Racial/Ethnic Group

Racial/Ethnic Groups	No. of Subjects	LYOPHILIZED % Subjects With Anti-PRP >0.15 mcg/mL	>1.0 mcg/mL	Anti-PRP GMT (mcg/mL)
Native American†	54	96	70	2.47
Caucasian	201	99	82	3.52
Hispanic	76	99	88	3.54
Black	23	100	96	5.40

* One month after the second dose
† Apache and Navajo

TABLE 4
Antibody Responses*
After Two Doses of Liquid PedvaxHIB Among Infants Initially Vaccinated at 2–3 Months of Age By Racial/Ethnic Group

Racial/Ethnic Groups	No. of Subjects	LIQUID % Subjects with Anti-PRP >0.15 mcg/mL	>1.0 mcg/mL	Anti-PRP GMT (mcg/mL)
Native American**	90	97	78	2.76
Caucasian	143	94	72	2.16
Hispanic	184	98	85	4.34
Black	18	100	94	7.58

* One month after the second dose
** Apache and Navajo

TABLE 5
Fever or Local Reactions in Subjects First Vaccinated at 2 to 6 Months of Age with Liquid PedvaxHIB*

Reaction	Post-Dose 1: No. of Subjects Evaluated	6 (hr) Percentage	24	48	Post-Dose 2: No. of Subjects Evaluated	6 (hr) Percentage	24	48
Fever** >38.3°C (≥101°F) Rectal	222	18.1	4.4	0.5	206	14.1	9.4	2.8
Erythema >2.5 cm diameter	674	2.2	1.0	0.5	562	1.6	1.1	0.4
Swelling >2.5 cm diameter	674	2.5	1.9	0.9	562	0.9	0.9	1.3

*DTP and OPV were administered concomitantly to most subjects.
**Fever was also measured by another method or reported as normal for an additional 345 infants after dose 1 and for an additional 249 infants after dose 2; however, these data are not included in this table.

CONTRAINDICATIONS

Hypersensitivity to any component of the vaccine or the diluent.

Persons who develop symptoms suggestive of hypersensitivity after an injection should not receive further injections of the vaccine.

PRECAUTIONS

General

As for any vaccine, adequate treatment provisions, including epinephrine, should be available for immediate use should an anaphylactoid reaction occur.

Special care should be taken to ensure that the injection does not enter a blood vessel.

It is important to use a separate sterile syringe and needle for each patient to prevent transmission of hepatitis B or other infectious agents from one person to another.

As with other vaccines, Liquid PedvaxHIB may not induce protective antibody levels immediately following vaccination.

As reported with Haemophilus b Polysaccharide Vaccine and another Haemophilus b Conjugate Vaccine, cases of Hib disease may occur in the week after vaccination, prior to the onset of the protective effects of the vaccines.

There is insufficient evidence that Liquid PedvaxHIB given immediately after exposure to natural *Haemophilus influenzae* type b will prevent illness.

The decision to administer or delay vaccination because of current or recent febrile illness depends on the severity of symptoms and on the etiology of the disease. The Advisory Committee on Immunization Practices (ACIP) has recommended that vaccination should be delayed during the course of an acute febrile illness. All vaccines can be administered to persons with minor illnesses such as diarrhea, mild upper-respiratory infection with or without low-grade fever, or other low-grade febrile illness. Persons with moderate or severe febrile illness should be vaccinated as soon as they have recovered from the acute phase of the illness.

If PedvaxHIB is used in persons with malignancies or those receiving immunosuppressive therapy or who are otherwise immunocompromised, the expected immune response may not be obtained.

Instructions to Healthcare Provider

The healthcare provider should determine the current health status and previous vaccination history of the vaccinee.

The healthcare provider should question the patient, parent, or guardian about reactions to a previous dose of PedvaxHIB or other Haemophilus b Conjugate Vaccines.

Information for Patients

The healthcare provider should provide the vaccine information required to be given with each vaccination to the patient, parent, or guardian.

The healthcare provider should inform the patient, parent, or guardian of the benefits and risks associated with vaccination. For risks associated with vaccination, see ADVERSE REACTIONS.

Patients, parents, and guardians should be instructed to report any serious adverse reactions to their healthcare provider who in turn should report such events to the U.S. Department of Health and Human Services through the Vaccine Adverse Event Reporting System (VAERS), 1-800-822-7967.

Laboratory Test Interactions

Sensitive tests (e.g., Latex Agglutination Kits) may detect PRP derived from the vaccine in urine of some vaccinees for at least 30 days following vaccination with lyophilized PedvaxHIB; in clinical studies with lyophilized PedvaxHIB, such children demonstrated normal immune response to the vaccine.

Carcinogenesis, Mutagenesis, Impairment of Fertility

Liquid PedvaxHIB has not been evaluated for carcinogenic or mutagenic potential, or potential to impair fertility.

Pregnancy

Pregnancy Category C: Animal reproduction studies have not been conducted with PedvaxHIB. Liquid PedvaxHIB is not recommended for use in individuals 6 years of age and older.

Continued on next page

Information on the Merck & Co., Inc., products listed on these pages is from the prescribing information in use October 1, 2004. For information, please call 1-800-NSC-MERCK [1-800-672-6372].

PedvaxHIB—Cont.

Pediatric Use
Safety and effectiveness in infants below the age of 2 months and in children 6 years of age and older have not been established. In addition, Liquid PedvaxHIB should not be used in infants younger than 6 weeks of age because this will lead to a reduced anti-PRP response and may lead to immune tolerance (impaired ability to respond to subsequent exposure to the PRP antigen). Liquid PedvaxHIB is not recommended for use in individuals 6 years of age and older because they are generally not a risk of Hib disease.
Geriatric Use
This vaccine is NOT recommended for use in adult populations.

ADVERSE REACTIONS

Liquid PedvaxHIB
In a multicenter clinical study (n=903) comparing the effects of Liquid PedvaxHIB with those of lyophilized PedvaxHIB, 1,699 doses of Liquid PedvaxHIB were administered to 678 healthy infants 2 to 6 months of age from the general U.S. population. DTP and OPV were administered concomitantly to most subjects. Both formulations of PedvaxHIB were generally well tolerated and no serious vaccine-related adverse reactions were reported.
During a three-day period following primary vaccination with Liquid PedvaxHIB in these infants, the most frequently reported (>1%) adverse reactions, without regard to causality, excluding those shown in TABLE 5, in decreasing order of frequency, were: irritability, sleepiness, injection site pain/soreness, injection site erythema (≤2.5 cm diameter, see also TABLE 5), injection site swelling/induration (≤2.5 cm diameter, see also TABLE 5), unusual high-pitched crying, prolonged crying (>4 hr), diarrhea, vomiting, crying, pain, otitis media, rash, and upper respiratory infection.
Selected objective observations reported by parents over a 48-hour period in these infants following primary vaccination with Liquid PedvaxHIB are summarized in TABLE 5.
[See table 5 on previous page]
Adverse reactions during a three-day period following administration of the booster dose were generally similar in type and frequency to those seen following primary vaccination.
Lyophilized PedvaxHIB
In The Protective Efficacy Study (see CLINICAL PHARMACOLOGY), 4,459 healthy Navajo infants 6 to 12 weeks of age received lyophilized PedvaxHIB or placebo. Most of these infants received DTP/OPV concomitantly. No differences were seen in the type and frequency of serious health problems expected in this Navajo population or in serious adverse experiences reported among those who received lyophilized PedvaxHIB and those who received placebo, and none was reported to be related to lyophilized PedvaxHIB. Only one serious reaction (tracheitis) was reported as possibly related to lyophilized PedvaxHIB and only one (diarrhea) as possibly related to placebo. Seizures occurred infrequently in both groups (9 occurred in vaccine recipients, 8 of whom also received DTP; 8 occurred in placebo recipients, 7 of whom also received DTP) and were not reported to be related to lyophilized PedvaxHIB.
In early clinical studies involving the administration of 8,086 doses of lyophilized PedvaxHIB alone to 5,027 healthy infants and children 2 months to 71 months of age, lyophilized PedvaxHIB was generally well tolerated. No serious adverse reactions were reported. In a subset of these infants, urticaria was reported in two children, and thrombocytopenia was seen in one child. A cause and effect relationship between these side effects and the vaccination has not been established.
Potential Adverse Reactions
The use of Haemophilus b Polysaccharide Vaccines and another Haemophilus b Conjugate Vaccine has been associated with the following additional adverse effects: early onset Hib disease and Guillain-Barré syndrome. A cause and effect relationship between these side effects and the vaccination was not established.
Post-Marketing Adverse Reactions
The following additional adverse reactions have been reported with the use of the lyophilized and liquid formulations of PedvaxHIB:
Hemic and Lymphatic System
Lymphadenopathy
Hypersensitivity
Rarely, angioedema
Nervous System
Febrile seizures
Skin
Sterile injection site abscess

DOSAGE AND ADMINISTRATION

Liquid PedvaxHIB
FOR INTRAMUSCULAR ADMINISTRATION
DO NOT INJECT INTRAVENOUSLY
If there is an interruption or delay between doses in the primary series, there is no need to repeat the series, but dosing should be continued at the next clinic visit. (See CONTRAINDICATIONS and PRECAUTIONS.)
2 to 14 Months of Age
Infants 2 to 14 months of age should receive a 0.5 mL dose of vaccine ideally beginning at 2 months of age followed by a 0.5 mL dose 2 months later (or as soon as possible thereafter). When the primary two-dose regimen is completed before 12 months of age, a booster dose is required (see below and TABLE 6). Infants born prematurely, regardless of birth weight, should be vaccinated at the same chronological age and according to the same schedule and precautions as full-term infants and children.
15 Months of Age and Older
Children 15 months of age and older previously unvaccinated against Hib disease should receive a single 0.5 mL dose of vaccine.
Booster Dose
In infants completing the primary two-dose regimen before 12 months of age, a booster dose (0.5 mL) should be administered at 12 to 15 months of age, but not earlier than 2 months after the second dose.
Vaccination regimens for Liquid PedvaxHIB by age group are outlined in TABLE 6.

TABLE 6
Vaccination Regimens for Liquid PedvaxHIB
By Age Groups

Age (Months) at First Dose	Primary	Age (Months) at Booster Dose
2–10	2 doses, 2 mo. apart	12–15
11–14	2 doses, 2 mo. apart	—
15–71	1 dose	—

Interchangeability
PedvaxHIB may be interchanged with other licensed Haemophilus b Conjugate Vaccines for the primary and booster doses. (See CLINICAL PHARMACOLOGY.)
Use with Other Vaccines
Results from clinical studies indicate that Liquid PedvaxHIB can be administered concomitantly with DTP, OPV, eIPV (enhanced inactivated poliovirus vaccine), VARIVAX [Varicella Virus Vaccine Live (Oka/Merck)], M-M-R II (Measles, Mumps, and Rubella Virus Vaccine Live) or RECOMBIVAX HB [Hepatitis B Vaccine (Recombinant)]. No impairment of immune response to these individually tested vaccine antigens was demonstrated.
The type, frequency and severity of adverse experiences observed in these studies with PedvaxHIB were similar to those seen with other vaccines when given alone. (See CLINICAL PHARMACOLOGY.)
In addition, a PRP-OMPC-containing product, COMVAX [Haemophilus b Conjugate (Meningococcal Protein Conjugate) and Hepatitis B (Recombinant) Vaccine], was given concomitantly with a booster dose of DTaP [diphtheria, tetanus, acellular pertussis] at approximately 15 months of age, using separate sites and syringes for injectable vaccines. No impairment of immune response to these individually tested vaccine antigens was demonstrated. COMVAX has also been administered concomitantly with the primary series of DTaP to a limited number of infants. PRP antibody responses are satisfactory for COMVAX, but immune responses are currently unavailable for DTaP (see Manufacturer's Product Circular for COMVAX). No serious vaccine-related adverse events were reported.
Parenteral drug products should be inspected visually for extraneous particulate matter and discoloration prior to administration whenever solution and container permit.
Liquid PedvaxHIB is a slightly opaque white suspension. (See DESCRIPTION.)
The vaccine should be used as supplied; no reconstitution is necessary.
Shake well before withdrawal and use. Thorough agitation is necessary to maintain suspension of the vaccine.
Inject 0.5 mL intramuscularly, preferably into the anterolateral thigh or the outer aspect of the upper arm. The buttocks should not be used for active vaccination of infants and children, because of the potential risk of injury to the sciatic nerve.

HOW SUPPLIED

Liquid PedvaxHIB is supplied as follows:
No. 4897—A box of 10 single-dose vials of liquid vaccine, **NDC** 0006-4897-00.
Storage
Store vaccine at 2–8°C (34–46°F).
DO NOT FREEZE.

9018902 Issued January 2001

PEPCID® Tablets ℞
(famotidine)

PEPCID® for Oral Suspension ℞
(famotidine)

DESCRIPTION

The active ingredient in PEPCID* (Famotidine), is a histamine H_2-receptor antagonist. Famotidine is *N* ′-(aminosulfonyl) -3- [[[2-[(diaminomethylene)amino] -4- thiazolyl] methyl]thio]propanimidamide. The empirical formula of famotidine is $C_8H_{15}N_7O_2S_3$ and its molecular weight is 337.43. Its structural formula is:

Famotidine is a white to pale yellow crystalline compound that is freely soluble in glacial acetic acid, slightly soluble in methanol, very slightly soluble in water, and practically insoluble in ethanol.
Each tablet for oral administration contains either 20 mg or 40 mg of famotidine and the following inactive ingredients: hydroxypropyl cellulose, hydroxypropyl methylcellulose, iron oxides, magnesium stearate, microcrystalline cellulose, corn starch, talc, titanium dioxide.
Each 5 mL of the oral suspension when prepared as directed contains 40 mg of famotidine and the following inactive ingredients: citric acid, flavors, microcrystalline cellulose and carboxymethylcellulose sodium, sucrose and xanthan gum. Added as preservatives are sodium benzoate 0.1%, sodium methylparaben 0.1%, and sodium propylparaben 0.02%.

*Registered trademark of MERCK & CO., INC.

CLINICAL PHARMACOLOGY IN ADULTS

GI Effects
PEPCID is a competitive inhibitor of histamine H_2-receptors. The primary clinically important pharmacologic activity of PEPCID is inhibition of gastric secretion. Both the acid concentration and volume of gastric secretion are suppressed by PEPCID, while changes in pepsin secretion are proportional to volume output.
In normal volunteers and hypersecretors, PEPCID inhibited basal and nocturnal gastric secretion, as well as secretion stimulated by food and pentagastrin. After oral administration, the onset of the antisecretory effect occurred within one hour; the maximum effect was dose-dependent, occurring within one to three hours. Duration of inhibition of secretion by doses of 20 and 40 mg was 10 to 12 hours.
Single evening oral doses of 20 and 40 mg inhibited basal and nocturnal acid secretion in all subjects; mean nocturnal gastric acid secretion was inhibited by 86% and 94%, respectively, for a period of at least 10 hours. The same doses given in the morning suppressed food-stimulated acid secretion in all subjects. The mean suppression was 76% and 84% respectively 3 to 5 hours after administration, and 25% and 30% respectively 8 to 10 hours after administration. In some subjects who received the 20 mg dose, however, the antisecretory effect was dissipated within 6–8 hours. There was no cumulative effect with repeated doses. The nocturnal intragastric pH was raised by evening doses of 20 and 40 mg of PEPCID to mean values of 5.0 and 6.4, respectively. When PEPCID was given after breakfast, the basal daytime interdigestive pH at 3 and 8 hours after 20 or 40 mg of PEPCID was raised to about 5.
PEPCID had little or no effect on fasting or postprandial serum gastrin levels. Gastric emptying and exocrine pancreatic function were not affected by PEPCID.
Other Effects
Systemic effects of PEPCID in the CNS, cardiovascular, respiratory or endocrine systems were not noted in clinical pharmacology studies. Also, no antiandrogenic effects were noted. (See ADVERSE REACTIONS.) Serum hormone levels, including prolactin, cortisol, thyroxine (T_4), and testosterone, were not altered after treatment with PEPCID.
Pharmacokinetics
PEPCID is incompletely absorbed. The bioavailability of oral doses is 40-45%. PEPCID Tablets and PEPCID for Oral Suspension are bioequivalent. Bioavailability may be slightly increased by food, or slightly decreased by antacids; however, these effects are of no clinical consequence. PEPCID undergoes minimal first-pass metabolism. After oral doses, peak plasma levels occur in 1-3 hours. Plasma levels after multiple doses are similar to those after single doses. Fifteen to 20% of PEPCID in plasma is protein bound. PEPCID has an elimination half-life of 2.5-3.5 hours. PEPCID is eliminated by renal (65-70%) and metabolic (30-35%) routes. Renal clearance is 250-450 mL/min, indicating some tubular excretion. Twenty-five to 30% of an oral dose and 65-70% of an intravenous dose are recovered in the urine as unchanged compound. The only metabolite identified in man is the S-oxide.
There is a close relationship between creatinine clearance values and the elimination half-life of PEPCID. In patients with severe renal insufficiency, i.e., creatinine clearance less than 10 mL/min, the elimination half-life of PEPCID may exceed 20 hours and adjustment of dose or dosing intervals in moderate and severe renal insufficiency may be necessary (see PRECAUTIONS, DOSAGE AND ADMINISTRATION).
In elderly patients, there are no clinically significant age-related changes in the pharmacokinetics of PEPCID. However, in elderly patients with decreased renal function, the clearance of the drug may be decreased (see PRECAUTIONS, *Geriatric Use*).
Clinical Studies
Duodenal Ulcer
In a U.S. multicenter, double-blind study in outpatients with endoscopically confirmed duodenal ulcer, orally administered PEPCID was compared to placebo. As shown in Table 1, 70% of patients treated with PEPCID 40 mg h.s. were healed by week 4.

Table 1
Outpatients with Endoscopically Confirmed Healed Duodenal Ulcers

	PEPCID 40 mg h.s. (N=89)	PEPCID 20 mg b.i.d. (N=84)	Placebo h.s. (N=97)
Week 2	**32%	**38%	17%
Week 4	**70%	**67%	31%

** Statistically significantly different than placebo (p< 0.001)

Patients not healed by week 4 were continued in the study. By week 8, 83% of patients treated with PEPCID had healed versus 45% of patients treated with placebo. The incidence of ulcer healing with PEPCID was significantly higher than with placebo at each time point based on proportion of endoscopically confirmed healed ulcers.

In this study, time to relief of daytime and nocturnal pain was significantly shorter for patients receiving PEPCID than for patients receiving placebo; patients receiving PEPCID also took less antacid than the patients receiving placebo.

Long-Term Maintenance Treatment of Duodenal Ulcers

PEPCID, 20 mg p.o. h.s. was compared to placebo h.s. as maintenance therapy in two double-blind, multicenter studies of patients with endoscopically confirmed healed duodenal ulcers. In the U.S. study the observed ulcer incidence within 12 months in patients treated with placebo was 2.4 times greater than in the patients treated with PEPCID. The 89 patients treated with PEPCID had a cumulative observed ulcer incidence of 23.4% compared to an observed ulcer incidence of 56.6% in the 89 patients receiving placebo (p<0.01). These results were confirmed in an international study where the cumulative observed ulcer incidence within 12 months in the 307 patients treated with PEPCID was 35.7%, compared to an incidence of 75.5% in the 325 patients treated with placebo (p<0.01).

Gastric Ulcer

In both a U.S. and an international multicenter, double-blind study in patients with endoscopically confirmed active benign gastric ulcer, orally administered PEPCID, 40 mg h.s., was compared to placebo h.s. Antacids were permitted during the studies, but consumption was not significantly different between the PEPCID and placebo groups. As shown in Table 2, the incidence of ulcer healing (dropouts counted as unhealed) with PEPCID was statistically significantly better than placebo at weeks 6 and 8 in the U.S. study, and at weeks 4, 6 and 8 in the international study, based on the number of ulcers that healed, confirmed by endoscopy.

Table 2
Patients with Endoscopically Confirmed Healed Gastric Ulcers

	U.S. Study		International Study	
	PEPCID 40 mg h.s. (N=74)	Placebo h.s. (N=75)	PEPCID 40 mg h.s. (N=149)	Placebo h.s. (N=145)
Week 4	45%	39%	†47%	31%
Week 6	†66%	44%	†65%	46%
Week 8	***78%	64%	†80%	54%

***† Statistically significantly better than placebo (p≤0.05, p≤0.01 respectively)

Time to complete relief of daytime and nighttime pain was statistically significantly shorter for patients receiving PEPCID than for patients receiving placebo; however, in neither study was there a statistically significant difference in the proportion of patients whose pain was relieved by the end of the study (week 8).

Gastroesophageal Reflux Disease (GERD)

Orally administered PEPCID was compared to placebo in a U.S. study that enrolled patients with symptoms of GERD and without endoscopic evidence of erosion or ulceration of the esophagus. PEPCID 20 mg b.i.d. was statistically significantly superior to 40 mg h.s. and to placebo in providing a successful symptomatic outcome, defined as moderate or excellent improvement of symptoms (Table 3).

Table 3
% Successful Symptomatic Outcome

	PEPCID 20 mg b.i.d. (N=154)	PEPCID 40 mg h.s. (N=149)	Placebo (N=73)
Week 6	82††	69	62

†† p≤0.01) vs Placebo

By two weeks of treatment, symptomatic success was observed in a greater percentage of patients taking PEPCID 20 mg b.i.d. compared to placebo (p≤0.01).

Symptomatic improvement and healing of endoscopically verified erosion and ulceration were studied in two additional trials. Healing was defined as complete resolution of all erosions or ulcerations visible with endoscopy. The U.S. study comparing PEPCID 40 mg p.o. b.i.d. to placebo and PEPCID 20 mg p.o. b.i.d. showed a significantly greater percentage of healing for PEPCID 40 mg b.i.d. at weeks 6 and 12 (Table 4).

Table 6
Pharmacokinetic Parameters[a] of Intravenous Famotidine

Age (N=number of patients)	Area Under the Curve (AUC) (ng-hr/mL)	Total Clearance (Cl) (L/hr/kg)	Volume of Distribution (V_d) (L/kg)	Elimination Half-life (T½) (hours)
0-1 month[c] (N=10)	NA	0.13 ± 0.06	1.4 ± 0.4	10.5 ± 5.4
0-3 months[d] (N=6)	2688 ± 847	0.21 ± 0.06	1.8 ± 0.3	8.1 ± 3.5
>3-12 months[d] (N=11)	1160 ± 474	0.49 ± 0.17	2.3 ± 0.7	4.5 ± 1.1
1-11 yrs (N=20)	1089 ± 834	0.54 ± 0.34	2.07 ± 1.49	3.38 ± 2.60
11-15 yrs (N=6)	1140 ± 320	0.48 ± 0.14	1.5 ± 0.4	2.3 ± 0.4
Adult (N=16)	1726[b]	0.39 ± 0.14	1.3 ± 0.2	2.83 ± 0.99

[a]Values are presented as means ± SD unless indicated otherwise.
[b]Mean value only.
[c]Single center study.
[d]Multicenter study.

Table 4
% Endoscopic Healing—U.S. Study

	PEPCID 40 mg b.i.d. (N=127)	PEPCID 20 mg b.i.d. (N=125)	Placebo (N=66)
Week 6	48†††,‡‡	32	18
Week 12	69†††,‡	54†††	29

††† p≤0.01 vs Placebo
‡ p≤0.05 vs PEPCID 20 mg b.i.d.
‡‡ p≤0.01 vs PEPCID 20 mg b.i.d.

As compared to placebo, patients who received PEPCID had faster relief of daytime and nighttime heartburn and a greater percentage of patients experienced complete relief of nighttime heartburn. These differences were statistically significant.

In the international study, when PEPCID 40 mg p.o. b.i.d. was compared to ranitidine 150 mg p.o. b.i.d., a statistically significantly greater percentage of healing was observed with PEPCID 40 mg b.i.d. at week 12 (Table 5). There was, however, no significant difference among treatments in symptom relief.

Table 5
% Endoscopic Healing—International Study

	PEPCID 40 mg b.i.d. (N=175)	PEPCID 20 mg b.i.d. (N=93)	Ranitidine 150 mg b.i.d. (N=172)
Week 6	48	52	42
Week 12	71‡‡‡	68	60

‡‡‡ p≤0.05 vs Ranitidine 150 mg b.i.d.

Pathological Hypersecretory Conditions (e.g., Zollinger-Ellison Syndrome, Multiple Endocrine Adenomas)

In studies of patients with pathological hypersecretory conditions such as Zollinger-Ellison Syndrome with or without multiple endocrine adenomas, PEPCID significantly inhibited gastric acid secretion and controlled associated symptoms. Orally administered doses from 20 to 160 mg q 6 h maintained basal acid secretion below 10 mEq/hr; initial doses were titrated to the individual patient need and subsequent adjustments were necessary with time in some patients. PEPCID was well tolerated at these high dose levels for prolonged periods (greater than 12 months) in eight patients, and there were no cases reported of gynecomastia, increased prolactin levels, or impotence which were considered to be due to the drug.

CLINICAL PHARMACOLOGY IN PEDIATRIC PATIENTS

Pharmacokinetics

Table 6 presents pharmacokinetic data from clinical trials and a published study in pediatric patients (<1 year of age; N=27) given famotidine I.V. 0.5 mg/kg and from published studies of small numbers of pediatric patients (1-15 years of age) given famotidine intravenously. Areas under the curve (AUCs) are normalized to a dose of 0.5 mg/kg I.V. for pediatric patients 1-15 years of age and compared with an extrapolated 40 mg intravenous dose in adults (extrapolation based on results obtained with a 20 mg I.V. adult dose).

[See table 6 above]

Plasma clearance is reduced and elimination half-life is prolonged in pediatric patients 0-3 months of age compared to older pediatric patients. The pharmacokinetic parameters for pediatric patients, ages >3 months-15 years, are comparable to those obtained for adults.

Bioavailability studies of 8 pediatric patients (11-15 years of age) showed a mean oral bioavailability of 0.5 compared to adult values of 0.42 to 0.49. Oral doses of 0.5 mg/kg achieved AUCs of 645 ± 249 ng-hr/mL and 580 ± 60 ng-hr/mL in pediatric patients <1 year of age (N=5) and in pediatric patients 11-15 years of age, respectively, compared to 482 ± 181 ng-hr/mL in adults treated with 40 mg orally.

Pharmacodynamics

Pharmacodynamics of famotidine were evaluated in 5 pediatric patients 2-13 years of age using the sigmoid E_{max} model. These data suggest that the relationship between serum concentration of famotidine and gastric acid suppression is similar to that observed in one study of adults (Table 7).

Table 7
Pharmacodynamics of famotidine using the sigmoid E_{max} model

	EC_{50} (ng/mL)*
Pediatric Patients	26 ± 13
Data from one study	
a) healthy adult subjects	26.5 ± 10.3
b) adult patients with upper GI bleeding	18.7 ± 10.8

*Serum concentration of famotidine associated with 50% maximum gastric acid reduction. Values are presented as means ± SD.

Five published studies (Table 8) examined the effect of famotidine on gastric pH and duration of acid suppression in pediatric patients. While each study had a different design, acid suppression data over time are summarized as follows:

[See table 8 at top of next page]

The duration of effect of famotidine I.V. 0.5 mg/kg on gastric pH and acid suppression was shown in one study to be longer in pediatric patients <1 month of age than in older pediatric patients. This longer duration of gastric acid suppression is consistent with the decreased clearance in pediatric patients <3 months of age (see Table 6).

INDICATIONS AND USAGE

PEPCID is indicated in:

1. *Short term treatment of active duodenal ulcer.* Most adult patients heal within 4 weeks; there is rarely reason to use PEPCID at full dosage for longer than 6 to 8 weeks. Studies have not assessed the safety of famotidine in uncomplicated active duodenal ulcer for periods of more than eight weeks.
2. *Maintenance therapy for duodenal ulcer patients at reduced dosage after healing of an active ulcer.* Controlled studies in adults have not extended beyond one year.
3. *Short term treatment of active benign gastric ulcer.* Most adult patients heal within 6 weeks. Studies have not assessed the safety or efficacy of famotidine in uncomplicated active benign gastric ulcer for periods of more than 8 weeks.
4. *Short term treatment of gastroesophageal reflux disease (GERD).* PEPCID is indicated for short term treatment of patients with symptoms of GERD (see CLINICAL PHARMACOLOGY IN ADULTS, *Clinical Studies*).
   PEPCID is also indicated for the short term treatment of esophagitis due to GERD including erosive or ulcerative disease diagnosed by endoscopy (see CLINICAL PHARMACOLOGY IN ADULTS, *Clinical Studies*).
5. *Treatment of pathological hypersecretory conditions (e.g., Zollinger-Ellison Syndrome, multiple endocrine adenomas)* (see CLINICAL PHARMACOLOGY IN ADULTS, *Clinical Studies*).

CONTRAINDICATIONS

Hypersensitivity to any component of these products. Cross sensitivity in this class of compounds has been observed. Therefore, PEPCID should not be administered to patients with a history of hypersensitivity to other H_2-receptor antagonists.

PRECAUTIONS

General

Symptomatic response to therapy with PEPCID does not preclude the presence of gastric malignancy.

Patients with Moderate or Severe Renal Insufficiency

Since CNS adverse effects have been reported in patients with moderate and severe renal insufficiency, longer intervals between doses or lower doses may need to be used in patients with moderate (creatinine clearance <50 mL/min)

Continued on next page

Information on the Merck & Co., Inc., products listed on these pages is from the prescribing information in use October 1, 2004. For information, please call 1-800-NSC-MERCK [1-800-672-6372].

Pepcid—Cont.

Table 8

Dosage	Route	Effect[a]	Number of Patients (age range)
0.5 mg/kg, single dose	I.V.	gastric pH >4 for 19.5 hours (17.3, 21.8)[c]	11 (5-19 days)
0.3 mg/kg, single dose	I.V.	gastric pH >3.5 for 8.7 ± 4.7[b] hours	6 (2-7 years)
0.4-0.8 mg/kg	I.V.	gastric pH >4 for 6-9 hours	18 (2-69 months)
0.5 mg/kg, single dose	I.V.	a >2 pH unit increase above baseline in gastric pH for >8 hours	9 (2-13 years)
0.5 mg/kg b.i.d.	I.V.	gastric pH >5 for 13.5 ± 1.8[b] hours	4 (6-15 years)
0.5 mg/kg b.i.d.	oral	gastric pH >5 for 5.0 ± 1.1[b] hours	4 (11-15 years)

[a]Values reported in published literature.
[b]Means ± SD.
[c]Mean (95% confidence interval).

or severe (creatinine clearance <10 mL/min) renal insufficiency to adjust for the longer elimination half-life of famotidine (see CLINICAL PHARMACOLOGY IN ADULTS and DOSAGE AND ADMINISTRATION).

Information for Patients

The patient should be instructed to shake the oral suspension vigorously for 5-10 seconds prior to each use. Unused constituted oral suspension should be discarded after 30 days.

Drug Interactions

No drug interactions have been identified. Studies with famotidine in man, in animal models, and *in vitro* have shown no significant interference with the disposition of compounds metabolized by the hepatic microsomal enzymes, e.g., cytochrome P450 system. Compounds tested in man include warfarin, theophylline, phenytoin, diazepam, aminopyrine and antipyrine. Indocyanine green as an index of hepatic drug extraction has been tested and no significant effects have been found.

Carcinogenesis, Mutagenesis, Impairment of Fertility

In a 106 week study in rats and a 92 week study in mice given oral doses of up to 2000 mg/kg/day (approximately 2500 times the recommended human dose for active duodenal ulcer), there was no evidence of carcinogenic potential for PEPCID.

Famotidine was negative in the microbial mutagen test (Ames test) using *Salmonella typhimurium* and *Escherichia coli* with or without rat liver enzyme activation at concentrations up to 10,000 mcg/plate. In *in vivo* studies in mice, with a micronucleus test and a chromosomal aberration test, no evidence of a mutagenic effect was observed.

In studies with rats given oral doses of up to 2000 mg/kg/day or intravenous doses of up to 200 mg/kg/day, fertility and reproductive performance were not affected.

Pregnancy

Pregnancy Category B

Reproductive studies have been performed in rats and rabbits at oral doses of up to 2000 and 500 mg/kg/day respectively and in both species at I.V. doses of up to 200 mg/kg/day, and have revealed no significant evidence of impaired fertility or harm to the fetus due to PEPCID. While no direct fetotoxic effects have been observed, sporadic abortions occurring only in mothers displaying marked decreased food intake were seen in some rabbits at oral doses of 200 mg/kg/day (250 times the usual human dose) or higher. There are, however, no adequate or well-controlled studies in pregnant women. Because animal reproductive studies are not always predictive of human response, this drug should be used during pregnancy only if clearly needed.

Nursing Mothers

Studies performed in lactating rats have shown that famotidine is secreted into breast milk. Transient growth depression was observed in young rats suckling from mothers treated with maternotoxic doses of at least 600 times the usual human dose. Famotidine is detectable in human milk. Because of the potential for serious adverse reactions in nursing infants from PEPCID, a decision should be made whether to discontinue nursing or discontinue the drug, taking into account the importance of the drug to the mother.

Pediatric Patients <1 year of age

Use of PEPCID in pediatric patients <1 year of age is supported by evidence from adequate and well-controlled studies of PEPCID in adults, and by the following studies in pediatric patients <1 year of age.

Two pharmacokinetic studies in pediatric patients <1 year of age (N=48) demonstrated that clearance of famotidine in patients >3 months to 1 year of age is similar to that seen in older pediatric patients (1-15 years of age) and adults. In contrast, pediatric patients 0-3 months of age had famotidine clearance values that were 2- to 4-fold less than those in older pediatric patients and adults. These studies also show that the mean bioavailability in pediatric patients <1 year of age after oral dosing is similar to older pediatric patients and adults. Pharmacodynamic data in pediatric patients 0-3 months of age suggest that the duration of acid suppression is longer compared with older pediatric patients, consistent with the longer famotidine half-life in pediatric patients 0-3 months of age. (See CLINICAL PHARMACOLOGY IN PEDIATRIC PATIENTS, *Pharmacokinetics* and *Pharmacodynamics*.)

In a double-blind, randomized, treatment-withdrawal study, 35 pediatric patients <1 year of age who were diagnosed as having gastroesophageal reflux disease were treated for up to 4 weeks with famotidine oral suspension (0.5 mg/kg/dose or 1 mg/kg/dose). Although an intravenous famotidine formulation was available, no patients were treated with intravenous famotidine in this study. Also, caregivers were instructed to provide conservative treatment including thickened feedings. Enrolled patients were diagnosed primarily by history of vomiting (spitting up) and irritability (fussiness). The famotidine dosing regimen was once daily for patients <3 months of age and twice daily for patients ≥3 months of age. After 4 weeks of treatment, patients were randomly withdrawn from the treatment and followed an additional 4 weeks for adverse events and symptomatology. Patients were evaluated for vomiting (spitting up), irritability (fussiness) and global assessments of improvement. The study patients ranged in age at entry from 1.3 to 10.5 months (mean 5.6 ± 2.9 months), 57% were female, 91% were white and 6% were black. Most patients (27/35) continued into the treatment-withdrawal phase of the study. Two patients discontinued famotidine due to adverse events. Most patients improved during the initial treatment phase of the study. Results of the treatment-withdrawal phase were difficult to interpret because of small numbers of patients. Of the 35 patients enrolled in the study, agitation was observed in 5 patients on famotidine that resolved when the medication was discontinued; agitation was not observed in patients on placebo (see ADVERSE REACTIONS, *Pediatric Patients*).

These studies suggest that a starting dose of 0.5 mg/kg/dose of famotidine oral suspension may be of benefit for the treatment of GERD for up to 4 weeks once daily in patients <3 months of age and twice daily in patients 3 months to <1 year of age; the safety and benefit of famotidine treatment beyond 4 weeks have not been established. Famotidine should be considered for the treatment of GERD only if conservative measures (e.g., thickened feedings) are used concurrently and if the potential benefit outweighs the risk.

Pediatric Patients 1-16 years of age

Use of PEPCID in pediatric patients 1-16 years of age is supported by evidence from adequate and well-controlled studies of PEPCID in adults, and by the following studies in pediatric patients: In published studies in small numbers of pediatric patients 1-15 years of age, clearance of famotidine was similar to that seen in adults. In pediatric patients 11-15 years of age, oral doses of 0.5 mg/kg were associated with a mean area under the curve (AUC) similar to that seen in adults treated orally with 40 mg. Similarly, in pediatric patients 1-15 years of age, intravenous doses of 0.5 mg/kg were associated with a mean AUC similar to that seen in adults treated intravenously with 40 mg. Limited published studies also suggest that the relationship between serum concentration and acid suppression is similar in pediatric patients 1-15 years of age as compared with adults. These studies suggest a starting dose for pediatric patients 1-16 years of age as follows:

Peptic ulcer—0.5 mg/kg/day p.o. at bedtime or divided b.i.d. up to 40 mg/day.

Gastroesophageal Reflux Disease with or without esophagitis including erosions and ulcerations—1.0 mg/kg/day p.o. divided b.i.d. up to 40 mg b.i.d.

While published uncontrolled studies suggest effectiveness of famotidine in the treatment of gastroesophageal reflux disease and peptic ulcer, data in pediatric patients are insufficient to establish percent response with dose and duration of therapy. Therefore, treatment duration (initially based on adult duration recommendations) and dose should be individualized based on clinical response and/or pH determination (gastric or esophageal) and endoscopy. Published uncontrolled clinical studies in pediatric patients have employed doses up to 1 mg/kg/day for peptic ulcer and 2 mg/kg/day for GERD with or without esophagitis including erosions and ulcerations.

Geriatric Use

Of the 4,966 subjects in clinical studies who were treated with famotidine, 488 subjects (9.8%) were 65 and older, and 88 subjects (1.7%) were greater than 75 years of age. No overall differences in safety or effectiveness were observed between these subjects and younger subjects. However, greater sensitivity of some older individuals cannot be ruled out.

No dosage adjustment is required based on age (see CLINICAL PHARMACOLOGY IN ADULTS, *Pharmacokinetics*). This drug is known to be substantially excreted by the kidney, and the risk of toxic reactions to this drug may be greater in patients with impaired renal function. Because elderly patients are more likely to have decreased renal function, care should be taken in dose selection, and it may be useful to monitor renal function. Dosage adjustment in the case of moderate or severe renal impairment is necessary (see PRECAUTIONS, *Patients with Moderate or Severe Renal Insufficiency* and DOSAGE AND ADMINISTRATION, *Dosage Adjustment for Patients with Moderate or Severe Renal Insufficiency*).

ADVERSE REACTIONS

The adverse reactions listed below have been reported during domestic and international clinical trials in approximately 2500 patients. In those controlled clinical trials in which PEPCID Tablets were compared to placebo, the incidence of adverse experiences in the group which received PEPCID Tablets, 40 mg at bedtime, was similar to that in the placebo group.

The following adverse reactions have been reported to occur in more than 1% of patients on therapy with PEPCID in controlled clinical trials, and may be causally related to the drug: headache (4.7%), dizziness (1.3%), constipation (1.2%) and diarrhea (1.7%).

The following other adverse reactions have been reported infrequently in clinical trials or since the drug was marketed. The relationship to therapy with PEPCID has been unclear in many cases. Within each category the adverse reactions are listed in order of decreasing severity:

Body as a Whole: fever, asthenia, fatigue

Cardiovascular: arrhythmia, AV block, palpitation

Gastrointestinal: cholestatic jaundice, liver enzyme abnormalities, vomiting, nausea, abdominal discomfort, anorexia, dry mouth

Hematologic: rare cases of agranulocytosis, pancytopenia, leukopenia, thrombocytopenia

Hypersensitivity: anaphylaxis, angioedema, orbital or facial edema, urticaria, rash, conjunctival injection

Musculoskeletal: musculoskeletal pain including muscle cramps, arthralgia

Nervous System/Psychiatric: grand mal seizure; psychic disturbances, which were reversible in cases for which follow-up was obtained, including hallucinations, confusion, agitation, depression, anxiety, decreased libido; paresthesia; insomnia; somnolence

Respiratory: bronchospasm

Skin: toxic epidermal necrolysis (very rare), alopecia, acne, pruritus, dry skin, flushing

Special Senses: tinnitus, taste disorder

Other: rare cases of impotence and rare cases of gynecomastia have been reported; however, in controlled clinical trials, the incidences were not greater than those seen with placebo.

The adverse reactions reported for PEPCID Tablets may also occur with PEPCID for Oral Suspension.

Pediatric Patients

In a clinical study in 35 pediatric patients <1 year of age with GERD symptoms [e.g., vomiting (spitting up), irritability (fussing)], agitation was observed in 5 patients on famotidine that resolved when the medication was discontinued.

OVERDOSAGE

There is no experience to date with deliberate overdosage. Oral doses of up to 640 mg/day have been given to adult patients with pathological hypersecretory conditions with no serious adverse effects. In the event of overdosage, treatment should be symptomatic and supportive. Unabsorbed material should be removed from the gastrointestinal tract, the patient should be monitored, and supportive therapy should be employed.

The oral LD_{50} of famotidine in male and female rats and mice was greater than 3000 mg/kg and the minimum lethal acute oral dose in dogs exceeded 2000 mg/kg. Famotidine did not produce overt effects at high oral doses in mice, rats, cats and dogs, but induced significant anorexia and growth depression in rabbits starting with 200 mg/kg/day orally. The intravenous LD_{50} of famotidine for mice and rats ranged from 254–563 mg/kg and the minimum lethal single I.V. dose in dogs was approximately 300 mg/kg. Signs of acute intoxication in I.V. treated dogs were emesis, restlessness, pallor of mucous membranes or redness of mouth and ears, hypotension, tachycardia and collapse.

DOSAGE AND ADMINISTRATION

Duodenal Ulcer

Acute Therapy: The recommended adult oral dosage for active duodenal ulcer is 40 mg once a day at bedtime. Most patients heal within 4 weeks; there is rarely reason to use PEPCID at full dosage for longer than 6 to 8 weeks. A regimen of 20 mg b.i.d. is also effective.

Maintenance Therapy: The recommended adult oral dose is 20 mg once a day at bedtime.

Benign Gastric Ulcer

Acute Therapy: The recommended adult oral dosage for active benign gastric ulcer is 40 mg once a day at bedtime.

Gastroesophageal Reflux Disease (GERD)

The recommended oral dosage for treatment of adult patients with symptoms of GERD is 20 mg b.i.d. for up to 6 weeks. The recommended oral dosage for the treatment of adult patients with esophagitis including erosions and ulcerations and accompanying symptoms due to GERD is 20 or 40 mg b.i.d. for up to 12 weeks (see CLINICAL PHARMACOLOGY IN ADULTS, *Clinical Studies*).

Dosage for Pediatric Patients <1 year of age Gastroesophageal Reflux Disease (GERD)

See PRECAUTIONS, *Pediatric Patients <1 year of age*.

The studies described in PRECAUTIONS, *Pediatric Patients <1 year of age* suggest the following starting doses in pediatric patients <1 year of age: *Gastroesophageal Reflux Disease (GERD)* - 0.5 mg/kg/dose of famotidine oral suspension for the treatment of GERD for up to 8 weeks once daily in patients <3 months of age and 0.5 mg/kg/dose twice daily in patients 3 months to <1 year of age. Patients should also be receiving conservative measures (e.g., thickened feedings). The use of intravenous famotidine in pediatric patients <1 year of age with GERD has not been adequately studied.

Dosage for Pediatric Patients 1-16 years of age

See PRECAUTIONS, *Pediatric Patients 1-16 years of age*. The studies described in PRECAUTIONS, *Pediatric Patients 1-16 years of age* suggest the following starting doses in pediatric patients 1-16 years of age:

Peptic ulcer—0.5 mg/kg/day p.o. at bedtime or divided b.i.d. up to 40 mg/day.

Gastroesophageal Reflux Disease with or without esophagitis including erosions and ulcerations—1.0 mg/kg/day p.o. divided b.i.d. up to 40 mg b.i.d.

While published uncontrolled studies suggest effectiveness of famotidine in the treatment of gastroesophageal reflux disease and peptic ulcer, data in pediatric patients *1-16 years of age* are insufficient to establish percent response with dose and duration of therapy. Therefore, treatment duration (initially based on adult duration recommendations) and dose should be individualized based on clinical response and/or pH determination (gastric or esophageal) and endoscopy. Published uncontrolled clinical studies in pediatric patients 1-16 years of age have employed doses up to 1 mg/kg/day for peptic ulcer and 2 mg/kg/day for GERD with or without esophagitis including erosions and ulcerations.

Pathological Hypersecretory Conditions (e.g., Zollinger-Ellison Syndrome, Multiple Endocrine Adenomas)

The dosage of PEPCID in patients with pathological hypersecretory conditions varies with the individual patient. The recommended adult oral starting dose for pathological hypersecretory conditions is 20 mg q 6 h. In some patients, a higher starting dose may be required. Doses should be adjusted to individual patient needs and should continue as long as clinically indicated. Doses up to 160 mg q 6 h have been administered to some adult patients with severe Zollinger-Ellison Syndrome.

Oral Suspension

PEPCID Oral Suspension may be substituted for PEPCID Tablets in any of the above indications. Each five mL contains 40 mg of famotidine after constitution of the powder with 46 mL of Purified Water as directed.

Directions for Preparing PEPCID Oral Suspension

Prepare suspension at time of dispensing. Slowly add 46 mL of Purified Water. Shake vigorously for 5–10 seconds immediately after adding the water and immediately before use.

Stability of PEPCID for Oral Suspension

Unused constituted oral suspension should be discarded after 30 days.

Concomitant Use of Antacids

Antacids may be given concomitantly if needed.

Dosage Adjustment for Patients with Moderate or Severe Renal Insufficiency

In adult patients with moderate (creatinine clearance <50 mL/min) or severe (creatinine clearance <10 mL/min) renal insufficiency, the elimination half-life of PEPCID is increased. For patients with severe renal insufficiency, it may exceed 20 hours, reaching approximately 24 hours in anuric patients. Since CNS adverse effects have been reported in patients with moderate and severe renal insufficiency, to avoid excess accumulation of the drug in patients with moderate or severe renal insufficiency, the dose of PEPCID may be reduced to half the dose or the dosing interval may be prolonged to 36–48 hours as indicated by the patient's clinical response.

Based on the comparison of pharmacokinetic parameters for PEPCID in adults and pediatric patients, dosage adjustment in pediatric patients with moderate or severe renal insufficiency should be considered.

HOW SUPPLIED

No. 3535—PEPCID Tablets, 20 mg, are beige colored, U-shaped, film-coated tablets coded MSD 963 on one side and PEPCID on the other. They are supplied as follows:

NDC 0006-0963-31 unit of use bottles of 30
NDC 0006-0963-94 unit of use bottles of 90
NDC 0006-0963-58 unit of use bottles of 100
NDC 0006-0963-28 unit dose package of 100
NDC 0006-0963-82 bottles of 1,000
NDC 0006-0963-87 bottles of 10,000
NDC 0006-0963-72 carton of 25 UNIBLISTER™ cards of 31 tablets each.

No. 3536—PEPCID Tablets, 40 mg, are light brownish-orange, U-shaped, film-coated tablets coded MSD 964 on one side and PEPCID on the other. They are supplied as follows:

NDC 0006-0964-31 unit of use bottles of 30
NDC 0006-0964-94 unit of use bottles of 90
NDC 0006-0964-58 unit of use bottles of 100
NDC 0006-0964-28 unit dose package of 100
NDC 0006-0964-82 bottles of 1,000
NDC 0006-0964-87 bottles of 10,000
NDC 0006-0964-72 carton of 25 UNIBLISTER™ cards of 31 tablets each.

No. 3538—PEPCID for Oral Suspension is a white to off-white powder containing 400 mg of famotidine for constitution. When constituted as directed, PEPCID for Oral Suspension is a smooth, mobile, off-white, homogeneous suspension with a cherry-banana-mint flavor, containing 40 mg of famotidine per 5 mL.

NDC 0006-3538-92, bottles containing 400 mg famotidine.

Storage

Store PEPCID Tablets at 25°C (77°F); excursions permitted to 15-30°C (59-86°F) [see USP Controlled Room Temperature].

Store PEPCID for Oral Suspension dry powder and suspension at 25°C (77°F); excursions permitted to 15-30°C (59-86°F) [see USP Controlled Room Temperature]. Suspension: Protect from freezing. Discard unused suspension after 30 days.

7825036 Issued June 2002

Shown in Product Identification Guide, page 323

PEPCID® Injection Premixed (Famotidine) ℞

PEPCID® Injection (Famotidine) ℞

DESCRIPTION

The active ingredient in PEPCID* (Famotidine) Injection Premixed and PEPCID (famotidine) Injection is a histamine H_2-receptor antagonist. Famotidine is *N*′-(aminosulfonyl)-3-[[[2-[(diaminomethylene)amino]-4-thiazolyl]methyl]thio]-propanimidamide. The empirical formula of famotidine is $C_8H_{15}N_7O_2S_3$ and its molecular weight is 337.43. Its structural formula is:

Famotidine is a white to pale yellow crystalline compound that is freely soluble in glacial acetic acid, slightly soluble in methanol, very slightly soluble in water, and practically insoluble in ethanol.

PEPCID Injection Premixed is supplied as a sterile solution, for intravenous use only, in plastic single dose containers. Each 50 mL of the premixed, iso-osmotic intravenous injection contains 20 mg famotidine, USP, and the following inactive ingredients: L-aspartic acid 6.8 mg, sodium chloride, USP, 450 mg, and Water for Injection. The pH ranges from 5.7 to 6.4 and may have been adjusted with additional L-aspartic acid or with sodium hydroxide.

The plastic container is fabricated from a specially designed multi-layer plastic (PL 2501). Solutions are in contact with the polyethylene layer of the container and can leach out certain chemical components of the plastic in very small amounts within the expiration period. The suitability and safety of the plastic have been confirmed in tests in animals according to the USP biological tests for plastic containers, as well as by tissue culture toxicity studies.

PEPCID (famotidine) Injection is supplied as a sterile concentrated solution for intravenous injection. Each mL of the solution contains 10 mg of famotidine and the following inactive ingredients: L-aspartic acid 4 mg, mannitol 20 mg, and Water for Injection q.s. 1 mL. The multidose injection also contains benzyl alcohol 0.9% added as preservative.

*Registered trademark of MERCK & CO., INC.

CLINICAL PHARMACOLOGY IN ADULTS

GI Effects

PEPCID is a competitive inhibitor of histamine H_2-receptors. The primary clinically important pharmacologic activity of PEPCID is inhibition of gastric secretion. Both the acid concentration and volume of gastric secretion are suppressed by PEPCID, while changes in pepsin secretion are proportional to volume output.

In normal volunteers and hypersecretors, PEPCID inhibited basal and nocturnal gastric secretion, as well as secretion stimulated by food and pentagastrin. After oral administration, the onset of the antisecretory effect occurred within one hour; the maximum effect was dose-dependent, occurring within one to three hours. Duration of inhibition of secretion by doses of 20 and 40 mg was 10 to 12 hours.

After intravenous administration, the maximum effect was achieved within 30 minutes. Single intravenous doses of 10 and 20 mg inhibited nocturnal secretion for a period of 10 to 12 hours. The 20 mg dose was associated with the longest duration of action in most subjects.

Single evening oral doses of 20 and 40 mg inhibited basal and nocturnal acid secretion in all subjects; mean nocturnal gastric acid secretion was inhibited by 86% and 94%, respectively, for a period of at least 10 hours. The same doses given in the morning suppressed food-stimulated acid secretion in all subjects. The mean suppression was 76% and 84% respectively, 3 to 5 hours after administration, and 25% and 30%, respectively, 8 to 10 hours after administration. In some subjects who received the 20 mg dose, however, the antisecretory effect was dissipated within 6-8 hours. There was no cumulative effect with repeated doses. The nocturnal intragastric pH was raised by evening doses of 20 and 40 mg of PEPCID to mean values of 5.0 and 6.4, respectively. When PEPCID was given after breakfast, the basal daytime interdigestive pH at 3 and 8 hours after 20 or 40 mg of PEPCID was raised to about 5.

PEPCID had little or no effect on fasting or postprandial serum gastrin levels. Gastric emptying and exocrine pancreatic function were not affected by PEPCID.

Other Effects

Systemic effects of PEPCID in the CNS, cardiovascular, respiratory or endocrine systems were not noted in clinical pharmacology studies. Also, no antiandrogenic effects were noted. (See ADVERSE REACTIONS.) Serum hormone levels, including prolactin, cortisol, thyroxine (T_4), and testosterone, were not altered after treatment with PEPCID.

Pharmacokinetics

Orally administered PEPCID is incompletely absorbed and its bioavailability is 40–45%. PEPCID undergoes minimal first-pass metabolism. After oral doses, peak plasma levels occur in 1-3 hours. Plasma levels after multiple doses are similar to those after single doses. Fifteen to 20% of PEPCID in plasma is protein bound. PEPCID has an elimination half-life of 2.5-3.5 hours. PEPCID is eliminated by renal (65-70%) and metabolic (30-35%) routes. Renal clearance is 250-450 mL/min, indicating some tubular excretion. Twenty-five to 30% of an oral dose and 65-70% of an intravenous dose are recovered in the urine as unchanged compound. The only metabolite identified in man is the S-oxide.

There is a close relationship between creatinine clearance values and the elimination half-life of PEPCID. In patients with severe renal insufficiency, i.e., creatinine clearance less than 10 mL/min, the elimination half-life of PEPCID may exceed 20 hours and adjustment of dose or dosing intervals in moderate and severe renal insufficiency may be necessary (see PRECAUTIONS, DOSAGE AND ADMINISTRATION).

In elderly patients, there are no clinically significant age-related changes in the pharmacokinetics of PEPCID. However, in elderly patients with decreased renal function, the clearance of the drug may be decreased (see PRECAUTIONS, *Geriatric Use*).

Clinical Studies

The majority of clinical study experience involved oral administration of PEPCID Tablets, and is provided herein for reference.

Duodenal Ulcer

In a U.S. multicenter, double-blind study in outpatients with endoscopically confirmed duodenal ulcer, orally administered PEPCID was compared to placebo. As shown in Table 1, 70% of patients treated with PEPCID 40 mg h.s. were healed by week 4.

Table 1
Outpatients with Endoscopically
Confirmed Healed Duodenal Ulcers

	PEPCID 40 mg h.s. (N=89)	PEPCID 20 mg b.i.d. (N=84)	Placebo h.s. (N=97)
Week 2	**32%	**38%	17%
Week 4	**70%	**67%	31%

** Statistically significantly different than placebo ($p < 0.001$)

Patients not healed by week 4 were continued in the study. By week 8, 83% of patients treated with PEPCID had healed versus 45% of patients treated with placebo. The incidence of ulcer healing with PEPCID was significantly higher than with placebo at each time point based on proportion of endoscopically confirmed healed ulcers.

In this study, time to relief of daytime and nocturnal pain was significantly shorter for patients receiving PEPCID than for patients receiving placebo; patients receiving PEPCID also took less antacid than the patients receiving placebo.

Long-Term Maintenance

Treatment of Duodenal Ulcers

PEPCID, 20 mg p.o. h.s. was compared to placebo h.s. as maintenance therapy in two double-blind, multicenter studies of patients with endoscopically confirmed healed duodenal ulcers. In the U.S. study the observed ulcer incidence within 12 months in patients treated with placebo was 2.4 times greater than in the patients treated with PEPCID. The 89 patients treated with PEPCID had a cumulative observed ulcer incidence of 23.4% compared to an observed ulcer incidence of 56.6% in the 89 patients receiving placebo ($p<0.01$). These results were confirmed in an international study where the cumulative observed ulcer incidence within 12 months in the 307 patients treated with PEPCID was 35.7%, compared to an incidence of 75.5% in the 325 patients treated with placebo ($p<0.01$).

Continued on next page

Information on the Merck & Co., Inc., products listed on these pages is from the prescribing information in use October 1, 2004. For information, please call 1-800-NSC-MERCK [1-800-672-6372].

Pepcid Injection—Cont.

Gastric Ulcer
In both a U.S. and an international multicenter, double-blind study in patients with endoscopically confirmed active benign gastric ulcer, orally administered PEPCID, 40 mg h.s., was compared to placebo h.s. Antacids were permitted during the studies, but consumption was not significantly different between the PEPCID and placebo groups. As shown in Table 2, the incidence of ulcer healing (dropouts counted as unhealed) with PEPCID was statistically significantly better than placebo at weeks 6 and 8 in the U.S. study, and at weeks 4, 6 and 8 in the international study, based on the number of ulcers that healed, confirmed by endoscopy.

Table 2
Patients with Endoscopically Confirmed Healed Gastric Ulcers

	U.S. Study		International Study	
	PEPCID 40 mg h.s. (N=74)	Placebo h.s. (N=75)	PEPCID 40 mg h.s. (N=149)	Placebo h.s. (N=145)
Week 4	45%	39%	†47%	31%
Week 6	†66%	44%	†65%	46%
Week 8	***78%	64%	†80%	54%

***,† Statistically significantly better than placebo (p≤0.05, p≤0.01 respectively)

Time to complete relief of daytime and nighttime pain was statistically significantly shorter for patients receiving PEPCID than for patients receiving placebo; however, in neither study was there a statistically significant difference in the proportion of patients whose pain was relieved by the end of the study (week 8).
Gastroesophageal Reflux Disease (GERD)
Orally administered PEPCID was compared to placebo in a U.S. study that enrolled patients with symptoms of GERD and without endoscopic evidence of erosion or ulceration of the esophagus. PEPCID 20 mg b.i.d. was statistically significantly superior to 40 mg h.s. and to placebo in providing a successful symptomatic outcome, defined as moderate or excellent improvement of symptoms (Table 3).

Table 3
% Successful Symptomatic Outcome

	PEPCID 20 mg b.i.d. (N=154)	PEPCID 40 mg h.s. (N=49)	Placebo (N=73)
Week 6	82††	69	62

†† p≤0.01 vs Placebo

By two weeks of treatment, symptomatic success was observed in a greater percentage of patients taking PEPCID 20 mg b.i.d. compared to placebo (p≤0.01).
Symptomatic improvement and healing of endoscopically verified erosion and ulceration were studied in two additional trials. Healing was defined as complete resolution of all erosions or ulcerations visible with endoscopy. The U.S. study comparing PEPCID 40 mg p.o. b.i.d. to placebo and PEPCID 20 mg p.o. b.i.d., showed a significantly greater percentage of healing for PEPCID 40 mg b.i.d. at weeks 6 and 12 (Table 4).

Table 4
% Endoscopic Healing—U.S. Study

	PEPCID 40 mg b.i.d. (N=127)	PEPCID 20 mg b.i.d. (N=125)	Placebo (N=66)
Week 6	48†††,‡‡	32	18
Week 12	69†††,‡	54†††	29

††† p≤0.01 vs Placebo
‡ p≤0.05 vs PEPCID 20 mg b.i.d.
‡‡ p≤0.01 vs PEPCID 20 mg b.i.d.

As compared to placebo, patients who received PEPCID had faster relief of daytime and nighttime heartburn and a greater percentage of patients experienced complete relief of nighttime heartburn. These differences were statistically significant.

In the international study, when PEPCID 40 mg p.o. b.i.d. was compared to ranitidine 150 mg p.o. b.i.d., a statistically significantly greater percentage of healing was observed with PEPCID 40 mg b.i.d. at week 12 (Table 5). There was, however, no significant difference among treatments in symptom relief.

Table 5
% Endoscopic Healing—International Study

	PEPCID 40 mg b.i.d. (N=175)	PEPCID 20 mg b.i.d. (N=93)	Ranitidine 150 mg b.i.d. (N=172)
Week 6	48	52	42
Week 12	71‡‡‡	68	60

‡‡‡ p≤0.05 vs Ranitidine 150 mg b.i.d.

Pathological Hypersecretory Conditions (e.g., Zollinger-Ellison Syndrome, Multiple Endocrine Adenomas)
In studies of patients with pathological hypersecretory conditions such as Zollinger-Ellison Syndrome with or without multiple endocrine adenomas, PEPCID significantly inhibited gastric acid secretion and controlled associated symptoms. Orally administered doses from 20 to 160 mg q 6 h maintained basal acid secretion below 10 mEq/hr; initial doses were titrated to the individual patient need and subsequent adjustments were necessary with time in some patients. PEPCID was well tolerated at these high dose levels for prolonged periods (greater than 12 months) in eight patients, and there were no cases reported of gynecomastia, increased prolactin levels, or impotence which were considered to be due to the drug.

CLINICAL PHARMACOLOGY IN PEDIATRIC PATIENTS

Pharmacokinetics
Table 6 presents pharmacokinetic data from clinical trials and a published study in pediatric patients (<1 year of age; N=27) given famotidine I.V. 0.5 mg/kg and from published studies of small numbers of pediatric patients (1-15 years of age) given famotidine intravenously. Areas under the curve (AUCs) are normalized to a dose of 0.5 mg/kg I.V. for pediatric patients 1-15 years of age and compared with an extrapolated 40 mg intravenous dose in adults (extrapolation based on results obtained with a 20 mg I.V. adult dose).
[See table 6 below]
Plasma clearance is reduced and elimination half-life is prolonged in pediatric patients 0-3 months of age compared to older pediatric patients. The pharmacokinetic parameters for pediatric patients, ages >3 months-15 years, are comparable to those obtained for adults.
Bioavailability studies of 8 pediatric patients (11-15 years of age) showed a mean oral bioavailability of 0.5 compared to adult values of 0.42 to 0.49. Oral doses of 0.5 mg/kg achieved AUCs of 645 ± 249 ng-hr/mL and 580 ± 60 ng-hr/mL in pediatric patients <1 year of age (N=5) and in pediatric patients 11-15 years of age, respectively, compared to 482 ± 181 ng-hr/mL in adults treated with 40 mg orally.
Pharmacodynamics
Pharmacodynamics of famotidine were evaluated in 5 pediatric patients 2-13 years of age using the sigmoid E_{max} model. These data suggest that the relationship between serum concentration of famotidine and gastric acid suppression is similar to that observed in one study of adults (Table 7).

Table 7
Pharmacodynamics of famotidine using the sigmoid E_{max} model

	EC_{50} (ng/mL)*
Pediatric Patients	26 ± 13
Data from one study	
a) healthy adult subjects	26.5 ± 10.3
b) adult patients with upper GI bleeding	18.7 ± 10.8

* Serum concentration of famotidine associated with 50% maximum gastric acid reduction. Values are presented as means ± SD.

Five published studies (Table 8) examined the effect of famotidine on gastric pH and duration of acid suppression in pediatric patients. While each study had a different design, acid suppression data over time are summarized as follows:
[See table at top of next page]
The duration of effect of famotidine I.V. 0.5 mg/kg on gastric pH and acid suppression was shown in one study to be longer in pediatric patients <1 month of age than in older pediatric patients. This longer duration of gastric acid suppression is consistent with the decreased clearance in pediatric patients <3 months of age (see Table 6).

INDICATIONS AND USAGE

PEPCID Injection Premixed, supplied as a premixed solution in plastic containers (PL 2501 Plastic), and PEPCID Injection, supplied as a concentrated solution for intravenous injection, are intended for intravenous use only. PEPCID Injection Premixed and PEPCID Injection are indicated in some hospitalized patients with pathological hypersecretory conditions or intractable ulcers, or as an alternative to the oral dosage forms for short term use in patients who are unable to take oral medication for the following conditions:
1. *Short term treatment of active duodenal ulcer.* Most adult patients heal within 4 weeks; there is rarely reason to use PEPCID at full dosage for longer than 6 to 8 weeks. Studies have not assessed the safety of famotidine in uncomplicated active duodenal ulcer for periods of more than eight weeks.
2. *Maintenance therapy for duodenal ulcer patients at reduced dosage after healing of an active ulcer.* Controlled studies in adults have not extended beyond one year.
3. *Short term treatment of active benign gastric ulcer.* Most adult patients heal within 6 weeks. Studies have not assessed the safety or efficacy of famotidine in uncomplicated active benign gastric ulcer for periods of more than 8 weeks.
4. *Short term treatment of gastroesophageal reflux disease (GERD).* PEPCID is indicated for short term treatment of patients with symptoms of GERD (see CLINICAL PHARMACOLOGY IN ADULTS, *Clinical Studies*).
PEPCID is also indicated for the short term treatment of esophagitis due to GERD including erosive or ulcerative disease diagnosed by endoscopy (see CLINICAL PHARMACOLOGY IN ADULTS, *Clinical Studies*).
5. *Treatment of pathological hypersecretory conditions (e.g., Zollinger-Ellison Syndrome, multiple endocrine adenomas)* (see CLINICAL PHARMACOLOGY IN ADULTS, *Clinical Studies*).

CONTRAINDICATIONS

Hypersensitivity to any component of these products. Cross sensitivity in this class of compounds has been observed. Therefore, PEPCID should not be administered to patients with a history of hypersensitivity to other H_2-receptor antagonists.

PRECAUTIONS

General
Symptomatic response to therapy with PEPCID does not preclude the presence of gastric malignancy.
Patients with Moderate or Severe Renal Insufficiency
Since CNS adverse effects have been reported in patients with moderate and severe renal insufficiency, longer intervals between doses or lower doses may need to be used in patients with moderate (creatinine clearance <50 mL/min) or severe (creatinine clearance <10 mL/min) renal insufficiency to adjust for the longer elimination half-life of famotidine (see CLINICAL PHARMACOLOGY IN ADULTS, DOSAGE AND ADMINISTRATION).
Drug Interactions
No drug interactions have been identified. Studies with famotidine in man, in animal models, and *in vitro* have shown no significant interference with the disposition of compounds metabolized by the hepatic microsomal enzymes, e.g., cytochrome P450 system. Compounds tested in man include warfarin, theophylline, phenytoin, diazepam, aminopyrine and antipyrine. Indocyanine green as an index of hepatic drug extraction has been tested and no significant effects have been found.
Carcinogenesis, Mutagenesis, Impairment of Fertility
In a 106 week study in rats and a 92 week study in mice given oral doses of up to 2000 mg/kg/day (approximately 2500 times the recommended human dose for active duodenal ulcer), there was no evidence of carcinogenic potential for PEPCID.
Famotidine was negative in the microbial mutagen test (Ames test) using *Salmonella typhimurium* and *Escherichia coli* with or without rat liver enzyme activation at concentrations up to 10,000 mcg/plate. In *in vivo* studies in mice, with a micronucleus test and a chromosomal aberration test, no evidence of a mutagenic effect was observed.
In studies with rats given oral doses of up to 2000 mg/kg/day or intravenous doses of up to 200 mg/kg/day fertility and reproductive performance were not affected.
Pregnancy
Pregnancy Category B
Reproductive studies have been performed in rats and rabbits at oral doses of up to 2000 and 500 mg/kg/day, respectively, and in both species at I.V. doses of up to 200 mg/kg/day, and have revealed no significant evidence of impaired fertility or harm to the fetus due to PEPCID. While no direct fetotoxic effects have been observed, sporadic abortions occurring only in mothers displaying marked decreased food intake were seen in some rabbits at oral doses of 200 mg/kg/

Table 6
Pharmacokinetic Parameters[a] of Intravenous Famotidine

Age (N=number of patients)	Area Under the Curve (AUC) (ng-hr/mL)	Total Clearance (Cl) (L/hr/kg)	Volume of Distribution (V_d) (L/kg)	Elimination Half-life ($T_{1/2}$) (hours)
0-1 month[c] (N=10)	NA	0.13 ± 0.06	1.4 ± 0.4	10.5 ± 5.4
0-3 months[d] (N=6)	2688 ± 847	0.21 ± 0.06	1.8 ± 0.3	8.1 ± 3.5
>3-12 months[d] (N=11)	1160 ± 474	0.49 ± 0.17	2.3 ± 0.7	4.5 ± 1.1
1-11 years (N=20)	1089 ± 834	0.54 ± 0.34	2.07 ± 1.49	3.38 ± 2.60
11-15 years (N=6)	1140 ± 320	0.48 ± 0.14	1.5 ± 0.4	2.3 ± 0.4
Adult (N=16)	1726[b]	0.39 ± 0.14	1.3 ± 0.2	2.83 ± 0.99

[a]Values are presented as means ± SD unless indicated otherwise.
[b]Mean value only.
[c]Single center study.
[d]Multicenter study.

day (250 times the usual human dose) or higher. There are, however, no adequate or well-controlled studies in pregnant women. Because animal reproductive studies are not always predictive of human response, this drug should be used during pregnancy only if clearly needed.

Nursing Mothers

Studies performed in lactating rats have shown that famotidine is secreted into breast milk. Transient growth depression was observed in young rats suckling from mothers treated with maternotoxic doses of at least 600 times the usual human dose. Famotidine is detectable in human milk. Because of the potential for serious adverse reactions in nursing infants from PEPCID, a decision should be made whether to discontinue nursing or discontinue the drug, taking into account the importance of the drug to the mother.

Pediatric Patients <1 year of age

Use of PEPCID in pediatric patients <1 year of age is supported by evidence from adequate and well-controlled studies of PEPCID in adults, and by the following studies in pediatric patients <1 year of age.

Two pharmacokinetic studies in pediatric patients <1 year of age (N=48) demonstrated that clearance of famotidine in patients >3 months to 1 year of age is similar to that seen in older pediatric patients (1-15 years of age) and adults. In contrast, pediatric patients 0-3 months of age had famotidine clearance values that were 2- to 4-fold less than those in older pediatric patients and adults. These studies also show that the mean bioavailability in pediatric patients <1 year of age after oral dosing is similar to older pediatric patients and adults. Pharmacodynamic data in pediatric patients 0-3 months of age suggest that the duration of acid suppression is longer compared with older pediatric patients, consistent with the longer famotidine half-life in pediatric patients 0-3 months of age. (See CLINICAL PHARMACOLOGY IN PEDIATRIC PATIENTS, *Pharmacokinetics* and *Pharmacodynamics*.)

In a double-blind, randomized, treatment-withdrawal study, 35 pediatric patients <1 year of age who were diagnosed as having gastroesophageal reflux disease were treated for up to 4 weeks with famotidine oral suspension (0.5 mg/kg/dose or 1 mg/kg/dose). Although an intravenous famotidine formulation was available, no patients were treated with intravenous famotidine in this study. Also, caregivers were instructed to provide conservative treatment including thickened feedings. Enrolled patients were diagnosed primarily by history of vomiting (spitting up) and irritability (fussiness). The famotidine dosing regimen was once daily for patients <3 months of age and twice daily for patients ≥3 months of age. After 4 weeks of treatment, patients were randomly withdrawn from the treatment and followed an additional 4 weeks for adverse events and symptomatology. Patients were evaluated for vomiting (spitting up), irritability (fussiness) and global assessments of improvement. The study patients ranged in age at entry from 1.3 to 10.5 months (mean 5.6 ± 2.9 months), 57% were female, 91% were white and 6% were black. Most patients (27/35) continued into the treatment withdrawal phase of the study. Two patients discontinued famotidine due to adverse events. Most patients improved during the initial treatment phase of the study. Results of the treatment withdrawal phase were difficult to interpret because of small numbers of patients. Of the 35 patients enrolled in the study, agitation was observed in 5 patients on famotidine that resolved when the medication was discontinued; agitation was not observed in patients on placebo (see ADVERSE REACTIONS, *Pediatric Patients*).

These studies suggest that a starting dose of 0.5 mg/kg/dose of famotidine oral suspension may be of benefit for the treatment of GERD for up to 4 weeks once daily in patients <3 months of age and twice daily in patients 3 months to <1 year of age; the safety and benefit of famotidine treatment beyond 4 weeks have not been established. Famotidine should be considered for the treatment of GERD only if conservative measures (e.g., thickened feedings) are used concurrently and if the potential benefit outweighs the risk.

Pediatric Patients 1-16 years of age

Use of PEPCID in pediatric patients 1-16 years of age is supported by evidence from adequate and well-controlled studies of PEPCID in adults, and by the following studies in pediatric patients: In published studies in small numbers of pediatric patients 1-15 years of age, clearance of famotidine was similar to that seen in adults. In pediatric patients 11-15 years of age, oral doses of 0.5 mg/kg were associated with a mean area under the curve (AUC) similar to that seen in adults treated orally with 40 mg. Similarly, in pediatric patients 1-15 years of age, intravenous doses of 0.5 mg/kg were associated with a mean AUC similar to that seen in adults treated intravenously with 40 mg. Limited published studies also suggest that the relationship between serum concentration and acid suppression is similar in pediatric patients 1-15 years of age as compared with adults. These studies suggest that the starting dose for pediatric patients 1-16 years of age is 0.25 mg/kg intravenously (injected over a period of not less than two minutes or as a 15 minute infusion) q 12 h up to 40 mg/day.

While published uncontrolled clinical studies suggest effectiveness of famotidine in the treatment of peptic ulcer, data in pediatric patients are insufficient to establish percent response with dose and duration of therapy. Therefore, treatment duration (initially based on adult duration recommendations) and dose should be individualized based on clinical response and/or gastric pH determination and endoscopy.

Table 8

Dosage	Route	Effect[a]	Number of Patients (age range)
0.5 mg/kg, single dose	I.V.	gastric pH >4 for 19.5 hours (17.3, 21.8)[c]	11 (5-19 days)
0.3 mg/kg, single dose	I.V.	gastric pH >3.5 for 8.7 ± 4.7[b] hours	6 (2-7 years)
0.4-0.8 mg/kg	I.V.	gastric pH >4 for 6-9 hours	18 (2-69 months)
0.5 mg/kg, single dose	I.V.	a >2 pH unit increase above baseline in gastric pH for >8 hours	9 (2-13 years)
0.5 mg/kg b.i.d.	I.V.	gastric pH >5 for 13.5 ± 1.8[b] hours	4 (6-15 years)
0.5 mg/kg b.i.d.	oral	gastric pH >5 for 5.0 ± 1.1[b] hours	4 (11-15 years)

[a]Values reported in published literature.
[b]Means ± SD.
[c]Mean (95% confidence interval).

Published uncontrolled studies in pediatric patients have demonstrated gastric acid suppression with doses up to 0.5 mg/kg intravenously q 12 h.

Geriatric Use

Of the 4,966 subjects in clinical studies who were treated with famotidine, 488 subjects (9.8%) were 65 and older, and 88 subjects (1.7%) were greater than 75 years of age. No overall differences in safety or effectiveness were observed between these subjects and younger subjects. However, greater sensitivity of some older patients cannot be ruled out.

No dosage adjustment is required based on age (see CLINICAL PHARMACOLOGY IN ADULTS, *Pharmacokinetics*). This drug is known to be substantially excreted by the kidney, and the risk of toxic reactions to this drug may be greater in patients with impaired renal function. Because elderly patients are more likely to have decreased renal function, care should be taken in dose selection, and it may be useful to monitor renal function. Dosage adjustment in the case of moderate or severe renal impairment is necessary (see PRECAUTIONS, *Patients with Moderate or Severe Renal Insufficiency* and DOSAGE AND ADMINISTRATION, *Dosage Adjustment for Patients with Moderate or Severe Renal Insufficiency*).

ADVERSE REACTIONS

The adverse reactions listed below have been reported during domestic and international clinical trials in approximately 2500 patients. In those controlled clinical trials in which PEPCID Tablets were compared to placebo, the incidence of adverse experiences in the group which received PEPCID Tablets, 40 mg at bedtime, was similar to that in the placebo group.

The following adverse reactions have been reported to occur in more than 1% of patients on therapy with PEPCID in controlled clinical trials, and may be causally related to the drug: headache (4.7%), dizziness (1.3%), constipation (1.2%) and diarrhea (1.7%).

The following other adverse reactions have been reported infrequently in clinical trials or since the drug was marketed. The relationship to therapy with PEPCID has been unclear in many cases. Within each category the adverse reactions are listed in order of decreasing severity:

Body as a Whole: fever, asthenia, fatigue
Cardiovascular: arrhythmia, AV block, palpitation
Gastrointestinal: cholestatic jaundice, liver enzyme abnormalities, vomiting, nausea, abdominal discomfort, anorexia, dry mouth
Hematologic: rare cases of agranulocytosis, pancytopenia, leukopenia, thrombocytopenia
Hypersensitivity: anaphylaxis, angioedema, orbital or facial edema, urticaria, rash, conjunctival injection
Musculoskeletal: musculoskeletal pain including muscle cramps, arthralgia
Nervous System/Psychiatric: grand mal seizure; psychic disturbances, which were reversible in cases for which follow-up was obtained, including hallucinations, confusion, agitation, depression, anxiety, decreased libido; paresthesia; insomnia; somnolence
Respiratory: bronchospasm
Skin: toxic epidermal necrolysis (very rare), alopecia, acne, pruritus, dry skin, flushing
Special Senses: tinnitus, taste disorder
Other: rare cases of impotence and rare cases of gynecomastia have been reported; however, in controlled clinical trials, the incidences were not greater than those seen with placebo.

The adverse reactions reported for PEPCID Tablets may also occur with PEPCID for Oral Suspension, PEPCID RPD Orally Disintegrating Tablets, PEPCID Injection Premixed or PEPCID Injection. In addition, transient irritation at the injection site has been observed with PEPCID Injection.

Pediatric Patients

In a clinical study in 35 pediatric patients <1 year of age with GERD symptoms [e.g., vomiting (spitting up), irritability (fussing)], agitation was observed in 5 patients on famotidine that resolved when the medication was discontinued.

OVERDOSAGE

There is no experience to date with deliberate overdosage. Oral doses of up to 640 mg/day have been given to adult patients with pathological hypersecretory conditions with no serious adverse effects. In the event of overdosage, treatment should be symptomatic and supportive. Unabsorbed material should be removed from the gastrointestinal tract, the patient should be monitored, and supportive therapy should be employed.

The intravenous LD_{50} of famotidine for mice and rats ranged from 254-563 mg/kg and the minimum lethal single I.V. dose in dogs was approximately 300 mg/kg. Signs of acute intoxication in I.V. treated dogs were emesis, restlessness, pallor of mucous membranes or redness of mouth and ears, hypotension, tachycardia and collapse. The oral LD_{50} of famotidine in male and female rats and mice was greater than 3000 mg/kg and the minimum lethal acute oral dose in dogs exceeded 2000 mg/kg. Famotidine did not produce overt effects at high oral doses in mice, rats, cats and dogs, but induced significant anorexia and growth depression in rabbits starting with 200 mg/kg/day orally.

DOSAGE AND ADMINISTRATION

In some hospitalized patients with pathological hypersecretory conditions or intractable ulcers, or in patients who are unable to take oral medication, PEPCID Injection Premixed or PEPCID Injection may be administered until oral therapy can be instituted.

The recommended dosage for PEPCID Injection Premixed and PEPCID Injection in adult patients is 20 mg intravenously q 12 h.

The doses and regimen for parenteral administration in patients with GERD have not been established.

Dosage for Pediatric Patients <1 year of age Gastroesophageal Reflux Disease (GERD)

See PRECAUTIONS, *Pediatric Patients <1 year of age*.

The studies described in PRECAUTIONS, *Pediatric Patients <1 year of age* suggest the following starting doses in pediatric patients <1 year of age: *Gastroesophageal Reflux Disease (GERD)* - 0.5 mg/kg/dose of famotidine oral suspension for the treatment of GERD for up to 8 weeks once daily in patients <3 months of age and 0.5 mg/kg/dose twice daily in patients 3 months to <1 year of age. Patients should also be receiving conservative measures (e.g., thickened feedings). The use of intravenous famotidine in pediatric patients <1 year of age with GERD has not been adequately studied.

Dosage for Pediatric Patients 1-16 years of age

See PRECAUTIONS, *Pediatric Patients 1-16 years of age*.

The studies described in PRECAUTIONS, *Pediatric Patients 1-16 years of age* suggest that the starting dose in pediatric patients 1-16 years of age is 0.25 mg/kg intravenously (injected over a period of not less than two minutes or as a 15-minute infusion) q 12 h up to 40 mg/day.

While published uncontrolled clinical studies suggest effectiveness of famotidine in the treatment of peptic ulcer, data in pediatric patients are insufficient to establish percent response with dose and duration of therapy. Therefore, treatment duration (initially based on adult duration recommendations) and dose should be individualized based on clinical response and/or gastric pH determination and endoscopy. Published uncontrolled studies in pediatric patients 1-16 years of age have demonstrated gastric acid suppression with doses up to 0.5 mg/kg intravenously q 12 h.

Dosage Adjustments for Patients with Moderate or Severe Renal Insufficiency

In adult patients with moderate (creatinine clearance <50 mL/min) or severe (creatinine clearance <10 mL/min) renal insufficiency, the elimination half-life of PEPCID is increased. For patients with severe renal insufficiency, it may exceed 20 hours, reaching approximately 24 hours in anuric patients. Since CNS adverse effects have been reported in patients with moderate and severe renal insufficiency, to avoid excess accumulation of the drug in patients with moderate or severe renal insufficiency, the dose of PEPCID Injection Premixed or PEPCID Injection may be reduced to half the dose, or the dosing interval may be prolonged to 36-48 hours as indicated by the patient's clinical response.

Based on the comparison of pharmacokinetic parameters for PEPCID in adults and pediatric patients, dosage adjustment in pediatric patients with moderate or severe renal insufficiency should be considered.

Continued on next page

Information on the Merck & Co., Inc., products listed on these pages is from the prescribing information in use October 1, 2004. For information, please call 1-800-NSC-MERCK [1-800-672-6372].

Pepcid Injection—Cont.

Pathological Hypersecretory Conditions (e.g., Zollinger-Ellison Syndrome, Multiple Endocrine Adenomas)
The dosage of PEPCID in patients with pathological hypersecretory conditions varies with the individual patient. The recommended adult intravenous dose is 20 mg q 12 h. Doses should be adjusted to individual patient needs and should continue as long as clinically indicated. In some patients, a higher starting dose may be required. Oral doses up to 160 mg q 6 h have been administered to some adult patients with severe Zollinger-Ellison Syndrome.
PEPCID Injection Premixed
PEPCID Injection Premixed, supplied in Galaxy[§] containers (PL 2501 Plastic), is a 50 mL iso-osmotic solution premixed with 0.9% sodium chloride for administration as an infusion over a 15–30 minute period. *This premixed solution is for intravenous use only using sterile equipment.*
Directions for Use of Galaxy® Containers
Check the container for minute leaks prior to use by squeezing the bag firmly. If leaks are found, discard solution as sterility may be impaired. Do not add supplementary medication. Do not use unless solution is clear and seal is intact.
CAUTION: Do not use plastic containers in series connections. Such use could result in air embolism due to residual air being drawn from the primary container before administration of the fluid from the secondary container is complete.
Preparation for administration:
1. Suspend container from eyelet support.
2. Remove plastic protector from outlet port at bottom of container.
3. Attach administration set. Refer to complete directions accompanying set.

To prepare PEPCID intravenous solutions, aseptically dilute 2 mL of PEPCID Injection (solution containing 10 mg/mL) with 0.9% Sodium Chloride Injection or other compatible intravenous solution (see *Stability, PEPCID Injection*) to a total volume of either 5 mL or 10 mL and inject over a period of not less than 2 minutes.
To prepare PEPCID intravenous infusion solutions, aseptically dilute 2 mL of PEPCID Injection with 100 mL of 5% dextrose or other compatible solution (see *Stability, PEPCID Injection*), and infuse over a 15-30 minute period.
Concomitant Use of Antacids
Antacids may be given concomitantly if needed.
Stability
Parenteral drug products should be inspected visually for particulate matter and discoloration prior to administration whenever solution and container permit.
PEPCID Injection Premixed
PEPCID Injection Premixed, as supplied premixed in 0.9% sodium chloride in Galaxy® containers (PL 2501 Plastic), is stable through the labeled expiration date when stored under the recommended conditions. (See HOW SUPPLIED, *Storage*).
PEPCID Injection
When added to or diluted with most commonly used intravenous solutions, e.g., Water for Injection, 0.9% Sodium Chloride Injection, 5% and 10% Dextrose Injection, or Lactated Ringer's Injection, diluted PEPCID Injection is physically and chemically stable (i.e., maintains at least 90% of initial potency) for 7 days at room temperature—see HOW SUPPLIED, *Storage.*
When added to or diluted with Sodium Bicarbonate Injection, 5%, PEPCID Injection at a concentration of 0.2 mg/mL (the recommended concentration of PEPCID intravenous infusion solutions) is physically and chemically stable (i.e., maintains at least 90% of initial potency) for 7 days at room temperature—see HOW SUPPLIED, *Storage.* However, a precipitate may form at higher concentrations of PEPCID Injection (>0.2 mg/mL) in Sodium Bicarbonate Injection, 5%.

[§] Galaxy® is a registered trademark of Baxter International Inc.

HOW SUPPLIED

FOR INTRAVENOUS USE ONLY
No. 3537—PEPCID (famotidine) Injection Premixed 20 mg per 50 mL is a clear, non-preserved, sterile solution premixed in a vehicle made iso-osmotic with Sodium Chloride, and is supplied as follows:
NDC 0006-3537-50, 50 mL single dose Galaxy® containers (PL 2501 Plastic).
No. 3539—PEPCID Injection 10 mg per 1 mL, is a non-preserved, clear, colorless solution and is supplied as follows:
NDC 0006-3539-04, 10 × 2 mL single dose vials
No. 3541—PEPCID Injection 10 mg per 1 mL, is a clear, colorless solution and is supplied as follows:
NDC 0006-3541-14, 4 mL vials
NDC 0006-3541-20, 20 mL vials
NDC 0006-3541-49, 10 ×20 mL vials.
Storage
Store PEPCID Injection Premixed in Galaxy® containers (PL 2501 Plastic) at room temperature (25°C, 77°F). Exposure of the premixed product to excessive heat should be avoided. Brief exposure to temperatures up to 35°C (95°F) does not adversely affect the product.
Store PEPCID Injection at 2-8°C (36-46°F). If solution freezes, bring to room temperature; allow sufficient time to solubilize all the components.
Although diluted PEPCID Injection has been shown to be physically and chemically stable for 7 days at room temperature, there are no data on the maintenance of sterility after dilution. Therefore, it is recommended that if not used immediately after preparation, diluted solutions of PEPCID Injection should be refrigerated and used within 48 hours (see DOSAGE AND ADMINISTRATION).
PEPCID (famotidine) Injection Premixed is manufactured for:
MERCK & CO., INC., West Point, PA 19486, USA
By:
BAXTER HEALTHCARE CORPORATION
Deerfield, Illinois 60015 USA
PEPCID (famotidine) Injection is manufactured by:
MERCK & CO., INC., West Point, PA 19486, USA
9042511 Issued June 2002

PNEUMOVAX® 23 ℞
(Pneumococcal Vaccine Polyvalent)

DESCRIPTION

PNEUMOVAX* 23 (Pneumococcal Vaccine Polyvalent) is a sterile, liquid vaccine for intramuscular or subcutaneous injection. It consists of a mixture of highly purified capsular polysaccharides from the 23 most prevalent or invasive pneumococcal types of *Streptococcus pneumoniae,* including the six serotypes that most frequently cause invasive drug-resistant pneumococcal infections among children and adults in the United States. (See Table 1.) The 23-valent vaccine accounts for at least 90% of pneumococcal blood isolates and at least 85% of all pneumococcal isolates from sites which are generally sterile as determined by ongoing surveillance of U.S. data.

*Registered trademark of MERCK & CO., Inc.

PNEUMOVAX 23 is manufactured according to methods developed by the MERCK Research Laboratories. Each 0.5 mL dose of vaccine contains 25 μg of each polysaccharide type dissolved in isotonic saline solution containing 0.25% phenol as preservative.
[See table 1 below]

CLINICAL PHARMACOLOGY

Pneumococcal infection is a leading cause of death throughout the world and a major cause of pneumonia, bacteremia, meningitis, and otitis media.
Strains of drug-resistant *S. pneumoniae* have become increasingly common in the United States and in other parts of the world. In some areas as many as 35% of pneumococcal isolates have been reported to be resistant to penicillin. Many penicillin-resistant pneumococci are also resistant to other antimicrobial drugs (e.g., erythromycin, trimethoprim-sulfamethoxazole and extended-spectrum cephalosporins); therefore emphasizing the importance of vaccine prophylaxis against pneumococcal disease.
Epidemiology
Pneumococcal infection causes approximately 40,000 deaths annually in the United States.
At least 500,000 cases of pneumococcal pneumonia are estimated to occur annually in the United States; *S. pneumoniae* accounts for approximately 25–35% of cases of community-acquired bacterial pneumonia in persons who require hospitalization.
Pneumococcal disease accounts for an estimated 50,000 cases of pneumococcal bacteremia annually in the United States. Some studies suggest the overall annual incidence of bacteremia to be approximately 15 to 30 cases/100,000 population with 50 to 83 cases/100,000 for persons 65 years of age and older and 160 cases/100,000 for children less than two years of age.
The incidence of pneumococcal bacteremia is as high as 1% (940 cases/100,000 population) among persons with acquired immunodeficiency syndrome (AIDS).
In the United States, the risk of acquiring bacteremia is lower among whites than among persons in some other racial/ethnic groups (i.e., blacks, Alaskan Natives, and American Indians).
Despite appropriate antimicrobial therapy and intensive medical care, the overall case-fatality rate for pneumococcal bacteremia is 15–20% among adults, and among elderly patients this rate is approximately 30–40%. An overall case-fatality rate of 36% was documented for adult inner-city residents who were hospitalized for pneumococcal bacteremia.
In the United States, pneumococcal disease accounts for an estimated 3,000 cases of meningitis annually. The estimated overall annual incidence of pneumococcal meningitis is approximately 1 to 2 cases per 100,000 population. The incidence of pneumococcal meningitis is highest among children six to 24 months and persons aged ≥ 65 years; rates for blacks are twice as high as those for whites or Hispanics.
Recurrent pneumococcal meningitis may occur in patients who have chronic cerebrospinal fluid leakage resulting from congenital lesions, skull fractures, or neurosurgical procedures.
Invasive pneumococcal disease (e.g., bacteremia or meningitis) and pneumonia cause high morbidity and mortality in spite of effective antimicrobial control by antibiotics. These effects of pneumococcal disease appear due to irreversible physiologic damage caused by the bacteria during the first 5 days following onset of illness, and occur irrespective of antimicrobial therapy. Vaccination offers an effective means of further reducing the mortality and morbidity of this disease.
Risk Factors
In addition to the very young and persons 65 years of age or older, patients with certain chronic conditions are at increased risk of developing pneumococcal infection and severe pneumococcal illness.
Patients with chronic cardiovascular diseases (e.g., congestive heart failure or cardiomyopathy), chronic pulmonary diseases (e.g., chronic obstructive pulmonary disease or emphysema), or chronic liver diseases (e.g., cirrhosis), diabetes mellitus, alcoholism or asthma (when it occurs with chronic bronchitis, emphysema, or long-term use of systemic corticosteroids) have an increased risk of pneumococcal disease. In adults, this population is generally immunocompetent.
Patients at high risk are those who have a decreased responsiveness to polysaccharide antigen or an increased rate of decline in serum antibody concentrations as a result of: immunosuppressive conditions (congenital immunodeficiency, human immunodeficiency virus [HIV] infection, leukemia, lymphoma, multiple myeloma, Hodgkin's disease, or generalized malignancy); organ or bone marrow transplantation; therapy with alkylating agents, antimetabolites, or systemic corticosteroids; chronic renal failure or nephrotic syndrome.
Patients at the highest risk of pneumococcal infection are those with functional or anatomic asplenia (e.g., sickle cell disease or splenectomy), because this condition leads to reduced clearance of encapsulated bacteria from the bloodstream. Children who have sickle cell disease or have had a splenectomy are at increased risk for fulminant pneumococcal sepsis associated with high mortality.
Immunogenicity
It has been established that the purified pneumococcal capsular polysaccharides induce antibody production and that such antibody is effective in preventing pneumococcal disease. Clinical studies have demonstrated the immunogenicity of each of the 23 capsular types when tested in polyvalent vaccines.
Studies with 12-, 14-, and 23-valent pneumococcal vaccines in children two years of age and older and in adults of all ages showed immunogenic responses. Protective capsular type-specific antibody levels generally develop by the third week following vaccination.
Bacterial capsular polysaccharides induce antibodies primarily by T-cell-independent mechanisms. Therefore, antibody response to most pneumococcal capsular types is generally poor or inconsistent in children aged < 2 years whose immune systems are immature.
Efficacy
The protective efficacy of pneumococcal vaccines containing 6 or 12 capsular polysaccharides was investigated in two controlled studies of young, healthy gold miners in South Africa, in whom there was a high attack rate for pneumococcal pneumonia and bacteremia. Capsular type-specific attack rates for pneumococcal pneumonia were observed for the period from 2 weeks through about 1 year after vaccination. Protective efficacy was 76% and 92%, respectively, in the two studies for the capsular types represented.
In similar studies carried out by Dr. R. Austrian and associates, using similar pneumococcal vaccines prepared for the National Institute of Allergy and Infectious Diseases, the reduction in pneumonia caused by the capsular types contained in the vaccines was 79%. Reduction in type-specific pneumococcal bacteremia was 82%.
A prospective study in France found pneumococcal vaccine to be 77% effective in reducing the incidence of pneumonia among nursing home residents.
In the United States, two postlicensure randomized controlled trials, in the elderly or patients with chronic medical conditions who received a multivalent polysaccharide vaccine, did not support the efficacy of the vaccine for nonbacteremic pneumonia. However, these studies may have lacked sufficient statistical power to detect a difference in the incidence of laboratory-confirmed, nonbacteremic pneumococcal pneumonia between the vaccinated and nonvaccinated study groups.
A meta-analysis of nine randomized controlled trials of pneumococcal vaccine concluded that pneumococcal vaccine

Table 1
23 Pneumococcal Capsular Types Included in
PNEUMOVAX 23

Nomenclature	Pneumococcal Types
Danish	1 2 3 4 5 6B** 7F 8 9N 9V** 10A 11A 12F 14** 15B 17F 18C 19F** 19A** 20 22F 23F** 33F

**These serotypes most frequently cause drug-resistant pneumococcal infections

is efficacious in reducing the frequency of nonbacteremic pneumococcal pneumonia among adults in low risk groups but not in high-risk groups. These studies may have been limited because of the lack of specific and sensitive diagnostic tests for nonbacteremic pneumococcal pneumonia. The pneumococcal polysaccharide vaccine is not effective for the prevention of common upper respiratory disease in children.

More recently, multiple, case-control studies have shown pneumococcal vaccine is effective in the prevention of serious pneumococcal disease, with point estimates of efficacy ranging from 56% to 81% in immunocompetent persons.

Only one case-control study did not document effectiveness against bacteremic disease possibly due to study limitations, including small sample size and incomplete ascertainment of vaccination status in patients. In addition, case-patients and persons who served as controls may not have been comparable regarding the severity of their underlying medical conditions, potentially creating a biased underestimate of vaccine effectiveness.

A serotype prevalence study, based on the Centers for Disease Control pneumococcal surveillance system, demonstrated 57% overall protective effectiveness against invasive infections caused by serotypes included in the vaccine in persons ≥ 6 years of age, 65–84% effectiveness among specific patient groups (e.g., persons with diabetes mellitus, coronary vascular disease, congestive heart failure, chronic pulmonary disease, and anatomic asplenia) and 75% effectiveness in immunocompetent persons aged ≥ 65 years of age. Vaccine effectiveness could not be confirmed for certain groups of immunocompromised patients; however, the study could not recruit sufficient numbers of unvaccinated patients from each disease group.

In an early study, vaccinated children and yound adults aged 2 to 25 years who had sickle cell disease, congenital asplenia, or undergone a splenectomy experienced significantly less bacteremic pneumococcal disease than patients who were not vaccinated.

Duration of Immunity

Following pneumococcal vaccination, serotype-specific antibody levels decline after 5–10 years. A more rapid decline in antibody levels may occur in some groups (e.g., children). Limited published data suggest that antibody levels may decline in the elderly > 60 years of age.

The Advisory Committee on Immunization Practices (ACIP) states that these findings indicate that revaccination may be needed to provide continued protection. (See INDICATIONS AND USAGE, *Revaccination*.)

The results from one epidemiologic study suggest that vaccination may provide protection for at least nine years after receipt of the initial dose. Decreasing estimates of effectiveness with increasing interval since vaccination, particularly among the very elderly (persons aged ≥ 85 years) have been reported.

INDICATIONS AND USAGE

PNEUMOVAX 23 is indicated for vaccination against pneumococcal disease caused by those pneumococcal types included in the vaccine. Effectiveness of the vaccine in the prevention of pneumococcal pneumonia and pneumococcal bacteremia has been demonstrated in controlled trials in South Africa, France and in case-control studies.

PNEUMOVAX 23 will not prevent disease caused by capsular types of pneumococcus other than those contained in the vaccine.

If it is known that a person has not received any pneumococcal vaccine or if earlier pneumococcal vaccination status is unknown, then persons in the categories listed below should be administered pneumococcal vaccine; however, if a person has received a primary dose of pneumococcal vaccine, before administering an additional dose of vaccine, please refer to the Revaccination section.

Vaccination with PNEUMOVAX 23 is recommended for selected individuals as follows:

Immunocompetent persons:

— routine vaccination for persons 50 years of age or older†

— persons aged ≥ 2 years with chronic cardiovascular disease (including congestive heart failure and cardiomyopathies), chronic pulmonary disease (including chronic obstructive pulmonary disease and emphysema), or diabetes mellitus

— persons aged ≥ 2 years with alcoholism, chronic liver disease (including cirrhosis) or cerebrospinal fluid leaks

— persons aged ≥ 2 years with functional or anatomic asplenia (including sickle cell disease and splenectomy)

— persons aged ≥ 2 years living in special environments or social settings (including Alaskan Natives and certain American Indian populations)

Immunocompromised persons:

— persons aged ≥ 2 years, including those with HIV infection, leukemia, lymphoma, Hodgkin's disease, multiple myeloma, generalized malignancy, chronic renal failure or nephrotic syndrome; those receiving immunosuppressive chemotherapy (including corticosteroids); and those who have received an organ or bone marrow transplant.

†NOTE: The ACIP recommends routine vaccination for immunocompetent persons 65 years of age and older.

Timing of Vaccination

Pneumococcal vaccine should be given at least two weeks before elective splenectomy, if possible.

For planning cancer chemotherapy or other immunosuppressive therapy (e.g., for patients with Hodgkin's disease or those who undergo organ or bone marrow transplantation), pneumococcal vaccination should be administered at least two weeks prior to the initiation of immunosuppressive therapy. Vaccination during chemotherapy or radiation therapy should be avoided. Based on literature reports, pneumococcal vaccine may be given as early as several months following completion of chemotherapy or radiation therapy for neoplastic disease. In Hodgkin's disease, immune response to vaccination may be impaired for two years or longer after intensive chemotherapy (with or without radiation). During the two years following the completion of chemotherapy or other immunosuppressive therapy, antibody responses improve in some patients as the interval between the end of treatment and pneumococcal vaccination increases.

Persons with asymptomatic or symptomatic HIV infection should be vaccinated as soon as possible after their diagnosis is confirmed.

Use With Other Vaccines

The ACIP states that pneumococcal vaccine may be administered at the same time as influenza vaccine (by separate injection in the other arm) without an increase in side effects or decreased antibody response to either vaccine. In contrast to pneumococcal vaccine, influenza vaccine is recommended annually, for appropriate populations.

Revaccination

Early studies have indicated that local reactions (i.e., arthus-type reactions) among adults receiving the second dose of 14–valent vaccine within 2 years after the first dose are more severe than those occurring after initial vaccination. However, subsequent studies have suggested that revaccination after intervals of ≥ 4 years is not associated with an increased incidence of adverse side effects.

Routine revaccination of immunocompetent persons previously vaccinated with 23–valent polysaccharide vaccine is not recommended. However, revaccination once is recommended for persons ≥ 2 years of age who are at highest risk of serious pneumococcal infection and those likely to have a rapid decline in pneumococcal antibody levels, provided that at least five years have passed since receipt of a first dose of pneumococcal vaccine.

The highest risk group includes persons with functional or anatomic asplenia (e.g., sickle cell disease or splenectomy), HIV infection, leukemia, lymphoma, Hodgkin's disease, multiple myeloma, generalized malignancy, chronic renal failure, nephrotic syndrome, or other conditions associated with immunosupression (e.g., organ or bone marrow transplantation), and those receiving immunosuppressive chemotherapy (including long-term systemic corticosteroids).

For children ≤ 10 years of age at revaccination and at highest risk of severe pneumococcal infection (e.g., children with functional or anatomic asplenia, including sickle cell disease or splenectomy or conditions associated with rapid antibody decline after initial vaccination including nephrotic syndrome, renal failure or renal transplantation), the ACIP recommends that revaccination may be considered three years after the previous dose.

If prior vaccination status is unknown for patients in the high risk group, patients should be given pneumococcal vaccine.

All persons ≥ 65 years of age who have not received vaccine within 5 years (and were < 65 years of age at the time of vaccination) should receive another dose of vaccine.

Because data are insufficient concerning the safety of pneumococcal vaccine when administered three or more times, revaccination following a second dose is not routinely recommended.

CONTRAINDICATIONS

Hypersensitivity to any component of the vaccine. Epinephrine injection (1:1000) must be immediately available should an acute anaphylactoid reaction occur due to any component of the vaccine.

WARNINGS

For planning cancer chemotherapy or other immunosuppressive therapy (e.g., for patients with Hodgkin's disease or those who undergo organ or bone marrow transplantation), the timing of the vaccination is critical. (See INDICATIONS AND USAGE, *Timing of Vaccination*.)

If the vaccine is used in persons receiving immunosuppressive therapy, the expected serum antibody response may not be obtained and potential impairment of future immune responses to pneumococcal antigens may occur. (See INDICATIONS AND USAGE, *Timing of Vaccination*.)

Intradermal administration may cause severe local reactions.

PRECAUTIONS

General

Caution and appropriate care should be exercised in administering PNEUMOVAX 23 to individuals with severely compromised cardiovascular and/or pulmonary function in whom a systemic reaction would pose a significant risk.

Any febrile respiratory illness or other active infection is reason for delaying use of PNEUMOVAX 23, except when, in the opinion of the physician, withholding the agent entails even greater risk.

In patients who require penicillin (or other antibiotic) prophylaxis against pneumococcal infection, such prophylaxis should not be discontinued after vaccination with PNEUMOVAX 23.

PNEUMOVAX 23 may not be effective in preventing pneumococcal meningitis in patients who have chronic cerebrospinal fluid (CSF) leakage resulting from congenital lesions, skull fractures, or neurosurgical procedures.

Routine revaccination of immunocompetent persons previously vaccinated with a 23–valent vaccine is not recommended. However, revaccination once is recommended for persons aged ≥ 2 years who are at highest risk for serious pneumococcal infections and those likely to have a rapid decline in pneumococcal antibody levels. (See INDICATIONS AND USAGE, *Revaccination*.)

Instructions to Healthcare Provider

The healthcare provider should determine the current health status and previous vaccination history of the vaccinee. (See INDICATIONS AND USAGE, *Revaccination*.)

The healthcare provider should question the patient, parent or guardian about reactions to a previous dose of PNEUMOVAX 23 or other pneumococcal vaccine.

Information for Patients

The healthcare provider should inform the patient, parent or guardian of the benefits and risks associated with vaccination. For risks associated with vaccination, see WARNINGS, PRECAUTIONS, and ADVERSE REACTIONS.

Patients, parents, and guardians should be instructed to report any serious adverse reactions to their healthcare provider who in turn should report such events to the vaccine manufacturer or the U.S. Department of Health and Human Services through the Vaccine Adverse Event Reporting System (VAERS), 1-800-822-7967.

Pregnancy

Pregnancy Category C: Animal reproduction studies have not been conducted with PNEUMOVAX 23. It is also not known whether PNEUMOVAX 23 can cause fetal harm when administered to a pregnant woman or can affect reproduction capacity. PNEUMOVAX 23 should be given to a pregnant woman only if clearly needed.

Nursing Mothers

It is not known whether this drug is excreted in human milk. Because many drugs are excreted in human milk, caution should be excercised when PNEUMOVAX 23 is administered to a nursing woman.

Pediatric Use

In general, children less than 2 years of age respond poorly to the capsular types of PNEUMOVAX 23 that are most often the cause of pneumococcal disease in this age group. (See CLINICAL PHARMACOLOGY, *Immunogenicity*.)

Safety and effectiveness in children below the age of 2 years have not been established. Accordingly, PNEUMOVAX 23 is not recommended in this age group.

Geriatric Use

Persons 65 years of age or older were enrolled in several clinical studies of PNEUMOVAX 23 that were conducted pre- and post-licensure. In the largest of these studies, the safety of PNEUMOVAX 23 in adults 65 years of age and older was compared to the safety of PNEUMOVAX 23 in adults 50 to 64 years of age. Of 1007 subjects enrolled in this study, 433 subjects were 65 to 74 years of age, and 195 subjects were 75 years of age or older. No overall difference in safety was observed between these subjects and younger subjects. However, since elderly individuals may not tolerate medical interventions as well as younger individuals, a higher frequency and/or a greater severity of reactions in some older individuals cannot be ruled out.

ADVERSE REACTIONS

The following adverse experiences have been reported with PNEUMOVAX 23 in clinical trials and/or post-marketing experience:

Local reactions at injection site including soreness, warmth, erythema, swelling and induration.‡ Very rarely, cellulitis-like reactions were reported. These cellulitis-like reactions, reported in post-marketing experience, show short onset time from vaccine administration and were transient in nature.

Fever ≤ 102°F.‡

‡Most common adverse experiences reported in clinical trials.

Other adverse experiences reported in clinical trials and/or in post-marketing experience include:

Body as a Whole

Cellulitis

Asthenia

Malaise

Fever (>102°F)

Digestive System

Nausea

Vomiting

Hematologic/Lymphatic

Lymphadenitis

Thrombocytopenia in patients with stabilized idiopathic thrombocytopenic purpura

Hemolytic anemia in patients who have had other hematologic disorders

Hypersensitivity

Anaphylactoid reactions

Serum Sickness

Angioneurotic edema

Continued on next page

Information on the Merck & Co., Inc., products listed on these pages is from the prescribing information in use October 1, 2004. For information, please call 1-800-NSC-MERCK [1-800-672-6372].

Pneumovax 23—Cont.

Musculoskeletal System
Arthralgia
Arthritis
Myalgia
Nervous System
Headache
Paresthesia
Radiculoneuropathy
Guillain-Barré Syndrome
Skin
Rash
Urticaria.

DOSAGE AND ADMINISTRATION

Do not inject intravenously or intradermally.
Parenteral drug products should be inspected visually for particulate matter and discoloration prior to administration, whenever solution and container permit. PNEUMOVAX 23 is a clear, colorless solution. The vaccine is used directly as supplied. No dilution or reconstitution is necessary. Phenol 0.25% has been added as a preservative. It is important to use a separate sterile syringe and needle for each individual patient to prevent transmission of infectious agents from one person to another.
Withdraw 0.5 mL from the vial using a sterile needle and syringe free of preservatives, antiseptics, and detergents.
Administer a single 0.5 mL dose of PNEUMOVAX 23 subcutaneously or intramuscularly (preferably in the deltoid muscle or lateral mid-thigh), with appropriate precautions to avoid intravascular administration.
Store unopened and opened vials at 2–8°C (36–46°F). All vaccines must be discarded after the expiration date.
Use With Other Vaccines
The ACIP states that pneumococcal vaccine may be administered at the same time as influenza vaccine (by separate injection in the other arm) without an increase in side effects or decreased antibody response to either vaccine. In contrast to pneumococcal vaccine, influenza vaccine is recommended annually, for appropriate populations.

HOW SUPPLIED

No. 4739 — PNEUMOVAX 23 is supplied as one 5-dose vial of liquid vaccine, color coded with a purple cap and stripe on the vial labels and cartons, **NDC** 0006-4739-00.
No. 4739 — PNEUMOVAX 23 is supplied as one 5-dose vial of liquid vaccine, in a box of 10 five-dose vials, color coded with a purple cap and stripe on the vial labels and cartons, **NDC** 0006-4739-50.
No. 4943 — PNEUMOVAX 23 is supplied as a single-dose vial of liquid vaccine, in a box of 10 single-dose vials, color coded with a purple cap and stripe on the vial labels and cartons, **NDC** 0006-4943-00.
7999821 Issued May 2004

PRIMAXIN® I.M. ℞

(Imipenem and Cilastatin for Injectable Suspension)

To reduce the development of drug-resistant bacteria and maintain the effectiveness of PRIMAXIN I.M.† and other antibacterial drugs, PRIMAXIN I.M. should be used only to treat or prevent infections that are proven or strongly suspected to be caused by bacteria.

For Intramuscular Injection Only

DESCRIPTION

PRIMAXIN† I.M. (Imipenem and Cilastatin for Injectable Suspension) is a formulation of imipenem (a thienamycin antibiotic) and cilastatin sodium (the inhibitor of the renal dipeptidase, dehydropeptidase I). PRIMAXIN I.M. is a potent broad spectrum antibacterial agent for intramuscular administration.
Imipenem (N-formimidoylthienamycin monohydrate) is a crystalline derivative of thienamycin, which is produced by *Streptomyces cattleya*. Its chemical name is [5*R* -[5α, 6α (*R* *)]]-6-(1-hydroxyethyl)-3-[[2-[(iminomethyl)amino] ethyl]thio]-7-oxo-1-azabicyclo [3.2.0] hept-2-ene-2-carboxylic acid monohydrate. It is an off-white, nonhygroscopic crystalline compound with a molecular weight of 317.37. It is sparingly soluble in water, and slightly soluble in methanol. Its empirical formula is $C_{12}H_{17}N_3O_4S{\cdot}H_2O$, and its structural formula is:

Cilastatin sodium is the sodium salt of a derivatized heptenoic acid. Its chemical name is [*R*- [*R**,*S**- (*Z*)]]-7-[(2-amino-2-carboxyethyl)thio]-2-[[(2, 2-dimethylcyclopropyl) carbonyl]amino]-2-heptenoic acid, monosodium salt. It is an off-white to yellowish-white, hygroscopic, amorphous compound with a molecular weight of 380.43. It is very soluble in water and in methanol. Its empirical formula is $C_{16}H_{25}N_2O_5SNa$, and its structural formula is:

PRIMAXIN I.M. 500 contains 32 mg of sodium (1.4 mEq) and PRIMAXIN I.M. 750 contains 48 mg of sodium (2.1 mEq). Prepared PRIMAXIN I.M. suspensions are white to light tan in color. Variations of color within this range do not affect the potency of the product.

† Registered trademark of MERCK & CO., Inc.

CLINICAL PHARMACOLOGY

Following intramuscular administrations of 500 or 750 mg doses of imipenem-cilastatin sodium in a 1:1 ratio with 1% lidocaine, peak plasma levels of imipenem antimicrobial activity occur within 2 hours and average 10 and 12 µg/mL, respectively. For cilastatin, peak plasma levels average 24 and 33 µg/mL, respectively, and occur within 1 hour. When compared to intravenous administration of imipenem-cilastatin sodium, imipenem is approximately 75% bioavailable following intramuscular administration while cilastatin is approximately 95% bioavailable. The absorption of imipenem from the IM injection site continues for 6 to 8 hours while that for cilastatin is essentially complete within 4 hours. This prolonged absorption of imipenem following the administration of the intramuscular formulation of imipenem-cilastatin sodium results in an effective plasma half-life of imipenem of approximately 2 to 3 hours and plasma levels of the antibiotic which remain above 2 µg/mL for at least 6 or 8 hours, following a 500 mg or 750 mg dose, respectively. This plasma profile for imipenem permits IM administration of the intramuscular formulation of imipenem-cilastatin sodium every 12 hours with no accumulation of cilastatin and only slight accumulation of imipenem.
A comparison of plasma levels of imipenem after a single dose of 500 mg or 750 mg of imipenem-cilastatin sodium (intravenous formulation) administered intravenously or of imipenem-cilastatin sodium (intramuscular formulation) diluted with 1% lidocaine and administered intramuscularly is as follows:

PLASMA CONCENTRATIONS OF IMIPENEM (µg/mL)

	500 MG		750 MG	
TIME	I.V.	I.M.	I.V.	I.M.
25 min	45.1	6.0	57.0	6.7
1 hr	21.6	9.4	28.1	10.0
2 hr	10.0	9.9	12.0	11.4
4 hr	2.6	5.6	3.4	7.3
6 hr	0.6	2.5	1.1	3.8
12 hr	ND**	0.5	ND**	0.8

** ND: Not Detectable (<0.3 µg/mL)

Imipenem urine levels remain above 10 µg/mL for the 12 hour dosing interval following the administration of 500 mg or 750 mg doses of the intramuscular formulation of imipenem-cilastatin sodium. Total urinary excretion of imipenem averages 50% while that for cilastatin averages 75% following either dose of the intramuscular formulation of imipenem-cilastatin sodium.
Imipenem, when administered alone, is metabolized in the kidneys by dehydropeptidase I resulting in relatively low levels in urine. Cilastatin sodium, an inhibitor of this enzyme, effectively prevents renal metabolism of imipenem so that when imipenem and cilastatin sodium are given concomitantly, increased levels of imipenem are achieved in the urine. The binding of imipenem to human serum proteins is approximately 20% and that of cilastatin is approximately 40%.
In a clinical study in which a 500 mg dose of the intramuscular formulation of imipenem-cilastatin sodium was administered to healthy subjects, the average peak level of imipenem in interstitial fluid (skin blister fluid) was approximately 5.0 µg/mL within 3.5 hours after administration.
Imipenem-cilastatin sodium is hemodialyzable. However, usefulness of this procedure in the overdosage setting is questionable. (See **OVERDOSAGE.**)
Microbiology
The bactericidal activity of imipenem results from the inhibition of cell wall synthesis. Its greatest affinity is for penicillin-binding proteins (PBPs) 1A, 1B, 2, 4, 5 and 6 of *Escherichia coli,* and 1A, 1B, 2, 4 and 5 of *Pseudomonas aeruginosa.* The lethal effect is related to binding to PBP 2 and PBP 1B.
Imipenem has a high degree of stability in the presence of beta-lactamases, including penicillinases and cephalosporinases produced by gram-negative and gram-positive bacteria. It is a potent inhibitor of beta-lactamases from certain gram-negative bacteria which are inherently resistant to many beta-lactam antibiotics, e.g., *Pseudomonas aeruginosa, Serratia* spp. and *Enterobacter* spp.
Imipenem has *in vitro* activity against a wide range of gram-positive and gram-negative organisms. Imipenem has been shown to be active against most strains of the following microorganisms, both *in vitro* and in clinical infections treated with the intramuscular formulation of imipenem-cilastatin sodium as described in the INDICATIONS AND USAGE section.
Gram-positive aerobes:
Staphylococcus aureus including penicillinase-producing strains
(NOTE: Methicillin-resistant staphylococci should be reported as resistant to imipenem.)
Group D streptococcus including *Enterococcus faecalis* (formerly *S. faecalis*)
(NOTE: Imipenem is inactive *in vitro* against *Enterococcus faecium* [formerly *S. faecium*].)
Streptococcus pneumoniae
Streptococcus pyogenes (Group A streptococci)
Streptococcus viridans group
Gram-negative aerobes:
Acinetobacter spp., including *A. calcoaceticus*
Citrobacter spp.
Enterobacter cloacae
Escherichia coli
Haemophilus influenzae
Klebsiella pneumoniae
Pseudomonas aeruginosa
(NOTE: Imipenem is inactive *in vitro* against *Xanthomonas (Pseudomonas) maltophilia* and *P. cepacia.*)
Gram-positive anaerobes:
Peptostreptococcus spp.
Gram-negative anaerobes:
Bacteroides spp., including
Bacteroides distasonis
Bacteroides intermedius (formerly *B. melaninogenicus intermedius)*
Bacteroides fragilis
Bacteroides thetaiotaomicron
Fusobacterium spp.
Imipenem exhibits *in vitro* minimal inhibitory concentrations (MICs) of 4 µg/mL or less against most (≥90%) strains of the following microorganisms; however, the safety and effectiveness of imipenem in treating clinical infections due to these microorganisms have not been established in adequate and well-controlled clinical trials.
Gram-positive aerobes:
Bacillus spp.
Listeria monocytogenes
Nocardia spp.
Group C streptococci
Group G streptococci
Gram-negative aerobes:
Aeromonas hydrophila
Alcaligenes spp.
Capnocytophaga spp.
Enterobacter agglomerans
Haemophilus ducreyi
Klebsiella oxytoca
Neisseria gonorrhoeae including penicillinase-producing strains
Pasteurella spp.
Proteus mirabilis
Providencia stuartii
Gram-positive anaerobes:
Clostridium perfringens
Gram-negative anaerobes:
Prevotella bivia
Prevotella disiens
Prevotella melaninogenica
Veillonella spp.
In vitro tests show imipenem to act synergistically with aminoglycoside antibiotics against some isolates of *Pseudomonas aeruginosa.*
Susceptibility Tests:
Dilution techniques:
Use a standardized dilution method[1] (broth, agar, microdilution) or equivalent with imipenem powder. The MIC values obtained should be interpreted according to the following criteria:

MIC (µg/mL)	Interpretation
≤4	Susceptible
8	Moderately Susceptible
≥16	Resistant

A report of "susceptible" indicates that the pathogen is likely to be inhibited by generally achievable blood levels. A report of "moderately susceptible" suggests that the organism would be susceptible if high dosage is used or if the infection is confined to tissues and fluids in which high antibiotic levels are attained. A report of "resistant" indicates that achievable concentrations are unlikely to be inhibitory and other therapy should be selected.
Standardized susceptibility test procedures require the use of laboratory control organisms. Standard imipenem powder should provide the following MIC values:

Organism	MIC (µg/mL)
E. coli ATCC 25922	0.06–0.25
S. aureus ATCC 29213	0.015–0.06
E. faecalis ATCC 29212	0.5–2.0
P. aeruginosa ATCC 27853	1.0–4.0

Diffusion techniques:
Quantitative methods that require measurement of zone diameters give the most precise estimate of antibiotic susceptibility. One such standard procedure[2], which has been recommended for use with disks to test susceptibility of organisms to imipenem, uses the 10-µg imipenem disk. Interpretation involves the correlation of the diameters obtained in the disk test with the minimum inhibitory concentration (MIC) for imipenem.
Reports from the laboratory giving results of the standard single-disk susceptibility test with a 10-µg imipenem disk should be interpreted according to the following criteria:

Zone Diameter (mm)	Interpretation
≥16	Susceptible
14–15	Moderately Susceptible
≤13	Resistant

Standardized procedures require the use of laboratory control organisms. The 10-µg imipenem disk should give the following zone diameters:

Organism	Zone Diameter (mm)
E. coli ATCC 25922	26–32
P. aeruginosa ATCC 27853	20–28

For anaerobic bacteria, the MIC of imipenem can be determined by agar or broth dilution (including microdilution) techniques.[3]
The MIC values obtained should be interpreted according to the following criteria:

MIC (µg/mL)	Interpretation
≤4	Susceptible
8	Moderately Susceptible
≥16	Resistant

INDICATIONS AND USAGE

PRIMAXIN I.M. is indicated for the treatment of serious infections (listed below) of mild to moderate severity for which intramuscular therapy is appropriate. **PRIMAXIN I.M. is not intended for the therapy of severe or life-threatening infections, including bacterial sepsis or endocarditis, or in instances of major physiological impairments such as shock.**
PRIMAXIN I.M. is indicated for the treatment of infections caused by susceptible strains of the designated microorganisms in the conditions listed below:

(1) **Lower respiratory tract infections,** including pneumonia and bronchitis as an exacerbation of COPD, caused by *Streptococcus pneumoniae* and *Haemophilus influenzae.*
(2) **Intra-abdominal infections,** including acute gangrenous or perforated appendicitis and appendicitis with peritonitis, caused by Group D streptococcus including *Enterococcus faecalis*; Streptococcus viridans* group*; *Escherichia coli; Klebsiella pneumoniae*; Pseudomonas aeruginosa*; Bacteroides* species including *B. fragilis, B. distasonis*, B. intermedius** and *B. thetaiotaomicron*; Fusobacterium* species and *Peptostreptococcus** species.
(3) **Skin and skin structure infections,** including abscesses, cellulitis, infected skin ulcers and wound infections caused by *Staphylococcus aureus* including penicillinase-producing strains; *Streptococcus pyogenes**; Group D streptococcus including *Enterococcus faecalis; Acinetobacter* species* including *A. calcoaceticus*; Citrobacter* species*; *Escherichia coli; Enterobacter cloacae; Klebsiella pneumoniae*; Pseudomonas aeruginosa** and *Bacteroides* species* including *B. fragilis**.
(4) **Gynecologic infections,** including postpartum endomyometritis, caused by Group D streptococcus including *Enterococcus faecalis*; Escherichia coli; Klebsiella pneumoniae*; Bacteroides intermedius**; and *Peptostreptococcus* species*.

As with other beta-lactam antibiotics, some strains of *Pseudomonas aeruginosa* may develop resistance fairly rapidly during treatment with PRIMAXIN I.M. During therapy of *Pseudomonas aeruginosa* infections, periodic susceptibility testing should be done when clinically appropriate.
To reduce the development of drug-resistant bacteria and maintain the effectiveness of PRIMAXIN I.M. and other antibacterial drugs, PRIMAXIN I.M. should be used only to treat or prevent infections that are proven or strongly suspected to be caused by susceptible bacteria. When culture and susceptibility information are available, they should be considered in selecting or modifying antibacterial therapy. In the absence of such data, local epidemiology and susceptibility patterns may contribute to the empiric selection of therapy.

*Efficacy for this organism in this organ system was studied in fewer than 10 infections.

CONTRAINDICATIONS

PRIMAXIN I.M. is contraindicated in patients who have shown hypersensitivity to any component of this product. Due to the use of lidocaine hydrochloride diluent, this product is contraindicated in patients with a known hypersensitivity to local anesthetics of the amide type and in patients with severe shock or heart block. (Refer to the package circular for lidocaine hydrochloride).

WARNINGS

SERIOUS AND OCCASIONALLY FATAL HYPERSENSITIVITY (anaphylactic) REACTIONS HAVE BEEN REPORTED IN PATIENTS RECEIVING THERAPY WITH BETA-LACTAMS. THESE REACTIONS ARE MORE LIKELY TO OCCUR IN INDIVIDUALS WITH A HISTORY OF SENSITIVITY TO MULTIPLE ALLERGENS. THERE HAVE BEEN REPORTS OF INDIVIDUALS WITH A HISTORY OF PENICILLIN HYPERSENSITIVITY WHO HAVE EXPERIENCED SEVERE REACTIONS WHEN TREATED WITH ANOTHER BETA-LACTAM. BEFORE INITIATING THERAPY WITH PRIMAXIN® I.M., CAREFUL INQUIRY SHOULD BE MADE CONCERNING PREVIOUS HYPERSENSITIVITY REACTIONS TO PENICILLINS, CEPHALOSPORINS, OTHER BETA-LACTAMS, AND OTHER ALLERGENS. IF AN ALLERGIC REACTION OCCURS, PRIMAXIN® SHOULD BE DISCONTINUED. **SERIOUS ANAPHYLACTIC REACTIONS REQUIRE IMMEDIATE EMERGENCY TREATMENT WITH EPINEPHRINE. OXYGEN, INTRAVENOUS STEROIDS, AND AIRWAY MANAGEMENT, INCLUDING INTUBATION, MAY ALSO BE ADMINISTERED AS INDICATED.**
Pseudomembranous colitis has been reported with nearly all antibacterial agents, including PRIMAXIN, and may range in severity from mild to life-threatening. Therefore, it is important to consider this diagnosis in patients who present with diarrhea subsequent to the administration of antibacterial agents.
Treatment with antibacterial agents alters the normal flora of the colon and may permit overgrowth of clostridia. Studies indicate that a toxin produced by *Clostridium difficile* is one primary cause of "antibiotic-associated colitis".
After the diagnosis of pseudomembranous colitis has been established, therapeutic measures should be initiated. Mild cases of pseudomembranous colitis usually respond to drug discontinuation alone. In moderate to severe cases, consideration should be given to management with fluids and electrolytes, protein supplementation and treatment with an antibacterial drug clinically effective against *C. difficile* colitis.
Lidocaine HCl —Refer to the package circular for lidocaine HCl.

PRECAUTIONS

General
CNS adverse experiences such as myoclonic activity, confusional states, or seizures have been reported with PRIMAXIN I.V. (Imipenem and Cilastatin for Injection). These experiences have occurred most commonly in patients with CNS disorders (e.g., brain lesions or history of seizures) who also have compromised renal function. However, there were reports in which there was no recognized or documented underlying CNS disorder. These adverse CNS effects have not been seen with PRIMAXIN I.M.; however, should they occur during treatment, PRIMAXIN I.M. should be discontinued. Anticonvulsant therapy should be continued in patients with a known seizure disorder.
As with other antibiotics, prolonged use of PRIMAXIN I.M. may result in overgrowth of nonsusceptible organisms. Repeated evaluation of the patient's condition is essential. If superinfection occurs during therapy, appropriate measures should be taken.
Prescribing PRIMAXIN I.M. in the absence of a proven or strongly suspected bacterial infection or a prophylactic indication is unlikely to provide benefit to the patient and increases the risk of the development of drug-resistant bacteria.
Caution should be taken to avoid inadvertent injection into a blood vessel. (See DOSAGE AND ADMINISTRATION.) For additional precautions, refer to the package circular for lidocaine HCl.
Information for Patients
Patients should be counseled that antibacterial drugs including PRIMAXIN I.M. should only be used to treat bacterial infections. They do not treat viral infections (e.g., the common cold). When PRIMAXIN I.M. is prescribed to treat a bacterial infection, patients should be told that although it is common to feel better early in the course of therapy, the medication should be taken exactly as directed. Skipping doses or not completing the full course of therapy may (1) decrease the effectiveness of the immediate treatment and (2) increase the likelihood that bacteria will develop resistance and will not be treatable by PRIMAXIN I.M. or other antibacterial drugs in the future.
Drug Interactions
Since concomitant administration of PRIMAXIN (Imipenem-Cilastatin Sodium) and probenecid results in only minimal increases in plasma levels of imipenem and plasma half-life, it is not recommended that probenecid be given with PRIMAXIN I.M.
PRIMAXIN I.M. should not be mixed with or physically added to other antibiotics. However, PRIMAXIN I.M. may be administered concomitantly with other antibiotics, such as aminoglycosides.
Carcinogenesis, Mutagenesis, Impairment of Fertility
Long term studies in animals have not been performed to evaluate carcinogenic potential of imipenem-cilastatin. Genetic toxicity studies were performed in a variety of bacterial and mammalian tests *in vivo* and *in vitro.* The tests used were: V79 mammalian cell mutagenesis assay (imipenem-cilastatin sodium alone and imipenem alone), Ames test (cilastatin sodium alone and imipenem alone), unscheduled DNA synthesis assay (imipenem-cilastatin sodium) and *in vivo* mouse cytogenetics test (imipenem-cilastatin sodium). None of these tests showed any evidence of genetic alterations.
Reproductive tests in male and female rats were performed with imipenem-cilastatin sodium at intravenous doses up to 80 mg/kg/day and at a subcutaneous dose of 320 mg/kg/day, 2.1 times*** the maximum recommended daily human dose of the intramuscular formulation (on a mg/m^2 body surface area basis). Slight decreases in live fetal body weight were restricted to the highest dosage level. No other adverse effects were observed on fertility, reproductive performance, fetal viability, growth, or postnatal development of pups.
Pregnancy: Teratogenic Effects
Pregnancy Category C: Teratology studies with cilastatin sodium at doses of 30, 100, and 300 mg/kg/day administered intravenously to rabbits and 40, 200, and 1000 mg/kg/day administered subcutaneously to rats, up to approximately 3.9 and 6.5 times*** the maximum recommended daily human dose (on a mg/m^2 body surface area basis) of the intramuscular formulation of PRIMAXIN (25 mg/kg/day) in the two species, respectively, showed no evidence of adverse effects on the fetus. No evidence of teratogenicity was observed in rabbits given imipenem at intravenous doses of 15, 30 or 60 mg/kg/day and rats given imipenem at intravenous doses of 225, 450, or 900 mg/kg/day, up to approximately 0.8 and 5.8 times*** the maximum recommended daily human dose (on a mg/m^2 body surface area basis) in the two species, respectively.
Teratology studies with imipenem-cilastatin sodium at intravenous doses of 20 and 80 and a subcutaneous dose of 320 mg/kg/day, approximately equal to (mice) and up to 2.1 times*** (rats) the maximum recommended daily intramuscular human dose (on a mg/m^2 body surface area basis) in pregnant rodents during the period of major organogenesis, revealed no evidence of teratogenicity.
Imipenem-cilastatin sodium, when administered to pregnant rabbits subcutaneously at dosages above the usual human dose of the intramuscular formulation (1000–1500 mg/day), caused body weight loss, diarrhea, and maternal deaths. When comparable doses of imipenem-cilastatin sodium were given to non-pregnant rabbits, body weight loss, diarrhea, and deaths were also observed. This intolerance is not unlike that seen with other beta-lactam antibiotics in this species and is probably due to alteration of gut flora.
A teratology study in pregnant cynomolgus monkeys given imipenem-cilastatin sodium at doses of 40 mg/kg/day (bolus intravenous injection) or 160 mg/kg/day (subcutaneous injection) resulted in maternal toxicity including emesis, inappetence, body weight loss, diarrhea, abortion and death in some cases. In contrast, no significant toxicity was observed when non-pregnant cynomolgus monkeys were given doses of imipenem-cilastatin sodium up to 180 mg/kg/day (subcutaneous injection). When doses of imipenem-cilastatin sodium (approximately 100 mg/kg/day or approximately 1.3 times*** the maximum recommended daily human dose of the intramuscular formulation) were administered to pregnant cynomolgus monkeys at an intraveous infusion rate which mimics human clinical use, there was minimal maternal intolerance (occasional emesis), no maternal deaths, no evidence of teratogenicity, but an increase in embryonic loss relative to the control groups.
No adverse effects on the fetus or on lactation were observed when imipenem-cilastatin sodium was administered subcutaneously to rats late in gestation at dosages up to 320 mg/kg/day, 2.1 times the maximum recommended daily human dose (on a mg/m^2 body surface area basis).
There are, however, no adequate and well-controlled studies in pregnant women. PRIMAXIN I.M. should be used during pregnancy only if the potential benefit justifies the potential risk to the mother and fetus.
Nursing Mothers
It is not known whether imipenem-cilastatin sodium or lidocaine HCl (diluent) is excreted in human milk. Because many drugs are excreted in human milk, caution should be exercised when PRIMAXIN I.M. is administered to a nursing woman.
Pediatric Use
Safety and effectiveness in pediatric patients below the age of 12 years have not been established.
Geriatric Use
Clinical studies of PRIMAXIN I.M. did not include sufficient numbers of subjects aged 65 and over to determine whether they respond differently from younger subjects; however, clinical studies of PRIMAXIN I.V. in a sufficient number of subjects aged 65 and over have not revealed overall differences in safety or effectiveness between these subjects and younger subjects (refer to the package circular for PRIMAXIN I.V.). Other reported clinical experience has not identified differences in responses between the elderly and younger patients. In general, dose selection for an elderly patient should be cautious, usually starting at the low end of the dosing range, reflecting the greater frequency of decreased hepatic, renal, or cardiac function, and of concomitant disease or other drug therapy.
This drug is known to be substantially excreted by the kidney, and the risk of toxic reactions to this drug may be greater in patients with impaired renal function. Because elderly patients are more likely to have decreased renal

Continued on next page

Information on the Merck & Co., Inc., products listed on these pages is from the prescribing information in use October 1, 2004. For information, please call 1-800-NSC-MERCK [1-800-672-6372].

Primaxin I.M.—Cont.

function, care should be taken in dose selection, and it may be useful to monitor renal function. Dosage adjustment in the case of renal impairment is necessary (see DOSAGE AND ADMINISTRATION, ADULTS WITH IMPAIRED RENAL FUNCTION).

*** Based on patient body surface area of 1.6 m^2 (weight of 60 kg).

ADVERSE REACTIONS

PRIMAXIN I.M.

In 686 patients in multiple dose clinical trials of PRIMAXIN I.M., the following adverse reactions were reported:

Local Adverse Reactions

The most frequent adverse local clinical reaction that was reported as possibly, probably or definitely related to therapy with PRIMAXIN I.M. was pain at the injection site (1.2%).

Systemic Adverse Reactions

The most frequently reported systemic adverse clinical reactions that were reported as possibly, probably, or definitely related to PRIMAXIN I.M. were nausea (0.6%), diarrhea (0.6%), vomiting (0.3%) and rash (0.4%).

Adverse Laboratory Changes

Adverse laboratory changes without regard to drug relationship that were reported during clinical trials were:

Hemic: decreased hemoglobin and hematocrit, eosinophilia, increased and decreased WBC, increased and decreased platelets, decreased erythrocytes, and increased prothrombin time.

Hepatic: increased AST, ALT, alkaline phosphatase, and bilirubin.

Renal: increased BUN and creatinine.

Urinalysis: presence of red blood cells, white blood cells, casts, and bacteria in the urine.

Potential ADVERSE EFFECTS:

In addition, a variety of adverse effects, not observed in clinical trials with PRIMAXIN I.M., have been reported with intravenous administration of PRIMAXIN I.V. (Imipenem and Cilastatin for Injection). Those listed below are to serve as alerting information to physicians.

Systemic Adverse Reactions

The most frequently reported systemic adverse clinical reactions that were reported as possibly, probably, or definitely related to PRIMAXIN I.V. (Imipenem and Cilastatin for Injection) were fever, hypotension, seizures (see PRECAUTIONS), dizziness, pruritus, urticaria, and somnolence.

Additional adverse systemic clinical reactions reported possibly, probably, or definitely drug related or reported since the drug was marketed are listed within each body system in order of decreasing severity: *Gastrointestinal:* pseudomembranous colitis (the onset of pseudomembranous colitis symptoms may occur during or after antibiotic treatment, see WARNINGS), hemorrhagic colitis, hepatitis, jaundice, gastroenteritis, abdominal pain, glossitis, tongue papillar hypertrophy, staining of the teeth and/or tongue, heartburn, pharyngeal pain, increased salivation; *Hematologic:* pancytopenia, bone marrow depression, thrombocytopenia, neutropenia, leukopenia, hemolytic anemia; *CNS:* encephalopathy, tremor, confusion, myoclonus, paresthesia, vertigo, headache, psychic disturbances including hallucinations; *Special Senses:* hearing loss, tinnitus, taste perversion; *Respiratory:* chest discomfort, dyspnea, hyperventilation, thoracic spine pain; *Cardiovascular:* palpitations, tachycardia; *Renal:* acute renal failure, oliguria/anuria, polyuria, urine discoloration; *Skin:* toxic epidermal necrolysis, Stevens-Johnson syndrome, erythema multiforme, angioneurotic edema, flushing, cyanosis, hyperhidrosis, skin texture changes, candidiasis, pruritus vulvae; *Body as a whole:* polyarthralgia, asthenia/weakness, drug fever.

Adverse Laboratory Changes

Adverse laboratory changes without regard to drug relationship that were reported during clinical trials or reported since the drug was marketed were:

Hepatic: increased LDH; *Hemic:* positive Coombs test, decreased neutrophils, agranulocytosis, increased monocytes, abnormal prothrombin time, increased lymphocytes, increased basophils; *Electrolytes:* decreased serum sodium, increased potassium, increased chloride; *Urinalysis:* presence of urine protein, urine bilirubin, and urine urobilinogen.

Lidocaine HCl —Refer to the package circular for lidocaine HCl.

OVERDOSAGE

The acute intravenous toxicity of imipenem-cilastatin sodium in a ratio of 1:1 was studied in mice at doses of 751 to 1359 mg/kg. Following drug administration, ataxia was rapidly produced and clonic convulsions were noted in about 45 minutes. Deaths occurred within 4–56 minutes at all doses. The acute intravenous toxicity of imipenem-cilastatin sodium was produced within 5–10 minutes in rats at doses of 771 to 1583 mg/kg. In all dosage groups, females had decreased activity, bradypnea and ptosis with clonic convulsions preceding death; in males, ptosis was seen at all dose levels while tremors and clonic convulsions were seen at all but the lowest dose (771 mg/kg). In another rat study, female rats showed ataxia, bradypnea and decreased activity in all but the lowest dose (550 mg/kg); deaths were preceded by clonic convulsions. Male rats showed tremors at all doses and clonic convulsions and ptosis were seen at the two highest doses (1130 and 1734 mg/kg). Deaths occurred between 6 and 88 minutes with doses of 771 to 1734 mg/kg.

In the case of overdosage, discontinue PRIMAXIN I.M., treat symptomatically, and institute supportive measures as required. Imipenem-cilastatin sodium is hemodialyzable. However, usefulness of this procedure in the overdosage setting is questionable.

DOSAGE AND ADMINISTRATION

PRIMAXIN I.M. is for intramuscular use only.

The dosage recommendations for PRIMAXIN I.M. represent the quantity of imipenem to be administered. An equivalent amount of cilastatin is also present.

Patients with lower respiratory tract infections, skin and skin structure infections, and gynecologic infections of mild to moderate severity may be treated with 500 mg or 750 mg administered every 12 hours depending on the severity of the infection.

Intra-abdominal infection may be treated with 750 mg every 12 hours.

[See table below]

Total daily IM dosages greater than 1500 mg per day are not recommended.

The dosage for any particular patient should be based on the location and severity of the infection, the susceptibility of the infecting pathogen(s), and renal function.

The duration of therapy depends upon the type and severity of the infection. Generally, PRIMAXIN I.M. should be continued for at least two days after the signs and symptoms of infection have resolved. Safety and efficacy of treatment beyond fourteen days have not been established.

PRIMAXIN I.M. should be administered by deep intramuscular injection into a large muscle mass (such as the gluteal muscles or lateral part of the thigh) with a 21 gauge 2" needle. Aspiration is necessary to avoid inadvertent injection into a blood vessel.

ADULTS WITH IMPAIRED RENAL FUNCTION

The safety and efficacy of PRIMAXIN I.M. have not been studied in patients with creatinine clearance of less than 20 mL/min/1.73m^2. Serum creatinine alone may not be a sufficiently accurate measure of renal function. Creatinine clearance (T_{cc}) may be estimated from the following equation:

$$T_{cc}\text{ (Males)} = \frac{\text{(wt. in kg) (140} - \text{age)}}{\text{(72) (creatinine in mg/dL)}}$$

$$T_{cc}\text{ (Females)} = 0.85 \times \text{above value}$$

PREPARATION FOR ADMINISTRATION

PRIMAXIN I.M. should be prepared for use with 1.0% lidocaine HCl solution††† (without epinephrine). PRIMAXIN I.M. 500 should be prepared with 2 mL and PRIMAXIN I.M. 750 with 3 mL of lidocaine HCl. Agitate to form a suspension, then withdraw and inject the entire contents of vial intramuscularly. The suspension of PRIMAXIN I.M. in lidocaine HCl should be used within one hour after preparation. **Note: The IM formulation is not for IV use.**

††† Refer to the package circular for lidocaine HCl for detailed information concerning CONTRAINDICATIONS, WARNINGS, PRECAUTIONS, and ADVERSE REACTIONS.

COMPATIBILITY AND STABILITY

Before reconsitution:

The dry powder should be stored at a temperature below 25°C (77°F).

Suspensions for IM Administration

Suspensions of PRIMAXIN I.M. are white to light tan in color. Variations of color within this range do not affect the potency of the product.

The suspension of PRIMAXIN I.M. in lidocaine HCl should be used within one hour after preparation.

PRIMAXIN I.M. should not be mixed with or physically added to other antibiotics. However, PRIMAXIN I.M. may be administered concomitantly but at separate sites with other antibiotics, such as aminoglycosides.

DOSAGE GUIDELINES

Type††/Location of Infection	Severity	Dosage Regimen
Lower respiratory tract Skin and skin structure Gynecologic	Mild/Moderate	500 or 750 mg q 12 h depending on the severity of infection
Intra-abdominal	Mild/Moderate	750 mg q 12 h

†† See INDICATIONS AND USAGE section.

HOW SUPPLIED

PRIMAXIN I.M. is supplied as a sterile powder mixture in vials for IM administration as follows:

No. 3582—500 mg imipenem equivalent and 500 mg cilastatin equivalent

NDC 0006-3582-75 in trays of 10 vials.

No. 3583—750 mg imipenem equivalent and 750 mg cilastatin equivalent

NDC 0006-3583-76 in trays of 10 vials.

REFERENCES

1. National Committee for Clinical Laboratory Standards, Methods for Dilution Antimicrobial Susceptibility Tests for Bacteria that Grow Aerobically—Fourth Edition. Approved Standard NCCLS Document M7-A4, Vol. 17, No. 2 NCCLS, Villanova, PA, 1997.
2. National Committee for Clinical Laboratory Standards, Performance Standards for Antimicrobial Disk Susceptibility Tests—Sixth Edition. Approved Standard NCCLS Document M2-A6, Vol. 17, No. 1 NCCLS, Villanova, PA, 1997.
3. National Committee for Clinical Laboratory Standards, Method for Antimicrobial Susceptibility Testing of Anaerobic Bacteria—Third Edition. Approved Standard NCCLS Document M11-A3, Vol. 13, No. 26 NCCLS, Villanova, PA, 1993.

7632911 Issued August 2003

PRIMAXIN® I.V. ℞

(Imipenem and Cilastatin for Injection)

To reduce the development of drug-resistant bacteria and maintain the effectiveness of PRIMAXIN I.V.† and other antibacterial drugs, PRIMAXIN I.V. should be used only to treat or prevent infections that are proven or strongly suspected to be caused by bacteria.

For Intravenous Injection Only

DESCRIPTION

PRIMAXIN† I.V. (Imipenem and Cilastatin for Injection) is a sterile formulation of imipenem (a thienamycin antibiotic) and cilastatin sodium (the inhibitor of the renal dipeptidase, dehydropeptidase I), with sodium bicarbonate added as a buffer. PRIMAXIN I.V. is a potent broad spectrum antibacterial agent for intravenous administration.

Imipenem (N-formimidoylthienamycin monohydrate) is a crystalline derivative of thienamycin, which is produced by *Streptomyces cattleya.* Its chemical name is (5*R* ,6*S*)-3-[[2-(formimidoylamino)ethyl]thio]-6-[(*R*)-1-hydroxyethyl]-7-oxo-1-azabicyclo[3.2.0]hept-2-ene-2-carboxylic acid monohydrate. It is an off-white, nonhygroscopic crystalline compound with a molecular weight of 317.37. It is sparingly soluble in water and slightly soluble in methanol. Its empirical formula is $C_{12}H_{17}N_3O_4S \cdot H_2O$, and its structural formula is:

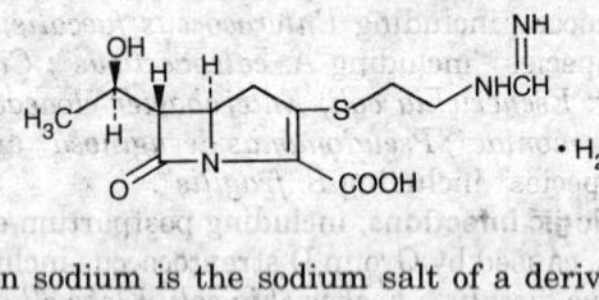

Cilastatin sodium is the sodium salt of a derivatized heptenoic acid. Its chemical name is sodium (*Z*)-7-[[(*R*)-2-amino-2-carboxyethyl]thio] -2- [(*S*) - 2,2- dimethylcyclopropanecarboxamido]-2-heptenoate. It is an off-white to yellowish-white, hygroscopic, amorphous compound with a molecular weight of 380.43. It is very soluble in water and in methanol. Its empirical formula is $C_{16}H_{25}N_2O_5S$ Na, and its structural formula is:

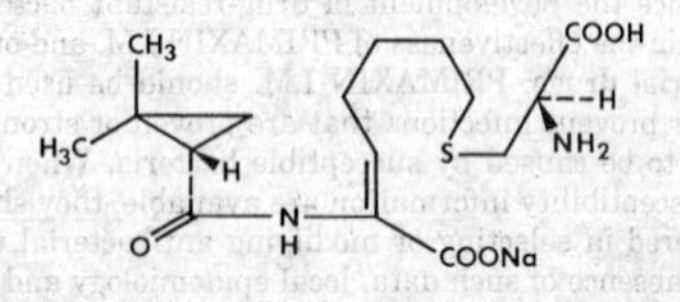

PRIMAXIN I.V. is buffered to provide solutions in the pH range of 6.5 to 8.5. There is no significant change in pH when solutions are prepared and used as directed. (See **COMPATIBILITY AND STABILITY**.) PRIMAXIN I.V. 250 contains 18.8 mg of sodium (0.8 mEq) and PRIMAXIN I.V. 500 contains 37.5 mg of sodium (1.6 mEq). Solutions of PRIMAXIN I.V. range from colorless to yellow. Variations of color within this range do not affect the potency of the product.

†Registered trademark of MERCK & CO., Inc.

CLINICAL PHARMACOLOGY

Adults

Intravenous Administration

Intravenous infusion of PRIMAXIN I.V. over 20 minutes results in peak plasma levels of imipenem antimicrobial activity that range from 14 to 24 μg/mL for the 250 mg dose, from 21 to 58 μg/mL for the 500 mg dose, and from 41 to 83 μg/mL for the 1000 mg dose. At these doses, plasma levels of imipenem antimicrobial activity decline to below 1 μg/mL or less in 4 to 6 hours. Peak plasma levels of cilastatin following a 20-minute intravenous infusion of PRIMAXIN I.V., range from 15 to 25 μg/mL for the 250 mg dose, from 31 to 49 μg/mL for the 500 mg dose, and from 56 to 88 μg/mL for the 1000 mg dose.

The plasma half-life of each component is approximately 1 hour. The binding of imipenem to human serum proteins is approximately 20% and that of cilastatin is approximately 40%. Approximately, 70% of the administered imipenem is recovered in the urine within 10 hours after which no further urinary excretion is detectable. Urine concentrations of imipenem in excess of 10 μg/mL can be maintained for up to 8 hours with PRIMAXIN I.V. at the 500-mg dose. Approximately, 70% of the cilastatin sodium dose is recovered in the urine within 10 hours of administration of PRIMAXIN I.V. No accumulation of imipenem/cilastatin in plasma or urine is observed with regimens administered as frequently as every 6 hours in patients with normal renal function.

In healthy elderly volunteers (65 to 75 years of age with normal renal function for their age), the pharmacokinetics of a single dose of imipenem 500 mg and cilastatin 500 mg administered intravenously over 20 minutes are consistent with those expected in subjects with slight renal impairment for which no dosage alteration is considered necessary. The mean plasma half-lives of imipenem and cilastatin are 91 ± 7.0 minutes and 69 ± 15 minutes, respectively. Multiple dosing has no effect on the pharmacokinetics of either imipenem or cilastatin, and no accumulation of imipenem/cilastatin is observed.

Imipenem, when administered alone, is metabolized in the kidneys by dehydropeptidase I resulting in relatively low levels in urine. Cilastatin sodium, an inhibitor of this enzyme, effectively prevents renal metabolism of imipenem so that when imipenem and cilastatin sodium are given concomitantly, fully adequate antibacterial levels of imipenem are achieved in the urine.

After a 1 gram dose of PRIMAXIN I.V., the following average levels of imipenem were measured (usually at 1 hour post-dose except where indicated) in the tissues and fluids listed:

Tissue or Fluid	n	Imipenem Level μg/mL or μg/g	Range
Vitreous Humor	3	3.4 (3.5 hours post dose)	2.88–3.6
Aqueous Humor	5	2.99 (2 hours post dose)	2.4–3.9
Lung Tissue	8	5.6 (median)	3.5–15.5
Sputum	1	2.1	—
Pleural	1	22.0	—
Peritoneal	12	23.9 S.D. ±5.3 (2 hours post dose)	—
Bile	2	5.3 (2.25 hours post dose)	4.6 to 6.0
CSF (uninflamed)	5	1.0 (4 hours post dose)	0.26–2.0
CSF (inflamed)	7	2.6 (2 hours post dose)	0.5–5.5
Fallopian Tubes	1	13.6	—
Endometrium	1	11.1	—
Myometrium	1	5.0	—
Bone	10	2.6	0.4–5.4
Interstitial Fluid	12	16.4	10.0–22.6
Skin	12	4.4	NA
Fascia	12	4.4	NA

[See table above]

Imipenem-cilastatin sodium is hemodialyzable. However, usefulness of this procedure in the overdosage setting is questionable. (See **OVERDOSAGE**.)

Microbiology

The bactericidal activity of imipenem results from the inhibition of cell wall synthesis. Its greatest affinity is for penicillin binding proteins (PBPs) 1A, 1B, 2, 4, 5 and 6 of *Escherichia coli*, and 1A, 1B, 2, 4 and 5 of *Pseudomonas aeruginosa*. The lethal effect is related to binding to PBP 2 and PBP 1B.

Imipenem has a high degree of stability in the presence of beta-lactamases, both penicillinases and cephalosporinases produced by gram-negative and gram-positive bacteria. It is a potent inhibitor of beta-lactamases from certain gram-negative bacteria which are inherently resistant to most beta-lactam antibiotics, e.g., *Pseudomonas aeruginosa*, *Serratia* spp., and *Enterobacter* spp.

Imipenem has *in vitro* activity against a wide range of gram-positive and gram-negative organisms. Imipenem has been shown to be active against most strains of the following microorganisms, both *in vitro* and in clinical infections treated with the intravenous formulation of imipenem-cilastatin sodium as described in the **INDICATIONS AND USAGE** section.

Gram-positive aerobes:
- *Enterococcus faecalis* (formerly *S. faecalis*)
  (NOTE: Imipenem is inactive *in vitro* against *Enterococcus faecium* [formerly *S. faecium*].)
- *Staphylococcus aureus* including penicillinase-producing strains
- *Staphylococcus epidermidis* including penicillinase-producing strains
  (NOTE: Methicillin-resistant staphylococci should be reported as resistant to imipenem.)
- *Streptococcus agalactiae* (Group B streptococci)
- *Streptococcus pneumoniae*
- *Streptococcus pyogenes*

Gram-negative aerobes:
- *Acinetobacter* spp.
- *Citrobacter* spp.
- *Enterobacter* spp.
- *Escherichia coli*
- *Gardnerella vaginalis*
- *Haemophilus influenzae*
- *Haemophilus parainfluenzae*
- *Klebsiella* spp.
- *Morganella morganii*
- *Proteus vulgaris*
- *Providencia rettgeri*
- *Pseudomonas aeruginosa*
  (NOTE: Imipenem is inactive *in vitro* against *Xanthomonas (Pseudomonas) maltophilia* and some strains of *P. cepacia*.)
- *Serratia* spp., including *S. marcescens*

Gram-positive anaerobes:
- *Bifidobacterium* spp.
- *Clostridium* spp.
- *Eubacterium* spp.
- *Peptococcus* spp.
- *Peptostreptococcus* spp.
- *Propionibacterium* spp.

Gram-negative anaerobes:
- *Bacteroides* spp., including *B. fragilis*
- *Fusobacterium* spp.

The following *in vitro* data are available, **but their clinical significance is unknown.**

Imipenem exhibits *in vitro* minimum inhibitory concentrations (MICs) of 4 μg/mL or less against most (≥90%) strains of the following microorganisms; however, the safety and effectiveness of imipenem in treating clinical infections due to these microorganisms have not been established in adequate and well-controlled clinical trials.

Gram-positive aerobes:
- *Bacillus* spp.
- *Listeria monocytogenes*
- *Nocardia* spp.
- *Staphylococcus saprophyticus*
- Group C streptococci
- Group G streptococci
- Viridans group streptococci

Gram-negative aerobes:
- *Aeromonas hydrophila*
- *Alcaligenes* spp.
- *Capnocytophaga* spp.
- *Haemophilus ducreyi*
- *Neisseria gonorrhoeae* including penicillinase-producing strains
- *Pasteurella* spp.
- *Providencia stuartii*

Gram-negative anaerobes:
- *Prevotella bivia*
- *Prevotella disiens*
- *Prevotella melaninogenica*
- *Veillonella* spp.

In vitro tests show imipenem to act synergistically with aminoglycoside antibiotics against some isolates of *Pseudomonas aeruginosa*.

Susceptibility Tests:

Measurement of MIC or minimum bactericidal concentration (MBC) and achieved antimicrobial compound concentrations may be appropriate to guide therapy in some infections. (See **CLINICAL PHARMACOLOGY** section for further information on drug concentrations achieved in infected body sites and other pharmacokinetic properties of this antimicrobial drug product.)

Dilution Techniques:

Quantitative methods that are used to determine MICs provide reproducible estimates of the susceptibility of bacteria to antimicrobial compounds. One such procedure uses a standardized dilution method[1] (broth, agar, or microdilution) or equivalent with imipenem powder.

The MIC values obtained should be interpreted according to the following criteria:

MIC (μg/mL)	Interpretation
≤4	Susceptible (S)
8	Intermediate (I)
≥16	Resistant (R)

A report of "Susceptible" indicates that the pathogen is likely to be inhibited by usually achievable concentrations of the antimicrobial compound in blood. A report of "Intermediate" indicates that the result should be considered equivocal, and, if the microorganism is not fully susceptible to alternative, clinically feasible drugs, the test should be repeated. This category implies possible clinical applicability in body sites where the drug is physiologically concentrated or in situations where high dosage of drug can be used. This category also provides a buffer zone that prevents small uncontrolled technical factors from causing major discrepancies in interpretation. A report of "Resistant" indicates that usually achievable concentrations of the antimicrobial compound in the blood are unlikely to be inhibitory and that other therapy should be selected.

Standardized susceptibility test procedures require the use of laboratory control microorganisms. Standard imipenem powder should provide the following MIC values:

Microorganism	MIC (μg/mL)
E. coli ATCC 25922	0.06–0.25
S. aureus ATCC 29213	0.015–0.06
E. faecalis ATCC 29212	0.5–2.0
P. aeruginosa ATCC 27853	1.0–4.0

Diffusion Techniques:

Quantitative methods that require measurement of zone diameters provide reproducible estimates of the susceptibility of bacteria to antimicrobial compounds. One such standardized procedure[2] that has been recommended for use with disks to test the susceptibility of microorganisms to imipenem uses the 10-μg imipenem disk. Interpretation involves correlation of the diameter obtained in the disk test with the MIC for imipenem.

Reports from the laboratory providing results of the standard single-disk susceptibility test with a 10-μg imipenem disk should be interpreted according to the following criteria:

Zone Diameter (mm)	Interpretation
≥16	Susceptible (S)
14–15	Intermediate (I)
≤13	Resistant (R)

Interpretation should be as stated above for results using dilution techniques.

Standardized susceptibility test procedures require the use of laboratory control microorganisms. The 10-μg imipenem disk should provide the following diameters in these laboratory test quality control strains:

Microorganism	Zone Diameter (mm)
E. coli ATCC 25922	26–32
P. aeruginosa ATCC 27853	20–28

Anaerobic techniques:

For anaerobic bacteria, the susceptibility to imipenem can be determined by the reference agar dilution method or by alternate standardized test methods.[3]

The MIC values obtained should be interpreted according to the following criteria:

MIC (μg/mL)	Interpretation
≤4	Susceptible (S)
8	Intermediate (I)
≥16	Resistant (R)

As with other susceptibility techniques, the use of laboratory control microorganisms is required. Standard imipenem powder should provide the following MIC values:

Reference Agar Dilution Testing:

Microorganism	MIC (μg/mL)
B. fragilis ATCC 25285	0.03–0.12
B. thetaiotaomicron ATCC 29741	0.06–0.25
E. lentum ATCC 43055	0.25–1.0

Broth Microdilution Testing:

Microorganism	MIC (μg/mL)
B. thetaiotaomicron ATCC 29741	0.06–0.25
E. lentum ATCC 43055	0.12–0.5

INDICATIONS AND USAGE

PRIMAXIN I.V. is indicated for the treatment of serious infections caused by susceptible strains of the designated microorganisms in the conditions listed below:

(1) **Lower respiratory tract infections.** *Staphylococcus aureus* (penicillinase-producing strains), *Acinetobacter* species, *Enterobacter* species, *Escherichia coli*, *Haemophilus influenzae*, *Haemophilus parainfluenzae**, *Klebsiella* species, *Serratia marcescens*

(2) **Urinary tract infections** (complicated and uncomplicated). *Enterococcus faecalis*, *Staphylococcus aureus*

Continued on next page

Information on the Merck & Co., Inc., products listed on these pages is from the prescribing information in use October 1, 2004. For information, please call 1-800-NSC-MERCK [1-800-672-6372].

Primaxin I.V.—Cont.

(penicillinase-producing strains)*, *Enterobacter* species, *Escherichia coli, Klebsiella* species, *Morganella morganii**, *Proteus vulgaris**, *Providencia rettgeri**, *Pseudomonas aeruginosa*

(3) **Intra-abdominal infections.** *Enterococcus faecalis, Staphylococcus aureus* (penicillinase-producing strains)*, *Staphylococcus epidermidis, Citrobacter* species, *Enterobacter* species, *Escherichia coli, Klebsiella* species, *Morganella morganii**, *Proteus* species, *Pseudomonas aeruginosa, Bifidobacterium* species, *Clostridium* species, *Eubacterium* species, *Peptococcus* species, *Peptostreptococcus* species, *Propionibacterium* species*, *Bacteroides* species including *B. fragilis, Fusobacterium* species

(4) **Gynecologic infections.** *Enterococcus faecalis, Staphylococcus aureus* (penicillinase-producing strains)*, *Staphylococcus epidermidis, Streptococcus agalactiae* (Group B streptococci), *Enterobacter* species*, *Escherichia coli, Gardnerella vaginalis, Klebsiella* species*, *Proteus* species, *Bifidobacterium* species*, *Peptococcus* species*, *Peptostreptococcus* species, *Propionibacterium* species*, *Bacteroides* species including *B. fragilis**

(5) **Bacterial septicemia.** *Enterococcus faecalis, Staphylococcus aureus* (penicillinase-producing strains), *Enterobacter* species, *Escherichia coli, Klebsiella* species, *Pseudomonas aeruginosa, Serratia* species*, *Bacteroides* species including *B. fragilis**

(6) **Bone and joint infections.** *Enterococcus faecalis, Staphylococcus aureus* (penicillinase-producing strains), *Staphylococcus epidermidis, Enterobacter* species, *Pseudomonas aeruginosa*

(7) **Skin and skin structure infections.** *Enterococcus faecalis, Staphylococcus aureus* (penicillinase-producing strains), *Staphylococcus epidermidis, Acinetobacter* species, *Citrobacter* species, *Enterobacter* species, *Escherichia coli, Klebsiella* species, *Morganella morganii, Proteus vulgaris, Providencia rettgeri**, *Pseudomonas aeruginosa, Serratia* species, *Peptococcus* species, *Peptostreptococcus* species, *Bacteroides* species including *B. fragilis, Fusobacterium* species*

(8) **Endocarditis.** *Staphylococcus aureus* (penicillinase-producing strains)

(9) **Polymicrobic infections.** PRIMAXIN I.V. is indicated for polymicrobic infections including those in which *S. pneumoniae* (pneumonia, septicemia), *S. pyogenes* (skin and skin structure), or nonpenicillinase-producing *S. aureus* is one of the causative organisms. However, monobacterial infections due to these organisms are usually treated with narrower spectrum antibiotics, such as penicillin G.

PRIMAXIN I.V. is not indicated in patients with meningitis because safety and efficacy have not been established.

For Pediatric Use information, See **PRECAUTIONS**, *Pediatric Use*, and **DOSAGE AND ADMINISTRATION** sections.

Because of its broad spectrum of bactericidal activity against gram-positive and gram-negative aerobic and anaerobic bacteria, PRIMAXIN I.V. is useful for the treatment of mixed infections and as presumptive therapy prior to the identification of the causative organisms.

Although clinical improvement has been observed in patients with cystic fibrosis, chronic pulmonary disease, and lower respiratory tract infections caused by *Pseudomonas aeruginosa,* bacterial eradication may not necessarily be achieved.

As with other beta-lactam antibiotics, some strains of *Pseudomonas aeruginosa* may develop resistance fairly rapidly during treatment with PRIMAXIN I.V. During therapy of *Pseudomonas aeruginosa* infections, periodic susceptibility testing should be done when clinically appropriate.

Infections resistant to other antibiotics, for example, cephalosporins, penicillin, and aminoglycosides, have been shown to respond to treatment with PRIMAXIN I.V.

To reduce the development of drug-resistant bacteria and maintain the effectiveness of PRIMAXIN I.V. and other antibacterial drugs, PRIMAXIN I.V. should be used only to treat or prevent infections that are proven or strongly suspected to be caused by susceptible bacteria. When culture and susceptibility information are available, they should be considered in selecting or modifying antibacterial therapy. In the absence of such data, local epidemiology and susceptibility patterns may contribute to the empiric selection of therapy.

*Efficacy for this organism in this organ system was studied in fewer than 10 infections.

CONTRAINDICATIONS

PRIMAXIN I.V. is contraindicated in patients who have shown hypersensitivity to any component of this product.

WARNINGS

SERIOUS AND OCCASIONALLY FATAL HYPERSENSITIVITY (ANAPHYLACTIC) REACTIONS HAVE BEEN REPORTED IN PATIENTS RECEIVING THERAPY WITH BETA-LACTAMS. THESE REACTIONS ARE MORE APT TO OCCUR IN PERSONS WITH A HISTORY OF SENSITIVITY TO MULTIPLE ALLERGENS.

THERE HAVE BEEN REPORTS OF PATIENTS WITH A HISTORY OF PENICILLIN HYPERSENSITIVITY WHO HAVE EXPERIENCED SEVERE HYPERSENSITIVITY REACTIONS WHEN TREATED WITH ANOTHER BETA-LACTAM. BEFORE INITIATING THERAPY WITH PRIMAXIN I.V., CAREFUL INQUIRY SHOULD BE MADE CONCERNING PREVIOUS HYPERSENSITIVITY REACTIONS TO PENICILLINS, CEPHALOSPORINS, OTHER BETA-LACTAMS, AND OTHER ALLERGENS. IF AN ALLERGIC REACTION OCCURS, PRIMAXIN SHOULD BE DISCONTINUED.

SERIOUS ANAPHYLACTIC REACTIONS REQUIRE IMMEDIATE EMERGENCY TREATMENT WITH EPINEPHRINE. OXYGEN, INTRAVENOUS STEROIDS, AND AIRWAY MANAGEMENT, INCLUDING INTUBATION, MAY ALSO BE ADMINISTERED AS INDICATED.

Seizures and other CNS adverse experiences, such as confusional states and myoclonic activity, have been reported during treatment with PRIMAXIN I.V. (See **PRECAUTIONS.**)

Pseudomembranous colitis has been reported with nearly all antibacterial agents, including imipenem-cilastatin sodium, and may range in severity from mild to life threatening. Therefore, it is important to consider this diagnosis in patients who present with diarrhea subsequent to the administration of antibacterial agents.

Treatment with antibacterial agents alters the normal flora of the colon and may permit overgrowth of clostridia. Studies indicate that a toxin produced by *Clostridium difficile* is one primary cause of "antibiotic-associated colitis".

After the diagnosis of pseudomembranous colitis has been established, therapeutic measures should be initiated. Mild cases of pseudomembranous colitis usually respond to drug discontinuation alone. In moderate to severe cases, consideration should be given to management with fluids and electrolytes, protein supplementation and treatment with an antibacterial drug clinically effective against *C. difficile* colitis.

PRECAUTIONS

General

CNS adverse experiences such as confusional states, myoclonic activity, and seizures have been reported during treatment with PRIMAXIN I.V., especially when recommended dosages were exceeded. These experiences have occurred most commonly in patients with CNS disorders (e.g., brain lesions or history of seizures) and/or compromised renal function. However, there have been reports of CNS adverse experiences in patients who had no recognized or documented underlying CNS disorder or compromised renal function.

When recommended doses were exceeded, adult patients with creatinine clearances of ≤20 mL/min/1.73 m^2, whether or not undergoing hemodialysis, had a higher risk of seizure activity than those without impairment of renal function. Therefore, close adherence to the dosing guidelines for these patients is recommended. (See **DOSAGE AND ADMINISTRATION.**)

Patients with creatinine clearances of ≤5 mL/min/1.73 m^2 should not receive PRIMAXIN I.V. unless hemodialysis is instituted within 48 hours.

For patients on hemodialysis, PRIMAXIN I.V. is recommended only when the benefit outweighs the potential risk of seizures.

Close adherence to the recommended dosage and dosage schedules is urged, especially in patients with known factors that predispose to convulsive activity. Anticonvulsant therapy should be continued in patients with known seizure disorders. If focal tremors, myoclonus, or seizures occur, patients should be evaluated neurologically, placed on anticonvulsant therapy if not already instituted, and the dosage of PRIMAXIN I.V. re-examined to determine whether it should be decreased or the antibiotic discontinued.

As with other antibiotics, prolonged use of PRIMAXIN I.V. may result in overgrowth of nonsusceptible organisms. Repeated evaluation of the patient's condition is essential. If superinfection occurs during therapy, appropriate measures should be taken.

Prescribing PRIMAXIN I.V. in the absence of a proven or strongly suspected bacterial infection or a prophylactic indication is unlikely to provide benefit to the patient and increases the risk of the development of drug-resistant bacteria.

Information for Patients

Patients should be counseled that antibacterial drugs including PRIMAXIN I.V. should only be used to treat bacterial infections. They do not treat viral infections (e.g., the common cold). When PRIMAXIN I.V. is prescribed to treat a bacterial infection, patients should be told that although it is common to feel better early in the course of therapy, the medication should be taken exactly as directed. Skipping doses or not completing the full course of therapy may (1) decrease the effectiveness of the immediate treatment and (2) increase the likelihood that bacteria will develop resistance and will not be treatable by PRIMAXIN I.V. or other antibacterial drugs in the future.

Laboratory Tests

While PRIMAXIN I.V. possesses the characteristic low toxicity of the beta-lactam group of antibiotics, periodic assessment of organ system functions, including renal, hepatic, and hematopoietic, is advisable during prolonged therapy.

Drug Interactions

Generalized seizures have been reported in patients who received ganciclovir and PRIMAXIN. These drugs should not be used concomitantly unless the potential benefits outweigh the risks.

Since concomitant administration of PRIMAXIN and probenecid results in only minimal increases in plasma levels of imipenem and plasma half-life, it is not recommended that probenecid be given with PRIMAXIN.

PRIMAXIN should not be mixed with or physically added to other antibiotics. However, PRIMAXIN may be administered concomitantly with other antibiotics, such as aminoglycosides.

Carcinogenesis, Mutagenesis, Impairment of Fertility

Long term studies in animals have not been performed to evaluate carcinogenic potential of imipenem-cilastatin. Genetic toxicity studies were performed in a variety of bacterial and mammalian tests in *in vivo* and *in vitro.* The tests used were: V79 mammalian cell mutagenesis assay (imipenem-cilastatin sodium alone and imipenem alone), Ames test (cilastatin sodium alone and imipenem alone), unscheduled DNA synthesis assay (imipenem-cilastatin sodium) and *in vivo* mouse cytogenetics test (imipenem-cilastatin sodium). None of these tests showed any evidence of genetic alterations.

Reproductive tests in male and female rats were performed with imipenem-cilastatin sodium at intravenous doses up to 80 mg/kg/day and at a subcutaneous dose of 320 mg/kg/day, approximately equal to the highest recommended human dose of the intravenous formulation (on a mg/m^2 body surface area basis). Slight decreases in live fetal body weight were restricted to the highest dosage level. No other adverse effects were observed on fertility, reproductive performance, fetal viability, growth or postnatal development of pups.

Pregnancy: Teratogenic Effects

Pregnancy Category C: Teratology studies with cilastatin sodium at doses of 30, 100, and 300 mg/kg/day administered intravenously to rabbits and 40, 200, and 1000 mg/kg/day administered subcutaneously to rats, up to approximately 1.9 and 3.2 times†† the maximum recommended daily human dose (on a mg/m^2 body surface area basis) of the intravenous formulation of imipenem-cilastatin sodium (50 mg/kg/day) in the two species, respectively, showed no evidence of adverse effect on the fetus. No evidence of teratogenicity was observed in rabbits given imipenem at intravenous doses of 15, 30 or 60 mg/kg/day and rats given imipenem at intravenous doses of 225, 450, or 900 mg/kg/day, up to approximately 0.4 and 2.9 times†† the maximum recommended daily human dose (on a mg/m^2 body surface area basis) in the two species, respectively.

Teratology studies with imipenem-cilastatin sodium at intravenous doses of 20 and 80, and a subcutaneous dose of 320 mg/kg/day, up to 0.5 times†† (mice) to approximately equal to (rats) the highest recommended daily intravenous human dose (on a mg/m^2 body surface area basis) in pregnant rodents during the period of major organogenesis, revealed no evidence of teratogenicity.

Imipenem-cilastatin sodium, when administered subcutaneously to pregnant rabbits at dosages equivalent to the usual human dose of the intravenous formulation and higher, (1000–4000 mg/day) caused body weight loss, diarrhea, and maternal deaths. When comparable doses of imipenem-cilastatin sodium were given to non-pregnant rabbits, body weight loss, diarrhea, and deaths were also observed. This intolerance is not unlike that seen with other beta-lactam antibiotics in this species and is probably due to alteration of gut flora.

A teratology study in pregnant cynomolgus monkeys given imipenem-cilastatin sodium at doses of 40 mg/kg/day (bolus intravenous injection) or 160 mg/kg/day (subcutaneous injection) resulted in maternal toxicity including emesis, inappetence, body weight loss, diarrhea, abortion, and death in some cases. In contrast, no significant toxicity was observed when non-pregnant cynomolgus monkeys were given doses of imipenem-cilastatin sodium up to 180 mg/kg/day (subcutaneous injection). When doses of imipenem-cilastatin sodium (approximately 100 mg/kg/day or approximately 0.6 times†† the maximum recommended daily human dose of the intravenous formulation) were administered to pregnant cynomolgus monkeys at an intravenous infusion rate which mimics human clinical use, there was minimal maternal intolerance (occasional emesis), no maternal deaths, no evidence of teratogenicity, but an increase in embryonic loss relative to control groups.

No adverse effects on the fetus or on lactation were observed when imipenem-cilastatin sodium was administered subcutaneously to rats late in gestation at dosages up to 320 mg/kg/day, approximately equal to the highest recommended human dose (on a mg/m^2 body surface area basis).

There are, however, no adequate and well-controlled studies in pregnant women. PRIMAXIN I.V. should be used during pregnancy only if the potential benefit justifies the potential risk to the mother and fetus.

Nursing Mothers

It is not known whether imipenem-cilastatin sodium is excreted in human milk. Because many drugs are excreted in human milk, caution should be exercised when PRIMAXIN I.V. is administered to a nursing woman.

Pediatric Use

Use of PRIMAXIN I.V. in pediatric patients, neonates to 16 years of age, is supported by evidence from adequate and well-controlled studies of PRIMAXIN I.V. in adults and by the following clinical studies and published literature in pediatric patients: Based on published studies of 178** pediatric patients ≥3 months of age (with non-CNS infections), the recommended dose of PRIMAXIN I.V. is 15–25 mg/kg/dose administered every six hours. Doses of 25 mg/kg/dose in patients 3 months to <3 years of age, and 15 mg/kg/dose in patients 3–12 years of age were associated with mean trough plasma concentrations of imipenem of 1.1±0.4 µg/mL and 0.6±0.2 µg/mL following multiple 60-

minute infusions, respectively; trough urinary concentrations of imipenem were in excess of 10 µg/mL for both doses. These doses have provided adequate plasma and urine concentrations for the treatment of non-CNS infections. Based on studies in adults, the maximum daily dose for treatment of infections with fully susceptible organisms is 2.0 g per day, and of infections with moderately susceptible organisms (primarily some strains of *P. aeruginosa*) is 4.0 g/day. (See Table 1, **DOSAGE AND ADMINISTRATION**.) Higher doses (up to 90 mg/kg/day in older children) have been used in patients with cystic fibrosis. (See **DOSAGE AND ADMINISTRATION**.)

Based on studies of 135*** pediatric patients ≤3 months of age (weighing ≥1,500 gms), the following dosage schedule is recommended for non-CNS infections:

<1 wk of age: 25 mg/kg every 12 hrs
1–4 wks of age: 25 mg/kg every 8 hrs
4 wks–3 mos. of age: 25 mg/kg every 6 hrs.

In a published dose-ranging study of smaller premature infants (670–1,890 gms) in the first week of life, a dose of 20 mg/kg q12h by 15–30 minutes infusion was associated with mean peak and trough plasma imipenem concentrations of 43 µg/mL and 1.7 µg/mL after multiple doses, respectively. However, moderate accumulation of cilastatin in neonates may occur following multiple doses of PRIMAXIN I.V. The safety of this accumulation is unknown.

PRIMAXIN I.V. is not recommended in pediatric patients with CNS infections because of the risk of seizures.

PRIMAXIN I.V. is not recommended in pediatric patients <30 kg with impaired renal function, as no data are available.

Geriatric Use

Of the approximately 3600 subjects ≥18 years of age in clinical studies of PRIMAXIN I.V., including postmarketing studies, approximately 2800 received PRIMAXIN I.V. Of the subjects who received PRIMAXIN I.V., data are available on approximately 800 subjects who were 65 and over, including approximately 300 subjects who were 75 and over. No overall differences in safety or effectiveness were observed between these subjects and younger subjects. Other reported clinical experience has not identified differences in responses between the elderly and younger patients, but greater sensitivity of some older individuals cannot be ruled out.

This drug is known to be substantially excreted by the kidney, and the risk of toxic reactions to this drug may be greater in patients with impaired renal function. Because elderly patients are more likely to have decreased renal function, care should be taken in dose selection, and it may be useful to monitor renal function.

No dosage adjustment is required based on age (see CLINICAL PHARMACOLOGY, *Adults*). Dosage adjustment in the case of renal impairment is necessary (see DOSAGE AND ADMINISTRATION, *Reduced Intravenous Schedule for Adults with Impaired Renal Function and/or Body Weight < 70 kg*).

†† Based on patient body surface area of 1.6 m^2 (weight of 60 kg).
** Two patients were less than 3 months of age.
*** One patient was greater than 3 months of age.

ADVERSE REACTIONS

Adults

PRIMAXIN I.V. is generally well tolerated. Many of the 1,723 patients treated in clinical trials were severely ill and had multiple background diseases and physiological impairments, making it difficult to determine causal relationship of adverse experiences to therapy with PRIMAXIN I.V.

Local Adverse Reactions

Adverse local clinical reactions that were reported as possibly, probably or definitely related to therapy with PRIMAXIN I.V. were:

Phlebitis/thrombophlebitis—3.1%
Pain at the injection site—0.7%
Erythema at the injection site—0.4%
Vein induration—0.2%
Infused vein infection—0.1%

Systemic Adverse Reactions

The most frequently reported systemic adverse clinical reactions that were reported as possibly, probably, or definitely related to PRIMAXIN I.V. were nausea (2.0%), diarrhea (1.8%), vomiting (1.5%), rash (0.9%), fever (0.5%), hypotension (0.4%), seizures (0.4%) (see **PRECAUTIONS**), dizziness (0.3%), pruritus (0.3%), urticaria (0.2%), somnolence (0.2%).

Additional adverse systemic clinical reactions reported as possibly, probably or definitely drug related occurring in less than 0.2% of the patients or reported since the drug was marketed are listed within each body system in order of decreasing severity: *Gastrointestinal* —pseudomembranous colitis (the onset of pseudomembranous colitis symptoms may occur during or after antibacterial treatment, see **WARNINGS**), hemorrhagic colitis, hepatitis, jaundice, gastroenteritis, abdominal pain, glossitis, tongue papillar hypertrophy, staining of the teeth and/or tongue, heartburn, pharyngeal pain, increased salivation; *Hematologic* —pancytopenia, bone marrow depression, thrombocytopenia, neutropenia, leukopenia, hemolytic anemia; *CNS* —encephalopathy, tremor, confusion, myoclonus, paresthesia, vertigo, headache, psychic disturbances including hallucinations; *Special Senses* —hearing loss, tinnitus, taste perversion; *Respiratory* —chest discomfort, dyspnea, hyperventilation, thoracic spine pain; *Cardiovascular* —palpitations, tachycardia; *Skin* —Stevens-Johnson syndrome, toxic epidermal necrolysis, erythema multiforme, angioneurotic edema, flushing, cyanosis, hyperhidrosis, skin texture changes, candidiasis, pruritus vulvae; *Body as a whole* —polyarthralgia, asthenia/weakness, drug fever; *Renal* —acute renal failure, oliguria/anuria, polyuria, urine discoloration. The role of PRIMAXIN I.V. in changes in renal function is difficult to assess, since factors predisposing to pre-renal azotemia or to impaired renal function usually have been present.

Patients ≥3 Months of Age With Normal Pretherapy but Abnormal During Therapy Laboratory Values

Laboratory Parameter	Abnormality			No. of Patients With Abnormalities/ No. of Patients With Lab Done	(%)
Hemoglobin	Age	<5 mos.:	<10 gm %	19/129	(14.7)
		6 mos.-12 yrs.:	<11.5 gm %		
Hematocrit	Age	<5 mos.:	<30 vol %	23/129	(17.8)
		6 mos.-12 yrs.:	<34.5 vol %		
Neutrophils		≤1000/mm^3 (absolute)		4/123	(3.3)
Eosinophils		≥7%		15/117	(12.8)
Platelet Count		≥500 ths/mm^3		16/119	(13.4)
Urine Protein		≥1		8/97	(8.2)
Serum Creatinine		>1.2 mg/dL		0/105	(0)
BUN		>22 mg/dL		0/108	(0)
AST (SGOT)		>36 IU/L		14/78	(17.9)
ALT (SGPT)		>30 IU/L		10/93	(10.8)

Adverse Laboratory Changes

Adverse laboratory changes without regard to drug relationship that were reported during clinical trials or reported since the drug was marketed were:

Hepatic: Increased ALT (SGPT), AST (SGOT), alkaline phosphatase, bilirubin and LDH
Hemic: Increased eosinophils, positive Coombs test, increased WBC, increased platelets, decreased hemoglobin and hematocrit, agranulocytosis, increased monocytes, abnormal prothrombin time, increased lymphocytes, increased basophils
Electrolytes: Decreased serum sodium, increased potassium, increased chloride
Renal: Increased BUN, creatinine
Urinalysis: Presence of urine protein, urine red blood cells, urine white blood cells, urine casts, urine bilirubin, and urine urobilinogen

Pediatric Patients

In studies of 178 pediatric patients ≥3 months of age, the following adverse events were noted:

The Most Common Clinical Adverse Experiences Without Regard to Drug Relationship (Patient Incidence >1%)

Adverse Experience	No. of Patients (%)
Digestive System	
Diarrhea	7* (3.9)
Gastroenteritis	2 (1.1)
Vomiting	2* (1.1)
Skin	
Rash	4 (2.2)
Irritation, I.V. site	2 (1.1)
Urogenital System	
Urine discoloration	2 (1.1)
Cardiovascular System	
Phlebitis	4 (2.2)

*One patient had both vomiting and diarrhea and is counted in each category.

In studies of 135 patients (newborn to 3 months of age), the following adverse events were noted:

The Most Common Clinical Adverse Experiences Without Regard to Drug Relationship (Patient Incidence >1%)

Adverse Experience	No. of Patients (%)
Digestive System	
Diarrhea	4 (3.0%)
Oral Candidiasis	2 (1.5%)
Skin	
Rash	2 (1.5%)
Urogenital System	
Oliguria/anuria	3 (2.2%)
Cardiovascular System	
Tachycardia	2 (1.5%)
Nervous System	
Convulsions	8 (5.9%)

[See table above]

Patients (<3 Months of Age) With Normal Pretherapy but Abnormal During Therapy Laboratory Values

Laboratory Parameter	No. of Patients With Abnormalities* (%)
Eosinophil Count ↑	11 (9.0%)
Hematocrit ↓	3 (2.0%)
Hematocrit ↑	1 (1.0%)
Platelet Count ↑	5 (4.0%)
Platelet Count ↓	2 (2.0%)
Serum Creatinine ↑	5 (5.0%)
Bilirubin ↑	3 (3.0%)
Bilirubin ↓	1 (1.0%)
AST (SGOT) ↑	5 (6.0%)
ALT (SGPT) ↑	3 (3.0%)
Serum Alkaline Phosphate ↑	2 (3.0%)

*The denominator used for percentages was the number of patients for whom the test was performed during or post-treatment and, therefore, varies by test.

Examination of published literature and spontaneous adverse event reports suggested a similar spectrum of adverse events in adult and pediatric patients.

OVERDOSAGE

The acute intravenous toxicity of imipenem-cilastatin sodium in a ratio of 1:1 was studied in mice at doses of 751 to 1359 mg/kg. Following drug administration, ataxia was rapidly produced and clonic convulsions were noted in about 45 minutes. Deaths occurred within 4–56 minutes at all doses.

The acute intravenous toxicity of imipenem-cilastatin sodium was produced within 5–10 minutes in rats at doses of 771 to 1583 mg/kg. In all dosage groups, females had decreased activity, bradypnea, and ptosis with clonic convulsions preceding death; in males, ptosis was seen at all dose levels while tremors and clonic convulsions were seen at all but the lowest dose (771 mg/kg). In another rat study, female rats showed ataxia, bradypnea, and decreased activity in all but the lowest dose (550 mg/kg); deaths were preceded by clonic convulsions. Male rats showed tremors at all doses and clonic convulsions, and ptosis were seen at the two highest doses (1130 and 1734 mg/kg). Deaths occurred between 6 and 88 minutes with doses of 771 to 1734 mg/kg.

In the case of overdosage, discontinue PRIMAXIN I.V., treat symptomatically, and institute supportive measures as required. Imipenem-cilastatin sodium is hemodialyzable. However, usefulness of this procedure in the overdosage setting is questionable.

DOSAGE AND ADMINISTRATION

Adults

The dosage recommendations for PRIMAXIN I.V. represent the quantity of imipenem to be administered. An equivalent amount of cilastatin is also present in the solution. Each 125 mg, 250 mg, or 500 mg dose should be given by intravenous administration over 20 to 30 minutes. Each 750 mg or 1000 mg dose should be infused over 40 to 60 minutes. In patients who develop nausea during the infusion, the rate of infusion may be slowed.

The total daily dosage for PRIMAXIN I.V. should be based on the type or severity of infection and given in equally divided doses based on consideration of degree of susceptibility of the pathogen(s), renal function, and body weight. Adult patients with impaired renal function, as judged by creatinine clearance ≤ 70 mL/min/1.73 m^2, require adjustment of dosage as described in the succeeding section of these guidelines.

Intravenous Dosage Schedule for Adults with Normal Renal Function and Body Weight ≥70 kg

Doses cited in Table I are based on a patient with normal renal function and a body weight of 70 kg. These doses should be used for a patient with a creatinine clearance of ≥71 mL/min/1.73 m^2 and a body weight of ≥70 kg. A reduction in dose must be made for a patient with a creatinine clearance ≤70 mL/min/1.73 m^2 and/or a body weight less than 70 kg. (See Tables II and III.)

Dosage regimens in column A of Table I are recommended for infections caused by fully susceptible organisms which

Continued on next page

Information on the Merck & Co., Inc., products listed on these pages is from the prescribing information in use October 1, 2004. For information, please call 1-800-NSC-MERCK [1-800-672-6372].

Primaxin I.V.—Cont.

represent the majority of pathogenic species. Dosage regimens in column B of Table I are recommended for infections caused by organisms with moderate susceptibility to imipenem, primarily some strains of *P. aeruginosa*.

TABLE I
INTRAVENOUS DOSAGE SCHEDULE FOR ADULTS WITH NORMAL RENAL FUNCTION AND BODY WEIGHT ≥ 70 kg

Type or Severity of Infection	A Fully susceptible organisms including gram-positive and gram-negative aerobes and anaerobes	B Moderately susceptible organisms, primarily some strains of *P. aeruginosa*
Mild	250 mg q6h (TOTAL DAILY DOSE=1.0g)	500 mg q6h (TOTAL DAILY DOSE=2.0g)
Moderate	500 mg q8h (TOTAL DAILY DOSE =1.5g) or 500 mg q6h (TOTAL DAILY DOSE=2.0g)	500 mg q6h (TOTAL DAILY DOSE=2.0g) or 1 g q8h (TOTAL DAILY DOSE=3.0g)
Severe, life threatening only	500 mg q6h (TOTAL DAILY DOSE=2.0g)	1 g q8h (TOTAL DAILY DOSE=3.0g) or 1 g q6h (TOTAL DAILY DOSE=4.0g)
Uncomplicated urinary tract infection	250 mg q6h (TOTAL DAILY DOSE=1.0g)	250 mg q6h (TOTAL DAILY DOSE=1.0g)
Complicated urinary tract infection	500 mg q6h (TOTAL DAILY DOSE=2.0g)	500 mg q6h (TOTAL DAILY DOSE=2.0g)

Due to the high antimicrobial activity of PRIMAXIN I.V., it is recommended that the maximum total daily dosage not exceed 50 mg/kg/day or 4.0 g/day, whichever is lower. There is no evidence that higher doses provide greater efficacy. However, patients over twelve years of age with cystic fibrosis and normal renal function have been treated with PRIMAXIN I.V. at doses up to 90 mg/kg/day in divided doses, not exceeding 4.0 g/day.

Reduced Intravenous Dosage Schedule for Adults with Impaired Renal Function and/or Body Weight <70 kg
Patients with creatinine clearance of ≤ 70 mL/min/1.73 m^2 and/or body weight less than 70 kg require dosage reduction of PRIMAXIN I.V. as indicated in the tables below. Creatinine clearance may be calculated from serum creatinine concentration by the following equation:

$$T_{cc} \text{ (Males)} = \frac{\text{(wt. in kg) (140 − age)}}{\text{(72) (creatinine in mg/dL)}}$$

$$T_{cc} \text{(Females)} = 0.85 \times \text{above value}$$

To determine the dose for adults with impaired renal function and/or reduced body weight:
1. Choose a total daily dose from Table I based on infection characteristics.
2. a) If the total daily dose is 1.0 g, 1.5 g, or 2.0 g, use the appropriate subsection of Table II and continue with step 3.
   b) If the total daily dose is 3.0 g or 4.0 g, use the appropriate subsection of Table III and continue with step 3.
3. From Table II or III:
   a) Select the body weight on the far left which is closest to the patient's body weight (kg).
   b) Select the patient's creatinine clearance category.
   c) Where the row and column intersect is the reduced dosage regimen.

[See table II above]
[See table III above]

Patients with creatinine clearances of 6 to 20 mL/min/1.73 m^2 should be treated with PRIMAXIN I.V. 125 mg or 250 mg every 12 hours for most pathogens. There may be an increased risk of seizures when doses of 500 mg every 12 hours are administered to these patients.
Patients with creatinine clearance ≤5 mL/min/1.73 m^2 should not receive PRIMAXIN I.V. unless hemodialysis is instituted within 48 hours. There is inadequate information to recommend usage of PRIMAXIN I.V. for patients undergoing peritoneal dialysis.

Hemodialysis
When treating patients with creatinine clearances of ≤5 mL/min/1.73 m^2 who are undergoing hemodialysis, use the dosage recommendations for patients with creatinine clearances of 6–20 mL/min/1.73 m^2. (See *Reduced Intravenous Dosage Schedule for Adults with Impaired Renal Function and/or Body Weight <70 kg.)* Both imipenem and cilastatin are cleared from the circulation during hemodialysis. The patient should receive PRIMAXIN I.V. after hemodialysis and at 12 hour intervals timed from the end of that hemodialysis session. Dialysis patients, especially those with background CNS disease, should be carefully monitored; for patients on hemodialysis, PRIMAXIN I.V. is recommended only when the benefit outweighs the potential risk of seizures. (See **PRECAUTIONS**.)

TABLE II
REDUCED INTRAVENOUS DOSAGE OF PRIMAXIN I.V. IN ADULT PATIENTS WITH IMPAIRED RENAL FUNCTION AND/OR BODY WEIGHT<70 kg

	If TOTAL DAILY DOSE from TABLE I is: 1.0 g/day				1.5 g/day				2.0 g/day			
and Body Weight (kg) is:	and creatinine clearance (mL/min/1.73m²) is: ≥71	41–70	21–40	6–20	and creatinine clearance (mL/min/1.73m²) is: ≥71	41–70	21–40	6–20	and creatinine clearance (mL/min/1.73m²) is: ≥71	41–70	21–40	6–20
	then the reduced dosage regimen (mg) is:				then the reduced dosage regimen (mg) is:				then the reduced dosage regimen (mg) is:			
≥70	250 q6h	250 q8h	250 q12h	250 q12h	500 q8h	250 q6h	250 q8h	250 q12h	500 q6h	500 q8h	250 q6h	250 q12h
60	250 q8h	125 q6h	250 q12h	125 q12h	250 q6h	250 q8h	250 q8h	250 q12h	500 q8h	250 q6h	250 q8h	250 q12h
50	125 q6h	125 q6h	125 q8h	125 q12h	250 q6h	250 q8h	250 q12h	250 q12h	250 q6h	250 q6h	250 q8h	250 q12h
40	125 q6h	125 q8h	125 q12h	125 q12h	250 q8h	125 q6h	125 q8h	125 q12h	250 q6h	250 q8h	250 q12h	250 q12h
30	125 q8h	125 q8h	125 q12h	125 q12h	125 q6h	125 q8h	125 q8h	125 q12h	250 q8h	125 q6h	125 q8h	125 q12h

TABLE III
REDUCED INTRAVENOUS DOSAGE OF PRIMAXIN I.V. IN ADULT PATIENTS WITH IMPAIRED RENAL FUNCTION AND/OR BODY WEIGHT<70 kg

	If TOTAL DAILY DOSE from TABLE I is: 3.0 g/day				4.0 g/day			
and Body Weight (kg) is:	and creatinine clearance (mL/min/1.73m²) is: ≥71	41–70	21–40	6–20	and creatinine clearance (mL/min/1.73m²) is: ≥71	41–70	21–40	6–20
	then the reduced dosage regimen (mg) is:				then the reduced dosage regimen (mg) is:			
≥70	1000 q8h	500 q6h	500 q8h	500 q12h	1000 q6h	750 q8h	500 q6h	500 q12h
60	750 q8h	500 q8h	500 q8h	500 q12h	1000 q8h	750 q8h	500 q8h	500 q12h
50	500 q6h	500 q8h	250 q6h	250 q12h	750 q8h	500 q6h	500 q8h	500 q12h
40	500 q8h	250 q6h	250 q8h	250 q12h	500 q6h	500 q8h	250 q6h	250 q12h
30	250 q6h	250 q8h	250 q8h	250 q12h	500 q8h	250 q6h	250 q8h	250 q12h

Pediatric Patients
See **PRECAUTIONS**, *Pediatric Patients.*
For pediatric patients ≥3 months of age, the recommended dose for non-CNS infections is 15–25 mg/kg/dose administered every six hours. Based on studies in adults, the maximum daily dose for treatment of infections with fully susceptible organisms is 2.0 g per day, and of infections with moderately susceptible organisms (primarily some strains of *P. aeruginosa*) is 4.0 g/day. Higher doses (up to 90 mg/kg/day in older children) have been used in patients with cystic fibrosis.
For pediatric patients ≤3 months of age (weighing ≥1,500 gms), the following dosage schedule is recommended for non-CNS infections:
  <1 wk of age: 25 mg/kg every 12 hrs
  1–4 wks of age: 25 mg/kg every 8 hrs
  4 wks–3 mos. of age: 25 mg/kg every 6 hrs.
Doses less than or equal to 500 mg should be given by intravenous infusion over 15 to 30 minutes. Doses greater than 500 mg should be given by intravenous infusion over 40 to 60 minutes.
PRIMAXIN I.V. is not recommended in pediatric patients with CNS infections because of the risk of seizures.
PRIMAXIN I.V. is not recommended in pediatric patients <30 kg with impaired renal function, as no data are available.

PREPARATION OF SOLUTION

Infusion Bottles
Contents of the infusion bottles of PRIMAXIN I.V. Powder should be restored with 100 mL of diluent (see list of diluents under **COMPATIBILITY AND STABILITY**) and shaken until a clear solution is obtained.
Vials
Contents of the vials must be suspended and transferred to 100 mL of an appropriate infusion solution.
A suggested procedure is to add approximately 10 mL from the appropriate infusion solution (see list of diluents under **COMPATIBILITY AND STABILITY**) to the vial. Shake well and transfer the resulting suspension to the infusion solution container.
Benzyl alcohol as a preservative has been associated with toxicity in neonates. While toxicity has not been demonstrated in pediatric patients greater than three months of age, small pediatric patients in this age range may also be at risk for benzyl alcohol toxicity. Therefore, diluents containing benzyl alcohol should not be used when PRIMAXIN I.V. is constituted for administration to pediatric patients in this age range.
CAUTION: THE SUSPENSION IS NOT FOR DIRECT INFUSION.
Repeat with an additional 10 mL of infusion solution to ensure complete transfer of vial contents to the infusion solution. **The resulting mixture should be agitated until clear.**
ADD-Vantage ®††† Vials
See separate INSTRUCTIONS FOR USE OF 'PRIMAXIN I.V.' IN ADD-Vantage® VIALS. PRIMAXIN I.V. in ADD-Vantage® vials should be reconstituted with ADD-Vantage® diluent containers containing 100 mL of either 0.9% Sodium Chloride Injection or 100 mL 5% Dextrose Injection.
MONOVIAL ®‡ Vials
See separate INSTRUCTIONS FOR USE OF 'PRIMAXIN I.V.' IN MONOVIAL® VIALS. PRIMAXIN I.V. in MONOVIAL® vials should be reconstituted using an appropriate diluent in an infusion bag, with a maximum port length of 14 mm.
The MONOVIAL vial is not compatible with the ADD-Vantage® diluent bags.

††† Registered trademark of Abbott Laboratories, Inc.
‡ Registered trademark of Becton Dickinson and Company.

COMPATIBILITY AND STABILITY

Before reconstitution:
The dry powder should be stored at a temperature below 25°C (77°F).
Reconstituted solutions:
Solutions of PRIMAXIN I.V. range from colorless to yellow. Variations of color within this range do not affect the potency of the product.
PRIMAXIN I.V., as supplied in single use infusion bottles, vials and MONOVIAL® vials and reconstituted with the following diluents (see **PREPARATION OF SOLUTION**), maintains satisfactory potency for 4 hours at room temperature or for 24 hours under refrigeration (5°C). Solutions of PRIMAXIN I.V. should not be frozen.
  0.9% Sodium Chloride Injection
  5% or 10% Dextrose Injection
  5% Dextrose and 0.9% Sodium Chloride Injection
  5% Dextrose Injection with 0.225% or 0.45% saline solution

5% Dextrose Injection with 0.15% potassium chloride solution

Mannitol 5% and 10%

PRIMAXIN I.V., as supplied in single dose ADD-Vantage® vials and reconstituted with the following diluents (see **PREPARATION OF SOLUTION**), maintains satisfactory potency for 4 hours at room temperature.

0.9% Sodium Chloride Injection

5% Dextrose Injection

PRIMAXIN I.V. should not be mixed with or physically added to other antibiotics. However, PRIMAXIN I.V. may be administered concomitantly with other antibiotics, such as aminoglycosides.

HOW SUPPLIED

PRIMAXIN I.V. is supplied as a sterile powder mixture in single dose containers including vials, infusion bottles, ADD-Vantage® vials, and MONOVIAL® vials containing imipenem (anhydrous equivalent) and cilastatin sodium as follows:

No. 3514—250 mg imipenem equivalent and 250 mg cilastatin equivalent and 10 mg sodium bicarbonate as a buffer **NDC** 0006-3514-58 in trays of 25 vials.

No. 3516—500 mg imipenem equivalent and 500 mg cilastatin equivalent and 20 mg sodium bicarbonate as a buffer **NDC** 0006-3516-59 in trays of 25 vials.

No. 3517—500 mg imipenem equivalent and 500 mg cilastatin equivalent and 20 mg sodium bicarbonate as a buffer **NDC** 0006-3517-75 in trays of 10 infusion bottles.

No. 3551 —250 mg imipenem equivalent and 250 mg cilastatin equivalent and 10 mg sodium bicarbonate as a buffer **NDC** 0006-3551-58 in trays of 25 ADD-Vantage® vials.

No. 3552 —500 mg imipenem equivalent and 500 mg cilastatin equivalent and 20 mg sodium bicarbonate as a buffer **NDC** 0006-3552-59 in trays of 25 ADD-Vantage® vials.

No. 3666 —500 mg imipenem equivalent and 500 mg cilastatin equivalent and 20 mg sodium bicarbonate as a buffer **NDC** 0006-3666-59 in trays of 25 MONOVIAL® vials.

REFERENCES

1. National Committee for Clinical Laboratory Standards, Methods for Dilution Antimicrobial Susceptibility Tests for Bacteria that Grow Aerobically—Fourth Edition. Approved Standard NCCLS Document M7–A4, Vol. 17, No. 2 NCCLS, Villanova, PA, 1997.
2. National Committee for Clinical Laboratory Standards, Performance Standards for Antimicrobial Disk Susceptibility Tests—Sixth Edition. Approved Standard NCCLS Document M2–A6, Vol. 17, No. 1 NCCLS, Villanova, PA, 1997.
3. National Committee for Clinical Laboratory Standards, Method for Antimicrobial Susceptibility Testing of Anaerobic Bacteria—Third Edition. Approved Standard NCCLS Document M11-A3, Vol. 13, No. 26 NCCLS, Villanova, PA, 1993.

7882128 Issued August 2003

PRINIVIL® Tablets ℞
(Lisinopril)

USE IN PREGNANCY

When used in pregnancy during the second and third trimesters, ACE inhibitors can cause injury and even death to the developing fetus. When pregnancy is detected, PRINIVIL should be discontinued as soon as possible. See WARNINGS, *Fetal/Neonatal Morbidity and Mortality.*

DESCRIPTION

PRINIVIL* (Lisinopril), a synthetic peptide derivative, is an oral long-acting angiotensin converting enzyme inhibitor. Lisinopril is chemically described as (*S*)-1-[N^2-(1-carboxy-3-phenylpropyl)-L-lysyl]-L-proline dihydrate. Its empirical formula is $C_{21}H_{31}N_3O_5{\cdot}2H_2O$ and its structural formula is:

Lisinopril is a white to off-white, crystalline powder, with a molecular weight of 441.52. It is soluble in water and sparingly soluble in methanol and practically insoluble in ethanol.

PRINIVIL is supplied as 2.5 mg, 5 mg, 10 mg, 20 mg and 40 mg tablets for oral administration. In addition to the active ingredient lisinopril, each tablet contains the following inactive ingredients: calcium phosphate, mannitol, magnesium stearate, and starch. The 10 mg, 20 mg and 40 mg tablets also contain iron oxide.

*Registered trademark of MERCK & CO., Inc.

CLINICAL PHARMACOLOGY

Mechanism of Action

Lisinopril inhibits angiotensin converting enzyme (ACE) in human subjects and animals. ACE is a peptidyl dipeptidase that catalyzes the conversion of angiotensin I to the vasoconstrictor substance, angiotensin II. Angiotensin II also stimulates aldosterone secretion by the adrenal cortex. The beneficial effects of lisinopril in hypertension and heart failure appear to result primarily from suppression of the renin-angiotensin-aldosterone system. Inhibition of ACE results in decreased plasma angiotensin II which leads to decreased vasopressor activity and to decreased aldosterone secretion. The latter decrease may result in a small increase of serum potassium. In hypertensive patients with normal renal function treated with PRINIVIL alone for up to 24 weeks, the mean increase in serum potassium was approximately 0.1 mEq/L; however, approximately 15 percent of patients had increases greater than 0.5 mEq/L and approximately six percent had a decrease greater than 0.5 mEq/L. In the same study, patients treated with PRINIVIL and hydrochlorothiazide for up to 24 weeks had a mean decrease in serum potassium of 0.1 mEq/L; approximately 4 percent of patients had increases greater than 0.5 mEq/L and approximately 12 percent had a decrease greater than 0.5 mEq/L. (See PRECAUTIONS.) Removal of angiotensin II negative feedback on renin secretion leads to increased plasma renin activity.

ACE is identical to kininase, an enzyme that degrades bradykinin. Whether increased levels of bradykinin, a potent vasodepressor peptide, play a role in the therapeutic effects of PRINIVIL remains to be elucidated.

While the mechanism through which PRINIVIL lowers blood pressure is believed to be primarily suppression of the renin-angiotensin-aldosterone system, PRINIVIL is antihypertensive even in patients with low-renin hypertension. Although PRINIVIL was antihypertensive in all races studied, Black hypertensive patients (usually a low-renin hypertensive population) had a smaller average response to monotherapy than non-Black patients.

Concomitant administration of PRINIVIL and hydrochlorothiazide further reduced blood pressure in Black and non-Black patients and any racial difference in blood pressure response was no longer evident.

Pharmacokinetics and Metabolism

Adult Patients: Following oral administration of PRINIVIL, peak serum concentrations of lisinopril occur within about 7 hours, although there was a trend to a small delay in time taken to reach peak serum concentrations in acute myocardial infarction patients. Declining serum concentrations exhibit a prolonged terminal phase which does not contribute to drug accumulation. This terminal phase probably represents saturable binding to ACE and is not proportional to dose. Lisinopril does not appear to be bound to other serum proteins.

Lisinopril does not undergo metabolism and is excreted unchanged entirely in the urine. Based on urinary recovery, the mean extent of absorption of lisinopril is approximately 25 percent, with large intersubject variability (6–60 percent) at all doses tested (5–80 mg). Lisinopril absorption is not influenced by the presence of food in the gastrointestinal tract. The absolute bioavailability of lisinopril is reduced to about 16 percent in patients with stable NYHA Class II-IV congestive heart failure, and the volume of distribution appears to be slightly smaller than that in normal subjects. The oral bioavailability of lisinopril in patients with acute myocardial infarction is similar to that in healthy volunteers.

Upon multiple dosing, lisinopril exhibits an effective half-life of accumulation of 12 hours.

Impaired renal function decreases elimination of lisinopril, which is excreted principally through the kidneys, but this decrease becomes clinically important only when the glomerular filtration rate is below 30 mL/min. Above this glomerular filtration rate, the elimination half-life is little changed. With greater impairment, however, peak and trough lisinopril levels increase, time to peak concentration increases and time to attain steady state is prolonged. Older patients, on average, have (approximately doubled) higher blood levels and area under the plasma concentration time curve (AUC) than younger patients. (See DOSAGE AND ADMINISTRATION.) Lisinopril can be removed by hemodialysis.

Studies in rats indicate that lisinopril crosses the blood-brain barrier poorly. Multiple doses of lisinopril in rats do not result in accumulation in any tissues. Milk of lactating rats contains radioactivity following administration of ^{14}C lisinopril. By whole body autoradiography, radioactivity was found in the placenta following administration of labeled drug to pregnant rats, but none was found in the fetuses.

Pediatric Patients: The pharmacokinetics of lisinopril were studied in 29 pediatric hypertensive patients between 6 years and 16 years with glomerular filtration rate >30 mL/min/1.73 m². After doses of 0.1 to 0.2 mg/kg, steady state peak plasma concentrations of lisinopril occurred within 6 hours and the extent of absorption based on urinary recovery was about 28%. These values are similar to those obtained previously in adults. The typical value of lisinopril oral clearance (systemic clearance/absolute bioavailability) in a child weighing 30 kg is 10 L/h, which increases in proportion to renal function.

Pharmacodynamics and Clinical Effects

Hypertension:

Adult Patients: Administration of PRINIVIL to patients with hypertension results in a reduction of supine and standing blood pressure to about the same extent with no compensatory tachycardia. Symptomatic postural hypotension is usually not observed although it can occur and should be anticipated in volume and/or salt-depleted patients. (See WARNINGS.) When given together with thiazide-type diuretics, the blood pressure lowering effects of the two drugs are approximately additive.

In most patients studied, onset of antihypertensive activity was seen at one hour after oral administration of an individual dose of PRINIVIL, with peak reduction of blood pressure achieved by six hours. Although an antihypertensive effect was observed 24 hours after dosing with recommended single daily doses, the effect was more consistent and the mean effect was considerably larger in some studies with doses of 20 mg or more than with lower doses. However, at all doses studied, the mean antihypertensive effect was substantially smaller 24 hours after dosing than it was six hours after dosing.

In some patients achievement of optimal blood pressure reduction may require two to four weeks of therapy.

The antihypertensive effects of PRINIVIL are maintained during long-term therapy. Abrupt withdrawal of PRINIVIL has not been associated with a rapid increase in blood pressure or a significant increase in blood pressure compared to pretreatment levels.

Two dose-response studies utilizing a once daily regimen were conducted in 438 mild to moderate hypertensive patients not on a diuretic. Blood pressure was measured 24 hours after dosing. An antihypertensive effect of PRINIVIL was seen with 5 mg in some patients. However, in both studies blood pressure reduction occurred sooner and was greater in patients treated with 10, 20, or 80 mg of PRINIVIL. In controlled clinical studies, PRINIVIL 20–80 mg has been compared in patients with mild to moderate hypertension to hydrochlorothiazide 12.5–50 mg and with atenolol 50–200 mg; and in patients with moderate to severe hypertension to metoprolol 100–200 mg. It was superior to hydrochlorothiazide in effects on systolic and diastolic blood pressure in a population that was 3/4 caucasian. PRINIVIL was approximately equivalent to atenolol and metoprolol in effects on diastolic blood pressure and had somewhat greater effects on systolic blood pressure.

PRINIVIL had similar effectiveness and adverse effects in younger and older (>65 years) patients. It was less effective in Blacks than in caucasians.

In hemodynamic studies in patients with essential hypertension, blood pressure reduction was accompanied by a reduction in peripheral arterial resistance with little or no change in cardiac output and in heart rate. In a study in nine hypertensive patients, following administration of PRINIVIL, there was an increase in mean renal blood flow that was not significant. Data from several small studies are inconsistent with respect to the effect of PRINIVIL on glomerular filtration rate in hypertensive patients with normal renal function, but suggest that changes, if any, are not large.

In patients with renovascular hypertension PRINIVIL has been shown to be well tolerated and effective in controlling blood pressure (see PRECAUTIONS).

Pediatric Patients: In a clinical study involving 115 hypertensive pediatric patients 6 to 16 years of age, patients who weighed <50 kg received either 0.625, 2.5, or 20 mg of lisinopril daily and patients who weighed ≥50 kg received either 1.25, 5, or 40 mg of lisinopril daily. At the end of 2 weeks, lisinopril administered once daily lowered trough blood pressure in a dose-dependent manner with consistent antihypertensive efficacy demonstrated at doses >1.25 mg (0.02 mg/kg). This effect was confirmed in a withdrawal phase, where the diastolic pressure rose by about 9 mmHg more in patients randomized to placebo than it did in patients who were randomized to remain on the middle and high doses of lisinopril. The dose-dependent antihypertensive effect of lisinopril was consistent across several demographic subgroups: age, Tanner stage, gender, race. In this study, lisinopril was generally well-tolerated.

In the above pediatric studies, lisinopril was given either as tablets or in a suspension for those children and infants who were unable to swallow tablets or who required a lower dose than is available in tablet form (see DOSAGE AND ADMINISTRATION, *Preparation of Suspension*).

Heart Failure: During baseline-controlled clinical trials, in patients receiving digitalis and diuretics, single doses of PRINIVIL resulted in decreases in pulmonary capillary wedge pressure, systemic vascular resistance and blood pressure accompanied by an increase in cardiac output and no change in heart rate.

In two placebo-controlled, 12-week clinical studies using doses of PRINIVIL up to 20 mg, PRINIVIL as adjunctive therapy to digitalis and diuretics improved the following signs and symptoms due to congestive heart failure: edema, rales, paroxysmal nocturnal dyspnea and jugular venous

Continued on next page

Information on the Merck & Co., Inc., products listed on these pages is from the prescribing information in use October 1, 2004. For information, please call 1-800-NSC-MERCK [1-800-672-6372].

Prinivil—Cont.

distention. In one of the studies beneficial response was also noted for: orthopnea, presence of third heart sound and the number of patients classified as NYHA Class III and IV. Exercise tolerance was also improved in this study. The effect of lisinopril on mortality in patients with heart failure has not been evaluated.
The once daily dosing for the treatment of congestive heart failure was the only dosage regimen used during clinical trial development and was determined by the measurement of hemodynamic responses.
Acute Myocardial Infarction: The Gruppo Italiano per lo Studio della Sopravvienza nell'Infarto Miocardico (GISSI-3) study was a multicenter, controlled, randomized, unblinded clinical trial conducted in 19,394 patients with acute myocardial infarction admitted to a coronary care unit. It was designed to examine the effects of short-term (6 week) treatment with lisinopril, nitrates, their combination, or no therapy on short-term (6 week) mortality and on long-term death and markedly impaired cardiac function. Patients presenting within 24 hours of the onset of symptoms who were hemodynamically stable were randomized, in a 2×2 factorial design, to six weeks of either
1) PRINIVIL alone (n = 4841),
2) nitrates alone (n = 4869),
3) PRINIVIL plus nitrates (n = 4841), or
4) open control (n = 4843).
All patients received routine therapies, including thrombolytics (72%), aspirin (84%), and a beta-blocker (31%), as appropriate, normally utilized in acute myocardial infarction (MI) patients.
The protocol excluded patients with hypotension (systolic blood pressure $\leq$100 mmHg), severe heart failure, cardiogenic shock and renal dysfunction (serum creatinine $>$2 mg/dL and/or proteinuria $>$500 mg/24 h). Doses of PRINIVIL were adjusted as necessary according to protocol. (See DOSAGE AND ADMINISTRATION.)
Study treatment was withdrawn at six weeks except where clinical conditions indicated continuation of treatment.
The primary outcomes of the trial were the overall mortality at six weeks and a combined endpoint at six months after the myocardial infarction, consisting of the number of patients who died, had late (day 4) clinical congestive heart failure, or had extensive left ventricular damage defined as ejection fraction $\leq$35%, or an akinetic-dyskinetic [A-D] score $\geq$45%. Patients receiving PRINIVIL (n = 9646) alone or with nitrates, had an 11 percent lower risk of death (2p [two-tailed] = 0.04) compared to patients receiving no PRINIVIL (n = 9672) (6.4 percent versus 7.2 percent, respectively) at six weeks. Although patients randomized to receive PRINIVIL for up to six weeks also fared numerically better on the combined endpoint at 6 months, the open nature of the assessment of heart failure, substantial loss of follow-up echocardiography, and substantial excess use of lisinopril between 6 weeks and 6 months in the group randomized to 6 weeks of lisinopril, preclude any conclusion about this endpoint.
Patients with acute myocardial infarction, treated with PRINIVIL had a higher (9.0 percent versus 3.7 percent, respectively) incidence of persistent hypotension (systolic blood pressure $<$90 mmHg for more than 1 hour) and renal dysfunction (2.4 percent versus 1.1 percent) in-hospital and at six weeks (increasing creatinine concentration to over 3 mg/dL or a doubling or more of the baseline serum creatinine concentration). See ADVERSE REACTIONS, *ACUTE MYOCARDIAL INFARCTION.*

INDICATIONS AND USAGE

Hypertension
PRINIVIL is indicated for the treatment of hypertension. It may be used alone as initial therapy or concomitantly with other classes of antihypertensive agents.
Heart Failure
PRINIVIL is indicated as adjunctive therapy in the management of heart failure in patients who are not responding adequately to diuretics and digitalis.
Acute Myocardial Infarction
PRINIVIL is indicated for the treatment of hemodynamically stable patients within 24 hours of acute myocardial infarction, to improve survival. Patients should receive, as appropriate, the standard recommended treatments such as thrombolytics, aspirin and beta-blockers.

In using PRINIVIL, consideration should be given to the fact that another angiotensin converting enzyme inhibitor, captopril, has caused agranulocytosis, particularly in patients with renal impairment or collagen vascular disease, and that available data are insufficient to show that PRINIVIL does not have a similar risk. (See WARNINGS.)
In considering use of PRINIVIL, it should be noted that in controlled clinical trials ACE inhibitors have an effect on blood pressure that is less in Black patients than in non-Blacks. In addition, it should be noted that Black patients receiving ACE inhibitors have been reported to have a higher incidence of angioedema compared to non-Blacks (see WARNINGS, *Anaphylactoid and Possibly Related Reactions, Angioedema*).

CONTRAINDICATIONS

PRINIVIL is contraindicated in patients who are hypersensitive to this product and in patients with a history of angioedema related to previous treatment with an angiotensin converting enzyme inhibitor and in patients with hereditary or idiopathic angioedema.

WARNINGS

Anaphylactoid and Possibly Related Reactions
Presumably because angiotensin converting enzyme inhibitors affect the metabolism of eicosanoids and polypeptides, including endogenous bradykinin, patients receiving ACE inhibitors (including PRINIVIL) may be subject to a variety of adverse reactions, some of them serious.
Head and Neck Angioedema: Angioedema of the face, extremities, lips, tongue, glottis and/or larynx has been reported in patients treated with angiotensin converting enzyme inhibitors, including PRINIVIL. This may occur at any time during treatment. ACE inhibitors have been associated with a higher rate of angioedema in Black than in non-Black patients. In such cases PRINIVIL should be promptly discontinued and appropriate therapy and monitoring should be provided until complete and sustained resolution of signs and symptoms has occurred. In instances where swelling has been confined to the face and lips the condition has generally resolved without treatment, although antihistamines have been useful in relieving symptoms. Angioedema associated with laryngeal edema may be fatal. **Where there is involvement of the tongue, glottis or larynx, likely to cause airway obstruction, appropriate therapy, e.g., subcutaneous epinephrine solution 1:1000 (0.3 mL to 0.5 mL) and/or measures necessary to ensure a patent airway, should be promptly provided.** (See ADVERSE REACTIONS.)
Patients with a history of angioedema unrelated to ACE inhibitor therapy may be at increased risk of angioedema while receiving an ACE inhibitor (see also INDICATIONS AND USAGE and CONTRAINDICATIONS).
Intestinal Angioedema: Intestinal angioedema has been reported in patients treated with ACE inhibitors. These patients presented with abdominal pain (with or without nausea or vomiting): in some cases there was no prior history of facial angioedema and C-1 esterase levels were normal. The angioedema was diagnosed by procedures including abdominal CT scan or ultrasound, or at surgery, and symptoms resolved after stopping the ACE inhibitor. Intestinal angioedema should be included in the differential diagnosis of patients on ACE inhibitors presenting with abdominal pain.
Anaphylactoid reactions during desensitization: Two patients undergoing desensitizing treatment with hymenoptera venom while receiving ACE inhibitors sustained life-threatening anaphylactoid reactions. In the same patients, these reactions were avoided when ACE inhibitors were temporarily withheld, but they reappeared upon inadvertent rechallenge.
Anaphylactoid reactions during membrane exposure: Sudden and potentially life-threatening anaphylactoid reactions have been reported in some patients dialyzed with high-flux membranes (e.g., AN69®) and treated concomitantly with an ACE inhibitor. In such patients, dialysis must be stopped immediately, and aggressive therapy for anaphylactoid reactions be initiated. Symptoms have not been relieved by antihistamines in these situations. In these patients, consideration should be given to using a different type of dialysis membrane or a different class of antihypertensive agent. Anaphylactoid reactions have also been reported in patients undergoing low-density lipoprotein apheresis with dextran sulfate absorption.
Hypotension
Excessive hypotension is rare in patients with uncomplicated hypertension treated with PRINIVIL alone.
Patients with heart failure given PRINIVIL commonly have some reduction in blood pressure with peak blood pressure reduction occurring 6 to 8 hours post dose, but discontinuation of therapy because of continuing symptomatic hypotension usually is not necessary when dosing instructions are followed; caution should be observed when initiating therapy. (See DOSAGE AND ADMINISTRATION.)
Patients at risk of excessive hypotension, sometimes associated with oliguria and/or progressive azotemia, and rarely with acute renal failure and/or death, include those with the following conditions or characteristics: heart failure with systolic blood pressure below 100 mmHg, hyponatremia, high dose diuretic therapy, recent intensive diuresis or increase in diuretic dose, renal dialysis, or severe volume and/or salt depletion of any etiology. It may be advisable to eliminate the diuretic (except in patients with heart failure), reduce the diuretic dose or increase salt intake cautiously before initiating therapy with PRINIVIL in patients at risk for excessive hypotension who are able to tolerate such adjustments. (See PRECAUTIONS, *Drug Interactions,* and ADVERSE REACTIONS.)
Patients with acute myocardial infarction in the GISSI-3 study had a higher (9.0 versus 3.7 percent) incidence of persistent hypotension (systolic blood pressure $<$90 mmHg for more than 1 hour) when treated with PRINIVIL. Treatment with PRINIVIL must not be initiated in acute myocardial infarction patients at risk of further serious hemodynamic deterioration after treatment with a vasodilator (e.g., systolic blood pressure of 100 mmHg or lower) or cardiogenic shock.
In patients at risk of excessive hypotension, therapy should be started under very close medical supervision and such patients should be followed closely for the first two weeks of treatment and whenever the dose of PRINIVIL and/or diuretic is increased. Similar considerations may apply to patients with ischemic heart or cerebrovascular disease, or in patients with acute myocardial infarction, in whom an excessive fall in blood pressure could result in a myocardial infarction or cerebrovascular accident.
If excessive hypotension occurs, the patient should be placed in the supine position and, if necessary, receive an intravenous infusion of normal saline. A transient hypotensive response is not a contraindication to further doses of PRINIVIL which usually can be given without difficulty once the blood pressure has stabilized. If symptomatic hypotension develops, a dose reduction or discontinuation of PRINIVIL or concomitant diuretic may be necessary.
Leukopenia/Neutropenia/Agranulocytosis
Another angiotensin converting enzyme inhibitor, captopril, has been shown to cause agranulocytosis and bone marrow depression, rarely in uncomplicated patients but more frequently in patients with renal impairment especially if they also have a collagen vascular disease. Available data from clinical trials of PRINIVIL are insufficient to show that PRINIVIL does not cause agranulocytosis at similar rates. Marketing experience has revealed rare cases of leukopenia/neutropenia and bone marrow depression in which a causal relationship to lisinopril cannot be excluded. Periodic monitoring of white blood cell counts in patients with collagen vascular disease and renal disease should be considered.
Hepatic Failure
Rarely, ACE inhibitors have been associated with a syndrome that starts with cholestatic jaundice and progresses to fulminant hepatic necrosis, and (sometimes) death. The mechanism of this syndrome is not understood. Patients receiving ACE inhibitors who develop jaundice or marked elevations of hepatic enzymes should discontinue the ACE inhibitor and receive appropriate medical follow-up.
Fetal/Neonatal Morbidity and Mortality
ACE inhibitors can cause fetal and neonatal morbidity and death when administered to pregnant women. Several dozen cases have been reported in the world literature. When pregnancy is detected, ACE inhibitors should be discontinued as soon as possible.
The use of ACE inhibitors during the second and third trimesters of pregnancy has been associated with fetal and neonatal injury, including hypotension, neonatal skull hypoplasia, anuria, reversible or irreversible renal failure, and death. Oligohydramnios has also been reported, presumably resulting from decreased fetal renal function; oligohydramnios in this setting has been associated with fetal limb contractures, craniofacial deformation, and hypoplastic lung development. Prematurity, intrauterine growth retardation, and patent ductus arteriosus have also been reported, although it is not clear whether these occurrences were due to the ACE-inhibitor exposure.
These adverse effects do not appear to have resulted from intrauterine ACE-inhibitor exposure that has been limited to the first trimester. Mothers whose embryos and fetuses are exposed to ACE inhibitors only during the first trimester should be so informed. Nonetheless, when patients become pregnant, physicians should make every effort to discontinue the use of PRINIVIL as soon as possible.
Rarely (probably less often than once in every thousand pregnancies), no alternative to ACE inhibitors will be found. In these rare cases, the mothers should be apprised of the potential hazards to their fetuses, and serial ultrasound examinations should be performed to assess the intraamniotic environment.
If oligohydramnios is observed, PRINIVIL should be discontinued unless it is considered lifesaving for the mother. Contraction stress testing (CST), a non-stress test (NST), or biophysical profiling (BPP) may be appropriate, depending upon the week of pregnancy. Patients and physicians should be aware, however, that oligohydramnios may not appear until after the fetus has sustained irreversible injury.
Infants with histories of *in utero* exposure to ACE inhibitors should be closely observed for hypotension, oliguria, and hyperkalemia. If oliguria occurs, attention should be directed toward support of blood pressure and renal perfusion. Exchange transfusion or dialysis may be required as means of reversing hypotension and/or substituting for disordered renal function. Lisinopril, which crosses the placenta, has been removed from neonatal circulation by peritoneal dialysis with some clinical benefit, and theoretically may be removed by exchange transfusion, although there is no experience with the latter procedure.
No teratogenic effects of lisinopril were seen in studies of pregnant mice, rats, and rabbits. On a body surface area basis, the doses used were up to 55 times, 33 times, and 0.15 times, respectively, the maximum recommended human daily dose (MRHDD).

PRECAUTIONS

General
Aortic Stenosis/Hypertrophic Cardiomyopathy: As with all vasodilators, lisinopril should be given with caution to patients with obstruction in the outflow tract of the left ventricle.
Impaired Renal Function: As a consequence of inhibiting the renin-angiotensin-aldosterone system, changes in renal function may be anticipated in susceptible individuals. In patients with severe congestive heart failure whose renal function may depend on the activity of the renin-angiotensin-aldosterone system, treatment with angiotensin converting enzyme inhibitors, including PRINIVIL, may be associated with oliguria and/or progressive azotemia and rarely with acute renal failure and/or death.

In hypertensive patients with unilateral or bilateral renal artery stenosis, increases in blood urea nitrogen and serum creatinine may occur. Experience with another angiotensin converting enzyme inhibitor suggests that these increases are usually reversible upon discontinuation of PRINIVIL and/or diuretic therapy. In such patients renal function should be monitored during the first few weeks of therapy.
Some patients with hypertension or heart failure with no apparent pre-existing renal vascular disease have developed increases in blood urea nitrogen and serum creatinine, usually minor and transient, especially when PRINIVIL has been given concomitantly with a diuretic. This is more likely to occur in patients with pre-existing renal impairment. Dosage reduction and/or discontinuation of the diuretic and/or PRINIVIL may be required.
Patients with acute myocardial infarction in the GISSI-3 study, treated with PRINIVIL, had a higher (2.4 percent versus 1.1 percent) incidence of renal dysfunction in-hospital and at six weeks (increasing creatinine concentration to over 3 mg/dL or a doubling or more of the baseline serum creatinine concentration). In acute myocardial infarction, treatment with PRINIVIL should be initiated with caution in patients with evidence of renal dysfunction, defined as serum creatinine concentration exceeding 2 mg/dL. If renal dysfunction develops during treatment with PRINIVIL (serum creatinine concentration exceeding 3 mg/dL or a doubling from the pre-treatment value) then the physician should consider withdrawal of PRINIVIL.
Evaluation of patients with hypertension, heart failure, or myocardial infarction should always include assessment of renal function. (See DOSAGE AND ADMINISTRATION.)
Hyperkalemia: In clinical trials hyperkalemia (serum potassium greater than 5.7 mEq/L) occurred in approximately 2.2 percent of hypertensive patients and 4.8 percent of patients with heart failure. In most cases these were isolated values which resolved despite continued therapy. Hyperkalemia was a cause of discontinuation of therapy in approximately 0.1 percent of hypertensive patients, 0.6 percent of patients with heart failure and 0.1 percent of patients with myocardial infarction. Risk factors for the development of hyperkalemia include renal insufficiency, diabetes mellitus, and the concomitant use of potassium-sparing diuretics, potassium supplements and/or potassium-containing salt substitutes, which should be used cautiously, if at all, with PRINIVIL. (See *Drug Interactions.*)
Cough: Presumably due to the inhibition of the degradation of endogenous bradykinin, persistent nonproductive cough has been reported with all ACE inhibitors, always resolving after discontinuation of therapy. ACE inhibitor-induced cough should be considered in the differential diagnosis of cough.
Surgery/Anesthesia: In patients undergoing major surgery or during anesthesia with agents that produce hypotension, PRINIVIL may block angiotensin II formation secondary to compensatory renin release. If hypotension occurs and is considered to be due to this mechanism, it can be corrected by volume expansion.
Information for Patients
Angioedema: Angioedema, including laryngeal edema, may occur at any time during treatment with angiotensin converting enzyme inhibitors, including lisinopril. Patients should be so advised and told to report immediately any signs or symptoms suggesting angioedema (swelling of face, extremities, eyes, lips, tongue, difficulty in swallowing or breathing) and to take no more drug until they have consulted with the prescribing physician.
Symptomatic Hypotension: Patients should be cautioned to report lightheadedness especially during the first few days of therapy. If actual syncope occurs, the patients should be told to discontinue the drug until they have consulted with the prescribing physician.
All patients should be cautioned that excessive perspiration and dehydration may lead to an excessive fall in blood pressure because of reduction in fluid volume. Other causes of volume depletion such as vomiting or diarrhea may also lead to a fall in blood pressure; patients should be advised to consult with their physician.
Hyperkalemia: Patients should be told not to use salt substitutes containing potassium without consulting their physician.
Leukopenia/Neutropenia: Patients should be told to report promptly any indication of infection (e.g., sore throat, fever) which may be a sign of leukopenia/neutropenia.
Pregnancy: Female patients of childbearing age should be told about the consequences of second- and third-trimester exposure to ACE inhibitors, and they should also be told that these consequences do not appear to have resulted from intrauterine ACE-inhibitor exposure that has been limited to the first trimester. These patients should be asked to report pregnancies to their physicians as soon as possible.
NOTE: As with many other drugs, certain advice to patients being treated with PRINIVIL is warranted. This information is intended to aid in the safe and effective use of this medication. It is not a disclosure of all possible adverse or intended effects.
Drug Interactions
Hypotension—Patients on Diuretic Therapy: Patients on diuretics, and especially those in whom diuretic therapy was recently instituted, may occasionally experience an excessive reduction of blood pressure after initiation of therapy with PRINIVIL. The possibility of hypotensive effects with PRINIVIL can be minimized by either discontinuing the diuretic or increasing the salt intake prior to initiation of

	Percent of Patients in Controlled Studies		
	PRINIVIL (n = 1349) Incidence (discontinuation)	PRINIVIL/ Hydrochlorothiazide (n = 629) Incidence (discontinuation)	Placebo (n = 207) Incidence (discontinuation)
Body As A Whole			
Fatigue	2.5 (0.3)	4.0 (0.5)	1.0 (0.0)
Asthenia	1.3 (0.5)	2.1 (0.2)	1.0 (0.0)
Orthostatic Effects	1.2 (0.0)	3.5 (0.2)	1.0 (0.0)
Cardiovascular			
Hypotension	1.2 (0.5)	1.6 (0.5)	0.5 (0.5)
Digestive			
Diarrhea	2.7 (0.2)	2.7 (0.3)	2.4 (0.0)
Nausea	2.0 (0.4)	2.5 (0.2)	2.4 (0.0)
Vomiting	1.1 (0.2)	1.4 (0.1)	0.5 (0.0)
Dyspepsia	0.9 (0.0)	1.9 (0.0)	0.0 (0.0)
Musculoskeletal			
Muscle Cramps	0.5 (0.0)	2.9 (0.8)	0.5 (0.0)
Nervous/Psychiatric			
Headache	5.7 (0.2)	4.5 (0.5)	1.9 (0.0)
Dizziness	5.4 (0.4)	9.2 (1.0)	1.9 (0.0)
Paresthesia	0.8 (0.1)	2.1 (0.2)	0.0 (0.0)
Decreased Libido	0.4 (0.1)	1.3 (0.1)	0.0 (0.0)
Vertigo	0.2 (0.1)	1.1 (0.2)	0.0 (0.0)
Respiratory			
Cough	3.5 (0.7)	4.6 (0.8)	1.0 (0.0)
Upper Respiratory Infection	2.1 (0.1)	2.7 (0.1)	0.0 (0.0)
Common Cold	1.1 (0.1)	1.3 (0.1)	0.0 (0.0)
Nasal Congestion	0.4 (0.1)	1.3 (0.1)	0.0 (0.0)
Influenza	0.3 (0.1)	1.1 (0.1)	0.0 (0.0)
Skin			
Rash	1.3 (0.4)	1.6 (0.2)	0.5 (0.5)
Urogenital			
Impotence	1.0 (0.4)	1.6 (0.5)	0.0 (0.0)

treatment with PRINIVIL. If it is necessary to continue the diuretic, initiate therapy with PRINIVIL at a dose of 5 mg daily, and provide close medical supervision after the initial dose until blood pressure has stabilized. (See WARNINGS, and DOSAGE AND ADMINISTRATION.) When a diuretic is added to the therapy of a patient receiving PRINIVIL, an additional antihypertensive effect is usually observed. Studies with ACE inhibitors in combination with diuretics indicate that the dose of the ACE inhibitor can be reduced when it is given with a diuretic. (See DOSAGE AND ADMINISTRATION.)
Non-steroidal Anti-inflammatory Agents: In some patients with compromised renal function who are being treated with non-steroidal anti-inflammatory drugs, the co-administration of lisinopril may result in a further deterioration of renal function. These effects are usually reversible.
Reports suggest that NSAIDs may diminish the antihypertensive effect of ACE inhibitors, including lisinopril. This interaction should be given consideration in patients taking NSAIDs concomitantly with ACE inhibitors.
In a study in 36 patients with mild to moderate hypertension where the antihypertensive effects of PRINIVIL alone were compared to PRINIVIL given concomitantly with indomethacin, the use of indomethacin was associated with a reduced antihypertensive effect, although the difference between the two regimens was not significant.
Other Agents: PRINIVIL has been used concomitantly with nitrates and/or digoxin without evidence of clinically significant adverse interactions. This included post myocardial infarction patients who were receiving intravenous or transdermal nitroglycerin. No clinically important pharmacokinetic interactions occurred when PRINIVIL was used concomitantly with propranolol or hydrochlorothiazide. The presence of food in the stomach does not alter the bioavailability of PRINIVIL.
Agents Increasing Serum Potassium: PRINIVIL attenuates potassium loss caused by thiazide-type diuretics. Use of PRINIVIL with potassium-sparing diuretics (e.g., spironolactone, triamterene, or amiloride), potassium supplements, or potassium-containing salt substitutes may lead to significant increases in serum potassium. Therefore, if concomitant use of these agents is indicated because of demonstrated hypokalemia, they should be used with caution and with frequent monitoring of serum potassium. Potassium sparing agents should generally not be used in patients with heart failure who are receiving PRINIVIL.
Lithium: Lithium toxicity has been reported in patients receiving lithium concomitantly with drugs which cause elimination of sodium, including ACE inhibitors. Lithium toxicity was usually reversible upon discontinuation of lithium and the ACE inhibitor. It is recommended that serum lithium levels be monitored frequently if PRINIVIL is administered concomitantly with lithium.
Carcinogenesis, Mutagenesis, Impairment of Fertility
There was no evidence of a tumorigenic effect when lisinopril was administered orally for 105 weeks to male and female rats at doses up to 90 mg/kg/day or for 92 weeks to male and female mice at doses up to 135 mg/kg/day. These doses are 10 times and 7 times, respectively, the maximum recommended human daily dose (MRHDD) when compared on a body surface area basis.
Lisinopril was not mutagenic in the Ames microbial mutagen test with or without metabolic activation. It was also negative in a forward mutation assay using Chinese hamster lung cells. Lisinopril did not produce single strand DNA breaks in an *in vitro* alkaline elution rat hepatocyte assay.
In addition, lisinopril did not produce increases in chromosomal aberrations in an *in vitro* test in Chinese hamster ovary cells or in an *in vivo* study in mouse bone marrow.
There were no adverse effects on reproductive performance in male and female rats treated with up to 300 mg/kg/day of lisinopril (33 times the MRHDD when compared on a body surface area basis).
Pregnancy
Pregnancy Categories C (first trimester) *and D* (second and third trimesters). See WARNINGS, *Fetal/Neonatal Morbidity and Mortality.*
Nursing Mothers
Milk of lactating rats contains radioactivity following administration of ^{14}C lisinopril. It is not known whether this drug is secreted in human milk. Because many drugs are secreted in human milk, and because of the potential for serious adverse reactions in nursing infants from ACE inhibitors, a decision should be made whether to discontinue nursing or discontinue PRINIVIL, taking into account the importance of the drug to the mother.
Pediatric Use
Antihypertensive effects of PRINIVIL have been established in hypertensive pediatric patients aged 6 to 16 years. There are no data on the effect of PRINIVIL on blood pressure in pediatric patients under the age of 6 or in pediatric patients with glomerular filtration rate <30 mL/min/1.73 m^2 (see CLINICAL PHARMACOLOGY, *Pharmacokinetics and Metabolism* and *Pharmacodynamics and Clinical Effects*, and DOSAGE AND ADMINISTRATION).

ADVERSE REACTIONS

PRINIVIL has been found to be generally well tolerated in controlled clinical trials involving 1969 patients with hypertension or heart failure. For the most part, adverse experiences were mild and transient.
HYPERTENSION
In clinical trials in patients with hypertension treated with PRINIVIL, discontinuation of therapy due to clinical adverse experiences occurred in 5.7 percent of patients. The overall frequency of adverse experiences could not be related to total daily dosage within the recommended therapeutic dosage range.
For adverse experiences occurring in greater than one percent of patients with hypertension treated with PRINIVIL or PRINIVIL plus hydrochlorothiazide in controlled clinical trials and more frequently with PRINIVIL and/or PRINIVIL plus hydrochlorothiazide than placebo, comparative incidence data are listed in the table below:
[See table above]
Chest pain and back pain were also seen but were more common on placebo than PRINIVIL.
HEART FAILURE
In patients with heart failure treated with PRINIVIL for up to four years, discontinuation of therapy due to clinical adverse experiences occurred in 11.0 percent of patients. In controlled studies in patients with heart failure, therapy

Continued on next page

Information on the Merck & Co., Inc., products listed on these pages is from the prescribing information in use October 1, 2004. For information, please call 1-800-NSC-MERCK [1-800-672-6372].

Prinivil—Cont.

was discontinued in 8.1 percent of patients treated with PRINIVIL for up to 12 weeks, compared to 7.7 percent of patients treated with placebo for 12 weeks.

The following table lists those adverse experiences which occurred in greater than one percent of patients with heart failure treated with PRINIVIL or placebo for up to 12 weeks in controlled clinical trials and more frequently on PRINIVIL than placebo.

	Controlled Trials	
	PRINIVIL (n=407) Incidence (discontinuation) 12 weeks	Placebo (n=155) Incidence (discontinuation) 12 weeks
Body As A Whole		
Chest Pain	3.4 (0.2)	1.3 (0.0)
Abdominal Pain	2.2 (0.7)	1.9 (0.0)
Cardiovascular		
Hypotension	4.4 (1.7)	0.6 (0.6)
Digestive		
Diarrhea	3.7 (0.5)	1.9 (0.0)
Nervous/Psychiatric		
Dizziness	11.8 (1.2)	4.5 (1.3)
Headache	4.4 (0.2)	3.9 (0.0)
Respiratory		
Upper Respiratory Infection	1.5 (0.0)	1.3 (0.0)
Skin		
Rash	1.7 (0.5)	0.6 (0.6)

Also observed at >1% with PRINIVIL but more frequent or as frequent on placebo than PRINIVIL in controlled trials were asthenia, angina pectoris, nausea, dyspnea, cough and pruritus.

Worsening of heart failure, anorexia, increased salivation, muscle cramps, back pain, myalgia, depression, chest sound abnormalities and pulmonary edema were also seen in controlled clinical trials, but were more common on placebo than PRINIVIL.

ACUTE MYOCARDIAL INFARCTION

In the GISSI-3 trial, in patients treated with PRINIVIL for six weeks following acute myocardial infarction, discontinuation of therapy occurred in 17.6 percent of patients.

Patients treated with PRINIVIL had a significantly higher incidence of hypotension and renal dysfunction compared with patients not taking PRINIVIL.

In the GISSI-3 trial, hypotension (9.7 percent), renal dysfunction (2.0 percent), cough (0.5 percent), post-infarction angina (0.3 percent), skin rash and generalized edema (0.01 percent), and angioedema (0.01 percent) resulted in withdrawal of treatment. In elderly patients treated with PRINIVIL, discontinuation due to renal dysfunction was 4.2 percent.

Other clinical adverse experiences occurring in 0.3 to 1.0 percent of patients with hypertension or heart failure treated with PRINIVIL in controlled trials and rarer, serious, possibly drug-related events reported in uncontrolled studies or marketing experience are listed below, and within each category, are in order of decreasing severity:

Body as a Whole: Anaphylactoid reactions (see WARNINGS, *Anaphylactoid and Possibly Related Reactions*), syncope, orthostatic effects, chest discomfort, pain, pelvic pain, flank pain, edema, facial edema, virus infection, fever, chills, malaise.

Cardiovascular: Cardiac arrest; myocardial infarction or cerebrovascular accident, possibly secondary to excessive hypotension in high risk patients (see WARNINGS, *Hypotension*); pulmonary embolism and infarction, arrhythmias (including ventricular tachycardia, atrial tachycardia, atrial fibrillation, bradycardia and premature ventricular contractions), palpitations, transient ischemic attacks, paroxysmal nocturnal dyspnea, orthostatic hypotension, decreased blood pressure, peripheral edema, vasculitis.

Digestive: Pancreatitis, hepatitis (hepatocellular or cholestatic jaundice) (see WARNINGS, *Hepatic Failure*), vomiting, gastritis, dyspepsia, heartburn, gastrointestinal cramps, constipation, flatulence, dry mouth.

Hematologic: Rare cases of bone marrow depression, hemolytic anemia, leukopenia/neutropenia, and thrombocytopenia.

Endocrine: Diabetes mellitus.

Metabolic: Weight loss, dehydration, fluid overload, gout, weight gain.

Musculoskeletal: Arthritis, arthralgia, neck pain, hip pain, low back pain, joint pain, leg pain, knee pain, shoulder pain, arm pain, lumbago.

Nervous System/Psychiatric: Stroke, ataxia, memory impairment, tremor, peripheral neuropathy (e.g., dysesthesia) spasm, paresthesia, confusion, insomnia, somnolence, hypersomnia, irritability, and nervousness.

Respiratory System: Malignant lung neoplasms, hemoptysis, pulmonary infiltrates, eosinophilic pneumonitis, bronchospasm, asthma, pleural effusion, pneumonia, bronchitis, wheezing, orthopnea, painful respiration, epistaxis, laryngitis, sinusitis, pharyngeal pain, pharyngitis, rhinitis, rhinorrhea.

Skin: Urticaria, alopecia, herpes zoster, photosensitivity, skin lesions, skin infections, pemphigus, erythema, flushing, diaphoresis. Other severe skin reactions (including toxic epidermal necrolysis and Stevens-Johnson syndrome) have been reported rarely; causal relationship has not been established.

Special Senses: Visual loss, diplopia, blurred vision, tinnitus, photophobia, taste disturbances.

Urogenital System: Acute renal failure, oliguria, anuria, uremia, progressive azotemia, renal dysfunction (see PRECAUTIONS and DOSAGE AND ADMINISTRATION), pyelonephritis, dysuria, urinary tract infection, breast pain.

Miscellaneous: A symptom complex has been reported which may include a positive ANA, an elevated erythrocyte sedimentation rate, arthralgia/arthritis, myalgia, fever, vasculitis, eosinophilia and leukocytosis. Rash, photosensitivity or other dermatological manifestations may occur alone or in combination with these symptoms.

Angioedema: Angioedema has been reported in patients receiving PRINIVIL (0.1%) with an incidence higher in Black than in non-Black patients. Angioedema associated with laryngeal edema may be fatal. If angioedema of the face, extremities, lips, tongue, glottis and/or larynx occurs, treatment with PRINIVIL should be discontinued and appropriate therapy instituted immediately. In rare cases, intestinal angioedema has been reported with angiotensin converting enzyme inhibitors including lisinopril. (See WARNINGS.)

Hypotension: In hypertensive patients, hypotension occurred in 1.2 percent and syncope occurred in 0.1 percent of patients. Hypotension or syncope was a cause for discontinuation of therapy in 0.5 percent of hypertensive patients. In patients with heart failure, hypotension occurred in 5.3 percent and syncope occurred in 1.8 percent of patients. These adverse experiences were causes for discontinuation of therapy in 1.8 percent of these patients. In patients treated with PRINIVIL for six weeks after acute myocardial infarction, hypotension (systolic blood pressure ≤100 mmHg) resulted in discontinuation of therapy in 9.7 percent of the patients. (See WARNINGS.)

Fetal/Neonatal Morbidity and Mortality: See WARNINGS, *Fetal/Neonatal Morbidity and Mortality.*

Pediatric Patients: No relevant differences between the adverse experience profile for pediatric patients and that previously reported for adult patients were identified.

Cough: See PRECAUTIONS, *Cough.*

Clinical Laboratory Test Findings

Serum Electrolytes: Hyperkalemia (see PRECAUTIONS), hyponatremia.

Creatinine, Blood Urea Nitrogen: Minor increases in blood urea nitrogen and serum creatinine, reversible upon discontinuation of therapy, were observed in about 2.0 percent of patients with essential hypertension treated with PRINIVIL alone. Increases were more common in patients receiving concomitant diuretics and in patients with renal artery stenosis. (See PRECAUTIONS.) Reversible minor increases in blood urea nitrogen and serum creatinine were observed in approximately 11.6 percent of patients with heart failure on concomitant diuretic therapy. Frequently, these abnormalities resolved when the dosage of the diuretic was decreased.

Hemoglobin and Hematocrit: Small decreases in hemoglobin and hematocrit (mean decreases of approximately 0.4 g percent and 1.3 vol percent, respectively) occurred frequently in patients treated with PRINIVIL but were rarely of clinical importance in patients without some other cause of anemia. In clinical trials, less than 0.1 percent of patients discontinued therapy due to anemia. Hemolytic anemia has been reported; a causal relationship to lisinopril cannot be excluded.

Liver Function Tests: Rarely, elevations of liver enzymes and/or serum bilirubin have occurred (see WARNINGS, *Hepatic Failure*).

In hypertensive patients, 2.0 percent discontinued therapy due to laboratory adverse experiences, principally elevations in blood urea nitrogen (0.6 percent), serum creatinine (0.5 percent) and serum potassium (0.4 percent). In the heart failure trials, 3.4 percent of patients discontinued therapy due to laboratory adverse experiences, 1.8 percent due to elevations in blood urea nitrogen and/or creatinine and 0.6 percent due to elevations in serum potassium. In the myocardial infarction trial, 2.0 percent of patients receiving PRINIVIL discontinued therapy due to renal dysfunction (increasing creatinine concentration to over 3 mg/dL or a doubling or more of the baseline serum creatinine concentration); less than 1.0 percent of patients discontinued therapy due to other laboratory adverse experiences: 0.1 percent with hyperkalemia and less than 0.1 percent with hepatic enzyme alterations.

OVERDOSAGE

Following a single oral dose of 20 g/kg, no lethality occurred in rats and death occurred in one of 20 mice receiving the same dose. The most likely manifestation of overdosage would be hypotension, for which the usual treatment would be intravenous infusion of normal saline solution.

Lisinopril can be removed by hemodialysis. (See WARNINGS, *Anaphylactoid reactions during membrane exposure.*)

DOSAGE AND ADMINISTRATION

Hypertension

Initial Therapy: In patients with uncomplicated essential hypertension not on diuretic therapy, the recommended initial dose is 10 mg once a day. Dosage should be adjusted according to blood pressure response. The usual dosage range is 20 to 40 mg per day administered in a single daily dose. The antihypertensive effect may diminish toward the end of the dosing interval regardless of the administered dose, but most commonly with a dose of 10 mg daily. This can be evaluated by measuring blood pressure just prior to dosing to determine whether satisfactory control is being maintained for 24 hours. If it is not, an increase in dose should be considered. Doses up to 80 mg have been used but do not appear to give a greater effect. If blood pressure is not controlled with PRINIVIL alone, a low dose of a diuretic may be added. Hydrochlorothiazide 12.5 mg has been shown to provide an additive effect. After the addition of a diuretic, it may be possible to reduce the dose of PRINIVIL.

Diuretic Treated Patients: In hypertensive patients who are currently being treated with a diuretic, symptomatic hypotension may occur occasionally following the initial dose of PRINIVIL. The diuretic should be discontinued, if possible, for two to three days before beginning therapy with PRINIVIL to reduce the likelihood of hypotension. (See WARNINGS.) The dosage of PRINIVIL should be adjusted according to blood pressure response. If the patient's blood pressure is not controlled with PRINIVIL alone, diuretic therapy may be resumed as described above.

If the diuretic cannot be discontinued, an initial dose of 5 mg should be used under medical supervision for at least two hours and until blood pressure has stabilized for at least an additional hour. (See WARNINGS and PRECAUTIONS, *Drug Interactions.*)

Concomitant administration of PRINIVIL with potassium supplements, potassium salt substitutes, or potassium-sparing diuretics may lead to increases of serum potassium (see PRECAUTIONS).

Dosage Adjustment in Renal Impairment: The usual dose of PRINIVIL (10 mg) is recommended for patients with a creatinine clearance > 30 mL/min (serum creatinine of up to approximately 3 mg/dL). For patients with creatinine clearance ≥ 10 mL/min ≤ 30 mL/min (serum creatinine ≥ 3 mg/dL), the first dose is 5 mg once daily. For patients with creatinine clearance < 10 mL/min (usually on hemodialysis) the recommended initial dose is 2.5 mg. The dosage may be titrated upward until blood pressure is controlled or to a maximum of 40 mg daily.

Renal Status	Creatinine-Clearance mL/min	Initial Dose mg/day
Normal Renal Function to Mild Impairment	> 30 mL/min	10 mg
Moderate to Severe Impairment	≥ 10 ≤ 30 mL/min	5 mg
Dialysis Patients**	< 10 mL/min	2.5 mg ***

** See WARNINGS, *Anaphylactoid reactions during membrane exposure.*

*** *Dosage or dosing interval should be adjusted depending on the blood pressure response.*

Heart Failure

PRINIVIL is indicated as adjunctive therapy with diuretics and (usually) digitalis. The recommended starting dose is 5 mg once a day.

When initiating treatment with lisinopril in patients with heart failure, the initial dose should be administered under medical observation, especially in those patients with low blood pressure (systolic blood pressure below 100 mmHg). The mean peak blood pressure lowering occurs six to eight hours after dosing. Observation should continue until blood pressure is stable. The concomitant diuretic dose should be reduced, if possible, to help minimize hypovolemia which may contribute to hypotension. (See WARNINGS and PRECAUTIONS, *Drug Interactions.*) The appearance of hypotension after the initial dose of PRINIVIL does not preclude subsequent careful dose titration with the drug, following effective management of the hypotension.

The usual effective dosage range is 5 to 20 mg per day administered as a single daily dose.

Dosage Adjustment in Patients with Heart Failure and Renal Impairment or Hyponatremia: In patients with heart failure who have hyponatremia (serum sodium <130 mEq/L) or moderate to severe renal impairment (creatinine clearance ≤30 mL/min or serum creatinine >3 mg/dL), therapy with PRINIVIL should be initiated at a dose of 2.5 mg once a day under close medical supervision. (See WARNINGS and PRECAUTIONS, *Drug Interactions.*)

Acute Myocardial Infarction

In hemodynamically stable patients within 24 hours of the onset of acute myocardial infarction, the first dose of PRINIVIL is 5 mg given orally, followed by 5 mg after 24 hours, 10 mg after 48 hours and then 10 mg of PRINIVIL once daily. Dosing should continue for six weeks. Patients should receive, as appropriate, the standard recommended treatments such as thrombolytics, aspirin and beta-blockers. Patients with a low systolic blood pressure (≤120 mmHg) when treatment is started or during the first 3 days after the infarct should be given a lower 2.5 mg oral dose of PRINIVIL (see WARNINGS). If hypotension occurs (systolic blood pressure ≤100 mmHg) a daily maintenance dose of 5 mg may be given with temporary reductions to 2.5 mg if needed. If prolonged hypotension occurs (systolic blood pressure <90 mmHg for more than 1 hour) PRINIVIL should be withdrawn. For patients who develop symptoms of heart failure, see DOSAGE AND ADMINISTRATION, *Heart Failure.*

Dosage Adjustment in Patients with Myocardial Infarction with Renal Impairment: In acute myocardial infarction, treatment with PRINIVIL should be initiated with caution in patients with evidence of renal dysfunction, defined as serum creatinine concentration exceeding 2 mg/dL. No evaluation of dosage adjustment in myocardial infarction patients with severe renal impairment has been performed.

Use in Elderly: In general, blood pressure response and adverse experiences were similar in younger and older patients given similar doses of PRINIVIL. Pharmacokinetic studies, however, indicate that maximum blood levels and area under the plasma concentration time curve (AUC) are doubled in older patients so that dosage adjustments should be made with particular caution.

Pediatric Hypertensive Patients ≥ 6 years of age

The usual recommended starting dose is 0.07 mg/kg once daily (up to 5 mg total). Dosage should be adjusted according to blood pressure response. Doses above 0.61 mg/kg (or in excess of 40 mg) have not been studied in pediatric patients. (See CLINICAL PHARMACOLOGY, *Pharmacokinetics and Metabolism* and *Pharmacodynamics and Clinical Effects.*)

PRINIVIL is not recommended in pediatric patients <6 years or in pediatric patients with glomerular filtration rate <30 mL/min/1.73 m^2 (see CLINICAL PHARMACOLOGY, *Pharmacokinetics and Metabolism, Pharmacodynamics and Clinical Effects* and PRECAUTIONS).

Preparation of Suspension (for 200 mL of a 1.0 mg/mL suspension)

Add 10 mL of Purified Water USP to a polyethylene terephthalate (PET) bottle containing ten 20-mg tablets of PRINIVIL and shake for at least one minute. Add 30 mL of Bicitra®** diluent and 160 mL of Ora-Sweet SF™*** to the concentrate in the PET bottle and gently shake for several seconds to disperse the ingredients. The suspension should be stored at or below 25°C (77°F) and can be stored for up to four weeks. Shake the suspension before each use.

**Registered trademark of Alza Corporation
***Trademark of Paddock Laboratories, Inc.

HOW SUPPLIED

No. 3658—Tablets PRINIVIL, 2.5 mg, are white, round flat-faced beveled edge compressed tablets, coded MSD on one side and 15 on the other. They are supplied as follows:
NDC 0006-0015-58 unit of use bottles of 100.

No. 3577—Tablets PRINIVIL, 5 mg, are white, shield shaped, scored, compressed tablets, with code MSD 19 on one side and PRINIVIL on the other. They are supplied as follows:
NDC 0006-0019-54 unit of use bottles of 90
NDC 0006-0019-82 bottles of 1,000
NDC 0006-0019-87 bottles of 10,000

No. 3578—Tablets PRINIVIL, 10 mg, are light yellow, shield shaped, compressed tablets, with code MSD 106 on one side and PRINIVIL on the other. They are supplied as follows:
NDC 0006-0106-54 unit of use bottles of 90
NDC 0006-0106-82 bottles of 1,000
NDC 0006-0106-87 bottles of 10,000

No. 3579—Tablets PRINIVIL, 20 mg, are peach, shield shaped, compressed tablets, with code MSD 207 on one side and PRINIVIL on the other. They are supplied as follows:
NDC 0006-0207-54 unit of use bottles of 90
NDC 0006-0207-82 bottles of 1,000
NDC 0006-0207-87 bottles of 10,000

No. 3580—Tablets PRINIVIL, 40 mg, are rose red, shield shaped, compressed tablets, with code MSD 237 on one side and PRINIVIL on the other. They are supplied as follows:
NDC 0006-0237-58 unit of use bottles of 100.

Storage

Store at controlled room temperature, 15–30°C (59–86°F), and protect from moisture.

Dispense in a tight container, if product package is subdivided.

7825249 Issued April 2003

Shown in Product Identification Guide, page 323

PRINZIDE® Tablets ℞
(Lisinopril-Hydrochlorothiazide)

USE IN PREGNANCY
When used in pregnancy during the second and third trimesters, ACE inhibitors can cause injury and even death to the developing fetus. When pregnancy is detected, PRINZIDE should be discontinued as soon as possible. See WARNINGS, *Pregnancy, Lisinopril, Fetal/Neonatal Morbidity and Mortality.*

DESCRIPTION

PRINZIDE* (Lisinopril-Hydrochlorothiazide) combines an angiotensin converting enzyme inhibitor, lisinopril, and a diuretic, hydrochlorothiazide.

Lisinopril, a synthetic peptide derivative, is an oral long-acting angiotensin converting enzyme inhibitor. It is chemically described as (*S*)-1-[*N*[2]-(1-carboxy-3-phenylpropyl)-L-lysyl]-L-proline dihydrate. Its empirical formula is $C_{21}H_{31}N_3O_5 \cdot 2H_2O$ and its structural formula is:

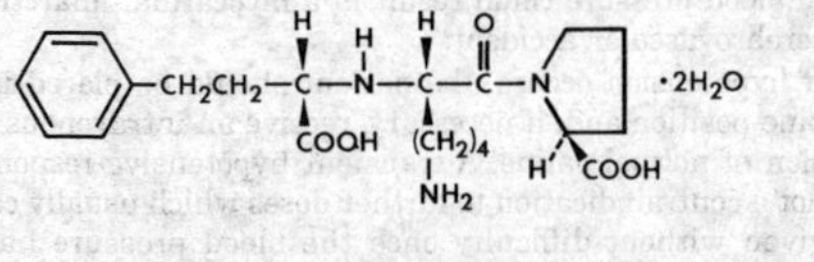

Lisinopril is a white to off-white, crystalline powder, with a molecular weight of 441.52. It is soluble in water, sparingly soluble in methanol, and practically insoluble in ethanol.

Hydrochlorothiazide is 6-chloro-3,4-dihydro-2*H*-1,2,4-benzothiadiazine-7-sulfonamide 1,1-dioxide. Its empirical formula is $C_7H_8ClN_3O_4S_2$ and its structural formula is:

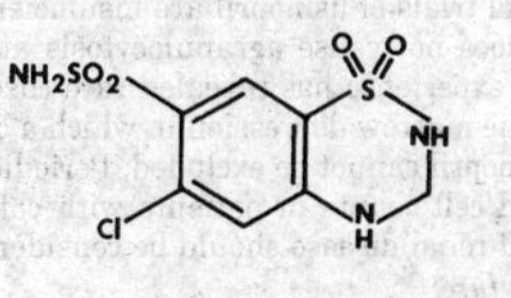

Hydrochlorothiazide is a white, or practically white, crystalline powder with a molecular weight of 297.73, which is slightly soluble in water, but freely soluble in sodium hydroxide solution.

PRINZIDE is available for oral use in three tablet combinations of lisinopril with hydrochlorothiazide: PRINZIDE 10-12.5, containing 10 mg lisinopril and 12.5 mg hydrochlorothiazide. PRINZIDE 20-12.5, containing 20 mg lisinopril and 12.5 mg hydrochlorothiazide and PRINZIDE 20-25, containing 20 mg lisinopril and 25 mg hydrochlorothiazide. Inactive ingredients are calcium phosphate, magnesium stearate, mannitol, and starch. PRINZIDE 10-12.5 also contains FD&C Blue #2 aluminum lake. PRINZIDE 20-12.5 and PRINZIDE 20-25 also contain iron oxide.

*Registered trademark of MERCK & CO., INC.

CLINICAL PHARMACOLOGY

Lisinopril-Hydrochlorothiazide

As a result of its diuretic effects, hydrochlorothiazide increases plasma renin activity, increases aldosterone secretion, and decreases serum potassium. Administration of lisinopril blocks the renin-angiotensin-aldosterone axis and tends to reverse the potassium loss associated with the diuretic.

In clinical studies, the extent of blood pressure reduction seen with the combination of lisinopril and hydrochlorothiazide was approximately additive. The PRINZIDE 10-12.5 combination worked equally well in black and white patients. The PRINZIDE 20-12.5 and PRINZIDE 20-25 combinations appeared somewhat less effective in black patients, but relatively few black patients were studied. In most patients, the antihypertensive effect of PRINZIDE was sustained for at least 24 hours.

In a randomized, controlled comparison, the main antihypertensive effects of PRINZIDE 20-12.5 and PRINZIDE 20-25 were similar, suggesting that many patients who respond adequately to the latter combination may be controlled with PRINZIDE 20-12.5. (See DOSAGE AND ADMINISTRATION.)

Concomitant administration of lisinopril and hydrochlorothiazide has little or no effect on the bioavailability of either drug. The combination tablet is bioequivalent to concomitant administration of the separate entities.

Lisinopril

Mechanism of Action

Lisinopril inhibits angiotensin-converting enzyme (ACE) in human subjects and animals. ACE is a peptidyl dipeptidase that catalyzes the conversion of angiotensin I to the vasoconstrictor substance, angiotensin II. Angiotensin II also stimulates aldosterone secretion by the adrenal cortex. Inhibition of ACE results in decreased plasma angiotensin II which leads to decreased vasopressor activity and to decreased aldosterone secretion. The latter decrease may result in a small increase of serum potassium. Removal of angiotensin II negative feedback on renin secretion leads to increased plasma renin activity. In hypertensive patients with normal renal function treated with lisinopril alone for up to 24 weeks, the mean increase in serum potassium was less than 0.1 mEq/L; however, approximately 15 percent of patients had increases greater than 0.5 mEq/L and approximately six percent had a decrease greater than 0.5 mEq/L. In the same study, patients treated with lisinopril plus a thiazide diuretic showed essentially no change in serum potassium. (See PRECAUTIONS.)

ACE is identical to kininase, an enzyme that degrades bradykinin. Whether increased levels of bradykinin, a potent vasodepressor peptide, play a role in the therapeutic effects of lisinopril remains to be elucidated.

While the mechanism through which lisinopril lowers blood pressure is believed to be primarily suppression of the renin-angiotensin-aldosterone system, lisinopril is antihypertensive even in patients with low-renin hypertension. Although lisinopril was antihypertensive in all races studied, black hypertensive patients (usually a low-renin hypertensive population) had a smaller average response to lisinopril monotherapy than non-black patients.

Pharmacokinetics and Metabolism

Following oral administration of lisinopril, peak serum concentrations occur within about 7 hours. Declining serum concentrations exhibit a prolonged terminal phase which does not contribute to drug accumulation. This terminal phase probably represents saturable binding to ACE and is not proportional to dose. Lisinopril does not appear to be bound to other serum proteins.

Lisinopril does not undergo metabolism and is excreted unchanged entirely in the urine. Based on urinary recovery, the mean extent of absorption of lisinopril is approximately 25 percent, with large intersubject variability (6–60 percent) at all doses tested (5–80 mg). Lisinopril absorption is not influenced by the presence of food in the gastrointestinal tract.

Upon multiple dosing, lisinopril exhibits an effective half-life of accumulation of 12 hours.

Impaired renal function decreases elimination of lisinopril, which is excreted principally through the kidneys, but this decrease becomes clinically important only when the glomerular filtration rate is below 30 mL/min. Above this glomerular filtration rate, the elimination half-life is little changed. With greater impairment, however, peak and trough lisinopril levels increase, time to peak concentration increases and time to attain steady state is prolonged. Older patients, on average, have (approximately doubled) higher blood levels and area under the plasma concentration time curve (AUC) than younger patients. (See DOSAGE AND ADMINISTRATION.) Lisinopril can be removed by hemodialysis.

Studies in rats indicate that lisinopril crosses the blood-brain barrier poorly. Multiple doses of lisinopril in rats do not result in accumulation in any tissues. However, milk of lactating rats contains radioactivity following administration of ^{14}C lisinopril. By whole body autoradiography, radioactivity was found in the placenta following administration of labeled drug to pregnant rats, but none was found in the fetuses.

Pharmacodynamics

Administration of lisinopril to patients with hypertension results in a reduction of supine and standing blood pressure to about the same extent with no compensatory tachycardia. Symptomatic postural hypotension is usually not observed although it can occur and should be anticipated in volume and/or salt-depleted patients. (See WARNINGS.)

In most patients studied, onset of antihypertensive activity was seen at one hour after oral administration of an individual dose of lisinopril, with peak reduction of blood pressure achieved by six hours.

In some patients achievement of optimal blood pressure reduction may require two to four weeks of therapy.

At recommended single daily doses, antihypertensive effects have been maintained for at least 24 hours after dosing, although the effect at 24 hours was substantially smaller than the effect six hours after dosing.

The antihypertensive effects of lisinopril have continued during long-term therapy. Abrupt withdrawal of lisinopril has not been associated with a rapid increase in blood pressure; nor with a significant overshoot of pretreatment blood pressure.

In hemodynamic studies in patients with essential hypertension, blood pressure reduction was accompanied by a reduction in peripheral arterial resistance with little or no change in cardiac output and in heart rate. In a study in nine hypertensive patients, following administration of lisinopril, there was an increase in mean renal blood flow that was not significant. Data from several small studies are inconsistent with respect to the effect of lisinopril on glomerular filtration rate in hypertensive patients with normal renal function, but suggest that changes, if any, are not large.

In patients with renovascular hypertension lisinopril has been shown to be well tolerated and effective in controlling blood pressure (see PRECAUTIONS).

Hydrochlorothiazide

The mechanism of the antihypertensive effect of thiazides is unknown. Thiazides do not usually affect normal blood pressure.

Hydrochlorothiazide is a diuretic and antihypertensive. It affects the distal renal tubular mechanism of electrolyte reabsorption. Hydrochlorothiazide increases excretion of sodium and chloride in approximately equivalent amounts. Natriuresis may be accompanied by some loss of potassium and bicarbonate.

After oral use diuresis begins within two hours, peaks in about four hours and lasts about 6 to 12 hours.

Hydrochlorothiazide is not metabolized but is eliminated rapidly by the kidney. When plasma levels have been followed for at least 24 hours, the plasma half-life has been observed to vary between 5.6 and 14.8 hours. At least 61 percent of the oral dose is eliminated unchanged within 24 hours. Hydrochlorothiazide crosses the placental but not the blood-brain barrier.

Continued on next page

Information on the Merck & Co., Inc., products listed on these pages is from the prescribing information in use October 1, 2004. For information, please call 1-800-NSC-MERCK [1-800-672-6372].

Prinzide—Cont.

INDICATIONS AND USAGE

PRINZIDE is indicated for the treatment of hypertension.

These fixed-dose combinations are not indicated for initial therapy (see DOSAGE AND ADMINISTRATION).

In using PRINZIDE, consideration should be given to the fact that an angiotensin converting enzyme inhibitor, captopril, has caused agranulocytosis, particularly in patients with renal impairment or collagen vascular disease, and that available data are insufficient to show that lisinopril does not have a similar risk. (See WARNINGS.)

In considering use of PRINZIDE, it should be noted that black patients receiving ACE inhibitors have been reported to have a higher incidence of angioedema compared to nonblacks. (See WARNINGS, *Angioedema.*)

CONTRAINDICATIONS

PRINZIDE is contraindicated in patients who are hypersensitive to any component of this product and in patients with a history of angioedema related to previous treatment with an angiotensin converting enzyme inhibitor and in patients with hereditary or idiopathic angioedema. Because of the hydrochlorothiazide component, this product is contraindicated in patients with anuria or hypersensitivity to other sulfonamide-derived drugs.

WARNINGS

General

Lisinopril

Anaphylactoid and Possibly Related Reactions:
Presumably because angiotensin-converting enzyme inhibitors affect the metabolism of eicosanoids and polypeptides, including endogenous bradykinin, patients receiving ACE inhibitors (including PRINZIDE) may be subject to a variety of adverse reactions, some of them serious.

Head and Neck Angioedema: Angioedema of the face, extremities, lips, tongue, glottis and/or larynx has been reported rarely in patients treated with angiotensin converting enzyme inhibitors, including lisinopril. This may occur at any time during treatment. In such cases PRINZIDE should be promptly discontinued and appropriate therapy and monitoring should be provided until complete and sustained resolution of signs and symptoms has occurred. In instances where swelling has been confined to the face and lips the condition has generally resolved without treatment, although antihistamines have been useful in relieving symptoms. Angioedema associated with laryngeal edema may be fatal. **Where there is involvement of the tongue, glottis or larynx, likely to cause airway obstruction, subcutaneous epinephrine solution 1:1000 (0.3 mL to 0.5 mL) and/or measures necessary to ensure a patent airway, should be promptly provided.** (See ADVERSE REACTIONS.)

Patients with a history of angioedema unrelated to ACE inhibitor therapy may be at increased risk of angioedema while receiving an ACE inhibitor (see also INDICATIONS AND USAGE and CONTRAINDICATIONS).

Intestinal Angioedema: Intestinal angioedema has been reported in patients treated with ACE inhibitors. These patients presented with abdominal pain (with or without nausea or vomiting); in some cases there was no prior history of facial angioedema and C-1 esterase levels were normal. The angioedema was diagnosed by procedures including abdominal CT scan or ultrasound, or at surgery, and symptoms resolved after stopping the ACE inhibitor. Intestinal angioedema should be included in the differential diagnosis of patients on ACE inhibitors presenting with abdominal pain.

Anaphylactoid reactions during desensitization: Two patients undergoing desensitizing treatment with hymenoptera venom while receiving ACE inhibitors sustained life-threatening anaphylactoid reactions. In the same patients, these reactions were avoided when ACE inhibitors were temporarily withheld, but they reappeared upon inadvertent rechallenge.

Anaphylactoid reactions during membrane exposure: Anaphylactoid reactions have been reported in patients dialyzed with high-flux membranes and treated concomitantly with an ACE inhibitor. Anaphylactoid reactions have also been reported in patients undergoing low-density lipoprotein apheresis with dextran sulfate absorption.

Hypotension and Related Effects:

Excessive hypotension was rarely seen in uncomplicated hypertensive patients but is a possible consequence of lisinopril use in salt/volume-depleted persons, such as those treated vigorously with diuretics or patients on dialysis. (See PRECAUTIONS, *Drug Interactions* and ADVERSE REACTIONS.)

Syncope has been reported in 0.8 percent of patients receiving PRINZIDE. In patients with hypertension receiving lisinopril alone, the incidence of syncope was 0.1 percent. The overall incidence of syncope may be reduced by proper titration of the individual components. (See PRECAUTIONS, *Drug Interactions,* ADVERSE REACTIONS and DOSAGE AND ADMINISTRATION.)

In patients with severe congestive heart failure, with or without associated renal insufficiency, excessive hypotension has been observed and may be associated with oliguria and/or progressive azotemia, and rarely with acute renal failure and/or death. Because of the potential fall in blood pressure in these patients, therapy should be started under very close medical supervision. Such patients should be followed closely for the first two weeks of treatment and whenever the dose of lisinopril and/or diuretic is increased. Similar considerations apply to patients with ischemic heart or cerebrovascular disease in whom an excessive fall in blood pressure could result in a myocardial infarction or cerebrovascular accident.

If hypotension occurs, the patient should be placed in supine position and, if necessary, receive an intravenous infusion of normal saline. A transient hypotensive response is not a contraindication to further doses which usually can be given without difficulty once the blood pressure has increased after volume expansion.

Neutropenia/Agranulocytosis:

Another angiotensin converting enzyme inhibitor, captopril, has been shown to cause agranulocytosis and bone marrow depression, rarely in uncomplicated patients but more frequently in patients with renal impairment, especially if they also have a collagen vascular disease. Available data from clinical trials of lisinopril are insufficient to show that lisinopril does not cause agranulocytosis at similar rates. Marketing experience has revealed rare cases of neutropenia and bone marrow depression in which a causal relationship to lisinopril cannot be excluded. Periodic monitoring of white blood cell counts in patients with collagen vascular disease and renal disease should be considered.

Hepatic Failure:

Rarely, ACE inhibitors have been associated with a syndrome that starts with cholestatic jaundice and progresses to fulminant hepatic necrosis, and (sometimes) death. The mechanism of this syndrome is not understood. Patients receiving ACE inhibitors who develop jaundice or marked elevations of hepatic enzymes should discontinue the ACE inhibitor and receive appropriate medical follow-up.

Hydrochlorothiazide

Thiazides should be used with caution in severe renal disease. In patients with renal disease, thiazides may precipitate azotemia. Cumulative effects of the drug may develop in patients with impaired renal function.

Thiazides should be used with caution in patients with impaired hepatic function or progressive liver disease, since minor alterations of fluid and electrolyte balance may precipitate hepatic coma.

Sensitivity reactions may occur in patients with or without a history of allergy or bronchial asthma.

The possibility of exacerbation or activation of systemic lupus erythematosus has been reported.

Lithium generally should not be given with thiazides (see PRECAUTIONS, *Drug Interactions, Lisinopril* and *Hydrochlorothiazide).*

Pregnancy

Lisinopril-Hydrochlorothiazide

Teratogenicity studies were conducted in mice and rats with up to 90 mg/kg/day of lisinopril in combination with 10 mg/kg/day of hydrochlorothiazide. This dose of lisinopril is 5 times (in mice) and 10 times (in rats) the maximum recommended human daily dose (MRHDD) when compared on a body surface area basis (mg/m^2); the dose of hydrochlorothiazide is 0.9 times (in mice) and 1.8 times (in rats) the MRHDD. Maternal or fetotoxic effects were not seen in mice with the combination. In rats decreased maternal weight gain and decreased fetal weight occurred down to 3/10 mg/kg/day (the lowest dose tested). Associated with the decreased fetal weight was a delay in fetal ossification. The decreased fetal weight and delay in fetal ossification were not seen in saline-supplemented animals given 90/10 mg/kg/day.

When used in pregnancy during the second and third trimesters, ACE inhibitors can cause injury and even death to the developing fetus. When pregnancy is detected, PRINZIDE should be discontinued as soon as possible. (See *Lisinopril, Fetal/Neonatal Morbidity and Mortality,* below.)

Lisinopril

Fetal/Neonatal Morbidity and Mortality: ACE inhibitors can cause fetal and neonatal morbidity and death when administered to pregnant women. Several dozen cases have been reported in the world literature. When pregnancy is detected, ACE inhibitors should be discontinued as soon as possible.

The use of ACE inhibitors during the second and third trimesters of pregnancy has been associated with fetal and neonatal injury, including hypotension, neonatal skull hypoplasia, anuria, reversible or irreversible renal failure, and death. Oligohydramnios has also been reported, presumably resulting from decreased fetal renal function; oligohydramnios in this setting has been associated with fetal limb contractures, craniofacial deformation, and hypoplastic lung development. Prematurity, intrauterine growth retardation, and patent ductus arteriosus have also been reported, although it is not clear whether these occurrences were due to the ACE-inhibitor exposure.

These adverse effects do not appear to have resulted from intrauterine ACE-inhibitor exposure that has been limited to the first trimester. Mothers whose embryos and fetuses are exposed to ACE inhibitors only during the first trimester should be so informed. Nonetheless, when patients become pregnant, physicians should make every effort to discontinue the use of PRINZIDE as soon as possible.

Rarely (probably less often than once in every thousand pregnancies), no alternative to ACE inhibitors will be found. In these rare cases, the mothers should be apprised of the potential hazards to their fetuses, and serial ultrasound examinations should be performed to assess the intraamniotic environment.

If oligohydramnios is observed, PRINZIDE should be discontinued unless it is considered lifesaving for the mother. Contraction stress testing (CST), a non-stress test (NST), or biophysical profiling (BPP) may be appropriate, depending upon the week of pregnancy. Patients and physicians should be aware, however, that oligohydramnios may not appear until after the fetus has sustained irreversible injury.

Infants with histories of *in utero* exposure to ACE inhibitors should be closely observed for hypotension, oliguria, and hyperkalemia. If oliguria occurs, attention should be directed toward support of blood pressure and renal perfusion. Exchange transfusion or dialysis may be required as means of reversing hypotension and/or substituting for disordered renal function. Lisinopril, which crosses the placenta, has been removed from neonatal circulation by peritoneal dialysis with some clinical benefit, and theoretically may be removed by exchange transfusion, although there is no experience with the latter procedure.

No teratogenic effects of lisinopril were seen in studies of pregnant mice, rats, and rabbits. On a body surface area basis, the doses used were up to 55 times, 33 times, and 0.15 times, respectively, the MRHDD.

Hydrochlorothiazide

Studies in which hydrochlorothiazide was orally administered to pregnant mice and rats during their respective periods of major organogenesis at doses up to 3000 and 1000 mg/kg/day, respectively, provided no evidence of harm to the fetus. These doses are more than 150 times the MRHDD on a body surface area basis. Thiazides cross the placental barrier and appear in cord blood. There is a risk of fetal or neonatal jaundice, thrombocytopenia and possibly other adverse reactions that have occurred in adults.

PRECAUTIONS

General

Lisinopril

Aortic Stenosis/Hypertrophic Cardiomyopathy: As with all vasodilators, lisinopril should be given with caution to patients with obstruction in the outflow tract of the left ventricle.

Impaired Renal Function: As a consequence of inhibiting the renin-angiotensin-aldosterone system, changes in renal function may be anticipated in susceptible individuals. In patients with severe congestive heart failure whose renal function may depend on the activity of the renin-angiotensin-aldosterone system, treatment with angiotensin converting enzyme inhibitors, including lisinopril, may be associated with oliguria and/or progressive azotemia and rarely with acute renal failure and/or death.

In hypertensive patients with unilateral or bilateral renal artery stenosis, increases in blood urea nitrogen and serum creatinine may occur. Experience with another angiotensin converting enzyme inhibitor suggests that these increases are usually reversible upon discontinuation of lisinopril and/ or diuretic therapy. In such patients renal function should be monitored during the first few weeks of therapy.

Some hypertensive patients with no apparent pre-existing renal vascular disease have developed increases in blood urea and serum creatinine, usually minor and transient, especially when lisinopril has been given concomitantly with a diuretic. This is more likely to occur in patients with pre-existing renal impairment. Dosage reduction of lisinopril and/or discontinuation of the diuretic may be required.

Evaluation of the hypertensive patient should always include assessment of renal function. (See DOSAGE AND ADMINISTRATION.)

Hyperkalemia: In clinical trials hyperkalemia (serum potassium greater than 5.7 mEq/L) occurred in approximately 1.4 percent of hypertensive patients treated with lisinopril plus hydrochlorothiazide. In most cases these were isolated values which resolved despite continued therapy. Hyperkalemia was not a cause of discontinuation of therapy. Risk factors for the development of hyperkalemia include renal insufficiency, diabetes mellitus, and the concomitant use of potassium-sparing diuretics, potassium supplements and/or potassium-containing salt substitutes, which should be used cautiously if at all with PRINZIDE. (See *Drug Interactions.*)

Cough: Presumably due to the inhibition of the degradation of endogenous bradykinin, persistent nonproductive cough has been reported with all ACE inhibitors, always resolving after discontinuation of therapy. ACE inhibitor-induced cough should be considered in the differential diagnosis of cough.

Surgery/Anesthesia: In patients undergoing major surgery or during anesthesia with agents that produce hypotension, lisinopril may block angiotensin II formation secondary to compensatory renin release. If hypotension occurs and is considered to be due to this mechanism, it can be corrected by volume expansion.

Hydrochlorothiazide

Periodic determination of serum electrolytes to detect possible electrolyte imbalance should be performed at appropriate intervals.

All patients receiving thiazide therapy should be observed for clinical signs of fluid or electrolyte imbalance: namely, hyponatremia, hypochloremic alkalosis, and hypokalemia. Serum and urine electrolyte determinations are particularly important when the patient is vomiting excessively or receiving parenteral fluids. Warning signs or symptoms of fluid and electrolyte imbalance, irrespective of cause, in-

clude dryness of mouth, thirst, weakness, lethargy, drowsiness, restlessness, confusion, seizures, muscle pains or cramps, muscular fatigue, hypotension, oliguria, tachycardia, and gastrointestinal disturbances such as nausea and vomiting.
Hypokalemia may develop, especially with brisk diuresis, when severe cirrhosis is present, or after prolonged therapy. Interference with adequate oral electrolyte intake will also contribute to hypokalemia. Hypokalemia may cause cardiac arrhythmia and may also sensitize or exaggerate the response of the heart to the toxic effects of digitalis (e.g., increased ventricular irritability). Because lisinopril reduces the production of aldosterone, concomitant therapy with lisinopril attenuates the diuretic-induced potassium loss (see *Drug Interactions, Agents Increasing Serum Potassium*).
Although any chloride deficit is generally mild and usually does not require specific treatment, except under extraordinary circumstances (as in liver disease or renal disease), chloride replacement may be required in the treatment of metabolic alkalosis.
Dilutional hyponatremia may occur in edematous patients in hot weather; appropriate therapy is water restriction, rather than administration of salt except in rare instances when the hyponatremia is life-threatening. In actual salt depletion, appropriate replacement is the therapy of choice.
Hyperuricemia may occur or frank gout may be precipitated in certain patients receiving thiazide therapy.
In diabetic patients dosage adjustments of insulin or oral hypoglycemic agents may be required. Hyperglycemia may occur with thiazide diuretics. Thus latent diabetes mellitus may become manifest during thiazide therapy.
The antihypertensive effects of the drug may be enhanced in the postsympathectomy patient.
If progressive renal impairment becomes evident consider withholding or discontinuing diuretic therapy.
Thiazides have been shown to increase the urinary excretion of magnesium; this may result in hypomagnesemia.
Thiazides may decrease urinary calcium excretion. Thiazides may cause intermittent and slight elevation of serum calcium in the absence of known disorders of calcium metabolism. Marked hypercalcemia may be evidence of hidden hyperparathyroidism. Thiazides should be discontinued before carrying out tests for parathyroid function.
Increases in cholesterol and triglyceride levels may be associated with thiazide diuretic therapy.

Information for Patients

Angioedema: Angioedema, including laryngeal edema, may occur at any time during treatment with angiotensin converting enzyme inhibitors, including lisinopril. Patients should be so advised and told to report immediately any signs or symptoms suggesting angioedema (swelling of face, extremities, eyes, lips, tongue, difficulty in swallowing or breathing) and to take no more drug until they have consulted with the prescribing physician.
Symptomatic Hypotension: Patients should be cautioned to report lightheadedness especially during the first few days of therapy. If actual syncope occurs, the patients should be told to discontinue the drug until they have consulted with the prescribing physician.
All patients should be cautioned that excessive perspiration and dehydration may lead to an excessive fall in blood pressure because of reduction in fluid volume. Other causes of volume depletion such as vomiting or diarrhea may also lead to a fall in blood pressure; patients should be advised to consult with their physician.
Hyperkalemia: Patients should be told not to use salt substitutes containing potassium without consulting their physician.
Neutropenia: Patients should be told to report promptly any indication of infection (e.g., sore throat, fever) which may be a sign of neutropenia.
Pregnancy: Female patients of childbearing age should be told about the consequences of second- and third-trimester exposure to ACE inhibitors, and they should also be told that these consequences do not appear to have resulted from intrauterine ACE-inhibitor exposure that has been limited to the first trimester. These patients should be asked to report pregnancies to their physicians as soon as possible.
NOTE: As with many other drugs, certain advice to patients being treated with PRINZIDE is warranted. This information is intended to aid in the safe and effective use of this medication. It is not a disclosure of all possible adverse or intended effects.

Drug Interactions

Lisinopril

Hypotension —Patients on Diuretic Therapy: Patients on diuretics, and especially those in whom diuretic therapy was recently instituted, may occasionally experience an excessive reduction of blood pressure after initiation of therapy with lisinopril. The possibility of hypotensive effects with lisinopril can be minimized by either discontinuing the diuretic or increasing the salt intake prior to initiation of treatment with lisinopril. If it is necessary to continue the diuretic, initiate therapy with lisinopril at a dose of 5 mg daily, and provide close medical supervision after the initial dose for at least two hours and until blood pressure has stabilized for at least an additional hour. (See WARNINGS and DOSAGE AND ADMINISTRATION.) When a diuretic is added to the therapy of a patient receiving lisinopril, an additional antihypertensive effect is usually observed. (See DOSAGE AND ADMINISTRATION.)
Non-steroidal Anti-inflammatory Agents: In some patients with compromised renal function who are being treated with non-steroidal anti-inflammatory drugs, the co-administration of lisinopril may result in a further deterioration of renal function. These effects are usually reversible.
Reports suggest that NSAIDs may diminish the antihypertensive effect of ACE-inhibitors, including lisinopril. The interaction should be given consideration in patients taking NSAIDs concomitantly with ACE-inhibitors.
Other Agents: Lisinopril has been used concomitantly with nitrates and/or digoxin without evidence of clinically significant adverse interactions. No meaningful clinically important pharmacokinetic interactions occurred when lisinopril was used concomitantly with propranolol, digoxin, or hydrochlorothiazide. The presence of food in the stomach does not alter the bioavailability of lisinopril.
Agents Increasing Serum Potassium: Lisinopril attenuates potassium loss caused by thiazide-type diuretics. Use of lisinopril with potassium-sparing diuretics (e.g., spironolactone, triamterene, or amiloride), potassium supplements, or potassium-containing salt substitutes may lead to significant increases in serum potassium. Therefore, if concomitant use of these agents is indicated, because of demonstrated hypokalemia, they should be used with caution and with frequent monitoring of serum potassium.
Lithium: Lithium toxicity has been reported in patients receiving lithium concomitantly with drugs which cause elimination of sodium, including ACE inhibitors. Lithium toxicity was usually reversible upon discontinuation of lithium and the ACE inhibitor. It is recommended that serum lithium levels be monitored frequently if lisinopril is administered concomitantly with lithium.

Hydrochlorothiazide

When administered concurrently the following drugs may interact with thiazide diuretics.
Alcohol, barbiturates, or narcotics —potentiation of orthostatic hypotension may occur.
Antidiabetic drugs (oral agents and insulin)—dosage adjustment of the antidiabetic drug may be required.
Other antihypertensive drugs —additive effect or potentiation.
Cholestyramine and colestipol resins —Absorption of hydrochlorothiazide is impaired in the presence of anionic exchange resins. Single doses of either cholestyramine or colestipol resins bind the hydrochlorothiazide and reduce its absorption from the gastrointestinal tract by up to 85 and 43 percent, respectively.
Corticosteroids, ACTH —intensified electrolyte depletion, particularly hypokalemia.
Pressor amines (e.g., norepinephrine) —possible decreased response to pressor amines but not sufficient to preclude their use.
Skeletal muscle relaxants, nondepolarizing (e.g., tubocurarine) —possible increased responsiveness to the muscle relaxant.
Lithium —should not generally be given with diuretics. Diuretic agents reduce the renal clearance of lithium and add a high risk of lithium toxicity. Refer to the package insert for lithium preparations before use of such preparations with PRINZIDE.
Non-steroidal Anti-inflammatory Drugs —In some patients, the administration of a non-steroidal anti-inflammatory agent can reduce the diuretic, natriuretic, and antihypertensive effects of loop, potassium-sparing and thiazide diuretics. Therefore, when PRINZIDE and non-steroidal anti-inflammatory agents are used concomitantly, the patient should be observed closely to determine if the desired effect of PRINZIDE is obtained.

Carcinogenesis, Mutagenesis, Impairment of Fertility

Lisinopril-Hydrochlorothiazide

Lisinopril in combination with hydrochlorothiazide was not mutagenic in a microbial mutagen test using *Salmonella typhimurium* (Ames test) or *Escherichia coli* with or without metabolic activation or in a forward mutation assay using Chinese hamster lung cells. Lisinopril-hydrochlorothiazide did not produce DNA single strand breaks in an *in vitro* alkaline elution rat hepatocyte assay. In addition, it did not produce increases in chromosomal aberrations in an *in vitro* test in Chinese hamster ovary cells or in an *in vivo* study in mouse bone marrow.

Lisinopril

There was no evidence of a tumorigenic effect when lisinopril was administered orally for 105 weeks to male and female rats at doses up to 90 mg/kg/day or for 92 weeks to male and female mice at doses up to 135 mg/kg/day. These doses are 10 times and 7 times, respectively, the maximum recommended human daily dose (MRHDD) when compared on a body surface area basis.
Lisinopril was not mutagenic in the Ames microbial mutagen test with or without metabolic activation. It was also negative in a forward mutation assay using Chinese hamster lung cells. Lisinopril did not produce single strand DNA breaks in an *in vitro* alkaline elution rat hepatocyte assay. In addition, lisinopril did not produce increases in chromosomal aberrations in an *in vitro* test in Chinese hamster ovary cells or in an *in vivo* study in mouse bone marrow.
There were no adverse effects on reproductive performance in male and female rats treated with up to 300 mg/kg/day of lisinopril (33 times the MRHDD when compared on a body surface area basis).

Hydrochlorothiazide

Two-year feeding studies in mice and rats conducted under the auspices of the National Toxicology Program (NTP) uncovered no evidence of a carcinogenic potential of hydrochlorothiazide in female mice at doses of up to approximately 600 mg/kg/day (53 times the MRHDD when compared on a body surface area basis) or in male and female rats at doses of up to approximately 100 mg/kg/day (18 times the MRHDD when compared on a body surface area basis). The NTP, however, found equivocal evidence for hepatocarcinogenicity in male mice.
Hydrochlorothiazide was not genotoxic *in vitro* in the Ames mutagenicity assay of *Salmonella typhimurium* strains TA 98, TA 100, TA 1535, TA 1537, and TA 1538 and in the Chinese Hamster Ovary (CHO) test for chromosomal aberrations, or *in vivo* in assays using mouse germinal cell chromosomes, Chinese hamster bone marrow chromosomes, and the *Drosophila* sex-linked recessive lethal trait gene. Positive test results were obtained only in the *in vitro* CHO Sister Chromatid Exchange (clastogenicity) and in the Mouse Lymphoma Cell (mutagenicity) assays, using concentrations of hydrochlorothiazide from 43 to 1300 μg/mL, and in the *Aspergillus nidulans* non-disjunction assay at an unspecified concentration.
Hydrochlorothiazide had no adverse effects on the fertility of mice and rats of either sex in studies wherein these species were exposed, via their diet, to doses of up to 100 and 4 mg/kg, respectively, prior to conception and throughout gestation. In mice and rats these doses are 9 times and 0.7 times, respectively, the MRHDD when compared on a body surface area basis.

Pregnancy

Pregnancy Categories C (first trimester) *and D* (second and third trimesters). See WARNINGS, *Pregnancy, Lisinopril, Fetal/Neonatal Morbidity and Mortality.*

Nursing Mothers

It is not known whether lisinopril is secreted in human milk. However, milk of lactating rats contains radioactivity following administration of ^{14}C lisinopril. In another study, lisinopril was present in rat milk at levels similar to plasma levels in the dams. Thiazides do appear in human milk. Because of the potential for serious reactions in nursing infants from ACE inhibitors and hydrochlorothiazide, a decision should be made whether to discontinue nursing or to discontinue PRINZIDE, taking into account the importance of the drug to the mother.

Pediatric Use

Safety and effectiveness in pediatric patients have not been established.

Geriatric Use

Clinical studies of PRINZIDE did not include sufficient numbers of subjects aged 65 and over to determine whether they respond differently from younger subjects. Other reported clinical experience has not identified differences in responses between the elderly and younger patients. In general, dose selection for an elderly patient should be cautious, usually starting at the low end of the dosing range, reflecting the greater frequency of decreased hepatic, renal, or cardiac function, and of concomitant disease or other drug therapy. In a multiple dose pharmacokinetic study in elderly versus young hypertensive patients using the lisinopril/hydrochlorothiazide combination, area under the plasma concentration time curve (AUC) increased approximately 120% for lisinopril and approximately 80% for hydrochlorothiazide in older patients.
This drug is known to be substantially excreted by the kidney, and the risk of toxic reactions to this drug may be greater in patients with impaired renal function. Because elderly patients are more likely to have decreased renal function, care should be taken in dose selection. Evaluation of the hypertensive patient should always include assessment of renal function. (See DOSAGE AND ADMINISTRATION.)

ADVERSE REACTIONS

PRINZIDE has been evaluated for safety in 930 patients, including 100 patients treated for 50 weeks or more.
In clinical trials with PRINZIDE no adverse experiences peculiar to this combination drug have been observed. Adverse experiences that have occurred have been limited to those that have been previously reported with lisinopril or hydrochlorothiazide.
The most frequent clinical adverse experiences in controlled trials (including open label extensions) with any combination of lisinopril and hydrochlorothiazide were: dizziness (7.5 percent), headache (5.2 percent), cough (3.9 percent), fatigue (3.7 percent) and orthostatic effects (3.2 percent), all of which were more common than in placebo-treated patients. Generally, adverse experiences were mild and transient in nature; but see WARNINGS regarding angioedema and excessive hypotension or syncope. Discontinuation of therapy due to adverse effects was required in 4.4 percent of patients, principally because of dizziness, cough, fatigue and muscle cramps.
Adverse experiences occurring in greater than one percent of patients treated with lisinopril plus hydrochlorothiazide in controlled clinical trials are shown below.
[See table at top of next page]

Continued on next page

Information on the Merck & Co., Inc., products listed on these pages is from the prescribing information in use October 1, 2004. For information, please call 1-800-NSC-MERCK [1-800-672-6372].

Prinzide—Cont.

Clinical adverse experiences occurring in 0.3 to 1.0 percent of patients in controlled trials included: *Body as a Whole:* Chest pain, abdominal pain, syncope, chest discomfort, fever, trauma, virus infection. *Cardiovascular:* Palpitation, orthostatic hypotension. *Digestive:* Gastrointestinal cramps, dry mouth, constipation, heartburn. *Musculoskeletal:* Back pain, shoulder pain, knee pain, back strain, myalgia, foot pain. *Nervous/Psychiatric:* Decreased libido, vertigo, depression, somnolence. *Respiratory:* Common cold, nasal congestion, influenza, bronchitis, pharyngeal pain, dyspnea, pulmonary congestion, chronic sinusitis, allergic rhinitis, pharyngeal discomfort. *Skin:* Flushing, pruritus, skin inflammation, diaphoresis. *Special Senses:* Blurred vision, tinnitus, otalgia. *Urogenital:* Urinary tract infection.

Angioedema: Angioedema has been reported in patients receiving PRINZIDE, with an incidence higher in black than in non-black patients. Angioedema associated with laryngeal edema may be fatal. If angioedema of the face, extremities, lips, tongue, glottis and/or larynx occurs, treatment with PRINZIDE should be discontinued and appropriate therapy instituted immediately. In rare cases, intestinal angioedema has been reported with angiotensin converting enzyme inhibitors including lisinopril. (See WARNINGS.)

Hypotension: In clinical trials, adverse effects relating to hypotension occurred as follows: hypotension (1.4), orthostatic hypotension (0.5), other orthostatic effects (3.2). In addition syncope occurred in 0.8 percent of patients. (See WARNINGS.)

Cough: See PRECAUTIONS, *Cough.*

Clinical Laboratory Test Findings

Serum Electrolytes: See PRECAUTIONS.

Creatinine, Blood Urea Nitrogen: Minor reversible increases in blood urea nitrogen and serum creatinine were observed in patients with essential hypertension treated with PRINZIDE. More marked increases have also been reported and were more likely to occur in patients with renal artery stenosis. (See PRECAUTIONS.)

Serum Uric Acid, Glucose, Magnesium, Cholesterol, Triglycerides and Calcium: See PRECAUTIONS.

Hemoglobin and Hematocrit: Small decreases in hemoglobin and hematocrit (mean decreases of approximately 0.5 g percent and 1.5 vol percent, respectively) occurred frequently in hypertensive patients treated with PRINZIDE but were rarely of clinical importance unless another cause of anemia coexisted. In clinical trials, 0.4 percent of patients discontinued therapy due to anemia.

Liver Function Tests: Rarely, elevations of liver enzymes and/or serum bilirubin have occurred (see WARNINGS, *Hepatic Failure*).

Other adverse reactions that have been reported with the individual components are listed below:

Lisinopril —In clinical trials adverse reactions which occurred with lisinopril were also seen with PRINZIDE. In addition, and since lisinopril has been marketed, the following adverse reactions have been reported with lisinopril and should be considered potential adverse reactions for PRINZIDE: *Body as a Whole:* Anaphylactoid reactions (see WARNINGS, *Anaphylactoid and Possibly Related Reactions),* malaise, edema, facial edema, pain, pelvic pain, flank pain, chills; *Cardiovascular:* Cardiac arrest, myocardial infarction or cerebrovascular accident, possibly secondary to excessive hypotension in high risk patients (see WARNINGS, *Hypotension),* pulmonary embolism and infarction, worsening of heart failure, arrhythmias (including tachycardia, ventricular tachycardia, atrial tachycardia, atrial fibrillation, bradycardia, and premature ventricular contractions), angina pectoris, transient ischemic attacks, paroxysmal nocturnal dyspnea, decreased blood pressure, peripheral edema, vasculitis; *Digestive:* Pancreatitis, hepatitis (hepatocellular or cholestatic jaundice) (see WARNINGS, *Hepatic Failure*), gastritis, anorexia, flatulence, increased salivation; *Endocrine:* Diabetes mellitus; *Hematologic:* Rare cases of neutropenia, thrombocytopenia, and bone marrow depression have been reported. Hemolytic anemia has been reported; a causal relationship to lisinopril cannot be excluded; *Metabolic:* Gout, weight loss, dehydration, fluid overload, weight gain; *Musculoskeletal:* Arthritis, arthralgia, neck pain, hip pain, joint pain, leg pain, arm pain, lumbago; *Nervous System/Psychiatric:* Ataxia, memory impairment, tremor, insomnia, stroke, nervousness, confusion, peripheral neuropathy (e.g., paresthesia, dysesthesia), spasm, hypersomnia, irritability; *Respiratory:* Malignant lung neoplasms, hemoptysis, pulmonary edema, pulmonary infiltrates, eosinophilic pneumonitis, bronchospasm, asthma, pleural effusion, pneumonia, wheezing, orthopnea, painful respiration, epistaxis, laryngitis, sinusitis, pharyngitis, rhinitis, rhinorrhea, chest sound abnormalities; *Skin:* Urticaria, alopecia, herpes zoster, photosensitivity, skin lesions, skin infections, pemphigus, erythema. Other severe skin reactions (including toxic epidermal necrolysis and Stevens-Johnson syndrome) have been reported rarely; causal relationship has not been established; *Speical Senses:* Visual loss, diplopia, photophobia, taste disturbances; *Urogenital:* Acute renal failure, oliguria, anuria, uremia, progressive azotemia, renal dysfunction (see PRECAUTIONS and DOSAGE AND ADMINISTRATION), pyelonephritis, dysuria, breast pain.

Miscellaneous: A symptom complex has been reported which may include a positive ANA, an elevated erythrocyte sedimentation rate, arthralgia/arthritis, myalgia, fever, vasculitis, leukocytosis, eosinophilia, photosensitivity, rash, and other dermatological manifestations.

	Percent of Patients in Controlled Studies	
	Lisinopril-Hydrochlorothiazide (n=930) Incidence (discontinuation)	Placebo (n=207) Incidence
Dizziness	7.5 (0.8)	1.9
Headache	5.2 (0.3)	1.9
Cough	3.9 (0.6)	1.0
Fatigue	3.7 (0.4)	1.0
Orthostatic Effects	3.2 (0.1)	1.0
Diarrhea	2.5 (0.2)	2.4
Nausea	2.2 (0.1)	2.4
Upper Respiratory Infection	2.2 (0.0)	0.0
Muscle Cramps	2.0 (0.4)	0.5
Asthenia	1.8 (0.2)	1.0
Paresthesia	1.5 (0.1)	0.0
Hypotension	1.4 (0.3)	0.5
Vomiting	1.4 (0.1)	0.5
Dyspepsia	1.3 (0.0)	0.0
Rash	1.2 (0.1)	0.5
Impotence	1.2 (0.3)	0.0

Fetal/Neonatal Morbidity and Mortality: See WARNINGS, *Pregnancy, Lisinopril, Fetal/Neonatal Morbidity and Mortality.*

Hydrochlorothiazide —Body as a Whole: Weakness; *Digestive:* Anorexia, gastric irritation, cramping, jaundice (intrahepatic cholestatic jaundice), pancreatitis, sialadenitis, constipation; *Hematologic:* Leukopenia, agranulocytosis, thrombocytopenia, aplastic anemia, hemolytic anemia; *Musculoskeletal:* Muscle spasm; *Nervous System/Psychiatric:* Restlessness; *Renal:* Renal failure, renal dysfunction, interstitial nephritis (see WARNINGS); *Skin:* Erythema multiforme including Stevens-Johnson syndrome, exfoliative dermatitis including toxic epidermal necrolysis, alopecia; *Special Senses:* Xanthopsia; *Hypersensitivity:* Purpura, photosensitivity, urticaria, necrotizing angiitis (vasculitis and cutaneous vasculitis), respiratory distress including pneumonitis and pulmonary edema, anaphylactic reactions.

OVERDOSAGE

No specific information is available on the treatment of overdosage with PRINZIDE. Treatment is symptomatic and supportive. Therapy with PRINZIDE should be discontinued and the patient observed closely. Suggested measures include induction of emesis and/or gastric lavage, and correction of dehydration, electrolyte imbalance and hypotension by established procedures.

Lisinopril

Following a single oral dose of 20 mg/kg, no lethality occurred in rats and death occurred in one of 20 mice receiving the same dose. The most likely manifestation of overdosage would be hypotension, for which the usual treatment would be intravenous infusion of normal saline solution.

Lisinopril can be removed by hemodialysis. (See WARNINGS, *Anaphylactoid reactions during membrane exposure.*)

Hydrochlorothiazide

Oral administration of a single oral dose of 10 mg/kg to mice and rats was not lethal. The most common signs and symptoms observed are those caused by electrolyte depletion (hypokalemia, hypochloremia, hyponatremia) and dehydration resulting from excessive diuresis. If digitalis has also been administered, hypokalemia may accentuate cardiac arrhythmias.

DOSAGE AND ADMINISTRATION

Lisinopril is an effective treatment of hypertension in once-daily doses of 10–80 mg, while hydrochlorothiazide is effective in doses of 12.5–50 mg. In clinical trials of lisinopril/hydrochlorothiazide combination therapy using lisinopril doses of 10–80 mg and hydrochlorothiazide doses of 6.25–50 mg, the antihypertensive response rates generally increased with increasing dose of either component.

The side effects (see WARNINGS) of lisinopril are generally rare and apparently independent of dose; those of hydrochlorothiazide are a mixture of dose-dependent phenomena (primarily hypokalemia) and dose-independent phenomena (e.g., pancreatitis), the former much more common than the latter. Therapy with any combination of lisinopril and hydrochlorothiazide will be associated with both sets of dose-independent side effects, but addition of lisinopril in clinical trials blunted the hypokalemia normally seen with diuretics.

To minimize dose-independent side effects, it is usually appropriate to begin combination therapy only after a patient has failed to achieve the desired effect with monotherapy.

Dose Titration Guided by Clinical Effect

A patient whose blood pressure is not adequately controlled with either lisinopril or hydrochlorothiazide monotherapy may be switched to PRINZIDE 10/12.5 or PRINZIDE 20/12.5. Further increases of either or both components could depend on clinical response. The hydrochlorothiazide dose should generally not be increased until 2–3 weeks have elapsed. Patients whose blood pressures are adequately controlled with 25 mg of daily hydrochlorothiazide, but who experience significant potassium loss with this regimen, may achieve similar or greater blood pressure control with less potassium loss if they are switched to PRINZIDE 10/12.5. Dosage higher than lisinopril 80 mg and hydrochlorothiazide 50 mg should not be used.

Replacement Therapy

The combination may be substituted for the titrated individual components.

Use in Renal Impairment

The usual regimens of therapy with PRINZIDE need not be adjusted as long as the patient's creatinine clearance is >30 mL /min/1.73 m^2 (serum creatinine approximately ≤3 mg/dL or 265 μmol/L. In patients with more severe renal impairment, loop diuretics are preferred to thiazides, so PRINZIDE is not recommended (see WARNINGS, *Anaphylactoid reactions during membrane exposure*).

HOW SUPPLIED

No. 3616—Tablets PRINZIDE 10-12.5 are blue hexagon-shaped tablets, coded MSD 145 on one side and PRINZIDE on the other. Each tablet contains 10 mg of lisinopril and 12.5 mg of hydrochlorothiazide. They are supplied as follows:

NDC 0006-0145-31 unit of use bottles of 30.
NDC 0006-0145-58 unit of use bottles of 100.

No. 3594—Tablets PRINZIDE 20-12.5 are yellow, round, fluted-edge tablets, coded MSD 140 on one side and PRINZIDE on the other. Each tablet contains 20 mg of lisinopril and 12.5 mg of hydrochlorothiazide. They are supplied as follows:

NDC 0006-0140-31 unit of use bottles of 30
NDC 0006-0140-58 unit of use bottles of 100.

No. 3595—Tablets PRINZIDE 20-25 are peach, round, fluted-edge tablets, coded MSD 142 on one side and PRINZIDE on the other. Each tablet contains 20 mg of lisinopril and 25 mg of hydrochlorothiazide. They are supplied as follows:

NDC 0006-0142-31 unit of use bottles of 30
NDC 0006-0142-58 unit of use bottles of 100.

Storage

Store at controlled room temperature. 15–30°C (59–86°F). Protect from excessive light and humidity.

Dispense in a well-closed container, if product package is subdivided.

7836336 Issued April 2003

Shown in Product Identification Guide, page 323

PROPECIA® ℞
(Finasteride)
Tablets, 1 mg

DESCRIPTION

PROPECIA* (finasteride), a synthetic 4-azasteroid compound, is a specific inhibitor of steroid Type II 5α-reductase, an intracellular enzyme that converts the androgen testosterone into 5α-dihydrotestosterone (DHT).

Finasteride is 4-azaandrost-1-ene-17-carboxamide,*N*-(1,1-dimethylethyl)-3-oxo-,(5α,17β)-. The empirical formula of finasteride is $C_{23}H_{36}N_2O_2$ and its molecular weight is 372.55. Its structural formula is:

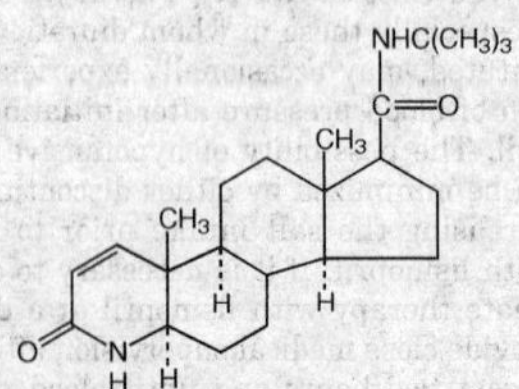

Finasteride is a white crystalline powder with a melting point near 250°C. It is freely soluble in chloroform and in lower alcohol solvents but is practically insoluble in water. PROPECIA tablets for oral administration are film-coated tablets that contain 1 mg of finasteride and the following inactive ingredients: lactose monohydrate, microcrystalline cellulose, pregelatinized starch, sodium starch glycolate, docusate sodium, magnesium stearate, hydroxypropyl methylcellulose 2910, hydroxypropyl cellulose, titanium dioxide, talc, yellow ferric oxide, and red ferric oxide.

*Registered trademark of MERCK & CO., INC.

CLINICAL PHARMACOLOGY

Finasteride is a competitive and specific inhibitor of Type II 5α-reductase, an intracellular enzyme that converts the androgen testosterone into DHT. Two distinct isozymes are found in mice, rats, monkeys, and humans: Type I and II. Each of these isozymes is differentially expressed in tissues and developmental stages. In humans, Type I 5α-reductase is predominant in the sebaceous glands of most regions of skin, including scalp, and liver. Type I 5α-reductase is responsible for approximately one-third of circulating DHT. The Type II 5α-reductase isozyme is primarily found in prostate, seminal vesicles, epididymides, and hair follicles as well as liver, and is responsible for two-thirds of circulating DHT.

In humans, the mechanism of action of finasteride is based on its preferential inhibition of the Type II isozyme. Using native tissues (scalp and prostate), *in vitro* binding studies examining the potential of finasteride to inhibit either isozyme revealed a 100-fold selectivity for the human Type II 5α-reductase over Type I isozyme (IC_{50}=500 and 4.2 nM for Type I and II, respectively). For both isozymes, the inhibition by finasteride is accompanied by reduction of the inhibitor to dihydrofinasteride and adduct formation with NADP+. The turnover for the enzyme complex is slow ($t_{1/2}$ approximately 30 days for the Type II enzyme complex and 14 days for the Type I complex).

Finasteride has no affinity for the androgen receptor and has no androgenic, antiandrogenic, estrogenic, antiestrogenic, or progestational effects. Inhibition of Type II 5α-reductase blocks the peripheral conversion of testosterone to DHT, resulting in significant decreases in serum and tissue DHT concentrations. Finasteride produces a rapid reduction in serum DHT concentration, reaching 65% suppression within 24 hours of oral dosing with a 1-mg tablet.

In men with male pattern hair loss (androgenetic alopecia), the balding scalp contains miniaturized hair follicles and increased amounts of DHT compared with hairy scalp. Administration of finasteride decreases scalp and serum DHT concentrations in these men. The relative contributions of these reductions to the treatment effect of finasteride have not been defined. By this mechanism, finasteride appears to interrupt a key factor in the development of androgenetic alopecia in those patients genetically predisposed.

A 48-week, placebo-controlled study designed to assess by phototrichogram the effect of PROPECIA on total and actively growing (anagen) scalp hairs in vertex baldness enrolled 212 men with androgenetic alopecia. At baseline and 48 weeks, total and anagen hair counts were obtained in a 1-cm^2 target area of the scalp. Men treated with PROPECIA showed increases from baseline in total and anagen hair counts of 7 hairs and 18 hairs, respectively, whereas men treated with placebo had decreases of 10 hairs and 9 hairs, respectively. These changes in hair counts resulted in a between-group difference of 17 hairs in total hair count ($p<0.001$) and 27 hairs in anagen hair count ($p<0.001$), and an improvement in the proportion of anagen hairs from 62% at baseline to 68% for men treated with PROPECIA.

Finasteride had no effect on circulating levels of cortisol, thyroid-stimulating hormone, or thyroxine, nor did it affect the plasma lipid profile (e.g., total cholesterol, low-density lipoproteins, high-density lipoproteins and triglycerides) or bone mineral density. In studies with finasteride, no clinically meaningful changes in luteinizing hormone (LH) or follicle-stimulating hormone (FSH) were detected. In healthy volunteers, treatment with finasteride did not alter the response of LH and FSH to gonadotropin-releasing hormone, indicating that the hypothalamic-pituitary-testicular axis was not affected. Mean circulating levels of testosterone and estradiol were increased by approximately 15% as compared to baseline in the first year of treatment, but these levels were within the physiologic range.

Pharmacokinetics

Following an oral dose of ^{14}C-finasteride in man, a mean of 39% (range, 32–46%) of the dose was excreted in the urine in the form of metabolites; 57% (range, 51–64%) was excreted in the feces. The major compound isolated from urine was the monocarboxylic acid metabolite; virtually no unchanged drug was recovered. The t-butyl side chain monohydroxylated metabolite has been isolated from plasma. These metabolites possessed no more than 20% of the 5α-reductase inhibitory activity of finasteride.

In a study in 15 healthy male subjects, the mean bioavailability of finasteride 1-mg tablets was 65% (range 26–170%), based on the ratio of AUC relative to a 5-mg intravenous dose infused over 60 minutes. Following intravenous infusion, mean plasma clearance was 165 mL/min (range, 70–279 mL/min) and mean steady-state volume of distribution was 76 liters (range, 44–96 liters). In a separate study, the bioavailability of finasteride was not affected by food.

Approximately 90% of circulating finasteride is bound to plasma proteins. Finasteride has been found to cross the blood-brain barrier.

There is a slow accumulation phase for finasteride after multiple dosing. At steady state following dosing with 1 mg/day, maximum finasteride plasma concentration averaged 9.2 ng/mL (range, 4.9–13.7 ng/mL) and was reached 1 to 2 hours postdose; $AUC_{(0-24\ hr)}$ was 53 ng·hr/mL (range, 20–154 ng·hr/mL) and mean terminal half-life of elimination was 4.8 hours (range, 3.3–13.4 hours).

Semen levels have been measured in 35 men taking finasteride 1 mg daily for 6 weeks. In 60% (21 of 35) of the samples, finasteride levels were undetectable. The mean finasteride level was 0.26 ng/mL and the highest level measured was 1.52 ng/mL. Using this highest semen level measured and assuming 100% absorption from a 5-mL ejaculate per day, human exposure through vaginal absorption would be up to 7.6 ng per day, which is 750 times lower than the exposure from the no-effect dose for developmental abnormalities in Rhesus monkeys (see PRECAUTIONS, *Pregnancy*).

The elimination rate of finasteride decreases somewhat with age. Mean terminal half-life is approximately 5–6 hours in men 18–60 years of age and 8 hours in men more than 70 years of age. These findings are of no clinical significance, and a reduction in dosage in the elderly is not warranted.

No dosage adjustment is necessary in patients with renal insufficiency. In patients with chronic renal impairment (creatinine clearance ranging from 9.0 to 55 mL/min), the values for AUC, maximum plasma concentration, half-life, and protein binding after a single dose of ^{14}C-finasteride were similar to those obtained in healthy volunteers. Urinary excretion of metabolites was decreased in patients with renal impairment. This decrease was associated with an increase in fecal excretion of metabolites. Plasma concentrations of metabolites were significantly higher in patients with renal impairment (based on a 60% increase in total radioactivity AUC). Furthermore, finasteride has been well tolerated in men with normal renal function receiving up to 80 mg/day for 12 weeks where exposure of these patients to metabolites would presumably be much greater.

Clinical Studies

Studies in Men

The efficacy of PROPECIA was demonstrated in men (88% Caucasian) with mild to moderate androgenetic alopecia (male pattern hair loss) between 18 and 41 years of age. In order to prevent seborrheic dermatitis which might confound the assessment of hair growth in these studies, all men, whether treated with finasteride or placebo, were instructed to use a specified, medicated, tar-based shampoo (Neutrogena T/Gel®** Shampoo) during the first 2 years of the studies.

There were three double-blind, randomized, placebo-controlled studies of 12-month duration. The two primary endpoints were hair count and patient self-assessment; the two secondary endpoints were investigator assessment and ratings of photographs. In addition, information was collected regarding sexual function (based on a self-administered questionnaire) and non-scalp body hair growth. The three studies were conducted in 1,879 men with mild to moderate, but not complete, hair loss. Two of the studies enrolled men with predominantly mild to moderate vertex hair loss (n=1,553). The third enrolled men having mild to moderate hair loss in the anterior midscalp area with or without vertex balding (n=326).

Studies in Men with Vertex Baldness

Of the men who completed the first 12 months of the two vertex baldness trials, 1,215 elected to continue in double-blind, placebo-controlled, 12-month extension studies. There were 547 men receiving PROPECIA for both the initial study and first extension periods (up to 2 years of treatment) and 60 men receiving placebo for the same periods. The extension studies were continued for 3 additional years, with 323 men on PROPECIA and 23 on placebo entering the fifth year of the study.

In order to evaluate the effect of discontinuation of therapy, there were 65 men who received PROPECIA for the initial 12 months followed by placebo in the first 12-month extension period. Some of these men continued in additional extension studies and were switched back to treatment with PROPECIA, with 32 men entering the fifth year of the study. Lastly, there were 543 men who received placebo for the initial 12 months followed by PROPECIA in the first 12-month extension period. Some of these men continued in additional extension studies receiving PROPECIA, with 290 men entering the fifth year of the study (see Figure below).

Hair counts were assessed by photographic enlargements of a representative area of active hair loss. In these two studies in men with vertex baldness, significant increases in hair count were demonstrated at 6 and 12 months in men treated with PROPECIA, while significant hair loss from baseline was demonstrated in those treated with placebo. At 12 months there was a 107-hair difference from placebo ($p<0.001$, PROPECIA [n=679] vs placebo [n=672]) within a 1-inch diameter circle (5.1 cm^2). Hair count was maintained in those men taking PROPECIA for up to 2 years, resulting in a 138-hair difference between treatment groups ($p<0.001$, PROPECIA [n=433] vs placebo [n=47]) within the same area. In men treated with PROPECIA, the maximum improvement in hair count compared to baseline was achieved during the first 2 years. Although the initial improvement was followed by a slow decline, hair count was maintained above baseline throughout the 5 years of the studies. Furthermore, because the decline in the placebo group was more rapid, the difference between treatment groups also continued to increase throughout the studies, resulting in a 277-hair difference ($p<0.001$, PROPECIA [n=219] vs placebo [n=15]) at 5 years (see Figure below).

Patients who switched from placebo to PROPECIA (n=425) had a decrease in hair count at the end of the initial 12-month placebo period, followed by an increase in hair count after 1 year of treatment with PROPECIA. This increase in hair count was less (56 hairs above original baseline) than the increase (91 hairs above original baseline) observed after 1 year of treatment in men initially randomized to PROPECIA. Although the increase in hair count, relative to when therapy was initiated, was comparable between these two groups, a higher absolute hair count was achieved in patients who were started on treatment with PROPECIA in the initial study. This advantage was maintained through the remaining 3 years of the studies. A change of treatment from PROPECIA to placebo (n=48) at the end of the initial 12 months resulted in reversal of the increase in hair count 12 months later, at 24 months (see Figure below).

At 12 months, 58% of men in the placebo group had further hair loss (defined as any decrease in hair count from baseline), compared with 14% of men treated with PROPECIA. In men treated for up to 2 years, 72% of men in the placebo group demonstrated hair loss, compared with 17% of men treated with PROPECIA. At 5 years, 100% of men in the placebo group demonstrated hair loss, compared with 35% of men treated with PROPECIA.

[See graphic above]

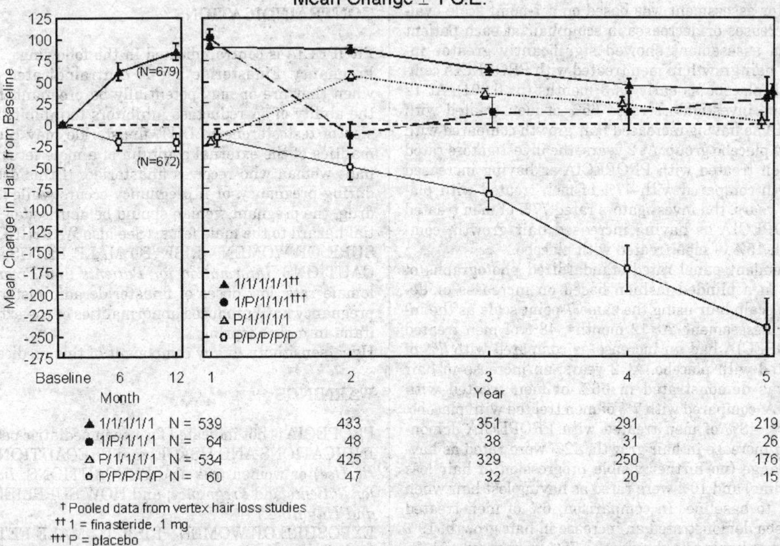

Patient self-assessment was obtained at each clinic visit from a self-administered questionnaire, which included questions on their perception of hair growth, hair loss, and appearance. This self-assessment demonstrated an increase in amount of hair, a decrease in hair loss, and improvement in appearance in men treated with PROPECIA. Overall improvement compared with placebo was seen as early as 3 months ($p<0.05$), with improvement maintained over 5 years.

Continued on next page

Information on the Merck & Co., Inc., products listed on these pages is from the prescribing information in use October 1, 2004. For information, please call 1-800-NSC-MERCK [1-800-672-6372].

Propecia—Cont.

Investigator assessment was based on a 7-point scale evaluating increases or decreases in scalp hair at each patient visit. This assessment showed significantly greater increases in hair growth in men treated with PROPECIA compared with placebo as early as 3 months ($p<0.001$). At 12 months, the investigators rated 65% of men treated with PROPECIA as having increased hair growth compared with 37% in the placebo group. At 2 years, the investigators rated 80% of men treated with PROPECIA as having increased hair growth compared with 47% of men treated with placebo. At 5 years, the investigators rated 77% of men treated with PROPECIA as having increased hair growth, compared with 15% of men treated with placebo.

An independent panel rated standardized photographs of the head in a blinded fashion based on increases or decreases in scalp hair using the same 7-point scale as the investigator assessment. At 12 months, 48% of men treated with PROPECIA had an increase as compared with 7% of men treated with placebo. At 2 years, an increase in hair growth was demonstrated in 66% of men treated with PROPECIA, compared with 7% of men treated with placebo. At 5 years, 48% of men treated with PROPECIA demonstrated an increase in hair growth, 42% were rated as having no change (no further visible progression of hair loss from baseline) and 10% were rated as having lost hair when compared to baseline. In comparison, 6% of men treated with placebo demonstrated an increase in hair growth, 19% were rated as having no change and 75% were rated as having lost hair when compared to baseline.

Other Results in Vertex Baldness Studies

A sexual function questionnaire was self-administered by patients participating in the two vertex baldness trials to detect more subtle changes in sexual function. At Month 12, statistically significant differences in favor of placebo were found in 3 of 4 domains (sexual interest, erections, and perception of sexual problems). However, no significant difference was seen in the question of overall satisfaction with sex life.

In one of the two vertex baldness studies, patients were questioned on non-scalp body hair growth. PROPECIA did not appear to affect non-scalp body hair.

Study in Men with Hair Loss in the Anterior Mid-Scalp Area

A study of 12-month duration, designed to assess the efficacy of PROPECIA in men with hair loss in the anterior mid-scalp area, also demonstrated significant increases in hair count compared with placebo. Increases in hair count were accompanied by improvements in patient self-assessment, investigator assessment, and ratings based on standardized photographs. Hair counts were obtained in the anterior mid-scalp area, and did not include the area of bitemporal recession or the anterior hairline.

Summary of Clinical Studies in Men

Clinical studies were conducted in men aged 18 to 41 with mild to moderate degrees of androgenetic alopecia. All men treated with PROPECIA or placebo received a tar-based shampoo (Neutrogena T/Gel®** Shampoo) during the first 2 years of the studies. Clinical improvement was seen as early as 3 months in the patients treated with PROPECIA and led to a net increase in scalp hair count and hair regrowth. In clinical studies for up to 5 years, treatment with PROPECIA slowed the further progression of hair loss observed in the placebo group. In general, the difference between treatment groups continued to increase throughout the 5 years of the studies.

Ethnic Analysis of Clinical Data from Men

In a combined analysis of the two studies on vertex baldness, mean hair count changes from baseline were 91 vs −19 hairs (PROPECIA vs placebo) among Caucasians (n=1,185), 49 vs −27 hairs among Blacks (n=84), 53 vs −38 hairs among Asians (n=17), 67 vs 5 hairs among Hispanics (n=45) and 67 vs −15 hairs among other ethnic groups (n=20). Patient self-assessment showed improvement across racial groups with PROPECIA treatment, except for satisfaction of the frontal hairline and vertex in Black men, who were satisfied overall.

Study in Women

In a study involving 137 postmenopausal women with androgenetic alopecia who were treated with PROPECIA (n=67) or placebo (n=70) for 12 months, effectiveness could not be demonstrated. There was no improvement in hair counts, patient self-assessment, investigator assessment, or ratings of standardized photographs in the women treated with PROPECIA when compared with the placebo group (see INDICATIONS AND USAGE).

**Registered trademark of Johnson & Johnson

INDICATIONS AND USAGE

PROPECIA is indicated for the treatment of male pattern hair loss (androgenetic alopecia) in **MEN ONLY**. Safety and efficacy were demonstrated in men between 18 to 41 years of age with mild to moderate hair loss of the vertex and anterior mid-scalp area (see CLINICAL PHARMACOLOGY, *Clinical Studies*).

Efficacy in bitemporal recession has not been established.

PROPECIA is not indicated in women (see CLINICAL PHARMACOLOGY, *Clinical Studies* and CONTRAINDICATIONS).

PROPECIA is not indicated in children (see PRECAUTIONS, *Pediatric Use*).

CONTRAINDICATIONS

PROPECIA is contraindicated in the following:

Pregnancy. Finasteride use is contraindicated in women when they are or may potentially be pregnant. Because of the ability of 5α-reductase inhibitors to inhibit the conversion of testosterone to DHT, finasteride may cause abnormalities of the external genitalia of a male fetus of a pregnant woman who receives finasteride. If this drug is used during pregnancy, or if pregnancy occurs while taking this drug, the pregnant woman should be apprised of the potential hazard to the male fetus. (See also WARNINGS, EXPOSURE OF WOMEN - RISK TO MALE FETUS; and PRECAUTIONS, *Information for Patients* and *Pregnancy*.) In female rats, low doses of finasteride administered during pregnancy have produced abnormalities of the external genitalia in male offspring.

Hypersensitivity to any component of this medication.

WARNINGS

PROPECIA is not indicated for use in pediatric patients (see INDICATIONS AND USAGE; and PRECAUTIONS, *Pediatric Use*) or women (see also PRECAUTIONS, *Information for Patients* and *Pregnancy*; and HOW SUPPLIED, *Storage and Handling*.)

EXPOSURE OF WOMEN - RISK TO MALE FETUS

Women should not handle crushed or broken PROPECIA tablets when they are pregnant or may potentially be pregnant because of the possibility of absorption of finasteride and the subsequent potential risk to a male fetus. PROPECIA tablets are coated and will prevent contact with the active ingredient during normal handling, provided that the tablets have not been broken or crushed. (See also CONTRAINDICATIONS; PRECAUTIONS, *Information for Patients* and *Pregnancy*; and HOW SUPPLIED, *Storage and Handling*.)

PRECAUTIONS

General

Caution should be used in the administration of PROPECIA in patients with liver function abnormalities, as finasteride is metabolized extensively in the liver.

Information for Patients

Women should not handle crushed or broken PROPECIA tablets when they are pregnant or may potentially be pregnant because of the possibility of absorption of finasteride and the subsequent potential risk to a male fetus. PROPECIA tablets are coated and will prevent contact with the active ingredient during normal handling, provided that the tablets have not been broken or crushed. (See also CONTRAINDICATIONS; WARNINGS, EXPOSURE OF WOMEN - RISK TO MALE FETUS; PRECAUTIONS, *Pregnancy*; and HOW SUPPLIED, *Storage and Handling*.)

Physicians should instruct their patients to promptly report any changes in their breasts such as lumps, pain or nipple discharge. Breast changes including breast enlargement, tenderness and neoplasm have been reported (see **ADVERSE REACTIONS**)

See also Patient Package Insert.

Drug/Laboratory Test Interactions

In clinical studies with PROPECIA in men 18–41 years of age, the mean value of serum prostate-specific antigen (PSA) decreased from 0.7 ng/mL at baseline to 0.5 ng/mL at Month 12. When finasteride is used in older men who have benign prostatic hyperplasia (BPH), PSA levels are decreased by approximately 50%. Until further information is gathered in men >41 years of age without BPH, consideration should be given to doubling the PSA level in men undergoing this test while taking PROPECIA.

Drug Interactions

No drug interactions of clinical importance have been identified. Finasteride does not appear to affect the cytochrome P450-linked drug metabolizing enzyme system. Compounds that have been tested in man include antipyrine, digoxin, propranolol, theophylline, and warfarin and no interactions were found.

Other concomitant therapy: Although specific interaction studies were not performed, finasteride doses of 1 mg or more were concomitantly used in clinical studies with acetaminophen, α-blockers, analgesics, angiotensin-converting enzyme (ACE) inhibitors, anticonvulsants, benzodiazepines, beta blockers, calcium-channel blockers, cardiac nitrates, diuretics, H_2 antagonists, HMG-CoA reductase inhibitors, prostaglandin synthetase inhibitors (NSAIDs), and quinolone anti-infectives without evidence of clinically significant adverse interactions.

Carcinogenesis, Mutagenesis, Impairment of Fertility

No evidence of a tumorigenic effect was observed in a 24-month study in Sprague-Dawley rats receiving doses of finasteride up to 160 mg/kg/day in males and 320 mg/kg/day in females. These doses produced respective systemic exposure in rats of 888 and 2,192 times those observed in man receiving the recommended human dose of 1 mg/day. All exposure calculations were based on calculated $AUC_{(0-24\ hr)}$ for animals and mean $AUC_{(0-24\ hr)}$ for man (0.05 μg·hr/mL).

In a 19-month carcinogenicity study in CD-1 mice, a statistically significant ($p \leq 0.05$) increase in the incidence of testicular Leydig cell adenomas was observed at a dose of 250 mg/kg/day (1,824 times the human exposure). In mice at a dose of 25 mg/kg/day (184 times the human exposure, estimated) and in rats at a dose of ≥40 mg/kg/day (312 times the human exposure) an increase in the incidence of Leydig cell hyperplasia was observed. A positive correlation between the proliferative changes in the Leydig cells and an increase in serum LH levels (2–3 fold above control) has been demonstrated in both rodent species treated with high doses of finasteride. No drug-related Leydig cell changes were seen in either rats or dogs treated with finasteride for 1 year at doses of 20 mg/kg/day and 45 mg/kg/day (240 and 2,800 times, respectively, the human exposure) or in mice treated for 19 months at a dose of 2.5 mg/kg/day (18.4 times the human exposure).

No evidence of mutagenicity was observed in an *in vitro* bacterial mutagenesis assay, a mammalian cell mutagenesis assay, or in an *in vitro* alkaline elution assay. In an *in vitro* chromosome aberration assay, when Chinese hamster ovary cells were treated with high concentrations (450–550 μmol) of finasteride, there was a slight increase in chromosome aberrations. These concentrations correspond to 18,000–22,000 times the peak plasma levels in man given a total dose of 1 mg. Further, the concentrations (450–550 μmol) used in *in vitro* studies are not achievable in a biological system. In an *in vivo* chromosome aberration assay in mice, no treatment-related increase in chromosome aberration was observed with finasteride at the maximum tolerated dose of 250 mg/kg/day (1,824 times the human exposure, estimated) as determined in the carcinogenicity studies.

In sexually mature male rabbits treated with finasteride at 80 mg/kg/day (4,344 times the estimated human exposure) for up to 12 weeks, no effect on fertility, sperm count, or ejaculate volume was seen. In sexually mature male rats treated with 80 mg/kg/day of finasteride (488 times the estimated human exposure), there were no significant effects on fertility after 6 or 12 weeks of treatment; however, when treatment was continued for up to 24 or 30 weeks, there was an apparent decrease in fertility, fecundity, and an associated significant decrease in the weights of the seminal vesicles and prostate. All these effects were reversible within 6 weeks of discontinuation of treatment. No drug-related effect on testes or on mating performance has been seen in rats or rabbits. This decrease in fertility in finasteride-treated rats is secondary to its effect on accessory sex organs (prostate and seminal vesicles) resulting in failure to form a seminal plug. The seminal plug is essential for normal fertility in rats but is not relevant in man.

Pregnancy

Teratogenic Effects: Pregnancy Category X

See CONTRAINDICATIONS.

PROPECIA is not indicated for use in women.

Administration of finasteride to pregnant rats at doses ranging from 100 μg/kg/day to 100 mg/kg/day (5–5,000 times the recommended human dose of 1 mg/day) resulted in dose-dependent development of hypospadias in 3.6 to 100% of male offspring. Pregnant rats produced male offspring with decreased prostatic and seminal vesicular weights, delayed preputial separation, and transient nipple development when given finasteride at ≥30 μg/kg/day (≥ 1.5 times the recommended human dose of 1 mg/day) and decreased anogenital distance when given finasteride at ≥3 μg/kg/day (one-fifth the recommended human dose of 1 mg/day). The critical period during which these effects can be induced in male rats has been defined to be days 16–17 of gestation. The changes described above are expected pharmacological effects of drugs belonging to the class of Type II 5α-reductase inhibitors and are similar to those reported in male infants with a genetic deficiency of Type II 5α-reductase. No abnormalities were observed in female offspring exposed to any dose of finasteride *in utero*.

No developmental abnormalities have been observed in first filial generation (F_1) male or female offspring resulting from mating finasteride-treated male rats (80 mg/kg/day; 488 times the human exposure) with untreated females. Administration of finasteride at 3 mg/kg/day (150 times the recommended human dose of 1 mg/day) during the late gestation and lactation period resulted in slightly decreased fertility in F_1 male offspring. No effects were seen in female offspring. No evidence of malformations has been observed in rabbit fetuses exposed to finasteride *in utero* from days 6–18 of gestation at doses up to 100 mg/kg/day (5000 times the recommended human dose of 1 mg/day). However, effects on male genitalia would not be expected since the rabbits were not exposed during the critical period of genital system development.

The *in utero* effects of finasteride exposure during the period of embryonic and fetal development were evaluated in the rhesus monkey (gestation days 20–100), a species more predictive of human development than rats or rabbits. Intravenous administration of finasteride to pregnant monkeys at doses as high as 800 ng/day (at least 750 times the highest estimated exposure of pregnant women to finasteride from semen of men taking 1 mg/day) resulted in no abnormalities in male fetuses. In confirmation of the relevance of the rhesus model for human fetal development, oral administration of a very high dose of finasteride (2 mg/kg/day; 100 times the recommended human dose of 1 mg/day or approximately 12 million times the highest estimated exposure to finasteride from semen of men taking 1 mg/day) to pregnant monkeys resulted in external genital abnormalities in male fetuses. No other abnormalities were observed in male fetuses and no finasteride-related abnormalities were observed in female fetuses at any dose.

Nursing Mothers
PROPECIA is not indicated for use in women.
It is not known whether finasteride is excreted in human milk.
Pediatric Use
PROPECIA is not indicated for use in pediatric patients. Safety and effectiveness in pediatric patients have not been established.
Geriatric Use
Clinical efficacy studies with PROPECIA did not include subjects aged 65 and over. Based on the pharmacokinetics of finasteride 5 mg, no dosage adjustment is necessary in the elderly for PROPECIA (see CLINICAL PHARMACOLOGY, *Pharmacokinetics*). However the efficacy of PROPECIA in the elderly has not been established.

ADVERSE REACTIONS

Clinical Studies for PROPECIA (finasteride 1 mg) in the Treatment of Male Pattern Hair Loss
In controlled clinical trials for PROPECIA of 12-month duration, 1.4% of the patients were discontinued due to adverse experiences that were considered to be possibly, probably or definitely drug-related (1.6% for placebo); 1.2% of patients on PROPECIA and 0.9% of patients on placebo discontinued therapy because of a drug-related sexual adverse experience. The following clinical adverse reactions were reported as possibly, probably or definitely drug-related in ≥1% of patients treated for 12 months with PROPECIA or placebo, respectively: decreased libido (1.8%, 1.3%), erectile dysfunction (1.3%, 0.7%) and ejaculation disorder (1.2%, 0.7%; primarily decreased volume of ejaculate:[0.8%, 0.4%]). Integrated analysis of clinical adverse experiences showed that during treatment with PROPECIA, 36 (3.8%) of 945 men had reported one or more of these adverse experiences as compared to 20 (2.1%) of 934 men treated with placebo (p=0.04). Resolution occurred in all men who discontinued therapy with PROPECIA due to these side effects and in most of those who continued therapy. The incidence of each of the above side effects decreased to ≤0.3% by the fifth year of treatment with PROPECIA.
In a study of finasteride 1 mg daily in healthy men, a median decrease in ejaculate volume of 0.3 mL (-11%) compared with 0.2 mL (−8%) for placebo was observed after 48 weeks of treatment. Two other studies showed that finasteride at 5 times the dosage of PROPECIA (5 mg daily) produced significant median decreases of approximately 0.5 mL (-25%) compared to placebo in ejaculate volume but this was reversible after discontinuation of treatment.
In the clinical studies with PROPECIA, the incidences for breast tenderness and enlargement, hypersensitivity reactions, and testicular pain in finasteride-treated patients were not different from those in patients treated with placebo.
Postmarketing Experience for PROPECIA (finasteride 1 mg)
Breast tenderness and enlargement; hypersensitivity reactions including rash, pruritus, urticaria, and swelling of the lips and face; and testicular pain.
Controlled Clinical Trials and Long-Term Open Extension Studies for PROSCAR (finasteride 5 mg) in the Treatment of Benign Prostatic Hyperplasia*
In controlled clinical trials for PROSCAR of 12-month duration, 1.3% of the patients were discontinued due to adverse experiences that were considered to be possibly, probably or definitely drug-related (0.9% for placebo); only one patient on PROSCAR (0.2%) and one patient on placebo (0.2%) discontinued therapy because of a drug-related sexual adverse experience. The following clinical adverse reactions were reported as possibly, probably or definitely drug-related in ≥1% of patients treated for 12 months with PROSCAR or placebo, respectively: erectile dysfunction (3.7%, 1.1%), decreased libido (3.3%, 1.6%) and decreased volume of ejaculate (2.8%, 0.9%). The adverse experience profiles for patients treated with finasteride 1 mg/day for 12 months and those maintained on PROSCAR for 24 to 48 months were similar to that observed in the 12-month controlled studies with PROSCAR. Sexual adverse experiences resolved with continued treatment in over 60% of patients who reported them.
The relationship between long-term use of finasteride and male breast neoplasia is currently unknown. During a 4- to 6-year placebo- and comparator-controlled study that enrolled 3047 men, there were 4 cases of breast cancer in men treated with PROSCAR but no cases in men not treated with PROSCAR. In another 4-year, placebo-controlled study that enrolled 3040 men, there were 2 cases of breast cancer in placebo-treated men, but no cases were reported in men treated with PROSCAR.
In a 7-year placebo-controlled trial that enrolled 18,882 healthy men, 9060 had prostate needle biopsy data available for analysis. In the PROSCAR group, 280 (6.4%) men had prostate cancer with Gleason scores of 7–10 detected on needle biopsy vs. 237 (5.1%) men in the placebo group. Of the total cases of prostate cancer diagnosed in this study, approximately 98% were classified as intracapsular (stage T1 or T2). The clinical significance of these findings is unknown.

OVERDOSAGE

In clinical studies, single doses of finasteride up to 400 mg and multiple doses of finasteride up to 80 mg/day for three months did not result in adverse reactions. Until further experience is obtained, no specific treatment for an overdose with finasteride can be recommended.
Significant lethality was observed in male and female mice at single oral doses of 1,500 mg/m² (500 mg/kg) and in female and male rats at single oral doses of 2,360 mg/m² (400 mg/kg) and 5,900 mg/m² (1,000 mg/kg), respectively.

DOSAGE AND ADMINISTRATION

The recommended dosage is 1 mg once a day.
PROPECIA may be administered with or without meals.
In general, daily use for three months or more is necessary before benefit is observed. Continued use is recommended to sustain benefit, which should be re-evaluated periodically. Withdrawal of treatment leads to reversal of effect within 12 months.

HOW SUPPLIED

No. 6642—PROPECIA tablets, 1 mg, are tan, octagonal, film-coated convex tablets with "stylized P" on one side and PROPECIA on the other. They are supplied as follows:
NDC 0006-0071-31 unit of use bottles of 30
NDC 0006-0071-61 ProPak®***- carton of 3 unit of use bottles of 30.
Storage and Handling
Store at room temperature, 15–30°C (59–86°F). Keep container closed and protect from moisture.
Women should not handle crushed or broken PROPECIA tablets when they are pregnant or may potentially be pregnant because of the possibility of absorption of finasteride and the subsequent potential risk to a male fetus. PROPECIA tablets are coated and will prevent contact with the active ingredient during normal handling, provided that the tablets are not broken or crushed. (See WARNINGS, EXPOSURE OF WOMEN - RISK TO MALE FETUS; and PRECAUTIONS, *Information for Patients* and *Pregnancy*.)

*** Registered trademark of MERCK & CO., Inc.
9328504 Issued October 2003

Patient Information about
PROPECIA® (Pro-pee-sha)
Generic name: finasteride
(fin-AS-tur-eyed)
PROPECIA is for use by MEN ONLY.**

Please read this leaflet before you start taking PROPECIA. Also, read the information included with PROPECIA each time you renew your prescription, just in case anything has changed. Remember, this leaflet does not take the place of careful discussions with your doctor. You and your doctor should discuss PROPECIA when you start taking your medication and at regular checkups.

** Registered trademark of MERCK & CO., Inc.

What is PROPECIA used for?
PROPECIA is used for the treatment of male pattern hair loss on the vertex and the anterior mid-scalp area.
PROPECIA is for use by **MEN ONLY** and should **NOT** be used by women or children.
What is male pattern hair loss?
Male pattern hair loss is a common condition in which men experience thinning of the hair on the scalp. Often, this results in a receding hairline and/or balding on the top of the head. These changes typically begin gradually in men in their 20s.
Doctors believe male pattern hair loss is due to heredity and is dependent on hormonal effects. Doctors refer to this type of hair loss as androgenetic alopecia.
Results of clinical studies:
For 12 months, doctors studied over 1800 men aged 18 to 41 with mild to moderate amounts of ongoing hair loss. Of these men, approximately 1200 with hair loss at the top of the head participated in additional extension studies, resulting in a total study time of up to five years. In general, men who took PROPECIA maintained or increased the number of visible scalp hairs and noticed improvement in their hair in the first year. Improvement, compared to the start of the study, was maintained through the remaining years of treatment. Hair counts in men who did not take PROPECIA continued to decrease.
In one study, patients were questioned on the growth of body hair. PROPECIA did not appear to affect hair in places other than the scalp.
Will PROPECIA work for me?
For most men, PROPECIA increases the number of scalp hairs in the first year of treatment, helping to fill in thin or balding areas of the scalp. In addition, men taking PROPECIA may note a slowing of hair loss. Although results will vary, generally you will not be able to grow back all of the hair you have lost. There is not sufficient evidence that PROPECIA works in the treatment of receding hairline in the temporal area on both sides of the head.
Male pattern hair loss occurs gradually over time. On average, healthy hair grows only about half an inch each month. Therefore, it will take time to see any effect.
You may need to take PROPECIA daily for three months or more before you see a benefit from taking PROPECIA. PROPECIA can only work over the long term if you continue taking it. If the drug has not worked for you in twelve months, further treatment is unlikely to be of benefit. If you stop taking PROPECIA, you will likely lose the hair you have gained within 12 months of stopping treatment. You should discuss this with your doctor.
PROPECIA is not effective in the treatment of hair loss due to androgenetic alopecia in postmenopausal women. PROPECIA should not be taken by women.
How should I take PROPECIA?
Follow your doctor's instructions.
- Take one tablet by mouth each day.
- You may take PROPECIA with or without food.
- If you forget to take PROPECIA, do not take an extra tablet. Just take the next tablet as usual.

PROPECIA will not work faster or better if you take it more than once a day.
Who should NOT take PROPECIA?
- PROPECIA is for the treatment of male pattern hair loss in **MEN ONLY** and should not be taken by women (see **A warning about PROPECIA and pregnancy**).
- PROPECIA should not be taken by children.
- Anyone allergic to any of the ingredients.

A warning about PROPECIA and pregnancy.
- **Women who are or may potentially be pregnant:**
  - **must not use PROPECIA**
  - **should not handle crushed or broken tablets of PROPECIA.**

If a woman who is pregnant with a male baby absorbs the active ingredient in PROPECIA, either by swallowing or through the skin, it may cause abnormalities of a male baby's sex organs. If a woman who is pregnant comes into contact with the active ingredient in PROPECIA, a doctor should be consulted. PROPECIA tablets are coated and will prevent contact with the active ingredient during normal handling, provided that the tablets are not broken or crushed.
What are the possible side effects of PROPECIA?
Like all prescription products, PROPECIA may cause side effects. In clinical studies, side effects from PROPECIA were uncommon and did not affect most men. A small number of men experienced certain sexual side effects. These men reported one or more of the following: less desire for sex; difficulty in achieving an erection; and, a decrease in the amount of semen. Each of these side effects occurred in less than 2% of men. These side effects went away in men who stopped taking PROPECIA. They also disappeared in most men who continued taking PROPECIA.
In general use, the following have been reported: allergic reactions including rash, itching, hives and swelling of the lips and face; problems with ejaculation; breast tenderness and enlargement; and testicular pain. You should promptly report to your doctor any changes in your breasts such as lumps, pain or nipple discharge. Tell your doctor promptly about these or any other unusual side effects.
- **PROPECIA can affect a blood test called PSA (Prostate-Specific Antigen) for the screening of prostate cancer. If you have a PSA test done, you should tell your doctor that you are taking PROPECIA.**

Storage and handling.
Keep PROPECIA in the original container and keep the container closed. Store it in a dry place at room temperature.
PROPECIA tablets are coated and will prevent contact with the active ingredient during normal handling, provided that the tablets are not broken or crushed.
Do not give your PROPECIA tablets to anyone else. It has been prescribed only for you. Keep PROPECIA and all medications out of the reach of children.
THIS LEAFLET PROVIDES A SUMMARY OF INFORMATION ABOUT PROPECIA. IF AFTER READING THIS LEAFLET YOU HAVE ANY QUESTIONS OR ARE NOT SURE ABOUT ANYTHING, ASK YOUR DOCTOR.
1-888-637-2522, Monday through Friday, 8:30 A.M. TO 7:00 P.M. (ET).
www.propecia.com
9329303 Issued October 2003

Shown in Product Identification Guide, page 323

PROSCAR® ℞
(Finasteride)
Tablets

DESCRIPTION

PROSCAR* (finasteride), a synthetic 4-azasteroid compound, is a specific inhibitor of steroid Type II 5α-reductase, an intracellular enzyme that converts the androgen testosterone into 5α-dihydrotestosterone (DHT).
Finasteride is 4-azaandrost-1-ene-17-carboxamide, *N*-(1,1-dimethylethyl)-3-oxo-,(5α,17β)-. The empirical formula of

Continued on next page

Information on the Merck & Co., Inc., products listed on these pages is from the prescribing information in use October 1, 2004. For information, please call 1-800-NSC-MERCK [1-800-672-6372].

Proscar—Cont.

finasteride is $C_{23}H_{36}N_2O_2$ and its molecular weight is 372.55. Its structural formula is:

Finasteride is a white crystalline powder with a melting point near 250°C. It is freely soluble in chloroform and in lower alcohol solvents, but is practically insoluble in water. PROSCAR (finasteride) tablets for oral administration are film-coated tablets that contain 5 mg of finasteride and the following inactive ingredients: hydrous lactose, microcrystalline cellulose, pregelatinized starch, sodium starch glycolate, hydroxypropyl cellulose LF, hydroxypropylmethyl cellulose, titanium dioxide, magnesium stearate, talc, docusate sodium, FD&C Blue 2 aluminum lake and yellow iron oxide.

*Registered trademark of MERCK & CO., Inc.

CLINICAL PHARMACOLOGY

The development and enlargement of the prostate gland is dependent on the potent androgen, 5α-dihydrotestosterone (DHT). Type II 5α-reductase metabolizes testosterone to DHT in the prostate gland, liver and skin. DHT induces androgenic effects by binding to androgen receptors in the cell nuclei of these organs.

Finasteride is a competitive and specific inhibitor of Type II 5α-reductase with which it slowly forms a stable enzyme complex. Turnover from this complex is extremely slow ($t_{1/2}$ ~ 30 days). This has been demonstrated both *in vivo* and *in vitro*. Finasteride has no affinity for the androgen receptor. In man, the 5α-reduced steroid metabolites in blood and urine are decreased after administration of finasteride.

In man, a single 5-mg oral dose of PROSCAR produces a rapid reduction in serum DHT concentration, with the maximum effect observed 8 hours after the first dose. The suppression of DHT is maintained throughout the 24-hour dosing interval and with continued treatment. Daily dosing of PROSCAR at 5 mg/day for up to 4 years has been shown to reduce the serum DHT concentration by approximately 70%. The median circulating level of testosterone increased by approximately 10–20% but remained within the physiologic range.

Adult males with genetically inherited Type II 5α-reductase deficiency also have decreased levels of DHT. Except for the associated urogenital defects present at birth, no other clinical abnormalities related to Type II 5α-reductase deficiency have been observed in these individuals. These individuals have a small prostate gland throughout life and do not develop BPH.

In patients with BPH treated with finasteride (1–100 mg/day) for 7–10 days prior to prostatectomy, an approximate 80% lower DHT content was measured in prostatic tissue removed at surgery, compared to placebo; testosterone tissue concentration was increased up to 10 times over pretreatment levels, relative to placebo. Intraprostatic content of prostate-specific antigen (PSA) was also decreased.

In healthy male volunteers treated with PROSCAR for 14 days, discontinuation of therapy resulted in a return of DHT levels to pretreatment levels in approximately 2 weeks. In patients treated for three months, prostate volume, which declined by approximately 20%, returned to close to baseline value after approximately three months of discontinuation of therapy.

Pharmacokinetics

Absorption

In a study of 15 healthy young subjects, the mean bioavailability of finasteride 5-mg tablets was 63% (range 34–108%), based on the ratio of area under the curve (AUC) relative to an intravenous (IV) reference dose. Maximum finasteride plasma concentration averaged 37 ng/mL (range, 27–49 ng/mL) and was reached 1–2 hours postdose. Bioavailability of finasteride was not affected by food.

Distribution

Mean steady-state volume of distribution was 76 liters (range, 44–96 liters). Approximately 90% of circulating finasteride is bound to plasma proteins. There is a slow accumulation phase for finasteride after multiple dosing. After dosing with 5 mg/day of finasteride for 17 days, plasma concentrations of finasteride were 47 and 54% higher than after the first dose in men 45–60 years old (n=12) and ≥70 years old (n=12), respectively. Mean trough concentrations after 17 days of dosing were 6.2 ng/mL (range, 2.4–9.8 ng/mL) and 8.1 ng/mL (range, 1.8–19.7 ng/mL), respectively, in the two age groups. Although steady state was not reached in this study, mean trough plasma concentration in another study in patients with BPH (mean age, 65 years) receiving 5 mg/day was 9.4 ng/mL (range, 7.1–13.3 ng/mL; n=22) after over a year of dosing.

Finasteride has been shown to cross the blood brain barrier but does not appear to distribute preferentially to the CSF. In 2 studies of healthy subjects (n=69) receiving PROSCAR 5 mg/day for 6–24 weeks, finasteride concentrations in semen ranged from undetectable (<0.1 ng/mL) to 10.54 ng/mL. In an earlier study using a less sensitive assay, finasteride concentrations in the semen of 16 subjects receiving PROSCAR 5 mg/day ranged from undetectable (<1.0 ng/mL) to 21 ng/mL. Thus, based on a 5-mL ejaculate volume, the amount of finasteride in semen was estimated to be 50- to 100-fold less than the dose of finasteride (5 µg) that had no effect on circulating DHT levels in men (see also PRECAUTIONS, *Pregnancy*).

Metabolism

Finasteride is extensively metabolized in the liver, primarily via the cytochrome P450 3A4 enzyme subfamily. Two metabolites, the t-butyl side chain monohydroxylated and monocarboxylic acid metabolites, have been identified that possess no more than 20% of the 5α-reductase inhibitory activity of finasteride.

Excretion

In healthy young subjects (n=15), mean plasma clearance of finasteride was 165 mL/min (range, 70–279 mL/min) and mean elimination half-life in plasma was 6 hours (range, 3–16 hours). Following an oral dose of ^{14}C-finasteride in man (n=6), a mean of 39% (range, 32–46%) of the dose was excreted in the urine in the form of metabolites; 57% (range, 51–64%) was excreted in the feces.

The mean terminal half-life of finasteride in subjects ≥ 70 years of age was approximately 8 hours (range, 6–15 hours; n=12), compared with 6 hours (range, 4–12 hours; n=12) in subjects 45–60 years of age. As a result, mean AUC (0–24 hr) after 17 days of dosing was 15% higher in subjects ≥ 70 years of age than in subjects 45–60 years of age (p=0.02).

Special Populations

Pediatric: Finasteride pharmacokinetics have not been investigated in patients <18 years of age.

Gender: Finasteride pharmacokinetics in women are not available.

Geriatric: No dosage adjustment is necessary in the elderly. Although the elimination rate of finasteride is decreased in the elderly, these findings are of no clinical significance. See also *Pharmacokinetics*, *Excretion*, PRECAUTIONS, *Geriatric Use* and DOSAGE AND ADMINISTRATION.

Race: The effect of race on finasteride pharmacokinetics has not been studied.

Renal Insufficiency: No dosage adjustment is necessary in patients with renal insufficiency. In patients with chronic renal impairment, with creatinine clearances ranging from 9.0 to 55 mL/min, AUC, maximum plasma concentration, half-life, and protein binding after a single dose of ^{14}C-finasteride were similar to values obtained in healthy volunteers. Urinary excretion of metabolites was decreased in patients with renal impairment. This decrease was associated with an increase in fecal excretion of metabolites. Plasma concentrations of metabolites were significantly higher in patients with renal impairment (based on a 60% increase in total radioactivity AUC). However, finasteride has been well tolerated in BPH patients with normal renal function receiving up to 80 mg/day for 12 weeks, where exposure of these patients to metabolites would presumably be much greater.

Hepatic Insufficiency: The effect of hepatic insufficiency on finasteride pharmacokinetics has not been studied. Caution should be used in the administration of PROSCAR in those patients with liver function abnormalities, as finasteride is metabolized extensively in the liver.

Drug Interactions (also see PRECAUTIONS, *Drug Interactions*)

No drug interactions of clinical importance have been identified. Finasteride does not appear to affect the cytochrome P450-linked drug metabolism enzyme system. Compounds that have been tested in man have included antipyrine, digoxin, propranolol, theophylline, and warfarin, and no clinically meaningful interactions were found.

Mean (SD) Noncompartmental Pharmacokinetic Parameters After Multiple Doses of 5 mg/day in Older Men

	Mean (± SD)	
	45-60 years old (n=12)	≥70 years old (n=12)
AUC (ng•hr/mL)	389 (98)	463 (186)
Peak Concentration (ng/mL)	46.2 (8.7)	48.4 (14.7)
Time to Peak (hours)	1.8 (0.7)	1.8 (0.6)
Half-Life (hours)*	6.0 (1.5)	8.2 (2.5)

*First-dose values; all other parameters are last-dose values

Mean (SD) Pharmacokinetic Parameters in Healthy Young Subjects (n=15)

	Mean (± SD)
Bioavailability	63% (34-108%)*
Clearance (mL/min)	165 (55)
Volume of Distribution (L)	76 (14)
Half-Life (hours)	6.2 (2.1)

*Range

[See table below]

Clinical Studies

PROSCAR 5 mg/day was initially evaluated in patients with symptoms of BPH and enlarged prostates by digital rectal examination in two 1-year, placebo-controlled, randomized, double-blind studies and their 5-year open extensions.

PROSCAR was further evaluated in the PROSCAR Long-Term Efficacy and Safety Study (PLESS), a double-blind randomized, placebo-controlled, 4-year, multicenter study. 3040 patients between the ages of 45 and 78, with moderate to severe symptoms of BPH and an enlarged prostate upon digital rectal examination, were randomized into the study (1524 to finasteride, 1516 to placebo) and 3016 patients were evaluable for efficacy. 1883 patients completed the 4-year study (1000 in the finasteride group, 883 in the placebo group).

Effect on Symptom Score

Symptoms were quantified using a score similar to the American Urological Association Symptom Score, which evaluated both obstructive symptoms (impairment of size and force of stream, sensation of incomplete bladder emptying, delayed or interrupted urination) and irritative symptoms (nocturia, daytime frequency, need to strain or push the flow of urine) by rating on a 0 to 5 scale for six symptoms and a 0 to 4 scale for one symptom, for a total possible score of 34.

Patients in PLESS, had moderate to severe symptoms at baseline (mean of approximately 15 points on a 0–34 point scale). Patients randomized to PROSCAR who remained on therapy for 4 years had a mean (± 1 SD) decrease in symptom score of 3.3 (± 5.8) points compared with 1.3 (± 5.6) points in the placebo group. (See Figure 1.) A statistically significant improvement in symptom score was evident at 1 year in patients treated with PROSCAR vs placebo (–2.3 vs –1.6), and this improvement continued through Year 4.

Figure 1
Symptom Score in PLESS

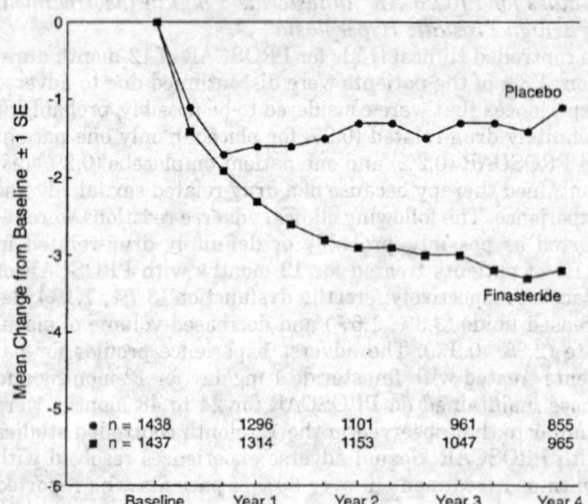

Results seen in earlier studies were comparable to those seen in PLESS. Although an early improvement in urinary symptoms was seen in some patients, a therapeutic trial of at least 6 months was generally necessary to assess whether a beneficial response in symptom relief had been achieved. The improvement in BPH symptoms was seen during the first year and maintained throughout an additional 5 years of open extension studies.

Effect on Acute Urinary Retention and the Need for Surgery

In PLESS, efficacy was also assessed by evaluating treatment failures. Treatment failure was prospectively defined as BPH related urological events or clinical deterioration, lack of improvement and/or the need for alternative therapy. BPH-related urological events were defined as urological surgical intervention and acute urinary retention requiring catheterization. Complete event information was available for 92% of the patients. The following table (Table 1) summarizes the results.

[See table 1 at top of next page]

Compared with placebo, PROSCAR was associated with a significantly lower risk for acute urinary retention or the need for BPH-related surgery [13.2% for placebo vs 6.6% for PROSCAR; 51% reduction in risk, 95% CI: (34 to 63%)]. Compared with placebo, PROSCAR was associated with a significantly lower risk for surgery [10.1% for placebo vs

4.6% for PROSCAR; 55% reduction in risk, 95% CI: (37 to 68%)] and with a significantly lower risk of acute urinary retention [6.6% for placebo vs 2.8% for PROSCAR; 57% reduction in risk, 95% CI: (34 to 72%)]; See Figures 2 and 3.

Figure 2
Percent of Patients Having Surgery for BPH, Including TURP

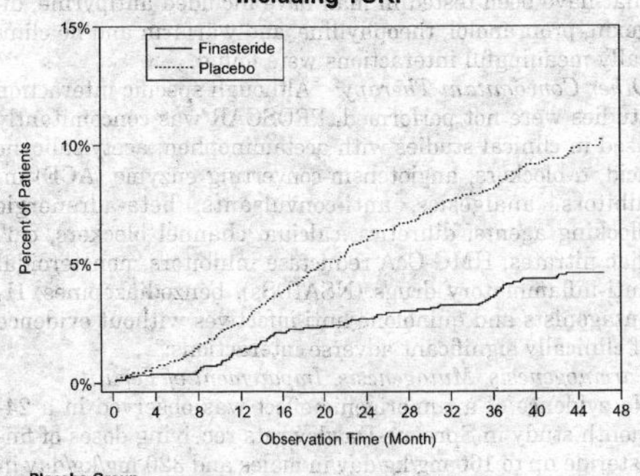

Placebo Group				
No. of events, cumulative	37	89	121	152
No. at risk, per year	1503	1454	1374	1314
Finasteride Group				
No. of events, cumulative	18	40	49	69
No. at risk, per year	1513	1483	1438	1410

Figure 3
Percent of Patients Developing Acute Urinary Retention (Spontaneous and Precipitated)

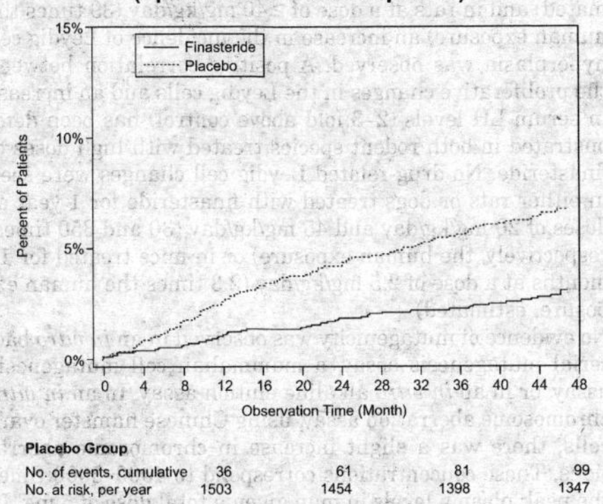

Placebo Group				
No. of events, cumulative	36	61	81	99
No. at risk, per year	1503	1454	1398	1347
Finasteride Group				
No. of events, cumulative	14	25	32	42
No. at risk, per year	1513	1487	1449	1421

Effect on Maximum Urinary Flow Rate

In the patients in PLESS who remained on therapy for the duration of the study and had evaluable urinary flow data, PROSCAR increased maximum urinary flow rate by 1.9 mL/sec compared with 0.2 mL/sec in the placebo group.

There was a clear difference between treatment groups in maximum urinary flow rate in favor of PROSCAR by month 4 (1.0 vs 0.3 mL/sec) which was maintained throughout the study. In the earlier 1-year studies, increase in maximum urinary flow rate was comparable to PLESS and was maintained through the first year and throughout an additional 5 years of open extension studies.

Effect on Prostate Volume

In PLESS, prostate volume was assessed yearly by magnetic resonance imaging (MRI) in a subset of patients. In patients treated with PROSCAR who remained on therapy, prostate volume was reduced compared with both baseline and placebo throughout the 4-year study. PROSCAR decreased prostate volume by 17.9% (from 55.9 cc at baseline to 45.8 cc at 4 years) compared with an increase of 14.1% (from 51.3 cc to 58.5 cc) in the placebo group (p<0.001). (See Figure 4.)

Results seen in earlier studies were comparable to those seen in PLESS. Mean prostate volume at baseline ranged between 40-50 cc. The reduction in prostate volume was seen during the first year and maintained throughout an additional five years of open extension studies.

Figure 4
Prostate Volume in PLESS

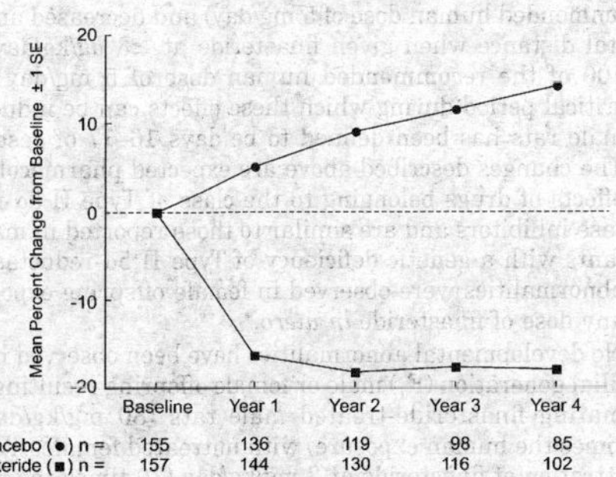

Placebo (●) n =	155	136	119	98	85
Finasteride (■) n =	157	144	130	116	102

Table 1
All Treatment Failures in PLESS

Event	Patients (%) * Placebo N=1503	Finasteride N=1513	Relative Risk**	95% CI	P Value**
All Treatment Failures	37.1	26.2	0.68	(0.57 to 0.79)	<0.001
Surgical Interventions for BPH	10.1	4.6	0.45	(0.32 to 0.63)	<0.001
Acute Urinary Retention Requiring Catheterization	6.6	2.8	0.43	(0.28 to 0.66)	<0.001
Two consecutive symptoms scores ≥20	9.2	6.7			
Bladder Stone	0.4	0.5			
Incontinence	2.1	1.7			
Renal Failure	0.5	0.6			
UTI	5.7	4.9			
Discontinuation due to worsening of BPH, lack of improvement, or to receive other medical treatment	21.8	13.3			

*patients with multiple events may be counted more than once for each type of event
**Hazard ratio based on log rank test

Table 2
Count and Percent Incidence of Primary Outcome Events by Treatment Group in MTOPS

Event	Treatment Group Placebo N=737 N (%)	Doxazosin N=756 N (%)	Finasteride N=768 N (%)	Combination N=786 N (%)	Total N=3047 N (%)
AUA 4-point rise	100 (13.6)	59 (7.8)	74 (9.6)	41 (5.2)	274 (9.0)
Acute urinary retention	18 (2.4)	13 (1.7)	6 (0.8)	4 (0.5)	41 (1.3)
Incontinence	8 (1.1)	11 (1.5)	9 (1.2)	3 (0.4)	31 (1.0)
Recurrent UTI/ urosepsis	2 (0.3)	2 (0.3)	0 (0.0)	1 (0.1)	5 (0.2)
Creatinine rise	0 (0.0)	0 (0.0)	0 (0.0)	0 (0.0)	0 (0.0)
Total events	128 (17.4)	85 (11.2)	89 (11.6)	49 (6.2)	351 (11.5)

Prostate Volume as a Predictor of Therapeutic Response

A meta-analysis combining 1-year data from seven double-blind, placebo-controlled studies of similar design, including 4491 patients with symptomatic BPH, demonstrated that, in patients treated with PROSCAR, the magnitude of symptom response and degree of improvement in maximum urinary flow rate were greater in patients with an enlarged prostate at baseline.

Medical Therapy of Prostatic Symptoms

The Medical Therapy of Prostatic Symptoms (MTOPS) Trial was a double-blind, randomized, placebo-controlled, multicenter, 4- to 6-year study (average 5 years) in 3047 men with symptomatic BPH, who were randomized to receive PROSCAR 5 mg/day (n=768), doxazosin 4 or 8 mg/day (n=756), the combination of PROSCAR 5 mg/day and doxazosin 4 or 8 mg/day (n=786), or placebo (n=737). All participants underwent weekly titration of doxazosin (or its placebo) from 1 to 2 to 4 to 8 mg/day. Only those who tolerated the 4 or 8 mg dose level were kept on doxazosin (or its placebo) in the study. The participant's final tolerated dose (either 4 mg or 8 mg) was administered beginning at end-Week 4. The final doxazosin dose was administered once per day, at bedtime.

The mean patient age at randomization was 62.6 years (±7.3 years). Patients were Caucasian (82%), African American (9%), Hispanic (7%), Asian (1%) or Native American (<1%). The mean duration of BPH symptoms was 4.7 years (±4.6 years). Patients had moderate to severe BPH symptoms at baseline with a mean AUA symptom score of approximately 17 out of 35 points. Mean maximum urinary flow rate was 10.5 mL/sec (±2.6 mL/sec). The mean prostate volume as measured by transrectal ultrasound was 36.3 mL (±20.1 mL). Prostate volume was ≤20 mL in 16% of patients, ≥50 mL in 18% of patients and between 21 and 40 mL in 66% of patients.

The primary endpoint was a composite measure of the first occurrence of any of the following five outcomes: a ≥4 point confirmed increase from baseline in symptom score, acute urinary retention, BPH-related renal insufficiency (creatinine rise), recurrent urinary tract infections or urosepsis, or incontinence. Compared to placebo, treatment with PROSCAR, doxazosin, or combination therapy resulted in a reduction in the risk of experiencing one of these five outcome events by 34% (p=0.002), 39% (p<0.001), and 67% (p<0.001), respectively. Combination therapy resulted in a significant reduction in the risk of the primary endpoint compared to treatment with PROSCAR alone (49%; p≤0.001) or doxazosin alone (46%; p≤0.001). (See Table 2.)

[See table 2 above]

The majority of the events (274 out of 351; 78%) was a confirmed ≥4 point increase in symptom score, referred to as symptom score progression. The risk of symptom score progression was reduced by 30% (p=0.016), 46% (p<0.001), and 64% (p<0.001) in patients treated with PROSCAR, doxazosin, or the combination, respectively, compared to patients treated with placebo (see Figure 5). Combination therapy significantly reduced the risk of symptom score progression compared to the effect of PROSCAR alone (p<0.001) and compared to doxazosin alone (p=0.037).

Figure 5
Cumulative Incidence of a 4-Point Rise in AUA Symptom Score by Treatment Group

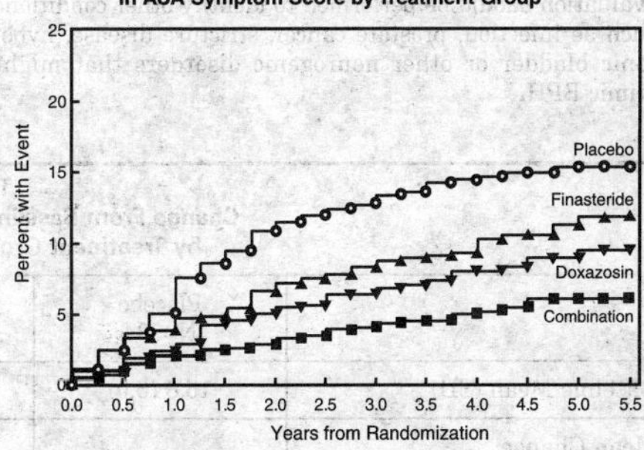

Treatment with PROSCAR, doxazosin or the combination of PROSCAR with doxazosin, reduced the mean symptom

Continued on next page

Information on the Merck & Co., Inc., products listed on these pages is from the prescribing information in use October 1, 2004. For information, please call 1-800-NSC-MERCK [1-800-672-6372].

Proscar—Cont.

score from baseline at year 4. Table 3 provides the mean change from baseline for AUA symptom score by treatment group for patients who remained on therapy for four years. [See table 3 below]

The results of MTOPS are consistent with the findings of the 4-year, placebo-controlled study PLESS (see CLINICAL PHARMACOLOGY, *Clinical Studies*) in that treatment with PROSCAR reduces the risk of acute urinary retention and the need for BPH-related surgery. In MTOPS, the risk of developing acute urinary retention was reduced by 67% in patients treated with PROSCAR compared to patients treated with placebo (0.8% for PROSCAR and 2.4% for placebo). Also, the risk of requiring BPH-related invasive therapy was reduced by 64% in patients treated with PROSCAR compared to patients treated with placebo (2.0% for PROSCAR and 5.4% for placebo).

Summary of Clinical Studies

The data from these studies, showing improvement in BPH-related symptoms, reduction in treatment failure (BPH-related urological events), increased maximum urinary flow rates, and decreasing prostate volume, suggest that PROSCAR arrests the disease process of BPH in men with an enlarged prostate.

INDICATIONS AND USAGE

PROSCAR is indicated for the treatment of symptomatic benign prostatic hyperplasia (BPH) in men with an enlarged prostate to:

— Improve symptoms
— Reduce the risk of acute urinary retention
— Reduce the risk of the need for surgery including transurethral resection of the prostate (TURP) and prostatectomy.

PROSCAR administered in combination with the alpha-blocker doxazosin is indicated to reduce the risk of symptomatic progression of BPH (a confirmed ≥4 point increase in AUA symptom score).

CONTRAINDICATIONS

PROSCAR is contraindicated in the following:

Hypersensitivity to any component of this medication.

Pregnancy. Finasteride use is contraindicated in women when they are or may potentially be pregnant. Because of the ability of Type II 5α-reductase inhibitors to inhibit the conversion of testosterone to DHT, finasteride may cause abnormalities of the external genitalia of a male fetus of a pregnant woman who receives finasteride. If this drug is used during pregnancy, or if pregnancy occurs while taking this drug, the pregnant woman should be apprised of the potential hazard to the male fetus. (See also WARNINGS, EXPOSURE OF WOMEN—RISK TO MALE FETUS and PRECAUTIONS, *Information for Patients* and *Pregnancy*.) In female rats, low doses of finasteride administered during pregnancy have produced abnormalities of the external genitalia in male offspring.

WARNINGS

PROSCAR is not indicated for use in pediatric patients (see PRECAUTIONS, *Pediatric Use*) or women (see also WARNINGS, EXPOSURE OF WOMEN—RISK TO MALE FETUS; PRECAUTIONS, *Information for Patients* and *Pregnancy*, and HOW SUPPLIED).

EXPOSURE OF WOMEN—RISK TO MALE FETUS

Women should not handle crushed or broken PROSCAR tablets when they are pregnant or may potentially be pregnant because of the possibility of absorption of finasteride and the subsequent potential risk to a male fetus. PROSCAR tablets are coated and will prevent contact with the active ingredient during normal handling, provided that the tablets have not been broken or crushed. (See CONTRAINDICATIONS; PRECAUTIONS, *Information for Patients* and *Pregnancy*, and HOW SUPPLIED).

PRECAUTIONS

General

Prior to initiating therapy with PROSCAR, appropriate evaluation should be performed to identify other conditions such as infection, prostate cancer, stricture disease, hypotonic bladder or other neurogenic disorders that might mimic BPH.

Patients with large residual urinary volume and/or severely diminished urinary flow should be carefully monitored for obstructive uropathy. These patients may not be candidates for finasteride therapy.

Caution should be used in the administration of PROSCAR in those patients with liver function abnormalities, as finasteride is metabolized extensively in the liver.

Effects on PSA and Prostate Cancer Detection

No clinical benefit has been demonstrated in patients with prostate cancer treated with PROSCAR. Patients with BPH and elevated PSA were monitored in controlled clinical studies with serial PSAs and prostate biopsies. In these BPH studies, PROSCAR did not appear to alter the rate of prostate cancer detection, and the overall incidence of prostate cancer was not significantly different in patients treated with PROSCAR or placebo.

PROSCAR causes a decrease in serum PSA levels by approximately 50% in patients with BPH, even in the presence of prostate cancer. This decrease is predictable over the entire range of PSA values, although it may vary in individual patients. Analysis of PSA data from over 3000 patients in PLESS confirmed that in typical patients treated with PROSCAR for six months or more, PSA values should be doubled for comparison with normal ranges in untreated men. This adjustment preserves the sensitivity and specificity of the PSA assay and maintains its ability to detect prostate cancer.

Any sustained increases in PSA levels while on PROSCAR should be carefully evaluated, including consideration of non-compliance to therapy with PROSCAR.

Percent free PSA (free to total PSA ratio) is not significantly decreased by PROSCAR. The ratio of free to total PSA remains constant even under the influence of PROSCAR. If clinicians elect to use percent free PSA as an aid in the detection of prostate cancer in men undergoing finasteride therapy, no adjustment to its value appears necessary.

Information for Patients

Women should not handle crushed or broken PROSCAR tablets when they are pregnant or may potentially be pregnant because of the possibility of absorption of finasteride and the subsequent potential risk to the male fetus (see CONTRAINDICATIONS; WARNINGS, EXPOSURE OF WOMEN—RISK TO MALE FETUS; PRECAUTIONS, *Pregnancy* and HOW SUPPLIED).

Physicians should inform patients that the volume of ejaculate may be decreased in some patients during treatment with PROSCAR. This decrease does not appear to interfere with normal sexual function. However, impotence and decreased libido may occur in patients treated with PROSCAR (see ADVERSE REACTIONS).

Physicians should instruct their patients to promptly report any changes in their breasts such as lumps, pain or nipple discharge. Breast changes including breast enlargement, tenderness and neoplasm have been reported (see ADVERSE REACTIONS).

Physicians should instruct their patients to read the patient package insert before starting therapy with PROSCAR and to reread it each time the prescription is renewed so that they are aware of current information for patients regarding PROSCAR.

Drug/Laboratory Test Interactions

In patients with BPH, PROSCAR has no effect on circulating levels of cortisol, estradiol, prolactin, thyroid-stimulating hormone, or thyroxine. No clinically meaningful effect was observed on the plasma lipid profile (i.e., total cholesterol, low density lipoproteins, high density lipoproteins and triglycerides) or bone mineral density. Increases of about 10% were observed in luteinizing hormone (LH) and follicle-stimulating hormone (FSH) in patients receiving PROSCAR, but levels remained within the normal range. In healthy volunteers, treatment with PROSCAR did not alter the response of LH and FSH to gonadotropin-releasing hormone indicating that the hypothalamic-pituitary-testicular axis was not affected.

Treatment with PROSCAR for 24 weeks to evaluate semen parameters in healthy male volunteers revealed no clinically meaningful effects on sperm concentration, mobility, morphology, or pH. A 0.6 mL (22.1%) median decrease in ejaculate volume with a concomitant reduction in total sperm per ejaculate, was observed. These parameters remained within the normal range and were reversible upon discontinuation of therapy with an average time to return to baseline of 84 weeks.

Drug Interactions

No drug interactions of clinical importance have been identified. Finasteride does not appear to affect the cytochrome P450-linked drug metabolizing enzyme system. Compounds that have been tested in man have included antipyrine, digoxin, propranolol, theophylline, and warfarin and no clinically meaningful interactions were found.

Other Concomitant Therapy: Although specific interaction studies were not performed, PROSCAR was concomitantly used in clinical studies with acetaminophen, acetylsalicylic acid, α-blockers, angiotensin-converting enzyme (ACE) inhibitors, analgesics, anti-convulsants, beta-adrenergic blocking agents, diuretics, calcium channel blockers, cardiac nitrates, HMG-CoA reductase inhibitors, nonsteroidal anti-inflammatory drugs (NSAIDSs), benzodiazepines, H_2 antagonists and quinolone anti-infectives without evidence of clinically significant adverse interactions.

Carcinogenesis, Mutagenesis, Impairment of Fertility

No evidence of a tumorigenic effect was observed in a 24-month study in Sprague-Dawley rats receiving doses of finasteride up to 160 mg/kg/day in males and 320 mg/kg/day in females. These doses produced respective systemic exposure in rats of 111 and 274 times those observed in man receiving the recommended human dose of 5 mg/day. All exposure calculations were based on calculated AUC (0–24hr) for animals and mean AUC (0–24 hr) for man (0.4 μg • hr/mL).

In a 19-month carcinogenicity study in CD-1 mice, a statistically significant ($p \leq 0.05$) increase in the incidence of testicular Leydig cell adenomas was observed at a dose of 250 mg/kg/day (228 times the human exposure). In mice at a dose of 25 mg/kg/day (23 times the human exposure, estimated) and in rats at a dose of ≥40 mg/kg/day (39 times the human exposure) an increase in the incidence of Leydig cell hyperplasia was observed. A positive correlation between the proliferative changes in the Leydig cells and an increase in serum LH levels (2–3 fold above control) has been demonstrated in both rodent species treated with high doses of finasteride. No drug-related Leydig cell changes were seen in either rats or dogs treated with finasteride for 1 year at doses of 20 mg/kg/day and 45 mg/kg/day (30 and 350 times, respectively, the human exposure) or in mice treated for 19 months at a dose of 2.5 mg/kg/day (2.3 times the human exposure, estimated).

No evidence of mutagenicity was observed in an *in vitro* bacterial mutagenesis assay, a mammalian cell mutagenesis assay, or in an *in vitro* alkaline elution assay. In an *in vitro* chromosome aberration assay, using Chinese hamster ovary cells, there was a slight increase in chromosome aberrations. These concentrations correspond to 4000–5000 times the peak plasma levels in man given a total dose of 5 mg. In an *in vivo* chromosome aberration assay in mice, no treatment-related increase in chromosome aberration was observed with finasteride at the maximum tolerated dose of 250 mg/kg/day (228 times the human exposure) as determined in the carcinogenicity studies.

In sexually mature male rabbits treated with finasteride at 80 mg/kg/day (543 times the human exposure) for up to 12 weeks, no effect on fertility, sperm count, or ejaculate volume was seen. In sexually mature male rats treated with 80 mg/kg/day of finasteride (61 times the human exposure), there were no significant effects on fertility after 6 or 12 weeks of treatment; however, when treatment was continued for up to 24 or 30 weeks, there was an apparent decrease in fertility, fecundity and an associated significant decrease in the weights of the seminal vesicles and prostate. All these effects were reversible within 6 weeks of discontinuation of treatment. No drug-related effect on testes or on mating performance has been seen in rats or rabbits. This decrease in fertility in finasteride-treated rats is secondary to its effect on accessory sex organs (prostate and seminal vesicles) resulting in failure to form a seminal plug. The seminal plug is essential for normal fertility in rats and is not relevant in man.

Pregnancy

Pregnancy Category X

See CONTRAINDICATIONS.

PROSCAR is not indicated for use in women.

Administration of finasteride to pregnant rats at doses ranging from 100 μg/kg/day to 100 mg/kg/day (1–1000 times the recommended human dose of 5 mg/day) resulted in dose-dependent development of hypospadias in 3.6 to 100% of male offspring. Pregnant rats produced male offspring with decreased prostatic and seminal vesicular weights, delayed preputial separation and transient nipple development when given finasteride at ≥30 μg/kg/day (≥3/10 of the recommended human dose of 5 mg/day) and decreased anogenital distance when given finasteride at ≥3 μg/kg/day (≥3/100 of the recommended human dose of 5 mg/day). The critical period during which these effects can be induced in male rats has been defined to be days 16–17 of gestation. The changes described above are expected pharmacological effects of drugs belonging to the class of Type II 5α-reductase inhibitors and are similar to those reported in male infants with a genetic deficiency of Type II 5α-reductase. No abnormalities were observed in female offspring exposed to any dose of finasteride *in utero*.

No developmental abnormalities have been observed in first filial generation (F_1) male or female offspring resulting from mating finasteride-treated male rats (80 mg/kg/day; 61 times the human exposure) with untreated females. Administration of finasteride at 3 mg/kg/day (30 times the recom-

Table 3
Change From Baseline in AUA Symptom Score by Treatment Group at Year 4 in MTOPS

	Placebo N=534	Doxazosin N=582	Finasteride N=565	Combination N=598
Baseline Mean (SD)	16.8 (6.0)	17.0 (5.9)	17.1 (6.0)	16.8 (5.8)
Mean Change AUA Symptom Score (SD)	−4.9 (5.8)	−6.6 (6.1)	−5.6 (5.9)	−7.4 (6.3)
Comparison to Placebo (95% CI)		−1.8 (−2.5, −1.1)	−0.7 (−1.4, 0.0)	−2.5 (−3.2, −1.8)
Comparison to Doxazosin alone (95% CI)				−0.7 (−1.4, 0.0)
Comparison to Finasteride alone (95% CI)				−1.8 (−2.5, −1.1)

mended human dose of 5 mg/day) during the late gestation and lactation period resulted in slightly decreased fertility in F_1 male offspring. No effects were seen in female offspring. No evidence of malformations has been observed in rabbit fetuses exposed to finasteride *in utero* from days 6–18 of gestation at doses up to 100 mg/kg/day (1000 times the recommended human dose of 5 mg/day). However, effects on male genitalia would not be expected since the rabbits were not exposed during the critical period of genital system development.

The *in utero* effects of finasteride exposure during the period of embryonic and fetal development were evaluated in the rhesus monkey (gestation days 20–100), a species more predictive of human development than rats or rabbits. Intravenous administration of finasteride to pregnant monkeys at doses as high as 800 ng/day (at least 60 to 120 times the highest estimated exposure of pregnant women to finasteride from semen of men taking 5 mg/day) resulted in no abnormalities in male fetuses. In confirmation of the relevance of the rhesus model for human fetal development, oral administration of a dose of finasteride (2 mg/kg/day; 20 times the recommended human dose of 5 mg/day or approximately 1–2 million times the highest estimated exposure to finasteride from semen of men taking 5 mg/day) to pregnant monkeys resulted in external genital abnormalities in male fetuses. No other abnormalities were observed in male fetuses and no finasteride-related abnormalities were observed in female fetuses at any dose.

Nursing Mothers

PROSCAR is not indicated for use in women.

It is not known whether finasteride is excreted in human milk.

Pediatric Use

PROSCAR is not indicated for use in pediatric patients. Safety and effectiveness in pediatric patients have not been established.

Geriatric Use

Of the total number of subjects included in PLESS, 1480 and 105 subjects were 65 and over and 75 and over, respectively. No overall differences in safety or effectiveness were observed between these subjects and younger subjects, and other reported clinical experience has not identified differences in responses between the elderly and younger patients. No dosage adjustment is necessary in the elderly (see CLINICAL PHARMACOLOGY, *Pharmacokinetics* and *Clinical Studies*).

ADVERSE REACTIONS

PROSCAR is generally well tolerated; adverse reactions usually have been mild and transient.

4-Year Placebo-Controlled Study

In PLESS, 1524 patients treated with PROSCAR and 1516 patients treated with placebo were evaluated for safety over a period of 4 years. The most frequently reported adverse reactions were related to sexual function. 3.7% (57 patients) treated with PROSCAR and 2.1% (32 patients) treated with placebo discontinued therapy as a result of adverse reactions related to sexual function, which are the most frequently reported adverse reactions.

Table 4 presents the only clinical adverse reactions considered possibly, probably or definitely drug related by the investigator, for which the incidence on PROSCAR was ≥1% and greater than placebo over the 4 years of the study. In years 2–4 of the study, there was no significant difference between treatment groups in the incidences of impotence, decreased libido and ejaculation disorder.

[See table 4 above]

TABLE 4
Drug-Related Adverse Experiences

	Year 1 (%)		Years 2, 3 and 4* (%)	
	Finasteride	Placebo	Finasteride	Placebo
Impotence	8.1	3.7	5.1	5.1
Decreased Libido	6.4	3.4	2.6	2.6
Decreased Volume of Ejaculate	3.7	0.8	1.5	0.5
Ejaculation Disorder	0.8	0.1	0.2	0.1
Breast Enlargement	0.5	0.1	1.8	1.1
Breast Tenderness	0.4	0.1	0.7	0.3
Rash	0.5	0.2	0.5	0.1

*Combined Years 2-4
N = 1524 and 1516, finasteride vs placebo, respectively

Phase III Studies and 5-Year Open Extensions

The adverse experience profile in the 1–year, placebo-controlled, Phase III studies, the 5-year open extensions, and PLESS were similar.

Medical Therapy of Prostatic Symptoms (MTOPS) Study

The incidence rates of drug-related adverse experiences reported by ≥2% of patients in any treatment group in the MTOPS Study are listed in Table 5.

The individual adverse effects which occurred more frequently in the combination group compared to either drug alone were: asthenia, postural hypotension, peripheral edema, dizziness, decreased libido, rhinitis, abnormal ejaculation, impotence and abnormal sexual function (see Table 5). Of these, the incidence of abnormal ejaculation in patients receiving combination therapy was comparable to the sum of the incidences of this adverse experience reported for the two monotherapies.

Combination therapy with finasteride and doxazosin was associated with no new clinical adverse experience.

Four patients in MTOPS reported the adverse exprience breast cancer. Three of these patients were on finasteride only and one was on combination therapy. (See ADVERSE REACTIONS, *Long-Term Data*.)

The MTOPS Study was not specifically designed to make statistical comparisons between groups for reported adverse experiences. In addition, direct comparisons of safety data between the MTOPS study and previous studies of the single agents may not be appropriate based upon differences in patient population, dosage or dose regimen, and other procedural and study design elements.

[See table 5 above]

Table 5
Incidence ≥ 2% in One or More Treatment Groups
Drug-Related Clinical Adverse Experiences in MTOPS

Adverse Experience	Placebo (N=737) (%)	Doxazosin 4 mg or 8 mg* (N=756) (%)	Finasteride (N=768) (%)	Combination (N=786) (%)
Body as a whole				
Asthenia	7.1	15.7	5.3	16.8
Headache	2.3	4.1	2.0	2.3
Cardiovascular				
Hypotension	0.7	3.4	1.2	1.5
Postural Hypotension	8.0	16.7	9.1	17.8
Metabolic and Nutritional				
Peripheral Edema	0.9	2.6	1.3	3.3
Nervous				
Dizziness	8.1	17.7	7.4	23.2
Libido Decreased	5.7	7.0	10.0	11.6
Somnolence	1.5	3.7	1.7	3.1
Respiratory				
Dyspnea	0.7	2.1	0.7	1.9
Rhinitis	0.5	1.3	1.0	2.4
Urogenital				
Abnormal Ejaculation	2.3	4.5	7.2	14.1
Gynecomastia	0.7	1.1	2.2	1.5
Impotence	12.2	14.4	18.5	22.6
Sexual Function Abnormal	0.9	2.0	2.5	3.1

*Doxazosin dose was achieved by weekly titration (1 to 2 to 4 to 8 mg). The final tolerated dose (4 mg or 8 mg) was administered at end-Week 4. Only those patients tolerating at least 4 mg were kept on doxazosin. The majority of patients received the 8-mg dose over the duration of the study.

Long-Term Data

There is no evidence of increased adverse experiences with increased duration of treatment with PROSCAR. New reports of drug-related sexual adverse experiences decreased with duration of therapy.

During the 4- to 6-year placebo- and comparator-controlled MTOPS study that enrolled 3047 men, there were 4 cases of breast cancer in men treated with finasteride but no cases in men not treated with finasteride. During the 4-year, placebo-controlled PLESS study that enrolled 3040 men, there were 2 cases of breast cancer in placebo-treated men, but no cases were reported in men treated with finasteride. The relationship between long-term use of finasteride and male breast neoplasia is currently unknown.

In a 7-year placebo-controlled trial that enrolled 18,882 healthy men, 9060 had prostate needle biopsy data available for analysis. In the PROSCAR group, 280 (6.4%) men had prostate cancer with Gleason scores of 7–10 detected on needle biopsy vs. 237 (5.1%) men in the placebo group. Of the total cases of prostate cancer diagnosed in this study, approximately 98% were classified as intracapsular (stage T1 or T2). The clinical significance of these findings is unknown. This information from the literature (Thompson IM, Goodman PJ, Tangen CM, et al. The influence of finasteride on the development of prostate cancer. *N Engl J Med* 2003; 349:213–22) is provided for considration by physicians when PROSCAR is used as indicated (see INDICATIONS AND USAGE). PROSCAR is not approved to reduce the risk of developing prostate cancer,

Post-Marketing Experience

The following additional adverse effects have been reported in post-marketing experience:

—hypersensitivity reactions, including pruritus, urticaria, and swelling of the lips and face

—testicular pain.

OVERDOSAGE

Patients have received single doses of PROSCAR up to 400 mg and multiple doses of PROSCAR up to 80 mg/day for three months without adverse effects. Until further experience is obtained, no specific treatment for an overdose with PROSCAR can be recommended.

Significant lethality was observed in male and female mice at single oral doses of 1500 mg/m^2 (500 mg/kg) and in female and male rats at single oral doses of 2360 mg/m^2 (400 mg/kg) and 5900 mg/m^2 (1000 mg/kg), respectively.

DOSAGE AND ADMINISTRATION

The recommended dose is 5 mg orally once a day.

PROSCAR can be administered alone or in combination with the alpha-blocker doxazosin (see CLINICAL PHARMACOLOGY, *Clinical Studies*).

PROSCAR may be administered with or without meals.

Continued on next page

Information on the Merck & Co., Inc., products listed on these pages is from the prescribing information in use October 1, 2004. For information, please call 1-800-NSC-MERCK [1-800-672-6372].

Proscar—Cont.

No dosage adjustment is necessary for patients with renal impairment or for the elderly (see CLINICAL PHARMACOLOGY, *Pharmacokinetics*).

HOW SUPPLIED

No. 3094—PROSCAR tablets 5 mg are blue, modified apple-shaped, film-coated tablets, with the code MSD 72 on one side and PROSCAR on the other. They are supplied as follows:

NDC 0006-0072-31 unit of use bottles of 30
NDC 0006-0072-58 unit of use bottles of 100
NDC 0006-0072-28 unit dose packages of 100
NDC 0006-0072-82 bottles of 1000.

Storage and Handling

Store at room temperatures below 30°C (86°F). Protect from light and keep container tightly closed.

Women should not handle crushed or broken PROSCAR tablets when they are pregnant or may potentially be pregnant because of the possibility of absorption of finasteride and the subsequent potential risk to a male fetus (see WARNINGS, EXPOSURE OF WOMEN—RISK TO MALE FETUS, and PRECAUTIONS, *Information for Patients* and *Pregnancy*).

9556708 Issued April 2004

Patient Information about PROSCAR® (Prahs-car)

Generic name: finasteride (fin-AS-tur-eyed)

PROSCAR* is for use by men only.

Please read this leaflet before you start taking PROSCAR. Also, read it each time you renew your prescription, just in case anything has changed. Remember, this leaflet does not take the place of careful discussions with your doctor. You and your doctor should discuss PROSCAR when you start taking your medication and at regular checkups.

---

*Registered trademark of MERCK & CO., INC.

Why your doctor has prescribed PROSCAR

Your doctor has prescribed PROSCAR because you have a medical condition called benign prostatic hyperplasia or BPH. This occurs only in men.

What is BPH?

BPH is an enlargement of the prostate gland. After age 50, most men develop enlarged prostates. The prostate is located below the bladder. As the prostate enlarges, it may slowly restrict the flow of urine. This can lead to symptoms such as:

- a weak or interrupted urinary stream
- a feeling that you cannot empty your bladder completely
- a feeling of delay or hesitation when you start to urinate
- a need to urinate often, especially at night
- a feeling that you must urinate right away.

In some men, BPH can lead to serious problems, including urinary tract infections, a sudden inability to pass urine (acute urinary retention), as well as the need for surgery.

Treatment options for BPH

There are three main treatment options for symptoms of BPH:

- **Program of monitoring or "Watchful Waiting".** If a man has an enlarged prostate gland and no symptoms or if his symptoms do not bother him, he and his doctor may decide on a program of monitoring which would include regular checkups, instead of medication or surgery.
- **Medication.** Your doctor may prescribe PROSCAR for BPH. See **"What PROSCAR does"** below.
- **Surgery.** Some patients may need surgery. Your doctor can suggest several different surgical procedures for BPH. Which procedure is best depends on your symptoms and medical condition.

There are two main treatment options to reduce the risk of serious problems due to BPH:

- **Medication.** Your doctor may prescribe PROSCAR for BPH. See **"What PROSCAR does"** below.
- **Surgery.** Some patients may need surgery. Your doctor can suggest several different surgical procedures for BPH. Which procedure is best depends on your symptoms and medical condition.

What PROSCAR does

PROSCAR lowers levels of a key hormone called DHT (dihydrotestosterone), which is a major cause of prostate growth. Lowering DHT leads to shrinkage of the enlarged prostate gland in most men. This can lead to gradual improvement in urine flow and symptoms over the next several months. PROSCAR will help reduce the risk of developing a sudden inability to pass urine and the need for surgery. However, since each case of BPH is different, you should know that:

- Even though the prostate shrinks, you may NOT notice an improvement in urine flow or symptoms.
- You may need to take PROSCAR for six (6) months or more to see whether it improves your symptoms.
- Therapy with PROSCAR may reduce your risk for a sudden inability to pass urine and the need for surgery.

What you need to know while taking PROSCAR

- **You must see your doctor regularly.** While taking PROSCAR, you must have regular checkups. Follow your doctor's advice about when to have these checkups.
- **About side effects.** Like all prescription drugs, PROSCAR may cause side effects. Side effects due to PROSCAR may include impotence (an inability to have an erection) or less desire for sex.
  Some men taking PROSCAR may have changes or problems with ejaculation, such as a decrease in the amount of semen released during sex. This decrease in the amount of semen does not appear to interfere with normal sexual function. In some cases these side effects went away while the patient continued to take PROSCAR.
  In addition, some men may have breast enlargement and/or tenderness. You should promptly report to your doctor any changes in your breasts such as lumps, pain or nipple discharge. Some men have reported allergic reactions such as rash, itching, hives, and swelling of the lips and face. Rarely, testicular pain has been reported.

You should discuss side effects with your doctor before taking PROSCAR and anytime you think you are having a side effect.

- **Checking for prostate cancer.** Your doctor has prescribed PROSCAR for symptomatic BPH and not for cancer—but a man can have BPH and prostate cancer at the same time. Doctors usually recommend that men be checked for prostate cancer once a year when they turn 50 (or 40 if a family member has had prostate cancer). These checks should continue while you take PROSCAR. PROSCAR is not a treatment for prostate cancer.
- **About Prostate-Specific Antigen (PSA).** Your doctor may have done a blood test called PSA. PROSCAR can alter PSA values. For more information, talk to your doctor.
- **A warning about PROSCAR and pregnancy.** PROSCAR is for use by MEN only.
  Women who are or may potentially be pregnant must not use PROSCAR. They should also not handle crushed or broken tablets of PROSCAR.
  If a woman who is pregnant with a male baby absorbs the active ingredient in PROSCAR after oral use or through the skin, it may cause the male baby to be born with abnormalities of the sex organs.
  PROSCAR tablets are coated and will prevent contact with the active ingredient during normal handling, provided that the tablets are not broken or crushed.

If a woman who is pregnant comes into contact with the active ingredient in PROSCAR, a doctor should be consulted. Remember, these warnings apply only when the woman is pregnant or could potentially be pregnant.

How to take PROSCAR

Follow your doctor's advice about how to take PROSCAR. You must take it every day. You may take it with or between meals. To avoid forgetting to take PROSCAR, it may be helpful to take it at the same time every day.

Your doctor may prescribe PROSCAR along with another medicine, an alpha-blocker called doxazosin, to help you better manage your BPH symptoms.

Do not share PROSCAR with anyone else; it was prescribed only for you.

Keep PROSCAR and all medicines out of the reach of children.

FOR MORE INFORMATION ABOUT 'PROSCAR' AND BPH, TALK WITH YOUR DOCTOR. IN ADDITION, TALK TO YOUR PHARMACIST OR OTHER HEALTH CARE PROVIDER.

7819309 Issued April 2004

Shown in Product Identification Guide, page 323

RECOMBIVAX HB® ℞

Hepatitis B Vaccine (Recombinant)

DESCRIPTION

RECOMBIVAX HB* Hepatitis B Vaccine (Recombinant) is a non-infectious subunit viral vaccine derived from Hepatitis B surface antigen (HBsAg) produced in yeast cells. A portion of the hepatitis B virus gene, coding for HBsAg, is cloned into yeast, and the vaccine for hepatitis B is produced from cultures of this recombinant yeast strain according to methods developed in the Merck Research Laboratories.

The antigen is harvested and purified from fermentation cultures of a recombinant strain of the yeast *Saccharomyces cerevisiae* containing the gene for the *adw* subtype of HBsAg. The fermentation process involves growth of *Saccharomyces cerevisiae* on a complex fermentation medium which consists of an extract of yeast, soy peptone, dextrose, amino acids and mineral salts. The HBsAg protein is released from the yeast cells by cell disruption and purified by a series of physical and chemical methods. The purified protein is treated in phosphate buffer with formaldehyde and then coprecipitated with alum (potassium aluminum sulfate) to form bulk vaccine adjuvanted with amorphous aluminum hydroxyphosphate sulfate. The vaccine contains no detectable yeast DNA but may contain not more than 1% yeast protein. The vaccine produced by the Merck method has been shown to be comparable to the plasma-derived vaccine in terms of animal potency (mouse, monkey, and chimpanzee) and protective efficacy (chimpanzee and human).

The vaccine against hepatitis B, prepared from recombinant yeast cultures, is free of association with human blood or blood products.

Each lot of hepatitis B vaccine is tested for sterility.

RECOMBIVAX HB is a sterile suspension for intramuscular injection. However, for persons at risk of hemorrhage following intramuscular injection, the vaccine may be administered subcutaneously. (See DOSAGE AND ADMINISTRATION).

RECOMBIVAX HB Hepatitis B Vaccine (Recombinant) is supplied in three formulations. (See HOW SUPPLIED.)

Pediatric/Adolescent Formulation (Without Preservative), 10 mcg/mL: each 0.5 mL dose contains 5 mcg of hepatitis B surface antigen.

Adult Formulation (Without Preservative), 10 mcg/mL: each 1 mL dose contains 10 mcg of hepatitis B surface antigen.

Dialysis Formulation (Without Preservative), 40 mcg/mL: each 1 mL dose contains 40 mcg of hepatitis B surface antigen.

All formulations contain approximately 0.5 mg of aluminum (provided as amorphous aluminum hydroxyphosphate sulfate, previously referred to as aluminum hydroxide) per mL of vaccine. In each formulation, hepatitis B surface antigen is adsorbed onto approximately 0.5 mg of aluminum (provided as amorphous aluminum hydroxyphosphate sulfate) per mL of vaccine. The vaccine is of the *adw* subtype. RECOMBIVAX HB is indicated for vaccination of persons at risk of infection from hepatitis B virus including all known subtypes. RECOMBIVAX HB Dialysis Formulation is indicated for vaccination of adult predialysis and dialysis patients against infection caused by all known subtypes of hepatitis B virus.

---

* Registered trademark of MERCK & CO., Inc.

CLINICAL PHARMACOLOGY

Hepatitis B virus is one of several hepatitis viruses that cause a systemic infection, with a major pathology in the liver. These include hepatitis A virus, hepatitis D virus, and hepatitis C and E viruses, previously referred to as non-A, non-B hepatitis viruses.

Hepatitis B virus is an important cause of viral hepatitis. There is no specific treatment for this disease. The incubation period for hepatitis B is relatively long; six weeks to six months may elapse between exposure and the onset of clinical symptoms. The prognosis following infection with hepatitis B virus is variable and dependent on at least three factors: (1) Age—Infants and younger children usually experience milder initial disease than older persons; (2) Dose of virus—The higher the dose, the more likely acute icteric hepatitis B will result; and, (3) Severity of associated underlying disease —underlying malignancy or pre-existing hepatic disease predisposes to increased morbidity and mortality.

Persistence of viral infection (the chronic hepatitis B virus carrier state) occurs in 5–10% of persons following acute hepatitis B, and occurs more frequently after initial anicteric hepatitis B than after initial icteric disease. Consequently, carriers of hepatitis B surface antigen (HBsAg) frequently give no history of having had recognized acute hepatitis. The Centers for Disease Control and Prevention (CDC) estimates that there are more than 300 million chronic carriers worldwide and 1.25 million chronic carriers of hepatitis B virus in the USA. Chronic carriers represent the largest human reservoir of hepatitis B virus.

Serious complications and sequelae of hepatitis B virus infection include massive hepatic necrosis, cirrhosis of the liver, and chronic active hepatitis. More than one million people worldwide die each year of hepatitis B-associated acute and chronic liver disease. In the United States, hepatitis B-virus-related acute and chronic liver disease causes approximately 4-5000 deaths annually.

Reduced Risk of Hepatocellular Carcinoma

Hepatocellular carcinoma is another serious complication of hepatitis B virus infection. Studies have demonstrated the link between chronic hepatitis B infection and hepatocellular carcinoma; 80% of primary liver cancers are caused by hepatitis B virus infection. The CDC has recognized hepatitis B vaccine as the first anti-cancer vaccine because it can prevent primary liver cancer.

There is also evidence that several diseases other than hepatitis have been associated with hepatitis B virus infection through an immunologic mechanism involving antigen-antibody complexes. Such diseases include a syndrome with rash, urticaria, and arthralgia resembling serum sickness; periarteritis nodosa; membranous glomerulonephritis; and infantile papular acrodermatitis.

Although the vehicles for transmission of the virus are often blood and blood products, viral antigen has also been found in tears, saliva, breast milk, urine, semen and vaginal secretions. Hepatitis B virus is capable of surviving at least a month on environmental surfaces exposed to body fluids containing hepatitis B virus. Infection may occur when hepatitis B virus, transmitted by infected body fluids, is implanted via mucous surfaces or percutaneously introduced through accidental or deliberate breaks in the skin.

Transmission of hepatitis B virus infection is often associated with close interpersonal contact with an infected individual and with crowded living conditions. In such circumstances, transmission by inoculation via routes other than overt percutaneous ones may be quite common. Perinatal transmission of hepatitis B infection from infected mother to child, at or shortly after birth, can occur if the mother is a hepatitis B surface antigen (HBsAg) carrier or if the mother has an acute hepatitis B infection in the third trimester. Infection in infancy by the hepatitis B virus usually leads to the chronic carrier state. Without prophylaxis, infants born to women whose sera are positive for both the hepatitis B surface antigen and the e antigen have an 85–90% likelihood of being infected and becoming a chronic carrier. Well-controlled studies have shown that administration of three 0.5 mL doses of Hepatitis B Immune Globulin (Human)-HBIG starting at birth is 75% effective in preventing establishment of the chronic carrier state in these infants during the first year of life. However, the protective effect of HBIG is transient.

Hepatitis B is endemic throughout the world and is a serious medical problem in population groups at increased risk. Because vaccination limited to high-risk individuals has failed to substantially lower the overall incidence of hepatitis B infection, both the Advisory Committee on Immunization Practices (ACIP) and the Committee on Infectious Diseases of the American Academy of Pediatrics (AAP) have also endorsed universal infant immunization as part of a comprehensive strategy for the control of hepatitis B infection. In addition, the ACIP also recommends hepatitis B vaccination for all infants and children born after November 21, 1991 and catch-up vaccination of children at high risk of infection (children <11 years of age in households of Pacific Islander ethnicity or of first generation immigrants/refugees from countries with an intermediate or high endemicity of infection). These advisory groups further recommend broad-based vaccination of adolescents. The ACIP recommends that all individuals not previously vaccinated with hepatitis B vaccine be vaccinated at 11–12 years of age with the age-appropriate dose of vaccine and that the vaccination schedule take into account the feasibility of delivering three doses of vaccine to this age group. In addition, older unvaccinated adolescents with identified risk factors for hepatitis B virus infection should also be vaccinated. Similarly, the AAP recommends that universal immunization of all adolescents should be implemented when resources permit with emphasis on those individuals in high-risk settings. A National Institutes of Health Consensus Development Conference Panel on the management of hepatitis C recommends the immunization of all hepatitis C virus (HCV) positive individuals with hepatitis B vaccine. (Refer to INDICATIONS AND USAGE.)

Numerous epidemiological studies have shown that persons who develop anti-HBs following active infection with the hepatitis B virus are protected against the disease on reexposure to the virus.

Clinical studies have shown that RECOMBIVAX HB when injected into the deltoid muscle induced protective levels of antibody in 96% of 1213 healthy adults who received the recommended 3-dose regimen. Antibody responses varied with age; a protective level of antibody was induced in 98% of 787 young adults 20–29 years of age, 94% of 249 adults 30–39 years of age and in 89% of 177 adults ≥ 40 years of age. Studies with hepatitis B vaccine derived from plasma have shown that a lower response rate (81%) to vaccine may be obtained if the vaccine is administered as a buttock injection. Seroconversion rates and geometric mean antibody titers were measured 1 to 2 months after the third dose. Multiple clinical studies have defined a protective antibody (anti-HBs) level as 1) 10 or more sample ratio units (SRU) as determined by radioimmunoassay or 2) a positive result as determined by enzyme immunoassay. Note: 10 SRU is comparable to 10 mIU/mL of antibody.

RECOMBIVAX HB was shown to be highly immunogenic in clinical studies involving infants, children, and adolescents. Three 5 mcg doses of vaccine induced a protective level of antibody in 100% of 92 infants, 99% of 129 children, and in 99% of 112 adolescents (see DOSAGE AND ADMINISTRATION).

The protective efficacy of three 5 mcg doses of RECOMBIVAX HB has been demonstrated in neonates born of mothers positive for both HBsAg and HBeAg (a core-associated antigenic complex which correlates with high infectivity). In a clinical study of infants who received one dose of HBIG at birth followed by the recommended three dose regimen of RECOMBIVAX HB, chronic infection had not occurred in 96% of 130 infants after nine months of follow-up. The estimated efficacy in prevention of chronic hepatitis B infection was 95% as compared to the infection rate in untreated historical controls. Significantly fewer neonates became chronically infected when given one dose of HBIG at birth followed by the recommended three dose regimen of RECOMBIVAX HB when compared to historical controls who received only a single dose of HBIG. Testing for HBsAg and anti-HBs is recommended at 12–15 months of age. If HBsAg is not detectable, and anti-HBs is present, the child has been protected.

As demonstrated in the above study, HBIG, when administered simultaneously with RECOMBIVAX HB at separate body sites, did not interfere with the induction of protective antibodies against hepatitis B virus elicited by the vaccine.

For adolescents (11 through 15 years of age), the immunogenicity of a two-dose regimen (10 mcg at 0 and 4–6 months) was compared with that of the standard three-dose regimen (5 mcg at 0, 1 and 6 months) in an open, randomized, multicenter study. The proportion of adolescents receiving the two-dose regimen who developed a protective level of antibody one month after the last dose (99% of 255 subjects) appears similar to that among adolescents who received the three-dose regimen (98% of 121 subjects). After adolescents (11 through 15 years of age) received the first 10-mcg dose of the two-dose regimen, the proportion who developed a protective level of antibody was approximately 72%.

In one published study, the seroprotection rates in individuals with chronic HCV infection given the standard regimen of RECOMBIVAX HB was approximately 70%. In a second published study of intravenous drug users given an accelerated schedule of RECOMBIVAX HB, infection with HCV did not affect the response to RECOMBIVAX HB.

As with other hepatitis B vaccines, the duration of the protective effect of RECOMBIVAX HB in healthy vaccinees is unknown at present, and the need for booster doses is not yet defined. However, long-term follow-up (5 to 9 years) of approximately 3000 high-risk vaccinees (infants of carrier mothers, male homosexuals, Alaskan Natives) who developed an anti-HBs titer of ≥10 mIU/mL when given a similar plasma-derived vaccine at intervals of 0, 1, and 6 months showed that no subjects developed clinically apparent hepatitis B infection and that 5 subjects developed antigenemia, even though up to half of the subjects failed to maintain a titer at this level. Persistence of vaccine-induced immunologic memory among healthy vaccinees who responded to a primary course of plasma-derived or recombinant hepatitis B vaccine has been demonstrated by an amnestic antibody response to a booster dose of RECOMBIVAX HB given 5–12 years later.

Predialysis and Dialysis Patients

Predialysis and dialysis adult patients respond less well to hepatitis B vaccines than do healthy individuals; however, vaccination of adult patients early in the course of their renal disease produces higher seroconversion rates than vaccination after dialysis has been initiated. In addition, the responses to these vaccines may be lower if the vaccine is administered as a buttock injection. When 40 mcg of Hepatitis B Vaccine (Recombinant) was administered in the deltoid muscle, 89% of 28 participants developed anti-HBs with 86% achieving levels ≥ 10 mIU/mL. However, when the same dosage of this vaccine was administered inappropriately either in the buttock or a combination of buttock and deltoid, 62% of 47 participants developed anti-HBs with 55% achieving levels of ≥ 10 mIU/mL.

A booster dose or revaccination with RECOMBIVAX HB Dialysis Formulation may be considered in predialysis/dialysis patients if the anti-HBs level is less than 10 mIU/mL.

Reports in the literature describe a more virulent form of hepatitis B associated with superinfections or coinfections by delta virus, an imcomplete RNA virus. Delta virus can only infect and cause illness in persons infected with hepatitis B virus since the delta agent requires a coat of HBsAg in order to become infectious. Therefore, persons immune to hepatitis B virus infection should also be immune to delta virus infection.

Interchangeability of Plasma-Derived and Recombinant Hepatitis B Vaccines

Although there have been no clinical studies in which a three-dose vaccine series was initiated with HEPTAVAX-B* (Hepatitis B Vaccine) and completed with RECOMBIVAX HB, or vice versa, extensive *in vitro* and *in vivo* studies have demonstrated that these two vaccines are immunologically comparable.

*Registered trademark of MERCK & CO., Inc.

INDICATIONS AND USAGE

RECOMBIVAX HB is indicated for vaccination against infection caused by all known subtypes of hepatitis B virus. **RECOMBIVAX HB Dialysis Formulation** is indicated for vaccination of adult predialysis and dialysis patients against infection caused by all known subtypes of hepatitis B virus.

Vaccination with RECOMBIVAX HB is recommended for:

1) Infants including those born to HBsAg positive mothers (high-risk infants).

2) Children born after November 21, 1991.

3) Adolescents (see CLINICAL PHARMACOLOGY).

4) Other persons of all ages in areas of high prevalence or those who are or may be at increased risk of infection with hepatitis B virus, such as:

- *Health Care Personnel*
  - Dentists and oral surgeons.
  - Physicians and surgeons.
  - Nurses.
  - Paramedical personnel and custodial staff who may be exposed to the virus via blood or other patient specimens.
  - Dental hygienists and dental nurses.
  - Laboratory personnel handling blood, blood products, and other patient specimens.
  - Dental, medical and nursing students.
- *Selected Patients and Patient Contacts*
  - Staff in hemodialysis units and hematology/oncology units.
  - Hemodialysis patients and patients with early renal failure before they require hemodialysis.
  - Patients requiring frequent and/or large volume blood transfusions or clotting factor concentrates (e.g., persons with hemophilia, thalassemia).
  - Individuals with hepatitis C virus infection.
  - Clients (residents) and staff of institutions for the mentally handicapped.
  - Classroom contacts of deinstitutionalized mentally handicapped persons who have persistent hepatitis B surface antigenemia and who show aggressive behavior.
  - Household and other intimate contacts of persons with persistent hepatitis B surface antigenemia.
- *Sub-populations with a known high incidence of the disease,* such as:
  - Alaskan Natives.
  - Pacific Islanders.
  - Refugees from areas where hepatitis B virus infection is endemic.
  - Adoptees from countries where hepatitis B virus infection is endemic.
- *International Travelers*
- *Military Personnel identified as being at increased risk*
- *Morticians and Embalmers*
- *Blood bank and plasma fractionation workers*
- *Persons at Increased Risk of the Disease Due to Their Sexual Practices,* such as:
  - Persons who have heterosexual activity with multiple partners.
  - Persons who repeatedly contract sexually transmitted diseases.
  - Homosexual and bisexual adolescent and adult men.
  - Female prostitutes.
- *Prisoners*
- *Injection drug users*

Neither dosage strength will prevent hepatitis caused by other agents, such as hepatitis A virus, hepatitis C virus, hepatitis E virus, or other viruses known to infect the liver.

Revaccination

See CLINICAL PHARMACOLOGY

Use with Other Vaccines

Results from clinical studies indicate that RECOMBIVAX HB can be administered concomitantly with DTP (Diphtheria, Tetanus and whole cell Pertussis), OPV (oral Poliomyelitis vaccine), M-M-R* II (Measles, Mumps, and Rubella Virus Vaccine Live), Liquid PedvaxHIB* [Haemophilus b Conjugate Vaccine (Meningococcal Protein Conjugate)] or a booster dose of DTaP [Diphtheria, Tetanus, acellular Pertussis], using separate sites and syringes for injectable vaccines. No impairment of immune response to individually tested vaccine antigens was demonstrated.

The type, frequency and severity of adverse experiences observed in these studies with RECOMBIVAX HB were similar to those seen when the other vaccines were given alone.

In addition, a HBsAg-containing product, COMVAX* [Haemophilus b Conjugate (Meningococcal Protein Conjugate) and Hepatitis B (Recombinant) Vaccine], was given concomitantly with eIPV (enhanced inactivated Poliovirus vaccine) or VARIVAX* [Varicella Virus Vaccine Live (Oka/Merck)], using separate sites and syringes for injectable vaccines. No impairment of immune response to these individually tested vaccine antigens was demonstrated. No serious vaccine-related adverse events were reported.

COMVAX has also been administered concomitantly with the primary series of DTaP to a limited number of infants. No serious vaccine-related adverse events were reported. Separate sites and syringes should be used for administration of injectable vaccines.

*Registered trademark of MERCK & CO., Inc.

CONTRAINDICATIONS

Hypersensitivity to yeast or any component of the vaccine.

WARNINGS

Patients who develop symptoms suggestive of hypersensitivity after an injection should not receive further injections of the vaccine (see CONTRAINDICATIONS).

Because of the long incubation period for hepatitis B, it is possible for unrecognized infection to be present at the time the vaccine is given. The vaccine may not prevent hepatitis B in such patients.

PRECAUTIONS

General

As with any percutaneous vaccine, epinephrine (1:1000) should be available for immediate use should an anaphylactoid reaction occur.

Any serious active infection including febrile illness is reason for delaying use of the vaccine except when in the opinion of the physician, withholding the vaccine entails a greater risk.

Caution and appropriate care should be exercised in administering the vaccine to individuals with severely compromised cardiopulmonary status or to others in whom a febrile or systemic reaction could pose a significant risk.

Instructions to Healthcare Provider

The healthcare provider should determine the current health status and previous vaccination history of the vaccinee.

The healthcare provider should question the patient, parent or guardian about reactions to a previous dose of RECOMBIVAX HB or other hepatitis B vaccines.

The healthcare provider must record in the patient's permanent record: the manufacturer, lot number, date of administration, and the name and address of the person administering the vaccine.

Injection of a blood vessel should be avoided.

Continued on next page

Information on the Merck & Co., Inc., products listed on these pages is from the prescribing information in use October 1, 2004. For information, please call 1-800-NSC-MERCK [1-800-672-6372].

Recombivax HB—Cont.

Information for Vaccine Recipients and Parents/Guardians
The healthcare provider should provide the vaccine information required to be given with each vaccination to the patient, parent or guardian.
The healthcare provider should inform the patient, parent or guardian of the benefits and risks associated with vaccination, as well as the importance of completing the immunization series. For risks associated with vaccination, see WARNINGS, PRECAUTIONS, and ADVERSE REACTIONS.
Patients, parents and guardians should be instructed to report any serious adverse reactions to their healthcare provider, who in turn should report such events to the U.S. Department of Health and Human Services through the Vaccine Adverse Event Reporting System (VAERS), 1-800-822-7967. The healthcare provider should inform the parent or guardian of the National Vaccine Injury Compensation Program (NVICP), 1-888-338-2382 or http://www.hrsa.dhhs.gov/bhpr/vicp.
Drug Interactions
There are no known drug interactions. (See INDICATIONS AND USAGE, *Use with Other Vaccines*.)
Carcinogenesis, Mutagenesis, Impairment of Fertility
RECOMBIVAX HB has not been evaluated for its carcinogenic or mutagenic potential, or its potential to impair fertility.
Pregnancy
Pregnancy Category C: Animal reproduction studies have not been conducted with the vaccine. It is also not known whether the vaccine can cause fetal harm when administered to a pregnant woman or can affect reproduction capacity. The vaccine should be given to a pregnant woman only if clearly needed.
Nursing Mothers
It is not known whether the vaccine is excreted in human milk. Because many drugs are excreted in human milk, cautions should be exercised when the vaccine is administered to a nursing woman.
Pediatric Use
RECOMBIVAX HB has been shown to be usually well-tolerated and highly immunogenic in infants and children of all ages. Newborns also respond well; maternally transferred antibodies do not interfere with the active immune response to the vaccine. See DOSAGE AND ADMINISTRATION for recommended pediatric dosage and for recommended dosage for infants born to HBsAg positive mothers. The safety and effectiveness of RECOMBIVAX HB Dialysis Formulation in children have not been established.
Geriatric Use
Clinical studies of RECOMBIVAX HB did not include sufficient numbers of subjects aged 65 and over to determine whether they respond differently from younger subjects. Other reports from the clinical literature indicate that hepatitis B vaccines are less immunogenic in adults aged 65 years or older than in younger individuals. No overall differences in safety were observed between these subjects and younger subjects.

ADVERSE REACTIONS

RECOMBIVAX HB and RECOMBIVAX HB Dialysis Formulation are generally well-tolerated. No serious adverse reactions attributable to the vaccine have been reported during the course of clinical trials. No adverse experiences were reported during clinical trials which could be related to changes in the titers of antibodies to yeast. As with any vaccine, there is the possibility that broad use of the vaccine could reveal adverse reactions not observed in clinical trials.
In three clinical studies, 434 doses of RECOMBIVAX HB, 5 mcg, were administered to 147 healthy infants and children (up to 10 years of age) who were monitored for 5 days after each dose. Injection site reactions and systemic complaints were reported following 0.2% and 10.4% of the injections, respectively. The most frequently reported systemic adverse reactions (>1% injections), in decreasing order of frequency, were irritability, fever (≥101°F oral equivalent), diarrhea, fatigue/weakness, diminished appetite, and rhinitis.
In a study that compared the three-dose regimen (5 mcg) with the two-dose regimen (10 mcg) of RECOMBIVAX HB in adolescents, the overall frequency of adverse reactions was generally similar.
In a group of studies, 3258 doses of RECOMBIVAX HB, 10 mcg, were administered to 1252 healthy adults who were monitored for 5 days after each dose. Injection site reactions and systemic complaints were reported following 17% and 15% of the injections, respectively. The following adverse reactions were reported:

Incidence Equal to or Greater Than 1% of Injections

LOCAL REACTION (INJECTION SITE)
Injection site reactions consisting principally of soreness, and including pain, tenderness, pruritus, erythema, ecchymosis, swelling, warmth, and nodule formation.
BODY AS A WHOLE
The most frequent systemic complaints include fatigue/weakness; headache; fever (≥100°F); and malaise.
DIGESTIVE SYSTEM
Nausea; and diarrhea
RESPIRATORY SYSTEM
Pharyngitis; and upper respiratory infection

Incidence Less than 1% of Injections

BODY AS A WHOLE
Sweating; achiness; sensation of warmth; lightheadedness; chills; and flushing
DIGESTIVE SYSTEM
Vomiting; abdominal pains/cramps; dyspepsia; and diminished appetite
RESPIRATORY SYSTEM
Rhinitis; influenza; and cough
NERVOUS SYSTEM
Vertigo/dizziness; and paresthesia
INTEGUMENTARY SYSTEM
Pruritus; rash (non-specified); angioedema; and urticaria
MUSCULOSKELETAL SYSTEM
Arthralgia including monoarticular; myalgia; back pain; neck pain; shoulder pain; and neck stiffness
HEMIC/LYMPHATIC SYSTEM
Lymphadenopathy
PSYCHIATRIC/BEHAVIORAL
Insomnia/Disturbed sleep
SPECIAL SENSES
Earache
UROGENITAL SYSTEM
Dysuria
CARDIOVASCULAR SYSTEM
Hypotension
Marketed Experience
The following additional adverse reactions have been reported with use of the marketed vaccine. In many instances, the relationship to the vaccine was unclear.
Hypersensitivity
Anaphylaxis and symptoms of immediate hypersensitivity reactions including rash, pruritus, urticaria, edema, angioedema, dyspnea, chest discomfort, bronchial spasm, palpitation, or symptoms consistent with a hypotensive episode have been reported within the first few hours after vaccination. An apparent hypersensitivity syndrome (serum-sickness-like) of delayed onset has been reported days to weeks after vaccination, including: arthralgia/arthritis (usually transient), fever, and dermatologic reactions such as urticaria, erythema multiforme, ecchymoses and erythema nodosum (See WARNINGS and PRECAUTIONS).
Digestive System
Elevation of liver enzymes; constipation
Nervous System
Guillain-Barré Syndrome; multiple sclerosis; exacerbation of multiple sclerosis; myelitis including transverse myelitis; seizure; febrile seizure; peripheral neuropathy including Bell's Palsy; radiculopathy; herpes zoster; migraine; muscle weakness; hypesthesia; encephalitis
Integumentary System
Stevens-Johnson Syndrome; petechiae
Musculoskeletal System
Arthritis
Hematologic
Increased erythrocyte sedimentation rate; thrombocytopenia
Immune System
Systemic lupus erythematosus (SLE); lupus-like syndrome; vasculitis
Psychiatric/Behavioral
Irritability; agitation; somnolence
Special Senses
Optic neuritis; tinnitus; conjunctivitis; visual disturbances
Cardiovascular System
Syncope; tachycardia.
The following adverse reaction has been reported with another Heaptitis B Vaccine (Recombinant) but not with RECOMBIVAX HB: keratitis.
Patients, parents and guardians should be instructed to report any serious adverse reactions to their healthcare provider, who in turn should report such events to the U.S. Department of Health and Human Services through the Vaccine Adverse Event Reporting System (VAERS), 1-800-822-7967.

DOSAGE AND ADMINISTRATION

Do not inject intravenously or intradermally.
RECOMBIVAX HB Hepatitis B Vaccine (Recombinant) DIALYSIS FORMULATION [(40 mcg/mL) (WITHOUT PRESERVATIVE)] IS INTENDED ONLY FOR ADULT PREDIALYSIS/DIALYSIS PATIENTS.
RECOMBIVAX HB Hepatitis B Vaccine (Recombinant) PEDIATRIC/ADOLESCENT (WITHOUT PRESERVATIVE) and ADULT FORMULATIONS (WITHOUT PRESERVATIVE) ARE NOT INTENDED FOR USE IN PREDIALYSIS/DIALYSIS PATIENTS.
Three-Dose Regimen
The vaccination regimen for each population consists of 3 doses of vaccine given according to the following schedule:
First dose: at elected date
Second dose: 1 month later
Third dose: 6 months after the first dose
For infants born of mothers who are HBsAg positive or mothers of unknown HBsAg status, treatment recommendations are described in the subsection titled: *Guidelines For Treatment of Infants Born of HBsAg Positive Mothers or Mothers of Unknown HBsAg Status.*
Two-Dose Regimen—Adolescents (11 through 15 years of age)
An alternate two-dose regimen is available for routine vaccination of adolescents (11 to 15 years of age). The regimen consists of two doses of vaccine (10 mcg) given according to the following schedule:
First injection: at elected date
Second dose: 4–6 months later
Table 1 summarizes the dose and formulation of RECOMBIVAX HB for specific populations, regardless of the risk of infection with hepatitis B virus.
[See table 1 below]

Table 1

Group	Dose/Regimen	Formulation	Color Code
Infants, Children, and Adolescents 0–19 years of age	5 mcg (0.5 mL) 3 × 5 mcg	Pediatric/Adolescent	Yellow
Adolescents◆ 11 through 15 years of age	10 mcg** (1.0 mL) 2 × 10 mcg	Adult	Green
Adults ≥20 years of age	10 mcg** (1.0 mL) 3 × 10 mcg	Adult	Green
Predialysis and Dialysis Patients†	40 mcg (1.0 mL) 3 × 40 mcg	Dialysis	Blue

** If the suggested formulation is not available, the appropriate dosage can be achieved from another formulation provided that the total volume of vaccine administered does not exceed 1 mL. However, the Dialysis Formulation may be used only for adult predialysis/dialysis patients.
◆ Adolescents (11 through 15 years of age) may receive either regimen: the 3 × 5 mcg (Pediatric/Adolescent Formulation) or the 2 × 10 mcg (Adult Formulation).
† See also recommendations for revaccination of predialysis and dialysis patients in DOSAGE AND ADMINISTRATION, *Revaccination.*

RECOMBIVAX HB is for intramuscular injection. The *deltoid muscle* is the preferred site for intramuscular injection in adults. Data suggests that injections given in the buttocks frequently are given into fatty tissue instead of into muscle. Such injections have resulted in a lower seroconversion rate than was expected. The *anterolateral thigh* is the recommended site for intramuscular injection in infants and young children.
For persons at risk of hemorrhage following intramuscular injection, RECOMBIVAX HB may be administered subcutaneously. However, when other aluminum-adsorbed vaccines have been administered subcutaneously, an increased incidence of local reactions including subcutaneous nodules has been observed. Therefore, subcutaneous administration should be used only in persons (e.g., hemophiliacs) who are at risk of hemorrhage following intramuscular injections.
The vaccine should be used as supplied; no dilution or reconstitution is necessary. The full recommended dose of the vaccine should be used.
For All Formulations: Since none of the formulations contain a preservative, once the single-dose vial has been penetrated, the withdrawn vaccine should be used promptly, and the vial must be discarded.
Shake well before use. Thorough agitation at the time of administration is necessary to maintain suspension of the vaccine.
Parenteral drug products should be inspected visually for particulate matter and discoloration prior to administration. After thorough agitation, the vaccine is a slightly opaque, white suspension.
Withdraw the recommended dose from the vial using a sterile needle and syringe free of preservatives, antiseptics, and detergents.
It is important to use a separate sterile syringe and needle for each individual patient to prevent transmission of hepatitis and other infectious agents from one person to another. Needles should be disposed of properly and should not be recapped.
Injection must be accomplished with a needle long enough to ensure intramuscular deposition of the vaccine.
Guidelines For Treatment of Infants Born of HBsAg Positive Mothers or Mothers of Unknown HBsAg Status
Each infant should receive three 5 mcg doses of RECOMBIVAX HB irrespective of the mother's HBsAg status (see Table 1). The ACIP recommends that if the mother is deter-

mined to be HBsAg positive within 7 days of delivery, the infant also should be given a dose of HBIG (0.5 mL) immediately. The first dose of RECOMBIVAX HB may be given at the same time as HBIG, but it should be administered in the opposite anterolateral thigh.

Revaccination

The duration of the protective effect of RECOMBIVAX HB in healthy vaccinees is unknown at present and the need for booster doses is not yet defined (see CLINICAL PHARMACOLOGY).

A booster dose or revaccination with RECOMBIVAX HB Dialysis Formulation (blue color code) may be considered in predialysis/dialysis patients if the anti-HBs level is less than 10 MIU/mL 1 to 2 months after the third dose. The ACIP recommends that the need for booster doses of vaccine should be assessed by annual antibody testing and a booster dose given when antibody levels decline to <10 mIU/mL.

Known or Presumed Exposure to HBsAg

There are no prospective studies directly testing the efficacy of a combination of HBIG and RECOMBIVAX HB in preventing clinical hepatitis B following percutaneous, ocular or mucous membrane exposure to hepatitis B virus. However, since most persons with such exposures (e.g., healthcare workers) are candidates for RECOMBIVAX HB and since combined HBIG plus vaccine is more efficacious than HBIG alone in perinatal exposures, the following guidelines are recommended for persons who have been exposed to hepatitis B virus such as through (1) percutaneous (needlestick), ocular, mucous membrane exposure to blood known or presumed to contain HBsAg, (2) human bites by known or presumed HBsAg carriers, that penetrate the skin, or (3) following intimate sexual contact with known or presumed HBsAg carriers.

HBIG (0.06 mL/kg) should be given intramuscularly as soon as possible after exposure and within 24 hours if possible. RECOMBIVAX HB (see dosage recommendation) should be given intramuscularly at a separate site within 7 days of exposure and second and third doses given one and six months, respectively, after the first dose.

HOW SUPPLIED

PEDIATRIC/ADOLESCENT FORMULATION (PRESERVATIVE-FREE)

No. 4980—RECOMBIVAX HB for use in infants, children, and adolescents is supplied as 5 mcg/0.5 mL of HBsAg in a 0.5 mL single-dose vial, color coded with a yellow cap and stripe on the vial labels and cartons and an orange banner on the vial labels and cartons stating "Preservative Free", **NDC** 0006-4980-00.

No. 4981—RECOMBIVAX HB for use in infants, children, and adolescents is supplied as 5 mcg/0.5 mL of HBsAg in a 0.5 mL single-dose vial, in a box of 10 single-dose vials, color coded with a yellow cap and stripe on the vial labels and cartons and an orange banner on the vial labels and cartons stating "Preservative Free", **NDC** 0006-4981-00.

ADULT FORMULATION (PRESERVATIVE FREE)

No. 4995—RECOMBIVAX HB for use in adults and adolescents (11 through 15 years of age) is supplied as 10 mcg/mL of HBsAg in a 1 mL single-dose vial, color coded with a green cap and stripe on the vial labels and cartons and an orange banner on the vial labels and cartons stating "Preservative Free", **NDC** 0006-4995-00.

No. 4995—RECOMBIVAX HB for use in adults and adolescents (11 through 15 years of age) is supplied as 10 mcg/mL of HBsAg in a 1 mL single-dose vial, in a box of 10 single-dose vials, color coded with a green cap and stripe on the vial labels and cartons and an orange banner on the vial labels and cartons stating "Preservative Free", **NDC** 0006-4995-41.

DIALYSIS FORMULATION (PRESERVATIVE FREE)

No. 4992—RECOMBIVAX HB Dialysis Formulation is supplied as 40 mcg/mL of HBsAg in a 1 mL single-dose vial, color coded with a blue cap and stripe on the vial labels and cartons and an orange banner on the vial labels and cartons stating "Preservative Free", **NDC** 0006-4992-00.

Storage

Store vials and syringes at 2–8°C (36°–46°F). Storage above or below the recommended temperature may reduce potency.

Do not freeze since freezing destroys potency.

7994327, Issued June 2004

SINGULAIR® Tablets, Chewable Tablets, and Oral Granules ℞
(montelukast sodium)

DESCRIPTION

Montelukast sodium, the active ingredient in SINGULAIR*, is a selective and orally active leukotriene receptor antagonist that inhibits the cysteinyl leukotriene $CysLT_1$ receptor.

Montelukast sodium is described chemically as [*R*-(*E*)]-1-[[[1-[3-[2-(7-chloro-2-quinolinyl)ethenyl]phenyl]-3-[2-(1-hydroxy-1-methylethyl)phenyl]propyl]thio]methyl]cyclopropaneacetic acid, monosodium salt.

The empirical formula is $C_{35}H_{35}ClNNaO_3S$, and its molecular weight is 608.18. The structural formula is:

Montelukast sodium is a hygroscopic, optically active, white to off-white powder. Montelukast sodium is freely soluble in ethanol, methanol, and water and practically insoluble in acetonitrile.

Each 10-mg film-coated SINGULAIR tablet contains 10.4 mg montelukast sodium, which is the equivalent to 10 mg of montelukast, and the following inactive ingredients: microcrystalline cellulose, lactose monohydrate, croscarmellose sodium, hydroxypropyl cellulose, and magnesium stearate. The film coating consists of: hydroxypropyl methylcellulose, hydroxypropyl cellulose, titanium dioxide, red ferric oxide, yellow ferric oxide, and carnauba wax.

Each 4-mg and 5-mg chewable SINGULAIR tablet contains 4.2 and 5.2 mg montelukast sodium, respectively, which are equivalent to 4 and 5 mg of montelukast, respectively. Both chewable tablets contain the following inactive ingredients: mannitol, microcrystalline cellulose, hydroxypropyl cellulose, red ferric oxide, croscarmellose sodium, cherry flavor, aspartame, and magnesium stearate.

Each packet of SINGULAIR 4-mg oral granules contains 4.2 mg montelukast sodium, which is equivalent to 4 mg of montelukast. The oral granule formulation contains the following inactive ingredients: mannitol, hydroxypropyl cellulose, and magnesium stearate.

*Registered trademark of MERCK & CO., Inc.

CLINICAL PHARMACOLOGY

Mechanism of Action

The cysteinyl leukotrienes (LTC_4, LTD_4, LTE_4) are products of arachidonic acid metabolism and are released from various cells, including mast cells and eosinophils. These eicosanoids bind to cysteinyl leukotriene (CysLT) receptors. The CysLT type-1 ($CysLT_1$) receptor is found in the human airway (including airway smooth muscle cells and airway macrophages) and on other pro-inflammatory cells (including eosinophils and certain myeloid stem cells). CysLTs have been correlated with the pathophysiology of asthma and allergic rhinitis. In asthma, leukotriene-mediated effects include airway edema, smooth muscle contraction, and altered cellular activity associated with the inflammatory process. In allergic rhinitis, CysLTs are released from the nasal mucosa after allergen exposure during both early- and late-phase reactions and are associated with symptoms of allergic rhinitis. Intranasal challenge with CysLTs has been shown to increase nasal airway resistance and symptoms of nasal obstruction. SINGULAIR has not been assessed in intranasal challenge studies. The clinical relevance of intranasal challenge studies is unknown.

Montelukast is an orally active compound that binds with high affinity and selectivity to the $CysLT_1$ receptor (in preference to other pharmacologically important airway receptors, such as the prostanoid, cholinergic, or β-adrenergic receptor). Montelukast inhibits physiologic actions of LTD_4 at the $CysLT_1$ receptor without any agonist activity.

Pharmacokinetics

Absorption

Montelukast is rapidly absorbed following oral administration. After administration of the 10-mg film-coated tablet to fasted adults, the mean peak montelukast plasma concentration (C_{max}) is achieved in 3 to 4 hours (T_{max}). The mean oral bioavailability is 64%. The oral bioavailability and C_{max} are not influenced by a standard meal in the morning.

For the 5-mg chewable tablet, the mean C_{max} is achieved in 2 to 2.5 hours after administration to adults in the fasted state. The mean oral bioavailability is 73% in the fasted state versus 63% when administered with a standard meal in the morning.

For the 4-mg chewable tablet, the mean C_{max} is achieved 2 hours after administration in pediatric patients 2 to 5 years of age in the fasted state.

The 4-mg oral granule formulation is bioequivalent to the 4-mg chewable tablet when administered to adults in the fasted state. The coadministration of the oral granule formulation with applesauce did not have a clinically significant effect on the pharmacokinetics of montelukast. A high fat meal in the morning did not affect the AUC of montelukast oral granules, however, the meal decreased C_{max} by 35% and prolonged T_{max} from 2.3 ± 1.0 hours to 6.4 ± 2.9 hours.

The safety and efficacy of SINGULAIR in patients with asthma were demonstrated in clinical trials in which the 10-mg film-coated tablet and 5-mg chewable tablet formulations were administered in the evening without regard to the time of food ingestion. The safety of SINGULAIR in patients with asthma was also demonstrated in clinical trials in which the 4-mg chewable tablet and 4-mg oral granule formulations were administered in the evening without regard to the time of food ingestion. The safety and efficacy of SINGULAIR in patients with seasonal allergic rhinitis were demonstrated in clinical trials in which the 10-mg film-coated tablet was administered in the morning or evening without regard to the time of food ingestion.

The comparative pharmacokinetics of montelukast when administered as two 5-mg chewable tablets versus one 10-mg film-coated tablet have not been evaluated.

Distribution

Montelukast is more than 99% bound to plasma proteins. The steady-state volume of distribution of montelukast averages 8 to 11 liters. Studies in rats with radiolabeled montelukast indicate minimal distribution across the blood-brain barrier. In addition, concentrations of radiolabeled material at 24 hours postdose were minimal in all other tissues.

Metabolism

Montelukast is extensively metabolized. In studies with therapeutic doses, plasma concentrations of metabolites of montelukast are undetectable at steady state in adults and pediatric patients.

In vitro studies using human liver microsomes indicate that cytochromes P450 3A4 and 2C9 are involved in the metabolism of montelukast. Clinical studies investigating the effect of known inhibitors of cytochromes P450 3A4 (e.g., ketoconazole, erythromycin) or 2C9 (e.g., fluconazole) on montelukast pharmacokinetics have not been conducted. Based on further *in vitro* results in human liver microsomes, therapeutic plasma concentrations of montelukast do not inhibit cytochromes P450 3A4, 2C9, 1A2, 2A6, 2C19, or 2D6 (see *Drug Interactions*).

Elimination

The plasma clearance of montelukast averages 45 mL/min in healthy adults. Following an oral dose of radiolabeled montelukast, 86% of the radioactivity was recovered in 5-day fecal collections and <0.2% was recovered in urine. Coupled with estimates of montelukast oral bioavailability, this indicates that montelukast and its metabolites are excreted almost exclusively via the bile.

In several studies, the mean plasma half-life of montelukast ranged from 2.7 to 5.5 hours in healthy young adults. The pharmacokinetics of montelukast are nearly linear for oral doses up to 50 mg. During once-daily dosing with 10-mg montelukast, there is little accumulation of the parent drug in plasma (14%).

Special Populations

Gender: The pharmacokinetics of montelukast are similar in males and females.

Elderly: The pharmacokinetic profile and the oral bioavailability of a single 10-mg oral dose of montelukast are similar in elderly and younger adults. The plasma half-life of montelukast is slightly longer in the elderly. No dosage adjustment in the elderly is required.

Race: Pharmacokinetic differences due to race have not been studied.

Hepatic Insufficiency: Patients with mild-to-moderate hepatic insufficiency and clinical evidence of cirrhosis had evidence of decreased metabolism of montelukast resulting in 41% (90% CI=7%, 85%) higher mean montelukast area under the plasma concentration curve (AUC) following a single 10-mg dose. The elimination of montelukast was slightly prolonged compared with that in healthy subjects (mean half-life, 7.4 hours). No dosage adjustment is required in patients with mild-to-moderate hepatic insufficiency. The pharmacokinetics of SINGULAIR in patients with more severe hepatic impairment or with hepatitis have not been evaluated.

Renal Insufficiency: Since montelukast and its metabolites are not excreted in the urine, the pharmacokinetics of montelukast were not evaluated in patients with renal insufficiency. No dosage adjustment is recommended in these patients.

Adolescents and Pediatric Patients: Pharmacokinetic studies evaluated the systemic exposure of the 4-mg oral granule formulation in pediatric patients 6 to 23 months of age, the 4-mg chewable tablets in pediatric patients 2 to 5 years of age, the 5-mg chewable tablets in pediatric patients 6 to 14 years of age, and the 10-mg film-coated tablets in young adults and adolescents ≥15 years of age.

The plasma concentration profile of montelukast following administration of the 10-mg film-coated tablet is similar in adolescents ≥15 years of age and young adults. The 10-mg film-coated tablet is recommended for use in patients ≥15 years of age.

The mean systemic exposure of the 4-mg chewable tablet in pediatric patients 2 to 5 years of age and the 5-mg chewable tablets in pediatric patients 6 to 14 years of age is similar to the mean systemic exposure of the 10-mg film-coated tablet in adults. The 5-mg chewable tablet should be used in pediatric patients 6 to 14 years of age and the 4-mg chewable tablet should be used in pediatric patients 2 to 5 years of age.

In children 6 to 11 months of age, the systemic exposure to montelukast and the variability of plasma montelukast concentrations were higher than those observed in adults. Based on population analyses, the mean AUC (4296 ng•hr/mL [range 1200 to 7153]) was 60% higher and the mean C_{max} (667 ng/mL [range 201 to 1058]) was 89% higher than those observed in adults (mean AUC 2689 ng•hr/mL [range 1521 to 4595]) and mean C_{max}

Continued on next page

Information on the Merck & Co., Inc., products listed on these pages is from the prescribing information in use October 1, 2004. For information, please call 1-800-NSC-MERCK [1-800-672-6372].

Singulair—Cont.

(353 ng/mL [range 180 to 548]). The systemic exposure in children 12 to 23 months of age was less variable, but was still higher than that observed in adults. The mean AUC (3574 ng•hr/mL [range 2229 to 5408]) was 33% higher and the mean C_{max} (562 ng/mL [range 296 to 814]) was 60% higher than those observed in adults. Safety and tolerability of montelukast in a single-dose pharmacokinetic study in 26 children 6 to 23 months of age were similar to that of patients two years and above (see ADVERSE REACTIONS). The 4-mg oral granule formulation should be used for pediatric patients 12 to 23 months of age. Since the 4-mg oral granule formulation is bioequivalent to the 4-mg chewable tablet, it can also be used as an alternative formulation to the 4-mg chewable tablet in pediatric patients 2 to 5 years of age.

Drug Interactions

Montelukast at a dose of 10 mg once daily dosed to pharmacokinetic steady state:

- did not cause clinically significant changes in the kinetics of a single intravenous dose of theophylline (predominantly a cytochrome P450 1A2 substrate).
- did not change the pharmacokinetic profile of warfarin (primarily a substrate of CYP 2C9, 3A4 and 1A2) or influence the effect of a single 30-mg oral dose of warfarin on prothrombin time or the INR (International Normalized Ratio).
- did not change the pharmacokinetic profile or urinary excretion of immunoreactive digoxin.
- did not change the plasma concentration profile of terfenadine (a substrate of CYP 3A4) or fexofenadine, its carboxylated metabolite, and did not prolong the QTc interval following co-administration with terfenadine 60 mg twice daily.

Montelukast at doses of ≥100 mg daily dosed to pharmacokinetic steady state:

- did not significantly alter the plasma concentrations of either component of an oral contraceptive containing norethindrone 1 mg/ethinyl estradiol 35 mcg.
- did not cause any clinically significant change in plasma profiles of prednisone or prednisolone following administration of either oral prednisone or intravenous prednisolone.

Phenobarbital, which induces hepatic metabolism, decreased the AUC of montelukast approximately 40% following a single 10-mg dose of montelukast. No dosage adjustment for SINGULAIR is recommended. It is reasonable to employ appropriate clinical monitoring when potent cytochrome P450 enzyme inducers, such as phenobarbital or rifampin, are co-administered with SINGULAIR.

Pharmacodynamics

Montelukast causes inhibition of airway cysteinyl leukotriene receptors as demonstrated by the ability to inhibit bronchoconstriction due to inhaled LTD_4 in asthmatics. Doses as low as 5 mg cause substantial blockage of LTD_4-induced bronchoconstriction. In a placebo-controlled, crossover study (n=12), SINGULAIR inhibited early- and late-phase bronchoconstriction due to antigen challenge by 75% and 57%, respectively.

The effect of SINGULAIR on eosinophils in the peripheral blood was examined in clinical trials. In patients with asthma aged 2 years and older who received SINGULAIR, a decrease in mean peripheral blood eosinophil counts ranging from 9% to 15% was noted, compared with placebo, over the double-blind treatment periods. In patients with seasonal allergic rhinitis aged 15 years and older who received SINGULAIR, a mean increase of 0.2% in peripheral blood eosinophil counts was noted, compared with a mean increase of 12.5% in placebo-treated patients, over the double-blind treatment periods; this reflects a mean difference of 12.3% in favor of SINGULAIR. The relationship between these observations and the clinical benefits of montelukast noted in the clinical trials is not known (see CLINICAL PHARMACOLOGY, *Clinical Studies*).

Clinical Studies – Asthma and Seasonal Allergic Rhinitis

GENERAL

There have been no clinical trials in asthmatics to evaluate the relative efficacy of morning versus evening dosing. The pharmacokinetics of montelukast are similar whether dosed in the morning or evening. Efficacy has been demonstrated for asthma when montelukast was administered in the evening without regard to time of food ingestion. Efficacy was demonstrated for seasonal allergic rhinitis when montelukast was administered in the morning or the evening without regard to time of food ingestion.

Clinical Studies – Asthma

ADULTS AND ADOLESCENTS 15 YEARS OF AGE AND OLDER

Clinical trials in adults and adolescents 15 years of age and older demonstrated there is no additional clinical benefit to montelukast doses above 10 mg once daily. This was shown in two chronic asthma trials using doses up to 200 mg once daily and in one exercise challenge study using doses up to 50 mg, evaluated at the end of the once-daily dosing interval.

The efficacy of SINGULAIR for the chronic treatment of asthma in adults and adolescents 15 years of age and older was demonstrated in two (U.S. and Multinational) similarly designed, randomized, 12-week, double-blind, placebo-controlled trials in 1576 patients (795 treated with SINGULAIR, 530 treated with placebo, and 251 treated with active control). The patients studied were mild and moderate, non-smoking asthmatics who required approximately 5 puffs of inhaled β-agonist per day on an "as-needed" basis. The patients had a mean baseline percent of predicted forced expiratory volume in 1 second (FEV_1) of 66% (approximate range, 40 to 90%). The co-primary endpoints in these trials were FEV_1 and daytime asthma symptoms. Secondary endpoints included morning and evening peak expiratory flow rates (AM PEFR, PM PEFR), rescue β-agonist requirements, nocturnal awakening due to asthma, and other asthma-related outcomes. In both studies after 12 weeks, a random subset of patients receiving SINGULAIR was switched to placebo for an additional 3 weeks of double-blind treatment to evaluate for possible rebound effects. The results of the U.S. trial on the primary endpoint, FEV_1, expressed as mean percent change from baseline, are shown in FIGURE 1.

FIGURE 1
FEV_1 Mean Percent Change from Baseline
(U.S. Trial)

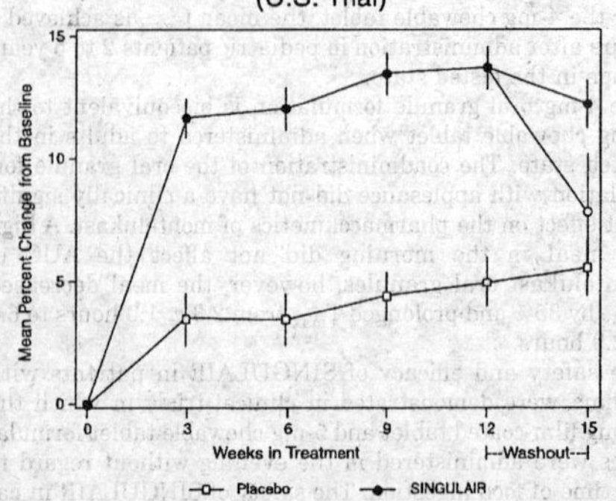

The effect of SINGULAIR on other primary and secondary endpoints is shown in TABLE 1 as combined analyses of the U.S. and Multinational trials.

[See table above]

In adult patients, SINGULAIR reduced "as-needed" β-agonist use by 26.1% from baseline compared with 4.6% for placebo. In patients with nocturnal awakenings of at least 2 nights per week, SINGULAIR reduced the nocturnal awakenings by 34% from baseline, compared with 15% for placebo (combined analysis).

SINGULAIR, compared with placebo, significantly improved other protocol-defined, asthma-related outcome measurements (see TABLE 2).

[See table 2 above]

In one of these trials, a non-U.S. formulation of inhaled beclomethasone dipropionate dosed at 200 mcg (two puffs of 100 mcg ex-valve) twice daily with a spacer device was included as an active control. Over the 12-week treatment period, the mean percentage change in FEV_1 over baseline for SINGULAIR and beclomethasone were 7.49% vs 13.3% (p<0.001) respectively, see FIGURE 2; and the change in daytime symptom scores was -0.49 vs -0.70 on a 0 to 6 scale (p<0.001) for SINGULAIR and beclomethasone, respectively. The percentages of individual patients treated with SINGULAIR or beclomethasone achieving any given percentage change in FEV_1 from baseline are shown in FIGURE 3.

FIGURE 2
FEV_1
Mean Percent Change From Baseline
(Multinational Trial)

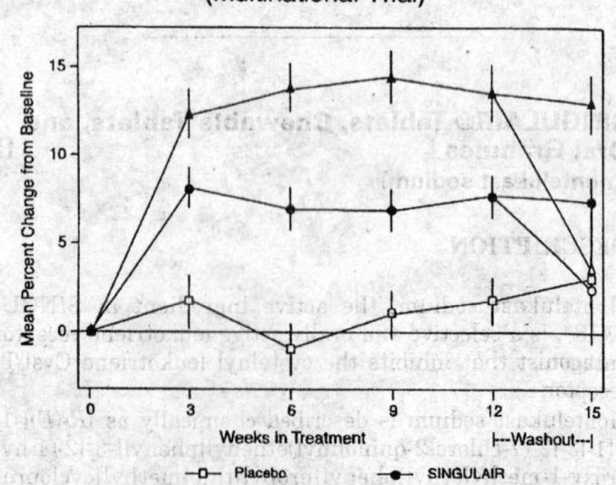

TABLE 1
Effect of SINGULAIR on Primary and Secondary Endpoints in Placebo-controlled Trials
(Combined Analyses - U.S. and Multinational Trials)

Endpoint	SINGULAIR		Placebo	
	Baseline	Mean Change from Baseline	Baseline	Mean Change from Baseline
Daytime Asthma Symptoms (0 to 6 scale)	2.43	-0.45*	2.45	-0.22
β-agonist (puffs per day)	5.38	-1.56*	5.55	-0.41
AM PEFR (L/min)	361.3	24.5*	364.9	3.3
PM PEFR (L/min)	385.2	17.9*	389.3	2.0
Nocturnal Awakenings (#/week)	5.37	-1.84*	5.44	-0.79

* p<0.001, compared with placebo

TABLE 2
Effect of SINGULAIR on Asthma-Related Outcome Measurements
(Combined Analyses - U.S. and Multinational Trials)

	SINGULAIR	Placebo
Asthma Attack* (% of patients)	11.6†	18.4
Oral Corticosteroid Rescue (% of patients)	10.7†	17.5
Discontinuation Due to Asthma (% of patients)	1.4‡	4.0
Asthma Exacerbations **(% of days)	12.8†	20.5
Asthma Control Days***(% of days)	38.5†	27.2
Physicians' Global Evaluation (score)§	1.77†	2.43
Patients' Global Evaluation (score)§§	1.60†	2.15

† p<0.001, compared with placebo
‡ p<0.01, compared with placebo

* Asthma Attack defined as utilization of health-care resources such as an unscheduled visit to a doctor's office, emergency room, or hospital; or treatment with oral, intravenous, or intramuscular corticosteroid.
** Asthma Exacerbation defined by specific clinically important decreases in PEFR, increase in β-agonist use, increases in day or nighttime symptoms, or the occurrence of an asthma attack.
*** An Asthma Control Day defined as a day without any of the following: nocturnal awakening, use of more than 2 puffs of β-agonist, or an asthma attack.
§ Physicians' evaluation of the patient's asthma, ranging from 0 to 6 ("very much better" through "very much worse," respectively).
§§ Patients' evaluation of asthma, ranging from 0 to 6 ("very much better" through "very much worse," respectively).

FIGURE 3
FEV_1
Distribution of Individual Patient Response
(Multinational Trial)

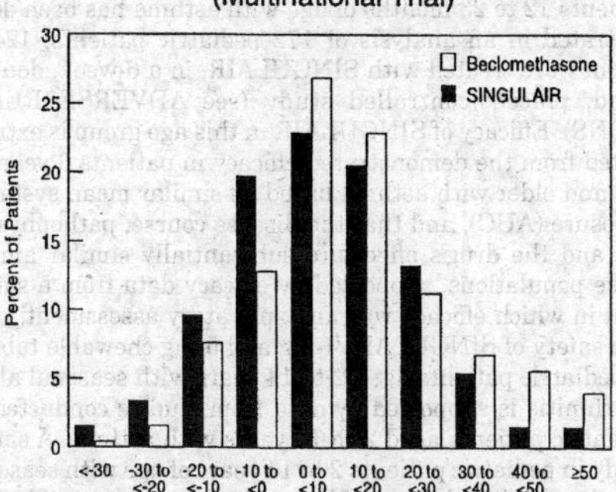

Onset of Action and Maintenance of Benefits
In each placebo-controlled trial in adults, the treatment effect of SINGULAIR, measured by daily diary card parameters, including symptom scores, "as-needed" β-agonist use, and PEFR measurements, was achieved after the first dose and was maintained throughout the dosing interval (24 hours). No significant change in treatment effect was observed during continuous once-daily evening administration in non-placebo-controlled extension trials for up to one year. Withdrawal of SINGULAIR in asthmatic patients after 12 weeks of continuous use did not cause rebound worsening of asthma.

PEDIATRIC PATIENTS 6 TO 14 YEARS OF AGE
The efficacy of SINGULAIR in pediatric patients 6 to 14 years of age was demonstrated in one 8-week double-blind, placebo-controlled trial in 336 patients (201 treated with SINGULAIR and 135 treated with placebo) using an inhaled β-agonist on an "as-needed" basis. The patients had a mean baseline percent predicted FEV_1 of 72% (approximate range, 45 to 90%) and a mean daily inhaled β-agonist requirement of 3.4 puffs of albuterol. Approximately 36% of the patients were on inhaled corticosteroids.
Compared with placebo, treatment with one 5-mg SINGULAIR chewable tablet daily, resulted in a significant improvement in mean morning FEV_1 percent change from baseline (8.7% in the group treated with SINGULAIR vs 4.2% change from baseline in the placebo group, $p<0.001$). There was a significant decrease in the mean percentage change in daily "as-needed" inhaled β-agonist use (11.7% decrease from baseline in the group treated with SINGULAIR vs 8.2% increase from baseline in the placebo group, $p<0.05$). This effect represents a mean decrease from baseline of 0.56 and 0.23 puffs per day for the montelukast and placebo groups, respectively. Subgroup analyses indicated that younger pediatric patients aged 6 to 11 had efficacy results comparable to those of the older pediatric patients aged 12 to 14.
SINGULAIR, one 5-mg chewable tablet daily at bedtime, significantly decreased the percent of days asthma exacerbations occurred (SINGULAIR 20.6% vs placebo 25.7%, $p \le 0.05$). (See TABLE 2 for definition of asthma exacerbation.) Parents' global asthma evaluations (parental evaluations of the patients' asthma, see TABLE 2 for definition of score) were significantly better with SINGULAIR compared with placebo (SINGULAIR 1.34 vs placebo 1.69, $p \le 0.05$).
Similar to the adult studies, no significant change in the treatment effect was observed during continuous once-daily administration in one open-label extension trial without a concurrent placebo group for up to 6 months.

PEDIATRIC PATIENTS 2 TO 5 YEARS OF AGE
The efficacy of SINGULAIR for the chronic treatment of asthma in pediatric patients 2 to 5 years of age was explored in a 12-week placebo-controlled safety and tolerability study in 689 patients, 461 of whom were treated with SINGULAIR. While the primary objective was to determine the safety and tolerability of SINGULAIR in this age group, the study included exploratory efficacy evaluations, including daytime and overnight asthma symptom scores, β-agonist use, oral corticosteroid rescue, and the physician's global evaluation. The findings of these exploratory efficacy evaluations, along with pharmacokinetics and extrapolation of efficacy data from older patients, support the overall conclusion that SINGULAIR is efficacious in the maintenance treatment of asthma in patients 2 to 5 years of age.

EFFECTS IN PATIENTS ON CONCOMITANT INHALED CORTICOSTEROIDS
Separate trials in adults evaluated the ability of SINGULAIR to add to the clinical effect of inhaled corticosteroids and to allow inhaled corticosteroid tapering when used concomitantly.
One randomized, placebo-controlled, parallel-group trial (n=226) enrolled stable asthmatic adults with a mean FEV_1 of approximately 84% of predicted who were previously maintained on various inhaled corticosteroids (delivered by metered-dose aerosol or dry powder inhalers). The types of inhaled corticosteroids and their mean baseline requirements included beclomethasone dipropionate (mean dose, 1203 mcg/day), triamcinolone acetonide (mean dose, 2004 mcg/day), flunisolide (mean dose, 1971 mcg/day), fluticasone propionate (mean dose, 1083 mcg/day), or budesonide (mean dose, 1192 mcg/day). Some of these inhaled corticosteroids were non-U.S.-approved formulations, and doses expressed may not be ex-actuator. The pre-study inhaled corticosteroid requirements were reduced by approximately 37% during a 5- to 7-week placebo run-in period designed to titrate patients toward their lowest effective inhaled corticosteroid dose. Treatment with SINGULAIR resulted in a further 47% reduction in mean inhaled corticosteroid dose compared with a mean reduction of 30% in the placebo group over the 12-week active treatment period ($p \le 0.05$). Approximately 40% of the montelukast-treated patients and 29% of the placebo-treated patients could be tapered off inhaled corticosteroids and remained off inhaled corticosteroids at the conclusion of the study (p=NS). It is not known whether the results of this study can be generalized to asthmatics who require higher doses of inhaled corticosteroids or systemic corticosteroids.

TABLE 3
Effects of SINGULAIR on Daytime Nasal Symptoms Score* in a Placebo- and Active-controlled Trial in Patients with Seasonal Allergic Rhinitis

Treatment Group (N)	Baseline Mean Score	Mean Change from Baseline	Difference Between Treatment and Placebo (95% CI) Least-Squares Mean
SINGULAIR 10 mg (344)	2.09	-0.39	-0.13[‡] (-0.21, -0.06)
Placebo (351)	2.10	-0.26	N.A.
Active Control[†] (Loratadine 10 mg) (599)	2.06	-0.46	-0.24[‡] (-0.31, -0.17)

*Average of individual scores of nasal congestion, rhinorrhea, nasal itching, sneezing as assessed by patients on a 0-3 categorical scale.
[†] The study was not designed for statistical comparison between SINGULAIR and the active control (loratadine).
[‡] Statistically different from placebo ($p \le 0.001$).

In another randomized, placebo-controlled, parallel-group trial (n=642) in a similar population of adult patients previously maintained, but not adequately controlled, on inhaled corticosteroids (beclomethasone 336 mcg/day), the addition of SINGULAIR to beclomethasone resulted in statistically significant improvements in FEV_1 compared with those patients who were continued on beclomethasone alone or those patients who were withdrawn from beclomethasone and treated with montelukast or placebo alone over the last 10 weeks of the 16-week, blinded treatment period. Patients who were randomized to treatment arms containing beclomethasone had statistically significantly better asthma control than those patients randomized to SINGULAIR alone or placebo alone as indicated by FEV_1, daytime asthma symptoms, PEFR, nocturnal awakenings due to asthma, and "as-needed" β-agonist requirements.
In adult asthmatic patients with documented aspirin sensitivity, nearly all of whom were receiving concomitant inhaled and/or oral corticosteroids, a 4-week randomized, parallel-group trial (n=80) demonstrated that SINGULAIR, compared with placebo, resulted in significant improvement in parameters of asthma control. The magnitude of effect of SINGULAIR in aspirin-sensitive patients was similar to the effect observed in the general population of asthmatic patients studied. The effect of SINGULAIR on the bronchoconstrictor response to aspirin or other non-steroidal anti-inflammatory drugs in aspirin-sensitive asthmatic patients has not been evaluated (see PRECAUTIONS, *General*).

EFFECTS ON EXERCISE-INDUCED BRONCHOCONSTRICTION (ADULTS AND PEDIATRIC PATIENTS)
In a 12-week, randomized, double-blind, parallel group study of 110 adult and adolescent asthmatics 15 years of age and older, with a mean baseline FEV_1 percent of predicted of 83% and with documented exercise-induced exacerbation of asthma, treatment with SINGULAIR, 10 mg, once daily in the evening, resulted in a statistically significant reduction in mean maximal percent fall in FEV_1 and mean time to recovery to within 5% of the pre-exercise FEV_1. Exercise challenge was conducted at the end of the dosing interval (i.e., 20 to 24 hours after the preceding dose). This effect was maintained throughout the 12-week treatment period indicating that tolerance did not occur. SINGULAIR did not, however, prevent clinically significant deterioration in maximal percent fall in FEV_1 after exercise (i.e., ≥20% decrease from pre-exercise baseline) in 52% of patients studied. In a separate crossover study in adults, a similar effect was observed after two once-daily 10-mg doses of SINGULAIR.
In pediatric patients 6 to 14 years of age, using the 5-mg chewable tablet, a 2-day crossover study demonstrated effects similar to those observed in adults when exercise challenge was conducted at the end of the dosing interval (i.e., 20 to 24 hours after the preceding dose).
SINGULAIR should not be used as monotherapy for the treatment and management of exercise-induced bronchospasm. Patients who have exacerbations of asthma after exercise should continue to use their usual regimen of inhaled β-agonists as prophylaxis and have available for rescue a short-acting inhaled β-agonist (see PRECAUTIONS, *General* and *Information for Patients*).

Clinical Studies – Seasonal Allergic Rhinitis
The efficacy of SINGULAIR tablets for the treatment of seasonal allergic rhinitis was investigated in 5 similarly designed, randomized, double-blind, parallel-group, placebo- and active-controlled (loratadine) trials conducted in North America. The 5 trials enrolled a total of 5029 patients, of whom 1799 were treated with SINGULAIR tablets. Patients were 15 to 82 years of age with a history of seasonal allergic rhinitis, a positive skin test to at least one relevant seasonal allergen, and active symptoms of seasonal allergic rhinitis at study entry.
The period of randomized treatment was 2 weeks in 4 trials and 4 weeks in one trial. The primary outcome variable was mean change from baseline in daytime nasal symptoms score (the average of individual scores of nasal congestion, rhinorrhea, nasal itching, sneezing) as assessed by patients on a 0-3 categorical scale.
Four of the five trials showed a significant reduction in daytime nasal symptoms scores with SINGULAIR 10 mg tablets compared with placebo. The efficacy results of one trial are shown below; the remaining three trials that demonstrated efficacy showed similar results. The mean changes from baseline in daytime nasal symptoms score in the treatment groups that received SINGULAIR tablets, loratadine and placebo are shown in TABLE 3.
[See table 3 above]

INDICATIONS AND USAGE

SINGULAIR is indicated for the prophylaxis and chronic treatment of asthma in adults and pediatric patients 12 months of age and older.
SINGULAIR is indicated for the relief of symptoms of seasonal allergic rhinitis in adults and pediatric patients 2 years of age and older.

CONTRAINDICATIONS

Hypersensitivity to any component of this product.

PRECAUTIONS

General
SINGULAIR is not indicated for use in the reversal of bronchospasm in acute asthma attacks, including status asthmaticus.
Patients should be advised to have appropriate rescue medication available. Therapy with SINGULAIR can be continued during acute exacerbations of asthma.
While the dose of inhaled corticosteroid may be reduced gradually under medical supervision, SINGULAIR should not be abruptly substituted for inhaled or oral corticosteroids.
SINGULAIR should not be used as monotherapy for the treatment and management of exercise-induced bronchospasm. Patients who have exacerbations of asthma after exercise should continue to use their usual regimen of inhaled β-agonists as prophylaxis and have available for rescue a short-acting inhaled β-agonist.
Patients with known aspirin sensitivity should continue avoidance of aspirin or non-steroidal anti-inflammatory agents while taking SINGULAIR. Although SINGULAIR is effective in improving airway function in asthmatics with documented aspirin sensitivity, it has not been shown to truncate bronchoconstrictor response to aspirin and other non-steroidal anti-inflammatory drugs in aspirin-sensitive asthmatic patients (see CLINICAL PHARMACOLOGY, *Clinical Studies*).

Eosinophilic Conditions
In rare cases, patients with asthma on therapy with SINGULAIR may present with systemic eosinophilia, sometimes presenting with clinical features of vasculitis consistent with Churg-Strauss syndrome, a condition which is often treated with systemic corticosteroid therapy. These events usually, but not always, have been associated with the reduction of oral corticosteroid therapy. Physicians should be alert to eosinophilia, vasculitic rash, worsening pulmonary symptoms, cardiac complications, and/or neuropathy presenting in their patients. A causal association between SINGULAIR and these underlying conditions has not been established (see ADVERSE REACTIONS).

Continued on next page

Information on the Merck & Co., Inc., products listed on these pages is from the prescribing information in use October 1, 2004. For information, please call 1-800-NSC-MERCK [1-800-672-6372].

Singulair—Cont.

Information for Patients

- Patients should be advised to take SINGULAIR daily as prescribed, even when they are asymptomatic, as well as during periods of worsening asthma, and to contact their physicians if their asthma is not well controlled.
- Patients should be advised that oral SINGULAIR is not for the treatment of acute asthma attacks. They should have appropriate short-acting inhaled β-agonist medication available to treat asthma exacerbations.
- Patients should be advised that, while using SINGULAIR, medical attention should be sought if short-acting inhaled bronchodilators are needed more often than usual, or if more than the maximum number of inhalations of short-acting bronchodilator treatment prescribed for a 24-hour period are needed.
- Patients receiving SINGULAIR should be instructed not to decrease the dose or stop taking any other antiasthma medications unless instructed by a physician.
- Patients who have exacerbations of asthma after exercise should be instructed to continue to use their usual regimen of inhaled β-agonists as prophylaxis unless otherwise instructed by their physician. All patients should have available for rescue a short-acting inhaled β-agonist.
- Patients with known aspirin sensitivity should be advised to continue avoidance of aspirin or non-steroidal anti-inflammatory agents while taking SINGULAIR.

Chewable Tablets

- *Phenylketonurics:* Phenylketonuric patients should be informed that the 4-mg and 5-mg chewable tablets contain phenylalanine (a component of aspartame), 0.674 and 0.842 mg per 4-mg and 5-mg chewable tablet, respectively.

Drug Interactions

SINGULAIR has been administered with other therapies routinely used in the prophylaxis and chronic treatment of asthma with no apparent increase in adverse reactions. In drug-interaction studies, the recommended clinical dose of montelukast did not have clinically important effects on the pharmacokinetics of the following drugs: theophylline, prednisone, prednisolone, oral contraceptives (norethindrone 1 mg/ethinyl estradiol 35 mcg), terfenadine, digoxin, and warfarin.

Although additional specific interaction studies were not performed, SINGULAIR was used concomitantly with a wide range of commonly prescribed drugs in clinical studies without evidence of clinical adverse interactions. These medications included thyroid hormones, sedative hypnotics, non-steroidal anti-inflammatory agents, benzodiazepines, and decongestants.

Phenobarbital, which induces hepatic metabolism, decreased the AUC of montelukast approximately 40% following a single 10-mg dose of montelukast. No dosage adjustment for SINGULAIR is recommended. It is reasonable to employ appropriate clinical monitoring when potent cytochrome P450 enzyme inducers, such as phenobarbital or rifampin, are co-administered with SINGULAIR.

Carcinogenesis, Mutagenesis, Impairment of Fertility

No evidence of tumorigenicity was seen in either a 2-year carcinogenicity study in Sprague-Dawley rats at oral gavage doses up to 200 mg/kg/day (estimated exposure was approximately 90 times the area under the plasma concentration versus time curve (AUC) for adults and children at the maximum recommended daily oral dose) or in a 92-week carcinogenicity study in mice at oral gavage doses up to 100 mg/kg/day (estimated exposure was approximately 30 times the AUC for adults and children at the maximum recommended daily oral dose.

Montelukast demonstrated no evidence of mutagenic or clastogenic activity in the following assays: the microbial mutagenesis assay, the V-79 mammalian cell mutagenesis assay, the alkaline elution assay in rat hepatocytes, the chromosomal aberration assay in Chinese hamster ovary cells, and in the *in vivo* mouse bone marrow chromosomal aberration assay.

In fertility studies in female rats, montelukast produced reductions in fertility and fecundity indices at an oral dose of 200 mg/kg (estimated exposure was approximately 70 times the AUC for adults at the maximum recommended daily oral dose). No effects on female fertility or fecundity were observed at an oral dose of 100 mg/kg (estimated exposure was approximately 20 times the AUC for adults at the maximum recommended daily oral dose). Montelukast had no effects on fertility in male rats at oral doses up to 800 mg/kg (estimated exposure was approximately 160 times the AUC for adults at the maximum recommended daily oral dose).

Pregnancy, Teratogenic Effects

Pregnancy Category B:

No teratogenicity was observed in rats at oral doses up to 400 mg/kg/day (estimated exposure was approximately 100 times the AUC for adults at the maximum recommended daily oral dose) and in rabbits at oral doses up to 300 mg/kg/day (estimated exposure was approximately 110 times the AUC for adults at the maximum recommended daily oral dose). Montelukast crosses the placenta following oral dosing in rats and rabbits. There are, however, no adequate and well-controlled studies in pregnant women. Because animal reproduction studies are not always predictive of human response, SINGULAIR should be used during pregnancy only if clearly needed.

Merck & Co., Inc. maintains a registry to monitor the pregnancy outcomes of women exposed to SINGULAIR while pregnant. Healthcare providers are encouraged to report any prenatal exposure to SINGULAIR by calling the Pregnancy Registry at (800) 986-8999.

Nursing Mothers

Studies in rats have shown that montelukast is excreted in milk. It is not known if montelukast is excreted in human milk. Because many drugs are excreted in human milk, caution should be exercised when SINGULAIR is given to a nursing mother.

Pediatric Use

Safety and efficacy of SINGULAIR have been established in adequate and well-controlled studies in pediatric patients with asthma 6 to 14 years of age. Safety and efficacy profiles in this age group are similar to those seen in adults. (See *Clinical Studies* and ADVERSE REACTIONS.)

The efficacy of SINGULAIR for the treatment of seasonal allergic rhinitis in pediatric patients 2 to 14 years of age is supported by extrapolation from the demonstrated efficacy in patients 15 years of age and older with seasonal allergic rhinitis as well as the assumption that the disease course, pathophysiology and the drug's effect are substantially similar among these populations.

The safety of SINGULAIR 4-mg chewable tablets in pediatric patients 2 to 5 years of age with asthma has been demonstrated by adequate and well-controlled data (see ADVERSE REACTIONS). Efficacy of SINGULAIR in this age group by extrapolation from the demonstrated efficacy in patients 6 years of age and older with asthma and is based on similar pharmacokinetic data, as well as the assumption that the disease course, pathophysiology and the drug's effect are substantially similar among these populations. Efficacy in this age group is supported by exploratory efficacy assessments from a large, well-controlled safety study conducted in patients 2 to 5 years of age.

The safety of SINGULAIR 4-mg oral granules in pediatric patients 12 to 23 months of age with asthma has been demonstrated in an analysis of 172 pediatric patients, 124 of whom were treated with SINGULAIR, in a 6-week, double-blind, placebo-controlled study (see ADVERSE REACTIONS). Efficacy of SINGULAIR in this age group is extrapolated from the demonstrated efficacy in patients 6 years of age and older with asthma based on similar mean systemic exposure (AUC), and that the disease course, pathophysiology and the drug's effect are substantially similar among these populations, supported by efficacy data from a safety trial in which efficacy was an exploratory assessment.

The safety of SINGULAIR 4-mg and 5-mg chewable tablets in pediatric patients aged 2 to 14 years with seasonal allergic rhinitis is supported by data from studies conducted in pediatric patients aged 2 to 14 years with asthma. A safety study in pediatric patients 2 to 14 years of age with seasonal allergic rhinitis demonstrated a similar safety profile (see ADVERSE REACTIONS).

The safety and effectiveness in pediatric patients below the age of 12 months have not been established. Long-term trials evaluating the effect of chronic administration of SINGULAIR on linear growth in pediatric patients have not been conducted.

Geriatric Use

Of the total number of subjects in clinical studies of montelukast, 3.5% were 65 years of age and over and 0.4% were 75 years of age and over. No overall differences in safety or effectiveness were observed between these subjects and younger subjects, and other reported clinical experience has not identified differences in responses between the elderly and younger patients, but greater sensitivity of some older individuals cannot be ruled out.

ADVERSE REACTIONS

Adults and Adolescents 15 Years of Age and Older with Asthma

SINGULAIR has been evaluated for safety in approximately 2600 adult and adolescent patients 15 years of age and older in clinical trials. In placebo-controlled clinical trials, the following adverse experiences reported with SINGULAIR occurred in greater than or equal to 1% of patients and at an incidence greater than that in patients treated with placebo, regardless of causality assessment:

[See table below]

The frequency of less common adverse events was comparable between SINGULAIR and placebo.

Cumulatively, 569 patients were treated with SINGULAIR for at least 6 months, 480 for one year, and 49 for two years in clinical trials. With prolonged treatment, the adverse experience profile did not significantly change.

Pediatric Patients 6 to 14 Years of Age with Asthma

SINGULAIR has been evaluated for safety in 321 pediatric patients 6 to 14 years of age. Cumulatively, 169 pediatric patients were treated with SINGULAIR for at least 6 months, and 121 for one year or longer in clinical trials. The safety profile of SINGULAIR in the 8-week, double-blind, pediatric efficacy trial was generally similar to the adult safety profile. In pediatric patients 6 to 14 years of age receiving SINGULAIR, the following events occurred with a frequency ≥2% and more frequently than in pediatric patients who received placebo, regardless of causality assessment: pharyngitis, influenza, fever, sinusitis, nausea, diarrhea, dyspepsia, otitis, viral infection, and laryngitis. The frequency of less common adverse events was comparable between SINGULAIR and placebo. With prolonged treatment, the adverse experience profile did not significantly change.

Pediatric Patients 2 to 5 Years of Age with Asthma

SINGULAIR has been evaluated for safety in 573 pediatric patients 2 to 5 years of age in single and multiple dose studies. Cumulatively, 426 pediatric patients 2 to 5 years of age were treated with SINGULAIR for at least 3 months, 230 for 6 months or longer, and 63 patients for one year or longer in clinical trials. SINGULAIR 4 mg administered once daily at bedtime was generally well tolerated in clinical trials. In pediatric patients 2 to 5 years of age receiving SINGULAIR, the following events occurred with a frequency ≥2% and more frequently than in pediatric patients who received placebo, regardless of causality assessment: fever, cough, abdominal pain, diarrhea, headache, rhinorrhea, sinusitis, otitis, influenza, rash, ear pain, gastroenteritis, eczema, urticaria, varicella, pneumonia, dermatitis, and conjunctivitis.

Pediatric Patients 12 to 23 Months of Age with Asthma

SINGULAIR has been evaluated for safety in 124 pediatric patients 12 to 23 months of age. The safety profile of SINGULAIR in a 6-week, double-blind, placebo-controlled clinical study was generally similar to the safety profile in adults and pediatric patients 2 to 14 years of age. SINGULAIR administered once daily at bedtime was generally well tolerated. In pediatric patients 12 to 23 months of age receiving SINGULAIR, the following events occurred with a frequency ≥2% and more frequently than in pediatric patients who received placebo, regardless of causality assessment: upper respiratory infection, wheezing; otitis media; pharyngitis, tonsillitis, cough; and rhinitis. The frequency of less common adverse events was comparable between SINGULAIR and placebo.

Adverse Experiences Occurring in ≥1% of Patients with an Incidence Greater than that in Patients Treated with Placebo, Regardless of Causality Assessment

	SINGULAIR 10 mg/day (%) (n=1955)	Placebo (%) (n=1180)
Body As A Whole		
Asthenia/fatigue	1.8	1.2
Fever	1.5	0.9
Pain, abdominal	2.9	2.5
Trauma	1.0	0.8
Digestive System Disorders		
Dyspepsia	2.1	1.1
Gastroenteritis, infectious	1.5	0.5
Pain, dental	1.7	1.0
Nervous System/Psychiatric		
Dizziness	1.9	1.4
Headache	18.4	18.1
Respiratory System Disorders		
Congestion, nasal	1.6	1.3
Cough	2.7	2.4
Influenza	4.2	3.9
Skin/Skin Appendages Disorder		
Rash	1.6	1.2
*Laboratory Adverse Experiences**		
ALT increased	2.1	2.0
AST increased	1.6	1.2
Pyuria	1.0	0.9

*Number of patients tested (SINGULAIR and placebo, respectively): ALT and AST, 1935, 1170; pyuria, 1924, 1159.

Adults and Adolescents 15 Years of Age and Older with Seasonal Allergic Rhinitis
SINGULAIR has been evaluated for safety in 2199 adult and adolescent patients 15 years of age and older in clinical trials. SINGULAIR administered once daily in the morning or in the evening was generally well tolerated with a safety profile similar to that of placebo. In placebo-controlled clinical trials, the following event was reported with SINGULAIR with a frequency ≥1% and at an incidence greater than placebo, regardless of causality assessment: upper respiratory infection, 1.9% of patients receiving SINGULAIR vs. 1.5% of patients receiving placebo. In a 4-week, placebo-controlled clinical study, the safety profile was consistent with that observed in 2-week studies. The incidence of somnolence was similar to that of placebo in all studies.
Pediatric Patients 2 to 14 Years of Age with Seasonal Allergic Rhinitis
SINGULAIR has been evaluated in 280 pediatric patients 2 to 14 years of age in a 2-week, multicenter, double-blind, placebo-controlled, parallel-group, safety study. SINGULAIR administered once daily in the evening was generally well tolerated with a safety profile similar to that of placebo. In this study, the following events occurred with a frequency ≥2% and at an incidence greater than placebo, regardless of causality assessment: headache, otitis media, pharyngitis, and upper respiratory infection.
Post-Marketing Experience
The following additional adverse reactions have been reported in post-marketing use: hypersensitivity reactions (including anaphylaxis, angioedema, pruritus, urticaria, and very rarely, hepatic eosinophilic infiltration), dream abnormalities and hallucinations, drowsiness, irritability, agitation including aggressive behavior, restlessness, insomnia, paraesthesia/hypoesthesia, and very rarely seizures; nausea, vomiting, dyspepsia, diarrhea, very rarely pancreatitis, and very rarely cholestatic hepatitis; arthralgia, myalgia including muscle cramps; increased bleeding tendency, bruising; palpitations; and edema.
In rare cases, patients with asthma on therapy with SINGULAIR may present with systemic eosinophilia, sometimes presenting with clinical features of vasculitis consistent with Churg-Strauss syndrome, a condition which is often treated with systemic corticosteroid therapy. These events usually, but not always, have been associated with the reduction of oral corticosteroid therapy. Physicians should be alert to eosinophilia, vasculitic rash, worsening pulmonary symptoms, cardiac complications, and/or neuropathy presenting in their patients. A causal association between SINGULAIR and these underlying conditions has not been established (see PRECAUTIONS, *Eosinophilic Conditions*).

OVERDOSAGE

No mortality occurred following single oral doses of montelukast up to 5000 mg/kg in mice (estimated exposure was approximately 250 times the AUC for adults and children at the maximum recommended daily oral dose) and rats (estimated exposure was approximately 170 times the AUC for adults and children at the maximum recommended daily oral dose).
No specific information is available on the treatment of overdosage with SINGULAIR. In chronic asthma studies, montelukast has been administered at doses up to 200 mg/day to adult patients for 22 weeks and, in short-term studies, up to 900 mg/day to patients for approximately a week without clinically important adverse experiences. In the event of overdose, it is reasonable to employ the usual supportive measures; e.g., remove unabsorbed material from the gastrointestinal tract, employ clinical monitoring, and institute supportive therapy, if required.
There have been reports of acute overdosage in pediatric patients in post-marketing experience and clinical studies of up to at least 150 mg/day with SINGULAIR. The clinical and laboratory findings observed were consistent with the safety profile in adults and older pediatric patients. There were no adverse experiences reported in the majority of overdosage reports. The most frequent adverse experiences observed were thirst, somnolence, mydriasis, hyperkinesia, and abdominal pain.
It is not known whether montelukast is removed by peritoneal dialysis or hemodialysis.

DOSAGE AND ADMINISTRATION

General Information
SINGULAIR should be taken once daily. For asthma, the dose should be taken in the evening. For seasonal allergic rhinitis, the time of administration may be individualized to suit patient needs.
Patients with both asthma and seasonal allergic rhinitis should take only one tablet daily in the evening.
Adults and Adolescents 15 Years of Age and Older with Asthma or Seasonal Allergic Rhinitis
The dosage for adults and adolescents 15 years of age and older is one 10-mg tablet daily.
Pediatric Patients 6 to 14 Years of Age with Asthma or Seasonal Allergic Rhinitis
The dosage for pediatric patients 6 to 14 years of age is one 5-mg chewable tablet daily. No dosage adjustment within this age group is necessary.
Pediatric Patients 2 to 5 Years of Age with Asthma or Seasonal Allergic Rhinitis
The dosage for pediatric patients 2 to 5 years of age is one 4-mg chewable tablet or one packet of 4-mg oral granules daily.
Pediatric Patients 12 to 23 Months of Age with Asthma
The dosage for pediatric patients 12 to 23 months of age is one packet of 4-mg oral granules daily to be taken in the evening. Safety and effectiveness in pediatric patients younger than 12 months of age have not been established.
Administration of SINGULAIR Oral Granules
SINGULAIR 4-mg oral granules can be administered either directly in the mouth, or mixed with a spoonful of cold or room temperature soft foods; based on stability studies, only applesauce, carrots, rice or ice cream should be used. The packet should not be opened until ready to use. After opening the packet, the full dose (with or without mixing with food) must be administered within 15 minutes. If mixed with food, SINGULAIR oral granules must not be stored for future use. Discard any unused portion. SINGULAIR oral granules are not intended to be dissolved in liquid for administration. However, liquids may be taken subsequent to administration. SINGULAIR oral granules can be administered without regard to the time of meals.

HOW SUPPLIED

No. 3841—SINGULAIR Oral Granules, 4 mg, are white granules with 500 mg net weight, packed in a child-resistant foil packet. They are supplied as follows:
NDC 0006-3841-30 unit of use carton with 30 packets.
No. 3796—SINGULAIR Tablets, 4 mg, are pink, oval biconvex-shaped chewable tablets, with code MRK 711 on one side and SINGULAIR on the other. They are supplied as follows:
NDC 0006-0711-31 unit of use high-density polyethylene (HDPE) bottles of 30 with a polypropylene child-resistant cap, an aluminum foil induction seal, and two silica gel desiccant canisters
NDC 0006-0711-54 unit of use high-density polyethylene (HDPE) bottles of 90 with a polypropylene child-resistant cap, an aluminum foil induction seal, and a silica gel desiccant canister
NDC 0006-0711-28 unit dose paper and aluminum foil-backed aluminum foil peelable blister packs of 100.
No. 3760—SINGULAIR Tablets, 5 mg, are pink, round, biconvex-shaped chewable tablets, with code MRK 275 on one side and SINGULAIR on the other. They are supplied as follows:
NDC 0006-0275-31 unit of use high-density polyethylene (HDPE) bottles of 30 with a polypropylene child-resistant cap, an aluminum foil induction seal, and two silica gel desiccant canisters
NDC 0006-0275-54 unit of use high-density polyethylene (HDPE) bottles of 90 with a polypropylene child-resistant cap, an aluminum foil induction seal, and a silica gel desiccant canister
NDC 0006-0275-28 unit dose paper and aluminum foil-backed aluminum foil peelable blister packs of 100.
No. 3761—SINGULAIR Tablets, 10 mg, are beige, rounded square-shaped, film-coated tablets, with code MRK 117 on one side and SINGULAIR on the other. They are supplied as follows:
NDC 0006-0117-31 unit of use high-density polyethylene (HDPE) bottles of 30 with a polypropylene child-resistant cap, an aluminum foil induction seal, and a silica gel desiccant canister
NDC 0006-0117-54 unit of use high-density polyethylene (HDPE) bottles of 90 with a polypropylene child-resistant cap, an aluminum foil induction seal, and a silica gel desiccant canister
NDC 0006-0117-28 unit dose paper and aluminum foil-backed aluminum foil peelable blister pack of 100.
NDC 0006-0117-80 bulk packaging high-density polyethylene (HDPE) bottles of 8000 with a non-child-resistant white plastic closure with a wax paper/pulp liner, an aluminum foil induction seal, and 25 silica gel desiccant canisters.
Storage
Store SINGULAIR 4-mg oral granules, 4-mg chewable tablets, 5-mg chewable tablets and 10-mg film-coated tablets at 25°C (77°F), excursions permitted to 15-30°C (59-86°F) [see USP Controlled Room Temperature]. Protect from moisture and light. Store in original package.
Storage for Bulk Bottles
Store bottle of 8000 SINGULAIR 10-mg film-coated tablets at 25°C (77°F), excursions permitted to 15-30°C (59-86°F) [see USP Controlled Room Temperature]. Protect from moisture and light. Store in original container. When product container is subdivided, repackage into a well-closed, light-resistant container. Entire contents must be repackaged immediately upon opening. Protect from moisture and light.

9088818 Issued April 2004

Patient Information

SINGULAIR® (SING-u-lair) Tablets, Chewable Tablets, and Oral Granules
Generic name: montelukast (mon-te-LOO-kast) sodium
Read this information before you start taking SINGULAIR®. Also, read the leaflet you get each time you refill SINGULAIR, since there may be new information in the leaflet since the last time you saw it. This leaflet does not take the place of talking with your doctor about your medical condition and/or your treatment.

What is SINGULAIR*?
- SINGULAIR is a medicine called a leukotriene receptor antagonist. It works by blocking substances in the body called leukotrienes. Blocking leukotrienes improves asthma and seasonal allergic rhinitis (also known as hay fever). SINGULAIR is not a steroid.

SINGULAIR is prescribed for the treatment of asthma and seasonal allergic rhinitis:

1. **Asthma.**
   SINGULAIR should be used for the long-term management of asthma in adults and children ages 12 months and older.
   Do not take SINGULAIR for the immediate relief of an asthma attack. If you get an asthma attack, you should follow the instructions your doctor gave you for treating asthma attacks. (See the end of this leaflet for more information about asthma.)
2. **Seasonal Allergic Rhinitis.**
   SINGULAIR is used to help control the symptoms of seasonal allergic rhinitis (sneezing, stuffy nose, runny nose, itching of the nose) in adults and children ages 2 years and older. (See the end of this leaflet for more information about seasonal allergic rhinitis.)

*Registered trademark of MERCK & CO., Inc.

Who should not take SINGULAIR?
Do not take SINGULAIR if you are allergic to SINGULAIR or any of its ingredients.
The active ingredient in SINGULAIR is montelukast sodium.
See the end of this leaflet for a list of all the ingredients in SINGULAIR.

What should I tell my doctor before I start taking SINGULAIR?
Tell your doctor about:
- **Pregnancy:** If you are pregnant or plan to become pregnant, SINGULAIR may not be right for you.
- **Breast-feeding:** If you are breast-feeding, SINGULAIR may be passed in your milk to your baby. You should consult your doctor before taking SINGULAIR if you are breast-feeding or intend to breast-feed.
- **Medical Problems or Allergies:** Talk about any medical problems or allergies you have now or had in the past.
- **Other Medicines:** Tell your doctor about all the medicines you take, including prescription and non-prescription medicines, and herbal supplements. Some medicines may affect how SINGULAIR works, or SINGULAIR may affect how your other medicines work.

How should I take SINGULAIR?
For adults and children 12 months of age and older with asthma:
- Take SINGULAIR once a day in the evening.
- Take SINGULAIR every day for as long as your doctor prescribes it, even if you have no asthma symptoms.
- You may take SINGULAIR with food or without food.
- If your asthma symptoms get worse, or if you need to increase the use of your inhaled rescue medicine for asthma attacks, call your doctor right away.
- **Do not take SINGULAIR for the immediate relief of an asthma attack.** If you get an asthma attack, you should follow the instructions your doctor gave you for treating asthma attacks.
- Always have your inhaled rescue medicine for asthma attacks with you.
- Do not stop taking or lower the dose of your other asthma medicines unless your doctor tells you to.
- If your doctor has prescribed a medicine for you to use before exercise, keep using that medicine unless your doctor tells you not to.

For adults and children 2 years of age and older with seasonal allergic rhinitis:
- Take SINGULAIR once a day, at about the same time each day.
- Take SINGULAIR every day for as long as your doctor prescribes it.
- You may take SINGULAIR with food or without food.

How should I give SINGULAIR oral granules to my child?
Do not open the packet until ready to use.
SINGULAIR 4-mg oral granules can be given either:
- directly in the mouth;

OR • mixed with a spoonful of one of the following soft foods at cold or room temperature: applesauce, mashed carrots, rice, or ice cream. Be sure that the entire dose is mixed with the food and that the child is given the entire spoonful of the mixture right away (with 15 minutes).

Continued on next page

Information on the Merck & Co., Inc., products listed on these pages is from the prescribing information in use October 1, 2004. For information, please call 1-800-NSC-MERCK [1-800-672-6372].

Singulair—Cont.

IMPORTANT: Never store any oral granule/food mixture for use at a later time. Throw away any unused portion.
Do not put SINGULAIR oral granules in liquid drink. However, your child may drink liquids after swallowing the SINGULAIR oral granules.

What is the daily dose of SINGULAIR for asthma or seasonal allergic rhinitis?

For Asthma (Take in the evening):

- One 10-mg tablet for adults and adolescents 15 years of age and older,
- One 5-mg chewable tablet for children 6 to 14 years of age,
- One 4-mg chewable tablet or one packet of 4-mg oral granules for children 2 to 5 years of age, or
- One packet of 4-mg oral granules for children 12 to 23 months of age.

For Seasonal Allergic Rhinitis (Take at about the same time each day):

- One 10-mg tablet for adults and adolescents 15 years of age and older,
- One 5-mg chewable tablet for children 6 to 14 years of age, or
- One 4-mg chewable tablet or one packet of 4-mg oral granules for children 2 to 5 years of age.

What should I avoid while taking SINGULAIR?

If you have asthma and if your asthma is made worse by aspirin, continue to avoid aspirin or other medicines called non-steroidal anti-inflammatory drugs while taking SINGULAIR.

What are the possible side effects of SINGULAIR?

The side effects of SINGULAIR are usually mild, and generally did not cause patients to stop taking their medicine. The side effects in patients treated with SINGULAIR were similar in type and frequency to side effects in patients who were given a placebo (a pill containing no medicine).

The most common side effects with SINGULAIR include:

- stomach pain
- stomach or intestinal upset
- heartburn
- tiredness
- fever
- stuffy nose
- cough
- flu
- upper respiratory infection
- dizziness
- headache
- rash

Less common side effects that have happened with SINGULAIR include (listed alphabetically):

agitation including aggressive behavior, allergic reactions (including swelling of the face, lips, tongue, and/or throat, which may cause trouble breathing or swallowing), hives, and itching, bad/vivid dreams, increased bleeding tendency, bruising, diarrhea, drowsiness, hallucinations (seeing things that are not there), hepatitis, indigestion, inflammation of the pancreas, irritability, joint pain, muscle aches and muscle cramps, nausea, palpitations, pins and needles/numbness, restlessness, seizures (convulsions or fits), swelling, trouble sleeping, and vomiting.

Rarely, asthmatic patients taking SINGULAIR have experienced a condition that includes certain symptoms that do not go away or that get worse. These occur usually, but not always, in patients who were taking steroid pills by mouth for asthma and those steroids were being slowly lowered or stopped. Although SINGULAIR has not been shown to cause this condition, **you must tell your doctor right away if you get one or more of these symptoms:**

- a feeling of pins and needles or numbness of arms or legs
- a flu-like illness
- rash
- severe inflammation (pain and swelling) of the sinuses (sinusitis)

These are not all the possible side effects of SINGULAIR. For more information ask your doctor or pharmacist.

Talk to your doctor if you think you have side effects from taking SINGULAIR.

General Information about the safe and effective use of SINGULAIR

Medicines are sometimes prescribed for conditions that are not mentioned in patient information leaflets. Do not use SINGULAIR for a condition for which it was not prescribed. Do not give SINGULAIR to other people even if they have the same symptoms you have. It may harm them. **Keep SINGULAIR and all medicines out of the reach of children.**

Store SINGULAIR at 25°C (77°F). Protect from moisture and light. Store in original package.

This leaflet summarizes information about SINGULAIR. If you would like more information, talk to your doctor. You can ask your pharmacist or doctor for information about SINGULAIR that is written for health professionals.

What are the ingredients in SINGULAIR?

Active ingredient: montelukast sodium

SINGULAIR chewable tablets contain aspartame, a source of phenylalanine.

Phenylketonurics: SINGULAIR 4-mg and 5-mg chewable tablets contain 0.674 and 0.842 mg phenylalanine, respectively.

Inactive ingredients:

- 4-mg oral granules: mannitol, hydroxypropyl cellulose, and magnesium stearate.
- 4-mg and 5-mg chewable tablets: mannitol, microcrystalline cellulose, hydroxypropyl cellulose, red ferric oxide, croscarmellose sodium, cherry flavor, aspartame, and magnesium stearate.
- 10-mg tablet: microcrystalline cellulose, lactose monohydrate, croscarmellose sodium, hydroxypropyl cellulose, magnesium stearate, hydroxypropyl methylcellulose, titanium dioxide, red ferric oxide, yellow ferric oxide, and carnauba wax.

What is asthma?

Asthma is a continuing (chronic) inflammation of the bronchial passageways which are the tubes that carry air from outside the body to the lungs.

Symptoms of asthma include:

- coughing
- wheezing
- chest tightness
- shortness of breath

What is seasonal allergic rhinitis?

- Seasonal allergic rhinitis, also known as hay fever, is an allergic response caused by pollens from trees, grasses and weeds.
- Symptoms of seasonal allergic rhinitis may include:
  - stuffy, runny, and/or itchy nose
  - sneezing

Rx Only

9094217 Issued April 2004

Shown in Product Identification Guide, page 324

STROMECTOL® Tablets ℞
(ivermectin)

DESCRIPTION

STROMECTOL* (Ivermectin) is a semisynthetic, anthelmintic agent for oral administration. Ivermectin is derived from the avermectins, a class of highly active broad-spectrum anti-parasitic agents isolated from the fermentation products of *Streptomyces avermitilis.* Ivermectin is a mixture containing at least 90% 5-*O*-demethyl-22,23-dihydroavermectin A_{1a} and less than 10% 5-*O*-demethyl-25-de(1-methylpropyl)-22,23-dihydro-25-(1-methylethyl)avermectin A_{1a}, generally referred to as 22,23-dihydroavermectin B_{1a} and B_{1b}, H_2B_{1a} and H_2B_{1b}, respectively. The respective empirical formulas are $C_{48}H_{74}O_{14}$ and $C_{47}H_{72}O_{14}$, with molecular weights of 875.10 and 861.07, respectively. The structural formulas are:

Component B_{1a}, $R=C_2H_5$ Component B_{1b}, $R=CH_3$

Ivermectin is a white to yellowish-white, nonhygroscopic, crystalline powder with a melting point of about 155°C. It is insoluble in water but is freely soluble in methanol and soluble in 95% ethanol.

STROMECTOL is available in 3-mg tablets and 6-mg scored tablets. Each tablet contains the following inactive ingredients: microcrystalline cellulose, pregelatinized starch, magnesium stearate, butylated hydroxyanisole, and citric acid powder (anhydrous).

* Registered trademark of MERCK & CO., Inc.

CLINICAL PHARMACOLOGY

Pharmacokinetics

Following oral administration of ivermectin, plasma concentrations are approximately proportional to the dose. In two studies, after single 12-mg doses of STROMECTOL (2×6 mg) in fasting healthy volunteers (representing a mean dose of 165 mcg/kg), the mean peak plasma concentrations of the major component (H_2B_{1a}) were 46.6 (±21.9) (range: 16.4–101.1) and 30.6 (±15.6) (range: 13.9–68.4) ng/mL, respectively, at approximately 4 hours after dosing. Ivermectin is metabolized in the liver, and ivermectin and/or its metabolites are excreted almost exclusively in the feces over an estimated 12 days, with less than 1% of the administered dose excreted in the urine. The plasma half-life of ivermectin in man is approximately 18 hours following oral administration.

The safety and pharmacokinetic properties of ivermectin were further assessed in a multiple-dose clinical pharmacokinetic study involving healthy volunteers. Subjects received oral doses of 30 to 120 mg (333 to 2000 mcg/kg) ivermectin in a fasted state or 30 mg (333 to 600 mcg/kg) ivermectin following a standard high-fat (48.6 g of fat) meal. Administration of 30 mg ivermectin following a high-fat meal resulted in an approximate 2.5-fold increase in bioavailability relative to administration of 30 mg ivermectin in the fasted state.

Microbiology

Ivermectin is a member of the avermectin class of broad-spectrum antiparasitic agents which have a unique mode of action. Compounds of the class bind selectively and with high affinity to glutamate-gated chloride ion channels which occur in invertebrate nerve and muscle cells. This leads to an increase in the permeability of the cell membrane to chloride ions with hyperpolarization of the nerve or muscle cell, resulting in paralysis and death of the parasite. Compounds of this class may also interact with other ligand-gated chloride channels, such as those gated by the neurotransmitter gamma-aminobutyric acid (GABA).

The selective activity of compounds of this class is attributable to the facts that some mammals do not have glutamate-gated chloride channels and that the avermectins have a low affinity for mammalian ligand-gated chloride channels. In addition, ivermectin does not readily cross the blood-brain barrier in humans.

Ivermectin is active against various life-cycle stages of many but not all nematodes. It is active against the tissue microfilariae of *Onchocerca volvulus* but not against the adult form. Its activity against *Strongyloides stercoralis* is limited to the intestinal stages.

Clinical Studies

Strongyloidiasis

Two controlled clinical studies using albendazole as the comparative agent were carried out in international sites where albendazole is approved for the treatment of strongyloidiasis of the gastrointestinal tract, and three controlled studies were carried out in the US and internationally using thiabendazole as the comparative agent. Efficacy, as measured by cure rate, was defined as the absence of larvae in at least two follow-up stool examinations 3 to 4 weeks post-therapy. Based on this criterion, efficacy was significantly greater for STROMECTOL (a single dose of 170 to 200 mcg/kg) than for albendazole (200 mg b.i.d. for 3 days). STROMECTOL administered as a single dose of 200 mcg/kg for 1 day was as efficacious as thiabendazole administered at 25 mg/kg b.i.d. for 3 days.

Summary of Cure Rates for Ivermectin Versus Comparative Agents in the Treatment of Strongyloidiasis

	Cure Rate* (%)	
	Ivermectin**	Comparative Agent
Albendazole *** Comparative		
International Study	24/26 (92)	12/22 (55)
WHO Study	126/152 (83)	67/149 (45)
Thiabendazole† Comparative		
International Study	9/14 (64)	13/15 (87)
US Studies	14/14 (100)	16/17 (94)

* Number and % of evaluable patients
** 170–200 mcg/kg
*** 200 mg b.i.d. for 3 days
† 25 mg/kg b.i.d. for 3 days

In one study conducted in France, a non-endemic area where there was no possibility of reinfection, several patients were observed to have recrudescence of *Strongyloides* larvae in their stool as long as 106 days following ivermectin therapy. Therefore, at least three stool examinations should be conducted over the three months following treatment to ensure eradication. If recrudescence of larvae is observed, retreatment with ivermectin is indicated. Concentration techniques (such as using a Baermann apparatus) should be employed when performing these stool examinations, as the number of *Strongyloides* larvae per gram of feces may be very low.

Onchocerciasis

The evaluation of STROMECTOL in the treatment of onchocerciasis is based on the results of clinical studies involving 1278 patients. In a double-blind, placebo-controlled study involving adult patients with moderate to severe onchocercal infection, patients who received a single dose of 150 mcg/kg STROMECTOL experienced an 83.2% and 99.5% decrease in skin microfilariae count (geometric mean) 3 days and 3 months after the dose, respectively. A marked reduction of > 90% was maintained for up to 12 months after the single dose. As with other microfilaricidal drugs, there was an increase in the microfilariae count in the anterior chamber of the eye at day 3 after treatment in some patients. However, at 3 and 6 months after the dose, a significantly greater percentage of patients treated with STROMECTOL had decreases in microfilariae count in the anterior chamber than patients treated with placebo.

In a separate open study involving pediatric patients ages 6 to 13 (n=103; weight range: 17–41 kg), similar decreases in skin microfilariae counts were observed for up to 12 months after dosing.

INDICATIONS AND USAGE

STROMECTOL is indicated for the treatment of the following infections:

Strongyloidiasis of the intestinal tract. STROMECTOL is indicated for the treatment of intestinal (i.e. nondisseminated) strongyloidiasis due to the nematode parasite *Strongyloides stercoralis.*

This indication is based on clinical studies of both comparative and open-label designs, in which from 64–100% of infected patients were cured following a single 200-mcg/kg dose of ivermectin. (See CLINICAL PHARMACOLOGY, *Clinical Studies.*)

Onchocerciasis. STROMECTOL is indicated for the treatment of onchocerciasis due to the nematode parasite *Onchocerca volvulus.*

This indication is based on randomized, double-blind, placebo-controlled and comparative studies conducted in 1427 patients in onchocerciasis-endemic areas of West Africa. The comparative studies used diethylcarbamazine citrate (DEC-C).

NOTE: STROMECTOL has no activity against adult *Onchocerca volvulus* parasites. The adult parasites reside in subcutaneous nodules which are infrequently palpable. Surgical excision of these nodules (nodulectomy) may be considered in the management of patients with onchocerciasis, since this procedure will eliminate the microfilariae-producing adult parasites.

CONTRAINDICATIONS

STROMECTOL is contraindicated in patients who are hypersensitive to any component of this product.

WARNINGS

Historical data have shown that microfilaricidal drugs, such as diethylcarbamazine citrate (DEC-C), might cause cutaneous and/or systemic reactions of varying severity (the Mazzotti reaction) and ophthalmological reactions in patients with onchocerciasis. These reactions are probably due to allergic and inflammatory responses to the death of microfilariae. Patients treated with STROMECTOL for onchocerciasis may experience these reactions in addition to clinical adverse reactions possibly, probably, or definitely related to the drug itself. (See ADVERSE REACTIONS, *Onchocerciasis.*)

The treatment of severe Mazzotti reactions has not been subjected to controlled clinical trials. Oral hydration, recumbency, intravenous normal saline, and/or parenteral corticosteroids have been used to treat postural hypotension. Antihistamines and/or aspirin have been used for most mild to moderate cases.

PRECAUTIONS

General

After treatment with microfilaricidal drugs, patients with hyperreactive onchodermatitis (sowda) may be more likely than others to experience severe advserse reactions, especially edema and aggravation of onchodermatitis.

Rarely, patients with onchocerciasis who are also heavily infected with *Loa loa* may develop a serious or even fatal encephalopathy either spontaneously or following treatment with an effective microfilaricide. In these patients, the following adverse experiences have also been reported: back pain, conjunctival hemorrhage, dyspnea, urinary and/or fecal incontinence, difficulty in standing/walking, mental status changes, confusion, lethargy, stupor, or coma. This syndrome has been seen very rarely following the use of ivermectin; a cause and effect relationship has not been established. In individuals who warrant treatment with ivermectin for any reason and have had significant exposure to Loa loa-endemic areas of West or Central Africa, pretreatment assessment for loiasis and careful posttreatment follow-up should be implemented.

Carcinogenesis, Mutagenesis, Impairment of Fertility

Long-term studies in animals have not been performed to evaluate the carcinogenic potential of ivermectin.

Ivermectin was not genotoxic *in vitro* in the Ames microbial mutagenicity assay of *Salmonella typhimurium* strains TA 1535, TA 1537, TA98, and TA100 with and without rat liver enzyme activation, the Mouse Lymphoma Cell Line L5178Y (cytotoxicity and mutagenicity) assays, or the unscheduled DNA synthesis assay in human fibroblasts.

Ivermectin had no adverse effects on the fertility in rats in studies at repeated doses of up to 3 times the maximum recommended human dose of 200 mcg/kg (on a mg/m^2/day basis).

Information for Patients

STROMECTOL should be taken on an empty stomach with water. (See CLINICAL PHARMACOLOGY, *Pharmacokinetics.*)

Strongyloidiasis: The patient should be reminded of the need for repeated stool examinations to document clearance of infection with *Strongyloides stercoralis.*

Onchocerciasis: The patient should be reminded that treatment with STROMECTOL does not kill the adult *Onchocerca* parasites, and therefore repeated follow-up and retreatment is usually required.

Pregnancy, Teratogenic Effects

Pregnancy Category C

Ivermectin has been shown to be teratogenic in mice, rats, and rabbits when given in repeated doses of 0.2, 8.1 and 4.5 times the maximum recommended human dose, respectively (on a mg/m^2/day basis). Teratogenicity was characterized in the three species tested by cleft palate; clubbed forepaws were additionally observed in rabbits. These developmental effects were found only at or near doses that were maternotoxic to the pregnant female. Therefore, ivermectin does not appear to be selectively fetotoxic to the developing fetus. There are, however, no adequate and well-controlled studies in pregnant women. Ivermectin should not be used during pregnancy since safety in pregnancy has not been established.

Nursing Mothers

STROMECTOL is excreted in human milk in low concentrations. Treatment of mothers who intend to breast-feed should only be undertaken when the risk of delayed treatment to the mother outweighs the possible risk to the newborn.

Pediatric Use

Safety and effectiveness in pediatric patients weighing less than 15 kg have not been established.

Geriatric Use

Clinical studies of STROMECTOL did not include sufficient numbers of subjects aged 65 and over to determine whether they respond differently from younger subjects. Other reported clinical experience has not identified differences in responses between the elderly and younger patients. In general, treatment of an elderly patient should be cautious, reflecting the greater frequency of decreased hepatic, renal, or cardiac function, and of concomitant disease or other drug therapy.

Strongyloidiasis in Immunocompromised Hosts

In immunocompromised (including HIV-infected) patients being treated for intestinal strongyloidiasis, repeated courses of therapy may be required. Adequate and well-controlled clinical studies have not been conducted in such patients to determine the optimal dosing regimen. Several treatments, i.e., at 2 week intervals, may be required, and cure may not be achievable. Control of extra-intestinal strongyloidiasis in these patients is difficult, and suppressive therapy, i.e., once per month may be helpful.

ADVERSE REACTIONS

Strongyloidiasis

In four clinical studies involving a total of 109 patients given either one or two doses of 170–200 mcg/kg of STROMECTOL, the following adverse reactions were reported as possibly, probably, or definitely related to STROMECTOL:

Body as a whole: asthenia/fatigue (0.9%), abdominal pain (0.9%)

Gastrointestinal: anorexia (0.9%), constipation (0.9%), diarrhea (1.8%), nausea (1.8%), vomiting (0.9%)

Nervous System / Psychiatric: dizziness (2.8%), somnolence (0.9%), vertigo (0.9%), tremor (0.9%)

Skin: pruritus (2.8%), rash (0.9%), and urticaria (0.9%)

In comparative trials, patients treated with STROMECTOL experienced more abdominal distention and chest discomfort than patients treated with albendazole. However, STROMECTOL was better tolerated than thiabendazole in comparative studies involving 37 patients treated with thiabendazole.

The Mazzotti-type and ophthalmologic reactions associated with the treatment of onchocerciasis or the disease itself would not be expected to occur in strongyloidiasis patients treated with STROMECTOL. (See ADVERSE REACTIONS, *Onchocerciasis.*)

Laboratory Test Findings

In clinical trials involving 109 patients given either one or two doses of 170–200 mcg/kg STROMECTOL, the following laboratory abnormalities were seen irrespective of drug relationship: elevation in ALT and/or AST (2%), decrease in leukocyte count (3%). Leukopenia and anemia were seen in one patient.

Onchocerciasis

In clinical trials involving 963 adult patients treated with 100 to 200 mcg/kg STROMECTOL, worsening of the following Mazzotti reactions during the first 4 days post-treatment were reported: arthralgia/synovitis (9.3%), axillary lymph node enlargement and tenderness (11.0% and 4.4%, respectively), cervical lymph node enlargement and tenderness (5.3% and 1.2%, respectively), inguinal lymph node enlargement and tenderness (12.6% and 13.9%, respectively), other lymph node enlargement and tenderness (3.0% and 1.9%, respectively), pruritus (27.5%), skin involvement including edema, papular and pustular or frank urticarial rash (22.7%), and fever (22.6%). (See WARNINGS.)

In clinical trials, ophthalmological conditions were examined in 963 adult patients before treatment, at day 3, and months 3 and 6 after treatment with 100 to 200 mcg/kg STROMECTOL. Changes observed were primarily deterioration from baseline 3 days post-treatment. Most changes either returned to baseline condition or improved over baseline severity at the month 3 and 6 visits. The percentages of patients with worsening of the following conditions at day 3, month 3 and 6, respectively, were: limbitis: 5.5%, 4.8%, and 3.5% and punctate opacity: 1.8%, 1.8%, and 1.4%. The corresponding percentages for patients treated with placebo were: limbitis: 6.2%, 9.9% and 9.4% and punctate opacity: 2.0%, 6.4% and 7.2%. (See WARNINGS.)

In clinical trials involving 963 adult patients who received 100 to 200 mcg/kg STROMECTOL, the following clinical adverse reactions were reported as possibly, probably, or definitely related to the drug in ≥ 1% of the patients: facial edema (1.2%), peripheral edema (3.2%), orthostatic hypotension (1.1%), and tachycardia (3.5%). Drug-related headache and myalgia occurred in < 1% of patients (0.2%, and 0.4%, respectively). However, these were the most common adverse experiences reported overall during these trials regardless of causality (22.3% and 19.7%, respectively).

A similar safety profile was observed in an open study in pediatric patients ages 6 to 13.

The following ophthalmological side effects do occur due to the disease itself but have also been reported after treatment with STROMECTOL: abnormal sensation in the eyes, eyelid edema, anterior uveitis, conjunctivitis, limbitis, keratitis, and chorioretinitis or choroiditis. These have rarely been severe or associated with loss of vision and have generally resolved without corticosteroid treatment.

Laboratory Test Findings

In controlled clinical trials, the following laboratory adverse experiences were reported as possibly, probably, or definitely related to the drug in ≥ 1% of the patients: eosinophilia (3%) and hemoglobin increase (1%).

Post-Marketing Experience for All Indications

The following adverse reactions have been reported since the drug was registered overseas: hypotension (mainly orthostatic hypotension), worsening of bronchial asthma, toxic epidermal necrolysis, and Stevens-Johnson syndrome.

OVERDOSAGE

Significant lethality was observed in mice and rats after single oral doses of 25 to 50 mg/kg and 40 to 50 mg/kg, respectively. No significant lethality was observed in dogs after single oral doses of up to 10 mg/kg. At these doses, the treatment related signs that were observed in these animals include ataxia, bradypnea, tremors, ptosis, decreased activity, emesis, and mydriasis.

In accidental intoxication with or significant exposure to unknown quantities of veterinary formulations of ivermectin in humans, either by ingestion, inhalation, injection, or exposure to body surfaces, the following adverse effects have been reported most frequently: rash, edema, headache, dizziness, asthenia, nausea, vomiting, and diarrhea. Other adverse effects that have been reported include: seizure, ataxia, dyspnea, abdominal pain, paresthesia, urticaria, and contact dermatitis.

In case of accidental poisoning, supportive therapy, if indicated, should include parenteral fluids and electrolytes, respiratory support (oxygen and mechanical ventilation if necessary) and pressor agents if clinically significant hypotension is present. Induction of emesis and/or gastric lavage as soon as possible, followed by purgatives and other routine anti-poison measures, may be indicated if needed to prevent absorption of ingested material.

DOSAGE AND ADMINISTRATION

Strongyloidiasis

The recommended dosage of STROMECTOL for the treatment of strongyloidiasis is a single oral dose designed to provide approximately 200 mcg of ivermectin per kg of body weight. See Table 1 for dosage guidelines. Patients should take tablets on an empty stomach with water. (See CLINICAL PHARMACOLOGY, *Pharmacokinetics*). In general, additional doses are not necessary. However, follow-up stool examinations should be performed to verify eradication of infection. (See CLINICAL PHARMACOLOGY, *Clinical Studies.*)

Table 1
Dosage Guidelines for
STROMECTOL for Strongyloidiasis

	Single Oral Dose	
Body Weight (kg)	Number of 3-mg Tablets	Number of 6-mg Tablets
15–24	1 tablet	1/2 tablet
25–35	2 tablets	1 tablet
36–50	3 tablets	1 1/2 tablets
51–65	4 tablets	2 tablets
66–79	5 tablets	2 1/2 tablets
≥80	200 mcg/kg	200 mcg/kg

Onchocerciasis

The recommended dosage of STROMECTOL for the treatment of onchocerciasis is a single oral dose designed to provide approximately 150 mcg of ivermectin per kg of body weight. See Table 2 for dosage guidelines. Patients should take tablets on an empty stomach with water. (See CLINICAL PHARMACOLOGY, *Pharmacokinetics*). In mass distribution campaigns in international treatment programs, the most commonly used dose interval is 12 months. For the treatment of individual patients, retreatment may be considered at intervals as short as 3 months.

Table 2
Dosage Guidelines for
STROMECTOL for Onchocerciasis

	Single Oral Dose	
Body Weight (kg)	Number of 3-mg Tablets	Number of 6-mg Tablets
15–25	1 tablet	1/2 tablet
26–44	2 tablets	1 tablet
45–64	3 tablets	1 1/2 tablets

Continued on next page

Information on the Merck & Co., Inc., products listed on these pages is from the prescribing information in use October 1, 2004. For information, please call 1-800-NSC-MERCK [1-800-672-6372].

Stromectol—Cont.

65–84	4 tablets	2 tablets
≥85	150 mcg/kg	150 mcg/kg

HOW SUPPLIED

No. 8107—Tablets STROMECTOL 6 mg are white, scored, round, flat, beveled-edged tablets coded MSD 139 on one side and scored on the other. They are supplied as follows:
NDC 0006-0139-10 unit dose packages of 10.
No. 8495—Tablets STROMECTOL 3 mg are white, round, flat, bevel-edged tablets coded MSD on one side and 32 on the other. They are supplied as follows:
NDC 0006-0032-20 unit dose packages of 20.
Storage
Store at temperatures below 30°C (86°F).
9032308 Issued February 2004

Shown in Product Identification Guide, page 324

SYPRINE® Capsules ℞
(Trientine Hydrochloride)

DESCRIPTION

Trientine hydrochloride is *N,N'* -bis (2-aminoethyl)-1,2-ethanediamine dihydrochloride. It is a white to pale yellow crystalline hygroscopic powder. It is freely soluble in water, soluble in methanol, slightly soluble in ethanol, and insoluble in chloroform and ether.
The empirical formula is $C_6H_{18}N_4{\cdot}2HCl$ with a molecular weight of 219.2. The structural formula is:

$$NH_2(CH_2)_2NH(CH_2)_2NH(CH_2)_2NH_2{\cdot}2HCl$$

Trientine hydrochloride is a chelating compound for removal of excess copper from the body. SYPRINE* (Trientine Hydrochloride) is available as 250 mg capsules for oral administration. Capsules SYPRINE contain gelatin, iron oxides, stearic acid, and titanium dioxide as inactive ingredients.

*Registered trademark of MERCK & CO., Inc.

CLINICAL PHARMACOLOGY

Introduction
Wilson's disease (hepatolenticular degeneration) is an autosomal inherited metabolic defect resulting in an inability to maintain a near-zero balance of copper. Excess copper accumulates possibly because the liver lacks the mechanism to excrete free copper into the bile. Hepatocytes store excess copper but when their capacity is exceeded copper is released into the blood and is taken up into extrahepatic sites. This condition is treated with a low copper diet and the use of chelating agents that bind copper to facilitate its excretion from the body.
Clinical Summary
Forty-one patients (18 male and 23 female) between the ages of 6 and 54 with a diagnosis of Wilson's disease and who were intolerant of d-penicillamine were treated in two separate studies with trientine hydrochloride. The dosage varied from 450 to 2400 mg per day. The average dosage required to achieve an optimal clinical response varied between 1000 mg and 2000 mg per day. The mean duration of trientine hydrochloride therapy was 48.7 months (range 2–164 months). Thirty-four of the 41 patients improved, 4 had no change in clinical global response, 2 were lost to follow-up and one showed deterioration in clinical condition. One of the patients who improved while on therapy with trientine hydrochloride experienced a recurrence of the symptoms of systemic lupus erythematosus which had appeared originally during therapy with penicillamine. Therapy with trientine hydrochloride was discontinued. No other adverse reactions, except iron deficiency, were noted among any of these 41 patients.
One investigator treated 13 patients with trientine hydrochloride following their development of intolerance to d-penicillamine. Retrospectively, he compared these patients to an additional group of 12 patients with Wilson's disease who were both tolerant of and controlled with d-penicillamine therapy, but who failed to continue any copper chelation therapy. The mean age at onset of disease of the latter group was 12 years as compared to 21 years for the former group. The trientine hydrochloride group received d-penicillamine for an average of 4 years as compared to an average of 10 years for the non-treated group.
Various laboratory parameters showed changes in favor of the patients treated with trientine hydrochloride. Free and total serum copper, SGOT, and serum bilirubin all showed mean increases over baseline in the untreated group which were significantly larger than with the patients treated with trientine hydrochloride. In the 13 patients treated with trientine hydrochloride, previous symptoms and signs relating to d-penicillamine intolerance disappeared in 8 patients, improved in 4 patients, and remained unchanged in one patient. The neurological status in the trientine hydrochloride group was unchanged or improved over baseline, whereas in the untreated group, 6 patients remained unchanged and 6 worsened. Kayser-Fleischer rings improved significantly during trientine hydrochloride treatment.

No. of Patients	Single Dose Treatment	Basal Excretion Rate (μg Cu + + /6hr)	Test-dose Excretion Rate (μg Cu + + /6hr)
6	Trientine, 1.2 g	19	234
4	Penicillamine, 500 mg	17	320

No. of Patients	Single Dose Treatment	Basal Excretion Rate (μg Cu + + /6hr)	Test-dose Excretion Rate (μg Cu + + /6hr)
8	Trientine, 1.2 g	71	1326
7	Penicillamine, 500 mg	68	1074

The clinical outcome of the two groups also differed markedly. Of the 13 patients on therapy with trientine hydrochloride (mean duration of therapy 4.1 years; range 1 to 13 years), all were alive at the data cutoff date, and in the non-treated group (mean years with no therapy 2.7 years; range 3 months to 9 years), 9 of the 12 died of hepatic disease.
Chelating Properties
Preclinical Studies
Studies in animals have shown that trientine hydrochloride has cupriuretic activities in both normal and copper-loaded rats. In general, the effects of trientine hydrochloride on urinary copper excretion are similar to those of equimolar doses of penicillamine, although in one study they were significantly smaller.
Human Studies
Renal clearance studies were carried out with penicillamine and trientine hydrochloride on separate occasions in selected patients treated with penicillamine for at least one year. Six-hour excretion rates of copper were determined off treatment and after a single dose of 500 mg of penicillamine or 1.2 g of trientine hydrochloride. The mean urinary excretion rates of copper were as follows:
[See first table above]
In patients *not* previously treated with chelating agents, a similar comparison was made:
[See second table above]
These results demonstrate that SYPRINE is effective as a cupriuretic agent in patients with Wilson's disease although on a molar basis it appears to be less potent or less effective than penicillamine. Evidence from a radio-labelled copper study indicates that the different cupriuretic effect between these two drugs could be due to a difference in selectivity of the drugs for different copper pools within the body.
Pharmacokinetics
Data on the pharmacokinetics of trientine hydrochloride are not available. Dosage adjustment recommendations are based upon clinical use of the drug (see DOSAGE AND ADMINISTRATION).

INDICATIONS AND USAGE

SYPRINE is indicated in the treatment of patients with Wilson's disease who are intolerant of penicillamine. Clinical experience with SYPRINE is limited and alternate dosing regimens have not been well-characterized; all endpoints in determining an individual patient's dose have not been well defined. SYPRINE and penicillamine cannot be considered interchangeable. SYPRINE should be used when continued treatment with penicillamine is no longer possible because of intolerable or life endangering side effects.
Unlike penicillamine, SYPRINE is not recommended in cystinuria or rheumatoid arthritis. The absence of a sulfhydryl moiety renders it incapable of binding cystine and, therefore, it is of no use in cystinuria. In 15 patients with rheumatoid arthritis, SYPRINE was reported not to be effective in improving any clinical or biochemical parameter after 12 weeks of treatment.
SYPRINE is not indicated for treatment of biliary cirrhosis.

CONTRAINDICATIONS

Hypersensitivity to this product.

WARNINGS

Patient experience with trientine hydrochloride is limited (see CLINICAL PHARMACOLOGY). Patients receiving SYPRINE should remain under regular medical supervision throughout the period of drug administration. Patients (especially women) should be closely monitored for evidence of iron deficiency anemia.

PRECAUTIONS

General
There are no reports of hypersensitivity in patients who have been administered trientine hydrochloride for Wilson's disease. However, there have been reports of asthma, bronchitis and dermatitis occurring after prolonged environmental exposure in workers who use trientine hydrochloride as a hardener of epoxy resins. Patients should be observed closely for signs of possible hypersensitivity.
Information for Patients
Patients should be directed to take SYPRINE on an empty stomach, at least one hour before meals or two hours after meals and at least one hour apart from any other drug, food, or milk. The capsules should be swallowed whole with water and should not be opened or chewed. Because of the potential for contact dermatitis, any site of exposure to the capsule contents should be washed with water promptly. For the first month of treatment, the patient should have his temperature taken nightly, and he should be asked to report any symptom such as fever or skin eruption.
Laboratory Tests
The most reliable index for monitoring treatment is the determination of free copper in the serum, which equals the difference between quantitatively determined total copper and ceruloplasmin-copper. Adequately treated patients will usually have less than 10 mcg free copper/dL of serum.
Therapy may be monitored with a 24 hour urinary copper analysis periodically (i.e., every 6–12 months). Urine must be collected in copper-free glassware. Since a low copper diet should keep copper absorption down to less than one milligram a day, the patient probably will be in the desired state of negative copper balance if 0.5 to 1.0 milligram of copper is present in a 24-hour collection of urine.
Drug Interactions
In general, mineral supplements should not be given since they may block the absorption of SYPRINE. However, iron deficiency may develop, especially in children and menstruating or pregnant women, or as a result of the low copper diet recommended for Wilson's disease. If necessary, iron may be given in short courses, but since iron and SYPRINE each inhibit absorption of the other, two hours should elapse between administration of SYPRINE and iron.
It is important that SYPRINE be taken on an empty stomach, at least one hour before meals or two hours after meals and at least one hour apart from any other drug, food, or milk. This permits maximum absorption and reduces the likelihood of inactivation of the drug by metal binding in the gastrointestinal tract.
Carcinogenesis, Mutagenesis, Impairment of Fertility
Data on carcinogenesis, mutagenesis, and impairment of fertility are not available.
Pregnancy
Pregnancy Category C. Trientine hydrochloride was teratogenic in rats at doses similar to the human dose. The frequencies of both resorptions and fetal abnormalities, including hemorrhage and edema, increased while fetal copper levels decreased when trientine hydrochloride was given in the maternal diets of rats. There are no adequate and well-controlled studies in pregnant women. SYPRINE should be used during pregnancy only if the potential benefit justifies the potential risk to the fetus.
Nursing Mothers
It is not known whether this drug is excreted in human milk. Because many drugs are excreted in human milk, caution should be exercised when SYPRINE is administered to a nursing mother.
Pediatric Use
Controlled studies of the safety and effectiveness of SYPRINE in pediatric patients have not been conducted. It has been used clinically in pediatric patients as young as 6 years with no reported adverse experiences.
Geriatric Use
Clinical studies of SYPRINE did not include sufficient numbers of subjects aged 65 and over to determine whether they respond differently from younger subjects. Other reported clinical experience is insufficient to determine differences in responses between the elderly and younger patients. In general, dose selection should be cautious, usually starting at the low end of the dosing range, reflecting the greater frequency of decreased hepatic, renal, or cardiac function, and of concomitant disease or other drug therapy.

ADVERSE REACTIONS

Clinical experience with SPYRINE has been limited. The following adverse reactions have been reported in a clinical study in patients with Wilson's disease who were on therapy with trientine hydrochloride: iron deficiency, systemic lupus erythematosus (see CLINICAL PHARMACOLOGY). In addition, the following adverse reactions have been reported in marketed use: dystonia, muscular spasm, myasthenia gravis.
SYPRINE is not indicated for treatment of biliary cirrhosis, but in one study of 4 patients treated with trientine hydrochloride for primary biliary cirrhosis, the following adverse reactions were reported: heartburn; epigastric pain and tenderness; thickening, fissuring and flaking of the skin; hypochromic microcytic anemia; acute gastritis; aphthoid ulcers; abdominal pain; melena; anorexia; malaise; cramps; muscle pain; weakness; rhabdomyolysis. A causal relationship of these reactions to drug therapy could not be rejected or established.

OVERDOSAGE

There is a report of an adult woman who ingested 30 grams of trientine hydrochloride without apparent ill effects. No other data on overdosage are available.

DOSAGE AND ADMINISTRATION

Systemic evaluation of dose and/or interval between dose has not been done. However, on limited clinical experience, the recommended initial dose of SYPRINE is 500–750 mg/day for pediatric patients and 750–1250 mg/day for adults given in divided doses two, three or four times daily. This may be increased to a maximum of 2000 mg/day for adults or 1500 mg/day for pediatric patients age 12 or under. The daily dose of SYPRINE should be increased only when the clinical response is not adequate or the concentration of free serum copper is persistently above 20 mcg/dL. Optimal long-term maintenance dosage should be determined at 6–12 month intervals (see PRECAUTIONS, *Laboratory Tests*).

It is important that SYPRINE be given on an empty stomach, at least one hour before meals or two hours after meals and at least one hour apart from any other drug, food, or milk. The capsules should be swallowed whole with water and should not be opened or chewed.

HOW SUPPLIED

No. 3408—Capsules SYPRINE, 250 mg, are light brown opaque capsules and are coded SYPRINE and MSD 661. They are supplied as follows:

NDC 0006-0661-68 in bottles of 100.

Storage

Keep container tightly closed.

Store at 2°–8°C (36°–46°F).

7664604 Issued January 2001

Shown in Product Identification Guide, page 324

TIMOLIDE® Tablets ℞
(Timolol Maleate-Hydrochlorothiazide)

DESCRIPTION

TIMOLIDE* (Timolol Maleate-Hydrochlorothiazide) is for the treatment of hypertension. It combines the antihypertensive activity of two agents: a non-selective beta-adrenergic receptor blocking agent (timolol maleate) and a diuretic (hydrochlorothiazide).

Timolol maleate is (*S*)-1-[(1, 1-dimethylethyl) amino]-3-[[4-(4-morpholinyl)-1, 2, 5-thiadiazol -3- yl] oxy]-2-propanol (*Z*)-2-butenedioate (1:1) salt. Its empirical formula is $C_{13}H_{24}N_4O_3S{\cdot}C_4H_4O_4$ and its structural formula is:

Timolol maleate has a molecular weight of 432.50. It is a white, odorless, crystalline powder which is soluble in water, methanol, and alcohol.

Hydrochlorothiazide is 6-chloro-3,4-dihydro-2*H* -1,2,4-benzothiadiazine-7-sulfonamide 1, 1- dioxide. Its empirical formula is $C_7H_8ClN_3O_4S_2$ and its structural formula is:

Hydrochlorothiazide has a molecular weight of 297.73. It is a white, or practically white, crystalline powder which is slightly soluble in water, but freely soluble in sodium hydroxide solution.

TIMOLIDE is supplied as tablets containing 10 mg of timolol maleate and 25 mg of hydrochlorothiazide for oral administration. Inactive ingredients are cellulose, FD&C Blue 2, magnesium stearate, and starch.

*Registered trademark of MERCK & CO., INC.

CLINICAL PHARMACOLOGY

TIMOLIDE

Timolol maleate and hydrochlorothiazide have been used singly and concomitantly for the treatment of hypertension. The antihypertensive effects of these agents are additive. The two components of TIMOLIDE have similar dosage schedules, and studies have shown that there is no interference with bioavailability when these agents are given together in the single combination tablet. Therefore, this combination provides a convenient formulation for the concomitant administration of these two entities.

In controlled clinical trials with TIMOLIDE in selected patients with mild to moderate essential hypertension, about 90 percent had a good to excellent response. In patients with more severe hypertension, TIMOLIDE may be administered with other antihypertensives such as ALDOMET* (Methyldopa) or a vasodilator.

Although the mechanisms of action of timolol maleate and hydrochlorothiazide in the treatment of hypertension have not been established, they are thought to be different; for example, hydrochlorothiazide increases plasma renin activity while timolol maleate reduces plasma renin activity.

Timolol Maleate

Timolol maleate is a $beta_1$ and $beta_2$ (non-selective) adrenergic receptor blocking agent that does not have significant intrinsic sympathomimetic, direct myocardial depressant, or local anesthetic activity.

Pharmacodynamics

Clinical pharmacology studies have confirmed the beta-adrenergic blocking activity as shown by (1) changes in resting heart rate and response of heart rate to changes in posture; (2) inhibition of isoproterenol-induced tachycardia; (3) alteration of the response to the Valsalva maneuver and amyl nitrite administration; and (4) reduction of heart rate and blood pressure changes on exercise.

Timolol maleate decreases the positive chronotropic, positive inotropic, bronchodilator, and vasodilator responses caused by beta-adrenergic receptor agonists. The magnitude of this decreased response is proportional to the existing sympathetic tone and the concentration of timolol maleate at receptor sites.

In normal volunteers, the reduction in heart rate response to a standard exercise was dose dependent over the test range of 0.5 to 20 mg, with a peak reduction at 2 hours of approximately 30% at higher doses.

Beta-adrenergic receptor blockade reduces cardiac output in both healthy subjects and patients with heart disease. In patients with severe impairment of myocardial function beta-adrenergic receptor blockade may inhibit the stimulatory effect of the sympathetic nervous system necessary to maintain adequate cardiac function.

Beta-adrenergic receptor blockade in the bronchi and bronchioles results in increased airway resistance from unopposed parasympathetic activity. Such an effect in patients with asthma or other bronchospastic conditions is potentially dangerous.

Clinical studies indicate that timolol maleate at a dosage of 20–60 mg/day reduces blood pressure without causing postural hypotension in most patients with essential hypertension. Administration of timolol maleate to patients with hypertension results initially in a decrease in cardiac output, little immediate change in blood pressure, and an increase in calculated peripheral resistance. With continued administration of timolol maleate blood pressure decreases within a few days, cardiac output usually remains reduced, and peripheral resistance falls toward pretreatment levels. Plasma volume may decrease or remain unchanged during therapy with timolol maleate. In the majority of patients with hypertension, timolol maleate also decreases plasma renin activity. Dosage adjustment to achieve optimal antihypertensive effect may require a few weeks. When therapy with timolol maleate is discontinued, the blood pressure tends to return to pretreatment levels gradually. In most patients the antihypertensive activity of timolol maleate is maintained with long-term therapy and is well tolerated.

The mechanism of the antihypertensive effects of beta-adrenergic receptor blocking agents is not established at this time. Possible mechanisms of action include reduction in cardiac output, reduction in plasma renin activity, and a central nervous system sympatholytic action.

Pharmacokinetics and Metabolism

Timolol maleate is rapidly and nearly completely absorbed (about 90%) following oral ingestion. Detectable plasma levels of timolol occur within one-half hour and peak plasma levels occur in about one to two hours. The drug half-life in plasma is approximately 4 hours and this is essentially unchanged in patients with moderate renal insufficiency. Timolol is partially metabolized by the liver and timolol and its metabolites are excreted by the kidney. Timolol is not extensively bound to plasma proteins; i.e., <10% by equilibrium dialysis and approximately 60% by ultrafiltration. An *in vitro* hemodialysis study, using ^{14}C timolol added to human plasma or whole blood, showed that timolol was readily dialyzed from these fluids; however, a study of patients with renal failure showed that timolol did not dialyze readily. Plasma levels following oral administration are about half those following intravenous administration indicating approximately 50% first pass metabolism. The level of beta sympathetic activity varies widely among individuals, and no simple correlation exists between the dose or plasma level of timolol maleate and its therapeutic activity. Therefore, objective clinical measurements such as reduction of heart rate and/or blood pressure should be used as guides in determining the optimal dosage for each patient.

Hydrochlorothiazide

Hydrochlorothiazide is a diuretic and antihypertensive agent. It affects the renal tubular mechanism of electrolyte reabsorption. Hydrochlorothiazide increases excretion of sodium and chloride in approximately equivalent amounts. Natriuresis may be accompanied by some loss of potassium and bicarbonate. The mechanism of the antihypertensive effect of thiazides may be related to the excretion and redistribution of body sodium. Hydrochlorothiazide usually does not cause clinically important changes in normal blood pressure.

*Registered trademark of MERCK & CO., INC.

INDICATIONS AND USAGE

TIMOLIDE is indicated for the treatment of hypertension. **This fixed combination drug is not indicated for initial therapy of hypertension. If the fixed combination represents the dose titrated to an individual patient's needs, it may be more convenient than the separate components.**

CONTRAINDICATIONS

TIMOLIDE is contraindicated in patients with bronchial asthma or with a history of bronchial asthma, or severe chronic obstructive pulmonary disease (see WARNINGS); sinus bradycardia; second and third degree atrioventricular block; overt cardiac failure (see WARNINGS); cardiogenic shock; anuria; hypersensitivity to this product or to sulfonamide-derived drugs.

WARNINGS

Cardiac Failure

Sympathetic stimulation may be essential for support of the circulation in individuals with diminished myocardial contractility, and its inhibition by beta-adrenergic receptor blockade may precipitate more severe failure. Although beta blockers should be avoided in overt congestive heart failure, they can be used, if necessary, with caution in patients with a history of failure who are well-compensated, usually with digitalis and diuretics. Both digitalis and timolol maleate slow AV conduction. If cardiac failure persists, therapy with TIMOLIDE should be withdrawn.

In Patients Without a History of Cardiac Failure continued depression of the myocardium with beta-blocking agents over a period of time can, in some cases, lead to cardiac failure. At the first sign or symptom of cardiac failure, patients receiving TIMOLIDE should be digitalized and/or be given additional diuretic therapy. Observe the patient closely. If cardiac failure continues, despite adequate digitalization and diuretic therapy, TIMOLIDE should be withdrawn.

Renal and Hepatic Disease and Electrolyte Disturbances

Since timolol maleate is partially metabolized in the liver and excreted mainly by the kidneys, dosage reductions may be necessary when hepatic and/or renal insufficiency is present.

Although the pharmacokinetics of timolol maleate are not greatly altered by renal impairment, marked hypotensive responses have been seen in patients with marked renal impairment undergoing dialysis after 20 mg doses. Dosing in such patients should therefore be especially cautious.

In patients with renal disease, thiazides may precipitate azotemia, and cumulative effects may develop in the presence of impaired renal function. If progressive renal impairment becomes evident, TIMOLIDE should be discontinued.

In patients with impaired hepatic function or progressive liver disease, even minor alterations in fluid and electrolyte balance may precipitate hepatic coma. Hepatic encephalopathy, manifested by tremors, confusion, and coma, has been reported in association with diuretic therapy including hydrochlorothiazide.

Exacerbation of Ischemic Heart Disease Following Abrupt Withdrawal —Hypersensitivity to catecholamines has been observed in patients withdrawn from beta blocker therapy; exacerbation of angina and, in some cases, myocardial infarction have occurred after *abrupt* discontinuation of such therapy. When discontinuing chronically administered timolol maleate, particularly in patients with ischemic heart disease, the dosage should be gradually reduced over a period of one to two weeks and the patient should be carefully monitored. If angina markedly worsens or acute coronary insufficiency develops, timolol maleate administration should be reinstituted promptly, at least temporarily, and other measures appropriate for the management of unstable angina should be taken. Patients should be warned against interruption or discontinuation of therapy without the physician's advice. Because coronary artery disease is common and may be unrecognized, it may be prudent not to discontinue timolol maleate therapy abruptly even in patients treated only for hypertension.

Obstructive Pulmonary Disease

PATIENTS WITH CHRONIC OBSTRUCTIVE PULMONARY DISEASE (e.g., CHRONIC BRONCHITIS, EMPHYSEMA) OF MILD OR MODERATE SEVERITY, BRONCHOSPASTIC DISEASE OR A HISTORY OF BRONCHOSPASTIC DISEASE (OTHER THAN BRONCHIAL ASTHMA OR A HISTORY OF BRONCHIAL ASTHMA, IN WHICH 'TIMOLIDE' IS CONTRAINDICATED, see CONTRAINDICATIONS), SHOULD IN GENERAL NOT RECEIVE BETA BLOCKERS, INCLUDING 'TIMOLIDE'. However, if TIMOLIDE is necessary in such patients, then the drug should be administered with caution since it may block bronchodilation produced by endogenous and exogenous catecholamine stimulation of $beta_2$ receptors.

Continued on next page

Information on the Merck & Co., Inc., products listed on these pages is from the prescribing information in use October 1, 2004. For information, please call 1-800-NSC-MERCK [1-800-672-6372].

Timolide—Cont.

Major Surgery
The necessity or desirability of withdrawal of beta-blocking therapy prior to major surgery is controversial. Beta-adrenergic receptor blockade impairs the ability of the heart to respond to beta-adrenergically mediated reflex stimuli. This may augment the risk of general anesthesia in surgical procedures. Some patients receiving beta-adrenergic receptor blocking agents have been subject to protracted severe hypotension during anesthesia. Difficulty in restarting and maintaining the heartbeat has also been reported. For these reasons, in patients undergoing elective surgery, some authorities recommend gradual withdrawal of beta-adrenergic receptor blocking agents.
If necessary during surgery, the effects of beta-adrenergic blocking agents may be reversed by sufficient doses of such agonists as isoproterenol, dopamine, dobutamine or levarterenol (see OVERDOSAGE).
Metabolic and Endocrine Effects
Beta-adrenergic blockade may mask certain clinical signs (e.g., tachycardia) of hyperthyroidism. Patients suspected of developing thyrotoxicosis should be managed carefully to avoid abrupt withdrawal of beta blockade which might precipitate a thyroid storm. Thiazides may decrease serum PBI levels without signs of thyroid disturbance.
Beta-adrenergic receptor blocking agents may mask the signs and symptoms of acute hypoglycemia. Therefore, TIMOLIDE should be administered with caution to patients subject to spontaneous hypoglycemia, or to diabetic patients (especially those with labile diabetes) who are receiving insulin or oral hypoglycemic agents. Insulin requirements in diabetic patients may be increased, decreased, or unchanged by thiazides. Diabetes mellitus which has been latent may become manifest during administration of thiazide diuretics.
Because calcium excretion is decreased by thiazides, TIMOLIDE should be discontinued before carrying out tests for parathyroid function. Pathologic changes in the parathyroid glands, with hypercalcemia and hypophosphatemia, have been observed in a few patients on prolonged thiazide therapy; however, the common complications of hyperparathyroidism such as renal lithiasis, bone resorption, and peptic ulceration have not been seen.
Hyperuricemia may occur or acute gout may be precipitated in certain patients receiving thiazide therapy.

PRECAUTIONS

General
Electrolyte and Fluid Balance Status: Periodic determination of serum electrolytes to detect possible electrolyte imbalance should be performed at appropriate intervals.
Patients should be observed for clinical signs of fluid or electrolyte imbalance, i.e., hyponatremia, hypochloremic alkalosis, and hypokalemia. Serum and urine electrolyte determinations are particularly important when the patient is vomiting excessively or receiving parenteral fluids. Warning signs or symptoms of fluid and electrolyte imbalance, irrespective of cause, include dryness of the mouth, thirst, weakness, lethargy, drowsiness, restlessness, confusion, seizures, muscle pains or cramps, muscular fatigue, hypotension, oliguria, tachycardia, and gastrointestinal disturbances such as nausea and vomiting.
Hypokalemia may develop, especially with brisk diuresis, when severe cirrhosis is present, or during concomitant use of corticosteroids or ACTH.
Interference with adequate oral electrolyte intake will also contribute to hypokalemia. Hypokalemia may cause cardiac arrhythmia and may also sensitize or exaggerate the response of the heart to the toxic effects of digitalis (e.g., increased ventricular irritability). Hypokalemia may be avoided or treated by use of potassium sparing diuretics or potassium supplements such as foods with a high potassium content.
Any chloride deficit during thiazide therapy is generally mild and usually does not require specific treatment except under extraordinary circumstances (as in liver disease or renal disease). Dilutional hyponatremia may occur in edematous patients in hot weather; appropriate therapy is water restriction rather than administration of salt except in rare instances when the hyponatremia is life threatening. In actual salt depletion, appropriate replacement is the therapy of choice.
Thiazides have been shown to increase urinary excretion of magnesium, which may result in hypomagnesemia.
Effects on Cholesterol and Triglyceride Levels:
Increases in cholesterol and triglyceride levels may be associated with thiazide diuretic therapy.
Muscle Weakness: Beta-adrenergic blockade has been reported to potentiate muscle weakness consistent with certain myasthenic symptoms (e.g., diplopia, ptosis, and generalized weakness). Timolol has been reported rarely to increase muscle weakness in some patients with myasthenia gravis or myasthenic symptoms.
Cerebrovascular Insufficiency: Because of potential effects of beta-adrenergic blocking agents relative to blood pressure and pulse, these agents should be used with caution in patients with cerebrovascular insufficiency. If signs or symptoms suggesting reduced cerebral blood flow are observed, consideration should be given to discontinuing these agents.

Drug Interactions
TIMOLIDE may potentiate the action of other antihypertensive agents used concomitantly. Close observation of the patient is recommended when TIMOLIDE is administered to patients receiving catecholamine-depleting drugs such as reserpine, because of possible additive effects and the production of hypotension and/or marked bradycardia, which may produce vertigo, syncope, or postural hypotension.
Blunting of the antihypertensive effect of beta-adrenoceptor blocking agents by non-steroidal anti-inflammatory drugs has been reported. In some patients, the administration of a non-steroidal anti-inflammatory agent can reduce the diuretic, natriuretic, and antihypertensive effects of loop, potassium-sparing and thiazide diuretics. Therefore, when TIMOLIDE and non-steroidal anti-inflammatory agents are used concomitantly, the patient should be observed closely to determine if the desired therapeutic effect has been obtained.
Literature reports suggest that oral calcium antagonists may be used in combination with beta-adrenergic blocking agents when heart function is normal, but should be avoided in patients with impaired cardiac function. Hypotension, AV conduction disturbances, and left ventricular failure have been reported in some patients receiving beta-adrenergic blocking agents when an oral calcium antagonist was added to the treatment regimen. Hypotension was more likely to occur if the calcium antagonist were a dihydropyridine derivative, e.g., nifedipine, while left ventricular failure and AV conduction disturbances were more likely to occur with either verapamil or diltiazem.
Intravenous calcium antagonists should be used with caution in patients receiving beta-adrenergic blocking agents.
The concomitant use of beta-adrenergic blocking agents with digitalis and either diltiazem or verapamil may have additive effects in prolonging AV conduction time.
Potentiated systemic beta-blockade (e.g., decreased heart rate) has been reported during combined treatment with quinidine and timolol, possibly because quinidine inhibits the metabolism of timolol via the P-450 enzyme, CYP2D6.
Beta adrenergic blocking agents may exacerbate the rebound hypertension which can follow the withdrawal of clonidine. If the two drugs are coadministered, the beta adrenergic blocking agent should be withdrawn several days before the gradual withdrawal of clonidine. If replacing clonidine by beta-blocker therapy, the introduction of beta adrenergic blocking agents should be delayed for several days after clonidine administration has stopped.
Risk from Anaphylactic Reaction: While taking beta-blockers, patients with a history of atopy or a history of severe anaphylactic reaction to a variety of allergens may be more reactive to repeated accidental, diagnostic, or therapeutic challenge with such allergens. Such patients may be unresponsive to the usual doses of epinephrine used to treat anaphylactic reactions.
In patients receiving thiazides, sensitivity reactions may occur with or without a history of allergy or bronchial asthma. The possible exacerbation or activation of systemic lupus erythematosus has been reported. The antihypertensive effects of thiazides may be enhanced in the post-sympathectomy patient.
Thiazides may decrease arterial responsiveness to norepinephrine. This diminution is not sufficient to preclude the therapeutic effectiveness of norepinephrine. Thiazides may increase the responsiveness to tubocurarine.
Lithium generally should not be given with diuretics because they reduce its renal clearance and add a high risk of lithium toxicity. Read circulars for lithium preparations before use of such preparations with TIMOLIDE.
Absorption of hydrochlorothiazide is impaired in the presence of anionic exchange resins. Single doses of either cholestyramine or colestipol resins bind the hydrochlorothiazide and reduce its absorption from the gastrointestinal tract by up to 85 and 43 percent, respectively.
Carcinogenesis, Mutagenesis, Impairment of Fertility
Carcinogenicity, mutagenicity, and fertility studies have not been conducted in animals with TIMOLIDE.
Timolol maleate: In a two-year study of timolol maleate in rats, there was a statistically significant increase in the incidence of adrenal pheochromocytomas in male rats administered 300 mg/kg/day (250 times** the maximum recommended daily human dose). Similar differences were not observed in rats administered doses equivalent to approximately 20 or 80 times** the maximum recommended daily human dose.
In a lifetime study in mice, there were statistically significant increases in the incidence of benign and malignant pulmonary tumors, benign uterine polyps and mammary adenocarcinoma in female mice at 500 mg/kg/day (approximately 400 times** the maximum recommended daily human dose), but not at 5 or 50 mg/kg/day. In a subsequent study in female mice, in which post-mortem examinations were limited to uterus and lungs, a statistically significant increase in the incidence of pulmonary tumors was again observed at 500 mg/kg/day.
The increased occurrence of mammary adenocarcinoma was associated with elevations of serum prolactin that occurred in female mice administered timolol at 500 mg/kg/day, but not at doses of 5 or 50 mg/kg/day. An increased incidence of mammary adenocarcinomas in rodents has been associated with administration of several other therapeutic agents which elevate serum prolactin, but no correlation between serum prolactin levels and mammary tumors has been established in man. Furthermore, in adult human female subjects who received oral dosages of up to 60 mg of timolol maleate, the maximum recommended daily human oral dosage, there were no clinically meaningful changes in serum prolactin.
Timolol maleate was devoid of mutagenic potential when evaluated *in vivo* (mouse) in the micronucleus test and cytogenetic assay (doses up to 800 mg/kg) and *in vitro* in a neoplastic cell transformation assay (up to 100 µg/mL). In Ames tests the highest concentrations of timolol employed, 5000 or 10,000 µg/plate, were associated with statistically significant elevations of revertants observed with tester strain TA100 (in seven replicate assays), but not in three additional strains. In the assays with tester strain TA100, no consistent dose response relationship was observed, nor did the ratio of test to control revertants reach 2. A ratio of 2 is usually considered the criterion for a positive Ames test.
Reproduction and fertility studies in rats showed no adverse effect on male or female fertility at doses up to 125 times** the maximum recommended daily human dose.
Hydrochlorothiazide: Two-year feeding studies in mice and rats conducted under the auspices of the National Toxicology Program (NTP) uncovered no evidence of a carcinogenic potential of hydrochlorothiazide in female mice (at doses of up to approximately 600 mg/kg/day) or in male and female rats (at doses of up to approximately 100 mg/kg/day). The NTP, however, found equivocal evidence for hepatocarcinogenicity in male mice.
Hydrochlorothiazide was not genotoxic *in vitro* in the Ames mutagenicity assay of *Salmonella typhimurium* strains TA 98, TA 100, TA 1535, TA 1537, and TA 1538 and in the Chinese Hamster Ovary (CHO) test for chromosomal aberrations, or *in vivo* in assays using mouse germinal cell chromosomes, Chinese hamster bone marrow chromosomes, and the *Drosophila* sex-linked recessive lethal trait gene. Positive test results were obtained only in the *in vitro* CHO Sister Chromatid Exchange (clastogenicity) and in the Mouse Lymphoma Cell (mutagenicity) assay, using concentrations of hydrochlorothiazide from 43 to 1300 µg/mL, and in the *Aspergillus nidulans* nondisjunction assay at an unspecified concentration.
Hydrochlorothiazide had no adverse effects on the fertility of mice and rats of either sex in studies wherein these species were exposed, via their diet, to doses of up to 100 and 4 mg/kg, respectively, prior to conception and throughout gestation.

** Based on patient weight of 50 kg

Pregnancy
Teratogenic Effects—Pregnancy Category C. Combinations of timolol maleate and hydrochlorothiazide were studied for teratogenic potential in the mouse and rabbit. The timolol maleate/hydrochlorothiazide combinations were administered orally to pregnant mice and pregnant rabbits at dosage levels of 1/2.5, 4/10, or 8/10 mg/kg/day. No teratogenic, embryotoxic, fetotoxic, or maternotoxic effects attributable to treatment were observed in either species. There are no adequate and well-controlled studies in pregnant women with TIMOLIDE. Because of the data listed below with the individual components, TIMOLIDE should be used during pregnancy only if the potential benefit justifies the potential risk to the fetus.
Timolol Maleate: Teratogenicity studies with timolol maleate in mice, rats and rabbits at doses up to 50 mg/kg/day (approximately 40 times** the maximum recommended daily human dose) showed no evidence of fetal malformations. Although delayed fetal ossification was observed at this dose in rats, there were no adverse effects on postnatal development of offspring. Doses of 1000 mg/kg/day (approximately 830 times** the maximum recommended daily human dose) were maternotoxic in mice and resulted in an increased number of fetal resorptions. Increased fetal resorptions were also seen in rabbits at doses of approximately 40 times** the maximum recommended daily human dose, in this case without apparent maternotoxicity.
Hydrochlorothiazide: Studies in which hydrochlorothiazide was orally administered to pregnant mice and rats during their respecitve periods of major organogenesis at doses up to 3000 and 1000 mg hydrochlorothiazide/kg, respectively, provided no evidence of harm to the fetus.
Nonteratogenic Effects.
Hydrochlorothiazide: TIMOLIDE contains hydrochlorothiazide. Thiazides cross the placental barrier and appear in cord blood. The possible hazards to the fetus include fetal or neonatal jaundice, thrombocytopenia, and possibly other adverse reactions which have occurred in the adult.

** Based on patient weight of 50 kg

Nursing Mothers
Timolol maleate and thiazides have been detected in human milk. Because of the potential for serious adverse reactions from timolol and hydrochlorothiazide in nursing infants, a decision should be made whether to discontinue nursing or to discontinue the drug, taking into account the importance of the drug to the mother.
Pediatric Use
Safety and effectiveness in pediatric patients have not been established.
Geriatric Use
Clinical studies of TIMOLIDE did not include sufficient numbers of subjects aged 65 and over to determine whether they respond differently from younger subjects. Other reported clinical experience has not identified differences in responses between the elderly and younger patients. In general, dose selection for an elderly patient should be cautious, usually starting at the low end of the dosing range, reflect-

ing the greater frequency of decreased hepatic, renal or cardiac function, and of concomitant disease or other drug therapy.

Both timolol and hydrochlorothiazide are known to be substantially excreted by the kidney, and the risk of toxic reactions to these drugs may be greater in patients with impaired renal function. Because elderly patients are more likely to have decreased renal function, care should be taken in dose selection, and it may be useful to monitor renal function. (See WARNINGS, *Renal and Hepatic Disease and Electrolyte Disturbances*.)

ADVERSE REACTIONS

TIMOLIDE is usually well tolerated in properly selected patients. Most adverse effects have been mild and transient. The adverse reactions listed in the following table were spontaneously reported and have been arranged into two groups: (1) incidence greater than 1%; and (2) incidence less than 1%. The incidence was obtained from clinical studies conducted in the United States (257 patients treated with TIMOLIDE).

Incidence Greater Than 1%	Incidence Less Than 1%
BODY AS A WHOLE	
fatigue/tiredness (1.9%)	chest pain
asthenia (1.9%)	headache
CARDIOVASCULAR	
hypotension (1.6%)	arrhythmia
bradycardia (1.2%)	syncope
	cardiac failure
DIGESTIVE SYSTEM	
none	diarrhea
	dyspepsia
	nausea
	gastrointestinal pain
	constipation
INTEGUMENTARY	
none	rash
	increased pigmentation
	dry mucous membranes
MUSCULOSKELETAL	
none	myalgia
NERVOUS SYSTEM	
dizziness (1.2%)	none
PSYCHIATRIC	
none	insomnia
	decreased libido
	nervousness
	confusion
	trouble concentrating
	somnolence
RESPIRATORY	
bronchial spasm (1.6%)	rales
dyspnea (1.2%)	
UROGENITAL	
none	renal colic

The following additional adverse effects have been reported in clinical experience with the drug: cerebral ischemia, cerebral vascular accident, gout, muscle cramps, oculogyric crisis, worsening of chronic obstructive pulmonary disease, earache, and impotence.

Other adverse reactions that have been reported with the individual components are listed below:

Timolol Maleate —Body as a Whole: extremity pain, decreased exercise tolerance, weight loss, fever; *Cardiovascular:* cardiac arrest, cerebral vascular accident, worsening of angina pectoris, sinoatrial block, AV block, worsening of arterial insufficiency, Raynaud's phenomenon, claudication, palpitations, vasodilatation, cold hands and feet, edema; *Digestive:* hepatomegaly, elevated liver function tests, vomiting; *Hematologic:* nonthrombocytopenic purpura; *Endocrine:* hyperglycemia, hypoglycemia; *Skin:* skin irritation, pruritus, sweating, alopecia; *Musculoskeletal:* arthralgia; *Nervous System:* local weakness, vertigo, paresthesia, increase in signs and symptoms of myasthenia gravis; *Psychiatric:* depression, nightmares, hallucinations; *Respiratory:* cough; *Special Senses:* visual disturbances, diplopia, ptosis, eye irritation, dry eyes, tinnitus; *Urogenital:* urination difficulties.

There have been reports of retroperitoneal fibrosis in patients receiving timolol maleate and in patients receiving other beta-adrenergic blocking agents. A causal relationship between this condition and therapy with beta-adrenergic blocking agents has not been established.

Hydrochlorothiazide —Body as a Whole: weakness; *Digestive:* anorexia, gastric irritation, vomiting, cramping, jaundice (intrahepatic cholestatic jaundice), pancreatitis, sialadenitis; *Nervous System/Psychiatric:* vertigo, paresthesias, restlessness; *Hematologic:* leukopenia, agranulocytosis, thrombocytopenia, aplastic anemia, hemolytic anemia; *Cardiovascular:* hypotension including orthostatic hypotension (may be aggravated by alcohol, barbiturates, narcotics or antihypertensive drugs); *Hypersensitivity:* purpura, photosensitivity, urticaria, necrotizing angiitis (vasculitis, cutaneous vasculitis), fever, respiratory distress including pneumonitis and pulmonary edema, anaphylactic reactions; *Metabolic:* hyperglycemia, glycosuria, hyperuricemia, electrolyte imbalance (see PRECAUTIONS); *Musculoskeletal:* muscle spasm; *Renal:* renal failure, renal dysfunction, interstitial nephritis (See WARNINGS); *Skin:* erythema multiforme including Stevens-Johnson syndrome, exfoliative dermatitis including toxic epidermal necrolysis, alopecia; *Special Senses:* transient blurred vision, xanthopsia.

Potential Adverse Effects: In addition, a variety of adverse effects not observed in clinical trials with timolol maleate, but reported with other beta-adrenergic blocking agents, should be considered potential adverse effects of timolol maleate: *Nervous System:* reversible mental depression progressing to catatonia; an acute reversible syndrome characterized by disorientation for time and place, short-term memory loss, emotional lability, slightly clouded sensorium, and decreased performance on neuropsychometrics; *Cardiovascular:* intensification of AV block (see CONTRAINDICATIONS); *Digestive:* mesenteric arterial thrombosis, ischemic colitis; *Hematologic:* agranulocytosis, thrombocytopenic purpura; *Allergic:* erythematous rash, fever combined with aching and sore throat, laryngospasm with respiratory distress; *Miscellaneous:* Peyronie's disease.

There have been reports of a syndrome comprising psoriasiform skin rash, conjunctivitis sicca, otitis, and sclerosing serositis attributed to the beta-adrenergic receptor blocking agent, practolol. This syndrome has not been reported with TIMOLIDE or BLOCADREN* (timolol maleate).

Clinical Laboratory Test Findings: Clinically important changes in standard laboratory parameters were rarely associated with the administration of TIMOLIDE. The changes in laboratory parameters were not progressive and usually were not associated with clinical manifestations. The most common changes were increases in serum triglycerides and uric acid and decreases in serum potassium and chloride. Decreases in HDL cholesterol have been reported.

*Registered trademark of MERCK & CO., INC.

OVERDOSAGE

No data are available with regard to overdosage with TIMOLIDE in humans.

Pretreatment of mice with hydrochlorothiazide (5 mg/kg) did not alter the LD_{50} of timolol (1320 mg/kg compared to 1300 mg/kg without pretreatment).

No specific information is available on the treatment of overdosage with TIMOLIDE, and no specific antidote is available. Treatment is symptomatic and supportive. Therapy with TIMOLIDE should be discontinued and the patient observed closely. Suggested measures include induction of emesis and/or gastric lavage, and correction of dehydration, electrolyte imbalance, and hypotension by established procedures.

Timolol Maleate

Overdosage has been reported with Tablets BLOCADREN* (timolol maleate). A 30-year-old female ingested 650 mg of BLOCADREN (maximum recommended daily dose—60 mg) and experienced second and third degree heart block. She recovered without treatment but approximately two months later developed irregular heartbeat, hypertension, dizziness, tinnitus, faintness, increased pulse rate and borderline first degree heart block.

The oral LD_{50} of the drug is 1190 and 900 mg/kg in female mice and female rats, respectively.

An *in vitro* hemodialysis study, using ^{14}C timolol added to human plasma or whole blood, showed that timolol was readily dialyzed from these fluids; however, a study of patients with renal failure showed that timolol did not dialyze readily.

The most common signs and symptoms to be expected with overdosage with a beta-adrenergic receptor blocking agent are symptomatic bradycardia, hypotension, bronchospasm, and acute cardiac failure. If overdosage occurs the following therapeutic measures should be considered:

(1) *Gastric lavage.*

(2) *Symptomatic bradycardia:* Use atropine sulfate intravenously in a dosage of 0.25 mg to 2 mg to induce vagal blockade. If bradycardia persists, intravenous isoproterenol hydrochloride should be administered cautiously. In refractory cases the use of a transvenous cardiac pacemaker may be considered.

(3) *Hypotension:* Use sympathomimetic pressor drug therapy, such as dopamine, dobutamine or levarterenol. In refractory cases the use of glucagon hydrochloride has been reported to be useful.

(4) *Bronchospasm:* Use isoproterenol hydrochloride. Additional therapy with aminophylline may be considered.

(5) *Acute cardiac failure:* Conventional therapy with digitalis, diuretics, and oxygen should be instituted immediately. In refractory cases the use of intravenous aminophylline is suggested. This may be followed, if necessary, by glucagon hydrochloride which has been reported to be useful.

(6) *Heart block (second or third degree):* Use isoproterenol hydrochloride or a transvenous cardiac pacemaker.

Hydrochlorothiazide

The most common signs and symptoms observed with hydrochlorothiazide overdosage are those caused by electrolyte depletion (hypokalemia, hypochloremia, hyponatremia) and dehydration resulting from excessive diuresis. If digitalis has also been administered, hypokalemia may accentuate cardiac arrhythmias.

*Registered trademark of MERCK & CO., INC.

DOSAGE AND ADMINISTRATION

The recommended starting and maintenance dosage is 1 tablet twice a day or 2 tablets once a day. Hydrochlorothiazide can be given at doses of 12.5 to 50 mg per day when used alone. If the antihypertensive response is not satisfactory, another nondiuretic antihypertensive agent may be added.

HOW SUPPLIED

No. 3373—Tablets TIMOLIDE 10-25 are light blue, flat, hexagonal-shaped, compressed tablets, with code MSD 67 on one side and TIMOLIDE on the other. Each tablet contains 10 mg of timolol maleate and 25 mg of hydrochlorothiazide. They are supplied as follows:

NDC 0006-0067-68 bottles of 100.

Storage

Store at controlled room temperature, 15–30°C (59–86°F). Keep container tightly closed. Protect from light.

7928435 Issued October 2003

Shown in Product Identification Guide, page 324

TIMOPTIC® ℞
0.25% and 0.5%
(Timolol Maleate Ophthalmic Solution)
Sterile Ophthalmic Solution

DESCRIPTION

TIMOPTIC* (timolol maleate ophthalmic solution) is a non-selective beta-adrenergic receptor blocking agent. Its chemical name is (-)-1-(*tert*-butylamino)-3-[(4-morpholino-1,2,5-thiadiazol-3-yl)oxy]-2-propanol maleate (1:1) (salt). Timolol maleate possesses an asymmetric carbon atom in its structure and is provided as the levo-isomer. The nominal optical rotation of timolol maleate is:

$$[\alpha]^{25°}_{405\ nm} \text{ in 1.0N HCl (C = 5\%)} = -12.2° \ (-11.7° \text{ to } -12.5°).$$

Its molecular formula is $C_{13}H_{24}N_4O_3S{\cdot}C_4H_4O_4$ and its structural formula is:

Timolol maleate has a molecular weight of 432.50. It is a white, odorless, crystalline powder which is soluble in water, methanol, and alcohol. TIMOPTIC is stable at room temperature.

TIMOPTIC Ophthalmic Solution is supplied as a sterile, isotonic, buffered, aqueous solution of timolol maleate in two dosage strengths: Each mL of TIMOPTIC 0.25% contains 2.5 mg of timolol (3.4 mg of timolol maleate). The pH of the solution is approximately 7.0, and the osmolarity is 274-328 mOsmol. Each mL of TIMOPTIC 0.5% contains 5 mg of timolol (6.8 mg of timolol maleate). Inactive ingredients: monobasic and dibasic sodium phosphate, sodium hydroxide to adjust pH, and water for injection. Benzalkonium chloride 0.01% is added as preservative.

*Registered trademark of MERCK & CO., INC.

CLINICAL PHARMACOLOGY

Mechanism of Action

Timolol maleate is a $beta_1$ and $beta_2$ (non-selective) adrenergic receptor blocking agent that does not have significant intrinsic sympathomimetic, direct myocardial depressant, or local anesthetic (membrane-stabilizing) activity.

Beta-adrenergic receptor blockade reduces cardiac output in both healthy subjects and patients with heart disease. In patients with severe impairment of myocardial function, beta-adrenergic receptor blockade may inhibit the stimulatory effect of the sympathetic nervous system necessary to maintain adequate cardiac function.

Beta-adrenergic receptor blockade in the bronchi and bronchioles results in increased airway resistance from unopposed parasympathetic activity. Such an effect in patients with asthma or other bronchospastic conditions is potentially dangerous.

TIMOPTIC Ophthalmic Solution, when applied topically on the eye, has the action of reducing elevated as well as normal intraocular pressure, whether or not accompanied by glaucoma. Elevated intraocular pressure is a major risk factor in the pathogenesis of glaucomatous visual field loss. The higher the level of intraocular pressure, the greater the likelihood of glaucomatous visual field loss and optic nerve damage.

Continued on next page

Information on the Merck & Co., Inc., products listed on these pages is from the prescribing information in use October 1, 2004. For information, please call 1-800-NSC-MERCK [1-800-672-6372].

Timoptic—Cont.

The onset of reduction in intraocular pressure following administration of TIMOPTIC can usually be detected within one-half hour after a single dose. The maximum effect usually occurs in one to two hours and significant lowering of intraocular pressure can be maintained for periods as long as 24 hours with a single dose. Repeated observations over a period of one year indicate that the intraocular pressure-lowering effect of TIMOPTIC is well maintained.

The precise mechanism of the ocular hypotensive action of TIMOPTIC is not clearly established at this time. Tonography and fluorophotometry studies in man suggest that its predominant action may be related to reduced aqueous formation. However, in some studies a slight increase in outflow facility was also observed.

Pharmacokinetics

In a study of plasma drug concentration in six subjects, the systemic exposure to timolol was determined following twice daily administration of TIMOPTIC 0.5%. The mean peak plasma concentration following morning dosing was 0.46 ng/mL and following afternoon dosing was 0.35 ng/mL.

Clinical Studies

In controlled multiclinic studies in patients with untreated intraocular pressures of 22 mmHg or greater, TIMOPTIC 0.25 percent or 0.5 percent administered twice a day produced a greater reduction in intraocular pressure than 1, 2, 3, or 4 percent pilocarpine solution administered four times a day or 0.5, 1, or 2 percent epinephrine hydrochloride solution administered twice a day.

In these studies, TIMOPTIC was generally well tolerated and produced fewer and less severe side effects than either pilocarpine or epinephrine. A slight reduction of resting heart rate in some patients receiving TIMOPTIC (mean reduction 2.9 beats/minute standard deviation 10.2) was observed.

INDICATIONS AND USAGE

Timoptic Ophthalmic Solution is indicated in the treatment of elevated intraocular pressure in patients with ocular hypertension or open-angle glaucoma.

CONTRAINDICATIONS

TIMOPTIC is contraindicated in patients with (1) bronchial asthma; (2) a history of bronchial asthma; (3) severe chronic obstructive pulmonary disease (see **WARNINGS**); (4) sinus bradycardia; (5) second or third degree atrioventricular block; (6) overt cardiac failure (see **WARNINGS**); (7) cardiogenic shock; or (8) hypersensitivity to any component of this product.

WARNINGS

As with many topically applied ophthalmic drugs, this drug is absorbed systemically.

The same adverse reactions found with systemic administration of beta-adrenergic blocking agents may occur with topical administration. For example, severe respiratory reactions and cardiac reactions, including death due to bronchospasm in patients with asthma, and rarely death in association with cardiac failure, have been reported following systemic or ophthalmic administration of timolol maleate (see CONTRAINDICATIONS).

Cardiac Failure

Sympathetic stimulation may be essential for support of the circulation in individuals with diminished myocardial contractility, and its inhibition by beta-adrenergic receptor blockade may precipitate more severe failure.

In Patients Without a History of Cardiac Failure continued depression of the myocardium with beta-blocking agents over a period of time can, in some cases, lead to cardiac failure. At the first sign or symptom of cardiac failure TIMOPTIC should be discontinued.

Obstructive Pulmonary Disease

Patients with chronic obstructive pulmonary disease (e.g., chronic bronchitis, emphysema) of mild or moderate severity, bronchospastic disease, or a history of bronchospastic disease (other than bronchial asthma or a history of bronchial asthma, in which TIMOPTIC is contraindicated [see **CONTRAINDICATIONS**]) should, in general, not receive beta-blockers, including TIMOPTIC.

Major Surgery

The necessity or desirability of withdrawal of beta-adrenergic blocking agents prior to major surgery is controversial. Beta-adrenergic receptor blockade impairs the ability of the heart to respond to beta-adrenergically mediated reflex stimuli. This may augment the risk of general anesthesia in surgical procedures. Some patients receiving beta-adrenergic receptor blocking agents have experienced protracted severe hypotension during anesthesia. Difficulty in restarting and maintaining the heartbeat has also been reported. For these reasons, in patients undergoing elective surgery, some authorities recommend gradual withdrawal of beta-adrenergic receptor blocking agents.

If necessary during surgery, the effects of beta-adrenergic blocking agents may be reversed by sufficient doses of adrenergic agonists.

Diabetes Mellitus

Beta-adrenergic blocking agents should be administered with caution in patients subject to spontaneous hypoglycemia or to diabetic patients (especially those with labile diabetes) who are receiving insulin or oral hypoglycemic agents. Beta-adrenergic receptor blocking agents may mask the signs and symptoms of acute hypoglycemia.

Thyrotoxicosis

Beta-adrenergic blocking agents may mask certain clinical signs (e.g., tachycardia) of hyperthyroidism. Patients suspected of developing thyrotoxicosis should be managed carefully to avoid abrupt withdrawal of beta-adrenergic blocking agents that might precipitate a thyroid storm.

PRECAUTIONS

General

Because of potential effects of beta-adrenergic blocking agents on blood pressure and pulse, these agents should be used with caution in patients with cerebrovascular insufficiency. If signs or symptoms suggesting reduced cerebral blood flow develop following initiation of therapy with TIMOPTIC, alternative therapy should be considered.

There have been reports of bacterial keratitis associated with the use of multiple dose containers of topical ophthalmic products. These containers had been inadvertently contaminated by patients who, in most cases, had a concurrent corneal disease or a disruption of the ocular epithelial surface. (See **PRECAUTIONS**, *Information for Patients.*)

Choroidal detachment after filtration procedures has been reported with the administration of aqueous suppressant therapy (e.g. timolol).

Angle-closure glaucoma: In patients with angle-closure glaucoma, the immediate objective of treatment is to reopen the angle. This requires constricting the pupil. Timolol maleate has little or no effect on the pupil. TIMOPTIC should not be used alone in the treatment of angle-closure glaucoma.

Anaphylaxis: While taking beta-blockers, patients with a history of atopy or a history of severe anaphylactic reactions to a variety of allergens may be more reactive to repeated accidental, diagnostic, or therapeutic challenge with such allergens. Such patients may be unresponsive to the usual doses of epinephrine used to treat anaphylactic reactions.

Muscle Weakness: Beta-adrenergic blockade has been reported to potentiate muscle weakness consistent with certain myasthenic symptoms (e.g., diplopia, ptosis, and generalized weakness). Timolol has been reported rarely to increase muscle weakness in some patients with myasthenia gravis or myasthenic symptoms.

Information for Patients

Patients should be instructed to avoid allowing the tip of the dispensing container to contact the eye or surrounding structures.

Patients should also be instructed that ocular solutions, if handled improperly, can become contaminated by common bacteria known to cause ocular infections. Serious damage to the eye and subsequent loss of vision may result from using contaminated solutions. (See **PRECAUTIONS**, *General.*)

Patients should also be advised that if they have ocular surgery or develop an intercurrent ocular condition (e.g., trauma or infection), they should immediately seek their physician's advice concerning the continued use of the present multidose container.

Patients with bronchial asthma, a history of bronchial asthma, severe chronic obstructive pulmonary disease, sinus bradycardia, second or third degree atrioventricular block, or cardiac failure should be advised not to take this product. (See **CONTRAINDICATIONS.**)

Patients should be advised that TIMOPTIC contains benzalkonium chloride which may be absorbed by soft contact lenses. Contact lenses should be removed prior to administration of the solution. Lenses may be reinserted 15 minutes following TIMOPTIC administration.

Drug Interactions

Although TIMOPTIC used alone has little or no effect on pupil size, mydriasis resulting from concomitant therapy with TIMOPTIC and epinephrine has been reported occasionally.

Beta-adrenergic blocking agents: Patients who are receiving a beta-adrenergic blocking agent orally and TIMOPTIC should be observed for potential additive effects of beta-blockade, both systemic and on intraocular pressure. The concomitant use of two topical beta-adrenergic blocking agents is not recommended.

Calcium antagonists: Caution should be used in the coadministration of beta-adrenergic blocking agents, such as TIMOPTIC, and oral or intravenous calcium antagonists because of possible atrioventricular conduction disturbances, left ventricular failure, and hypotension. In patients with impaired cardiac function, coadministration should be avoided.

Catecholamine-depleting drugs: Close observation of the patient is recommended when a beta blocker is administered to patients receiving catecholamine-depleting drugs such as reserpine, because of possible additive effects and the production of hypotension and/or marked bradycardia, which may result in vertigo, syncope, or postural hypotension.

Digitalis and calcium antagonists: The concomitant use of beta-adrenergic blocking agents with digitalis and calcium antagonists may have additive effects in prolonging atrioventricular conduction time.

Quinidine: Potentiated systemic beta-blockade (e.g., decreased heart rate) has been reported during combined treatment with quinidine and timolol, possibly because quinidine inhibits the metabolism of timolol via the P-450 enzyme, CYP2D6.

Clonidine: Oral beta-adrenergic blocking agents may exacerbate the rebound hypertension which can follow the withdrawal of clonidine. There have been no reports of exacerbation of rebound hypertension with ophthalmic timolol maleate.

Injectable epinephrine: (See **PRECAUTIONS**, *General, Anaphylaxis*)

Carcinogenesis, Mutagenesis, Impairment of Fertility

In a two-year oral study of timolol maleate administered orally to rats, there was a statistically significant increase in the incidence of adrenal pheochromocytomas in male rats administered 300 mg/kg/day (approximately 42,000 times the systemic exposure following the maximum recommended human ophthalmic dose). Similar difference were not observed in rats administered oral doses equivalent to approximately 14,000 times the maximum recommended human ophthalmic dose.

In a lifetime oral study in mice, there were statistically significant increases in the incidence of benign and malignant pulmonary tumors, benign uterine polyps and mammary adenocarcinomas in female mice at 500 mg/kg/day, (approximately 71,000 times the systemic exposure following the maximum recommended human ophthalmic dose), but not at 5 or 50 mg/kg/day (approximately 700 or 7,000, respectively, times the systemic exposure following the maximum recommended human ophthalmic dose). In a subsequent study in female mice, in which post-mortem examinations were limited to the uterus and the lungs, a statistically significant increase in the incidence of pulmonary tumors was again observed at 500 mg/kg/day.

The increased occurrence of mammary adenocarcinomas was associated with elevations in serum prolactin which occurred in female mice administered oral timolol at 500 mg/kg/day, but not at doses of 5 or 50 mg/kg/day. An increased incidence of mammary adenocarcinomas in rodents has been associated with administration of several other therapeutic agents that elevate serum prolactin, but no correlation between serum prolactin levels and mammary tumors has been established in humans. Furthermore, in adult human female subjects who received oral dosages of up to 60 mg of timolol maleate (the maximum recommended human oral dosage), there were no clinically meaningful changes in serum prolactin.

Timolol maleate was devoid of mutagenic potential when tested *in vivo* (mouse) in the micronucleus test and cytogenetic assay (doses up to 800 mg/kg) and *in vitro* in a neoplastic cell transformation assay (up to 100 mcg/mL). In Ames tests the highest concentrations of timolol employed, 5000 or 10,000 mcg/plate, were associated with statistically significant elevations of revertants observed with tester strain TA100 (in seven replicate assays), but not in the remaining three strains. In the assays with tester strain TA100, no consistent dose response relationship was observed, and the ratio of test to control revertants did not reach 2. A ratio of 2 is usually considered the criterion for a positive Ames test.

Reproduction and fertility studies in rats demonstrated no adverse effect on male or female fertility at doses up to 21,000 times the systemic exposure following the maximum recommended human ophthalmic dose.

Pregnancy:

Teratogenic Effects—Pregnancy Category C. Teratogenicity studies with timolol in mice, rats, and rabbits at oral doses up to 50 mg/kg/day (7,000 times the systemic exposure following the maximum recommended human ophthalmic dose) demonstrated no evidence of fetal malformations. Although delayed fetal ossification was observed at this dose in rats, there were no adverse effects on postnatal development of offspring. Doses of 1000 mg/kg/day (142,000 times the systemic exposure following the maximum recommended human ophthalmic dose) were maternotoxic in mice and resulted in an increased number of fetal resorptions. Increased fetal resorptions were also seen in rabbits at doses of 14,000 times the systemic exposure following the maximum recommended human ophthalmic dose, in this case without apparent maternotoxicity.

There are no adequate and well-controlled studies in pregnant women. TIMOPTIC should be used during pregnancy only if the potential benefit justifies the potential risk to the fetus.

Nursing Mothers

Timolol maleate has been detected in human milk following oral and ophthalmic drug administration. Because of the potential for serious adverse reactions from TIMOPTIC in nursing infants, a decision should be made whether to discontinue nursing or to discontinue the drug, taking into account the importance of the drug to the mother.

Pediatric Use

Safety and effectiveness in pediatric patients have not been established.

Geriatric Use

No overall differences in safety or effectiveness have been observed between elderly and younger patients.

ADVERSE REACTIONS

The most frequently reported adverse experiences have been burning and stinging upon instillation (approximately one in eight patients).

The following additional adverse experiences have been reported less frequently with ocular administration of this or other timolol maleate formulations:

BODY AS A WHOLE

Headache, asthenia/fatigue, and chest pain.

CARDIOVASCULAR

Bradycardia, arrhythmia, hypotension, hypertension, syncope, heart block, cerebral vascular accident, cerebral ische-

mia, cardiac failure, worsening of angina pectoris, palpitation, cardiac arrest, pulmonary edema, edema, claudication, Raynaud's phenomenon, and cold hands and feet.
DIGESTIVE
Nausea, diarrhea, dyspepsia, anorexia, and dry mouth.
IMMUNOLOGIC
Systemic lupus erythematosus.
NERVOUS SYSTEM/PSYCHIATRIC
Dizziness, increase in signs and symptoms of myasthenia gravis, paresthesia, somnolence, insomnia, nightmares, behavioral changes and psychic disturbances including depression, confusion, hallucinations, anxiety, disorientation, nervousness, and memory loss.
SKIN
Alopecia and psoriasiform rash or exacerbation of psoriasis.
HYPERSENSITIVITY
Signs and symptoms of systemic allergic reactions, including anaphylaxis, angioedema, urticaria, and localized and generalized rash.
RESPIRATORY
Bronchospasm (predominantly in patients with pre-existing bronchospastic disease), respiratory failure, dyspnea, nasal congestion, cough and upper respiratory infections.
ENDOCRINE
Masked symptoms of hypoglycemia in diabetic patients (see **WARNINGS**).
SPECIAL SENSES
Signs and symptoms of ocular irritation including conjunctivitis, blepharitis, keratitis, ocular pain, discharge (e.g., crusting), foreign body sensation, itching and tearing, and dry eyes; ptosis; decreased corneal sensitivity; cystoid macular edema; visual disturbances including refractive changes and diplopia; pseudopemphigoid; choroidal detachment following filtration surgery (see **PRECAUTIONS**, *General*); and tinnitus.
UROGENITAL
Retroperitoneal fibrosis, decreased libido, impotence, and Peyronie's disease.
The following additional adverse effects have been reported in clinical experience with ORAL timolol maleate or other ORAL beta-blocking agents and may be considered potential effects of ophthalmic timolol maleate: *Allergic:* Erythematous rash, fever combined with aching and sore throat, laryngospasm with respiratory distress; *Body as a Whole:* Extremity pain, decreased exercise tolerance, weight loss; *Cardiovascular:* Worsening of arterial insufficiency, vasodilatation; *Digestive:* Gastrointestinal pain, hepatomegaly, vomiting, mesenteric arterial thrombosis, ischemic colitis; *Hematologic:* Nonthrombocytopenic purpura; thrombocytopenic purpura, agranulocytosis; *Endocrine:* Hyperglycemia, hypoglycemia; *Skin:* Pruritus, skin irritation, increased pigmentation, sweating; *Musculoskeletal:* Arthralgia; *Nervous System/Psychiatric:* Vertigo, local weakness, diminished concentration, reversible mental depression progressing to catatonia, and acute reversible syndrome characterized by disorientation for time and place, emotional lability, slightly clouded sensorium, and decreased performance on neuropsychometrics; *Respiratory:* Rales, bronchial obstruction; *Urogenital:* Urination difficulties.

OVERDOSAGE

There have been reports of inadvertent overdosage with TIMOPTIC Ophthalmic Solution resulting in systemic effects similar to those seen with systemic beta-adrenergic blocking agents such as dizziness, headache, shortness of breath, bradycardia, bronchospasm, and cardiac arrest (see also ADVERSE REACTIONS).
Overdosage has been reported with Tablets BLOCADREN* (timolol maleate tablets). A 30 year old female ingested 650 mg of BLOCADREN (maximum recommended oral daily dose is 60 mg) and experienced second and third degree heart block. She recovered without treatment but approximately two months later developed irregular heartbeat, hypertension, dizziness, tinnitus, faintness, increased pulse rate, and borderline first degree heart block.
An *in vitro* hemodialysis study, using ^{14}C timolol added to human plasma or whole blood, showed that timolol was readily dialyzed from these fluids; however, a study of patients with renal failure showed that timolol did not dialyze readily.

*Registered trademark of MERCK & CO., INC.

DOSAGE AND ADMINISTRATION

TIMOPTIC Ophthalmic Solution is available in concentrations of 0.25 and 0.5 percent. The usual starting dose is one drop of 0.25 percent TIMOPTIC in the affected eye(s) twice a day. If the clinical response is not adequate, the dosage may be changed to one drop of 0.5 percent solution in the affected eye(s) twice a day.
Since in some patients the pressure-lowering response to TIMOPTIC may require a few weeks to stabilize, evaluation should include a determination of intraocular pressure after approximately 4 weeks of treatment with TIMOPTIC.
If the intraocular pressure is maintained at satisfactory levels, the dosage schedule may be changed to one drop once a day in the affected eye(s). Because of diurnal variations in intraocular pressure, satisfactory response to the once-a-day dose is best determined by measuring the intraocular pressure at different times during the day.
Dosages above one drop of 0.5 percent TIMOPTIC twice a day generally have not been shown to produce further reduction in intraocular pressure. If the patient's intraocular

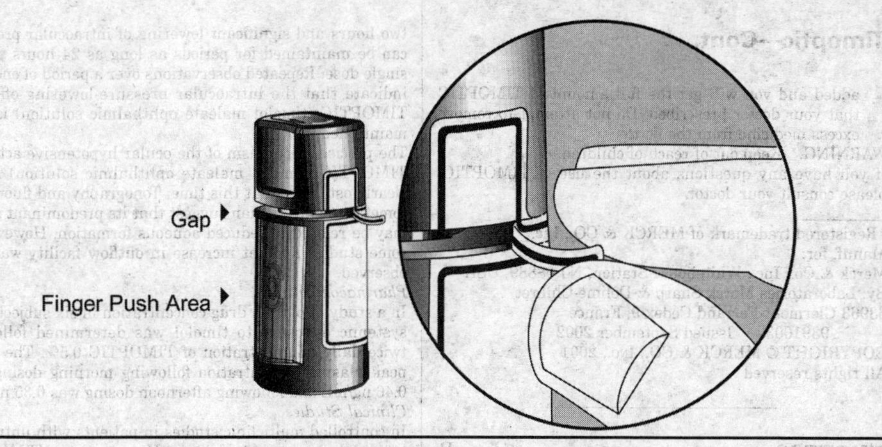

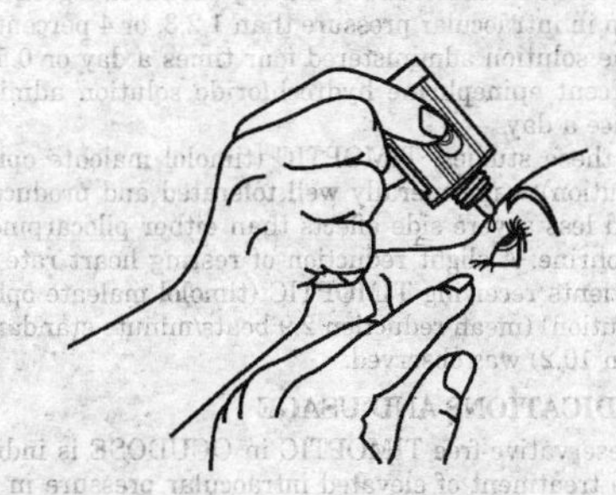

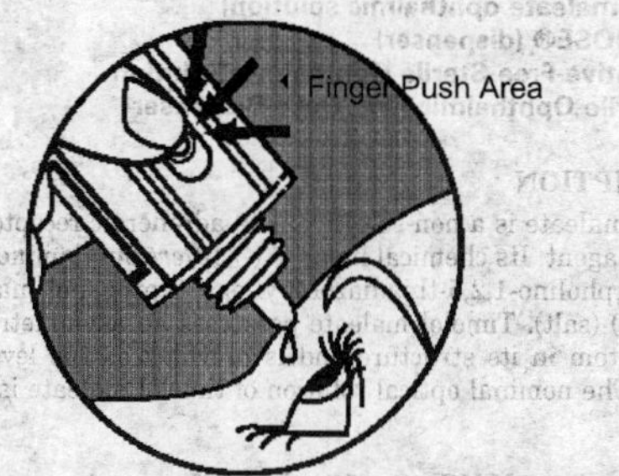

pressure is still not at a satisfactory level on this regimen, concomitant therapy with other agent(s) for lowering intraocular pressure can be instituted. The concomitant use of two topical beta-adrenergic blocking agents is not recommended. (See PRECAUTIONS, *Drug Interactions, Beta-adrenergic blocking agents.*)

HOW SUPPLIED

Sterile Ophthalmic Solution TIMOPTIC is a clear, colorless to light yellow solution.
No. 8895—TIMOPTIC Ophthalmic Solution, 0.25% timolol equivalent, is supplied in an OCUMETER®* PLUS container, a translucent, natural HDPE plastic ophthalmic dispenser with a white polystyrene cap with color coded label, and a controlled drop tip as follows:
NDC 0006-8895-35, 5 mL in a 7.5 mL bottle
NDC 0006-8895-36, 10 mL in an 18 mL bottle.
No. 8896—TIMOPTIC Ophthalmic Solution, 0.5% timolol equivalent, is supplied in an OCUMETER®* PLUS container, a translucent, natural HDPE plastic ophthalmic dispenser with a white polystyrene cap with color coded label, and a controlled drop tip as follows:
NDC 0006-8896-35, 5 mL in a 7.5 mL bottle
NDC 0006-8896-36, 10 mL in an 18 mL bottle.

Storage

Store at room temperature, 15–30°C (59–86°F). Protect from freezing. Protect from light.

*Registered trademark of MERCK & CO., INC.

INSTRUCTIONS FOR USE

Please follow these instructions carefully when using TIMOPTIC*. Use TIMOPTIC as prescribed by your doctor.

1. If you use other topically applied ophthalmic medications, they should be administered at least 10 minutes before or after TIMOPTIC.
2. Wash hands before each use.
3. Before using the medication for the first time, be sure the Safety Strip on the front of the bottle is unbroken. A gap between the bottle and the cap is normal for an unopened bottle.

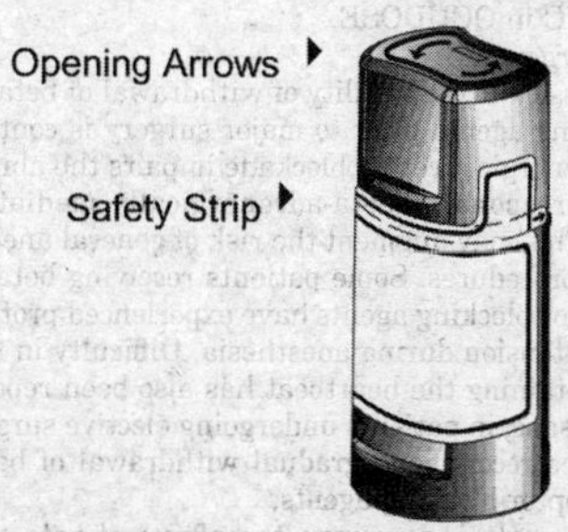

4. Tear off the Safety Strip to break the seal. [See first figure above]
5. To open the bottle, unscrew the cap by turning as indicated by the arrows.

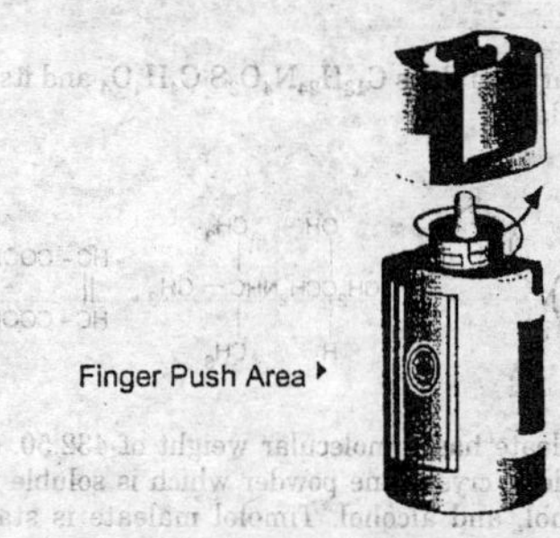

6. Tilt your head back and pull your lower eyelid down slightly to form a pocket between your eyelid and your eye.

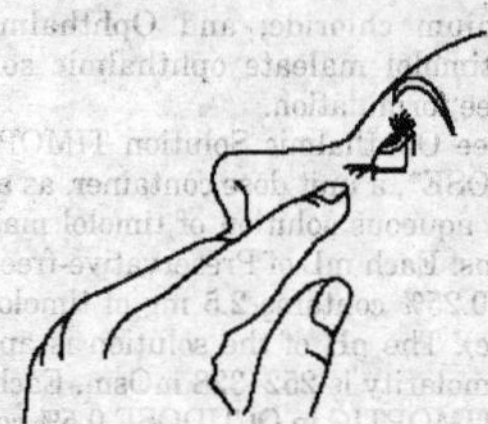

7. Invert the bottle, and press lightly with the thumb or index finger over the "Finger Push Area" (as shown) until a single drop is dispensed into the eye as directed by your doctor.
[See second figure above]
DO NOT TOUCH YOUR EYE OR EYELID WITH THE DROPPER TIP.
Ophthalmic medications, if handled improperly, can become contaminated by common bacteria known to cause eye infections. Serious damage to the eye and subsequent loss of vision may result from using contaminated ophthalmic medications. If you think your medication may be contaminated, or if you develop an eye infection, contact your doctor immediately concerning continued use of this bottle.
8. Repeat steps 6 & 7 with the other eye if instructed to do so by your doctor.
9. Replace the cap by turning until it is firmly touching the bottle. Do not overtighten the cap.
10. The dispenser tip is designed to provide a pre-measured drop; therefore, do NOT enlarge the hole of the dispenser tip.
11. After you have used all doses, there will be some TIMOPTIC left in the bottle. You should not be concerned since an extra amount of TIMOPTIC has been

Continued on next page

Information on the Merck & Co., Inc., products listed on these pages is from the prescribing information in use October 1, 2004. For information, please call 1-800-NSC-MERCK [1-800-672-6372].

Timoptic—Cont.

added and you will get the full amount of TIMOPTIC that your doctor prescribed. Do not attempt to remove excess medicine from the bottle.

WARNING: Keep out of reach of children.

If you have any questions about the use of TIMOPTIC, please consult your doctor.

*Registered trademark of MERCK & CO., Inc.

Manuf. for:
Merck & Co., Inc., Whitehouse Station, NJ 08889, USA
By: Laboratories Merck Sharp & Dohme-Chibret
63963 Clermont-Ferrand Cedex 9, France
9391003 Issued September 2002

TIMOPTIC® ℞
0.25% and 0.5%
(timolol maleate ophthalmic solution)
in OCUDOSE® (dispenser)
Preservative-Free Sterile Ophthalmic Solution
in a Sterile Ophthalmic Unit Dose Dispenser

DESCRIPTION

Timolol maleate is a non-selective beta-adrenergic receptor blocking agent. Its chemical name is (-)-1-(*tert*-butylamino)-3-[(4-morpholino-1,2,5-thiadiazol-3-yl)oxy]-2-propanol maleate (1:1) (salt). Timolol maleate possesses an asymmetric carbon atom in its structure and is provided as the levo-isomer. The nominal optical rotation of timolol maleate is

$$[\alpha]^{25°}_{405\ nm} \text{ in 1.0N HCl (C = 5\%)} = -12.2° \ (-11.7° \text{ to } -12.5°).$$

Its molecular formula is $C_{13}H_{24}N_4O_3S{\cdot}C_4H_4O_4$ and its structural formula is:

Timolol maleate has a molecular weight of 432.50. It is a white, odorless, crystalline powder which is soluble in water, methanol, and alcohol. Timolol maleate is stable at room temperature.

Timolol maleate ophthalmic solution is supplied in two formulations: Ophthalmic Solution TIMOPTIC* (timolol maleate ophthalmic solution), which contains the preservative benzalkonium chloride; and Ophthalmic Solution TIMOPTIC* (timolol maleate ophthalmic solution), the preservative-free formulation.

Preservative-free Ophthalmic Solution TIMOPTIC is supplied in OCUDOSE*, a unit dose container, as a sterile, isotonic, buffered, aqueous solution of timolol maleate in two dosage strengths: Each mL of Preservative-free TIMOPTIC in OCUDOSE 0.25% contains 2.5 mg of timolol (3.4 mg of timolol maleate). The pH of the solution is approximately 7.0, and the osmolarity is 252–328 mOsm. Each mL of Preservative-free TIMOPTIC in OCUDOSE 0.5% contains 5 mg of timolol (6.8 mg of timolol maleate). Inactive ingredients: monobasic and dibasic sodium phosphate, sodium hydroxide to adjust pH, and water for injection.

*Registered trademark of MERCK & CO., INC.

CLINICAL PHARMACOLOGY

Mechanism of Action

Timolol maleate is a $beta_1$ and $beta_2$ (non-selective) adrenergic receptor blocking agent that does not have significant intrinsic sympathomimetic, direct myocardial depressant, or local anesthetic (membrane-stabilizing) activity.

Beta-adrenergic receptor blockade reduces cardiac output in both healthy subjects and patients with heart disease. In patients with severe impairment of myocardial function beta-adrenergic receptor blockade may inhibit the stimulatory effect of the sympathetic nervous system necessary to maintain adequate cardiac function.

Beta-adrenergic receptor blockade in the bronchi and bronchioles results in increased airway resistance from unopposed parasympathetic activity. Such an effect in patients with asthma or other bronchospastic conditions is potentially dangerous.

TIMOPTIC (timolol maleate ophthalmic solution), when applied topically on the eye, has the action of reducing elevated as well as normal intraocular pressure, whether or not accompanied by glaucoma. Elevated intraocular pressure is a major risk factor in the pathogenesis of glaucomatous visual field loss. The higher the level of intraocular pressure, the greater the likelihood of glaucomatous visual field loss and optic nerve damage.

The onset of reduction in intraocular pressure following administration of TIMOPTIC (timolol maleate ophthalmic solution) can usually be detected within one-half hour after a single dose. The maximum effect usually occurs in one to two hours and significant lowering of intraocular pressure can be maintained for periods as long as 24 hours with a single dose. Repeated observations over a period of one year indicate that the intraocular pressure-lowering effect of TIMOPTIC (timolol maleate ophthalmic solution) is well maintained.

The precise mechanism of the ocular hypotensive action of TIMOPTIC (timolol maleate ophthalmic solution) is not clearly established at this time. Tonography and fluorophotometry studies in man suggest that its predominant action may be related to reduced aqueous formation. However, in some studies a slight increase in outflow facility was also observed.

Pharmacokinetics

In a study of plasma drug concentration in six subjects, the systemic exposure to timolol was determined following twice daily administration of TIMOPTIC 0.5%. The mean peak plasma concentration following morning dosing was 0.46 ng/mL and following afternoon dosing was 0.35 ng/mL.

Clinical Studies

In controlled multiclinic studies in patients with untreated intraocular pressures of 22 mmHg or greater, TIMOPTIC (timolol maleate ophthalmic solution) 0.25 percent or 0.5 percent administered twice a day produced a greater reduction in intraocular pressure than 1,2,3, or 4 percent pilocarpine solution administered four times a day or 0.5, 1, or 2 percent epinephrine hydrochloride solution administered twice a day.

In these studies, TIMOPTIC (timolol maleate ophthalmic solution) was generally well tolerated and produced fewer and less severe side effects than either pilocarpine or epinephrine. A slight reduction of resting heart rate in some patients receiving TIMOPTIC (timolol maleate ophthalmic solution) (mean reduction 2.9 beats/minute standard deviation 10.2) was observed.

INDICATIONS AND USAGE

Preservative-free TIMOPTIC in OCUDOSE is indicated in the treatment of elevated intraocular pressure in patients with ocular hypertension or open-angle glaucoma.

Preservative-free TIMOPTIC in OCUDOSE may be used when a patient is sensitive to the preservative in TIMOPTIC (timolol maleate ophthalmic solution), benzalkonium chloride, or when use of a preservative-free topical medication is advisable.

CONTRAINDICATIONS

Preservative-free TIMOPTIC in OCUDOSE is contraindicated in patients with (1) bronchial asthma; (2) a history of bronchial asthma; (3) severe chronic obstructive pulmonary disease (see **WARNINGS**); (4) sinus bradycardia; (5) second or third degree atrioventricular block; (6) overt cardiac failure (see **WARNINGS**); (7) cardiogenic shock; or (8) hypersensitivity to any component of this product.

WARNINGS

As with many topically applied ophthalmic drugs, this drug is absorbed systemically.

The same adverse reactions found with systemic administration of beta-adrenergic blocking agents may occur with topical administration. For example, severe respiratory reactions and cardiac reactions, including death due to bronchospasm in patients with asthma, and rarely death in association with cardiac failure, have been reported following systemic or ophthalmic administration of timolol maleate (see CONTRAINDICATIONS).

Cardiac Failure

Sympathetic stimulation may be essential for support of the circulation in individuals with diminished myocardial contractility, and its inhibition by beta-adrenergic receptor blockade may precipitate more severe failure.

In Patients Without a History of Cardiac Failure continued depression of the myocardium with beta-blocking agents over a period of time can, in some cases, lead to cardiac failure. At the first sign or symptom of cardiac failure Preservative-free TIMOPTIC in OCUDOSE should be discontinued.

Obstructive Pulmonary Disease

Patients with chronic obstructive pulmonary disease (e.g., chronic bronchitis, emphysema) of mild or moderate severity, bronchospastic disease, or a history of bronchospastic disease (other than bronchial asthma or a history of bronchial asthma, in which TIMOPTIC in OCUDOSE is contraindicated [see **CONTRAINDICATIONS**]) should, in general, not receive beta-blockers, including Preservative-free TIMOPTIC in OCUDOSE.

Major Surgery

The necessity or desirability of withdrawal of beta-adrenergic blocking agents prior to major surgery is controversial. Beta-adrenergic receptor blockade impairs the ability of the heart to respond to beta-adrenergically mediated reflex stimuli. This may augment the risk of general anesthesia in surgical procedures. Some patients receiving beta-adrenergic receptor blocking agents have experienced protracted severe hypotension during anesthesia. Difficulty in restarting and maintaining the heartbeat has also been reported. For these reasons, in patients undergoing elective surgery, some authorities recommend gradual withdrawal of beta-adrenergic receptor blocking agents.

If necessary during surgery, the effects of beta-adrenergic blocking agents may be reversed by sufficient doses of adrenergic agonists.

Diabetes Mellitus

Beta-adrenergic blocking agents should be administered with caution in patients subject to spontaneous hypoglycemia or to diabetic patients (especially those with labile diabetes) who are receiving insulin or oral hypoglycemic agents. Beta-adrenergic receptor blocking agents may mask the signs and symptoms of acute hypoglycemia.

Thyrotoxicosis

Beta-adrenergic blocking agents may mask certain clinical signs (e.g., tachycardia) of hyperthyroidism. Patients suspected of developing thyrotoxicosis should be managed carefully to avoid abrupt withdrawal of beta-adrenergic blocking agents that might precipitate a thyroid storm.

PRECAUTIONS

General

Because of potential effects of beta-adrenergic blocking agents on blood pressure and pulse, these agents should be used with caution in patients with cerebrovascular insufficiency. If signs or symptoms suggesting reduced cerebral blood flow develop following initiation of therapy with Preservative-free TIMOPTIC in OCUDOSE, alternative therapy should be considered.

Choroidal detachment after filtration procedures has been reported with the administration of aqueous suppressant therapy (e.g. timolol).

Angle-closure glaucoma: In patients with angle-closure glaucoma, the immediate objective of treatment is to reopen the angle. This requires constricting the pupil. Timolol maleate has little or no effect on the pupil. TIMOPTIC in OCUDOSE should not be used alone in the treatment of angle-closure glaucoma.

Anaphylaxis: While taking beta-blockers, patients with a history of atopy or a history of severe anaphylactic reactions to a variety of allergens may be more reactive to repeated accidental, diagnostic, or therapeutic challenge with such allergens. Such patients may be unresponsive to the usual doses of epinephrine used to treat anaphylactic reactions.

Muscle Weakness: Beta-adrenergic blockade has been reported to potentiate muscle weakness consistent with certain myasthenic symptoms (e.g., diplopia, ptosis, and generalized weakness). Timolol has been reported rarely to increase muscle weakness in some patients with myasthenia gravis or myasthenic symptoms.

Information for Patients

Patients should be instructed about the use of Preservative-free TIMOPTIC in OCUDOSE.

Since sterility cannot be maintained after the individual unit is opened, patients should be instructed to use the product immediately after opening, and to discard the individual unit and any remaining contents immediately after use.

Patients with bronchial asthma, a history of bronchial asthma, severe chronic obstructive pulmonary disease, sinus bradycardia, second or third degree atrioventricular block, or cardiac failure should be advised not to take this product. (See **CONTRAINDICATIONS**.)

Drug Interactions

Although TIMOPTIC (timolol maleate ophthalmic solution) used alone has little or no effect on pupil size, mydriasis resulting from concomitant therapy with TIMOPTIC (timolol maleate ophthalmic solution) and epinephrine has been reported occasionally.

Beta-adrenergic blocking agents: Patients who are receiving a beta-adrenergic blocking agent orally and Preservative-free TIMOPTIC in OCUDOSE should be observed for potential additive effects of beta-blockade, both systemic and on intraocular pressure. The concomitant use of two topical beta-adrenergic blocking agents is not recommended.

Calcium antagonists: Caution should be used in the coadministration of beta-adrenergic blocking agents, such as Preservative-free TIMOPTIC in OCUDOSE, and oral or intravenous calcium antagonists, because of possible atrioventricular conduction disturbances, left ventricular failure, and hypotension. In patients with impaired cardiac function, coadministration should be avoided.

Catecholamine-depleting drugs: Close observation of the patient is recommended when a beta blocker is administered to patients receiving catecholamine-depleting drugs such as reserpine, because of possible additive effects and the production of hypotension and/or marked bradycardia, which may result in vertigo, syncope, or postural hypotension.

Digitalis and calcium antagonists: The concomitant use of beta-adrenergic blocking agents with digitalis and calcium antagonists may have additive effects in prolonging atrioventricular conduction time.

Quinidine: Potentiated systemic beta-blockade (e.g., decreased heart rate) has been reported during combined treatment with quinidine and timolol, possibly because quinidine inhibits the metabolism of timolol via the P-450 enzyme, CYP2D6.

Clonidine: Oral beta-adrenergic blocking agents may exacerbate the rebound hypertension which can follow the withdrawal of clonidine. There have been no reports of exacerbation of rebound hypertension with ophthalmic timolol maleate.

Injectable epinephrine: (See **PRECAUTIONS**, *General, Anaphylaxis)*

Carcinogenesis, Mutagenesis, Impairment of Fertility

In a two-year oral study of timolol maleate administered orally to rats, there was a statistically significant increase in the incidence of adrenal pheochromocytomas in male rats administered 300 mg/kg/day (approximately 42,000 times the systemic exposure following the maximum recommended human ophthalmic dose). Similar differences were not observed in rats administered oral doses equivalent to approximately 14,000 times the maximum recommended human ophthalmic dose.

In a lifetime oral study in mice, there were statistically significant increases in the incidence of benign and malignant pulmonary tumors, benign uterine polyps and mammary adenocarcinomas in female mice at 500 mg/kg/day (approximately 71,000 times the systemic exposure following the maximum recommended human ophthalmic dose), but not at 5 or 50 mg/kg/day (approximately 700 or 7,000 times, respectively, the systemic exposure following the maximum recommended human ophthalmic dose). In a subsequent study in female mice, in which post-mortem examinations were limited to the uterus and the lungs, a statistically significant increase in the incidence of pulmonary tumors was again observed at 500 mg/kg/day.

The increased occurrence of mammary adenocarcinomas was associated with elevations in serum prolactin which occurred in female mice administered oral timolol at 500 mg/kg/day, but not at doses of 5 or 50 mg/kg/day. An increased incidence of mammary adenocarcinomas in rodents has been associated with administration of several other therapeutic agents that elevate serum prolactin, but no correlation between serum prolactin levels and mammary tumors has been established in humans. Furthermore, in adult human female subjects who received oral dosages of up to 60 mg of timolol maleate (the maximum recommended human oral dosage), there were no clinically meaningful changes in serum prolactin.

Timolol maleate was devoid of mutagenic potential when tested *in vivo* (mouse) in the micronucleus test and cytogenetic assay (doses up to 800 mg/kg) and *in vitro* in a neoplastic cell transformation assay (up to 100 mcg/mL). In Ames tests the highest concentrations of timolol employed, 5000 or 10,000 mcg/plate, were associated with statistically significant elevations of revertants observed with tester strain TA 100 (in seven replicate assays), but not in the remaining three strains. In the assays with tester strain TA 100, no consistent dose response relationship was observed, and the ratio of test to control revertants did not reach 2. A ratio of 2 is usually considered the criterion for a positive Ames test.

Reproduction and fertility studies in rats demonstrated no adverse effect on male or female fertility at doses up to 21,000 times the systemic exposure following the maximum recommended human ophthalmic dose.

Pregnancy:

Teratogenic Effects—Pregnancy Category C. Teratogenicity studies with timolol in mice, rats and rabbits at oral doses up to 50 mg/kg/day (7,000 times the systemic exposure following the maximum recommended human ophthalmic dose) demonstrated no evidence of fetal malformations. Although delayed fetal ossification was observed at this dose in rats, there were no adverse effects on postnatal development of offspring. Doses of 1000 mg/kg/day (142,000 times the systemic exposure following the maximum recommended human ophthalmic dose) were maternotoxic in mice and resulted in an increased number of fetal resorptions. Increased fetal resorptions were also seen in rabbits at doses of 14,000 times the systemic exposure following the maximum recommended human ophthalmic dose, in this case without apparent maternotoxicity.

There are no adequate and well-controlled studies in pregnant women. Preservative-free TIMOPTIC in OCUDOSE should be used during pregnancy only if the potential benefit justifies the potential risk to the fetus.

Nursing Mothers

Timolol maleate has been detected in human milk following oral and ophthalmic drug administration. Because of the potential for serious adverse reactions from timolol in nursing infants, a decision should be made whether to discontinue nursing or to discontinue the drug, taking into account the importance of the drug to the mother.

Pediatric Use

Safety and effectiveness in pediatric patients have not been established.

Geriatric Use

No overall differences in safety or effectiveness have been observed between elderly and younger patients.

ADVERSE REACTIONS

The most frequently reported adverse experiences have been burning and stinging upon instillation (approximately one in eight patients).

The following additional adverse experiences have been reported less frequently with ocular administration of this or other timolol maleate formulations:

BODY AS A WHOLE

Headache, asthenia/fatigue, chest pain.

CARDIOVASCULAR

Bradycardia, arrhythmia, hypotension, hypertension, syncope, heart block, cerebral vascular accident, cerebral ischemia, cardiac failure, worsening of angina pectoris, palpitation, cardiac arrest, pulmonary edema, edema, claudication, Raynaud's phenomenon, and cold hands and feet.

DIGESTIVE

Nausea, diarrhea. dyspepsia, anorexia, and dry mouth.

IMMUNOLOGIC

Systemic lupus erythematosus.

NERVOUS SYSTEM/PSYCHIATRIC

Dizziness, increase in signs and symptoms of myasthenia gravis, paresthesia, somnolence, insomnia, nightmares, behavioral changes and psychic disturbances including depression, confusion, hallucinations, anxiety, disorientation, nervousness, and memory loss.

SKIN

Alopecia and psoriasiform rash or exacerbation of psoriasis.

HYPERSENSITIVITY

Signs and symptoms of systemic allergic reactions, including anaphylaxis, angioedema, urticaria, and localized and generalized rash.

RESPIRATORY

Bronchospasm (predominantly in patients with pre-existing bronchospastic disease), respiratory failure, dyspnea, nasal congestion, cough and upper respiratory infections.

ENDOCRINE

Masked symptoms of hypoglycemia in diabetic patients (see **WARNINGS**).

SPECIAL SENSES

Signs and symptoms of ocular irritation including conjunctivitis, blepharitis, keratitis, ocular pain, discharge (e.g., crusting), foreign body sensation, itching and tearing, and dry eyes; ptosis; decreased corneal sensitivity; cystoid macular edema; visual disturbances including refractive changes and diplopia; pseudopemphigoid; choroidal detachment following filtration surgery (see **PRECAUTIONS**, *General*); and tinnitus.

UROGENITAL

Retroperitoneal fibrosis, decreased libido, impotence, and Peyronie's disease.

The following additional adverse effects have been reported in clinical experience with ORAL timolol maleate or other ORAL beta blocking agents, and may be considered potential effects of ophthalmic timolol maleate: *Allergic:* Erythematous rash, fever combined with aching and sore throat, laryngospasm with respiratory distress; *Body as a Whole:* Extremity pain, decreased exercise tolerance, weight loss; *Cardiovascular:* Worsening of arterial insufficiency, vasodilatation; *Digestive:* Gastrointestinal pain, hepatomegaly, vomiting, mesenteric arterial thrombosis, ischemic colitis; *Hematologic:* Nonthrombocytopenic purpura; thrombocytopenic purpura; agranulocytosis; *Endocrine:* Hyperglycemia, hypoglycemia; *Skin:* Pruritus, skin irritation, increased pigmentation, sweating; *Musculoskeletal:* Arthralgia; *Nervous System/Psychiatric:* Vertigo, local weakness, diminished concentration, reversible mental depression progressing to catatonia, an acute reversible syndrome characterized by disorientation for time and place, emotional lability, slightly clouded sensorium, and decreased performance on neuropsychometrics; *Respiratory:* Rales, bronchial obstruction; *Urogenital:* Urination difficulties.

OVERDOSAGE

There have been reports of inadvertent overdosage with Ophthalmic Solution TIMOPTIC (timolol maleate ophthalmic solution) resulting in systemic effects similar to those seen with systemic beta-adrenergic blocking agents such as dizziness, headache, shortness of breath, bradycardia, bronchospasm, and cardiac arrest (see also **ADVERSE REACTIONS**).

Overdosage has been reported with Tablets BLOCADREN* (timolol maleate tablets). A 30 year old female ingested 650 mg of BLOCADREN (maximum recommended oral daily dose is 60 mg) and experienced second and third degree heart block. She recovered without treatment but approximately two months later developed irregular heartbeat, hypertension, dizziness, tinnitus, faintness, increased pulse rate, and borderline first degree heart block.

An *in vitro* hemodialysis study, using ^{14}C timolol added to human plasma or whole blood, showed that timolol was readily dialyzed from these fluids; however, a study of patients with renal failure showed that timolol did not dialyze readily.

* Registered trademark of MERCK & CO., INC.

DOSAGE AND ADMINISTRATION

Preservative-free TIMOPTIC in OCUDOSE is a sterile solution that does not contain a preservative. The solution from one individual unit is to be used immediately after opening for administration to one or both eyes. Since sterility cannot be guaranteed after the individual unit is opened, the remaining contents should be discarded immediately after administration.

Preservative-free TIMOPTIC in OCUDOSE is available in concentrations of 0.25 and 0.5 percent. The usual starting dose is one drop of 0.25 percent Preservative-free TIMOPTIC in OCUDOSE in the affected eye(s) administered twice a day. Apply enough gentle pressure on the individual container to obtain a single drop of solution. If the clinical response is not adequate, the dosage may be changed to one drop of 0.5 percent solution in the affected eye(s) administered twice a day.

Since in some patients the pressure-lowering response to Preservative-free TIMOPTIC in OCUDOSE may require a few weeks to stabilize, evaluation should include a determination of intraocular pressure after approximately 4 weeks of treatment with Preservative-free TIMOPTIC in OCUDOSE.

If the intraocular pressure is maintained at satisfactory levels, the dosage schedule may be changed to one drop once a day in the affected eye(s). Because of diurnal variations in intraocular pressure, satisfactory response to the once-a-day dose is best determined by measuring the intraocular pressure at different times during the day.

Dosages above one drop of 0.5 percent TIMOPTIC (timolol maleate ophthalmic solution) twice a day generally have not been shown to produce further reduction in intraocular pressure. If the patient's intraocular pressure is still not at a satisfactory level on this regimen, concomitant therapy with other agent(s) for lowering intraocular pressure can be instituted taking into consideration that the preparation(s) used concomitantly may contain one or more preservatives. The concomitant use of two topical beta-adrenergic blocking agents is not recommended. (See **PRECAUTIONS,** ***Drug Interactions, Beta-adrenergic blocking agents.***)

HOW SUPPLIED

Preservative-free Sterile Ophthalmic Solution TIMOPTIC in OCUDOSE is a clear, colorless to light yellow solution.

No. 9689—Preservative-free TIMOPTIC, 0.25% timolol equivalent, is supplied in OCUDOSE, a clear low density polyethylene unit dose container. Each individual unit contains 0.2 mL of solution, and is available in a foil laminate overwrapped pouch as follows:

NDC 0006-9689-60; 60 Individual Unit Doses

No. 9690—Preservative-free TIMOPTIC, 0.5% timolol equivalent, is supplied in OCUDOSE, a clear low density polyethylene unit dose container. Each individual unit contains 0.2 mL of solution, and is available in a foil laminate overwrapped pouch as follows:

NDC 0006-9690-60; 60 Individual Unit Doses

Storage

Store at room temperature, 15–30°C (59–86°F). Protect from freezing. Protect from light.

Because evaporation can occur through the unprotected polyethylene unit dose container and prolonged exposure to direct light can modify the product, the unit dose container should be kept in the protective foil overwrap and used within one month after the foil package has been opened.

Manuf. for:
Merck & Co., Inc., Whitehouse Station, NJ 08889, USA
By: Laboratories Merck Sharp & Dohme-Chibret
63963 Clermont-Ferrand Cedex 9, France
9351204 Issued September 2002

TIMOPTIC-XE® ℞

0.25% and 0.5%
(timolol maleate ophthalmic gel forming solution)
Sterile Ophthalmic Gel Forming Solution

DESCRIPTION

TIMOPTIC-XE* (timolol maleate ophthalmic gel forming solution) is a non-selective beta-adrenergic receptor blocking agent. Its chemical name is (-)-1-(*tert*-butyl-amino)-3-[(4-morpholino-1,2,5-thiadiazol-3-yl)oxy]-2-propanol maleate (1:1) (salt). Timolol maleate possesses an asymmetric carbon atom in its structure and is provided as the levo-isomer. The optical rotation of timolol maleate is:

$[\alpha]^{25°}_{405\ nm}$ in 1.0N HCl (C=5%) = −12.2° (−11.7° to −12.5°).

Its molecular formula is $C_{13}H_{24}N_4O_3S \cdot C_4H_4O_4$ and its structural formula is:

Timolol maleate has a molecular weight of 432.50. It is a white, odorless, crystalline powder which is soluble in water, methanol, and alcohol.

TIMOPTIC-XE Sterile Ophthalmic Gel Forming Solution is supplied as a sterile, isotonic, buffered, aqueous solution of timolol maleate in two dosage strengths. The pH of the solution is approximately 7.0, and the osmolarity is 260–330 mOsm. Each mL of TIMOPTIC-XE 0.25% contains 2.5 mg of timolol (3.4 mg of timolol maleate). Each mL of TIMOPTIC-XE 0.5% contains 5 mg of timolol (6.8 mg of timolol maleate). Inactive ingredients: GELRITE* gellan gum, tromethamine, mannitol, and water for injection. Preservative: benzododecinium bromide 0.012%.

GELRITE is a purified anionic heteropolysaccharide derived from gellan gum. An aqueous solution of GELRITE, in the presence of a cation, has the ability to gel. Upon contact

Continued on next page

Information on the Merck & Co., Inc., products listed on these pages is from the prescribing information in use October 1, 2004. For information, please call 1-800-NSC-MERCK [1-800-672-6372].

Timoptic-XE—Cont.

with the precorneal tear film, TIMOPTIC-XE forms a gel that is subsequently removed by the flow of tears.

* Registered trademark of MERCK & CO., INC.

CLINICAL PHARMACOLOGY

Mechanism of Action

Timolol maleate is a $beta_1$ and $beta_2$ (non-selective) adrenergic receptor blocking agent that does not have significant intrinsic sympathomimetic, direct myocardial depressant, or local anesthetic (membrane-stabilizing) activity.

TIMOPTIC-XE, when applied topically on the eye, has the action of reducing elevated, as well as normal intraocular pressure, whether or not accompanied by glaucoma. Elevated intraocular pressure is a major risk factor in the pathogenesis of glaucomatous visual field loss and optic nerve damage.

The precise mechanism of the ocular hypotensive action of TIMOPTIC-XE is not clearly established at this time. Tonography and fluorophotometry studies of TIMOPTIC* (timolol maleate ophthalmic solution) in man suggest that its predominant action may be related to reduced aqueous formation. However, in some studies, a slight increase in outflow facility was also observed.

Beta-adrenergic receptor blockade reduces cardiac output in both healthy subjects and patients with heart disease. In patients with severe impairment of myocardial function beta-adrenergic receptor blockade may inhibit the stimulatory effect of the sympathetic nervous system necessary to maintain adequate cardiac function.

Beta-adrenergic receptor blockade in the bronchi and bronchioles results in increased airway resistance from unopposed parasympathetic activity. Such an effect in patients with asthma or other bronchospastic conditions is potentially dangerous.

Pharmacokinetics

In a study of plasma drug concentration in six subjects, the systemic exposure to timolol was determined following once daily administration of TIMOPTIC-XE 0.5% in the morning. The mean peak plasma concentration following this morning dose was 0.28 ng/mL.

Clinical Studies

In controlled, double-masked, multicenter clinical studies, comparing TIMOPTIC-XE 0.25% to TIMOPTIC 0.25% and TIMOPTIC-XE 0.5% to TIMOPTIC 0.5%, TIMOPTIC-XE administered once a day was shown to be equally effective in lowering intraocular pressure as the equivalent concentration of TIMOPTIC administered twice a day. The effect of timolol in lowering intraocular pressure was evident for 24 hours with a single dose of TIMOPTIC-XE. Repeated observations over a period of six months indicate that the intraocular pressure-lowering effect of TIMOPTIC-XE was consistent. The results from the largest U.S. and international clinical trials comparing TIMOPTIC-XE 0.5% to TIMOPTIC 0.5% are shown in Figure 1.

Figure 1

Mean IOP and Std Deviation (mm Hg) by Treatment Group

U.S. Study

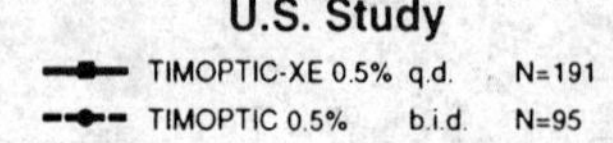

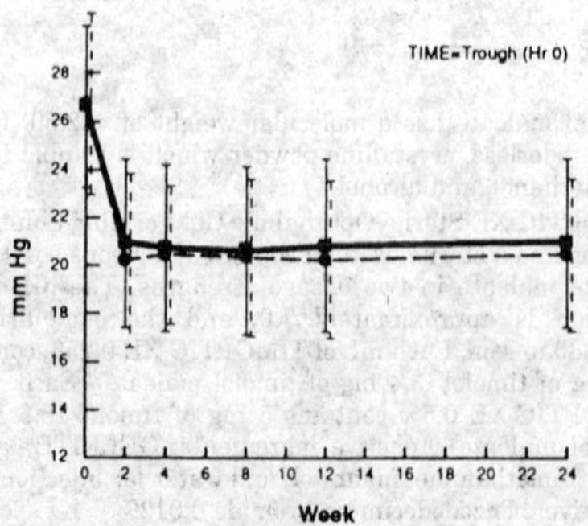

[See first figure at top of next column]
[See second figure at top of next column]
[See third figure in next column]

TIMOPTIC-XE administered once daily had a safety profile similar to that of an equivalent concentration of TIMOPTIC administered twice daily. Due to the physical characteristics of the formulation, there was a higher incidence of transient blurred vision in patients administered TIMOPTIC-XE. A slight reduction in resting heart rate was observed in some patients receiving TIMOPTIC-XE 0.5% (mean reduction 24

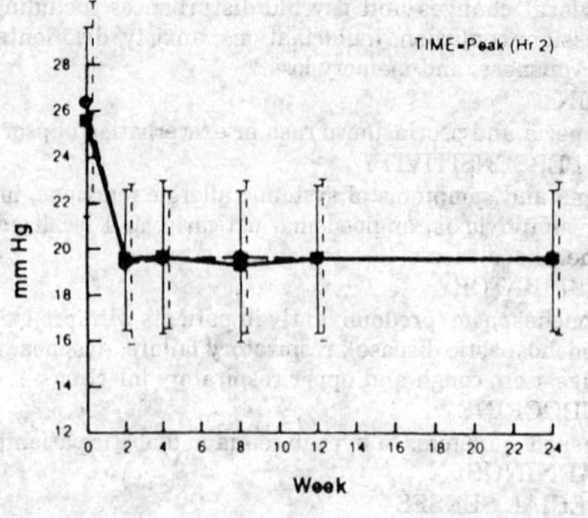

International Study

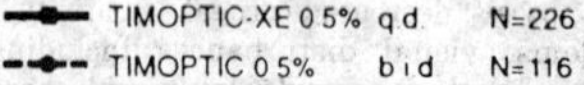

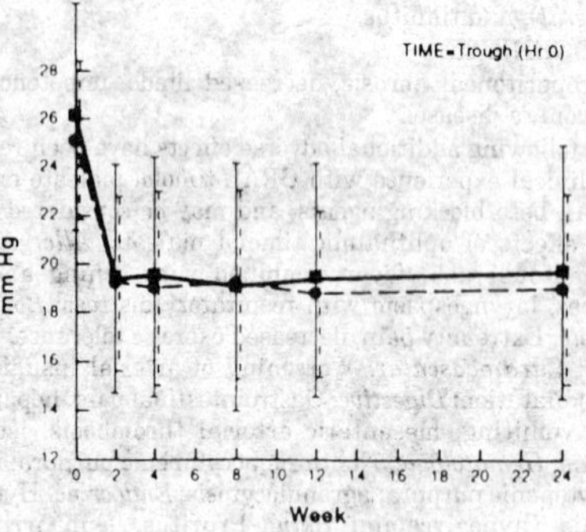

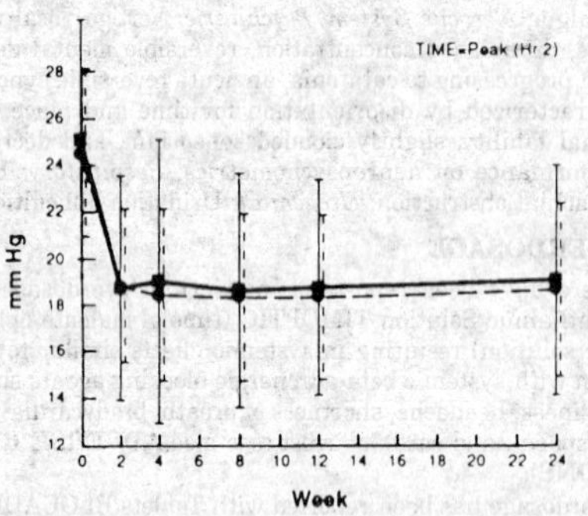

hours post-dose 0.8 beats/minute, mean reduction 2 hours post-dose 3.8 beats/minute). (See **ADVERSE REACTIONS.**)

TIMOPTIC-XE has not been studied in patients wearing contact lenses.

* Registered trademark of MERCK & CO., INC.

INDICATIONS AND USAGE

TIMOPTIC-XE Sterile Ophthalmic Gel Forming Solution is indicated in the treatment of elevated intraocular pressure in patients with ocular hypertension or open-angle glaucoma.

CONTRAINDICATIONS

TIMOPTIC-XE is contraindicated in patients with (1) bronchial asthma; (2) a history of bronchial asthma; (3) severe chronic obstructive pulmonary disease (see **WARNINGS**); (4) sinus bradycardia; (5) second or third degree atrioventricular block; (6) overt cardiac failure (see **WARNINGS**); (7) cardiogenic shock; or (8) hypersensitivity to any component of this product.

WARNINGS

As with many topically applied ophthalmic drugs, this drug is absorbed systemically.

The same adverse reactions found with systemic administration of beta-adrenergic blocking agents may occur with topical ophthalmic administration. For example, severe respiratory reactions and cardiac reactions, including death due to bronchospasm in patients with asthma, and rarely death in association with cardiac failure, have been reported following systemic or ophthalmic administration of timolol maleate. (See CONTRAINDICATIONS.)

Cardiac Failure

Sympathetic stimulation may be essential for support of the circulation in individuals with diminished myocardial contractility, and its inhibition by beta-adrenergic receptor blockade may precipitate more severe failure.

In Patients Without a History of Cardiac Failure, continued depression of the myocardium with beta-blocking agents over a period of time can, in some cases, lead to cardiac failure. At the first sign or symptom of cardiac failure, TIMOPTIC-XE should be discontinued.

Obstructive Pulmonary Disease

Patients with chronic obstructive pulmonary disease (e.g., chronic bronchitis, emphysema) of mild or moderate severity, bronchospastic disease, or a history of bronchospastic disease (other than bronchial asthma or a history of bronchial asthma, in which TIMOPTIC-XE is contraindicated [see **CONTRAINDICATIONS**]) should, in general, not receive beta-blockers, including TIMOPTIC-XE.

Major Surgery

The necessity or desirability of withdrawal of beta-adrenergic blocking agents prior to major surgery is controversial. Beta-adrenergic receptor blockade impairs the ability of the heart to respond to beta-adrenergically mediated reflex stimuli. This may augment the risk of general anesthesia in surgical procedures. Some patients receiving beta-adrenergic receptor blocking agents have experienced protracted, severe hypotension during anesthesia. Difficulty in restarting and maintaining the heartbeat has also been reported. For these reasons, in patients undergoing elective surgery, some authorities recommend gradual withdrawal of beta-adrenergic receptor blocking agents.

If necessary during surgery, the effects of beta-adrenergic blocking agents may be reversed by sufficient doses of adrenergic agonists.

Diabetes Mellitus

Beta-adrenergic blocking agents should be administered with caution in patients subject to spontaneous hypoglycemia or to diabetic patients (especially those with labile diabetes) who are receiving insulin or oral hypoglycemic agents. Beta-adrenergic receptor blocking agents may mask the signs and symptoms of acute hypoglycemia.

Thyrotoxicosis

Beta-adrenergic blocking agents may mask certain clinical signs (e.g., tachycardia) of hyperthyroidism. Patients suspected of developing thyrotoxicosis should be managed carefully to avoid abrupt withdrawal of beta-adrenergic blocking agents that might precipitate a thyroid storm.

PRECAUTIONS

General

Because of potential effects of beta-adrenergic blocking agents on blood pressure and pulse, these agents should be used with caution in patients with cerebrovascular insufficiency. If signs or symptoms suggesting reduced cerebral blood flow develop following initiation of therapy with TIMOPTIC-XE, alternative therapy should be considered.

There have been reports of bacterial keratitis associated with the use of multiple dose containers of topical ophthalmic products. These containers had been inadvertently contaminated by patients who, in most cases, had a concurrent corneal disease or a disruption of the ocular epithelial surface. (See **PRECAUTIONS,** *Information for Patients.*)

Choroidal detachment after filtration procedures has been reported with the administration of aqueous suppressant therapy (e.g. timolol).

Angle-closure glaucoma: In patients with angle-closure glaucoma, the immediate objective of treatment is to reopen the angle. This may require constricting the pupil. Timolol maleate has little or no effect on the pupil. TIMOPTIC-XE should not be used alone in the treatment of angle-closure glaucoma.

Anaphylaxis: While taking beta-blockers, patients with a history of atopy or a history of severe anaphylactic reactions to a variety of allergens may be more reactive to repeated accidental, diagnostic, or therapeutic challenge with such allergens. Such patients may be unresponsive to the usual doses of epinephrine used to treat anaphylactic reactions.

Muscle Weakness: Beta-adrenergic blockade has been reported to potentiate muscle weakness consistent with certain myasthenic symptoms (e.g., diplopia, ptosis, and generalized weakness). Timolol has been reported rarely to increase muscle weakness in some patients with myasthenia gravis or myasthenic symptoms.

Information for Patients

Patients should be instructed to avoid allowing the tip of the dispensing container to contact the eye or surrounding structures.

Patients should also be instructed that ocular solutions, if handled improperly or if the tip of the dispensing container contacts the eye or surrounding structures, can become contaminated by common bacteria known to cause ocular infections. Serious damage to the eye and subsequent loss of vision may result from using contaminated solutions. (See **PRECAUTIONS,** *General.*)

Patients should also be advised that if they have ocular surgery or develop an intercurrent ocular condition (e.g., trauma or infection), they should immediately seek their physician's advice concerning the continued use of the present multidose container.

Patients should be instructed to invert the closed container and shake once before each use. It is not necessary to shake the container more than once.

Patients requiring concomitant topical ophthalmic medications should be instructed to administer these at least 10 minutes before instilling TIMOPTIC-XE.

Patients with bronchial asthma, a history of bronchial asthma, severe chronic obstructive pulmonary disease, sinus bradycardia, second or third degree atrioventricular block, or cardiac failure should be advised not to take this product. (See **CONTRAINDICATIONS.**)

Transient blurred vision, generally lasting from 30 seconds to 5 minutes, following instillation, and potential visual disturbances may impair the ability to perform hazardous tasks such as operating machinery or driving a motor vehicle.

Drug Interactions

Beta-adrenergic blocking agents: Patients who are receiving a beta-adrenergic blocking agent orally and TIMOPTIC-XE should be observed for potential additive effects of beta-blockade, both systemic and on intraocular pressure. The concomitant use of two topical beta-adrenergic blocking agents is not recommended.

Calcium antagonists: Caution should be used in the coadministration of beta-adrenergic blocking agents, such as TIMOPTIC-XE, and oral or intravenous calcium antagonists because of possible atrioventricular conduction disturbances, left ventricular failure, or hypotension. In patients with impaired cardiac function, coadministration should be avoided.

Catecholamine-depleting drugs: Close observation of the patient is recommended when a beta blocker is administered to patients receiving catecholamine-depleting drugs such as reserpine, because of possible additive effects and the production of hypotension and/or marked bradycardia, which may result in vertigo, syncope, or postural hypotension.

Digitalis and calcium antagonists: The concomitant use of beta-adrenergic blocking agents with digitalis and calcium antagonists may have additive effects in prolonging atrioventricular conduction time.

Quinidine: Potentiated systemic beta-blockade (e.g., decreased heart rate) has been reported during combined treatment with quinidine and timolol, possibly because quinidine inhibits the metabolism of timolol via the P-450 enzyme, CYP2D6.

Clonidine: Oral beta-adrenergic blocking agents may exacerbate the rebound hypertension which can follow the withdrawal of clonidine. There have been no reports of exacerbation of rebound hypertension with ophthalmic timolol maleate.

Injectable epinephrine: (See **PRECAUTIONS,** *General, Anaphylaxis*)

Carcinogenesis, Mutagenesis, Impairment of Fertility

In a two-year study of timolol maleate administered orally to rats, there was a statistically significant increase in the incidence of adrenal pheochromocytomas in male rats administered 300 mg/kg/day (approximately 42,000 times the systemic exposure following the maximum recommended human ophthalmic dose). Similar differences were not observed in rats administered oral doses equivalent to approximately 14,000 times the maximum recommended human ophthalmic dose.

In a lifetime oral study in mice, there were statistically significant increases in the incidence of benign and malignant pulmonary tumors, benign uterine polyps, and mammary adenocarcinomas in female mice at 500 mg/kg/day (approximately 71,000 times the systemic exposure following the maximum recommended human ophthalmic dose), but not at 5 or 50 mg/kg/day (approximately 700 or 7,000, respectively, times the systemic exposure following the maximum recommended human ophthalmic dose). In a subsequent study in female mice, in which post-mortem examinations were limited to the uterus and the lungs, a statistically significant increase in the incidence of pulmonary tumors was again observed at 500 mg/kg/day.

The increased occurrence of mammary adenocarcinomas was associated with elevations in serum prolactin, which occurred in female mice administered oral timolol at 500 mg/kg/day, but not at oral doses of 5 or 50 mg/kg/day. An increased incidence of mammary adenocarcinomas in rodents has been associated with administration of several other therapeutic agents that elevate serum prolactin, but no correlation between serum prolactin levels and mammary tumors has been established in humans. Furthermore, in adult human female subjects who received oral dosages of up to 60 mg of timolol maleate (the maximum recommended human oral dosage), there were no clinically meaningful changes in serum prolactin.

Timolol maleate was devoid of mutagenic potential when tested *in vivo* (mouse) in the micronucleus test and cytogenetic assay (doses up to 800 mg) and *in vitro* in a neoplastic cell transformation assay (up to 100 mcg/mL). In Ames tests, the highest concentrations of timolol employed, 5,000 or 10,000 mcg/plate, were associated with statistically significant elevations of revertants observed with tester strain TA100 (in seven replicate assays), but not in the remaining three strains. In the assays with tester strain TA100, no consistent dose response relationship was observed, and the ratio of test to control revertants did not reach 2. A ratio of 2 is usually considered the criterion for a positive Ames test.

Reproduction and fertility studies in rats demonstrated no adverse effect on male or female fertility at doses up to 21,000 times the systemic exposure following the maximum recommended human ophthalmic dose.

Pregnancy:

Teratogenic Effects—Pregnancy Category C. Teratogenicity studies with timolol in mice and rabbits at oral doses up to 50 mg/kg/day (7,000 times the systemic exposure following the maximum recommended human ophthalmic dose) demonstrated no evidence of fetal malformations. Although delayed fetal ossification was observed at this dose in rats, there were no adverse effects on postnatal development of offspring. Doses of 1000 mg/kg/day (142,000 times the systemic exposure following the maximum recommended human ophthalmic dose) were maternotoxic in mice and resulted in an increased number of fetal resorptions. Increased fetal resorptions were also seen in rabbits at doses of 14,000 times the systemic exposure following the maximum recommended human ophthalmic dose, in this case without apparent maternotoxicity.

There are no adequate and well-controlled studies in pregnant women. TIMOPTIC-XE should be used during pregnancy only if the potential benefit justifies the potential risk to the fetus.

Nursing Mothers

Timolol maleate has been detected in human milk following oral and ophthalmic drug administration. Because of the potential for serious adverse reactions from TIMOPTIC-XE in nursing infants, a decision should be made whether to discontinue nursing or to discontinue the drug, taking into account the importance of the drug to the mother.

Pediatric Use

Safety and effectiveness in pediatric patients have not been established.

Geriatric Use

No overall differences in safety or effectiveness have been observed between elderly and younger patients.

ADVERSE REACTIONS

In clinical trials, transient blurred vision upon instillation of the drop was reported in approximately one in three patients (lasting from 30 seconds to 5 minutes). Less than 1% of patients discontinued from the studies due to blurred vision. The frequency of patients reporting burning and stinging upon instillation was comparable between TIMOPTIC-XE and TIMOPTIC (approximately one in eight patients).

Adverse experiences reported in 1–5% of patients were:

Ocular: Pain, conjunctivitis, discharge (e.g. crusting), foreign body sensation, itching and tearing;

Systemic: Headache, dizziness, and upper respiratory infections.

The following additional adverse experiences have been reported with the ocular administration of this or other timolol maleate formulations:

BODY AS A WHOLE

Asthenia/fatigue, and chest pain.

CARDIOVASCULAR

Bradycardia, arrhythmia, hypotension, hypertension, syncope, heart block, cerebral vascular accident, cerebral ischemia, cardiac failure, worsening of angina pectoris, palpitation, cardiac arrest, pulmonary edema, edema, claudication, Raynaud's phenomenon, and cold hands and feet.

DIGESTIVE

Nausea, diarrhea, dyspepsia, anorexia, and dry mouth.

IMMUNOLOGIC

Systemic lupus erythematosus.

NERVOUS SYSTEM/PSYCHIATRIC

Increase in signs and symptoms of myasthenia gravis, paresthesia, somnolence, insomnia, nightmares, behavioral changes and psychic disturbances including depression, confusion, hallucinations, anxiety, disorientation, nervousness, and memory loss.

SKIN

Alopecia and psoriasiform rash or exacerbation of psoriasis.

HYPERSENSITIVITY

Signs and symptoms of systemic allergic reactions including anaphylaxis, angioedema, urticaria, localized and generalized rash.

RESPIRATORY

Bronchospasm (predominantly in patients with preexisting bronchospastic disease), respiratory failure, dyspnea, nasal congestion, and cough.

ENDOCRINE

Masked symptoms of hypoglycemia in diabetic patients (see **WARNINGS**).

SPECIAL SENSES

Signs and symptoms of ocular irritation including blepharitis, keratitis, and dry eyes; ptosis; decreased corneal sensitivity; cystoid macular edema; visual disturbances including refractive changes and diplopia; pseudopemphigoid; choroidal detachment following filtration surgery (see **PRECAUTIONS,** *General*); and tinnitus.

UROGENITAL

Retroperitoneal fibrosis, decreased libido, impotence, and Peyronie's disease.

The following additional adverse effects have been reported in clinical experience with ORAL timolol maleate or other ORAL beta-blocking agents and may be considered potential effects of ophthalmic timolol maleate: *Allergic:* Erythematous rash, fever combined with aching and sore throat, laryngospasm with respiratory distress; *Body as a Whole:* Extremity pain, decreased exercise tolerance, weight loss; *Cardiovascular:* Worsening of arterial insufficiency, vasodilatation; *Digestive:* Gastrointestinal pain, hepatomegaly, vomiting, mesenteric arterial thrombosis, ischemic colitis; *Hematologic:* Nonthrombocytopenic purpura, thrombocytopenic purpura, agranulocytosis; *Endocrine:* Hyperglycemia, hypoglycemia; *Skin:* Pruritus, skin irritation, increased pigmentation, sweating; *Musculoskeletal:* Arthralgia; *Nervous System/Psychiatric:* Vertigo, local weakness, diminished concentration, reversible mental depression progressing to catatonia, an acute reversible syndrome characterized by disorientation for time and place, emotional lability, slightly clouded sensorium, and decreased performance on neuropsychometrics; *Respiratory:* Rales, bronchial obstruction; *Urogenital:* Urination difficulties.

OVERDOSAGE

No data are available in regard to human overdosage with or accidental oral ingestion of TIMOPTIC-XE.

There have been reports of inadvertent overdosage with TIMOPTIC Ophthalmic Solution resulting in systemic effects similar to those seen with systemic beta-adrenergic blocking agents such as dizziness, headache, shortness of breath, bradycardia, bronchospasm, and cardiac arrest (see also **ADVERSE REACTIONS**).

Overdosage has been reported with Tablets BLOCADREN* (timolol maleate tablets). A 30 year old female ingested 650 mg of BLOCADREN (maximum recommended oral daily dose is 60 mg) and experienced second and third degree heart block. She recovered without treatment but approximately two months later developed irregular heartbeat, hypertension, dizziness, tinnitus, faintness, increased pulse rate, and borderline first degree heart block.

An *in vitro* hemodialysis study, using ^{14}C timolol added to human plasma or whole blood, showed that timolol was readily dialyzed from these fluids; however, a study of patients with renal failure showed that timolol did not dialyze readily.

*Registered trademark of MERCK & CO., Inc.

DOSAGE AND ADMINISTRATION

Patients should be instructed to invert the closed container and shake once before each use. It is not necessary to shake the container more than once. Other topically applied ophthalmic medications should be administered at least 10 minutes before TIMOPTIC-XE. (See **PRECAUTIONS,** *Information for Patients* and accompanying INSTRUCTIONS FOR USE.)

TIMOPTIC-XE Sterile Ophthalmic Gel Forming Solution is available in concentrations of 0.25% and 0.5%. The dose is one drop of TIMOPTIC-XE (either 0.25% or 0.5%) in the affected eye(s) once a day.

Because in some patients the pressure-lowering response to TIMOPTIC-XE may require a few weeks to stabilize, evaluation should include a determination of intraocular pressure after approximately 4 weeks of treatment with TIMOPTIC-XE.

Dosages higher than one drop of 0.5% TIMOPTIC-XE once a day have not been studied. If the patient's intraocular pressure is still not at a satisfactory level on this regimen, concomitant therapy can be considered. The concomitant use of two topical beta-adrenergic blocking agents is not recommended. (See **PRECAUTIONS,** *Drug Interactions, Beta-adrenergic blocking agents.*)

When patients have been switched from therapy with TIMOPTIC administered twice daily to TIMOPTIC-XE administered once daily, the ocular hypotensive effect has remained consistent.

HOW SUPPLIED

TIMOPTIC-XE Sterile Ophthalmic Gel Forming Solution is a colorless to nearly colorless, slightly opalescent, and slightly viscous solution.

No. 3557—TIMOPTIC-XE Sterile Ophthalmic Gel Forming Solution, 0.25% timolol equivalent, is supplied in OCUMETER*, a white, opaque, LDPE, plastic, ophthalmic dispenser with a controlled drop tip and color coded polypropylene cap as follows:

NDC 0006-3557-32, 2.5 mL in a 5 mL bottle
NDC 0006-3557-03, 5 mL in a 7.5 mL bottle.

No. 3558—TIMOPTIC-XE Sterile Ophthalmic Gel Forming Solution, 0.5% timolol equivalent, is supplied in OCUMETER, a white, opaque, LDPE, plastic, ophthalmic dispenser with a controlled drop tip and color coded polypropylene cap as follows:

NDC 0006-3558-32, 2.5 mL in a 5 mL bottle
NDC 0006-3558-03, 5 mL in a 7.5 mL bottle.

Storage

Store between 15° and 25°C (59° and 77°F). **AVOID FREEZING.** Protect from light.

TIMOPTIC-XE®
0.25% AND 0.5%
(timolol maleate ophthalmic gel forming solution)

INSTRUCTIONS FOR USE

Please follow these instructions carefully when using TIMOPTIC-XE*. Use TIMOPTIC-XE as prescribed by your doctor.

1. If you use other topically applied ophthalmic medications, they should be administered at least 10 minutes before TIMOPTIC-XE.
2. Wash hands before each use.

Continued on next page

Information on the Merck & Co., Inc., products listed on these pages is from the prescribing information in use October 1, 2004. For information, please call 1-800-NSC-MERCK [1-800-672-6372].

Timoptic-XE—Cont.

3. Invert the closed bottle and shake ONCE before each use. (It is not necessary to shake the bottle more than once.)

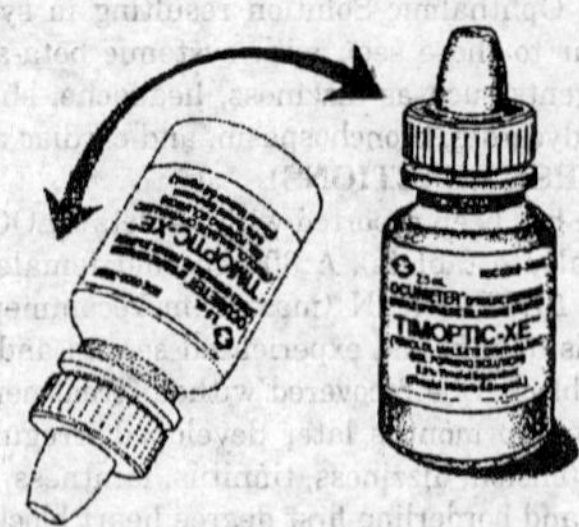

4. Remove the cap from the bottle carefully so that the dispenser tip does not touch anything. Place the cap in a clean, dry area.
5. Hold the bottle between the thumb and index finger. Use the index finger of the other hand to pull down the lower eyelid to form a pocket for the eye drop. Tilt your head back.

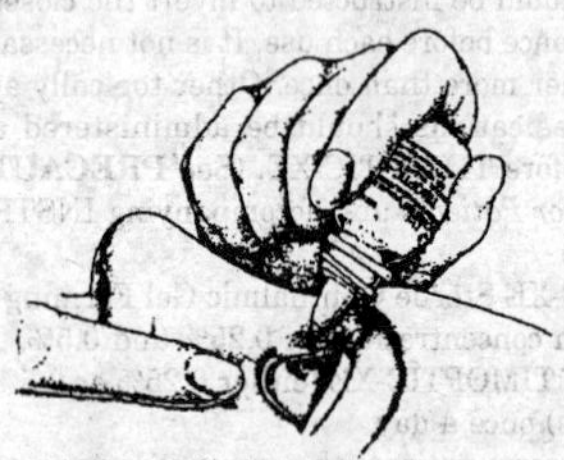

6. Place the dispenser tip close to your eye and gently squeeze the bottle to administer one drop. Remove pressure after a single drop has been released. If instructed, repeat steps 5 and 6 in the other eye.
DO NOT ALLOW THE DISPENSER TIP TO TOUCH THE EYE OR SURROUNDING AREAS.
Ophthalmic medications, if handled improperly, can become contaminated by common bacteria known to cause eye infections. Serious damage to the eye and subsequent loss of vision may result from using contaminated ophthalmic medications. If you think your medication may be contaminated, or you develop an eye infection, contact your doctor immediately concerning continued use of this bottle.
7. Replace the cap. Store the bottle at room temperature in an upright position in a clean area.
8. The dispenser tip is designed to provide a pre-measured drop; therefore, do NOT enlarge the hole of the dispenser.
9. Do NOT wash the tip of the dispenser with water, soap, or any other cleaner.

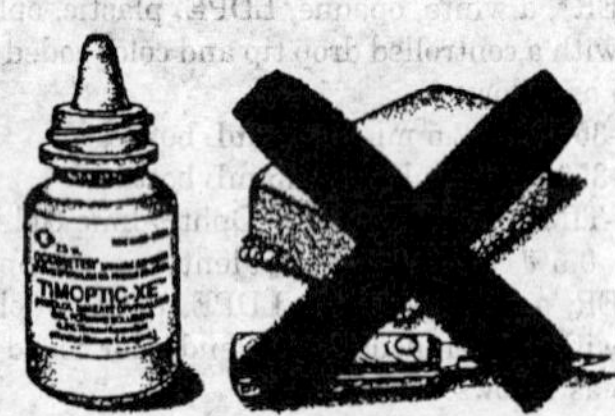

WARNING: Keep out of reach of children.
If you have any questions about the use of TIMOPTIC-XE, please consult your doctor.

*Registered trademark of MERCK & CO., Inc.

9028714 Issued September 2002

TRUSOPT® ℞

Sterile Ophthalmic Solution 2%
(dorzolamide hydrochloride ophthalmic solution)

DESCRIPTION

TRUSOPT* (dorzolamide hydrochloride ophthalmic solution) is a carbonic anhydrase inhibitor formulated for topical ophthalmic use.
Dorzolamide hydrochloride is described chemically as: (4*S*-*trans*)-4-(ethylamino)-5,6-dihydro-6-methyl-4*H*-thieno [2,3-*b*]thiopyran-2-sulfonamide 7,7-dioxide monohydrochloride. Dorzolamide hydrochloride is optically active. The specific rotation is

$\alpha_{405}^{25°}$ (C =1, water) = ~ −17°.

Its empirical formula is $C_{10}H_{16}N_2O_4S_3{\cdot}HCl$ and its structural formula is:

Dorzolamide hydrochloride has a molecular weight of 360.9 and a melting point of about 264°C. It is a white to off-white, crystalline powder, which is soluble in water and slightly soluble in methanol and ethanol.
TRUSOPT Sterile Ophthalmic Solution is supplied as a sterile, isotonic, buffered, slightly viscous, aqueous solution of dorzolamide hydrochloride. The pH of the solution is approximately 5.6, and the osmolarity is 260–330 mOsM. Each mL of TRUSOPT 2% contains 20 mg dorzolamide (22.3 mg of dorzolamide hydrochloride). Inactive ingredients are hydroxyethyl cellulose, mannitol, sodium citrate dihydrate, sodium hydroxide (to adjust pH) and water for injection. Benzalkonium chloride 0.0075% is added as a preservative.

*Registered trademark of MERCK & CO., Inc.

CLINICAL PHARMACOLOGY

Mechanism of Action
Carbonic anhydrase (CA) is an enzyme found in many tissues of the body including the eye. It catalyzes the reversible reaction involving the hydration of carbon dioxide and the dehydration of carbonic acid. In humans, carbonic anhydrase exists as a number of isoenzymes, the most active being carbonic anhydrase II (CA-II), found primarily in red blood cells (RBCs), but also in other tissues. Inhibition of carbonic anhydrase in the ciliary processes of the eye decreases aqueous humor secretion, presumably by slowing the formation of bicarbonate ions with subsequent reduction in sodium and fluid transport. The result is a reduction in intraocular pressure (IOP).
TRUSOPT Ophthalmic Solution contains dorzolamide hydrochloride, an inhibitor of human carbonic anhydrase II. Following topical ocular administration, TRUSOPT reduces elevated intraocular pressure. Elevated intraocular pressure is a major risk factor in the pathogenesis of optic nerve damage and glaucomatous visual field loss.
Pharmacokinetics/Pharmacodynamics
When topically applied, dorzolamide reaches the systemic circulation. To assess the potential for systemic carbonic anhydrase inhibition following topical administration, drug and metabolite concentrations in RBCs and plasma and carbonic anhydrase inhibition in RBCs were measured. Dorzolamide accumulates in RBCs during chronic dosing as a result of binding to CA-II. The parent drug forms a single N-desethyl metabolite, which inhibits CA-II less potently than the parent drug but also inhibits CA-I. The metabolite also accumulates in RBCs where it binds primarily to CA-I. Plasma concentrations of dorzolamide and metabolite are generally below the assay limit of quantitation (15nM). Dorzolamide binds moderately to plasma proteins (approximately 33%). Dorzolamide is primarily excreted unchanged in the urine; the metabolite also is excreted in urine. After dosing is stopped, dorzolamide washes out of RBCs nonlinearly, resulting in a rapid decline of drug concentration initially, followed by a slower elimination phase with a half-life of about four months.
To simulate the systemic exposure after long-term topical ocular administration, dorzolamide was given orally to eight healthy subjects for up to 20 weeks. The oral dose of 2 mg b.i.d. closely approximates the amount of drug delivered by topical ocular administration of TRUSOPT 2% t.i.d. Steady state was reached within 8 weeks. The inhibition of CA-II and total carbonic anhydrase activities was below the degree of inhibition anticipated to be necessary for a pharmacological effect on renal function and respiration in healthy individuals.
Clinical Studies
The efficacy of TRUSOPT was demonstrated in clinical studies in the treatment of elevated intraocular pressure in patients with glaucoma or ocular hypertension (baseline IOP ≥23 mmHg). The IOP-lowering effect of TRUSOPT was approximately 3 to 5 mmHg throughout the day and this was consistent in clinical studies of up to one year duration. The efficacy of TRUSOPT when dosed less frequently than three times a day (alone or in combination with other products) has not been established.
In a one year clinical study, the effect of TRUSOPT 2% t.i.d. on the corneal endothelium was compared to that of betaxolol ophthalmic solution b.i.d. and timolol maleate ophthalmic solution 0.5% b.i.d. There were no statistically significant differences between groups in corneal endothelial cell counts or in corneal thickness measurements. There was a mean loss of approximately 4% in the endothelial cell counts for each group over the one year period.

INDICATIONS AND USAGE

TRUSOPT Ophthalmic Solution is indicated in the treatment of elevated intraocular pressure in patients with ocular hypertension or open-angle glaucoma.

CONTRAINDICATIONS

TRUSOPT is contraindicated in patients who are hypersensitive to any component of this product.

WARNINGS

TRUSOPT is a sulfonamide and although administered topically is absorbed systemically. Therefore, the same types of adverse reactions that are attributable to sulfonamides may occur with topical administration with TRUSOPT. Fatalities have occurred, although rarely, due to severe reactions to sulfonamides including Stevens-Johnson syndrome, toxic epidermal necrolysis, fulminant hepatic necrosis, agranulocytosis, aplastic anemia, and other blood dyscrasias. Sensitization may recur when a sulfonamide is readministered irrespective of the route of administration. If signs of serious reactions or hypersensitivity occur, discontinue the use of this preparation.

PRECAUTIONS

General
The management of patients with acute angle-closure glaucoma requires therapeutic interventions in addition to ocular hypotensive agents. TRUSOPT has not been studied in patients with acute angle-closure glaucoma.
TRUSOPT has not been studied in patients with severe renal impairment (CrCl < 30 mL/min). Because TRUSOPT and its metabolite are excreted predominantly by the kidney, TRUSOPT is not recommended in such patients.
TRUSOPT has not been studied in patients with hepatic impairment and should therefore be used with caution in such patients.
In clinical studies, local ocular adverse effects, primarily conjunctivitis and lid reactions, were reported with chronic administration of TRUSOPT. Many of these reactions had the clinical appearance and course of an allergic-type reaction that resolved upon discontinuation of drug therapy. If such reactions are observed, TRUSOPT should be discontinued and the patient evaluated before considering restarting the drug. (See **ADVERSE REACTIONS**.)
There is a potential for an additive effect on the known systemic effects of carbonic anhydrase inhibition in patients receiving an oral carbonic anhydrase inhibitor and TRUSOPT. The concomitant administration of TRUSOPT and oral carbonic anhydrase inhibitors is not recommended.
There have been reports of bacterial keratitis associated with the use of multiple dose containers of topical ophthalmic products. These containers had been inadvertently contaminated by patients who, in most cases, had a concurrent corneal disease or a disruption of the ocular epithelial surface.
Choroidal detachment has been reported with administration of aqueous suppressant therapy (e.g., dorzolamide) after filtration procedures.
Information for Patients
TRUSOPT is a sulfonamide and although administered topically is absorbed systemically. Therefore the same types of adverse reactions that are attributable to sulfonamides may occur with topical administration. Patients should be advised that if serious or unusual reactions or signs of hypersensitivity occur, they should discontinue the use of the product (see **WARNINGS**).
Patients should be advised that if they develop any ocular reactions, particularly conjunctivitis and lid reactions, they should discontinue use and seek their physician's advice.
Patients should be instructed to avoid allowing the tip of the dispensing container to contact the eye or surrounding structures.
Patients should also be instructed that ocular solutions, if handled improperly or if the tip of the dispensing container contacts the eye or surrounding structures, can become contaminated by common bacteria known to cause ocular infections. Serious damage to the eye and subsequent loss of vision may result from using contaminated solutions.
Patients also should be advised that if they have ocular surgery or develop an intercurrent ocular condition (e.g., trauma or infection), they should immediately seek their physician's advice concerning the continued use of the present multidose container.
If more than one topical ophthalmic drug is being used, the drugs should be administered at least ten minutes apart.
Patients should be advised that TRUSOPT contains benzalkonium chloride which may be absorbed by soft contact lenses. Contact lenses should be removed prior to administration of the solution. Lenses may be reinserted 15 minutes following TRUSOPT administration.
Drug Interactions
Although acid-base and electrolyte disturbances were not reported in the clinical trials with TRUSOPT, these disturbances have been reported with oral carbonic anhydrase inhibitors and have, in some instances, resulted in drug interactions (e.g., toxicity associated with high-dose salicylate therapy). Therefore, the potential for such drug interactions should be considered in patients receiving TRUSOPT.
Carcinogenesis, Mutagenesis, Impairment of Fertility
In a two-year study of dorzolamide hydrochloride administered orally to male and female Sprague-Dawley rats, urinary bladder papillomas were seen in male rats in the highest dosage group of 20 mg/kg/day (250 times the recommended human ophthalmic dose). Papillomas were not seen in rats given oral doses equivalent to approximately 12 times the recommended human ophthalmic dose. No treatment-related tumors were seen in a 21-month study in female and male mice given oral doses up to 75 mg/kg/day (~900 times the recommended human ophthalmic dose).

The increased incidence of urinary bladder papillomas seen in the high-dose male rats is a class-effect of carbonic anhydrase inhibitors in rats. Rats are particularly prone to developing papillomas in response to foreign bodies, compounds causing crystalluria, and diverse sodium salts.

No changes in bladder urothelium were seen in dogs given oral dorzolamide hydrochloride for one year at 2 mg/kg/day (25 times the recommended human ophthalmic dose) or monkeys dosed topically to the eye at 0.4 mg/kg/day (~5 times the recommended human ophthalmic dose) for one year.

The following tests for mutagenic potential were negative: (1) *in vivo* (mouse) cytogenetic assay; (2) *in vitro* chromosomal aberration assay; (3) alkaline elution assay; (4) V-79 assay; and (5) Ames test.

In reproduction studies of dorzolamide hydrochloride in rats, there were no adverse effects on the reproductive capacity of males or females at doses up to 188 or 94 times, respectively, the recommended human ophthalmic dose.

Pregnancy

Teratogenic Effects. Pregnancy Category C. Developmental toxicity studies with dorzolamide hydrochloride in rabbits at oral doses of ≥2.5 mg/kg/day (31 times the recommended human ophthalmic dose) revealed malformations of the vertebral bodies. These malformations occurred at doses that caused metabolic acidosis with decreased body weight gain in dams and decreased fetal weights. No treatment-related malformations were seen at 1.0 mg/kg/day (13 times the recommended human ophthalmic dose). There are no adequate and well-controlled studies in pregnant women. TRUSOPT should be used during pregnancy only if the potential benefit justifies the potential risk to the fetus.

Nursing Mothers

In a study of dorzolamide hydrochloride in lactating rats, decreases in body weight gain of 5 to 7% in offspring at an oral dose of 7.5 mg/kg/day (94 times the recommended human ophthalmic dose) were seen during lactation. A slight delay in postnatal development (incisor eruption, vaginal canalization and eye openings), secondary to lower fetal body weight, was noted.

It is not known whether this drug is excreted in human milk. Because many drugs are excreted in human milk and because of the potential for serious adverse reactions in nursing infants from TRUSOPT, a decision should be made whether to discontinue nursing or to discontinue the drug, taking into account the importance of the drug to the mother.

Pediatric Use

Safety and IOP-lowering effects of TRUSOPT have been demonstrated in pediatric patients in a 3-month, multicenter, double-masked, active-treatment-controlled trial.

Geriatric Use

No overall differences in safety and effectiveness have been observed between elderly and younger patients.

ADVERSE REACTIONS

Controlled clinical trials: The most frequent adverse events associated with TRUSOPT were ocular burning, stinging, or discomfort immediately following ocular administration (approximately one-third of patients). Approximately one-quarter of patients noted a bitter taste following administration. Superficial punctate keratitis occurred in 10–15% of patients and signs and symptoms of ocular allergic reaction in approximately 10%. Events occurring in approximately 1–5% of patients were conjunctivitis and lid reactions (see PRECAUTIONS, *General*), blurred vision, eye redness, tearing, dryness, and photophobia. Other ocular events and systemic events were reported infrequently, including headache, nausea, asthenia/fatigue; and, rarely, skin rashes, urolithiasis, and iridocyclitis.

In a 3-month, double-masked, active-treatment-controlled, multicenter study in pediatric patients, the adverse experience profile of TRUSOPT was comparable to that seen in adult patients.

Clinical practice: The following adverse events have occurred either at low incidence (<1%) during clinical trials or have been reported during the use of TRUSOPT in clinical practice where these events were reported voluntarily from a population of unknown size and frequency of occurrence cannot be determined precisely. They have been chosen for inclusion based on factors such as seriousness, frequency of reporting, possible causal connection to TRUSOPT, or a combination of these factors: signs and symptoms of systemic allergic reactions including angioedema, bronchospasm, pruritus, and urticaria; dizziness, paresthesia; ocular pain, transient myopia, choroidal detachment following filtration surgery, eyelid crusting; dyspnea; contact dermatitis, epistaxis, dry mouth and throat irritation.

OVERDOSAGE

Electrolyte imbalance, development of an acidotic state, and possible central nervous system effects may occur. Serum electrolyte levels (particularly potassium) and blood pH levels should be monitored.

DOSAGE AND ADMINISTRATION

The dose is one drop of TRUSOPT Ophthalmic Solution in the affected eye(s) three times daily.

TRUSOPT may be used concomitantly with other topical ophthalmic drug products to lower intraocular pressure. If more than one topical ophthalmic drug is being used, the drugs should be administered at least ten minutes apart.

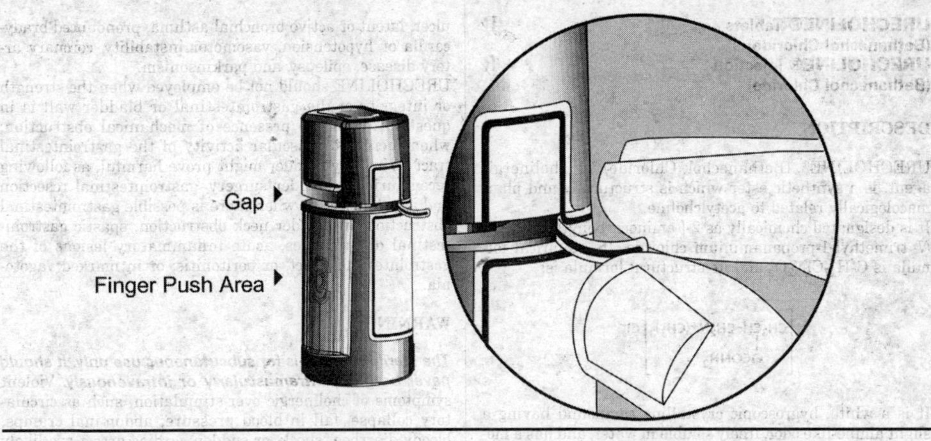

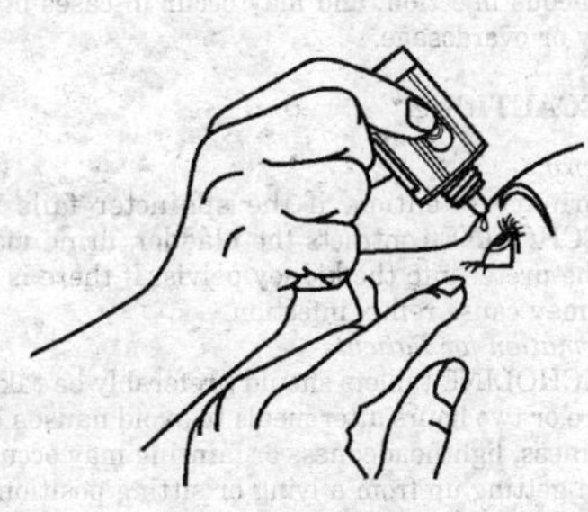

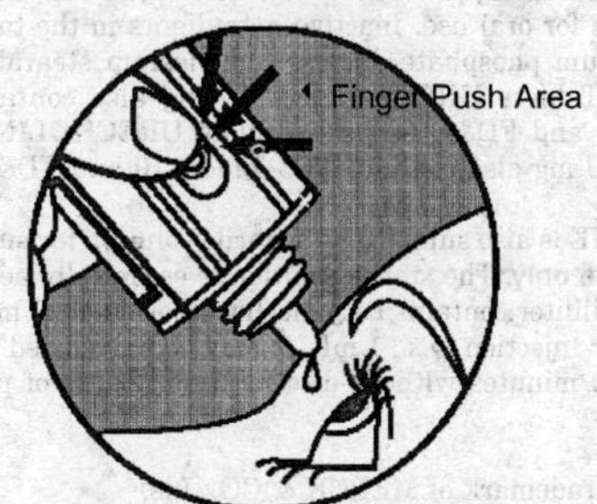

HOW SUPPLIED

TRUSOPT Ophthalmic Solution is a slightly opalescent, nearly colorless, slightly viscous solution.

No. 3519—TRUSOPT Ophthalmic Solution 2% is supplied in OCUMETER®* PLUS container, a white, opaque, plastic ophthalmic dispenser with a controlled drop tip as follows:

NDC 0006-3519-35, 5 mL

NDC 0006-3519-36, 10 mL.

Storage

Store TRUSOPT Ophthalmic Solution at 15–30°C (59–86°F). Protect from light.

*Registered trademark of MERCK & CO., Inc.

INSTRUCTIONS FOR USE

Please follow these instructions carefully when using TRUSOPT*. Use TRUSOPT as prescribed by your doctor.

1. If you use other topically applied ophthalmic medications, they should be administered at least 10 minutes before or after TRUSOPT.
2. Wash hands before each use.
3. Before using the medication for the first time, be sure the Safety Strip on the front of the bottle is unbroken. A gap between the bottle and the cap is normal for an unopened bottle.

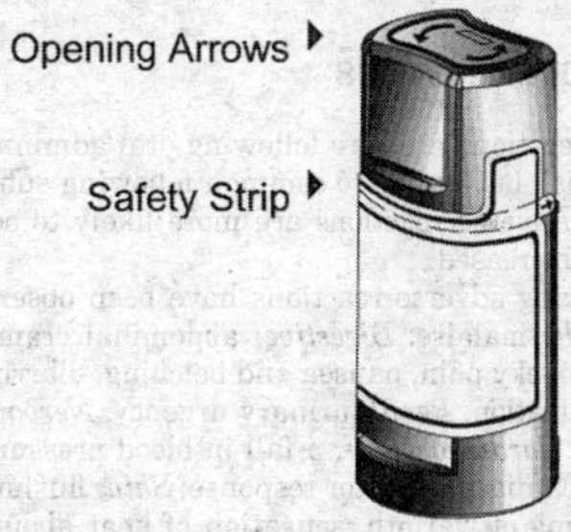

4. Tear off the Safety Strip to break the seal. [See first figure above]
5. To open the bottle, unscrew the cap by turning as indicated by the arrows.

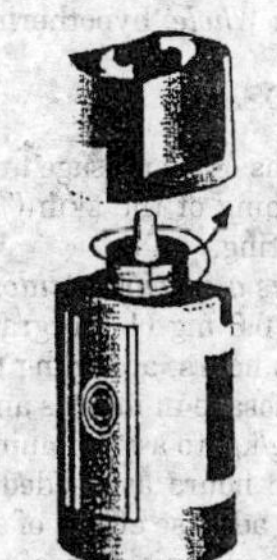

6. Tilt your head back and pull your lower eyelid down slightly to form a pocket between your eyelid and your eye.

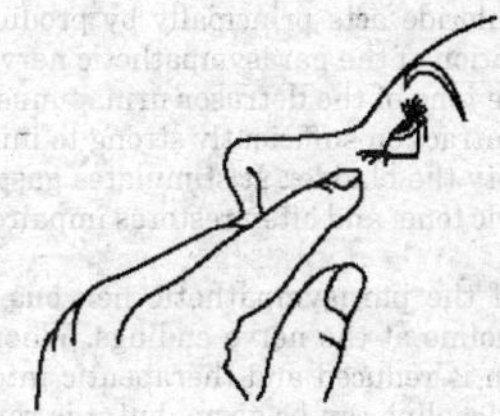

7. Invert the bottle, and press lightly with the thumb or index finger over the "Finger Push Area" (as shown) until a single drop is dispensed into the eye as directed by your doctor.
   [See second figure above]
   DO NOT TOUCH YOUR EYE OR EYELID WITH THE DROPPER TIP.
   Ophthalmic medications, if handled improperly, can become contaminated by common bacteria known to cause eye infections. Serious damage to the eye and subsequent loss of vision may result from using contaminated ophthalmic medications. If you think your medication may be contaminated, or if you develop an eye infection, contact your doctor immediately concerning continued use of this bottle.
8. Repeat steps 6 & 7 with the other eye if instructed to do so by your doctor.
9. Replace the cap by turning until it is firmly touching the bottle. Do not overtighten the cap.
10. The dispenser tip is designed to provide a pre-measured drop; therefore, do NOT enlarge the hole of the dispenser tip.
11. After you have used all doses, there will be some TRUSOPT left in the bottle. You should not be concerned since an extra amount of TRUSOPT has been added and you will get the full amount of TRUSOPT that your doctor prescribed. Do not attempt to remove excess medicine from the bottle.

WARNING: Keep out of reach of children.

If you have any questions about the use of TRUSOPT, please consult your doctor.

*Registered trademark of MERCK & CO., Inc.

Manuf. for:
Merck & Co., Inc., Whitehouse Station, NJ 08889, USA
By: Laboratoires Merck Sharp & Dohme-Chibret
63963 Clermont-Ferrand Cedex 9, France

9368204 Issued April 2004

Shown in Product Identification Guide, page 105

Continued on next page

Information on the Merck & Co., Inc., products listed on these pages is from the prescribing information in use October 1, 2004. For information, please call 1-800-NSC-MERCK [1-800-672-6372].

URECHOLINE® Tablets ℞
(Bethanechol Chloride)
URECHOLINE® Injection ℞
(Bethanechol Chloride)

DESCRIPTION

URECHOLINE* (Bethanechol Chloride), a cholinergic agent, is a synthetic ester which is structurally and pharmacologically related to acetylcholine.
It is designated chemically as 2-[(aminocarbonyl)oxy]-*N, N, N*- trimethyl-1-propanaminium chloride. Its empirical formula is $C_7H_{17}ClN_2O_2$ and its structural formula is:

$$\left[\begin{array}{l} CH_3CH-CH_2N^+(CH_3)_3 \\ \quad | \\ \quad OCONH_2 \end{array}\right] Cl^-$$

It is a white, hygroscopic crystalline compound having a slight amine-like odor, freely soluble in water, and has a molecular weight of 196.68.
URECHOLINE is supplied as 5 mg, 10 mg, 25 mg, and 50 mg tablets for oral use. Inactive ingredients in the tablets are calcium phosphate, lactose, magnesium stearate, and starch. Tablets URECHOLINE 10 mg also contain FD&C Red 3 and FD&C Red 40. Tablets URECHOLINE 25 mg and 50 mg also contain D&C Yellow 10 and FD&C Yellow 6.
URECHOLINE is also supplied as a sterile solution **for subcutaneous use only.** The sterile solution is essentially neutral. Each milliliter contains bethanechol chloride, 5.15 mg, and Water for Injection, q.s., 1 mL. It may be autoclaved at 120° C for 20 minutes without discoloration or loss of potency.

*Registered trademark of MERCK & CO., INC.

CLINICAL PHARMACOLOGY

Bethanechol chloride acts principally by producing the effects of stimulation of the parasympathetic nervous system. It increases the tone of the detrusor urinae muscle, usually producing a contraction sufficiently strong to initiate micturition and empty the bladder. It stimulates gastric motility, increases gastric tone, and often restores impaired rhythmic peristalsis.
Stimulation of the parasympathetic nervous system releases acetylcholine at the nerve endings. When spontaneous stimulation is reduced and therapeutic intervention is required, acetylcholine can be given, but it is rapidly hydrolyzed by cholinesterase, and its effects are transient. Bethanechol chloride is not destroyed by cholinesterase and its effects are more prolonged than those of acetylcholine.
Effects on the GI and urinary tracts sometimes appear within 30 minutes after oral administration of bethanechol chloride, but more often 60–90 minutes are required to reach maximum effectiveness. Following oral administration, the usual duration of action of bethanechol is one hour, although large doses (300–400 mg) have been reported to produce effects for up to six hours. Subcutaneous injection produces a more intense action on bladder muscle than does oral administration of the drug.
Because of the selective action of bethanechol, nicotinic symptoms of cholinergic stimulation are usually absent or minimal when orally or subcutaneously administered in therapeutic doses, while muscarinic effects are prominent. Muscarinic effects usually occur within 5–15 minutes after subcutaneous injection, reach a maximum in 15–30 minutes, and disappear within two hours. Doses that stimulate micturition and defecation and increase peristalsis do not ordinarily stimulate ganglia or voluntary muscles. Therapeutic test doses in normal human subjects have little effect on heart rate, blood pressure, or peripheral circulation.
Bethanechol chloride does not cross the blood-brain barrier because of its charged quaternary amine moiety. The metabolic fate and mode of excretion of the drug have not been elucidated.
A clinical study** was conducted on the relative effectiveness of oral and subcutaneous doses of bethanechol chloride on the stretch response of bladder muscle in patients with urinary retention. Results showed that 5 mg of the drug given subcutaneously stimulated a response that was more rapid in onset and of larger magnitude than an oral dose of 50 mg, 100 mg, or 200 mg. All the oral doses, however, had a longer duration of effect than the subcutaneous dose. Although the 50 mg oral dose caused little change in intravesical pressure in this study, this dose has been found in other studies to be clinically effective in the rehabilitation of patients with decompensated bladders.

**Diokno, A. C.; Lapides, J., Urol. *10:* 23–24, July 1977.

INDICATIONS AND USAGE

For the treatment of acute postoperative and postpartum nonobstructive (functional) urinary retention and for neurogenic atony of the urinary bladder with retention.

CONTRAINDICATIONS

Hypersensitivity to URECHOLINE tablets or to any component of URECHOLINE injection, hyperthyroidism, peptic ulcer, latent or active bronchial asthma, pronounced bradycardia or hypotension, vasomotor instability, coronary artery disease, epilepsy, and parkinsonism.
URECHOLINE should not be employed when the strength or integrity of the gastrointestinal or bladder wall is in question, or in the presence of mechanical obstruction; when increased muscular activity of the gastrointestinal tract or urinary bladder might prove harmful, as following recent urinary bladder surgery, gastrointestinal resection and anastomosis, or when there is possible gastrointestinal obstruction; in bladder neck obstruction, spastic gastrointestinal disturbances, acute inflammatory lesions of the gastrointestinal tract, or peritonitis; or in marked vagotonia.

WARNING

The sterile solution is for subcutaneous use only. It should never be given intramuscularly or intravenously. Violent symptoms of cholinergic over-stimulation, such as circulatory collapse, fall in blood pressure, abdominal cramps, bloody diarrhea, shock, or sudden cardiac arrest are likely to occur if the drug is given by either of these routes. Although rare, these same symptoms have occurred after subcutaneous injection, and may occur in cases of hypersensitivity or overdosage.

PRECAUTIONS

General
In urinary retention, if the sphincter fails to relax as URECHOLINE contracts the bladder, urine may be forced up the ureter into the kidney pelvis. If there is bacteriuria, this may cause reflux infection.
Information for Patients
URECHOLINE tablets should preferably be taken one hour before or two hours after meals to avoid nausea or vomiting. Dizziness, lightheadedness or fainting may occur, especially when getting up from a lying or sitting position.
Drug Interactions
Special care is required if this drug is given to patients receiving ganglion blocking compounds because a critical fall in blood pressure may occur. Usually, severe abdominal symptoms appear before there is such a fall in the blood pressure.
Carcinogenesis, Mutagenesis, Impairment of Fertility
Long-term studies in animals have not been performed to evaluate the effects upon fertility, mutagenic or carcinogenic potential of URECHOLINE.
Pregnancy
Pregnancy Category C. Animal reproduction studies have not been conducted with URECHOLINE. It is also not known whether URECHOLINE can cause fetal harm when administered to a pregnant woman or can affect reproduction capacity. URECHOLINE should be given to a pregnant woman only if clearly needed.
Nursing Mothers
It is not known whether this drug is secreted in human milk. Because many drugs are secreted in human milk and because of the potential for serious adverse reactions from URECHOLINE in nursing infants, a decision should be made whether to discontinue nursing or to discontinue the drug, taking into account the importance of the drug to the mother.
Pediatric Use
Safety and effectiveness in pediatric patients have not been established.

ADVERSE REACTIONS

Adverse reactions are rare following oral administration of bethanechol, but are more common following subcutaneous injection. Adverse reactions are more likely to occur when dosage is increased.
The following adverse reactions have been observed: *Body as a Whole:* malaise; *Digestive:* abdominal cramps or discomfort, colicky pain, nausea and belching, diarrhea, borborygmi, salivation; *Renal:* urinary urgency; *Nervous System:* headache; *Cardiovascular:* a fall in blood pressure with reflex tachycardia, vasomotor response; *Skin:* flushing producing a feeling of warmth, sensation of heat about the face, sweating; *Respiratory:* bronchial constriction, asthmatic attacks; *Special Senses:* lacrimation, miosis.
Causal Relationship Unknown: The following adverse reactions have been reported, and a causal relationship to therapy with URECHOLINE has not been established: *Body as a Whole:* hypothermia: *Nervous System:* seizures.

OVERDOSAGE

Early signs of overdosage are abdominal discomfort, salivation, flushing of the skin ("hot feeling"), sweating, nausea and vomiting.
Atropine is a specific antidote. The recommended dose for adults is 0.6 mg (1/100 grain). Repeat doses can be given every two hours, according to clinical response. The recommended dosage in infants and children up to 12 years of age is 0.01 mg/kg (to a maximum single dose of 0.4 mg) repeated every two hours as needed until the desired effect is obtained, or adverse effects of atropine preclude further usage. Subcutaneous injection of atropine is preferred except in emergencies when the intravenous route may be employed.
When URECHOLINE is administered subcutaneously, a syringe containing a dose of atropine sulfate should always be available to treat symptoms of toxicity.
The oral LD_{50} of bethanechol chloride is 1510 mg/kg in the mouse.

DOSAGE AND ADMINISTRATION

Dosage and route of administration must be individualized, depending on the type and severity of the condition to be treated.
Preferably give the drug when the stomach is empty. If taken soon after eating, nausea and vomiting may occur.
Oral—The usual adult dosage is 10 to 50 mg three or four times a day. The minimum effective dose is determined by giving 5 or 10 mg initially and repeating the same amount at hourly intervals until satisfactory response occurs or until a maximum of 50 mg has been given. The effects of the drug sometimes appear within 30 minutes and usually within 60 to 90 minutes. They persist for about an hour.
Subcutaneous—The usual dose is 1 mL (5.15 mg), although some patients respond satisfactorily to as little as 0.5 mL (2.575 mg). The minimum effective dose is determined by injecting 0.5 mL (2.575 mg) initially and repeating the same amount at 15 to 30 minute intervals to a maximum of four doses until satisfactory response is obtained, unless disturbing reactions appear. The minimum effective dose may be repeated thereafter three or four times a day as required.
Rarely, single doses up to 2 mL (10.30 mg) may be required. Such large doses may cause severe reactions and should be used only after adequate trial of single doses of 0.5 to 1 mL (2.575 to 5.15 mg) has established that smaller doses are not sufficient.
URECHOLINE is usually effective in 5 to 15 minutes after subcutaneous injection.
If necessary, the effects of the drug can be abolished promptly by atropine (see OVERDOSAGE).
Parenteral drug products should be inspected visually for particulate matter and discoloration prior to administration, whenever solution and container permit.

HOW SUPPLIED

Tablets URECHOLINE are round, compressed tablets, scored on one side. They are supplied as follows:
No. 7785—5 mg, white in color, coded MSD 403 on one side and URECHOLINE on the other.
NDC 0006-0403-68 in bottles of 100.
No. 7787—10 mg, pink in color, coded MSD 412 on one side and URECHOLINE on the other.
NDC 0006-0412-68 in bottles of 100
(6505-00-616-7856 10 mg 100's).
No. 7788—25 mg, yellow in color, coded MSD 457 on one side and URECHOLINE on the other.
NDC 0006-0457-68 in bottles of 100
(6505-00-912-7440 25 mg, 100's).
No. 7790 — 50 mg, yellow in color, coded MSD 460 on one side and URECHOLINE on the other.
NDC 0006-0460-68 in bottles of 100.
No. 7786—Injection URECHOLINE, 5.15 mg per mL, is a clear, colorless solution, and is supplied as follows:
NDC 0006-7786-29 in box of 6 × 1 mL vials
(6505-00-616-8947 in box of 6 × 1 mL vials).
Storage
Store Tablets URECHOLINE in a tightly-closed container. Avoid storage at temperatures above 40°C (104°F).
Avoid storage of Injection URECHOLINE at temperatures below −20°C (−4°F) and above 40°C (104°F).
7875834 Issued August 1997

Shown in Product Identification Guide, page 324

VAQTA® ℞
(Hepatitis A Vaccine, Inactivated)

DESCRIPTION

VAQTA* [Hepatitis A Vaccine, Inactivated] is an inactivated whole virus vaccine derived from hepatitis A virus (HAV) grown in cell culture in human MRC-5 diploid fibroblasts. It contains inactivated virus of a strain which was originally derived by further serial passage of a proven attenuated strain. The virus is grown, harvested, purified by a combination of physical and high performance liquid chromatographic techniques developed at the Merck Research Laboratories, formalin inactivated, and then adsorbed onto amorphous aluminum hydroxyphosphate sulfate. One milliliter of the vaccine contains approximately 50 units (U) of hepatitis A virus antigen, which is purified and formulated without a preservative. Within the limits of current assay variability, the 50U dose of VAQTA contains less than 0.1 mcg of a non-viral protein, less than 4×10^{-6} mcg of DNA, less than 10^{-4} mcg of bovine albumin, and less than 0.8 mcg of formaldehyde. Other process chemical residuals are less than 10 parts per billion (ppb).
VAQTA is a sterile suspension for intramuscular injection. VAQTA is supplied in two formulations:
Pediatric/Adolescent Formulation: each 0.5 mL dose contains approximately 25U of hepatitis A virus antigen adsorbed onto approximately 0.225 mg of aluminum provided as amorphous aluminum hydroxyphosphate sulfate, and 35 mcg of sodium borate as a pH stabilizer, in 0.9% sodium chloride.
Adult Formulation: each 1 mL dose contains approximately 50U of hepatitis A virus antigen adsorbed onto ap-

proximately 0.45 mg of aluminum provided as amorphous aluminum hydroxyphosphate sulfate, and 70 mcg of sodium borate as a pH stabilizer, in 0.9% sodium chloride.

*Registered trademark of MERCK & CO., Inc.

CLINICAL PHARMACOLOGY

Hepatitis A Disease

Hepatitis A virus is one of several hepatitis viruses that cause a systemic infection with pathology in the liver. The incubation period ranges from approximately 20 to 50 days. While the course of the disease is generally benign and does not result in chronic hepatitis, infection with hepatitis A virus remains an important cause of morbidity and occasional fulminant hepatitis and death.

Hepatitis A is transmitted most often by the fecal-oral route, with infection occurring primarily within private households. Common-source outbreaks due to contaminated food and water supplies have occurred following consumption of certain foods such as raw shellfish, and uncooked foods prepared by an infected food-handler or otherwise contaminated prior to ingestion (salads, sandwiches, frozen raspberries, etc.). Bloodborne transmission, while uncommon, is possible via blood transfusion, contaminated blood products, or from needles shared with an infected viremic individual. Sexual transmission has also been reported.

The disease burden due to hepatitis A in the United States has been estimated to be approximately 143,000 infections per year, of which 75,800 result in clinical hepatitis A disease, 11,400 hospitalizations, and 80 deaths due to fulminant hepatitis. Worldwide, it has been estimated that 1.4 million cases are reported annually. The clinical manifestations of hepatitis A infection often pass unrecognized in children ≤2 years of age whereas overt hepatitis A develops in the majority of infected older children and adults. Symptoms and signs of hepatitis A infection are similar to those associated with other types of viral hepatitis and include anorexia, nausea, fever/chills, jaundice, dark urine, light-colored stools, abdominal pain, malaise, and fatigue.

Clinical Trials

Clinical trials conducted worldwide with several formulations of the vaccine in 9421 healthy individuals ranging from 2 to 85 years of age have demonstrated that VAQTA is highly immunogenic and generally well tolerated.

Protection from hepatitis A disease has been shown to be related to the presence of antibody; an anamnestic antibody response occurs in healthy individuals with a history of infection who are subsequently re-exposed to hepatitis A virus. Similarly, protection after vaccination with VAQTA has been associated with the onset of serconversion (≥10 mIU/mL of hepatitis A antibody, measured by a modification of the HAVAB** radioimmunoassay [RIA]) and with an anamnestic antibody response following booster vaccination with VAQTA.

**Trademark of Abbott Laboratories

Post-marketing Safety Study

In a post-marketing short-term safety surveillance study, conducted at a large health maintenance organization in the United States, a total of 42,110 individuals ≥2 years of age received 1 or 2 doses of VAQTA (13,735 children/adolescent and 28,375 adult subjects). Safety was passively monitored by electronic search of the automated medical records database for emergency room and outpatient visits, hospitalizations, and deaths. Medical charts were reviewed when indicated. There was no serious, vaccine-related, adverse event identified among the 42,110 vaccine recipients in this study. Diarrhea/gastroenteritis, resulting in outpatient visits, was determined by the investigator to be the only vaccine-related nonserious adverse event in the study. There was no vaccine-related, adverse event identified that had not been reported in earlier clinical trials with VAQTA. (See ADVERSE REACTIONS, *Post-marketing Safety Study*.)

Immunology

In combined clinical studies, 97% of 1230 healthy children and adolescents 2 through 18 years of age seroconverted with a geometric mean titer (GMT) of 43 mIU/mL within 4 weeks after a single ~25U/0.5 mL intramuscular dose of VAQTA. Similarly, 95% of 1411 adults ≥19 years of age seroconverted with a GMT of 37 mIU/mL within 4 weeks after a single ~50U/1.0 mL intramuscular dose of VAQTA. Furthermore, at 2 weeks post-vaccination, 69% (n=744) of adults seroconverted with a GMT of 16 mIU/mL after a single dose of VAQTA. Immune memory was demonstrated by an anamnestic antibody response in individuals who received either a ~25U/0.5 mL or ~50U/1.0 mL booster dose (see *Persistence*).

A ~50U/1.0 mL intramuscular dose of VAQTA also was evaluated at four weeks post primary dose in healthy adolescents (18 years of age); 94% of 17 adolescents seroconverted with a GMT of 40 mIU/mL. In individuals 18 years of age, the GMT following a ~50 U/1.0 mL booster dose was greater than the GMT following a ~25U/0.5 mL booster dose. Both doses were immunogenic and were generally well tolerated. (See DOSAGE AND ADMINISTRATION.)

While a study evaluating VAQTA alone in a post-exposure setting has not been conducted, the concurrent use of VAQTA (~50U) and immune globulin (IG, 0.06 mL/kg) was evaluated in a clinical study involving healthy adults 18 to 39 years of age. Table 1 provides seroconversion rates and GMT at 4 and 24 weeks after the first dose in each treatment group and at one month after a booster dose of VAQTA (administered at 24 weeks).

Table 2
Children/Adolescents
Seroconversion Rates (%) and Geometric Mean Titers (GMT) for Cohorts of Initially Seronegative Vaccinees at the Time of the Booster (~25U) and 4 Weeks Later

Months Following Initial ~25U Dose	Cohort* (n=960) 0 and 6 Months	Cohort* (n=35) 0 and 12 Months	Cohort* (n=39) 0 and 18 Months
	Seroconversion Rate GMT (mIU/mL) (95% CI)		
6	97% 107 (98, 117)		
7	100% 10433 (9681, 11243)		
12	—	91% 48 (33, 71)	—
13	—	100% 12308 (9337, 16226)	—
18	—		90% 50 (28, 89)
19	—		100% 9591 (7613, 12082)

*Blood samples were taken at prebooster and postbooster time points.

Table 1
Seroconversion Rates (%) and Geometric Mean Titers (GMT) after Vaccination with VAQTA plus IG, VAQTA Alone, and IG Alone

	VAQTA plus IG	VAQTA	IG
Weeks	Seroconversion Rate GMT (mIU/mL)		
4	100% 42 (n=129)	96% 38 (n=135)	87% 19 (n=30)
24	92% 83 (n=125)	97%* 137* (n=132)	0% Undetectable† (n=28)
28	100% 4872 (n=114)	100% 6498 (n=128)	N/A

† Undetectable is defined as <10mIU/mL.
*The seroconversion rate and the GMT in the group receiving VAQTA alone were significantly higher than in the group receiving VAQTA plus IG (p=0.05, p<0.001, respectively).
N/A = Not Applicable

Efficacy

A very high degree of protection has been demonstrated after a single dose of VAQTA in children and adolescents. The protective efficacy, immunogenicity and safety of VAQTA were evaluated in a randomized, double-blind, placebo-controlled study involving 1037 susceptible healthy children and adolescents 2 through 16 years of age in a U.S. community with recurrent outbreaks of hepatitis A (The Monroe Efficacy Study). Each child received an intramuscular dose of VAQTA (~25U) or placebo. Among those individuals who were initially seronegative (by modified HAVAB), seroconversion was achieved in >99% of vaccine recipients within 4 weeks after vaccination. The onset of seroconversion following a single dose of VAQTA was shown to parallel the onset of protection against clinical hepatitis A disease.

Because of the long incubation period of the disease (approximately 20 to 50 days, or longer in children), the primary endpoint was based on clinically confirmed cases*** of hepatitis A occurring ≥50 days after vaccination in order to exclude any children incubating the infection before vaccination. In subjects who were initially seronegative, the protective efficacy of a single dose of VAQTA was observed to be 100% with 21 cases of clinically confirmed hepatitis A occurring in the placebo group and none in the vaccine group (p<0.001). A secondary endpoint was pre-defined as the number of clinically confirmed cases of hepatitis A ≥30 days. With this secondary endpoint, 28 cases of clinically confirmed hepatitis A occurred in the placebo group while none occurrred in the vaccine group ≥30 days after vaccination. In addition, it was observed in this trial that no cases of clinically confirmed hepatitis A occurred in the vaccine group after day 16.† Following demonstration of protection with a single dose and termination of the study, a booster dose was administered to a subset of vaccinees 6, 12, or 18 months after the primary dose.

*** The clinical case definition included all of the following occurring at the same time: 1) one or more typical clinical signs or symptoms of hepatitis A (e.g., jaundice, malaise, fever ≥38.3°C), 2) elevation of hepatitis A IgM antibody (HAVAB-M), 3) elevation of alanine transferase (ALT) ≥2 times the upper limit of normal.
† One vaccine did not meet the pre-defined criteria for clinically confirmed hepatitis A but did have positive hepatitis A IgM and borderline liver enzyme (ALT) elevations on days 34, 50, and 58 after vaccination with mild clinical symptoms observed on days 49 and 50.

Persistence

The total duration of the protective effect of VAQTA in healthy vaccinees is unknown at present. However, seropositivity was shown to persist up to 18 months after a single ~25U dose in a cohort of 35 out of 39 children and adolescents who participated in The Monroe Efficacy Study; 95% of this cohort responded anamnestically following a booster at 18 months. To date, no cases of clinically confirmed hepatitis A disease ≥50 days after vaccination have occurred in those vaccinees from The Monroe Efficacy Study monitored for up to 6 years.

The effectiveness of VAQTA for use in community outbreak control has been demonstrated by the fact that, although cases of imported infection have occurred, the study community has remained free of outbreaks. In contrast, three nearby sister communities to Monroe have continued to experience outbreaks.

In adults, seropositivity has been shown to persist up to 18 months after a single ~50U dose. Persistence of immunologic memory was demonstrated with an anamnestic antibody response to a booster dose of ~25U given 6 to 18 months after the primary dose in children and adolescents (Table 2), and to a booster dose of ~50U given 6 to 18 months after the primary dose to adults (Table 3).

[See table 2 above]

[See table 3 at top of next page]

In a clinical study involving healthy children and adolescents who received two doses (~25U) of VAQTA, detectable levels of anti-HAV antibodies (≥10 mIU/mL) were present in 100% of subjects for up to 6 years postvaccination. In subjects who received VAQTA at 0 and 6 months, the GMT was 819 mIU/mL (n=175) at 2.5 to 3.5 years and 505 mIU/mL (n=174) at 5 to 6 years postvaccination. In subjects who received VAQTA at 0 and 12 months, the GMT was 2224 mIU/mL (n=49) at 2.5 to 3.5 years and 1191 mIU/mL (n=47) at 5 to 6 years postvaccination. In subjects who received VAQTA at 0 and 18 months, the GMT was 2501 mIU/mL (n=53) at 2.5 to 3.5 years and 1500 mIU/mL (n=53) at 5 to 6 years postvaccination.

In studies of healthy adults who received two doses (~50U) of VAQTA at 0 and 6 months, the hepatitis A antibody response to date has been shown to persist up to 6 years. Detectable levels of anti-HAV antibodies (≥10 mIU/mL) were present in 100% (378/378) of subjects with a GMT of 1734 mIU/mL at 1 year, 99.2% (252/254) of subjects with a GMT of 687 mIU/mL at 2 to 3 years, 99.1% (219/221) of subjects with a GMT of 605 mIU/mL at 4 years, and 99.4% (170/171) of subjects with a GMT of 684 mIU/mL at 6 years postvaccination.

Studies in healthy children, adolescents and adults are ongoing to evaluate longer-term antibody persistence and the need, if any, for additional booster doses.

Interchangeability of the Booster Dose

A clinical study in 537 healthy adults, 18 to 83 years of age, evaluated the immune response to a booster dose of VAQTA and HAVRIX‡ (hepatitis A vaccine, inactivated) given at 6 or 12 months following an initial dose of HAVRIX. When VAQTA was given as a booster dose following HAVRIX, the vaccine produced an adequate immune response (see Table

Continued on next page

Information on the Merck & Co., Inc., products listed on these pages is from the prescribing information in use October 1, 2004. For information, please call 1-800-NSC-MERCK [1-800-672-6372].

Vaqta—Cont.

4) and was generally well tolerated. (See DOSAGE AND ADMINISTRATION, *Interchangability of the Booster Dose.*)
[See table 4 at right]

‡Registered trademark of SmithKline Beecham

Use With Other Vaccines

A controlled clinical study was conducted with 240 healthy adults, 18 to 54 years of age, who were randomized to receive either VAQTA, typhoid and yellow fever vaccines concomitantly at separate injection sites, typhoid and yellow fever vaccines concomitantly at separate injection sites, or VAQTA alone. The seropositivity rate for hepatitis A when VAQTA, typhoid and yellow fever vaccines were administered concomitantly was generally similar to when VAQTA was given alone. The antibody response rates for typhoid and yellow fever were adequate when typhoid and yellow fever vaccines were administered concomitantly with and without VAQTA. The GMTs for hepatitis A when VAQTA, typhoid and yellow fever vaccines were administered concomitantly were reduced when compared to VAQTA alone. Following receipt of the booster dose of VAQTA, the GMTs for hepatitis A in these two groups were observed to be comparable. The concomitant administration of these three vaccines at separate injection sites was generally well tolerated. (See INDICATIONS AND USAGE, *Use With Other Vaccines* and DOSAGE AND ADMINISTRATION, *Use With Other Vaccines.*)

INDICATIONS AND USAGE

VAQTA is indicated for active pre-exposure prophylaxis against disease caused by hepatitis A virus in persons 2 years of age and older. Primary immunization should be given at least 2 weeks prior to expected exposure to HAV. Individuals who are or will be at increased risk of infection by HAV include:

TRAVELERS

Persons traveling to areas of higher endemicity for hepatitis A. These areas include, but are not limited to, Africa, Asia (except Japan), the Mediterranean basin, Eastern Europe, the Middle East, Central and South America, Mexico, and parts of the Caribbean. Current CDC (Centers for Disease Control and Prevention) advisories should be consulted with regard to specific locales.

MILITARY PERSONNEL

PEOPLE LIVING, IN, OR RELOCATING TO, AREAS OF HIGH ENDEMICITY

CERTAIN ETHNIC AND GEOGRAPHIC POPULATIONS THAT EXPERIENCE CYCLIC HEPATITIS A EPIDEMICS SUCH AS:

Native peoples of Alaska and the Americas.

OTHERS

Persons engaging in high-risk sexual activity (such as homosexually active males); users of illicit injectable drugs; residents of a community experiencing an outbreak of hepatitis A.

Hemophiliacs and other recipients of therapeutic blood products (see PRECAUTIONS and DOSAGE AND ADMINISTRATION).

Persons who test positive for hepatitis C virus and have diagnosed liver disease.

Although the epidemiology of hepatitis A does not permit the identification of other specific populations at high risk of disease, outbreaks of hepatitis A or exposure to hepatitis A virus have been described in a variety of populations in which VAQTA may be useful:

— Certain institutional workers (e.g., caretakers for the developmentally challenged)
— Employees of child day-care centers
— Laboratory workers who handle live hepatitis A virus
— Handlers of primate animals that may be harboring HAV

PEOPLE EXPOSED TO HEPATITIS A

For those requiring both immediate and long-term protection, VAQTA may be administered concomitantly with IG.

Revaccination

See DOSAGE AND ADMINISTRATION, *DOSAGE.*

Use With Other Vaccines

VAQTA may be given concomitantly at separate injection sites with typhoid and yellow fever vaccines. The GMTs for hepatitis A when VAQTA, typhoid and yellow fever vaccines were administered concomitantly were reduced when compared to VAQTA alone. Following receipt of the booster dose of VAQTA, the GMTs for hepatitis A in these two groups were observed to be comparable. (See CLINICAL PHARMACOLOGY, *Use With Other Vaccines* and DOSAGE AND ADMINISTRATION, *Use With Other Vaccines.*)

The Advisory Committee on Immunization Practices has stated that limited data from studies conducted among adults indicate that simultaneous administration of hepatitis A vaccine with diphtheria, poliovirus (oral and inactivated), tetanus, oral typhoid, cholera, Japanese encephalitis, rabies, or yellow fever vaccine does not decrease the immune response to either vaccine or increase the frequency of reported adverse events. Studies indicate that hepatitis B vaccine can be administered with VAQTA without affecting immunogenicity or increasing the frequency of adverse events.

Use With Immune Globulin

For individuals requiring either post-exposure prophylaxis or combined immediate and longer-term protection (e.g., travelers departing on short notice to endemic areas),

Table 3
Adults
Seroconversion Rates (%) and Geometric Mean Titers (GMT) for a Cohort of Vaccinees at the Time of the Booster (~50U) and 4 Weeks Later

Months Following Initial ~50U Dose	Cohort* (n=1201) 0 and 6 Months	Cohort*(n=91) 0 and 12 Months	Cohort* (n=84) 0 and 18 Months
		Seroconversion Rate GMT (mIU/mL) (95% CI)	
6	98% 139 (129, 149)	—	—
7	100% 5987 (5561, 6445)		
12	—	93% 107 (78, 146)	
13	—	98% 4896 (3589, 6679)	—
18	—	—	96% 120 (88, 164)
19	—	—	100% 6043 (4687, 7793)

*Blood samples were taken at prebooster and postbooster time points.

Table 4
VAQTA Versus HAVRIX
Seropositivity Rate, Booster Response Rate† and Geometric Mean Titer at 4 Weeks Postbooster

First Dose	Booster Dose	Seropositivity Rate	Booster Response Rate†	Geometric Mean Titer
HAVRIX 1440 EL.U.	VAQTA 50 U	99.7% (n=313)	86.1% (n=310)	3272 (n=313)
HAVRIX 1440 EL.U.	HAVRIX 1440 EL.U.	99.3% (n=151)	80.1% (n=151)	2423 (n=151)

† Booster Response Rate is defined as greater than or equal to a tenfold rise from prebooster to postbooster titer and postbooster titer ≥100 mIU/mL.

VAQTA may be administered concomitantly with IG using separate sites and syringes (see CLINICAL PHARMACOLOGY and DOSAGE AND ADMINISTRATION).

VAQTA IS NOT RECOMMENDED FOR USE IN INFANTS YOUNGER THAN 2 YEARS OF AGE SINCE DATA ON USE IN THIS AGE GROUP ARE NOT CURRENTLY AVAILABLE.

CONTRAINDICATIONS

Hypersensitivity to any component of the vaccine.

WARNINGS

Individuals who develop symptoms suggestive of hypersensitivity after an injection of VAQTA should not receive further injections of the vaccine (see CONTRAINDICATIONS).

If VAQTA is used in individuals with malignancies or those receiving immunosuppressive therapy or who are otherwise immunocompromised, the expected immune response may not be obtained.

PRECAUTIONS

General

VAQTA will not prevent hepatitis caused by infectious agents other than hepatitis A virus. Because of the long incubation period (approximately 20 to 50 days) for hepatitis A, it is possible for unrecognized hepatitis A infection to be present at the time the vaccine is given. The vaccine may not prevent hepatitis A in such individuals.

As with any vaccine, adequate treatment provisions, including epinephrine, should be available for immediate use should an anaphylactic or anaphylactoid reaction occur.

VAQTA should be administered with caution to people with bleeding disorders who are at risk of hemorrhage following intramuscular injection (see DOSAGE AND ADMINISTRATION).

As with any vaccine, vaccination with VAQTA may not result in a protective response in all susceptible vaccinees.

An acute infection or febrile illness may be reason for delaying use of VAQTA except when, in the opinion of the physician, withholding the vaccine entails a greater risk.

Carcinogenesis, Mutagenesis, Impairment of Fertility

VAQTA has not been evaluated for its carcinogenic or mutagenic potential, or its potential to impair fertility.

Pregnancy

Pregnancy Category C: Animal reproduction studies have not been conducted with VAQTA. It is also not known whether VAQTA can cause fetal harm when administered to a pregnant woman or can affect reproduction capacity. VAQTA should be given to a pregnant woman only if clearly needed.

Nursing Mothers

It is not known whether VAQTA is excreted in human milk. Because many drugs are excreted in human milk, caution should be exercised when VAQTA is administered to a woman who is breast feeding.

Pediatric Use

VAQTA has been shown to be generally well tolerated and highly immunogenic in individuals 2 through 18 years of age. See DOSAGE AND ADMINISTRATION for the recommended dosage schedule.

Safety and effectiveness in infants below 2 years of age have not been established.

Geriatric Use

Of the total number of adults in clinical studies of VAQTA, conducted pre- and post-licensure, 68 were 65 years of age or older, 10 of whom were 75 years of age or older. No overall differences in safety and immunogenicity were observed between these subjects and younger subjects; however, greater sensitivity of some older individuals cannot be ruled out. In a large post-marketing safety study in 42,110 individuals, ≥2 years of age, 4769 were 65 years of age or older, 1073 of whom were 75 years of age or older. There were no adverse experiences judged by the investigator to be vaccine related in the geriatric study population. Other reported clinical experience has not identified differences in responses between the elderly and younger subjects.

ADVERSE REACTIONS

VAQTA is generally well tolerated; adverse reactions usually are mild and transient.

Clinical Studies

In combined clinical trials, 16,252 doses of VAQTA were administered to 9181 healthy children, adolescents, and adults. VAQTA was generally well tolerated.

No serious vaccine-related adverse experiences were observed during clinical trials.

The Monroe Efficacy Study

In this study, 1037 healthy children and adolescents, 2 through 16 years of age, received a primary dose of ~25U of hepatitis A vaccine and a booster 6, 12, or 18 months later, or placebo. Subjects were observed during a 5-day period for fever and local complaints and during a 14-day period for systemic complaints. Injection-site complaints, generally mild and transient, were the most frequently reported complaints. Table 5 summarizes the local and systemic complaints (≥1%) reported in this study, without regard to causality. There were no significant differences in the rates of any complaints between vaccine and placebo recipients after Dose 1.

[See table 5 at top of next page]

Children/Adolescents—2 through 18 Years of Age

In combined clinical trials (including Monroe Efficacy Study participants) involving 2615 healthy children and adolescents who received one or more ~25U doses of hepatitis A vaccine, fever and local complaints were observed during a 5-day period following vaccination and systemic complaints during a 14-day period following vaccination. Injection-site complaints, generally mild and transient, were the most frequently reported complaints. Listed below are the complaints (≥1%) reported, without regard to causality, in decreasing order of frequency within each body system.

LOCALIZED INJECTION-SITE REACTIONS
Pain (18.7%); tenderness (16.9%); warmth (8.6%); erythema (7.5%); swelling (7.3%); ecchymosis (1.3%).
BODY AS A WHOLE
Fever (≥102°F, Oral) (3.1%); abdominal pain (1.6%).
DIGESTIVE SYSTEM
Diarrhea (1.0%); vomiting (1.0%).
NERVOUS SYSTEM/PSYCHIATRIC
Headache (2.3%).
RESPIRATORY SYSTEM
Pharyngitis (1.5%); upper respiratory infection (1.1%); cough (1.0%).
LABORATORY FINDINGS
Very few laboratory abnormalities were reported and included isolated reports of elevated liver function tests, eosinophilia, and increased urine protein.
Adults—19 Years of Age and Older
In combined clinical trials involving 1512 healthy adults who received one or more ~50U doses of hepatitis A vaccine, fever and local complaints were observed during a 5-day period following vaccination and systemic complaints during a 14-day period following vaccination. Injection-site complaints, generally mild and transient, were the most frequently reported complaints. Listed below are the complaints (≥1%) reported, without regard to causality, in decreasing order of frequency within each body system.
LOCALIZED INJECTION-SITE REACTIONS
Tenderness (52.7%); pain (51.1%); warmth (17.4%); swelling (13.8%); erythema (13.1%); ecchymosis (1.5%); pain/soreness (1.2%).
BODY AS A WHOLE
Asthenia/fatigue (3.9%); fever (2.7%); abdominal pain (1.3%).
DIGESTIVE SYSTEM
Diarrhea (2.5%); nausea (2.3%).
MUSCULOSKELETAL SYSTEM
Myalgia (1.9%); arm pain (1.3%); back pain (1.1%); stiffness (1.0%).
NERVOUS SYSTEM/PSYCHIATRIC
Headache (16.0%).
RESPIRATORY SYSTEM
Pharyngitis (2.7%); upper respiratory infection (2.7%); nasal congestion (1.1%).
UROGENITAL SYSTEM
Menstruation disorder (1.1%).
Allergic Reactions
Local and/or systemic allergic reactions that occurred in <1% of children/adolescents or adults in clinical trials regardless of causality included:
LOCAL
Injection site pruritus and/or rash.
SYSTEMIC
Bronchial constriction; asthma; wheezing; edema/swelling; rash; generalized erythema; urticaria; pruritus; eye irritation/itching; dermatitis. (See CONTRAINDICATIONS and WARNINGS.)
As with any vaccine, there is the possibility that use of VAQTA in very large populations might reveal adverse experiences not observed in clinical trials.
Marketed Experience
The following additional adverse reactions have been reported with use of the marketed vaccine.
NERVOUS SYSTEM
Very rarely, Guillain-Barré syndrome, cerebellar ataxia.
HEMIC and LYMPHATIC SYSTEM
Very rarely, thrombocytopenia.
Post-marketing Safety Study
In a post-marketing safety study, a total of 42,110 people ≥2 years of age received 1 or 2 doses of VAQTA. There was no serious, vaccine-related, adverse event identified among the 42,110 vaccine recipients in this study. There was no vaccine-related, adverse event identified that had not been reported in earlier clinical trials with VAQTA. Diarrhea/gastroenteritis, resulting in outpatient visits (in adults), was determined by the investigator to be the only vaccine-related nonserious adverse event in the study. VAQTA was generally well tolerated in this study. (See CLINICAL PHARMACOLOGY, *Post-marketing Safety Study.*)

DOSAGE AND ADMINISTRATION

Do not inject intravenously, intradermally, or subcutaneously.
VAQTA is for intramuscular injection. The *deltoid muscle* is the preferred site for intramuscular injection.
DOSAGE
The vaccination regimen consists of one primary dose and one booster dose for healthy children, adolescents, and adults, as follows:
Pediatric/Adolescent
Individuals 2 through 18 years of age should receive a single 0.5 mL (~25U) dose of vaccine at elected date and a booster dose of 0.5 mL (~25U) 6 to 18 months later.
A 1.0 mL (~50U) dose also was evaluated in individuals 18 years of age and was found to be immunogenic and generally well tolerated. (See CLINICAL PHARMACOLOGY, *Immunology*.)
Adult
Adults 19 years of age and older should receive a single 1.0 mL (~50U) dose of vaccine at elected date and a booster dose of 1.0 mL (~50U) 6 to 18 months later.
For all age groups, a booster dose is recommended anytime between 6 and 18 months after the administration of the primary dose in order to elicit a high antibody titer.

Table 5
Local and Systemic Complaints (≥1%) in Healthy Children and Adolescents from The Monroe Efficacy Study

Reaction	VAQTA Dose 1*	VAQTA Booster	Placebo*†
Injection-Site Complaints			
Pain	6.4% (33/515)	3.4% (16/475)	6.3% (32/510)
Tenderness	4.9% (25/515)	1.7% (8/475)	6.1% (31/510)
Erythema	1.9% (10/515)	0.8% (4/475)	1.8% (9/510)
Swelling	1.7% (9/515)	1.5% (7/475)	1.6% (8/510)
Warmth	1.7% (9/515)	0.6% (3/475)	1.6% (8/510)
Systemic Complaints			
Abdominal Pain	1.2% (6/519)	1.1% (5/475)	1.0% (5/518)
Pharyngitis	1.2% (6/519)	0% (0/475)	0.8% (4/518)
Headache	0.4% (2/519)	0.8% (4/475)	1.0% (5/518)

*No statistically significant differences between the two groups.
† Second injection of placebo not administered because code for the trial was broken.

Interchangeability of the Booster Dose
A booster dose of VAQTA may be given at 6 to 12 months following the initial dose of other inactivated hepatitis A vaccines (e.g., HAVRIX). (See CLINICAL PHARMACOLOGY, *Interchangeability of Booster Dose.*)
Use With Other Vaccines
VAQTA may be given concomitantly with typhoid and yellow fever vaccines. The GMTs for hepatitis A when VAQTA, typhoid and yellow fever vaccines were administered concomitantly were reduced when compared to VAQTA alone. Following receipt of the booster dose of VAQTA, the GMTs for hepatitis A in these two groups were observed to be comparable. Data on concomitatnt use with other vaccines are limited. Separate injection sites and syringes should be used for concomitant administration of injectable vaccines. (See CLINICAL PHARMACOLOGY, *Use With Other Vaccines* and INDICATIONS AND USAGE, *Use With Other Vaccines.*)
Use With Immune Globulin
VAQTA may be administered concomitantly with IG using separate sites and syringes. The vaccination regimen for VAQTA should be followed as stated above. Consult the manufacturer's product circular for the appropriate dosage of IG. A booster dose of VAQTA should be administered at the appropriate time as outlined above.
ADMINISTRATION
Known or Presumed Exposure to HAV/Travel to Endemic Areas
For individuals requiring either post-exposure prophylaxis or combined immediate and longer term protection (e.g., travelers departing on short notice to endemic areas), VAQTA may be administered concomitantly with IG using separate sites and syringes (see CLINICAL PHARMACOLOGY and DOSAGE AND ADMINISTRATION, *Use With Immune Globulin*).
Injection must be accomplished with a needle long enough to ensure intramuscular deposition of the vaccine. The Advisory Committee on Immunization Practices (ACIP) has recommended that "For all intramuscular injections, the needle should be long enough to reach the muscle mass and prevent vaccine from seeping into subcutaneous tissue, but not so long as to endanger underlying neurovascular structure or bone." For toddlers and older children they further state that "...the deltoid may be used if the muscle mass is adequate. The needle size can range from 22 to 25 gauge and from 5/8 to 1¼ inches, based on the size of the muscle...the anterolateral thigh may be used, but the needle should be longer—generally ranging from 7/8 to 1¼ inches". For adults they state that "...the deltoid is recommended for routine intramuscular vaccination among adults... The suggested needle size is 1 to 1½ inches and from 20 to 25 gauge."
For individuals with bleeding disorders who are at risk of hemorrhage following intramuscular injection, the ACIP recommends that when any intramuscular vaccine is indicated for such patients, "...it should be administered intramuscularly if, in the opinion of a physician familiar with the patient's bleeding risk, the vaccine can be administered with reasonable safety by this route. If the patient receives antihemophilia or other similar therapy, intramuscular vaccination can be scheduled shortly after such therapy is administered. A fine needle (≤23 gauge) can be used for the vaccination and firm pressure applied to the site (without rubbing) for at least two minutes. The patient or family should be instructed concerning the risk of hematoma from the injection."
The vaccine should be used as supplied; no reconstitution is necessary.
Shake well before withdrawal and use. Thorough agitation is necessary to maintain suspension of the vaccine. Discard if the suspension does not appear homogenous.
Parenteral drug products should be inspected visually for extraneous particulate matter and discoloration prior to administration whenever solution and container permit. After thorough agitation, VAQTA is a slightly opaque, white suspension.
It is important to use a separate sterile syringe and needle for each individual to prevent transmission of infectious agents from one person to another.

HOW SUPPLIED

PEDIATRIC/ADOLESCENT FORMULATION
Vials
No. 4831—VAQTA for pediatric/adolescent use is supplied as 25U/0.5 mL of hepatitis A virus protein in a 0.5 mL single-dose vial, **NDC** 0006-4831-00.
No. 4831—VAQTA for pediatric/adolescent use is supplied as 25U/0.5 mL of hepatitis A virus protein in a 0.5 mL single-dose vial, in a box of 5 single-dose vials, **NDC** 0006-4831-38.
No. 4831—VAQTA for pediatric/adolescent use is supplied as 25U/0.5 mL of hepatitis A virus protein in a 0.5 mL single-dose vial, in a box of 10 single-dose vials, **NDC** 0006-4831-41.
Syringes
No. 4845—VAQTA for pediatric/adolescent use is supplied as 25U/0.5 mL of hepatitis A virus protein in a 0.5 mL single-dose prefilled syringe, with a 5/8 needle, **NDC** 0006-4845-00.
No. 4845—VAQTA for pediatric/adolescent use is supplied as 25U/0.5 mL of hepatitis A virus protein in a 0.5 mL single-dose prefilled syringe, with a 5/8 inch needle, in a box of 5 single-dose prefilled syringes, with 5/8 inch needles, **NDC** 0006-4845-38.
ADULT FORMULATION
Vials
No. 4841—VAQTA for adult use is supplied as 50U/1 mL of hepatitis A virus protein in a 1 mL single-dose vial, **NDC** 0006-4841-00.
No. 4841—VAQTA for adult use is supplied as 50U/1 mL of hepatitis A virus protein in a 1 mL single-dose vial, in a box of 5 single-dose vials, **NDC** 0006-4841-38.
No. 4841—VAQTA for adult use is supplied as 50U/1 mL of hepatitis A virus protein in a 1 mL single-dose vial, in a box of 10 single-dose vials, **NDC** 0006-4841-41.
Syringes
No. 4844—VAQTA for adult use is supplied as 50U/1 mL of hepatitis A virus protein in a 1 mL single-dose prefilled syringe, with a one inch needle, **NDC** 0006-4844-00.
No. 4844—VAQTA for adult use is supplied as 50U/1 mL of hepatitis A virus protein in a 1 mL single-dose prefilled syringe, with a one inch needle, in a box of 5 single-dose, prefilled syringes, with one inch needles, **NDC** 0006-4844-38.
Storage
Store vaccine at 2-8°C (36-46°F).
DO NOT FREEZE since freezing destroys potency.
Manuf. and Dist. by:
MERCK & CO., INC., Whitehouse Station, NJ 08889, USA
Syringes of VAQTA are also filled by:
Evans Vaccines Ltd.
Gaskill Road, Speke, Liverpool L24 9GR, England
9413405 Issued January 2004

VARIVAX® ℞
[Varicella Virus Vaccine Live (Oka/Merck)]

DESCRIPTION

VARIVAX* [Varicella Virus Vaccine Live (Oka/Merck)] is a preparation of the Oka/Merck strain of live, attenuated var-

Continued on next page

Information on the Merck & Co., Inc., products listed on these pages is from the prescribing information in use October 1, 2004. For information, please call 1-800-NSC-MERCK [1-800-672-6372].

Varivax—Cont.

icella virus. The virus was initially obtained from a child with natural varicella, then introduced into human embryonic lung cell cultures, adapted to and propagated in embryonic guinea pig cell cultures and finally propagated in human diploid cell cultures (WI-38). Further passage of the virus for varicella vaccine was performed at Merck Research Laboratories (MRL) in human diploid cell cultures (MRC-5) that were free of adventitious agents. This live, attenuated varicella vaccine is a lyophilized preparation containing sucrose, phosphate, glutamate, and processed gelatin as stabilizers.

VARIVAX, when reconstituted as directed, is a sterile preparation for subcutaneous administration. Each 0.5 mL dose contains the following: a minimum of 1350 PFU (plaque forming units) of Oka/Merck varicella virus when reconstituted and stored at room temperature for 30 minutes, approximately 25 mg of sucrose, 12.5 mg hydrolyzed gelatin, 3.2 mg sodium chloride, 0.5 mg monosodium L-glutamate, 0.45 mg of sodium phosphate dibasic, 0.08 mg of potassium phosphate monobasic, 0.08 mg of potassium chloride; residual components of MRC-5 cells including DNA and protein; and trace quantities of sodium phosphate monobasic, EDTA, neomycin, and fetal bovine serum. The product contains no preservative.

To maintain potency, the lyophilized vaccine must be kept frozen at an average temperature of −15°C (+5°F) or colder and must be used before the expiration date (see HOW SUPPLIED, *Stability* and *Storage*). Storage in any freezer (e.g., chest, frost-free) that reliably maintains an average temperature of −15°C (+5°F) or colder and has a separate sealed freezer door is acceptable.

*Registered trademark of MERCK & CO., Inc.

CLINICAL PHARMACOLOGY

Varicella is a highly communicable disease in children, adolescents, and adults caused by the varicella-zoster virus. The disease usually consists of 300 to 500 maculopapular and/or vesicular lesions accompanied by a fever (oral temperature ≥100°F) in up to 70% of individuals. Approximately 3.5 million cases of varicella occurred annually from 1980–1994 in the United States with the peak incidence occurring in children five to nine years of age. The incidence rate of chickenpox in the total population was 8.3–9.1% per year in children 1–9 years of age before licensure of VARIVAX. The attack rate of natural varicella following household exposure among healthy susceptible children was shown to be 87% in unvaccinated populations. Although it is generally a benign, self-limiting disease, varicella may be associated with serious complications (e.g., bacterial superinfection, pneumonia, encephalitis, Reye's Syndrome), and/or death.

Evaluation of Clinical Efficacy Afforded by VARIVAX

Clinical Data in Children

In combined clinical trials of VARIVAX at doses ranging from 1,000–17,000 PFU, the majority of subjects who received VARIVAX and were exposed to wild-type virus were either completely protected from chickenpox or developed a milder form (for clinical description see below) of the disease. The protective efficacy of VARIVAX was evaluated in three different ways: 1) by comparing chickenpox rates in vaccinees versus historical controls, 2) by assessment of protection from disease following household exposure, and 3) by a placebo-controlled, double-blind clinical trial.

In early clinical trials, a total of 4240 children 1 to 12 years of age received 1000–1625 PFU of attenuated virus per dose of VARIVAX and have been followed for up to nine years post single-dose vaccination. In this group there was considerable variation in chickenpox rates among studies and study sites, and much of the reported data was acquired by passive follow-up. It was observed that 0.3%–3.8% of vaccinees per year reported chickenpox (called breakthrough cases). This represents an approximate 83% (95% confidence interval [CI], 82%, 84%) decrease from the age-adjusted expected incidence rates in susceptible subjects over this same period. In those who developed breakthrough chickenpox postvaccination, the majority experienced mild disease (median of the maximum number of lesions <50). In one study, a total of 47% (27/58) of breakthrough cases had <50 lesions compared with 8% (7/92) in unvaccinated individuals, and 7% (4/58) of breakthrough cases had >300 lesions compared with 50% (46/92) in unvaccinated individuals.

Among a subset of vaccinees who were actively followed in these early trials for up to nine years postvaccination, 179 individuals had household exposure to chickenpox. There were no reports of breakthrough chickenpox in 84% (150/179) of exposed children, while 16% (29/179) reported a mild form of chickenpox (38% [11/29] of the cases with a maximum total number of <50 lesions; no individuals with >300 lesions). This represents an 81% reduction in the expected number of varicella cases utilizing the historical attack rate of 87% following household exposure to chickenpox in unvaccinated individuals in the calculation of efficacy.

In later clinical trials with the current vaccine, a total of 1164 children 1 to 12 years of age received 2900–9000 PFU of attenuated virus per dose of VARIVAX and have been actively followed for up to six years post single-dose vaccination. It was observed that 0.2%–2.4% of vaccinees per year reported breakthrough chickenpox for up to six years post single-dose vaccination. This represents an approximate 93% (95% CI, 92%, 95%) decrease from the age-adjusted expected incidence rates in susceptible subjects over the same period. In those who developed breakthrough chickenpox postvaccination, the majority experienced mild disease with the median of the maximum total number of lesions <50. The severity of reported breakthrough chickenpox, as measured by number of lesions and maximum temperature, appeared not to increase with time since vaccination.

Among a subset of vaccinees who were actively followed in these later trials for up to five years postvaccination, 64 individuals were exposed to an unvaccinated individual with wild-type chickenpox in a household setting. There were no reports of breakthrough chickenpox in 91% (58/64) of exposed children, while 9% (6/64) reported a mild form of chickenpox (maximum total number of lesions <50, ranging from 6 to 40 lesions). This represents an 89% reduction in the expected number of varicella cases utilizing the historical attack rate of 87% following household exposure to chickenpox in unvaccinated individuals in the calculation of efficacy.

Although no placebo-controlled trial was carried out with VARIVAX using the current vaccine, a placebo-controlled trial was conducted using a formulation containing 17,000 PFU per dose. In this trial, a single dose of VARIVAX protected 96–100% of children against chickenpox over a two-year period. The study enrolled healthy individuals 1 to 14 years of age (n=491 vaccine, n=465 placebo). In the first year, 8.5% of placebo recipients contracted chickenpox, while no vaccine recipient did, for a calculated protection rate of 100% during the first varicella season. In the second year, when only a subset of individuals agreed to remain in the blinded study (n=163 vaccine, n=161 placebo), 96% protective efficacy was calculated for the vaccine group as compared to placebo.

There are insufficient data to assess the rate of protection against the complications of chickenpox (e.g., encephalitis, hepatitis, pneumonia) in children.

Clinical Data in Adolescents and Adults

In early clinical trials, a total of 796 adolescents and adults received 905–1230 PFU of attenuated virus per dose of VARIVAX and have been followed for up to six years following 2-dose vaccination. A total of 50 clinical varicella cases were reported >42 days following 2-dose vaccination. Based on passive follow-up, the annual chickenpox breakthrough event rate ranged from <0.1% to 1.9%. The median of the maximum total number of lesions ranged from 15 to 42 per year.

Although no placebo-controlled trial was carried out in adolescents and adults, the protective efficacy of VARIVAX was determined by evaluation of protection when vaccinees received 2 doses of VARIVAX 4 or 8 weeks apart and were subsequently exposed to chickenpox in a household setting. Among the subset of vaccinees who were actively followed in these early trials for up to six years, 76 individuals had household exposure to chickenpox. There were no reports of breakthrough chickenpox in 83% (63/76) of exposed vaccinees, while 17% (13/76) reported a mild form of chickenpox. Among 13 vaccinated individuals who developed breakthrough chickenpox after a household exposure, 62% (8/13) of the cases reported maximum total number of lesions <50, while no individual reported >75 lesions. The attack rate of unvaccinated adults exposed to a single contact in a household has not been previously studied. Utilizing the previously reported historical attack rate of 87% for natural varicella following household exposure to chickenpox among unvaccinated children in the calculation of efficacy, this represents an approximate 80% reduction in the expected number of cases in the household setting.

In later clinical trials, a total of 220 adolescents and adults received 3315–9000 PFU of attenuated virus per dose of VARIVAX and have been actively followed for up to six years following 2-dose vaccination. A total of 3 clinical varicella cases were reported >42 days following 2-dose vaccination. Two cases reported <50 lesions and none reported >75. The annual chickenpox breakthrough event rate ranged from 0% to 1.2%. Among the subset of vaccinees who were actively followed in these later trials for up to five years, 16 individuals were exposed to an unvaccinated individual with wild-type chickenpox in a household setting. There were no reports of breakthrough chickenpox among the exposed vaccinees.

There are insufficient data to assess the rate of protection of VARIVAX against the serious complications of chickenpox in adults (e.g., encephalitis, hepatitis, pneumonitis) and during pregnancy (congenital varicella syndrome).

Immunogenicity of VARIVAX

Clinical trials with several formulations of the vaccine containing attenuated virus ranging from 1000 to 17,000 PFU per dose have demonstrated that VARIVAX induces detectable immune responses in a high proportion of individuals and is generally well tolerated in healthy individuals ranging from 12 months to 55 years of age.

Seroconversion as defined by the acquisition of any detectable varicella antibodies (gpELISA >0.3, a highly sensitive assay which is not commercially available) was observed in 97% of vaccinees at approximately 4–6 weeks postvaccination in 6889 susceptible children 12 months to 12 years of age. Rates of breakthrough disease were significantly lower among children with varicella antibody titers ≥5 compared to children with titers <5. Titers ≥5 were induced in approximately 76% of children vaccinated with a single dose of vaccine at 1000–17,000 PFU per dose. In a multicenter study involving susceptible adolescents and adults 13 years of age and older, two doses of VARIVAX administered four to eight weeks apart induced a seroconversion rate (gpELISA >0.3) of approximately 75% in 539 individuals four weeks after the first dose and of 99% in 479 individuals four weeks after the second dose. The average antibody response in vaccinees who received the second dose eight weeks after the first dose was higher than that in those, who received the second dose four weeks after the first dose. In another multicenter study involving adolescents and adults, two doses of VARIVAX administered eight weeks apart induced a seroconversion rate (gpELISA >0.3) of 94% in 142 individuals six weeks after the first dose and 99% in 122 individuals six weeks after the second dose.

VARIVAX also induces cell-mediated immune responses in vaccinees. The relative contributions of humoral immunity and cell-mediated immunity to protection from chickenpox are unknown.

Persistence of Immune Response

In clinical studies involving healthy children who received 1 dose of vaccine, detectable varicella antibodies (gpELISA >0.6 units) were present in 99.0% (3886/3926) at 1 year, 99.3% (1555/1566) at 2 years, 98.6% (1106/1122) at 3 years, and 99.4% (1168/1175) at 4 years, 99.2% (737/743) at 5 years, 100% (142/142) at 6 years, 97.4% (38/39) at 7 years, 100% (34/34) at 8 years, and 100% (16/16) at 10 years postvaccination.

In clinical studies involving healthy adolescents and adults who received 2 doses of vaccine, detectable varicella antibodies (gpELISA >0.6 units) were present in 97.9% (568/580) at 1 year, 97.1% (34/35) at 2 years, 100% (144/144) at 3 years, 97.0% (98/101) at 4 years, 97.4% (76/78) at 5 years, and 100% (34/34) at 6 years postvaccination.

A boost in antibody levels has been observed in vaccinees following exposure to natural varicella which could account for the apparent long-term persistence of antibody levels after vaccination in these studies. The duration of protection from varicella obtained using VARIVAX in the absence of wild-type boosting is unknown. VARIVAX also induces cell-mediated immune responses in vaccinees. The relative contributions of humoral immunity and cell-mediated immunity to protection from chickenpox are unknown.

Transmission

In the placebo-controlled trial, transmission of vaccine virus was assessed in household settings (during the 8-week post-vaccination period) in 416 susceptible placebo recipients who were household contacts of 445 vaccine recipients. Of the 416 placebo recipients, three developed chickenpox and seroconverted, nine reported a varicella-like rash and did not seroconvert, and six had no rash but seroconverted. If vaccine virus transmission occurred, it did so at a very low rate and possibly without recognizable clinical disease in contacts. These cases may represent either natural varicella from community contacts or a low incidence of transmission of vaccine virus from vaccinated contacts (see PRECAUTIONS, *Transmission*). Postmarketing experience suggests that transmission of vaccine virus may occur rarely between healthy vaccinees who develop a varicella-like rash and healthy susceptible contacts. Transmission of vaccine virus from vaccinees without a varicella-like rash has been reported but has not been confirmed.

Herpes Zoster

Overall, 9454 healthy children (12 months to 12 years of age) and 1648 adolescents and adults (13 years of age and older) have been vaccinated with Oka/Merck live attenuated varicella vaccine in clinical trials. Eight cases of herpes zoster have been reported in children during 42,556 person years of follow-up in clinical trials, resulting in a calculated incidence of at least 18.8 cases per 100,000 person years. The completeness of this reporting has not been determined. One case of herpes zoster has been reported in the adolescent and adult age group during 5410 person years of follow-up in clinical trials resulting in a calculated incidence of 18.5 cases per 100,000 person years.

All nine cases were mild and without sequelae. Two cultures (one child and one adult) obtained from vesicles were positive for wild-type varicella zoster virus as confirmed by restriction endonuclease analysis. The long-term effect of VARIVAX on the incidence of herpes zoster, particularly in those vaccinees exposed to natural varicella, is unknown at present.

In children, the reported rate of zoster in vaccine recipients appears not to exceed that previously determined in a population-based study of healthy children who had experienced natural varicella. The incidence of zoster in adults who have had natural varicella infection is higher than that in children.

Reye's Syndrome

Reye's Syndrome has occurred in children and adolescents following natural varicella infection, the majority of whom had received salicylates. In clinical studies in healthy children and adolescents in the United States, physicians advised varicella vaccine recipients not to use salicylates for six weeks after vaccination. There were no reports of Reye's Syndrome in varicella vaccine recipients during these studies.

Studies with Other Vaccines

In combined clinical studies involving 1080 children 12 to 36 months of age, 653 received VARIVAX and M-M-R* II (Measles, Mumps, and Rubella Virus Vaccine Live) concomitantly at separate sites and 427 received the vaccines six weeks apart. Seroconversion rates and antibody levels were comparable between the two groups at approximately six weeks post-vaccination to each of the virus vaccine components. No differences were noted in adverse reactions reported in those who received VARIVAX concomitantly with M-M-R II at separate sites and those who received VARIVAX and M-M-R II at different times (see PRECAUTIONS, *Drug Interactions, Use with Other Vaccines*).

In a clinical study involving 318 children 12 months to 42 months of age, 160 received an investigational vaccine (a formulation combining measles, mumps, rubella, and varicella in one syringe) concomitantly with booster doses of DTaP (diphtheria, tetanus, acellular pertussis) and OPV (oral poliovirus vaccine) while 144 received M-M-R II concomitantly with booster doses of DTaP and OPV followed by VARIVAX 6 weeks later. At six weeks postvaccination, seroconversion rates for measles, mumps, rubella, and varicella and the percentage of vaccinees whose titers were boosted for diphtheria, tetanus, pertussis, and polio were comparable between the two groups, but anti-varicella levels were decreased when the investigational vaccine containing varicella was administered concomitantly with DTaP. No clinically significant differences were noted in adverse reactions between the two groups.

In another clinical study involving 307 children 12 to 18 months of age, 150 received an investigational vaccine (a formulation combining measles, mumps, rubella, and varicella in one syringe) concomitantly with a booster dose of PedvaxHIB* [Haemophilus b Conjugate Vaccine (Meningococcal Protein Conjugate)] while 130 received M-M-R II concomitantly with a booster dose of PedvaxHIB followed by VARIVAX 6 weeks later. At six weeks postvaccination, seroconversion rates for measles, mumps, rubella, and varicella, and geometric mean titers for PedvaxHIB were comparable between the two groups, but anti-varicella levels were decreased when the investigational vaccine containing varicella was administered concomitantly with PedvaxHIB. No clinically significant differences in adverse reactions were seen between the two groups.

In a clinical study involving 609 children 12 to 23 months of age, 305 received VARIVAX, M-M-R II, and TETRAMUNE** (*Haemophilus influenzae* type b, diphtheria, tetanus, and pertussis vaccines) concomitantly at separate sites, and 304 received M-M-R II and TETRAMUNE concomitantly at separate sites, followed by VARIVAX 6 weeks later. At six weeks postvaccination, seroconversion rates for measles, mumps, rubella and varicella were similar between the two groups. Postvaccination GMTs for all antigens were similar in both treatment groups except for varicella, which was lower when VARIVAX was administered concomitantly with M-M-R II and TETRAMUNE, but within the range of GMTs seen in previous clinical experience when VARIVAX was administered alone. At 1 year postvaccination, GMTs for measles, mumps, rubella, varicella and *Haemophilus influenzae* type b were similar between the two groups. All three vaccines were well tolerated regardless of whether they were administered concomitantly at separate sites or 6 weeks apart. There were no clinically important differences in reaction rates when the three vaccines were administered concomitantly versus 6 weeks apart.

In a clinical study involving 822 children 12 to 15 months of age, 410 received COMVAX* [Haemophilus b Conjugate (Meningococcal Protein Conjugate) and Hepatitis B (Recombinant) vaccine], M-M-R II, and VARIVAX concomitantly at separate sites, and 412 received COMVAX followed by M-M-R II and VARIVAX given concomitantly at separate sites, 6 weeks later. At six weeks postvaccination, the immune responses for the subjects who received the concomitant injections of COMVAX, M-M-R II, and VARIVAX were similar to those of the subjects who received COMVAX followed 6 weeks later by M-M-R II and VARIVAX with respect to all antigens administered. All three vaccines were generally well tolerated regardless of whether they were administered concomitantly at separate sites or 6 weeks apart. There were no clinically important differences in reaction rates when the three vaccines were administered concomitantly versus 6 weeks apart.

VARIVAX is recommended for subcutaneous administration. However, during clinical trials, some children received VARIVAX intramuscularly resulting in seroconversion rates similar to those in children who received the vaccine by the subcutaneous route. Persistence of antibody and efficacy in those receiving intramuscular injections have not been defined.

*Registered trademark of MERCK & Co., Inc.
**Registered trademark of Lederle Laboratories

INDICATIONS AND USAGE

VARIVAX is indicated for vaccination against varicella in individuals 12 months of age and older.

Revaccination

The duration of protection of VARIVAX is unknown at present and the need for booster doses is not defined. However, a boost in antibody levels has been observed in vaccinees following exposure to natural varicella as well as following a booster dose of VARIVAX administered four to six years postvaccination.

In a highly vaccinated population, immunity for some individuals may wane due to lack of exposure to natural varicella as a result of shifting epidemiology. Post-marketing surveillance studies are ongoing to evaluate the need and timing for booster vaccination.

Vaccination with VARIVAX may not result in protection of all healthy, susceptible children, adolescents, and adults (see CLINICAL PHARMACOLOGY).

Table 1
Fever, Local Reactions, or Rashes (%) in Children 0 to 42 Days Postvaccination

Reaction	N	Post Dose 1	Peak Occurrence in Postvaccination Days
Fever ≥102°F (39°C) Oral	8827	14.7%	0-42
Injection-site complaints (pain/soreness, swelling and/or erythema, rash, pruritus, hematoma, induration, stiffness)	8916	19.3%	0–2
Varicella-like rash (injection site)	8916	3.4%	8–19
Median number of lesions		2	
Varicella-like rash (generalized)	8916	3.8%	5–26
Median number of lesions		5	

CONTRAINDICATIONS

A history of hypersensitivity to any component of the vaccine, including gelatin.

A history of anaphylactoid reaction to neomycin (each dose of reconstituted vaccine contains trace quantities of neomycin).

Individuals with blood dyscrasias, leukemia, lymphomas of any type, or other malignant neoplasms affecting the bone marrow or lymphatic systems.

Individuals receiving immunosuppressive therapy. Individuals who are on immunosuppressant drugs are more susceptible to infections than healthy individuals. Vaccination with live attenuated varicella vaccine can result in a more extensive vaccine-associated rash or disseminated disease in individuals on immunosuppressant doses of corticosteroids.

Individuals with primary and acquired immunodeficiency states, including those who are immunosuppressed in association with AIDS or other clinical manifestations of infection with human immunodeficiency virus; cellular immune deficiencies; and hypogammaglobulinemic and dysgammaglobulinemic states.

A family history of congenital or hereditary immunodeficiency, unless the immune competence of the potential vaccine recipient is demonstrated.

Active untreated tuberculosis.

Any febrile respiratory illness or other active febrile infection.

Pregnancy; the possible effects of the vaccine on fetal development are unknown at this time. However, natural varicella is known to sometimes cause fetal harm. If vaccination of postpubertal females is undertaken, pregnancy should be avoided for three months following vaccination. (See PRECAUTIONS, *Pregnancy*).

PRECAUTIONS

General

Adequate treatment provisions, including epinephrine injection (1:1000), should be available for immediate use should an anaphylactoid reaction occur.

The duration of protection from varicella infection after vaccination with VARIVAX is unknown.

It is not known whether VARIVAX given immediately after exposure to natural varicella virus will prevent illness.

Vaccination should be deferred for at least 5 months following blood or plasma transfusions, or administration of immune globulin or varicella zoster immune globulin (VZIG).

Following administration of VARIVAX, any immune globulin including VZIG should not be given for 2 months thereafter unless its use outweighs the benefits of vaccination.

Vaccine recipients should avoid use of salicylates for 6 weeks after vaccination with VARIVAX as Reye's Syndrome has been reported following the use of salicylates during natural varicella infection (see CLINICAL PHARMACOLOGY, *Reye's Syndrome*).

The safety and efficacy of VARIVAX have not been established in children and young adults who are known to be infected with human immunodeficiency viruses with and without evidence of immunosuppression (see also CONTRAINDICATIONS).

Care is to be taken by the health care provider for safe and effective use of VARIVAX.

The health care provider should question the patient, parent, or guardian about reactions to a previous dose of VARIVAX or a similar product.

The health care provider should obtain the previous immunization history of the vaccinee.

VARIVAX should not be injected into a blood vessel.

Vaccination should be deferred in patients with a family history of congenital or hereditary immunodeficiency until the patient's own immune system has been evaluated.

A separate sterile needle and syringe should be used for administration of each dose of VARIVAX to prevent transfer of infectious diseases.

Needles should be disposed of properly and should not be recapped.

Transmission

Post-marketing experience suggests that transmission of vaccine virus may occur rarely between healthy vaccinees who develop a varicella-like rash and healthy susceptible contacts. Transmission of vaccine virus from vaccinees without a varicella-like rash has been reported but has not been confirmed.

Therefore, vaccine recipients should attempt to avoid, whenever possible, close association with susceptible high-risk individuals for up to six weeks. In circumstances where contact with high-risk individuals is unavoidable, the potential risk of transmission of vaccine virus should be weighed against the risk of acquiring and transmitting natural varicella virus. Susceptible high-risk individuals include:

- immunocompromised individuals
- pregnant women without documented history of chickenpox or laboratory evidence of prior infection
- newborn infants of mothers without documented history of chickenpox or laboratory evidence of prior infection

Information for Patients

The health care provider should inform the patient, parent or guardian of the benefits and risks of VARIVAX.

Patients, parents, or guardians should be instructed to report any adverse reactions to the health care provider.

The U.S. Department of Health and Human Services has established a Vaccine Adverse Event Reporting System (VAERS) to accept all reports of suspected adverse events after the administration of any vaccine, including but not limited to the reporting of events required by the National Childhood Vaccine Injury Act of 1986. The VAERS toll-free number for VAERS forms and information is 1-800-822-7967.

Pregnancy should be avoided for three months following vaccination.

Drug Interactions

See PRECAUTIONS, *General,* regarding the administration of immune globulins, salicylates, and transfusions.

Drug Interactions, Use with Other Vaccines

Results from clinical studies indicate that VARIVAX can be administered concomitantly with M-M-R II, COMVAX, or TETRAMUNE (see CLINICAL PHARMACOLOGY, *Studies with Other Vaccines*).

Limited data from an experimental product containing varicella vaccine suggest that VARIVAX can be administered concomitantly with DTaP and PedvaxHIB using separate sites and syringes (see CLINICAL PHARMACOLOGY, *Studies with Other Vaccines*). However, there are no data relating to simultaneous administration of VARIVAX with DTP or OPV.

Carcinogenesis, Mutagenesis, Impairment of Fertility

VARIVAX has not been evaluated for its carcinogenic or mutagenic potential, or its potential to impair fertility.

Pregnancy

Pregnancy Category C: Animal reproduction studies have not been conducted with VARIVAX. It is also not known whether VARIVAX can cause fetal harm when administered to a pregnant woman or can affect reproduction capacity. Therefore, VARIVAX should not be administered to pregnant females; furthermore, pregnancy should be avoided for three months following vaccination (see CONTRAINDICATIONS).

Merck & Co., Inc. maintains a Pregnancy Registry to monitor fetal outcomes of pregnant women exposed to VARIVAX. Patients and healthcare providers are encouraged to report any exposure to VARIVAX during pregnancy by calling (800) 986-8999.

Nursing Mothers

It is not known whether varicella vaccine virus is secreted in human milk. Therefore, because some viruses are secreted in human milk, caution should be exercised if VARIVAX is administered to a nursing woman.

Geriatric Use

Clinical studies of VARIVAX did not include sufficient numbers of seronegative subjects aged 65 and over to determine whether they respond differently from younger subjects. Other reported clinical experience has not identified differences in responses between the elderly and younger subjects.

Pediatric Use

No clinical data are available on safety or efficacy of VARIVAX in children less than one year of age, and administration to infants under twelve months of age is not recommended.

Continued on next page

Information on the Merck & Co., Inc., products listed on these pages is from the prescribing information in use October 1, 2004. For information, please call 1-800-NSC-MERCK [1-800-672-6372].

Varivax—Cont.

ADVERSE REACTIONS

In clinical trials, VARIVAX was administered to 11,102 healthy children, adolescents, and adults. VARIVAX was generally well tolerated.

In a double-blind placebo controlled study among 914 healthy children and adolescents who were serologically confirmed to be susceptible to varicella, the only adverse reactions that occurred at a significantly ($p<0.05$) greater rate in vaccine recipients than in placebo recipients were pain and redness at the injection site.

Children 1 to 12 Years of Age

In clinical trials involving healthy children monitored for up to 42 days after a single dose of VARIVAX, the frequency of fever, injection-site complaints, or rashes were reported as follows:

[See table 1 at top of previous page]

In addition, the most frequently (≥1%) reported adverse experiences, without regard to causality, are listed in decreasing order of frequency: upper respiratory illness, cough, irritability/nervousness, fatigue, disturbed sleep, diarrhea, loss of appetite, vomiting, otitis, diaper rash/contact rash, headache, teething, malaise, abdominal pain, other rash, nausea, eye complaints, chills, lymphadenopathy, myalgia, lower respiratory illness, allergic reactions (including allergic rash, hives), stiff neck, heat rash/prickly heat, arthralgia, eczema/dry skin/dermatitis, constipation, itching.

Pneumonitis has been reported rarely (<1%) in children vaccinated with VARIVAX; a causal relationship has not been established.

Febrile seizures have occurred rarely (<0.1%) in children vaccinated with VARIVAX; a causal relationship has not been established.

Adolescents and Adults 13 Years of Age and Older

In clinical trials involving healthy adolescents and adults, the majority of whom received two doses of VARIVAX and were monitored for up to 42 days after any dose, the frequency of fever, injection-site complaints, or rashes were reported as follows:

[See table 2 below]

In addition, the most frequently (≥1%) reported adverse experiences, without regard to causality, are listed in decreasing order of frequency: upper respiratory illness, headache, fatigue, cough, myalgia, disturbed sleep, nausea, malaise, diarrhea, stiff neck, irritability/nervousness, lymphadenopathy, chills, eye complaints, abdominal pain, loss of appetite, arthralgia, otitis, itching, vomiting, other rashes, constipation, lower respiratory illness, allergic reactions (including allergic rash, hives), contact rash, cold/canker sore.

As with any vaccine, there is the possibility that broad use of the vaccine could reveal adverse reactions not observed in clinical trials.

The following additional adverse reactions have been reported since the vaccine has been marketed:

Body as a Whole

Anaphylaxis in individuals with or without an allergic history.

Hemic and Lymphatic System

Thrombocytopenia.

Nervous/Psychiatric

Encephalitis; cerebrovascular accident; transverse myelitis; Guillain-Barré syndrome; Bell's palsy; ataxia; non-febrile seizures; dizziness; paresthesia.

Respiratory

Pharyngitis; Pneumonia/Pneumonitis.

Skin

Stevens-Johnson syndrome; erythema multiforme; Henoch-Schönlein purpura; secondary bacterial infections of skin and soft tissue, including impetigo and cellulitis; herpes zoster.

DOSAGE AND ADMINISTRATION

FOR SUBCUTANEOUS ADMINISTRATION

Do not inject intravenously

Children 12 months to 12 years of age should receive a single 0.5 mL dose administered subcutaneously.

Adolescents and adults 13 years of age and older should receive a 0.5 mL dose administered subcutaneously at elected date and a second 0.5 mL dose 4 to 8 weeks later.

VARIVAX is for subcutaneous administration. The outer aspect of the upper arm (deltoid) is the preferred site of injection.

VARIVAX **SHOULD BE STORED FROZEN** at an average temperature of −15°C (+5°F) or colder until it is reconstituted for injection (see HOW SUPPLIED, *Storage*). Any freezer (e.g. chest, frost-free) that reliably maintains an average temperature of −15°C and has a separate sealed freezer door is acceptable for storing VARIVAX. The diluent should be stored separately at room temperature or in the refrigerator. To reconstitute the vaccine, first withdraw 0.7 mL of diluent into the syringe to be used for reconstitution. Inject all the diluent in the syringe into the vial of lyophilized vaccine and gently agitate to mix thoroughly. Withdraw the entire contents into a syringe and inject the total volume (about 0.5 mL) of reconstituted vaccine subcutaneously, preferably into the outer aspect of the upper arm (deltoid) or the anterolateral thigh. **IT IS RECOMMENDED THAT THE VACCINE BE ADMINISTERED IMMEDIATELY AFTER RECONSTITUTION, TO MINIMIZE LOSS OF POTENCY. DISCARD IF RECONSTITUTED VACCINE IS NOT USED WITHIN 30 MINUTES.**

CAUTION: A sterile syringe free of preservatives, antiseptics, and detergents should be used for each injection and/or reconstitution of VARIVAX because these substances may inactivate the vaccine virus.

It is important to use a separate sterile syringe and needle for each patient to prevent transmission of infectious agents from one individual to another.

To reconstitute the vaccine, use only the Merck sterile diluent supplied with VARIVAX, M-M-R II, or the component vaccines of M-M-R II, since it is free of preservatives or other anti-viral substances which might inactivate the vaccine virus.

Do not freeze reconstituted vaccine.

Do not give immune globulin including Varicella Zoster Immune Globulin concurrently with VARIVAX (see also PRECAUTIONS).

Parenteral drug products should be inspected visually for particulate matter and discoloration prior to administration, whenever solution and container permit. VARIVAX when reconstituted is a clear, colorless to pale yellow liquid.

HOW SUPPLIED

No. 4826/4309—VARIVAX is supplied as follows: (1) a single-dose vial of lyophilized vaccine, **NDC** 0006-4826-00 (package A); and (2) a box of 10 vials of diluent (package B).

No. 4827/4309—VARIVAX is supplied as follows: (1) a box of 10 single-dose vials of lyophilized vaccine (package A), **NDC** 0006-4827-00; and (2) a box of 10 vials of diluent (package B).

Stability

VARIVAX retains a potency level of 1500 PFU or higher per dose for at least 24 months in a frost-free freezer with an average temperature of −15°C (+5°F) or colder.

VARIVAX has a minimum potency level of approximately 1350 PFU 30 minutes after reconstitution at room temperature (20-25°C, 68-77°F).

Prior to reconstitution, VARIVAX retains potency when stored for up to 72 continuous hours at refrigerator temperature (2-8°C, 36-46°F).

For information regarding stability under conditions other than those recommended, call 1-800-9-VARIVAX.

Storage

During shipment, to ensure that there is no loss of potency, the vaccine must be maintained at a temperature of −20°C (−4°F) or colder.

Before reconstitution, store the lyophilized vaccine in a freezer at an average temperature of −15°C (+5°F) or colder. Any freezer (e.g. chest, frost-free) that reliably maintains an average temperature of −15°C and has a separate sealed freezer door is acceptable for storing VARIVAX.

VARIVAX may be stored at refrigerator temperature (2-8°C, 36-46°F) for up to 72 continuous hours prior to reconstitution. Vaccine stored at 2-8°C which is not used within 72 hours of removal from −15°C storage should be discarded.

Before reconstitution, protect from light.

The diluent should be stored separately at room temperature (20-25°C, 68-77°F), or in the refrigerator.

7999911 Issued December 2003

Table 2
Fever, Local Reactions, or Rashes (%) in Adolescents and Adults 0 to 42 Days Postvaccination

Reaction	N	Post Dose 1	Peak Occurrence in Postvaccination Days	N	Post Dose 2	Peak Occurrence in Postvaccination Days
Fever ≥100°F (37.7°C) Oral	1584	10.2%	14-27	956	9.5%	0-42
Injection-site complaints (soreness, erythema, swelling, rash, pruritus, pyrexia, hematoma, induration, numbness)	1606	24.4%	0–2	955	32.5%	0–2
Varicella-like rash (injection site)	1606	3%	6–20	955	1%	0–6
Median number of lesions		2			2	
Varicella-like rash (generalized)	1606	5.5%	7–21	955	0.9%	0–23
Median number of lesions		5			5.5	

VASERETIC* Tablets ℞

(enalapril maleate-hydrochlorothiazide)

Distributed by Biovail Pharmaceuticals, Inc.
Morrisville, NC 27560
To make additional inquiries or to report an adverse event, please contact Biovail Pharmaceuticals, Inc. at 1-866-276-1030.

*Registered trademark of Biovail Pharmaceuticals, Inc.

VASERETIC® Tablets ℞

(enalapril maleate-hydrochlorothiazide)

USE IN PREGNANCY

When used in pregnancy during the second and third trimesters, ACE inhibitors can cause injury and even death to the developing fetus. When pregnancy is detected, VASERETIC should be discontinued as soon as possible. See WARNINGS, *Pregnancy, Enalapril Maleate, Fetal/Neonatal Morbidity and Mortality.*

DESCRIPTION

VASERETIC* (Enalapril Maleate-Hydrochlorothiazide) combines an angiotensin converting enzyme inhibitor, enalapril maleate, and a diuretic, hydrochlorothiazide.

Enalapril maleate is the maleate salt of enalapril, the ethyl ester of a long-acting angiotensin converting enzyme inhibitor, enalaprilat. Enalapril maleate is chemically described as (*S*)-1-[*N*-[1-(ethoxycarbonyl)-3-phenylpropyl]-L-alanyl]-L-proline, (*Z*)-2-butenedioate salt (1:1). Its empirical formula is $C_{20}H_{28}N_2O_5 \cdot C_4H_4O_4$, and its structural formula is:

Enalapril maleate is a white to off-white crystalline powder with a molecular weight of 492.53. It is sparingly soluble in water, soluble in ethanol, and freely soluble in methanol.

Enalapril is a pro-drug; following oral administration, it is bioactivated by hydrolysis of the ethyl ester to enalaprilat, which is the active angiotensin converting enzyme inhibitor.

Hydrochlorothiazide is 6-chloro-3,4-dihydro-2*H*-1,2,4-benzothiadiazine-7-sulfonamide 1,1-dioxide. Its empirical formula is $C_7H_8ClN_3O_4S_2$ and its structural formula is:

It is a white, or practically white, crystalline powder with a molecular weight of 297.74, which is slightly soluble in water, but freely soluble in sodium hydroxide solution.

VASERETIC is available in two tablet combinations of enalapril maleate with hydrochlorothiazide: VASERETIC 5–12.5, containing 5 mg enalapril maleate and 12.5 mg hydrochlorothiazide and VASERETIC 10–25, containing 10 mg enalapril maleate and 25 mg hydrochlorothiazide. Inactive ingredients are: iron oxides, lactose, magnesium stearate, starch and other ingredients.

*Registered trademark of MERCK & CO., INC.

CLINICAL PHARMACOLOGY

As a result of its diuretic effects, hydrochlorothiazide increases plasma renin activity, increases aldosterone secretion, and decreases serum potassium. Administration of enalapril maleate blocks the renin-angiotensin-aldosterone axis and tends to reverse the potassium loss associated with the diuretic.

In clinical studies, the extent of blood pressure reduction seen with the combination of enalapril maleate and hydrochlorothiazide was approximately additive. The antihypertensive effect of VASERETIC was usually sustained for at least 24 hours.

Concomitant administration of enalapril maleate and hydrochlorothiazide has little, or no effect on the bioavailability of either drug. The combination tablet is bioequivalent to concomitant administration of the separate entities.

Enalapril Maleate

Mechanism of Action: Enalapril, after hydrolysis to enalaprilat, inhibits angiotensin-converting enzyme (ACE) in human subjects and animals. ACE is a peptidyl dipeptidase that catalyzes the conversion of angiotensin I to the vasoconstrictor substance, angiotensin II. Angiotensin II also stimulates aldosterone secretion by the adrenal cortex. Inhibition of ACE results in decreased plasma angiotensin II, which leads to decreased vasopressor activity and to decreased aldosterone secretion. Although the latter decrease is small, it results in small increases of serum potassium. In hypertensive patients treated with enalapril maleate alone for up to 48 weeks, mean increases in serum potassium of approximately 0.2 mEq/L were observed. In patients treated with enalapril maleate plus a thiazide diuretic, there was essentially no change in serum potassium. (See PRECAUTIONS.) Removal of angiotensin II negative feedback on renin secretion leads to increased plasma renin activity.

ACE is identical to kininase, an enzyme that degrades bradykinin. Whether increased levels of bradykinin, a potent vasodepressor peptide, play a role in the therapeutic effects of enalapril remains to be elucidated.

While the mechanism through which enalapril lowers blood pressure is believed to be primarily suppression of the renin-angiotensin-aldosterone system, enalapril is antihypertensive even in patients with low-renin hypertension. Although enalapril was antihypertensive in all races studied, black hypertensive patients (usually a low-renin hypertensive population) had a smaller average response to enalapril maleate monotherapy than non-black patients. In contrast, hydrochlorothiazide was more effective in black patients than enalapril. Concomitant administration of enalapril maleate and hydrochlorothiazide was equally effective in black and non-black patients.

Pharmacokinetics and Metabolism: Following oral administration of enalapril maleate, peak serum concentrations of enalapril occur within about one hour. Based on urinary recovery, the extent of absorption of enalapril is approximately 60 percent. Enalapril absorption is not influenced by the presence of food in the gastrointestinal tract. Following absorption, enalapril is hydrolyzed to enalaprilat, which is a more potent angiotensin converting enzyme inhibitor than enalapril; enalaprilat is poorly absorbed when administered orally. Peak serum concentrations of enalaprilat occur three to four hours after an oral dose of enalapril maleate. Excretion of enalaprilat and enalapril is primarily renal. Approximately 94 percent of the dose is recovered in the urine and feces as enalaprilat or enalapril. The principal components in urine are enalaprilat, accounting for about 40 percent of the dose, and intact enalapril. There is no evidence of metabolites of enalapril, other than enalaprilat.

The serum concentration profile of enalaprilat exhibits a prolonged terminal phase, apparently representing a small fraction of the administered dose that has been bound to ACE. The amount bound does not increase with dose, indicating a saturable site of binding. The effective half-life for accumulation of enalaprilat following multiple doses of enalapril maleate is 11 hours.

The disposition of enalapril and enalaprilat in patients with renal insufficiency is similar to that in patients with normal renal function until the glomerular filtration rate is 30 mL/min or less. With glomerular filtration rate ≤30 mL/min, peak and trough enalaprilat levels increase, time to peak concentration increases and time to steady state may be delayed. The effective half-life of enalaprilat following multiple doses of enalapril maleate is prolonged at this level of renal insufficiency. Enalaprilat is dialyzable at the rate of 62 mL/min.

Studies in dogs indicate that enalapril crosses the blood-brain barrier poorly, if at all; enalaprilat does not enter the brain. Multiple doses of enalapril maleate in rats do not result in accumulation in any tissues. Milk of lactating rats contains radioactivity following administration of ^{14}C enalapril maleate. Radioactivity was found to cross the placenta following administration of labeled drug to pregnant hamsters.

Pharmacodynamics: Administration of enalapril maleate to patients with hypertension of severity ranging from mild to severe results in a reduction of both supine and standing blood pressure usually with no orthostatic component. Symptomatic postural hypotension is infrequent with enalapril alone but it can be anticipated in volume-depleted patients, such as patients treated with diuretics. In clinical trials with enalapril and hydrochlorothiazide administered concurrently, syncope occurred in 1.3 percent of patients. (See WARNINGS and DOSAGE AND ADMINISTRATION.)

In most patients studied, after oral administration of a single dose of enalapril maleate, onset of antihypertensive activity was seen at one hour with peak reduction of blood pressure achieved by four to six hours.

At recommended doses, antihypertensive effects of enalapril maleate monotherapy have been maintained for at least 24 hours. In some patients the effects may diminish toward the end of the dosing interval; this was less frequently observed with concomitant administration of enalapril maleate and hydrochlorothiazide.

Achievement of optimal blood pressure reduction may require several weeks of enalapril therapy in some patients.

The antihypertensive effects of enalapril have continued during long term therapy. Abrupt withdrawal of enalapril has not been associated with a rapid increase in blood pressure.

In hemodynamic studies in patients with essential hypertension, blood pressure reduction produced by enalapril was accompanied by a reduction in peripheral arterial resistance with an increase in cardiac output and little or no change in heart rate. Following administration of enalapril maleate, there is an increase in renal blood flow; glomerular filtration rate is usually unchanged. The effects appear to be similar in patients with renovascular hypertension.

In a clinical pharmacology study, indomethacin or sulindac was administered to hypertensive patients receiving enalapril maleate. In this study there was no evidence of a blunting of the antihypertensive action of enalapril maleate. (See PRECAUTIONS, *Drug Interactions, Enalapril Maleate.*)

Hydrochlorothiazide

The mechanism of the antihypertensive effect of thiazides is unknown. Thiazides do not usually affect normal blood pressure. Hydrochlorothiazide is a diuretic and antihypertensive. It affects the distal renal tubular mechanism of electrolyte reabsorption. Hydrochlorothiazide increases excretion of sodium and chloride in approximately equivalent amounts. Natriuresis may be accompanied by some loss of potassium and bicarbonate. After oral use diuresis begins within two hours, peaks in about four hours and lasts about 6 to 12 hours. Hydrochlorothiazide is not metabolized but is eliminated rapidly by the kidney. When plasma levels have been followed for at least 24 hours, the plasma half-life has been observed to vary between 5.6 and 14.8 hours. At least 61 percent of the oral dose is eliminated unchanged within 24 hours. Hydrochlorothiazide crosses the placental but not the blood-brain barrier.

INDICATIONS AND USAGE

VASERETIC is indicated for the treatment of hypertension. These fixed dose combinations are not indicated for initial treatment (see DOSAGE AND ADMINISTRATION).

In using VASERETIC, consideration should be given to the fact that another angiotensin converting enzyme inhibitor, captopril, has caused agranulocytosis, particularly in patients with renal impairment or collagen vascular disease, and that available data are insufficient to show that enalapril does not have a similar risk. (See WARNINGS.)

In considering use of VASERETIC, it should be noted that black patients receiving ACE inhibitors have been reported to have a higher incidence of angioedema compared to non-blacks. (See WARNINGS, *Angioedema.*)

CONTRAINDICATIONS

VASERETIC is contraindicated in patients who are hypersensitive to any component of this product and in patients with a history of angioedema related to previous treatment with an angiotensin converting enzyme inhibitor and in patients with hereditary or idiopathic angioedema. Because of the hydrochlorothiazide component, this product is contraindicated in patients with anuria or hypersensitivity to other sulfonamide-derived drugs.

WARNINGS

General

Enalapril Maleate

Hypotension: Excessive hypotension was rarely seen in uncomplicated hypertensive patients but is a possible consequence of enalapril use in severely salt/volume depleted persons such as those treated vigorously with diuretics or patients on dialysis.

Syncope has been reported in 1.3 percent of patients receiving VASERETIC. In patients receiving enalapril alone, the incidence of syncope is 0.5 percent. The overall incidence of syncope may be reduced by proper titration of the individual components. (See PRECAUTIONS, *Drug Interactions,* ADVERSE REACTIONS and DOSAGE AND ADMINISTRATION.)

In patients with severe congestive heart failure, with or without associated renal insufficiency, excessive hypotension has been observed and may be associated with oliguria and/or progressive azotemia, and rarely with acute renal failure and/or death. Because of the potential fall in blood pressure in these patients, therapy should be started under very close medical supervision. Such patients should be followed closely for the first two weeks of treatment and whenever the dose of enalapril and/or diuretic is increased. Similar considerations may apply to patients with ischemic heart or cerebrovascular disease, in whom an excessive fall in blood pressure could result in a myocardial infarction or cerebrovascular accident.

If hypotension occurs, the patient should be placed in the supine position and, if necessary, receive an intravenous infusion of normal saline. A transient hypotensive response is not a contraindication to further doses, which usually can be given without difficulty once the blood pressure has increased after volume expansion.

Anaphylactoid and Possibly Related Reactions:

Presumably because angiotensin-converting enzyme inhibitors affect the metabolism of eicosanoids and polypeptides, including endogenous bradykinin, patients receiving ACE inhibitors (including VASERETIC) may be subject to a variety of adverse reactions, some of them serious.

Angioedema: Angioedema of the face, extremities, lips, tongue, glottis and/or larynx has been reported in patients treated with angiotensin converting enzyme inhibitors, including enalapril. This may occur at any time during treatment. In such cases VASERETIC should be promptly discontinued and appropriate therapy and monitoring should be provided until complete and sustained resolution of signs and symptoms has occurred. In instances where swelling has been confined to the face and lips the condition has generally resolved without treatment, although antihistamines have been useful in relieving symptoms. Angioedema associated with laryngeal edema may be fatal. **Where there is involvement of the tongue, glottis or larynx, likely to cause airway obstruction, appropriate therapy, e.g., subcutaneous epinephrine solution 1:1000 (0.3 mL to 0.5 mL) and/or measures necessary to ensure a patent airway, should be promptly provided.** (See ADVERSE REACTIONS.)

Patients with a history of angioedema unrelated to ACE inhibitor therapy may be at increased risk of angioedema while receiving an ACE inhibitor (see also INDICATIONS AND USAGE and CONTRAINDICATIONS).

Anaphylactoid reactions during desensitization: Two patients undergoing desensitizing treatment with hymenoptera venom while receiving ACE inhibitors sustained life-threatening anaphylactoid reactions. In the same patients, these reactions were avoided when ACE inhibitors were temporarily withheld, but they reappeared upon inadvertent rechallenge.

Anaphylactoid reactions during membrane exposure: Anaphylactoid reactions have been reported in patients dialyzed with high-flux membranes and treated concomitantly with an ACE inhibitor. Anaphylactoid reactions have also been reported in patients undergoing low-density lipoprotein apheresis with dextran sulfate absorption.

Neutropenia/Agranulocytosis: Another angiotensin converting enzyme inhibitor, captopril, has been shown to cause agranulocytosis and bone marrow depression, rarely in uncomplicated patients but more frequently in patients with renal impairment especially if they also have a collagen vascular disease. Available data from clinical trials of enalapril are insufficient to show that enalapril does not cause agranulocytosis at similar rates. Marketing experience has revealed cases of neutropenia or agranulocytosis in which a causal relationship to enalapril cannot be excluded. Periodic monitoring of white blood cell counts in patients with collagen vascular disease and renal disease should be considered.

Hepatic Failure: Rarely, ACE inhibitors have been associated with a syndrome that starts with cholestatic jaundice and progresses to fulminant hepatic necrosis, and (sometimes) death. The mechanism of this syndrome is not understood. Patients receiving ACE inhibitors who develop jaundice or marked elevations of hepatic enzymes should discontinue the ACE inhibitor and receive appropriate medical follow-up.

Hydrochlorothiazide

Thiazides should be used with caution in severe renal disease. In patients with renal disease, thiazides may precipitate azotemia. Cumulative effects of the drug may develop in patients with impaired renal function.

Thiazides should be used with caution in patients with impaired hepatic function or progressive liver disease, since minor alterations of fluid and electrolyte balance may precipitate hepatic coma.

Sensitivity reactions may occur in patients with or without a history of allergy or bronchial asthma.

The possibility of exacerbation or activation of systemic lupus erythematosus has been reported.

Lithium generally should not be given with thiazides (see PRECAUTIONS, *Drug Interactions, Enalapril Maleate* and *Hydrochlorothiazide*).

Pregnancy

Enalapril-Hydrochlorothiazide

There was no teratogenicity in mice given up to 30 mg/kg/day or in rats given up to 90 mg/kg/day of enalapril in combination with 10 mg/kg/day of hydrochlorothiazide. These doses of enalapril are 4.3 and 26 times (mice and rats, respectively) the maximum recommended human daily dose (MRHDD) when compared on a body surface area basis (mg/m^2); the dose of hydrochlorothiazide is 0.8 times (in mice) and 1.6 times (in rats) the MRHDD. At these doses, fetotoxicity expressed as a decrease in average fetal weight occurred in both species. No fetotoxicity occurred at lower doses; 30/10 mg/kg/day of enalapril-hydrochlorothiazide in rats and 10/10 mg/kg/day of enalapril-hydrochlorothiazide in mice.

When used in pregnancy during the second and third trimesters, ACE inhibitors can cause injury and even death to the developng fetus. When pregnancy is detected, VASERETIC should be discontinued as soon as possible. (See *Enalapril Maleate, Fetal/Neonatal Morbidity and Mortality,* below.)

Enalapril Maleate

Fetal/Neonatal Morbidity and Mortality: ACE inhibitors can cause fetal and neonatal morbidity and death when administered to pregnant women. Several dozen cases have been reported in the world literature. When pregnancy is detected, ACE inhibitors should be discontinued as soon as possible.

The use of ACE inhibitors during the second and third trimesters of pregnancy has been associated with fetal and neonatal injury, including hypotension, neonatal skull hypoplasia, anuria, reversible or irreversible renal failure, and death. Oligohydramnios has also been reported, presumably resulting from decreased fetal renal function; oligohydramnios in this setting has been associated with fetal limb contractures, craniofacial deformation, and hypoplastic lung development. Prematurity, intrauterine growth retardation,

Continued on next page

Information on the Merck & Co., Inc., products listed on these pages is from the prescribing information in use October 1, 2004. For information, please call 1-800-NSC-MERCK [1-800-672-6372].

Vaseretic—Cont.

and patent ductus arteriosus have also been reported, although it is not clear whether these occurrences were due to the ACE-inhibitor exposure.
These adverse effects do not appear to have resulted from intrauterine ACE-inhibitor exposure that has been limited to the first trimester. Mothers whose embryos and fetuses are exposed to ACE inhibitors only during the first trimester should be so informed. Nonetheless, when patients become pregnant, physicians should make every effort to discontinue the use of VASERETIC as soon as possible.
Rarely (probably less often than once in every thousand pregnancies), no alternative to ACE inhibitors will be found. In these rare cases, the mothers should be apprised of the potential hazards to their fetuses, and serial ultrasound examinations should be performed to assess the intraamniotic environment.
If oligohydramnios is observed, VASERETIC should be discontinued unless it is considered lifesaving for the mother. Contraction stress testing (CST), a non-stress test (NST), or biophysical profiling (BPP) may be appropriate, depending upon the week of pregnancy. Patients and physicians should be aware, however, that oligohydramnios may not appear until after the fetus has sustained irreversible injury.
Infants with histories of *in utero* exposure to ACE inhibitors should be closely observed for hypotension, oliguria, and hyperkalemia. If oliguria occurs, attention should be directed toward support of blood pressure and renal perfusion. Exchange transfusion or dialysis may be required as means of reversing hypotension and/or substituting for disordered renal functon. Enalapril, which crosses the placenta, has been removed from neonatal circulation by peritoneal dialysis with some clinical benefit, and theoretically may be removed by exchange transfusion, although there is no experience with the latter procedure.
No teratogenic effects of enalapril were seen in studies of pregnant rats and rabbits. On a body surface area basis, the doses were 57 times and 12 times, respectively, the MRHDD.
Hydrochlorothiazide
Studies in which hydrochlorothiazide was orally administered to pregnant mice and rats during their respective periods of major organogenesis at doses up to 3000 and 1000 mg/kg/day, respectively, provided no evidence of harm to the fetus. These doses are more than 150 times the MRHDD on a body surface area basis. Thiazides cross the placental barrier and appear in cord blood. There is a risk of fetal or neonatal jaundice, thrombocytopenia, and possibly other adverse reactions that have occurred in adults.

PRECAUTIONS

General
Enalapril Maleate
Aortic Stenosis/Hypertrophic Cardiomyopathy: As with all vasodilators, enalapril should be given with caution to patients with obstruction in the outflow tract of the left ventricle.
Impaired Renal Function: As a consequence of inhibiting the renin-angiotensin-aldosterone system, changes in renal function may be anticipated in susceptible individuals. In patients with severe congestive heart failure whose renal function may depend on the activity of the renin-angiotensin-aldosterone system, treatment with angiotensin converting enzyme inhibitors, including enalapril, may be associated with oliguria and/or progressive azotemia and rarely with acute renal failure and/or death.
In clinical studies in hypertensive patients with unilateral or bilateral renal artery stenosis, increases in blood urea nitrogen and serum creatinine were observed in 20 percent of patients. These increases were almost always reversible upon discontinuation of enalapril and/or diuretic therapy. In such patients renal function should be monitored during the first few weeks of therapy.
Some patients with hypertension or heart failure with no apparent pre-existing renal vascular disease have developed increases in blood urea and serum creatinine, usually minor and transient, especially when enalapril has been given concomitantly with a diuretic. This is more likely to occur in patients with pre-existing renal impairment. Dosage reduction of enalapril and/or discontinuation of the diuretic may be required.
Evaluation of the hypertensive patient should always include assessment of renal function.
Hyperkalemia: Elevated serum potassium (greater than 5.7 mEq/L) was observed in approximately one percent of hypertensive patients in clinical trials treated with enalapril alone. In most cases these were isolated values which resolved despite continued therapy, although hyperkalemia was a cause of discontinuation of therapy in 0.28 percent of hypertensive patients. Hyperkalemia was less frequent (approximately 0.1 percent) in patients treated with enalapril plus hydrochlorothiazide. Risk factors for the development of hyperkalemia include renal insufficiency, diabetes mellitus, and the concomitant use of potassium-sparing diuretics, potassium supplements and/or potassium-containing salt substitutes, which should be used cautiously, if at all, with enalapril. (See *Drug Interactions.*)
Cough: Presumably due to the inhibition of the degradation of endogenous bradykinin, persistent nonproductive cough has been reported with all ACE inhibitors, always resolving after discontinuation of therapy. ACE inhibitor-induced cough should be considered in the differential diagnosis of cough.
Surgery/Anesthesia: In patients undergoing major surgery or during anesthesia with agents that produce hypotension, enalapril may block angiotensin II formation secondary to compensatory renin release. If hypotension occurs and is considered to be due to this mechanism, it can be corrected by volume expansion.
Hydrochlorothiazide
Periodic determination of serum electrolytes to detect possible electrolyte imbalance should be performed at appropriate intervals. All patients receiving thiazide therapy should be observed for clinical signs of fluid or electrolyte imbalance: namely hyponatremia, hypochloremic alkalosis, and hypokalemia. Serum and urine electrolyte determinations are particularly important when the patient is vomiting excessively or receiving parenteral fluids. Warning signs or symptoms of fluid and electrolyte imbalance, irrespective of cause, include dryness of mouth, thirst, weakness, lethargy, drowsiness, restlessness, confusion, seizures, muscle pains or cramps, muscular fatigue, hypotension, oliguria, tachycardia, and gastrointestinal disturbances such as nausea and vomiting.
Hypokalemia may develop, especially with brisk diuresis, when severe cirrhosis is present, or after prolonged therapy. Interference with adequate oral electrolyte intake will also contribute to hypokalemia. Hypokalemia may cause cardiac arrhythmia and may also sensitize or exaggerate the response of the heart to the toxic effects of digitalis (e.g., increased ventricular irritability). Because enalapril reduces the production of aldosterone, concomitant therapy with enalapril attenuates the diuretic-induced potassium loss (see *Drug Interactions, Agents Increasing Serum Potassium*).
Although any chloride deficit is generally mild and usually does not require specific treatment except under extraordinary circumstances (as in liver disease or renal disease), chloride replacement may be required in the treatment of metabolic alkalosis.
Dilutional hyponatremia may occur in edematous patients in hot weather; appropriate therapy is water restriction, rather than administration of salt except in rare instances when the hyponatremia is life-threatening. In actual salt depletion, appropriate replacement is the therapy of choice.
Hyperuricemia may occur or frank gout may be precipitated in certain patients receiving thiazide therapy.
In diabetic patients dosage adjustments of insulin or oral hypoglycemic agents may be required. Hyperglycemia may occur with thiazide diuretics. Thus latent diabetes mellitus may become manifest during thiazide therapy.
The antihypertensive effects of the drug may be enhanced in the postsympathectomy patient.
If progressive renal impairment becomes evident consider withholding or discontinuing diuretic therapy.
Thiazides have been shown to increase the urinary excretion of magnesium; this may result in hypomagnesemia.
Thiazides may decrease urinary calcium excretion. Thiazides may cause intermittent and slight elevation of serum calcium in the absence of known disorders of calcium metabolism. Marked hypercalcemia may be evidence of hidden hyperparathyroidism. Thiazides should be discontinued before carrying out tests for parathyroid function.
Increases in cholesterol and triglyceride levels may be associated with thiazide diuretic therapy.
Information for Patients
Angioedema: Angioedema, including laryngeal edema, may occur at any time during treatment with angiotensin converting enzyme inhibitors, including enalapril. Patients should be so advised and told to report immediately any signs or symptoms suggesting angioedema (swelling of face, extremities, eyes, lips, tongue, difficulty in swallowing or breathing) and to take no more drug until they have consulted with the prescribing physician.
Hypotension: Patients should be cautioned to report lightheadedness especially during the first few days of therapy. If actual syncope occurs, the patients should be told to discontinue the drug until they have consulted with the prescribing physician.
All patients should be cautioned that excessive perspiration and dehydration may lead to an excessive fall in blood pressure because of reduction in fluid volume. Other causes of volume depletion such as vomiting or diarrhea may also lead to a fall in blood pressure; patients should be advised to consult with the physician.
Hyperkalemia: Patients should be told not to use salt substitutes containing potassium without consulting their physician.
Neutropenia: Patients should be told to report promptly any indication of infection (e.g., sore throat, fever) which may be a sign of neutropenia.
Pregnancy: Female patients of childbearing age should be told about the consequences of second- and third-trimester exposure to ACE inhibitors, and they should also be told that these consequences do not appear to have resulted from intrauterine ACE-inhibitor exposure that has been limited to the first trimester. These patients should be asked to report pregnancies to their physicians as soon as possible.
NOTE: As with many other drugs, certain advice to patients being treated with VASERETIC is warranted. This information is intended to aid in the safe and effective use of this medication. It is not a disclosure of all possible adverse or intended effects.
Drug Interactions
Enalapril Maleate
Hypotension—Patients on Diuretic Therapy: Patients on diuretics and especially those in whom diuretic therapy was recently instituted, may occasionally experience an excessive reduction of blood pressure after initiation of therapy with enalapril. The possibility of hypotensive effects with enalapril can be minimized by either discontinuing the diuretic or increasing the salt intake prior to initiation of treatment with enalapril. If it is necessary to continue the diuretic, provide medical supervision for at least two hours and until blood pressure has stabilized for at least an additional hour. (See WARNINGS, and DOSAGE AND ADMINISTRATION.)
Agents Causing Renin Release: The antihypertensive effect of enalapril is augmented by antihypertensive agents that cause renin release (e.g., diuretics).
Non-steroidal Anti-inflammatory Agents: In some patients with compromised renal function who are being treated with non-steroidal anti-inflammatory drugs, the coadministration of enalapril may result in a further deterioration of renal function. These effects are usually reversible.
In a clinical pharmacology study, indomethacin or sulindac was administered to hypertensive patients receiving enalapril maleate. In this study there was no evidence of a blunting of the antihypertensive action of enalapril maleate. However, reports suggest that NSAIDs may diminish the antihypertensive effect of ACE inhibitors. This interaction should be given consideration in patients taking NSAIDs concomitantly with ACE inhibitors.
Other Cardiovascular Agents: Enalapril has been used concomitantly with beta adrenergic-blocking agents, methyldopa, nitrates, calcium-blocking agents, hydralazine and prazosin without evidence of clinically significant adverse interactions.
Agents Increasing Serum Potassium: Enalapril attenuates diuretic-induced potassium loss. Potassium-sparing diuretics (e.g., spironolactone, triamterene, or amiloride), potassium supplements, or potassium-containing salt substitutes may lead to significant increases in serum potassium. Therefore, if concomitant use of these agents is indicated because of demonstrated hypokalemia they should be used with caution and with frequent monitoring of serum potassium.
Lithium: Lithium toxicity has been reported in patients receiving lithium concomitantly with drugs which cause elimination of sodium, including ACE inhibitors. A few cases of lithium toxicity have been reported in patients receiving concomitant enalapril and lithium and were reversible upon discontinuation of both drugs. It is recommended that serum lithium levels be monitored frequently if enalapril is administered concomitantly with lithium.
Hydrochlorothiazide
When administered concurrently the following drugs may interact with thiazide diuretics:
Alcohol, barbiturates, or narcotics—potentiation of orthostatic hypotension may occur.
Antidiabetic drugs (oral agents and insulin)—dosage adjustment of the antidiabetic drug may be required.
Other antihypertensive drugs—additive effect or potentiation.
Cholestyramine and colestipol resins—Absorption of hydrochlorothiazide is impaired in the presence of anionic exchange resins. Single doses of either cholestyramine or colestipol resins bind the hydrochlorothiazide and reduce its absorption from the gastrointestinal tract by up to 85 and 43 percent, respectively.
Corticosteroids, ACTH—intensified electrolyte depletion, particularly hypokalemia.
Pressor amines (e.g., norepinephrine)—possible decreased response to pressor amines but not sufficient to preclude their use.
Skeletal muscle relaxants, nondepolarizing (e.g., tubocurarine)—possible increased responsiveness to the muscle relaxant.
Lithium—should not generally be given with diuretics. Diuretic agents reduce the renal clearance of lithium and add a high risk of lithium toxicity. Refer to the package insert for lithium preparations before use of such preparations with VASERETIC.
Non-steroidal Anti-inflammatory Drugs—In some patients, the administration of a non-steroidal anti-inflammatory agent can reduce the diuretic, natriuretic, and antihypertensive effects of loop, potassium-sparing and thiazide diuretics. Therefore, when VASERETIC and non-steroidal anti-inflammatory agents are used concomitantly, the patient should be observed closely to determine if the desired effect of the diuretic is obtained.
Carcinogenesis, Mutagenesis, Impairment of Fertility
Enalapril in combination with hydrochlorothiazide was not mutagenic in the Ames microbial mutagen test with or without metabolic activation. Enalapril-hydrochlorothiazide did not produce DNA single strand breaks in an *in vitro* alkaline elution assay in rat hepatocytes or chromosomal aberrations in an *in vivo* mouse bone marrow assay.
Enalapril Maleate
There was no evidence of a tumorigenic effect when enalapril was administered for 106 weeks to male and female rats at doses up to 90 mg/kg/day or for 94 weeks to male and female mice at doses up to 90 and 180 mg/kg/day, respectively. These doses are 26 times (in rats and female mice) and 13 times (in male mice) the maximum recommended human daily dose (MRHDD) when compared on a body surface area basis.

Neither enalapril maleate nor the active diacid was mutagenic in the Ames microbial mutagen test with or without metabolic activation. Enalapril was also negative in the following genotoxicity studies: rec-assay, reverse mutation assay with *E. coli*, sister chromatid exchange with cultured mammalian cells, and the micronucleus test with mice, as well as in an *in vivo* cytogenic study using mouse bone marrow.

There were no adverse effects on reproductive performance of male and female rats treated with up to 90 mg/kg/day of enalapril (26 times the MRHDD when compared on a body surface area basis).

Hydrochlorothiazide

Two year feeding studies in mice and rats conducted under the auspices of the National Toxicology Program (NTP) uncovered no evidence of a carcinogenic potential of hydrochlorothiazide in female mice at doses up to approximately 600 mg/kg/day (53 times the MRHDD when compared on a body surface area basis) or in male and female rats at doses up to approximately 100 mg/kg/day (18 times the MRHDD when compared on a body surface area basis). The NTP, however, found equivocal evidence for hepatocarcinogenicity in male mice.

Hydrochlorothiazide was not genotoxic *in vitro* in the Ames mutagenicity assay of *Salmonella typhimurium* strains TA 98, TA 100, TA 1535, TA 1537, and TA 1538 and in the Chinese Hamster Ovary (CHO) test for chromosomal aberrations, or *in vivo* in assays using mouse germinal cell chromosomes, Chinese hamster bone marrow chromosomes, and the *Drosophila* sex-linked recessive lethal trait gene. Positive test results were obtained only in the *in vitro* CHO Sister Chromatid Exchange (clastogenicity) and in the Mouse Lymphoma Cell (mutagenicity) assays, using concentrations of hydrochlorothiazide from 43 to 1300 µg/mL, and in the *Aspergillus nidulans* non-disjunction assay at an unspecified concentration.

Hydrochlorothiazide had no adverse effects on the fertility of mice and rats of either sex in studies wherein these species were exposed, via their diet, to doses of up to 100 and 4 mg/kg, respectively, prior to mating and throughout gestation. In mice and rats these doses are 9 times and 0.7 times, respectively, the MRHDD when compared on a body surface area basis.

Pregnancy

Pregnancy Categories C (first trimester) *and D* (second and third trimesters). See WARNINGS, *Pregnancy, Enalapril Maleate, Fetal/Neonatal Morbidity and Mortality.*

Nursing Mothers

Enalapril, enalaprilat, and hydrochlorothiazide have been detected in human breast milk. Because of the potential for serious reactions in nursing infants from either drug, a decision should be made whether to discontinue nursing or to discontinue VASERETIC, taking into account the importance of the drug to the mother.

Pediatric Use

Safety and effectiveness in pediatric patients have not been established.

ADVERSE REACTIONS

VASERETIC has been evaluated for safety in more than 1500 patients, including over 300 patients treated for one year or more. In clinical trials with VASERETIC no adverse experiences peculiar to this combination drug have been observed. Adverse experiences that have occurred, have been limited to those that have been previously reported with enalapril or hydrochlorothiazide.

The most frequent clinical adverse experiences in controlled trials were: dizziness (8.6 percent), headache (5.5 percent), fatigue (3.9 percent) and cough (3.5 percent). Generally, adverse experiences were mild and transient in nature. Adverse experiences occurring in greater than two percent of patients treated with VASERETIC in controlled clinical trials are shown below.

	Percent of Patients in Controlled Studies	
	VASERETIC (n=1580) Incidence (discontinuation)	Placebo (n=230) Incidence
Dizziness	8.6 (0.7)	4.3
Headache	5.5 (0.4)	9.1
Fatigue	3.9 (0.8)	2.6
Cough	3.5 (0.4)	0.9
Muscle Cramps	2.7 (0.2)	0.9
Nausea	2.5 (0.4)	1.7
Asthenia	2.4 (0.3)	0.9
Orthostatic Effects	2.3 (<0.1)	0.0
Impotence	2.2 (0.5)	0.5
Diarrhea	2.1 (<0.1)	1.7

Clinical adverse experiences occurring in 0.5 to 2.0 percent of patients in controlled trials included: *Body As A Whole:* Syncope, chest pain, abdominal pain; *Cardiovascular:* Orthostatic hypotension, palpitation, tachycardia; *Digestive:* Vomiting, dyspepsia, constipation, flatulence, dry mouth; *Nervous/Psychiatric:* Insomnia, nervousness, paresthesia, somnolence, vertigo; *Skin:* Pruritus, rash; *Other:* Dyspnea, gout, back pain, arthralgia, diaphoresis, decreased libido, tinnitus, urinary tract infection.

Angioedema: Angioedema has been reported in patients receiving VASERETIC, with an incidence higher in black than in non-black patients. Angioedema associated with laryngeal edema may be fatal. If angioedema of the face, extremities, lips, tongue, glottis and/or larynx occurs, treatment with VASERETIC should be discontinued and appropriate therapy instituted immediately. (See WARNINGS.)

Hypotension: In clinical trials, adverse effects relating to hypotension occurred as follows: hypotension (0.9 percent), orthostatic hypotension (1.5 percent), other orthostatic effects (2.3 percent). In addition syncope occurred in 1.3 percent of patients. (See WARNINGS.)

Cough: See PRECAUTIONS, *Cough.*

Clinical Laboratory Test Findings

Serum Electrolytes: See PRECAUTIONS.

Creatinine, Blood Urea Nitrogen: In controlled clinical trials minor increases in blood urea nitrogen and serum creatinine, reversible upon discontinuation of therapy, were observed in about 0.6 percent of patients with essential hypertension treated with VASERETIC. More marked increases have been reported in other enalapril experience. Increases are more likely to occur in patients with renal artery stenosis. (See PRECAUTIONS.)

Serum Uric Acid, Glucose, Magnesium, and Calcium: See PRECAUTIONS.

Hemoglobin and Hematocrit: Small decreases in hemoglobin and hematocrit (mean decreases of approximately 0.3 g percent and 1.0 vol percent, respectively) occur frequently in hypertensive patients treated with VASERETIC but are rarely of clinical importance unless another cause of anemia coexists. In clinical trials, less than 0.1 percent of patients discontinued therapy due to anemia.

Liver Function Tests: Rarely, elevations of liver enzymes and/or serum bilirubin have occurred (see WARNINGS, *Hepatic Failure*).

Other adverse reactions that have been reported with the individual components are listed below and, within each category, are in order of decreasing severity.

Enalapril Maleate —Enalapril has been evaluated for safety in more than 10,000 patients. In clinical trials adverse reactions which occurred with enalapril were also seen with VASERETIC. However, since enalapril has been marketed, the following adverse reactions have been reported: *Body As A Whole:* Anaphylactoid reactions (see WARNINGS, *Anaphylactoid reactions during membrane exposure*); *Cardiovascular:* Cardiac arrest; myocardial infarction or cerebrovascular accident, possibly secondary to excessive hypotension in high risk patients (see WARNINGS, *Hypotension*); pulmonary embolism and infarction; pulmonary edema; rhythm disturbances including atrial tachycardia and bradycardia, atrial fibrillation; hypotension; angina pectoris, Raynaud's phenomenon; *Digestive:* Ileus, pancreatitis, hepatic failure, hepatitis (hepatocellular [proven on rechallenge] or cholestatic jaundice) (see WARNINGS, *Hepatic Failure*), melena, anorexia, glossitis, stomatitis, dry mouth; *Hematologic:* Rare cases of neutropenia, thrombocytopenia and bone marrow depression. Hemolytic anemia, including cases of hemolysis in patients with G-6-PD deficiency, has been reported; a causal relationship to enalapril cannot be excluded. *Nervous System/Psychiatric:* Depression, confusion, ataxia, peripheral neuropathy (e.g., paresthesia, dysesthesia), dream abnormality; *Urogenital:* Renal failure, oliguria, renal dysfunction, (see PRECAUTIONS and DOSAGE AND ADMINISTRATION), flank pain, gynecomastia; *Respiratory:* Pulmonary infiltrates, eosinophilic pneumonitis, bronchospasm, pneumonia, bronchitis, rhinorrhea, sore throat and hoarseness, asthma, upper respiratory infection; *Skin:* Exfoliative dermatitis, toxic epidermal necrolysis, Stevens-Johnson syndrome, herpes zoster, erythema multiforme, urticaria, pemphigus, alopecia, flushing, photosensitivity; *Special Senses:* Blurred vision, taste alteration, anosmia, conjunctivitis, dry eyes, tearing.

Miscellaneous: A symptom complex has been reported which may include some or all of the following: a positive ANA, an elevated erythrocyte sedimentation rate, arthralgia/arthritis, myalgia/myositis, fever, serositis, vasculitis, leukocytosis, eosinophilia, photosensitivity, rash and other dermatologic manifestations.

Fetal/Neonatal Morbidity and Mortality: See WARNINGS, *Pregnancy, Enalapril Maleate, Fetal/Neonatal Morbidity and Mortality.*

Hydrochlorothiazide—Body as a Whole: Weakness; *Digestive:* Pancreatitis, jaundice (intrahepatic cholestatic jaundice), sialadenitis, cramping, gastric irritation, anorexia; *Hematologic:* Aplastic anemia, agranulocytosis, leukopenia, hemolytic anemia, thrombocytopenia; *Hypersensitivity:* Purpura, photosensitivity, urticaria, necrotizing angiitis (vasculitis and cutaneous vasculitis), fever, respiratory distress including pneumonitis and pulmonary edema, anaphylactic reactions; *Musculoskeletal:* Muscle spasm; *Nervous system/Psychiatric:* Restlessness; *Renal:* Renal failure, renal dysfunction, interstitial nephritis (see WARNINGS); *Skin:* Erythema multiforme including Stevens-Johnson syndrome, exfoliative dermatitis including toxic epidermal necrolysis, alopecia; *Special Senses:* Transient blurred vision, xanthopsia.

OVERDOSAGE

No specific information is available on the treatment of overdosage with VASERETIC. Treatment is symptomatic and supportive. Therapy with VASERETIC should be discontinued and the patient observed closely. Suggested measures include induction of emesis and/or gastric lavage, and correction of dehydration, electrolyte imbalance and hypotension by established procedures.

Enalapril Maleate —Single oral doses of enalapril above 1,000 mg/kg and ≥1,775 mg/kg were associated with lethality in mice and rats, respectively. The most likely manifestation of overdosage would be hypotension, for which the usual treatment would be intravenous infusion of normal saline solution. Enalaprilat may be removed from general circulation by hemodialysis and has been removed from neonatal circulation by peritoneal dialysis. (See WARNINGS, *Anaphylactoid reactions during membrane exposure.*)

Hydrochlorothiazide —Lethality was not observed after administration of an oral dose of 10 g/kg to mice and rats. The most common signs and symptoms observed are those caused by electrolyte depletion (hypokalemia, hypochloremia, hyponatremia) and dehydration resulting from excessive diuresis. If digitalis has also been administered, hypokalemia may accentuate cardiac arrhythmias.

DOSAGE AND ADMINISTRATION

Enalapril and hydrochlorothiazide are effective treatments for hypertension. The usual dosage range of enalapril is 10 to 40 mg per day administered in a single or two divided doses; hydrochlorothiazide is effective in doses of 12.5 to 50 mg daily. The side effects (see WARNINGS) of enalapril are generally rare and apparently independent of dose; those of hydrochlorothiazide are a mixture of dose-dependent phenomena (primarily hypokalemia) and dose-independent phenomena (e.g., pancreatitis), the former much more common than the latter. Therapy with any combination of enalapril and hydrochlorothiazide will be associated with both sets of dose-independent side effects but the addition of enalapril in clinicial trials blunted the hypokalemia normally seen with diuretics. To minimize dose-independent side effects, it is usually appropriate to begin combination therapy only after a patient has failed to achieve the desired effect with monotherapy.

Dose Titration Guided by Clinical Effect: A patient whose blood pressure is not adequately controlled with either enalapril or hydrochlorothiazide monotherapy may be given VASERETIC 5–12.5 or VASERETIC 10–25. Further increases of enalapril, hydrochlorothiazide or both depend on clinical response. The hydrochlorothiazide dose should generally not be increased until 2–3 weeks have elapsed. In general, patients do not require doses in excess of 20 mg of enalapril or 50 mg of hydrochlorothiazide. The daily dosage should not exceed four tablets of VASERETIC 5–12.5 or two tablets of VASERETIC 10–25.

Replacement Therapy: The combination may be substituted for the titrated components.

Use in Renal Impairment: The usual regimens of therapy with VASERETIC need not be adjusted as long as the patient's creatinine clearance is >30 mL/min/1.73 m^2 (serum creatinine approximately ≤3 mg/dL or 265 µmol/L). In patients with more severe renal impairment, loop diuretics are preferred to thiazides, so enalapril maleate-hydrochlorothiazide is not recommended (see WARNINGS, *Anaphylactoid reactions during membrane exposure*).

Use in Elderly: Clinical studies in VASERETIC did not include sufficient numbers of patients aged 65 and over to determine whether they respond differently from younger patients. In general, dose selection for an elderly patient should be cautious, usually starting at the low end of the dosing range.

HOW SUPPLIED

No. 3644—Tablets VASERETIC 5-12.5 are green, squared capsule-shaped compressed tablets, coded MSD on one side and 173 on the other. Each tablet contains 5 mg of enalapril maleate and 12.5 mg of hydrochlorothiazide. They are supplied as follows:

NDC 0006-0173-68 bottles of 100 (with desiccant).

No. 3418—Tablets VASERETIC 10-25, are rust, squared capsule-shaped, compressed tablets, coded MSD 720 on one side and VASERETIC on the other. Each tablet contains 10 mg of enalapril maleate and 25 mg of hydrochlorothiazide. They are supplied as follows:

NDC 0006-0720-68 bottles of 100 (with desiccant).

Storage

Store below 30°C (86°F) and avoid transient temperatures above 50°C (122°F). Keep container tightly closed. Protect from moisture.

Dispense in a tight container, if product package is subdivided.

7843635 Issued January 2001

Shown in Product Identification Guide, page 324

Continued on next page

Information on the Merck & Co., Inc., products listed on these pages is from the prescribing information in use October 1, 2004. For information, please call 1-800-NSC-MERCK [1-800-672-6372].

VASOTEC* I.V. Injection ℞
(enalaprilat)
Distributed by Biovail Pharmaceuticals, Inc.
Morrisville, NC 27560
To make additional inquiries or to report an adverse event, please contact Biovail Pharmaceuticals, Inc. at 1-866-276-1030.

*Registered trademark of Biovail Pharmaceuticals, Inc.

VASOTEC® I.V. Injection ℞
(enalaprilat)

USE IN PREGNANCY
When used in pregnancy during the second and third trimesters, ACE inhibitors can cause injury and even death to the developing fetus. When pregnancy is detected, VASOTEC I.V. should be discontinued as soon as possible. See WARNINGS, *Fetal/Neonatal Morbidity and Mortality.*

DESCRIPTION

VASOTEC* I.V. (Enalaprilat) is a sterile aqueous solution for intravenous administration. Enalaprilat is an angiotensin converting enzyme inhibitor. It is chemically described as (*S*)-1-[*N*-(1-carboxy-3-phenylpropyl)-L-alanyl]-L-proline dihydrate. Its empirical formula is $C_{18}H_{24}N_2O_5 \cdot 2H_2O$ and its structural formula is:

[structural formula: C6H5–CH2CH2–C(H)(COOH)–N(H)–C(H)(CH3)–C(=O)–N(pyrrolidine-COOH) · 2H2O]

Enalaprilat is a white to off-white, crystalline powder with a molecular weight of 384.43. It is sparingly soluble in methanol and slightly soluble in water.
Each milliliter of VASOTEC I.V. contains 1.25 mg enalaprilat (anhydrous equivalent); sodium chloride to adjust tonicity; sodium hydroxide to adjust pH; water for injection, q.s.; with benzyl alcohol, 9 mg, added as a preservative.

*Registered trademark of MERCK & CO., INC.

CLINICAL PHARMACOLOGY

Enalaprilat, an angiotensin-converting enzyme (ACE) inhibitor when administered intravenously, is the active metabolite of the orally administered pro-drug, enalapril maleate. Enalaprilat is poorly absorbed orally.

Mechanism of Action
Intravenous enalaprilat, or oral enalapril, after hydrolysis to enalaprilat, inhibits ACE in human subjects and animals. ACE is a peptidyl dipeptidase that catalyzes the conversion of angiotensin I to the vasoconstrictor substance, angiotensin II. Angiotensin II also stimulates aldosterone secretion by the adrenal cortex. Inhibition of ACE results in decreased plasma angiotensin II, which leads to decreased vasopressor activity and to decreased aldosterone secretion. Although the latter decrease is small, it results in small increases of serum potassium. In hypertensive patients treated with enalapril alone for up to 48 weeks, mean increases in serum potassium of approximately 0.2 mEq/L were observed. In patients treated with enalapril plus a thiazide diuretic, there was essentially no change in serum potassium. (See PRECAUTIONS.) Removal of angiotensin II negative feedback on renin secretion leads to increased plasma renin activity.
ACE is identical to kininase, an enzyme that degrades bradykinin. Whether increased levels of bradykinin, a potent vasodepressor peptide, play a role in the therapeutic effects of enalaprilat remains to be elucidated.
While the mechanism through which enalaprilat lowers blood pressure is believed to be primarily suppression of the renin-angiotensin-aldosterone system, enalaprilat has antihypertensive activity even in patients with low-renin hypertension. In clinical studies, black hypertensive patients (usually a low-renin hypertensive population) had a smaller average response to enalaprilat monotherapy than non-black patients.

Pharmacokinetics and Metabolism
Following intravenous administration of a single dose, the serum concentration profile of enalaprilat is polyexponential with a prolonged terminal phase, apparently representing a small fraction of the administered dose that has been bound to ACE. The amount bound does not increase with dose, indicating a saturable site of binding. The effective half-life for accumulation of enalaprilat, as determined from oral administration of multiple doses of enalapril maleate, is approximately 11 hours. Excretion of enalaprilat is primarily renal with more than 90 percent of an administered dose recovered in the urine as unchanged drug within 24 hours. Enalaprilat is poorly absorbed following oral administration.
The disposition of enalaprilat in patients with renal insufficiency is similar to that in patients with normal renal function until the glomerular filtration rate is 30 mL/min or less. With glomerular filtration rate ≤30 mL/min, peak and trough enalaprilat levels increase, time to peak concentration increases and time to steady state may be delayed. The effective half-life of enalaprilat is prolonged at this level of renal insufficiency. (See DOSAGE AND ADMINISTRATION.) Enalaprilat is dialyzable at the rate of 62 mL/min. Studies in dogs indicate that enalaprilat does not enter the brain, and that enalapril crosses the blood-brain barrier poorly, if at all. Multiple doses of enalapril maleate in rats do not result in accumulation in any tissues. Milk in lactating rats contains radioactivity following administration of ^{14}C enalapril maleate. Radioactivity was found to cross the placenta following administration of labeled drug to pregnant hamsters.

Pharmacodynamics
VASOTEC I.V. results in the reduction of both supine and standing systolic and diastolic blood pressure, usually with no orthostatic component. Symptomatic postural hypotension is therefore infrequent, although it might be anticipated in volume-depleted patients (see WARNINGS). The onset of action usually occurs within fifteen minutes of administration with the maximum effect occurring within one to four hours. The abrupt withdrawal of enalaprilat has not been associated with a rapid increase in blood pressure.
The duration of hemodynamic effects appears to be dose-related. However, for the recommended dose, the duration of action in most patients is approximately six hours.
Following administration of enalapril, there is an increase in renal blood flow; glomerular filtration rate is usually unchanged. The effects appear to be similar in patients with renovascular hypertension.
In a clinical pharmacology study, indomethacin or sulindac was administered to hypertensive patients receiving enalapril maleate. In this study there was no evidence of a blunting of the antihypertensive action of enalapril maleate. (See PRECAUTIONS, *Drug Interactions.*)

INDICATIONS AND USAGE

VASOTEC I.V. is indicated for the treatment of hypertension when oral therapy is not practical.
VASOTEC I.V. has been studied with only one other antihypertensive agent, furosemide, which showed approximately additive effects on blood pressure. Enalapril, the pro-drug of enalaprilat, has been used extensively with a variety of other antihypertensive agents, without apparent difficulty except for occasional hypotension.
In using VASOTEC I.V., consideration should be given to the fact that another angiotensin converting enzyme inhibitor, captopril, has caused agranulocytosis, particularly in patients with renal impairment or collagen vascular disease, and that available data are insufficient to show that VASOTEC I.V. does not have a similar risk. (See WARNINGS.)
In considering use of VASOTEC I.V., it should be noted that in controlled clinical trials ACE inhibitors have an effect on blood pressure that is less in black patients than in non-blacks. In addition, it should be noted that black patients receiving ACE inhibitors have been reported to have a higher incidence of angioedema compared to non-blacks. (See WARNINGS, *Angioedema.*)

CONTRAINDICATIONS

VASOTEC I.V. is contraindicated in patients who are hypersensitive to any component of this product and in patients with a history of angioedema related to previous treatment with an angiotensin converting enzyme inhibitor and in patients with hereditary or idiopathic angioedema.

WARNINGS

Hypotension
Excessive hypotension is rare in uncomplicated hypertensive patients but is a possible consequence of the use of enalaprilat especially in severely salt/volume depleted persons such as those treated vigorously with diuretics or patients on dialysis. Patients at risk for excessive hypotension, sometimes associated with oliguria and/or progressive azotemia, and rarely with acute renal failure and/or death, include those with the following conditions or characteristics: heart failure, hyponatremia, high dose diuretic therapy, recent intensive diuresis or increase in diuretic dose, renal dialysis, or severe volume and/or salt depletion of any etiology. It may be advisable to eliminate the diuretic, reduce the diuretic dose or increase salt intake cautiously before initiating therapy with VASOTEC I.V. in patients at risk for excessive hypotension who are able to tolerate such adjustment. (See PRECAUTIONS, *Drug Interactions,* ADVERSE REACTIONS, and DOSAGE AND ADMINISTRATION.) In patients with heart failure, with or without associated renal insufficiency, excessive hypotension has been observed and may be associated with oliguria and/or progressive azotemia, and rarely with acute renal failure and/or death. Because of the potential for an excessive fall in blood pressure especially in these patients, therapy should be followed closely whenever the dose of enalaprilat is adjusted and/or diuretic is increased. Similar consideration may apply to patients with ischemic heart or cerebrovascular disease, in whom an excessive fall in blood pressure could result in a myocardial infarction or cerebrovascular accident.
If hypotension occurs, the patient should be placed in the supine position and, if necessary, receive an intravenous infusion of normal saline. A transient hypotensive response is not a contraindication to further doses, which usually can be given without difficulty once the blood pressure has increased after volume expansion.

Anaphylactoid and Possibly Related Reactions
Presumably because angiotensin-converting enzyme inhibitors affect the metabolism of eicosanoids and polypeptides, including endogenous bradykinin, patients receiving ACE inhibitors (including VASOTEC I.V.) may be subject to a variety of adverse reactions, some of them serious.
Angioedema: Angioedema of the face, extremities, lips, tongue, glottis and/or larynx has been reported in patients treated with angiotensin converting enzyme inhibitors, including enalaprilat. This may occur at any time during treatment. In such cases VASOTEC I.V. should be promptly discontinued and appropriate therapy and monitoring should be provided until complete and sustained resolution of signs and symptoms has occurred. In instances where swelling has been confined to the face and lips the condition has generally resolved without treatment, although antihistamines have been useful in relieving symptoms. Angioedema associated with laryngeal edema may be fatal. **Where there is involvement of the tongue, glottis or larynx, likely to cause airway obstruction, appropriate therapy, e.g., subcutaneous epinephrine solution 1:1000 (0.3 mL to 0.5 mL) and/or measures necessary to ensure a patent airway, should be promptly provided.** (See ADVERSE REACTIONS.)
Patients with a history of angioedema unrelated to ACE inhibitor therapy may be at increased risk of angioedema while receiving an ACE inhibitor (see also INDICATIONS AND USAGE and CONTRAINDICATIONS).
Anaphylactoid reactions during desensitization: Two patients undergoing desensitizing treatment with hymenoptera venom while receiving ACE inhibitors sustained life-threatening anaphylactoid reactions. In the same patients, these reactions were avoided when ACE inhibitors were temporarily withheld, but they reappeared upon inadvertent rechallenge.
Anaphylactoid reactions during membrane exposure: Anaphylactoid reactions have been reported in patients dialyzed with high-flux membranes and treated concomitantly with an ACE inhibitor. Anaphylactoid reactions have also been reported in patients undergoing low-density lipoprotein apheresis with dextran sulfate absorption.

Neutropenia/Agranulocytosis
Another angiotensin converting enzyme inhibitor, captopril, has been shown to cause agranulocytosis and bone marrow depression, rarely in uncomplicated patients but more frequently in patients with renal impairment especially if they also have a collagen vascular disease. Available data from clinical trials of enalapril are insufficient to show that enalapril does not cause agranulocytosis in similar rates. Marketing experience has revealed cases of neutropenia, or agranulocytosis in which a causal relationship to enalapril cannot be excluded. Periodic monitoring of white blood cell counts in patients with collagen vascular disease and renal disease should be considered.

Hepatic Failure
Rarely, ACE inhibitors have been associated with a syndrome that starts with cholestatic jaundice and progresses to fulminant hepatic necrosis, and (sometimes) death. The mechanism of this syndrome is not understood. Patients receiving ACE inhibitors who develop jaundice or marked elevations of hepatic enzymes should discontinue the ACE inhibitor and receive appropriate medical follow-up.

Fetal/Neonatal Morbidity and Mortality
ACE inhibitors can cause fetal and neonatal morbidity and death when administered to pregnant women. Several dozen cases have been reported in the world literature. When pregnancy is detected, ACE inhibitors should be discontinued as soon as possible.
The use of ACE inhibitors during the second and third trimesters of pregnancy has been associated with fetal and neonatal injury, including hypotension, neonatal skull hypoplasia, anuria, reversible or irreversible renal failure, and death. Oligohydramnios has also bee reported, presumably resulting from decreased fetal renal function: oligohydramnois in this setting has been associated with fetal limb contractures, craniofacial deformation, and hypoplastic lung development. Prematurity, intrauterine growth retardation, and patent ductus arteriosus have also been reported, although it is not clear whether these occurrences were due to the ACE-inhibitor exposure.
These adverse effects do not appear to have resulted from intrauterine ACE-inhibitor exposure that has been limited to the first trimester. Mothers whose embryos and fetuses are exposed to ACE inhibitors only during the first trimester should be so informed. Nonetheless, when patients become pregnant, physicians should make every effort to discontinue the use of VASOTEC I.V. as soon as possible.
Rarely (probably less often than once in every thousand pregnancies), no alternative to ACE inhibitors will be found. In these rare cases, the mothers should be apprised of the potential hazards to their fetuses, and serial ultrasound examinations should be performed to assess the intraamniotic environment.
If oligohydramnois is observed, VASOTEC I.V. should be discontinued unless it is considered lifesaving for the mother. Contraction stress testing (CST), a non-stress test (NST), or biophysical profiling (BPP) may be appropriate, depending upon the week of pregnancy. Patients and physi-

cians should be aware, however, that oligohydramnois may not appear until after the fetus has sustained irreversible injury.

Infants with histories of *in utero* exposure to ACE inhibitors should be closely observed for hypotension, oliguria, and hyperkalemia. If oliguria occurs, attention should be directed toward support of blood pressure and renal perfusion. Exchange transfusion or dialysis may be required as means of reversing hypotension and/or substituting for disordered renal function. Enalapril, which crosses the placenta, has been removed from neonatal circulation by peritoneal dialysis with some clinical benefit, and theoretically may be removed by exchange transfusion, although there is no experience with the latter procedure.

No teratogenic effects of oral enalapril were seen in studies of pregnant rats and rabbits. On a body surface area basis, the doses used were 57 times and 12 times, respectively, the maximum recommended human daily dose (MRHDD).

PRECAUTIONS

General

Aortic Stenosis/Hypertrophic Cardiomyopathy: As with all vasodilators, enalapril should be given with caution to patients with obstruction in the outflow tract of the left ventricle.

Impaired Renal Function: As a consequence of inhibiting the renin-angiotensin-aldosterone system, changes in renal function may be anticipated in susceptible individuals. In patients with severe heart failure whose renal function may depend on the activity of the renin-angiotensin-aldosterone system, treatment with angiotensin converting enzyme inhibitors, including enalapril or enalaprilat, may be associated with oliguria and/or progressive azotemia and rarely with acute renal failure and/or death.

In clinical studies in hypertensive patients with unilateral or bilateral renal artery stenosis, increases in blood urea nitrogen and serum creatinine were observed in 20 percent of patients receiving enalapril. These increases were almost always reversible upon discontinuation of enalapril or enalaprilat and/or diuretic therapy. In such patients renal function should be monitored during the first few weeks of therapy.

Some hypertensive patients with no apparent pre-existing renal vascular disease have developed increases in blood urea and serum creatinine, usually minor and transient, especially when enalaprilat has been given concomitantly with a diuretic. This is more likely to occur in patients with pre-existing renal impairment. Dosage reduction of enalaprilat and/or discontinuation of the diuretic may be required.

Evaluation of the hypertensive patient should always include assessment of renal function. (See DOSAGE AND ADMINISTRATION.)

Hyperkalemia: Elevated serum potassium (greater than 5.7 mEq/L) was observed in approximately one percent of hypertensive patients in clinical trials receiving enalapril. In most cases these were isolated values which resolved despite continued therapy. Hyperkalemia was a cause of discontinuation of therapy in 0.28 percent of hypertensive patients. Risk factors for the development of hyperkalemia include renal insufficiency, diabetes mellitus, and the concomitant use of potassium-sparing agents or potassium supplements, which should be used cautiously, if at all, with VASOTEC I.V. (See *Drug Interactions.*)

Cough: Presumably due to the inhibition of the degradation of endogenous bradykinin, persistent nonproductive cough has been reported with all ACE inhibitors, always resolving after discontinuation of therapy. ACE inhibitor-induced cough should be considered in the differential diagnosis of cough.

Surgery/Anesthesia: In patients undergoing major surgery or during anesthesia with agents that produce hypotension, enalapril may block angiotensin II formation secondary to compensatory renin release. If hypotension occurs and is considered to be due to this mechanism, it can be corrected by volume expansion.

Drug Interactions

Hypotension—Patients on Diuretic Therapy: Patients on diuretics and especially those in whom diuretic therapy was recently instituted, may occasionally experience an excessive reduction of blood pressure after initiation of therapy with enalaprilat. The possibility of hypotensive effects with enalaprilat can be minimized by administration of an intravenous infusion of normal saline, discontinuing the diuretic or increasing the salt intake prior to initiation of treatment with enalaprilat. If it is necessary to continue the diuretic, provide close medical supervision for at least one hour after the initial dose of enalaprilat. (See WARNINGS.)

Agents Causing Renin Release: The antihyertensive effect of VASOTEC I.V. appears to be augmented by antihypertensive agents that cause renin release (e.g., diuretics.)

Non-steroidal Anti-inflammatory Agents: In some patients with compromised renal function who are being treated with non-steroidal anti-inflammatory drugs, the co-administration of enalapril may result in a further deterioration of renal function. These effects are usually reversible.

In a clinical pharmacology study, indomethacin or sulindac was administered to hypertensive patients receiving enalapril maleate. In this study there was no evidence of a blunting of the antihypertensive action of enalapril maleate. However, reports suggest that NSAIDs may diminish the antihypertensive effect of ACE-inhibitors. This interaction should be given consideration in patients taking NSAIDs concomitantly with ACE-inhibitors.

Other Cardiovascular Agents: VASOTEC I.V. has been used concomitantly with digitalis, beta adrenergic-blocking agents, methyldopa, nitrates, calcium-blocking agents, hydralazine and prazosin without evidence of clinically significant adverse interactions.

Agents Increasing Serum Potassium: VASOTEC I.V. attenuates potassium loss caused by thiazide-type diuretics. Potassium-sparing diuretics (e.g., spironolactone, triamterene, or amiloride), potassium supplements, or potassium-containing salt substitutes may lead to significant increases in serum potassium. Therefore, if concomitant use of these agents is indicated because of demonstrated hypokalemia, they should be used with caution and with frequent monitoring of serum potassium.

Lithium: Lithium toxicity has been reported in patients receiving lithium concomitantly with drugs which cause elimination of sodium, including ACE inhibitors. A few cases of lithium toxicity have been reported in patients receiving concomitant enalapril and lithium and were reversible upon discontinuation of both drugs. It is recommended that serum lithium levels be monitored frequently if enalapril is administered concomitantly with lithium.

Carcinogenesis, Mutagenesis, Impairment of Fertility

Carcinogenicity studies have not been done with VASOTEC I.V.

VASOTEC I.V. is the bioactive form of its ethyl ester, enalapril maleate. There was no evidence of a tumorigenic effect when enalapril was administered for 106 weeks to male and female rats at doses up to 90 mg/kg/day or for 94 weeks to male and female mice at doses up to 90 and 180 mg/kg/day, respectively. These doses are 26 times (in rats and female mice) and 13 times (in male mice) the maximum recommended human daily dose (MRHDD) when compared on a body surface area basis.

VASOTEC I.V. was not mutagenic in the Ames microbial mutagen test with or without metabolic activation. Enalapril showed no drug-related changes in the following genotoxicity studies: rec-assay, reverse mutation assay with *E. coli,* sister chromatid exchange with cultured mammalian cells, the micronucleus test with mice, and in an *in vivo* cytogenic study using mouse bone marrow. There were no adverse effects on reproductive performance of male and female rats treated with up to 90 mg/kg/day of enalapril (26 times the MRHDD when compared on a body surface area basis).

Pregnancy

Pregnancy Categories C (first trimester) and *D* (second and third trimesters). See WARNINGS, *Fetal/Neonatal Morbidity and Mortality.*

Nursing Mothers

Enalapril and enalaprilat have been detected in human breast milk. Because of the potential for serious adverse reactions in nursing infants from enalapril, a decision should be made whether to discontinue nursing or to discontinue VASOTEC I.V., taking into account the importance of the drug to the mother.

Pediatric Use

Safety and effectiveness in pediatric patients have not been established.

ADVERSE REACTIONS

VASOTEC I.V. has been found to be generally well tolerated in controlled clinical trials involving 349 patients (168 with hypertension, 153 with congestive heart failure and 28 with coronary artery disease). The most frequent clinically significant adverse experience was hypotension (3.4 percent), occurring in eight patients (5.2 percent) with congestive heart failure, three (1.8 percent) with hypertension and one with coronary artery disease. Other adverse experiences occurring in greater than one percent of patients were: headache (2.9 percent) and nausea (1.1 percent).

Adverse experiences occurring in 0.5 to 1.0 percent of patients in controlled clinical trials included: myocardial infarction, fatigue, dizziness, fever, rash and constipation.

Angioedema: Angioedema has been reported in patients receiving enalaprilat, with an incidence higher in black than in non-black patients. Angioedema associated with laryngeal edema may be fatal. If angioedema of the face, extremities, lips, tongue, glottis and/or larynx occurs, treatment with enalaprilat should be discontinued and appropriate therapy instituted immediately. (See WARNINGS.)

Cough: See PRECAUTIONS, *Cough.*

Enalapril Maleate

Since enalapril is converted to enalaprilat, those adverse experiences associated with enalapril might also be expected to occur with VASOTEC I.V.

The following adverse experiences have been reported with enalapril and, within each category, are listed in order of decreasing severity.

Body As A Whole: Syncope, orthostatic effects, anaphylactoid reactions (see WARNINGS, *Anaphylactoid reactions during membrane exposure*), chest pain, abdominal pain, asthenia.

Cardiovascular: Cardiac arrest; myocardial infarction or cerebrovascular accident, possibly secondary to excessive hypotension in high risk patients (see WARNINGS, *Hypotension*); pulmonary embolism and infarction; pulmonary edema; rhythm disturbances including atrial tachycardia and bradycardia; atrial fibrillation; orthostatic hypotension; angina pectoris; palpitation, Raynaud's phenomenon.

Digestive: Ileus, pancreatitis, hepatic failure, hepatitis (hepatocellular [proven on rechallenge] or cholestatic jaundice) (see WARNINGS, *Hepatic Failure*), melena, diarrhea, vomiting, dyspepsia, anorexia, glossitis, stomatitis, dry mouth.

Hematologic: Rare cases of neutropenia, thrombocytopenia and bone marrow depression.

Musculoskeletal: Muscle cramps.

Nervous/Psychiatric: Depression, vertigo, confusion, ataxia, somnolence, insomnia, nervousness, peripheral neuropathy (e.g. paresthesia, dysesthesia), dream abnormality.

Respiratory: Bronchospasm, dyspnea, pneumonia, bronchitis, cough, rhinorrhea, sore throat and hoarseness, asthma, upper respiratory infection, pulmonary infiltrates, eosinophilic pneumonitis.

Skin: Exfoliative dermatitis, toxic epidermal necrolysis, Stevens-Johnson syndrome, pemphigus, herpes zoster, erythema multiforme, urticaria, pruritus, alopecia, flushing, diaphoresis, photosensitivity.

Special Senses: Blurred vision, taste alteration, anosmia, tinnitus, conjunctivitis, dry eyes, tearing.

Urogenital: Renal failure, oliguria, renal dysfunction (see PRECAUTIONS and DOSAGE AND ADMINISTRATION), urinary tract infection, flank pain, gynecomastia, impotence.

Miscellaneous: A symptom complex has been reported which may include some or all of the following: a positive ANA, an elevated erythrocyte sedimentation rate, arthralgia/arthritis, myalgia/myositis, fever, serositis, vasculitis, leukocytosis, eosinophilia, photosensitivity, rash and other dermatologic manifestations.

Hypotension: Combining the results of clinical trials in patients with hypertension or congestive heart failure, hypotension (including postural hypotension, and other orthostatic effects) was reported in 2.3 percent of patients following the initial dose of enalapril or during extended therapy. In the hypertensive patients, hypotension occurred in 0.9 percent and syncope occurred in 0.5 percent of patients. Hypotension or syncope was a cause for discontinuation of therapy in 0.1 percent of hypertensive patients. (See WARNINGS.)

Fetal/Neonatal Morbidity and Mortality: See WARNINGS, *Fetal/Neonatal Morbidity and Mortality.*

Clinical Laboratory Test Findings

Serum Electrolytes: Hyperkalemia (see PRECAUTIONS), hyponatremia.

Creatinine, Blood Urea Nitrogen: In controlled clinical trials minor increases in blood urea nitrogen and serum creatinine, reversible upon discontinuation of therapy, were observed in about 0.2 percent of patients with essential hypertension treated with enalapril alone. Increases are more likely to occur in patients receiving concomitant diuretics or in patients with renal artery stenosis. (See PRECAUTIONS.)

Hematology: Small decreases in hemoglobin and hematocrit (mean decreases of approximately 0.3 g percent and 1.0 vol percent, respectively) occur frequently in hypertensive patients treated with enalapril but are rarely of clinical importance unless another cause of anemia coexists. In clinical trials, less than 0.1 percent of patients discontinued therapy due to anemia. Hemolytic anemia, including cases of hemolysis in patients with G-6-PD deficiency, has been reported; a causal relationship to enalapril cannot be excluded.

Liver Function Tests: Elevations of liver enzymes and/or serum bilirubin have occurred (see WARNINGS, *Hepatic Failure*).

OVERDOSAGE

In clinical studies, some hypertensive patients received a maximum dose of 80 mg of enalaprilat intravenously over a fifteen minute period. At this high dose, no adverse effects beyond those as associated with the recommended dosages were observed.

A single intravenous dose of ≤ 4167 mg/kg of enalaprilat was associated with lethality in female mice. No lethality occurred after an intravenous dose of 3472 mg/kg.

The most likely manifestation of overdosage would be hypotension, for which the usual treatment would be intravenous infusion of normal saline solution.

Enalaprilat may be removed from general circulation by hemodialysis and has been removed from neonatal circulation by peritoneal dialysis. (See WARNINGS, *Anaphylactoid reactions during membrane exposure.*)

DOSAGE AND ADMINISTRATION

FOR INTRAVENOUS ADMINISTRATION ONLY

The dose in hypertension is 1.25 mg every six hours administered intravenously over a five minute period. A clinical response is usually seen within 15 minutes. Peak effects after the first dose may not occur for up to four hours after dosing. The peak effects of the second and subsequent doses may exceed those of the first.

Continued on next page

Information on the Merck & Co., Inc., products listed on these pages is from the prescribing information in use October 1, 2004. For information, please call 1-800-NSC-MERCK [1-800-672-6372].

Vasotec I.V.—Cont.

No dosage regimen for VASOTEC I.V. has been clearly demonstrated to be more effective in treating hypertension than 1.25 mg every six hours. However, in controlled clinical studies in hypertension, doses as high as 5 mg every six hours were well tolerated for up to 36 hours. There has been inadequate experience with doses greater than 20 mg per day.
In studies of patients with hypertension, VASOTEC I.V. has not been administered for periods longer than 48 hours. In other studies, patients have received VASOTEC I.V. for as long as seven days.
The dose for patients being converted to VASOTEC I.V. from oral therapy for hypertension with enalapril maleate is 1.25 mg every six hours. For conversion from intravenous to oral therapy, the recommended initial dose of Tablets VASOTEC (Enalapril Maleate) is 5 mg once a day with subsequent dosage adjustments as necessary.
Patients on Diuretic Therapy
For patients on diuretic therapy the recommended starting dose for hypertension is 0.625 mg administered intravenously over a five minute period. A clinical response is usually seen within 15 minutes. Peak effects after the first dose may not occur for up to four hours after dosing, although most of the effect is usually apparent within the first hour. If after one hour there is an inadequate clinical response, the 0.625 mg dose may be repeated. Additional doses of 1.25 mg may be administered at six hour intervals.
For conversion from intravenous to oral therapy, the recommended initial dose of Tablets VASOTEC (Enalapril Maleate) for patients who have responded to 0.625 mg of enalaprilat every six hours is 2.5 mg once a day with subsequent dosage adjustment as necessary.
Dosage Adjustment in Renal Impairment
The usual dose of 1.25 mg of enalaprilat every six hours is recommended for patients with a creatinine clearance >30 mL/min (serum creatinine of up to approximately 3 mg/dL). For patients with creatinine clearance ≤30 mL/min (serum creatinine ≥3 mg/dL), the initial dose is 0.625 mg. (See WARNINGS.)
If after one hour there is an inadequate clinical response, the 0.625 mg dose may be repeated. Additional doses of 1.25 mg may be administered at six hour intervals.
For dialysis patients, see below, *Patients at Risk of Excessive Hypotension.*
For conversion from intravenous to oral therapy, the recommended initial dose of Tablets VASOTEC (Enalapril Maleate) is 5 mg once a day for patients with creatinine clearance >30 mL/min and 2.5 mg once daily for patients with creatinine clearance ≤30 mL/min. Dosage should then be adjusted according to blood pressure response.
Patients at Risk of Excessive Hypotension
Hypertensive patients at risk of excessive hypotension include those with the following concurrent conditions or characteristics: heart failure, hyponatremia, high dose diuretic therapy, recent intensive diuresis or increase in diuretic dose, renal dialysis, or severe volume and/or salt depletion of any etiology (see WARNINGS). Single doses of enalaprilat as low as 0.2 mg have produced excessive hypotension in normotensive patients with these diagnoses. Because of the potential for an extreme hypotensive response in these patients, therapy should be started under very close medical supervision. The starting dose should be no greater than 0.625 mg administered intravenously over a period of no less than five minutes and preferably longer (up to one hour).
Patients should be followed closely whenever the dose of enalaprilat is adjusted and/or diuretic is increased.
Administration
VASOTEC I.V. should be administered as a slow intravenous infusion, as indicated above, over at least five minutes. It may be administered as provided or diluted with up to 50 mL of a compatible diluent.
Parenteral drug products should be inspected visually for particulate matter and discoloration prior to use whenever solution and container permit.
Compatibility and Stability
VASOTEC I.V. as supplied and mixed with the following intravenous diluents has been found to maintain full activity for 24 hours at room temperature:
5 percent Dextrose Injection
0.9 percent Sodium Chloride Injection
0.9 percent Sodium Chloride Injection in 5 percent Dextrose
5 percent Dextrose in Lactated Ringer's Injection
McGaw ISOLYTE* E.

*Registered trademark of American Hospital Supply Corporation.

HOW SUPPLIED

No. 3824—VASOTEC I.V., 1.25 mg per mL, is a clear, colorless solution and is supplied in vials containing 1 mL and 2 mL.
NDC 0006-3824-01, 1 mL vials
NDC 0006-3824-04, 2 mL vials.
Storage
Store at 25°C (77°F); excursions permitted to 15–30°C (59–86°F) [see USP Controlled Room Temperature].
7875732 Issued November 2001

VASOTEC* Tablets ℞
(enalapril maleate)
Distributed by Biovail Pharmaceuticals, Inc.
Morrisville, NC 27560
To make additional inquiries or to report an adverse event, please contact Biovail Pharmaceuticals, Inc. at 1-866-276-1030.

*Registered trademark of Biovail Pharmaceuticals, Inc.

VIOXX® ℞
[vi-oks]
(rofecoxib tablets and oral suspension)

DESCRIPTION

VIOXX* (rofecoxib) is described chemically as 4-[4-(methylsulfonyl)phenyl]-3-phenyl-2(*5H*)-furanone. It has the following chemical structure:

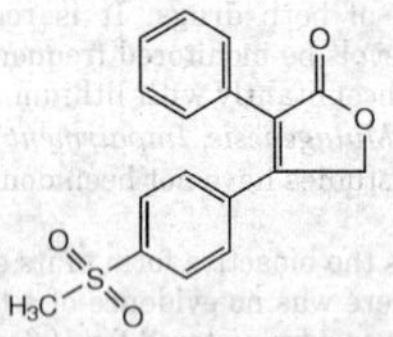

Rofecoxib is a white to off-white to light yellow powder. It is sparingly soluble in acetone, slightly soluble in methanol and isopropyl acetate, very slightly soluble in ethanol, practically insoluble in octanol, and insoluble in water. The empirical formula for rofecoxib is $C_{17}H_{14}O_4S$, and the molecular weight is 314.36.
Each tablet of VIOXX for oral administration contains either 12.5 mg, 25 mg, or 50 mg of rofecoxib and the following inactive ingredients: croscarmellose sodium, hydroxypropyl cellulose, lactose, magnesium stearate, microcrystalline cellulose, and yellow ferric oxide. The 50 mg tablets also contain red ferric oxide.
Each 5 mL of the oral suspension contains either 12.5 or 25 mg of rofecoxib and the following inactive ingredients: citric acid (monohydrate), sodium citrate (dihydrate), sorbitol solution, strawberry flavor, xanthan gum, and purified water. Added as preservatives are sodium methylparaben 0.13% and sodium propylparaben 0.02%.

* Registered trademark of MERCK & CO., Inc., Whitehouse Station, New Jersey, USA

CLINICAL PHARMACOLOGY

Mechanism of Action
VIOXX is a nonsteroidal anti-inflammatory drug (NSAID) that exhibits anti-inflammatory, analgesic, and antipyretic activities in animal models. The mechanism of action of VIOXX is believed to be due to inhibition of prostaglandin synthesis, via inhibition of cyclooxygenase-2 (COX-2). At therapeutic concentrations in humans, VIOXX does not inhibit the cyclooxygenase-1 (COX-1) isoenzyme. Studies to elucidate the mechanism of action of VIOXX in the acute treatment of migraine have not been conducted.
Pharmacokinetics
Absorption
The mean oral bioavailability of VIOXX at therapeutically recommended doses of 12.5, 25, and 50 mg is approximately 93%. The area under the curve (AUC) and peak plasma level (C_{max}) following a single 25-mg dose were 3286 (±843) ng•hr/mL and 207 (±111) ng/mL, respectively. Both C_{max} and AUC are roughly dose proportional across the clinical dose range. At doses greater than 50 mg, there is a less than proportional increase in C_{max} and AUC, which is thought to be due to the low solubility of the drug in aqueous media. The plasma concentration-time profile exhibited multiple peaks. The median time to maximal concentration (T_{max}), as assessed in nine pharmacokinetic studies, is 2 to 3 hours. Individual T_{max} values in these studies ranged between 2 to 9 hours. This may not reflect rate of absorption as T_{max} may occur as a secondary peak in some individuals. With multiple dosing, steady-state conditions are reached by Day 4. The $AUC_{0\text{-}24hr}$ and C_{max} at steady state after multiple doses of 25 mg rofecoxib was 4018 (±1140) ng•hr/mL and 321 (±104) ng/mL, respectively. The accumulation factor based on geometric means was 1.67.
VIOXX Tablets 12.5 mg and 25 mg are bioequivalent to VIOXX Oral Suspension 12.5 mg/5 mL and 25 mg/5 mL, respectively.
Food and Antacid Effects
Food had no significant effect on either the peak plasma concentration (C_{max}) or extent of absorption (AUC) of rofecoxib when VIOXX Tablets were taken with a high fat meal. The time to peak plasma concentration (T_{max}), however, was delayed by 1 to 2 hours. The food effect on the suspension formulation has not been studied. VIOXX tablets can be administered without regard to timing of meals. There was a 13% and 8% decrease in AUC when VIOXX was administered with calcium carbonate antacid and magnesium/aluminum antacid to elderly subjects, respectively. There was an approximate 20% decrease in C_{max} of rofecoxib with either antacid.
Distribution
Rofecoxib is approximately 87% bound to human plasma protein over the range of concentrations of 0.05 to 25 mcg/mL. The apparent volume of distribution at steady state (V_{dss}) is approximately 91 L following a 12.5-mg dose and 86 L following a 25-mg dose.
Rofecoxib has been shown to cross the placenta in rats and rabbits, and the blood-brain barrier in rats.
Metabolism
Metabolism of rofecoxib is primarily mediated through reduction by cytosolic enzymes. The principal metabolic products are the cis-dihydro and trans-dihydro derivatives of rofecoxib, which account for nearly 56% of recovered radioactivity in the urine. An additional 8.8% of the dose was recovered as the glucuronide of the hydroxy derivative, a product of oxidative metabolism. The biotransformation of rofecoxib and this metabolite is reversible in humans to a limited extent (<5%). These metabolites are inactive as COX-1 or COX-2 inhibitors.
Cytochrome P450 plays a minor role in metabolism of rofecoxib. Inhibition of CYP 3A activity by administration of ketoconazole 400 mg daily does not affect rofecoxib disposition. However, induction of general hepatic metabolic activity by administration of the non-specific inducer rifampin 600 mg daily produces a 50% decrease in rofecoxib plasma concentrations. (Also see *Drug Interactions.*)
Excretion
Rofecoxib is eliminated predominantly by hepatic metabolism with little (<1%) unchanged drug recovered in the urine. Following a single radiolabeled dose of 125 mg, approximately 72% of the dose was excreted into the urine as metabolites and 14% in the feces as unchanged drug.
The plasma clearance after 12.5- and 25-mg doses was approximately 141 and 120 mL/min, respectively. Higher plasma clearance was observed at doses below the therapeutic range, suggesting the presence of a saturable route of metabolism (i.e., non-linear elimination). The effective half-life (based on steady-state levels) was approximately 17 hours.
Special Populations
Gender
The pharmacokinetics of rofecoxib are comparable in men and women.
Geriatric
After a single dose of 25 mg VIOXX in elderly subjects (over 65 years old) a 34% increase in AUC was observed as compared to the young subjects. Dosage adjustment in the elderly is not necessary; however, therapy with VIOXX should be initiated at the lowest recommended dose.
Pediatric
VIOXX has not been investigated in patients below 18 years of age.
Race
Meta-analysis of pharmacokinetic studies has suggested a slightly (10-15%) higher AUC of rofecoxib in Blacks and Hispanics as compared to Caucasians. No dosage adjustment is necessary on the basis of race.
Hepatic Insufficiency
A single-dose pharmacokinetic study in mild (Child-Pugh score ≤6) hepatic insufficiency patients indicated that rofecoxib AUC was similar between these patients and healthy subjects. A pharmacokinetic study in patients with moderate (Child-Pugh score 7-9) hepatic insufficiency indicated that mean rofecoxib plasma concentrations were higher (mean AUC: 55%; mean C_{max}: 53%) relative to healthy subjects. Since patients with hepatic insufficiency are prone to fluid retention and hemodynamic compromise, the maximum recommended chronic dose of VIOXX for patients with moderate hepatic insufficiency is 12.5 mg daily. (See PRECAUTIONS, *Hepatic Effects* and DOSAGE AND ADMINISTRATION, *Hepatic Insufficiency.*) Patients with severe hepatic insufficiency have not been studied.
Renal Insufficiency
In a study (N=6) of patients with end stage renal disease undergoing dialysis, peak rofecoxib plasma levels and AUC declined 18% and 9%, respectively, when dialysis occurred four hours after dosing. When dialysis occurred 48 hours after dosing, the elimination profile of rofecoxib was unchanged. While renal insufficiency does not influence the pharmacokinetics of rofecoxib, use of VIOXX in advanced renal disease is not recommended. (See WARNINGS, *Advanced Renal Disease.*)
Drug Interactions (Also see PRECAUTIONS, *Drug Interactions.*)
General
In human studies the potential for rofecoxib to inhibit or induce CYP 3A4 activity was investigated in studies using the intravenous erythromycin breath test and the oral midazolam test. No significant difference in erythromycin demethylation was observed with rofecoxib (75 mg daily) compared to placebo, indicating no induction of hepatic CYP 3A4. A 30% reduction of the AUC of midazolam was observed with rofecoxib (25 mg daily). This reduction is most likely due to increased first pass metabolism through induction of intestinal CYP 3A4 by rofecoxib. *In vitro* studies in rat hepatocytes also suggest that rofecoxib might be a mild inducer for CYP 3A4.
Drug interaction studies with the recommended doses of rofecoxib have identified potentially significant interactions with rifampin, theophylline, and warfarin. Patients receiving these agents with VIOXX should be appropriately monitored. Drug interaction studies do not support the potential for clinically important interactions between antacids or cimetidine with rofecoxib. Similar to experience with other

nonsteroidal anti-inflammatory drugs (NSAIDs), studies with rofecoxib suggest the potential for interaction with ACE inhibitors. The effects of rofecoxib on the pharmacokinetics and/or pharmacodynamics of ketoconazole, prednisone/prednisolone, oral contraceptives, and digoxin have been studied *in vivo* and clinically important interactions have not been found.

CLINICAL STUDIES

Osteoarthritis (OA)

VIOXX has demonstrated significant reduction in joint pain compared to placebo. VIOXX was evaluated for the treatment of the signs and symptoms of OA of the knee and hip in placebo- and active-controlled clinical trials of 6 to 86 weeks duration that enrolled approximately 3900 patients. In patients with OA, treatment with VIOXX 12.5 mg and 25 mg once daily resulted in improvement in patient and physician global assessments and in the WOMAC (Western Ontario and McMaster Universities) osteoarthritis questionnaire, including pain, stiffness, and functional measures of OA. In six studies of pain accompanying OA flare, VIOXX provided a significant reduction in pain at the first determination (after one week in one study, after two weeks in the remaining five studies); this continued for the duration of the studies. In all OA clinical studies, once daily treatment in the morning with VIOXX 12.5 and 25 mg was associated with a significant reduction in joint stiffness upon first awakening in the morning. At doses of 12.5 and 25 mg, the effectiveness of VIOXX was shown to be comparable to ibuprofen 800 mg TID and diclofenac 50 mg TID for treatment of the signs and symptoms of OA. The ibuprofen studies were 6-week studies; the diclofenac studies were 12-month studies in which patients could receive additional arthritis medication during the last 6 months.

Rheumatoid Arthritis (RA)

VIOXX has demonstrated significant reduction of joint tenderness/pain and joint swelling compared to placebo. VIOXX was evaluated for the treatment of the signs and symptoms of RA in two 12-week placebo- and active-controlled clinical trials that enrolled a total of approximately 2,000 patients. VIOXX was shown to be superior to placebo on all primary endpoints (number of tender joints, number of swollen joints, patient and physician global assessments of disease activity). In addition, VIOXX was shown to be superior to placebo using the American College of Rheumatology 20% (ACR20) Responder Index, a composite of clinical, laboratory, and functional measures of RA. VIOXX 25 mg once daily and naproxen 500 mg twice daily showed generally similar effects in the treatment of RA. A 50-mg dose once daily of VIOXX was also studied; however, no additional efficacy was seen compared to the 25-mg dose.

Analgesia, including Dysmenorrhea

In acute analgesic models of post-operative dental pain, post-orthopedic surgical pain, and primary dysmenorrhea, VIOXX relieved pain that was rated by patients as moderate to severe. The analgesic effect (including onset of action) of a single 50-mg dose of VIOXX was generally similar to 550 mg of naproxen sodium or 400 mg of ibuprofen. In single-dose post-operative dental pain studies, the onset of analgesia with a single 50-mg dose of VIOXX occurred within 45 minutes. In a multiple-dose study of post-orthopedic surgical pain in which patients received VIOXX or placebo for up to 5 days, 50 mg of VIOXX once daily was effective in reducing pain. In this study, patients on VIOXX consumed a significantly smaller amount of additional analgesic medication than patients treated with placebo (1.5 versus 2.5 doses per day of additional analgesic medication for VIOXX and placebo, respectively).

Migraine with or without aura

The efficacy of VIOXX in the acute treatment of migraine headaches was demonstrated in two double-blind, placebo-controlled, outpatient trials. Doses of 25 and 50 mg were compared to placebo in the treatment of one migraine attack. A second dose of VIOXX was not allowed in either trial. In these controlled short-term studies, patients were predominantly female (88%) and Caucasian (84%), with a mean age of 40 years (range 18 to 78). Patients were instructed to treat a moderate to severe headache. Headache relief, defined as a reduction in headache severity from moderate or severe pain to mild or no pain, was assessed up to 2 hours after dosing. Associated symptoms such as nausea, photophobia, and phonophobia were also assessed. Maintenance of relief was assessed for up to 24 hours post-dose. Other medication, with the exception of NSAIDs (including COX-2 inhibitors) or combination medications that contained NSAIDs, was permitted from 2 hours after the dose of study medication. The frequency and time to use of additional medications were also recorded.

In both placebo-controlled trials, the percentage of patients achieving headache relief 2 hours after treatment was significantly greater among patients receiving VIOXX at all doses compared to those who received placebo (Table 1). There were no statistically significant differences between the 25- and the 50-mg dose groups in either trial.

[See table 1 above]

Note that, in general, comparisons of results obtained in different clinical studies conducted under different conditions by different investigators with different samples of patients are ordinarily unreliable for purposes of quantitative comparison.

Table 1
Percentage of Patients with Headache Relief (Mild or No Headache) 2 hours Following Treatment

Trial	VIOXX 25 mg	VIOXX 50 mg	Placebo
1	54%* (n=176)	57%* (n=187)	34% (n=175)
2	60%* (n=187)	62%* (n=188)	30% (n=187)

*p<0.0001 vs. placebo

Table 2
VIGOR-Summary of Patients with Gastrointestinal Safety Events[1]
COMPARISON TO NAPROXEN

GI Safety Endpoints	VIOXX 50 mg daily (N=4047)[2] n[3] (Cumulative Rate[4])	Naproxen 1000 mg daily (N=4029)[2] n[3] (Cumulative Rate[4])	Relative Risk of VIOXX compared to naproxen[5]	95% CI[5]
PUBs	56 (1.80)	121 (3.87)	0.46*	(0.33, 0.64)
Complicated PUBs	16 (0.52)	37 (1.22)	0.43*	(0.24, 0.78)

[1]As confirmed by an independent committee blinded to treatment,
[2]N=Patients randomized,
[3]n=Patients with events,
[4]Kaplan-Meier cumulative rate at end of study when at least 500 patients remained (approx. 10 1/2 months),
[5]Based on Cox proportional hazard model
*p-value ≤0.005 for relative risk compared to naproxen

The estimated probability of achieving initial headache relief within 2 hours following treatment is depicted in Figure 1.

Figure 1
Estimated Probability of Achieving Initial Headache Relief within 2 Hours

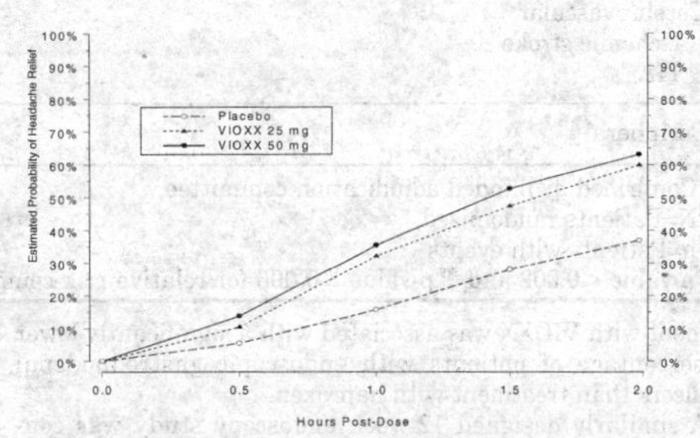

Figure 1 shows the Kaplan-Meier plot of the probability over time of obtaining headache relief (no or mild pain) following treatment with VIOXX or placebo. The plot is based on pooled data from the 2 placebo-controlled, outpatient trials in adults providing evidence of efficacy. Patients taking additional medication or not achieving headache relief prior to 2 hours were censored at 2 hours.

There was a decreased incidence of migraine-associated nausea, photophobia and phonophobia in VIOXX treated patients compared to placebo. The estimated probability of taking other medication for migraine over the 24 hours following initial dose of study treatment is summarized in Figure 2.

Figure 2
Estimated Probability of Patients Taking Additional Medication for Migraines over the 24 Hours Following the Initial Dose of Study Treatment

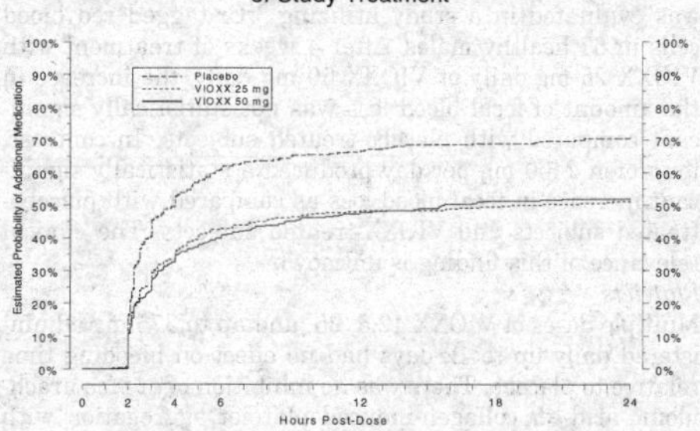

This Kaplan-Meier plot is based on pooled data obtained in 2 placebo-controlled outpatient trials. Patients not using additional medications were censored at 24 hours. The plot includes both patients who had headache relief at 2 hours and those who had no response to the initial dose. Additional medication was not allowed within 2 hours postdose.

VIOXX was effective regardless of presence of aura, gender, race, age, presence of menses or dysmenorrhea. Similarly, the concomitant use of common migraine prophylactic drugs (e.g., beta-blockers, calcium channel blockers, tricyclic antidepressants) or oral contraceptives did not affect efficacy. VIOXX was also effective whether or not there was a history of prior response to NSAIDs.

Special Studies

The following special studies were conducted to evaluate the comparative safety of VIOXX.

VIOXX GI Clinical Outcomes Research (VIGOR Study)

Study Design

The VIGOR study was designed to evaluate the comparative GI safety of VIOXX 50 mg once daily (twice the highest dose recommended for chronic use in OA and RA) versus naproxen 500 mg twice daily (common therapeutic dose). The general safety and tolerability of VIOXX 50 mg once daily versus naproxen 500 mg twice daily was also studied. VIGOR was a randomized, double-blind study (median duration of 9 months) in 8076 patients with rheumatoid arthritis (RA) requiring chronic NSAID therapy (mean age 58 years). Patients were not permitted to use concomitant aspirin or other antiplatelet drugs. Patients with a recent history of myocardial infarction or stroke and patients deemed to require low-dose aspirin for cardiovascular prophylaxis were to be excluded from the study. Fifty-six percent of patients used concomitant oral corticosteroids. The GI safety endpoints (confirmed by a blinded adjudication committee) included:

PUBs-symptomatic ulcers, upper GI perforation, obstruction, major or minor upper GI bleeding.

Complicated PUBs (a subset of PUBs)-upper GI perforation, obstruction or major upper GI bleeding.

Study Results

Gastrointestinal Safety in VIGOR

The VIGOR study showed a significant reduction in the risk of development of PUBs, including complicated PUBs in patients taking VIOXX compared to naproxen (see Table 2).

[See table 2 above]

The risk reduction for PUBs and complicated PUBs for VIOXX compared to naproxen (approximately 50%) was maintained in patients with or without the following risk factors for developing a PUB (Kaplan-Meier cumulative rate of PUBs at approximately 10 1/2 months, VIOXX versus naproxen, respectively): with a prior PUB (5.12, 11.47); without a prior PUB (1.54, 3.27); age 65 or older (2.83, 6.49); or younger than 65 years of age (1.48, 3.01). A similar risk reduction for PUBs and complicated PUBs (approximately 50%) was also maintained in patients with or without *Helicobacter pylori* infection or concomitant corticosteroid use.

Other Safety Findings: Cardiovascular Safety

The VIGOR study showed a higher incidence of adjudicated serious cardiovascular thrombotic events in patients treated with VIOXX 50 mg once daily as compared to patients treated with naproxen 500 mg twice daily (see Table 3). This finding was largely due to a difference in the incidence of myocardial infarction between the groups. (See Table 4.) (See PRECAUTIONS, *Cardiovascular Effects*.) Adjudicated serious cardiovascular events (confirmed by a blinded adjudication committee) included: sudden death, myocardial infarction, unstable angina, ischemic stroke, transient ischemic attack and peripheral venous and arterial thromboses.

[See table 3 at top of next page]
[See table 4 at top of next page]

For cardiovascular data from 2 long-term placebo-controlled studies, see PRECAUTIONS, *Cardiovascular Effects*.

Upper Endoscopy in Patients with Osteoarthritis and Rheumatoid Arthritis

The VIGOR study described above compared clinically relevant outcomes. Several studies summarized below have utilized scheduled endoscopic evaluations to assess the occurrence of asymptomatic ulcers in individual patients taking VIOXX or a comparative agent. The results of outcomes studies, such as VIGOR, are more clinically relevant than the results of endoscopy studies (see CLINICAL STUDIES, *Special Studies, VIGOR*).

Continued on next page

Information on the Merck & Co., Inc., products listed on these pages is from the prescribing information in use October 1, 2004. For information, please call 1-800-NSC-MERCK [1-800-672-6372].

Vioxx—Cont.

Two identical (U.S. and Multinational) endoscopy studies in a total of 1516 patients were conducted to compare the percentage of patients who developed endoscopically detectable gastroduodenal ulcers with VIOXX 25 mg daily or 50 mg daily, ibuprofen 2400 mg daily, or placebo. Entry criteria for these studies permitted enrollment of patients with active *Helicobacter pylori* infection, baseline gastroduodenal erosions, prior history of an upper gastrointestinal perforation, ulcer, or bleed (PUB), and/or age ≥65 years. However, patients receiving aspirin (including low-dose aspirin for cardiovascular prophylaxis) were not enrolled in these studies. Patients who were 50 years of age and older with osteoarthritis and who had no ulcers at baseline were evaluated by endoscopy after weeks 6, 12, and 24 of treatment. The placebo-treatment group was discontinued at week 16 by design.

Treatment with VIOXX 25 mg daily or 50 mg daily was associated with a significantly lower percentage of patients with endoscopic gastroduodenal ulcers than treatment with ibuprofen 2400 mg daily. See Figures 3 and 4 for the results of these studies.

Figure 3

COMPARISON TO IBUPROFEN

Life-Table Cumulative Incidence Rate of Gastroduodenal Ulcers ≥ 3 mm (Intention-to-Treat)**

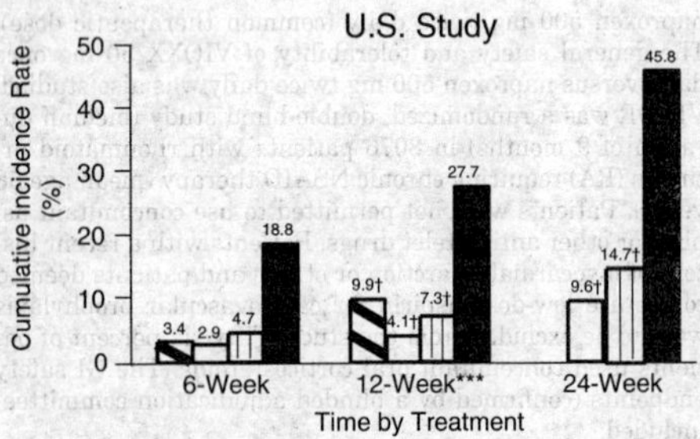

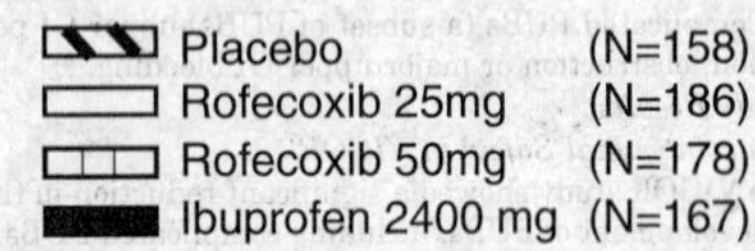

† p < 0.001 versus ibuprofen 2400 mg
** Results of analyses using a ≥ 5mm gastroduodenal ulcer endpoint were consistent.
*** The primary endpoint was the cumulative incidence of gastroduodenal ulcer at 12 weeks.

Figure 4

COMPARISON TO IBUPROFEN

Life-Table Cumulative Incidence Rate of Gastroduodenal Ulcers ≥ 3 mm (Intention-to-Treat)**

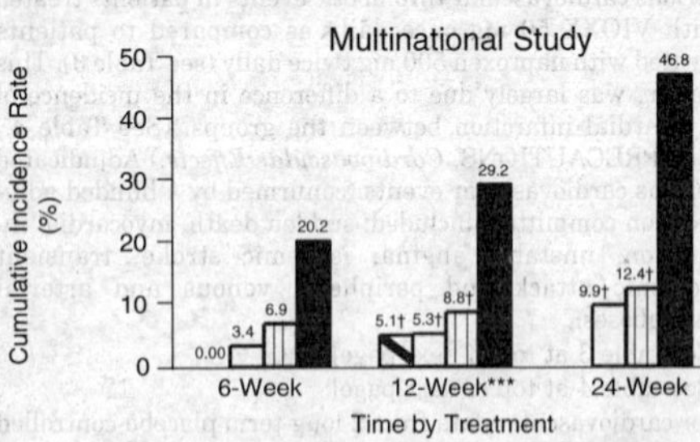

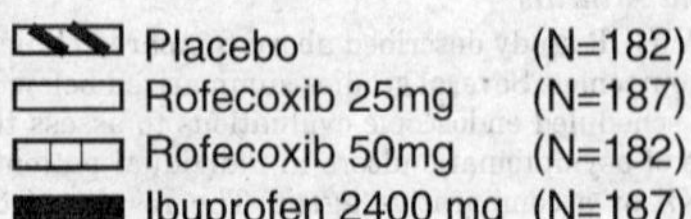

† p < 0.001 versus ibuprofen 2400 mg
** Results of analyses using a ≥ 5mm gastroduodenal ulcer endpoint were consistent.
*** The primary endpoint was the cumulative incidence of gastroduodenal ulcer at 12 weeks.

In a similarly designed 12-week endoscopy study in RA patients treated with VIOXX 50 mg once daily (twice the highest dose recommended for chronic use in OA and RA) or naproxen 1000 mg daily (common therapeutic dose), treatment with VIOXX was associated with a significantly lower percentage of patients with endoscopic gastroduodenal ulcers than treatment with naproxen.

Table 3
VIGOR-Summary of Patients with Serious Cardiovascular Thrombotic Adverse Events[1] Over Time
COMPARISON TO NAPROXEN

Treatment Group	Patients Randomized		4 Months[2]	8 Months[3]	10 ½ months[4]
VIOXX 50 mg	4047	Total number of events	17	29	45
		Cumulative Rate†	0.46%	0.82%	1.81%*
Naproxen 1000 mg	4029	Total number of events	9	15	19
		Cumulative Rate†	0.23%	0.43%	0.60%

[1]Confirmed by blinded adjudication committee,
[2]Number of patients remaining after 4 months were 3405 and 3395 for VIOXX and naproxen respectively,
[3]Number of patients remaining after 8 months were 2806 and 2798 for VIOXX and naproxen respectively,
[4]Number of patients remaining were 531 and 514 for VIOXX and naproxen respectively.
†Kaplan-Meier cumulative rate.
*p-value <0.002 for the overall relative risk compared to naproxen by Cox proportional hazard model

Table 4
VIGOR-Serious Cardiovascular Thrombotic Adverse Events[1]

	VIOXX 50 mg N[2]=4047 n[3]	**Naproxen 1000 mg N[2]=4029 n[3]**
Any CV thrombotic event	45 *	19
Cardiac events	28**	10
Fatal MI/Sudden death	5	4
Non-fatal MI	18**	4
Unstable angina	5	2
Cerebrovascular	11	8
Ischemic stroke	9	8
TIA	2	0
Peripheral	6	1

[1]Confirmed by blinded adjudication committee,
[2]N=Patients randomized,
[3]n=Patients with events
*p-value <0.002 and **p-value ≤0.006 for relative risk compared to naproxen by Cox proportional hazard model

A similarly designed 12-week endoscopy study was conducted in OA patients treated with low-dose enteric coated aspirin 81 mg daily, low-dose enteric coated aspirin 81 mg plus VIOXX 25 mg daily, ibuprofen 2400 mg daily, or placebo. There was no difference in the cumulative incidence of endoscopic gastroduodenal ulcers in patients taking low-dose aspirin plus VIOXX 25 mg as compared to those taking ibuprofen 2400 mg daily alone. Patients taking low-dose aspirin plus ibuprofen were not studied. (See PRECAUTIONS, *Drug Interactions, Aspirin.*)

Serious clinically significant upper GI bleeding has been observed in patients receiving VIOXX in controlled trials, albeit infrequently (see WARNINGS, *Gastrointestinal (GI) Effects - Risk of GI Ulceration, Bleeding, and Perforation*).

Assessment of Fecal Occult Blood Loss in Healthy Subjects

Occult fecal blood loss associated with VIOXX 25 mg daily, VIOXX 50 mg daily, ibuprofen 2400 mg per day, and placebo was evaluated in a study utilizing ^{51}Cr-tagged red blood cells in 67 healthy males. After 4 weeks of treatment with VIOXX 25 mg daily or VIOXX 50 mg daily, the increase in the amount of fecal blood loss was not statistically significant compared with placebo-treated subjects. In contrast, ibuprofen 2400 mg per day produced a statistically significant increase in fecal blood loss as compared with placebo-treated subjects and VIOXX-treated subjects. The clinical relevance of this finding is unknown.

Platelets

Multiple doses of VIOXX 12.5, 25, and up to 375 mg administered daily up to 12 days had no effect on bleeding time relative to placebo. There was no inhibition of *ex vivo* arachidonic acid- or collagen-induced platelet aggregation with 12.5, 25, and 50 mg of VIOXX.

Because of its lack of platelet effects, VIOXX is not a substitute for aspirin for cardiovascular prophylaxis. (See PRECAUTIONS, *Cardiovascular Effects.*)

INDICATIONS AND USAGE

VIOXX is indicated:
For relief of the signs and symptoms of osteoarthritis.
For relief of the signs and symptoms of rheumatoid arthritis in adults.
For the management of acute pain in adults.
For the treatment of primary dysmenorrhea.
For the acute treatment of migraine attacks with or without aura in adults.
The safety and effectiveness of VIOXX have not been established for cluster headache, which is present in an older, predominantly male, population.

CONTRAINDICATIONS

VIOXX is contraindicated in patients with known hypersensitivity to rofecoxib or any other component of VIOXX.

VIOXX should not be given to patients who have experienced asthma, urticaria, or allergic-type reactions after taking aspirin or other NSAIDs. Severe, rarely fatal, anaphylactic-like reactions to NSAIDs have been reported in such patients (see WARNINGS, *Anaphylactoid Reactions* and PRECAUTIONS, *Preexisting Asthma*).

WARNINGS

Gastrointestinal (GI) Effects - Risk of GI Ulceration, Bleeding, and Perforation

Serious gastrointestinal toxicity such as bleeding, ulceration, and perforation of the stomach, small intestine or large intestine, can occur at any time, with or without warning symptoms, in patients treated with nonsteroidal anti-inflammatory drugs (NSAIDs). Minor upper gastrointestinal problems, such as dyspepsia, are common and may also occur at any time during NSAID therapy. Therefore, physicians and patients should remain alert for ulceration and bleeding, even in the absence of previous GI tract symptoms. Patients should be informed about the signs and/or symptoms of serious GI toxicity and the steps to take if they occur. The utility of periodic laboratory monitoring has not been demonstrated, nor has it been adequately assessed. Only one in five patients who develop a serious upper GI adverse event on NSAID therapy is symptomatic. It has been demonstrated that upper GI ulcers, gross bleeding or perforation, caused by NSAIDs, appear to occur in approximately 1% of patients treated for 3-6 months, and in about 2-4% of patients treated for one year. These trends continue thus, increasing the likelihood of developing a serious GI event at some time during the course of therapy. However, even short-term therapy is not without risk.

Although the risk of GI toxicity is not completely eliminated with VIOXX, the results of the VIOXX GI outcomes research (VIGOR) study demonstrate that in patients treated with VIOXX, the risk of GI toxicity with VIOXX 50 mg once daily is significantly less than with naproxen 500 mg twice daily. (See CLINICAL STUDIES, *Special Studies, VIGOR.*)

NSAIDs should be prescribed with extreme caution in patients with a prior history of ulcer disease or gastrointestinal bleeding. Most spontaneous reports of fatal GI events are in elderly or debilitated patients and therefore special care should be taken in treating this population. **To minimize the potential risk for an adverse GI event, the lowest effective dose should be used for the shortest possible duration.** For high risk patients, alternate therapies that do not involve NSAIDs should be considered.

Previous studies have shown that patients with a *prior history of peptic ulcer disease and/or gastrointestinal bleeding* and who use NSAIDs, have a greater than 10-fold higher risk for developing a GI bleed than patients with neither of these risk factors. In addition to a past history of ulcer disease, pharmacoepidemiological studies have identified several other co-therapies or co-morbid conditions that may increase the risk for GI bleeding such as: treatment with oral corticosteroids, treatment with anticoagulants, longer duration of NSAID therapy, smoking, alcoholism, older age, and poor general health status.

Anaphylactoid Reactions

As with NSAIDs in general, anaphylactoid reactions have occurred in patients without known prior exposure to VIOXX. In post-marketing experience, rare cases of anaphylactic/anaphylactoid reactions and angioedema have been reported in patients receiving VIOXX. VIOXX should not be given to patients with the aspirin triad. This symptom complex typically occurs in asthmatic patients who experience rhinitis with or without nasal polyps, or who exhibit severe, potentially fatal bronchospasm after taking aspirin or other NSAIDs (see CONTRAINDICATIONS and PRECAUTIONS, *Preexisting Asthma*). Emergency help should be sought in cases where an anaphylactoid reaction occurs.

Advanced Renal Disease

Treatment with VIOXX is not recommended in patients with advanced renal disease. If VIOXX therapy must be initiated, close monitoring of the patient's kidney function is advisable (see PRECAUTIONS, *Renal Effects*).

Pregnancy

In late pregnancy VIOXX should be avoided because it may cause premature closure of the ductus arteriosus.

PRECAUTIONS

General

VIOXX cannot be expected to substitute for corticosteroids or to treat corticosteroid insufficiency. Abrupt discontinuation of corticosteroids may lead to exacerbation of corticosteroid-responsive illness. Patients on prolonged corticosteroid therapy should have their therapy tapered slowly if a decision is made to discontinue corticosteroids.

The pharmacological activity of VIOXX in reducing inflammation, and possibly fever, may diminish the utility of these diagnostic signs in detecting infectious complications of presumed noninfectious, painful conditions.

Cardiovascular Effects

The information below should be taken into consideration and caution should be exercised when VIOXX is used in patients with a medical history of ischemic heart disease.

In VIGOR, a study in 8076 patients (mean age 58; VIOXX n=4047, naproxen n=4029) with a median duration of exposure of 9 months, the risk of developing a serious cardiovascular thrombotic event was significantly higher in patients treated with VIOXX 50 mg once daily (n=45) as compared to patients treated with naproxen 500 mg twice daily (n=19). In VIGOR, mortality due to cardiovascular thrombotic events (7 vs 6, VIOXX vs naproxen, respectively) was similar between the treatment groups. (See CLINICAL STUDIES, *Special Studies, VIGOR, Other Safety Findings: Cardiovascular Safety*.) In a placebo-controlled database derived from 2 studies with a total of 2142 elderly patients (mean age 75; VIOXX n=1067, placebo n=1075) with a median duration of exposure of approximately 14 months, the number of patients with serious cardiovascular thrombotic events was 21 vs 35 for patients treated with VIOXX 25 mg once daily versus placebo, respectively. In these same 2 placebo-controlled studies, mortality due to cardiovascular thrombotic events was 8 vs 3 for VIOXX versus placebo, respectively. The significance of the cardiovascular findings from these 3 studies (VIGOR and 2 placebo-controlled studies) is unknown. Prospective studies specifically designed to compare the incidence of serious CV events in patients taking VIOXX versus NSAID comparators or placebo have not been performed.

Because of its lack of platelet effects, VIOXX is not a substitute for aspirin for cardiovascular prophylaxis. Therefore, in patients taking VIOXX, antiplatelet therapies should not be discontinued and should be considered in patients with an indication for cardiovascular prophylaxis. (See CLINICAL STUDIES, *Special Studies, Platelets;* PRECAUTIONS, *Drug Interactions, Aspirin.*) Prospective, long-term studies on concomitant administration of VIOXX and aspirin evaluating cardiovascular outcomes have not been conducted.

Fluid Retention, Edema, and Hypertension

Fluid retention, edema, and hypertension have been reported in some patients taking VIOXX. In clinical trials of VIOXX at daily doses of 25 mg in patients with rheumatoid arthritis the incidence of hypertension was twice as high in patients treated with VIOXX as compared to patients treated with naproxen 1000 mg daily. Clinical trials with VIOXX at daily doses of 12.5 and 25 mg in patients with osteoarthritis have shown effects on hypertension and edema similar to those observed with comparator NSAIDs; these occurred with an increased frequency with chronic use of VIOXX at daily doses of 50 mg. (See ADVERSE REACTIONS.) VIOXX should be used with caution, and should be introduced at the lowest recommended dose in patients with fluid retention, hypertension, or heart failure.

Renal Effects

Long-term administration of NSAIDs has resulted in renal papillary necrosis and other renal injury. Renal toxicity has also been seen in patients in whom renal prostaglandins have a compensatory role in the maintenance of renal perfusion. In these patients, administration of a nonsteroidal anti-inflammatory drug may cause a dose-dependent reduction in prostaglandin formation and, secondarily, in renal blood flow, which may precipitate overt renal decompensation. Patients at greatest risk of this reaction are those with impaired renal function, heart failure, liver dysfunction, those taking diuretics and ACE inhibitors, and the elderly. Discontinuation of NSAID therapy is usually followed by recovery to the pretreatment state.

Caution should be used when initiating treatment with VIOXX in patients with considerable dehydration. It is advisable to rehydrate patients first and then start therapy with VIOXX. Caution is also recommended in patients with pre-existing kidney disease (see WARNINGS, *Advanced Renal Disease*).

Hepatic Effects

Borderline elevations of one or more liver tests may occur in up to 15% of patients taking NSAIDs, and notable elevations of ALT or AST (approximately three or more times the upper limit of normal) have been reported in approximately 1% of patients in clinical trials with NSAIDs. These laboratory abnormalities may progress, may remain unchanged, or may be transient with continuing therapy. Rare cases of severe hepatic reactions, including jaundice and fatal fulminant hepatitis, liver necrosis and hepatic failure (some with fatal outcome) have been reported with NSAIDs, including VIOXX. In controlled clinical trials of VIOXX, the incidence of borderline elevations of liver tests at doses of 12.5 and 25 mg daily was comparable to the incidence observed with ibuprofen and lower than that observed with diclofenac. In placebo-controlled trials, approximately 0.5% of patients taking rofecoxib (12.5 or 25 mg QD) and 0.1% of patients taking placebo had notable elevations of ALT or AST.

A patient with symptoms and/or signs suggesting liver dysfunction, or in whom an abnormal liver test has occurred, should be monitored carefully for evidence of the development of a more severe hepatic reaction while on therapy with VIOXX. The maximum recommended chronic daily dose in patients with moderate hepatic insufficiency is 12.5 mg daily. Use of VIOXX is not recommended in patients with severe hepatic insufficiency (see CLINICAL PHARMACOLOGY, *Special Populations* and DOSAGE AND ADMINISTRATION, *Hepatic Insufficiency*). If clinical signs and symptoms consistent with liver disease develop, or if systemic manifestations occur (e.g., eosinophilia, rash, etc.), VIOXX should be discontinued.

Hematological Effects

Anemia is sometimes seen in patients receiving VIOXX. In placebo-controlled trials, there were no significant differences observed between VIOXX and placebo in clinical reports of anemia. Patients on long-term treatment with VIOXX should have their hemoglobin or hematocrit checked if they exhibit any signs or symptoms of anemia or blood loss. VIOXX does not generally affect platelet counts, prothrombin time (PT), or partial thromboplastin time (PTT), and does not inhibit platelet aggregation at indicated dosages (see CLINICAL STUDIES, *Special Studies, Platelets*).

Preexisting Asthma

Patients with asthma may have aspirin-sensitive asthma. The use of aspirin in patients with aspirin-sensitive asthma has been associated with severe bronchospasm which can be fatal. Since cross reactivity, including bronchospasm, between aspirin and other nonsteroidal anti-inflammatory drugs has been reported in such aspirin-sensitive patients, VIOXX should not be administered to patients with this form of aspirin sensitivity and should be used with caution in patients with preexisting asthma.

Information for Patients

Physicians should instruct their patients to read the patient package insert before starting therapy with VIOXX and to reread it each time the prescription is renewed in case any information has changed.

VIOXX can cause discomfort and, rarely, more serious side effects, such as gastrointestinal bleeding, which may result in hospitalization and even fatal outcomes. Although serious GI tract ulcerations and bleeding can occur without warning symptoms, patients should be alert for the signs and symptoms of ulcerations and bleeding, and should ask for medical advice when observing any indicative signs or symptoms. Patients should be apprised of the importance of this follow-up. For additional gastrointestinal safety information see CLINICAL STUDIES, *Special Studies, VIGOR* and WARNINGS, *Gastrointestinal (GI) Effects - Risk of GI Ulceration, Bleeding and Perforation*. Patients should be informed that VIOXX is not a substitute for aspirin for cardiovascular prophylaxis because of its lack of effect on platelets. For additional cardiovascular safety information see CLINICAL STUDIES, *Special Studies, VIGOR* and PRECAUTIONS, *Cardiovascular Effects*.

Patients should promptly report signs or symptoms of gastrointestinal ulceration or bleeding, skin rash, unexplained weight gain, edema or chest pain to their physicians.

Patients should be informed of the warning signs and symptoms of hepatotoxicity (e.g., nausea, fatigue, lethargy, pruritus, jaundice, right upper quadrant tenderness, and "flu-like" symptoms). If these occur, patients should be instructed to stop therapy and seek immediate medical therapy.

Patients should also be instructed to seek immediate emergency help in the case of an anaphylactoid reaction (see WARNINGS).

In late pregnancy VIOXX should be avoided because it may cause premature closure of the ductus arteriosus.

Laboratory Tests

Because serious GI tract ulcerations and bleeding can occur without warning symptoms, physicians should monitor for signs or symptoms of GI bleeding.

Drug Interactions

ACE inhibitors: Reports suggest that NSAIDs may diminish the antihypertensive effect of Angiotensin Converting Enzyme (ACE) inhibitors. In patients with mild to moderate hypertension, administration of 25 mg daily of VIOXX with the ACE inhibitor benazepril, 10 to 40 mg for 4 weeks, was associated with an average increase in mean arterial pressure of about 3 mm Hg compared to ACE inhibitor alone. This interaction should be given consideration in patients taking VIOXX concomitantly with ACE inhibitors.

Aspirin: Concomitant administration of low-dose aspirin with VIOXX may result in an increased rate of GI ulceration or other complications, compared to use of VIOXX alone. In a 12-week endoscopy study conducted in OA patients there was no difference in the cumulative incidence of endoscopic gastroduodenal ulcers in patients taking low-dose (81 mg) enteric coated aspirin plus VIOXX 25 mg daily, as compared to those taking ibuprofen 2400 mg daily alone. Patients taking low-dose aspirin plus ibuprofen were not studied. (See CLINICAL STUDIES, *Special Studies, Upper Endoscopy in Patients with Osteoarthritis and Rheumatoid Arthritis*.)

At steady state, VIOXX 50 mg once daily had no effect on the anti-platelet activity of low-dose (81 mg once daily) aspirin, as assessed by *ex vivo* platelet aggregation and serum TXB2 generation in clotting blood. Because of its lack of platelet effects, VIOXX is not a substitute for aspirin for cardiovascular prophylaxis. Therefore, in patients taking VIOXX, antiplatelet therapies should not be discontinued and should be considered in patients with an indication for cardiovascular prophylaxis. (See CLINICAL STUDIES, *Special Studies, Platelets* and PRECAUTIONS, *Cardiovascular Effects*.) Prospective, long-term studies on concomitant administration of VIOXX and aspirin have not been conducted.

Cimetidine: Co-administration with high doses of cimetidine [800 mg twice daily] increased the C_{max} of rofecoxib by 21%, the $AUC_{0-120hr}$ by 23% and the $t_{1/2}$ by 15%. These small changes are not clinically significant and no dose adjustment is necessary.

Digoxin: Rofecoxib 75 mg once daily for 11 days does not alter the plasma concentration profile or renal elimination of digoxin after a single 0.5 mg oral dose.

Furosemide: Clinical studies, as well as post-marketing observations, have shown that NSAIDs can reduce the natriuretic effect of furosemide and thiazides in some patients. This response has been attributed to inhibition of renal prostaglandin synthesis.

Ketoconazole: Ketoconazole 400 mg daily did not have any clinically important effect on the pharmacokinetics of rofecoxib.

Lithium: NSAIDs have produced an elevation of plasma lithium levels and a reduction in renal lithium clearance. In post-marketing experience there have been reports of increases in plasma lithium levels. Thus, when VIOXX and lithium are administered concurrently, subjects should be observed carefully for signs of lithium toxicity.

Methotrexate: VIOXX 12.5, 25, and 50 mg, each dose administered once daily for 7 days, had no effect on the plasma concentration of methotrexate as measured by AUC_{0-24hr} in patients receiving single weekly methotrexate doses of 7.5 to 20 mg for rheumatoid arthritis. At higher than recommended doses, VIOXX 75 mg administered once daily for 10 days increased plasma concentrations by 23% as measured by AUC_{0-24hr} in patients receiving methotrexate 7.5 to 15 mg/week for rheumatoid arthritis. At 24 hours postdose, a similar proportion of patients treated with methotrexate alone (94%) and subsequently treated with methotrexate co-administered with 75 mg of rofecoxib (88%) had methotrexate plasma concentrations below the measurable limit (5 ng/mL). Standard monitoring of methotrexate-related toxicity should be continued if VIOXX and methotrexate are administered concomitantly.

Oral Contraceptives: Rofecoxib did not have any clinically important effect on the pharmacokinetics of ethinyl estradiol and norethindrone.

Prednisone/prednisolone: Rofecoxib did not have any clinically important effect on the pharmacokinetics of prednisolone or prednisone.

Rifampin: Co-administration of VIOXX with rifampin 600 mg daily, a potent inducer of hepatic metabolism, produced an approximate 50% decrease in rofecoxib plasma concentrations. Therefore, a starting daily dose of 25 mg of VIOXX should be considered for the treatment of osteoarthritis when VIOXX is co-administered with potent inducers of hepatic metabolism.

Theophylline: VIOXX 12.5, 25, and 50 mg administered once daily for 7 days increased plasma theophylline concentrations ($AUC_{(0-\infty)}$) by 38 to 60% in healthy subjects administered a single 300-mg dose of theophylline. Adequate monitoring of theophylline plasma concentrations should be considered when therapy with VIOXX is initiated or changed in patients receiving theophylline.

These data suggest that rofecoxib may produce a modest inhibition of cytochrome P450 (CYP) 1A2. Therefore, there is a potential for an interaction with other drugs that are metabolized by CYP 1A2 (e.g., amitriptyline, tacrine, and zileuton).

Warfarin: Anticoagulant activity should be monitored, particularly in the first few days after initiating or changing VIOXX therapy in patients receiving warfarin or similar

Continued on next page

Information on the Merck & Co., Inc., products listed on these pages is from the prescribing information in use October 1, 2004. For information, please call 1-800-NSC-MERCK [1-800-672-6372].

Vioxx—Cont.

agents, since these patients are at an increased risk of bleeding complications. In single and multiple dose studies in healthy subjects receiving both warfarin and rofecoxib, prothrombin time (measured as INR) was increased by approximately 8% to 11%. In post-marketing experience, bleeding events have been reported, predominantly in the elderly, in association with increases in prothrombin time in patients receiving VIOXX concurrently with warfarin.

Carcinogenesis, Mutagenesis, Impairment of Fertility

Rofecoxib was not carcinogenic in mice given oral doses up to 30 mg/kg (male) and 60 mg/kg (female) (approximately 5- and 2-fold the human exposure at 25 and 50 mg daily based on AUC_{0-24}) and in male and female rats given oral doses up to 8 mg/kg (approximately 6- and 2-fold the human exposure at 25 and 50 mg daily based on AUC_{0-24}) for two years. Rofecoxib was not mutagenic in an Ames test or in a V-79 mammalian cell mutagenesis assay, nor clastogenic in a chromosome aberration assay in Chinese hamster ovary (CHO) cells, in an *in vitro* and an *in vivo* alkaline elution assay, or in an *in vivo* chromosomal aberration test in mouse bone marrow.

Rofecoxib did not impair male fertility in rats at oral doses up to 100 mg/kg (approximately 20- and 7-fold human exposure at 25 and 50 mg daily based on the AUC_{0-24}) and rofecoxib had no effect on fertility in female rats at doses up to 30 mg/kg (approximately 19- and 7-fold human exposure at 25 and 50 mg daily based on AUC_{0-24}).

Pregnancy

Teratogenic effects: Pregnancy Category C.

Rofecoxib was not teratogenic in rats at doses up to 50 mg/kg/day (approximately 28- and 10-fold human exposure at 25 and 50 mg daily based on AUC_{0-24}). There was a slight, non-statistically significant increase in the overall incidence of vertebral malformations only in the rabbit at doses of 50 mg/kg/day (approximately 1- or <1-fold human exposure at 25 and 50 mg daily based on AUC_{0-24}). There are no studies in pregnant women. VIOXX should be used during pregnancy only if the potential benefit justifies the potential risk to the fetus.

Nonteratogenic effects

Rofecoxib produced peri-implantation and post-implantation losses and reduced embryo/fetal survival in rats and rabbits at oral doses ≥10 and ≥75 mg/kg/day, respectively (approximately 9- and 3-fold [rats] and 2- and <1-fold [rabbits] human exposure based on the AUC_{0-24} at 25 and 50 mg daily). These changes are expected with inhibition of prostaglandin synthesis and are not the result of permanent alteration of female reproductive function. There was an increase in the incidence of postnatal pup mortality in rats at ≥5 mg/kg/day (approximately 5- and 2-fold human exposure at 25 and 50 mg daily based on AUC_{0-24}). In studies in pregnant rats administered single doses of rofecoxib, there was a treatment-related decrease in the diameter of the ductus arteriosus at all doses used (3-300 mg/kg: 3 mg/kg is approximately 2- and <1-fold human exposure at 25 or 50 mg daily based on AUC_{0-24}). As with other drugs known to inhibit prostaglandin synthesis, use of VIOXX during the third trimester of pregnancy should be avoided.

Labor and delivery

Rofecoxib produced no evidence of significantly delayed labor or parturition in females at doses 15 mg/kg in rats (approximately 10- and 3-fold human exposure as measured by the AUC_{0-24} at 25 and 50 mg). The effects of VIOXX on labor and delivery in pregnant women are unknown.

Merck & Co., Inc. maintains a registry to monitor the pregnancy outcomes of women exposed to VIOXX while pregnant. Healthcare providers are encouraged to report any prenatal exposure to VIOXX by calling the **Pregnancy Registry at (800) 986-8999.**

Nursing mothers

Rofecoxib is excreted in the milk of lactating rats at concentrations similar to those in plasma. There was an increase in pup mortality and a decrease in pup body weight following exposure of pups to milk from dams administered VIOXX during lactation. The dose tested represents an approximate 18- and 6-fold human exposure at 25 and 50 mg based on AUC_{0-24}. It is not known whether this drug is excreted in human milk. Because many drugs are excreted in human milk and because of the potential for serious adverse reactions in nursing infants from VIOXX, a decision should be made whether to discontinue nursing or to discontinue the drug, taking into account the importance of the drug to the mother.

Pediatric Use

Safety and effectiveness in pediatric patients below the age of 18 years have not been evaluated.

Geriatric Use

Of the patients who received VIOXX in osteoarthritis clinical trials, 1455 were 65 years of age or older. This included 460 patients who were 75 years or older, and in one of these studies, 174 patients who were 80 years or older. No substantial differences in safety and effectiveness were observed between these subjects and younger subjects. Greater sensitivity of some older individuals cannot be ruled out. As with other NSAIDs, including those that selectively inhibit COX-2, there have been more spontaneous post-marketing reports of fatal GI events and acute renal failure in the elderly than in younger patients. Dosage adjustment in the elderly is not necessary; however, therapy with VIOXX should be initiated at the lowest recommended dose.

ADVERSE REACTIONS

Osteoarthritis

Approximately 3600 patients with osteoarthritis were treated with VIOXX; approximately 1400 patients received VIOXX for 6 months or longer and approximately 800 patients for one year or longer. The following table of adverse experiences lists all adverse events, regardless of causality, occurring in at least 2% of patients receiving VIOXX in nine controlled studies of 6-week to 6-month duration conducted in patients with OA at the therapeutically recommended doses (12.5 and 25 mg), which included a placebo and/or positive control group.

[See table below]

In the OA studies, the following spontaneous adverse events occurred in >0.1% to 1.9% of patients treated with VIOXX regardless of causality:

Clinical Adverse Experiences occurring in ≥ 2.0% of Patients Treated with VIOXX in OA Clinical Trials

	Placebo	VIOXX 12.5 or 25 mg daily	Ibuprofen 2400 mg daily	Diclofenac 150 mg daily
	(N = 783)	(N = 2829)	(N = 847)	(N = 498)
Body As A Whole/Site Unspecified				
Abdominal Pain	4.1	3.4	4.6	5.8
Asthenia/Fatigue	1.0	2.2	2.0	2.6
Dizziness	2.2	3.0	2.7	3.4
Influenza-Like Disease	3.1	2.9	1.5	3.2
Lower Extremity Edema	1.1	3.7	3.8	3.4
Upper Respiratory Infection	7.8	8.5	5.8	8.2
Cardiovascular System				
Hypertension	1.3	3.5	3.0	1.6
Digestive System				
Diarrhea	6.8	6.5	7.1	10.6
Dyspepsia	2.7	3.5	4.7	4.0
Epigastric Discomfort	2.8	3.8	9.2	5.4
Heartburn	3.6	4.2	5.2	4.6
Nausea	2.9	5.2	7.1	7.4
Eyes, Ears, Nose, And Throat				
Sinusitis	2.0	2.7	1.8	2.4
Musculoskeletal System				
Back Pain	1.9	2.5	1.4	2.8
Nervous System				
Headache	7.5	4.7	6.1	8.0
Respiratory System				
Bronchitis	0.8	2.0	1.4	3.2
Urogenital System				
Urinary Tract Infection	2.7	2.8	2.5	3.6

Body as a Whole: abdominal distension, abdominal tenderness, abscess, chest pain, chills, contusion, cyst, diaphragmatic hernia, fever, fluid retention, flushing, fungal infection, infection, laceration, pain, pelvic pain, peripheral edema, postoperative pain, syncope, trauma, upper extremity edema, viral syndrome.

Cardiovascular System: angina pectoris, atrial fibrillation, bradycardia, hematoma, irregular heartbeat, palpitation, premature ventricular contraction, tachycardia, venous insufficiency.

Digestive System: acid reflux, aphthous stomatitis, constipation, dental caries, dental pain, digestive gas symptoms, dry mouth, duodenal disorder, dysgeusia, esophagitis, flatulence, gastric disorder, gastritis, gastroenteritis, hematochezia, hemorrhoids, infectious gastroenteritis, oral infection, oral lesion, oral ulcer, vomiting.

Eyes, Ears, Nose, and Throat: allergic rhinitis, blurred vision, cerumen impaction, conjunctivitis, dry throat, epistaxis, laryngitis, nasal congestion, nasal secretion, ophthalmic injection, otic pain, otitis, otitis media, pharyngitis, tinnitus, tonsillitis.

Immune System: allergy, hypersensitivity, insect bite reaction.

Metabolism and Nutrition: appetite change, hypercholesterolemia, weight gain.

Musculoskeletal System: ankle sprain, arm pain, arthralgia, back strain, bursitis, cartilage trauma, joint swelling, muscular cramp, muscular disorder, muscular weakness, musculoskeletal pain, musculoskeletal stiffness, myalgia, osteoarthritis, tendinitis, traumatic arthropathy, wrist fracture.

Nervous System: hypesthesia, insomnia, median nerve neuropathy, migraine, muscular spasm, paresthesia, sciatica, somnolence, vertigo.

Psychiatric: anxiety, depression, mental acuity decreased.

Respiratory System: asthma, cough, dyspnea, pneumonia, pulmonary congestion, respiratory infection.

Skin and Skin Appendages: abrasion, alopecia, atopic dermatitis, basal cell carcinoma, blister, cellulitis, contact dermatitis, herpes simplex, herpes zoster, nail unit disorder, perspiration, pruritus, rash, skin erythema, urticaria, xerosis.

Urogenital System: breast mass, cystitis, dysuria, menopausal symptoms, menstrual disorder, nocturia, urinary retention, vaginitis.

The following serious adverse events have been reported rarely (estimated <0.1%) in patients taking VIOXX, regardless of causality. Cases reported only in the post-marketing experience are indicated in italics.

Cardiovascular: cerebrovascular accident, congestive heart failure, deep venous thrombosis, *hypertensive crisis*, myocardial infarction, *pulmonary edema*, pulmonary embolism, transient ischemic attack, unstable angina.

Gastrointestinal: cholecystitis, colitis, colonic malignant neoplasm, *duodenal perforation*, duodenal ulcer, *esophageal ulcer, gastric perforation, gastric ulcer*, gastrointestinal bleeding, *hepatic failure, hepatitis*, intestinal obstruction, *jaundice*, pancreatitis.

Hemic and lymphatic: agranulocytosis, aplastic anemia, leukopenia, lymphoma, *pancytopenia, thrombocytopenia.*

Immune System: anaphylactic/anaphylactoid reaction, angioedema, bronchospasm, hypersensitivity vasculitis.

Metabolism and nutrition: hyponatremia.

Nervous System: aseptic meningitis, epilepsy aggravated.

Psychiatric: confusion, hallucinations.

Skin and Skin Appendages: photosensitivity reactions, severe skin reactions, including Stevens-Johnson syndrome and toxic epidermal necrolysis.

Urogenital System: acute renal failure, breast malignant neoplasm, *hyperkalemia, interstitial nephritis,* prostatic malignant neoplasm, urolithiasis, *worsening chronic renal failure.*

In 1-year controlled clinical trials and in extension studies for up to 86 weeks (approximately 800 patients treated with VIOXX for one year or longer), the adverse experience profile was qualitatively similar to that observed in studies of shorter duration.

Rheumatoid Arthritis

Approximately 1,100 patients were treated with VIOXX in the Phase III rheumatoid arthritis efficacy studies. These studies included extensions of up to 1 year. The adverse experience profile was generally similar to that reported in the osteoarthritis studies. In studies of at least three months, the incidence of hypertension in RA patients receiving the 25 mg once daily dose of VIOXX was 10.0% and the incidence of hypertension in patients receiving naproxen 500 mg twice daily was 4.7%.

Analgesia, including primary dysmenorrhea

Approximately one thousand patients were treated with VIOXX in analgesia studies. All patients in post-dental surgery pain studies received only a single dose of study medication. Patients in primary dysmenorrhea studies may have taken up to 3 daily doses of VIOXX, and those in the post-orthopedic surgery pain study were prescribed 5 daily doses of VIOXX.

The adverse experience profile in the analgesia studies was generally similar to those reported in the osteoarthritis studies. The following additional adverse experience, which occurred at an incidence of at least 2% of patients treated with VIOXX, was observed in the post-dental pain surgery studies: post-dental extraction alveolitis (dry socket).

Migraine with or without aura

Approximately 750 patients were treated with a single dose of VIOXX 25 mg or 50 mg in two single-attack migraine studies. Approximately 460 patients in the 3-month extension phase of one study treated up to 8 (average 3) migraine attacks per month. In single attack studies, the following adverse events were more frequent in the VIOXX treatment groups (25 mg and 50 mg) compared to the placebo group, and occurred at an incidence of at least 2% of patients treated: dizziness, nausea, somnolence and dyspepsia. In the 3-month extension phase of one study, the following adverse events occurred at an incidence of at least 2% of patients treated in the VIOXX treatment groups (25 mg and 50 mg): dizziness, dry mouth, nausea, and vomiting.

Clinical Studies in OA and RA with VIOXX 50 mg (Twice the highest dose recommended for chronic use)

In OA and RA clinical trials which contained VIOXX 12.5 or 25 mg as well as VIOXX 50 mg, VIOXX 50 mg QD was associated with a higher incidence of gastrointestinal symptoms (abdominal pain, epigastric pain, heartburn, nausea and vomiting), lower extremity edema, hypertension, serious* adverse experiences and discontinuation due to clinical adverse experiences compared to the recommended chronic doses of 12.5 and 25 mg (see DOSAGE AND ADMINISTRATION).

*adverse experience that resulted in death, permanent or substantial disability, hospitalization, congenital anomaly, or cancer, was immediately life threatening, was due to an overdose, or was thought by the investigator to require intervention to prevent one of the above outcomes

OVERDOSAGE

No overdoses of VIOXX were reported during clinical trials. Administration of single doses of VIOXX 1000 mg to 6 healthy volunteers and multiple doses of 250 mg/day for 14 days to 75 healthy volunteers did not result in serious toxicity.

In the event of overdose, it is reasonable to employ the usual supportive measures, e.g., remove unabsorbed material from the gastrointestinal tract, employ clinical monitoring, and institute supportive therapy, if required.

Rofecoxib is not removed by hemodialysis; it is not known whether rofecoxib is removed by peritoneal dialysis.

DOSAGE AND ADMINISTRATION

VIOXX is administered orally. The lowest dose of VIOXX should be sought for each patient.

Osteoarthritis

The recommended starting dose of VIOXX is 12.5 mg once daily. Some patients may receive additional benefit by increasing the dose to 25 mg once daily. The maximum recommended daily dose is 25 mg.

Rheumatoid Arthritis

The recommended dose is 25 mg once daily. The maximum recommended daily dose is 25 mg.

Management of Acute Pain and Treatment of Primary Dysmenorrhea

The recommended dose of VIOXX is 50 mg once daily. The maximum recommended daily dose is 50 mg. Use of VIOXX for more than 5 days in management of pain has not been studied. Chronic use of VIOXX 50 mg daily is not recommended. (See ADVERSE REACTIONS, *Clinical Studies in OA and RA with VIOXX 50 mg*).

Acute Treatment of Migraine Attacks with or without aura

The recommended starting dose of VIOXX is 25 mg once daily. Some patients may receive additional benefit with 50 mg as compared to 25 mg. The maximum recommended daily dose is 50 mg. The safety of treating more than 5 migraine attacks in any given month has not been established. Chronic daily use of VIOXX for the acute treatment of migraine is not recommended.

Hepatic Insufficiency

Because of significant increases in both AUC and C_{max} in patients with moderate hepatic impairment (Child-Pugh score: 7-9), the maximum recommended chronic daily dose is 12.5 mg. (See CLINICAL PHARMACOLOGY, *Special Populations*). The efficacy of 12.5 mg in rheumatoid arthritis patients with moderate hepatic insufficiency has not been studied.

VIOXX Tablets may be taken with or without food.

Oral Suspension

VIOXX Oral Suspension 12.5 mg/5 mL or 25 mg/5 mL may be substituted for VIOXX Tablets 12.5 or 25 mg, respectively, in any of the above indications. Shake before using.

HOW SUPPLIED

No. 3810 — Tablets VIOXX, 12.5 mg, are cream/off-white, round, shallow cup tablets engraved MRK 74 on one side and VIOXX on the other. They are supplied as follows:
NDC 0006-0074-31 unit of use bottles of 30
NDC 0006-0074-28 unit dose packages of 100
NDC 0006-0074-68 bottles of 100
NDC 0006-0074-82 bottles of 1000
NDC 0006-0074-80 bottles of 8000.

No. 3834 — Tablets VIOXX, 25 mg, are yellow, round tablets engraved MRK 110 on one side and VIOXX on the other. They are supplied as follows:
NDC 0006-0110-31 unit of use bottles of 30
NDC 0006-0110-28 unit dose packages of 100
NDC 0006-0110-68 bottles of 100
NDC 0006-0110-82 bottles of 1000
NDC 0006-0110-80 bottles of 8000.

No. 3835 — Tablets VIOXX, 50 mg, are orange, round tablets engraved MRK 114 on one side and VIOXX on the other. They are supplied as follows:
NDC 0006-0114-31 unit of use bottles of 30
NDC 0006-0114-28 unit dose packages of 100
NDC 0006-0114-68 bottles of 100
NDC 0006-0114-74 bottles of 500
NDC 0006-0114-81 bottles of 4000.

No. 3784 — Oral Suspension VIOXX, 12.5 mg/5 mL, is an opaque, white to faint yellow suspension with a strawberry flavor that is easily resuspended upon shaking.
NDC 0006-3784-64 unit of use bottles containing 150 mL (12.5 mg/5 mL).

No. 3785 — Oral Suspension VIOXX, 25 mg/5 mL, is an opaque, white to faint yellow suspension with a strawberry flavor that is easily resuspended upon shaking.
NDC 0006-3785-64 unit of use bottles containing 150 mL (25 mg/5 mL).

Storage

VIOXX Tablets:
Store at 25°C (77°F), excursions permitted to 15-30°C (59-86°F). [See USP Controlled Room Temperature.]

VIOXX Oral Suspension:
Store at 25°C (77°F), excursions permitted to 15-30°C (59-86°F). [See USP Controlled Room Temperature.]

Rx only

MERCK & CO., INC., Whitehouse Station, NJ 08889, USA
9556416 Issued March 2004

Patient Information about VIOXX® (rofecoxib tablets and oral suspension) VIOXX® (pronounced "VI-ox") for Osteoarthritis, Rheumatoid Arthritis, Pain and Migraine Attacks

Generic name: rofecoxib ("ro-fa-COX-ib")

You should read this information before you start taking VIOXX*. Also, read the leaflet each time you refill your prescription, in case any information has changed. This leaflet provides only a summary of certain information about VIOXX. Your doctor or pharmacist can give you an additional leaflet that is written for health professionals that contains more complete information. This leaflet does not take the place of careful discussions with your doctor. You and your doctor should discuss VIOXX when you start taking your medicine and at regular checkups.

*Registered trademark of MERCK & CO., Inc.

What is VIOXX?

VIOXX is a prescription medicine called a COX-2 selective, nonsteroidal anti-inflammatory drug (NSAID).

VIOXX is used in adults for:
- relief of the pain and inflammation (swelling and soreness) of osteoarthritis (arthritis from wear and tear on your bones and your joints)
- relief of the pain and inflammation of rheumatoid arthritis in adults (arthritis caused by a condition where your immune system attacks your joints)
- management of short-term pain
- treatment of menstrual pain (pain during women's monthly periods)
- treatment of migraine headache attacks with or without aura.

VIOXX has not been studied in children under the age of 18.

Who should not take VIOXX?

Do not take VIOXX if you:
- have had an allergic reaction such as asthma attacks (wheezing), hives, or swelling of the throat and face to aspirin or other medicines called non-steroidal anti-inflammatory drugs (NSAIDs). There are many NSAID medicines. Ask your doctor or pharmacist for a list of medicines that contain NSAIDs if you are not sure.
- are allergic to rofecoxib, the active ingredient of VIOXX, or to any other ingredients in VIOXX. See the end of this leaflet for a complete list of ingredients in VIOXX.

What should I tell my doctor before and during treatment with VIOXX?

Tell your doctor about all your medical conditions including if you have or have had:
- an allergic to reaction to aspirin or other NSAIDs
- asthma (a small number of patients with asthma have reactions to aspirin or other NSAIDs)
- stomach problems such as ulcers or bleeding
- kidney disease
- liver disease
- angina (chest pain), a heart attack, or a blocked artery in your heart
- heart failure
- high blood pressure

Tell your doctor if you are:
- pregnant or plan to become pregnant. VIOXX may harm your unborn baby if you take it in late pregnancy. If you take VIOXX while you are pregnant, ask your doctor how you can be on the VIOXX Pregnancy Registry.
- breast-feeding or plan to breast-feed. It is not known if VIOXX passes into your milk and if it can harm your baby. You should discuss with your doctor whether or not to take VIOXX if you are breast-feeding.

Tell your doctor about:
- any other medical problems or allergies you have now or have had.
- all the medicines you take including prescription and non-prescription medicines, vitamins, and herbal supplements.

Tell your doctor right away if you develop:
- serious stomach problems such as ulcer or bleeding symptoms (for instance, stomach burning, vomiting blood, or if there is blood in your bowel movement or it is black and sticky like tar, which are signs of possible stomach bleeding).
- unexplained weight gain or swelling of the legs, feet, and/or hands.
- skin rash or allergic reactions. If you have a severe allergic reaction, get medical help right away.

How should I take VIOXX?
- Take VIOXX exactly as prescribed by your doctor. Your dose will depend on the condition being treated and other medical problems you may have. Do not change your dose of VIOXX or take extra doses unless your doctor has told you to.
- You can take VIOXX with or without food.
- If you miss a dose of VIOXX by a few hours, take it as soon as you remember. If it is close to your next dose, do NOT take the missed dose.
- If you take too much VIOXX, call your doctor, pharmacist, or poison control center right away.

Can I take VIOXX with other medicines?

Tell your doctor about all of the other medicines you are taking or plan to take while you are on VIOXX, even other medicines that you can get without a prescription, including vitamins and herbal supplements. VIOXX and certain other medicines can affect each other causing serious side effects. Keep a list of the medicines you take. Show the list to your doctors and pharmacists each time you get a new medicine. They will tell you if it is safe to take VIOXX with other medicines. Your doctor may want to check that your medicines are working properly together. Especially tell your doctor if you are taking:
- or have taken warfarin (Coumadin®) or any other similar blood thinner within the past 10 days
- theophylline (a medicine used to treat asthma)
- rifampin (an antibiotic)
- ACE inhibitors (medicines used for high blood pressure and heart failure)
- lithium (a medicine used to treat a certain type of depression).

VIOXX cannot take the place of aspirin for prevention of heart attack or stroke. If you take both aspirin and VIOXX, you may have a higher chance of serious stomach problems than if you take VIOXX alone. If you are taking aspirin for prevention of heart attack or stroke, you should not stop taking aspirin without talking to your doctor.

What are the possible side effects of VIOXX?

Serious but rare side effects that have been reported in patients taking VIOXX and/or related medicines have included:
- Serious allergic reactions including swelling of the face, lips, tongue, and/or throat which may cause difficulty breathing or swallowing, hives, wheezing, or shock (loss of blood pressure and consciousness) can occur. These may require treatment right away. Severe skin reactions have also been reported.
- Serious stomach problems, such as stomach and intestinal bleeding, can occur with or without warning symptoms. These problems, if severe, could lead to hospitalization or death. Although this happens rarely, you should watch for signs (for instance, stomach burning, vomiting blood, or if there is blood in your bowel movement or it is black and sticky like tar) that you may have this serious side effect and tell your doctor right away.
- Heart attacks and other serious events, such as blood clots in your body, have been reported in patients taking VIOXX.
- Serious kidney problems can occur, including acute (sudden) kidney failure and worsening of chronic kidney failure.
- Severe liver problems, including hepatitis, jaundice and liver failure, can occur in patients taking NSAIDs, including VIOXX. Tell your doctor if you develop symptoms of liver problems. These include nausea, tiredness, itching, pain in the right upper abdomen, yellow skin or eyes, and flu-like symptoms.

Your doctor may do blood tests and check you for problems that may happen during treatment with VIOXX.

In addition, the following side effects have been reported: anxiety, blurred vision, colitis, confusion, constipation, decreased levels of sodium in the blood, depression, fluid in the lungs, hair loss, hallucinations, increased levels of potassium in the blood, insomnia, low blood cell counts, menstrual disorder, palpitations, pancreatitis, ringing in the ears, severe increase in blood pressure, skin reactions caused by sunlight, tingling sensation, unusual headache with stiff neck (aseptic meningitis), vertigo, worsening of epilepsy.

More common, but less serious side effects reported with VIOXX have included the following:
Respiratory infections
Headache
Dizziness
Diarrhea
Nausea, vomiting and upset stomach
Heartburn

Continued on next page

Information on the Merck & Co., Inc., products listed on these pages is from the prescribing information in use October 1, 2004. For information, please call 1-800-NSC-MERCK [1-800-672-6372].

Vioxx—Cont.

Stomach pain
Swelling of the legs and/or feet
High blood pressure
Back pain
Tiredness
Urinary tract infection.

These are not all the side effects reported with VIOXX. Do not rely on this leaflet alone for information about side effects. Your doctor or pharmacist can discuss with you a more complete list of side effects. Any time you have a medical problem you think may be related to VIOXX, talk to your doctor.

How should I store VIOXX?

- Store VIOXX at room temperature, 59° to 86°F (15° to 30°C).
- Safely throw away VIOXX that is out of date or no longer needed.
- Keep VIOXX and all medicines out of the reach of children.

What else should I know about VIOXX?

This leaflet provides a summary of certain information about VIOXX. If you have any questions or concerns about VIOXX, osteoarthritis, rheumatoid arthritis, pain or migraine attacks, talk to your health professional. Your doctor or pharmacist can give you an additional leaflet that is written for health professionals. This leaflet is also available at www.vioxx.com.

Medicines are sometimes prescribed for conditions other than those described in patient information leaflets. Do not use VIOXX for a condition for which it was not prescribed. Do not give VIOXX to other people even if they have the same symptoms you have. It may harm them.

What are the ingredients in VIOXX?

Active Ingredient: rofecoxib
Inactive Ingredients:
Oral suspension: citric acid (monohydrate), sodium citrate (dihydrate), sorbitol solution, strawberry flavor, xanthan gum, sodium methylparaben, sodium propylparaben.
Tablets: croscarmellose sodium, hydroxypropyl cellulose, lactose, magnesium stearate, microcrystalline cellulose, and yellow ferric oxide.

Rx Only

9183914 Issued March 2004
MERCK & CO., Inc.
Whitehouse Station, NJ 08889, USA

Shown in Product Identification Guide, page 324

ZOCOR® Tablets ℞
[*zō'kōr*]
(simvastatin)

DESCRIPTION

ZOCOR[1] (simvastatin) is a lipid-lowering agent that is derived synthetically from a fermentation product of *Aspergillus terreus*. After oral ingestion, simvastatin, which is an inactive lactone, is hydrolyzed to the corresponding β-hydroxyacid form. This is an inhibitor of 3-hydroxy-3-methylglutaryl-coenzyme A (HMG-CoA) reductase. This enzyme catalyzes the conversion of HMG-CoA to mevalonate, which is an early and rate-limiting step in the biosynthesis of cholesterol.

Simvastatin is butanoic acid, 2,2-dimethyl-,1,2,3,7,8,8a-hexahydro-3,7-dimethyl-8-[2-(tetrahydro-4-hydroxy-6-oxo-2*H*-pyran-2-yl)-ethyl]-1-naphthalenyl ester, [1S-[1α,3α,7β, 8β(2*S**,4*S**),-8aβ]]. The empirical formula of simvastatin is $C_{25}H_{38}O_5$ and its molecular weight is 418.57. Its structural formula is:

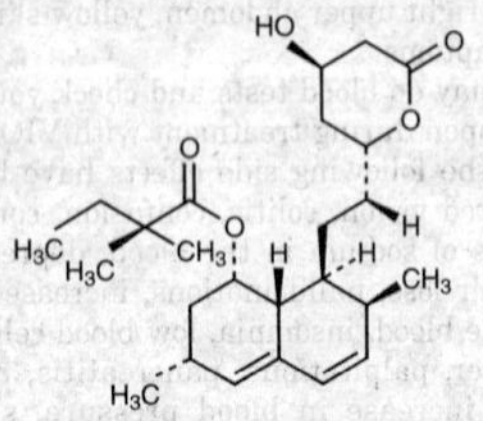

Simvastatin is a white to off-white, nonhygroscopic, crystalline powder that is practically insoluble in water, and freely soluble in chloroform, methanol and ethanol.

Tablets ZOCOR for oral administration contain either 5 mg, 10 mg, 20 mg, 40 mg or 80 mg of simvastatin and the following inactive ingredients: cellulose, hydroxypropyl cellulose, hydroxypropyl methylcellulose, iron oxides, lactose, magnesium stearate, starch, talc, titanium dioxide and other ingredients. Butylated hydroxyanisole is added as a preservative.

---

[1] Registered trademark of MERCK & CO., Inc.

CLINICAL PHARMACOLOGY

The involvement of low-density lipoprotein cholesterol (LDL-C) in atherogenesis has been well-documented in clinical and pathological studies, as well as in many animal experiments. Epidemiological studies have established that elevated plasma levels of total cholesterol (total-C), LDL-C, and apolipoprotein B (Apo B) promote human atherosclerosis and are risk factors for developing cardiovascular disease, while increased levels of high-density lipoprotein cholesterol (HDL-C) and its transport complex, Apo A-I, are associated with decreased cardiovascular risk. High plasma triglycerides (TG) and cholesterol-enriched TG-rich lipoproteins, including very-low-density lipoproteins (VLDL), intermediate-density lipoproteins (IDL), and remnants, can also promote atherosclerosis. Elevated plasma TG are frequently found in a triad with low HDL-C and small LDL particles, as well as in association with non-lipid metabolic risk factors for CHD. As such, total plasma TG has not consistently been shown to be an independent risk factor for CHD. Furthermore, the independent effect of raising HDL-C or lowering TG on the risk of coronary and cardiovascular morbidity and mortality has not been determined.

In the Scandinavian Simvastatin Survival Study (4S), the effect of improving lipoprotein levels with ZOCOR on total mortality was assessed in 4,444 patients with CHD and baseline total cholesterol (total-C) 212-309 mg/dL (5.5-8.0 mmol/L). The patients were followed for a median of 5.4 years. In this multicenter, randomized, double-blind, placebo-controlled study, ZOCOR significantly reduced the risk of mortality by 30% (11.5% vs 8.2%, placebo vs ZOCOR); of CHD mortality by 42% (8.5% vs 5.0%); and of having a hospital-verified non-fatal myocardial infarction by 37% (19.6% vs 12.9%). Furthermore, ZOCOR significantly reduced the risk for undergoing myocardial revascularization procedures (coronary artery bypass grafting or percutaneous transluminal coronary angioplasty) by 37% (17.2% vs 11.4%) [see CLINICAL PHARMACOLOGY, *Clinical Studies*].

ZOCOR has been shown to reduce both normal and elevated LDL-C concentrations. LDL is formed from very-low-density lipoprotein (VLDL) and is catabolized predominantly by the high-affinity LDL receptor. The mechanism of the LDL-lowering effect of ZOCOR may involve both reduction of VLDL cholesterol concentration, and induction of the LDL receptor, leading to reduced production and/or increased catabolism of LDL-C. Apo B also falls substantially during treatment with ZOCOR. As each LDL particle contains one molecule of Apo B, and since in patients with predominant elevations in LDL-C (without accompanying elevation in VLDL) little Apo B is found in other lipoproteins, this strongly suggests that ZOCOR does not merely cause cholesterol to be lost from LDL, but also reduces the concentration of circulating LDL particles. In addition, ZOCOR reduces VLDL and TG and increases HDL-C. The effects of ZOCOR on Lp(a), fibrinogen, and certain other independent biochemical risk markers for CHD are unknown.

ZOCOR is a specific inhibitor of HMG-CoA reductase, the enzyme that catalyzes the conversion of HMG-CoA to mevalonate. The conversion of HMG-CoA to mevalonate is an early step in the biosynthetic pathway for cholesterol.

Pharmacokinetics

Simvastatin is a lactone that is readily hydrolyzed *in vivo* to the corresponding β-hydroxyacid, a potent inhibitor of HMG-CoA reductase. Inhibition of HMG-CoA reductase is the basis for an assay in pharmacokinetic studies of the β-hydroxyacid metabolites (active inhibitors) and, following base hydrolysis, active plus latent inhibitors (total inhibitors) in plasma following administration of simvastatin.

Following an oral dose of ^{14}C-labeled simvastatin in man, 13% of the dose was excreted in urine and 60% in feces. The latter represents absorbed drug equivalents excreted in bile, as well as any unabsorbed drug. Plasma concentrations of total radioactivity (simvastatin plus ^{14}C-metabolites) peaked at 4 hours and declined rapidly to about 10% of peak by 12 hours postdose. Absorption of simvastatin, estimated relative to an intravenous reference dose, in each of two animal species tested, averaged about 85% of an oral dose. In animal studies, after oral dosing, simvastatin achieved substantially higher concentrations in the liver than in non-target tissues. Simvastatin undergoes extensive first-pass extraction in the liver, its primary site of action, with subsequent excretion of drug equivalents in the bile. As a consequence of extensive hepatic extraction of simvastatin (estimated to be > 60% in man), the availability of drug to the general circulation is low. In a single-dose study in nine healthy subjects, it was estimated that less than 5% of an oral dose of simvastatin reaches the general circulation as active inhibitors. Following administration of simvastatin tablets, the coefficient of variation, based on between-subject variability, was approximately 48% for the area under the concentration-time curve (AUC) for total inhibitory activity in the general circulation.

Both simvastatin and its β-hydroxyacid metabolite are highly bound (approximately 95%) to human plasma proteins. Animal studies have not been performed to determine whether simvastatin crosses the blood-brain and placental barriers. However, when radiolabeled simvastatin was administered to rats, simvastatin-derived radioactivity crossed the blood-brain barrier.

The major active metabolites of simvastatin present in human plasma are the β-hydroxyacid of simvastatin and its 6′-hydroxy, 6′-hydroxymethyl, and 6′-exomethylene derivatives. Peak plasma concentrations of both active and total inhibitors were attained within 1.3 to 2.4 hours postdose. While the recommended therapeutic dose range is 5 to 80 mg/day, there was no substantial deviation from linearity of AUC of inhibitors in the general circulation with an increase in dose to as high as 120 mg. Relative to the fasting state, the plasma profile of inhibitors was not affected when simvastatin was administered immediately before an American Heart Association recommended low-fat meal.

In a study including 16 elderly patients between 70 and 78 years of age who received ZOCOR 40 mg/day, the mean plasma level of HMG-CoA reductase inhibitory activity was increased approximately 45% compared with 18 patients between 18-30 years of age. Clinical study experience in the elderly (n=1522), suggests that there were no overall differences in safety between elderly and younger patients (see PRECAUTIONS, *Geriatric Use*).

Kinetic studies with another reductase inhibitor, having a similar principal route of elimination, have suggested that for a given dose level higher systemic exposure may be achieved in patients with severe renal insufficiency (as measured by creatinine clearance).

In a study of 12 healthy volunteers, simvastatin at the 80-mg dose had no effect on the metabolism of the probe cytochrome P450 isoform 3A4 (CYP3A4) substrates midazolam and erythromycin. This indicates that simvastatin is not an inhibitor of CYP3A4, and, therefore, is not expected to affect the plasma levels of other drugs metabolized by CYP3A4.

The risk of myopathy is increased by high levels of HMG-CoA reductase inhibitory activity in plasma. Potent inhibitors of CYP3A4 can raise the plasma levels of HMG-CoA reductase inhibitory activity and increase the risk of myopathy (see WARNINGS, *Myopathy/Rhabdomyolysis* and PRECAUTIONS, *Drug Interactions*).

Simvastatin is a substrate for CYP3A4 (see PRECAUTIONS, *Drug Interactions*). Grapefruit juice contains one or more components that inhibit CYP3A4 and can increase the plasma concentrations of drugs metabolized by CYP3A4. In one study[2], 10 subjects consumed 200 mL of double-strength grapefruit juice (one can of frozen concentrate diluted with one rather than 3 cans of water) three times daily for 2 days and an additional 200 mL double-strength grapefruit juice together with, and 30 and 90 minutes following, a single dose of 60 mg simvastatin on the third day. This regimen of grapefruit juice resulted in mean increases in the concentration (as measured by the area under the concentration-time curve) of active and total HMG-CoA reductase inhibitory activity [measured using a radioenzyme inhibition assay both before (for active inhibitors) and after (for total inhibitors) base hydrolysis] of 2.4-fold and 3.6-fold, respectively, and of simvastatin and its β-hydroxyacid metabolite [measured using a chemical assay — liquid chromatography/tandem mass spectrometry] of 16-fold and 7-fold, respectively. In a second study, 16 subjects consumed one 8 oz glass of single-strength grapefruit juice (one can of frozen concentrate diluted with 3 cans of water) with breakfast for 3 consecutive days and a single dose of 20 mg simvastatin in the evening of the third day. This regimen of grapefruit juice resulted in a mean increase in the plasma concentration (as measured by the area under the concentration-time curve) of active and total HMG-CoA reductase inhibitory activity [using a validated enzyme inhibition assay different from that used in the first[2] study, both before (for active inhibitors) and after (for total inhibitors) base hydrolysis] of 1.13-fold and 1.18-fold, respectively, and of simvastatin and its β-hydroxyacid metabolite [measured using a chemical assay — liquid chromatography/tandem mass spectrometry] of 1.88-fold and 1.31-fold, respectively. The effect of amounts of grapefruit juice between those used in these two studies on simvastatin pharmacokinetics has not been studied.

---

[2] Lilja JJ, Kivisto KT, Neuvonen PJ. Clin Pharmacol Ther 1998;64(5):477-83.

Clinical Studies in Adults

Reductions in Risk of CHD Mortality and Cardiovascular Events

In 4S, the effect of therapy with ZOCOR on total mortality was assessed in 4,444 patients with CHD and baseline total cholesterol 212-309 mg/dL (5.5-8.0 mmol/L). In this multicenter, randomized, double-blind, placebo-controlled study, patients were treated with standard care, including diet, and either ZOCOR 20-40 mg/day (n=2,221) or placebo (n=2,223) for a median duration of 5.4 years. After six weeks of treatment with ZOCOR the median (25th and 75th percentile) changes in LDL-C, TG, and HDL-C were -39% (-46, -31%), -19% (-31, 0%), and 6% (-3, 17%). Over the course of the study, treatment with ZOCOR led to mean reductions in total-C, LDL-C and TG of 25%, 35%, and 10%, respectively, and a mean increase in HDL-C of 8%. ZOCOR significantly reduced the risk of mortality by 30%, (p=0.0003, 182 deaths in the ZOCOR group vs 256 deaths in the placebo group). The risk of CHD mortality was significantly reduced by 42% (p=0.00001, 111 vs 189 deaths). There was no statistically significant difference between groups in non-cardiovascular mortality. ZOCOR also significantly decreased the risk of having major coronary events (CHD mortality plus hospital-verified and silent non-fatal myocardial infarction [MI]) by 34% (p<0.00001, 431 vs 622 patients with one or more events). The risk of having a hospital-verified non-fatal MI was reduced by 37%. ZOCOR significantly reduced the risk for undergoing myocardial revascularization procedures (coronary artery bypass grafting or percutaneous transluminal coronary angioplasty) by 37%, (p<0.00001, 252 vs 383 patients). Furthermore, ZOCOR significantly reduced the risk of fatal plus non-fatal cerebrovascular events (combined stroke and transient ischemic attacks) by 28% (p=0.033, 75 vs 102 patients). ZOCOR reduced the risk of major coronary events to a similar extent across the range of baseline total and LDL cholesterol levels. Because there were only 53 female deaths, the effect of ZOCOR on mortality in women could not be adequately assessed. However, ZOCOR significantly lessened the risk of having major coronary events by 34% (60 vs 91 women with one or more event). The randomization was stratified by angina alone (21% of each treatment group) or a previous MI. Because there were only 57 deaths among the patients with angina alone at baseline, the effect of ZOCOR on mortality in this subgroup could not be adequately assessed. However, trends in reduced coronary mortality, major coronary events and revascularization procedures were consistent between this group and the total study cohort. Additionally, in this study, 1,021 of the patients were 65 and older. Cholesterol reduction with simvastatin resulted in similar decreases in relative risk for total mortality, CHD mortality, and major coronary events in these elderly patients, compared with younger patients.

The Heart Protection Study (HPS) was a large, multi-center, placebo-controlled, double-blind study with a mean duration of 5 years conducted in 20,536 patients (10,269 on ZOCOR 40 mg and 10,267 on placebo). Patients were allocated to treatment using a covariate adaptive method[3] which took into account the distribution of 10 important baseline characteristics of patients already enrolled and minimized the imbalance of those characteristics across the groups. Patients had a mean age of 64 years (range 40-80 years), were 97% Caucasian and were at high risk of developing a major coronary event because of existing coronary heart disease (65%), diabetes (Type 2, 26%; Type 1, 3%), history of stroke or other cerebrovascular disease (16%), peripheral vessel disease (33%), or hypertension in males 65 years of age and older (6%). At baseline, 3,421 patients (17%) had LDL-C levels below 100 mg/dL, of whom 953 (5%) had LDL-C levels below 80 mg/dL; 7,068 patients (34%) had levels between 100 and 130 mg/dL; and 10,047 patients (49%) had levels greater than 130 mg/dL.

[3] D.R. Taves, Minimization: a new method of assigning patients to treatment and control groups. Clin. Pharmacol. Ther. **15** (1974), pp. 443-453

The HPS results showed that ZOCOR 40 mg/day significantly reduced: total and CHD mortality; non-fatal myocardial infarctions, stroke, and revascularization procedures (coronary and non-coronary) (see Table 1).

[See table 1 at right]

Two composite endpoints were defined in order to have sufficient events to assess relative risk reductions across a range of baseline characteristics (see Figure 1). A composite of major coronary events (MCE) was comprised of CHD mortality and non-fatal MI (analyzed by time-to-first event; 898 patients treated with ZOCOR had events and 1,212 patients on placebo had events). A composite of major vascular events (MVE) was comprised of MCE, stroke and revascularization procedures including coronary, peripheral and other non-coronary procedures (analyzed by time-to-first event; 2,033 patients treated with ZOCOR had events and 2,585 patients on placebo had events). Significant relative risk reductions were observed for both composite endpoints (27% for MCE and 24% for MVE, p<0.0001). Furthermore, treatment with ZOCOR produced significant relative risk reductions for all components of the composite endpoints. The risk reductions produced by ZOCOR in both MCE and MVE were evident and consistent regardless of cardiovascular disease related medical history at study entry (i.e., CHD alone; or peripheral vascular disease, cerebrovascular disease, diabetes or treated hypertension, with or without CHD), gender, age, creatinine levels up to the entry limit of 2.3 mg/dL, baseline levels of LDL-C, HDL-C, apolipoprotein B and A-1, baseline concomitant cardiovascular medications (i.e., aspirin, beta blockers, or calcium channel blockers), smoking status, alcohol intake, or obesity. Diabetics showed risk reductions for MCE and MVE due to ZOCOR treatment regardless of baseline HbA1c levels or obesity with the greatest effects seen for diabetics without CHD.

[See figure 1 above]

[See second table above]

Angiographic Studies

In the Multicenter Anti-Atheroma Study, the effect of simvastatin on atherosclerosis was assessed by quantitative coronary angiography in hypercholesterolemic patients with coronary heart disease. In this randomized, double-blind, controlled study, patients were treated with simvastatin 20 mg/day or placebo. Angiograms were evaluated at baseline, two and four years. The co-primary study endpoints were mean change per-patient in minimum and mean lumen diameters, indicating focal and diffuse disease, respectively. Simvastatin significantly slowed the progression of lesions as measured in the Year 4 angiogram by both parameters, as well as by change in percent diameter stenosis. In addition, simvastatin significantly decreased the proportion of patients with new lesions and with new total occlusions.

Modifications of Lipid Profiles

Primary Hypercholesterolemia (Fredrickson type IIa and IIb)

ZOCOR has been shown to be highly effective in reducing total-C and LDL-C in heterozygous familial and non-familial forms of hypercholesterolemia and in mixed hyperlipidemia. A marked response was seen within 2 weeks, and the maximum therapeutic response occurred within 4-6 weeks. The response was maintained during chronic therapy. Furthermore, improving lipoprotein levels with ZOCOR improved survival in patients with CHD and hypercholesterolemia treated with 20-40 mg/day for a median of 5.4 years.

TABLE 1
Summary of Heart Protection Study Results

Endpoint	ZOCOR (N=10,269) n (%)†	Placebo (N=10,267) n (%)†	Risk Reduction (%) (95% CI)	p-Value
Primary				
Mortality	1,328 (12.9)	1,507 (14.7)	13 (6-19)	p=0.0003
CHD mortality	587 (5.7)	707 (6.9)	18 (8-26)	p=0.0005
Secondary				
Non-fatal MI	357 (3.5)	574 (5.6)	38 (30-46)	p<0.0001
Stroke	444 (4.3)	585 (5.7)	25 (15-34)	p<0.0001
Tertiary				
Coronary revascularization	513 (5)	725 (7.1)	30 (22-38)	p<0.0001
Peripheral and other non-coronary revascularization	450 (4.4)	532 (5.2)	16 (5-26)	p=0.006

† n = number of patients with indicated event

Figure 1
The Effects of Treatment with ZOCOR on Major Vascular Events and Major Coronary Events in HPS

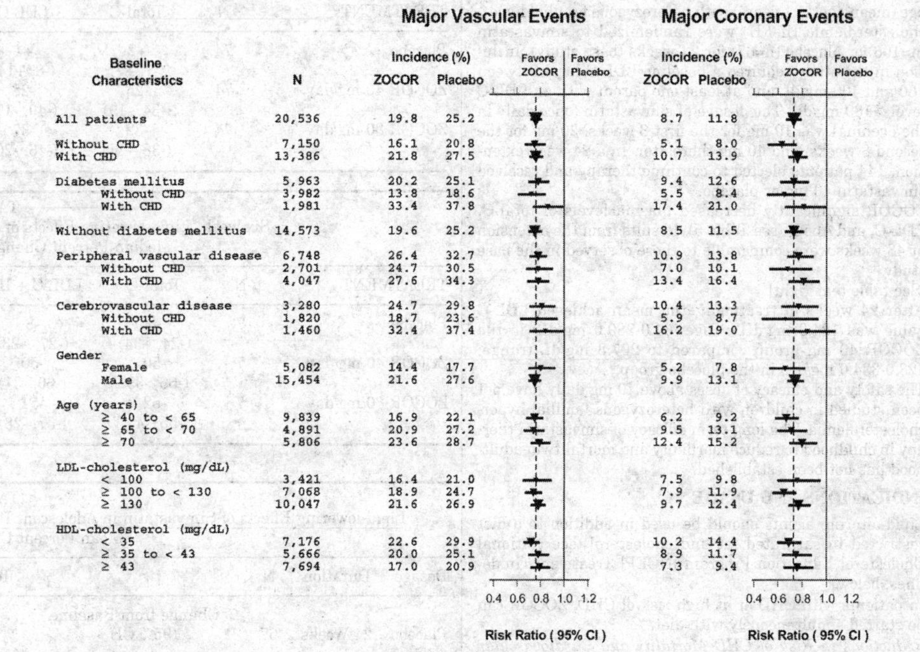

Baseline Characteristics	N	Major Vascular Events Incidence (%) ZOCOR	Major Vascular Events Incidence (%) Placebo	Major Coronary Events Incidence (%) ZOCOR	Major Coronary Events Incidence (%) Placebo
All patients	20,536	19.8	25.2	8.7	11.8
Without CHD	7,150	16.1	20.8	5.1	8.0
With CHD	13,386	21.8	27.5	10.7	13.9
Diabetes mellitus	5,963	20.2	25.1	9.4	12.6
Without CHD	3,982	13.8	18.6	5.5	8.4
With CHD	1,981	33.4	37.8	17.4	21.0
Without diabetes mellitus	14,573	19.6	25.2	8.5	11.5
Peripheral vascular disease	6,748	26.4	32.7	10.9	13.8
Without CHD	2,701	24.7	30.5	7.0	10.1
With CHD	4,047	27.6	34.3	13.4	16.4
Cerebrovascular disease	3,280	24.7	29.8	10.4	13.3
Without CHD	1,820	18.7	23.6	5.9	8.7
With CHD	1,460	32.4	37.4	16.2	19.0
Gender					
Female	5,082	14.4	17.7	5.2	7.8
Male	15,454	21.6	27.6	9.9	13.1
Age (years)					
≥ 40 to < 65	9,839	16.9	22.1	6.2	9.2
≥ 65 to < 70	4,891	20.9	27.2	9.5	13.1
≥ 70	5,806	23.6	28.7	12.4	15.2
LDL-cholesterol (mg/dL)					
< 100	3,421	16.4	21.0	7.5	9.8
≥ 100 to < 130	7,068	18.9	24.7	7.9	11.9
≥ 130	10,047	21.6	26.9	9.7	12.4
HDL-cholesterol (mg/dL)					
< 35	7,176	22.6	29.9	10.2	14.4
≥ 35 to < 43	5,666	20.0	25.1	8.9	11.7
≥ 43	7,694	17.0	20.9	7.3	9.4

Favors ZOCOR | Favors Placebo
0.4 0.6 0.8 1.0 1.2
Risk Ratio (95% CI)

N= number of patients in each subgroup. The inverted triangles are point estimates of the relative risk, with their 95% confidence intervals represented as a line. The area of a triangle is proportional to the number of patients with MVE or MCE in the subgroup relative to the number with MVE or MCE, respectively, in the entire study population. The vertical solid line represents a relative risk of one. The vertical dashed line represents the point estimate of relative risk in the entire study population.

In a multicenter, double-blind, placebo-controlled, dose-response study in patients with familial or non-familial hypercholesterolemia, ZOCOR given as a single dose in the evening (the recommended dosing) was similarly effective as when given on a twice-daily basis. ZOCOR consistently and significantly decreased total-C, LDL-C, total-C/HDL-C ratio, and LDL-C/HDL-C ratio. ZOCOR also decreased TG and increased HDL-C.

The results of studies depicting the mean response to simvastatin in patients with primary hypercholesterolemia and combined (mixed) hyperlipidemia are presented in Table 2.

[See table 2 at top of next page]

In the Upper Dose Comparative Study, the mean reduction in LDL-C was 47% at the 80-mg dose. Of the 664 patients randomized to 80 mg, 475 patients with plasma TG ≤ 200 mg/dL had a median reduction in TG of 21%, while in 189 patients with TG > 200 mg/dL, the median reduction in TG was 36%. In these studies, patients with TG > 350 mg/dL were excluded.

In the Multi-Center Combined Hyperlipidemia Study, a randomized, 3-period crossover study, 130 patients with combined hyperlipidemia (LDL-C>130 mg/dL and TG: 300-700 mg/dL) were treated with placebo, ZOCOR 40, and 80 mg/day for 6 weeks. In a dose-dependent manner ZOCOR 40 and 80 mg/day, respectively, decreased mean LDL-C by 29 and 36% (placebo: +2%) and median TG levels by 28 and 33% (placebo: 4%), and increased mean HDL-C by 13 and 16% (placebo: 3%) and apolipoprotein A-I by 8 and 11% (placebo: 4%).

Hypertriglyceridemia (Fredrickson type IV)

The results of a subgroup analysis in 74 patients with type IV hyperlipidemia from a 130-patient, double-blind, placebo-controlled, 3-period crossover study are presented in Table 3. The median baseline values (mg/dL) for the patients in this study were: total-C = 254, LDL-C = 135, HDL-C = 36, TG = 404, VLDL-C = 83, and non-HDL-C = 215.

[See table 3 on next page]

Dysbetalipoproteinemia (Fredrickson type III)

The results of a subgroup analysis in 7 patients with type III hyperlipidemia (dysbetalipoproteinemia) (apo E2/2) (VLDL-C/TG>0.25) from a 130-patient, double-blind, placebo-controlled, 3-period crossover study are presented in Table 4. In this study the median baseline values (mg/dL) were: total-C = 324, LDL-C = 121, HDL-C = 31, TG = 411, VLDL-C = 170, and non-HDL-C = 291.

[See table 4 on next page]

Homozygous Familial Hypercholesterolemia

In a controlled clinical study, 12 patients 15-39 years of age with homozygous familial hypercholesterolemia received simvastatin 40 mg/day in a single dose or in 3 divided doses, or 80 mg/day in 3 divided doses. Eleven of the 12 patients had reductions in LDL-C. In those patients with reductions, the mean LDL-C changes for the 40- and 80-mg doses were 14% (range 8% to 23%, median 12%) and 30% (range 14% to

Continued on next page

Zocor—Cont.

46%, median 29%), respectively. One patient had an increase of 15% in LDL-C. Another patient with absent LDL-C receptor function had an LDL-C reduction of 41% with the 80-mg dose.

Endocrine Function

In clinical studies, simvastatin did not impair adrenal reserve or significantly reduce basal plasma cortisol concentration. Small reductions from baseline in basal plasma testosterone in men were observed in clinical studies with simvastatin, an effect also observed with other inhibitors of HMG-CoA reductase and the bile acid sequestrant cholestyramine. There was no effect on plasma gonadotropin levels. In a placebo-controlled, 12-week study there was no significant effect of simvastatin 80 mg on the plasma testosterone response to human chorionic gonadotropin (hCG). In another 24-week study, simvastatin 20-40 mg had no detectable effect on spermatogenesis. In 4S, in which 4,444 patients were randomized to simvastatin 20-40 mg/day or placebo for a median duration of 5.4 years, the incidence of male sexual adverse events in the two treatment groups was not significantly different. Because of these factors, the small changes in plasma testosterone are unlikely to be clinically significant. The effects, if any, on the pituitary-gonadal axis in pre-menopausal women are unknown.

Clinical Studies in Adolescents

In a double-blind, placebo-controlled study, 175 patients (99 adolescent boys and 76 post-menarchal girls) 10-17 years of age (mean age 14.1 years) with heterozygous familial hypercholesterolemia (heFH) were randomized to simvastatin (n=106) or placebo (n=67) for 24 weeks (base study). Inclusion in the study required a baseline LDL-C level between 160 and 400 mg/dL and at least one parent with an LDL-C level >189 mg/dL. The dosage of simvastatin (once daily in the evening) was 10 mg for the first 8 weeks, 20 mg for the second 8 weeks, and 40 mg thereafter. In a 24-week extension, 144 patients elected to continue therapy and received simvastatin 40 mg or placebo.

ZOCOR significantly decreased plasma levels of total-C, LDL-C, and Apo B (see Table 5). Results from the extension at 48 weeks were comparable to those observed in the base study.

[See table 5 at right]

After 24 weeks of treatment, the mean achieved LDL-C value was 124.9 mg/dL (range: 64.0-289.0 mg/dL) in the ZOCOR 40 mg group compared to 207.8 mg/dL (range: 128.0-334.0 mg/dL) in the placebo group.

The safety and efficacy of doses above 40 mg daily have not been studied in children with heterozygous familial hypercholesterolemia. The long-term efficacy of simvastatin therapy in childhood to reduce morbidity and mortality in adulthood has not been established.

INDICATIONS AND USAGE

Lipid-altering agents should be used in addition to a diet restricted in saturated fat and cholesterol (see National Cholesterol Education Program [NCEP] Treatment Guidelines, below).

In patients with CHD or at high risk of CHD, ZOCOR can be started simultaneously with diet.

Reductions in Risk of CHD Mortality and Cardiovascular Events

In patients at high risk of coronary events because of existing coronary heart disease, diabetes, peripheral vessel disease, history of stroke or other cerebrovascular disease, ZOCOR is indicated to:

- Reduce the risk of total mortality by reducing CHD deaths.
- Reduce the risk of non-fatal myocardial infarction and stroke.
- Reduce the need for coronary and non-coronary revascularization procedures.

Patients with Hypercholesterolemia Requiring Modifications of Lipid Profiles

ZOCOR is indicated to:

- Reduce elevated total-C, LDL-C, Apo B, and TG, and to increase HDL-C in patients with primary hypercholesterolemia (heterozygous familial and nonfamilial) and mixed dyslipidemia (Fredrickson types IIa and IIb[4]).
- Treat patients with hypertriglyceridemia (Fredrickson type IV hyperlipidemia).
- Treat patients with primary dysbetalipoproteinemia (Fredrickson type III hyperlipidemia).
- Reduce total-C and LDL-C in patients with homozygous familial hypercholesterolemia as an adjunct to other lipid-lowering treatments (e.g., LDL apheresis) or if such treatments are unavailable.

Adolescent Patients with Heterozygous Familial Hypercholesterolemia (HeFH)

ZOCOR is indicated as an adjunct to diet to reduce total-C, LDL-C, and Apo B levels in adolescent boys and girls who are at least one year post-menarche, 10-17 years of age, with heterozygous familial hypercholesterolemia, if after an adequate trial of diet therapy the following findings are present:

1. LDL cholesterol remains ≥190 mg/dL; or
2. LDL cholesterol remains ≥160 mg/dL and
   - There is a positive family history of premature cardiovascular disease (CVD) or
   - Two or more other CVD risk factors are present in the adolescent patient

TABLE 2
Mean Response in Patients with Primary Hypercholesterolemia and Combined (mixed) Hyperlipidemia
(Mean Percent Change from Baseline After 6 to 24 Weeks)

TREATMENT	N	TOTAL-C	LDL-C	HDL-C	TG†
Lower Dose Comparative Study (Mean % Change at Week 6)					
ZOCOR 5 mg q.p.m.	109	-19	-26	10	-12
ZOCOR 10 mg q.p.m.	110	-23	-30	12	-15
Scandinavian Simvastatin Survival Study (Mean % Change at Week 6)					
Placebo	2223	-1	-1	0	-2
ZOCOR 20 mg q.p.m.	2221	-28	-38	8	-19
Upper Dose Comparative Study (Mean % Change Averaged at Weeks 18 and 24)					
ZOCOR 40 mg q.p.m.	433	-31	-41	9	-18
ZOCOR 80 mg q.p.m.	664	-36	-47	8	-24
Multi-Center Combined Hyperlipidemia Study (Mean % Change at Week 6)					
Placebo	125	1	2	3	-4
ZOCOR 40 mg q.p.m.	123	-25	-29	13	-28
ZOCOR 80 mg q.p.m.	124	-31	-36	16	-33

† median percent change

TABLE 3
Six-week, Lipid-lowering Effects of Simvastatin in Type IV Hyperlipidemia
Median Percent Change (25th and 75th percentile) from Baseline

TREATMENT	N	Total-C	LDL-C	HDL-C	TG	VLDL-C	Non-HDL-C
Placebo	74	+2 (-7, +7)	+1 (-8, +14)	+3 (-3, +10)	-9 (-25, +13)	-7 (-25, +11)	+1 (-9, +8)
ZOCOR 40 mg/day	74	-25 (-34, -19)	-28 (-40, -17)	+11 (+5, +23)	-29 (-43, -16)	-37 (-54,-23)	-32 (-42, -23)
ZOCOR 80 mg/day	74	-32 (-38, -24)	-37 (-46, -26)	+15 (+5, +23)	-34 (-45, -18)	-41 (-57, -28)	-38 (-49,-32)

TABLE 4
Six-week, Lipid-lowering Effects of Simvastatin in Type III Hyperlipidemia
Median Percent Change (min,max) from Baseline

TREATMENT	N	Total-C	LDL-C + IDL	HDL-C	TG	VLDL-C+IDL	Non-HDL-C
Placebo	7	-8 (-24, +34)	-8 (-27, +23)	-2 (-21, +16)	+4 (-22, +90)	-4 (-28, +78)	-8 (-26, -39)
ZOCOR 40 mg/day	7	-50 (-66, -39)	-50 (-60, -31)	+7 (-8, +23)	-41 (-74, -16)	-58 (-90, -37)	-57 (-72, -44)
ZOCOR 80 mg/day	7	-52 (-55, -41)	-51 (-57, -28)	+7 (-5, +29)	-38 (-58, +2)	-60 (-72, -39)	-59 (-61, -46)

TABLE 5
Lipid-lowering Effects of Simvastatin in Adolescent Patients with Heterozygous Familial Hypercholesterolemia
(Mean Percent Change from Baseline)

Dosage	Duration	N		Total-C	LDL-C	HDL-C	TG†	Apo B
Placebo	24 Weeks	67	% Change from Baseline (95% CI)	1.6 (-2.2, 5.3)	1.1 (-3.4, 5.5)	3.6 (-0.7, 8.0)	-3.2 (-11.8, 5.4)	-0.5 (-4.7, 3.6)
			Mean baseline, mg/dL (SD)	278.6 (51.8)	211.9 (49.0)	46.9 (11.9)	90.0 (50.7)	186.3 (38.1)
ZOCOR	24 Weeks	106	% Change from Baseline (95% CI)	-26.5 (-29.6, -23.3)	-36.8 (-40.5, -33.0)	8.3 (4.6, 11.9)	-7.9 (-15.8, 0.0)	-32.4 (-35.9, -29.0)
			Mean baseline, mg/dL (SD)	270.2 (44.0)	203.8 (41.5)	47.7 (9.0)	78.3 (46.0)	179.9 (33.8)

† median percent change

The minimum goal of treatment in pediatric and adolescent patients is to achieve a mean LDL-C <130 mg/dL. The optimal age at which to initiate lipid-lowering therapy to decrease the risk of symptomatic adulthood CAD has not been determined.

General Recommendations

Prior to initiating therapy with simvastatin, secondary causes for hypercholesterolemia (e.g., hypothyroidism, nephrotic syndrome, dysproteinemias, obstructive liver disease, other drug therapy, alcoholism) should be excluded, and a lipid profile performed to measure total-C, HDL-C, and TG. For patients with TG less than 400 mg/dL (<4.5 mmol/L), LDL-C can be estimated using the following equation:

$$\text{LDL-C} = \text{total-C} - [(0.20 \times \text{TG}) + \text{HDL-C}]$$

For TG levels >400 mg/dL (>4.5 mmol/L), this equation is less accurate and LDL-C concentrations should be determined by ultracentrifugation. In many hypertriglyceridemic patients, LDL-C may be low or normal despite elevated total-C. In such cases, ZOCOR is not indicated.

Lipid determinations should be performed at intervals of no less than four weeks and dosage adjusted according to the patient's response to therapy.

The NCEP Treatment Guidelines are summarized in Table 6:

[See table 6 at top of next page]

After the LDL-C goal has been achieved, if the TG is still ≥200 mg/dL, non-HDL-C (total-C minus HDL-C) becomes a secondary target of therapy. Non-HDL-C goals are set 30 mg/dL higher than LDL-C goals for each risk category.

At the time of hospitalization for an acute coronary event, consideration can be given to initiating drug therapy at discharge if the LDL-C is ≥ 130 mg/dL (see NCEP Treatment Guidelines, above).

The NCEP classification of cholesterol levels in pediatric patients with a familial history of either hypercholesterolemia or premature cardiovascular disease is summarized in Table 7.

TABLE 7
NCEP Classification of Cholesterol Levels in Pediatric Patients with a Familial History of Either HeFH or Premature CVD

Category	Total-C (mg/dL)	LDL-C (mg/dL)
Acceptable	<170	<110
Borderline	170-199	110-129
High	≥200	≥130

Since the goal of treatment is to lower LDL-C, the NCEP recommends that LDL-C levels be used to initiate and assess treatment response. Only if LDL-C levels are not available, should the total-C be used to monitor therapy.

ZOCOR is indicated to reduce elevated LDL-C and TG levels in patients with Type IIb hyperlipidemia (where hypercholesterolemia is the major abnormality). However, it has not been studied in conditions where the major abnormality is elevation of chylomicrons (i.e., hyperlipidemia Fredrickson types I and V).[4]

[4]Classification of Hyperlipoproteinemias

Type	Lipoproteins elevated	Lipid Elevations major	minor
I (rare)	chylomicrons	TG	↑→C
IIa	LDL	C	—
IIb	LDL, VLDL	C	TG
III (rare)	IDL	C/TG	—
IV	VLDL	TG	↑→C
V (rare)	chylomicrons, VLDL	TG	↑→C

C = cholesterol, TG = triglycerides,
LDL = low-density lipoprotein,
VLDL = very-low-density lipoprotein,
IDL = intermediate-density lipoprotein.

CONTRAINDICATIONS

Hypersensitivity to any component of this medication.

Active liver disease or unexplained persistent elevations of serum transaminases (see WARNINGS).

Pregnancy and lactation. Atherosclerosis is a chronic process and the discontinuation of lipid-lowering drugs during pregnancy should have little impact on the outcome of long-term therapy of primary hypercholesterolemia. Moreover, cholesterol and other products of the cholesterol biosynthesis pathway are essential components for fetal development, including synthesis of steroids and cell membranes. Because of the ability of inhibitors of HMG-CoA reductase such as ZOCOR to decrease the synthesis of cholesterol and possibly other products of the cholesterol biosynthesis pathway, ZOCOR is contraindicated during pregnancy and in nursing mothers. **ZOCOR should be administered to women of childbearing age only when such patients are highly unlikely to conceive.** If the patient becomes pregnant while taking this drug, ZOCOR should be discontinued immediately and the patient should be apprised of the potential hazard to the fetus (see PRECAUTIONS, *Pregnancy*).

WARNINGS

Myopathy/Rhabdomyolysis

Simvastatin, like other inhibitors of HMG-CoA reductase, occasionally causes myopathy manifested as muscle pain, tenderness or weakness with creatine kinase (CK) above 10× the upper limit of normal (ULN). Myopathy sometimes takes the form of rhabdomyolysis with or without acute renal failure secondary to myoglobinuria, and rare fatalities have occurred. The risk of myopathy is increased by high levels of HMG-CoA reductase inhibitory activity in plasma.

- **The risk of myopathy/rhabdomyolysis is increased by concomitant use of simvastatin with the following:**

  Potent inhibitors of CYP3A4: Cyclosporine, itraconazole, ketoconazole, erythromycin, clarithromycin, HIV protease inhibitors, nefazodone, or large quantities of grapefruit juice (>1 quart daily), particularly with higher doses of simvastatin (see below; CLINICAL PHARMACOLOGY, *Pharmacokinetics*; PRECAUTIONS, *Drug Interactions, CYP3A4 Interactions*).

  Other drugs:

  Gemfibrozil particularly with higher doses of simvastatin (see below; PRECAUTIONS, *Drug Interactions, Interactions with lipid-lowering drugs that can cause myopathy when given alone*; DOSAGE AND ADMINISTRATION).

  Other lipid-lowering drugs (other fibrates or ≥1 g/day of niacin) that can cause myopathy when given alone (see below; PRECAUTIONS, *Drug Interactions, Interactions with lipid-lowering drugs that can cause myopathy when given alone*).

  Amiodarone or verapamil with higher doses of simvastatin (see below; PRECAUTIONS, *Drug Interactions, Other drug interactions*). In an ongoing clinical trial, myopathy has been reported in 6% of patients receiving simvastatin 80 mg and amiodarone. In an analysis of clinical trials involving 25,248 patients treated with simvastatin 20 to 80 mg, the incidence of myopathy was higher in patients receiving verapamil and simvastatin (4/635; 0.63%) than in patients taking simvastatin without a calcium channel blocker (13/21,224; 0.061%).

- **The risk of myopathy/rhabdomyolysis is dose related.** The incidence in clinical trials, in which patients were carefully monitored and some interacting drugs were excluded, has been approximately 0.02% at 20 mg, 0.07% at 40 mg and 0.3% at 80 mg.

Consequently:

1. Use of simvastatin concomitantly with itraconazole, ketoconazole, erythromycin, clarithromycin, HIV protease inhibitors, nefazodone, or large quantities of grapefruit juice (>1 quart daily) should be avoided. If treatment with itraconazole, ketoconazole, erythromycin, or clarithromycin is unavoidable, therapy with simvastatin should be suspended during the course of treatment. Concomitant use with other medicines labeled as having a potent inhibitory effect on CYP3A4 at therapeutic doses should be avoided unless the benefits of combined therapy outweigh the increased risk.

2. The dose of simvastatin should not exceed 10 mg daily in patients receiving concomitant medication with gemfibrozil. The combined use of simvastatin with gemfibrozil should be avoided, unless the benefits are likely to outweigh the increased risks of this drug combination. Caution should be used when prescribing other lipid-lowering drugs (other fibrates or lipid-lowering doses (≥1 g/day) of niacin) with simvastatin, as these agents can cause myopathy when given alone. **The benefit of further alterations in lipid levels by the combined use of simvastatin with fibrates or niacin should be carefully weighed against the potential risks of these combinations.** Addition of fibrates or niacin to simvastatin typically provides little additional reduction in LDL-C, but further reductions of TG and further increases in HDL-C may be obtained.

TABLE 6
NCEP Treatment Guidelines:
LDL-C Goals and Cutpoints for Therapeutic Lifestyle Changes and Drug Therapy in Different Risk Categories

Risk Category	LDL Goal (mg/dL)	LDL Level at Which to Initiate Therapeutic Lifestyle Changes (mg/dL)	LDL Level at Which to Consider Drug Therapy (mg/dL)
CHD† or CHD risk equivalents (10-year risk >20%)	<100	≥100	≥130 (100-129: drug optional)‡
2+ Risk factors (10-year risk ≤20%)	<130	≥130	10-year risk 10-20%: ≥130 10-year risk <10%: ≥160
0-1 Risk factor§	<160	≥160	≥190 (160-189: LDL-lowering drug optional)

†CHD, coronary heart disease

‡Some authorities recommend use of LDL-lowering drugs in this category if an LDL-C level of <100 mg/dL cannot be achieved by therapeutic lifestyle changes. Others prefer use of drugs that primarily modify triglycerides and HDL-C, e.g., nicotinic acid or fibrate. Clinical judgment also may call for deferring drug therapy in this subcategory.

§Almost all people with 0-1 risk factor have a 10-year risk <10%; thus, 10-year risk assessment in people with 0-1 risk factor is not necessary.

3. The dose of simvastatin should not exceed 10 mg daily in patients receiving concomitant medication with cyclosporine. The benefits of the use of simvastatin in patients receiving cyclosporine should be carefully weighed against the risks of this combination.

4. The dose of simvastatin should not exceed 20 mg daily in patients receiving concomitant medication with amiodarone or verapamil. The combined use of simvastatin at doses higher than 20 mg daily with amiodarone or verapamil should be avoided unless the clinical benefit is likely to outweigh the increased risk of myopathy.

5. All patients starting therapy with simvastatin, or whose dose of simvastatin is being increased, should be advised of the risk of myopathy and told to report promptly any unexplained muscle pain, tenderness or weakness. Simvastatin therapy should be discontinued immediately if myopathy is diagnosed or suspected. The presence of these symptoms, and/or a CK level >10 times the ULN indicates myopathy. In most cases, when patients were promptly discontinued from treatment, muscle symptoms and CK increases resolved. Periodic CK determinations may be considered in patients starting therapy with simvastatin or whose dose is being increased, but there is no assurance that such monitoring will prevent myopathy.

6. Many of the patients who have developed rhabdomyolysis on therapy with simvastatin have had complicated medical histories, including renal insufficiency usually as a consequence of long-standing diabetes mellitus. Such patients merit closer monitoring. Therapy with simvastatin should be temporarily stopped a few days prior to elective major surgery and when any major medical or surgical condition supervenes.

Liver Dysfunction

Persistent increases (to more than 3× the ULN) in serum transaminases have occurred in approximately 1% of patients who received simvastatin in clinical studies. When drug treatment was interrupted or discontinued in these patients, the transaminase levels usually fell slowly to pretreatment levels. The increases were not associated with jaundice or other clinical signs or symptoms. There was no evidence of hypersensitivity.

In 4S (see CLINICAL PHARMACOLOGY, *Clinical Studies*), the number of patients with more than one transaminase elevation to > 3× ULN, over the course of the study, was not significantly different between the simvastatin and placebo groups (14 [0.7%] vs. 12 [0.6%]). Elevated transaminases resulted in the discontinuation of 8 patients from therapy in the simvastatin group (n=2,221) and 5 in the placebo group (n=2,223). Of the 1,986 simvastatin treated patients in 4S with normal liver function tests (LFTs) at baseline, only 8 (0.4%) developed consecutive LFT elevations to > 3× ULN and/or were discontinued due to transaminase elevations during the 5.4 years (median follow-up) of the study. Among these 8 patients, 5 initially developed these abnormalities within the first year. All of the patients in this study received a starting dose of 20 mg of simvastatin; 37% were titrated to 40 mg.

In 2 controlled clinical studies in 1,105 patients, the 12-month incidence of persistent hepatic transaminase elevation without regard to drug relationship was 0.9% and 2.1% at the 40- and 80-mg dose, respectively. No patients developed persistent liver function abnormalities following the initial 6 months of treatment at a given dose.

It is recommended that liver function tests be performed before the initiation of treatment, and thereafter when clinically indicated. Patients titrated to the 80-mg dose should receive an additional test prior to titration, 3 months after titration to the 80-mg dose, and periodically thereafter (e.g., semiannually) for the first year of treatment. Patients who develop increased transaminase levels should be monitored with a second liver function evaluation to confirm the finding and be followed thereafter with frequent liver function tests until the abnormality(ies) return to normal. Should an increase in AST or ALT of 3× ULN or greater persist, withdrawal of therapy with ZOCOR is recommended.

The drug should be used with caution in patients who consume substantial quantities of alcohol and/or have a past history of liver disease. Active liver diseases or unexplained transaminase elevations are contraindications to the use of simvastatin.

As with other lipid-lowering agents, moderate (less than 3× ULN) elevations of serum transaminases have been reported following therapy with simvastatin. These changes appeared soon after initiation of therapy with simvastatin, were often transient, were not accompanied by any symptoms and did not require interruption of treatment.

PRECAUTIONS

General

Simvastatin may cause elevation of CK and transaminase levels (see WARNINGS and ADVERSE REACTIONS). This should be considered in the differential diagnosis of chest pain in a patient on therapy with simvastatin.

Information for Patients

Patients should be advised about substances they should not take concomitantly with simvastatin and be advised to report promptly unexplained muscle pain, tenderness, or weakness (see list below and WARNINGS, *Myopathy/Rhabdomyolysis*). Patients should also be advised to inform other physicians prescribing a new medication that they are taking ZOCOR.

Drug Interactions

CYP3A4 Interactions

Simvastatin is metabolized by CYP3A4 but has no CYP3A4 inhibitory activity; therefore it is not expected to affect the plasma concentrations of other drugs metabolized by CYP3A4. Potent inhibitors of CYP3A4 (below) increase the risk of myopathy by reducing the elimination of simvastatin.

See WARNINGS, *Myopathy/Rhabdomyolysis*, and CLINICAL PHARMACOLOGY, *Pharmacokinetics*.

Itraconazole
Ketoconazole
Erythromycin
Clarithromycin
HIV protease inhibitors
Nefazodone
Cyclosporine
Large quantities of grapefruit juice (>1 quart daily)

Interactions with lipid-lowering drugs that can cause myopathy when given alone

See WARNINGS, *Myopathy/Rhabdomyolysis*.

The risk of myopathy is increased by gemfibrozil (**see DOSAGE AND ADMINISTRATION**) and to a lesser extent by other fibrates and niacin (nicotinic acid) (≥1 g/day).

Other drug interactions

Amiodarone or Verapamil: The risk of myopathy/rhabdomyolysis is increased by concomitant administration of amiodarone or verapamil (see WARNINGS, *Myopathy/Rhabdomyolysis*).

Propranolol: In healthy male volunteers there was a significant decrease in mean C_{max}, but no change in AUC, for simvastatin total and active inhibitors with concomitant administration of single doses of ZOCOR and propranolol. The clinical relevance of this finding is unclear. The pharmacokinetics of the enantiomers of propranolol were not affected.

Digoxin: Concomitant administration of a single dose of digoxin in healthy male volunteers receiving simvastatin resulted in a slight elevation (less than 0.3 ng/mL) in digoxin concentrations in plasma (as measured by a radioimmunoassay) compared to concomitant administration of placebo and digoxin. Patients taking digoxin should be monitored appropriately when simvastatin is initiated.

Warfarin: In two clinical studies, one in normal volunteers and the other in hypercholesterolemic patients, simvastatin

Continued on next page

Information on the Merck & Co., Inc., products listed on these pages is from the prescribing information in use October 1, 2004. For information, please call 1-800-NSC-MERCK [1-800-672-6372].

Zocor—Cont.

20-40 mg/day modestly potentiated the effect of coumarin anticoagulants: the prothrombin time, reported as International Normalized Ratio (INR), increased from a baseline of 1.7 to 1.8 and from 2.6 to 3.4 in the volunteer and patient studies, respectively. With other reductase inhibitors, clinically evident bleeding and/or increased prothrombin time has been reported in a few patients taking coumarin anticoagulants concomitantly. In such patients, prothrombin time should be determined before starting simvastatin and frequently enough during early therapy to insure that no significant alteration of prothrombin time occurs. Once a stable prothrombin time has been documented, prothrombin times can be monitored at the intervals usually recommended for patients on coumarin anticoagulants. If the dose of simvastatin is changed or discontinued, the same procedure should be repeated. Simvastatin therapy has not been associated with bleeding or with changes in prothrombin time in patients not taking anticoagulants.

CNS Toxicity

Optic nerve degeneration was seen in clinically normal dogs treated with simvastatin for 14 weeks at 180 mg/kg/day, a dose that produced mean plasma drug levels about 12 times higher than the mean plasma drug level in humans taking 80 mg/day.

A chemically similar drug in this class also produced optic nerve degeneration (Wallerian degeneration of retinogeniculate fibers) in clinically normal dogs in a dose-dependent fashion starting at 60 mg/kg/day, a dose that produced mean plasma drug levels about 30 times higher than the mean plasma drug level in humans taking the highest recommended dose (as measured by total enzyme inhibitory activity). This same drug also produced vestibulocochlear Wallerian-like degeneration and retinal ganglion cell chromatolysis in dogs treated for 14 weeks at 180 mg/kg/day, a dose that resulted in a mean plasma drug level similar to that seen with the 60 mg/kg/day dose.

CNS vascular lesions, characterized by perivascular hemorrhage and edema, mononuclear cell infiltration of perivascular spaces, perivascular fibrin deposits and necrosis of small vessels were seen in dogs treated with simvastatin at a dose of 360 mg/kg/day, a dose that produced mean plasma drug levels that were about 14 times higher than the mean plasma drug levels in humans taking 80 mg/day. Similar CNS vascular lesions have been observed with several other drugs of this class.

There were cataracts in female rats after two years of treatment with 50 and 100 mg/kg/day (22 and 25 times the human AUC at 80 mg/day, respectively) and in dogs after three months at 90 mg/kg/day (19 times) and at two years at 50 mg/kg/day (5 times).

Carcinogenesis, Mutagenesis, Impairment of Fertility

In a 72-week carcinogenicity study, mice were administered daily doses of simvastatin of 25, 100, and 400 mg/kg body weight, which resulted in mean plasma drug levels approximately 1, 4, and 8 times higher than the mean human plasma drug level, respectively (as total inhibitory activity based on AUC) after an 80-mg oral dose. Liver carcinomas were significantly increased in high-dose females and mid- and high-dose males with a maximum incidence of 90% in males. The incidence of adenomas of the liver was significantly increased in mid- and high-dose females. Drug treatment also significantly increased the incidence of lung adenomas in mid- and high-dose males and females. Adenomas of the Harderian gland (a gland of the eye of rodents) were significantly higher in high-dose mice than in controls. No evidence of a tumorigenic effect was observed at 25 mg/kg/day.

In a separate 92-week carcinogenicity study in mice at doses up to 25 mg/kg/day, no evidence of a tumorigenic effect was observed (mean plasma drug levels were 1 times higher than humans given 80 mg simvastatin as measured by AUC).

In a two-year study in rats at 25 mg/kg/day, there was a statistically significant increase in the incidence of thyroid follicular adenomas in female rats exposed to approximately 11 times higher levels of simvastatin than in humans given 80 mg simvastatin (as measured by AUC).

A second two-year rat carcinogenicity study with doses of 50 and 100 mg/kg/day produced hepatocellular adenomas and carcinomas (in female rats at both doses and in males at 100 mg/kg/day). Thyroid follicular cell adenomas were increased in males and females at both doses; thyroid follicular cell carcinomas were increased in females at 100 mg/kg/day. The increased incidence of thyroid neoplasms appears to be consistent with findings from other HMG-CoA reductase inhibitors. These treatment levels represented plasma drug levels (AUC) of approximately 7 and 15 times (males) and 22 and 25 times (females) the mean human plasma drug exposure after an 80 milligram daily dose.

No evidence of mutagenicity was observed in a microbial mutagenicity (Ames) test with or without rat or mouse liver metabolic activation. In addition, no evidence of damage to genetic material was noted in an *in vitro* alkaline elution assay using rat hepatocytes, a V-79 mammalian cell forward mutation study, an *in vitro* chromosome aberration study in CHO cells, or an *in vivo* chromosomal aberration assay in mouse bone marrow.

There was decreased fertility in male rats treated with simvastatin for 34 weeks at 25 mg/kg body weight (4 times the maximum human exposure level, based on AUC, in patients receiving 80 mg/day); however, this effect was not observed during a subsequent fertility study in which simvastatin was administered at this same dose level to male rats for 11 weeks (the entire cycle of spermatogenesis including epididymal maturation). No microscopic changes were observed in the testes of rats from either study. At 180 mg/kg/day, (which produces exposure levels 22 times higher than those in humans taking 80 mg/day based on surface area, mg/m^2), seminiferous tubule degeneration (necrosis and loss of spermatogenic epithelium) was observed. In dogs, there was drug-related testicular atrophy, decreased spermatogenesis, spermatocytic degeneration and giant cell formation at 10 mg/kg/day, (approximately 2 times the human exposure, based on AUC, at 80 mg/day). The clinical significance of these findings is unclear.

Pregnancy

Pregnancy Category X

See CONTRAINDICATIONS.

Safety in pregnant women has not been established.

Simvastatin was not teratogenic in rats at doses of 25 mg/kg/day or in rabbits at doses up to 10 mg/kg daily. These doses resulted in 3 times (rat) or 3 times (rabbit) the human exposure based on mg/m^2 surface area. However, in studies with another structurally-related HMG-CoA reductase inhibitor, skeletal malformations were observed in rats and mice.

Rare reports of congenital anomalies have been received following intrauterine exposure to HMG-CoA reductase inhibitors. In a review[5] of approximately 100 prospectively followed pregnancies in women exposed to ZOCOR or another structurally related HMG-CoA reductase inhibitor, the incidences of congenital anomalies, spontaneous abortions and fetal deaths/stillbirths did not exceed what would be expected in the general population. The number of cases is adequate only to exclude a 3- to 4-fold increase in congenital anomalies over the background incidence. In 89% of the prospectively followed pregnancies, drug treatment was initiated prior to pregnancy and was discontinued at some point in the first trimester when pregnancy was identified. As safety in pregnant women has not been established and there is no apparent benefit to therapy with ZOCOR during pregnancy (see CONTRAINDICATIONS), treatment should be immediately discontinued as soon as pregnancy is recognized. ZOCOR should be administered to women of childbearing potential only when such patients are highly unlikely to conceive and have been informed of the potential hazards.

[5] Manson, J.M., Freyssinges, C., Ducrocq, M.B., Stephenson, W.P., Postmarketing Surveillance of Lovastatin and Simvastatin Exposure During Pregnancy, *Reproductive Toxicology*, 10(6):439-446, 1996.

Nursing Mothers

It is not known whether simvastatin is excreted in human milk. Because a small amount of another drug in this class is excreted in human milk and because of the potential for serious adverse reactions in nursing infants, women taking simvastatin should not nurse their infants (see CONTRAINDICATIONS).

Pediatric Use

Safety and effectiveness of simvastatin in patients 10-17 years of age with heterozygous familial hypercholesterolemia have been evaluated in a controlled clinical trial in adolescent boys and in girls who were at least 1 year post-menarche. Patients treated with simvastatin had an adverse experience profile generally similar to that of patients treated with placebo. **Doses greater than 40 mg have not been studied in this population.** In this limited controlled study, there was no detectable effect on growth or sexual maturation in the adolescent boys or girls, or any effect on menstrual cycle length in girls. See CLINICAL PHARMACOLOGY, *Clinical Studies in Adolescents;* ADVERSE REACTIONS, *Adolescent Patients;* and DOSAGE AND ADMINISTRATION, *Adolescents (10-17 years of age) with Heterozygous Familial Hypercholesterolemia.* Adolescent females should be counseled on appropriate contraceptive methods while on simvastatin therapy (see CONTRAINDICATIONS and PRECAUTIONS, *Pregnancy*). Simvastatin has not been studied in patients younger than 10 years of age, nor in pre-menarchal girls.

Geriatric Use

A pharmacokinetic study with simvastatin showed the mean plasma level of HMG-CoA reductase inhibitory activity to be approximately 45% higher in elderly patients between 70-78 years of age compared with patients between 18-30 years of age. In 4S, 1,021 (23%) of 4,444 patients were 65 or older. In 4S, lipid-lowering efficacy was at least as great in elderly patients compared with younger patients. In this study, ZOCOR significantly reduced total mortality and CHD mortality in elderly patients with a history of CHD. In HPS, 52% of patients were elderly (4,891 patients 65-69 years and 5,806 patients 70 years or older). The relative risk reductions of CHD death, non-fatal MI, coronary and non-coronary revascularization procedures, and stroke were similar in older and younger patients (see CLINICAL PHARMACOLOGY). In HPS, among 32,145 patients entering the active run-in period, there were 2 cases of myopathy/rhabdomyolysis; these patients were aged 67 and 73. Of the 7 cases of myopathy/rhabdomyolysis among 10,269 patients allocated to simvastatin, 4 were aged 65 or more (at baseline), of whom one was over 75. There were no overall differences in safety between older and younger patients in either 4S or HPS.

ADVERSE REACTIONS

In the pre-marketing controlled clinical studies and their open extensions (2,423 patients with mean duration of follow-up of approximately 18 months), 1.4% of patients were discontinued due to adverse experiences attributable to ZOCOR. Adverse reactions have usually been mild and transient. ZOCOR has been evaluated for serious adverse reactions in more than 21,000 patients and is generally well tolerated.

Clinical Adverse Experiences

In Adults

Adverse experiences occurring in adults at an incidence of 1% or greater in patients treated with ZOCOR, regardless of causality, in controlled clinical studies are shown in Table 8. [See table 8 at left]

TABLE 8
Adverse Experiences in Clinical Studies Incidence 1 Percent or Greater, Regardless of Causality

	ZOCOR (N = 1,583) %	Placebo (N = 157) %	Cholestyramine (N = 179) %
Body as a Whole			
Abdominal pain	3.2	3.2	8.9
Asthenia	1.6	2.5	1.1
Gastrointestinal			
Constipation	2.3	1.3	29.1
Diarrhea	1.9	2.5	7.8
Dyspepsia	1.1	—	4.5
Flatulence	1.9	1.3	14.5
Nausea	1.3	1.9	10.1
Nervous System/Psychiatric			
Headache	3.5	5.1	4.5
Respiratory			
Upper respiratory infection	2.1	1.9	3.4

Scandinavian Simvastatin Survival Study

Clinical Adverse Experiences

In 4S (see CLINICAL PHARMACOLOGY, *Clinical Studies*) involving 4,444 patients treated with 20-40 mg/day of ZOCOR (n=2,221) or placebo (n=2,223), the safety and tolerability profiles were comparable between groups over the median 5.4 years of the study. The clinical adverse experiences reported as possibly, probably, or definitely drug-related in ≥ 0.5% in either treatment group are shown in Table 9.

TABLE 9
Drug-Related Clinical Adverse Experiences in 4S Incidence 0.5 Percent or Greater

	ZOCOR (N = 2,221) %	Placebo (N = 2,223) %
Body as a Whole		
Abdominal pain	0.9	0.9
Gastrointestinal		
Diarrhea	0.5	0.3
Dyspepsia	0.6	0.5
Flatulence	0.9	0.7
Nausea	0.4	0.6
Musculoskeletal		
Myalgia	1.2	1.3
Skin		
Eczema	0.8	0.8
Pruritus	0.5	0.4
Rash	0.6	0.6
Special Senses		
Cataract	0.5	0.8

Heart Protection Study

Clinical Adverse Experiences

In HPS (see CLINICAL PHARMACOLOGY, *Clinical Studies*), involving 20,536 patients treated with ZOCOR 40 mg/day (n=10,269) or placebo (n=10,267), the safety profiles were comparable between patients treated with ZOCOR and patients treated with placebo over the mean 5 years of the study. In this large trial, only serious adverse events and discontinuations due to any adverse events were recorded. Discontinuation rates due to adverse experiences were comparable (4.8% in patients treated with ZOCOR compared with 5.1% in patients treated with placebo). The incidence of myopathy/rhabdomyolysis was <0.1% in patients treated with ZOCOR.

The following effects have been reported with drugs in this class. Not all the effects listed below have necessarily been associated with simvastatin therapy.

Skeletal: muscle cramps, myalgia, myopathy, rhabdomyolysis, arthralgias.

Neurological: dysfunction of certain cranial nerves (including alteration of taste, impairment of extra-ocular movement, facial paresis), tremor, dizziness, vertigo, memory loss, paresthesia, peripheral neuropathy, peripheral nerve palsy, psychic disturbances, anxiety, insomnia, depression.

Hypersensitivity Reactions: An apparent hypersensitivity syndrome has been reported rarely which has included one or more of the following features: anaphylaxis, angioedema, lupus erythematous-like syndrome, polymyalgia rheumatica, dermatomyositis, vasculitis, purpura, thrombocytopenia, leukopenia, hemolytic anemia, positive ANA, ESR increase, eosinophilia, arthritis, arthralgia, urticaria, asthenia, photosensitivity, fever, chills, flushing, malaise, dyspnea, toxic epidermal necrolysis, erythema multiforme, including Stevens-Johnson syndrome.

Gastrointestinal: pancreatitis, hepatitis, including chronic active hepatitis, cholestatic jaundice, fatty change in liver, and, rarely, cirrhosis, fulminant hepatic necrosis, and hepatoma; anorexia, vomiting.

Skin: alopecia, pruritus. A variety of skin changes (e.g., nodules, discoloration, dryness of skin/mucous membranes, changes to hair/nails) have been reported.

Reproductive: gynecomastia, loss of libido, erectile dysfunction.

Eye: progression of cataracts (lens opacities), ophthalmoplegia.

Laboratory Abnormalities: elevated transaminases, alkaline phosphatase, γ-glutamyl transpeptidase, and bilirubin; thyroid function abnormalities.

Laboratory Tests

Marked persistent increases of serum transaminases have been noted (see WARNINGS, *Liver Dysfunction*). About 5% of patients had elevations of CK levels of 3 or more times the normal value on one or more occasions. This was attributable to the noncardiac fraction of CK. Muscle pain or dysfunction usually was not reported (see WARNINGS, *Myopathy/Rhabdomyolysis*).

Concomitant Lipid-Lowering Therapy

In controlled clinical studies in which simvastatin was administered concomitantly with cholestyramine, no adverse reactions peculiar to this concomitant treatment were observed. The adverse reactions that occurred were limited to those reported previously with simvastatin or cholestyramine. The combined use of simvastatin at doses exceeding 10 mg/day with gemfibrozil should be avoided (see WARNINGS, *Myopathy/Rhabdomyolysis*).

Adolescent Patients (ages 10-17 years)

In a 48-week, controlled study in adolescent boys and girls who were at least 1 year post-menarche, 10-17 years of age with heterozygous familial hypercholesterolemia (n=175), the safety and tolerability profile of the group treated with ZOCOR (10-40 mg daily) was generally similar to that of the group treated with placebo, with the most common adverse experiences observed in both groups being upper respiratory infection, headache, abdominal pain, and nausea (see CLINICAL PHARMACOLOGY, *Clinical Studies in Adolescents*, and PRECAUTIONS, *Pediatric Use*).

OVERDOSAGE

Significant lethality was observed in mice after a single oral dose of 9 g/m^2. No evidence of lethality was observed in rats or dogs treated with doses of 30 and 100 g/m^2, respectively. No specific diagnostic signs were observed in rodents. At these doses the only signs seen in dogs were emesis and mucoid stools.

A few cases of overdosage with ZOCOR have been reported; the maximum dose taken was 3.6 g. All patients recovered without sequelae. Until further experience is obtained, no specific treatment of overdosage with ZOCOR can be recommended.

The dialyzability of simvastatin and its metabolites in man is not known at present.

DOSAGE AND ADMINISTRATION

The patient should be placed on a standard cholesterol-lowering diet. In patients with CHD or at high risk of CHD, ZOCOR can be started simultaneously with diet. The dosage should be individualized according to the goals of therapy and the patient's response. (For the treatment of adult dyslipidemia, see NCEP Treatment Guidelines. For the reduction in risks of major coronary events, see CLINICAL PHARMACOLOGY, *Clinical Studies in Adults*.) The dosage range is 5-80 mg/day (see below).

The recommended usual starting dose is 20 to 40 mg once a day in the evening. For patients at high risk for a CHD event due to existing coronary heart disease, diabetes, peripheral vessel disease, history of stroke or other cerebrovascular disease, the recommended starting dose is 40 mg/day. Lipid determinations should be performed after 4 weeks of therapy and periodically thereafter. See below for dosage recommendations in special populations (i.e., homozygous familial hypercholesterolemia, adolescents and renal insufficiency) or for patients receiving concomitant therapy (i.e., cyclosporine, amiodarone, verapamil, or gemfibrozil).

Patients with Homozygous Familial Hypercholesterolemia

The recommended dosage for patients with homozygous familial hypercholesterolemia is ZOCOR 40 mg/day in the evening or 80 mg/day in 3 divided doses of 20 mg, 20 mg, and an evening dose of 40 mg. ZOCOR should be used as an adjunct to other lipid-lowering treatments (e.g., LDL apheresis) in these patients or if such treatments are unavailable.

Adolescents (10-17 years of age) with Heterozygous Familial Hypercholesterolemia

The recommended usual starting dose is 10 mg once a day in the evening. The recommended dosing range is 10-40 mg/day; the maximum recommended dose is 40 mg/day. Doses should be individualized according to the recommended goal of therapy (see NCEP Pediatric Panel Guidelines[6] and CLINICAL PHARMACOLOGY). Adjustments should be made at intervals of 4 weeks or more.

Concomitant Lipid-Lowering Therapy

ZOCOR is effective alone or when used concomitantly with bile-acid sequestrants. If ZOCOR is used in combination with gemfibrozil, the dose of ZOCOR should not exceed 10 mg/day (see WARNINGS, *Myopathy/Rhabdomyolysis* and PRECAUTIONS, *Drug Interactions*).

Patients taking Cyclosporine

In patients taking cyclosporine concomitantly with ZOCOR (see WARNINGS, *Myopathy/Rhabdomyolysis*), therapy should begin with 5 mg/day and should not exceed 10 mg/day.

Patients taking Amiodarone or Verapamil

In patients taking amiodarone or verapamil concomitantly with ZOCOR, the dose should not exceed 20 mg/day (see WARNINGS, *Myopathy/Rhabdomyolysis* and PRECAUTIONS, *Drug Interactions, Other drug interactions*).

Patients with Renal Insufficiency

Because ZOCOR does not undergo significant renal excretion, modification of dosage should not be necessary in patients with mild to moderate renal insufficiency. However, caution should be exercised when ZOCOR is administered to patients with severe renal insufficiency; such patients should be started at 5 mg/day and be closely monitored (see CLINICAL PHARMACOLOGY, *Pharmacokinetics* and WARNINGS, *Myopathy/Rhabdomyolysis*).

[6] National Cholesterol Education Program (NCEP): Highlights of the Report of the Expert Panel on Blood Cholesterol Levels in Children and Adolescents. *Pediatrics.* 89(3): 495-501. 1992.

HOW SUPPLIED

No. 3588 — Tablets ZOCOR 5 mg are buff, shield-shaped, film-coated tablets, coded MSD 726 on one side and ZOCOR on the other. They are supplied as follows:

NDC 0006-0726-31 unit of use bottles of 30
NDC 0006-0726-61 unit of use bottles of 60
NDC 0006-0726-54 unit of use bottles of 90
NDC 0006-0726-28 unit dose packages of 100
NDC 0006-0726-82 bottles of 1000.

No. 3589 — Tablets ZOCOR 10 mg are peach, shield-shaped, film-coated tablets, coded MSD 735 on one side and ZOCOR on the other. They are supplied as follows:

NDC 0006-0735-31 unit of use bottles of 30
NDC 0006-0735-54 unit of use bottles of 90
NDC 0006-0735-28 unit dose packages of 100
NDC 0006-0735-82 bottles of 1000
NDC 0006-0735-87 bottles of 10,000.

No. 3590 — Tablets ZOCOR 20 mg are tan, shield-shaped, film-coated tablets, coded MSD 740 on one side and ZOCOR on the other. They are supplied as follows:

NDC 0006-0740-31 unit of use bottles of 30
NDC 0006-0740-61 unit of use bottles of 60
NDC 0006-0740-54 unit of use bottles of 90
NDC 0006-0740-28 unit dose packages of 100
NDC 0006-0740-82 bottles of 1000
NDC 0006-0740-87 bottles of 10,000.

No. 3591 — Tablets ZOCOR 40 mg are brick red, shield-shaped, film-coated tablets, coded MSD 749 on one side and ZOCOR on the other. They are supplied as follows:

NDC 0006-0749-31 unit of use bottles of 30
NDC 0006-0749-61 unit of use bottles of 60
NDC 0006-0749-54 unit of use bottles of 90
NDC 0006-0749-28 unit dose packages of 100
NDC 0006-0749-82 bottles of 1000.

No. 6577 — Tablets ZOCOR 80 mg are brick red, capsule-shaped, film-coated tablets, coded 543 on one side and 80 on the other. They are supplied as follows:

NDC 0006-0543-31 unit of use bottles of 30
NDC 0006-0543-61 unit of use bottles of 60
NDC 0006-0543-54 unit of use bottles of 90
NDC 0006-0543-28 unit dose packages of 100
NDC 0006-0543-82 bottles of 1000.

Storage

Store between 5-30°C (41-86°F).

Tablets ZOCOR (simvastatin) 5 mg, 10 mg, 20 mg, and 40 mg are manufactured by:
MERCK & CO., INC.
Whitehouse Station, NJ 08889, USA
Tablets ZOCOR (simvastatin) 80 mg are manufactured for:
MERCK & CO., INC.
Whitehouse Station, NJ 08889, USA
By:
MERCK SHARP & DOHME LTD,
Cramlington, Northumberland, UK NE23 3JU
9556646, Issued February 2004

Shown in Product Identification Guide, page 324

Merck/Schering-Plough Pharmaceuticals

PO BOX 1000
UG4B–75A
351 N. SUMNEYTOWN PIKE
NORTH WALES, PA 19454

For Product and Service Information, Medical Information, and Adverse Drug Experience Reporting:

Call: Merck/Schering-Plough National Service Center
Monday through Friday, 8:00 AM to 7:00 PM (ET)
866-637-2501

Fax: 800-637-2568

For 24-hour emergency information, healthcare professionals should call:

Merck/Schering-Plough National Service Center at 866-637-2501

For Product Ordering,

Call: Order Management Center
Monday through Friday, 8:00 AM to 7:00 PM (ET)
800-637-2579

VYTORIN™ 10/10 ℞
(EZETIMIBE 10 MG/SIMVASTATIN 10 MG TABLETS)
VYTORIN™ 10/20 ℞
(EZETIMIBE 10 MG/SIMVASTATIN 20 MG TABLETS)
VYTORIN™ 10/40 ℞
(EZETIMIBE 10 MG/SIMVASTATIN 40 MG TABLETS)
VYTORIN™ 10/80 ℞
(EZETIMIBE 10 MG/SIMVASTATIN 80 MG TABLETS)

[*vī-tŏr-in*]

DESCRIPTION

VYTORIN contains ezetimibe, a selective inhibitor of intestinal cholesterol and related phytosterol absorption, and simvastatin, a 3-hydroxy-3-methylglutaryl-coenzyme A (HMG-CoA) reductase inhibitor.

The chemical name of ezetimibe is 1-(4-fluorophenyl)-3(R)-[3-(4-fluorophenyl)-3(S)-hydroxypropyl]- 4(S)-(4-hydroxyphenyl)-2-azetidinone. The empirical formula is $C_{24}H_{21}F_2NO_3$ and its molecular weight is 409.4.

Ezetimibe is a white, crystalline powder that is freely to very soluble in ethanol, methanol, and acetone and practically insoluble in water. Its structural formula is:

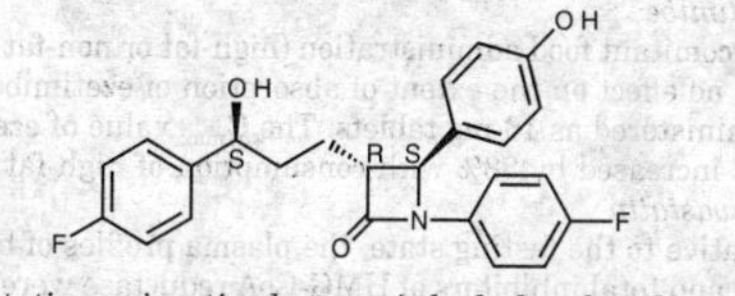

Simvastatin, an inactive lactone, is hydrolyzed to the corresponding β-hydroxyacid form, which is an inhibitor of HMG-CoA reductase. Simvastatin is butanoic acid, 2,2-dimethyl, 1,2,3,7,8,8a-hexahydro-3,7- dimethyl-8-[2-(tetrahydro-4-hydroxy-6-oxo-2*H*-pyran-2-yl)-ethyl]-1-naphthalenyl ester, [1*S*- [1α,3α,7β,8β(2*S**,4*S**),-8aβ]]. The empirical formula of simvastatin is $C_{25}H_{38}O_5$ and its molecular weight is 418.57.

Simvastatin is a white to off-white, nonhygroscopic, crystalline powder that is practically insoluble in water, and freely soluble in chloroform, methanol and ethanol. Its structural formula is:

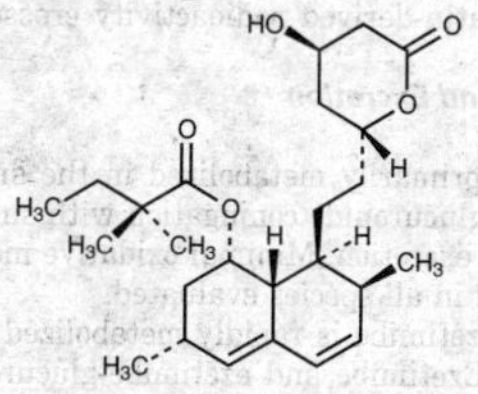

VYTORIN is available for oral use as tablets containing 10 mg of ezetimibe, and 10 mg of simvastatin (VYTORIN 10/10), 20 mg of simvastatin (VYTORIN 10/20), 40 mg of simvastatin (VYTORIN 10/40), or 80 mg of simvastatin (VYTORIN 10/80). Each tablet contains the following inactive ingredients: butylated hydroxyanisole NF, citric acid monohydrate USP, croscarmellose sodium NF, hydroxypropyl methylcellulose USP, lactose monohydrate NF, magnesium stearate NF, microcrystalline cellulose NF, and propyl gallate NF.

CLINICAL PHARMACOLOGY

Background

Clinical studies have demonstrated that elevated levels of total cholesterol (total-C), low-density lipoprotein cholesterol (LDL-C) and apolipoprotein B (Apo B), the major pro-

Continued on next page

Vytorin—Cont.

tein constituent of LDL, promote human atherosclerosis. In addition, decreased levels of high-density lipoprotein cholesterol (HDL-C) are associated with the development of atherosclerosis. Epidemiologic studies have established that cardiovascular morbidity and mortality vary directly with the level of total-C and LDL-C and inversely with the level of HDL-C. Like LDL, cholesterol-enriched triglyceride-rich lipoproteins, including very-low-density lipoproteins (VLDL), intermediate-density lipoproteins (IDL), and remnants, can also promote atherosclerosis. The independent effect of raising HDL-C or lowering triglycerides (TG) on the risk of coronary and cardiovascular morbidity and mortality has not been determined.

Mode of Action

VYTORIN

Plasma cholesterol is derived from intestinal absorption and endogenous synthesis. VYTORIN contains ezetimibe and simvastatin, two lipid-lowering compounds with complementary mechanisms of action. VYTORIN reduces elevated total-C, LDL-C, Apo B, TG, and non-HDL-C, and increases HDL-C through dual inhibition of cholesterol absorption and synthesis.

Ezetimibe

Ezetimibe reduces blood cholesterol by inhibiting the absorption of cholesterol by the small intestine. In a 2-week clinical study in 18 hypercholesterolemic patients, ezetimibe inhibited intestinal cholesterol absorption by 54%, compared with placebo. Ezetimibe had no clinically meaningful effect on the plasma concentrations of the fat-soluble vitamins A, D, and E and did not impair adrenocortical steroid hormone production.

Ezetimibe localizes and appears to act at the brush border of the small intestine and inhibits the absorption of cholesterol, leading to a decrease in the delivery of intestinal cholesterol to the liver. This causes a reduction of hepatic cholesterol stores and an increase in clearance of cholesterol from the blood; this distinct mechanism is complementary to that of HMG-CoA reductase inhibitors (see CLINICAL STUDIES).

Simvastatin

Simvastatin reduces cholesterol by inhibiting the conversion of HMG-CoA to mevalonate, an early step in the biosynthetic pathway for cholesterol. In addition, simvastatin reduces VLDL and TG and increases HDL-C.

Pharmacokinetics

Absorption

VYTORIN

VYTORIN is bioequivalent to coadministered ezetimibe and simvastatin.

Ezetimibe

After oral administration, ezetimibe is absorbed and extensively conjugated to a pharmacologically active phenolic glucuronide (ezetimibe-glucuronide).

Effect of Food on Oral Absorption

Ezetimibe

Concomitant food administration (high-fat or non-fat meals) had no effect on the extent of absorption of ezetimibe when administered as 10-mg tablets. The C_{max} value of ezetimibe was increased by 38% with consumption of high-fat meals.

Simvastatin

Relative to the fasting state, the plasma profiles of both active and total inhibitors of HMG-CoA reductase were not affected when simvastatin was administered immediately before an American Heart Association recommended low-fat meal.

Distribution

Ezetimibe

Ezetimibe and ezetimibe-glucuronide are highly bound (>90%) to human plasma proteins.

Simvastatin

Both simvastatin and its β-hydroxyacid metabolite are highly bound (approximately 95%) to human plasma proteins. When radiolabeled simvastatin was administered to rats, simvastatin-derived radioactivity crossed the blood-brain barrier.

Metabolism and Excretion

Ezetimibe

Ezetimibe is primarily metabolized in the small intestine and liver via glucuronide conjugation with subsequent biliary and renal excretion. Minimal oxidative metabolism has been observed in all species evaluated.

In humans, ezetimibe is rapidly metabolized to ezetimibe-glucuronide. Ezetimibe and ezetimibe-glucuronide are the major drug-derived compounds detected in plasma, constituting approximately 10 to 20% and 80 to 90% of the total drug in plasma, respectively. Both ezetimibe and ezetimibe-glucuronide are slowly eliminated from plasma with a half-life of approximately 22 hours for both ezetimibe and ezetimibe-glucuronide. Plasma concentration-time profiles exhibit multiple peaks, suggesting enterohepatic recycling. Following oral administration of ^{14}C-ezetimibe (20 mg) to human subjects, total ezetimibe (ezetimibe + ezetimibe-glucuronide) accounted for approximately 93% of the total radioactivity in plasma. After 48 hours, there were no detectable levels of radioactivity in the plasma.

Approximately 78% and 11% of the administered radioactivity were recovered in the feces and urine, respectively, over a 10-day collection period. Ezetimibe was the major component in feces and accounted for 69% of the administered dose, while ezetimibe-glucuronide was the major component in urine and accounted for 9% of the administered dose.

Simvastatin

Simvastatin is a lactone that is readily hydrolyzed *in vivo* to the corresponding β-hydroxyacid, a potent inhibitor of HMG-CoA reductase. Inhibition of HMG-CoA reductase is a basis for an assay in pharmacokinetic studies of the β-hydroxyacid metabolites (active inhibitors) and, following base hydrolysis, active plus latent inhibitors (total inhibitors) in plasma following administration of simvastatin. The major active metabolites of simvastatin present in human plasma are the β-hydroxyacid of simvastatin and its 6′- hydroxy, 6′-hydroxymethyl, and 6′-exomethylene derivatives.

Plasma concentrations of total radioactivity (simvastatin plus ^{14}C-metabolites) peaked at 4 hours and declined rapidly to about 10% of peak by 12 hours postdose. Simvastatin undergoes extensive first-pass extraction in the liver, its primary site of action, with subsequent excretion of drug equivalents in the bile. As a consequence of extensive hepatic extraction of simvastatin (estimated to be >60% in man), the availability of drug to the general circulation is low.

Following an oral dose of ^{14}C-labeled simvastatin in man, 13% of the dose was excreted in urine and 60% in feces. The latter represents absorbed drug equivalents excreted in bile, as well as any unabsorbed drug.

In a single-dose study in nine healthy subjects, it was estimated that less than 5% of an oral dose of simvastatin reaches the general circulation as active inhibitors.

Special Populations

Geriatric Patients

Ezetimibe

In a multiple-dose study with ezetimibe given 10 mg once daily for 10 days, plasma concentrations for total ezetimibe were about 2-fold higher in older (≥65 years) healthy subjects compared to younger subjects.

Simvastatin

In a study including 16 elderly patients between 70 and 78 years of age who received simvastatin 40 mg/day, the mean plasma level of HMG-CoA reductase inhibitory activity was increased approximately 45% compared with 18 patients between 18–30 years of age.

Pediatric Patients

Ezetimibe

In a multiple-dose study with ezetimibe given 10 mg once daily for 7 days, the absorption and metabolism of ezetimibe were similar in adolescents (10 to 18 years) and adults. Based on total ezetimibe, there are no pharmacokinetic differences between adolescents and adults. Pharmacokinetic data in the pediatric population <10 years of age are not available.

Gender

Ezetimibe

In a multiple-dose study with ezetimibe given 10 mg once daily for 10 days, plasma concentrations for total ezetimibe were slightly higher (<20%) in women than in men.

Race

Ezetimibe

Based on a meta-analysis of multiple-dose pharmacokinetic studies, there were no pharmacokinetic differences between Blacks and Caucasians. There were too few patients in other racial or ethnic groups to permit further pharmacokinetic comparisons.

Hepatic Insufficiency

Ezetimibe

After a single 10-mg dose of ezetimibe, the mean exposure (based on area under the curve [AUC]) to total ezetimibe was increased approximately 1.7-fold in patients with mild hepatic insufficiency (Child-Pugh score 5 to 6), compared to healthy subjects. The mean AUC values for total ezetimibe and ezetimibe increased approximately 3- to 4-fold and 5- to 6-fold, respectively, in patients with moderate (Child-Pugh score 7 to 9) or severe hepatic impairment (Child-Pugh score 10 to 15). In a 14-day, multiple-dose study (10 mg daily) in patients with moderate hepatic insufficiency, the mean AUC for total ezetimibe and ezetimibe increased approximately 4-fold compared to healthy subjects.

Renal Insufficiency

Ezetimibe

After a single 10-mg dose of ezetimibe in patients with severe renal disease (n=8; mean CrCl ≤30 mL/min/1.73 m^2), the mean AUC for total ezetimibe and ezetimibe increased approximately 1.5-fold, compared to healthy subjects (n=9).

Simvastatin

Pharmacokinetic studies with another statin having a similar principal route of elimination to that of simvastatin have suggested that for a given dose level higher systemic exposure may be achieved in patients with severe renal insufficiency (as measured by creatinine clearance).

***Drug Interactions* (See also PRECAUTIONS, *Drug Interactions*)**

No clinically significant pharmacokinetic interaction was seen when ezetimibe was coadministered with simvastatin. Specific pharmacokinetic drug interaction studies with VYTORIN have not been performed.

Cytochrome P450: Ezetimibe had no significant effect on a series of probe drugs (caffeine, dextromethorphan, tolbutamide, and IV midazolam) known to be metabolized by cytochrome P450 (1A2, 2D6, 2C8/9 and 3A4) in a "cocktail" study of twelve healthy adult males. This indicates that ezetimibe is neither an inhibitor nor an inducer of these cytochrome P450 isozymes, and it is unlikely that ezetimibe will affect the metabolism of drugs that are metabolized by these enzymes.

In a study of 12 healthy volunteers, simvastatin at the 80-mg dose had no effect on the metabolism of the probe cytochrome P450 isoform 3A4 (CYP3A4) substrates midazolam and erythromycin. This indicates that simvastatin is not an inhibitor of CYP3A4, and, therefore, is not expected to affect the plasma levels of other drugs metabolized by CYP3A4.

Simvastatin is a substrate for CYP3A4. Potent inhibitors of CYP3A4 can raise the plasma levels of HMG-CoA reductase inhibitory activity and increase the risk of myopathy. (See WARNINGS, *Myopathy/Rhabdomyolysis* and PRECAUTIONS, *Drug Interactions*.)

Antacids: In a study of twelve healthy adults, a single dose of antacid (Supralox™ 20 mL) administration had no significant effect on the oral bioavailability of total ezetimibe, ezetimibe-glucuronide, or ezetimibe based on AUC values. The C_{max} value of total ezetimibe was decreased by 30%.

Cholestyramine: In a study of forty healthy hypercholesterolemic (LDL-C ≥130 mg/dL) adult subjects, concomitant cholestyramine (4 g twice daily) administration decreased the mean AUC of total ezetimibe and ezetimibe approximately 55% and 80%, respectively.

Cyclosporine: In a study of eight post-renal transplant patients with mildly impaired or normal renal function (creatinine clearance of >50 mL/min), stable doses of cyclosporine (75 to 150 mg twice daily) increased the mean AUC and C_{max} values of total ezetimibe 3.4-fold (range 2.3- to 7.9-fold) and 3.9-fold (range 3.0- to 4.4-fold), respectively, compared to a historical healthy control population (n=17). In a different study, a renal transplant patient with severe renal insufficiency (creatinine clearance of 13.2 mL/min/1.73 m^2) who was receiving multiple medications, including cyclosporine, demonstrated a 12-fold greater exposure to total ezetimibe compared to healthy subjects.

Fenofibrate: In a study of thirty-two healthy hypercholesterolemic (LDL-C ≥130 mg/dL) adult subjects, concomitant fenofibrate (200 mg once daily) administration increased the mean C_{max} and AUC values of total ezetimibe approximately 64% and 48%, respectively. Pharmacokinetics of fenofibrate were not significantly affected by ezetimibe (10 mg once daily).

Gemfibrozil: In a study of twelve healthy adult males, concomitant administration of gemfibrozil (600 mg twice daily) significantly increased the oral bioavailability of total ezetimibe by a factor of 1.7. Ezetimibe (10 mg once daily) did not significantly affect the bioavailability of gemfibrozil.

Grapefruit Juice: Grapefruit juice contains one or more components that inhibit CYP3A4 and can increase the plasma concentrations of drugs metabolized by CYP3A4. In one study[1], 10 subjects consumed 200 mL of double-strength grapefruit juice (one can of frozen concentrate diluted with one rather than 3 cans of water) three times daily for 2 days and an additional 200 mL double-strength grapefruit juice together with, and 30 and 90 minutes following, a single dose of 60 mg simvastatin on the third day. This regimen of grapefruit juice resulted in mean increases in the concentration (as measured by the area under the concentration-time curve) of active and total HMG-CoA reductase inhibitory activity [measured using a radioenzyme inhibition assay both before (for active inhibitors) and after (for total inhibitors) base hydrolysis] of 2.4-fold and 3.6-fold, respectively, and of simvastatin and its β-hydroxyacid metabolite [measured using a chemical assay — liquid chromatography/tandem mass spectrometry] of 16-fold and 7-fold, respectively. In a second study, 16 subjects consumed one 8 oz glass of single-strength grapefruit juice (one can of frozen concentrate diluted with 3 cans of water) with breakfast for 3 consecutive days and a single dose of 20 mg simvastatin in the evening of the third day. This regimen of grapefruit juice resulted in a mean increase in the plasma concentration (as measured by the area under the concentration-time curve) of active and total HMG-CoA reductase inhibitory activity [using a validated enzyme inhibition assay different from that used in the first[1] study, both before (for active inhibitors) and after (for total inhibitors) base hydrolysis] of 1.13-fold and 1.18-fold, respectively, and of simvastatin and its β-hydroxyacid metabolite [measured using a chemical assay — liquid chromatography/tandem mass spectrometry] of 1.88-fold and 1.31-fold, respectively. The effect of amounts of grapefruit juice between those used in these two studies on simvastatin pharmacokinetics has not been studied.

[1] Lilja JJ, Kivisto KT, Neuvonen PJ. Clin Pharmacol Ther 1998;64(5):477-83.

ANIMAL PHARMACOLOGY

Ezetimibe

The hypocholesterolemic effect of ezetimibe was evaluated in cholesterol-fed Rhesus monkeys, dogs, rats, and mouse models of human cholesterol metabolism. Ezetimibe was found to have an ED_{50} value of 0.5 μg/kg/day for inhibiting the rise in plasma cholesterol levels in monkeys. The ED_{50} values in dogs, rats, and mice were 7, 30, and 700 μg/kg/day, respectively. These results are consistent with ezetimibe being a potent cholesterol absorption inhibitor.

In a rat model, where the glucuronide metabolite of ezetimibe (ezetimibe-glucuronide) was administered intraduodenally, the metabolite was as potent as ezetimibe in inhibiting the absorption of cholesterol, suggesting that the glucuronide metabolite had activity similar to the parent drug.

In 1-month studies in dogs given ezetimibe (0.03-300 mg/kg/day), the concentration of cholesterol in gallbladder bile increased ~2- to 4-fold. However, a dose of 300 mg/kg/day administered to dogs for one year did not result in gallstone formation or any other adverse hepatobiliary effects. In a 14-day study in mice given ezetimibe (0.3-5 mg/kg/day) and fed a low-fat or cholesterol-rich diet, the concentration of cholesterol in gallbladder bile was either unaffected or reduced to normal levels, respectively.

A series of acute preclinical studies was performed to determine the selectivity of ezetimibe for inhibiting cholesterol absorption. Ezetimibe inhibited the absorption of ^{14}C-cholesterol with no effect on the absorption of triglycerides, fatty acids, bile acids, progesterone, ethyl estradiol, or the fat-soluble vitamins A and D.

In 4- to 12-week toxicity studies in mice, ezetimibe did not induce cytochrome P450 drug metabolizing enzymes. In toxicity studies, a pharmacokinetic interaction of ezetimibe with HMG-CoA reductase inhibitors (parents or their active hydroxy acid metabolites) was seen in rats, dogs, and rabbits.

CLINICAL STUDIES

Primary Hypercholesterolemia

VYTORIN

VYTORIN reduces total-C, LDL-C, Apo B, TG, and non-HDL-C, and increases HDL-C in patients with hypercholesterolemia. Maximal to near maximal response is generally achieved within 2 weeks and maintained during chronic therapy.

VYTORIN is effective in men and women with hypercholesterolemia. Experience in non-Caucasians is limited and does not permit a precise estimate of the magnitude of the effects of VYTORIN.

In a multicenter, double-blind, placebo-controlled, 12-week trial, 1528 hypercholesterolemic patients were randomized to one of ten treatment groups: placebo, ezetimibe (10 mg), simvastatin (10 mg, 20 mg, 40 mg, or 80 mg), or VYTORIN (10/10, 10/20, 10/40, or 10/80).

When patients receiving VYTORIN were compared to those receiving all doses of simvastatin, VYTORIN significantly lowered total-C, LDL-C, Apo B, TG, and non-HDL-C. The effects of VYTORIN on HDL-C were similar to the effects seen with simvastatin. Further analysis showed VYTORIN significantly increased HDL-C compared with placebo. (See Table 1.) The lipid response to VYTORIN was similar in patients with TG levels greater than or less than 200 mg/dL.

[See table 1 at right]

In a multicenter, double-blind, controlled, 23-week study, 710 patients with known CHD or CHD risk equivalents, as defined by the NCEP ATP III guidelines, and an LDL-C ≥130 mg/dL were randomized to one of four treatment groups: coadministered ezetimibe and simvastatin equivalent to VYTORIN (10/10, 10/20, and 10/40), or simvastatin 20 mg. Patients not reaching an LDL-C <100 mg/dL had their simvastatin dose titrated at 6-week intervals to a maximal dose of 80 mg.

At Week 5, the LDL-C reductions with VYTORIN 10/10, 10/20, or 10/40 were significantly larger than with simvastatin 20 mg (see Table 2).

Table 2
Response to VYTORIN after 5 Weeks in Patients with CHD or CHD Risk Equivalents and an LDL-C ≥130 mg/dL

	Simvastatin 20 mg	VYTORIN 10/10	VYTORIN 10/20	VYTORIN 10/40
N	253	251	109	97
Mean baseline LDL-C	174	165	167	171
Percent change LDL-C	−38	−47	−53	−59

In a multicenter, double-blind, 24-week, forced titration study, 788 patients with primary hypercholesterolemia, who had not met their NCEP ATP III target LDL-C goal, were randomized to receive coadministered ezetimibe and simvastatin equivalent to VYTORIN (10/10 and 10/20) or atorvastatin 10 mg. For all three treatment groups, the dose of the statin was titrated at 6-week intervals to 80 mg. At each pre-specified dose comparison, VYTORIN lowered LDL-C to a greater degree than atorvastatin (see Table 3).

[See table 3 at right]

In a multicenter, double-blind, 24-week trial, 214 patients with type 2 diabetes mellitus treated with thiazolidinediones (rosiglitazone or pioglitazone) for a minimum of 3 months and simvastatin 20 mg for a minimum of 6 weeks, were randomized to receive either simvastatin 40 mg or the coadministered active ingredients equivalent to VYTORIN 10/20. The median LDL-C and HbA1c levels at baseline were 89 mg/dL and 7.1%, respectively.

VYTORIN 10/20 was significantly more effective than doubling the dose of simvastatin to 40 mg. The median percent changes from baseline for VYTORIN vs simvastatin were: LDL-C -25% and -5%; total-C -16% and -5%; Apo B -19% and -5%; and non-HDL-C -23% and -5%. Results for HDL-C and TG between the two treatment groups were not significantly different.

Ezetimibe

In two multicenter, double-blind, placebo-controlled, 12-week studies in 1719 patients with primary hypercholesterolemia, ezetimibe significantly lowered total-C (-13%), LDL-C (-19%), Apo B (-14%), and TG (-8%), and increased HDL-C (+3%) compared to placebo. Reduction in LDL-C was consistent across age, sex, and baseline LDL-C.

Table 1
Response to VYTORIN in Patients with Primary Hypercholesterolemia
(Mean[a] % Change from Untreated Baseline[b])

Treatment (Daily Dose)	N	Total-C	LDL-C	Apo B	HDL-C	TG[a]	Non-HDL-C
Pooled data (All VYTORIN doses)[c]	609	−38	−53	−42	+7	−24	−49
Pooled data (All simvastatin doses)[c]	622	−28	−39	−32	+7	−21	−36
Ezetimibe 10 mg	149	−13	−19	−15	+5	−11	−18
Placebo	148	−1	−2	0	0	−2	−2
VYTORIN by dose							
10/10	152	−31	−45	−35	+8	−23	−41
10/20	156	−36	−52	−41	+10	−24	−47
10/40	147	−39	−55	−44	+6	−23	−51
10/80	154	−43	−60	−49	+6	−31	−56
Simvastatin by dose							
10 mg	158	−23	−33	−26	+5	−17	−30
20 mg	150	−24	−34	−28	+7	−18	−32
40 mg	156	−29	−41	−33	+8	−21	−38
80 mg	158	−35	−49	−39	+7	−27	−45

[a] For triglycerides, median % change from baseline
[b] Baseline - on no lipid-lowering drug
[c] VYTORIN doses pooled (10/10-10/80) significantly reduced total-C, LDL-C, Apo B, TG, and non-HDL-C compared to simvastatin, and significantly increased HDL-C compared to placebo.

Table 3
Response to VYTORIN and Atorvastatin in Patients with Primary Hypercholesterolemia
(Mean[a] % Change from Untreated Baseline[b])

Treatment	N	Total-C	LDL-C	Apo B	HDL-C	TG[a]	Non-HDL-C
Week 6							
Atorvastatin 10 mg[c]	262	−28	−37	−32	+5	−23	−35
VYTORIN 10/10[d]	263	−34[f]	−46[f]	−38[f]	+8[f]	−26	−43[f]
VYTORIN 10/20[e]	263	−36[f]	−50[f]	−41[f]	+10[f]	−25	−46[f]
Week 12							
Atorvastatin 20 mg	246	−33	−44	−38	+7	−28	−42
VYTORIN 10/20	250	−37[f]	−50[f]	−41[f]	+9	−28	−46[f]
VYTORIN 10/40	252	−39[f]	−54[f]	−45[f]	+12[f]	−31	−50[f]
Week 18							
Atorvastatin 40 mg	237	−37	−49	−42	+8	−31	−47
VYTORIN 10/40[g]	482	−40[f]	−56[f]	−45[f]	+11[f]	−32	−52[f]
Week 24							
Atorvastatin 80 mg	228	−40	−53	−45	+6	−35	−50
VYTORIN 10/80[g]	459	−43[f]	−59[f]	−49[f]	+12[f]	−35	−55[f]

[a] For triglycerides, median % change from baseline
[b] Baseline - on no lipid-lowering drug
[c] Atorvastatin: 10 mg start dose titrated to 20 mg, 40 mg, and 80 mg through Weeks 6, 12, 18, and 24
[d] VYTORIN: 10/10 start dose titrated to 10/20, 10/40, and 10/80 through Weeks 6, 12, 18, and 24
[e] VYTORIN: 10/20 start dose titrated to 10/40, 10/40, and 10/80 through Weeks 6, 12, 18, and 24
[f] p≤0.05 for difference with atorvastatin in the specified week
[g] Data pooled for common doses of VYTORIN at Weeks 18 and 24.

Simvastatin

In two large, placebo-controlled clinical trials, the Scandinavian Simvastatin Survival Study (N=4,444 patients) and the Heart Protection Study (N=20,536 patients), the effects of treatment with simvastatin were assessed in patients at high risk of coronary events because of existing coronary heart disease, diabetes, peripheral vessel disease, history of stroke or other cerebrovascular disease. Simvastatin was proven to reduce: the risk of total mortality by reducing CHD deaths; the risk of non-fatal myocardial infarction and stroke; and the need for coronary and non-coronary revascularization procedures.

No incremental benefit of VYTORIN on cardiovascular morbidity and mortality over and above that demonstrated for simvastatin has been established.

Homozygous Familial Hypercholesterolemia (HoFH)

A double-blind, randomized, 12-week study was performed in patients with a clinical and/or genotypic diagnosis of HoFH. Data were analyzed from a subgroup of patients (n=14) receiving simvastatin 40 mg at baseline. Increasing the dose of simvastatin from 40 to 80 mg (n=5) produced a reduction of LDL-C of 13% from baseline on simvastatin 40 mg. Coadministered ezetimibe and simvastatin equivalent to VYTORIN (10/40 and 10/80 pooled, n=9), produced a reduction of LDL-C of 23% from baseline on simvastatin 40 mg. In those patients coadministered ezetimibe and simvastatin equivalent to VYTORIN (10/80, n=5), a reduction of LDL-C of 29% from baseline on simvastatin 40 mg was produced.

INDICATIONS AND USAGE

Primary Hypercholesterolemia

VYTORIN is indicated as adjunctive therapy to diet for the reduction of elevated total-C, LDL-C, Apo B, TG, and non-HDL-C, and to increase HDL-C in patients with primary (heterozygous familial and non- familial) hypercholesterolemia or mixed hyperlipidemia.

Homozygous Familial Hypercholesterolemia (HoFH)

VYTORIN is indicated for the reduction of elevated total-C and LDL-C in patients with homozygous familial hypercholesterolemia, as an adjunct to other lipid-lowering treatments (e.g., LDL apheresis) or if such treatments are unavailable.

Therapy with lipid-altering agents should be a component of multiple risk-factor intervention in individuals at increased risk for atherosclerotic vascular disease due to hypercholesterolemia. Lipid- altering agents should be used in addition to an appropriate diet (including restriction of saturated fat and cholesterol) and when the response to diet and other non-pharmacological measures has been inadequate. (See NCEP Adult Treatment Panel (ATP) III Guidelines, summarized in Table 4.)

Continued on next page

Vytorin—Cont.

[See table 4 below]

Prior to initiating therapy with VYTORIN, secondary causes for dyslipidemia (i.e., diabetes, hypothyroidism, obstructive liver disease, chronic renal failure, and drugs that increase LDL-C and decrease HDL-C [progestins, anabolic steroids, and corticosteroids]), should be excluded or, if appropriate, treated. A lipid profile should be performed to measure total-C, LDL-C, HDL-C and TG. For TG levels >400 mg/dL (>4.5 mmol/L), LDL-C concentrations should be determined by ultracentrifugation.

At the time of hospitalization for an acute coronary event, lipid measures should be taken on admission or within 24 hours. These values can guide the physician on initiation of LDL-lowering therapy before or at discharge.

CONTRAINDICATIONS

Hypersensitivity to any component of this medication.

Active liver disease or unexplained persistent elevations in serum transaminases (see WARNINGS, *Liver Enzymes*).

Pregnancy and lactation. Atherosclerosis is a chronic process and the discontinuation of lipid-lowering drugs during pregnancy should have little impact on the outcome of long-term therapy of primary hypercholesterolemia. Moreover, cholesterol and other products of the cholesterol biosynthesis pathway are essential components for fetal development, including synthesis of steroids and cell membranes. Because of the ability of inhibitors of HMG-CoA reductase such as simvastatin to decrease the synthesis of cholesterol and possibly other products of the cholesterol biosynthesis pathway, VYTORIN is contraindicated during pregnancy and in nursing mothers. **VYTORIN should be administered to women of childbearing age only when such patients are highly unlikely to conceive.** If the patient becomes pregnant while taking this drug, VYTORIN should be discontinued immediately and the patient should be apprised of the potential hazard to the fetus (see PRECAUTIONS, *Pregnancy*).

WARNINGS

Myopathy/Rhabdomyolysis

In clinical trials, there was no excess of myopathy or rhabdomyolysis associated with ezetimibe compared with the relevant control arm (placebo or HMG-CoA reductase inhibitor alone). However, myopathy and rhabdomyolysis are known adverse reactions to HMG-CoA reductase inhibitors and other lipid-lowering drugs. In clinical trials, the incidence of CK >10 X the upper limit of normal [ULN] was 0.2% for VYTORIN.

Simvastatin, like other inhibitors of HMG-CoA reductase, occasionally causes myopathy manifested as muscle pain, tenderness or weakness with creatine kinase above 10 X ULN. Myopathy sometimes takes the form of rhabdomyolysis with or without acute renal failure secondary to myoglobinuria, and rare fatalities have occurred. The risk of myopathy is increased by high levels of HMG-CoA reductase inhibitory activity in plasma.

- **Because VYTORIN contains simvastatin, the risk of myopathy/rhabdomyolysis is increased by concomitant use of VYTORIN with the following:**

Potent inhibitors of CYP3A4: Cyclosporine, itraconazole, ketoconazole, erythromycin, clarithromycin, HIV protease inhibitors, nefazodone, or large quantities of grapefruit juice (>1 quart daily), particularly with higher doses of VYTORIN (see CLINICAL PHARMACOLOGY, *Pharmacokinetics*; PRECAUTIONS, *Drug Interactions, CYP3A4 Interactions*).

Other drugs:

Gemfibrozil, particularly with higher doses of VYTORIN (see CLINICAL PHARMACOLOGY, *Pharmacokinetics*; PRECAUTIONS, *Drug Interactions, Interactions with lipid-lowering drugs that can cause myopathy when given alone*).

Other lipid-lowering drugs (other fibrates or ≥1 g/day of niacin) that can cause myopathy when given alone (see PRECAUTIONS, *Drug Interactions, Interactions with lipid-lowering drugs that can cause myopathy when given alone*).

Amiodarone or verapamil with higher doses of VYTORIN (see PRECAUTIONS, *Drug Interactions, Other drug interactions*). In an ongoing clinical trial, myopathy has been reported in 6% of patients receiving simvastatin 80 mg and amiodarone. In an analysis of clinical trials involving 25,248 patients treated with simvastatin 20 to 80 mg, the incidence of myopathy was higher in patients receiving verapamil and simvastatin (4/635; 0.63%) than in patients taking simvastatin without a calcium channel blocker (13/21,224; 0.061%).

- **The risk of myopathy/rhabdomyolysis is dose related for simvastatin.** The incidence in clinical trials, in which patients were carefully monitored and some interacting drugs were excluded, has been approximately 0.02% at 20 mg, 0.07% at 40 mg and 0.3% at 80 mg.

Consequently:

1. **Use of VYTORIN concomitantly with itraconazole, ketoconazole, erythromycin, clarithromycin, HIV protease inhibitors, nefazodone, or large quantities of grapefruit juice (>1 quart daily) should be avoided.** If treatment with itraconazole, ketoconazole, erythromycin, or clarithromycin is unavoidable, therapy with VYTORIN should be suspended during the course of treatment. Concomitant use with other medicines labeled as having a potent inhibitory effect on CYP3A4 at therapeutic doses should be avoided unless the benefits of combined therapy outweigh the increased risk.
2. There is an increased risk of myopathy when simvastatin is used concomitantly with gemfibrozil or other fibrates; the safety and effectiveness of ezetimibe administered with fibrates have not been established. **Therefore, the concomitant use of VYTORIN and fibrates should be avoided.** (See PRECAUTIONS, *Drug Interactions, Other Drug Interactions, Fibrates.*)
3. Caution should be used when prescribing lipid-lowering doses (≥1 g/day) of niacin with VYTORIN, as niacin can cause myopathy when given alone. **The benefit of further alterations in lipid levels by the combined use of VYTORIN with niacin should be carefully weighed against the potential risks of this drug combination.**
4. **The dose of VYTORIN should not exceed 10/10 mg daily in patients receiving concomitant medication with cyclosporine.** The benefits of the use of VYTORIN in patients receiving cyclosporine should be carefully weighed against the risks of this combination. **(See PRECAUTIONS, *Drug Interactions, Other Drug Interactions, Cyclosporine.*)**
5. **The dose of VYTORIN should not exceed 10/20 mg daily in patients receiving concomitant medication with amiodarone or verapamil. The combined use of VYTORIN at doses higher than 10/20 mg daily with amiodarone or verapamil should be avoided unless the clinical benefit is likely to outweigh the increased risk of myopathy.**
6. **All patients starting therapy with VYTORIN, or whose dose of VYTORIN is being increased, should be advised of the risk of myopathy and told to report promptly any unexplained muscle pain, tenderness or weakness. VYTORIN therapy should be discontinued immediately if myopathy is diagnosed or suspected.** The presence of these symptoms, and/or a CK level >10 times the ULN indicates myopathy. In most cases, when patients were promptly discontinued from simvastatin treatment, muscle symptoms and CK increases resolved. Periodic CK determinations may be considered in patients starting therapy with VYTORIN or whose dose is being increased, but there is no assurance that such monitoring will prevent myopathy.
7. Many of the patients who have developed rhabdomyolysis on therapy with simvastatin have had complicated medical histories, including renal insufficiency usually as a consequence of long-standing diabetes mellitus. Such patients taking VYTORIN merit closer monitoring. Therapy with VYTORIN should be temporarily stopped a few days prior to elective major surgery and when any major medical or surgical condition supervenes.

Liver Enzymes

In three placebo-controlled, 12-week trials, the incidence of consecutive elevations (≥3 X ULN) in serum transaminases was 1.7% overall for patients treated with VYTORIN and appeared to be dose-related with an incidence of 2.6% for patients treated with VYTORIN 10/80. In controlled long-term (48-week) extensions, which included both newly-treated and previously-treated patients, the incidence of consecutive elevations (≥3 X ULN) in serum transaminases was 1.8% overall and 3.6% for patients treated with VYTORIN 10/80. These elevations in transaminases were generally asymptomatic, not associated with cholestasis, and returned to baseline after discontinuation of therapy or with continued treatment.

It is recommended that liver function tests be performed before the initiation of treatment with VYTORIN, and thereafter when clinically indicated. Patients titrated to the 10/80-mg dose should receive an additional test prior to titration, 3 months after titration to the 10/80-mg dose, and periodically thereafter (e.g., semiannually) for the first year of treatment. Patients who develop increased transaminase levels should be monitored with a second liver function evaluation to confirm the finding and be followed thereafter with frequent liver function tests until the abnormality(ies) return to normal. Should an increase in AST or ALT of 3 X ULN or greater persist, withdrawal of therapy with VYTORIN is recommended.

VYTORIN should be used with caution in patients who consume substantial quantities of alcohol and/or have a past history of liver disease. Active liver diseases or unexplained persistent transaminase elevations are contraindications to the use of VYTORIN.

PRECAUTIONS

Information for Patients

Patients should be advised about substances they should not take concomitantly with VYTORIN and be advised to report promptly unexplained muscle pain, tenderness, or weakness (see list below and WARNINGS, *Myopathy/Rhabdomyolysis*). Patients should also be advised to inform other physicians prescribing a new medication that they are taking VYTORIN.

Hepatic Insufficiency

Due to the unknown effects of the increased exposure to ezetimibe in patients with moderate or severe hepatic insufficiency, VYTORIN is not recommended in these patients. (See CLINICAL PHARMACOLOGY, *Pharmacokinetics, Special Populations.*)

***Drug Interactions* (See also CLINICAL PHARMACOLOGY, Drug Interactions)**

VYTORIN

CYP3A4 Interactions

Potent inhibitors of CYP3A4 (below) increase the risk of myopathy by reducing the elimination of the simvastatin component of VYTORIN.

See WARNINGS, *Myopathy/Rhabdomyolysis*, and CLINICAL PHARMACOLOGY, *Pharmacokinetics, Drug Interactions.*

Itraconazole
Ketoconazole
Erythromycin
Clarithromycin
HIV protease inhibitors
Nefazodone
Cyclosporine
Large quantities of grapefruit juice (>1 quart daily)

Interactions with lipid-lowering drugs that can cause myopathy when given alone

See WARNINGS, *Myopathy/Rhabdomyolysis*.

The risk of myopathy is increased by gemfibrozil and to a lesser extent by other fibrates and niacin (nicotinic acid) (≥1 g/day).

Other drug interactions

Amiodarone or Verapamil: The risk of myopathy/rhabdomyolysis is increased by concomitant administration of amiodarone or verapamil (see WARNINGS, *Myopathy/Rhabdomyolysis*).

Cholestyramine: Concomitant cholestyramine administration decreased the mean AUC of total ezetimibe approximately 55%. The incremental LDL-C reduction due to adding VYTORIN to cholestyramine may be reduced by this interaction.

Cyclosporine: Caution should be exercised when initiating VYTORIN in patients treated with cyclosporine due to increased exposure to ezetimibe. This exposure may be greater in patients with severe renal insufficiency. In patients treated with cyclosporine, the potential effects of the increased exposure to ezetimibe from concomitant use should be carefully weighed against the benefits of alter-

Table 4
Summary of NCEP ATP III Guidelines

Risk Category	LDL Goal (mg/dL)	LDL Level at Which to Initiate Therapeutic Lifestyle Changes[a] (mg/dL)	LDL level at Which to Consider Drug Therapy (mg/dL)
CHD or CHD risk equivalents[b] (10-year risk >20%)[c]	<100	≥100	≥130 (100-129: drug optional)[d]
2+ Risk factors[e] (10-year risk ≤20%)[c]	<130	≥130	10-year risk 10–20%: ≥130[c] 10-year risk <10%: ≥160[c]
0–1 Risk factor[f]	<160	≥160	≥190 (160–189: LDL-lowering drug optional)

[a] Therapeutic lifestyle changes include: 1) dietary changes: reduced intake of saturated fats (<7% of total calories) and cholesterol (<200 mg per day), and enhancing LDL lowering with plant stanols/sterols (2 g/d) and increased viscous (soluble) fiber (10–25 g/d), 2) weight reduction, and 3) increased physical activity.

[b] CHD risk equivalents comprise: diabetes, multiple risk factors that confer a 10-year risk for CHD >20%, and other clinical forms of atherosclerotic disease (peripheral arterial disease, abdominal aortic aneurysm and symptomatic carotid artery disease).

[c] Risk assessment for determining the 10-year risk for developing CHD is carried out using the Framingham risk scoring. Refer to JAMA, May 16, 2001; 285 (19): 2486–2497, or the NCEP website (http://www.nhlbi.nih.gov) for more details.

[d] Some authorities recommend use of LDL-lowering drugs in this category if an LDL cholesterol <100 mg/dL cannot be achieved by therapeutic lifestyle changes. Others prefer use of drugs that primarily modify triglycerides and HDL, e.g., nicotinic acid or fibrate. Clinical judgment also may call for deferring drug therapy in this subcategory.

[e] Major risk factors (exclusive of LDL cholesterol) that modify LDL goals include cigarette smoking, hypertension (BP ≥140/90 mm Hg or on anti-hypertensive medication), low HDL cholesterol (<40 mg/dL), family history of premature CHD (CHD in male first-degree relative <55 years; CHD in female first-degree relative <65 years), age (men ≥45 years; women ≥55 years). HDL cholesterol ≥60 mg/dL counts as a "negative" risk factor; its presence removes one risk factor from the total count.

[f] Almost all people with 0-1 risk factor have a 10-year risk <10%; thus, 10-year risk assessment in people with 0-1 risk factor is not necessary.

ations in lipid levels provided by ezetimibe. In a pharmacokinetic study in post-renal transplant patients with mildly impaired or normal renal function (creatinine clearance of >50 mL/min), concomitant cyclosporine administration increased the mean AUC and C_{max} of total ezetimibe 3.4-fold (range 2.3- to 7.9-fold) and 3.9-fold (range 3.0- to 4.4-fold), respectively. In a separate study, the total ezetimibe exposure increased 12-fold in one renal transplant patient with severe renal insufficiency receiving multiple medications, including cyclosporine. (See CLINICAL PHARMACOLOGY, *Drug Interactions* and WARNINGS, *Myopathy/Rhabdomyolysis.*)

Digoxin: Concomitant administration of a single dose of digoxin in healthy male volunteers receiving simvastatin resulted in a slight elevation (less than 0.3 ng/mL) in plasma digoxin concentrations compared to concomitant administration of placebo and digoxin. Patients taking digoxin should be monitored appropriately when VYTORIN is initiated.

Fibrates: The safety and effectiveness of VYTORIN administered with fibrates have not been established.

Fibrates may increase cholesterol excretion into the bile, leading to cholelithiasis. In a preclinical study in dogs, ezetimibe increased cholesterol in the gallbladder bile (see ANIMAL PHARMACOLOGY). Coadministration of VYTORIN with fibrates is not recommended until use in patients is studied. (See WARNINGS, *Myopathy/Rhabdomyolysis.*)

Warfarin: Simvastatin 20-40 mg/day modestly potentiated the effect of coumarin anticoagulants: the prothrombin time, reported as International Normalized Ratio (INR), increased from a baseline of 1.7 to 1.8 and from 2.6 to 3.4 in a normal volunteer study and in a hypercholesterolemic patient study, respectively. With other statins, clinically evident bleeding and/or increased prothrombin time has been reported in a few patients taking coumarin anticoagulants concomitantly. In such patients, prothrombin time should be determined before starting VYTORIN and frequently enough during early therapy to insure that no significant alteration of prothrombin time occurs. Once a stable prothrombin time has been documented, prothrombin times can be monitored at the intervals usually recommended for patients on coumarin anticoagulants. If the dose of VYTORIN is changed or discontinued, the same procedure should be repeated. Simvastatin therapy has not been associated with bleeding or with changes in prothrombin time in patients not taking anticoagulants.

Ezetimibe

Fenofibrate: In a pharmacokinetic study, concomitant fenofibrate administration increased total ezetimibe concentrations approximately 1.5-fold.

Gemfibrozil: In a pharmacokinetic study, concomitant gemfibrozil administration increased total ezetimibe concentrations approximately 1.7-fold.

Simvastatin

Propranolol: In healthy male volunteers there was a significant decrease in mean C_{max}, but no change in AUC, for simvastatin total and active inhibitors with concomitant administration of single doses of simvastatin and propranolol. The clinical relevance of this finding is unclear. The pharmacokinetics of the enantiomers of propranolol were not affected.

CNS Toxicity

Optic nerve degeneration was seen in clinically normal dogs treated with simvastatin for 14 weeks at 180 mg/kg/day, a dose that produced mean plasma drug levels about 12 times higher than the mean plasma drug level in humans taking 80 mg/day.

A chemically similar drug in this class also produced optic nerve degeneration (Wallerian degeneration of retinogeniculate fibers) in clinically normal dogs in a dose-dependent fashion starting at 60 mg/kg/day, a dose that produced mean plasma drug levels about 30 times higher than the mean plasma drug level in humans taking the highest recommended dose (as measured by total enzyme inhibitory activity). This same drug also produced vestibulocochlear Wallerian-like degeneration and retinal ganglion cell chromatolysis in dogs treated for 14 weeks at 180 mg/kg/day, a dose that resulted in a mean plasma drug level similar to that seen with the 60 mg/kg/day dose.

CNS vascular lesions, characterized by perivascular hemorrhage and edema, mononuclear cell infiltration of perivascular spaces, perivascular fibrin deposits and necrosis of small vessels were seen in dogs treated with simvastatin at a dose of 360 mg/kg/day, a dose that produced mean plasma drug levels that were about 14 times higher than the mean plasma drug levels in humans taking 80 mg/day. Similar CNS vascular lesions have been observed with several other drugs of this class.

There were cataracts in female rats after two years of treatment with 50 and 100 mg/kg/day (22 and 25 times the human AUC at 80 mg/day, respectively) and in dogs after three months at 90 mg/kg/day (19 times) and at two years at 50 mg/kg/day (5 times).

Carcinogenesis, Mutagenesis, Impairment of Fertility

VYTORIN

No animal carcinogenicity or fertility studies have been conducted with the combination of ezetimibe and simvastatin. The combination of ezetimibe with simvastatin did not show evidence of mutagenicity *in vitro* in a microbial mutagenicity (Ames) test with *Salmonella typhimurium* and *Escherichia coli* with or without metabolic activation. No evidence of clastogenicity was observed *in vitro* in a chromosomal aberration assay in human peripheral blood lymphocytes with ezetimibe and simvastatin with or without metabolic activation. There was no evidence of genotoxicity at doses up to 600 mg/kg with the combination of ezetimibe and simvastatin (1:1) in the *in vivo* mouse micronucleus test.

Ezetimibe

A 104-week dietary carcinogenicity study with ezetimibe was conducted in rats at doses up to 1500 mg/kg/day (males) and 500 mg/kg/day (females) (~20 times the human exposure at 10 mg daily based on AUC_{0-24hr} for total ezetimibe). A 104-week dietary carcinogenicity study with ezetimibe was also conducted in mice at doses up to 500 mg/kg/day (>150 times the human exposure at 10 mg daily based on AUC_{0-24hr} for total ezetimibe). There were no statistically significant increases in tumor incidences in drug-treated rats or mice.

No evidence of mutagenicity was observed *in vitro* in a microbial mutagenicity (Ames) test with *Salmonella typhimurium* and *Escherichia coli* with or without metabolic activation. No evidence of clastogenicity was observed *in vitro* in a chromosomal aberration assay in human peripheral blood lymphocytes with or without metabolic activation. In addition, there was no evidence of genotoxicity in the *in vivo* mouse micronucleus test.

In oral (gavage) fertility studies of ezetimibe conducted in rats, there was no evidence of reproductive toxicity at doses up to 1000 mg/kg/day in male or female rats (~7 times the human exposure at 10 mg daily based on AUC_{0-24hr} for total ezetimibe).

Simvastatin

In a 72-week carcinogenicity study, mice were administered daily doses of simvastatin of 25, 100, and 400 mg/kg body weight, which resulted in mean plasma drug levels approximately 1, 4, and 8 times higher than the mean human plasma drug level, respectively (as total inhibitory activity based on AUC) after an 80-mg oral dose. Liver carcinomas were significantly increased in high-dose females and mid- and high-dose males with a maximum incidence of 90% in males. The incidence of adenomas of the liver was significantly increased in mid- and high-dose females. Drug treatment also significantly increased the incidence of lung adenomas in mid- and high-dose males and females. Adenomas of the Harderian gland (a gland of the eye of rodents) were significantly higher in high-dose mice than in controls. No evidence of a tumorigenic effect was observed at 25 mg/kg/day.

In a separate 92-week carcinogenicity study in mice at doses up to 25 mg/kg/day, no evidence of a tumorigenic effect was observed (mean plasma drug levels were 1 times higher than humans given 80 mg simvastatin as measured by AUC).

In a two-year study in rats at 25 mg/kg/day, there was a statistically significant increase in the incidence of thyroid follicular adenomas in female rats exposed to approximately 11 times higher levels of simvastatin than in humans given 80 mg simvastatin (as measured by AUC).

A second two-year rat carcinogenicity study with doses of 50 and 100 mg/kg/day produced hepatocellular adenomas and carcinomas (in female rats at both doses and in males at 100 mg/kg/day). Thyroid follicular cell adenomas were increased in males and females at both doses; thyroid follicular cell carcinomas were increased in females at 100 mg/kg/day. The increased incidence of thyroid neoplasms appears to be consistent with findings from other HMG-CoA reductase inhibitors. These treatment levels represented plasma drug levels (AUC) of approximately 7 and 15 times (males) and 22 and 25 times (females) the mean human plasma drug exposure after an 80 milligram daily dose.

No evidence of mutagenicity was observed in a microbial mutagenicity (Ames) test with or without rat or mouse liver metabolic activation. In addition, no evidence of damage to genetic material was noted in an *in vitro* alkaline elution assay using rat hepatocytes, a V-79 mammalian cell forward mutation study, an *in vitro* chromosome aberration study in CHO cells, or an *in vivo* chromosomal aberration assay in mouse bone marrow.

There was decreased fertility in male rats treated with simvastatin for 34 weeks at 25 mg/kg body weight (4 times the maximum human exposure level, based on AUC, in patients receiving 80 mg/day); however, this effect was not observed during a subsequent fertility study in which simvastatin was administered at this same dose level to male rats for 11 weeks (the entire cycle of spermatogenesis including epididymal maturation). No microscopic changes were observed in the testes of rats from either study. At 180 mg/kg/day, (which produces exposure levels 22 times higher than those in humans taking 80 mg/day based on surface area, mg/m^2), seminiferous tubule degeneration (necrosis and loss of spermatogenic epithelium) was observed. In dogs, there was drug-related testicular atrophy, decreased spermatogenesis, spermatocytic degeneration and giant cell formation at 10 mg/kg/day, (approximately 2 times the human exposure, based on AUC, at 80 mg/day). The clinical significance of these findings is unclear.

Pregnancy

Pregnancy Category: X

See CONTRAINDICATIONS.

VYTORIN

As safety in pregnant women has not been established, treatment should be immediately discontinued as soon as pregnancy is recognized. VYTORIN should be administered to women of child-bearing potential only when such patients are highly unlikely to conceive and have been informed of the potential hazards.

Ezetimibe

In oral (gavage) embryo-fetal development studies of ezetimibe conducted in rats and rabbits during organogenesis, there was no evidence of embryolethal effects at the doses tested (250, 500, 1000 mg/kg/day). In rats, increased incidences of common fetal skeletal findings (extra pair of thoracic ribs, unossified cervical vertebral centra, shortened ribs) were observed at 1000 mg/kg/day (~10 times the human exposure at 10 mg daily based on AUC_{0-24hr} for total ezetimibe). In rabbits treated with ezetimibe, an increased incidence of extra thoracic ribs was observed at 1000 mg/kg/day (150 times the human exposure at 10 mg daily based on AUC_{0-24hr} for total ezetimibe). Ezetimibe crossed the placenta when pregnant rats and rabbits were given multiple oral doses.

Multiple-dose studies of ezetimibe coadministered with HMG-CoA reductase inhibitors (statins) in rats and rabbits during organogenesis result in higher ezetimibe and statin exposures. Reproductive findings occur at lower doses in coadministration therapy compared to monotherapy.

Simvastatin

Simvastatin was not teratogenic in rats at doses of 25 mg/kg/day or in rabbits at doses up to 10 mg/kg daily. These doses resulted in 3 times (rat) or 3 times (rabbit) the human exposure based on mg/m^2 surface area. However, in studies with another structurally-related HMG-CoA reductase inhibitor, skeletal malformations were observed in rats and mice.

Rare reports of congenital anomalies have been received following intrauterine exposure to HMG-CoA reductase inhibitors. In a review[2] of approximately 100 prospectively followed pregnancies in women exposed to simvastatin or another structurally related HMG-CoA reductase inhibitor, the incidences of congenital anomalies, spontaneous abortions and fetal deaths/stillbirths did not exceed what would be expected in the general population. The number of cases is adequate only to exclude a 3- to 4-fold increase in congenital anomalies over the background incidence. In 89% of the prospectively followed pregnancies, drug treatment was initiated prior to pregnancy and was discontinued at some point in the first trimester when pregnancy was identified.

Labor and Delivery

The effects of VYTORIN on labor and delivery in pregnant women are unknown.

Nursing Mothers

In rat studies, exposure to ezetimibe in nursing pups was up to half of that observed in maternal plasma. It is not known whether ezetimibe or simvastatin are excreted into human breast milk. Because a small amount of another drug in the same class as simvastatin is excreted in human milk and because of the potential for serious adverse reactions in nursing infants, women who are nursing should not take VYTORIN (see CONTRAINDICATIONS).

Pediatric Use

VYTORIN

There are insufficient data for the safe and effective use of VYTORIN in pediatric patients. (See *Ezetimibe* and *Simvastatin* below.)

Ezetimibe

The pharmacokinetics of ezetimibe in adolescents (10 to 18 years) have been shown to be similar to that in adults. Treatment experience with ezetimibe in the pediatric population is limited to 4 patients (9 to 17 years) with homozygous sitosterolemia and 5 patients (11 to 17 years) with HoFH. Treatment with ezetimibe in children (<10 years) is not recommended.

Simvastatin

Safety and effectiveness of simvastatin in patients 10–17 years of age with heterozygous familial hypercholesterolemia have been evaluated in a controlled clinical trial in adolescent boys and in girls who were at least 1 year post-menarche. Patients treated with simvastatin had an adverse experience profile generally similar to that of patients treated with placebo. **Doses greater than 40 mg have not been studied in this population.** In this limited controlled study, there was no detectable effect on growth or sexual maturation in the adolescent boys or girls, or any effect on menstrual cycle length in girls. Adolescent females should be counseled on appropriate contraceptive methods while on therapy with simvastatin (see CONTRAINDICATIONS and PRECAUTIONS, *Pregnancy*). Simvastatin has not been studied in patients younger than 10 years of age, nor in pre-menarchal girls.

Geriatric Use

Of the patients who received VYTORIN in clinical studies, 792 were 65 and older (this included 176 who were 75 and older). The safety of VYTORIN was similar between these patients and younger patients. Greater sensitivity of some older individuals cannot be ruled out. (See CLINICAL PHARMACOLOGY, *Special Populations* and ADVERSE REACTIONS.)

[2] Manson, J.M., Freyssinges, C., Ducrocq, M.B., Stephenson, W.P., Postmarketing Surveillance of Lovastatin and Simvastatin Exposure During Pregnancy, *Reproductive Toxicology*, 10(6):439–446, 1996.

ADVERSE REACTIONS

VYTORIN has been evaluated for safety in more than 3800 patients in clinical trials. VYTORIN was generally well tolerated.

Table 5 summarizes the frequency of clinical adverse experiences reported in ≥2% of patients treated with VYTORIN

Continued on next page

Vytorin—Cont.

(n=1236) and at an incidence greater than placebo regardless of causality assessment from three similarly designed, placebo-controlled trials.
[See table 5 below]

Ezetimibe

Other adverse experiences reported with ezetimibe in placebo-controlled studies, regardless of causality assessment: *Body as a whole – general disorders:* fatigue; *Gastrointestinal system disorders:* abdominal pain, diarrhea; *Infection and infestations:* infection viral, pharyngitis, sinusitis; *Musculoskeletal system disorders:* arthralgia, back pain; *Respiratory system disorders:* coughing.

Post-marketing Experience

The following adverse reactions have been reported in post-marketing experience, regardless of causality assessment: Hypersensitivity reactions, including angioedema and rash; pancreatitis; nausea; cholelithiasis; cholecystitis.

Simvastatin

Other adverse experiences reported with simvastatin in placebo-controlled clinical studies, regardless of causality assessment: *Body as a whole – general disorders:* asthenia; *Eye disorders:* cataract; *Gastrointestinal system disorders:* abdominal pain, constipation, diarrhea, dyspepsia, flatulence, nausea; *Skin and subcutaneous tissue disorders:* eczema, pruritus, rash.

The following effects have been reported with other HMG-CoA reductase inhibitors. Not all the effects listed below have necessarily been associated with simvastatin therapy.

Musculoskeletal system disorders: muscle cramps, myalgia, myopathy, rhabdomyolysis, arthralgias.

Nervous system disorders: dysfunction of certain cranial nerves (including alteration of taste, impairment of extraocular movement, facial paresis), tremor, dizziness, memory loss, paresthesia, peripheral neuropathy, peripheral nerve palsy, psychic disturbances.

Ear and labyrinth disorders: vertigo.

Psychiatric disorders: anxiety, insomnia, depression, loss of libido.

Hypersensitivity Reactions: An apparent hypersensitivity syndrome has been reported rarely which has included one or more of the following features: anaphylaxis, angioedema, lupus erythematous-like syndrome, polymyalgia rheumatica, dermatomyositis, vasculitis, purpura, thrombocytopenia, leukopenia, hemolytic anemia, positive ANA, ESR increase, eosinophilia, arthritis, arthralgia, urticaria, asthenia, photosensitivity, fever, chills, flushing, malaise, dyspnea, toxic epidermal necrolysis, erythema multiforme, including Stevens-Johnson syndrome.

Gastrointestinal system disorders: pancreatitis, vomiting.

Hepatobiliary disorders: hepatitis, including chronic active hepatitis, cholestatic jaundice, fatty change in liver, and, rarely, cirrhosis, fulminant hepatic necrosis, and hepatoma.

Metabolism and nutrition disorders: anorexia.

Skin and subcutaneous tissue disorders: alopecia, pruritus. A variety of skin changes (e.g., nodules, discoloration, dryness of skin/mucous membranes, changes to hair/nails) have been reported.

Reproductive system and breast disorders: gynecomastia, erectile dysfunction.

Eye disorders: progression of cataracts (lens opacities), ophthalmoplegia.

Laboratory Abnormalities: elevated transaminases, alkaline phosphatase, γ-glutamyl transpeptidase, and bilirubin; thyroid function abnormalities.

Laboratory Tests

Marked persistent increases of serum transaminases have been noted (see WARNINGS, *Liver Enzymes*). About 5% of patients taking simvastatin had elevations of CK levels of 3 or more times the normal value on one or more occasions. This was attributable to the noncardiac fraction of CK. Muscle pain or dysfunction usually was not reported (see WARNINGS, *Myopathy/Rhabdomyolysis*).

Concomitant Lipid-Lowering Therapy

In controlled clinical studies in which simvastatin was administered concomitantly with cholestyramine, no adverse reactions peculiar to this concomitant treatment were observed. The adverse reactions that occurred were limited to those reported previously with simvastatin or cholestyramine.

Adolescent Patients (ages 10–17 years)

In a 48-week controlled study in adolescent boys and girls who were at least 1 year post-menarche, 10–17 years of age with heterozygous familial hypercholesterolemia (n=175), the safety and tolerability profile of the group treated with simvastatin (10–40 mg daily) was generally similar to that of the group treated with placebo, with the most common adverse experiences observed in both groups being upper respiratory infection, headache, abdominal pain, and nausea (see CLINICAL PHARMACOLOGY, *Special Populations* and PRECAUTIONS, *Pediatric Use*).

OVERDOSAGE

VYTORIN

No specific treatment of overdosage with VYTORIN can be recommended. In the event of an overdose, symptomatic and supportive measures should be employed.

Ezetimibe

In clinical studies, administration of ezetimibe, 50 mg/day to 15 healthy subjects for up to 14 days, or 40 mg/day to 18 patients with primary hypercholesterolemia for up to 56 days, was generally well tolerated.

A few cases of overdosage have been reported; most have not been associated with adverse experiences. Reported adverse experiences have not been serious.

Simvastatin

A few cases of overdosage with simvastatin have been reported; the maximum dose taken was 3.6 g. All patients recovered without sequelae.

The dialyzability of simvastatin and its metabolites in man is not known at present.

DOSAGE AND ADMINISTRATION

The patient should be placed on a standard cholesterol-lowering diet before receiving VYTORIN and should continue on this diet during treatment with VYTORIN. The dosage should be individualized according to the baseline LDL-C level, the recommended goal of therapy, and the patient's response. (See NCEP Adult Treatment Panel (ATP) III Guidelines, summarized in Table 4.) VYTORIN should be taken as a single daily dose in the evening, with or without food.

The dosage range is 10/10 mg/day through 10/80 mg/day. The recommended usual starting dose is 10/20 mg/day. Initiation of therapy with 10/10 mg/day may be considered for patients requiring less aggressive LDL-C reductions. Patients who require a larger reduction in LDL-C (greater than 55%) may be started at 10/40 mg/day. After initiation or titration of VYTORIN, lipid levels may be analyzed after 2 or more weeks and dosage adjusted, if needed. See below for dosage recommendations for patients receiving certain concomitant therapies and for those with renal insufficiency.

Patients with Homozygous Familial Hypercholesterolemia

The recommended dosage for patients with homozygous familial hypercholesterolemia is VYTORIN 10/40 mg/day or 10/80 mg/day in the evening. VYTORIN should be used as an adjunct to other lipid-lowering treatments (e.g., LDL apheresis) in these patients or if such treatments are unavailable.

Patients with Hepatic Insufficiency

No dosage adjustment is necessary in patients with mild hepatic insufficiency (see PRECAUTIONS, *Hepatic Insufficiency*).

Patients with Renal Insufficiency

No dosage adjustment is necessary in patients with mild or moderate renal insufficiency. However, for patients with severe renal insufficiency, VYTORIN should not be started unless the patient has already tolerated treatment with simvastatin at a dose of 5 mg or higher. Caution should be exercised when VYTORIN is administered to these patients and they should be closely monitored (see CLINICAL PHARMACOLOGY, *Pharmacokinetics* and WARNINGS, *Myopathy/Rhabdomyolysis*).

Geriatric Patients

No dosage adjustment is necessary in geriatric patients (see CLINICAL PHARMACOLOGY, *Special Populations*).

Coadministration with Bile Acid Sequestrants

Dosing of VYTORIN should occur either ≥2 hours before or ≥4 hours after administration of a bile acid sequestrant (see PRECAUTIONS, *Drug Interactions*).

Patients taking Cyclosporine

Caution should be exercised when initiating VYTORIN in the setting of cyclosporine. In patients taking cyclosporine, VYTORIN should not be started unless the patient has already tolerated treatment with simvastatin at a dose of 5 mg or higher. The dose of VYTORIN should not exceed 10/10 mg/day.

Patients taking Amiodarone or Verapamil

In patients taking amiodarone or verapamil concomitantly with VYTORIN, the dose should not exceed 10/20 mg/day (see WARNINGS, *Myopathy/Rhabdomyolysis* and PRECAUTIONS, *Drug Interactions, Other drug interactions*).

HOW SUPPLIED

No. 3873 — Tablets VYTORIN 10/10 are white to off-white capsule-shaped tablets with code "311" on one side.
They are supplied as follows:
NDC 66582-311-31 bottles of 30
NDC 66582-311-54 bottles of 90
NDC 66582-311-82 bottles of 1000 (If repackaged in blisters, then opaque or light-resistant blisters should be used.)
NDC 66582-311-28 unit dose packages of 100.

No. 3874 — Tablets VYTORIN 10/20 are white to off-white capsule-shaped tablets with code "312" on one side.
They are supplied as follows:
NDC 66582-312-31 bottles of 30
NDC 66582-312-54 bottles of 90
NDC 66582-312-82 bottles of 1000 (If repackaged in blisters, then opaque or light-resistant blisters should be used.)
NDC 66582-312-28 unit dose packages of 100.

No. 3875 — Tablets VYTORIN 10/40 are white to off-white capsule-shaped tablets with code "313" on one side.
They are supplied as follows:
NDC 66582-313-31 bottles of 30
NDC 66582-313-54 bottles of 90
NDC 66582-313-74 bottles of 500 (If repackaged in blisters, then opaque or light-resistant blisters should be used.)
NDC 66582-313-52 unit dose packages of 50.

No. 3876 — Tablets VYTORIN 10/80 are white to off-white capsule-shaped tablets with code "315" on one side.
They are supplied as follows:
NDC 66582-315-31 bottles of 30
NDC 66582-315-54 bottles of 90
NDC 66582-315-74 bottles of 500 (If repackaged in blisters, then opaque or light-resistant blisters should be used.)
NDC 66582-315-52 unit dose packages of 50.

Storage

Store at 20–25°C (68–77°F). [See USP Controlled Room Temperature.] Keep container tightly closed.

9619600
Issued July 2004
Printed in USA
MERCK/Schering-Plough Pharmaceuticals
Manufactured for:
MERCK/Schering-Plough Pharmaceuticals
North Wales, PA 19454, USA
By:
MSD Technology Singapore Pte. Ltd.
Singapore 637766

VYTORIN™ (ezetimibe/simvastatin) Tablets

Patient Information about VYTORIN (VI-tor-in)

Generic name: ezetimibe/simvastatin tablets

Read this information carefully before you start taking VYTORIN. Review this information each time you refill your prescription for VYTORIN as there may be new information. This information does not take the place of talking with your doctor about your medical condition or your treatment. If you have any questions about VYTORIN, ask your doctor. Only your doctor can determine if VYTORIN is right for you.

What is VYTORIN?

VYTORIN contains two cholesterol-lowering medications, ezetimibe and simvastatin, available as a tablet in four strengths:

— VYTORIN 10/10 (ezetimibe 10 mg/simvastatin 10 mg)
— VYTORIN 10/20 (ezetimibe 10 mg/simvastatin 20 mg)
— VYTORIN 10/40 (ezetimibe 10 mg/simvastatin 40 mg)
— VYTORIN 10/80 (ezetimibe 10 mg/simvastatin 80 mg)

VYTORIN is a medicine used to lower levels of total cholesterol, LDL (bad) cholesterol, and fatty substances called triglycerides in the blood. In addition, VYTORIN raises levels of HDL (good) cholesterol. It is used for patients who cannot control their cholesterol levels by diet alone. You should stay on a cholesterol-lowering diet while taking this medicine.

VYTORIN works to reduce your cholesterol in two ways. It reduces the cholesterol absorbed in your digestive tract, as well as the cholesterol your body makes by itself. VYTORIN does not help you lose weight.

For more information about cholesterol, see the section called "What should I know about high cholesterol?"

Who should not take VYTORIN?

Do not take VYTORIN:

- If you are allergic to ezetimibe or simvastatin, the active ingredients in VYTORIN, or to the inactive ingredients. For a list of inactive ingredients, see the "Inactive ingredients" section at the end of this information sheet.
- If you have active liver disease or repeated blood tests indicating possible liver problems.

Table 5*

Clinical Adverse Events Occurring in ≥2% of Patients Treated with VYTORIN and at an Incidence Greater than Placebo, Regardless of Causality

Body System/Organ Class Adverse Event	Placebo (%) n=311	Ezetimibe 10 mg (%) n=302	Simvastatin** (%) n=1234	VYTORIN** (%) n=1236
Body as a whole – general disorders				
Headache	6.4	6.0	5.9	6.8
Infection and infestations				
Influenza	1.0	1.0	1.9	2.6
Upper respiratory tract infection	2.6	5.0	5.0	3.9
Musculoskeletal and connective tissue disorders				
Myalgia	2.9	2.3	2.6	3.5
Pain in extremity	1.3	3.0	2.0	2.3

*Includes two placebo-controlled combination studies in which the active ingredients equivalent to VYTORIN were coadministered and one placebo-controlled study in which VYTORIN was administered.
**All doses.

- If you are pregnant, or think you may be pregnant, or planning to become pregnant or breast-feeding.

VYTORIN is not recommended for use in children under 10 years of age.

What should I tell my doctor before and while taking VYTORIN?

Tell your doctor right away if you experience unexplained muscle pain, tenderness, or weakness. This is because on rare occasions, muscle problems can be serious, including muscle breakdown resulting in kidney damage.

The risk of muscle breakdown is greater at higher doses of VYTORIN.

The risk of muscle breakdown is greater in patients with kidney problems.

Taking VYTORIN with certain substances can increase the risk of muscle problems. It is particularly important to tell your doctor if you are taking any of the following:

- cyclosporine
- antifungal agents (such as itraconazole or ketoconazole)
- fibric acid derivatives (such as gemfibrozil, bezafibrate, or fenofibrate)
- the antibiotics erythromycin and clarithromycin
- HIV protease inhibitors (such as indinavir, nelfinavir, ritonavir, and saquinavir)
- the antidepressant nefazodone
- amiodarone (a drug used to treat an irregular heartbeat)
- verapamil (a drug used to treat high blood pressure, chest pain associated with heart disease, or other heart conditions)
- large doses (≥1 g/day) of niacin or nicotinic acid
- large quantities of grapefruit juice (>1 quart daily)

It is also important to tell your doctor if you are taking coumarin anticoagulants (drugs that prevent blood clots, such as warfarin).

Tell your doctor about any prescription and nonprescription medicines you are taking or plan to take, including natural or herbal remedies.

Tell your doctor about all your medical conditions including allergies.

Tell your doctor if you:

- drink substantial quantities of alcohol or ever had liver problems. VYTORIN may not be right for you.
- are pregnant or plan to become pregnant. Do not use VYTORIN if you are pregnant, trying to become pregnant or suspect that you are pregnant. If you become pregnant while taking VYTORIN, stop taking it and contact your doctor immediately.
- are breast-feeding. Do not use VYTORIN if you are breast-feeding.

Tell other doctors prescribing a new medication that you are taking VYTORIN.

How should I take VYTORIN?

Your doctor has prescribed your dose of VYTORIN. The available doses of VYTORIN are 10/10, 10/20, 10/40, and 10/80. The usual daily starting dose is VYTORIN 10/20.

- Take VYTORIN once a day, in the evening, with or without food.
- Try to take VYTORIN as prescribed. If you miss a dose, do not take an extra dose. Just resume your usual schedule.
- Continue to follow a cholesterol-lowering diet while taking VYTORIN. Ask your doctor if you need diet information.
- Keep taking VYTORIN unless your doctor tells you to stop. If you stop taking VYTORIN, your cholesterol may rise again.

What should I do in case of an overdose?

Contact your doctor immediately.

What are the possible side effects of VYTORIN?

See your doctor regularly to check your cholesterol level and to check for side effects. Your doctor may do blood tests to check your liver before you start taking VYTORIN and during treatment.

In clinical studies patients reported the following common side effects while taking VYTORIN: headache and muscle pain (see What should I tell my doctor before and while taking VYTORIN?).

The following side effects have been reported in general use with either ezetimibe or simvastatin tablets (tablets that contain the active ingredients of VYTORIN):

- allergic reactions including swelling of the face, lips, tongue, and/or throat that may cause difficulty in breathing or swallowing (which may require treatment right away), and rash; inflammation of the pancreas; nausea; gallstones; inflammation of the gallbladder.

Tell your doctor if you are having these or any other medical problems while on VYTORIN. This is not a complete list of side effects. For a complete list, ask your doctor or pharmacist.

What should I know about high cholesterol?

Cholesterol is a type of fat found in your blood. Cholesterol comes from two sources. It is produced by your body and it comes from the food you eat. Your total cholesterol is made up of both LDL and HDL cholesterol.

LDL cholesterol is called "bad" cholesterol because it can build up in the wall of your arteries and form plaque. Over time, plaque build-up can cause a narrowing of the arteries. This narrowing can slow or block blood flow to your heart, brain, and other organs. High LDL cholesterol is a major cause of heart disease and stroke.

HDL cholesterol is called "good" cholesterol because it keeps the bad cholesterol from building up in the arteries.

Triglycerides also are fats found in your body.

General Information about VYTORIN

Medicines are sometimes prescribed for conditions that are not mentioned in patient information leaflets. Do not use VYTORIN for a condition for which it was not prescribed. Do not give VYTORIN to other people, even if they have the same condition you have. It may harm them.

This summarizes the most important information about VYTORIN. If you would like more information, talk with your doctor. You can ask your pharmacist or doctor for information about VYTORIN that is written for health professionals. For additional information, visit the following web site: vytorin.com.

Inactive ingredients:

Butylated hydroxyanisole NF, citric acid monohydrate USP, croscarmellose sodium NF, hydroxypropyl methylcellulose USP, lactose monohydrate NF, magnesium stearate NF, microcrystalline cellulose NF, and propyl gallate NF.

9621000 Issued July 2004

Manufactured for:
Merck/Schering-Plough Pharmaceuticals
North Wales, PA 19454, USA
By:
MSD Technology Singapore Pte. Ltd.
Singapore 637766

ZETIA® ℞

[*zĕt' ē ă*]
(ezetimibe)
TABLETS

DESCRIPTION

ZETIA (ezetimibe) is in a class of lipid-lowering compounds that selectively inhibits the intestinal absorption of cholesterol and related phytosterols. The chemical name of ezetimibe is 1-(4-fluorophenyl)-3(R)-[3-(4-fluorophenyl)-3(S)-hydroxypropyl]-4(S)-(4-hydroxyphenyl)-2-azetidinone. The empirical formula is $C_{24}H_{21}F_2NO_3$. Its molecular weight is 409.4 and its structural formula is:

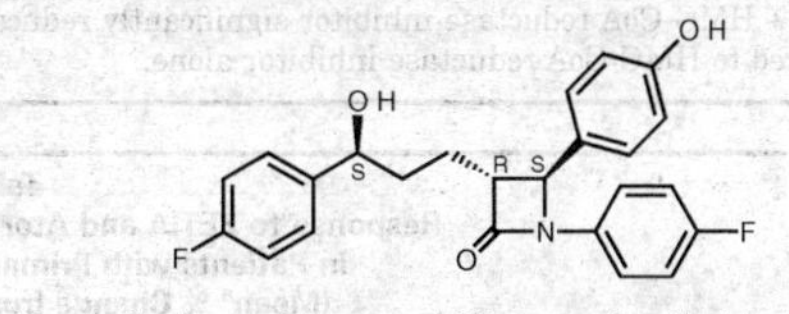

Ezetimibe is a white, crystalline powder that is freely to very soluble in ethanol, methanol, and acetone and practically insoluble in water. Ezetimibe has a melting point of about 163°C and is stable at ambient temperature. ZETIA is available as a tablet for oral administration containing 10 mg of ezetimibe and the following inactive ingredients: croscarmellose sodium NF, lactose monohydrate NF, magnesium stearate NF, microcrystalline cellulose NF, povidone USP, and sodium lauryl sulfate NF.

CLINICAL PHARMACOLOGY

Background

Clinical studies have demonstrated that elevated levels of total cholesterol (total-C), low density lipoprotein cholesterol (LDL-C) and apolipoprotein B (Apo B), the major protein constituent of LDL, promote human atherosclerosis. In addition, decreased levels of high density lipoprotein cholesterol (HDL-C) are associated with the development of atherosclerosis. Epidemiologic studies have established that cardiovascular morbidity and mortality vary directly with the level of total-C and LDL-C and inversely with the level of HDL-C. Like LDL, cholesterol-enriched triglyceride-rich lipoproteins, including very-low-density lipoproteins (VLDL), intermediate-density lipoproteins (IDL), and remnants, can also promote atherosclerosis. The independent effect of raising HDL-C or lowering triglycerides (TG) on the risk of coronary and cardiovascular morbidity and mortality has not been determined.

ZETIA reduces total-C, LDL-C, Apo B, and TG, and increases HDL-C in patients with hypercholesterolemia. Administration of ZETIA with an HMG-CoA reductase inhibitor is effective in improving serum total-C, LDL-C, Apo B, TG, and HDL-C beyond either treatment alone. The effects of ezetimibe given either alone or in addition to an HMG-CoA reductase inhibitor on cardiovascular morbidity and mortality have not been established.

Mode of Action

Ezetimibe reduces blood cholesterol by inhibiting the absorption of cholesterol by the small intestine. In a 2-week clinical study in 18 hypercholesterolemic patients, ZETIA inhibited intestinal cholesterol absorption by 54%, compared with placebo. ZETIA had no clinically meaningful effect on the plasma concentrations of the fat-soluble vitamins A, D, and E (in a study of 113 patients), and did not impair adrenocortical steroid hormone production (in a study of 118 patients).

The cholesterol content of the liver is derived predominantly from three sources. The liver can synthesize cholesterol, take up cholesterol from the blood from circulating lipoproteins, or take up cholesterol absorbed by the small intestine. Intestinal cholesterol is derived primarily from cholesterol secreted in the bile and from dietary cholesterol.

Ezetimibe has a mechanism of action that differs from those of other classes of cholesterol-reducing compounds (HMG-CoA reductase inhibitors, bile acid sequestrants [resins], fibric acid derivatives, and plant stanols).

Ezetimibe does not inhibit cholesterol synthesis in the liver, or increase bile acid excretion. Instead, ezetimibe localizes and appears to act at the brush border of the small intestine and inhibits the absorption of cholesterol, leading to a decrease in the delivery of intestinal cholesterol to the liver. This causes a reduction of hepatic cholesterol stores and an increase in clearance of cholesterol from the blood; this distinct mechanism is complementary to that of HMG-CoA reductase inhibitors (see CLINICAL STUDIES).

Pharmacokinetics

Absorption

After oral administration, ezetimibe is absorbed and extensively conjugated to a pharmacologically active phenolic glucuronide (ezetimibe-glucuronide). After a single 10-mg dose of ZETIA to fasted adults, mean ezetimibe peak plasma concentrations (C_{max}) of 3.4 to 5.5 ng/mL were attained within 4 to 12 hours (T_{max}). Ezetimibe-glucuronide mean C_{max} values of 45 to 71 ng/mL were achieved between 1 and 2 hours (T_{max}). There was no substantial deviation from dose proportionality between 5 and 20 mg. The absolute bioavailability of ezetimibe cannot be determined, as the compound is virtually insoluble in aqueous media suitable for injection. Ezetimibe has variable bioavailability; the coefficient of variation, based on inter-subject variability, was 35 to 60% for AUC values.

Effect of Food on Oral Absorption

Concomitant food administration (high fat or non-fat meals) had no effect on the extent of absorption of ezetimibe when administered as ZETIA 10-mg tablets. The C_{max} value of ezetimibe was increased by 38% with consumption of high fat meals. ZETIA can be administered with or without food.

Distribution

Ezetimibe and ezetimibe-glucuronide are highly bound (>90%) to human plasma proteins.

Metabolism and Excretion

Ezetimibe is primarily metabolized in the small intestine and liver via glucuronide conjugation (a phase II reaction) with subsequent biliary and renal excretion. Minimal oxidative metabolism (a phase I reaction) has been observed in all species evaluated.

In humans, ezetimibe is rapidly metabolized to ezetimibe-glucuronide. Ezetimibe and ezetimibe-glucuronide are the major drug-derived compounds detected in plasma, constituting approximately 10 to 20% and 80 to 90% of the total drug in plasma, respectively. Both ezetimibe and ezetimibe-glucuronide are slowly eliminated from plasma with a half-life of approximately 22 hours for both ezetimibe and ezetimibe-glucuronide. Plasma concentration-time profiles exhibit multiple peaks, suggesting enterohepatic recycling.

Following oral administration of ^{14}C-ezetimibe (20 mg) to human subjects, total ezetimibe (ezetimibe + ezetimibe-glucuronide) accounted for approximately 93% of the total radioactivity in plasma. After 48 hours, there were no detectable levels of radioactivity in the plasma.

Approximately 78% and 11% of the administered radioactivity were recovered in the feces and urine, respectively, over a 10-day collection period. Ezetimibe was the major component in feces and accounted for 69% of the administered dose, while ezetimibe-glucuronide was the major component in urine and accounted for 9% of the administered dose.

Special Populations

Geriatric Patients

In a multiple dose study with ezetimibe given 10 mg once daily for 10 days, plasma concentrations for total ezetimibe were about 2-fold higher in older (≥65 years) healthy subjects compared to younger subjects.

Pediatric Patients

In a multiple dose study with ezetimibe given 10 mg once daily for 7 days, the absorption and metabolism of ezetimibe were similar in adolescents (10 to 18 years) and adults. Based on total ezetimibe, there are no pharmacokinetic differences between adolescents and adults. Pharmacokinetic data in the pediatric population <10 years of age are not available.

Gender

In a multiple dose study with ezetimibe given 10 mg once daily for 10 days, plasma concentrations for total ezetimibe were slightly higher (<20%) in women than in men.

Race

Based on a meta-analysis of multiple-dose pharmacokinetic studies, there were no pharmacokinetic differences between Blacks and Caucasians. There were too few patients in other racial or ethnic groups to permit further pharmacokinetic comparisons.

Hepatic Insufficiency

After a single 10-mg dose of ezetimibe, the mean area under the curve (AUC) for total ezetimibe was increased approximately 1.7-fold in patients with mild hepatic insufficiency (Child-Pugh score 5 to 6), compared to healthy subjects. The mean AUC values for total ezetimibe and ezetimibe were increased approximately 3- to 4-fold and 5- to 6-fold, respectively, in patients with moderate (Child-Pugh score 7 to 9) or severe hepatic impairment (Child-Pugh score 10 to 15). In a 14-day, multiple-dose study (10 mg daily) in patients with moderate hepatic insufficiency, the mean AUC values for total ezetimibe and ezetimibe were increased approximately 4-fold on Day 1 and Day 14 compared to healthy subjects. Due to the unknown effects of the increased exposure to ezetimibe in patients with moderate or severe hepatic insuf-

Continued on next page

Zetia—Cont.

ficiency, ZETIA is not recommended in these patients (see CONTRAINDICATIONS and PRECAUTIONS, *Hepatic Insufficiency*).

Renal Insufficiency

After a single 10-mg dose of ezetimibe in patients with severe renal disease (n=8; mean CrCl ≤30 mL/min/1.73 m^2), the mean AUC values for total ezetimibe, ezetimibe-glucuronide, and ezetimibe were increased approximately 1.5-fold, compared to healthy subjects (n=9).

Drug Interactions (See also PRECAUTIONS, *Drug Interactions*)

ZETIA had no significant effect on a series of probe drugs (caffeine, dextromethorphan, tolbutamide, and IV midazolam) known to be metabolized by cytochrome P450 (1A2, 2D6, 2C8/9 and 3A4) in a "cocktail" study of twelve healthy adult males. This indicates that ezetimibe is neither an inhibitor nor an inducer of these cytochrome P450 isozymes, and it is unlikely that ezetimibe will affect the metabolism of drugs that are metabolized by these enzymes.

Warfarin: Concomitant administration of ezetimibe (10 mg once daily) had no significant effect on bioavailability of warfarin and prothrombin time in a study of twelve healthy adult males.

Digoxin: Concomitant administration of ezetimibe (10 mg once daily) had no significant effect on the bioavailability of digoxin and the ECG parameters (HR, PR, QT, and QTc intervals) in a study of twelve healthy adult males.

Gemfibrozil: In a study of twelve healthy adult males, concomitant administration of gemfibrozil (600 mg twice daily) significantly increased the oral bioavailability of total ezetimibe by a factor of 1.7. Ezetimibe (10 mg once daily) did not significantly affect the bioavailability of gemfibrozil.

Oral Contraceptives: Co-administration of ezetimibe (10 mg once daily) with oral contraceptives had no significant effect on the bioavailability of ethinyl estradiol or levonorgestrel in a study of eighteen healthy adult females.

Cimetidine: Multiple doses of cimetidine (400 mg twice daily) had no significant effect on the oral bioavailability of ezetimibe and total ezetimibe in a study of twelve healthy adults.

Antacids: In a study of twelve healthy adults, a single dose of antacid (Supralox™ 20 mL) administration had no significant effect on the oral bioavailability of total ezetimibe, ezetimibe-glucuronide, or ezetimibe based on AUC values. The C_{max} value of total ezetimibe was decreased by 30%.

Glipizide: In a study of twelve healthy adult males, steady-state levels of ezetimibe (10 mg once daily) had no significant effect on the pharmacokinetics and pharmacodynamics of glipizide. A single dose of glipizide (10 mg) had no significant effect on the exposure to total ezetimibe or ezetimibe.

HMG-CoA Reductase Inhibitors: In studies of healthy hypercholesterolemic (LDL-C ≥130 mg/dL) adult subjects, concomitant administration of ezetimibe (10 mg once daily) had no significant effect on the bioavailability of either lovastatin, simvastatin, pravastatin, atorvastatin, or fluvastatin. No significant effect on the bioavailability of total ezetimibe and ezetimibe was demonstrated by either lovastatin (20 mg once daily), pravastatin (20 mg once daily), atorvastatin (10 mg once daily), or fluvastatin (20 mg once daily).

Fenofibrate: In a study of thirty-two healthy hypercholesterolemic (LDL-C ≥130 mg/dL) adult subjects, concomitant fenofibrate (200 mg once daily) administration increased the mean C_{max} and AUC values of total ezetimibe approximately 64% and 48%, respectively. Pharmacokinetics of fenofibrate were not significantly affected by ezetimibe (10 mg once daily).

Cholestyramine: In a study of forty healthy hypercholesterolemic (LDL-C ≥130 mg/dL) adult subjects, concomitant cholestyramine (4 g twice daily) administration decreased the mean AUC values of total ezetimibe and ezetimibe approximately 55% and 80%, respectively.

Cyclosporine: In a study of eight post-renal transplant patients with mildly impaired or normal renal function (creatinine clearance of >50 mL/min), stable doses of cyclosporine (75 to 150 mg twice daily) increased the mean AUC and C_{max} values of total ezetimibe 3.4-fold (range 2.3- to 7.9-fold) and 3.9-fold (range 3.0- to 4.4-fold), respectively, compared to a historical healthy control population (n=17). In a different study, a renal transplant patient with severe renal insufficiency (creatinine clearance of 13.2 mL/min/1.73 m^2) who was receiving multiple medications, including cyclosporine, demonstrated a 12-fold greater exposure to total ezetimibe compared to healthy subjects.

ANIMAL PHARMACOLOGY

The hypocholesterolemic effect of ezetimibe was evaluated in cholesterol-fed Rhesus monkeys, dogs, rats, and mouse models of human cholesterol metabolism. Ezetimibe was found to have an ED_{50} value of 0.5 μg/kg/day for inhibiting the rise in plasma cholesterol levels in monkeys. The ED_{50} values in dogs, rats, and mice were 7, 30, and 700 μg/kg/day, respectively. These results are consistent with ZETIA being a potent cholesterol absorption inhibitor.

In a rat model, where the glucuronide metabolite of ezetimibe (SCH 60663) was administered intraduodenally, the metabolite was as potent as the parent compound (SCH 58235) in inhibiting the absorption of cholesterol, suggesting that the glucuronide metabolite had activity similar to the parent drug.

Table 1
Response to ZETIA in Patients with Primary Hypercholesterolemia
(Mean[a] % Change from Untreated Baseline[b])

Treatment group		N	Total-C	LDL-C	Apo B	TG[a]	HDL-C
Study 1[c]	Placebo	205	+1	+1	-1	-1	-1
	Ezetimibe	622	-12	-18	-15	-7	+1
Study 2[c]	Placebo	226	+1	+1	-1	+2	-2
	Ezetimibe	666	-12	-18	-16	-9	+1
Pooled Data[c] (Studies 1 & 2)	Placebo	431	0	+1	-2	0	-2
	Ezetimibe	1288	-13	-18	-16	-8	+1

[a] For triglycerides, median % change from baseline
[b] Baseline - on no lipid-lowering drug
[c] ZETIA significantly reduced total-C, LDL-C, Apo B, and TG, and increased HDL-C compared to placebo.

Table 2
Response to Addition of ZETIA to On-going HMG-CoA Reductase Inhibitor Therapy[a] in Patients with Hypercholesterolemia
(Mean[b] % Change from Treated Baseline[c])

Treatment (Daily Dose)	N	Total-C	LDL-C	Apo B	TG[b]	HDL-C
On-going HMG-CoA reductase inhibitor +Placebo[d]	390	-2	-4	-3	-3	+1
On-going HMG-CoA reductase inhibitor +ZETIA[d]	379	-17	-25	-19	-14	+3

[a] Patients receiving each HMG-CoA reductase inhibitor: 40% atorvastatin, 31% simvastatin, 29% others (pravastatin, fluvastatin, cerivastatin, lovastatin)
[b] For triglycerides, median % change from baseline
[c] Baseline - on an HMG-CoA reductase inhibitor alone.
[d] ZETIA + HMG-CoA reductase inhibitor significantly reduced total-C, LDL-C, Apo B, and TG, and increased HDL-C compared to HMG-CoA reductase inhibitor alone.

Table 3
Response to ZETIA and Atorvastatin Initiated Concurrently in Patients with Primary Hypercholesterolemia
(Mean[a] % Change from Untreated Baseline[b])

Treatment (Daily Dose)	N	Total-C	LDL-C	Apo B	TG[a]	HDL-C
Placebo	60	+4	+4	+3	-6	+4
ZETIA	65	-14	-20	-15	-5	+4
Atorvastatin 10 mg	60	-26	-37	-28	-21	+6
ZETIA + Atorvastatin 10 mg	65	-38	-53	-43	-31	+9
Atorvastatin 20 mg	60	-30	-42	-34	-23	+4
ZETIA + Atorvastatin 20 mg	62	-39	-54	-44	-30	+9
Atorvastatin 40 mg	66	-32	-45	-37	-24	+4
ZETIA + Atorvastatin 40 mg	65	-42	-56	-45	-34	+5
Atorvastatin 80 mg	62	-40	-54	-46	-31	+3
ZETIA + Atorvastatin 80 mg	63	-46	-61	-50	-40	+7
Pooled data (All Atorvastatin Doses)[c]	248	-32	-44	-36	-24	+4
Pooled data (All ZETIA + Atorvastatin Doses)[c]	255	-41	-56	-45	-33	+7

[a] For triglycerides, median % change from baseline
[b] Baseline - on no lipid-lowering drug
[c] ZETIA + all doses of atorvastatin pooled (10-80 mg) significantly reduced total-C, LDL-C, Apo B, and TG, and increased HDL-C compared to all doses of atorvastatin pooled (10-80 mg).

In 1-month studies in dogs given ezetimibe (0.03-300 mg/kg/day), the concentration of cholesterol in gallbladder bile increased ~2- to 4-fold. However, a dose of 300 mg/kg/day administered to dogs for one year did not result in gallstone formation or any other adverse hepatobiliary effects. In a 14-day study in mice given ezetimibe (0.3-5 mg/kg/day) and fed a low-fat or cholesterol-rich diet, the concentration of cholesterol in gallbladder bile was either unaffected or reduced to normal levels, respectively.

A series of acute preclinical studies was performed to determine the selectivity of ZETIA for inhibiting cholesterol absorption. Ezetimibe inhibited the absorption of ^{14}C-cholesterol with no effect on the absorption of triglycerides, fatty acids, bile acids, progesterone, ethyl estradiol, or the fat-soluble vitamins A and D.

In 4- to 12-week toxicity studies in mice, ezetimibe did not induce cytochrome P450 drug metabolizing enzymes. In toxicity studies, a pharmacokinetic interaction of ezetimibe with HMG-CoA reductase inhibitors (parents or their active hydroxy acid metabolites) was seen in rats, dogs, and rabbits.

CLINICAL STUDIES

Primary Hypercholesterolemia

ZETIA reduces total-C, LDL-C, Apo B, and TG, and increases HDL-C in patients with hypercholesterolemia. Maximal to near maximal response is generally achieved within 2 weeks and maintained during chronic therapy.

ZETIA is effective in patients with hypercholesterolemia, in men and women, in younger and older patients, alone or administered with an HMG-CoA reductase inhibitor. Experience in pediatric and adolescent patients (ages 9 to 17) has been limited to patients with homozygous familial hypercholesterolemia (HoFH) or sitosterolemia.

Experience in non-Caucasians is limited and does not permit a precise estimate of the magnitude of the effects of ZETIA.

Monotherapy

In two, multicenter, double-blind, placebo-controlled, 12-week studies in 1719 patients with primary hypercholesterolemia, ZETIA significantly lowered total-C, LDL-C, Apo B, and TG, and increased HDL-C compared to placebo (see Table 1). Reduction in LDL-C was consistent across age, sex, and baseline LDL-C.

[See table 1 at top of previous page]

Combination with HMG-CoA Reductase Inhibitors

ZETIA Added to On-going HMG-CoA Reductase Inhibitor Therapy

In a multicenter, double-blind, placebo-controlled, 8-week study, 769 patients with primary hypercholesterolemia, known coronary heart disease or multiple cardiovascular risk factors who were already receiving HMG-CoA reductase inhibitor monotherapy, but who had not met their NCEP ATP II target LDL-C goal were randomized to receive either ZETIA or placebo in addition to their on-going HMG-CoA reductase inhibitor therapy.

ZETIA, added to on-going HMG-CoA reductase inhibitor therapy, significantly lowered total-C, LDL-C, Apo B, and TG, and increased HDL-C compared with an HMG-CoA reductase inhibitor administered alone (see Table 2). LDL-C reductions induced by ZETIA were generally consistent across all HMG-CoA reductase inhibitors.

[See table 2 at top of previous page]

ZETIA Initiated Concurrently with an HMG-CoA Reductase Inhibitor

In four, multicenter, double-blind, placebo-controlled, 12-week trials, in 2382 hypercholesterolemic patients, ZETIA or placebo was administered alone or with various doses of atorvastatin, simvastatin, pravastatin, or lovastatin.

When all patients receiving ZETIA with an HMG-CoA reductase inhibitor were compared to all those receiving the corresponding HMG-CoA reductase inhibitor alone, ZETIA significantly lowered total-C, LDL-C, Apo B, and TG, and, with the exception of pravastatin, increased HDL-C compared to the HMG-CoA reductase inhibitor administered alone. LDL-C reductions induced by ZETIA were generally consistent across all HMG-CoA reductase inhibitors. (See footnote c, Tables 3 to 6.)

[See table 3 on previous page]

[See table 4 above]

[See table 5 at right]

[See table 6 at top of next page]

Homozygous Familial Hypercholesterolemia (HoFH)

A study was conducted to assess the efficacy of ZETIA in the treatment of HoFH. This double-blind, randomized, 12-week study enrolled 50 patients with a clinical and/or genotypic diagnosis of HoFH, with or without concomitant LDL apheresis, already receiving atorvastatin or simvastatin (40 mg). Patients were randomized to one of three treatment groups, atorvastatin or simvastatin (80 mg), ZETIA administered with atorvastatin or simvastatin (40 mg), or ZETIA administered with atorvastatin or simvastatin (80 mg). Due to decreased bioavailability of ezetimibe in patients concomitantly receiving cholestyramine (see PRECAUTIONS), ezetimibe was dosed at least 4 hours before or after administration of resins. Mean baseline LDL-C was 341 mg/dL in those patients randomized to atorvastatin 80 mg or simvastatin 80 mg alone and 316 mg/dL in the group randomized to ZETIA plus atorvastatin 40 or 80 mg or simvastatin 40 or 80 mg. ZETIA, administered with atorvastatin or simvastatin (40 and 80 mg statin groups, pooled), significantly reduced LDL-C (21%) compared with increasing the dose of simvastatin or atorvastatin monotherapy from 40 to 80 mg (7%). In those treated with ZETIA plus 80 mg atorvastatin or with ZETIA plus 80 mg simvastatin, LDL-C was reduced by 27%.

Homozygous Sitosterolemia (Phytosterolemia)

A study was conducted to assess the efficacy of ZETIA in the treatment of homozygous sitosterolemia. In this multicenter, double-blind, placebo-controlled, 8-week trial, 37 patients with homozygous sitosterolemia with elevated plasma sitosterol levels (>5 mg/dL) on their current therapeutic regimen (diet, bile-acid-binding resins, HMG-CoA reductase inhibitors, ileal bypass surgery and/or LDL apheresis), were randomized to receive ZETIA (n=30) or placebo (n=7). Due to decreased bioavailability of ezetimibe in patients concomitantly receiving cholestyramine (see PRECAUTIONS), ezetimibe was dosed at least 2 hours before or 4 hours after resins were administered. Excluding the one subject receiving LDL apheresis, ZETIA significantly lowered plasma sitosterol and campesterol, by 21% and 24% from baseline, respectively. In contrast, patients who received placebo had increases in sitosterol and campesterol of 4% and 3% from baseline, respectively. For patients treated with ZETIA, mean plasma levels of plant sterols were reduced progressively over the course of the study. The effects of reducing plasma sitosterol and campesterol on reducing the risks of cardiovascular morbidity and mortality have not been established.

Reductions in sitosterol and campesterol were consistent between patients taking ZETIA concomitantly with bile acid sequestrants (n=8) and patients not on concomitant bile acid sequestrant therapy (n=21).

Table 4
Response to ZETIA and Simvastatin Initiated Concurrently in Patients with Primary Hypercholesterolemia (Mean[a] % Change from Untreated Baseline[b])

Treatment (Daily Dose)	N	Total-C	LDL-C	Apo B	TG[a]	HDL-C
Placebo	70	-1	-1	0	+2	+1
ZETIA	61	-13	-19	-14	-11	+5
Simvastatin 10 mg	70	-18	-27	-21	-14	+8
ZETIA + Simvastatin 10 mg	67	-32	-46	-35	-26	+9
Simvastatin 20 mg	61	-26	-36	-29	-18	+6
ZETIA + Simvastatin 20 mg	69	-33	-46	-36	-25	+9
Simvastatin 40 mg	65	-27	-38	-32	-24	+6
ZETIA + Simvastatin 40 mg	73	-40	-56	-45	-32	+11
Simvastatin 80 mg	67	-32	-45	-37	-23	+8
ZETIA + Simvastatin 80 mg	65	-41	-58	-47	-31	+8
Pooled data (All Simvastatin Doses)[c]	263	-26	-36	-30	-20	+7
Pooled data (All ZETIA + Simvastatin Doses)[c]	274	-37	-51	-41	-29	+9

[a] For triglycerides, median % change from baseline
[b] Baseline - on no lipid-lowering drug
[c] ZETIA + all doses of simvastatin pooled (10-80 mg) significantly reduced total-C, LDL-C, Apo B, and TG, and increased HDL-C compared to all doses of simvastatin pooled (10-80 mg).

Table 5
Response to ZETIA and Pravastatin Initiated Concurrently in Patients with Primary Hypercholesterolemia (Mean[a] % Change from Untreated Baseline[b])

Treatment (Daily Dose)	N	Total-C	LDL-C	Apo B	TG[a]	HDL-C
Placebo	65	0	-1	-2	-1	+2
ZETIA	64	-13	-20	-15	-5	+4
Pravastatin 10 mg	66	-15	-21	-16	-14	+6
ZETIA + Pravastatin 10 mg	71	-24	-34	-27	-23	+8
Pravastatin 20 mg	69	-15	-23	-18	-8	+8
ZETIA + Pravastatin 20 mg	66	-27	-40	-31	-21	+8
Pravastatin 40 mg	70	-22	-31	-26	-19	+6
ZETIA + Pravastatin 40 mg	67	-30	-42	-32	-21	+8
Pooled data (All Pravastatin Doses)[c]	205	-17	-25	-20	-14	+7
Pooled data (All ZETIA + Pravastatin Doses)[c]	204	-27	-39	-30	-21	+8

[a] For triglycerides, median % change from baseline
[b] Baseline - on no lipid-lowering drug
[c] ZETIA + all doses of pravastatin pooled (10-40 mg) significantly reduced total-C, LDL-C, Apo B, and TG compared to all doses of pravastatin pooled (10-40 mg).

INDICATIONS AND USAGE

Primary Hypercholesterolemia

Monotherapy

ZETIA, administered alone, is indicated as adjunctive therapy to diet for the reduction of elevated total-C, LDL-C, and Apo B in patients with primary (heterozygous familial and non-familial) hypercholesterolemia.

Combination therapy with HMG-CoA reductase inhibitors

ZETIA, administered in combination with an HMG-CoA reductase inhibitor, is indicated as adjunctive therapy to diet for the reduction of elevated total-C, LDL-C, and Apo B in patients with primary (heterozygous familial and non-familial) hypercholesterolemia.

Homozygous Familial Hypercholesterolemia (HoFH)

The combination of ZETIA and atorvastatin or simvastatin, is indicated for the reduction of elevated total-C and LDL-C levels in patients with HoFH, as an adjunct to other lipid-lowering treatments (e.g., LDL apheresis) or if such treatments are unavailable.

Homozygous Sitosterolemia

ZETIA is indicated as adjunctive therapy to diet for the reduction of elevated sitosterol and campesterol levels in patients with homozygous familial sitosterolemia.

Therapy with lipid-altering agents should be a component of multiple risk-factor intervention in individuals at increased risk for atherosclerotic vascular disease due to hypercholesterolemia. Lipid-altering agents should be used in addition to an appropriate diet (including restriction of saturated fat and cholesterol) and when the response to diet and other non-pharmacological measures has been inadequate. (See NCEP Adult Treatment Panel (ATP) III Guidelines, summarized in Table 7.)

[See table 7 at top of next page]

Prior to initiating therapy with ZETIA, secondary causes for dyslipidemia (i.e., diabetes, hypothyroidism, obstructive liver disease, chronic renal failure, and drugs that increase

Continued on next page

Zetia—Cont.

LDL-C and decrease HDL-C [progestins, anabolic steroids, and corticosteroids]), should be excluded or, if appropriate, treated. A lipid profile should be performed to measure total-C, LDL-C, HDL-C and TG. For TG levels >400 mg/dL (>4.5 mmol/L), LDL-C concentrations should be determined by ultracentrifugation.

At the time of hospitalization for an acute coronary event, lipid measures should be taken on admission or within 24 hours. These values can guide the physician on initiation of LDL-lowering therapy before or at discharge.

CONTRAINDICATIONS

Hypersensitivity to any component of this medication.

The combination of ZETIA with an HMG-CoA reductase inhibitor is contraindicated in patients with active liver disease or unexplained persistent elevations in serum transaminases.

All HMG-CoA reductase inhibitors are contraindicated in pregnant and nursing women. When ZETIA is administered with an HMG-CoA reductase inhibitor in a woman of childbearing potential, refer to the pregnancy category and product labeling for the HMG-CoA reductase inhibitor. (See PRECAUTIONS, *Pregnancy*.)

PRECAUTIONS

Concurrent administration of ZETIA with a specific HMG-CoA reductase inhibitor should be in accordance with the product labeling for that HMG-CoA reductase inhibitor.

Liver Enzymes

In controlled clinical monotherapy studies, the incidence of consecutive elevations (≥3 × the upper limit of normal [ULN]) in serum transaminases was similar between ZETIA (0.5%) and placebo (0.3%).

In controlled clinical combination studies of ZETIA initiated concurrently with an HMG-CoA reductase inhibitor, the incidence of consecutive elevations (≥3 × ULN) in serum transaminases was 1.3% for patients treated with ZETIA administered with HMG-CoA reductase inhibitors and 0.4% for patients treated with HMG-CoA reductase inhibitors alone. These elevations in transaminases were generally asymptomatic, not associated with cholestasis, and returned to baseline after discontinuation of therapy or with continued treatment. When ZETIA is co-administered with an HMG-CoA reductase inhibitor, liver function tests should be performed at initiation of therapy and according to the recommendations of the HMG-CoA reductase inhibitor.

Skeletal Muscle

In clinical trials, there was no excess of myopathy or rhabdomyolysis associated with ZETIA compared with the relevant control arm (placebo or HMG-CoA reductase inhibitor alone). However, myopathy and rhabdomyolysis are known adverse reactions to HMG-CoA reductase inhibitors and other lipid-lowering drugs. In clinical trials, the incidence of CPK >10 X ULN was 0.2% for ZETIA vs 0.1% for placebo, and 0.1% for ZETIA co-administered with an HMG-CoA reductase inhibitor vs 0.4% for HMG-CoA reductase inhibitors alone.

Hepatic Insufficiency

Due to the unknown effects of the increased exposure to ezetimibe in patients with moderate or severe hepatic insufficiency, ZETIA is not recommended in these patients. (See CLINICAL PHARMACOLOGY, *Special Populations*.)

Drug Interactions (See also CLINICAL PHARMACOLOGY, *Drug Interactions*)

Cholestyramine: Concomitant cholestyramine administration decreased the mean AUC of total ezetimibe approximately 55%. The incremental LDL-C reduction due to adding ezetimibe to cholestyramine may be reduced by this interaction.

Fibrates: The safety and effectiveness of ezetimibe administered with fibrates have not been established.

Fibrates may increase cholesterol excretion into the bile, leading to cholelithiasis. In a preclinical study in dogs, ezetimibe increased cholesterol in the gallbladder bile (see ANIMAL PHARMACOLOGY). Co-administration of ZETIA with fibrates is not recommended until use in patients is studied.

Fenofibrate: In a pharmacokinetic study, concomitant fenofibrate administration increased total ezetimibe concentrations approximately 1.5-fold.

Gemfibrozil: In a pharmacokinetic study, concomitant gemfibrozil administration increased total ezetimibe concentrations approximately 1.7-fold.

HMG-CoA Reductase Inhibitors: No clinically significant pharmacokinetic interactions were seen when ezetimibe was co-administered with atorvastatin, simvastatin, pravastatin, lovastatin, or fluvastatin.

Cyclosporine: Caution should be exercised when initiating ezetimibe in patients treated with cyclosporine due to increased exposure to ezetimibe. This exposure may be greater in patients with severe renal insufficiency. In patients treated with cyclosporine, the potential effects of the increased exposure to ezetimibe from concomitant use should be carefully weighed against the benefits of alterations in lipid levels provided by ezetimibe. In a pharmacokinetic study in post-renal transplant patients with mildly impaired or normal renal function (creatinine clearance of >50 mL/min), concomitant cyclosporine administration increased the mean AUC and C_{max} of total ezetimibe 3.4-fold (range 2.3- to 7.9-fold) and 3.9-fold (range 3.0- to 4.4-fold), respectively. In a separate study, the total ezetimibe exposure increased 12-fold in one renal transplant patient with severe renal insufficiency receiving multiple medications, including cyclosporine (see CLINICAL PHARMACOLOGY, *Drug Interactions*).

Table 6
Response to ZETIA and Lovastatin Initiated Concurrently in Patients with Primary Hypercholesterolemia (Mean[a] % Change from Untreated Baseline[b])

Treatment (Daily Dose)	N	Total-C	LDL-C	Apo B	TG[a]	HDL-C
Placebo	64	+1	0	+1	+6	0
ZETIA	72	-13	-19	-14	-5	+3
Lovastatin 10 mg	73	-15	-20	-17	-11	+5
ZETIA + Lovastatin 10 mg	65	-24	-34	-27	-19	+8
Lovastatin 20 mg	74	-19	-26	-21	-12	+3
ZETIA + Lovastatin 20 mg	62	-29	-41	-34	-27	+9
Lovastatin 40 mg	73	-21	-30	-25	-15	+5
ZETIA + Lovastatin 40 mg	65	-33	-46	-38	-27	+9
Pooled data (All Lovastatin Doses)[c]	220	-18	-25	-21	-12	+4
Pooled data (All ZETIA + Lovastatin Doses)[c]	192	-29	-40	-33	-25	+9

[a] For triglycerides, median % change from baseline

[b] Baseline - on no lipid-lowering drug

[c] ZETIA + all doses of lovastatin pooled (10-40 mg) significantly reduced total-C, LDL-C, Apo B, and TG, and increased HDL-C compared to all doses of lovastatin pooled (10-40 mg).

Table 7
Summary of NCEP ATP III Guidelines

Risk Category	LDL Goal (mg/dL)	LDL Level at Which to Initiate Therapeutic Lifestyle Changes[a] (mg/dL)	LDL level at Which to Consider Drug Therapy (mg/dL)
CHD or CHD risk equivalents[b] (10-year risk >20%)[c]	<100	≥100	≥130 (100-129: drug optional)[d]
2+ Risk factors[e] (10-year risk ≤20%)[c]	<130	≥130	10-year risk 10-20%: ≥130[c] 10-year risk <10%: ≥160[c]
0-1 Risk factor[f]	<160	≥160	≥190 (160-189: LDL-lowering drug optional)

[a] Therapeutic lifestyle changes include: 1) dietary changes: reduced intake of saturated fats (<7% of total calories) and cholesterol (<200 mg per day), and enhancing LDL lowering with plant stanols/sterols (2 g/d) and increased viscous (soluble) fiber (10-25 g/d), 2) weight reduction, and 3) increased physical activity.

[b] CHD risk equivalents comprise: diabetes, multiple risk factors that confer a 10-year risk for CHD >20%, and other clinical forms of atherosclerotic disease (peripheral arterial disease, abdominal aortic aneurysm and symptomatic carotid artery disease).

[c] Risk assessment for determining the 10-year risk for developing CHD is carried out using the Framingham risk scoring. Refer to JAMA, May 16, 2001; 285 (19): 2486-2497, or the NCEP website (http://www.nhlbi.nih.gov) for more details.

[d] Some authorities recommend use of LDL-lowering drugs in this category if an LDL cholesterol <100 mg/dL cannot be achieved by therapeutic lifestyle changes. Others prefer use of drugs that primarily modify triglycerides and HDL, e.g., nicotinic acid or fibrate. Clinical judgment also may call for deferring drug therapy in this subcategory.

[e] Major risk factors (exclusive of LDL cholesterol) that modify LDL goals include cigarette smoking, hypertension (BP ≥140/90 mm Hg or on anti-hypertensive medication), low HDL cholesterol (<40 mg/dL), family history of premature CHD (CHD in male first-degree relative <55 years; CHD in female first-degree relative <65 years), age (men ≥45 years; women ≥55 years). HDL cholesterol ≥60 mg/dL counts as a "negative" risk factor; its presence removes one risk factor from the total count.

[f] Almost all people with 0-1 risk factor have a 10-year risk <10%; thus, 10-year risk assessment in people with 0-1 risk factor is not necessary.

Carcinogenesis, Mutagenesis, Impairment of Fertility

A 104-week dietary carcinogenicity study with ezetimibe was conducted in rats at doses up to 1500 mg/kg/day (males) and 500 mg/kg/day (females) (~20 times the human exposure at 10 mg daily based on $AUC_{0\text{-}24hr}$ for total ezetimibe). A 104-week dietary carcinogenicity study with ezetimibe was also conducted in mice at doses up to 500 mg/kg/day (>150 times the human exposure at 10 mg daily based on $AUC_{0\text{-}24hr}$ for total ezetimibe). There were no statistically significant increases in tumor incidences in drug-treated rats or mice.

No evidence of mutagenicity was observed *in vitro* in a microbial mutagenicity (Ames) test with *Salmonella typhimurium* and *Escherichia coli* with or without metabolic activation. No evidence of clastogenicity was observed *in vitro* in a chromosomal aberration assay in human peripheral blood lymphocytes with or without metabolic activation. In addition, there was no evidence of genotoxicity in the *in vivo* mouse micronucleus test.

In oral (gavage) fertility studies of ezetimibe conducted in rats, there was no evidence of reproductive toxicity at doses up to 1000 mg/kg/day in male or female rats (~7 times the human exposure at 10 mg daily based on $AUC_{0\text{-}24hr}$ for total ezetimibe).

Pregnancy

Pregnancy Category: C

There are no adequate and well-controlled studies of ezetimibe in pregnant women. Ezetimibe should be used during pregnancy only if the potential benefit justifies the risk to the fetus.

In oral (gavage) embryo-fetal development studies of ezetimibe conducted in rats and rabbits during organogenesis, there was no evidence of embryolethal effects at the doses tested (250, 500, 1000 mg/kg/day). In rats, increased incidences of common fetal skeletal findings (extra pair of thoracic ribs, unossified cervical vertebral centra, shortened ribs) were observed at 1000 mg/kg/day (~10 times the human exposure at 10 mg daily based on $AUC_{0\text{-}24hr}$ for total ezetimibe). In rabbits treated with ezetimibe, an increased incidence of extra thoracic ribs was observed at 1000 mg/kg/day (150 times the human exposure at 10 mg daily based on $AUC_{0\text{-}24hr}$ for total ezetimibe). Ezetimibe crossed the placenta when pregnant rats and rabbits were given multiple oral doses.

Multiple dose studies of ezetimibe given in combination with HMG-CoA reductase inhibitors (statins) in rats and rabbits during organogenesis result in higher ezetimibe and statin exposures. Reproductive findings occur at lower doses in combination therapy compared to monotherapy.

All HMG-CoA reductase inhibitors are contraindicated in pregnant and nursing women. When ZETIA is administered with an HMG-CoA reductase inhibitor in a woman of child-

bearing potential, refer to the pregnancy category and product labeling for the HMG-CoA reductase inhibitor. (See CONTRAINDICATIONS.)

Labor and Delivery
The effects of ZETIA on labor and delivery in pregnant women are unknown.

Nursing Mothers
In rat studies, exposure to total ezetimibe in nursing pups was up to half of that observed in maternal plasma. It is not known whether ezetimibe is excreted into human breast milk; therefore, ZETIA should not be used in nursing mothers unless the potential benefit justifies the potential risk to the infant.

Pediatric Use
The pharmacokinetics of ZETIA in adolescents (10 to 18 years) have been shown to be similar to that in adults. Treatment experience with ZETIA in the pediatric population is limited to 4 patients (9 to 17 years) in the sitosterolemia study and 5 patients (11 to 17 years) in the HoFH study. Treatment with ZETIA in children (<10 years) is not recommended. (See CLINICAL PHARMACOLOGY, *Special Populations*.)

Geriatric Use
Of the patients who received ZETIA in clinical studies, 948 were 65 and older (this included 206 who were 75 and older). The effectiveness and safety of ZETIA were similar between these patients and younger subjects. Greater sensitivity of some older individuals cannot be ruled out. (See CLINICAL PHARMACOLOGY, *Special Populations*, and ADVERSE REACTIONS.)

ADVERSE REACTIONS

ZETIA has been evaluated for safety in more than 4700 patients in clinical trials. Clinical studies of ZETIA (administered alone or with an HMG-CoA reductase inhibitor) demonstrated that ZETIA was generally well tolerated. The overall incidence of adverse events reported with ZETIA was similar to that reported with placebo, and the discontinuation rate due to adverse events was also similar for ZETIA and placebo.

Monotherapy
Adverse experiences reported in ≥2% of patients treated with ZETIA and at an incidence greater than placebo in placebo-controlled studies of ZETIA, regardless of causality assessment, are shown in Table 8.

Table 8*
Clinical Adverse Events Occurring in ≥2% of Patients Treated with ZETIA and at an Incidence Greater than Placebo, Regardless of Causality

Body System/Organ Class Adverse Event	Placebo (%) n = 795	ZETIA 10 mg (%) n = 1691
Body as a whole – general disorders		
Fatigue	1.8	2.2
Gastro-intestinal system disorders		
Abdominal pain	2.8	3.0
Diarrhea	3.0	3.7
Infection and infestations		
Infection viral	1.8	2.2
Pharyngitis	2.1	2.3
Sinusitis	2.8	3.6
Musculo-skeletal system disorders		
Arthralgia	3.4	3.8
Back pain	3.9	4.1
Respiratory system disorders		
Coughing	2.1	2.3

*Includes patients who received placebo or ZETIA alone reported in Table 9.

The frequency of less common adverse events was comparable between ZETIA and placebo.

Combination with an HMG-CoA Reductase Inhibitor
ZETIA has been evaluated for safety in combination studies in more than 2000 patients.
In general, adverse experiences were similar between ZETIA administered with HMG-CoA reductase inhibitors and HMG-CoA reductase inhibitors alone. However, the frequency of increased transaminases was slightly higher in patients receiving ZETIA administered with HMG-CoA reductase inhibitors than in patients treated with HMG-CoA reductase inhibitors alone. (See PRECAUTIONS, *Liver Enzymes*.)
Clinical adverse experiences reported in ≥2% of patients and at an incidence greater than placebo in four placebo-controlled trials where ZETIA was administered alone or initiated concurrently with various HMG-CoA reductase inhibitors, regardless of causality assessment, are shown in Table 9.
[See table 9 above]

Table 9*
Clinical Adverse Events occurring in ≥2% of Patients and at an Incidence Greater than Placebo, Regardless of Causality, in ZETIA/Statin Combination Studies

Body System/Organ Class Adverse Event	Placebo (%) n=259	ZETIA 10 mg (%) n=262	All Statins** (%) n=936	ZETIA + All Statins** (%) n=925
Body as a whole – general disorders				
Chest pain	1.2	3.4	2.0	1.8
Dizziness	1.2	2.7	1.4	1.8
Fatigue	1.9	1.9	1.4	2.8
Headache	5.4	8.0	7.3	6.3
Gastro-intestinal system disorders				
Abdominal pain	2.3	2.7	3.1	3.5
Diarrhea	1.5	3.4	2.9	2.8
Infection and infestations				
Pharyngitis	1.9	3.1	2.5	2.3
Sinusitis	1.9	4.6	3.6	3.5
Upper respiratory tract infection	10.8	13.0	13.6	11.8
Musculo-skeletal system disorders				
Arthralgia	2.3	3.8	4.3	3.4
Back pain	3.5	3.4	3.7	4.3
Myalgia	4.6	5.0	4.1	4.5

*Includes four placebo-controlled combination studies in which ZETIA was initiated concurrently with an HMG-CoA reductase inhibitor.
**All Statins = all doses of all HMG-CoA reductase inhibitors.

Post-marketing Experience
The following adverse reactions have been reported in post-marketing experience, regardless of causality assessment: Hypersensitivity reactions, including angioedema and rash; pancreatitis; nausea; cholelithiasis; cholecystitis.

OVERDOSAGE

In clinical studies, administration of ezetimibe, 50 mg/day to 15 healthy subjects for up to 14 days, or 40 mg/day to 18 patients with primary hypercholesterolemia for up to 56 days, was generally well tolerated.
A few cases of overdosage with ZETIA have been reported; most have not been associated with adverse experiences. Reported adverse experiences have not been serious. In the event of an overdose, symptomatic and supportive measures should be employed.

DOSAGE AND ADMINISTRATION

The patient should be placed on a standard cholesterol-lowering diet before receiving ZETIA and should continue on this diet during treatment with ZETIA.
The recommended dose of ZETIA is 10 mg once daily. ZETIA can be administered with or without food.
ZETIA may be administered with an HMG-CoA reductase inhibitor for incremental effect. For convenience, the daily dose of ZETIA may be taken at the same time as the HMG-CoA reductase inhibitor, according to the dosing recommendations for the HMG-CoA reductase inhibitor.

Patients with Hepatic Insufficiency
No dosage adjustment is necessary in patients with mild hepatic insufficiency (see PRECAUTIONS, *Hepatic Insufficiency*).

Patients with Renal Insufficiency
No dosage adjustment is necessary in patients with renal insufficiency (see CLINICAL PHARMACOLOGY, *Special Populations*).

Geriatric Patients
No dosage adjustment is necessary in geriatric patients (see CLINICAL PHARMACOLOGY, *Special Populations*).

Co-administration with Bile Acid Sequestrants
Dosing of ZETIA should occur either ≥2 hours before or ≥4 hours after administration of a bile acid sequestrant (see PRECAUTIONS, *Drug Interactions*).

HOW SUPPLIED

No. 3861 - Tablets ZETIA, 10 mg, are white to off-white, capsule-shaped tablets debossed with "414" on one side. They are supplied as follows:
NDC 66582-414-31 bottles of 30
NDC 66582-414-54 bottles of 90
NDC 66582-414-74 bottles of 500
NDC 66582-414-28 unit dose packages of 100.

Storage
Store at 25°C (77°F); excursions permitted to 15-30°C (59-86°F). [See USP Controlled Room Temperature.] Protect from moisture.

25751868T
REV 04
Issued August 2004
Printed in USA.
Manufactured for:
Merck/Schering-Plough Pharmaceuticals
North Wales, PA 19454, USA
By:
Schering Corporation
Kenilworth, NJ 07033, USA
or
Merck & Co., Inc.
Whitehouse Station, NJ 08889, USA

ZETIA® (ezetimibe) Tablets
Patient Information about ZETIA (zĕt'-ē-ă)
Generic name: ezetimibe (ĕ-zĕt'-ĕ-mīb)
Read this information carefully before you start taking ZETIA and each time you get more ZETIA. There may be new information. This information does not take the place of talking with your doctor about your medical condition or your treatment. If you have any questions about ZETIA, ask your doctor. Only your doctor can determine if ZETIA is right for you.

What is ZETIA?
ZETIA is a medicine used to lower levels of total cholesterol and LDL (bad) cholesterol in the blood. It is used for patients who cannot control their cholesterol levels by diet alone. It can be used by itself or with other medicines to treat high cholesterol. You should stay on a cholesterol-lowering diet while taking this medicine.
ZETIA works to reduce the amount of cholesterol your body absorbs. ZETIA does not help you lose weight.
For more information about cholesterol, see the "What should I know about high cholesterol?" section that follows.

Who should not take ZETIA?
- Do not take ZETIA if you are allergic to ezetimibe, the active ingredient in ZETIA, or to the inactive ingredients. For a list of inactive ingredients, see the "Inactive ingredients" section that follows.
- If you have active liver disease, do not take ZETIA while taking cholesterol-lowering medicines called statins.
- If you are pregnant or breast-feeding, do not take ZETIA while taking a statin.

What should I tell my doctor before and while taking ZETIA?
Tell your doctor about any prescription and non-prescription medicines you are taking or plan to take, including natural or herbal remedies.
Tell your doctor about all your medical conditions including allergies.
Tell your doctor if you:
- ever had liver problems. ZETIA may not be right for you.
- are pregnant or plan to become pregnant. Your doctor will decide if ZETIA is right for you.
- are breast-feeding. We do not know if ZETIA can pass to your baby through your milk. Your doctor will decide if ZETIA is right for you.
- experience unexplained muscle pain, tenderness, or weakness.

How should I take ZETIA?
- Take ZETIA once a day, with or without food. It may be easier to remember to take your dose if you do it at the same time every day, such as with breakfast, dinner, or at bedtime. If you also take another medicine to reduce your cholesterol, ask your doctor if you can take them at the same time.
- If you forget to take ZETIA, take it as soon as you remember. However, do not take more than one dose of ZETIA a day.
- Continue to follow a cholesterol-lowering diet while taking ZETIA. Ask your doctor if you need diet information.
- Keep taking ZETIA unless your doctor tells you to stop. It is important that you keep taking ZETIA even if you do not feel sick.

See your doctor regularly to check your cholesterol level and to check for side effects. Your doctor may do blood tests to check your liver before you start taking ZETIA with a statin and during treatment.

What are the possible side effects of ZETIA?
In clinical studies patients reported few side effects while taking ZETIA. These included stomach pain and feeling tired.
Additionally, the following side effects have been reported in general use: allergic reactions (which may require treatment right away) including swelling of the face, lips, tongue, and/or throat that may cause difficulty in breathing or swallowing, and rash; inflammation of the pancreas; nausea; gallstones; inflammation of the gallbladder.
Tell your doctor if you are have these or any other medical problems while on ZETIA. For a complete list of side effects, ask your doctor or pharmacist.

What should I know about high cholesterol?
Cholesterol is a type of fat found in your blood. Your total cholesterol is made up of LDL and HDL cholesterol.
LDL cholesterol is called "bad" cholesterol because it can build up in the wall of your arteries and form plaque. Over time, plaque build-up can cause a narrowing of the arteries.

Continued on next page

Zetia—Cont.

This narrowing can slow or block blood flow to your heart, brain, and other organs. High LDL cholesterol is a major cause of heart disease and stroke.
HDL cholesterol is called "good" cholesterol because it keeps the bad cholesterol from building up in the arteries.
Triglycerides also are fats found in your blood.

General Information about ZETIA

Medicines are sometimes prescribed for conditions that are not mentioned in patient information leaflets. Do not use ZETIA for a condition for which it was not prescribed. Do not give ZETIA to other people, even if they have the same condition you have. It may harm them.
This summarizes the most important information about ZETIA. If you would like more information, talk with your doctor. You can ask your pharmacist or doctor for information about ZETIA that is written for health professionals.

Inactive ingredients:

Croscarmellose sodium, lactose monohydrate, magnesium stearate, microcrystalline cellulose, povidone, and sodium lauryl sulfate.
25751760T
REV 04
Issued August 2004
Manufactured for:
Merck/Schering-Plough Pharmaceuticals
North Wales, PA 19454, USA
By:
Schering Corporation
Kenilworth, NJ 07033, USA
or
Merck & Co., Inc.
Whitehouse Station, NJ 08889, USA

Shown in Product Identification Guide, page 324

Mericon Industries, Inc.

8819 N. PIONEER ROAD
PEORIA, IL 61615

Direct Inquiries to:
William R. Connelly
(309) 693-2150
FAX: (309) 693-2158

BIOTIN OTC

[*'bī-ō-tĭn*]
biotin supplement–high potency

ACTIVE INGREDIENTS

Biotin 5 mg

DIRECTIONS

Take one capsule daily or as directed by your physician.

HOW SUPPLIED

Biotin is supplied as capsules in bottles of 120.
NDC 00394-0130-12

FLORICAL® OTC

[*flor ĭ cal*]
(fluoride and calcium supplement)

ACTIVE INGREDIENTS

Florical® contains 3.75 mg fluoride (as sodium fluoride), 145 mg calcium (as calcium carbonate)

DIRECTIONS

Take one tablet or capsule daily, or as recommended by physician.

HOW SUPPLIED

Florical® is supplied as tablets or capsules in bottles of 100 or 500.
NDC 00394-0102-02 (Capsules 100's)
NDC 00394-0102-05 (Capsules 500's)
NDC 00394-0100-02 (Tablets 100's)
NDC 00394-0100-05 (Tablets 500's)

MONOCAL® OTC

[*mon ō cal*]
(fluoride and calcium supplement)

ACTIVE INGREDIENTS

Monocal® contains 3 mg fluoride (as monofluorophosphate) and 250 mg calcium (as calcium carbonate)

DIRECTIONS

Take one tablet daily, or as recommended by physician.

HOW SUPPLIED

Monocal® is supplied as tablets in bottles of 100 & 500.
NDC 00394-0105-02
NDC 00394-0105-05

Merz Pharmaceuticals

DIVISION OF MERZ, INC.
4215 TUDOR LANE (27410)
P.O. Box 18806
GREENSBORO, NC 27419

Direct Inquiries to:
Medical/Regulatory Affairs
(336) 856-2003

FAX: (336) 856-0107

For Medical Information Contact:
In Emergencies:
Medical/Regulatory Affairs
(336) 856-2003
FAX: (336) 856-0107

APPEAREX® OTC

(biotin 2.5 mg)

DESCRIPTION AND MECHANISM OF ACTION

Appearex® is a biotin preparation (2.5 mg) available for oral administration as a small, easy-to-swallow tablet. Each Appearex® tablet contains as its active ingredient 2.5 mg of biotin, a dose clinically proven to improve nail strength and quality.[1–4] Inactive ingredients include lactose monohydrate, cornstarch, povidone (K25), and magnesium stearate. Biotin is a water-soluble vitamin component of the vitamin B complex. As an essential nutrient, biotin acts as a coenzyme for the body's carboxylation reactions and is a factor in maintaining healthy muscle, hair, nails, and skin. Its molecular formula is $C_{10}H_{16}N_2O_3S$, and its molecular weight is 244.308. It has the following structural formula:

The presumed mechanism of action by which Appearex® affects brittle nails is via the pharmacologic effects of biotin on all keratin structures. Biotin stimulates the differentiation of epidermal cells and is involved in keratinization. It is also believed that biotin increases the quantity of keratin matrix proteins in the nail, thereby improving keratin structure.[3,5]

PHARMACOKINETICS

ABSORPTION AND TRANSPORT:
Biotin is efficiently absorbed in the small intestine sodium-mediated carrier transport.[6,7] Once absorbed, 80% of biotin is free, and the remaining 20% is bound to plasma proteins.[8] Cellular entry of biotin occurs by both diffusion and sodium-dependent transport.
DEGRADATION AND EXCRETION:
About 43% of biotin is excreted unchanged in the urine.[9] The remainder is excreted as degradation products including bisnorbiotin (30%), biotin sulfoxide (11%), and other small amounts of biotin sulfone, bisnorbiotin methylketone, and tetranorbiotin sulfoxide.[10]

ADVERSE REACTIONS

Adverse reactions associated with biotin supplementation are rare in the medical literature; however, urticaria and gastrointestinal upset have been reported. As with any oral treatment, if patients experience any adverse reactions or side effects, they should inform their physicians immediately and discontinue use.

DRUG INTERACTIONS

The anticonvulsants carbamazepine, phenytoin, Phenobarbital, and primidone may accelerate biotin metabolism, leading to a reduction in available biotin. Chronic use of these drugs has been associated with decreased plasma concentrations of biotin.[11,12]
The use of antibiotics may reduce the contribution of biotin made by bacteria within the large intestine.

PRECAUTIONS AND WARNINGS

Pregnant women and nursing mothers should consult their physicians before taking this product. Appearex® should not be used in patients with known allergy or hypersensitivity to any of its ingredients.

TOXICITY

No toxic effects have been reported, even at higher doses.[13]

INDICATION AND USAGE

Appearex® is recommended for first-line treatment of weak, brittle, splitting, or soft nails.
Appearex® therapy should be taken regularly as directed to maintain strong, healthy nails. Clinical improvement is generally realized within 3 to 6 months.[1–3] Cessation of therapy may result in deterioration of nail health within 6 to 9 months.

CONTRAINDICATION

Appearex® is contraindicated in patients allergic or hypersensitive to any of its ingredients.

DOSAGE AND ADMINISTRATION

Recommended treatment for adults is 1 tablet taken daily with water. For use in children under 12 years of age, consult a physician for guidance regarding proper dosing and administration.

HOW SUPPLIED

One Appearex® package contains 30 tablets (1 month's supply) enclosed in blister packs.

SUMMARY

Appearex®, for the treatment of weak, brittle, splitting, or soft nails, is pharmaceutical grade oral biotin that restores nail quality by promoting keratinization. It has been clinically proven to increase nail plate thickness, smooth brittle nail ridges, and improve overall nail quality. As a water-soluble essential vitamin the biotin in Appearex® is safe and well tolerated. For patients with brittle nails, one Appearex® tablet taken daily provides the additional biotin needed to manage onychoschizia/onychorrhexis.

These statements have not been evaluated by the Food and Drug Administration. This product is not intended to diagnose, treat, cure, or prevent any disease.

REFERENCES

1. Hochman LG, Scher RK, Meyerson MS. Brittle nails: response to daily biotin supplementation. *Cutis.* 1993;51:303–305.
2. Floersheim GL. Treatment of brittle nails with biotin [in German]. *Z Hautkr.* 1989;64:41–48.
3. Gehring W. Effect of biotin on poor nail quality: a placebo-controlled double-blind clinical study [in German]. *Aktuelle Dermatol.* 1996;22:20–25.
4. Colombo VE, Gerber F, Bronhofer M, Floersheim GL. Treatment of brittle fingernails and onychoschizia with biotin: scanning electron microscopy. *J Am Acad Dermatol.* 1990;23:1127–1132.
5. Schmidt KH. Comparison of the operating mechanisms of different ingredients for treatment of brittle nails [in German]. *Z Hautkr.* 1993;68:517–520.
6. Stipanuk MH. *Biochemical and Physiological Aspects of Human Nutrition.* Philadelphia, Pa: WB Saunders Co; 2000;529–540.
7. Zempleni J, Mock DM. Bioavailability of biotin given orally to humans in pharmacologic doses. *Am J Clin Nutr.* 1999; 69:504–508.
8. Mock DM, Malik MI. Distribution of biotin in human plasma: most of the biotin is not bound to protein. *Am J Clin Nutr.* 1992;56:427–432.
9. Mock DM, Lankford GL, Cazin JJr. Biotin and biotin analogs in human urine: biotin accounts for only half of the total. *J Nutr.* 1993;123;1844–1851.
10. Zempleni J, McCormick DB, Mock DM. Identification of biotin sulfone bisnorbiotin methyl ketone, and tetranorbiotin-1-sulfoxide in human urine. *Am J Clin Nutr.* 1997;65:508–511.
11. Mock DM, Dyken ME. Biotin catabolism is accelerated in adults receiving long-term therapy with anticonvulsants. *Neurology.* 1997;49:1444–1447.
12. Mock DM, Mock NI, Nelson RP, Lombard KA. Disturbances in biotin metabolism in children undergoing long-term anticonvulsant therapy. *J Pediatr Gastroenterol Nutr.* 1998;16:245–250.
13. Marcus R, Coulston AM. Water-soluble vitamins. In: Hardman JG, Limbird LE, Gilman AG, eds. *Goodman and Gilman's the Pharmacologic Basis of Therapeutics.* 10th ed. New York, NY: McGraw-Hill Medical Publishing Division; 2001:1753–1771.

70-2062-00 Rev 06/04

ELDERTONIC® OTC

(Multi-vitamin)

INDICATIONS

B-complex vitamins with minerals for nutritional supplementation.

DOSAGE

Adults: one tablespoon three times daily just before meals.

WARNING

Do not exceed recommended dosage unless directed by a physician.

USAGE IN PREGNANCY

Safe use of this product in pregnancy has not been established.

CAUTION

Keep out of the reach of children.

HOW SUPPLIED

ELDERTONIC is available in 16 fl. oz. bottles: #0259-0351-16.

Supplement Facts

Serving Size 1 tablespoon (15 mL)
Servings Per Container 31

	Amount Per Serving	% Daily Value
Calories	35	
Total Carbohydrates	5g	1%*
Sugar	4g	†
Thiamin HCl (Vitamin B1)	0.5mg	33%
Riboflavin (Vitamin B2)	0.6mg	33%
Niacin	7mg	33%
Vitamin B6	0.7mg	33%
Vitamin B12	2mcg	33%
Pantothenic Acid	3mg	33%
Magnesium	0.7mg	< 1%
Zinc	5mg	33%
Manganese	0.7mg	33%

*Percent daily value based on a 2000 calorie diet
†Daily value not established Alcohol content 13.5%

Other ingredients: sherry wine, sucrose, sorbitol, FD&C red #40, purified water
30-1113-01 Rev. 08/03

ERYGEL® ℞
ERYTHROMYCIN
TOPICAL GEL USP 2%
Rx Only
For Dermatologic Use Only-Not for Ophthalmic Use-

DESCRIPTION

ERYGEL® Topical Gel contains erythromycin ((3R*, 4S*, 5S*, 6R*, 7R*, 9R*, 11R*, 12R*, 13S*, 14R*)-4-[(2, 6-Dideoxy-3-*C*-methyl-3-*O*-methyl-α-L-*ribo*-hexopyranosyl)oxy]-14-ethyl-7, 12, 13-trihydroxy-3, 5, 7, 9, 11, 13-hexamethyl-6-[[3, 4, 6,-trideoxy-3-(dimethylamino)-β-D-*xylo*-hexopyranosyl] oxy] oxacyclotetradecane-2, 10-dione), for topical dermatological use. Erythromycin is a macrolide antibiotic produced from a strain of *Saccaropolyspora erythraea* (formerly *Streptomyces erythreus*). It is a base and readily forms salts with acids.
Chemically, erythromycin is $C_{37}H_{67}NO_{13}$. It has the following structural formula:

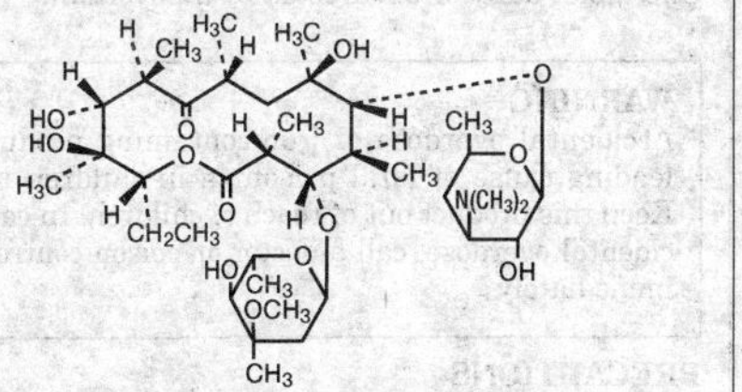

Erythromycin has a molecular weight of 733.94. It is a white or slightly yellow, odorless or practically odorless, bitter crystalline powder. Erythromycin is very soluble in very polar organic solvents such as alcohols, acetone, chloroform, acetonitrile and ethyl acetate. It is moderately soluble in less polar solvents such as ether, dichloroethylene and amyl acetate. It is slightly soluble in nonpolar solvents such as hexane. It is very poorly soluble in water.
Each gram of ERYGEL® Topical Gel contains 20 mg of erythromycin, USP in a base of alcohol 92% and hydroxypropyl cellulose.

CLINICAL PHARMACOLOGY

The exact mechanism by which erythromycin reduces lesions of acne vulgaris is not fully known; however, the effect appears to be due in part to the antibacterial activity of the drug.

MICROBIOLOGY

Erythromycin acts by inhibition of protein synthesis in susceptible organisms by reversibly binding to 50S ribosomal subunits, thereby inhibiting translocation of aminoacyl transfer-RNA and inhibiting polypeptide synthesis. Antagonism has been demonstrated *in vitro* between erythromycin, lincomycin, chloramphenicol, and clindamycin.

INDICATIONS AND USAGE

ERYGEL® Topical Gel is indicated for the topical treatment of acne vulgaris.

CONTRAINDICATIONS

ERYGEL® Topical Gel is contraindicated in those individuals who have shown hypersensitivity to any of its components.

WARNINGS

Pseudomembranous colitis has been reported with nearly all antibacterial agents, including erythromycin, and may range in severity from mild to life-threatening. Therefore, it is important to consider this diagnosis in patients who present with diarrhea subsequent to the administration of antibacterial agents.
Treatment with antibacterial agents alters the normal flora of the colon and may permit overgrowth of clostridia. Studies indicate that a toxin produced by *Clostridium difficile* is one primary cause of "antibiotic-associated colitis".
After the diagnosis of pseudomembranous colitis has been established, therapeutic measures should be initiated. Mild cases of pseudomembranous colitis usually respond to drug discontinuation alone. In moderate to severe cases, consideration should be given to management with fluids and electrolytes, protein supplementation and treatment with an antibacterial drug clinically effective against *C. difficile* colitis.

PRECAUTIONS

General: For topical use only; not for ophthalmic use. Concomitant topical acne therapy should be used with caution because a possible cumulative irritancy effect may occur, especially with the use of peeling, desquamating or abrasive agents.
The use of antibiotic agents may be associated with the overgrowth of antibiotic-resistant organisms. If this occurs, discontinue use and take appropriate measures.
Avoid contact with eyes and all mucous membranes.
Information For Patients: Patients using ERYGEL® Topical Gel should receive the following information and instructions:

1. This medication is to be used as directed by the physician. It is for external use only. Avoid contact with the eyes, nose, mouth, and all mucous membranes.
2. This medication should not be used for any disorder other than that for which it was prescribed.
3. Patients should not use any other topical acne medication unless otherwise directed by their physician.
4. Patients should report to their physician any signs of local adverse reactions.

Carcinogenesis, mutagenesis, impairment of fertility: No animal studies have been performed to evaluate carcinogenic and mutagenic potential or effects on fertility of topical erythromycin. However, long-term (2-year) oral studies in rats with erythromycin ethylsuccinate and erythromycin base did not provide evidence of tumorigenicity. There was no apparent effect on male or female fertility in rats fed erythromycin (base) at levels up to 0.25% of diet.
Pregnancy: Teratogenic effects: Pregnancy Category B: There was no evidence of teratogenicity or any other adverse effect on reproduction in female rats fed erythromycin base (up to 0.25% of diet) prior to and during mating, during gestation and through weaning of two successive litters. There are, however, no adequate and well-controlled studies in pregnant women. Because animal reproduction studies are not always predictive of human response, this drug should be used in pregnancy only if clearly needed. Erythromycin has been reported to cross the placental barrier in humans, but fetal plasma levels are generally low.
Nursing women: It is not known whether erythromycin is excreted in human milk following topical application. However, erythromycin is excreted in human milk following oral and parenteral erythromycin administration. Therefore, caution should be exercised when erythromycin is administered to a nursing woman.
Pediatric Use: Safety and effectiveness in pediatric patients have not been established.

ADVERSE REACTIONS

In controlled clinical trials, the incidence of burning associated with ERYGEL® Topical Gel was approximately 25%. The following additional local adverse reactions have been reported occasionally: peeling, dryness, itching, erythema, and oiliness. Irritation of the eyes and tenderness of the skin have also been reported with the topical use of erythromycin. A generalized urticarial reaction, possibly related to the use of erythromycin, which required systemic steroid therapy has been reported.

DOSAGE AND ADMINISTRATION

ERYGEL® Topical Gel should be applied sparingly as a thin film to affected area(s) once or twice a day after the skin is thoroughly cleansed and patted dry. If there has been no improvement after 6 to 8 weeks, or if the condition becomes worse, treatment should be discontinued, and the physician should be reconsulted. Spread the medication lightly rather than rubbing it in. There are no data directly comparing the safety and efficacy of b.i.d. versus q.d. dosing.

HOW SUPPLIED

ERYGEL® (Erythromycin Topical Gel USP) 2% is supplied in plastic tubes in the following sizes:
30g - NDC 0259-4312-30 and 60 g - NDC 0259-4312-60.

Note: FLAMMABLE. Keep away from heat and flame. Store and dispense in original container. Keep tube tightly closed. Store between 15° and 25°C (59° and 77°F).
Manufactured for: **Merz Pharmaceuticals, Greensboro, NC 27410**
70-2057-00 Rev 10/01

MEDERMA® OTC
[*mə-der-mă*]
allium cepa
Skin Care for Scars™

DESCRIPTION

HELPS THE APPEARANCE OF SCARS RESULTING FROM: Surgery, Burns, Injury, Acne, Stretch Marks
Mederma® is a topical gel formulated to benefit anyone with new scars or existing scars. Mederma® is a greaseless, pleasant-smelling topical gel that not only helps scars appear softer and smoother, but also offers convenience, ease of use and affordability.

INGREDIENTS

Water (Purified), PEG-4, Allium Cepa (Onion) Bulb Extract, Xanthan Gum, Allantoin, Fragrance, Methylparaben, Sorbic Acid.

DOSAGE AND ADMINISTRATION

Gently massage Mederma® into the scar or stretch marks 3 to 4 times daily. Mederma should be used for 8 weeks on new scars and 2–6 months on existing scars and stretch marks.
NOT INTENDED FOR USE ON OPEN WOUNDS
FOR TOPICAL USE ONLY

STORAGE

Store at room temperature

HOW SUPPLIED

Mederma® is supplied in 20g (#0259-03032-1) and 50g (#0259-03035-2) tubes. The 20g tube will last approximately 3 months when treating a scar up to 3 inches in length. The 50g tube will last approximately 3 months when treating a scar 8 to 10 inches in length.
30-2065-01 Rev. 06/04
Manufactured for: Merz Pharmaceuticals, Greensboro, NC 27410

NAFTIN® ℞
(naftifine hydrochloride) 1%
Cream
℞ only

DESCRIPTION

NAFTIN® Cream, 1% contains the synthetic, broad-spectrum, antifungal agent naftifine hydrochloride.
NAFTIN® Cream, 1% is for topical use only.
Chemical Name: (E)-N-Cinnamyl-N-methyl-1-naphthalenemethyl-amine hydrochloride. Naftifine hydrochloride has an empirical formula of $C_{21}H_{21}N{\cdot}HCl$ and a molecular weight of 323.86.

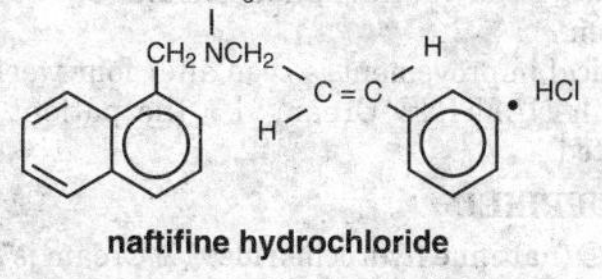

naftifine hydrochloride

Active Ingredient: Naftifine hydrochloride 1%
Inactive Ingredients: benzyl alcohol, cetyl alcohol, cetyl esters wax, isopropyl myristate, polysorbate 60, purified water, sodium hydroxide, sorbitan monostearate, and stearyl alcohol. Hydrochloric acid may be added to adjust pH.

CLINICAL PHARMACOLOGY

Naftifine hydrochloride is a synthetic allylamine derivative. The following *in vitro* data are available, but their clinical significance is unknown. Naftifine hydrochloride has been shown to exhibit fungicidal activity *in vitro* against a broad spectrum of organisms including *Trichophyton rubrum, Trichophyton mentagrophytes, Trichophyton tonsurans, Epidermophyton floccosum, Microsporum canis, Microsporum audouini,* and *Microsporum gypseum;* and fungistatic activity against *Candida* species, including *Candida albicans.* NAFTIN® Cream, 1% has only been shown to be clinically effective against the disease entities listed in the INDICATIONS AND USAGE section.
Although the exact mechanism of action against fungi is not known, naftifine hydrochloride appears to interfere with sterol biosynthesis by inhibiting the enzyme squalene 2,3-epoxidase. This inhibition of enzyme activity results in decreased amounts of sterols, especially ergosterol, and a corresponding accumulation of squalene in the cells.
Pharmacokinetics: *In vitro* and *in vivo* bioavailability studies have demonstrated that naftifine penetrates the stratum corneum in sufficient concentration to inhibit the growth of dermatophytes.

Continued on next page

Naftin Cream—Cont.

Following a single topical application of 1% naftifine cream to the skin of healthy subjects, systemic absorption of naftifine was approximately 6% of the applied dose. Naftifine and/or its metabolites are excreted via the urine and feces with a half-life of approximately two to three days.

INDICATIONS AND USAGE

NAFTIN® Cream, 1% is indicated for the topical treatment of tinea pedis, tinea cruris and tinea corporis caused by the organisms *Tricophyton rubrum, Tricophyton mentagrophytes,* and *Epidermophyton floccosum.*

CONTRAINDICATIONS

NAFTIN® Cream, 1% is contraindicated in individuals who have shown hypersensitivity to any of its components.

WARNING

NAFTIN® Cream, 1% is for topical use only and not for ophthalmic use.

PRECAUTIONS

General: NAFTIN® Cream, 1% is for external use only. If irritation or sensitivity develops with the use of NAFTIN® Cream 1%, treatment should be discontinued and appropriate therapy instituted. Diagnosis of the disease should be confirmed either by direct microscopic examination of a mounting of infected tissue in a solution of potassium hydroxide or by culture on an appropriate medium.

Information for patients: The patient should be told to:

1. Avoid the use of occlusive dressings or wrappings unless otherwise directed by the physician.
2. Keep NAFTIN® Cream, 1% away from the eyes, nose, mouth and other mucous membranes.

Carcinogenesis, mutagenesis, impairment of fertility: Long-term animal studies to evaluate the carcinogenic potential of NAFTIN® Cream, 1% have not been performed. *In vitro* and animal studies have not demonstrated any mutagenic effect or effect on fertility.

Pregnancy: Teratogenic Effects: Pregnancy Category B: Reproduction studies have been performed in rats and rabbits (via oral administration) at doses 150 times or more the topical human dose and have revealed no significant evidence of impaired fertility or harm to the fetus due to naftifine. There are, however, no adequate and well-controlled studies in pregnant women. Because animal reproduction studies are not always predictive of human response, this drug should be used during pregnancy only if clearly needed.

Nursing mothers: It is not known whether this drug is excreted in human milk. Because many drugs are excreted in human milk, caution should be exercised when NAFTIN® Cream, 1% is administered to a nursing woman.

Pediatric use: Safety and effectiveness in pediatric patients have not been established.

ADVERSE REACTIONS

During clinical trials with NAFTIN® Cream 1%, the incidence of adverse reactions was as follows: burning/stinging (6%), dryness (3%), erythema (2%), itching (2%), local irritation (2%).

DOSAGE AND ADMINISTRATION

A sufficient quantity of NAFTIN® Cream, 1% should be gently massaged into the affected and surrounding skin areas once a day. The hands should be washed after application.

If no clinical improvement is seen after four weeks of treatment with NAFTIN® Cream, 1% the patient should be reevaluated.

HOW SUPPLIED

NAFTIN® (naftifine hydrochloride) 1% Cream is supplied in collapsible tubes in the following sizes.

15 g-NDC-0259-4126-15
30 g-NDC-0259-4126-30
60 g-NDC-0259-4126-60
60 g (4×15 g)-NDC-0259-4126-04

Note: Store below 30°C (86°F).

Manufactured for: Merz Pharmaceuticals,
Greensboro, NC 27410

30-1364-00 Rev 4/04

NAFTIN® ℞
(naftifine hydrochloride) 1%
Gel
℞ only

DESCRIPTION

NAFTIN® Gel, 1% contains the synthetic, broad-spectrum, antifungal agent naftifine hydrochloride.

NAFTIN® Gel, 1% is for topical use only.

Chemical Name: (E)-N-Cinnamyl-N-methyl-1-naphthalene-methylamine hydrochloride. Naftifine hydrochloride has an empirical formula of $C_{21}H_{21}N{\cdot}HCl$ and a molecular weight of 323.86.

[See chemical structure at top of next column]

Contains:

Active Ingredient: Naftifine hydrochloride 1%

Inactive Ingredients: polysorbate 80, carbomer 934P, diisopropanolamine, edetate disodium, alcohol (52% v/v), and purified water.

naftifine hydrochloride

CLINICAL PHARMACOLOGY

Naftifine hydrochloride is a synthetic allylamine derivative. The following *in vitro* data are available but their clinical significance is unknown. Naftifine hydrochloride has been shown to exhibit fungicidal activity *in vitro* against a broad spectrum of organisms including *Trichophyton rubrum, Trichophyton mentagrophytes, Trichophyton tonsurans, Epidermophyton floccosum,* and *Microsporum canis, Microsporum audouini,* and *Microsporum gypseum;* and fungistatic activity against *Candida* species including *Candida albicans.* NAFTIN® Gel, 1% has only been shown to be clinically effective against the disease entities listed in the INDICATIONS AND USAGE section.

Although the exact mechanism of action against fungi is not known, naftifine hydrochloride appears to interfere with sterol biosynthesis by inhibiting the enzyme squalene 2,3-epoxidase. This inhibition of enzyme activity results in decreased amounts of sterols, especially ergosterol, and a corresponding accumulation of squalene in the cells.

Pharmacokinetics: *In vitro* and *in vivo* bioavailability studies have demonstrated that naftifine penetrates the stratum corneum in sufficient concentration to inhibit the growth of dermatophytes.

Following single topical application of ^{3}H-labeled naftifine gel 1% to the skin of healthy subjects, up to 4.2% of the applied dose was absorbed. Naftifine and/or its metabolites are excreted via the urine and feces with a half-life of approximately two to three days.

INDICATION AND USAGE

NAFTIN® Gel, 1% is indicated for the topical treatment of tinea pedis, tinea cruris and tinea corporis caused by the organisms *Trichophyton rubrum, Trichophyton mentagrophytes, Trichophyton tonsurans** and *Epidermophyton floccosum.**

*Efficacy for this organism in this organ system was studied in fewer than 10 infections.

CONTRAINDICATIONS

NAFTIN® Gel, 1% is contraindicated in individuals who have shown hypersensitivity to any of its components.

WARNINGS

NAFTIN® Gel, 1% is for topical use only and not for ophthalmic use.

PRECAUTIONS

General: NAFTIN® Gel, 1% is for external use only. If irritation or sensitivity develop with the use of NAFTIN® Gel, 1%, treatment should be discontinued and appropriate therapy instituted. Diagnosis of the disease should be confirmed either by direct microscopic examination of a mounting of infected tissue in a solution of potassium hydroxide or by culture on an appropriate medium.

Information for patients:

The patient should be told to:

1. Avoid the use of occlusive dressings or wrappings unless otherwise directed by the physician.
2. Keep NAFTIN® Gel, 1% away from the eyes, nose, mouth and other mucous membranes.

Carcinogenesis, mutagenesis, impairment of fertility: Long-term studies to evaluate the carcinogenic potential of NAFTIN® Gel, 1% have not been performed. *In vitro* and animal studies have not demonstrated any mutagenic effect or effect on fertility.

Pregnancy: Teratogenic Effects: Pregnancy Category B: Reproduction studies have been performed in rats and rabbits (via oral administration) at doses 150 times or more than the topical human dose and have revealed no evidence of impaired fertility or harm to the fetus due to naftifine. There are, however, no adequate and well-controlled studies in pregnant women. Because animal reproduction studies are not always predictive of human response, this drug should be used during pregnancy only if clearly needed.

Nursing mothers: It is not known whether this drug is excreted in human milk. Because many drugs are excreted in human milk, caution should be exercised when NAFTIN® Gel, 1% is administered to a nursing woman.

Pediatric use: Safety and effectiveness in pediatric patients have not been established.

ADVERSE REACTIONS

During clinical trials with NAFTIN® Gel, 1%, the incidence of adverse reactions was as follows: burning/stinging (5.0%), itching (1.0%), erythema (0.5%), rash (0.5%), skin tenderness (0.5%).

DOSAGE AND ADMINISTRATION

A sufficient quantity of NAFTIN® Gel, 1% should be gently massaged into the affected and surrounding skin areas twice a day, in the morning and evening. The hands should be washed after application.

If no clinical improvement is seen after four weeks of treatment with NAFTIN® Gel, 1%, the patient should be reevaluated.

HOW SUPPLIED

NAFTIN® (naftifine hydrochloride) is supplied in collapsible tubes in the following sizes:

20 g-NDC-0259-4770-20
40 g-NDC-0259-4770-40
60 g-NDC-0259-4770-60

Note: Store at room temperature.

Manufactured for: Merz Pharmaceuticals,
Greensboro, NC 27410

30-1365-00 Rev 4/04

NU-IRON® 150 CAPSULES OTC
(polysaccharide-iron complex)

Each NU-IRON 150 Capsule contains:
Iron (elemental) .... 150 mg.
(as a Polysaccharide Iron Complex)

> **WARNING**
> Accidental overdose of iron-containing products is a leading cause of fatal poisoning in children under 6. Keep this product out of reach of children. In case of accidental overdose, call a doctor or poison control center immediately.

INDICATIONS

For treatment of uncomplicated iron deficiency anemia.

CONTRAINDICATIONS

Hemochromatosis, hemosiderosis or a known hypersensitivity to any of the ingredients.

DOSAGE

ADULTS: One or two NU-IRON® 150 Capsules daily.
CHILDREN: consult physician.

HOW SUPPLIED

NU-IRON® 150 CAPSULES in packages of 100 (10 blister cards): #0259-0291-01.

Non-USP

Distributed by Merz Pharmaceuticals, Greensboro, NC 27410

Store at controlled room temperature, 15°–30°C (59°–86°F)

40-0291-10 Rev. 10/99

NU-IRON® V ℞
Polysaccharide-iron complex and multi-vitamin

DESCRIPTION

EACH MAROON FILM-COATED TABLET CONTAINS:

Iron (Elemental) 60 mg (as a POLYSACCHARIDE-IRON COMPLEX); Folic Acid 1 mg; Ascorbic Acid 50 mg (as sodium ascorbate); Cyanocobalamin (Vitamin B_{12}) 3 mcg; Vitamin A 4,000 I.U.; Vitamin D_2 400 I.U.; Thiamine Mononitrate 3 mg; Riboflavin 3 mg; Pyridoxine Hydrochloride 2 mg; Niacinamide 10 mg; Calcium Carbonate 312 mg

DOSAGE

One tablet daily or as directed by a physician.

> **WARNING**
> Accidental overdose of iron-containing products is a leading cause of fatal poisoning in children under 6. Keep this product out of reach of children. In case of accidental overdose, call a doctor or poison control center immediately.

PRECAUTIONS

The use of folic acid in patients having or who may develop pernicious anemia involves the hazard of treating the anemia characteristic of the disease while permitting progressive development of combined system disease of the spinal cord. Parenteral Vitamin B_{12} is the drug of choice in pernicious anemia and should be used in patients receiving folic acid unless pernicious anemia has been ruled out.

INDICATIONS

For the prevention and/or treatment of dietary vitamin and iron deficiencies.

CONTRAINDICATIONS

Sensitivity to any of the ingredients.

℞ only.

TABLETS ARE INDIVIDUALLY SEALED. IF SEAL IS BROKEN DO NOT USE.

NDC 0259-0331-01

Store at controlled room temperature, 15°–30°C (59°–86°F).

Non-USP

Distributed By:
MERZ PHARMACEUTICALS
GREENSBORO, NC 27410

40-0331-10 Rev. 6/98

SEDAPAP® TABLETS ℞
(Butalbital and Acetaminophen Tablets)
50 mg/650 mg

DESCRIPTION

Butalbital and acetaminophen is supplied in tablet form for oral administration.

Butalbital (5-allyl-5-isobutylbarbituric acid), a slightly bitter, white, odorless, crystalline powder, is a short to intermediate-acting barbiturate. It has the following structural formula:

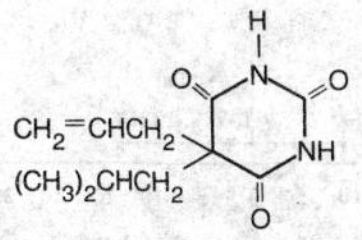

$C_{11}H_{16}N_2O_3$ MW = 224.26

Acetaminophen (4′-hydroxyacetanalide), a slightly bitter, white, odorless, crystalline powder, is a non-opiate, non-salicylate analgesic and antipyretic. It has the following structural formula:

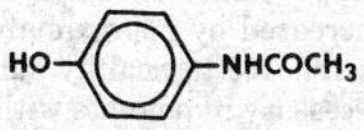

$C_8H_9NO_2$ MW = 151.16

Each Sedapap Tablet contains:
Butalbital .... 50 mg
(Warning: May be habit forming)
Acetaminophen .... 650 mg

In addition, each tablet contains the following inactive ingredients: colloidal silicon dioxide, croscarmellose sodium, crospovidone, microcrystalline cellulose, povidone, pregelatinized starch and stearic acid.

CLINICAL PHARMACOLOGY

This combination drug product is intended as a treatment for tension headache.

It consists of a fixed combination of butalbital, and acetaminophen. The role each component plays in the relief of the complex of symptoms known as tension headache is not completely understood.

Pharmacokinetics: The behavior of the individual components is described below.

Butalbital: Butalbital is well absorbed from the gastrointestinal tract and is expected to distribute to most tissues in the body. Barbiturates in general may appear in breast milk and readily cross the placental barrier. They are bound to plasma and tissue proteins to a varying degree and binding increases directly as a function of lipid solubility.

Elimination of butalbital is primarily via the kidney (59% to 88% of the dose) as unchanged drug or metabolites. The plasma half-life is about 35 hours. Urinary excretion products include parent drug (about 3.6% of the dose), 5-isobutyl-5-(2,3-dihydroxypropyl) barbituric acid (about 24% of the dose), 5-allyl-5(3-hydroxy-2-methyl-1-propyl) barbituric acid (about 4.8% of the dose), products with the barbituric acid ring hydrolyzed with excretion of urea (about 14% of the dose), as well as unidentified materials. Of the material excreted in the urine, 32% is conjugated.

See OVERDOSAGE for toxicity information.

Acetaminophen: Acetaminophen is rapidly absorbed from the gastrointestinal tract and is distributed throughout most body tissues. The plasma half-life is 1.25 to 3 hours, but may be increased by liver damage and following overdosage. Elimination of acetaminophen is principally by liver metabolism (conjugation) and subsequent renal excretion of metabolites. Approximately 85% of an oral dose appears in the urine within 24 hours of administration, most as the glucuronide conjugate, with small amounts of other conjugates and unchanged drug.

See OVERDOSAGE for toxicity information.

INDICATIONS AND USAGE

Butalbital and Acetaminophen Tablets are indicated for the relief of the symptom complex of tension (or muscle contraction) headache.

Evidence supporting the efficacy and safety of this combination product in the treatment of multiple recurrent headaches is unavailable. Caution in this regard is required because butalbital is habit-forming and potentially abusable.

CONTRAINDICATIONS

This product is contraindicated under the following conditions:

- Hypersensitivity or intolerance to any component of this product.
- Patients with porphyria.

WARNINGS

Butalbital is habit-forming and potentially abusable. Consequently, the extended use of this product is not recommended.

PRECAUTIONS

General: Butalbital and Acetaminophen Tablets should be prescribed with caution in certain special-risk patients, such as the elderly or debilitated, and those with severe impairment of renal or hepatic function, or acute abdominal conditions.

Information for Patients: This product may impair mental and/or physical abilities required for the performance of potentially hazardous tasks such as driving a car or operating machinery. Such tasks should be avoided while taking this product.

Alcohol and other CNS depressants may produce an additive CNS depression, when taken with this combination product, and should be avoided.

Butalbital may be habit-forming. Patients should take the drug only for as long as it is prescribed, in the amounts prescribed, and no more frequently than prescribed.

Laboratory Tests: In patients with severe hepatic or renal disease, effects of therapy should be monitored with serial liver and/or renal function tests.

Drug Interactions: The CNS effects of butalbital may be enhanced by monoamine oxidase (MAO) inhibitors.

Butalbital and acetaminophen may enhance the effects of: other narcotic analgesics, alcohol, general anesthetics, tranquilizers such as chlordiazepoxide, sedative-hypnotics, or other CNS depressants, causing increased CNS depression.

Drug/Laboratory Test Interactions: Acetaminophen may produce false-positive test results for urinary 5-hydroxyindoleacetic acid.

Carcinogenesis, Mutagenesis, Impairment of Fertility: No adequate studies have been conducted in animals to determine whether acetaminophen or butalbital have a potential for carcinogenesis, mutagenesis or impairment of fertility.

Pregnancy: *Teratogenic Effects:* Pregnancy Category C: Animal reproduction studies have not been conducted with this combination product. It is also not known whether butalbital and acetaminophen can cause fetal harm when administered to a pregnant woman or can affect reproduction capacity. This product should be given to a pregnant woman only when clearly needed.

Nonteratogenic Effects: Withdrawal seizures were reported in a two-day-old male infant whose mother had taken butalbital-containing drug during the last two months of pregnancy. Butalbital was found in the infant's serum. The infant was given phenobarbital 5 mg/kg, which was tapered without further seizure or other withdrawal symptoms.

Nursing Mothers: Barbiturates and acetaminophen are excreted in breast milk in small amounts, but the significance of their effects on nursing infants is not known. Because of potential for serious adverse reactions in nursing infants from butalbital and acetaminophen, a decision should be made whether to discontinue nursing or to discontinue the drug, taking into account the importance of the drug to the mother.

Pediatric Use: Safety and effectiveness in pediatric patients below the age of 12 have not been established.

ADVERSE REACTIONS

Frequently Observed: The most frequently reported adverse reactions are drowsiness, lightheadedness, dizziness, sedation, shortness of breath, nausea, vomiting, abdominal pain, and intoxicated feeling.

Infrequently Observed: All adverse events tabulated below are classified as infrequent.

Central Nervous: headache, shaky feeling, tingling, agitation, fainting, fatigue, heavy eyelids, high energy, hot spells, numbness, sluggishness, seizure. Mental confusion, excitement or depression can also occur due to intolerance, particularly in elderly or debilitated patients, or due to overdosage of butalbital.

Autonomic Nervous: dry mouth, hyperhidrosis.

Gastrointestinal: difficulty swallowing, heartburn, flatulence, constipation.

Cardiovascular: tachycardia.

Musculoskeletal: leg pain, muscle fatigue.

Genitourinary: diuresis.

Miscellaneous: pruritus, fever, earache, nasal congestion, tinnitus, euphoria, allergic reactions.

Several cases of dermatological reactions, including toxic epidermal necrolysis and erythema multiforme, have been reported.

The following adverse drug events may be borne in mind as a potential effect of the components of this product. Potential effects of high dosage are listed in the OVERDOSAGE section.

Acetaminophen: allergic reactions, rash, thrombocytopenia, agranulocytosis.

DRUG ABUSE AND DEPENDENCE

Abuse and Dependence: Butalbital: *Barbiturates may be habit-forming:* Tolerance, psychological dependence, and physical dependence may occur especially following prolonged use of high doses of barbiturates. The average daily dose for the barbiturate addict is usually about 1500 mg. As tolerance to barbiturates develops, the amount needed to maintain the same level of intoxication increases; tolerance to a fatal dosage, however, does not increase more than twofold. As this occurs, the margin between an intoxication dosage and fatal dosage becomes smaller. The lethal dose of a barbiturate is far less if alcohol is also ingested. Major withdrawal symptoms (convulsions and delirium) may occur within 16 hours and last up to 5 days after abrupt cessation of these drugs. Intensity of withdrawal symptoms gradually declines over a period of approximately 15 days. Treatment of barbiturate dependence consists of cautious and gradual withdrawal of the drug. Barbiturate-dependent patients can be withdrawn by using a number of different withdrawal regimens. One method involves initiating treatment at the patient's regular dosage level and gradually decreasing the daily dosage as tolerated by the patient.

OVERDOSAGE

Following an acute overdosage of butalbital and acetaminophen, toxicity may result from the barbiturate or the acetaminophen.

Signs and Symptoms: Toxicity from barbiturate poisoning include drowsiness, confusion, and coma; respiratory depression; hypotension; and hypovolemic shock.

In acetaminophen overdosage: dose-dependent, potentially fatal hepatic necrosis is the most serious adverse effect. Renal tubular necroses, hypoglycemic coma and thrombocytopenia may also occur. Early symptoms following a potentially hepatotoxic overdose may include: nausea, vomiting, diaphoresis and general malaise. Clinical and laboratory evidence of hepatic toxicity may not be apparent until 48 to 72 hours post-ingestion. In adults hepatic toxicity has rarely been reported with acute overdoses of less than 10 grams, or fatalities with less than 15 grams.

Treatment: A single or multiple overdose with this combination product is a potentially lethal polydrug overdose, and consultation with a regional poison control center is recommended.

Immediate treatment includes support of cardiorespiratory function and measures to reduce drug absorption. Vomiting should be induced mechanically, or with syrup of ipecac, if the patient is alert (adequate pharyngeal and laryngeal reflexes). Oral activated charcoal (1 g/kg) should follow gastric emptying. The first dose should be accompanied by an appropriate cathartic. If repeated doses are used, the cathartic might be included with alternate doses as required. Hypotension is usually hypovolemic and should respond to fluids. Pressors should be avoided. A cuffed endotracheal tube should be inserted before gastric lavage of the unconscious patient and, when necessary, to provide assisted respiration. If renal function is normal, forced diuresis may aid in the elimination of the barbiturate. Alkalinization of the urine increases renal excretion of some barbiturates, especially phenobarbital.

Meticulous attention should be given to maintaining adequate pulmonary ventilation. In severe cases of intoxication, peritoneal dialysis, or preferably hemodialysis may be considered. If hypoprothrombinemia occurs due to acetaminophen overdose, vitamin K should be administered intravenously.

If the dose of acetaminophen may have exceeded 140 mg/kg, acetylcysteine should be administered as early as possible. Serum acetaminophen levels should be obtained, since levels four or more hours following ingestion help predict acetaminophen toxicity. Do not await acetaminophen assay results before initiating treatment. Hepatic enzymes should be obtained initially, and repeated at 24-hour intervals.

Methemoglobinemia over 30% should be treated with methylene blue by slow intravenous administration.

Toxic Doses (for adults):
Butalbital: toxic dose 1 g (20 tablets)
Acetaminophen: toxic dose 10 g (15 tablets)

DOSAGE AND ADMINISTRATION

Oral: One table every four hours as needed. Total daily dosage should not exceed 6 tablets.

Extended and repeated use of this product is not recommended because of the potential for physical dependence.

HOW SUPPLIED

SEDAPAP® TABLETS (Butalbital and Acetaminophen Tablets) 50 mg/650 mg are supplied in bottles of 100 tablets, NDC 0259-0392-01. Each tablet contains butalbital 50 mg (Warning: May be habit forming) and acetaminophen 650 mg. Tablets are uncoated, white, capsule-shaped and are debossed "MP" score "392" on one side.

Storage: Protect from light and moisture. Store at controlled room temperature, 15° - 30°C (59° - 86°F).

Dispense in a tight, light-resistant container with a child-resistant closure.

CAUTION: Federal law prohibits dispensing without prescription.

MFG. FOR:
MERZ PHARMACEUTICALS
Greensboro, NC 27407

Rev. 07/01 Code 805A00

IDENTIFICATION PROBLEM?
Turn to the **Product Identification Guide,** where you'll find more than 1600 products pictured in actual size and full color.

Methapharm, Inc.
11772 WEST SAMPLE ROAD
SUITE 101
CORAL SPRINGS, FLORIDA 33065

Direct Inquiries to:
(800) 287-7686
FAX: (877) 718-9222
www.methapharm.com
sales@methapharm.com

PROVOCHOLINE® ℞
brand of
methacholine chloride
POWDER FOR INHALATION
NOT FOR INJECTION

DESCRIPTION
Provocholine® (methacholine chloride powder for inhalation) is a parasympathomimetic (cholinergic) bronchoconstrictor agent to be administered in solution only, by inhalation for diagnostic purposes. Each 20 mL vial contains 100 mg of methacholine chloride powder which is to be reconstituted with 0.9% sodium chloride injection containing 0.4% phenol (pH 7.0).
Chemically, methacholine chloride (the active ingredient) is 1-propanaminium, 2-(acetyloxy)-*N,N,N*,-trimethyl,-chloride. It is a white to practically white deliquescent compound, soluble in water. Methacholine chloride has an empirical formula of $C_8H_{18}ClNO_2$, a calculated molecular weight of 195.69, and the following structural formula:

$$\left[CH_3COOCHCH_2N^{+}(CH_3)_3 \atop \quad | \atop \quad CH_3 \right] Cl^{-}$$

HOW SUPPLIED
20 mL amber vials containing 100 mg of methacholine chloride powder which are to be reconstituted with 0.9% sodium chloride injection containing 0.4% phenol (pH 7.0)—boxes of 12 (NDC 64281-100-12) or boxes of 6 (NDC 64281-100-06). Store the powder at 59° to 86°F (15° to 30°C). Refrigerate the reconstituted solutions (dilutions 25 mg/mL – 0.25 mg/mL) at 36° to 46°F (2° to 8°C) for not more than 2 weeks. Dilution 0.025 mg/mL must be prepared on the day of the challenge.

MGI Pharma, Inc.
5775 WEST OLD SHAKOPEE ROAD
SUITE 100
BLOOMINGTON, MN 55437-3174

For Medical Information Contact:
Generally:
Medical Information
800-562-5580
FAX: (952) 346-4800

Customer Service
(800) 562-4531
FAX: (952) 346-4800

ALOXI™ ℞
[a-lŏk-sē]
(palonosetron hydrochloride)
injection

DESCRIPTION
ALOXI[1] (palonosetron hydrochloride) is an antiemetic and antinauseant agent. It is a selective serotonin subtype 3 (5-HT_3) receptor antagonist with a strong binding affinity for this receptor. Chemically, palonosetron hydrochloride is: (3aS)-2-[(S)-1-Azabicyclo[2.2.2]oct-3-yl]-2,3,3a,4,5,6-hexahydro-1-oxo-1*H*benz[*de*]isoquinoline hydrochloride. The empirical formula is $C_{19}H_{24}N_2O \bullet HCl$, with a molecular weight of 332.87. Palonosetron hydrochloride exists as a single isomer and has the following structural formula:

• HCl

Palonosetron hydrochloride is a white to off-white crystalline powder. It is freely soluble in water, soluble in propylene glycol, and slightly soluble in ethanol and 2-propanol. ALOXI injection is a sterile, clear, colorless, non-pyrogenic, isotonic, buffered solution for intravenous administration. Each 5-ml vial of ALOXI injection contains 0.25 mg palonosetron base as hydrochloride, 207.5 mg mannitol, disodium edetate and citrate buffer in water for intravenous administration. The pH of the solution is 4.5 to 5.5.

Table 1: Prevention of Acute Nausea and Vomiting (0-24 hours): Complete Response Rates

Chemo-therapy	Study	Treatment Group	N [a]	% with Complete Response	p-value [b]	97.5% Confidence Interval Aloxi minus Comparator [c]
Moderately Emetogenic	1	Aloxi 0.25 mg	189	81	0.009	[2%, 23%]
		Ondansetron 32 mg IV	185	69		
	2	Aloxi 0.25 mg	189	63	NS	[-2%, 22%]
		Dolasetron 100 mg IV	191	53		
Highly Emetogenic	3	Aloxi 0.25 mg	223	59	NS	[-9%, 13%]
		Ondansetron 32 mg IV	221	57		

-10 -5 0 5 10 15 20 25 30 35
Difference in Complete Response Rates

a Intent-to-treat cohort
b 2-sided Fisher's exact test. Significance level at α=0.025.
c These studies were designed to show non-inferiority. A lower bound greater than –15% demonstrates non-inferiority between Aloxi and comparator.

[1] Pending trademark of Helsinn Healthcare SA, Lugano, Switzerland

CLINICAL PHARMACOLOGY
Pharmacodynamics
Palonosetron is a selective 5-HT_3 receptor antagonist with a strong binding affinity for this receptor and little or no affinity for other receptors.
Cancer chemotherapy may be associated with a high incidence of nausea and vomiting, particularly when certain agents, such as cisplatin, are used. 5-HT_3 receptors are located on the nerve terminals of the vagus in the periphery and centrally in the chemoreceptor trigger zone of the area postrema. It is thought that chemotherapeutic agents produce nausea and vomiting by releasing serotonin from the enterochromaffin cells of the small intestine and that the released serotonin then activates 5-HT_3 receptors located on vagal afferents to initiate the vomiting reflex.
The effect of palonosetron on blood pressure, heart rate, and ECG parameters including QTc were comparable to ondansetron and dolasetron in clinical trials. In non-clinical studies palonosetron possesses the ability to block ion channels involved in ventricular de- and re-polarization and to prolong action potential duration. In clinical trials, the dose-response relationship to the QTc interval has not been fully evaluated.
Pharmacokinetics
After intravenous dosing of palonosetron in healthy subjects and cancer patients, an initial decline in plasma concentrations is followed by a slow elimination from the body. Mean maximum plasma concentration (C_{max}) and area under the concentration-time curve ($AUC_{0-\infty}$) are generally dose-proportional over the dose range of 0.3–90 μg/kg in healthy subjects and in cancer patients. Following single IV dose of palonosetron at 3 μg/kg (or 0.21 mg/70 kg) to six cancer patients, mean (±SD) maximum plasma concentration was estimated to be 5.6 ± 5.5 ng/mL and mean AUC was 35.8 ± 20.9 ng hr/mL.
Distribution
Palonosetron has a volume of distribution of approximately 8.3 ± 2.5 L/kg. Approximately 62% of palonosetron is bound to plasma proteins.
Metabolism
Palonosetron is eliminated by multiple routes with approximately 50% metabolized to form two primary metabolites: N-oxide-palonosetron and 6-S-hydroxy-palonosetron. These metabolites each have less than 1% of the 5-HT_3 receptor antagonist activity of palonosetron. *In vitro* metabolism studies have suggested that CYP2D6 and to a lesser extent, CYP3A and CYP1A2 are involved in the metabolism of palonosetron. However, clinical pharmacokinetic parameters are not significantly different between poor and extensive metabolizers of CYP2D6 substrates.
Elimination
After a single intravenous dose of 10 μg/kg [^{14}C]-palonosetron, approximately 80% of the dose was recovered within 144 hours in the urine with palonosetron representing approximately 40% of the administered dose. In healthy subjects the total body clearance of palonosetron was 160 ± 35 mL/h/kg and renal clearance was 66.5±18.2 mL/h/kg. Mean terminal elimination half-life is approximately 40 hours.
Special Populations
Geriatrics
Population PK analysis and clinical safety and efficacy data did not reveal any differences between cancer patients ≥ 65 years of age and younger patients (18 to 64 years). No dose adjustment is required for these patients.
Race
Intravenous palonosetron pharmacokinetics was characterized in twenty-four healthy Japanese subjects over the dose range of 3–90 μg/kg. Total body clearance was 25% higher in Japanese subjects compared to Whites, however, no dose adjustment is required. The pharmacokinetics of palonosetron in Blacks has not been adequately characterized.
Renal Impairment
Mild to moderate renal impairment does not significantly affect palonosetron pharmacokinetic parameters. Total systemic exposure increased by approximately 28% in severe renal impairment relative to healthy subjects. Dosage adjustment is not necessary in patients with any degree of renal impairment.
Hepatic Impairment
Hepatic impairment does not significantly affect total body clearance of palonosetron compared to the healthy subjects. Dosage adjustment is not necessary in patients with any degree of hepatic impairment.
Drug-Drug Interactions
Palonosetron is eliminated from the body through both renal excretion and metabolic pathways with the latter mediated via multiple CYP enzymes. Further *in vitro* studies indicated that palonosetron is not an inhibitor of CYP1A2, CYP2A6, CYP2B6, CYP2C9, CYP2D6, CYP2E1 and CYP3A4/5 (CYP2C19 was not investigated) nor does it induce the activity of CYP1A2, CYP2D6, or CYP3A4/5. Therefore the potential for clinically significant drug interactions with palonosetron appears to be low.
A study in healthy volunteers involving single-dose IV palonosetron (0.75 mg) and steady state oral metoclopramide (10 mg four times daily) demonstrated no significant pharmacokinetic interaction.
In controlled clinical trials, ALOXI injection has been safely administered with corticosteroids, analgesics, antiemetics/antinauseants, antispasmodics and anticholinergic agents.
Palonosetron did not inhibit the antitumor activity of the five chemotherapeutic agents tested (cisplatin, cyclophosphamide, cytarabine, doxorubicin and mitomycin C) in murine tumor models.

CLINICAL STUDIES
Efficacy of single-dose palonosetron injection in preventing acute and delayed nausea and vomiting induced by both moderately and highly emetogenic chemotherapy was studied in three Phase 3 trials and one Phase 2 trial. In these double-blind studies, complete response rates (no emetic episodes and no rescue medication) and other efficacy parameters were assessed through at least 120 hours after administration of chemotherapy. The safety and efficacy of palonosetron in repeated courses of chemotherapy was also studied.
Moderately Emetogenic Chemotherapy
Two Phase 3, double-blind trials involving 1132 patients compared single-dose IV ALOXI with either single-dose IV ondansetron (study 1) or dolasetron (study 2) given 30 minutes prior to moderately emetogenic chemotherapy including carboplatin, cisplatin ≤ 50 mg/m^2, cyclophosphamide < 1500 mg/m^2, doxorubicin > 25 mg/m^2, epirubicin, irinotecan, and methotrexate > 250 mg/m^2. Concomitant corticosteroids were not administered prophylactically in study 1 and were only used by 4–6% of patients in study 2. The majority of patients in these studies were women (77%), White (65%) and naïve to previous chemotherapy (54%). The mean age was 55 years.
Highly Emetogenic Chemotherapy
A Phase 2, double-blind, dose-ranging study evaluated the efficacy of single-dose IV palonosetron from 0.3 to 90 μg/kg (equivalent to < 0.1 mg to 6 mg fixed dose) in 161 chemotherapy-naïve adult cancer patients receiving highly-emetogenic chemotherapy (either cisplatin ≥ 70 mg/m^2 or cyclophosphamide > 1100 mg/m^2). Concomitant corticosteroids were not administered prophylactically. Analysis of data from this trial indicates that 0.25 mg is the lowest effective dose in preventing acute nausea and vomiting induced by highly emetogenic chemotherapy.
A Phase 3, double-blind trial involving 667 patients compared single-dose IV ALOXI with single-dose IV ondansetron (study 3) given 30 minutes prior to highly emetogenic chemotherapy including cisplatin ≥ 60 mg/m^2, cyclophosphamide > 1500 mg/m^2, and dacarbazine. Corticosteroids were co-administered prophylactically before chemotherapy in 67% of patients. Of the 667 patients, 51% were women, 60% White, and 59% naïve to previous chemotherapy. The mean age was 52 years.

Efficacy Results

The antiemetic activity of ALOXI was evaluated during the acute phase (0-24 hours) [Table 1], delayed phase (24-120 hours) [Table 2], and overall phase (0-120 hours) [Table 3] post-chemotherapy in Phase 3 trials.

[See table 1 at top of previous page]

These studies show that ALOXI was effective in the prevention of acute nausea and vomiting associated with initial and repeat courses of moderately and highly emetogenic cancer chemotherapy. In study 3, efficacy was greater when prophylactic corticosteroids were administered concomitantly. Clinical superiority over other 5-HT3 receptor antagonists has not been adequately demonstrated in the acute phase.

[See table 2 at right]

These studies show that ALOXI was effective in the prevention of delayed nausea and vomiting associated with initial and repeat courses of moderately emetogenic chemotherapy.

[See table 3 at right]

These studies show that ALOXI was effective in the prevention of nausea and vomiting throughout the 120 hours (5 days) following initial and repeat courses of moderately emetogenic cancer chemotherapy.

INDICATIONS AND USAGE

ALOXI is indicated for:

1) the prevention of acute nausea and vomiting associated with initial and repeat courses of moderately and highly emetogenic cancer chemotherapy, and
2) the prevention of delayed nausea and vomiting associated with initial and repeat courses of moderately emetogenic cancer chemotherapy.

CONTRAINDICATIONS

ALOXI is contraindicated in patients known to have hypersensitivity to the drug or any of its components.

PRECAUTIONS

General

Hypersensitivity reactions may occur in patients who have exhibited hypersensitivity to other selective 5-HT_3 receptor antagonists.

Although palonosetron has been safely administered to 192 patients with pre-existing cardiac impairment in the Phase 3 studies, ALOXI should be administered with caution in patients who have or may develop prolongation of cardiac conduction intervals, particularly QTc. These include patients with hypokalemia or hypomagnesemia, patients taking diuretics with potential for inducing electrolyte abnormalities, patients with congenital QT syndrome, patients taking anti-arrhythmic drugs or other drugs which lead to QT prolongation, and cumulative high dose anthracycline therapy. In 3 pivotal trials, ECGs were obtained at baseline and 24 hours after subjects received palonosetron or a comparator drug. In a subset of patients ECGs were also obtained 15 minutes following dosing. The percentage of patients (< 1%) with changes in QT and QTc intervals (either absolute values of > 500 msec or changes of > 60 msec from baseline) was similar to that seen with the comparator drugs.

Drug Interactions

Palonosetron is eliminated from the body through both renal excretion and metabolic pathways. Therefore, the potential for clinically significant drug interactions with palonosetron appears to be low (See CLINICAL PHARMACOLOGY, Drug-Drug Interactions section).

Carcinogenesis, Mutagenesis, Impairment of Fertility

In a 104-week carcinogenicity study in CD-1 mice, animals were treated with oral doses of palonosetron at 10, 30 and 60 mg/kg/day. Treatment with palonosetron was not tumorigenic. The highest tested dose produced a systemic exposure to palonosetron (Plasma AUC) of about 150 to 289 times the human exposure (AUC= 29.8 ng•h/ml) at the recommended intravenous dose of 0.25 mg. In a 104-week carcinogenicity study in Sprague-Dawley rats, male and female rats were treated with oral doses of 15, 30 and 60 mg/kg/day and 15, 45 and 90 mg/kg/day, respectively. The highest doses produced a systemic exposure to palonosetron (Plasma AUC) of 137 and 308 times the human exposure at the recommended dose. Treatment with palonosetron produced increased incidences of adrenal benign pheochromocytoma and combined benign and malignant pheochromocytoma, increased incidences of pancreatic Islet cell adenoma and combined adenoma and carcinoma and pituitary adenoma in male rats. In female rats, it produced hepatocellular adenoma and carcinoma and increased the incidences of thyroid C-cell adenoma and combined adenoma and carcinoma.

Palonosetron was not genotoxic in the Ames test, the Chinese hamster ovarian cell (CHO/HGPRT) forward mutation test, the ex vivo hepatocyte unscheduled DNA synthesis (UDS) test or the mouse micronucleus test. It was, however, positive for clastogenic effects in the Chinese hamster ovarian (CHO) cell chromosomal aberration test.

Palonosetron at oral doses up to 60 mg/kg/day (about 1894 times the recommended human intravenous dose based on body surface area) was found to have no effect on fertility and reproductive performance of male and female rats.

Pregnancy. Teratogenic Effects: Category B

Teratology studies have been performed in rats at oral doses up to 60 mg/kg/day (1894 times the recommended human intravenous dose based on body surface area) and rabbits at oral doses up to 60 mg/kg/day (3789 times the recommended human intravenous dose based on body surface area) and have revealed no evidence of impaired fertility or harm to the fetus due to palonosetron. There are, however, no adequate and well-controlled studies in pregnant women. Because animal reproduction studies are not always predictive of human response, palonosetron should be used during pregnancy only if clearly needed.

Table 2: Prevention of Delayed Nausea and Vomiting (24-120 hours): Complete Response Rates

Chemo-therapy	Study	Treatment Group	N [a]	% with Complete Response	p-value [b]	97.5% Confidence Interval Aloxi minus Comparator [c]
Moderately Emetogenic	1	Aloxi 0.25 mg	189	74	<0.001	[8%, 30%]
		Ondansetron 32 mg IV	185	55		
	2	Aloxi 0.25 mg	189	54	0.004	[3%, 27%]
		Dolasetron 100 mg IV	191	39		

-10 -5 0 5 10 15 20 25 30 35
Difference in Complete Response Rates

a Intent-to-treat cohort
b 2-sided Fisher's exact test. Significance level at α=0.025.
c These studies were designed to show non-inferiority. A lower bound greater than –15% demonstrates non-inferiority between Aloxi and comparator.

Table 3: Prevention of Overall Nausea and Vomiting (0-120 hours): Complete Response Rates

Chemo-therapy	Study	Treatment Group	N [a]	% with Complete Response	p-value [b]	97.5% Confidence Interval Aloxi minus Comparator [c]
Moderately Emetogenic	1	Aloxi 0.25 mg	189	69	<0.001	[7%, 31%]
		Ondansetron 32 mg IV	185	50		
	2	Aloxi 0.25 mg	189	46	0.021	[0%, 24%]
		Dolasetron 100 mg IV	191	34		

-10 -5 0 5 10 15 20 25 30 35
Difference in Complete Response Rates

a Intent-to-treat cohort
b 2-sided Fisher's exact test. Significance level at α=0.025.
c These studies were designed to show non-inferiority. A lower bound greater than –15% demonstrates non-inferiority between Aloxi and comparator.

Table 4: Adverse Reactions from Chemotherapy-Induced Nausea and Vomiting Studies ≥ 2% in any Treatment Group

Event	ALOXI 0.25 mg (N=633)	Ondansetron 32 mg IV (N=410)	Dolasetron 100 mg IV (N=194)
Headache	60 (9%)	34 (8%)	32 (16%)
Constipation	29 (5%)	8 (2%)	12 (6%)
Diarrhea	8 (1%)	7 (2%)	4 (2%)
Dizziness	8 (1%)	9 (2%)	4 (2%)
Fatigue	3 (< 1%)	4 (1%)	4 (2%)
Abdominal Pain	1 (< 1%)	2 (< 1%)	3 (2%)
Insomnia	1 (< 1%)	3 (1%)	3 (2%)

Labor and Delivery

Palonosetron has not been administered to patients undergoing labor and delivery, so its effects on the mother or child are unknown.

Nursing Mothers

It is not known whether palonosetron is excreted in human milk. Because many drugs are excreted in human milk and because of the potential for serious adverse reactions in nursing infants and the potential for tumorigenicity shown for palonosetron in the rat carcinogenicity study, a decision should be made whether to discontinue nursing or to discontinue the drug, taking into account the importance of the drug to the mother.

Pediatric Use

Safety and effectiveness in patients below the age of 18 years have not been established.

Geriatric Use

Of the 1374 adult cancer patients in clinical studies of palonosetron, 316 (23%) were ≥ 65 years old, while 71 (5%) were ≥ 75 years old. No overall differences in safety or effectiveness were observed between these subjects and the younger subjects but greater sensitivity in some older individuals cannot be ruled out. No dose adjustments or special monitoring are required for geriatric patients.

ADVERSE REACTIONS

In clinical trials for the prevention of nausea and vomiting induced by moderately or highly emetogenic chemotherapy, 1374 adult patients received palonosetron. Adverse reactions were similar in frequency and severity with ALOXI and ondansetron or dolasetron. Following is a listing of all adverse reactions reported by ≥ 2% of patients in these trials (Table 4).

[See table 4 above]

In other studies, 2 subjects experienced severe constipation following a single palonosetron dose of approximately 0.75 mg, three times the recommended dose. One patient received a 10 μg/kg oral dose in a post-operative nausea and vomiting study and one healthy subject received a 0.75 mg IV dose in a pharmacokinetic study.

In clinical trials, the following infrequently reported adverse reactions, assessed by investigators as treatment-related or causality unknown, occurred following administration of ALOXI to adult patients receiving concomitant cancer chemotherapy:

Cardiovascular: 1%: non-sustained tachycardia, bradycardia, hypotension, < 1%: hypertension, myocardial ischemia, extrasystoles, sinus tachycardia, sinus arrhythmia, supraventricular extrasystoles and QT prolongation. In many cases, the relationship to ALOXI was unclear.

Dermatological: < 1%: allergic dermatitis, rash.

Hearing and Vision: < 1% motion sickness, tinnitus, eye irritation and amblyopia.

Gastrointestinal System: 1%: diarrhea, < 1%: dyspepsia, abdominal pain, dry mouth, hiccups and flatulence.

General: 1%: weakness, < 1%: fatigue, fever, hot flash, flu-like syndrome.

Liver: < 1%: transient, asymptomatic increases in AST and/or ALT and bilirubin. These changes occurred predominantly in patients receiving highly emetogenic chemotherapy.

Metabolic: 1%: hyperkalemia, < 1%: electrolyte fluctuations, hyperglycemia, metabolic acidosis, glycosuria, appetite decrease, anorexia.

Musculoskeletal: < 1%: arthralgia.

Nervous System: 1%: dizziness, < 1%: somnolence, insomnia, hypersomnia, paresthesia.

Psychiatric: 1%: anxiety, < 1%: euphoric mood.

Urinary System: < 1%: urinary retention.

Vascular: < 1%: vein discoloration, vein distention.

Continued on next page

Aloxi—Cont.

OVERDOSAGE

There is no known antidote to ALOXI. Overdose should be managed with supportive care. Fifty adult cancer patients were administered palonosetron at a dose of 90 µg/kg (equivalent to 6 mg fixed dose) as part of a dose ranging study. This is approximately 25 times the recommended dose of 0.25 mg. This dose group had a similar incidence of adverse events compared to the other dose groups and no dose response effects were observed. Dialysis studies have not been performed, however, due to the large volume of distribution, dialysis is unlikely to be an effective treatment for palonosetron overdose. A single intravenous dose of palonosetron at 30 mg/kg (947 and 474 times the human dose for rats and mice, respectively, based on body surface area) was lethal to rats and mice. The major signs of toxicity were convulsions, gasping, pallor, cyanosis and collapse.

DOSAGE AND ADMINISTRATION

Dosage for Adults

The recommended dosage of ALOXI is 0.25 mg administered as a single dose approximately 30 minutes before the start of chemotherapy. Repeated dosing of ALOXI™ within a seven day interval is not recommended because the safety and efficacy of frequent (consecutive or alternate day) dosing in patients has not been evaluated.

Use in Geriatric Patients and in Patients with Impaired Renal or Hepatic Function

No dosage adjustment is recommended.

Dosage for Pediatric Patients

A recommended intravenous dosage has not been established for pediatric patients.

Administration

ALOXI is to be infused intravenously over 30 seconds. ALOXI should not be mixed with other drugs. Flush the infusion line with normal saline before and after administration of ALOXI.

Stability

Parenteral drug products should be inspected visually for particulate matter and discoloration before administration, whenever solution and container permit.

HOW SUPPLIED

ALOXI (palonosetron hydrochloride), 0.25 mg (free base) in 5 ml, is supplied as a single-use sterile, clear, colorless solution in glass vials ready for intravenous injection.
Store at controlled temperature of 20-25°C (68°F-77°F). Excursions permitted to 15-30°C (59-86°F). Protect from freezing. Protect from light.
NDC Number 58063-797-25
Prescribing information as of July 2003
Mfd by Cardinal Health, Albuquerque, NM, USA and Helsinn Birex Pharmaceuticals, Dublin, Ireland
Mfd for Helsinn Healthcare SA, Switzerland
Distributed by MGI PHARMA, INC., Bloomington, MN, U.S.A.

HEXALEN® capsules ℞

[hĕx'-ă-lĕn]
(altretamine)
HEXALEN®
(altretamine)
CAPSULES 50 mg

> **WARNINGS**
> 1. **HEXALEN® should only be given under the supervision of a physician experienced in the use of antineoplastic agents.**
> 2. **Peripheral blood counts should be monitored at least monthly, prior to the initiation of each course of HEXALEN, and as clinically indicated (see Adverse Reactions).**
> 3. **Because of the possibility of HEXALEN-related neurotoxicity, neurologic examination should be performed regularly during HEXALEN administration (see Adverse Reactions).**

DESCRIPTION

HEXALEN (altretamine), is a synthetic cytotoxic antineoplastic s-triazine derivative. HEXALEN capsules contain 50 mg of altretamine for oral administration. Inert ingredients include lactose, anhydrous and calcium stearate. Altretamine, known chemically as N,N,N',N',N",N"-hexamethyl-1,3,5-triazine-2,4,6-triamine, has the following structural formula:

$(CH_3)_2N$ — $N(CH_3)_2$ — $N(CH_3)_2$

Its empirical formula is $C_9H_{18}N_6$ with a molecular weight of 210.28. Altretamine is a white crystalline powder, melting at 172° ± 1°C. Altretamine is practically insoluble in water but is increasingly soluble at pH 3 and below.

CLINICAL PHARMACOLOGY

The precise mechanism by which HEXALEN exerts its cytotoxic effect is unknown, although a number of theoretical possibilities have been studied. Structurally, HEXALEN resembles the alkylating agent triethylenemelamine, yet *in vitro* tests for alkylating activity of HEXALEN and its metabolites have been negative. HEXALEN has been demonstrated to be efficacious for certain ovarian tumors resistant to classical alkylating agents. Metabolism of altretamine is a requirement for cytotoxicity. Synthetic monohydroxymethylmelamines, and products of altretamine metabolism, *in vitro* and *in vivo*, can form covalent adducts with tissue macromolecules including DNA, but the relevance of these reactions to antitumor activity is unknown.
HEXALEN is well-absorbed following oral administration in humans, but undergoes rapid and extensive demethylation in the liver, producing variation in altretamine plasma levels. The principal metabolites are pentamethylmelamine and tetramethylmelamine.
Pharmacokinetic studies were performed in a limited number of patients and should be considered preliminary. After oral administration of HEXALEN to 11 patients with advanced ovarian cancer in doses of 120–300 mg/m^2, peak plasma levels (as measured by gas-chromatographic assay) were reached between 0.5 and 3 hours, varying from 0.2 to 20.8 mg/l. Half-life of the β-phase of elimination ranged from 4.7 to 10.2 hours. Altretamine and metabolites show binding to plasma proteins. The free fractions of altretamine, pentamethylmelamine and tetramethylmelamine are 6%, 25% and 50%, respectively.
Following oral administration of ^{14}C-ring-labeled altretamine (4 mg/kg), urinary recovery of radioactivity was 61% at 24 hours and 90% at 72 hours. Human urinary metabolites were N-demethylated homologues of altretamine with <1% unmetabolized altretamine excreted at 24 hours.
After intraperitoneal administration of ^{14}C-ring-labeled altretamine to mice, tissue distribution was rapid in all organs, reaching a maximum at 30 minutes. The excretory organs (liver and kidney) and the small intestine showed high concentrations of radioactivity, whereas relatively low concentrations were found in other organs, including the brain.
There have been no formal pharmacokinetic studies in patients with compromised hepatic and/or renal function, though HEXALEN has been administered both concurrently and following nephrotoxic drugs such as cisplatin.
HEXALEN (altretamine) has been administered in 4 divided doses, with meals and at bedtime, though there is no pharmacokinetic data on this schedule nor information from formal interaction studies about the effect of food on its bioavailability or pharmacokinetics.
In two studies in patients with persistent or recurrent ovarian cancer following first-line treatment with cisplatin and/or alkylating agent-based combinations, HEXALEN was administered as a single agent for 14 or 21 days of a 28 day cycle. In the 51 patients with measurable or evaluable disease, there were 6 clinical complete responses, 1 pathologic complete response, and 2 partial responses for an overall response rate of 18%. The duration of these responses ranged from 2 months in a patient with a palpable pelvic mass to 36 months in a patient who achieved a pathologic complete response. In some patients, tumor regression was associated with improvement in symptoms and performance status.

INDICATIONS AND USAGE

HEXALEN is indicated for use as a single agent in the palliative treatment of patients with persistent or recurrent ovarian cancer following first-line therapy with a cisplatin and/or alkylating agent-based combination.

CONTRAINDICATIONS

HEXALEN is contraindicated in patients who have shown hypersensitivity to it. HEXALEN should not be employed in patients with preexisting severe bone marrow depression or severe neurologic toxicity. HEXALEN has been administered safely, however, to patients heavily pretreated with cisplatin and/or akylating agents, including patients with preexisting cisplatin neuropathies. Careful monitoring of neurologic function in these patients is essential.

WARNINGS

See boxed Warnings.
Concurrent administration of HEXALEN and antidepressants of the monoamine oxidase (MAO) inhibitor class may cause severe orthostatic hypotension. Four patients, all over 60 years of age, were reported to have experienced symptomatic hypotension after 4 to 7 days of concomitant therapy with HEXALEN and MAO inhibitors.
HEXALEN causes mild to moderate myelosuppression and neurotoxicity. Blood counts and a neurologic examination should be performed prior to the initiation of each course of therapy and the dose of HEXALEN adjusted as clinically indicated (see Dosage and Administration).

Pregnancy: Category D

HEXALEN has been shown to be embryotoxic and teratogenic in rats and rabbits when given at doses 2 and 10 times the human dose. HEXALEN may cause fetal damage when administered to a pregnant woman. If HEXALEN is used during pregnancy, or if the patient becomes pregnant while taking the drug, the patient should be apprised of the potential hazard to the fetus. Women of childbearing potential should be advised to avoid becoming pregnant.

PRECAUTIONS

General

Neurologic examination should be performed regularly (see Adverse Reactions).

Laboratory Tests

Peripheral blood counts should be monitored at least monthly, prior to the initiation of each course of HEXALEN, and as clinically indicated (see Adverse Reactions).

Drug Interactions

Concurrent administration of HEXALEN and antidepressants of the MAO inhibitor class may cause severe orthostatic hypotension (see Warnings section). Cimetidine, an inhibitor of microsomal drug metabolism, increased altretamine's half-life and toxicity in a rat model.
Data from a randomized trial of HEXALEN and cisplatin plus or minus pyridoxine in ovarian cancer indicated that pyridoxine significantly reduced neurotoxicity; however, it adversely affected response duration suggesting that pyridoxine should not be administered with HEXALEN and/or cisplatin (1).

Carcinogenesis, Mutagenesis and Impairment of Fertility

The carcinogenic potential of HEXALEN has not been studied in animals, but drugs with similar mechanisms of action have been shown to be carcinogenic. HEXALEN was weakly mutagenic when tested in strain TA100 of *Salmonella typhimurium*. HEXALEN administered to female rats 14 days prior to breeding through the gestation period had no adverse effect on fertility, but decreased postnatal survival at 120 mg/m^2/day and was embryocidal at 240 m/m^2/day. Administration of 120 mg/m^2/day HEXALEN to male rats for 60 days prior to mating resulted in testicular atrophy, reduced fertility and a possible dominant lethal mutagenic effect. Male rats treated with HEXALEN at 450 mg/m^2/day for 10 days had decreased spermatogenesis, atrophy of testes, seminal vesicles and ventral prostate.

Pregnancy

Pregnancy Category D: see Warnings section.

Nursing Mothers

It is not known whether altretamine is excreted in human milk. Because there is a possibility of toxicity in nursing infants secondary to HEXALEN treatment of the mother, it is recommended that breast feeding be discontinued if the mother is treated with HEXALEN.

Pediatric Use

The safety and effectiveness of HEXALEN in children have not been established.

ADVERSE REACTIONS

Gastrointestinal

With continuous high-dose daily HEXALEN, nausea and vomiting of gradual onset occur frequently. Although in most instances these symptoms are controllable with antiemetics, at times the severity requires HEXALEN dose reduction or, rarely, discontinuation of HEXALEN therapy. In some instances, a tolerance of these symptoms develops after several weeks of therapy. The incidence and severity of nausea and vomiting are reduced with moderate-dose administration of HEXALEN. In 2 clinical studies of single-agent HEXALEN utilizing a moderate, intermittent dose and schedule, only 1 patient (1%) discontinued HEXALEN due to severe nausea and vomiting.

Neurotoxicity

Peripheral neuropathy and central nervous system symptoms (mood disorders, disorders of consciousness, ataxia, dizziness, vertigo) have been reported. They are more likely to occur in patients receiving continuous high-dose daily HEXALEN (altretamine) than moderate-dose HEXALEN administered on an intermittent schedule. Neurologic toxicity has been reported to be reversible when therapy is discontinued. Data from a randomized trial of HEXALEN and cisplatin plus or minus pyridoxine in ovarian cancer indicated that pyridoxine significantly reduced neurotoxicity; however, it adversely affected response duration suggesting that pyridoxine should not be administered with HEXALEN and/or cisplatin (1).

Hematologic

HEXALEN causes mild to moderate dose-related myelosuppression. Leukopenia below 3000 WBC/mm^3 occurred in <15% of patients on a variety of intermittent or continuous dose regimens. Less than 1% had leukopenia below 1000 WBC/mm^3. Thrombocytopenia below 50,000 platelets/mm^3 was seen in <10% of patients. When given in doses of 8–12 mg/kg/day over a 21 day course, nadirs of leukocyte and platelet counts were reached by 3–4 weeks, and normal counts were regained by 6 weeks. With continuous administration at doses of 6–8 mg/kg/day, nadirs are reached in 6–8 weeks (median).
Data in the following table are based on the experience of 76 patients with ovarian cancer previously treated with a cisplatin-based combination regimen who received single-agent HEXALEN. In one study, HEXALEN, 260 mg/m^2/day, was administered for 14 days of a 28 day cycle. In another study, HEXALEN, 6–8 mg/kg/day, was administered for 21 days of a 28 day cycle.

ADVERSE EXPERIENCES IN 76 PREVIOUSLY TREATED OVARIAN CANCER PATIENTS RECEIVING SINGLE-AGENT HEXALEN

Adverse Experiences	% Patients	
Gastrointestinal		
Nausea and Vomiting	33	
Mild to Moderate		32
Severe		1
Increased Alkaline Phosphatase	9	

Neurologic	
Peripheral Sensory Neuropathy	31
Mild	22
Moderate to Severe	9
Anorexia and Fatigue	1
Seizures	1
Hematologic	
Leukopenia	5
WBC 2000–2999/mm^3	4
WBC <2000/mm^3	1
Thrombocytopenia	9
Platelets 75,000–99,000/mm^3	6
Platelets <75,000/mm^3	3
Anemia	33
Mild	20
Moderate to Severe	13
Renal	
Serum Creatinine 1.6–3.75 mg/dl	7
BUN	9
25–40 mg%	5
41–60 mg%	3
>60 mg%	1

Additional adverse reaction information is available from 13 single-agent altretamine studies (total of 1014 patients) conducted under the auspices of the National Cancer Institute. The treated patients had a variety of tumors and many were heavily pretreated with other chemotherapies; most of these trials utilized high, continuous daily doses of altretamine (6–12 mg/kg/day). In general, adverse reaction experiences were similar in the two trials described above. Additional toxicities, not reported in the above table, included hepatic toxicity, skin rash, pruritus and alopecia, each occurring in <1% of patients.

OVERDOSAGE

No case of acute overdosage in humans has been described. The oral LD50 dose in rats was 1050 mg/kg and 437 mg/kg in mice.

DOSAGE AND ADMINISTRATION

HEXALEN (altretamine) is administered orally. Doses are calculated on the basis of body surface area.

HEXALEN may be administered either for 14 or 21 consecutive days in a 28 day cycle at a dose of 260 mg/m^2/day. The total daily dose should be given as 4 divided oral doses after meals and at bedtime. There is no pharmacokinetic information supporting this dosing regimen and the effect of food on HEXALEN bioavailability or pharmacokinetics has not been evaluated.

HEXALEN should be temporarily discontinued (for 14 days or longer) and subsequently restarted at 200 mg/m^2/day for any of the following situations:

1) Gastrointestinal intolerance unresponsive to symptomatic measures;
2) White blood count <2000/mm^3 or granulocyte count <1000/mm^3;
3) Platelet count <75,000/mm^3;
4) Progressive neurotoxicity.

If neurologic symptoms fail to stabilize on the reduced dose schedule, HEXALEN should be discontinued indefinitely.

Procedures to proper handling and disposal of anticancer drugs should be considered. Several guidelines on this subject have been published (2–8). There is no general agreement that all of the procedures recommended in the guidelines are necessary or appropriate.

HOW SUPPLIED

HEXALEN is available in 50 mg clear, hard gelatin capsules imprinted with the following inscription: USB 001.

Bottles of 100 capsules (NDC 58063-0001-70)

Store at controlled room temperature 15° to 30°C (59° to 86°F).

REFERENCES

1. Wiernik PH, et al. Hexamethylmelamine and Low or Moderate Dose Cisplatin With or Without Pyridoxine for Treatment of Advanced Ovarian Carcinoma: A Study of the Eastern Cooperative Oncology Group. *Cancer Investigation* 10(1): 1–9, 1992.
2. ONS Clinical Practice Committee. Cancer Chemotherapy Guidelines and Recommendations for Practice. Pittsburgh, Pa: Oncology Nursing Society; 1999:32–41.
3. Recommendations for the Safe Handling of Cytotoxic Drugs. NIH Publication 92-2621. NIH: Division of Safety, Clinical Center Pharmacy Department and Cancer Nursing Service, 1992. U.S. Department of Health and Human Services, Public Health Service, National Institutes of Health.
4. AMA Council on Scientific Affairs. Guidelines for Handling Parenteral Antineoplastics. *Journal of the American Medical Association* 1985;253:1590–1591.
5. National Study Commission on Cytotoxic Exposure. Recommendations for Handling Cytotoxic Agents, 1987. Available from Louis P. Jeffrey, Chairman, National Study Commission on Cytotoxic Exposure. Massachusetts College of Pharmacy and Allied Health Sciences, 179 Longwood Avenue, Boston, MA 02115.
6. Clinical Oncological Society of Australia. Guidelines and Recommendations for Safe Handling of Antineoplastic Agents. *Medical Journal of Australia* 1983;1:426–428.
7. Jones RB, Frank R, Mass T. Safe Handling of Chemotherapeutic Agents: A Report from the Mount Sinai Medical Center.—*A Cancer Journal for Clinicians* 1983;33:258–263.
8. American Society of Hospital Pharmacists. ASHP Technical Assistance Bulletin on Handling Cytotoxic and Hazardous Drugs. *Am J of Hosp Pharm_* 1990;47:1033–1049.
9. Controlling Occupational Exposure to Hazardous Drugs. (OSHA Work Practice Guidelines). *Am J of Health Syst Pharm.* 1996;53:1669–1685.

Revised SEPTEMBER 2001

Manufactured for:
MGI®
PHARMA
MGI PHARMA, INC.
Bloomington, MN 55437

SALAGEN® TABLETS ℞

[sal' ə jen]
(pilocarpine hydrochloride)

DESCRIPTION

SALAGEN® Tablets contain pilocarpine hydrochloride, a cholinergic agonist for oral use. Pilocarpine hydrochloride is a hygroscopic, odorless, bitter tasting white crystal or powder which is soluble in water and alcohol and virtually insoluble in most non-polar solvents. Pilocarpine hydrochloride, with a chemical name of (3*S*-*cis*)-2(3*H*)-Furanone, 3-ethyldihydro-4-[(1-methyl-1*H*-imidazol-5-yl)methyl] monohydrochloride, has a molecular weight of 244.72.

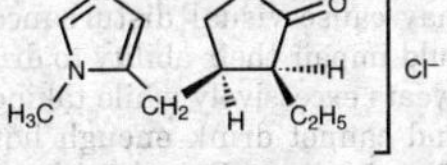

Each 5 mg SALAGEN® Tablet for oral administration contains 5 mg of pilocarpine hydrochloride. Inactive ingredients in the tablet, the tablet's film coating, and polishing are: carnauba wax, hydroxypropyl methylcellulose, microcrystalline cellulose, stearic acid, titanium dioxide and other ingredients.

Each 7.5 mg SALAGEN® Tablet for oral administration contains 7.5 mg of pilocarpine hydrochloride. Inactive ingredients in the tablet, the tablet's film coating, and polishing are: carnauba wax, hydroxypropyl methylcellulose, microcrystalline cellulose, stearic acid, titanium dioxide, FD&C blue #2 aluminum lake, and other ingredients.

CLINICAL PHARMACOLOGY

Pharmacodynamics: Pilocarpine is a cholinergic parasympathomimetic agent exerting a broad spectrum of pharmacologic effects with predominant muscarinic action. Pilocarpine, in appropriate dosage, can increase secretion by the exocrine glands. The sweat, salivary, lacrimal, gastric, pancreatic, and intestinal glands and the mucous cells of the respiratory tract may be stimulated. When applied topically to the eye as a single dose it causes miosis, spasm of accommodation, and may cause a transitory rise in intraocular pressure followed by a more persistent fall. Dose-related smooth muscle stimulation of the intestinal tract may cause increased tone, increased motility, spasm, and tenesmus. Bronchial smooth muscle tone may increase. The tone and motility of urinary tract, gallbladder, and biliary duct smooth muscle may be enhanced. Pilocarpine may have paradoxical effects on the cardiovascular system. The expected effect of a muscarinic agonist is vasodepression, but administration of pilocarpine may produce hypertension after a brief episode of hypotension. Bradycardia and tachycardia have both been reported with use of pilocarpine.

In a study of 12 healthy male volunteers there was a dose-related increase in unstimulated salivary flow following single 5 and 10 mg oral doses of SALAGEN® Tablets. This effect of pilocarpine on salivary flow was time-related with an onset at 20 minutes and a peak effect at 1 hour with a duration of 3 to 5 hours (See **Pharmacokinetics** section).

Head & Neck Cancer Patients: In a 12 week randomized, double-blind, placebo-controlled study in 207 patients (placebo, N=65; 5 mg, N=73; 10 mg, N=69), increases from baseline (means 0.072 and 0.112 mL/min, ranges -0.690 to 0.728 and -0.380 to 1.689) of whole saliva flow for the 5 mg (63%) and 10 mg (90%) tablet, respectively, were seen 1 hour after the first dose of SALAGEN® Tablets. Increases in unstimulated parotid flow were seen following the first dose (means 0.025 and 0.046 mL/min, ranges 0 to 0.414 and -0.070 to 1.002 mL/min for the 5 and 10 mg dose, respectively). In this study, no correlation existed between the amount of increase in salivary flow and the degree of symptomatic relief.

Sjogren's Syndrome Patients: In two 12 week randomized, double-blind, placebo-controlled studies in 629 patients (placebo, N=253; 2.5 mg, N=121; 5 mg, N=255; 5-7.5 mg, N=114), the ability of SALAGEN® Tablets to stimulate saliva production was assessed. In these trials using varying doses of SALAGEN® Tablets (2.5-7.5 mg), the rate of saliva production was plotted against time. An Area Under the Curve (AUC) representing the total amount of saliva produced during the observation interval was calculated. Relative to placebo, an increase in the amount of saliva being produced was observed following the first dose of SALAGEN® Tablets and was maintained throughout the duration (12 weeks) of the trials in an approximate dose response fashion (See **Clinical Studies** section).

Pharmacokinetics: In a multiple-dose pharmacokinetic study in male volunteers following 2 days of 5 or 10 mg of oral pilocarpine hydrochloride tablets given at 8 a.m., noontime, and 6 p.m., the mean elimination half-life was 0.76 hours for the 5 mg dose and 1.35 hours for the 10 mg dose. T_{max} values were 1.25 hours and 0.85 hours. C_{max} values were 15 ng/mL and 41 ng/mL. The AUC trapezoidal values were 33 h(ng/mL) and 108 h(ng/mL), respectively, for the 5 and 10 mg doses following the last 6 hour dose.

Pharmacokinetics in elderly male volunteers (N=11) were comparable to those in younger men. In five healthy elderly female volunteers, the mean C_{max} and AUC were approximately twice that of elderly males and young normal male volunteers.

When taken with a high fat meal by 12 healthy male volunteers, there was a decrease in the rate of absorption of pilocarpine from SALAGEN® Tablets. Mean $T_{max's}$ were 1.47 and 0.87 hours, and mean $C_{max's}$ were 51.8 and 59.2 ng/mL for fed and fasted, respectively.

Limited information is available about the metabolism and elimination of pilocarpine in humans. Inactivation of pilocarpine is thought to occur at neuronal synapses and probably in plasma. Pilocarpine and its minimally active or inactive degradation products, including pilocarpic acid, are excreted in the urine. Pilocarpine does not bind to human or rat plasma proteins over a concentration range of 5 to 25,000 ng/mL. The effect of pilocarpine on plasma protein binding of other drugs has not been evaluated.

In patients with mild to moderate hepatic impairment (N=12), administration of a single 5 mg dose resulted in a 30% decrease in total plasma clearance and a doubling of exposure (as measured by AUC). Peak plasma levels were also increased by about 30% and half-life was increased to 2.1 hrs.

There were no significant differences in the pharmacokinetics of oral pilocarpine in volunteer subjects (N=8) with renal insufficiency (mean creatinine clearances 25.4 mL/min; range 9.8-40.8 mL/min) compared to the pharmacokinetics previously observed in normal volunteers.

CLINICAL STUDIES

Head & Neck Cancer Patients: A 12 week randomized, double-blind, placebo-controlled study in 207 patients (142 men, 65 women) was conducted in patients whose mean age was 58.5 years with a range of 19 to 77; the racial distribution was Caucasian 95%, Black 4%, and other 1%. In this population, a statistically significant improvement in mouth dryness occurred in the 5 and 10 mg SALAGEN® Tablet treated patients compared to placebo treated patients. The 5 and 10 mg treated patients could not be distinguished. (See **Pharmacodynamics** section for flow study details.)

Another 12 week, double-blind, randomized, placebo-controlled study was conducted in 162 patients whose mean age was 57.8 years with a range of 27 to 80; the racial distribution was Caucasian 88%, Black 10%, and other 2%. The effects of placebo were compared to 2.5 mg three times a day of SALAGEN® Tablets for 4 weeks followed by adjustment to 5 mg three times a day and 10 mg three times a day. Lowering of the dose was necessary because of adverse events in 3 of 67 patients treated with 5 mg of SALAGEN® Tablets and in 7 of 66 patients treated with 10 mg of SALAGEN® Tablets. After 4 weeks of treatment, 2.5 mg of SALAGEN® Tablets three times a day was comparable to placebo in relieving dryness. In patients treated with 5 mg and 10 mg of SALAGEN® Tablets, the greatest improvement in dryness was noted in patients with no measurable salivary flow at baseline.

In both studies, some patients noted improvement in the global assessment of their dry mouth, speaking without liquids, and a reduced need for supplemental oral comfort agents.

In the two placebo-controlled clinical trials, the most common adverse events related to drug, and increasing in rate as dose increases, were sweating, nausea, rhinitis, diarrhea, chills, flushing, urinary frequency, dizziness, and asthenia. The most common adverse experience causing withdrawal from treatment was sweating (5 mg t.i.d. ≤1%; 10 mg t.i.d. =12%).

Sjogren's Syndrome Patients: Two separate studies were conducted in patients with primary or secondary Sjogren's Syndrome. In both studies, the majority of patients best fit the European criteria for having primary Sjogren's Syndrome. ["Criteria for the Classification of Sjogren's Syndrome" (Vitali C, Bombardieri S, Moutsopoulos HM, et al: Preliminary criteria for the classification of Sjogren's Syndrome. *Arthritis Rheum.* 1993;36:340-347.)]

A 12-week, randomized, double-blind, parallel-group, placebo-controlled study was conducted in 256 patients (14 men, 242 women) whose mean age was 57 years with a range of 24 to 85 years. The racial distribution was as follows: Caucasian 91%, Black 6%, and other 3%.

The effects of placebo were compared with those of SALAGEN® Tablets 5 mg four times a day (20 mg/day) for 6 weeks. At 6 weeks, the patients' dosage was increased from 5 mg SALAGEN® Tablets q.i.d. to 7.5 mg q.i.d. The data collected during the first 6 weeks of the trial were evaluated for safety and efficacy, and the data of the second 6 weeks of the trial were used to provide additional evidence of safety. After 6 weeks of treatment, statistically significant global improvement of dry mouth was observed compared to pla-

Continued on next page

Salagen—Cont.

cebo. "Global improvement" is defined as a score of 55 mm or more on a 100 mm visual analogue scale in response to the question, "Please rate your present condition of dry mouth (xerostomia) compared with your condition at the start of this study. Consider the changes to your dry mouth and other symptoms related to your dry mouth that have occurred since you have taken this medication." Patients' assessments of specific dry mouth symptoms such as severity of dry mouth, mouth discomfort, ability to speak without water, ability to sleep without drinking water, ability to swallow food without drinking, and a decreased use of saliva substitutes were found to be consistent with the significant global improvement described.

Another 12 week randomized, double-blind, parallel-group, placebo-controlled study was conducted in 373 patients (16 men, 357 women) whose mean age was 55 years with a range of 21 to 84. The racial distribution was Caucasian 80%, Oriental 14%, Black 2%, and 4% of other origin. The treatment groups were 2.5 mg pilocarpine tablets, 5 mg SALAGEN® Tablets, and placebo. All treatments were administered on a four times a day regimen.

After 12 weeks of treatment, statistically significant global improvement of dry mouth was observed at a dose of 5 mg compared with placebo. The 2.5 mg (10mg/day) group was not significantly different than placebo. However, a subgroup of patients with rheumatoid arthritis tended to improve in global assessments at both the 2.5 mg q.i.d. (9 patients) and 5 mg q.i.d. (16 patients) dose (10-20 mg/day). The clinical significance of this finding is unknown.

Patients' assessments of specific dry mouth symptoms such as severity of dry mouth, mouth discomfort, ability to sleep without drinking water, and decreased use of saliva substitutes were also found to be consistent with the significant global improvement described when measured after 6 weeks and 12 weeks of SALAGEN® Tablets use.

INDICATIONS AND USAGE

SALAGEN® Tablets are indicated for 1) the treatment of symptoms of dry mouth from salivary gland hypofunction caused by radiotherapy for cancer of the head and neck; and 2) the treatment of symptoms of dry mouth in patients with Sjogren's Syndrome.

CONTRAINDICATIONS

SALAGEN® Tablets are contraindicated in patients with uncontrolled asthma, known hypersensitivity to pilocarpine, and when miosis is undesirable, e.g., in acute iritis and in narrow-angle (angle closure) glaucoma.

WARNINGS

Cardiovascular Disease: Patients with significant cardiovascular disease may be unable to compensate for transient changes in hemodynamics or rhythm induced by pilocarpine. Pulmonary edema has been reported as a complication of pilocarpine toxicity from high ocular doses given for acute angle-closure glaucoma. Pilocarpine should be administered with caution in and under close medical supervision of patients with significant cardiovascular disease.

Ocular: Ocular formulations of pilocarpine have been reported to cause visual blurring which may result in decreased visual acuity, especially at night and in patients with central lens changes, and to cause impairment of depth perception. Caution should be advised while driving at night or performing hazardous activities in reduced lighting.

Pulmonary Disease: Pilocarpine has been reported to increase airway resistance, bronchial smooth muscle tone, and bronchial secretions. Pilocarpine hydrochloride should be administered with caution to and under close medical supervision in patients with controlled asthma, chronic bronchitis, or chronic obstructive pulmonary disease requiring pharmacotherapy.

PRECAUTIONS

General: Pilocarpine toxicity is characterized by an exaggeration of its parasympathomimetic effects. These may include: headache, visual disturbance, lacrimation, sweating, respiratory distress, gastrointestinal spasm, nausea, vomiting, diarrhea, atrioventricular block, tachycardia, bradycardia, hypotension, hypertension, shock, mental confusion, cardiac arrhythmia, and tremors.

The dose-related cardiovascular pharmacologic effects of pilocarpine include hypotension, hypertension, bradycardia, and tachycardia.

Pilocarpine should be administered with caution to patients with known or suspected cholelithiasis or biliary tract disease. Contractions of the gallbladder or biliary smooth muscle could precipitate complications including cholecystitis, cholangitis, and biliary obstruction.

Pilocarpine may increase ureteral smooth muscle tone and could theoretically precipitate renal colic (or "ureteral reflux"), particularly in patients with nephrolithiasis.

Cholinergic agonists may have dose-related central nervous system effects. This should be considered when treating patients with underlying cognitive or psychiatric disturbances.

Hepatic Insufficiency: Based on decreased plasma clearance observed in patients with moderate hepatic impairment, the starting dose in these patients should be 5 mg twice daily, followed by adjustment based on therapeutic response and tolerability. Patients with mild hepatic insufficiency (Child-Pugh score of 5-6) do not require dosage reductions. To date, pharmacokinetic studies in subjects with severe hepatic impairment (Child-Pugh score of 10-15) have not been carried out. The use of pilocarpine in these patients is not recommended.

Child-Pugh scoring system for Hepatic impairment

Clinical and Biochemical Measurements	Points Scored for Increasing Abnormality		
	1	2	3
Encephalopathy (grade)*	None	1 and 2	3 and 4
Ascites	Absent	Slight	Moderate
Bilirubin (mg. per 100 mL)	1-2	2-3	>3
Albumin (g. per 100 mL)	3-5	2.8-3.5	<2.8
Prothrombin Time (sec. Prolonged)	1-4	4-6	>6
For Primary Biliary Cirrhosis:- Bilirubin (mg. per 100 mL)	1-4	4-10	>10

*According to grading of Trey C, Burns D, and Saunders S. Treatment of hepatic coma by exchange blood transfusion. *N Engl J Med.* 1966;274:473-481.

Reference: Pugh, RNH, Murray-Lyon IM, Dawson JL, Pietroni, MC, Williams R. Transection of the oesophagus for bleeding oesophageal varices. *Brit J Surg.* 1973;60:646-9.

Information for Patients: Patients should be informed that pilocarpine may cause visual disturbances, especially at night, that could impair their ability to drive safely.

If a patient sweats excessively while taking pilocarpine hydrochloride and cannot drink enough liquid, the patient should consult a physician. Dehydration may develop.

Drug Interactions: Pilocarpine should be administered with caution to patients taking beta-adrenergic antagonists because of the possibility of conduction disturbances. Drugs with parasympathomimetic effects administered concurrently with pilocarpine would be expected to result in additive pharmacologic effects. Pilocarpine might antagonize the anticholinergic effects of drugs used concomitantly. These effects should be considered when anticholinergic properties may be contributing to the therapeutic effect of concomitant medication (e.g., atropine, inhaled ipratropium).

While no formal drug interaction studies have been performed, the following concomitant drugs were used in at least 10% of patients in either or both Sjogren's efficacy studies: acetylsalicylic acid, artificial tears, calcium, conjugated estrogens, hydroxychloroquine sulfate, ibuprofen, levothyroxine sodium, medroxyprogesterone acetate, methotrexate, multivitamins, naproxen, omeprazole, paracetamol, and prednisone.

Carcinogenesis, Mutagenesis, Impairment of Fertility: Lifetime oral carcinogenicity studies were conducted in CD-1 mice and Sprague-Dawley rats. Pilocarpine did not induce tumors in mice at any dosage studied (up to 30 mg/kg/day, which yielded a systemic exposure approximately 50 times larger than the maximum systemic exposure observed clinically). In rats, a dosage of 18 mg/kg/day, which yielded a systemic exposure approximately 100 times larger than the maximum systemic exposure observed clinically, resulted in a statistically significant increase in the incidence of benign pheochromocytomas in both males and females, and a statistically significant increase in the incidence of hepatocellular adenomas in female rats. The tumorigenicity observed in rats was observed only at a large multiple of the maximum labeled clinical dose, and may not be relevant to clinical use.

No evidence that pilocarpine has the potential to cause genetic toxicity was obtained in a series of studies that included: 1) bacterial assays (*Salmonella* and *E. coli*) for reverse gene mutations; 2) an *in vitro* chromosome aberration assay in a Chinese hamster ovary cell line; 3) an *in vitro* chromosome aberration assay (micronucleus test) in mice; and 4) a primary DNA damage assay (unscheduled DNA synthesis) in rat hepatocyte primary cultures.

Oral administration of pilocarpine to male and female rats at a dosage of 18 mg/kg/day, which yielded a systemic exposure approximately 100 times larger than the maximum systemic exposure observed clinically, resulted in impaired reproductive function, including reduced fertility, decreased sperm motility, and morphologic evidence of abnormal sperm. It is unclear whether the reduction in fertility was due to effects on male animals, female animals, or both males and females. In dogs, exposure to pilocarpine at a dosage of 3 mg/kg/day (approximately 3 times the maximum recommended human dose when compared on the basis of body surface area (mg/m^2) estimates) for six months resulted in evidence of impaired spermatogenesis. The data obtained in these studies suggest that pilocarpine may impair the fertility of male and female humans. SALAGEN® Tablets should be administered to individuals who are attempting to conceive a child only if the potential benefit justifies potential impairment of fertility.

Pregnancy: Teratogenic Effects

Pregnancy Category C: Pilocarpine was associated with a reduction in the mean fetal body weight and an increase in the incidence of skeletal variations when given to pregnant rats at a dosage of 90 mg/kg/day (approximately 26 times the maximum recommended dose for a 50 kg human when compared on the basis of body surface area (mg/m^2) estimates). These effects may have been secondary to maternal toxicity. In another study, oral administration of pilocarpine to female rats during gestation and lactation at a dosage of 36 mg/kg/day (approximately 10 times the maximum recommended dose for a 50 kg human when compared on the basis of body surface area (mg/m^2) estimates) resulted in an increased incidence of stillbirths; decreased neonatal survival and reduced mean body weight of pups were observed at dosages of 18 mg/kg/day (approximately 5 times the maximum recommended dose for a 50 kg human when compared on the basis of body surface area (mg/m^2) estimates) and above. There are no adequate and well-controlled studies in pregnant women. SALAGEN® Tablets should be used during pregnancy only if the potential benefit justifies the potential risk to the fetus.

Nursing Mothers: It is not known whether this drug is excreted in human milk. Because many drugs are excreted in human milk and because of the potential for serious adverse reactions in nursing infants from SALAGEN® Tablets, a decision should be made whether to discontinue nursing or to discontinue the drug, taking into account the importance of the drug to the mother.

Pediatric Use: Safety and effectiveness in pediatric patients have not been established.

Geriatric Use: Head & Neck Cancer Patients: In the placebo-controlled clinical trials (See **Clinical Studies** section) the mean age of patients was approximately 58 years (range 19 to 80). Of these patients, 97/369 (61/217 receiving pilocarpine) were over the age of 65 years. In the healthy volunteer studies, 15/150 subjects were over the age of 65 years. In both study populations, the adverse events reported by those over 65 years and those 65 years and younger were comparable. Of the 15 elderly volunteers (5 women, 10 men), the 5 women had higher $C_{max's}$ and AUC's than the men. (See **Pharmacokinetics** section.)

Sjogren's Syndrome Patients: In the placebo-controlled clinical trials (See **Clinical Studies** section), the mean age of patients was approximately 55 years (range 21 to 85). The adverse events reported by those over 65 years and those 65 years and younger were comparable except for notable trends for urinary frequency, diarrhea, and dizziness (See **ADVERSE REACTIONS** section).

ADVERSE REACTIONS

Head & Neck Cancer Patients: In controlled studies, 217 patients received pilocarpine, of whom 68% were men and 32% were women. Race distribution was 91% Caucasian, 8% Black, and 1% of other origin. Mean age was approximately 58 years. The majority of patients were between 50 and 64 years (51%), 33% were 65 years and older and 16% were younger than 50 years of age.

The most frequent adverse experiences associated with SALAGEN® Tablets were a consequence of the expected pharmacologic effects of pilocarpine.

Adverse Event	Pilocarpine HCl 10 mg t.i.d. (30 mg/day) N=121	Pilocarpine HCl 5 mg t.i.d. (15 mg/day) N=141	Placebo (t.i.d.) N=152
Sweating	68%	29%	9%
Nausea	15	6	4
Rhinitis	14	5	7
Diarrhea	7	4	5
Chills	15	3	<1
Flushing	13	8	3
Urinary Frequency	12	9	7
Dizziness	12	5	4
Asthenia	12	6	3

In addition, the following adverse events (≥3% incidence) were reported at dosages of 15-30 mg/day in the controlled clinical trials:

Adverse Event	Pilocarpine HCl 5-10 mg t.i.d. (15-30 mg/day) N=212	Placebo (t.i.d.) N=152
Headache	11%	8%
Dyspepsia	7	5
Lacrimation	6	8
Edema	5	4
Abdominal Pain	4	4
Amblyopia	4	2

Vomiting	4	1
Pharyngitis	3	8
Hypertension	3	1

The following events were reported with treated head and neck cancer patients at incidences of 1% to 2% at dosages of 7.5 to 30 mg/day: abnormal vision, conjunctivitis, dysphagia, epistaxis, myalgias, pruritus, rash, sinusitis, tachycardia, taste perversion, tremor, voice alteration.

The following events were reported rarely in treated head and neck cancer patients (<1%):

Causal relation is unknown.

Body as a whole: body odor, hypothermia, mucous membrane abnormality

Cardiovascular: bradycardia, ECG abnormality, palpitations, syncope

Digestive: anorexia, increased appetite, esophagitis, gastrointestinal disorder, tongue disorder

Hematologic: leukopenia, lymphadenopathy

Nervous: anxiety, confusion, depression, abnormal dreams, hyperkinesia, hypesthesia, nervousness, paresthesias, speech disorder, twitching

Respiratory: increased sputum, stridor, yawning

Skin: seborrhea

Special senses: deafness, eye pain, glaucoma

Urogenital: dysuria, metrorrhagia, urinary impairment

In long-term treatment were two patients with underlying cardiovascular disease of whom one experienced a myocardial infarct and another an episode of syncope. The association with drug is uncertain.

Sjogren's Syndrome Patients: In controlled studies, 376 patients received pilocarpine, of whom 5% were men and 95% were women. Race distribution was 84% Caucasian, 9% Oriental, 3% Black, and 4% of other origin. Mean age was 55 years. The majority of patients were between 40 and 69 years (70%), 16% were 70 years and older and 14% were younger than 40 years of age. Of these patients, 161/629 (89/376 receiving pilocarpine) were over the age of 65 years. The adverse events reported by those over 65 years and those 65 years and younger were comparable except for notable trends for urinary frequency, diarrhea, and dizziness. The incidences of urinary frequency and diarrhea in the elderly were about double those of the non-elderly. The incidence of dizziness was about three times as high in the elderly as in the non-elderly. These adverse experiences were not considered to be serious. In the 2 placebo-controlled studies, the most common adverse events related to drug use were sweating, urinary frequency, chills, and vasodilatation (flushing). The most commonly reported reason for patient discontinuation of treatment was sweating. Expected pharmacologic effects of pilocarpine include the following adverse experiences associated with SALAGEN® Tablets:

Adverse Event	Pilocarpine HCl 5 mg q.i.d. (20 mg/day) N=255	Placebo (q.i.d.) N=253
Sweating	40%	7%
Urinary Frequency	10	4
Nausea	9	9
Flushing	9	2
Rhinitis	7	8
Diarrhea	6	7
Chills	4	2
Increased Salivation	3	0
Asthenia	2	2

In addition, the following adverse events (≥3% incidence) were reported at dosages of 20 mg/day in the controlled clinical trials:

Adverse Event	Pilocarpine HCl 5 mg q.i.d. (20 mg/day) N=255	Placebo (q.i.d.) N=253
Headache	13%	19%
Flu Syndrome	9	9
Dyspepsia	7	7
Dizziness	6	7
Pain	4	2
Sinusitis	4	5
Abdominal Pain	3	4
Vomiting	3	1
Pharyngitis	2	5
Rash	2	3
Infection	2	6

The following events were reported in Sjogren's patients at incidences of 1% to 2% at dosing of 20 mg/day: accidental injury, allergic reaction, back pain, blurred vision, constipation, increased cough, edema, epistaxis, face edema, fever, flatulence, glossitis, lab test abnormalities, including chemistry, hematology, and urinalysis, myalgia, palpitation, pruritus, somnolence, stomatitis, tachycardia, tinnitus, urinary incontinence, urinary tract infection, and vaginitis.

The following events were reported rarely in treated Sjogren's patients (<1%) at dosing of 10-30 mg/day: Causal relation is unknown.

Body as a whole: chest pain, cyst, death, moniliasis, neck pain, neck rigidity, photosensitivity reaction

Cardiovascular: angina pectoris, arrhythmia, ECG abnormality, hypotension, hypertension, intracranial hemorrhage, migraine, myocardial infarction

Digestive: anorexia, bilirubinemia, cholelithiasis, colitis, dry mouth, eructation, gastritis, gastroenteritis, gastrointestinal disorder, gingivitis, hepatitis, abnormal liver function tests, melena, nausea & vomiting, pancreatitis, parotid gland enlargement, salivary gland enlargement, sputum increased, taste loss, tongue disorder, tooth disorder

Hematologic: hematuria, lymphadenopathy, abnormal platelets, thrombocythemia, thrombocytopenia, thrombosis, abnormal WBC

Metabolic and Nutritional: peripheral edema, hypoglycemia

Musculoskeletal: arthralgia, arthritis, bone disorder, spontaneous bone fracture, pathological fracture, myasthenia, tendon disorder, tenosynovitis

Nervous: aphasia, confusion, depression, abnormal dreams, emotional lability, hyperkinesia, hypesthesia, insomnia, leg cramps, nervousness, parethesias, abnormal thinking, tremor

Respiratory: bronchitis, dyspnea, hiccup, laryngismus, laryngitis, pneumonia, viral infection, voice alteration

Skin: alopecia, contact dermatitis, dry skin, eczema, erythema nodosum, exfoliative dermatitis, herpes simplex, skin ulcer, vesiculobullous rash

Special Senses: cataract, conjunctivitis, dry eyes, ear disorder, ear pain, eye disorder, eye hemorrhage, glaucoma, lacrimation disorder, retinal disorder, taste perversion, abnormal vision

Urogenital: breast pain, dysuria, mastitis, menorrhagia, metrorrhagia, ovarian disorder, pyuria, salpingitis, urethral pain, urinary urgency, vaginal hemorrhage, vaginal moniliasis

The following adverse experiences have been reported rarely with ocular pilocarpine: A-V block, agitation, ciliary congestion, confusion, delusion, depression, dermatitis, middle ear disturbance, eyelid twitching, malignant glaucoma, iris cysts, macular hole, shock, and visual hallucination.

MANAGEMENT OF OVERDOSE: Fatal overdosage with pilocarpine has been reported in the scientific literature at doses presumed to be greater than 100 mg in two hospitalized patients. 100 mg of pilocarpine is considered potentially fatal. Overdosage should be treated with atropine titration (0.5 mg to 1.0 mg given subcutaneously or intravenously) and supportive measures to maintain respiration and circulation. Epinephrine (0.3 mg to 1.0 mg, subcutaneously or intramuscularly) may also be of value in the presence of severe cardiovascular depression or bronchoconstriction. It is not known if pilocarpine is dialyzable.

DOSAGE AND ADMINISTRATION

Regardless of the indication, the starting dose in patients with moderate hepatic impairment should be 5 mg twice daily, followed by adjustment based on therapeutic response and tolerability. Patients with mild hepatic insufficiency do not require dosage reductions. The use of pilocarpine in patients with severe hepatic insufficiency is not recommended. If needed, refer to the *Hepatic Insufficiency* subsection of the **Precautions** section of this label for definitions of mild, moderate and severe hepatic impairment.

Head & Neck Cancer Patients: The recommended initial dose of SALAGEN® Tablets is 5 mg taken three times a day. Dosage should be titrated according to therapeutic response and tolerance. The usual dosage range is up to 15-30 mg per day. (Not to exceed 10 mg per dose.) Although early improvement may be realized, at least 12 weeks of uninterrupted therapy with SALAGEN® Tablets may be necessary to assess whether a beneficial response will be achieved. The incidence of the most common adverse events increases with dose. The lowest dose that is tolerated and effective should be used for maintenance.

Sjogren's Syndrome Patients: The recommended dose of SALAGEN® Tablets is 5 mg taken four times a day. Efficacy was established by 6 weeks of use.

HOW SUPPLIED

SALAGEN® Tablets, 5 mg, are white, film coated, debossed round tablets, coded SAL 5. Each tablet contains 5 mg pilocarpine hydrochloride. They are supplied as follows:

NDC 58063-705-10 bottles of 100

Store up to 25°C (77°F); excursions permitted to 15°-30°C (59°-86°F).

SALAGEN® Tablets, 7.5 mg, are blue, film coated, debossed round tablets, coded SAL 7.5. Each tablet contains 7.5 mg pilocarpine hydrochloride. They are supplied as follows:

NDC 58063-775-10 bottles of 100

Store up to 25°C (77°F); excursions permitted to 15°-30°C (59°-86°F).

Manufactured by: IN-10619/Y

Patheon YM Inc.,

Toronto, Ontario, M3B 1Y5

For:

MGI PHARMA, INC., Bloomington, MN 55437

SALAGEN® is a registered trademark of **MGI PHARMA, INC.**

43-5025-008 2/04

Millennium Pharmaceuticals, Inc.

40 LANDSDOWNE STREET
CAMBRIDGE, MA 02139

Direct Inquiries to:
Ph. 1-800-589-9005

INTEGRILIN® ℞

[*ĭn-tĕg'-rĭl-in*]

(eptifibatide)

Injection

For Intravenous Administration

DESCRIPTION

Eptifibatide is a cyclic heptapeptide containing six amino acids and one mercaptopropionyl (des-amino cysteinyl) residue. An interchain disulfide bridge is formed between the cysteine amide and the mercaptopropionyl moieties. Chemically it is N^6-(aminoiminomethyl)-N^2-(3-mercapto-1-oxopropyl-L-lysylglycyl-L-α-aspartyl-L-tryptophyl-L-prolyl-L-cysteinamide, cyclic (1→6)-disulfide. Eptifibatide binds to the platelet receptor glycoprotein (GP) IIb/IIIa of human platelets and inhibits platelet aggregation.

The eptifibatide peptide is produced by solution-phase peptide synthesis, and is purified by preparative reverse-phase liquid chromatography and lyophilized. The structural formula is:

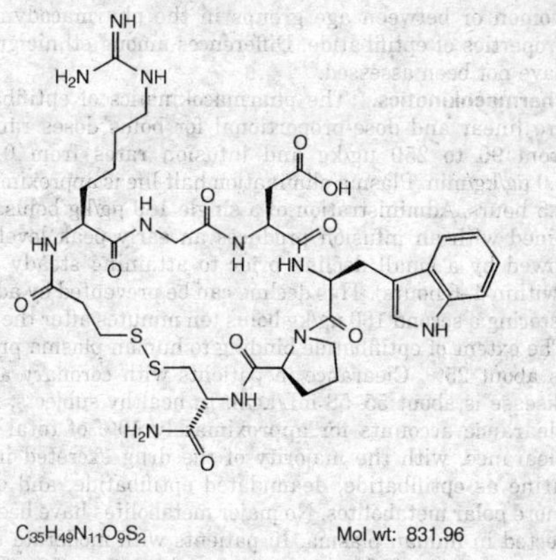

$C_{35}H_{49}N_{11}O_9S_2$ Mol wt: 831.96

INTEGRILIN (eptifibatide) Injection is a clear, colorless, sterile, non-pyrogenic solution for intravenous (IV) use. Each 10-mL vial contains 2 mg/mL of eptifibatide and each 100-mL vial contains either 0.75 mg/mL or 2 mg/mL of eptifibatide. Each vial of either size also contains 5.25 mg/mL citric acid and sodium hydroxide to adjust the pH to 5.35.

CLINICAL PHARMACOLOGY

Mechanism of Action. Eptifibatide reversibly inhibits platelet aggregation by preventing the binding of fibrinogen, von Willebrand factor, and other adhesive ligands to GP IIb/IIIa. When administered intravenously, eptifibatide inhibits *ex vivo* platelet aggregation in a dose- and concentration-dependent manner. Platelet aggregation inhibition is reversible following cessation of the eptifibatide infusion; this is thought to result from dissociation of eptifibatide from the platelet.

Pharmacodynamics. Infusion of eptifibatide into baboons caused a dose-dependent inhibition of *ex vivo* platelet aggregation, with complete inhibition of aggregation achieved at infusion rates greater than 5.0 μg/kg/min. In a baboon model that is refractory to aspirin and heparin, doses of eptifibatide that inhibit aggregation prevented acute thrombosis with only a modest prolongation (2- to 3-fold) of the bleeding time. Platelet aggregation in dogs was also inhibited by infusions of eptifibatide, with complete inhibition at

Continued on next page

Integrilin—Cont.

2.0 μg/kg/min. This infusion dose completely inhibited canine coronary thrombosis induced by coronary artery injury (Folts model).
Human pharmacodynamic data were obtained in healthy subjects and in patients presenting with unstable angina (UA) or non-ST-segment elevation myocardial infarction (NSTEMI) and/or undergoing percutaneous coronary interventions. Studies in healthy subjects enrolled only males; patient studies enrolled approximately one third women. In these studies, eptifibatide inhibited *ex vivo* platelet aggregation induced by adenosine diphosphate (ADP) and other agonists in a dose- and concentration-dependent manner. The effect of eptifibatide was observed immediately after administration of a 180 μg/kg intravenous bolus. Table 1 shows the effects of dosing regimens of eptifibatide used in the IMPACT II and PURSUIT studies on *ex vivo* platelet aggregation induced by 20 μM ADP in PPACK-anticoagulated platelet-rich plasma and on bleeding time. The effects of the dosing regimen used in ESPRIT on platelet aggregation have not been studied.

Table 1
Platelet Inhibition and Bleeding Time

	IMPACT II 135/0.5*	PURSUIT 180/2.0**
Inhibition of platelet aggregation 15 min. after bolus	69%	84%
Inhibition of platelet aggregation at steady state	40–50%	>90%
Bleeding-time prolongation at steady state	<5×	<5×
Inhibition of platelet aggregation 4h after infusion discontinuation	<30%	<50%
Bleeding-time prolongation 6h after infusion discontinuation	1×	1.4×

*135 μg/kg bolus followed by a continuous infusion of 0.5 μg/kg/min
**180 μg/kg bolus followed by a continuous infusion of 2.0 μg/kg/min

The eptifibatide dosing regimen used in the ESPRIT study included two 180 μg/kg bolus doses given ten minutes apart combined with a continuous 2.0 μg/kg/min infusion.
When administered alone, eptifibatide has no measurable effect on prothrombin time (PT) or activated partial thromboplastin time (aPTT). (See also PRECAUTIONS: Drug Interactions).
There were no important differences between men and women or between age groups in the pharmacodynamic properties of eptifibatide. Differences among ethnic groups have not been assessed.
Pharmacokinetics. The pharmacokinetics of eptifibatide are linear and dose-proportional for bolus doses ranging from 90 to 250 μg/kg and infusion rates from 0.5 to 3.0 μg/kg/min. Plasma elimination half-life is approximately 2.5 hours. Administration of a single 180 μg/kg bolus combined with an infusion produces an early peak level, followed by a small decline prior to attaining steady state (within 4–6 hours). This decline can be prevented by administering a second 180 μg/kg bolus ten minutes after the first. The extent of eptifibatide binding to human plasma protein is about 25%. Clearance in patients with coronary artery disease is about 55–58 mL/kg/h. In healthy subjects, renal clearance accounts for approximately 50% of total body clearance, with the majority of the drug excreted in the urine as eptifibatide, deamidated eptifibatide, and other, more polar metabolites. No major metabolites have been detected in human plasma. In patients with moderate to severe renal insufficiency (creatinine clearance <50 mL/min using the Cockroft-Gault equation), the clearance of eptifibatide is reduced by approximately 50% and steady-state plasma levels approximately doubled (see WARNINGS, DOSAGE AND ADMINISTRATION).
Special Populations. Patients in clinical studies were older (range 20 to 94 years) than those in the clinical pharmacology studies. Elderly patients with coronary artery disease demonstrated higher plasma levels and lower total body clearance of eptifibatide when given the same dose as younger patients. Limited data are available on lighter weight (<50 kg) patients over 75 years of age.
No studies have been conducted in patients with hepatic impairment.
Males and females have not demonstrated any clinically significant differences in the pharmacokinetics of eptifibatide.

CLINICAL STUDIES

Eptifibatide was studied in three placebo-controlled, randomized studies. PURSUIT evaluated patients with acute coronary syndromes: unstable angina (UA) or non-ST-segment myocardial infarction (NSTEMI). Two other studies, ESPRIT and IMPACT II, evaluated patients about to undergo a percutaneous coronary intervention (PCI). Patients underwent primarily balloon angioplasty in IMPACT II and intracoronary stent placement, with or without angioplasty, in ESPRIT.

Non-ST-segment Elevation Acute Coronary Syndrome
Non-ST-segment elevation acute coronary syndrome is defined as prolonged (≥10 minutes) symptoms of cardiac ischemia within the previous 24 hours associated with either ST-segment changes (elevation between 0.6 mm and 1 mm or depression >0.5 mm), T-wave inversion (>1 mm), or positive CK-MB. This definition includes "unstable angina" and "NSTEMI" but excludes myocardial infarction that is associated with Q waves or greater degrees of ST-segment elevation.

PURSUIT (Platelet Glycoprotein IIb/IIIa in Unstable Angina: Receptor Suppression Using INTEGRILIN Therapy)
PURSUIT was a 726-center, 27-country, double-blind, randomized, placebo-controlled study in 10,948 patients presenting with UA or NSTEMI. Patients could be enrolled only if they had experienced cardiac ischemia at rest (≥10 minutes) within the previous 24 hours and had either ST-segment changes (elevations between 0.6 mm and 1 mm or depression >0.5 mm), T-wave inversion (>1 mm), or increased CK-MB. Important exclusion criteria included a history of bleeding diathesis, evidence of abnormal bleeding within the previous 30 days, uncontrolled hypertension, major surgery within the previous 6 weeks, stroke within the previous 30 days, any history of hemorrhagic stroke, serum creatinine >2.0 mg/dL, dependency on renal dialysis, or platelet count <100,000/mm^3.
Patients were randomized to either placebo, eptifibatide 180 μg/kg bolus followed by a 2.0 μg/kg/min infusion (180/2.0), or eptifibatide 180 μg/kg bolus followed by a 1.3 μg/kg/min infusion (180/1.3). The infusion was continued for 72 hours, until hospital discharge, or until the time of coronary artery bypass grafting (CABG), whichever occurred first, except that if PCI was performed, the eptifibatide infusion was continued for 24 hours after the procedure, allowing for a duration of infusion up to 96 hours.
The lower-infusion-rate arm was stopped after the first interim analysis when the two active-treatment arms appeared to have the same incidence of bleeding.
Patient age ranged from 20 to 94 (mean 63) years, and 65% were male. The patients were 89% Caucasian, 6% Hispanic, and 5% Black, recruited in the United States and Canada (40%), Western Europe (39%), Eastern Europe (16%), and Latin America (5%).
This was a "real world" study; each patient was managed according to the usual standards of the investigational site; frequencies of angiography, PCI, and CABG therefore differed widely from site to site and from country to country. Of the patients in PURSUIT, 13% were managed with PCI during drug infusion, of whom 50% received intracoronary stents; 87% were managed medically (without PCI during drug infusion).
The majority of patients received aspirin (75–325 mg once daily). Heparin was administered intravenously or subcutaneously, at the physician's discretion, most commonly as an intravenous bolus of 5000 U followed by a continuous infusion of 1000 U/h. For patients weighing less than 70 kg, the recommended heparin bolus dose was 60 U/kg followed by a continuous infusion of 12 U/kg/h. A target aPTT of 50–70 seconds was recommended. A total of 1250 patients underwent PCI within 72 hours after randomization, in which case they received intravenous heparin to maintain an activated clotting time (ACT) of 300–350 seconds.
The primary endpoint of the study was the occurrence of death from any cause or new myocardial infarction (MI) (evaluated by a blinded Clinical Endpoints Committee) within 30 days of randomization.
Compared to placebo, eptifibatide administered as a 180 μg/kg bolus followed by a 2.0 μg/kg/min infusion significantly (p=0.042) reduced the incidence of endpoint events (see Table 2). The reduction in the incidence of endpoint events in patients receiving eptifibatide was evident early during treatment, and this reduction was maintained through at least 30 days (see Figure 1). Table 2 also shows the incidence of the components of the primary endpoint, death (whether or not preceded by an MI) and new MI in surviving patients at 30 days.
[See table 2 below]

Table 2
Clinical Events in The PURSUIT Study

Death or MI	Placebo (n = 4739) n (%)	Eptifibatide (180/2.0) (n = 4722) n (%)	p-value
3 days	359 (7.6%)	279 (5.9%)	0.001
7 days	552 (11.6%)	477 (10.1%)	0.016
30 days			
Death or MI (Primary Endpoint)	745 (15.7%)	672 (14.2%)	0.042
Death	177 (3.7%)	165 (3.5%)	
Nonfatal MI	568 (12.0%)	507 (10.7%)	

Figure 1
Kaplan-Meier Plot of Time to Death or Myocardial Infarction Within 30 Days of Randomization

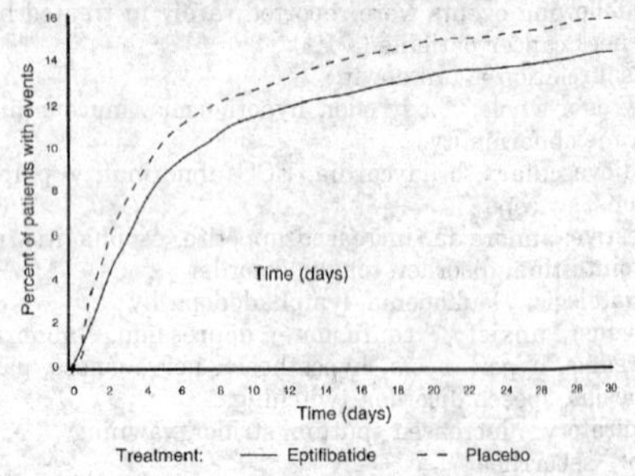

Treatment with eptifibatide prior to determination of patient management strategy reduced clinical events regardless of whether patients ultimately underwent diagnostic catheterization, revascularization (i.e., PCI or CABG surgery) or continued to receive medical management alone. Table 3 shows the incidence of death or MI within 72 hours.

Table 3
Clinical Events (Death or MI) in the PURSUIT Study Within 72 Hours of Randomization

	Placebo	Eptifibatide 180/2.0
Overall Patient Population	n=4739	n=4722
- At 72 hours	7.6%	5.9%
Patients undergoing early PCI	n=631	n=619
- Pre-procedure (nonfatal MI only)	5.5%	1.8%
- At 72 hours	14.4%	9.0%
Patients not undergoing early PCI	n=4108	n=4103
- At 72 hours	6.5%	5.4%

All of the effect of eptifibatide was established within 72 hours (during the period of drug infusion), regardless of management strategy. Moreover, for patients undergoing early PCI, a reduction in events was evident prior to the procedure.
Follow-up data were available through 165 days for 10,611 patients enrolled in the PURSUIT trial (96.9 percent of the initial enrollment). This follow-up included 4,566 patients who received eptifibatide at the 180/2.0 dose. As reported by the investigators, the occurrence of death from any cause or new myocardial infarction for patients followed for at least 165 days was reduced from 13.6 percent with placebo to 12.1 percent with eptifibatide 180/2.0.

Percutaneous Coronary Intervention

IMPACT II (INTEGRILIN to Minimize Platelet Aggregation and Prevent Coronary Thrombosis II)
IMPACT II was a multi-center, double-blind, randomized, placebo-controlled study conducted in the United States in 4010 patients undergoing PCI. Major exclusion criteria included a history of bleeding diathesis, major surgery within 6 weeks of treatment, gastrointestinal bleeding within 30 days, any stroke or structural CNS abnormality, uncontrolled hypertension, PT >1.2 times control, hematocrit <30%, platelet count <100,000/mm^3, and pregnancy.
Patient age ranged from 24 to 89 (mean 60) years, and 75% were male. The patients were 92% Caucasian, 5% Black, and 3% Hispanic. Forty-one percent of the patients underwent PCI for ongoing ACS. Patients were randomly assigned to one of three treatment regimens, each incorporating a bolus dose initiated immediately prior to PCI followed by a continuous infusion lasting 20–24 hours: 1) 135 μg/kg bolus followed by a continuous infusion of 0.5 μg/kg/min of eptifibatide (135/0.5); 2) 135 μg/kg bolus followed by a continuous infusion of 0.75 μg/kg/min of eptifibatide (135/0.75); or 3) a matching placebo bolus followed by a matching placebo continuous infusion. Each patient received aspirin and an intravenous heparin bolus of 100 U/kg, with additional bolus infusions of up to 2000 additional units of heparin every 15 minutes to maintain an activated clotting time (ACT) of 300–350 seconds.
The primary endpoint was the composite of death, MI, or urgent revascularization, analyzed at 30 days after randomization in all patients who received at least one dose of study drug.
As shown in Table 4, each eptifibatide regimen reduced the rate of death, MI, or urgent intervention, although at 30 days, this finding was statistically significant only in the lower-dose eptifibatide group. As in the PURSUIT study, the effects of eptifibatide were seen early and persisted throughout the 30-day period.
[See table 4 at top of next page]

ESPRIT (Enhanced Suppression of the Platelet IIb/IIIa Receptor with INTEGRILIN Therapy)

The ESPRIT study was a multi-center, double-blind, randomized, placebo-controlled study conducted in the United States and Canada that enrolled 2064 patients undergoing elective or urgent PCI with intended intracoronary stent placement. Exclusion criteria included MI within the previous 24 hours, ongoing chest pain, administration of any oral anti-platelet or oral anticoagulant other than aspirin within 30 days of PCI (although loading doses of thienopyridine on the day of PCI were encouraged), planned PCI of a saphenous vein graft or subsequent "staged" PCI, prior stent placement in the target lesion, PCI within the previous 90 days, a history of bleeding diathesis, major surgery within 6 weeks of treatment, gastrointestinal bleeding within 30 days, any stroke or structural CNS abnormality, uncontrolled hypertension, PT >1.2 times control, hematocrit <30%, platelet count <100,000/mm^3, and pregnancy.

Patient age ranged from 24 to 93 (mean 62) years and 73% of patients were male. The study enrolled 90% Caucasian, 5% African American, 2% Hispanic and 1% Asian patients. Patients received a wide variety of stents. Patients were randomized either to placebo or eptifibatide administered as an intravenous bolus of 180 µg/kg followed immediately by a continuous infusion of 2.0 µg/kg/min, and a second bolus of 180 µg/kg administered 10 minutes later (180/2.0/180). Eptifibatide infusion was continued for 18–24 hours after PCI or until hospital discharge, whichever came first. Each patient received at least one dose of aspirin (162–325 mg) and 60 U/kg of heparin as a bolus (not to exceed 6000 Units) if not already receiving a heparin infusion. Additional boluses of heparin (10–40 U/kg) could be administered in order to reach a target ACT between 200 and 300 seconds.

The primary endpoint of the ESPRIT study was the composite of death, MI, urgent target vessel revascularization (UTVR) and "bailout" to open label eptifibatide due to a thrombotic complication of PCI (TBO) (e.g., visible thrombus, "no reflow", or abrupt closure) at 48 hours. MI, UTVR and TBO were evaluated by a blinded Clinical Events Committee.

As shown in Table 5, the incidence of the primary endpoint and selected secondary endpoints was significantly reduced in patients who received eptifibatide. A treatment benefit in patients who received eptifibatide was seen by 48 hours and at the end of the 30-day observation period.

[See table 5 at right]

The need for thrombotic "bailout" was significantly reduced with eptifibatide at 48 hours (2.1% for placebo, 1.0% for eptifibatide; p=0.029). Consistent with previous studies of GP IIb/IIIa inhibitors, most of the benefit achieved acutely with eptifibatide was in the reduction of MI. Eptifibatide reduced the occurrence of MI at 48 hours from 9.0% for placebo to 5.4% (p=0.0015) and maintained that effect with significance at 30 days.

Follow-up (12 month) mortality data were available for 2024 patients (1017 on eptifibatide) enrolled in the ESPRIT trial (98.1% of the initial enrollment). Twelve-month clinical event data were available for 1964 patients (988 on eptifibatide) representing 95.2% of the initial enrollment. As shown in Table 6, the treatment effect of eptifibatide seen at 48 hours and 30 days appeared preserved at 6 months and 1 year. Most of the benefit was in reduction of MI.

[See table 6 at right]

Table 4
Clinical Events in the IMPACT II Study

	Placebo n (%)	Eptifibatide (135/0.5) n (%)	Eptifibatide (135/0.75) n (%)
Patients	1285	1300	1286
Abrupt Closure	65 (5.1%)	36 (2.8%)	43 (3.3%)
p-value vs. placebo		0.003	0.030
Death, MI, or Urgent Intervention			
24 hours	123 (9.6%)	86 (6.6%)	89 (6.9%)
p-value vs. placebo		0.006	0.014
48 hours	131 (10.2%)	99 (7.6%)	102 (7.9%)
p-value vs. placebo		0.021	0.045
30 days (primary endpoint)	149 (11.6%)	118 (9.1%)	128 (10.0%)
p-value vs. placebo		0.035	0.179
Death or MI			
30 days	110 (8.6%)	89 (6.8%)	95 (7.4%)
p-value vs. placebo		0.102	0.272
6 months	151 (11.9%)*	136 (10.6%)*	130 (10.3%)*
p-value vs. placebo		0.297	0.182

*Kaplan-Meier estimate of event rate.

Table 5
Clinical Events in the ESPRIT Study

	Placebo (n=1024)	Eptifibatide 180/2.0/180 (n=1040)	Relative Risk (95% CI)	p-Value
Death, MI, Urgent Target Vessel Revascularization, or Thrombotic "Bailout"				
48 Hours (primary endpoint)	108 (10.5%)	69 (6.6%)	0.629 (0.471, 0.840)	0.0015
30 Days	120 (11.7%)	78 (7.5%)	0.640 (0.488, 0.840)	0.0011
Death, MI, or Urgent Target Vessel Revascularization				
48 Hours	95 (9.3%)	62 (6.0%)	0.643 (0.472, 0.875)	0.0045
30 Days (key secondary endpoint)	107 (10.4%)	71 (6.8%)	0.653 (0.490, 0.871)	0.0034
Death or MI				
48 Hours	94 (9.2%)	57 (5.5%)	0.597 (0.435, 0.820)	0.0013
30 Days	104 (10.2%)	66 (6.3%)	0.625 (0.465, 0.840)	0.0016

Table 6
Clinical Events at 6 months and 1 year in the ESPRIT Study

	Placebo (n=1024)	Eptifibatide 180/2.0/180 (n=1040)	Hazard Ratio (95% CI)
Death, MI, or Target Vessel Revascularization			
6 Months	187 (18.5%)	146 (14.3%)	0.744 (0.599, 0.924)
1 Year	222 (22.1%)	178 (17.5%)	0.762 (0.626, 0.929)
Death, MI			
6 Months	117 (11.5%)	77 (7.4%)	0.631 (0.473, 0.841)
1 Year	126 (12.4%)	83 (8.0%)	0.630 (0.478, 0.832)

Percentages are Kaplan-Meier event rates.

INDICATIONS AND USAGE

INTEGRILIN is indicated:

- For the treatment of patients with acute coronary syndrome (unstable angina/non-ST-segment elevation myocardial infarction) including patients who are to be managed medically and those undergoing percutaneous coronary intervention (PCI). In this setting, INTEGRILIN has been shown to decrease the rate of a combined endpoint of death or new myocardial infarction.
- For the treatment of patients undergoing PCI, including those undergoing intracoronary stenting. In this setting, INTEGRILIN has been shown to decrease the rate of a combined endpoint of death, new myocardial infarction, or need for urgent intervention.

In the IMPACT II, PURSUIT and ESPRIT studies of eptifibatide, most patients received heparin and aspirin, as described in CLINICAL TRIALS.

CONTRAINDICATIONS

Treatment with eptifibatide is contraindicated in patients with:

- A history of bleeding diathesis, or evidence of active abnormal bleeding within the previous 30 days.
- Severe hypertension (systolic blood pressure >200 mm Hg or diastolic blood pressure >110 mm Hg) not adequately controlled on antihypertensive therapy.
- Major surgery within the preceding 6 weeks.
- History of stroke within 30 days or any history of hemorrhagic stroke.
- Current or planned administration of another parenteral GP IIb/IIIa inhibitor.
- Dependency on renal dialysis.
- Known hypersensitivity to any component of the product.

WARNINGS

Bleeding. Bleeding is the most common complication encountered during eptifibatide therapy. Administration of eptifibatide is associated with an increase in major and minor bleeding, as classified by the criteria of the Thrombolysis in Myocardial Infarction Study group (TIMI), (see ADVERSE REACTIONS). Most major bleeding associated with eptifibatide has been at the arterial access site for cardiac catheterization or from the gastrointestinal or genitourinary tract.

In patients undergoing percutaneous coronary interventions, patients receiving eptifibatide experience an increased incidence of major bleeding compared to those receiving placebo without a significant increase in transfusion requirement. Special care should be employed to minimize the risk of bleeding among these patients (see PRECAUTIONS). If bleeding cannot be controlled with pressure, infusion of eptifibatide and concomitant heparin should be stopped immediately.

Renal Insufficiency. Approximately 50% of eptifibatide is cleared by the kidney in patients with normal renal function. Total drug clearance is decreased by approximately 50% and steady-state plasma eptifibatide concentrations are doubled in patients with an estimated creatinine clearance <50 mL/min (using the Cockroft-Gault equation). Therefore, the infusion dose should be reduced to 1 µg/kg-min in such patients. If an estimated creatinine clearance is not available, the infusion dose should be reduced in patients with a serum creatinine >2 mg/dL (see DOSAGE AND ADMINISTRATION section). There has been no clinical experience in patients dependent on dialysis.

Platelet Count <100,000/mm^3. Because it is an inhibitor of platelet aggregation, caution should be exercised when administering eptifibatide to patients with a platelet count <100,000/mm^3; there has been no clinical experience with eptifibatide initiated in patients with a platelet count <100,000/mm^3.

PRECAUTIONS

Bleeding Precautions

Care of the Femoral Artery Access Site in Patients Undergoing Percutaneous Coronary Intervention (PCI). In patients undergoing PCI, treatment with eptifibatide is associated with an increase in major and minor bleeding at the site of arterial sheath placement. After PCI, eptifibatide infusion should be continued until hospital discharge or up to 18–24 hours, whichever comes first. Heparin use is discouraged after the PCI procedure. Early sheath removal is encouraged while eptifibatide is being infused. Prior to removing the sheath, it is recommended that heparin be discontinued for 3–4 hours and an aPTT of <45 seconds or ACT <150 seconds be achieved. In any case, both heparin and eptifibatide should be discontinued and sheath hemostasis should be achieved at least 2–4 hours before hospital discharge.

Use of Thrombolytics, Anticoagulants, and Other Antiplatelet Agents. In the IMPACT II, PURSUIT and ESPRIT studies, eptifibatide was used concomitantly with unfractionated heparin and aspirin (see CLINICAL STUDIES). In the ESPRIT study, clopidogrel or ticlopidine were used routinely starting the day of PCI. Because eptifibatide inhibits platelet aggregation, caution should be employed when it is used with other drugs that affect hemostasis, including **thrombolytics, oral anticoagulants, non-steroidal anti-inflammatory drugs,** and **dipyridamole.** To avoid potentially additive pharmacologic effects, concomitant treatment with **other inhibitors of platelet receptor GP IIb/IIIa** should be avoided.

There is only a small experience with concomitant use of eptifibatide and **thrombolytics.** In a study of 180 patients with acute myocardial infarction (AMI), eptifibatide (in regimens up to a bolus of 180 µg/kg followed by a continuous infusion of 0.75 µg/kg/min for 24 hours) was administered concomitantly with the approved "accelerated" regimen of alteplase, a thrombolytic agent. The studied regimens of eptifibatide did not increase the incidence of major bleeding or transfusion compared to the incidence seen when alteplase was given alone.

In the IMPACT II study, 15 patients received a thrombolytic agent in conjunction with the 135/0.5 dosing regimen, 2 of whom experienced a major bleed. In the PURSUIT study, 40 patients who received eptifibatide at the 180/2.0 dosing regimen received a thrombolytic agent, 10 of whom experienced a major bleed.

In another AMI study involving 181 patients, eptifibatide (in regimens up to a bolus of 180 µg/kg followed by a continuous infusion of up to 2.0 µg/kg/min for up to 72 hours) was administered concomitantly with streptokinase (1.5

Continued on next page

Integrilin—Cont.

million units over 60 minutes), another thrombolytic agent. At the highest studied infusion rates (1.3 µg/kg/min and 2.0 µg/kg/min), eptifibatide was associated with an increase in the incidence of bleeding and transfusions compared to the incidence seen when streptokinase was given alone. These limited data on the use of eptifibatide in patients receiving thrombolytic agents do not allow an estimate of the bleeding risk associated with concomitant use of thrombolytics. Systemic thrombolytic therapy should be used with caution in patients who have received eptifibatide.

Minimization of Vascular and Other Trauma. Arterial and venous punctures, intramuscular injections, and the use of urinary catheters, nasotracheal intubation, and nasogastric tubes should be minimized. When obtaining intravenous access, non-compressible sites (e.g., subclavian or jugular veins) should be avoided.

Laboratory Tests. Before infusion of eptifibatide, the following laboratory tests should be performed to identify pre-existing hemostatic abnormalities: hematocrit or hemoglobin, platelet count, serum creatinine, and PT/aPTT. In patients undergoing PCI, the activated clotting time (ACT) should also be measured.

Maintaining Target aPTT and ACT. The aPTT should be maintained between 50 and 70 seconds unless PCI is to be performed. In patients treated with heparin, bleeding can be minimized by close monitoring of the aPTT. Table 7 displays the risk of major bleeding according to the maximum aPTT attained within 72 hours in the PURSUIT study.

[See table 7 at right]

The ESPRIT study stipulated a target ACT of 200 to 300 seconds during PCI. Patients receiving eptifibatide 180/2.0/180 (mean ACT 284 seconds) experienced an increased incidence of bleeding relative to placebo (mean ACT 276 seconds), primarily at the femoral artery access site. At these lower ACTs, bleeding was less than previously reported with eptifibatide in the PURSUIT and IMPACT II studies.

The aPTT or ACT should be checked prior to arterial sheath removal. The sheath should not be removed unless the aPTT is <45 seconds or the ACT is <150 seconds.

Thrombocytopenia. If the patient experiences a confirmed platelet decrease to <100,000/mm^3, INTEGRILIN and heparin should be discontinued and the condition appropriately monitored and treated.

Drug Interactions. Enoxaparin dosed as a 1.0 mg/kg subcutaneous injection q12h for four doses did not alter the pharmacokinetics of eptifibatide or the level of platelet aggregation in healthy adults.

Geriatric Use. The PURSUIT and IMPACT II clinical studies enrolled patients up to the age of 94 years (45% were age 65 and over; 12% were age 75 and older). There was no apparent difference in efficacy between older and younger patients treated with eptifibatide. The incidence of bleeding complications was higher in the elderly in both placebo and eptifibatide groups, and the incremental risk of eptifibatide-associated bleeding was greater in the older patients. No dose adjustment was made for elderly patients, but patients over 75 years of age had to weigh at least 50 kg to be enrolled in the PURSUIT study; no such limitation was stipulated in the ESPRIT study (see also ADVERSE REACTIONS).

Carcinogenesis, Mutagenesis, Impairment of Fertility. No long-term studies in animals have been performed to evaluate the carcinogenic potential of eptifibatide. Eptifibatide was not genotoxic in the Ames test, the mouse lymphoma cell (L 5178Y, TK$^{+/-}$) forward mutation test, the human lymphocyte chromosome aberration test, or the mouse micronucleus test. Administered by continuous intravenous infusion at total daily doses up to 72 mg/kg/day (about 4 times the recommended maximum daily human dose on a body surface area basis), eptifibatide had no effect on fertility and reproductive performance of male and female rats.

Pregnancy. Pregnancy Category B. Teratology studies have been performed by continuous intravenous infusion of eptifibatide in pregnant rats at total daily doses of up to 72 mg/kg/day (about 4 times the recommended maximum daily human dose on a body surface area basis) and in pregnant rabbits at total daily doses of up to 36 mg/kg/day (also about 4 times the recommended maximum daily human dose on a body surface area basis). These studies revealed no evidence of harm to the fetus due to eptifibatide. There are, however, no adequate and well-controlled studies in pregnant women with eptifibatide. Because animal reproduction studies are not always predictive of human response, eptifibatide should be used during pregnancy only if clearly needed.

Pediatric Use. Safety and effectiveness of eptifibatide in pediatric patients have not been studied.

Nursing Mothers. It is not known whether eptifibatide is excreted in human milk. Because many drugs are excreted in human milk, caution should be exercised when eptifibatide is administered to a nursing mother.

ADVERSE REACTIONS

A total of 16,782 patients were treated in the Phase III clinical trials (PURSUIT, ESPRIT and IMPACT II). These 16,782 patients had a mean age of 62 years (range 20 to 94 years). Eighty-nine percent of the patients were Caucasian, with the remainder being predominantly Black (5%) and Hispanic (5%). Sixty-eight percent were men. Because of the different regimens used in PURSUIT, IMPACT II and ESPRIT, data from the three studies were not pooled.

Table 7
Major Bleeding by Maximal aPTT Within 72 Hours in the PURSUIT Study

	Placebo n (%)	Eptifibatide 180/1.3* n (%)	Eptifibatide 180/2.0 n (%)
Maximum aPTT (seconds)			
<50	44/721(6.1%)	21/244(8.6%)	44/743(5.9%)
50–70 (recommended)	92/908(10.1%)	28/259(10.8%)	99/883(11.2%)
>70	281/2786(10.1%)	99/891(11.1%)	345/2811(12.3%)

*Administered only until the first interim analysis

Table 8
Bleeding Events and Transfusions in the PURSUIT, ESPRIT and IMPACT II Studies

PURSUIT	Placebo n (%)	Eptifibatide 180/1.3* n (%)	Eptifibatide 180/2.0 n (%)
Patients	4696	1472	4679
Major bleeding[a]	425 (9.3%)	152 (10.5%)	498 (10.8%)
Minor bleeding[a]	347 (7.6%)	152 (10.5%)	604 (13.1%)
Requiring Transfusions[b]	490 (10.4%)	188 (12.8%)	601 (12.8%)
ESPRIT	**Placebo n (%)**	**Eptifibatide 180/2.0/180 n (%)**	
Patients	1024	1040	
Major bleeding[a]	4 (0.4%)	13 (1.3%)	
Minor bleeding[a]	18 (2.0%)	29 (3.0%)	
Requiring Transfusions[b]	11 (1.1%)	16 (1.5%)	
IMPACT II	**Placebo n (%)**	**Eptifibatide 135/0.5 n (%)**	**Eptifibatide 135/0.75 n (%)**
Patients	1285	1300	1286
Major bleeding[a]	55 (4.5%)	55 (4.4%)	58 (4.7%)
Minor bleeding[a]	115 (9.3%)	146 (11.7%)	177 (14.2%)
Requiring Transfusions[b]	66 (5.1%)	71 (5.5%)	74 (5.8%)

Note: denominator is based on patients for whom data are available
* Administered only until the first interim analysis
[a] For major and minor bleeding, patients are counted only once according to the most severe classification.
[b] Includes transfusions of whole blood, packed red blood cells, fresh frozen plasma, cryoprecipitate, platelets, and autotransfusion during the initial hospitalization.

Table 9
Major Bleeding by Procedures in the PURSUIT Study

	Placebo n (%)	Eptifibatide 180/1.3* n (%)	Eptifibatide 180/2.0 n (%)
Patients	4577	1451	4604
Overall Incidence of Major Bleeding	425 (9.3%)	152 (10.5%)	498 (10.8%)
Breakdown by Procedure:			
CABG	375 (8.2%)	123 (8.5%)	377 (8.2%)
Angioplasty without CABG	27 (0.6%)	16 (1.1%)	64 (1.4%)
Angiography without angioplasty or CABG	11 (0.2%)	7 (0.5%)	29 (0.6%)
Medical Therapy Only	12 (0.3%)	6 (0.4%)	28 (0.6%)

Denominators are based on the total number of patients whose TIMI classification was resolved.
*Administered only until the first interim analysis

Bleeding. The incidences of bleeding events and transfusions in the PURSUIT, IMPACT II and ESPRIT studies are shown in Table 8. Bleeding was classified as major or minor by the criteria of the TIMI study group. Major bleeding events consisted of intracranial hemorrhage and other bleeding that led to decreases in hemoglobin greater than 5 g/dL. Minor bleeding events included spontaneous gross hematuria, spontaneous hematemesis, other observed blood loss with a hemoglobin decrease of more than 3 g/dL, and other hemoglobin decreases that were greater than 4 g/dL but less than 5 g/dL. In patients who received transfusions, the corresponding loss in hemoglobin was estimated through an adaptation period of the method of Landefeld *et al.*

[See table 8 above]

The majority of major bleeding events in the ESPRIT study occurred at the vascular access site (1 and 8 patients, or 0.1% and 0.8% in the placebo and eptifibatide groups, respectively). Bleeding at "other" locations occurred in 0.2% and 0.4% of patients, respectively.

In the PURSUIT study, the greatest increase in major bleeding in eptifibatide-treated patients compared to placebo was also associated with bleeding at the femoral artery access site (2.8% versus 1.3%). Oropharyngeal (primarily gingival), genito-urinary, gastrointestinal, and retroperitoneal bleeding were also seen more commonly in eptifibatide-treated patients compared to placebo-treated patients. Among patients experiencing a major bleed in the IMPACT II study, an increase in bleeding on eptifibatide versus placebo was observed only for the femoral artery access site (3.2% versus 2.8%).

Table 9 displays the incidence of TIMI major bleeding according to the cardiac procedures carried out in the PURSUIT study. The most common bleeding complications were related to cardiac revascularization (CABG-related or femoral artery access site bleeding). A corresponding table for ESPRIT is not presented as every patient underwent PCI in the ESPRIT study and only 11 patients underwent CABG.

[See table 9 above]

In the PURSUIT and ESPRIT studies, the risk of major bleeding with eptifibatide increased as patient weight decreased. This relationship was most apparent for patients weighing less than 70 kg.

Bleeding adverse events resulting in discontinuation of study drug were more frequent among patients receiving eptifibatide than placebo (4.6% versus 0.9% in ESPRIT, 8% versus 1% in PURSUIT, 3.5% versus 1.9% in IMPACT II).

Intracranial Hemorrhage and Stroke. Intracranial hemorrhage was rare in the PURSUIT, IMPACT II and ESPRIT clinical studies. In the PURSUIT study, 3 patients in the placebo group, 1 patient in the group treated with eptifibatide 180/1.3 and 5 patients in the group treated with eptifibatide 180/2.0 experienced a hemorrhagic stroke. The overall incidence of stroke was 0.5% in patients receiving eptifibatide 180/1.3, 0.7% in patients receiving eptifibatide 180/2.0, and 0.8% in placebo patients.

In the IMPACT II study, intracranial hemorrhage was experienced by 1 patient treated with eptifibatide 135/0.5, 2 patients treated with eptifibatide 135/0.75 and 2 patients in the placebo group. The overall incidence of stroke was 0.5% in patients receiving eptifibatide 135/0.5, 0.7% in patients receiving eptifibatide 135/0.75 and 0.7% in the placebo group.

In the ESPRIT study, there were 3 hemorrhagic strokes, 1 in the placebo group and 2 in the eptifibatide group. In addition there was 1 case of cerebral infarction in the eptifibatide group.

Thrombocytopenia. In the PURSUIT and IMPACT II studies, the incidence of thrombocytopenia (<100,000/mm^3 or ≥50% reduction from baseline) and the incidence of platelet transfusions were similar between patients treated with eptifibatide and placebo. In the ESPRIT study, the incidence was 0.6% in the placebo group and 1.2% in the eptifibatide group.

Allergic Reactions. In the PURSUIT study, anaphylaxis was reported in 7 patients receiving placebo (0.15%) and 7 patients receiving eptifibatide 180/2.0 (0.16%). In the IMPACT II study, anaphylaxis was reported in 1 patient (0.08%) on placebo and in no patients on eptifibatide. In the IMPACT II study, 2 patients (1 patient (0.04%) receiving eptifibatide and 1 patient (0.08%) receiving placebo) discontinued study drug because of allergic reactions. In the ESPRIT study, there were no cases of anaphylaxis reported. There were 3 patients who suffered an allergic reaction, 1 on placebo and 2 on eptifibatide. In addition, 1 patient in the placebo group was diagnosed with urticaria.

The potential for development of antibodies to eptifibatide has been studied in 433 subjects. Eptifibatide was non-antigenic in 412 patients receiving a single administration of eptifibatide (135 µg/kg bolus followed by a continuous infusion of either 0.5 µg/kg/min or 0.75 µg/kg/min), and in 21 subjects to whom eptifibatide (135 µg/kg bolus followed by a continuous infusion of 0.75 µg/kg/min) was administered twice, 28 days apart. In both cases, plasma for antibody detection was collected approximately 30 days after each dose. The development of antibodies to eptifibatide at higher doses has not been evaluated.

Other Adverse Reactions. In the PURSUIT and ESPRIT studies, the incidence of serious non-bleeding adverse events was similar in patients receiving placebo or eptifibatide (19% and 19%, respectively in PURSUIT; 6% and 7%, respectively in ESPRIT). In PURSUIT, the only serious non-bleeding adverse event that occurred at a rate of at least 1% and was more common with eptifibatide than placebo (7% versus 6%) was hypotension. Most of the serious non-bleeding events consisted of cardiovascular events typical of an unstable angina population. In the IMPACT II study, serious non-bleeding events that occurred in greater than 1% of patients were uncommon and similar in incidence between placebo- and eptifibatide-treated patients.

Discontinuation of study drug due to adverse events other than bleeding was uncommon in the PURSUIT, IMPACT II and ESPRIT studies, with no single event occurring in >0.5% of the study population (except for "other" in the ESPRIT study). In the PURSUIT study, non-bleeding adverse events leading to discontinuation occurred in the eptifibatide and placebo groups in the following body systems with an incidence of ≥0.1%: cardiovascular system (0.3% and 0.3%), digestive system (0.1% and 0.1%), hemic/lymphatic system (0.1% and 0.1%), nervous system (0.3% and 0.4%), urogenital system (0.1% and 0.1%), and whole body system (0.2% and 0.2%). In the ESPRIT study, the following non-bleeding adverse events leading to discontinuation occurred in the eptifibatide and placebo groups with an incidence of ≥0.1%: "other" (1.2% and 1.1%). In the IMPACT II study, non-bleeding adverse events leading to discontinuation occurred in the 135/0.5 eptifibatide and placebo groups in the following body systems with an incidence of ≥0.1%: whole body (0.3% and 0.1%), cardiovascular system (1.4% and 1.4%), digestive system (0.2% and 0%), hemic/lymphatic system (0.2% and 0%), nervous system (0.3% and 0.2%), and respiratory system (0.1% and 0.1%).

Post-Marketing Experience. The following adverse events have been reported in post-marketing experience, primarily with eptifibatide in combination with heparin and aspirin: cerebral, GI and pulmonary hemorrhage. Fatal bleeding events have been reported.

OVERDOSAGE

There has been only limited experience with overdosage of eptifibatide. There were 8 patients in the IMPACT II study, 9 patients in the PURSUIT study and no patient in the ESPRIT study who received bolus doses and/or infusion doses more than double those called for in the protocols. None of these patients experienced an intracranial bleed or other major bleeding.

Eptifibatide was not lethal to rats, rabbits, or monkeys when administered by continuous intravenous infusion for 90 minutes at a total dose of 45 mg/kg (about 2 to 5 times the recommended maximum daily human dose on a body surface area basis). Symptoms of acute toxicity were loss of righting reflex, dyspnea, ptosis, and decreased muscle tone in rabbits and petechial hemorrhages in the femoral and abdominal areas of monkeys.

From *in vitro* studies, eptifibatide is not extensively bound to plasma proteins and thus may be cleared from plasma by dialysis.

INTEGRILIN Dosing Charts by Weight

Patient Weight		180 µg/kg Bolus Volume	2.0 µg/kg/min Infusion Volume		1.0 µg/kg/min Infusion Volume	
(kg)	(lb)	(from 2 mg/mL vial)	(from 2 mg/mL 100-mL vial)	(from 0.75 mg/mL 100-mL vial)	(from 2 mg/mL 100-mL vial)	(from 0.75 mg/mL 100-mL vial)
37–41	81–91	3.4 mL	2.0 mL/h	6.0 mL/h	1.0 mL/h	3.0 mL/h
42–46	92–102	4.0 mL	2.5 mL/h	7.0 mL/h	1.3 mL/h	3.5 mL/h
47–53	103–117	4.5 mL	3.0 mL/h	8.0 mL/h	1.5 mL/h	4.0 mL/h
54–59	118–130	5.0 mL	3.5 mL/h	9.0 mL/h	1.8 mL/h	4.5 mL/h
60–65	131–143	5.6 mL	3.8 mL/h	10.0 mL/h	1.9 mL/h	5.0 mL/h
66–71	144–157	6.2 mL	4.0 mL/h	11.0 mL/h	2.0 mL/h	5.5 mL/h
72–78	158–172	6.8 mL	4.5 mL/h	12.0 mL/h	2.3 mL/h	6.0 mL/h
79–84	173–185	7.3 mL	5.0 mL/h	13.0 mL/h	2.5 mL/h	6.5 mL/h
85–90	186–198	7.9 mL	5.3 mL/h	14.0 mL/h	2.7 mL/h	7.0 mL/h
91–96	199–212	8.5 mL	5.6 mL/h	15.0 mL/h	2.8 mL/h	7.5 mL/h
97–103	213–227	9.0 mL	6.0 mL/h	16.0 mL/h	3.0 mL/h	8.0 mL/h
104–109	228–240	9.5 mL	6.4 mL/h	17.0 mL/h	3.2 mL/h	8.5 mL/h
110–115	241–253	10.2 mL	6.8 mL/h	18.0 mL/h	3.4 mL/h	9.0 mL/h
116–121	254–267	10.7 mL	7.0 mL/h	19.0 mL/h	3.5 mL/h	9.5 mL/h
>121	>267	11.3 mL	7.5 mL/h	20.0 mL/h	3.7 mL/h	10.0 mL/h

DOSAGE AND ADMINISTRATION

The safety and efficacy of eptifibatide has been established in clinical studies that employed concomitant use of heparin and aspirin. Different dose regimens of eptifibatide were used in the major clinical studies. (See CLINICAL STUDIES.)

Acute Coronary Syndrome

The recommended adult dosage of eptifibatide in patients with acute coronary syndrome and normal renal function is an intravenous bolus of 180 µg/kg as soon as possible following diagnosis, followed by a continuous infusion of 2.0 µg/kg/min until hospital discharge or initiation of CABG surgery, up to 72 hours. If a patient is to undergo a percutaneous coronary intervention (PCI) while receiving eptifibatide, the infusion should be continued up to hospital discharge, or for up to 18–24 hours after the procedure, whichever comes first, allowing for up to 96 hours of therapy.

The recommended adult dosage of eptifibatide in patients with acute coronary syndrome with an estimated creatinine clearance (using the Cockroft-Gault equation)* < 50 mL/min or, if creatinine clearance is not available, a serum creatinine > 2.0 mg/dL, is an intravenous bolus of 180 µg/kg as soon as possible following diagnosis, immediately followed by a continuous infusion of 1.0 µg/kg-min.

Percutaneous Coronary Intervention (PCI)

The recommended adult dosage of eptifibatide in patients with normal renal function is an intravenous bolus of 180 µg/kg administered immediately before the initiation of PCI followed by a continuous infusion of 2.0 µg/kg/min and a second 180 µg/kg bolus 10 minutes after the first bolus. Infusion should be continued until hospital discharge, or for up to 18 to 24 hours, whichever comes first. A minimum of 12 hours of infusion is recommended.

The recommended adult dose of eptifibatide in patients with an estimated clearance (using the Cockroft-Gault equation)* <50 mL/min or, if creatinine clearance is not available, a serum creatinine >2.0 mg/dL, is an intravenous bolus of 180 µg/kg administered immediately before the initiation of the procedure, immediately followed by a continuous infusion of 1.0 µg/kg-min and a second 180 µg/kg bolus administered 10 minutes after the first.

In patients who undergo coronary artery bypass graft surgery, eptifibatide infusion should be discontinued prior to surgery.

*Using the Cockroft-Gault equation, creatinine clearance is calculated as:

Males: $\dfrac{(140\text{–age})\ (\text{body wt in kg})}{72\ (\text{serum creatinine})}$

Females: $\dfrac{(140\text{–age})\ (\text{body wt in kg})\ (0.85)}{72\ (\text{serum creatinine})}$

Aspirin and Heparin Dosing Recommendations

In the clinical trials that showed eptifibatide to be effective, most patients received concomitant aspirin and heparin. The recommended aspirin and heparin doses to be used are as follows:

Acute Coronary Syndrome

Aspirin:

160–325 mg po initially and daily thereafter

Heparin:

Target aPTT 50–70 seconds during medical management

- If weight ≥70 kg, 5000 U bolus followed by infusion of 1000 U/hr.
- If weight <70 kg, 60 U/kg bolus followed by infusion of 12 U/kg/hr.

Target ACT 200–300 seconds during PCI

- If heparin is initiated prior to PCI, additional boluses during PCI to maintain an ACT target of 200–300 seconds.
- Heparin infusion after the PCI is discouraged.

PCI

Aspirin:

160–325 mg po 1–24 hours prior to PCI and daily thereafter

Heparin:

Target ACT 200–300 seconds

- 60 U/kg bolus initially in patients not treated with heparin within 6 hours prior to PCI.
- Additional boluses during PCI to maintain ACT within target.
- Heparin infusion after the PCI is strongly discouraged.

Patients requiring thrombolytic therapy should have eptifibatide infusions stopped.

Instructions for Administration

1. Like other parenteral drug products, INTEGRILIN solutions should be inspected visually for particulate matter and discoloration prior to administration, whenever solution and container permit.
2. INTEGRILIN may be administered in the same intravenous line as alteplase, atropine, dobutamine, heparin, lidocaine, meperidine, metoprolol, midazolam, morphine, nitroglycerin, or verapamil. INTEGRILIN should not be administered through the same intravenous line as furosemide.
3. INTEGRILIN may be administered in the same IV line with 0.9% NaCl or 0.9% NaCl/5% dextrose. With either vehicle, the infusion may also contain up to 60 mEq/L of potassium chloride. No incompatibilities have been observed with intravenous administration sets. No compatibility studies have been performed with PVC bags.
4. The bolus dose(s) of INTEGRILIN should be withdrawn from the 10-mL vial into a syringe. The bolus dose(s) should be administered by IV push.
5. Immediately following the bolus dose administration, a continuous infusion of INTEGRILIN should be initiated. When using an intravenous infusion pump, INTEGRILIN should be administered undiluted directly from the 100-mL vial. The 100-mL vial should be spiked with a vented infusion set. Care should be taken to center the spike within the circle on the stopper top.

INTEGRILIN is to be administered by volume according to patient weight. Patients should receive INTEGRILIN according to the following table:

[See table above]

HOW SUPPLIED

INTEGRILIN (eptifibatide) Injection is supplied as a sterile solution in 10-mL vials containing 20 mg of eptifibatide (NDC 0085-1177-01) and 100-mL vials containing either 75 mg of eptifibatide (NDC 0085-1136-01) or 200 mg of eptifibatide (NDC 0085-1177-02).

Vials should be stored refrigerated at 2–8°C (36–46°F). Vials may be transferred to room temperature storage* for a period not to exceed 2 months. Upon transfer, vial cartons must be marked by the dispensing pharmacist with a "DISCARD BY" date (2 months from the transfer date or the labeled expiration date, whichever comes first).

Do not use beyond the labeled expiration date. Protect from light until administration. Discard any unused portion left in the vial.

* USP controlled Room Temperature: 25°C (77°F) with excursions permitted between 15–30°C (59–86°F).

Rx only

INTEGRILIN is a registered trademark of Millennium Pharmaceuticals, Inc.

Marketed By:

Millennium Pharmaceuticals, Inc.
Cambridge, MA 02139
and
Schering Corporation
Kenilworth, NJ 07033

Distributed By:

Schering Corporation
Kenilworth, NJ 07033

Issued June 2003
Rev 9

Shown in Product Identification Guide, page 324

VELCADE®

℞

[*vĕl′-kād*]
(bortezomib)
for Injection
PRESCRIBING INFORMATION

DESCRIPTION

VELCADE® (bortezomib) for Injection is an antineoplastic agent available for intravenous injection (IV) use only. Each

Continued on next page

Velcade—Cont.

single dose vial contains 3.5 mg of bortezomib as a sterile lyophilized powder. Inactive ingredient: 35 mg mannitol, USP.
Bortezomib is a modified dipeptidyl boronic acid. The product is provided as a mannitol boronic ester which, in reconstituted form, consists of the mannitol ester in equilibrium with its hydrolysis product, the monomeric boronic acid. The drug substance exists in its cyclic anhydride form as a trimeric boroxine.
The chemical name for bortezomib, the monomeric boronic acid, is [(1R)-3-methyl-1-[[(2S)-1-oxo-3-phenyl-2-[(pyrazinylcarbonyl) amino]propyl]amino]butyl] boronic acid.
Bortezomib has the following chemical structure:

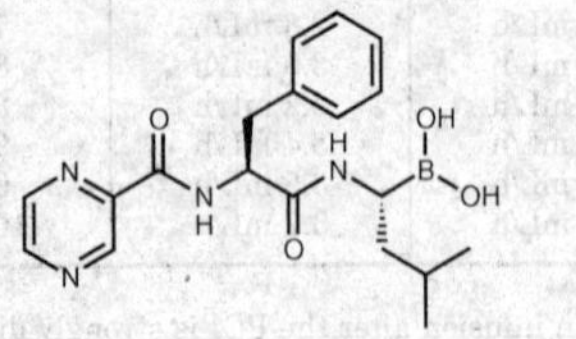

The molecular weight is 384.24. The molecular formula is: $C_{19}H_{25}BN_4O_4$. The solubility of bortezomib, as the monomeric boronic acid, in water is 3.3-3.8 mg/mL in a pH range of 2–6.5.

CLINICAL PHARMACOLOGY

Mechanism of Action

Bortezomib is a reversible inhibitor of the chymotrypsin-like activity of the 26S proteasome in mammalian cells. The 26S proteasome is a large protein complex that degrades ubiquitinated proteins. The ubiquitin-proteasome pathway plays an essential role in regulating the intracellular concentration of specific proteins, thereby maintaining homeostasis within cells. Inhibition of the 26S proteasome prevents this targeted proteolysis which can affect multiple signaling cascades within the cell. This disruption of normal homeostatic mechanisms can lead to cell death. Experiments have demonstrated that bortezomib is cytotoxic to a variety of cancer cell types *in vitro*. Bortezomib causes a delay in tumor growth *in vivo* in nonclinical tumor models, including multiple myeloma.

Pharmacokinetics

Following intravenous administration of 1.3 mg/m^2 dose, the median estimated maximum plasma concentration of bortezomib was 509 ng/mL (range=109-1300 ng/mL) in eight patients with multiple myeloma and creatinine clearance values ranging from 31-169 mL/min. The mean elimination half-life of bortezomib after first dose ranged from 9 to 15 hours at doses ranging from 1.45 to 2.00 mg/m^2 in patients with advanced malignancies. The pharmacokinetics of bortezomib as a single agent have not been fully characterized at the recommended dose in multiple myeloma patients.

Distribution

The distribution volume of bortezomib as a single agent was not assessed at the recommended dose in patients with multiple myeloma. The binding of bortezomib to human plasma proteins averaged 83% over the concentration range of 100-1000 ng/mL.

Metabolism

In vitro studies with human liver microsomes and human cDNA-expressed cytochrome P450 isozymes indicate that bortezomib is primarily oxidatively metabolized via cytochrome P450 enzymes, 3A4, 2D6, 2C19, 2C9, and 1A2. The major metabolic pathway is deboronation to form two deboronated metabolites that subsequently undergo hydroxylation to several metabolites. Deboronated-bortezomib metabolites are inactive as 26S proteasome inhibitors. Pooled plasma data from 8 patients at 10 min and 30 min after dosing indicate that the plasma levels of metabolites are low compared to the parent drug.

Elimination

The pathways of elimination of bortezomib have not been characterized in humans.

Special Populations

Age, Gender, and Race: The effects of age, gender, and race on the pharmacokinetics of bortezomib have not been evaluated.

Hepatic Impairment: No pharmacokinetic studies were conducted with bortezomib in patients with hepatic impairment (**see PRECAUTIONS**).

Renal Impairment: No pharmacokinetic studies were conducted with bortezomib in patients with renal impairment. Clinical studies included patients with creatinine clearances values ranging from 13.8 to 220 mL/min (**see PRECAUTIONS**).

Pediatric: There are no pharmacokinetic data in pediatric patients.

Drug Interactions

No formal drug interaction studies have been conducted with bortezomib.
In vitro studies with human liver microsomes indicate that bortezomib is a substrate of cytochrome P450 3A4, 2D6, 2C19, 2C9, and 1A2 (**see PRECAUTIONS**).
Bortezomib is a poor inhibitor of human liver microsome cytochrome P450 1A2, 2C9, 2D6, and 3A4, with IC$_{50}$ values of >30 µM (>11.5 µg/mL). Bortezomib may inhibit 2C19 activity (IC$_{50}$ = 18 µM, 6.9 µg/mL) and increase exposure to drugs that are substrates for this enzyme.

Table 1: Summary of Patient Population and Disease Characteristics*

	N = 202
Patient Characteristics	
Median age in years (range)	59 (34, 84)
Gender: male/female	60%/40%
Race: caucasian/black/other	81%/10%/8%
Karnofsky Performance Status score ≤70	20%
Hemoglobin <100 g/L	44%
Platelet count <75 × 10^9/L	21%
Disease Characteristics	
Type of myeloma (%): IgG/IgA/Light chain	60%/24%/14%
Median β2-microglobulin (mg/L)	3.5
Median creatinine clearance (mL/min)	73.9
Abnormal cytogenetics	35%
Chromosome 13 deletion	15%
Median Duration of Multiple Myeloma Since Diagnosis in Years	4.0
Previous Therapy	
Any prior steroids, e.g., dexamethasone, VAD	99%
Any prior alkylating agents, e.g., MP, VBMCP	92%
Any prior anthracyclines, e.g., VAD, mitoxantrone	81%
Any prior thalidomide therapy	83%
Received at least 2 of the above	98%
Received at least 3 of the above	92%
Received all 4 of the above	66%
Any prior stem cell transplant/other high-dose therapy	64%
Prior experimental or other types of therapy	44%

* Based on number of patients with baseline data available

Table 2: Summary of Disease Outcomes

Response Analyses (VELCADE monotherapy) N = 188	**N (%)**	**(95% CI)**
Overall Response Rate (Bladé) (CR + PR)	52 (27.7%)	(21, 35)
Complete Response (CR)[1]	5 (2.7%)	(1, 6)
Partial Response (PR)[2]	47 (25%)	(19, 32)
Clinical Remission (SWOG)[3]	33 (17.6%)	(12, 24)
Kaplan-Meier Estimated Median Duration of Response (95% CI)	365 Days	(224, NE)

[1] **Complete Response** required 100% disappearance of the original monoclonal protein from blood and urine on at least 2 determinations at least 6 weeks apart by immunofixation, and <5% plasma cells in the bone marrow on at least two determinations for a minimum of six weeks, stable bone disease and calcium.
[2] **Partial Response** requires ≥50% reduction in serum myeloma protein and ≥90% reduction of urine myeloma protein on at least 2 occasions for a minimum of at least 6 weeks, stable bone disease and calcium.
[3] **Clinical Remission (SWOG)** required ≥75% reduction in serum myeloma protein and/or ≥90% reduction of urine myeloma protein on at least 2 occasions for a minimum of at least 6 weeks, stable bone disease and calcium.

Bortezomib did not induce the activities of cytochrome P450 3A4 and 1A2 in primary cultured human hepatocytes.

CLINICAL STUDIES

Clinical Study in Relapsed and Refractory Multiple Myeloma

The safety and efficacy of VELCADE were evaluated in an open-label, single-arm, multicenter study of 202 patients who had received at least 2 prior therapies and demonstrated disease progression on their most recent therapy. The median number of prior therapies was six. Baseline patient and disease characteristics are summarized in **Table 1**.
An IV bolus injection of VELCADE 1.3 mg/m^2/dose was administered twice weekly for 2 weeks, followed by a 10-day rest period (21 day treatment cycle) for a maximum of 8 treatment cycles. The study employed dose modifications for toxicity (**see DOSAGE AND ADMINISTRATION**). Patients who experienced a response to VELCADE treatment were allowed to continue VELCADE treatment in an extension study.
[See table 1 above]
Responses to VELCADE alone are shown in **Table 2**. Response rates to VELCADE alone were determined by an independent review committee (IRC) based on criteria published by Bladé and others.[1] Complete response required <5% plasma cells in the marrow, 100% reduction in M protein, and a negative immunofixation test (IF$^-$). Response rates using the SWOG criteria are also shown. SWOG response required a ≥75% reduction in serum myeloma protein and/or ≥90% urine protein.[2] A total of 188 patients were evaluated for response; 9 patients with nonmeasurable disease could not be evaluated for response by the IRC. Five patients were excluded from the efficacy analyses because they had minimal prior therapy.
Ninety-eight percent of study patients received a starting dose of 1.3 mg/m^2. Twenty-eight percent of these patients received a dose of 1.3 mg/m^2 throughout the study, while 33% of patients who started at a dose of 1.3 mg/m^2 had to have their dose reduced during the study. Sixty-three percent of patients had at least one dose held during the study. In general, patients who had a confirmed CR received 2 additional cycles of VELCADE treatment beyond confirmation. The mean number of cycles administered was six.
The median time to response was 38 days (range 30 to 127 days).
The median survival of all patients enrolled was 16 months (range <1 to 18+ months).
[See table 2 above]
In this study, the response rate to VELCADE was independent of the number and types of prior therapies. There was a decreased likelihood of response in patients with either >50% plasma cells or abnormal cytogenetics in the bone marrow. Responses were seen in patients with chromosome 13 abnormalities.
A small dose-response study was performed in 54 patients with multiple myeloma who received a 1.0 mg/m^2/dose or a 1.3 mg/m^2/dose twice weekly for two out of three weeks. A single complete response was seen at each dose, and there were overall (CR + PR) response rates of 30% (8/27) at 1.0 mg/m^2 and 38% (10/26) at 1.3 mg/m^2.

INDICATIONS AND USAGE

VELCADE® (bortezomib) for Injection is indicated for the treatment of multiple myeloma patients who have received at least two prior therapies and have demonstrated disease progression on the last therapy.
The effectiveness of VELCADE is based on response rates (**see CLINICAL STUDIES section**). There are no controlled trials demonstrating a clinical benefit, such as an improvement in survival.

CONTRAINDICATIONS

VELCADE is contraindicated in patients with hypersensitivity to bortezomib, boron or mannitol.

WARNINGS

VELCADE should be administered under the supervision of a physician experienced in the use of antineoplastic therapy.

Pregnancy Category D

Women of childbearing potential should avoid becoming pregnant while being treated with VELCADE.
Bortezomib was not teratogenic in nonclinical developmental toxicity studies in rats and rabbits at the highest dose tested (0.075 mg/kg; 0.5 mg/m^2 in the rat and 0.05 mg/kg; 0.6 mg/m^2 in the rabbit) when administered during organogenesis. These dosages are approximately half the clinical dose of 1.3 mg/m^2 based on body surface area.
Pregnant rabbits given bortezomib during organogenesis at a dose of 0.05 mg/kg (0.6 mg/m^2) experienced significant post-implantation loss and decreased number of live fetuses. Live fetuses from these litters also showed significant decreases in fetal weight. The dose is approximately 0.5 times the clinical dose of 1.3 mg/m^2 based on body surface area.
No placental transfer studies have been conducted with bortezomib. There are no adequate and well-controlled studies in pregnant women. If VELCADE is used during pregnancy, or if the patient becomes pregnant while receiving this drug, the patient should be apprised of the potential hazard to the fetus.

PRECAUTIONS

Peripheral Neuropathy: VELCADE treatment causes a peripheral neuropathy that is predominantly sensory, although cases of mixed sensori-motor neuropathy have also been reported. Patients with pre-existing symptoms (numbness, pain or a burning feeling in the feet or hands) and/or signs of peripheral neuropathy may experience worsening during treatment with VELCADE. Patients should be monitored for symptoms of neuropathy, such as a burning sensation, hyperesthesia, hypoesthesia, paresthesia, discomfort or neuropathic pain. Patients experiencing new or worsening peripheral neuropathy may require change in the dose and schedule of VELCADE (**see DOSAGE AND ADMINISTRATION**). Limited follow-up data regarding the outcome of peripheral neuropathy are available. Of the patients who experienced treatment emergent neuropathy more than 70% had previously been treated with neurotoxic agents and more than 80% of these patients had signs or symptoms of peripheral neuropathy at baseline (**also see ADVERSE REACTIONS**).

Hypotension: VELCADE treatment can cause orthostatic/postural hypotension in about 12% of patients. These events are observed throughout therapy. Caution should be used when treating patients with a history of syncope, patients receiving medications known to be associated with hypotension, and patients who are dehydrated. Management of orthostatic/postural hypotension may include adjustment of antihypertensive medications, hydration, or administration of mineralocorticoids.

Heart Failure: Acute development or exacerbation of congestive heart failure has been seen in patients with risk factors for or existing heart disease. Such patients should be closely monitored.

Laboratory Tests: Complete blood counts (CBC) should be frequently monitored throughout treatment with VELCADE.

Gastrointestinal Adverse Events: VELCADE treatment can cause nausea, diarrhea, constipation, and vomiting (**see ADVERSE REACTIONS**) sometimes requiring use of antiemetics and antidiarrheals. Fluid and electrolyte replacement should be administered to prevent dehydration.

Thrombocytopenia: Thrombocytopenia, which was reported in 43% of patients throughout therapy, was maximal at Day 11 and typically recovered by the next cycle. On average, the pattern of platelet count decrease and recovery remained consistent over the 8 cycle study period and there was no evidence of cumulative thrombocytopenia. The mean platelet count nadir measured was approximately 40% of baseline. The severity of thrombocytopenia related to pretreatment platelet count is shown in **Table 3**. Platelet counts should be monitored prior to each dose of VELCADE. VELCADE therapy should be held when the platelet count is <25,000/μL and reinitiated at a reduced dose. Transfusions may be used at the discretion of the physician. There have been reports of gastrointestinal and intracerebral hemorrhage in association with VELCADE induced thrombocytopenia (**see DOSAGE AND ADMINISTRATION and ADVERSE REACTIONS**).

Table 3: The Severity of Thrombocytopenia Related to Pre-Treatment Platelet Count

Pre-treatment Platelet Count	Number of Patients (N=228)	Number of Patients with Platelet Count <10,000/μL
≥ 75,000/μL	186	1 (1%)
≥ 50,000/μL - < 75,000/μL	15	2 (13%)
≥ 10,000/μL - < 50,000/μL	27	8 (30%)

Tumor Lysis Syndrome: Because VELCADE is a cytotoxic agent and can rapidly kill malignant cells the complications of tumor lysis syndrome may occur. The patients at risk of tumor lysis syndrome are those with high tumor burden prior to treatment. These patients should be monitored closely and appropriate precautions taken.

Patients with Hepatic Impairment

Bortezomib is metabolized by liver enzymes and bortezomib's clearance may decrease in patients with hepatic impairment. These patients should be closely monitored for toxicities when treated with VELCADE (**see CLINICAL PHARMACOLOGY/Pharmacokinetics-Special Populations**).

Patients with Renal Impairment

No clinical information is available on the use of VELCADE in patients with creatinine clearance values less than 13 mL/min and patients on hemodialysis. These patients should be closely monitored for toxicities when treated with VELCADE (**see CLINICAL PHARMACOLOGY/Pharmacokinetics-Special Populations**).

Animal Toxicity Findings

Cardiovascular toxicity

Studies in monkeys showed that administration of dosages approximately twice the recommended clinical dose resulted in heart rate elevations, followed by profound progressive hypotension, bradycardia, and death 12-14 hours post dose. Doses ≥1.2 mg/m^2 induced dose proportional changes in cardiac parameters. Bortezomib has been shown to distribute to most tissues in the body, including the myocardium. In a repeated dosing toxicity study in the monkey, myocardial hemorrhage, inflammation, and necrosis were also observed.

Table 4: Most Commonly Reported (≥10% Overall) Adverse Events (N = 228)

Adverse Event	All Patients (N = 228) [n (%)] All Events	Grade 3 Events	Grade 4 Events
Asthenic conditions	149 (65)	42 (18)	1 (<1)
Nausea	145 (64)	13 (6)	0
Diarrhea	116 (51)	16 (7)	2 (<1)
Appetite decreased	99 (43)	6 (3)	0
Constipation	97 (43)	5 (2)	0
Thrombocytopenia	97 (43)	61 (27)	7 (3)
Peripheral neuropathy	84 (37)	31 (14)	0
Pyrexia	82 (36)	9 (4)	0
Vomiting	82 (36)	16 (7)	1 (<1)
Anemia	74 (32)	21 (9)	0
Headache	63 (28)	8 (4)	0
Insomnia	62 (27)	3 (1)	0
Arthralgia	60 (26)	11 (5)	0
Pain in limb	59 (26)	16 (7)	0
Edema	58 (25)	3 (1)	0
Neutropenia	55 (24)	30 (13)	6 (3)
Paresthesia and dysesthesia	53 (23)	6 (3)	0
Dyspnea	50 (22)	7 (3)	1 (<1)
Dizziness (excluding vertigo)	48 (21)	3 (1)	0
Rash	47 (21)	1 (<1)	0
Dehydration	42 (18)	15 (7)	0
Upper respiratory tract infection	41 (18)	0	0
Cough	39 (17)	1 (<1)	0
Bone pain	33 (14)	5 (2)	0
Anxiety	32 (14)	0	0
Myalgia	32 (14)	5 (2)	0
Back pain	31 (14)	9 (4)	0
Muscle cramps	31 (14)	1 (<1)	0
Dyspepsia	30 (13)	0	0
Abdominal pain	29 (13)	5 (2)	0
Dysgeusia	29 (13)	1 (<1)	0
Hypotension	27 (12)	8 (4)	0
Rigors	27 (12)	1 (<1)	0
Herpes zoster	26 (11)	2 (<1)	0
Pruritus	26 (11)	0	0
Vision blurred	25 (11)	1 (<1)	0
Pneumonia	23 (10)	12 (5)	0

Chronic Administration

In animal studies at a dose and schedule similar to that recommended for patients (twice weekly dosing for 2 weeks followed by 1 week rest) toxicities observed included severe anemia and thrombocytopenia, gastrointestinal, neurological and lymphoid system toxicities. Neurotoxic effects of bortezomib in animal studies included axonal swelling and degeneration in peripheral nerves, dorsal spinal roots, and tracts of the spinal cord. Additionally, multifocal hemorrhage and necrosis in the brain, eye, and heart were observed.

Information for Patients

Physicians are advised to discuss the following with patients to whom VELCADE will be administered.

Effects on Ability to Drive or Operate Machinery or Impairment of Mental Ability: Since VELCADE may be associated with fatigue, dizziness, syncope, orthostatic/postural hypotension, diplopia or blurred vision, patients should be cautious when operating machinery, including automobiles.

Pregnancy/Nursing: Patients should be advised to use effective contraceptive measures to prevent pregnancy and to avoid breast feeding during treatment with VELCADE.

Dehydration/Hypotension: Since patients receiving VELCADE therapy may experience vomiting and/or diarrhea, patients should be advised regarding appropriate measures to avoid dehydration. Patients should be instructed to seek medical advice if they experience symptoms of dizziness, light headedness or fainting spells.

Concomitant Medications: Patients should be cautioned about the use of concomitant medications that may be associated with peripheral neuropathy (such as amiodarone, anti-virals, isoniazid, nitrofurantoin, or statins), or with a decrease in blood pressure.

Peripheral Neuropathy: Patients should be instructed to contact their physician if they experience new or worsening symptoms of peripheral neuropathy (**see PRECAUTIONS and DOSAGE AND ADMINISTRATION**).

Drug Interactions

No formal drug interaction studies have been conducted with VELCADE.

In vitro studies with human liver microsomes indicate that bortezomib is a substrate for cytochrome P450 3A4, 2D6, 2C19, 2C9, and 1A2. Patients who are concomitantly receiving VELCADE and drugs that are inhibitors or inducers of cytochrome P450 3A4 should be closely monitored for either toxicities or reduced efficacy (**see CLINICAL PHARMACOLOGY/Pharmacokinetics-Drug Interactions**).

During clinical trials, hypoglycemia and hyperglycemia were reported in diabetic patients receiving oral hypoglycemics. Patients on oral antidiabetic agents receiving VELCADE treatment may require close monitoring of their blood glucose levels and adjustment of the dose of their antidiabetic medication.

Drug Laboratory Test Interactions

None known.

Carcinogenesis, Mutagenesis, Impairment of Fertility

Carcinogenicity studies have not been conducted with bortezomib.

Bortezomib showed clastogenic activity (structural chromosomal aberrations) in the *in vitro* chromosomal aberration assay using Chinese hamster ovary cells. Bortezomib was not genotoxic when tested in the *in vitro* mutagenicity assay (Ames test) and *in vivo* micronucleus assay in mice.

Fertility studies with bortezomib were not performed but evaluation of reproductive tissues has been performed in the general toxicity studies. In the 6-month rat toxicity study, degenerative effects in the ovary were observed at doses ≥0.3 mg/m^2 (one-fourth of the recommended clinical dose), and degenerative changes in the testes occurred at 1.2 mg/m^2. VELCADE could have a potential effect on either male or female fertility.

Pregnancy Category D (see WARNINGS)

Nursing Mothers

It is not known whether bortezomib is excreted in human milk. Because many drugs are excreted in human milk and because of the potential for serious adverse reactions in nursing infants from VELCADE, women should be advised against breast feeding while being treated with VELCADE.

Pediatric Use

The safety and effectiveness of VELCADE in children has not been established.

Geriatric Use

Of the 202 patients enrolled, 35% were 65 years of age or older. Nineteen percent (19%) of patients aged 65 years or older experienced responses versus 32% in patients under the age of 65. Across the 256 patients analyzed for safety, the incidence of Grade 3 or 4 events reported was 74%, 80%, and 85% for patients ≤50 years, 51 to 65 years, and >65 years, respectively.

ADVERSE REACTIONS

The two studies described (**see CLINICAL STUDIES**) evaluated 228 patients with multiple myeloma receiving VELCADE 1.3 mg/m^2/dose twice weekly for 2 weeks followed by a 10-day rest period (21 day treatment cycle length) for a maximum of 8 treatment cycles.

The most commonly reported adverse events were asthenic conditions (including fatigue, malaise and weakness) (65%), nausea (64%), diarrhea (51%), appetite decreased (including anorexia) (43%), constipation (43%), thrombocytopenia (43%), peripheral neuropathy (including peripheral sensory neuropathy and peripheral neuropathy aggravated) (37%), pyrexia (36%), vomiting (36%), and anemia (32%). Fourteen percent of patients experienced at least one episode of grade 4 toxicity, with the most common toxicity being thrombocytopenia (3%) and neutropenia (3%).

Serious Adverse Events (SAEs): Serious Adverse Events are defined as any event, regardless of causality, that: results in death, is life-threatening, requires hospitalization or prolongs a current hospitalization, results in a significant disability or is deemed to be an important medical event. A total of 113 (50%) of the 228 patients experienced SAEs during the studies. The most commonly reported SAEs included pyrexia (7%), pneumonia (7%), diarrhea (6%), vomiting (5%), dehydration (5%), and nausea (4%).

Continued on next page

Velcade—Cont.

Adverse events thought by the investigator to be drug-related and leading to discontinuation occurred in 18% of patients. The reasons for discontinuation included peripheral neuropathy (5%), thrombocytopenia (4%), diarrhea (2%), and fatigue (2%).

Two deaths were reported and considered by the investigator to be possibly related to study drug: one case of cardiopulmonary arrest and one case of respiratory failure.

The most common adverse events are shown in **Table 4**. All adverse events occurring at ≥10% are included. In the single arm studies conducted it is often not possible to distinguish adverse events that are drug-caused and those that reflect the patient's underlying disease. See discussion of specific adverse reactions following **Table 4**.

[See table 4 at top of previous page]

Asthenic conditions (fatigue, malaise, weakness)

Asthenia was reported in 65% of patients and was predominantly reported as Grade 1 or 2. The first onset of fatigue was most often reported during the 1st and 2nd cycles of therapy. Asthenia was Grade 3 for 18% of patients. Two percent of patients discontinued treatment due to fatigue.

Gastrointestinal Events

The majority of patients experienced gastrointestinal adverse events during the studies, including nausea, diarrhea, constipation, and vomiting. Grade 3 or 4 gastrointestinal events occurred in 21% of patients and were considered serious in 13% of patients. Vomiting and diarrhea each were of Grade 3 severity in 7% of patients and were Grade 4 in <1%. Five percent of patients discontinued due to gastrointestinal events. Appetite decreased (anorexia) was reported as an adverse event for 43% of patients. The incidence of Grade 3 decreased appetite was 3%.

Thrombocytopenia

Thrombocytopenia was reported during treatment with VELCADE for 43% of patients. The thrombocytopenia was characterized by a dose related decrease in platelet count during the VELCADE dosing period (days 1 to 11) and a return towards baseline during the rest period (days 12 to 21) in each treatment cycle. The mean platelet count nadir measured was approximately 40% of baseline. The platelet count was <50,000/µL and <10,000/µL for 27% and 3%, respectively, of patients. Four percent (4%) of patients discontinued VELCADE treatment due to thrombocytopenia of any grade.

Peripheral Sensory Neuropathy

Events reported as peripheral neuropathy, peripheral sensory neuropathy, and peripheral neuropathy aggravated occurred in 37% of patients. Peripheral neuropathy was Grade 3 for 14% of patients with no Grade 4 events. New onset or worsening of existing neuropathy was noted throughout the cycles of treatment. Six percent (6%) of patients discontinued VELCADE due to neuropathy. More than 80% of all study patients had signs or symptoms of peripheral neuropathy at baseline evaluation. The incidence of Grade 3 neuropathy was 5% (2 of 41 patients) in patients without baseline neuropathy. Symptoms may improve or return to baseline in some patients upon discontinuation of VELCADE. The complete time-course of this toxicity has not been fully characterized.

Pyrexia

Pyrexia (>38°C) was reported as an adverse event for 36% of patients and was assessed as Grade 3 in 4% of patients.

Neutropenia

Neutropenia occurred in 24% of patients and was grade 3 in 13% and grade 4 in 3%. The incidence of febrile neutropenia was <1%.

Hypotension

Hypotension (including reports of orthostatic hypotension) was reported in 12% of patients. Most events were Grade 1 or 2 in severity. Grade 3 hypotension occurred in 4% of patients; no patient experienced Grade 4 hypotension. Patients developing orthostatic hypotension did not have evidence of orthostatic hypotension at study entry; half had pre-existing hypertension and one third had evidence of peripheral neuropathy. Doses of antihypertensive medications may need to be adjusted in patients receiving VELCADE. Four percent of patients experienced hypotension, including orthostatic hypotension, and had a concurrent syncopal event.

Serious Adverse Events from Clinical Studies

In approximately 580 patients, the following serious adverse events (not described above) were reported, considered at least possibly related to study medication, in at least one patient treated with VELCADE administered as monotherapy or in combination with other chemotherapeutics. These studies were conducted in patients with hematological malignancies and in solid tumors.

Blood and lymphatic system disorders: Disseminated intravascular coagulation

Cardiac disorders: Atrial fibrillation aggravated, atrial flutter, cardiac amyloidosis, cardiac arrest, cardiac failure congestive, myocardial ischemia, myocardial infarction, pericardial effusion, pulmonary edema, ventricular tachycardia

Gastrointestinal disorders: Ascites, dysphagia, fecal impaction, gastritis hemorrhagic, gastrointestinal hemorrhage, hematemesis, ileus paralytic, large intestinal obstruction, paralytic intestinal obstruction, small intestinal obstruction, large intestinal perforation, stomatitis, melena, pancreatitis acute

Table 5: Recommended Dose Modification for VELCADE-related Neuropathic Pain and/or Peripheral Sensory Neuropathy

Severity of Peripheral Neuropathy Signs and Symptoms	Modification of Dose and Regimen
Grade 1 (paresthesias and/or loss of reflexes) without pain or loss of function	No action
Grade 1 with pain or Grade 2 (interfering with function but not with activities of daily living)	Reduce VELCADE to 1.0 mg/m^2
Grade 2 with pain or Grade 3 (interfering with activities of daily living)	Withhold VELCADE therapy until toxicity resolves. When toxicity resolves reinitiate with a reduced dose of VELCADE at 0.7 mg/m^2 and change treatment schedule to once per week.
Grade 4 (Permanent sensory loss that interferes with function	Discontinue VELCADE

NCI Common Toxicity Criteria website – http://ctep.info.nih.gov/reporting/ctc.html

Hepatobiliary: Hyperbilirubinemia, portal vein thrombosis

Immune system disorders: Anaphylactic reaction, drug hypersensitivity, immune complex mediated hypersensitivity

Infections and Infestations: Bacteremia

Injury, poisoning and procedural complications: Skeletal fracture, subdural hematoma

Metabolism and nutrition disorders: Hypocalcemia, hyperuricemia, hypokalemia, hyponatremia, tumor lysis syndrome

Nervous system: Ataxia, coma, dizziness, dysarthria, dysautonomia, cranial palsy, grand mal convulsion, hemorrhagic stroke, motor dysfunction, spinal cord compression, transient ischemic attack

Psychiatric: Agitation, confusion, psychotic disorder, suicidal ideation

Renal and urinary: Calculus renal, bilateral hydronephrosis, bladder spasm, hematuria urinary incontinence, urinary retention, renal failure (acute and chronic), glomerular nephritis proliferative

Respiratory, thoracic and mediastinal: Acute respiratory distress syndrome, atelectasis, chronic obstructive airways disease exacerbated, dysphagia, dyspnea, dyspnea exertional, epistaxis, hemoptysis, hypoxia, lung infiltration, pleural effusion, pneumonitis, respiratory distress, respiratory failure

Vascular: Cerebrovascular accident, deep venous thrombosis, peripheral embolism, pulmonary embolism

OVERDOSAGE

Cardiovascular safety pharmacology studies in monkeys show that lethal IV doses are associated with decreases in blood pressure, increases in heart rate, increases in contractility, and ultimately terminal hypotension. In monkeys, doses of 3.0 mg/m^2 and greater (approximately twice the recommended clinical dose) resulted in progressive hypotension starting at 1 hour and progressing to death by 12 to 14 hours following drug administration.

No cases of overdosage with VELCADE were reported during clinical trials. Single doses of up to 2.0 mg/m^2 per week have been administered in adults. In the event of overdosage, patient's vital signs should be monitored and appropriate supportive care given to maintain blood pressure and body temperature (**see PRECAUTIONS and DOSAGE AND ADMINISTRATION**).

There is no known specific antidote for VELCADE overdosage.

DOSAGE AND ADMINISTRATION

The recommended dose of VELCADE is 1.3 mg/m^2/dose administered as a bolus intravenous injection twice weekly for two weeks (days 1, 4, 8, and 11) followed by a 10-day rest period (days 12–21) (**see CLINICAL STUDIES section for a description of dose administration during the trials**).

This 3-week period is considered a treatment cycle. At least 72 hours should elapse between consecutive doses of VELCADE.

Dose Modification and Reinitiation of Therapy

VELCADE therapy should be withheld at the onset of any Grade 3 non-hematological or Grade 4 hematological toxicities excluding neuropathy as discussed below (**see PRECAUTIONS**). Once the symptoms of the toxicity have resolved, VELCADE therapy may be reinitiated at a 25% reduced dose (1.3 mg/m^2/dose reduced to 1.0 mg/m^2/dose; 1.0 mg/m^2/dose reduced to 0.7 mg/m^2/dose). The following table contains the recommended dose modification for the management of patients who experience VELCADE-related neuropathic pain and/or peripheral sensory neuropathy (**Table 5**). Patients with pre-existing severe neuropathy should be treated with VELCADE only after careful risk/benefit assessment.

[See table 5 above]

Administration Precautions: VELCADE is an antineoplastic. Caution should be used during handling and preparation. Proper aseptic technique should be used. Use of gloves and other protective clothing to prevent skin contact is recommended. In clinical trials, local skin irritation was reported in 5% of patients, but extravasation of VELCADE was not associated with tissue damage.

Reconstitution/Preparation for Intravenous Administration: Prior to use, the contents of each vial must be reconstituted with 3.5 mL of normal (0.9%) saline, Sodium Chloride Injection, USP. The reconstituted product should be a clear and colorless solution.

Parenteral drug products should be inspected visually for particulate matter and discoloration prior to administration whenever solution and container permit. If any discoloration or particulate matter is observed, the reconstituted product should not be used.

Stability: Unopened vials of VELCADE are stable until the date indicated on the package when stored in the original package protected from light.

VELCADE contains no antimicrobial preservative. When reconstituted as directed, VELCADE may be stored at 25°C (77°F); excursions permitted from 15 to 30°C (59 to 86°F) [see USP Controlled Room Temperature]. Reconstituted VELCADE should be administered within eight hours of preparation. The reconstituted material may be stored in the original vial and/or the syringe prior to administration. The product may be stored for up to three hours in a syringe, however total storage time for the reconstituted material must not exceed eight hours when exposed to normal indoor lighting.

HOW SUPPLIED

VELCADE (bortezomib) for Injection is supplied as individually cartoned 10 mL vials containing 3.5 mg of bortezomib as a white to off-white cake or powder.

NDC 63020-049-01

3.5 mg single dose vial

STORAGE

Unopened vials may be stored at controlled room temperature 25°C (77°F); excursions permitted from 15 to 30°C (59 to 86°F) [see USP Controlled Room Temperature]. Retain in original package to protect from light.

Caution: ℞ **only**

U.S. Patents: 5,780,454; 6,083,903; 6,297,217

Distributed and Marketed by:

Millennium Pharmaceuticals, Inc.

40 Landsdowne Street

Cambridge, MA 02139

MILLENNIUM™

Issued April 2004 Rev 1

REFERENCES

1. Bladé J, Samson D, Reece D, Apperley J, Bjorkstrand B, Gahrton G et al. Criteria for evaluating disease response and progression in patients with multiple myeloma treated by high-dose therapy and haematopoietic stem cell transplantation. Myeloma Subcommittee of the EBMT. European Group for Blood and Marrow Transplant. *British Journal of Haematology* 1998;102(5):1115-1123. **2.** Salmon SE, Haut A, Bonnet JD, Amare M, Weick JK, Durie BG et al. Alternating combination chemotherapy and levamisole improves survival in multiple myeloma: a Southwest Oncology Group Study. *Journal of Clinical Oncology* 1983;1(8):453-461.

PATIENT INFORMATION

VELCADE is intended for use under the guidance and supervision of a health care professional. Please discuss the possibility of the following side effects with your doctor:

Effects on Ability to Drive or Operate Machinery or Impairment of Mental Ability:

VELCADE may be associated with fatigue, dizziness, lightheadedness, fainting or blurred vision. Please exercise caution or avoid operating machinery, including automobiles, following use of VELCADE.

Pregnancy/Nursing:

Please use effective contraceptive measures to prevent pregnancy and avoid breast feeding during treatment with VELCADE.

Dehydration/Hypotension:

Following the use of VELCADE therapy, you may experience vomiting and/or diarrhea. Drink plenty of fluids. Speak with your doctor if these symptoms occur about what you should do to control or manage these symptoms.

If you experience symptoms of dizziness or light-headedness, consult a healthcare professional. Seek immediate medical attention if you experience fainting spells.

Concomitant Medications:

Please speak with your doctor about any other medication you are currently taking. Your doctor will want to be aware of any other medications.

Peripheral Neuropathy:
Contact your doctor if you experience new or worsening symptoms of peripheral neuropathy such as numbness, pain, or a burning feeling in the feet or hands.

Millennium Pharmaceuticals, Inc.
40 Landsdowne Street
Cambridge, MA 02139
MILLENNIUM™

Issued April 2004 Rev 1
Shown in Product Identification Guide, page 324

Mission Pharmacal Company

10999 IH 10 WEST, SUITE 1000
SAN ANTONIO, TX 78230-1355

Direct Inquiries to:
PO Box 786099
San Antonio, TX 78278–6099
TOLL FREE: (800) 292-7364
(210) 696-8400
FAX: (210) 696-6010
For Medical Emergencies Contact:
Mary Ann Walter at (210) 696-8400

CALCET® OTC
[kăl 'sĕt]
Calcium-Vit. D Dietary Supplement

HOW SUPPLIED
CALCET® is supplied as yellow, rectangular shaped, coated tablets in bottles of 100 (UPC 0178–0251–01).

CALCET® PLUS OTC
[kăl 'sĕt]
Calcium-Iron-Zinc-Multivitamin

WARNING: Accidental overdose of **iron-containing** products is a leading cause of fatal poisoning in children under 6. Keep this product out of reach of children. In case of accidental overdose, call a doctor or poison control center immediately.

HOW SUPPLIED
CALCET PLUS is supplied as white, modified oval shaped, coated tablets in bottles of 60 (UPC 0178-0252-60).

CALCIBIND® ℞
[kal 'sĕ-bīnd]
Cellulose Sodium Phosphate Oral Powder

DESCRIPTION
Cellulose Sodium Phosphate (CSP), the active ingredient in CALCIBIND®, is a synthetic compound made by phosphorylation of cellulose and has the following structural formula:

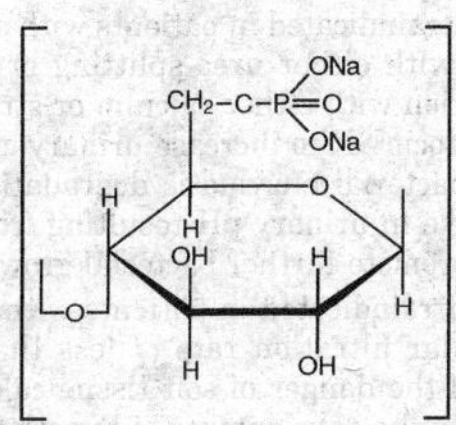

Where n indicates the degree of polymerization and has an average value of approximately 3000. The molecular weight of CSP monomer is 286.1 and the average molecular weight of the polymer is 858,000.
It has an inorganic bound phosphate of 31–36%, free phosphate of 3.5%, sodium content of approximately 11% and a calcium binding capacity of 1.8 mmol of Ca per gram of the oral powder. It has excellent ion exchange properties, the sodium ion exchanging for calcium. When taken orally, CSP binds calcium, the complex of calcium and cellulose phosphate being excreted in feces. The dosage of CALCIBIND® is powder for oral administration.

HOW SUPPLIED
CALCIBIND®, NDC 0178-0255-30, is available for oral administration in bottles of 300 grams of CSP, cream colored, bulk powder.

CITRACAL® 250 MG + D OTC
[sĭ' trə-kăl]
Ultradense® calcium citrate-Vitamin D dietary supplement

INGREDIENTS
Calcium (as Ultradense® calcium citrate) 250 mg., polyethylene glycol, citric acid, microcrystalline cellulose, polyvinyl alcohol-part hydrolyzed, croscarmellose sodium, color added, magnesium silicate, magnesium stearate, vitamin D_3 (62.5 IU).

HOW SUPPLIED
CITRACAL® 250 MG + D is supplied as white, modified rectangle shaped, coated tablets in bottles of 150 (UPC 0178-0837-15).

CITRACAL® Ⓤ OTC
[sĭ'trə-kăl]
Ultradense® calcium citrate dietary supplement

INGREDIENTS
Calcium (as Ultradense® calcium citrate) 200 mg., polyethylene glycol, croscarmellose sodium, polyvinyl alcohol-part hydrolyzed, color added, magnesium silicate, magnesium stearate.

SENSITIVE PATIENTS
CITRACAL® contains no wheat, barley, yeast or rye; is sugar, dairy and gluten free.

ONE TABLET PROVIDES
200 mg. calcium (elemental), equaling 20% of the U.S. recommended daily value for adults and children 4 or more years of age.

DIRECTIONS
Take 1 to 2 tablets two times daily or as recommended by a physician, pharmacist or health professional.
Store at room temperature.

HOW SUPPLIED
CITRACAL® is supplied as white, barrel shaped, coated tablets in bottles of 100 (UPC 0178-0800-01), and bottles of 200 (UPC 0178-0800-20).
Ⓤ = Kosher Parvae approved by Orthodox Union.

CITRACAL® Caplets + D OTC
[sĭ'trə-kăl]
Ultradense® calcium citrate - vitamin D dietary supplement

INGREDIENTS
Calcium (as Ultradense® calcium citrate) 315 mg., polyethylene glycol, croscarmellose sodium, polyvinyl alcohol-part hydrolyzed, color added, magnesium silicate, magnesium stearate, vitamin D_3 (200IU).

HOW SUPPLIED
CITRACAL® Caplets + D are supplied as white, arc rectangle shaped, coated tablets in bottles of 60 (UPC 0178-0815-60); bottles of 120 (UPC 0178-0815-12), and bottles of 180 (UPC 0178-0815-18).

CITRACAL® PLUS OTC
[sĭ' trə-kăl]
Ultradense® calcium citrate-Vitamin D-multi-mineral dietary supplement

Ingredients: Calcium (as Ultradense® calcium citrate) 250 mg., polyethylene glycol, magnesium oxide, povidone, croscarmellose sodium, polyvinyl alcohol-part hydrolyzed, hydroxypropyl methylcellulose, color added, pyridoxine hydrochloride, zinc oxide, magnesium silicate, sodium borate, manganese gluconate, copper gluconate, magnesium stearate, maltodextrin, vitamin D_3 (125 IU).

HOW SUPPLIED
CITRACAL® PLUS is supplied as white, arc rectangle shaped, coated tablets in bottles of 150 (UPC 0178-0825-15).

CITRACAL® PRENATAL Rx ℞
[sĭ'trə-kăl]
PRENATAL VITAMINS AND MINERALS

DESCRIPTION
Citracal Prenatal Rx is a scored, white, modified oval shaped multivitamin/multimineral tablet. The tablet is embossed "CITRACAL" on one side and "PN RX" on the other side.
Each tablet contains:

Vitamin A (Vitamin A palmitate)	2700 IU
Vitamin C (Ascorbic acid)	120 mg
Calcium (Calcium citrate)	125 mg
Iron (Carbonyl iron, Ferrous gluconate)	27 mg
Vitamin D_3 (Cholecalciferol)	400 IU
Vitamin E (dl-alpha tocopheryl acetate)	30 IU
Thiamin (Vitamin B_1)	3 mg
Riboflavin (Vitamin B_2)	3.4 mg
Niacinamide (Vitamin B_3)	20 mg
Pyridoxine HCl (Vitamin B_6)	20 mg
Folic Acid	1 mg
Iodine (Potassium iodide)	150 mcg
Zinc (Zinc oxide)	25 mg
Copper (Cupric oxide)	2 mg
Docusate Sodium	50 mg

INDICATIONS
CITRACAL PRENATAL Rx is a multivitamin/multimineral prescription drug indicated for use in improving the nutritional status of women prior to conception, throughout pregnancy, and in the postnatal period for both lactating and nonlactating mothers.

CONTRAINDICATIONS
This product is contraindicated in patients with a known hypersensitivity to any of the ingredients.

WARNING
Accidental overdose of iron-containing products is a leading cause of fatal poisoning in children under 6. KEEP THIS PRODUCT OUT OF THE REACH OF CHILDREN. In case of accidental overdose, call a doctor or poison control center immediately.

Folic acid alone is improper therapy in the treatment of pernicious anemia and other megaloblastic anemias where Vitamin B_{12} is deficient.

NOTICE
Contact with moisture may produce surface discoloration or erosion of the tablet.

PRECAUTIONS
Folic acid in doses above 0.1 mg may obscure pernicious anemia in that hematologic remission can occur while neurological manifestations progress.

ADVERSE REACTIONS
Allergic sensitization has been reported following both oral and parenteral administration of folic acid.

DOSAGE AND ADMINISTRATION
One tablet daily or as directed by a physician.

HOW SUPPLIED
Bottles of 100 tablets (NDC 0178-0852-01)
DISPENSE IN A TIGHT, LIGHT-RESISTANT CONTAINER AS DEFINED BY THE USP/NF WITH A CHILD-RESISTANT CLOSURE.
Store at controlled room temperature.
U.S. Patent 4,814,177 Other Patent(s) pending
REV. 008010

FOSFREE® OTC
[fos 'frē]
Calcium—Iron—Multivitamin

WARNING: Accidental overdose of **iron-containing** products is a leading cause of fatal poisoning in children under 6. KEEP THIS PRODUCT OUT OF REACH OF CHILDREN. In case of accidental overdose, call a doctor or poison control center immediately. If you are pregnant or nursing a baby, seek the advice of a health professional before using this product.

HOW SUPPLIED
FOSFREE® is supplied as yellow, modified oval shaped, coated tablets in bottles of 60 (UPC 0178-0031-60) and bottles of 120 (UPC 0178-0031-12).

IROMIN®-G OTC
[i 'rō-min]
Hematinic plus vitamins, calcium and folic acid Dietary Supplement

WARNING: Accidental overdose of **iron-containing** products is a leading cause of fatal poisoning in children under 6. Keep this product out of reach of children. In case of accidental overdose, call a doctor or poison control center immediately.

HOW SUPPLIED
IROMIN-G® is supplied as red, rectangular shaped coated tablets in bottles of 100 (UPC 0178-0081-01).

Continued on next page

LITHOSTAT® ℞
[*lith 'o-stat*]
Acetohydroxamic Acid (AHA)

DESCRIPTION

Acetohydroxamic acid (AHA) is a stable, synthetic compound derived from hydroxylamine and ethyl acetate. Its molecular structure is similar to urea:

$$H_3C-C(=O)-N(H)-OH$$

ACETOHYDROXAMIC ACID (AHA)

AHA is weakly acidic, highly soluble in water, and chelates metals - notably iron. The molecular weight is 75.068. AHA has a pKa of 9.32 and a melting point of 89–91°C. AHA is a urease inhibitor. Available as 250 mg tablets.

HOW SUPPLIED

LITHOSTAT®, NDC 0178-0500-01, is available for oral administration as 250 mg white, round tablets, embossed with "MPC 500" on one side, in unit of use packages of 100 tablets.

MISSION PRENATAL DIETARY SUPPLEMENT SERIES

MISSION® PRENATAL
Vitamins—Iron—Calcium—0.4 mg. Folic Acid
UPC 0178-0132-01

MISSION® PRENATAL F.A.
Vitamins—Iron—Calcium—Zinc—0.8 mg. Folic Acid
UPC 0178-0153-01

MISSION® PRENATAL H.P.
Vitamins—Iron—Calcium—0.8 mg. Folic Acid
UPC 0178-0161-01

WARNING: Accidental overdose of **iron-containing** products is a leading cause of fatal poisoning in children under 6. Keep this product out of reach of children. In case of accidental overdose, call a doctor or poison control center immediately.

HOW SUPPLIED

MISSION® PRENATAL is supplied as salmon, rectangular-shaped, coated tablets in bottles of 100.
MISSION® PRENATAL F.A. is supplied as blue, rectangular-shaped, coated tablets in bottles of 100.
MISSION® PRENATAL H.P. is supplied as green, rectangular-shaped, coated tablets in bottles of 100.

MISSION PHARMACAL UROLOGICALS

THERA-GESIC® OTC
[*thĕr 'ə-jē-zik*]
TOPICAL ANALGESIC CREME

ACTIVE INGREDIENTS	PURPOSE:
Menthol 1%	Analgesic
Methyl Salicylate 15%	Counterirritant

USE

Temporary relief of minor aches and pains of muscles and joints associated with: Arthritis, simple backaches, strains, bruises, sprains.

WARNINGS

For external use only. Use only as directed. Avoid contact with eyes or mucous membranes.

Do not bandage tightly Do not bandage, wrap or cover until after washing the areas where THERA-GESIC has been applied.

Do not use

- immediately after shower or bath
- if skin is sensitive to oil of wintergreen (methyl salicylate)
- on wounds or damaged skin

Ask a doctor before use

- for children under 2 and through 12 years of age
- if prone or sensitive to allergic reactions from aspirin or salicylate

When using this product

- discontinue use if skin irritation develops, or redness is present
- do not swallow
- do not use a heating pad after application of THERA-GESIC

Stop use and ask a doctor if condition worsens, or if symptoms persist for more than 7 days or clear up and occur again within a few days.

If pregnant or breast-feeding, ask a health professional before use.

Keep out of reach of children to avoid accidental poisoning. If swallowed, get medical help or contact a Poison Control Center right away.

DIRECTIONS

Adults and children 12 or more years of age: Apply thin layers of crème into and around the sore or painful area, not more than 3 to 4 times daily. The number of thin layers controls the intensity of the action of THERA-GESIC. One thin layer provides a mild effect, two thin layers provide a strong effect and three thin layers provide a very strong effect. SEE WARNINGS.

OTHER INFORMATION: Once THERA-GESIC has penetrated the skin, the area may be washed, leaving it dry, clean and fragrance-free without decreasing the effectiveness of the product. Avoid contact with clothing or other surfaces. Store at 20–25° C (68–77° F).

INACTIVE INGREDIENTS: Carbomer 934, Dimethicone, Glycerine, Methylparaben, Propylparaben, Sodium Lauryl Sulfate, Trolamine, Water.

HOW SUPPLIED:

NDC 0178-0320-03	3 oz. tube
NDC 0178-0320-05	5 oz. tube

THERA-GESIC® PLUS OTC
[*thĕr" ə-jē' zik*]
Topical Analgesic Creme

Active Ingredients	Purpose:
Methyl Salicylate 25%	Topical Analgesic
Menthol 4%	Topical Analgesic

WARNINGS

For external use only. Use only as directed. Avoid contact with eyes or mucous membranes. **Do not bandage tightly, wrap or cover until after washing the areas where THERA-GESIC® PLUS has been applied.**

INACTIVE INGREDIENTS

Aloe Vera, Carbomer 980, Dimethicone, Glycerine, Methylparaben, Propylparaben, Sodium Lauryl Sulfate, Trolamine, Water.

HOW SUPPLIED

NDC 0178-0350-03	3 oz. tube
NDC 0178-0350-05	5 oz. tube

Rev. 004040

[For all other information, see listing for THERA-GESIC®.]

THIOLA® ℞
[*thi-ól-a*]
Tiopronin Tablets

DESCRIPTION

THIOLA® (Tiopronin) is a reducing and complexing thiol compound. Tiopronin is N-(2-Mercaptopropionyl) glycine and has the following structure:

$$CH_3-CH(SH)-CONHCH_2-COOH$$

Tiopronin has the empirical formula $C_5H_9NO_3S$ and a molecular weight of 163.20. In this drug product tiopronin exists as a dl racemic mixture.

Tiopronin is a white crystalline powder which is freely soluble in water.

HOW SUPPLIED

THIOLA®, NDC 0178-0900-01, is available for oral administration as 100 mg. round, white, sugar coated tablets, imprinted with "MPC 900" on one side, in bottles of 100 tablets each.

UROCIT®-K ℞
[*yu 'ro-cĭt kay*]
Potassium Citrate

DESCRIPTION

Urocit®-K is a citrate salt of potassium. Its empirical formula is $K_3C_6H_5O_7 \cdot H_2O$, and its structural formula is:

$$HO-C(CH_2-COOK)(COOK)(CH_2-COOK) \cdot H_2O$$

Potassium citrate is a white granular powder that is soluble in water at 154 g/100 ml, almost insoluble in alcohol, and insoluble in organic solvents.

Urocit®-K is supplied as wax matrix tablets, containing 5 mEq (540 mg) potassium citrate and 10 mEq (1080 mg) potassium citrate each, for oral administration.

CLINICAL PHARMACOLOGY

When Urocit®-K is given orally, the metabolism of absorbed citrate produces an alkaline load. The induced alkaline load in turn increases urinary pH and raises urinary citrate by augmenting citrate clearance without measurably altering ultrafilterable serum citrate. Thus, Urocit®-K therapy appears to increase urinary citrate principally by modifying the renal handling of citrate, rather than by increasing the filtered load of citrate. The increased filtered load of citrate may play some role, however, as in small comparisons of oral citrate and oral bicarbonate, citrate had a greater effect on urinary citrate.

In addition to raising urinary pH and citrate, Urocit®-K increases urinary potassium by approximately the amount contained in the medication. In some patients, Urocit®-K causes a transient reduction in urinary calcium.

The changes induced by Urocit®-K produce a urine that is less conducive to the crystallization of stone-forming salts (calcium oxalate, calcium phosphate and uric acid). Increased citrate in the urine, by complexing with calcium, decreases calcium ion activity and thus the saturation of calcium oxalate. Citrate also inhibits the spontaneous nucleation of calcium oxalate and calcium phosphate (brushite).

The increase in urinary pH also decreases calcium ion activity by increasing calcium complexation to dissociated anions. The rise in urinary pH also increases the ionization of uric acid to more soluble urate ion.

Urocit®-K therapy does not alter the urinary saturation of calcium phosphate, since the effect of increased citrate complexation of calcium is opposed by the rise in pH-dependent dissociation of phosphate. Calcium phosphate stones are more stable in alkaline urine.

In the setting of normal renal function, the rise in urinary citrate following a single dose begins by the first hour and lasts for 12 hours. With multiple doses the rise in citrate excretion reaches its peak by the third day and averts the normally wide circadian fluctuation in urinary citrate, thus maintaining urinary citrate at a higher, more constant level throughout the day. When the treatment is withdrawn, urinary citrate begins to decline toward the pre-treatment level on the first day.

The rise in citrate excretion is directly dependent on the Urocit®-K dosage. Following long-term treatment, Urocit®-K at a dosage of 60 mEq/day raises urinary citrate by approximately 400 mg/day and increases urinary pH by approximately 0.7 units.

In patients with severe renal tubular acidosis or chronic diarrheal syndrome where urinary citrate may be very low (<100 mg/day), Urocit®-K may be relatively ineffective in raising urinary citrate. A higher dose of Urocit®-K may therefore be required to produce a satisfactory citraturic response. In patients with renal tubular acidosis in whom urinary pH may be high, Urocit®-K produces a relatively small rise in urinary pH.

INDICATIONS AND USAGE

Potassium citrate is indicated for the management of renal tubular acidosis (RTA) with calcium stones, hypocitraturic calcium oxalate nephrolithiasis of any etiology, and uric acid lithiasis with or without calcium stones.

CONTRAINDICATIONS

Urocit®-K is contraindicated in patients with hyperkalemia (or who have conditions predisposing them to hyperkalemia), as a further rise in serum potassium concentration may produce cardiac arrest. Such conditions include: chronic renal failure, uncontrolled diabetes mellitus, acute dehydration, strenuous physical exercise in unconditioned individuals, adrenal insufficiency, extensive tissue breakdown, or the administration of a potassium-sparing agent (such as triamterene, spironolactone or amiloride).

Urocit®-K is contraindicated in patients in whom there is cause for arrest or delay in tablet passage through the gastrointestinal tract, such as those suffering from delayed gastric emptying, esophageal compression, intestinal obstruction or stricture or those taking anticholinergic medication. Because of its ulcerogenic potential, Urocit®-K should not be given to patients with peptic ulcer disease.

Urocit®-K is contraindicated in patients with active urinary tract infection (with either urea-splitting or other organisms, in association with either calcium or struvite stones). The ability of Urocit®-K to increase urinary citrate may be attenuated by bacterial enzymatic degradation of citrate. Moreover, the rise in urinary pH resulting from Urocit®-K therapy might promote further bacterial growth.

Urocit®-K is contraindicated in patients with renal insufficiency (glomerular filtration rate of less than 0.7 ml/kg/min), because of the danger of soft tissue calcification and increased risk for the development of hyperkalemia.

WARNINGS

HYPERKALEMIA: In patients with impaired mechanisms for excreting potassium, Urocit®-K administration can produce hyperkalemia and cardiac arrest. Potentially fatal hyperkalemia can develop rapidly and be asymptomatic. The use of Urocit®-K in patients with chronic renal failure, or any other condition which impairs potassium excretion such as severe myocardial damage or heart failure, should be avoided.

INTERACTION WITH POTASSIUM-SPARING DIURETICS

Concomitant administration of Urocit®-K and a potassium-sparing diuretic (such as triamterene, spironolactone or amiloride) should be avoided, since the simultaneous administration of these agents can produce severe hyperkalemia.

GASTROINTESTINAL LESIONS

Because of reports of upper gastrointestinal mucosal lesions following administration of potassium chloride (wax-matrix), and endoscopic examination of the upper gastrointestinal mucosa was performed in 30 normal volunteers after they had taken glycopyrrolate 2 mg. p.o. t.i.d., Urocit®-K 95 mEq/day, wax-matrix potassium chloride 96 mEq/day or wax matrix placebo, in thrice daily schedule in the fasting state for one week. Urocit®-K and the wax-matrix formulation of potassium chloride were indistinguishable but both were significantly more irritating than the wax-matrix placebo. In a subsequent similar study, lesions were less severe when glycopyrrolate was omitted.

Solid dosage forms of potassium chloride have produced stenotic and/or ulcerative lesions of the small bowel and deaths. These lesions are caused by a high local concentration of potassium ions in the region of the dissolving tablets, which injured the bowel. In addition, perhaps because wax-matrix preparations are not enteric-coated and release some of their potassium content in the stomach, there have been reports of upper gastrointestinal bleeding associated with these products. The frequency of gastrointestinal lesions with wax-matrix potassium chloride products is estimated at one per 100,000 patient-years. Experience with Urocit®-K is limited, but a similar frequency of gastrointestinal lesions should be anticipated.

If there is severe vomiting, abdominal pain or gastro-intestinal bleeding, Urocit®-K should be discontinued immediately and the possibility of bowel perforation or obstruction investigated.

PRECAUTIONS

Information For Patients:

Physicians should consider reminding the patient of the following:

To take each dose without crushing, chewing or sucking the tablet.

To take this medicine only as directed. This is especially important if the patient is also taking both diuretics and digitalis preparations.

To check with physician if there is trouble swallowing tablets or if the tablet seems to stick in the throat.

To check with the doctor at once if tarry stools or other evidence of gastrointestinal bleeding is noticed.

Laboratory Tests: Regular serum potassium determinations are recommended. Careful attention should be paid to acid-base balance, other serum electrolyte levels, the electrocardiogram, and the clinical status of the patient, particularly in the presence of cardiac disease, renal disease or acidosis.

Drug Interactions: POTASSIUM-SPARING DIURETICS: See WARNINGS section.

DRUGS THAT SLOW GASTROINTESTINAL TRANSIT TIME (such as anticholinergics) can be expected to increase the gastrointestinal irritation produced by potassium salts. (See CONTRAINDICATIONS section).

Carcinogenesis, Mutagenesis, Impairment Of Fertility: Long-term carcinogenicity studies in animals have not been performed.

Pregnancy Category C: Animal reproduction studies have not been conducted with Urocit®-K. It is also not known whether Urocit®-K can cause fetal harm when administered to a pregnant woman or can affect reproduction capacity. Urocit®-K should be given to a pregnant woman only if clearly needed.

Nursing Mothers: The normal potassium ion content of human milk is about 13 mEq/l. It is not known if Urocit®-K has an effect on this content. Caution should be exercised when Urocit®-K is administered to a nursing woman.

Pediatric Use: Safety and effectiveness in children have not been established.

ADVERSE REACTIONS

Some patients may develop minor gastrointestinal complaints during Urocit®-K therapy, such as abdominal discomfort, vomiting, diarrhea, loose bowel movements or nausea. These symptoms are due to the irritation of the gastrointestinal tract, and may be alleviated by taking the dose with meals or snack, or by reducing the dosage. Patients may find intact matrices in feces. (See also CONTRAINDICATIONS, WARNINGS)

OVERDOSAGE

The administration of potassium salts to persons without predisposing conditions for hyperkalemia (see CONTRAINDICATIONS) rarely causes serious hyperkalemia at recommended dosages. It is important to recognize that hyperkalemia is usually asymptomatic and may be manifested only by an increased serum potassium concentration and characteristic electrocardiographic changes (peaking of T-wave, loss of P-wave, depression of S-T segment and prolongation of the QT interval). Late manifestations include muscle paralysis and cardiovascular collapse from cardiac arrest.

Treatment measures for hyperkalemia include the following: (1) elimination of potassium-rich foods, medications containing potassium, and of potassium-sparing diuretics, (2) intravenous administration of 300–500 ml/hr of 10% dextrose solution containing 10–20 units of insulin/1000 ml, (3) correction of acidosis, if present, with intravenous sodium bicarbonate, and (4) use of exchange resins, hemodialysis or peritoneal dialysis.

In treating hyperkalemia, it should be recalled that in patients who have been stabilized on digitalis, too rapid a lowering of the serum potassium concentration can produce digitalis toxicity.

DOSAGE AND ADMINISTRATION

Treatment with Urocit®-K should be added to a regimen that limits salt intake (avoidance of foods with high salt content and of added salt at the table) and encourages high fluid intake (urine volume should be at least two liters per day). The objective of treatment with Urocit®-K is to provide Urocit®-K in sufficient dosage to restore normal urinary citrate (greater than 320 mg/day and as close to the normal mean of 640 mg/day as possible), and to increase urinary pH to a level of 6.0 to 7.0.

In patients with severe hypocitraturia (urinary citrate of less than 150 mg/day), therapy should be initiated at a dosage of 60 mEq/day (20 mEq three times/day or 15 mEq four times/day with meals or within 30 minutes after meals or bedtime snack). In patients with mild-moderate hypocitraturia (>150 mg/day), Urocit®-K should be initiated at a dosage of 30 mEq/day (10 mEq three times/day with meals).

Twenty-four hour urinary citrate and/or urinary pH measurements should be used to determine the adequacy of the initial dosage and to evaluate the effectiveness of any dosage change. In addition, urinary citrate and/or pH should be measured every four months.

Doses of Urocit®-K greater than 100 mEq/day have not been studied and should be avoided.

Serum electrolytes (sodium, potassium, chloride and carbon dioxide), serum creatinine, and complete blood count should be monitored every four months. Treatment should be discontinued if there is hyperkalemia, a significant rise in serum creatinine, or a significant fall in blood hematocrit or hemoglobin.

HOW SUPPLIED

Urocit®-K is available for oral administration in tablet form in the following sizes: (NDC 0178-0600-01) 5 mEq potassium citrate and (NDC 0178-0610-01) 10 mEq potassium citrate, packaged in bottles of 100 each. Urocit®-K 5 mEq tablets are uncoated, modified ball-shaped, and tan to yellowish in color. Each 5 mEq tablet is debossed MPC 600 on one side and blank on the other side. Urocit®-K 10 mEq tablets are uncoated, elliptical-shaped, and tan to yellowish in color. Each 10 mEq tablet is debossed with 610 on one side and MISSION on the other side.

Store in tight container.

Rev. 003030

Monarch Pharmaceuticals

Please see King Pharmaceuticals, Inc.

Montiff, Inc, Don Tyson's Advanced Nutraceuticals

3205 SANTA MONICA BLVD.
SANTA MONICA, CA 90404

Direct Inquiries to:
Customer Service
Tel. (310-582–8938)
FAX (310-582-8939)
(Toll free 877-820-4883)
E-mail: montiffinc@aol.com

TRYPTOPHAN Serotonin precursor	OTC –NDC # 65883-477-14 Bottles of 100 -500mg/cap
NEURO-BALANCE Catecholamine precursor	OTC –NDC # 65883-070-12 Bottles of 80 –620mg/cap
VASO-LENE Source for Nitric Oxide Endothelial support	OTC –NDC# 65883-340-12 Bottles of 60 - 425 mg/ cap
PURE L-ARGININE HCL Precursor to Nitric Oxide	OTC- NDC# 685883-502-14 Bottles of 100 - 500 mg./cap
ULTRA CARNITINE L-Carnitine Fummarate + N-Acetyl-L-Carnitine Cardiovascular support	OCT –NDC#65883-350-10 Bottles of 30 – 300mg/cap
PURE D-PHENYL-RELIEF Enhances endorphin production	OTC – NDC# 65883-410-11 Bottles of 50 –500 mg/cap
KARNO-LIFE L-Carnosine Inhibits glycosylation	OTC –NDC#65883-668-13 Bottles of 90-200mg/cap
VITA-MINZ PLUS Vitamin-Mineral-Complex	OTC –NDC#65883-110-15 Bottles 120 capsules
B-LONG Sustained B-Complex	OTC-NDC# 85883-140-12 Bottles of 60 sustained tab
SUPER ANTIOXIDANT FORMULA Antioxidant preparation	OTC-NDC# 65883-210-12 Bottles of 60 capsules
CO-Q 10 PLUS Co-enz. Q 10 + Vit. E Myocardial support	OTC- NDC#85883-383-10 Bottles of 30-100 mg + 100 IU/sg
ATP Adenosine Triphosphate Myocardial support	OTC-NDC#65883-381-13 Bottles of 90 –25 mg/enteric tab
PROST-8-PALMETTO Prostate support-BHP	OTC-NDC#65883-365-12 Bottles of 60-160mg/sg
CALCIUM PLUS Calcium/Vit.D/Ipriflavone	OTC-NDC#65883-151-15 Bottles of 120-312mg/tab

ALL-BASIC OTC

DESCRIPTION

20 L-Crystalline Amino acid formula—helps reverse negative nitrogen balance.

CONTAINS: 677mg. L-Crystalline amino acids including neurotransmitter precursors, sulfur and branched chain amino acids plus Alpha Lipoic Acid.

COMPOSITION

L-Lysine HCL, L-Isoleucine, L-Glutamine, L-Tyrosine, L-Threonine, L-Alanine, L-Leucine, L-Histidine, L-Arginine HCL, L-Aspartic Acid, L-Valine, Omithine Alpha Ketoglutarate, L-Methionine, L-Cystine, L-Glutamic Acid, Glycine, L-Phenylalanine, N-Acetyl-L-Tyrosine, L-Serine, L-Proline, Alpha Lipoic Acid

USAGE AND ADMINISTRATION

2–3 capsules t.i.d. a half-hour before meals

HOW SUPPLIED

Bottles of 100–687mg/cap OTC –NDC # 65883-010-14

GLUCA-BALANCE OTC

DESCRIPTION

14 L-Crystalline amino acid formula—700mg/cap-for mental stamina. For adults and children 12 years or older. High in glycogenic amino acids plus L-Alanyl-Glutamine and L-Glycyl-L-Glutamine.

CONTENTS

L-Lysine HCL, L-Isoleucine, L-Glutamine, L-Tyrosine, L-Threonine, L-Alanine, L-Leucine, L-Histidine, L-Arginine HCL, L-Aspartic Acid, L-Valine, L-Methionine, L-Cystine, L-Glutamic Acid, Glycine, L-Phenylalanine, N-Acetyl-L-Tyrosine, L-Serine, L-Proline -plus Ornithine Alpha Ketoglutarate, and Di-peptides; L-Alanyl-L-Glutamine and L-Glycyl-L-Glutamine.

DOSAGE AND ADMINISTRATION

2–4 capsules b.i.d. between meals

HOW SUPPLIED

Bottles of 100–700mg/cap OTC—NDC #65883-050-14

Mylan Pharmaceuticals Inc.

781 CHESTNUT RIDGE ROAD
P.O. BOX 4310
MORGANTOWN, WV 26504-4310

Direct Inquiries to:
(304) 599-2595
For Medical Information Contact:
Clinical Research Department
877-446-3679
877 4INFO-RX
Sales and Ordering:
Sales Department
(800) RX-MYLAN

The following list of Mylan products is provided to facilitate identification. It includes the color(s) and identification codes for all tablets and capsules.

PRODUCT GENERIC NAME Description *Color(s)*	**IDENTIFICATION CODE** (Front/Back*)
ACEBUTOLOL HYDROCHLORIDE Capsules, USP, 200 mg ℞ *Med. Orange & Med. Orange*	MYLAN 1200
ACEBUTOLOL HYDROCHLORIDE Capsules, USP, 400 mg ℞ *Med. Orange & Med. Orange*	MYLAN 1400
ACYCLOVIR Capsules, USP, 200 mg ℞ *Lavender & Lavender*	MYLAN 2200
ACYCLOVIR Tablets, USP, 400 mg ℞ *White*	M253/Blank
ACYCLOVIR Tablets, USP, 800 mg ℞ *White*	MYLAN/302

Continued on next page

Mylan-Product List—Cont.

ALBUTEROL M255/Blank
Tablets, USP, 2 mg ℞
White

ALBUTEROL M572/Blank
Tablets, USP, 4 mg ℞
White

ALLOPURINOL M31/Blank
Tablets, USP, 100 mg ℞
White

ALLOPURINOL M71/Blank
Tablets, USP, 300 mg ℞
White

ALPRAZOLAM MYLAN A/Scored
Tablets, USP, 0.25 mg CIV/℞
White

ALPRAZOLAM MYLAN A3/Scored
Tablets, USP, 0.5 mg CIV/℞
Peach

ALPRAZOLAM MYLAN A1/Scored
Tablets, USP, 1 mg CIV/℞
Blue

ALPRAZOLAM MYLAN A4/Scored
Tablets, USP, 2 mg CIV/℞
White

AMILORIDE HYDROCHLORIDE and HYDROCHLOROTHIAZIDE M577/Blank
Tablets, USP, 5 mg/50 mg ℞
Lt. Orange

AMITRIPTYLINE HYDROCHLORIDE M77/Blank
Tablets, USP, 10 mg ℞
White

AMITRIPTYLINE HYDROCHLORIDE M51/Blank
Tablets, USP, 25 mg ℞
Lt. Green

AMITRIPTYLINE HYDROCHLORIDE M36/Blank
Tablets, USP, 50 mg ℞
Brown

AMITRIPTYLINE HYDROCHLORIDE M37/Blank
Tablets, USP, 75 mg ℞
Blue

AMITRIPTYLINE HYDROCHLORIDE M38/Blank
Tablets, USP, 100 mg ℞
Orange

AMITRIPTYLINE HYDROCHLORIDE M39/Blank
Tablets, USP, 150 mg ℞
Flesh

ATENOLOL M/A2
Tablets, USP, 25 mg ℞
White

ATENOLOL M/231
Tablets, USP, 50 mg ℞
White

ATENOLOL M/757
Tablets, USP, 100 mg ℞
White

ATENOLOL and CHLORTHALIDONE M63/Blank
Tablets, USP, 50 mg/25 mg ℞
White

ATENOLOL and CHLORTHALIDONE M64/Blank
Tablets, USP, 100 mg/25 mg ℞
White

BENAZEPRIL HYDROCHLORIDE M/441
Tablets, 5 mg ℞
White

BENAZEPRIL HYDROCHLORIDE M/443
Tablets, 10 mg ℞
White

BENAZEPRIL HYDROCHLORIDE M444/Blank
Tablets, 20 mg ℞
White

BENAZEPRIL HYDROCHLORIDE M447/Blank
Tablets, 40 mg ℞
White

BENAZEPRIL HYDROCHLORIDE and HYDROCHLOROTHIAZIDE M725/Scored
Tablets, 5 mg/6.25 mg ℞
Beige

BENAZEPRIL HYDROCHLORIDE and HYDROCHLOROTHIAZIDE M735/Blank
Tablets, 10 mg/12.5 mg ℞
Beige

BENAZEPRIL HYDROCHLORIDE and HYDROCHLOROTHIAZIDE M745/Blank
Tablets, 20 mg/12.5 mg ℞
Beige

BENAZEPRIL HYDROCHLORIDE and HYDROCHLOROTHIAZIDE M775/Blank
Tablets, 20 mg/25 mg ℞
Beige

BISOPROLOL FUMARATE and HYDROCHLOROTHIAZIDE M/501
Tablets, 2.5 mg/6.25 mg ℞
Orange

BISOPROLOL FUMARATE and HYDROCHLOROTHIAZIDE M/503
Tablets, 5 mg/6.25 mg ℞
Blue

BISOPROLOL FUMARATE and HYDROCHLOROTHIAZIDE M/505
Tablets, 10 mg/6.25 mg ℞
White

BUMETANIDE E128/Blank
Tablets, USP, 0.5 mg ℞
Lt. Green

BUMETANIDE E129/Blank
Tablets, USP, 1 mg ℞
Yellow

BUMETANIDE E130/Blank
Tablets, USP, 2 mg ℞
Peach

BUPROPION HYDROCHLORIDE M/433
Tablets, USP, 75 mg ℞
Peach

BUPROPION HYDROCHLORIDE M/435
Tablets, USP, 100 mg ℞
Lt. Blue

BUSPIRONE HYDROCHLORIDE MB1/Blank
Tablets, USP, 5 mg ℞
White

BUSPIRONE HYDROCHLORIDE MB2/Blank
Tablets, USP, 10 mg ℞
White

BUSPIRONE HYDROCHLORIDE MB3/555 (Trisect)
Tablets, USP, 15 mg ℞
White

BUSPIRONE HYDROCHLORIDE MB4/10 10 10 (Trisect)
Tablets, USP, 30 mg ℞
White

BUTORPHANOL TARTRATE —
Nasal Spray, 10 mg/mL CIV/℞

CAPTOPRIL MC1/Scored
Tablets, USP, 12.5 mg ℞
White

CAPTOPRIL MC2/(Quadrisect)
Tablets, USP, 25 mg ℞
White

CAPTOPRIL MC3/Blank
Tablets, USP, 50 mg ℞
White

CAPTOPRIL MC4/Blank
Tablets, USP, 100 mg ℞
White

CAPTOPRIL and HYDROCHLOROTHIAZIDE M81/Scored
Tablets, USP, 25 mg/15 mg ℞
White

CAPTOPRIL and HYDROCHLOROTHIAZIDE M84/Scored
Tablets, USP, 50 mg/15 mg ℞
White

CAPTOPRIL and HYDROCHLOROTHIAZIDE M83/Scored
Tablets, USP, 25 mg/25 mg ℞
Peach

CAPTOPRIL and HYDROCHLOROTHIAZIDE M86/Scored
Tablets, USP, 50 mg/25 mg ℞
Peach

CARBIDOPA and LEVODOPA MYLAN/88
Extended-release Tablets, 25 mg/100 mg ℞
Purple

CARBIDOPA and LEVODOPA MYLAN/94
Extended-release Tablets, 50 mg/200 mg ℞
Purple

CEFACLOR —
Powders for Oral Suspension, USP, 125 mg/5 mL ℞

CEFACLOR —
Powders for Oral Suspension, USP, 187 mg/5 mL ℞

CEFACLOR —
Powders for Oral Suspension, USP, 250 mg/5 mL ℞

CEFACLOR —
Powders for Oral Suspension, USP, 375 mg/5 mL ℞

CHLORDIAZEPOXIDE and AMITRIPTYLINE HYDROCHLORIDE MYLAN/211
Tablets, USP, 5 mg/12.5 mg CIV/℞
Green

CHLORDIAZEPOXIDE and AMITRIPTYLINE HYDROCHLORIDE MYLAN/277
Tablets, USP, 10 mg/25 mg CIV/℞
White

CHLOROTHIAZIDE M50/Blank
Tablets, USP, 250 mg ℞
White

CHLOROTHIAZIDE MYLAN 162/Blank
Tablets, USP, 500 mg ℞
White

CHLORPROPAMIDE MYLAN 197/100
Tablets, USP, 100 mg ℞
Green

CHLORPROPAMIDE MYLAN 210/250
Tablets, USP, 250 mg ℞
Green

CHLORTHALIDONE M35/Blank
Tablets, USP, 25 mg ℞
Lt. Yellow

CHLORTHALIDONE M75/Blank
Tablets, USP, 50 mg ℞
Lt. Green

CIMETIDINE M/53
Tablets, USP, 200 mg ℞
Green

CIMETIDINE M/317
Tablets, USP, 300 mg ℞
Green

CIMETIDINE M/372
Tablets, USP, 400 mg ℞
Green

CIMETIDINE M541/Blank
Tablets, USP, 800 mg ℞
Green

CIPROFLOXACIN 322/M
Tablets, USP, 250 mg ℞
Orange

CIPROFLOXACIN 323/MYLAN
Tablets, USP, 500 mg ℞
Orange

CIPROFLOXACIN 324/MYLAN
Tablets, USP, 750 mg ℞
Orange

CLOMIPRAMINE HYDROCHLORIDE MYLAN 3025
Capsules, USP, 25 mg ℞
Medium Orange & Flesh

CLOMIPRAMINE HYDROCHLORIDE MYLAN 3050
Capsules, USP, 50 mg ℞
Yellow & Flesh

CLOMIPRAMINE HYDROCHLORIDE MYLAN 3075
Capsules, USP, 75 mg ℞
Swedish Orange & Flesh

CLONAZEPAM M/C13
Tablets, USP, 0.5 mg CIV/℞
Yellow

CLONAZEPAM M/C14
Tablets, USP, 1 mg CIV/℞
Lt. Green

CLONAZEPAM M/C15
Tablets, USP, 2 mg CIV/℞
White

CLONIDINE HYDROCHLORIDE MYLAN 152/Blank
Tablets, USP, 0.1 mg ℞
White

CLONIDINE HYDROCHLORIDE MYLAN 186/Blank
Tablets, USP, 0.2 mg ℞
White

CLONIDINE HYDROCHLORIDE MYLAN 199/Blank
Tablets, USP, 0.3 mg ℞
White

CLORAZEPATE DIPOTASSIUM M30/Blank
Tablets, USP, 3.75 mg CIV/℞
Blue

CLORAZEPATE DIPOTASSIUM M40/Blank
Tablets, USP, 7.5 mg CIV/℞
Peach

CLORAZEPATE DIPOTASSIUM M70/Blank
Tablets, USP, 15 mg CIV/℞
White

CLOZAPINE M/C7
Tablets, USP, 25 mg ℞
Peach

CLOZAPINE M/C11
Tablets, USP, 100 mg ℞
Green

CYCLOBENZAPRINE HYDROCHLORIDE M/751
Tablets, USP, 10 mg ℞
Butterscotch-Yellow

CYSTAGON® MYLAN/CYSTAGON 50
(Cysteamine Bitartrate)
Capsules, 50 mg ℞
White & White

CYSTAGON® MYLAN/CYSTAGON 150
(Cysteamine Bitartrate)
Capsules, 150 mg ℞
White & White

DIAZEPAM MYLAN 271/Scored
Tablets, USP, 2 mg CIV/℞
White

DIAZEPAM MYLAN 345/Scored
Tablets, USP, 5 mg CIV/℞
Orange

DIAZEPAM MYLAN 477/Scored
Tablets, USP, 10 mg CIV/℞
Green

DICLOFENAC POTASSIUM M/D5
Tablets, 50 mg ℞
White

DICLOFENAC SODIUM M355/Blank
Extended-release Tablets, 100 mg ℞
Yellow

DICYCLOMINE HYDROCHLORIDE MYLAN 1610
Capsules, USP, 10 mg ℞
Lt. Blue & Lt. Blue

DICYCLOMINE HYDROCHLORIDE MD6/Blank
Tablets, USP, 20 mg ℞
Blue

DILTIAZEM HYDROCHLORIDE MYLAN 5220
Extended-release Capsules, USP (once-a-day), 120 mg ℞
Lt. Pink & Flesh

DILTIAZEM HYDROCHLORIDE MYLAN 5280
Extended-release Capsules, USP (once-a-day), 180 mg ℞
Lavender & Flesh

DILTIAZEM HYDROCHLORIDE MYLAN 5340
Extended-release Capsules, USP (once-a-day), 240 mg ℞
Lt. Blue & Flesh

DILTIAZEM HYDROCHLORIDE MYLAN 6060
Extended-release Capsules, USP (twice-a-day), 60 mg ℞
Coral & White

DILTIAZEM HYDROCHLORIDE MYLAN 6090
Extended-release Capsules, USP (twice-a-day), 90 mg ℞
Coral & Ivory

DILTIAZEM HYDROCHLORIDE MYLAN 6120
Extended-release Capsules, USP (twice-a-day), 120 mg ℞
Coral & Coral

DILTIAZEM HYDROCHLORIDE M23/Blank
Tablets, USP, 30 mg ℞
White
DILTIAZEM HYDROCHLORIDE M45/Scored
Tablets, USP, 60 mg ℞
White
DILTIAZEM HYDROCHLORIDE M135/Scored
Tablets, USP, 90 mg ℞
White
DILTIAZEM HYDROCHLORIDE M525/Scored
Tablets, USP, 120 mg ℞
White
DIPHENOXYLATE HYDROCHLORIDE M15/Blank
and ATROPINE SULFATE
Tablets, USP, 2.5 mg/0.025 mg ©/℞
White
DOXAZOSIN MESYLATE MD9/Scored
Tablets, 1 mg ℞
White
DOXAZOSIN MESYLATE MD10/Scored
Tablets, 2 mg ℞
Pink
DOXAZOSIN MESYLATE MD11/Scored
Tablets, 4 mg ℞
Blue
DOXAZOSIN MESYLATE MD12/Scored
Tablets, 8 mg ℞
Purple
DOXEPIN HYDROCHLORIDE MYLAN 1049
Capsules, USP, 10 mg ℞
Buff & Buff
DOXEPIN HYDROCHLORIDE MYLAN 3125
Capsules, USP, 25 mg ℞
Ivory & White
DOXEPIN HYDROCHLORIDE MYLAN 4250
Capsules, USP, 50 mg ℞
Ivory & Ivory
DOXEPIN HYDROCHLORIDE MYLAN 5375
Capsules, USP, 75 mg ℞
Bright Lt. Green & Bright Lt. Green
DOXEPIN HYDROCHLORIDE MYLAN 6410
Capsules, USP, 100 mg ℞
Bright Lt. Green & White
ENALAPRIL MALEATE M/712
and HYDROCHLOROTHIAZIDE
Tablets, USP, 5 mg /12.5 mg ℞
White
ENALAPRIL MALEATE M/723
and HYDROCHLOROTHIAZIDE
Tablets, USP, 10 mg/25 mg ℞
White
ENALAPRIL MALEATE ME15/Scored
Tablets, USP, 2.5 mg ℞
White
ENALAPRIL MALEATE ME16/Scored
Tablets, USP, 5 mg ℞
White
ENALAPRIL MALEATE ME17/Scored
Tablets, USP, 10 mg ℞
Lt. Blue
ENALAPRIL MALEATE ME18/Scored
Tablets, USP, 20 mg ℞
Med. Blue
ERYTHROMYCIN ETHYLSUCCINATE M400/Blank
Tablets, USP, 400 mg ℞
Beige
ERYTHROMYCIN STEARATE MYLAN 106/250
Tablets, USP, 250 mg ℞
Yellow
ERYTHROMYCIN STEARATE MYLAN 107/500
Tablets, USP, 500 mg ℞
Yellow
ESTRADIOL M/E3
Tablets, USP, 0.5 mg ℞
White to Off-White
ESTRADIOL M/E4
Tablets, USP, 1 mg ℞
Pink
ESTRADIOL M/E5
Tablets, USP, 2 mg ℞
Pale Blue
ESTRADIOL TRANSDERMAL
SYSTEM Estradiol
Patches, 0.05 mg/day ℞ 0.05 mg/day
Flesh
ESTRADIOL TRANSDERMAL
SYSTEM Estradiol
Patches, 0.1 mg/day ℞ 0.1 mg/day
Flesh
ESTROPIPATE ME7/Blank
Tablets, USP, 0.75 mg ℞
Yellow
ESTROPIPATE ME8/Blank
Tablets, USP, 1.5 mg ℞
Peach
ETODOLAC MYLAN/237
Tablets, USP, 400 mg ℞
White
ETODOLAC MYLAN/242
Tablets, USP, 500 mg ℞
Pink
ETOPOSIDE E50
Capsules, USP, 50 mg ℞
Dark Pink

FAMOTIDINE MF1/Blank
Tablets, USP, 20 mg ℞
Yellow
FAMOTIDINE MF2/Blank
Tablets, USP, 40 mg ℞
Green
FENOPROFEN CALCIUM M471/Scored
Tablets, USP, 600 mg ℞
Lt. Orange
FLECAINIDE ACETATE M/8505
Tablets, 50 mg ℞
White
FLECAINIDE ACETATE M/8510
Tablets, 100 mg ℞
White
FLECAINIDE ACETATE M/8515
Tablets, 150 mg ℞
White
FLUOXETINE MYLAN 4210
Capsules, USP, 10 mg ℞
White Opaque & Flesh Opaque
FLUOXETINE MYLAN 4220
Capsules, USP, 20 mg ℞
Lt. Turquoise Blue Opaque & Flesh Opaque
FLUPHENAZINE HYDROCHLORIDE M/4
Tablets, USP, 1 mg ℞
White
FLUPHENAZINE HYDROCHLORIDE M/9
Tablets, USP, 2.5 mg ℞
Yellow
FLUPHENAZINE HYDROCHLORIDE M/74
Tablets, USP, 5 mg ℞
Lt. Green
FLUPHENAZINE HYDROCHLORIDE M/97
Tablets, USP, 10 mg ℞
Orange
FLURAZEPAM HYDROCHLORIDE MYLAN 4415
Capsules, USP, 15 mg ©/℞
White & Powder Blue
FLURAZEPAM HYDROCHLORIDE MYLAN 4430
Capsules, USP, 30 mg ©/℞
Powder Blue & Powder Blue
FLURBIPROFEN M76/Blank
Tablets, USP, 50 mg ℞
Beige
FLURBIPROFEN M93/Blank
Tablets, USP, 100 mg ℞
Beige
FLUVOXAMINE MALEATE M407/Blank
Tablets, 25 mg ℞
Orange
FLUVOXAMINE MALEATE M412/Scored
Tablets, 50 mg ℞
Orange
FLUVOXAMINE MALEATE M414/Scored
Tablets, 100 mg ℞
Orange
FUROSEMIDE M2/Blank
Tablets, USP, 20 mg ℞
White
FUROSEMIDE MYLAN 216/40
Tablets, USP, 40 mg ℞
White
FUROSEMIDE MYLAN 232/80
Tablets, USP, 80 mg ℞
White
GLIPIZIDE MYLAN G1/Blank
Tablets, USP, 5 mg ℞
White
GLIPIZIDE MYLAN G2/Blank
Tablets, USP, 10 mg ℞
White
GLYBURIDE M113/Blank
Tablets, USP (micronized), 1.5 mg ℞
White
GLYBURIDE M125/Blank
Tablets, USP (micronized), 3 mg ℞
Lt. Yellow
GLYBURIDE M142/Blank
Tablets, USP (micronized), 6 mg ℞
Lt. Green
GUANFACINE M/G4
Tablets, USP, 1 mg ℞
White
GUANFACINE M/G5
Tablets, USP, 2 mg ℞
Blue
HALOPERIDOL MYLAN 351/Scored
Tablets, USP, 0.5 mg ℞
Orange
HALOPERIDOL MYLAN 257/Scored
Tablets, USP, 1 mg ℞
Orange
HALOPERIDOL MYLAN 214/Scored
Tablets, USP, 2 mg ℞
Orange
HALOPERIDOL MYLAN 327/Scored
Tablets, USP, 5 mg ℞
Orange
HYDROCHLOROTHIAZIDE MYLAN 810
Capsules, 12.5 mg ℞
White

HYDROXYCHLOROQUINE SULFATE M/373
Tablets, USP, 200 mg ℞
White
INDAPAMIDE M/69
Tablets, USP, 1.25 mg ℞
Pink
INDAPAMIDE M/80
Tablets, USP, 2.5 mg ℞
White
INDOMETHACIN MYLAN 143
Capsules, USP, 25 mg ℞
Lt. Green & Lt. Green
INDOMETHACIN MYLAN 147
Capsules, USP, 50 mg ℞
Lt. Green & Lt. Green
KETOCONAZOLE M261/Blank
Tablets, USP, 200 mg ℞
White
KETOPROFEN MYLAN 8200
Extended-release Capsules, 200 mg ℞
Blue Green & Iron Gray
KETOPROFEN MYLAN 4070
Capsules, 50 mg ℞
Lt. Celery & Lt. Celery
KETOPROFEN MYLAN 5750
Capsules, 75 mg ℞
Lt. Aqua & Lt. Aqua
KETOROLAC TROMETHAMINE M134
Tablets, USP, 10 mg ℞
White
LEVOTHYROXINE SODIUM L4/M
Tablets, USP, 25 mcg ℞
Orange
LEVOTHYROXINE SODIUM L5/M
Tablets, USP, 50 mcg ℞
White
LEVOTHYROXINE SODIUM L6/M
Tablets, USP, 75 mcg ℞
Violet
LEVOTHYROXINE SODIUM L7/M
Tablets, USP, 88 mcg ℞
Olive
LEVOTHYROXINE SODIUM L8/M
Tablets, USP, 100 mcg ℞
Yellow
LEVOTHYROXINE SODIUM L9/M
Tablets, USP, 112 mcg ℞
Rose
LEVOTHYROXINE SODIUM L10/M
Tablets, USP, 125 mcg ℞
Gray
LEVOTHYROXINE SODIUM L11/M
Tablets, USP, 150 mcg ℞
Blue
LEVOTHYROXINE SODIUM L12/M
Tablets, USP, 175 mcg ℞
Lilac
LEVOTHYROXINE SODIUM L13/M
Tablets, USP, 200 mcg ℞
Pink
LEVOTHYROXINE SODIUM L14/M
Tablets, USP, 300 mcg ℞
Green
LISINOPRIL LH1/M
and HYDROCHLOROTHIAZIDE
Tablets, 10 mg/12.5 mg ℞
White
LISINOPRIL LH2/M
and HYDROCHLOROTHIAZIDE
Tablets, 20 mg/12.5 mg ℞
Yellow
LISINOPRIL LH3/M
and HYDROCHLOROTHIAZIDE
Tablets, 20 mg/25 mg ℞
Green
LISINOPRIL L22/M
Tablets, USP, 2.5 mg ℞
Blue
LISINOPRIL ML23/M
Tablets, USP, 5 mg ℞
Peach
LISINOPRIL L24/M
Tablets, USP, 10 mg ℞
White
LISINOPRIL L25/M
Tablets, USP, 20 mg ℞
Yellow
LISINOPRIL L27/M
Tablets, USP, 30 mg ℞
Blue
LISINOPRIL L26/M
Tablets, USP, 40 mg ℞
Green
LOPERAMIDE HYDROCHLORIDE MYLAN 2100
Capsules, USP, 2 mg ℞
Lt. Brown & Lt. Brown
LORAZEPAM M/321
Tablets, USP, 0.5 mg ©/℞
White

Continued on next page

Mylan-Product List—Cont.

LORAZEPAM MYLAN 457/Blank
Tablets, USP, 1 mg CIV/℞
White

LORAZEPAM MYLAN 777/Blank
Tablets, USP, 2 mg CIV/℞
White

LOVASTATIN ML19/Blank
Tablets, USP, 10 mg ℞
White to Off-White

LOVASTATIN ML20/Blank
Tablets, USP, 20 mg ℞
Yellow

LOVASTATIN ML21/Blank
Tablets, USP, 40 mg ℞
Pink

MAPROTILINE HYDROCHLORIDE M/60
Tablets, USP, 25 mg ℞
White

MAPROTILINE HYDROCHLORIDE M/87
Tablets, USP, 50 mg ℞
Blue

MAPROTILINE HYDROCHLORIDE M/92
Tablets, USP, 75 mg ℞
White

MECLOFENAMATE SODIUM MYLAN 2150
Capsules, USP, 50 mg ℞
Coral & Coral

MECLOFENAMATE SODIUM MYLAN 3000
Capsules, USP, 100 mg ℞
Coral & White

METFORMIN HYDROCHLORIDE M/234
Tablets, 500 mg ℞
White

METFORMIN HYDROCHLORIDE M/240
Tablets, 850 mg ℞
White

METFORMIN HYDROCHLORIDE M244/Scored
Tablets, 1000 mg ℞
White

METHOTREXATE M14/Blank
Tablets, USP, 2.5 mg ℞
Orange

METHYCLOTHIAZIDE M29/Blank
Tablets, USP, 5 mg ℞
Blue

METHYLDOPA MYLAN/611
Tablets, USP, 250 mg ℞
Beige

METHYLDOPA MYLAN/421
Tablets, USP, 500 mg ℞
Beige

METHYLDOPA MYLAN/507
and HYDROCHLOROTHIAZIDE
Tablets, USP, 250 mg/15 mg ℞
Green

METHYLDOPA MYLAN/711
and HYDROCHLOROTHIAZIDE
Tablets, USP, 250 mg/25 mg ℞
Green

METOLAZONE M/172
Tablets, USP, 2.5 mg ℞
Peach

METOPROLOL TARTRATE M18/Scored
Tablets, USP, 25 mg ℞
White

METOPROLOL TARTRATE M32/Scored
Tablets, USP, 50 mg ℞
Pink

METOPROLOL TARTRATE M47/Scored
Tablets, USP, 100 mg ℞
Lt. Blue

MIDODRINE HYDROCHLORIDE MH1/M
Tablets, 2.5 mg ℞
White to off-white

MIDODRINE HYDROCHLORIDE MH2/M
Tablets, 5 mg ℞
White to off-white

MIDODRINE HYDROCHLORIDE MH3/M
Tablets, 10 mg ℞
White to off-white

MIRTAZAPINE M515/Scored
Tablets, 15 mg ℞
Beige

MIRTAZAPINE M530/Scored
Tablets, 30 mg ℞
Beige

MIRTAZAPINE M545/Blank
Tablets, 45 mg ℞
Beige

NADOLOL M28/Blank
Tablets, USP, 20 mg ℞
Yellow

NADOLOL M171/Blank
Tablets, USP, 40 mg ℞
Yellow

NADOLOL M132/Blank
Tablets, USP, 80 mg ℞
Yellow

NAPROXEN MYLAN/377
Tablets, USP, 250 mg ℞
White

NAPROXEN MYLAN/555
Tablets, USP, 375 mg ℞
White

NAPROXEN MYLAN/451
Tablets, USP, 500 mg ℞
White

NAPROXEN SODIUM M/537
Tablets, USP, 275 mg ℞
Lt. Blue

NAPROXEN SODIUM MYLAN/733
Tablets, USP, 550 mg ℞
Lt. Blue

NEFAZODONE HYDROCHLORIDE N52/M
Tablets, 100 mg ℞
White

NEFAZODONE HYDROCHLORIDE N53/M
Tablets, 150 mg ℞
White

NEFAZODONE HYDROCHLORIDE N54/M
Tablets, 200 mg ℞
White

NEFAZODONE HYDROCHLORIDE N55/M
Tablets, 250 mg ℞
White

NICARDIPINE HYDROCHLORIDE MYLAN 1020
Capsules, 20 mg ℞
Med. Blue Green & Ivory

NICARDIPINE HYDROCHLORIDE MYLAN 1430
Capsules, 30 mg ℞
Bluish Green & Rich Yellow

NIFEDIPINE M475/Blank
Extended-release Tablets, 30 mg ℞
Pink

NIFEDIPINE M482/Blank
Extended-release Tablets, 60 mg ℞
Pink

NIFEDIPINE M495/Blank
Extended-release Tablets, 90 mg ℞
Pink

NITROFURANTOIN (Macrocrystals) MYLAN 1650
Capsules, USP, 50 mg ℞
Lt. Brown & Lt. Brown

NITROFURANTOIN (Macrocrystals) MYLAN 1700
Capsules, USP, 100 mg ℞
Gray & Gray

NITROFURANTOIN MYLAN 3422
(Monohydrate/Macrocrystals)
Capsules, 100 mg ℞
Lt. gray & Lt. brown

NITROGLYCERIN TRANSDERMAL SYSTEM Nitroglycerin 0.1 mg/hr
Patches, 0.1 mg ℞
Translucent

NITROGLYCERIN TRANSDERMAL SYSTEM Nitroglycerin 0.2 mg/hr
Patches, 0.2 mg ℞
Translucent

NITROGLYCERIN TRANSDERMAL SYSTEM Nitroglycerin 0.4 mg/hr
Patches, 0.4 mg ℞
Translucent

NITROGLYCERIN TRANSDERMAL SYSTEM Nitroglycerin 0.6 mg/hr
Patches, 0.6 mg ℞
Translucent

NIZATIDINE MYLAN 5150
Capsules, USP, 150 mg ℞
Lavender & Lt. Lavender

NIZATIDINE MYLAN 5300
Capsules, USP, 300 mg ℞
Lavender & Lavender

NORTRIPTYLINE HYDROCHLORIDE MYLAN 1410
Capsules, USP, 10 mg ℞
Swedish Orange & Swedish Orange

NORTRIPTYLINE HYDROCHLORIDE MYLAN 2325
Capsules, USP, 25 mg ℞
Orange & Swedish Orange

NORTRIPTYLINE HYDROCHLORIDE MYLAN 3250
Capsules, USP, 50 mg ℞
Yellow & Swedish Orange

NORTRIPTYLINE HYDROCHLORIDE MYLAN 4175
Capsules, USP, 75 mg ℞
Brown & Swedish Orange

OMEPRAZOLE MYLAN 5211
Delayed-release Capsules, 10 mg ℞
Dark Green & Dark Green

OMEPRAZOLE MYLAN 6150
Delayed-release Capsules, 20 mg ℞
Dark Green & Blue-Green

ORPHENADRINE CITRATE M/3358
Extended-release Tablets, 100 mg ℞
White

ORPHENADRINE CITRATE, M3354/Blank
ASPIRIN and CAFFEINE
Tablets, 25 mg/385 mg/30 mg ℞
White & Yellow

ORPHENADRINE CITRATE, M3356/Blank
ASPIRIN and CAFFEINE
Tablets, 50 mg/770 mg/60 mg ℞
White & Yellow

OXAPROZIN 11/77 MYLAN
Tablets, 600 mg ℞
White

PACLITAXEL —
Injection, 30 mg/5 mL (6 mg/mL) ℞

PENTOXIFYLLINE MYLAN/357
Extended-release Tablets, 400 mg ℞
Lavender

PERPHENAZINE and AMITRIPTYLINE MYLAN/330
HYDROCHLORIDE
Tablets, USP, 2 mg/10 mg ℞
White

PERPHENAZINE and AMITRIPTYLINE MYLAN/442
HYDROCHLORIDE
Tablets, USP, 2 mg/25 mg ℞
Purple

PERPHENAZINE and AMITRIPTYLINE MYLAN/727
HYDROCHLORIDE
Tablets, USP, 4 mg/10 mg ℞
Blue

PERPHENAZINE and AMITRIPTYLINE MYLAN/574
HYDROCHLORIDE
Tablets, USP, 4 mg/25 mg ℞
Orange

PERPHENAZINE and AMITRIPTYLINE MYLAN/73
HYDROCHLORIDE
Tablets, USP, 4 mg/50 mg ℞
Purple

EXTENDED PHENYTOIN SODIUM MYLAN 1560
Capsules, USP, 100 mg ℞
Lt. Lavender & White

PINDOLOL M52/Blank
Tablets, USP, 5 mg ℞
White

PINDOLOL M127/Blank
Tablets, USP, 10 mg ℞
White

PIROXICAM MYLAN 1010
Capsules, USP, 10 mg ℞
Dark Green & Olive

PIROXICAM MYLAN 2020
Capsules, USP, 20 mg ℞
Medium Green & Medium Green

PRAZOSIN HYDROCHLORIDE MYLAN 1101
Capsules, USP, 1 mg ℞
Dark Green & Lt. Brown

PRAZOSIN HYDROCHLORIDE MYLAN 2302
Capsules, USP, 2 mg ℞
Brown & Lt. Brown

PRAZOSIN HYDROCHLORIDE MYLAN 3205
Capsules, USP, 5 mg ℞
Lt. Blue & Lt. Brown

PROBENECID MYLAN 156/500
Tablets, USP, 500 mg ℞
Yellow

PROCHLORPERAZINE MALEATE M/P1
Tablets, USP, 5 mg ℞
Maroon

PROCHLORPERAZINE MALEATE M/P2
Tablets, USP, 10 mg ℞
Maroon

PROPOXYPHENE HYDROCHLORIDE, MYLAN 131
ASPIRIN and CAFFEINE
Capsules, USP, 65 mg/389 mg/32.4 mg CIV/℞
Gray & Red

PROPOXYPHENE HYDROCHLORIDE MYLAN 129
Capsules, USP, 65 mg CIV/℞
Pink & Pink

PROPOXYPHENE HYDROCHLORIDE MYLAN/130
and ACETAMINOPHEN
Tablets, USP, 65 mg/650 mg CIV/℞
Orange

PROPOXYPHENE NAPSYLATE MYLAN/155
and ACETAMINOPHEN
Tablets, USP, 100 mg/650 mg CIV/℞
Pink

PROPOXYPHENE NAPSYLATE MYLAN/1155
and ACETAMINOPHEN
Tablets, USP, 100 mg/650 mg CIV/℞
White

PROPRANOLOL HYDROCHLORIDE MYLAN 182/10
Tablets, USP, 10 mg ℞
Orange

PROPRANOLOL HYDROCHLORIDE MYLAN 183/20
Tablets, USP, 20 mg ℞
Blue

PROPRANOLOL HYDROCHLORIDE MYLAN 184/40
Tablets, USP, 40 mg ℞
Green

PROPRANOLOL HYDROCHLORIDE MYLAN 185/80
Tablets, USP, 80 mg ℞
Yellow

PROPRANOLOL HYDROCHLORIDE and HYDROCHLOROTHIAZIDE MYLAN 731/Scored
Tablets, USP, 40 mg/25 mg ℞
White

PROPRANOLOL HYDROCHLORIDE and HYDROCHLOROTHIAZIDE MYLAN 347/Scored
Tablets, USP, 80 mg/25 mg ℞
White

SELEGILINE HYDROCHLORIDE MYLAN 2252
Capsules, 5 mg ℞
Blue Opaque & Aqua Blue Opaque

SELEGILINE HYDROCHLORIDE S/5
Tablets, 5 mg ℞
White

SOTALOL HYDROCHLORIDE M305/Blank
Tablets, USP, 80 mg ℞
Lt. Orange

SOTALOL HYDROCHLORIDE M310/Blank
Tablets, USP, 120 mg ℞
Lt. Orange

SOTALOL HYDROCHLORIDE M314/Blank
Tablets, USP, 160 mg ℞
Lt. Orange

SPIRONOLACTONE M146/Blank
Tablets, USP, 25 mg ℞
White

SPIRONOLACTONE M243/Scored
Tablets, USP, 50 mg ℞
White

SPIRONOLACTONE M437/Scored
Tablets, USP, 100 mg ℞
White

SPIRONOLACTONE and HYDROCHLOROTHIAZIDE M41/Blank
Tablets, USP, 25 mg/25 mg ℞
Ivory

SULINDAC MYLAN/427
Tablets, USP, 150 mg ℞
Yellow-Orange

SULINDAC MYLAN 531/Blank
Tablets, USP, 200 mg ℞
Yellow-Orange

TAMOXIFEN CITRATE M/144
Tablets, USP, 10 mg ℞
White

TAMOXIFEN CITRATE M/274
Tablets, USP, 20 mg ℞
White to Off-White

TEMAZEPAM MYLAN 4010
Capsules, USP, 15 mg CIV/℞
Peach & Peach

TEMAZEPAM MYLAN 5050
Capsules, USP, 30 mg CIV/℞
Yellow & Yellow

TERAZOSIN HYDROCHLORIDE MYLAN 2260
Capsules, 1 mg ℞
Rich Yellow & Lt. Lavender

TERAZOSIN HYDROCHLORIDE MYLAN 2264
Capsules, 2 mg ℞
Black & Lt. Lavender

TERAZOSIN HYDROCHLORIDE MYLAN 2268
Capsules, 5 mg ℞
Iron Gray & Lt. Lavender

TERAZOSIN HYDROCHLORIDE MYLAN 1570
Capsules, 10 mg ℞
Lt. Lavender & Lt. Lavender

TETRACYCLINE HYDROCHLORIDE MYLAN 101
Capsules, USP, 250 mg ℞
Med. Orange & Yellow

TETRACYCLINE HYDROCHLORIDE MYLAN 102
Capsules, USP, 500 mg ℞
Black & Yellow

THIORIDAZINE HYDROCHLORIDE M54/10
Tablets, USP, 10 mg ℞
Orange

THIORIDAZINE HYDROCHLORIDE M58/25
Tablets, USP, 25 mg ℞
Orange

THIORIDAZINE HYDROCHLORIDE M59/50
Tablets, USP, 50 mg ℞
Orange

THIORIDAZINE HYDROCHLORIDE M61/100
Tablets, USP, 100 mg ℞
Orange

THIOTHIXENE MYLAN 1001
Capsules, USP, 1 mg ℞
Caramel & Powder Blue

THIOTHIXENE MYLAN 2002
Capsules, USP, 2 mg ℞
Caramel & Yellow

THIOTHIXENE MYLAN 3005
Capsules, USP, 5 mg ℞
Caramel & White

THIOTHIXENE MYLAN 5010
Capsules, USP, 10 mg ℞
Caramel & Peach

TIMOLOL MALEATE M55/Blank
Tablets, USP, 5 mg ℞
Green

TIMOLOL MALEATE M221/Blank
Tablets, USP, 10 mg ℞
Green

TIMOLOL MALEATE M715/Blank
Tablets, USP, 20 mg ℞
Green

TIZANIDINE HYDROCHLORIDE M 722/scored
Tablets, 2 mg ℞
White to Off-White

TIZANIDINE HYDROCHLORIDE M 724/Quadrisect Scored
Tablets, 4 mg ℞
White to Off-White

TOLAZAMIDE MYLAN 217/250
Tablets, USP, 250 mg ℞
White

TOLAZAMIDE MYLAN 551/Blank
Tablets, USP, 500 mg ℞
White

TOLBUTAMIDE M13/Blank
Tablets, USP, 500 mg ℞
White

TOLMETIN SODIUM MYLAN 5200
Capsules, USP, 400 mg ℞
Lt. Blue & Lt. Blue

TOLMETIN SODIUM M313/Blank
Tablets, USP, 600 mg ℞
Beige

TRAMADOL HYDROCHLORIDE M/T7
Tablets, 50 mg ℞
White

TRIAMTERENE and HYDROCHLOROTHIAZIDE MYLAN 2537
Capsules, USP, 37.5 mg/25 mg ℞
Olive & Rich Yellow

TRIAMTERENE and HYDROCHLOROTHIAZIDE MYLAN/TH1
Tablets, USP, 37.5 mg/25 mg ℞
Green

TRIAMTERENE and HYDROCHLOROTHIAZIDE MYLAN/TH2
Tablets, USP, 75 mg/50 mg ℞
Yellow

TRIFLUOPERAZINE HYDROCHLORIDE M/T3
Tablets, USP, 1 mg ℞
White

TRIFLUOPERAZINE HYDROCHLORIDE M/T4
Tablets, USP, 2 mg ℞
White

TRIFLUOPERAZINE HYDROCHLORIDE M/T5
Tablets, USP, 5 mg ℞
Lavender

TRIFLUOPERAZINE HYDROCHLORIDE M/T6
Tablets, USP, 10 mg ℞
Lavender

VERAPAMIL HYDROCHLORIDE MYLAN 512/Blank
Tablets, USP, 80 mg ℞
White

VERAPAMIL HYDROCHLORIDE MYLAN 772/Blank
Tablets, USP, 120 mg ℞
White

VERAPAMIL HYDROCHLORIDE MYLAN 6320
Extended-release Capsules, 120 mg ℞
Bluish Green & White

VERAPAMIL HYDROCHLORIDE MYLAN 6380
Extended-release Capsules, 180 mg ℞
Bluish Green & Lt. Green

VERAPAMIL HYDROCHLORIDE MYLAN 6440
Extended-release Capsules, 240 mg ℞
Bluish Green & Bluish Green

VERAPAMIL HYDROCHLORIDE MYLAN/244
Extended-release Tablets, USP, 120 mg ℞
Blue

VERAPAMIL HYDROCHLORIDE M312/Blank
Extended-release Tablets, USP, 180 mg ℞
Blue

VERAPAMIL HYDROCHLORIDE M411/Blank
Extended-release Tablets, USP, 240 mg ℞
Blue

*Front/Back Side for Tablets or Both Cap and Body for Capsules.

CAPTOPRIL TABLETS, USP ℞

12.5 mg, 25 mg, 50 mg and 100 mg

USE IN PREGNANCY

When used in pregnancy during the second and third trimesters, ACE inhibitors can cause injury and even death to the developing fetus. When pregnancy is detected, captopril should be discontinued as soon as possible. **See WARNINGS: Fetal/Neonatal Morbidity and Mortality.**

DESCRIPTION

Captopril is a specific competitive inhibitor of angiotensin I-converting enzyme (ACE), the enzyme responsible for the conversion of angiotensin I to angiotensin II.

Captopril is designated chemically as 1-[(2S)-3-mercapto-2-methylpropionyl]-L-proline (MW 217.29).

Captopril is a white to off-white crystalline powder that may have a slight sulfurous odor; it is soluble in water (approx. 160 mg/mL), methanol, and ethanol and sparingly soluble in chloroform and ethyl acetate.

The structural formula is:

$C_9H_{15}NO_3S$

Each tablet for oral administration contains 12.5 mg, 25 mg, 50 mg or 100 mg of captopril and the following inactive ingredients: anhydrous lactose, colloidal silicon dioxide, crospovidone, microcrystalline cellulose and stearic acid.

CLINICAL PHARMACOLOGY

Mechanism of Action: The mechanism of action of captopril has not yet been fully elucidated. Its beneficial effects in hypertension and heart failure appear to result primarily from suppression of the renin-angiotensin-aldosterone system. However, there is no consistent correlation between renin levels and response to the drug. Renin, an enzyme synthesized by the kidneys, is released into the circulation where it acts on a plasma globulin substrate to produce angiotensin I, a relatively inactive decapeptide. Angiotensin I is then converted by angiotensin converting enzyme (ACE) to angiotensin II, a potent endogenous vasoconstrictor substance. Angiotensin II also stimulates aldosterone secretion from the adrenal cortex, thereby contributing to sodium and fluid retention.

Captopril prevents the conversion of angiotensin I to angiotensin II by inhibition of ACE, a peptidyldipeptide carboxy hydrolase. This inhibition has been demonstrated in both healthy human subjects and in animals by showing that the elevation of blood pressure caused by exogenously administered angiotensin I was attenuated or abolished by captopril. In animal studies, captopril did not alter the pressor responses to a number of other agents, including angiotensin II and norepinephrine, indicating specificity of action.

ACE is identical to "bradykininase", and captopril may also interfere with the degradation of the vasodepressor peptide, bradykinin. Increased concentrations of bradykinin or prostaglandin E_2 may also have a role in the therapeutic effect of captopril.

Inhibition of ACE results in decreased plasma angiotensin II and increased plasma renin activity (PRA), the latter resulting from loss of negative feedback on renin release caused by reduction in angiotensin II. The reduction of angiotensin II leads to decreased aldosterone secretion, and, as a result, small increases in serum potassium may occur along with sodium and fluid loss.

The antihypertensive effects persist for a longer period of time than does demonstrable inhibition of circulating ACE. It is not known whether the ACE present in vascular endothelium is inhibited longer than the ACE in circulating blood.

Pharmacokinetics: After oral administration of therapeutic doses of captopril, rapid absorption occurs with peak blood levels at about one hour. The presence of food in the gastrointestinal tract reduces absorption by about 30 to 40 percent; captopril therefore should be given one hour before meals. Based on carbon-14 labeling, average minimal absorption is approximately 75 percent. In a 24-hour period, over 95 percent of the absorbed dose is eliminated in the urine; 40 to 50 percent is unchanged drug; most of the remainder is the disulfide dimer of captopril and captopril-cysteine disulfide.

Approximately 25 to 30 percent of the circulating drug is bound to plasma proteins. The apparent elimination half-life for total radioactivity in blood is probably less than 3 hours. An accurate determination of half-life of unchanged captopril is not, at present, possible, but it is probably less than 2 hours. In patients with renal impairment, however, retention of captopril occurs (see DOSAGE AND ADMINISTRATION).

Pharmacodynamics: Administration of captopril results in a reduction of peripheral arterial resistance in hypertensive patients with either no change, or an increase, in cardiac output. There is an increase in renal blood flow following administration of captopril and glomerular filtration rate is usually unchanged.

Reductions of blood pressure are usually maximal 60 to 90 minutes after oral administration of an individual dose of captopril. The duration of effect is dose related. The reduction in blood pressure may be progressive, so to achieve maximal therapeutic effects, several weeks of therapy may be required. The blood pressure lowering effects of captopril and thiazide-type diuretics are additive. In contrast, captopril and beta-blockers have a less than additive effect.

Blood pressure is lowered to about the same extent in both standing and supine positions. Orthostatic effects and tachycardia are infrequent but may occur in volume-depleted patients. Abrupt withdrawal of captopril has not been associated with a rapid increase in blood pressure.

In patients with heart failure, significantly decreased peripheral (systemic vascular) resistance and blood pressure (afterload), reduced pulmonary capillary wedge pressure (preload) and pulmonary vascular resistance, increased cardiac output, and increased exercise tolerance time (ETT) have been demonstrated. These hemodynamic and clinical effects occur after the first dose and appear to persist for the duration of therapy. Placebo controlled studies of 12 weeks duration in patients who did not respond adequately to diuretics and digitalis show no tolerance to beneficial effects on ETT; open studies, with exposure up to 18 months in some cases, also indicate that ETT benefit is maintained. Clinical improvement has been observed in some patients where acute hemodynamic effects were minimal.

The Survival and Ventricular Enlargement (SAVE) study was a multicenter, randomized, double-blind, placebo-controlled trial conducted in 2,231 patients (age 21 to 79 years) who survived the acute phase of a myocardial infarction and did not have active ischemia. Patients had left ventricular dysfunction (LVD), defined as a resting left ventricular ejection fraction ≤40%, but at the time of randomization were not sufficiently symptomatic to require ACE inhibitor therapy for heart failure. About half of the patients had had symptoms of heart failure in the past. Patients were given a test dose of 6.25 mg oral captopril and were randomized within 3 to 16 days post-infarction to receive either captopril or placebo in addition to conventional therapy. Captopril was initiated at 6.25 mg or 12.5 mg tid and after two weeks titrated to a target maintenance dose of 50 mg tid. About 80% of patients were receiving the target dose at the

Continued on next page

Captopril—Cont.

end of the study. Patients were followed for a minimum of two years and for up to five years, with an average follow-up of 3.5 years.

Baseline blood pressure was 113/70 mm Hg and 112/70 mm Hg for the placebo and captopril groups, respectively. Blood pressure increased slightly in both treatment groups during the study and was somewhat lower in the captopril group (119/74 vs. 125/77 mm Hg at 1 yr).

Therapy with captopril improved long-term survival and clinical outcomes compared to placebo. The risk reduction for all cause mortality was 19% (P = 0.02) and for cardiovascular death was 21% (P = 0.014). Captopril treated subjects had 22% (P = 0.034) fewer first hospitalizations for heart failure. Compared to placebo, 22% fewer patients receiving captopril developed symptoms of overt heart failure. There was no significant difference between groups in total hospitalizations for all cause (2056 placebo; 2036 captopril).

In a multicenter study, a marketed brand of captopril tablets, USP were well tolerated in the presence of other therapies such as aspirin, beta blockers, nitrates, vasodilators, calcium antagonists and diuretics.

Studies in rats and cats indicate that captopril does not cross the blood-brain barrier to any significant extent.

INDICATIONS AND USAGE

Hypertension: Captopril tablets are indicated for the treatment of hypertension.

In using captopril, consideration should be given to the risk of neutropenia/agranulocytosis (see WARNINGS).

Captopril may be used as initial therapy for patients with normal renal function, in whom the risk is relatively low. In patients with impaired renal function, particularly those with collagen vascular disease, captopril should be reserved for hypertensives who have either developed unacceptable side effects on other drugs, or have failed to respond satisfactorily to drug combinations.

Captopril is effective alone and in combination with other antihypertensive agents, especially thiazide-type diuretics. The blood pressure lowering effects of captopril and thiazides are approximately additive.

Heart Failure: Captopril tablets, USP are indicated in the treatment of congestive heart failure usually in combination with diuretics and digitalis. The beneficial effect of captopril in heart failure does not require the presence of digitalis, however, most controlled clinical trial experience with captopril has been in patients receiving digitalis, as well as diuretic treatment.

Left Ventricular Dysfunction After Myocardial Infarction: Captopril tablets, USP are indicated to improve survival following myocardial infarction in clinically stable patients with left ventricular dysfunction manifested as an ejection fraction $\leq$ 40% and to reduce the incidence of overt heart failure and subsequent hospitalizations for congestive heart failure in these patients.

In considering use of captopril tablets, USP it should be noted that in controlled trials ACE inhibitors have an effect on blood pressure that is less in black patients than in non-blacks. In addition, ACE inhibitors (for which adequate data are available) cause a higher rate of angioedema in black than in non-black patients (see WARNINGS: Angioedema).

CONTRAINDICATIONS

Captopril tablets, USP are contraindicated in patients who are hypersensitive to this product or any other angiotensin-converting enzyme inhibitor (e.g., a patient who has experienced angioedema during therapy with any other ACE inhibitor).

WARNINGS

Anaphylactoid and Possibly Related Reactions: Presumably because angiotensin-converting enzyme inhibitors affect the metabolism of eicosanoids and polypeptides, including endogenous bradykinin, patients receiving ACE inhibitors (including captopril) may be subject to a variety of adverse reactions, some of them serious.

Angioedema: Angioedema involving the extremities, face, lips, mucous membranes, tongue, glottis or larynx has been seen in patients treated with ACE inhibitors, including captopril. If angioedema involves the tongue, glottis or larynx, airway obstruction may occur and be fatal. Emergency therapy, including but not necessarily limited to, subcutaneous administration of a 1:1000 solution of epinephrine should be promptly instituted.

Swelling confined to the face, mucous membranes of the mouth, lips and extremities has usually resolved with discontinuation of captopril; some cases required medical therapy. (See PRECAUTIONS: Information for Patients and ADVERSE REACTIONS.)

Anaphylactoid Reactions During Desensitization: Two patients undergoing desensitizing treatment with hymenoptera venom while receiving ACE inhibitors sustained life-threatening anaphylactoid reactions. In the same patients, these reactions were avoided when ACE inhibitors were temporarily withheld, but they reappeared upon inadvertent rechallenge.

Anaphylactoid Reactions During Membrane Exposure: Anaphylactoid reactions have been reported in patients dialyzed with high-flux membranes and treated concomitantly with an ACE inhibitor. Anaphylactoid reactions have also been reported in patients undergoing low-density lipoprotein apheresis with dextran sulfate absorption.

Neutropenia/Agranulocytosis: Neutropenia (< 1000/mm^3) with myeloid hypoplasia has resulted from use of captopril. About half of the neutropenic patients developed systemic or oral cavity infections or other features of the syndrome of agranulocytosis.

The risk of neutropenia is dependent on the clinical status of the patient:

In clinical trials in patients with hypertension who have normal renal function (serum creatinine less than 1.6 mg/dL and no collagen vascular disease), neutropenia has been seen in one patient out of over 8,600 exposed.

In patients with some degree of renal failure (serum creatinine at least 1.6 mg/dL) but no collagen vascular disease, the risk of neutropenia in clinical trials was about 1 per 500, a frequency over 15 times that for uncomplicated hypertension. Daily doses of captopril were relatively high in these patients, particularly in view of their diminished renal function. In foreign marketing experience in patients with renal failure, use of allopurinol concomitantly with captopril has been associated with neutropenia but this association has not appeared in U.S. reports.

In patients with collagen vascular diseases (e.g., systemic lupus erythematosus, scleroderma) and impaired renal function, neutropenia occurred in 3.7 percent of patients in clinical trials.

While none of the over 750 patients in formal clinical trials of heart failure developed neutropenia, it has occurred during the subsequent clinical experience. About half of the reported cases had serum creatinine $\geq$ 1.6 mg/dL and more than 75 percent were in patients also receiving procainamide. In heart failure, it appears that the same risk factors for neutropenia are present.

The neutropenia has usually been detected with in three months after captopril was started. Bone marrow examinations in patients with neutropenia consistently showed myeloid hypoplasia, frequently accompanied by erythroid hypoplasia and decreased numbers of megakaryocytes (e.g., hypoplastic bone marrow and pancytopenia); anemia and thrombocytopenia were sometimes seen.

In general, neutrophils returned to normal in about two weeks after captopril was discontinued, and serious infections were limited to clinically complex patients. About 13 percent of the cases of neutropenia have ended fatally, but almost all fatalities were in patients with serious illness, having collagen vascular disease, renal failure, heart failure or immunosuppressant therapy, or a combination of these complicating factors.

Evaluation of the hypertensive or heart failure patient should always include assessment of renal function.

If captopril is used in patients with impaired renal function, white blood cell and differential counts should be evaluated prior to starting treatment and at approximately two-week intervals for about three months, then periodically.

In patients with collagen vascular disease or who are exposed to other drugs known to affect the white cells or immune response, particularly when there is impaired renal function, captopril should be used only after an assessment of benefit and risk, and then with caution.

All patients treated with captopril should be told to report any signs of infection (e.g., sore throat, fever). If infection is suspected, white cell counts should be performed without delay.

Since discontinuation of captopril and other drugs has generally led to prompt return of the white count to normal, upon confirmation of neutropenia (neutrophil count < 1000/mm^3) the physician should withdraw captopril and closely follow the patient's course.

Proteinuria: Total urinary proteins greater than 1 g per day were seen in about 0.7 percent of patients receiving captopril. About 90 percent of affected patients had evidence of prior renal disease or received relatively high doses of captopril (in excess of 150 mg/day), or both. The nephrotic syndrome occurred in about one-fifth of proteinuric patients. In most cases, proteinuria subsided or cleared within six months whether or not captopril was continued. Parameters of renal function, such as BUN and creatinine, were seldom altered in the patients with proteinuria.

Hypotension: Excessive hypotension was rarely seen in hypertensive patients but is a possible consequence of captopril use in salt/volume depleted persons (such as those treated vigorously with diuretics), patients with heart failure or those patients undergoing renal dialysis. (See PRECAUTIONS: Drug Interactions.)

In heart failure, where the blood pressure was either normal or low, transient decreases in mean blood pressure greater than 20 percent were recorded in about half of the patients. This transient hypotension is more likely to occur after any of the first several doses and is usually well tolerated, producing either no symptoms or brief mild lightheadedness, although in rare instances it has been associated with arrhythmia or conduction defects. Hypotension was the reason for discontinuation of drug in 3.6 percent of patients with heart failure.

BECAUSE OF THE POTENTIAL FALL IN BLOOD PRESSURE IN THESE PATIENTS, THERAPY SHOULD BE STARTED UNDER VERY CLOSE MEDICAL SUPERVISION. A starting dose of 6.25 or 12.5 mg tid may minimize the hypotensive effect. Patients should be followed closely for the first two weeks of treatment and whenever the dose of captopril and/or diuretic is increased. In patients with heart failure, reducing the dose of diuretic, if feasible, may minimize the fall in blood pressure.

Hypotension is not *per se* a reason to discontinue captopril. Some decrease of systemic blood pressure is a common and desirable observation upon initiation of captopril treatment in heart failure. The magnitude of the decrease is greatest early in the course of treatment; this effect stabilizes within a week or two, and generally returns to pretreatment levels, without a decrease in therapeutic efficacy, within two months.

Fetal/Neonatal Morbidity and Mortality: ACE inhibitors can cause fetal and neonatal morbidity and death when administered to pregnant women. Several dozen cases have been reported in the world literature. When pregnancy is detected, ACE inhibitors should be discontinued as soon as possible.

The use of ACE inhibitors during the second and third trimesters of pregnancy has been associated with fetal and neonatal injury, including hypotension, neonatal skull hypoplasia, anuria, reversible or irreversible renal failure, and death. Oligohydramnios has also been reported, presumably resulting from decreased fetal renal function; oligohydramnios in this setting has been associated with fetal limb contractures, craniofacial deformation, and hypoplastic lung development. Prematurity, intrauterine growth retardation, and patent ductus arteriosus have also been reported, although it is not clear whether these occurrences were due to the ACE-inhibitor exposure.

These adverse effects do not appear to have resulted from intrauterine ACE-inhibitor exposure that has been limited to the first trimester. Mothers whose embryos and fetuses are exposed to ACE inhibitors only during the first trimester should be so informed. Nonetheless, when patients become pregnant, physicians should make every effort to discontinue the use of captopril as soon as possible.

Rarely (probably less often than once in every thousand pregnancies), no alternative to ACE inhibitors will be found. In these rare cases, the mothers should be apprised of the potential hazards to their fetuses, and serial ultrasound examinations should be performed to assess the intra-amniotic environment.

If oligohydramnios is observed, captopril should be discontinued unless it is considered life-saving for the mother. Contraction stress testing (CST), a non-stress test (NST), or biophysical profiling (BPP) may be appropriate, depending upon the week of pregnancy. Patients and physicians should be aware, however, that oligohydramnios may not appear until after the fetus has sustained irreversible injury.

Infants with histories of *in utero* exposure to ACE inhibitors should be closely observed for hypotension, oliguria, and hyperkalemia. If oliguria occurs, attention should be directed toward support of blood pressure and renal perfusion. Exchange transfusion or dialysis may be required as a means of reversing hypotension and/or substituting for disordered renal function. While captopril may be removed from the adult circulation by hemodialysis, there is inadequate data concerning the effectiveness of hemodialysis for removing it from the circulation of neonates or children. Peritoneal dialysis is not effective for removing captopril; there is no information concerning exchange transfusion for removing captopril from the general circulation.

When captopril was given to rabbits at doses about 0.8 to 70 times (on a mg/kg basis) the maximum recommended human dose, low incidences of craniofacial malformations were seen. No teratogenic effects of captopril were seen in studies of pregnant rats and hamsters. On a mg/kg basis, the doses used were up to 150 times (in hamsters) and 625 times (in rats) the maximum recommended human dose.

Hepatic Failure: Rarely, ACE inhibitors have been associated with a syndrome that starts with cholestatic jaundice and progresses to fulminant hepatic necrosis and (sometimes) death. The mechanism of this syndrome is not understood. Patients receiving ACE inhibitors who develop jaundice or marked elevations of hepatic enzymes should discontinue the ACE inhibitor and receive appropriate medical follow-up.

PRECAUTIONS

General: ***Impaired Renal Function:*** *Hypertension:* Some patients with renal disease, particularly those with severe renal artery stenosis have developed increases in BUN and serum creatinine after reduction of blood pressure with captopril. Captopril dosage reduction and/or discontinuation of diuretic may be required. For some of these patients, it may not be possible to normalize blood pressure and maintain adequate renal perfusion.

Heart Failure: About 20 percent of patients develop stable elevations of BUN and serum creatinine greater than 20 percent above normal or baseline upon long-term treatment with captopril. Less than 5 percent of patients, generally those with severe preexisting renal disease, required discontinuation of treatment due to progressively increasing creatinine; subsequent improvement probably depends upon the severity of the underlying renal disease.

See CLINICAL PHARMACOLOGY, DOSAGE AND ADMINISTRATION, ADVERSE REACTIONS: Altered Laboratory Findings.

Hyperkalemia: Elevations in serum potassium have been observed in some patients treated with ACE inhibitors, including captopril. When treated with ACE inhibitors, patients at risk for the development of hyperkalemia include those with: renal insufficiency; diabetes mellitus; and those using concomitant potassium-sparing diuretics, potassium supplements or potassium-containing salt substitutes; or other drugs associated with increases in serum potassium. (See PRECAUTIONS: Information for Patients and Drug Interactions; ADVERSE REACTIONS: Altered Laboratory Findings.)

Cough: Presumably due to the inhibition of the degradation of endogenous bradykinin, persistent nonproductive cough has been reported with all ACE inhibitors, always resolving after discontinuation of therapy. ACE inhibitor-induced cough should be considered in the differential diagnosis of cough.

Valvular Stenosis: There is concern, on theoretical grounds, that patients with aortic stenosis might be at particular risk of decreased coronary perfusion when treated with vasodilators because they do not develop as much afterload reduction as others.

Surgery/Anesthesia: In patients undergoing major surgery or during anesthesia with agents that produce hypotension, captopril will block angiotensin II formation secondary to compensatory renin release. If hypotension occurs and is considered to be due to this mechanism, it can be corrected by volume expansion.

Hemodialysis: Recent clinical observations have shown an association of hypersensitivity-like (anaphylactoid) reactions during hemodialysis with high-flux dialysis membranes (e.g., AN69) in patients receiving ACE inhibitors. In these patients, consideration should be given to using a different type of dialysis membrane or a different class of medication. (See WARNINGS: Anaphylactoid Reactions During Membrane Exposure.)

Information For Patients: Patients should be advised to immediately report to their physician any signs or symptoms suggesting angioedema (e.g., swelling of face, eyes, lips, tongue, larynx and extremities; difficulty in swallowing or breathing; hoarseness) and to discontinue therapy. (See WARNINGS: Angioedema.)

Patients should be told to report promptly any indication of infection (e.g., sore throat, fever), which may be a sign of neutropenia, or of progressive edema which might be related to proteinuria and nephrotic syndrome.

All patients should be cautioned that excessive perspiration and dehydration may lead to an excessive fall in blood pressure because of reduction in fluid volume. Other causes of volume depletion such as vomiting or diarrhea may also lead to a fall in blood pressure; patients should be advised to consult with the physician.

Patients should be advised not to use potassium-sparing diuretics, potassium supplements or potassium-containing salt substitutes without consulting their physician. (See PRECAUTIONS: General and Drug Interactions; ADVERSE REACTIONS.)

Patients should be warned against interruption or discontinuation of medication unless instructed by the physician. Heart failure patients on captopril therapy should be cautioned against rapid increases in physical activity.

Patients should be informed that captopril should be taken one hour before meals (see DOSAGE AND ADMINISTRATION).

Pregnancy: Female patients of childbearing age should be told about the consequences of second- and third-trimester exposure to ACE inhibitors, and they should also be told that these consequences do not appear to have resulted from intrauterine ACE-inhibitor exposure that has been limited to the first trimester. These patients should be asked to report pregnancies to their physicians as soon as possible.

Drug Interactions: *Hypotension-Patients on Diuretic Therapy:* Patients on diuretics and especially those in whom diuretic therapy was recently instituted, as well as those on severe dietary salt restriction or dialysis, may occasionally experience a precipitous reduction of blood pressure usually within the first hour after receiving the initial dose of captopril.

The possibility of hypotensive effects with captopril can be minimized by either discontinuing the diuretic or increasing the salt intake approximately one week prior to initiation of treatment with captopril or initiating therapy with small doses (6.25 or 12.5 mg). Alternatively, provide medical supervision for at least one hour after the initial dose. If hypotension occurs, the patient should be placed in a supine position and, if necessary, receive an intravenous infusion of normal saline. This transient hypotensive response is not a contraindication to further doses which can be given without difficulty once the blood pressure has increased after volume expansion.

Agents Having Vasodilator Activity: Data on the effect of concomitant use of other vasodilators in patients receiving captopril for heart failure are not available; therefore, nitroglycerin or other nitrates (as used for management of angina) or other drugs having vasodilator activity should, if possible, be discontinued before starting captopril. If resumed during captopril therapy, such agents should be administered cautiously, and perhaps at lower dosage.

Agents Causing Renin Release: Captopril's effect will be augmented by antihypertensive agents that cause renin release. For example, diuretics (e.g., thiazides) may activate the renin-angiotensin-aldosterone system.

Agents Affecting Sympathetic Activity: The sympathetic nervous system may be especially important in supporting blood pressure in patients receiving captopril alone or with diuretics. Therefore, agents affecting sympathetic activity (e.g., ganglionic blocking agents or adrenergic neuron blocking agents) should be used with caution. Beta-adrenergic blocking drugs add some further antihypertensive effect to captopril, but the overall response is less than additive.

Agents Increasing Serum Potassium: Since captopril decreases aldosterone production, elevation of serum potassium may occur. Potassium-sparing diuretics such as spironolactone, triamterene, or amiloride, or potassium supplements should be given only for documented hypokalemia, and then with caution, since they may lead to a significant increase of serum potassium. Salt substitutes containing potassium should also be used with caution.

Inhibitors of Endogenous Prostaglandin Synthesis: It has been reported that indomethacin may reduce the antihypertensive effect of captopril, especially in cases of low renin hypertension. Other nonsteroidal anti-inflammatory agents (e.g., aspirin) may also have this effect.

Lithium: Increased serum lithium levels and symptoms of lithium toxicity have been reported in patients receiving concomitant lithium and ACE inhibitor therapy. These drugs should be co-administered with caution and frequent monitoring of serum lithium levels is recommended. If a diuretic is also used, it may increase the risk of lithium toxicity.

Cardiac Glycosides: In a study of young healthy male subjects no evidence of a direct pharmacokinetic captopril-digoxin interaction could be found.

Loop Diuretics: Furosemide administered concurrently with captopril does not alter the pharmacokinetics of captopril in renally impaired hypertensive patients.

Allopurinol: In a study of healthy male volunteers no significant pharmacokinetic interaction occurred when captopril and allopurinol were administered concomitantly for 6 days.

Drug/Laboratory Test Interactions: Captopril may cause a false-positive urine test for acetone.

Carcinogenesis, Mutagenesis and Impairment of Fertility: Two-year studies with doses of 50 to 1350 mg/kg/day in mice and rats failed to show any evidence of carcinogenic potential. The high dose in these studies is 150 times the maximum recommended human dose of 450 mg, assuming a 50 kg subject. On a body-surface-area basis, the high doses for mice and rats are 13 and 26 times the maximum recommended human dose, respectively.

Studies in rats have revealed no impairment of fertility.

Animal Toxicology: Chronic oral toxicity studies were conducted in rats (2 years), dogs (47 weeks; 1 year), mice (2 years), and monkeys (1 year). Significant drug-related toxicity included effects on hematopoiesis, renal toxicity, erosion/ulceration of the stomach, and variation of retinal blood vessels.

Reductions in hemoglobin and/or hematocrit values were seen in mice, rats, and monkeys at doses 50 to 150 times the maximum recommended human dose (MRHD) of 450 mg, assuming a 50 kg subject. On a body-surface-area basis, these doses are 5 to 25 times maximum recommended human dose (MRHD). Anemia, leukopenia, thrombocytopenia, and bone marrow suppression occurred in dogs at doses 8 to 30 times MRHD on a body-weight basis (4 to 15 times MRHD on a surface-area basis). The reductions in hemoglobin and hematocrit values in rats and mice were only significant at 1 year and returned to normal with continued dosing by the end of the study. Marked anemia was seen at all dose levels (8 to 30 times MRHD) in dogs, whereas moderate to marked leukopenia was noted only at 15 and 30 times MRHD and thrombocytopenia at 30 times MRHD. The anemia could be reversed upon discontinuation of dosing. Bone marrow suppression occurred to a varying degree, being associated only with dogs that died or were sacrificed in a moribund condition in the 1 year study. However, in the 47-week study at a dose 30 times MRHD, bone marrow suppression was found to be reversible upon continued drug administration.

Captopril caused hyperplasia of the juxtaglomerular apparatus of the kidneys in mice and rats at doses 7 to 200 times MRHD on a body-weight basis (0.6 to 35 times MRHD on a surface-area basis); in monkeys at 20 to 60 times MRHD on a body-weight basis (7 to 20 times MRHD on a surface-area basis); and in dogs at 30 times MRHD on a body-weight basis (15 times MRHD on a surface-area basis).

Gastric erosions/ulcerations were increased in incidence in male rats at 20 to 200 times MRHD on a body-weight basis (3.5 and 35 times MRHD on a surface-area basis); in dogs at 30 times MRHD on a body-weight basis (15 times MRHD on a surface-area basis); and in monkeys at 65 times MRHD on a body-weight basis (20 times MRHD on a surface-area basis). Rabbits developed gastric and intestinal ulcers when given oral doses approximately 30 times MRHD on a body-weight basis (10 times MRHD on a surface-area basis) for only 5 to 7 days.

In the two-year rat study, irreversible and progressive variations in the caliber of retinal vessels (focal sacculations and constrictions) occurred at all dose levels (7 to 200 times MRHD) on a body-weight basis; 1 to 35 times MRHD on a surface-area basis in a dose-related fashion. The effect was first observed in the 88th week of dosing, with a progressively increased incidence thereafter, even after cessation of dosing.

Pregnancy Categories C (first trimester) and D (second and third trimesters): See WARNINGS: Fetal/Neonatal Morbidity and Mortality.

Nursing Mothers: Concentrations of captopril in human milk are approximately one percent of those in maternal blood. Because of the potential for serious adverse reactions in nursing infants from captopril, a decision should be made whether to discontinue nursing or to discontinue the drug, taking into account the importance of captopril to the mother. (See PRECAUTIONS: Pediatric Use.)

Pediatric Use: Safety and effectiveness in pediatric patients have not been established. There is limited experience reported in the literature with the use of captopril in the pediatric population; dosage, on a weight basis, was generally reported to be comparable to or less than that used in adults.

Infants, especially newborns, may be more susceptible to the adverse hemodynamic effects of captopril. Excessive, prolonged and unpredictable decreases in blood pressure and associated complications, including oliguria and seizures, have been reported.

Captopril should be used in pediatric patients only if other measures for controlling blood pressure have not been effective.

ADVERSE REACTIONS

Reported incidences are based on clinical trials involving approximately 7000 patients.

Renal: About one of 100 patients developed proteinuria (see WARNINGS).

Each of the following has been reported in approximately 1 to 2 of 1000 patients and are of uncertain relationship to drug use: renal insufficiency, renal failure, nephrotic syndrome, polyuria, oliguria, and urinary frequency.

Hematologic: Neutropenia/agranulocytosis has occurred (see WARNINGS). Cases of anemia, thrombocytopenia, and pancytopenia have been reported.

Dermatologic: Rash, often with pruritus, and sometimes with fever, arthralgia, and eosinophilia, occurred in about 4 to 7 (depending on renal status and dose) of 100 patients, usually during the first four weeks of therapy. It is usually maculopapular, and rarely urticarial. The rash is usually mild and disappears within a few days of dosage reduction, short-term treatment with an antihistaminic agent, and/or discontinuing therapy; remission may occur even if captopril is continued. Pruritus, without rash, occurs in about 2 of 100 patients. Between 7 and 10 percent of patients with skin rash have shown an eosinophilia and/or positive ANA titers. A reversible associated pemphigoid-like lesion, and photosensitivity, have also been reported.

Flushing or pallor has been reported in 2 to 5 of 1000 patients.

Cardiovascular: Hypotension may occur; see WARNINGS and PRECAUTIONS (Drug Interactions) for discussion of hypotension with captopril therapy.

Tachycardia, chest pain, and palpitations have each been observed in approximately 1 of 100 patients.

Angina pectoris, myocardial infarction, Raynaud's syndrome, and congestive heart failure have each occurred in 2 to 3 of 1000 patients.

Dysgeusia: Approximately 2 to 4 (depending on renal status and dose) of 100 patients developed a diminution or loss of taste perception. Taste impairment is reversible and usually self-limited (2 to 3 months) even with continued drug administration. Weight loss may be associated with the loss of taste.

Angioedema: Angioedema involving the extremities, face, lips, mucous membranes, tongue, glottis or larynx has been reported in approximately one in 1000 patients. Angioedema involving the upper airways has caused fatal airway obstruction. (See WARNINGS: Angioedema and PRECAUTIONS: Information for Patients.)

Cough: Cough has been reported in 0.5 to 2% of patients treated with captopril in clinical trials (see PRECAUTIONS: General: *Cough*).

The following have been reported in about 0.5 to 2 percent of patients but did not appear at increased frequency compared to placebo or other treatments used in controlled trials: gastric irritation, abdominal pain, nausea, vomiting, diarrhea, anorexia, constipation, aphthous ulcers, peptic ulcer, dizziness, headache, malaise, fatigue, insomnia, dry mouth, dyspnea, alopecia, paresthesias.

Other clinical adverse effects reported since the drug was marketed are listed below by body system. In this setting, an incidence or causal relationship cannot be accurately determined.

Body as a Whole: Anaphylactoid reactions (see WARNINGS: Anaphylactoid and Possible Related Reactions and PRECAUTIONS: Hemodialysis.)

General: Asthenia, gynecomastia.

Cardiovascular: Cardiac arrest, cerebrovascular accident/insufficiency, rhythm disturbances, orthostatic hypotension, syncope.

Dermatologic: Bullous pemphigus, erythema multiforme (including Stevens-Johnson syndrome), exfoliative dermatitis.

Gastrointestinal: Pancreatitis, glossitis, dyspepsia.

Hematologic: Anemia, including aplastic and hemolytic.

Hepatobiliary: Jaundice, hepatitis, including rare cases of necrosis, cholestasis.

Metabolic: Symptomatic hyponatremia.

Musculoskeletal: Myalgia, myasthenia.

Nervous/Psychiatric: Ataxia, confusion, depression, nervousness, somnolence.

Respiratory: Bronchospasm, eosinophilic pneumonitis, rhinitis.

Special Senses: Blurred vision.

Urogenital: Impotence.

As with other ACE inhibitors, a syndrome has been reported which may include: fever, myalgia, arthralgia, interstitial nephritis, vasculitis, rash or other dermatologic manifestations, eosinophilia and an elevated ESR.

Fetal/Neonatal Morbidity and Mortality: See WARNINGS: Fetal/Neonatal Morbidity and Mortality.

Continued on next page

Captopril—Cont.

Altered Laboratory Findings: ***Serum Electrolytes:*** *Hyperkalemia:* small increases in serum potassium, especially in patients with renal impairment (see PRECAUTIONS).
Hyponatremia: particularly in patients receiving a low sodium diet or concomitant diuretics.
BUN/Serum Creatinine: Transient elevations of BUN or serum creatinine especially in volume or salt depleted patients or those with renovascular hypertension may occur. Rapid reduction of longstanding or markedly elevated blood pressure can result in decreases in the glomerular filtration rate and, in turn, lead to increases in BUN or serum creatinine.
Hematologic: A positive ANA has been reported.
Liver Function Tests: Elevations of liver transaminases, alkaline phosphatase, and serum bilirubin have occurred.

OVERDOSAGE

Correction of hypotension would be of primary concern. Volume expansion with an intravenous infusion of normal saline is the treatment of choice for restoration of blood pressure.
While captopril may be removed from the adult circulation by hemodialysis, there is inadequate data concerning the effectiveness of hemodialysis for removing it from the circulation of neonates or children. Peritoneal dialysis is not effective for removing captopril; there is no information concerning exchange transfusion for removing captopril from the general circulation.

DOSAGE AND ADMINISTRATION

Captopril should be taken one hour before meals. Dosage must be individualized.
Hypertension: Initiation of therapy requires consideration of recent antihypertensive drug treatment, the extent of blood pressure elevation, salt restriction, and other clinical circumstances. If possible, discontinue the patient's previous antihypertensive drug regimen for one week before starting captopril.
The initial dose of captopril is 25 mg bid or tid. If satisfactory reduction of blood pressure has not been achieved after one or two weeks, the dose may be increased to 50 mg bid or tid. Concomitant sodium restriction may be beneficial when captopril is used alone.
The dose of captopril in hypertension usually does not exceed 50 mg tid. Therefore, if the blood pressure has not been satisfactorily controlled after one to two weeks at this dose, (and the patient is not already receiving a diuretic), a modest dose of a thiazide-type diuretic (e.g., hydrochlorothiazide, 25 mg daily), should be added. The diuretic dose may be increased at one- to two-week intervals until its highest usual antihypertensive dose is reached.
If captopril is being started in a patient already receiving a diuretic, captopril therapy should be initiated under close medical supervision (see WARNINGS and PRECAUTIONS [Drug Interactions] regarding hypotension), with dosage and titration of captopril as noted above.
If further blood pressure reduction is required, the dose of captopril may be increased to 100 mg bid or tid and then, if necessary, to 150 mg bid or tid (while continuing the diuretic). The usual dose range is 25 to 150 mg bid or tid. A maximum daily dose of 450 mg captopril should not be exceeded.
For patients with severe hypertension (e.g., accelerated or malignant hypertension), when temporary discontinuation of current antihypertensive therapy is not practical or desirable, or when prompt titration to more normotensive blood pressure levels is indicated, diuretic should be continued but other current antihypertensive medication stopped and captopril dosage promptly initiated at 25 mg bid or tid, under close medical supervision.
When necessitated by the patient's clinical condition, the daily dose of captopril may be increased every 24 hours or less under continuous medical supervision until a satisfactory blood pressure response is obtained or the maximum dose of captopril is reached. In this regimen, addition of a more potent diuretic, e.g., furosemide, may also be indicated.
Beta-blockers may also be used in conjunction with captopril therapy (see PRECAUTIONS: Drug Interactions), but the effects of the two drugs are less than additive.
Heart Failure: Initiation of therapy requires consideration of recent diuretic therapy and the possibility of severe salt/volume depletion. In patients with either normal or low blood pressure, who have been vigorously treated with diuretics and who may be hyponatremic and/or hypovolemic, a starting dose of 6.25 or 12.5 mg tid may minimize the magnitude or duration of the hypotensive effect (see WARNINGS: Hypotension); for these patients, titration to the usual daily dosage can then occur within the next several days.
For most patients the usual initial daily dosage is 25 mg tid. After a dose of 50 mg tid is reached, further increases in dosage should be delayed, where possible, for at least two weeks to determine if a satisfactory response occurs. Most patients studied have had a satisfactory clinical improvement at 50 or 100 mg tid. A maximum daily dose of 450 mg of captopril should not be exceeded.
Captopril should generally be used in conjunction with a diuretic and digitalis. Captopril therapy must be initiated under very close medical supervision.
Left Ventricular Dysfunction After Myocardial Infarction: The recommended dose for long-term use in patients following a myocardial infarction is a target maintenance dose of 50 mg tid.
Therapy may be initiated as early as three days following a myocardial infarction. After a single dose of 6.25 mg, captopril therapy should be initiated at 12.5 mg tid. Captopril should then be increased to 25 mg tid during the next several days and to a target dose of 50 mg tid over the next several weeks as tolerated (see CLINICAL PHARMACOLOGY).
Captopril may be used in patients treated with other post-myocardial infarction therapies, e.g., thrombolytics, aspirin, beta-blockers.
Dosage Adjustment in Renal Impairment: Because captopril is excreted primarily by the kidneys, excretion rates are reduced in patients with impaired renal function. These patients will take longer to reach steady-state captopril levels and will reach higher steady-state levels for a given daily dose than patients with normal renal function. Therefore, these patients may respond to smaller or less frequent doses.
Accordingly, for patients with significant renal impairment, initial daily dosage of captopril should be reduced, and smaller increments utilized for titration, which should be quite slow (one- to two-week intervals). After the desired therapeutic effect has been achieved, the dose should be slowly back-titrated to determine the minimal effective dose. When concomitant diuretic therapy is required, a loop diuretic (e.g., furosemide), rather than a thiazide diuretic, is preferred in patients with severe renal impairment. (See WARNINGS: Anaphylactoid Reactions During Membrane Exposure and PRECAUTIONS: Hemodialysis.)

HOW SUPPLIED

Captopril tablets, USP are available containing 12.5 mg, 25 mg, 50 mg or 100 mg of captopril.
The 12.5 mg tablets are white, partially scored (both sides), oval tablets marked with **M** to the left of the score and **C1** to the right of the score on one side. They are available as follows:

NDC 0378-3007-01
bottles of 100 tablets
NDC 0378-3007-10
bottles of 1000 tablets

The 25 mg tablets are white, quadrisect scored, round tablets marked with **M** over **C2** on the non-scored side. They are available as follows:

NDC 0378-3012-01
bottles of 100 tablets
NDC 0378-3012-10
bottles of 1000 tablets

The 50 mg tablets are white, scored, round tablets marked with **M** over **C3** on the scored side. They are available as follows:

NDC 0378-3017-01
bottles of 100 tablets
NDC 0378-3017-10
bottles of 1000 tablets

The 100 mg tablets are white, scored, round tablets marked with **M** over **C4** on the scored side. They are available as follows:

NDC 0378-3022-01
bottles of 100 tablets

Captopril tablets, USP may exhibit a slight sulfurous odor. Bottles contain a desiccant-charcoal canister.
STORE AT CONTROLLED ROOM TEMPERATURE 15°–30°C (59°–86°F).
PROTECT FROM MOISTURE.
Dispense in a tight container using a child-resistant closure.
Mylan Pharmaceuticals Inc.
Morgantown, WV 26505

REVISED SEPTEMBER 1999
CAPT:R8

FUROSEMIDE TABLETS, USP 20 mg, 40 mg and 80 mg ℞

WARNING: Furosemide is a potent diuretic which, if given in excessive amounts, can lead to a profound diuresis with water and electrolyte depletion. Therefore, careful medical supervision is required, and dose and dose schedule must be adjusted to the individual patient's needs. (See "DOSAGE AND ADMINISTRATION".)

DESCRIPTION

Furosemide is a diuretic which is an anthranilic acid derivative. Chemically, it is 4-chloro-*N*-furfuryl-5-sulfamoylanthranilic acid. Furosemide is a white to slightly yellow odorless, crystalline powder. It is practically insoluble in water, sparingly soluble in alcohol, freely soluble in dilute alkali solutions and insoluble in dilute acids.
The structural formula is as follows:

COOH, NHCH₂, O, H_2NS, O, O, Cl

$C_{12}H_{11}ClN_2O_5S$
M.W. 330.75

Each tablet for oral administration contains 20 mg, 40 mg or 80 mg of furosemide and the following inactive ingredients: colloidal silicon dioxide, lactose monohydrate, microcrystalline cellulose, pregelatinized starch and stearic acid. Furosemide Tablets, USP 20 mg, 40 mg and 80 mg meet *USP DISSOLUTION TEST 1.*

CLINICAL PHARMACOLOGY

Investigations into the mode of action of furosemide have utilized micropuncture studies in rats, stop flow experiments in dogs, and various clearance studies in both humans and experimental animals. It has been demonstrated that furosemide inhibits primarily the reabsorption of sodium and chloride not only in the proximal and distal tubules but also in the loop of Henle. The high degree of efficacy is largely due to this unique site of action. The action on the distal tubule is independent of any inhibitory effect on carbonic anhydrase and aldosterone.
Recent evidence suggests that furosemide glucuronide is the only or at least the major biotransformation product of furosemide in man. Furosemide is extensively bound to plasma proteins, mainly to albumin. Plasma concentrations ranging from 1 to 400 µg/mL are 91 to 99% bound in healthy individuals. The unbound fraction averages 2.3 to 4.1% at therapeutic concentrations.
The onset of diuresis following oral administration is within one hour. The peak effect occurs within the first or second hour. The duration of diuretic effect is 6 to 8 hours.
In fasted normal men, the mean bioavailability of furosemide from furosemide tablets and furosemide oral solution has been shown to be about 60% of that from an intravenous injection of the drug. Although furosemide is more rapidly absorbed from the oral solution than from the tablet, peak plasma levels and area under the plasma concentration-time curves do not differ significantly. Peak plasma concentrations of furosemide increase with increasing dose but times-to-peak do not differ among doses. The terminal half-life of furosemide is approximately 2 hours.
Significantly more furosemide is excreted in urine following the IV injection than after the tablet or oral solution. There are no significant differences between the two oral formulations in the amount of unchanged drug excreted in urine.

INDICATIONS AND USAGE

Edema: Furosemide is indicated in adults, infants, and children for the treatment of edema associated with congestive heart failure, cirrhosis of the liver, and renal disease, including the nephrotic syndrome. Furosemide is particularly useful when an agent with greater diuretic potential is desired.
Hypertension: Oral furosemide may be used in adults for the treatment of hypertension alone or in combination with other antihypertensive agents. Hypertensive patients who cannot be adequately controlled with thiazides will probably also not be adequately controlled with furosemide alone.

CONTRAINDICATIONS

Furosemide is contraindicated in patients with anuria and in patients with a history of hypersensitivity to furosemide.

WARNINGS

In patients with hepatic cirrhosis and ascites, furosemide therapy is best initiated in the hospital. In hepatic coma and in states of electrolyte depletion, therapy should not be instituted until the basic condition is improved. Sudden alteration of fluid and electrolyte balance in patients with cirrhosis may precipitate hepatic coma; therefore, strict observation is necessary during the period of diuresis. Supplemental potassium chloride and, if required, an aldosterone antagonist are helpful in preventing hypokalemia and metabolic alkalosis.
If increasing azotemia and oliguria occur during treatment of severe progressive renal disease, furosemide should be discontinued.
Cases of tinnitus and reversible or irreversible hearing impairment have been reported. Usually, reports indicate that furosemide ototoxicity is associated with rapid injection, severe renal impairment, doses exceeding several times the usual recommended dose, or concomitant therapy with aminoglycoside antibiotics, ethacrynic acid, or other ototoxic drugs. If the physician elects to use high dose parenteral therapy, controlled intravenous infusion is advisable (for adults, an infusion rate not exceeding 4 mg furosemide per minute has been used).

PRECAUTIONS

General: Excessive diuresis may cause dehydration and blood volume reduction with circulatory collapse and possible vascular thrombosis and embolism, particularly in elderly patients. As with any effective diuretic, electrolyte depletion may occur during furosemide therapy, especially in patients receiving higher doses and a restricted salt intake. Hypokalemia may develop with furosemide, especially with brisk diuresis, inadequate oral electrolyte intake, when cirrhosis is present or during concomitant use of corticosteroids or ACTH. Digitalis therapy may exaggerate metabolic effects of hypokalemia, especially myocardial effects.
All patients receiving furosemide therapy should be observed for these signs or symptoms of fluid or electrolyte imbalance (hyponatremia, hypochloremic alkalosis, hypokalemia, hypomagnesemia or hypocalcemia): dryness of mouth, thirst, weakness, lethargy, drowsiness, restlessness, muscle pains or cramps, muscular fatigue, hypotension, oliguria, tachycardia, arrhythmia, or gastrointestinal disturbances such as nausea and vomiting.

Increases in blood glucose and alterations in glucose tolerance tests (with abnormalities of the fasting and 2-hour postprandial sugar) have been observed, and rarely, precipitation of diabetes mellitus has been reported.
Asymptomatic hyperuricemia can occur and gout may rarely be precipitated.
Patients allergic to sulfonamides may also be allergic to furosemide.
The possibility exists of exacerbation or activation of systemic lupus erythematosus.
As with many other drugs, patients should be observed regularly for the possible occurrence of blood dyscrasias, liver or kidney damage or other idiosyncratic reactions.
Information for Patients: Patients receiving furosemide should be advised that they may experience symptoms from excessive fluid and/or electrolyte losses. The postural hypotension that sometimes occurs can usually be managed by getting up slowly. Potassium supplements and/or dietary measures may be needed to control or avoid hypokalemia.
Patients with diabetes mellitus should be told that furosemide may increase blood glucose levels and thereby affect urine glucose tests. The skin of some patients may be more sensitive to the effects of sunlight while taking furosemide.
Hypertensive patients should avoid medications that may increase blood pressure, including over-the-counter products for appetite suppression and cold symptoms.
Laboratory Tests: Serum electrolytes, (particularly potassium), CO_2, creatinine and BUN should be determined frequently during the first few months of furosemide therapy and periodically thereafter. Serum and urine electrolyte determinations are particularly important when the patient is vomiting profusely or receiving parenteral fluids. Abnormalities should be corrected or the drug temporarily withdrawn. Other medications may also influence serum electrolytes.
Reversible elevations of BUN may occur and are associated with dehydration which should be avoided, particularly in patients with renal insufficiency.
Urine and blood glucose should be checked periodically in diabetics receiving furosemide, even in those suspected of latent diabetes.
Furosemide may lower serum levels of calcium (rarely cases of tetany have been reported) and magnesium. Accordingly, serum levels of these electrolytes should be determined periodically.
Drug Interactions: Furosemide may increase the ototoxic potential of aminoglycoside antibiotics, especially in the presence of impaired renal function. Except in life threatening situations, avoid this combination.
Furosemide should not be used concomitantly with ethacrynic acid because of the possibility of ototoxicity.
Patients receiving high doses of salicylates concomitantly with furosemide, as in rheumatic disease, may experience salicylate toxicity at lower doses because of competitive renal excretory sites.
Furosemide has a tendency to antagonize the skeletal muscle relaxing effects of tubocurarine and may potentiate the action of succinylcholine.
Lithium generally should not be given with diuretics because they reduce lithium's renal clearance and add a high risk of lithium toxicity.
Furosemide may add to or potentiate the therapeutic effect of other antihypertensive drugs. Potentiation occurs with ganglionic or peripheral adrenergic blocking drugs.
Furosemide may decrease arterial responsiveness to norepinephrine. However, norepinephrine may still be used effectively.
Simultaneous administration of sucralfate and furosemide tablets may reduce the natriuretic and antihypertensive effects of furosemide. Patients receiving both drugs should be observed closely to determine if the desired diuretic and/or antihypertensive effect of furosemide is achieved. The intake of furosemide and sucralfate should be separated by at least two hours.
One study in six subjects demonstrated that the combination of furosemide and acetylsalicylic acid temporarily reduced creatinine clearance in patients with chronic renal insufficiency. There are case reports of patients who developed increased BUN, serum creatinine and serum potassium levels, and weight gain when furosemide was used in conjunction with NSAIDs.
Literature reports indicate that coadministration of indomethacin may reduce the natriuretic and antihypertensive effects of furosemide in some patients by inhibiting prostaglandin synthesis. Indomethacin may also affect plasma renin levels, aldosterone excretion and renin profile evaluation. Patients receiving both indomethacin and furosemide should be observed closely to determine if the desired diuretic and/or antihypertensive effect of furosemide is achieved.
Carcinogenesis, Mutagenesis, Impairment of Fertility: Furosemide was tested for carcinogenicity by oral administration in one strain of mice and one strain of rats. A small but significantly increased incidence of mammary gland carcinomas occurred in female mice at a dose 17.5 times the maximum human dose of 600 mg. There were marginal increases in uncommon tumors in male rats at a dose of 15 mg/kg (slightly greater than the maximum human dose) but not at 30 mg/kg.
Furosemide was devoid of mutagenic activity in various strains of *Salmonella typhimurium* when tested in the presence or absence of an *in vitro* metabolic activation system, and questionably positive for gene mutation in mouse lymphoma cells in the presence of rat liver S9 at the highest dose tested. Furosemide did not induce sister chromatid exchange in human cells *in vitro*, but other studies on chromosomal aberrations in human cells *in vitro* gave conflicting results. In Chinese hamster cells it induced chromosomal damage but was questionably positive for sister chromatid exchange. Studies on the induction by furosemide of chromosomal aberrations in mice were inconclusive. The urine of rats treated with this drug did not induce gene conversion in *Saccharomyces cerevisiae*.
Furosemide produced no impairment of fertility in male or female rats at 100 mg/kg/day (the maximum effective diuretic dose in the rat and 8 times the maximal human dose of 600 mg/day).
Pregnancy: *Teratogenic Effects. Pregnancy Category C:* Furosemide has been shown to cause unexplained maternal deaths and abortions in rabbits at 2, 4 and 8 times the maximal recommended human dose. There are no adequate and well-controlled studies in pregnant women. Furosemide should be used during pregnancy only if the potential benefit justifies the potential risk to the fetus.
The effects of furosemide on embryonic and fetal development and on pregnant dams were studied in mice, rats, and rabbits.
Furosemide caused unexplained maternal deaths and abortions in the rabbit at the lowest dose of 25 mg/kg (two times the maximal recommended human dose of 600 mg/day). In another study, a dose of 50 mg/kg (four times the maximal recommended human dose of 600 mg/day) also caused maternal deaths and abortions when administered to rabbits between Days 12 and 17 of gestation. In a third study, none of the pregnant rabbits survived a dose of 100 mg/kg. Data from the above studies indicate fetal lethality that can precede maternal deaths.
The results of the mouse study and one of the three rabbit studies also showed an increased incidence and severity of hydronephrosis (distention of the renal pelvis and in some cases of the ureters) in fetuses derived from the treated dams as compared with the incidence in fetuses from the control group.
Nursing Mothers: Because it appears in breast milk, caution should be exercised when furosemide is administered to a nursing mother.

ADVERSE REACTIONS

Adverse reactions are categorized below by organ system and listed by decreasing severity.

Gastrointestinal System Reactions

1. pancreatitis
2. jaundice (intrahepatic cholestatic jaundice)
3. anorexia
4. oral and gastric irritation
5. cramping
6. diarrhea
7. constipation
8. nausea
9. vomiting

Systemic Hypersensitivity Reactions

1. systemic vasculitis
2. interstitial nephritis
3. necrotizing angiitis

Central Nervous System Reactions

1. tinnitus and hearing loss
2. paresthesias
3. vertigo
4. dizziness
5. headache
6. blurred vision
7. xanthopsia

Hematologic Reactions

1. aplastic anemia (rare)
2. thrombocytopenia
3. agranulocytosis (rare)
4. hemolytic anemia
5. leukopenia
6. anemia

Dermatologic-Hypersensitivity Reactions

1. exfoliative dermatitis
2. erythema multiforme
3. purpura
4. photosensitivity
5. urticaria
6. rash
7. pruritus

Cardiovascular Reaction

Orthostatic hypotension may occur and may be aggravated by alcohol, barbiturates, or narcotics.

Other Reactions

1. hyperglycemia
2. glycosuria
3. hyperuricemia
4. muscle spasm
5. weakness
6. restlessness
7. urinary bladder spasm
8. thrombophlebitis
9. fever

Whenever adverse reactions are moderate or severe, furosemide dosage should be reduced or therapy withdrawn.

OVERDOSAGE

The principal signs and symptoms of overdosage with furosemide are dehydration, blood volume reduction, hypotension, electrolyte imbalance, hypokalemia and hypochloremic alkalosis, and are extensions of its diuretic action.
The acute toxicity of furosemide has been determined in mice, rats, and dogs. In all three, the oral LD_{50} exceeded 1000 mg/kg body weight while the intravenous LD_{50} ranged from 300 to 680 mg/kg. The acute intragastric toxicity in neonatal rats is 7 to 10 times that of adult rats.
The concentration of furosemide in biological fluid associated with toxicity or death is not known.
Treatment of overdosage is supportive and consists of replacement of excessive fluid and electrolyte losses. Serum electrolytes, carbon dioxide level and blood pressure should be determined frequently. Adequate drainage must be assured in patients with urinary bladder outlet obstruction (such as prostatic hypertrophy).
Hemodialysis does not accelerate furosemide elimination.

DOSAGE AND ADMINISTRATION

Edema: Therapy should be individualized according to patient response to gain maximal therapeutic response and to determine the minimal dose needed to maintain that response.
Adults: The usual initial dose of furosemide is 20 to 80 mg given as a single dose. Ordinarily a prompt diuresis ensues. If needed, the same dose can be administered 6 to 8 hours later or the dose may be increased. The dose may be raised by 20 to 40 mg and given not sooner than 6 to 8 hours after the previous dose until the desired diuretic effect has been obtained. This individually determined single dose should then be given once or twice daily (e.g., at 8 am and 2 pm). The dose of furosemide may be carefully titrated up to 600 mg/day in patients with clinically severe edematous states.
Edema may be most efficiently and safely mobilized by giving furosemide on 2 to 4 consecutive days each week.
When doses exceeding 80 mg/day are given for prolonged periods, careful clinical observation and laboratory monitoring are particularly advisable. (See PRECAUTIONS: Laboratory Tests.)
Infants and Children: The usual initial dose of oral furosemide in infants and children is 2 mg/kg body weight, given as a single dose. If the diuretic response is not satisfactory after the initial dose, dosage may be increased by 1 or 2 mg/kg no sooner than 6 to 8 hours after the previous dose. Doses greater than 6 mg/kg body weight are not recommended. For maintenance therapy in infants and children, the dose should be adjusted to the minimum effective level. For ease of administration, and to allow maximum flexibility in dosing, the use of Furosemide Oral Solution is suggested.
Hypertension: Therapy should be individualized according to the patient's response to gain maximal therapeutic response and to determine the minimal dose needed to maintain that therapeutic response.
Adults: The usual initial dose of furosemide for hypertension is 80 mg, usually divided into 40 mg twice a day. Dosage should then be adjusted according to response. If response is not satisfactory, add other antihypertensive agents.
Changes in blood pressure must be carefully monitored when furosemide is used with other antihypertensive drugs, especially during initial therapy. To prevent excessive drop in blood pressure, the dosage of other agents should be reduced by at least 50 percent when furosemide is added to the regimen. As the blood pressure falls under the potentiating effect of furosemide, a further reduction in dosage or even discontinuation of other antihypertensive drugs may be necessary.

HOW SUPPLIED

The 20 mg tablets are white, round, unscored, flat-bevel-edged tablets debossed with **M2**. They are available as follows:

NDC 0378-0208-01
bottles of 100 tablets
NDC 0378-0208-10
bottles of 1000 tablets

The 40 mg tablets are white, round, scored, flat-bevel-edged tablets debossed with **MYLAN** over **216** on one side and **40** on the other side. They are available as follows:

NDC 0378-0216-01
bottles of 100 tablets
NDC 0378-0216-10
bottles of 1000 tablets

The 80 mg tablets are white, round, scored, flat-bevel-edged tablets debossed with **MYLAN** over **232** on one side and **80** on the other side. They are available as follows:

NDC 0378-0232-01
bottles of 100 tablets
NDC 0378-0232-05
bottles of 500 tablets

STORE AT CONTROLLED ROOM TEMPERATURE 15°–30°C (59°–86°F).

PROTECT FROM LIGHT.

Dispense in a tight, light-resistant container using a child-resistant closure. Exposure to light may cause slight discoloration. Discolored tablets should not be dispensed.

Continued on next page

Furosemide—Cont.

MYLAN®
Mylan Pharmaceuticals Inc.
Morgantown, WV 26505

REVISED OCTOBER 2002
FUR:R25

INDAPAMIDE TABLETS, USP ℞
1.25 mg and 2.5 mg

DESCRIPTION

Indapamide is an oral antihypertensive/diuretic. Its molecule contains both a polar sulfamoyl chlorobenzamide moiety and a lipid-soluble methylindoline moiety. It differs chemically from the thiazides in that it does not possess the thiazide ring system and contains only one sulfonamide group. The chemical name of indapamide is 4-Chloro-N-(2-methyl-1-indolinyl)-3- Sulfamoylbenzamide, and its molecular weight is 365.84. The compound is a weak acid, pK_a=8.8, and is soluble in aqueous solutions of strong bases. It is a white to yellow-white crystalline (tetragonal) powder.

H_3C Cl— —CO—NH—N SO_2NH_2

$C_{16}H_{16}ClN_3O_3S$

Each tablet, for oral administration, contains 1.25 mg or 2.5 mg of indapamide and the following inactive ingredients: anhydrous lactose, colloidal silicon dioxide, hypromellose, magnesium stearate, microcrystalline cellulose, polydextrose, polyethylene glycol, pregelatinized starch, sodium lauryl sulfate, and titanium dioxide. Additionally, the 1.25 mg product contains glyceryl triacetate and D&C Red No. 30 Aluminum Lake and the 2.5 mg product contains triacetin.

CLINICAL PHARMACOLOGY

Indapamide is the first of a new class of antihypertensive/diuretics, the indolines. It has been reported that the oral administration of 2.5 mg (two 1.25 mg tablets) of indapamide to male subjects produced peak concentrations of approximately 115 ng/mL of the drug in the blood within two hours. It has been reported that the oral administration of 5 mg (two 2.5 mg tablets) of indapamide to healthy male subjects produced peak concentrations of approximately 260 ng/mL of the drug in the blood within two hours. A minimum of 70% of a single oral dose is eliminated by the kidneys and an additional 23% by the gastrointestinal tract, probably including the biliary route. The half-life of indapamide in whole blood is approximately 14 hours.

Indapamide is preferentially and reversibly taken up by the erythrocytes in the peripheral blood. The whole blood/plasma ratio is approximately 6:1 at the time of peak concentration and decreases to 3.5:1 at eight hours. From 71 to 79% of the indapamide in plasma is reversibly bound to plasma proteins.

Indapamide is an extensively metabolized drug, with only about 7% of the total dose administered, recovered in the urine as unchanged drug during the first 48 hours after administration. The urinary elimination of ^{14}C-labeled indapamide and metabolites is biphasic with a terminal half-life of excretion of total radioactivity of 26 hours.

In a parallel design double-blind, placebo controlled trial in hypertension, daily doses of indapamide between 1.25 mg and 10 mg produced dose-related antihypertensive effects. Doses of 5 and 10 mg were not distinguishable from each other although each was differentiated from placebo and 1.25 mg indapamide. At daily doses of 1.25 mg, 5 mg and 10 mg, a mean decrease of serum potassium of 0.28, 0.61 and 0.76 mEq/L, respectively, was observed and uric acid increased by about 0.69 mg/100 mL.

In other parallel design, dose-ranging clinical trials in hypertension and edema, daily doses of indapamide between 0.5 and 5 mg produced dose-related effects. Generally, doses of 2.5 and 5 mg were not distinguishable from each other although each was differentiated from placebo and from 0.5 or 1 mg indapamide. At daily doses of 2.5 and 5 mg a mean decrease of serum potassium of 0.5 and 0.6 mEq/Liter, respectively, was observed and uric acid increased by about 1 mg/100 mL.

At these doses, the effects of indapamide on blood pressure and edema are approximately equal to those obtained with conventional doses of other antihypertensive/diuretics.

In hypertensive patients, daily doses of 1.25, 2.5 and 5 mg of indapamide have no appreciable cardiac inotropic or chronotropic effect. The drug decreases peripheral resistance, with little or no effect on cardiac output, rate or rhythm. Chronic administration of indapamide to hypertensive patients has little or no effect on glomerular filtration rate or renal plasma flow.

Indapamide had an antihypertensive effect in patients with varying degrees of renal impairment, although in general, diuretic effects declined as renal function decreased.

In a small number of controlled studies, indapamide taken with other antihypertensive drugs such as hydralazine, propranolol, guanethidine and methyldopa, appeared to have the additive effect typical of thiazide-type diuretics.

TABLE 1: Adverse Reactions from Studies of 1.25 mg

Incidence ≥ 5%	Incidence < 5%*
BODY AS A WHOLE	
Headache	Asthenia
Infection	Flu Syndrome
Pain	Abdominal Pain
Back Pain	Chest Pain
GASTROINTESTINAL SYSTEM	
	Constipation
	Diarrhea
	Dyspepsia
	Nausea
METABOLIC SYSTEM	
	Peripheral Edema
CENTRAL NERVOUS SYSTEM	
Dizziness	Nervousness
	Hypertonia
RESPIRATORY SYSTEM	
Rhinitis	Cough
	Pharyngitis
	Sinusitis
SPECIAL SENSES	
	Conjunctivitis

*OTHER
All other clinical adverse reactions occurred at an incidence of < 1%.

INDICATIONS AND USAGE

Indapamide tablets are indicated for the treatment of hypertension, alone or in combination with other antihypertensive drugs.

Indapamide tablets are also indicated for the treatment of salt and fluid retention associated with congestive heart failure.

Usage in Pregnancy: The routine use of diuretics in an otherwise healthy woman is inappropriate and exposes mother and fetus to unnecessary hazard (see PRECAUTIONS below).

Diuretics do not prevent development of toxemia of pregnancy, and there is no satisfactory evidence that they are useful in the treatment of developed toxemia.

Edema during pregnancy may arise from pathological causes or from the physiologic and mechanical consequences of pregnancy. Indapamide is indicated in pregnancy when edema is due to pathologic causes, just as it is in the absence of pregnancy (however, see PRECAUTIONS below). Dependent edema in pregnancy, resulting from restriction of venous return by the expanded uterus, is properly treated through elevation of the lower extremities and use of support hose; use of diuretics to lower intravascular volume in this case is illogical and unnecessary. There is hypervolemia during normal pregnancy which is not harmful to either the fetus or the mother (in the absence of cardiovascular disease), but which is associated with edema, including generalized edema in the majority of pregnant women. If this edema produces discomfort, increased recumbency will often provide relief. In rare instances, this edema may cause extreme discomfort which is not relieved by rest. In these cases, a short course of diuretics may provide relief and may be appropriate.

CONTRAINDICATIONS

Anuria. Known hypersensitivity to indapamide or to other sulfonamide-derived drugs.

WARNINGS

Severe cases of hyponatremia, accompanied by hypokalemia, have been reported with recommended doses of indapamide. This occurred primarily in elderly females. This appears to be dose-related. Also a large case-controlled pharmacoepidemiology study indicates that there is an increased risk of hyponatremia with indapamide 2.5 mg and 5 mg doses. Hyponatremia considered possibly clinically significant (less than 125 mEq/L) has not been observed in clinical trials with the 1.25 mg dosage (see PRECAUTIONS). Thus patients should be started at the 1.25 mg dose and maintained at the lowest possible dose. (See DOSAGE AND ADMINISTRATION.)

Hypokalemia occurs commonly with diuretics (see ADVERSE REACTIONS, Hypokalemia), and electrolyte monitoring is essential, particularly in patients who would be at increased risk from hypokalemia, such as those with cardiac arrhythmias or who are receiving concomitant cardiac glycosides.

In general, diuretics should not be given concomitantly with lithium because they reduce its renal clearance and add a high risk of lithium toxicity. Read prescribing information for lithium preparations before use of such concomitant therapy.

PRECAUTIONS

General: ***1. Hypokalemia, Hyponatremia, and Other Fluid and Electrolyte Imbalances:*** Periodic determinations of serum electrolytes should be performed at appropriate intervals. In addition, patients should be observed for clinical signs of fluid or electrolyte imbalance, such as hyponatremia, hypochloremic alkalosis, or hypokalemia. Warning signs include dry mouth, thirst, weakness, fatigue, lethargy, drowsiness, restlessness, muscle pains or cramps, hypotension, oliguria, tachycardia, and gastrointestinal disturbance. Electrolyte determinations are particularly important in patients who are vomiting excessively or receiving parenteral fluids, in patients subject to electrolyte imbalance (including those with heart failure, kidney disease, and cirrhosis), and in patients on a salt-restricted diet.

The risk of hypokalemia secondary to diuresis and natriuresis is increased when larger doses are used, when the diuresis is brisk, when severe cirrhosis is present and during concomitant use of corticosteroids or ACTH. Interference with adequate oral intake of electrolytes will also contribute to hypokalemia. Hypokalemia can sensitize or exaggerate the response of the heart to the toxic effects of digitalis, such as increase ventricular irritability.

Dilutional hyponatremia may occur in edematous patients; the appropriate treatment is restriction of water rather than administration of salt, except in rare instances when the hyponatremia is life threatening. However, in actual salt depletion, appropriate replacement is the treatment of choice. Any chloride deficit that may occur during treatment is generally mild and usually does not require specific treatment except in extraordinary circumstances as in liver or renal disease. Thiazide-like diuretics have been shown to increase the urinary excretion of magnesium; this may result in hypomagnesemia.

2. Hyperuricemia and Gout: Serum concentrations of uric acid increased by an average of 0.69 mg/100 mL in patients treated with indapamide 1.25 mg, and by an average of 1 mg/100 mL in patients treated with indapamide 2.5 mg and 5 mg, and frank gout may be precipitated in certain patients receiving indapamide (see ADVERSE REACTIONS below). Serum concentrations of uric acid should, therefore, be monitored periodically during treatment.

3. Renal Impairment: Indapamide, like the thiazides, should be used with caution in patients with severe renal disease, as reduced plasma volume may exacerbate or precipitate azotemia. If progressive renal impairment is observed in a patient receiving indapamide, withholding or discontinuing diuretic therapy should be considered. Renal function tests should be performed periodically during treatment with indapamide.

4. Impaired Hepatic Function: Indapamide, like the thiazides, should be used with caution in patients with impaired hepatic function or progressive liver disease, since minor alterations of fluid and electrolyte balance may precipitate hepatic coma.

5. Glucose Tolerance: Latent diabetes may become manifest and insulin requirements in diabetic patients may be altered during thiazide administration. A mean increase in glucose of 6.47 mg/dL was observed in patients treated with indapamide 1.25 mg, which was not considered clinically significant in these trials. Serum concentrations of glucose should be monitored routinely during treatment with indapamide.

6. Calcium Excretion: Calcium excretion is decreased by diuretics pharmacologically related to indapamide. After six to eight weeks of indapamide 1.25 mg treatment and in long-term studies of hypertensive patients, with higher doses of indapamide, however, serum concentrations of calcium increased only slightly with indapamide. Prolonged treatment with drugs pharmacologically related to indapamide may in rare instances be associated with hypercalcemia and hypophosphatemia secondary to physiologic changes in the parathyroid gland; however, the common complications of hyperparathyroidism, such as renal lithiasis, bone resorption, and peptic ulcer, have not been seen. Treatment should be discontinued before tests for parathyroid function are performed. Like the thiazides, indapamide may decrease serum PBI levels without signs of thyroid disturbance.

7. Interaction with Systemic Lupus Erythematosus: Thiazides have exacerbated or activated systemic lupus erythematosus and this possibility should be considered with indapamide as well.

Drug Interactions:

1. Other Antihypertensives: Indapamide may add to or potentiate the action of other antihypertensive drugs. In limited controlled trials that compared the effect of indapamide combined with other antihypertensive drugs with the effect of the other drugs administered alone, there was no notable change in the nature or frequency of adverse reactions associated with the combined therapy.

2. Lithium: See WARNINGS.

3. Post-Sympathectomy Patient: The antihypertensive effect of the drug may be enhanced in the postsympathectomized patient.
4. Norepinephrine: Indapamide, like the thiazides, may decrease arterial responsiveness to norepinephrine; but this diminution is not sufficient to preclude effectiveness of the pressor agent for the therapeutic use.
Carcinogenesis, Mutagenesis, Impairment of Fertility: Both mouse and rat lifetime carcinogenicity studies were conducted. There was no significant difference in the incidence of tumors between the indapamide-treated animals and the control groups.
Pregnancy: *Teratogenic Effects.* Pregnancy Category B: Reproduction studies have been performed in rats, mice and rabbits at doses up to 6,250 times the therapeutic human dose and have revealed no evidence of impaired fertility or harm to the fetus due to indapamide. Postnatal development in rats and mice was unaffected by pretreatment of parent animals during gestation. There are, however, no adequate and well-controlled studies in pregnant women. Moreover, diuretics are known to cross the placental barrier and appear in cord blood. Because animal reproduction studies are not always predictive of human response, this drug should be used during pregnancy only if clearly needed. There may be hazards associated with this use such as fetal or neonatal jaundice, thrombocytopenia, and possibly other adverse reactions that have occurred in the adult.
Nursing Mothers: It is not known whether this drug is excreted in human milk. Because most drugs are excreted in human milk, if use of this drug is deemed essential, the patient should stop nursing.
Pediatric Use: Safety and effectiveness of indapamide in pediatric patients have not been established.

ADVERSE REACTIONS

Most adverse effects have been mild and transient.
The clinical adverse reactions listed in Table 1 represent data from Phase II/III placebo-controlled studies (306 patients given indapamide 1.25 mg). The clinical adverse reactions listed in Table 2 represent data from Phase II placebo-controlled studies and long-term controlled clinical trials (426 patients given indapamide 2.5 mg or 5 mg). The reactions are arranged into two groups: 1) a cumulative incidence equal to or greater than 5%; 2) a cumulative incidence less than 5%. Reactions are counted regardless of relation to drug.
[See table 1 at top of previous page]
Approximately 4% of patients given indapamide 1.25 mg compared to 5% of the patients given placebo discontinued treatment in the trials of up to eight weeks because of adverse reactions.
In controlled clinical trials of six to eight weeks in duration, 20% of patients receiving indapamide 1.25 mg, 61% of patients receiving indapamide 5 mg, and 80% of patients receiving indapamide 10 mg had at least one potassium value below 3.4 mEq/L. In the indapamide 1.25 mg group, about 40% of those patients who reported hypokalemia as a laboratory adverse event returned to normal serum potassium values without intervention. Hypokalemia with concomitant clinical signs or symptoms occurred in 2% of patients receiving indapamide 1.25 mg.
[See table 2 above]
Because most of these data are from long-term studies (up to 40 weeks of treatment), it is probable that many of the adverse experiences reported are due to causes other than the drug. Approximately 10% of patients given indapamide discontinued treatment in long-term trials because of reactions either related or unrelated to the drug.
Hypokalemia with concomitant clinical signs or symptoms occurred in 3% of patients receiving indapamide 2.5 mg q.d. and 7% of patients receiving indapamide 5 mg q.d. In long-term controlled clinical trials comparing the hypokalemic effects of daily doses of indapamide and hydrochlorothiazide, however, 47% of patients receiving indapamide 2.5 mg, 72% of patients receiving indapamide 5 mg, and 44% of patients receiving hydrochlorothiazide 50 mg had at least one potassium value (out of a total of 11 taken during the study) below 3.5 mEq/L. In the indapamide 2.5 mg group, over 50% of those patients returned to normal serum potassium values without intervention.
In clinical trials of six to eight weeks, the mean changes in selected values were as shown in the tables below.
[See second table at right]
No patients receiving indapamide 1.25 mg experienced hyponatremia considered possibly clinically significant (< 125 mEq/L).
Indapamide had no adverse effects on lipids.
[See third table at right]
The following reactions have been reported with clinical usage of indapamide: jaundice (intrahepatic cholestatic jaundice), hepatitis, pancreatitis, and abnormal liver function tests. These reactions were reversible with discontinuance of the drug.
Also reported are erythema multiforme, Stevens-Johnson Syndrome, bullous eruptions, purpura, photosensitivity, fever, pneumonitis, anaphylactic reactions, agranulocytosis, leukopenia, thrombocytopenia and aplastic anemia. Other adverse reactions reported with antihypertensive/diuretics are necrotizing angiitis, respiratory distress, sialadenitis, xanthopsia.

OVERDOSAGE

Symptoms of overdosage includes nausea, vomiting, weakness, gastrointestinal disorders and disturbances of electrolyte balance. In severe instances, hypotension and depressed respiration may be observed. If this occurs, support of respiration and cardiac circulation should be instituted. There is no specific antidote. An evacuation of the stomach is recommended by emesis and gastric lavage after which the electrolyte and fluid balance should be evaluated carefully.

TABLE 2: Adverse Reactions from Studies of 2.5 mg and 5 mg

Incidence ≥ 5%	Incidence < 5%
CENTRAL NERVOUS SYSTEM/NEUROMUSCULAR	
Headache	Lightheadedness
Dizziness	Drowsiness
Fatigue, weakness, loss of energy, lethargy, tiredness, or malaise	Vertigo
Muscle cramps or spasm, numbness of the extremities	Insomnia
Nervousness, tension, anxiety, irritability, or agitation	Depression
	Blurred vision
GASTROINTESTINAL SYSTEM	
	Constipation
	Nausea
	Vomiting
	Diarrhea
	Gastric irritation
	Abdominal pain or cramps
	Anorexia
CARDIOVASCULAR SYSTEM	
	Orthostatic hypotension
	Premature ventricular contractions
	Irregular heart beat
	Palpitations
GENITOURINARY SYSTEM	
	Frequency of urination
	Nocturia
	Polyuria
DERMATOLOGIC/HYPERSENSITIVITY	
	Rash
	Hives
	Pruritus
	Vasculitis
OTHER	
	Impotence or reduced libido
	Rhinorrhea
	Flushing
	Hyperuricemia
	Hyperglycemia
	Hyponatremia
	Hypochloremia
	Increase in serum urea nitrogen (BUN) or creatinine
	Glycosuria
	Weight loss
	Dry mouth
	Tingling of extremities

MEAN CHANGES FROM BASELINE AFTER 8 WEEKS OF TREATMENT
1.25 mg

	Serum Electrolytes (mEq/L)			Serum Uric Acid (mg/dL)	BUN (mg/dL)
	Potassium	Sodium	Chloride		
Indapamide 1.25 mg (n=255–257)	−0.28	−0.63	−2.60	0.69	1.46
Placebo (n=263–266)	0.00	−0.11	−0.21	0.06	0.06

MEAN CHANGES FROM BASELINE AFTER 40 WEEKS OF TREATMENT
2.5 mg and 5 mg

	Serum Electrolytes (mEq/L)			Serum Uric Acid (mg/dL)	BUN (mg/dL)
	Potassium	Sodium	Chloride		
Indapamide 2.5 mg (n=76)	−0.4	−0.6	−3.6	0.7	−0.1
Indapamide 5 mg (n=81)	−0.6	−0.7	−5.1	1.1	1.4

DOSAGE AND ADMINISTRATION

Hypertension: The adult starting indapamide dose for hypertension is 1.25 mg as a single daily dose taken in the morning. If the response to 1.25 mg is not satisfactory after four weeks, the daily dose may be increased to 2.5 mg taken once daily. If the response to 2.5 mg is not satisfactory after four weeks, the daily dose may be increased to 5 mg taken once daily, but adding another antihypertensive should be considered.
Edema of Congestive Heart Failure: The adult starting indapamide dose for edema of congestive heart failure is 2.5 mg as a single daily dose taken in the morning. If the response to 2.5 mg is not satisfactory after one week, the daily dose may be increased to 5 mg taken once daily.
If the antihypertensive response to indapamide is insufficient, indapamide may be combined with other antihypertensive drugs, with careful monitoring of blood pressure. It is recommended that the usual dose of other agents be reduced by 50% during initial combination therapy. As the blood pressure response becomes evident, further dosage adjustments may be necessary.
In general, doses of 5 mg and larger have not appeared to provide additional effects on blood pressure or heart failure, but are associated with a greater degree of hypokalemia. There is minimal clinical trial experience in patients with doses greater than 5 mg once a day.

HOW SUPPLIED

Indapamide Tablets, USP are available containing 1.25 mg and 2.5 mg of indapamide.
The 1.25 mg tablets are pink film-coated, unscored, round, biconvex, beveled edge tablets debossed with **M** on one side of the tablet and **69** on the other side. They are available as follows:

NDC 0378-0069-01
bottles of 100 tablets
NDC 0378-0069-05
bottles of 500 tablets

The 2.5 mg tablets are white film-coated, unscored, round, biconvex, beveled edge tablets debossed with **M** on one side of the tablet and **80** on the other side. They are available as follows:

NDC 0378-0080-01
bottles of 100 tablets
NDC 0378-0080-10
bottles of 1000 tablets

STORE AT CONTROLLED ROOM TEMPERATURE 15°–30°C (59°–86°F).

Continued on next page

Indapamide—Cont.

AVOID EXCESSIVE HEAT.
Dispense in a tight container as defined in the USP using a child-resistant closure.
Mylan Pharmaceuticals Inc.
Morgantown, WV 26505

REVISED JULY 2003
INDAP:R5

NADOLOL TABLETS, USP ℞
20 mg, 40 mg and 80 mg

DESCRIPTION

Nadolol is a synthetic nonselective beta-adrenergic receptor blocking agent designated chemically as 1-(*tert*-butylamino)-3-[(5,6,7,8-tetrahydro-*cis*-6,7-dihydroxy-1-naphthyl)oxy]-2-propanol. Its structural formula is:

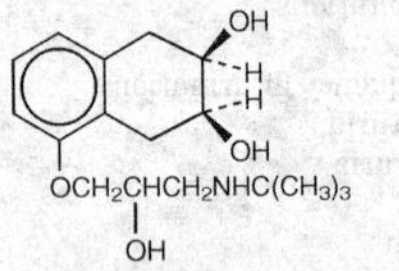

$C_{17}H_{27}NO_4$
M.W. 309.41

Nadolol is a white crystalline powder. It is freely soluble in ethanol, soluble in hydrochloric acid, slightly soluble in water and in chloroform, and very slightly soluble in sodium hydroxide.
Each tablet for oral administration contains 20 mg, 40 mg or 80 mg of nadolol and the following inactive ingredients: croscarmellose sodium, lactose (anhydrous), magnesium stearate, microcrystalline cellulose, sodium lauryl sulfate, and D&C Yellow #10 Aluminum Lake.

CLINICAL PHARMACOLOGY

Nadolol is a nonselective beta-adrenergic receptor blocking agent. Clinical pharmacology studies have demonstrated beta-blocking activity by showing (1) reduction in heart rate and cardiac output at rest and on exercise, (2) reduction of systolic and diastolic blood pressure at rest and on exercise, (3) inhibition of isoproterenol-induced tachycardia, and (4) reduction of reflex orthostatic tachycardia.
Nadolol specifically competes with beta-adrenergic receptor agonists for available beta receptor sites; it inhibits both the $beta_1$ receptors located chiefly in cardiac muscle and the $beta_2$ receptors located chiefly in the bronchial and vascular musculature, inhibiting the chronotropic, inotropic, and vasodilator responses to beta-adrenergic stimulation proportionately. Nadolol has no intrinsic sympathomimetic activity and, unlike some other beta-adrenergic blocking agents, nadolol has little direct myocardial depressant activity and does not have an anesthetic-like membrane-stabilizing action. Animal and human studies show that nadolol slows the sinus rate and depresses AV conduction. In dogs, only minimal amounts of nadolol were detected in the brain relative to amounts in blood and other organs and tissues. Nadolol has low lipophilicity as determined by octanol/water partition coefficient, a characteristic of certain beta-blocking agents that has been correlated with the limited extent to which these agents cross the blood-brain barrier, their low concentration in the brain, and low incidence of CNS-related side effects.
In controlled clinical studies, nadolol at doses of 40 to 320 mg/day has been shown to decrease both standing and supine blood pressure, the effect persisting for approximately 24 hours after dosing.
The mechanism of the antihypertensive effects of beta-adrenergic receptor blocking agents has not been established; however, factors that may be involved include (1) competitive antagonism of catecholamines at peripheral (non-CNS) adrenergic neuron sites (especially cardiac) leading to decreased cardiac output, (2) a central effect leading to reduced tonic-sympathetic nerve outflow to the periphery, and (3) suppression of renin secretion by blockade of the beta-adrenergic receptors responsible for renin release from the kidneys.
While cardiac output and arterial pressure are reduced by nadolol therapy, renal hemodynamics are stable, with preservation of renal blood flow and glomerular filtration rate.
By blocking catecholamine-induced increases in heart rate, velocity and extent of myocardial contraction, and blood pressure, nadolol generally reduces the oxygen requirements of the heart at any given level of effort, making it useful for many patients in the long-term management of angina pectoris. On the other hand, nadolol can increase oxygen requirements by increasing left ventricular fiber length and end diastolic pressure, particularly in patients with heart failure.
Although beta-adrenergic receptor blockade is useful in treatment of angina and hypertension, there are also situations in which sympathetic stimulation is vital. For example, in patients with severely damaged hearts, adequate ventricular function may depend on sympathetic drive. Beta-adrenergic blockade may worsen AV block by preventing the necessary facilitating effects of sympathetic activity on conduction. $Beta_2$-adrenergic blockade results in passive bronchial constriction by interfering with endogenous adrenergic bronchodilator activity in patients subject to bronchospasm and may also interfere with exogenous bronchodilators in such patients.
Absorption of nadolol after oral dosing is variable, averaging about 30%. Peak serum concentrations of nadolol usually occur in 3 to 4 hours after oral administration and the presence of food in the gastrointestinal tract does not affect the rate or extent of nadolol absorption. Approximately 30% of the nadolol present in serum is reversibly bound to plasma protein.
Unlike many other beta-adrenergic blocking agents, nadolol is not metabolized by the liver and is excreted unchanged, principally by the kidneys.
The half-life of therapeutic doses of nadolol is about 20 to 24 hours, permitting once-daily dosage. Because nadolol is excreted predominantly in the urine, its half-life increases in renal failure (see PRECAUTIONS and DOSAGE AND ADMINISTRATION). Steady-state serum concentrations of nadolol are attained in 6 to 9 days with once-daily dosage in persons with normal renal function. Because of variable absorption and different individual responsiveness, the proper dosage must be determined by titration.
Exacerbation of angina and, in some cases, myocardial infarction and ventricular dysrhythmias have been reported after abrupt discontinuation of therapy with beta-adrenergic blocking agents in patients with coronary artery disease. Abrupt withdrawal of these agents in patients without coronary artery disease has resulted in transient symptoms, including tremulousness, sweating, palpitation, headache, and malaise. Several mechanisms have been proposed to explain these phenomena, among them increased sensitivity to catecholamines because of increased numbers of beta receptors.

INDICATIONS AND USAGE

Angina Pectoris: Nadolol Tablets are indicated for the long-term management of patients with angina pectoris.
Hypertension: Nadolol Tablets are indicated in the management of hypertension; it may be used alone or in combination with other antihypertensive agents, especially thiazide-type diuretics.

CONTRAINDICATIONS

Nadolol Tablets are contraindicated in bronchial asthma, sinus bradycardia and greater than first degree conduction block, cardiogenic shock, and overt cardiac failure (see WARNINGS).

WARNINGS

Cardiac Failure: Sympathetic stimulation may be a vital component supporting circulatory function in patients with congestive heart failure, and its inhibition by beta-blockade may precipitate more severe failure. Although beta-blockers should be avoided in overt congestive heart failure, if necessary, they can be used with caution in patients with a history of failure who are well compensated, usually with digitalis and diuretics. Beta-adrenergic blocking agents do not abolish the inotropic action of digitalis on heart muscle.
IN PATIENTS WITHOUT A HISTORY OF HEART FAILURE, continued use of beta-blockers can, in some cases, lead to cardiac failure. Therefore, at the first sign or symptom of heart failure, the patient should be digitalized and/or treated with diuretics, and the response observed closely, or nadolol should be discontinued (gradually, if possible).

Exacerbation of Ischemic Heart Disease Following Abrupt Withdrawal: Hypersensitivity to catecholamines has been observed in patients withdrawn from beta-blocker therapy; exacerbation of angina and, in some cases, myocardial infarction have occurred after *abrupt* discontinuation of such therapy. When discontinuing chronically administered nadolol, particularly in patients with ischemic heart disease, the dosage should be gradually reduced over a period of 1 to 2 weeks and the patient should be carefully monitored. If angina markedly worsens or acute coronary insufficiency develops, nadolol administration should be reinstituted promptly, at least temporarily, and other measures appropriate for the management of unstable angina should be taken. Patients should be warned against interruption or discontinuation of therapy without the physician's advice. Because coronary artery disease is common and may be unrecognized, it may be prudent not to discontinue nadolol therapy abruptly even in patients treated only for hypertension.

Nonallergic Bronchospasm (e.g., chronic bronchitis, emphysema): PATIENTS WITH BRONCHOSPASTIC DISEASES SHOULD IN GENERAL NOT RECEIVE BETA-BLOCKERS. Nadolol should be administered with caution since it may block bronchodilation produced by endogenous or exogenous catecholamine stimulation of $beta_2$ receptors.
Major Surgery: Because beta-blockade impairs the ability of the heart to respond to reflex stimuli and may increase the risks of general anesthesia and surgical procedures, resulting in protracted hypotension or low cardiac output, it has generally been suggested that such therapy should be withdrawn several days prior to surgery. Recognition of the increased sensitivity to catecholamines of patients recently withdrawn from beta-blocker therapy, however, has made this recommendation controversial. If possible, beta-blockers should be withdrawn well before surgery takes place. In the event of emergency surgery, the anesthesiologist should be informed that the patient is on beta-blocker therapy. The effects of nadolol can be reversed by administration of beta-receptor agonists such as isoproterenol, dopamine, dobutamine, or norepinephrine. Difficulty in restarting and maintaining the heart beat has also been reported with beta-adrenergic receptor blocking agents.
Diabetes and Hypoglycemia: Beta-adrenergic blockade may prevent the appearance of premonitory signs and symptoms (e.g., tachycardia and blood pressure changes) of acute hypoglycemia. This is especially important with labile diabetics. Beta-blockade also reduces the release of insulin in response to hyperglycemia; therefore, it may be necessary to adjust the dose of antidiabetic drugs.
Thyrotoxicosis: Beta-adrenergic blockade may mask certain clinical signs (e.g., tachycardia) of hyperthyroidism. Patients suspected of developing thyrotoxicosis should be managed carefully to avoid abrupt withdrawal of beta-adrenergic blockade which might precipitate a thyroid storm.

PRECAUTIONS

Impaired Renal Function: Nadolol should be used with caution in patients with impaired renal function. (See DOSAGE AND ADMINISTRATION.)
Information for Patients: Patients, especially those with evidence of coronary artery insufficiency, should be warned against interruption or discontinuation of nadolol therapy without the physician's advice. Although cardiac failure rarely occurs in properly selected patients, patients being treated with beta-adrenergic blocking agents should be advised to consult the physician at the first sign or symptom of impending failure. The patient should also be advised of a proper course in the event of an inadvertently missed dose.
Drug Interactions: When administered concurrently, the following drugs may interact with beta-adrenergic receptor blocking agents:
Anesthetics, general: Exaggeration of the hypotension induced by general anesthetics (see WARNINGS, Major Surgery).
Antidiabetic drugs (oral agents and insulin): Hypoglycemia or hyperglycemia; adjust dosage of antidiabetic drug accordingly (see WARNINGS, Diabetes and Hypoglycemia).
Catecholamine-depleting drugs (e.g., reserpine): Additive effect; monitor closely for evidence of hypotension and/or excessive bradycardia (e.g., vertigo, syncope, postural hypotension).
Response to Treatment for Anaphylactic Reaction: While taking beta-blockers, patients with a history of severe anaphylactic reaction to a variety of allergens may be more reactive to repeated challenge, either accidental, diagnostic, or therapeutic. Such patients may be unresponsive to the usual doses of epinephrine used to treat allergic reaction.
Carcinogenesis, Mutagenesis, Impairment of Fertility: In chronic oral toxicologic studies (1 to 2 years) in mice, rats, and dogs, nadolol did not produce any significant toxic effects. In 2-year oral carcinogenic studies in rats and mice, nadolol did not produce any neoplastic, preneoplastic, or nonneoplastic pathologic lesions. In fertility and general reproductive performance studies in rats, nadolol caused no adverse effects.
Pregnancy Category C: In animal reproduction studies with nadolol, evidence of embryo- and fetotoxicity was found in rabbits, but not in rats or hamsters, at doses 5 to 10 times greater (on a mg/kg basis) than the maximum indicated human dose. No teratogenic potential was observed in any of these species.
There are no adequate and well-controlled studies in pregnant women. Nadolol should be used during pregnancy only if the potential benefit justifies the potential risk to the fetus. Neonates whose mothers are receiving nadolol at parturition have exhibited bradycardia, hypoglycemia, and associated symptoms.
Nursing Mothers: Nadolol is excreted in human milk. Because of the potential for adverse effects in nursing infants, a decision should be made whether to discontinue nursing or to discontinue therapy taking into account the importance of nadolol to the mother.
Pediatric Use: Safety and effectiveness in children have not been established.

ADVERSE REACTIONS

Most adverse effects have been mild and transient and have rarely required withdrawal of therapy.
Cardiovascular: Bradycardia with heart rates of less than 60 beats per minute occurs commonly, and heart rates below 40 beats per minute and/or symptomatic bradycardia were seen in about 2 of 100 patients. Symptoms of peripheral vascular insufficiency, usually of the Raynaud type, have occurred in approximately 2 of 100 patients. Cardiac failure, hypotension, and rhythm/conduction disturbances have each occurred in about 1 of 100 patients. Single instances of first degree and third degree heart block have been reported; intensification of AV block is a known effect of beta-blockers (see also CONTRAINDICATIONS, WARNINGS, and PRECAUTIONS).
Central Nervous System: Dizziness or fatigue has been reported in approximately 2 of 100 patients; paresthesias, sedation, and change in behavior have each been reported in approximately 6 of 1000 patients.
Respiratory: Bronchospasm has been reported in approximately 1 of 1000 patients (see CONTRAINDICATIONS and WARNINGS).
Gastrointestinal: Nausea, diarrhea, abdominal discomfort, constipation, vomiting, indigestion, anorexia, bloating, and flatulence have been reported in 1 to 5 of 1000 patients.
Miscellaneous: Each of the following has been reported in 1 to 5 of 1000 patients: rash; pruritus; headache; dry mouth,

eyes, or skin; impotence or decreased libido; facial swelling; weight gain; slurred speech; cough; nasal stuffiness; sweating; tinnitus; blurred vision. Reversible alopecia has been reported infrequently.

The following adverse reactions have been reported in patients taking nadolol and/or other beta-adrenergic blocking agents, but no causal relationship to nadolol has been established.

Central Nervous System: Reversible mental depression progressing to catatonia; visual disturbances; hallucinations; an acute reversible syndrome characterized by disorientation for time and place, short-term memory loss, emotional lability with slightly clouded sensorium, and decreased performance on neuropsychometrics.

Gastrointestinal: Mesenteric arterial thrombosis; ischemic colitis; elevated liver enzymes.

Hematologic: Agranulocytosis; thrombocytopenic or nonthrombocytopenic purpura.

Allergic: Fever combined with aching and sore throat; laryngospasm; respiratory distress.

Miscellaneous: Pemphigoid rash; hypertensive reaction in patients with pheochromocytoma; sleep disturbances; Peyronie's disease.

The oculomucocutaneous syndrome associated with the beta-blocker practolol has not been reported with nadolol.

OVERDOSAGE

Nadolol can be removed from the general circulation by hemodialysis.

In addition to gastric lavage, the following measures should be employed, as appropriate. In determining the duration of corrective therapy, note must be taken of the long duration of the effect of nadolol.

Excessive Bradycardia: Administer atropine (0.25 to 1.0 mg). If there is no response to vagal blockade, administer isoproterenol cautiously.

Cardiac Failure: Administer a digitalis glycoside and diuretic. It has been reported that glucagon may also be useful in this situation.

Hypotension: Administer vasopressors, e.g., epinephrine or norepinephrine. (There is evidence that epinephrine may be the drug of choice.)

Bronchospasm: Administer a beta$_2$-stimulating agent and/or a theophylline derivative.

DOSAGE AND ADMINISTRATION

DOSAGE MUST BE INDIVIDUALIZED. NADOLOL MAY BE ADMINISTERED WITHOUT REGARD TO MEALS.

Angina Pectoris: The usual initial dose is 40 mg nadolol once daily. Dosage may be gradually increased in 40 to 80 mg increments at 3- to 7-day intervals until optimum clinical response is obtained or there is pronounced slowing of the heart rate. The usual maintenance dose is 40 or 80 mg administered once daily. Doses up to 160 or 240 mg administered once daily may be needed.

The usefulness and safety in angina pectoris of dosages exceeding 240 mg per day have not been established. If treatment is to be discontinued, reduce the dosage gradually over a period of one to two weeks (see WARNINGS).

Hypertension: The usual initial dose is 40 mg nadolol once daily, whether it is used alone or in addition to diuretic therapy. Dosage may be gradually increased in 40 to 80 mg increments until optimum blood pressure reduction is achieved. The usual maintenance dose is 40 or 80 mg administered once daily. Doses up to 240 or 320 mg administered once daily may be needed.

Dosage Adjustment in Renal Failure: Absorbed nadolol is excreted principally by the kidneys and, although nonrenal elimination does occur, dosage adjustments are necessary in patients with renal impairment. The following dose intervals are recommended:

Creatinine Clearance (mL/min/1.73^2)	Dosage Interval (hours)
>50	24
31-50	24-36
10-30	24-48
<10	40-60

HOW SUPPLIED

Nadolol Tablets are available containing 20 mg, 40 mg or 80 mg of nadolol, USP.

The 20 mg tablets are yellow, round, beveled edge, scored tablets debossed with **M** above the score and **28** below the score on one side of the tablet and blank on the other side. They are available as follows:

NDC 0378-0028-01
bottles of 100 tablets

The 40 mg tablets are yellow, round, beveled edge, scored tablets debossed with **M** above the score and **171** below the score on one side of the tablet and blank on the other side. They are available as follows:

NDC 0378-1171-01
bottles of 100 tablets
NDC 0378-1171-10
bottles of 1000 tablets

The 80 mg tablets are yellow, round, beveled edge, scored tablets debossed with **M** above the score and **132** below the score on one side of the tablet and blank on the other side. They are available as follows:

NDC 0378-1132-01
bottles of 100 tablets
NDC 0378-1132-10
bottles of 1000 tablets

Store at 20° to 25°C (68° to 77°F). [See USP for Controlled Room Temperature.]

Protect from light.

Dispense in a tight, light-resistant container using a child-resistant closure.

MYLAN®
Mylan Pharmaceuticals Inc.
Morgantown, WV 26505

REVISED FEBRUARY 2004
NAD:R8

THIORIDAZINE HYDROCHLORIDE TABLETS, USP ℞

10 mg, 25 mg, 50 mg and 100 mg

WARNING

THIORIDAZINE HAS BEEN SHOWN TO PROLONG THE QTc INTERVAL IN A DOSE RELATED MANNER, AND DRUGS WITH THIS POTENTIAL, INCLUDING THIORIDAZINE, HAVE BEEN ASSOCIATED WITH TORSADE DE POINTES-TYPE ARRHYTHMIAS AND SUDDEN DEATH. DUE TO ITS POTENTIAL FOR SIGNIFICANT, POSSIBLY LIFE-THREATENING, PROARRHYTHMIC EFFECTS, THIORIDAZINE SHOULD BE RESERVED FOR USE IN THE TREATMENT OF SCHIZOPHRENIC PATIENTS WHO FAIL TO SHOW AN ACCEPTABLE RESPONSE TO ADEQUATE COURSES OF TREATMENT WITH OTHER ANTIPSYCHOTIC DRUGS, EITHER BECAUSE OF INSUFFICIENT EFFECTIVENESS OR THE INABILITY TO ACHIEVE AN EFFECTIVE DOSE DUE TO INTOLERABLE ADVERSE EFFECTS FROM THOSE DRUGS. (SEE WARNINGS, CONTRAINDICATIONS, AND INDICATIONS).

DESCRIPTION

Thioridazine hydrochloride is 2-methylmercapto-10-[2-(N-methyl-2-piperidyl) ethyl] phenothiazine. Its structural formula, molecular weight and molecular formula are:

CH_3 N CH_2—CH_2 N • HCl SCH_3 S

$C_{21}H_{26}N_2S_2$ • HCl M.Wt.: 407.05

Thioridazine hydrochloride is available as tablets for oral administration containing 10 mg, 25 mg, 50 mg or 100 mg. Each tablet for oral administration contains the following inactive ingredients: colloidal silicon dioxide, croscarmellose sodium, hydroxypropyl cellulose, hypromellose, magnesium stearate, microcrystalline cellulose, polyethylene glycol, sodium lauryl sulfate, titanium dioxide and FD&C Yellow #6 Aluminum Lake.

CLINICAL PHARMACOLOGY

The basic pharmacological activity of thioridazine is similar to that of other phenothiazines, but is associated with minimal extrapyramidal stimulation.

However, thioridazine has been shown to prolong the QTc interval in a dose-dependent fashion. This effect may increase the risk of serious, potentially fatal, ventricular arrhythmias, such as torsade de pointes-type arrhythmias. Due to this risk, thioridazine is indicated only for schizophrenic patients who have not been responsive to or cannot tolerate other antipsychotic agents (see WARNINGS and CONTRAINDICATIONS). However, the prescriber should be aware that thioridazine has not been systematically evaluated in controlled trials in treatment refractory schizophrenic patients and its efficacy in such patients is unknown.

INDICATIONS AND USAGE

Thioridazine is indicated for the management of schizophrenic patients who fail to respond adequately to treatment with other antipsychotic drugs. Due to the risk of significant, potentially life-threatening, proarrhythmic effects with thioridazine treatment, thioridazine should be used only in patients who have failed to respond adequately to treatment with appropriate courses of other antipsychotic drugs, either because of insufficient effectiveness or the inability to achieve an effective dose due to intolerable adverse effects from those drugs. Consequently, before initiating treatment with thioridazine, it is strongly recommended that a patient be given at least 2 trials, each with a different antipsychotic drug product, at an adequate dose, and for an adequate duration (see WARNINGS and CONTRAINDICATIONS).

However, the prescriber should be aware that thioridazine has not been systematically evaluated in controlled trials in treatment refractory schizophrenic patients and its efficacy in such patients is unknown.

CONTRAINDICATIONS

Thioridazine use should be avoided in combination with other drugs that are known to prolong the QTc interval and in patients with congenital long QT syndrome or a history of cardiac arrhythmias.

Reduced cytochrome P450 2D6 isozyme activity drugs that inhibit this isozyme (e.g., fluoxetine and paroxetine) and certain other drugs (e.g., fluvoxamine, propranolol, and pindolol) appear to appreciably inhibit the metabolism of thioridazine. The resulting elevated levels of thioridazine would be expected to augment the prolongation of the QTc interval associated with thioridazine and may increase the risk of serious, potentially fatal, cardiac arrhythmias, such as torsade de pointes-type arrhythmias. Such an increased risk may result also from the additive effect of coadministering thioridazine with other agents that prolong the QTc interval. Therefore, thioridazine is contraindicated with these drugs as well as in patients, comprising about 7% of the normal population, who are known to have a genetic defect leading to reduced levels of activity of P450 2D6 (see WARNINGS and PRECAUTIONS).

In common with other phenothiazines, thioridazine is contraindicated in severe central nervous system depression or comatose states from any cause including drug induced central nervous system depression (see WARNINGS). It should also be noted that hypertensive or hypotensive heart disease of extreme degree is a contraindication of phenothiazine administration.

WARNINGS

Potential for Proarrhythmic Effects: DUE TO THE POTENTIAL FOR SIGNIFICANT, POSSIBLY LIFE-THREATENING, PROARRHYTHMIC EFFECTS WITH THIORIDAZINE TREATMENT, THIORIDAZINE SHOULD BE RESERVED FOR USE IN THE TREATMENT OF SCHIZOPHRENIC PATIENTS WHO FAIL TO SHOW AN ACCEPTABLE RESPONSE TO ADEQUATE COURSES OF TREATMENT WITH OTHER ANTIPSYCHOTIC DRUGS, EITHER BECAUSE OF INSUFFICIENT EFFECTIVENESS OR THE INABILITY TO ACHIEVE AN EFFECTIVE DOSE DUE TO INTOLERABLE ADVERSE EFFECTS FROM THOSE DRUGS. CONSEQUENTLY, BEFORE INITIATING TREATMENT WITH THIORIDAZINE, IT IS STRONGLY RECOMMENDED THAT A PATIENT BE GIVEN AT LEAST TWO TRIALS, EACH WITH A DIFFERENT ANTIPSYCHOTIC DRUG PRODUCT, AT AN ADEQUATE DOSE, AND FOR AN ADEQUATE DURATION. THIORIDAZINE HAS NOT BEEN SYSTEMATICALLY EVALUATED IN CONTROLLED TRIALS IN THE TREATMENT OF REFRACTORY SCHIZOPHRENIC PATIENTS AND ITS EFFICACY IN SUCH PATIENTS IS UNKNOWN.

A crossover study in nine healthy males comparing single doses of thioridazine 10 mg and 50 mg with placebo demonstrated a dose-related prolongation of the QTc interval. The mean maximum increase in QTc interval following the 50 mg dose was about 23 msec; greater prolongation may be observed in the clinical treatment of unscreened patients.

Prolongation of the QTc interval has been associated with the ability to cause torsade de pointes-type arrhythmias, a potentially fatal polymorphic ventricular tachycardia, and sudden death. There are several published case reports of torsade de pointes and sudden death associated with thioridazine treatment. A causal relationship between these events and thioridazine therapy has not been established but, given the ability of thioridazine to prolong the QTc interval, such a relationship is possible.

Certain circumstances may increase the risk of torsade de pointes and/or sudden death in association with the use of drugs that prolong the QTc interval, including 1) bradycardia, 2) hypokalemia, 3) concomitant use of other drugs that prolong the QTc interval, 4) presence of congenital prolongation of the QT interval, and 5) for thioridazine in particular, its use in patients with reduced activity of P450 2D6 or its co-administration with drugs that may inhibit P450 2D6 or by some other mechanism interfere with the clearance of thioridazine (see CONTRAINDICATIONS and PRECAUTIONS).

It is recommended that patients being considered for thioridazine treatment have a baseline ECG performed and serum potassium levels measured. Serum potassium should be normalized before initiating treatment and patients with a QTc interval greater than 450 msec should not receive thioridazine treatment. It may also be useful to periodically monitor ECG's and serum potassium during thioridazine treatment, especially during a period of dose adjustment. Thioridazine should be discontinued in patients who are found to have a QTc interval over 500 msec.

Patients taking thioridazine who experience symptoms that may be associated with the occurrence of torsade de pointes (e.g., dizziness, palpitations, or syncope) may warrant further cardiac evaluation; in particular, Holter monitoring should be considered.

Tardive Dyskinesia: Tardive dyskinesia, a syndrome consisting of potentially irreversible, involuntary, dyskinetic movements may develop in patients treated with antipsychotic drugs. Although the prevalence of the syndrome appears to be highest among the elderly, especially elderly women, it is impossible to rely upon prevalence estimates to predict, at the inception of antipsychotic treatment, which patients are likely to develop the syndrome. Whether antipsychotic drug products differ in their potential to cause tardive dyskinesia is unknown.

Both the risk of developing the syndrome and the likelihood that it will become irreversible are believed to increase as the duration of treatment and the total cumulative dose of antipsychotic drugs administered to the patient increase.

Continued on next page

Thioridazine HCl—Cont.

However, the syndrome can develop, although much less commonly, after relatively brief treatment periods at low doses.
There is no known treatment for established cases of tardive dyskinesia, although the syndrome may remit, partially or completely, if antipsychotic treatment is withdrawn. Antipsychotic treatment itself, however, may suppress (or partially suppress) the signs and symptoms of the syndrome and thereby may possibly mask the underlying disease process. The effect that symptomatic suppression has upon the long-term course of the syndrome is unknown.
Given these considerations, antipsychotics should be prescribed in a manner that is most likely to minimize the occurrence of tardive dyskinesia. Chronic antipsychotic treatment should generally be reserved for patients who suffer from a chronic illness that, 1) is known to respond to antipsychotic drugs, and, 2) for whom alternative, equally effective, but potentially less harmful treatments are *not* available or appropriate. In patients who do require chronic treatment, the smallest dose and the shortest duration of treatment producing a satisfactory clinical response should be sought. The need for continued treatment should be reassessed periodically.
If signs and symptoms of tardive dyskinesia appear in a patient on antipsychotics, drug discontinuation should be considered. However, some patients may require treatment despite the presence of the syndrome.
(For further information about the description of tardive dyskinesia and its clinical detection, please refer to the sections on Information for Patients and ADVERSE REACTIONS.)
It has been suggested in regard to phenothiazines in general, that people who have demonstrated a hypersensitivity reaction (e.g., blood dyscrasias, jaundice) to one may be more prone to demonstrate a reaction to others. Attention should be paid to the fact that phenothiazines are capable of potentiating central nervous system depressants (e.g., anesthetics, opiates, alcohol, etc.) as well as atropine and phosphorus insecticides. Physicians should carefully consider benefit versus risk when treating less severe disorders.
Reproductive studies in animals and clinical experience to date have failed to show a teratogenic effect with thioridazine. However, in view of the desirability of keeping the administration of all drugs to a minimum during pregnancy, thioridazine should be given only when the benefits derived from treatment exceed the possible risks to mother and fetus.
Neuroleptic Malignant Syndrome (NMS): A potentially fatal symptom complex sometimes referred to as Neuroleptic Malignant Syndrome (NMS) has been reported in association with antipsychotic drugs. Clinical manifestations of NMS are hyperpyrexia, muscle rigidity, altered mental status, and evidence of autonomic instability (irregular pulse or blood pressure, tachycardia, diaphoresis, and cardiac dysrhythmias).
The diagnostic evaluation of patients with this syndrome is complicated. In arriving at a diagnosis, it is important to identify cases where the clinical presentation includes both serious medical illness (e.g., pneumonia, systemic infection, etc.) and untreated or inadequately treated extrapyramidal signs and symptoms (EPS). Other important considerations in the differential diagnosis include central anticholinergic toxicity, heat stroke, drug fever, and primary central nervous system (CNS) pathology.
The management of NMS should include, 1) immediate discontinuation of antipsychotic drugs and other drugs not essential to concurrent therapy, 2) intensive symptomatic treatment and medical monitoring, and 3) treatment of any concomitant serious medical problems for which specific treatments are available. There is no general agreement about specific pharmacological treatment regimens for uncomplicated NMS.
If a patient requires antipsychotic drug treatment after recovery from NMS, the potential reintroduction of drug therapy should be carefully considered. The patient should be carefully monitored, since recurrences of NMS have been reported.
Central Nervous System Depressants: As in the case of other phenothiazines, thioridazine is capable of potentiating central nervous system depressants (e.g., alcohol, anesthetics, barbiturates, narcotics, opiates, other psychoactive drugs, etc.) as well as atropine and phosphorus insecticides. Severe respiratory depression and respiratory arrest have been reported when a patient was given a phenothiazine and a concomitant high dose of a barbiturate.

PRECAUTIONS

Leukopenia and/or agranulocytosis and convulsive seizures have been reported but are infrequent. In schizophrenic patients with epilepsy, anticonvulsant medication should be maintained during treatment with thioridazine. Pigmentary retinopathy, which has been observed primarily in patients taking larger than recommended doses, is characterized by diminution of visual acuity, brownish coloring of vision, and impairment of night vision; examination of the fundus discloses deposits of pigment. The possibility of this complication may be reduced by remaining within the recommended limits of dosage.
Where patients are participating in activities requiring complete mental alertness (e.g., driving) it is advisable to administer the phenothiazines cautiously and to increase the dosage gradually. Female patients appear to have a greater tendency to orthostatic hypotension than male patients. The administration of epinephrine should be avoided in the treatment of drug-induced hypotension in view of the fact that phenothiazines may induce a reversed epinephrine effect on occasion. Should a vasoconstrictor be required, the most suitable are levarterenol and phenylephrine.
Antipsychotic drugs elevate prolactin levels; the elevation persists during chronic administration. Tissue culture experiments indicate that approximately one-third of human breast cancers are prolactin dependent *in vitro*, a factor of potential importance if the prescription of these drugs is contemplated in a patient with a previously detected breast cancer. Although disturbances such as galactorrhea, amenorrhea, gynecomastia, and impotence have been reported, the clinical significance of elevated serum prolactin levels is unknown for most patients. An increase in mammary neoplasms has been found in rodents after chronic administration of neuroleptic drugs. Neither clinical studies nor epidemiologic studies conducted to date, however, have shown an association between chronic administration of these drugs and mammary tumorigenesis; the available evidence is considered too limited to be conclusive at this time.
Drug Interactions: Reduced cytochrome P450 2D6 isozyme activity, drugs which inhibit this isozyme (e.g., fluoxetine and paroxetine), and certain other drugs (e.g., fluvoxamine, propranolol, and pindolol) appear to appreciably inhibit the metabolism of thioridazine. The resulting elevated levels of thioridazine would be expected to augment the prolongation of the QTc interval associated with thioridazine and may increase the risk of serious, potentially fatal, cardiac arrhythmias, such as torsade de pointes-type arrhythmias. Such an increased risk may result also from the additive effect of coadministering thioridazine with other agents that prolong the QTc interval. Therefore, thioridazine is contraindicated with these drugs as well as in patients, comprising about 7% of the normal population, who are known to have a genetic defect leading to reduced levels of activity of P450 2D6 (see WARNINGS and CONTRAINDICATIONS).
Drugs That Inhibit Cytochrome P450 2D6: In a study of 19 healthy male subjects, which included 6 slow and 13 rapid hydroxylators of debrisoquin, a single 25 mg oral dose of thioridazine produced a 2.4-fold higher C_{max} and a 4.5-fold higher AUC for thioridazine in the slow hydroxylators compared to rapid hydroxylators. The rate of debrisoquin hydroxylation is felt to depend on the level of cytochrome P450 2D6 isozyme activity. Thus, this study suggests that drugs that inhibit P450 2D6 or the presence of reduced activity levels of this isozyme will produce elevated plasma levels of thioridazine. Therefore, the co-administration of drugs that inhibit P450 2D6 with thioridazine and the use of thioridazine in patients known to have reduced activity of P450 2D6 are contraindicated.
Drugs That Reduce the Clearance of Thioridazine Through Other Mechanisms: *Fluvoxamine:* The effect of fluvoxamine (25 mg b.i.d. for one week) on thioridazine steady state concentration was evaluated in 10 male in-patients with schizophrenia. Concentrations of thioridazine and its two active metabolites, mesoridazine and sulforidazine, increased three-fold following co-administration of fluvoxamine. Fluvoxamine and thioridazine should not be co-administered.
Propranolol: Concurrent administration of propranolol (100 to 800 mg daily) has been reported to produce increases in plasma levels of thioridazine (approximately 50% to 400%) and its metabolites (approximately 80% to 300%). Propranolol and thioridazine should not be co-administered.
Pindolol: Concurrent administration of pindolol and thioridazine have resulted in moderate, dose-related increases in the serum levels of thioridazine and two of its metabolites, as well as higher than expected serum pindolol levels. Pindolol and thioridazine should not be coadministered.
Drugs That Prolong the QTc Interval: There are no studies of the co-administration of thioridazine and other drugs that prolong the QTc interval. However, it is expected that such co-administration would produce additive prolongation of the QTc interval and, thus, such use is contraindicated.
Information for Patients: Patients should be informed that thioridazine has been associated with potentially fatal heart rhythm disturbances. The risk of such events may be increased when certain drugs are given together with thioridazine. Therefore, patients should inform the prescriber that they are receiving thioridazine treatment before taking any new medication.
Given the likelihood that some patients exposed chronically to antipsychotics will develop tardive dyskinesia, it is advised that all patients in whom chronic use is contemplated be given, if possible, full information about this risk. The decision to inform patients and/or their guardians must obviously take into account the clinical circumstances and the competency of the patient to understand the information provided.
Pediatric Use: See DOSAGE AND ADMINISTRATION: Pediatric Patients.

ADVERSE REACTIONS

In the recommended dosage ranges with thioridazine hydrochloride most side effects are mild and transient.
Central Nervous System: Drowsiness may be encountered on occasion, especially where large doses are given early in treatment. Generally, this effect tends to subside with continued therapy or a reduction in dosage. Pseudoparkinsonism and other extrapyramidal symptoms may occur but are infrequent. Nocturnal confusion, hyperactivity, lethargy, psychotic reactions, restlessness, and headache have been reported but are extremely rare.
Autonomic Nervous System: Dryness of mouth, blurred vision, constipation, nausea, vomiting, diarrhea, nasal stuffiness, and pallor have been seen.
Endocrine System: Galactorrhea, breast engorgement, amenorrhea, inhibition of ejaculation, and peripheral edema have been described.
Skin: Dermatitis and skin eruptions of the urticarial type have been observed infrequently. Photosensitivity is extremely rare.
Cardiovascular System: Thioridazine produces a dose related prolongation of the QTc interval, which is associated with the ability to cause torsade de pointes-type arrhythmias, a potentially fatal polymorphic ventricular tachycardia, and sudden death (see WARNINGS). Both torsade de pointes-type arrhythmias and sudden death have been reported in association with thioridazine. A causal relationship between these events and thioridazine therapy has not been established but, given the ability of thioridazine to prolong the QTc interval, such a relationship is possible. Other ECG changes have been reported (see Phenothiazine Derivatives: *Cardiovascular Effects*).
Other: Rare cases described as parotid swelling have been reported following administration of thioridazine.
Post Introduction Reports: These are voluntary reports of adverse events temporally associated with thioridazine that were received since marketing, and there may be no causal relationship between thioridazine use and these events: priapism.
Phenothiazine Derivatives: It should be noted that efficacy, indications, and untoward effects have varied with the different phenothiazines. It has been reported that old age lowers the tolerance for phenothiazines. The most common neurological side effects in these patients are parkinsonism and akathisia. There appears to be an increased risk of agranulocytosis and leukopenia in the geriatric population. The physician should be aware that the following have occurred with one or more phenothiazines and should be considered whenever one of these drugs is used:
Autonomic Reactions: Miosis, obstipation, anorexia, paralytic ileus.
Cutaneous Reactions: Erythema, exfoliative dermatitis, contact dermatitis.
Blood Dyscrasias: Agranulocytosis, leukopenia, eosinophilia, thrombocytopenia, anemia, aplastic anemia, pancytopenia.
Allergic Reactions: Fever, laryngeal edema, angioneurotic edema, asthma.
Hepatotoxicity: Jaundice, biliary stasis.
Cardiovascular Effects: Changes in the terminal portion of the electrocardiogram to include prolongation of the QT interval, depression and inversion of the T wave, and the appearance of a wave tentatively identified as a bifid T wave or a U wave have been observed in patients receiving phenothiazines, including thioridazine. To date, these appear to be due to altered repolarization, not related to myocardial damage, and reversible. Nonetheless, significant prolongation of the QT interval has been associated with serious ventricular arrhythmias and sudden death (see WARNINGS). Hypotension, rarely resulting in cardiac arrest, has been reported.
Extrapyramidal Symptoms: Akathisia, agitation, motor restlessness, dystonic reactions, trismus, torticollis, opisthotonus, oculogyric crises, tremor, muscular rigidity, akinesia.
Tardive Dyskinesia: Chronic use of antipsychotics may be associated with the development of tardive dyskinesia. The salient features of this syndrome are described in the WARNINGS section and subsequently.
The syndrome is characterized by involuntary choreoathetoid movements which variously involve the tongue, face, mouth, lips, or jaw (e.g., protrusion of the tongue, puffing of cheeks, puckering of the mouth, chewing movements), trunk, and extremities. The severity of the syndrome and the degree of impairment produced vary widely.
The syndrome may become clinically recognizable either during treatment, upon dosage reduction, or upon withdrawal of treatment. Movements may decrease in intensity and may disappear altogether if further treatment with antipsychotics is withheld. It is generally believed that reversibility is more likely after short rather than long-term antipsychotic exposure. Consequently, early detection of tardive dyskinesia is important. To increase the likelihood of detecting the syndrome at the earliest possible time, the dosage of antipsychotic drug should be reduced periodically (if clinically possible) and the patient observed for signs of the disorder. This maneuver is critical, for antipsychotic drugs may mask the signs of the syndrome.
Neuroleptic Malignant Syndrome (NMS): Chronic use of antipsychotics may be associated with the development of Neuroleptic Malignant Syndrome. The salient features of this syndrome are described in the WARNINGS section and subsequently. Clinical manifestations of NMS are hyperpyrexia, muscle rigidity, altered mental status, and evidence of autonomic instability (irregular pulse or blood pressure, tachycardia, diaphoresis, and cardiac dysrhythmias).
Endocrine Disturbances: Menstrual irregularities, altered libido, gynecomastia, lactation, weight gain, edema. False positive pregnancy tests have been reported.
Urinary Disturbances: Retention, incontinence.
Others: Hyperpyrexia. Behavioral effects suggestive of a paradoxical reaction have been reported. These include ex-

citement, bizarre dreams, aggravation of psychoses, and toxic confusional states. More recently, a peculiar skin-eye syndrome has been recognized as a side effect following long-term treatment with phenothiazines. This reaction is marked by progressive pigmentation of areas of the skin or conjunctiva and/or accompanied by discoloration of the exposed sclera and cornea. Opacities of the anterior lens and cornea described as irregular or stellate in shape have also been reported. Systemic lupus erythematosus-like syndrome.

OVERDOSAGE

Many of the symptoms observed are extensions of the side effects described under ADVERSE REACTIONS. Thioridazine can be toxic in overdose, with cardiac toxicity being of particular concern. Frequent ECG and vital sign monitoring of overdosed patients is recommended. Observation for several days may be required because of the risk of delayed effects.

Signs and Symptoms: Effects and clinical complications of acute overdose involving phenothiazines may include:

Cardiovascular: Cardiac arrhythmias, hypotension, shock, ECG changes, increased QT and PR intervals, non-specific ST and T wave changes, bradycardia, sinus tachycardia, atrioventricular block, ventricular tachycardia, ventricular fibrillation, Torsade de pointes, myocardial depression.

Central Nervous System: Sedation, extrapyramidal effects, confusion, agitation, hypothermia, hyperthermia, restlessness, seizures, areflexia, coma.

Autonomic Nervous System: Mydriasis, miosis, dry skin, dry mouth, nasal congestion, urinary retention, blurred vision.

Respiratory: Respiratory depression, apnea, pulmonary edema.

Gastrointestinal: Hypomotility, constipation, ileus.

Renal: Oliguria, uremia.

Toxic dose and blood concentration ranges for the phenothiazines have not been firmly established. It has been suggested that the toxic blood concentration range for thioridazine begins at 1 mg/dL, and 2 to 8 mg/dL is the lethal concentration range.

Treatment: An airway must be established and maintained. Adequate oxygenation and ventilation must be ensured.

Cardiovascular monitoring should commence immediately and should include continuous electrocardiographic monitoring to detect possible arrhythmias. Treatment may include one or more of the following therapeutic interventions: correction of electrolyte abnormalities and acid-base balance, lidocaine, phenytoin, isoproterenol, ventricular pacing, and defibrillation. Disopyramide, procainamide, and quinidine may produce additive QT-prolonging effects when administered to patients with acute overdosage of thioridazine and should be avoided (see WARNINGS and CONTRAINDICATIONS). Caution must be exercised when administering lidocaine, as it may increase the risk of developing seizures.

Treatment of hypotension may require intravenous fluids and vasopressors. Phenylephrine, levarterenol, or metaraminol are the appropriate pressor agents for use in the management of refractory hypotension. The potent α adrenergic blocking properties of the phenothiazines makes the use of vasopressors with mixed α and β adrenergic agonist properties inappropriate, including epinephrine and dopamine. Paradoxical vasodilation may result. In addition, it is reasonable to expect that the α adrenergic-blocking properties of bretylium might be additive to those of thioridazine, resulting in problematic hypotension.

In managing overdosage, the physician should always consider the possibility of multiple drug involvement. Gastric lavage and repeated doses of activated charcoal should be considered. Induction of emesis is less preferable to gastric lavage because of the risk of dystonia and the potential for aspiration of vomitus. Emesis should not be induced in patients expected to deteriorate rapidly, or those with impaired consciousness.

Acute extrapyramidal symptoms may be treated with diphenhydramine hydrochloride or benztropine mesylate.

Avoid the use of barbiturates when treating seizures, as they may potentiate phenothiazine-induced respiratory depression.

Forced diuresis, hemoperfusion, hemodialysis and manipulation of urine pH are of unlikely benefit in the treatment of phenothiazine overdose due to their large volume of distribution and extensive plasma protein binding.

Up-to-date information about the treatment of overdose can often be obtained from a certified Regional Poison Control Center. Telephone numbers of certified Regional Poison Control Centers are listed in the Physicians' Desk Reference®**.

DOSAGE AND ADMINISTRATION

Since thioridazine is associated with a dose-related prolongation of the QTc interval, which is a potentially life-threatening event, its use should be reserved for schizophrenic patients who fail to respond adequately to treatment with other antipsychotic drugs. Dosage must be individualized and the smallest effective dosage should be determined for each patient (see INDICATIONS and WARNINGS).

Adults: The usual starting dose for adult schizophrenic patients is 50 to 100 mg three times a day, with a gradual increment to a maximum of 800 mg daily if necessary. Once effective control of symptoms has been achieved, the dosage may be reduced gradually to determine the minimum maintenance dose. The total daily dosage ranges from 200 to 800 mg, divided into two to four doses.

Pediatric Patients: For pediatric patients with schizophrenia who are unresponsive to other agents, the recommended initial dose is 0.5 mg/kg/day given in divided doses. Dosage may be increased gradually until optimum therapeutic effect is obtained or the maximum dose of 3 mg/kg/day has been reached.

HOW SUPPLIED

Thioridazine Hydrochloride Tablets, USP are available containing 10 mg, 25 mg, 50 mg or 100 mg of thioridazine hydrochloride.

The 10 mg tablets are orange, round, unscored, film-coated tablets debossed with **M54** on one side and **10** on the other side. They are available as follows:

NDC 0378-0612-01
bottles of 100 tablets
NDC 0378-0612-10
bottles of 1000 tablets

The 25 mg tablets are orange, round, unscored, film-coated tablets debossed with **M58** on one side and **25** on the other side. They are available as follows:

NDC 0378-0614-01
bottles of 100 tablets
NDC 0378-0614-10
bottles of 1000 tablets

The 50 mg tablets are orange, round, unscored, film-coated tablets debossed with **M59** on one side and **50** on the other side. They are available as follows:

NDC 0378-0616-01
bottles of 100 tablets
NDC 0378-0616-10
bottles of 1000 tablets

The 100 mg tablets are orange, round, unscored, film-coated tablets debossed with **M61** on one side and **100** on the other side. They are available as follows:

NDC 0378-0618-01
bottles of 100 tablets
NDC 0378-0618-10
bottles of 1000 tablets

STORE AT CONTROLLED ROOM TEMPERATURE 15°–30°C (59°–86°F). PROTECT FROM LIGHT.

Dispense in a tight, light-resistant container using a child-resistant closure.

**Trademark of Medical Economics Company, Inc.

Mylan Pharmaceuticals Inc.
Morgantown, WV 26505

REVISED JULY 2003
THIO:R12AQ

THIOTHIXENE CAPSULES, USP ℞

1 mg, 2 mg, 5 mg and 10 mg

DESCRIPTION

Thiothixene is a thioxanthene derivative. Specifically, it is the *cis* isomer of N,N-dimethyl-9-[3-(4-methyl-1-piperazinyl)-propylidene] thioxanthene-2-sulfonamide. It may be represented by the following structural formula:

The thioxanthenes differ from the phenothiazines by the replacement of nitrogen in the central ring with a carbon-linked side chain fixed in space in a rigid structural configuration. An N,N-dimethyl sulfonamide functional group is bonded to the thioxanthene nucleus.

Each capsule contains 1 mg, 2 mg, 5 mg or 10 mg of thiothixene and the following inactive ingredients: colloidal silicon dioxide, croscarmellose sodium (Type A), gelatin, magnesium stearate, microcrystalline cellulose, powdered cellulose, pregelatinized starch, sodium lauryl sulfate, titanium dioxide and other inactive ingredients. The following coloring agents are employed:

1 mg - FD&C Blue #1, D&C Red #28, FD&C Red #40, FD&C Yellow #6
2 mg - FD&C Blue #1, FD&C Red #40, FD&C Yellow #6, D&C Yellow #10
5 mg - FD&C Blue #1, FD&C Red #40, FD&C Yellow #6
10 mg - FD&C Blue #1, FD&C Red #40, FD&C Yellow #6

CLINICAL PHARMACOLOGY

Thiothixene is an antipsychotic of the thioxanthene series. Thiothixene possesses certain chemical and pharmacological similarities to the piperazine phenothiazines and differences from the aliphatic group of phenothiazines.

INDICATIONS AND USAGE

Thiothixene is effective in the management of schizophrenia. Thiothixene has not been evaluated in the management of behavioral complications in patients with mental retardation.

CONTRAINDICATIONS

Thiothixene is contraindicated in patients with circulatory collapse, comatose states, central nervous system depression due to any cause, and blood dyscrasias. Thiothixene is contraindicated in individuals who have shown hypersensitivity to the drug. It is not known whether there is a cross sensitivity between the thioxanthenes and the phenothiazine derivatives, but this possibility should be considered.

WARNINGS

Tardive Dyskinesia: Tardive dyskinesia, a syndrome consisting of potentially irreversible, involuntary, dyskinetic movements may develop in patients treated with antipsychotic drugs. Although the prevalence of the syndrome appears to be highest among the elderly, especially elderly women, it is impossible to rely upon prevalence estimates to predict, at the inception of antipsychotic treatment, which patients are likely to develop the syndrome. Whether antipsychotic drug products differ in their potential to cause tardive dyskinesia is unknown.

Both the risk of developing the syndrome and the likelihood that it will become irreversible are believed to increase as the duration of treatment and the total cumulative dose of antipsychotic drugs administered to the patient increase. However, the syndrome can develop, although much less commonly, after relatively brief treatment periods at low doses.

There is no known treatment for established cases of tardive dyskinesia, although the syndrome may remit, partially or completely, if antipsychotic treatment is withdrawn. Antipsychotic treatment, itself, however, may suppress (or partially suppress) the signs and symptoms of the syndrome and thereby may possibly mask the underlying disease process. The effect that symptomatic suppression has upon the long-term course of the syndrome is unknown.

Given these considerations, antipsychotics should be prescribed in a manner that is most likely to minimize the occurrence of tardive dyskinesia. Chronic antipsychotic treatment should generally be reserved for patients who suffer from a chronic illness that, 1) is known to respond to antipsychotic drugs, and 2) for whom alternative, equally effective, but potentially less harmful treatments are not available or appropriate. In patients who do require chronic treatment, the smallest dose and the shortest duration of treatment producing a satisfactory clinical response should be sought. The need for continued treatment should be reassessed periodically.

If signs and symptoms of tardive dyskinesia appear in a patient on antipsychotics, drug discontinuation should be considered. However, some patients may require treatment despite the presence of the syndrome.

(For further information about the description of tardive dyskinesia and its clinical detection, please refer to Information for Patients in the PRECAUTIONS section, and to the ADVERSE REACTIONS section.)

Neuroleptic Malignant Syndrome (NMS): A potentially fatal symptom complex sometimes referred to as Neuroleptic Malignant Syndrome (NMS) has been reported in association with antipsychotic drugs. Clinical manifestations of NMS are hyperpyrexia, muscle rigidity, altered mental status and evidence of autonomic instability (irregular pulse or blood pressure, tachycardia, diaphoresis, and cardiac dysrhythmias).

The diagnostic evaluation of patients with this syndrome is complicated. In arriving at a diagnosis, it is important to identify cases where the clinical presentation includes both serious medical illness (e.g., pneumonia, systemic infection, etc.) and untreated or inadequately treated extrapyramidal signs and symptoms (EPS). Other important considerations in the differential diagnosis include central anticholinergic toxicity, heat stroke, drug fever and primary central nervous system (CNS) pathology.

The management of NMS should include 1) immediate discontinuation of antipsychotic drugs and other drugs not essential to concurrent therapy, 2) intensive symptomatic treatment and medical monitoring, and 3) treatment of any concomitant serious medical problems for which specific treatments are available. There is no general agreement about specific pharmacological treatment regimens for uncomplicated NMS.

If a patient requires antipsychotic drug treatment after recovery from NMS, the potential reintroduction of drug therapy should be carefully considered. The patient should be carefully monitored, since recurrences of NMS have been reported.

Usage in Pregnancy: Safe use of thiothixene during pregnancy has not been established. Therefore, this drug should be given to pregnant patients only when, in the judgment of the physician, the expected benefits from the treatment exceed the possible risks to mother and fetus. Animal reproduction studies and clinical experience to date have not demonstrated any teratogenic effects.

In the animal reproduction studies with thiothixene, there was some decrease in conception rate and litter size, and an increase in resorption rate in rats and rabbits. Similar findings have been reported with other psychotropic agents. After repeated oral administration of thiothixene to rats (5 to 15 mg/kg/day), rabbits (3 to 50 mg/kg/day), and monkeys (1 to 3 mg/kg/day) before and during gestation, no teratogenic effects were seen.

Usage in Children: The use of thiothixene in children under 12 years of age is not recommended because safe conditions for its use have not been established.

Continued on next page

Thiothixene—Cont.

As is true with many CNS drugs, thiothixene may impair the mental and/or physical abilities required for the performance of potentially hazardous tasks such as driving a car or operating machinery, especially during the first few days of therapy. Therefore, the patient should be cautioned accordingly.
As in the case of other CNS-acting drugs, patients receiving thiothixene should be cautioned about the possible additive effects (which may include hypotension) with CNS depressants and with alcohol.

PRECAUTIONS

An antiemetic effect was observed in animal studies with thiothixene; since this effect may also occur in man, it is possible that thiothixene may mask signs of overdosage of toxic drugs and may obscure conditions such as intestinal obstruction and brain tumor.
In consideration of the known capability of thiothixene and certain other psychotropic drugs to precipitate convulsions, extreme caution should be used in patients with a history of convulsive disorders or those in a state of alcohol withdrawal, since it may lower the convulsive threshold. Although thiothixene potentiates the actions of the barbiturates, the dosage of the anticonvulsant therapy should not be reduced when thiothixene is administered concurrently.
Though exhibiting rather weak anticholinergic properties, thiothixene should be used with caution in patients who might be exposed to extreme heat or who are receiving atropine or related drugs.
Use with caution in patients with cardiovascular disease.
Caution as well as careful adjustment of the dosages is indicated when thiothixene is used in conjunction with other CNS depressants.
Also, careful observation should be made for pigmentary retinopathy, and lenticular pigmentation (fine lenticular pigmentation has been noted in a small number of patients treated with thiothixene for prolonged periods). Blood dyscrasias (agranulocytosis, pancytopenia, thrombocytopenic purpura), and liver damage (jaundice, biliary stasis), have been reported with related drugs.
Antipsychotic drugs elevate prolactin levels; the elevation persists during chronic administration. Tissue culture experiments indicate that approximately one-third of human breast cancers are prolactin dependent *in vitro*, a factor of potential importance if the prescription of these drugs is contemplated in a patient with a previously detected breast cancer. Although disturbances such as galactorrhea, amenorrhea, gynecomastia, and impotence have been reported, the clinical significance of elevated serum prolactin levels is unknown for most patients. An increase in mammary neoplasms has been found in rodents after chronic administration of antipsychotic drugs. Neither clinical studies nor epidemiologic studies conducted to date, however, have shown an association between chronic administration of these drugs and mammary tumorigenesis; the available evidence is considered too limited to be conclusive at this time.
Information for Patients: Given the likelihood that some patients exposed chronically to antipsychotics will develop tardive dyskinesia, it is advised that all patients in whom chronic use is contemplated be given, if possible, full information about this risk. The decision to inform patients and/or their guardians must obviously take into account the clinical circumstances and the competency of the patient to understand the information provided.

ADVERSE REACTIONS:

NOTE: Not all of the following adverse reactions have been reported with thiothixene. However, since thiothixene has certain chemical and pharmacologic similarities to the phenothiazines, all of the known side effects and toxicity associated with phenothiazine therapy should be borne in mind when thiothixene is used.
Cardiovascular Effects: Tachycardia, hypotension, lightheadedness, and syncope. In the event hypotension occurs, epinephrine should not be used as a pressor agent since a paradoxical further lowering of blood pressure may result. Nonspecific EKG changes have been observed in some patients receiving thiothixene. These changes are usually reversible and frequently disappear on continued thiothixene therapy. The incidence of these changes is lower than that observed with some phenothiazines. The clinical significance of these changes is not known.
CNS Effects: Drowsiness, usually mild, may occur although it usually subsides with continuation of thiothixene therapy. The incidence of sedation appears similar to that of the piperazine group of phenothiazines but less than that of certain aliphatic phenothiazines. Restlessness, agitation and insomnia have been noted with thiothixene. Seizures and paradoxical exacerbation of psychotic symptoms have occurred with thiothixene infrequently.
Hyperreflexia has been reported in infants delivered from mothers having received structurally related drugs.
In addition, phenothiazine derivatives have been associated with cerebral edema and cerebrospinal fluid abnormalities.
Extrapyramidal symptoms, such as pseudoparkinsonism, akathisia and dystonia have been reported. Management of these extrapyramidal symptoms depends upon the type and severity. Rapid relief of acute symptoms may require the use of an injectable antiparkinson agent. More slowly emerging symptoms may be managed by reducing the dosage of thiothixene and/or administering an oral antiparkinson agent.
Persistent Tardive Dyskinesia: As with all antipsychotic agents, tardive dyskinesia may appear in some patients on long-term therapy or may occur after drug therapy has been discontinued. The syndrome is characterized by rhythmical involuntary movements of the tongue, face, mouth or jaw (e.g., protrusion of tongue, puffing of cheeks, puckering of mouth, chewing movements). Sometimes these may be accompanied by involuntary movements of extremities.
Since early detection of tardive dyskinesia is important, patients should be monitored on an ongoing basis. It has been reported that fine vermicular movement of the tongue may be an early sign of the syndrome. If this or any other presentation of the syndrome is observed, the clinician should consider possible discontinuation of antipsychotic medication. (See WARNINGS.)
Hepatic Effects: Elevations of serum transaminase and alkaline phosphatase, usually transient, have been infrequently observed in some patients. No clinically confirmed cases of jaundice attributable to thiothixene have been reported.
Hematologic Effects: As is true with certain other psychotropic drugs, leukopenia and leucocytosis which are usually transient, can occur occasionally with thiothixene. Other antipsychotic drugs have been associated with agranulocytosis, eosinophilia, hemolytic anemia, thrombocytopenia and pancytopenia.
Allergic Reactions: Rash, pruritus, urticaria, photosensitivity and rare cases of anaphylaxis have been reported with thiothixene. Undue exposure to sunlight should be avoided. Although not experienced with thiothixene, exfoliative dermatitis and contact dermatitis (in nursing personnel) have been reported with certain phenothiazines.
Endocrine Disorders: Lactation, moderate breast enlargement and amenorrhea have occurred in a small percentage of females receiving thiothixene. If persistent, this may necessitate a reduction in dosage or the discontinuation of therapy. Phenothiazines have been associated with false positive pregnancy tests, gynecomastia, hypoglycemia, hyperglycemia and glycosuria.
Autonomic Effects: Dry mouth, blurred vision, nasal congestion, constipation, increased sweating, increased salivation and impotence have occurred infrequently with thiothixene therapy. Phenothiazines have been associated with miosis, mydriasis, and adynamic ileus.
Other Adverse Reactions: Hyperpyrexia, anorexia, nausea, vomiting, diarrhea, increase in appetite and weight, weakness or fatigue, polydipsia, and peripheral edema.
Although not reported with thiothixene, evidence indicates there is a relationship between phenothiazine therapy and the occurrence of a systemic lupus erythematosus-like syndrome.
Neuroleptic Malignant Syndrome (NMS): Please refer to the text regarding NMS in the WARNINGS section.
NOTE: Sudden deaths have occasionally been reported in patients who have received certain phenothiazine derivatives. In some cases the cause of death was apparently cardiac arrest or asphyxia due to failure of the cough reflex. In others, the cause could not be determined nor could it be established that death was due to phenothiazine administration.

OVERDOSAGE

Manifestations include muscular twitching, drowsiness and dizziness. Symptoms of gross overdosage may include CNS depression, rigidity, weakness, torticollis, tremor, salivation, dysphagia, hypotension, disturbances of gait, or coma.
Treatment: Essentially symptomatic and supportive. Early gastric lavage is helpful. Keep patient under careful observation and maintain an open airway, since involvement of the extrapyramidal system may produce dysphagia and respiratory difficulty in severe overdosage. If hypotension occurs, the standard measures for managing circulatory shock should be used (I.V. fluids and/or vasoconstrictors).
If a vasoconstrictor is needed, norepinephrine and phenylephrine are the most suitable drugs. Other pressor agents, including epinephrine, are not recommended, since phenothiazine derivatives may reverse the usual pressor action of these agents and cause further lowering of blood pressure.
If CNS depression is marked, symptomatic treatment is indicated. Extrapyramidal symptoms may be treated with antiparkinson drugs.
There are no data on the use of peritoneal or hemodialysis, but they are known to be of little value in phenothiazine intoxication.

DOSAGE AND ADMINISTRATION

Dosage of thiothixene should be individually adjusted depending on the chronicity and severity of the schizophrenia.
In general, small doses should be used initially and gradually increased to the optimal effective level, based on patient response.
Some patients have been successfully maintained on once-a-day thiothixene therapy.
The use of thiothixene in children under 12 years of age is not recommended because safe conditions for its use have not been established.
In milder conditions, an initial dose of 2 mg three times daily. If indicated, a subsequent increase to 15 mg/day total daily dose is often effective.
In more severe conditions, an initial dose of 5 mg twice daily.
The usual optimal dose is 20 to 30 mg daily. If indicated, an increase to 60 mg/day total daily dose is often effective. Exceeding a total daily dose of 60 mg rarely increases the beneficial response.

HOW SUPPLIED

Thiothixene Capsules, USP are available containing 1 mg, 2 mg, 5 mg or 10 mg of thiothixene.
The 1 mg product is a caramel and powder blue capsule imprinted in black ink with **MYLAN 1001** on both body and cap. It is available as follows:

NDC 0378-1001-01
bottles of 100 capsules

The 2 mg product is a caramel and yellow capsule imprinted in black ink with **MYLAN 2002** on both body and cap. It is available as follows:

NDC 0378-2002-01
bottles of 100 capsules
NDC 0378-2002-10
bottles of 1000 capsules

The 5 mg product is a caramel and white capsule imprinted in black ink with **MYLAN 3005** on both body and cap. It is available as follows:

NDC 0378-3005-01
bottles of 100 capsules
NDC 0378-3005-10
bottles of 1000 capsules

The 10 mg product is a caramel and peach capsule imprinted in black ink with **MYLAN 5010** on both body and cap. It is available as follows:

NDC 0378-5010-01
bottles of 100 capsules
NDC 0378-5010-10
bottles of 1000 capsules

Store at 20° to 25°C (68° to 77°F). [See USP for Controlled Room Temperature.]
PROTECT FROM LIGHT.
Dispense in a tight, light-resistant container as defined in the USP using a child-resistant closure.
Mylan Pharmaceuticals Inc.
Morgantown, WV 26505

REVISED OCTOBER 2003
THTX:R16

Mylan Bertek Pharmaceuticals Inc.

530 DAVIS DRIVE
RESEARCH TRIANGLE PARK, NC 27709

Direct Inquiries to:
(888) 523-7835
Fax: (919) 993-5910

Other Products Available:
NITREK® ℞

ACTICIN® ℞

[act' ĭ cĭn]
(permethrin) Cream 5%
℞ only

DESCRIPTION

Acticin (permethrin) Cream 5% is a topical scabicidal agent for the treatment of infestation with *Sarcoptes scabiei* (scabies). It is available in an off-white, vanishing cream base. Acticin Cream is for topical use only.
Structural Formula:

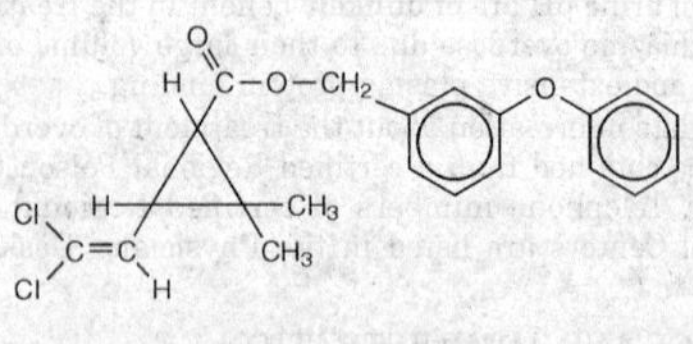

Chemical Name: The permethrin used is an approximate 1:3 mixture of the cis and trans isomers of the pyrethroid 3-(2,2-dichloroethenyl)-2,2-dimethylcyclopropane carboxylic acid, (3-phenoxyphenyl) methyl ester. Permethrin has a molecular formula of $C_{21}H_{20}Cl_2O_3$ and a molecular weight of 391.29. It is a yellow to light orange-brown, low melting solid or viscous liquid.
Each gram of Acticin Cream 5% contains permethrin 50 mg (5%) and the inactive ingredients butylated hydroxytoluene, carbomer 934P, coconut oil, glycerin, glyceryl stearate, isopropyl myristate, lanolin alcohols, light mineral oil, polyox-

yethylene cetyl ethers, purified water, and sodium hydroxide. Formaldehyde 1 mg (0.1%) is added as a preservative.

CLINICAL PHARMACOLOGY

Permethrin, a pyrethroid, is active against a broad range of pests including lice, ticks, fleas, mites, and other arthropods. It acts on the nerve cell membrane to disrupt the sodium channel current by which the polarization of the membrane is regulated. Delayed repolarization and paralysis of the pests are the consequences of this disturbance.

Permethrin is rapidly metabolized by ester hydrolysis to inactive metabolites which are excreted primarily in the urine. Although the amount of permethrin absorbed after a single application of the 5% cream has not been determined precisely, data from studies with ^{14}C-labeled permethrin and absorption studies of the cream applied to patients with moderate to severe scabies indicate it is 2% or less of the amount applied.

INDICATIONS AND USAGE

Acticin Cream 5% is indicated for the treatment of infestation with *Sarcoptes scabiei* (scabies).

CONTRAINDICATIONS

Permethrin cream is contraindicated in patients with known hypersensitivity to any of its components, to any synthetic pyrethroid or pyrethrin.

WARNINGS

If hypersensitivity to permethrin cream occurs, discontinue use.

PRECAUTIONS

General: Scabies infestation is often accompanied by pruritis, edema and erythema. Treatment with permethrin cream may temporarily exacerbate these conditions.

Information for Patients: Patients with scabies should be advised that itching, mild burning and/or stinging may occur after application of permethrin cream. In clinical trials, approximately 75% of patients treated with permethrin cream who continued to manifest pruritis at 2 weeks had cessation by 4 weeks. If irritation persists, they should consult their physician. Permethrin cream may be very mildly irritating to the eyes. Patients should be advised to avoid contact with eyes during application and to flush with water immediately if permethrin cream gets in the eyes.

Carcinogenesis, Mutagenesis, Impairment of Fertility: Six carcinogenicity bioassays were evaluated with permethrin, three each in rats and mice. No tumorigenicity was seen in the rat studies. However, species-specific increases in pulmonary adenomas, a common benign tumor of mice of high spontaneous background incidence, were seen in the three mouse studies. In one of these studies there was an increased incidence of pulmonary alveolar-cell carcinomas and benign liver adenomas only in female mice when permethrin was given in their food at a concentration of 5000 ppm. Mutagenicity assays, which give useful correlative data for interpreting results from carcinogenicity bioassays in rodents, were negative. Permethrin showed no evidence of mutagenic potential in a battery of *in vitro* and *in vivo* genetic toxicity studies.

Permethrin did not have any adverse effect on reproductive function at a dose of 180 mg/kg/day orally in a three-generation rat study.

Pregnancy: ***Teratogenic Effects:*** Pregnancy Category B: Reproduction studies have been performed in mice, rats, and rabbits (200 to 400 mg/kg/day orally) and have revealed no evidence of impaired fertility or harm to the fetus due to permethrin. There are, however, no adequate and well-controlled studies in pregnant women. Because animal reproduction studies are not always predictive of human response, this drug should be used during pregnancy only if clearly needed.

Nursing Mothers: It is not known whether this drug is excreted in human milk. Because many drugs are excreted in human milk and because of the evidence for tumorigenic potential of permethrin in animal studies, consideration should be given to discontinuing nursing temporarily or withholding the drug while the mother is nursing.

Pediatric Use: Permethrin cream is safe and effective in pediatric patients two months of age and older. Safety and effectiveness in pediatric patients less than two months of age have not been established.

Geriatric Use: Clinical studies of permethrin cream did not identify sufficient numbers of subjects aged 65 and over to allow a definitive statement regarding whether elderly subjects respond differently from younger subjects. Other reported clinical experience has not identified differences in responses between the elderly and younger patients. This drug is known to be substantially excreted by the kidney. However, since topical permethrin is metabolized in the liver and excreted in the urine as inactive metabolites, there does not appear to be an increased risk of toxic reactions in patients with impaired renal function when used as labeled.

ADVERSE REACTIONS

In clinical trials, generally mild and transient burning and stinging followed application with permethrin cream in 10% of patients and was associated with the severity of infestation. Pruritis was reported in 7% of patients at various times post-application. Erythema, numbness, tingling, and rash were reported in 1 to 2% or less of patients (see PRECAUTIONS: General).

OVERDOSAGE

No instance of accidental ingestion of permethrin cream has been reported. If ingested, gastric lavage and general supportive measures should be employed.

DOSAGE AND ADMINISTRATION

Adults and children: Thoroughly massage Acticin (permethrin) Cream into the skin from the head to the soles of the feet. Scabies rarely infests the scalp of adults, although the hairline, neck, temple, and forehead may be infested in infants and geriatric patients. Usually 30 grams is sufficient for an average adult. The cream should be removed by washing (shower or bath) after 8 to 14 hours. Infants should be treated on the scalp, temple and forehead. ONE APPLICATION IS GENERALLY CURATIVE.

Patients may experience persistent pruritus after treatment. This is rarely a sign of treatment failure and is not an indication for retreatment. Demonstrable living mites after 14 days indicate that retreatment is necessary.

HOW SUPPLIED

Acticin (permethrin) Cream 5% (wt./wt.) is supplied in 60g tubes.

NDC Code	Strength	Quantity
62794-131-06	5%	60 g

Store at room temperature 15°–25°C (59°–77°F).

Distributed by: BERTEK PHARMACEUTICALS INC. Research Triangle Park, NC 27709

Manufactured by: Alpharma USPD Inc. Baltimore, MD 21244

PN402.01C ACT-01
Rev. 11/02 VC2289

Shown in Product Identification Guide, page 324

AMNESTEEM® ℞
[*ăm-nĕ-stēm*]
(isotretinoin)
10 mg, 20 mg, 40 mg Capsules
℞ Only

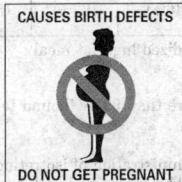

CONTRAINDICATIONS AND WARNINGS

Amnesteem capsules must not be used by females who are pregnant. Although not every fetus exposed to isotretinoin has resulted in a deformed child, there is an extremely high risk that a deformed infant can result if pregnancy occurs while taking isotretinoin capsules in any amount even for short periods of time. Potentially any fetus exposed during pregnancy can be affected. Presently, there are no accurate means of determining, after isotretinoin exposure, which fetus has been affected and which fetus has not been affected.

Major human fetal abnormalities related to isotretinoin administration in females have been documented. There is an increased risk of spontaneous abortion. In addition, premature births have been reported.

Documented external abnormalities include: skull abnormality; ear abnormalities (including anotia, micropinna, small or absent external auditory canals); eye abnormalities (including microphthalmia); facial dysmorphia; cleft palate. Documented internal abnormalities include: CNS abnormalities (including cerebral abnormalities, cerebellar malformation, hydrocephalus, microcephaly, cranial nerve deficit); cardiovascular abnormalities; thymus gland abnormality; parathyroid hormone deficiency. In some cases death has occurred with certain of the abnormalities previously noted.

Cases of IQ scores less than 85 with or without obvious CNS abnormalities have also been reported.

Amnesteem is contraindicated in females of childbearing potential unless the patient meets all of the following conditions:

- **Must NOT be pregnant or breast-feeding.**
- **Must be capable of complying with the mandatory contraceptive measures required for Amnesteem therapy and understand behaviors associated with an increased risk of pregnancy.**
- **Must be reliable in understanding and carrying out instructions.**

Amnesteem must be prescribed under the System to Prevent Isotretinoin-Related Issues of Teratogenicity™ (S.P.I.R.I.T.™).

To prescribe Amnesteem, the prescriber must obtain a supply of yellow self-adhesive isotretinoin qualification stickers. To obtain these stickers:

1) Read the booklet entitled System to Prevent Isotretinoin-Related Issues of Teratogenicity (S.P.I.R.I.T.) Guide to Best Practices.

2) Sign and return the completed S.P.I.R.I.T. Letter of Understanding containing the following Prescriber Checklist:

- **I know the risk and severity of fetal injury/birth defects from isotretinoin**
- **I know how to diagnose and treat the various presentations of acne**
- **I know the risk factors for unplanned pregnancy and the effective measures for avoidance of unplanned pregnancy**
- **It is the informed patient's responsibility to avoid pregnancy during Amnesteem therapy and for 1 month after stopping Amnesteem. To help patients have the knowledge and tools to do so: Before beginning treatment of female patients with Amnesteem I will refer for expert, detailed pregnancy prevention counseling and prescribing, reimbursed by Bertek Pharmaceuticals Inc., OR I have the expertise to perform this function and elect to do so**
- **I understand, and will properly use throughout the Amnesteem treatment course, the S.P.I.R.I.T. procedures for Amnesteem, including monthly pregnancy avoidance counseling, pregnancy testing and use of the yellow self-adhesive isotretinoin qualification stickers**

3) To use the yellow self-adhesive isotretinoin qualification stickers: Amnesteem should not be prescribed or dispensed to any patient (male or female) without a yellow self-adhesive isotretinoin qualification sticker.

For female patients, the yellow self-adhesive isotretinoin qualification sticker signifies that she:

- **Must have had 2 negative urine or serum pregnancy tests with a sensitivity of at least 25 mIU/mL before receiving the initial Amnesteem prescription. The first test (a screening test) is obtained by the prescriber when the decision is made to pursue qualification of the patient for Amnesteem. The second pregnancy test (a confirmation test) should be done during the first 5 days of the menstrual period immediately preceding the beginning of Amnesteem therapy. For patients with amenorrhea, the second test should be done at least 11 days after the last act of unprotected sexual intercourse (without using 2 effective forms of contraception). Each month of therapy, the patient must have a negative result from a urine or serum pregnancy test. A pregnancy test must be repeated every month prior to the female patient receiving each prescription.**
- **Must have selected and have committed to use 2 forms of effective contraception simultaneously, at least 1 of which must be a primary form, unless absolute abstinence is the chosen method, or the patient has undergone a hysterectomy. Patients must use 2 forms of effective contraception for at least 1 month prior to initiation of Amnesteem therapy, during Amnesteem therapy, and for 1 month after discontinuing Amnesteem therapy. Counseling about contraception and behaviors associated with an increased risk of pregnancy must be repeated on a monthly basis.**

Effective forms of contraception include both primary and secondary forms of contraception. Primary forms of contraception include: tubal ligation, partner's vasectomy, intrauterine devices, birth control pills, and topical/injectable/implantable/insertable hormonal birth control products. Secondary forms of contraception include diaphragms, latex condoms, and cervical caps; each must be used with a spermicide.

Any birth control method can fail. Therefore, it is critically important that women of childbearing potential use 2 effective forms of contraception simultaneously. A drug interaction that decreases effectiveness of hormonal contraceptives has not been entirely ruled out for isotretinoin. Although hormonal contraceptives are highly effective, there have been reports of pregnancy from women who have used oral contraceptives, as well as topical/injectable/implantable/insertable hormonal birth control products. These reports occurred while these patients were taking isotretinoin. These reports are more frequent for women who use only a single method of contraception. Patients must receive written warnings about the rates of possible contraception failure (included in patient education kits).

Prescribers are advised to consult the package insert of any medication administered concomitantly with hormonal contraceptives, since some medications may decrease the effectiveness of these birth control products.

Patients should be prospectively cautioned not to self-medicate with the herbal supplement St. John's Wort because a possible interaction has been suggested with hormonal contraceptives based on reports of breakthrough bleeding on oral contraceptives shortly after starting St. John's Wort. Pregnancies have been reported by users of combined hormonal contraceptives who also used some form of St. John's Wort (see PRECAUTIONS).

- **Must have signed a Patient Information/Consent form that contains warnings about the risk of potential birth defects if the fetus is exposed to isotretinoin.**
- **Must have been informed of the purpose and importance of participating in the Isotretinoin Survey and have been given the opportunity to enroll (see PRECAUTIONS).**

Continued on next page

Amnesteem—Cont.

The yellow self-adhesive isotretinoin qualification sticker documents that the female patient is qualified, and includes the date of qualification, patient gender, cut-off date for filling the prescription, and up to a 30-day supply limit with no refills.

These yellow self-adhesive isotretinoin qualification stickers should also be used for male patients.

If a pregnancy does occur during treatment of a woman with Amnesteem, the prescriber and patient should discuss the desirability of continuing the pregnancy. Prescribers are strongly encouraged to report all cases of pregnancy to Bertek Medical Services @ 1-800-809-8237 where a Bertek Pregnancy Prevention Initiative Specialist will be available to discuss Bertek pregnancy information, or prescribers may contact the Food and Drug Administration MedWatch Program @ 1-800-FDA-1088.

Amnesteem should be prescribed only by prescribers who have demonstrated special competence in the diagnosis and treatment of severe recalcitrant nodular acne, are experienced in the use of systemic retinoids, have read the S.P.I.R.I.T. Guide to Best Practices, signed and returned the completed S.P.I.R.I.T. Letter of Understanding, and obtained yellow self-adhesive isotretinoin qualification stickers. Amnesteem should not be prescribed or dispensed without a yellow self-adhesive isotretinoin qualification sticker.

INFORMATION FOR PHARMACISTS:

AMNESTEEM MUST ONLY BE DISPENSED:

- **IN NO MORE THAN A 30-DAY SUPPLY**
- **ONLY ON PRESENTATION OF AN ISOTRETINOIN CAPSULES PRESCRIPTION WITH A YELLOW SELF-ADHESIVE ISOTRETINOIN QUALIFICATION STICKER**
- **WITHIN 7 DAYS OF THE QUALIFICATION DATE**
- **REFILLS REQUIRE A NEW PRESCRIPTION WITH A YELLOW SELF-ADHESIVE ISOTRETINOIN QUALIFICATION STICKER**
- **NO TELEPHONE OR COMPUTERIZED PRESCRIPTIONS ARE PERMITTED.**

AN AMNESTEEM MEDICATION GUIDE MUST BE GIVEN TO THE PATIENT EACH TIME AMNESTEEM IS DISPENSED, AS REQUIRED BY LAW. THIS AMNESTEEM MEDICATION GUIDE IS AN IMPORTANT PART OF THE RISK MANAGEMENT PROGRAM FOR THE PATIENT.

[See table 1 below]

DESCRIPTION

Isotretinoin, a retinoid, is available as Amnesteem in 10 mg, 20 mg and 40 mg soft gelatin capsules for oral administration. Each capsule contains yellow wax, butylated hydroxyanisole, edetate disodium, hydrogenated vegetable oil, and soybean oil. Gelatin capsules contain glycerin, with the following dye systems: 10 mg – red iron oxide paste and black ink; 20 mg – red iron oxide paste, yellow iron oxide paste, titanium dioxide and black ink; 40 mg – red iron oxide paste, yellow iron oxide paste, titanium dioxide, and black ink.

Chemically, isotretinoin is 13-*cis*-retinoic acid and is related to both retinoic acid and retinol (vitamin A). It is a yellow to orange crystalline powder with a molecular weight of 300.44. The structural formula is:

COOH

CLINICAL PHARMACOLOGY

Isotretinoin is a retinoid, which when administered in pharmacologic dosages of 0.5 to 1.0 mg/kg/day (see **DOSAGE AND ADMINISTRATION**), inhibits sebaceous gland function and keratinization. The exact mechanism of action of isotretinoin is unknown.

Nodular Acne

Clinical improvement in nodular acne patients occurs in association with a reduction in sebum secretion. The decrease in sebum secretion is temporary and is related to the dose and duration of treatment with isotretinoin capsules, and reflects a reduction in sebaceous gland size and an inhibition of sebaceous gland differentiation.[1]

Pharmacokinetics

Absorption

Due to its high lipophilicity, oral absorption of isotretinoin is enhanced when given with a high-fat meal. In a crossover study, 74 healthy adult subjects received a single 80 mg oral dose (2 × 40 mg capsules) of isotretinoin under fasted and fed conditions. Both peak plasma concentration (C_{max}) and the total exposure (AUC) of isotretinoin were more than doubled following a standardized high-fat meal when compared with isotretinoin given under fasted conditions (see Table 2 below). The observed elimination half-life was unchanged. This lack of change in half-life suggests that food increases the bioavailability of isotretinoin without altering its disposition. The time to peak concentration (T_{max}) was also increased with food and may be related to a longer absorption phase. Therefore, isotretinoin capsules should always be taken with food (see **DOSAGE AND ADMINISTRATION**). Clinical studies have shown that there is no difference in the pharmacokinetics of isotretinoin between patients with nodular acne and healthy subjects with normal skin.

Table 2. Pharmacokinetic Parameters of Isotretinoin Mean (%CV), N=74

Isotretinoin 2 × 40 mg Capsules	$AUC_{0-\infty}$ (ng·hr/mL)	C_{max} (ng/mL)	T_{max} (hr)	$t_{1/2}$ (hr)
Fed*	10,004 (22%)	862 (22%)	5.3 (77%)	21 (39%)
Fasted	3,703 (46%)	301 (63%)	3.2 (56%)	21 (30%)

*Eating a standardized high-fat meal

Distribution

Isotretinoin is more than 99.9% bound to plasma proteins, primarily albumin.

Metabolism

Following oral administration of isotretinoin, at least three metabolites have been identified in human plasma: 4-*oxo*-isotretinoin, retinoic acid (tretinoin), and 4-*oxo*-retinoic acid (4-*oxo*-tretinoin). Retinoic acid and 13-*cis*-retinoic acid are geometric isomers and show reversible interconversion. The administration of one isomer will give rise to the other. Isotretinoin is also irreversibly oxidized to 4-*oxo*-isotretinoin, which forms its geometric isomer 4-*oxo*-tretinoin.

After a single 80 mg oral dose of isotretinoin capsules to 74 healthy adult subjects, concurrent administration of food increased the extent of formation of all metabolites in plasma when compared to the extent of formation under fasted conditions.

All of these metabolites possess retinoid activity that is in some in vitro models more than that of the parent isotretinoin. However, the clinical significance of these models is unknown. After multiple oral dose administration of isotretinoin to adult cystic acne patients (≥ 18 years), the exposure of patients to 4-*oxo*-isotretinoin at steady-state under fasted and fed conditions was approximately 3.4 times higher than that of isotretinoin.

In vitro studies indicate that the primary P450 isoforms involved in isotretinoin metabolism are 2C8, 2C9, 3A4, and 2B6. Isotretinoin and its metabolites are further metabolized into conjugates, which are then excreted in urine and feces.

Elimination

Following oral administration of an 80 mg dose of ^{14}C-isotretinoin as a liquid suspension, ^{14}C-activity in blood declined with a half-life of 90 hours. The metabolites of isotretinoin and any conjugates are ultimately excreted in the feces and urine in relatively equal amounts (total of 65% to 83%). After a single 80 mg oral dose of isotretinoin to 74 healthy adult subjects under fed conditions, the mean ± SD elimination half-lives ($t_{1/2}$) of isotretinoin and 4-*oxo*-isotretinoin were 21.0 ± 8.2 hours and 24.0 ± 5.3 hours, respectively. After both single and multiple doses, the observed accumulation ratios of isotretinoin ranged from 0.90 to 5.43 in patients with cystic acne.

Special Patient Populations

Pediatric Patients

Pediatric pharmacokinetic information related to the use of isotretinoin after single and multiple doses is approved for Hoffman La-Roche's isotretinoin capsules. However, due to Hoffman La-Roche's marketing exclusivity rights, this drug product is not labeled for pediatric use.

INDICATIONS AND USAGE

Severe Recalcitrant Nodular Acne

Amnesteem is indicated for the treatment of severe recalcitrant nodular acne. Nodules are inflammatory lesions with a diameter of 5 mm or greater. The nodules may become suppurative or hemorrhagic. "Severe," by definition[2], means "many" as opposed to "few or several" nodules. Because of significant adverse effects associated with its use, Amnesteem should be reserved for patients with severe nodular acne who are unresponsive to conventional therapy, including systemic antibiotics. In addition, Amnesteem is indicated only for those females who are not pregnant, because isotretinoin can cause severe birth defects (see boxed CONTRAINDICATIONS AND WARNINGS).

A single course of therapy for 15 to 20 weeks has been shown to result in complete and prolonged remission of disease in many patients.[1,3,4] If a second course of therapy is needed, it should not be initiated until at least 8 weeks after completion of the first course, because experience has shown that patients may continue to improve while off isotretinoin. The optimal interval before retreatment has not been defined for patients who have not completed skeletal growth (see WARNINGS: Skeletal: Bone Mineral Density, Hyperostosis and Premature Epiphyseal Closure).

CONTRAINDICATIONS

Pregnancy: Category X. See boxed CONTRAINDICATIONS AND WARNINGS.

Allergic Reactions

Amnesteem is contraindicated in patients who are hypersensitive to this medication or to any of its components.

WARNINGS

Psychiatric Disorders

Isotretinoin may cause depression, psychosis and, rarely, suicidal ideation, suicide attempts, suicide, and aggressive and/or violent behaviors. Discontinuation of isotretinoin capsules therapy may be insufficient; further evaluation may be necessary. No mechanism of action has been established for these events (see ADVERSE REACTIONS: Psychiatric). Prescribers should read the brochure, Recognizing Psychiatric Disorders in Adolescents and Young Adults: Guide for Prescribers of Amnesteem.

Pseudotumor Cerebri

Isotretinoin use has been associated with a number of cases of pseudotumor cerebri (benign intracranial hypertension), some of which involved concomitant use of tetracyclines. Concomitant treatment with tetracyclines should therefore be avoided. Early signs and symptoms of pseudotumor cerebri include papilledema, headache, nausea and vomiting, and visual disturbances. Patients with these symptoms should be screened for papilledema and, if present, they should be told to discontinue Amnesteem immediately and be referred to a neurologist for further diagnosis and care (see ADVERSE REACTIONS: Neurological).

Pancreatitis

Acute pancreatitis has been reported in patients with either elevated or normal serum triglyceride levels. **In rare instances, fatal hemorrhagic pancreatitis has been reported.** Amnesteem should be stopped if hypertriglyceridemia cannot be controlled at an acceptable level or if symptoms of pancreatitis occur.

Lipids

Elevations of serum triglycerides in excess of 800 mg/dL have been reported in patients treated with isotretinoin. Marked elevations of serum triglycerides were reported in approximately 25% of patients receiving isotretinoin in clinical trials. In addition, approximately 15% developed a decrease in high-density lipoproteins and about 7% showed an increase in cholesterol levels. In clinical trials, the effects on triglycerides, HDL, and cholesterol were reversible upon cessation of isotretinoin therapy. Some patients have been able to reverse triglyceride elevation by reduction in weight, restriction of dietary fat and alcohol, and reduction in dose while continuing isotretinoin.[5]

Blood lipid determinations should be performed before Amnesteem is given and then at intervals until the lipid response to isotretinoin is established, which usually occurs within 4 weeks. Especially careful consideration must be given to risk/benefit for patients who may be at high risk during Amnesteem therapy (patients with diabetes, obesity, increased alcohol intake, lipid metabolism disorder or familial history of lipid metabolism disorder). If Amnesteem therapy is instituted, more frequent checks of serum values for lipids and/or blood sugar are recommended (see PRECAUTIONS: Laboratory Tests).

The cardiovascular consequences of hypertriglyceridemia associated with isotretinoin capsules are unknown.

Table 1. Use of Pregnancy Tests and Isotretinoin Qualification Stickers for Patients

Patient Type	Pregnancy Test Required	Qualification Date	Isotretinoin Qualification Sticker Necessary	Dispense Within 7 Days of Qualification Date
All Males	**No**	**Date Prescription Written**	**Yes**	**Yes**
Females of Childbearing Potential	**Yes**	**Date Sample Taken for Confirmatory Negative Pregnancy Test**	**Yes**	**Yes**
Females* Not of Childbearing Potential	**No**	**Date Prescription Written**	**Yes**	**Yes**

***Females who have had a hysterectomy or who are postmenopausal are not considered to be of childbearing potential.**

Animal Studies: In rats given 8 or 32 mg/kg/day of isotretinoin (1.3 to 5.3 times the recommended clinical dose of 1.0 mg/kg/day after normalization for total body surface area) for 18 months or longer, the incidences of focal calcification, fibrosis and inflammation of the myocardium, calcification of coronary, pulmonary and mesenteric arteries, and metastatic calcification of the gastric mucosa were greater than in control rats of similar age. Focal endocardial and myocardial calcifications associated with calcification of the coronary arteries were observed in two dogs after approximately 6 to 7 months of treatment with isotretinoin at a dosage of 60 to 120 mg/kg/day (30 to 60 times the recommended clinical dose of 1.0 mg/kg/day, respectively, after normalization for total body surface area).

Hearing Impairment

Impaired hearing has been reported in patients taking isotretinoin; in some cases, the hearing impairment has been reported to persist after therapy has been discontinued. Mechanism(s) and causality for this event have not been established. Patients who experience tinnitus or hearing impairment should discontinue Amnesteem treatment and be referred for specialized care for further evaluation (see ADVERSE REACTIONS: Special Senses).

Hepatotoxicity

Clinical hepatitis considered to be possibly or probably related to isotretinoin therapy has been reported. Additionally, mild to moderate elevations of liver enzymes have been observed in approximately 15% of individuals treated during clinical trials, some of which normalized with dosage reduction or continued administration of the drug. If normalization does not readily occur or if hepatitis is suspected during treatment with Amnesteem, the drug should be discontinued and the etiology further investigated.

Inflammatory Bowel Disease

Isotretinoin has been associated with inflammatory bowel disease (including regional ileitis) in patients without a prior history of intestinal disorders. In some instances, symptoms have been reported to persist after isotretinoin treatment has been stopped. Patients experiencing abdominal pain, rectal bleeding or severe diarrhea should discontinue Amnesteem immediately (see ADVERSE REACTIONS: Gastrointestinal).

Skeletal

Bone Mineral Density

Effects of multiple courses of isotretinoin on the developing musculoskeletal system are unknown. There is some evidence that long-term, high-dose, or multiple courses of therapy with isotretinoin have more of an effect than a single course of therapy on the musculoskeletal system. In an open-label clinical trial (N=217) of a single course of therapy with isotretinoin for severe recalcitrant nodular acne, bone density measurements at several skeletal sites were not significantly decreased (lumbar spine change >−4% and total hip change >−5%) or were increased in the majority of patients. One patient had a decrease in lumbar spine bone mineral density >4% based on unadjusted data. Sixteen (7.9%) patients had decreases in lumbar spine bone mineral density >4%, and all the other patients (92%) did not have significant decreases or had increases (adjusted for body mass index). Nine patients (4.5%) had a decrease in total hip bone mineral density >5% based on unadjusted data. Twenty-one (10.6%) patients had decreases in total hip bone mineral density >5%, and all the other patients (89%) did not have significant decreases or had increases (adjusted for body mass index). Follow-up studies performed in 8 of the patients with decreased bone mineral density for up to 11 months thereafter demonstrated increasing bone density in 5 patients at the lumbar spine, while the other 3 patients had lumbar spine bone density measurements below baseline values. Total hip bone mineral densities remained below baseline (range -1.6% to -7.6%) in 5 of 8 patients (62.5%).

In a separate open-label extension study of 10 patients, ages 13-18 years, who started a second course of isotretinoin 4 months after the first course, two patients showed a decrease in mean lumbar spine bone mineral density up to 3.25% (see PRECAUTIONS: Pediatric Use).

Spontaneous reports of osteoporosis, osteopenia, bone fractures, and delayed healing of bone fractures have been seen in the isotretinoin population. While causality to isotretinoin has not been established, an effect cannot be ruled out. Longer term effects have not been studied. It is important that Amnesteem be given at the recommended doses for no longer than the recommended duration.

Hyperostosis

A high prevalence of skeletal hyperostosis was noted in clinical trials for disorders of keratinization with a mean dose of 2.24 mg/kg/day. Additionally, skeletal hyperostosis was noted in 6 of 8 patients in a prospective study of disorders of keratinization.[6] Minimal skeletal hyperostosis and calcification of ligaments and tendons have also been observed by x-ray in prospective studies of nodular acne patients treated with a single course of therapy at recommended doses. The skeletal effects of multiple isotretinoin capsules treatment courses for acne are unknown.

In a clinical study of 217 pediatric patients (12 to 17 years) with severe recalcitrant nodular acne, hyperostosis was not observed after 16 to 20 weeks of treatment with approximately 1 mg/kg/day of isotretinoin given in two divided doses. Hyperostosis may require a longer time frame to appear. The clinical course and significance remain unknown.

Premature Epiphyseal Closure

There are spontaneous reports of premature epiphyseal closure in acne patients receiving recommended doses of isotretinoin. The effect of multiple courses of isotretinoin capsules treatment on epiphyseal closure are unknown.

Vision Impairment

Visual problems should be carefully monitored. All Amnesteem patients experiencing visual difficulties should discontinue Amnesteem treatment and have an ophthalmological examination (see ADVERSE REACTIONS: Special Senses).

Corneal Opacities

Corneal opacities have occurred in patients receiving isotretinoin for acne and more frequently when higher drug dosages were used in patients with disorders of keratinization. The corneal opacities that have been observed in clinical trial patients treated with isotretinoin have either completely resolved or were resolving at follow-up 6 to 7 weeks after discontinuation of the drug (see ADVERSE REACTIONS: Special Senses).

Decreased Night Vision

Decreased night vision has been reported during isotretinoin therapy and in some instances the event has persisted after therapy was discontinued. Because the onset in some patients was sudden, patients should be advised of this potential problem and warned to be cautious when driving or operating any vehicle at night.

PRECAUTIONS

The Amnesteem Pregnancy Prevention Risk Management Programs consist of the *System to Prevent Isotretinoin-Related Issues of Teratogenicity* (S.P.I.R.I.T.) and the Amnesteem Pregnancy Prevention Initiative. S.P.I.R.I.T. should be followed for prescribing Amnesteem with the goal of preventing fetal exposure to isotretinoin. It consists of: 1) reading the booklet entitled *System to Prevent Isotretinoin-Related Issues of Teratogenicity* (S.P.I.R.I.T.) *Guide to Best Practices*, 2) signing and returning the completed S.P.I.R.I.T. *Letter of Understanding* containing the Prescriber Checklist, 3) a yellow self-adhesive isotretinoin qualification sticker to be affixed to the prescription page. In addition, the patient education material, *A Personal Guide to Your Prescription*, should be used with each patient. The following further describes each component:

1) The S.P.I.R.I.T. *Guide to Best Practices* includes: isotretinoin teratogenic potential, information on pregnancy testing, specific information about effective contraception, the limitations of contraceptive methods and behaviors associated with an increased risk of contraceptive failure and pregnancy, the methods to evaluate pregnancy risk, and the method to complete a qualified Amnesteem prescription.
2) The S.P.I.R.I.T. *Letter of Understanding* attests that Amnesteem prescribers understand that isotretinoin is a teratogen, have read the S.P.I.R.I.T. *Guide to Best Practices*, understand their responsibilities in preventing exposure of pregnant females to isotretinoin and the procedures for qualifying female patients as defined in the boxed CONTRAINDICATIONS AND WARNINGS.
   The Prescriber Checklist attests that Amnesteem prescribers know the risk and severity of injury/birth defects from isotretinoin; know how to diagnose and treat the various presentations of acne; know the risk factors for unplanned pregnancy and the effective measures for avoidance; will refer the patient for, or provide, detailed pregnancy prevention counseling to help the patient have knowledge and tools needed to fulfill their ultimate responsibility to avoid becoming pregnant; understand and properly use throughout the isotretinoin capsules treatment course, the revised risk management procedures, including monthly pregnancy avoidance counseling, pregnancy testing, and use of qualified prescriptions with the yellow self-adhesive isotretinoin qualification sticker.
3) The yellow self-adhesive isotretinoin qualification sticker is used as documentation that the prescriber has qualified the female patient according to the qualification criteria (see boxed CONTRAINDICATIONS AND WARNINGS).
4) Amnesteem Pregnancy Prevention Initiative is a systematic approach to comprehensive patient education about their responsibilities and includes education for contraception compliance and reinforcement of educational messages. The Amnesteem Pregnancy Prevention Initiative includes information on the risks and benefits of isotretinoin which is linked to the Amnesteem Medication Guide dispensed by pharmacists with each prescription.
   Male and female patients are provided with separate booklets. Each booklet contains information on Amnesteem therapy, including precautions and warnings, an Informed Consent/Patient Agreement form, and a toll-free line which provides Amnesteem information in English and Spanish.
   The booklet for male patients, *A Personal Guide to Your Prescription for Men*, also includes information about male reproduction, a warning not to share Amnesteem with others or to donate blood during Amnesteem therapy and for 1 month following discontinuation of Amnesteem.
   The booklet for female patients, *A Personal Guide to Your Prescription for Women*, also includes a referral program that offers females free contraception counseling, reimbursed by Bertek Pharmaceuticals Inc., by a reproductive specialist; a second Patient Information/Consent form concerning birth defects, obtaining her consent to be treated within this agreement; an enrollment form for the *Isotretinoin Survey;* and a qualification checklist affirming the conditions under which female patients may receive Amnesteem. In addition, there is information on the types of contraceptive methods, the selection and use of appropriate, effective contraception, and the rates of possible contraceptive failure; a toll-free contraception counseling line; and patient education videos — the video *Don't Risk It: The importance of preventing pregnancy while you're taking Amnesteem®*, and the video *Birth Defects and Amnesteem®: Things You Should Know.*

General

Although an effect of isotretinoin on bone loss is not established, physicians should use caution when prescribing Amnesteem to patients with a genetic predisposition for age-related osteoporosis, a history of childhood osteoporosis conditions, osteomalacia, or other disorders of bone metabolism. This would include patients diagnosed with anorexia nervosa and those who are on chronic drug therapy that causes drug-induced osteoporosis/osteomalacia and/or affects vitamin D metabolism, such as systemic corticosteroids and any anticonvulsant.

Patients may be at increased risk when participating in sports with repetitive impact where the risks of spondylolisthesis with and without pars fractures and hip growth plate injuries in early and late adolescence are known. There are spontaneous reports of fractures and/or delayed healing in patients while on treatment with isotretinoin or following cessation of treatment with isotretinoin while involved in these activities. While causality to isotretinoin has not been established, an effect cannot be ruled out.

Information for Patients and Prescribers

- Patients should be instructed to read the Medication Guide supplied as required by law when isotretinoin capsules are dispensed. The complete text of the Medication Guide is reprinted at the end of this document. For additional information, patients should also read the *Patient Product Information, Important Information Concerning Your Treatment with Amnesteem.* All patients should sign the Informed Consent/Patient Agreement.
- Females of childbearing potential should be instructed that they must not be pregnant when Amnesteem therapy is initiated, and that they should use 2 forms of effective contraception 1 month before starting Amnesteem, while taking Amnesteem, and for 1 month after Amnesteem has been stopped. They should also sign a consent form prior to beginning Amnesteem therapy. They should be given an opportunity to enroll in the *Isotretinoin Survey* and to review the patient videotapes provided by Bertek Pharmaceuticals Inc. to the prescriber. The videos include information about contraception, the most common reasons that contraception fails, and the importance of using 2 forms of effective contraception when taking teratogenic drugs and comprehensive information about types of potential birth defects which could occur if a woman who is pregnant takes isotretinoin at any time during pregnancy. Female patients should be seen by their prescribers monthly and have a urine or serum pregnancy test performed each month during treatment to confirm negative pregnancy status before another Amnesteem prescription is written (see boxed CONTRAINDICATIONS AND WARNINGS).
- Isotretinoin is found in the semen of male patients taking isotretinoin capsules, but the amount delivered to a female partner would be about 1 million times lower than an oral dose of 40 mg. While the no-effect limit for isotretinoin-induced embryopathy is unknown, 20 years of postmarketing reports include 4 with isolated defects compatible with features of retinoid exposed fetuses. None of these cases had the combination of malformations characteristic of retinoid exposure, and all had other possible explanations for the defects observed.
- Patients may report mental health problems or family history of psychiatric disorders. These reports should be discussed with the patient and/or the patient's family. A referral to a mental health professional may be necessary. The physician should consider whether or not Amnesteem therapy is appropriate in this setting (see WARNINGS: Psychiatric Disorders).
- Patients should be informed that they must not share Amnesteem with anyone else because of the risk of birth defects and other serious adverse events.
- Patients should not donate blood during therapy and for 1 month following discontinuance of the drug because the blood might be given to a pregnant woman whose fetus must not be exposed to isotretinoin.
- Patients should be reminded to take Amnesteem with a meal (see DOSAGE AND ADMINISTRATION). To decrease the risk of esophageal irritation, patients should swallow the capsules with a full glass of liquid.
- Patients should be informed that transient exacerbation (flare) of acne has been seen, generally during the initial period of therapy.
- Wax epilation and skin resurfacing procedures (such as dermabrasion, laser) should be avoided during Amnesteem therapy and for at least 6 months thereafter due to the possibility of scarring (see ADVERSE REACTIONS: Skin and Appendages).
- Patients should be advised to avoid prolonged exposure to UV rays or sunlight.
- Patients should be informed that they may experience decreased tolerance to contact lenses during and after therapy.
- Patients should be informed that approximately 16% of patients treated with isotretinoin in a clinical trial devel-

Continued on next page

Amnesteem—Cont.

oped musculoskeletal symptoms (including arthralgia) during treatment. In general, these symptoms were mild to moderate, but occasionally required discontinuation of the drug. Transient pain in the chest has been reported less frequently. In the clinical trial, these symptoms generally cleared rapidly after discontinuation of isotretinoin, but in some cases persisted (see ADVERSE REACTIONS: Musculoskeletal). There have been rare postmarketing reports of rhabdomyolysis, some associated with strenuous physical activity (see Laboratory Tests: CPK)

- Pediatric patients and their caregivers should be informed that approximately 29% (104/358) of pediatric patients treated with isotretinoin developed back pain. Back pain was severe in 13.5% (14/104) of the cases and occurred at a higher frequency in female than male patients. Arthralgias were experienced in 22% (79/358) of pediatric-patients. Arthralgias were severe in 7.6% (6/79) of patients. Appropriate evaluation of the musculoskeletal system should be done in patients who present with these symptoms during or after a course of isotretinoin. Consideration should be given to discontinuation of isotretinoin if any significant abnormality is found.
- Neutropenia and rare cases of agranulocytosis have been reported. Amnesteem should be discontinued if clinically significant decreases in white cell counts occur.

Hypersensitivity

Anaphylactic reactions and other allergic reactions have been reported. Cutaneous allergic reactions and serious cases of allergic vasculitis, often with purpura (bruises and red patches) of the extremities and extracutaneous involvement (including renal) have been reported. Severe allergic reaction necessitates discontinuation of therapy and appropriate medical management.

Drug Interactions

- *Vitamin A:* Because of the relationship of isotretinoin to vitamin A, patients should be advised against taking vitamin supplements containing vitamin A to avoid additive toxic effects.
- *Tetracyclines:* Concomitant treatment with isotretinoin and tetracyclines should be avoided because isotretinoin use has been associated with a number of cases of pseudotumor cerebri (benign intracranial hypertension), some of which involved concomitant use of tetracyclines.
- *Micro-dosed Progesterone Preparations:* Micro-dosed progesterone preparations ("minipills" that do not contain an estrogen) may be an inadequate method of contraception during isotretinoin capsules therapy. Although other hormonal contraceptives are highly effective, there have been reports of pregnancy from women who have used combined oral contraceptives, as well as topical/injectable/implantable/insertable hormonal birth control products. These reports are more frequent for women who use only a single method of contraception. It is not known if hormonal contraceptives differ in their effectiveness when used with isotretinoin. Therefore, it is critically important for women of childbearing potential to select and commit to use 2 forms of effective contraception simultaneously, at least 1 of which must be a primary form, unless absolute abstinence is the chosen method, or the patient has undergone a hysterectomy (see boxed CONTRAINDICATIONS AND WARNINGS).
- *Phenytoin:* Isotretinoin has not been shown to alter the pharmacokinetics of phenytoin in a study in seven healthy volunteers. These results are consistent with the in vitro finding that neither isotretinoin nor its metabolites induce or inhibit the activity of the CYP 2C9 human hepatic P450 enzyme. Phenytoin is known to cause osteomalacia. No formal clinical studies have been conducted to assess if there is an interactive effect on bone loss between phenytoin and isotretinoin. Therefore, caution should be exercised when using these drugs together.
- *Systemic Corticosteroids:* Systemic corticosteroids are known to cause osteoporosis. No formal clinical studies have been conducted to assess if there is an interactive effect on bone loss between systemic corticosteroids and isotretinoin. Therefore, caution should be exercised when using these drugs together.

Prescribers are advised to consult the package insert of medication administered concomitantly with hormonal contraceptives, since some medications may decrease the effectiveness of these birth control products. **Isotretinoin use is associated with depression in some patients (See WARNINGS: Psychiatric Disorders and ADVERSE REACTIONS: Psychiatric).** Patients should be prospectively cautioned not to self-medicate with the herbal supplement St. John's Wort because a possible interaction has been suggested with hormonal contraceptives based on reports of breakthrough bleeding on oral contraceptives shortly after starting St. John's Wort. Pregnancies have been reported by users of combined hormonal contraceptives who also used some form of St. John's Wort.

Laboratory Tests

Pregnancy Test

Female patients of childbearing potential must have negative results from 2 urine or serum pregnancy tests with a sensitivity of at least 25 mIU/mL before receiving the initial Amnesteem prescription. The first test is obtained by the prescriber when the decision is made to pursue qualification of the patient for Amnesteem (a screening test). The second pregnancy test (a confirmation test) should be done during the first 5 days of the menstrual period immediately preceding the beginning of Amnesteem therapy. For patients with amenorrhea, the second test should be done at least 11 days after the last act of unprotected sexual intercourse (without using 2 effective forms of contraception).

Each month of therapy, the patient must have a negative result from a urine or serum pregnancy test. A pregnancy test must be repeated each month prior to the female patient receiving each prescription.

- *Lipids:* Pretreatment and follow-up blood lipids should be obtained under fasting conditions. After consumption of alcohol, at least 36 hours should elapse before these determinations are made. It is recommended that these tests be performed at weekly or biweekly intervals until the lipid response to isotretinoin is established. The incidence of hypertriglyceridemia is 1 patient in 4 on isotretinoin therapy (see WARNINGS: Lipids).
- *Liver Function Tests:* Since elevations of liver enzymes have been observed during clinical trials, and hepatitis has been reported, pretreatment and follow-up liver function tests should be performed at weekly or biweekly intervals until the response to isotretinoin has been established (see WARNINGS: Hepatotoxicity).
- *Glucose:* Some patients receiving isotretinoin have experienced problems in the control of their blood sugar. In addition, new cases of diabetes have been diagnosed during isotretinoin therapy, although no causal relationship has been established.
- *CPK:* Some patients undergoing vigorous physical activity while on isotretinoin therapy have experienced elevated CPK levels; however, the clinical significance is unknown. There have been rare postmarketing reports of rhabdomyolysis, some associated with strenuous physical activity. In a clinical trial of 217 pediatric patients (12 to 17 years) with severe recalcitrant nodular acne, transient elevations in CPK were observed in 12% of patients, including those undergoing strenuous physical activity in association with reported musculoskeletal adverse events such as back pain, arthralgia, limb injury, or muscle sprain. In these patients, approximately half of the CPK elevations returned to normal within 2 weeks and half returned to normal within 4 weeks. No cases of rhabdomyolysis were reported in this trial.

Carcinogenesis, Mutagenesis and Impairment of Fertility

In male and female Fischer 344 rats given oral isotretinoin at dosages of 8 or 32 mg/kg/day (1.3 to 5.3 times the recommended clinical dose of 1.0 mg/kg/day, respectively, after normalization for total body surface area) for greater than 18 months, there was a dose-related increased incidence of pheochromocytoma relative to controls. The incidence of adrenal medullary hyperplasia was also increased at the higher dosage in both sexes. The relatively high level of spontaneous pheochromocytomas occurring in the male Fischer 344 rat makes it an equivocal model for study of this tumor; therefore, the relevance of this tumor to the human population is uncertain.

The Ames test was conducted with isotretinoin in two laboratories. The results of the tests in one laboratory were negative while in the second laboratory a weakly positive response (less than 1.6 × background) was noted in *S. typhimurium* TA100 when the assay was conducted with metabolic activation. No dose-response effect was seen and all other strains were negative. Additionally, other tests designed to assess genotoxicity (Chinese hamster cell assay, mouse micronucleus test, *S. cerevisiae* D7 assay, in vitro clastogenesis assay with human-derived lymphocytes, and unscheduled DNA synthesis assay) were all negative.

In rats, no adverse on gonadal function, fertility, conception rate, gestation or parturition were observed at oral dosages of isotretinoin of 2, 8 or 32 mg/kg/day (0.3, 1.3 or 5.3 times the recommended clinical dose of 1.0 mg/kg/day, respectively, after normalization for total body surface area).

In dogs, testicular atrophy was noted after treatment with oral isotretinoin for approximately 30 weeks at dosages of 20 or 60 mg/kg/day (10 or 30 times the recommended clinical dose of 1.0 mg/kg/day, respectively, after normalization for total body surface area). In general, there was microscopic evidence for appreciable depression of spermatogenesis but some sperm were observed in all testes examined and in no instance were completely atrophic tubules seen. In studies of 66 men, 30 of whom were patients with nodular acne under treatment with oral isotretinoin, no significant changes were noted in the count or motility of spermatozoa in the ejaculate. In a study of 50 men (ages 17 to 32 years) receiving isotretinoin therapy for nodular acne, no significant effects were seen on ejaculate volume, sperm count, total sperm motility, morphology or seminal plasma fructose.

Pregnancy: Category X. See boxed CONTRAINDICATIONS AND WARNINGS.

Nursing Mothers

It is not known whether this drug is excreted in human milk. Because of the potential for adverse effects, nursing mothers should not receive isotretinoin capsules.

Pediatric Use

The use of isotretinoin in pediatric patients less than 12 years of age has not been studied. The use of isotretinoin for the treatment of severe recalcitrant nodular acne in pediatric patients ages 12 to 17 years should be given careful consideration, especially for those patients where a known metabolic or structural bone disease exists (see PRECAUTIONS: General).

Evidence supporting the use of isotretinoin in this age group for severe recalcitrant nodular acne is approved for Hoffman La-Roche's isotretinoin capsules. However, due to Hoffman La-Roche's marketing exclusivity rights, this drug is not labeled for pediatric use.

In studies with isotretinoin, adverse reactions reported in pediatric patients were similar to those described in adults except for the increased incidence of back pain and arthralgia (both of which were sometimes severe) and myalgia in pediatric patients (see ADVERSE REACTIONS).

In an open-label clinical trial (N=217) of a single course of therapy with isotretinoin for severe recalcitrant nodular acne, bone density measurements at several skeletal sites were not significantly decreased (lumbar spine change >−4% and total hip change >−5%) or were increased in the majority of patients. One patient had a decrease in lumbar spine bone mineral density >4% based on unadjusted data. Sixteen (7.9%) patients had decreases in lumbar spine bone mineral density >4%, and all the other patients (92%) did not have significant decreases or had increases (adjusted for body mass index). Nine patients (4.5%) had a decrease in total hip bone mineral density >5% based on unadjusted data. Twenty-one (10.6%) patients had decreases in total hip bone mineral density >5%, and all the other patients (89%) did not have significant decreases or had increases (adjusted for body mass index). Follow-up studies performed in 8 of the patients with decreased bone mineral density for up to 11 months thereafter demonstrated increasing bone density in 5 patients at the lumbar spine, while the other 3 patients had lumbar spine bone density measurements below baseline values. Total hip bone mineral densities remained below baseline (range –1.6% to –7.6%) in 5 of 8 patients (62.5%).

In a separate open-label extension study of 10 patients, ages 13-18 years, who started a second course of isotretinoin 4 months after the first course, two patients showed a decrease in mean lumbar spine bone mineral density up to 3.25% (See WARNINGS: Skeletal: Bone Mineral Density).

Geriatric Use

Clinical studies of isotretinoin did not include sufficient number of subjects aged 65 years and over to determine whether they respond differently from younger subjects. Although reported clinical experience has not identified differences in responses between the elderly and younger patients, effects of aging might be expected to increase some risks associated with isotretinoin therapy (see WARNINGS and PRECAUTIONS).

ADVERSE REACTIONS

Clinical Trials and Postmarketing Surveillance

The adverse reactions listed below reflect the experience from investigational studies of isotretinoin, and the postmarketing experience. The relationship of some of these events to isotretinoin therapy is unknown. Many of the side effects and adverse reactions seen in patients receiving isotretinoin are similar to those described in patients taking very high doses of vitamin A (dryness of the skin and mucous membranes, e.g., of the lips, nasal passage, and eyes).

Dose Relationship

Cheilitis and hypertriglyceridemia are usually dose related. Most adverse reactions reported in clinical trials were reversible when therapy was discontinued; however, some persisted after cessation of therapy (see WARNINGS and ADVERSE REACTIONS).

Body as a Whole

allergic reactions, including vasculitis, systemic hypersensitivity (see PRECAUTIONS: Hypersensitivity), edema, fatigue, lymphadenopathy, weight loss

Cardiovascular

palpitation, tachycardia, vascular thrombotic disease, stroke

Endocrine/Metabolic

hypertriglyceridemia (see WARNINGS: Lipids), alterations in blood sugar levels (see PRECAUTIONS: Laboratory Tests)

Gastrointestinal

inflammatory bowel disease (see WARNINGS: Inflammatory Bowel Disease), hepatitis (see WARNINGS: Hepatotoxicity), pancreatitis (see WARNINGS: Lipids), bleeding and inflammation of the gums, colitis, esophagitis/esophageal ulceration, ileitis, nausea, other nonspecific gastrointestinal symptoms

Hematologic

allergic reactions (see PRECAUTIONS: Hypersensitivity), anemia, thrombocytopenia, neutropenia, rare reports of agranulocytosis (see PRECAUTIONS: Information for Patients and Prescribers). See PRECAUTIONS: Laboratory Tests for other hematological parameters.

Musculoskeletal

skeletal hyperostosis, calcification of tendons and ligaments, premature epiphyseal closure, decreases in bone mineral density (see WARNINGS: Skeletal), musculoskeletal symptoms (sometimes severe) including back pain and arthralgia (see PRECAUTIONS: Information for Patients and Prescribers), transient pain in the chest (see PRECAUTIONS: Information for Patients and Prescribers), arthritis, tendonitis, other types of bone abnormalities, elevations of CPK/rare reports of rhabdomyolysis (see PRECAUTIONS: Laboratory Tests).

Neurological

pseudotumor cerebri (see WARNINGS: Pseudotumor Cerebri), dizziness, drowsiness, headache, insomnia, lethargy, malaise, nervousness, paresthesias, seizures, stroke, syncope, weakness

Psychiatric
suicidal ideation, suicide attempts, suicide, depression, psychosis, aggression, violent behaviors (see WARNINGS: Psychiatric Disorders), emotional instability
Of the patients reporting depression, some reported that the depression subsided with discontinuation of therapy and recurred with reinstitution of therapy.
Reproductive System
abnormal menses
Respiratory
bronchospasms (with or without a history of asthma), respiratory infection, voice alteration
Skin and Appendages
acne fulminans, alopecia (which in some cases persists), bruising, cheilitis (dry lips), dry mouth, dry nose, dry skin, epistaxis, eruptive xanthomas[7] flushing, fragility of skin, hair abnormalities, hirsutism, hyperpigmentation and hypopigmentation, infections (including disseminated herpes simplex), nail dystrophy, paronychia, peeling of palms and soles, photoallergic/photosensitizing reactions, pruritus, pyogenic granuloma, rash (including facial erythema, seborrhea, and eczema), sunburn susceptibility increased, sweating, urticaria, vasculitis (including Wegener's granulomatosis; see PRECAUTIONS: Hypersensitivity), abnormal wound healing (delayed healing or exuberant granulation tissue with crusting; see PRECAUTIONS: Information for Patients and Prescribers)
Special Senses:
Hearing: hearing impairment (see WARNINGS: Hearing Impairment), tinnitus
Vision: corneal opacities (see WARNINGS: Corneal Opacities), decreased night vision which may persist (see WARNINGS: Decreased Night Vision), cataracts, color vision disorder, conjunctivitis, dry eyes, eyelid inflammation, keratitis, optic neuritis, photophobia, visual disturbances
Urinary System
glomerulonephritis (see PRECAUTIONS: Hypersensitivity), nonspecific urogenital findings (see PRECAUTIONS: Laboratory Tests for other urological parameters)

Laboratory
Elevation of plasma triglycerides (see WARNINGS: Lipids), decrease in serum high-density lipoprotein (HDL) levels, elevations of serum cholesterol during treatment
Increased alkaline phosphatase, SGOT (AST), SGPT (ALT), GGTP or LDH (see WARNINGS: Hepatotoxicity)
Elevation of fasting blood sugar, elevations of CPK (see PRECAUTIONS: Laboratory Tests), hyperuricemia
Decreases in red blood cell parameters, decreases in white blood cell counts (including severe neutropenia and rare reports of agranulocytosis; see PRECAUTIONS: Information for Patients and Prescribers), elevated sedimentation rates, elevated platelet counts, thrombocytopenia
White cells in the urine, proteinuria, microscopic or gross hematuria

OVERDOSAGE

The oral LD_{50} of isotretinoin is greater than 4000 mg/kg in rats and mice (>600 times the recommended clinical dose of 1.0 mg/kg/day after normalization of the rat dose for total body surface area and >300 times the recommended clinical dose of 1.0 mg/kg/day after normalization of the mouse dose for total body surface area) and is approximately 1960 mg/kg in rabbits (653 times the recommended clinical dose of 1.0 mg/kg/day after normalization for total body surface area). In humans, overdosage has been associated with vomiting, facial flushing, cheilosis, abdominal pain, headache, dizziness, and ataxia. All symptoms quickly resolved without apparent residual effects.
Isotretinoin causes serious birth defects at any dosage (see boxed CONTRAINDICATIONS AND WARNINGS). Females of childbearing potential who present with isotretinoin overdose must be evaluated for pregnancy. Patients who are pregnant should receive counseling about the risks to the fetus, as described in the boxed CONTRAINDICATIONS AND WARNINGS. Non-pregnant patients must be warned to avoid pregnancy for at least one month and receive contraceptive counseling as described in the boxed CONTRAINDICATIONS AND WARNINGS. Educational materials for such patients can be obtained by calling Bertek Pharmaceuticals Inc. Because an overdose would be expected to result in higher levels of isotretinoin in semen than found during a normal treatment course, male patients should use a condom, or avoid reproductive sexual activity with a female who is or might become pregnant, for 30 days after the overdose. All patients with isotretinoin overdose should not donate blood for at least 30 days.

DOSAGE AND ADMINISTRATION

Amnesteem should be administered with a meal (see PRECAUTIONS: Information for Patients and Prescribers).
The recommended dosage range for Amnesteem is 0.5 to 1.0 mg/kg/day given in two divided doses with food for 15 to 20 weeks. In studies comparing 0.1, 0.5, and 1.0 mg/kg/day[8], it was found that all dosages provided initial clearing of disease, but there was a greater need for retreatment with the lower dosages. During treatment, the dose may be adjusted according to response of the disease and/or the appearance of clinical side effects — some of which may be dose related. Adult patients whose disease is very severe with scarring or is primarily manifested on the trunk may require dose adjustments up to 2.0 mg/kg/day, as tolerated. Failure to take Amnesteem with food will significantly decrease absorption. Before upward dose adjustments are made, the patient should be questioned about their compliance with food instructions.

Table 3. Amnesteem Dosing by Body Weight (Based on Administration with Food)

Body Weight		Total mg/day		
kilograms	pounds	0.5 mg/kg	1 mg/kg	2 mg/kg*
40	88	20	40	80
50	110	25	50	100
60	132	30	60	120
70	154	35	70	140
80	176	40	80	160
90	198	45	90	180
100	220	50	100	200

* See DOSAGE AND ADMINISTRATION: the recommended dosage range is 0.5 to 1.0 mg/kg/day.

The safety of once daily dosing with Amnesteem has not been established. Once daily dosing is **not** recommended.
If the total nodule count has been reduced by more than 70% prior to completing 15 to 20 weeks of treatment, the drug may be discontinued. After a period of 2 months or more off therapy, and if warranted by persistent or recurring severe nodular acne, a second course of therapy may be initiated. The optimal interval before retreatment has not been defined for patients who have not completed skeletal growth. Long-term use of Amnesteem, even in low doses, has not been studied, and is not recommended. It is important that Amnesteem be given at the recommended doses for no longer than the recommended duration. The effect of long-term use of Amnesteem on bone loss is unknown (see WARNINGS: Skeletal: Bone Mineral Density, Hyperostosis, and Premature Epiphyseal Closure).
Contraceptive measures must be followed for any subsequent course of therapy (see boxed CONTRAINDICATIONS AND WARNINGS).
[See table 3 above]

Information for Pharmacists

Amnesteem must only be dispensed in no more than a 30-day supply and only on presentation of an isotretinoin prescription with a yellow self-adhesive isotretinoin qualification sticker within 7 days of the qualification date. **REFILLS REQUIRE A NEW WRITTEN PRESCRIPTION WITH A YELLOW SELF-ADHESIVE ISOTRETINOIN QUALIFICATION STICKER WITHIN 7 DAYS OF THE QUALIFICATION DATE.** No telephone or computerized prescriptions are permitted.
An Amnesteem Medication Guide must be given to the patient each time Amnesteem is dispensed, as required by law. This Amnesteem Medication Guide is an important part of the risk management program for the patient.

HOW SUPPLIED

Soft gelatin capsules, 10 mg (reddish brown), imprinted I10.
– Cartons of 30 containing 3 Prescription Paks of 10 capsules NDC 62794-611-93
– Cartons of 100 containing 10 Prescription Paks of 10 capsules NDC 62794-611-88
Soft gelatin capsules, 20 mg (reddish brown and cream), imprinted I20.
– Cartons of 30 containing 3 Prescription Paks of 10 capsules NDC 62794-612-93
– Cartons of 100 containing 10 Prescription Paks of 10 capsules NDC 62794-612-88
Soft gelatin capsules, 40 mg (orange-brown), imprinted I40.
– Cartons of 30 containing 3 Prescription Paks of 10 capsules NDC 62794-614-93
– Cartons of 100 containing 10 Prescription Paks of 10 capsules NDC 62794-614-88

Storage
Store at controlled room temperature (59° to 86°F, 15° to 30°C). Protect from light.

REFERENCES

1. Peck GL, Olsen TG, Yoder FW, et al. Prolonged remissions of cystic and conglobate acne with 13-*cis*-retinoic acid. *N Engl J Med* 300:329-333, 1979.
2. Pochi PE, Shalita AR, Strauss JS, Webster SB. Report of the consensus conference on acne classification. *J Am Acad Dermatol* 24: 495-500, 1991.
3. Farrell LN, Strauss JS, Stranieri AM. The treatment of severe cystic acne with 13-*cis*-retinoic acid: evaluation of sebum production and the clinical response in a multiple-dose trial. *J Am Acad Dermatol* 3:602-611, 1980.
4. Jones H, Blanc D, Cunliffe WJ. 13-*cis*-retinoic acid and acne. *Lancet* 2:1048-1049, 1980.
5. Katz RA, Jorgensen H, Nigra TP. Elevation of serum triglyceride levels from oral isotretinoin in disorders of keratinization. *Arch Dermatol* 116:1369-1372, 1980.
6. Ellis CN, Madison KC, Pennes DR, Martel W, Voorhees JJ. Isotretinoin therapy is associated with early skeletal radiographic changes. *J Am Acad Dermatol* 10:1024-1029, 1984.
7. Dicken CH, Connolly SM. Eruptive xanthomas associated with isotretinoin (13-*cis*-retinoic acid). *Arch Dermatol* 116:951-952, 1980.
8. Strauss JS, Rapini RP, Shalita AR, et al. Isotretinoin therapy for acne: results of a multicenter dose-response study. *J Am Acad Dermatol* 10:490-496, 1984.

PATIENT INFORMATION/CONSENT (FOR FEMALE PATIENTS CONCERNING BIRTH DEFECTS)

To be completed by the patient, her parent/guardian* and signed by her prescriber.

Read each item below and initial in the space provided to show that you understand each item and agree to follow your prescriber's instructions. **Do not sign this consent and do not take Amnesteem® (isotretinoin) if there is anything that you do not understand.**
*A parent or guardian of a minor patient (under age 18) must also read and initial each item before signing the consent.

____
(Patient's Name)

1. I understand that there is a very high risk that my unborn baby could have severe birth defects if I am pregnant or become pregnant while taking isotretinoin capsules in any amount even for short periods of time. This is why I must not be pregnant while taking Amnesteem.
Initial: _____
2. I understand that I must not take Amnesteem® (isotretinoin) if I am pregnant.
Initial: _____
3. I understand that I must not get pregnant during the entire time of my treatment and for 1 month after the end of my treatment with Amnesteem.
Initial: _____
4. I understand that I must avoid sexual intercourse completely, or I must use 2 separate, effective forms of birth control (contraception) **at the same time.** The only exception is if I have had surgery to remove the womb (a hysterectomy).
Initial: _____
5. I understand that birth control pills and topical/injectable/implantable/insertable hormonal birth control products are among the most effective forms of birth control. However, any form of birth control can fail. Therefore, I must use 2 different methods at the same time, every time I have sexual intercourse, even if 1 of the methods I choose is birth control pills or topical/injectable/implantable/insertable hormonal birth control.
Initial: _____
6. I will talk with my prescriber about any drugs or herbal products I plan to take during my Amnesteem treatment because hormonal birth control methods (for example, birth control pills) may not work if I am taking certain drugs or herbal products (for example, St. John's Wort).
Initial: _____
7. I understand that the following are considered effective forms of birth control:
Primary: Tubal ligation (tying my tubes), partner's vasectomy, birth control pills, topical/injectable/ implantable/insertable hormonal birth control products, and an IUD (intrauterine device).
Secondary: Diaphragms, latex condoms, and cervical caps. Each must be used with a spermicide, which is a special cream or jelly that kills sperm.
I understand that at least 1 of my 2 methods of birth control must be a primary method.
Initial: _____
8. I understand that I may receive a free contraceptive (birth control) counseling session from a doctor or other family planning expert. My Amnesteem prescriber can give me an Amnesteem Patient Referral Form for this free consultation.
Initial: _____
9. I understand that I must begin using the birth control methods I have chosen as described above at least 1 month before I start taking Amnesteem.
Initial: _____
10. I understand that I cannot get a prescription for Amnesteem unless I have 2 negative pregnancy test results. The first pregnancy test should be done when my prescriber decides to prescribe Amnesteem. The second pregnancy test should be done during the first 5 days of my menstrual period right before starting Amnesteem therapy, or as instructed by my prescriber. I will then have 1 pregnancy test every month during my Amnesteem therapy.
Initial: _____

Continued on next page

Amnesteem—Cont.

11. I understand that I should not start taking Amnesteem until I am sure that I am not pregnant and have negative results from 2 pregnancy tests.
Initial: _____
12. I have read and understand the materials my prescriber has given to me, including the *Patient Product Information, Important Information Concerning Your Treatment with Amnesteem.* My prescriber gave me and asked me to watch the videos about contraception. I was told about a confidential counseling line that I may call for more information about birth control. I have received information on emergency contraception (birth control).
Initial: _____
13. I understand that I must stop taking Amnesteem right away and inform my prescriber if I get pregnant, miss my menstrual period, stop using birth control, or have sexual intercourse without using my 2 birth control methods at any time.
Initial: _____
14. My prescriber gave me information about the confidential *Isotretinoin Survey* and explained to me how important it is to take part in the *Isotretinoin Survey*.
Initial: _____
15. I understand that the yellow self-adhesive isotretinoin qualification sticker on my prescription for isotretinoin capsules means that I am qualified to receive an Amnesteem prescription, because I:
   - have had 2 negative urine or serum pregnancy tests before receiving the initial Amnesteem prescription. I must have a negative result from a urine or serum pregnancy test repeated each month prior to my receiving each subsequent prescription.
   - have selected and committed to use 2 forms of effective contraception simultaneously, at least 1 of which must be a primary form, unless absolute abstinence is the chosen method, or I have undergone a hysterectomy. I must use 2 forms of contraception for at least 1 month prior to initiation of isotretinoin capsules therapy, during therapy, and for 1 month after discontinuing therapy. I must receive counseling, repeated on a monthly basis, about contraception and behaviors associated with an increased risk of pregnancy.
   - have signed a Patient Information/Consent form that contains warnings about the risk of potential birth defects if I am pregnant or become pregnant and my unborn baby is exposed to isotretinoin.
   - have been informed of the purpose and importance of participating in the *Isotretinoin Survey* and given the opportunity to enroll.

Initial: _____

My prescriber has answered all my questions about Amnesteem and I understand that it is my responsibility not to get pregnant during Amnesteem treatment or for 1 month after I stop taking Amnesteem.
Initial: _____

I now authorize my prescriber _______________ to begin my treatment with Amnesteem.

Patient Signature: _______________ Date

Parent/Guardian Signature (if under age 18): _______________ Date

Please print: Patient Name and Address _______________

Telephone _______________

I have fully explained to the patient, _______________, the nature and purpose of the treatment described above and the risks to females of childbearing potential. I have asked the patient if she has any questions regarding her treatment with Amnesteem and have answered those questions to the best of my ability.

Prescriber Signature: _______________ Date

INFORMED CONSENT/PATIENT AGREEMENT (FOR ALL PATIENTS):

To be completed by patient
(parent or guardian if patient is under 18)
and signed by the prescriber.

Read each item below and initial in the space provided if you understand each item and agree to follow your prescriber's instructions. A parent or guardian of a patient under age 18 must also read and understand each item before signing the agreement.

Do not sign this agreement and do not take Amnesteem® (isotretinoin) if there is anything that you do not understand about all the information you have received about using Amnesteem.

1. I, _______________,
(Patient's Name)
understand that Amnesteem is a medicine used to treat severe nodular acne that cannot be cleared up by any other acne treatments, including antibiotics. In severe nodular acne, many red, swollen, tender lumps form in the skin. If untreated, severe nodular acne can lead to permanent scars.
Initials: _____
2. My prescriber has told me about my choices for treating my acne.
Initials: _____
3. I understand that there are serious side effects that may happen while I am taking isotretinoin capsules. These have been explained to me. These side effects include serious birth defects in babies of pregnant females. (Note: There is a second Informed Consent form for female patients concerning birth defects.)
Initials: _____
4. I understand that some patients, while taking isotretinoin or soon after stopping isotretinoin, have become depressed or developed other serious mental problems. Symptoms of these problems include sad, "anxious" or empty mood, irritability, anger, loss of pleasure or interest in social or sports activities, sleeping too much or too little, changes in weight or appetite, school or work performance going down, or trouble concentrating. Some patients taking isotretinoin have had thoughts about hurting themselves or putting an end to their own lives (suicidal thoughts). Some people tried to end their own lives. And some people have ended their own lives. There were reports that some of these people did not appear depressed. There have been reports of patients on isotretinoin becoming aggressive or violent. No one knows if isotretinoin caused these behaviors or if they would have happened even if the person did not take isotretinoin. Some people have had other signs of depression while taking isotretinoin (see #7 below).
Initials: _____
5. Before I start taking Amnesteem, I agree to tell my prescriber if, to the best of my knowledge, I have **ever** had symptoms of depression (see #7 below), been psychotic, attempted suicide, had any other mental problems, or take medicine for any of these problems. Being psychotic means having a loss of contact with reality, such as hearing voices or seeing things that are not there.
Initials: _____
6. Before I start taking Amnesteem, I agree to tell my prescriber if, to the best of my knowledge, anyone in my family has ever had symptoms of depression, been psychotic, attempted suicide, or had any other serious mental problems.
Initials: _____
7. Once I start taking Amnesteem, I agree to stop using Amnesteem and tell my prescriber right away if any of the following happen. I:
   - Start to feel sad or have crying spells
   - Lose interest in activities I once enjoyed
   - Sleep too much or have trouble sleeping
   - Become more irritable, angry, or aggressive than usual (for example, temper outbursts, thoughts of violence)
   - Have a change in my appetite or body weight
   - Have trouble concentrating
   - Withdraw from my friends or family
   - Feel like I have no energy
   - Have feelings of worthlessness or inappropriate guilt
   - Start having thoughts about hurting myself or taking my own life (suicidal thoughts)

   Initials: _____
8. **I agree to return to see my prescriber every month I take Amnesteem to get a new prescription for Amnesteem, to check my progress, and to check for signs of side effects.**
Initials: _____
9. Amnesteem will be prescribed just for me — I will not share Amnesteem with other people because it may cause serious side effects, including birth defects.
Initials: _____
10. I will not give blood while taking Amnesteem or for 1 month after I stop taking Amnesteem. I understand that if someone who is pregnant gets my donated blood, her baby may be exposed to isotretinoin and may be born with serious birth defects.
Initials: _____
11. I have read the *Patient Product Information, Important Information Concerning Your Treatment with Amnesteem,* and other materials my provider gave me containing important safety information about Amnesteem. I understand all the information I received.
Initials: _____
12. My prescriber and I have decided I should take Amnesteem. I understand that each of my Amnesteem prescriptions must have a yellow self-adhesive isotretinoin qualification sticker on it. I understand that I can stop taking Amnesteem at any time. I agree to tell my prescriber if I stop taking Amnesteem.
Initials: _____

I now authorize my prescriber _______________ to begin my treatment with Amnesteem.

Patient Signature: _______________ Date

Parent/Guardian Signature (if under age 18): _______________ Date

Patient Name (print) _______________

Patient Address _______________

Telephone _______________

I have:

- fully explained to the patient, _______________, the nature and purpose of Amnesteem treatment, including its benefits and risks
- given the patient the appropriate educational materials, *A Personal Guide to Your Prescription,* for Amnesteem and asked the patient if he/she has any questions regarding his/her treatment with Amnesteem
- answered those questions to the best of my ability
- placed the yellow self-adhesive isotretinoin qualification sticker on the prescription.

Prescriber Signature: _______________ Date

MEDICATION GUIDE

Read this Medication Guide every time you get a prescription or a refill for Amnesteem (am nes team). There may be new information. This information does not take the place of talking with your prescriber (doctor or other health care provider).

What is the most important information I should know about Amnesteem?

Amnesteem® (isotretinoin) is used to treat a type of severe acne (nodular acne) that has not been helped by other treatments, including antibiotics. However, isotretinoin can cause serious side effects. Before starting Amnesteem, discuss with your prescriber how bad your acne is, the possible benefits of Amnesteem, and its possible side effects, to decide if Amnesteem is right for you. Your prescriber will ask you to read and sign a form or forms indicating you understand some of the serious risks of Amnesteem.

Possible serious side effects of taking isotretinoin capsules include *birth defects* and *mental disorders*.

1. **Birth defects. Isotretinoin can cause birth defects (deformed babies) if taken by a pregnant woman.** It can also cause miscarriage (losing the baby before birth), premature (early) birth, or death of the baby. Do not take Amnesteem if you are pregnant or plan to become pregnant while you are taking Amnesteem. Do not get pregnant for 1 month after you stop taking Amnesteem. Also, if you get pregnant while taking Amnesteem, stop taking it right away and call your prescriber.
   All females should read the section in this Medication Guide "What are the important warnings for females taking Amnesteem?"
2. **Mental problems and suicide.** Some patients, while taking isotretinoin capsules or soon after stopping isotretinoin capsules, have become depressed or developed other serious mental problems. Symptoms of these problems include sad, "anxious" or empty mood, irritability, anger, loss of pleasure or interest in social or sports activities, sleeping too much or too little, changes in weight or appetite, school or work performance going down, or trouble concentrating. Some patients taking isotretinoin capsules have had thoughts about hurting themselves or putting an end to their own lives (suicidal thoughts). Some people tried to end their own lives. And some people have ended their own lives. There were reports that some of these people did not appear depressed. There have been reports of patients on isotretinoin becoming aggressive or violent. No one knows if isotretinoin capsules caused these behaviors or if they would have happened even if the person did not take isotretinoin capsules.
   All patients should read the section in this Medication Guide "What are the signs of mental problems?"
   For other possible serious side effects of isotretinoin capsules, see "What are the possible side effects of Amnesteem?" in this Medication Guide.

What are the important warnings for females taking Amnesteem?

You must not become pregnant while taking Amnesteem, or for 1 month after you stop taking Amnesteem. Isotretinoin can cause severe birth defects in babies of women who take it while they are pregnant, even if they take isotretinoin capsules for only a short time. **There is an extremely high risk that your baby will be deformed or will die** if you are pregnant while taking isotretinoin capsules. Taking isotretinoin capsules also increases the chance of miscarriage and premature births.

Female patients will not get their first prescription for Amnesteem unless there is proof they have had 2 negative pregnancy tests. The first test must be done when your prescriber decides to prescribe Amnesteem. The second pregnancy test must be done during the first 5 days of the menstrual period right before starting Amnesteem therapy, or as instructed by your prescriber. Each month of treatment, you must have a negative result from a urine or serum pregnancy test. Female patients cannot get another prescription for Amnesteem unless there is proof that they have had a negative pregnancy test.

A yellow self-adhesive isotretinoin qualification sticker on your prescription indicates to the pharmacist that you are qualified by your prescriber to get Amnesteem.

While you are taking Amnesteem, you **must** use effective birth control. **You must use 2 separate effective forms of birth control at the same time** for at least 1 month before starting Amnesteem, while you take it, and for 1 month after you stop taking it. You can either discuss effective birth control methods with your prescriber or go for a free visit to discuss birth control with another physician or family planning expert. Your prescriber can arrange this free visit, which will be paid for by Bertek Pharmaceuticals Inc.

You must use 2 separate forms of effective birth control because any method, including birth control pills and sterilization, can fail. There are only 2 reasons you would not need to use 2 separate methods of effective birth control:

1. You have had your womb removed by surgery (a hysterectomy).
2. You are absolutely certain you will not have genital-to-genital sexual contact with a male before, during, and for 1 month after isotretinoin capsules treatment.

If you have sex at any time without using 2 forms of effective birth control, get pregnant, or miss your period, stop using Amnesteem and call your prescriber right away.

All patients should read the rest of this Medication Guide.

What are the signs of mental problems?
Tell your prescriber if, to the best of your knowledge, you or someone in your family has ever had any mental illness, including depression, suicidal behavior, or psychosis. Psychosis means a loss of contact with reality, such as hearing voices or seeing things that are not there. Also, tell your prescriber if you take medicines for any of these problems.

Stop using Amnesteem and tell your prescriber right away if you:

- Start to feel sad or have crying spells
- Lose interest in activities you once enjoyed
- Sleep too much or have trouble sleeping
- Become more irritable, angry, or aggressive than usual (for example, temper outbursts, thoughts of violence)
- Have a change in your appetite or body weight
- Have trouble concentrating
- Withdraw from your friends or family
- Feel like you have no energy
- Have feelings of worthlessness or inappropriate guilt
- Start having thoughts about hurting yourself or taking your own life (suicidal thoughts)

What is Amnesteem?
Amnesteem is used to treat the most severe form of acne (nodular acne) that cannot be cleared up by any other acne treatments, including antibiotics. In severe nodular acne, many red, swollen, tender lumps form in the skin. These can be the size of pencil erasers or larger. If untreated, nodular acne can lead to permanent scars. However, because isotretinoin can have serious side effects, you should talk with your prescriber about all of the possible treatments for your acne, and whether Amnesteem's possible benefits outweigh its possible risks.

Who should not take Amnesteem?

- **Do not take Amnesteem if you are pregnant, plan to become pregnant, or become pregnant during Amnesteem treatment.** Isotretinoin causes severe birth defects. All females should read the section "What are the important warnings for females taking Amnesteem?" for more information and warnings about Amnesteem and pregnancy.
- Do not take Amnesteem unless you completely understand its possible risks and are willing to follow all of the instructions in this Medication Guide.

Tell your prescriber if you or someone in your family has had any kind of mental problems, asthma, liver disease, diabetes, heart disease, osteoporosis (bone loss), weak bones, anorexia nervosa (an eating disorder where people eat too little), or any other important health problems. Tell your prescriber about any food or drug allergies you have had in the past. These problems do not necessarily mean you cannot take Amnesteem, but your prescriber needs this information to discuss if isotretinoin capsules are right for you.

How should I take Amnesteem?

- You will get no more than a 30-day supply of Amnesteem at a time, to be sure you check in with your prescriber each month to discuss side effects.
- Your prescription should have a special yellow self-adhesive sticker attached to it. The sticker is YELLOW. If your prescription does not have this yellow self-adhesive sticker, call your prescriber. The pharmacy should not fill your prescription unless it has the yellow self-adhesive sticker.
- The amount of Amnesteem you take has been specially chosen for you and may change during treatment.
- You will take Amnesteem 2 times a day with a meal, unless your prescriber tells you otherwise. Swallow your Amnesteem with a full glass of liquid. This will help prevent the medication inside the capsule from irritating the lining of your esophagus (connection between mouth and stomach). For the same reason, do not chew or suck on the capsule.
- If you miss a dose, just skip that dose. Do **not** take 2 doses the next time.
- You should return to your prescriber as directed to make sure you don't have signs of serious side effects. Because some of isotretinoin's serious side effects show up in blood tests, some of these visits may involve blood tests (monthly visits for female patients should always include a urine or serum pregnancy test).

What should I avoid while taking Amnesteem?

- **Do not get pregnant** while taking Amnesteem. See "What is the most important information I should know about Amnesteem?" and "What are the important warnings for females taking Amnesteem?"
- **Do not breast feed** while taking Amnesteem and for 1 month after stopping Amnesteem. We do not know if isotretinoin can pass through your milk and harm the baby.
- **Do not give blood** while you take Amnesteem and for 1 month after stopping Amnesteem. If someone who is pregnant gets your donated blood, her baby may be exposed to isotretinoin and may be born with birth defects.
- **Do not take vitamin A** supplements. Vitamin A in high doses has many of the same side effects as isotretinoin. Taking both together may increase your chance of getting side effects.
- **Do not have cosmetic procedures to smooth your skin, including waxing, dermabrasion, or laser procedures, while you are using Amnesteem and for at least 6 months after you stop.** Isotretinoin can increase your chance of scarring from these procedures. Check with your prescriber for advice about when you can have cosmetic procedures.
- **Avoid sunlight and ultraviolet lights** as much as possible. Tanning machines use ultraviolet lights. Isotretinoin may make your skin more sensitive to light.
- **Do not use birth control pills that do not contain estrogen ("minipills").** They may not work while you take Amnesteem. Ask your prescriber or pharmacist if you are not sure what type you are using.
- **Talk with your doctor if you plan to take other drugs or herbal products.** This is especially important for patients using birth control pills and other hormonal types of birth control because the birth control may not work as effectively if you are taking certain drugs or herbal products. You should not take the herbal supplement St. John's Wort because this herbal supplement may make birth control pills not work as effectively.
- **Talk with your doctor if you are currently taking an oral or injected corticosteroid or anticonvulsant (seizure) medication prior to using Amnesteem.** These drugs may weaken your bones.
- **Do not share Amnesteem with other people.** It can cause birth defects and other serious health problems.
- **Do not take Amnesteem with antibiotics unless you talk to your prescriber.** For some antibiotics, you may have to stop taking Amnesteem until the antibiotic treatment is finished. Use of both drugs together can increase the chances of getting increased pressure in the brain.

What are the possible side effects of Amnesteem?

Amnesteem has possible serious side effects

- **Isotretinoin capsules can cause birth defects, premature births, and death in babies** whose mothers took isotretinoin capsules while they were pregnant. See "What is the most important information I should know about Amnesteem?" and "What are the important warnings for females taking Amnesteem?"
- **Serious mental health problems.** See "What is the most important information I should know about Amnesteem?"
- **Serious brain problems.** Isotretinoin capsules can increase the pressure in your brain. This can lead to permanent loss of sight, or in rare cases, death. Stop taking Amnesteem and call your prescriber right away if you get any of these signs of increased brain pressure: bad headache, blurred vision, dizziness, nausea, or vomiting. Also, some patients taking isotretinoin capsules have had seizures (convulsions) or stroke.
- **Abdomen (stomach area) problems.** Certain symptoms may mean that your internal organs are being damaged. These organs include the liver, pancreas, bowel (intestines), and esophagus (connection between mouth and stomach). If your organs are damaged, they may not get better even after you stop taking isotretinoin capsules. Stop taking Amnesteem and call your prescriber if you get severe stomach, chest or bowel pain, trouble swallowing or painful swallowing, new or worsening heartburn, diarrhea, rectal bleeding, yellowing of your skin or eyes, or dark urine.
- **Bone and muscle problems.** Isotretinoin may affect bones, muscles, and ligaments and cause pain in your joints or muscles. Tell your prescriber if you plan vigorous physical activity during treatment with isotretinoin. Tell your prescriber if you develop pain, particularly back pain or joint pain. There are reports that some patients have had stunted growth after taking isotretinoin for acne as directed. There are also some reports of broken bones or reduced healing of broken bones after taking isotretinoin for acne as directed. No one knows if taking isotretinoin for acne will affect your bones. If you have a broken bone, tell your provider that you are taking isotretinoin. Muscle weakness with or without pain can be a sign of serious muscle damage. If this happens, stop taking Amnesteem and call your prescriber right away.
- **Hearing problems.** Some people taking isotretinoin have developed hearing problems. It is possible that hearing loss can be permanent. Stop using Amnesteem and call your prescriber if your hearing gets worse or if you have ringing in your ears.
- **Vision problems.** While taking isotretinoin you may develop a sudden inability to see in the dark, so driving at night can be dangerous. This condition usually clears up after you stop taking isotretinoin, but it may be permanent. Other serious eye effects can occur. Stop taking Amnesteem and call your prescriber right away if you have any problems with your vision or dryness of the eyes that is painful or constant.
- **Lipid (fats and cholesterol in blood) problems.** Many people taking isotretinoin develop high levels of cholesterol and other fats in their blood. This can be a serious problem. Return to your prescriber for blood tests to check your lipids and to get any needed treatment. These problems generally go away when isotretinoin capsules treatment is finished.
- **Allergic reactions.** In some people, isotretinoin can cause serious allergic reactions. Stop taking Amnesteem and get emergency care right away if you develop hives, a swollen face or mouth, or have trouble breathing. Stop taking Amnesteem and call your prescriber if you develop a fever, rash, or red patches or bruises on your legs.
- **Signs of other possibly serious problems.** Isotretinoin may cause other problems. Tell your prescriber if you have trouble breathing (shortness of breath), are fainting, are very thirsty or urinate a lot, feel weak, have leg swelling, convulsions, slurred speech, problems moving, or any other serious or unusual problems. Frequent urination and thirst can be signs of blood sugar problems.

Serious permanent problems do not happen often. However, because the symptoms listed above may be signs of serious problems, if you get these symptoms, stop taking Amnesteem and call your prescriber. If not treated, they could lead to serious health problems. Even if these problems are treated, they may not clear up after you stop taking Amnesteem.

Amnesteem has less serious possible side effects
The common less serious side effects of Amnesteem are dry skin, chapped lips, dry eyes, and dry nose that may lead to nosebleeds. People who wear contact lenses may have trouble wearing them while taking Amnesteem and after therapy. Sometimes, people's acne may get worse for a while. They should continue taking Amnesteem unless told to stop by their prescriber.

These are not all of isotretinoin's possible side effects. Your prescriber or pharmacist can give you more detailed information that is written for health care professionals.

This Medication Guide is only a summary of some important information about Amnesteem. Medicines are sometimes prescribed for purposes other than those listed in a Medication Guide. If you have any concerns or questions about Amnesteem, ask your prescriber. Do not use Amnesteem for a condition for which it was not prescribed.

Active Ingredient: Isotretinoin.

Inactive ingredients: yellow wax, butylated hydroxyanisole, edetate disodium, hydrogenated vegetable oil, and soybean oil. Gelatin capsules contain glycerin, with the following dye systems: 10 mg — red iron oxide paste and black ink; 20 mg — red iron oxide paste, yellow iron oxide paste, titanium dioxide, and black ink; 40 mg — red iron oxide paste, yellow iron oxide paste, titanium dioxide, and black ink.

This Medication Guide has been approved by the U.S. Food and Drug Administration.

Rx only

Distributed by:
Bertek Pharmaceuticals Inc.
Research Triangle Park, NC 27709

BKISO:R2 May 2004

Shown in Product Identification Guide, page 324

APOKYN™ ℞
[*ă-pō-kĭn*]
(apomorphine hydrochloride injection)
10 mg/mL
For Subcutaneous Use Only
Not for IV Use
℞ only

DESCRIPTION

APOKYN™ (apomorphine hydrochloride, USP) is a non-ergoline dopamine agonist. Apomorphine hydrochloride is chemically designated as 6aβ-Aporphine-10,11-diol hydrochloride hemihydrate with a molecular formula of $C_{17}H_{17}NO_2 \bullet HCl \bullet 1/2H_2O$. Its structural formula and molecular weight are:

M.W. 312.79

Apomorphine hydrochloride appears as minute, white or grayish-white glistening crystals or as white powder that is soluble in water at 80°C.

APOKYN™ 10 mg/mL is a clear, colorless, sterile solution for subcutaneous injection and is available in 2 mL ampules and 3 mL cartridges. Each mL of solution contains 10 mg of apomorphine hydrochloride, USP as apomorphine hydrochloride hemihydrate and 1 mg of sodium metabisulfite, NF in water for injection, USP. In addition, each mL of solution may contain sodium hydroxide, NF and/or hydrochloric acid, NF to adjust the pH of the solution. In addition, the cartridges contain 5 mg/mL of benzyl alcohol.

CLINICAL PHARMACOLOGY

Mechanism of Action: APOKYN is a non-ergoline dopamine agonist with high *in vitro* binding affinity for the dopamine D_4 receptor (K_i = 4.4 nM), moderate affinity for the dopamine D_2, D_3, and D_5 (K_i = 35-83, 26, and 15 nM, respectively), and adrenergic α_{1D}, α_{2B}, α_{2C} (K_i = 65, 66, and 36 nM, respectively) receptors, and low affinity for the dopamine D_1, serotonin $5HT_{1A}$, $5HT_{2A}$, $5HT_{2B}$, and $5HT_{2C}$ (K_i = 370, 120, 120, 130, and 100 nM, respectively) receptors. Apomorphine exhibits no affinity for the adrenergic β_1 and β_2 or histamine H_1 receptors (K_i > 10,000 nM).

The precise mechanism of action of APOKYN as a treatment for Parkinson's disease is unknown, although it is believed to be due to stimulation of post-synaptic dopamine D_2-type receptors within the caudate-putamen in the brain. Apomorphine has been shown to improve motor function in an animal model of Parkinson's disease. In particular, apomorphine attenuates the motor deficits induced by lesions in the ascending nigrostriatal dopaminergic pathway with the neurotoxin 1-methyl-4-phenyl-1,2,3,6-tetrahydropyridine (MPTP) in primates.

Continued on next page

Apokyn—Cont.

Pharmacokinetics: ***Absorption:*** Apomorphine hydrochloride is a lipophilic compound that is rapidly absorbed (time to peak concentration ranges from 10 to 60 minutes) following subcutaneous administration into the abdominal wall. After subcutaneous administration, apomorphine appears to have bioavailability equal to that of an intravenous administration. Apomorphine exhibits linear pharmacokinetics over a dose range of 2 to 8 mg following a single subcutaneous injection of apomorphine into the abdominal wall in patients with idiopathic Parkinson's disease.

Distribution: The plasma-to-whole blood apomorphine concentration ratio is equal to one. Mean (range) apparent volume of distribution was 218L (123 – 404 L). Maximum concentrations in cerebrospinal fluid (CSF) are less than 10% of maximum plasma concentrations and occur 10 to 20 minutes later.

Metabolism and Elimination: The mean apparent clearance (range) is 223 L/hr (125 – 401 L/hr) and the mean terminal elimination half-life is about 40 minutes (range about 30 to 60 minutes).

The route of metabolism in humans is not known. Potential routes of metabolism in humans include sulfation, N-demethylation, glucuronidation and oxidation. In vitro, apomorphine undergoes rapid autooxidation.

Special Populations: The clearance of apomorphine does not appear to be influenced by age, gender, weight, duration of Parkinson's disease, levodopa dose or duration of therapy.

Hepatic Impairment: In a study comparing subjects with hepatic impairment (moderately impaired as determined by the Child-Pugh classification method) to healthy matched volunteers, the $AUC_{0-\infty}$ and C_{max} values were increased by approximately 10% and 25%, respectively, following a single subcutaneous administration of apomorphine into the abdominal wall. Studies in subjects with severe hepatic impairment have not been conducted (see PRECAUTIONS and DOSAGE AND ADMINISTRATION).

Renal Impairment: In a study comparing renally-impaired subjects (moderately impaired as determined by estimated creatinine clearance) to healthy matched volunteers, the $AUC_{0-\infty}$ and C_{max} values were increased by approximately 16% and 50%, respectively, following a single subcutaneous administration of apomorphine into the abdominal wall. The mean time to peak concentrations and the mean terminal half-life of apomorphine were unaffected by the renal status of the individual. Studies in subjects with severe renal impairment have not been conducted. The starting dose for patients with mild or moderate renal impairment should be reduced (see PRECAUTIONS and DOSAGE AND ADMINISTRATION).

Drug-Drug Interactions: ***Carbidopa/levodopa:*** Levodopa pharmacokinetics were unchanged when subcutaneous apomorphine and levodopa were co-administrated in patients. However, motor response differences were significant. The threshold levodopa concentration necessary for an improved motor response was reduced significantly, leading to an increased duration of effect without a change in the maximal response to levodopa therapy.

Other Drugs Eliminated Via Hepatic Metabolism: Based upon an *in vitro* study, cytochrome P450 enzymes play a minor role in the metabolism of apomorphine. *In vitro* studies have also demonstrated that drug interactions are unlikely due to apomorphine acting as a substrate, an inhibitor, or an inducer of cytochrome P450 enzymes.

COMT Interactions: A pharmacokinetic interaction of apomorphine with catechol-O-methyl transferase (COMT) inhibitors or drugs metabolized by this route is unlikely since apomorphine appears not to be metabolized by COMT.

Clinical Studies: The effectiveness of APOKYN in the acute symptomatic treatment of the recurring episodes of hypomobility, "off" episodes ("end-of-dose wearing off" and unpredictable "on/off" episodes), associated with advanced Parkinson's disease was established in three randomized, controlled trials. On average, patients participating in these trials had Parkinson's disease for 11.3 years and were being treated with L-dopa and at least one other agent, usually an oral dopamine agonist. One of the three studies was conducted in patients who did not have prior exposure to apomorphine and two were conducted in patients with at least 3 months of apomorphine use immediately prior to study enrollment. Almost all patients without prior exposure to apomorphine began taking an antiemetic (trimethobenzamide) three days prior to starting apomorphine. After exposure to apomorphine, 50% of patients were able to discontinue use of a concomitant antiemetic, on average 2 months after initiating apomorphine.

Change in Part III (Motor Examination) of the Unified Parkinson's Disease Rating Scale (UPDRS) served as the primary outcome assessment measure in each study. Part III of the UPDRS contains 14 items designed to assess the severity of the cardinal motor findings (e.g., tremor, rigidity, bradykinesia, postural instability, etc.) in patients with Parkinson's disease.

The first trial used a parallel design, randomizing 29 patients with advanced Parkinson's disease to subcutaneous apomorphine or placebo in a 2:1 ratio. Patients had no prior exposure to apomorphine. In an office setting, hypomobility was allowed to occur by withholding the patients' Parkinson's disease medications overnight. The following morning, patients (in a hypomobile state) were started in a blinded fashion on study treatment (placebo or 2 mg of apomorphine) and redosed at increasing doses, after at least 2 hours, until a therapeutic response approximately equivalent to the individual patient's response to their usual dose of levodopa was observed (or until 10 mg apomorphine or placebo equivalent was given). At each redosing, study drug was increased by 2 mg or 0.2 mL (to 4 mg, 6 mg, 8 mg, or 10 mg of apomorphine) or placebo equivalent. Of the 20 patients assigned to apomorphine, 18 achieved a therapeutic response at about 20 minutes that was approximately equivalent to the therapeutic response to a usual dose of levodopa. The average apomorphine dose was 5.4 mg (3 patients on 2 mg, 7 on 4 mg, 5 on 6 mg, 3 on 8 mg, and 2 on 10 mg). In contrast, of the 9 patients assigned to placebo, none reached such a therapeutic response. The mean changes-from-baseline for UPDRS Part III scores at the best dose were 23.9 and 0.1 for the apomorphine and placebo respectively ($p < 0.0001$).

The second trial used a crossover design, randomizing 17 patients who had been using apomorphine for at least 3 months. Patients received their usual morning doses of Parkinson's disease medications and were followed until hypomobility occurred, at which time they received either a single dose of apomorphine (at their usual dose) or placebo. Their UPDRS Part III scores were then evaluated over time. The average dose of apomorphine was 4 mg (2 patients on 2 mg, 9 on 3 mg, 2 on 4 mg, and 1 each on 4.5 mg, 5 mg, 8 mg, and 10 mg). On average, the mean changes-from-baseline UPDRS Part III scores at 20 minutes were 20.0 and 3.0 points for the apomorphine and placebo groups respectively ($p < 0.0001$).

The third trial used a parallel design, randomizing 62 patients who had been using apomorphine for at least 3 months. Patients were randomized in a 2:1 (active: placebo) ratio to one of four groups and were dosed once. The groups were: apomorphine at the usual dose, placebo at a volume matching the usual apomorphine dose, apomorphine at the usual dose + 2 mg (0.2 mL), or placebo at a volume matching the usual apomorphine dose + 0.2 mL. Patients received their usual morning doses of Parkinson's disease medications and were followed until hypomobility occurred, at which time they received the randomized treatment. The mean changes-from-baseline for UPDRS Part III scores at 20 minutes post dosing were 24.2 and 7.4 points for the pooled apomorphine groups and the pooled placebo groups, respectively ($p < 0.0001$). The figure below describes the mean change in UPDRS Motor Scores over time after pooled apomorphine and pooled placebo administration.

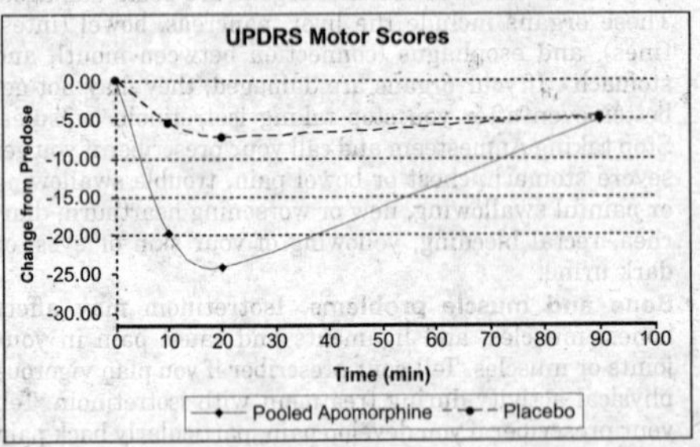

In this third trial, comparing patients randomized to apomorphine at the usual dose (mean dose about 4.5 mg) and patients randomized to apomorphine + 2 mg (mean dose about 6 mg), the mean changes-from-baseline for UPDRS Part III scores at 20 minutes post dosing were 24 and 25, respectively. This suggests that patients chronically treated at a dose of 4 mg might derive little additional benefit from a dose increment of 2 mg. There was an increased incidence of adverse events in patients randomized to apomorphine + 2 mg.

INDICATIONS AND USAGE

APOKYN™ (apomorphine hydrochloride injection) is indicated for the acute, intermittent treatment of hypomobility, "off" episodes ("end-of-dose wearing off" and unpredictable "on/off" episodes) associated with advanced Parkinson's disease. APOKYN has been studied as an adjunct to other medications (see CLINICAL PHARMACOLOGY: Clinical Trials).

CONTRAINDICATIONS

Based on reports of profound hypotension and loss of consciousness when apomorphine was administered with ondansetron, the concomitant use of apomorphine with drugs of the $5HT_3$ antagonist class (including, for example, ondansetron, granisetron, dolasetron, palonosetron, and alosetron) is contraindicated.

APOKYN is contraindicated in patients who have demonstrated hypersensitivity to the drug or its ingredients (notably sodium metabisulfite).

WARNINGS

Avoid Intravenous Administration: Serious adverse events (such as intravenous crystallization of apomorphine, leading to thrombus formation and pulmonary embolism) have followed the intravenous administration of apomorphine. Consequently, apomorphine should not be administered intravenously.

General: The significant adverse events described below have been reported in association with the use of subcutaneous apomorphine, but almost all of them occurred during open-label, uncontrolled studies. In the development program, the controlled trial data involved relatively few patients, and examined primarily the effects of single doses. Because the background rate of many of these events in a population of patients with advanced Parkinson's disease is unknown, it is difficult to assess the role of apomorphine in their causation.

Nausea and Vomiting: At the recommended doses of apomorphine, severe nausea and vomiting can be expected. Because of this, in domestic clinical studies, 98% of all patients were treated with the antiemetic trimethobenzamide for three days prior to beginning apomorphine and were then encouraged to continue trimethobenzamide for at least 6 weeks. Among 522 patients treated, 262 (50%) discontinued trimethobenzamide while continuing apomorphine. The average time to discontinuation of trimethobenzamide was about 2 months (range: 1 day to 33 months). For the 262 patients who discontinued trimethobenzamide, 249 patients continued apomorphine without trimethobenzamide for a duration of follow-up that averaged 1 year (range: 0-3 years). Even with the use of trimethobenzamide in clinical trials, 31% of the patients experienced nausea and 11% of the patients experienced vomiting. In clinical trials, 3% of the patients discontinued apomorphine due to nausea and 2% discontinued due to vomiting.

In the domestic development of apomorphine, there was no experience with antiemetics other than trimethobenzamide. Some antiemetics with anti-dopaminergic actions have the potential to worsen the clinical state of patients with Parkinson's disease and should be avoided.

Syncope: In clinical studies, about 2% of patients experienced syncope.

QT Prolongation and Potential for Proarrhythymic Effects: In a study in which patients received increasing single doses of apomorphine from 2 to 10 mg (if tolerated) as well as placebo, the mean difference in QTc between apomorphine and placebo, as measured by Holter monitor, was 0 msec at 4 mg, 1 msec at 6 mg, and 7 msec at 8 mg. Too few patients received a 10 mg dose to be able to adequately characterize the change in QTc interval at that dose. In a controlled trial in which patients were administered placebo or a single dose of apomorphine (mean dose of 5.2 mg; range of 2-10 mg, with 30 of 35 patients receiving a dose of 6 mg or less), the mean difference between apomorphine and placebo in the change in QTc was about 3 msec at 20 and 90 minutes. In the entire database, 2 patients (one at 2 and 6 mg, one at 6 mg) exhibited large QTc increments (> 60 msecs from pre-dose) and had QTc intervals greater than 500 msecs acutely after dosing. Doses of 6 mg or less thus are associated with minimal increases in QTc. Doses greater than 6 mg do not provide additional clinical benefit and are not recommended.

Some drugs that prolong the QT/QTc interval have been associated with the occurrence of torsades de pointes and with sudden unexplained death. The relationship of QT prolongation to torsades de pointes is clearest for larger increases (20 msec and greater), but it is possible that smaller QT/QTc prolongations may also increase risk, or increase it in susceptible individuals, such as those with hypokalemia, hypomagnesemia, bradycardia, concomitant use of other drugs that prolong the QTc interval, or genetic predisposition (e.g., congenital prolongation of the QT interval). Although torsades de pointes has not been observed in association with the use of apomorphine at recommended doses in premarketing studies, experience is too limited to rule out an increased risk. Palpitations and syncope may signal the occurrence of an episode of torsades de pointes.

Caution is recommended when administering apomorphine to patients with the risk factors described above.

Symptomatic Hypotension: Dopamine agonists may cause orthostatic hypotension at any time, especially during dose escalation. Parkinson's disease patients, in addition, may have an impaired capacity to respond to an orthostatic challenge. For these reasons, Parkinson's disease patients being treated with dopaminergic agonists ordinarily require careful monitoring for signs and symptoms of orthostatic hypotension, especially during dose escalation, and should be informed of this risk.

Apomorphine causes dose-related decreases in systolic (SBP) and diastolic blood pressure (DBP). Dose-dependent mean decrements in SBP ranged from 5 mm Hg after 2 mg to 16 mm Hg after 10 mg. Dose-dependent mean decrements in DBP ranged from 3 mm Hg after 2 mg to 8 mm Hg after 10 mg. These changes were observed at 10 minutes, appeared to peak at about 20 minutes after dosing, and persisted up to at least 90 minutes post-dosing. Patients undergoing titration of apomorphine showed an increased incidence (from 4% pre-dose to 18% post-dose) of systolic orthostatic hypotension (≥ 20 mmHg decrease) when evaluated at various times after in-office dosing. A small number of patients developed severe systolic orthostatic hypotension (≥ 30 mmHg decrease and systolic BP ≤ 90 mmHg) after subcutaneous apomorphine injection.

In clinical trials of apomorphine in patients with advanced Parkinson's disease, 59 of 550 patients (11%) had orthostatic hypotension, hypotension, and/or syncope. These events were considered serious in 4 patients (< 1%) and resulted in withdrawal of apomorphine in 10 patients (2%). These events occurred both with initial dosing and during long-term treatment. Whether or not hypotension contributed to other significant adverse events seen (e.g., falls), is unknown.

The effects of apomorphine on blood pressure may be increased by the concomitant use of alcohol, antihypertensive medications, and vasodilators (especially nitrates). Alcohol should be avoided when using Apokyn and extra caution should be exercised if Apokyn must be administered with concomitant antihypertensive medications and/or vasodilators (see PRECAUTIONS: Drug Interactions and Information for Patients).

Falls: Patients with Parkinson's disease (PD) are at risk of falling due to the underlying postural instability and concomitant autonomic instability seen in some patients with PD, and from syncope caused by the blood pressure lowering effects of the drugs used to treat PD. Subcutaneous apomorphine might increase the risk of falling by simultaneously lowering blood pressure and altering mobility (see WARNINGS: Symptomatic Hypotension; PRECAUTIONS: Dyskinesias).

In clinical trials, 30% of patients had events that could reasonably be considered falls and about 5% of patients had falls that were considered serious. Because these data were obtained in open, uncontrolled studies, and given the unknown background rate of falls in a population of patients with advanced Parkinson's disease, it is impossible to definitively assess the contribution of apomorphine to these events.

Hallucinations: During clinical development, hallucinations were reported by 14% of the patients. Hallucinations resulted in discontinuation of apomorphine in 1% of patients.

Falling Asleep During Activities of Daily Living: There have been reports in the literature of patients treated with apomorphine subcutaneous injections who suddenly fell asleep without prior warning of sleepiness while engaged in activities of daily living. It is clear that somnolence is commonly associated with APOKYN and many clinical experts believe that falling asleep while engaged in activities of daily living always occurs in a setting of pre-existing somnolence even if patients do not give such a history. Prescribers should therefore continually reassess patients for drowsiness or sleepiness, especially since some of the events occur well after the start of treatment. Prescribers should also be aware that patients may not acknowledge drowsiness or sleepiness until directly questioned about drowsiness or sleepiness during specific activities.

Before initiating treatment with APOKYN, patients should be advised of the possibility that they may develop drowsiness and specifically asked about factors that could increase the risk with APOKYN, such as concomitant sedating medications and the presence of sleep disorders. If a patient develops significant daytime sleepiness or episodes of falling asleep during activities that require active participation (e.g., conversations, eating, etc.), APOKYN should ordinarily be discontinued. If a decision is made to continue APOKYN, patients should be advised not to drive and to avoid other potentially dangerous activities. There is insufficient information to determine whether dose reduction will eliminate episodes of falling asleep while engaged in activities of daily living.

Coronary Events: During clinical development, 4% of patients treated with apomorphine experienced angina, myocardial infarction, cardiac arrest and/or sudden death; some cases of angina and myocardial infarction occurred in close proximity to apomorphine dosing (within 2 hours), while other cases of cardiac arrest and sudden death were observed at times unrelated to dosing. Apomorphine has been shown to reduce resting systolic and diastolic blood pressure and, as such, it has the potential to exacerbate coronary (and cerebral) ischemia. Extra caution should be used in prescribing apomorphine for patients with known cardiovascular and cerebrovascular disease. If patients develop signs and symptoms of coronary or cerebral ischemia, the continued use of apomorphine should be carefully reevaluated.

Contains Sulfite: APOKYN contains sodium metabisulfite, a sulfite that may cause allergic-type reactions, including anaphylactic symptoms and life-threatening or less severe asthmatic episodes in certain susceptible people. The overall prevalence of sulfite sensitivity in the general population is unknown and probably low. Sulfite sensitivity is seen more frequently in asthmatic than in non-asthmatic people.

Injection Site Reactions: Among the 550 patients treated with apomorphine subcutaneous injections during development, 26% of patients complained of injection site reactions, including bruising (16%), granuloma (4%), and pruritus (2%). There was a limited experience (both for overall numbers of patients as well as the total number of injections per patient) with apomorphine injections in controlled trials. In this limited controlled experience, the number of injection site reactions reported by patients receiving apomorphine was similar to that reported by patients receiving placebo.

Potential for Abuse: There are rare reports of apomorphine abuse by patients with Parkinson's disease in other countries. These cases are characterized by increasingly frequent dosing leading to hallucinations, dyskinesia, and abnormal behavior. Psychosexual stimulation with increased libido is believed to underlie these cases. Prescribers should be vigilant for evidence that patients are abusing apomorphine, such as use out of proportion to motor signs (see DRUG ABUSE AND DEPENDENCE).

PRECAUTIONS

Dyskinesias: Apomorphine may cause dyskinesia or exacerbate preexisting dyskinesia. During clinical development, dyskinesia or worsening of dyskinesia was reported in 24% of patients. Overall, 2% of patients withdrew from studies due to dyskinesias.

Events Reported with Dopaminergic Therapy: Although the events enumerated below have not been reported in association with the use of apomorphine, they are associated with the use of other dopaminergic drugs.

Withdrawal-emergent Hyperpyrexia and Confusion: Although not reported with apomorphine, a symptom complex resembling the neuroleptic malignant syndrome (characterized by elevated temperature, muscular rigidity, altered consciousness, and autonomic instability), with no other obvious etiology, has been reported in association with rapid dose reduction, withdrawal of, or changes in antiparkinsonian therapy.

Fibrotic Complications: Cases of retroperitoneal fibrosis, pulmonary infiltrates, pleural effusion, pleural thickening, and cardiac valvulopathy have been reported in some patients treated with ergot-derived dopaminergic agents. While these complications may resolve when the drug is discontinued, complete resolution does not always occur. Although these adverse events are believed to be related to the ergoline structure of these compounds, whether other, nonergot derived dopamine agonists can cause them is unknown.

Priapism: Apomorphine may cause prolonged painful erections in some patients. During clinical development, painful erections were reported by 3 of 361 males (< 1%), and one patient withdrew from apomorphine therapy because of priapism. Although no patients in the clinical development program required surgical intervention, severe priapism may require surgical intervention.

Hepatic Impairment: Caution should be exercised when administrating apomorphine to patients with mild and moderate hepatic impairment due to the increased C_{max} and AUC in these patients. Studies of subjects with severe hepatic impairment have not been conducted (see CLINICAL PHARMACOLOGY and DOSAGE AND ADMINISTRATION).

Renal Impairment: The starting dose should be reduced to 1 mg when administrating apomorphine to patients with mild or moderate renal impairment because the C_{max} and AUC are increased in these patients. Studies in subjects with severe renal impairment have not been conducted (see CLINICAL PHARMACOLOGY and DOSAGE AND ADMINISTRATION).

Retinal Pathology in Albino Rats: Retinal degeneration has been observed in albino rats treated with dopamine agonists for prolonged periods (generally during 2-year carcinogenicity studies). This lesion has also been observed when albino rats were exposed to these agents for shorter periods under higher intensity light exposures. Similar changes have not been observed in 2-year carcinogenicity studies in albino mice or in rats or monkeys treated for 1 year. APOKYN has not been tested in carcinogenicity studies, but based on its mechanism of action it would be expected to cause similar toxicity. The significance of this effect in humans has not been established, but cannot be disregarded because disruption of a mechanism that is universally present in vertebrates (e.g., disk shedding) may be involved.

Information for Patients: APOKYN is intended only for subcutaneous injection and must not be given intravenously. Patients and caregivers should be urged to read the attached Patient Package Insert and Directions for Use of the ampule and dosing pen. Patients should be instructed to use APOKYN only as prescribed. Patients and/or caregivers who are advised to administer APOKYN in medically unsupervised situations should receive instruction on the proper use of the product from the physician or other suitably qualified health care professional and then observed during the initial dosing.

In particular, patients and caregivers must receive detailed instruction in the use of the dosing pen, with particular attention paid to two issues: 1) Patients need to be aware that the drug is dosed in milliliters, not milligrams. Patients should be particularly cautioned that a dose of 1 mg is represented on the dosing pen as 0.1 mL, and not as 1.0 (the latter representing a dose of 10 mg). It is critical that patients and caregivers be made to understand this distinction to prevent potentially life-threatening overdose if a dose of 1 mg is prescribed. 2) Patients and caregivers must be informed that it is possible to dial in their usual dose of apomorphine even though the cartridge may contain less than that amount of drug. In this case, they will receive only a partial dose with the injection, and the amount left to inject will appear in the dosing window. To complete the correct dose, patients/caregivers will need to "re-arm" the device and dial in the correct amount of the remaining dose. If at all possible, this situation should be avoided, and patients and caregivers should be alerted to the fact that there may be insufficient drug left in the cartridge to deliver a complete dose (for example, patients and caregivers should be urged to keep records of how many doses they have delivered for each cartridge, so that they can replace any cartridge that has an inadequate amount of drug remaining).

Patients should be instructed to rotate the injection site and to observe proper aseptic technique.

Patients should be informed that hallucinations can occur. Patients should be advised that they may develop postural (orthostatic) hypotension with or without symptoms such as dizziness, nausea, syncope, and sometimes sweating. Hypotension and/or orthostatic symptoms may occur more frequently during initial therapy or with an increase in dose at any time (cases have been seen after months of treatment). Accordingly, patients should be cautioned against rising rapidly after sitting or lying down, especially if they have been sitting or lying for prolonged periods, and especially at the initiation of treatment with APOKYN. Alcohol, antihypertensive medications, and vasodilating medications may potentiate the hypotensive effect of apomorphine (see WARNINGS: Symptomatic Hypotension; PRECAUTIONS: Drug Interactions).

Patients should be alerted to the potential sedating effects of APOKYN, including somnolence and the possibility of falling asleep while engaged in activities of daily living. Since somnolence is a frequent adverse event with potentially serious consequences, patients should neither drive a car nor engage in other potentially dangerous activities until they have gained sufficient experience with APOKYN to gauge whether or not it affects their mental and/or motor performance adversely. Patients should be advised that if increased somnolence or episodes of falling asleep during activities of daily living (e.g., watching television, passenger in a car, etc.) are experienced at any time during treatment, they should not drive or participate in potentially dangerous activities until they have contacted their physician. Because of possible additive effects, caution should be advised when patients are taking other sedating medications or alcohol in combination with APOKYN.

Because apomorphine has not been evaluated for effects on reproduction and embryo-fetal development, patients should be advised to notify their physicians if they become pregnant or intend to become pregnant (see PRECAUTIONS: Pregnancy).

Because of the possibility that apomorphine may be excreted in breast milk, patients should be advised to notify their physicians if they intend to breast-feed.

Rare cases of abuse (use of apomorphine significantly in excess of prescribed frequency) have been reported. Apomorphine abuse may be associated with inappropriate sexual behavior.

Drug Interactions

$5HT_3$ Antagonists: Based on reports of profound hypotension and loss of consciousness when apomorphine was administered with ondansetron, the concomitant use of apomorphine with drugs of the $5HT_3$ antagonist class (including, for example, ondansetron, granisetron, dolasetron, palonosetron, and alosetron) is contraindicated (see Contraindications).

Antihypertensive Medications and Vasodilators: The following adverse events were experienced more commonly in patients receiving concomitant antihypertensive medications or vasodilators (n = 94) compared to patients not receiving these concomitant drugs (n = 456): hypotension 10% vs 4%, myocardial infarction 3% vs 1%, serious pneumonia 5% vs 3%, serious falls 9% vs 3%, and bone and joint injuries 6% vs 2%. The mechanism underlying many of these events is unknown, but may represent increased hypotension (see WARNINGS: Symptomatic Hypotension).

Dopamine Antagonists: Since apomorphine is a dopamine agonist, it is possible that dopamine antagonists, such as the neuroleptics (phenothiazines, butyrophenones, thioxanthenes) or metoclopramide, may diminish the effectiveness of APOKYN. Patients with major psychotic disorders, treated with neuroleptics, should be treated with dopamine agonists only if the potential benefits outweigh the risks.

Drugs Prolonging the QT/QTc Interval: Caution should be exercised when prescribing apomorphine concomitantly with drugs that prolong the QT/QTc interval (see WARNINGS: QT Prolongation and Potential for Proarrhythmic Effects).

Drug/Laboratory Test Interactions: There are no known interactions between APOKYN and laboratory tests.

Carcinogenesis, Mutagenesis, Impairment of Fertility: Carcinogenicity studies have not been conducted with APOKYN.

Apomorphine was mutagenic in the *in vitro* bacterial Ames test and the *in vitro* mammalian mouse lymphoma assay. Apomorphine was also clastogenic in the *in vitro* chromosomal aberration assay in human lymphocytes and the *in vitro* mouse lymphoma assay. Apomorphine was negative in the *in vivo* micronucleus assay in mice. In a published fertility study in male rats, an adverse effect on fertility was observed at a dose of 2 mg/kg administered subcutaneously (0.6 times the MRHD in a mg/m^2 basis). A significant decrease in testis weight was observed in a 39-week study in cynomolgus monkey at subcutaneous doses of 1.0 and 1.5 mg/kg (0.6 and 1 times the MRHD on a mg/m^2 basis).

Pregnancy: Pregnancy Category C: Reproduction studies have not been conducted with apomorphine. It is also not known whether apomorphine can cause fetal harm when administered to a pregnant woman or can affect reproductive capacity. Apomorphine should be given to a pregnant woman only if clearly needed.

Nursing Mothers: It is not known whether apomorphine is excreted in human milk. Because many drugs are excreted in human milk and because of the potential for serious adverse reactions in nursing infants from apomorphine, a decision should be made as to whether to discontinue nursing or to discontinue the drug, taking into account the importance of the drug to the mother.

Pediatric Use: The safety and efficacy of APOKYN in pediatric patients has not been established.

Geriatric Use: In the apomorphine clinical development program, there were 239 patients less than 65 years of age and 311 who were 65 years of age or older. Adverse events were about equally common in older and younger patients (90 vs 87%), but with older patients more likely to experience confusion and hallucinations. Serious adverse events

Continued on next page

Apokyn—Cont.

(life-threatening events or events resulting in hospitalization and/or increased disability) were also more common in older patients (27 vs 17%), with older patients more likely to fall (experiencing bone and joint injuries), have cardiovascular events, develop respiratory disorders, and have gastrointestinal events. Older patients were more likely to discontinue apomorphine treatment as a result of adverse events (29 vs 21%).

ADVERSE EVENTS

Adverse Event Incidence in Controlled Clinical Studies: APOKYN™ has been administered to 550 Parkinson's disease patients who were taking some form of L-Dopa along with other Parkinson's disease medications. Eighty-six percent of patients were taking a concomitant dopamine agonist. All patients had some degree of spontaneously occurring hypomobility ("off episodes") at baseline. Adverse events were recorded by the clinical investigators using terminology of their own choosing. To provide a meaningful estimate of the proportion of individuals having adverse events, similar types of events were grouped into a smaller number of standardized categories using MEDRA dictionary terminology.

The most common adverse events seen in controlled trials were yawning, dyskinesias, nausea and/or vomiting, somnolence, dizziness, rhinorrhea, hallucinations, edema, chest pain, increased sweating, flushing, and pallor.

The most extensive experience with apomorphine in randomized, controlled trials comes from a multicenter randomized placebo-controlled parallel group trial conducted in apomorphine-naïve PD patients treated for up to 4 weeks (Table 1). Individual apomorphine doses in this trial ranged from 2-10 mg, optimized to achieve control of symptoms comparable to each patient's response to his or her usual dose of L-dopa. The prescriber should be aware that these figures cannot be used to predict the incidence of adverse events in the course of usual medical practice where patient characteristics and other factors differ from those that prevailed in the clinical studies. Similarly, the cited frequencies cannot be compared with figures obtained from other clinical investigations involving different treatments, uses, and investigators. However, the cited figures do provide the prescribing physician with some basis for estimating the relative contribution of drug and nondrug factors to the adverse-event incidence rate in the population studied.

[See table 1 below]

Other Adverse Events Observed During All Phase 2/3 Clinical Trials: APOKYN has been administered to 550 patients; 89% had at least one adverse event (AE). The most common AEs in addition to those in Table 1 (occurring in at least 5% of the patients and at least plausibly related to treatment) in descending order were injection site complaint, fall, arthralgia, insomnia, headache, depression, urinary tract infection, anxiety, congestive heart failure, limb pain, back pain, Parkinson's disease aggravated, pneumonia, confusion, sweating increased, dyspnea, fatigue, ecchymosis, constipation, diarrhea, weakness, and dehydration.

DRUG ABUSE AND DEPENDENCE

Potential for Abuse: A rarely reported motivation for apomorphine abuse (escalation of dose beyond prescribed frequency) is the use of apomorphine to attempt to avoid all symptoms of all "off" events when "off" events occur frequently. A second, rarely reported, motivation for apomorphine abuse is a psychosexual reaction related to the stimulation of penile erection and increase in libido. Adverse events that have been reported in males with overuse include frequent penile erections, atypical sexual behavior, heightened libido, dyskinesias, agitation, confusion, and depression. No studies have been conducted to evaluate the potential for dependence when apomorphine is used as acute (rescue) treatment of "off" episodes in the patients with "on/off" or "wearing-off" effects associated with late stage Parkinson's disease.

OVERDOSAGE

Intermittent Injection: A report of an accidental overdose of 25 mg injected subcutaneously in a 62 year old man was published in Journal of Neurology, Neurosurgery, and Psychiatry (1990), Vol. 53, pp. 96-102. After 3 minutes, the patient felt nauseated and lost consciousness for 20 minutes. Afterwards, he was alert with a heart rate 40/minute and a supine blood pressure of 90/50. He recovered completely within an hour.

DOSAGE AND ADMINISTRATION

The prescribed dose of APOKYN should always be expressed in mL to avoid confusion and doses greater than 0.6 mL (6 mg) are not recommended. Patients and caregivers must receive detailed instructions in the preparation and injection of doses, with particular attention paid to the correct use of the dosing pen (see PRECAUTIONS: Information for Patients).

APOKYN™ is indicated for subcutaneous administration only. APOKYN should not be initiated without use of a concomitant antiemetic (see WARNINGS: Nausea and Vomiting). Most antiemetic experience is with trimethobenzamide and this should generally be used. Trimethobenzamide (300 mg tid orally) should be started 3 days prior to the initial dose of apomorphine and continued at least during the first two months of therapy.

Based on reports of profound hypotension and loss of consciousness when apomorphine was administered with ondansetron, the concomitant use of apomorphine with drugs of the $5HT_3$ antagonist class (including, for example, ondansetron, granisetron, dolasetron, palonosetron, and alosetron) is contraindicated (see CONTRAINDICATIONS).

The dose of Apokyn must be titrated on the basis of effectiveness and tolerance, starting at 0.2 mL (2 mg) and up to a maximum recommended dose of 0.6 mL (6 mg) as follows:

Patients in an "off" state should be given a 0.2 mL (2 mg) test dose in a setting where blood pressure can be closely monitored by medical personnel. Both supine and standing blood pressure should be checked predose and at 20, 40, and 60 minutes post dose. Patients who develop clinically significant orthostatic hypotension in response to this test dose of apomorphine should not be considered candidates for treatment with APOKYN. If the patient tolerates the 0.2 mL (2 mg) dose, and responds, the starting dose should be 0.2 mL (2 mg) used on an as needed basis to treat existing "off" episodes. If needed, the dose can be increased in 0.1 mL (1 mg) increments every few days on an outpatient basis.

Beyond this, the general principle guiding dosing (described in detail below) is to determine a dose (0.3 mL or 0.4 mL) that the patient will tolerate as a test dose under monitored conditions, and then begin an outpatient dosing trial (periodically assessing both efficacy and tolerability) using a dose 0.1 mL (1 mg) lower than the tolerated test dose.

For patients who tolerate the test dose of 0.2 mL (2 mg) but achieve no response, a dose of 0.4 mL (4 mg) may be administered at the next observed "off" period, but no sooner than 2 hours after the initial test dose of 0.2 mL (2 mg). Both supine and standing blood pressure should be checked predose and at 20, 40, and 60 minutes post dose. If the patient tolerates a test dose of 0.4 mL (4 mg) the starting dose should be 0.3 mL (3 mg) used on an as needed basis to treat existing "off" episodes. If needed, the dose can be increased in 0.1 mL (1 mg) increments every few days on an outpatient basis. If a patient does not tolerate a test dose of 0.4 mL (4 mg), a test dose of 0.3 mL (3 mg) may be administered during a separate "off" period, no sooner than 2 hours after the test dose of 0.4 mL (4 mg). Both supine and standing blood pressure should be checked predose and at 20, 40, and 60 minutes post dose. If the patient tolerates the 0.3 mL (3 mg) test dose, the starting dose should be 0.2 mL (2 mg) used on an as needed basis to treat existing "off" episodes. If needed, and the 0.2 mL (2 mg) dose is tolerated, the dose can be increased to 0.3 mL (3 mg) after a few days. In such a patient, the dose should ordinarily not be increased to 0.4 mL (4 mg) on an out-patient basis.

Most patients studied in the apomorphine development program responded to 0.3 mL to 0.6 mL (3 mg to 6 mg). There is no evidence from controlled trials that doses greater than 0.6 mL (6 mg) give an increased effect and these doses are not recommended. The average frequency of dosing was 3 times per day in the development program, and there is limited experience with single doses greater than 0.6 mL (6 mg), dosing more than 5 times per day and with total daily doses greater than 2.0 mL (20 mg).

If a single dose of apomorphine is ineffective for a particular "off" period, a second dose should not be given for that "off" episode. The efficacy of a second dose for a single "off" episode has not been systematically studied and the safety of redosing has not been characterized.

Patients who have a significant interruption in therapy (more than a week) should be restarted on a 0.2 mL (2 mg) dose and gradually titrated to effect. When dosing patients with mild and moderate hepatic impairment, caution should be exercised due to the increased C_{max} and AUC in these patients (see CLINICAL PHARMACOLOGY and PRECAUTIONS).

For patients with mild and moderate renal impairment, the testing dose and subsequently the starting dose should be reduced to 0.1 mL (1 mg) (see CLINICAL PHARMACOLOGY and PRECAUTIONS).

Patients should be instructed to administer apomorphine as described in the Patient Instruction Leaflets.

HOW SUPPLIED

APOKYN™ (10 mg/mL) containing apomorphine hydrochloride (as apomorphine hydrochloride hemihydrate), USP is supplied as a clear, colorless, sterile, solution in 2 mL glass ampules and 3 mL cartridges. The 3 mL glass cartridges are used with a manual reusable, multiple dose injector pen. The pen can deliver doses up to 1.0 mL in 0.02 mL increments. The pen is provided in a package with six needles and a carrying case.

The 2 mL glass ampules are provided as follows:
NDC 62794-256-98
Cartons of five 2 mL ampules
Manufactured for Mylan Bertek Pharmaceuticals by:
Draxis Pharma Inc.
Kirkland, Quebec, Canada H9H 4J4
The 3 mL glass cartridges are provided as follows:
NDC 62794-255-37
Cartons of five 3 mL cartridges
Manufactured for Mylan Bertek Pharmaceuticals by:
Vetter Pharma-Fertigung GmbH & Co. KG
88212 Ravensburg, Germany
The injector pen is manufactured for Mylan Bertek Pharmaceuticals by:
Becton, Dickinson and Company
Franklin Lakes, NJ 07417
or
Becton Dickinson Europe
11, Rue Aristide Berges
B.P. 4, 38800 Le Pont–De-Claix, France
Store at 25°C (77°F)
Excursions permitted to 15 to 30°C (59 to 86°F)
[See USP Controlled Room Temperature]
MYLAN BERTEK PHARMACEUTICALS INC.
RESEARCH TRIANGLE PARK, NC 27709-4149
REVISED APRIL 2004
MBAPO:R1P

Patient Information

APOKYN™
(apomorphine hydrochloride injection)
APOKYN™ (AY-po-kin)
(apomorphine hydrochloride injection)

Read the Patient Information that comes with APOKYN before you start taking it and each time you get a refill. There may be new information. Share this information with your caregiver. This leaflet does not take the place of talking with your doctor about your medical condition or treatment. If you or your caregiver do not understand the information, or have any questions about APOKYN, talk with your doctor or pharmacist.

What is APOKYN?

APOKYN is used by injection, as needed, only to treat loss of control of body movements in people with advanced Parkinson's disease (PD). This condition is also called hypomobility or "off" episodes. An "off" episode may include symptoms such as muscle stiffness, slow movements, and difficulty starting movements. APOKYN may improve your ability to control your movements when it is used during an "off" episode. This may help you walk, talk, or move around easier. APOKYN is not used to prevent "off" episodes. APOKYN does not take the place of your other medicines for PD.

Who should not take APOKYN?

Do not take APOKYN if you are:

- **allergic to APOKYN or to any of its ingredients.** The active ingredient is apomorphine hydrochloride. **APOKYN also contains a sulfite called metabisulfite.** Sulfites can cause severe, life-threatening allergic reactions in some people, especially in people with asthma. Tell your doctor if you have had an allergic reaction to

Table 1
Summary of Adverse Events Occurring in Two or More Patients

Adverse Event	APOMORPHINE n = 20		PLACEBO n = 9	
	N	%	N	%
Any Adverse Reaction	17	85	8	89
Yawning	8	40	0	0
Dyskinesias	7	35	1	11
Drowsiness or Somnolence	7	35	0	0
Nausea and/or Vomiting	6	30	1	11
Dizziness or Postural Hypotension	4	20	0	0
Rhinorrhea	4	20	0	0
Chest Pain/Pressure/Angina	3	15	1	11
Hallucination or Confusion	2	10	0	0
Edema/Swelling of Extremities	2	10	0	0

any "sulfa" containing medicines. See the end of this leaflet for a complete list of ingredients in APOKYN.

- **being treated with certain drugs to treat nausea and vomiting or irritable bowel syndrome. These medications (including, for example, ondansetron, granisetron, dolasetron, palonosetron, and alosetron) are called $5HT_3$ antagonists or blockers. People taking this type of drug together with apomorphine have had severely low blood pressure and lost consciousness or "blacked out."**

APOKYN has not been studied in children.

Before using APOKYN, tell your doctor

- **about all your medical conditions including if you:**
  - **have dizziness**
  - **have fainting spells**
  - **have low blood pressure**
  - **have asthma**
  - **are allergic to sulfites or sulfa medicines**
  - **have liver problems**
  - **have kidney problems**
  - **have heart problems**
  - **have had a stroke or other brain problems**
  - **have a mental problem called a major psychotic disorder**
  - **drink alcohol**
  - **are pregnant or planning to become pregnant.** It is not known if APOKYN can harm your unborn baby.
  - **are breastfeeding.** It is not known if APOKYN passes into your milk and if it can harm your baby. You should choose to either use APOKYN or breastfeed, but not both.
- **about all the medicines you take, including prescription and nonprescription medicines, vitamins, and herbal supplements.** APOKYN and certain other medicines interact with each other, causing serious side effects. This happens especially when you take APOKYN with certain medicines called "vasodilators" and some other medications that lower blood pressure, or take medicines that make you sleepy. Keep a list of all the medicines you take. Your doctor or pharmacist will tell you if you can take APOKYN with your other medicines.

How should I take APOKYN?

Read the APOKYN "Instructions for Use" for complete instructions on preparing and giving an injection of APOKYN. **Do not inject APOKYN unless you and your caregiver have been taught the right way and both of you understand all the directions.** Ask your doctor if you do not understand something.

Use APOKYN exactly as prescribed by your doctor. APOKYN should be injected just under the skin (i.e., subcutaneously), and not into a vein. Your doctor must show you and your caregiver how to inject APOKYN before you start using it. Your doctor will prescribe APOKYN that comes in either:

- small glass containers (ampules) that must be used with a tuberculin syringe, or
- prefilled glass cartridges that are used with a special multiple-dose injector pen

Talk to your doctor about which of these is best for your use.

- Your doctor will tell you what dose of APOKYN to use and how often you should take it. Your doctor will also tell you how to change your dose of APOKYN, if needed. Do not change your dose of APOKYN or use it more often unless your doctor has told you to.
- Choose an injection site on your stomach area, upper arm, or upper leg. Change your injection site each time APOKYN is used. This will lower your chances of having a skin reaction at the site where you inject APOKYN. Do not inject APOKYN into an area of skin that is sore, red, infected or damaged.
- **Never reuse needles with your APOKYN Injections.** Use a new needle with each injection.
- Only use APOKYN that is clear and colorless. Do not use APOKYN that is cloudy, green, or contains particles. Call your pharmacy for a replacement.
- Your doctor will usually prescribe another medicine called an "antiemetic", to take when you are using APOKYN. Antiemetic medicines help to lessen the symptoms of nausea and vomiting that can happen with APOKYN.
- If you take too much APOKYN, you may experience more side effects than usual and they may be stronger than usual. If you are experiencing more side effects or stronger side effects than you commonly have, you should contact your physician immediately. If you are unable to contact your physician, you should have someone take you to the Emergency Room. It is a good idea to discuss this potential problem with your physician at the time that you start APOKYN.

What should I avoid while taking APOKYN?

- **Do not take APOKYN with any of these drugs: ondansetron, dolasetron, granisetron, palonosetron, and alosetron or any drug of the $5HT_3$ antagonist class or group.**
- **Do not drink alcohol while you are taking APOKYN.** Alcohol used with APOKYN can cause worse side effects.
- **Do not take medicines that make you sleepy while you are taking APOKYN.**
- **Do not drive a car, operate machinery, or do anything that might put you at risk of getting hurt until you know how APOKYN affects you.** APOKYN may cause dizziness or fainting. Tell your doctor if you get dizzy or faint with APOKYN.
- **Do not change your body position too fast.** Get up slowly from sitting or lying. APOKYN can lower your blood pressure and cause dizziness or fainting.

What are the possible side effects of APOKYN?

- **heart problems.** If you develop shortness of breath, fast heartbeat, or chest pain while taking APOKYN, call your doctor right away or get emergency help.
- **severe nausea and vomiting.** Severe nausea and vomiting can happen with APOKYN. Talk to your doctor about medicines you can take to help prevent nausea and vomiting. Some patients may stop having nausea and vomiting with APOKYN after using it for some time. Some patients will keep having nausea and vomiting with APOKYN. Tell your doctor if this is a problem for you.
- **sleepiness or falling asleep during the day.** Some patients treated with APOKYN may get sleepy during the day or fall asleep without warning while doing everyday activities such as talking, eating, or driving a car. **Tell your doctor if you (or your caregiver) see either of these effects.**
- **falls.** The changes that occur with PD, and the effects of some PD medicines, can increase the risk of falling. APOKYN can also increase this risk.
- **sudden uncontrolled movements** (dyskinesias). Some people with PD may get sudden, uncontrolled movements after treatment with some PD medicines used to treat PD. APOKYN can cause or worsen this effect.
- **dizziness.** APOKYN can lower your blood pressure and cause dizziness. This effect usually happens when APOKYN treatment is started or when the APOKYN dose is increased. With dizziness, there may also be other symptoms such as nausea, fainting, and sometimes sweating. Do **not** get up too fast from sitting or after lying down, especially if you have been sitting or lying down for a long period of time. Tell your doctor if dizziness is a problem for you.
- **hallucinations.** APOKYN may cause hallucinations (seeing or hearing things that are not real) in some people. Call your doctor right away if you get hallucinations with APOKYN.
- **depression.** Some people get depression while taking APOKYN. Call your doctor right away if you get depression with APOKYN.
- **headache.** APOKYN can cause headaches. If these become severe or do not go away, call your doctor.
- **injection site reactions.** Soreness, redness, pain, bruising or swelling, or itching may happen at the injection site. Changing the injection site with each injection, and putting ice on the injection site before and after injections, may help lower these effects.

APOKYN can also cause yawning, a runny nose, and swelling of your hands, arms, legs, and feet.

Talk to your doctor about any side effects that bother you or that don't go away.

These are not all the side effects with APOKYN. For more information, ask your doctor or pharmacist.

How should I store APOKYN?

- Store APOKYN ampules and cartridges at room temperature, 77°F (25°C). Syringes can be filled from the APOKYN ampules the night before use and stored in the refrigerator until the next day.
- When traveling, keep the ampules, cartridges, and prefilled syringes at 59 to 86°F (15 to 30°C).
- **Keep APOKYN and all medicines out of the reach of children.**

General informatiom about APOKYN.

Medicines are sometimes prescribed for conditions that are not mentioned in patient information leaflets. Do not use APOKYN for a condition for which it was not prescribed. Do not give APOKYN to other people, even if they have the same symptoms you have. It may harm them.

This leaflet summarizes the most important information about APOKYN. If you would like more information, talk with your doctor. You can ask your pharmacist or doctor for information about APOKYN that is written for health professionals. You can also call 1-877-727-6596 or visit www.apokyn.com for more information.

What are the ingredients in APOKYN?

Active ingredient: apomorphine hydrochloride, USP

Inactive ingredients: sodium metabisulfate, NF, water for injection, USP. It may also contain sodium hydroxide, NF and/or hydrochloric acid, NF. The cartridges also contain benzyl alcohol.

MYLAN BERTEK PHARMACEUTICALS INC.
RESEARCH TRIANGLE PARK, NC 27709-4149

REVISED APRIL 2004
MBPLAPO:R1

Shown in Product Identification Guide, page 324

AVITA® ℞

[ă vēt' ă]
(tretinoin cream)
CREAM, 0.025%
For Topical Use Only

DESCRIPTION

AVITA® Cream, a topical retinoid, contains tretinoin 0.025% by weight in a hydrophilic cream vehicle of stearic acid, polyolprepolymer-2, isopropyl myristate, polyoxyl 40 stearate, propylene glycol, stearyl alcohol, xanthan gum, sorbic acid, butylated hydroxytoluene, and purified water. Chemically, tretinoin is all-trans-retinoic acid (C20H28O2; molecular weight 300.44 vitamin A acid) and has the following structural formula:

[structural formula: H_3C, CH_3, CH_3, CH_3, COOH, CH_3]

CLINICAL PHARMACOLOGY

Although the exact mode of action of tretinoin is unknown, current evidence suggests that topical tretinoin decreases cohesiveness of follicular epithelial cells with decreased microcomedo formation. Additionally, tretinoin stimulates mitotic activity and increased turnover of follicular epithelial cells causing extrusion of the comedones.

Pharmacokinetics:
In vitro and in vivo pharmacokinetic studies with AVITA® Cream indicate that less than 0.3% of the topically applied dose is bioavailable. Circulating plasma levels of both tretinoin and isotretinoin are only slightly elevated above those found in healthy normal controls.

CLINICAL STUDIES

In one vehicle-controlled clinical trial, AVITA® (tretinoin cream) Cream 0.025%, applied once daily was more effective than vehicle in the treatment of facial acne vulgaris of mild to moderate severity. Percent reductions in lesion count after treatment for 12 weeks in this study are shown in the following table:

	AVITA® Cream, 0.025%	Vehicle Cream
	N=75	N=58
Noninflammatory Lesions	45%	27%
Inflammatory Lesions	46%	32%
Total Lesions	46%	28%

N=Number of Subjects

INDICATIONS AND USAGE

AVITA® Cream is indicated for topical application in the treatment of acne vulgaris. The safety and efficacy of this product in the treatment of other disorders have not been established.

CONTRAINDICATIONS

The product should not be used if there is hypersensitivity to any of the ingredients.

PRECAUTIONS

General: If a reaction suggesting sensitivity or chemical irritation occurs, use of the medication should be discontinued. Exposure to sunlight, including sunlamps, should be minimized during the use of AVITA® Cream, and patients with sunburn should be advised not to use the product until fully recovered because of heightened susceptibility to sunlight as a result of the use of tretinoin. Patients who may be required to have considerable sun exposure due to occupation and those with inherent sensitivity to the sun should exercise particular caution. Use of sunscreen products and protective clothing over treated areas is recommended when exposure cannot be avoided. Weather extremes, such as wind or cold, also may be irritating to patients under treatment with tretinoin.

AVITA® Cream should be kept away from the eyes, the mouth, the paranasal creases, and mucous membranes. Topical use may induce severe local erythema and peeling at the site of application. If the degree of local irritation warrants, patients should be directed to temporarily use the medication less frequently, discontinue use temporarily, or discontinue use altogether. Efficacy at reduced frequencies of application has not been established. Tretinoin has been reported to cause severe irritation on eczematous skin and should be used with utmost caution in patients with this condition.

Information for Patients: See attached Patient Package Insert.

Drug Interactions: Concomitant topical medication, medicated or abrasive soaps and cleansers, soaps and cosmetics that have a strong drying effect, and products with high concentrations of alcohol, astringents, spices or lime should be used with caution because of possible interaction with tretinoin. Particular caution should be exercised in using preparations containing sulfur, resorcinol, or salicylic acid with AVITA® Cream. It also is advisable to "rest" a patient's skin until the effects of such preparations subside before use of AVITA® Cream is begun.

Carinogenesis Mutagenesis and Impairment of Fertility:
In a life-time dermal study in CD-1 mice with another tretinoin cream, at 100 and 200 times the average recommended human topical clinical dose, a few skin tumors in the female mice and liver tumors in male mice were observed. The biological significance of these findings is not clear because they occurred at doses that exceeded the dermal maximally tolerated dose (MTD) of tretinoin and because they were within the background natural occurrence rate for these tumors in this strain of mice. There was no

Continued on next page

Avita Cream—Cont.

evidence of carcinogenic potential when tretinoin was administered topically at a dose five times the average recommended human topical clinical dose. For purposes of comparisons of the animal exposure to human exposure, the "recommended human topical clinical dose" is defined as 1.0 g of 0.025% AVITA® Cream applied daily to a 50 kg person. In a chronic, two-year bioassay of vitamin A acid in mice performed by Tsubura and Yamamoto, generalized amyloid deposition was reported in all vitamin A treated groups in the basal layer of the skin. In CD-1 mice, a similar study reported hyalinization at the treated skin sites and the incidence of this finding was 0/50, 3/50, 3/50, and 2/50 in male mice and 1/50, 0/50, 4/50, and 2/50 in female mice from the vehicle control, 0.25 mg/kg, 0.5 mg/kg, and 1 mg/kg groups, respectively.
Studies in hairless albino mice suggest that tretinoin may enhance the tumorigenic potential of carcinogenic doses of UVB and UVA light from a solar simulator. In other studies, when lightly pigmented hairless mice treated with tretinoin were exposed to carcinogenic doses of UVA/UVB light, the incidence and rate of development of skin tumors were either reduced or no effect was seen. Due to significantly different experimental conditions, no strict comparison of these disparate data is possible at this time. Although the significance of these studies to humans is not clear, patients should minimize exposure to sun.
The mutagenic potential of tretinoin was evaluated in the Ames assay and in the *in vivo* mouse micronucleus assay, both of which were negative.
Dermal Segment I and III studies with AVITA® Cream have not been performed in any species. In oral Segment I and Segment III studies in rats with tretinoin, decreased survival of neonates and growth retardation were observed at doses in excess of 2 mg/kg/day (> 400 times the average recommended human topical clinical dose).
Pregnancy: Pregnancy Category C.
Teratogenic Effects: Oral tretinoin has been shown to be teratogenic in rats, mice, rabbits, hamsters, and subhuman primates. It was teratogenic and fetotoxic in rats when given orally in doses 1000 times the average recommended human topical clinical dose. However, variations in teratogenic doses among various strains of rats have been reported. In the cynomolgus monkey, which metabolically is closer to humans for tretinoin than other species examined, fetal malformations were reported at oral doses of 10 mg/kg/day or greater, but none were observed at 5 mg/kg/day (1000 times the average recommended human topical clinical dose), although increased skeletal variations were observed at all doses. Dose-related increased embryolethality and abortion were reported. Similar results have also been reported in pigtail macaques.
Topical tretinoin in animal teratogenicity tests has generated equivocal results. There is evidence for teratogenicity (shortened or kinked tail) of topical tretinoin in Wistar rats at doses greater than 1 mg/kg/day (200 times the recommended human topical clinical dose). Anomalies (humerus: short 13%, bent 6%; os parietal incompletely ossified 14%) have also been reported in rats when 10 mg/kg/day was dermally applied.
Topical tretinoin (AVITA® Cream, 0.1%) has been shown to be teratogenic in rabbits when given in doses 91 times the topical human dose for cream (assuming a 50 mg adult applies 1.0 g of 0.1% cream topically). In this study, increased incidence of cleft palate and hydrocephaly was reported in the tretinoin-treated animals.
There are other reports, in New Zealand White rabbits with doses of approximately 80 times the recommended human topical clinical dose, of an increased incidence of domed head and hydrocephaly, typical of retinoid induced fetal malformations in this species.
When given subcutaneously to rabbits, tretinoin was teratogenic at 2 mg/kg/day but not at 1 mg/kg/day. These doses are approximately 400 and 200 times, respectively, the human topical dose of tretinoin cream, 0.025% (assuming a 50 kg adult applies 1.0 g of 0.025% cream topically).
In contrast, several well-controlled animal studies have shown that dermally applied tretinoin was not teratogenic at doses of 100 and 200 times the recommended human topical clinical dose, in rats and rabbits, respectively.
With widespread use of any drug, a small number of birth defect reports associated temporally with the administration of the drug would be expected by chance alone. Thirty cases of temporally associated congenital malformations have been reported during two decades of clinical use of another formulation of topical tretinoin (Retin-A). Although no definite pattern of teratogenicity and no causal association have been established from these cases, five of the reports describe the rare birth defect category, holoprosencephaly (defects associated with incomplete midline development of the forebrain). The significance of these spontaneous reports in terms of risk to the fetus is not known.
Nonteratogenic Effects: Dermal tretinoin has been shown to be fetotoxic in rabbits when administered in doses 100 times the recommended topical human clinical dose. Oral tretinoin has been shown to be fetotoxic in rats when administered in doses 500 times the recommended topical human clinical dose. There are, however, no adequate and well-controlled studies in pregnant women. AVITA® Cream should not be used during pregnancy.
Nursing Mothers: It is not known whether this drug is excreted in human milk. Because many drugs are excreted in human milk, caution should be exercised when AVITA® Cream is administered to a nursing woman.

ADVERSE REACTIONS

The skin of certain sensitive individuals may become excessively red, edematous, blistered, or crusted. If these effects occur, the medication should either be discontinued until the integrity of the skin is restored, or the medication dosing frequency should be adjusted temporarily to a level the patient can tolerate. However, efficacy has not been established for lower dosing frequencies. True contact allergy to topical tretinoin is rarely encountered. Temporary hyper- or hypopigmentation has been reported with repeated application of AVITA® Cream. Some individuals have been reported to have heightened susceptiblity to sunlight while under treatment with AVITA® Cream. Adverse effects of AVITA® Cream have been reversible upon discontinuation of therapy (see Dosage and Administration Section).

OVERDOSAGE

If medication is applied excessively, no more rapid or better results will be obtained and marked redness, peeling, or discomfort may occur. Oral ingestion of the drug may lead to the same side effects as those associated with excessive oral intake of vitamin A.

DOSAGE AND ADMINISTRATION

AVITA® Cream should be applied once a day, in the evening, to the skin where acne lesions appear, using enough to cover the entire affected area lightly. Application may cause a transient feeling of warmth or slight stinging. In cases where it has been necessary to temporarily discontinue therapy or reduce the frequency of applications, therapy may be resumed or frequency of application increased when the patients become able to tolerate the treatment. Alterations of dose frequency should be closely monitored by careful observation of the clinical therapeutic response and skin tolerance. Efficacy has not been established for less than once-daily dosing frequencies.
During the early weeks of therapy, an apparent increase in number and exacerbation of inflammatory acne lesions may occur. This is due, in part, to the action of the medication on deep, previously unseen lesions and should not be considered a reason to discontinue therapy. Therapeutic results should be noticed after two to three weeks but more than six weeks of therapy may be required before definite beneficial effects are seen. Patients treated with AVITA® Cream may use cosmetics, but the areas to be treated should be cleansed thoroughly before the medication is applied (see Precautions Section).

HOW SUPPLIED

AVITA® (tretinoin cream) Cream, 0.025% is supplied as:

NDC Code	Strength	Quantity
62794-141-02	0.025%	20 g
62794-141-03	0.025%	45 g

Storage Conditions: Store below 30°C (86°F); avoid freezing.
Rx Only
BERTEK PHARMACEUTICALS INC.
Research Triangle Park, NC 27709-4149
Revised January 2002 023.1

Remove this portion before dispensing
AVITA®
(tretinoin cream)
CREAM, 0.025%

PATIENT INSTRUCTIONS
Acne Treatment
IMPORTANT
Read Directions Carefully Before Using
THIS LEAFLET TELLS YOU ABOUT AVITA® (TRETINOIN) CREAM ACNE TREATMENT AS PRESCRIBED BY YOUR PHYSICIAN. THIS PRODUCT IS TO BE USED ONLY ACCORDING TO YOUR DOCTOR'S INSTRUCTIONS, AND IT SHOULD NOT BE APPLIED TO OTHER AREAS OF THE BODY OR TO OTHER GROWTHS OR LESIONS. THE SAFETY AND EFFECTIVENESS OF THIS PRODUCT IN OTHER DISORDERS HAVE NOT BEEN EVALUATED. IF YOU HAVE ANY QUESTIONS, BE SURE TO ASK YOUR DOCTOR.

PRECAUTIONS

The effects of the sun on your skin. As you know, overexposure to natural sunlight or the artificial sunlight of a sunlamp can cause sunburn. Overexposure to the sun over many years may cause premature aging of the skin and even skin cancer. The chances of these effects occurring will vary depending on skin type, the climate and the care taken to avoid overexposure to the sun. Therapy with AVITA® Cream may make your skin more susceptible to sunburn and other adverse effects of the sun, so unprotected exposure to natural or artificial sunlight should be minimized.
Laboratory findings. *When laboratory mice are exposed to artificial sunlight, they often develop skin tumors. These sunlight-induced tumors may appear more quickly and in greater number if the mouse is also topically treated with the active ingredient in AVITA® Cream, tretinoin. In some studies, under different conditions, however, when mice treated with tretinoin were exposed to artificial sunlight, the incidence and rate of development of skin tumors was reduced. There is no evidence to date that tretinoin alone will cause the development of skin tumors in either laboratory animals or humans. However, investigations in this area are continuing.*
Use caution in the sun. When outside, even on hazy days, areas treated with AVITA® Cream should be protected. An effective sunscreen should be used any time you are outside (consult your physician for a recommendation of an SPF level which will provide you with the necessary high level of protection). For extended sun exposure, protective clothing, like a hat, should be worn. Do not use artificial sunlamps while you are using AVITA® Cream. If you do become sunburned, stop your therapy with AVITA® Cream until your skin has recovered.
Avoid excessive exposure to wind or cold. Extremes of climate tend to dry or burn normal skin. Skin treated with AVITA® Cream may be more vulnerable to these extremes. Your physician can recommend ways to manage your acne treatment under such conditions.
Possible problems. The skin of certain sensitive individuals may become excessively red, swollen, blistered, or crusted. If you are experiencing severe or persistent irritation, discontinue the use of AVITA® Cream and consult your physician.
There have been reports that, in some patients, areas treated with AVITA® Cream developed a temporary increase or decrease in the amount of skin pigment (color) present.
Use other medication only on your physician's advice. Only your physician knows which other medications may be helpful during treatment and will recommend them to you if necessary. Follow the physician's instructions carefully. In addition, you should avoid preparations that may dry or irritate your skin. These preparations may include certain astringents, toiletries containing alcohol, spices or lime, or certain medicated soaps, shampoos, and hair permanent solutions. Do not allow anyone else to use this medication.
Do not use other medications with AVITA® Cream which are not recommended by your doctor. The medications you have used in the past might cause unnecessary redness or peeling.
If you are pregnant, think you are pregnant, or are nursing an infant: No studies have been conducted in humans to establish the safety of AVITA® Cream in pregnant women. If you are pregnant, think you are pregnant, or are nursing a baby, consult your physician before using this medication.

AND WHILE YOU'RE ON AVITA® THERAPY
Use a mild non-medicated soap. Avoid frequent washings and harsh scrubbing. Acne isn't caused by dirt, so no matter how hard you scrub, you can't wash it away. Washing too frequently or scrubbing too roughly may at times actually make your acne worse. Wash your skin gently with a mild, bland soap. Two or three times a day should be sufficient. Pat skin dry with a towel. Let the face dry 20 to 30 minutes before applying AVITA® Cream. Remember, excessive irritation such as rubbing, too much washing, use of other medications not suggested by your physician, etc., may worsen your acne.

HOW TO USE AVITA® (TRETINOIN) CREAM
To get the best results with AVITA® Cream therapy, it is necessary to use it properly. Forget about the instructions given for other products and the advice of friends. Just stick to the special plan your doctor has laid out for you and be patient. Remember, when AVITA® Cream is used properly, many users see improvement by 12 weeks. AGAIN, FOLLOW INSTRUCTIONS – BE PATIENT – DON'T START AND STOP THERAPY ON YOUR OWN – IF YOU HAVE QUESTIONS, ASK YOUR DOCTOR.
To help you use the medication correctly, keep these simple instructions in mind.

- AVITA® Cream should be applied once a day, in the evening, or as directed by our physician, to the skin where acne lesions appear, using enough to cover the entire affected area lightly. First, wash with a mild soap and dry your skin gently. WAIT 20 to 30 MINUTES BEFORE APPLYING MEDICATION; it is important for skin to be completely dry in order to minimize possible irritation.
- It is better not to use more than the amount suggested by your physician or to apply more frequently than instructed. Too much may irritate the skin, waste medication, and won't give faster or better results.
- Keep the medication away from the corners of the nose, mouth, eyes, and open wounds. *Spread away from these areas when applying.*
- *Cream:* Squeeze about a half inch or less of medications onto the fingertip. While that should be enough for your whole face, after you have had some experience with the medication you may find you need slightly more or less to do the job. The medication should become invisible almost immediately. If it is still visible, you are using too much. Cover the affected area lightly with AVITA® Cream by first dabbing it on your forehead, chin, and both cheeks, then spreading it over the entire affected area. Smooth gently into the skin.
- If needed, you may apply a moisturizer or a moisturizer with sunscreen that will not aggravate your acne (noncomedogenic) in the morning after you wash.

WHAT TO EXPECT WITH YOUR NEW TREATMENT
AVITA® Cream works deep inside your skin and this takes time. You cannot make AVITA® Cream work any faster by applying more than one dose each day, but an excess amount of AVITA® Cream may irritate your skin. Be patient.
There may be some discomfort or peeling during the early days of treatment. Some patients also notice that their skin begins to take on a blush.
These reactions do not happen to everyone. If they do, it is just skin adjusting to AVITA® Cream and this usually sub-

sides within two to four weeks. These reactions can usually be minimized by following instructions carefully. Should the effects become excessively troublesome, consult your doctor.
BY THREE TO SIX WEEKS, some patients notice an appearance of new blemishes (papules and pustules). At this stage it is important to continue using AVITA® Cream.
If AVITA® Cream is going to have a beneficial effect for you, you should notice an improvement in your appearance by 6 to 12 weeks of therapy. Don't be discouraged if you see no immediate improvement. Don't stop treatment at the first signs of improvement.
Once your acne is under control you should continue regular application of AVITA® Cream until your physician instructs otherwise.

BERTEK PHARMACEUTICALS INC.
Research Triangle Park, NC 27709-4149
Revised January 2002

Shown in Product Identification Guide, page 324

AVITA® ℞
[*ă vēt' ă*]
(tretinoin gel)
GEL, 0.025%
For Topical Use Only

DESCRIPTION

AVITA® Gel, a topical retinoid, contains tretinoin 0.025% by weight in a gel vehicle of butylated hydroxytoluene, hydroxypropyl cellulose, polyolprepolymer-2, and ethanol (denatured with *tert*-butyl alcohol and brucine sulfate) 83% w/w. Chemically, tretinoin is all-*trans*-retinoic acid ($C_{20}H_{28}O_2$; molecular weight 300.44 vitamin A acid) and has the following structural formula:

CLINICAL PHARMACOLOGY

Although the exact mode of action of tretinoin is unknown, current evidence suggests that topical tretinoin decreases cohesiveness of follicular epithelial cells with decreased microcomedo formation. Additionally, tretinoin stimulates mitotic activity and increased turnover of follicular epithelial cells causing extrusion of the comedones.

Pharmacokinetics:
In vitro and in vivo pharmacokinetic studies with AVITA® Gel indicate that less than 0.3% of the topically applied dose is bioavailable. Circulating plasma levels of both tretinoin and isotretinoin are only slightly elevated above those found in healthy normal controls.

CLINICAL STUDIES

In two large vehicle-controlled clinical trials, AVITA® (tretinoin gel) Gel 0.025%, applied once daily was more effective than vehicle in the treatment of facial acne vulgaris of mild to moderate severity. Percent reductions in lesion counts after treatment for 12 weeks in these studies are shown in the following Tables:

Study 1	AVITA® Gel, 0.025%	Vehicle Gel
	N = 198	N= 204
Noninflammatory Lesions	-36%	-27%
Inflammatory Lesions	-35%	-25%
Total Lesions	-36%	-27%

Study 2	AVITA® Gel, 0.025%	Vehicle Gel
	N = 58	N= 58
Noninflammatory Lesions	-42%	-26%
Inflammatory Lesions	-38%	-23%
Total Lesions	-41%	-26%

N = Number of Subjects

INDICATIONS AND USAGE

AVITA® Gel is indicated for topical application in the treatment of acne vulgaris. The safety and efficacy of this product in the treatment of other disorders have not been established.

CONTRAINDICATIONS

The product should not be used if there is hypersensitivity to any of the ingredients.

WARNINGS

GELS ARE FLAMMABLE. Note: Keep away from heat and flame. Keep tube tightly closed.

PRECAUTIONS

General: If a reaction suggesting sensitivity or chemical irritation occurs, use of the medication should be discontinued. Exposure to sunlight, including sunlamps, should be minimized during the use of AVITA® Gel, and patients with sunburn should be advised not to use the product until fully recovered because of heightened susceptibility to sunlight as a result of the use of tretinoin. Patients who may be required to have considerable sun exposure due to occupation and those with inherent sensitivity to the sun should exercise particular caution. Use of sunscreen products and protective clothing over treated areas is recommended when exposure cannot be avoided. Weather extremes, such as wind or cold, also may be irritating to patients under treatment with tretinoin.
AVITA® Gel should be kept away from the eyes, the mouth, the paranasal creases, and mucous membranes. Topical use may induce severe local erythema and peeling at the site of application. If the degree of local irritation warrants, patients should be directed to temporarily use the medication less frequently, discontinue use temporarily, or discontinue use altogether. Efficacy at reduced frequencies of application has not been established. Tretinoin has been reported to cause severe irritation on eczematous skin and should be used with utmost caution in patients with this condition.

Information for Patients: See attached Patient Package Insert.

Drug Interactions: Concomitant topical medication, medicated or abrasive soaps and cleansers, soaps and cosmetics that have a strong drying effect, and products with high concentrations of alcohol, astringents, spices or lime should be used with caution because of possible interaction with tretinoin. Particular caution should be exercised in using preparations containing sulfur, resorcinol, or salicylic acid with AVITA® Gel. It also is advisable to "rest" a patient's skin until the effects of such preparations subside before use of AVITA® Gel is begun.

Carcinogenesis Mutagenesis and Impairment of Fertility: In a life-time dermal study in CD-1 mice with another tretinoin gel, at 100 and 200 times the average recommended human topical clinical dose, a few skin tumors in the female mice and liver tumors in male mice were observed. The biological significance of these findings is not clear because they occurred at doses that exceeded the dermal maximally tolerated dose (MTD) of tretinoin and because they were within the background natural occurrence rate for these tumors in this strain of mice. There was no evidence of carcinogenic potential when tretinoin was administered topically at a dose 5 times the average recommended human topical clinical dose. For purposes of comparisons of the animal exposure to human exposure, the "recommended human topical clinical dose" is defined as 1.0 g of 0.025% AVITA® Gel applied daily to a 50 kg person. In a chronic, two-year bioassay of Vitamin A acid in mice performed by Tsubura and Yamamoto, generalized amyloid deposition was reported in all Vitamin A treated groups in the basal layer of the skin. In CD-1 mice, a similar study reported hyalinization at the treated skin sites and the incidence of this finding was 0/50, 3/50, 3/50, and 2/50 in male mice and 1/50, 0/50, 4/50, and 2/50 in female mice from the vehicle control, 0.25 mg/kg, 0.5 mg/kg, and 1 mg/kg groups, respectively.
Studies in hairless albino mice suggest that tretinoin may enhance the tumorigenic potential of carcinogenic doses of UVB and UVA light from a solar simulator. In other studies, when lightly pigmented hairless mice treated with tretinoin were exposed to carcinogenic doses of UVA/UVB light, the incidence and rate of development of skin tumors were either reduced or no effect was seen. Due to significantly different experimental conditions, no strict comparison of these disparate data is possible at this time. Although the significance of these studies to humans is not clear, patients should minimize exposure to sun.
The mutagenic potential of tretinoin was evaluated in the Ames assay and in the *in vivo* mouse micronucleus assay, both of which were negative.
Dermal Segment I and III studies with AVITA® Gel have not been performed in any species. In oral Segment I and Segment III studies in rats with tretinoin, decreased survival of neonates and growth retardation were observed at doses in excess of 2 mg/kg/day (> 400 times the average recommended human topical clinical dose).

Pregnancy: Pregnancy Category C.

Teratogenic Effects: Oral tretinoin has been shown to be teratogenic in rats, mice, rabbits, hamsters, and subhuman primates. It was teratogenic and fetotoxic in rats when given orally in doses 1000 times the average recommended human topical clinical dose. However, variations in teratogenic doses among various strains of rats have been reported. In the cynomolgus monkey, which metabolically is closer to humans for tretinoin than other species examined, fetal malformations were reported at oral doses of 10 mg/kg/day or greater, but none were observed at 5 mg/kg/day (1000 times the average recommended human topical clinical dose), although increased skeletal variations were observed at all doses. Dose-related increased embryolethality and abortion were reported. Similar results have also been reported in pigtail macaques.
Topical tretinoin in animal teratogenicity tests has generated equivocal results. There is evidence for teratogenicity (shortened or kinked tail) of topical tretinoin in Wistar rats at doses greater than 1 mg/kg/day (200 times the recommended human topical clinical dose). Anomalies (humerus: short 13%, bent 6%; os parietal incompletely ossified 14%) have also been reported in rats when 10 mg/kg/day was dermally applied.
Topical tretinoin (AVITA® Gel, 0.025%) has been shown to be teratogenic in rabbits when given in doses 364 times the topical human dose for gel (assuming a 50 kg adult applies 1.0 g of 0.025% gel topically). In this study, increased incidence of cleft palate and hydrocephaly was reported in the tretinoin-treated animals.
There are other reports, in New Zealand White rabbits with doses of approximately 80 times the recommended human topical clinical dose, of an increased incidence of domed head and hydrocephaly, typical of retinoid-induced fetal malformations in this species.
When given subcutaneously to rabbits, tretinoin was teratogenic at 2 mg/kg/day but not at 1 mg/kg/day. These doses are approximately 400 and 200 times, respectively, the human topical dose of tretinoin gel, 0.025% (assuming a 50 kg adult applies 1.0 g of 0.025% gel topically).
In contrast, several well-controlled animal studies have shown that dermally applied tretinoin was not teratogenic at doses of 100 and 200 times the recommended human topical clinical dose, in rats and rabbits, respectively.
With widespread use of any drug, a small number of birth defect reports associated temporally with the administration of the drug would be expected by chance alone. Thirty cases of temporally associated congenital malformations have been reported during two decades of clinical use of another formulation of topical tretinoin (Retin A). Although no definite pattern of teratogenicity and no causal association have been established from these cases, 5 of the reports describe the rare birth defect category, holoprosencephaly (defects associated with incomplete midline development of the forebrain). The significance of these spontaneous reports in terms of risk to the fetus is not known.

Nonteratogenic Effects: Dermal tretinoin has been shown to be fetotoxic in rabbits when administered in doses 100 times the recommended topical human clinical dose. Oral tretinoin has been shown to be fetotoxic in rats when administered in doses 500 times the recommended topical human clinical dose. There are, however, no adequate and well-controlled studies in pregnant women. AVITA® Gel should not be used during pregnancy.

Nursing Mothers: It is not known whether this drug is excreted in human milk, caution should be exercised when AVITA® Gel is administered to a nursing woman.

ADVERSE REACTIONS

The skin of certain sensitive individuals may become excessively red, edematous, blistered, or crusted. If these effects occur, the medication should either be discontinued until the integrity of the skin is restored, or the medication dosing frequency should be adjusted temporarily to a level the patient can tolerate. However, efficacy has not been established for lower dosing frequencies. True contact allergy to topical tretinoin is rarely encountered. Temporary hyper- or hypopigmentation has been reported with repeated application of AVITA® Gel. Some individuals have been reported to have heightened susceptibility to sunlight while under treatment with AVITA® Gel. Adverse effects of AVITA® Gel have been reversible upon discontinuation of therapy (see Dosage and Administration Section).

OVERDOSAGE

If medication is applied excessively, no more rapid or better results will be obtained and marked redness, peeling, or discomfort may occur. Oral ingestion of the drug may lead to the same side effects as those associated with excessive oral intake of Vitamin A.

DOSAGE AND ADMINISTRATION

AVITA® Gel should be applied once a day, in the evening, to the skin where acne lesions appear, using enough to cover the entire affected area lightly. Application may cause a transient feeling of warmth or slight stinging. In cases where it has been necessary to temporarily discontinue therapy or reduce the frequency of application, therapy may be resumed or frequency of application increased when the patients become able to tolerate the treatment. Alterations of dose frequency should be closely monitored by careful observation of the clinical therapeutic response and skin tolerance. Efficacy has not been established for less than once-daily dosing frequencies.
During the early weeks of therapy, an *apparent* increase in number and exacerbation of inflammatory acne lesions may occur. This is due, in part, to the action of the medication on deep, previously unseen lesions and should not be considered a reason to discontinue therapy. Therapeutic results should be noticed after two to three weeks, but more than six weeks of therapy may be required before definite beneficial effects are seen. Patients treated with AVITA® Gel may use cosmetics, but the areas to be treated should be cleansed thoroughly before the medication is applied (see Precautions Section).

HOW SUPPLIED

AVITA® (tretinoin gel) Gel, 0.025% is supplied as:

NDC Code	Strength	Quantity
62794-140-02	0.025%	20 g
62794-140-03	0.025%	45 g

Storage Conditions: Store below 30°C (86°F); avoid freezing.
Rx only
BERTEK PHARMACEUTICALS INC.
Research Triangle Park, NC 27709-4149

Revised November 2001 022.1

Continued on next page

Avita Gel—Cont.

Remove this portion before dispensing
AVITA®
(tretinoin gel)
GEL, 0.025%

PATIENT INSTRUCTIONS
Acne Treatment
IMPORTANT
Read Directions Carefully
Before Using

THIS LEAFLET TELLS YOU ABOUT AVITA® (TRETINOIN) ACNE TREATMENT AS PRESCRIBED BY YOUR PHYSICIAN. THIS PRODUCT IS TO BE USED ONLY ACCORDING TO YOUR DOCTOR'S INSTRUCTIONS, AND IT SHOULD NOT BE APPLIED TO OTHER AREAS OF THE BODY OR TO OTHER GROWTHS OR LESIONS. THE SAFETY AND EFFECTIVENESS OF THIS PRODUCT IN OTHER DISORDERS HAVE NOT BEEN EVALUATED. IF YOU HAVE ANY QUESTIONS, BE SURE TO ASK YOUR DOCTOR.

WARNINGS

GELS ARE FLAMMABLE. Note: Keep away from heat and flame. Keep tube tightly closed.

PRECAUTIONS

The effects of the sun on your skin. As you know, overexposure to natural sunlight or the artificial sunlight of a sunlamp can cause sunburn. Overexposure to the sun over many years may cause premature aging of the skin and even skin cancer. The chances of the these effects occurring will vary depending on skin type, the climate and the care taken to avoid overexposure to the sun. Therapy with AVITA® Gel may make your skin more susceptible to sunburn and other adverse effects of the sun, so unprotected exposure to natural or artificial sunlight should be minimized.

Laboratory findings. *When laboratory mice are exposed tc artificial sunlight, they often develop skin tumors. These sunlight-induced tumors may appear more quickly and in greater number if the mouse is also topically treated with the active ingredient in AVITA® Gel, tretinoin. In some studies, under different conditions, however, when mice treated with tretinoin were exposed to artificial sunlight, the incidence and rate of development of skin tumors were reduced. There is no evidence to date that tretinoin alone will cause the development of skin tumors in either laboratory animals or humans. However, investigations in this area are continuing.*

Use caution in the sun. When outside, even on hazy days, areas treated with AVITA® Gel should be protected. An effective sunscreen should be used any time you are outside (consult your physician for a recommendation of an SPF level which will provide you with the necessary high level of protection). For extended sun exposure, protective clothing, like a hat, should be worn. Do not use artificial sunlamps while you are using AVITA® Gel. If you do become sunburned, stop your therapy with AVITA® Gel until your skin has recovered.

Avoid excessive exposure to wind or cold. Extremes of climate tend to dry or burn normal skin. Skin treated with AVITA® Gel may be more vulnerable to these extremes. Your physician can recommend ways to manage your acne treatment under such conditions.

Possible problems. The skin of certain sensitive individuals may become excessively red, swollen, blistered, or crusted. If you are experiencing severe or persistent irritation, discontinue the use of AVITA® Gel and consult your physician.

There have been reports that, in some patients, areas treated with AVITA® Gel developed a temporary increase or decrease in the amount of skin pigment (color) present.

Use other medication only on your physician's advice. Only your physician knows which other medications may be helpful during treatment and will recommend them to you if necessary. Follow the physician's instructions carefully. In addition, you should avoid preparations that may dry or irritate your skin. These preparations may include certain astringents, toiletries containing alcohol, spices or lime, or certain medicated soaps, shampoos, and hair permanent solutions. Do not allow anyone else to use this medication.

Do no use other medications with AVITA® Gel which are not recommended by your doctor. The medications you have used in the past might cause unnecessary redness or peeling.

If you are pregnant, think you are pregnant, or are nursing an infant: No studies have been conducted in humans to establish the safety of AVITA® Gel in pregnant women. If you are pregnant, think you are pregnant, or are nursing a baby, consult your physician before using this medication.

AND WHILE YOU'RE ON AVITA® THERAPY

Use a mild non-mediated soap. Avoid frequent washings and harsh scrubbing. Acne isn't caused by dirt, so no matter how hard you scrub, you can't wash it away. Washing too frequently or scrubbing too roughly may at times actually make your acne worse. Wash your skin gently with a mild, bland soap. Two or three times a day should be sufficient. Pat skin dry with a towel. Let the face dry 20 to 30 minutes before applying AVITA® Gel. Remember, excessive irritation such as rubbing, too much washing, use of other medications not suggested by your physician, etc., may worsen your acne.

HOW TO USE AVITA® (TRETINOIN) GEL

To get the best results with AVITA® Gel therapy, it is necessary to use it properly. Forget about the instructions given for other products and the advice of friends. Just stick to the special plan your doctor has laid out of you and be patient. Remember, when AVITA® Gel is *used properly*, many users see improvement by 12 weeks. AGAIN, FOLLOW INSTRUCTIONS – BE PATIENT – DON'T START AND STOP THERAPY ON YOUR OWN – IF YOU HAVE QUESTIONS, ASK YOUR DOCTOR.

To help you use the medication correctly, keep these simple instructions in mind.

- AVITA® Gel should be applied once a day, in the evening, or as directed by your physician, to the skin where acne lesions appear, using enough to cover the entire affected area lightly. First, wash with a mild soap and dry your skin gently. WAIT 20 to 30 MINUTES BEFORE APPLYING MEDICATION; it is important for skin to be completely dry in order to minimize possible irritation.
- It is better not to use more than the amount suggested by your physician or to apply more frequently than instructed. Too much may irritate the skin, waste medication, and won't give faster or better results.
- Keep the medication away from the corners of the nose, mouth, eyes, and open wounds. *Spread away from these areas when applying.*
- *Gel:* Squeeze about a half inch or less of medication onto the fingertip. While that should be enough for your whole face, after you have had some experience with the medication you may find you need slightly more or less to do the job. The medication should become invisible almost immediately. If it is still visible, or if dry flaking occurs from the gel *within a minute or so* you are using too much. Cover the affected area lightly with AVITA® Gel by first dabbing it on your forehead, chin, and both cheeks, then spreading it over the entire affected area. Smooth gently into the skin.
- If needed, you may apply a moisturizer or a moisturizer with sunscreen that will not aggravate your acne (noncomedogenic) in the morning after you wash.

WHAT TO EXPECT WITH YOUR NEW TREATMENT

AVITA® Gel works deep inside your skin and this takes time. You cannot make AVITA® Gel work any faster by applying more than one dose each day, but an excess amount of AVITA® Gel may irritate your skin. Be patient.

There may be some discomfort or peeling during the early days of treatment. Some patients also notice that their skin begins to take on a blush.

These reactions do not happen to everyone. If they do, it is just your skin adjusting to AVITA® Gel and this usually subsides within two to four weeks. These reactions can usually be minimized by following instructions carefully. Should the effects become excessively troublesome, consult your doctor.

BY THREE TO SIX WEEKS, some patients notice an appearance of new blemishes (papules and pustules). At this stage it is important to continue using AVITA® Gel.

If AVITA® Gel is going to have a beneficial effect for you, you should notice an improvement in your appearance by 6 to 12 weeks of therapy. Don't be discouraged if you see no immediate improvement. Don't stop treatment at the first signs of improvement.

Once your acne is under control you should continue regular application of AVITA® Gel until your physician instructs otherwise.

BERTEK PHARMACEUTICALS INC
Research Triangle Park, NC 27709-4149

Revised November 2001 Printed in U.S.A.

Shown in Product Identification Guide, page 324

CLORPRES® ℞

[klŏr prĕs]
(Clonidine Hydrochloride and Chlorthalidone)
TABLETS, USP
0.1 mg/15 mg, 0.2 mg/15 mg and 0.3 mg/15 mg

DESCRIPTION

CLORPRES® is a combination of clonidine hydrochloride (a centrally acting antihypertensive agent) and chlorthalidone (a diuretic). CLORPRES® is available as tablets for oral administration in three dosage strengths: 0.1 mg/15 mg, 0.2 mg/15 mg and 0.3 mg/15 mg of clonidine hydrochloride/chlorthalidone, respectively.

The inactive ingredients are ammonium chloride, colloidal silicon dioxide, croscarmellose sodium (Type A), magnesium stearate, microcrystalline cellulose, sodium lauryl sulfate, D&C yellow #10.

Clonidine Hydrochloride: Clonidine hydrochloride is an imidazoline derivative and exists as a mesomeric compound. The chemical name is 2-[(2,6-dichlorophenyl)imino]imidazoline monohydrochloride. The following are the structural formula, molecular formula and molecular weight:

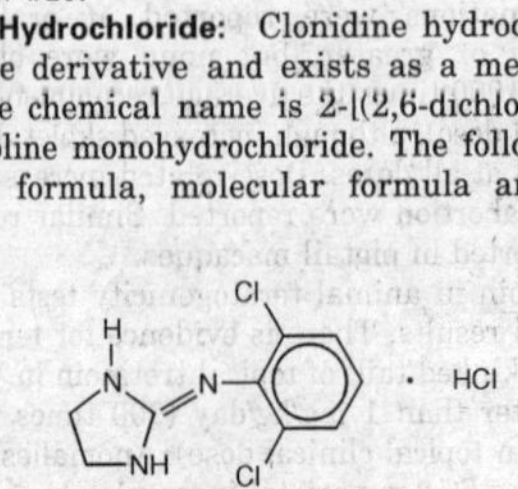

$C_9H_9Cl_2N_3 \cdot HCl$
M.W. 266.56

Clonidine hydrochloride is an odorless, bitter, white crystalline substance soluble in water and alcohol.

Chlorthalidone: Chlorthalidone is a monosulfamyl diuretic that differs chemically from thiazide diuretics in that a double ring system is incorporated in its structure. It is 2-chloro-5-(1-hydroxy-3-oxo-1-isoindolinyl) benzenesulfonamide with the following structural formula, molecular formula and molecular weight:

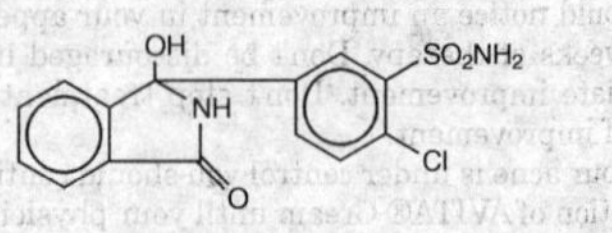

$C_{14}H_{11}ClN_2O_4S$
M.W. 338.76

Chlorthalidone is practically insoluble in water, in ether and in chloroform; soluble in methanol; slightly soluble in alcohol.

CLINICAL PHARMACOLOGY

CLORPRES®: Clorpres produces a more pronounced antihypertensive response than occurs after either clonidine hydrochloride or chlorthalidone alone in equivalent doses.

Clonidine Hydrochloride: Clonidine hydrochloride acts relatively rapidly. The patient's blood pressure declines within 30 to 60 minutes after an oral dose, the maximum decrease occurring within 2 to 4 hours. The plasma level of clonidine hydrochloride peaks in approximately 3 to 5 hours and the plasma half-life ranges from 12 to 16 hours. The half-life increases up to 41 hours in patients with severe impairment of renal function. Following oral administration about 40 to 60% of the absorbed dose is recovered in the urine as unchanged drug in 24 hours. About 50% of the absorbed dose is metabolized in the liver.

Clonidine stimulates alpha-adrenoreceptors in the brain stem, resulting in reduced sympathetic outflow from the central nervous system and a decrease in peripheral resistance, renal vascular resistance, heart rate, and blood pressure. Renal blood flow and glomerular filtration rate remain essentially unchanged. Normal postural reflexes are intact and therefore orthostatic symptoms are mild and infrequent.

Acute studies with clonidine hydrochloride in humans have demonstrated a moderate reduction (15 to 20%) of cardiac output in the supine position with no change in the peripheral resistance; at a 45° tilt there is a smaller reduction in cardiac output and a decrease of peripheral resistance. During long-term therapy, cardiac output tends to return to control values, while peripheral resistance remains decreased. Slowing of the pulse rate has been observed in most patients given clonidine but the drug does not alter normal hemodynamic response to exercise.

Other studies in patients have provided evidence of a reduction in plasma renin activity and in the excretion of aldosterone and catecholamines, but the exact relationship of these pharmacologic actions to the antihypertensive effect has not been fully elucidated.

Clonidine acutely stimulates growth hormone release in both children and adults, but does not produce a chronic elevation of growth hormone with long-term use.

Tolerance may develop in some patients, necessitating a reevaluation of therapy.

Chlorthalidone: Chlorthalidone is a long-acting oral diuretic with antihypertensive activity. Its diuretic action commences a mean of 2.6 hours after dosing and continues for up to 72 hours. The drug produces diuresis with increased excretion of sodium and chloride. The diuretic effects of chlorthalidone and the benzothiadiazine (thiazide) diuretics appear to arise from similar mechanisms and the maximal effect of chlorthalidone and the thiazides appears to be similar. The site of action appears to be the distal convoluted tubule of the nephron. The diuretic effects of chlorthalidone lead to decreased extracellular fluid volume, plasma volume, cardiac output, total exchangeable sodium, glomerular filtration rate, and renal plasma flow. Although the mechanism of action of chlorthalidone and related drugs is not wholly clear, sodium and water depletion appear to provide a basis for its antihypertensive effect. Like the thiazide diuretics, chlorthalidone produces dose-related reductions in serum potassium levels, elevations in serum uric acid and blood glucose, and it can lead to decreased sodium and chloride levels.

The mean plasma half-life of chlorthalidone is about 40 to 60 hours. It is eliminated primarily as unchanged drug in the urine. Non-renal routes of elimination have yet to be clarified. In the blood, approximately 75% of the drug is bound to plasma proteins.

INDICATIONS AND USAGE

CLORPRES® (clonidine hydrochloride USP/chlorthalidone USP) is indicated in the treatment of hypertension. **This fixed combination drug is not indicated for initial therapy of hypertension. Hypertension requires therapy titrated to the individual patient. If the fixed combination represents the dosage so determined, its use may be more convenient in patient management. The treatment of hypertension is not static, but must be reevaluated as conditions in each patient warrant.**

CONTRAINDICATIONS

Anuria: CLORPRES® is contraindicated in patients with known hypersensitivity to chlorthalidone or other sulfonamide-derived drugs.

WARNINGS

Chlorthalidone should be used with caution in severe renal disease. In patients with renal disease, chlorthalidone or related drugs may precipitate azotemia. Cumulative effects of the drug may develop in patients with impaired renal function. Chlorthalidone should be used with caution in patients with impaired hepatic function or progressive liver disease, because minor alterations of fluid and electrolyte balance may precipitate hepatic coma.

Sensitivity reactions may occur in patients with a history of allergy or bronchial asthma.

The possibility of exacerbation or activation of systemic lupus erythematosus has been reported with thiazide diuretics which are structurally related to chlorthalidone. However, systemic lupus erythematosus has not been reported following chlorthalidone administration.

PRECAUTIONS

Clonidine Hydrochloride: ***General:*** In patients who have developed localized contact sensitization to transdermal clonidine, substitution of oral clonidine hydrochloride therapy may be associated with the development of a generalized skin rash.

In patients who develop an allergic reaction from transdermal clonidine that extends beyond the local patch site (such as generalized skin rash, urticaria or angioedema), oral clonidine hydrochloride substitution may elicit a similar reaction.

As with all antihypertensive therapy, clonidine hydrochloride should be used with caution in patients with severe coronary insufficiency, recent myocardial infarction, cerebrovascular disease or chronic renal failure.

Withdrawal: Patients should be instructed not to discontinue therapy without consulting their physician. Sudden cessation of clonidine treatment has resulted in subjective symptoms such as nervousness, agitation and headache, accompanied or followed by a rapid rise in blood pressure and elevated catecholamine concentrations in the plasma, but such occurrences have usually been associated with previous administration of high oral doses (exceeding 1.2 mg/day) and/or with continuation of concomitant beta-blocker therapy. Rare instances of hypertensive encephalopathy and death have been reported. When discontinuing therapy with clonidine hydrochloride, the physician should reduce the dose gradually over 2 to 4 days to avoid withdrawl symptomatology.

An excessive rise in blood pressure following clonidine hydrochloride discontinuance can be reversed by administration of oral clonidine or by intravenous phentolamine. If therapy is to be discontinued in patients receiving beta-blockers and clonidine concurrently, beta-blockers should be discontinued several days before the gradual withdrawal of clonidine hydrochloride.

Perioperative Use: Administration of clonidine hydrochloride should be continued to within four hours of surgery and resumed as soon as possible thereafter. The blood pressure should be carefully monitored and appropriate measures instituted to control it as necessary.

Information for Patients: Patients who engage in potentially hazardous activities, such as operating machinery or driving, should be advised of a potential sedative effect of clonidine. Patients should be cautioned against interruption of clonidine hydrochloride therapy without a physician's advice.

Drug Interactions: If a patient receiving clonidine hydrochloride is also taking tricyclic antidepressants, the effect of clonidine may be reduced, thus necessitating an increase in dosage. Clonidine hydrochloride may enhance the CNS-depressive effects of alcohol, barbiturates or other sedatives. Amitriptyline in combination with clonidine enhances the manifestation of corneal lesions in rats (see Ocular Toxicity).

Ocular Toxicity: In several studies, oral clonidine hydrochloride produced a dose-dependent increase in the incidence and severity of spontaneously occurring retinal degeneration in albino rats treated for six months or longer. Tissue distribution studies in dogs and monkeys revealed that clonidine hydrochloride was concentrated in the choroid of the eye. In view of the retinal degeneration observed in rats, eye examinations were performed in 908 patients prior to the start of clonidine hydrochloride therapy, who were then examined periodically thereafter. In 353 of these 908 patients, examinations were performed for periods of 24 months or longer. Except for some dryness of the eyes, no drug-related abnormal ophthalmologic findings were recorded and clonidine hydrochloride did not alter retinal function as shown by specialized tests such as the electroretinogram and macular dazzle.

In rats, clonidine hydrochloride in combination with amitriptyline produced corneal lesions within 5 days.

Carcinogenesis, Mutagenesis, Impairment of Fertility: In a 132-week (fixed concentration) dietary administration study in rats, clonidine hydrochloride administered at 32 to 46 times the maximum recommended daily human oral dose was unassociated with evidence of carcinogenic potential.

Fertility of male or female rats was unaffected by clonidine hydrochloride doses as high as 150 mcg/kg or about 3 times the maximum recommended daily human oral dose (MRDHD). Fertility of female rats did, however, appear to be affected (in another experiment) at dose levels of 500 to 2000 mcg/kg or 10 to 40 times the MRDHD.

Usage in Pregnancy: *Teratogenic Effect. Pregnancy Category C:* Reproduction studies performed in rabbits at doses up to approximately 3 times the maximum recommended daily human dose (MRDHD) of clonidine hydrochloride have revealed no evidence of teratogenic or embryotoxic potential. In rats however, doses as low as 1/3 the MRDHD were associated with increased resorptions in a study in which dams were treated continuously from 2 months prior to mating. Increased resorptions were not associated with treatment at the same or at higher dose levels (up to 3 times the MRDHD) when dams were treated days 6 to 15 of gestation. Increased resorptions were observed at much higher levels (40 times the MRDHD) in rats and mice treated days 1 to 14 of gestation (lowest dose employed in that study was 500 mcg/kg). There are, however, no adequate and well-controlled studies in pregnant women. Because animal reproduction studies are not always predictive of human response, this drug should be used during pregnancy only if clearly needed.

Nursing Mothers: As clonidine hydrochloride is excreted in human milk, caution should be exercised when it is administered to a nursing woman.

Pediatric Use: Safety and effectiveness in the pediatric population have not been established.

Chlorthalidone: ***General:*** Hypokalemia and other electrolyte abnormalities, including hyponatremia and hypochloremic alkalosis, are common in patients receiving chlorthalidone. These abnormalities are dose-related but may occur even at the lowest marketed doses of chlorthalidone. Serum electrolytes should be determined before initiating therapy and at periodic intervals during therapy. Serum and urine electrolyte determinations are particularly important when the patient is vomiting excessively or receiving parenteral fluids. All patients taking chlorthalidone should be observed for clinical signs of electrolyte imbalance, including dryness of mouth, thirst, weakness, lethargy, drowsiness, restlessness, muscle pains or cramps, muscular fatigue, hypotension, oliguria, tachycardia, palpitations and gastrointestinal disturbances, such as nausea and vomiting. Digitalis therapy may exaggerate metabolic effects of hypokalemia especially with reference to myocardial activity.

Any chloride deficit is generally mild and usually does not require specific treatment except under extraordinary circumstances (as in liver disease or renal disease). Dilutional hyponatremia may occur in edematous patients in hot weather: appropriate therapy is water restriction rather than administration of salt, except in rare instances when the hyponatremia is life-threatening. In cases of actual salt depletion, appropriate replacement is the therapy of choice.

Uric Acid: Hyperuricemia may occur or frank gout may be precipitated in certain patients receiving chlorthalidone.

Other: Increases in serum glucose may occur and latent diabetes mellitus may become manifest during chlorthalidone therapy (see PRECAUTIONS: Chlorthalidone: Drug Interactions). Chlorthalidone and related drugs may decrease serum PBI levels without signs of thyroid disturbance.

Information for Patients: Patients should inform their doctor if they have: 1) had an allergic reaction to chlorthalidone or other diuretics or have asthma 2) kidney disease 3) liver disease 4) gout 5) systemic lupus erythematosus, or 6) been taking other drugs such as cortisone, digitalis, lithium carbonate, or drugs for diabetes.

Patients should be cautioned to contact their physician if they experience any of the following symptoms of potassium loss: excess thirst, tiredness, drowsiness, restlessness, muscle pains or cramps, nausea, vomiting or increased heart rate or pulse.

Patients should also be cautioned that taking alcohol can increase the chance of dizziness occurring.

Laboratory Tests: Periodic determination of serum electrolytes to detect possible electrolyte imbalance should be performed at appropriate intervals.

All patients receiving chlorthalidone should be observed for clinical signs of fluid or electrolyte imbalance: namely, hyponatremia, hypochloremic alkalosis and hypokalemia. Serum and urine electrolyte determinations are particularly important when the patient is vomiting excessively or receiving parenteral fluids.

Drug Interactions: Chlorthalidone may add to or potentiate the action of other antihypertensive drugs. Insulin requirements in diabetic patients may be increased, decreased or unchanged. Higher dosage of oral hypoglycemic agents may be required. Chlorthalidone and related drugs may increase the responsiveness to tubocurarine. Chlorthalidone and related drugs may decrease arterial responsiveness to norepinephrine. This diminution is not sufficient to preclude effectiveness of the pressor agent for therapeutic use. Lithium renal clearance is reduced by chlorthalidone, increasing the risk of lithium toxicity.

Drug/Laboratory Test Interactions: Chlorthalidone and related drugs may decrease serum PBI levels without signs of thyroid disturbance.

Carcinogenesis, Mutagenesis, Impairment of Fertility: No information is available.

Usage in Pregnancy: *Teratogenic Effects. Pregnancy Category B:* Reproduction studies have been performed in the rat and the rabbit at doses up to 420 times the human dose and have revealed no evidence of harm to the fetus due to chlorthalidone. There are, however, no adequate and well-controlled studies in pregnant women. Because animal reproduction studies are not always predictive of human response, this drug should be used during pregnancy only if clearly needed.

Non-Teratogenic Effects: Thiazides cross the placental barrier and appear in cord blood. The use of chlorthalidone and related drugs in pregnant women requires that the anticipated benefits of the drug be weighed against possible hazards to the fetus. These hazards include fetal or neonatal jaundice, thrombocytopenia, and possibly other adverse reactions that have occurred in the adult.

Nursing Mothers: Thiazides are excreted in human milk. Because of the potential for serious adverse reactions in nursing infants from chlorthalidone, a decision should be made whether to discontinue nursing or to discontinue the drug, taking into account the importance of the drug to the mother.

Pediatric Use: Safety and effectiveness in the pediatric population have not been established.

ADVERSE REACTIONS

CLORPRES® is generally well tolerated. Most adverse effects are mild and tend to diminish with continued therapy. The most frequent (which appear to be dose-related) are dry mouth, occurring in about 40 of 100 patients; drowsiness, about 33 in 100; dizziness, about 16 in 100; constipation and sedation, each about 10 in 100.

In addition to the reactions listed above, certain less frequent adverse experiences, which are shown below, have also been reported in patients receiving the component drugs of CLORPRES® but in many cases patients were receiving concomitant medication and a causal relationship has not been established:

Clonidine Hydrochloride: ***Gastrointestinal:*** Nausea and vomiting, about 5 in 100 patients; anorexia and malaise, each about 1 in 100; mild transient abnormalities in liver function tests, about 1 in 100; rare reports of hepatitis; parotitis, rarely.

Metabolic: Weight gain, about 1 in 100 patients; gynecomastia, about 1 in 1000, transient elevation of blood glucose or serum creatine phosphokinase, rarely.

Central Nervous System: Nervousness and agitation, about 3 in 100 patients; mental depression, about 1 in 100; headache, about 1 in 100; insomnia, about 5 in 1000. Vivid dreams or nightmares, other behavioral changes, restlessness, anxiety, visual and auditory hallucinations and delirium have been reported.

Cardiovascular: Orthostatic symptoms, about 3 in 100 patients; palpitations and tachycardia, and bradycardia, each about 5 in 1000. Raynaud's phenomenon, congestive heart failure, and electrocardiographic abnormalities, i.e., conduction disturbances and arrhythmias, have been reported rarely. Rare cases of sinus bradycardia and atrioventricular block have been reported, both with and without the use of concomitant digitalis.

Dermatological: Rash, about 1 in 100 patients; pruritus, about 7 in 1000; hives, angioneurotic edema and urticaria, about 5 in 1000, alopecia, about 2 in 1000.

Genitourinary: Decreased sexual activity, impotence and loss of libido, about 3 in 100 patients; nocturia, about 1 in 100; difficulty in micturition, about 2 in 1000; urinary retention, about 1 in 1000.

Other: Weakness, about 10 in 100 patients; fatigue, about 4 in 100; discontinuation syndrome, about 1 in 100; muscle or joint pain, about 6 in 1000 and cramps of the lower limbs, about 3 in 1000. Dryness, burning of the eyes, blurred vision, dryness of the nasal mucosa, pallor, weakly positive Coombs' test, increased sensitivity to alcohol and fever have been reported.

Chlorthalidone: ***Gastrointestinal:*** Anorexia, gastric irritation, nausea, vomiting, cramping, diarrhea, constipation, jaundice (intrahepatic cholestatic jaundice), pancreatitis.

Central Nervous System: Dizziness, vertigo, paresthesias, headache, xanthopsia.

Hematologic: Leukopenia, agranulocytosis, thrombocytopenia, aplastic anemia.

Dermatologic-Hypersensitivity: Purpura, photosensitivity, rash, urticaria, necrotizing angiitis (vasculitis) (cutaneous vasculitis), Lyell's syndrome (toxic epidermal necrolysis).

Cardiovascular: Orthostatic hypotension may occur and may be aggravated by alcohol, barbiturates or narcotics.

Other Adverse Reactions: Hyperglycemia, glycosuria, hyperuricemia, muscle spasm, weakness, restlessness, impotence.

Whenever adverse reactions are moderate or severe, chlorthalidone dosage should be reduced or therapy withdrawn.

OVERDOSAGE

Clonidine Hydrochloride: The signs and symptoms of clonidine hydrochloride overdosage include hypotension, bradycardia, lethargy, irritability, weakness, somnolence, diminished or absent reflexes, miosis, vomiting and hypoventilation. With large overdoses, reversible cardiac conduction defects or arrhythmias, apnea, seizures and transient hypertension have been reported. The oral LD_{50} of clonidine in rats was 465 mg/kg, and in mice 206 mg/kg.

The general treatment of clonidine hydrochloride overdosage may include intravenous fluids as indicated. Bradycardia can be treated with intravenous atropine sulfate and hypotension with dopamine infusion in addition to intravenous fluids. Hypertension, associated with overdosage, has been treated with intravenous furosemide or diazoxide or alpha-blocking agents such as phentolamine. Tolazoline, an alpha-blocker, in intravenous doses of 10 mg at 30-minute intervals, may reverse clonidine's effects if other efforts fail. Routine hemodialysis is of limited benefit, since a maximum of 5% of circulating clonidine is removed.

In a patient who ingested 100 mg clonidine hydrochloride, plasma clonidine levels were 60 ng/mL (one hour), 190 ng/mL (1.5 hours), 370 ng/mL (two hours) and

Continued on next page

Clorpres—Cont.

120 ng/mL (5.5 and 6.5 hours). This patient developed hypertension followed by hypotension, bradycardia, apnea, hallucinations, semicoma, and premature ventricular contractions. The patient fully recovered after intensive treatment.

Chlorthalidone: Symptoms of acute overdosage include nausea, weakness, dizziness and disturbances of electrolyte balance. The oral LD_{50} of the drug in the mouse and the rat is more than 25,000 mg/kg body weight. The minimum lethal dose (MLD) in humans has not been established. There is no specific antidote but gastric lavage is recommended, followed by supportive treatment. Where necessary, this may include intravenous dextrose-saline with potassium, administered with caution.

DOSAGE AND ADMINISTRATION

The dosage must be determined by individual titration. (See INDICATIONS AND USAGE.)

Chlorthalidone is usually initiated at a dose of 25 mg once daily and may be increased to 50 mg if the response is insufficient after a suitable trial.

Clonidine hydrochloride is usually initiated at a dose of 0.1 mg twice daily. Elderly patients may benefit from a lower initial dose. Further increments of 0.1 mg/day may be made if necessary until the desired response is achieved. The therapeutic doses most commonly employed have ranged from 0.2 to 0.6 mg per day in divided doses.

One CLORPRES® (clonidine hydrochloride/chlorthalidone) Tablet administered once or twice daily can be used to administer a minimum of 0.1 mg clonidine hydrochloride and 15 mg chlorthalidone to a maximum of 0.6 mg clonidine hydrochloride and 30 mg chlorthalidone.

HOW SUPPLIED

CLORPRES® (clonidine hydrochloride and chlorthalidone) Tablets, USP are available containing:

0.1 mg clonidine hydrochloride, USP and 15 mg chlorthalidone, USP

or

0.2 mg clonidine hydrochloride, USP and 15 mg chlorthalidone, USP

or

0.3 mg clonidine hydrochloride, USP and 15 mg chlorthalidone, USP

The 0.1 mg/15 mg product is a yellow, round, scored tablet debossed with M1. They are available as follows:

NDC 62794-001-01
bottles of 100 tablets

The 0.2 mg/15 mg product is a yellow, round, scored tablet debossed with M27. They are available as follows:

NDC 62794-027-01
bottles of 100 tablets

The 0.3 mg/15 mg product is a yellow, round, scored tablet debossed with M72. They are available as follows:

NDC 62794-072-01
bottles of 100 tablets

STORE AT CONTROLLED ROOM TEMPERATURE 15° to 30° C (59° to 86°F).[See USP]

AVOID EXCESSIVE HUMIDITY.

Dispense in tight, light-resistant container as defined in the USP using a child-resistant closure.

Rx only

BERTEK PHARMACEUTICALS INC.
Research Triangle Park, NC 27709-4149

REVISED November 2002
BKCLCH:R3

Shown in Product Identification Guide, page 324

CLOZAPINE TABLETS, USP ℞

25 mg and 100 mg

℞ only

Prescribing Information: Before prescribing clozapine, the physician should be thoroughly familiar with the details of this prescribing information.

WARNING:

1. AGRANULOCYTOSIS: BECAUSE OF A SIGNIFICANT RISK OF AGRANULOCYTOSIS, A POTENTIALLY LIFE-THREATENING ADVERSE EVENT, CLOZAPINE SHOULD BE RESERVED FOR USE IN THE TREATMENT OF SEVERELY ILL SCHIZOPHRENIC PATIENTS WHO FAIL TO SHOW AN ACCEPTABLE RESPONSE TO ADEQUATE COURSES OF STANDARD ANTIPSYCHOTIC DRUG TREATMENT.

PATIENTS BEING TREATED WITH CLOZAPINE MUST HAVE A BASELINE WHITE BLOOD CELL (WBC) AND DIFFERENTIAL COUNT BEFORE INITIATION OF TREATMENT AS WELL AS REGULAR WBC COUNTS DURING TREATMENT AND FOR 4 WEEKS AFTER DISCONTINUATION OF TREATMENT.

CLOZAPINE IS AVAILABLE ONLY THROUGH A DISTRIBUTION SYSTEM THAT ENSURES MONITORING OF WBC COUNTS ACCORDING TO THE SCHEDULE DESCRIBED BELOW PRIOR TO DELIVERY OF THE NEXT SUPPLY OF MEDICATION. (SEE WARNINGS.)

2. SEIZURES: SEIZURES HAVE BEEN ASSOCIATED WITH THE USE OF CLOZAPINE. DOSE APPEARS TO BE AN IMPORTANT PREDICTOR OF SEIZURE, WITH A GREATER LIKELIHOOD AT HIGHER CLOZAPINE DOSES. CAUTION SHOULD BE USED WHEN ADMINISTERING CLOZAPINE TO PATIENTS HAVING A HISTORY OF SEIZURES OR OTHER PREDISPOSING FACTORS. PATIENTS SHOULD BE ADVISED NOT TO ENGAGE IN ANY ACTIVITY WHERE SUDDEN LOSS OF CONSCIOUSNESS COULD CAUSE SERIOUS RISK TO THEMSELVES OR OTHERS. (SEE WARNINGS.)

3. MYOCARDITIS: ANALYSES OF POSTMARKETING SAFETY DATABASES SUGGEST THAT CLOZAPINE IS ASSOCIATED WITH AN INCREASED RISK OF FATAL MYOCARDITIS, ESPECIALLY DURING, BUT NOT LIMITED TO, THE FIRST MONTH OF THERAPY. IN PATIENTS IN WHOM MYOCARDITIS IS SUSPECTED, CLOZAPINE TREATMENT SHOULD BE PROMPTLY DISCONTINUED. (SEE WARNINGS.)

4. OTHER ADVERSE CARDIOVASCULAR AND RESPIRATORY EFFECTS: ORTHOSTATIC HYPOTENSION, WITH OR WITHOUT SYNCOPE, CAN OCCUR WITH CLOZAPINE TREATMENT. RARELY, COLLAPSE CAN BE PROFOUND AND BE ACCOMPANIED BY RESPIRATORY AND/OR CARDIAC ARREST. ORTHOSTATIC HYPOTENSION IS MORE LIKELY TO OCCUR DURING INITIAL TITRATION IN ASSOCIATION WITH RAPID DOSE ESCALATION. IN PATIENTS WHO HAVE HAD EVEN A BRIEF INTERVAL OFF CLOZAPINE, i.e., 2 OR MORE DAYS SINCE THE LAST DOSE, TREATMENT SHOULD BE STARTED WITH 12.5 mg ONCE OR TWICE DAILY. (SEE WARNINGS and DOSAGE AND ADMINISTRATION.)

SINCE COLLAPSE, RESPIRATORY ARREST AND CARDIAC ARREST DURING INITIAL TREATMENT HAS OCCURRED IN PATIENTS WHO WERE BEING ADMINISTERED BENZODIAZEPINES OR OTHER PSYCHOTROPIC DRUGS, CAUTION IS ADVISED WHEN CLOZAPINE IS INITIATED IN PATIENTS TAKING A BENZODIAZEPINE OR ANY OTHER PSYCHOTROPIC DRUG. (SEE WARNINGS.)

DESCRIPTION

Clozapine, an atypical antipsychotic drug, is a tricyclic dibenzodiazepine derivative, 8-chloro-11-(4-methyl-1-piperazinyl)-5*H*-dibenzo [*b,e*] [1,4] diazepine. Clozapine's structural formula, molecular formula, and molecular weight are as follows:

$C_{18}H_{19}ClN_4$
M.W. 326.83

Clozapine is a yellow, crystalline powder, very slightly soluble in water.

Clozapine tablets, for oral administration, are available containing 25 mg and 100 mg of clozapine. In addition, each tablet contains the following inactive ingredients: colloidal silicon dioxide, crospovidone, lactose (monohydrate), magnesium stearate, microcrystalline cellulose, and sodium lauryl sulfate. In addition, the 25 mg tablet contains FD&C red #40 lake and the 100 mg tablet contains FD&C blue #2 lake.

CLINICAL PHARMACOLOGY

Pharmacodynamics: Clozapine is classified as an 'atypical' antipsychotic drug because its profile of binding to dopamine receptors and its effects on various dopamine mediated behaviors differ from those exhibited by more typical antipsychotic drug products. In particular, although clozapine does interfere with the binding of dopamine at D_1, D_2, D_3 and D_5 receptors, and has a high affinity for the D_4 receptor, it does not induce catalepsy nor inhibit apomorphine-induced stereotypy. This evidence, consistent with the view that clozapine is preferentially more active at limbic than at striatal dopamine receptors, may explain the relative freedom of clozapine from extrapyramidal side effects. Clozapine also acts as an antagonist at adrenergic, cholinergic, histaminergic and serotonergic receptors.

Absorption, Distribution, Metabolism and Excretion: In man, clozapine tablets (25 mg and 100 mg) are equally bioavailable relative to a clozapine solution. Following a dosage of 100 mg b.i.d., the average steady state peak plasma concentration was 319 ng/mL (range: 102 to 771 ng/mL), occurring at the average of 2.5 hours (range: 1 to 6 hours) after dosing. The average minimum concentration at steady state was 122 ng/mL (range: 41 to 343 ng/mL), after 100 mg b.i.d. dosing. Food does not appear to affect the systemic bioavailability of clozapine. Thus, clozapine may be administered with or without food.

Clozapine is approximately 97% bound to serum proteins. The interaction between clozapine and other highly protein-bound drugs has not been fully evaluated but may be important. (See PRECAUTIONS.)

Clozapine is almost completely metabolized prior to excretion and only trace amounts of unchanged drug are detected in the urine and feces. Approximately 50% of the administered dose is excreted in the urine and 30% in the feces. The demethylated, hydroxylated and N-oxide derivatives are components in both urine and feces. Pharmacological testing has shown the desmethyl metabolite to have only limited activity, while the hydroxylated and N-oxide derivatives were inactive.

The mean elimination half-life of clozapine after a single 75 mg dose was 8 hours (range: 4 to 12 hours), compared to a mean elimination half-life, after achieving steady state with 100 mg b.i.d. dosing, of 12 hours (range: 4 to 66 hours). A comparison of single-dose and multiple-dose administration of clozapine showed that the elimination half-life increased significantly after multiple dosing relative to that after single-dose administration, suggesting the possibility of concentration dependent pharmacokinetics. However, at steady state, linearly dose-proportional changes with respect to AUC (area under the curve), peak and minimum clozapine plasma concentrations were observed after administration of 37.5 mg, 75 mg, and 150 mg b.i.d.

Human Pharmacology: In contrast to more typical antipsychotic drugs, clozapine therapy produces little or no prolactin elevation.

As is true of more typical antipsychotic drugs, clinical EEG studies have shown that clozapine increases delta and theta activity and slows dominant alpha frequencies. Enhanced synchronization occurs, and sharp wave activity and spike and wave complexes may also develop. Patients, on rare occasions, may report an intensification of dream activity during clozapine therapy. REM sleep was found to be increased to 85% of the total sleep time. In these patients, the onset of REM sleep occurred almost immediately after falling asleep.

INDICATIONS AND USAGE

Clozapine is indicated for the management of severely ill schizophrenic patients who fail to respond adequately to standard drug treatment for schizophrenia. Because of the significant risk of agranulocytosis and seizure associated with its use, clozapine should be used only in patients who have failed to respond adequately to treatment with appropriate courses of standard drug treatments for schizophrenia, either because of insufficient effectiveness or the inability to achieve an effective dose due to intolerable adverse effects from those drugs. (See WARNINGS.)

The effectiveness of clozapine in a treatment resistant schizophrenic population was demonstrated in a 6-week study comparing clozapine and chlorpromazine. Patients meeting DSM-III criteria for schizophrenia and having a mean BPRS total score of 61 were demonstrated to be treatment resistant by history and by open, prospective treatment with haloperidol before entering into the double-blind phase of the study. The superiority of clozapine to chlorpromazine was documented in statistical analyses employing both categorical and continuous measures of treatment effect.

Because of the significant risk of agranulocytosis and seizure, events which both present a continuing risk over time, the extended treatment of patients failing to show an acceptable level of clinical response should ordinarily be avoided. In addition, the need for continuing treatment in patients exhibiting beneficial clinical responses should be periodically re-evaluated.

CONTRAINDICATIONS

Clozapine is contraindicated in patients with a previous hypersensitivity to clozapine or any other component of this drug, in patients with myeloproliferative disorders, uncontrolled epilepsy, or a history of clozapine induced agranulocytosis or severe granulocytopenia. As with more typical antipsychotic drugs, clozapine is contraindicated in severe central nervous system depression or comatose states from any cause.

Clozapine should not be used simultaneously with other agents having a well-known potential to cause agranulocytosis or otherwise suppress bone marrow function. The mechanism of clozapine induced agranulocytosis is unknown; nonetheless, it is possible that causative factors may interact synergistically to increase the risk and/or severity of bone marrow suppression.

WARNINGS

General: BECAUSE OF THE SIGNIFICANT RISK OF AGRANULOCYTOSIS, A POTENTIALLY LIFE-THREATENING ADVERSE EVENT (SEE FOLLOWING), CLOZAPINE SHOULD BE RESERVED FOR USE IN THE TREATMENT OF SEVERELY ILL SCHIZOPHRENIC PATIENTS WHO FAIL TO SHOW AN ACCEPTABLE RESPONSE TO ADEQUATE COURSES OF STANDARD DRUG TREATMENT FOR SCHIZOPHRENIA, EITHER BECAUSE OF INSUFFICIENT EFFECTIVENESS OR THE INABILITY TO ACHIEVE AN EFFECTIVE DOSE DUE TO INTOLERABLE ADVERSE EFFECTS FROM THOSE DRUGS. CONSEQUENTLY, BEFORE INITIATING TREATMENT WITH CLOZAPINE, IT IS STRONGLY RECOMMENDED THAT A PATIENT BE GIVEN AT LEAST 2 TRIALS, EACH WITH A DIFFERENT STANDARD DRUG PRODUCT FOR SCHIZOPHRENIA, AT AN ADEQUATE DOSE, AND FOR AN ADEQUATE DURATION.

PATIENTS WHO ARE BEING TREATED WITH CLOZAPINE MUST HAVE A BASELINE WHITE BLOOD CELL (WBC) AND DIFFERENTIAL COUNT BEFORE INITIATION OF TREATMENT, AND A WBC COUNT EVERY WEEK FOR THE FIRST SIX MONTHS. THEREAFTER, IF ACCEPTABLE WBC COUNTS (WBC greater than or equal to 3, 000/mm³ ANC ≥ 1500/mm³) HAVE BEEN MAINTAINED DURING THE FIRST 6 MONTHS OF CONTINUOUS THERAPY, WBC COUNTS CAN BE MONITORED EVERY OTHER WEEK. WBC COUNTS MUST BE MONITORED WEEKLY FOR AT LEAST 4 WEEKS AFTER THE DISCONTINUATION OF CLOZAPINE.

CLOZAPINE IS AVAILABLE ONLY THROUGH A DISTRIBUTION SYSTEM THAT ENSURES MONITORING OF WBC COUNTS ACCORDING TO THE SCHEDULE DESCRIBED BELOW PRIOR TO DELIVERY OF THE NEXT SUPPLY OF MEDICATION.

Agranulocytosis: Agranulocytosis, defined as an absolute neutrophil count (ANC) of less than 500/mm^3, has been estimated to occur in association with clozapine use at a cumulative incidence at 1 year of approximately 1.3%, based on the occurrence of 15 US cases out of 1743 patients exposed to clozapine during its clinical testing prior to domestic marketing. All of these cases occurred at a time when the need for close monitoring of WBC counts was already recognized. This reaction could prove fatal if not detected early and therapy interrupted. Of the 149 cases of agranulocytosis reported worldwide in association with clozapine use as of December 31, 1989, 32% were fatal. However, few of these deaths occurred since 1977, at which time the knowledge of clozapine induced agranulocytosis became more widespread, and close monitoring of WBC counts more widely practiced. Nevertheless, it is unknown at present what the case fatality rate will be for clozapine induced agranulocytosis, despite strict adherence to the required frequency of monitoring. In the U.S., under a weekly WBC monitoring system with clozapine, there have been 585 cases of agranulocytosis as of August 21, 1997; 19 were fatal. During this period 150,409 patients received clozapine. A hematologic risk analysis was conducted based upon the available information in the Clozapine National Registry (CNR) for U.S. patients. Based upon a cut-off date of April 30, 1995, the incidence rates of agranulocytosis based upon a weekly monitoring schedule, rose steeply during the first two months of therapy, peaking in the third month. Among clozapine patients who continued the drug beyond the third month, the weekly incidence of agranulocytosis fell to a substantial degree, so that by the sixth month the weekly incidence of agranulocytosis was reduced to 3 per 1000 person-years. After six months, the weekly incidence of agranulocytosis declines still further, however, never reaches zero. It should be noted that any type of reduction in the frequency of monitoring WBC counts may result in an increase incidence of agranulocytosis.

Because of the substantial risk for developing agranulocytosis in association with clozapine use, which may persist over an extended period of time, patients must have a blood sample drawn for a WBC count before initiation of treatment with clozapine, and must have subsequent WBC counts done at least weekly for the first 6 months of continuous treatment. If WBC counts remain acceptable (WBC greater than or equal to 3000/mm^3, ANC $\geq$ 1500/mm^3) during this period, WBC counts may be monitored every other week thereafter. After the discontinuation of clozapine, weekly WBC counts should be continued for an additional 4 weeks.

If a patient is on clozapine therapy for less than 6 months with no abnormal blood events and there is a break on therapy which is less than or equal to 1 month, then patients can continue where they left off with weekly WBC testing for 6 months. When this 6 month period has been completed, the frequency of WBC count monitoring can be reduced to every other week. If a patient is on clozapine therapy for less than 6 months with no abnormal blood events and there is a break on therapy which is greater than 1 month, then patients should be tested weekly for an additional 6 month period before bi-weekly testing is initiated. If a patient is on clozapine therapy for less than 6 months and experiences an abnormal blood event as described below but remains a rechallengeable patient (patients cannot be reinitiated on clozapine therapy if WBC counts fall below 2000/mm^3 or the ANC falls below 1000/mm^3 during clozapine therapy), the patient must re-start the 6 month period of weekly WBC monitoring at day 0.

If a patient is on clozapine therapy for 6 months or longer with no abnormal blood events and there is a break on therapy which is 1 year or less, then the patient can continue WBC count monitoring every other week if clozapine therapy is reinitiated. If a patient is on clozapine therapy for 6 months or longer with no abnormal blood events and there is a break on therapy which is greater than 1 year, then, if clozapine therapy is reinitiated, the patient must have WBC counts monitored weekly for an additional 6 months. If a patient is on clozapine therapy for 6 months or longer and subsequently has an abnormal blood event, but remains a rechallengeable patient, then the patient must re-start weekly WBC count monitoring until an additional 6 months of clozapine therapy has been received. The distribution of clozapine is contingent upon performance of the required blood tests.

Treatment should not be initiated if the WBC count is less than 3500/mm^3, or if the patient has a history of a myeloproliferative disorder, or previous clozapine induced agranulocytosis or granulocytopenia. Patients should be advised to report immediately the appearance of lethargy, weakness, fever, sore throat or any other signs of infection. If, after the initiation of treatment, the total WBC count has dropped below 3500/mm^3 or it has dropped by a substantial amount from baseline, even if the count is above 3500/mm^3, or if immature forms are present, a repeat WBC count and a differential count should be done. A substantial drop is defined as a single drop of 3,000 or more in the WBC count or a cumulative drop of 3,000 or more within 3 weeks. If subsequent WBC counts and the differential count reveal a total WBC count between 3000 and 3500/mm^3 and an ANC above 1500/mm^3, twice weekly WBC counts and differential counts should be performed.

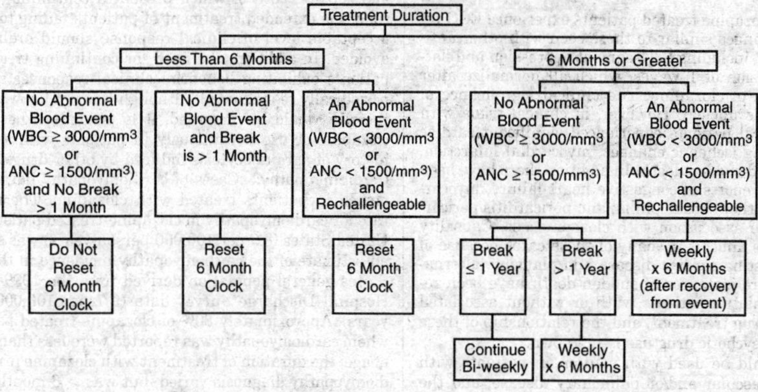

If the total WBC count falls below 3000/mm^3 or the ANC below 1500/mm^3, clozapine therapy should be interrupted, WBC count and differential should be performed daily, and patients should be carefully monitored for flu-like symptoms or other symptoms suggestive of infection. Clozapine therapy may be resumed if no symptoms of infection develop, and if the total WBC count returns to levels above 3000/mm^3 and the ANC returns to levels above 1500/mm^3. However, in this event, twice weekly WBC counts and differential counts should continue until total WBC counts return to levels above 3500/mm^3.

If the total WBC count falls below 2000/mm^3 or the ANC falls below 1000/mm^3, bone marrow aspiration should be considered to ascertain granulopoietic status. Protective isolation with close observation may be indicated if granulopoiesis is determined to be deficient. Should evidence of infection develop, the patient should have appropriate cultures performed and an appropriate antibiotic regimen instituted.

Patients whose total WBC counts fall below 2000/mm^3, or ANCs below 1000/mm^3 during clozapine therapy should have daily WBC count and differential. These patients should not be rechallenged with clozapine. Patients discontinued from clozapine therapy due to significant WBC suppression have been found to develop agranulocytosis upon rechallenge, often with a shorter latency on re-exposure. To reduce the chances of rechallenge occurring in patients who have experienced significant bone marrow suppression during clozapine therapy, a single, national master file will be maintained confidentially.

Except for evidence of significant bone marrow suppression during initial clozapine therapy, there are no established risk factors, based on world-wide experience, for the development of agranulocytosis in association with clozapine use. However, a disproportionate number of the US cases of agranulocytosis occurred in patients of Jewish background compared to the overall proportion of such patients exposed during domestic development of clozapine. Most of the US cases occurred within 4 to 10 weeks of exposure, but neither dose nor duration is a reliable predictor of this problem. No patient characteristics have been clearly linked to the development of agranulocytosis in association with clozapine use, but agranulocytosis associated with other antipsychotic drugs has been reported to occur with a greater frequency in women, the elderly and in patients who are cachectic or have serious underlying medical illness; such patients may also be at particular risk with clozapine.

To reduce the risk of agranulocytosis developing undetected, clozapine is available only through a distribution system that ensures monitoring of WBC counts according to the schedule described above prior to delivery of the next supply of medication.

[See figure above]

Eosinophilia: In clinical trials, 1% of patients developed eosinophilia, which, in rare cases, can be substantial. If a differential count reveals a total eosinophil count above 4,000/mm^3, clozapine therapy should be interrupted until the eosinophil count falls below 3,000/mm^3.

Seizures: Seizure has been estimated to occur in association with clozapine use at a cumulative incidence at one year of approximately 5%, based on the occurrence of one or more seizures in 61 of 1743 patients exposed to clozapine during its clinical testing prior to domestic marketing (i.e., a crude rate of 3.5%). Dose appears to be an important predictor of seizure, with a greater likelihood of seizure at the higher clozapine doses used.

Caution should be used in administering clozapine to patients having a history of seizures or other predisposing factors. Because of the substantial risk of seizure associated with clozapine use, patients should be advised not to engage in any activity where sudden loss of consciousness could cause serious risk to themselves or others, e.g., the operation of complex machinery, driving an automobile, swimming, climbing, etc.

Myocarditis: Post-marketing surveillance data from four countries that employ hematological monitoring of clozapine-treated patients revealed: 30 reports of myocarditis with 17 fatalities in 205,493 U.S. patients (August 2001); 7 reports of myocarditis with 1 fatality in 15,600 Canadian patients (April 2001); 30 reports of myocarditis with 8 fatalities in 24,108 U.K. patients (August 2001); 15 reports of myocarditis with 5 fatalities in 8,000 Australian patients (March 1999). These reports represent an incidence of 5, 16.3, 43.2, and 96.6 cases/100,000 patient years, respectively. The number of fatalities represent an incidence of 2.8, 2.3, 11.5, and 32.2 cases/100,000 patient years, respectively.

The overall incidence rate of myocarditis in patients with schizophrenia treated with antipsychotic agents is unknown. However, for the established market economies (WHO), the incidence of myocarditis is 0.3 cases/100,000 patient years and the fatality rate is 0.2 cases/100,000 patient years. Therefore, the rate of myocarditis in clozapine-treated patients appears to be 17 to 322 times greater than the general population and is associated with an increased risk of fatal myocarditis that is 14 to 161 times greater than the general population.

The total reports of myocarditis for these four countries was 82 of which 51 (62%) occurred within the first month of clozapine treatment, 25 (31%) occurred after the first month of therapy and 6 (7%) were unknown. The median duration of treatment was 3 weeks. Of 5 patients rechallenged with clozapine, 3 had a recurrence of myocarditis. Of the 82 reports, 31 (38%) were fatal and 25 patients who died had evidence of myocarditis at autopsy. These data also suggest that the incidence of fatal myocarditis may be highest during the first month of therapy.

Therefore, the possibility of myocarditis should be considered in patients receiving clozapine who present with unexplained fatigue, dyspnea, tachypnea, fever, chest pain, palpitations, other signs or symptoms of heart failure, or electrocardiographic findings such as ST-T wave abnormalities or arrhythmias. It is not known whether eosinophilia is a reliable predictor of myocarditis. Tachycardia, which has been associated with clozapine treatment, has also been noted as a presenting sign in patients with myocarditis. Therefore, tachycardia during the first month of therapy warrants close monitoring for other signs of myocarditis.

Prompt discontinuation of clozapine treatment is warranted upon suspicion of myocarditis. Patients with clozapine-related myocarditis should not be rechallenged with clozapine.

Other Adverse Cardiovascular and Respiratory Effects: Orthostatic hypotension with or without syncope can occur with clozapine treatment and may represent a continuing risk in some patients. Rarely (approximately 1 case per 3,000 patients), collapse can be profound and be accompanied by respiratory and/or cardiac arrest. Orthostatic hypotension is more likely to occur during initial titration in association with rapid dose escalation and may even occur on first dose. In one report, initial doses as low as 12.5 mg were associated with collapse and respiratory arrest. When restarting patients who have had even a brief interval off clozapine, i.e., 2 days or more since the last dose, it is recommended that treatment be reinitiated with one-half of a 25 mg tablet (12.5 mg) once or twice daily (see **DOSAGE AND ADMINISTRATION**).

Some of the cases of collapse/respiratory arrest/cardiac arrest during initial treatment occurred in patients who were being administered benzodiazepines; similar events have been reported in patients taking other psychotropic drugs or even clozapine by itself. Although it has not been established that there is an interaction between clozapine and benzodiazepines or other psychotropics, caution is advised when clozapine is initiated in patients taking a benzodiazepine or any other psychotropic drug.

Tachycardia, which may be sustained, has also been observed in approximately 25% of patients taking clozapine, with patients having an average increase in pulse rate of 10 to 15 bpm. The sustained tachycardia is not simply a reflex response to hypotension, and is present in all positions monitored. Either tachycardia or hypotension may pose a serious risk for an individual with compromised cardiovascular function.

Continued on next page

Clozapine—Cont.

A minority of clozapine treated patients experience ECG repolarization changes similar to those seen with other antipsychotic drugs, including S-T segment depression and flattening or inversion of T waves, which all normalize after discontinuation of clozapine. The clinical significance of these changes is unclear. However, in clinical trials with clozapine, several patients experienced significant cardiac events, including ischemic changes, myocardial infarction, arrhythmias and sudden death. In addition there have been postmarketing reports of congestive heart failure, myocarditis, with or without eosinophilia, and pericarditis/pericardial effusions in association with clozapine use. Causality assessment was difficult in many of these cases because of serious pre-existing cardiac disease and plausible alternative causes. Rare instances of sudden death have been reported in psychiatric patients, with or without associated antipsychotic drug treatment, and the relationship of these events to antipsychotic drug use is unknown.

Clozapine should be used with caution in patients with known cardiovascular and/or pulmonary disease, and the recommendation for gradual titration of dose should be carefully observed.

Neuroleptic Malignant Syndrome (NMS): A potentially fatal symptom complex sometimes referred to as Neuroleptic Malignant Syndrome (NMS) has been reported in association with antipsychotic drugs. Clinical manifestations of NMS are hyperpyrexia, muscle rigidity, altered mental status and evidence of autonomic instability (irregular pulse or blood pressure, tachycardia, diaphoresis, and cardiac dysrhythmias).

The diagnostic evaluation of patients with this syndrome is complicated. In arriving at a diagnosis, it is important to identify cases where the clinical presentation includes both serious medical illness (e.g., pneumonia, systemic infection, etc.) and untreated or inadequately treated extrapyramidal signs and symptoms (EPS). Other important considerations in the differential diagnosis include central anticholinergic toxicity, heat stroke, drug fever and primary central nervous system (CNS) pathology.

The management of NMS should include 1) immediate discontinuation of antipsychotic drugs and other drugs not essential to concurrent therapy, 2) intensive symptomatic treatment and medical monitoring, and 3) treatment of any concomitant serious medical problems for which specific treatments are available. There is no general agreement about specific pharmacological treatment regimens for uncomplicated NMS.

If a patient requires antipsychotic drug treatment after recovery from NMS, the potential reintroduction of drug therapy should be carefully considered. The patient should be carefully monitored, since recurrences of NMS have been reported.

There have been several reported cases of NMS in patients receiving clozapine alone or in combination with lithium or other CNS-active agents.

Tardive Dyskinesia: A syndrome consisting of potentially irreversible, involuntary, dyskinetic movements may develop in patients treated with antipsychotic drugs. Although the prevalence of the syndrome appears to be highest among the elderly, especially elderly women, it is impossible to rely upon prevalence estimates to predict, at the inception of treatment, which patients are likely to develop the syndrome.

There are several reasons for predicting that clozapine may be different from other antipsychotic drugs in its potential for inducing tardive dyskinesia, including the preclinical finding that it has a relatively weak dopamine blocking effect and the clinical finding of a virtual absence of certain acute extrapyramidal symptoms, e.g., dystonia. A few cases of tardive dyskinesia have been reported in patients on clozapine who had been previously treated with other antipsychotic agents, so that a causal relationship cannot be established. There have been no reports of tardive dyskinesia directly attributable to clozapine alone. Nevertheless, it cannot be concluded, without more extended experience, that clozapine is incapable of inducing this syndrome.

Both the risk of developing the syndrome and the likelihood that it will become irreversible are believed to increase as the duration of treatment and the total cumulative dose of antipsychotic drugs administered to the patient increase. However, the syndrome can develop, although much less commonly, after relatively brief treatment periods at low doses. There is no known treatment for established cases of tardive dyskinesia, although the syndrome may remit, partially or completely, if antipsychotic drug treatment is withdrawn. Antipsychotic drug treatment, itself, however, may suppress (or partially suppress) the signs and symptoms of the syndrome and thereby may possibly mask the underlying process. The effect that symptom suppression has upon the long-term course of the syndrome is unknown.

Given these considerations, clozapine should be prescribed in a manner that is most likely to minimize the occurrence of tardive dyskinesia. As with any antipsychotic drug, chronic clozapine use should be reserved for patients who appear to be obtaining substantial benefit from the drug. In such patients, the smallest dose and the shortest duration of treatment should be sought. The need for continued treatment should be reassessed periodically.

If signs and symptoms of tardive dyskinesia appear in a patient on clozapine, drug discontinuation should be considered. However, some patients may require treatment with clozapine despite the presence of the syndrome.

PRECAUTIONS

General: Because of the significant risk of agranulocytosis and seizure, both of which present a continuing risk over time, the extended treatment of patients failing to show an acceptable level of clinical response should ordinarily be avoided. In addition, the need for continuing treatment in patients exhibiting beneficial clinical responses should be periodically re-evaluated. Although it is not known whether the risk would be increased, it is prudent either to avoid clozapine or use it cautiously in patients with a previous history of agranulocytosis induced by other drugs.

Cardiomyopathy: Cases of cardiomyopathy have been reported in patients treated with clozapine. The reporting rate for cardiomyopathy in clozapine-treated patients in the United States (8.9 per 100,000 person-years) was similar to an estimate of the cardiomyopathy incidence in the United States general population derived from the 1999 National Hospital Discharge Survey data (9.7 per 100,000 person-years). Approximately 80% of clozapine-treated patients in whom cardiomyopathy was reported were less than 50 years of age; the duration of treatment with clozapine prior to cardiomyopathy diagnosis varied, but was > 6 months in 65% of the reports. Dilated cardiomyopathy was most frequently reported, although a large percentage of reports did not specify the type of cardiomyopathy. Signs and symptoms suggestive of cardiomyopathy, particularly exertional dyspnea, fatigue, orthopnea, paroxysmal nocturnal dyspnea, and peripheral edema should alert the clinician to perform further investigations. If the diagnosis of cardiomyopathy is confirmed, the prescriber should discontinue clozapine unless the benefit to the patient clearly outweighs the risk.

Fever: During clozapine therapy, patients may experience transient temperature elevations above 100.4°F (38°C), with the peak incidence within the first 3 weeks of treatment. While this fever is generally benign and self limiting, it may necessitate discontinuing patients from treatment. On occasion, there may be an associated increase or decrease in WBC count. Patients with fever should be carefully evaluated to rule out the possibility of an underlying infectious process or the development of agranulocytosis. In the presence of high fever, the possibility of Neuroleptic Malignant Syndrome (NMS) must be considered. There have been several reports of NMS in patients receiving clozapine, usually in combination with lithium or other CNS-active drugs. [See WARNINGS: Neuroleptic Malignant Syndrome (NMS).]

Pulmonary Embolism: The possibility of pulmonary embolism should be considered in patients receiving clozapine who present with deep vein thrombosis, acute dyspnea, chest pain or with other respiratory signs and symptoms. As of December 31, 1993 there were 18 cases of fatal pulmonary embolism in association with clozapine therapy in users 10 to 54 years of age. Based upon the extent of use observed in the Clozapine National Registry, the mortality rate associated with pulmonary embolus was 1 death per 3450 person-years of use. This rate was about 27.5 times higher than that in the general population of a similar age and gender (95% Confidence Interval; 17.1, 42.2). Deep vein thrombosis has also been observed in association with clozapine therapy. Whether pulmonary embolus can be attributed to clozapine or some characteristic(s) of its users is not clear, but the occurrence of deep vein thrombosis or respiratory symptomatology should suggest its presence.

Hyperglycemia: Severe hyperglycemia, sometimes leading to ketoacidosis, has been reported during clozapine treatment in patients with no prior history of hyperglycemia. While a causal relationship to clozapine use has not been definitively established, glucose levels normalized in most patients after discontinuation of clozapine, and a rechallenge in one patient produced a recurrence of hyperglycemia. The effect of clozapine on glucose metabolism in patients with diabetes mellitus has not been studied. The possibility of impaired glucose tolerance should be considered in patients receiving clozapine who develop symptoms of hyperglycemia, such as polydipsia, polyuria, polyphagia, and weakness. In patients with significant treatment-emergent hyperglycemia, the discontinuation of clozapine should be considered.

Hepatitis: Caution is advised in patients using clozapine who have concurrent hepatic disease. Hepatitis has been reported in both patients with normal and pre-existing liver function abnormalities. In patients who develop nausea, vomiting, and/or anorexia during clozapine treatment, liver function tests should be performed immediately. If the elevation of these values is clinically relevant or if symptoms of jaundice occur, treatment with clozapine should be discontinued.

Anticholinergic Toxicity: ***Eye:*** Clozapine has potent anticholinergic effects and care should be exercised in using this drug in the presence of narrow angle glaucoma.

Gastrointestinal: Clozapine use has been associated with varying degrees of impairment of intestinal peristalsis, ranging from constipation to intestinal obstruction, fecal impaction and paralytic ileus (see ADVERSE REACTIONS). On rare occasions, these cases have been fatal. Constipation should be initially treated by ensuring adequate hydration, and use of ancillary therapy such as bulk laxatives. Consultation with a gastroenterologist is advisable in more serious cases.

Prostate: Clozapine has potent anticholinergic effects and care should be exercised in using this drug in the presence of prostatic enlargement.

Interference with Cognitive and Motor Performance: Because of initial sedation, clozapine may impair mental and/or physical abilities, especially during the first few days of therapy. The recommendations for gradual dose escalation should be carefully adhered to, and patients cautioned about activities requiring alertness.

Use in Patients with Concomitant Illness: Clinical experience with clozapine in patients with concomitant systemic diseases is limited. Nevertheless, caution is advisable in using clozapine in patients with renal or cardiac disease.

Use in Patients Undergoing General Anesthesia: Caution is advised in patients being administered general anesthesia because of the CNS effects of clozapine. Check with the anesthesiologist regarding continuation of clozapine therapy in a patient scheduled for surgery.

Information for Patients: Physicians are advised to discuss the following issues with patients for whom they prescribe clozapine:

— Patients who are to receive clozapine should be warned about the significant risk of developing agranulocytosis. They should be informed that weekly blood tests are required for the first 6 months, if acceptable WBC counts (WBC greater than or equal to 3000/mm^3, ANC ≥ 1500/mm^3) have been maintained during the first 6 months of continuous therapy, then WBC counts can be monitored every other week in order to monitor for the occurrence of agranulocytosis, and that clozapine tablets will be made available only through a special program designed to ensure the required blood monitoring. Patients should be advised to report immediately the appearance of lethargy, weakness, fever, sore throat, malaise, mucous membrane ulceration or other possible signs of infection. Particular attention should be paid to any flu-like complaints or other symptoms that might suggest infection.

— Patients should be informed of the significant risk of seizure during clozapine treatment, and they should be advised to avoid driving and any other potentially hazardous activity while taking clozapine.

— Patients should be advised of the risk of orthostatic hypotension, especially during the period of initial dose titration.

— Patients should be informed that if they stop taking clozapine for more than 2 days, they should not restart their medication at the same dosage, but should contact their physician for dosing instructions.

— Patients should notify their physician if they are taking, or plan to take, any prescription or over-the-counter drugs or alcohol.

— Patients should notify their physician if they become pregnant or intend to become pregnant during therapy.

— Patients should not breast feed an infant if they are taking clozapine.

Drug Interactions: The risks of using clozapine in combination with other drugs have not been systematically evaluated.

Pharmacodynamic-related Interactions: The mechanism of clozapine induced agranulocytosis is unknown; nonetheless, the possibility that causative factors may interact synergistically to increase the risk and/or severity of bone marrow suppression warrants consideration. Therefore, clozapine should not be used with other agents having a well-known potential to suppress bone marrow function.

Given the primary CNS effects of clozapine, caution is advised in using it concomitantly with other CNS-active drugs or alcohol.

Orthostatic hypotension in patients taking clozapine can, in rare cases (approximately 1 case per 3,000 patients), be accompanied by profound collapse and respiratory and/or cardiac arrest. Some of the cases of collapse/respiratory arrest/cardiac arrest during initial treatment occurred in patients who were being administered benzodiazepines; similar events have been reported in patients taking other psychotropic drugs or even clozapine by itself. Although it has not been established that there is an interaction between clozapine and benzodiazepines or other psychotropics, caution is advised when clozapine is initiated in patients taking a benzodiazepine or any other psychotropic drug.

Clozapine may potentiate the hypotensive effects of antihypertensive drugs and the anticholinergic effects of atropine-type drugs. The administration of epinephrine should be avoided in the treatment of drug induced hypotension because of a possible reverse epinephrine effect.

Pharmacokinetic-related Interactions: Clozapine is a substrate for many CYP 450 isozymes, in particular 1A2, 2D6, and 3A4. The risk of metabolic interactions caused by an effect on an individual isoform is therefore minimized. Nevertheless, caution should be used in patients receiving concomitant treatment with other drugs which are either inhibitors or inducers of these enzymes.

Concomitant administration of drugs known to induce cytochrome P450 enzymes may decrease the plasma levels of clozapine. Phenytoin, nicotine, and rifampin may decrease clozapine plasma levels, resulting in a decrease in effectiveness of a previously effective clozapine dose.

Concomitant administration of drugs known to inhibit the activity of cytochrome P450 isozymes may increase the plasma levels of clozapine. Cimetidine, caffeine, and erythromycin may increase plasma levels of clozapine, potentially resulting in adverse effects. Although concomitant use of clozapine and carbamazepine is not recommended, it should be noted that discontinuation of concomitant carbamazepine administration may result in an increase in clozapine plasma levels.

In a study of schizophrenic patients who received clozapine under steady state conditions, fluvoxamine or paroxetine was added in 16 and 14 patients, respectively. After 14 days of co-administration, mean trough concentrations of clozapine and its metabolites, *N*-desmethylclozapine and clozapine *N*-oxide, were elevated with fluvoxamine by about three-fold compared to baseline concentrations. Paroxetine produced only minor changes in the levels of clozapine and its metabolites. However, other published reports describe modest elevations (less than two-fold) of clozapine and metabolite concentrations when clozapine was taken with paroxetine, fluoxetine, and sertraline. Therefore, such combined treatment should be approached with caution and patients should be monitored closely when clozapine is combined with these drugs, particularly with fluvoxamine. A reduced clozapine dose should be considered.

A subset (3% to 10%) of the population has reduced activity of certain drug metabolizing enzymes such as the cytochrome P450 isozyme P450 2D6. Such individuals are referred to as "poor metabolizers" of drugs such as debrisoquin, dextromethorphan, the tricyclic antidepressants, and clozapine. These individuals may develop higher than expected plasma concentrations of clozapine when given usual doses. In addition, certain drugs that are metabolized by this isozyme, including many antidepressants (clozapine, selective serotonin reuptake inhibitors, and others), may inhibit the activity of this isozyme, and thus may make normal metabolizers resemble poor metabolizers with regard to concomitant therapy with other drugs metabolized by this enzyme system, leading to drug interaction.

Concomitant use of clozapine with other drugs metabolized by cytochrome P450 2D6 may require lower doses than usually prescribed for either clozapine or the other drug. Therefore, co-administration of clozapine with other drugs that are metabolized by this isozyme, including antidepressants, phenothiazines, carbamazepine, and Type 1C antiarrhythmics (e.g., propafenone, flecainide and encainide), or that inhibit this enzyme (e.g., quinidine), should be approached with caution.

Carcinogenesis, Mutagenesis, Impairment of Fertility: No carcinogenic potential was demonstrated in long-term studies in mice and rats at doses approximately 7 times the typical human dose on a mg/kg basis. Fertility in male and female rats was not adversely affected by clozapine. Clozapine did not produce genotoxic or mutagenic effects when assayed in appropriate bacterial and mammalian tests.

Pregnancy: *Teratogenic Effects. Pregnancy Category B:* Reproduction studies have been performed in rats and rabbits at doses of approximately 2 to 4 times the human dose and have revealed no evidence of impaired fertility or harm to the fetus due to clozapine. There are, however, no adequate and well-controlled studies in pregnant women. Because animal reproduction studies are not always predictive of human response, and in view of the desirability of keeping the administration of all drugs to a minimum during pregnancy, this drug should be used only if clearly needed.

Nursing Mothers: Animal studies suggest that clozapine may be excreted in breast milk and have an effect on the nursing infant. Therefore, women receiving clozapine should not breast feed.

Pediatric Use: Safety and effectiveness in pediatric patients have not been established.

Geriatric Use: Clinical Studies of clozapine did not include sufficient numbers of subjects aged 65 and over to determine whether they respond differently from younger subjects.

Orthostatic hypotension can occur with clozapine treatment and tachycardia, which may be sustained, has been observed in about 25% of patients taking clozapine (see WARNINGS: Adverse Cardiovascular and Respiratory Effects). Elderly patients, particularly those with compromised cardiovascular functioning, may be more susceptible to these effects.

Also, elderly patients may be particularly susceptible to the anticholinergic effects of clozapine, such as urinary retention and constipation. (See PRECAUTIONS: Anticholinergic Toxicity.)

Dose selection for an elderly patient should be cautious, reflecting the greater frequency of decreased hepatic, renal, or cardiac function, and of concomitant disease or other drug therapy. Other reported clinical experience does suggest that the prevalence of tardive dyskinesia appears to be highest among the elderly, especially elderly women (see WARNINGS: Tardive Dyskinesia).

ADVERSE REACTIONS

Associated with Discontinuation of Treatment: Sixteen percent of 1080 patients who received clozapine in premarketing clinical trials discontinued treatment due to an adverse event, including both those that could be reasonably attributed to clozapine treatment and those that might more appropriately be considered intercurrent illness. The more common events considered to be causes of discontinuation included: CNS, primarily drowsiness/sedation, seizures, dizziness/syncope; cardiovascular, primarily tachycardia, hypotension and ECG changes; gastrointestinal, primarily nausea/vomiting; hematologic, primarily leukopenia/granulocytopenia/agranulocytosis; and fever. None of the events enumerated accounts for more than 1.7% of all discontinuations attributed to adverse clinical events.

Commonly Observed: Adverse events observed in association with the use of clozapine in clinical trials at an incidence of greater than 5% were: central nervous system complaints, including drowsiness/sedation, dizziness/vertigo, headache and tremor; autonomic nervous system complaints, including salivation, sweating, dry mouth and visual disturbances; cardiovascular findings, including tachycardia, hypotension and syncope; and gastrointestinal complaints, including constipation and nausea; and fever. Complaints of drowsiness/sedation tend to subside with continued therapy or dose reduction. Salivation may be profuse, especially during sleep, but may be diminished with dose reduction.

Incidence in Clinical Trials: The following table enumerates adverse events that occurred at a frequency of 1% or greater among clozapine patients who participated in clinical trials. These rates are not adjusted for duration of exposure.

Treatment-Emergent Adverse Experience Incidence Among Patients Taking Clozapine in Clinical Trials (N = 842) (Percentage of Patients Reporting)

Body System Adverse Events[a]	Percent
Central Nervous System	
Drowsiness/Sedation	39
Dizziness/Vertigo	19
Headache	7
Tremor	6
Syncope	6
Disturbed sleep/Nightmares	4
Restlessness	4
Hypokinesia/Akinesia	4
Agitation	4
Seizures (convulsions)	3[b]
Rigidity	3
Akathisia	3
Confusion	3
Fatigue	2
Insomnia	2
Hyperkinesia	1
Weakness	1
Lethargy	1
Ataxia	1
Slurred speech	1
Depression	1
Epileptiform movements/Myoclonic jerks	1
Anxiety	1
Cardiovascular	
Tachycardia	25[b]
Hypotension	9
Hypertension	4
Chest pain/Angina	1
ECG Change/Cardiac abnormality	1
Gastrointestinal	
Constipation	14
Nausea	5
Abdominal discomfort/Heartburn	4
Nausea/Vomiting	3
Vomiting	3
Diarrhea	2
Liver test abnormality	1
Anorexia	1
Urogenital	
Urinary abnormalities	2
Incontinence	1
Abnormal ejaculation	1
Urinary urgency/frequency	1
Urinary retention	1
Autonomic Nervous System	
Salivation	31
Sweating	6
Dry mouth	6
Visual disturbances	5
Integumentary (Skin)	
Rash	2
Musculoskeletal	
Muscle weakness	1
Pain (back, neck, legs)	1
Muscle spasm	1
Muscle pain, ache	1
Respiratory	
Throat discomfort	1
Dyspnea, shortness of breath	1
Nasal congestion	1
Hemic/Lymphatic	
Leukopenia/Decreased WBC/Neutropenia	3
Agranulocytosis	1[b]
Eosinophilia	1
Miscellaneous	
Fever	5
Weight gain	4
Tongue numb/sore	1

[a] Events reported by at least 1% of clozapine patients are included.

[b] Rate based on population of approximately 1700 exposed during premarket clinical evaluation of clozapine.

Other Events Observed During the Premarketing Evaluation of Clozapine: This section reports additional, less frequent adverse events which occurred among the patients taking clozapine in clinical trials. Various adverse events were reported as part of the total experience in these clinical studies; a causal relationship to clozapine treatment cannot be determined in the absence of appropriate controls in some of the studies. The table above enumerates adverse events that occurred at a frequency of at least 1% of patients treated with clozapine. The list below includes all additional adverse experiences reported as being temporally associated with the use of the drug which occurred at a frequency less than 1%, enumerated by organ system.

Central Nervous System: loss of speech, amentia, tics, poor coordination, delusions/hallucinations, involuntary movement, stuttering, dysarthria, amnesia/memory loss, histrionic movements, libido increase or decrease, paranoia, shakiness, Parkinsonism, and irritability.

Cardiovascular System: edema, palpitations, phlebitis/thrombophlebitis, cyanosis, premature ventricular contraction, bradycardia, and nose bleed.

Gastrointestinal System: abdominal distention, gastroenteritis, rectal bleeding, nervous stomach, abnormal stools, hematemesis, gastric ulcer, bitter taste, and eructation.

Urogenital System: dysmenorrhea, impotence, breast pain/discomfort, and vaginal itch/infection.

Autonomic Nervous System: numbness, polydipsia, hot flashes, dry throat, and mydriasis.

Integumentary (Skin): pruritus, pallor, eczema, erythema, bruise, dermatitis, petechiae, and urticaria.

Musculoskeletal System: twitching and joint pain.

Respiratory System: coughing, pneumonia/pneumonia-like symptoms, rhinorrhea, hyperventilation, wheezing, bronchitis, laryngitis, and sneezing.

Hemic and Lymphatic System: anemia and leukocytosis.

Miscellaneous: chills/chills with fever, malaise, appetite increase, ear disorder, hypothermia, eyelid disorder, bloodshot eyes, and nystagmus.

Postmarketing Clinical Experience: Postmarketing experience has shown an adverse experience profile similar to that presented above. Voluntary reports of adverse events temporally associated with clozapine not mentioned above that have been received since market introduction and that may have no causal relationship with the drug include the following:

Central Nervous System: delirium; EEG abnormal; exacerbation of psychosis; myoclonus; overdose; paresthesia; possible mild cataplexy; and status epilepticus.

Cardiovascular System: atrial or ventricular fibrillation and periorbital edema.

Gastrointestinal System: acute pancreatitis; dysphagia; fecal impaction; intestinal obstruction/paralytic ileus; and salivary gland swelling.

Hepatobiliary System: cholestasis; hepatitis; and jaundice.

Hepatic System: cholestasis.

Urogenital System: acute interstitial nephritis and priapism.

Integumentary (Skin): hypersensitivity reactions: photosensitivity, vasculitis, erythema multiforme, and Stevens-Johnson Syndrome.

Musculoskeletal System: myasthenic syndrome and rhabdomyolysis.

Respiratory System: aspiration and pleural effusion.

Hemic and Lymphatic System: deep vein thrombosis; elevated hemoglobin/hematocrit; ESR increased; pulmonary embolism; sepsis; thrombocytosis; and thrombocytopenia.

Vision Disorders: narrow angle glaucoma.

Miscellaneous: CPK elevation; hyperglycemia; hyperuricemia; hyponatremia; and weight loss.

DRUG ABUSE AND DEPENDENCE

Physical and psychological dependence have not been reported or observed in patients taking clozapine.

OVERDOSAGE

Human Experience: The most commonly reported signs and symptoms associated with clozapine overdose are: altered states of consciousness, including drowsiness, delirium and coma; tachycardia; hypotension; respiratory depression or failure; hypersalivation. Aspiration pneumonia and cardiac arrhythmias have also been reported. Seizures have occurred in a minority of reported cases. Fatal overdoses have been reported with clozapine, generally at doses above 2500 mg. There have also been reports of patients recovering from overdoses well in excess of 4 g.

Management of Overdose: Establish and maintain an airway; ensure adequate oxygenation and ventilation. Activated charcoal, which may be used with sorbitol, may be as or more effective than emesis or lavage, and should be considered in treating overdosage. Cardiac and vital signs monitoring is recommended along with general symptomatic and supportive measures. Additional surveillance should be continued for several days because of the risk of delayed effects. Avoid epinephrine and derivatives when treating hypotension, and quinidine and procainamide when treating cardiac arrhythmia.

There are no specific antidotes for clozapine. Forced diuresis, dialysis, hemoperfusion and exchange transfusion are unlikely to be of benefit.

In managing overdosage, the physician should consider the possibility of multiple drug involvement.

Continued on next page

Clozapine—Cont.

Up-to-date information about the treatment of overdose can often be obtained from a certified Regional Poison Control Center. Telephone numbers of certified Poison Control Centers are listed in the Physicians' Desk Reference®.*

DOSAGE AND ADMINISTRATION

Upon initiation of clozapine therapy, up to a 1 week supply of additional clozapine tablets may be provided to the patient to be held for emergencies (e.g., weather, holidays).

Initial Treatment: It is recommended that treatment with clozapine begin with one-half of a 25 mg tablet (12.5 mg) once or twice daily and then be continued with daily dosage increments of 25 to 50 mg/day, if well-tolerated, to achieve a target dose of 300 to 450 mg/day by the end of 2 weeks. Subsequent dosage increments should be made no more than once or twice weekly, in increments not to exceed 100 mg. Cautious titration and a divided dosage schedule are necessary to minimize the risks of hypotension, seizure, and sedation.

In the multicenter study that provides primary support for the effectiveness of clozapine in patients resistant to standard antipsychotic drug treatment, patients were titrated during the first 2 weeks up to a maximum dose of 500 mg/day, on a t.i.d. basis, and were then dosed in a total daily dose range of 100 to 900 mg/day, on a t.i.d. basis thereafter, with clinical response and adverse effects as guides to correct dosing.

Therapeutic Dose Adjustment: Daily dosing should continue on a divided basis as an effective and tolerable dose level is sought. While many patients may respond adequately at doses between 300 to 600 mg/day, it may be necessary to raise the dose to the 600 to 900 mg/day range to obtain an acceptable response. [Note: In the multicenter study providing the primary support for the superiority of clozapine in treatment resistant patients, the mean and median clozapine doses were both approximately 600 mg/day.]

Because of the possibility of increased adverse reactions at higher doses, particularly seizures, patients should ordinarily be given adequate time to respond to a given dose level before escalation to a higher dose is contemplated.

Clozapine can cause EEG changes, including the occurrence of spike and wave complexes. It lowers the seizures threshold in a dose-dependent manner and may induce myoclonic jerks or generalized seizures. These symptoms may be likely to occur with rapid dose increase and in patients with pre-existing epilepsy. In this case, the dose should be reduced and, if necessary, anticonvulsant treatment initiated. Dosing should not exceed 900 mg/day.

Because of the significant risk of agranulocytosis and seizure, events which both present a continuing risk over time, the extended treatment of patients failing to show an acceptable level of clinical response should ordinarily be avoided.

Maintenance Treatment: While the maintenance effectiveness of clozapine in schizophrenia is still under study, the effectiveness of maintenance treatment is well established for many other antipsychotic drugs. It is recommended that responding patients be continued on clozapine, but at the lowest level needed to maintain remission. Because of the significant risk associated with the use of clozapine, patients should be periodically reassessed to determine the need for maintenance treatment.

Discontinuation of Treatment: In the event of planned termination of clozapine therapy, gradual reduction in dose is recommended over a 1 to 2 week period. However, should a patient's medical condition require abrupt discontinuation (e.g., leukopenia), the patient should be carefully observed for the recurrence of psychotic symptoms and symptoms related to cholinergic rebound such as headache, nausea, vomiting, and diarrhea.

Reinitiation of Treatment in Patients Previously Discontinued: When restarting patients who have had even a brief off clozapine, i.e., 2 days or more since the last dose, it is recommended that treatment be reinitiated with one-half of a 25 mg tablet (12.5 mg) once or twice daily (see WARNINGS). If that dose is well tolerated, it may be feasible to titrate patients back to a therapeutic dose more quickly than is recommended for initial treatment. However, any patient who has previously experienced respiratory or cardiac arrest with initial dosing, but was then able to be successfully titrated to a therapeutic dose, should be re-titrated with extreme caution after even 24 hours of discontinuation.

Certain additional precautions seem prudent when reinitiating treatment. The mechanisms underlying clozapine induced adverse reactions are unknown. It is conceivable, however, that re-exposure of a patient might enhance the risk of an untoward event's occurrence and increase its severity. Such phenomena, for example, occur when immune mediated mechanisms are responsible. Consequently, during the reinitiation of treatment, additional caution is advised. Patients discontinued for WBC counts below $2000/mm^3$ or an ANC below $1000/mm^3$ must *not* be re-started on clozapine. (See WARNINGS.)

HOW SUPPLIED

Clozapine Tablets USP, 25 mg and 100 mg are available as follows:

The 25 mg tablets are round, peach, scored, biconvex tablets with **C** to the left of the score and **7** to the right of the score on one side of the tablet and **M** on the other side. They are available as follows:

NDC 0378-0825-01
bottles of 100 tablets

The 100 mg tablets are round, green, scored, biconvex tablets with **C11** above the score and blank below the score on one side of the tablet and **M** on the other side. They are available as follows:

NDC 0378-0860-01
bottles of 100 tablets
NDC 0378-0860-05
bottles of 500 tablets

STORE AT ROOM TEMPERATURE 15° TO 30°C (59° TO 86°F).

Dispense in a tight, light-resistant container as defined in the USP using a child-resistant closure.

Drug dispensing should not ordinarily exceed a weekly supply. If a patient is eligible for WBC testing every other week, then a two week supply of clozapine can be dispensed. Dispensing should be contingent upon the results of a WBC count.

*Trademark of Medical Economics Company, Inc.

MYLAN®
Mylan Pharmaceuticals Inc.
Morgantown, WV 26505

REVISED JANUARY 2003
CLOZ:R6

DIGITEK®
(digoxin tablets, USP) ℞

℞ only

DESCRIPTION

DIGITEK (digoxin) is one of the cardiac (or digitalis) glycosides, a closely related group of drugs having in common specific effects on the myocardium. These drugs are found in a number of plants. Digoxin is extracted from the leaves of *Digitalis lanata.* The term "digitalis" is used to designate the whole group of glycosides. The glycosides are composed of two portions: a sugar and a cardenolide (hence "glycosides").

Digoxin is described chemically as (3 β, 5 β, 12 β)-3-[(*O*-2,6-dideoxy-β-*D*-*ribo*-hexopyranosyl-(1→4)-*O*-2,6-dideoxy-β-*D*-*ribo*-hexopyranosyl-(1→4)-2,6-dideoxy-β-*D*-*ribo*-hexopyranosyl)oxy]-12,14-dihydroxy-card-20(22)-enolide. Its molecular formula is $C_{41}H_{64}O_{14}$, its molecular weight is 780.94, and the structural formula shown:

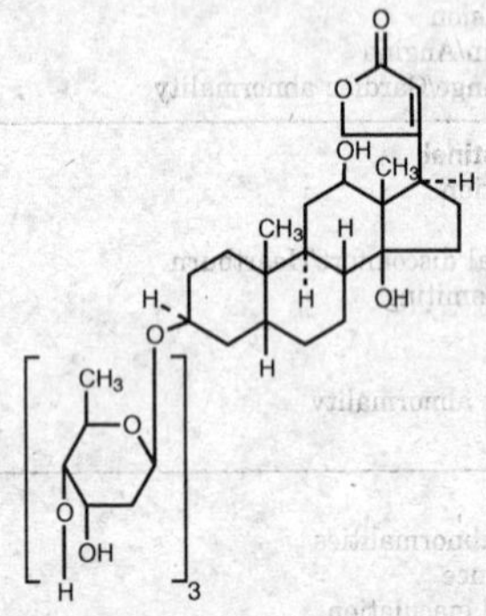

Digoxin exists as odorless white crystals that melt with decomposition above 230°C. The drug is practically insoluble in water and in ether; slightly soluble in diluted (50%) alcohol and in chloroform; and freely soluble in pyridine.

DIGITEK is supplied as 125-mcg (0.125-mg) or 250-mcg (0.25-mg) tablets for oral administration. Each tablet contains the labeled amount of digoxin USP and the following inactive ingredients: corn starch, croscarmellose sodium, microcrystalline cellulose, pregelatinized starch, lactose monohydrate and anhydrous lactose, silicon dioxide and stearic acid. In addition, the 125-mcg (0.125-mg) tablet contains D&C Yellow No. 10 Aluminum Lake.

CLINICAL PHARMACOLOGY

Mechanism of Action: Digoxin inhibits sodium-potassium ATPase, an enzyme that regulates the quantity of sodium and potassium inside cells. Inhibition of the enzyme leads to an increase in the intracellular concentration of sodium and thus (by stimulation of sodium-calcium exchange) an increase in the intracellular concentration of calcium. The beneficial effects of digoxin result from direct actions on cardiac muscle, as well as indirect actions on the cardiovascular system mediated by effects on the autonomic nervous system. The autonomic effects include: (1) a vagomimetic action, which is responsible for the effects of digoxin on the sinoatrial and atrioventricular (AV) nodes; and (2) baroreceptor sensitization, which results in increased afferent inhibitory activity and reduced activity of the sympathetic nervous system and renin-angiotensin system for any given increment in mean arterial pressure. The pharmacologic consequences of these direct and indirect effects are: (1) an increase in the force and velocity of myocardial systolic contraction (positive inotropic action); (2) a decrease in the degree of activation of the sympathetic nervous system and renin-angiotensin system (neurohormonal deactivating effect); and (3) slowing of the heart rate and decreased conduction velocity through the AV node (vagomimetic effect).

The effects of digoxin in heart failure are mediated by its positive inotropic and neurohormonal deactivating effects, whereas the effects of the drug in atrial arrhythmias are related to its vagomimetic actions. In high doses, digoxin increases sympathetic outflow from the central nervous system (CNS). This increase in sympathetic activity may be an important factor in digitalis toxicity.

Pharmacokinetics: ***Absorption:*** Following oral administration, peak serum concentrations of digoxin occur at 1 to 3 hours. Absorption of digoxin from digoxin tablets has been demonstrated to be 60% to 80% complete compared to an identical intravenous dose of digoxin (absolute bioavailability) or Digoxin Solution in Capsules (relative bioavailability). When digoxin tablets are taken after meals, the rate of absorption is slowed, but the total amount of digoxin absorbed is usually unchanged. When taken with meals high in bran fiber, however, the amount absorbed from an oral dose may be reduced. Comparisons of the systemic availability and equivalent doses for oral preparations of digoxin are shown in Table 1:

Table 1: Comparisons of the Systemic Availability and Equivalent Doses for Oral Preparations of Digoxin

Product	Absolute Bio-availability	Equivalent Doses (mcg)* Among Dosage Forms			
Digoxin Tablets	60-80%	62.5	125	250	500
Digoxin Pediatric Elixir	70-85%	62.5	125	250	500
Digoxin Solution in Capsules	90-100%	50	100	200	400
Digoxin Injection/IV	100%	50	100	200	400

*For example, 125-mcg Digoxin Tablets equivalent to 125 mcg Digoxin Pediatric Elixir equivalent to 100 mcg Digoxin Solution in Capsules equivalent to 100 mcg Digoxin Injection/IV.

In some patients, orally administered digoxin is converted to inactive reduction products (e.g., dihydrodigoxin) by colonic bacteria in the gut. Data suggest that one in ten patients treated with digoxin tablets will degrade 40% or more of the ingested dose. As a result, certain antibiotics may increase the absorption of digoxin in such patients. Although inactivation of these bacteria by antibiotics is rapid, the serum digoxin concentration will rise at a rate consistent with the elimination half-life of digoxin. The magnitude of rise in serum digoxin concentration relates to the extent of bacterial inactivation, and may be as much as two-fold in some cases.

Distribution: Following drug administration, a 6-to 8-hour tissue distribution phase is observed. This is followed by a much more gradual decline in the serum concentration of the drug, which is dependent on the elimination of digoxin from the body. The peak height and slope of the early portion (absorption/distribution phases) of the serum concentration-time curve are dependent upon the route of administration and the absorption characteristics of the formulation. Clinical evidence indicates that the early high serum concentrations do not reflect the concentration of digoxin at its site of action, but that with chronic use, the steady-state post-distribution serum concentrations are in equilibrium with tissue concentrations and correlate with pharmacologic effects. In individual patients, these post-distribution serum concentrations may be useful in evaluating therapeutic and toxic effects (see DOSAGE AND ADMINISTRATION: Serum Digoxin Concentrations).

Digoxin is concentrated in tissues and therefore has a large apparent volume of distribution. Digoxin crosses both the blood-brain barrier and the placenta. At delivery, the serum digoxin concentration in the newborn is similar to the serum concentration in the mother. Approximately 25% of digoxin in the plasma is bound to protein. Serum digoxin concentrations are not significantly altered by large changes in fat tissue weight, so that its distribution space correlates best with lean (i.e., ideal) body weight, not total body weight.

Metabolism: Only a small percentage (16%) of a dose of digoxin is metabolized. The end metabolites, which include 3 β-digoxigenin, 3-keto-digoxigenin, and their glucuronide and sulfate conjugates, are polar in nature and are postulated to be formed via hydrolysis, oxidation, and conjugation. The metabolism of digoxin is not dependent upon the cytochrome P-450 system, and digoxin is not known to induce or inhibit the cytochrome P-450 system.

Excretion: Elimination of digoxin follows first-order kinetics (that is, the quantity of digoxin eliminated at any time is proportional to the total body content). Following intravenous administration to healthy volunteers, 50% to 70% of a digoxin dose is excreted unchanged in the urine. Renal excretion of digoxin is proportional to glomerular filtration rate and is largely independent of urine flow. In healthy volunteers with normal renal function, digoxin has a half-life of 1.5 to 2 days. The half-life in anuric patients is prolonged to 3.5 to 5 days. Digoxin is not effectively removed from the body by dialysis, exchange transfusion, or during cardiopulmonary bypass because most of the drug is bound to tissue and does not circulate in the blood.

Special Populations: Race differences in digoxin pharmacokinetics have not been formally studied. Because digoxin is primarily eliminated as unchanged drug via the kidney and because there are no important differences in creatinine clearance among races, pharmacokinetic differences due to race are not expected.

The clearance of digoxin can be primarily correlated with renal function as indicated by creatinine clearance. The Cockcroft and Gault formula for estimation of creatinine clearance includes age, body weight, and gender. A table that provides the usual daily maintenance dose requirements of digoxin tablets based on creatinine clearance (per 70 kg) is presented in the DOSAGE AND ADMINISTRATION section.

Plasma digoxin concentration profiles in patients with acute hepatitis generally fell within the range of profiles in a group of healthy subjects.

Pharmacodynamic and Clinical Effects: The times to onset of pharmacologic effect and to peak effect of preparations of digoxin are shown in Table 2:

Table 2: Times to Onset of Pharmacologic Effect and to Peak Effect of Preparations of Digoxin

Product	Time to Onset of Effect*	Time to Peak Effect*
Digoxin Tablets	0.5-2 hours	2-6 hours
Digoxin Pediatric Elixir	0.5-2 hours	2-6 hours
Digoxin Solution in Capsules	0.5-2 hours	2-6 hours
Digoxin Injection/IV	5-30 minutes†	1-4 hours

*Documented for ventricular response rate in atrial fibrillation, inotropic effects and electrocardiographic changes.
† Depending upon rate of infusion.

Hemodynamic effects: Digoxin produces hemodynamic improvement in patients with heart failure. Short- and long-term therapy with the drug increases cardiac output and lowers pulmonary artery pressure, pulmonary capillary wedge pressure, and systemic vascular resistance. These hemodynamic effects are accompanied by an increase in the left ventricular ejection fraction and a decrease in end-systolic and end-diastolic dimensions.

Chronic Heart Failure: Two 12-week, double-blind, placebo-controlled studies enrolled 178 (RADIANCE trial) and 88 (PROVED trial) patients with NYHA class II or III heart failure previously treated with digoxin, a diuretic, and an ACE inhibitor (RADIANCE only) and randomized them to placebo or treatment with digoxin. Both trials demonstrated better preservation of exercise capacity in patients randomized to digoxin. Continued treatment with digoxin reduced the risk of developing worsening heart failure, as evidenced by heart failure-related hospitalizations and emergency care and the need for concomitant heart failure therapy. The larger study also showed treatment-related benefits in NYHA class and patients' global assessment. In the smaller trial, these trended in favor of a treatment benefit.

The Digitalis Investigation Group (DIG) main trial was a multicenter, randomized, double-blind, placebo-controlled mortality study of 6,801 patients with heart failure and left ventricular ejection fraction ≤0.45. At randomization, 67% were NYHA class I or II, 71% had heart failure of ischemic etiology, 44% had been receiving digoxin, and most were receiving concomitant ACE inhibitor (94%) and diuretic (82%). Patients were randomized to placebo or digoxin, the dose of which was adjusted for the patient's age, sex, lean body weight, and serum creatinine (see DOSAGE AND ADMINISTRATION), and followed for up to 58 months (median 37 months). The median daily dose prescribed was 0.25 mg. Overall all-cause mortality was 35% with no difference between groups (95% confidence limits for relative risk of 0.91 to 1.07). Digoxin was associated with a 25% reduction in the number of hospitalizations for heart failure, a 28% reduction in the risk of a patient having at least one hospitalization for heart failure, and a 6.5% reduction in total hospitalizations (for any cause).

Use of digoxin was associated with a trend in reduction in time to all-cause death or hospitalization. The trend was evident in subgroups of patients with mild heart failure as well as more severe disease, as shown in Table 3. Although the effect on all-cause death or hospitalization was not statistically significant, much of the apparent benefit derived from effects on mortality and hospitalization attributed to heart failure.

[See table 3 above]

Table 3: Subgroup Analyses of Mortality and Hospitalization During the First Two Years Following Randomization.

	n	Risk of All Cause Mortality or All Cause Hospitalization* Placebo	Digoxin	Relative risk†
All Patients (EF ≤0.45)	6801	604	593	0.94 (0.88-1.00)
NYHA I/II	4571	549	541	0.96 (0.89-1.04)
EF 0.25-0.45	4543	568	571	0.99 (0.91-1.07)
CTR ≤ 0.55	4455	561	563	0.98 (0.91-1.06)
NYHA III/IV	2224	719	696	0.88 (0.80-0.97)
EF<0.25	2258	677	637	0.84 (0.76-0.93)
CTR>0.55	2346	687	650	0.85 (0.77-0.94)
EF>0.45‡	987	571	585	1.04 (0.88-1.23)
	n	Risk of HF Related Mortality or HF Related Hospitalization* Placebo	Digoxin	Relative risk†
All Patients (EF≤0.45)	6801	294	217	0.69 (0.63-0.76)
NYHA I/II	4571	242	178	0.70 (0.62-0.80)
EF 0.25-0.45	4543	244	190	0.74 (0.66-0.84)
CTR≤0.55	4455	239	180	0.71 (0.63-0.81)
NYHA III/IV	2224	402	295	0.65 (0.57-0.75)
EF <0.25	2258	394	270	0.61 (0.53-0.71)
CTR >0.55	2346	398	287	0.65 (0.57-0.75)
EF >0.45‡	987	179	136	0.72 (0.53-0.99)

*Number of patients with an event during the first 2 years per 1000 randomized patients.
† Relative risk (95% confidence interval).
‡ DIG Ancillary Study.

In situations where there is no statistically significant benefit of treatment evident from a trial's primary endpoint, results pertaining to a secondary end-point should be interpreted cautiously.

Chronic Atrial Fibrillation: In patients with chronic atrial fibrillation, digoxin slows rapid ventricular response rate in linear dose-response fashion from 0.25 to 0.75 mg/day. Digoxin should not be used for the treatment of multifocal atrial tachycardia.

INDICATIONS AND USAGE

Heart Failure: DIGITEK is indicated for the treatment of mild to moderate heart failure. Digoxin increases left ventricular ejection fraction and improves heart failure symptoms as evidenced by exercise capacity and heart failure-related hospitalizations and emergency care, while having no effect on mortality. Where possible, digoxin should be used with a diuretic and an angiotensin-converting enzyme inhibitor, but an optimal order for starting these three drugs cannot be specified.

Atrial Fibrillation: DIGITEK is indicated for the control of ventricular response rate in patients with chronic atrial fibrillation.

CONTRAINDICATIONS

Digitalis glycosides are contraindicated in patients with ventricular fibrillation or in patients with a known hypersensitivity to digoxin. A hypersensitivity reaction to other digitalis preparations usually constitutes a contraindication to digoxin.

WARNINGS

Sinus Node Disease and AV Block: Because digoxin slows sinoatrial and AV conduction, the drug commonly prolongs the PR interval. The drug may cause severe sinus bradycardia or sinoatrial block in patients with pre-existing sinus node disease and may cause advanced or complete heart block in patients with pre-existing incomplete AV block. In such patients consideration should be given to the insertion of a pacemaker before treatment with digoxin.

Accessory AV Pathway (Wolff-Parkinson-White Syndrome): After intravenous digoxin therapy, some patients with paroxysmal atrial fibrillation or flutter and a coexisting accessory AV pathway have developed increased antegrade conduction across the accessory pathway bypassing the AV node, leading to a very rapid ventricular response or ventricular fibrillation. Unless conduction down the accessory pathway has been blocked (either pharmacologically or by surgery), digoxin should not be used in such patients. The treatment of paroxysmal supraventricular tachycardia in such patients is usually direct-current cardioversion.

Use in Patients with Preserved Left Ventricular Systolic Function: Patients with certain disorders involving heart failure associated with preserved left ventricular ejection fraction may be particularly susceptible to toxicity of the drug. Such disorders include restrictive cardiomyopathy, constrictive pericarditis, amyloid heart disease, and acute cor pulmonale. Patients with idiopathic hypertrophic subaortic stenosis may have worsening of the outflow obstruction due to the inotropic effects of digoxin.

PRECAUTIONS

Use in Patients with Impaired Renal Function: Digoxin is primarily excreted by the kidneys; therefore, patients with impaired renal function require smaller than usual maintenance doses of digoxin (see DOSAGE AND ADMINISTRATION). Because of the prolonged elimination half-life, a longer period of time is required to achieve an initial or new steady-state serum concentration in patients with renal impairment than in patients with normal renal function. If appropriate care is not taken to reduce the dose of digoxin, such patients are at high risk for toxicity, and toxic effects will last longer in such patients than in patients with normal renal function.

Use in Patients with Electrolyte Disorders: In patients with hypokalemia or hypomagnesemia, toxicity may occur despite serum digoxin concentrations below 2 ng/mL, because potassium or magnesium depletion sensitizes the myocardium to digoxin. Therefore, it is desirable to maintain normal serum potassium and magnesium concentrations in patients being treated with digoxin. Deficiencies of these electrolytes may result from malnutrition, diarrhea, or prolonged vomiting, as well as the use of the following drugs or procedures: diuretics, amphotericin B, corticosteroids, antacids, dialysis, and mechanical suction of gastrointestinal secretions.

Hypercalcemia from any cause predisposes the patient to digitalis toxicity. Calcium, particularly when administered rapidly by the intravenous route, may produce serious arrhythmias in digitalized patients. On the other hand, hypocalcemia can nullify the effects of digoxin in humans; thus, digoxin may be ineffective until serum calcium is restored to normal. These interactions are related to the fact that digoxin affects contractility and excitability of the heart in a manner similar to that of calcium.

Use in Thyroid Disorders and Hypermetabolic States: Hypothyroidism may reduce the requirements for digoxin. Heart failure and/or atrial arrhythmias resulting from hypermetabolic or hyperdynamic states (e.g., hyperthyroidism, hypoxia, or arteriovenous shunt) are best treated by addressing the underlying condition. Atrial arrhythmias associated with hypermetabolic states are particularly resistant to digoxin treatment. Care must be taken to avoid toxicity if digoxin is used.

Use in Patients with Acute Myocardial Infarction: Digoxin should be used with caution in patients with acute myocardial infarction. The use of inotropic drugs in some patients in this setting may result in undesirable increases in myocardial oxygen demand and ischemia.

Use During Electrical Cardioversion: It may be desirable to reduce the dose of digoxin for 1 to 2 days prior to electrical cardioversion of atrial fibrillation to avoid the induction of ventricular arrhythmias, but physicians must consider the consequences of increasing the ventricular response if digoxin is withdrawn. If digitalis toxicity is suspected, elective cardioversion should be delayed. If it is not prudent to

Continued on next page

Digitek—Cont.

delay cardioversion, the lowest possible energy level should be selected to avoid provoking ventricular arrhythmias.

Laboratory Test Monitoring: Patients receiving digoxin should have their serum electrolytes and renal function (serum creatinine concentrations) assessed periodically; the frequency of assessments will depend on the clinical setting. For discussion of serum digoxin concentrations, see DOSAGE AND ADMINISTRATION section.

Drug Interactions: Potassium-depleting *diuretics* are a major contributing factor to digitalis toxicity. *Calcium*, particularly if administered rapidly by the intravenous route, may produce serious arrhythmias in digitalized patients. *Quinidine, verapamil, amiodarone, propafenone, indomethacin, itraconazole, alprazolam, and spironolactone* raise the serum digoxin concentration due to a reduction in clearance and/or in volume of distribution of the drug, with the implication that digitalis intoxication may result. *Erythromycin* and *clarithromycin* (and possibly other *macrolide antibiotics*) and *tetracycline* may increase digoxin absorption in patients who inactivate digoxin by bacterial metabolism in the lower intestine, so that digitalis intoxication may result (see CLINICAL PHARMACOLOGY: Absorption). *Propantheline* and *diphenoxylate*, by decreasing gut motility, may increase digoxin absorption. *Antacids, kaolin-pectin, sulfasalazine, neomycin, cholestyramine,* certain *anticancer drugs,* and *metoclopramide* may interfere with intestinal digoxin absorption, resulting in unexpectedly low serum concentrations. *Rifampin* may decrease serum digoxin concentration, especially in patients with renal dysfunction, by increasing the non-renal clearance of digoxin. There have been inconsistent reports regarding the effects of other drugs [e.g., *quinine, penicillamine*] on serum digoxin concentration. *Thyroid* administration to a digitalized, hypothyroid patient may increase the dose requirement of digoxin. Concomitant use of digoxin and *sympathomimetics* increases the risk of cardiac arrhythmias. *Succinylcholine* may cause a sudden extrusion of potassium from muscle cells, and may thereby cause arrhythmias in digitalized patients. Although beta-adrenergic blockers or calcium channel blockers and digoxin may be useful in combination to control atrial fibrillation, their additive effects on AV node conduction can result in advanced or complete heart block.

Due to the considerable variability of these interactions, the dosage of digoxin should be individualized when patients receive these medications concurrently. Furthermore, caution should be exercised when combining digoxin with any drug that may cause a significant deterioration in renal function, since a decline in glomerular filtration or tubular secretion may impair the excretion of digoxin.

Drug/Laboratory Test Interactions: The use of therapeutic doses of digoxin may cause prolongation of the PR interval and depression of the ST segment on the electrocardiogram. Digoxin may produce false positive ST-T changes on the electrocardiogram during exercise testing. These electrophysiologic effects reflect an expected effect of the drug and are not indicative of toxicity.

Carcinogenesis, Mutagenesis, Impairment of Fertility: There have been no long-term studies performed in animals to evaluate carcinogenic potential, nor have studies been conducted to assess the mutagenic potential of digoxin or its potential to affect fertility.

Pregnancy: ***Teratogenic Effects:*** Pregnancy Category C. Animal reproduction studies have not been conducted with digoxin. It is also not known whether digoxin can cause fetal harm when administered to a pregnant woman or can affect reproductive capacity. Digoxin should be given to a pregnant woman only if clearly needed.

Nursing Mothers: Studies have shown that digoxin concentrations in the mother's serum and milk are similar. However, the estimated exposure of a nursing infant to digoxin via breast feeding will be far below the usual infant maintenance dose. Therefore, this amount should have no pharmacologic effect upon the infant. Nevertheless, caution should be exercised when digoxin is administered to a nursing woman.

Pediatric Use: Newborn infants display considerable variability in their tolerance to digoxin. Premature and immature infants are particularly sensitive to the effects of digoxin, and the dosage of the drug must not only be reduced but must be individualized according to their degree of maturity. Digitalis glycosides can cause poisoning in children due to accidental ingestion.

Geriatric Use: The majority of clinical experience gained with digoxin has been in the elderly population. This experience has not identified differences in response or adverse effects between the elderly and younger patients. However, this drug is known to be substantially excreted by the kidney, and the risk of toxic reactions to this drug may be greater in patients with impaired renal function. Because elderly patients are more likely to have decreased renal function, care should be taken in dose selection, which should be based on renal function, and it may be useful to monitor renal function (see DOSAGE AND ADMINISTRATION).

ADVERSE REACTIONS

In general, the adverse reactions of digoxin are dose-dependent and occur at doses higher than those needed to achieve a therapeutic effect. Hence, adverse reactions are less common when digoxin is used within the recommended dose range or therapeutic serum concentration range and when there is careful attention to concurrent medications and conditions.

Because some patients may be particularly susceptible to side effects with digoxin, the dosage of the drug should always be selected carefully and adjusted as the clinical condition of the patient warrants. In the past, when high doses of digoxin were used and little attention was paid to clinical status or concurrent medications, adverse reactions to digoxin were more frequent and severe. Cardiac adverse reactions accounted for about one-half, gastrointestinal disturbances for about one-fourth, and CNS and other toxicity for about one-fourth of these adverse reactions. However, available evidence suggests that the incidence and severity of digoxin toxicity has decreased substantially in recent years. In recent controlled clinical trials, in patients with predominantly mild to moderate heart failure, the incidence of adverse experiences was comparable in patients taking digoxin and in those taking placebo. In a large mortality trial, the incidence of hospitalization for suspected digoxin toxicity was 2% in patients taking digoxin compared to 0.9% in patients taking placebo. In this trial, the most common manifestations of digoxin toxicity included gastrointestinal and cardiac disturbances; CNS manifestations were less common.

Adults: ***Cardiac:*** Therapeutic doses of digoxin may cause heart block in patients with pre-existing sinoatrial or AV conduction disorders; heart block can be avoided by adjusting the dose of digoxin. Prophylactic use of a cardiac pacemaker may be considered if the risk of heart block is considered unacceptable. High doses of digoxin may produce a variety of rhythm disturbances, such as first-degree, second-degree (Wenckebach), or third-degree heart block (including asystole); atrial tachycardia with block; AV dissociation; accelerated junctional (nodal) rhythm; unifocal or multiform ventricular premature contractions (especially bigeminy or trigeminy); ventricular tachycardia; and ventricular fibrillation. Digoxin produces PR prolongation and ST segment depression which should not by themselves be considered digoxin toxicity. Cardiac toxicity can also occur at therapeutic doses in patients who have conditions which may alter their sensitivity to digoxin (see WARNINGS and PRECAUTIONS).

Gastrointestinal: Digoxin may cause anorexia, nausea, vomiting and diarrhea. Rarely, the use of digoxin has been associated with abdominal pain, intestinal ischemia, and hemorrhagic necrosis of the intestines.

CNS: Digoxin can produce visual disturbances (blurred or yellow vision), headache, weakness, dizziness, apathy, confusion and mental disturbances (such as anxiety, depression, delirium, and hallucination).

Other: Gynecomastia has been occasionally observed following the prolonged use of digoxin. Thrombocytopenia and maculopapular rash and other skin reactions have been rarely observed.

The following table summarizes the incidence of those adverse experiences listed above for patients treated with digoxin tablets or placebo from two randomized, double-blind, placebo-controlled withdrawal trials. Patients in these trials were also receiving diuretics with or without angiotensin-converting enzyme inhibitors. These patients have been stable on digoxin, and were randomized to digoxin or placebo. The results shown in Table 4 reflect the experience in patients following dosage titration with the use of serum digoxin concentrations and careful follow-up. These adverse experiences are consistent with results from a large, placebo-controlled mortality trial (DIG trial) wherein over half the patients were not receiving digoxin prior to enrollment.

Table 4: Adverse Experiences in Two Parallel, Double-Blind, Placebo-Controlled Withdrawal Trials (Number of Patients Reporting)

Adverse Experience	Digoxin Patients (n=123)	Placebo Patients (n=125)
Cardiac		
Palpitation	1	4
Ventricular extrasystole	1	1
Tachycardia	2	1
Heart arrest	1	1
Gastrointestinal		
Anorexia	1	4
Nausea	4	2
Vomiting	2	1
Diarrhea	4	1
Abdominal pain	0	6
CNS		
Headache	4	4
Dizziness	6	5
Mental disturbances	5	1
Other		
Rash	2	1
Death	4	3

Infants and Children: The side effects of digoxin in infants and children differ from those seen in adults in several respects. Although digoxin may produce anorexia, nausea, vomiting, diarrhea, and CNS disturbances in young patients, these are rarely the initial symptoms of overdosage. Rather, the earliest and most frequent manifestation of excessive dosing with digoxin in infants and children is the appearance of cardiac arrhythmias, including sinus bradycardia. In children, the use of digoxin may produce any arrhythmia. The most common are conduction disturbances or supraventricular tachyarrhythmias, such as atrial tachycardia (with or without block) and junctional (nodal) tachycardia. Ventricular arrhythmias are less common. Sinus bradycardia may be a sign of impending digoxin intoxication, especially in infants, even in the absence of first-degree heart block. Any arrhythmia or alteration in cardiac conduction that develops in a child taking digoxin should be assumed to be caused by digoxin, until further evaluation proves otherwise.

OVERDOSAGE

Treatment of Adverse Reactions Produced by Overdosage: Digoxin should be temporarily discontinued until the adverse reaction resolves. Every effort should also be made to correct factors that may contribute to the adverse reaction (such as electrolyte disturbances or concurrent medications). Once the adverse reaction has resolved, therapy with digoxin may be reinstituted, following a careful reassessment of dose.

Withdrawal of digoxin may be all that is required to treat the adverse reaction. However, when the primary manifestation of digoxin overdosage is a cardiac arrhythmia, additional therapy may be needed.

If the rhythm disturbance is a symptomatic bradyarrhythmia or heart block, consideration should be given to the reversal of toxicity with DIGIBIND® [Digoxin Immune Fab (Ovine)] (see below), the use of atropine, or the insertion of a temporary cardiac pacemaker. However, asymptomatic bradycardia or heart block related to digoxin may require only temporary withdrawal of the drug and cardiac monitoring of the patient.

If the rhythm disturbance is a ventricular arrhythmia, consideration should be given to the correction of electrolyte disorders, particularly if hypokalemia (see below) or hypomagnesemia is present. DIGIBIND® [Digoxin Immune Fab (Ovine)] is a specific antidote for digoxin and may be used to reverse potentially life-threatening ventricular arrhythmias due to digoxin overdosage.

Administration of Potassium: Every effort should be made to maintain the serum potassium concentration between 4 and 5.5 mmol/L. Potassium is usually administered orally, but when correction of the arrhythmia is urgent and the serum potassium concentration is low, potassium may be administered cautiously by the intravenous route. The electrocardiogram should be monitored for any evidence of potassium toxicity (e.g., peaking of T waves) and to observe the effect on the arrhythmia. Potassium salts may be dangerous in patients who manifest bradycardia or heart block due to digoxin (unless primarily related to supraventricular tachycardia) and in the setting of massive digitalis overdosage (see Massive Digitalis Overdosage subsection).

Massive Digitalis Overdosage: Manifestations of life-threatening toxicity include ventricular tachycardia or ventricular fibrillation, or progressive bradyarrhythmias, or heart block. The administration of more than 10 mg of digoxin in a previously healthy adult or more than 4 mg in a previously healthy child, or a steady-state serum concentration greater than 10 ng/mL often results in cardiac arrest.

DIGIBIND® [Digoxin Immune Fab (Ovine)] should be used to reverse the toxic effects of ingestion of a massive overdose. The decision to administer DIGIBIND® [Digoxin Immune Fab (Ovine)] to a patient who has ingested a massive dose of digoxin but who has not yet manifested life-threatening toxicity should depend on the likelihood that life-threatening toxicity will occur (see above).

Patients with massive digitalis ingestion should receive large doses of activated charcoal to prevent absorption and bind digoxin in the gut during enteroenteric recirculation. Emesis or gastric lavage may be indicated especially if ingestion has occurred within 30 minutes of the patient's presentation at the hospital. Emesis should not be induced in patients who are obtunded. If a patient presents more than 2 hours after ingestion or already has toxic manifestations, it may be unsafe to induce vomiting or attempt passage of a gastric tube, because such maneuvers may induce an acute vagal episode that can worsen digitalis-related arrhythmias.

Severe digitalis intoxication can cause a massive shift of potassium from inside to outside the cell, leading to life-threatening hyperkalemia. The administration of potassium supplements in the setting of massive intoxication may be hazardous and should be avoided. Hyperkalemia caused by massive digitalis toxicity is best treated with DIGIBIND® [Digoxin Immune Fab (Ovine)]; initial treatment with glucose and insulin may also be required if hyperkalemia itself is acutely life-threatening.

DOSAGE AND ADMINISTRATION

General: Recommended dosages of digoxin may require considerable modification because of individual sensitivity of the patient to the drug, the presence of associated conditions, or the use of concurrent medications. In selecting a dose of digoxin, the following factors must be considered:

1. The body weight of the patient. Doses should be calculated based upon lean (i.e., ideal) body weight.
2. The patient's renal function, preferably evaluated on the basis of estimated creatinine clearance.
3. The patient's age. Infants and children require different doses of digoxin than adults. Also, advanced age may be

indicative of diminished renal function even in patients with normal serum creatinine concentration (i.e., below 1.5 mg/dL)

4. Concomitant disease states, concurrent medications, or other factors likely to alter the pharmacokinetic or pharmacodynamic profile of digoxin (see PRECAUTIONS).

Serum Digoxin Concentrations: In general, the dose of digoxin used should be determined on clinical grounds. However, measurement of serum digoxin concentrations can be helpful to the clinician in determining the adequacy of digoxin therapy and in assigning certain probabilities to the likelihood of digoxin intoxication. About two-thirds of adults considered adequately digitalized (without evidence of toxicity) have serum digoxin concentrations ranging from 0.8 to 2 ng/mL. However, digoxin may produce clinical benefits even at serum concentrations below this range. About two-thirds of adult patients with clinical toxicity have serum digoxin concentrations greater than 2 ng/mL. However, since one third of patients with clinical toxicity have concentrations less than 2 ng/mL, values below 2 ng/mL do not rule out the possibility that a certain sign or symptom is related to digoxin therapy. Rarely, there are patients who are unable to tolerate digoxin at serum concentrations below 0.8 ng/mL. Consequently, the serum concentration of digoxin should always be interpreted in the overall clinical context, and an isolated measurement should not be used alone as the basis for increasing or decreasing the dose of the drug.

To allow adequate time for equilibration of digoxin between serum and tissue, sampling of serum concentrations should be done just before the next scheduled dose of the drug. If this is not possible, sampling should be done at least 6 to 8 hours after the last dose, regardless of the route of administration or the formulation used. On a once-daily dosing schedule, the concentration of digoxin will be 10% to 25% lower when sampled at 24 versus 8 hours, depending upon the patient's renal function. On a twice-daily dosing schedule, there will be only minor differences in serum digoxin concentrations whether sampling is done at 8 or 12 hour after a dose.

If a discrepancy exists between the reported serum concentration and the observed clinical response, the clinician should consider the following possibilities:

1. Analytical problems in the assay procedure.
2. Inappropriate serum sampling time.
3. Administration of a digitalis glycoside other than digoxin.
4. Conditions (described in WARNINGS and PRECAUTIONS) causing an alteration in the sensitivity of the patient to digoxin.
5. Serum digoxin concentration may decrease acutely during periods of exercise without any associate change in clinical efficacy due to increased binding of digoxin to skeletal muscle.

Heart Failure: ***Adults:*** Digitalization may be accomplished by either of two general approaches that vary in dosage and frequency of administration, but reach the same endpoint in terms of total amount of digoxin accumulated in the body.

1. If rapid digitalization is considered medically appropriate, it may be achieved by administering a loading dose based upon projected peak digoxin body stores. Maintenance dose can be calculated as a percentage of the loading dose.
2. More gradual digitalization may be obtained by beginning an appropriate maintenance dose, thus allowing digoxin body stores to accumulate slowly. Steady-state serum digoxin concentrations will be achieved in approximately five half-lives of the drug for the individual patient. Depending upon the patient's renal function, this will take between 1 and 3 weeks.

Rapid Digitalization with a Loading Dose: Peak digoxin body stores of 8 to 12 mcg/kg should provide therapeutic effect with minimum risk of toxicity in most patients with heart failure and normal sinus rhythm. Because of altered digoxin distribution and elimination, projected peak body stores for patients with renal insufficiency should be conservative (i.e., 6 to 10 mcg/kg) [see PRECAUTIONS].

The loading dose should be administered in several portions, with roughly half the total given as the first dose. Additional fractions of this planned total dose may be given at 6- to 8-hour intervals, **with careful assessment of clinical response before each additional dose.**

If the patient's clinical response necessitates a change from the calculated loading dose of digoxin, then calculation of the maintenance dose should be based upon the amount actually given.

A single initial dose of 500 to 750 mcg (0.5 to 0.75 mg) of digoxin tablets usually produces a detectable effect in 0.5 to 2 hours that becomes maximal in 2 to 6 hours. Additional doses of 125 to 375 mcg (0.125 to 0.375 mg) may be given cautiously at 6- to 8-hour intervals until clinical evidence of an adequate effect is noted. The usual amount of digoxin tablets that a 70-kg patient requires to achieve 8 to 12 mcg/kg peak body stores is 750 to 1,250 mcg (0.75 to 1.25 mg).

Digoxin Injection is frequently used to achieve rapid digitalization, with conversion to digoxin tablets or Digoxin Solution in Capsules for maintenance therapy. If patients are switched from intravenous to oral digoxin formulations, allowances must be made for differences in bioavailability when calculating maintenance dosages (see table, CLINICAL PHARMACOLOGY).

Maintenance Dosing: The doses of digoxin used in controlled trials in patients with heart failure have ranged from 125 to 500 mcg (0.125 to 0.5 mg) once daily. In these studies, the digoxin dose has been generally titrated according to the patient's age, lean body weight, and renal function. Therapy is generally initiated at a dose of 250 mcg (0.25 mg) once daily in patients under age 70 with good renal function, at a dose of 125 mcg (0.125 mg) once daily in patients over age 70 or with impaired renal function, and at a dose of 62.5 mcg (0.0625 mg) in patients with marked renal impairment. Doses may be increased every 2 weeks according to clinical response.

Table 5: Usual Daily Maintenance Dose Requirements (mcg) of Digoxin for Estimated Peak Body Stores of 10 mcg/kg

Corrected Ccr (mL/min per 70 kg)*	Lean Body Weight kg / lb	50 / 110	60 / 132	70 / 154	80 / 176	90 / 198	100 / 220	Number of Days Before Steady-State Achieved†
0		62.5‡	125	125	125	187.5	187.5	22
10		125	125	125	187.5	187.5	187.5	19
20		125	125	187.5	187.5	187.5	250	16
30		125	187.5	187.5	187.5	250	250	14
40		125	187.5	187.5	250	250	250	13
50		187.5	187.5	250	250	250	250	12
60		187.5	187.5	250	250	250	375	11
70		187.5	250	250	250	250	375	10
80		187.5	250	250	250	375	375	9
90		187.5	250	250	250	375	500	8
100		250	250	250	375	375	500	7

*Ccr is creatinine clearance, corrected to 70 kg body weight or 1.73 m^2 body surface area. *For adults,* if only serum creatinine concentrations (Scr) are available, a Ccr (corrected to 70 kg body weight) may be estimated in men as (140-Age)/Scr. For women, this result should be multiplied by 0.85.

Note: This equation cannot be used for estimating creatinine clearance in infants or children.

† If no loading dose administered.

‡ 62.5 mcg = 0.0625 mg

In a subset of approximately 1,800 patients enrolled in the DIG trial (wherein dosing was based on an algorithm similar to that in Table 5) the mean (±SD) serum digoxin concentrations at 1 month and 12 months were 1.01 ± 0.47 ng/mL and 0.97 ± 0.43 ng/mL, respectively.

The maintenance dose should be based upon the percentage of the peak body stores lost each day through elimination. The following formula has had wide clinical use:

Maintenance Dose = Peak Body Stores (i.e., Loading Dose) × % Daily Loss/100

Where: % Daily Loss = 14 + Ccr/5

(Ccr is creatinine clearance, corrected to 70 kg body weight or 1.73 m^2 body surface area.)

Table 5 provides average daily maintenance dose requirements of digoxin tablets for patients with heart failure based upon lean body weight and renal function:

[See table 5 above]

Example: Based on the above table, a patient in heart failure with an estimated lean body weight of 70 kg and a Ccr of 60 mL/min, should be given a dose of 250 mcg (0.25 mg) daily of digoxin tablets, usually taken after the morning meal. If no loading dose is administered, steady-state serum concentrations in this patient should be anticipated at approximately 11 days.

Infants and Children: In general, divided daily dosing is recommended for infants and young children (under age 10). In the newborn period, renal clearance of digoxin is diminished and suitable dosage adjustments must be observed. This is especially pronounced in the premature infant. Beyond the immediate newborn period, children generally require proportionally larger doses than adults on the basis of body weight or body surface area. Children over 10 years of age require adult dosages in proportion to their body weight. Some researchers have suggested that infants and young children tolerate slightly higher serum concentrations than do adults.

Daily maintenance doses for each age group are given in Table 6 and should provide therapeutic effects with minimum risk of toxicity in most patients with heart failure and normal sinus rhythm. These recommendations assume the presence of normal renal function:

Table 6: Daily Maintenance Doses in Children with Normal Renal Function

Age	Daily Maintenance Dose (mcg/kg)
2 to 5 years	10 to 15
5 to 10 years	7 to 10
Over 10 years	3 to 5

In children with renal disease, digoxin must be carefully titrated based upon clinical response.

It cannot be overemphasized that both the adult and pediatric dosage guidelines provided are based upon average patient response and substantial individual variation can be expected. Accordingly, ultimate dosage selection must be based upon clinical assessment of the patient.

Atrial Fibrillation: Peak digoxin body stores larger than the 8 to 12 mcg/kg required for most patients with heart failure and normal sinus rhythm have been used for control of ventricular rate in patients with atrial fibrillation. Doses of digoxin used for the treatment of chronic atrial fibrillation should be titrated to the minimum dose that achieves the desired ventricular rate control without causing undesirable side effects. Data are not available to establish the appropriate resting or exercise target rates that should be achieved.

Dosage Adjustment When Changing Preparations: The difference in bioavailability between Digoxin injection or Digoxin Solution in Capsules and Digoxin Pediatric Elixir or digoxin tablets must be considered when changing patients from one dosage form to another.

Doses of 100 mcg (0.1 mg) and 200 mcg (0.2 mg) of Digoxin Solution in Capsules are approximately equivalent to 125-mcg (0.125-mg) and 250-mcg (0.25-mg) doses of digoxin tablets and Pediatric Elixir, respectively. (see table in CLINICAL PHARMACOLOGY: Pharmacokinetics).

HOW SUPPLIED

DIGITEK® (digoxin tablets, USP) 125 mcg (0.125 mg) are yellow, round tablets, and imprinted with **B 145** on the scored side of the tablet. They are available as follows:

NDC 62794-145-01
bottles of 100 tablets
NDC 62794-145-10
bottles of 1000 tablets
NDC 62794-145-56
bottles of 5000 tablets

DIGITEK™ (digoxin tablets, USP) 250 mcg (0.25 mg) are white, round tablets, and imprinted with **B 146** on the scored side of the tablet. They are available as follows:

NDC 62794-146-01
bottles of 100 tablets
NDC 62794-146-10
bottles of 1000 tablets
NDC 62794-146-56
bottles of 5000 tablets

Store at 15° to 25°C (59° to 77°F) in a dry place and protect from light.

Dispense in a tight, light-resistant container as defined in the USP.

REVISED NOVEMBER 2000
BKDGTK:R4
8070-02

Distributed by:
BERTEK PHARMACEUTICALS INC.
Sugar Land, TX 77478 USA
Manufactured by:
AMIDE PHARMACEUTICAL, INC.
101 East Main Street, Little Falls, NJ 07424 USA

GRANULEX

℞

℞ Only

DESCRIPTION

GRANULEX is an aerosol spray. Each gram of **GRANULEX** contains: 0.12 mg trypsin USP, 87.0 mg balsam peru, 788.0 mg castor oil USP, an emulsifier and propellants (water dispersible).

INDICATIONS AND USAGE

GRANULEX is indicated for the treatment of varicose ulcers, dehiscent wounds, decubital ulcers, sunburn and debridement of eschar. It is also used for wound healing.

GRANULEX will relieve pain and promote healing; debrides eschar and necrotic tissue physiologically; stimulates vascular bed; improves epithelization by reducing premature epithelial dessication and cornification; reduces odor from malodorous necrotic wounds.

DIRECTIONS

Shake well before spraying. Hold upright and approximately 12 inches from the area to be treated. Press valve and coat wound rapidly. Wound may be left unbandaged or a wet dressing may be applied. Apply twice daily or as often as necessary. To remove, wash gently with water. When applied to sensitive area, a temporary stinging sensation may be noted.

WARNING

Do not use on fresh arterial clots. Avoid spraying in eyes. Flammable, do not expose to fire or open flame. Contents under pressure. Do not puncture or incinerate. Do not store

Continued on next page

Granulex—Cont.

at temperature above 120°F. Keep out of reach of children. Use only as directed. Intentional misuse by deliberately concentrating and inhaling the contents can be harmful or fatal.

NDC Code	Net Weight
62794-002-50	2 oz. (56.7g)
62794-002-51	4 oz. (113.4g)

Inert propellant 25% of total content.
BERTEK PHARMACEUTICALS INC.
Morgantown, WV 26505

KRISTALOSE™ ℞

[*krĭs' tă lōsĕ*]
(LACTULOSE)
For Oral Solution

DESCRIPTION

KRISTALOSE™ (LACTULOSE) is a synthetic disaccharide in the form of crystals for reconstitution prior to use for oral administration. Each 10 g of lactulose contains less than 0.3 g galactose and lactose as a total sum. The pH range is 3.0 to 7.0

Lactulose is a colonic acidifier which promotes laxation.

The chemical name for lactulose is 4-O-β-D-Galactopyranosyl-D-fructofuranose. It has the following structural formula:

The molecular formula is $C_{12}H_{22}O_{11}$. The molecular weight is 342.30. It is freely soluble in water.

CLINICAL PHARMACOLOGY

KRISTALOSE™ (LACTULOSE) is poorly absorbed from the gastrointestinal tract and no enzyme capable of hydrolysis of this disaccharide is present in human gastrointestinal tissue. As a result, oral doses of lactulose reach the colon virtually unchanged. In the colon, lactulose is broken down primarily to lactic acid, and also to small amounts of formic and acetic acids, by the action of colonic bacteria, which results in an increase in osmotic pressure and slight acidification of the colonic contents. This in turn causes an increase in stool water content and softens the stool.

Since lactulose does not exert its effect until it reaches the colon, and since transit time through the colon may be slow, 24 to 48 hours may be required to produce desired bowel movement.

Lactulose given orally to man and experimental animals resulted in only small amounts reaching the blood. Urinary excretion has been determined to be 3% or less and is essentially complete within 24 hours.

INDICATIONS AND USAGE

KRISTALOSE™ (LACTULOSE) For Oral Solution is indicated for the treatment of constipation. In patients with a history of chronic constipation, lactulose therapy increases the number of bowel movements per day and the number of days on which bowel movements occur.

CONTRAINDICATIONS

Since KRISTALOSE™ (LACTULOSE) For Oral Solution contains galactose (less than 0.3 g/10 g as a total sum with lactose), it is contraindicated in patients who require a low galactose diet.

WARNINGS

A theoretical hazard may exist for patients being treated with lactulose who may be required to undergo electrocautery procedures during proctoscopy or colonoscopy. Accumulation of H_2 gas in significant concentration in the presence of an electrical spark may result in an explosive reaction. Although this complication has not been reported with lactulose, patients on lactulose therapy undergoing such procedures should have a thorough bowel cleansing with a non-fermentable solution. Insufflation of CO_2 as an additional safeguard may be pursued but is considered to be a redundant measure.

PRECAUTIONS

General

Since KRISTALOSE™ (LACTULOSE) For Oral Solution contains galactose and lactose (less than 0.3 g/10 g as a total sum), it should be used with caution in diabetics.

Information for patients

In the event that an unusual diarrheal condition occurs, contact your physician.

Laboratory Tests

Elderly, debilitated patients who receive lactulose for more than six months should have serum electrolytes (potassium, chloride, carbon dioxide) measured periodically.

Drug Interactions

Results of preliminary studies in humans and rats suggest that nonabsorbable antacids given concurrently with lactulose may inhibit the desired lactulose-induced drop in colonic pH. Therefore, a possible lack of desired effect of treatment should be taken into consideration before such drugs are given concomitantly with lactulose.

Carcinogenesis, Mutagenesis, Impairment of Fertility

There are no known human data on long-term potential for carcinogenicity, mutagenicity, or impairment of fertility.

There are no known animal data on long-term potential for mutagenicity.

Administration of lactulose syrup in the diet of mice for 18 months in concentrations of 3 and 10 percent (v/w) did not produce any evidence of carcinogenicity.

In studies in mice, rats, and rabbits, doses of lactulose syrup up to 6 or 12 mL/kg/day produced no deleterious effects in breeding, conception, or parturition.

Pregnancy

Teratogenic Effects

Pregnancy Category B

Reproduction studies have been performed in mice, rats, and rabbits at doses up to 3 or 6 times the usual human oral dose and have revealed no evidence of impaired fertility or harm to the fetus due to lactulose. There are, however, no adequate and well-controlled studies in pregnant women. Because animal reproduction studies are not always predictive of human response, this drug should be used during pregnancy only if clearly needed.

Nursing Mothers

It is not known whether this drug is excreted in human milk. Because many drugs are excreted in human milk, caution should be exercised when lactulose is administered to a nursing woman.

Pediatric Use

Safety and effectiveness in pediatric patients have not been established.

ADVERSE REACTIONS

Precise frequency data are not available.

Initial dosing may produce flatulence and intestinal cramps, which are usually transient. Excessive dosage can lead to diarrhea with potential complications such as loss of fluids, hypokalemia, and hypernatremia.

Nausea and vomiting have been reported.

OVERDOSAGE

Signs and Symptoms

There have been no reports of accidental overdosage. In the event of overdosage, it is expected that diarrhea and abdominal cramps would be the major symptoms. Medication should be terminated.

Oral LD_{50}

The acute oral LD_{50} of the drug is 48.8 mL/kg in mice and greater than 30 mL/kg in rats.

Dialysis

Dialysis data are not available for lactulose. Its molecular similarity to sucrose, however, would suggest that it should be dialyzable.

DOSAGE AND ADMINISTRATION

The usual adult dosage is 10 g to 20 g of lactulose daily. The dose may be increased to 40 g daily if necessary. Twenty-four to 48 hours may be required to produce a normal bowel movement.

DIRECTIONS FOR PREPARATION

Dissolve contents of packet in half a glass (4 ounces) of water.

When Lactulose for Oral Solution is dissolved in water, the resulting solution may be colorless to a slightly pale yellow color.

HOW SUPPLIED

KRISTALOSE™ (LACTULOSE) For Oral Solution is available in single dose packets of 10 g (NDC 62794-501-17) and single dose packets of 20 g (NDC 62794-502-17). The packets are supplied as follows:

NDC 62794-501-93	Carton of thirty 10 g packets
NDC 62794-502-93	Carton of thirty 20 g packets

STORE AT ROOM TEMPERATURE, 15°–30°C (59°–86°F).

Distributed by
BERTEK PHARMACEUTICALS INC.
Sugar Land, TX 77478
Manufactured by
Inalco S.p.A.
Milan, Italy

089.1
REVISED OCTOBER 2003

MAXZIDE® and MAXZIDE®-25 MG TABLETS ℞

[*măx 'zīde*]
BRAND OF (TRIAMTERENE AND HYDROCHLOROTHIAZIDE)

DESCRIPTION

MAXZIDE® (triamterene and hydrochlorothiazide) combines triamterene, a potassium-conserving diuretic, with the natriuretic agent, hydrochlorothiazide.

Each MAXZIDE® tablet contains:

Triamterene, USP	75 mg
Hydrochlorothiazide, USP	50 mg

Each MAXZIDE®-25 MG tablet contains:

Triamterene, USP	37.5 mg
Hydrochlorothiazide, USP	25 mg

MAXZIDE® and MAXZIDE®-25 MG tablets for oral administration contain the following inactive ingredients: Colloidal Silicon Dioxide, Croscarmellose Sodium, Magnesium Stearate, Microcrystalline Cellulose, Powdered Cellulose, Sodium Lauryl Sulfate and D&C Yellow #10. MAXZIDE®-25 MG tablets also contain FD&C Blue #1.

Triamterene is 2,4,7-triamino-6-phenylpteridine. Triamterene is practically insoluble in water, benzene, chloroform, ether and dilute alkali hydroxides. It is soluble in formic acid and sparingly soluble in methoxyethanol. Triamterene is very slightly soluble in acetic acid, alcohol and dilute mineral acids. Its molecular weight is 253.27. Its structural formula is:

Hydrochlorothiazide is 6-chloro-3,4-dihydro-2*H*-1,2,4, benzothiadiazine-7-sulfonamide 1,1-dioxide. Hydrochlorothiazide is slightly soluble in water and freely soluble in sodium hydroxide solution, n-butylamine and dimethylformamide. It is sparingly soluble in methanol and insoluble in ether, chloroform and dilute mineral acids. Its molecular weight is 297.73. Its structural formula is:

CLINICAL PHARMACOLOGY

MAXZIDE (triamterene and hydrochlorothiazide) is a diuretic, antihypertensive drug product, principally due to its hydrochlorothiazide component; the triamterene component of MAXZIDE reduces the excessive potassium loss which may occur with hydrochlorothiazide use.

Hydrochlorothiazide

Hydrochlorothiazide is a diuretic and antihypertensive agent. It blocks the renal tubular absorption of sodium and chloride ions. This natriuresis and diuresis is accompanied by a secondary loss of potassium and bicarbonate. Onset of hydrochlorothiazide's diuretic effect occurs within two hours and the peak action takes place in four hours. Diuretic activity persists for approximately six to twelve hours.

The exact mechanism of hydrochlorothiazide's antihypertensive action is not known although it may relate to the excretion and redistribution of body sodium. Hydrochlorothiazide does not affect normal blood pressure. Following oral administration, peak hydrochlorothiazide plasma levels are attained in approximately two hours. It is excreted rapidly and unchanged in the urine.

Well-controlled studies have demonstrated that doses of hydrochlorothiazide as low as 25 mg given once daily are effective in treating hypertension, but the dose response has not been clearly established.

Triamterene

Triamterene is a potassium-conserving (antikaliuretic) diuretic with relatively weak natriuretic properties. It exerts its diuretic effect on the distal renal tubule to inhibit the reabsorption of sodium in exchange for potassium and hydrogen. With this action, triamterene increases sodium excretion and reduces the excessive loss of potassium and hydrogen associated with hydrochlorothiazide. Triamterene is not a competitive antagonist of the mineralocorticoids and its potassium-conserving effect is observed in patients with Addison's disease, i.e., without aldosterone. Triamterene's onset and duration of activity is similar to hydrochlorothiazide. No predictable antihypertensive effect has been demonstrated with triamterene.

Triamterene is rapidly absorbed following oral administration. Peak plasma levels are achieved within one hour after dosing. Triamterene is primarily metabolized to the sulfate conjugate of hydroxytriamterene. Both the plasma and urine levels of this metabolite greatly exceed triamterene levels.

The amount of triamterene added to 50 mg of hydrochlorothiazide in MAXZIDE tablets was determined from steady-state dose response evaluations in which various doses of liquid preparations of triamterene were administered to hypertensive persons who developed hypokalemia with hydrochlorothiazide (50 mg given once daily). Single daily doses of 75 mg triamterene resulted in greater increases in serum potassium than lower doses (25 mg and 50 mg), while doses greater than 75 mg of triamterene resulted in no additional elevations in serum potassium levels. The amount of triamterene added to the 25 mg of hydrochlorothiazide in MAXZIDE-25 MG tablets was also determined from steady-state dose response evaluations in which various doses of liquid preparations of triamterene were administered to hypertensive persons who developed hypokalemia with hydrochlorothiazide (25 mg given once daily). Single daily doses of 37.5 mg triamterene resulted in greater increases in serum potassium than a lower dose (25 mg), while doses greater than 37.5 mg of triamterene, i.e., 75 and 100 mg, resulted in no additional elevations in serum potassium levels. The dose response relationship of triamterene was also evaluated in patients rendered hypokalemic by hydrochlorothiazide given 25 mg twice daily. Triamterene given twice daily increased serum potassium levels in a dose-related fashion. However, the combination of triamterene and hydrochlorothiazide given twice daily also appeared to produce an increased frequency of elevation in serum BUN and creatinine levels. The largest increases in serum potassium, BUN and creatinine in this study were observed with 50 mg of triamterene given twice daily, the largest dose tested. Ordinarily, triamterene does not entirely compensate for the kaliuretic effect of hydrochlorothiazide and some patients may remain hypokalemic while receiving triamterene and hydrochlorothiazide. In some individuals, however, it may induce hyperkalemia (see WARNINGS).

The triamterene and hydrochlorothiazide components of MAXZIDE and MAXZIDE-25 MG are well absorbed and are bioequivalent to liquid preparations of the individual components administered orally. Food does not influence the absorption of triamterene or hydrochlorothiazide from MAXZIDE or MAXZIDE-25 MG tablets. The hydrochlorothiazide component of MAXZIDE is bioequivalent to single entity hydrochlorothiazide tablet formulations.

INDICATIONS AND USAGE

This fixed combination drug is not indicated for the initial therapy of edema or hypertension except in individuals in whom the development of hypokalemia cannot be risked.

1. MAXZIDE (triamterene and hydrochlorothiazide) is indicated for the treatment of hypertension or edema in patients who develop hypokalemia on hydrochlorothiazide alone.
2. MAXZIDE is also indicated for those patients who require a thiazide diuretic and in whom the development of hypokalemia cannot be risked (e.g., patients on concomitant digitalis preparations, or with a history of cardiac arryhthmias, etc.).

MAXZIDE may be used alone or in combination with other antihypertensive drugs, such as beta-blockers. Since MAXZIDE (triamterene and hydrochlorothiazide) may enhance the actions of these drugs, dosage adjustments may be necessary.

Usage In Pregnancy

The routine use of diuretics in an otherwise healthy woman is inappropriate and exposes mother and fetus to unnecessary hazard. Diuretics do not prevent development of toxemia of pregnancy, and there is no satisfactory evidence that they are useful in the treatment of developed toxemia. Edema during pregnancy may arise from pathological causes or from the physiologic and mechanical consequences of pregnancy. Thiazides are indicated in pregnancy when edema is due to pathologic causes, just as they are in absence of pregnancy. Dependent edema in pregnancy, resulting from restriction of venous return by the expanded uterus, is properly treated through elevation of the lower extremities and use of support hose; use of diuretics to lower intravascular volume in this case is illogical and unnecessary. There is hypervolemia during normal pregnancy which is harmful to neither the fetus nor the mother (in the absence of cardiovascular disease), but which is associated with edema, including generalized edema, in the majority of pregnant women. If this edema produces discomfort, increased recumbency will often provide relief. In rare instances, this edema may cause extreme discomfort which is not relieved by rest. In these cases, a short course of diuretics may provide relief and may be appropriate.

CONTRAINDICATIONS

Hyperkalemia

MAXZIDE (triamterene and hydrochlorothiazide) should not be used in the presence of elevated serum potassium levels (greater than or equal to 5.5 mEq/liter). If hyperkalemia develops, this drug should be discontinued and a thiazide alone should be substituted.

Antikaliuretic Therapy or Potassium Supplementation

MAXZIDE should not be given to patients receiving other potassium-conserving agents such as spironolactone, amiloride HCl or other formulations containing triamterene. Concomitant potassium supplementation in the form of medication, potassium-containing salt substitute or potassium-enriched diets should also not be used.

Impaired Renal Function

MAXZIDE is contraindicated in patients with anuria, acute and chronic renal insufficiency or significant renal impairment.

Hypersensitivity

MAXZIDE should not be used in patients who are hypersensitive to triamterene or hydrochlorothiazide or other sulfonamide-derived drugs.

WARNINGS

Hyperkalemia

Abnormal elevation of serum potassium levels (greater than or equal to 5.5 mEq/liter) can occur with all potassium-conserving diuretic combinations, including MAXZIDE. Hyperkalemia is more likely to occur in patients with renal impairment, diabetes (even without evidence of renal impairment), or elderly or severely ill patients. Since uncorrected hyperkalemia may be fatal, serum potassium levels must be monitored at frequent intervals especially in patients first receiving MAXZIDE, when dosages are changed or with any illness that may influence renal function.

If hyperkalemia is suspected, (warning signs include paresthesias, muscular weakness, fatigue, flaccid paralysis of the extremities, bradycardia and shock) an electrocardiogram (ECG) should be obtained. However, it is important to monitor serum potassium levels because mild hyperkalemia may not be associated with ECG changes.

If hyperkalemia is present, MAXZIDE (triamterene and hydrochlorothiazide) should be discontinued immediately and a thiazide alone should be substituted. If the serum potassium exceeds 6.5 mEq/liter, more vigorous therapy is required. The clinical situation dictates the procedures to be employed. These include the intravenous administration of calcium chloride solution, sodium bicarbonate solution and/or the oral or parenteral administration of glucose with a rapid-acting insulin preparation. Cationic exchange resins such as sodium polystyrene sulfonate may be orally or rectally administered. Persistent hyperkalemia may require dialysis.

The development of hyperkalemia associated with potassium-sparing diuretics is accentuated in the presence of renal impairment (see CONTRAINDICATIONS). Patients with mild renal functional impairment should not receive this drug without frequent and continuing monitoring of serum electrolytes. Cumulative drug effects may be observed in patients with impaired renal function. The renal clearances of hydrochlorothiazide and the pharmacologically active metabolite of triamterene, the sulfate ester of hydroxytriamterene, have been shown to be reduced and the plasma levels increased following MAXZIDE (triamterene and hydrochlorothiazide) administration to elderly patients and patients with impaired renal function.

Hyperkalemia has been reported in diabetic patients with the use of potassium-conserving agents even in the absence of apparent renal impairment. Accordingly, MAXZIDE (triamterene and hydrochlorothiazide) should be avoided in diabetic patients. If it is employed, serum electrolytes must be frequently monitored.

Because of the potassium-sparing properties of angiotensin-converting enzyme (ACE) inhibitors, MAXZIDE should be used cautiously, if at all, with these agents (see PRECAUTIONS, Drug Interactions).

Metabolic or Respiratory Acidosis

Potassium-conserving therapy should also be avoided in severely ill patients in whom respiratory or metabolic acidosis may occur. Acidosis may be associated with rapid elevations in serum potassium levels. If MAXZIDE is employed, frequent evaluations of acid/base balance and serum electrolytes are necessary.

PRECAUTIONS

General

Electrolyte Imbalance and BUN Increases

Patients receiving MAXZIDE (triamterene and hydrochlorothiazide) should be carefully monitored for fluid or electrolyte imbalances, i.e., hyponatremia, hypochloremic alkalosis, hypokalemia and hypomagnesemia. Determination of serum electrolytes to detect possible electrolyte imbalance should be performed at appropriate intervals. Serum and urine electrolyte determinations are especially important and should be frequently performed when the patient is vomiting or receiving parenteral fluids. Warning signs or symptoms of fluid and electrolyte imbalance include: dryness of mouth, thirst, weakness, lethargy, drowsiness, restlessness, muscle pains or cramps, muscular fatigue, hypotension, oliguria, tachycardia and gastrointestinal disturbances such as nausea and vomiting.

Any chloride deficit during thiazide therapy is generally mild and usually does not require any specific treatment except under extraordinary circumstances (as in liver disease or renal disease). Dilutional hyponatremia may occur in edematous patients in hot weather; appropriate therapy is water restriction, rather than administration of salt, except in rare instances when the hyponatremia is life threatening. In actual salt depletion, appropriate replacement is the therapy of choice.

Hypokalemia may develop with thiazide therapy, especially with brisk diuresis, when severe cirrhosis is present, or during concomitant use of corticosteroids, ACTH, amphotericin B or after prolonged thiazide therapy. However, hypokalemia of this type is usually prevented by the triamterene component of MAXZIDE (triamterene and hydrochlorothiazide).

Interference with adequate oral electrolyte intake will also contribute to hypokalemia. Hypokalemia can sensitize or exaggerate the response of the heart to the toxic effects of digitalis (e.g., increased ventricular irritability).

MAXZIDE (triamterene and hydrochlorothiazide) may produce an elevated blood urea nitrogen level (BUN), creatinine level or both. This is probably not the result of renal toxicity but is secondary to a reversible reduction of the glomerular filtration rate or a depletion of the intravascular fluid volume. Elevations in BUN and creatinine levels may be more frequent in patients receiving divided dose diuretic therapy. Periodic BUN and creatinine determinations should be made especially in elderly patients, patients with suspected or confirmed hepatic disease or renal insufficiencies. If azotemia increases, MAXZIDE (triamterene and hydrochlorothiazide) should be discontinued.

Hepatic Coma

MAXZIDE should be used with caution in patients with impaired hepatic function or progressive liver disease, since minor alterations of fluid and electrolyte balance may precipitate hepatic coma.

Renal Stones

Triamterene has been reported in renal stones in association with other calculus components. MAXZIDE should be used with caution in patients with histories of renal lithiasis.

Folic Acid Deficiency

Triamterene is a weak folic acid antagonist and may contribute to the appearance of megaloblastosis in instances where folic acid stores are decreased. In such patients, periodic blood elevations are recommended.

Hyperuricemia

Hyperuricemia may occur or acute gout may be precipitated in certain patients receiving thiazide therapy.

Metabolic and Endocrine Effects

The thiazides may decrease serum PBI levels without signs of thyroid disturbance.

Calcium excretion is decreased by thiazides. Pathological changes in the parathyroid gland with hypercalcemia and hypophosphatemia have been observed in a few patients on prolonged thiazide therapy. The common complications of hyperparathyroidism such as renal lithiasis, bone resorption, and peptic ulceration have not been seen. Thiazides should be discontinued before carrying out tests for parathyroid function.

Insulin requirements in diabetic patients may be increased, decreased or unchanged. Diabetes mellitus which has been latent may become manifest during thiazide administration.

Hypersensitivity

Sensitivity reactions to thiazides may occur in patients with or without a history of allergy or bronchial asthma.

Possible exacerbation or activation of systemic lupus erythematosus by thiazides has been reported.

Drug Interactions

Thiazides may add to or potentiate the action of other antihypertensive drugs.

The thiazides may decrease arterial responsiveness to norepinephrine. This diminution is not sufficient to preclude effectiveness of the pressor agent for therapeutic use. Thiazides have also been shown to increase the responsiveness to tubocurarine.

Lithium generally should not be given with diuretics because they reduce its renal clearance and add a high risk of lithium toxicity. Refer to the package insert on lithium before use of such concomitant therapy.

Acute renal failure has been reported in a few patients receiving indomethacin and formulations containing triamterene and hydrochlorothiazide. Caution is therefore advised when administering nonsteroidal anti-inflammatory agents with MAXZIDE (triamterene and hydrochlorothiazide).

Potassium-sparing agents should be used very cautiously, if at all, in conjunction with angiotensin-converting enzyme (ACE) inhibitors due to a greatly increased risk of hyperkalemia. Serum potassium should be monitored frequently.

Drug/Laboratory Test Interactions

Triamterene and quinidine have similar fluorescence spectra; thus MAXZIDE (triamterene and hydrochlorothiazide) may interfere with the measurement of quinidine.

Carcinogenesis, Mutagenesis, Impairment of Fertility:

Carcinogenesis: Long term studies with MAXZIDE, the triamterene/hydrochlorothiazide combination, have not been conducted.

Triamterene: In studies conducted under the auspices of the National Toxicology Program, groups of rats were fed diets containing 0, 150, 300 or 600 ppm triamterene, and groups of mice were fed diets containing 0, 100, 200 or 400 ppm triamterene. Male and female rats exposed to the highest tested concentration received triamterene at about 25 and 30 mg/kg/day, respectively. Male and female mice exposed to the highest tested concentration received triamterene at about 45 and 60 mg/kg/day, respectively.

There was an increased incidence of hepatocellular neoplasia (primarily adenomas) in male and female mice at the highest dosage level. These doses represent 7.5X and 10X the MRHD of 300 mg/kg (or 6 mg/kg/day based on a 50 kg patient) for male and female mice, respectively when based on body-weight and 0.7X and 0.9X the MRHD when based on body-surface area. Although hepatocellular neoplasia (exclusively adenomas) in the rat study was limited to triamterene-exposed males, incidence was not dose-dependent and there was no statistically significant difference from control incidence at any dose level.

Hydrochlorothiazide: Two-year feeding studies in mice and rats, conducted under the auspices of the National Toxicology Program (NTP), treated mice and rats with doses of hydrochlorothiazide up to 600 and 100 mg/kg/day, respectively. On a body-weight basis, these doses are 600 times (in mice) and 100 times (in rats) the Maximum Recommended Human Dose (MRHD) for the hydrochlorothiazide component of MAXZIDE (50 mg/day or 1.0 mg/kg/day based on a 50 kg patient). On the basis of body-surface area, these doses are 56 times (in mice) and 21 times (in rats) the MRHD. These studies uncovered no evidence of carcinogenic potential of hydrochlorothiazide in rats or female mice, but there was equivocal evidence of hepatocarcinogenicity in male mice.

Mutagenesis: Studies of the mutagenic potential of MAXZIDE, the triamterene/hydrochlorothiazide combination, have not been performed.

Continued on next page

Maxzide/Maxzide-25—Cont.

Triamterene: Triamterene was not mutagenic in bacteria (*S. typhimurium* strains TA 98, TA 100, TA 1535 or TA 1537) with or without metabolic activation. It did not induce chromosomal aberrations in Chinese hamster ovary (CHO) cells *in vitro* with or without metabolic activation, but it did induce sister chromatid exchanges in CHO cells *in vitro* with and without metabolic activation.

Hydrochlorothiazide: Hydrochlorothiazide was not genotoxic in *in vitro* assays using strains TA 98, TA 100, TA 1535, TA 1537 and TA 1538 of *Salmonella typhimurium* (the Ames test), in the Chinese hamster ovary (CHO) test for chromosomal aberrations, or in *in vivo* assays using mouse germinal cell chromosomes, Chinese hamster bone marrow chromosomes, and the *Drosophila* sex-linked recessive lethal trait gene. Positive test results were obtained in the *in vitro* CHO sister chromatid exchange (clastogenicity) test, and in the mouse lymphoma cell (mutagenicity) assays, using concentrations of hydrochlorothiazide of 43-1300 mcg/mL. Positive test results were also obtained in the *Aspergillus nidulans* nondisjunction assay using an unspecified concentration of hydrochlorothiazide.

Impairment of Fertility: Studies of the effects of MAXZIDE, the triamterene/hydrochlorothiazide combination, or of triamterene alone on animal reproductive function have not been conducted.

Hydrochlorothiazide: Hydrochlorothiazide had no adverse effects on the fertility of mice and rats of either sex in studies wherein these species were exposed, via their diet, to doses of up to 100 and 4 mg/kg/day, respectively, prior to mating and throughout gestation. Corresponding multiples of the MRHD are 100 (mice) and 4 (rats) on the basis of body-weight and 9.4 (mice) and 0.8 (rats) on the basis of body-surface area.

Pregnancy Category C

Teratogenic Effects:

MAXZIDE: Animal reproduction studies to determine the potential for fetal harm by MAXZIDE have not been conducted. Nevertheless, a One Generation Study in the rat approximated MAXZIDE's composition by using a 1:1 ratio of triamterene to hydrochlorothiazide (30:30 mg/kg/day). There was no evidence of teratogenicity at those doses that were, on a body- weight basis, 15 and 30 times, respectively, the MRHD, and, on the basis of body-surface area, 3.1 and 6.2 times, respectively, the MRHD.

The safe use of MAXZIDE in pregnancy has not been established since there are no adequate and well-controlled studies with MAXZIDE in pregnant women. MAXZIDE should be used during pregnancy only if the potential benefit justifies the risk to the fetus.

Triamterene: Reproduction studies have been performed in rats at doses as high as 20 times the Maximum Recommended Human Dose (MRHD) on the basis of body-weight, and 6 times the MRHD on the basis of body-surface area without evidence of harm to the fetus due to triamterene. Because animal reproduction studies are not always predictive of human response, this drug should be used during pregnancy only if clearly needed.

Hydrochlorothiazide: Hydrochlorothiazide was orally administered to pregnant mice and rats during respective periods of major organogenesis at doses up to 3000 and 1000 mg/kg/day, respectively. At these doses, which are multiples of the MRHD equal to 3000 for mice and 1000 for rats, based on body-weight, and equal to 282 for mice and 206 for rats, based on body-surface area, there was no evidence of harm to the fetus. There are, however, no adequate and well-controlled studies in pregnant women. Because animal reproduction studies are not always predictive of human response, this drug should be used during pregnancy only if clearly needed.

Nonteratogenic Effects: Thiazides and triamterene have been shown to cross the placental barrier and appear in cord blood. The use of thiazides and triamterene in pregnant women requires that the anticipated benefits be weighed against possible hazards to the fetus. These hazards include fetal or neonatal jaundice, pancreatitis, thrombocytopenia, and possibly other adverse reactions that have occurred in the adult.

Nursing Mothers Thiazides and triamterene in combination have not been studied in nursing mothers. Triamterene appears in animal milk and this may occur in humans. Thiazides are excreted in human breast milk. If use of the combination drug product is deemed essential, the patient should stop nursing.

Pediatric Use: Safety and effectiveness in pediatric patients have not been established.

ADVERSE REACTIONS

Side effects observed in association with the use of MAXZIDE, other combination products containing triamterene/hydrochlorothiazide, and products containing triamterene or hydrochlorothiazide include the following:

Gastrointestinal: jaundice (intrahepatic cholestatic jaundice), pancreatitis, nausea, appetite disturbance, taste alteration, vomiting, diarrhea, constipation, anorexia, gastric irritation, cramping.

Central Nervous System: drowsiness and fatigue, insomnia, headache, dizziness, dry mouth, depression, anxiety, vertigo, restlessness, paresthesias.

Cardiovascular: tachycardia, shortness of breath and chest pain, orthostatic hypotension (may be aggravated by alcohol, barbiturates or narcotics).

Renal: acute renal failure, acute interstitial nephritis, renal stones composed of triamterene in association with other calculus materials, urine discoloration.

Hematologic: leukopenia, agranulocytosis, thrombocytopenia, aplastic anemia, hemolytic anemia and megaloblastosis.

Ophthalmic: xanthopsia, transient blurred vision.

Hypersensitivity: anaphylaxis, photosensitivity, rash, urticaria, purpura, necrotizing angiitis (vasculitis, cutaneous vasculitis), fever, respiratory distress including pneumonitis.

Other: muscle cramps and weakness, decreased sexual performance and sialadenitis.

Whenever adverse reactions are moderate to severe, therapy should be reduced or withdrawn.

Altered Laboratory Findings:

Serum Electrolytes: hyperkalemia, hypokalemia, hyponatremia, hypomagnesemia, hypochloremia (see WARNINGS, PRECAUTIONS).

Creatinine, Blood Urea Nitrogen: Reversible elevations in BUN and serum creatinine have been observed in hypertensive patients treated with MAXZIDE.

Glucose: hyperglycemia, glycosuria and diabetes mellitus (see PRECAUTIONS).

Serum Uric Acid, PBI and Calcium: (see PRECAUTIONS).

Other: Elevated liver enzymes have been reported in patients receiving MAXZIDE.

OVERDOSAGE

No specific data are available regarding MAXZIDE (triamterene and hydrochlorothiazide) overdosage in humans and no specific antidote is available.

Fluid and electrolyte imbalances are the most important concern. Excessive doses of the triamterene component may elicit hyperkalemia, dehydration, nausea, vomiting and weakness and possibly hypotension. Overdosing with hydrochlorothiazide has been associated with hypokalemia, hypochloremia, hyponatremia, dehydration, lethargy (may progress to coma) and gastrointestinal irritation. Treatment is symptomatic and supportive. Therapy with MAXZIDE (triamterene and hydrochlorothiazide) should be discontinued. Induce emesis or institute gastric lavage. Monitor serum electrolyte levels and fluid balance. Institute supportive measures as required to maintain hydration, electrolyte balance, respiratory, cardiovascular and renal function.

DOSAGE AND ADMINISTRATION

The usual dose of MAXZIDE-25 MG is one or two tablets daily, given as a single dose, with appropriate monitoring of serum potassium (see WARNINGS). The usual dose of MAXZIDE is one tablet daily, with appropriate monitoring of serum potassium (see WARNINGS). There is no experience with the use of more than one MAXZIDE tablet daily or more than two MAXZIDE-25 MG tablets daily. Clinical experience with the administration of two MAXZIDE-25 MG tablets daily in divided doses (rather than as a single dose) suggests an increased risk of electrolyte imbalance and renal dysfunction.

Patients receiving 50 mg of hydrochlorothiazide who become hypokalemic may be transferred to MAXZIDE (triamterene and hydrochlorothiazide) directly. Patients receiving 25 mg hydrochlorothiazide who become hypokalemic may be transferred to MAXZIDE-25 MG (37.5 mg triamterene/25 mg hydrochlorothiazide) directly.

In patients requiring hydrochlorothiazide therapy and in whom hypokalemia cannot be risked therapy may be initiated with MAXZIDE-25 MG. If an optimal blood pressure response is not obtained with MAXZIDE-25 MG, the dose should be increased to two MAXZIDE-25 MG tablets daily as a single dose, or one MAXZIDE tablet daily. If blood pressure still is not controlled, another antihypertensive agent may be added (see PRECAUTIONS, Drug Interactions).

Clinical studies have shown that patients taking less bioavailable formulations of triamterene and hydrochlorothiazide in daily doses of 25-50 mg hydrochlorothiazide and 50-100 mg triamterene may be safely changed to one MAXZIDE-25 MG tablet daily. All patients changed from less bioavailable formulations to MAXZIDE should be monitored clinically and for serum potassium after the transfer.

HOW SUPPLIED

MAXZIDE® (triamterene and hydrochlorothiazide) tablets are bowtie-shaped, flat-faced beveled, light yellow tablets, engraved with MAXZIDE on one side and scored on the other with B on the left and M8 on the right of the score. Each tablet contains 75 mg of triamterene, USP and 50 mg of hydrochlorothiazide, USP. They are supplied as follows:

NDC 62794-460-01—Bottle of 100 with CRC

NDC 62794-460-05—Bottle of 500

NDC 62794-460-88—Unit Dose 10 × 10s

MAXZIDE®-25 MG (triamterene and hydrochlorothiazide) tablets are bowtie-shaped, flat-faced beveled, light green tablets, engraved with MAXZIDE on one side and scored on the other with B on the left and M9 on the right of the score. Each tablet contains 37.5 mg of triamterene, USP and 25 mg of hydrochlorothiazide, USP. They are supplied as follows:

NDC 62794-464-01—Bottle of 100 with CRC

NDC 62794-464-05—Bottle of 500

NDC 62794-464-88—Unit Dose 10 × 10s

STORE AT CONTROLLED ROOM TEMPERATURE 15-30°C (59-86°F).

PROTECT FROM LIGHT.

Dispense in a tight, light-resistant, child-resistant container.

BERTEK PHARMACEUTICALS INC.
Research Triangle Park, N.C. 27709-4149

Revised December 2002
BKMAX-R6

Shown in Product Identification Guide, page 324

MENTAX® ℞

[*mĕn-tax*]

(butenafine HCl) Cream, 1%

Rx Only

DESCRIPTION

Mentax® Cream, 1%, contains the synthetic antifungal agent, butenafine hydrochloride. Butenafine is a member of the class of antifungal compounds known as benzylamines which are structurally related to the allylamines.

Butenafine HCl is designated chemically as N-4-*tert*-butylbenzyl-N-methyl-1-naphthalenemethylamine hydrochloride. The compound has the empirical formula $C_{23}H_{27}N \bullet HCl$, a molecular weight of 353.93, and the following structural formula:

Butenafine HCl is a white, odorless, crystalline powder. It is freely soluble in methanol, ethanol, and chloroform, and slightly soluble in water. Each gram of Mentax® Cream, 1%, contains 10 mg of butenafine HCl in a white cream base of purified water USP, propylene glycol dicaprylate, glycerin USP, cetyl alcohol NF, glyceryl monostearate SE, white petrolatum USP, stearic acid NF, polyoxyethylene (23) cetyl ether, benzyl alcohol NF, diethanolamine NF, and sodium benzoate NF.

CLINICAL PHARMACOLOGY

Pharmacokinetics

In one study conducted in healthy subjects for 14 days, 6 grams of Mentax® Cream, 1%, was applied once daily to the dorsal skin (3,000 cm^2) of 7 subjects, and 20 grams of the cream was applied once daily to the arms, trunk and groin areas (10,000 cm^2) of another 12 subjects. After 14 days of topical applications, the 6-gram dose group yielded a mean peak plasma butenafine HCl concentration, Cmax, of 1.4 ± 0.8 ng/mL, occurring at a mean time to the peak plasma concentration, Tmax, of 15 ± 8 hours, and a mean area under the plasma concentration-time curve, $AUC_{0\text{-}24\ hrs}$ of 23.9 ± 11.3 ng-hr/mL. For the 20-gram dose group, the mean Cmax was 5.0 ± 2.0 ng/mL, occurring at a mean Tmax of 6 ± 6 hours, and the mean $AUC_{0\text{-}24\ hrs}$ was 87.8 ± 45.3 ng-hr/mL. A biphasic decline of plasma butenafine HCl concentrations was observed with the half-lives estimated to be 35 hours and > 150 hours, respectively.

At 72 hours after the last dose application, the mean plasma concentrations decreased to 0.3 ± 0.2 ng/mL for the 6-gram dose group and 1.1 ± 0.9 ng/mL for the 20-gram dose group. Low levels of butenafine HCl remained in the plasma 7 days after the last dose application (mean: 0.1 ± 0.2 ng/mL for the 6-gram dose group, and 0.7 ± 0.5 ng/mL for the 20-gram dose group). The total amount (or % dose) of butenafine HCl absorbed through the skin into the systemic circulation has not been quantitated. It was determined that the primary metabolite in urine was formed through hydroxylation at the terminal *t*-butyl side-chain.

In 11 patients with tinea pedis, butenafine HCl cream, 1%, was applied by the patients to cover the affected and immediately surrounding skin area once daily for 4 weeks, and a single blood sample was collected between 10 and 20 hours following dosing at 1, 2 and 4 weeks after treatment. The plasma butenafine HCl concentration ranged from undetectable to 0.3 ng/mL.

In 24 patients with tinea cruris, butenafine HCl cream, 1%, was applied by the patients to cover the affected and immediately surrounding skin area once daily for 2 weeks (mean average daily dose: 1.3 ± 0.2 g). A single blood sample was collected between 0.5 and 65 hours after the last dose, and the plasma butenafine HCl concentration ranged from undetectable to 2.52 ng/mL (mean ± SD: 0.91 ± 0.15 ng/mL). Four weeks after cessation of treatment, the plasma butenafine HCl concentration ranged from undetectable to 0.28 ng/mL.

Microbiology

Butenafine HCl is a benzylamine derivative with a mode of action similar to that of the allylamine class of antifungal drugs. Butenafine HCl is hypothesized to act by inhibiting the epoxidation of squalene, thus blocking the biosynthesis of ergosterol, an essential component of fungal cell membranes. The benzylamine derivatives, like the allylamines, act at an earlier step in the ergosterol biosynthesis pathway than the azole class of antifungal drugs. Depending on the concentration of the drug and the fungal species tested, butenafine HCl may be fungicidal or fungistatic *in vitro*. However, the clinical significance of these *in vitro* data are unknown.

Butenafine HCl has been shown to be active against most strains of the following microorganisms, both *in vitro* and in clinical infections as described in the INDICATIONS AND USAGE section:

Epidermophyton floccosum
Malassezia furfur
Trichophyton mentagrophytes
Trichophyton rubrum
Trichophyton tonsurans

CLINICAL STUDIES

Tinea (pityriasis) versicolor

In the following data presentations, patients with tinea (pityriasis) versicolor were studied. The term **"Negative Mycology"** is defined as absence of hyphae in a KOH preparation of skin scrapings, i.e., no fungal forms seen or the presence of yeast cells (blastospores) only. The term **"Effective Treatment"** is defined as Negative Mycology plus total signs and symptoms score (on a scale from zero to three) for erythema, scaling, and pruritus equal to or less than 1 at Week 8. The term **"Complete Cure"** refers to patients who had negative mycology plus sign/symptoms score of zero for erythema, scaling, and pruritus.

Two separate studies compared Mentax® Cream to vehicle applied once daily for 2 weeks in the treatment of tinea (pityriasis) versicolor. Patients were treated for 2 weeks and were evaluated at the following weeks post-treatment: 2 (Week 4) and 6 (Week 8). All subjects with a positive baseline KOH and who were dispensed medications were included in the "intent-to-treat" analysis shown in the table below. Statistical significance (Mentax® vs. vehicle) was achieved for Effective Treatment, but not Complete Cure at 6 weeks post-treatment in Study 31. Marginal statistical significance (p=0.051) (Mentax® vs. vehicle) was achieved for Effective Treatment, but not Complete Cure at 6 weeks post-treatment in Study 32. Data from these two controlled studies are presented in the table below.

[See table above]

Proportion (%) of responders in pivotal clinical trials (all randomized patients)

Patient Response Category	Week@	Study 31		Study 32	
		Butenafine	Vehicle	Butenafine	Vehicle
Complete Cure*	2	41/87 (47%)	11/40 (28%)	29/85 (34%)	12/41 (29%)
	4	43/86 (50%)	15/42 (36%)	36/83 (43%)	13/41 (32%)
	8	44/87 (51%)	15/42 (36%)	30/86 (35%)	10/43 (23%)
Effective Treatment**	2	56/87 (64%)	16/40 (40%)	46/85 (54%)	16/41 (39%)
	4	50/86 (58%)	19/42 (45%)	45/83 (54%)	16/41 (39%)
	8	48/87 (55%)	15/42 (36%)	37/86 (43%)	11/43 (26%)
Negative Mycology***	2	57/87 (66%)	20/40 (50%)	57/85 (67%)	21/41 (51%)
	4	51/86 (59%)	20/42 (48%)	52/83 (63%)	18/41 (44%)
	8	48/87 (55%)	15/42 (36%)	43/86 (50%)	12/43 (28%)

@ Week 2 (end of treatment), Week 4 (2 weeks post-treatment), and Week 8 (6 weeks post-treatment)
* Negative Mycology plus absence of erythema, scaling, and pruritus
** Negative Mycology plus no or minimal involvement of erythema, scaling or pruritus
*** Absence of hyphae in a KOH preparation of skin scrapings, i.e., no fungal forms seen or the presence of yeast cells (blastospores) only.

Tinea (pityriasis) versicolor is a superficial, chronically recurring infection of the glabrous skin caused by *Malassezia furfur* (formerly *Pityrosporum orbiculare*). The commensal organism is part of the normal skin flora. In susceptible individuals the condition may give rise to hyperpigmented or hypopigmented patches on the trunk which may extend to the neck, arms and upper thighs.

Treatment of the infection may not immediately result in restoration of pigment of the affected sites. Normalization of pigment following successful therapy is variable and may take months, depending upon individual skin type and incidental sun exposure. The rate of recurrence of infection is variable.

INDICATIONS AND USAGE

Mentax® (butenafine HCl) Cream, 1% is indicated for the topical treatment of the dermatologic infection, tinea (pityriasis) versicolor due to *M. furfur* (formerly *P. orbiculare*).

Butenafine HCl cream was not studied in immunocompromised patients. (See **DOSAGE AND ADMINISTRATION**).

CONTRAINDICATIONS

Mentax® (butenafine HCl) Cream, 1%, is contraindicated in individuals who have known or suspected sensitivity to Mentax® Cream, 1%, or any of its components.

WARNINGS

Mentax® (butenafine HCl) Cream, 1%, is not for ophthalmic, oral, or intravaginal use.

PRECAUTIONS

General

Mentax® Cream, 1%, is for external use only. If irritation or sensitivity develops with the use of Mentax® Cream, 1%, treatment should be discontinued and appropriate therapy instituted. Diagnosis of the disease should be confirmed either by culture on an appropriate medium, [except *M. furfur* (formerly *P. orbiculare*)] or by direct microscopic examination of infected superficial epidermal tissue in a solution of potassium hydroxide.

Patients who are known to be sensitive to allylamine antifungals should use Mentax® (butenafine HCl) Cream, 1%, with caution, since cross-reactivity may occur.

Use Mentax® Cream, 1%, as directed by the physician, and avoid contact with the eyes, nose, mouth, and other mucous membranes.

Information for Patients

The patient should be instructed to:

1. Use Mentax® Cream, 1%, as directed by the physician. The hands should be washed after applying the medication to the affected area(s). Avoid contact with the eyes, nose, mouth, and other mucous membranes. Mentax® Cream, 1%, is for external use only.
2. Dry the affected area(s) thoroughly before application, if you wish to apply Mentax® Cream, 1%, after bathing.
3. Use the medication for the full treatment time recommended by the physician, even though symptoms may have improved.
   Notify the physician if there is no improvement after the end of the prescribed treatment period, or sooner, if the condition worsens (see below).
4. Inform the physician if the area of application shows signs of increased irritation, redness, itching, burning, blistering, swelling, or oozing.
5. Avoid the use of occlusive dressings unless otherwise directed by the physician.
6. Do not use this medication for any disorder other than that for which it was prescribed.

Drug Interactions

Potential drug interactions between Mentax® (butenafine HCl) Cream, 1%, and other drugs have not been systematically evaluated.

Carcinogenesis, Mutagenesis, Impairment of Fertility

Long-term studies to evaluate the carcinogenic potential of Mentax® Cream, 1%, have not been conducted. Two *in vitro* assays (bacterial reverse mutation test and chromosome aberration test in Chinese hamster lymphocytes) and one *in vivo* study (rat micronucleus bioassay) revealed no mutagenic or clastogenic potential for butenafine.

In subcutaneous fertility studies conducted in rats at dose levels up to 25 mg/kg/day (0.5 times the maximum recommended dose in humans for tinea versicolor based on body surface area comparisons), butenafine did not produce any adverse effects on male or female fertility.

Pregnancy

Teratogenic Effects: Pregnancy Category C

Subcutaneous doses of butenafine (dose levels up to 25 mg/kg/day administered during organogenesis) (equivalent to 0.5 times the maximum recommended dose in humans for tinea versicolor based on body surface area comparisons) were not teratogenic in rats. In an oral embryofetal developmental study in rabbits (dose levels up to 400 mg butenafine HCl/kg/day administered during organogenesis) (equivalent to 16 times the maximum recommended dose in humans for tinea versicolor based on body surface area comparisons), no treatment-related external, visceral, skeletal malformations or variations were observed.

In an oral peri- and post-natal developmental study in rats (dose levels up to 125 mg butenafine HCl/kg/day) (equivalent to 2.5 times the maximum recommended dose in humans for tinea versicolor based on body surface area comparisons), no treatment-related effects on postnatal survival, development of the F1 generation or their subsequent maturation and fertility were observed.

There are, however, no adequate and well-controlled studies that have been conducted with topically applied butenafine in pregnant women. Because animal reproduction studies are not always predictive human response, this drug should be used during pregnancy only if clearly needed.

Nursing Mothers

It is not known if butenafine HCl is excreted in human milk. Because many drugs are excreted in human milk, caution should be exercised in prescribing Mentax® Cream, 1%, to a nursing woman.

Pediatric Use

Safety and efficacy in pediatric patients below the age of 12 years have not been studied, since tinea versicolor is uncommon in patients below the age of 12 years.

ADVERSE REACTIONS

In controlled clinical trials, 9 (approximately 1%) of 815 patients treated with Mentax® Cream, 1%, reported adverse events related to the skin. These included burning/stinging, itching and worsening of the condition. No patient treated with Mentax® Cream, 1%, discontinued treatment due to an adverse event. In the vehicle-treated patients, two of 718 patients discontinued because of treatment site adverse events, one of which was severe burning/stinging and itching at the site of application.

In uncontrolled clinical trials, the most frequently reported adverse events in patients treated with Mentax® Cream, 1%, were: contact dermatitis, erythema, irritation, and itching, each occurring in less than 2% of patients.

In provocative testing in over 200 subjects, there was no evidence of allergic contact sensitization for either cream or vehicle base for Mentax® Cream 1%.

OVERDOSAGE

Overdosage of butenafine HCl in humans has not been reported to date.

DOSAGE AND ADMINISTRATION

Patients with tinea (pityriasis) versicolor should apply Mentax® once daily for two weeks. Sufficient Mentax® Cream should be applied to cover affected areas and immediately surrounding skin of patients with tinea versicolor. If a patient shows no clinical improvement after the treatment period, the diagnosis and therapy should be reviewed.

HOW SUPPLIED

Mentax® (butenafine HCl) Cream, 1%, is supplied in tubes in the following sizes:

15-gram tube (NDC 62794-151-02)
30-gram tube (NDC 62794-151-03)

STORE BETWEEN 5°C and 30°C (41° and 86°F).

BERTEK PHARMACEUTICALS INC. June 2003
Research Triangle Park, NC 27709-4149 029.3
Patent # 5,021,458

Shown in Product Identification Guide, page 324

PHENYTEK™ CAPSULES ℞

(extended phenytoin sodium capsules, USP)
200 mg and 300 mg
℞ only

DESCRIPTION

PHENYTEK™ (phenytoin sodium) is an antiepileptic drug. Phenytoin sodium is related to the barbiturates in chemical structure, but has a five-membered ring. The chemical name is 5,5-Diphenylhydantoin sodium salt, having a molecular weight of 274.25 and having the following structural formula and molecular formula:

$C_{15}H_{11}N_2NaO_2$

Each PHENYTEK™ CAPSULE, (extended phenytoin sodium capsule, USP) for oral administration, contains 200 mg or 300 mg of phenytoin sodium. Each capsule also contains the following inactive ingredients: black iron oxide, colloidal silicon dioxide, D&C yellow no. 10 aluminum lake, FD&C blue #1, FD&C blue no. 1 aluminum lake, FD&C blue no. 2 aluminum lake, FD&C red no. 40 aluminum lake, gelatin, hydroxyethyl cellulose, magnesium oxide, magnesium stearate, microcrystalline cellulose, pharmaceutical glaze, povidone, propylene glycol, silicon dioxide, sodium lauryl sulfate and titanium dioxide. Product *in vivo* performance is characterized by a slow and extended rate of absorption with peak blood concentrations expected in 4 to 12 hours as contrasted to prompt phenytoin sodium capsules, USP with a rapid rate of absorption with peak blood concentration expected in 1½ to 3 hours.

PHENYTEK™ CAPSULES, 200 mg and 300 mg meet USP *Dissolution Test* 3.

CLINICAL PHARMACOLOGY

Phenytoin is an antiepileptic drug which can be useful in the treatment of epilepsy. The primary site of action appears to be the *motor cortex* where spread of *seizure* activity is inhibited. Possibly by promoting sodium efflux from neurons, phenytoin tends to stabilize the threshold against hyperexcitability caused by excessive stimulation or environmental changes capable of reducing membrane sodium gradient. This includes the reduction of posttetanic potentiation at synapses. Loss of posttetanic potentiation prevents

Continued on next page

Phenytek—Cont.

cortical seizure foci from detonating adjacent cortical areas. Phenytoin reduces the maximal activity of brain stem centers responsible for the tonic phase of tonic-clonic (grand mal) seizures.
The plasma half-life in man after oral administration of phenytoin averages 22 hours, with a range of 7 to 42 hours. Steady-state therapeutic levels are achieved at least 7 to 10 days (5 to 7 half-lives) after initiation of therapy with recommended doses of 300 mg/day.
When serum level determinations are necessary, they should be obtained at least 5 to 7 half-lives after treatment initiation, dosage change, or addition or subtraction of another drug to the regimen so that equilibrium or steady-state will have been achieved. Trough levels provide information about clinically effective serum level range and confirm patient compliance and are obtained just prior to the patient's next scheduled dose. Peak levels indicate an individual's threshold for emergence of dose-related side effects and are obtained at the time of expected peak concentration. For extended phenytoin sodium capsules peak serum levels occur 4 to 12 hours after administration.
Optimum control without clinical signs of toxicity occurs more often with serum levels between 10 and 20 mcg/mL, although some mild cases of tonic-clonic (grand mal) epilepsy may be controlled with lower serum levels of phenytoin.
In most patients maintained at a steady dosage, stable phenytoin serum levels are achieved. There may be wide interpatient variability in phenytoin serum levels with equivalent dosages. Patients with unusually low levels may be noncompliant or hypermetabolizers of phenytoin. Unusually high levels result from liver disease, congenital enzyme deficiency, or drug interactions which result in metabolic interference. The patient with large variations in phenytoin plasma levels, despite standard doses, presents a difficult clinical problem. Serum level determinations in such patients may be particularly helpful. As phenytoin is highly protein bound, free phenytoin levels may be altered in patients whose protein binding characteristics differ from normal.
Most of the drug is excreted in the bile as inactive metabolites which are then reabsorbed from the intestinal tract and excreted in the urine. Urinary excretion of phenytoin and its metabolites occurs partly with glomerular filtration but more importantly by tubular secretion. Because phenytoin is hydroxylated in the liver by an enzyme system which is saturable at high plasma levels, small incremental doses may increase the half-life and produce very substantial increases in serum levels, when these are in the upper range. The steady-state level may be disproportionately increased, with resultant intoxication, from an increase in dosage of 10% or more.

INDICATIONS AND USAGE

PHENYTEK™ CAPSULES (extended phenytoin sodium capsules, USP) are indicated for the control of generalized tonic-clonic (grand mal) and complex partial (psychomotor, temporal lobe) seizures and prevention and treatment of seizures occurring during or following neurosurgery.
Phenytoin serum level determinations may be necessary for optimal dosage adjustments (see DOSAGE AND ADMINISTRATION and CLINICAL PHARMACOLOGY sections).

CONTRAINDICATIONS

Phenytoin is contraindicated in those patients with a history of hypersensitivity to phenytoin or other hydantoins.

WARNINGS

Abrupt withdrawal of phenytoin in epileptic patients may precipitate status epilepticus. When, in the judgment of the clinician, the need for dosage reduction, discontinuation, or substitution of alternative antiepileptic medication arises, this should be done gradually. However, in the event of an allergic or hypersensitivity reaction, more rapid substitution of alternative therapy may be necessary. In this case, alternative therapy should be an anticonvulsant drug not belonging to the hydantoin chemical class.
There have been a number of reports suggesting a relationship between phenytoin and the development of lymphadenopathy (local or generalized) including benign lymph node hyperplasia, pseudolymphoma, lymphoma, and Hodgkin's Disease. Although a cause and effect relationship has not been established, the occurrence of lymphadenopathy indicates the need to differentiate such a condition from other types of lymph node pathology. Lymph node involvement may occur with or without symptoms and signs resembling serum sickness, e.g., fever, rash, and liver involvement.
In all cases of lymphadenopathy, follow-up observation for an extended period is indicated and every effort should be made to achieve seizure control using alternative antiepileptic drugs.
Acute alcoholic intake may increase phenytoin serum levels while chronic alcoholic use may decrease serum levels.
In view of isolated reports associating phenytoin with exacerbation of porphyria, caution should be exercised in using this medication in patients suffering from this disease.
Usage in Pregnancy: A number of reports suggests an association between the use of antiepileptic drugs by women with epilepsy and a higher incidence of birth defects in children born to these women. Data are more extensive with respect to phenytoin and phenobarbital, but these are also the most commonly prescribed antiepileptic drugs; less systematic or anecdotal reports suggest a possible similar association with the use of all known antiepileptic drugs.
The reports suggesting a higher incidence of birth defects in children of drug-treated epileptic women cannot be regarded as adequate to prove a definite cause and effect relationship. There are intrinsic methodologic problems in obtaining adequate data on drug teratogenicity in humans; genetic factors or the epileptic condition itself may be more important than drug therapy in leading to birth defects. The great majority of mothers on antiepileptic medication deliver normal infants. It is important to note that antiepileptic drugs should not be discontinued in patients in whom the drug is administered to prevent major seizures, because of the strong possibility of precipitating status epilepticus with attendant hypoxia and threat to life. In individual cases where the severity and frequency of the seizure disorder are such that the removal of medication does not pose a serious threat to the patient, discontinuation of the drug may be considered prior to and during pregnancy, although it cannot be said with any confidence that even minor seizures do not pose some hazard to the developing embryo or fetus. The prescribing physician will wish to weigh these considerations in treating or counseling epileptic women of childbearing potential.
In addition to the reports of increased incidence of congenital malformation, such as cleft lip/palate and heart malformations in children of women receiving phenytoin and other antiepileptic drugs, there have more recently been reports of a fetal hydantoin syndrome. This consists of prenatal growth deficiency, microcephaly, and mental deficiency in children born to mothers who have received phenytoin, barbiturates, alcohol, or trimethadione. However, these features are all interrelated and are frequently associated with intrauterine growth retardation from other causes.
There have been isolated reports of malignancies, including neuroblastoma, in children whose mothers received phenytoin during pregnancy.
An increase in seizure frequency during pregnancy occurs in a high proportion of patients, because of altered phenytoin absorption or metabolism. Periodic measurement of serum phenytoin levels is particularly valuable in the management of a pregnant epileptic patient as a guide to an appropriate adjustment of dosage. However, postpartum restoration of the original dosage will probably be indicated.
Neonatal coagulation defects have been reported within the first 24 hours in babies born to epileptic mothers receiving phenobarbital and/or phenytoin. Vitamin K has been shown to prevent or correct this defect and has been recommended to be given to the mother before delivery and to the neonate after birth.

PRECAUTIONS

General: The liver is the chief site of biotransformation of phenytoin; patients with impaired liver function, elderly patients, or those who are gravely ill may show early signs of toxicity.
A small percentage of individuals who have been treated with phenytoin have been shown to metabolize the drug slowly. Slow metabolism may be due to limited enzyme availability and lack of induction; it appears to be genetically determined.
Phenytoin should be discontinued if a skin rash appears (see WARNINGS section regarding drug discontinuation). If the rash is exfoliative, purpuric, or bullous, or if lupus erythematosus, Stevens-Johnson syndrome, or toxic epidermal necrolysis is suspected, use of this drug should not be resumed and alternative therapy should be considered. (See ADVERSE REACTIONS section.) If the rash is of a milder type (measles-like or scarlatiniform), therapy may be resumed after the rash has completely disappeared. If the rash recurs upon reinstitution of therapy, further phenytoin medication is contraindicated.
Phenytoin and other hydantoins are contraindicated in patients who have experienced phenytoin hypersensitivity. Additionally, caution should be exercised if using structurally similar compounds (e.g., barbiturates, succinamides, oxazolidinediones and other related compounds) in these same patients.
Hyperglycemia, resulting from the drug's inhibitory effects on insulin release, has been reported. Phenytoin may also raise the serum glucose level in diabetic patients.
Osteomalacia has been associated with phenytoin therapy and is considered to be due to phenytoin's interference with Vitamin D metabolism.
Phenytoin is not indicated for seizures due to hypoglycemic or other metabolic causes. Appropriate diagnostic procedures should be performed as indicated.
Phenytoin is not effective for absence (petit mal) seizures. If tonic-clonic (grand mal) and absence (petit mal) seizures are present, combined drug therapy is needed.
Serum levels of phenytoin sustained above the optimal range may produce confusional states referred to as "delirium," "psychosis," or "encephalopathy," or rarely irreversible cerebellar dysfunction. Accordingly, at the first sign of acute toxicity, plasma levels are recommended. Dose reduction of phenytoin therapy is indicated if plasma levels are excessive; if symptoms persist, termination is recommended. (See WARNINGS section.)
Information for Patients: Patients taking phenytoin should be advised of the importance of adhering strictly to the prescribed dosage regimen, and of informing the physician of any clinical condition in which it is not possible to take the drug orally as prescribed, e.g., surgery, etc.
Patients should also be cautioned on the use of other drugs or alcoholic beverages without first seeking the physician's advice.
Patients should be instructed to call their physician if skin rash develops.
The importance of good dental hygiene should be stressed in order to minimize the development of gingival hyperplasia and its complications.
Laboratory Tests: Phenytoin serum level determinations may be necessary to achieve optimal dosage adjustments.
Drug Interactions: There are many drugs which may increase or decrease phenytoin levels or which phenytoin may affect. Serum level determinations for phenytoin are especially helpful when possible drug interactions are suspected. The most commonly occurring drug interactions are listed below.

1. Drugs which may increase phenytoin serum levels include: acute alcohol intake, amiodarone, chloramphenicol, chlordiazepoxide, diazepam, dicumarol, disulfiram, estrogens, ethosuximide, H_2-antagonists, halothane, isoniazid, methylphenidate, phenothiazines, phenylbutazone, salicylates, succinamides, sulfonamides, tolbutamide, trazodone.
2. Drugs which may decrease phenytoin levels include: carbamazepine, chronic alcohol abuse, reserpine, and sucralfate. Moban® brand of molindone hydrochloride contains calcium ions which interfere with the absorption of phenytoin. Ingestion times of phenytoin and antacid preparations containing calcium should be staggered in patients with low serum phenytoin levels to prevent absorption problems.
3. Drugs which may either increase or decrease phenytoin serum levels include: phenobarbital, sodium valproate, and valproic acid. Similarly, the effect of phenytoin on phenobarbital, valproic acid and sodium valproate serum levels is unpredictable.
4. Although not a true drug interaction, tricyclic antidepressants may precipitate seizures in susceptible patients and phenytoin dosage may need to be adjusted.
5. Drugs whose efficacy is impaired by phenytoin include: corticosteroids, coumarin anticoagulants, digitoxin, doxycycline, estrogens, furosemide, oral contraceptives, quinidine, rifampin, theophylline, vitamin D.

Drug/Laboratory Test Interactions: Phenytoin may cause decreased serum levels of protein-bound iodine (PBI). It may also produce lower than normal values for dexamethasone or metyrapone tests. Phenytoin may cause increased serum levels of glucose, alkaline phosphatase, and gamma glutamyl transpeptidase (GGT).
Carcinogenesis: See WARNINGS section for information on carcinogenesis.
Pregnancy: See WARNINGS section.
Nursing Mothers: Infant breast feeding is not recommended for women taking this drug because phenytoin appears to be secreted in low concentrations in human milk.

ADVERSE REACTIONS

Central Nervous System: The most common manifestations encountered with phenytoin therapy are referable to this system and are usually dose-related. These include nystagmus, ataxia, slurred speech, decreased coordination, and mental confusion. Dizziness, insomnia, transient nervousness, motor twitchings, and headaches have also been observed. There have also been rare reports of phenytoin induced dyskinesias, including chorea, dystonia, tremor and asterixis, similar to those induced by phenothiazine and other neuroleptic drugs.
A predominantly sensory peripheral polyneuropathy has been observed in patients receiving long-term phenytoin therapy.
Gastrointestinal System: Nausea, vomiting, constipation, toxic hepatitis and liver damage.
Integumentary System: Dermatological manifestations sometimes accompanied by fever have included scarlatiniform or morbilliform rashes. A morbilliform rash (measles-like) is the most common; other types of dermatitis are seen more rarely. Other more serious forms which may be fatal have included bullous, exfoliative or purpuric dermatitis, lupus erythematosus, Stevens-Johnson syndrome, and toxic epidermal necrolysis (see PRECAUTIONS section).
Hemopoietic System: Hemopoietic complications, some fatal, have occasionally been reported in association with administration of phenytoin. These have included thrombocytopenia, leukopenia, granulocytopenia, agranulocytosis, and pancytopenia with or without bone marrow suppression. While macrocytosis and megaloblastic anemia have occurred, these conditions usually respond to folic acid therapy. Lymphadenopathy including benign lymph node hyperplasia, pseudolymphoma, lymphoma, and Hodgkin's Disease have been reported (see WARNINGS section).
Connective Tissue System: Coarsening of the facial features, enlargement of the lips, gingival hyperplasia, hypertrichosis, and Peyronie's Disease.
Cardiovascular: Periarteritis nodosa.
Immunologic: Hypersensitivity syndrome (which may include, but is not limited to, symptoms such as arthralgias, eosinophilia, fever, liver dysfunction, lymphadenopathy or rash), systemic lupus erythematosus, and immunoglobulin abnormalities.

OVERDOSAGE

The lethal dose in children is not known. The lethal dose in adults is estimated to be 2 to 5 grams. The initial symptoms are nystagmus, ataxia, and dysarthria. Other signs are tremor, hyperreflexia, lethargy, slurred speech, nausea, vomiting. The patient may become comatose and hypotensive. Death is due to respiratory and circulatory depression. There are marked variations among individuals with respect to phenytoin plasma levels where toxicity may occur. Nystagmus, on lateral gaze, usually appears at 20 mcg/mL, ataxia at 30 mcg/mL, dysarthria and lethargy appear when the plasma concentration is over 40 mcg/mL, but as high a concentration as 50 mcg/mL has been reported without evidence of toxicity. As much as 25 times the therapeutic dose has been taken to result in a serum concentration over 100 mcg/mL with complete recovery.

Treatment: Treatment is nonspecific since there is no known antidote.

The adequacy of the respiratory and circulatory systems should be carefully observed and appropriate supportive measures employed. Hemodialysis can be considered since phenytoin is not completely bound to plasma proteins. Total exchange transfusion has been used in the treatment of severe intoxication in children.

In acute overdosage, the possibility of other CNS depressants, including alcohol, should be borne in mind.

DOSAGE AND ADMINISTRATION

Serum concentrations should be monitored in changing from extended phenytoin sodium capsules, USP, to prompt phenytoin sodium capsules, USP, and from the sodium salt to the free acid form.

PHENYTEK™ CAPSULES (extended phenytoin sodium capsules, USP) are formulated with the sodium salt of phenytoin. Because there is approximately an 8% increase in drug content with the free acid form over that of the sodium salt, dosage adjustments and serum level monitoring may be necessary when switching from a product formulated with the free acid to a product formulated with the sodium salt and vice versa.

General: Dosage should be individualized to provide maximum benefit. In some cases, serum blood level determinations may be necessary for optimal dosage adjustments—the clinically effective serum level is usually 10 to 20 mcg/mL. With recommended dosage, a period of seven to ten days may be required to achieve steady-state blood levels with phenytoin and changes in dosage (increase or decrease) should not be carried out at intervals shorter than seven to ten days.

Adult Dosage: *Divided Daily Dosage:* Patients who have received no previous treatment may be started on one 100 mg extended phenytoin sodium capsule three times daily and the dosage then adjusted to suit individual requirements. For most adults, the satisfactory maintenance dosage will be one 100 mg capsule three to four times a day. An increase up to one 200 mg PHENYTEK™ three times a day may be made, if necessary.

Once-A-Day Dosage: In adults, if seizure control is established with divided doses of three 100 mg extended phenytoin sodium capsules daily, once-a-day dosage with 300 mg PHENYTEK™ may be considered. Studies comparing divided doses of 300 mg with a single daily dose of this quantity indicated absorption, peak plasma levels, biologic half-life, difference between peak and minimum values, and urinary recovery were equivalent. Once-a-day dosage offers a convenience to the individual patient or to nursing personnel for institutionalized patients and is intended to be used only for patients requiring this amount of drug daily. A major problem in motivating noncompliant patients may also be lessened when the patient can take this drug once a day. However, patients should be cautioned not to miss a dose, inadvertently.

Only extended phenytoin sodium capsules are recommended for once-a-day dosing. Inherent differences in dissolution characteristics and resultant absorption rates of phenytoin due to different manufacturing procedures and/or dosage forms preclude such recommendation for other phenytoin products. When a change in the dosage form or brand is prescribed, careful monitoring of phenytoin serum levels should be carried out.

Loading Dose: Some authorities have advocated use of an oral loading dose of phenytoin in adults who require rapid steady-state serum levels and where intravenous administration is not desirable. This dosing regimen should be reserved for patients in a clinic or hospital setting where phenytoin serum levels can be closely monitored. Patients with a history of renal or liver disease should not receive the oral loading regimen.

Initially, one gram of phenytoin capsules is divided into 3 doses (400 mg, 300 mg, 300 mg) and administered at two-hour intervals. Normal maintenance dosage is then instituted 24 hours after the loading dose, with frequent serum level determinations.

Pediatric Dosage: Initially, 5 mg/kg/day in two or three equally divided doses, with subsequent dosage individualized to a maximum of 300 mg daily. A recommended daily maintenance dosage is usually 4 to 8 mg/kg. Children over 6 years old may require the minimum adult dose (300 mg/day).

HOW SUPPLIED

PHENYTEK™ CAPSULES (extended phenytoin sodium capsules, USP) are available containing 200 mg or 300 mg of phenytoin sodium.

The 200 mg capsule has a dark blue opaque cap and a blue opaque body. The hard-shell gelatin capsule is filled with two white to off-white round, beveled edge tablets. The capsule is rectified radially printed with **BERTEK** over **670** in black ink on both the cap and the body.

They are available as follows:

NDC 62794-670-93
bottles of 30 capsules
NDC 62794-670-01
bottles of 100 capsules

The 300 mg capsule has a blue opaque cap and a blue opaque body. The hard-shell gelatin capsule is filled with three white to off-white round, beveled edge tablets. The capsule is rectified radially printed with **BERTEK** over **750** in black ink on both the cap and the body. They are available as follows:

NDC 62794-750-93
bottles of 30 capsules
NDC 62794-750-01
bottles of 100 capsules

STORE AT CONTROLLED ROOM TEMPERATURE 15° TO 30°C (59° TO 86°F) [See USP].
PROTECT FROM LIGHT AND MOISTURE.

Dispense in a tight, light-resistant container as defined in the USP using a child-resistant closure.

BERTEK PHARMACEUTICALS INC.
Research Triangle Park
NC 27709-4149

REVISED JUNE 2003
BKPHTK:R5

Shown in Product Identification Guide, page 324

SULFAMYLON® CREAM ℞

Brand of MAFENIDE ACETATE CREAM, USP
Topical Antibacterial Agent for Adjunctive Therapy in Second- and Third-Degree Burns

DESCRIPTION

SULFAMYLON Cream is a soft, white, nonstaining, water-miscible, anti-infective cream for topical administration to burn wounds.

SULFAMYLON Cream spreads easily, and can be washed off readily with water. It has a slight acetic odor. Each gram of SULFAMYLON Cream contains mafenide acetate equivalent to 85 mg of the base. The cream vehicle consists of cetyl alcohol, stearyl alcohol, cetyl esters wax, polyoxyl 40 stearate, polyoxyl 8 stearate, glycerin, and water, with methylparaben, propylparaben, sodium metabisulfite, and edetate disodium as preservatives.

Chemically, mafenide acetate is α-Amino-ρ-toluenesulfonamide monoacetate and has the following structural formula:

$H_2NO_2S-C_6H_4-CH_2NH_2 \cdot CH_3COOH$

CLINICAL PHARMACOLOGY

SULFAMYLON Cream, applied topically, produces a marked reduction in the bacterial population present in the avascular tissues of second- and third-degree burns. Reduction in bacterial growth after application of SULFAMYLON Cream has also been reported to permit spontaneous healing of deep partial-thickness burns, and thus prevent conversion of burn wounds from partial thickness to full thickness. It should be noted, however, that delayed eschar separation has occurred in some cases.

Absorption and Metabolism. Applied topically, SULFAMYLON Cream diffuses through devascularized areas, is absorbed, and rapidly converted to a metabolite (ρ-carboxybenzenesulfonamide) which is cleared through the kidneys. SULFAMYLON is active in the presence of pus and serum, and its activity is not altered by changes in the acidity of the environment.

Antibacterial Activity. SULFAMYLON exerts bacteriostatic action against many gram-negative and gram-positive organisms, including *Pseudomonas aeruginosa* and certain strains of anaerobes.

INDICATIONS AND USAGE

SULFAMYLON Cream is a topical agent indicated for adjunctive therapy of patients with second- and third-degree burns.

CONTRAINDICATIONS

SULFAMYLON is contraindicated in patients who are hypersensitive to it. It is not known whether there is cross sensitivity to other sulfonamides.

WARNINGS

Fatal hemolytic anemia with disseminated intravascular coagulation, presumably related to a glucose-6-phosphate dehydrogenase deficiency, has been reported following therapy with SULFAMYLON Cream.

Contains sodium metabisulfite, a sulfite that may cause allergic-type reactions including anaphylactic symptoms and life-threatening or less severe asthmatic episodes in certain susceptible people. The overall prevalence of sulfite sensitivity in the general population is unknown and probably low. Sulfite sensitivity is seen more frequently in asthmatic than in nonasthmatic people.

PRECAUTIONS

SULFAMYLON and its metabolite, ρ-carboxybenzenesulfonamide, inhibit carbonic anhydrase, which may result in metabolic acidosis, usually compensated by hyperventilation. In the presence of impaired renal function, high blood levels of SULFAMYLON and its metabolite may exaggerate the carbonic anhydrase inhibition. Therefore, close monitoring of acid-base balance is necessary, particularly in patients with extensive second-degree or partial thickness burns and in those with pulmonary or renal dysfunction. Some burn patients treated with SULFAMYLON Cream have also been reported to manifest an unexplained syndrome of marked hyperventilation with resulting respiratory alkalosis (slightly alkaline blood pH, low arterial pCO_2, and decreased total CO_2); change in arterial pO_2 is variable. The etiology and significance of these findings are unknown. Mafenide acetate cream should be used with caution in burn patients with acute renal failure.

SULFAMYLON Cream should be administered with caution to patients with history of hypersensitivity to mafenide. It is not known whether there is cross sensitivity to other sulfonamides.

Fungal colonization in and below the eschar may occur concomitantly with reduction of bacterial growth in the burn wound. However, fungal dissemination through the infected burn wound is rare.

Carcinogenesis, Mutagenesis, Impairment of Fertility. No long-term animal studies have been performed to evaluate the drug's potential in these areas.

Pregnancy Category C. Animal reproduction studies have not been conducted with SULFAMYLON. It is also not known whether SULFAMYLON can cause fetal harm when administered to a pregnant woman or can affect reproduction capacity. Therefore, the preparation is not recommended for the treatment of women of childbearing potential, unless the burned area covers more than 20% of the total body surface, or the need for the therapeutic benefit of SULFAMYLON Cream is, in the physician's judgment, greater than the possible risk to the fetus.

Nursing Mothers. It is not known whether mafenide acetate is excreted in human milk. Because many drugs are excreted in human milk and because of the potential for serious adverse reaction in nursing infants from SULFAMYLON, a decision should be made whether to discontinue nursing or to discontinue the drug, taking into account the importance of the drug to the mother.

Pediatric Use. Same as for adults. (See DOSAGE AND ADMINISTRATION.)

ADVERSE REACTIONS

It is frequently difficult to distinguish between an adverse reaction to SULFAMYLON Cream and the effect of a severe burn. A single case of bone marrow depression and a single case of an acute attack of porphyria have been reported following therapy with SULFAMYLON Cream. Fatal hemolytic anemia with disseminated intravascular coagulation, presumably related to a glucose-6-phosphate dehydrogenase deficiency, has been reported following therapy with SULFAMYLON Cream.

Dermatologic: The most frequently reported reaction was pain on application or a burning sensation. Rare occurrences are excoriation of new skin, and bleeding of skin.

Allergic: Rash, itching, facial edema, swelling, hives, blisters, erythema, and eosinophilia.

Respiratory: Tachypnea or hyperventilation, decrease in arterial pCO_2.

Metabolic: Acidosis, increase in serum chloride.

Accidental ingestion of SULFAMYLON Cream has been reported to cause diarrhea.

DOSAGE AND ADMINISTRATION

Prompt institution of appropriate measures for controlling shock and pain is of prime importance. The burn wounds are then cleansed and debrided, and SULFAMYLON Cream is applied with a sterile gloved hand. Satisfactory results can be achieved with application of the cream once or twice daily, to a thickness of approximately 1/16 inch; thicker application is not recommended. The burned areas should be covered with SULFAMYLON Cream at all times. Therefore, whenever necessary, the cream should be reapplied to any areas from which it has been removed (eg, by patient activity). The routine of administration can be accomplished in minimal time, since dressings usually are not required. If individual patient demands make them necessary, however, only a thin layer of dressing should be used.

When feasible, the patient should be bathed daily, to aid in debridement. A whirlpool bath is particularly helpful, but the patient may be bathed in bed or in a shower.

The duration of therapy with SULFAMYLON Cream depends on each patient's requirements. Treatment is usually continued until healing is progressing well or until the burn site is ready for grafting. SULFAMYLON Cream *should not be withdrawn from the therapeutic regimen while there is the possibility of infection.* However, if allergic manifestations occur during treatment with SULFAMYLON Cream, discontinuation of treatment should be considered.

If acidosis occurs and becomes difficult to control, particularly in patients with pulmonary dysfunction, discontinuing therapy with SULFAMYLON Cream for 24 to 48 hours while continuing fluid therapy may aid in restoring acid-base balance.

HOW SUPPLIED

16 ounce Plastic Jar (453.6 g)—NDC 62794-101-54
4 oz. Tube (113.4 g)—NDC 62794-101-51
2 oz. Tube (56.7 g)—NDC 62794-101-50

Continued on next page

Sulfamylon Cream—Cont.

Avoid exposure to excessive heat (temperatures above 104°F or 40°C).
Rx only
BERTEK PHARMACEUTICALS INC.
Research Triangle Park, NC 27709-4149
December 2002
030.1

SULFAMYLON® ℞
(Mafenide Acetate, USP)
FOR 5% TOPICAL SOLUTION
℞ only (sterile)

DESCRIPTION

Mafenide acetate, USP is a synthetic antimicrobial agent designated chemically as α-amino-*p*-toluenesulfonamide monoacetate. It has the following structural formula:

H_2NO_2S–⟨benzene ring⟩–$CH_2NH_2 \cdot CH_3COOH$

$C_7H_{10}N_2O_2S \bullet C_2H_4O_2$
M.W. 246.29

Mafenide acetate, USP is a white, crystalline powder which is freely soluble in water.
SULFAMYLON® For 5% Topical Solution is provided in packets containing 50 g of sterile mafenide acetate to be reconstituted in 1000 mL of Sterile Water for Irrigation, USP or 0.9% Sodium Chloride Irrigation, USP. After mixing, the solution contains 5% w/v of mafenide acetate. The solution is an antimicrobial preparation suitable for topical administration. **The solution is not for injection.** The reconstituted solution may be held up to 28 days after preparation if stored in unopened containers. ONCE A CONTAINER IS OPENED, ANY UNUSED PORTION SHOULD BE DISCARDED AFTER 48 HOURS. Store the reconstituted solution at 20° to 25°C (68° to 77°F). Limited storage periods at 15° to 30°C (59° to 86°F) are acceptable.

CLINICAL PHARMACOLOGY

Mechanism of Action: The mechanism of action of mafenide is not known, but is different from that of the sulfonamides. Mafenide is not antagonized by pABA, serum, pus or tissue exudates, and there is no correlation between bacterial sensitivities to mafenide and to the sulfonamides. Its activity is not altered by changes in the acidity of the environment. The osmolality of the 5% topical solution is approximately 340 mOsm/kg.
Absorption and Metabolism: Applied topically, mafenide acetate diffuses through devascularized areas. Approximately 80% of a mafenide acetate dose is delivered to burned tissue over four hours following topical application of the 5% solution. Following application of mafenide acetate cream and solution, peak mafenide concentrations in human burned skin tissue occur at two and four hours, respectively. Peak tissue concentrations are similar following administration of the solution or cream. Once absorbed, mafenide is rapidly converted to an inactive metabolite (p-carboxybenzenesulfonamide) which is cleared through the kidneys. Clinical studies have shown that when applied topically to burns as an 11.2% mafenide acetate cream, blood levels of the parent drug peaked at 2 hours following application, ranging from 26 to 197 μg/mL for single doses of 14 to 77 g of mafenide acetate. Metabolite levels peaked at 3 hours, ranging from 10 to 340 μg/mL. Twenty-four hours after application, combined parent and metabolite blood levels had fallen to pretreatment levels.
Antimicrobial Activity: Mafenide acetate exerts broad bacteriostatic action against many gram-negative and gram-positive organisms, including *Pseudomonas aeruginosa* and certain strains of anaerobes.
***In Vitro* Cytotoxicity:** Data from *in vitro* studies on cell culture suggests that mafenide acetate may have a deleterious effect on human keratinocytes. The clinical significance of this information is unknown.

INDICATIONS AND USAGE

SULFAMYLON® For 5% Topical Solution is indicated for use as an adjunctive topical antimicrobial agent to control bacterial infection when used under moist dressings over meshed autografts on excised burn wounds.

CONTRAINDICATIONS

SULFAMYLON® For 5% Topical Solution is contraindicated in patients who are hypersensitive to mafenide acetate. It is not known whether there is cross sensitivity to other sulfonamides.

WARNINGS

Fatal hemolytic anemia with disseminated intravascular coagulation, presumably related to a glucose-6-phosphate dehydrogenase deficiency, has been reported following therapy with mafenide acetate.

PRECAUTIONS

General: Mafenide acetate and its metabolite, p-carboxybenzenesulfonamide, inhibit carbonic anhydrase, which may result in metabolic acidosis, usually compensated by hyperventilation. In the presence of impaired renal function, high blood levels of mafenide acetate and its metabolite may exaggerate the carbonic anhydrase inhibition. Therefore, close monitoring of acid-base balance is necessary, particularly in patients with extensive second-degree or partial thickness burns and in those with pulmonary or renal dysfunction. Some burn patients treated with mafenide acetate have also been reported to manifest an unexplained syndrome of masked hyperventilation with resulting respiratory alkalosis (slightly alkaline blood pH, low arterial pCO_2, and decreased total CO_2); change in arterial pO_2 is variable. The etiology and significance of these findings are unknown.
Mafenide acetate should be used with caution in burn patients with acute renal failure.
Fungal colonization may occur concomitantly with reduction of bacterial growth in the burn wound. However, systemic fungal infection through the infected burn wound is rare.
Carcinogenesis, Mutagenesis, Impairment of Fertility: No long-term animal studies have been performed to evaluate the carcinogenic potential of mafenide acetate, however, the drug did not induce mutations in L5178Y mouse lymphoma cells at the TK locus.
Animal studies have not been performed to evaluate the potential effects of mafenide acetate on fertility.
Pregnancy: ***Teratogenic Effects. Pregnancy Category C:*** A teratology study performed in rats using oral doses of up to 600 mg/kg/day revealed no evidence of harm to the fetus due to mafenide acetate. There are no adequate data regarding the potential reproductive toxicity of mafenide acetate in a non-rodent species, nor are there adequate and well-controlled studies in pregnant women. Mafenide acetate should be used during pregnancy only if the potential benefit justifies the potential risk to the fetus.
Nursing Mothers: It is not known whether mafenide acetate is excreted in human milk. Because many drugs are excreted in human milk and because of the potential for serious adverse reactions in nursing infants from mafenide acetate, a decision should be made whether to discontinue nursing or to discontinue the drug, taking into account the importance of the drug to the mother.
Pediatric Use: The safety and effectiveness of SULFAMYLON® For 5% Topical Solution have been established in the age groups 3 months to 16 years.
Geriatric Use: No studies have been conducted to specifically examine the effects of mafenide acetate on burn wounds in geriatric patients.

ADVERSE REACTIONS

In the clinical setting of severe burns, it is often difficult to distinguish between an adverse reaction to mafenide acetate and burn sequelae. In a clinical study of pediatric patients with acute burns requiring autografts who received SULFAMYLON® 5% SOLUTION in addition to double antibiotic solution (DAB) wound therapy (neomycin sulfate 40 mg and polymyxin B 200,000 units/liter), the incidence of rash (4.6%) and itching (2.8%) in the group which received SULFAMYLON® 5% Solution was not different from that experienced with DAB dressings alone (5.7% and 1.3%, respectively).
From other clinical settings, a single case of bone marrow depression and a single case of an acute attack of porphyria have been reported following therapy with mafenide acetate. Fatal hemolytic anemia with disseminated intravascular coagulation, presumably related to a glucose-6-phosphate dehydrogenase deficiency, has been reported following therapy with mafenide acetate. The following adverse reactions have been reported with topical mafenide acetate therapy:
Dermatologic and Allergic: Pain or burning sensation, rash and pruritus (often localized to the area covered by the wound dressing), erythema, skin maceration from prolonged wet dressings, facial edema, swelling, hives, blisters, eosinophilia.
Respiratory or Metabolic: Tachypnea, hyperventilation, decrease in pCO_2, metabolic acidosis, increase in serum chloride.

OVERDOSAGE

Single oral doses of 2000 mg/kg of mafenide acetate as a 5% solution did not cause mortality or clinical symptoms of toxicity in rats.

DOSAGE AND ADMINISTRATION

SULFAMYLON® For 5% Topical Solution: *Directions for Preparation of the Solution:* SULFAMYLON® (mafenide acetate, USP) For 5% Topical Solution is supplied as a sterile powder and is to be reconstituted with Sterile Water for Irrigation, USP or 0.9% Sodium Chloride Irrigation, USP. Aseptic techniques should be observed during preparation of the solution. Pre-measured quantities of 50 g of mafenide acetate powder are provided in sterile packets. The entire quantity of SULFAMYLON® should be emptied into a suitable container which contains 1000 mL of Sterile Water for Irrigation, USP or 0.9% Sodium Chloride Irrigation, USP and mixed until completely dissolved. The reconstituted solution may be held up to 28 days after preparation if stored in unopened containers. ONCE A CONTAINER IS OPENED, ANY UNUSED PORTION SHOULD BE DISCARDED AFTER 48 HOURS. Store the reconstituted solution at 20° to 25°C (68° to 77°F). Limited storage periods at 15° to 30°C (59° to 86°F) are acceptable. **Not for Injection—For Topical Use Only.**

Directions for Use of the Solution: The grafted area should be covered with one layer of fine mesh gauze. An eight-ply burn dressing should be cut to the size of the graft and wetted with SULFAMYLON® 5% SOLUTION using an irrigation syringe and/or irrigation tubing until leaking is noticeable. If irrigation tubing is used, the tubing should be placed over the burn dressing in contact with the wound and covered with a second piece of eight-ply dressing. The irrigation dressing should be secured with a bolster dressing and wrapped as appropriate. The gauze dressing should be kept wet. In clinical studies, this has been accomplished by irrigating with a syringe or injecting the solution into the irrigation tubing every 4 hours or as necessary. If irrigation tubing is not used, the gauze dressing may be moistened every 6–8 hours or as necessary to keep wet.
Wound dressings may be left undisturbed, except for the irrigations, for up to five days. Additional soaks may be initiated until graft take is complete. Maceration of skin may result from wet dressings applied for intervals as short as 24 hours. Treatment is usually continued until autograft vascularization occurs and healing is progressing (typically occurring in about 5 days). Safety and effectiveness have not been established for longer than 5 days for an individual grafting procedure.
If allergic manifestations occur during treatment with SULFAMYLON® 5% SOLUTION, discontinuation of treatment should be considered. If acidosis occurs and becomes difficult to control, particularly in patients with pulmonary dysfunction, discontinuing the soaks with the mafenide acetate solution for 24 to 48 hours may aid in restoring acid-base balance (see PRECAUTIONS section). Dressing changes and monitoring the site for bacterial growth during this interruption should be adjusted accordingly.

HOW SUPPLIED

SULFAMYLON® (mafenide acetate, USP) For 5% Topical Solution is available in packets (NDC 62794-111-17) containing 50 g of sterile mafenide acetate to be prepared using 1000 mL Sterile Water for Irrigation, USP or 0.9% Sodium Chloride Irrigation, USP. (See DOSAGE AND ADMINISTRATION: SULFAMYLON® For 5% Topical Solution: *Directions for Preparation of the Solution.*) The packets are supplied as follows:
Carton of five 50 g packets
NDC 62794-111-98
Recommended Storage:
Packets—Store PACKETS in a dry place at room temperature 15° to 30°C (59° to 86°F).
Prepared Solution—Store SOLUTION at 20° to 25°C (68° to 77°F) with excursions permitted to 15° to 30°C (59° to 86°F). [See USP Controlled Room Temperature.]
The solution may be held for up to 28 days if stored in unopened containers.
ONCE A CONTAINER IS OPENED, ANY UNUSED SOLUTION MUST BE DISCARDED WITHIN 48 HOURS.
Distributed By: Bertek Pharmaceuticals Inc.
Morgantown, WV 26505
BERTEK PHARMACEUTICALS INC.
BKSFMN:R6
REVISED JULY 2001

Nabi® Biopharmaceuticals

5800 PARK OF COMMERCE BLVD., N.W.
BOCA RATON, FL 33487

For Medical Information Contact:
Generally:
Customer Service
(800) 458-4244
561-989-5783
(800) 4-WINRHO (494-6746)
(800) 685-5579 - Medical
FAX: 561-989-5722
In Emergencies:
Customer Service
(800) 458-4244
(800) 4WINRHO (494-6746)
FAX: 561-989-5722

ALOPRIM™ ℞
[al'-ō-prim]
(allopurinol sodium)
for Injection
For Intravenous Infusion Only

DESCRIPTION

ALOPRIM (allopurinol sodium) for Injection is the brand name for allopurinol, a xanthine oxidase inhibitor. ALOPRIM (allopurinol sodium) for Injection is a sterile solution for intravenous infusion only. It is available in vials as the sterile lyophilized sodium salt of allopurinol equivalent to 500 mg of allopurinol. ALOPRIM (allopurinol sodium) for Injection contains no preservatives.
The chemical name for allopurinol sodium is 1,5-dihydro-4*H*-pyrazolo[3,4-*d*]pyrimidin-4-one monosodium salt. It is a white amorphous mass with a molecular weight of 158.09

and molecular formula $C_5H_3N_4NaO$. The structural formula is:

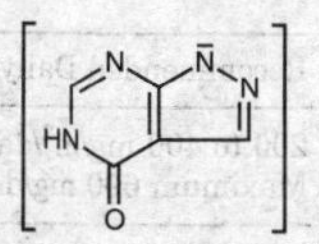

The pKa of allopurinol sodium is 9.31.

CLINICAL PHARMACOLOGY

Allopurinol acts on purine catabolism without disrupting the biosynthesis of purines. It reduces the production of uric acid by inhibiting the biochemical reactions immediately preceding its formation. The degree of this decrease is dose dependent.

Allopurinol is a structural analogue of the natural purine base, hypoxanthine. It is an inhibitor of xanthine oxidase, the enzyme responsible for the conversion of hypoxanthine to xanthine and of xanthine to uric acid, the end product of purine metabolism in man. Allopurinol is metabolized to the corresponding xanthine analogue, oxypurinol (alloxanthine), which also is an inhibitor of xanthine oxidase.

Reutilization of both hypoxanthine and xanthine for nucleotide and nucleic acid synthesis is markedly enhanced when their oxidations are inhibited by allopurinol and oxypurinol. This reutilization does not disrupt normal nucleic acid anabolism, however, because feedback inhibition is an integral part of purine biosynthesis. As a result of xanthine oxidase inhibition, the serum concentration of hypoxanthine plus xanthine in patients receiving allopurinol for treatment of hyperuricemia is usually in the range of 0.3 to 0.4 mg/dL compared to a normal level of approximately 0.15 mg/dL. A maximum of 0.9 mg/dL of these oxypurines has been reported when the serum urate was lowered to less than 2 mg/dL by high doses of allopurinol. These values are far below the saturation levels, at which point their precipitation would be expected to occur (above 7 mg/dL).

The renal clearance of hypoxanthine and xanthine is at least 10 times greater than that of uric acid. The increased xanthine and hypoxanthine in the urine have not been accompanied by problems of nephrolithiasis. There are isolated case reports of xanthine crystalluria in patients who were treated with oral allopurinol.

The action of oral allopurinol differs from that of uricosuric agents, which lower the serum uric acid level by increasing urinary excretion of uric acid. Allopurinol reduces both the serum and urinary uric acid levels by inhibiting the formation of uric acid. The use of allopurinol to block the formation of urates avoids the hazard of increased renal excretion of uric acid posed by uricosuric drugs.

PHARMACOKINETICS: Following intravenous administration in six healthy male and female subjects, allopurinol was rapidly eliminated from the systemic circulation primarily via oxidative metabolism to oxypurinol, with no detectable plasma concentration of allopurinol after 5 hours post dosing. Approximately 12% of the allopurinol intravenous dose was excreted unchanged, 76% excreted as oxypurinol, and the remaining dose excreted as riboside conjugates in the urine. The rapid conversion of allopurinol to oxypurinol was not significantly different after repeated allopurinol dosing. Oxypurinol was present in systemic circulation in much higher concentrations and for a much longer period than allopurinol; thus, it is generally believed that the pharmacological action of allopurinol is mediated via oxypurinol. Oxypurinol was primarily eliminated unchanged in urine by glomerular filtration and tubular reabsorption, with a net renal clearance of about 30 mL/min.

To compare the pharmacokinetics of allopurinol and oxypurinol between intravenous (i.v.) and oral (p.o.) administration of ALOPRIM (allopurinol sodium) for Injection, a well-controlled, four-way crossover study was conducted in 16 male healthy volunteers. ALOPRIM (allopurinol sodium) for Injection was administered via an intravenous infusion over 30 minutes. Pharmacokinetic parameter estimates of allopurinol (mean ± S.D.) following single i.v. and p.o. administration of ALOPRIM (allopurinol sodium) for Injection are summarized as follows:

[See first table above]

Oxypurinol was measurable in the plasma within 10 to 15 minutes following the administration of ALOPRIM (allopurinol sodium) for Injection. Pharmacokinetic parameter estimates of oxypurinol following i.v. and p.o. administration of ALOPRIM (allopurinol sodium) for Injection are shown below:

[See second table above]

In general, the ratio of the area under the plasma concentration vs time curve ($AUC_{0-\infty}$) between oxypurinol and allopurinol was in the magnitude of 30 to 40. The C_{max} and $AUC_{0-\infty}$ for both allopurinol and oxypurinol following i.v. administration of ALOPRIM (allopurinol sodium) for Injection were dose proportional in the dose range of 100 to 300 mg. The half-life of allopurinol and oxypurinol was not influenced by the route of ALOPRIM (allopurinol sodium) for Injection administration. Oral and intravenous administration of ALOPRIM (allopurinol sodium) for Injection at equal doses produced nearly superimposable oxypurinol plasma concentration vs time profiles, and the relative bioavailability of oxypurinol ($F_{relative}$) was approximately 100%. Thus, the pharmacokinetics and plasma profiles of oxypurinol, the major pharmacological component derived from allopurinol, are similar after intravenous and oral administration of ALOPRIM (allopurinol sodium) for Injection.

Administration of ALOPRIM™ (allopurinol sodium) for Injection

Allopurinol Parameters	100 mg i.v.	300 mg i.v.	100 mg p.o.*	300 mg p.o.
C_{max} (μg/mL)	1.58 ± 0.22	5.12 ± 0.82	0.53 ± 0.10	1.35 ± 0.49
T_{max} (hr)	0.50	0.50	1.00 ± 0.39	1.67 ± 0.96
T 1/2 (hr)	1.00 ± 0.46	1.21 ± 0.33	0.98 ± 0.43	1.32 ± 0.32
$AUC_{0\to\infty}$ (hr•μg/mL)	1.99 ± 0.63	7.10 ± 1.28	1.03 ± 0.24	3.69 ± 0.96
CL (mL/min/kg)	12.2 ± 3.11	9.94 ± 2.36		
V_{SS} (L/kg)†	0.84 ± 0.13	0.87 ± 0.13		
$F_{absolute}$ (%)††			48.8 ± 19.7	52.7 ± 13.1

*n=7
†Volume of Distribution (Steady-State)
††Absolute Bioavailability

Administration of ALOPRIM™ (allopurinol sodium) for Injection

Oxypurinol Parameters	100 mg i.v.	300 mg i.v.	100 mg p.o.	300 mg p.o.
C_{max} (μg/mL)	2.20 ± 0.31	6.18 ± 0.78	2.36 ± 0.30	6.36 ± 0.83
T_{max} (hr)	3.89 ±1.41	4.16 ± 1.2	3.10 ± 1.49	4.13 ± 1.35
T 1/2 (hr)	24.1 ± 5.4	23.5 ± 4.5	24.9 ± 8.4	23.7 ± 3.4
$AUC_{0\to\infty}$ (hr•μg/mL)	80 ± 24	231 ± 54	83 ± 22	245 ± 49
$F_{relative}$ (%)*			107 ± 25	108 ± 9

*Relative Bioavailability

Clinical Trials: A compassionate plea trial was conducted from 1977 through 1989 in which 718 evaluable patients with malignancies requiring treatment with cytotoxic chemotherapy, but who were unable to ingest or retain oral medication, received i.v. ALOPRIM (allopurinol sodium) for Injection in the U.S. Of these patients, 411 had established hyperuricemia and 307 had normal serum urate levels at the time that treatment was initiated. Normal serum uric acid levels were achieved in 68% (reduction of serum uric acid was documented in 93%) of the former, and were maintained throughout chemotherapy in 97% of the latter. Because of the study design, it was not possible to assess the impact of the treatment upon the clinical outcome of the patient groups.

INDICATIONS AND USAGE

ALOPRIM (allopurinol sodium) for Injection is indicated for the management of patients with leukemia, lymphoma, and solid tumor malignancies who are receiving cancer therapy which causes elevations of serum and urinary uric acid levels and who cannot tolerate oral therapy.

CONTRAINDICATIONS

Patients who have developed a severe reaction to allopurinol should not be restarted on the drug.

WARNINGS

ALLOPURINOL SHOULD BE DISCONTINUED AT THE FIRST APPEARANCE OF SKIN RASH OR OTHER SIGNS WHICH MAY INDICATE AN ALLERGIC REACTION. In some instances with oral allopurinol, a skin rash may be followed by more severe hypersensitivity reactions such as exfoliative, urticarial, and purpuric lesions as well as Stevens-Johnson syndrome (erythema multiforme exudativum), and/or generalized vasculitis, irreversible hepatotoxicity and, on rare occasions, death.

In patients receiving mercaptopurine or azathioprine, the concomitant administration of 300 to 600 mg of ALOPRIM (allopurinol sodium) for Injection per day will require a reduction in dose to approximately one-third to one-fourth of the usual dose of mercaptopurine or azathioprine. Subsequent adjustment of doses of mercaptopurine or azathioprine should be made on the basis of therapeutic response and the appearance of toxic effects (see PRECAUTIONS: Drug Interactions).

A few cases of reversible clinical hepatotoxicity have been noted in patients taking oral allopurinol, and in some patients asymptomatic rises in serum alkaline phosphatase or serum transaminase have been observed. If anorexia, weight loss, or pruritus develop in patients on allopurinol, evaluation of liver function should be part of their diagnostic workup. In patients with pre-existing liver disease, periodic liver function tests are recommended during the early stages of therapy.

Due to the occasional occurrence of drowsiness, patients should be alerted to the need for due precaution when engaging in activities where alertness is mandatory.

The occurrence of hypersensitivity reactions to allopurinol may be increased in patients with decreased renal function receiving thiazides and allopurinol concurrently. Thus, in patients with decreased renal function, such combinations should be administered with caution.

PRECAUTIONS

General: A fluid intake sufficient to yield a daily urinary output of at least two liters in adults and the maintenance of a neutral or, preferably, slightly alkaline urine are desirable to (1) avoid the theoretical possibility of formation of xanthine calculi under the influence of allopurinol therapy and (2) help prevent renal precipitation of urates in patients receiving concomitant uricosuric agents.

A few patients with pre-existing renal disease or poor urate clearance have shown a rise in BUN during allopurinol administration, although a decrease in BUN has also been observed. In patients with hyperuricemia due to malignancy, the vast majority of changes in renal function are attributable to the underlying malignancy rather than to therapy with allopurinol. Concurrent conditions such as multiple myeloma and congestive myocardial disease were present among those patients whose renal function deteriorated after allopurinol was begun. Renal failure is rarely associated with hypersensitivity reactions to allopurinol.

Patients with decreased renal function do require lower doses of allopurinol. Patients should be carefully observed during the early stages of allopurinol administration so that the dosage can be appropriately adjusted for renal function. In patients with severely impaired renal function or decreased urate clearance, the half-life of oxypurinol in the plasma is greatly prolonged. Patients should be treated with the lowest effective dose, in order to minimize possible side effects. The appropriate dose of ALOPRIM (allopurinol sodium) for Injection for patients with a creatinine clearance ≤10 mL/min is 100 mg per day. For patients with a creatinine clearance between 10 and 20 mL/min, a dose of 200 mg per day is recommended. With extreme renal impairment (creatinine clearance less than 3 mL/min), the interval between doses may also need to be extended.

Bone marrow suppression has been reported in patients receiving allopurinol; however, most of these patients were receiving concomitant medications with the known potential to cause such an effect. The suppression has occurred from as early as 6 weeks to as long as 6 years after the initiation of allopurinol therapy.

Laboratory Tests: The correct dosage and schedule for maintaining the serum uric acid within the normal range is best determined by using the serum uric acid as an index. In patients with pre-existing liver disease, periodic liver function tests are recommended during the early stages of therapy (see WARNINGS).

Allopurinol and its primary active metabolite, oxypurinol, are eliminated by the kidneys; therefore, changes in renal function have a profound effect on dosage. In patients with decreased renal function, or who have concurrent illnesses which can affect renal function such as hypertension and diabetes mellitus, periodic laboratory parameters of renal function, particularly BUN and serum creatinine or creatinine clearance, should be performed and the patient's allopurinol dosage reassessed.

The prothrombin time should be reassessed periodically in the patients receiving dicumarol who are given allopurinol.

Drug Interactions: The following drug interactions were observed in some patients undergoing treatment with oral allopurinol. Although the pattern of use for oral allopurinol includes longer term therapy, particularly for gout and renal calculi, the experience gained may be relevant.

Mercaptopurine/Azathioprine: Allopurinol inhibits the enzymatic oxidation of mercaptopurine and azathioprine to 6-thiouric acid. This oxidation, which is catalyzed by xanthine oxidase, inactivates mercaptopurine. Therefore, the concomitant administration of 300 to 600 mg of oral allopurinol per day will require a reduction in dose to approximately one-third to one-fourth of the usual dose of mercaptopurine or azathioprine. Subsequent adjustment of doses of mercaptopurine or azathioprine should be made on the basis of therapeutic response and the appearance of toxic effects.

Dicumarol: It has been reported that allopurinol prolongs the half-life of the anticoagulant, dicumarol. Consequently, prothrombin time should be reassessed periodically in patients receiving both drugs. The clinical basis of this drug interaction has not been established.

Uricosuric Agents: Since the excretion of oxypurinol is similar to that of urate, uricosuric agents, which increase the excretion of urate, are also likely to increase the excretion of oxypurinol. As a result, the concomitant administration of uricosuric agents decreases the inhibition of xanthine oxidase by oxypurinol and increases the urinary excretion of uric acid.

Thiazide Diuretics: Reports that the concomitant administration of allopurinol and thiazide diuretics contributed to increased allopurinol toxicity were reviewed; a causal mech-

Continued on next page

Aloprim—Cont.

anism or cause-and-effect relationship was not found. Renal function should be monitored in patients on thiazide diuretics and allopurinol (see WARNINGS).

Ampicillin/Amoxicillin: An increase in the frequency of skin rash has been reported among patients receiving ampicillin or amoxicillin concurrently with allopurinol compared to patients who are not receiving both drugs. The cause of this reaction has not been established.

Cytotoxic Agents: Enhanced bone marrow suppression by cyclophosphamide and other cytotoxic agents has been reported among patients with neoplastic disease, except leukemia, in the presence of allopurinol. However, in a well-controlled study of patients with lymphoma on combination therapy, allopurinol did not increase the marrow toxicity of patients treated with cyclophosphamide, doxorubicin, bleomycin, procarbazine, and/or mechlorethamine.

Chlorpropamide: The half-life of chlorpropamide in the plasma may be prolonged by allopurinol, since allopurinol and chlorpropamide may compete for excretion in the renal tubule. The risk of hypoglycemia secondary to this mechanism may be increased if allopurinol and chlorpropamide are given concomitantly in the presence of renal insufficiency.

Cyclosporin: Reports indicate that cyclosporine levels may be increased during concomitant treatment with ALOPRIM (allopurinol sodium) for Injection. Monitoring of cyclosporine levels and possible adjustment of cyclosporine dosage should be considered when these drugs are co-administered.

Drug/Laboratory Test Interactions: Allopurinol is not known to alter the accuracy of laboratory tests.

Carcinogenesis, Mutagenesis and Impairment of Fertility:

Carcinogenesis: Allopurinol was administered at doses up to 20 mg/kg/day to mice and rats for the majority of their life span. No evidence of carcinogenicity was seen in either mice or rats (at doses about 1/6 or 1/3 the recommended human dose on a mg/m^2 basis, respectively).

Mutagenesis: Allopurinol administered intravenously to rats (50 mg/kg) was not incorporated into rapidly replicating intestinal DNA. No evidence of clastogenicity was observed in an in vivo micronucleus test in rats, or in lymphocytes taken from patients treated with allopurinol (mean duration of treatment 40 months), or in an in vitro assay with human lymphocytes.

Impairment of Fertility: Allopurinol oral doses of 20 mg/kg/day had no effect on male or female fertility in rats or rabbits (about 1/3 or 1/2 the human dose on a mg/m^2 basis, respectively).

Pregnancy: *Teratogenic Effects:* Pregnancy Category C. There was no evidence of fetotoxicity or teratogenicity in rats or rabbits treated during the period of organogenesis with oral allopurinol at doses up to 200 mg/kg/day and up to 100 mg/kg/day, respectively (about three times the human dose on a mg/m^2 basis). However, there is a published report in pregnant mice that single intraperitoneal doses of 50 or 100 mg/kg (about 1/3 or 3/4 the human dose on a mg/m^2 basis) of allopurinol on gestation days 10 or 13 produced significant increases in fetal deaths and teratogenic effects (cleft palate, harelip, and digital defects). It is uncertain whether these findings represented a fetal effect or an effect secondary to maternal toxicity. There are, however, no adequate or well-controlled studies in pregnant women. Because animal reproduction studies are not always predictive of human response, this drug should be used during pregnancy only if the potential benefit justifies the potential risk to the fetus.

Experience with allopurinol during human pregnancy has been limited partly because women of reproductive age rarely require treatment with allopurinol. Two unpublished reports and one published paper describe women giving birth to normal offspring after receiving oral allopurinol during pregnancy. There have been no pregnancies reported in patients receiving ALOPRIM (allopurinol sodium) for Injection, but it is assumed that the same risks would apply.

Nursing Mothers: Allopurinol and oxypurinol have been found in the milk of a mother who was receiving allopurinol. Since the effect of allopurinol on the nursing infant is unknown, caution should be exercised when allopurinol is administered to a nursing woman.

Pediatric Use: Clinical data are available on approximately 200 pediatric patients treated with ALOPRIM (allopurinol sodium) for Injection. The efficacy and safety profile observed in this patient population were similar to that observed in adults (see INDICATIONS and DOSAGE AND ADMINISTRATION).

Geriatric Use: Clinical studies of ALOPRIM (allopurinol sodium) for Injection did not include sufficient numbers of patients aged 65 and over to determine whether they respond differently than younger patients. Other reported clinical experience has not identified differences in responses between the elderly and younger patients. In general, dose selection for an elderly patient should be cautious, usually starting at the low end of the dosing range, reflecting the greater frequency of decreased hepatic, renal, or cardiac function, and of concomitant disease or other drug therapy.

ADVERSE REACTIONS

In an uncontrolled, compassionate plea protocol, 125 of 1,378 patients reported a total of 301 adverse reactions while receiving ALOPRIM (allopurinol sodium) for Injection. Most of the patients had advanced malignancies or serious underlying diseases and were taking multiple concomitant medications. Side effects directly attributable to ALOPRIM (allopurinol sodium) for Injection were reported in 19 patients. Fifteen of these adverse experiences were allergic in nature (rash, eosinophilia, local injection site reaction). One adverse experience of severe diarrhea and one incidence of nausea were also reported as being possibly attributable to ALOPRIM (allopurinol sodium) for Injection. Two patients had serious adverse experiences (decreased renal function and generalized seizure) reported as being possibly attributable to ALOPRIM (allopurinol sodium) for Injection.

A listing of the adverse reactions regardless of causality reported from clinical trials follows:

Incidence Greater Than 1%:

Cutaneous/Dermatologic:	rash (1.5%)
Genitourinary:	renal failure/insufficiency (1.2%)
Gastrointestinal:	nausea (1.3%), vomiting (1.2%)

Incidence Less Than 1%:

Body as Whole:	fever, pain, chills, alopecia, infection, sepsis, enlarged abdomen, mucositis/pharyngitis, blast crisis, cellulitis, hypervolemia
Cardiovascular:	heart failure, cardiorespiratory arrest, hypertension, pulmonary embolus, hypotension, decreased venous pressure, flushing, headache, stroke, septic shock, cardiovascular disorder, ECG abnormality, hemorrhage, bradycardia, thrombophlebitis, ventricular fibrillation
Cutaneous/Dermatologic;	urticaria, pruritus, local injection site reaction
Gastrointestinal:	diarrhea, gastrointestinal bleeding, hyperbilirubinemia, splenomegaly, hepatomegaly, intestinal obstruction, jaundice, flatulence, constipation, liver failure, proctitis
Genitourinary:	hematuria, increased creatinine, oliguria, kidney function abnormality, urinary tract infection
Hematologic:	leukopenia, marrow aplasia, thrombocytopenia, eosinophilia, neutropenia, anemia, pancytopenia, ecchymosis, bone marrow suppression, disseminated intravascular coagulation
Metabolic:	hypocalcemia, hyperphosphatemia, hypokalemia, hyperuricemia, electrolyte abnormality, hypercalcemia, hyperglycemia, hypernatremia, hyponatremia, metabolic acidosis, edema, glycosuria, hyperkalemia, lactic acidosis, water intoxication, hypomagnesemia
Neurologic:	seizure, status epilepticus, myoclonus, twitching, agitation, mental status changes, cerebral infarction, coma, dystonia, paralysis, tremor
Pulmonary:	respiratory failure/insufficiency, ARDS, increased respiration rate, apnea
Musculoskeletal:	arthralgia
Other:	hypotonia, diaphoresis, tumor lysis syndrome

The most frequent adverse reaction to oral allopurinol is skin rash. Skin reactions can be severe and sometimes fatal. Therefore, treatment with ALOPRIM (allopurinol sodium) for Injection should be discontinued immediately if a rash develops (see WARNINGS). For further details on hypersensitivity reactions to treatment with oral allopurinol, refer to the package insert for allopurinol tablets.

OVERDOSAGE

Massive overdosing or acute poisoning by ALOPRIM (allopurinol sodium) for Injection has not been reported.

In mice, the minimal lethal dose is 45 mg/kg given intravenously or 500 mg/kg orally (about 1/3 or 4 times the usual human dose on a mg/m^2 basis). Hypoactivity was observed with these doses. In rats, the minimum lethal dose is 100 mg/kg i.v., and 5000 mg/kg orally (about 1.5 and 75 times the usual human dose on a mg/m^2 basis).

In the management of overdosage, there is no specific antidote for ALOPRIM (allopurinol sodium) for Injection. There has been no clinical experience in the management of a patient who has taken massive amounts of allopurinol.

Both allopurinol and oxypurinol are dialyzable; however, the usefulness of hemodialysis or peritoneal dialysis in the management of an overdose of ALOPRIM (allopurinol sodium) for Injection is unknown.

DOSAGE AND ADMINISTRATION

Children and Adults: The dosage of ALOPRIM (allopurinol sodium) for Injection to lower serum uric acid to normal or near-normal varies with the severity of the disease. The amount and frequency of dosage for maintaining the serum uric acid just within the normal range is best determined by using the serum uric acid level as an index. In adults, in one clinical trial, doses over 600 mg a day did not appear to be more effective. The recommended daily dose of ALOPRIM (allopurinol sodium) for Injection is as follows:

	Recommended Daily Dose
Adult:	200 to 400 mg/m^2/day Maximum 600 mg/day
Child:	Starting Dose 200 mg/m^2/day

Hydration: A fluid intake sufficient to yield a daily urinary output of at least two liters in adults and the maintenance of a neutral or, preferably, slightly alkaline urine are desirable.

Impaired Renal Function: The dose of ALOPRIM (allopurinol sodium) for Injection should be reduced in patients with impaired renal function to avoid accumulation of allopurinol and its metabolites:

Creatinine Clearance	Recommended Daily Dose
10 to 20 mL/min	200 mg/day
3 to 10 mL/min	100 mg/day
<3 mL/min	100 mg/day at extended intervals

Administration: In both adults and children, the daily dose can be given as single infusion or in equally divided infusions at 6-, 8-, or 12- hour intervals at the recommended final concentration of not greater than 6 mg/mL (see Preparation of Solution). The rate of infusion depends on the volume of infusate. Whenever possible, therapy with ALOPRIM (allopurinol sodium) for Injection should be initiated 24 to 48 hours before the start of chemotherapy known to cause tumor cell lysis (including adrenocortico steroids).

ALOPRIM (allopurinol sodium) for Injection should not be mixed with or administered through the same intravenous port with agents which are incompatible in solution with ALOPRIM (allopurinol sodium) for Injection (see Preparation of Solution).

Preparation of Solution: ALOPRIM (allopurinol sodium) for Injection must be reconstituted and diluted. The contents of each 30 mL vial should be dissolved with 25 mL of Sterile Water for Injection. Reconstitution yields a clear, almost colorless solution with no more than a slight opalescence. This concentrated solution has a pH of 11.1 to 11.8. It should be diluted to the desired concentration with 0.9% Sodium Chloride Injection or 5% Dextrose for Injection. Sodium bicarbonate-containing solutions should not be used. A final concentration of no greater than 6 mg/mL is recommended. The solution should be stored at 20° to 25°C (68° to 77°F) and administration should begin within 10 hours after reconstitution. Do not refrigerate the reconstituted and/or diluted product.

Parenteral drug products should be inspected visually for particulate matter and discoloration prior to administration, whenever solution and container permit. Do not use this product if particulate matter or discoloration is present. The following table lists drugs that are physically incompatible in solution with ALOPRIM (allopurinol sodium) for Injection.

Drugs That are Physically Incompatible in Solution with ALOPRIM™ (allopurinol solution) for Injection

Amikacin sulfate	Hydroxyzine HCl
Amphoterecin B	Idarubicin HCl
Carmustine	Imipenem-cilastatin sodium
Cefotaxime sodium	Mechlorethamine HCl
Chlorpromazine HCl	Meperidine HCl
Cimetidine HCl	Metoclopramide HCl
Clindamycin phosphate	Methylprednisolone sodium succinate
Cytarabine	Minocycline HCl
Dacarbazine	Nalbuphine HCl
Daunorubicin HCl	Netilmicin sulfate
Diphenhydramine HCl	Ondansetron HCl
Doxorubicin HCl	Prochlorperazine edisylate
Doxycycline hyclate	Promethazine HCl
Droperidol	Sodium bicarbonate
Floxuridine	Streptozocin
Gentamicin sulfate	Tobramycin sulfate
Haloperidol lactate	Vinorelbine tartrate

HOW SUPPLIED

STERILE SINGLE USE VIAL FOR INTRAVENOUS INFUSION.

ALOPRIM (allopurinol sodium) for Injection, 30 mL flint glass vials with rubber stoppers each containing allopurinol sodium equivalent to 500 mg of allopurinol (white lyophilized powder), box of 1 (NDC 59730-5601-1). Store unreconstituted powder at 25°C (77°F); excursions permitted to 15°–30°C (59°–86°F) [see USP controlled room temperature].

Distributed by:
Nabi Biopharmaceuticals
Boca Raton, FL 33487
Toll Free: 1-800-327-7106
Manufactured by:
DSM Pharmaceuticals, Inc.
Greenville, NC 27834
February 2003 650374

Shown in Product Identification Guide, page 324

PHOSLO® Tablets ℞

[*phos "lō '*]

(Calcium Acetate)

PHOSLO® GelCaps

(Calcium Acetate)

DESCRIPTION

Tablets: Each white round tablet (stamped "BRA200") contains 667 mg of calcium acetate, USP (anhydrous; $Ca(CH_3COO)_2$; MW=158.17 grams) equal to 169 mg (8.45 mEq) calcium, and 10 mg of the inert binder, polyethylene glycol 8000 NF.

PhosLo Tablets (calcium acetate) are administered orally for the control of hyperphosphatemia in end stage renal failure.

Gelcaps: Each opaque gelcap with a blue cap and white body is spin printed in blue and white ink with "PhosLo®" printed on the cap and "667 mg" printed on the body. Each gelcap contains 667 mg calcium acetate, USP (anhydrous; $Ca(CH_3COO)_2$; MW=158.17 grams) equal to 169 mg (8.45 mEq) calcium, and 10 mg of the inert binder, polyethylene glycol 8000 NF. The gelatin cap and body have the following inactive ingredients: FD&C blue #1, D&C red #28, titanium dioxide, USP and gelatin, USP.

PhosLo Gelcaps (calcium acetate) are administered orally for the control of hyperphosphatemia in end stage renal failure.

CLINICAL PHARMACOLOGY

Patients with advanced renal insufficiency (creatinine clearance less than 30 ml/min) exhibit phosphate retention and some degree of hyperphosphatemia. The retention of phosphate plays a pivotal role in causing secondary hyperparathyroidism associated with osteodystrophy, and soft-tissue calcification. The mechanism by which phosphate retention leads to hyperparathyroidism is not clearly delineated. Therapeutic efforts directed toward the control of hyperphosphatemia include reduction in the dietary intake of phosphate, inhibition of absorption of phosphate in the intestine with phosphate binders, and removal of phosphate from the body by more efficient methods of dialysis. The rate of removal of phosphate by dietary manipulation or by dialysis is insufficient. Dialysis patients absorb 40% to 80% of dietary phosphorus. Therefore, the fraction of dietary phosphate absorbed from the diet needs to be reduced by using phosphate binders in most renal failure patients on maintenance dialysis. Calcium acetate (PhosLo) when taken with meals combines with dietary phosphate to form insoluble calcium phosphate which is excreted in the feces. Maintenance of serum phosphorus below 6.0 mg/dl is generally considered as a clinically acceptable outcome of treatment with phosphate binders. PhosLo is highly soluble at neutral pH, making the calcium readily available for binding to phosphate in the proximal small intestine.

Orally administered calcium acetate from pharmaceutical dosage forms has been demonstrated to be systemically absorbed up to approximately 40% under fasting conditions and up to approximately 30% under nonfasting conditions. This range represents data from both healthy subjects and renal dialysis patients under various conditions.

INDICATIONS AND USAGE

PhosLo is indicated for the control of hyperphosphatemia in end stage renal failure and does not promote aluminum absorption.

CONTRAINDICATIONS

Patients with hypercalcemia.

WARNINGS

Patients with end stage renal failure may develop hypercalcemia when given calcium with meals. No other calcium supplements should be given concurrently with PhosLo.

Progressive hypercalcemia due to overdose of PhosLo may be severe as to require emergency measures. Chronic hypercalcemia may lead to vascular calcification, and other soft-tissue calcification. The serum calcium level should be monitored twice weekly during the early dose adjustment period. **The serum calcium times phosphate (CaXP) product should not be allowed to exceed 66.** Radiographic evaluation of suspect anatomical region may be helpful in early detection of soft-tissue calcification.

PRECAUTIONS

General: Excessive dosage of PhosLo induces hypercalcemia; therefore, early in the treatment during dosage adjustment serum calcium should be determined twice weekly. Should hypercalcemia develop, the dosage should be reduced or the treatment discontinued immediately depending on the severity of hypercalcemia. PhosLo should not be given to patients on digitalis, because hypercalcemia may precipitate cardiac arrhythmias. PhosLo therapy should always be started at low dose and should not be increased without careful monitoring of serum calcium. An estimate of daily dietary calcium intake should be made initially and the intake adjusted as needed. Serum phosphorus should also be determined periodically.

Information for the patient: The patient should be informed about compliance with dosage instructions, adherence to instructions about diet and avoidance of the use of nonprescription antacids. Patients should be informed about the symptoms of hypercalcemia (See ADVERSE REACTIONS section).

Drug Interactions: PhosLo may decrease the bioavailability of tetracyclines.

Carcinogenesis, Mutagenesis, Impairment of Fertility: Long term animal studies have not been performed to evaluate the carcinogenic potential, mutagenicity, or effect on fertility of PhosLo.

Pregnancy: Teratogenic Effects: Category C. Animal reproduction studies have not been conducted with PhosLo. It is also not known whether PhosLo can cause fetal harm when administered to a pregnant woman or can affect reproduction capacity. PhosLo should be given to a pregnant woman only if clearly needed.

Pediatric Use: Safety and effectiveness in pediatric patients have not been established.

Geriatric Use: Of the total number of subjects in clinical studies of PhosLo (n=91), 25 percent were 65 and over, while 7 percent were 75 and over. No overall differences in safety or effectiveness were observed between these subjects and younger subjects, and other reported clinical experience has not identified differences in responses between the elderly and younger patients, but greater sensitivity of some older individuals cannot be ruled out.

ADVERSE REACTIONS

In clinical studies, patients have occasionally experienced nausea during PhosLo therapy. Hypercalcemia may occur during treatment with PhosLo. Mild hypercalcemia (Ca> 10.5mg/dl) may be asymptomatic or manifest itself as constipation, anorexia, nausea and vomiting. More severe hypercalcemia (Ca> 12mg/dl) is associated with confusion, delirium, stupor and coma. Mild hypercalcemia is easily controlled by reducing the PhosLo dose or temporarily discontinuing therapy. Severe hypercalcemia can be treated by acute hemodialysis and discontinuing PhosLo therapy. Decreasing dialysate calcium concentration could reduce the incidence and severity of PhosLo induced hypercalcemia. The long-term effect of PhosLo on the progression of vascular or soft-tissue calcification has not been determined.

Isolated cases of pruritus have been reported which may represent allergic reactions.

OVERDOSAGE

Administration of PhosLo in excess of the appropriate daily dosage can cause severe hypercalcemia (See ADVERSE REACTIONS section).

DOSAGE AND ADMINISTRATION

Tablets: The recommended initial dose of PhosLo for the adult dialysis patient is 2 tablets with each meal. The dosage may be increased gradually to bring the serum value below 6 mg/dl, as long as hypercalcemia does not develop. Most patients require 3–4 tablets with each meal.

Gelcaps: The recommended initial dose of PhosLo for the adult dialysis patient is 2 gelcaps with each meal. The dosage may be increased gradually to bring the serum phosphate value below 6 mg/dl, as long as hypercalcemia does not develop. Most patients require 3–4 gelcaps with each meal.

HOW SUPPLIED

Tablets: In tablet form for oral administration. Each white round tablet contains 667 mg of calcium acetate (anhydrous $Ca(CH_3COO)_2$; MW=158.17 grams) equal to 169 mg (8.45 mEq) calcium, and 10 mg of the inert binder, polyethylene glycol 8000 NF.

Gelcaps: A white and blue gelcap for oral administration containing 667 mg calcium acetate (anhydrous $Ca(CH_3COO)_2$; MW=158.17 grams) equal to 169 mg (8.45 mEq) calcium.

Tablets NDC 59730-6401-01
Gelcaps NDC 59730-6402-01

STORAGE

Store at 25°C (77°F); excursions permitted to 15–30°C (59–86°F). See USP "Controlled Room Temperature".

Rx only

Manufactured for Nabi Biopharmaceuticals
Nabi® Biopharmaceuticals
5800 PARK OF COMMERCE BLVD., N.W.
BOCA RATON, FL 33487

8/03

Shown in Product Identification Guide, page 324

HEPATITIS B IMMUNE GLOBULIN (HUMAN) ℞
NABI-HB®

Solvent/Detergent Treated and Filtered

DESCRIPTION

Hepatitis B Immune Globulin (Human), Nabi-HB, is a sterile solution of immunoglobulin (5 ± 1% protein) containing antibodies to hepatitis B surface antigen (anti-HBs). It is prepared from plasma donated by individuals with high titers of anti-HBs. The plasma is processed using a modified Cohn 6 / Oncley 9 cold-alcohol fractionation process[1,2] with two added viral reduction steps described below. Nabi-HB is formulated in 0.075 M sodium chloride, 0.15 M glycine, and 0.01% polysorbate 80, at pH 6.2. The product is supplied as a nonturbid sterile liquid in single dose vials and appears as clear to opalescent. It contains no preservative and is intended for single use by the intramuscular route only.

The manufacturing steps for Nabi-HB are designed to reduce the risk of transmission of viral disease. The solvent/detergent treatment step, using tri-*n*-butyl phosphate and Triton® X-100, is effective in inactivating known enveloped viruses such as hepatitis B virus (HBV), hepatitis C virus (HCV), and human immunodeficiency virus (HIV) [3]. Virus filtration, using a Planova® 35 nm Virus Filter, is effective in reducing some known enveloped and non-enveloped viruses[4]. The inactivation and reduction of known enveloped and non-enveloped model viruses were validated in laboratory studies as summarized in the following table:

[See table 1 at top of next page]

Product potency is expressed in international units (IU) by comparison to the World Health Organization (WHO) standard. Each milliliter (mL) of product contains greater than 312 IU anti-HBs. The potency of each milliliter of Nabi-HB exceeds the potency of anti-HBs in a U.S. reference hepatitis B immune globulin (FDA). The U.S. reference has been tested by Nabi® Biopharmaceuticals against the WHO standard and found to be equal to 208 IU/mL.

CLINICAL PHARMACOLOGY

Hepatitis B Immune Globulin (Human) products provide passive immunization for individuals exposed to the hepatitis B virus as evidenced by a reduction in the attack rate of hepatitis B following use[6-9].

Clinical studies[10,11] conducted prior to 1983 with hepatitis B immune globulins similar to Nabi-HB indicate the advantage of simultaneous administration of hepatitis B vaccine and Hepatitis B Immune Globulin (Human). The Centers for Disease Control and Prevention Advisory Committee on Immunization Practices (ACIP) advises that the combination prophylaxis be provided in certain instances of exposure based upon the increased efficacy found with that regimen in neonates[12]. Cases of hepatitis B are rarely seen following exposure to HBV in persons with preexisting anti-HBs. However, no prospective studies have been performed on the efficacy of concurrent hepatitis B vaccine and Hepatitis B Immune Globulin (Human) administration following parenteral exposure, mucous membrane contact, or oral ingestion in adults.

Infants born to HBsAg-positive mothers are at risk of being infected with HBV and becoming chronic carriers[13]. The risk is especially great if the mother is also HBeAg-positive[14]. Studies conducted with hepatitis B immune globulins similar to Nabi-HB indicated that for an infant with perinatal exposure to an HBsAg-positive and HBeAg-positive mother, a regimen combining one dose of Hepatitis B Immune Globulin (Human) at birth with the hepatitis B vaccine series started soon after birth is 85-98% effective in preventing development of the HBV carrier state[15-17]. Regimens involving either multiple doses of Hepatitis B Immune Globulin (Human) alone or the vaccine series alone have a 70-90% efficacy, while a single dose of Hepatitis B Immune Globulin (Human) alone has 50% efficacy[18].

Since infants have close contact with primary caregivers and they have a higher risk of becoming HBV carriers after acute HBV infection, prophylaxis of an infant less than 12 months of age with Hepatitis B Immune Globulin (Human) and hepatitis B vaccine is indicated if the mother or primary caregiver has acute HBV infection[19].

Sexual partners of HBsAg-positive persons are at increased risk of acquiring HBV infection. A single dose of Hepatitis B Immune Globulin (Human) is 75% effective if administered within two weeks of the last sexual exposure to a person with acute hepatitis B[19].

Pharmacokinetics

Pharmacokinetics trials[20] of Nabi-HB, Hepatitis B Immune Globulin (Human), given intramuscularly to 50 healthy volunteers demonstrated pharmacokinetic parameters similar to those reported by Scheiermann and Kuwert[21]. The half-life for Nabi-HB was 23.1 ± 5.5 days. The clearance rate was 0.35 ± 0.12 L/day and the volume of distribution was 11.2 ± 3.4 L.

Maximum concentration of Nabi-HB was reached in 6.5 ± 4.3 days. The maximum concentration of anti-HBs and the area under the time-concentration curve achieved by Nabi-HB were bioequivalent to that of another licensed Hepatitis B Immune Globulin (Human) when compared in the same pharmacokinetics trial. Comparability of pharmacokinetics between Nabi-HB and a commercially available hepatitis B immunoglobulin indicate that similar efficacy of Nabi-HB should be inferred.

INDICATIONS AND USAGE

Nabi-HB, Hepatitis B Immune Globulin (Human), is indicated for treatment of acute exposure to blood containing

Continued on next page

Nabi-HB—Cont.

HBsAg, perinatal exposure of infants born to HBsAg-positive mothers, sexual exposure to HBsAg-positive persons and household exposure to persons with acute HBV infection in the following settings:

- Acute Exposure to Blood Containing HBsAg
  Following either parenteral exposure (needlestick, bite, sharps), direct mucous membrane contact (accidental splash), or oral ingestion (pipetting accident), involving HBsAg-positive materials such as blood, plasma, or serum.
- Perinatal Exposure of Infants Born to HBsAg-positive Mothers
  Infants born to mothers positive for HBsAg with or without HBeAg[12].
- Sexual Exposure to HBsAg-positive Persons
  Sexual partners of HBsAg-positive persons.
- Household Exposure to Persons with Acute HBV Infection
  Infants less than 12 months old whose mother or primary caregiver is positive for HBsAg. Other household contacts with an identifiable blood exposure to the index patient.

Nabi-HB is indicated for intramuscular use only.

CONTRAINDICATIONS

Individuals known to have had an anaphylactic or severe systemic reaction to human globulin should not receive Nabi-HB, Hepatitis B Immune Globulin (Human), or any other human immune globulin. Nabi-HB contains less than 100 micrograms per mL IgA. Individuals who are deficient in IgA may have the potential to develop IgA antibodies and have an anaphylactoid reaction. The physician must weigh the potential benefit of treatment with Nabi-HB against the potential for hypersensitivity reactions.

WARNINGS

In patients who have severe thrombocytopenia or any coagulation disorder that would contraindicate intramuscular injections, Nabi-HB, Hepatitis B Immune Globulin (Human), should be given only if the expected benefits outweigh the potential risks.

Nabi-HB is made from human plasma. Products made from human plasma may contain infectious agents, e.g., viruses, and theoretically, the Creutzfeldt-Jakob disease (CJD) agent. The risk that such products can transmit an infectious agent has been reduced by screening plasma donors for prior exposure to certain viruses, by testing for the presence of certain current viral infections, and by inactivating and/or reducing certain viruses. The Nabi-HB manufacturing process includes a solvent/detergent treatment step (using tri-*n*-butyl phosphate and Triton® X-100) that is effective in inactivating known enveloped viruses such as HBV, HCV, and HIV. Nabi-HB is filtered using a Planova® 35 nm Virus Filter that is effective in reducing the levels of some enveloped and non-enveloped viruses. These two processes are designed to increase product safety. Despite these measures, such products can still potentially transmit disease. There is also the possibility that unknown infectious agents may be present in such products. ALL infections thought by a physician possibly to have been transmitted by this product should be reported by the physician or other health care provider to Nabi® Biopharmaceuticals at 1-800-458-4244. The physician should discuss the risks and benefits of this product with the patient.

PRECAUTIONS

General

Nabi-HB, Hepatitis B Immune Globulin (Human), must be administered only intramuscularly for post-exposure prophylaxis. The preferred sites for intramuscular injections are the anterolateral aspect of the upper thigh and the deltoid muscle. If the buttock is used due to the volume to be injected, the central region should be avoided; only the upper, outer quadrant should be used, and the needle should be directed anterior (i.e., not inferior or perpendicular to the skin) to minimize the possibility of involvement with the sciatic nerve[22].

The 50 healthy volunteers who received Nabi-HB in pharmacokinetic studies were followed for 84 days for possible development of anti-HCV antibodies. No subject seroconverted.

Drug Interactions

Vaccination with live virus vaccines should be deferred until approximately three months after administration of Nabi-HB, Hepatitis B Immune Globulin (Human). It may be necessary to revaccinate persons who received Nabi-HB shortly after live virus vaccination.

There are no available data on concomitant use of Nabi-HB and other drugs; therefore, Nabi-HB should not be mixed with other drugs.

Pregnancy Category C

Animal reproduction studies have not been conducted with Nabi-HB. It is also not known whether Nabi-HB can cause fetal harm when administered to a pregnant woman or can affect a woman's ability to conceive. Nabi-HB should be given to a pregnant woman only if clearly indicated.

Nursing Mothers

It is not known whether this drug is excreted in human milk. Because many drugs are excreted in human milk, caution should be exercised when Nabi-HB is administered to a nursing mother.

Table 1 Log Reduction of Test Viruses[5]

			Test Virus		
	HIV	BVD	PRV	EMC	PPV
Model Virus:	HIV	HCV	HBV	Hepatitis A	PVB19
Envelope/Genome:	yes/RNA	yes/RNA	yes/DNA	no/RNA	no/DNA
Manufacturing Step					
Precipitation of Cohn Fraction III	> 5.9	3.6	3.7	4.4	3.9
Cuno Filtration	NT	NT	NT	> 6.6	5.4
Solvent/Detergent	> 4.2	> 6.9	> 6.4	NT	NT
Nanofiltration	> 7.4	> 6.9	> 5.7	3.0	0.7*
Cumulative	> 17.5	> 17.4	> 15.8	> 14.0	9.3

BVD = Bovine Viral Diarrhea Virus
EMC = Encephalomyocarditis Virus
HIV = Human Immunodeficiency Virus
PVB19 = Parvovirus B19
PPV = Porcine Parvovirus
PRV = Pseudorabies Virus
NT = not tested
* Value not included in cumulative clearance

Table 2 Recommendations for Hepatitis B Prophylaxis Following Percutaneous or Permucosal Exposure[12]

	Exposed Person	
Source	Unvaccinated	Vaccinated
HBsAg-positive	1. Hepatitis B Immune Globulin (Human) X 1 immediately* 2. Initiate HB vaccine series†	1. Test exposed person for anti-HBs 2. If inadequate antibody‡, Hepatitis B Immune Globulin (Human) X 1 immediately plus either HB vaccine booster dose or second dose of Hepatitis B Immune Globulin (Human) one month later§
Known Source - High Risk for HBsAg-positive	1. Initiate HB vaccine series 2. Test source for HBsAg. If positive, Hepatitis B Immune Globulin (Human) X 1	1. Test source for HBsAg only if exposed is vaccine nonresponder; if source is HBsAg-positive, give Hepatitis B Immune Globulin (Human) X 1 immediately plus either HB vaccine booster dose or second dose of Hepatitis B Immune Globulin (Human) one month later§
Known Source - Low Risk for HBsAg-positive	Initiate HB vaccine series	Nothing required
Unknown Source	Initiate HB vaccine series	Nothing required

* Hepatitis B Immune Globulin (Human) dose of 0.06 mL/kg IM.
† See manufacturers' recommendation for appropriate dose.
‡ Less than 10 mIU/mL anti-HBs by radioimmunoassay, negative by enzyme immunoassay.
§ Two doses of Hepatitis B Immune Globulin (Human) is preferred if no response after at least four doses of vaccine.

Pediatric Use

Safety and effectiveness in the pediatric population have not been established for Nabi-HB. However, the safety and effectiveness of similar hepatitis B immune globulins have been demonstrated in infants and children[12].

Geriatric Use

Clinical studies of Nabi-HB did not include sufficient numbers of subjects aged 65 and over to determine whether they respond differently than younger subjects. Other reported clinical experience has not identified differences in responses between the elderly and younger patients.

ADVERSE REACTIONS

Fifty male and female volunteers received Nabi-HB, Hepatitis B Immune Globulin (Human), intramuscularly in pharmacokinetics trials[20]. The number of patients with reactions related to the administration of Nabi-HB included local reactions such as erythema 6 (12%) and ache 2 (4%) at the injection site, as well as systemic reactions such as headache 7 (14%), myalgia 5 (10%), malaise 3 (6%), nausea 2 (4%), and vomiting 1 (2%). The majority (92%) of reactions were reported as mild. The following adverse events were reported in the pharmacokinetics trials and were considered probably related to Nabi-HB: elevated alkaline phosphatase 2 (4%), ecchymosis 1 (2%), joint stiffness 1 (2%), elevated AST 1 (2%), decreased WBC 1 (2%), and elevated creatinine 1 (2%). All adverse events were mild in intensity. There were no serious adverse events.

No anaphylactic reactions with Nabi-HB have been reported. However, these reactions, although rare, have been reported following the injection of human immune globulins[23].

OVERDOSAGE

Although no data are available, clinical experience reported with other human immune globulins suggests that the only manifestations of overdose with Nabi-HB, Hepatitis B Immune Globulin (Human), would be pain and tenderness at the injection site.

DOSAGE AND ADMINISTRATION

This product is for intramuscular use only. The use of this product by the intravenous route is not indicated. Parenteral drug products should be inspected visually for particulate matter and discoloration prior to administration.

It is important to use a separate vial, sterile syringe, and needle for each individual patient, in order to prevent transmission of infectious agents from one person to another. **Any vial of Nabi-HB, Hepatitis B Immune Globulin (Human) that has been entered should be used promptly. Do not reuse or save for future use. This product contains no preservative; therefore, partially used vials should be discarded immediately.**

Hepatitis B Immune Globulin (Human) may be administered at the same time (but at a different site), or up to one month preceding hepatitis B vaccination without impairing the active immune response to hepatitis B vaccine[11].

- Acute Exposure to Blood Containing HBsAg
  Table 2 summarizes prophylaxis for percutaneous (needlestick, bite, sharps), ocular, or mucous membrane exposure to blood according to the source of exposure and vaccination status of the exposed person. For greatest effectiveness, passive prophylaxis with Hepatitis B Immune Globulin (Human) should be given as soon as possible after exposure, as its value after seven days following exposure is unclear[12]. An injection of 0.06 mL/kg of body weight should be administered intramuscularly as soon as possible after exposure and within 24 hours, if possible. Consult the hepatitis B vaccine package insert for dosage information regarding the vaccine.
  For persons who refuse hepatitis B vaccine or are known non-responders to vaccine, a second dose of Hepatitis B Immune Globulin (Human) should be given one month after the first dose[12].
  [See table 2 above]
- Prophylaxis of Infants Born to Mothers who are Positive for HBsAg with or without HBeAg
  Table 3 contains the recommended schedule of hepatitis B prophylaxis for infants born to mothers that are either known to be positive for HBsAg or have not been screened. Infants born to mothers known to be HBsAg-positive should receive 0.5 mL Hepatitis B Immune Globulin (Human) after physiologic stabilization of the infant and preferably within 12 hours of birth. The hepatitis B vaccine series should be initiated simultaneously, if not contraindicated, with the first dose of the vaccine given concurrently with the Hepatitis B Immune Globulin (Human), but at a different site. Subsequent doses of the vaccine should be administered in accordance with the recommendations of the manufacturer.
  Women admitted for delivery, who were not screened for HBsAg during the prenatal period, should be tested. While test results are pending, the newborn infant should receive hepatitis B vaccine within 12 hours of birth (see manufacturers' recommendations for dose). If the mother is later found to be HBsAg-positive, the infant should receive 0.5 mL Hepatitis B Immune Globulin (Human) as soon as possible and within seven days of birth; however, the efficacy of Hepatitis B Immune Globulin (Human) ad-

ministered after 48 hours of age is not known[10,19]. Testing for HBsAg and anti-HBs is recommended at 12-15 months of age. If HBsAg is not detectable and anti-HBs is present, the child has been protected[12].

Table 3 Recommended Schedule of Hepatitis B Immunoprophylaxis to Prevent Perinatal Transmission of Hepatitis B Virus Infection [19]

	Age of Infant	
Administer	Infant Born to mother known to be HBsAg-positive	Infant born to mother not screened for HBsAg
First Vaccination*	Birth (within 12 hours)	Birth (within 12 hours)
Hepatitis B Immune Globulin (Human)†	Birth (within 12 hours)	If mother is found to be HBsAg-positive, administer dose to infant as soon as possible, not later than 1 week after birth
Second Vaccination*	1 month	1-2 months
Third Vaccination*	6 months‡	6 months‡

* See manufacturers' recommendations for appropriate dose.
† 0.5 mL administered IM at a site different from that used for the vaccine.
‡ See ACIP recommendation.

- Sexual Exposure to HBsAg-positive Persons
All susceptible persons whose sexual partners have acute hepatitis B infection should receive a single dose of Hepatitis B Immune Globulin (Human) (0.06 mL/kg) and should begin the hepatitis B vaccine series, if not contraindicated, within 14 days of the last sexual contact or if sexual contact with the infected person will continue. Administering the vaccine with Hepatitis B Immune Globulin (Human) may improve the efficacy of post exposure treatment. The vaccine has the added advantage of conferring long-lasting protection[19].
- Household Exposure to Persons with Acute HBV Infection
Prophylaxis of an infant less than 12 months of age with 0.5 mL Hepatitis B Immune Globulin (Human) and hepatitis B vaccine is indicated if the mother or primary caregiver has acute HBV infection. Prophylaxis of other household contacts of persons with acute HBV infection is not indicated unless they had an identifiable blood exposure to the index patient, such as by sharing toothbrushes or razors. Such exposures should be treated like sexual exposures. If the index patient becomes an HBV carrier, all household contacts should receive hepatitis B vaccine[19].

HOW SUPPLIED

Nabi-HB, Hepatitis B Immune Globulin (Human), is supplied as:

NDC Number	Contents
59730-4202-1 59730-4204-1	a carton containing a 1 mL dose in a single-use vial (>312 IU) and package insert
59730-4203-1 59730-4205-1	a carton containing a 5 mL dose in a single-use vial (>1560 IU) and package insert

STORAGE

Refrigerate between 2 to 8 °C (36 to 46 °F). Do not freeze. Do not use after expiration date. Use within 6 hours after the vial has been entered.

REFERENCES

1. Cohn E.J., Strong W.L., Mulford D.J., Ashworth J.N., Melin M., Taylor H.L. Preparation and Properties of Serum and Plasma Proteins IV. A system for the separation into fractions of the protein and lipoprotein components of biological tissues and fluids. *J Am Chem Soc* 1946, 68: 459-475.
2. Oncley J.L, Melin M, Richert D.A, Cameron J. W, Gross P.M. The separation of antibodies, isoagglutinins, prothrombin, plasminogen and b1-lipoproteins into subfractions of human plasma. *J Am Chem Soc* 1949, 71: 541-550.
3. Horowitz B: Investigations into the application of tri(*n*-butyl)phosphate/detergent mixtures to blood derivatives. Morgenthaler J (ed): *Virus Inactivation in Plasma Products, Curr Stud Hematol Blood Transfus* 1989; 56: 83-96.
4. Burnouf T: Value of virus filtration as method for improving the safety of plasma products. *Vox Sang* 1996; 70:235-236.
5. Unpublished data on file, Viral Validation Study Reports, Nabi® Biopharmaceuticals.
6. Grady GF, and Lee VA: Hepatitis B immune globulin - prevention of hepatitis from accidental exposure among medical personnel. *N Engl J Med* 1975; 293:1067-1070.
7. Seeff LB, *et al.*: Type B hepatitis after needle-stick exposure: Prevention with hepatitis B immune globulin. *Ann Int Med* 1978; 88:285-293.
8. Krugman S, and Giles JP: Viral hepatitis, type B (MS-2-strain). Further observations on natural history and prevention. *N Engl J Med* 1973; 288:755-760.
9. Hoofnagle JH, *et al.*: Passive - active immunity from hepatitis B immune globulin. *Ann Int Med* 1979; 91:813-818.
10. Beasley RP, *et al.*: Efficacy of hepatitis B immune globulin for prevention of perinatal transmission of the hepatitis B virus carrier state: Final report of a randomized double-blind, placebo - controlled trial. *Hepatology* 1983; 3:135-141.
11. Szmuness W, *et al.*: Passive active immunisation against hepatitis B: Immunogenicity studies in adult Americans. *Lancet* 1981; 1:575-577.
12. Centers for Disease Control: Recommendations for protection against viral hepatitis. Recommendations of the Immunization Practices Advisory Committee (ACIP). *MMWR* 1985; 34(22):313-335.
13. Shiraki Y, *et al.*: Hepatitis B surface antigen and chronic hepatitis in infants born to asymptomatic carrier mothers. *Am J Dis Child* 1977; 131:644-647.
14. Beasley RP, *et al.*: The e antigen and vertical transmission of hepatitis B surface antigen. *Am J Epidemiol* 1977; 105:94-98.
15. Wong VCW, *et al.*: Prevention of the HBsAg carrier state in newborn infants of mothers who are chronic carriers of HBsAg and HBeAg by administration of hepatitis B vaccine and hepatitis B immunoglobulin: Double-blind randomized placebo-controlled study. *Lancet* 1984; 1:921-926.
16. Poovorawan Y, *et al.*: Long term hepatitis B vaccine in infants born to hepatitis B e antigen positive mothers. *Archives of Diseases in Childhood* 1997; 77:F47-F51.
17. Stevens CE, *et al.*: Perinatal Hepatitis B virus transmission in the United States: Prevention by passive-active immunization. *JAMA* 1985; 253:1740-1745.
18. Jhaveri R, *et al.*: High titer multiple dose therapy with HBIG in newborn infants of HBsAg positive mothers. *J Pediatr* 1980; 97:305-308.
19. Centers for Disease Control: Hepatitis B virus: A comprehensive strategy for eliminating transmission in the United States through universal childhood vaccination. Recommendations of the Immunization Practices Advisory Committee (ACIP). *MMWR* 1991; 40(13):1-25.
20. Data on file, Nabi® Biopharmaceuticals
21. Scheiermann N, Kuwert EK: Uptake and elimination of hepatitis B immunoglobulins after intramuscular application in man. *Develop Biol Standard* 1983; 54:347.
22. Centers for Disease Control: General recommendations on immunization. Recommendations of the Advisory Committee on Immunization Practices (ACIP). *MMWR* 1994; 43:1-38.
23. Ellis EF, Henney CS: Adverse reactions following administration of human gamma globulin. *J Allerg* 1969; 43:45-54.

Manufactured by:
Nabi® Biopharmaceuticals
Boca Raton, FL 33487
U.S. License No. 1687
June 2003

3-683-1118

Shown in Product Identification Guide, page 324

WINRHO SDF® ℞

[win' rō s d f]

Rh_o(D) Immune Globulin Intravenous (Human)

DESCRIPTION

Rh_o(D) Immune Globulin Intravenous (Human) (Rh_o(D) IGIV) – WinRho SDF® – is a sterile, freeze-dried gamma globulin (IgG) fraction containing antibodies to the Rh_o(D) antigen (D antigen). WinRho SDF® is prepared from human plasma by an anion-exchange column chromatography method.[1-3] The manufacturing process includes a solvent detergent treatment step (using tri-n-butyl phosphate and Triton® X-100) that is effective in inactivating lipid enveloped viruses such as hepatitis B, hepatitis C, and HIV.[4] WinRho SDF® is filtered using a Planova™ 35 nm Virus Filter which has been validated to be effective in the removal of some nonlipid enveloped viruses.[5-6] These two processes are designed to increase product safety by reducing the risk of transmission of enveloped and nonenveloped viruses, respectively.

The product potency is expressed in international units by comparison to the World Health Organization (WHO) standard. A 300 µg (1,500 International Unit [IU]*) vial contains sufficient anti-Rh_o(D) to effectively suppress the immunizing potential of approximately 17 mL of Rh_o(D) (D-positive) red blood cells (RBCs). This product contains approximately 5 µg/mL IgA.

The product is stabilized with 0.1 M glycine, 0.04 M sodium chloride, and 0.01% polysorbate 80. It contains no preservative.

Treatment of ITP

For use in the treatment of immune thrombocytopenic purpura (ITP), WinRho SDF® **must be administered intravenously.**

Suppression of Rh Isoimmunization

For use in the suppression of Rh isoimmunization, WinRho SDF® may be administered either intramuscularly or intravenously.

*In the past, a full dose of Rh_o(D) Immune Globulin (Human) has traditionally been referred to as a "300 µg" dose. Potency and dosing recommendations are now expressed in IU by comparison to the WHO anti-Rh_o(D) standard. The conversion of "µg" to "IU" is 1 µg = 5 IU.

CLINICAL PHARMACOLOGY

Treatment of ITP

WinRho SDF®, Rh_o(D) Immune Globulin Intravenous (Human), has been shown to increase platelet counts in non-splenectomized, Rh_o(D) positive patients with ITP. Platelet counts usually rise within one to two days and peak within seven to 14 days after initiation of therapy. The duration of response is variable; however, the average duration is approximately 30 days. The mechanism of action is not completely understood, but is thought to be due to the formation of anti-Rh_o(D) (anti-D)-coated RBC complexes resulting in Fc receptor blockade, thus sparing antibody-coated platelets.[7-8]

Suppression of Rh Isoimmunization

WinRho SDF® is used to suppress the immune response of non-sensitized Rh_o(D) negative individuals following exposure to Rh_o(D) positive RBCs by fetomaternal hemorrhage during delivery of an Rh_o(D) positive infant, abortion (spontaneous or induced), amniocentesis, abdominal trauma, or mismatched transfusion.[9-11] The mechanism of action is not completely understood.

WinRho SDF®, when administered within 72 hours of a full-term delivery of an Rh_o(D) positive infant by an Rh_o(D) negative mother, will reduce the incidence of Rh isoimmunization from 12-13% to 1-2%. The 1-2% is, for the most part, due to isoimmunization during the last trimester of pregnancy. When treatment is given both antenatally at 28 weeks gestation and postpartum, the Rh immunization rate drops to about 0.1%.[12-15]

When 120 µg (600 IU) of Rh_o(D) IGIV is administered to pregnant women, passive anti-Rh_o(D) antibodies are not detectable in the circulation for more than six weeks and therefore a dose of 300 µg (1,500 IU) should be used for antenatal administration.

In a clinical study with Rh_o(D) negative volunteers (nine males and one female), Rh_o(D) positive red cells were completely cleared from the circulation within eight hours of intravenous administration of Rh_o(D) IGIV. There was no indication of Rh isoimmunization of these subjects at six months after the clearance of the Rh_o(D) positive red cells.

Pharmacokinetics - IM versus IV Administration

In a clinical study involving Rh_o(D) negative volunteers, two subjects received 120 µg (600 IU) Rh_o(D) IGIV by intravenous (IV) administration and two subjects received this dose by intramuscular (IM) administration. Peak levels (36 to 48 ng/mL) were reached within two hours of IV administration and peak levels (18 to 19 ng/mL) were reached at five to 10 days after IM administration. The calculated areas under the curve were the same for both routes of administration. The $t_{1/2}$ for anti-Rh_o(D) was about 24 days following IV administration and about 30 days following IM administration.

INDICATIONS AND CLINICAL USE

Treatment of ITP

WinRho SDF®, Rh_o(D) Immune Globulin Intravenous (Human), is recommended for the treatment of non-splenectomized, Rh_o(D) positive

- children with chronic or acute ITP,
- adults with chronic ITP, or
- children and adults with ITP secondary to HIV infection

in clinical situations requiring an increase in platelet count to prevent excessive hemorrhage. The safety and efficacy of WinRho have not been evaluated in clinical trials for patients with non-ITP causes of thrombocytopenia or in previously splenectomized patients.

Suppression of Rh Isoimmunization

Pregnancy and Other Obstetric Conditions

WinRho SDF® is recommended for the suppression of Rh isoimmunization in non-sensitized, Rh_o(D) negative (D-negative) women within 72 hours after spontaneous or induced abortions, amniocentesis, chorionic villus sampling, ruptured tubal pregnancy, abdominal trauma or transplacental hemorrhage or in the normal course of pregnancy unless the blood type of the fetus or father is known to be Rh_o(D) negative. In the case of maternal bleeding due to threatened abortion, WinRho SDF® should be administered as soon as possible. Suppression of Rh isoimmunization reduces the likelihood of hemolytic disease in an Rh_o(D) positive fetus in present and future pregnancies.

The criteria for an Rh-incompatible pregnancy requiring administration of WinRho SDF® at 28 weeks gestation and within 72 hours after delivery are:

- the mother must be Rh_o(D) negative,
- the mother is carrying a child whose father is either Rh_o(D) positive or Rh_o(D) unknown,
- the baby is either Rh_o(D) positive or Rh_o(D) unknown, and
- the mother must not be previously sensitized to the Rh_o(D) factor.

Transfusion

WinRho SDF®, Rh_o(D) Immune Globulin Intravenous (Human), is recommended for the suppression of Rh isoimmunization in Rh_o(D) negative female children and female adults in their childbearing years transfused with Rh_o(D)

Continued on next page

WinRho SDF—Cont.

positive RBCs or blood components containing Rh_o(D) positive RBCs. Treatment should be initiated within 72 hours of exposure. Treatment should be given (without preceding exchange transfusion) only if the transfused Rh_o(D) positive blood represents less than 20% of the total circulating red cells. A 300 µg (1,500 IU) dose will suppress the immunizing potential of approximately 17 mL of Rh_o(D) positive RBCs.

CLINICAL TRIALS

Treatment of ITP

Efficacy was documented in four subgroups of patients with ITP:

Childhood Chronic ITP

In an open-label, single arm, multicenter study, 24 non-splenectomized, Rh_o(D) positive children with ITP of greater than six months duration were treated initially with 50 µg/kg (250 IU/kg) Rh_o(D) Immune Globulin Intravenous (Human) (25 µg/kg (125 IU/kg) on days 1 and 2, with subsequent doses ranging from 25 to 55 µg/kg (125 to 275 IU/kg)). Response was defined as a platelet increase to at least 50,000/mm^3 and a doubling of the baseline. Nineteen of 24 patients responded for an overall response rate of 79%, an overall mean peak platelet count of 229,400/mm^3 (range 43,300 to 456,000), and a mean duration of response of 36.5 days (range 6 to 84).[16–17]

Childhood Acute ITP

A multicenter, randomized, controlled trial comparing Rh_o(D) IGIV to high dose and low dose Immune Globulin Intravenous (Human) and prednisone was conducted in 146 non-splenectomized, Rh_o(D) positive children with acute ITP and platelet counts less than 20,000/mm^3. Of 38 patients receiving Rh_o(D) IGIV (25 µg/kg (125 IU/kg) on days 1 and 2), 32 patients (84%) responded (platelet count $\geq$ 50,000/mm^3) with a mean peak platelet count of 319,500/mm^3 (range 61,000 to 892,000), with no statistically significant differences compared to other treatment arms. The mean times to achieving $\geq$ 20,000/mm^3 or $\geq$ 50,000/mm^3 platelets for patients receiving Rh_o(D) IGIV were 1.9 and 2.8 days, respectively. When comparing the different therapies for time to platelet count $\geq$ 20,000/mm^3 or $\geq$ 50,000/mm^3, no statistically significant differences among treatment groups were detected, with a range of 1.3 to 1.9 days and 2.0 to 3.2 days, respectively.[18–19]

Adult Chronic ITP

Twenty-four non-splenectomized, Rh_o(D) positive adults with ITP of greater than six months duration and platelet counts < 30,000/mm^3 or requiring therapy were enrolled in a single-arm, open-label trial and treated with 20 to 75 µg/kg (100 to 375 IU/kg) Rh_o(D) IGIV (mean dose 46.2 µg/kg (231 IU/kg)). Twenty-one of 24 patients responded (increase $\geq$ 20,000/mm^3) during the first two courses of therapy for an overall response rate of 88% with a mean peak platelet count of 92,300/mm^3 (range 8,000 to 229,000).[20–21]

ITP Secondary to HIV Infection

Eleven children and 52 adults, who were non-splenectomized and Rh_o(D) positive, with all Walter Reed classes of HIV infection and ITP, with initial platelet counts of $\leq$ 30,000/mm^3 or requiring therapy, were treated with 20 to 75 µg/kg (100 to 375 IU/kg) Rh_o(D) IGIV in an open label trial. Rh_o(D) IGIV was administered for an average of 7.3 courses (range 1 to 57) over a mean period of 407 days (range 6 to 1,952). Fifty-seven of 63 patients responded (increase $\geq$ 20,000/mm^3) during the first six courses of therapy for an overall response rate of 90%. The overall mean change in platelet count for six courses was 60,900/mm^3 (range -2,000 to 565,000), and the mean peak platelet count was 81,700/mm^3 (range 16,000 to 593,000).[21–23]

Suppression of Rh Isoimmunization

The pivotal study[24] supporting this indication was conducted in 1,186 non-sensitized, Rh_o(D) negative pregnant women in cases in which the blood types of the fathers were either Rh_o(D) positive or unknown. Rh_o(D) IGIV was administered according to one of three regimens: 1) 93 women received 120 µg (600 IU) at 28 weeks; 2) 131 women received 240 µg (1200 IU) each at 28 and 34 weeks; 3) 962 women received 240 µg (1200 IU) at 28 weeks. All women received a postnatal administration of 120 µg (600 IU) if the newborn was found to be Rh_o(D) positive. Of 1,186 women who received antenatal Rh_o(D) IGIV, 806 were given Rh_o(D) IGIV postnatally following the delivery of an Rh_o(D) positive infant, of which 325 women underwent testing at six months after delivery for evidence of Rh isoimmunization. Of these 325 women, 23 would have been expected to display signs of Rh isoimmunization; however, none was observed ($p < 0.001$ in a Chi-square test of significance of difference between observed and expected isoimmunization in the absence of Rh_o(D) IGIV).

CONTRAINDICATIONS

Treatment of ITP and Suppression of Rh Isoimmunization

Individuals known to have had an anaphylactic or severe systemic reaction to human globulin should not receive WinRho SDF®, Rh_o(D) Immune Globulin Intravenous (Human), or any other Immune Globulin (Human). WinRho SDF® contains trace amounts of IgA (approximately 5 µg/mL). Individuals who are deficient in IgA may have the potential for developing IgA antibodies and have anaphylactic reactions. The physician must weigh the potential benefit of treatment with WinRho SDF® against the potential for hypersensitivity reactions.

WARNINGS

WinRho SDF®, Rh_o(D) Immune Globulin Intravenous (Human), is made from human plasma. Products made from human plasma may carry a risk of transmitting infectious agents, e.g., viruses and theoretically, the Creutzfeldt-Jakob disease (CJD) agent. The risk that such products will transmit an infectious agent has been reduced by screening plasma donors for prior exposure to certain viruses, by testing for the presence of certain current virus infections, and by inactivating and/or removing certain viruses. The WinRho SDF® manufacturing process includes a solvent detergent treatment step (using tri-n-butyl phosphate and Triton® X-100) that is effective in inactivating lipid enveloped viruses such as hepatitis B, hepatitis C, and HIV. WinRho SDF® is filtered using a Planova™ 35 nm Virus Filter that is effective in reducing the level of some non-lipid enveloped viruses such as hepatitis A. These two processes are designed to increase product safety by reducing the risk of transmission of lipid enveloped and non-lipid enveloped viruses, respectively. Despite these measures, such products can still potentially transmit disease. There is also the possibility that unknown infectious agents may be present in such products. ALL infections thought by a physician possibly to have been transmitted by this product should be reported by the physician or other healthcare provider to the distributor, Nabi® Biopharmaceuticals at 1-800-4WINRHO (1-800-494-6746). The physician should discuss the risks and benefits of this product with the patient.

Treatment of ITP

WinRho SDF® **must be administered via the intravenous route** for the treatment of ITP as its efficacy has not been established by the intramuscular or subcutaneous routes. WinRho SDF® should not be administered to Rh_o(D) negative or splenectomized individuals as its efficacy in these patients has not been demonstrated.

Suppression of Rh Isoimmunization

For the suppression of Rh isoimmunization in the mother, do not administer to the infant.

PRECAUTIONS

WinRho SDF®, Rh_o(D) Immune Globulin Intravenous (Human), should not be administered as immunoglobulin replacement therapy for immune globulin deficiency syndromes.

Treatment of ITP

Following administration of WinRho SDF®, Rh_o(D) positive ITP patients should be monitored for signs and/or symptoms of intravascular hemolysis (IVH), clinically compromising anemia, and renal insufficiency.

If patients are to be transfused, Rh_o(D) negative red blood cells (PRBCs) should be used so as not to exacerbate ongoing IVH. Platelet products may contain up to 5.0 mL of RBCs, thus caution should likewise be exercised if platelets from Rh_o(D) positive donors are transfused.

If the patient has a lower than normal hemoglobin level (less than 10 g/dL), a reduced dose of 25 to 40 µg/kg (125 to 200 IU/kg) should be given to minimize the risk of increasing the severity of anemia in the patient. WinRho SDF® must be used with extreme caution in patients with a hemoglobin level that is less than 8 g/dL due to the risk of increasing the severity of the anemia (See DOSAGE AND ADMINISTRATION, Treatment of ITP).

Suppression of Rh Isoimmunization

WinRho SDF® should not be administered to Rh_o(D) negative individuals who are Rh immunized as evidenced by an indirect antiglobulin (Coombs') test revealing the presence of anti-Rh_o(D) (anti-D) antibody.

A large fetomaternal hemorrhage late in pregnancy or following delivery may cause a weak mixed field positive D^u test result. Such an individual should be assessed for a large fetomaternal hemorrhage and the dose of WinRho SDF® adjusted accordingly. WinRho SDF® should be administered if there is any doubt about the mother's blood type.

Laboratory Tests

In addition to anti-D, WinRho SDF® contains trace amounts of anti-A, anti-B, anti-C and anti-E antibodies.

Treatment of ITP

Passively acquired anti-A, anti-B, anti-C, and anti-E blood group antibodies may be detectable in direct and indirect antiglobulin (Coombs') tests obtained following WinRho SDF®, Rh_o(D) Immune Globulin Intravenous (Human), administration. Interpretation of direct and indirect antiglobulin tests must be made in the context of the patient's underlying clinical condition and supporting laboratory data.

Suppression of Rh Isoimmunization

The presence of passively administered anti-Rh_o(D) in maternal or fetal blood can lead to a positive direct antiglobulin (Coombs') test. If there is an uncertainty about the mother's Rh group or immune status, WinRho SDF® should be administered to the mother.

Drug Interactions

Treatment of ITP and Suppression of Rh Isoimmunization

Administration of WinRho SDF® concomitantly with other drugs has not been evaluated. Other antibodies contained in WinRho SDF® may interfere with the response to live virus vaccines such as measles, mumps, polio or rubella. Therefore, immunization with live vaccines should not be given within 3 months after WinRho SDF® administration.

Refer to Dosage and Administration section for information on drug compatibility.

Pregnancy Category C

Treatment of ITP and Suppression of Rh Isoimmunization

Animal reproduction studies have not been conducted with WinRho SDF®. It is not known whether WinRho SDF® can cause fetal harm when administered to a pregnant woman or can affect reproductive capacity. WinRho SDF® should be given to a pregnant woman only if clearly needed.

ADVERSE REACTIONS

Treatment of ITP

In clinical trials of subjects (n=161) with childhood acute ITP, adults and children with chronic ITP, and adults and children with ITP secondary to HIV, 60/848 (7%) of infusions were associated with at least one adverse event that was considered to be related to the study medication. The most common adverse events were headache (19 infusions; 2%), chills (14 infusions; <2%), and fever (nine infusions; 1%). All are expected adverse events associated with infusions of immunoglobulins.

WinRho SDF®, Rh_o(D) Immune Globulin Intravenous (Human), is administered to Rh_o(D) positive patients with ITP. Therefore, side effects related to the destruction of Rh_o(D) positive red blood cells, most notably a decreased hemoglobin, can be expected. In four clinical trials of patients treated with the recommended initial intravenous dose of 50 µg/kg (250 IU/kg), the mean maximum decrease in hemoglobin was 1.70 g/dL (range: +0.40 to -6.1 g/dL). At a reduced dose, ranging from 25 to 40 µg/kg (125 to 200 IU/kg), the mean maximum decrease in hemoglobin was 0.81 g/dL (range: +0.65 to -1.9 g/dL). Only 5/137 (3.7%) of patients had a maximum decrease in hemoglobin of greater than 4 g/dL (range 4.2 to 6.1 g/dL).

In most cases, the RBC destruction is believed to occur in the spleen. However, signs and symptoms consistent with IVH, including back pain, shaking chills, and/or hemoglobinuria, have been reported, occurring within 4 hours of WinRho administration. IVH-related complications that have been reported include death (four cases reported between May 1996 and April 1999), acute onset or exacerbation of anemia, and acute onset or exacerbation of renal insufficiency. One patient died from complications secondary to IVH-induced exacerbation of anemia after administration of WinRho for treatment of ITP. Although the primary cause of death in the other three ITP patients treated with WinRho was related to underlying disease, the extent to which IVH-related clinical complications exacerbated their conditions and contributed to their deaths is unknown.

The mean maximum decrease in hemoglobin in patients who were not transfused with PRBCs was 3.7 g/dL (range: 0.0-7.6 g/dL). Transfusions for treatment-associated anemia were administered within hours to days of the onset of IVH and consisted of between 1-6 units of PRBCs. Acute renal insufficiency was noted within 2 to 48 hours of the onset of IVH. The mean maximum increase in serum creatinine was 3.5 mg/dL (range: 0.8-10.3 mg/dL) and occurred within 2-9 days. The renal insufficiency in all surviving patients resolved with medical management, including dialysis, within 4-23 days.

The etiology of IVH following WinRho administration is unknown. No known risk factors associated with this adverse event have yet been identified from among those examined, which included age, gender, pre-treatment renal function, pre-treatment hemoglobin, concomitantly administered PRBCs, or WinRho dose.

Suppression of Rh Isoimmunization

Adverse reactions to Rh_o(D) Immune Globulin Intravenous (Human) are infrequent in Rh_o(D) negative individuals. In the clinical trial[24] of 1,186 Rh_o(D) negative pregnant women, no adverse events were attributed to Rh_o(D) IGIV. Discomfort and slight swelling at the site of injection and slight elevation in temperature have been reported in a small number of cases. A post-marketing survey conducted since the Canadian licensure of Rh_o(D) IGIV in 1980 for this indication included data obtained from 31,059 injections (25,068 for routine Rh prophylaxis and 5,991 following abortions, amniocentesis, chorionic villus sampling and antepartum hemorrhage). There were 9,905 Rh_o(D) negative women who delivered Rh_o(D) positive infants, almost all of whom had received antenatal as well as postnatal prophylaxis. Of the patients followed in this survey, there were 26 reported treatment failures that resulted in the development of Rh_o(D) antibodies. There were no adverse experiences related to Rh_o(D) IGIV reported in this survey.

General Adverse Reactions

In addition to the adverse reactions described above, the following have been reported infrequently in clinical trials and/or postmarketing experience, in patients treated for ITP or the suppression of Rh isoimmunization, and are thought to be temporally associated with WinRho SDF®, Rh_o(D) Immune Globulin Intravenous (Human), use: asthenia, abdominal or back pain, hypotension, pallor, diarrhea, increased LDH, arthralgia, myalgia, dizziness, hyperkinesia, somnolence, vasodilation, pruritus, rash, and sweating.

As is the case with all drugs of this nature, there is a remote chance of an idiosyncratic or anaphylactic reaction with WinRho SDF® in individuals with hypersensitivity to blood products.

SYMPTOMS AND TREATMENT OF OVERDOSAGE

Treatment of ITP and Suppression of Rh Isoimmunization

There are no reports of known overdoses in patients being treated for Rh isoimmunization or ITP. In clinical studies with nonpregnant Rh_o(D) positive patients with ITP (n=141) treated with 120 to 6,500 µg (600 to 32,500 IU) of Rh_o(D) IGIV, there were no signs or symptoms that warranted medical intervention. However, these same doses were associated with a mild, transient hemolytic anemia.

DOSAGE AND ADMINISTRATION

Treatment of ITP and Suppression of Rh Isoimmunization

WinRho SDF®, Rh_o(D) Immune Globulin Intravenous (Human), should be reconstituted only with the accompanying vial of Sterile Diluent (0.8% sodium chloride, 10mM sodium phosphate). It should not be administered concurrently with other products.

Reconstitution

Intravenous Administration

Aseptically reconstitute the product shortly before use with 2.5 mL of Sterile Diluent for 120 µg (600 IU) and 300 µg (1,500 IU) and 8.5 mL of Sterile Diluent for 1,000 µg (5,000 IU) (see the next table). Discard unused portion of diluent. Inject the diluent slowly onto the inside wall of the vial and gently swirl until dissolved. **Do not shake**.

Intramuscular Administration

Aseptically reconstitute the product shortly before use with 1.25 mL of Sterile Diluent for 120 µg (600 IU) and 300 µg (1,500 IU) and 8.5 mL of Sterile Diluent for 1,000 µg (5,000 IU) (see the next table). Inject the diluent slowly onto the inside wall of the vial and gently swirl until dissolved. **Do not shake**.

Reconstitution of WinRho SDF®

Vial Size	Volume of Diluent to be Added to Vial
Intravenous Injection	—
120 µg (600 IU)	2.5 mL
300 µg (1,500 IU)	2.5 mL
1,000 µg (5,000 IU)	8.5 mL
Intramuscular Injection	—
120 µg (600 IU)	1.25 mL
300 µg (1,500 IU)	1.25 mL
1,000 µg (5,000 IU)	8.5 mL*

* To be administered into several sites

Injection

Parenteral products such as WinRho SDF® should be inspected for particulate matter and discoloration prior to administration. Use the product within 12 hours of reconstitution. Discard any unused portion.

Intravenous Administration

Infuse the entire dose into a suitable vein over three to five minutes. WinRho SDF® should be administered separately from other drugs.

Intramuscular Administration

Administer into the deltoid muscle of the upper arm or the anterolateral aspects of the upper thigh. Due to the risk of sciatic nerve injury, the gluteal region should not be used as a routine injection site. If the gluteal region is used, use only the upper, outer quadrant.

Treatment of ITP

WinRho SDF®, Rh_o(D) Immune Globulin Intravenous (Human), **must be given by intravenous administration** for the treatment of ITP.

Initial Dosing: After confirming that the patient is Rh_o(D) positive, an initial dose of 50 µg/kg (250 IU/kg) body weight, given as a single injection, is recommended for the treatment of ITP. The initial dose may be administered in two divided doses given on separate days, if desired. If the patient has a hemoglobin level that is less than 10 g/dL, a reduced dose of 25 to 40 µg/kg (125 to 200 IU/kg) should be given to minimize the risk of increasing the severity of anemia in the patient. All patients should be monitored to determine clinical response by assessing platelet counts, red cell counts, hemoglobin, and reticulocyte levels (See PRECAUTIONS, *Treatment of ITP*).

Subsequent Dosing: If subsequent therapy is required to elevate platelet counts, an intravenous dose of 25 to 60 µg/kg (125 to 300 IU/kg) body weight of WinRho SDF® is recommended. The frequency and dose used in maintenance therapy should be determined by the patient's clinical response by assessing platelet counts, red cell counts, hemoglobin, and reticulocyte levels.

If patient responded to initial dose with a satisfactory increase in platelets:

Maintenance Therapy:

Dosing (25-60 µg/kg (125-300 IU/kg)) individualized based on platelet and Hgb levels.

If patient did not respond to initial dose, administer a subsequent dose based on Hgb:

If Hgb between 8-10 g/dL, redose between 25-40 µg/kg (125-200 IU/kg).

If Hgb >10 g/dL, redose between 50-60 µg/kg (250-300 IU/kg).

If Hgb <8 g/dL, use with caution.

The following equations are provided to determine the dosage and number of vials needed for the treatment of ITP:

- weight in lbs. / 2.2083 = weight in kg
- weight in kg × selected µg (IU) dosing level = dosage
- dosage / vial size = number of vials needed

Suppression of Rh Isoimmunization

WinRho SDF® may be given by intravenous or intramuscular administration for the suppression of Rh isoimmunization.

Pregnancy

The same dosage, as described below, is to be administered by either the intramuscular or intravenous routes.

A 300 µg (1,500 IU) dose of WinRho SDF® should be administered at 28 weeks gestation. If WinRho SDF® is administered early in the pregnancy, it is recommended that WinRho SDF® be administered at 12-week intervals in order to maintain an adequate level of passively acquired anti-Rh.

A 120 µg (600 IU) dose should be administered as soon as possible after delivery of a confirmed Rh_o(D) positive baby and normally no later than 72 hours after delivery. In the event that the Rh status of the baby is not known at 72 hours, WinRho SDF® should be administered to the mother at 72 hours after delivery. If more than 72 hours have elapsed, WinRho SDF® should not be withheld, but administered as soon as possible up to 28 days after delivery.

Other Obstetric Conditions

The same dosage, as described below, is to be administered by either the intramuscular or intravenous routes.

A 120 µg (600 IU) dose of WinRho SDF® should be administered immediately after abortion, amniocentesis (after 34 weeks gestation) or any other manipulation late in pregnancy (after 34 weeks gestation) associated with increased risk of Rh isoimmunization. Administration should take place within 72 hours after the event.

A 300 µg (1,500 IU) dose of WinRho SDF® should be administered immediately after amniocentesis before 34 weeks gestation or after chorionic villus sampling. This dose should be repeated every 12 weeks while the woman is pregnant. In the case of threatened abortion, WinRho SDF® should be administered as soon as possible.

Obstetric Indications and Recommended Dose

Indication	Dose (Administer IM or IV)
Pregnancy:	
• 28 weeks gestation	300 µg (1,500 IU)
• Postpartum (if newborn Rh positive)	120 µg (600 IU)
Obstetric Conditions:	
• Threatened abortion at any time	300 µg (1,500 IU)
• Amniocentesis and chorionic villus sampling before 34 weeks gestation	300 µg (1,500 IU)
• Abortion, amniocentesis, or any other manipulation after 34 weeks gestation	120 µg (600 IU)

Transfusion

WinRho SDF® should be administered within 72 hours after exposure for treatment of incompatible blood transfusions or massive fetal hemorrhage.

Transfusion Indication and Recommended Dose

Route of Administration	WinRho SDF® Dose	
	If exposed to Rh_o(D) Positive Whole Blood:	If exposed to Rh_o(D) Positive Red Blood Cells:
Intravenous	9 µg (45 IU)/ mL blood	18 µg (90 IU)/ mL cells
Intramuscular	12 µg (60 IU)/ mL blood	24 µg (120 IU)/ mL cells

Administer 600 µg (3,000 IU) **every 8 hours via the intravenous route,** until the total dose, calculated from the above table, is administered.

Administer 1,200 µg (6,000 IU) **every 12 hours via the intramuscular route,** until the total dose, calculated from the above table, is administered.

HOW SUPPLIED

WinRho SDF®, Rh_o(D) Immune Globulin Intravenous (Human), is available in packages containing:

NDC Number	Contents
60492-0021-1	A box containing a single dose vial of 120 µg (600 IU) anti-Rh_o(D) IGIV, a single dose vial of Sterile Diluent, and a package insert
60492-0023-1	A box containing a single dose vial of 300 µg (1,500 IU) anti-Rh_o(D) IGIV, a single dose vial of Sterile Diluent, and a package insert
60492-0024-1	A box containing a single dose vial of 1,000 µg (5,000 IU) anti-Rh_o(D) IGIV, a single dose vial of Sterile Diluent, and a package insert

STORAGE

Store at 2 to 8 °C (35 to 46 °F). Do not freeze. Do not use after expiration date.

If the reconstituted product is not used immediately, store it at room temperature for no longer than 12 hours. Do not freeze the reconstituted product. Discard the product if not administered within 12 hours.

Rx Only

REFERENCES

1. Bowman, JM, et al.: Low protein Rh immune globulin (Rh IgG)-purity, stability, activity and prophylactic value. *Vox Sang* 1973; 24:301-316.
2. Bowman, JM, et al.: WinRho: Rh immune globulin prepared by ion exchange for intravenous use. *Can. Med. Assoc. J.* 1980; 123:1121-1125.
3. Friesen, AD, et al.: Column ion-exchange preparation and characterization of an Rh immune globulin (WinRho) for intravenous use. *J. Appl. Biochem.* 1981; 3:164-175.
4. Horowitz, B: Investigations into the application of tri(n-butyl)phosphate/detergent mixtures to blood derivatives. Morgenthaler J (ed): *Virus Inactivation in Plasma Products, Curr. Stud. Hematol. Blood. Transfus.* 1989; 56:83-96.
5. Information on file at Cangene Corporation.
6. Burnouf, T: Value of virus filtration as a method for improving the safety of plasma products. *Vox Sang.* 1996; 70:235-236.
7. Ballow, M: Mechanisms of action of intravenous immunoglobulin therapy and potential use in autoimmune connective tissue diseases. *Cancer.* 1991; 68:1430-1436.
8. Kniker, WT: Immunosuppressive agents, γ-globulin, immunomodulation, immunization, and apheresis. *J. Aller. Clin. Immunol.* 1989; 84:1104-1106.
9. Chown, B, et al.: The effect of anti-D IgG on D-positive recipients. *Can. Med. Assoc. J.* 1970; 102:1161-1164.
10. Bowman, JM and Chown, B: Prevention of Rh immunization after massive Rh-positive transfusion. *Can. Med. Assoc. J.* 1968; 99:385-388.
11. Bowman, JM: Suppression of Rh isoimmunization: a review. *Obstet. & Gynec.* 1978; 52:385-393.
12. Bowman, JM, et al.: Rh isoimmunization during pregnancy: antenatal prophylaxis. *Can. Med. Assoc. J.* 1978; 118:623-627.
13. Bowman, JM, and Pollock, JM: Antenatal prophylaxis of Rh isoimmunization: 28 weeks'-gestation service program. *Can. Med. Assoc. J.* 1978; 118:627-630.
14. Bowman, JM, and Pollock, JM: Failures of intravenous Rh immune globulin prophylaxis: An analysis of the reasons for such failures. *Trans. Med. Rev.* 1987; 1:101-11
15. Bowman, JM: Antenatal suppression of Rh alloimmunization. *Clin Obstet. & Gynec.* 1991; 34:296-303.
16. Unpublished data on file, CITP Report, May 1993.
17. Andrew, M, et al.: A multicenter study of the treatment of childhood chronic idiopathic thrombocytopenic purpura with anti-D. *J Pediatrics* 120:522-527, 1992.
18. Unpublished data on file, AITP Report, May 1993.
19. Blanchette, V, et al.: Randomised trial of intravenous immunoglobulin G, intravenous anti-D, and oral prednisone in childhood acute immune thrombocytopenic purpura. *Lancet* 344:703-707, 1994.
20. Unpublished data on file, BITP-2 Report, May 1993.
21. Bussel, JB, et al.: Intravenous anti-D treatment of immune thrombocytopenic purpura: Analysis of efficacy, toxicity, and mechanism of effect. *Blood* 77:1884-1893, 1991.
22. Unpublished data on file, BITP-1 Report, May 1993.
23. Bussel, JB, et al.: IV anti-D treatment of ITP: Results in 210 cases. Abstract, *The American Society of Hematology,* Anaheim, CA, December, 1992.
24. Unpublished data on file, WR3 Report, May 1993.

Manufactured by:
Cangene Corporation
Winnipeg, Canada R3T 5Y3
U.S. License No. 1201
Distributed by:
Nabi® Biopharmaceuticals
Boca Raton, FL 33487
To report adverse events contact
Nabi® Biopharmaceuticals at
1-800-327-7106

Triton® is a trademark of Rohm & Haas Company
Planova™ is a trademark of Asahi Kasei Kogyo Kabushiki Kaisha Corporation.
Date of Revision: Oct./2003
Part No. 07.0205.10

Shown in Product Identification Guide, page 324

Novartis Consumer Health, Inc.

200 KIMBALL DRIVE
PARSIPPANY, NJ 07054-0622

Direct Inquiries to:
Consumer & Professional Affairs
(800) 452-0051
FAX: (800) 635-2801
or write to 445 STATE STREET
FREMONT, MI 49413-0001

DENAVIR® ℞

[den-a-v r]
brand of
penciclovir cream, 1%
For Dermatologic Use Only
Rx only
Prescribing Information

DESCRIPTION

Denavir contains penciclovir, an antiviral agent active against herpes viruses. *Denavir* is available for topical administration as a 1% white cream. Each gram of *Denavir* contains 10 mg of penciclovir and the following inactive ingredients: cetomacrogol 1000 BP, cetostearyl alcohol, mineral oil, propylene glycol, purified water and white petrolatum.

Chemically, penciclovir is known as 9-[4-hydroxy-3-(hydroxymethyl) butyl]guanine. Its molecular formula is $C_{10}H_{15}N_5O_3$; its molecular weight is 253.26. It is a synthetic acyclic guanine derivative and has the following structure:

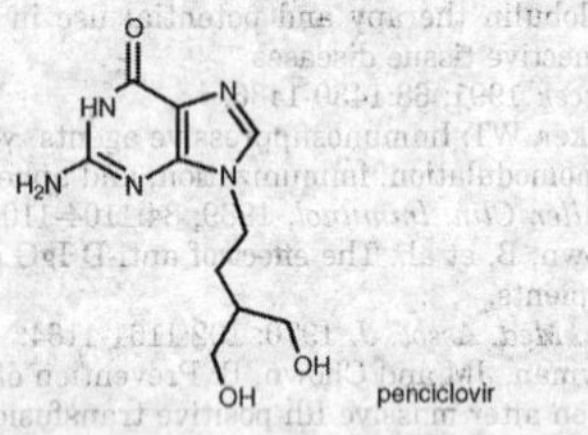

penciclovir

Penciclovir is a white to pale yellow solid. At 20°C it has a solubility of 0.2 mg/mL in methanol, 1.3 mg/mL in propylene glycol, and 1.7 mg/mL in water. In aqueous buffer (pH 2) the solubility is 10.0 mg/mL. Penciclovir is not hygroscopic. Its partition coefficient in n-octanol/water at pH 7.5 is 0.024 (logP = -1.62).

CLINICAL PHARMACOLOGY

Microbiology

Mechanism of Antiviral Activity: The antiviral compound penciclovir has *in vitro* inhibitory activity against herpes simplex virus types 1 (HSV-1) and 2 (HSV-2). In cells infected with HSV-1 or HSV-2, viral thymidine kinase phosphorylates penciclovir to a monophosphate form which, in turn, is converted to penciclovir triphosphate by cellular kinases. *In vitro* studies demonstrate that penciclovir triphosphate inhibits HSV polymerase competitively with deoxyguanosine triphosphate. Consequently, herpes viral DNA synthesis and, therefore, replication are selectively inhibited.

Antiviral Activity In Vitro and In Vivo: In cell culture studies, penciclovir has antiviral activity against HSV-1 and HSV-2. Sensitivity test results, expressed as the concentration of the drug required to inhibit growth of the virus by 50% (IC_{50}) or 99% (IC_{99}) in cell culture, vary depending upon a number of factors, including the assay protocols. See Table 1.

[See table 1 below]

Drug Resistance: Penciclovir-resistant mutants of HSV can result from qualitative changes in viral thymidine kinase or DNA polymerase. The most commonly encountered acyclovir-resistant mutants that are deficient in viral thymidine kinase are also resistant to penciclovir.

Pharmacokinetics

Measurable penciclovir concentrations were not detected in plasma or urine of healthy male volunteers (n=12) following single or repeat application of the 1% cream at a dose of 180 mg penciclovir daily (approximately 67 times the estimated usual clinical dose).

Pediatric Patients: The systemic absorption of penciclovir following topical administration has not been evaluated in patients <18 years of age.

CLINICAL TRIALS

Denavir was studied in two double-blind, placebo (vehicle)-controlled trials for the treatment of recurrent herpes labialis in which otherwise healthy adults were randomized to either *Denavir* or placebo. Therapy was to be initiated by the subjects within 1 hour of noticing signs or symptoms and continued for 4 days, with application of study medication every 2 hours while awake. In both studies, the mean duration of lesions was approximately one-half-day shorter in the subjects treated with *Denavir* (N=1,516) as compared to subjects treated with placebo (N=1,541) (approximately 4.5 days versus 5 days, respectively). The mean duration of lesion pain was also approximately one-half-day shorter in the *Denavir* group compared to the placebo group.

INDICATIONS AND USAGE

Denavir (penciclovir cream) is indicated for the treatment of recurrent herpes labialis (cold sores) in adults and children 12 years of age and older.

CONTRAINDICATIONS

Denavir is contraindicated in patients with known hypersensitivity to the product or any of its components.

PRECAUTIONS

General

Denavir should only be used on herpes labialis on the lips and face. Because no data are available, application to human mucous membranes is not recommended. Particular care should be taken to avoid application in or near the eyes since it may cause irritation. Lesions that do not improve or that worsen on therapy should be evaluated for secondary bacterial infection. The effect of *Denavir* has not been established in immunocompromised patients.

Information for Patients

Denavir is a prescription topical cream for the treatment of cold sores (recurrent herpes labialis) that occur on the face and lips. It is not a cure for cold sores and not all patients respond to it. Do not use if you are allergic to *Denavir* (penciclovir) or any of the ingredients in *Denavir* cream. Before you use *Denavir*, tell your doctor if you are pregnant, planning to become pregnant, or are breast-feeding.

Directions: Wash your hands. Your face should be clean and dry. Apply a layer of *Denavir* cream to cover only the cold sore area or the area of tingling (or other symptoms) before the cold sore appears. Rub in the cream until it disappears. Apply the cream every 2 hours during waking hours for 4 days. Even though *Denavir* works at the blister stage, treatment should be started at the earliest sign of a cold sore (i.e. tingling, redness, itching, or bump). Wash your hands with soap and water after using *Denavir* cream. Store *Denavir* cream at room temperature (59°-86°F). Keep out of reach of children.

Possible side effects: *Denavir* cream was well tolerated in clinical studies in patients with cold sores. The most frequently reported side effect was headache. Common skin-related side effects of *Denavir* cream are application site reactions, local anesthesia, taste perversion, and rash.

Carcinogenesis, Mutagenesis, Impairment of Fertility

In clinical trials, systemic drug exposure following the topical administration of penciclovir cream was negligible, as the penciclovir content of all plasma and urine samples was below the limit of assay detection (0.1 mcg/mL and 10 mcg/mL, respectively). However, for the purpose of inter-species dose comparisons presented in the following sections, an assumption of 100% absorption of penciclovir from the topically applied product has been used. Based on use of the maximal recommended topical dose of penciclovir of 0.05 mg/kg/day and an assumption of 100% absorption, the maximum theoretical plasma $AUC_{0\text{-}24\ hrs}$ for penciclovir is approximately 0.129 mcg.hr/mL.

Carcinogenesis: Two-year carcinogenicity studies were conducted with famciclovir (the oral prodrug of penciclovir) in rats and mice. An increase in the incidence of mammary adenocarcinoma (a common tumor in female rats of the strain used) was seen in female rats receiving 600 mg/kg/day (approximately 395× the maximum theoretical human exposure to penciclovir following application of the topical product, based on area under the plasma concentration curve comparisons [24 hr. AUC]). No increases in tumor incidence were seen among male rats treated at doses up to 240 mg/kg/day (approximately 190× the maximum theoretical human AUC for penciclovir), or in male and female mice at doses up to 600 mg/kg/day (approximately 100× the maximum theoretical human AUC for penciclovir).

Mutagenesis: When tested *in vitro*, penciclovir did not cause an increase in gene mutation in the Ames assay using multiple strains of *S. typhimurium* or *E. coli* (at up to 20,000 mcg/plate), nor did it cause an increase in unscheduled DNA repair in mammalian HeLa S3 cells (at up to 5,000 mcg/mL). However, an increase in clastogenic responses was seen with penciclovir in the L5178Y mouse lymphoma cell assay (at doses ≥1000 mcg/mL) and, in human lymphocytes incubated *in vitro* at doses ≥250 mcg/mL. When tested *in vivo*, penciclovir caused an increase in micronuclei in mouse bone marrow following the intravenous administration of doses ≥500 mg/kg (≥810× the maximum human dose, based on body surface area conversion).

Impairment of Fertility: Testicular toxicity was observed in multiple animal species (rats and dogs) following repeated intravenous administration of penciclovir (160 mg/kg/day and 100 mg/kg/day, respectively, approximately 1155 and 3255× the maximum theoretical human AUC). Testicular changes seen in both species included atrophy of the seminiferous tubules and reductions in epididymal sperm counts and/or an increased incidence of sperm with abnormal morphology or reduced motility. Adverse testicular effects were related to an increasing dose or duration of exposure to penciclovir. No adverse testicular or reproductive effects (fertility and reproductive function) were observed in rats after 10 to 13 weeks dosing at 80 mg/kg/day, or testicular effects in dogs after 13 weeks dosing at 30 mg/kg/day (575 and 845× the maximum theoretical human AUC, respectively). Intravenously administered penciclovir had no effect on fertility or reproductive performance in female rats at doses of up to 80 mg/kg/day (260× the maximum human dose [BSA]).

There was no evidence of any clinically significant effects on sperm count, motility or morphology in 2 placebo-controlled clinical trials of Famvir® (famciclovir [the oral prodrug of penciclovir], 250 mg b.i.d.; n=66) in immunocompetent men with recurrent genital herpes, when dosing and follow-up were maintained for 18 and 8 weeks, respectively (approximately 2 and 1 spermatogenic cycles in the human).

Pregnancy

Teratogenic Effects-Pregnancy Category B. No adverse effects on the course and outcome of pregnancy or on fetal development were noted in rats and rabbits following the intravenous administration of penciclovir at doses of 80 and 60 mg/kg/day, respectively (estimated human equivalent doses of 13 and 18 mg/kg/day for the rat and rabbit, respectively, based on body surface area conversion; the body surface area doses being 260 and 355× the maximum recommended dose following topical application of the penciclovir cream). There are, however, no adequate and well-controlled studies in pregnant women. Because animal reproduction studies are not always predictive of human response, penciclovir should be used during pregnancy only if clearly needed.

Nursing Mothers

There is no information on whether penciclovir is excreted in human milk after topical administration. However, following oral administration of famciclovir (the oral prodrug of penciclovir) to lactating rats, penciclovir was excreted in breast milk at concentrations higher than those seen in the plasma. Therefore, a decision should be made whether to discontinue the drug, taking into account the importance of the drug to the mother. There are no data on the safety of penciclovir in newborns.

Pediatric Use

An open-label, uncontrolled trial with penciclovir cream 1% was conducted in 102 patients, ages 12–17 years, with recurrent herpes labialis. The frequency of adverse events was generally similar to the frequency previously reported for adult patients. Safety and effectiveness in pediatric patients less than 12 years of age have not been established.

Geriatric Use

In 74 patients ≥ 65 years of age, the adverse events profile was comparable to that observed in younger patients.

ADVERSE REACTIONS

In two double-blind, placebo-controlled trials, 1516 patients were treated with *Denavir* (penciclovir cream) and 1541 with placebo. The most frequently reported adverse event was headache, which occurred in 5.3% of the patients treated with *Denavir* and 5.8% of the placebo-treated patients. The rates of reported local adverse reactions are shown in Table 2 below. One or more local adverse reactions were reported by 2.7% of the patients treated with *Denavir* and 3.9% of placebo-treated patients.

Table 2—Local Adverse Reactions Reported in Phase III Trials

	Penciclovir n=1516 %	Placebo n=1541 %
Application site reaction	1.3	1.8
Hypesthesia/Local anesthesia	0.9	1.4
Taste perversion	0.2	0.3
Pruritus	0.0	0.3
Pain	0.0	0.1
Rash (erythematous)	0.1	0.1
Allergic reaction	0.0	0.1

Two studies, enrolling 108 healthy subjects, were conducted to evaluate the dermal tolerance of 5% penciclovir cream (a 5-fold higher concentration than the commercial formulation) compared to vehicle using repeated occluded patch

Table 1

Method of Assay	Virus Type	Cell Type	IC50 (mcg/mL)	IC99 (mcg/mL)
Plaque Reduction	HSV-1 (c.i.)	MRC-5	0.2–0.6	
	HSV-1 (c.i.)	WISH	0.04–0.5	
	HSV-2 (c.i.)	MRC-5	0.9–2.1	
	HSV-2 (c.i.)	WISH	0.1–0.8	
Virus Yield Reduction	HSV-1 (c.i.)	MRC-5		0.4-0.5
	HSV-2 (c.i.)	MRC-5		0.6-0.7
DNA Synthesis Inhibition	HSV-1 (SC16)	MRC-5	0.04	
	HSV-2 (MS)	MRC-5	0.05	

(c.i.) = clinical isolates. The latent state of any herpes virus is not known to respond to any antiviral therapy.

testing methodology. The 5% penciclovir cream induced mild erythema in approximately one-half of the subjects exposed, an irritancy profile similar to the vehicle control in terms of severity and proportion of subjects with a response. No evidence of sensitization was observed.

Post-Marketing Experience

The following events have been identified from worldwide post-marketing use of *Denavir* in treatment of recurrent herpes labialis (cold sores) in adults. These events have been chosen for inclusion due to a combination of their seriousness, frequency of reporting, or potential causal connections to *Denavir* cream.

General: Headache, oral/pharyngeal edema, parosmia.

Skin: Application site reactions, aggravated condition, decreased therapeutic response, erythematous rash, local edema, pain, paresthesia, pruritus, skin discoloration and urticaria.

OVERDOSAGE

Since penciclovir is poorly absorbed following oral administration, adverse reactions related to penciclovir ingestion are unlikely. There is no information on overdose.

DOSAGE AND ADMINISTRATION

Denavir should be applied every 2 hours during waking hours for a period of 4 days. Treatment should be started as early as possible (i.e., during the prodrome or when lesions appear).

HOW SUPPLIED

Denavir is supplied in a 1.5 gram tube containing 10 mg of penciclovir per gram.

NDC 0067-6024-15

Store at controlled room temperature, 20°-25°C (68°-77°F) [see USP].

QUESTIONS? call **1-800-452-0051** 24 hours a day, 7 days a week.

October 2003

Manufactured by Novartis Pharma GmbH, Wehr, Germany for

Novartis Consumer Health, Inc.

Parsippany, NJ 07054-0622

©2004 Novartis

US 830935 - 494302/1

42010B

EX•LAX® LAXATIVE OTC

Ex•Lax Maximum Strength Pills
Ex•Lax Regular Strength Pills
Ex•Lax Chocolated Pieces
Ex•Lax Milk of Magnesia
Ex•Lax Ultra Pills

(See PDR For Nonprescription Drugs and Dietary Supplements™)

GAS–X® OTC

REGULAR STRENGTH CHEWABLE TABLETS
EXTRA STRENGTH CHEWABLE TABLETS
EXTRA STRENGTH SOFTGELS
MAXIMUM STRENGTH SOFTGELS
EXTRA STRENGTH GAS-X® WITH MAALOX® CHEWABLE TABLETS
EXTRA STRENGTH GAS-X® WITH MAALOX® SOFTGELS

(See PDR For Nonprescription Drugs and Dietary Supplements™.)

LAMISIL[AT]® CREAM OTC
LAMISIL[AT]® SPRAY PUMP

(See PDR for Nonprescription Drugs and Dietary Supplements™)

MAALOX® OTC

Regular Strength
Liquid Antacid/Anti-Gas

Liquids
- Cooling Mint
- Smooth Cherry

DESCRIPTION

Maalox® Antacid/Anti-Gas, a balanced combination of magnesium and aluminum hydroxides plus simethicone, is an Antacid/Anti-Gas product to provide relief of acid indigestion, heartburn, sour stomach, upset stomach associated with these symptoms, and relief of pressure and bloating commonly referred to as gas.

[See first table above]

Uses: For the relief of
- acid indigestion
- heartburn
- sour stomach
- upset stomach associated with these symptoms
- bloating and pressure commonly referred to as gas

Active Ingredients	Maalox Suspension 5 mL teaspoon	Purpose
Aluminum Hydroxide (equivalent to dried gel, USP)	200 mg	Antacid
Magnesium Hydroxide	200 mg	Antacid
Simethicone	20 mg	Antigas

Active Ingredients	Maximum Strength Maalox® Max® Antacid/Anti-Gas Per Tsp. (5 mL)	Purpose
Aluminum Hydroxide (equivalent to dried gel, USP)	400 mg	antacid
Magnesium Hydroxide	400 mg	antacid
Simethicone	40 mg	antigas

Inactive Ingredients: butylparaben, carboxymethylcellulose sodium, flavor, hypromellose, microcrystalline cellulose, propylparaben, purified water, saccharin sodium, sorbitol.

	Maalox® Suspension Per 2 Tsp. (10 mL) (Minimum Recommended Dosage)
Acid neutralizing capacity	19.4 mEq

WARNINGS

Ask a doctor before use if you have kidney disease

Ask a doctor or pharmacist before use if you are taking a prescription drug. Antacids may interact with certain prescription drugs.

Stop use and ask a doctor if symptoms last for more than 2 weeks

Keep out of reach of children.

DIRECTIONS

- shake well before using
- Adults/children 12 years and older: take 2 to 4 teaspoonsful four times a day or as directed by a physician
- do not take more than 16 teaspoonsful in 24 hours or use the maximum dosage for more than 2 weeks.
- Children under 12 years: consult a physician

PROFESSIONAL LABELING INDICATIONS

As an antacid for symptomatic relief of hyperacidity associated with the diagnosis of peptic ulcer, gastritis, peptic esophagitis, gastric hyperacidity, or hiatal hernia. As an antiflatulent to alleviate the symptoms of gas, including postoperative gas pain.

WARNINGS

Prolonged use of aluminum-containing antacids in patients with renal failure may result in or worsen dialysis osteomalacia. Elevated tissue aluminum levels contribute to the development of the dialysis encephalopathy and osteomalacia syndromes. Small amounts of aluminum are absorbed from the gastrointestinal tract and renal excretion of aluminum is impaired in renal failure. Aluminum is not well removed by dialysis because it is bound to albumin and transferrin, which do not cross dialysis membranes. As a result, aluminum is deposited in bone, and dialysis osteomalacia may develop when large amounts of aluminum are ingested orally by patients with impaired renal function.

Aluminum forms insoluble complexes with phosphate in the gastrointestinal tract, thus decreasing phosphate absorption. Prolonged use of aluminum-containing antacids by normophosphatemic patients may result in hypophosphatemia if phosphate intake is not adequate. In its more severe forms, hypophosphatemia can lead to anorexia, malaise, muscle weakness, and osteomalacia.

Advantages: In addition to the fast acting antacid ingredients, Aluminum Hydroxide and Magnesium Hydroxide, MAALOX® Regular Strength Antacid/Antigas contains the powerful antigas ingredient, simethicone, to provide concurrent fast relief from discomfort associated with gas.

HOW SUPPLIED

Maalox® Regular Strength Cooling Mint Suspension is available in plastic bottles of 5 oz. (148 mL), 12 oz. (355 mL) and 26 oz. (769 mL)

Maalox® Regular Strength Smooth Cherry Suspension is available in plastic bottles of 12 oz. (355 mL)

MAALOX® MAX® MAXIMUM STRENGTH ANTACID/ANTI-GAS Liquid OTC

Oral Suspension Antacid/Anti-Gas

Liquids
- ☐ Lemon
- ☐ Cherry
- ☐ Mint
- ☐ Vanilla Crème
- ☐ Wild Berry

DESCRIPTION

MAALOX® Max® Maximum Strength Antacid/Anti-Gas, a balanced combination of magnesium and aluminum hydroxides plus simethicone, is an antacid/anti-gas product to provide symptomatic relief of acid indigestion, heartburn, sour stomach, upset stomach associated with these symptoms and relief of pressure and bloating commonly referred to as gas.

COMPOSITION

To provide symptomatic relief of hyperacidity plus alleviation of gas symptoms, each teaspoonful contains:

[See second table above]

Uses: For the relief of
- acid indigestion
- heartburn
- sour stomach
- upset stomach associated with these symptoms
- bloating and pressure commonly referred to as gas

Inactive Ingredients: butylparaben, carboxymethylcellulose sodium, D&C Yellow #10 (Lemon Flavor only), flavor, hypromellose, microcrystalline cellulose, potassium citrate, propylparaben, purified water, saccharin sodium, sorbitol.

WARNINGS

Ask a doctor before use if you have kidney disease.

Ask a doctor or pharmacist before use if you are taking a prescription drug. Antacids may interact with certain prescription drugs.

Stop use and ask a doctor if symptoms last for more than 2 weeks

Keep out of reach of children.

DIRECTIONS

- shake well before using
- Adults/children 12 years and older: take 2 to 4 teaspoonsful four times a day or as directed by a physician
- do not take more than 12 teaspoonsful in 24 hours or use the maximum dosage for more than 2 weeks.
- Children under 12 years: consult a physician

To aid in establishing proper dosage schedules, the following information is provided:

MAALOX® Max® Maximum Strength Antacid/Anti-Gas	Per 2 Tsp. (10 mL) (Minimum Recommended Dosage)
Acid neutralizing capacity	38.8 mEq

Continued on next page

Maalox Max Antacid/Anti-Gas—Cont.

PROFESSIONAL LABELING

INDICATIONS

As an antacid for symptomatic relief of hyperacidity associated with the diagnosis of peptic ulcer, gastritis, peptic esophagitis, gastric hyperacidity, or hiatal hernia. As an antiflatulent to alleviate the symptoms of gas, including postoperative gas pain.

WARNINGS

Prolonged use of aluminum-containing antacids in patients with renal failure may result in or worsen dialysis osteomalacia. Elevated tissue aluminum levels contribute to the development of the dialysis encephalopathy and osteomalacia syndromes. Small amounts of aluminum are absorbed from the gastrointestinal tract and renal excretion of aluminum is impaired in renal failure. Aluminum is not well removed by dialysis because it is bound to albumin and transferrin, which do not cross dialysis membranes. As a result, aluminum is deposited in bone, and dialysis osteomalacia may develop when large amounts of aluminum are ingested orally by patients with impaired renal function.
Aluminum forms insoluble complexes with phosphate in the gastrointestinal tract, thus decreasing phosphate absorption. Prolonged use of aluminum-containing antacids by normophosphatemic patients may result in hypophosphatemia if phosphate intake is not adequate. In its more severe forms, hypophosphatemia can lead to anorexia, malaise, muscle weakness, and osteomalacia.
Advantages: In addition to the fast acting antacid ingredients, Aluminum Hydroxide and Magnesium Hydroxide, MAALOX® Max® Maximum Strength Antacid/Antigas contains the powerful antigas ingredient, simethicone, to provide concurrent fast relief from discomfort associated with gas.

HOW SUPPLIED

MAALOX® MAX® MAXIMUM STRENGTH ANTACID/ANTI-GAS Liquid
Oral Suspension Antacid/Anti-Gas
Maalox® Max® **Lemon** is available in plastic bottles of 5 fl. oz. (148 mL), 12 fl. oz. (355 mL), and 26 fl. oz. (769 mL).
Maalox® Max® **Cherry** is available in plastic bottles of 12 fl. oz. (355 mL) and 26 fl. oz. (769 mL).
Maalox® Max® **Mint** is available in plastic bottles of 12 fl. oz. (355 mL) and 26 fl. oz. (769 mL).
Maalox® Max® **Vanilla Crème** is available in Plastic Bottles of 12 fl. oz. (355 mL).
Maalox® Max® **Wild Berry** is available in Plastic Bottles of 12 fl. oz. (355 mL).

Quick Dissolve OTC
MAALOX® MAX® Maximum Strength

Antacid/Antigas.
Calcium Carbonate and Simethicone
Chewable Tablets
Assorted, Lemon and Wild Berry
Flavors. Quick Dissolving Tablets

Drug Facts:
MAALOX® Max Maximum Strength
Active Ingredients:
(in each tablet) **Purpose:**
Calcium carbonate
1000 mg .... Antacid
Simethicone 60 mg .... Antigas

USES

For the relief of
- acid indigestion
- heartburn
- sour stomach
- upset stomach associated with these symptoms
- bloating and pressure commonly referred to as gas

WARNINGS

Allergy Alert: contains FD&C Yellow #5 aluminum lake (tartrazine) as a color additive (In Lemon, Assorted)
Ask a doctor or pharmacist before use if you are: presently taking a prescription drug. Antacids may interact with certain prescription drugs.
Stop use and ask a doctor if: symptoms last for more than 2 weeks.
Keep out of reach of children.

DIRECTIONS

- Chew 1 to 2 tablets as symptoms occur or as directed by a physician
- do not take more than 8 tablets in a 24-hour period or use the maximum dosage for more than 2 weeks except under the advice and supervision of a physician

Other Information:
- store at controlled room temperature 20–25°C (68–77°F)
- keep tightly closed and dry
- Acid neutralizing capacity (per 2 tablets) is 34mEq.

INACTIVE INGREDIENTS

Acesulfame K, colloidal silicon dioxide, croscarmellose sodium, dextrose, FD&C Red #40 aluminum lake, FD&C Yellow #5 aluminum lake, FD&C Yellow #6 aluminum lake, flavors, magnesium stearate, maltodextrin, mannitol, pregelatinized starch.

HOW SUPPLIED

Maalox® Max® Lemon — Plastic Bottles of 35 and 65 Tablets.
Maalox® Max® Wild Berry — Plastic Bottles of 35 and 65 Tablets.
Maalox® Max® Assorted — Plastic Bottles of 35, 65 and 90 tablets.
Questions? call 1-800-452-0051 24 hours a day, 7 days a week.

Quick Dissolve OTC
MAALOX® Regular Strength Antacid. Calcium Carbonate Chewable Tablets

Assorted, Lemon and Wild Berry flavors. Quick Dissolving Tablets

Drug Facts:
MAALOX® Regular Strength

Active Ingredient **Purpose:**
(in each tablet)
Calcium carbonate
600 mg .... Antacid

USES

For the relief of
- acid indigestion
- heartburn
- sour stomach
- upset stomach associated with these symptoms

WARNINGS

Ask a doctor or pharmacist before use if you are: presently taking a prescription drug. Antacids may interact with certain prescription drugs
Stop use and ask a doctor if symptoms last for more than 2 weeks.
Keep out of reach of children.

DIRECTIONS

- Chew 1 to 2 tablets as symptoms occur or as directed by a physician
- do not take more than 12 tablets in a 24-hour period or use the maximum dosage for more than 2 weeks except under the advice and supervision of a physician

Other Information:
- Phenylketonurics: Contains Phenylalanine, .5 mg per tablet
- store at controlled room temperature 20–25°C (68–77°F)
- keep tightly closed and dry
- Acid neutralizing capacity (per 2 tablets) is 21.6 mEq.

INACTIVE INGREDIENTS

Aspartame, colloidal silicon dioxide, croscarmellose sodium, D&C Red #30 aluminum lake, D&C Yellow #10 aluminum lake, dextrose, FD&C Blue #1 aluminum lake, flavors, magnesium stearate, maltodextrin, mannitol, pregelatinized starch.

HOW SUPPLIED

Maalox® Regular Strength Lemon — Plastic Bottles of 85 Tablets.
Maalox® Regular Strength Wild Berry — Plastic Bottles of 45 Tablets.
Maalox® Regular Strength Assorted — Plastic Bottles of 85 Tablets.
Questions? call 1-800-452-0051 24 hours a day, 7 days a week.

Overnight Relief OTC
PERDIEM®

(Sennosides)
Stimulant laxative

Drug Facts

Active ingredient (in each pill) **Purpose**
Sennosides, USP, 15 mg .... Stimulant Laxative

USES

- relieves occasional constipation (irregularity)
- generally produces bowel movement in 6 to 12 hours

WARNINGS

Do not use laxative products when abdominal pain, nausea, or vomiting are present
Ask a doctor or pharmacist before use if you
- have noticed a sudden change in bowel habits that persists over a period of 2 weeks
- are taking any other drug. Take this product 2 or more hours before or after other drugs.
  Laxatives may affect how other drugs work.

When using this product • do not use for a period longer than 1 week
Stop use and ask a doctor if • rectal bleeding or failure to have a bowel movement occur after use of a laxative. These may be signs of a serious condition.
If pregnant or breast-feeding, ask a health care professional before use.
Keep out of reach of children. In case of overdose, get medical help or contact a Poison Control Center right away.

DIRECTIONS

- swallow (pill)s with a glass of water
- swallow (pill)s whole, do not crush, break or chew

adults and children 12 years of age and over	take 2 pills once or twice daily
children 6 to under 12 years of age	take 1 pill once or twice daily
children under 6 years of age	consult a doctor

OTHER INFORMATION

- very low sodium
- protect from moisture
- store at controlled room temperature 20–25°C (68–77°F)

INACTIVE INGREDIENTS

acacia, alginic acid, black iron oxide, carnauba wax, colloidal silicon dioxide, D&C yellow #10 aluminum lake, dibasic calcium phosphate, magnesium stearate, methylparaben, microcrystalline cellulose, potassium hydroxide, povidone, pregelatinized starch, propylene glycol, propylparaben, red iron oxide, shellac, sodium benzoate, sodium lauryl sulfate, starch, stearic acid, sucrose, talc, titanium dioxide, yellow iron oxide
Questions? call **1-800-452-0051** 24 hours a day, 7 days a week.

HOW SUPPLIED

Bottles of 60 Pills.

The Perdiem® Guarantee: When taken at bedtime, Perdiem® is guaranteed to work gently, effectively or your money back. Return product to Novartis, attention Consumer Affairs, for full refund.

Tamper Evident Feature: Protective printed inner seal beneath cap. If missing or damaged, do not use contents.

NDC 0067-6025-60

THERAFLU® OTC

- Cold & Sore Throat Hot Liquid Medicine
- Cold & Cough Hot Liquid Medicine
- Severe Cold Hot Liquid Medicine
- Severe Cold non-drowsy Hot Liquid Medicine
- Flu & Sore Throat Hot Liquid Medicine
- Severe Cold & Cough Hot Liquid Medicine
- Flu & Chest Congestion non-drowsy
- Severe Cold Caplets
- Severe Cold non-drowsy Caplets

(See PDR for Nonprescription Drugs and Dietary Supplements)

TRANSDERM SCŌP® ℞

[trans-derm scōpe]
scopolamine 1.5 mg

Transdermal Therapeutic System

Programmed to deliver *in-vivo* approximately
1.0 mg of scopolamine over 3 days

DESCRIPTION

The Transderm Scōp (transdermal scopolamine) system is a circular flat patch designed for continuous release of scopolamine following application to an area of intact skin on the head, behind the ear. Each system contains 1.5 mg of scopolamine base. Scopolamine is α-(hydroxymethyl) benzeneacetic acid 9-methyl-3-oxa-9-azatricyclo $[3.3.1.0^{2,4}]$ non-7-yl ester. The empirical formula is $C_{17}H_{21}NO_4$ and its structural formula is

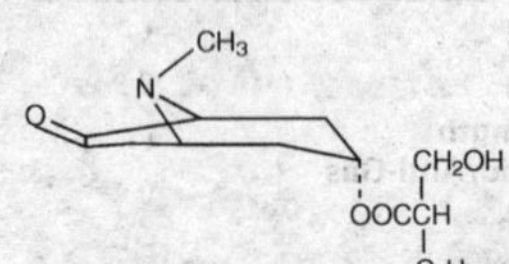

Scopolamine is a viscous liquid that has a molecular weight of 303.35 and a pKa of 7.55–7.81. The Transderm Scōp system is a film 0.2 mm thick and 2.5 cm^2, with four layers. Proceeding from the visible surface towards the surface attached to the skin, these layers are: (1) a backing layer of tan-colored, aluminized, polyester film; (2) a drug reservoir of scopolamine, light mineral oil, and polyisobutylene; (3) a microporous polypropylene membrane that controls the rate of delivery of scopolamine from the system to the skin surface; and (4) an adhesive formulation of mineral oil, polyisobutylene, and scopolamine. A protective peel strip of siliconized polyester, which covers the adhesive layer, is removed before the system is used. The inactive components, light mineral oil (12.4 mg) and polyisobutylene (11.4 mg), are not released from the system.

Cross section of the system:

Backing Layer
Drug Reservoir
Rate-Controlling Membrane
Contact Adhesive
Protective Peel Strip

CLINICAL PHARMACOLOGY

Pharmacology

The sole active agent of Transderm Scōp is scopolamine, a belladonna alkaloid with well-known pharmacological properties. It is an anticholinergic agent which acts: i) as a competitive inhibitor at postganglionic muscarinic receptor sites of the parasympathetic nervous system, and ii) on smooth muscles that respond to acetylcholine but lack cholinergic innervation. It has been suggested that scopolamine acts in the central nervous system (CNS) by blocking cholinergic transmission from the vestibular nuclei to higher centers in the CNS and from the reticular formation to the vomiting center[1,2]. Scopolamine can inhibit the secretion of saliva and sweat, decrease gastrointestinal secretions and motility, cause drowsiness, dilate the pupils, increase heart rate, and depress motor function[2].

Pharmacokinetics

Scopolamine's activity is due to the parent drug. The pharmacokinetics of scopolamine delivered via the system are due to the characteristics of both the drug and dosage form. The system is programmed to deliver *in-vivo* approximately 1.0 mg of scopolamine at an approximately constant rate to the systemic circulation over 3 days. Upon application to the post-auricular skin, an initial priming dose of scopolamine is released from the adhesive layer to saturate skin binding sites. The subsequent delivery of scopolamine to the blood is determined by the rate controlling membrane and is designed to produce stable plasma levels in a therapeutic range. Following removal of the used system, there is some degree of continued systemic absorption of scopolamine bound in the skin layers.

Absorption: Scopolamine is well-absorbed percutaneously. Following application to the skin behind the ear, circulating plasma levels are detected within 4 hours with peak levels being obtained, on average, within 24 hours. The average plasma concentration produced is 87 pg/mL for free scopolamine and 354 pg/mL for total scopolamine (free + conjugates).

Distribution: The distribution of scopolamine is not well characterized. It crosses the placenta and the blood brain barrier and may be reversibly bound to plasma proteins.

Metabolism: Although not well characterized, scopolamine is extensively metabolized and conjugated with less than 5% of the total dose appearing unchanged in the urine.

Elimination: The exact elimination pattern of scopolamine has not been determined. Following patch removal, plasma levels decline in a log linear fashion with an observed half-life of 9.5 hours. Less than 10% of the total dose is excreted in the urine as parent and metabolites over 108 hours.

Clinical Results: In 195 adult subjects of different racial origins who participated in clinical efficacy studies at sea or in a controlled motion environment, there was a 75% reduction in the incidence of motion-induced nausea and vomiting[3].

In two pivotal clinical efficacy studies in 391 adult female patients undergoing cesarean section or gynecological surgery with anesthesia and opiate analgesia, 66% of those treated with Transderm Scōp (compared to only 46% of those receiving placebo) reported no retching/vomiting within the 24-hour period following administration of anesthesia/opiate analgesia. When the need for additional antiemetic medication was assessed during the same period, there was no need for medication in 76% of patients treated with Transderm Scōp as compared to 59% of placebo-treated patients[4,5].

INDICATIONS AND USAGE

Transderm Scōp is indicated in adults for prevention of nausea and vomiting associated with motion sickness and recovery from anesthesia and surgery. The patch should be applied only to skin in the postauricular area.

CONTRAINDICATIONS

Transderm Scōp is contraindicated in persons who are hypersensitive to the drug scopolamine or to other belladonna alkaloids, or to any ingredient or component in the formulation or delivery system, or in patients with angle-closure (narrow angle) glaucoma.

WARNINGS

Glaucoma therapy in patients with chronic open-angle (wide-angle) glaucoma should be monitored and may need to be adjusted during Transderm Scōp use, as the mydriatic effect of scopolamine may cause an increase in intraocular pressure.

Transderm Scōp should not be used in children and should be used with caution in the elderly. See PRECAUTIONS.

Since drowsiness, disorientation, and confusion may occur with the use of scopolamine, patients should be warned of the possibility and cautioned against engaging in activities that require mental alertness, such as driving a motor vehicle or operating dangerous machinery.

Rarely, idiosyncratic reactions may occur with ordinary therapeutic doses of scopolamine. The most serious of these that have been reported are: acute toxic psychosis, including confusion, agitation, rambling speech, hallucinations, paranoid behaviors, and delusions.

PRECAUTIONS

General

Scopolamine should be used with caution in patients with pyloric obstruction or urinary bladder neck obstruction. Caution should be exercised when administering and antiemetic or antimuscarinic drug to patients suspected of having intestinal obstruction.

Transderm Scōp should be used with caution in the elderly or in individuals with impaired liver or kidney functions because of the increased likelihood of CNS effects.

Caution should be exercised in patients with a history of seizures or psychosis, since scopolamine can potentially aggravate both disorders.

Information for Patients

Since scopolamine can cause temporary dilation of the pupils and blurred vision if it comes in contact with the eyes, patients should be strongly advised to wash their hands thoroughly with soap and water immediately after handling the patch. In addition, it is important that used patches be disposed of properly to avoid contact with children or pets. Patients should be advised to remove the patch immediately and promptly contact a physician in the unlikely event that they experience symptoms of acute narrow-angle glaucoma (pain and reddening of the eyes, accompanied by dilated pupils). Patients should also be instructed to remove the patch if they develop any difficulties in urinating.

Patients who expect to participate in underwater sports should be cautioned regarding the potentially disorienting effects of scopolamine. A patient brochure is available.

Drug Interactions

The absorption of oral medications may be decreased during the concurrent use of scopolamine because of decreased gastric motility and delayed gastric emptying.

Scopolamine should be used with care in patients taking other drugs that are capable of causing CNS effects such as sedatives, tranquilizers, or alcohol. Special attention should be paid to potential interactions with drugs having anticholinergic properties; e.g., other belladonna alkaloids, antihistamines (including meclizine), tricyclic antidepressants, and muscle relaxants.

Laboratory Test Interactions

Scopolamine will interfere with the gastric secretion test.

Carcinogenesis, Mutagenesis, Impairment of Fertility

No long-term studies in animals have been completed to evaluate the carcinogenic potential of scopolamine. The mutagenic potential of scopolamine has not been evaluated. Fertility studies were performed in female rats and revealed no evidence of impaired fertility or harm to the fetus due to scopolamine hydrobromide administered by daily subcutaneous injection. Maternal body weights were reduced in the highest-dose group (plasma level approximately 500 times the level achieved in humans using a transdermal system).

Pregnancy Category C

Teratogenic studies were performed in pregnant rats and rabbits with scopolamine hydrobromide administered by daily intravenous injection. No adverse effects were recorded in rats. Scopolamine hydrobromide has been shown to have a marginal embryotoxic effect in rabbits when administered by daily intravenous injection at doses producing plasma levels approximately 100 times the level achieved in humans using a transdermal system. During a clinical study among women undergoing cesarean section treated with Transderm Scōp in conjunction with epidural anesthesia and opiate analgesia, no evidence of CNS depression was found in the newborns. There are no other adequate and well-controlled studies in pregnant women. Other than in the adjunctive use for delivery by cesarean section, Transderm Scōp should be used in pregnancy only if the potential benefit justifies the potential risk to the fetus.

Nursing Mothers

Because scopolamine is excreted in human milk, caution should be exercised when Transderm Scōp is administered to a nursing woman.

Labor and Delivery

Scopolamine administered parenterally at higher doses than the dose delivered by Transderm Scōp does not increase the duration of labor, nor does it affect uterine contractions. Scopolamine does cross the placenta.

Pediatric Use

The safety and effectiveness of Transderm Scōp in children has not been established. Children are particularly susceptible to the side effects of belladonna alkaloids. Transderm Scōp should not be used in children because it is not known whether this system will release an amount of scopolamine that could produce serious adverse effects in children.

ADVERSE DRUG EXPERIENCES

The adverse reactions for Transderm Scōp are provided separately for patients with motion sickness and with post-operative nausea and vomiting.

Motion Sickness: In motion sickness clinical studies of Transderm Scōp, the most frequent adverse reaction was dryness of the mouth. This occurred in about two thirds of patients on drug. A less frequent adverse drug reaction was drowsiness, which occurred in less than one sixth of patients on drug. Transient impairment of eye accommodation, including blurred vision and dilation of the pupils, was also observed.

Post-operative Nausea and Vomiting: In a total of five clinical studies in which Transderm Scōp was administered perioperatively to a total of 461 patients and safety was assessed, dry mouth was the most frequently reported adverse drug experience, which occurred in approximately 29% of patients on drug. Dizziness was reported by approximately 12% of patients on drug[6].

Postmarketing and Other Experience: In addition to the adverse experiences reported during clinical testing of Transderm Scōp, the following are spontaneously reported adverse events from postmarketing experience. Because the reports cite events reported spontaneously from worldwide postmarketing experience, frequency of events and the role of Transderm Scōp in their causation cannot be reliably determined: acute angle-closure (narrow-angle) glaucoma; confusion; difficulty urinating; dry, itchy, or conjunctival injection of eyes; restlessness; hallucinations; memory disturbances; rashes and erythema; and transient changes in heart rate.

Drug Withdrawal/Post-Removal Symptoms: Symptoms such as dizziness, nausea, vomiting, and headache occur following abrupt discontinuation of antimuscarinics. Similar symptoms, including disturbances of equilibrium, have been reported in some patients following discontinuation of use of the Transderm Scōp system. These symptoms usually do not appear until 24 hours or more after the patch has been removed. Some symptoms may be related to adaptation from a motion environment to a motion-free environment. More serious symptoms including muscle weakness, bradycardia and hypotension may occur following discontinuation of Transderm Scōp.

OVERDOSAGE

Because strategies for the management of drug overdose continually evolve, it is strongly recommended that a poison control center be connected to obtain up-to-date information regarding the management of Transderm Scōp patch overdose. The prescriber should be mindful that antidotes used routinely in the past may no longer be considered optimal treatment. For example, physostigmine, used more or less routinely in the past, is seldom recommended for the routine management of anticholinergic syndromes.

Until up-to-date authoritative advice is obtained, routine supportive measures should be directed to maintaining adequate respiratory and cardiac function.

The signs and symptoms of anticholinergic toxicity include: lethargy, somnolence, coma, confusion, agitation, hallucinations, convulsion, visual disturbance, dry flushed skin, dry mouth, decreased bowel sounds, urinary retention, tachycardia, hypertension, and supraventricular arrhythmias.

Most cases of toxicity involving the use of the product will resolve with simple removal of the patch. Serious symptomatic cases of overdosage involving multiple patch applications and/or ingestion may be managed by initially ensuring the patient has an adequate airway, and supporting respiration and circulation. This should be rapidly followed by removal of all patches from the skin and the mouth. If there is evidence of patch ingestion, gastric lavage, endoscopic removal of swallowed patches, or administration of activated charcoal should be considered, as indicated by the clinical situation. In any case where there is serious overdosage or signs of evolving acute toxicity, continuous monitoring of vital signs and ECG, establishment of intravenous access, and administration of oxygen are all recommended. The symptoms of overdose/toxicity due to scopolamine should be carefully distinguished from the occasionally observed syndrome of withdrawal (see Drug Withdrawal/Post Removal Symptoms). Although mental confusion and dizziness may be observed with both acute toxicity and withdrawal, other characteristic findings differ: tachyarrhythmias, dry skin, and decreased bowel sounds suggest anticholinergic toxicity, while bradycardia, headache, nausea and abdominal cramps, and sweating suggest post-removal withdrawal. Obtaining a careful history is crucial to making the correct diagnosis.

DOSAGE AND ADMINISTRATION

Initiation of Therapy: To prevent the nausea and vomiting associated with motion sickness, one Transderm Scōp patch (programmed to deliver approximately 1.0 mg of scopolamine over 3 days) should be applied to the hairless area behind one ear at least 4 hours before the antiemetic effect is required. To prevent post operative nausea and vomiting, the patch should be applied the evening before scheduled surgery. To minimize exposure of the newborn baby to the drug, apply the patch one hour prior to cesarean section. Only one patch should be worn at any time. Do not cut the patch.

Handling: After the patch is applied on dry skin behind the ear, the hands should be washed thoroughly with soap and water and dried. Upon removal, the patch should be discarded. To prevent any traces of scopolamine from coming into direct contact with the eyes, the hands and the application site should be washed thoroughly with soap and water and dried. (A patient brochure is available).

Continuation of Therapy: Should the patch become displaced, it should be discarded, and a fresh one placed on the hairless area behind the other ear. For motion sickness, if therapy is required for longer than 3 days, the first patch should be removed and a fresh one placed on the hairless area behind the other ear. For perioperative use, the patch should be kept in place for 24 hours following surgery at which time it should be removed and discarded.

HOW SUPPLIED

The Transderm Scōp system is a tan-colored circular patch, 2.5 cm^2, on a clear, oversized, hexagonal peel strip, which is removed prior to use.

Continued on next page

Transderm Scōp—Cont.

Each Transderm Scōp system contains 1.5 mg of scopolamine and is programmed to deliver *in-vivo* approximately 1.0 mg of scopolamine over 3 days. Transderm Scōp is available in packages of four patches. Each patch is foil wrapped. Patient instructions are included.

1 Package (4 patches) NDC 0067-4345-04

The system should be stored at controlled room temperature between 20°C and 25°C (68°F and 77°F).

CAUTION

Federal law prohibits dispensing without prescription.

REFERENCES

1. McEvoy, G.K. (ed.); AHSF Drug Information; American Society of Hospital Pharmacists, Bethesda, MD, pp. 608–611 (1990).
2. Gilman, A.G. et al (ed.); The pharmacological Basis of Therapeutics (8th Ed.); Pergamon Press, New York, NY, pp. 150–165 (1990).
3. Pharmacokinetic clinical data on file.
4. Kotelko, D.M. et al; "Transdermal scopolamine decreases nausea and vomiting following cesarean section in patients receiving epidural morphine". Anesthesiology 71(5): 675–678 (1989).
5. Bailey, P.L. et al; "Transdermal scopolamine reduces nausea and vomiting after outpatient laparoscopy". Anesthesiology 72(6): 977–980 (1990).
6. Clinical safety data on file.

Mfd by: ALZA Corporation
Mountain View, CA 94043
Distributed by:
Novartis Consumer Health, Inc.
Parsippany, NJ 07054-0622

REV 06/02

Please read this instruction sheet carefully before opening the system package.

Information for the Patient
TRANSDERM SCŌP®
Generic Name: scopolamine, pronounced skoe-POL-a-meen
Transdermal Therapeutic System

The Transderm Scōp system helps to prevent the nausea and vomiting of motion sickness for up to 3 days. It is a round adhesive patch that you place behind your ear several hours before you travel. It also helps to prevent the nausea and vomiting associated with the use of anesthesia and certain analgesics used during or after many types of surgery. If the patch is to be used in conjunction with schedule surgery, it is applied the evening before surgery. For cesarean section, the patch is applied one hour prior to surgery to minimize exposure of the unborn child to the drug. Wear only one patch at any time.

Be sure to wash your hands thoroughly with soap and water immediately after handling the patch, so that any drug that might get on your hands will not come into contact with your eyes.

Avoid drinking alcohol while using Transderm Scōp. Also, be careful about driving or operating any machinery while using the system because the drug might make you drowsy.

DO NOT USE TRANSDERM SCŌP IF YOU ARE ALLERGIC TO SCOPOLAMINE

TRANSDERM SCŌP SHOULD NOT BE USED IN CHILDREN AND SHOULD BE USED WITH CAUTION IN THE ELDERLY.

How The Transderm Scōp System Works

A group of nerve fibers deep inside the ear helps people keep their balance. For some people, the motion of ships, airplanes, trains, automobiles, and buses increases the activity of these nerve fibers. This increased activity causes the dizziness, nausea, and vomiting of motion sickness. People may have one, some, or all of these symptoms.

Transderm Scōp contains the drug scopolamine, which helps reduce the activity of the nerve fibers in the inner ear. When a Transderm Scōp patch is placed on the skin behind one of the ears, scopolamine passes through the skin and into the bloodstream. One patch may be kept in place for 3 days if needed.

It has been suggested that Transderm Scōp when used to reduce nausea and vomiting associated with surgical anesthesia or analgesia, acts on the same nerve fibers that are affected when the product is taken for motion sickness.

Precautions

Before using Transderm Scōp be sure to tell your doctor if you:

- Are pregnant or nursing (or plan to become pregnant)
- Have (or have had) glaucoma (increased pressure in the eyeball) or a predisposition to glaucoma
- Have (or have had) any metabolic, heart, liver, kidney, or other serious medical conditions
- Have any obstructions of the stomach or intestine
- Have any trouble urinating due to prostate enlargement or any bladder obstruction
- Have any allergy or have had a reaction such as a skin rash or redness to any drug, especially scopolamine, or chemical or food substance

Any of these conditions could make Transderm Scōp unsuitable for you. Also tell your doctor if you are taking any other medicines.

In the unlikely event that you experience pain in the eye and reddened whites of the eye while wearing the patch, which may be accompanied by widening of the pupil and blurred vision, remove the patch immediately and consult your doctor. As indicated below under **Side Effects**, widening of the pupils and blurred vision without pain or reddened whites of the eye is usually temporary and not serious.

Transderm Scōp should not be used in children. The safety of its use in children has not been determined. Children and the elderly may be particularly sensitive to the effects of scopolamine.

Side Effects

The most common side effect experienced by people using Transderm Scōp is dryness of the mouth. This occurs in about two thirds of the people. A less frequent side effect is drowsiness, which occurs in less than one sixth of the people. Temporary blurring or vision and dilation (widening) of the pupils may occur, especially if the drug is on your hands and comes in contact with the eyes. On infrequent occasions, disorientation, memory disturbances, dizziness, restlessness, hallucinations, confusion, difficulty urinating, skin rashes or redness, temporary changes in heart rate such as palpitations, dry itchy, or reddened whites of the eyes, and eye pain have been reported. If these effects do occur, remove the patch and call your doctor. Since drowsiness, disorientation, and confusion may occur with the use of scopolamine, be careful driving or operating any dangerous machinery, especially when you first start using the drug system.

In addition, if you plan to participate in underwater sports while wearing the patch, you should discuss with your doctor the potentially disorienting effects of scopolamine.

Eye Effects: Temporary blurring of vision and dilation (widening) of the pupils may occur, especially if the drug is on your fingers or hands and comes into contact with the eyes. Dry, itchy, or reddened whites of the eye and eye pain have been reported infrequently. In the unlikely event that you experience pain in the eye and reddened whites of the eye, which may be accompanied by widening of the pupil and blurred vision, remove the patch and consult your doctor promptly. Widening of the pupils and blurred vision without pain, or reddened whites of the eye, is usually temporary and not serious.

Drug Withdrawal/Post-Removal Symptoms: Symptoms such as dizziness, nausea, vomiting, headache, and disturbances of equilibrium have been reported by some people following discontinuation of use of the Transderm Scōp patch. These symptoms have occurred most often in people who have used the patches for more than 3 days, and frequently do not appear until 24 hours or more after the patch has been removed. These symptoms may be associated with adaptation from a motion environment to a motion-free environment. It is recommended that you consult with your doctor if these symptoms persist.

How to Use Transderm Scōp

Transderm Scōp should be stored at controlled room temperature between 20°C and 25°C (68°F and 77°F) until you are ready to use it.

1. For the prevention of motion sickness, plan to apply one Transderm Scōp patch at least 4 hours before you need it. If the patch is to be used in conjunction with scheduled surgery, it is applied the evening before surgery. For cesarean section, the patch is applied one hour prior to surgery to minimize exposure of the unborn child to the drug. **Wear only one patch at any time.** Do not cut the patch.
2. Select a hairless area of skin behind one ear, taking care to avoid any cuts or irritations. Wipe the area with a clean, dry tissue.
3. Cut along the dotted line and remove the patch (Figure 1).

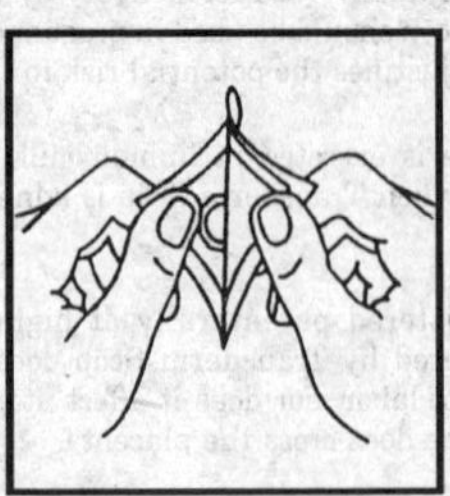

(Figure 1)

4. Remove the clear plastic six-sided backing from the round patch. Try not to touch the adhesive surface on the patch with your hands (Figure 2).

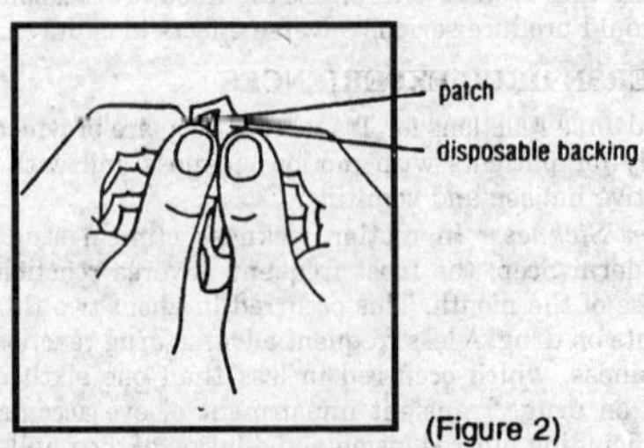

(Figure 2)

5. Firmly apply the adhesive surface (metallic side) to the dry area of skin behind the ear so that the tan-colored side is showing (Figure 3). Make good contact, especially around the edge. Once you have placed the patch behind your ear, do not move it for as long as you want to use it (e.g., up to 3 days for prevention of motion sickness).

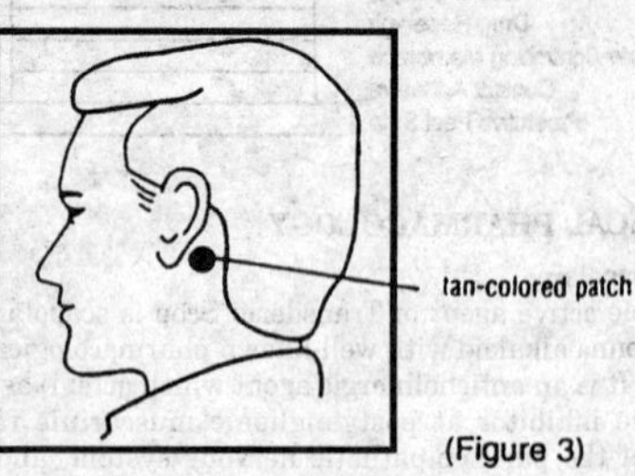

(Figure 3)

6. *Important:* **After the patch is in place, be sure to wash your hands thoroughly with soap and water to remove any scopolamine. If this drug were to come into contact with your eyes, it could cause temporary blurring of vision and dilation (widening) of the pupils (the dark circles in the center of your eyes). Unless accompanied by eye pain and reddened whites of the eyes (see Precautions), this is not serious and your pupils should return to normal.**
7. If the patch is being used to prevent the nausea and vomiting of motion sickness, remove the patch after 3 days and throw it away. (You may remove it sooner if you are no longer concerned about motion sickness). If the patch is being used to prevent nausea and vomiting associated with anesthesia or analgesia, the patch should be kept in place for 24 hours following surgery at which time it should be removed and discarded. After removing the patch, be sure to wash your hands and the area behind your ear thoroughly with soap and water. Since the patch will still contain some active ingredient after use, and to avoid accidental contact or ingestion by children or pets, fold the used patch in half with the sticky side together and dispose in the trash out of the reach of children and pets.
8. If you wish to control the nausea and vomiting of motion sickness for longer than 3 days, remove the first patch after 3 days and place a new one behind the other ear, repeating instructions 2 through 7.
9. Keep the patch dry, if possible, to prevent it from falling off. Limited contact with water, however, as in bathing or swimming, will not affect the system. In the unlikely event that the patch falls off, throw it away and put a new one behind the other ear.
10. Please inform your doctor if you are taking other medications, including over-the-counter medications.

This presents a summary of information about Transderm Scōp. If you would like more information or if you have any questions, ask your doctor or pharmacist. A more technical leaflet is available, written for your doctor. If you would like to read the leaflet, ask your pharmacist to show you a copy. You may need the help of your doctor or pharmacist to understand some of the information.

Mfd. by: ALZA Corporation
Mountain View, CA 94043
Distributed by:
Novartis Consumer Health, Inc.
Parsippany, NJ 07054-0622

(Rev. 6/02)

Shown in Product Identification Guide, page 324

Novartis Ophthalmics, Inc.

Novartis Pharmaceutical Corporation
ONE HEALTH PLAZA
EAST HANOVER, NJ 07936

Customer Response Department
(888) NOW-NOVARTIS [888-669-6682]
http://www.novartis.com

VISUDYNE® ℞
[*vĭs-ŭ-dīn*]
(verteporfin for injection)
Rx only

The following prescribing information is based on official labeling in effect July 2004

DESCRIPTION

VISUDYNE® (verteporfin for injection) is a light activated drug used in photodynamic therapy. The finished drug product is a lyophilized dark green cake. Verteporfin is a 1:1 mixture of two regioisomers (I and II), represented by the following structures:

[See graphic at top of next page]

The chemical names for the verteporfin regioisomers are: 9-methyl (I) and 13-methyl (II) *trans*-(±)-18-ethenyl-4,4a-dihydro-3,4-bis(methoxycarbonyl)-4a,8,14,19-tetramethyl-23*H*, 25*H*-benzo[*b*]porphine-9,13-dipropanoate

The molecular formula is $C_{41}H_{42}N_4O_8$ with a molecular weight of approximately 718.8.

Each mL of reconstituted VISUDYNE contains:
ACTIVE: Verteporfin, 2 mg
INACTIVES: Lactose, egg phosphatidylglycerol, dimyristoyl phosphatidylcholine, ascorbyl palmitate and butylated hydroxytoluene

CLINICAL PHARMACOLOGY

Mechanism of Action

VISUDYNE therapy is a two-stage process requiring administration of both verteporfin for injection and nonthermal red light.

Verteporfin is transported in the plasma primarily by lipoproteins. Once verteporfin is activated by light in the presence of oxygen, highly reactive, short-lived singlet oxygen and reactive oxygen radicals are generated. Light activation of verteporfin results in local damage to neovascular endothelium, resulting in vessel occlusion. Damaged endothelium is known to release procoagulant and vasoactive factors through the lipo-oxygenase (leukotriene) and cyclo-oxygenase (eicosanoids such as thromboxane) pathways, resulting in platelet aggregation, fibrin clot formation and vasoconstriction. Verteporfin appears to somewhat preferentially accumulate in neovasculature, including choroidal neovasculature. However, animal models indicate that the drug is also present in the retina. Therefore, there may be collateral damage to retinal structures following photoactivation including the retinal pigmented epithelium and outer nuclear layer of the retina. The temporary occlusion of choroidal neovascularization (CNV) following VISUDYNE therapy has been confirmed in humans by fluorescein angiography.

Pharmacokinetics

Following intravenous infusion, verteporfin exhibits a bi-exponential elimination with a terminal elimination half-life of approximately 5-6 hours. The extent of exposure and the maximal plasma concentration are proportional to the dose between 6 and 20 mg/m^2. At the intended dose, pharmacokinetic parameters are not significantly affected by gender.

Verteporfin is metabolized to a small extent to its diacid metabolite by liver and plasma esterases. NADPH-dependent liver enzyme systems (including the cytochrome P450 isozymes) do not appear to play a role in the metabolism of verteporfin. Elimination is by the fecal route, with less than 0.01% of the dose recovered in urine.

In a study of patients with mild hepatic insufficiency (defined as having two abnormal hepatic function tests at enrollment), AUC and C_{max} were not significantly different from the control group, half-life however was significantly increased by approximately 20%.

Clinical Studies

Age-Related Macular Degeneration (AMD)

Two adequate and well-controlled, double-masked, placebo-controlled, randomized studies were conducted in patients with classic-containing subfoveal CNV secondary to age-related macular degeneration. A total of 609 patients (VISUDYNE 402, placebo 207) were enrolled in these two studies. During these studies, retreatment was allowed every 3 months if fluorescein angiograms showed any recurrence or persistence of leakage. The placebo control (sham treatment) consisted of intravenous administration of Dextrose 5% in Water, followed by light application identical to that used for VISUDYNE therapy.

The difference between treatment groups statistically favored VISUDYNE at the 1-year and 2-year analyses for visual acuity endpoints.

The subgroup of patients with predominantly classic CNV lesions was more likely to exhibit a treatment benefit (N=242; VISUDYNE 159, placebo 83). Predominantly classic CNV lesions were defined as those in which the classic component comprised 50% or more of the area of the entire lesion. For the primary efficacy endpoint (percentage of patients who lost less than 3 lines of visual acuity), these patients showed a difference of approximately 28% between treatment groups at both Months 12 and 24 (67% for VISUDYNE patients compared to 40% for placebo patients, at Month 12; and 59% for VISUDYNE patients compared to 31% for placebo patients, at Month 24). Severe vision loss (≥6 lines of visual acuity from baseline) was experienced by 12% of VISUDYNE-treated patients compared to 34% of placebo-treated patients at Month 12, and by 15% of VISUDYNE-treated patients compared to 36% of placebo-treated patients at Month 24.

Patients with predominantly classic CNV lesions that did not contain occult CNV exhibited the greatest benefit (N=134; VISUDYNE 90, placebo 44). At 1 year, these patients demonstrated a 49% difference between treatment groups when assessed by the <3 lines-lost definition (77% vs. 27%).

Older patients (≥75 years), patients with dark irides, patients with occult lesions or patients with less than 50% classic CNV were less likely to benefit from VISUDYNE therapy.

The safety and efficacy of VISUDYNE beyond 2 years have not been demonstrated.

Pathologic Myopia

One adequate and well-controlled, double-masked, placebo-controlled, randomized study was conducted in patients with subfoveal CNV secondary to pathologic myopia. A total of 120 patients (VISUDYNE 81, placebo 39) were enrolled in the study. The treatment dosing and retreatments were the same as in the AMD studies. The difference between treatment groups statistically favored VISUDYNE at the 1-year analysis but not at the 2-year analysis for visual acuity endpoints. For the primary efficacy endpoint (percentage of patients who lost less than 3 lines of visual acuity), patients at the 1-year time point showed a difference of approximately 19% between treatment groups (86% for VISUDYNE patients compared to 67% for placebo patients). However, by the 2-year timepoint, the effect was no longer statistically significant (79% for VISUDYNE patients compared to 72% for placebo patients).

Presumed Ocular Histoplasmosis

One open-label study was conducted in patients with subfoveal CNV secondary to presumed ocular histoplasmosis. A total of 26 patients were treated with VISUDYNE in the study. The treatment dosing and retreatments for VISUDYNE were the same as in the AMD studies. VISUDYNE-treated patients compare favorably with historical control data demonstrating a reduction in the number of episodes of severe visual acuity loss (>6 lines of loss).

[Structural formulas I and II of verteporfin regioisomers: rings A, B, C, D; substituents $CH_3O-C(=O)$, CH_3, vinyl, $CH_3O-C(=O)-$, OH, HO, OCH_3]

I II

INDICATIONS AND USAGE

VISUDYNE therapy is indicated for the treatment of patients with predominantly classic subfoveal choroidal neovascularization due to age-related macular degeneration, pathologic myopia or presumed ocular histoplasmosis. There is insufficient evidence to indicate VISUDYNE for the treatment of predominantly occult subfoveal choroidal neovascularization.

CONTRAINDICATIONS

VISUDYNE is contraindicated for patients with porphyria or a known hypersensitivity to any component of this preparation.

WARNINGS

Following injection with VISUDYNE, care should be taken to avoid exposure of skin or eyes to direct sunlight or bright indoor light for 5 days. In the event of extravasation during infusion, the extravasation area must be thoroughly protected from direct light until the swelling and discoloration have faded in order to prevent the occurrence of a local burn which could be severe. If emergency surgery is necessary within 48 hours after treatment, as much of the internal tissue as possible should be protected from intense light.

Patients who experience severe decrease of vision of 4 lines or more within 1 week after treatment should not be retreated, at least until their vision completely recovers to pretreatment levels and the potential benefits and risks of subsequent treatment are carefully considered by the treating physician.

Use of incompatible lasers that do not provide the required characteristics of light for the photoactivation of VISUDYNE could result in incomplete treatment due to partial photoactivation of VISUDYNE, overtreatment due to overactivation of VISUDYNE, or damage to surrounding normal tissue.

PRECAUTIONS

General

Standard precautions should be taken during infusion of VISUDYNE to avoid extravasation. Examples of standard precautions include, but are not limited to:

- A free-flowing intravenous (IV) line should be established before starting VISUDYNE infusion and the line should be carefully monitored.
- Due to the possible fragility of vein walls of some elderly patients, it is strongly recommended that the largest arm vein possible, preferably antecubital, be used for injection.
- Small veins in the back of the hand should be avoided.

If extravasation does occur, the infusion should be stopped immediately and cold compresses applied *(see Warnings)*.

VISUDYNE therapy should be considered carefully in patients with moderate to severe hepatic impairment or biliary obstruction since there is no clinical experience with verteporfin in such patients.

There is no clinical data related to the use of VISUDYNE in anesthetized patients. At a >10-fold higher dose given by bolus injection to sedated or anesthetized pigs, verteporfin caused severe hemodynamic effects, including death, probably as a result of complement activation. These effects were diminished or abolished by pretreatment with antihistamine and they were not seen in conscious non-sedated pigs. VISUDYNE resulted in a concentration-dependent increase in complement activation in human blood *in vitro*. At 10 µg/mL (approximately 5 times the expected plasma concentration in human patients), there was mild to moderate complement activation. At ≥100 µg/mL, there was significant complement activation. Signs [chest pain, syncope, dyspnea, and flushing] consistent with complement activation have been observed in <1% of patients administered VISUDYNE. Patients should be supervised during VISUDYNE infusion.

Information for Patients

Patients who receive VISUDYNE will become temporarily photosensitive after the infusion. Patients should wear a wrist band to remind them to avoid direct sunlight for 5 days. During that period, patients should avoid exposure of unprotected skin, eyes or other body organs to direct sunlight or bright indoor light. Sources of bright light include, but are not limited to, tanning salons, bright halogen lighting and high power lighting used in surgical operating rooms or dental offices. Prolonged exposure to light from light-emitting medical devices such as pulse oximeters should also be avoided for 5 days following VISUDYNE administration.

If treated patients must go outdoors in daylight during the first 5 days after treatment, they should protect all parts of their skin and their eyes by wearing protective clothing and dark sunglasses. UV sunscreens are not effective in protecting against photosensitivity reactions because photoactivation of the residual drug in the skin can be caused by visible light.

Patients should not stay in the dark and should be encouraged to expose their skin to ambient indoor light, as it will help inactivate the drug in the skin through a process called photobleaching.

Drug Interactions

Drug interaction studies in humans have not been conducted with VISUDYNE.

Verteporfin is rapidly eliminated by the liver, mainly as unchanged drug. Metabolism is limited and occurs by liver and plasma esterases. Microsomal cytochrome P450 does not appear to play a role in verteporfin metabolism.

Based on the mechanism of action of verteporfin, many drugs used concomitantly could influence the effect of VISUDYNE therapy. Possible examples include the following:

Calcium channel blockers, polymyxin B or radiation therapy could enhance the rate of VISUDYNE uptake by the vascular endothelium. Other photosensitizing agents (e.g., tetracyclines, sulfonamides, phenothiazines, sulfonylurea hypoglycemic agents, thiazide diuretics and griseofulvin) could increase the potential for skin photosensitivity reactions. Compounds that quench active oxygen species or scavenge radicals, such as dimethyl sulfoxide, β-carotene, ethanol, formate and mannitol, would be expected to decrease VISUDYNE activity. Drugs that decrease clotting, vasoconstriction or platelet aggregation, e.g., thromboxane A_2 inhibitors, could also decrease the efficacy of VISUDYNE therapy.

Carcinogenesis, Mutagenesis, Impairment of Fertility

No studies have been conducted to evaluate the carcinogenic potential of verteporfin.

Photodynamic therapy (PDT) as a class has been reported to result in DNA damage including DNA strand breaks, alkali-labile sites, DNA degradation, and DNA-protein cross links which may result in chromosomal aberrations, sister chromatid exchanges (SCE), and mutations. In addition, other photodynamic therapeutic agents have been shown to increase the incidence of SCE in Chinese hamster ovary (CHO) cells irradiated with visible light and in Chinese hamster lung fibroblasts irradiated with near UV light, increase mutations and DNA-protein cross-linking in mouse L5178 cells, and increase DNA-strand breaks in malignant human cervical carcinoma cells, but not in normal cells. Verteporfin was not evaluated in these latter systems. It is not known how the potential for DNA damage with PDT agents translates into human risk.

No effect on male or female fertility has been observed in rats following intravenous administration of verteporfin for injection up to 10 mg/kg/day (approximately 60-and 40-fold human exposure at 6 mg/m^2 based on AUC_{inf} in male and female rats, respectively).

Pregnancy

Teratogenic Effects: Pregnancy Category C.

Rat fetuses of dams administered verteporfin for injection intravenously at ≥10 mg/kg/day during organogenesis (approximately 40-fold human exposure at 6 mg/m^2 based on AUC_{inf} in female rats) exhibited an increase in the incidence of anophthalmia/microphthalmia. Rat fetuses of dams administered 25 mg/kg/day (approximately 125 fold the human exposure at 6 mg/m^2 based on AUC_{inf} in female rats) had an increased incidence of wavy ribs and anophthalmia/microphthalmia.

In pregnant rabbits, a decrease in body weight gain and food consumption was observed in animals that received

Continued on next page

Visudyne—Cont.

verteporfin for injection intravenously at ≥10 mg/kg/day during organogenesis. The no observed adverse effect level (NOAEL) for maternal toxicity was 3 mg/kg/day (approximately 7-fold human exposure at 6 mg/m² based on body surface area). There were no teratogenic effects observed in rabbits at doses up to 10 mg/kg/day.

There are no adequate and well-controlled studies in pregnant women. VISUDYNE should be used during pregnancy only if the benefit justifies the potential risk to the fetus.

Nursing Mothers

It is not known whether verteporfin for injection is excreted in human milk. Because many drugs are excreted in human milk, caution should be exercised when VISUDYNE is administered to a woman who is nursing.

Pediatric Use

Safety and effectiveness in pediatric patients have not been established.

Geriatric Use

Approximately 90% of the patients treated with VISUDYNE in the clinical efficacy trials were over the age of 65. A reduced treatment effect was seen with increasing age.

ADVERSE REACTIONS

The most frequently reported adverse events to VISUDYNE are headaches, injection site reactions (including extravasation and rashes) and visual disturbances (including blurred vision, decreased visual acuity and visual field defects). These events occurred in approximately 10-30% of patients.

The following events, listed by Body System, were reported more frequently with VISUDYNE therapy than with placebo therapy and occurred in 1-10% of patients:

Ocular Treatment Site:	Blepharitis, cataracts, conjunctivitis/conjunctival injection, dry eyes, ocular itching, severe vision loss with or without subretinal or vitreous hemorrhage
Body as a Whole:	Asthenia, back pain (primarily during infusion), fever, flu syndrome, photosensitivity reactions
Cardiovascular:	Atrial fibrillation, hypertension, peripheral vascular disorder, varicose veins
Dermatologic:	Eczema
Digestive:	Constipation, gastrointestinal cancers, nausea
Hemic and Lymphatic:	Anemia, white blood cell count decreased, white blood cell count increased
Hepatic:	Elevated liver function tests
Metabolic/Nutritional:	Albuminuria, creatinine increased
Musculoskeletal:	Arthralgia, arthrosis, myasthenia
Nervous System:	Hypesthesia, sleep disorder, vertigo
Respiratory:	Cough, pharyngitis, pneumonia
Special Senses:	Cataracts, decreased hearing, diplopia, lacrimation disorder
Urogenital:	Prostatic disorder

Severe vision decrease, equivalent of 4 lines or more, within 7 days after treatment has been reported in 1-5% of patients. Partial recovery of vision was observed in some patients. Photosensitivity reactions usually occurred in the form of skin sunburn following exposure to sunlight. The higher incidence of back pain in the VISUDYNE group occurred primarily during infusion.

The following adverse events have occurred either at low incidence (<1%) during clinical trials or have been reported during the use of VISUDYNE in clinical practice where these events were reported voluntarily from a population of unknown size and frequency of occurrence cannot be determined precisely. They have been chosen for inclusion based on factors such as seriousness, frequency of reporting, possible causal connection to VISUDYNE, or a combination of these factors:

Ocular Treatment Site:	Retinal detachment (nonrhegmatogenous), retinal or choroidal vessel nonperfusion
Non-ocular Events:	Chest pain and other musculoskeletal pain during infusion, hypersensitivity reactions (which can be severe), syncope, severe allergic reactions with dyspnea and flushing, and vaso-vagal reactions.

OVERDOSAGE

Overdose of drug and/or light in the treated eye may result in nonperfusion of normal retinal vessels with the possibility of severe decrease in vision that could be permanent. An overdose of drug will also result in the prolongation of the period during which the patient remains photosensitive to bright light. In such cases, it is recommended to extend the photosensitivity precautions for a time proportional to the overdose.

DOSAGE AND ADMINISTRATION

A course of VISUDYNE therapy is a two-step process requiring administration of both drug and light.

The first step is the intravenous infusion of VISUDYNE. The second step is the activation of VISUDYNE with light from a nonthermal diode laser.

The physician should re-evaluate the patient every 3 months and if choroidal neovascular leakage is detected on fluorescein angiography, therapy should be repeated.

Lesion Size Determination

The greatest linear dimension (GLD) of the lesion is estimated by fluorescein angiography and color fundus photography. All classic and occult CNV, blood and/or blocked fluorescence, and any serous detachments of the retinal pigment epithelium should be included for this measurement. Fundus cameras with magnification within the range of 2.4-2.6X are recommended. The GLD of the lesion on the fluorescein angiogram must be corrected for the magnification of the fundus camera to obtain the GLD of the lesion on the retina.

Spot Size Determination

The treatment spot size should be 1000 microns larger than the GLD of the lesion on the retina to allow a 500 micron border, ensuring full coverage of the lesion. The maximum spot size used in the clinical trials was 6400 microns.

The nasal edge of the treatment spot must be positioned at least 200 microns from the temporal edge of the optic disc, even if this will result in lack of photoactivation of CNV within 200 microns of the optic nerve.

VISUDYNE Administration

Reconstitute each vial of VISUDYNE with 7 mL of sterile Water for Injection to provide 7.5 mL containing 2 mg/mL. Reconstituted VISUDYNE must be protected from light and used within 4 hours. It is recommended that reconstituted VISUDYNE be inspected visually for particulate matter and discoloration prior to administration. Reconstituted VISUDYNE is an opaque dark green solution.

The volume of reconstituted VISUDYNE required to achieve the desired dose of 6 mg/m² body surface area is withdrawn from the vial and diluted with 5% Dextrose for Injection to a total infusion volume of 30 mL. The full infusion volume is administered intravenously over 10 minutes at a rate of 3 mL/minute, using an appropriate syringe pump and in-line filter. The clinical studies were conducted using a standard infusion line filter of 1.2 microns.

Precautions should be taken to prevent extravasation at the injection site. If extravasation occurs, protect the site from light *(See Precautions)*.

Light Administration

Initiate 689 nm wavelength laser light delivery to the patient 15 minutes after the start of the 10-minute infusion with VISUDYNE.

Photoactivation of VISUDYNE is controlled by the total light dose delivered. In the treatment of choroidal neovascularization, the recommended light dose is 50 J/cm² of neovascular lesion administered at an intensity of 600 mW/cm². This dose is administered over 83 seconds.

Light dose, light intensity, ophthalmic lens magnification factor and zoom lens setting are important parameters for the appropriate delivery of light to the predetermined treatment spot. Follow the laser system manuals for procedure set up and operation.

The laser system must deliver a stable power output at a wavelength of 689±3 nm. Light is delivered to the retina as a single circular spot via a fiber optic and a slit lamp, using a suitable ophthalmic magnification lens.

The following laser systems have been tested for compatibility with VISUDYNE and are approved for delivery of a stable power output at a wavelength of 689±3 nm:

Coherent Opal Photoactivator laser console and modified Coherent LaserLink adapter,
Manufactured by Lumenis, Inc., Santa Clara, CA
Zeiss VISULAS 690s laser and VISULINK PDT/U adapter,
Manufactured by Carl Zeiss Inc., Thornwood, NY.

Concurrent Bilateral Treatment

The controlled trials only allowed treatment of one eye per patient. In patients who present with eligible lesions in both eyes, physicians should evaluate the potential benefits and risks of treating both eyes concurrently. If the patient has already received previous VISUDYNE therapy in one eye with an acceptable safety profile, both eyes can be treated concurrently after a single administration of VISUDYNE. The more aggressive lesion should be treated first, at 15 minutes after the start of infusion. Immediately at the end of light application to the first eye, the laser settings should be adjusted to introduce the treatment parameters for the second eye, with the same light dose and intensity as for the first eye, starting no later than 20 minutes from the start of infusion.

In patients who present for the first time with eligible lesions in both eyes without prior VISUDYNE therapy, it is prudent to treat only one eye (the most aggressive lesion) at the first course. One week after the first course, if no significant safety issues are identified, the second eye can be treated using the same treatment regimen after a second VISUDYNE infusion. Approximately 3 months later, both eyes can be evaluated and concurrent treatment following a new VISUDYNE infusion can be started if both lesions still show evidence of leakage.

HOW SUPPLIED

VISUDYNE is supplied in a single use glass vial with a gray bromobutyl stopper and aluminum flip-off cap. It contains a lyophilized cake with 15 mg verteporfin. The product is intended for intravenous injection only.

Spills and Disposal

Spills of VISUDYNE should be wiped up with a damp cloth. Skin and eye contact should be avoided due to the potential for photosensitivity reactions upon exposure to light. Use of rubber gloves and eye protection is recommended. All materials should be disposed of properly.

Accidental Exposure

Because of the potential to induce photosensitivity reactions, it is important to avoid contact with the eyes and skin during preparation and administration of VISUDYNE. Any exposed person must be protected from bright light *(See Warnings)*.

NDC 58768-150-15

Store VISUDYNE between 20°C and 25°C (68°F-77°F).

Manufactured by:
Parkedale Pharmaceuticals, Inc.
Rochester, MI 48307
or
Cardinal Health
Albuquerque, NM 87107
For:
QLT PhotoTherapeutics, Inc.
Seattle, WA 98101
Co-developed and Distributed by:
Novartis Ophthalmics, Inc.
Duluth, GA 30097
Effective: April, 2003
I6154-E (April, 2003)

VOLTAREN OPHTHALMIC® ℞

[vol-ta-ren]

(diclofenac sodium ophthalmic solution) 0.1%
Sterile Ophthalmic Solution
Rx only

Prescribing Information

The following prescribing information is based on official labeling in effect July 2004.

DESCRIPTION

Voltaren Ophthalmic (diclofenac sodium ophthalmic solution) 0.1% solution is a sterile, topical, non-steroidal, anti-inflammatory product for ophthalmic use. Diclofenac sodium is designated chemically as 2-[(2,6-dichlorophenyl)amino] benzeneacetic acid, monosodium salt, with an empirical formula of $C_{14}H_{10}Cl_2NO_2Na$. The structural formula of diclofenac sodium is:

O
NaOCCH2 Cl
NH
Cl

Voltaren Ophthalmic is available as a sterile solution which contains diclofenac sodium 0.1% (1 mg/mL).

Inactive Ingredients: polyoxyl 35 castor oil, Boric acid, tromethamine, sorbic acid (2 mg/mL), edetate disodium (1 mg/mL), and purified water.

Diclofenac sodium is a faintly yellow-white to light-beige, slightly hygroscopic crystalline powder. It is freely soluble in methanol, sparingly soluble in water, very slightly soluble in acetonitrile, and insoluble in chloroform and in 0.1N hydrochloric acid. Its molecular weight is 318.14. Voltaren Ophthalmic 0.1% is an iso-osmotic solution with an osmolality of about 300 mOsmol/1000 g, buffered at approximately pH 7.2. Voltaren Ophthalmic solution has a faint characteristic odor of castor oil.

CLINICAL PHARMACOLOGY

Pharmacodynamics

Diclofenac sodium is one of a series of phenylacetic acids that has demonstrated anti-inflammatory and analgesic properties in pharmacological studies. It is thought to inhibit the enzyme cyclooxygenase, which is essential in the biosynthesis of prostaglandins.

Animal Studies

Prostaglandins have been shown in many animal models to be mediators of certain kinds of intraocular inflammation. In studies performed in animal eyes, prostaglandins have been shown to produce disruption of the blood-aqueous humor barrier, vasodilation, increased vascular permeability, leukocytosis, and increased intraocular pressure.

Pharmacokinetics

Results from a bioavailability study established that plasma levels of diclofenac following ocular instillation of two drops of Voltaren Ophthalmic to each eye were below the limit of quantification (10 ng/mL) over a 4-hour period. This study suggests that limited, if any, systemic absorption occurs with Voltaren Ophthalmic.

Clinical Trials

Postoperative Anti-Inflammatory Effects

In two double-masked, controlled, efficacy studies of postoperative inflammation, a total of 206 cataract patients were treated with Voltaren Ophthalmic and 103 patients were treated with vehicle placebo. Voltaren Ophthalmic was favored over vehicle placebo over a 2-week period for the clinical assessments of inflammation as measured by anterior chamber cells and flare.

In double-masked, controlled studies of corneal refractive surgery (radial keratotomy (RK) and laser photorefractive keratectomy (PRK)) patients were treated with Voltaren Ophthalmic and/or vehicle placebo. The efficacy of Voltaren Ophthalmic given before and shortly after surgery was favored over vehicle placebo during the 6-hour period following surgery for the clinical assessments of pain and photophobia. Patients were permitted to use a hydrogel soft contact lens with Voltaren Ophthalmic for up to three days after PRK.

INDICATIONS AND USAGE

Voltaren Ophthalmic is indicated for the treatment of postoperative inflammation in patients who have undergone cataract extraction and for the temporary relief of pain and photophobia in patients undergoing corneal refractive surgery.

CONTRAINDICATIONS

Voltaren Ophthalmic is contraindicated in patients who are hypersensitive to any component of the medication.

WARNINGS

The refractive stability of patients undergoing corneal refractive procedures and treated with Voltaren has not been established. Patients should be monitored for a year following use in this setting.

With some nonsteroidal anti-inflammatory drugs, there exists the potential for increased bleeding time due to interference with thrombocyte aggregation. There have been reports that ocularly applied nonsteroidal anti-inflammatory drugs may cause increased bleeding of ocular tissues (including hyphemas) in conjunction with ocular surgery.

There is the potential for cross-sensitivity to acetylsalicylic acid, phenylacetic acid derivatives, and other nonsteroidal anti-inflammatory agents. Therefore, caution should be used when treating individuals who have previously exhibited sensitivities to these drugs.

PRECAUTIONS

General

All topical nonsteroidal anti-inflammatory drugs (NSAIDs) may slow or delay healing. Topical corticosteroids are also known to slow or delay healing. Concomitant use of topical NSAIDs and topical steroids may increase the potential for healing problems.

Use of topical NSAIDs may result in keratitis. In some susceptible patients continued use of topical NSAIDs may result in epithelial breakdown, corneal thinning, corneal infiltrates, corneal erosion, corneal ulceration, and corneal perforation. These events may be sight threatening. Patients with evidence of corneal epithelial breakdown should immediately discontinue use of topical NSAIDs and should be closely monitored for corneal health.

Postmarketing experience with topical NSAIDs suggests that patients experiencing complicated ocular surgeries, corneal denervation, corneal epithelial defects, diabetes mellitus, ocular surface disease (e.g., dry eye syndrome), rheumatoid arthritis, or repeat ocular surgeries within a short period-of-time may be at increased risk for corneal adverse events, which may become sight threatening. Topical NSAIDs should be used with caution in these patients.

Postmarketing experience with topical NSAIDs also suggests that use more than 24 hours prior to surgery or use beyond 14 days post surgery may increase patient risk for occurrence and severity of corneal adverse events.

It is recommended that Voltaren Ophthalmic, like other NSAIDs, be used with caution in patients with known bleeding tendencies or who are receiving other medications which may prolong bleeding time.

Results from clinical studies indicate that Voltaren Ophthalmic has no significant effect upon ocular pressure. However, elevations in intraocular pressure may occur following cataract surgery.

Information for Patients

Except for the use of a bandage hydrogel soft contact lens during the first 3 days following refractive surgery, Voltaren Ophthalmic should not be used by patients currently wearing soft contact lenses due to adverse events that have occurred in other circumstances.

Carcinogenesis, Mutagenesis, Impairment of Fertility

Long-term carcinogenicity studies in rats given Voltaren in oral doses up to 2 mg/kg/day (approximately 500 times the human topical ophthalmic dose) revealed no significant increases in tumor incdence. A 2-year carcinogenicity study conducted in mice employing oral Voltaren up to 2 mg/kg/day did not reveal any oncogenic potential. Voltaren did not show mutagenic potential in various mutagenicity studies including the Ames test. Voltaren administered to male and female rats at 4 mg/kg/day (approximately 1000 times the human topical ophthalmic dose) did not affect fertility.

Geriatric Use

No overall differences in safety or effectiveness have been observed between elderly and younger adult patients.

PREGNANCY

Teratogenic Effects

Pregnancy Category C. Reproduction studies performed in mice at oral doses up to 5,000 times (20 mg/kg/day) and in rats and rabbits at oral doses up to 2,500 times (10 mg/kg/day) the human topical dose have revealed no evidence of teratogenicity due to Voltaren despite the induction of maternal toxicity and fetal toxicity. In rats, maternally toxic doses were associated with dystocia, prolonged gestation, reduced fetal weights and growth, and reduced fetal survival. Voltaren has been shown to cross the placental barrier in mice and rats.

There are, however, no adequate and well-controlled studies in pregnant women. Because animal reproduction studies are not always predictive of human response, this drug should be used during pregnancy only if clearly needed.

Non-teratogenic Effects

Because of the known effects of prostaglandin biosynthesis-inhibiting drugs on the fetal cardiovascular system (closure of ductus arteriosus), the use of Voltaren Ophthalmic during late pregnancy should be avoided.

Pediatric Use

Safety and effectiveness in pediatric patients have not been established.

ADVERSE REACTIONS

Clinical Practice: The following events have been identified during postmarketing use of topical diclofenac sodium ophthalmic solution, 0.1% in clinical practice. Because they are reported voluntarily from a population of unknown size, estimates of frequency cannot be made. The events, which have been chosen for inclusion due to either their seriousness, frequency of reporting, possible causal connection to topical diclofenac sodium ophthalmic solution, 0.1%, or a combination of these factors, include corneal erosion, corneal infiltrates, corneal perforation, corneal thinning, corneal ulceration, epithelial breakdown, and superficial punctate keratitis, (see *PRECAUTIONS, General*)

Ocular: Transient burning and stinging were reported in approximately 15% of patients across studies with the use of Voltaren Ophthalmic. In cataract surgery studies, keratitis was reported in up to 28% of patients receiving Voltaren Ophthalmic, although in many of these cases keratitis was initially noted prior to the initiation of treatment. Elevated intraocular pressure following cataract surgery was reported in approximately 15% of patients undergoing cataract surgery. Lacrimation complaints were reported in approximately 30% of case studies undergoing incisional refractive surgery.

The following adverse reactions were reported in approximately 5% or less of the patients: abnormal vision, acute elevated IOP, blurred vision, conjunctivitis, corneal deposits, corneal edema, corneal opacity, corneal lesions, discharge, eyelid swelling, injection, iritis, irritation, itching, lacrimation disorder and ocular allergy.

Systemic: The following adverse reactions were reported in 3% or less of the patients: abdominal pain, asthenia, chills, dizziness, facial edema, fever, headache, insomnia, nausea, pain, rhinitis, viral infection, and vomiting.

OVERDOSAGE

Overdosage will not ordinarily cause acute problems. If Voltaren Ophthalmic is accidentally ingested, fluids should be taken to dilute the medication.

DOSAGE AND ADMINISTRATION

Cataract Surgery: One drop of Voltaren Ophthalmic should be applied to the affected eye, 4 times daily beginning 24 hours after cataract surgery and continuing throughout the first 2 weeks of the post operative period.

Corneal Refractive Surgery: One or two drops of Voltaren Ophthalmic should be applied to the operative eye within the hour prior to corneal refractive surgery. Within 15 minutes after surgery, one or two drops should be applied to the operative eye and continued 4 times daily for up to 3 days.

HOW SUPPLIED

Voltaren Ophthalmic 0.1% (1 mg/mL) Sterile Solution is supplied in a low density polyethylene (LDPE) white bottle with a LDPE Dropper Tip and Polypropylene grey closure. The 2.5 mL fill is supplied in a 7.5 mL size bottle. The 5.0 mL fill is supplied in a 10.0 mL size bottle.

Bottles of 2.5 mL	NDC 58768-100-02
Bottles of 5 mL	NDC 58768-100-05

Store at 15°C to 25°C (59° to 77°F).

Dispense in original, unopened container only.

Printed in Canada

Made in Canada. Manufactured for:

Novartis Ophthalmics, Duluth, Georgia 30097

CS 665635G September, 2003

ZADITOR™ ℞

[za-di-tor]

Ketotifen Fumarate Ophthalmic Solution, 0.025%

Rx only

Prescribing Information

The following prescribing information is based on official labeling in effect July 2004.

DESCRIPTION

ZADITOR™ is a sterile ophthalmic solution containing ketotifen for topical administration to the eyes. Ketotifen fumarate is a finely crystalline powder with an empirical formula of $C_{23}H_{23}NO_5S$ and a molecular weight of 425.50.

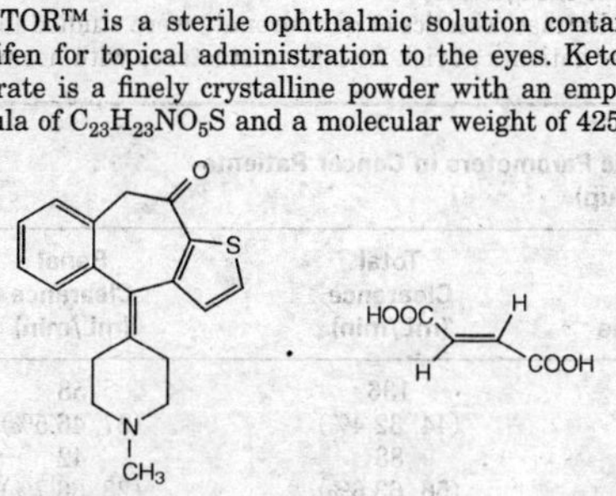

Established Name

ketotifen fumarate ophthalmic solution

CHEMICAL NAME

4-(1-Methyl-4-piperidylidene)-4*H*-benzo[4,5]cyclohepta[1,2-*b*] thiophen-10(9*H*)-one hydrogen fumarate

Each mL of ZADITOR™ contains:

Active: 0.345 mg ketotifen fumarate equivalent to 0.25 mg ketotifen.

Inactives: glycerol, sodium hydroxide/hydrochloric acid (to adjust pH) and purified water.

Preservative: benzalkonium chloride 0.01%. It has a pH of 4.4 to 5.8 and an osmolality of 210-300 mOsm/kg.

CLINICAL PHARMACOLOGY

Ketotifen is a relatively selective, non-competitive histamine antagonist (H1-receptor) and mast cell stabilizer. Ketotifen inhibits the release of mediators from cells involved in hypersensitivity reactions. Decreased chemotaxis and activation of eosinophils has also been demonstrated. Ketotifen has been shown to have little systemic exposure following topical ocular administration. A study conducted with 15 healthy volunteers dosed bilaterally with ketotifen fumarate ophthalmic solution twice daily for 14 days demonstrated plasma concentrations generally below the quantitation limit of assay (< 20 pg/mL).

In human conjunctival allergen challenge studies, ZADITOR™ was significantly more effective than placebo in preventing ocular itching associated with allergic conjunctivitis. The action of ketotifen occurs rapidly with an effect seen within minutes after administration.

INDICATIONS AND USAGE

ZADITOR™ (ketotifen fumarate ophthalmic solution) is indicated for the temporary prevention of itching of the eye due to allergic conjunctivitis.

CONTRAINDICATIONS

ZADITOR™ is contraindicated in persons with a known hypersensitivity to any component of this product.

WARNINGS

For topical ophthalmic use only. Not for injection or oral use.

PRECAUTIONS

Information for patients

To prevent contaminating the dropper tip and solution, care should be taken not to touch the eyelids or surrounding areas with the dropper tip of the bottle. Keep the bottle tightly closed when not in use. Patients should be advised not to wear a contact lens if their eye is red. ZADITOR™ should not be used to treat contact lens related irritation. The preservative in ZADITOR™, benzalkonium chloride, may be absorbed by soft contact lenses. Patients who wear soft contact lenses and whose eyes are not red, should be instructed to wait at least ten minutes after instilling ZADITOR™ before they insert their contact lenses.

Carcinogenesis, Mutagenesis, Impairment of Fertility

Ketotifen fumarate was determined to be non-mutagenic in a battery of *in vitro* and *in vivo* mutagenicity assays including: Ames test, *in vitro* chromosomal aberration test with V79 Chinese hamster cells, *in vivo* micronucleus assay in mouse, and mouse dominant lethal test.

Treatment of male rats with oral doses of ketotifen ≥ 10 mg/kg/day orally [6,667 times the maximum recommended human ocular dose of 0.0015 mg/kg/day on a mg/kg basis (MRHOD)] for 70 days prior to mating resulted in mortality and a decrease in fertility. Treatment with ketotifen did not impair fertility in female rats receiving up to 50 mg/kg/day of ketotifen orally (33,333 times the MRHOD) for 15 days prior to mating.

Pregnancy: Pregnancy Category C

Oral treatment of pregnant rabbits during organogenesis with 45 mg/kg/day of ketotifen (30,000 times the MRHOD) resulted in an increased incidence of retarded ossification of the sternebrae. However, no effects were observed in rabbits treated with up to 15 mg/kg/day (10,000 times the MRHOD). Similar treatment of rats during organogenesis with 100 mg/kg/day of ketotifen (66,667 times the MRHOD) did not reveal any biologically relevant effects.

Oral treatment of pregnant rats (up to 100 mg/kg/day or 66,667 times the MRHOD) and rabbits (up to 45 mg/kg/day or 30,000 times the MRHOD) during organogenesis did not result in any biologically relevant embryofetal toxicity. In the offspring of the rats that received ketotifen orally from day 15 of pregnancy to day 21 post partum at 50 mg/kg/day (33,333 times the MRHOD), a maternally toxic treatment protocol, the incidence of postnatal mortality was slightly increased, and body weight gain during the first four days post partum was slightly decreased.

Nursing Mothers

Ketotifen fumarate has been identified in breast milk in rats following oral administration. It is not known whether topical ocular administration could result in sufficient systemic absorption to produce detectable quantities in breast milk. Nevertheless, caution should be exercised when ketotifen fumarate is administered to a nursing mother.

Pediatric Use

Safety and effectiveness in pediatric patients below the age of 3 years have not been established.

ADVERSE REACTIONS

In controlled clinical studies, conjunctival injection, headaches, and rhinitis were reported at an incidence of 10 to 25%. The occurrence of these side effects was generally mild. Some of these events were similar to the underlying ocular disease being studied.

The following ocular and non-ocular adverse reactions were reported at an incidence of less than 5%:

Continued on next page

Zaditor—Cont.

Ocular: Allergic reactions, burning or stinging, conjunctivitis, discharge, dry eyes, eye pain, eyelid disorder, itching, keratitis, lacrimation disorder, mydriasis, photophobia, and rash.
Non-Ocular: Flu syndrome, pharyngitis.

OVERDOSAGE

Oral ingestion of the contents of a 5 mL bottle would be equivalent to 1.725 mg of ketotifen fumarate. Clinical results have shown no serious signs or symptoms after the ingestion of up to 20 mg of ketotifen fumarate.

DOSAGE AND ADMINISTRATION

The recommended dose is one drop in the affected eye(s) twice daily, every 8 to 12 hours.

HOW SUPPLIED

ZADITOR 5 mL .... NDC 58768-102-05
is supplied in a white Polypropylene (PP) 7.5 cc container with a PP dropper tip and closure.
ZADITOR 1 mL .... NDC 58768-102-99
is supplied in a white Low Density Polypropylene (LDPE) 3.0 cc container with a LDPE dropper tip and PP closure.

STORAGE
Store at 4°-25°C (39°-77°F)
Made in Canada by CIBA Vision Sterile Mfg.
for Novartis Ophthalmics
Duluth, GA 30097
I6137-E October, 2002
Shown in Product Identification Guide, page 324

Novartis Pharmaceuticals Corporation

Novartis Pharmaceuticals Corporation
One Health Plaza
East Hanover, NJ 07936
(for branded products)

For Information Contact *(branded products)*:
Customer Response Department
(888) NOW-NOVARTIS [888-669-6682]

http: //www.novartis.com

AREDIA® ℞

[ă-rē-dēă]
(pamidronate disodium for injection)
For Intravenous Infusion
Rx only

Prescribing Information
The following prescribing information is based on official labeling in effect July 2004.

DESCRIPTION

Aredia, pamidronate disodium (APD), is a bone-resorption inhibitor available in 30-mg or 90-mg vials for intravenous administration. Each 30-mg, and 90-mg vial contains, respectively, 30 mg and 90 mg of sterile, lyophilized pamidronate disodium and 470 mg and 375 mg of mannitol, USP. The pH of a 1% solution of pamidronate disodium in distilled water is approximately 8.3. Aredia, a member of the group of chemical compounds known as bisphosphonates, is an analog of pyrophosphate. Pamidronate disodium is designated chemically as phosphonic acid (3-amino-1-hydroxypropylidene) bis-, disodium salt, pentahydrate, (APD), and its structural formula is

$$PO_3HNa$$
$$NH_2-CH_2-CH_2-C-OH \bullet 5H_2O$$
$$PO_3HNa$$

Pamidronate disodium is a white-to-practically-white powder. It is soluble in water and in 2N sodium hydroxide, sparingly soluble in 0.1N hydrochloric acid and in 0.1N acetic acid, and practically insoluble in organic solvents. Its molecular formula is $C_3H_9NO_7P_2Na_2 \bullet 5H_2O$ and its molecular weight is 369.1.

Inactive Ingredients. Mannitol, USP, and phosphoric acid (for adjustment to pH 6.5 prior to lyophilization).

CLINICAL PHARMACOLOGY

The principal pharmacologic action of Aredia is inhibition of bone resorption. Although the mechanism of antiresorptive action is not completely understood, several factors are thought to contribute to this action. Aredia adsorbs to calcium phosphate (hydroxyapatite) crystals in bone and may directly block dissolution of this mineral component of bone. *In vitro* studies also suggest that inhibition of osteoclast activity contributes to inhibition of bone resorption. In animal studies, at doses recommended for the treatment of hypercalcemia, Aredia inhibits bone resorption apparently without inhibiting bone formation and mineralization. Of relevance to the treatment of hypercalcemia of malignancy is the finding that Aredia inhibits the accelerated bone resorption that results from osteoclast hyperactivity induced by various tumors in animal studies.

Pharmacokinetics
Cancer patients (n=24) who had minimal or no bony involvement were given an intravenous infusion of 30, 60, or 90 mg of Aredia over 4 hours and 90 mg of Aredia over 24 hours *(Table 1)*.

Distribution
The mean ± SD body retention of pamidronate was calculated to be 54 ± 16% of the dose over 120 hours.

Metabolism
Pamidronate is not metabolized and is exclusively eliminated by renal excretion.

Excretion
After administration of 30, 60, and 90 mg of Aredia over 4 hours, and 90 mg of Aredia over 24 hours, an overall mean ± SD of 46 ± 16% of the drug was excreted unchanged in the urine within 120 hours. Cumulative urinary excretion was linearly related to dose. The mean ± SD elimination half-life is 28 ± 7 hours. Mean ± SD total and renal clearances of pamidronate were 107 ± 50 mL/min and 49 ± 28 mL/min, respectively. The rate of elimination from bone has not been determined.

Special Populations
There are no data available on the effects of age, gender, or race on the pharmacokinetics of pamidronate.

Pediatric
Pamidronate is not labeled for use in the pediatric population.

Renal Insufficiency
The pharmacokinetics of pamidronate were studied in cancer patients (n=19) with normal and varying degrees of renal impairment. Each patient received a single 90-mg dose of Aredia infused over 4 hours. The renal clearance of pamidronate in patients was found to closely correlate with creatinine clearance *(see Figure 1)*. A trend toward a lower percentage of drug excreted unchanged in urine was observed in renally impaired patients. Adverse experiences noted were not found to be related to changes in renal clearance of pamidronate. Given the recommended dose, 90 mg infused over 4 hours, excessive accumulation of pamidronate in renally impaired patients is not anticipated if Aredia is administered on a monthly basis.

Figure 1: Pamidronate renal clearance as a function of creatinine clearance in patients with normal and impaired renal function. The lines are the mean prediction line and 95% confidence intervals.

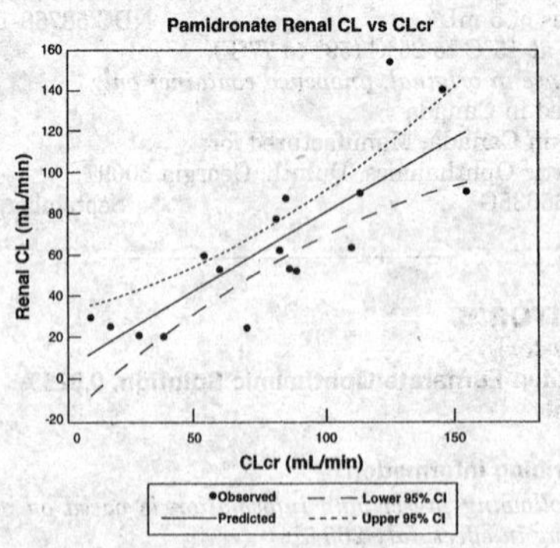

Hepatic Insufficiency
The pharmacokinetics of pamidronate were studied in male cancer patients at risk for bone metastases with normal hepatic function (n=6) and mild to moderate hepatic dysfunction (n=7). Each patient received a single 90-mg dose of Aredia infused over 4 hours. Although there was a statistically significant difference in the pharmacokinetics between patients with normal and impaired hepatic function, the difference was not considered clinically relevant. Patients with hepatic impairment exhibited higher mean AUC (53%) and C_{max} (29%), and decreased plasma clearance (33%) values. Nevertheless, pamidronate was still rapidly cleared from the plasma. Drug levels were not detectable in patients by 12 to 36 hours after drug infusion. Because Aredia is administered on a monthly basis, drug accumulation is not expected. No changes in Aredia dosing regimen are recommended for patients with mild to moderate abnormal hepatic function. Aredia has not been studied in patients with severe hepatic impairment.

Drug-Drug Interactions
There are no human pharmacokinetic data for drug interactions with Aredia.
[See table 1 below]
After intravenous administration of radiolabeled in rats, approximately 50%-60% of the compound was rapidly adsorbed by bone and slowly eliminated from the body by the kidneys. In rats given 10 mg/kg bolus injections of radiolabeled Aredia, approximately 30% of the compound was found in the liver shortly after administration and was then redistributed to bone or eliminated by the kidneys over 24-48 hours. Studies in rats injected with radiolabeled Aredia showed that the compound was rapidly cleared from the circulation and taken up mainly by bones, liver, spleen, teeth, and tracheal cartilage. Radioactivity was eliminated from most soft tissues within 1-4 days; was detectable in liver and spleen for 1 and 3 months, respectively; and remained high in bones, trachea, and teeth for 6 months after dosing. Bone uptake occurred preferentially in areas of high bone turnover. The terminal phase of elimination half-life in bone was estimated to be approximately 300 days.

Pharmacodynamics
Serum phosphate levels have been noted to decrease after administration of Aredia, presumably because of decreased release of phosphate from bone and increased renal excretion as parathyroid hormone levels, which are usually suppressed in hypercalcemia associated with malignancy, return toward normal. Phosphate therapy was administered in 30% of the patients in response to a decrease in serum phosphate levels. Phosphate levels usually returned toward normal within 7–10 days.
Urinary calcium/creatinine and urinary hydroxyproline/creatinine ratios decrease and usually return to within or below normal after treatment with Aredia. These changes occur within the first week after treatment, as do decreases in serum calcium levels, and are consistent with an antiresorptive pharmacologic action.

Hypercalcemia of Malignancy
Osteoclastic hyperactivity resulting in excessive bone resorption is the underlying pathophysiologic derangement in metastatic bone disease and hypercalcemia of malignancy. Excessive release of calcium into the blood as bone is resorbed results in polyuria and gastrointestinal disturbances, with progressive dehydration and decreasing glomerular filtration rate. This, in turn, results in increased renal resorption of calcium, setting up a cycle of worsening systemic hypercalcemia. Correction of excessive bone resorption and adequate fluid administration to correct volume deficits are therefore essential to the management of hypercalcemia.
Most cases of hypercalcemia associated with malignancy occur in patients who have breast cancer; squamous-cell tumors of the lung or head and neck; renal-cell carcinoma; and certain hematologic malignancies, such as multiple myeloma and some types of lymphomas. A few less-common malignancies, including vasoactive intestinal-peptide-producing tumors and cholangiocarcinoma, have a high incidence of hypercalcemia as a metabolic complication. Patients who have hypercalcemia of malignancy can generally be divided into two groups, according to the pathophysiologic mechanism involved.
In humoral hypercalcemia, osteoclasts are activated and bone resorption is stimulated by factors such as parathyroid-hormone-related protein, which are elaborated by the tumor and circulate systemically. Humoral hypercalcemia usually occurs in squamous-cell malignancies of the lung or head and neck or in genitourinary tumors such as renal-cell carcinoma or ovarian cancer. Skeletal metastases may be absent or minimal in these patients.
Extensive invasion of bone by tumor cells can also result in hypercalcemia due to local tumor products that stimulate bone resorption by osteoclasts. Tumors commonly associated with locally mediated hypercalcemia include breast cancer and multiple myeloma.
Total serum calcium levels in patients who have hypercalcemia of malignancy may not reflect the severity of hypercalcemia, since concomitant hypoalbuminemia is commonly present. Ideally, ionized calcium levels should be used to diagnose and follow hypercalcemic conditions; however, these are not commonly or rapidly available in many clinical situations. Therefore, adjustment of the total serum calcium value for differences in albumin levels is often used in place of measurement of ionized calcium; several nomograms are in use for this type of calculation *(see DOSAGE AND ADMINISTRATION)*.

Clinical Trials
In one double-blind clinical trial, 52 patients who had hypercalcemia of malignancy were enrolled to receive 30 mg,

Table 1
Mean (SD, CV%) Pamidronate Pharmacokinetic Parameters in Cancer Patients
(n=6 for each group)

Dose (infusion rate)	Maximum Concentration (µg/mL)	Percent of dose excreted in urine	Total Clearance (mL/min)	Renal Clearance (mL/min)
30 mg (4 hrs)	0.73 (0.14, 19.1%)	43.9 (14.0, 31.9%)	136 (44, 32.4%)	58 (27, 46.5%)
60 mg (4 hrs)	1.44 (0.57, 39.6%)	47.4 (47.4, 54.4%)	88 (56, 63.6%)	42 (28, 66.7%)
90 mg (4 hrs)	2.61 (0.74, 28.3%)	45.3 (25.8, 56.9%)	103 (37, 35.9%)	44 (16, 36.4%)
90 mg (24 hrs)	1.38 (1.97, 142.7%)	47.5 (10.2, 21.5%)	101 (58, 57.4%)	52 (42, 80.8%)

60 mg, or 90 mg of Aredia as a single 24-hour intravenous infusion if their corrected serum calcium levels were ≥12.0 mg/dL after 48 hours of saline hydration.
The mean baseline-corrected serum calcium for the 30-mg, 60-mg, and 90-mg groups were 13.8 mg/dL, 13.8 mg/dL, and 13.3 mg/dL, respectively.
The majority of patients (64%) had decreases in albumin-corrected serum calcium levels by 24 hours after initiation of treatment. Mean-corrected serum calcium levels at days 2-7 after initiation of treatment with Aredia were significantly reduced from baseline in all three dosage groups. As a result, by 7 days after initiation of treatment with Aredia, 40%, 61%, and 100% of the patients receiving 30 mg, 60 mg, and 90 mg of Aredia, respectively, had normal-corrected serum calcium levels. Many patients (33%-53%) in the 60-mg and 90-mg dosage groups continued to have normal-corrected serum calcium levels, or a partial response (≥15% decrease of corrected serum calcium from baseline), at day 14.
In a second double-blind, controlled clinical trial, 65 cancer patients who had corrected serum calcium levels of ≥12.0 mg/dL after at least 24 hours of saline hydration were randomized to receive either 60 mg of Aredia as a single 24-hour intravenous infusion or 7.5 mg/kg of etidronate disodium as a 2-hour intravenous infusion daily for 3 days. Thirty patients were randomized to receive Aredia and 35 to receive etidronate disodium.
The mean baseline-corrected serum calcium for the Aredia 60-mg and etidronate disodium groups were 14.6 mg/dL and 13.8 mg/dL, respectively.
By day 7, 70% of the patients in the Aredia group and 41% of the patients in the etidronate disodium group had normal-corrected serum calcium levels (P<0.05). When partial responders (≥15% decrease of serum calcium from baseline) were also included, the response rates were 97% for the Aredia group and 65% for the etidronate disodium group (P<0.01). Mean-corrected serum calcium for the Aredia and etidronate disodium groups decreased from baseline values to 10.4 and 11.2 mg/dL, respectively, on day 7. At day 14, 43% of patients in the Aredia group and 18% of patients in the etidronate disodium group still had normal-corrected serum calcium levels, or maintenance of a partial response. For responders in the Aredia and etidronate disodium groups, the median duration of response was similar (7 and 5 days, respectively). The time course of effect on corrected serum calcium is summarized in the following table.

Change in Corrected Serum Calcium by Time from Initiation of Treatment

Time (hr)	Mean Change from Baseline in Corrected Serum Calcium (mg/dL)		
	Aredia®	Etidronate Disodium	P-Value[1]
Baseline	14.6	13.8	
24	-0.3	-0.5	
48	-1.5	-1.1	
72	-2.6	-2.0	
96	-3.5	-2.0	<0.01
168	-4.1	-2.5	<0.01

[1]Comparison between treatment groups

In a third multicenter, randomized, parallel double-blind trial, a group of 69 cancer patients with hypercalcemia was enrolled to receive 60 mg of Aredia as a 4- or 24-hour infusion, which was compared to a saline treatment group. Patients who had a corrected serum calcium level of ≥12.0 mg/dL after 24 hours of saline hydration were eligible for this trial.
The mean baseline-corrected serum calcium levels for Aredia 60-mg 4-hour infusion, Aredia 60-mg 24-hour infusion, and saline infusion were 14.2 mg/dL, 13.7 mg/dL, and 13.7 mg/dL, respectively.
By day 7 after initiation of treatment, 78%, 61%, and 22% of the patients had normal-corrected serum calcium levels for the 60-mg 4-hour infusion, 60-mg 24-hour infusion, and saline infusion, respectively. At day 14, 39% of the patients in the Aredia 60-mg 4-hour infusion group and 26% of the patients in the Aredia 60-mg 24-hour infusion group had normal-corrected serum calcium levels or maintenance of a partial response.
For responders, the median duration of complete responses was 4 days and 6.5 days for Aredia 60-mg 4-hour infusion and Aredia 60-mg 24-hour infusion, respectively.
In all three trials, patients treated with Aredia had similar response rates in the presence or absence of bone metastases. Concomitant administration of furosemide did not affect response rates.
Thirty-two patients who had recurrent or refractory hypercalcemia of malignancy were given a second course of 60 mg of Aredia over a 4- or 24-hour period. Of these, 41% showed a complete response and 16% showed a partial response to the retreatment, and these responders had about a 3-mg/dL fall in mean-corrected serum calcium levels 7 days after retreatment.
In a fourth multicenter, randomized, double-blind trial, 103 patients with cancer and hypercalcemia (corrected serum calcium ≥12.0 mg/dL) received 90 mg of Aredia as a 2-hour infusion. The mean baseline corrected serum calcium was 14.0 mg/dL. Patients were not required to receive IV hydration prior to drug administration, but all subjects did receive at least 500 mL of IV saline hydration concomitantly with the pamidronate infusion. By Day 10 after drug infusion, 70% of patients had normal corrected serum calcium levels (<10.8 mg/dL).

	Breast Cancer Patients Receiving Chemotherapy						Breast Cancer Patients Receiving Hormonal Therapy					
	Any SRE		Radiation		Fractures		Any SRE		Radiation		Fractures	
	A	P	A	P	A	P	A	P	A	P	A	P
N	185	195	185	195	185	195	182	189	182	189	182	189
Skeletal Morbidity Rate (#SRE/year) Mean	2.5	3.7	0.8	1.3	1.6	2.2	2.4	3.6	0.6	1.2	1.6	2.2
P-Value	<.001		<.001[†]		.018[†]		.021		.013[†]		.040[†]	
Proportion of patients having an SRE	46%	65%	28%	45%	36%	49%	55%	63%	31%	40%	45%	55%
P-Value	<.001		<.001[†]		.014[†]		.094		.058[†]		.054[†]	
Median Time to SRE (months)	13.9	7.0	NR**	14.2	25.8	13.3	10.9	7.4	NR**	23.4	20.6	12.8
P-Value	<.001		<.001[†]		.009[†]		.118		.016[†]		.113[†]	

[†]Fractures and radiation to bone were two of several secondary endpoints. The statistical significance of these analyses may be overestimated since numerous analyses were performed.
**NR = Not Reached.

Paget's Disease
Paget's disease of bone (osteitis deformans) is an idiopathic disease characterized by chronic, focal areas of bone destruction complicated by concurrent excessive bone repair, affecting one or more bones. These changes result in thickened but weakened bones that may fracture or bend under stress. Signs and symptoms may be bone pain, deformity, fractures, neurological disorders resulting from cranial and spinal nerve entrapment and from spinal cord and brain stem compression, increased cardiac output to the involved bone, increased serum alkaline phosphatase levels (reflecting increased bone formation) and/or urine hydroxyproline excretion (reflecting increased bone resorption).
Clinical Trials
In one double-blind clinical trial, 64 patients with moderate to severe Paget's disease of bone were enrolled to receive 5 mg, 15 mg, or 30 mg of Aredia as a single 4-hour infusion on 3 consecutive days, for total doses of 15 mg, 45 mg, and 90 mg of Aredia.
The mean baseline serum alkaline phosphatase levels were 1409 U/L, 983 U/L, and 1085 U/L, and the mean baseline urine hydroxyproline/creatinine ratios were 0.25, 0.19, and 0.19 for the 15-mg, 45-mg, and 90-mg groups, respectively.
The effects of Aredia on serum alkaline phosphatase (SAP) and urine hydroxyproline/creatinine ratios (UOHP/C) are summarized in the following table:

Percent of Patients With Significant % Decreases in SAP and UOHP/C

	SAP			UOHP/C		
% Decrease	15 mg	45 mg	90 mg	15 mg	45 mg	90 mg
≥50	26	33	60	15	47	72
≥30	40	65	83	35	57	85

The median maximum percent decreases from baseline in serum alkaline phosphatase and urine hydroxyproline/creatinine ratios were 25%, 41%, and 57%, and 25%, 47%, and 61% for the 15-mg, 45-mg, and 90-mg groups, respectively. The median time to response (≥50% decrease) for serum alkaline phosphatase was approximately 1 month for the 90-mg group, and the response duration ranged from 1 to 372 days.
No statistically significant differences between treatment groups, or statistically significant changes from baseline were observed for the bone pain response, mobility, and global evaluation in the 45-mg and 90-mg groups. Improvement in radiologic lesions occurred in some patients in the 90-mg group.
Twenty-five patients who had Paget's disease were retreated with 90 mg of Aredia. Of these, 44% had a ≥50% decrease in serum alkaline phosphatase from baseline after treatment, and 39% had a ≥50% decrease in urine hydroxyproline/creatinine ratio from baseline after treatment.
Osteolytic Bone Metastases of Breast Cancer and Osteolytic Lesions of Multiple Myeloma
Osteolytic bone metastases commonly occur in patients with multiple myeloma or breast cancer. These cancers demonstrate a phenomenon known as osteotropism, meaning they possess an extraordinary affinity for bone. The distribution of osteolytic bone metastases in these cancers is predominantly in the axial skeleton, particularly the spine, pelvis, and ribs, rather than the appendicular skeleton, although lesions in the proximal femur and humerus are not uncommon. This distribution is similar to the red bone marrow in which slow blood flow possibly assists attachment of metastatic cells. The surface-to-volume ratio of trabecular bone is much higher than cortical bone, and therefore disease processes tend to occur more floridly in trabecular bone than at sites of cortical tissue.
These bone changes can result in patients having evidence of osteolytic skeletal destruction leading to severe bone pain that requires either radiation therapy or narcotic analgesics (or both) for symptomatic relief. These changes also cause pathologic fractures of bone in both the axial and appendicular skeleton. Axial skeletal fractures of the vertebral bodies may lead to spinal cord compression or vertebral body collapse with significant neurologic complications. Also, patients may experience episode(s) of hypercalcemia.
Clinical Trials
In a double-blind, randomized, placebo-controlled trial, 392 patients with advanced multiple myeloma were enrolled to receive Aredia or placebo in addition to their underlying antimyeloma therapy to determine the effect of Aredia on the occurrence of skeletal-related events (SREs). SREs were defined as episodes of pathologic fractures, radiation therapy to bone, surgery to bone, and spinal cord compression. Patients received either 90 mg of Aredia or placebo as a monthly 4-hour intravenous infusion for 9 months. Of the 392 patients, 377 were evaluable for efficacy (196 Aredia, 181 placebo). The proportion of patients developing any SRE was significantly smaller in the Aredia group (24% vs 41%, P<0.001), and the mean skeletal morbidity rate (#SRE/year) was significantly smaller for Aredia patients than for placebo patients (mean: 1.1 vs 2.1, P<.02). The times to the first SRE occurrence, pathologic fracture, and radiation to bone were significantly longer in the Aredia group (P=.001, .006, and .046, respectively). Moreover, fewer Aredia patients suffered any pathologic fracture (17% vs 30%, P=.004) or needed radiation to bone (14% vs 22%, P=.049).
In addition, decreases in pain scores from baseline occurred at the last measurement for those Aredia patients with pain at baseline (P=.026) but not in the placebo group. At the last measurement, a worsening from baseline was observed in the placebo group for the Spitzer quality of life variable (P<.001) and ECOG performance status (P<.011) while there was no significant deterioration from baseline in these parameters observed in Aredia-treated patients.*
After 21 months, the proportion of patients experiencing any skeletal event remained significantly smaller in the Aredia group than the placebo group (P=.015). In addition, the mean skeletal morbidity rate (#SRE/year) was 1.3 vs 2.2 for Aredia patients vs placebo patients (P=.008), and time to first SRE was significantly longer in the Aredia group compared to placebo (P=.016). Fewer Aredia patients suffered vertebral pathologic fractures (16% vs 27%, P=.005). Survival of all patients was not different between treatment groups.
Two double-blind, randomized, placebo-controlled trials compared the safety and efficacy of 90 mg of Aredia infused over 2 hours every 3 to 4 weeks for 24 months to that of placebo in preventing SREs in breast cancer patients with osteolytic bone metastases who had one or more predominantly lytic metastases of at least 1 cm in diameter: one in patients being treated with antineoplastic chemotherapy and the second in patients being treated with hormonal antineoplastic therapy at trial entry.
382 patients receiving chemotherapy were randomized, 185 to Aredia and 197 to placebo. 372 patients receiving hormonal therapy were randomized, 182 to Aredia and 190 to placebo. All but three patients were evaluable for efficacy. Patients were followed for 24 months of therapy or until they went off study. Median duration of follow-up was 13 months in patients receiving chemotherapy and 17 months in patients receiving hormone therapy. Twenty-five percent of the patients in the chemotherapy study and 37% of the patients in the hormone therapy study received Aredia for 24 months. The efficacy results are shown in the table below:
[See first table above]
Bone lesion response was radiographically assessed at baseline and at 3, 6, and 12 months. The complete + partial response rate was 33% in Aredia patients and 18% in placebo patients treated with chemotherapy (P=.001). No difference was seen between Aredia and placebo in hormonally-treated patients.
Pain and analgesic scores, ECOG performance status and Spitzer quality of life index were measured at baseline and

Continued on next page

Aredia—Cont.

periodically during the trials. The changes from baseline to the last measurement carried forward are shown in the following table:
[See table below]

INDICATIONS AND USAGE

Hypercalcemia of Malignancy
Aredia, in conjunction with adequate hydration, is indicated for the treatment of moderate or severe hypercalcemia associated with malignancy, with or without bone metastases. Patients who have either epidermoid or non-epidermoid tumors respond to treatment with Aredia. Vigorous saline hydration, an integral part of hypercalcemia therapy, should be initiated promptly and an attempt should be made to restore the urine output to about 2 L/day throughout treatment. Mild or asymptomatic hypercalcemia may be treated with conservative measures (i.e., saline hydration, with or without loop diuretics). Patients should be hydrated adequately throughout the treatment, but overhydration, especially in those patients who have cardiac failure, must be avoided. Diuretic therapy should not be employed prior to correction of hypovolemia. The safety and efficacy of Aredia in the treatment of hypercalcemia associated with hyperparathyroidism or with other non-tumor-related conditions has not been established.

Paget's Disease
Aredia is indicated for the treatment of patients with moderate to severe Paget's disease of bone. The effectiveness of Aredia was demonstrated primarily in patients with serum alkaline phosphatase ≥3 times the upper limit of normal. Aredia therapy in patients with Paget's disease has been effective in reducing serum alkaline phosphatase and urinary hydroxyproline levels by ≥50% in at least 50% of patients, and by ≥30% in at least 80% of patients. Aredia therapy has also been effective in reducing these biochemical markers in patients with Paget's disease who failed to respond, or no longer responded to other treatments.

Osteolytic Bone Metastases of Breast Cancer and Osteolytic Lesions of Multiple Myeloma
Aredia is indicated, in conjunction with standard antineoplastic therapy, for the treatment of osteolytic bone metastases of breast cancer and osteolytic lesions of multiple myeloma. The Aredia treatment effect appeared to be smaller in the study of breast cancer patients receiving hormonal therapy than in the study of those receiving chemotherapy, however, overall evidence of clinical benefit has been demonstrated *(see CLINICAL PHARMACOLOGY, Osteolytic Bone Metastases of Breast Cancer and Osteolytic Lesions of Multiple Myeloma, Clinical Trials section).*

CONTRAINDICATIONS

Aredia is contraindicated in patients with clinically significant hypersensitivity to Aredia or other bisphosphonates.

WARNINGS

DUE TO THE RISK OF CLINICALLY SIGNIFICANT DETERIORATION IN RENAL FUNCTION, WHICH MAY PROGRESS TO RENAL FAILURE, SINGLE DOSES OF AREDIA SHOULD NOT EXCEED 90 MG *(see DOSAGE AND ADMINISTRATION for appropriate infusion durations).*
Bisphosphonates, including Aredia, have been associated with renal toxicity manifested as deterioration of renal function and potential renal failure.
Patients who receive Aredia should have serum creatinine assessed prior to each treatment. Patients treated with Aredia for bone metastases should have the dose withheld if renal function has deteriorated. *(See DOSAGE AND ADMINISTRATION.)*
In both rats and dogs, nephropathy has been associated with intravenous (bolus and infusion) administration of Aredia.
Two 7-day intravenous infusion studies were conducted in the dog wherein Aredia was given for 1, 4, or 24 hours at doses of 1-20 mg/kg for up to 7 days. In the first study, the compound was well tolerated at 3 mg/kg (1.7 × highest recommended human dose [HRHD] for a single intravenous infusion) when administered for 4 or 24 hours, but renal findings such as elevated BUN and creatinine levels and renal tubular necrosis occurred when 3 mg/kg was infused for 1 hour and at doses of ≥10 mg/kg. In the second study, slight renal tubular necrosis was observed in 1 male at 1 mg/kg when infused for 4 hours. Additional findings included elevated BUN levels in several treated animals and renal tubular dilation and/or inflammation at ≥1 mg/kg after each infusion time.
Aredia was given to rats at doses of 2, 6, and 20 mg/kg and to dogs at doses of 2, 4, 6, and 20 mg/kg as a 1-hour infusion, once a week, for 3 months followed by a 1-month recovery period. In rats, nephrotoxicity was observed at ≥6 mg/kg and included increased BUN and creatinine levels and tubular degeneration and necrosis. These findings were still present at 20 mg/kg at the end of the recovery period. In dogs, moribundity/death and renal toxicity occurred at 20 mg/kg as did kidney findings of elevated BUN and creatinine levels at ≥6 mg/kg and renal tubular degeneration at ≥4 mg/kg. The kidney changes were partially reversible at 6 mg/kg. In both studies, the dose level that produced no adverse renal effects was considered to be 2 mg/kg (1.1 × HRHD for a single intravenous infusion).

PREGNANCY: AREDIA SHOULD NOT BE USED DURING PREGNANCY
Aredia may cause fetal harm when administered to a pregnant woman. *(See PRECAUTIONS, Pregnancy Category D.)* There are no studies in pregnant women using Aredia. If the patient becomes pregnant while taking this drug, the patient should be apprised of the potential harm to the fetus. Women of childbearing potential should be advised to avoid becoming pregnant.
Studies conducted in young rats have reported the disruption of dental dentine formation following single- and multi-dose administration of bisphosphonates. The clinical significance of these findings is unknown.

PRECAUTIONS

General
Standard hypercalcemia-related metabolic parameters, such as serum levels of calcium, phosphate, magnesium, and potassium, should be carefully monitored following initiation of therapy with Aredia. Cases of asymptomatic hypophosphatemia (12%), hypokalemia (7%), hypomagnesemia (11%), and hypocalcemia (5%-12%), were reported in Aredia-treated patients. Rare cases of symptomatic hypocalcemia (including tetany) have been reported in association with Aredia therapy. If hypocalcemia occurs, short-term calcium therapy may be necessary. In Paget's disease of bone, 17% of patients treated with 90 mg of Aredia showed serum calcium levels below 8 mg/dL.

Renal Insufficiency
Aredia is excreted intact primarily via the kidney, and the risk of renal adverse reactions may be greater in patients with impaired renal function. Patients who receive Aredia should have serum creatinine assessed prior to each treatment. In patients receiving Aredia for bone metastases, who show evidence of deterioration in renal function, Aredia treatment should be withheld until renal function returns to baseline *(see WARNINGS and DOSAGE AND ADMINISTRATION).*
Aredia has not been tested in patients who have class Dc renal impairment (creatinine >5.0 mg/dL), and has been tested in few multiple myeloma patients with serum creatinine ≥3.0 mg/dL. *(See also CLINICAL PHARMACOLOGY, Pharmacokinetics.)* For the treatment of bone metastases, the use of Aredia in patients with severe renal impairment is not recommended. In other indications, clinical judgment should determine whether the potential benefit outweighs the potential risk in such patients.

Laboratory Tests
Patients who receive Aredia should have serum creatinine assessed prior to each treatment. Serum calcium, electrolytes, phosphate, magnesium, and CBC, differential, and hematocrit/hemoglobin must be closely monitored in patients treated with Aredia. Patients who have preexisting anemia, leukopenia, or thrombocytopenia should be monitored carefully in the first 2 weeks following treatment.

Drug Interactions
Concomitant administration of a loop diuretic had no effect on the calcium-lowering action of Aredia.
Caution is indicated when Aredia is used with other potentially nephrotoxic drugs.

Carcinogenesis, Mutagenesis, Impairment of Fertility
In a 104-week carcinogenicity study (daily oral administration) in rats, there was a positive dose response relationship for benign adrenal pheochromocytoma in males (P <0.00001). Although this condition was also observed in females, the incidence was not statistically significant. When the dose calculations were adjusted to account for the limited oral bioavailability of Aredia in rats, the lowest daily dose associated with adrenal pheochromocytoma was similar to the intended clinical dose. Adrenal pheochromocytoma was also observed in low numbers in the control animals and is considered a relatively common spontaneous neoplasm in the rat. Aredia (daily oral administration) was not carcinogenic in an 80-week study in mice.
Aredia was nonmutagenic in six mutagenicity assays: Ames test, *Salmonella* and *Escherichia*/liver-microsome test, nucleus-anomaly test, sister-chromatid-exchange study, point-mutation test, and micronucleus test in the rat.
In rats, decreased fertility occurred in first-generation offspring of parents who had received 150 mg/kg of Aredia orally; however, this occurred only when animals were mated with members of the same dose group. Aredia has not been administered intravenously in such a study.

Pregnancy Category D *(See WARNINGS)*
There are no adequate and well-controlled studies in pregnant women.
Bolus intravenous studies conducted in rats and rabbits determined that Aredia produces maternal toxicity and embryo/fetal effects when given during organogenesis at doses of 0.6 to 8.3 times the highest recommended human dose for a single intravenous infusion. As it has been shown that Aredia can cross the placenta in rats and has produced marked maternal and nonteratogenic embryo/fetal effects in rats and rabbits, it should not be given to women during pregnancy.
Bisphosphonates are incorporated into the bone matrix, from where they are gradually released over periods of weeks to years. The extent of bisphosphonate incorporation into adult bone, and hence, the amount available for release back into the systemic circulation, is directly related to the total dose and duration of bisphosphonate use. Although there are no data on fetal risk in humans, bisphosphonates do cause fetal harm in animals, and animal data suggest that uptake of bisphosphonates into fetal bone is greater than into maternal bone. Therefore, there is a theoretical risk of fetal harm (e.g., skeletal and other abnormalities) if a woman becomes pregnant after completing a course of bisphosphonate therapy. The impact of variables such as time between cessation of bisphosphonate therapy to conception, the particular bisphosphonate used, and the route of administration (intravenous versus oral) on this risk has not been established.

Nursing Mothers
It is not known whether Aredia is excreted in human milk. Because many drugs are excreted in human milk, caution should be exercised when Aredia is administered to a nursing woman.

Pediatric Use
Safety and effectiveness of Aredia in pediatric patients have not been established.

ADVERSE REACTIONS

Clinical Studies

Hypercalcemia of Malignancy
Transient mild elevation of temperature by at least 1°C was noted 24 to 48 hours after administration of Aredia in 34% of patients in clinical trials. In the saline trial, 18% of patients had a temperature elevation of at least 1°C 24 to 48 hours after treatment.
Drug-related local soft-tissue symptoms (redness, swelling or induration and pain on palpation) at the site of catheter insertion were most common in patients treated with 90 mg of Aredia. Symptomatic treatment resulted in rapid resolution in all patients.
Rare cases of uveitis, iritis, scleritis, and episcleritis have been reported, including one case of scleritis, and one case of uveitis upon separate rechallenges.
Five of 231 patients (2%) who received Aredia during the four U.S. controlled hypercalcemia clinical studies were reported to have had seizures, 2 of whom had preexisting seizure disorders. None of the seizures were considered to be drug-related by the investigators. However, a possible relationship between the drug and the occurrence of seizures cannot be ruled out. It should be noted that in the saline arm 1 patient (4%) had a seizure.
There are no controlled clinical trials comparing the efficacy and safety of 90 mg Aredia over 24 hours to 2 hours in patients with hypercalcemia of malignancy. However, a comparison of data from separate clinical trials suggests that the overall safety profile in patients who received 90 mg Aredia over 24 hours is similar to those who received 90 mg Aredia over 2 hours. The only notable differences observed were an increase in the proportion of patients in the Aredia 24 hour group who experienced fluid overload and electrolyte/mineral abnormalities.
At least 15% of patients treated with Aredia for hypercalcemia of malignancy also experienced the following adverse events during a clinical trial:
General: Fluid overload, generalized pain
Cardiovascular: Hypertension
Gastrointestinal: Abdominal pain, anorexia, constipation, nausea, vomiting
Genitourinary: Urinary tract infection
Musculoskeletal: Bone pain
Laboratory abnormality: Anemia, hypokalemia, hypomagnesemia, hypophosphatemia
Many of these adverse experiences may have been related to the underlying disease state. The following table lists the adverse experiences considered to be treatment-related during comparative, controlled U.S. trials.
[See table at top of next page]

Paget's Disease
Transient mild elevation of temperature >1°C above pretreatment baseline was noted within 48 hours after completion of treatment in 21% of the patients treated with 90 mg of Aredia in clinical trials.

Mean Change (Δ) from Baseline at Last Measurement

	Breast Cancer Patients Receiving Chemotherapy					Breast Cancer Patients Receiving Hormonal Therapy				
	Aredia®		Placebo		A vs P	Aredia®		Placebo		A vs P
	N	Mean Δ	N	Mean Δ	P-Value*	N	Mean Δ	N	Mean Δ	P-Value*
Pain Score	175	+0.93	183	+1.69	.050	173	+0.50	179	+1.60	.007
Analgesic Score	175	+0.74	183	+1.55	.009	173	+0.90	179	+2.28	<.001
ECOG PS	178	+0.81	186	+1.19	.002	175	+0.95	182	+0.90	.773
Spitzer QOL	177	-1.76	185	-2.21	.103	173	-1.86	181	-2.05	.409

Decreases in pain, analgesic scores and ECOG PS, and increases in Spitzer QOL indicate an improvement from baseline.

*The statistical significance of analyses of these secondary endpoints of pain, quality of life, and performance status in all three trials may be overestimated since numerous analyses were performed.

Drug-related musculoskeletal pain and nervous system symptoms (dizziness, headache, paresthesia, increased sweating) were more common in patients with Paget's disease treated with 90 mg of Aredia than in patients with hypercalcemia of malignancy treated with the same dose.
Adverse experiences considered to be related to trial drug, which occurred in at least 5% of patients with Paget's disease treated with 90 mg of Aredia in two U.S. clinical trials, were fever, nausea, back pain, and bone pain.
At least 10% of all Aredia-treated patients with Paget's disease also experienced the following adverse experiences during clinical trials:
Cardiovascular: Hypertension
Musculoskeletal: Arthrosis, bone pain
Nervous system: Headache
Most of these adverse experiences may have been related to the underlying disease state.

Osteolytic Bone Metastases of Breast Cancer and Osteolytic Lesions of Multiple Myeloma

The most commonly reported (>15%) adverse experiences occurred with similar frequencies in the Aredia and placebo treatment groups, and most of these adverse experiences may have been related to the underlying disease state or cancer therapy.
[See table at top of next page]
Of the toxicities commonly associated with chemotherapy, the frequency of vomiting, anorexia, and anemia were slightly more common in the Aredia patients whereas stomatitis and alopecia occurred at a frequency similar to that in placebo patients. In the breast cancer trials, mild elevations of serum creatinine occurred in 18.5% of Aredia patients and 12.3% of placebo patients. Mineral and electrolyte disturbances, including hypocalcemia, were reported rarely and in similar percentages of Aredia-treated patients compared with those in the placebo group. The reported frequencies of hypocalcemia, hypokalemia, hypophosphatemia, and hypomagnesemia for Aredia-treated patients were 3.3%, 10.5%, 1.7%, and 4.4%, respectively, and for placebo-treated patients were 1.2%, 12%, 1.7%, and 4.5%, respectively. In previous hypercalcemia of malignancy trials, patients treated with Aredia (60 or 90 mg over 24 hours) developed electrolyte abnormalities more frequently *(see ADVERSE REACTIONS, Hypercalcemia of Malignancy).*
Arthralgias and myalgias were reported slightly more frequently in the Aredia group than in the placebo group (13.6% and 26% vs 10.8% and 20.1%, respectively).
In multiple myeloma patients, there were five Aredia-related serious and unexpected adverse experiences. Four of these were reported during the 12-month extension of the multiple myeloma trial. Three of the reports were of worsening renal function developing in patients with progressive multiple myeloma or multiple myeloma-associated amyloidosis. The fourth report was the adult respiratory distress syndrome developing in a patient recovering from pneumonia and acute gangrenous cholecystitis. One Aredia-treated patient experienced an allergic reaction characterized by swollen and itchy eyes, runny nose, and scratchy throat within 24 hours after the sixth infusion.
In the breast cancer trials, there were four Aredia-related adverse experiences, all moderate in severity, that caused a patient to discontinue participation in the trial. One was due to interstitial pneumonitis, another to malaise and dyspnea. One Aredia patient discontinued the trial due to a symptomatic hypocalcemia. Another Aredia patient discontinued therapy due to severe bone pain after each infusion, which the investigator felt was trial-drug-related.

Renal Toxicity

In a study of the safety and efficacy of Aredia 90 mg (2 hour infusion) versus Zometa 4 mg (15 minute infusion) in bone metastases patients with multiple myeloma or breast cancer, renal deterioration was defined as an increase in serum creatinine of 0.5 mg/dL for patients with normal baseline creatinine (<1.4 mg/dL) or an increase of 1.0 mg/dL for patients with an abnormal baseline creatinine (≥1.4 mg/dL). The following are data on the incidence of renal deterioration in patients in this trial. *See Table below.*

Incidence of Renal Function Deterioration in Multiple Myeloma and Breast Cancer Patients with Normal and Abnormal Serum Creatinine at Baseline*

Patient Population/ Baseline Creatinine	Aredia® 90 mg/2 hours		Zometa® 4 mg/15 minutes	
	n/N	**(%)**	**n/N**	**(%)**
Normal	20/246	(8.1%)	23/246	(9.3%)
Abnormal	2/22	(9.1%)	1/26	(3.8%)
Total	22/268	(8.2%)	24/272	(8.8%)

*Patients were randomized following the 15-minute infusion amendment for the Zometa arm.

Post-Marketing Experience

Rare instances of allergic manifestations have been reported, including hypotension, dyspnea, or angioedema, and, very rarely, anaphylactic shock. Aredia is contraindicated in patients with clinically significant hypersensitivity to Aredia or other bisphosphonates *(see CONTRAINDICATIONS).*
Cases of osteonecrosis (primarily of the jaws) have been reported since market introduction. Osteonecrosis of the jaws has other well documented multiple risk factors. It is not possible to determine if these events are related to Aredia or other bisphosphonates, to concomitant drugs or other therapies (e.g., chemotherapy, radiotherapy, corticosteroid), to patient's underlying disease, or to other comorbid risk factors (e.g., anemia, infection, preexisting oral disease).

Treatment-Related Adverse Experiences Reported in Three U.S. Controlled Clinical Trials

	Percent of Patients				
	Aredia®			Etidronate Disodium	Saline
	60 mg over 4 hr	60 mg over 24 hr	90 mg over 24 hr	7.5 mg/kg × 3 days	
	N=23	N=73	N=17	N=35	N=23
General					
Edema	0	1	0	0	0
Fatigue	0	0	12	0	0
Fever	26	19	18	9	0
Fluid overload	0	0	0	6	0
Infusion-site reaction	0	4	18	0	0
Moniliasis	0	0	6	0	0
Rigors	0	0	0	0	4
Gastrointestinal					
Abdominal pain	0	1	0	0	0
Anorexia	4	1	12	0	0
Constipation	4	0	6	3	0
Diarrhea	0	1	0	0	0
Dyspepsia	4	0	0	0	0
Gastrointestinal hemorrhage	0	0	6	0	0
Nausea	4	0	18	6	0
Stomatitis	0	1	0	3	0
Vomiting	4	0	0	0	0
Respiratory					
Dyspnea	0	0	0	3	0
Rales	0	0	6	0	0
Rhinitis	0	0	6	0	0
Upper respiratory infection	0	3	0	0	0
CNS					
Anxiety	0	0	0	0	4
Convulsions	0	0	0	3	0
Insomnia	0	1	0	0	0
Nervousness	0	0	0	0	4
Psychosis	4	0	0	0	0
Somnolence	0	1	6	0	0
Taste perversion	0	0	0	3	0
Cardiovascular					
Atrial fibrillation	0	0	6	0	4
Atrial flutter	0	1	0	0	0
Cardiac failure	0	1	0	0	0
Hypertension	0	0	6	0	4
Syncope	0	0	6	0	0
Tachycardia	0	0	6	0	4
Endocrine					
Hypothyroidism	0	0	6	0	0
Hemic and Lymphatic					
Anemia	0	0	6	0	0
Leukopenia	4	0	0	0	0
Neutropenia	0	1	0	0	0
Thrombocytopenia	0	1	0	0	0
Musculoskeletal					
Myalgia	0	1	0	0	0
Urogenital					
Uremia	4	0	0	0	0
Laboratory Abnormalities					
Hypocalcemia	0	1	12	0	0
Hypokalemia	4	4	18	0	0
Hypomagnesemia	4	10	12	3	4
Hypophosphatemia	0	9	18	3	0
Abnormal liver function	0	0	0	3	0

OVERDOSAGE

There have been several cases of drug maladministration of intravenous Aredia in hypercalcemia patients with total doses of 225 mg to 300 mg given over 2 ½ to 4 days. All of these patients survived, but they experienced hypocalcemia that required intravenous and/or oral administration of calcium. **Single doses of Aredia should not exceed 90 mg and the duration of the intravenous infusion should be no less than 2 hours. *(See WARNINGS.)***
In addition, one obese woman (95 kg) who was treated with 285 mg of Aredia/day for 3 days experienced high fever (39.5°C), hypotension (from 170/90 mmHg to 90/60 mmHg), and transient taste perversion, noted about 6 hours after the first infusion. The fever and hypotension were rapidly corrected with steroids.
If overdosage occurs, symptomatic hypocalcemia could also result; such patients should be treated with short-term intravenous calcium.

DOSAGE AND ADMINISTRATION

Hypercalcemia of Malignancy

Consideration should be given to the severity of as well as the symptoms of hypercalcemia. Vigorous saline hydration alone may be sufficient for treating mild, asymptomatic hypercalcemia. Overhydration should be avoided in patients who have potential for cardiac failure. In hypercalcemia associated with hematologic malignancies, the use of glucocorticoid therapy may be helpful.

Moderate Hypercalcemia

The recommended dose of Aredia in moderate hypercalcemia (corrected serum calcium* of approximately 12-13.5 mg/dL) is 60 to 90 mg given as a SINGLE-DOSE, intravenous infusion over 2 to 24 hours. Longer infusions (i.e., >2 hours) may reduce the risk for renal toxicity, particularly in patients with preexisting renal insufficiency.

Severe Hypercalcemia

The recommended dose of Aredia in severe hypercalcemia (corrected serum calcium* >13.5 mg/dL) is 90 mg given as a SINGLE-DOSE, intravenous infusion over 2 to 24 hours. Longer infusions (i.e., >2 hours) may reduce the risk for renal toxicity, particularly in patients with preexisting renal insufficiency.

*Albumin-corrected serum calcium (CCa,mg/dL) = serum calcium, mg/dL + 0.8 (4.0-serum albumin, g/dL).

Retreatment

A limited number of patients have received more than one treatment with Aredia for hypercalcemia. Retreatment with Aredia, in patients who show complete or partial response initially, may be carried out if serum calcium does not return to normal or remain normal after initial treatment. **It is recommended that a minimum of 7 days elapse before retreatment, to allow for full response to the initial dose.** The dose and manner of retreatment is identical to that of the initial therapy.

Paget's Disease

The recommended dose of Aredia in patients with moderate to severe Paget's disease of bone is 30 mg daily, administered as a 4-hour infusion on 3 consecutive days for a total dose of 90 mg.

Retreatment

A limited number of patients with Paget's disease have received more than one treatment of Aredia in clinical trials. When clinically indicated, patients should be retreated at the dose of initial therapy.

Continued on next page

Commonly Reported Adverse Experiences in Three U.S. Controlled Clinical Trials

	Aredia® 90 mg over 4 hours	Placebo	Aredia® 90 mg over 2 hours	Placebo	All Aredia® 90 mg	Placebo
	N=205 %	N=187 %	N=367 %	N=386 %	N=572 %	N=573 %
General						
Asthenia	16.1	17.1	25.6	19.2	22.2	18.5
Fatigue	31.7	28.3	40.3	28.8	37.2	29.0
Fever	38.5	38.0	38.1	32.1	38.5	34.0
Metastases	1.0	3.0	31.3	24.4	20.5	17.5
Pain	13.2	11.8	15.0	18.1	14.3	16.1
Digestive System						
Anorexia	17.1	17.1	31.1	24.9	26.0	22.3
Constipation	28.3	31.7	36.0	38.6	33.2	35.1
Diarrhea	26.8	26.8	29.4	30.6	28.5	29.7
Dyspepsia	17.6	13.4	18.3	15.0	22.6	17.5
Nausea	35.6	37.4	63.5	59.1	53.5	51.8
Pain Abdominal	19.5	16.0	24.3	18.1	22.6	17.5
Vomiting	16.6	19.8	46.3	39.1	35.7	32.8
Hemic and Lymphatic						
Anemia	47.8	41.7	39.5	36.8	42.5	38.4
Granulocytopenia	20.5	15.5	19.3	20.5	19.8	18.8
Thrombocytopenia	16.6	17.1	12.5	14.0	14.0	15.0
Musculoskeletal System						
Arthralgias	10.7	7.0	15.3	12.7	13.6	10.8
Myalgia	25.4	15.0	26.4	22.5	26.0	20.1
Skeletal Pain	61.0	71.7	70.0	75.4	66.8	74.0
CNS						
Anxiety	7.8	9.1	18.0	16.8	14.3	14.3
Headache	24.4	19.8	27.2	23.6	26.2	22.3
Insomnia	17.1	17.2	25.1	19.4	22.2	19.0
Respiratory System						
Coughing	26.3	22.5	25.3	19.7	25.7	20.6
Dyspnea	22.0	21.4	35.1	24.4	30.4	23.4
Pleural Effusion	2.9	4.3	15.0	9.1	10.7	7.5
Sinusitis	14.6	16.6	16.1	10.4	15.6	12.0
Upper Respiratory Tract Infection	32.2	28.3	19.6	20.2	24.1	22.9
Urogenital System						
Urinary Tract Infection	15.6	9.1	20.2	17.6	18.5	15.6

Aredia—Cont.

Osteolytic Bone Lesions of Multiple Myeloma

The recommended dose of Aredia in patients with osteolytic bone lesions of multiple myeloma is 90 mg administered as a 4-hour infusion given on a monthly basis.

Patients with marked Bence-Jones proteinuria and dehydration should receive adequate hydration prior to Aredia infusion.

Limited information is available on the use of Aredia in multiple myeloma patients with a serum creatinine ≥3.0 mg/dL.

Patients who receive Aredia should have serum creatinine assessed prior to each treatment. Treatment should be withheld for renal deterioration. In a clinical study, renal deterioration was defined as follows:

- For patients with normal baseline creatinine, increase of 0.5 mg/dL.
- For patients with abnormal baseline creatinine, increase of 1.0 mg/dL.

In this clinical study, Aredia treatment was resumed only when the creatinine returned to within 10% of the baseline value.

The optimal duration of therapy is not yet known, however, in a study of patients with myeloma, final analysis after 21 months demonstrated overall benefits *(see CLINICAL TRIALS section).*

Osteolytic Bone Metastases of Breast Cancer

The recommended dose of Aredia in patients with osteolytic bone metastases is 90 mg administered over a 2-hour infusion given every 3-4 weeks.

Aredia has been frequently used with doxorubicin, fluorouracil, cyclophosphamide, methotrexate, mitoxantrone, vinblastine, dexamethasone, prednisone, melphalan, vincristine, megesterol, and tamoxifen. It has been given less frequently with etoposide, cisplatin, cytarabine, paclitaxel, and aminoglutethimide.

Patients who receive Aredia should have serum creatinine assessed prior to each treatment. Treatment should be withheld for renal deterioration. In a clinical study, renal deterioration was defined as follows:

- For patients with normal baseline creatinine, increase of 0.5 mg/dL.
- For patients with abnormal baseline creatinine, increase of 1.0 mg/dL.

In this clinical study, Aredia treatment was resumed only when the creatinine returned to within 10% of the baseline value.

The optimal duration of therapy is not known, however, in two breast cancer studies, final analyses performed after 24 months of therapy demonstrated overall benefits *(see CLINICAL TRIALS section).*

Preparation of Solution

Reconstitution

Aredia is reconstituted by adding 10 mL of Sterile Water for Injection, USP, to each vial, resulting in a solution of 30 mg/10 mL or 90 mg/10 mL. The pH of the reconstituted solution is 6.0-7.4. The drug should be completely dissolved before the solution is withdrawn.

Method of Administration

DUE TO THE RISK OF CLINICALLY SIGNIFICANT DETERIORATION IN RENAL FUNCTION, WHICH MAY PROGRESS TO RENAL FAILURE, SINGLE DOSES OF AREDIA SHOULD NOT EXCEED 90 MG. *(SEE WARNINGS.)*

There must be strict adherence to the intravenous administration recommendations for Aredia in order to decrease the risk of deterioration in renal function.

Hypercalcemia of Malignancy

The daily dose must be administered as an intravenous infusion over at least 2 to 24 hours for the 60-mg and 90-mg doses. The recommended dose should be diluted in 1000 mL of sterile 0.45% or 0.9% Sodium Chloride, USP, or 5% Dextrose Injection, USP. This infusion solution is stable for up to 24 hours at room temperature.

Paget's Disease

The recommended daily dose of 30 mg should be diluted in 500 mL of sterile 0.45% or 0.9% Sodium Chloride, USP, or 5% Dextrose Injection, USP, and administered over a 4-hour period for 3 consecutive days.

Osteolytic Bone Metastases of Breast Cancer

The recommended dose of 90 mg should be diluted in 250 mL of sterile 0.45% or 0.9% Sodium Chloride, USP, or 5% Dextrose Injection, USP, and administered over a 2-hour period every 3-4 weeks.

Osteolytic Bone Lesions of Multiple Myeloma

The recommended dose of 90 mg should be diluted in 500 mL of sterile 0.45% or 0.9% Sodium Chloride, USP, or 5% Dextrose Injection, USP, and administered over a 4-hour period on a monthly basis.

Aredia must not be mixed with calcium-containing infusion solutions, such as Ringer's solution, and should be given in a single intravenous solution and line separate from all other drugs.

Note: **Parenteral drug products should be inspected visually for particulate matter and discoloration prior to administration, whenever solution and container permit.**

Aredia reconstituted with Sterile Water for Injection may be stored under refrigeration at 2°C-8°C (36°F-46°F) for up to 24 hours.

HOW SUPPLIED

Vials - 90 mg - each contains 90 mg of sterile, lyophilized pamidronate disodium and 470 mg of mannitol, USP.

Carton of 4 vials .... NDC 0083-2601-04

Vials - 90 mg - each contains 90 mg of sterile, lyophilized pamidronate disodium and 375 mg of mannitol, USP.

Carton of 1 vial .... NDC 0083-2609-01

Do not store above 30°C (86°F).

T2003-83

REV: OCTOBER 2003 Printed in U.S.A. 89002607

Novartis Pharmaceuticals Corporation
East Hanover, New Jersey 07936

© Novartis

Shown in Product Identification Guide, page 324

CATAFLAM® ℞

[kăt-ă-flăm]

(diclofenac potassium immediate-release) tablets
Tablets of 50 mg
Rx only

Prescribing Information

The following prescribing information is based on official labeling in effect August 2003.

DESCRIPTION

Cataflam® (diclofenac potassium immediate-release tablets), is a benzeneacetic acid derivative. Cataflam is available as immediate-release Tablets of 50 mg (light brown) for oral administration. The chemical name is 2-[(2,6-dichlorophenyl)amino] benzeneacetic acid, monopotassium salt. The molecular weight is 334.25. Its molecular formula is $C_{14}H_{10}Cl_2NKO_2$, and it has the following structural formula

CH_2COO K
NH
Cl Cl

The inactive ingredients in Cataflam include: calcium phosphate, colloidal silicon dioxide, iron oxides, magnesium stearate, microcrystalline cellulose, polyethylene glycol, povidone, sodium starch glycolate, maize starch, sucrose, talc, titanium dioxide.

CLINICAL PHARMACOLOGY

Pharmacodynamics

Cataflam® (diclofenac potassium immediate-release tablets) is a nonsteroidal anti-inflammatory drug (NSAID) that exhibits anti-inflammatory, analgesic, and antipyretic activities in animal models. The mechanism of action of Cataflam, like that of other NSAIDs, is not completely understood but may be related to prostaglandin synthetase inhibition.

Pharmacokinetics

Absorption

Diclofenac is 100% absorbed after oral administration compared to IV administration as measured by urine recovery. However, due to first-pass metabolism, only about 50% of the absorbed dose is systemically available (see Table 1). In some fasting volunteers, measurable plasma levels are observed within 10 minutes of dosing with Cataflam. Peak plasma levels are achieved approximately 1 hour in fasting normal volunteers, with a range of .33 to 2 hours. Food has no significant effect on the extent of diclofenac absorption. However, there is usually a delay in the onset of absorption and a reduction in peak plasma levels of approximately 30%.

Table 1. Pharmacokinetic Parameters for Diclofenac

PK Parameter	Normal Healthy Adults (20–52 yrs.)	
	Mean	Coefficient of Variation (%)
Absolute Bioavailability (%) [N = 7]	55	40
T_{max} (hr) [N = 65]	1.0	76
Oral Clearance (CL/F; mL/min) [N = 61]	622	21
Renal Clearance (% unchanged drug in urine) [N = 7]	<1	—
Apparent Volume of Distribution (V/F; L/kg) [N = 61]	1.3	33
Terminal Half-life (hr) [N = 48]	1.9	29

Distribution

The apparent volume of distribution (V/F) of diclofenac potassium is 1.3 L/kg.

Diclofenac is more than 99% bound to human serum proteins, primarily to albumin. Serum protein binding is constant over the concentration range (0.15-105 µg/mL) achieved with recommended doses.

Diclofenac diffuses into and out of the synovial fluid. Diffusion into the joint occurs when plasma levels are higher than those in the synovial fluid, after which the process reverses and synovial fluid levels are higher than plasma levels. It is not known whether diffusion into the joint plays a role in the effectiveness of diclofenac.

Metabolism

Five diclofenac metabolites have been identified in human plasma and urine. The metabolites include 4′-hydroxy-, 5-hydroxy-, 3′-hydroxy-, 4′,5-dihydroxy- and 3′-hydroxy-4′-methoxy diclofenac. In patients with renal dysfunction, peak concentrations of metabolites 4′-hydroxy-and 5-hydroxy-diclofenac were approximately 50% and 4% of the parent compound after single oral dosing compared to 27% and 1% in normal healthy subjects. However, diclofenac metabolites undergo further glucuronidation and sulfation followed by biliary excretion.

One diclofenac metabolite 4′-hydroxy-diclofenac has very weak pharmacologic activity.

Excretion

Diclofenac is eliminated through metabolism and subsequent urinary and biliary excretion of the glucuronide and the sulfate conjugates of the metabolites. Little or no free unchanged diclofenac is excreted in the urine. Approximately 65% of the dose is excreted in the urine and approximately 35% in the bile as conjugates of unchanged diclofenac plus metabolites. Because renal elimination is not a significant pathway of elimination for unchanged diclofenac, dosing adjustment in patients with mild to moderate renal dysfunction is not necessary. The terminal half-life of unchanged diclofenac is approximately 2 hours.

Special Populations

Pediatric: The pharmacokinetics of Cataflam has not been investigated in pediatric patients.

Race: Pharmacokinetics differences due to race have not been identified.

Hepatic Insufficiency: Hepatic metabolism accounts for almost 100% of Cataflam elimination, so patients with hepatic disease may require reduced doses of Cataflam compared to patients with normal hepatic function.

Renal Insufficiency: Diclofenac pharmacokinetics has been investigated in subjects with renal insufficiency. No differences in the pharmacokinetics of diclofenac have been detected in studies of patients with renal impairment. In patients with renal impairment (inulin clearance 60-90, 30-60, and <30 mL/min; N=6 in each group), AUC values and elimination rate were comparable to those in healthy subjects.

INDICATIONS AND USAGE

Cataflam® (diclofenac potassium immediate-release tablets) is indicated:

- For treatment of primary dysmenorrhea
- For relief of mild to moderate pain
- For relief of signs and symptoms of osteoarthritis
- For relief of signs and symptoms of rheumatoid arthritis

CONTRAINDICATIONS

Cataflam® (diclofenac potassium immediate-release tablets) is contraindicated in patients with known hypersensitivity to diclofenac. Cataflam should not be given to patients who have experienced asthma, urticaria, or allergic-type reactions after taking aspirin or other NSAIDs. Severe, rarely fatal, anaphylactic-like reactions to NSAIDs have been reported in such patients (see WARNINGS - Anaphylactoid Reactions, and PRECAUTIONS - Preexisting Asthma).

WARNINGS

Gastrointestinal (GI) Effects - Risk of GI Ulceration, Bleeding, and Perforation:

Serious gastrointestinal toxicity such as inflammation, bleeding, ulceration, and perforation of the stomach, small intestine or large intestine, can occur at any time, with or without warning symptoms, in patients treated with nonsteroidal anti-inflammatory drugs (NSAIDs). Minor upper gastrointestinal problems, such as dyspepsia, are common and may also occur at any time during NSAID therapy. Therefore, physicians and patients should remain alert for ulceration and bleeding even in the absence of previous GI tract symptoms. Patients should be informed about the signs and/or symptoms of serious GI toxicity and the steps to take if they occur. The utility of periodic laboratory monitoring has not been demonstrated, nor has it been adequately assessed. Only one in five patients, who develop a serious upper GI adverse event on NSAID therapy, is symptomatic. It has been demonstrated that upper GI ulcers, gross bleeding or perforation, caused by NSAIDs, appear to occur in approximately 1% of patients treated for 3-6 months, and in about 2%-4% of patients treated for one year. These trends continue thus, increasing the likelihood of developing a serious GI event at some time during the course of therapy. However, even short term therapy is not without risk.

NSAIDs should be prescribed with extreme caution in those with a prior history of ulcer disease or gastrointestinal bleeding. Most spontaneous reports of fatal GI events are in elderly or debilitated patients and therefore special care should be taken in treating this population. **To minimize the potential risk for an adverse GI event, the lowest effective dose should be used for the shortest possible duration.** For high risk patients, alternate therapies that do not involve NSAIDs should be considered.

Studies have shown that patients with *a prior history of peptic ulcer disease and/or gastrointestinal bleeding* and who use NSAIDs, have a greater than 10-fold risk for developing a GI bleed than patients with neither of these risk factors. In addition to a past history of ulcer disease, pharmacoepidemiological studies have identified several other co-therapies or co-morbid conditions that may increase the risk for GI bleeding such as: treatment with oral corticosteroids, treatment with anticoagulants, longer duration of NSAID therapy, smoking, alcoholism, older age, and poor general health status.

Anaphylactoid Reactions

As with other NSAIDs, anaphylactoid reactions may occur in patients without known prior exposure to Cataflam® (diclofenac potassium immediate-release tablets). Cataflam should not be given to patients with the aspirin triad. This symptom complex typically occurs in asthmatic patients who experience rhinitis with or without nasal polyps, or who exhibit severe, potentially fatal bronchospasm after taking aspirin or other NSAIDs. (See CONTRAINDICATIONS and PRECAUTIONS - Preexisting Asthma.) Emergency help should be sought in cases where an anaphylactoid reaction occurs.

Advanced Renal Disease

In cases with advanced kidney disease, treatment with Cataflam is not recommended. If NSAID therapy, however, must be initiated, close monitoring of the patient's kidney function is advisable (see PRECAUTIONS - Renal Effects).

Pregnancy

In late pregnancy, as with other NSAIDs, Cataflam should be avoided because it may cause premature closure of the ductus arteriosus.

PRECAUTIONS

General

Cataflam® (diclofenac potassium immediate-release tablets) cannot be expected to substitute for corticosteroids or to treat corticosteroid insufficiency. Abrupt discontinuation of corticosteroids may lead to disease exacerbation. Patients on prolonged corticosteroid therapy should have their therapy tapered slowly if a decision is made to discontinue corticosteroids.

The pharmacological activity of Cataflam in reducing fever and inflammation may diminish the utility of these diagnostic signs in detecting complications of presumed noninfectious, painful conditions.

Hepatic Effects

Borderline elevations of one or more liver tests may occur in up to 15% of patients taking NSAIDs including Cataflam. These laboratory abnormalities may progress, may remain unchanged, or may be transient with continued therapy. Based on this experience, in patients on chronic treatment with Cataflam, periodic monitoring of transaminases is recommended (see PRECAUTIONS - Laboratory Tests). Notable elevations of ALT or AST (three or more times the upper limit of normal) have been reported in approximately 2%-4% of patients, including marked elevations (eight or more times the upper limit of normal) in about 1% of patients in clinical trials with diclofenac. In addition, rare cases of severe hepatic reactions, including jaundice and fatal fulminant hepatitis, liver necrosis and hepatic failure, some of them with fatal outcomes have been reported.

A patient with symptoms and/or signs suggesting liver dysfunction, or in whom an abnormal liver test has occurred, should be evaluated for evidence of the development of a more severe hepatic reaction while on therapy with Cataflam. If clinical signs and symptoms consistent with liver disease develop, or if systemic manifestations occur (e.g., eosinophilia, rash, etc.), Cataflam should be discontinued.

Renal Effects

Caution should be used when initiating treatment with Cataflam in patients with considerable dehydration. It is advisable to rehydrate patients first and then start therapy with Cataflam. Caution is also recommended in patients with pre-existing kidney disease (see WARNINGS - Advanced Renal Disease).

As with other NSAIDs, long-term administration of diclofenac has resulted in renal papillary necrosis and other renal medullary changes. Renal toxicity has also been seen in patients in which renal prostaglandins have a compensatory role in the maintenance of renal perfusion. In these patients, administration of a nonsteroidal anti-inflammatory drug may cause a dose-dependent reduction in prostaglandin formation and, secondarily, in renal blood flow, which may precipitate overt renal decompensation. Patients at greatest risk of this reaction are those with impaired renal function, heart failure, liver dysfunction, those taking diuretics and ACE inhibitors, and the elderly. Discontinuation of nonsteroidal anti-inflammatory drug therapy is usually followed by recovery to the pretreatment state.

Cataflam metabolites are eliminated primarily by the kidneys. The extent to which the metabolites may accumulate in patients with renal failure has not been studied. As with other NSAIDs, metabolites of which are excreted by the kidney, patients with significantly impaired renal function should be more closely monitored.

Hematological Effects

Anemia is sometimes seen in patients receiving NSAIDs, including Cataflam. This may be due to fluid retention, GI loss, or an incompletely described effect upon erythropoiesis. Patients on long-term treatment with NSAIDs, including Cataflam, should have their hemoglobin or hematocrit checked if they exhibit any signs or symptoms of anemia.

All drugs which inhibit the biosynthesis of prostaglandins may interfere to some extent with platelet function and vascular responses to bleeding.

NSAIDs inhibit platelet aggregation and have been shown to prolong bleeding time in some patients. Unlike aspirin, their effect on platelet function is quantitatively less, of shorter duration, and reversible. Cataflam does not generally affect platelet counts, prothrombin time (PT), or partial thromboplastin time (PTT). Patients receiving Cataflam who may be adversely affected by alterations in platelet function, such as those with coagulation disorders or patients receiving anticoagulants, should be carefully monitored.

Fluid Retention and Edema

Fluid retention and edema have been observed in some patients taking NSAIDs. Therefore, as with other NSAIDs, Cataflam should be used with caution in patients with fluid retention, hypertension, or heart failure.

Preexisting Asthma

Patients with asthma may have aspirin-sensitive asthma. The use of aspirin in patients with aspirin-sensitive asthma has been associated with severe bronchospasm which can be fatal. Since cross-reactivity, including bronchospasm, between aspirin and other nonsteroidal anti-inflammatory drugs has been reported in such aspirin-sensitive patients, Cataflam should not be administered to patients with this form of aspirin sensitivity and should be used with caution in all patients with preexisting asthma.

Information for Patients

Cataflam, like other drugs of its class, can cause discomfort and, rarely, more serious side effects, such as gastrointestinal bleeding, which may result in hospitalization and even fatal outcomes. Although serious GI tract ulcerations and bleeding can occur without warning symptoms, patients should be alert for the signs and symptoms of ulcerations and bleeding, and should ask for medical advice when observing any indicative sign or symptoms. Patients should be apprised of the importance of this follow-up (see WARNINGS - Risk of Gastrointestinal Ulceration, Bleeding and Perforation).

Patients should report to their physicians signs or symptoms of gastrointestinal ulceration or bleeding, skin rash, weight gain, or edema.

Patients should be informed of the warning signs and symptoms of hepatotoxicity (e.g., nausea, fatigue, lethargy, pruritus, jaundice, right upper quadrant tenderness, and "flu-like" symptoms). If these occur, patients should be instructed to stop therapy and seek immediate medical therapy.

Patients should also be instructed to seek immediate emergency help in the case of an anaphylactoid reaction (see WARNINGS).

In late pregnancy, as with other NSAIDs, Cataflam should be avoided because it will cause premature closure of the ductus arteriosus.

Laboratory Tests

Patients on long-term treatment with NSAIDs, should have their CBC and a chemistry profile (including transaminases) checked periodically. If clinical signs and symptoms consistent with liver or renal disease develop, systemic manifestations occur (e.g., eosinophilia, rash, etc.) or if abnormal liver tests persist or worsen, Cataflam should be discontinued.

Drug Interactions

Aspirin: When Cataflam is administered with aspirin, its protein binding is reduced. The clinical significance of this interaction is not known; however, as with other NSAIDs, concomitant administration of diclofenac and aspirin is not generally recommended because of the potential of increased adverse effects.

Methotrexate: NSAIDs have been reported to competitively inhibit methotrexate accumulation in rabbit kidney slices. This may indicate that they could enhance the toxicity of methotrexate. Caution should be used when NSAIDs are administered concomitantly with methotrexate.

Cyclosporine: Cataflam, like other NSAIDs, may affect renal prostaglandins and increase the toxicity of certain drugs. Therefore, concomitant therapy with Cataflam may increase cyclosporine's nephrotoxicity. Caution should be used when Cataflam is administered concomitantly with cyclosporine.

ACE-inhibitors: Reports suggest that NSAIDs may diminish the antihypertensive effect of ACE-inhibitors. This interaction should be given consideration in patients taking NSAIDs concomitantly with ACE-inhibitors.

Furosemide: Clinical studies, as well as post-marketing observations, have shown that Cataflam can reduce the natriuretic effect of furosemide and thiazides in some patients. This response has been attributed to inhibition of renal prostaglandin synthesis. During concomitant therapy with NSAIDs, the patient should be observed closely for signs of renal failure (see PRECAUTIONS - Renal Effects), as well as to assure diuretic efficacy.

Lithium: NSAIDs have produced an elevation of plasma lithium levels and a reduction in renal lithium clearance. The mean minimum lithium concentration increased 15% and the renal clearance was decreased by approximately 20%. These effects have been attributed to inhibition of renal prostaglandin synthesis by the NSAID. Thus, when NSAIDs and lithium are administered concurrently, subjects should be observed carefully for signs of lithium toxicity.

Warfarin: The effects of warfarin and NSAIDs on GI bleeding are synergistic, such that users of both drugs together have a risk of serious GI bleeding higher than users of either drug alone.

Pregnancy

Teratogenic Effects: Pregnancy Category C Reproductive studies conducted in rats and rabbits have not demonstrated evidence of developmental abnormalities. However, animal reproduction studies are not always predictive of human response. There are no adequate and well-controlled studies in pregnant women.

Nonteratogenic Effects: Because of the known effects of nonsteroidal anti-inflammatory drugs on the fetal cardiovascular system (closure of ductus arteriosus), use during pregnancy (particularly late pregnancy) should be avoided.

Labor and Delivery

In rat studies with NSAIDs, as with other drugs known to inhibit prostaglandin synthesis, an increased incidence of

Continued on next page

Cataflam—Cont.

dystocia, delayed parturition, and decreased pup survival occurred. The effects of Cataflam on labor and delivery in pregnant women are unknown.

Nursing Mothers

It is not known whether this drug is excreted in human milk. Because many drugs are excreted in human milk and because of the potential for serious adverse reactions in nursing infants from Cataflam, a decision should be made whether to discontinue nursing or to discontinue the drug, taking into account the importance of the drug to the mother.

Pediatric Use

Safety and effectiveness in pediatric patients have not been established.

Geriatric Use

As with any NSAIDs, caution should be exercised in treating the elderly (65 years and older).

ADVERSE REACTIONS

In 718 patients treated for shorter periods, i.e., 2 weeks or less, with Cataflam® (diclofenac potassium immediate-release tablets), adverse reactions were reported one-half to one-tenth as frequently as by patients treated for longer periods. In a 6-month, double-blind trial comparing Cataflam (N=196) versus Voltaren® (diclofenac sodium delayed-release tablets) (N=197) versus ibuprofen (N=197), adverse reactions were similar in nature and frequency.

In patients taking Cataflam or other NSAIDs, the most frequently reported adverse experiences occurring in approximately 1%-10% of patients are:

Gastrointestinal experiences including: abdominal pain, constipation, diarrhea, dyspepsia, flatulence, gross bleeding/perforation, heartburn, nausea, GI ulcers (gastric/duodenal) and vomiting.

Abnormal renal function, anemia, dizziness, edema, elevated liver enzymes, headaches, increased bleeding time, pruritus, rashes and tinnitus.

Additional adverse experiences reported occasionally include:

Body as a Whole: fever, infection, sepsis

Cardiovascular System: congestive heart failure, hypertension, tachycardia, syncope

Digestive System: dry mouth, esophagitis, gastric/peptic ulcers, gastritis, gastrointestinal bleeding, glossitis, hematemesis, hepatitis, jaundice

Hemic and Lymphatic System: ecchymosis, eosinophilia, leukopenia, melena, purpura, rectal bleeding, stomatitis, thrombocytopenia

Metabolic and Nutritional: weight changes

Nervous System: anxiety, asthenia, confusion, depression, dream abnormalities, drowsiness, insomnia, malaise, nervousness, paresthesia, somnolence, tremors, vertigo

Respiratory System: asthma, dyspnea

Skin and Appendages: alopecia, photosensitivity, sweating increased

Special Senses: blurred vision

Urogenital System: cystitis, dysuria, hematuria, interstitial nephritis, oliguria/polyuria, proteinuria, renal failure

Other adverse reactions, which occur rarely are:

Body as a Whole: anaphylactic reactions, appetite changes, death

Cardiovascular System: arrhythmia, hypotension, myocardial infarction, palpitations, vasculitis

Digestive System: colitis, eructation, liver failure, pancreatitis

Hemic and Lymphatic System: agranulocytosis, hemolytic anemia, aplastic anemia, lymphadenopathy, pancytopenia

Metabolic and Nutritional: hyperglycemia

Nervous System: convulsions, coma, hallucinations, meningitis

Respiratory System: respiratory depression, pneumonia

Skin and Appendages: angioedema, toxic epidermal necrolysis, erythema multiforme, exfoliative dermatitis, Stevens-Johnson syndrome, urticaria

Special Senses: conjunctivitis, hearing impairment.

OVERDOSAGE

Symptoms following acute NSAID overdoses are usually limited to lethargy, drowsiness, nausea, vomiting, and epigastric pain, which are generally reversible with supportive care. Gastrointestinal bleeding can occur. Hypertension, acute renal failure, respiratory depression and coma may occur, but are rare. Anaphylactoid reactions have been reported with therapeutic ingestion of NSAIDs, and may occur following an overdose.

Patients should be managed by symptomatic and supportive care following an NSAID overdose. There are no specific antidotes. Emesis and/or activated charcoal (60 to 100 g in adults, 1 to 2 g/kg in children) and/or osmotic cathartic may be indicated in patients seen within 4 hours of ingestion with symptoms or following a large overdose (5 to 10 times the usual dose). Forced diuresis, alkalinization of urine, hemodialysis, or hemoperfusion may not be useful due to high protein binding.

DOSAGE AND ADMINISTRATION

As with other NSAIDs, the lowest dose should be sought for each patient. Therefore, after observing the response to initial therapy with Cataflam® (diclofenac potassium immediate-release tablets), the dose and frequency should be adjusted to suit an individual patient's needs.

For treatment of pain or primary dysmenorrhea the recommended dosage is 50 mg t.i.d. With experience, physicians may find that in some patients an initial dose of 100 mg of Cataflam, followed by 50-mg doses, will provide better relief.

For the relief of osteoarthritis the recommended dosage is 100-150 mg/day in divided doses, 50 mg b.i.d. or t.i.d.

For the relief of rheumatoid arthritis the recommended dosage is 150-200 mg/day in divided doses, 50 mg t.i.d. or q.i.d. Different formulations of diclofenac [Voltaren® (diclofenac sodium enteric-coated tablets); Voltaren®-XR (diclofenac sodium extended-release tablets); Cataflam® (diclofenac potassium immediate-release tablets)] are not necessarily bioequivalent even if the milligram strength is the same.

HOW SUPPLIED

Cataflam Immediate-Release Tablets

50 mg – light brown, round, biconvex, sugar-coated tablets (imprinted Cataflam on one side and 50 on the other side in black ink)

Bottles of 100 .... NDC 0028-0151-01

Do not store above 30°C (86°F).

Dispense in tight container (USP).

REV: OCTOBER 2002 T2002-44
89020601

NOVARTIS

Manufactured by:
Patheon Whitby Inc.
Whitby, Ontario, Canada L1N 525 for
Novartis Pharmaceuticals Corporation
East Hanover, NJ 07936

Shown in Product Identification Guide, page 324

CLOZARIL® ℞

[klō-ză-rĭl]

(clozapine) Tablets

Rx only

The following prescribing information is based on official labeling in effect July 2004

Prescribing Information

Before prescribing CLOZARIL® (clozapine), the physician should be thoroughly familiar with the details of this prescribing information.

WARNING

1. AGRANULOCYTOSIS

BECAUSE OF A SIGNIFICANT RISK OF AGRANULOCYTOSIS, A POTENTIALLY LIFE-THREATENING ADVERSE EVENT, CLOZARIL® (CLOZAPINE) SHOULD BE RESERVED FOR USE IN (1) THE TREATMENT OF SEVERELY ILL PATIENTS WITH SCHIZOPHRENIA WHO FAIL TO SHOW AN ACCEPTABLE RESPONSE TO ADEQUATE COURSES OF STANDARD ANTIPSYCHOTIC DRUG TREATMENT, OR (2) FOR REDUCING THE RISK OF RECURRENT SUICIDAL BEHAVIOR IN PATIENTS WITH SCHIZOPHRENIA OR SCHIZOAFFECTIVE DISORDER WHO ARE JUDGED TO BE AT RISK OF RE-EXPERIENCING SUICIDAL BEHAVIOR.

PATIENTS BEING TREATED WITH CLOZAPINE MUST HAVE A BASELINE WHITE BLOOD CELL (WBC) AND DIFFERENTIAL COUNT BEFORE INITIATION OF TREATMENT AS WELL AS REGULAR WBC COUNTS DURING TREATMENT AND FOR 4 WEEKS AFTER DISCONTINUATION OF TREATMENT.

CLOZAPINE IS AVAILABLE ONLY THROUGH A DISTRIBUTION SYSTEM THAT ENSURES MONITORING OF WBC COUNTS ACCORDING TO THE SCHEDULE DESCRIBED BELOW PRIOR TO DELIVERY OF THE NEXT SUPPLY OF MEDICATION. *(SEE WARNINGS.)*

2. SEIZURES

SEIZURES HAVE BEEN ASSOCIATED WITH THE USE OF CLOZAPINE. DOSE APPEARS TO BE AN IMPORTANT PREDICTOR OF SEIZURE, WITH A GREATER LIKELIHOOD AT HIGHER CLOZAPINE DOSES. CAUTION SHOULD BE USED WHEN ADMINISTERING CLOZAPINE TO PATIENTS HAVING A HISTORY OF SEIZURES OR OTHER PREDISPOSING FACTORS. PATIENTS SHOULD BE ADVISED NOT TO ENGAGE IN ANY ACTIVITY WHERE SUDDEN LOSS OF CONSCIOUSNESS COULD CAUSE SERIOUS RISK TO THEMSELVES OR OTHERS. *(SEE WARNINGS.)*

3. MYOCARDITIS

ANALYSES OF POST-MARKETING SAFETY DATABASES SUGGEST THAT CLOZAPINE IS ASSOCIATED WITH AN INCREASED RISK OF FATAL MYOCARDITIS, ESPECIALLY DURING, BUT NOT LIMITED TO, THE FIRST MONTH OF THERAPY. IN PATIENTS IN WHOM MYOCARDITIS IS SUSPECTED, CLOZAPINE TREATMENT SHOULD BE PROMPTLY DISCONTINUED. *(SEE WARNINGS.)*

4. OTHER ADVERSE CARDIOVASCULAR AND RESPIRATORY EFFECTS

ORTHOSTATIC HYPOTENSION, WITH OR WITHOUT SYNCOPE, CAN OCCUR WITH CLOZAPINE TREATMENT. RARELY, COLLAPSE CAN BE PROFOUND AND BE ACCOMPANIED BY RESPIRATORY AND/OR CARDIAC ARREST. ORTHOSTATIC HYPOTENSION IS MORE LIKELY TO OCCUR DURING INITIAL TITRATION IN ASSOCIATION WITH RAPID DOSE ESCALATION. IN PATIENTS WHO HAVE HAD EVEN A BRIEF INTERVAL OFF CLOZAPINE, i.e., 2 OR MORE DAYS SINCE THE LAST DOSE, TREATMENT SHOULD BE STARTED WITH 12.5 MG ONCE OR TWICE DAILY. *(SEE WARNINGS and DOSAGE AND ADMINISTRATION.)*

SINCE COLLAPSE, RESPIRATORY ARREST AND CARDIAC ARREST DURING INITIAL TREATMENT HAS OCCURRED IN PATIENTS WHO WERE BEING ADMINISTERED BENZODIAZEPINES OR OTHER PSYCHOTROPIC DRUGS, CAUTION IS ADVISED WHEN CLOZAPINE IS INITIATED IN PATIENTS TAKING A BENZODIAZEPINE OR ANY OTHER PSYCHOTROPIC DRUG. *(SEE WARNINGS.)*

DESCRIPTION

CLOZARIL® (clozapine), an atypical antipsychotic drug, is a tricyclic dibenzodiazepine derivative, 8-chloro-11-(4-methyl-1-piperazinyl)-5*H*-dibenzo [*b,e*] [1,4] diazepine.

The structural formula is

$C_{18}H_{19}ClN_4$ Mol. wt. 326.83

CLOZARIL is available in pale yellow tablets of 25 mg and 100 mg for oral administration.

25 mg and 100 mg Tablets

Active Ingredient: clozapine is a yellow, crystalline powder, very slightly soluble in water.

Inactive Ingredients: colloidal silicon dioxide, lactose, magnesium stearate, povidone, starch (corn), and talc.

CLINICAL PHARMACOLOGY

Pharmacodynamics

CLOZARIL® (clozapine) is classified as an 'atypical' antipsychotic drug because its profile of binding to dopamine receptors and its effects on various dopamine mediated behaviors differ from those exhibited by more typical antipsychotic drug products. In particular, although CLOZARIL does interfere with the binding of dopamine at D_1, D_2, D_3 and D_5 receptors, and has a high affinity for the D_4 receptor, it does not induce catalepsy nor inhibit apomorphine-induced stereotypy. This evidence, consistent with the view that CLOZARIL is preferentially more active at limbic than at striatal dopamine receptors, may explain the relative freedom of CLOZARIL from extrapyramidal side effects.

CLOZARIL also acts as an antagonist at adrenergic, cholinergic, histaminergic and serotonergic receptors.

Absorption, Distribution, Metabolism and Excretion

In man, CLOZARIL tablets (25 mg and 100 mg) are equally bioavailable relative to a clozapine solution. Following a dosage of 100 mg b.i.d., the average steady state peak plasma concentration was 319 ng/mL (range: 102-771 ng/mL), occurring at the average of 2.5 hours (range: 1-6 hours) after dosing. The average minimum concentration at steady state was 122 ng/mL (range: 41-343 ng/mL), after 100 mg b.i.d. dosing. Food does not appear to affect the systemic bioavailability of CLOZARIL. Thus, CLOZARIL may be administered with or without food.

Clozapine is approximately 97% bound to serum proteins. The interaction between CLOZARIL and other highly protein-bound drugs has not been fully evaluated but may be important. *(See PRECAUTIONS.)*

Clozapine is almost completely metabolized prior to excretion and only trace amounts of unchanged drug are detected in the urine and feces. Approximately 50% of the administered dose is excreted in the urine and 30% in the feces. The demethylated, hydroxylated and N-oxide derivatives are components in both urine and feces. Pharmacological testing has shown the desmethyl metabolite to have only limited activity, while the hydroxylated and N-oxide derivatives were inactive.

The mean elimination half-life of clozapine after a single 75 mg dose was 8 hours (range: 4-12 hours), compared to a mean elimination half-life, after achieving steady state with 100 mg b.i.d. dosing, of 12 hours (range: 4-66 hours). A comparison of single-dose and multiple-dose administration of clozapine showed that the elimination half-life increased significantly after multiple dosing relative to that after single-dose administration, suggesting the possibility of concentration dependent pharmacokinetics. However, at steady state, linearly dose-proportional changes with respect to AUC (area under the curve), peak and minimum clozapine plasma concentrations were observed after administration of 37.5 mg, 75 mg, and 150 mg b.i.d.

Human Pharmacology

In contrast to more typical antipsychotic drugs, CLOZARIL therapy produces little or no prolactin elevation.

As is true of more typical antipsychotic drugs, clinical EEG studies have shown that CLOZARIL increases delta and theta activity and slows dominant alpha frequencies. Enhanced synchronization occurs, and sharp wave activity and spike and wave complexes may also develop. Patients, on rare occasions, may report an intensification of dream activity during CLOZARIL therapy. REM sleep was found to be increased to 85% of the total sleep time. In these patients, the onset of REM sleep occurred almost immediately after falling asleep.

Clinical Trial Data (Reducing the Risk of Recurrent Suicidal Behavior in Patients with Schizophrenia or Schizoaffective Disorder Who are Judged to be at Risk of Re-experiencing Suicidal Behavior)

The effectiveness of CLOZARIL in reducing the risk of recurrent suicidal behavior was assessed in the International Suicide Prevention Trial (InterSePT™), which was a prospective, randomized, international, parallel-group comparison of CLOZARIL vs. Zyprexa®* (olanzapine) in patients with schizophrenia or schizoaffective disorder (DSM-IV) who were judged to be at risk for re-experiencing suicidal behavior. Only about one-fourth of these patients (27%) were considered resistant to standard antipsychotic drug treatment, and the remainder were not. Patients met one of the following criteria:

— They had attempted suicide within the 3 years prior to their baseline evaluation.
— They had been hospitalized to prevent a suicide attempt within the 3 years prior to their base-line evaluation.
— They demonstrated moderate-to-severe suicidal ideation with a depressive component within 1 week prior to their baseline evaluation.
— They demonstrated moderate-to-severe suicidal ideation accompanied by command hallucinations to do self-harm within 1 week prior to their baseline evaluation.

Dosing regimens for each treatment group were determined by individual investigators and were individualized by patient. Dosing was flexible, with a dose range of 200-900 mg/day for CLOZARIL and 5-20 mg/day for Zyprexa. For the 956 patients who received CLOZARIL or Zyprexa in this study, there was extensive use of concomitant psychotropics: 84% with antipsychotics; 65% with anxiolytics; 53% with antidepressants, and 28% with mood stabilizers. There was significantly greater use of concomitant psychotropic medications among the patients in the Zyprexa group.

The primary efficacy measure was time to (1) a significant suicide attempt, including a completed suicide, (2) hospitalization due to imminent suicide risk (including increased level of surveillance for suicidality for patients already hospitalized), or (3) worsening of suicidality severity as demonstrated by "much worsening" or "very much worsening" from baseline in the Clinical Global Impression of Severity of Suicidality as assessed by the Blinded Psychiatrist (CGI-SS-BP) scale. A determination of whether or not a reported event met criterion 1 or 2 above was made by the Suicide Monitoring Board (SMB, a group of experts blinded to patient data).

A total of 980 patients were randomized to the study and 956 received study medication. Sixty-two percent of the patients were diagnosed with schizophrenia, and the remainder (38%) were diagnosed with schizoaffective disorder. Only about one-fourth of the total patient population (27%) was identified as "treatment resistant" at baseline. There were more males than females in the study (61% of all patients were male). The mean age of patients entering the study was 37 years (range 18-69). Most patients were Caucasian (71%), 15% were Black, 1% were Oriental, and 13% were classified as being of "other" races.

Data from this study indicate that CLOZARIL had a statistically significant longer delay in the time to recurrent suicidal behavior in comparison with Zyprexa. This result should be interpreted only as evidence of the effectiveness of CLOZARIL in delaying time to recurrent suicidal behavior, and not a demonstration of the superior efficacy of CLOZARIL over Zyprexa.

The probability of experiencing (1) a significant suicide attempt, including a completed suicide, or (2) hospitalization due to imminent suicide risk (including increased level of surveillance for suicidality for patients already hospitalized) was lower for CLOZARIL patients than for Zyprexa patients at Week 104: CLOZARIL 24% vs. Zyprexa 32%; 95% C.I. of the difference: 2%, 14% (Figure 1).

Figure 1
Kaplan-Meier Estimates of Cumulative Probability of a Significant Suicide Attempt or Hospitalization to Prevent Suicide.

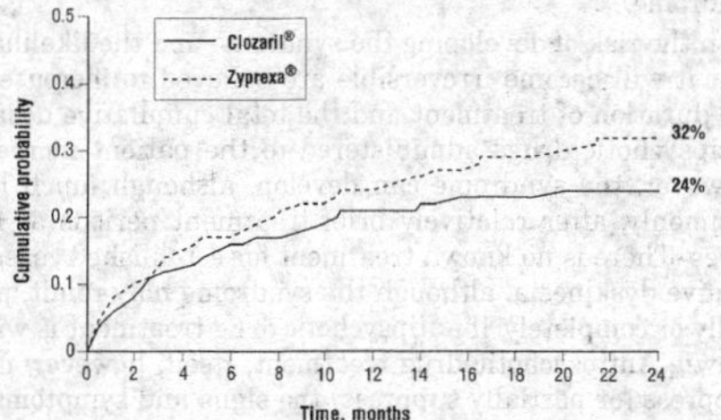

INDICATIONS AND USAGE

Treatment-Resistant Schizophrenia

CLOZARIL® (clozapine) is indicated for the management of severely ill schizophrenic patients who fail to respond adequately to standard drug treatment for schizophrenia. Because of the significant risk of agranulocytosis and seizure associated with its use, CLOZARIL should be used only in patients who have failed to respond adequately to treatment with appropriate courses of standard drug treatments for schizophrenia, either because of insufficient effectiveness or the inability to achieve an effective dose due to intolerable adverse effects from those drugs. *(See WARNINGS.)*

The effectiveness of CLOZARIL in a treatment resistant schizophrenic population was demonstrated in a 6-week study comparing CLOZARIL and chlorpromazine. Patients meeting DSM-III criteria for schizophrenia and having a mean BPRS total score of 61 were demonstrated to be treatment resistant by history and by open, prospective treatment with haloperidol before entering into the double-blind phase of the study. The superiority of CLOZARIL to chlorpromazine was documented in statistical analyses employing both categorical and continuous measures of treatment effect.

Because of the significant risk of agranulocytosis and seizure, events which both present a continuing risk over time, the extended treatment of patients failing to show an acceptable level of clinical response should ordinarily be avoided. In addition, the need for continuing treatment in patients exhibiting beneficial clinical responses should be periodically re-evaluated.

Reduction in the Risk of Recurrent Suicidal Behavior in Schizophrenia or Schizoaffective Disorders

CLOZARIL is indicated for reducing the risk of recurrent suicidal behavior in patients with schizophrenia or schizoaffective disorder who are judged to be at chronic risk for re-experiencing suicidal behavior, based on history and recent clinical state. Suicidal behavior refers to actions by a patient that puts him/herself at risk for death.

The effectiveness of CLOZARIL in reducing the risk of recurrent suicidal behavior was demonstrated over a 2-year treatment period in the InterSePT Trial *(see Clinical Trial Data under CLINICAL PHARMACOLOGY)*. Therefore, CLOZARIL treatment to reduce the risk of suicidal behavior should be continued for at least 2 years *(see DOSAGE AND ADMINISTRATION)*.

The prescriber should be aware that a majority of patients in both treatment groups in InterSePT received other treatments as well to reduce suicide risk, such as antidepressants and other medications, hospitalization, and/or psychotherapy. The contributions of these additional measures are unknown.

CONTRAINDICATIONS

CLOZARIL® (clozapine) is contraindicated in patients with a previous hypersensitivity to clozapine or any other component of this drug, in patients with myeloproliferative disorders, uncontrolled epilepsy, or a history of CLOZARIL induced agranulocytosis or severe granulocytopenia. As with more typical antipsychotic drugs, CLOZARIL is contraindicated in severe central nervous system depression or comatose states from any cause.

CLOZARIL should not be used simultaneously with other agents having a well-known potential to cause agranulocytosis or otherwise suppress bone marrow function. The mechanism of CLOZARIL induced agranulocytosis is unknown; nonetheless, it is possible that causative factors may interact synergistically to increase the risk and/or severity of bone marrow suppression.

WARNINGS

General

BECAUSE OF THE SIGNIFICANT RISK OF AGRANULOCYTOSIS, A POTENTIALLY LIFE-THREATENING ADVERSE EVENT *(SEE FOLLOWING)*, CLOZARIL® (CLOZAPINE) SHOULD BE RESERVED FOR USE IN (1) THE TREATMENT OF SEVERELY ILL PATIENTS WITH SCHIZOPHRENIA WHO FAIL TO SHOW AN ACCEPTABLE RESPONSE TO ADEQUATE COURSES OF STANDARD DRUG TREATMENT FOR SCHIZOPHRENIA, EITHER BECAUSE OF INSUFFICIENT EFFECTIVENESS OR THE INABILITY TO ACHIEVE AN EFFECTIVE DOSE DUE TO INTOLERABLE ADVERSE EFFECTS FROM THOSE DRUGS, OR (2) FOR REDUCING THE RISK OF RECURRENT SUICIDAL BEHAVIOR IN PATIENTS WITH SCHIZOPHRENIA OR SCHIZOAFFECTIVE DISORDER WHO ARE JUDGED TO BE AT RISK OF RE-EXPERIENCING SUICIDAL BEHAVIOR. CONSEQUENTLY, UNLESS THE PATIENT IS AT RISK FOR RECURRENT SUICIDAL BEHAVIOR, BEFORE INITIATING TREATMENT WITH CLOZARIL, IT IS STRONGLY RECOMMENDED THAT A PATIENT BE GIVEN AT LEAST 2 TRIALS, EACH WITH A DIFFERENT STANDARD DRUG PRODUCT FOR SCHIZOPHRENIA, AT AN ADEQUATE DOSE, AND FOR AN ADEQUATE DURATION.

PATIENTS WHO ARE BEING TREATED WITH CLOZARIL MUST HAVE A BASELINE WHITE BLOOD CELL (WBC) AND DIFFERENTIAL COUNT BEFORE INITIATION OF TREATMENT, AND A WBC COUNT EVERY WEEK FOR THE FIRST SIX MONTHS. THEREAFTER, IF ACCEPTABLE WBC COUNTS (WBC ≥3000/MM^3, ANC ≥1500/MM^3) HAVE BEEN MAINTAINED DURING THE FIRST 6 MONTHS OF CONTINUOUS THERAPY, WBC COUNTS CAN BE MONITORED EVERY OTHER WEEK. WBC COUNTS MUST BE MONITORED WEEKLY FOR AT LEAST 4 WEEKS AFTER THE DISCONTINUATION OF CLOZARIL.

CLOZARIL IS AVAILABLE ONLY THROUGH A DISTRIBUTION SYSTEM THAT ENSURES MONITORING OF WBC COUNTS ACCORDING TO THE SCHEDULE DESCRIBED BELOW PRIOR TO DELIVERY OF THE NEXT SUPPLY OF MEDICATION.

Agranulocytosis

Agranulocytosis, defined as an absolute neutrophil count (ANC) of less than 500/mm^3, has been estimated to occur in association with CLOZARIL use at a cumulative incidence at 1 year of approximately 1.3%, based on the occurrence of 15 U.S. cases out of 1,743 patients exposed to CLOZARIL during its clinical testing prior to domestic marketing. All of these cases occurred at a time when the need for close monitoring of WBC counts was already recognized. This reaction could prove fatal if not detected early and therapy interrupted. Of the 149 cases of agranulocytosis reported worldwide in association with CLOZARIL use as of December 31, 1989, 32% were fatal. However, few of these deaths occurred since 1977, at which time the knowledge of CLOZARIL induced agranulocytosis became more widespread, and close monitoring of WBC counts more widely practiced. Nevertheless, it is unknown at present what the case fatality rate will be for CLOZARIL induced agranulocytosis, despite strict adherence to the required frequency of monitoring. In the U.S., under a weekly WBC monitoring system with CLOZARIL, there have been 585 cases of agranulocytosis as of August 21, 1997; 19 were fatal. During this period 150,409 patients received CLOZARIL. A hematologic risk analysis was conducted based upon the available information in the Clozaril® National Registry (CNR) for U.S. patients. Based upon a cut-off date of April 30, 1995, the incidence rates of agranulocytosis based upon a weekly monitoring schedule, rose steeply during the first two months of therapy, peaking in the third month. Among CLOZARIL patients who continued the drug beyond the third month, the weekly incidence of agranulocytosis fell to a substantial degree, so that by the sixth month the weekly incidence of agranulocytosis was reduced to 3 per 1,000 person-years. After six months, the weekly incidence of agranulocytosis declines still further, however, never reaches zero. It should be noted that any type of reduction in the frequency of monitoring WBC counts may result in an increased incidence of agranulocytosis.

Because of the substantial risk for developing agranulocytosis in association with CLOZARIL use, which may persist over an extended period of time, patients must have a blood sample drawn for a WBC count before initiation of treatment with CLOZARIL, and must have subsequent WBC counts done at least weekly for the first 6 months of continuous treatment. If WBC counts remain acceptable (WBC ≥3000/mm^3, ANC ≥1500/mm^3) during this period, WBC counts may be monitored every other week thereafter. After the discontinuation of CLOZARIL, weekly WBC counts should be continued for an additional 4 weeks.

If a patient is on CLOZARIL therapy for less than 6 months with no abnormal blood events and there is a break on therapy which is less than or equal to 1 month, then patients can continue where they left off with weekly WBC testing for 6 months. When this 6-month period has been completed, the frequency of WBC count monitoring can be reduced to every other week. If a patient is on CLOZARIL therapy for less than 6 months with no abnormal blood events and there is a break on therapy which is greater than 1 month, then patients should be tested weekly for an additional 6-month period before biweekly testing is initiated. If a patient is on CLOZARIL therapy for less than 6 months and experiences an abnormal blood event as described below but remains a rechallengeable patient (patients cannot be reinitiated on CLOZARIL therapy if WBC counts fall below 2000/mm^3 or the ANC falls below 1000/mm^3 during CLOZARIL therapy), the patient must restart the 6-month period of weekly WBC monitoring at Day 0.

If a patient is on CLOZARIL therapy for 6 months or longer with no abnormal blood events and there is a break on therapy which is 1 year or less, then the patient can continue WBC count monitoring every other week if CLOZARIL therapy is reinitiated. If a patient is on CLOZARIL therapy for 6 months or longer with no abnormal blood events and there is a break on therapy which is greater than 1 year, then, if CLOZARIL therapy is reinitiated, the patient must have WBC counts monitored weekly for an additional 6 months. If a patient is on CLOZARIL therapy for 6 months or longer and subsequently has an abnormal blood event, but remains a rechallengeable patient, then the patient must restart weekly WBC count monitoring until an additional 6 months of CLOZARIL therapy has been received. The distribution of CLOZARIL is contingent upon performance of the required blood tests.

Treatment should not be initiated if the WBC count is less than 3500/mm^3, or if the patient has a history of a myeloproliferative disorder, or previous CLOZARIL induced agranulocytosis or granulocytopenia. Patients should be advised to report immediately the appearance of lethargy, weakness, fever, sore throat or any other signs of infection. If, after the initial treatment, the total WBC count has dropped below 3500/mm^3 or it has dropped by a substantial amount from baseline, even if the count is above 3500/mm^3, or if immature forms are present, a repeat WBC count and a differential count should be done. A substantial drop is defined as a single drop of 3,000 or more in the WBC count or a cumulative drop of 3,000 or more within 3 weeks. If subsequent WBC counts and the differential count reveal a total WBC count between 3000 and 3500/mm^3 and an ANC above 1500/mm^3, twice weekly WBC counts and differential counts should be performed. If the total WBC count falls below 3000/mm^3 or the ANC below 1500/mm^3, CLOZARIL therapy should be interrupted, WBC count and differential should be performed daily, and patients should be carefully monitored for flu-like symptoms or other symptoms suggestive of infection. CLOZARIL therapy may be resumed if no symptoms of infection develop, and if the total WBC count returns to levels above 3000/mm^3 and the ANC returns to levels above 1500/mm^3. However, in this event, twice-weekly WBC counts and differential counts should continue until total WBC counts return to levels above 3500/mm^3.

Continued on next page

Clozaril—Cont.

If the total WBC count falls below 2000/mm^3 or the ANC falls below 1000/mm^3, bone marrow aspiration should be considered to ascertain granulopoietic status. Protective isolation with close observation may be indicated if granulopoiesis is determined to be deficient. Should evidence of infection develop, the patient should have appropriate cultures performed and an appropriate antibiotic regimen instituted.

Patients whose total WBC counts fall below 2000/mm^3, or ANCs below 1000/mm^3 during CLOZARIL therapy should have daily WBC count and differential. These patients should not be rechallenged with CLOZARIL. Patients discontinued from CLOZARIL therapy due to significant WBC suppression have been found to develop agranulocytosis upon rechallenge, often with a shorter latency on re-exposure. To reduce the chances of rechallenge occurring in patients who have experienced significant bone marrow suppression during CLOZARIL therapy, a single, national master file will be maintained confidentially.

Except for evidence of significant bone marrow suppression during initial CLOZARIL therapy, there are no established risk factors, based on world-wide experience, for the development of agranulocytosis in association with CLOZARIL use. However, a disproportionate number of the U.S. cases of agranulocytosis occurred in patients of Jewish background compared to the overall proportion of such patients exposed during domestic development of CLOZARIL. Most of the U.S. cases occurred within 4-10 weeks of exposure, but neither dose nor duration is a reliable predictor of this problem. No patient characteristics have been clearly linked to the development of agranulocytosis in association with CLOZARIL use, but agranulocytosis associated with other antipsychotic drugs has been reported to occur with a greater frequency in women, the elderly and in patients who are cachectic or have serious underlying medical illness; such patients may also be at particular risk with CLOZARIL.

To reduce the risk of agranulocytosis developing undetected, CLOZARIL is available only through a distribution system that ensures monitoring of WBC counts according to the schedule described above prior to delivery of the next supply of medication.

Interrupted Therapy (WBC <3000/mm^3 ANC <1500/mm^3) for Bi-Weekly Monitoring

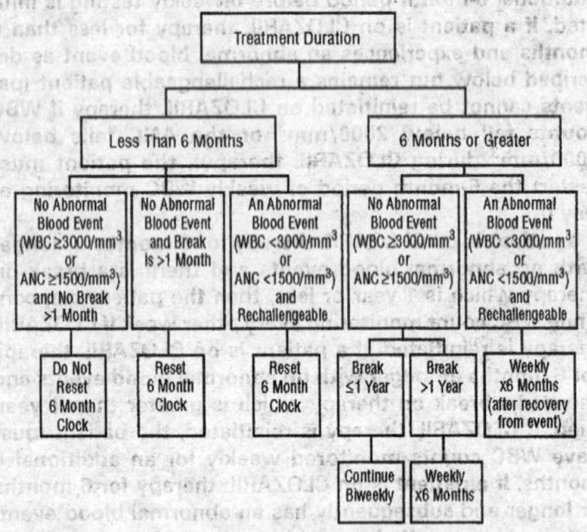

Eosinophilia

In clinical trials, 1% of patients developed eosinophilia, which, in rare cases, can be substantial. If a differential count reveals a total eosinophil count above 4000/mm^3, CLOZARIL therapy should be interrupted until the eosinophil count falls below 3000/mm^3.

Seizures

Seizure has been estimated to occur in association with CLOZARIL use at a cumulative incidence at one year of approximately 5%, based on the occurrence of one or more seizures in 61 of 1,743 patients exposed to CLOZARIL during its clinical testing prior to domestic marketing (i.e., a crude rate of 3.5%). Dose appears to be an important predictor of seizure, with a greater likelihood of seizure at the higher CLOZARIL doses used.

Caution should be used in administering CLOZARIL to patients having a history of seizures or other predisposing factors. Because of the substantial risk of seizure associated with CLOZARIL use, patients should be advised not to engage in any activity where sudden loss of consciousness could cause serious risk to themselves or others, e.g., the operation of complex machinery, driving an automobile, swimming, climbing, etc.

Myocarditis

Post-marketing surveillance data from four countries that employ hematological monitoring of clozapine-treated patients revealed: 30 reports of myocarditis with 17 fatalities in 205,493 U.S. patients (August 2001); 7 reports of myocarditis with 1 fatality in 15,600 Canadian patients (April 2001); 30 reports of myocarditis with 8 fatalities in 24,108 U.K. patients (August 2001); 15 reports of myocarditis with 5 fatalities in 8,000 Australian patients (March 1999). These reports represent an incidence of 5.0, 16.3, 43.2, and 96.6 cases/100,000 patient-years, respectively. The number of fatalities represent an incidence of 2.8, 2.3, 11.5, and 32.2 cases/100,000 patient-years, respectively.

The overall incidence rate of myocarditis in patients with schizophrenia treated with antipsychotic agents is unknown. However, for the established market economies (WHO), the incidence of myocarditis is 0.3 cases/100,000 patient-years and the fatality rate is 0.2 cases/100,000 patient-years. Therefore, the rate of myocarditis in clozapine-treated patients appears to be 17-322 times greater than the general population and is associated with an increased risk of fatal myocarditis that is 14-161 times greater than the general population.

The total reports of myocarditis for these four countries was 82 of which 51 (62%) occurred within the first month of clozapine treatment, 25 (31%) occurred after the first month of therapy and 6 (7%) were unknown. The median duration of treatment was 3 weeks. Of 5 patients rechallenged with clozapine, 3 had a recurrence of myocarditis. Of the 82 reports, 31 (38%) were fatal and 25 patients who died had evidence of myocarditis at autopsy. These data also suggest that the incidence of fatal myocarditis may be highest during the first month of therapy.

Therefore, the possibility of myocarditis should be considered in patients receiving CLOZARIL who present with unexplained fatigue, dyspnea, tachypnea, fever, chest pain, palpitations, other signs or symptoms of heart failure, or electrocardiographic findings such as ST-T wave abnormalities or arrhythmias. It is not known whether eosinophilia is a reliable predictor of myocarditis. Tachycardia, which has been associated with CLOZARIL treatment, has also been noted as a presenting sign in patients with myocarditis. Therefore, tachycardia during the first month of therapy warrants close monitoring for other signs of myocarditis.

Prompt discontinuation of CLOZARIL treatment is warranted upon suspicion of myocarditis. Patients with clozapine-related myocarditis should not be rechallenged with CLOZARIL.

Other Adverse Cardiovascular and Respiratory Effects

Orthostatic hypotension with or without syncope can occur with CLOZARIL treatment and may represent a continuing risk in some patients. Rarely (approximately 1 case per 3,000 patients), collapse can be profound and be accompanied by respiratory and/or cardiac arrest. Orthostatic hypotension is more likely to occur during initial titration in association with rapid dose escalation and may even occur on first dose. In one report, initial doses as low as 12.5 mg were associated with collapse and respiratory arrest. When restarting patients who have had even a brief interval off CLOZARIL, i.e., 2 days or more since the last dose, it is recommended that treatment be reinitiated with one-half of a 25 mg tablet (12.5 mg) once or twice daily. *(See DOSAGE AND ADMINISTRATION.)*

Some of the cases of collapse/respiratory arrest/cardiac arrest during initial treatment occurred in patients who were being administered benzodiazepines; similar events have been reported in patients taking other psychotropic drugs or even CLOZARIL by itself. Although it has not been established that there is an interaction between CLOZARIL and benzodiazepines or other psychotropics, caution is advised when clozapine is initiated in patients taking a benzodiazepine or any other psychotropic drug.

Tachycardia, which may be sustained, has also been observed in approximately 25% of patients taking CLOZARIL, with patients having an average increase in pulse rate of 10-15 bpm. The sustained tachycardia is not simply a reflex response to hypotension, and is present in all positions monitored. Either tachycardia or hypotension may pose a serious risk for an individual with compromised cardiovascular function.

A minority of CLOZARIL treated patients experience ECG repolarization changes similar to those seen with other anti-psychotic drugs, including S-T segment depression and flattening or inversion of T waves, which all normalize after discontinuation of CLOZARIL. The clinical significance of these changes is unclear. However, in clinical trials with CLOZARIL, several patients experienced significant cardiac events, including ischemic changes, myocardial infarction, arrhythmias and sudden death. In addition there have been post-marketing reports of congestive heart failure, pericarditis, and pericardial effusions. Causality assessment was difficult in many of these cases because of serious preexisting cardiac disease and plausible alternative causes. Rare instances of sudden death have been reported in psychiatric patients, with or without associated antipsychotic drug treatment, and the relationship of these events to antipsychotic drug use is unknown.

CLOZARIL should be used with caution in patients with known cardiovascular and/or pulmonary disease, and the recommendation for gradual titration of dose should be carefully observed.

Hyperglycemia and Diabetes Mellitus

Hyperglycemia, in some cases extreme and associated with ketoacidosis or hyperosmolar coma or death, has been reported in patients treated with atypical antipsychotics including CLOZARIL. Assessment of the relationship between atypical antipsychotic use and glucose abnormalities is complicated by the possibility of an increased background risk of diabetes mellitus in patients with schizophrenia and the increasing incidence of diabetes mellitus in the general population. Given these confounders, the relationship between atypical antipsychotic use and hyperglycemia-related adverse events is not completely understood. However, epidemiological studies suggest an increased risk of treatment-emergent hyperglycemia-related adverse events in patients treated with the atypical antipsychotics. Precise risk estimates for hyperglycemia-related adverse events in patients treated with atypical antipsychotics are not available.

Patients with an established diagnosis of diabetes mellitus who are started on atypical antipsychotics should be monitored regularly for worsening of glucose control. Patients with risk factors for diabetes mellitus (e.g., obesity, family history of diabetes) who are starting treatment with atypical antipsychotics should undergo fasting blood glucose testing at the beginning of treatment and periodically during treatment. Any patient treated with atypical antipsychotics should be monitored for symptoms of hyperglycemia including polydipsia, polyuria, polyphagia, and weakness. Patients who develop symptoms of hyperglycemia during treatment with atypical antipsychotics should undergo fasting blood glucose testing. In some cases, hyperglycemia has resolved when the atypical antipsychotic was discontinued; however, some patients required continuation of anti-diabetic treatment despite discontinuation of the suspect drug.

Neuroleptic Malignant Syndrome (NMS)

A potentially fatal symptom complex sometimes referred to as Neuroleptic Malignant Syndrome (NMS) has been reported in association with antipsychotic drugs. Clinical manifestations of NMS are hyperpyrexia, muscle rigidity, altered mental status and evidence of autonomic instability (irregular pulse or blood pressure, tachycardia, diaphoresis, and cardiac dysrhythmias).

The diagnostic evaluation of patients with this syndrome is complicated. In arriving at a diagnosis, it is important to identify cases where the clinical presentation includes both serious medical illness (e.g., pneumonia, systemic infection, etc.) and untreated or inadequately treated extrapyramidal signs and symptoms (EPS). Other important considerations in the differential diagnosis include central anticholinergic toxicity, heat stroke, drug fever and primary central nervous system (CNS) pathology.

The management of NMS should include 1) immediate discontinuation of antipsychotic drugs and other drugs not essential to concurrent therapy, 2) intensive symptomatic treatment and medical monitoring, and 3) treatment of any concomitant serious medical problems for which specific treatments are available. There is no general agreement about specific pharmacological treatment regimens for uncomplicated NMS.

If a patient requires antipsychotic drug treatment after recovery from NMS, the potential reintroduction of drug therapy should be carefully considered. The patient should be carefully monitored, since recurrences of NMS have been reported.

There have been several reported cases of NMS in patients receiving CLOZARIL alone or in combination with lithium or other CNS-active agents.

Tardive Dyskinesia

A syndrome consisting of potentially irreversible, involuntary, dyskinetic movements may develop in patients treated with antipsychotic drugs. Although the prevalence of the syndrome appears to be highest among the elderly, especially elderly women, it is impossible to rely upon prevalence estimates to predict, at the inception of treatment, which patients are likely to develop the syndrome.

There are several reasons for predicting that CLOZARIL may be different from other antipsychotic drugs in its potential for inducing tardive dyskinesia, including the preclinical finding that it has a relatively weak dopamine-blocking effect and the clinical finding of a virtual absence of certain acute extrapyramidal symptoms, e.g., dystonia. A few cases of tardive dyskinesia have been reported in patients on CLOZARIL who had been previously treated with other antipsychotic agents, so that a causal relationship cannot be established. There have been no reports of tardive dyskinesia directly attributable to CLOZARIL alone. Nevertheless, it cannot be concluded, without more extended experience, that CLOZARIL is incapable of inducing this syndrome.

Both the risk of developing the syndrome and the likelihood that it will become irreversible are believed to increase as the duration of treatment and the total cumulative dose of antipsychotic drugs administered to the patient increase. However, the syndrome can develop, although much less commonly, after relatively brief treatment periods at low doses. There is no known treatment for established cases of tardive dyskinesia, although the syndrome may remit, partially or completely, if antipsychotic drug treatment is withdrawn. Antipsychotic drug treatment, itself, however, may suppress (or partially suppress) the signs and symptoms of the syndrome and thereby may possibly mask the underlying process. The effect that symptom suppression has upon the long-term course of the syndrome is unknown.

Given these considerations, CLOZARIL should be prescribed in a manner that is most likely to minimize the occurrence of tardive dyskinesia. As with any antipsychotic drug, chronic CLOZARIL use should be reserved for patients who appear to be obtaining substantial benefit from the drug. In such patients, the smallest dose and the shortest duration of treatment should be sought. The need for continued treatment should be reassessed periodically.

If signs and symptoms of tardive dyskinesia appear in a patient on CLOZARIL, drug discontinuation should be considered. However, some patients may require treatment with CLOZARIL despite the presence of the syndrome.

PRECAUTIONS

General

Because of the significant risk of agranulocytosis and seizure, both of which present a continuing risk over time, the extended treatment of patients failing to show an acceptable level of clinical response should ordinarily be avoided. In addition, the need for continuing treatment in patients exhibiting beneficial clinical responses should be periodically re-evaluated. Although it is not known whether the risk would be increased, it is prudent either to avoid CLOZARIL® (clozapine) or use it cautiously in patients with a previous history of agranulocytosis induced by other drugs.

Cardiomyopathy

Cases of cardiomyopathy have been reported in patients treated with clozapine. The reporting rate for cardiomyopathy in clozapine-treated patients in the U.S. (8.9 per 100,000 person-years) was similar to an estimate of the cardiomyopathy incidence in the U.S. general population derived from the 1999 National Hospital Discharge Survey data (9.7 per 100,000 person-years). Approximately 80% of clozapine-treated patients in whom cardiomyopathy was reported were less than 50 years of age; the duration of treatment with clozapine prior to cardiomyopathy diagnosis varied, but was >6 months in 65% of the reports. Dilated cardiomyopathy was most frequently reported, although a large percentage of reports did not specify the type of cardiomyopathy. Signs and symptoms suggestive of cardiomyopathy, particularly exertional dyspnea, fatigue, orthopnea, paroxysmal nocturnal dyspnea, and peripheral edema should alert the clinician to perform further investigations. If the diagnosis of cardiomyopathy is confirmed, the prescriber should discontinue clozapine unless the benefit to the patient clearly outweighs the risk.

Fever

During CLOZARIL therapy, patients may experience transient temperature elevations above 100.4°F (38°C), with the peak incidence within the first 3 weeks of treatment. While this fever is generally benign and self limiting, it may necessitate discontinuing patients from treatment. On occasion, there may be an associated increase or decrease in WBC count. Patients with fever should be carefully evaluated to rule out the possibility of an underlying infectious process or the development of agranulocytosis. In the presence of high fever, the possibility of Neuroleptic Malignant Syndrome (NMS) must be considered. There have been several reports of NMS in patients receiving CLOZARIL, usually in combination with lithium or other CNS-active drugs. *(See Neuroleptic Malignant Syndrome [NMS], under WARNINGS.)*

Pulmonary Embolism

The possibility of pulmonary embolism should be considered in patients receiving CLOZARIL who present with deep vein thrombosis, acute dyspnea, chest pain or with other respiratory signs and symptoms. As of December 31, 1993 there were 18 cases of fatal pulmonary embolism in association with CLOZARIL therapy in users 10-54 years of age. Based upon the extent of use observed in the Clozaril® National Registry, the mortality rate associated with pulmonary embolus was 1 death per 3,450 person-years of use. This rate was about 27.5 times higher than that in the general population of a similar age and gender (95% Confidence Interval; 17.1, 42.2). Deep vein thrombosis has also been observed in association with CLOZARIL therapy. Whether pulmonary embolus can be attributed to CLOZARIL or some characteristic(s) of its users is not clear, but the occurrence of deep vein thrombosis or respiratory symptomatology should suggest its presence.

Hepatitis

Caution is advised in patients using CLOZARIL who have concurrent hepatic disease. Hepatitis has been reported in both patients with normal and pre-existing liver function abnormalities. In patients who develop nausea, vomiting, and/or anorexia during CLOZARIL treatment, liver function tests should be performed immediately. If the elevation of these values is clinically relevant or if symptoms of jaundice occur, treatment with CLOZARIL should be discontinued.

Anticholinergic Toxicity

Eye: CLOZARIL has potent anticholinergic effects and care should be exercised in using this drug in the presence of narrow angle glaucoma.

Gastrointestinal: CLOZARIL use has been associated with varying degrees of impairment of intestinal peristalsis, ranging from constipation to intestinal obstruction, fecal impaction and paralytic ileus *(see ADVERSE REACTIONS)*. On rare occasions, these cases have been fatal. Constipation should be initially treated by ensuring adequate hydration, and use of ancillary therapy such as bulk laxatives. Consultation with a gastroenterologist is advisable in more serious cases.

Prostate: CLOZARIL has potent anticholinergic effects and care should be exercised in using this drug in the presence of prostatic enlargement.

Interference with Cognitive and Motor Performance

Because of initial sedation, CLOZARIL may impair mental and/or physical abilities, especially during the first few days of therapy. The recommendations for gradual dose escalation should be carefully adhered to, and patients cautioned about activities requiring alertness.

Use in Patients with Concomitant Illness

Clinical experience with CLOZARIL in patients with concomitant systemic diseases is limited. Nevertheless, caution is advisable in using CLOZARIL in patients with renal or cardiac disease.

Use in Patients Undergoing General Anesthesia

Caution is advised in patients being administered general anesthesia because of the CNS effects of CLOZARIL. Check with the anesthesiologist regarding continuation of CLOZARIL therapy in a patient scheduled for surgery.

Information for Patients

Physicians are advised to discuss the following issues with patients for whom they prescribe CLOZARIL:

— Patients who are to receive CLOZARIL should be warned about the significant risk of developing agranulocytosis. They should be informed that weekly blood tests are required for the first 6 months, if acceptable WBC counts (WBC ≥3000/mm^3, ANC ≥1500/mm^3) have been maintained during the first 6 months of continuous therapy, then WBC counts can be monitored every other week in order to monitor for the occurrence of agranulocytosis, and that CLOZARIL tablets will be made available only through a special program designed to ensure the required blood monitoring. Patients should be advised to report immediately the appearance of lethargy, weakness, fever, sore throat, malaise, mucous membrane ulceration or other possible signs of infection. Particular attention should be paid to any flu-like complaints or other symptoms that might suggest infection.

— Patients should be informed of the significant risk of seizure during CLOZARIL treatment, and they should be advised to avoid driving and any other potentially hazardous activity while taking CLOZARIL.

— Patients should be advised of the risk of orthostatic hypotension, especially during the period of initial dose titration.

— Patients should be informed that if they stop taking CLOZARIL for more than 2 days, they should not restart their medication at the same dosage, but should contact their physician for dosing instructions.

— Patients should notify their physician if they are taking, or plan to take, any prescription or over-the-counter drugs or alcohol.

— Patients should notify their physician if they become pregnant or intend to become pregnant during therapy.

— Patients should not breast-feed an infant if they are taking CLOZARIL.

Drug Interactions

The risks of using CLOZARIL in combination with other drugs have not been systematically evaluated.

Pharmacodynamic-Related Interactions: The mechanism of CLOZARIL induced agranulocytosis is unknown; nonetheless, the possibility that causative factors may interact synergistically to increase the risk and/or severity of bone marrow suppression warrants consideration. Therefore, CLOZARIL should not be used with other agents having a well-known potential to suppress bone marrow function.

Given the primary CNS effects of CLOZARIL, caution is advised in using it concomitantly with other CNS-active drugs or alcohol.

Orthostatic hypotension in patients taking clozapine can, in rare cases (approximately 1 case per 3,000 patients), be accompanied by profound collapse and respiratory and/or cardiac arrest. Some of the cases of collapse/respiratory arrest/cardiac arrest during initial treatment occurred in patients who were being administered benzodiazepines; similar events have been reported in patients taking other psychotropic drugs or even CLOZARIL by itself. Although it has not been established that there is an interaction between CLOZARIL and benzodiazepines or other psychotropics, caution is advised when clozapine is initiated in patients taking a benzodiazepine or any other psychotropic drug.

CLOZARIL may potentiate the hypotensive effects of antihypertensive drugs and the anticholinergic effects of atropine-type drugs. The administration of epinephrine should be avoided in the treatment of drug induced hypotension because of a possible reverse epinephrine effect.

Pharmacokinetic-Related Interactions: Clozapine is a substrate for many CYP 450 isozymes, in particular 1A2, 2D6, and 3A4. The risk of metabolic interactions caused by an effect on an individual isoform is therefore minimized. Nevertheless, caution should be used in patients receiving concomitant treatment with other drugs that are either inhibitors or inducers of these enzymes.

Concomitant administration of drugs known to induce cytochrome P450 enzymes may decrease the plasma levels of clozapine. Phenytoin, nicotine, and rifampin may decrease CLOZARIL plasma levels, resulting in a decrease in effectiveness of a previously effective CLOZARIL dose.

Concomitant administration of drugs known to inhibit the activity of cytochrome P450 isozymes may increase the plasma levels of clozapine. Cimetidine, caffeine, and erythromycin may increase plasma levels of CLOZARIL, potentially resulting in adverse effects. Although concomitant use of CLOZARIL and carbamazepine is not recommended, it should be noted that discontinuation of concomitant carbamazepine administration may result in an increase in CLOZARIL plasma levels.

In a study of schizophrenic patients who received clozapine under steady state conditions, fluvoxamine or paroxetine was added in 16 and 14 patients, respectively. After 14 days ofco-administration, meantroughconcentrationsofclozapine and its metabolites, *N*-desmethylclozapine and clozapine *N*-oxide, were elevated with fluvoxamine by about three-fold compared to baseline concentrations. Paroxetine produced only minor changes in the levels of clozapine and its metabolites. However, other published reports describe modest elevations (less than two-fold) of clozapine and metabolite concentrations when clozapine was taken with paroxetine, fluoxetine, and sertraline. Therefore, such combined treatment should be approached with caution and patients should be monitored closely when CLOZARIL is combined with these drugs, particularly with fluvoxamine. A reduced CLOZARIL dose should be considered.

A subset (3%-10%) of the population has reduced activity of certain drug metabolizing enzymes such as the cytochrome P450 isozyme P450 2D6. Such individuals are referred to as "poor metabolizers" of drugs such as debrisoquin, dextromethorphan, the tricyclic antidepressants, and clozapine. These individuals may develop higher than expected plasma concentrations of clozapine when given usual doses. In addition, certain drugs that are metabolized by this isozyme, including many antidepressants (clozapine, selective serotonin reuptake inhibitors, and others), may inhibit the activity of this isozyme, and thus may make normal metabolizers resemble poor metabolizers with regard to concomitant therapy with other drugs metabolized by this enzyme system, leading to drug interaction.

Concomitant use of clozapine with other drugs metabolized by cytochrome P450 2D6 may require lower doses than usually prescribed for either clozapine or the other drug. Therefore, co-administration of clozapine with other drugs that are metabolized by this isozyme, including antidepressants, phenothiazines, carbamazepine, and Type 1C antiarrhythmics (e.g., propafenone, flecainide and encainide), or that inhibit this enzyme (e.g., quinidine), should be approached with caution.

Carcinogenesis, Mutagenesis, Impairment of Fertility

No carcinogenic potential was demonstrated in long-term studies in mice and rats at doses approximately 7 times the typical human dose on a mg/kg basis. Fertility in male and female rats was not adversely affected by clozapine. Clozapine did not produce genotoxic or mutagenic effects when assayed in appropriate bacterial and mammalian tests.

Pregnancy Category B

Reproduction studies have been performed in rats and rabbits at doses of approximately 2-4 times the human dose and have revealed no evidence of impaired fertility or harm to the fetus due to clozapine. There are, however, no adequate and well-controlled studies in pregnant women. Because animal reproduction studies are not always predictive of human response, and in view of the desirability of keeping the administration of all drugs to a minimum during pregnancy, this drug should be used only if clearly needed.

Nursing Mothers

Animal studies suggest that clozapine may be excreted in breast milk and have an effect on the nursing infant. Therefore, women receiving CLOZARIL should not breast-feed.

Pediatric Use

Safety and effectiveness in pediatric patients have not been established.

Geriatric Use

Clinical studies of clozapine did not include sufficient numbers of subjects age 65 and over to determine whether they respond differently from younger subjects.

Orthostatic hypotension can occur with CLOZARIL treatment and tachycardia, which may be sustained, has been observed in about 25% of patients taking CLOZARIL *(see BOXED WARNING, Other Adverse Cardiovascular and Respiratory Effects)*. Elderly patients, particularly those with compromised cardiovascular functioning, may be more susceptible to these effects.

Also, elderly patients may be particularly susceptible to the anticholinergic effects of CLOZARIL, such as urinary retention and constipation. *(See PRECAUTIONS, Anticholinergic Toxicity.)*

Dose selection for an elderly patient should be cautious, reflecting the greater frequency of decreased hepatic, renal, or cardiac function, and of concomitant disease or other drug therapy. Other reported clinical experience does suggest that the prevalence of tardive dyskinesia appears to be highest among the elderly, especially elderly women. *(See WARNINGS, Tardive Dyskinesia.)*

ADVERSE REACTIONS

Associated with Discontinuation of Treatment

Sixteen percent of 1,080 patients who received CLOZARIL® (clozapine) in pre-marketing clinical trials discontinued treatment due to an adverse event, including both those that could be reasonably attributed to CLOZARIL treatment and those that might more appropriately be considered intercurrent illness. The more common events considered to be causes of discontinuation included: CNS, primarily drowsiness/sedation, seizures, dizziness/syncope; cardiovascular, primarily tachycardia, hypotension and ECG changes; gastrointestinal, primarily nausea/vomiting; hematologic, primarily leukopenia/granulocytopenia/agranulocytosis; and fever. None of the events enumerated accounts for more than 1.7% of all discontinuations attributed to adverse clinical events.

Commonly Observed

Adverse events observed in association with the use of CLOZARIL in clinical trials at an incidence of greater than 5% were: central nervous system complaints, including drowsiness/sedation, dizziness/vertigo, headache and tremor; autonomic nervous system complaints, including salivation, sweating, dry mouth and visual disturbances; cardiovascular findings, including tachycardia, hypotension and syncope; and gastrointestinal complaints, including constipation and nausea; and fever. Complaints of drowsi-

Continued on next page

Clozaril—Cont.

ness/sedation tend to subside with continued therapy or dose reduction. Salivation may be profuse, especially during sleep, but may be diminished with dose reduction.

Incidence in Clinical Trials

The following table enumerates adverse events that occurred at a frequency of 1% or greater among CLOZARIL patients who participated in clinical trials. These rates are not adjusted for duration of exposure.

Treatment-Emergent Adverse Experience Incidence Among Patients Taking CLOZARIL® (clozapine) in Clinical Trials (excluding the InterSePT™ Study) (N = 842) (Percentage of Patients Reporting)

Body System / Adverse Event[a]	Percent
Central Nervous System	
Drowsiness/Sedation	39
Dizziness/Vertigo	19
Headache	7
Tremor	6
Syncope	6
Disturbed sleep/Nightmares	4
Restlessness	4
Hypokinesia/Akinesia	4
Agitation	4
Seizures (convulsions)	3[b]
Rigidity	3
Akathisia	3
Confusion	3
Fatigue	2
Insomnia	2
Hyperkinesia	1
Weakness	1
Lethargy	1
Ataxia	1
Slurred speech	1
Depression	1
Epileptiform movements/Myoclonic jerks	1
Anxiety	1
Cardiovascular	
Tachycardia	25[b]
Hypotension	9
Hypertension	4
Chest pain/Angina	1
ECG change/Cardiac abnormality	1
Gastrointestinal	
Constipation	14
Nausea	5
Abdominal discomfort/Heartburn	4
Nausea/Vomiting	3
Vomiting	3
Diarrhea	2
Liver test abnormality	1
Anorexia	1
Urogenital	
Urinary abnormalities	2
Incontinence	1
Abnormal ejaculation	1
Urinary urgency/frequency	1
Urinary retention	1
Autonomic Nervous System	
Salivation	31
Sweating	6
Dry mouth	6
Visual disturbances	5
Integumentary (Skin)	
Rash	2
Musculoskeletal	
Muscle weakness	1
Pain (back, neck, legs)	1
Muscle spasm	1
Muscle pain, ache	1
Respiratory	
Throat discomfort	1
Dyspnea, shortness of breath	1
Nasal congestion	1
Hemic/Lymphatic	
Leukopenia/Decreased WBC/Neutropenia	3
Agranulocytosis	1[b]
Eosinophilia	1
Miscellaneous	
Fever	5
Weight gain	4
Tongue numb/sore	1

[a] Events reported by at least 1% of CLOZARIL patients are included.

[b] Rate based on population of approximately 1,700 exposed during pre-market clinical evaluation of CLOZARIL.

The following table enumerates adverse events that occurred at a frequency of 10% for either treatment group in patients who took at least 1 dose of study medication during their participation in InterSePT, which was an adequate and well-controlled 2-year study evaluating the efficacy of CLOZARIL relative to Zyprexa in reducing the risk of emergent suicidal behavior in patients with schizophrenia or schizoaffective disorder. These rates are not adjusted for duration of exposure.

[See table below]

Other Events Observed During the Pre-marketing Evaluation of CLOZARIL® (clozapine)

This section reports additional, less frequent adverse events which occurred among the patients taking CLOZARIL in clinical trials. Various adverse events were reported as part of the total experience in these clinical studies; a causal relationship to CLOZARIL treatment cannot be determined in the absence of appropriate controls in some of the studies. The table above enumerates adverse events that occurred at a frequency of at least 1% of patients treated with CLOZARIL. The list below includes all additional adverse experiences reported as being temporally associated with the use of the drug which occurred at a frequency less than 1%, enumerated by organ system.

Central Nervous System: loss of speech, amentia, tics, poor coordination, delusions/hallucinations, involuntary movement, stuttering, dysarthria, amnesia/memory loss, histrionic movements, libido increase or decrease, paranoia, shakiness, Parkinsonism, and irritability.

Cardiovascular System: edema, palpitations, phlebitis/thrombophlebitis, cyanosis, premature ventricular contraction, bradycardia, and nose bleed.

Gastrointestinal System: abdominal distention, gastroenteritis, rectal bleeding, nervous stomach, abnormal stools, hematemesis, gastric ulcer, bitter taste, and eructation.

Urogenital System: dysmenorrhea, impotence, breast pain/discomfort, and vaginal itch/infection.

Autonomic Nervous System: numbness, polydipsia, hot flashes, dry throat, and mydriasis.

Integumentary (Skin): pruritus, pallor, eczema, erythema, bruise, dermatitis, petechiae, and urticaria.

Musculoskeletal System: twitching and joint pain.

Respiratory System: coughing, pneumonia/pneumonia-like symptoms, rhinorrhea, hyperventilation, wheezing, bronchitis, laryngitis, and sneezing.

Hemic and Lymphatic System: anemia and leukocytosis.

Miscellaneous: chills/chills with fever, malaise, appetite increase, ear disorder, hypothermia, eyelid disorder, bloodshot eyes, and nystagmus.

Post-marketing Clinical Experience

Post-marketing experience has shown an adverse experience profile similar to that presented above. Voluntary reports of adverse events temporally associated with CLOZARIL not mentioned above that have been received since market introduction and that may have no causal relationship with the drug include the following:

Central Nervous System: delirium; EEG abnormal; exacerbation of psychosis; myoclonus; overdose; paresthesia; possible mild cataplexy; and status epilepticus.

Cardiovascular System: atrial or ventricular fibrillation and periorbital edema.

Gastrointestinal System: acute pancreatitis; dysphagia; fecal impaction; intestinal obstruction/paralytic ileus; and salivary gland swelling.

Hepatobiliary System: cholestasis; hepatitis; jaundice.

Hepatic System: cholestasis.

Urogenital System: acute interstitial nephritis and priapism.

Integumentary (Skin): hypersensitivity reactions: photosensitivity, vasculitis, erythema multiforme, and Stevens-Johnson Syndrome.

Musculoskeletal System: myasthenic syndrome and rhabdomyolysis.

Respiratory System: aspiration and pleural effusion.

Hemic and Lymphatic System: deep vein thrombosis; elevated hemoglobin/hematocrit; ESR increased; pulmonary embolism; sepsis; thrombocytosis; and thrombocytopenia.

Vision Disorders: narrow angle glaucoma.

Miscellaneous: CPK elevation; hyperglycemia; hyperuricemia; hyponatremia; and weight loss.

DRUG ABUSE AND DEPENDENCE

Physical and psychological dependence have not been reported or observed in patients taking CLOZARIL® (clozapine).

OVERDOSAGE

Human Experience

The most commonly reported signs and symptoms associated with CLOZARIL® (clozapine) overdose are: altered states of consciousness, including drowsiness, delirium and coma; tachycardia; hypotension; respiratory depression or failure; hypersalivation. Aspiration pneumonia and cardiac arrhythmias have also been reported. Seizures have occurred in a minority of reported cases. Fatal overdoses have been reported with CLOZARIL, generally at doses above 2500 mg. There have also been reports of patients recovering from overdoses well in excess of 4 g.

Management of Overdose

Establish and maintain an airway; ensure adequate oxygenation and ventilation. Activated charcoal, which may be used with sorbitol, may be as or more effective than emesis or lavage, and should be considered in treating overdosage. Cardiac and vital signs monitoring is recommended along with general symptomatic and supportive measures. Additional surveillance should be continued for several days because of the risk of delayed effects. Avoid epinephrine and derivatives when treating hypotension, and quinidine and procainamide when treating cardiac arrhythmia.

There are no specific antidotes for CLOZARIL. Forced diuresis, dialysis, hemoperfusion and exchange transfusion are unlikely to be of benefit.

In managing overdosage, the physician should consider the possibility of multiple drug involvement.

Up-to-date information about the treatment of overdose can often be obtained from a certified Regional Poison Control Center. Telephone numbers of certified Poison Control Centers are listed in the Physicians' Desk Reference®.**

DOSAGE AND ADMINISTRATION

Treatment-Resistant Schizophrenia

Upon initiation of CLOZARIL® (clozapine) therapy, up to a 1 week supply of additional CLOZARIL tablets may be provided to the patient to be held for emergencies (e.g., weather, holidays).

Initial Treatment: It is recommended that treatment with CLOZARIL begin with one-half of a 25 mg tablet (12.5 mg) once or twice daily and then be continued with daily dosage increments of 25-50 mg/day, if well tolerated, to achieve a target dose of 300-450 mg/day by the end of 2 weeks. Subsequent dosage increments should be made no more than once or twice weekly, in increments not to exceed 100 mg. Cautious titration and a divided dosage schedule are necessary to minimize the risks of hypotension, seizure, and sedation.

In the multicenter study that provides primary support for the effectiveness of CLOZARIL in patients resistant to standard drug treatment for schizophrenia, patients were titrated during the first 2 weeks up to a maximum dose of 500 mg/day, on a t.i.d. basis, and were then dosed in a total daily dose range of 100-900 mg/day, on a t.i.d. basis thereafter, with clinical response and adverse effects as guides to correct dosing.

Therapeutic Dose Adjustment: Daily dosing should continue on a divided basis as an effective and tolerable dose level is sought. While many patients may respond adequately at doses between 300-600 mg/day, it may be necessary to raise the dose to the 600-900 mg/day range to obtain an acceptable response. (Note: In the multicenter study providing the primary support for the superiority of CLOZARIL in treatment-resistant patients, the mean and median CLOZARIL doses were both approximately 600 mg/day.)

Because of the possibility of increased adverse reactions at higher doses, particularly seizures, patients should ordinarily be given adequate time to respond to a given dose level before escalation to a higher dose is contemplated.

CLOZARIL can cause EEG changes, including the occurrence of spike and wave complexes. It lowers the seizures

Treatment-Emergent Adverse Experience Incidence[1] Among Patients Taking CLOZARIL® (clozapine) or Zyprexa® (olanzapine) in the InterSePT™ Study (Percentage of Patients Reporting)

	Clozaril® N = 479 % Reporting	Zyprexa® N = 477 % Reporting
Adverse Events		
Salivary hypersecretion	48%	6%
Somnolence	46%	25%
Weight increased	31%	56%
Dizziness (excluding vertigo)	27%	12%
Constipation	25%	10%
Insomnia NEC	20%	33%
Nausea	17%	10%
Vomiting NOS	17%	9%
Dyspepsia	14%	8%

[1] AEs are listed by frequency in Clozaril group, and included in the table are those for which the risk ratio of Clozaril over Zyprexa or of Zyprexa over Clozaril was greater than 1.5.

NEC - not elsewhere classified

NOS - not otherwise classified

threshold in a dose-dependent manner and may induce myoclonic jerks or generalized seizures. These symptoms may be likely to occur with rapid dose increase and in patients with pre-existing epilepsy. In this case, the dose should be reduced and, if necessary, anticonvulsant treatment initiated.

Dosing should not exceed 900 mg/day.

Because of the significant risk of agranulocytosis and seizure, events which both present a continuing risk over time, the extended treatment of patients failing to show an acceptable level of clinical response should ordinarily be avoided.

Maintenance Treatment: While the maintenance effectiveness of CLOZARIL in schizophrenia is still under study, the effectiveness of maintenance treatment is well established for many other drugs used to treat schizophrenia. It is recommended that responding patients be continued on CLOZARIL, but at the lowest level needed to maintain remission. Because of the significant risk associated with the use of CLOZARIL, patients should be periodically reassessed to determine the need for maintenance treatment.

Discontinuation of Treatment: In the event of planned termination of CLOZARIL therapy, gradual reduction in dose is recommended over a 1-2 week period. However, should a patient's medical condition require abrupt discontinuation (e.g., leukopenia), the patient should be carefully observed for the recurrence of psychotic symptoms and symptoms related to cholinergic rebound such as headache, nausea, vomiting, and diarrhea.

Reinitiation of Treatment in Patients Previously Discontinued: When restarting patients who have had even a brief interval off CLOZARIL, i.e., 2 days or more since the last dose, it is recommended that treatment be reinitiated with one-half of a 25 mg tablet (12.5 mg) once or twice daily *(see WARNINGS)*. If that dose is well tolerated, it may be feasible to titrate patients back to a therapeutic dose more quickly than is recommended for initial treatment. However, any patient who has previously experienced respiratory or cardiac arrest with initial dosing, but was then able to be successfully titrated to a therapeutic dose, should be re-titrated with extreme caution after even 24 hours of discontinuation.

Certain additional precautions seem prudent when reinitiating treatment. The mechanisms underlying CLOZARIL induced adverse reactions are unknown. It is conceivable, however, that re-exposure of a patient might enhance the risk of an untoward event's occurrence and increase its severity. Such phenomena, for example, occur when immune mediated mechanisms are responsible. Consequently, during the reinitiation of treatment, additional caution is advised. Patients discontinued for WBC counts below 2000/mm^3 or an ANC below 1000/mm^3 must *not* be restarted on CLOZARIL. *(See WARNINGS.)*

Reducing the Risk of Recurrent Suicidal Behavior in Patients with Schizophrenia or Schizoaffective Disorder

The dosage and administration recommendations outlined above regarding the use of CLOZARIL in patients with treatment-resistant schizophrenia should also be followed when treating patients with schizophrenia or schizoaffective disorder at risk for recurrent suicidal behavior.

The InterSePT study demonstrated the efficacy of CLOZARIL in treatment of patients with schizophrenia or schizoaffective disorder at risk for recurrent suicidal behavior where the mean daily dose was about 300 mg (range 12.5 to 900 mg).

Patients previously treated with other antipsychotics were cross-titrated to CLOZARIL over a one-month interval; the dose of the previous antipsychotic was gradually decreased simultaneous with a gradual increase in CLOZARIL dose over the first month of the study. Patients on depot antipsychotic medication began CLOZARIL after one full dosing interval since the last injection.

Recommendations to Reduce the Risk of Recurrent Suicidal Behavior in Patients Who Otherwise Previously Responded to Treatment of Schizophrenia or Schizoaffective Disorder with Another Antipsychotic Medication: The results of the InterSePT study demonstrated that, for a 2-year treatment period, the probability of a suicide attempt or a hospitalization due to imminent suicide risk is stable at approximately 24% after one year of treatment with CLOZARIL (Figure 1, Clinical Trial Data Section) A course of treatment with CLOZARIL of at least 2 years is therefore recommended in order to maintain the reduction of risk for suicidal behavior. After 2 years, it is recommended that the patient's risk of suicidal behavior be assessed. If the physician's assessment indicates that a significant risk for suicidal behavior is still present, treatment with CLOZARIL should be continued. Thereafter, the decision to continue treatment with CLOZARIL should be revisited at regular intervals, based on thorough assessments of the patient's risk for suicidal behavior during treatment. If the physician determines that the patient is no longer at risk for suicidal behavior, treatment with CLOZARIL may be discontinued *(see recommendations above regarding discontinuation of treatment)* and treatment of the underlying disorder with an antipsychotic medication to which the patient has previously responded may be resumed.

HOW SUPPLIED

CLOZARIL® (clozapine) is available as 25 mg and 100 mg round, pale-yellow, uncoated tablets with a facilitated score on one side.

CLOZARIL® (clozapine) Tablets

25 mg

Engraved with "CLOZARIL" once on the periphery of one side.

Engraved with a facilitated score and "25" once on the other side.

Bottle of 100 .... NDC 0078-0126-05
Bottle of 500 .... NDC 0078-0126-08
Unit dose packages of 100: 2 × 5 strips,
10 blisters per strip .... NDC 0078-0126-06

100 mg

Engraved with "CLOZARIL" once on the periphery of one side.

Engraved with a facilitated score and "100" once on the other side.

Bottle of 100 .... NDC 0078-0127-05
Bottle of 500 .... NDC 0078-0127-08
Unit dose packages of 100: 2 × 5 strips,
10 blisters per strip .... NDC 0078-0127-06

Store and Dispense

Storage temperature should not exceed 86°F (30°C). Drug dispensing should not ordinarily exceed a weekly supply. If a patient is eligible for WBC testing every other week, then a two-week supply of CLOZARIL can be dispensed. Dispensing should be contingent upon the results of a WBC count.

*Zyprexa® (olanzapine) is a registered trademark of Eli Lilly and Company.
**Trademark of Medical Economics Company, Inc.

T2003-88
REV: DECEMBER 2003 Printed in U.S.A 89004512
Novartis Pharmaceuticals Corporation
East Hanover, New Jersey 07936
©Novartis

Shown in Product Identification Guide, page 324

COMBIPATCH® ℞

[kŏm-bĭ-păch]

(estradiol/norethindrone acetate transdermal system)

Rx only

Prescribing Information

The following prescribing information is based on official labeling in effect July 2004.

WARNING

Estrogens and progestins should not be used for the prevention of cardiovascular disease.

The Women's Health Initiative (WHI) study reported increased risks of myocardial infarction, stroke, invasive breast cancer, pulmonary emboli, and deep vein thrombosis in postmenopausal women during five years of treatment with conjugated equine estrogens (CE 0.625 mg) combined with medroxyprogesterone acetate (MPA 2.5 mg) relative to placebo *(see CLINICAL PHARMACOLOGY, Clinical Studies)*. Other doses of conjugated estrogens with medroxyprogesterone, and other combinations of estrogens and progestins were not studied in the WHI and, in the absence of comparable data, these risks should be assumed to be similar. Because of these risks, estrogens with or without progestins should be prescribed at the lowest effective doses and for the shortest duration consistent with treatment goals and risks for the individual woman.

DESCRIPTION

CombiPatch® estradiol/norethindrone acetate transdermal system) is an adhesive-based matrix transdermal patch designed to release both estradiol and norethindrone acetate (NETA), a progestational agent, continuously upon application to intact skin.

Two systems are available, providing the following delivery rates of estradiol and norethindrone acetate.

[See table below]

Estradiol USP (estradiol) is a white to creamy white, odorless, crystalline powder, chemically described as estra-1,3,5(10)-triene-3,17β-diol. The molecular weight of estradiol is 272.39 and the molecular formula is $C_{18}H_{24}O_2$.

Norethindrone acetate USP is a white to creamy white, odorless, crystalline powder, chemically described as 17-hydroxy-19-nor-17α-pregn-4-en-20-yn-3-one acetate. The molecular weight of norethindrone acetate is 340.47 and the molecular formula is $C_{22}H_{28}O_3$.

The structural formulas for estradiol and norethindrone acetate are

[See chemical structures at top of next column]

CombiPatch transdermal systems are comprised of three layers. Proceeding from the visible surface toward the surface attached to the skin, these layers are (1) a translucent

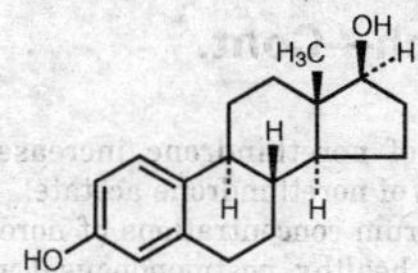

Estradiol

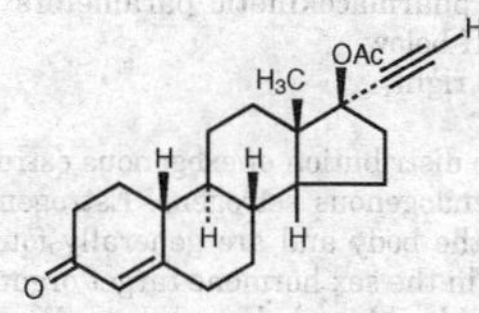

Norethindrone Acetate

polyolefin film backing, (2) an adhesive layer containing estradiol, norethindrone acetate, acrylic adhesive, silicone adhesive, oleyl alcohol, oleic acid NF, povidone USP and dipropylene glycol, and (3) a polyester release protective liner, which is attached to the adhesive surface and must be removed before the system can be used.

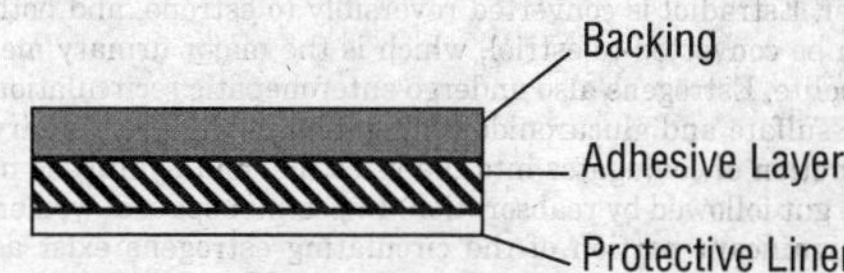

The active components of the system are estradiol USP and norethindrone acetate USP. The remaining components of the system are pharmacologically inactive.

CLINICAL PHARMACOLOGY

Endogenous estrogens are largely responsible for the development and maintenance of the female reproductive system and secondary sexual characteristics. Although circulating estrogens exist in a dynamic equilibrium of metabolic interconversions, estradiol is the principal intracellular human estrogen and is substantially more potent than its metabolites, estrone and estriol at the receptor level. The primary source of estrogen in normally cycling adult women is the ovarian follicle, which secretes 70 to 500 µg of estradiol daily, depending on the phase of the menstrual cycle. After menopause, most endogenous estrogen is produced by conversion of androstenedione, secreted by the adrenal cortex, to estrone by peripheral tissues. Thus, estrone and the sulfate conjugated form, estrone sulfate, are the most abundant circulating estrogens in postmenopausal women.

Estrogens act through binding to nuclear receptors in estrogen-responsive tissues. To date, two estrogen receptors have been identified. These vary in proportion from tissue to tissue.

Circulating estrogens modulate the pituitary secretion of the gonadotropins, luteinizing hormone (LH), and follicle stimulating hormone (FSH) through a negative feedback mechanism. Estrogens act to reduce the elevated levels of these hormones seen in postmenopausal women.

Pharmacokinetics

Absorption

Estradiol: Estrogens used in hormone therapy are well absorbed through the skin, mucous membranes, and gastrointestinal tract. Administration of CombiPatch every three to four days in postmenopausal women produces average steady-state estradiol serum concentrations of 45 to 50 pg/mL, which are equivalent to the normal ranges observed at the early follicular phase in premenopausal women. These concentrations are achieved within 12 to 24 hours following CombiPatch application. Minimal fluctuations in serum estradiol concentrations are observed following CombiPatch application, indicating consistent hormone delivery over the application interval.

In one study, serum concentrations of estradiol were measured in 40 healthy, postmenopausal women throughout three consecutive CombiPatch applications to the abdomen (each dose was applied for three 3.5-day periods). The corresponding pharmacokinetic parameters are summarized in Table I below.

[See table I at top of next page]

Norethindrone: Progestins used in hormone therapy are well absorbed through the skin, mucous membranes, and gastrointestinal tract. Norethindrone steady-state concentrations are attained within 24 hours of application of the CombiPatch transdermal delivery systems. Minimal fluctuations in serum norethindrone concentrations are observed following CombiPatch treatment, indicating consistent hormone delivery over the application interval. Serum

Continued on next page

System Size	Estradiol (mg)	NETA[1] (mg)	Nominal Delivery Rate[2] (mg per day) Estradiol/NETA
9 sq cm round	0.62	2.7	0.05/0.14
16 sq cm round	0.51	4.8	0.05/0.25

[1] NETA = norethindrone acetate.
[2] Based on *in vivo/in vitro* flux data, delivery of both components per day via skin of average permeability (interindividual variation in skin permeability is approximately 20%).

CombiPatch—Cont.

concentrations of norethindrone increase linearly with increasing doses of norethindrone acetate.

In one study, serum concentrations of norethindrone were measured in 40 healthy, postmenopausal women throughout three consecutive CombiPatch applications to the abdomen (each dose was applied for three 3.5-day periods). The corresponding pharmacokinetic parameters are summarized in Table II below.

[See table II at right]

Distribution

Estradiol: The distribution of exogenous estrogens is similar to that of endogenous estrogens. Estrogens are widely distributed in the body and are generally found in higher concentrations in the sex hormone target organs. Estrogens circulate in the blood largely bound to sex hormone binding globulin (SHBG) and albumin.

Norethindrone: In plasma, norethindrone is bound approximately 90% to SHBG and albumin.

Metabolism

Estradiol: Exogenous estrogens are metabolized in the same manner as endogenous estrogens. Circulating estrogens exist in a dynamic equilibrium of metabolic interconversions. These transformations take place mainly in the liver. Estradiol is converted reversibly to estrone, and both can be converted to estriol, which is the major urinary metabolite. Estrogens also undergo enterohepatic recirculation via sulfate and glucuronide conjugation in the liver, biliary secretion of conjugates into the intestine, and hydrolysis in the gut followed by reabsorption. In postmenopausal women a significant portion of the circulating estrogens exist as sulfate conjugates, especially estrone sulfate, which serves as a circulating reservoir for the formation of more active estrogens. Transdermally delivered estradiol is metabolized only to a small extent by the skin and bypasses the first-pass effect seen with orally administered estrogen products. Therapeutic estradiol serum levels with lower circulating levels of estrone and estrone conjugates are achieved with smaller transdermal doses (daily and total) as compared to oral therapy.

Norethindrone: Norethindrone acetate is hydrolyzed to the active moiety, norethindrone, in most tissues including skin and blood. Norethindrone is primarily metabolized in the liver; however, transdermal administration significantly decreases metabolism because hepatic first-pass effect is avoided.

Excretion

Estradiol: Estradiol, estrone and estriol are excreted in the urine along with glucuronide and sulfate conjugates. Estradiol has a short elimination half-life of approximately two to three hours; therefore, a rapid decline in serum levels is observed after the CombiPatch estradiol/norethindrone acetate transdermal system is removed. Within four to eight hours serum estradiol concentrations return to untreated, postmenopausal levels (<20 pg/mL).

Concentration data from Phase II and III studies indicate that the pharmacokinetics of estradiol did not change over time, suggesting no evidence of the accumulation of estradiol following extended patch wear periods (up to one year).

Norethindrone: The elimination half-life of norethindrone is reported to be six to eight hours. Norethindrone serum concentrations diminish rapidly and are less than 50 pg/mL within 48 hours after removal of the CombiPatch transdermal delivery system.

Concentration data from Phase II and III studies indicate that the pharmacokinetics of norethindrone did not change over time, suggesting no evidence of the accumulation of norethindrone following extended patch wear periods (up to one year).

Special Populations

CombiPatch has been studied only in postmenopausal women.

Drug Interactions

In vitro and *in vivo* studies have shown that estrogens are metabolized partially by cytochrome P450 3A4 (CYP3A4). Therefore, inducers or inhibitors of CYP3A4 may affect estrogen drug metabolism. Inducers of CYP3A4 such as St. John's Wort preparations (Hypericum perforatum), phenobarbital, carbamazepine and rifampin may reduce plasma concentrations of estrogens, possibly resulting in a decrease in therapeutic effects and/or changes in the uterine bleeding profile. Inhibitors of CYP3A4 such as erythromycin, clarithromycin, ketoconazole, itraconazole, ritonavir and grapefruit juice may increase plasma concentrations of estrogens and may result in side effects.

Adhesion

Averaging across six clinical trials lasting three months to one year, of 1,287 patients treated, CombiPatch transdermal systems completely adhered to the skin nearly 90% of the time over the 3- to 4-day wear period. Less than 2% of the patients required reapplication or replacement of systems due to lifting or detachment. Only two patients (0.2%) discontinued therapy during clinical trials due to adhesion failure.

CLINICAL STUDIES

In two clinical trials designed to assess the degree of relief of moderate to severe vasomotor symptoms in postmenopausal women (n=332), CombiPatch was administered for three 28-day cycles in *Continuous Combined* or *Continuous Sequential* treatment regimens versus placebo. In the *Continuous Combined* regimen, CombiPatch was applied throughout the three cycles, replacing the system twice weekly. In the *Continuous Sequential* regimen, an estradiol-only transdermal system (Vivelle® 0.05 mg) was applied twice weekly during the first 14 days of a 28-day cycle; CombiPatch was applied for the remaining 14 days of the cycle and replaced twice weekly, as well. The mean number of hot flushes at baseline were 10 to 11 per day and 11 to 12 per day in the *Continuous Combined* and *Continuous Sequential* regimen trials, respectively. The mean number and intensity of daily hot flushes (intent-to-treat population) was significantly reduced from baseline to endpoint with either the *Continuous Combined* or *Continuous Sequential* administration of CombiPatch at all doses as compared to placebo (intent-to-treat population). *[See tables below.]*

[See third table above]
[See fourth table above]

The use of unopposed estrogen therapy has been associated with an increased risk of endometrial hyperplasia, a possible precursor of endometrial adenocarcinoma. Progestins counter the estrogenic effects by decreasing the number of nuclear estradiol receptors and suppressing epithelial DNA synthesis in endometrial tissue.

Clinical studies indicate that the addition of a progestin to an estrogen regimen at least 12 days per cycle reduces the incidence of endometrial hyperplasia and the potential risk of adenocarcinoma in women with intact uteri. The addition of a progestin to an estrogen regimen has not been shown to interfere with the efficacy of estrogen therapy for its approved indications.

CombiPatch was effective in reducing the incidence of estrogen-induced endometrial hyperplasia after one year of therapy in two Phase II clinical trials. Nine hundred fifty-five (955) postmenopausal women (with intact uteri) were treated with (i) a continuous regimen of CombiPatch alone (*Continuous Combined* regimen), (ii) a sequential regimen with an estradiol-only (Vivelle 0.05 mg) transdermal system followed by a CombiPatch transdermal system (*Continuous Sequential* regimen), or (iii) continuous regimen with an estradiol-only transdermal system (Vivelle 0.05 mg). The incidence of endometrial hyperplasia (primary endpoint) was significantly less after one year of therapy with either CombiPatch regimen than with the estradiol-only transdermal system. The tables below summarize these results (intent-to-treat populations).

Table I
Mean (SD) Serum Estradiol and Estrone Concentrations (pg/mL) at Steady-State [Uncorrected for Baseline Levels]

System Size	Dose Estradiol/NETA (mg per day)	C_{max}	C_{min}	C_{avg}
Estradiol				
9 sq cm	0.05/0.14	71 (32)	27 (17)	45 (21)
16 sq cm	0.05/0.25	71 (30)	37 (17)	50 (21)
Estrone				
9 sq cm	0.05/0.14	72 (23)	49 (19)	54 (19)
16 sq cm	0.05/0.25	78 (22)	58 (22)	60 (18)

Table II
Mean (SD) Serum Norethindrone Concentrations (pg/mL) at Steady-State

System Size	Dose Estradiol/NETA (mg per day)	C_{max}	C_{min}	C_{avg}
9 sq cm	0.05/0.14	617 (341)	386 (137)	489 (244)
16 sq cm	0.05/0.25	1,060 (543)	686 (306)	840 (414)

Adjusted Mean Change In the Number of Hot Flushes and Daily Intensity of Hot Flushes per Day in CombiPatch® *Continuous Combined* Transdermal Therapy

	CombiPatch® Continuous Combined		Placebo
Adjusted Mean Change from Baseline[1]	0.05/0.14 mg per day[2] n = 57	0.05/0.25 mg per day[2] n = 52	n = 51
Number of Hot Flushes[3]	-9.3[5]	-8.9[5]	-6.2
Daily Intensity of Hot Flushes[3,4]	-4.6[5,6]	-5.0[5]	-2.8[7]

[1] Means were adjusted for imbalance among treatment groups and investigators (least squares mean from ANOVA).
[2] Represents the milligrams of estradiol/norethindrone acetate delivered daily by each system.
[3] Population represents those patients who had baseline and endpoint observations.
[4] The intensity of hot flushes was evaluated on a scale of 0 to 9 (none = 0, mild = 1-3, moderate = 4-6, severe = 7-9).
[5] P value versus placebo = <0.001.
[6] Total number of patients with available data is 56.
[7] Total number of patients with available data is 50.

Adjusted Mean Change In the Number of Hot Flushes and Daily Intensity of Hot Flushes per Day in CombiPatch® *Continuous Sequential* Transdermal Therapy

	CombiPatch® Continuous Sequential		Placebo
Adjusted Mean Change from Baseline[1]	0.05/0.14 mg per day[2] n = 54	0.05/0.25 mg per day[2] n = 59	n = 53
Number of Hot Flushes[3]	-9.3[5]	-9.5[5]	-5.5
Daily Intensity of Hot Flushes[3,4]	-4.4[5]	-4.5[5]	-2.1

[1] Means were adjusted for imbalance among treatment groups and investigators (least squares mean from ANOVA).
[2] Represents the milligrams of estradiol/norethindrone acetate delivered daily by each system.
[3] Population represents those patients who had baseline and endpoint observations.
[4] The intensity of hot flushes was evaluated on a scale of 0 to 9 (none = 0, mild = 1-3, moderate = 4-6, severe = 7-9).
[5] P value versus placebo = <0.001.

Incidence of Endometrial Hyperplasia in a *Continuous Combined* CombiPatch® Regimen

	CombiPatch® Continuous Combined 0.05/0.14 mg per day[1]	CombiPatch® Continuous Combined 0.05/0.25 mg per day[1]	Vivelle® Continuous 0.05 mg per day
No. of Patients with Biopsies[2]	123	98	103
No. (%) of Patients with Hyperplasia	1 (<1%)[3]	1 (1%)[3,4]	39 (38%)[5]

[1] Represents milligrams of estradiol/NETA delivered daily by each system.
[2] Biopsy after 12 cycles of treatment or hyperplasia before cycle 12.
[3] Comparison of continuous combined regimen versus estradiol-only patch was significant (p value <0.001).
[4] This patient had hyperplasia at baseline.
[5] One of 39 patients had hyperplasia in an endometrial polyp.

[See fifth table on previous page]
[See first table at right]
With the *Continuous Combined* regimen, of the women treated with CombiPatch and who completed the one-year study, the incidence of cumulative amenorrhea (the absence of bleeding or spotting during a 28-day cycle and sustained to the end of the study) increased over time. The incidence of amenorrhea from cycle 10 through 12 was 53% and 39% for the CombiPatch 0.05/0.14 mg per day and CombiPatch 0.05/0.25 mg per day treatment groups, respectively. Women who experienced bleeding, usually characterized it as light (intensity of 1.3 on a scale of 1 to 4) with a duration of four and six days for the CombiPatch 0.05/0.14 mg per day and CombiPatch 0.05/0.25 mg per day treatment groups, respectively.

Incidence of Cumulative Amenorrhea* in CombiPatch® *Continuous Combined* Transdermal Therapy by Cycle over a One-Year Period (Intent-to-Treat Population)

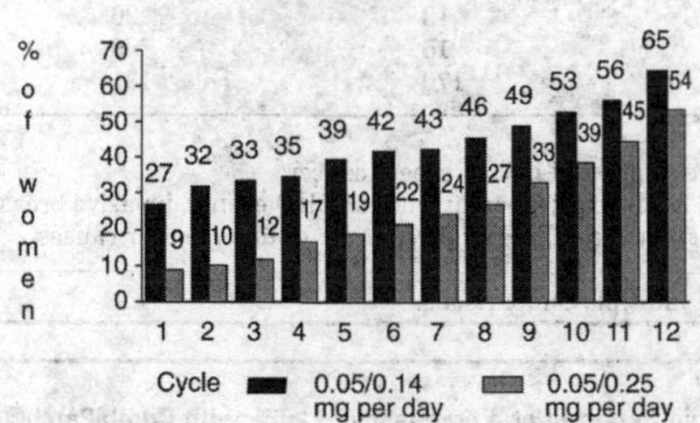

*Cumulative amenorrhea is defined as the absence of bleeding for the duration of a 28-day cycle and sustained to the end of the study.

Information Regarding Lipid Effects

In the CE/MPA substudy of the WHI (n=16,608 predominantly healthy postmenopausal women) hormone therapy lowered the level of low-density lipoprotein (LDL) cholesterol and increased the level of high-density lipoprotein (HDL), yet an increased risk of coronary heart disease events was observed. Therefore, estrogens and progestins should not be used for the prevention of cardiovascular disease. *(See BOXED WARNING and CLINICAL PHARMACOLOGY, Clinical Studies.)*

The results of clinical trials conducted in a 90% Caucasian population at low risk for cardiovascular disease showed that compared to Vivelle (an estrogen-alone treatment), CombiPatch demonstrated significantly greater reductions in total cholesterol (TC) concentrations. Mean high density lipoprotein-cholesterol (HDL-C) values, however, decreased after one year of CombiPatch therapy whereas they were noted to increase in Vivelle users. Shifts in mean TC/HDL-C were minimal after one year of therapy in both Vivelle and CombiPatch treatment groups. Decreases in triglycerides were observed in both CombiPatch regimens.

The following tables summarize lipid parameters from these two clinical trials in 955 postmenopausal women (with intact uteri) after one year of therapy. Subjects were treated with (i) a continuous regimen of CombiPatch alone (*Continuous Combined* regimen), (ii) a sequential CombiPatch regimen consisting of an estradiol-only (Vivelle 0.05 mg) transdermal system followed by a CombiPatch transdermal system (*Continuous Sequential* regimen), or (iii) a continuous regimen with an estradiol-only transdermal system (Vivelle 0.05 mg). The values below represent mean percent change from baseline in patients with data at baseline and one year.
[See second table above]
[See third table above]

Women's Health Initiative Studies

A substudy of the Women's Health Initiative (WHI) enrolled a total of 16,608 predominantly healthy postmenopausal women (average age of 63 years, range 50 to 79, 83.9% White, 6.5% Black, 5.5% Hispanic) to assess the risks and benefits of the use of 0.625 mg conjugated equine estrogens (CE) per day alone and of 0.625 mg conjugated equine estrogens plus 2.5 mg medroxyprogesterone acetate (MPA) per day compared to placebo in the prevention of certain chronic diseases. The primary endpoint was the incidence of coronary heart disease (CHD) (nonfatal myocardial infarction and CHD death), with invasive breast cancer as the primary adverse outcome studied. A "global index" included the earliest occurrence of CHD, invasive breast cancer, stroke, pulmonary embolism (PE), endometrial cancer, colorectal cancer, hip fracture, or death due to other cause. The study did not evaluate the effects of CE or CE/MPA on menopausal symptoms.

The CE/MPA substudy was stopped early because, according to the predefined stopping rule, the increased risk of breast cancer and cardiovascular events exceeded the specified benefits included in the "global index." Results of the CE/MPA substudy, which included 16,608 women (average age of 63 years, range 50 to 79, 83.9% White, 6.5% Black, 5.5% Hispanic), after an average follow-up of 5.2 years are presented in Table III below.
[See table III at top of next page]
For those outcomes included in the "global index," absolute excess risks per 10,000 person-years in the group treated with CE/MPA were seven more CHD events, eight more strokes, eight more PEs, and eight more invasive breast cancers, while absolute risk reductions per 10,000 person-years were six fewer colorectal cancers and five fewer hip fractures. The absolute excess risk of events included in the "global index" was 19 per 10,000 person-years. There was no difference between the groups in terms of all-cause mortality *(see BOXED WARNING, WARNINGS, and PRECAUTIONS.)*

Incidence of Endometrial Hyperplasia in a *Continuous Sequential* CombiPatch® Regimen

	CombiPatch® Continuous Sequential 0.05/0.14 mg per day[1]	CombiPatch® Continuous Sequential 0.05/0.25 mg per day[1]	Vivelle® Continuous 0.05 mg per day
No. of Patients with Biopsies[2]	117	114	115
No. (%) of Patients with Hyperplasia	1 (<1%)[3,4]	1 (<1%)[3,5]	23 (20%)

[1] Represents milligrams of estradiol/NETA delivered daily by each system.
[2] Biopsy after 12 cycles of treatment or hyperplasia before cycle 12.
[3] Comparison of continuous sequential regimen versus estradiol-only patch was significant (p value <0.001).
[4] This patient had hyperplasia at baseline.
[5] This patient had hyperplasia in an endometrial polyp.

Lipid Profile Values, Adjusted Mean Percent Change from Baseline after One Year of *Continuous Combined* CombiPatch® Transdermal Therapy

Lipid Parameter (%)	CombiPatch® Continuous Combined 0.05/0.14 mg per day[1] n = 122	CombiPatch® Continuous Combined 0.05/0.25 mg per day[1] n = 99	Vivelle® Continuous 0.05 mg per day n = 79
Total Cholesterol	-5.4%[2]	-8.6%[3]	-2.0%
HDL-C	-3.1%[3]	-9.1%[3]	+7.3%
LDL-C	-4.6%[4]	-7.6%[5]	-3.4%
Triglycerides	-4.6%	-9.5%	-6.7%

[1] Represents milligrams of estradiol/NETA delivered daily by each system.
[2] Comparison with estradiol-only patch was significant (p <0.05).
[3] Comparison with estradiol-only patch was significant (p <0.001).
[4] Total number of patients with available data is 121.
[5] Total number of patients with available data is 97.

Lipid Profile Values, Adjusted Mean Percent Change from Baseline after One Year of *Continuous Sequential* CombiPatch® Transdermal Therapy

Lipid Parameter (%)	CombiPatch® Continuous Sequential 0.05/0.14 mg per day[1] n = 117	CombiPatch® Continuous Sequential 0.05/0.25 mg per day[1] n = 115	Vivelle® Continuous 0.05 mg per day n = 105
Total Cholesterol	-4.1%[2]	-9.0%[3]	-1.0%
HDL-C	-4.7%[3]	-8.9%[3]	+0.9%
LDL-C	-1.2%[4]	-6.8%[2,5]	-2.0%[6]
Triglycerides	-8.2%[3]	-14.1%[3]	+13.2%

[1] Represents milligrams of estradiol/NETA delivered daily by each system.
[2] Comparison with estradiol-only patch was significant (p <0.05).
[3] Comparison with estradiol-only patch was significant (p <0.001).
[4] Total number of patients with available data is 116.
[5] Total number of patients with available data is 114.
[6] Total number of patients with available data is 103.

INDICATIONS AND USAGE

In women with an intact uterus, CombiPatch is indicated for the following:

- Treatment of moderate to severe vasomotor symptoms associated with the menopause.
- Treatment of moderate to severe symptoms of vulvar and vaginal atrophy associated with the menopause. When prescribing solely for the treatment of symptoms of vulvar and vaginal atrophy, topical vaginal products should be considered.
- Treatment of hypoestrogenism due to hypogonadism, castration, or primary ovarian failure.

CONTRAINDICATIONS

Estrogens/progestins combined should not be used in women under any of the following conditions:

- Undiagnosed abnormal genital bleeding.
- Known, suspected, or history of cancer of the breast.
- Known or suspected estrogen-dependent neoplasia.
- Active deep vein thrombosis, pulmonary embolism or history of these conditions.
- Active or recent (e.g., within the past year) arterial thromboembolic disease (e.g., stroke, myocardial infarction).
- CombiPatch should not be used in patients with known hypersensitivity to its ingredients.
- Known or suspected pregnancy. There is no indication for CombiPatch in pregnancy. There appears to be little or no increased risk of birth defects in women who have used estrogens and progestins from oral contraceptives inadvertently during early pregnancy *(see PRECAUTIONS)*.

WARNINGS

See BOXED WARNING.

Cardiovascular Disorders

Estrogen/progestin therapy has been associated with an increased risk of cardiovascular events such as myocardial infarction and stroke, as well as venous thrombosis and pulmonary embolism (venous thromboembolism or VTE). Should any of these occur or be suspected, estrogens/progestins should be discontinued immediately.

Risk factors for cardiovascular disease (e.g., hypertension, diabetes mellitus, tobacco use, hypercholesterolemia, and obesity) should be managed appropriately.

Coronary Heart Disease and Stroke

In the CE/MPA substudy of the Women's Health Initiative study (WHI), an increased risk of coronary heart disease (CHD) events (defined as nonfatal myocardial infarction and CHD death) was observed in women receiving CE/MPA compared to women receiving placebo (37 versus 30 per 10,000 person-years). The increase in risk was observed in year one and persisted *(see CLINICAL PHARMACOLOGY, Clinical Studies)*.

In the same substudy of WHI, an increased risk of stroke was observed in women receiving CE/MPA compared to women receiving placebo (29 versus 21 per 10,000 person-years). The increase in risk was observed after the first year and persisted.

In postmenopausal women with documented heart disease (n = 2,763, average age 66.7 years) a controlled clinical trial of secondary prevention of cardiovascular disease (Heart and Estrogen/Progestin Replacement Study; HERS) treatment with CE/MPA-0.625 mg/2.5 mg per day demonstrated no cardiovascular benefit. During an average follow-up of 4.1 years, treatment with CE/MPA did not reduce the overall rate of CHD events in postmenopausal women with established coronary heart disease. There were more CHD events in the CE/MPA-treated group than in the placebo group in year one, but not during the subsequent years. Two thousand three hundred and twenty-one women from the original HERS trial agreed to participate in an open label extension of HERS, HERS II. Average follow-up in HERS II was an additional 2.7 years, for a total of 6.8 years overall. Rates of CHD events were comparable among women in the CE/MPA group and in the placebo group in HERS, HERS II, and overall.

Large doses of estrogen (5 mg conjugated estrogens per day), comparable to those used to treat cancer of the pros-

Continued on next page

CombiPatch—Cont.

tate and breast, have been shown in a large prospective clinical trial in men to increase the risks of nonfatal myocardial infarction, pulmonary embolism, and thrombophlebitis. These risks cannot necessarily be extrapolated from men to women or from unopposed estrogen to combination estrogen/progestin therapy. However, to avoid the theoretical cardiovascular risk associated with high estrogen doses, the dose for estrogen therapy should not exceed the lowest effective dose.

Venous Thromboembolism (VTE)

In the CE/MPA substudy of WHI, a 2-fold greater rate of VTE, including deep venous thrombosis and pulmonary embolism, was observed in women receiving CE/MPA compared to women receiving placebo. The rate of VTE was 34 per 10,000 woman-years in the CE/MPA group compared to 16 per 10,000 woman-years in the placebo group. The increase in VTE risk was observed during the first year and persisted. *(See CLINICAL PHARMACOLOGY, Clinical Studies.)*

If feasible, estrogens should be discontinued at least four to six weeks before surgery of the type associated with an increased risk of thromboembolism, or during periods of prolonged immobilization.

Malignant Neoplasms

Breast Cancer

Estrogen/progestin therapy in postmenopausal women has been associated with an increased risk of breast cancer. In the CE/MPA substudy of the Women's Health Initiative study (WHI), a 26% increase of invasive breast cancer (38 versus 30 per 10,000 woman-years) after an average of 5.2 years of treatment was observed in women receiving CE/MPA compared to women receiving placebo. The increased risk of breast cancer became apparent after four years on CE/MPA. The women reporting prior postmenopausal use of estrogen and/or estrogen with progestin had a higher relative risk for breast cancer associated with CE/MPA than those who had never used these hormones. *(See CLINICAL PHARMACOLOGY, Clinical Studies.)*

Epidemiologic studies have reported an increased risk of breast cancer in association with increasing duration of postmenopausal treatment with estrogens with or without a progestin. This association was reanalyzed in original data from 51 studies that involved various doses and types of estrogens, with and without progestins. In the reanalysis, an increased risk of having breast cancer diagnosed became apparent after about five years of continued treatment, and subsided after treatment had been discontinued for five years or longer. Some later studies have suggested that postmenopausal treatment with estrogens and progestin increase the risk of breast cancer more than treatment with estrogen alone.

A postmenopausal woman without a uterus who requires estrogen should receive estrogen-alone therapy, and should not be exposed unnecessarily to progestins. All postmenopausal women should receive yearly breast exams by a health care provider and perform monthly breast self-examinations. In addition, mammography examinations should be scheduled as suggested by providers based on patient age and risk factors.

Endometrial Cancer

The reported endometrial cancer risk among users of unopposed estrogen is about 2- to 12-fold or greater than in non-users, and appears dependent on duration of treatment and on estrogen dose. Most studies show no significant increased risk associated with the use of estrogens for less than one year. The greatest risk appears to be associated with prolonged use with increased risks of 15- to 24-fold for five to ten years or more and this risk has been shown to persist for at least 8 to 15 years after estrogen therapy is discontinued.

Clinical surveillance of all women taking estrogen/progestin combinations is important. Adequate diagnostic measures, including endometrial sampling when indicated, should be undertaken to rule out malignancy in all cases of undiagnosed persistent or recurring abnormal vaginal bleeding. There is no evidence that the use of natural estrogens results in a different endometrial risk profile than synthetic estrogens of equivalent estrogen dose.

Gallbladder Disease

A 2- to 4-fold increase in the risk of gallbladder disease requiring surgery in postmenopausal women receiving estrogens has been reported.

Hypercalcemia

Administration of estrogen may lead to severe hypercalcemia in patients with breast cancer and bone metastases. If this occurs, the drug should be stopped and appropriate measures taken to reduce the serum calcium level.

Visual Abnormalities

Retinal vascular thrombosis has been reported in patients receiving estrogens. Discontinue medication pending examination if there is sudden partial or complete loss of vision, or a sudden onset of proptosis, diplopia, or migraine. If examination reveals papilledema or retinal vascular lesions, estrogens should be discontinued.

PRECAUTIONS

General

Addition of a Progestin When a Woman Has Not Had a Hysterectomy

Studies of the addition of a progestin for 10 or more days of a cycle of estrogen administration, or daily with estrogen in

Table III
Relative and Absolute Risk Seen in the CE/MPA Substudy of WHI[a]

Event[c]	Relative Risk CE/MPA vs. Placebo at 5.2 Years (95% CI*)	Placebo n = 8102	CE/MPA n = 8506
		Absolute Risk per 10,000 Person-Years	
CHD Events	1.29 (1.02-1.63)	30	37
Non-fatal MI	1.32 (1.02-1.72)	23	30
CHD Death	1.18 (0.70-1.97)	6	7
Invasive Breast Cancer[b]	1.26 (1.00-1.59)	30	38
Stroke	1.41 (1.07-1.85)	21	29
Pulmonary Embolism	2.13 (1.39-3.25)	8	16
Colorectal Cancer	0.63 (0.43-0.92)	16	10
Endometrial Cancer	0.83 (0.47-1.47)	6	5
Hip Fracture	0.66 (0.45-0.98)	15	10
Death Due to Causes Other than the Events Above	0.92 (0.74-1.14)	40	37
Global Index[c]	1.15 (1.03-1.28)	151	170
Deep Vein Thrombosis[d]	2.07 (1.49-2.87)	13	26
Vertebral Fractures[d]	0.66 (0.44-0.98)	15	9
Other Osteoporotic Fractures[d]	0.77 (0.69-0.86)	170	131

[a] Adapted from JAMA, 2002: 288: 321-333.
[b] Includes metastatic and non-metastatic breast cancer with the exception of *in situ* breast cancer.
[c] A subset of the events was combined in a "global index," defined as the earliest occurrence of CHD events, invasive breast cancer, stroke, pulmonary embolism, endometrial cancer, colorectal cancer, hip fracture, or death due to other causes.
[d] Not included in global index.
*Nominal confidence intervals unadjusted for multiple looks and multiple comparisons.

Table IV
All Treatment Emergent Study Events Regardless of Relationship Reported at a Frequency of ≥5% with CombiPatch®
VASOMOTOR SYMPTOM STUDIES

	CombiPatch® 0.05/0.14 mg per day[1] n = 113	CombiPatch® 0.05/0.25 mg per day[1] n = 112	Placebo n = 107
Body as a Whole	46%	48%	41%
Abdominal Pain	7%	6%	4%
Accidental Injury	4%	5%	8%
Asthenia	8%	12%	4%
Back Pain	11%	9%	5%
Flu Syndrome	9%	5%	7%
Headache	18%	20%	20%
Pain	6%	4%	9%
Digestive	19%	23%	24%
Diarrhea	4%	5%	7%
Dyspepsia	1%	5%	5%
Flatulence	4%	5%	4%
Nausea	11%	8%	7%
Nervous	16%	28%	28%
Depression	3%	5%	9%
Insomnia	3%	6%	7%
Nervousness	3%	5%	1%
Respiratory	24%	38%	26%
Pharyngitis	4%	10%	2%
Respiratory Disorder	7%	12%	7%
Rhinitis	7%	13%	9%
Sinusitis	4%	9%	9%
Skin and Appendages	8%	17%	16%
Application Site Reaction	2%	6%	4%
Urogenital	54%	63%	28%
Breast Pain	25%	31%	7%
Dysmenorrhea	20%	21%	5%
Leukorrhea	5%	5%	3%
Menstrual Disorder	6%	12%	2%
Papanicolaou Smear Suspicious	8%	4%	5%
Vaginitis	6%	13%	5%

[1]Represents milligrams of estradiol/NETA delivered daily by each system.

a continuous regimen, have reported a lowered incidence of endometrial hyperplasia than would be induced by estrogen treatment alone. Endometrial hyperplasia may be a precursor to endometrial cancer.

There are, however, possible risks that may be associated with the use of progestins with estrogens compared to estrogen-alone regimens. These include a possible increased risk of breast cancer.

Elevated Blood Pressure

In a small number of case reports, substantial increases in blood pressure have been attributed to idiosyncratic reactions to estrogens. In a large, randomized, placebo-controlled clinical trial, a generalized effect of estrogen therapy on blood pressure was not seen. Blood pressure should be monitored at regular intervals with estrogen use.

Familial Hyperlipoproteinemia

In patients with familial defects of lipoprotein metabolism, estrogen therapy may be associated with elevations of plasma triglycerides leading to pancreatitis and other complications.

Impaired Liver Function

Although transdermally administered estrogen therapy avoids first-pass hepatic metabolism, estrogens may be poorly metabolized in patients with impaired liver function. For patients with a history of cholestatic jaundice associated with past estrogen use or with pregnancy, caution should be exercised and in the case of recurrence, medication should be discontinued.

Hypothyroidism

Estrogen administration leads to increased thyroid-binding globulin (TBG) levels. Patients with normal thyroid function can compensate for the increased TBG by making more thyroid hormone, thus maintaining free T_4 and T_3 serum concentrations in the normal range. Patients dependent on thyroid hormone replacement therapy who are also receiving estrogens may require increased doses of their thyroid replacement therapy. These patients should have their thyroid function monitored in order to maintain their free thyroid hormone levels in an acceptable range.

Fluid Retention

Because estrogens may cause some degree of fluid retention, conditions which might be influenced by this factor, such as asthma, epilepsy, migraine, and cardiac or renal dysfunction, warrant careful observation when estrogens are prescribed.

Hypocalcemia

Estrogens should be used with caution in individuals with severe hypocalcemia.

Ovarian Cancer

Use of estrogen-only products, in particular for ten or more years, has been associated with an increased risk of ovarian cancer in some epidemiological studies. Other studies did not show a significant association. Data are insufficient to determine whether there is an increased risk with estrogen/progestin combination therapy in postmenopausal women.

Exacerbation of Endometriosis

Endometriosis may be exacerbated with administration of estrogen therapy.

Exacerbation of Other Conditions

Estrogens may cause an exacerbation of asthma, diabetes mellitus, epilepsy, migraine or porphyria and should be used with caution in women with these conditions.

Patient Information

Physicians are advised to discuss the **Patient Information** leaflet with patients for whom they prescribe CombiPatch.

Laboratory Tests

Estrogen administration should be initiated at the lowest dose for the approved indication and then guided by clinical response, rather than by serum hormone levels (e.g., estradiol, FSH).

Drug/Laboratory Test Interactions

- Accelerated prothrombin time, partial thromboplastin time, and platelet aggregation time; increased platelet count; increased factors II, VII antigen, VIII antigen, VIII coagulant activity, IX, X, XII, VII-X complex, II-VII-X complex; and beta-thromboglobulin; decreased levels of anti-factor Xa and antithrombin III; decreased antithrombin III activity; increased levels of fibrinogen and fibrinogen activity; increased plasminogen antigen and activity.
- Increased thyroid-binding globulin (TBG) leading to increased circulating total thyroid hormone, as measured by protein-bound iodine (PBI), T_4 levels (by column or by radioimmunoassay) or T_3 levels by radioimmunoassay. T_3 resin uptake is decreased, reflecting the elevated TBG. Free T_4 and free T_3 concentrations are unaltered. Patients on thyroid replacement therapy may require higher doses of thyroid hormone.
- Other binding proteins may be elevated in serum (i.e., corticosteroid binding globulin (CBG), sex hormone-binding globulin (SHBG), leading to increased circulating corticosteroids and sex steroids, respectively. Free or biologically active hormone concentrations are unchanged. Other plasma proteins may be increased (angiotensinogen/renin substrate, alpha-1-antitrypsin, ceruloplasmin).
- Increased plasma HDL and HDL-2 subfraction concentrations, reduced LDL cholesterol concentration, increased triglycerides levels.
- Impaired glucose tolerance.
- Reduced response to metyrapone test.

Carcinogenesis, Mutagenesis, Impairment of Fertility

Long-term continuous administration of natural and synthetic estrogens in certain animal species increases the frequency of carcinomas of the breast, uterus, cervix, vagina, testis, and liver. *(See BOXED WARNING, CONTRAINDICATIONS and WARNINGS.)*

Norethindrone acetate was not mutagenic in a battery of *in vitro* or *in vivo* genetic toxicity assays.

Pregnancy

Estrogens and progestins should not be used during pregnancy. *(See CONTRAINDICATIONS.)*

Nursing Mothers

Estrogen administration to nursing mothers has been shown to decrease the quantity and quality of the milk. Detectable amounts of estrogens and progestins have been identified in the milk of mothers receiving this drug. Caution should be exercised when CombiPatch is administered to a nursing mother.

ADVERSE REACTIONS

See BOXED WARNING, WARNINGS and *PRECAUTIONS*.

Because clinical trials are conducted under widely varying conditions, adverse reaction rates observed in the clinical trials of a drug cannot be directly compared to rates in the clinical trials of another drug and may not reflect the rates observed in practice. The adverse reaction information from clinical trials does, however, provide a basis for identifying the adverse events that appear to be related to drug use and for approximating rates.

[See table IV on previous page]

[See table V above]

Table V.
All Treatment Emergent Study Events Regardless of Relationship Reported at a Frequency of ≥5% with CombiPatch®
ENDOMETRIAL HYPERPLASIA STUDIES

	CombiPatch® 0.05/0.14 mg per day[1] n = 325	CombiPatch® 0.05/0.25 mg per day[1] n = 312	Vivelle® 0.05 mg per day n = 318
Body as a Whole	61%	60%	59%
Abdominal Pain	12%	14%	16%
Accidental Injury	10%	11%	8%
Asthenia	10%	13%	11%
Back Pain	15%	14%	13%
Flu Syndrome	14%	10%	7%
Headache	25%	17%	21%
Infection	5%	3%	3%
Pain	19%	15%	13%
Digestive	42%	32%	31%
Constipation	2%	5%	3%
Diarrhea	14%	9%	7%
Dyspepsia	8%	6%	5%
Flatulence	7%	5%	6%
Nausea	8%	12%	11%
Tooth Disorder	6%	4%	1%
Metabolic and Nutritional Disorders	12%	13%	11%
Peripheral edema	6%	6%	5%
Musculoskeletal	17%	17%	15%
Arthralgia	6%	6%	5%
Nervous	33%	30%	28%
Depression	8%	9%	8%
Dizziness	6%	7%	5%
Insomnia	8%	6%	4%
Nervousness	5%	6%	3%
Respiratory	45%	43%	40%
Bronchitis	5%	3%	4%
Pharyngitis	9%	9%	8%
Respiratory Disorder	13%	9%	13%
Rhinitis	19%	22%	17%
Sinusitis	10%	12%	12%
Skin and Appendages	38%	37%	31%
Acne	4%	5%	4%
Application Site Reaction	20%	23%	17%
Rash	6%	5%	3%
Urogenital	71%	79%	74%
Breast Enlargement	2%	7%	2%
Breast Pain	34%	48%	40%
Dysmenorrhea	30%	31%	19%
Leukorrhea	10%	8%	9%
Menorrhagia	2%	5%	9%
Menstrual Disorder	17%	19%	14%
Vaginal Hemorrhage	3%	6%	12%
Vaginitis	9%	13%	13%

[1] Represents milligrams of estradiol/NETA delivered daily by each system.

OVERDOSAGE

Overdosage with this dosage form is unlikely. Overdosage may cause nausea, and withdrawal bleeding may occur in females. Serious ill effects have not been reported following acute ingestion of large doses of estrogen/progestin-containing oral contraceptives by young children. In the event of a possible overdosage, the system should be removed immediately and medical attention sought.

DOSAGE AND ADMINISTRATION

Use of estrogen alone or in combination with a progestin, should be limited to the shortest duration consistent with treatment goals and risks for the individual woman. Patients should be reevaluated periodically as clinically appropriate (e.g., 3-month to 6-month intervals) to determine whether treatment is still necessary *(see BOXED WARNING and WARNINGS)*. For women who have a uterus, adequate diagnostic measures, such as endometrial sampling, when indicated, should be undertaken to rule out malignancy in cases of undiagnosed persistent or recurring abnormal vaginal bleeding.

Initiation of Therapy

Treatment of postmenopausal symptoms is usually initiated during the menopausal stage when vasomotor symptoms occur. Patients should be started at the lowest dose.

Women not currently using continuous estrogen or combination estrogen/progestin therapy may start therapy with CombiPatch at any time. However, women currently using continuous estrogen or combination estrogen/progestin therapy should complete the current cycle of therapy, before initiating CombiPatch therapy. Women often experience withdrawal bleeding at the completion of the cycle. The first day of this bleeding would be an appropriate time to begin CombiPatch therapy.

Therapeutic Regimens

Combination estrogen/progestin regimens are indicated for women with an intact uterus. Two CombiPatch (estradiol/NETA) transdermal delivery systems are available: 0.05 mg estradiol with 0.14 mg NETA per day (9 sq cm) and 0.05 mg estradiol with 0.25 mg NETA per day (16 sq cm). The lowest effective dose should be used. For all regimens, women should be reevaluated at 3- to 6-month intervals to determine if changes in hormone therapy or if continued hormone therapy is appropriate.

Continuous Combined Regimen

A CombiPatch 0.05 mg estradiol/0.14 mg NETA per day (9 sq cm) matrix transdermal system is worn continuously on the lower abdomen. Additionally, a dose of 0.05 mg estradiol/0.25 mg NETA (16 sq cm system) is available if a greater progestin dose is desired. A new system should be applied twice weekly during a 28-day cycle. Irregular bleeding may occur particularly in the first six months, but generally decreases with time, and often to an amenorrheic state.

Continuous Sequential Regimen

CombiPatch can be applied as a sequential regimen in combination with an estradiol-only transdermal delivery system.

In this treatment regimen, an 0.05 mg per day (nominal delivery rate) estradiol transdermal system (Vivelle) is worn for the first 14 days of a 28-day cycle, replacing the system twice weekly according to product directions. For the remaining 14 days of the 28-day cycle, CombiPatch 0.05 mg estradiol/0.14 mg NETA per day (9 sq cm) transdermal system should be applied to the lower abdomen. Additionally, a dose of 0.05 mg estradiol/0.25 mg NETA (16 sq cm system) is available if a greater progestin dose is desired. The CombiPatch system should be replaced twice weekly during this period in the cycle. Women should be advised that monthly withdrawal bleeding often occurs.

Application of the System

Site Selection

CombiPatch should be placed on a smooth (fold-free), clean, dry area of the skin on the lower abdomen. **CombiPatch should not be applied to or near the breasts.** The area selected should not be oily (which can impair adherence of the system), damaged, or irritated. The waistline should be avoided, since tight clothing may rub the system off or modify drug delivery. The sites of application must be rotated, with an interval of at least one week allowed between applications to the same site.

Application

After opening the pouch, remove one side of the protective liner, taking care not to touch the adhesive part of the transdermal delivery system with the fingers. Immediately apply the transdermal delivery system to a smooth (fold-free) area of skin on the lower abdomen. Remove the second side of the protective liner and press the system firmly in place with the hand for at least 10 seconds, making sure there is good contact, especially around the edges.

Care should be taken that the system does not become dislodged during bathing and other activities. If a system should fall off, the same system may be reapplied to another area of the lower abdomen. If necessary, a new transdermal system may be applied, in which case, the original treatment schedule should be continued. **Only one system should be worn at any one time during the 3- to 4-day dosing interval.**

Once in place, the transdermal system should not be exposed to the sun for prolonged periods of time.

Removal of the System

Removal of the system should be done carefully and slowly to avoid irritation of the skin. Should any adhesive remain on the skin after removal of the system, allow the area to dry for 15 minutes. Then gently rub the area with an oil-based cream or lotion to remove the adhesive residue.

HOW SUPPLIED

CombiPatch® estradiol/norethindrone acetate transdermal delivery system is available in:

[See first table at top of next page]

Storage Conditions

Prior to dispensing to the patient, store refrigerated 2-8°C (36-46°F). After dispensing to the patient, CombiPatch can be stored at room temperature below 25°C (77°F) for up to six months. *For the Pharmacist:* When CombiPatch is dispensed to the patient, place an expiration date on the label. The date should not exceed either six months from the date of sale or the expiration date, whichever comes first.

Store the systems in the **sealed** foil pouch.

Do not store the system in areas where extreme temperatures can occur.

Keep out of the reach of children.

REV: JULY 2004 T2004-55

Vivelle® is a registered trademark of Novartis Pharmaceuticals Corporation.

Continued on next page

CombiPatch—Cont.

System Size	Nominal Delivery Rate* Estradiol / Norethindrone Acetate	Presentation	NDC	Markings
9 sq cm	0.05/0.14 mg per day	8 systems per carton	0078-0377-42	CombiPatch 0.05/0.14 mg per day
		Cartons of 3 patient packs of 8 systems	0078-0377-45	
16 sq cm	0.05/0.25 mg per day	8 systems per carton	0078-0378-42	CombiPatch 0.05/0.25 mg per day
		Cartons of 3 patient packs of 8 systems	0078-0378-45	

*Nominal delivery rate described. See DESCRIPTION for more details regarding drug delivery.

Patient Information

CombiPatch®

(estradiol/norethindrone acetate transdermal system)

Rx only

Read this PATIENT INFORMATION before you start taking CombiPatch® (estradiol/norethindrone acetate transdermal system) and read all the information that you get each time you refill CombiPatch. There may be new information. This information does not take the place of talking to your health care provider about your medical condition or your treatment.

What is the most important information I should know about CombiPatch (a combination of estrogen and progestin hormones)?

- Do not use estrogens and progestins to prevent heart disease, heart attacks, or strokes.

Using estrogens and progestins may increase your chances of getting heart attacks, strokes, breast cancer, and blood clots. You and your health care provider should talk regularly about whether you still need treatment with CombiPatch and whether you are taking the lowest dose that works for you.

What is CombiPatch®?

CombiPatch is a medicine that contains two kinds of hormones, estrogen and progestin. CombiPatch, when applied to the skin on your lower abdomen, releases small amounts of these two hormones every day. These hormones travel through your skin into your bloodstream. The first hormone, estradiol, is an estrogen, the same hormone that your ovaries produced before menopause. The second hormone is norethindrone acetate (abbreviated as NETA), a progestin similar to the progesterone hormones your body used to produce naturally.

CombiPatch is available in two round sizes:

[See second table above]

System Size	Amount of Each Drug in Each System Estradiol/NETA (mg)	Amount of Each Drug Released Every Day Estradiol/NETA (mg per day)
9 sq cm	0.62/2.7	0.05/0.14
16 sq cm	0.51/4.8	0.05/0.25

What is CombiPatch® used for?

CombiPatch is used after the menopause to:

- **Reduce moderate to severe hot flashes.**

  Estrogens are hormones made by a woman's ovaries. The ovaries normally stop making estrogens when a woman is between 45 and 55 years old. This drop in body estrogen levels causes the "Change of life" or menopause (the end of monthly menstrual periods). Sometimes, both ovaries are removed during an operation before natural menopause takes place. The sudden drop in estrogen levels causes "surgical menopause."

  When the estrogen levels begin dropping, some women develop very uncomfortable symptoms, such as feelings of warmth in the face, neck, and chest or sudden strong feelings of heat and sweating ("hot flashes" or "hot flushes"). In some women the symptoms are mild, and they will not need estrogens. In other women, symptoms can be more severe. You and your health care provider should talk regularly about whether you still need treatment with CombiPatch.
- **Treat moderate to severe dryness, itching and burning in or around the vagina.**

  You and your health care provider should talk regularly about whether you still need treatment with CombiPatch to control these problems.
- **Treat certain conditions in which a young woman's ovaries do not produce enough estrogens naturally.**

Who should not take CombiPatch®?

Do not take CombiPatch if you have had your uterus removed (hysterectomy). CombiPatch contains a progestin to decrease the chances of getting cancer of the uterus. If you do not have a uterus, you do not need a progestin and you should not take CombiPatch.

Do not start taking CombiPatch if you:

- **Have unusual vaginal bleeding.**
- **Currently have or have had certain cancers.** Estrogens may increase the chances of getting certain types of cancers, including cancer of the breast or uterus. If you have or had cancer, talk with your health care provider about whether you should take CombiPatch.
- **Had a stroke or heart attack in the recent past (for example in the past year).**
- **Currently have or have had blood clots.**
- **Are allergic to CombiPatch or any of its ingredients.** See the end of this leaflet for a list of ingredients in CombiPatch.
- **Think you may be, or know that you are, pregnant.**

Tell your health care provider:

- **If you are breast-feeding.** The hormones in CombiPatch can pass into your milk.
- **About all of your medical problems.** Your health care provider may need to check you more carefully if you have certain conditions such as asthma (wheezing), epilepsy (seizures), migraine, endometriosis, or problems with your heart, liver, thyroid, kidneys, or have high calcium levels in your blood.
- **About all the medicines you take,** including prescription and nonprescription medicines, vitamins, and herbal supplements. Some medicines may affect how CombiPatch works. CombiPatch may also affect how other medicines work.
- **If you are going to have surgery or will be on bed rest.** You may need to stop taking estrogens.

How should I use CombiPatch®?

Estrogens should be used only as long as needed and at the lowest possible dose that works. You and your health care provider should talk regularly (for example every 3 to 6 months) about whether you still need treatment with CombiPatch.

CombiPatch is a thin, opaque, plastic patch that sticks to the skin. Each patch is sealed in a pouch that protects it until you are ready to put it on. Do not open the pouch or remove a patch until just before you apply it.

How often should you apply CombiPatch®?

- Put on a new CombiPatch every 3 to 4 days, according to your health care provider's instructions.
- Wear the patch all the time until it is time to replace it with a new patch.
- **Change the patch on the same days each week.** Your CombiPatch package contains a calendar checklist to help you remember a schedule. Mark the 2-day schedule you plan to follow.
- **Only one CombiPatch should be worn at any one time.**

Where do you apply CombiPatch®?

CombiPatch® (estradiol/norethindrone acetate transdermal system) should be placed on the lower abdomen (below the panty line).

For best results, choose:

- A smooth (fold-free), clean, dry area of skin.
- An area that has been freshly washed and dried well (free of oils, lotions or powders that could keep the patch from sticking well to your skin).
- An area that has no cuts, rashes, or other skin problems.

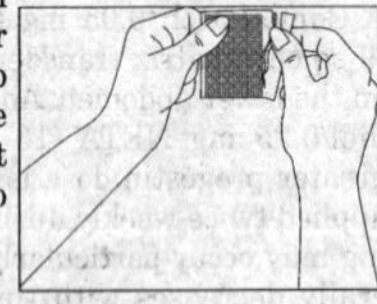

Every time you put on a new CombiPatch, move to a different area on your lower abdomen than used before. The same area should not be used again for at least 1 week.

Do not put CombiPatch on or near your breasts. You should not put CombiPatch on the waistline, since tight clothing may rub off the patch. To avoid disturbing the patch it may help to choose an area where your underwear will cover it all the time.

How do you apply CombiPatch®?

- Each CombiPatch is sealed in its own protective pouch. Tear open this pouch at the slit (do not use scissors) and remove the patch. The pouch should not be opened until you are ready to put the patch on.

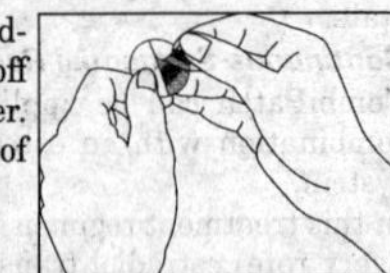

- A protective liner covers the adhesive side of the patch. Peel off one side of the protective liner. Do not touch the sticky part of the patch with your fingers.

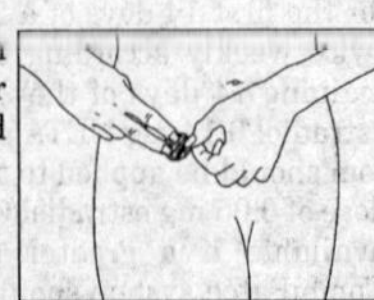

- Put the sticky side of the patch on an area of skin on your lower abdomen. Peel off the second side of the protective liner.

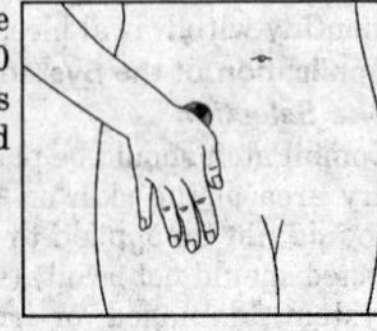

- Press the patch firmly in place with your hand for about 10 seconds. Make sure there is good contact, especially around the edges.

When changing CombiPatch, peel off the used patch slowly. Fold the used patch in half (sticky sides together) and throw it in the trash. **Please remember to keep CombiPatch out of the reach of children.**

If any adhesive remains on your skin after removal of the patch, let the area dry for 15 minutes. Then gently rub the area with an oil-based cream or lotion to remove the adhesive from your skin.

What if you forget to put on a new CombiPatch®?

If you are currently wearing a patch, remove it and put on a new patch in a different area of your lower abdomen. Then go back to changing the patch on the same days each week.

Can you wear CombiPatch® when bathing, swimming, or in the sun?

- Bathing, swimming, or showering should not affect the patch. Make sure that the patch does not loosen during these activities.
- The patch should not be exposed to the sun for long periods of time. Once in place, make sure that the patch is covered by your clothing (but remember not to apply CombiPatch on or near your breasts).

What should I do if CombiPatch® comes off?

Most women find that CombiPatch seldom comes off. But if a patch should fall off, the same patch may be put on a different area of the lower abdomen (make sure you are choosing a clean, dry, lotion-free area of skin). If the patch will not stick completely to your skin, put a new CombiPatch on a different area of the lower abdomen. No matter what day this happens, go back to changing the patch on the same days each week.

What are the possible side effects of estrogens?

Less common but serious side effects include:

— Breast cancer
— Cancer of the uterus
— Stroke
— Stroke
— Heart attack
— Blood clots
— Gallbladder disease
— Ovarian cancer

These are some of the warning signs of serious side effects:

— Breast lumps
— Unusual vaginal bleeding
— Dizziness and faintness
— Changes in speech
— Changes in speech
— Severe headaches
— Chest pain
— Shortness of breath
— Pains in your legs
— Changes in vision
— Vomiting

Call your health care provider right away if you get any of these warning signs, or any other unusual symptom that concerns you.

Common side effects include:

— Headache
— Breast pain
— Irregular vaginal bleeding or spotting
— Stomach/abdominal cramps, bloating
— Nausea and vomiting
— Hair loss

Other side effects include:

— High blood pressure
— Liver problems
— High blood sugar. Taking oral medicines that have an estrogen and/or progestin in them may have effects on blood sugar levels. This may make a diabetic condition worse. Similar blood sugar effects have not been reported in women who used estradiol/NETA skin patches, such as CombiPatch.
— Fluid retention
— Enlargement of benign tumors of the uterus ("fibroids")
— Vaginal yeast infection

Other side effects of CombiPatch are possible. For more information, ask your health care provider or pharmacist.

What can I do to lower my chances of a serious side effect with CombiPatch®?

- Talk with your health care provider regularly about whether you should continue taking CombiPatch.
- See your health care provider right away if you get vaginal bleeding while taking CombiPatch.

- Have a breast exam and mammogram (breast X-ray) every year unless your health care provider tells you something else. If members of your family have had breast cancer or if you have ever had breast lumps or an abnormal mammogram, you may need to have breast exams more often.
- If you have high blood pressure, high cholesterol (fat in the blood), diabetes, are overweight, or if you use tobacco, you may have higher chances for getting heart disease. Ask your health care provider for ways to lower your chances for getting heart disease.

General information about the safe and effective use of CombiPatch®

Medicines are sometimes prescribed for conditions that are not mentioned in patient information leaflets. Do not take CombiPatch for conditions for which it was not prescribed. Do not give CombiPatch to other people, even if they have the same symptoms you have. It may harm them. **Keep CombiPatch out of the reach of children.**

This leaflet provides a summary of the most important information about CombiPatch. If you would like more information, talk with your health care provider or pharmacist. You can ask for information about CombiPatch that is written for health professionals. You can get more information by calling the toll free number 888-NOW-NOVA (888-669-6682).

What are the ingredients in CombiPatch®?

CombiPatch transdermal systems are comprised of three layers. Proceeding from the visible surface toward the surface attached to the skin, these layers are (1) a translucent polyolefin film backing, (2) an adhesive layer containing estradiol, norethindrone acetate, acrylic adhesive, silicone adhesive, oleyl alcohol, NF (Phase 1 system) or oleic acid NF (Phase 2 system), povidone USP and dipropylene glycol, and (3) a polyester release protective liner, which is attached to the adhesive surface and must be removed before the system can be used. The active components of the system are estradiol USP and norethindrone acetate USP. The remaining components of the system are pharmacologically inactive.

Where should you store CombiPatch®?

Each CombiPatch is sealed in its own pouch. To protect the medication, store the patch in the pouch until you are ready to use it.

Before CombiPatch was sold to you, the pharmacist stored the package in the refrigerator. **You can store CombiPatch at room temperature, below 77°F (25°C).** The patch sticks best to your skin when stored at room temperature. For best results, DO NOT store CombiPatch patches in the refrigerator or in areas where the temperature can become extreme (very high or very low), such as in DIRECT SUNLIGHT or in a car.

Keep this and all medicines out of the reach of children.

T2004-56
T2004-55/T2004-56
REV: JULY 2004 89012905
101932-4

Manufactured by:
Noven Pharmaceuticals Inc.
Miami, FL 33186
Distributed by:
Novartis Pharmaceuticals Corp.
East Hanover, NJ 07936
©Novartis

COMTAN® ℞

[cŏm-tăn]
(entacapone) Tablets
Rx only

Prescribing Information

The following prescribing information is based on official labeling in effect July, 2003.

DESCRIPTION

Comtan® (entacapone) is available as tablets containing 200-mg entacapone.

Entacapone is an inhibitor of catechol-*O*-methyltransferase (COMT), used in the treatment of Parkinson's Disease as an adjunct to levodopa/carbidopa therapy. It is a nitrocatechol-structured compound with a relative molecular mass of 305.29. The chemical name of entacapone is (E)-2-cyano-3-(3,4-dihydroxy-5-nitrophenyl)-N,N-diethyl-2-propenamide. Its empirical formula is $C_{14}H_{15}N_3O_5$ and its structural formula is:

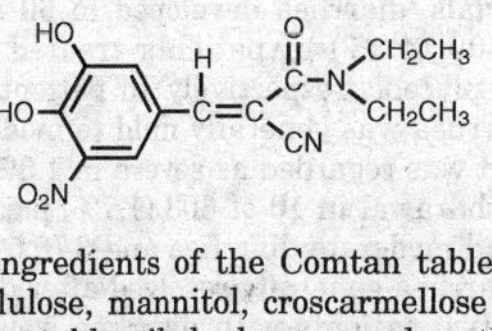

The inactive ingredients of the Comtan tablet are microcrystalline cellulose, mannitol, croscarmellose sodium, hydrogenated vegetable oil, hydroxypropyl methylcellulose, polysorbate 80, glycerol 85%, sucrose, magnesium stearate, yellow iron oxide, red oxide, and titanium dioxide.

CLINICAL PHARMACOLOGY

Mechanism of Action

Entacapone is a selective and reversible inhibitor of catechol-*O*-methyltransferase (COMT).

Table 1. Nordic Study

	Baseline	Change from Baseline at Month 6*	p-value vs. placebo
Primary Measure from Home Diary (from an 18-hour Diary Day)			
Hours of Awake Time "On"			
Placebo	9.2	+0.1	—
Comtan	9.3	+1.5	<0.001
Duration of "On" time after first AM dose (hrs)			
Placebo	2.2	0.0	—
Comtan	2.1	+0.2	<0.05
Secondary Measures from Home Diary (from an 18-hour Diary Day)			
Hours of Awake Time "Off"			
Placebo	5.3	0.0	—
Comtan	5.5	-1.3	<0.001
Proportion of Awake Time "On" * (%)**			
Placebo	63.8	+0.6	—
Comtan	62.7	+9.3	<0.001
Levodopa Total Daily Dose (mg)			
Placebo	705	+14	—
Comtan	701	-87	<0.001
Frequency of Levodopa Daily Intakes			
Placebo	6.1	+0.1	—
Comtan	6.2	-0.4	<0.001
Other Secondary Measures			
	Baseline	Change from Baseline at Month 6	p-value vs. placebo
Investigator's Global (overall) % Improved**			
Placebo	—	28	—
Comtan	—	56	<0.01
Patient's Global (overall) % Improved**			
Placebo	—	22	—
Comtan	—	39	N.S.‡
UPDRS Total			
Placebo	37.4	-1.1	—
Comtan	38.5	-4.8	<0.01
UPDRS Motor			
Placebo	24.6	-0.7	—
Comtan	25.5	-3.3	<0.05
UPDRS ADL			
Placebo	11.0	-0.4	—
Comtan	11.2	-1.8	<0.05

* Mean; the month 6 values represent the average of weeks 8, 16, and 24, by protocol-defined outcome measure.
** At least one category change at endpoint.
*** Not an endpoint for this study but primary endpoint in the North American Study.
‡ Not significant.

In mammals, COMT is distributed throughout various organs with the highest activities in the liver and kidney. COMT also occurs in the heart, lung, smooth and skeletal muscles, intestinal tract, reproductive organs, various glands, adipose tissue, skin, blood cells, and neuronal tissues, especially in glial cells. COMT catalyzes the transfer of the methyl group of S-adenosyl-L-methionine to the phenolic group of substrates that contain a catechol structure. Physiological substrates of COMT include dopa, catecholamines (dopamine, norepinephrine, and epinephrine) and their hydroxylated metabolites. The function of COMT is the elimination of biologically active catechols and some other hydroxylated metabolites. In the presence of a decarboxylase inhibitor, COMT becomes the major metabolizing enzyme for levodopa, catalyzing the metabolism to 3-methoxy-4-hydroxy-L-phenylalanine (3-OMD) in the brain and periphery.

The mechanism of action of entacapone is believed to be through its ability to inhibit COMT and alter the plasma pharmacokinetics of levodopa. When entacapone is given in conjunction with levodopa and an aromatic amino acid decarboxylase inhibitor, such as carbidopa, plasma levels of levodopa are greater and more sustained than after administration of levodopa and an aromatic amino acid decarboxylase inhibitor alone. It is believed that at a given frequency of levodopa administration, these more sustained plasma levels of levodopa result in more constant dopaminergic stimulation in the brain, leading to greater effects on the signs and symptoms of Parkinson's Disease. The higher levodopa levels also lead to increased levodopa adverse effects, sometimes requiring a decrease in the dose of levodopa.

In animals, while entacapone enters the CNS to a minimal extent, it has been shown to inhibit central COMT activity. In humans, entacapone inhibits the COMT enzyme in peripheral tissues. The effects of entacapone on central COMT activity in humans have not been studied.

Pharmacodynamics

COMT Activity in Erythrocytes: Studies in healthy volunteers have shown that entacapone reversibly inhibits human erythrocyte catechol-*O*-methyltransferase (COMT) activity after oral administration. There was a linear correlation between entacapone dose and erythrocyte COMT inhibition, the maximum inhibition being 82% following an 800-mg single dose. With a 200-mg single dose of entacapone, maximum inhibition of erythrocyte COMT activity is on average 65% with a return to baseline level within 8 hours.

Effect on the Pharmacokinetics of Levodopa and its Metabolites

When 200 mg entacapone is administered together with levodopa/carbidopa, it increases the area under the curve (AUC) of levodopa by approximately 35% and the elimination half-life of levodopa is prolonged from 1.3 h-2.4 h. In general, the average peak levodopa plasma concentration and the time of its occurrence (T_{max} of 1 hour) are unaffected. The onset of effect occurs after the first administration and is maintained during long-term treatment. Studies in Parkinson's Disease patients suggest that the maximal effect occurs with 200-mg entacapone. Plasma levels of 3-OMD are markedly and dose-dependently decreased by entacapone when given with levodopa/carbidopa.

Pharmacokinetics of Entacapone

Entacapone pharmacokinetics are linear over the dose range of 5 mg-800 mg, and are independent of levodopa/carbidopa coadministration. The elimination of entacapone is biphasic, with an elimination half-life of 0.4 h-0.7 h based on the β-phase and 2.4 h based on the γ-phase. The γ-phase accounts for approximately 10% of the total AUC. The total body clearance after i.v. administration is 850 mL/min. After a single 200-mg dose of Comtan (entacapone), the C_{max} is approximately 1.2 µg/mL.

Absorption: Entacapone is rapidly absorbed, with a T_{max} of approximately 1 hour. The absolute bioavailability following oral administration is 35%. Food does not affect the pharmacokinetics of entacapone.

Distribution: The volume of distribution of entacapone at steady state after i.v. injection is small (20 L). Entacapone does not distribute widely into tissues due to its high plasma protein binding. Based on *in vitro* studies, the plasma protein binding of entacapone is 98% over the concentration range of 0.4-50 µg/mL. Entacapone binds mainly to serum albumin.

Metabolism and Elimination: Entacapone is almost completely metabolized prior to excretion, with only a very small amount (0.2% of dose) found unchanged in urine. The main metabolic pathway is isomerization to the *cis*-isomer, followed by direct glucuronidation of the parent and *cis*-isomer; the glucuronide conjugate is inactive. After oral administration of a ^{14}C-labeled dose of entacapone, 10% of labeled parent and metabolite is excreted in urine and 90% in feces.

Continued on next page

Comtan—Cont.

Special Populations: Entacapone pharmacokinetics are independent of age. No formal gender studies have been conducted. Racial representation in clinical trials was largely limited to Caucasians (there were only 4 blacks in one US trial and no Asians in any of the clinical trials); no conclusions can therefore be reached about the effect of Comtan on groups other than Caucasian.

Hepatic Impairment: A single 200-mg dose of entacapone, without levodopa/dopa decarboxylase inhibitor coadministration, showed approximately twofold higher AUC and C_{max} values in patients with a history of alcoholism and hepatic impairment (n=10) compared to normal subjects (n=10). All patients had biopsy-proven liver cirrhosis caused by alcohol. According to Child-Pugh grading 7 patients with liver disease had mild hepatic impairment and 3 patients had moderate hepatic impairment. As only about 10% of the entacapone dose is excreted in urine as parent compound and conjugated glucuronide, biliary excretion appears to be the major route of excretion of this drug. Consequently, entacapone should be administered with care to patients with biliary obstruction.

Renal Impairment: The pharmacokinetics of entacapone have been investigated after a single 200-mg entacapone dose, without levodopa/dopa decarboxylase inhibitor coadministration, in a specific renal impairment study. There were three groups: normal subjects (n=7; creatinine clearance >1.12 mL/sec/1.73 m^2), moderate impairment (n=10; creatinine clearance ranging from 0.60-0.89 mL/sec/1.73 m^2), and severe impairment (n=7; creatinine clearance ranging from 0.20-0.44 mL/sec/1.73 m^2). No important effects of renal function on the pharmacokinetics of entacapone were found.

Drug Interactions: See PRECAUTIONS, *Drug Interactions.*

Clinical Studies

The effectiveness of Comtan (entacapone) as an adjunct to levodopa in the treatment of Parkinson's Disease was established in three 24-week multicenter, randomized, double-blind placebo-controlled trials in patients with Parkinson's Disease. In two of these trials, the patients' disease was "fluctuating", i.e., was characterized by documented periods of "On" (periods of relatively good functioning) and "Off" (periods of relatively poor functioning), despite optimum levodopa therapy. There was also a withdrawal period following 6 months of treatment. In the third trial patients were not required to have been experiencing fluctuations. Prior to the controlled part of the trials, patients were stabilized on levodopa for 2-4 weeks. Comtan has not been systematically evaluated in patients who do not experience fluctuations.

In the first two studies to be described, patients were randomized to receive placebo or entacapone 200 mg administered concomitantly with each dose of levodopa/carbidopa (up to 10 times daily, but averaging 4-6 doses per day). The formal double-blind portion of both trials was 6 months long. Patients recorded the time spent in the "On" and "Off" states in home diaries periodically throughout the duration of the trial. In one study, conducted in the Nordic countries, the primary outcome measure was the total mean time spent in the "On" state during an 18-hour diary recorded day (6 AM to midnight). In the other study, the primary outcome measure was the proportion of awake time spent over 24 hours in the "On" state.

In addition to the primary outcome measure, the amount of time spent in the "Off" state was evaluated, and patients were also evaluated by subparts of the Unified Parkinson's Disease Rating Scale (UPDRS), a frequently used multi-item rating scale intended to assess mentation (Part I), activities of daily living (Part II), motor function (Part III), complications of therapy (Part IV), and disease staging (Part V & VI); an investigator's and patient's global assessment of clinical condition, a 7-point subjective scale designed to assess global functioning in Parkinson's Disease; and the change in daily levodopa/carbidopa dose.

In one of the studies, 171 patients were randomized in 16 centers in Finland, Norway, Sweden, and Denmark (Nordic study), all of whom received concomitant levodopa plus dopa-decarboxylase inhibitor (either levodopa/carbidopa or levodopa/benserazide). In the second trial, 205 patients were randomized in 17 centers in North America (US and Canada); all patients received concomitant levodopa/carbidopa.

The following tables display the results of these two trials:

[See table 1 at top of previous page]

[See table 2 above]

Effects on "On" time did not differ by age, sex, weight, disease severity at baseline, levodopa dose and concurrent treatment with dopamine agonists or selegiline.

Withdrawal of entacapone: In the North American study, abrupt withdrawal of entacapone, without alteration of the dose of levodopa/carbidopa, resulted in a significant worsening of fluctuations, compared to placebo. In some cases, symptoms were slightly worse than at baseline, but returned to approximately baseline severity within two weeks following levodopa dose increase on average by 80 mg. In the Nordic study, similarly, a significant worsening of parkinsonian symptoms was observed after entacapone withdrawal, as assessed two weeks after drug withdrawal. At this phase, the symptoms were approximately at baseline severity following levodopa dose increase by about 50 mg.

In the third placebo controlled trial, a total of 301 patients were randomized in 32 centers in Germany and Austria. In this trial, as in the other two trials, entacapone 200 mg was administered with each dose of levodopa/dopa decarboxylase inhibitor (up to 10 times daily) and UPDRS Parts II and III and total daily "On" time were the primary measures of effectiveness. The following results were seen for the primary measures, as well as for some secondary measures:

[See table 3 at top of next page]

Table 2. North American Study

Primary Measure from Home Diary (for a 24-hour Diary Day)	Baseline	Change from Baseline at Month 6*	p-value vs. placebo
Percent of Awake Time "On"			
Placebo	60.8	+2.0	—
Comtan	60.0	+6.7	<0.05
Secondary Measures from Home Diary (for a 24-hour Diary Day)			
Hours of Awake Time "Off"			
Placebo	6.6	-0.3	—
Comtan	6.8	-1.2	<0.01
Hours of Awake Time "On"			
Placebo	10.3	+0.4	—
Comtan	10.2	+1.0	N.S.‡
Levodopa Total Daily Dose (mg)			
Placebo	758	+19	—
Comtan	804	-93	<0.001
Frequency of Levodopa Daily Intakes			
Placebo	6.0	+0.2	—
Comtan	6.2	0.0	N.S.‡
Other Secondary Measures	**Baseline**	**Change from Baseline at Month 6**	**p-value vs. placebo**
Investigator's Global (overall) % Improved**			
Placebo	—	21	—
Comtan	—	34	<0.05
Patient's Global (overall) % Improved**			
Placebo	—	20	—
Comtan	—	31	<0.05
UPDRS Total***			
Placebo	35.6	+2.8	—
Comtan	35.1	-0.6	<0.05
UPDRS Motor***			
Placebo	22.6	+1.2	—
Comtan	22.0	-0.9	<0.05
UPDRS ADL***			
Placebo	11.7	+1.1	—
Comtan	11.9	0.0	<0.05

*Mean; the month 6 values represent the average of weeks 8, 16, and 24, by protocol-defined outcome measure.
** At least one category change at endpoint.
*** Score change at endpoint similarly to the Nordic Study.
‡ Not significant.

INDICATIONS

Comtan (entacapone) is indicated as an adjunct to levodopa/carbidopa to treat patients with idiopathic Parkinson's Disease who experience the signs and symptoms of end-of-dose "wearing-off" *(see CLINICAL PHARMACOLOGY, Clinical Studies).*

Comtan's effectiveness has not been systematically evaluated in patients with idiopathic Parkinson's Disease who do not experience end-of-dose "wearing-off".

CONTRAINDICATIONS

Comtan (entacapone) tablets are contraindicated in patients who have demonstrated hypersensitivity to the drug or its ingredients.

WARNINGS

Monoamine oxidase (MAO) and COMT are the two major enzyme systems involved in the metabolism of catecholamines. It is theoretically possible, therefore, that the combination of Comtan (entacapone) and a non-selective MAO inhibitor (e.g., phenelzine and tranylcypromine) would result in inhibition of the majority of the pathways responsible for normal catecholamine metabolism. For this reason, patients should ordinarily not be treated concomitantly with Comtan and a non-selective MAO inhibitor.

Entacapone can be taken concomitantly with a selective MAO-B inhibitor (e.g., selegiline).

Drugs Metabolized by Catechol-*O*-methyltransferase (COMT)

When a single 400-mg dose of entacapone was given together with intravenous isoprenaline (isoproterenol) and epinephrine without coadministered levodopa/dopa decarboxylase inhibitor, the overall mean maximal changes in heart rate during infusion were about 50% and 80% higher than with placebo, for isoprenaline and epinephrine, respectively.

Therefore, drugs known to be metabolized by COMT, such as isoproterenol, epinephrine, norepinephrine, dopamine, dobutamine, alpha-methyldopa, apomorphine, isoetherine, and bitolterol should be administered with caution in patients receiving entacapone regardless of the route of administration (including inhalation), as their interaction may result in increased heart rates, possibly arrhythmias, and excessive changes in blood pressure.

Ventricular tachycardia was noted in one 32-year-old healthy male volunteer in an interaction study after epinephrine infusion and oral entacapone administration. Treatment with propranolol was required. A causal relationship to entacapone administration appears probable but cannot be attributed with certainty.

PRECAUTIONS

Hypotension/Syncope

Dopaminergic therapy in Parkinson's Disease patients has been associated with orthostatic hypotension. Entacapone enhances levodopa bioavailability and, therefore, might be expected to increase the occurrence of orthostatic hypotension. In Comtan (entacapone) clinical trials, however, no differences from placebo were seen for measured orthostasis or symptoms of orthostasis. Orthostatic hypotension was documented at least once in 2.7% and 3.0% of the patients treated with 200 mg Comtan and placebo, respectively. A total of 4.3% and 4.0% of the patients treated with 200 mg Comtan and placebo, respectively, reported orthostatic symptoms at some time during their treatment and also had at least one episode of orthostatic hypotension documented (however, the episode of orthostatic symptoms itself was not accompanied by vital sign measurements). Neither baseline treatment with dopamine agonists or selegiline, nor the presence of orthostasis at baseline, increased the risk of orthostatic hypotension in patients treated with Comtan compared to patients on placebo.

In the large controlled trials, approximately 1.2% and 0.8% of 200 mg entacapone and placebo patients, respectively, reported at least one episode of syncope. Reports of syncope were generally more frequent in patients in both treatment groups who had an episode of documented hypotension (although the episodes of syncope, obtained by history, were themselves not documented with vital sign measurement).

Diarrhea

In clinical trials, diarrhea developed in 60 of 603 (10.0%) and 16 of 400 (4.0%) of patients treated with 200 mg Comtan and placebo, respectively. In patients treated with Comtan, diarrhea was generally mild to moderate in severity (8.6%) but was regarded as severe in 1.3%. Diarrhea resulted in withdrawal in 10 of 603 (1.7%) patients, 7 (1.2%) with mild and moderate diarrhea and 3 (0.5%) with severe diarrhea. Diarrhea generally resolved after discontinuation of Comtan. Two patients with diarrhea were hospitalized. Typically, diarrhea presents within 4-12 weeks after entacapone is started, but it may appear as early as the first week and as late as many months after the initiation of treatment.

Hallucinations

Dopaminergic therapy in Parkinson's Disease patients has been associated with hallucinations. In clinical trials, hallucinations developed in approximately 4.0% of patients treated with 200 mg Comtan or placebo. Hallucinations led to drug discontinuation and premature withdrawal from clinical trials in 0.8% and 0% of patients treated with 200 mg Comtan and placebo, respectively. Hallucinations led to hospitalization in 1.0% and 0.3% of patients in the 200 mg Comtan and placebo groups, respectively.

Dyskinesia

Comtan may potentiate the dopaminergic side effects of levodopa and may cause and/or exacerbate preexisting dyskinesia. Although decreasing the dose of levodopa may ameliorate this side effect, many patients in controlled trials continued to experience frequent dyskinesias despite a reduction in their dose of levodopa. The rates of withdrawal for dyskinesia were 1.5% and 0.8% for 200 mg Comtan and placebo, respectively.

Other Events Reported With Dopaminergic Therapy

The events listed below are rare events known to be associated with the use of drugs that increase dopaminergic activity, although they are most often associated with the use of direct dopamine agonists.

Rhabdomyolysis: Cases of severe rhabdomyolysis have been reported with Comtan use. The complicated nature of these cases makes it impossible to determine what role, if any, Comtan played in their pathogenesis. Severe prolonged motor activity including dyskinesia may account for rhabdomyolysis. One case, however, included fever and alteration of consciousness. It is therefore possible that the rhabdomyolysis may be a result of the syndrome described in Hyperpyrexia and Confusion *(see PRECAUTIONS, Other Events Reported With Dopaminergic Therapy)*.

Hyperpyrexia and Confusion: Cases of a symptom complex resembling the neuroleptic malignant syndrome characterized by elevated temperature, muscular rigidity, altered consciousness, and elevated CPK have been reported in association with the rapid dose reduction or withdrawal of other dopaminergic drugs. Several cases with similar signs and symptoms have been reported in association with Comtan therapy, although no information about dose manipulation is available. The complicated nature of these cases makes it difficult to determine what role, if any, Comtan may have played in their pathogenesis. No cases have been reported following the abrupt withdrawal or dose reduction of entacapone treatment during clinical studies.

Prescribers should exercise caution when discontinuing entacapone treatment. When considered necessary, withdrawal should proceed slowly. If a decision is made to discontinue treatment with Comtan, recommendations include monitoring the patient closely and adjusting other dopaminergic treatments as needed. This syndrome should be considered in the differential diagnosis for any patient who develops a high fever or severe rigidity. Tapering Comtan has not been systematically evaluated.

Fibrotic Complications: Cases of retroperitoneal fibrosis, pulmonary infiltrates, pleural effusion, and pleural thickening have been reported in some patients treated with ergot derived dopaminergic agents. These complications may resolve when the drug is discontinued, but complete resolution does not always occur. Although these adverse events are believed to be related to the ergoline structure of these compounds, whether other, nonergot derived drugs (e.g., entacapone) that increase dopaminergic activity can cause them is unknown. It should be noted that the expected incidence of fibrotic complications is so low that even if entacapone caused these complications at rates similar to those attributable to other dopaminergic therapies, it is unlikely that it would have been detected in a cohort of the size exposed to entacapone. Four cases of pulmonary fibrosis were reported during clinical development of entacapone; three of these patients were also treated with pergolide and one with bromocriptine. The duration of treatment with entacapone ranged from 7-17 months.

Renal Toxicity

In a 1 year toxicity study, entacapone (plasma exposure 20 times that in humans receiving the maximum recommended daily dose of 1600 mg) caused an increased incidence in male rats of nephrotoxicity that was characterized by regenerative tubules, thickening of basement membranes, infiltration of mononuclear cells and tubular protein casts. These effects were not associated with changes in clinical chemistry parameters, and there is no established method for monitoring for the possible occurrence of these lesions in humans. Although this toxicity could represent a species-specific effect, there is not yet evidence that this is so.

Hepatic Impairment

Patients with hepatic impairment should be treated with caution. The AUC and C_{max} of entacapone approximately doubled in patients with documented liver disease compared to controls. (See CLINICAL PHARMACOLOGY, Pharmacokinetics of Entacapone and DOSAGE AND ADMINISTRATION).

Information for Patients

Patients should be instructed to take Comtan only as prescribed.

Patients should be informed that hallucinations can occur.

Patients should be advised that they may develop postural (orthostatic) hypotension with or without symptoms such as dizziness, nausea, syncope, and sweating. Hypotension may occur more frequently during initial therapy. Accordingly, patients should be cautioned against rising rapidly after sitting or lying down, especially if they have been doing so for prolonged periods, and especially at the initiation of treatment with Comtan.

Table 3. German-Austrian Study

	Baseline	Change from Baseline at Month 6	p-value vs. placebo (LOCF)
Primary Measures			
UPDRS ADL*			
Placebo	12.0	+0.5	—
Comtan	12.4	-0.4	<0.05
UPDRS Motor*			
Placebo	24.1	+0.1	—
Comtan	24.9	-2.5	<0.05
Hours of Awake Time "On" (Home diary)**			
Placebo	10.1	+0.5	—
Comtan	10.2	+1.1	N.S.‡
Secondary Measures			
	Baseline	**Change from Baseline at Month 6**	**p-value vs. placebo**
UPDRS Total*			
Placebo	37.7	+0.6	—
Comtan	39.0	-3.4	<0.05
Percent of Awake Time "On" (Home diary)**			
Placebo	59.8	+3.5	—
Comtan	62.0	+6.5	N.S.‡
Hours of Awake Time "Off" (Home diary)**			
Placebo	6.8	-0.6	—
Comtan	6.3	-1.2	0.07
Levodopa Total Daily Dose (mg)*			
Placebo	572	+4	—
Comtan	566	-35	N.S.‡
Frequency of Levodopa Daily Intake*			
Placebo	5.6	+0.2	—
Comtan	5.4	0.0	<0.01
Global (overall) % Improved***			
Placebo	—	34	
Comtan	—	38	N.S.‡

*Total population; score change at endpoint.
** Fluctuating population, with 5-10 doses; score change at endpoint.
*** Total population; at least one category change at endpoint.
‡ Not significant.

Patients should be advised that they should neither drive a car nor operate other complex machinery until they have gained sufficient experience on Comtan to gauge whether or not it affects their mental and/or motor performance adversely. Because of the possible additive sedative effects, caution should be used when patients are taking other CNS depressants in combination with Comtan.

Patients should be informed that nausea may occur, especially at the initiation of treatment with Comtan.

Patients should be advised of the possibility of an increase in dyskinesia.

Patients should be advised that treatment with entacapone may cause a change in the color of their urine (a brownish orange discoloration) that is not clinically relevant. In controlled trials, 10% of patients treated with Comtan reported urine discoloration compared to 0% of placebo patients.

Although Comtan has not been shown to be teratogenic in animals, it is always given in conjunction with levodopa/carbidopa, which is known to cause visceral and skeletal malformations in the rabbit. Accordingly, patients should be advised to notify their physicians if they become pregnant or intend to become pregnant during therapy (see PRECAUTIONS, Pregnancy).

Entacapone is excreted into maternal milk in rats. Because of the possibility that entacapone may be excreted into human maternal milk, patients should be advised to notify their physicians if they intend to breastfeed or are breastfeeding an infant.

Laboratory Tests

Comtan is a chelator of iron. The impact of entacapone on the body's iron stores is unknown; however, a tendency towards decreasing serum iron concentrations was noted in clinical trials. In a controlled clinical study serum ferritin levels (as marker of iron deficiency and subclinical anemia) were not changed with entacapone compared to placebo after one year of treatment and there was no difference in rates of anemia or decreased hemoglobin levels.

Special Populations

Patients with hepatic impairment should be treated with caution (see INDICATIONS, DOSAGE AND ADMINISTRATION).

Drug Interactions

In vitro studies of human CYP enzymes showed that entacapone inhibited the CYP enzymes 1A2, 2A6, 2C9, 2C19, 2D6, 2E1 and 3A only at very high concentrations (IC50 from 200 to over 1000 µM; an oral 200 mg dose achieves a highest level of approximately 5 µM in people); these enzymes would therefore not be expected to be inhibited in clinical use.

Protein Binding

Entacapone is highly protein bound (98%). *In vitro* studies have shown no binding displacement between entacapone and other highly bound drugs, such as warfarin, salicylic acid, phenylbutazone, and diazepam.

Drugs Metabolized by Catechol-*O*-methyltransferase (COMT)

See WARNINGS.

Hormone levels

Levodopa is known to depress prolactin secretion and increase growth hormone levels. Treatment with entacapone coadministered with levodopa/dopa decarboxylase inhibitor does not change these effects.

Effect of Entacapone on the Metabolism of Other Drugs

See WARNINGS regarding concomitant use of Comtan and non-selective MAO inhibitors.

No interaction was noted with the MAO-B inhibitor selegiline in two multiple-dose interaction studies when entacapone was coadministered with a levodopa/dopa decarboxylase inhibitor (n=29). More than 600 Parkinson's Disease patients in clinical trials have used selegiline in combination with entacapone and levodopa/dopa decarboxylase inhibitor.

As most entacapone excretion is via the bile, caution should be exercised when drugs known to interfere with biliary excretion, glucuronidation, and intestinal beta-glucuronidase are given concurrently with entacapone. These include probenecid, cholestyramine, and some antibiotics (e.g., erythromycin, rifampicin, ampicillin and chloramphenicol).

No interaction with the tricyclic antidepressant imipramine was shown in a single-dose study with entacapone without coadministered levodopa/dopa-decarboxylase inhibitor.

Carcinogenesis

Two-year carcinogenicity studies of entacapone were conducted in mice and rats. Rats were treated once daily by oral gavage with entacapone doses of 20, 90, or 400 mg/kg. An increased incidence of renal tubular adenomas and carcinomas was found in male rats treated with the highest dose of entacapone. Plasma exposures (AUC) associated with this dose were approximately 20 times higher than estimated plasma exposures of humans receiving the maximum recommended daily dose of entacapone (MRDD = 1600 mg). Mice were treated once daily by oral gavage with doses of 20, 100 or 600 mg/kg of entacapone (0.05, 0.3, and 2 times the MRDD for humans on a mg/m^2 basis). Because of a high incidence of premature mortality in mice receiving the highest dose of entacapone, the mouse study is not an adequate assessment of carcinogenicity. Although no treatment related tumors were observed in animals receiving the lower doses, the carcinogenic potential of entacapone has not been fully evaluated. The carcinogenic potential of entacapone administered in combination with levodopa/carbidopa has not been evaluated.

Mutagenesis

Entacapone was mutagenic and clastogenic in the *in vitro* mouse lymphoma/thymidine kinase assay in the presence and absence of metabolic activation, and was clastogenic in cultured human lymphocytes in the presence of metabolic activation. Entacapone, either alone or in combination with

Continued on next page

Comtan—Cont.

levodopa/carbidopa, was not clastogenic in the *in vivo* mouse micronucleus test or mutagenic in the bacterial reverse mutation assay (Ames test).

Impairment of Fertility

Entacapone did not impair fertility or general reproductive performance in rats treated with up to 700 mg/kg/day (plasma AUCs 28 times those in humans receiving the MRDD). Delayed mating, but no fertility impairment, was evident in female rats treated with 700 mg/kg/day of entacapone.

Pregnancy

Pregnancy Category C. In embryofetal development studies, entacapone was administered to pregnant animals throughout organogenesis at doses of up to 1000 mg/kg/day in rats and 300 mg/kg/day in rabbits. Increased incidences of fetal variations were evident in litters from rats treated with the highest dose, in the absence of overt signs of maternal toxicity. The maternal plasma drug exposure (AUC) associated with this dose was approximately 34 times the estimated plasma exposure in humans receiving the maximum recommended daily dose (MRDD) of 1600 mg. Increased frequencies of abortions and late/total resorptions and decreased fetal weights were observed in the litters of rabbits treated with maternotoxic doses of 100 mg/kg/day (plasma AUCs 0.4 times those in humans receiving the MRDD) or greater. There was no evidence of teratogenicity in these studies.

However, when entacapone was administered to female rats prior to mating and during early gestation, an increased incidence of fetal eye anomalies (macrophthalmia, microphthalmia, anophthalmia) was observed in the litters of dams treated with doses of 160 mg/kg/day (plasma AUCs 7 times those in humans receiving the MRDD) or greater, in the absence of maternotoxicity. Administration of up to 700 mg/kg/day (plasma AUCs 28 times those in humans receiving the MRDD) to female rats during the latter part of gestation and throughout lactation, produced no evidence of developmental impairment in the offspring.

Entacapone is always given concomitantly with levodopa/carbidopa, which is known to cause visceral and skeletal malformations in rabbits. The teratogenic potential of entacapone in combination with levodopa/carbidopa was not assessed in animals.

There is no experience from clinical studies regarding the use of Comtan in pregnant women. Therefore, Comtan should be used during pregnancy only if the potential benefit justifies the potential risk to the fetus.

Nursing Women

In animal studies, entacapone was excreted into maternal rat milk.

It is not known whether entacapone is excreted in human milk. Because many drugs are excreted in human milk, caution should be exercised when entacapone is administered to a nursing woman.

Pediatric Use

There is no identified potential use of entacapone in pediatric patients.

ADVERSE REACTIONS

During the pre-marketing development of entacapone, 1450 patients with Parkinson's Disease were treated with entacapone. Included were patients with fluctuating symptoms, as well as those with stable responses to levodopa therapy. All patients received concomitant treatment with levodopa preparations, however, and were similar in other clinical aspects.

The most commonly observed adverse events (>5%) in the double-blind, placebo-controlled trials (N=1003) associated with the use of Comtan (entacapone) and not seen at an equivalent frequency among the placebo-treated patients were: dyskinesia/hyperkinesia, nausea, urine discoloration, diarrhea, and abdominal pain.

Approximately 14% of the 603 patients given entacapone in the double-blind, placebo-controlled trials discontinued treatment due to adverse events compared to 9% of the 400 patients who received placebo. The most frequent causes of discontinuation in decreasing order are: psychiatric reasons (2% vs. 1%), diarrhea (2% vs. 0%), dyskinesia/hyperkinesia (2% vs. 1%), nausea (2% vs. 1%), abdominal pain (1% vs. 0%), and aggravation of Parkinson's Disease symptoms (1% vs. 1%).

Adverse Event Incidence in Controlled Clinical Studies

Table 4 lists treatment emergent adverse events that occurred in at least 1% of patients treated with entacapone participating in the double-blind, placebo-controlled studies and that were numerically more common in the entacapone group, compared to placebo. In these studies, either entacapone or placebo was added to levodopa/carbidopa (or levodopa/benserazide).

[See table 4 below]

The prescriber should be aware that these figures cannot be used to predict the incidence of adverse events in the course of usual medical practice where patient characteristics and other factors differ from those that prevailed in the clinical studies. Similarly, the cited frequencies cannot be compared with figures obtained from other clinical investigations involving different treatments, uses, and investigators. The cited figures do, however, provide the prescriber with some basis for estimating the relative contribution of drug and nondrug factors to the adverse events observed in the population studied.

Effects of gender and age on adverse reactions

No differences were noted in the rate of adverse events attributable to entacapone by age or gender.

DRUG ABUSE AND DEPENDENCE

Comtan (entacapone) is not a controlled substance. Animal studies to evaluate the drug abuse and potential dependence have not been conducted. Although clinical trials have not revealed any evidence of the potential for abuse, tolerance or physical dependence, systematic studies in humans designed to evaluate these effects have not been performed.

OVERDOSAGE

There have been no reported cases of either accidental or intentional overdose with entacapone tablets. However, COMT inhibition by entacapone treatment is dose-dependent. A massive overdose of Comtan (entacapone) may theoretically produce a 100% inhibition of the COMT enzyme in people, thereby preventing the metabolism of endogenous and exogenous catechols.

The highest single dose of entacapone administered to humans was 800 mg, resulting in a plasma concentration of 14.1 µg/mL. The highest daily dose given to humans was 2400 mg, administered in one study as 400 mg six times daily with levodopa/carbidopa for 14 days in 15 Parkinson's Disease patients, and in another study as 800 mg t.i.d. for 7 days in 8 healthy volunteers. At this daily dose, the peak plasma concentrations of entacapone averaged 2.0 µg/mL (at 45 min., compared to 1.0 and 1.2 µg/mL with 200 mg entacapone at 45 min.). Abdominal pain and loose stools were the most commonly observed adverse events during this study. Daily doses as high as 2000 mg Comtan have been administered as 200 mg 10 times daily with levodopa/carbidopa or levodopa/benserazide for at least 1 year in 10 patients, for at least 2 years in 8 patients and for at least 3 years in 7 patients. Overall, however, clinical experience with daily doses above 1600 mg is limited.

The range of lethal plasma concentrations of entacapone based on animal data was 80-130 µg/mL in mice. Respiratory difficulties, ataxia, hypoactivity, and convulsions were observed in mice after high oral (gavage) doses.

Management of Overdose

Management of Comtan overdose is symptomatic; there is no known antidote to Comtan. Hospitalization is advised, and general supportive care is indicated. There is no experience with hemodialysis or hemoperfusion, but these procedures are unlikely to be of benefit, because Comtan is highly bound to plasma proteins. An immediate gastric lavage and repeated doses of charcoal over time may hasten the elimination of Comtan by decreasing its absorption/reabsorption from the GI tract. The adequacy of the respiratory and circulatory systems should be carefully monitored and appropriate supportive measures employed. The possibility of drug interactions, especially with catechol-structured drugs, should be borne in mind.

DOSAGE AND ADMINISTRATION

The recommended dose of Comtan (entacapone) is one 200 mg tablet administered concomitantly with each levodopa/carbidopa dose to a maximum of 8 times daily (200 mg × 8 = 1600 mg per day). Clinical experience with daily doses above 1600 mg is limited.

Comtan should always be administered in association with levodopa/carbidopa. Entacapone has no antiparkinsonian effect of its own.

In clinical trials, the majority of patients required a decrease in daily levodopa dose if their daily dose of levodopa had been ≥800 mg or if patients had moderate or severe dyskinesias before beginning treatment.

To optimize an individual patient's response, reductions in daily levodopa dose or extending the interval between doses may be necessary. In clinical trials, the average reduction in daily levodopa dose was about 25% in those patients requiring a levodopa dose reduction. (More than 58% of patients with levodopa doses above 800 mg daily required such a reduction.)

Comtan can be combined with both the immediate and sustained-release formulations of levodopa/carbidopa.

Comtan may be taken with or without food (see CLINICAL PHARMACOLOGY).

Patients With Impaired Hepatic Function: Patients with hepatic impairment should be treated with caution. The AUC and C_{max} of entacapone approximately doubled in patients with documented liver disease, compared to controls. However, these studies were conducted with single-dose entacapone without levodopa/dopa decarboxylase inhibitor coadministration, and therefore the effects of liver disease on the kinetics of chronically administered entacapone have not been evaluated (see CLINICAL PHARMACOLOGY, Pharmacokinetics of Entacapone).

Withdrawing Patients from Comtan: Rapid withdrawal or abrupt reduction in the Comtan dose could lead to emergence of signs and symptoms of Parkinson's Disease (see CLINICAL PHARMACOLOGY, Clinical Studies), and may lead to Hyperpyrexia and Confusion, a symptom complex resembling the neuroleptic malignant syndrome (see PRECAUTIONS, Other Events Reported With Dopaminergic Therapy). This syndrome should be considered in the differential diagnosis for any patient who develops a high fever or severe rigidity. If a decision is made to discontinue treatment with Comtan, patients should be monitored closely and other dopaminergic treatments should be adjusted as needed. Although tapering Comtan has not been systematically evaluated, it seems prudent to withdraw patients slowly if the decision to discontinue treatment is made.

HOW SUPPLIED

Comtan (entacapone) is supplied as 200-mg film-coated tablets for oral administration. The oval-shaped tablets are brownish-orange, unscored, and embossed "COMTAN" on one side. Tablets are provided in HDPE containers as follows:

Bottles of 100 .... NDC 0078-0327-05

Table 4
Summary of Patients with Adverse Events after Start of Trial Drug Administration
At least 1% in Comtan® (entacapone) group and > Placebo

SYSTEM ORGAN CLASS Preferred term	Comtan (n = 603) % of patients	Placebo (n = 400) % of patients
SKIN AND APPENDAGES DISORDERS		
Sweating increased	2	1
MUSCULOSKELETAL SYSTEM DISORDERS		
Back pain	2	1
CENTRAL & PERIPHERAL NERVOUS SYSTEM DISORDERS		
Dyskinesia	25	15
Hyperkinesia	10	5
Hypokinesia	9	8
Dizziness	8	6
SPECIAL SENSES, OTHER DISORDERS		
Taste perversion	1	0
PSYCHIATRIC DISORDERS		
Anxiety	2	1
Somnolence	2	0
Agitation	1	0
GASTROINTESTINAL SYSTEM DISORDERS		
Nausea	14	8
Diarrhea	10	4
Abdominal pain	8	4
Constipation	6	4
Vomiting	4	1
Mouth dry	3	0
Dyspepsia	2	1
Flatulence	2	0
Gastritis	1	0
Gastrointestinal disorders nos	1	0
RESPIRATORY SYSTEM DISORDERS		
Dyspnea	3	1
PLATELET, BLEEDING & CLOTTING DISORDERS		
Purpura	2	1
URINARY SYSTEM DISORDERS		
Urine discoloration	10	0
BODY AS A WHOLE – GENERAL DISORDERS		
Back pain	4	2
Fatigue	6	4
Asthenia	2	1
RESISTANCE MECHANISM DISORDERS		
Infection bacterial	1	0

Store at 25°C (77°F) excursions permitted to 15°-30°C (59°-86° F).
[See USP Controlled Room Temperature.]
Comtan (entacapone) tablets are manufactured by Orion Corporation, Orion Pharma (Espoo, Finland) and marketed by Novartis Pharmaceuticals Corporation (East Hanover, N.J. 07936, U.S.A.).
REV: MARCH 2000 T2000-10
89005303
Shown in Product Identification Guide, page 324

DESFERAL® ℞

[dĕs-fər-ăl]
(deferoxamine mesylate for injection USP)
Vials
Rx only

Prescribing Information
The following prescribing information is based on official labeling in effect July 2004.

DESCRIPTION

Desferal, deferoxamine mesylate USP, is an iron-chelating agent, available in vials for intramuscular, subcutaneous, and intravenous administration. Desferal is supplied as vials containing 500 mg and 2 g of deferoxamine mesylate USP in sterile, lyophilized form. Deferoxamine mesylate is *N*-[5-[3-[(5-aminopentyl)hydroxycarbamoyl]propionamido]pentyl]-3-[[5-(*N*-hydroxyacetamido)pentyl]carbamoyl]propionohydroxamic acid monomethanesulfonate (salt), and its structural formula is

$$H_2N(CH_2)_5N(OH)C(=O)(CH_2)_2C(=O)NH(CH_2)_5N(OH)C(=O)(CH_2)_2C(=O)NH(CH_2)_5N(OH)C(=O)CH_3 \cdot CH_3SO_3H$$

Deferoxamine mesylate USP is a white to off-white powder. It is freely soluble in water and slightly soluble in methanol. Its molecular weight is 656.79.

CLINICAL PHARMACOLOGY

Desferal chelates iron by forming a stable complex that prevents the iron from entering into further chemical reactions. It readily chelates iron from ferritin and hemosiderin but not readily from transferrin; it does not combine with the iron from cytochromes and hemoglobin. Desferal does not cause any demonstrable increase in the excretion of electrolytes or trace metals. Theoretically, 100 parts by weight of Desferal is capable of binding approximately 8.5 parts by weight of ferric iron.
Desferal is metabolized principally by plasma enzymes, but the pathways have not yet been defined. The chelate is readily soluble in water and passes easily through the kidney, giving the urine a characteristic reddish color. Some is also excreted in the feces via the bile.

INDICATIONS AND USAGE

Desferal is indicated for the treatment of acute iron intoxication and of chronic iron overload due to transfusion-dependent anemias.

Acute Iron Intoxication
Desferal is an adjunct to, and not a substitute for, standard measures used in treating acute iron intoxication, which may include the following: induction of emesis with syrup of ipecac; gastric lavage; suction and maintenance of a clear airway; control of shock with intravenous fluids, blood, oxygen, and vasopressors; and correction of acidosis.

Chronic Iron Overload
Desferal can promote iron excretion in patients with secondary iron overload from multiple transfusions (as may occur in the treatment of some chronic anemias, including thalassemia). Long-term therapy with Desferal slows accumulation of hepatic iron and retards or eliminates progression of hepatic fibrosis.
Iron mobilization with Desferal is relatively poor in patients under the age of 3 years with relatively little iron overload. The drug should ordinarily not be given to such patients unless significant iron mobilization (e.g., 1 mg or more of iron per day) can be demonstrated.
Desferal is not indicated for the treatment of primary hemochromatosis, since phlebotomy is the method of choice for removing excess iron in this disorder.

CONTRAINDICATIONS

Desferal is contraindicated in patients with severe renal disease or anuria, since the drug and the iron chelate are excreted primarily by the kidney. *(See WARNINGS).*

WARNINGS

Ocular and auditory disturbances have been reported when Desferal was administered over prolonged periods of time, at high doses, or in patients with low ferritin levels. The ocular disturbances observed have been blurring of vision; cataracts after prolonged administration in chronic iron overload; decreased visual acuity including visual loss, visual defects, scotoma; impaired peripheral, color, and night vision; optic neuritis, cataracts, corneal opacities, and retinal pigmentary abnormalities. The auditory abnormalities reported have been tinnitus and hearing loss including high frequency sensorineural hearing loss. In most cases, both ocular and auditory disturbances were reversible upon immediate cessation of treatment *(see PRECAUTIONS/Information for Patients and ADVERSE REACTIONS/Special Senses).*
Visual acuity tests, slit-lamp examinations, funduscopy and audiometry are recommended periodically in patients treated for prolonged periods of time. Toxicity is more likely to be reversed if symptoms or test abnormalities are detected early.
High doses of Desferal and concomitant low ferritin levels have also been associated with growth retardation. After reduction of Desferal dose, growth velocity may partially resume to pretreatment rates *(see PRECAUTIONS/Pediatric Use).*
Adult respiratory distress syndrome, also reported in children, has been described following treatment with excessively high intravenous doses of Desferal in patients with acute iron intoxication or thalassemia.

PRECAUTIONS

General
Flushing of the skin, urticaria, hypotension, and shock have occurred in a few patients when Desferal was administered by rapid intravenous injection. THEREFORE, DESFERAL SHOULD BE GIVEN INTRAMUSCULARLY OR BY SLOW SUBCUTANEOUS OR INTRAVENOUS INFUSION.
Iron overload increases susceptibility of patients to *Yersinia enterocolitica* and *Yersinia pseudotuberculosis* infections. In some rare cases, treatment with Desferal has enhanced this susceptibility, resulting in generalized infections by providing this bacteria with a siderophore otherwise missing. In such cases, Desferal treatment should be discontinued until the infection is resolved.
In patients receiving Desferal, rare cases of mucormycosis, some with a fatal outcome, have been reported. If any of the suspected signs or symptoms occur, Desferal should be discontinued, mycological tests carried out and appropriate treatment instituted immediately.
In patients with severe chronic iron overload, impairment of cardiac function has been reported following concomitant treatment with Desferal and high doses of vitamin C (more than 500 mg daily in adults). The cardiac dysfunction was reversible when vitamin C was discontinued. The following precautions should be taken when vitamin C and Desferal are to be used concomitantly:

- Vitamin C supplements should not be given to patients with cardiac failure.
- Start supplemental vitamin C only after an initial month of regular treatment with Desferal.
- Give vitamin C only if the patient is receiving Desferal regularly, ideally soon after setting up the infusion pump.
- Do not exceed a daily vitamin C dose of 200 mg in adults, given in divided doses.
- Clinical monitoring of cardiac function is advisable during such combined therapy.

In patients with aluminum-related encephalopathy, high doses of Desferal may exacerbate neurological dysfunction (seizures), probably owing to an acute increase in circulating aluminum. Desferal may precipitate the onset of dialysis dementia. Treatment with Desferal in the presence of aluminum overload may result in decreased serum calcium and aggravation of hyperparathyroidism.

Drug Interactions
Vitamin C: Patients with iron overload usually become vitamin C deficient, probably because iron oxidizes the vitamin. As an adjuvant to iron chelation therapy, vitamin C in doses up to 200 mg for adults may be given in divided doses, starting after an initial month of regular treatment with Desferal *(see PRECAUTIONS).* Vitamin C increases availability of iron for chelation. In general, 50 mg daily suffices for children under 10 years old and 100 mg daily for older children. Larger doses of vitamin C fail to produce any additional increase in excretion of iron complex.
Prochlorperazine: Concurrent treatment with Desferal and prochlorperazine, a phenothiazine derivative, may lead to temporary impairment of consciousness.
Gallium-67: Imaging results may be distorted because of the rapid urinary excretion of Desferal-bound gallium-67. Discontinuation of Desferal 48 hours prior to scintigraphy is advisable.

Information for Patients
Patients experiencing dizziness or other nervous system disturbances, or impairment of vision or hearing, should refrain from driving or operating potentially hazardous machines *(see ADVERSE REACTIONS).*
Patients should be informed that occasionally their urine may show a reddish discoloration.

Carcinogenesis, Mutagenesis, Impairment of Fertility
Long-term carcinogenicity studies in animals have not been performed with Desferal.
Cytotoxicity may occur, since Desferal has been shown to inhibit DNA synthesis *in vitro.*

Pregnancy Category C
Delayed ossification in mice and skeletal anomalies in rabbits were observed after Desferal was administered in daily doses up to 4.5 times the maximum daily human dose. No adverse effects were observed in similar studies in rats.
There are no adequate and well-controlled studies in pregnant women. Desferal should be used during pregnancy only if the potential benefit justifies the potential risk to the fetus.

Nursing Mothers
It is not known whether this drug is excreted in human milk. Because many drugs are excreted in human milk, caution should be exercised when Desferal is administered to a nursing woman.

Pediatric Use
Pediatric patients receiving Desferal should be monitored for body weight and growth every 3 months.
Safety and effectiveness in pediatric patients under the age of 3 years have not been established *(see INDICATIONS AND USAGE, WARNINGS, PRECAUTIONS/Drug Interactions/Vitamin C, and ADVERSE REACTIONS).*

ADVERSE REACTIONS

The following adverse reactions have been observed, but there are not enough data to support an estimate of their frequency.
At the Injection Site: localized irritation, pain, burning, swelling, induration, infiltration, pruritus, erythema, wheal formation, eschar, crust, vesicles, local edema. Injection site reactions may be associated with systemic allergic reactions *(see Body as a Whole, below).*
Hypersensitivity Reactions and Systemic Allergic Reactions: generalized rash, urticaria, anaphylactic reaction with or without shock, angioedema.
Body as a Whole: Local injection site reactions may be accompanied by systemic reactions like arthralgia, fever, headache, myalgia, nausea, vomiting, abdominal pain, or asthma.
Rare infections with *Yersinia* and *Mucormycosis* have been reported in association with Desferal use *(see PRECAUTIONS).*
Cardiovascular: hypotension, shock.
Digestive: abdominal discomfort, diarrhea, nausea, vomiting.
Hematologic: blood dyscrasia (e.g., cases of thrombocytopenia and/or leukopenia have been reported. A causal relationship has not been clearly established).
Musculoskeletal: Leg cramps. Growth retardation and bone changes (e.g., metaphyseal dysplasia) are common in chelated patients given doses above 60 mg/kg, especially those who begin iron chelation in the first three years of life. If doses are kept to 40 mg/kg or below, the risk may be reduced *(see WARNINGS, PRECAUTIONS/Pediatric Use).*
Nervous system: neurological disturbances including dizziness, peripheral sensory, motor, or mixed neuropathy, paresthesias; exacerbation or precipitation of aluminum-related dialysis encephalopathy *(see PRECAUTIONS/Information for Patients).*
Special Senses: High-frequency sensorineural hearing loss and/or tinnitus are uncommon if dosage guidelines are not exceeded and if dose is reduced when ferritin levels decline. Visual disturbances are rare if dosage guidelines are not exceeded. These may include decreased acuity, blurred vision, loss of vision, dyschromatopsia, night blindness, visual field defects, scotoma, retinopathy (pigmentary degeneration), optic neuritis, and cataracts *(see WARNINGS).*
Respiratory: acute respiratory distress syndrome (with dyspnea, cyanosis, and/or interstitial infiltrates) *(see WARNINGS).*
Skin: very rare generalized rash.
Urogenital: dysuria, impaired renal function *(see CONTRAINDICATIONS).*

OVERDOSAGE

Acute Toxicity
Intravenous LD_{50}s (mg/kg): mice, 287; rats, 329.

Signs and Symptoms
Inadvertent administration of an overdose or inadvertent intravenous bolus administration/rapid intravenous infusion may be associated with hypotension, tachycardia and gastrointestinal disturbances; acute but transient loss of vision, aphasia, agitation, headache, nausea, pallor, CNS depression including coma, bradycardia and acute renal failure have been reported.

Treatment
There is no specific antidote. Desferal should be discontinued and appropriate symptomatic measures undertaken. Desferal is readily dialyzable.

DOSAGE AND ADMINISTRATION

Preparation of Solution
Desferal is preferably dissolved by adding 5 mL of Sterile Water for Injection to each 500 mg vial or 20 mL of Sterile Water for Injection to each 2 g vial. The reconstituted Desferal solution is isotonic, clear and colorless to slightly yellowish at the recommended concentration of 10%.
In clinical situations requiring a smaller volume of solution (e.g., intramuscular injection), Desferal may be dissolved by adding 2 mL of Sterile Water for Injection to each 500 mg vial or 8 mL of Sterile Water for Injection to each 2 g vial. This concentration may produce a stronger yellow-colored solution. The drug should be completely dissolved before the solution is withdrawn.
Preparation of the above reconstituted solutions results in a final volume that is greater than the specified volume of Sterile Water added.
Note: **Parenteral drug products should be inspected visually for particulate matter and discoloration prior to administration, whenever solution and container permit.**
Desferal reconstituted with Sterile Water for Injection **IS FOR SINGLE USE ONLY.**
The product should be used immediately after reconstitution (commencement of treatment within 3 hours) for microbiological safety. When reconstitution is carried out under validated aseptic conditions (in a sterile laminar flow hood using aseptic technique), the product may be stored at room temperature for a maximum period of 24 hours before use.

Continued on next page

Desferal—Cont.

Do not refrigerate reconstituted solution. Reconstituting Desferal in solvents or under conditions other than indicated may result in precipitation. Turbid solutions should not be used.

Acute Iron Intoxication

Intramuscular Administration

This route is preferred and should be used for ALL PATIENTS NOT IN SHOCK.

Dosage. See Preparation of Solution above. A dose of 1000 mg should be administered initially. This may be followed by 500 mg every 4 hours for two doses. Depending upon the clinical response, subsequent doses of 500 mg may be administered every 4-12 hours. The total amount administered should not exceed 6000 mg in 24 hours.

Intravenous Administration

THIS ROUTE SHOULD BE USED ONLY FOR PATIENTS IN A STATE OF CARDIOVASCULAR COLLAPSE AND THEN ONLY BY SLOW INFUSION. THE RATE OF INFUSION SHOULD NOT EXCEED 15 MG/KG/HR FOR THE FIRST 1000 MG ADMINISTERED. SUBSEQUENT IV DOSING, IF NEEDED, MUST BE AT A SLOWER RATE, NOT TO EXCEED 125 MG/HR.

Dosage. See Preparation of Solution, above.

The reconstituted solution is added to physiologic saline, glucose in water, or Ringer's lactate solution.

An initial dose of 1000 mg should be administered at a rate NOT TO EXCEED 15 mg/kg/hr. This may be followed by 500 mg over 4 hours for two doses. Depending upon the clinical response, subsequent doses of 500 mg may be administered over 4-12 hours. The total amount administered should not exceed 6000 mg in 24 hours.

As soon as the clinical condition of the patient permits, intravenous administration should be discontinued and the drug should be administered intramuscularly.

Chronic Iron Overload

The more effective of the following routes of administration must be chosen on an individual basis for each patient.

Intramuscular Administration

See Preparation of Solution above. A daily dose of 500-1000 mg should be administered intramuscularly. In addition, 2000 mg should be administered intravenously with each unit of blood transfused; however, Desferal should be administered separately from the blood. The rate of intravenous infusion must not exceed 15 mg/kg/hr. The total daily dose should not exceed 1000 mg in the absence of a transfusion, or 6000 mg even if transfused three or more units of blood or packed red blood cells.

Subcutaneous Administration

See Preparation of Solution above. A daily dose of 1000-2000 mg (20-40 mg/kg/day) should be administered over 8-24 hours, utilizing a small portable pump capable of providing continuous mini-infusion. The duration of infusion must be individualized. In some patients, as much iron will be excreted after a short infusion of 8-12 hours as with the same dose given over 24 hours.

HOW SUPPLIED

Vials—each containing 500 mg of sterile, lyophilized deferoxamine mesylate

Cartons of 4 vials .... NDC 0083-3801-04

Vials—each containing 2 g of sterile, lyophilized deferoxamine mesylate

Cartons of 4 vials .... NDC 0078-0347-51

Do not store above 25°C (77°F).

T2002-75

REV: OCTOBER 2002 Printed in U.S.A. 89003406

Manufactured by:
Novartis Pharma Stein AG
Schaffhauserstrasse
CH-4332 Stein, Switzerland

Distributed by:
Novartis Pharmaceuticals Corporation
East Hanover, New Jersey 07936
©Novartis

DIOVAN® ℞

[dī-ō-văn]
(valsartan)
Tablets
Rx only

Prescribing Information

The following prescribing information is based on official labeling in effect July 2004.

USE IN PREGNANCY
When used in pregnancy during the second and third trimesters, drugs that act directly on the renin-angiotensin system can cause injury and even death to the developing fetus. When pregnancy is detected, Diovan should be discontinued as soon as possible.
See ***WARNINGS: Fetal/Neonatal Morbidity and Mortality.***

DESCRIPTION

Diovan® (valsartan) is a nonpeptide, orally active, and specific angiotensin II antagonist acting on the AT_1 receptor subtype.

Valsartan is chemically described as *N*-(1-oxopentyl)-*N*-[[2'-(1*H*-tetrazol-5-yl) [1,1'-biphenyl]-4-yl]methyl]-L-valine. Its empirical formula is $C_{24}H_{29}N_5O_3$, its molecular weight is 435.5, and its structural formula is

Valsartan is a white to practically white fine powder. It is soluble in ethanol and methanol and slightly soluble in water.

Diovan is available as tablets for oral administration, containing 40 mg, 80 mg, 160 mg or 320 mg of valsartan. The inactive ingredients of the tablets are colloidal silicon dioxide, crospovidone, hydroxypropyl methylcellulose, iron oxides (yellow, black and/or red), magnesium stearate, microcrystalline cellulose, polyethylene glycol 8000, and titanium dioxide.

CLINICAL PHARMACOLOGY

Mechanism of Action

Angiotensin II is formed from angiotensin I in a reaction catalyzed by angiotensin-converting enzyme (ACE, kininase II). Angiotensin II is the principal pressor agent of the renin-angiotensin system, with effects that include vasoconstriction, stimulation of synthesis and release of aldosterone, cardiac stimulation, and renal reabsorption of sodium. Valsartan blocks the vasoconstrictor and aldosterone-secreting effects of angiotensin II by selectively blocking the binding of angiotensin II to the AT_1 receptor in many tissues, such as vascular smooth muscle and the adrenal gland. Its action is therefore independent of the pathways for angiotensin II synthesis.

There is also an AT_2 receptor found in many tissues, but AT_2 is not known to be associated with cardiovascular homeostasis. Valsartan has much greater affinity (about 20,000-fold) for the AT_1 receptor than for the AT_2 receptor. The increased plasma levels of angiotensin II following AT_1 receptor blockade with valsartan may stimulate the unblocked AT_2 receptor. The primary metabolite of valsartan is essentially inactive with an affinity for the AT_1 receptor about one 200th that of valsartan itself.

Blockade of the renin-angiotensin system with ACE inhibitors, which inhibit the biosynthesis of angiotensin II from angiotensin I, is widely used in the treatment of hypertension. ACE inhibitors also inhibit the degradation of bradykinin, a reaction also catalyzed by ACE. Because valsartan does not inhibit ACE (kininase II), it does not affect the response to bradykinin. Whether this difference has clinical relevance is not yet known. Valsartan does not bind to or block other hormone receptors or ion channels known to be important in cardiovascular regulation.

Blockade of the angiotensin II receptor inhibits the negative regulatory feedback of angiotensin II on renin secretion, but the resulting increased plasma renin activity and angiotensin II circulating levels do not overcome the effect of valsartan on blood pressure.

Pharmacokinetics

Valsartan peak plasma concentration is reached 2 to 4 hours after dosing. Valsartan shows bi-exponential decay kinetics following intravenous administration, with an average elimination half-life of about 6 hours. Absolute bioavailability for Diovan is about 25% (range 10%-35%). Food decreases the exposure (as measured by AUC) to valsartan by about 40% and peak plasma concentration (C_{max}) by about 50%. AUC and C_{max} values of valsartan increase approximately linearly with increasing dose over the clinical dosing range. Valsartan does not accumulate appreciably in plasma following repeated administration.

Metabolism and Elimination

Valsartan, when administered as an oral solution, is primarily recovered in feces (about 83% of dose) and urine (about 13% of dose). The recovery is mainly as unchanged drug, with only about 20% of dose recovered as metabolites. The primary metabolite, accounting for about 9% of dose, is valeryl 4-hydroxy valsartan. The enzyme(s) responsible for valsartan metabolism have not been identified but do not seem to be CYP 450 isozymes.

Following intravenous administration, plasma clearance of valsartan is about 2 L/h and its renal clearance is 0.62 L/h (about 30% of total clearance).

Distribution

The steady state volume of distribution of valsartan after intravenous administration is small (17 L), indicating that valsartan does not distribute into tissues extensively. Valsartan is highly bound to serum proteins (95%), mainly serum albumin.

Special Populations

Pediatric: The pharmacokinetics of valsartan have not been investigated in patients < 18 years of age.

Geriatric: Exposure (measured by AUC) to valsartan is higher by 70% and the half-life is longer by 35% in the elderly than in the young. No dosage adjustment is necessary (*see DOSAGE AND ADMINISTRATION*).

Gender: Pharmacokinetics of valsartan does not differ significantly between males and females.

Heart Failure: The average time to peak concentration and elimination half-life of valsartan in heart failure patients are similar to that observed in healthy volunteers. AUC and C_{max} values of valsartan increase linearly and are almost proportional with increasing dose over the clinical dosing range (40 to 160 mg twice a day). The average accumulation factor is about 1.7. The apparent clearance of valsartan following oral administration is approximately 4.5 L/h. Age does not affect the apparent clearance in heart failure patients.

Renal Insufficiency: There is no apparent correlation between renal function (measured by creatinine clearance) and exposure (measured by AUC) to valsartan in patients with different degrees of renal impairment. Consequently, dose adjustment is not required in patients with mild-to-moderate renal dysfunction. No studies have been performed in patients with severe impairment of renal function (creatinine clearance < 10 mL/min). Valsartan is not removed from the plasma by hemodialysis. In the case of severe renal disease, exercise care with dosing of valsartan (*see DOSAGE AND ADMINISTRATION*).

Hepatic Insufficiency: On average, patients with mild-to-moderate chronic liver disease have twice the exposure (measured by AUC values) to valsartan of healthy volunteers (matched by age, sex and weight). In general, no dosage adjustment is needed in patients with mild-to-moderate liver disease. Care should be exercised in patients with liver disease (*see DOSAGE AND ADMINISTRATION*).

Pharmacodynamics and Clinical Effects

Hypertension

Valsartan inhibits the pressor effect of angiotensin II infusions. An oral dose of 80 mg inhibits the pressor effect by about 80% at peak with approximately 30% inhibition persisting for 24 hours. No information on the effect of larger doses is available.

Removal of the negative feedback of angiotensin II causes a 2- to 3-fold rise in plasma renin and consequent rise in angiotensin II plasma concentration in hypertensive patients. Minimal decreases in plasma aldosterone were observed after administration of valsartan; very little effect on serum potassium was observed.

In multiple-dose studies in hypertensive patients with stable renal insufficiency and patients with renovascular hypertension, valsartan had no clinically significant effects on glomerular filtration rate, filtration fraction, creatinine clearance, or renal plasma flow.

In multiple-dose studies in hypertensive patients, valsartan had no notable effects on total cholesterol, fasting triglycerides, fasting serum glucose, or uric acid.

The antihypertensive effects of Diovan were demonstrated principally in 7 placebo-controlled, 4- to 12-week trials (one in patients over 65) of dosages from 10 to 320 mg/day in patients with baseline diastolic blood pressures of 95-115. The studies allowed comparison of once-daily and twice-daily regimens of 160 mg/day; comparison of peak and trough effects; comparison (in pooled data) of response by gender, age, and race; and evaluation of incremental effects of hydrochlorothiazide.

Administration of valsartan to patients with essential hypertension results in a significant reduction of sitting, supine, and standing systolic and diastolic blood pressure, usually with little or no orthostatic change.

In most patients, after administration of a single oral dose, onset of antihypertensive activity occurs at approximately 2 hours, and maximum reduction of blood pressure is achieved within 6 hours. The antihypertensive effect persists for 24 hours after dosing, but there is a decrease from peak effect at lower doses (40 mg) presumably reflecting loss of inhibition of angiotensin II. At higher doses, however (160 mg), there is little difference in peak and trough effect. During repeated dosing, the reduction in blood pressure with any dose is substantially present within 2 weeks, and maximal reduction is generally attained after 4 weeks. In long-term follow-up studies (without placebo control), the effect of valsartan appeared to be maintained for up to two years. The antihypertensive effect is independent of age, gender or race. The latter finding regarding race is based on pooled data and should be viewed with caution, because antihypertensive drugs that affect the renin-angiotensin system (that is, ACE inhibitors and angiotensin-II blockers) have generally been found to be less effective in low-renin hypertensives (frequently blacks) than in high-renin hypertensives (frequently whites). In pooled, randomized, controlled trials of Diovan that included a total of 140 blacks and 830 whites, valsartan and an ACE-inhibitor control were generally at least as effective in blacks as whites. The explanation for this difference from previous findings is unclear.

Abrupt withdrawal of valsartan has not been associated with a rapid increase in blood pressure.

The blood pressure lowering effect of valsartan and thiazide-type diuretics are approximately additive.

The 7 studies of valsartan monotherapy included over 2,000 patients randomized to various doses of valsartan and about 800 patients randomized to placebo. Doses below 80 mg were not consistently distinguished from those of placebo at trough, but doses of 80, 160 and 320 mg produced dose-related decreases in systolic and diastolic blood pressure, with the difference from placebo of approximately 6-9/3-5 mmHg at 80-160 mg and 9/6 mmHg at 320 mg. In a

controlled trial the addition of HCTZ to valsartan 80 mg resulted in additional lowering of systolic and diastolic blood pressure by approximately 6/3 and 12/5 mmHg for 12.5 and 25 mg of HCTZ, respectively, compared to valsartan 80 mg alone.
Patients with an inadequate response to 80 mg once daily were titrated to either 160 mg once daily or 80 mg twice daily, which resulted in a comparable response in both groups.
In controlled trials, the antihypertensive effect of once-daily valsartan 80 mg was similar to that of once-daily enalapril 20 mg or once-daily lisinopril 10 mg.
There was essentially no change in heart rate in valsartan-treated patients in controlled trials.

Heart Failure

The Valsartan Heart Failure Trial (Val-HeFT) was a multinational, double-blind study in which 5,010 patients with NYHA class II (62%) to IV (2%) heart failure and LVEF < 40%, on baseline therapy chosen by their physicians, were randomized to placebo or valsartan (titrated from 40 mg twice daily to the highest tolerated dose or 160 mg twice daily) and followed for a mean of about 2 years. Although Val-HeFT's primary goal was to examine the effect of valsartan when added to an ACE inhibitor, about 7% were not receiving an ACE inhibitor. Other background therapy included diuretics (86%), digoxin (67%), and beta-blockers (36%). The population studied was 80% male, 46% 65 years or older and 89% Caucasian. At the end of the trial, patients in the valsartan group had a blood pressure that was 4 mmHg systolic and 2 mmHg diastolic lower than the placebo group. There were two primary end points, both assessed as time to first event: all-cause mortality and heart failure morbidity, the latter defined as all-cause mortality, sudden death with resuscitation, hospitalization for heart failure, and the need for intravenous inotropic or vasodilatory drugs for at least 4 hours. These results are summarized in the table below.
[See first table above]
Although the overall morbidity result favored valsartan, this result was largely driven by the 7% of patients not receiving an ACE inhibitor, as shown in the following table.
[See second table above]
The modest favorable trend in the group receiving an ACE inhibitor was largely driven by the patients receiving less than the recommended dose of ACE inhibitor. Thus, there is little evidence of further clinical benefit when valsartan is added to an adequate dose of ACE inhibitor.
Secondary end points in the subgroup not receiving ACE inhibitors were as follows.
[See third table above]
In patients not receiving an ACE inhibitor, valsartan-treated patients had an increase in ejection fraction and reduction in left ventricular internal diastolic diameter (LVIDD).
Concomitant use of an ACE inhibitor, a beta-blocker, and valsartan was associated with a worse outcome for heart failure morbidity, as shown in the following table.
[See fourth table above]
It is not known if this is a reproducible effect or a chance occurrence. The use of a beta-blocker did not appear to influence the effect of valsartan in patients not receiving an ACE inhibitor.
Effects were generally consistent across subgroups defined by age and gender for the population of patients not receiving an ACE inhibitor. The number of black patients was small and does not permit a meaningful assessment in this subset of patients.

	Placebo (N=2,499)	Valsartan (N=2,511)	Hazard Ratio (95% CI*)	Nominal p-value
All-cause mortality	484 (19.4%)	495 (19.7%)	1.02 (0.90-1.15)	0.80
HF morbidity	801 (32.1%)	723 (28.8%)	0.87 (0.79-0.97)	0.009

* CI = Confidence Interval

	Without ACE Inhibitor		With ACE Inhibitor	
	Placebo (N=181)	Valsartan (N=185)	Placebo (N=2,318)	Valsartan (N=2,326)
Events (%)	77 (42.5%)	46 (24.9%)	724 (31.2%)	677 (29.1%)
Hazard ratio (95% CI)	0.51 (0.35, 0.73)		0.92 (0.82, 1.02)	
p-value	0.0002		0.0965	

	Placebo (N=181)	Valsartan (N=185)	Hazard ratio (95% CI)
Components of HF morbidity			
All-cause mortality	49 (27.1%)	32 (17.3%)	0.59 (0.37, 0.91)
Sudden death with resuscitation	2 (1.1%)	1 (0.5%)	0.47 (0.04, 5.20)
CHF therapy	1 (0.6%)	0 (0.0%)	–
CHF hospitalization	48 (26.5%)	24 (13.0%)	0.43 (0.27, 0.71)
Cardiovascular mortality	40 (22.1%)	29 (15.7%)	0.65 (0.40, 1.05)
Non-fatal morbidity	49 (27.1%)	24 (13.0%)	0.42 (0.26, 0.69)

	Placebo (N=816)	Valsartan (N=794)	Hazard ratio (95% CI)
Heart failure morbidity	179 (21.9%)	202 (25.4%)	1.18 (0.97, 1.45)
All-cause mortality	97 (11.9%)	129 (16.2%)	1.42 (1.09, 1.85)

INDICATIONS AND USAGE

Hypertension

Diovan® (valsartan) is indicated for the treatment of hypertension. It may be used alone or in combination with other antihypertensive agents.

Heart Failure

Diovan is indicated for the treatment of heart failure (NYHA class II-IV) in patients who are intolerant of angiotensin converting enzyme inhibitors. In a controlled clinical trial, Diovan significantly reduced hospitalizations for heart failure. There is no evidence that Diovan provides added benefits when it is used with an adequate dose of an ACE inhibitor. *(See CLINICAL PHARMACOLOGY, Pharmacodynamics and Clinical Effects, Heart Failure for details.)*

CONTRAINDICATIONS

Diovan® (valsartan) is contraindicated in patients who are hypersensitive to any component of this product.

WARNINGS

Fetal/Neonatal Morbidity and Mortality

Drugs that act directly on the renin-angiotensin system can cause fetal and neonatal morbidity and death when administered to pregnant women. Several dozen cases have been reported in the world literature in patients who were taking angiotensin-converting enzyme inhibitors. When pregnancy is detected, Diovan® (valsartan) should be discontinued as soon as possible.
The use of drugs that act directly on the renin-angiotensin system during the second and third trimesters of pregnancy has been associated with fetal and neonatal injury, including hypotension, neonatal skull hypoplasia, anuria, reversible or irreversible renal failure, and death. Oligohydramnios has also been reported, presumably resulting from decreased fetal renal function; oligohydramnios in this setting has been associated with fetal limb contractures, craniofacial deformation, and hypoplastic lung development. Prematurity, intrauterine growth retardation, and patent ductus arteriosus have also been reported, although it is not clear whether these occurrences were due to exposure to the drug.
These adverse effects do not appear to have resulted from intrauterine drug exposure that has been limited to the first trimester. Mothers whose embryos and fetuses are exposed to an angiotensin II receptor antagonist only during the first trimester should be so informed. Nonetheless, when patients become pregnant, physicians should advise the patient to discontinue the use of valsartan as soon as possible.
Rarely (probably less often than once in every thousand pregnancies), no alternative to a drug acting on the renin-angiotensin system will be found. In these rare cases, the mothers should be apprised of the potential hazards to their fetuses, and serial ultrasound examinations should be performed to assess the intra-amniotic environment.
If oligohydramnios is observed, valsartan should be discontinued unless it is considered life-saving for the mother. Contraction stress testing (CST), a nonstress test (NST), or biophysical profiling (BPP) may be appropriate, depending upon the week of pregnancy. Patients and physicians should be aware, however, that oligohydramnios may not appear until after the fetus has sustained irreversible injury.
Infants with histories of *in utero* exposure to an angiotensin II receptor antagonist should be closely observed for hypotension, oliguria, and hyperkalemia. If oliguria occurs, attention should be directed toward support of blood pressure and renal perfusion. Exchange transfusion or dialysis may be required as means of reversing hypotension and/or substituting for disordered renal function.
No teratogenic effects were observed when valsartan was administered to pregnant mice and rats at oral doses up to 600 mg/kg/day and to pregnant rabbits at oral doses up to 10 mg/kg/day. However, significant decreases in fetal weight, pup birth weight, pup survival rate, and slight delays in developmental milestones were observed in studies in which parental rats were treated with valsartan at oral, maternally toxic (reduction in body weight gain and food consumption) doses of 600 mg/kg/day during organogenesis or late gestation and lactation. In rabbits, fetotoxicity (i.e., resorptions, litter loss, abortions, and low body weight) associated with maternal toxicity (mortality) was observed at doses of 5 and 10 mg/kg/day. The no observed adverse effect doses of 600, 200 and 2 mg/kg/day in mice, rats and rabbits represent 9, 6, and 0.1 times, respectively, the maximum recommended human dose on a mg/m^2 basis. (Calculations assume an oral dose of 320 mg/day and a 60-kg patient.)

Hypotension

Excessive hypotension was rarely seen (0.1%) in patients with uncomplicated hypertension treated with Diovan alone. In patients with an activated renin-angiotensin system, such as volume- and/or salt-depleted patients receiving high doses of diuretics, symptomatic hypotension may occur. This condition should be corrected prior to administration of Diovan, or the treatment should start under close medical supervision.
If excessive hypotension occurs, the patient should be placed in the supine position and, if necessary, given an intravenous infusion of normal saline. A transient hypotensive response is not a contraindication to further treatment, which usually can be continued without difficulty once the blood pressure has stabilized.

Hypotension in Heart Failure Patients

Caution should be observed when initiating therapy in patients with heart failure. Patients with heart failure given Diovan commonly have some reduction in blood pressure, but discontinuation of therapy because of continuing symptomatic hypotension usually is not necessary when dosing instructions are followed. In controlled trials, the incidence of hypotension in valsartan-treated patients was 5.5% compared to 1.8% in placebo-treated patients.

PRECAUTIONS

General

Impaired Hepatic Function: As the majority of valsartan is eliminated in the bile, patients with mild-to-moderate hepatic impairment, including patients with biliary obstructive disorders, showed lower valsartan clearance (higher AUCs). Care should be exercised in administering Diovan® (valsartan) to these patients.

Impaired Renal Function—Hypertension: In studies of ACE inhibitors in hypertensive patients with unilateral or bilateral renal artery stenosis, increases in serum creatinine or blood urea nitrogen have been reported. In a 4-day trial of valsartan in 12 hypertensive patients with unilateral renal artery stenosis, no significant increases in serum creatinine or blood urea nitrogen were observed. There has been no long-term use of Diovan in patients with unilateral or bilateral renal artery stenosis, but an effect similar to that seen with ACE inhibitors should be anticipated.

Impaired Renal Function—Heart Failure: As a consequence of inhibiting the renin-angiotensin-aldosterone system, changes in renal function may be anticipated in susceptible individuals. In patients with severe heart failure whose renal function may depend on the activity of the renin-angiotensin-aldosterone system, treatment with angiotensin-converting enzyme inhibitors and angiotensin receptor antagonists has been associated with oliguria and/or progressive azotemia and (rarely) with acute renal failure and/or death. Similar outcomes have been reported with Diovan.
Some patients with heart failure have developed increases in blood urea nitrogen, serum creatinine, and potassium. These effects are usually minor and transient, and they are more likely to occur in patients with pre-existing renal impairment. Dosage reduction and/or discontinuation of the diuretic and/or Diovan may be required. In the Valsartan Heart Failure Trial, in which 93% of patients were on concomitant ACE inhibitors, treatment was discontinued for elevations in creatinine or potassium (total of 1.0% on valsartan vs. 0.2% on placebo). Evaluation of patients with heart failure should always include assessment of renal function.

Concomitant Therapy in Patients with Heart Failure: In patients with heart failure, concomitant use of Diovan, an ACE inhibitor, and a beta blocker is not recommended. In the Valsartan Heart Failure Trial, this triple combination was associated with an unfavorable heart failure outcome *(see CLINICAL PHARMACOLOGY, Pharmacodynamics and Clinical Effects, Heart Failure).*

Information for Patients

Pregnancy: Female patients of childbearing age should be told about the consequences of second- and third-trimester exposure to drugs that act on the renin-angiotensin system,

Continued on next page

Diovan—Cont.

and they should also be told that these consequences do not appear to have resulted from intrauterine drug exposure that has been limited to the first trimester. These patients should be asked to report pregnancies to their physicians as soon as possible.

Drug Interactions

No clinically significant pharmacokinetic interactions were observed when valsartan was coadministered with amlodipine, atenolol, cimetidine, digoxin, furosemide, glyburide, hydrochlorothiazide, or indomethacin. The valsartan-atenolol combination was more antihypertensive than either component, but it did not lower the heart rate more than atenolol alone.

Coadministration of valsartan and warfarin did not change the pharmacokinetics of valsartan or the time-course of the anticoagulant properties of warfarin.

CYP 450 Interactions: The enzyme(s) responsible for valsartan metabolism have not been identified but do not seem to be CYP 450 isozymes. The inhibitory or induction potential of valsartan on CYP 450 is also unknown.

As with other drugs that block angiotensin II or its effects, concomitant use of potassium sparing diuretics (e.g., spironolactone, triamterene, amiloride), potassium supplements, or salt substitutes containing potassium may lead to increases in serum potassium and in heart failure patients to increases in serum creatinine.

Carcinogenesis, Mutagenesis, Impairment of Fertility

There was no evidence of carcinogenicity when valsartan was administered in the diet to mice and rats for up to 2 years at doses up to 160 and 200 mg/kg/day, respectively. These doses in mice and rats are about 2.6 and 6 times, respectively, the maximum recommended human dose on a mg/m^2 basis. (Calculations assume an oral dose of 320 mg/day and a 60-kg patient.)

Mutagenicity assays did not reveal any valsartan-related effects at either the gene or chromosome level. These assays included bacterial mutagenicity tests with *Salmonella* (Ames) and *E coli;* a gene mutation test with Chinese hamster V79 cells; a cytogenetic test with Chinese hamster ovary cells; and a rat micronucleus test.

Valsartan had no adverse effects on the reproductive performance of male or female rats at oral doses up to 200 mg/kg/day. This dose is 6 times the maximum recommended human dose on a mg/m^2 basis. (Calculations assume an oral dose of 320 mg/day and a 60-kg patient.)

Pregnancy

Pregnancy Categories C (first trimester) and D (second and third trimesters)

See WARNINGS, Fetal/Neonatal Morbidity and Mortality.

Nursing Mothers

It is not known whether valsartan is excreted in human milk, but valsartan was excreted in the milk of lactating rats. Because of the potential for adverse effects on the nursing infant, a decision should be made whether to discontinue nursing or discontinue the drug, taking into account the importance of the drug to the mother.

Pediatric Use

Safety and effectiveness in pediatric patients have not been established.

Geriatric Use

In the controlled clinical trials of valsartan, 1,214 (36.2%) of hypertensive patients treated with valsartan were ≥ 65 years and 265 (7.9%) were ≥ 75 years. No overall difference in the efficacy or safety of valsartan was observed in this patient population, but greater sensitivity of some older individuals cannot be ruled out.

Of the 2,511 patients with heart failure randomized to valsartan in the Valsartan Heart Failure Trial, 45% (1,141) were 65 years of age or older. There were no notable differences in efficacy or safety between older and younger patients.

ADVERSE REACTIONS

Hypertension

Diovan® (valsartan) has been evaluated for safety in more than 4,000 patients, including over 400 treated for over 6 months, and more than 160 for over 1 year. Adverse experiences have generally been mild and transient in nature and have only infrequently required discontinuation of therapy. The overall incidence of adverse experiences with Diovan was similar to placebo.

The overall frequency of adverse experiences was neither dose-related nor related to gender, age, race, or regimen. Discontinuation of therapy due to side effects was required in 2.3% of valsartan patients and 2.0% of placebo patients. The most common reasons for discontinuation of therapy with Diovan were headache and dizziness.

The adverse experiences that occurred in placebo-controlled clinical trials in at least 1% of patients treated with Diovan and at a higher incidence in valsartan (n=2,316) than placebo (n=888) patients included viral infection (3% vs. 2%), fatigue (2% vs. 1%), and abdominal pain (2% vs. 1%).

Headache, dizziness, upper respiratory infection, cough, diarrhea, rhinitis, sinusitis, nausea, pharyngitis, edema, and arthralgia occurred at a more than 1% rate but at about the same incidence in placebo and valsartan patients.

In trials in which valsartan was compared to an ACE inhibitor with or without placebo, the incidence of dry cough was significantly greater in the ACE-inhibitor group (7.9%) than in the groups who received valsartan (2.6%) or placebo (1.5%). In a 129-patient trial limited to patients who had had dry cough when they had previously received ACE inhibitors, the incidences of cough in patients who received valsartan, HCTZ, or lisinopril were 20%, 19%, and 69% respectively ($p < 0.001$).

Dose-related orthostatic effects were seen in less than 1% of patients. An increase in the incidence of dizziness was observed in patients treated with Diovan 320 mg (8%) compared to 10 to 160 mg (2% to 4%).

Diovan has been used concomitantly with hydrochlorothiazide without evidence of clinically important adverse interactions.

Other adverse experiences that occurred in controlled clinical trials of patients treated with Diovan (> 0.2% of valsartan patients) are listed below. It cannot be determined whether these events were causally related to Diovan.

Body as a Whole: Allergic reaction and asthenia

Cardiovascular: Palpitations

Dermatologic: Pruritus and rash

Digestive: Constipation, dry mouth, dyspepsia, and flatulence

Musculoskeletal: Back pain, muscle cramps, and myalgia

Neurologic and Psychiatric: Anxiety, insomnia, paresthesia, and somnolence

Respiratory: Dyspnea

Special Senses: Vertigo

Urogenital: Impotence

Other reported events seen less frequently in clinical trials included chest pain, syncope, anorexia, vomiting, and angioedema.

Heart Failure

The adverse experience profile of Diovan in heart failure patients was consistent with the pharmacology of the drug and the health status of the patients. In the Valsartan Heart Failure Trial, comparing valsartan in total daily doses up to 320 mg (n=2,506) to placebo (n=2,494), 10% of valsartan patients discontinued for adverse events vs. 7% of placebo patients.

The table shows adverse events in double-blind short-term heart failure trials, including the first 4 months of the Valsartan Heart Failure Trial, with an incidence of at least 2% that were more frequent in valsartan-treated patients than in placebo-treated patients. All patients received standard drug therapy for heart failure, frequently as multiple medications, which could include diuretics, digitalis, beta-blockers, or ACE inhibitors.

	Valsartan (n=3,282)	Placebo (n=2,740)
Dizziness	17%	9%
Hypotension	7%	2%
Diarrhea	5%	4%
Arthralgia	3%	2%
Fatigue	3%	2%
Back Pain	3%	2%
Dizziness, postural	2%	1%
Hyperkalemia	2%	1%
Hypotension, postural	2%	1%

Other adverse events with an incidence greater than 1% and greater than placebo included headache NOS, nausea, renal impairment NOS, syncope, blurred vision, upper abdominal pain and vertigo. (NOS = not otherwise specified).

From the long term data in the Valsartan Heart Failure Trial, there did not appear to be any significant adverse events not previously identified.

Post-Marketing Experience

The following additional adverse reactions have been reported in post-marketing experience:

Hypersensitivity: There are rare reports of angioedema;

Digestive: Elevated liver enzymes and very rare reports of hepatitis;

Renal: renal function;

Clinical Laboratory Tests: Hyperkalemia;

Dermatologic: Alopecia.

Clinical Laboratory Test Findings

In controlled clinical trials, clinically important changes in standard laboratory parameters were rarely associated with administration of Diovan.

Creatinine: Minor elevations in creatinine occurred in 0.8% of patients taking Diovan and 0.6% given placebo in controlled clinical trials of hypertensive patients. In heart failure trials, greater than 50% increases in creatinine were observed in 3.9% of Diovan-treated patients compared to 0.9% of placebo-treated patients.

Hemoglobin and Hematocrit: Greater than 20% decreases in hemoglobin and hematocrit were observed in 0.4% and 0.8%, respectively, of Diovan patients, compared with 0.1% and 0.1% in placebo-treated patients. One valsartan patient discontinued treatment for microcytic anemia.

Liver function tests: Occasional elevations (greater than 150%) of liver chemistries occurred in Diovan-treated patients. Three patients (< 0.1%) treated with valsartan discontinued treatment for elevated liver chemistries.

Neutropenia: Neutropenia was observed in 1.9% of patients treated with Diovan and 0.8% of patients treated with placebo.

Serum Potassium: In hypertensive patients, greater than 20% increases in serum potassium were observed in 4.4% of Diovan-treated patients compared to 2.9% of placebo-treated patients. In heart failure patients, greater than 20% increases in serum potassium were observed in 10.0% of Diovan-treated patients compared to 5.1% of placebo-treated patients.

Blood Urea Nitrogen (BUN): In heart failure trials, greater than 50% increases in BUN were observed in 16.6% of Diovan-treated patients compared to 6.3% of placebo-treated patients.

OVERDOSAGE

Limited data are available related to overdosage in humans. The most likely manifestations of overdosage would be hypotension and tachycardia; bradycardia could occur from parasympathetic (vagal) stimulation. If symptomatic hypotension should occur, supportive treatment should be instituted.

Valsartan is not removed from the plasma by hemodialysis. Valsartan was without grossly observable adverse effects at single oral doses up to 2000 mg/kg in rats and up to 1000 mg/kg in marmosets, except for salivation and diarrhea in the rat and vomiting in the marmoset at the highest dose (60 and 37 times, respectively, the maximum recommended human dose on a mg/m^2 basis). (Calculations assume an oral dose of 320 mg/day and a 60-kg patient.)

DOSAGE AND ADMINISTRATION

Hypertension

The recommended starting dose of Diovan® (valsartan) is 80 mg or 160 mg once daily when used as monotherapy in patients who are not volume-depleted. Patients requiring greater reductions may be started at the higher dose. Diovan may be used over a dose range of 80 mg to 320 mg daily, administered once-a-day.

The antihypertensive effect is substantially present within 2 weeks and maximal reduction is generally attained after 4 weeks. If additional antihypertensive effect is required over the starting dose range, the dose may be increased to a maximum of 320 mg or a diuretic may be added. Addition of a diuretic has a greater effect than dose increases beyond 80 mg.

No initial dosage adjustment is required for elderly patients, for patients with mild or moderate renal impairment, or for patients with mild or moderate liver insufficiency. Care should be exercised with dosing of Diovan in patients with hepatic or severe renal impairment.

Diovan may be administered with other antihypertensive agents.

Diovan may be administered with or without food.

Heart Failure

The recommended starting dose of Diovan is 40 mg twice daily. Uptitration to 80 mg and 160 mg twice daily should be done to the highest dose, as tolerated by the patient. Consideration should be given to reducing the dose of concomitant diuretics. The maximum daily dose administered in clinical trials is 320 mg in divided doses.

Concomitant use with an ACE inhibitor and a beta blocker is not recommended.

HOW SUPPLIED

Diovan® (valsartan) is available as tablets containing valsartan 40 mg, 80 mg, 160 mg, or 320 mg. All strengths are packaged in bottles and unit dose blister packages (10 strips of 10 tablets) as described below.

40 mg tablets are round and slightly convex with bevelled edges. 80 mg, 160 mg, and 320 mg tablets are almond-shaped with bevelled edges. All tablets are unscored.

[See table below]

Store at 25°C (77°F); excursions permitted to 15-30°C (59-86°F)

[see USP Controlled Room Temperature].

Protect from moisture.

Dispense in tight container (USP).

Tablet	Color	Deboss		NDC 0078-XXXX-XX		
		Side 1	Side 2	Bottle of 30	Bottle of 90	Blister
40 mg	Yellow	NVR	DO	0376-15	–	0376-06
80 mg	Pale red	NVR	DV	–	0358-34	0358-06
160 mg	Grey-orange	NVR	DX	–	0359-34	0359-06
320 mg	Dark grey-violet	NVR	DXL	–	0360-34	0360-06

T2003-71

REV: NOVEMBER 2003 PRINTED IN U.S.A. 89004209

Distributed by:

Novartis Pharmaceuticals Corporation

East Hanover, New Jersey 07936

Shown in Product Identification Guide, page 325

DIOVAN HCT® ℞
[*dī-o-văn*]
(valsartan and hydrochlorothiazide, USP)
Combination Tablets
80 mg/12.5 mg
160 mg/12.5 mg
160 mg/25 mg

Rx only

Prescribing Information
The following prescribing information is based on official labeling in effect July 2004.

USE IN PREGNANCY
When used in pregnancy during the second and third trimesters, drugs that act directly on the renin-angiotensin system can cause injury and even death to the developing fetus. When pregnancy is detected, Diovan HCT should be discontinued as soon as possible. *See* ***WARNINGS: Fetal/Neonatal Morbidity and Mortality.***

DESCRIPTION

Diovan HCT® (valsartan and hydrochlorothiazide, USP) is a combination of valsartan, an orally active, specific angiotensin II antagonist acting on the AT_1 receptor subtype, and hydrochlorothiazide, a diuretic.
Valsartan, a nonpeptide molecule, is chemically described as *N*-(1-oxopentyl)-*N*-[[2′-(1*H*-tetrazol-5-yl)[1,1′-biphenyl]-4-yl]methyl]-L-Valine. Its empirical formula is $C_{24}H_{29}N_5O_3$, its molecular weight is 435.5, and its structural formula is

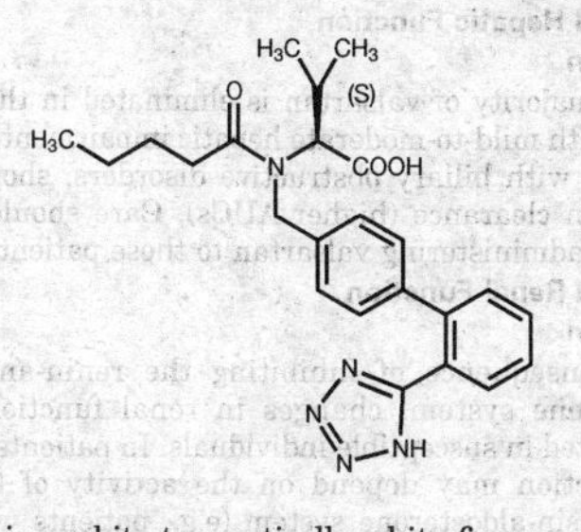

Valsartan is a white to practically white fine powder. It is soluble in ethanol and methanol and slightly soluble in water.
Hydrochlorothiazide USP is a white, or practically white, practically odorless, crystalline powder. It is slightly soluble in water; freely soluble in sodium hydroxide solution, in *n*-butylamine, and in dimethylformamide; sparingly soluble in methanol; and insoluble in ether, in chloroform, and in dilute mineral acids. Hydrochlorothiazide is chemically described as 6-chloro-3,4-dihydro-2*H*-1,2,4-benzothiadiazine-7-sulfonamide 1,1-dioxide. Hydrochlorothiazide is a thiazide diuretic. Its empirical formula is $C_7H_8ClN_3O_4S_2$, its molecular weight is 297.73, and its structural formula is

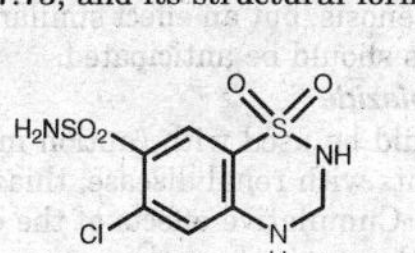

Diovan HCT tablets are formulated for oral administration to contain valsartan and hydrochlorothiazide, USP 80/12.5 mg, 160/12.5 mg and 160/25 mg. The inactive ingredients of the tablets are colloidal silicon dioxide, crospovidone, hydroxypropyl methylcellulose, iron oxides, magnesium stearate, microcrystalline cellulose, polyethylene glycol, talc, and titanium dioxide.

CLINICAL PHARMACOLOGY

Mechanism of Action
Angiotensin II is formed from angiotensin I in a reaction catalyzed by angiotensin-converting enzyme (ACE, kininase II). Angiotensin II is the principal pressor agent of the renin-angiotensin system, with effects that include vasoconstriction, stimulation of synthesis and release of aldosterone, cardiac stimulation, and renal reabsorption of sodium. Valsartan blocks the vasoconstrictor and aldosterone-secreting effects of angiotensin II by selectively blocking the binding of angiotensin II to the AT_1 receptor in many tissues, such as vascular smooth muscle and the adrenal gland. Its action is therefore independent of the pathways for angiotensin II synthesis.
There is also an AT_2 receptor found in many tissues, but AT_2 is not known to be associated with cardiovascular homeostasis. Valsartan has much greater affinity (about 20,000-fold) for the AT_1 receptor than for the AT_2 receptor. The primary metabolite of valsartan is essentially inactive with an affinity for the AT_1 receptor about one 200th that of valsartan itself.
Blockade of the renin-angiotensin system with ACE inhibitors, which inhibit the biosynthesis of angiotensin II from angiotensin I, is widely used in the treatment of hypertension. ACE inhibitors also inhibit the degradation of bradykinin, a reaction also catalyzed by ACE. Because valsartan does not inhibit ACE (kininase II) it does not affect the response to bradykinin. Whether this difference has clinical relevance is not yet known. Valsartan does not bind to or block other hormone receptors or ion channels known to be important in cardiovascular regulation.
Blockade of the angiotensin II receptor inhibits the negative regulatory feedback of angiotensin II on renin secretion, but the resulting increased plasma renin activity and angiotensin II circulating levels do not overcome the effect of valsartan on blood pressure.
Hydrochlorothiazide is a thiazide diuretic. Thiazides affect the renal tubular mechanisms of electrolyte reabsorption, directly increasing excretion of sodium and chloride in approximately equivalent amounts. Indirectly, the diuretic action of hydrochlorothiazide reduces plasma volume, with consequent increases in plasma renin activity, increases in aldosterone secretion, increases in urinary potassium loss, and decreases in serum potassium. The renin-aldosterone link is mediated by angiotensin II, so coadministration of an angiotensin II receptor antagonist tends to reverse the potassium loss associated with these diuretics.
The mechanism of the antihypertensive effect of thiazides is unknown.

Pharmacokinetics
Valsartan
Valsartan peak plasma concentration is reached 2 to 4 hours after dosing. Valsartan shows bi-exponential decay kinetics following intravenous administration, with an average elimination half-life of about 6 hours. Absolute bioavailability for the capsule formulation is about 25% (range 10%-35%). Food decreases the exposure (as measured by AUC) to valsartan by about 40% and peak plasma concentration (C_{max}) by about 50%. AUC and C_{max} values of valsartan increase approximately linearly with increasing dose over the clinical dosing range. Valsartan does not accumulate appreciably in plasma following repeated administration.

Metabolism and Elimination
Valsartan
Valsartan, when administered as an oral solution, is primarily recovered in feces (about 83% of dose) and urine (about 13% of dose). The recovery is mainly as unchanged drug, with only about 20% of dose recovered as metabolites. The primary metabolite, accounting for about 9% of dose, is valeryl 4-hydroxy valsartan. The enzyme(s) responsible for valsartan metabolism have not been identified but do not seem to be CYP 450 isozymes.
Following intravenous administration, plasma clearance of valsartan is about 2 L/h and its renal clearance is 0.62 L/h (about 30% of total clearance).
Hydrochlorothiazide
Hydrochlorothiazide is not metabolized but is eliminated rapidly by the kidney. At least 61% of the oral dose is eliminated as unchanged drug within 24 hours. The elimination half-life is between 5.8 and 18.9 hours.

Distribution
Valsartan
The steady state volume of distribution of valsartan after intravenous administration is small (17 L), indicating that valsartan does not distribute into tissues extensively. Valsartan is highly bound to serum proteins (95%), mainly serum albumin.
Hydrochlorothiazide
Hydrochlorothiazide crosses the placental but not the blood-brain barrier and is excreted in breast milk.

Special Populations
Pediatric: The pharmacokinetics of valsartan have not been investigated in patients <18 years of age.
Geriatric: Exposure (measured by AUC) to valsartan is higher by 70% and the half-life is longer by 35% in the elderly than in the young. No dosage adjustment is necessary *(see DOSAGE AND ADMINISTRATION)*.
Gender: Pharmacokinetics of valsartan does not differ significantly between males and females.
Race: Pharmacokinetic differences due to race have not been studied.
Renal Insufficiency: There is no apparent correlation between renal function (measured by creatinine clearance) and exposure (measured by AUC) to valsartan in patients with different degrees of renal impairment. Consequently, dose adjustment is not required in patients with mild-to-moderate renal dysfunction. No studies have been performed in patients with severe impairment of renal function (creatinine clearance <10 mL/min). Valsartan is not removed from the plasma by hemodialysis. In the case of severe renal disease, exercise care with dosing of valsartan *(see DOSAGE AND ADMINISTRATION)*.
Thiazide diuretics are eliminated by the kidney, with a terminal half-life of 5-15 hours. In a study of patients with impaired renal function (mean creatinine clearance of 19 mL/min), the half-life of hydrochlorothiazide elimination was lengthened to 21 hours.
Hepatic Insufficiency: On average, patients with mild-to-moderate chronic liver disease have twice the exposure (measured by AUC values) to valsartan of healthy volunteers (matched by age, sex and weight). In general, no dosage adjustment is needed in patients with mild-to-moderate liver disease. Care should be exercised in patients with liver disease *(see DOSAGE AND ADMINISTRATION)*.

Pharmacodynamics and Clinical Effects
Valsartan—Hydrochlorothiazide
In controlled clinical trials including over 1500 patients, 730 patients were exposed to valsartan (80 and 160 mg) and concomitant hydrochlorothiazide (12.5 and 25 mg). A factorial trial compared the combinations of 80/12.5 mg, 80/25 mg, 160/12.5 mg and 160/25 mg with their respective components and placebo. The combination of valsartan and hydrochlorothiazide resulted in additive placebo-adjusted decreases in systolic and diastolic blood pressure at trough of 15-21/8-11 mmHg at 80/12.5 mg to 160/25 mg, compared to 7-10/4-6 mmHg for valsartan 80 mg to 160 mg and 6-10/3-5 mmHg for hydrochlorothiazide 12.5 mg to 25 mg, alone.
In another controlled trial the addition of hydrochlorothiazide to valsartan 80 mg resulted in additional lowering of systolic and diastolic blood pressure by approximately 6/3 and 12/5 mmHg for 12.5 mg and 25 mg of hydrochlorothiazide, respectively, compared to valsartan 80 mg alone.
The maximal antihypertensive effect was attained 4 weeks after the initiation of therapy, the first time point at which blood pressure was measured in these trials.
In long-term follow-up studies (without placebo control) the effect of the combination of valsartan and hydrochlorothiazide appeared to be maintained for up to two years. The antihypertensive effect is independent of age or gender. The overall response to the combination was similar for black and non-black patients.
There was essentially no change in heart rate in patients treated with the combination of valsartan and hydrochlorothiazide in controlled trials.
Valsartan
Valsartan inhibits the pressor effect of angiotensin II infusions. An oral dose of 80 mg inhibits the pressor effect by about 80% at peak with approximately 30% inhibition persisting for 24 hours. No information on the effect of larger doses is available.
Removal of the negative feedback of angiotensin II causes a 2- to 3-fold rise in plasma renin and consequent rise in angiotensin II plasma concentration in hypertensive patients. Minimal decreases in plasma aldosterone were observed after administration of valsartan; very little effect on serum potassium was observed.
In multiple-dose studies in hypertensive patients with stable renal insufficiency and patients with renovascular hypertension, valsartan had no clinically significant effects on glomerular filtration rate, filtration fraction, creatinine clearance, or renal plasma flow.
In multiple-dose studies in hypertensive patients, valsartan had no notable effects on total cholesterol, fasting triglycerides, fasting serum glucose, or uric acid.
The antihypertensive effects of valsartan were demonstrated principally in 7 placebo-controlled, 4- to 12-week trials (one in patients over 65) of dosages from 10 to 320 mg/day in patients with baseline diastolic blood pressures of 95-115. The studies allowed comparison of once-daily and twice-daily regimens of 160 mg/day; comparison of peak and trough effects; comparison (in pooled data) of response by gender, age, and race; and evaluation of incremental effects of hydrochlorothiazide.
Administration of valsartan to patients with essential hypertension results in a significant reduction of sitting, supine, and standing systolic and diastolic blood pressure, usually with little or no orthostatic change.
In most patients, after administration of a single oral dose, onset of antihypertensive activity occurs at approximately 2 hours, and maximum reduction of blood pressure is achieved within 6 hours. The antihypertensive effect persists for 24 hours after dosing, but there is a decrease from peak effect at lower doses (40 mg) presumably reflecting loss of inhibition of angiotensin II. At higher doses, however (160 mg), there is little difference in peak and trough effect. During repeated dosing, the reduction in blood pressure with any dose is substantially present within 2 weeks, and maximal reduction is generally attained after 4 weeks. In long-term follow-up studies (without placebo control) the effect of valsartan appeared to be maintained for up to two years. The antihypertensive effect is independent of age, gender or race. The latter finding regarding race is based on pooled data and should be viewed with caution, because antihypertensive drugs that affect the renin-angiotensin system (that is, ACE inhibitors and angiotensin-II blockers) have generally been found to be less effective in low-renin hypertensives (frequently blacks) than in high-renin hypertensives (frequently whites). In pooled, randomized, controlled trials of Diovan that included a total of 140 blacks and 830 whites, valsartan and an ACE-inhibitor control were generally at least as effective in blacks as whites. The explanation for this difference from previous findings is unclear.
Abrupt withdrawal of valsartan has not been associated with a rapid increase in blood pressure.
The 7 studies of valsartan monotherapy included over 2000 patients randomized to various doses of valsartan and about 800 patients randomized to placebo. Doses below 80 mg were not consistently distinguished from those of placebo at trough, but doses of 80, 160 and 320 mg produced dose-related decreases in systolic and diastolic blood pressure, with the difference from placebo of approximately 6-9/3-5 mmHg at 80-160 mg and 9/6 mmHg at 320 mg.
Patients with an inadequate response to 80 mg once daily were titrated to either 160 mg once daily or 80 mg twice daily, which resulted in a comparable response in both groups.
In controlled trials, the antihypertensive effect of once daily valsartan 80 mg was similar to that of once daily enalapril 20 mg or once daily lisinopril 10 mg.
There was essentially no change in heart rate in valsartan-treated patients in controlled trials.

Continued on next page

Diovan HCT—Cont.

Hydrochlorothiazide

After oral administration of hydrochlorothiazide, diuresis begins within 2 hours, peaks in about 4 hours and lasts about 6 to 12 hours.

INDICATIONS AND USAGE

Diovan HCT® (valsartan and hydrochlorothiazide, USP) is indicated for the treatment of hypertension. This fixed dose combination is not indicated for initial therapy *(see DOSAGE AND ADMINISTRATION).*

CONTRAINDICATIONS

Diovan HCT® (valsartan and hydrochlorothiazide, USP) is contraindicated in patients who are hypersensitive to any component of this product.

Because of the hydrochlorothiazide component, this product is contraindicated in patients with anuria or hypersensitivity to other sulfonamide-derived drugs.

WARNINGS

Fetal/Neonatal Morbidity and Mortality

Drugs that act directly on the renin-angiotensin system can cause fetal and neonatal morbidity and death when administered to pregnant women. Several dozen cases have been reported in the world literature in patients who were taking angiotensin-converting enzyme inhibitors. When pregnancy is detected, Diovan HCT® (valsartan and hydrochlorothiazide, USP) should be discontinued as soon as possible.

The use of drugs that act directly on the renin-angiotensin system during the second and third trimesters of pregnancy has been associated with fetal and neonatal injury, including hypotension, neonatal skull hypoplasia, anuria, reversible or irreversible renal failure, and death. Oligohydramnios has also been reported, presumably resulting from decreased fetal renal function; oligohydramnios in this setting has been associated with fetal limb contractures, craniofacial deformation, and hypoplastic lung development. Prematurity, intrauterine growth retardation, and patent ductus arteriosus have also been reported, although it is not clear whether these occurrences were due to exposure to the drug.

These adverse effects do not appear to have resulted from intrauterine drug exposure that has been limited to the first trimester.

Mothers whose embryos and fetuses are exposed to an angiotensin II receptor antagonist only during the first trimester should be so informed. Nonetheless, when patients become pregnant, physicians should advise the patient to discontinue the use of Diovan HCT as soon as possible.

Rarely (probably less often than once in every thousand pregnancies), no alternative to a drug acting on the renin-angiotensin system will be found. In these rare cases, the mothers should be apprised of the potential hazards to their fetuses, and serial ultrasound examinations should be performed to assess the intraamniotic environment.

If oligohydramnios is observed, Diovan HCT should be discontinued unless it is considered life-saving for the mother. Contraction stress testing (CST), a nonstress test (NST), or biophysical profiling (BPP) may be appropriate, depending upon the week of pregnancy. Patients and physicians should be aware, however, that oligohydramnios may not appear until after the fetus has sustained irreversible injury.

Infants with histories of *in utero* exposure to an angiotensin II receptor antagonist should be closely observed for hypotension, oliguria, and hyperkalemia. If oliguria occurs, attention should be directed toward support of blood pressure and renal perfusion. Exchange transfusion or dialysis may be required as means of reversing hypotension and/or substituting for disordered renal function.

Valsartan—Hydrochlorothiazide in Animals

There was no evidence of teratogenicity in mice, rats, or rabbits treated orally with valsartan at doses up to 600, 100 and 10 mg/kg/day, respectively, in combination with hydrochlorothiazide at doses up to 188, 31 and 3 mg/kg/day. These non-teratogenic doses in mice, rats and rabbits, respectively, represent 18, 7 and 1 times the maximum recommended human dose (MRHD) of valsartan and 38, 13 and 2 times the MRHD of hydrochlorothiazide on a mg/m^2 basis. (Calculations assume an oral dose of 160 mg/day valsartan in combination with 25 mg/day hydrochlorothiazide and a 60-kg patient.)

Fetotoxicity was observed in association with maternal toxicity in rats and rabbits at valsartan doses of ≥200 and 10 mg/kg/day, respectively, in combination with hydrochlorothiazide doses of ≥63 and 3 mg/kg/day. Fetotoxicity in rats was considered to be related to decreased fetal weights and included fetal variations of sternebrae, vertebrae, ribs and/or renal papillae. Fetotoxicity in rabbits included increased numbers of late resorptions with resultant increases in total resorptions, postimplantation losses and decreased number of live fetuses. The no observed adverse effect doses in mice, rats and rabbits for valsartan were 600, 100 and 3 mg/kg/day, respectively, in combination with hydrochlorothiazide doses of 188, 31 and 1 mg/kg/day. These no adverse effect doses in mice, rats and rabbits, respectively, represent 5, 1.5 and 0.06 times the MRHD of valsartan and 38, 13 and 0.5 times the MRHD of hydrochlorothiazide on a mg/m^2 basis. (Calculations assume an oral dose of 160 mg/day valsartan in combination with 25 mg/day hydrochlorothiazide and a 60-kg patient.)

Valsartan in Animals

No teratogenic effects were observed when valsartan was administered to pregnant mice and rats at oral doses up to 600 mg/kg/day and to pregnant rabbits at oral doses up to 10 mg/kg/day. However, significant decreases in fetal weight, pup birth weight, pup survival rate, and slight delays in developmental milestones were observed in studies in which parental rats were treated with valsartan at oral, maternally toxic (reduction in body weight gain and food consumption) doses of 600 mg/kg/day during organogenesis or late gestation and lactation. In rabbits, fetotoxicity (i.e., resorptions, litter loss, abortions, and low body weight) associated with maternal toxicity (mortality) was observed at doses of 5 and 10 mg/kg/day. The no observed adverse effect doses of 600, 200 and 2 mg/kg/day in mice, rats and rabbits represent 18, 12 and 0.2 times, respectively, the maximum recommended human dose on a mg/m^2 basis. (Calculations assume an oral dose of 160 mg/day and a 60-kg patient.)

Hydrochlorothiazide in Animals

Under the auspices of the National Toxicology Program, pregnant mice and rats that received hydrochlorothiazide via gavage at doses up to 3000 and 1000 mg/kg/day, respectively, on gestation days 6 through 15 showed no evidence of teratogenicity. These doses of hydrochlorothiazide in mice and rats represent 608 and 405 times, respectively, the maximum recommended human dose on a mg/m^2 basis. (Calculations assume an oral dose of 25 mg/day and a 60-kg patient.)

Intrauterine exposure to thiazide diuretics is associated with fetal or neonatal jaundice, thrombocytopenia, and possibly other adverse reactions that have occurred in adults.

Hypotension in Volume- and/or Salt-Depleted Patients

Excessive reduction of blood pressure was rarely seen (0.5%) in patients with uncomplicated hypertension treated with Diovan HCT. In patients with an activated renin-angiotensin system, such as volume- and/or salt-depleted patients receiving high doses of diuretics, symptomatic hypotension may occur. This condition should be corrected prior to administration of Diovan HCT, or the treatment should start under close medical supervision.

If hypotension occurs, the patient should be placed in the supine position and, if necessary, given an intravenous infusion of normal saline. A transient hypotensive response is not a contraindication to further treatment, which usually can be continued without difficulty once the blood pressure has stabilized.

Hydrochlorothiazide

Impaired Hepatic Function

Thiazide diuretics should be used with caution in patients with impaired hepatic function or progressive liver disease, since minor alterations of fluid and electrolyte balance may precipitate hepatic coma.

Hypersensitivity Reaction

Hypersensitivity reactions to hydrochlorothiazide may occur in patients with or without a history of allergy or bronchial asthma, but are more likely in patients with such a history.

Systemic Lupus Erythematosus

Thiazide diuretics have been reported to cause exacerbation or activation of systemic lupus erythematosus.

Lithium Interaction

Lithium generally should not be given with thiazides *(see PRECAUTIONS, Drug Interactions Hydrochlorothiazide, Lithium).*

PRECAUTIONS

Serum Electrolytes

Valsartan—Hydrochlorothiazide

In the controlled trials of various doses of the combination of valsartan and hydrochlorothiazide the incidence of hypertensive patients who developed hypokalemia (serum potassium <3.5 mEq/L) was 4.5%; the incidence of hyperkalemia (serum potassium >5.7 mEq/L) was 0.3%. Two patients (0.3%) discontinued from a trial for decreases in serum potassium.

In controlled clinical trials of Diovan HCT® (valsartan and hydrochlorothiazide, USP), the average change in serum potassium was near zero in subjects who received Diovan HCT 160/12.5 mg, but the average subject who received Diovan HCT 80/12.5 mg, 80/25 mg or 160/25 mg experienced a mild reduction in serum potassium.

In clinical trials, the opposite effects of valsartan (80 or 160 mg) and hydrochlorothiazide (12.5 mg) on serum potassium approximately balanced each other in many patients. In other patients, one or the other effect may be dominant. Periodic determinations of serum electrolytes to detect possible electrolyte imbalance should be performed at appropriate intervals.

Hydrochlorothiazide

All patients receiving thiazide therapy should be observed for clinical signs of fluid or electrolyte imbalance: hyponatremia, hypochloremic alkalosis, and hypokalemia. Serum and urine electrolyte determinations are particularly important when the patient is vomiting excessively or receiving parenteral fluids. Warning signs or symptoms of fluid and electrolyte imbalance, irrespective of cause, include dryness of mouth, thirst, weakness, lethargy, drowsiness, restlessness, confusion, seizures, muscle pains or cramps, muscular fatigue, hypotension, oliguria, tachycardia, and gastrointestinal disturbances such as nausea and vomiting.

Hypokalemia may develop, especially with brisk diuresis, when severe cirrhosis is present, or after prolonged therapy. Interference with adequate oral electrolyte intake will also contribute to hypokalemia. Hypokalemia may cause cardiac arrhythmia and may also sensitize or exaggerate the response of the heart to the toxic effects of digitalis (e.g., increased ventricular irritability).

Although any chloride deficit is generally mild and usually does not require specific treatment except under extraordinary circumstances (as in liver disease or renal disease), chloride replacement may be required in the treatment of metabolic alkalosis.

Dilutional hyponatremia may occur in edematous patients in hot weather; appropriate therapy is water restriction, rather than administration of salt except in rare instances when the hyponatremia is life-threatening. In actual salt depletion, appropriate replacement is the therapy of choice.

Hyperuricemia may occur or frank gout may be precipitated in certain patients receiving thiazide therapy.

In diabetic patients dosage adjustments of insulin or oral hypoglycemic agents may be required. Hyperglycemia may occur with thiazide diuretics. Thus latent diabetes mellitus may become manifest during thiazide therapy.

The antihypertensive effects of the drug may be enhanced in the post-sympathectomy patient.

If progressive renal impairment becomes evident, consider withholding or discontinuing diuretic therapy.

Thiazides have been shown to increase the urinary excretion of magnesium; this may result in hypomagnesemia.

Thiazides may decrease urinary calcium excretion. Thiazides may cause intermittent and slight elevation of serum calcium in the absence of known disorders of calcium metabolism. Marked hypercalcemia may be evidence of hidden hyperparathyroidism. Thiazides should be discontinued before carrying out tests for parathyroid function.

Increases in cholesterol and triglyceride levels may be associated with thiazide diuretic therapy.

Impaired Hepatic Function

Valsartan

As the majority of valsartan is eliminated in the bile, patients with mild-to-moderate hepatic impairment, including patients with biliary obstructive disorders, showed lower valsartan clearance (higher AUCs). Care should be exercised in administering valsartan to these patients.

Impaired Renal Function

Valsartan

As a consequence of inhibiting the renin-angiotensin-aldosterone system, changes in renal function may be anticipated in susceptible individuals. In patients whose renal function may depend on the activity of the renin-angiotensin-aldosterone system (e.g., patients with severe congestive heart failure), treatment with angiotensin-converting enzyme inhibitors and angiotensin receptor antagonists has been associated with oliguria and/or progressive azotemia and (rarely) with acute renal failure and/or death. Similar outcomes have been reported with Diovan.

In studies of ACE inhibitors in patients with unilateral or bilateral renal artery stenosis, increases in serum creatinine or blood urea nitrogen have been reported. In a 4-day trial of valsartan in 12 patients with unilateral renal artery stenosis, no significant increases in serum creatinine or blood urea nitrogen were observed. There has been no long-term use of valsartan in patients with unilateral or bilateral renal artery stenosis, but an effect similar to that seen with ACE inhibitors should be anticipated.

Hydrochlorothiazide

Thiazides should be used with caution in severe renal disease. In patients with renal disease, thiazides may precipitate azotemia. Cumulative effects of the drug may develop in patients with impaired renal function.

Information for Patients

Pregnancy: Female patients of childbearing age should be told about the consequences of second- and third-trimester exposure to drugs that act on the renin-angiotensin system, and they should also be told that these consequences do not appear to have resulted from intrauterine drug exposure that has been limited to the first trimester. These patients should be asked to report pregnancies to their physicians as soon as possible.

Symptomatic Hypotension: A patient receiving Diovan HCT should be cautioned that lightheadedness can occur, especially during the first days of therapy, and that it should be reported to the prescribing physician. The patients should be told that if syncope occurs, Diovan HCT should be discontinued until the physician has been consulted.

All patients should be cautioned that inadequate fluid intake, excessive perspiration, diarrhea, or vomiting can lead to an excessive fall in blood pressure, with the same consequences of lightheadedness and possible syncope.

Potassium Supplements: A patient receiving Diovan HCT should be told not to use potassium supplements or salt substitutes containing potassium without consulting the prescribing physician.

Drug Interactions

Valsartan

No clinically significant pharmacokinetic interactions were observed when valsartan was coadministered with amlodipine, atenolol, cimetidine, digoxin, furosemide, glyburide, hydrochlorothiazide, or indomethacin. The valsartan-atenolol combination was more antihypertensive than either component, but it did not lower the heart rate more than atenolol alone.

Coadministration of valsartan and warfarin did not change the pharmacokinetics of valsartan or the time-course of the anticoagulant properties of warfarin.

CYP 450 Interactions: The enzyme(s) responsible for valsartan metabolism have not been identified but do not seem to be CYP 450 isozymes. The inhibitory or induction potential of valsartan on CYP 450 is also unknown.

Hydrochlorothiazide

When administered concurrently the following drugs may interact with thiazide diuretics:

Alcohol, barbiturates, or narcotics—Potentiation of orthostatic hypotension may occur.

Antidiabetic drugs (oral agents and insulin)—Dosage adjustment of the antidiabetic drug may be required.

Other antihypertensive drugs—Additive effect or potentiation.

Cholestyramine and colestipol resins—Absorption of hydrochlorothiazide is impaired in the presence of anionic exchange resins. Single doses of either cholestyramine or colestipol resins bind the hydrochlorothiazide and reduce its absorption from the gastrointestinal tract by up to 85% and 43% respectively.

Corticosteroids, ACTH—Intensified electrolyte depletion, particularly hypokalemia.

Pressor amines (e.g., norepinephrine)—Possible decreased response to pressor amines but not sufficient to preclude their use.

Skeletal muscle relaxants, nondepolarizing (e.g., tubocurarine)—Possible increased responsiveness to the muscle relaxant.

Lithium—Should not generally be given with diuretics. Diuretic agents reduce the renal clearance of lithium and add a high risk of lithium toxicity. Refer to the package insert for lithium preparations before use of such preparations with Diovan HCT.

Non-steroidal anti-inflammatory Drugs—In some patients, the administration of a non-steroidal anti-inflammatory agent can reduce the diuretic, natriuretic, and antihypertensive effects of loop, potassium-sparing and thiazide diuretics. Therefore, when Diovan HCT and non-steroidal anti-inflammatory agents are used concomitantly, the patient should be observed closely to determine if the desired effect of the diuretic is obtained.

Carcinogenesis, Mutagenesis, Impairment of Fertility

Valsartan—Hydrochlorothiazide

No carcinogenicity, mutagenicity or fertility studies have been conducted with the combination of valsartan and hydrochlorothiazide. However, these studies have been conducted for valsartan as well as hydrochlorothiazide alone. Based on the preclinical safety and human pharmacokinetic studies, there is no indication of any adverse interaction between valsartan and hydrochlorothiazide.

Valsartan

There was no evidence of carcinogenicity when valsartan was administered in the diet to mice and rats for up to 2 years at doses up to 160 and 200 mg/kg/day, respectively. These doses in mice and rats are about 5 and 12 times, respectively, the maximum recommended human dose on a mg/m^2 basis. (Calculations assume an oral dose of 160 mg/day and a 60-kg patient.)

Mutagenicity assays did not reveal any valsartan-related effects at either the gene or chromosome level. These assays included bacterial mutagenicity tests with *Salmonella* (Ames) and *E coli;* a gene mutation test with Chinese hamster V79 cells; a cytogenetic test with Chinese hamster ovary cells; and a rat micronucleus test.

Valsartan had no adverse effects on the reproductive performance of male or female rats at oral doses up to 200 mg/kg/day. This dose is about 12 times the maximum recommended human dose on a mg/m^2 basis. (Calculations assume an oral dose of 160 mg/day and a 60-kg patient.)

Hydrochlorothiazide

Two-year feeding studies in mice and rats conducted under the auspices of the National Toxicology Program (NTP) uncovered no evidence of a carcinogenic potential of hydrochlorothiazide in female mice (at doses of up to approximately 600 mg/kg/day) or in male and female rats (at doses of up to approximately 100 mg/kg/day). The NTP, however, found equivocal evidence for hepatocarcinogenicity in male mice. Hydrochlorothiazide was not genotoxic *In Vitro* in the Ames mutagenicity assay of Salmonella Typhimurium strains TA 98, TA 100, TA 1535, TA 1537, and TA 1538 and in the Chinese Hamster Ovary (CHO) test for chromosomal aberrations, or *In Vivo* in assays using mouse germinal cell chromosomes, Chinese hamster bone marrow chromosomes, and the Drosophila sex-linked recessive lethal trait gene. Positive test results were obtained only in the *In Vitro* CHO Sister Chromatid Exchange (clastogenicity) and in the Mouse Lymphoma Cell (mutagenicity) assays, using concentrations of hydrochlorothiazide from 43 to 1300 mcgm/mL, and in the Aspergillus Nidulans non-disjunction assay at an unspecified concentration.

Hydrochlorothiazide had no adverse effects on the fertility of mice and rats of either sex in studies wherein these species were exposed, via their diet, to doses of up to 100 and 4 mg/kg, respectively, prior to mating and throughout gestation.

Pregnancy Categories C (first trimester) and D (second and third trimesters)

See WARNINGS Fetal/Neonatal Morbidity and Mortality.

Nursing Mothers

It is not known whether valsartan is excreted in human milk, but valsartan was excreted in the milk of lactating rats. Thiazides appear in human milk. Because of the potential for adverse effects on the nursing infant, a decision should be made whether to discontinue nursing or discontinue the drug, taking into account the importance of the drug to the mother.

Pediatric Use

Safety and effectiveness in pediatric patients have not been established.

Geriatric Use

In the controlled clinical trials of Diovan HCT, 117 (16%) of patients treated with valsartan-hydrochlorothiazide were ≥65 years and 16 (2.2%) were ≥75 years. No overall difference in the efficacy or safety of valsartan-hydrochlorothiazide was observed between these patients and younger patients, but greater sensitivity of some older individuals cannot be ruled out.

ADVERSE REACTIONS

Diovan HCT® (valsartan and hydrochlorothiazide, USP) has been evaluated for safety in more than 1,300 patients, including over 360 treated for over 6 months, and 170 for over 1 year. Adverse experiences have generally been mild and transient in nature and have only infrequently required discontinuation of therapy. The overall incidence of adverse experiences with Diovan HCT was comparable to placebo.

The overall frequency of adverse experiences was neither dose-related nor related to gender, age or race. In controlled clinical trials, discontinuation of therapy due to side effects was required in 3.6% of valsartan-hydrochlorothiazide patients and 4.3% of placebo patients. The most common reasons for discontinuation of therapy with Diovan HCT were headache, fatigue and dizziness.

The adverse experiences that occurred in controlled clinical trials in at least 2% of patients treated with Diovan HCT and at a higher incidence in valsartan-hydrochlorothiazide (n=730) than placebo (n=93) patients included dizziness (9% vs 7%), viral infection (3% vs 1%), fatigue (5% vs 1%), pharyngitis (3% vs 1%), coughing (3% vs 0%) and diarrhea (3% vs 0%).

Headache, upper respiratory infection, sinusitis, back pain and chest pain occurred at a more than 2% rate but at about the same incidence in placebo and valsartan-hydrochlorothiazide patients.

Dose-related orthostatic effects were seen in less than 1% of patients. A dose-related increase in the incidence of dizziness was observed in patients treated with Diovan HCT from 80/12.5 mg (6%) to 160/25 mg (16%).

Other adverse experiences that have been reported with valsartan-hydrochlorothiazide (>0.2% of valsartan-hydrochlorothiazide patients in controlled clinical trials) without regard to causality, are listed below:

Body as a Whole: Allergic reaction, anaphylaxis, asthenia, and dependent edema.

Cardiovascular: Palpitations, syncope, and tachycardia.

Dermatologic: Flushing, rash, sunburn, and increased sweating.

Digestive: Increased appetite, constipation, dyspepsia, flatulence, dry mouth, nausea, abdominal pain, and vomiting.

Metabolic: Dehydration and gout.

Musculoskeletal: Arthralgia, muscle cramps, muscle weakness, arm pain, and leg pain.

Neurologic and Psychiatric: Anxiety, depression, insomnia, decreased libido, paresthesia, and somnolence.

Respiratory: Bronchospasm, dyspnea, and epistaxis.

Special Senses: Tinnitus, vertigo, and abnormal vision.

Urogenital: Dysuria, impotence, micturition frequency, and urinary tract infection.

Valsartan

In trials in which valsartan was compared to an ACE inhibitor with or without placebo, the incidence of dry cough was significantly greater in the ACE inhibitor group (7.9%) than in the groups who received valsartan (2.6%) or placebo (1.5%). In a 129-patient trial limited to patients who had had dry cough when they had previously received ACE inhibitors, the incidences of cough in patients who received valsartan, hydrochlorothiazide, or lisinopril were 20%, 19%, 69% respectively ($p < 0.001$).

Other reported events seen less frequently in clinical trials included chest pain, syncope, anorexia, vomiting, and angioedema.

Post-Marketing Experience

The following additional adverse reactions have been reported in post-marketing experience:

Hypersensitivity: There are rare reports of angioedema;

Digestive: Elevated liver enzymes and very rare reports of hepatitis;

Renal: Impaired Renal Function;

Clinical Laboratory Tests: Hyperkalemia;

Dermatologic: Alopecia.

Hydrochlorothiazide

Other adverse experiences that have been reported with hydrochlorothiazide, without regard to causality, are listed below:

Body as a Whole: weakness;

Digestive: pancreatitis, jaundice (intrahepatic cholestatic jaundice), sialadenitis, cramping, gastric irritation;

Hematologic: aplastic anemia, agranulocytosis, leukopenia, hemolytic anemia, thrombocytopenia;

Hypersensitivity: purpura, photosensitivity, urticaria, necrotizing angiitis (vasculitis and cutaneous vasculitis), fever, respiratory distress including pneumonitis and pulmonary edema, anaphylactic reactions;

Metabolic: hyperglycemia, glycosuria, hyperuricemia;

Musculoskeletal: muscle spasm;

Nervous System/Psychiatric: restlessness;

Renal: renal failure, renal dysfunction, interstitial nephritis;

Skin: erythema multiforme including Stevens-Johnson syndrome, exfoliative dermatitis including toxic epidermal necrolysis;

Special Senses: transient blurred vision, xanthopsia.

Clinical Laboratory Test Findings

In controlled clinical trials, clinically important changes in standard laboratory parameters were rarely associated with administration of Diovan HCT.

Creatinine: Minor elevations in creatinine occurred in 1.4% of patients taking Diovan HCT and 1.1% given placebo in controlled clinical trials.

Hemoglobin and Hematocrit: Greater than 20% decreases in hemoglobin and hematocrit were observed in 0.1% and 1.0%, respectively, of Diovan HCT patients, compared with 0.0% in placebo-treated patients.

Liver Function Tests: Occasional elevations (greater than 150%) of liver chemistries occurred in Diovan HCT-treated patients.

Neutropenia: Neutropenia was observed in 0.6% of patients treated with Diovan HCT and 0.0% of patients treated with placebo.

Serum Electrolytes: *See PRECAUTIONS.*

OVERDOSAGE

Valsartan—Hydrochlorothiazide

Limited data are available related to overdosage in humans. The most likely manifestations of overdosage would be hypotension and tachycardia; bradycardia could occur from parasympathetic (vagal) stimulation. If symptomatic hypotension should occur, supportive treatment should be instituted.

Valsartan is not removed from the plasma by dialysis.

The degree to which hydrochlorothiazide is removed by hemodialysis has not been established. The most common signs and symptoms observed in patients are those caused by electrolyte depletion (hypokalemia, hypochloremia, hyponatremia) and dehydration resulting from excessive diuresis. If digitalis has also been administered, hypokalemia may accentuate cardiac arrhythmias.

In rats and marmosets, single oral doses of valsartan up to 1524 and 762 mg/kg in combination with hydrochlorothiazide at doses up to 476 and 238 mg/kg, respectively, were very well tolerated without any treatment-related effects. These no adverse effect doses in rats and marmosets, respectively, represent 93 and 56 times the maximum recommended human dose (MRHD) of valsartan and 188 and 113 times the MRHD of hydrochlorothiazide on a mg/m^2 basis. (Calculations assume an oral dose of 160 mg/day valsartan in combination with 25 mg/day hydrochlorothiazide and a 60-kg patient.)

Valsartan

Valsartan was without grossly observable adverse effects at single oral doses up to 2000 mg/kg in rats and up to 1000 mg/kg in marmosets, except for salivation and diarrhea in the rat and vomiting in the marmoset at the highest dose (31 and 18 times, respectively, the maximum recommended human dose on a mg/m^2 basis). (Calculations assume an oral dose of 160 mg/day and a 60-kg patient.)

Hydrochlorothiazide

The oral LD_{50} of hydrochlorothiazide is greater than 10 g/kg in both mice and rats, which represents 2027 and 4054 times, respectively, the maximum recommended human dose on a mg/m^2 basis. (Calculations assume an oral dose of 25 mg/day and a 60-kg patient.)

DOSAGE AND ADMINISTRATION

The recommended starting dose of valsartan is 80 mg or 160 mg once daily when used as monotherapy in patients who are not volume depleted. Patients requiring greater reductions may be started at the higher dose. Valsartan may be used over a dose range of 80 mg to 320 mg daily, administered once-a-day. Hydrochlorothiazide is effective in doses of 12.5 to 50 mg once daily, and can be given at doses of 12.5 mg to 25 mg as Diovan HCT® (valsartan and hydrochlorothiazide, USP).

To minimize dose-independent side effects, it is usually appropriate to begin combination therapy only after a patient has failed to achieve the desired effect with monotherapy.

The side effects *(see WARNINGS)* of valsartan are generally rare and apparently independent of dose; those of hydrochlorothiazide are a mixture of dose-dependent phenomena (primarily hypokalemia) and dose-independent phenomena (e.g., pancreatitis), the former much more common than the latter. Therapy with any combination of valsartan and hydrochlorothiazide will be associated with both sets of dose-independent side effects.

Replacement Therapy: The combination may be substituted for the titrated components.

Dose Titration by Clinical Effect: Diovan HCT tablets contain valsartan and hydrochlorothiazide, 80/12.5 mg, 160/12.5 mg and 160/25 mg. A patient whose blood pressure is not adequately controlled with valsartan monotherapy *(see above)* may add hydrochlorothiazide by switching to Diovan HCT (valsartan 80 mg/hydrochlorothiazide 12.5 mg or valsartan 160 mg/hydrochlorothiazide 12.5 mg) once daily. If blood pressure remains uncontrolled after about 3-4 weeks of therapy, either valsartan or both components may be increased depending on clinical response. There are no studies evaluating doses of valsartan greater than 160 mg in combination with hydrochlorothiazide 25 mg.

Continued on next page

Diovan HCT—Cont.

A patient whose blood pressure is inadequately controlled by 25 mg once daily of hydrochlorothiazide, or is controlled but who experiences hypokalemia with this regimen, may be switched to Diovan HCT (valsartan 80 mg/hydrochlorothiazide 12.5 mg or valsartan 160 mg/hydrochlorothiazide 12.5 mg) once daily, reducing the dose of hydrochlorothiazide without reducing the overall expected antihypertensive response. The clinical response to Diovan HCT should be subsequently evaluated and if blood pressure remains uncontrolled after 3-4 weeks of therapy, the dose may be titrated up to valsartan 160 mg/hydrochlorothiazide 25 mg.
The maximal antihypertensive effect is attained about 4 weeks after initiation of therapy.

Patients with Renal Impairment: The usual regimens of therapy with Diovan HCT may be followed as long as the creatinine clearance is >30 mL/min. In patients with more severe renal impairment, loop diuretics are preferred to thiazides, so Diovan HCT is not recommended.

Patients with Hepatic Impairment: Care should be exercised with dosing of Diovan HCT in patients with hepatic impairment.

Other: No initial dosage adjustment is required for elderly patients.
Diovan HCT may be administered with other antihypertensive agents.
Diovan HCT may be administered with or without food.

HOW SUPPLIED

Diovan HCT® (valsartan and hydrochlorothiazide, USP) is available as tablets containing valsartan/hydrochlorothiazide 80/12.5 mg, 160/12.5 mg and 160/25 mg. All strengths are packaged in bottles of 90 tablets and unit dose blister packages.

80/12.5 mg Tablet – Light orange, ovaloid with slightly convex faces debossed CG on one side HGH on the other side.
Bottles of 90 .... NDC 0078-0314-34
Unit Dose (blister pack) .... NDC 0078-0314-06
Box of 100 (strips of 10)

160/12.5 mg Tablet – Dark red, ovaloid with slightly convex faces debossed CG on one side HHH on the other side.
Bottles of 90 .... NDC 0078-0315-34
Unit Dose (blister pack) .... NDC 0078-0315-06
Box of 100 (strips of 10)

160/25 mg Tablet – Brown orange, ovaloid with slightly convex faces debossed NVR on one side HXH on the other side.
Bottles of 90 .... NDC 0078-0383-34
Unit Dose (blister pack) .... NDC 0078-0383-06
Box of 100 (strips of 10)

Store at 25°C (77°F); excursions permitted to 15-30°C (59-86°F)
[see USP Controlled Room Temperature].
Protect from moisture.
Dispense in tight container (USP).

T2003-74

REV: NOVEMBER 2003 Printed in U.S.A.
Distributed by:
Novartis Pharmaceuticals Corporation
East Hanover, New Jersey 07936
©Novartis

Shown in Product Identification Guide, page 325

ELIDEL® ℞

[ĕl-ĭ-dĕl]
(pimecrolimus) Cream 1%
FOR DERMATOLOGIC USE ONLY
NOT FOR OPHTHALMIC USE
Rx only

Prescribing Information

The following prescribing information is based on official labeling in effect July 2003.

DESCRIPTION

Elidel® (pimecrolimus) Cream 1% contains the compound pimecrolimus, the 33-epi-chloro-derivative of the macrolactam ascomycin.
Chemically, pimecrolimus is (1R,9S,12S,13R,14S,17R,18E, 21S,23S,24R,25S,27R)-12-[(1E)-2-[(1R,3R,4S)-4-chloro-3-methoxycyclohexyl]-1-methylvinyl]-17-ethyl-1,14-dihydroxy-23,25-dimethoxy-13,19,21,27-tetramethyl-11,28-dioxa-4-aza-tricyclo[22.3.1.$0^{4,9}$]octacos-18-ene-2,3,10,16-tetraone.
The compound has the empirical formula $C_{43}H_{68}ClNO_{11}$ and the molecular weight of 810.47. The structural formula is

Pimecrolimus is a white to off-white fine crystalline powder. It is soluble in methanol and ethanol and insoluble in water. Each gram of Elidel Cream 1% contains 10 mg of pimecrolimus in a whitish cream base of benzyl alcohol, cetyl alcohol, citric acid, mono- and di-glycerides, oleyl alcohol, propylene glycol, sodium cetostearyl sulphate, sodium hydroxide, stearyl alcohol, triglycerides, and water.

CLINICAL PHARMACOLOGY

Mechanism of Action/Pharmacodynamics

The mechanism of action of pimecrolimus in atopic dermatitis is not known. While the following have been observed, the clinical significance of these observations in atopic dermatitis is not known. It has been demonstrated that pimecrolimus binds with high affinity to macrophilin-12 (FKBP-12) and inhibits the calcium-dependent phosphatase, calcineurin. As a consequence, it inhibits T cell activation by blocking the transcription of early cytokines. In particular, pimecrolimus inhibits at nanomolar concentrations Interleukin-2 and interferon gamma (Th1-type) and Interleukin-4 and Interleukin-10 (Th2-type) cytokine synthesis in human T cells. In addition, pimecrolimus prevents the release of inflammatory cytokines and mediators from mast cells *in vitro* after stimulation by antigen/IgE.

Pharmacokinetics

Absorption

In adult patients being treated for atopic dermatitis [13%-62% Body Surface Area (BSA) involvement] for periods up to a year, blood concentrations of pimecrolimus are routinely either at or below the limit of quantification of the assay (< 0.5 ng/mL). In those subjects with detectable blood levels they are routinely < 2 ng/mL and show no sign of drug accumulation with time. Because of the low systemic absorption of pimecrolimus following topical application the calculation of standard pharmacokinetic measures such as AUC, C_{max}, $T_{1/2}$, et cetera cannot be reliably done.

Distribution

In vitro studies of the protein binding of pimecrolimus indicate that it is 74%-87% bound to plasma proteins.

Metabolism

Following the administration of a single oral radiolabeled dose of pimecrolimus numerous circulating O-demethylation metabolites were seen. Studies with human liver microsomes indicate that pimecrolimus is metabolized *in vitro* by the CYP3A sub-family of metabolizing enzymes. No evidence of skin mediated drug metabolism was identified *in vivo* using the minipig or *in vitro* using stripped human skin.

Elimination

Based on the results of the aforementioned radiolabeled study, following a single oral dose of pimecrolimus ~81% of the administered radioactivity was recovered, primarily in the feces (78.4%) as metabolites. Less than 1% of the radioactivity found in the feces was due to unchanged pimecrolimus.

Special Populations

Pediatrics

The systemic exposure to pimecrolimus from Elidel® (pimecrolimus) Cream 1% was investigated in 26 pediatric patients with atopic dermatitis (20%-69% BSA involvement) between the ages of 2-14 yrs. Following twice daily application for three weeks, blood concentrations of pimecrolimus were consistently low (< 3 ng/mL), with the majority of the blood samples being below the limit of quantification (0.5 ng/mL). However, the children (20 children out of the total 23 children investigated) had at least one detectable blood level as compared to the adults (13 adults out of the total 25 adults investigated) over a 3-week treatment period. Due to the low and erratic nature of the blood levels observed, no correlation could be made between amount of cream, degree of BSA involvement, and blood concentrations. In general, the blood concentrations measured in adult atopic dermatitis patients were comparable to those seen in the pediatric population.
In a second group of 22 pediatric patients aged 3-23 months with 10%-92% BSA involvement, a higher proportion of detectable blood levels was seen ranging from 0.1 ng/mL to 2.6 ng/mL (limit of quantification 0.1 ng/mL). This increase in the absolute number of positive blood levels may be due to the larger surface area to body mass ratio seen in these younger subjects. In addition, a higher incidence of upper respiratory symptoms/infections was also seen relative to the older age group in the PK studies. At this time a causal relationship between these findings and Elidel use cannot be ruled out. Use of Elidel in this population is not recommended *(see Pediatric Use)*.

Renal Insufficiency

The effect of renal insufficiency on the pharmacokinetics of topically administered pimecrolimus has not been evaluated. Given the very low systemic exposure of pimecrolimus via the topical route, no change in dosing is required.

Hepatic Insufficiency

The effect of hepatic insufficiency on the pharmacokinetics of topically administered pimecrolimus has not been evaluated. Given the very low systemic exposure of pimecrolimus via the topical route, no change in dosing is required.

CLINICAL STUDIES

Three randomized, double-blind, vehicle-controlled, multicenter, Phase 3 studies were conducted in 1335 pediatric patients ages 3 months-17 years old to evaluate Elidel® (pimecrolimus) Cream 1% for the treatment of mild to moderate atopic dermatitis. Two of the three trials support the use of Elidel Cream in patients 2 years and older with mild to moderate atopic dermatitis *(see Pediatric Use)*. Three other trials provided additional data regarding the safety of Elidel Cream in the treatment of atopic dermatitis. Two of these other trials were vehicle-controlled with optional sequential use of a medium potency topical corticosteroid in pediatric patients and one trial was an active comparator trial in adult patients with atopic dermatitis *(see Pediatric Use and ADVERSE REACTIONS)*.
Two identical 6-week, randomized, vehicle-controlled, multi-center, Phase 3 trials were conducted to evaluate Elidel Cream for the treatment of mild to moderate atopic dermatitis. A total of 403 pediatric patients 2-17 years old were included in the studies. The male/female ratio was approximately 50% and 29% of the patients were African American. At study entry, 59% of patients had moderate disease and the mean body surface area (BSA) affected was 26%. About 75% of patients had atopic dermatitis affecting the face and/or neck region. In these studies, patients applied either Elidel Cream or vehicle cream twice daily to 5% to 96% of their BSA for up to 6 weeks. At endpoint, based on the physician's global evaluation of clinical response, 35% of patients treated with Elidel Cream were clear or almost clear of signs of atopic dermatitis compared to only 18% of vehicle-treated patients. More Elidel patients (57%) had mild or no pruritus at 6 weeks compared to vehicle patients (34%). The improvement in pruritus occurred in conjunction with the improvement of the patients' atopic dermatitis.
In these two 6-week studies of Elidel, the combined efficacy results at endpoint are as follows:

	% Patients	
	Elidel® (N=267)	Vehicle (N=136)
Global Assessment		
Clear	28 (10%)	5 (4%)
Clear or Almost Clear	93 (35%)	25 (18%)
Clear to Mild Disease	180 (67%)	55 (40%)

In the two pediatric studies that independently support the use of Elidel Cream in mild to moderate atopic dermatitis, a significant treatment effect was seen by day 15. Of the key signs of atopic dermatitis, erythema, infiltration/papulation, lichenification, and excoriations, erythema and infiltration/papulation were reduced at day 8 when compared to vehicle.
The following graph depicts the time course of improvement in the percent body surface area affected as a result of treatment with Elidel Cream in 2-17 year olds.

Figure 1
Body Surface Area Over Time

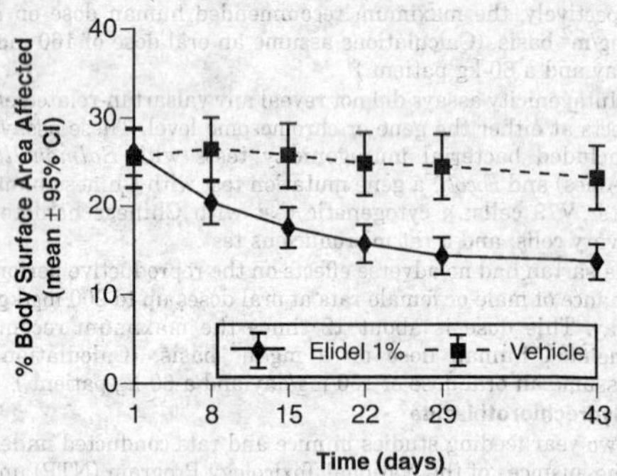

The following graph shows the time course of improvement in erythema as a result of treatment with Elidel Cream in 2-17 year olds.

Figure 2
Mean Erythema Over Time

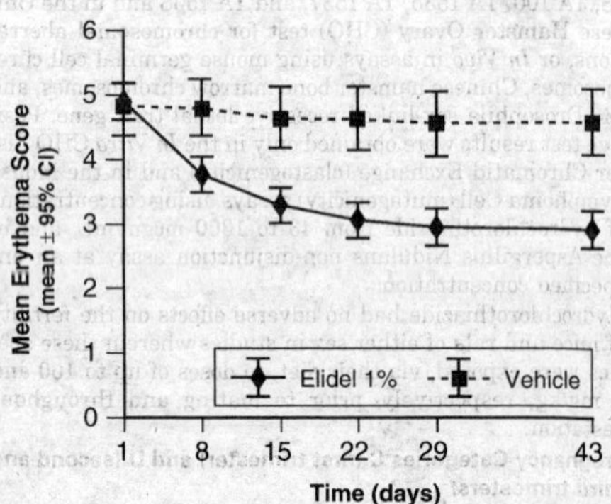

INDICATIONS AND USAGE

Elidel® (pimecrolimus) Cream 1% is indicated for short-term and intermittent long-term therapy in the treatment of *mild to moderate* atopic dermatitis in non-immunocompromised patients 2 years of age and older, in whom the use of alternative, conventional therapies is deemed inadvisable because of potential risks, or in the treatment of patients who are not adequately responsive to or intolerant of alternative, conventional therapies *(see DOSAGE AND ADMINISTRATION)*.

CONTRAINDICATIONS

Elidel® (pimecrolimus) Cream 1% is contraindicated in individuals with a history of hypersensitivity to pimecrolimus or any of the components of the cream.

PRECAUTIONS

General

Elidel® (pimecrolimus) Cream 1% should not be applied to areas of active cutaneous viral infections.

Studies have not evaluated the safety and efficacy of Elidel Cream in the treatment of clinically infected atopic dermatitis. Before commencing treatment with Elidel Cream, clinical infections at treatment sites should be cleared.

While patients with atopic dermatitis are predisposed to superficial skin infections including eczema herpeticum (Kaposi's varicelliform eruption), treatment with Elidel Cream may be associated with an increased risk of varicella zoster virus infection (chicken pox or shingles), herpes simplex virus infection, or eczema herpeticum. In the presence of these skin infections, the balance of risks and benefits associated with Elidel Cream use should be evaluated.

In clinical studies, 14 cases of lymphadenopathy (0.9%) were reported while using Elidel Cream. These cases of lymphadenopathy were usually related to infections and noted to resolve upon appropriate antibiotic therapy. Of these 14 cases, the majority had either a clear etiology or were known to resolve. Patients who receive Elidel Cream and who develop lymphadenopathy should have the etiology of their lymphadenopathy investigated. In the absence of a clear etiology for the lymphadenopathy, or in the presence of acute infectious mononucleosis, discontinuation of Elidel Cream should be considered. Patients who develop lymphadenopathy should be monitored to ensure that the lymphadenopathy resolves.

In clinical studies, 15 cases of skin papilloma or warts (1%) were observed in patients using Elidel Cream. The youngest patient was age 2 and the oldest was age 12. In cases where there is worsening of skin papillomas or they do not respond to conventional therapy, discontinuation of Elidel Cream should be considered until complete resolution of the warts is achieved.

The enhancement of ultraviolet carcinogenicity is not necessarily dependent on phototoxic mechanisms. Despite the absence of observed phototoxicity in humans *(see ADVERSE REACTIONS)*, Elidel Cream shortened the time to skin tumor formation in an animal photo-carcinogenicity study *(see Carcinogenesis, Mutagenesis, Impairment of Fertility)*. Therefore, it is prudent for patients to minimize or avoid natural or artificial sunlight exposure.

The use of Elidel Cream in patients with Netherton's Syndrome is not recommended due to the potential for increased systemic absorption of pimecrolimus.

There are no data to support use of Elidel in immunocompromised patients.

The use of Elidel Cream may cause local symptoms such as skin burning. Localized symptoms are most common during the first few days of Elidel Cream application and typically improve as the lesions of atopic dermatitis resolve. Most application site reactions lasted no more than 5 days, were mild to moderate in severity, and started within 1-5 days of treatment. *(See ADVERSE REACTIONS.)*

Information for Patients

Patients using Elidel should receive the following information and instructions:

- Patients should use Elidel Cream as directed by the physician. Elidel Cream is for external use on the skin only. As with any topical medication, patients or caregivers should wash hands after application if hands are not an area for treatment.
- Patients should minimize or avoid exposure to natural or artificial sunlight (tanning beds or UVA/B treatment) while using Elidel Cream.
- Patients should not use this medication for any disorder other than that for which it was prescribed.
- Patients should report any signs or symptoms of adverse reactions to their physician.
- Therapy should be discontinued after signs and symptoms of atopic dermatitis have resolved. Treatment with Elidel should be resumed at the first signs or symptoms of recurrence.
- Use of Elidel may cause reactions at the site of application such as a mild to moderate feeling of warmth and/or sensation of burning. Patients should see a physician if an application site reaction is severe or persists for more than 1 week.
- The patient should contact the physician if no improvement in the atopic dermatitis is seen following 6 weeks of treatment, or if at any time the condition worsens.

Drug Interactions

Potential interactions between Elidel and other drugs, including immunizations, have not been systematically evaluated. Due to the very low blood levels of pimecrolimus detected in some patients after topical application, systemic drug interactions are not expected, but cannot be ruled out. The concomitant administration of known CYP3A family of inhibitors in patients with widespread and/or erythrodermic disease should be done with caution. Some examples of such drugs are erythromycin, itraconazole, ketoconazole, fluconazole, calcium channel blockers and cimetidine.

Carcinogenesis, Mutagenesis, Impairment of Fertility

In a 2-year rat dermal carcinogenicity study using Elidel Cream, a statistically significant increase in the incidence of follicular cell adenoma of the thyroid was noted in low, mid and high dose male animals compared to vehicle and saline control male animals. Follicular cell adenoma of the thyroid was noted in the dermal rat carcinogenicity study at the lowest dose of 2 mg/kg/day [0.2% pimecrolimus cream; 1.5× the Maximum Recommended Human Dose (MRHD) based on AUC comparisons]. No increase in the incidence of follicular cell adenoma of the thyroid was noted in the oral carcinogenicity study in male rats up to 10 mg/kg/day (66× MRHD based on AUC comparisons). However, oral studies may not reflect continuous exposure or the same metabolic profile as by the dermal route. In a mouse dermal carcinogenicity study using pimecrolimus in an ethanolic solution, no increase in incidence of neoplasms was observed in the skin or other organs up to the highest dose of 4 mg/kg/day (0.32% pimecrolimus in ethanol) 27× MRHD based on AUC comparisons. However, lymphoproliferative changes (including lymphoma) were noted in a 13 week repeat dose dermal toxicity study conducted in mice using pimecrolimus in an ethanolic solution at a dose of 25 mg/kg/day (47× MRHD based on AUC comparisons). No lymphoproliferative changes were noted in this study at a dose of 10 mg/kg/day (17× MRHD based on AUC comparison). However, the latency time to lymphoma formation was shortened to 8 weeks after dermal administration of pimecrolimus dissolved in ethanol at a dose of 100 mg/kg/day (179-217× MRHD based on AUC comparisons).

In a mouse oral (gavage) carcinogenicity study, a statistically significant increase in the incidence of lymphoma was noted in high dose male and female animals compared to vehicle control male and female animals. Lymphomas were noted in the oral mouse carcinogenicity study at a dose of 45 mg/kg/day (258-340× MRHD based on AUC comparisons). No drug-related tumors were noted in the mouse oral carcinogenicity study at a dose of 15 mg/kg/day (60-133× MRHD based on AUC comparisons). In an oral (gavage) rat carcinogenicity study, a statistically significant increase in the incidence of benign thymoma was noted in 10 mg/kg/day pimecrolimus treated male and female animals compared to vehicle control treated male and female animals. In addition, a significant increase in the incidence of benign thymoma was noted in another oral (gavage) rat carcinogenicity study in 5 mg/kg/day pimecrolimus treated male animals compared to vehicle control treated male animals. No drug-related tumors were noted in the rat oral carcinogenicity study at a dose of 1 mg/kg/day male animals (1.1× MRHD based on AUC comparisons) and at a dose of 5 mg/kg/day for female animals (21× MRHD based on AUC comparisons).

In a 52-week dermal photo-carcinogenicity study, the median time to onset of skin tumor formation was decreased in hairless mice following chronic topical dosing with concurrent exposure to UV radiation (40 weeks of treatment followed by 12 weeks of observation) with the Elidel Cream vehicle alone. No additional effect on tumor development beyond the vehicle effect was noted with the addition of the active ingredient, pimecrolimus, to the vehicle cream.

A battery of *in vitro* genotoxicity tests, including Ames assay, mouse lymphoma L5178Y assay, and chromosome aberration test in V79 Chinese hamster cells and an *in vivo* mouse micronucleus test revealed no evidence for a mutagenic or clastogenic potential for the drug.

An oral fertility and embryofetal developmental study in rats revealed estrus cycle disturbances, post-implantation loss and reduction in litter size at the 45 mg/kg/day dose (38× MRHD based on AUC comparisons). No effect on fertility in female rats was noted at 10 mg/kg/day (12× MRHD based on AUC comparisons). No effect on fertility in male rats was noted at 45 mg/kg/day (23× MRHD based on AUC comparisons), which was the highest dose tested in this study.

Pregnancy

Teratogenic Effects: Pregnancy Category C

There are no adequate and well-controlled studies of topically administered pimecrolimus in pregnant women. The experience with Elidel Cream when used by pregnant women is too limited to permit assessment of the safety of its use during pregnancy.

In dermal embryofetal developmental studies, no maternal or fetal toxicity was observed up to the highest practicable doses tested, 10 mg/kg/day (1% pimecrolimus cream) in rats (0.14× MRHD based on body surface area) and 10 mg/kg/day (1% pimecrolimus cream) in rabbits (0.65× MRHD based on AUC comparisons). The 1% pimecrolimus cream was administered topically for 6 hours/day during the period of organogenesis in rats and rabbits (gestational days 6-21 in rats and gestational days 6-20 in rabbits).

A combined oral fertility and embryofetal developmental study was conducted in rats and an oral embryofetal developmental study was conducted in rabbits. Pimecrolimus was administered during the period of organogenesis (2 weeks prior to mating until gestational day 16 in rats, gestational days 6-18 in rabbits) up to dose levels of 45 mg/kg/day in rats and 20 mg/kg/day in rabbits. In the absence of maternal toxicity, indicators of embryofetal toxicity (post-implantation loss and reduction in litter size) were noted at 45 mg/kg/day (38× MRHD based on AUC comparisons) in the oral fertility and embryofetal developmental study conducted in rats. No malformations in the fetuses were noted at 45 mg/kg/day (38× MRHD based on AUC comparisons) in this study. No maternal toxicity, embryotoxicity or teratogenicity were noted in the oral rabbit embryofetal developmental toxicity study at 20 mg/kg/day (3.9× MRHD based on AUC comparisons), which was the highest dose tested in this study.

An oral peri- and post-natal developmental study was conducted in rats. Pimecrolimus was administered from gestational day 6 through lactational day 21 up to a dose level of 40 mg/kg/day. Only 2 of 22 females delivered live pups at the highest dose of 40 mg/kg/day. Postnatal survival, development of the F1 generation, their subsequent maturation and fertility were not affected at 10 mg/kg/day (12× MRHD based on AUC comparisons), the highest dose evaluated in this study.

Pimecrolimus was transferred across the placenta in oral rat and rabbit embryofetal developmental studies.

There are, however, no adequate and well-controlled studies in pregnant women. Because animal reproduction studies are not always predictive of human response, this drug should be used only if clearly needed during pregnancy.

Nursing Mothers

It is not known whether this drug is excreted in human milk. Because of the potential for serious adverse reactions in nursing infants from pimecrolimus, a decision should be made whether to discontinue nursing or to discontinue the drug, taking into account the importance of the drug to the mother.

Pediatric Use

Elidel Cream may be used in pediatric patients 2 years of age and older. Three Phase 3 pediatric studies were conducted involving 1114 patients 2-17 years of age. Two studies were 6-week randomized vehicle-controlled studies with a 20-week open-label phase and one was a vehicle-controlled long-term (up to 1 year) safety study with the option for sequential topical corticosteroid use. Of these patients 542 (49%) were 2-6 years of age. In the short-term studies, 11% of Elidel patients did not complete these studies and 1.5% of Elidel patients discontinued due to adverse events. In the one-year study, 32% of Elidel patients did not complete this study and 3% of Elidel patients discontinued due to adverse events. Most discontinuations were due to unsatisfactory therapeutic effect.

The most common local adverse event in the short-term studies of Elidel Cream in pediatric patients ages 2-17 was application site burning (10% vs. 13% vehicle); the incidence in the long-term study was 9% Elidel vs. 7% vehicle *(see ADVERSE REACTIONS)*. Adverse events that were more frequent (> 5%) in patients treated with Elidel Cream compared to vehicle were headache (14% vs. 9%) in the short-term trial. Nasopharyngitis (26% vs. 21%), influenza (13% vs. 4%), pharyngitis (8% vs. 3%), viral infection (7% vs. 1%), pyrexia (13% vs. 5%), cough (16% vs. 11%), and headache (25% vs. 16%) were increased over vehicle in the 1-year safety study *(see ADVERSE REACTIONS)*. In 843 patients ages 2-17 years treated with Elidel Cream, 9 (0.8%) developed eczema herpeticum (5 on Elidel Cream alone and 4 on Elidel Cream used in sequence with corticosteroids). In 211 patients on vehicle alone, there were no cases of eczema herpeticum. The majority of adverse events were mild to moderate in severity.

Elidel Cream is not recommended for use in pediatric patients below the age of 2 years. Two Phase 3 studies were conducted involving 436 infants age 3 months - 23 months. One 6-week randomized vehicle-controlled study with a 20-week open-label phase and one long term safety study were conducted. In the 6-week study, 11% of Elidel and 48% of vehicle patients did not complete this study; no patient in either group discontinued due to adverse events. Infants on Elidel Cream had an increased incidence of some adverse events compared to vehicle. In the 6-week vehicle-controlled study these adverse events included pyrexia (32% vs. 13% vehicle), URI (24% vs. 14%), nasopharyngitis (15% vs. 8%), gastroenteritis (7% vs. 3%), otitis media (4% vs. 0%), and diarrhea (8% vs. 0%). In the open-label phase of the study, for infants who switched to Elidel Cream from vehicle, the incidence of the above-cited adverse events approached or equaled the incidence of those patients who remained on Elidel Cream. In the 6-month safety data, 16% of Elidel and 35% of vehicle patients discontinued early and 1.5% of Elidel and 0% of vehicle patients discontinued due to adverse events. Infants on Elidel Cream had a greater incidence of some adverse events as compared to vehicle. These included pyrexia (30% vs. 20%), URI (21% vs. 17%), cough (15% vs. 9%), hypersensitivity (8% vs. 2%), teething (27% vs. 22%), vomiting (9% vs. 4%), rhinitis (13% vs. 9%), viral rash (4% vs. 0%), rhinorrhea (4% vs. 0%), and wheezing (4% vs. 0%).

The effects of Elidel Cream on the developing immune system in infants are unknown.

Geriatric Use

Nine (9) patients ≥ 65 years old received Elidel Cream in Phase 3 studies. Clinical studies of Elidel did not include sufficient numbers of patients aged 65 and over to assess efficacy and safety.

ADVERSE REACTIONS

In human dermal safety studies, Elidel® (pimecrolimus) Cream 1% did not induce contact sensitization, phototoxicity, or photoallergy, nor did it show any cumulative irritation.

In a one-year safety study in pediatric patients age 2-17 years old involving sequential use of Elidel Cream and a

Continued on next page

Elidel—Cont.

topical corticosteroid, 43% of Elidel patients and 68% of vehicle patients used corticosteroids during the study. Corticosteroids were used for more than 7 days by 34% of Elidel patients and 54% of vehicle patients. An increased incidence of impetigo, skin infection, superinfection (infected atopic dermatitis), rhinitis, and urticaria were found in the patients that had used Elidel Cream and topical corticosteroid sequentially as compared to Elidel Cream alone.

In 3 randomized, double-blind vehicle-controlled pediatric studies and one active-controlled adult study, 843 and 328 patients respectively, were treated with Elidel Cream. In these clinical trials, 48 (4%) of the 1171 Elidel patients and 13 (3%) of 408 vehicle-treated patients discontinued therapy due to adverse events. Discontinuations for AEs were primarily due to application site reactions, and cutaneous infections. The most common application site reaction was application site burning, which occurred in 8%-26% of patients treated with Elidel Cream.

The following table depicts the incidence of adverse events pooled across the 2 identically designed 6-week studies with their open label extensions and the 1-year safety study for pediatric patients ages 2-17. Data from the adult active-controlled study is also included in this table. Adverse events are listed regardless of relationship to study drug. [See table below]

Treatment Emergent Adverse Events (≥ 1%) in Elidel® Treatment Groups

	Pediatric Patients* Vehicle-Controlled (6 weeks)		Pediatric Patients* Open-Label (20 weeks)	Pediatric Patients* Vehicle-Controlled (1 year)		Adult Active Comparator (1 year)
	Elidel® Cream (N=267) N (%)	Vehicle (N=136) N (%)	Elidel® Cream (N=335) N (%)	Elidel® Cream (N=272) N (%)	Vehicle (N=75) N (%)	Elidel® Cream (N=328) N (%)
At least 1 AE	182 (68.2%)	97 (71.3%)	240 (72.0%)	230 (84.6%)	56 (74.7%)	256 (78.0%)
Infections and Infestations						
Upper Respiratory Tract Infection NOS	38 (14.2%)	18 (13.2%)	65 (19.4%)	13 (4.8%)	6 (8.0%)	14 (4.3%)
Nasopharyngitis	27 (10.1%)	10 (7.4%)	32 (19.6%)	72 (26.5%)	16 (21.3%)	25 (7.6%)
Skin Infection NOS	8 (3.0%)	9 (5.1%)	18 (5.4%)	6 (2.2%)	3 (4.0%)	21 (6.4%)
Influenza	8 (3.0%)	1 (0.7%)	22 (6.6%)	36 (13.2%)	3 (4.0%)	32 (9.8%)
Ear Infection NOS	6 (2.2%)	2 (1.5%)	19 (5.7%)	9 (3.3%)	1 (1.3%)	2 (0.6%)
Otitis Media	6 (2.2%)	1 (0.7%)	10 (3.0%)	8 (2.9%)	4 (5.3%)	2 (0.6%)
Impetigo	5 (1.9%)	3 (2.2%)	12 (3.6%)	11 (4.0%)	4 (5.3%)	8 (2.4%)
Bacterial Infection	4 (1.5%)	3 (2.2%)	4 (1.2%)	3 (1.1%)	0	6 (1.8%)
Folliculitis	3 (1.1%)	1 (0.7%)	3 (0.9%)	6 (2.2%)	3 (4.0%)	20 (6.1%)
Sinusitis	3 (1.1%)	1 (0.7%)	11 (3.3%)	6 (2.2%)	1 (1.3%)	2 (0.6%)
Pneumonia NOS	3 (1.1%)	1 (0.7%)	5 (1.5%)	0	1 (1.3%)	1 (0.3%)
Pharyngitis NOS	2 (0.7%)	2 (1.5%)	3 (0.9%)	22 (8.1%)	2 (2.7%)	3 (0.9%)
Pharyngitis Streptococcal	2 (0.7%)	2 (1.5%)	10 (3.0%)	0	<1%	0
Molluscum Contagiosum	2 (0.7%)	0	4 (1.2%)	5 (1.8%)	0	0
Staphylococcal Infection	1 (0.4%)	5 (3.7%)	7 (2.1%)	0	<1%	3 (0.9%)
Bronchitis NOS	1 (0.4%)	3 (2.2%)	4 (1.2%)	29 (10.7%)	6 (8.0%)	8 (2.4%)
Herpes Simplex	1 (0.4%)	0	4 (1.2%)	9 (3.3%)	2 (2.7%)	13 (4.0%)
Tonsillitis NOS	1 (0.4%)	0	3 (0.9%)	17 (6.3%)	0	2 (0.6%)
Viral Infection NOS	2 (0.7%)	1 (0.7%)	1 (0.3%)	18 (6.6%)	1 (1.3%)	0
Gastroenteritis NOS	0	3 (2.2%)	2 (0.6%)	20 (7.4%)	2 (2.7%)	6 (1.8%)
Chickenpox	2 (0.7%)	0	3 (0.9%)	8 (2.9%)	3 (4.0%)	1 (0.3%)
Skin Papilloma	1 (0.4%)	0	2 (0.6%)	9 (3.3%)	<1%	0
Tonsillitis Acute NOS	0	0	0	7 (2.6%)	0	0
Upper Respiratory Tract Infection Viral NOS	1 (0.4%)	0	3 (0.9%)	4 (1.5%)	0	1 (0.3%)
Herpes Simplex Dermatitis	0	0	1 (0.3%)	4 (1.5%)	0	2 (0.6%)
Bronchitis Acute NOS	0	0	0	4 (1.5%)	0	0
Eye Infection NOS	0	0	0	3 (1.1%)	<1%	1 (0.3%)
General Disorders and Administration Site Conditions						
Application Site Burning	28 (10.4%)	17 (12.5%)	5 (1.5%)	23 (8.5%)	5 (6.7%)	85 (25.9%)
Pyrexia	20 (7.5%)	12 (8.8%)	41 (12.2%)	34 (12.5%)	4 (5.3%)	4 (1.2%)
Application Site Reaction NOS	8 (3.0%)	7 (5.1%)	7 (2.1%)	9 (3.3%)	2 (2.7%)	48 (14.6%)
Application Site Irritation	8 (3.0%)	8 (5.9%)	3 (0.9%)	1 (0.4%)	3 (4.0%)	21 (6.4%)
Influenza Like Illness	1 (0.4%)	0	2 (0.6%)	5 (1.8%)	2 (2.7%)	6 (1.8%)
Application Site Erythema	1 (0.4%)	0	0	6 (2.2%)	0	7 (2.1%)
Application Site Pruritus	3 (1.1%)	2 (1.5%)	2 (0.6%)	5 (1.8%)	0	18 (5.5%)
Respiratory, Thoracic and Mediastinal Disorders						
Cough	31 (11.6%)	11 (8.1%)	31 (9.3%)	43 (15.8%)	8 (10.7%)	8 (2.4%)
Nasal Congestion	7 (2.6%)	2 (1.5%)	6 (1.8%)	4 (1.5%)	1 (1.3%)	2 (0.6%)
Rhinorrhea	5 (1.9%)	1 (0.7%)	3 (0.9%)	1 (0.4%)	1 (1.3%)	0
Asthma Aggravated	4 (1.5%)	3 (2.2%)	13 (3.9%)	3 (1.1%)	1 (1.3%)	0
Sinus Congestion	3 (1.1%)	1 (0.7%)	2 (0.6%)	<1%	<1%	3 (0.9%)
Rhinitis	1 (0.4%)	0	5 (1.5%)	12 (4.4%)	5 (6.7%)	7 (2.1%)
Wheezing	1 (0.4%)	1 (0.7%)	4 (1.2%)	2 (0.7%)	<1%	0
Asthma NOS	2 (0.7%)	1 (0.7%)	11 (3.3%)	10 (3.7%)	2 (2.7%)	8 (2.4%)
Epistaxis	0	1 (0.7%)	0	9 (3.3%)	1 (1.3%)	1 (0.3%)
Dyspnea NOS	0	0	0	5 (1.8%)	1 (1.3%)	2 (0.6%)
Gastrointestinal Disorders						
Abdominal Pain Upper	11 (4.1%)	6 (4.4%)	10 (3.0%)	15 (5.5%)	5 (6.7%)	1 (0.3%)
Sore Throat	9 (3.4%)	5 (3.7%)	15 (5.4%)	22 (8.1%)	4 (5.3%)	12 (3.7%)
Vomiting NOS	8 (3.0%)	6 (4.4%)	14 (4.2%)	18 (6.6%)	6 (8.0%)	2 (0.6%)
Diarrhea NOS	3 (1.1%)	1 (0.7%)	2 (0.6%)	21 (7.7%)	4 (5.3%)	7 (2.1%)
Nausea	1 (0.4%)	3 (2.2%)	4 (1.2%)	11 (4.0%)	5 (6.7%)	6 (1.8%)
Abdominal Pain NOS	1 (0.4%)	1 (0.7%)	5 (1.5%)	12 (4.4%)	3 (4.0%)	1 (0.3%)
Toothache	1 (0.4%)	1 (0.7%)	2 (0.6%)	7 (2.6%)	1 (1.3%)	2 (0.6%)
Constipation	1 (0.4%)	0	2 (0.6%)	10 (3.7%)	<1%	0
Loose Stools	0	1 (0.7%)	4 (1.2%)	<1%	<1%	0
Reproductive System and Breast Disorders						
Dysmenorrhea	3 (1.1%)	0	5 (1.5%)	3 (1.1%)	1 (1.3%)	4 (1.2%)
Eye Disorders						
Conjunctivitis NEC	2 (0.7%)	1 (0.7%)	7 (2.1%)	6 (2.2%)	3 (4.0%)	10 (3.0%)
Skin & Subcutaneous Tissue Disorders						
Urticaria	3 (1.1%)	0	1 (0.3%)	1 (0.4%)	<1%	3 (0.9%)
Acne NOS	0	1 (0.7%)	1 (0.3%)	4 (1.5%)	<1%	6 (1.8%)
Immune System Disorders						
Hypersensitivity NOS	11 (4.1%)	6 (4.4%)	16 (4.8%)	14 (5.1%)	1 (1.3%)	11 (3.4%)
Injury and Poisoning						
Accident NOS	3 (1.1%)	1 (0.7%)	1 (0.3%)	<1%	1 (1.3%)	0
Laceration	2 (0.7%)	1 (0.7%)	5 (1.5%)	<1%	<1%	0
Musculoskeletal, Connective Tissue and Bone Disorders						
Back Pain	1 (0.4%)	2 (1.5%)	1 (0.3%)	<1%	0	6 (1.8%)
Arthralgias	0	0	1 (0.3%)	3 (1.1%)	1 (1.3%)	5 (1.5%)
Ear and Labyrinth Disorders						
Earache	2 (0.7%)	1 (0.7%)	0	8 (2.9%)	2 (2.7%)	0
Nervous System Disorders						
Headache	37 (13.9%)	12 (8.8%)	38 (11.3%)	69 (25.4%)	12 (16.0%)	23 (7.0%)

*Ages 2-17 years

OVERDOSAGE

There has been no experience of overdose with Elidel® (pimecrolimus) Cream 1%. No incidents of accidental ingestion have been reported. If oral ingestion occurs, medical advice should be sought.

DOSAGE AND ADMINISTRATION

Apply a thin layer of Elidel® (pimecrolimus) Cream 1% to the affected skin twice daily and rub in gently and completely. Elidel may be used on all skin surfaces, including the head, neck, and intertriginous areas.

Elidel should be used twice daily for as long as signs and symptoms persist. Treatment should be discontinued if resolution of disease occurs. If symptoms persist beyond 6 weeks, the patient should be re-evaluated.

The safety of Elidel Cream under occlusion, which may promote systemic exposure, has not been evaluated. **Elidel Cream should not be used with occlusive dressings.**

HOW SUPPLIED

Elidel® (pimecrolimus) Cream 1% is available in tubes of 15 grams, 30 grams, 60 grams, and 100 grams.

15 gram tube .... NDC 0078-0375-40
30 gram tube .... NDC 0078-0375-46
60 gram tube .... NDC 0078-0375-49
100 gram tube .... NDC 0078-0375-63

Store at 25°C (77°F); excursions permitted to 15°C-30°C (59°F-86°F). Do not freeze.

Manufactured by:
Novartis Pharma GmbH
Wehr, Germany
Distributed by:
Novartis Pharmaceuticals Corp.
East Hanover, NJ 07936

T2003-01
REV: APRIL 2003 89012002
492362/1 US

EXELON® ℞

[ĕx ′ ə-lŏn]
(rivastigmine tartrate)
Capsules
Rx only

Prescribing Information

The following prescribing information is based on official labeling in effect July 2004.

DESCRIPTION

Exelon® (rivastigmine tartrate) is a reversible cholinesterase inhibitor and is known chemically as (S)-N-Ethyl-N-methyl-3-[1-(dimethylamino)ethyl]-phenyl carbamate hydrogen-(2R,3R)-tartrate. Rivastigmine tartrate is commonly referred to in the pharmacological literature as SDZ ENA 713 or ENA 713. It has an empirical formula of $C_{14}H_{22}N_2O_2 \bullet C_4H_6O_6$ (hydrogen tartrate salt – hta salt) and a molecular weight of 400.43 (hta salt). Rivastigmine tartrate is a white to off-white, fine crystalline powder that is very soluble in water, soluble in ethanol and acetonitrile, slightly soluble in n-octanol and very slightly soluble in ethyl acetate. The distribution coefficient at 37°C in n-octanol/phosphate buffer solution pH 7 is 3.0.

Exelon is supplied as capsules containing rivastigmine tartrate, equivalent to 1.5, 3, 4.5 and 6 mg of rivastigmine base for oral administration. Inactive ingredients are hydroxypropyl methylcellulose, magnesium stearate, microcrystalline cellulose, and silicon dioxide. Each hard-gelatin capsule contains gelatin, titanium dioxide and red and/or yellow iron oxides.

CLINICAL PHARMACOLOGY

Mechanism of Action

Pathological changes in Dementia of the Alzheimer type involve cholinergic neuronal pathways that project from the basal forebrain to the cerebral cortex and hippocampus. These pathways are thought to be intricately involved in memory, attention, learning, and other cognitive processes. While the precise mechanism of rivastigmine's action is unknown, it is postulated to exert its therapeutic effect by enhancing cholinergic function. This is accomplished by increasing the concentration of acetylcholine through reversible inhibition of its hydrolysis by cholinesterase. If this proposed mechanism is correct, Exelon's effect may lessen as the disease process advances and fewer cholinergic neurons remain functionally intact. There is no evidence that rivastigmine alters the course of the underlying dementing process. After a 6-mg dose of rivastigmine, anticholinesterase activity is present in CSF for about 10 hours, with a maximum inhibition of about 60% five hours after dosing.

In vitro and *in vivo* studies demonstrate that the inhibition of cholinesterase by rivastigmine is not affected by the concomitant administration of memantine, an N-methyl-D-aspartate receptor antagonist.

Clinical Trial Data

The effectiveness of Exelon® (rivastigmine tartrate) as a treatment for Alzheimer's Disease is demonstrated by the results of two randomized, double-blind, placebo-controlled clinical investigations in patients with Alzheimer's Disease [diagnosed by NINCDS-ADRDA and DSM-IV criteria, Mini-Mental State Examination (MMSE) ≥10 and ≤26, and the Global Deterioration Scale (GDS)]. The mean age of patients participating in Exelon trials was 73 years with a range of 41-95. Approximately 59% of patients were women and 41% were men. The racial distribution was Caucasian 87%, Black 4% and Other races 9%.

Study Outcome Measures: In each study, the effectiveness of Exelon was evaluated using a dual outcome assessment strategy.

The ability of Exelon to improve cognitive performance was assessed with the cognitive subscale of the Alzheimer's Disease Assessment Scale (ADAS-cog), a multi item instrument that has been extensively validated in longitudinal cohorts of Alzheimer's Disease patients. The ADAS-cog examines selected aspects of cognitive performance including elements of memory, orientation, attention, reasoning, language and praxis. The ADAS-cog scoring range is from 0 to 70, with higher scores indicating greater cognitive impairment. Elderly normal adults may score as low as 0 or 1, but it is not unusual for non-demented adults to score slightly higher.

The patients recruited as participants in each study had mean scores on ADAS-cog of approximately 23 units, with a range from 1 to 61. Experience gained in longitudinal studies of ambulatory patients with mild to moderate Alzheimer's Disease suggest that they gain 6-12 units a year on the ADAS-cog. Lesser degrees of change, however, are seen in patients with very mild or very advanced disease because the ADAS-cog is not uniformly sensitive to change over the course of the disease. The annualized rate of decline in the placebo patients participating in Exelon trials was approximately 3-8 units per year.

The ability of Exelon to produce an overall clinical effect was assessed using a Clinician's Interview Based Impression of Change that required the use of caregiver information, the CIBIC-Plus. The CIBIC-Plus is not a single instrument and is not a standardized instrument like the ADAS-cog. Clinical trials for investigational drugs have used a variety of CIBIC formats, each different in terms of depth and structure. As such, results from a CIBIC-Plus reflect clinical experience from the trial or trials in which it was used and can not be compared directly with the results of CIBIC-Plus evaluations from other clinical trials. The CIBIC-Plus used in the Exelon trials was a structured instrument based on a comprehensive evaluation at baseline and subsequent time-points of three domains: patient cognition, behavior and functioning, including assessment of activities of daily living. It represents the assessment of a skilled clinician using validated scales based on his/her observation at interviews conducted separately with the patient and the caregiver familiar with the behavior of the patient over the interval rated. The CIBIC-Plus is scored as a seven point categorical rating, ranging from a score of 1, indicating "markedly improved," to a score of 4, indicating "no change" to a score of 7, indicating "marked worsening." The CIBIC-Plus has not been systematically compared directly to assessments not using information from caregivers (CIBIC) or other global methods.

U.S. Twenty-Six-Week Study

In a study of 26 weeks duration, 699 patients were randomized to either a dose range of 1-4 mg or 6-12 mg of Exelon per day or to placebo, each given in divided doses. The 26-week study was divided into a 12-week forced dose titration phase and a 14-week maintenance phase. The patients in the active treatment arms of the study were maintained at their highest tolerated dose within the respective range.

Effects on the ADAS-cog: Figure 1 illustrates the time course for the change from baseline in ADAS-cog scores for all three dose groups over the 26 weeks of the study. At 26 weeks of treatment, the mean differences in the ADAS-cog change scores for the Exelon-treated patients compared to the patients on placebo were 1.9 and 4.9 units for the 1-4 mg and 6-12 mg treatments, respectively. Both treatments were statistically significantly superior to placebo and the 6-12 mg/day range was significantly superior to the 1-4 mg/day range.

[See figure 1 at top of next column]

Figure 2 illustrates the cumulative percentages of patients from each of the three treatment groups who had attained at least the measure of improvement in ADAS-cog score shown on the X axis. Three change scores, (7-point and 4-point reductions from baseline or no change in score) have been identified for illustrative purposes, and the percent of patients in each group achieving that result is shown in the inset table.

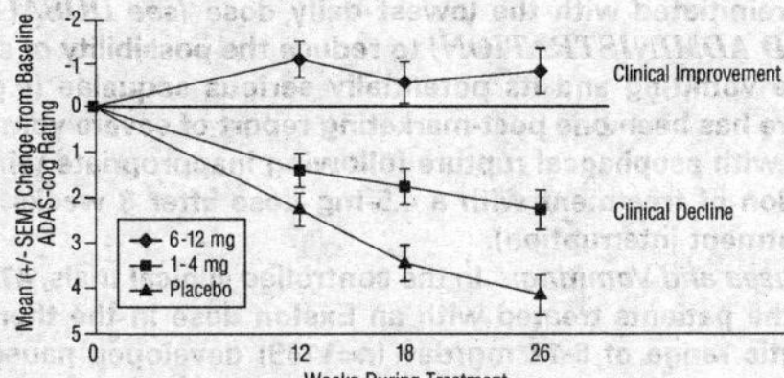

Figure 1: Time-course of the Change from Baseline in ADAS-cog Score for Patients Completing 26 Weeks of Treatment

The curves demonstrate that both patients assigned to Exelon and placebo have a wide range of responses, but that the Exelon groups are more likely to show the greater improvements. A curve for an effective treatment would be shifted to the left of the curve for placebo, while an ineffective or deleterious treatment would be superimposed upon, or shifted to the right of the curve for placebo, respectively.

Figure 2: Cumulative Percentage of Patients Completing 26 Weeks of Double-blind Treatment with Specified Changes from Baseline ADAS-cog Scores. The Percentages of Randomized Patients who Completed the Study were: Placebo 84%, 1-4 mg 85%, and 6-12 mg 65%.

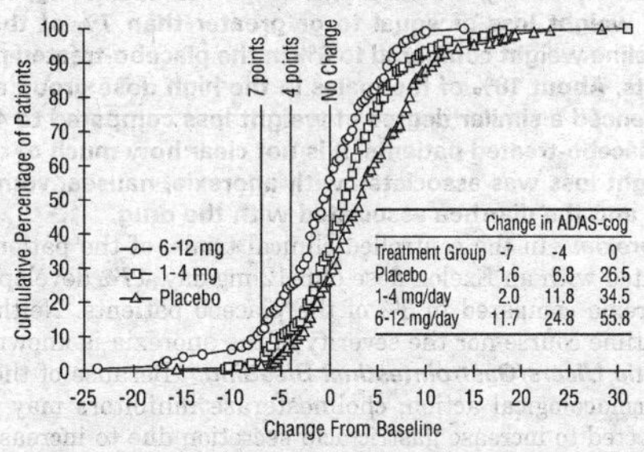

Effects on the CIBIC-Plus: Figure 3 is a histogram of the frequency distribution of CIBIC-Plus scores attained by patients assigned to each of the three treatment groups who completed 26 weeks of treatment. The mean Exelon-placebo differences for these groups of patients in the mean rating of change from baseline were 0.32 units and 0.35 units for 1-4 mg and 6-12 mg of Exelon, respectively. The mean ratings for the 6-12 mg/day and 1-4 mg/day groups were statistically significantly superior to placebo. The differences between the 6-12 mg/day and the 1-4 mg/day groups were statistically significant.

Figure 3: Frequency Distribution of CIBIC-Plus Scores at Week 26

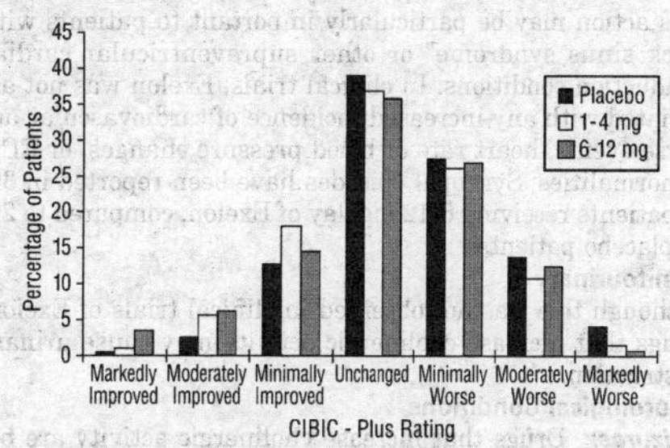

Global Twenty-Six-Week Study

In a second study of 26 weeks duration, 725 patients were randomized to either a dose range of 1-4 mg or 6-12 mg of Exelon per day or to placebo, each given in divided doses. The 26-week study was divided into a 12-week forced dose titration phase and a 14-week maintenance phase. The patients in the active treatment arms of the study were maintained at their highest tolerated dose within the respective range.

Effects on the ADAS-cog: Figure 4 illustrates the time course for the change from baseline in ADAS-cog scores for all three dose groups over the 26 weeks of the study. At 26 weeks of treatment, the mean differences in the ADAS-cog change scores for the Exelon-treated patients compared to the patients on placebo were 0.2 and 2.6 units for the 1-4 mg and 6-12 mg treatments, respectively. The 6-12 mg/day group was statistically significantly superior to placebo, as well as to the 1-4 mg/day group. The difference between the 1-4 mg/day group and placebo was not statistically significant.

Figure 4: Time-course of the Change from Baseline in ADAS-cog Score for Patients Completing 26 Weeks of Treatment

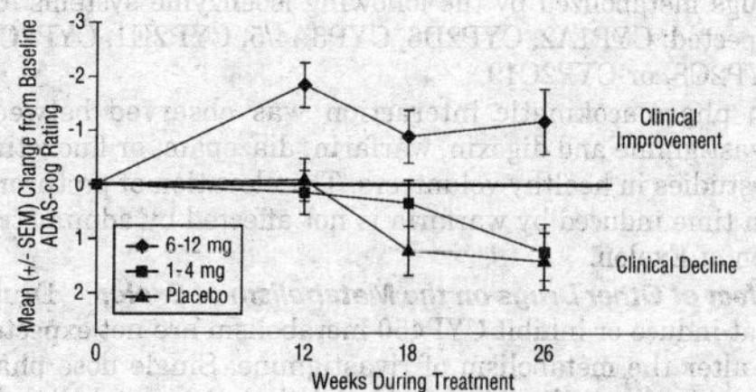

Figure 5 illustrates the cumulative percentages of patients from each of the three treatment groups who had attained at least the measure of improvement in ADAS-cog score shown on the X axis. Similar to the U.S. 26-week study, the curves demonstrate that both patients assigned to Exelon and placebo have a wide range of responses, but that the 6-12 mg/day Exelon group is more likely to show the greater improvements.

Figure 5: Cumulative Percentage of Patients Completing 26 Weeks of Double-blind Treatment with Specified Changes from Baseline ADAS-cog Scores. The Percentages of Randomized Patients who Completed the Study were: Placebo 87%, 1-4 mg 86%, and 6-12 mg 67%.

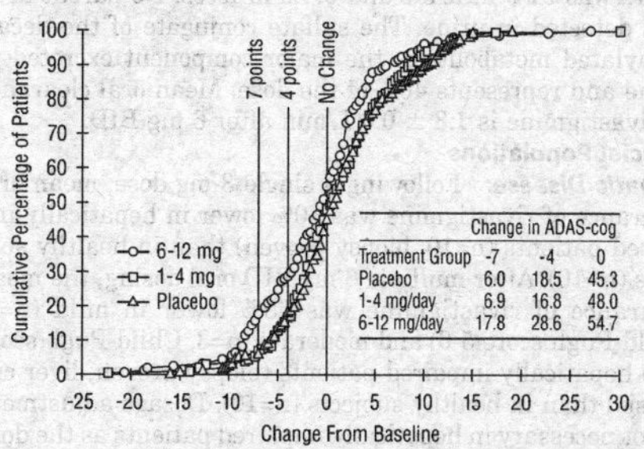

Effects on the CIBIC-Plus: Figure 6 is a histogram of the frequency distribution of CIBIC-Plus scores attained by patients assigned to each of the three treatment groups who completed 26 weeks of treatment. The mean Exelon-placebo differences for these groups of patients for the mean rating of change from baseline were 0.14 units and 0.41 units for 1-4 mg and 6-12 mg of Exelon, respectively. The mean ratings for the 6-12 mg/day group was statistically significantly superior to placebo. The comparison of the mean ratings for the 1-4 mg/day group and placebo group was not statistically significant.

Figure 6: Frequency Distribution of CIBIC-Plus Scores at Week 26

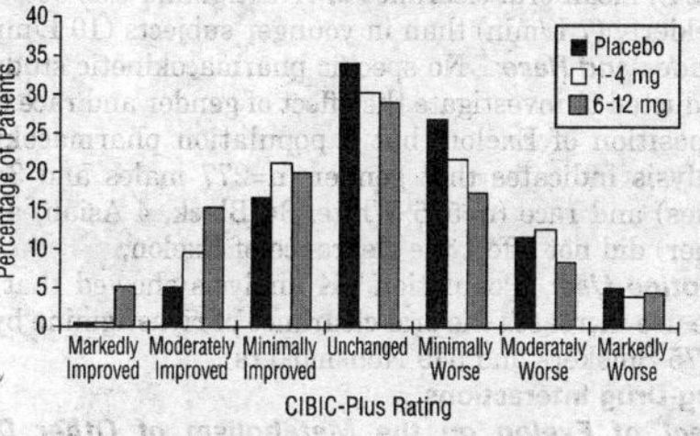

U.S. Fixed Dose Study

In a study of 26 weeks duration, 702 patients were randomized to doses of 3, 6, or 9 mg/day of Exelon or to placebo, each given in divided doses. The fixed-dose study design, which included a 12-week forced titration phase and a 14-week maintenance phase, led to a high dropout rate in the 9 mg/day group because of poor tolerability. At 26 weeks of treatment, significant differences were observed for the ADAS-cog mean change from baseline for the 9 mg/day and 6 mg/day groups, compared to placebo. No significant differences were observed between any of the Exelon dose groups and placebo for the analysis of the CIBIC-Plus mean rating of change. Although no significant differences were observed between Exelon treatment groups, there was a trend toward numerical superiority with higher doses.

Age, Gender and Race

Patient's age, gender, or race did not predict clinical outcome to Exelon treatment.

Pharmacokinetics

Rivastigmine is well absorbed with absolute bioavailability of about 40% (3-mg dose). It shows linear pharmacokinetics up to 3 mg BID but is non-linear at higher doses. Doubling the dose from 3 to 6 mg BID results in a 3-fold increase in AUC. The elimination half-life is about 1.5 hours, with most elimination as metabolites via the urine.

Absorption: Rivastigmine is rapidly and completely absorbed. Peak plasma concentrations are reached in approximately 1 hour. Absolute bioavailability after a 3-mg dose is about 36%. Administration of Exelon with food delays absorption (t_{max}) by 90 min, lowers C_{max} by approximately 30% and increases AUC by approximately 30%.

Distribution: Rivastigmine is widely distributed throughout the body with a volume of distribution in the range of 1.8-2.7 L/kg. Rivastigmine penetrates the blood brain barrier, reaching CSF peak concentrations in 1.4-2.6 hours. Mean AUC_{1-12hr} ratio of CSF/plasma averaged 40 ± 0.5% following 1-6 mg BID doses.

Rivastigmine is about 40% bound to plasma proteins at concentrations of 1-400 ng/mL, which cover the therapeutic concentration range. Rivastigmine distributes equally between blood and plasma with a blood-to-plasma partition ratio of 0.9 at concentrations ranging from 1-400 ng/mL.

Continued on next page

Exelon Capsules—Cont.

Metabolism: Rivastigmine is rapidly and extensively metabolized, primarily via cholinesterase-mediated hydrolysis to the decarbamylated metabolite. Based on evidence from *in vitro* and animal studies the major cytochrome P450 isozymes are minimally involved in rivastigmine metabolism. Consistent with these observations is the finding that no drug interactions related to cytochrome P450 have been observed in humans *(see Drug-Drug Interactions)*.

Elimination: The major pathway of elimination is via the kidneys. Following administration of ^{14}C-rivastigmine to 6 healthy volunteers total recovery of radioactivity over 120 hours was 97% in urine and 0.4% in feces. No parent drug was detected in urine. The sulfate conjugate of the decarbamylated metabolite is the major component excreted in urine and represents 40% of the dose. Mean oral clearance of rivastigmine is 1.8 ± 0.6 L/min after 6 mg BID.

Special Populations

Hepatic Disease: Following a single 3-mg dose, mean oral clearance of rivastigmine was 60% lower in hepatically impaired patients (n=10, biopsy proven) than in healthy subjects (n=10). After multiple 6 mg BID oral dosing, the mean clearance of rivastigmine was 65% lower in mild (n=7, Child-Pugh score 5-6) and moderate (n=3, Child-Pugh score 7-9) hepatically impaired patients (biopsy proven, liver cirrhosis) than in healthy subjects (n=10). Dosage adjustment is not necessary in hepatically impaired patients as the dose of drug is individually titrated to tolerability.

Renal Disease: Following a single 3-mg dose, mean oral clearance of rivastigmine is 64% lower in moderately impaired renal patients (n=8, GFR=10-50 mL/min) than in healthy subjects (n=10, GFR≥60 mL/min); Cl/F=1.7 L/min (cv=45%) and 4.8 L/min (cv=80%), respectively. In severely impaired renal patients (n=8, GFR<10 mL/min), mean oral clearance of rivastigmine is 43% higher than in healthy subjects (n=10, GFR≥60 mL/min); Cl/F=6.9 L/min and 4.8 L/min, respectively. For unexplained reasons, the severely impaired renal patients had a higher clearance of rivastigmine than moderately impaired patients. However, dosage adjustment may not be necessary in renally impaired patients as the dose of the drug is individually titrated to tolerability.

Age: Following a single 2.5 mg oral dose to elderly volunteers (>60 years of age, n=24) and younger volunteers (n=24), mean oral clearance of rivastigmine was 30% lower in elderly (7 L/min) than in younger subjects (10 L/min).

Gender and Race: No specific pharmacokinetic study was conducted to investigate the effect of gender and race on the disposition of Exelon, but a population pharmacokinetic analysis indicates that gender (n=277 males and 348 females) and race (n=575 White, 34 Black, 4 Asian, and 12 Other) did not affect the clearance of Exelon.

Nicotine Use: Population PK analysis showed that nicotine use increases the oral clearance of rivastigmine by 23% (n=75 Smokers and 549 Nonsmokers).

Drug-Drug Interactions

Effect of Exelon on the Metabolism of Other Drugs: Rivastigmine is primarily metabolized through hydrolysis by esterases. Minimal metabolism occurs via the major cytochrome P450 isoenzymes. Based on *in vitro* studies, no pharmacokinetic drug interactions with drugs metabolized by the following isoenzyme systems are expected: CYP1A2, CYP2D6, CYP3A4/5, CYP2E1, CYP2C9, CYP2C8, or CYP2C19.

No pharmacokinetic interaction was observed between rivastigmine and digoxin, warfarin, diazepam, or fluoxetine in studies in healthy volunteers. The elevation of prothrombin time induced by warfarin is not affected by administration of Exelon.

Effect of Other Drugs on the Metabolism of Exelon: Drugs that induce or inhibit CYP450 metabolism are not expected to alter the metabolism of rivastigmine. Single dose pharmacokinetic studies demonstrated that the metabolism of rivastigmine is not significantly affected by concurrent administration of digoxin, warfarin, diazepam, or fluoxetine.

Population PK analysis with a database of 625 patients showed that the pharmacokinetics of rivastigmine were not influenced by commonly prescribed medications such as antacids (n=77), antihypertensives (n=72), β-blockers (n=42), calcium channel blockers (n=75), antidiabetics (n=21), nonsteroidal anti-inflammatory drugs (n=79), estrogens (n=70), salicylate analgesics (n=177), antianginals (n=35), and antihistamines (n=15). In addition, in clinical trials, no increased risk of clinically relevant untoward effects was observed in patients treated concomitantly with Exelon and these agents.

INDICATIONS AND USAGE

Exelon® (rivastigmine tartrate) is indicated for the treatment of mild to moderate dementia of the Alzheimer's type.

CONTRAINDICATIONS

Exelon® (rivastigmine tartrate) is contraindicated in patients with known hypersensitivity to rivastigmine, other carbamate derivatives or other components of the formulation *(see DESCRIPTION)*.

WARNINGS

Gastrointestinal Adverse Reactions

Exelon® (rivastigmine tartrate) use is associated with significant gastrointestinal adverse reactions, including nausea and vomiting, anorexia, and weight loss. For this reason, patients should always be started at a dose of 1.5 mg BID and titrated to their maintenance dose. If treatment is interrupted for longer than several days, treatment should be reinitiated with the lowest daily dose *(see DOSAGE AND ADMINISTRATION)* to reduce the possibility of severe vomiting and its potentially serious sequelae (e.g., there has been one post-marketing report of severe vomiting with esophageal rupture following inappropriate reinitiation of treatment with a 4.5-mg dose after 8 weeks of treatment interruption).

Nausea and Vomiting: **In the controlled clinical trials, 47% of the patients treated with an Exelon dose in the therapeutic range of 6-12 mg/day (n=1189) developed nausea (compared with 12% in placebo). A total of 31% of Exelon-treated patients developed at least one episode of vomiting (compared with 6% for placebo). The rate of vomiting was higher during the titration phase (24% vs. 3% for placebo) than in the maintenance phase (14% vs. 3% for placebo). The rates were higher in women than men. Five percent of patients discontinued for vomiting, compared to less than 1% for patients on placebo. Vomiting was severe in 2% of Exelon-treated patients and was rated as mild or moderate each in 14% of patients. The rate of nausea was higher during the titration phase (43% vs. 9% for placebo) than in the maintenance phase (17% vs. 4% for placebo).**

Weight Loss: **In the controlled trials, approximately 26% of women on high doses of Exelon (greater than 9 mg/day) had weight loss of equal to or greater than 7% of their baseline weight compared to 6% in the placebo-treated patients. About 18% of the males in the high dose group experienced a similar degree of weight loss compared to 4% in placebo-treated patients. It is not clear how much of the weight loss was associated with anorexia, nausea, vomiting, and the diarrhea associated with the drug.**

Anorexia: In the controlled clinical trials, of the patients treated with an Exelon dose of 6-12 mg/day, 17% developed anorexia compared to 3% of the placebo patients. Neither the time course nor the severity of the anorexia is known.

Peptic Ulcers/Gastrointestinal Bleeding: Because of their pharmacological action, cholinesterase inhibitors may be expected to increase gastric acid secretion due to increased cholinergic activity. Therefore, patients should be monitored closely for symptoms of active or occult gastrointestinal bleeding, especially those at increased risk for developing ulcers, e.g., those with a history of ulcer disease or those receiving concurrent nonsteroidal anti-inflammatory drugs (NSAIDS). Clinical studies of Exelon have shown no significant increase, relative to placebo, in the incidence of either peptic ulcer disease or gastrointestinal bleeding.

Anesthesia

Exelon as a cholinesterase inhibitor, is likely to exaggerate succinylcholine-type muscle relaxation during anesthesia.

Cardiovascular Conditions

Drugs that increase cholinergic activity may have vagotonic effects on heart rate (e.g., bradycardia). The potential for this action may be particularly important to patients with "sick sinus syndrome" or other supraventricular cardiac conduction conditions. In clinical trials, Exelon was not associated with any increased incidence of cardiovascular adverse events, heart rate or blood pressure changes, or ECG abnormalities. Syncopal episodes have been reported in 3% of patients receiving 6-12 mg/day of Exelon, compared to 2% of placebo patients.

Genitourinary

Although this was not observed in clinical trials of Exelon, drugs that increase cholinergic activity may cause urinary obstruction.

Neurological Conditions

Seizures: Drugs that increase cholinergic activity are believed to have some potential for causing seizures. However, seizure activity also may be a manifestation of Alzheimer's Disease.

Pulmonary Conditions

Like other drugs that increase cholinergic activity, Exelon should be used with care in patients with a history of asthma or obstructive pulmonary disease.

PRECAUTIONS

Information for Patients and Caregivers

Caregivers should be advised of the high incidence of nausea and vomiting associated with the use of the drug along with the possibility of anorexia and weight loss. Caregivers should be encouraged to monitor for these adverse events and inform the physician if they occur. It is critical to inform caregivers that if therapy has been interrupted for more than several days, the next dose should not be administered until they have discussed this with the physician.

Drug-Drug Interactions

Effect of Exelon® (rivastigmine tartrate) on the Metabolism of Other Drugs: Rivastigmine is primarily metabolized through hydrolysis by esterases. Minimal metabolism occurs via the major cytochrome P450 isoenzymes. Based on *in vitro* studies, no pharmacokinetic drug interactions with drugs metabolized by the following isoenzyme systems are expected: CYP1A2, CYP2D6, CYP3A4/5, CYP2E1, CYP2C9, CYP2C8, or CYP2C19.

No pharmacokinetic interaction was observed between rivastigmine and digoxin, warfarin, diazepam, or fluoxetine in studies in healthy volunteers. The elevation of prothrombin time induced by warfarin is not affected by administration of Exelon.

Effect of Other Drugs on the Metabolism of Exelon: Drugs that induce or inhibit CYP450 metabolism are not expected to alter the metabolism of rivastigmine. Single dose pharmacokinetic studies demonstrated that the metabolism of rivastigmine is not significantly affected by concurrent administration of digoxin, warfarin, diazepam, or fluoxetine.

Population PK analysis with a database of 625 patients showed that the pharmacokinetics of rivastigmine were not influenced by commonly prescribed medications such as antacids (n=77), antihypertensives (n=72), β-blockers (n=42), calcium channel blockers (n=75), antidiabetics (n=21), nonsteroidal anti-inflammatory drugs (n=79), estrogens (n=70), salicylate analgesics (n=177), antianginals (n=35), and antihistamines (n=15).

Use with Anticholinergics: Because of their mechanism of action, cholinesterase inhibitors have the potential to interfere with the activity of anticholinergic medications.

Use with Cholinomimetics and Other Cholinesterase Inhibitors: A synergistic effect may be expected when cholinesterase inhibitors are given concurrently with succinylcholine, similar neuromuscular blocking agents or cholinergic agonists such as bethanechol.

Carcinogenesis, Mutagenesis, Impairment of Fertility

In carcinogenicity studies conducted at dose levels up to 1.1 mg-base/kg/day in rats and 1.6 mg-base/kg/day in mice, rivastigmine was not carcinogenic. These dose levels are approximately 0.9 times and 0.7 times the maximum recommended human daily dose of 12 mg/day on a mg/m^2 basis. Rivastigmine was clastogenic in two *in vitro* assays in the presence, but not the absence, of metabolic activation. It caused structural chromosomal aberrations in V79 Chinese hamster lung cells and both structural and numerical (polyploidy) chromosomal aberrations in human peripheral blood lymphocytes. Rivastigmine was not genotoxic in three *in vitro* assays: the Ames test, the unscheduled DNA synthesis (UDS) test in rat hepatocytes (a test for induction of DNA repair synthesis), and the HGPRT test in V79 Chinese hamster cells. Rivastigmine was not clastogenic in the *in vivo* mouse micronucleus test.

Rivastigmine had no effect on fertility or reproductive performance in the rat at dose levels up to 1.1 mg-base/kg/day. This dose is approximately 0.9 times the maximum recommended human daily dose of 12 mg/day on a mg/m^2 basis.

Pregnancy

Pregnancy Category B: Reproduction studies conducted in pregnant rats at doses up to 2.3 mg-base/kg/day (approximately 2 times the maximum recommended human dose on a mg/m^2 basis) and in pregnant rabbits at doses up to 2.3 mg-base/kg/day (approximately 4 times the maximum recommended human dose on a mg/m^2 basis) revealed no evidence of teratogenicity. Studies in rats showed slightly decreased fetal/pup weights, usually at doses causing some maternal toxicity; decreased weights were seen at doses which were several fold lower than the maximum recommended human dose on a mg/m^2 basis. There are no adequate or well-controlled studies in pregnant women. Because animal reproduction studies are not always predictive of human response, Exelon should be used during pregnancy only if the potential benefit justifies the potential risk to the fetus.

Nursing Mothers

It is not known whether rivastigmine is excreted in human breast milk. Exelon has no indication for use in nursing mothers.

Pediatric Use

There are no adequate and well-controlled trials documenting the safety and efficacy of Exelon in any illness occurring in children.

ADVERSE REACTIONS

Adverse Events Leading to Discontinuation

The rate of discontinuation due to adverse events in controlled clinical trials of Exelon® (rivastigmine tartrate) was 15% for patients receiving 6-12 mg/day compared to 5% for patients on placebo during forced weekly dose titration. While on a maintenance dose, the rates were 6% for patients on Exelon compared to 4% for those on placebo.

The most common adverse events leading to discontinuation, defined as those occurring in at least 2% of patients and at twice the incidence seen in placebo patients, are shown in Table 1.

[See table 1 at top of next page]

Most Frequent Adverse Clinical Events Seen in Association with the Use of Exelon

The most common adverse events, defined as those occurring at a frequency of at least 5% and twice the placebo rate, are largely predicted by Exelon's cholinergic effects. These include nausea, vomiting, anorexia, dyspepsia, and asthenia.

Gastrointestinal Adverse Reactions: Exelon use is associated with significant nausea, vomiting, and weight loss *(see WARNINGS)*.

Adverse Events Reported in Controlled Trials

Table 2 lists treatment emergent signs and symptoms that were reported in at least 2% of patients in placebo-controlled trials and for which the rate of occurrence was greater for patients treated with Exelon doses of 6-12 mg/day than for those treated with placebo. The prescriber should be aware that these figures cannot be used to predict the frequency of adverse events in the course of usual medical practice when patient characteristics and other factors may differ from those prevailing during clinical studies. Similarly, the cited frequencies cannot be directly compared with figures obtained from other clinical investigations involving different treatments, uses, or investigators. An inspection of these frequencies, however, does provide the pre-

Table 1
Most Frequent Adverse Events Leading to Withdrawal from Clinical Trials during Titration and Maintenance in Patients Receiving 6-12 mg/day Exelon® Using a Forced Dose Titration

Study Phase	Titration		Maintenance		Overall	
	Placebo (n=868)	Exelon ≥6-12 mg/day (n=1,189)	Placebo (n=788)	Exelon ≥6-12 mg/day (n=987)	Placebo (n=868)	Exelon ≥6-12 mg/day (n=1,189)
Event/% Discontinuing						
Nausea	<1	8	<1	1	1	8
Vomiting	<1	4	<1	1	<1	5
Anorexia	0	2	<1	1	<1	3
Dizziness	<1	2	<1	1	<1	2

scriber with one basis by which to estimate the relative contribution of drug and non-drug factors to the adverse event incidences in the population studied.
In general, adverse reactions were less frequent later in the course of treatment.
No systematic effect of race or age could be determined on the incidence of adverse events in the controlled studies.
Nausea, vomiting and weight loss were more frequent in women than men.

Table 2
Adverse Events Reported in Controlled Clinical Trials in at Least 2% of Patients Receiving Exelon® (6-12 mg/day) and at a Higher Frequency than Placebo-treated Patients

Body System/Adverse Event	Placebo (n=868)	Exelon (6-12 mg/day) (n=1,189)
Percent of Patients with any Adverse Event	79	92
Autonomic Nervous System		
Sweating increased	1	4
Syncope	2	3
Body as a Whole		
Accidental Trauma	9	10
Fatigue	5	9
Asthenia	2	6
Malaise	2	5
Influenza-like Symptoms	2	3
Weight Decrease	<1	3
Cardiovascular Disorders, General		
Hypertension	2	3
Central and Peripheral Nervous System		
Dizziness	11	21
Headache	12	17
Somnolence	3	5
Tremor	1	4
Gastrointestinal System		
Nausea	12	47
Vomiting	6	31
Diarrhea	11	19
Anorexia	3	17
Abdominal Pain	6	13
Dyspepsia	4	9
Constipation	4	5
Flatulence	2	4
Eructation	1	2
Psychiatric Disorders		
Insomnia	7	9
Confusion	7	8
Depression	4	6
Anxiety	3	5
Hallucination	3	4
Aggressive Reaction	2	3
Resistance Mechanism Disorders		
Urinary Tract Infection	6	7
Respiratory System		
Rhinitis	3	4

Other adverse events observed at a rate of 2% or more on Exelon 6-12 mg/day but at a greater or equal rate on placebo were chest pain, peripheral edema, vertigo, back pain, arthralgia, pain, bone fracture, agitation, nervousness, delusion, paranoid reaction, upper respiratory tract infections, infection (general), coughing, pharyngitis, bronchitis, rash (general), urinary incontinence.

Other Adverse Events Observed During Clinical Trials
Exelon has been administered to over 5,297 individuals during clinical trials worldwide. Of these, 4,326 patients have been treated for at least 3 months, 3,407 patients have been treated for at least 6 months, 2,150 patients have been treated for 1 year, 1,250 have been treated for 2 years, and 168 have been treated for over 3 years. With regard to exposure to the highest dose, 2,809 patients were exposed to doses of 10-12 mg, 2,615 patients treated for 3 months, 2,328 patients treated for 6 months, 1,378 patients treated for 1 year, 917 patients treated for 2 years, and 129 treated for over 3 years.
Treatment emergent signs and symptoms that occurred during 8 controlled clinical trials and 9 open-label trials in North America, Western Europe, Australia, South Africa, and Japan were recorded as adverse events by the clinical investigators using terminology of their own choosing. To provide an overall estimate of the proportion of individuals having similar types of events, the events were grouped into a smaller number of standardized categories using a modified WHO dictionary, and event frequencies were calculated across all studies. These categories are used in the listing below. The frequencies represent the proportion of 5,297 patients from these trials who experienced that event while receiving Exelon. All adverse events occurring in at least 6 patients (approximately 0.1%) are included, except for those already listed elsewhere in labeling, WHO terms too general to be informative, relatively minor events, or events unlikely to be drug caused. Events are classified by body system and listed using the following definitions: frequent adverse events – those occurring in at least 1/100 patients; infrequent adverse events – those occurring in 1/100 to 1/1000 patients. These adverse events are not necessarily related to Exelon treatment and in most cases were observed at a similar frequency in placebo-treated patients in the controlled studies.

Autonomic Nervous System: *Infrequent:* Cold clammy skin, dry mouth, flushing, increased saliva.
Body as a Whole: *Frequent:* Accidental trauma, fever, edema, allergy, hot flushes, rigors. *Infrequent:* Edema periorbital or facial, hypothermia, edema, feeling cold, halitosis.
Cardiovascular System: *Frequent:* Hypotension, postural hypotension, cardiac failure.
Central and Peripheral Nervous System: *Frequent:* Abnormal gait, ataxia, paraesthesia, convulsions. *Infrequent:* Paresis, apraxia, aphasia, dysphonia, hyperkinesia, hyperreflexia, hypertonia, hypoesthesia, hypokinesia, migraine, neuralgia, nystagmus, peripheral neuropathy.
Endocrine System: *Infrequent:* Goitre, hypothyroidism.
Gastrointestinal System: *Frequent:* Fecal incontinence, gastritis. *Infrequent:* Dysphagia, esophagitis, gastric ulcer, gastritis, gastroesophageal reflux, GI hemorrhage, hernia, intestinal obstruction, melena, rectal hemorrhage, gastroenteritis, ulcerative stomatitis, duodenal ulcer, hematemesis, gingivitis, tenesmus, pancreatitis, colitis, glossitis.
Hearing and Vestibular Disorders: *Frequent:* Tinnitus.
Heart Rate and Rhythm Disorders: *Frequent:* Atrial fibrillation, bradycardia, palpitation. *Infrequent:* AV block, bundle branch block, sick sinus syndrome, cardiac arrest, supraventricular tachycardia, extrasystoles, tachycardia.
Liver and Biliary System Disorders: *Infrequent:* Abnormal hepatic function, cholecystitis.
Metabolic and Nutritional Disorders: *Frequent:* Dehydration, hypokalemia. *Infrequent:* Diabetes mellitus, gout, hypercholesterolemia, hyperlipemia, hypoglycemia, cachexia, thirst, hyperglycemia, hyponatremia.
Musculoskeletal Disorders: *Frequent:* Arthritis, leg cramps, myalgia. *Infrequent:* Cramps, hernia, muscle weakness.
Myo-, Endo-, Pericardial and Valve Disorders: *Frequent:* Angina pectoris, myocardial infarction.
Platelet, Bleeding, and Clotting Disorders: *Frequent:* Epistaxis. *Infrequent:* Hematoma, thrombocytopenia, purpura.
Psychiatric Disorders: *Frequent:* Paranoid reaction, confusion. *Infrequent:* Abnormal dreaming, amnesia, apathy, delirium, dementia, depersonalization, emotional lability, impaired concentration, decreased libido, personality disorder, suicide attempt, increased libido, neurosis, suicidal ideation, psychosis.
Red Blood Cell Disorders: *Frequent:* Anemia. *Infrequent:* Hypochromic anemia.
Reproductive Disorders (Female & Male): *Infrequent:* Breast pain, impotence, atrophic vaginitis.
Resistance Mechanism Disorders: *Infrequent:* Cellulitis, cystitis, herpes simplex, otitis media.
Respiratory System: *Infrequent:* Bronchospasm, laryngitis, apnea.
Skin and Appendages: *Frequent:* Rashes of various kinds (maculopapular, eczema, bullous, exfoliative, psoriaform, erythematous). *Infrequent:* Alopecia, skin ulceration, urticaria, dermatitis contact.
Special Senses: *Infrequent:* Perversion of taste, loss of taste.
Urinary System Disorders: *Frequent:* Hematuria. *Infrequent:* Albuminuria, oliguria, acute renal failure, dysuria, micturition urgency, nocturia, polyuria, renal calculus, urinary retention.
Vascular (extracardiac) Disorders: *Infrequent:* Hemorrhoids, peripheral ischemia, pulmonary embolism, thrombosis, thrombophlebitis deep, aneurysm, hemorrhage intracranial.
Vision Disorders: *Frequent:* Cataract. *Infrequent:* Conjunctival hemorrhage, blepharitis, diplopia, eye pain, glaucoma.
White Cell and Resistance Disorders: *Infrequent:* Lymphadenopathy, leukocytosis.

Post-Introduction Reports
Voluntary reports of adverse events temporally associated with Exelon that have been received since market introduction that are not listed above, and that may or may not be causally related to the drug include the following:
Skin and Appendages: Stevens-Johnson syndrome.

OVERDOSAGE

Because strategies for the management of overdose are continually evolving, it is advisable to contact a Poison Control Center to determine the latest recommendations for the management of an overdose of any drug.
As Exelon® (rivastigmine tartrate) has a short plasma half-life of about one hour and a moderate duration of acetylcholinesterase inhibition of 8-10 hours, it is recommended that in cases of asymptomatic overdoses, no further dose of Exelon should be administered for the next 24 hours.
As in any case of overdose, general supportive measures should be utilized. Overdosage with cholinesterase inhibitors can result in cholinergic crisis characterized by severe nausea, vomiting, salivation, sweating, bradycardia, hypotension, respiratory depression, collapse and convulsions. Increasing muscle weakness is a possibility and may result in death if respiratory muscles are involved. Atypical responses in blood pressure and heart rate have been reported with other drugs that increase cholinergic activity when coadministered with quaternary anticholinergics such as glycopyrrolate. Due to the short half-life of Exelon, dialysis (hemodialysis, peritoneal dialysis, or hemofiltration) would not be clinically indicated in the event of an overdose.
In overdoses accompanied by severe nausea and vomiting, the use of antiemetics should be considered. In a documented case of a 46 mg overdose with Exelon, the patient experienced vomiting, incontinence, hypertension, psychomotor retardation, and loss of consciousness. The patient fully recovered within 24 hours and conservative management was all that was required for treatment.

DOSAGE AND ADMINISTRATION

The dosage of Exelon® (rivastigmine tartrate) shown to be effective in controlled clinical trials is 6-12 mg/day, given as twice a day dosing (daily doses of 3 to 6 mg BID). There is evidence from the clinical trials that doses at the higher end of this range may be more beneficial.
The starting dose of Exelon is 1.5 mg twice a day (BID). If this dose is well tolerated, after a minimum of two weeks of treatment, the dose may be increased to 3 mg BID. Subsequent increases to 4.5 mg BID and 6 mg BID should be attempted after a minimum of 2 weeks at the previous dose. If adverse effects (e.g., nausea, vomiting, abdominal pain, loss of appetite) cause intolerance during treatment, the patient should be instructed to discontinue treatment for several doses and then restart at the same or next lower dose level. If treatment is interrupted for longer than several days, treatment should be reinitiated with the lowest daily dose and titrated as described above *(see WARNINGS)*. The maximum dose is 6mg BID (12 mg/day).
Exelon should be taken with meals in divided doses in the morning and evening.

HOW SUPPLIED

Exelon® (rivastigmine tartrate) capsules equivalent to 1.5 mg, 3 mg, 4.5 mg, or 6 mg of rivastigmine base are available as follows:
1.5 mg Capsule – yellow, "Exelon 1,5 mg" is printed in red on the body of the capsule.
Bottles of 60 .... NDC 0078-0323-44
Bottles of 500 .... NDC 0078-0323-08
Unit Dose (blister pack)
Box of 100 (strips of 10) .... NDC 0078-0323-06
3 mg Capsule – orange, "Exelon 3 mg" is printed in red on the body of the capsule.
Bottles of 60 .... NDC 0078-0324-44
Bottles of 500 .... NDC 0078-0324-08
Unit Dose (blister pack)
Box of 100 (strips of 10) .... NDC 0078-0324-06
4.5 mg Capsule – red, "Exelon 4,5 mg" is printed in white on the body of the capsule.
Bottles of 60 .... NDC 0078-0325-44
Bottles of 500 .... NDC 0078-0325-08
Unit Dose (blister pack)
Box of 100 (strips of 10) .... NDC 0078-0325-06
6 mg Capsule – orange and red, "Exelon 6 mg" is printed in red on the body of the capsule.
Bottles of 60 .... NDC 0078-0326-44
Bottles of 500 .... NDC 0078-0326-08
Unit Dose (blister pack)
Box of 100 (strips of 10) .... NDC 0078-0326-06
Store below 77°F (25°C) in a tight container.

T2004-47
REV: JUNE 2004 Printed in U.S.A. 89007405
Manufactured by:
Novartis Farmacéutica S.A.
08210 Barberà del Vallès
Barcelona, Spain
Distributed by:
Novartis Pharmaceuticals Corporation
East Hanover, New Jersey 07936
©Novartis

Shown in Product Identification Guide, page 325

Continued on next page

EXELON® ℞

[ĕx' ə-lŏn]
(rivastigmine tartrate)
Oral Solution
Rx only

Prescribing Information

The following prescribing information is based on official labeling in effect July 2004.

DESCRIPTION

Exelon® (rivastigmine tartrate) is a reversible cholinesterase inhibitor and is known chemically as (S)-N-Ethyl-N-methyl-3-[1-(dimethylamino)ethyl]-phenyl carbamate hydrogen-(2R,3R)-tartrate. Rivastigmine tartrate is commonly referred to in the pharmacological literature as SDZ ENA 713 or ENA 713. It has an empirical formula of $C_{14}H_{22}N_2O_2 \cdot C_4H_6O_6$ (hydrogen tartrate salt – hta salt) and a molecular weight of 400.43 (hta salt). Rivastigmine tartrate is a white to off-white, fine crystalline powder that is very soluble in water, soluble in ethanol and acetonitrile, slightly soluble in n-octanol and very slightly soluble in ethyl acetate. The distribution coefficient at 37°C in n-octanol/phosphate buffer solution pH 7 is 3.0.

Exelon Oral Solution is supplied as a solution containing rivastigmine tartrate, equivalent to 2 mg/mL of rivastigmine base for oral administration. Inactive ingredients are citric acid, D&C yellow #10, purified water, sodium benzoate and sodium citrate.

CLINICAL PHARMACOLOGY

Mechanism of Action

Pathological changes in Dementia of the Alzheimer type involve cholinergic neuronal pathways that project from the basal forebrain to the cerebral cortex and hippocampus. These pathways are thought to be intricately involved in memory, attention, learning, and other cognitive processes. While the precise mechanism of rivastigmine's action is unknown, it is postulated to exert its therapeutic effect by enhancing cholinergic function. This is accomplished by increasing the concentration of acetylcholine through reversible inhibition of its hydrolysis by cholinesterase. If this proposed mechanism is correct, Exelon's effect may lessen as the disease process advances and fewer cholinergic neurons remain functionally intact. There is no evidence that rivastigmine alters the course of the underlying dementing process. After a 6-mg dose of rivastigmine, anticholinesterase activity is present in CSF for about 10 hours, with a maximum inhibition of about 60% five hours after dosing.

In vitro and *in vivo* studies demonstrate that the inhibition of cholinesterase by rivastigmine is not affected by the concomitant administration of memantine, an N-methyl-D-aspartate receptor antagonist.

Clinical Trial Data

The effectiveness of Exelon® (rivastigmine tartrate) as a treatment for Alzheimer's Disease is demonstrated by the results of two randomized, double-blind, placebo-controlled clinical investigations in patients with Alzheimer's Disease [diagnosed by NINCDS-ADRDA and DSM-IV criteria, Mini-Mental State Examination (MMSE) ≥10 and ≤26, and the Global Deterioration Scale (GDS)]. The mean age of patients participating in Exelon trials was 73 years with a range of 41-95. Approximately 59% of patients were women and 41% were men. The racial distribution was Caucasian 87%, Black 4% and Other races 9%.

Study Outcome Measures: In each study, the effectiveness of Exelon was evaluated using a dual outcome assessment strategy.

The ability of Exelon to improve cognitive performance was assessed with the cognitive subscale of the Alzheimer's Disease Assessment Scale (ADAS-cog), a multi-item instrument that has been extensively validated in longitudinal cohorts of Alzheimer's Disease patients. The ADAS-cog examines selected aspects of cognitive performance including elements of memory, orientation, attention, reasoning, language and praxis. The ADAS-cog scoring range is from 0 to 70, with higher scores indicating greater cognitive impairment. Elderly normal adults may score as low as 0 or 1, but it is not unusual for non-demented adults to score slightly higher.

The patients recruited as participants in each study had mean scores on ADAS-cog of approximately 23 units, with a range from 1 to 61. Experience gained in longitudinal studies of ambulatory patients with mild to moderate Alzheimer's Disease suggest that they gain 6-12 units a year on the ADAS-cog. Lesser degrees of change, however, are seen in patients with very mild or very advanced disease because the ADAS-cog is not uniformly sensitive to change over the course of the disease. The annualized rate of decline in the placebo patients participating in Exelon trials was approximately 3-8 units per year.

The ability of Exelon to produce an overall clinical effect was assessed using a Clinician's Interview Based Impression of Change that required the use of caregiver information, the CIBIC-Plus. The CIBIC-Plus is not a single instrument and is not a standardized instrument like the ADAS-cog. Clinical trials for investigational drugs have used a variety of CIBIC formats, each different in terms of depth and structure. As such, results from a CIBIC-Plus reflect clinical experience from the trial or trials in which it was used and can not be compared directly with the results of CIBIC-Plus evaluations from other clinical trials. The CIBIC-Plus used in the Exelon trials was a structured instrument based on a comprehensive evaluation at baseline and subsequent time-points of three domains: patient cognition, behavior and functioning, including assessment of activities of daily living. It represents the assessment of a skilled clinician using validated scales based on his/her observation at interviews conducted separately with the patient and the caregiver familiar with the behavior of the patient over the interval rated. The CIBIC-Plus is scored as a seven point categorical rating, ranging from a score of 1, indicating "markedly improved," to a score of 4, indicating "no change" to a score of 7, indicating "marked worsening." The CIBIC-Plus has not been systematically compared directly to assessments not using information from caregivers (CIBIC) or other global methods.

U.S. Twenty-Six-Week Study

In a study of 26 weeks duration, 699 patients were randomized to either a dose range of 1-4 mg or 6-12 mg of Exelon per day or to placebo, each given in divided doses. The 26-week study was divided into a 12-week forced dose titration phase and a 14-week maintenance phase. The patients in the active treatment arms of the study were maintained at their highest tolerated dose within the respective range.

Effects on the ADAS-cog: Figure 1 illustrates the time course for the change from baseline in ADAS-cog scores for all three dose groups over the 26 weeks of the study. At 26 weeks of treatment, the mean differences in the ADAS-cog change scores for the Exelon-treated patients compared to the patients on placebo were 1.9 and 4.9 units for the 1-4 mg and 6-12 mg treatments, respectively. Both treatments were statistically significantly superior to placebo and the 6-12 mg/day range was significantly superior to the 1-4 mg/day range.

Figure 1: Time-course of the Change from Baseline in ADAS-cog Score for Patients Completing 26 Weeks of Treatment

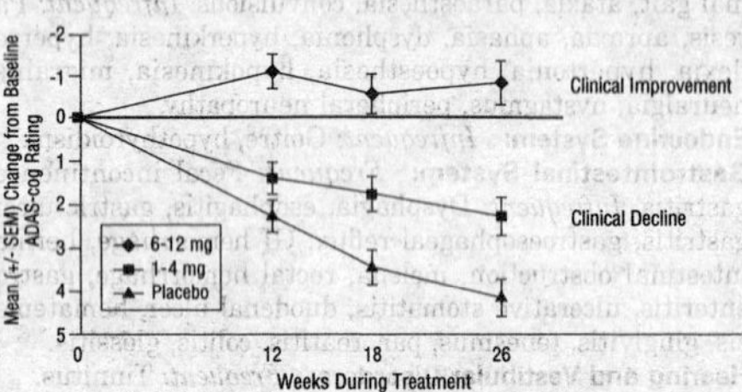

Figure 2 illustrates the cumulative percentages of patients from each of the three treatment groups who had attained at least the measure of improvement in ADAS-cog score shown on the X axis. Three change scores, (7-point and 4-point reductions from baseline or no change in score) have been identified for illustrative purposes, and the percent of patients in each group achieving that result is shown in the inset table.

The curves demonstrate that both patients assigned to Exelon and placebo have a wide range of responses, but that the Exelon groups are more likely to show the greater improvements. A curve for an effective treatment would be shifted to the left of the curve for placebo, while an ineffective or deleterious treatment would be superimposed upon, or shifted to the right of the curve for placebo, respectively.

Figure 2: Cumulative Percentage of Patients Completing 26 Weeks of Double-blind Treatment with Specified Changes from Baseline ADAS-cog Scores. The Percentages of Randomized Patients who Completed the Study were: Placebo 84%, 1-4 mg 85%, and 6-12 mg 65%.

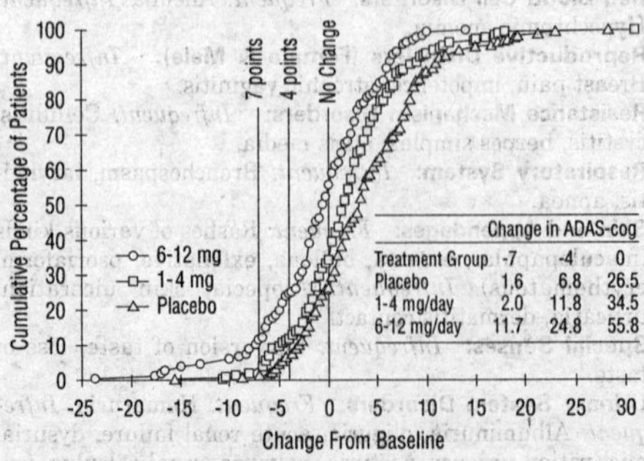

Effects on the CIBIC-Plus: Figure 3 is a histogram of the frequency distribution of CIBIC-Plus scores attained by patients assigned to each of the three treatment groups who completed 26 weeks of treatment. The mean Exelon-placebo differences for these groups of patients in the mean rating of change from baseline were 0.32 units and 0.35 units for 1-4 mg and 6-12 mg of Exelon, respectively. The mean ratings for the 6-12 mg/day and 1-4 mg/day groups were statistically significantly superior to placebo. The differences between the 6-12 mg/day and the 1-4 mg/day groups were statistically significant.

Figure 3: Frequency Distribution of CIBIC-Plus Scores at Week 26

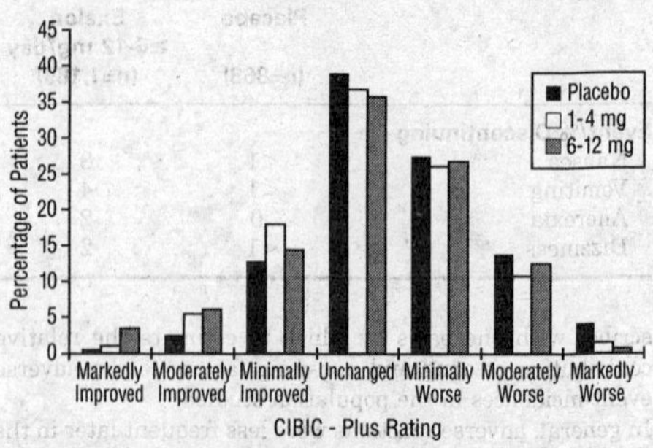

Global Twenty-Six-Week Study

In a second study of 26 weeks duration, 725 patients were randomized to either a dose range of 1-4 mg or 6-12 mg of Exelon per day or to placebo, each given in divided doses. The 26-week study was divided into a 12-week forced dose titration phase and a 14-week maintenance phase. The patients in the active treatment arms of the study were maintained at their highest tolerated dose within the respective range.

Effects on the ADAS-cog: Figure 4 illustrates the time course for the change from baseline in ADAS-cog scores for all three dose groups over the 26 weeks of the study. At 26 weeks of treatment, the mean differences in the ADAS-cog change scores for the Exelon-treated patients compared to the patients on placebo were 0.2 and 2.6 units for the 1-4 mg and 6-12 mg treatments, respectively. The 6-12 mg/day group was statistically significantly superior to placebo, as well as to the 1-4 mg/day group. The difference between the 1-4 mg/day group and placebo was not statistically significant.

Figure 4: Time-course of the Change from Baseline in ADAS-cog Score for Patients Completing 26 Weeks of Treatment

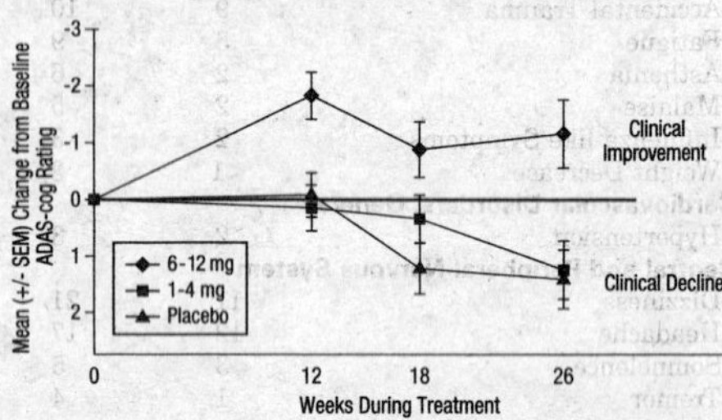

Figure 5 illustrates the cumulative percentages of patients from each of the three treatment groups who had attained at least the measure of improvement in ADAS-cog score shown on the X axis. Similar to the U.S. 26-week study, the curves demonstrate that both patients assigned to Exelon and placebo have a wide range of responses, but that the 6-12 mg/day Exelon group is more likely to show the greater improvements.

Figure 5: Cumulative Percentage of Patients Completing 26 Weeks of Double-blind Treatment with Specified Changes from Baseline ADAS-cog Scores. The Percentages of Randomized Patients who Completed the Study were: Placebo 87%, 1-4 mg 86%, and 6-12 mg 67%.

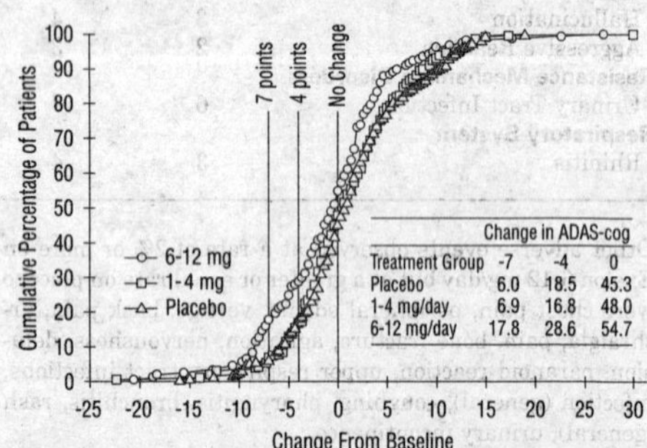

Effects on the CIBIC-Plus: Figure 6 is a histogram of the frequency distribution of CIBIC-Plus scores attained by patients assigned to each of the three treatment groups who completed 26 weeks of treatment. The mean Exelon-placebo differences for these groups of patients for the mean rating of change from baseline were 0.14 units and 0.41 units for 1-4 mg and 6-12 mg of Exelon, respectively. The mean ratings for the 6-12 mg/day group was statistically significantly superior to placebo. The comparison of the mean ratings for the 1-4 mg/day group and placebo group was not statistically significant.

[See figure 6 at top of next column]

U.S. Fixed Dose Study

In a study of 26 weeks duration, 702 patients were randomized to doses of 3, 6, or 9 mg/day of Exelon or to placebo, each given in divided doses. The fixed-dose study design, which included a 12-week forced titration phase and a 14-

Figure 6: Frequency Distribution of CIBIC-Plus Scores at Week 26

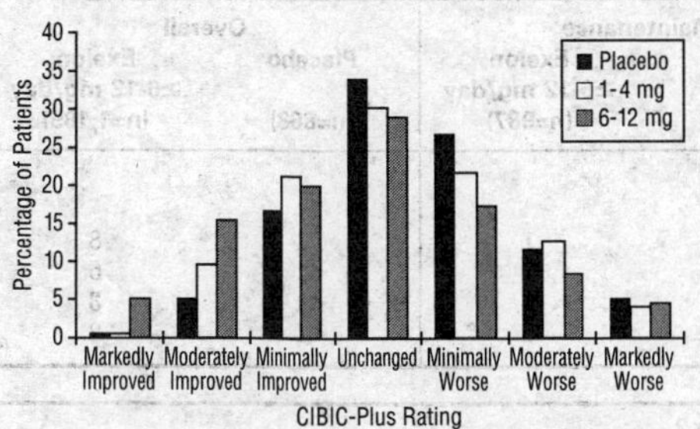

week maintenance phase, led to a high dropout rate in the 9 mg/day group because of poor tolerability. At 26 weeks of treatment, significant differences were observed for the ADAS-cog mean change from baseline for the 9 mg/day and 6 mg/day groups, compared to placebo. No significant differences were observed between any of the Exelon dose groups and placebo for the analysis of the CIBIC-Plus mean rating of change. Although no significant differences were observed between Exelon treatment groups, there was a trend toward numerical superiority with higher doses.

Age, Gender and Race: Patient's age, gender, or race did not predict clinical outcome to Exelon treatment.

Pharmacokinetics

Rivastigmine is well absorbed with absolute bioavailability of about 40% (3-mg dose). It shows linear pharmacokinetics up to 3 mg BID but is non-linear at higher doses. Doubling the dose from 3 to 6 mg BID results in a 3-fold increase in AUC. The elimination half-life is about 1.5 hours, with most elimination as metabolites via the urine.

Absorption: Rivastigmine is rapidly and completely absorbed. Peak plasma concentrations are reached in approximately 1 hour. Absolute bioavailability after a 3-mg dose is about 36%. Administration of Exelon with food delays absorption (t_{max}) by 90 min, lowers C_{max} by approximately 30% and increases AUC by approximately 30%.

Distribution: Rivastigmine is widely distributed throughout the body with a volume of distribution in the range of 1.8-2.7 L/kg. Rivastigmine penetrates the blood brain barrier, reaching CSF peak concentrations in 1.4-2.6 hours. Mean $AUC_{1\text{-}12hr}$ ratio of CSF/plasma averaged 40 ± 0.5% following 1-6 mg BID doses.

Rivastigmine is about 40% bound to plasma proteins at concentrations of 1-400 ng/mL, which cover the therapeutic concentration range. Rivastigmine distributes equally between blood and plasma with a blood-to-plasma partition ratio of 0.9 at concentrations ranging from 1-400 ng/mL.

Metabolism: Rivastigmine is rapidly and extensively metabolized, primarily via cholinesterase-mediated hydrolysis to the decarbamylated metabolite. Based on evidence from *in vitro* and animal studies the major cytochrome P450 isozymes are minimally involved in rivastigmine metabolism. Consistent with these observations is the finding that no drug interactions related to cytochrome P450 have been observed in humans *(see Drug-Drug Interactions)*.

Elimination: The major pathway of elimination is via the kidneys. Following administration of ^{14}C-rivastigmine to 6 healthy volunteers total recovery of radioactivity over 120 hours was 97% in urine and 0.4% in feces. No parent drug was detected in urine. The sulfate conjugate of the decarbamylated metabolite is the major component excreted in urine and represents 40% of the dose. Mean oral clearance of rivastigmine is 1.8 ± 0.6 L/min after 6 mg BID.

Special Populations

Hepatic Disease: Following a single 3-mg dose, mean oral clearance of rivastigmine was 60% lower in hepatically impaired patients (n=10, biopsy proven) than in healthy subjects (n=10). After multiple 6 mg BID oral dosing, the mean clearance of rivastigmine was 65% lower in mild (n=7, Child-Pugh score 5-6) and moderate (n=3, Child-Pugh score 7-9) hepatically impaired patients (biopsy proven, liver cirrhosis) than in healthy subjects (n=10). Dosage adjustment is not necessary in hepatically impaired patients as the dose of drug is individually titrated to tolerability.

Renal Disease: Following a single 3-mg dose, mean oral clearance of rivastigmine is 64% lower in moderately impaired renal patients (n=8, GFR=10-50 mL/min) than in healthy subjects (n=10, GFR≥60 mL/min); Cl/F=1.7 L/min (cv=45%) and 4.8 L/min (cv=80%), respectively. In severely impaired renal patients (n=8, GFR<10 mL/min), mean oral clearance of rivastigmine is 43% higher than in healthy subjects (n=10, GFR≥60 mL/min); Cl/F=6.9 L/min and 4.8 L/min, respectively. For unexplained reasons, the severely impaired renal patients had a higher clearance of rivastigmine than moderately impaired patients. However, dosage adjustment may not be necessary in renally impaired patients as the dose of the drug is individually titrated to tolerability.

Age: Following a single 2.5 mg oral dose to elderly volunteers (>60 years of age, n=24) and younger volunteers (n=24), mean oral clearance of rivastigmine was 30% lower in elderly (7 L/min) than in younger subjects (10 L/min).

Gender and Race: No specific pharmacokinetic study was conducted to investigate the effect of gender and race on the disposition of Exelon, but a population pharmacokinetic analysis indicates that gender (n=277 males and 348 females) and race (n=575 White, 34 Black, 4 Asian, and 12 Other) did not affect the clearance of Exelon.

Nicotine Use: Population PK analysis showed that nicotine use increases the oral clearance of rivastigmine by 23% (n=75 Smokers and 549 Nonsmokers).

Drug-Drug Interactions

Effect of Exelon on the Metabolism of Other Drugs: Rivastigmine is primarily metabolized through hydrolysis by esterases. Minimal metabolism occurs via the major cytochrome P450 isoenzymes. Based on *in vitro* studies, no pharmacokinetic drug interactions with drugs metabolized by the following isoenzyme systems are expected: CYP1A2, CYP2D6, CYP3A4/5, CYP2E1, CYP2C9, CYP2C8, or CYP2C19.

No pharmacokinetic interaction was observed between rivastigmine and digoxin, warfarin, diazepam, or fluoxetine in studies in healthy volunteers. The elevation of prothrombin time induced by warfarin is not affected by administration of Exelon.

Effect of Other Drugs on the Metabolism of Exelon: Drugs that induce or inhibit CYP450 metabolism are not expected to alter the metabolism of rivastigmine. Single dose pharmacokinetic studies demonstrated that the metabolism of rivastigmine is not significantly affected by concurrent administration of digoxin, warfarin, diazepam, or fluoxetine.

Population PK analysis with a database of 625 patients showed that the pharmacokinetics of rivastigmine were not influenced by commonly prescribed medications such as antacids (n=77), antihypertensives (n=72), β-blockers (n=42), calcium channel blockers (n=75), antidiabetics (n=21), nonsteroidal anti-inflammatory drugs (n=79), estrogens (n=70), salicylate analgesics (n=177), antianginals (n=35), and antihistamines (n=15). In addition, in clinical trials, no increased risk of clinically relevant untoward effects was observed in patients treated concomitantly with Exelon and these agents.

INDICATIONS AND USAGE

Exelon® (rivastigmine tartrate) is indicated for the treatment of mild to moderate dementia of the Alzheimer's type.

CONTRAINDICATIONS

Exelon® (rivastigmine tartrate) is contraindicated in patients with known hypersensitivity to rivastigmine, other carbamate derivatives or other components of the formulation *(see DESCRIPTION)*.

WARNINGS

Gastrointestinal Adverse Reactions

Exelon® (rivastigmine tartrate) use is associated with significant gastrointestinal adverse reactions, including nausea and vomiting, anorexia, and weight loss. For this reason, patients should always be started at a dose of 1.5 mg BID and titrated to their maintenance dose. If treatment is interrupted for longer than several days, treatment should be reinitiated with the lowest daily dose *(see DOSAGE AND ADMINISTRATION)* to reduce the possibility of severe vomiting and its potentially serious sequelae (e.g., there has been one post-marketing report of severe vomiting with esophageal rupture following inappropriate reinitiation of treatment with a 4.5-mg dose after 8 weeks of treatment interruption).

Nausea and Vomiting: **In the controlled clinical trials, 47% of the patients treated with an Exelon dose in the therapeutic range of 6-12 mg/day (n=1189) developed nausea (compared with 12% in placebo). A total of 31% of Exelon-treated patients developed at least one episode of vomiting (compared with 6% for placebo). The rate of vomiting was higher during the titration phase (24% vs. 3% for placebo) than in the maintenance phase (14% vs. 3% for placebo). The rates were higher in women than men. Five percent of patients discontinued for vomiting, compared to less than 1% for patients on placebo. Vomiting was severe in 2% of Exelon-treated patients and was rated as mild or moderate each in 14% of patients. The rate of nausea was higher during the titration phase (43% vs. 9% for placebo) than in the maintenance phase (17% vs. 4% for placebo).**

Weight Loss: **In the controlled trials, approximately 26% of women on high doses of Exelon (greater than 9 mg/day) had weight loss of equal to or greater than 7% of their baseline weight compared to 6% in the placebo-treated patients. About 18% of the males in the high dose group experienced a similar degree of weight loss compared to 4% in placebo-treated patients. It is not clear how much of the weight loss was associated with anorexia, nausea, vomiting, and the diarrhea associated with the drug.**

Anorexia: In the controlled clinical trials, of the patients treated with an Exelon dose of 6-12 mg/day, 17% developed anorexia compared to 3% of the placebo patients. Neither the time course or the severity of the anorexia is known.

Peptic Ulcers/Gastrointestinal Bleeding: Because of their pharmacological action, cholinesterase inhibitors may be expected to increase gastric acid secretion due to increased cholinergic activity. Therefore, patients should be monitored closely for symptoms of active or occult gastrointestinal bleeding, especially those at increased risk for developing ulcers, e.g., those with a history of ulcer disease or those receiving concurrent non-steroidal anti-inflammatory drugs (NSAIDS). Clinical studies of Exelon have shown no significant increase, relative to placebo, in the incidence of either peptic ulcer disease or gastrointestinal bleeding.

Anesthesia

Exelon as a cholinesterase inhibitor, is likely to exaggerate succinylcholine-type muscle relaxation during anesthesia.

Cardiovascular Conditions

Drugs that increase cholinergic activity may have vagotonic effects on heart rate (e.g., bradycardia). The potential for this action may be particularly important to patients with "sick sinus syndrome" or other supraventricular cardiac conduction conditions. In clinical trials, Exelon was not associated with any increased incidence of cardiovascular adverse events, heart rate or blood pressure changes, or ECG abnormalities. Syncopal episodes have been reported in 3% of patients receiving 6-12 mg/day of Exelon, compared to 2% of placebo patients.

Genitourinary

Although this was not observed in clinical trials of Exelon, drugs that increase cholinergic activity may cause urinary obstruction.

Neurological Conditions

Seizures: Drugs that increase cholinergic activity are believed to have some potential for causing seizures. However, seizure activity also may be a manifestation of Alzheimer's Disease.

Pulmonary Conditions

Like other drugs that increase cholinergic activity, Exelon should be used with care in patients with a history of asthma or obstructive pulmonary disease.

PRECAUTIONS

Information for Patients and Caregivers

Caregivers should be advised of the high incidence of nausea and vomiting associated with the use of the drug along with the possibility of anorexia and weight loss. Caregivers should be encouraged to monitor for these adverse events and inform the physician if they occur. It is critical to inform caregivers that if therapy has been interrupted for more than several days, the next dose should not be administered until they have discussed this with the physician.

Caregivers should be instructed in the correct procedure for administering Exelon® (rivastigmine tartrate) Oral Solution. In addition, they should be informed of the existence of an Instruction Sheet (included with the product) describing how the solution is to be administered. They should be urged to read this sheet prior to administering Exelon Oral Solution. Caregivers should direct questions about the administration of the solution to either their physician or pharmacist.

Drug-Drug Interactions

Effect of Exelon® on the Metabolism of Other Drugs: Rivastigmine is primarily metabolized through hydrolysis by esterases. Minimal metabolism occurs via the major cytochrome P450 isoenzymes. Based on *in vitro* studies, no pharmacokinetic drug interactions with drugs metabolized by the following isoenzyme systems are expected: CYP1A2, CYP2D6, CYP3A4/5, CYP2E1, CYP2C9, CYP2C8, or CYP2C19.

No pharmacokinetic interaction was observed between rivastigmine and digoxin, warfarin, diazepam, or fluoxetine in studies in healthy volunteers. The elevation of prothrombin time induced by warfarin is not affected by administration of Exelon.

Effect of Other Drugs on the Metabolism of Exelon: Drugs that induce or inhibit CYP450 metabolism are not expected to alter the metabolism of rivastigmine. Single dose pharmacokinetic studies demonstrated that the metabolism of rivastigmine is not significantly affected by concurrent administration of digoxin, warfarin, diazepam, or fluoxetine.

Population PK analysis with a database of 625 patients showed that the pharmacokinetics of rivastigmine were not influenced by commonly prescribed medications such as antacids (n=77), antihypertensives (n=72), β-blockers (n=42), calcium channel blockers (n=75), antidiabetics (n=21), nonsteroidal anti-inflammatory drugs (n=79), estrogens (n=70), salicylate analgesics (n=177), antianginals (n=35), and antihistamines (n=15).

Use with Anticholinergics: Because of their mechanism of action, cholinesterase inhibitors have the potential to interfere with the activity of anticholinergic medications.

Use with Cholinomimetics and Other Cholinesterase Inhibitors: A synergistic effect may be expected when cholinesterase inhibitors are given concurrently with succinylcholine, similar neuromuscular blocking agents or cholinergic agonists such as bethanechol.

Carcinogenesis, Mutagenesis, Impairment of Fertility

In carcinogenicity studies conducted at dose levels up to 1.1 mg-base/kg/day in rats and 1.6 mg-base/kg/day in mice, rivastigmine was not carcinogenic. These dose levels are approximately 0.9 times and 0.7 times the maximum recommended human daily dose of 12 mg/day on a mg/m^2 basis.

Rivastigmine was clastogenic in two *in vitro* assays in the presence, but not the absence, of metabolic activation. It caused structural chromosomal aberrations in V79 Chinese hamster lung cells and both structural and numerical (polyploidy) chromosomal aberrations in human peripheral blood lymphocytes. Rivastigmine was not genotoxic in three *in vitro* assays: the Ames test, the unscheduled DNA synthesis (UDS) test in rat hepatocytes (a test for induction of DNA repair synthesis), and the HGPRT test in V79 Chinese hamster cells. Rivastigmine was not clastogenic in the *in vivo* mouse micronucleus test.

Rivastigmine had no effect on fertility or reproductive performance in the rat at dose levels up to 1.1 mg-base/kg/day.

Continued on next page

Exelon Oral Solution—Cont.

This dose is approximately 0.9 times the maximum recommended human daily dose of 12 mg/day on a mg/m² basis.

Pregnancy

Pregnancy Category B: Reproduction studies conducted in pregnant rats at doses up to 2.3 mg-base/kg/day (approximately 2 times the maximum recommended human dose on a mg/m² basis) and in pregnant rabbits at doses up to 2.3 mg-base/kg/day (approximately 4 times the maximum recommended human dose on a mg/m² basis) revealed no evidence of teratogenicity. Studies in rats showed slightly decreased fetal/pup weights, usually at doses causing some maternal toxicity; decreased weights were seen at doses which were several fold lower than the maximum recommended human dose on a mg/m² basis. There are no adequate or well-controlled studies in pregnant women. Because animal reproduction studies are not always predictive of human response, Exelon should be used during pregnancy only if the potential benefit justifies the potential risk to the fetus.

Nursing Mothers

It is not known whether rivastigmine is excreted in human breast milk. Exelon has no indication for use in nursing mothers.

Pediatric Use

There are no adequate and well-controlled trials documenting the safety and efficacy of Exelon in any illness occurring in children.

ADVERSE REACTIONS

Adverse Events Leading to Discontinuation

The rate of discontinuation due to adverse events in controlled clinical trials of Exelon® (rivastigmine tartrate) was 15% for patients receiving 6-12 mg/day compared to 5% for patients on placebo during forced weekly dose titration. While on a maintenance dose, the rates were 6% for patients on Exelon compared to 4% for those on placebo.

The most common adverse events leading to discontinuation, defined as those occurring in at least 2% of patients and at twice the incidence seen in placebo patients, are shown in Table 1.

[See table 1 above]

Table 1
Most Frequent Adverse Events Leading to Withdrawal from Clinical Trials during Titration and Maintenance in Patients Receiving 6-12 mg/day Exelon® Using a Forced Dose Titration

Study Phase	Titration		Maintenance		Overall	
	Placebo (n=868)	Exelon ≥6-12 mg/day (n=1,189)	Placebo (n=788)	Exelon ≥6-12 mg/day (n=987)	Placebo (n=868)	Exelon ≥6-12 mg/day (n=1,189)
Event/% Discontinuing						
Nausea	<1	8	<1	1	1	8
Vomiting	<1	4	<1	1	<1	5
Anorexia	0	2	<1	1	<1	3
Dizziness	<1	2	<1	1	<1	2

Most Frequent Adverse Clinical Events Seen in Association with the Use of Exelon

The most common adverse events, defined as those occurring at a frequency of at least 5% and twice the placebo rate, are largely predicted by Exelon's cholinergic effects. These include nausea, vomiting, anorexia, dyspepsia, and asthenia.

Gastrointestinal Adverse Reactions

Exelon use is associated with significant nausea, vomiting, and weight loss *(see WARNINGS)*.

Adverse Events Reported in Controlled Trials

Table 2 lists treatment emergent signs and symptoms that were reported in at least 2% of patients in placebo-controlled trials and for which the rate of occurrence was greater for patients treated with Exelon doses of 6-12 mg/day than for those treated with placebo. The prescriber should be aware that these figures cannot be used to predict the frequency of adverse events in the course of usual medical practice when patient characteristics and other factors may differ from those prevailing during clinical studies. Similarly, the cited frequencies cannot be directly compared with figures obtained from other clinical investigations involving different treatments, uses, or investigators. An inspection of these frequencies, however, does provide the prescriber with one basis by which to estimate the relative contribution of drug and non-drug factors to the adverse event incidences in the population studied.

In general, adverse reactions were less frequent later in the course of treatment.

No systematic effect of race or age could be determined on the incidence of adverse events in the controlled studies. Nausea, vomiting and weight loss were more frequent in women than men.

[See table 2 above]

Table 2
Adverse Events Reported in Controlled Clinical Trials in at Least 2% of Patients Receiving Exelon® (6-12 mg/day) and at a Higher Frequency than Placebo-treated Patients

Body System/Adverse Event	Placebo (n=868)	Exelon (6-12 mg/day) (n=1,189)
Percent of Patients with any Adverse Event	79	92
Autonomic Nervous System		
Sweating increased	1	4
Syncope	2	3
Body as a Whole		
Accidental Trauma	9	10
Fatigue	5	9
Asthenia	2	6
Malaise	2	5
Influenza-like Symptoms	2	3
Weight Decrease	<1	3
Cardiovascular Disorders, General		
Hypertension	2	3
Central and Peripheral Nervous System		
Dizziness	11	21
Headache	12	17
Somnolence	3	5
Tremor	1	4
Gastrointestinal System		
Nausea	12	47
Vomiting	6	31
Diarrhea	11	19
Anorexia	3	17
Abdominal Pain	6	13
Dyspepsia	4	9
Constipation	4	5
Flatulence	2	4
Eructation	1	2
Psychiatric Disorders		
Insomnia	7	9
Confusion	7	8
Depression	4	6
Anxiety	3	5
Hallucination	3	4
Aggressive Reaction	2	3
Resistance Mechanism Disorders		
Urinary Tract Infection	6	7
Respiratory System		
Rhinitis	3	4

Other adverse events observed at a rate of 2% or more on Exelon 6-12 mg/day but at a greater or equal rate on placebo were chest pain, peripheral edema, vertigo, back pain, arthralgia, pain, bone fracture, agitation, nervousness, delusion, paranoid reaction, upper respiratory tract infections, infection (general), coughing, pharyngitis, bronchitis, rash (general), urinary incontinence.

Other Adverse Events Observed During Clinical Trials

Exelon has been administered to over 5,297 individuals during clinical trials worldwide. Of these, 4,326 patients have been treated for at least 3 months, 3,407 patients have been treated for at least 6 months, 2,150 patients have been treated for 1 year, 1,250 have been treated for 2 years, and 168 have been treated for over 3 years. With regard to exposure to the highest dose, 2,809 patients were exposed to doses of 10-12 mg, 2,615 patients treated for 3 months, 2,328 patients treated for 6 months, 1,378 patients treated for 1 year, 917 patients treated for 2 years, and 129 treated for over 3 years.

Treatment emergent signs and symptoms that occurred during 8 controlled clinical trials and 9 open-label trials in North America, Western Europe, Australia, South Africa, and Japan were recorded as adverse events by the clinical investigators using terminology of their own choosing. To provide an overall estimate of the proportion of individuals having similar types of events, the events were grouped into a smaller number of standardized categories using a modified WHO dictionary, and event frequencies were calculated across all studies. These categories are used in the listing below. The frequencies represent the proportion of 5,297 patients from these trials who experienced that event while receiving Exelon. All adverse events occurring in at least 6 patients (approximately 0.1%) are included, except for those already listed elsewhere in labeling, WHO terms too general to be informative, relatively minor events, or events unlikely to be drug caused. Events are classified by body system and listed using the following definitions: frequent adverse events – those occurring in at least 1/100 patients; infrequent adverse events – those occurring in 1/100 to 1/1,000 patients. These adverse events are not necessarily related to Exelon treatment and in most cases were observed at a similar frequency in placebo-treated patients in the controlled studies.

Autonomic Nervous System: *Infrequent:* Cold clammy skin, dry mouth, flushing, increased saliva.

Body as a Whole: *Frequent:* Accidental trauma, fever, edema, allergy, hot flushes, rigors. *Infrequent:* Edema periorbital or facial, hypothermia, edema, feeling cold, halitosis.

Cardiovascular System: *Frequent:* Hypotension, postural hypotension, cardiac failure.

Central and Peripheral Nervous System: *Frequent:* Abnormal gait, ataxia, paraesthesia, convulsions. *Infrequent:* Paresis, apraxia, aphasia, dysphonia, hyperkinesia, hyperreflexia, hypertonia, hypoesthesia, hypokinesia, migraine, neuralgia, nystagmus, peripheral neuropathy.

Endocrine System: *Infrequent:* Goitre, hypothyroidism.

Gastrointestinal System: *Frequent:* Fecal incontinence, gastritis. *Infrequent:* Dysphagia, esophagitis, gastric ulcer, gastritis, gastroesophageal reflux, GI hemorrhage, hernia, intestinal obstruction, melena, rectal hemorrhage, gastroenteritis, ulcerative stomatitis, duodenal ulcer, hematemesis, gingivitis, tenesmus, pancreatitis, colitis, glossitis.

Hearing and Vestibular Disorders: *Frequent:* Tinnitus.

Heart Rate and Rhythm Disorders: *Frequent:* Atrial fibrillation, bradycardia, palpitation. *Infrequent:* AV block, bundle branch block, sick sinus syndrome, cardiac arrest, supraventricular tachycardia, extrasystoles, tachycardia.

Liver and Biliary System Disorders: *Infrequent:* Abnormal hepatic function, cholecystitis.

Metabolic and Nutritional Disorders: *Frequent:* Dehydration, hypokalemia. *Infrequent:* Diabetes mellitus, gout, hypercholesterolemia, hyperlipemia, hypoglycemia, cachexia, thirst, hyperglycemia, hyponatremia.

Musculoskeletal Disorders: *Frequent:* Arthritis, leg cramps, myalgia. *Infrequent:* Cramps, hernia, muscle weakness.

Myo-, Endo-, Pericardial and Valve Disorders: *Frequent:* Angina pectoris, myocardial infarction.

Platelet, Bleeding, and Clotting Disorders: *Frequent:* Epistaxis. *Infrequent:* Hematoma, thrombocytopenia, purpura.

Psychiatric Disorders: *Frequent:* Paranoid reaction, confusion. *Infrequent:* Abnormal dreaming, amnesia, apathy, delirium, dementia, depersonalization, emotional lability, impaired concentration, decreased libido, personality disorder, suicide attempt, increased libido, neurosis, suicidal ideation, psychosis.

Red Blood Cell Disorders: *Frequent:* Anemia. *Infrequent:* Hypochromic anemia.

Reproductive Disorders (Female & Male): *Infrequent:* Breast pain, impotence, atrophic vaginitis.

Resistance Mechanism Disorders: *Infrequent:* Cellulitis, cystitis, herpes simplex, otitis media.

Respiratory System: *Infrequent:* Bronchospasm, laryngitis, apnea.

Skin and Appendages: *Frequent:* Rashes of various kinds (maculopapular, eczema, bullous, exfoliative, psoriaform, erythematous). *Infrequent:* Alopecia, skin ulceration, urticaria, dermatitis contact.

Special Senses: *Infrequent:* Perversion of taste, loss of taste.

Urinary System Disorders: *Frequent:* Hematuria. *Infrequent:* Albuminuria, oliguria, acute renal failure, dysuria, micturition urgency, nocturia, polyuria, renal calculus, urinary retention.

Vascular (extracardiac) Disorders: *Infrequent:* Hemorrhoids, peripheral ischemia, pulmonary embolism, thrombosis, thrombophlebitis deep, aneurysm, hemorrhage intracranial.
Vision Disorders: *Frequent:* Cataract. *Infrequent:* Conjunctival hemorrhage, blepharitis, diplopia, eye pain, glaucoma.
White Cell and Resistance Disorders: *Infrequent:* Lymphadenopathy, leukocytosis.
Post-Introduction Reports
Voluntary reports of adverse events temporally associated with Exelon that have been received since market introduction that are not listed above, and that may or may not be causally related to the drug include the following:
Skin and Appendages: Stevens-Johnson syndrome.

OVERDOSAGE

Because strategies for the management of overdose are continually evolving, it is advisable to contact a Poison Control Center to determine the latest recommendations for the management of an overdose of any drug.
As Exelon® (rivastigmine tartrate) has a short plasma half-life of about one hour and a moderate duration of acetylcholinesterase inhibition of 8-10 hours, it is recommended that in cases of asymptomatic overdoses, no further dose of Exelon should be administered for the next 24 hours.
As in any case of overdose, general supportive measures should be utilized. Overdosage with cholinesterase inhibitors can result in cholinergic crisis characterized by severe nausea, vomiting, salivation, sweating, bradycardia, hypotension, respiratory depression, collapse and convulsions. Increasing muscle weakness is a possibility and may result in death if respiratory muscles are involved. Atypical responses in blood pressure and heart rate have been reported with other drugs that increase cholinergic activity when co-administered with quaternary anticholinergics such as glycopyrrolate. Due to the short half-life of Exelon, dialysis (hemodialysis, peritoneal dialysis, or hemofiltration) would not be clinically indicated in the event of an overdose.
In overdoses accompanied by severe nausea and vomiting, the use of antiemetics should be considered. In a documented case of a 46 mg overdose with Exelon, the patient experienced vomiting, incontinence, hypertension, psychomotor retardation, and loss of consciousness. The patient fully recovered within 24 hours and conservative management was all that was required for treatment.

DOSAGE AND ADMINISTRATION

The dosage of Exelon® (rivastigmine tartrate) shown to be effective in controlled clinical trials is 6-12 mg/day, given as twice a day dosing (daily doses of 3 to 6 mg BID). There is evidence from the clinical trials that doses at the higher end of this range may be more beneficial.
The starting dose of Exelon is 1.5 mg twice a day (BID). If this dose is well tolerated, after a minimum of two weeks of treatment, the dose may be increased to 3 mg BID. Subsequent increases to 4.5 mg BID and 6 mg BID should be attempted after a minimum of 2 weeks at the previous dose. If adverse effects (e.g., nausea, vomiting, abdominal pain, loss of appetite) cause intolerance during treatment, the patient should be instructed to discontinue treatment for several doses and then restart at the same or next lower dose level. If treatment is interrupted for longer than several days, treatment should be reinitiated with the lowest daily dose and titrated as described above *(see WARNINGS)*. The maximum dose is 6 mg BID (12 mg/day).
Exelon should be taken with meals in divided doses in the morning and evening.
Recommendations for Administration: Caregivers should be instructed in the correct procedure for administering Exelon Oral Solution. In addition, they should be directed to the Instruction Sheet (included with the product) describing how the solution is to be administered. Caregivers should direct questions about the administration of the solution to either their physician or pharmacist *(see PRECAUTIONS: Information for Patients and Caregivers)*.
Patients should be instructed to remove the oral dosing syringe provided in its protective case, and using the provided syringe, withdraw the prescribed amount of Exelon Oral Solution from the container. Each dose of Exelon Oral Solution may be swallowed directly from the syringe or first mixed with a small glass of water, cold fruit juice or soda. Patients should be instructed to stir and drink the mixture.
Exelon Oral Solution and Exelon Capsules may be interchanged at equal doses.

HOW SUPPLIED

Exelon® (rivastigmine tartrate) Oral Solution is supplied as 120 mL of a clear, yellow solution (2 mg/mL base) in a 4 ounce USP Type III amber glass bottle with a child-resistant 28 mm cap, 0.5 mm foam liner, dip tube and self-aligning plug. The oral solution is packaged with a dispenser set which consists of an assembled oral dosing syringe that allows dispensing a maximum volume of 3 mL corresponding to a 6 mg dose, with a plastic tube container.
Bottles of 120 mL .... NDC 0078-0339-31
Store below 77°F (25°C) in an upright position and protect from freezing.
When Exelon Oral Solution is combined with cold fruit juice or soda, the mixture is stable at room temperature for up to 4 hours.

Exelon® (rivastigmine tartrate) Oral Solution
Instructions for Use

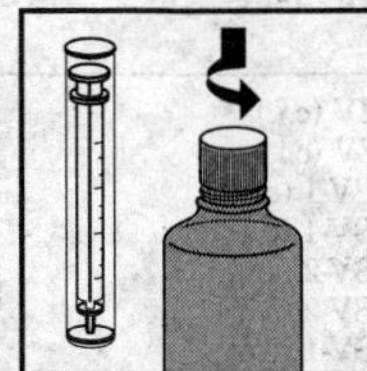

1. Remove oral dosing syringe from its protective case.
Push down and twist child resistant closure to open bottle.

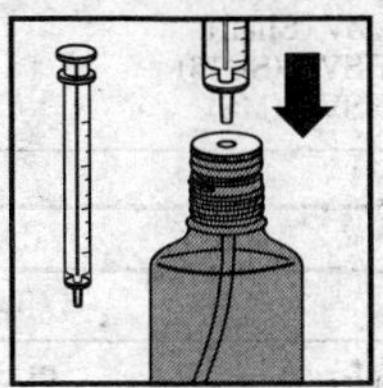

2. Insert tip of syringe into opening of white stopper.

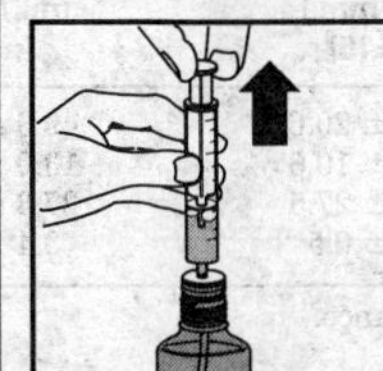

3. While holding the syringe, pull the plunger up to the level (see markings on side of syringe) that equals the dose prescribed by your doctor.

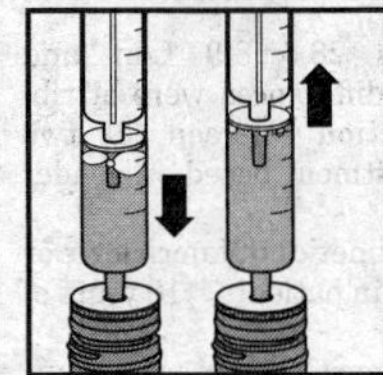

4. Before removing syringe containing prescribed dose from bottle, push out large bubbles by moving plunger up and down a few times. After the **large** bubbles are gone, pull the plunger again to the level that equals the dose prescribed by your doctor. Do not worry about a few tiny bubbles. This will not affect your dose in any way.
Remove the syringe from the bottle.

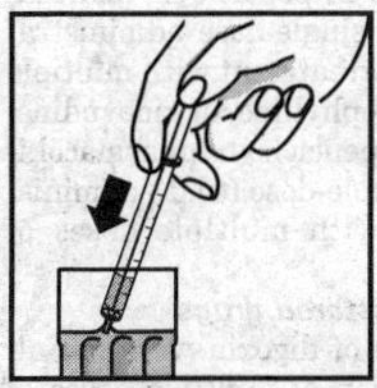

5. You may swallow Exelon Oral Solution directly from the syringe or mix with a small glass of water, cold fruit juice or soda. If mixing with water, juice or soda, be sure to stir completely and to drink the entire mixture. DO NOT MIX WITH OTHER LIQUIDS.

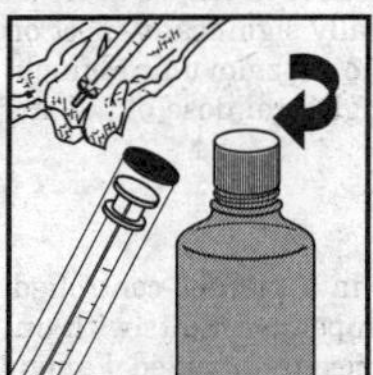

6. After use, wipe outside of syringe with a clean tissue and put it back into its case.
Close bottle using child resistant closure.

Store Exelon Oral Solution at room temperature (below 77°F) in an upright position. Do not place in freezer.

(86000501 4/00)
T2004-48
REV: JUNE 2004 Printed in U.S.A. 89009403
416242
Manufactured by:
Novartis Consumer Health, Incorporated
Lincoln, Nebraska 68517
Distributed by:
Novartis Pharmaceuticals Corporation
East Hanover, New Jersey 07936

FAMVIR® ℞
[făm-vәr]
(famciclovir)
Tablets
Rx only

Prescribing Information
The following prescribing information is based on official labeling in effect July 2004.

DESCRIPTION

Famvir® (famciclovir) contains famciclovir, an orally administered prodrug of the antiviral agent penciclovir. Chemically, famciclovir is known as 2-[2-(2-amino-9*H*-purin-9-yl)ethyl]-1,3-propanediol diacetate. Its molecular formula is $C_{14}H_{19}N_5O_4$; its molecular weight is 321.3. It is a synthetic acyclic guanine derivative and has the following structure
[See chemical structure at top of next column]

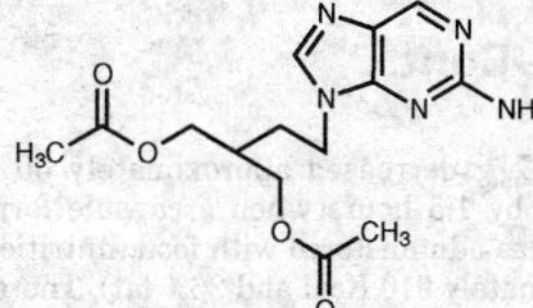
famciclovir

Famciclovir is a white to pale yellow solid. It is freely soluble in acetone and methanol, and sparingly soluble in ethanol and isopropanol. At 25°C famciclovir is freely soluble (>25% w/v) in water initially, but rapidly precipitates as the sparingly soluble (2%-3% w/v) monohydrate. Famciclovir is not hygroscopic below 85% relative humidity. Partition coefficients are: octanol/water (pH 4.8) *P*=1.09 and octanol/phosphate buffer (pH 7.4) *P*=2.08.
Tablets for Oral Administration: Each white, film-coated tablet contains famciclovir. The 125-mg and 250-mg tablets are round; the 500-mg tablets are oval. Inactive ingredients consist of hydroxypropyl cellulose, hydroxypropyl methylcellulose, lactose, magnesium stearate, polyethylene glycols, sodium starch glycolate and titanium dioxide.

MICROBIOLOGY

Mechanism of Antiviral Activity: Famciclovir undergoes rapid biotransformation to the active antiviral compound penciclovir, which has inhibitory activity against herpes simplex virus types 1 (HSV-1) and 2 (HSV-2) and varicella zoster virus (VZV). In cells infected with HSV-1, HSV-2 or VZV, viral thymidine kinase phosphorylates penciclovir to a monophosphate form that, in turn, is converted to penciclovir triphosphate by cellular kinases. *In vitro* studies demonstrate that penciclovir triphosphate inhibits HSV-2 DNA polymerase competitively with deoxyguanosine triphosphate. Consequently, herpes viral DNA synthesis and, therefore, replication are selectively inhibited.
Penciclovir triphosphate has an intracellular half-life of 10 hours in HSV-1-, 20 hours in HSV-2- and 7 hours in VZV-infected cells cultured *in vitro;* however, the clinical significance is unknown.
Antiviral Activity *In Vitro* and *In Vivo*: In cell culture studies, penciclovir has antiviral activity against the following herpes viruses (listed in decreasing order of potency): HSV-1, HSV-2 and VZV. Sensitivity test results, expressed as the concentration of the drug required to inhibit the growth of the virus by 50% (IC_{50}) or 99% (IC_{99}) in cell culture, vary greatly depending upon a number of factors, including the assay protocols, and in particular the cell type used. *See Table 1.*
[See table 1 at top of next page]
Drug Resistance: Penciclovir-resistant mutants of HSV and VZV can result from mutations in the viral thymidine kinase (TK) and DNA polymerase genes. Mutations in the viral TK gene may lead to complete loss of TK activity (TK negative), reduced levels of TK activity (TK partial), or alteration in the ability of viral TK to phosphorylate the drug without an equivalent loss in the ability to phosphorylate thymidine (TK altered). The most commonly encountered acyclovir-resistant mutants that are TK negative are also resistant to penciclovir. The possibility of viral resistance to penciclovir should be considered in patients who fail to respond or experience recurrent viral shedding during therapy.

CLINICAL PHARMACOLOGY

Pharmacokinetics
Absorption and Bioavailability: Famciclovir is the diacetyl 6-deoxy analog of the active antiviral compound penciclovir. Following oral administration, little or no famciclovir is detected in plasma or urine.
The absolute bioavailability of famciclovir is 77±8% as determined following the administration of a 500-mg famciclovir oral dose and a 400-mg penciclovir intravenous dose to 12 healthy male subjects.
Penciclovir concentrations increased in proportion to dose over a famciclovir dose range of 125 mg to 750 mg administered as a single dose. Single oral-dose administration of 125-mg, 250-mg or 500-mg famciclovir to healthy male volunteers across 17 studies gave the following pharmacokinetic parameters:

Table 2

Dose	$AUC_{(0\text{-}inf)}$ † (mcg hr/mL)	C_{max} ‡ (mcg/mL)	T_{max} § (h)
125 mg	2.24	0.8	0.9
250 mg	4.48	1.6	0.9
500 mg	8.95	3.3	0.9

†$AUC_{(0\text{-}inf)}$ (mcg hr/mL)=area under the plasma concentration-time profile extrapolated to infinity.
‡C_{max} (mcg/mL)=maximum observed plasma concentration.
§T_{max} (h)=time to C_{max}.

Following single oral-dose administration of 500-mg famciclovir to seven patients with herpes zoster, the mean ± SD AUC, C_{max}, and T_{max} were 12.1±1.7 mcg hr/mL, 4.0±0.7 mcg/mL, and 0.7±0.2 hours, respectively. The AUC of penciclovir was approximately 35% greater in patients with herpes zoster as compared to healthy volunteers. Some of this difference may be due to differences in renal function between the two groups.
There is no accumulation of penciclovir after the administration of 500-mg famciclovir t.i.d. for 7 days.

Continued on next page

Famvir—Cont.

Penciclovir C_{max} decreased approximately 50% and T_{max} was delayed by 1.5 hours when a capsule formulation of famciclovir was administered with food (nutritional content was approximately 910 Kcal and 26% fat). There was no effect on the extent of availability (AUC) of penciclovir. There was an 18% decrease in C_{max} and a delay in T_{max} of about 1 hour when famciclovir was given 2 hours after a meal as compared to its administration 2 hours before a meal. Because there was no effect on the extent of systemic availability of penciclovir, it appears that Famvir® (famciclovir) can be taken without regard to meals.

Distribution: The volume of distribution (Vd_{β}) was 1.08±0.17 L/kg in 12 healthy male subjects following a single intravenous dose of penciclovir at 400 mg administered as a 1-hour intravenous infusion.

Penciclovir is <20% bound to plasma proteins over the concentration range of 0.1 to 20 mcg/mL. The blood/plasma ratio of penciclovir is approximately 1.

Metabolism: Following oral administration, famciclovir is deacetylated and oxidized to form penciclovir. Metabolites that are inactive include 6-deoxy penciclovir, monoacetylated penciclovir, and 6-deoxy monoacetylated penciclovir (5%, <0.5% and <0.5% of the dose in the urine, respectively). Little or no famciclovir is detected in plasma or urine.

An *in vitro* study using human liver microsomes demonstrated that cytochrome P450 does not play an important role in famciclovir metabolism. The conversion of 6-deoxy penciclovir to penciclovir is catalyzed by aldehyde oxidase.

Elimination: Approximately 94% of administered radioactivity was recovered in urine over 24 hours (83% of the dose was excreted in the first 6 hours) after the administration of 5 mg/kg radiolabeled penciclovir as a 1-hour infusion to three healthy male volunteers. Penciclovir accounted for 91% of the radioactivity excreted in the urine.

Following the oral administration of a single 500-mg dose of radiolabeled famciclovir to three healthy male volunteers, 73% and 27% of administered radioactivity were recovered in urine and feces over 72 hours, respectively. Penciclovir accounted for 82% and 6-deoxy penciclovir accounted for 7% of the radioactivity excreted in the urine. Approximately 60% of the administered radiolabeled dose was collected in urine in the first 6 hours.

After intravenous administration of penciclovir in 48 healthy male volunteers, mean ± S.D. total plasma clearance of penciclovir was 36.6±6.3 L/hr (0.48±0.09 L/hr/kg). Penciclovir renal clearance accounted for 74.5±8.8% of total plasma clearance.

Renal clearance of penciclovir following the oral administration of a single 500-mg dose of famciclovir to 109 healthy male volunteers was 27.7±7.6 L/hr.

The plasma elimination half-life of penciclovir was 2.0±0.3 hours after intravenous administration of penciclovir to 48 healthy male volunteers and 2.3±0.4 hours after oral administration of 500-mg famciclovir to 124 healthy male volunteers. The half-life in seven patients with herpes zoster was 3.0±1.1 hours.

HIV-Infected Patients: Following oral administration of a single dose of 500-mg famciclovir (the oral prodrug of penciclovir) to HIV-positive patients, the pharmacokinetic parameters of penciclovir were comparable to those observed in healthy subjects.

Renal Insufficiency: Apparent plasma clearance, renal clearance, and the plasma-elimination rate constant of penciclovir decreased linearly with reductions in renal function. After the administration of a single 500-mg famciclovir oral dose (n=27) to healthy volunteers and to volunteers with varying degrees of renal insufficiency (CL_{CR} ranged from 6.4 to 138.8 mL/min.), the following results were obtained (Table 3):

[See table 3 above]

In a multiple-dose study of famciclovir conducted in subjects with varying degrees of renal impairment (n=18), the pharmacokinetics of penciclovir were comparable to those after single doses.

A dosage adjustment is recommended for patients with renal insufficiency *(see DOSAGE AND ADMINISTRATION).*

Hepatic Insufficiency: Well-compensated chronic liver disease (chronic hepatitis [n=6], chronic ethanol abuse [n=8], or primary biliary cirrhosis [n=1]) had no effect on the extent of availability (AUC) of penciclovir following a single dose of 500-mg famciclovir. However, there was a 44% decrease in penciclovir mean maximum plasma concentration and the time to maximum plasma concentration was increased by 0.75 hours in patients with hepatic insufficiency compared to normal volunteers. No dosage adjustment is recommended for patients with well-compensated hepatic impairment. The pharmacokinetics of penciclovir have not been evaluated in patients with severe uncompensated hepatic impairment.

Elderly Subjects: Based on cross-study comparisons, mean penciclovir AUC was 40% larger and penciclovir renal clearance was 22% lower after the oral administration of famciclovir in elderly volunteers (n=18, age 65 to 79 years) compared to younger volunteers. Some of this difference may be due to differences in renal function between the two groups.

Gender: The pharmacokinetics of penciclovir were evaluated in 18 healthy male and 18 healthy female volunteers after single-dose oral administration of 500-mg famciclovir. AUC of penciclovir was 9.3±1.9 mcg hr/mL and 11.1±2.1 mcg hr/mL in males and females, respectively.

Table 1

Method of Assay	Virus Type	Cell Type	IC_{50} (mcg/mL)	IC_{99}
Plaque Reduction	VZV (c.i.)	MRC-5	5.0 ± 3.0	
	VZV (c.i.)	Hs68	0.9 ± 0.4	
	HSV-1 (c.i.)	MRC-5	0.2 – 0.6	
	HSV-1 (c.i.)	WISH	0.04 – 0.5	
	HSV-2 (c.i.)	MRC-5	0.9 – 2.1	
	HSV-2 (c.i.)	WISH	0.1 – 0.8	
Virus Yield Reduction	HSV-1 (c.i.)	MRC-5		0.4 – 0.5
	HSV-2 (c.i.)	MRC-5		0.6 – 0.7
DNA Synthesis Inhibition	VZV (Ellen)	MRC-5	0.1	
	HSV-1 (SC16)	MRC-5	0.04	
	HSV-2 (MS)	MRC-5	0.05	

(c.i.) = clinical isolates.

Table 3

Parameter (mean ± S.D.)	CL_{CR}† ≥60 (mL/min.) (n=15)	CL_{CR} 40-59 (mL/min.) (n=5)	CL_{CR} 20-39 (mL/min.) (n=4)	CL_{CR} <20 (mL/min.) (n=3)
CL_{CR} (mL/min)	88.1 ± 20.6	49.3 ± 5.9	26.5 ± 5.3	12.7 ± 5.9
CL_R (L/hr)	30.1 ± 10.6	13.0 ± 1.3‡	4.2 ± 0.9	1.6 ± 1.0
CL/F§ (L/hr)	66.9 ± 27.5	27.3 ± 2.8	12.8 ± 1.3	5.8 ± 2.8
Half-life (hr)	2.3 ± 0.5	3.4 ± 0.7	6.2 ± 1.6	13.4 ± 10.2

†CL_{CR} is measured creatinine clearance.
‡n=4.
§CL/F consists of bioavailability factor and famciclovir to penciclovir conversion factor.

Penciclovir renal clearance was 28.5±8.9 L/hr and 21.8±4.3 L/hr, respectively. These differences were attributed to differences in renal function between the two groups. No famciclovir dosage adjustment based on gender is recommended.

Pediatric Patients: The pharmacokinetics of famciclovir or penciclovir have not been evaluated in patients <18 years of age.

Race: The pharmacokinetics of famciclovir or penciclovir with respect to race have not been evaluated.

Drug Interactions

Effects on penciclovir

No clinically significant alterations in penciclovir pharmacokinetics were observed following single-dose administration of 500-mg famciclovir after pre-treatment with multiple doses of allopurinol, cimetidine, theophylline, or zidovudine. No clinically significant effect on penciclovir pharmacokinetics was observed following multiple-dose (t.i.d.) administration of famciclovir (500 mg) with multiple doses of digoxin.

Effects of famciclovir on co-administered drugs

The steady-state pharmacokinetics of digoxin were not altered by concomitant administration of multiple doses of famciclovir (500 mg t.i.d.). No clinically significant effect on the pharmacokinetics of zidovudine or zidovudine glucuronide was observed following a single oral dose of 500-mg famciclovir.

CLINICAL TRIALS

Herpes Zoster

Famvir® (famciclovir) was studied in a placebo-controlled, double-blind trial of 419 immunocompetent adults with uncomplicated herpes zoster. Comparisons included Famvir 500 mg t.i.d., Famvir 750 mg t.i.d., or placebo. Treatment was begun within 72 hours of initial lesion appearance and therapy was continued for 7 days.

The median time to full crusting in Famvir-treated patients was 5 days compared to 7 days in placebo-treated patients. The times to full crusting, loss of vesicles, loss of ulcers, and loss of crusts were shorter for Famvir 500 mg-treated patients than for placebo-treated patients in the overall study population. The effects of Famvir were greater when therapy was initiated within 48 hours of rash onset; it was also more pronounced in patients 50 years of age or older. Among the 65.2% of patients with at least one positive viral culture, Famvir-treated patients had a shorter median duration of viral shedding than placebo-treated patients (1 day and 2 days, respectively).

There were no overall differences in the duration of pain before rash healing between Famvir- and placebo-treated groups. In addition, there was no difference in the incidence of pain after rash healing (postherpetic neuralgia) between the treatment groups. In the 186 patients (44.4% of total study population) who did develop postherpetic neuralgia, the median duration of postherpetic neuralgia was shorter in patients treated with Famvir 500 mg than in those treated with placebo (63 days and 119 days, respectively). No additional efficacy was demonstrated with higher doses of Famvir.

A double-blind controlled trial in 545 immunocompetent adults with uncomplicated herpes zoster treated within 72 hours of initial lesion appearance compared three doses of Famvir to acyclovir 800 mg 5 times per day. Times to full lesion crusting and times to loss of acute pain were comparable for all groups and there were no statistically significant differences in the time to loss of postherpetic neuralgia between Famvir- and acyclovir-treated groups.

Herpes Simplex Infections

Recurrent Genital Herpes: In two placebo-controlled trials, 626 immunocompetent adults with a recurrence of genital herpes were treated with Famvir 125 mg b.i.d. (n=160), Famvir 250 mg b.i.d. (n=169), Famvir 500 mg b.i.d. (n=154) or placebo (n=143) for 5 days. Treatment was initiated within 6 hours of either symptom onset or lesion appearance. In the two studies combined, the median time to healing in Famvir 125 mg-treated patients was 4 days compared to 5 days in placebo-treated patients and the median time to cessation of viral shedding was 1.8 vs. 3.4 days in Famvir 125-mg and placebo-recipients, respectively. The median time to loss of all symptoms was 3.2 days in Famvir 125 mg-treated patients vs. 3.8 days in placebo-treated patients. No additional efficacy was demonstrated with higher doses of Famvir.

Suppression of Recurrent Genital Herpes: 934 immunocompetent adults with a history of 6 or more recurrences per year were randomized into two double-blind, 1-year, placebo-controlled trials. Comparisons included Famvir 125 mg t.i.d., 250 mg b.i.d., 250 mg t.i.d. and placebo. At one year, 60% to 65% of patients were still receiving Famvir and 25% were receiving placebo treatment. Patient reported recurrence rates for the 250 mg b.i.d. dose at 6 and 12 months as shown in Table 4.

Table 4

	Recurrence Rates at 6 Months		Recurrence Rates at 12 Months	
	Famvir® 250 mg b.i.d. (n=236)	Placebo (n=233)	Famvir® 250 mg b.i.d. (n=236)	Placebo (n=233)
Recurrence-free	39%	10%	29%	6%
Recurrences†	47%	74%	53%	78%
Lost to Follow-up‡	14%	16%	17%	16%

† Based on patient reported data; not necessarily confirmed by a physician.
‡ Patients recurrence-free at time of last contact prior to withdrawal.

Famvir-treated patients had approximately 1/5 the median number of recurrences as compared to placebo-treated patients.

Higher doses of Famvir were not associated with an increase in efficacy.

Recurrent Mucocutaneous Herpes Simplex Infection in HIV-Infected Patients: A randomized, double-blind, multicenter study compared famciclovir 500 mg twice daily for 7 days (n=150) with oral acyclovir 400 mg 5 times daily for 7 days (n=143) in HIV-infected patients with recurrent mucocutaneous HSV infection treated within 48 hours of lesion onset. Approximately 40% of patients had a CD_4 count below 200 cells/mm^3, 54% of patients had anogenital lesions and [illegible] had orolabial lesions. Famciclovir therapy was comparable to oral acyclovir in reducing new lesion formation and in time to complete healing.

INDICATIONS AND USAGE

Herpes Zoster: Famvir® (famciclovir) is indicated for the treatment of acute herpes zoster (shingles).

Herpes Simplex Infections: Famvir is indicated for:

- treatment or suppression of recurrent genital herpes in immunocompetent patients.
- treatment of recurrent mucocutaneous herpes simplex infections in HIV-infected patients.

CONTRAINDICATIONS

Famvir® (famciclovir) is contraindicated in patients with known hypersensitivity to the product, its components, and Denavir® (penciclovir cream).

PRECAUTIONS

General

The efficacy of Famvir® (famciclovir) has not been established for initial episode genital herpes infection, ophthalmic zoster, disseminated zoster or in immunocompromised patients with herpes zoster.

Dosage adjustment is recommended when administering Famvir to patients with creatinine clearance values <60 mL/min. *(See DOSAGE AND ADMINISTRATION)*. In patients with underlying renal disease who have received inappropriately high doses of Famvir for their level of renal function, acute renal failure has been reported.

Information for Patients

Patients should be informed that Famvir is not a cure for genital herpes. There are no data evaluating whether Famvir will prevent transmission of infection to others. As genital herpes is a sexually transmitted disease, patients should avoid contact with lesions or intercourse when lesions and/or symptoms are present to avoid infecting partners. Genital herpes can also be transmitted in the absence of symptoms through asymptomatic viral shedding. If medical management of recurrent episodes is indicated, patients should be advised to initiate therapy at the first sign or symptom.

Drug Interactions

Concurrent use with probenecid or other drugs significantly eliminated by active renal tubular secretion may result in increased plasma concentrations of penciclovir.

The conversion of 6-deoxy penciclovir to penciclovir is catalyzed by aldehyde oxidase. Interactions with other drugs metabolized by this enzyme could potentially occur.

Carcinogenesis, Mutagenesis, Impairment of Fertility

Famciclovir was administered orally unless otherwise stated.

Carcinogenesis: Two-year dietary carcinogenicity studies with famciclovir were conducted in rats and mice. An increase in the incidence of mammary adenocarcinoma (a common tumor in animals of this strain) was seen in female rats receiving the high dose of 600 mg/kg/day (1.5 to 9.0× the human systemic exposure at the recommended daily oral doses of 500 mg t.i.d., 250 mg b.i.d., or 125 mg b.i.d. based on area under the plasma concentration curve comparisons [24 hr AUC] for penciclovir). No increases in tumor incidence were reported in male rats treated at doses up to 240 mg/kg/day (0.9 to 5.4× the human AUC), or in male and female mice at doses up to 600 mg/kg/day (0.4 to 2.4× the human AUC).

Mutagenesis: Famciclovir and penciclovir (the active metabolite of famciclovir) were tested for genotoxic potential in a battery of *in vitro* and *in vivo* assays. Famciclovir and penciclovir were negative in *in vitro* tests for gene mutations in bacteria (*S. typhimurium* and *E. coli*) and unscheduled DNA synthesis in mammalian HeLa 83 cells (at doses up to 10,000 and 5,000 mcg/plate, respectively). Famciclovir was also negative in the L5178Y mouse lymphoma assay (5000 mcg/mL), the *in vivo* mouse micronucleus test (4800 mg/kg), and rat dominant lethal study (5000 mg/kg). Famciclovir-induced increases in polyploidy in human lymphocytes *in vitro* in the absence of chromosomal damage (1200 mcg/mL). Penciclovir was positive in the L5178Y mouse lymphoma assay for gene mutation/chromosomal aberrations, with and without metabolic activation (1000 mcg/mL). In human lymphocytes, penciclovir caused chromosomal aberrations in the absence of metabolic activation (250 mcg/mL).

Penciclovir caused an increased incidence of micronuclei in mouse bone marrow *in vivo* when administered intravenously at doses highly toxic to bone marrow (500 mg/kg), but not when administered orally.

Impairment of Fertility: Testicular toxicity was observed in rats, mice, and dogs following repeated administration of famciclovir or penciclovir. Testicular changes included atrophy of the seminiferous tubules, reduction in sperm count, and/or increased incidence of sperm with abnormal morphology or reduced motility. The degree of toxicity to male reproduction was related to dose and duration of exposure. In male rats, decreased fertility was observed after 10 weeks of dosing at 500 mg/kg/day (1.9 to 11.4× the human AUC). The no observable effect level for sperm and testicular toxicity in rats following chronic administration (26 weeks) was 50 mg/kg/day (0.2 to 1.2× the human systemic exposure based on AUC comparisons). Testicular toxicity was observed following chronic administration to mice (104 weeks) and dogs (26 weeks) at doses of 600 mg/kg/day (0.4 to 2.4× the human AUC) and 150 mg/kg/day (1.7 to 10.2× the human AUC), respectively.

Famciclovir had no effect on general reproductive performance or fertility in female rats at doses up to 1000 mg/kg/day (3.6 to 21.6× the human AUC).

Two placebo-controlled studies in a total of 130 otherwise healthy men with a normal sperm profile over an 8-week baseline period and recurrent genital herpes receiving oral Famvir (250 mg b.i.d.) (n=66) or placebo (n=64) therapy for 18 weeks showed no evidence of significant effects on sperm count, motility or morphology during treatment or during an 8-week follow-up.

Pregnancy

Teratogenic Effects–Pregnancy Category B: Famciclovir was tested for effects on embryo-fetal development in rats and rabbits at oral doses up to 1000 mg/kg/day (approximately 3.6 to 21.6× and 1.8 to 10.8× the human systemic exposure to penciclovir based on AUC comparisons for the rat and rabbit, respectively) and intravenous doses of 360 mg/kg/day in rats (2 to 12× the human dose based on body surface area [BSA] comparisons) or 120 mg/kg/day in rabbits (1.5 to 9.0× the human dose [BSA]). No adverse effects were observed on embryo-fetal development. Similarly, no adverse effects were observed following intravenous administration of penciclovir to rats (80 mg/kg/day, 0.4 to 2.6× the human dose [BSA]) or rabbits (60 mg/kg/day, 0.7 to 4.2× the human dose [BSA]). There are, however, no adequate and well-controlled studies in pregnant women. Because animal reproduction studies are not always predictive of human response, famciclovir should be used during pregnancy only if the benefit to the patient clearly exceeds the potential risk to the fetus.

Pregnancy Exposure Registry: To monitor maternal-fetal outcomes of pregnant women exposed to Famvir, Novartis Pharmaceuticals Corporation maintains a Famvir Pregnancy Registry. Physicians are encouraged to register their patients by calling (888) 669-6682.

Nursing Mothers

Following oral administration of famciclovir to lactating rats, penciclovir was excreted in breast milk at concentrations higher than those seen in the plasma. It is not known whether it is excreted in human milk. There are no data on the safety of Famvir in infants.

Usage in Children

Safety and efficacy in children under the age of 18 years have not been established.

Geriatric Use

Of 816 patients with herpes zoster in clinical studies who were treated with Famvir, 248 (30.4%) were ≥65 years of age and 103 (13%) were ≥75 years of age. No overall differences were observed in the incidence or types of adverse events between younger and older patients.

ADVERSE REACTIONS

Immunocompetent Patients

The safety of Famvir® (famciclovir) has been evaluated in clinical studies involving 816 Famvir-treated patients with herpes zoster (Famvir, 250 mg t.i.d. to 750 mg t.i.d.); 528 Famvir-treated patients with recurrent genital herpes (Famvir, 125 mg b.i.d. to 500 mg t.i.d.); and 1,197 patients with recurrent genital herpes treated with Famvir as suppressive therapy (125 mg q.d. to 250 mg t.i.d.) of which 570 patients received Famvir (open-labeled and/or double-blind) for at least 10 months. Table 5 lists selected adverse events.

[See table 5 above]

Table 5
Selected Adverse Events Reported by ≥2% of Patients in Placebo-controlled Famvir® (famciclovir) Trials*

	Incidence					
	Herpes Zoster		Recurrent Genital Herpes		Genital Herpes-Suppression	
Event	Famvir® (n=273) %	Placebo (n=146) %	Famvir® (n=640) %	Placebo (n=225) %	Famvir® (n=458) %	Placebo (n=63) %
Nervous System						
Headache	22.7	17.8	23.6	16.4	39.3	42.9
Paresthesia	2.6	0.0	1.3	0.0	0.9	0.0
Migraine	0.7	0.7	1.3	0.4	3.1	0.0
Gastrointestinal						
Nausea	12.5	11.6	10.0	8.0	7.2	9.5
Diarrhea	7.7	4.8	4.5	7.6	9.0	9.5
Vomiting	4.8	3.4	1.3	0.9	3.1	1.6
Flatulence	1.5	0.7	1.9	2.2	4.8	1.6
Abdominal Pain	1.1	3.4	3.9	5.8	7.9	7.9
Body as a Whole						
Fatigue	4.4	3.4	6.3	4.4	4.8	3.2
Skin and Appendages						
Pruritus	3.7	2.7	0.9	0.0	2.2	0.0
Rash	0.4	0.7	0.6	0.4	3.3	1.6
Reproductive Female						
Dysmenorrhea	0.0	0.7	2.2	1.3	7.6	6.3

*Patients may have entered into more than one clinical trial.

The following adverse events have been reported during post-approval use of Famvir: urticaria, hallucinations and confusion (including delirium, disorientation, confusional state, occurring predominantly in the elderly). Because these adverse events are reported voluntarily from a population of unknown size, estimates of frequency cannot be made. Table 6 lists selected laboratory abnormalities in genital herpes suppression trials.

Table 6
Selected Laboratory Abnormalities in Genital Herpes Suppression Studies*

Parameter	Famvir® (n=660)† %	Placebo (n=210)† %
Anemia (<0.8 × NRL)	0.1	0.0
Leukopenia (<0.75 × NRL)	1.3	0.9
Neutropenia (<0.8 × NRL)	3.2	1.5
AST (SGOT) (>2 × NRH)	2.3	1.2
ALT (SGPT) (>2 × NRH)	3.2	1.5
Total Bilirubin (>1.5 × NRH)	1.9	1.2
Serum Creatinine (>1.5 × NRH)	0.2	0.3
Amylase (>1.5 × NRH)	1.5	1.9
Lipase (>1.5 × NRH)	4.9	4.7

*Percentage of patients with laboratory abnormalities that were increased or decreased from baseline and were outside of specified ranges.

†n values represent the minimum number of patients assessed for each laboratory parameter.

NRH = Normal Range High.

NRL = Normal Range Low.

Table 7

Indication and Normal Dosage Regimen	Creatinine Clearance (mL/min.)	Adjusted Dosage Regimen Dose (mg)	Dosing Interval
Herpes Zoster			
500 mg every 8 hours	>60	500	every 8 hours
	40–59	500	every 12 hours
	20–39	500	every 24 hours
	<20	250	every 24 hours
	HD*	250	following each dialysis
Recurrent Genital Herpes			
125 mg every 12 hours	≥40	125	every 12 hours
	20–39	125	every 24 hours
	<20	125	every 24 hours
	HD*	125	following each dialysis
Suppression of Recurrent Genital Herpes			
250 mg every 12 hours	≥40	250	every 12 hours
	20–39	125	every 12 hours
	<20	125	every 24 hours
	HD*	125	following each dialysis
Recurrent Orolabial and Genital Herpes Simplex Infection in HIV-Infected Patients			
500 mg every 12 hours	≥40	500	every 12 hours
	20–39	500	every 24 hours
	<20	250	every 24 hours
	HD*	250	following each dialysis

*Hemodialysis

Continued on next page

Famvir—Cont.

HIV-Infected Patients

In HIV-infected patients, the most frequently reported adverse events for famciclovir (500 mg twice daily; n=150) and acyclovir (400 mg, 5×/day; n=143), respectively, were headache (16.7% vs. 15.4%), nausea (10.7% vs. 12.6%), diarrhea (6.7% vs. 10.5%), vomiting (4.7% vs. 3.5%), fatigue (4.0% vs. 2.1%), and abdominal pain (3.3% vs. 5.6%).

OVERDOSAGE

Appropriate symptomatic and supportive therapy should be given. Penciclovir is removed by hemodialysis *(see PRECAUTIONS, General).*

DOSAGE AND ADMINISTRATION

Herpes Zoster

The recommended dosage is 500 mg every 8 hours for 7 days. Therapy should be initiated promptly as soon as herpes zoster is diagnosed. No data are available on efficacy of treatment started greater than 72 hours after rash onset.

Herpes Simplex Infections

Recurrent genital herpes: The recommended dosage is 125 mg twice daily for 5 days. Initiate therapy at the first sign or symptom if medical management of a genital herpes recurrence is indicated. The efficacy of Famvir® (famciclovir) has not been established when treatment is initiated more than 6 hours after onset of symptoms or lesions.

Suppression of recurrent genital herpes: The recommended dosage is 250 mg twice daily for up to 1 year. The safety and efficacy of Famvir therapy beyond 1 year of treatment have not been established.

HIV-Infected Patients

For recurrent orolabial or genital herpes simplex infection, the recommended dosage is 500 mg twice daily for 7 days. In patients with reduced renal function, dosage reduction is recommended *(see PRECAUTIONS, General).*

[See table 7 at top of previous page]

Administration with Food

When famciclovir was administered with food, penciclovir C_{max} decreased approximately 50%. Because the systemic availability of penciclovir (AUC) was not altered, it appears that Famvir may be taken without regard to meals.

HOW SUPPLIED

Famvir® (famciclovir) is supplied as film-coated tablets as follows:

125 mg in bottles of 30; 250 mg in bottles of 30; and 500 mg in bottles of 30 and Single Unit Packages of 50 (intended for institutional use only).

Famvir 125 mg tablet:

White round film-coated, biconvex, beveled edges, debossed with "FAMVIR" on one side and "125" on the other.

125 mg 30's .... NDC 0078-0366-15

Famvir 250 mg tablet:

White round film-coated, biconvex, beveled edges, debossed with "FAMVIR" on one side and "250" on the other.

250 mg 30's .... NDC 0078-0367-15

Famvir 500 mg tablet:

White oval film-coated, biconvex, beveled edges, debossed with "FAMVIR" on one side and "500" on the other.

500 mg 30's .... NDC 0078-0368-15

500 mg SUP 50's .... NDC 0078-0368-64

Store at 25°C (77°F); excursions permitted to 15-30°C (59-86°F)

[see USP Controlled Room Temperature].

T2004-06

REV: MARCH 2004 89011404

Manufactured by:

Novartis Farmacéutica S.A.

08210 Barberà del Vallès

Barcelona, Spain

Distributed by:

Novartis Pharmaceuticals Corp.

East Hanover, NJ 07936

©Novartis

FEMARA® ℞

[fĕm-ara]

(letrozole tablets)

2.5 mg Tablets

℞ only

Prescribing Information

The following prescribing information is based on official labeling in effect July 2003.

DESCRIPTION

Femara® (letrozole tablets) for oral administration contains 2.5 mg of letrozole, a nonsteroidal aromatase inhibitor (inhibitor of estrogen synthesis). It is chemically described as 4,4'-(1H-1,2,4-Triazol-1-ylmethylene)dibenzonitrile, and its structural formula is

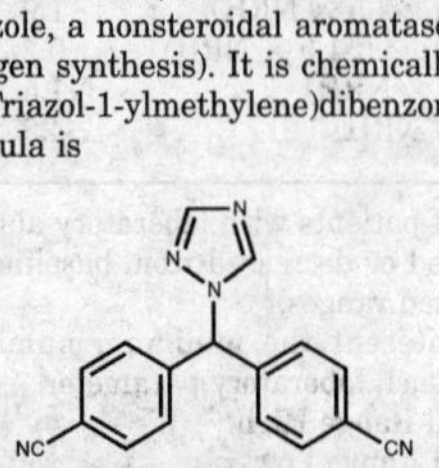

Letrozole is a white to yellowish crystalline powder, practically odorless, freely soluble in dichloromethane, slightly soluble in ethanol, and practically insoluble in water. It has a molecular weight of 285.31, empirical formula $C_{17}H_{11}N_5$, and a melting range of 184°C-185°C.

Femara® (letrozole tablets) is available as 2.5 mg tablets for oral administration.

Inactive Ingredients: Colloidal silicon dioxide, ferric oxide, hydroxypropyl methylcellulose, lactose monohydrate, magnesium stearate, maize starch, microcrystalline cellulose, polyethylene glycol, sodium starch glycolate, talc, and titanium dioxide.

CLINICAL PHARMACOLOGY

Mechanism of Action: The growth of some cancers of the breast is stimulated or maintained by estrogens. Treatment of breast cancer thought to be hormonally responsive (i.e., estrogen and/or progesterone receptor positive or receptor unknown) has included a variety of efforts to decrease estrogen levels (ovariectomy, adrenalectomy, hypophysectomy) or inhibit estrogen effects (antiestrogens and progestational agents). These interventions lead to decreased tumor mass or delayed progression of tumor growth in some women.

In postmenopausal women, estrogens are mainly derived from the action of the aromatase enzyme, which converts adrenal androgens (primarily androstenedione and testosterone) to estrone and estradiol. The suppression of estrogen biosynthesis in peripheral tissues and in the cancer tissue itself can therefore be achieved by specifically inhibiting the aromatase enzyme.

Letrozole is a nonsteroidal competitive inhibitor of the aromatase enzyme system; it inhibits the conversion of androgens to estrogens. In adult nontumor- and tumor-bearing female animals, letrozole is as effective as ovariectomy in reducing uterine weight, elevating serum LH, and causing the regression of estrogen-dependent tumors. In contrast to ovariectomy, treatment with letrozole does not lead to an increase in serum FSH. Letrozole selectively inhibits gonadal steroidogenesis but has no significant effect on adrenal mineralocorticoid or glucocorticoid synthesis.

Letrozole inhibits the aromatase enzyme by competitively binding to the heme of the cytochrome P450 subunit of the enzyme, resulting in a reduction of estrogen biosynthesis in all tissues. Treatment of women with letrozole significantly lowers serum estrone, estradiol and estrone sulfate and has not been shown to significantly affect adrenal corticosteroid synthesis, aldosterone synthesis, or synthesis of thyroid hormones.

Pharmacokinetics: Letrozole is rapidly and completely absorbed from the gastrointestinal tract and absorption is not affected by food. It is metabolized slowly to an inactive metabolite whose glucuronide conjugate is excreted renally, representing the major clearance pathway. About 90% of radiolabeled letrozole is recovered in urine. Letrozole's terminal elimination half-life is about 2 days and steady-state plasma concentration after daily 2.5 mg dosing is reached in 2-6 weeks. Plasma concentrations at steady-state are 1.5 to 2 times higher than predicted from the concentrations measured after a single dose, indicating a slight non-linearity in the pharmacokinetics of letrozole upon daily administration of 2.5 mg. These steady-state levels are maintained over extended periods, however, and continuous accumulation of letrozole does not occur. Letrozole is weakly protein bound and has a large volume of distribution (approximately 1.9 L/kg).

Metabolism and Excretion: Metabolism to a pharmacologically-inactive carbinol metabolite (4,4'-methanol-bisbenzonitrile) and renal excretion of the glucuronide conjugate of this metabolite is the major pathway of letrozole clearance. Of the radiolabel recovered in urine, at least 75% was the glucuronide of the carbinol metabolite, about 9% was two unidentified metabolites, and 6% was unchanged letrozole.

In human microsomes with specific CYP isozyme activity, CYP3A4 metabolized letrozole to the carbinol metabolite while CYP2A6 formed both this metabolite and its ketone analog. In human liver microsomes, letrozole strongly inhibited CYP2A6 and moderately inhibited CYP2C19.

Special Populations: ***Pediatric, Geriatric and Race:*** In the study populations (adults ranging in age from 35 to >80 years), no change in pharmacokinetic parameters was observed with increasing age. Differences in letrozole pharmacokinetics between adult and pediatric populations have not been studied. Differences in letrozole pharmacokinetics due to race have not been studied.

Renal Insufficiency: In a study of volunteers with varying renal function (24-hour creatinine clearance: 9-116 mL/min), no effect of renal function on the pharmacokinetics of single doses of 2.5 mg of Femara® (letrozole tablets) was found. In addition, in a study of 347 patients with advanced breast cancer, about half of whom received 2.5 mg Femara and half 0.5 mg Femara, renal impairment (calculated creatinine clearance: 20-50 mL/min) did not affect steady-state plasma letrozole concentration.

Hepatic Insufficiency: In a study of subjects with mild to moderate non-metastatic hepatic dysfunction (e.g., cirrhosis, Child-Pugh classification A and B), the mean AUC values of the volunteers with moderate hepatic impairment were 37% higher than in normal subjects, but still within the range seen in subjects without impaired function. In a pharmacokinetics study, subjects with liver cirrhosis and severe hepatic impairment (Child-Pugh classification C, which included bilirubins about 2-11 times ULN with minimal to severe ascites) had two-fold increase in exposure (AUC) and 47% reduction in systemic clearance. Breast cancer patients with severe hepatic impairment are thus expected to be exposed to higher levels of letrozole than patients with normal liver function receiving similar doses of this drug. *(See DOSAGE AND ADMINISTRATION, Hepatic Impairment.)*

Drug/Drug Interactions: A pharmacokinetic interaction study with cimetidine showed no clinically significant effect on letrozole pharmacokinetics. An interaction study with warfarin showed no clinically significant effect of letrozole on warfarin pharmacokinetics. In *in-vitro* experiments, letrozole showed no significant inhibition in the metabolism of diazepam. Similarly, no significant inhibition of letrozole metabolism by diazepam was observed.

Coadministration of Femara and tamoxifen 20 mg daily resulted in a reduction of letrozole plasma levels of 38% on average. Clinical experience in the second-line breast cancer pivotal trials indicates that the therapeutic effect of Femara therapy is not impaired if Femara is administered immediately after tamoxifen.

There is no clinical experience to date on the use of Femara in combination with other anticancer agents.

Pharmacodynamics: In postmenopausal patients with advanced breast cancer, daily doses of 0.1 mg to 5 mg Femara suppress plasma concentrations of estradiol, estrone, and

Table 1
Selected Study Population Demographics

Baseline Status	Femara® N=458	tamoxifen N=458	Baseline Status	Femara® N=458	tamoxifen N=458
Stage of Disease			**Previous Antiestrogen Therapy**		
IIIB	6%	7%	Adjuvant	19%	18%
IV	93%	92%	None	81%	82%
Receptor Status			**Dominant Site of Disease**		
ER and PgR Positive	38%	41%	Soft Tissue	25%	25%
ER or PgR Positive	26%	26%	Bone	32%	29%
Both Unknown	34%	33%	Viscera	43%	46%
ER⁻ or PgR⁻ / Other Unknown	<1%	0			

Table 2
Results

	Femara® 2.5 mg N=453	tamoxifen 20 mg N=454	Hazard or Odds Ratio (95% CI) p-value (2-sided)
Median Time to Progression	9.4 months	6.0 months	0.72 (0.62, 0.83)[1] P<0.0001
Objective Response Rate (CR + PR)	145 (32%)	95 (21%)	1.77 (1.31, 2.39)[2] P=0.0002
(CR)	42 (9%)	15 (3%)	2.99 (1.63, 5.47)[2] P=0.0004
Duration of Objective Response Median	18 months (N=145)	16 months (N=95)	
Overall Survival	35 months (N=458)	32 months (N=458)	P=0.5136[3]

[1]Hazard ratio
[2]Odds ratio
[3]Overall logrank test

estrone sulfate by 75%–95% from baseline with maximal suppression achieved within two-three days. Suppression is dose-related, with doses of 0.5 mg and higher giving many values of estrone and estrone sulfate that were below the limit of detection in the assays. Estrogen suppression was maintained throughout treatment in all patients treated at 0.5 mg or higher.

Letrozole is highly specific in inhibiting aromatase activity. There is no impairment of adrenal steroidogenesis. No clinically-relevant changes were found in the plasma concentrations of cortisol, aldosterone, 11-deoxycortisol, 17-hydroxy-progesterone, ACTH or in plasma renin activity among postmenopausal patients treated with a daily dose of Femara 0.1 mg to 5 mg. The ACTH stimulation test performed after 6 and 12 weeks of treatment with daily doses of 0.1, 0.25, 0.5, 1, 2.5, and 5 mg did not indicate any attenuation of aldosterone or cortisol production. Glucocorticoid or mineralocorticoid supplementation is, therefore, not necessary.

No changes were noted in plasma concentrations of androgens (androstenedione and testosterone) among healthy postmenopausal women after 0.1, 0.5, and 2.5 mg single doses of Femara or in plasma concentrations of androstenedione among postmenopausal patients treated with daily doses of 0.1 mg to 5 mg. This indicates that the blockade of estrogen biosynthesis does not lead to accumulation of androgenic precursors. Plasma levels of LH and FSH were not affected by letrozole in patients, nor was thyroid function as evaluated by TSH levels, T3 uptake, and T4 levels.

Clinical Studies: ***First-Line Breast Cancer:*** A randomized, double-blinded, multinational trial compared Femara 2.5 mg with tamoxifen 20 mg in 916 postmenopausal patients with locally advanced (Stage IIIB or locoregional recurrence not amenable to treatment with surgery or radiation) or metastatic breast cancer. Time to progression (TTP) was the primary endpoint of the trial. Selected baseline characteristics for this study are shown in Table 1.

[See table 1 at top of previous page]

Femara was superior to tamoxifen in TTP and rate of objective tumor response *(see Table 2).*

Table 2 summarizes the results of the trial, with a total median follow-up of approximately 32 months. (All analyses are unadjusted and use 2-sided P-values.)

[See table 2 at top of previous page]

Figure 1 shows the Kaplan-Meier curves for TTP.

Figure 1
Kaplan-Meier Estimates of Time to Progression (Tamoxifen Study)

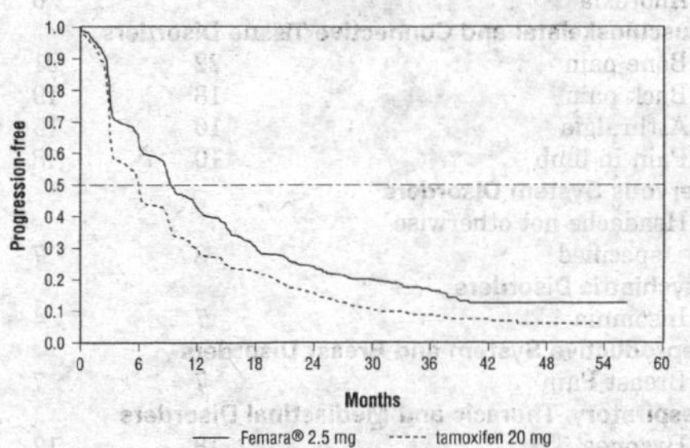

Table 3 shows results in the subgroup of women who had received prior antiestrogen adjuvant therapy, Table 4, results by disease site and Table 5, the results by receptor status.

[See table 3 above]
[See table 4 above]
[See table 5 above]

Figure 2 shows the Kaplan-Meier curves for survival.

Figure 2
Survival by Randomized Treatment Arm

Legend: Randomized letrozole: n=458, events 57%, median overall survival 35 months (95% CI 32 to 38 months) Randomized tamoxifen: n=458, events 57%, median overall survival 32 months (95% CI 28 to 37 months) Overall logrank P=0.5136 (i.e., there was no significant difference between treatment arms in overall survival).

The median overall survival was 35 months for the letrozole group and 32 months for the tamoxifen group, with a P value 0.5136.

Study design allowed patients to crossover upon progression to the other therapy. Approximately 50% of patients crossed over to the opposite treatment arm and almost all patients who crossed over had done so by 36 months. The median time to crossover was 17 months (Femara to tamoxifen) and

Table 3
Efficacy in Patients Who Received Prior Antiestrogen Therapy

Variable	Femara® 2.5 mg N = 84	tamoxifen 20 mg N = 83
Median Time to Progression (95% CI)	8.9 months (6.2, 12.5)	5.9 months (3.2, 6.2)
Hazard Ratio for TTP (95% CI)	0.60 (0.43, 0.84)	
Objective Response Rate (CR + PR)	22 (26%)	7 (8%)
Odds Ratio for Response (95% CI)	3.85 (1.50, 9.60)	

Hazard ratio less than 1 or odds ratio greater than 1 favors letrozole; hazard ratio greater than 1 or odds ratio less than 1 favors tamoxifen.

Table 4
Efficacy by Disease Site

	Femara® 2.5 mg	tamoxifen 20 mg		Femara® 2.5 mg	tamoxifen 20 mg
Dominant Disease Site			**Bone:**		
Soft Tissue:	N=113	N=115	Objective Response Rate	23%	15%
Median TTP	12.1 months	6.4 months			
Objective Response Rate	50%	34%	**Viscera:**	N=195	N=208
			Median TTP	8.3 months	4.6 months
Bone:	N=145	N=131			
Median TTP	9.5 months	6.3 months	Objective Response Rate	28%	17%

Table 5
Efficacy by Receptor Status

Variable	Femara® 2.5	tamoxifen 20 mg
Receptor Positive	N=294	N=305
Median Time to Progression (95% CI)	9.4 months (8.9, 11.8)	6.0 months (5.1, 8.5)
Hazard Ratio for TTP (95% CI)	0.69 (0.58, 0.83)	
Objective Response Rate (CR+PR)	97 (33%)	66 (22%)
Odds Ratio for Response (95% CI)	1.78 (1.20, 2.60)	
Receptor Unknown	N=159	N=149
Median Time to Progression (95% CI)	9.2 months (6.1, 12.3)	6.0 months (4.1, 6.4)
Hazard Ratio for TTP (95% CI)	0.77 (0.60, 0.99)	
Objective Response Rate (CR+PR)	48 (30%)	29 (20%)
Odds Ratio for Response (95% CI)	1.79 (1.10, 3.00)	

Hazard ratio less than 1 or odds ratio greater then 1 favors letrozole; hazard ratio greater then 1 or odds ratio less than 1 favors tamoxifen.

13 months (tamoxifen to Femara). In patients who did not crossover to the opposite treatment arm, median survival was 35 months with Femara (n=219, 95% CI 29 to 43 months) vs. 20 months with tamoxifen (n=229, 95% CI 16 to 26 months).

Second-Line Breast Cancer: Femara was initially studied at doses of 0.1 mg to 5.0 mg daily in six non-comparative Phase I/II trials in 181 postmenopausal estrogen/progesterone receptor positive or unknown advanced breast cancer patients previously treated with at least antiestrogen therapy. Patients had received other hormonal therapies and also may have received cytotoxic therapy. Eight (20%) of forty patients treated with Femara 2.5 mg daily in Phase I/II trials achieved an objective tumor response (complete or partial response).

Two large randomized controlled multinational (predominantly European) trials were conducted in patients with advanced breast cancer who had progressed despite antiestrogen therapy. Patients were randomized to Femara 0.5 mg daily, Femara 2.5 mg daily, or a comparator (megestrol acetate 160 mg daily in one study; and aminoglutethimide 250 mg b.i.d. with corticosteroid supplementation in the other study). In each study over 60% of the patients had received therapeutic antiestrogens, and about one-fifth of these patients had had an objective response. The megestrol acetate controlled study was double-blind; the other study was open label. Selected baseline characteristics for each study are shown in Table 6.

Table 6
Selected Study Population Demographics

Parameter	megestrol acetate study	amino-glutethimide study
No. of Participants	552	557
Receptor Status		
ER/PR Positive	57%	56%
ER/PR Unknown	43%	44%
Previous Therapy		
Adjuvant Only	33%	38%
Therapeutic ± Adj.	66%	62%
Sites of Disease		
Soft Tissue	56%	50%
Bone	50%	55%
Viscera	40%	44%

Confirmed objective tumor response (complete response plus partial response) was the primary endpoint of the trials. Responses were measured according to the Union Internationale Contre le Cancer (UICC) criteria and verified by independent, blinded review. All responses were confirmed by a second evaluation 4-12 weeks after the documentation of the initial response.

Table 7 shows the results for the first trial, with a minimum follow-up of 15 months, that compared Femara 0.5 mg, Femara 2.5 mg, and megestrol acetate 160 mg daily. (All analyses are unadjusted.)

[See table 7 at top of next page]

The Kaplan-Meier Curve for progression for the megestrol acetate study is shown in Figure 3.

Figure 3
Kaplan-Meier Estimates of Time to Progression (Megestrol Acetate Study)

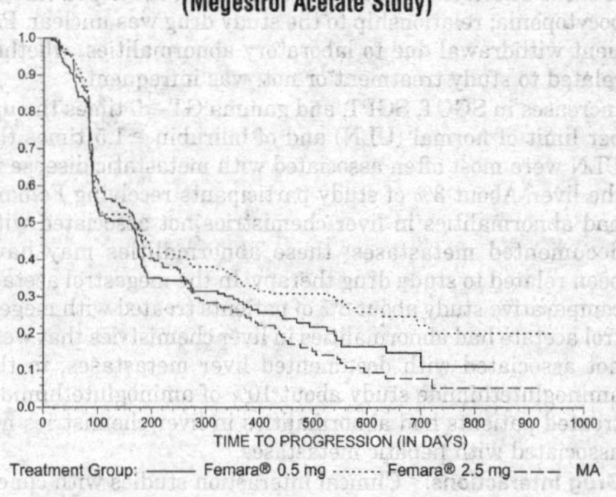

The results for the study comparing Femara to aminoglutethimide, with a minimum follow-up of nine months, are shown in Table 8. (Unadjusted analyses are used.)

[See table 8 at top of next page]

The Kaplan-Meier Curve for progression for the aminoglutethimide study is shown in Figure 4.

[See figure 4 at top of next column]

INDICATIONS AND USAGE

Femara® (letrozole tablets) is indicated for first-line treatment of postmenopausal women with hormone receptor positive or hormone receptor unknown locally advanced or metastatic breast cancer. Femara is also indicated for the

Continued on next page

Femara—Cont.

Figure 4
Kaplan-Meier Estimates of Time to Progression (Aminoglutethimide Study)

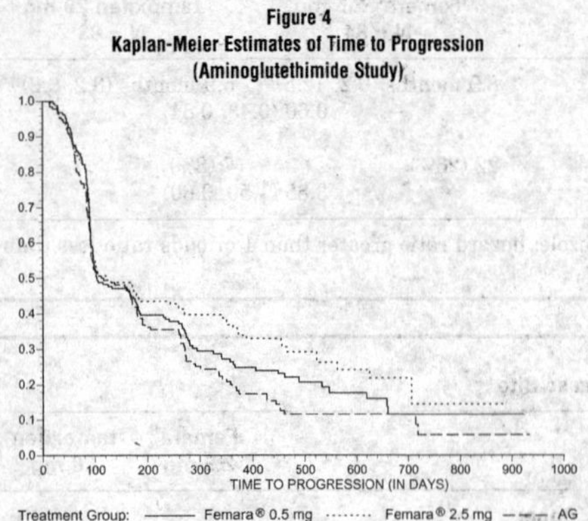

treatment of advanced breast cancer in postmenopausal women with disease progression following antiestrogen therapy.

CONTRAINDICATIONS

Femara® (letrozole tablets) is contraindicated in patients with known hypersensitivity to Femara or any of its excipients.

WARNINGS

Pregnancy: Letrozole may cause fetal harm when administered to pregnant women. Studies in rats at doses equal to or greater than 0.003 mg/kg (about 1/100 the daily maximum recommended human dose on a mg/m^2 basis) administered during the period of organogenesis, have shown that letrozole is embryotoxic and fetotoxic, as indicated by intrauterine mortality, increased resorption, increased postimplantation loss, decreased numbers of live fetuses and fetal anomalies including absence and shortening of renal papilla, dilation of ureter, edema and incomplete ossification of frontal skull and metatarsals. Letrozole was teratogenic in rats. A 0.03 mg/kg dose (about 1/10 the daily maximum recommended human dose on a mg/m^2 basis) caused fetal domed head and cervical/centrum vertebral fusion.

Letrozole is embryotoxic at doses equal to or greater than 0.002 mg/kg and fetotoxic when administered to rabbits at 0.02 mg/kg (about 1/100,000 and 1/10,000 the daily maximum recommended human dose on a mg/m^2 basis, respectively). Fetal anomalies included incomplete ossification of the skull, sternebrae, and fore- and hindlegs.

There are no studies in pregnant women. Femara® (letrozole tablets) is indicated for postmenopausal women. If there is exposure to letrozole during pregnancy, the patient should be apprised of the potential hazard to the fetus and potential risk for loss of the pregnancy.

PRECAUTIONS

Since fatigue and dizziness have been observed with the use of Femara® (letrozole tablets) and somnolence was uncommonly reported, caution is advised when driving or using machinery.

Laboratory Tests: No dose-related effect of Femara on any hematologic or clinical chemistry parameter was evident. Moderate decreases in lymphocyte counts, of uncertain clinical significance, were observed in some patients receiving Femara 2.5 mg. This depression was transient in about half of those affected. Two patients on Femara developed thrombocytopenia; relationship to the study drug was unclear. Patient withdrawal due to laboratory abnormalities, whether related to study treatment or not, was infrequent.

Increases in SGOT, SGPT, and gamma GT ≥5 times the upper limit of normal (ULN) and of bilirubin ≥1.5 times the ULN were most often associated with metastatic disease in the liver. About 3% of study participants receiving Femara had abnormalities in liver chemistries not associated with documented metastases; these abnormalities may have been related to study drug therapy. In the megestrol acetate comparative study about 8% of patients treated with megestrol acetate had abnormalities in liver chemistries that were not associated with documented liver metastases; in the aminoglutethimide study about 10% of aminoglutethimide-treated patients had abnormalities in liver chemistries not associated with hepatic metastases.

Drug Interactions: Clinical interaction studies with cimetidine and warfarin indicated that the coadministration of Femara with these drugs does not result in clinically-significant drug interactions. *(See CLINICAL PHARMACOLOGY.)*

Coadministration of Femara and tamoxifen 20 mg daily resulted in a reduction of letrozole plasma levels by 38% on average.There is no clinical experience to date on the use of Femara in combination with other anticancer agents.

Hepatic Insufficiency: Subjects with cirrhosis and severe hepatic dysfunction *(see CLINICAL PHARMACOLOGY, Special Populations)* who were dosed with 2.5 mg of Femara experienced approximately twice the exposure to letrozole as healthy volunteers with normal liver function. Therefore, a dose reduction is recommended for this patient population. The effect of hepatic impairment on Femara exposure in cancer patients with elevated bilirubin levels has not been determined. *(See DOSAGE AND ADMINISTRATION.)*

Table 7
Megestrol Acetate Study Results

	Femara® 0.5 mg N=188	Femara® 2.5 mg N=174	megestrol acetate N=190
Objective Response (CR + PR)	22 (11.7%)	41 (23.6%)	31 (16.3%)
Median Duration of Response	552 days	(Not reached)	561 days
Median Time to Progression	154 days	170 days	168 days
Median Survival	633 days	730 days	659 days
Odds Ratio for Response	Femara 2.5: Femara 0.5 = 2.33 (95% CI: 1.32, 4.17); P=0.004*		Femara 2.5: megestrol = 1.58 (95% CI: 0.94, 2.66); P=0.08*
Relative Risk of Progression	Femara 2.5: Femara 0.5 = 0.81 (95% CI: 0.63, 1.03); P=0.09*		Femara 2.5: megestrol = 0.77 (95% CI: 0.60, 0.98); P=0.03*

*two-sided P-value

Table 8
Aminoglutethimide Study Results

	Femara® 0.5 N=193	Femara® 2.5 N=185	aminoglutethimide N=179
Objective Response (CR + PR)	34 (17.6%)	34 (18.4%)	22 (12.3%)
Median Duration of Response	619 days	706 days	450 days
Median Time to Progression	103 days	123 days	112 days
Median Survival	636 days	792 days	592 days
Odds Ratio for Response	Femara 2.5: Femara 0.5 = 1.05 (95% CI: 0.62, 1.79); P=0.85*		Femara 2.5: aminoglutethimide=1.61 (95% CI: 0.90, 2.87); P=0.11*
Relative Risk of Progression	Femara 2.5: Femara 0.5 = 0.86 (95% CI: 0.68, 1.11); P=0.25*		Femara 2.5: aminoglutethimide=0.74 (95% CI: 0.57, 0.94); P=0.02*

*two-sided P-value

Table 9
Percentage (%) of Patients with Adverse Events

Adverse Experience	Femara® 2.5 mg (N=455) %	tamoxifen 20 mg (N=455) %
General Disorders		
Fatigue	13	13
Chest pain	8	9
Edema peripheral	5	6
Pain not otherwise specified	5	7
Weakness	6	4
Investigations		
Weight decreased	7	5
Vascular Disorders		
Hot flushes	19	16
Hypertension	8	4
Gastrointestinal Disorders		
Nausea	17	17
Constipation	10	11
Diarrhea	8	4
Vomiting	7	8
Infections/Infestations		
Influenza	6	4
Urinary tract infection not otherwise specified	6	3

Adverse Experience	Femara® 2.5 mg (N=455) %	tamoxifen 20 mg (N=455) %
Injury, Poisoning and Procedural Complications		
Post-mastectomy lymphedema	7	7
Metabolism and Nutrition Disorders		
Anorexia	4	6
Musculoskeletal and Connective Tissue Disorders		
Bone pain	22	21
Back pain	18	19
Arthralgia	16	15
Pain in limb	10	8
Nervous System Disorders		
Headache not otherwise specified	8	7
Psychiatric Disorders		
Insomnia	7	4
Reproductive System and Breast Disorders		
Breast Pain	7	7
Respiratory, Thoracic and Mediastinal Disorders		
Dyspnea	18	17
Cough	13	13
Chest wall pain	6	6

Drug/Laboratory Test-Interactions: None observed.

Carcinogenesis, Mutagenesis, Impairment of Fertility: A conventional carcinogenesis study in mice at doses of 0.6 to 60 mg/kg/day (about one to 100 times the daily maximum recommended human dose on a mg/m^2 basis) administered by oral gavage for up to 2 years revealed a dose-related increase in the incidence of benign ovarian stromal tumors. The incidence of combined hepatocellular adenoma and carcinoma showed a significant trend in females when the high dose group was excluded due to low survival. In a separate study, plasma AUC_{0-12hr} levels in mice at 60 mg/kg/day were 55 times higher than the AUC_{0-24hr} level in breast cancer patients at the recommended dose. The carcinogenicity study in rats at oral doses of 0.1 to 10 mg/kg/day (about 0.4 to 40 times the daily maximum recommended human dose on a mg/m^2 basis) for up to 2 years also produced an increase in the incidence of benign ovarian stromal tumors at 10 mg/kg/day. Ovarian hyperplasia was observed in females at doses equal to or greater than 0.1 mg/kg/day. At 10 mg/kg/day, plasma AUC_{0-24hr} levels in rats were 80 times higher than the level in breast cancer patients at the recommended dose.

Letrozole was not mutagenic in *in vitro* tests (Ames and E.coli bacterial tests) but was observed to be a potential clastogen in *in vitro* assays (CHO K1 and CCL 61 Chinese hamster ovary cells). Letrozole was not clastogenic *in vivo* (micronucleus test in rats).

Studies to investigate the effect of letrozole on fertility have not been conducted; however, repeated dosing caused sexual inactivity in females and atrophy of the reproductive tract in males and females at doses of 0.6, 0.1 and 0.03 mg/kg in mice, rats and dogs, respectively (about one, 0.4 and 0.4 the daily maximum recommended human dose on a mg/m^2 basis, respectively).

Pregnancy: ***Pregnancy Category D*** *(see WARNINGS).*

Nursing Mothers: It is not known if letrozole is excreted in human milk. Because many drugs are excreted in human milk, caution should be exercised when letrozole is administered to a nursing woman *(see WARNINGS and PRECAUTIONS).*

Pediatric Use: The safety and effectiveness in pediatric patients have not been established.

Geriatric Use: The median age of patients in all studies of first-line and second-line treatment for breast cancer was 64–65 years. About 1/3 of the patients were ≥70 years old. In the first-line study patients ≥70 years of age experienced longer time to tumor progression and higher response rates than patients <70.

ADVERSE REACTIONS

Femara® (letrozole tablets) was generally well tolerated across all studies as first-line and second-line treatment for breast cancer and adverse reaction rates were similar in both settings.

First-Line Breast Cancer: A total of 455 patients was treated for a median time of exposure of 11 months. The incidence of adverse experiences was similar for Femara and tamoxifen. The most frequently reported adverse experiences were bone pain, hot flushes, back pain, nausea, arthralgia and dyspnea. Discontinuations for adverse experiences other than progression of tumor occurred in 10/455 (2%) of patients on Femara and in 15/455 (3%) of patients on tamoxifen.

Adverse events, regardless of relationship to study drug, that were reported in at least 5% of the patients treated with Femara 2.5 mg or tamoxifen 20 mg in the first-line treatment study are shown in Table 9.

[See table 9 above]

Other less frequent (≤2%) adverse experiences considered consequential for both treatment groups, included peripheral thromboembolic events, cardiovascular events, and cerebrovascular events. Peripheral thromboembolic events in-

Table 10
Percentage (%) of Patients with Adverse Events

Adverse Experience	Pooled Femara® 2.5 mg (N=359) %	Pooled Femara® 0.5 mg (N=380) %	megestrol acetate 160 mg (N=189) %	aminoglutethimide 500 mg (N=178) %
Body as a Whole				
Fatigue	8	6	11	3
Chest pain	6	3	7	3
Peripheral edema[1]	5	5	8	3
Asthenia	4	5	4	5
Weight increase	2	2	9	3
Cardiovascular				
Hypertension	5	7	5	6
Digestive System				
Nausea	13	15	9	14
Vomiting	7	7	5	9
Constipation	6	7	9	7
Diarrhea	6	5	3	4
Pain-abdominal	6	5	9	8
Anorexia	5	3	5	5
Dyspepsia	3	4	6	5
Infections/Infestations				
Viral infection	6	5	6	3
Lab Abnormality				
Hypercholesterolemia	3	3	0	6
Musculoskeletal System				
Musculoskeletal[2]	21	22	30	14
Arthralgia	8	8	8	3
Nervous System				
Headache	9	12	9	7
Somnolence	3	2	2	9
Dizziness	3	5	7	3
Respiratory System				
Dyspnea	7	9	16	5
Coughing	6	5	7	5
Skin and Appendages				
Hot flushes	6	5	4	3
Rash[3]	5	4	3	12
Pruritus	1	2	5	3

[1] Includes peripheral edema, leg edema, dependent edema, edema
[2] Includes musculoskeletal pain, skeletal pain, back pain, arm pain, leg pain
[3] Includes rash, erythematous rash, maculopapular rash, psoriaform rash, vesicular rash

cluded venous thrombosis, thrombophlebitis, portal vein thrombosis and pulmonary embolism. Cardiovascular events included angina, myocardial infarction, myocardial ischemia, and coronary heart disease. Cerebrovascular events included transient ischemic attacks, thrombotic or hemorrhagic strokes and development of hemiparesis.

Second-Line Breast Cancer: Femara was generally well tolerated in two controlled clinical trials.

Study discontinuations in the megestrol acetate comparison study for adverse events other than progression of tumor occurred in 5/188 (2.7%) of patients on Femara 0.5 mg, in 4/174 (2.3%) of the patients on Femara 2.5 mg, and in 15/190 (7.9%) of patients on megestrol acetate. There were fewer thromboembolic events at both Femara doses than on the megestrol acetate arm (2 of 362 patients or 0.6% vs. 9 of 190 patients or 4.7%). There was also less vaginal bleeding (1 of 362 patients or 0.3% vs. 6 of 190 patients or 3.2%) on letrozole than on megestrol acetate. In the aminoglutethimide comparison study, discontinuations for reasons other than progression occurred in 6/193 (3.1%) of patients on 0.5 mg Femara, 7/185 (3.8%) of patients on 2.5 mg Femara, and 7/178 (3.9%) of patients on aminoglutethimide.

Comparisons of the incidence of adverse events revealed no significant differences between the high and low dose Femara groups in either study. Most of the adverse events observed in all treatment groups were mild to moderate in severity and it was generally not possible to distinguish adverse reactions due to treatment from the consequences of the patient's metastatic breast cancer, the effects of estrogen deprivation, or intercurrent illness.

Adverse events, regardless of relationship to study drug, that were reported in at least 5% of the patients treated with Femara 0.5 mg, Femara 2.5 mg, megestrol acetate, or aminoglutethimide in the two controlled trials are shown in Table 10.

[See table 10 above]

Other less frequent (<5%) adverse experiences considered consequential and reported in at least 3 patients treated with Femara, included hypercalcemia, fracture, depression, anxiety, pleural effusion, alopecia, increased sweating and vertigo.

OVERDOSAGE

Isolated cases of Femara® (letrozole tablets) overdose have been reported. In these instances, the highest single dose ingested was 62.5 mg or 25 tablets. While no serious adverse events were reported in these cases, because of the limited data available, no firm recommendations for treatment can be made. However, emesis could be induced if the patient is alert. In general, supportive care and frequent monitoring of vital signs are also appropriate. In single dose studies the highest dose used was 30 mg, which was well tolerated; in multiple dose trials, the largest dose of 10 mg was well tolerated.

Lethality was observed in mice and rats following single oral doses that were equal to or greater than 2000 mg/kg (about 4000 to 8000 times the daily maximum recommended human dose on a mg/m^2 basis); death was associated with reduced motor activity, ataxia and dyspnea. Lethality was observed in cats following single IV doses that were equal to or greater than 10 mg/kg (about 50 times the daily maximum recommended human dose on a mg/m^2 basis); death was preceded by depressed blood pressure and arrhythmias.

DOSAGE AND ADMINISTRATION

Adult and Elderly Patients: The recommended dose of Femara® (letrozole tablets) is one 2.5 mg tablet administered once a day, without regard to meals. Treatment with Femara should continue until tumor progression is evident. No dose adjustment is required for elderly patients. Patients treated with Femara do not require glucocorticoid or mineralocorticoid replacement therapy.

Renal Impairment: *(See CLINICAL PHARMACOLOGY.)* No dosage adjustment is required for patients with renal impairment if creatinine clearance is ≥10 mL/min.

Hepatic Impairment: No dosage adjustment is recommended for patients with mild to moderate hepatic impairment, although letrozole blood concentrations were modestly increased in subjects with moderate hepatic impairment due to cirrhosis. The dose of letrozole in patients with cirrhosis and severe hepatic dysfunction should be reduced by 50% *(see CLINICAL PHARMACOLOGY)*. The recommended dose of Femara® (letrozole tablets) for such patients is 2.5 mg administered every other day. The effect of hepatic impairment on Femara exposure in noncirrhotic cancer patients with elevated bilirubin levels has not been determined. *(See CLINICAL PHARMACOLOGY.)*

HOW SUPPLIED

2.5 mg tablets – dark yellow, film-coated, round, slightly biconvex, with beveled edges (imprinted with the letters FV on one side and CG on the other side).

Packaged in HDPE bottles with a safety screw cap.

Bottles of 30 tablets .... NDC 0078-0249-15

Store at 25°C (77°F); excursions permitted to 15°C-30°C (59°F-86°F). [See USP Controlled Room Temperature].

T2003-10

REV: FEBRUARY 2003 89010303

Novartis Pharmaceuticals Corporation
East Hanover, New Jersey 07936
©Novartis

Shown in Product Identification Guide, page 325

FOCALIN™ Ⓒ℞
[fōk' ă-lĭn]
dexmethylphenidate hydrochloride
tablets
Rx only

Prescribing Information
The following prescribing information is based on official labeling in effect July 2003.

DESCRIPTION

Focalin™ (dexmethylphenidate hydrochloride) is the *d-threo*-enantiomer of racemic methylphenidate hydrochloride, which is a 50/50 mixture of the *d-threo* and *l-threo*-enantiomers. Focalin is a central nervous system (CNS) stimulant, available in three tablet strengths. Each tablet contains dexmethylphenidate hydrochloride 2.5, 5, or 10 mg for oral administration. Dexmethylphenidate hydrochloride is methyl α-phenyl-2-piperidineacetate hydrochloride, (R,R')-(+)-. Its empirical formula is $C_{14}H_{19}NO_2$•HCl.

Its molecular weight is 269.77 and its structural formula is

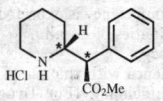

Note: * = asymmetric carbon centers

Dexmethylphenidate hydrochloride is a white to off white powder. Its solutions are acid to litmus. It is freely soluble in water and in methanol, soluble in alcohol, and slightly soluble in chloroform and in acetone.

Focalin also contains the following inert ingredients: pregelatinized starch, lactose monohydrate, sodium starch glycolate, microcrystalline cellulose, magnesium stearate, and FD&C Blue No.1 #5516 aluminum lake (2.5 mg tablets), D&C Yellow Lake #10 (5 mg tablets); the 10 mg tablet contains no dye.

CLINICAL PHARMACOLOGY

Pharmacodynamics

Dexmethylphenidate hydrochloride is a central nervous system stimulant. Focalin, the more pharmacologically active enantiomer of the *d*- and *l*-enantiomers, is thought to block the reuptake of norepinephrine and dopamine into the presynaptic neuron and increase the release of these monoamines into the extraneuronal space. The mode of therapeutic action in Attention Deficit Hyperactivity Disorder (ADHD) is not known.

Pharmacokinetics

Absorption

Dexmethylphenidate hydrochloride is readily absorbed following oral administration of Focalin. In patients with ADHD, plasma dexmethylphenidate concentrations increase rapidly, reaching a maximum in the fasted state at about 1 to 1½ hours post-dose. No differences in the pharmacokinetics of Focalin were noted following single and repeated twice daily dosing, thus indicating no significant drug accumulation in children with ADHD.

When given to children as capsules in single doses of 2.5 mg, 5 mg, and 10 mg, C_{max} and $AUC_{0\text{-}inf}$ of dexmethylphenidate were proportional to dose. In the same study, plasma dexmethylphenidate levels were comparable to those achieved following single *dl-threo*-methylphenidate HCl doses given as capsules in twice the total mg amount (equimolar with respect to Focalin).

Food Effects

In a single dose study conducted in adults, coadministration of 2 × 10 mg Focalin with a high fat breakfast resulted in a dexmethylphenidate t_{max} of 2.9 hours post-dose as compared to 1.5 hours post-dose when given in a fasting state. C_{max} and $AUC_{0\text{-}inf}$ were comparable in both the fasted and non-fasted states.

Distribution

Plasma dexmethylphenidate concentrations in children decline exponentially following oral administration of Focalin.

Metabolism and Excretion

In humans, dexmethylphenidate is metabolized primarily to *d*-α-phenyl-piperidine acetic acid (also known as *d*-ritalinic acid) by de-esterification. This metabolite has little or no pharmacological activity. There is little or no *in vivo* interconversion to the *l-threo*-enantiomer, based on a finding of minute levels of *l-threo*-methylphenidate being detectable in a few samples in only 2 of 58 children and adults. After oral dosing of radiolabeled racemic methylphenidate in humans, about 90% of the radioactivity was recovered in urine. The main urinary metabolite was ritalinic acid, accountable for approximately 80% of the dose.

In vitro studies showed that dexmethylphenidate did not inhibit cytochrome P450 isoenzymes.

The mean plasma elimination half-life of dexmethylphenidate is approximately 2.2 hours.

Special Populations

Gender

Pharmacokinetic parameters were similar for boys and girls (mean age 10 years).

In a single dose study conducted in adults, the mean dexmethylphenidate $AUC_{0\text{-}inf}$ values (adjusted for body weight) following single 2 × 10 mg doses of Focalin were 25%-35% higher in adult female volunteers (n=6) compared to male volunteers (n=9). Both t_{max} and $t_{½}$ were comparable for males and females.

Race

There is insufficient experience with the use of Focalin to detect ethnic variations in pharmacokinetics.

Age

The pharmacokinetics of dexmethylphenidate after Focalin administration have not been studied in children less than 6 years of age. When single doses of Focalin were given to children between the ages of 6 to 12 years and healthy adult

Continued on next page

Focalin—Cont.

volunteers, C_{max} of dexmethylphenidate was similar, however, children showed somewhat lower AUCs compared to the adults.

Renal Insufficiency

There is no experience with the use of Focalin in patients with renal insufficiency. After oral administration of radiolabeled racemic methylphenidate in humans, methylphenidate was extensively metabolized and approximately 80% of the radioactivity was excreted in the urine in the form of ritalinic acid. Since very little unchanged drug is excreted in the urine, renal insufficiency is expected to have little effect on the pharmacokinetics of Focalin.

Hepatic Insufficiency

There is no experience with the use of Focalin in patients with hepatic insufficiency. (For Drug Interactions, see PRECAUTIONS.)

Clinical Studies

Focalin was evaluated in two double-blind, parallel-group, placebo-controlled trials in untreated or previously treated patients aged 6 to 17 years old with a DSM-IV diagnosis of Attention Deficit Hyperactivity Disorder (ADHD). Both studies included all three subtypes of ADHD, i.e., Combined Type, Predominantly Inattentive Type, or Predominantly Hyperactive-Impulsive Type. While both children and adolescents were included, the sample was predominantly children, thus, the findings are most pertinent to this age group. In both studies, the primary comparison of interest was Focalin *versus* placebo.

Focalin (5, 10, or 20 mg/day total dose), *dl-threo*-methylphenidate HCl (10, 20, or 40 mg/day total dose), and placebo were compared in a multicenter, 4-week, parallel group study in n=132 patients. Patients took the study medication twice daily, 3.5 to 5.5 hours between doses. Treatment was initiated with the lowest dose, and doses could be doubled at weekly intervals, depending on clinical response and tolerability, up to the maximum dose. The change from baseline to week 4 of the averaged score (an average of two ratings during the week) of the teacher's version of the SNAP-ADHD Rating Scale, a scale for assessing ADHD symptoms, was the primary outcome. Patients treated with Focalin showed a statistically significant improvement in symptom scores from baseline over patients who received placebo.

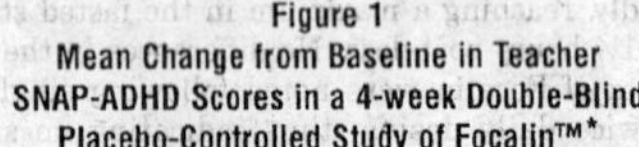

Figure 1
Mean Change from Baseline in Teacher SNAP-ADHD Scores in a 4-week Double-Blind Placebo-Controlled Study of Focalin™*

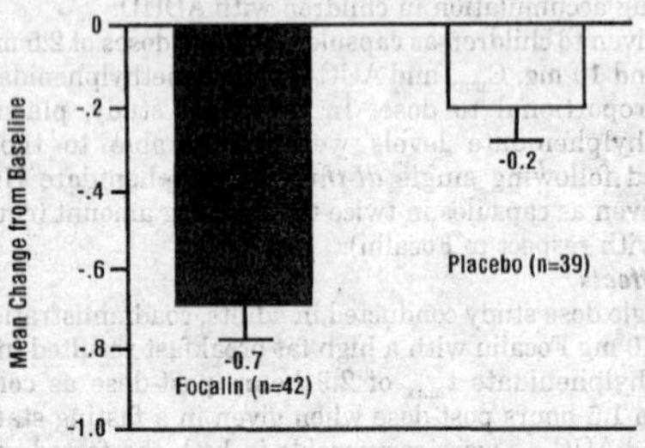

*Figure 1: Error bars represent the standard error of the mean.

The other study, involving n=75 patients, was a multicenter, placebo-controlled, double-blind, 2-week treatment withdrawal study in children who were responders during a 6-week, open label initial treatment period. Children took study medication twice a day separated by a 3.5 to 5.5 hour interval. The primary outcome was proportion of treatment failures at the end of the 2-week withdrawal phase, where treatment failure was defined as a rating of 6 (much worse) or 7 (very much worse) on the Investigator Clinical Global Impression - Improvement (CGI-I). Patients continued on Focalin showed a statistically significant lower rate of failure over patients who received placebo.

Figure 2
Percent of Treatment Failures following a 2-week Double-Blind Placebo-Controlled Withdrawal of Focalin™

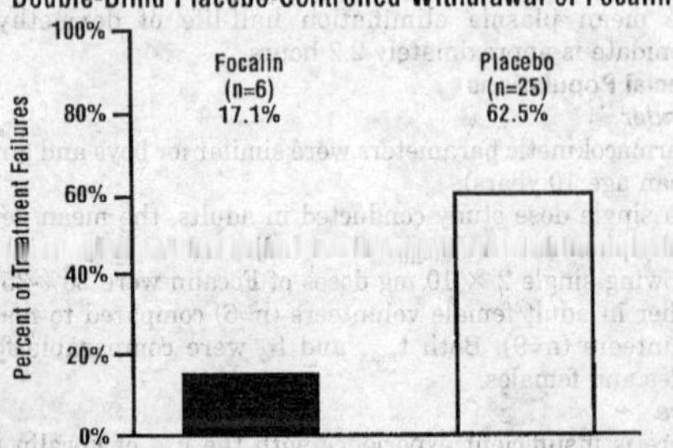

INDICATION AND USAGE

Focalin is indicated for the treatment of Attention Deficit Hyperactivity Disorder (ADHD).

The efficacy of Focalin in the treatment of ADHD was established in two controlled trials of patients aged 6 to 17 years of age who met DSM-IV criteria for ADHD (see Clinical Studies).

A diagnosis of ADHD (DSM-IV) implies the presence of hyperactive-impulsive or inattentive symptoms that cause impairment and were present before age 7 years. The symptoms must cause clinically significant impairment, e.g., in social, academic, or occupational functioning; and be present in two or more settings, e.g., school (or work) and at home. The symptoms must not be better accounted for by another mental disorder. For the inattentive type, at least six of the following symptoms must have persisted for at least 6 months: lack of attention to details/careless mistakes; lack of sustained attention; poor listener; failure to follow through on tasks; poor organization; avoids tasks requiring sustained mental effort; loses things; easily distracted; forgetful. For the Hyperactive-Impulsive Type, at least six of the following symptoms must have persisted for at least 6 months: fidgeting/squirming; leaving seat; inappropriate running/climbing; difficulty with quiet activities; "on the go," excessive talking; blurting answers; can't wait turn; intrusive. The Combined Type requires both inattentive and hyperactive-impulsive criteria to be met.

Special Diagnostic Considerations

Specific etiology of this syndrome is unknown, and there is no single diagnostic test. Adequate diagnosis requires the use not only of medical but of special psychological, educational, and social resources. Learning may or may not be impaired. The diagnosis must be based upon a complete history and evaluation of the child and not solely on the presence of the required number of DSM-IV characteristics.

Need for Comprehensive Treatment Program

Focalin is indicated as an integral part of a total treatment program for ADHD that may include other measures (psychological, educational, social) for patients with this syndrome. Drug treatment may not be indicated for all patients with this syndrome. Stimulants are not intended for use in the patient who exhibits symptoms secondary to environmental factors and/or other primary psychiatric disorders, including psychosis. Appropriate educational placement is essential and psychosocial intervention is often helpful. When remedial measures alone are insufficient, the decision to prescribe stimulant medication will depend upon the physician's assessment of the chronicity and severity of the patient's symptoms.

Long-term Use

The effectiveness of Focalin for long-term use, i.e., for more than 6 weeks, has not been systematically evaluated in controlled trials. Therefore, the physician who elects to use Focalin for extended periods should periodically re-evaluate the long-term usefulness of the drug for the individual patient (see DOSAGE AND ADMINISTRATION).

CONTRAINDICATIONS

Agitation

Focalin is contraindicated in patients with marked anxiety, tension, and agitation, since the drug may aggravate these symptoms.

Hypersensitivity to Methylphenidate

Focalin is contraindicated in patients known to be hypersensitive to methylphenidate or other components of the product.

Glaucoma

Focalin is contraindicated in patients with glaucoma.

Tics

Focalin is contraindicated in patients with motor tics or with a family history or diagnosis of Tourette's syndrome (see ADVERSE REACTIONS).

Monoamine Oxidase Inhibitors

Focalin is contraindicated during treatment with monoamine oxidase inhibitors, and also within a minimum of 14 days following discontinuation of a monoamine oxidase inhibitor (hypertensive crises may result).

WARNINGS

Depression

Focalin should not be used to treat severe depression.

Fatigue

Focalin should not be used for the prevention or treatment of normal fatigue states.

Long-Term Suppression of Growth

Sufficient data on safety of long-term use of Focalin in children are not yet available. Although a causal relationship has not been established, suppression of growth (i.e., weight gain and/or height) has been reported with the long-term use of stimulants in children. Therefore, patients requiring long-term therapy should be carefully monitored. Patients who are not growing or gaining weight as expected should have their treatment interrupted.

Psychosis

Clinical experience suggests that in psychotic children, administration of methylphenidate may exacerbate symptoms of behavior disturbance and thought disorder.

Seizures

There is some clinical evidence that methylphenidate may lower the convulsive threshold in patients with prior history of seizures, in patients with prior EEG abnormalities in the absence of a history of seizures, and, very rarely, in the absence of a history of seizures and no prior EEG evidence of seizures. In the presence of seizures, the drug should be discontinued.

Hypertension and Other Cardiovascular Conditions

Use cautiously in patients with hypertension. Blood pressure should be monitored at appropriate intervals in all patients taking Focalin, especially those with hypertension. In the placebo controlled studies, the mean pulse increase was 2-5 bpm for both Focalin and racemic methylphenidate compared to placebo, with mean increases of systolic and diastolic blood pressure of 2-3 mmHg, compared to placebo. Therefore, caution is indicated in treating patients whose underlying medical conditions might be compromised by increases in blood pressure or heart rate, e.g., those with pre-existing hypertension, heart failure, recent myocardial infarction, or hyperthyroidism.

Visual Disturbance

Symptoms of visual disturbances have been encountered in rare cases following use of methylphenidate. Difficulties with accommodation and blurring of vision have been reported.

Use in Children Under 6 Years of Age

Focalin should not be used in children under 6 years, since safety and efficacy in this age group have not been established.

DRUG DEPENDENCE: Focalin should be given cautiously to patients with a history of drug dependence or alcoholism. Chronic, abusive use can lead to marked tolerance and psychological dependence with varying degrees of abnormal behavior. Frank psychotic episodes can occur, especially with parenteral abuse. Careful supervision is required during drug withdrawal from abusive use since severe depression may occur. Withdrawal following chronic therapeutic use may unmask symptoms of the underlying disorder that may require follow-up.

PRECAUTIONS

Hematologic Monitoring

Periodic CBC, differential, and platelet counts are advised during prolonged therapy.

Information for Patients

Patient information is printed at the end of this insert. To assure safe and effective use of Focalin, the information and instructions provided in the patient information section should be discussed with patients.

Drug Interactions

Methylphenidate may decrease the effectiveness of drugs used to treat hypertension. Because of possible effects on blood pressure, Focalin should be used cautiously with pressor agents.

Human pharmacologic studies have shown that racemic methylphenidate may inhibit the metabolism of coumarin anticoagulants, anticonvulsants (e.g., phenobarbital, phenytoin, primidone), and some antidepressants (tricyclics and selective serotonin reuptake inhibitors). Downward dose adjustments of these drugs may be required when given concomitantly with methylphenidate. It may be necessary to adjust the dosage and monitor plasma drug concentration (or, in the case of coumarin, coagulation times), when initiating or discontinuing concomitant methylphenidate.

Serious adverse events have been reported in concomitant use with clonidine, although no causality for the combination has been established. The safety of using methylphenidate in combination with clonidine or other centrally acting alpha-2 agonists has not been systematically evaluated.

Carcinogenesis, Mutagenesis, and Impairment of Fertility

Lifetime carcinogenicity studies have not been carried out with dexmethylphenidate. In a lifetime carcinogenicity study carried out in B6C3F1 mice, racemic methylphenidate caused an increase in hepatocellular adenomas, and in males only, an increase in hepatoblastomas at a daily dose of approximately 60 mg/kg/day. Hepatoblastoma is a relatively rare rodent malignant tumor type. There was no increase in total malignant hepatic tumors. The mouse strain used is sensitive to the development of hepatic tumors, and the significance of these results to humans is unknown.

Racemic methylphenidate did not cause any increase in tumors in a lifetime carcinogenicity study carried out in F344 rats; the highest dose used was approximately 45 mg/kg/day.

In a 24-week study of racemic methylphenidate in the transgenic mouse strain p53+/-, which is sensitive to genotoxic carcinogens, there was no evidence of carcinogenicity. Mice were fed diets containing the same concentrations as in the lifetime carcinogenicity study; the high-dose group was exposed to 60-74 mg/kg/day of racemic methylphenidate.

Dexmethylphenidate was not mutagenic in the *in vitro* Ames reverse mutation assay, the *in vitro* mouse lymphoma cell forward mutation assay, or the *in vivo* mouse bone marrow micronucleus test.

Racemic methylphenidate was not mutagenic in the *in vitro* Ames reverse mutation assay or the *in vitro* mouse lymphoma cell forward mutation assay, and was negative *in vivo* in the mouse bone marrow micronucleus assay. However, sister chromatid exchanges and chromosome aberrations were increased, indicative of a weak clastogenic response, in an *in vitro* assay of racemic methylphenidate in cultured Chinese Hamster Ovary (CHO) cells.

Racemic methylphenidate did not impair fertility in male or female mice that were fed diets containing the drug in an 18-week Continuous Breeding study. The study was conducted at doses of up to 160 mg/kg/day.

Pregnancy

Pregnancy Category C

In studies conducted in rats and rabbits, dexmethylphenidate was administered orally at doses of up to 20 and 100 mg/kg/day, respectively, during the period of organogenesis. No evidence of teratogenic activity was found in either the rat or rabbit study; however, delayed fetal skeletal ossification was observed at the highest dose level in rats. When dexmethylphenidate was administered to rats throughout pregnancy and lactation at doses of up to 20 mg/kg/day, postweaning body weight gain was decreased in male offspring at the highest dose, but no other effects on postnatal development were observed. At the highest doses tested, plasma levels (AUCs) of dexmethylphenidate in pregnant rats and rabbits were approximately 5 and 1 times, respectively, those in adults dosed with the maximum recommended human dose of 20 mg/day.

Racemic methylphenidate has been shown to have teratogenic effects in rabbits when given in doses of 200 mg/kg/day throughout organogenesis.

Adequate and well-controlled studies in pregnant women have not been conducted. Focalin should be used during pregnancy only if the potential benefit justifies the potential risk to the fetus.

Nursing Mothers

It is not known whether dexmethylphenidate is excreted in human milk. Because many drugs are excreted in human milk, caution should be exercised if Focalin is administered to a nursing woman.

Pediatric Use

The safety and efficacy of Focalin in children under 6 years old have not been established. Long-term effects of Focalin in children have not been well established (see WARNINGS).

ADVERSE REACTIONS

The pre-marketing development program for Focalin included exposures in a total of 696 participants in clinical trials (684 patients, 12 healthy adult subjects). These participants received Focalin 5, 10, or 20 mg/day. The 684 ADHD patients (ages 6 to 17 years) were evaluated in two controlled clinical studies, two clinical pharmacology studies, and two uncontrolled long-term safety studies. Safety data on all patients are included in the discussion that follows. Adverse reactions were assessed by collecting adverse events, and results of physical examinations, vital sign and body weight measurements, and laboratory analyses.

Adverse events during exposure were primarily obtained by general inquiry and recorded by clinical investigators using terminology of their own choosing. Consequently, it is not possible to provide a meaningful estimate of the proportion of individuals experiencing adverse events without first grouping similar types of events into a smaller number of standardized event categories. In the tables and tabulations that follow, standard COSTART dictionary terminology has been used to classify reported adverse events.

The stated frequencies of adverse events represent the proportion of individuals who experienced, at least once, a treatment-emergent adverse event of the type listed. An event was considered treatment emergent if it occurred for the first time or worsened while receiving therapy following baseline evaluation.

Adverse Findings in Clinical Trials with Focalin

Adverse Events Associated with Discontinuation of Treatment

No Focalin-treated patients discontinued due to adverse events in two placebo-controlled trials. Overall, 50 of 684 children treated with Focalin (7.3%) experienced an adverse event that resulted in discontinuation. The most common reasons for discontinuation were twitching (described as motor or vocal tics), anorexia, insomnia, and tachycardia (approximately 1% each).

Adverse Events Occurring at an Incidence of 5% or More Among Focalin-Treated Patients

Table 1 enumerates treatment-emergent adverse events for two, placebo-controlled, parallel group trials in children with ADHD at Focalin doses of 5, 10, and 20 mg/day. The table includes only those events that occurred in 5% or more of patients treated with Focalin where the incidence in patients treated with Focalin was at least twice the incidence in placebo-treated patients. The prescriber should be aware that these figures cannot be used to predict the incidence of adverse events in the course of usual medical practice where patient characteristics and other factors differ from those which prevailed in the clinical trials. Similarly, the cited frequencies cannot be compared with figures obtained from other clinical investigations involving different treatments, uses, and investigators. The cited figures, however, do provide the prescribing physician with some basis for estimating the relative contribution of drug and non-drug factors to the adverse event incidence rate in the population studied.

Table 1
Treatment-Emergent Adverse Events[1] Occurring During Double-Blind Treatment in Clinical Trials of Focalin™

Body System	Preferred Term	Focalin (n=79)	Placebo (n=82)
Body as a Whole			
	Abdominal Pain	15%	6%
	Fever	5%	1%
Digestive System			
	Anorexia	6%	1%
	Nausea	9%	1%

[1]Events, regardless of causality, for which the incidence for patients treated with Focalin was at least 5% and twice the incidence among placebo-treated patients. Incidence has been rounded to the nearest whole number.

Adverse Events with Other Methylphenidate HCl Products

Nervousness and insomnia are the most common adverse reactions reported with other methylphenidate products. In children, loss of appetite, abdominal pain, weight loss during prolonged therapy, insomnia, and tachycardia may occur more frequently; however, any of the other adverse reactions listed below may also occur.

Other reactions include:

Cardiac: angina, arrhythmia, palpitations, pulse increased or decreased

Gastrointestinal: nausea

Immune: hypersensitivity reactions including skin rash, urticaria, fever, arthralgia, exfoliative dermatitis, erythema multiforme with histopathological findings of necrotizing vasculitis, and thrombocytopenic purpura

Nervous System: dizziness, drowsiness, dyskinesia, headache, rare reports of Tourette's syndrome, toxic psychosis

Vascular: blood pressure increased or decreased, cerebral arteritis and/or occlusion

Although a definite causal relationship has not been established, the following have been reported in patients taking methylphenidate:

Blood/lymphatic: leukopenia and/or anemia

Hepatobiliary: abnormal liver function, ranging from transaminase elevation to hepatic coma

Psychiatric: transient depressed mood

Skin/subcutaneous: scalp hair loss

Very rare reports of neuroleptic malignant syndrome (NMS) have been received, and, in most of these, patients were concurrently receiving therapies associated with NMS. In a single report, a ten year old boy who had been taking methylphenidate for approximately 18 months experienced an NMS-like event within 45 minutes of ingesting his first dose of venlafaxine. It is uncertain whether this case represented a drug-drug interaction, a response to either drug alone, or some other cause.

In children, loss of appetite, abdominal pain, weight loss during prolonged therapy, insomnia, and tachycardia may occur more frequently; however, any of the other adverse reactions listed above may also occur.

DRUG ABUSE AND DEPENDENCE

Controlled Substance Class

Focalin, like other methylphenidate products, is classified as a Schedule II controlled substance by Federal regulation.

Abuse, Dependence, and Tolerance

See WARNINGS for boxed warning containing drug abuse and dependence information.

OVERDOSAGE

Signs and Symptoms

Signs and symptoms of acute methylphenidate overdosage, resulting principally from overstimulation of the CNS and from excessive sympathomimetic effects, may include the following: vomiting, agitation, tremors, hyperreflexia, muscle twitching, convulsions (may be followed by coma), euphoria, confusion, hallucinations, delirium, sweating, flushing, headache, hyperpyrexia, tachycardia, palpitations, cardiac arrhythmias, hypertension, mydriasis, and dryness of mucous membranes.

Recommended Treatment

Treatment consists of appropriate supportive measures. The patient must be protected against self-injury and against external stimuli that would aggravate overstimulation already present. Gastric contents may be evacuated by gastric lavage as indicated. Before performing gastric lavage, control agitation and seizures if present and protect the airway. Other measures to detoxify the gut include administration of activated charcoal and a cathartic. Intensive care must be provided to maintain adequate circulation and respiratory exchange; external cooling procedures may be required for hyperpyrexia.

Efficacy of peritoneal dialysis for Focalin overdosage has not been established.

Poison Control Center

As with the management of all overdosage, the possibility of multiple drug ingestion should be considered. The physician may wish to consider contacting a poison control center for up-to-date information on the management of overdosage with methylphenidate.

DOSAGE AND ADMINISTRATION

Focalin is administered twice daily, at least 4 hours apart. Focalin may be administered with or without food.

Dosage should be individualized according to the needs and responses of the patient.

Patients New to Methylphenidate

The recommended starting dose of Focalin for patients who are not currently taking racemic methylphenidate, or for patients who are on stimulants other than methylphenidate, is 5 mg/day (2.5 mg twice daily).

Dosage may be adjusted in 2.5 to 5 mg increments to a maximum of 20 mg/day (10 mg twice daily). In general, dosage adjustments may proceed at approximately weekly intervals.

Patients Currently Using Methylphenidate

For patients currently using methylphenidate, the recommended starting dose of Focalin is half the dose of racemic methylphenidate. The maximum recommended dose is 20 mg/day (10 mg twice daily).

Maintenance/Extended Treatment

There is no body of evidence available from controlled trials to indicate how long the patient with ADHD should be treated with Focalin. It is generally agreed, however, that pharmacological treatment of ADHD may be needed for extended periods. Nevertheless, the physician who elects to use Focalin for extended periods in patients with ADHD should periodically re-evaluate the long-term usefulness of the drug for the individual patient with periods off medication to assess the patient's functioning without pharmacotherapy. Improvement may be sustained when the drug is either temporarily or permanently discontinued.

Dose Reduction and Discontinuation

If paradoxical aggravation of symptoms or other adverse events occur, the dosage should be reduced, or, if necessary, the drug should be discontinued.

If improvement is not observed after appropriate dosage adjustment over a 1-month period, the drug should be discontinued.

HOW SUPPLIED

Tablets, D-shaped, embossed "D" on upper convex face and dosage strength on lower convex face

2.5 mg Tablets - blue
Bottles of 100 .... NDC 0078-0380-05

5 mg Tablets - yellow
Bottles of 100 .... NDC 0078-0381-05

10 mg Tablets - white
Bottles of 100 .... NDC 0078-0382-05

Store at 25°C (77°F); excursions permitted 15°C-30°C (59°F-86°F).
[see USP Controlled Room Temperature]
Protect from light and moisture.

REFERENCE

American Psychiatric Association. Diagnosis and Statistical Manual of Mental Disorders. 4th ed. Washington DC: American Psychiatric Association 1994.

REV: NOVEMBER 2001 T2001-85

INFORMATION FOR PATIENTS TAKING FOCALIN™, OR FOR THEIR PARENTS OR CAREGIVERS

Focalin™ Ⓒ II
dexmethylphenidate hydrochloride tablets
Rx only

This information for patients or their parents or caregivers is about Focalin, a medication intended for the treatment of Attention Deficit Hyperactivity Disorder (ADHD).

Please read this before you start taking Focalin. It is not intended to replace your doctor's instructions or advice. If you have any questions about this material or about Focalin, be sure to talk to your doctor or pharmacist.

What is Focalin?

Focalin is a central nervous system stimulant for the treatment of Attention Deficit Hyperactivity Disorder (ADHD). Dexmethylphenidate hydrochloride, the active ingredient of Focalin, is also found in methylphenidate, a central nervous system stimulant that has been used to treat ADHD for more than 30 years. Focalin is available in a D-shaped tablet form, 2.5 mg, 5 mg, and 10 mg, and is intended to be used in doses of 5 to 20 mg per day, given as divided doses, as directed by your doctor.

What is Attention Deficit Hyperactivity Disorder (ADHD)?

Attention Deficit Hyperactivity Disorder (ADHD) is a disorder characterized by symptoms of inattentiveness and/or hyperactivity-impulsivity inappropriate to the patient's age which interfere with functioning in two or more settings (e.g., school and home). Symptoms of inattention may include not paying attention, making careless mistakes, not listening, not finishing tasks, not following directions, and being easily distracted. Symptoms of hyperactivity-impulsiveness may include fidgeting, talking excessively, running around at inappropriate times, and interrupting others. Some patients have more symptoms of hyperactivity and impulsiveness while others have more symptoms of inattentiveness. Some patients have both types of symptoms. Symptoms must be present for at least 6 months to be certain of the diagnosis.

How Does Focalin work?

Focalin (dexmethylphenidate hydrochloride) is rapidly absorbed into the bloodstream and acts for a period of several hours. Focalin helps to increase attention and decrease impulsiveness and hyperactivity in patients with ADHD.

Before Focalin Treatment

It is very important that ADHD be accurately diagnosed and that the need for medication be carefully assessed. It is important to remember that Focalin is only part of the overall management of ADHD. Parents, teachers, physicians and other professionals are part of a team that must work together.

Before Focalin treatment, your doctor should be made aware of any current or past physical or mental problems. Tell your doctor if there is a history of drug or alcohol abuse, depression, psychosis, epilepsy or seizure disorders, high blood pressure, glaucoma, facial tics (involuntary movements), or a family history of Tourette's syndrome.

Both your doctor and your pharmacist should also be informed of all medicines that you are taking, even if these drugs are not taken on a regular basis and are available without prescription. Your doctor will decide whether you can take Focalin with other medicines. Methylphenidate is known to interact with a number of other drugs. These include medicines to treat depression, such as monoamine oxidase inhibitors; to control seizures; and to thin blood. Sometimes these interactions may require a change in dosage, or occasionally stopping one of the drugs involved.

Tell your doctor if you are pregnant or nursing a baby.

Continued on next page

Focalin—Cont.

Who Should Not Take Focalin?
You should NOT take Focalin if:
- You have significant anxiety, tension, or agitation since Focalin may make these conditions worse.
- You are allergic to methylphenidate or any of the other ingredients in Focalin.
- You have glaucoma, an eye disease.
- You have tics or Tourette's syndrome, or a family history of Tourette's syndrome.
- You are taking a monoamine oxidase inhibitor, a type of drug, or have discontinued a monoamine oxidase inhibitor in the last 14 days.

Talk to your doctor if you believe any of these conditions apply to you.

How Should I Take Focalin?
Take the dose prescribed by your doctor. Your doctor may adjust the amount of drug you take until it is right for you. From time to time, your doctor may interrupt your treatment to check your symptoms while you are not taking the drug.

What are the Possible Side Effects of Focalin?
In the clinical studies with patients using Focalin, the most common side effects were stomach pain, fever, decreased appetite, and nausea. Other side effects seen with Focalin include vomiting, dizziness, sleeplessness, nervousness, tics, allergic reactions, increased blood pressure and psychosis (abnormal thinking or hallucinations).
This is not a complete list of possible side effects. Ask your doctor about other side effects. If you develop any side effect, talk to your doctor.

What Must I Discuss with my Doctor before Taking Focalin?
Talk to your doctor ***before*** taking Focalin if you:
- Are being treated for depression or have symptoms of depression such as feelings of sadness, worthlessness, and hopelessness.
- Have motion tics (hard-to-control, repeated twitching of any parts of your body) or verbal tics (hard-to-control repeating of sounds or words).
- Have someone in your family with motion tics, verbal tics, or Tourette's syndrome.
- Have abnormal thoughts or visions, hear abnormal sounds, or have been diagnosed with psychosis.
- Have had seizures (convulsions, epilepsy) or abnormal EEGs (electroencephalograms).
- Have high blood pressure.
- Have an abnormal heart rate or rhythm.

Tell your doctor ***immediately*** if you develop any of the above conditions or symptoms while taking Focalin.

Can I Take Focalin with Other Medicines?
Tell your doctor about ***all*** medicines that you are taking. Your doctor should decide whether you can take Focalin with other medicines. These include:
- Other medicines that a doctor has prescribed.
- Medicines that you buy yourself without a prescription.
- Any herbal remedies that you may be taking.

You should not take Focalin with monoamine oxidase (MAO) inhibitors.
While on Focalin, do not start taking a new medicine or herbal remedy before checking with your doctor.
Focalin may change the way your body reacts to certain medicines. These include medicines used to treat depression, prevent seizures, or prevent blood clots (commonly called "blood thinners"). Your doctor may need to change your dose of these medicines if you are taking them with Focalin.

Other Important Safety Information
Abuse of Focalin can lead to dependence.
Tell your doctor if you have ever abused or been dependent on alcohol or drugs, or if you are now abusing or dependent on alcohol or drugs.
Before taking Focalin, tell your doctor if you are pregnant or plan on becoming pregnant. If you take Focalin, it may be in your breast milk. Tell your doctor if you are nursing a baby.
Tell your doctor if you have blurred vision when taking Focalin.
Slower growth (weight gain and/or height) has been reported with long-term use of methylphenidate in children. Your doctor will be carefully watching your height and weight. If you are not growing or gaining weight as your doctor expects, your doctor may stop your Focalin treatment.
Call your doctor ***immediately*** if you take more than the amount of Focalin prescribed by your doctor.

What Else Should I Know about Focalin?
Focalin has not been studied in children under 6 years of age.
Focalin may be a part of your overall treatment for ADHD. Your doctor may also recommend that you have counseling or other therapy.
As with all medicines, never share Focalin with anyone else and take only the number of Focalin tablets prescribed by your doctor.
Focalin may be taken at the same time as food or with no food. Focalin should be stored in a safe place at room temperature (between 59°F - 86°F). Do not store this medicine in hot, damp, or humid places.
Keep the container of Focalin in a safe place, away from high-traffic areas where other people could have accidental or unauthorized access to the medication. Keep track of the number of tablets so that you will know if any are missing. Sadly, someone who has easy access to Focalin may be able to give the tablets to others or misuse the medication.

Keep Out of the Reach of Children

REV: NOVEMBER 2001 T2001-86
Printed in U.S.A. T2001-85/T2001-86
Code 888B00 89013602
Manufactured for:
Novartis Pharmaceuticals Corporation
East Hanover, NJ 07936
By:
Mikart, Inc.
Atlanta, GA 30318

Shown in Product Identification Guide, page 325

GLEEVEC® ℞
[glē-vĕk]
(imatinib mesylate)
Tablets
Rx only

Prescribing Information
The following prescribing information is based on official labeling in effect September 2004.

DESCRIPTION
Gleevec® (imatinib mesylate) film-coated tablets contain imatinib mesylate equivalent to 100 mg or 400 mg of imatinib free base. Imatinib mesylate is designated chemically as 4-[(4-Methyl-1-piperazinyl)methyl]-N-[4-methyl-3-[[4-(3-pyridinyl)-2-pyrimidinyl]amino]-phenyl]benzamide methanesulfonate and its structural formula is

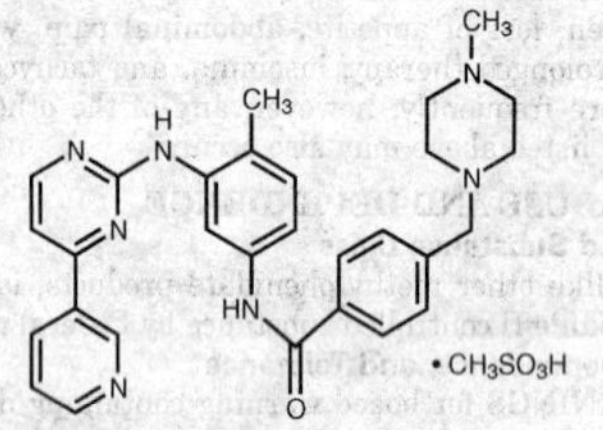

Imatinib mesylate is a white to off-white to brownish or yellowish tinged crystalline powder. Its molecular formula is $C_{29}H_{31}N_7O \bullet CH_4SO_3$ and its molecular weight is 589.7. Imatinib mesylate is soluble in aqueous buffers ≤ pH 5.5 but is very slightly soluble to insoluble in neutral/alkaline aqueous buffers. In non-aqueous solvents, the drug substance is freely soluble to very slightly soluble in dimethyl sulfoxide, methanol and ethanol, but is insoluble in n-octanol, acetone and acetonitrile.
Inactive Ingredients: colloidal silicon dioxide (NF); crospovidone (NF); hydroxypropyl methylcellulose (USP); magnesium stearate (NF); and microcrystalline cellulose (NF). *Tablet coating:* ferric oxide, red (NF); ferric oxide, yellow (NF); hydroxypropyl methylcellulose (USP); polyethylene glycol (NF) and talc (USP).

CLINICAL PHARMACOLOGY
Mechanism of Action
Imatinib mesylate is a protein-tyrosine kinase inhibitor that inhibits the Bcr-Abl tyrosine kinase, the constitutive abnormal tyrosine kinase created by the Philadelphia chromosome abnormality in chronic myeloid leukemia (CML). It inhibits proliferation and induces apoptosis in Bcr-Abl positive cell lines as well as fresh leukemic cells from Philadelphia chromosome positive chronic myeloid leukemia. In colony formation assays using *ex vivo* peripheral blood and bone marrow samples, imatinib shows inhibition of Bcr-Abl positive colonies from CML patients.
In vivo, it inhibits tumor growth of Bcr-Abl transfected murine myeloid cells as well as Bcr-Abl positive leukemia lines derived from CML patients in blast crisis.
Imatinib is also an inhibitor of the receptor tyrosine kinases for platelet-derived growth factor (PDGF) and stem cell factor (SCF), c-kit, and inhibits PDGF- and SCF-mediated cellular events. *In vitro,* imatinib inhibits proliferation and induces apoptosis in gastrointestinal stromal tumor (GIST) cells, which express an activating c-kit mutation.

Pharmacokinetics
The pharmacokinetics of Gleevec® (imatinib mesylate) have been evaluated in studies in healthy subjects and in population pharmacokinetic studies in over 900 patients. Imatinib is well absorbed after oral administration with C_{max} achieved within 2-4 hours post-dose. Mean absolute bioavailability is 98%. Following oral administration in healthy volunteers, the elimination half-lives of imatinib and its major active metabolite, the N-desmethyl derivative, are approximately 18 and 40 hours, respectively. Mean imatinib AUC increases proportionally with increasing doses ranging from 25 mg-1000 mg. There is no significant change in the pharmacokinetics of imatinib on repeated dosing, and accumulation is 1.5- to 2.5-fold at steady state when Gleevec is dosed once daily. At clinically relevant concentrations of imatinib, binding to plasma proteins in *in vitro* experiments is approximately 95%, mostly to albumin and α_1-acid glycoprotein.
The pharmacokinetics of Gleevec are similar in CML and GIST patients.

Metabolism and Elimination
CYP3A4 is the major enzyme responsible for metabolism of imatinib. Other cytochrome P450 enzymes, such as CYP1A2, CYP2D6, CYP2C9, and CYP2C19, play a minor role in its metabolism. The main circulating active metabolite in humans is the N-demethylated piperazine derivative, formed predominantly by CYP3A4. It shows *in vitro* potency similar to the parent imatinib. The plasma AUC for this metabolite is about 15% of the AUC for imatinib. The plasma protein binding of the N-demethylated metabolite CGP71588 is similar to that of the parent compound.
Elimination is predominately in the feces, mostly as metabolites. Based on the recovery of compound(s) after an oral ^{14}C-labeled dose of imatinib, approximately 81% of the dose was eliminated within 7 days, in feces (68% of dose) and urine (13% of dose). Unchanged imatinib accounted for 25% of the dose (5% urine, 20% feces), the remainder being metabolites.
Typically, clearance of imatinib in a 50-year-old patient weighing 50 kg is expected to be 8 L/h, while for a 50-year-old patient weighing 100 kg the clearance will increase to 14 L/h. However, the inter-patient variability of 40% in clearance does not warrant initial dose adjustment based on body weight and/or age but indicates the need for close monitoring for treatment-related toxicity.

Special Populations
Pediatric: As in adult patients, imatinib was rapidly absorbed after oral administration in pediatric patients, with a C_{max} of 2-4 hours. Apparent oral clearance was similar to adult values (11.0 L/hr/m² in children vs. 10.0 L/hr/m² in adults), as was the half-life (14.8 hours in children vs. 17.1 hr in adults). Dosing in children at both 260 mg/m² and 340 mg/m² achieved an AUC similar to the 400-mg dose in adults. The comparison of $AUC_{(0\text{-}24)}$ on Day 8 vs. Day 1 at 260 mg/m² and 340 mg/m² dose levels revealed a 1.5- and 2.2-fold drug accumulation, respectively, after repeated once-daily dosing. Mean imatinib AUC did not increase proportionally with increasing dose.
Hepatic Insufficiency: No clinical studies were conducted with Gleevec in patients with impaired hepatic function.
Renal Insufficiency: No clinical studies were conducted with Gleevec in patients with decreased renal function (studies excluded patients with serum creatinine concentration more than 2 times the upper limit of the normal range). Imatinib and its metabolites are not significantly excreted via the kidney.

Drug-Drug Interactions
CYP3A4 Inhibitors: There was a significant increase in exposure to imatinib (mean C_{max} and AUC increased by 26% and 40%, respectively) in healthy subjects when Gleevec was co-administered with a single dose of ketoconazole (a CYP3A4 inhibitor). (See PRECAUTIONS.)
CYP3A4 Substrates: Gleevec increased the mean C_{max} and AUC of simvastatin (CYP3A4 substrate) by 2- and 3.5-fold, respectively, indicating an inhibition of CYP3A4 by Gleevec. (See PRECAUTIONS.)
CYP3A4 Inducers: Pretreatment of 14 healthy volunteers with multiple doses of rifampin, 600 mg daily for 8 days, followed by a single 400-mg dose of Gleevec, increased Gleevec oral-dose clearance by 3.8-fold (90% confidence interval = 3.5- to 4.3-fold), which represents mean decreases in C_{max} $AUC_{(0\text{-}24)}$ and $AUC_{(0\text{-}\infty)}$ by 54%, 68% and 74%, of the respective values without rifampin treatment. (See PRECAUTIONS and DOSAGE AND ADMINISTRATION.)
In Vitro Studies of CYP Enzyme Inhibition: Human liver microsome studies demonstrated that Gleevec is a potent competitive inhibitor of CYP2C9, CYP2D6, and CYP3A4/5 with K_i values of 27, 7.5 and 8 µM, respectively. Gleevec is likely to increase the blood level of drugs that are substrates of CYP2C9, CYP2D6 and CYP3A4/5. (See PRECAUTIONS.)

CLINICAL STUDIES
Chronic Myeloid Leukemia
Chronic Phase, Newly Diagnosed: An open-label, multicenter, international randomized Phase 3 study has been conducted in patients with newly diagnosed Philadelphia chromosome positive (Ph+) chronic myeloid leukemia (CML) in chronic phase. This study compared treatment with either single-agent Gleevec® (imatinib mesylate) or a combination of interferon-alfa (IFN) plus cytarabine (Ara-C). Patients were allowed to cross over to the alternative treatment arm if they failed to show a complete hematologic response (CHR) at 6 months, a major cytogenetic response (MCyR) at 12 months, or if they lost a CHR or MCyR. Patients with increasing WBC or severe intolerance to treatment were also allowed to cross over to the alternative treatment arm with the permission of the study monitoring committee (SMC). In the Gleevec arm, patients were treated initially with 400 mg daily. In the IFN arm, patients were treated with a target dose of IFN of 5 MIU/m²/day subcutaneously in combination with subcutaneous Ara-C 20 mg/m²/day for 10 days/month.
A total of 1106 patients were randomized from 177 centers in 16 countries, 553 to each arm. Baseline characteristics were well balanced between the two arms. Median age was 51 years (range 18-70 years), with 21.9% of patients ≥60 years of age. There were 59% males and 41% females; 89.9% Caucasian and 4.7% Black patients. With a median follow-up of 14 and 13 months for Gleevec and IFN, respectively, 90% of patients randomized to Gleevec were still receiving first-line treatment. Due to discontinuations and cross-overs, only 30% of patients randomized to IFN were still on first-line treatment. In the IFN arm, withdrawal of consent (13.4%) was the most frequent reason for discon-

tinuation of first-line therapy, and the most frequent reason for cross-over to the Gleevec arm was severe intolerance to treatment (22.8%).

The primary efficacy endpoint of the study was progression-free survival (PFS). The final analysis of progression-free survival was planned after 5 years, however, the reported analysis was conducted at one year after the last patient was randomized to the study. Progression was defined as any of the following events: progression to accelerated phase or blast crisis, death, loss of CHR or MCyR, or in patients not achieving a CHR an increasing WBC despite appropriate therapeutic management. The protocol specified that the progression analysis would compare the intent to treat (ITT) population: patients randomized to receive Gleevec were compared with patients randomized to receive interferon. Patients that crossed over prior to progression were not censored at the time of cross-over, and events that occurred in these patients following cross-over were attributed to the original randomized treatment. A total of 218 patients crossed over from the interferon arm to the Gleevec arm, and 7 patients crossed over from the Gleevec arm to the interferon arm. The estimated rate of progression-free survival at 12 months in the ITT population was 97.2% in the Gleevec arm and 80.3% in the control arm. (Figure 1.) The estimated rate of patients free of progression to accelerated phase (AP) or blast crisis (BC) at 12 months was 98.5% in the Gleevec arm compared to the 93.1% in the IFN arm. (Figure 2.) There were 11 and 20 deaths reported in the Gleevec and IFN arm, respectively.

Figure 1 Time to Progression (ITT Principle)

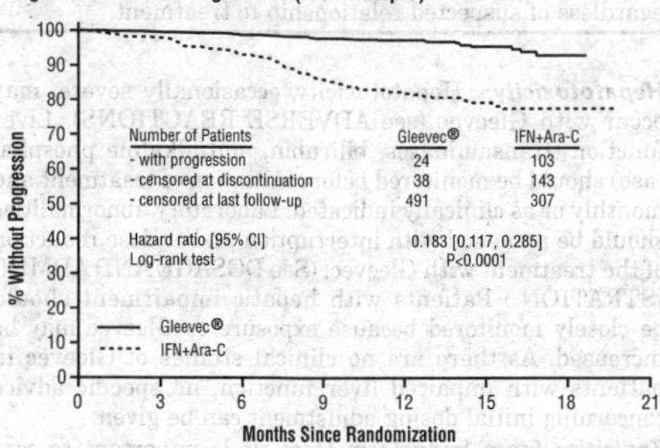

Figure 2 Time to Progression to AP or BC (ITT Principle)

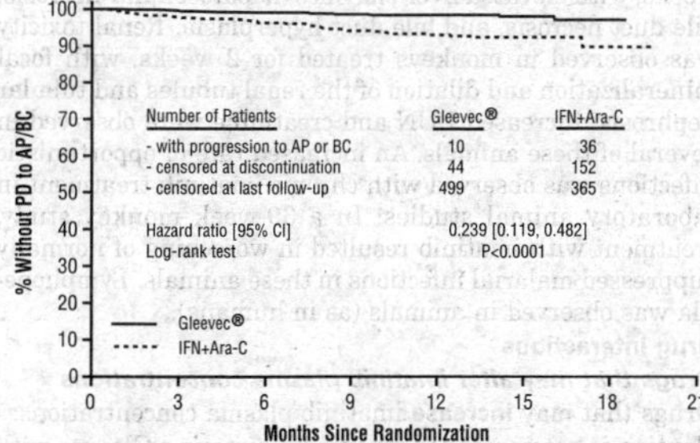

Major cytogenetic response, hematologic response, time to accelerated phase or blast crisis and survival were main secondary endpoints. Response data are shown in Table 1. Complete hematologic response, major cytogenetic response and complete cytogenetic response were also statistically significantly higher in the Gleevec arm compared to the IFN + Ara-C arm.

[See table 1 above]

Physical, functional, and treatment-specific biologic response modifier scales from the FACT-BRM (Functional Assessment of Cancer Therapy - Biologic Response Modifier) instrument were used to assess patient-reported general effects of interferon toxicity in 1067 patients with CML in chronic phase. After one month of therapy to six months of therapy, there was a 13%-21% decrease in median index from baseline in patients treated with interferon, consistent with increased symptoms of interferon toxicity. There was no apparent change from baseline in median index for patients treated with Gleevec.

Late Chronic Phase CML and Advanced Stage CML: Three international, open-label, single-arm Phase 2 studies were conducted to determine the safety and efficacy of Gleevec in patients with Ph+ CML: 1) in the chronic phase after failure of IFN therapy, 2) in accelerated phase disease, or 3) in myeloid blast crisis. About 45% of patients were women and 6% were Black. In clinical studies 38%-40% of patients were ≥60 years of age and 10%-12% of patients were ≥70 years of age.

Chronic Phase, Prior Interferon-Treatment: 532 patients were treated at a starting dose of 400 mg; dose escalation to 600 mg was allowed. The patients were distributed in three main categories according to their response to prior interferon: failure to achieve (within 6 months), or loss of a complete hematologic response (29%), failure to achieve (within 1 year) or loss of a major cytogenetic response (35%), or intolerance to interferon (36%). Patients had received a median of 14 months of prior IFN therapy at doses $\geq 25 \times 10^6$ IU/week and were all in late chronic phase, with a median time from diagnosis of 32 months. Effectiveness was evaluated on the basis of the rate of hematologic response and by bone marrow exams to assess the rate of major cytogenetic response (up to 35% Ph+ metaphases) or complete cytogenetic response (0% Ph+ metaphases). Median duration of treatment was 29 months with 81% of patients treated for ≥24 months (maximum = 31.5 months). Efficacy results are reported in Table 2. Confirmed major cytogenetic response rates were higher in patients with IFN intolerance (66%) and cytogenetic failure (64%), than in patients with hematologic failure (47%). Hematologic response was achieved in 98% of patients with cytogenetic failure, 94% of patients with hematologic failure, and 92% of IFN–intolerant patients.

Accelerated Phase: 235 patients with accelerated phase disease were enrolled. These patients met one or more of the following criteria: ≥15%-<30% blasts in PB or BM; ≥30% blasts + promyelocytes in PB or BM; ≥20% basophils in PB; and $<100 \times 10^9$/L platelets. The first 77 patients were started at 400 mg, with the remaining 158 patients starting at 600 mg.

Effectiveness was evaluated primarily on the basis of the rate of hematologic response, reported as either complete hematologic response, no evidence of leukemia (i.e., clearance of blasts from the marrow and the blood, but without a full peripheral blood recovery as for complete responses), or return to chronic phase CML. Cytogenetic responses were also evaluated. Median duration of treatment was 18 months with 45% of patients treated for ≥24 months (maximum = 35 months). Efficacy results are reported in Table 2. Response rates in accelerated phase CML were higher for the 600-mg dose group than for the 400-mg group: hematologic response (75% vs. 64%), confirmed and unconfirmed major cytogenetic response (31% vs. 19%).

Myeloid Blast Crisis: 260 patients with myeloid blast crisis were enrolled. These patients had ≥30% blasts in PB or BM and/or extramedullary involvement other than spleen or liver; 95 (37%) had received prior chemotherapy for treatment of either accelerated phase or blast crisis ("pretreated patients") whereas 165 (63%) had not ("untreated patients"). The first 37 patients were started at 400 mg; the remaining 223 patients were started at 600 mg.

Effectiveness was evaluated primarily on the basis of rate of hematologic response, reported as either complete hematologic response, no evidence of leukemia, or return to chronic phase CML using the same criteria as for the study in accelerated phase. Cytogenetic responses were also assessed. Median duration of treatment was 4 months with 21% of patients treated for ≥12 months and 10% for ≥24 months (maximum = 35 months). Efficacy results are reported in Table 2. The hematologic response rate was higher in untreated patients than in treated patients (36% vs. 22%, respectively) and in the group receiving an initial dose of 600 mg rather than 400 mg (33% vs. 16%). The confirmed and unconfirmed major cytogenetic response rate was also higher for the 600-mg dose group than for the 400-mg group (17% vs. 8%).

[See table 2 above]

The median time to hematologic response was 1 month. In late chronic phase CML, with a median time from diagnosis of 32 months, an estimated 87.8% of patients who achieved MCyR maintain their response 2 years after achieving their initial response. After 2 years of treatment, an estimated 85.4% of patients were free of progression to AP or BC, and estimated overall survival was 90.8% [88.3, 93.2]. In accelerated phase, median duration of hematologic response was 28.8 months for patients with an initial dose of 600 mg (16.5 months for 400 mg, p=0.0035). An estimated 63.8% of patients who achieved MCyR were still in response 2 years after achieving initial response. The median survival was 20.9 [13.1, 34.4] months for the 400-mg group and was not yet reached for the 600-mg group (p=0.0097). An estimated 46.2% [34.7, 57.7] vs. 65.8% [58.4, 73.3] of patients were still alive after 2 years of treatment in the 400-mg vs. 600-mg dose groups, respectively (p=0.0088). In blast crisis, the estimated median duration of hematologic response is 10 months. An estimated 27.2% [16.8, 37.7] of hematologic responders maintained their response 2 years after achieving their initial response. Median survival was 6.9 [5.8, 8.6] months, and an estimated 18.3% [13.4, 23.3] of all patients with blast crisis were alive 2 years after start of study.

Efficacy results were similar in men and women and in patients younger and older than age 65. Responses were seen in Black patients, but there were too few Black patients to allow a quantitative comparison.

Pediatric CML: One open-label, single-arm study enrolled 14 pediatric patients with Ph+ chronic phase CML recurrent after stem cell transplant or resistant to alpha interferon therapy. Patients ranged in age from 3 to 20 years old;

Continued on next page

Table 1 Response in Newly Diagnosed CML Study (First-Line)

(Best Response Rates)	Gleevec® n=553	IFN+Ara-C n=553
Hematologic Response[1]		
CHR Rate n (%)	522 (94.4%)*	302 (54.6%)*
[95% CI]	[92.1%, 96.2%]	[50.4%, 58.8%]
Cytogenetic Response[2]		
Major Cytogenetic Response n (%)	419 (75.8%)*	67 (12.1%)*
[95% CI]	[72.0%, 79.3%]	[9.5%, 15.1%]
Unconfirmed[3]	82.6%*	20.3%*
Complete Cytogenetic Response n (%)	297 (53.7%)*	15 (2.7%)*
Unconfirmed[3]	67.8%*	7.4%*

*p<0.001, Fischer's exact test

[1] **Hematologic response criteria (all responses to be confirmed after ≥4 weeks):** WBC$<10 \times 10^9$/L, platelet $<450 \times 10^9$/L, myelocyte + metamyelocyte <5% in blood, no blasts and promyelocytes in blood, basophils <20%, no extramedullary involvement.

[2] **Cytogenetic response criteria (confirmed after ≥4 weeks):** complete (0% Ph+ metaphases) or partial (1%-35%). A major response (0%-35%) combines both complete and partial responses.

[3] Unconfirmed cytogenetic response is based on a single bone marrow cytogenetic evaluation, therefore unconfirmed complete or partial cytogenetic responses might have had a lesser cytogenetic response on a subsequent bone marrow evaluation.

Table 2 Response in CML Studies

	Chronic Phase IFN Failure (n=532)	Accelerated Phase (n=235)	Myeloid Blast Crisis (n=260)
		600 mg n=158	600 mg n=223
	400 mg	400 mg n=77	400 mg n=37
		% of patients [$CI_{95\%}$]	
Hematologic Response[1]	**95% [92.3-96.3]**	**71% [64.8-76.8]**	**31% [25.2-36.8]**
Complete Hematologic Response (CHR)	95%	38%	7%
No evidence of Leukemia (NEL)	Not applicable	13%	5%
Return to Chronic Phase (RTC)	Not applicable	20%	18%
Major Cytogenetic Response[2]	**60% [55.3-63.8]**	**21% [16.2-27.1]**	**7% [4.5-11.2]**
(Unconfirmed[3])	(65%)	(27%)	(15%)
Complete[4] (Unconfirmed[3])	39% (47%)	16% (20%)	2% (7%)

[1]**Hematologic response criteria (all responses to be confirmed after ≥4 weeks):**

CHR: Chronic phase study [WBC $<10 \times 10^9$/L, platelet $<450 \times 10^9$/L, myelocytes + metamyelocytes <5% in blood, no blasts and promyelocytes in blood, basophils <20%, no extramedullary involvement] and in the accelerated and blast crisis studies [ANC $\geq 1.5 \times 10^9$/L, platelets $\geq 100 \times 10^9$/L, no blood blasts, BM blasts <5% and no extramedullary disease]

NEL: same criteria as for CHR but ANC $\geq 1 \times 10^9$/L and platelets $\geq 20 \times 10^9$/L (accelerated and blast crisis studies)

RTC: <15% blasts BM and PB, <30% blasts + promyelocytes in BM and PB, <20% basophils in PB, no extramedullary disease other than spleen and liver (accelerated and blast crisis studies).

BM=bone marrow, PB=peripheral blood

[2] **Cytogenetic response criteria (confirmed after ≥4 weeks):** complete (0% Ph+ metaphases) or partial (1%-35%). A major response (0%-35%) combines both complete and partial responses.

[3] Unconfirmed cytogenetic response is based on a single bone marrow cytogenetic evaluation, therefore unconfirmed complete or partial cytogenetic responses might have had a lesser cytogenetic response on a subsequent bone marrow evaluation.

[4] Complete cytogenetic response confirmed by a second bone marrow cytogenetic evaluation performed at least one month after the initial bone marrow study.

Gleevec—Cont.

3 were 3-11 years old, 9 were 12-18 years old, and 2 were >18 years old. Patients were treated at doses of 260 mg/m²/day (n=3), 340 mg/m²/day (n=4), 440 mg/m²/day (n=5) and 570 mg/m²/day (n=2). In the 13 patients for whom cytogenetic data are available, 4 achieved a major cytogenetic response, 7 achieved a complete cytogenetic response, and 2 had minimal cytogenetic response. At the recommended dose of 260 mg/m²/day, 2 of 3 patients achieved a complete cytogenetic response. Cytogenetic response rate was similar at all dose levels.

In a second study, 2 of 3 patients with Ph+ chronic phase CML resistant to alpha interferon achieved a complete cytogenetic response at doses of 242 and 257 mg/m²/day.

Gastrointestinal Stromal Tumors

One open-label, multinational study was conducted in patients with unresectable or metastatic malignant gastrointestinal stromal tumors (GIST). In this study 147 patients were enrolled and randomized to receive either 400 mg or 600 mg orally q.d. for up to 24 months. The study was not powered to show a statistically significant difference in response rates between the two dose groups. Patients ranged in age from 18 to 83 years old and had a pathologic diagnosis of Kit-positive unresectable and/or metastatic malignant GIST. Immunohistochemistry was routinely performed with Kit antibody (A-4502, rabbit polyclonal antiserum, 1:100; DAKO Corporation, Carpinteria, CA) according to analysis by an avidin-biotin-peroxidase complex method after antigen retrieval.

The primary outcome of the study was objective response rate. Tumors were required to be measurable at entry in at least one site of disease, and response characterization was based on Southwestern Oncology Group (SWOG) criteria. Results are shown in Table 3.

Table 3 Tumor Response in GIST Study

Total Patients	N	Confirmed Partial Response N (%)	95% Confidence Interval
400 mg Daily	73	24 (33%)	22%, 45%
600 mg Daily	74	32 (43%)	32%, 55%
Total	147	56 (38%)	30%, 46%

A statistically significant difference in response rates between the two dose groups was not demonstrated. At the time of interim analysis, when the median follow-up was less than 7 months, 55 of 56 patients with a confirmed partial response (PR) had a maintained PR. The data were too immature to determine a meaningful response duration. No responses were observed in 12 patients with progressive disease on 400 mg daily whose doses were increased to 600 mg daily.

INDICATIONS AND USAGE

Gleevec® (imatinib mesylate) is indicated for the treatment of newly diagnosed adult patients with Philadelphia chromosome positive chronic myeloid leukemia (CML) in chronic phase. Follow-up is limited.

Gleevec is also indicated for the treatment of patients with Philadelphia chromosome positive chronic myeloid leukemia (CML) in blast crisis, accelerated phase, or in chronic phase after failure of interferon-alpha therapy. Gleevec is also indicated for the treatment of pediatric patients with Ph+ chronic phase CML whose disease has recurred after stem cell transplant or who are resistant to interferon-alpha therapy. There are no controlled trials in pediatric patients demonstrating a clinical benefit, such as improvement in disease-related symptoms or increased survival.

Gleevec is also indicated for the treatment of patients with Kit (CD117) positive unresectable and/or metastatic malignant gastrointestinal stromal tumors (GIST). (See CLINICAL STUDIES, Gastrointestinal Stromal Tumors.) The effectiveness of Gleevec in GIST is based on objective response rate (see CLINICAL STUDIES). There are no controlled trials demonstrating a clinical benefit, such as improvement in disease-related symptoms or increased survival.

CONTRAINDICATIONS

Use of Gleevec® (imatinib mesylate) is contraindicated in patients with hypersensitivity to imatinib or to any other component of Gleevec.

WARNINGS

Pregnancy

Women of childbearing potential should be advised to avoid becoming pregnant.

Imatinib mesylate was teratogenic in rats when administered during organogenesis at doses ≥100 mg/kg, approximately equal to the maximum clinical dose of 800 mg/day (based on body surface area). Teratogenic effects included exencephaly or encephalocele, absent/reduced frontal and absent parietal bones. Female rats administered doses ≥45 mg/kg (approximately one-half the maximum human dose of 800 mg/day, based on body surface area) also experienced significant post-implantation loss as evidenced by either early fetal resorption or stillbirths, nonviable pups and early pup mortality between postpartum Days 0 and 4. At doses higher than 100 mg/kg, total fetal loss was noted in all animals. Fetal loss was not seen at doses ≤30 mg/kg (one-third the maximum human dose of 800 mg).

Table 4 Adverse Experiences Reported in Newly Diagnosed CML Clinical Trial (≥10% of all patients)[(1)]

Preferred Term	All Grades Gleevec® N=551 (%)	All Grades IFN+Ara-C N=533 (%)	CTC Grades 3/4 Gleevec® N=551 (%)	CTC Grades 3/4 IFN+Ara-C N=533 (%)
Fluid Retention	54.1	10.1	0.9	0.9
– Superficial Edema	53.2	8.8	0.9	0.4
– Other Fluid Retention Events	3.4	1.5	0	0.6
Nausea	42.5	60.8	0.4	5.1
Muscle Cramps	35.4	9.9	1.1	0.2
Musculoskeletal Pain	33.6	40.5	2.7	7.7
Rash	31.9	25.0	2.0	2.1
Fatigue	30.7	64.7	1.1	24.0
Diarrhea	30.3	40.9	1.3	3.2
Headache	28.5	41.8	0.4	3.2
Joint Pain	26.7	38.3	2.2	6.8
Abdominal Pain	23.4	22.9	2.0	3.6
Myalgia	20.9	38.6	1.5	8.1
Nasopharyngitis	19.2	7.7	0	0.2
Hemorrhage	18.9	19.9	0.7	1.3
Dyspepsia	15.1	9.0	0	0.8
Vomiting	14.7	26.6	0.9	3.4
Pharyngolaryngeal Pain	14.2	11.4	0.2	0
Dizziness	13.2	23.1	0.5	3.4
Cough	12.5	21.6	0.2	0.6
Upper Respiratory Tract Infection	12.5	7.9	0.2	0.4
Pyrexia	11.8	38.6	0.5	2.8
Weight Increased	11.6	1.5	0.7	0.2
Insomnia	11.4	18.4	0	2.3

(1) All adverse events occurring in ≥10% of patients are listed regardless of suspected relationship to treatment.

Male and female rats were exposed *in utero* to a maternal imatinib mesylate dose of 45 mg/kg (approximately one-half the maximum human dose of 800 mg) from Day 6 of gestation and through milk during the lactation period. These animals then received no imatinib exposure for nearly 2 months. Body weights were reduced from birth until terminal sacrifice in these rats. Although fertility was not affected, fetal loss was seen when these male and female animals were then mated.

There are no adequate and well-controlled studies in pregnant women. If Gleevec® (imatinib mesylate) is used during pregnancy, or if the patient becomes pregnant while taking (receiving) Gleevec, the patient should be apprised of the potential hazard to the fetus.

PRECAUTIONS

General

Dermatologic Toxicities: Bullous dermatologic reactions, including erythema multiforme and Stevens-Johnson syndrome, have been reported with use of Gleevec® (imatinib mesylate). In some cases reported during post-marketing surveillance, a recurrent dermatologic reaction was observed upon rechallenge. Several foreign post-marketing reports have described cases in which patients tolerated the reintroduction of Gleevec therapy after resolution or improvement of the bullous reaction. In these instances, Gleevec was resumed at a dose lower than that at which the reaction occurred and some patients also received concomitant treatment with corticosteroids or antihistamines.

Fluid Retention and Edema: Gleevec is often associated with edema and occasionally serious fluid retention (see ADVERSE REACTIONS). Patients should be weighed and monitored regularly for signs and symptoms of fluid retention. An unexpected rapid weight gain should be carefully investigated and appropriate treatment provided. The probability of edema was increased with higher Gleevec dose and age >65 years in the CML studies. Severe superficial edema was reported in 0.9% of newly diagnosed CML patients taking Gleevec, and in 2%-6% of other adult CML patients taking Gleevec. In addition, other severe fluid retention (e.g., pleural effusion, pericardial effusion, pulmonary edema, and ascites) events were reported in 2%-6% of other adult CML patients taking Gleevec. Severe superficial edema and severe fluid retention (pleural effusion, pulmonary edema and ascites) were reported in 1%-6% of patients taking Gleevec for GIST.

There have been post-marketing reports, including fatalities, of cardiac tamponade, cerebral edema, increased intracranial pressure, and papilledema in patients treated with Gleevec.

GI Irritation: Gleevec is sometimes associated with GI irritation. Gleevec should be taken with food and a large glass of water to minimize this problem.

Hemorrhage: In the newly diagnosed CML trial, 0.7% of patients had grade 3/4 hemorrhage. In the GIST clinical trial seven patients (5%), four in the 600-mg dose group and three in the 400-mg dose group, had a total of eight events of CTC grade 3/4 - gastrointestinal (GI) bleeds (3 patients), intra-tumoral bleeds (3 patients) or both (1 patient). Gastrointestinal tumor sites may have been the source of GI bleeds.

Hematologic Toxicity: Treatment with Gleevec is associated with anemia, neutropenia, and thrombocytopenia. Complete blood counts should be performed weekly for the first month, biweekly for the second month, and periodically thereafter as clinically indicated (for example, every 2-3 months). In CML, the occurrence of these cytopenias is dependent on the stage of disease and is more frequent in patients with accelerated phase CML or blast crisis than in patients with chronic phase CML. (See DOSAGE AND ADMINISTRATION.)

Hepatotoxicity: Hepatotoxicity, occasionally severe, may occur with Gleevec (see ADVERSE REACTIONS). Liver function (transaminases, bilirubin, and alkaline phosphatase) should be monitored before initiation of treatment and monthly or as clinically indicated. Laboratory abnormalities should be managed with interruption and/or dose reduction of the treatment with Gleevec. (See DOSAGE AND ADMINISTRATION.) Patients with hepatic impairment should be closely monitored because exposure to Gleevec may be increased. As there are no clinical studies of Gleevec in patients with impaired liver function, no specific advice concerning initial dosing adjustment can be given.

Toxicities From Long-Term Use: It is important to consider potential toxicities suggested by animal studies, specifically, *liver and kidney toxicity and immunosuppression.* Severe liver toxicity was observed in dogs treated for 2 weeks, with elevated liver enzymes, hepatocellular necrosis, bile duct necrosis, and bile duct hyperplasia. Renal toxicity was observed in monkeys treated for 2 weeks, with focal mineralization and dilation of the renal tubules and tubular nephrosis. Increased BUN and creatinine were observed in several of these animals. An increased rate of opportunistic infections was observed with chronic imatinib treatment in laboratory animal studies. In a 39-week monkey study, treatment with imatinib resulted in worsening of normally suppressed malarial infections in these animals. Lymphopenia was observed in animals (as in humans).

Drug Interactions

Drugs that may alter imatinib plasma concentrations

Drugs that may **increase** imatinib plasma concentrations: Caution is recommended when administering Gleevec with inhibitors of the CYP3A4 family (e.g., ketoconazole, itraconazole, erythromycin, clarithromycin). Substances that inhibit the cytochrome P450 isoenzyme (CYP3A4) activity may decrease metabolism and increase imatinib concentrations. There is a significant increase in exposure to imatinib when Gleevec is coadministered with ketoconazole (CYP3A4 inhibitor).

Drugs that may **decrease** imatinib plasma concentrations: Substances that are inducers of CYP3A4 activity may increase metabolism and decrease imatinib plasma concentrations. Co-medications that induce CYP3A4 (e.g., dexamethasone, phenytoin, carbamazepine, rifampin, phenobarbital or St. John's Wort) may significantly reduce exposure to Gleevec. Pretreatment of healthy volunteers with multiple doses of rifampin followed by a single dose of Gleevec, increased Gleevec oral-dose clearance by 3.8-fold, which significantly ($p<0.05$) decreased mean C_{max} and $AUC_{(0-\infty)}$. In patients where rifampin or other CYP3A4 inducers are indicated, alternative therapeutic agents with less enzyme induction potential should be considered. (See CLINICAL PHARMACOLOGY and DOSAGE AND ADMINISTRATION.)

Drugs that may have their plasma concentration altered by Gleevec

Gleevec increases the mean C_{max} and AUC of simvastatin (CYP3A4 substrate) 2- and 3.5-fold, respectively, suggesting an inhibition of the CYP3A4 by Gleevec. Particular caution is recommended when administering Gleevec with CYP3A4 substrates that have a narrow therapeutic window (e.g., cyclosporine or pimozide). Gleevec will increase plasma concentration of other CYP3A4 metabolized drugs (e.g., triazolo-benzodiazepines, dihydropyridine calcium channel blockers, certain HMG-CoA reductase inhibitors, etc.).

Because *warfarin* is metabolized by CYP2C9 and CYP3A4, patients who require anticoagulation should receive low-molecular weight or standard heparin.

In vitro, Gleevec inhibits the cytochrome P450 isoenzyme CYP2D6 activity at similar concentrations that affect CYP3A4 activity. Systemic exposure to substrates of

CYP2D6 is expected to be increased when coadministered with Gleevec. No specific studies have been performed and caution is recommended.

In vitro, Gleevec inhibits acetaminophen O-glucuronidation (K_i value of 58.5 μM) at therapeutic levels. Systemic exposure to acetaminophen is expected to be increased when coadministered with Gleevec. No specific studies in humans have been performed and caution is recommended.

Carcinogenesis, Mutagenesis, Impairment of Fertility

Carcinogenicity studies have not been performed with imatinib mesylate.

Positive genotoxic effects were obtained for imatinib in an *in vitro* mammalian cell assay (Chinese hamster ovary) for clastogenicity (chromosome aberrations) in the presence of metabolic activation. Two intermediates of the manufacturing process, which are also present in the final product, are positive for mutagenesis in the Ames assay. One of these intermediates was also positive in the mouse lymphoma assay. Imatinib was not genotoxic when tested in an *in vitro* bacterial cell assay (Ames test), an *in vitro* mammalian cell assay (mouse lymphoma) and an *in vivo* rat micronucleus assay.

In a study of fertility, in male rats dosed for 70 days prior to mating, testicular and epididymal weights and percent motile sperm were decreased at 60 mg/kg, approximately three-fourths the maximum clinical dose of 800 mg/day, based on body surface area. This was not seen at doses ≤20 mg/kg (one-fourth the maximum human dose of 800 mg). When female rats were dosed 14 days prior to mating and through to gestational Day 6, there was no effect on mating or on number of pregnant females.

In female rats dosed with imatinib mesylate at 45 mg/kg (approximately one-half the maximum human dose of 800 mg, based on body surface area) from gestational Day 6 until the end of lactation, red vaginal discharge was noted on either gestational Day 14 or 15.

Pregnancy

Pregnancy Category D. (See WARNINGS.)

Nursing Mothers

It is not known whether imatinib mesylate or its metabolites are excreted in human milk. However, in lactating female rats administered 100 mg/kg, a dose approximately equal to the maximum clinical dose of 800 mg/day based on body surface area, imatinib and its metabolites were extensively excreted in milk. Concentration in milk was approximately three-fold higher than in plasma. It is estimated that approximately 1.5% of a maternal dose is excreted into milk, which is equivalent to a dose to the infant of 30% the maternal dose per unit body weight. Because many drugs are excreted in human milk and because of the potential for serious adverse reactions in nursing infants, women should be advised against breast-feeding while taking Gleevec.

Pediatric Use

Gleevec safety and efficacy have been demonstrated only in children with Ph+ chronic phase CML with recurrence after stem cell transplantation or resistance to interferon-alpha therapy. There are no data in children under 3 years of age.

Geriatric Use

In the CML clinical studies, approximately 40% of patients were older than 60 years and 10% were older than 70 years. In the study of patients with newly diagnosed CML, 22% of patients were 60 years of age or older. No difference was observed in the safety profile in patients older than 65 years as compared to younger patients, with the exception of a higher frequency of edema. (See PRECAUTIONS.) The efficacy of Gleevec was similar in older and younger patients. In the GIST study, 29% of patients were older than 60 years and 10% of patients were older than 70 years. No obvious differences in the safety or efficacy profile were noted in patients older than 65 years as compared to younger patients, but the small number of patients does not allow a formal analysis.

ADVERSE REACTIONS

Chronic Myeloid Leukemia

The majority of Gleevec-treated patients experienced adverse events at some time. Most events were of mild-to-moderate grade, but drug was discontinued for drug-related adverse events in 4% of patients in chronic phase, 5% in accelerated phase and 5% in blast crisis.

The most frequently reported drug-related adverse events were edema, nausea and vomiting, muscle cramps, musculoskeletal pain, diarrhea and rash (Table 4 for newly diagnosed CML, Table 5 for other CML patients). Edema was most frequently periorbital or in lower limbs and was managed with diuretics, other supportive measures, or by reducing the dose of Gleevec® (imatinib mesylate). (See DOSAGE AND ADMINISTRATION.) The frequency of severe superficial edema was 0.9%-6%.

A variety of adverse events represent local or general fluid retention including pleural effusion, ascites, pulmonary edema and rapid weight gain with or without superficial edema. These events appear to be dose related, were more common in the blast crisis and accelerated phase studies (where the dose was 600 mg/day), and are more common in the elderly. These events were usually managed by interrupting Gleevec treatment and with diuretics or other appropriate supportive care measures. However, a few of these events may be serious or life threatening, and one patient with blast crisis died with pleural effusion, congestive heart failure, and renal failure.

Adverse events, regardless of relationship to study drug, that were reported in at least 10% of the patients treated in the Gleevec studies are shown in Tables 4 and 5.

Table 5 Adverse Experiences Reported in Other CML Clinical Trials (≥10% of all patients in any trial)[(1)]

Preferred Term	Myeloid Blast Crisis (n=260) % All Grades	Grade 3/4	Accelerated Phase (n=235) % All Grades	Grade 3/4	Chronic Phase, IFN Failure (n=532) % All Grades	Grade 3/4
Fluid Retention	72	11	76	6	69	4
– Superficial Edema	66	6	74	3	67	2
– Other Fluid Retention Events[(2)]	22	6	15	4	7	2
Nausea	71	5	73	5	63	3
Muscle Cramps	28	1	47	0.4	62	2
Vomiting	54	4	58	3	36	2
Diarrhea	43	4	57	5	48	3
Hemorrhage	53	19	49	11	30	2
– CNS Hemorrhage	9	7	3	3	2	1
– Gastrointestinal Hemorrhage	8	4	6	5	2	0.4
Musculoskeletal Pain	42	9	49	9	38	2
Fatigue	30	4	46	4	48	1
Skin Rash	36	5	47	5	47	3
Pyrexia	41	7	41	8	21	2
Arthralgia	25	5	34	6	40	1
Headache	27	5	32	2	36	0.6
Abdominal Pain	30	6	33	4	32	1
Weight Increased	5	1	17	5	32	7
Cough	14	0.8	27	0.9	20	0
Dyspepsia	12	0	22	0	27	0
Myalgia	9	0	24	2	27	0.2
Nasopharyngitis	10	0	17	0	22	0.2
Asthenia	18	5	21	5	15	0.2
Dyspnea	15	4	21	7	12	0.9
Upper Respiratory Tract Infection	3	0	12	0.4	19	0
Anorexia	14	2	17	2	7	0
Night Sweats	13	0.8	17	1	14	0.2
Constipation	16	2	16	0.9	9	0.4
Dizziness	12	0.4	13	0	16	0.2
Pharyngitis	10	0	12	0	15	0
Insomnia	10	0	14	0	14	0.2
Pruritus	8	1	14	0.9	14	0.8
Hypokalemia	13	4	9	2	6	0.8
Pneumonia	13	7	10	7	4	1
Anxiety	8	0.8	12	0	8	0.4
Liver Toxicity	10	5	12	6	6	3
Rigors	10	0	12	0.4	10	0
Chest Pain	7	2	10	0.4	11	0.8
Influenza	0.8	0.4	6	0	11	0.2
Sinusitis	4	0.4	11	0.4	9	0.4

(1) All adverse events occurring in ≥10% of patients are listed regardless of suspected relationship to treatment.

(2) Other fluid retention events include pleural effusion, ascites, pulmonary edema, pericardial effusion, anasarca, edema aggravated, and fluid retention not otherwise specified.

Table 6 Lab Abnormalities in Newly Diagnosed CML Trial

CTC Grades	Gleevec® N=551 % Grade 3	Grade 4	IFN+Ara-C N=533 % Grade 3	Grade 4
Hematology Parameters				
- Neutropenia*	11.4	2.2	20.3	4.3
- Thrombocytopenia*	6.9	0.2	15.8	0.6
- Anemia	2.7	0.4	4.1	0.2
Biochemistry Parameters				
- Elevated Creatinine	0	0	0.4	0
- Elevated Bilirubin	0.2	0.5	0.2	0
- Elevated Alkaline Phosphatase	0.2	0	0.8	0
- Elevated SGOT (AST)	2.9	0.2	3.8	0.4
- Elevated SGPT (ALT)	3.1	0.4	5.6	0

*p<0.001 (difference in grade 3 plus 4 abnormalities between the two treatment groups)

[See table 4 at top of previous page]

[See table 5 above]

Hematologic Toxicity

Cytopenias, and particularly neutropenia and thrombocytopenia, were a consistent finding in all studies, with a higher frequency at doses ≥750 mg (Phase 1 study). However, the occurrence of cytopenias in CML patients was also dependent on the stage of the disease.

In patients with newly diagnosed CML, cytopenias were less frequent than in the other CML patients (see Tables 6 and 7). The frequency of grade 3 or 4 neutropenia and thrombocytopenia was between 2- and 3-fold higher in blast crisis and accelerated phase compared to chronic phase (see Tables 6 and 7). The median duration of the neutropenic and thrombocytopenic episodes varied from 2 to 3 weeks, and from 2 to 4 weeks, respectively.

These events can usually be managed with either a reduction of the dose or an interruption of treatment with Gleevec, but in rare cases require permanent discontinuation of treatment.

Hepatotoxicity

Severe elevation of transaminases or bilirubin occurred in 3%-6% (see Table 5) and were usually managed with dose reduction or interruption (the median duration of these episodes was approximately one week). Treatment was discontinued permanently because of liver laboratory abnormalities in less than 1% of patients. However, one patient, who was taking acetaminophen regularly for fever, died of acute liver failure.

Adverse Reactions in Pediatric Population

The overall safety profile of pediatric patients treated with Gleevec in 39 children studied was similar to that found in studies with adult patients, except that musculoskeletal pain was less frequent (20.5%) and peripheral edema was not reported.

Adverse Effects in Other Subpopulations

In older patients (≥65 years old), with the exception of edema, where it was more frequent, there was no evidence of an increase in the incidence or severity of adverse events. In women there was an increase in the frequency of neutropenia, as well as grade 1/2 superficial edema, headache, nausea, rigors, vomiting, rash, and fatigue. No differences were seen related to race but the subsets were too small for proper evaluation.

[See table 6 above]

[See table 7 at top of next page]

Gastrointestinal Stromal Tumors

The majority of Gleevec-treated patients experienced adverse events at some time. The most frequently reported adverse events were edema, nausea, diarrhea, abdominal

Continued on next page

Gleevec—Cont.

pain, muscle cramps, fatigue, and rash. Most events were of mild-to-moderate severity. Drug was discontinued for adverse events in 6 patients (8%) in both dose levels studied. Superficial edema, most frequently periorbital or lower extremity edema, was managed with diuretics, other supportive measures, or by reducing the dose of Gleevec® (imatinib mesylate). (See DOSAGE AND ADMINISTRATION.) Severe (CTC grade 3/4) superficial edema was observed in 3 patients (2%), including face edema in one patient. Grade 3/4 pleural effusion or ascites was observed in 3 patients (2%).

Adverse events, regardless of relationship to study drug, that were reported in at least 10% of the patients treated with Gleevec are shown in Table 8. No major differences were seen in the severity of adverse events between the 400-mg or 600-mg treatment groups, although overall incidence of diarrhea, muscle cramps, headache, dermatitis, and edema was somewhat higher in the 600-mg treatment group.

[See table 8 at right]

Clinically relevant or severe abnormalities of routine hematologic or biochemistry laboratory values are presented in Table 9.

[See table 9 at right]

Additional Data from Multiple Clinical Trials

The following less common (estimated 1%-10%), infrequent (estimated 0.1%-1%), and rare (estimated less than 0.1%) adverse events have been reported during clinical trials of Gleevec. These events are included based on clinical relevance.

Cardiovascular: *Infrequent:* cardiac failure, tachycardia, hypertension, hypotension, flushing, peripheral coldness
Rare: pericarditis

Clinical Laboratory Tests: *Infrequent:* blood CPK increased, blood LDH increased

Dermatologic: *Less common:* dry skin, alopecia
Infrequent: exfoliative dermatitis, bullous eruption, nail disorder, skin pigmentation changes, photosensitivity reaction, purpura, psoriasis
Rare: vesicular rash, Stevens-Johnson syndrome, acute generalized exanthematous pustulosis

Digestive: *Less common:* abdominal distention, gastroesophageal reflux, mouth ulceration
Infrequent: gastric ulcer, gastroenteritis, gastritis
Rare: colitis, ileus/intestinal obstruction, pancreatitis

General Disorders and Administration Site Conditions:
Rare: tumor necrosis

Hematologic: *Infrequent:* pancytopenia
Rare: aplastic anemia

Hypersensitivity: *Rare:* angioedema

Infections: *Infrequent:* sepsis, herpes simplex, herpes zoster

Metabolic and Nutritional: *Infrequent:* hypophosphatemia, dehydration, gout, appetite disturbances, weight decreased
Rare: hyperkalemia, hyponatremia

Musculoskeletal: *Less common:* joint swelling
Infrequent: sciatica, joint and muscle stiffness

Nervous System/Psychiatric: *Less common:* paresthesia
Infrequent: depression, anxiety, syncope, peripheral neuropathy, somnolence, migraine, memory impairment
Rare: increased intracranial pressure, cerebral edema (including fatalities), confusion, convulsions

Renal: *Infrequent:* renal failure, urinary frequency, hematuria

Reproductive: *Infrequent:* breast enlargement, menorrhagia, sexual dysfunction

Respiratory: *Rare:* interstitial pneumonitis, pulmonary fibrosis

Special Senses: *Less common:* conjunctivitis, vision blurred
Infrequent: conjunctival hemorrhage, dry eye, vertigo, tinnitus
Rare: macular edema, papilledema, retinal hemorrhage, glaucoma, vitreous hemorrhage

Vascular Disorders: *Rare:* thrombosis/embolism

OVERDOSAGE

Experience with doses greater than 800 mg is limited. In the event of overdosage, the patient should be observed and appropriate supportive treatment given. An oral dose of 1200 mg/m^2/day, approximately 2.5 times the human dose of 800 mg, based on body surface area, was not lethal to rats following 14 days of administration. A dose of 3600 mg/m^2/day, approximately 7.5 times the human dose of 800 mg, was lethal to rats after 7-10 administrations, due to general deterioration of the animals with secondary degenerative histological changes in many tissues.

DOSAGE AND ADMINISTRATION

Therapy should be initiated by a physician experienced in the treatment of patients with chronic myeloid leukemia or gastrointestinal stromal tumors.

The recommended dosage of Gleevec® (imatinib mesylate) is 400 mg/day for adult patients in chronic phase CML and 600 mg/day for adult patients in accelerated phase or blast crisis. The recommended Gleevec dosage is 260 mg/m^2/day for children with Ph+ chronic phase CML recurrent after stem cell transplant or who are resistant to interferon-alpha therapy. The recommended dosage of Gleevec is 400 mg/day or 600 mg/day for adult patients with unresectable and/or metastatic, malignant GIST.

The prescribed dose should be administered orally, with a meal and a large glass of water. Doses of 400 mg or 600 mg should be administered once daily, whereas a dose of 800 mg should be administered as 400 mg twice a day.

In children, Gleevec treatment can be given as a once-daily dose or alternatively the daily dose may be split into two - once in the morning and once in the evening. There is no experience with Gleevec treatment in children under 3 years of age.

For patients unable to swallow the film-coated tablets, the tablets may be dispersed in a glass of water or apple juice. The required number of tablets should be placed in the appropriate volume of beverage (approximately 50 mL for a 100-mg tablet, and 200 mL for a 400-mg tablet) and stirred with a spoon. The suspension should be administered immediately after complete disintegration of the tablet(s).

Treatment may be continued as long as there is no evidence of progressive disease or unacceptable toxicity.

In CML, a dose increase from 400 mg to 600 mg in adult patients with chronic phase disease, or from 600 mg to 800 mg (given as 400 mg twice daily) in adult patients in accelerated phase or blast crisis may be considered in the absence of severe adverse drug reaction and severe non-leukemia related neutropenia or thrombocytopenia in the following circumstances: disease progression (at any time); failure to achieve a satisfactory hematologic response after at least 3 months of treatment; failure to achieve a cytogenetic response after 6-12 months of treatment; or loss of a previously achieved hematologic or cytogenetic response. In children with chronic phase CML, daily doses can be increased under circumstances similar to those leading to an increase in adult chronic phase disease, from 260 mg/m^2/day to 340 mg/m^2/day, as clinically indicated.

Table 7 Lab Abnormalities in Other CML Clinical Trials

	Myeloid Blast Crisis (n=260) 600 mg n=223 400 mg n=37 %		Accelerated Phase (n=235) 600 mg n=158 400 mg n=77 %		Chronic Phase, IFN Failure (n=532) 400 mg %	
CTC Grades	Grade 3	Grade 4	Grade 3	Grade 4	Grade 3	Grade 4
Hematology Parameters						
- Neutropenia	16	48	23	36	27	9
- Thrombocytopenia	30	33	31	13	21	<1
- Anemia	42	11	34	7	6	1
Biochemistry Parameters						
- Elevated Creatinine	1.5	0	1.3	0	0.2	0
- Elevated Bilirubin	3.8	0	2.1	0	0.6	0
- Elevated Alkaline Phosphatase	4.6	0	5.5	0.4	0.2	0
- Elevated SGOT (AST)	1.9	0	3.0	0	2.3	0
- Elevated SGPT (ALT)	2.3	0.4	4.3	0	2.1	0

CTC grades: neutropenia (grade 3 ≥0.5-1.0 × 10^9/L), grade 4 <0.5 × 10^9/L), thrombocytopenia (grade 3 ≥10-50 × 10^9/L, grade 4 <10 × 10^9/L), anemia (hemoglobin ≥65-80 g/L, grade 4 <65 g/L), elevated creatinine (grade 3 >3-6 × upper limit normal range [ULN], grade 4 >6 × ULN), elevated bilirubin (grade 3 >3-10 × ULN, grade 4 >10 × ULN), elevated alkaline phosphatase (grade 3 >5-20 × ULN, grade 4 >20 × ULN), elevated SGOT or SGPT (grade 3 >5-20 × ULN, grade 4 >20 × ULN)

Table 8 Adverse Experiences Reported in GIST Trial (≥10% of all patients at either dose)(1)

	All CTC Grades Initial Dose (mg/day)		CTC Grade 3/4 Initial Dose (mg/day)	
Preferred Term	400 mg (n=73) %	600 mg (n=74) %	400 mg (n=73) %	600 mg (n=74) %
Fluid retention	71	76	6	3
- Superficial Edema	71	76	4	0
- Pleural Effusion or Ascites	6	4	1	3
Diarrhea	56	60	1	4
Nausea	53	56	3	3
Fatigue	33	38	1	0
Muscle Cramps	30	41	0	0
Abdominal Pain	37	37	7	3
Skin Rash	26	38	3	3
Headache	25	35	0	0
Vomiting	22	23	1	3
Musculoskeletal Pain	19	11	3	0
Flatulence	16	23	0	0
Any Hemorrhage	18	19	5	8
- Tumor Hemorrhage	1	4	1	4
- Cerebral Hemorrhage	1	0	1	0
- GI Tract Hemorrhage	6	4	4	1
Nasopharyngitis	12	14	0	0
Pyrexia	12	5	0	0
Insomnia	11	11	0	0
Back Pain	11	10	1	0
Lacrimation Increased	6	11	0	0
Upper Respiratory Tract Infection	6	11	0	0
Taste Disturbance	1	14	0	0

(1) All adverse events occurring in ≥10% of patients are listed regardless of suspected relationship to treatment.

Table 9 Laboratory Abnormalities in GIST Trial

	400 mg (n=73) %		600 mg (n=74) %	
CTC Grades	Grade 3	Grade 4	Grade 3	Grade 4
Hematology Parameters				
- Anemia	3	0	4	1
- Thrombocytopenia	0	0	1	0
- Neutropenia	3	3	5	4
Biochemistry Parameters				
- Elevated Creatinine	0	1	3	0
- Reduced Albumin	3	0	4	0
- Elevated Bilirubin	1	0	1	3
- Elevated Alkaline Phosphatase	0	0	1	0
- Elevated SGOT (AST)	3	0	1	1
- Elevated SGPT (ALT)	3	0	4	0

CTC grades: neutropenia (grade 3 ≥0.5-1.0 × 10^9/L, grade 4 <0.5 × 10^9/L), thrombocytopenia (grade 3 ≥10-50 × 10^9/L, grade 4 <10 × 10^9/L), anemia (grade 3 ≥65-80 g/L, grade 4 <65 g/L), elevated creatinine (grade 3 >3-6 × upper limit normal range [ULN], grade 4 >6 × ULN), elevated bilirubin (grade 3 >3-10 × ULN, grade 4 >10 × ULN), elevated alkaline phosphatase, SGOT or SGPT (grade 3 >5-20 × ULN, grade 4 >20 × ULN), albumin (grade 3 <20 g/L)

Table 10 Dose Adjustments for Neutropenia and Thrombocytopenia

Chronic Phase CML (starting dose 400 mg[1]) or GIST (starting dose either 400 mg or 600 mg)	ANC $<1.0 \times 10^9$/L and/or Platelets $<50 \times 10^9$/L	1. Stop Gleevec until ANC $\geq 1.5 \times 10^9$/L and platelets $\geq 75 \times 10^9$/L 2. Resume treatment with Gleevec at the original starting dose of 400 mg[1] or 600 mg 3. If recurrence of ANC $<1.0 \times 10^9$/L and/or platelets $<50 \times 10^9$/L, repeat step 1 and resume Gleevec at a reduced dose (300 mg[2] if starting dose was 400 mg[1], 400 mg if starting dose was 600 mg)
Accelerated Phase CML and Blast Crisis (starting dose 600 mg)	[3]ANC $<0.5 \times 10^9$/L and/or Platelets $<10 \times 10^9$/L	1. Check if cytopenia is related to leukemia (marrow aspirate or biopsy) 2. If cytopenia is unrelated to leukemia, reduce dose of Gleevec to 400 mg 3. If cytopenia persists 2 weeks, reduce further to 300 mg 4. If cytopenia persists 4 weeks and is still unrelated to leukemia, stop Gleevec until ANC $\geq 1 \times 10^9$/L and platelets $\geq 20 \times 10^9$/L and then resume treatment at 300 mg

[1]or 260 mg/m² in children
[2]or 200 mg/m² in children
[3]occurring after at least 1 month of treatment

Dosage of Gleevec should be increased by at least 50%, and clinical response should be carefully monitored, in patients receiving Gleevec with a potent CYP3A4 inducer such as rifampin or phenytoin.

For daily dosing of 800 mg and above, dosing should be accomplished using the 400-mg tablet to reduce exposure to iron. Patients at a total dose of 1200 mg daily may have an increased susceptibility to excess iron. If routine blood sampling indicates sustained increases in iron levels, attempts to lower other sources of iron exposure should be undertaken.

Dose Adjustment for Hepatotoxicity and Other Non-Hematologic Adverse Reactions

If a severe non-hematologic adverse reaction develops (such as severe hepatotoxicity or severe fluid retention), Gleevec should be withheld until the event has resolved. Thereafter, treatment can be resumed as appropriate depending on the initial severity of the event.

If elevations in bilirubin $>3 \times$ institutional upper limit of normal (IULN) or in liver transaminases $>5 \times$ IULN occur, Gleevec should be withheld until bilirubin levels have returned to a $<1.5 \times$ IULN and transaminase levels to $<2.5 \times$ IULN. In adults, treatment with Gleevec may then be continued at a reduced daily dose (i.e., 400 mg to 300 mg or 600 mg to 400 mg). In children, daily doses can be reduced under the same circumstances from 260 mg/m²/day to 200 mg/m²/day or from 340 mg/m/day to 260 mg/m²/day, respectively.

Dose Adjustment for Hematologic Adverse Reactions

Dose reduction or treatment interruptions for severe neutropenia and thrombocytopenia are recommended as indicated in Table 10.

[See table 10 above]

HOW SUPPLIED

Each film-coated tablet contains 100 mg or 400 mg of imatinib free base.

100 mg Tablets

Very dark yellow to brownish orange film-coated tablets, round, biconvex with bevelled edges debossed with "NVR" on one side and "SA" with score on the other side.

Bottles of 100 tablets .... NDC 0078-0401-05

400 mg Tablets

Very dark yellow to brownish orange film-coated tablets, ovaloid, biconvex with bevelled edges, debossed with "NVR" on one side and "SL" on the other side.

Bottles of 30 tablets .... NDC 0078-0402-15

Storage

Store at 25°C (77°F); excursions permitted to 15-30°C (59-86°F) [see USP Controlled Room Temperature]. Protect from moisture.

Dispense in a tight container, USP.

T2004-61
REV: JULY 2004 Printed in U.S.A. 5000021
Manufactured by:
Novartis Pharma Stein AG
Stein, Switzerland
Distributed by:
Novartis Pharmaceuticals Corporation
East Hanover, New Jersey 07936
©NOVARTIS

Shown in Product Identification Guide, page 325

LAMISIL® ℞

[la″mə′səl]

(terbinafine hydrochloride tablets)

Tablets

Rx only

Prescribing Information

The following prescribing information is based on official labeling in effect July 2004.

DESCRIPTION

LAMISIL® (terbinafine hydrochloride tablets) Tablets contain the synthetic allylamine antifungal compound terbinafine hydrochloride.

Chemically, terbinafine hydrochloride is (E)-*N*-(6,6-dimethyl-2-hepten-4-ynyl)-*N*-methyl-1-naphthalenemethanamine hydrochloride. The empirical formula $C_{21}H_{26}ClN$ with a molecular weight of 327.90, and the following structural formula:

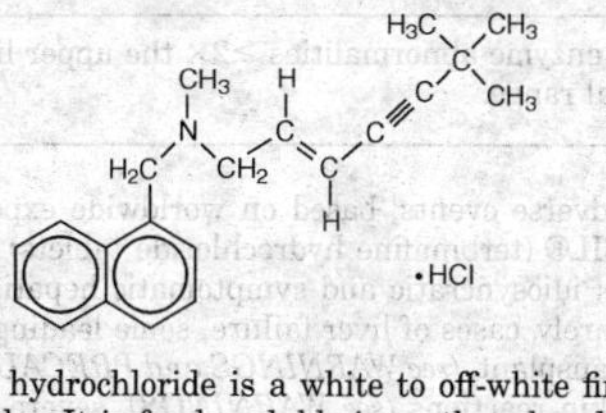

Terbinafine hydrochloride is a white to off-white fine crystalline powder. It is freely soluble in methanol and methylene chloride, soluble in ethanol, and slightly soluble in water.

Each tablet contains:

Active Ingredients: terbinafine hydrochloride (equivalent to 250 mg base)

Inactive Ingredients: colloidal silicon dioxide, NF; hydroxypropyl methylcellulose, USP; magnesium stearate, NF; microcrystalline cellulose, NF; sodium starch glycolate, NF

CLINICAL PHARMACOLOGY

Pharmacokinetics

Following oral administration, terbinafine is well absorbed (>70%) and the bioavailability of LAMISIL® (terbinafine hydrochloride tablets) Tablets as a result of first-pass metabolism is approximately 40%. Peak plasma concentrations of 1 µg/mL appear within 2 h after a single 250 mg dose; the AUC (area under the curve) is approximately 4.56 µg·h/mL. An increase in the AUC of terbinafine of less than 20% is observed when LAMISIL® is administered with food. No clinically relevant age-dependent changes in steady-state plasma concentrations of terbinafine have been reported. In patients with renal impairment (creatinine clearance ≤50 mL/min) or hepatic cirrhosis, the clearance of terbinafine is decreased by approximately 50% compared to normal volunteers. No effect of gender on the blood levels of terbinafine was detected in clinical trials. In plasma, terbinafine is >99% bound to plasma proteins and there are no specific binding sites. At steady-state, in comparison to a single dose, the peak concentration of terbinafine is 25% higher and plasma AUC increases by a factor of 2.5; the increase in plasma AUC is consistent with an effective half-life of ~36 hours. Terbinafine is distributed to the sebum and skin. A terminal half-life of 200-400 h may represent the slow elimination of terbinafine from tissues such as skin and adipose. Prior to excretion, terbinafine is extensively metabolized. No metabolites have been identified that have antifungal activity similar to terbinafine. Approximately 70% of the administered dose is eliminated in the urine.

Microbiology

Terbinafine hydrochloride is a synthetic allylamine derivative. Terbinafine hydrochloride is hypothesized to act by inhibiting squalene epoxidase, thus blocking the biosynthesis of ergosterol, an essential component of fungal cell membranes. *In vitro*, mammalian squalene epoxidase is only inhibited at higher (4000 fold) concentrations than is needed for inhibition of the dermatophyte enzyme. Depending on the concentration of the drug and the fungal species test *in vitro*, terbinafine hydrochloride may be fungicidal. However, the clinical significance of *in vitro* data is unknown.

Terbinafine has been shown to be active against most strains of the following microorganisms both *in vitro* and in clinical infections as described in the *INDICATIONS AND USAGE* section:

Trichophyton mentagrophytes
Trichophyton rubrum

The following *in vitro* data are available, but their clinical significance is unknown. *In vitro*, terbinafine exhibits satisfactory MIC's against most strains of the following microorganisms; however, the safety and efficacy of terbinafine in treating clinical infections due to these microorganisms have not been established in adequate and well-controlled clinical trials:

Candida albicans
Epidermophyton floccosum
Scopulariopsis brevicaulis

CLINICAL STUDIES

The efficacy of LAMISIL® (terbinafine hydrochloride tablets) Tablets in the treatment of onychomycosis is illustrated by the response of patients with toenail and/or fingernail infections who participated in three US/Canadian placebo-controlled clinical trials.

Results of the first toenail study, as assessed at week 48 (12 weeks of treatment with 36 weeks follow-up after completion of therapy), demonstrated mycological cure, defined as simultaneous occurrence of negative KOH plus negative culture, in 70% of patients. Fifty-nine percent (59%) of patients experienced effective treatment (mycological cure plus 0% nail involvement or >5mm of new unaffected nail growth); 38% of patients demonstrated mycological cure plus clinical cure (0% nail involvement).

In a second toenail study of dermatophytic onychomycosis, in which non-dermatophytes were also cultured, similar efficacy against the dermatophytes was demonstrated. The pathogenic role of the non-dermatophytes cultured in the presence of dermatophytic onychomycosis has not been established. The clinical significance of this association is unknown.

Results of the fingernail study, as assessed at week 24 (6 weeks of treatment with 18 weeks follow-up after completion of therapy), demonstrated mycological cure in 79% of patients, effective treatment in 75% of the patients, and mycological cure plus clinical cure in 59% of the patients.

The mean time to overall success was approximately 10 months for the first toenail study and 4 months for the fingernail study. In the first toenail study, for patients evaluated at least six months after achieving clinical cure and at least one year after completing LAMISIL® therapy, the clinical relapse rate was approximately 15%.

INDICATIONS AND USAGE

LAMISIL® (terbinafine hydrochloride tablets) Tablets are indicated for the treatment of onychomycosis of the toenail or fingernail due to dermatophytes (tinea unguium) *(see DOSAGE AND ADMINISTRATION* and *CLINICAL STUDIES).*

Prior to initiating treatment, appropriate nail specimens for laboratory testing (KOH preparation, fungal culture, or nail biopsy) should be obtained to confirm the diagnosis of onychomycosis.

CONTRAINDICATIONS

LAMISIL® (terbinafine hydrochloride tablets) Tablets are contraindicated in individuals with hypersensitivity to terbinafine or to any other ingredients of the formulation.

WARNINGS

Rare cases of liver failure, some leading to death or liver transplant, have occurred with the use of LAMISIL® (terbinafine hydrochloride tablets) Tablets for the treatment of onychomycosis in individuals with and without pre-existing liver disease.

In the majority of liver cases reported in association with LAMISIL® use, the patients had serious underlying systemic conditions and an uncertain causal association with LAMISIL®. The severity of hepatic events and/or their outcome may be worse in patients with active or chronic liver disease *(see PRECAUTIONS).* Treatment with LAMISIL® Tablets should be discontinued if biochemical or clinical evidence of liver injury develops *(see PRECAUTIONS below).*

There have been isolated reports of serious skin reactions (e.g., Stevens-Johnson Syndrome and toxic epidermal necrolysis). If progressive skin rash occurs, treatment with LAMISIL® should be discontinued.

PRECAUTIONS

General

LAMISIL® (terbinafine hydrochloride tablets) Tablets are not recommended for patients with chronic or active liver disease. Before prescribing LAMISIL® Tablets, pre-existing liver disease should be assessed. Hepatotoxicity may occur in patients with and without pre-existing liver disease. Pretreatment serum transaminase (ALT and AST) tests are advised for all patients before taking LAMISIL® Tablets. Patients prescribed LAMISIL® Tablets should be warned to report immediately to their physician any symptoms of persistent nausea, anorexia, fatigue, vomiting, right upper abdominal pain or jaundice, dark urine or pale stools *(see WARNINGS).* Patients with these symptoms should discontinue taking oral terbinafine, and the patient's liver function should be immediately evaluated.

In patients with renal impairment (creatinine clearance ≤50 mL/min), the use of LAMISIL® has not been adequately studied, and therefore, is not recommended *(see CLINICAL PHARMACOLOGY, Pharmacokinetics).*

During post-marketing experience, precipitation and exacerbation of cutaneous and systemic lupus erythemato-

Continued on next page

Lamisil—Cont.

sus have been reported infrequently in patients taking LAMISIL®. LAMISIL® therapy should be discontinued in patients with clinical signs and symptoms suggestive of lupus erythematosus.

Changes in the ocular lens and retina have been reported following the use of LAMISIL® (terbinafine hydrochloride tablets) Tablets in controlled trials. The clinical significance of these changes is unknown.

Transient decreases in absolute lymphocyte counts (ALC) have been observed in controlled clinical trials. In placebo-controlled trials, 8/465 LAMISIL®-treated patients (1.7%) and 3/137 placebo-treated patients (2.2%) had decreases in ALC to below 1000/mm^3 on two or more occasions. The clinical significance of this observation is unknown. However, in patients with known or suspected immunodeficiency, physicians should consider monitoring complete blood counts in individuals using LAMISIL® therapy for greater than six weeks.

Isolated cases of severe neutropenia have been reported. These were reversible upon discontinuation of LAMISIL®, with or without supportive therapy. If clinical signs and symptoms suggestive of secondary infection occur, a complete blood count should be obtained. If the neutrophil count is ≤1,000 cells/mm^3, LAMISIL® should be discontinued and supportive management started.

Drug Interactions

In vivo studies have shown that terbinafine is an inhibitor of the CYP450 2D6 isozyme. Coadministration of LAMISIL® with drugs predominantly metabolized by the CYP450 2D6 isozyme (e.g., tricyclic antidepressants, selective serotonin reuptake inhibitors, beta-blockers and monoamine oxidase inhibitors Type B) should be done with careful monitoring and may require a reduction in dose of the 2D6-metabolized drug. In a study to assess the effects of terbinafine on desipramine in healthy volunteers characterized as normal metabolizers, the administration of terbinafine resulted in a 2-fold increase in C_{max} and a 5-fold increase in AUC. In this study, these effects were shown to persist at the last observation at 4 weeks after discontinuation of LAMISIL®.

In vitro studies with human liver microsomes showed that terbinafine does not inhibit the metabolism of tolbutamide, ethinylestradiol, ethoxycoumarin, and cyclosporine.

In vivo drug-drug interaction studies conducted in healthy volunteer subjects showed that terbinafine does not affect the clearance of antipyrine or digoxin. Terbinafine decreases the clearance of caffeine by 19%. Terbinafine increases the clearance of cyclosporine by 15%.

There have been spontaneous reports of increase or decrease in prothrombin times in patients concomitantly taking oral terbinafine and warfarin, however, a causal relationship between LAMISIL® Tablets and these changes has not been established.

Terbinafine clearance is increased 100% by rifampin, a CYP450 enzyme inducer, and decreased 33% by cimetidine, a CYP450 enzyme inhibitor. Terbinafine clearance is unaffected by cyclosporine.

There is no information available from adequate drug-drug interaction studies with the following classes of drugs: oral contraceptives, hormone replacement therapies, hypoglycemics, theophyllines, phenytoins, thiazide diuretics, and calcium channel blockers.

Carcinogenesis, Mutagenesis, Impairment of Fertility

In a 28-month oral carcinogenicity study in rats, an increase in the incidence of liver tumors was observed in males at the highest dose tested, 69 mg/kg/day [2× the Maximum Recommended Human Dose (MRHD) based on AUC comparisons of the parent terbinafine]; however, even though dose-limiting toxicity was not achieved at the highest tested dose, higher doses were not tested.

The results of a variety of *in vitro* (mutations in *E. coli* and *S. typhimurium*, DNA repair in rat hepatocytes, mutagenicity in Chinese hamster fibroblasts, chromosome aberration and sister chromatid exchanges in Chinese hamster lung cells), and *in vivo* (chromosome aberration in Chinese hamsters, micronucleus test in mice) genotoxicity tests gave no evidence of a mutagenic or clastogenic potential. Oral reproduction studies in rats at doses up to 300 mg/kg/day (approximately 12× the MRHD based on body surface area comparisons, BSA) did not reveal any specific effects on fertility or other reproductive parameters. Intravaginal application of terbinafine hydrochloride at 150 mg/day in pregnant rabbits did not increase the incidence of abortions or premature deliveries nor affect fetal parameters.

Pregnancy

Pregnancy Category B: Oral reproduction studies have been performed in rabbits and rats at doses up to 300 mg/kg/day (12× to 23× the MRHD, in rabbits and rats, respectively, based on BSA) and have revealed no evidence of impaired fertility or harm to the fetus due to terbinafine. There are, however, no adequate and well-controlled studies in pregnant women. Because animal reproduction studies are not always predictive of human response, and because treatment of onychomycosis can be postponed until after pregnancy is completed, it is recommended that LAMISIL® not be initiated during pregnancy.

Nursing Mothers

After oral administration, terbinafine is present in breast milk of nursing mothers. The ratio of terbinafine in milk to plasma is 7:1. Treatment with LAMISIL® is not recommended in nursing mothers.

Pediatric Use

The safety and efficacy of LAMISIL® have not been established in pediatric patients.

ADVERSE REACTIONS

The most frequently reported adverse events observed in the three US/Canadian placebo-controlled trials are listed in the table below. The adverse events reported encompass gastrointestinal symptoms (including diarrhea, dyspepsia, and abdominal pain), liver test abnormalities, rashes, urticaria, pruritus, and taste disturbances. In general, the adverse events were mild, transient, and did not lead to discontinuation from study participation.

	Adverse Event		Discontinuation	
	LAMISIL® (%) n=465	Placebo (%) n=137	LAMISIL® (%) n=465	Placebo (%) n=137
Headache	12.9	9.5	0.2	0.0
Gastrointestinal Symptoms:				
Diarrhea	5.6	2.9	0.6	0.0
Dyspepsia	4.3	2.9	0.4	0.0
Abdominal Pain	2.4	1.5	0.4	0.0
Nausea	2.6	2.9	0.2	0.0
Flatulence	2.2	2.2	0.0	0.0
Dermatological Symptoms:				
Rash	5.6	2.2	0.9	0.7
Pruritus	2.8	1.5	0.2	0.0
Urticaria	1.1	0.0	0.0	0.0
Liver Enzyme Abnormalities*	3.3	1.4	0.2	0.0
Taste Disturbance	2.8	0.7	0.2	0.0
Visual Disturbance	1.1	1.5	0.9	0.0

*Liver enzyme abnormalities ≥2× the upper limit of the normal range.

Rare adverse events, based on worldwide experience with LAMISIL® (terbinafine hydrochloride tablets) Tablets use, include: idiosyncratic and symptomatic hepatic injury and more rarely, cases of liver failure, some leading to death or liver transplant, *(see WARNINGS and PRECAUTIONS)*, serious skin reactions *(see WARNINGS)*, severe neutropenia *(see PRECAUTIONS)*, thrombocytopenia, angioedema and allergic reactions (including anaphylaxis). Precipitation and exacerbation of cutaneous and systemic lupus erythematosus have been reported infrequently in patients taking LAMISIL®. Uncommonly, LAMISIL® may cause taste disturbance (including taste loss) which usually recovers within several weeks after discontinuation of the drug. There have been isolated reports of prolonged (greater than one year) taste disturbance. Rarely, taste disturbances associated with oral terbinafine have been reported to be severe enough to result in decreased food intake leading to significant and unwanted weight loss.

Other adverse reactions which have been reported include malaise, fatigue, vomiting, arthralgia, myalgia, and hair loss.

Clinical adverse effects reported spontaneously since the drug was marketed include altered prothrombin time (prolongation and reduction) in patients concomitantly treated with warfarin and LAMISIL® Tablets and agranulocytosis (rare).

OVERDOSAGE

Clinical experience regarding overdose with LAMISIL® (terbinafine hydrochloride tablets) Tablets is limited. Doses up to 5 grams (20 times the therapeutic daily dose) have been taken without inducing serious adverse reactions. The symptoms of overdose included nausea, vomiting, abdominal pain, dizziness, rash, frequent urination, and headache.

DOSAGE AND ADMINISTRATION

LAMISIL® (terbinafine hydrochloride tablets) Tablets, one 250 mg tablet, should be taken once daily for 6 weeks by patients with fingernail onychomycosis. LAMISIL®, one 250 mg tablet, should be taken once daily for 12 weeks by patients with toenail onychomycosis. The optimal clinical effect is seen some months after mycological cure and cessation of treatment. This is related to the period required for outgrowth of healthy nail.

HOW SUPPLIED

LAMISIL®
(terbinafine hydrochloride tablets)
Tablets

Supplied as white to yellow-tinged white circular, bi-convex, bevelled tablets containing 250 mg of terbinafine imprinted with "LAMISIL" in circular form on one side and code "250" on the other.

Bottles of 100 tablets .... NDC 0078-0179-05
Bottles of 30 tablets .... NDC 0078-0179-15

Store tablets below 25°C (77°F); in a tight container. Protect from light.

ANIMAL TOXICOLOGY

A wide range of *in vivo* studies in mice, rats, dogs, and monkeys, and *in vitro* studies using rat, monkey, and human hepatocytes suggest that peroxisome proliferation in the liver is a rat-specific finding. However, other effects, including increased liver weights and APTT, occurred in dogs and monkeys at doses giving Css trough levels of the parent terbinafine 2-3× those seen in humans at the MRHD. Higher doses were not tested.

REV: MARCH 2004

T2004-21
89006805
2343-25-04A

Manufactured by:
Patheon Inc.
Whitby Operations
Whitby, Ontario Canada L1N 5Z5
Distributed by:
Novartis Pharmaceuticals Corporation
East Hanover, New Jersey 07936
©Novartis

Shown in Product Identification Guide, page 325

LESCOL® ℞

[lĕs-kōl]
(fluvastatin sodium)
Capsules

LESCOL® XL

(fluvastatin sodium)
Extended-Release Tablets
Rx only

Prescribing Information

The following prescribing information is based on official labeling in effect July 2003.

DESCRIPTION

Lescol® (fluvastatin sodium), is a water-soluble cholesterol lowering agent which acts through the inhibition of 3-hydroxy-3-methylglutaryl-coenzyme A (HMG-CoA) reductase. Fluvastatin sodium is [*R**,*S**-(E)]-(±)-7-[3-(4-fluorophenyl)-1-(1-methylethyl)-1*H*-indol-2-yl]-3,5-dihydroxy-6-heptenoic acid, monosodium salt. The empirical formula of fluvastatin sodium is $C_{24}H_{25}FNO_4 \cdot Na$, its molecular weight is 433.46 and its structural formula is:

F, OH, OH, O, O-, Na+, N, H_3C, CH_3

$C_{24}H_{25}FNO_4 \cdot Na$ Mol. wt. 433.46

This molecular entity is the first entirely synthetic HMG-CoA reductase inhibitor, and is in part structurally distinct from the fungal derivatives of this therapeutic class.

Fluvastatin sodium is a white to pale yellow, hygroscopic powder soluble in water, ethanol and methanol. Lescol is supplied as capsules containing fluvastatin sodium, equivalent to 20 mg or 40 mg of fluvastatin, for oral administration. Lescol® XL (fluvastatin sodium) is supplied as extended-release tablets containing fluvastatin sodium, equivalent to 80 mg of fluvastatin, for oral administration.

Active Ingredient: fluvastatin sodium

Inactive Ingredients in capsules: gelatin, magnesium stearate, microcrystalline cellulose, pregelatinized starch (corn), red iron oxide, sodium lauryl sulfate, talc, titanium dioxide, yellow iron oxide, and other ingredients.

Capsules may also include: benzyl alcohol, black iron oxide, butylparaben, carboxymethylcellulose sodium, edetate calcium disodium, methylparaben, propylparaben, silicon dioxide and sodium propionate.

Inactive Ingredients in extended-release tablets: microcrystalline cellulose, hydroxypropyl cellulose, hydroxypropyl methyl cellulose, potassium bicarbonate, povidone, magnesium stearate, iron oxide yellow, titanium dioxide and polyethylene glycol 8000.

CLINICAL PHARMACOLOGY

A variety of clinical studies have demonstrated that elevated levels of total cholesterol (Total-C), low density lipoprotein cholesterol (LDL-C), triglycerides (TG) and apolipoprotein B (a membrane transport complex for LDL-C) promote human atherosclerosis. Similarly, decreased levels of HDL-cholesterol (HDL-C) and its transport complex, apolipoprotein A, are associated with the development of atherosclerosis. Epidemiologic investigations have established that cardiovascular morbidity and mortality vary directly with the level of Total-C and LDL-C and inversely with the level of HDL-C.

Like LDL, cholesterol enriched triglyceride-rich lipoproteins, including VLDL, IDL and remnants, can also promote atherosclerosis. Elevated plasma triglycerides are frequently found in a triad with low HDL-C levels and small LDL particles, as well as in association with non-lipid metabolic risk factors for coronary heart disease. As such, total plasma TG has not consistently been shown to be an independent risk factor for CHD. Furthermore, the independent effect of raising HDL or lowering TG on the risk of coronary and cardiovascular morbidity and mortality has not been determined.

In patients with hypercholesterolemia and mixed dyslipidemia, treatment with Lescol® (fluvastatin sodium) or

Lescol® XL (fluvastatin sodium) reduced Total-C, LDL-C, apolipoprotein B, and triglycerides while producing an increase in HDL-C. Increases in HDL-C are greater in patients with low HDL-C (<35 mg/dL). Neither agent had a consistent effect on either Lp(a) or fibrinogen. The effect of Lescol or Lescol XL induced changes in lipoprotein levels, including reduction of serum cholesterol, on cardiovascular mortality has not been determined.

Mechanism of Action

Lescol is a competitive inhibitor of HMG-CoA reductase, which is responsible for the conversion of 3-hydroxy-3-methylglutaryl-coenzyme A (HMG-CoA) to mevalonate, a precursor of sterols, including cholesterol. The inhibition of cholesterol biosynthesis reduces the cholesterol in hepatic cells, which stimulates the synthesis of LDL receptors and thereby increases the uptake of LDL particles. The end result of these biochemical processes is a reduction of the plasma cholesterol concentration.

Pharmacokinetics/Metabolism

Oral Absorption

Fluvastatin is absorbed rapidly and completely following oral administration of the capsule, with peak concentrations reached in less than 1 hour. Following administration of a 10 mg dose, the absolute bioavailability is 24% (range 9%-50%). Administration with food reduces the rate but not the extent of absorption. At steady-state, administration of fluvastatin with the evening meal results in a two-fold decrease in C_{max} and more than two-fold increase in t_{max} as compared to administration 4 hours after the evening meal. No significant differences in extent of absorption or in the lipid-lowering effects were observed between the two administrations. After single or multiple doses above 20 mg, fluvastatin exhibits saturable first-pass metabolism resulting in higher-than-expected plasma fluvastatin concentrations.

Fluvastatin has two optical enantiomers, an active 3R,5S and an inactive 3S,5R form. *In vivo* studies showed that stereo-selective hepatic binding of the active form occurs during the first pass resulting in a difference in the peak levels of the two enantiomers, with the active to inactive peak concentration ratio being about 0.7. The approximate ratio of the active to inactive approaches unity after the peak is seen and thereafter the two enantiomers decline with the same half-life. After an intravenous administration, bypassing the first-pass metabolism, the ratios of the enantiomers in plasma were similar throughout the concentration-time profiles.

Fluvastatin administered as Lescol XL 80 mg tablets reaches peak concentration in approximately 3 hours under fasting conditions, after a low-fat meal, or 2.5 hours after a low-fat meal. The mean relative bioavailability of the XL tablet is approximately 29% (range: 9%-66%) compared to that of the Lescol immediate release capsule administered under fasting conditions. Administration of a high fat meal delayed the absorption (T_{max}: 6H) and increased the bioavailability of the XL tablet by approximately 50%. Once Lescol XL begins to be absorbed, fluvastatin concentrations rise rapidly. The maximum concentration seen after a high fat meal is much less than the peak concentration following a single dose or twice daily dose of the 40 mg Lescol capsule. Overall variability in the pharmacokinetics of Lescol XL is large (42%-64% CV for C_{max} and AUC), and especially so after a high fat meal (63%-89% for C_{max} and AUC). Intrasubject variability in the pharmacokinetics of Lescol XL under fasting conditions (about 25% for C_{max} and AUC) tends to be much smaller as compared to the overall variability. Multiple peaks in plasma fluvastatin concentrations have been observed after Lescol XL administration.

Distribution

Fluvastatin is 98% bound to plasma proteins. The mean volume of distribution (VDss) is estimated at 0.35 L/kg. The parent drug is targeted to the liver and no active metabolites are present systemically. At therapeutic concentrations, the protein binding of fluvastatin is not affected by warfarin, salicylic acid and glyburide.

Metabolism

Fluvastatin is metabolized in the liver, primarily via hydroxylation of the indole ring at the 5- and 6-positions. N-dealkylation and beta-oxidation of the side-chain also occurs. The hydroxy metabolites have some pharmacologic activity, but do not circulate in the blood. Both enantiomers of fluvastatin are metabolized in a similar manner.

In vitro studies demonstrated that fluvastatin undergoes oxidative metabolism, predominantly via 2C9 isozyme systems (75%). Other isozymes that contribute to fluvastatin metabolism are 2C8 (~5%) and 3A4 (~20%). *(See PRECAUTIONS: Drug Interactions Section).*

Elimination

Fluvastatin is primarily (about 90%) eliminated in the feces as metabolites, with less than 2% present as unchanged drug. Urinary recovery is about 5%. After a radiolabeled dose of fluvastatin, the clearance was 0.8 L/h/kg. Following multiple oral doses of radiolabeled compound, there was no accumulation of fluvastatin; however, there was a 2.3 fold accumulation of total radioactivity.

Steady-state plasma concentrations show no evidence of accumulation of fluvastatin following immediate release capsule administration of up to 80 mg daily, as evidenced by a beta-elimination half-life of less than 3 hours. However, under conditions of maximum rate of absorption (i.e., fasting) systemic exposure to fluvastatin is increased 33% to 53% compared to a single 20 mg or 40 mg dose of the immediate release capsule. Following once daily administration of the 80 mg Lescol XL tablet for 7 days, systemic exposure to fluvastatin is increased (20%-30%) compared to a single dose of

Table 1
Single-Dose and Steady-State Pharmacokinetic Parameters

	C_{max} (ng/mL) mean ± SD (range)	AUC (ng·h/mL) mean ± SD (range)	t_{max} (hr) mean ± SD (range)	CL/F (L/hr) mean ± SD (range)	$t_{1/2}$ (hr) mean ± SD (range)
Capsules					
20 mg single dose (n=17)	166±106 (48.9-517)	207±65 (111-288)	0.9±0.4 (0.5-2.0)	107±38.1 (69.5-181)	2.5±1.7 (0.5-6.6)
20 mg twice daily (n=17)	200±86 (71.8-366)	275±111 (91.6-467)	1.2±0.9 (0.5-4.0)	87.8±45 (42.8-218)	2.8±1.7 (0.9-6.0)
40 mg single dose (n=16)	273±189 (72.8-812)	456±259 (207-1221)	1.2±0.7 (0.75-3.0)	108±44.7 (32.8-193)	2.7±1.3 (0.8-5.9)
40 mg twice daily (n=16)	432±236 (119-990)	697±275 (359-1559)	1.2±0.6 (0.5-2.5)	64.2±21.1 (25.7-111)	2.7±1.3 (0.7-5.0)
Extended-Release Tablets 80 mg single dose (n=24)					
80 mg single dose fasting (n=24)	126±53 (37-242)	579±341 (144-1760)	3.2±2.6 (1-12)	–	
80 mg single dose, fed-state high fat meal (n=24)	183±163 (21-733)	861±632 (199-3132)	6 (2-24)		
Extended-Release Tablets 80 mg following 7 days dosing (steady-state) (n=11)					
80 mg once daily fasting (n=11)	102±42 (43.9-181)	630±326 (247-1406)	2.6±0.91 (1.5-4)	–	

Table 2
Median Percent Change in Lipid Parameters from Baseline to Week 24 Endpoint
All Placebo-Controlled Studies (Lescol®) and Active Controlled Trials (Lescol® XL)

	Total Chol.		TG		LDL		Apo B		HDL	
Dose	**N**	**% Δ**	**N**	**% Δ**	**N**	**% Δ**	**N**	**% Δ**	**N**	**% Δ**
All Patients										
Lescol 20 mg[1]	747	-17	747	-12	747	-22	114	-19	747	+3
Lescol 40 mg[1]	748	-19	748	-14	748	-25	125	-18	748	+4
Lescol 40 mg twice daily[1]	257	-27	257	-18	257	-36	232	-28	257	+6
Lescol XL 80 mg[2]	750	-25	750	-19	748	-35	745	-27	750	+7
Baseline TG ≥200 mg/dL										
Lescol 20 mg[1]	148	-16	148	-17	148	-22	23	-19	148	+6
Lescol 40 mg[1]	179	-18	179	-20	179	-24	47	-18	179	+7
Lescol 40 mg twice daily[1]	76	-27	76	-23	76	-35	69	-28	76	+9
Lescol XL 80 mg[2]	239	-25	239	-25	237	-33	235	-27	239	+11

[1]Data for Lescol from 12 placebo controlled trials
[2]Data for Lescol XL 80 mg tablet from three 24 week controlled trials

the 80 mg Lescol XL tablet. Terminal half-life of Lescol XL was about 9 hours as a result of the slow-release formulation.

Single-dose and steady-state pharmacokinetic parameters in 33 subjects with hypercholesterolemia for the capsules and in 35 healthy subjects for the extended-release tablets are summarized below:

[See table 1 above]

Special Populations

Renal Insufficiency: No significant (<6%) renal excretion of fluvastatin occurs in humans.

Hepatic Insufficiency: Fluvastatin is subject to saturable first-pass metabolism/sequestration by the liver and is eliminated primarily via the biliary route. Therefore, the potential exists for drug accumulation in patients with hepatic insufficiency. Caution should therefore be exercised when fluvastatin sodium is administered to patients with a history of liver disease or heavy alcohol ingestion *(see WARNINGS).*

Fluvastatin AUC and C_{max} values increased by about 2.5 fold in hepatic insufficiency patients. This result was attributed to the decreased presystemic metabolism due to hepatic dysfunction. The enantiomer ratios of the two isomers of fluvastatin in hepatic insufficiency patients were comparable to those observed in healthy subjects.

Age: Plasma levels of fluvastatin are not affected by age.

Gender: Women tend to have slightly higher (but statistically insignificant) fluvastatin concentrations than men for the immediate release capsule. This is most likely due to body weight differences, as adjusting for body weight decreases the magnitude of the differences seen. For Lescol XL, there are 67% and 77% increases in systemic availability for women over men under fasted and high fat meal conditions.

Pediatric: No data are available. Fluvastatin is not indicated for use in the pediatric population.

CLINICAL STUDIES

Hypercholesterolemia (heterozygous familial and non familial) and Mixed Dyslipidemia

In 12 placebo-controlled studies in patients with Type IIa or IIb hyperlipoproteinemia, Lescol® (fluvastatin sodium) alone was administered to 1621 patients in daily dose regimens of 20 mg, 40 mg, and 80 mg (40 mg twice daily) for at least 6 weeks duration. After 24 weeks of treatment, daily doses of 20 mg, 40 mg, and 80 mg (40 mg twice daily) resulted in median LDL-C reductions of 22% (n=747), 25% (n=748) and 36% (n=257), respectively. Lescol treatment produced dose-related reductions in Apo B and in triglycerides and increases in HDL-C. The median (25th, 75th percentile) percent changes from baseline in HDL-C after 12 weeks of treatment with Lescol at daily doses of 20 mg, 40 mg and 80 mg (40 mg twice daily) were +2 (-4,+10), +5 (-2,+12), and +4 (-3,+12), respectively. In a subgroup of patients with primary mixed dyslipidemia, defined as baseline TG levels ≥200 mg/dL, treatment with Lescol also produced significant decreases in Total-C, LDL-C, TG and Apo B and variable increases in HDL-C. The median (25th, 75th percentile) percent changes from baseline in HDL-C after 12 weeks of treatment with Lescol at daily doses of 20 mg, 40 mg and 80 mg (40 mg twice daily) in this population were +4 (-2,+12), +8 (+1,+15), and +4 (-3,+13), respectively.

In a long-term open-label free titration study, after 96 weeks LDL-C decreases of 25% (20 mg, n=68), 31% (40 mg, n=298) and 34% (80 mg, n=209) were seen. No consistent effect on Lp(a) was observed.

Lescol® XL (fluvastatin sodium) Extended-Release Tablets have been studied in five controlled studies of patients with Type IIa or IIb hyperlipoproteinemia. Lescol XL was administered to over 900 patients in trials from 4 to 26 weeks in duration. In the three largest of these studies, Lescol XL given as a single daily dose of 80 mg significantly reduced Total-C, LDL-C, TG and Apo B. Therapeutic response is well established within two weeks, and a maximum response is achieved within four weeks. After four weeks of therapy, the median decrease in LDL-C was 38% and at week 24 endpoint the median LDL-C decrease was 35%. Significant increases in HDL-C were also observed. The median (25th and 75th percentile) percent changes from baseline in HDL-C for Lescol XL were +7(+0,+15) after 24 weeks of treatment.

[See table 2 above]

In patients with primary mixed dyslipidemia (Fredrickson Type IIb) as defined by baseline plasma triglycerides levels ≥200 mg/dL, Lescol XL 80 mg produced a median reduction in triglycerides of 25%. In these patients, Lescol XL 80 mg produced median (25th and 75th percentile) percent change from baseline in HDL-C of +11(+3,+20). Significant decreases in Total-C, LDL-C, and Apo B were also achieved. In these studies, patients with triglycerides >400 mg/dL were excluded.

Reduction in the Risk of Recurrent Cardiac Events

In the Lescol Intervention Prevention Study, the effect of Lescol 40 mg administered twice daily on the risk of recurrent cardiac events (time to first occurrence of cardiac death, nonfatal myocardial infarction, or revascularization) was assessed in 1677 patients with coronary heart disease who had undergone a percutaneous coronary intervention (PCI) procedure (mean time from PCI to randomization=3 days). In this multicenter, randomized, double-blind, placebo-controlled study, patients were treated with dietary/lifestyle counseling and either Lescol 40 mg (n=844) or pla-

Continued on next page

Lescol/Lescol XL—Cont.

cebo (n=833) given twice daily for a median of 3.9 years. The study population was 84% male, 98% Caucasian, with 37% >65 years of age. At baseline patients had total cholesterol between 100 and 367 mg/dL (mean 201 mg/dL), LDL-C between 42 and 243 mg/dL (mean 132 mg/dL), triglycerides between 15 and 270 mg/dL (mean 70 mg/dL) and HDL-C between 8 and 174 mg/dL (mean 39 mg/dL).

Lescol significantly reduced the risk of recurrent cardiac events *(Figure 1)* by 22% (p=0.013, 181 patients in the Lescol group vs. 222 patients in the placebo group). Revascularization procedures comprised the majority of the initial recurrent cardiac events (143 revascularization procedures in the Lescol group and 171 in the placebo group). Consistent trends in risk reduction were observed in patients >65 years of age.

[See figure 1 at right]

Outcome data for the Lescol Intervention Prevention Study are shown in Figure 2. After exclusion of revascularization procedures (CABG and repeat PCI) occurring within the first 6 months of the initial procedure involving the originally instrumented site, treatment with Lescol was associated with a 32% (p=0.002) reduction in risk of late revascularization procedures (CABG or PCI occurring at the original site >6 months after the initial procedure, or at another site).

[See figure 2 at right]

Atherosclerosis

In the Lipoprotein and Coronary Atherosclerosis Study (LCAS), the effect of Lescol therapy on coronary atherosclerosis was assessed by quantitative coronary angiography (QCA) in patients with coronary artery disease and mild to moderate hypercholesterolemia (baseline LDL-C range 115-190 mg/dL). In this randomized double-blind, placebo controlled trial, 429 patients were treated with conventional measures (Step 1 AHA Diet) and either Lescol 40 mg/day or placebo. In order to provide treatment to patients receiving placebo with LDL-C levels ≥160 mg/dL at baseline, adjunctive therapy with cholestyramine was added after week 12 to all patients in the study with baseline LDL-C values of ≥160 mg/dL. These baseline levels were present in 25% of the study population. Quantitative coronary angiograms were evaluated at baseline and 2.5 years in 340 (79%) angiographic evaluable patients.

Lescol significantly slowed the progression of coronary atherosclerosis. Compared to placebo, Lescol significantly slowed the progression of lesions as measured by within-patient per-lesion change in minimum lumen diameter (MLD), the primary endpoint *(see Figure 3 below)*, percent diameter stenosis *(Figure 4)*, and the formation of new lesions (13% of all fluvastatin patients versus 22% of all placebo patients). Additionally, a significant difference in favor of Lescol was found between all fluvastatin and all placebo patients in the distribution among the three categories of definite progression, definite regression, and mixed or no change. Beneficial angiographic results (change in MLD) were independent of patients' gender and consistent across a range of baseline LDL-C levels.

Figure 3
Change in Minimum Lumen Diameter (mm)

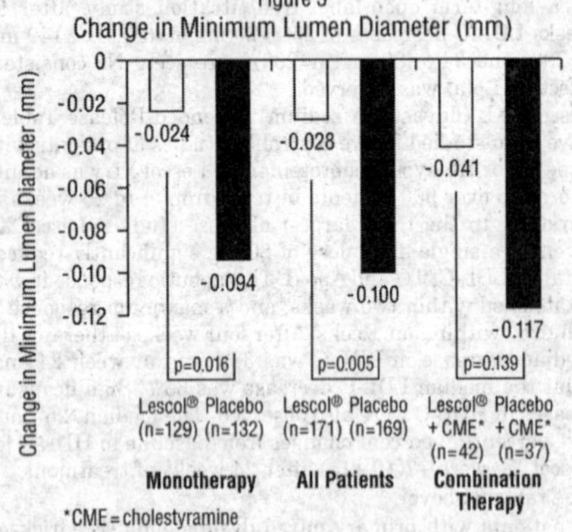

*CME = cholestyramine

[See figure 4 at right]

INDICATIONS AND USAGE

Therapy with lipid-altering agents should be used in addition to a diet restricted in saturated fat and cholesterol *(see National Cholesterol Education Program (NCEP) Treatment Guidelines, below)*.

Hypercholesterolemia (heterozygous familial and non familial) and Mixed Dyslipidemia

Lescol® (fluvastatin sodium) and Lescol® XL (fluvastatin sodium) are indicated to reduce elevated total cholesterol (Total-C), LDL-C, TG and Apo B levels, and to increase HDL-C in patients with primary hypercholesterolemia and mixed dyslipidemia (Fredrickson Type IIa and IIb) whose response to dietary restriction of saturated fat and cholesterol and other nonpharmacological measures has not been adequate.

Secondary Prevention of Coronary Events

In patients with coronary heart disease, Lescol and Lescol XL are indicated to reduce the risk of undergoing coronary revascularization procedures.

Figure 1
Primary Endpoint – Recurrent Cardiac Events (Cardiac Death, Nonfatal MI or Revascularization Procedure) (ITT Population)

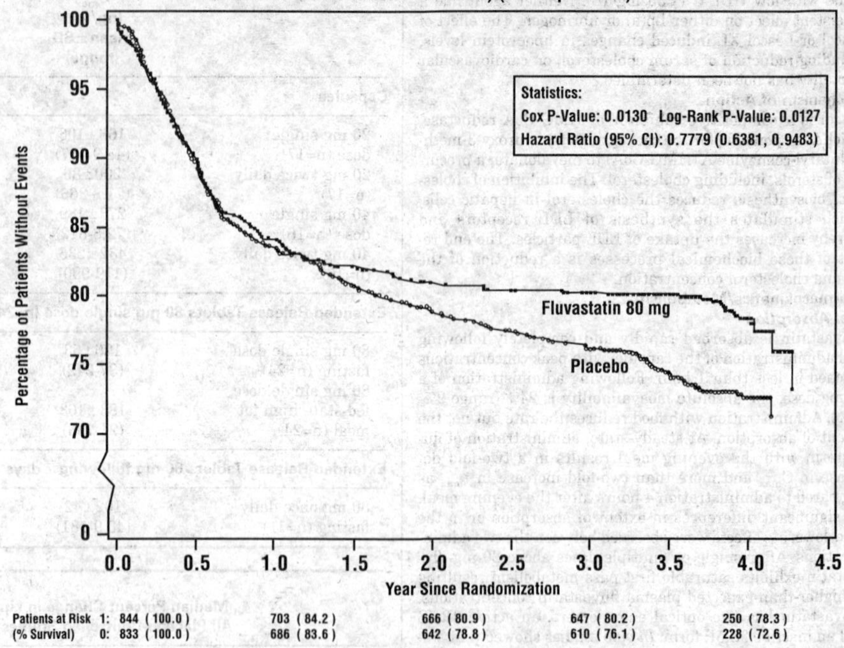

Figure 2
Lescol® Intervention Prevention Study – Primary and Secondary Endpoints

Event	Incidence* Lescol® n (%) N=844	Placebo n (%) N=833	Risk Reduction % (95% CI)
Primary Endpoint, Recurrent Cardiac			
Events (as a first event)	181 (21.4)	222 (26.7)	22 (5, 36)
Cardiac Death	8 (0.9)	18 (2.2)	—
Nonfatal MI	30 (3.4)	33 (4.0)	—
Revascularization	143 (16.2)	171 (20.5)	—
Secondary Endpoints (any time during the study)			
Cardiac Death	13 (1.5)	24 (2.9)	47 (-5, 79)
Nonfatal MI	30 (3.6)	38 (4.6)	22 (-27, 52)
Revascularization	167 (19.8)	193 (23.2)	17 (-2, 33)
Late Revascularization**	111 (13.2)	151 (18.1)	32 (13, 47)
Noncardiac Death	23 (2.7)	25 (3.0)	16 (-49, 52)

Cox Risk Ratio (95% CI): 0.00 0.25 0.50 0.75 1.00 1.25 1.50 — ← Favors Lescol® | Favors placebo →

*Number of patients with events

**Excludes revascularization procedures of the target lesion within the first 6 months of the initial procedure

Figure 4
Change in % Diameter Stenosis

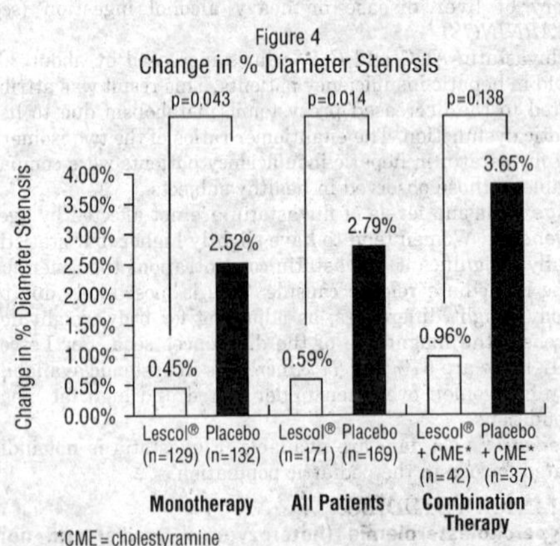

*CME = cholestyramine

Atherosclerosis

Lescol and Lescol XL are also indicated to slow the progression of coronary atherosclerosis in patients with coronary heart disease as part of a treatment strategy to lower total and LDL cholesterol to target levels.

Therapy with lipid-altering agents should be considered only after secondary causes for hyperlipidemia such as poorly controlled diabetes mellitus, hypothyroidism, nephrotic syndrome, dysproteinemias, obstructive liver disease, other medication, or alcoholism, have been excluded.

Prior to initiation of fluvastatin sodium, a lipid profile should be performed to measure Total-C, HDL-C and TG. For patients with TG <400 mg/dL (<4.5 mmol/L), LDL-C can be estimated using the following equation:

$$\text{LDL-C} = \text{Total-C} - \text{HDL-C} - 1/5\ \text{TG}$$

For TG levels >400 mg/dL (>4.5 mmol/L), this equation is less accurate and LDL-C concentrations should be determined by ultracentrifugation. In many hypertriglyceridemic patients LDL-C may be low or normal despite elevated Total-C. In such cases, Lescol is not indicated.

Lipid determinations should be performed at intervals of no less than 4 weeks and dosage adjusted according to the patient's response to therapy.

The National Cholesterol Education Program (NCEP) Treatment Guidelines are summarized below:

[See table 3 at top of next page]

After the LDL-C goal has been achieved, if the TG is still ≥200 mg/dL, non-HDL-C (total-C minus HDL-C) becomes a secondary target of therapy. Non-HDL-C goals are set 30 mg/dL higher than LDL-C goals for each risk category.

At the time of hospitalization for an acute coronary event, consideration can be given to initiating drug therapy at discharge if the LDL-C level is ≥130 mg/dL (NCEP-ATP II).

Since the goal of therapy is to lower LDL-C, the NCEP recommends that the LDL-C levels be used to initiate and assess treatment response. Only if LDL-C levels are not available, should the Total-C be used to monitor therapy.

[See table 4 at top of next page]

Neither Lescol nor Lescol XL have been studied in conditions where the major abnormality is elevation of chylomicrons, VLDL, or IDL (i.e., hyperlipoproteinemia Types I, III, IV, or V).

CONTRAINDICATIONS

Hypersensitivity to any component of this medication. Lescol® (fluvastatin sodium) and Lescol® XL (fluvastatin sodium) are contraindicated in patients with active liver disease or unexplained, persistent elevations in serum transaminases *(see WARNINGS)*.

Pregnancy and Lactation

Atherosclerosis is a chronic process and discontinuation of lipid-lowering drugs during pregnancy should have little impact on the outcome of long-term therapy of primary hypercholesterolemia. Cholesterol and other products of cholesterol biosynthesis are essential components for fetal development (including synthesis of steroids and cell membranes). Since HMG-CoA reductase inhibitors decrease cholesterol synthesis and possibly the synthesis of other biologically active substances derived from cholesterol, they may cause fetal harm when administered to pregnant women. Therefore, HMG-CoA reductase inhibitors are contraindicated during pregnancy and in nursing mothers. **Fluvastatin sodium should be administered to women of childbearing age only when such patients are highly unlikely to conceive and have been informed of the potential hazards.** If the patient becomes pregnant while taking this class of drug, therapy should be discontinued and the patient apprised of the potential hazard to the fetus.

WARNINGS

Liver Enzymes

Biochemical abnormalities of liver function have been associated with HMG-CoA reductase inhibitors and other lipid-lowering agents. Approximately 1.1% of patients treated with Lescol® (fluvastatin sodium) capsules in worldwide trials developed dose-related, persistent elevations of transaminase levels to more than 3 times the upper limit of normal. Fourteen of these patients (0.6%) were discontinued from therapy. In all clinical trials, a total of 33/2969 patients (1.1%) had persistent transaminase elevations with an average fluvastatin exposure of approximately 71.2 weeks; 19 of these patients (0.6%) were discontinued. The majority of patients with these abnormal biochemical findings were asymptomatic.

In a pooled analysis of all placebo-controlled studies in which Lescol capsules were used, persistent transaminase elevations (>3 times the upper limit of normal [ULN] on two consecutive weekly measurements) occurred in 0.2%, 1.5%, and 2.7% of patients treated with 20, 40, and 80 mg (titrated to 40 mg twice daily) Lescol capsules, respectively. Ninety-one percent of the cases of persistent liver function test abnormalities (20 of 22 patients) occurred within 12 weeks of therapy and in all patients with persistent liver function test abnormalities there was an abnormal liver function test present at baseline or by week 8.

In the pooled analysis of the 24-week controlled trials, persistent transaminase elevation occurred in 1.9%, 1.8% and 4.9% of patients treated with Lescol® XL (fluvastatin sodium) 80 mg, Lescol 40 mg and Lescol 40 mg twice daily, respectively. In 13 of 16 patients treated with Lescol XL the abnormality occurred within 12 weeks of initiation of treatment with Lescol XL 80 mg.

It is recommended that liver function tests be performed before the initiation of therapy and at 12 weeks following initiation of treatment or elevation in dose. Patients who develop transaminase elevations or signs and symptoms of liver disease should be monitored to confirm the finding and should be followed thereafter with frequent liver function tests until the levels return to normal. Should an increase in AST or ALT of three times the upper limit of normal or greater persist (found on two consecutive occasions) withdrawal of fluvastatin sodium therapy is recommended.

Active liver disease or unexplained transaminase elevations are contraindications to the use of Lescol and Lescol XL *(see CONTRAINDICATIONS)*. Caution should be exercised when fluvastatin sodium is administered to patients with a history of liver disease or heavy alcohol ingestion *(see CLINICAL PHARMACOLOGY: Pharmacokinetics/Metabolism)*. Such patients should be closely monitored.

Skeletal Muscle

Rhabdomyolysis with renal dysfunction secondary to myoglobinuria has been reported with fluvastatin and with other drugs in this class. Myopathy, defined as muscle aching or muscle weakness in conjunction with increases in creatine phosphokinase (CPK) values to greater than 10 times the upper limit of normal, has been reported.

Myopathy should be considered in any patients with diffuse myalgias, muscle tenderness or weakness, and/or marked elevation of CPK. Patients should be advised to report promptly unexplained muscle pain, tenderness or weakness, particularly if accompanied by malaise or fever. Fluvastatin sodium therapy should be discontinued if markedly elevated CPK levels occur or myopathy is diagnosed or suspected. Fluvastatin sodium therapy should also be temporarily withheld in any patient experiencing an acute or serious condition predisposing to the development of renal failure secondary to rhabdomyolysis, e.g., sepsis; hypotension; major surgery; trauma; severe metabolic, endocrine, or electrolyte disorders; or uncontrolled epilepsy.

The risk of myopathy and or rhabdomyolysis during treatment with HMG-CoA reductase inhibitors has been reported to be increased if therapy with either cyclosporine, gemfibrozil, erythromycin, or niacin is administered concurrently. Myopathy was not observed in a clinical trial in 74 patients involving patients who were treated with fluvastatin sodium together with niacin.

Table 3

NCEP Treatment Guidelines: LDL-C Goals and Cutpoints for Therapeutic Lifestyle Changes and Drug Therapy in Different Risk Categories

Risk Category	LDL Goal (mg/dL)	LDL Level at Which to Initiate Therapeutic Lifestyle Changes (mg/dL)	LDL Level at Which to Consider Drug Therapy (mg/dL)
CHD† or CHD risk equivalents (10-year risk >20%)	<100	≥100	≥130 (100-129; drug optional)††
2+ Risk factors (10-year risk (<20%)	<130	≥130	10-year risk 10%-20%: ≥130 10-year risk <10%: ≥160
0-1 Risk factor†††	<160	≥160	≥190 (160-189: LDL-lowering drug optional)

†CHD, coronary heart disease

††Some authorities recommend use of LDL-lowering drugs in this category if an LDL-C level of <100mg/dL cannot be achieved by therapeutic lifestyle changes. Others prefer use of drugs that primarily modify triglycerides and HDL-C, e.g., nicotinic acid or fibrate. Clinical judgement also may call for deferring drug therapy in this subcategory.

†††Almost all people with 0-1 risk factor have 10-year risk <10%; thus, 10-year risk assessment in people with 0-1 risk factor is not necessary.

Table 4

Classification of Hyperlipoproteinemias

Type	Lipoproteins Elevated	Lipid Elevations: Major	Lipid Elevations: Minor
I (rare)	Chylomicrons	TG	↑ → C
IIa	LDL	C	
IIb	LDL, VLDL	C	TG
III (rare)	IDL	C/TG	
IV	VLDL	TG	↑ → C
V (rare)	Chylomicrons, VLDL	TG	↑ → C

C = cholesterol, TG = triglycerides, LDL = low density lipoprotein, VLDL = very low density lipoprotein, IDL = intermediate density lipoprotein

Uncomplicated myalgia has been observed infrequently in patients treated with Lescol at rates indistinguishable from placebo.

The use of fibrates alone may occasionally be associated with myopathy. The combined use of HMG-CoA reductase inhibitors and fibrates should generally be avoided.

PRECAUTIONS

General

Before instituting therapy with Lescol® (fluvastatin sodium) or Lescol® XL (fluvastatin sodium), an attempt should be made to control hypercholesterolemia with appropriate diet, exercise, and weight reduction in obese patients, and to treat other underlying medical problems *(see INDICATIONS AND USAGE)*.

The HMG-CoA reductase inhibitors may cause elevation of creatine phosphokinase and transaminase levels *(see WARNINGS and ADVERSE REACTIONS)*. This should be considered in the differential diagnosis of chest pain in a patient on therapy with fluvastatin sodium.

Homozygous Familial Hypercholesterolemia

HMG-CoA reductase inhibitors are reported to be less effective in patients with rare homozygous familial hypercholesterolemia, possibly because these patients have few functional LDL receptors.

Information for Patients

Patients should be advised to report promptly unexplained muscle pain, tenderness or weakness, particularly if accompanied by malaise or fever.

Women should be informed that if they become pregnant while receiving Lescol or Lescol XL the drug should be discontinued immediately to avoid possible harmful effects on a developing fetus from a relative deficit of cholesterol and biological products derived from cholesterol. In addition, Lescol or Lescol XL should not be taken during nursing. *(See CONTRAINDICATIONS.)*

Drug Interactions

The below listed drug interaction information is derived from studies using immediate release fluvastatin. Similar studies have not been conducted using the Lescol XL tablet.

Immunosuppressive Drugs, Gemfibrozil, Niacin (Nicotinic Acid), Erythromycin *(See WARNINGS: Skeletal Muscle)*.

In vitro data indicate that fluvastatin metabolism involves multiple Cytochrome P450 (CYP) isozymes. CYP2C9 isoenzyme is primarily involved in the metabolism of fluvastatin (~75%), while CYP2C8 and CYP3A4 isoenzymes are involved to a much less extent, i.e. ~5% and ~20%, respectively. If one pathway is inhibited in the elimination process of fluvastatin other pathways may compensate.

In vivo drug interaction studies with CYP3A4 inhibitors/substrates such as cyclosporine, erythromycin, and itraconazle result in minimal changes in the pharmacokinetics of fluvastatin, confirming less involvement of CYP3A4 isozyme. Concomitant administration of fluvastatin and phenytoin increased the levels of phenytoin and fluvastatin, suggesting predominant involvement of CYP2C9 in fluvastatin metabolism.

Niacin/Propranolol: Concomitant administration of immediate release fluvastatin sodium with niacin or propranolol has no effect on the bioavailability of fluvastatin sodium.

Cholestyramine: Administration of immediate release fluvastatin sodium concomitantly with, or up to 4 hours after cholestyramine, results in fluvastatin decreases of more than 50% for AUC and 50%-80% for C_{max}. However, administration of immediate release fluvastatin sodium 4 hours after cholestyramine resulted in a clinically significant additive effect compared with that achieved with either component drug.

Cyclosporine: Plasma cyclosporine levels remain unchanged when fluvastatin (20 mg daily) was administered concurrently in renal transplant recipients on stable cyclosporine regimens. Fluvastatin AUC increased 1.9 fold, and C_{max} increased 1.3 fold compared to historical controls.

Digoxin: In a crossover study involving 18 patients chronically receiving digoxin, a single 40 mg dose of immediate release fluvastatin had no effect on digoxin AUC, but had an 11% increase in digoxin C_{max} and small increase in digoxin urinary clearance.

Erythromycin: Erythromycin (500 mg, single dose) did not affect steady-state plasma levels of fluvastatin (40 mg daily).

Itraconazole: Concomitant administration of fluvastatin (40 mg) and itraconazole (100 mg daily × 4 days) does not affect plasma itraconazole or fluvastatin levels.

Gemfibrozil: There is no change in either fluvastatin (20 mg twice daily) or gemfibrozil (600 mg twice daily) plasma levels when these drugs are co-administered.

Phenytoin: Single morning dose administration of phenytoin (300 mg extended release) increased mean steady-state fluvastatin (40 mg) C_{max} by 27% and AUC by 40% whereas fluvastatin increased the mean phenytoin C_{max} by 5% and AUC by 20%. Patients on phenytoin should continue to be monitored appropriately when fluvastatin therapy is initiated or when the fluvastatin dosage is changed.

Diclofenac: Concurrent administration of fluvastatin (40 mg) increased the mean C_{max} and AUC of diclofenac by 60% and 25% respectively.

Tolbutamide: In healthy volunteers, concurrent administration of either single or multiple daily doses of fluvastatin sodium (40 mg) with tolbutamide (1 g) did not affect the plasma levels of either drug to a clinically significant extent.

Glibenclamide (Glyburide): In glibenclamide-treated NIDDM patients (n=32), administration of fluvastatin (40 mg twice daily for 14 days) increased the mean C_{max}, AUC, and $t_{½}$ of glibenclamide approximately 50%, 69% and 121%, respectively. Glibenclamide (5-20 mg daily) increased the mean C_{max} and AUC of fluvastatin by 44% and 51%, respectively. In this study there were no changes in glucose, insulin and C-peptide levels. However, patients on concomitant therapy with glibenclamide (glyburide) and fluvastatin should continue to be monitored appropriately when their fluvastatin dose is increased to 40 mg twice daily.

Losartan: Concomitant administration of fluvastatin with losartan has no effect on the bioavailability of either losartan or its active metabolite.

Cimetidine/Ranitidine/Omeprazole: Concomitant administration of immediate release fluvastatin sodium with ci-

Continued on next page

Lescol/Lescol XL—Cont.

metidine, ranitidine and omeprazole results in a significant increase in the fluvastatin C_{max} (43%, 70% and 50%, respectively) and AUC (24%-33%), with an 18%-23% decrease in plasma clearance.

Rifampicin: Administration of immediate release fluvastatin sodium to subjects pretreated with rifampicin results in significant reduction in C_{max} (59%) and AUC (51%), with a large increase (95%) in plasma clearance.

Warfarin: *In vitro* protein binding studies demonstrated no interaction at therapeutic concentrations. Concomitant administration of a single dose of warfarin (30 mg) in young healthy males receiving immediate release fluvastatin sodium (40 mg/day × 8 days) resulted in no elevation of racemic warfarin concentration. There was also no effect on prothrombin complex activity when compared to concomitant administration of placebo and warfarin. However, bleeding and/or increased prothrombin times have been reported in patients taking coumarin anticoagulants concomitantly with other HMG-CoA reductase inhibitors. Therefore, patients receiving warfarin-type anticoagulants should have their prothrombin times closely monitored when fluvastatin sodium is initiated or the dosage of fluvastatin sodium is changed.

Endocrine Function

HMG-CoA reductase inhibitors interfere with cholesterol synthesis and lower circulating cholesterol levels and, as such, might theoretically blunt adrenal or gonadal steroid hormone production.

Fluvastatin exhibited no effect upon non-stimulated cortisol levels and demonstrated no effect upon thyroid metabolism as assessed by TSH. Small declines in total testosterone have been noted in treated groups, but no commensurate elevation in LH occurred, suggesting that the observation was not due to a direct effect upon testosterone production. No effect upon FSH in males was noted. Due to the limited number of premenopausal females studied to date, no conclusions regarding the effect of fluvastatin upon female sex hormones may be made.

Two clinical studies in patients receiving fluvastatin at doses up to 80 mg daily for periods of 24 to 28 weeks demonstrated no effect of treatment upon the adrenal response to ACTH stimulation. A clinical study evaluated the effect of fluvastatin at doses up to 80 mg daily for 28 weeks upon the gonadal response to HCG stimulation. Although the mean total testosterone response was significantly reduced ($p<0.05$) relative to baseline in the 80 mg group, it was not significant in comparison to the changes noted in groups receiving either 40 mg of fluvastatin or placebo.

Patients treated with fluvastatin sodium who develop clinical evidence of endocrine dysfunction should be evaluated appropriately. Caution should be exercised if an HMG-CoA reductase inhibitor or other agent used to lower cholesterol levels is administered to patients receiving other drugs (e.g., ketoconazole, spironolactone, or cimetidine) that may decrease the levels of endogenous steroid hormones.

CNS Toxicity

CNS effects, as evidenced by decreased activity, ataxia, loss of righting reflex, and ptosis were seen in the following animal studies: the 18-month mouse carcinogenicity study at 50 mg/kg/day, the 6-month dog study at 36 mg/kg/day, the 6-month hamster study at 40 mg/kg/day, and in acute, high-dose studies in rats and hamsters (50 mg/kg), rabbits (300 mg/kg) and mice (1500 mg/kg). CNS toxicity in the acute high-dose studies was characterized (in mice) by conspicuous vacuolation in the ventral white columns of the spinal cord at a dose of 5000 mg/kg and (in rat) by edema with separation of myelinated fibers of the ventral spinal tracts and sciatic nerve at a dose of 1500 mg/kg. CNS toxicity, characterized by periaxonal vacuolation, was observed in the medulla of dogs that died after treatment for 5 weeks with 48 mg/kg/day; this finding was not observed in the remaining dogs when the dose level was lowered to 36 mg/kg/day. CNS vascular lesions, characterized by perivascular hemorrhages, edema, and mononuclear cell infiltration of perivascular spaces, have been observed in dogs treated with other members of this class. No CNS lesions have been observed after chronic treatment for up to 2 years with fluvastatin in the mouse (at doses up to 350 mg/kg/day), rat (up to 24 mg/kg/day), or dog (up to 16 mg/kg/day).

Prominent bilateral posterior Y suture lines in the ocular lens were seen in dogs after treatment with 1, 8, and 16 mg/kg/day for 2 years.

Carcinogenesis, Mutagenesis, Impairment of Fertility

A 2-year study was performed in rats at dose levels of 6, 9, and 18-24 (escalated after 1 year) mg/kg/day. These treatment levels represented plasma drug levels of approximately 9, 13, and 26-35 times the mean human plasma drug concentration after a 40 mg oral dose. A low incidence of forestomach squamous papillomas and 1 carcinoma of the forestomach at the 24 mg/kg/day dose level was considered to reflect the prolonged hyperplasia induced by direct contact exposure to fluvastatin sodium rather than to a systemic effect of the drug. In addition, an increased incidence of thyroid follicular cell adenomas and carcinomas was recorded for males treated with 18-24 mg/kg/day. The increased incidence of thyroid follicular cell neoplasm in male rats with fluvastatin sodium appears to be consistent with findings from other HMG-CoA reductase inhibitors. In contrast to other HMG-CoA reductase inhibitors, no hepatic adenomas or carcinomas were observed.

The carcinogenicity study conducted in mice at dose levels of 0.3, 15 and 30 mg/kg/day revealed, as in rats, a statistically significant increase in forestomach squamous cell papillomas in males and females at 30 mg/kg/day and in females at 15 mg/kg/day. These treatment levels represented plasma drug levels of approximately 0.05, 2, and 7 times the mean human plasma drug concentration after a 40 mg oral dose.

No evidence of mutagenicity was observed *in vitro*, with or without rat-liver metabolic activation, in the following studies: microbial mutagen tests using mutant strains of *Salmonella typhimurium* or *Escherichia coli;* malignant transformation assay in BALB/3T3 cells; unscheduled DNA synthesis in rat primary hepatocytes; chromosomal aberrations in V79 Chinese Hamster cells; HGPRT V79 Chinese Hamster cells. In addition, there was no evidence of mutagenicity *in vivo* in either a rat or mouse micronucleus test.

In a study in rats at dose levels for females of 0.6, 2 and 6 mg/kg/day and at dose levels for males of 2, 10 and 20 mg/kg/day, fluvastatin sodium had no adverse effects on the fertility or reproductive performance.

Seminal vesicles and testes were small in hamsters treated for 3 months at 20 mg/kg/day (approximately three times the 40 milligram human daily dose based on surface area, mg/m²). There was tubular degeneration and aspermatogenesis in testes as well as vesiculitis of seminal vesicles. Vesiculitis of seminal vesicles and edema of the testes were also seen in rats treated for 2 years at 18 mg/kg/day (approximately 4 times the human C_{max} achieved with a 40 milligram daily dose).

Pregnancy

Pregnancy Category X

See CONTRAINDICATIONS.

Fluvastatin sodium produced delays in skeletal development in rats at doses of 12 mg/kg/day and in rabbits at doses of 10 mg/kg/day. Malaligned thoracic vertebrae were seen in rats at 36 mg/kg, a dose that produced maternal toxicity. These doses resulted in 2 times (rat at 12 mg/kg) or 5 times (rabbit at 10 mg/kg) the 40 mg human exposure based on mg/m² surface area. A study in which female rats were dosed during the third trimester at 12 and 24 mg/kg/day resulted in maternal mortality at or near term and postpartum. In addition, fetal and neonatal lethality were apparent. No effects on the dam or fetus occurred at 2 mg/kg/day. A second study at levels of 2, 6, 12 and 24 mg/kg/day confirmed the findings in the first study with neonatal mortality beginning at 6 mg/kg. A modified Segment III study was performed at dose levels of 12 or 24 mg/kg/day with or without the presence of concurrent supplementation with mevalonic acid, a product of HMG-CoA reductase which is essential for cholesterol biosynthesis. The concurrent administration of mevalonic acid completely prevented the maternal and neonatal mortality but did not prevent low body weights in pups at 24 mg/kg on days 0 and 7 postpartum. Therefore, the maternal and neonatal lethality observed with fluvastatin sodium reflect its exaggerated pharmacologic effect during pregnancy. There are no data with fluvastatin sodium in pregnant women. However, rare reports of congenital anomalies have been received following intrauterine exposure to other HMG-CoA reductase inhibitors. There has been one report of severe congenital bony deformity, tracheo-esophageal fistula, and anal atresia (VATER association) in a baby born to a woman who took another HMG-CoA reductase inhibitor with dextroamphetamine sulfate during the first trimester of pregnancy. **Lescol or Lescol XL should be administered to women of child-bearing potential only when such patients are highly unlikely to conceive and have been informed of the potential hazards.** If a woman becomes pregnant while taking Lescol or Lescol XL, the drug should be discontinued and the patient advised again as to the potential hazards to the fetus.

Nursing Mothers

Based on preclinical data, drug is present in breast milk in a 2:1 ratio (milk:plasma). Because of the potential for serious adverse reactions in nursing infants, nursing women should not take Lescol or Lescol XL *(see CONTRAINDICATIONS).*

Pediatric Use

Safety and effectiveness in individuals less than 18 years old have not been established. Treatment in patients less than 18 years of age is not recommended at this time.

Geriatric Use

The effect of age on the pharmacokinetics of immediate release fluvastatin sodium was evaluated. Results indicate that for the general patient population plasma concentrations of fluvastatin sodium do not vary as a function of age. *(See also CLINICAL PHARMACOLOGY: Pharmacokinetics/Metabolism.)* Elderly patients (≥65 years of age) demonstrated a greater treatment response in respect to LDL-C, Total-C and LDL/HDL ratio than patients <65 years of age.

ADVERSE REACTIONS

In all clinical studies of Lescol® (fluvastatin sodium), 1.0% (32/2969) of fluvastatin-treated patients were discontinued due to adverse experiences attributed to study drug (mean exposure approximately 16 months ranging in duration from 1 to >36 months). This results in an exposure adjusted rate of 0.8% (32/4051) per patient year in fluvastatin patients in controlled studies compared to an incidence of 1.1% (4/355) in placebo patients. Adverse reactions have usually been of mild to moderate severity.

In controlled clinical studies, 3.9% (36/912) of patients treated with Lescol® XL (fluvastatin sodium) 80 mg discontinued due to adverse events (causality not determined).

Clinically relevant adverse experiences occurring in the Lescol and Lescol XL controlled studies with a frequency >2%, regardless of causality, include the following:

Table 5
Clinically Relevant Adverse Experiences Occurring in >2% Patients in Lescol® and Lescol® XL Controlled Studies

Adverse Event	Lescol®[1] (%) (N=2326)	Placebo[1] (%) (N=960)	Lescol® XL[2] (%) (N=912)
Musculoskeletal			
Myalgia	5.0	4.5	3.8
Arthritis	2.1	2.0	1.3
Arthropathy	NA	NA	3.2
Respiratory			
Sinusitis	2.6	1.9	3.5
Bronchitis	1.8	1.0	2.6
Gastrointestinal			
Dyspepsia	7.9	3.2	3.5
Diarrhea	4.9	4.2	3.3
Abdominal Pain	4.9	3.8	3.7
Nausea	3.2	2.0	2.5
Flatulence	2.6	2.5	1.4
Psychiatric Disorders			
Insomnia	2.7	1.4	0.8
Genitourinary			
Urinary Tract Infection	1.6	1.1	2.7
Miscellaneous			
Headache	8.9	7.8	4.7
Influenza-Like Symptoms	5.1	5.7	7.1
Accidental Trauma	5.1	4.8	4.2
Fatigue	2.7	2.3	1.6
Allergy	2.3	2.2	1.0

[1] Controlled trials with Lescol Capsules (20 and 40 mg daily and 40 mg twice daily)
[2] Controlled trials with Lescol XL 80 mg Tablets

The following effects have been reported with drugs in this class. Not all the effects listed below have necessarily been associated with fluvastatin sodium therapy.

Skeletal: muscle cramps, myalgia, myopathy, rhabdomyolysis, arthralgias.

Neurological: dysfunction of certain cranial nerves (including alteration of taste, impairment of extra-ocular movement, facial paresis), tremor, dizziness, vertigo, memory loss, paresthesia, peripheral neuropathy, peripheral nerve palsy, psychic disturbances, anxiety, insomnia, depression.

Hypersensitivity Reactions: An apparent hypersensitivity syndrome has been reported rarely which has included one or more of the following features: anaphylaxis, angioedema, lupus erythematosus-like syndrome, polymyalgia rheumatica, vasculitis, purpura, thrombocytopenia, leukopenia, hemolytic anemia, positive ANA, ESR increase, eosinophilia, arthritis, arthralgia, urticaria, asthenia, photosensitivity, fever, chills, flushing, malaise, dyspnea, toxic epidermal necrolysis, erythema multiforme, including Stevens-Johnson syndrome.

Gastrointestinal: pancreatitis, hepatitis, including chronic active hepatitis, cholestatic jaundice, fatty change in liver, and, rarely, cirrhosis, fulminant hepatic necrosis, and hepatoma; anorexia, vomiting.

Skin: alopecia, pruritus. A variety of skin changes (e.g., nodules, discoloration, dryness of skin/mucous membranes, changes to hair/nails) have been reported.

Reproductive: gynecomastia, loss of libido, erectile dysfunction.

Eye: progression of cataracts (lens opacities), ophthalmoplegia.

Laboratory Abnormalities: elevated transaminases, alkaline phosphatase, γ-glutamyl transpeptidase, and bilirubin; thyroid function abnormalities.

Concomitant Therapy

Fluvastatin sodium has been administered concurrently with cholestyramine and nicotinic acid. No adverse reactions unique to the combination or in addition to those previously reported for this class of drugs alone have been reported. Myopathy and rhabdomyolysis (with or without acute renal failure) have been reported when another HMG-CoA reductase inhibitor was used in combination with immunosuppressive drugs, gemfibrozil, erythromycin, or lipid-lowering doses of nicotinic acid. Concomitant therapy with HMG-CoA reductase inhibitors and these agents is generally not recommended. *(See WARNINGS, Skeletal Muscle.)*

OVERDOSAGE

The approximate oral LD_{50} is greater than 2 g/kg in mice and greater than 0.7 g/kg in rats.

The maximum single oral dose of Lescol® (fluvastatin sodium) capsules received by healthy volunteers was 80 mg. No clinically significant adverse experiences were seen at this dose. The maximum dose administered with an extended-release formulation was 640 mg for two weeks. This dose was not well tolerated and produced a variety of GI complaints and an increase in transaminase values (i.e., SGOT and SGPT).

There has been a single report of 2 children, one 2 years old and the other 3 years of age, either of whom may have possibly ingested fluvastatin sodium. The maximum amount of fluvastatin sodium that could have been ingested was 80 mg (4 × 20 mg capsules). Vomiting was induced by ipecac in both children and no capsules were noted in their emesis. Neither child experienced any adverse symptoms and both recovered from the incident without problems.

Should an accidental overdose occur, treat symptomatically and institute supportive measures as required. The dialyzability of fluvastatin sodium and of its metabolites in humans is not known at present.

Information about the treatment of overdose can often be obtained from a certified Regional Poison Control Center. Telephone numbers of certified Regional Poison Control Centers are listed in the Physicians' Desk Reference®.*

DOSAGE AND ADMINISTRATION

The patient should be placed on a standard cholesterol-lowering diet before receiving Lescol® (fluvastatin sodium) or Lescol® XL (fluvastatin sodium) and should continue on this diet during treatment with Lescol or Lescol XL. *(See NCEP Treatment Guidelines for details on dietary therapy.)*

For patients requiring LDL-C reduction to a goal of ≥25%, the recommended starting dose is 40 mg as one capsule, 80 mg as one Lescol XL tablet administered as a single dose in the evening or 80 mg in divided doses of the 40 mg capsule given twice daily. For patients requiring LDL-C reduction to a goal of <25% a starting dose of 20 mg may be used. The recommended dosing range is 20-80 mg/day. Lescol or Lescol XL may be taken without regard to meals, since there are no apparent differences in the lipid-lowering effects of fluvastatin sodium administered with the evening meal or 4 hours after the evening meal. Since the maximal reductions in LDL-C of a given dose are seen within 4 weeks, periodic lipid determinations should be performed and dosage adjustment made according to the patient's response to therapy and established treatment guidelines. The therapeutic effect of Lescol or Lescol XL is maintained with prolonged administration.

Concomitant Therapy

Lipid-lowering effects on total cholesterol and LDL cholesterol are additive when immediate release Lescol is combined with a bile-acid binding resin or niacin. When administering a bile-acid resin (e.g., cholestyramine) and fluvastatin sodium, Lescol should be administered at bedtime, at least 2 hours following the resin to avoid a significant interaction due to drug binding to resin. *(See also ADVERSE REACTIONS: Concomitant Therapy.)*

Dosage in Patients with Renal Insufficiency

Since fluvastatin sodium is cleared hepatically with less than 6% of the administered dose excreted into the urine, dose adjustments for mild to moderate renal impairment are not necessary. Fluvastatin has not been studied at doses greater than 40 mg in patients with severe renal impairment; therefore caution should be exercised when treating such patients at higher doses.

HOW SUPPLIED

Lescol® (fluvastatin sodium) Capsules

20 mg

Brown and light brown imprinted twice with "⚠" and "20" on one half and "LESCOL" and the Lescol® (fluvastatin sodium) logo twice on the other half of the capsule.

Bottles of 30 capsules .... (NDC 0078-0176-15)
Bottles of 100 capsules .... (NDC 0078-0176-05)

40 mg

Brown and gold imprinted twice with "⚠" and "40" on one half and "LESCOL" and the Lescol® (fluvastatin sodium) logo twice on the other half of the capsule.

Bottles of 30 capsules .... (NDC 0078-0234-15)
Bottles of 100 capsules .... (NDC 0078-0234-05)

Lescol® XL (fluvastatin sodium) Extended-Release Tablets

80 mg

Yellow, round, slightly biconvex film-coated tablet with beveled edges debossed with "Lescol XL" on one side and "80" on the other.

Bottles of 30 tablets .... (NDC 0078-0354-15)
Bottle of 100 tablets .... (NDC 0078-0354-05)

Store and Dispense

Store at 25°C (77°F); excursions permitted to 15°C-30°C (59°F-86°F). [See USP Controlled Room Temperature]. Dispense in a tight container. Protect from light.

*Trademark of Medical Economics Company, Inc.

Distributed by:
Novartis Pharmaceuticals Corporation
East Hanover, New Jersey 07936

T2003-40

REV: MAY 2003
©Novartis

Shown in Product Identification Guide, page 325

LOTENSIN® ℞

[lō-tĕn-sĭn]
(benazepril hydrochloride)
Tablets
Rx only

Prescribing Information

The following prescribing information is based on official labeling in effect July 2004.

Use in Pregnancy

When used in pregnancy during the second and third trimesters, ACE inhibitors can cause injury and even death to the developing fetus. When pregnancy is detected, Lotensin should be discontinued as soon as possible. See **WARNINGS, Fetal/Neonatal Morbidity and Mortality.**

DESCRIPTION

Benazepril hydrochloride is a white to off-white crystalline powder, soluble (>100 mg/mL) in water, in ethanol, and in methanol. Its chemical name is 3-[[1-(ethoxy-carbonyl)-3-phenyl-(1S)-propyl]amino]-2,3,4,5-tetrahydro-2-oxo-1*H*-1-(3S)-benzazepine-1-acetic acid monohydrochloride; its structural formula is

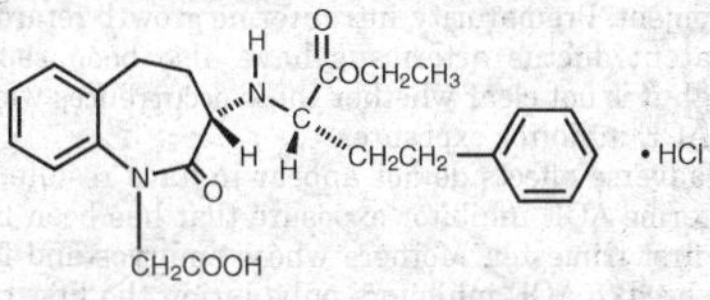

Its empirical formula is $C_{24}H_{28}N_2O_5$•HCl, and its molecular weight is 460.96.

Benazeprilat, the active metabolite of benazepril, is a non-sulfhydryl angiotensin-converting enzyme inhibitor. Benazepril is converted to benazeprilat by hepatic cleavage of the ester group.

Lotensin is supplied as tablets containing 5 mg, 10 mg, 20 mg, and 40 mg of benazepril hydrochloride for oral administration. The inactive ingredients are colloidal silicon dioxide, crospovidone, hydrogenated castor oil (5-mg, 10-mg, and 20-mg tablets), hypromellose, iron oxides, lactose, magnesium stearate (40-mg tablets), microcrystalline cellulose, polysorbate 80, propylene glycol (5-mg and 40-mg tablets), starch, talc, and titanium dioxide.

CLINICAL PHARMACOLOGY

Mechanism of Action

Benazepril and benazeprilat inhibit angiotensin-converting enzyme (ACE) in human subjects and animals. ACE is a peptidyl dipeptidase that catalyzes the conversion of angiotensin I to the vasoconstrictor substance, angiotensin II. Angiotensin II also stimulates aldosterone secretion by the adrenal cortex.

Inhibition of ACE results in decreased plasma angiotensin II, which leads to decreased vasopressor activity and to decreased aldosterone secretion. The latter decrease may result in a small increase of serum potassium. Hypertensive patients treated with Lotensin alone for up to 52 weeks had elevations of serum potassium of up to 0.2 mEq/L. Similar patients treated with Lotensin and hydrochlorothiazide for up to 24 weeks had no consistent changes in their serum potassium (see PRECAUTIONS).

Removal of angiotensin II negative feedback on renin secretion leads to increased plasma renin activity. In animal studies, benazepril had no inhibitory effect on the vasopressor response to angiotensin II and did not interfere with the hemodynamic effects of the autonomic neurotransmitters acetylcholine, epinephrine, and norepinephrine.

ACE is identical to kininase, an enzyme that degrades bradykinin. Whether increased levels of bradykinin, a potent vasodepressor peptide, play a role in the therapeutic effects of Lotensin remains to be elucidated.

While the mechanism through which benazepril lowers blood pressure is believed to be primarily suppression of the renin-angiotensin-aldosterone system, benazepril has an antihypertensive effect even in patients with low-renin hypertension (see INDICATIONS AND USAGE).

Pharmacokinetics and Metabolism

Following oral administration of Lotensin, peak plasma concentrations of benazepril are reached within 0.5-1.0 hours. The extent of absorption is at least 37% as determined by urinary recovery and is not significantly influenced by the presence of food in the GI tract.

Cleavage of the ester group (primarily in the liver) converts benazepril to its active metabolite, benazeprilat. Peak plasma concentrations of benazeprilat are reached 1-2 hours after drug intake in the fasting state and 2-4 hours after drug intake in the nonfasting state. The serum protein binding of benazepril is about 96.7% and that of benazeprilat about 95.3%, as measured by equilibrium dialysis; on the basis of in vitro studies, the degree of protein binding should be unaffected by age, hepatic dysfunction, or concentration (over the concentration range of 0.24-23.6 μmol/L).

Benazepril is almost completely metabolized to benazeprilat, which has much greater ACE inhibitory activity than benazepril, and to the glucuronide conjugates of benazepril and benazeprilat. Only trace amounts of an administered dose of Lotensin can be recovered in the urine as unchanged benazepril, while about 20% of the dose is excreted as benazeprilat, 4% as benazepril glucuronide, and 8% as benazeprilat glucuronide.

The kinetics of benazepril are approximately dose-proportional within the dosage range of 10-80 mg.

In adults, the effective half-life of accumulation of benazeprilat following multiple dosing of benazepril hydrochloride is 10-11 hours. Thus, steady-state concentrations of benazeprilat should be reached after 2 or 3 doses of benazepril hydrochloride given once daily.

The kinetics did not change, and there was no significant accumulation during chronic administration (28 days) of once-daily doses between 5 mg and 20 mg. Accumulation ratios based on AUC and urinary recovery of benazeprilat were 1.19 and 1.27, respectively.

Benazepril and benazeprilat are cleared predominantly by renal excretion in healthy subjects with normal renal function. Nonrenal (i.e., biliary) excretion accounts for approximately 11%-12% of benazeprilat excretion in healthy subjects. In patients with renal failure, biliary clearance may compensate to an extent for deficient renal clearance.

In patients with renal insufficiency, the disposition of benazepril and benazeprilat in patients with mild-to-moderate renal insufficiency (creatinine clearance >30 mL/min) is similar to that in patients with normal renal function. In patients with creatinine clearance ≤30 mL/min, peak benazeprilat levels and the initial (alpha phase) half-life increase, and time to steady state may be delayed (see DOSAGE AND ADMINISTRATION).

When dialysis was started two hours after ingestion of 10 mg of benazepril, approximately 6% of benazeprilat was removed in 4 hours of dialysis. The parent compound, benazepril, was not detected in the dialysate.

In patients with hepatic insufficiency (due to cirrhosis), the pharmacokinetics of benazeprilat are essentially unaltered.

The pharmacokinetics of benazepril and benazeprilat do not appear to be influenced by age.

In pediatric patients, (N=45) hypertensive, age 6 to 16 years, given multiple daily doses of Lotensin (0.1 to 0.5 mg/kg), the clearance of benazeprilat for children 6 to 12 years old was 0.35 L/hr/kg, more than twice that of healthy adults receiving a single dose of 10 mg (0.13 L/hr/kg). In adolescents, it was 0.17 L/hr/kg, 27% higher than that of healthy adults. The terminal elimination half-life of benazeprilat in pediatric patients was around 5 hours, one third that observed in adults.

Pharmacodynamics

Single and multiple doses of 10 mg or more of Lotensin cause inhibition of plasma ACE activity by at least 80%-90% for at least 24 hours after dosing. Pressor responses to exogenous angiotensin I were inhibited by 60%-90% (up to 4 hours post-dose) at the 10-mg dose.

Hypertension

Adult

Administration of Lotensin to patients with mild-to-moderate hypertension results in a reduction of both supine and standing blood pressure to about the same extent with no compensatory tachycardia. Symptomatic postural hypotension is infrequent, although it can occur in patients who are salt- and/or volume-depleted (see WARNINGS).

In single-dose studies, Lotensin lowered blood pressure within 1 hour, with peak reductions achieved 2-4 hours after dosing. The antihypertensive effect of a single dose persisted for 24 hours. In multiple-dose studies, once-daily doses of 20-80 mg decreased seated pressure (systolic/diastolic) 24 hours after dosing by about 6 -12 /4-7 mmHg. The trough values represent reductions of about 50% of that seen at peak.

Four dose-response studies using once-daily dosing were conducted in 470 mild-to-moderate hypertensive patients not using diuretics. The minimal effective once-daily dose of Lotensin was 10 mg; but further falls in blood pressure, especially at morning trough, were seen with higher doses in the studied dosing range (10-80 mg). In studies comparing the same daily dose of Lotensin given as a single morning dose or as a twice-daily dose, blood pressure reductions at the time of morning trough blood levels were greater with the divided regimen.

During chronic therapy, the maximum reduction in blood pressure with any dose is generally achieved after 1-2 weeks. The antihypertensive effects of Lotensin have continued during therapy for at least two years. Abrupt withdrawal of Lotensin has not been associated with a rapid increase in blood pressure.

In patients with mild-to-moderate hypertension, Lotensin 10-20 mg was similar in effectiveness to captopril, hydrochlorothiazide, nifedipine SR, and propranolol.

The antihypertensive effects of Lotensin were not appreciably different in patients receiving high- or low-sodium diets.

In hemodynamic studies in dogs, blood pressure reduction was accompanied by a reduction in peripheral arterial resistance, with an increase in cardiac output and renal blood flow and little or no change in heart rate. In normal human volunteers, single doses of benazepril caused an increase in renal blood flow but had no effect on glomerular filtration rate.

Use of Lotensin in combination with thiazide diuretics gives a blood-pressure-lowering effect greater than that seen with either agent alone. By blocking the renin-angiotensin-aldosterone axis, administration of Lotensin tends to reduce the potassium loss associated with the diuretic.

Pediatric

In a clinical study of 107 pediatric patients, 7 to 16 years of age, with either systolic or diastolic pressure above the 95th percentile, patients were given 0.1 or 0.2 mg/kg then titrated up to 0.3 or 0.6 mg/kg with a maximum dose of 40 mg once daily. After four weeks of treatment, the 85 patients whose blood pressure was reduced on therapy were then randomized to either placebo or benazepril and were followed up for an additional two weeks. At the end of two weeks, blood pressure (both systolic and diastolic) in chil-

Continued on next page

Lotensin—Cont.

dren withdrawn to placebo rose by 4 to 6 mmHg more than in children on benazepril. No dose-response was observed for the three doses.

INDICATIONS AND USAGE

Lotensin is indicated for the treatment of hypertension. It may be used alone or in combination with thiazide diuretics.
In using Lotensin, consideration should be given to the fact that another angiotensin-converting enzyme inhibitor, captopril, has caused agranulocytosis, particularly in patients with renal impairment or collagen-vascular disease. Available data are insufficient to show that Lotensin does not have a similar risk (see WARNINGS).
Black patients receiving ACE-inhibitors have been reported to have a higher incidence of angioedema compared to nonblacks. It should also be noted that in controlled clinical trials ACE inhibitors have an effect on blood pressure that is less in black patients than in nonblacks.

CONTRAINDICATIONS

Lotensin is contraindicated in patients who are hypersensitive to this product or to any other ACE inhibitor.

WARNINGS

Anaphylactoid and Possibly Related Reactions
Presumably because angiotensin-converting enzyme inhibitors affect the metabolism of eicosanoids and polypeptides, including endogenous bradykinin, patients receiving ACE inhibitors (including Lotensin) may be subject to a variety of adverse reactions, some of them serious.
Head and Neck Angioedema: Angioedema of the face, extremities, lips, tongue, glottis, and larynx has been reported in patients treated with angiotensin-converting enzyme inhibitors. In U.S. clinical trials, symptoms consistent with angioedema were seen in none of the subjects who received placebo and in about 0.5% of the subjects who received Lotensin. Angioedema associated with laryngeal edema can be fatal. If laryngeal stridor or angioedema of the face, tongue, or glottis occurs, treatment with Lotensin should be discontinued and appropriate therapy instituted immediately. **Where there is involvement of the tongue, glottis, or larynx, likely to cause airway obstruction, appropriate therapy, e.g., subcutaneous epinephrine injection 1:1000 (0.3 mL to 0.5 mL) should be promptly administered (see ADVERSE REACTIONS).**
Intestinal Angioedema: Intestinal angioedema has been reported in patients treated with ACE inhibitors. These patients presented with abdominal pain (with or without nausea or vomiting); in some cases there was no prior history of facial angioedema and C-1 esterase levels were normal. The angioedema was diagnosed by procedures including abdominal CT scan or ultrasound, or at surgery, and symptoms resolved after stopping the ACE inhibitor. Intestinal angioedema should be included in the differential diagnosis of patients on ACE inhibitors presenting with abdominal pain.
Anaphylactoid Reactions During Desensitization: Two patients undergoing desensitizing treatment with hymenoptera venom while receiving ACE inhibitors sustained life-threatening anaphylactoid reactions. In the same patients, these reactions were avoided when ACE inhibitors were temporarily withheld, but they reappeared upon inadvertent rechallenge.
Anaphylactoid Reactions During Membrane Exposure: Anaphylactoid reactions have been reported in patients dialyzed with high-flux membranes and treated concomitantly with an ACE inhibitor. Anaphylactoid reactions have also been reported in patients undergoing low-density lipoprotein apheresis with dextran sulfate absorption (a procedure dependent upon devices not approved in the United States).
Hypotension
Lotensin can cause symptomatic hypotension. Like other ACE inhibitors, benazepril has been only rarely associated with hypotension in uncomplicated hypertensive patients. Symptomatic hypotension is most likely to occur in patients who have been volume- and/or salt-depleted as a result of prolonged diuretic therapy, dietary salt restriction, dialysis, diarrhea, or vomiting. Volume- and/or salt-depletion should be corrected before initiating therapy with Lotensin.
In patients with congestive heart failure, with or without associated renal insufficiency, ACE inhibitor therapy may cause excessive hypotension, which may be associated with oliguria or azotemia and, rarely, with acute renal failure and death. In such patients, Lotensin therapy should be started under close medical supervision; they should be followed closely for the first 2 weeks of treatment and whenever the dose of benazepril or diuretic is increased.
If hypotension occurs, the patient should be placed in a supine position, and, if necessary, treated with intravenous infusion of physiological saline. Lotensin treatment usually can be continued following restoration of blood pressure and volume.
Neutropenia/Agranulocytosis
Another angiotensin-converting enzyme inhibitor, captopril, has been shown to cause agranulocytosis and bone marrow depression, rarely in uncomplicated patients, but more frequently in patients with renal impairment, especially if they also have a collagen-vascular disease such as systemic lupus erythematosus or scleroderma. Available data from clinical trials of benazepril are insufficient to show that benazepril does not cause agranulocytosis at similar rates. Monitoring of white blood cell counts should be considered in patients with collagen-vascular disease, especially if the disease is associated with impaired renal function.
Fetal/Neonatal Morbidity and Mortality
ACE inhibitors can cause fetal and neonatal morbidity and death when administered to pregnant women. Several dozen cases have been reported in the world literature. When pregnancy is detected, ACE inhibitors should be discontinued as soon as possible.
The use of ACE inhibitors during the second and third trimesters of pregnancy has been associated with fetal and neonatal injury, including hypotension, neonatal skull hypoplasia, anuria, reversible or irreversible renal failure, and death. Oligohydramnios has also been reported, presumably resulting from decreased fetal renal function; oligohydramnios in this setting has been associated with fetal limb contractures, craniofacial deformation, and hypoplastic lung development. Prematurity, intrauterine growth retardation, and patent ductus arteriosus have also been reported, although it is not clear whether these occurrences were due to the ACE inhibitor exposure.
These adverse effects do not appear to have resulted from intrauterine ACE inhibitor exposure that has been limited to the first trimester. Mothers whose embryos and fetuses are exposed to ACE inhibitors only during the first trimester should be so informed. Nonetheless, when patients become pregnant, physicians should make every effort to discontinue the use of benazepril as soon as possible.
Rarely (probably less often than once in every thousand pregnancies), no alternative to ACE inhibitors will be found. In these rare cases, the mothers should be apprised of the potential hazards to their fetuses, and serial ultrasound examinations should be performed to assess the intraamniotic environment.
If oligohydramnios is observed, benazepril should be discontinued unless it is considered life-saving for the mother. Contraction stress testing (CST), a nonstress test (NST), or biophysical profiling (BPP) may be appropriate, depending upon the week of pregnancy. Patients and physicians should be aware, however, that oligohydramnios may not appear until after the fetus has sustained irreversible injury.
Infants with histories of in utero exposure to ACE inhibitors should be closely observed for hypotension, oliguria, and hyperkalemia. If oliguria occurs, attention should be directed toward support of blood pressure and renal perfusion. Exchange transfusion or dialysis may be required as means of reversing hypotension and/or substituting for disordered renal function. Benazepril, which crosses the placenta, can theoretically be removed from the neonatal circulation by these means; there are occasional reports of benefit from these maneuvers with another ACE inhibitor, but experience is limited.
No teratogenic effects of Lotensin were seen in studies of pregnant rats, mice, and rabbits. On a mg/m^2 basis, the doses used in these studies were 60 times (in rats), 9 times (in mice), and more than 0.8 times (in rabbits) the maximum recommended human dose (assuming a 50-kg woman). On a mg/kg basis these multiples are 300 times (in rats), 90 times (in mice), and more than 3 times (in rabbits) the maximum recommended human dose.
Hepatic Failure
Rarely, ACE inhibitors have been associated with a syndrome that starts with cholestatic jaundice and progresses to fulminant hepatic necrosis and (sometimes) death. The mechanism of this syndrome is not understood. Patients receiving ACE inhibitors who develop jaundice or marked elevations of hepatic enzymes should discontinue the ACE inhibitor and receive appropriate medical follow-up.

PRECAUTIONS

General
Impaired Renal Function: As a consequence of inhibiting the renin-angiotensin-aldosterone system, changes in renal function may be anticipated in susceptible individuals. In patients with severe congestive heart failure whose renal function may depend on the activity of the renin-angiotensin-aldosterone system, treatment with angiotensin-converting enzyme inhibitors, including Lotensin, may be associated with oliguria and/or progressive azotemia and (rarely) with acute renal failure and/or death. In a small study of hypertensive patients with renal artery stenosis in a solitary kidney or bilateral renal artery stenosis, treatment with Lotensin was associated with increases in blood urea nitrogen and serum creatinine; these increases were reversible upon discontinuation of Lotensin or diuretic therapy, or both. When such patients are treated with ACE inhibitors, renal function should be monitored during the first few weeks of therapy. Some hypertensive patients with no apparent preexisting renal vascular disease have developed increases in blood urea nitrogen and serum creatinine, usually minor and transient, especially when Lotensin has been given concomitantly with a diuretic. This is more likely to occur in patients with preexisting renal impairment. Dosage reduction of Lotensin and/or discontinuation of the diuretic may be required. **Evaluation of the hypertensive patient should always include assessment of renal function (see DOSAGE AND ADMINISTRATION).**
Hyperkalemia: In clinical trials, hyperkalemia (serum potassium at least 0.5 mEq/L greater than the upper limit of normal) occurred in approximately 1% of hypertensive patients receiving Lotensin. In most cases, these were isolated values which resolved despite continued therapy. Risk factors for the development of hyperkalemia include renal insufficiency, diabetes mellitus, and the concomitant use of potassium-sparing diuretics, potassium supplements, and/or potassium-containing salt substitutes, which should be used cautiously, if at all, with Lotensin (see Drug Interactions).
Cough: Presumably due to the inhibition of the degradation of endogenous bradykinin, persistent nonproductive cough has been reported with all ACE inhibitors, always resolving after discontinuation of therapy. ACE inhibitor-induced cough should be considered in the differential diagnosis of cough.
Impaired Liver Function: In patients with hepatic dysfunction due to cirrhosis, levels of benazeprilat are essentially unaltered (see WARNINGS, Hepatic Failure).
Surgery/Anesthesia: In patients undergoing surgery or during anesthesia with agents that produce hypotension, benazepril will block the angiotensin II formation that could otherwise occur secondary to compensatory renin release. Hypotension that occurs as a result of this mechanism can be corrected by volume expansion.
Information for Patients
Pregnancy: Female patients of childbearing age should be told about the consequences of second- and third-trimester exposure to ACE inhibitors, and they should also be told that these consequences do not appear to have resulted from intrauterine ACE inhibitor exposure that has been limited to the first trimester. These patients should be asked to report pregnancies to their physicians as soon as possible.
Angioedema: Angioedema, including laryngeal edema, can occur at any time with treatment with ACE inhibitors. Patients should be so advised and told to report immediately any signs or symptoms suggesting angioedema (swelling of face, eyes, lips, or tongue, or difficulty in breathing) and to take no more drug until they have consulted with the prescribing physician.
Symptomatic Hypotension: Patients should be cautioned that lightheadedness can occur, especially during the first days of therapy, and it should be reported to the prescribing physician. Patients should be told that if syncope occurs, Lotensin should be discontinued until the prescribing physician has been consulted.
All patients should be cautioned that inadequate fluid intake or excessive perspiration, diarrhea, or vomiting can lead to an excessive fall in blood pressure, with the same consequences of lightheadedness and possible syncope.
Hyperkalemia: Patients should be told not to use potassium supplements or salt substitutes containing potassium without consulting the prescribing physician.
Neutropenia: Patients should be told to promptly report any indication of infection (e.g., sore throat, fever), which could be a sign of neutropenia.
Drug Interactions
Diuretics: Patients on diuretics, especially those in whom diuretic therapy was recently instituted, may occasionally experience an excessive reduction of blood pressure after initiation of therapy with Lotensin. The possibility of hypotensive effects with Lotensin can be minimized by either discontinuing the diuretic or increasing the salt intake prior to initiation of treatment with Lotensin. If this is not possible, the starting dose should be reduced (see DOSAGE AND ADMINISTRATION).
Potassium Supplements and Potassium-Sparing Diuretics: Lotensin can attenuate potassium loss caused by thiazide diuretics. Potassium-sparing diuretics (spironolactone, amiloride, triamterene, and others) or potassium supplements can increase the risk of hyperkalemia. Therefore, if concomitant use of such agents is indicated, they should be given with caution, and the patient's serum potassium should be monitored frequently.
Oral Anticoagulants: Interaction studies with warfarin and acenocoumarol failed to identify any clinically important effects on the serum concentrations or clinical effects of these anticoagulants.
Lithium: Increased serum lithium levels and symptoms of lithium toxicity have been reported in patients receiving ACE inhibitors during therapy with lithium. These drugs should be coadministered with caution, and frequent monitoring of serum lithium levels is recommended. If a diuretic is also used, the risk of lithium toxicity may be increased.
Other: No clinically important pharmacokinetic interactions occurred when Lotensin was administered concomitantly with hydrochlorothiazide, chlorthalidone, furosemide, digoxin, propranolol, atenolol, naproxen, or cimetidine. Lotensin has been used concomitantly with beta-adrenergic-blocking agents, calcium-channel-blocking agents, diuretics, digoxin, and hydralazine, without evidence of clinically important adverse interactions. Benazepril, like other ACE inhibitors, has had less than additive effects with beta-adrenergic blockers, presumably because both drugs lower blood pressure by inhibiting parts of the renin-angiotensin system.
Carcinogenesis, Mutagenesis, Impairment of Fertility
No evidence of carcinogenicity was found when benazepril was administered to rats and mice for up to two years at doses of up to 150 mg/kg/day. When compared on the basis of body weights, this dose is 110 times the maximum recommended human dose. When compared on the basis of body surface areas, this dose is 18 and 9 times (rats and mice, respectively) the maximum recommended human dose (calculations assume a patient weight of 60 kg). No mutagenic activity was detected in the Ames test in bacteria (with or without metabolic activation), in an in vitro test for forward mutations in cultured mammalian cells, or in a nucleus anomaly test. In doses of 50-500 mg/kg/day (6-60 times the

maximum recommended human dose based on mg/m^2 comparison and 37-375 times the maximum recommended human dose based on a mg/kg comparison), Lotensin had no adverse effect on the reproductive performance of male and female rats.

Pregnancy Categories C (first trimester) and D (second and third trimesters)

See WARNINGS, Fetal/Neonatal Morbidity and Mortality.

Nursing Mothers

Minimal amounts of unchanged benazepril and of benazeprilat are excreted into the breast milk of lactating women treated with benazepril. A newborn child ingesting entirely breast milk would receive less than 0.1% of the mg/kg maternal dose of benazepril and benazeprilat.

Geriatric Use

Of the total number of patients who received benazepril in U.S. clinical studies of Lotensin, 18% were 65 or older while 2% were 75 or older. No overall differences in effectiveness or safety were observed between these patients and younger patients, and other reported clinical experience has not identified differences in responses between the elderly and younger patients, but greater sensitivity of some older individuals cannot be ruled out.

Benazepril and benazeprilat are substantially excreted by the kidney. Because elderly patients are more likely to have decreased renal function, care should be taken in dose selection, and it may be useful to monitor renal function.

Pediatric Use

The antihypertensive effects of Lotensin have been evaluated in a double-blind study in pediatric patients 7 to 16 years of age (see CLINICAL PHARMACOLOGY: Pharmacodynamics, Hypertension). The pharmacokinetics of Lotensin have been evaluated in pediatric patients 6 to 16 years of (see CLINICAL PHARMACOLOGY: Pharmacokinetics and Metabolism). Lotensin was generally well tolerated and adverse effects were similar to those described in adults. (See ADVERSE REACTIONS: *Pediatric Patients*).

Treatment with Lotensin is not recommended in pediatric patients less than 6 years of age (see ADVERSE REACTIONS), and in children with glomerular filtration rate <30 mL/min as there are insufficient data available to support a dosing recommendation in these groups. (See CLINICAL PHARMACOLOGY: In *pediatric patients* and DOSAGE AND ADMINISTRATION.)

ADVERSE REACTIONS

Lotensin has been evaluated for safety in over 6000 patients with hypertension; over 700 of these patients were treated for at least one year. The overall incidence of reported adverse events was comparable in Lotensin and placebo patients.

The reported side effects were generally mild and transient, and there was no relation between side effects and age, duration of therapy, or total dosage within the range of 2 to 80 mg. Discontinuation of therapy because of a side effect was required in approximately 5% of U.S. patients treated with Lotensin and in 3% of patients treated with placebo.

The most common reasons for discontinuation were headache (0.6%) and cough (0.5%) (see PRECAUTIONS, Cough).

The side effects considered possibly or probably related to study drug that occurred in U.S. placebo-controlled trials in more than 1% of patients treated with Lotensin are shown below.

PATIENTS IN U.S. PLACEBO-CONTROLLED STUDIES

	LOTENSIN (N=964)		PLACEBO (N=496)	
	N	%	N	%
Headache	60	6.2	21	4.2
Dizziness	35	3.6	12	2.4
Fatigue	23	2.4	11	2.2
Somnolence	15	1.6	2	0.4
Postural Dizziness	14	1.5	1	0.2
Nausea	13	1.3	5	1.0
Cough	12	1.2	5	1.0

Other adverse experiences reported in controlled clinical trials (in less than 1% of benazepril patients), and rarer events seen in postmarketing experience, include the following (in some, a causal relationship to drug use is uncertain):

Cardiovascular: Symptomatic hypotension was seen in 0.3% of patients, postural hypotension in 0.4%, and syncope in 0.1%; these reactions led to discontinuation of therapy in 4 patients who had received benazepril monotherapy and in 9 patients who had received benazepril with hydrochlorothiazide (see PRECAUTIONS and WARNINGS). Other reports included angina pectoris, palpitations, and peripheral edema.

Renal: Of hypertensive patients with no apparent preexisting renal disease, about 2% have sustained increases in serum creatinine to at least 150% of their baseline values while receiving Lotensin, but most of these increases have disappeared despite continuing treatment. A much smaller fraction of these patients (less than 0.1%) developed simultaneous (usually transient) increases in blood urea nitrogen and serum creatinine.

Fetal/Neonatal Morbidity and Mortality: See WARNINGS, Fetal/Neonatal Morbidity and Mortality.

Angioedema: Angioedema has been reported in patients receiving ACE inhibitors. During clinical trials in hypertensive patients with benazepril, 0.5% of patients experienced edema of the lips or face without other manifestations of angioedema. Angioedema associated with laryngeal edema and/or shock may be fatal. If angioedema of the face, extremities, lips, tongue, or glottis and/or larynx occurs, treatment with Lotensin should be discontinued and appropriate therapy instituted immediately (see WARNINGS).

Dermatologic: Stevens-Johnson syndrome, pemphigus, apparent hypersensitivity reactions (manifested by dermatitis, pruritus, or rash), photosensitivity, and flushing.

Gastrointestinal: Pancreatitis, constipation, gastritis, vomiting, and melena.

Hematologic: Thrombocytopenia and hemolytic anemia.

Neurologic and Psychiatric: Anxiety, decreased libido, hypertonia, insomnia, nervousness, and paresthesia.

Other: Asthma, bronchitis, dyspnea, sinusitis, urinary tract infection, infection, arthritis, impotence, alopecia, arthralgia, myalgia, asthenia, and sweating.

Another potentially important adverse experience, eosinophilic pneumonitis, has been attributed to other ACE inhibitors.

Pediatric Patients: The adverse experience profile for pediatric patients appears to be similar that seen in adult patients. Infants below the age of 1 year should not be given ACE inhibitors due to concerns over possible effects on kidney development.

The long-term effects of benazepril on growth and development have not been studied.

Clinical Laboratory Test Findings

Creatinine and Blood Urea Nitrogen: Of hypertensive patients with no apparent preexisting renal disease, about 2% have sustained increases in serum creatinine to at least 150% of their baseline values while receiving Lotensin, but most of these increases have disappeared despite continuing treatment. A much smaller fraction of these patients (less than 0.1%) developed simultaneous (usually transient) increases in blood urea nitrogen and serum creatinine. None of these increases required discontinuation of treatment. Increases in these laboratory values are more likely to occur in patients with renal insufficiency or those pretreated with a diuretic and, based on experience with other ACE inhibitors, would be expected to be especially likely in patients with renal artery stenosis (see PRECAUTIONS, General).

Potassium: Since benazepril decreases aldosterone secretion, elevation of serum potassium can occur. Potassium supplements and potassium-sparing diuretics should be given with caution, and the patient's serum potassium should be monitored frequently (see PRECAUTIONS).

Hemoglobin: Decreases in hemoglobin (a low value and a decrease of 5 g/dL) were rare, occurring in only 1 of 2,014 patients receiving Lotensin alone and in 1 of 1,357 patients receiving Lotensin plus a diuretic. No U.S. patients discontinued treatment because of decreases in hemoglobin.

Other (causal relationships unknown): Clinically important changes in standard laboratory tests were rarely associated with Lotensin administration. Elevations of uric acid, blood glucose, serum bilirubin, and liver enzymes (see WARNINGS) have been reported, as have scattered incidents of hyponatremia, electrocardiographic changes, leukopenia, eosinophilia, and proteinuria. In U.S. trials, less than 0.5% of patients discontinued treatment because of laboratory abnormalities.

OVERDOSAGE

Single oral doses of 3 g/kg benazepril were associated with significant lethality in mice. Rats, however, tolerated single oral doses of up to 6 g/kg. Reduced activity was seen at 1 g/kg in mice and at 5 g/kg in rats. Human overdoses of benazepril have not been reported, but the most common manifestation of human benazepril overdosage is likely to be hypotension.

Laboratory determinations of serum levels of benazepril and its metabolites are not widely available, and such determinations have, in any event, no established role in the management of benazepril overdose.

No data are available to suggest physiological maneuvers (e.g., maneuvers to change the pH of the urine) that might accelerate elimination of benazepril and its metabolites. Benazepril is only slightly dialyzable, but dialysis might be considered in overdosed patients with severely impaired renal function (see WARNINGS).

Angiotensin II could presumably serve as a specific antagonist-antidote in the setting of benazepril overdose, but angiotensin II is essentially unavailable outside of scattered research facilities. Because the hypotensive effect of benazepril is achieved through vasodilation and effective hypovolemia, it is reasonable to treat benazepril overdose by infusion of normal saline solution.

DOSAGE AND ADMINISTRATION

Hypertension

Adults

The recommended initial dose for patients not receiving a diuretic is 10 mg once-a-day. The usual maintenance dosage range is 20-40 mg per day administered as a single dose or in two equally divided doses. A dose of 80 mg gives an increased response, but experience with this dose is limited. The divided regimen was more effective in controlling trough (pre-dosing) blood pressure than the same dose given as a once-daily regimen. Dosage adjustment should be based on measurement of peak (2-6 hours after dosing) and trough responses. If a once-daily regimen does not give adequate trough response, an increase in dosage or divided administration should be considered. If blood pressure is not controlled with Lotensin alone, a diuretic can be added. Total daily doses above 80 mg have not been evaluated.

Concomitant administration of Lotensin with potassium supplements, potassium salt substitutes, or potassium-sparing diuretics can lead to increases of serum potassium (see PRECAUTIONS).

In patients who are currently being treated with a diuretic, symptomatic hypotension occasionally can occur following the initial dose of Lotensin. To reduce the likelihood of hypotension, the diuretic should, if possible, be discontinued two to three days prior to beginning therapy with Lotensin (see WARNINGS). Then, if blood pressure is not controlled with Lotensin alone, diuretic therapy should be resumed.

If the diuretic cannot be discontinued, an initial dose of 5 mg Lotensin should be used to avoid excessive hypotension.

Pediatrics

In children, doses of Lotensin between 0.1 and 0.6 mg/kg once daily have been studied, and doses greater than 0.1 mg/kg were shown to reduce blood pressure (see Pharmacodynamics). Based on this, the recommended starting dose of Lotensin is 0.2 mg/kg once per day as monotherapy. Doses above 0.6 mg/kg (or in excess of 40 mg daily) have not been studied in pediatric patients.

For pediatric patients who cannot swallow tablets, or for whom the calculated dosage (mg/kg) does not correspond to the available tablet strengths for Lotensin, follow the suspension preparation instructions below to administer benazepril HCl as a suspension.

Treatment with Lotensin is not advised for children below the age of 6 years (see PRECAUTIONS, PEDIATRICS) and in pediatric patients with glomerular filtration rate <30 mL, as there are insufficient data available to support a dosing recommendation in these groups.

For Hypertensive Patients with Renal Impairment

For patients with a creatinine clearance < 30 mL/min/ 1.73 m^2 (serum creatinine > 3 mg/dL), the recommended initial dose is 5 mg Lotensin once daily. Dosage may be titrated upward until blood pressure is controlled or to a maximum total daily dose of 40 mg (see WARNINGS).

Preparation of Suspension (for 150 mL of a 2 mg/mL suspension)

Add 75 mL of Ora-Plus®* oral suspending vehicle to an amber polyethylene terephthalate (PET) bottle containing fifteen Lotensin 20 mg tablets, and shake for at least 2 minutes. Allow the suspension to stand for a minimum of 1 hour. After the standing time, shake the suspension for a minimum of 1 additional minute. Add 75 mL of Ora-Sweet®* oral syrup vehicle to the bottle and shake the suspension to disperse the ingredients. The suspension should be refrigerated at 2-8 °C (36-46°F) and can be stored for up to 30 days in the PET bottle with a child-resistant screw-cap closure. Shake the suspension before each use.

*Ora-Plus® and Ora-Sweet® are registered trademarks of Paddock Laboratories, Inc. Ora-Plus® contains carrageenan, calcium sulfate, citric acid, methylparaben, microcrystalline cellulose, carboxymethylcellulose sodium, potassium sorbate, simethicone, sodium phosphate monobasic, xanthan gum, and water. Ora-Sweet® contains citric acid, berry citrus flavorant, glycerin, methylparaben, potassium sorbate, sodium phosphate monobasic, sorbitol, sucrose, and water.

HOW SUPPLIED

Lotensin is available in tablets of 5 mg, 10 mg, 20 mg, and 40 mg, packaged with a desiccant in bottles of 90 and 100 tablets. Lotensin is also supplied in blister packages (1 tablet/blister), in unit dose boxes containing 10 strips of 10 blisters each.

Each tablet is imprinted with LOTENSIN on one side and the tablet strength ("5," "10," "20," or "40") on the other.

The National Drug Codes for the various packages are:

[See table above]

Dose	Tablet Color	Bottle of 90	Bottle of 100	Unit Dose of 100
5 mg	light yellow	NDC 0083-0059-90	NDC 0083-0059-30	NDC 0083-0059-32
10 mg	dark yellow	NDC 0083-0063-90	NDC 0083-0063-30	NDC 0083-0063-32
20 mg	pink	NDC 0083-0079-90	NDC 0083-0079-30	NDC 0083-0079-32
40 mg	dark rose	NDC 0083-0094-90	NDC 0083-0094-30	NDC 0083-0094-32

Storage: Do not store above 30°C (86°F). Protect from moisture.

Dispense in tight container (USP).

T2004-32

REV: MAY 2004 Printed in U.S.A. 89008508

NOVARTIS

Manufactured by:
Novartis Pharmaceuticals Corporation
Suffern, New York 10901

Distributed by:
Novartis Pharmaceuticals Corporation
East Hanover, New Jersey 07936

Shown in Product Identification Guide, page 325

Continued on next page

LOTENSIN HCT® ℞

[lō-tĕn-sĭn]

(benazepril hydrochloride and hydrochlorothiazide USP)

Combination Tablets

5 mg/6.25 mg

10 mg/12.5 mg

20 mg/12.5 mg

20 mg/25 mg

Rx only

Prescribing Information

The following prescribing information is based on official labeling in effect October 2003.

USE IN PREGNANCY

When used in pregnancy during the second and third trimesters, ACE inhibitors can cause injury and even death to the developing fetus. When pregnancy is detected, Lotensin HCT should be discontinued as soon as possible. See **WARNINGS, Fetal/Neonatal Morbidity and Mortality.**

DESCRIPTION

Benazepril hydrochloride is a white to off-white crystalline powder, soluble (>100 mg/mL) in water, in ethanol, and in methanol. Benazepril hydrochloride's chemical name is 3-[[1-(ethoxycarbonyl)-3-phenyl-(1S)-propyl]amino]-2,3,4,5-tetrahydro-2-oxo-1*H*-1-(3S)-benzazepine-1-acetic acid monohydrochloride; its structural formula is

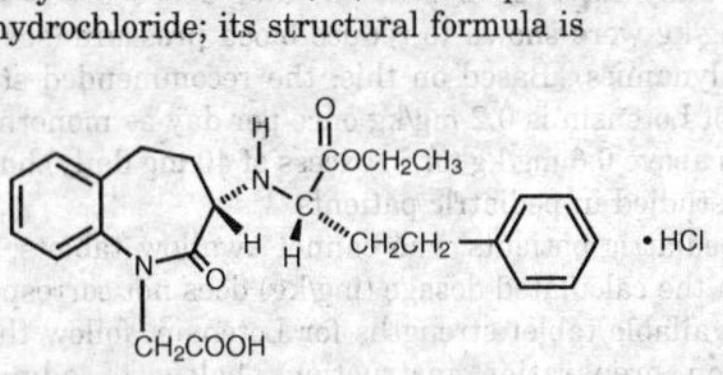

Its empirical formula is $C_{24}H_{28}N_2O_5$•HCl, and its molecular weight is 460.96.

Benazeprilat, the active metabolite of benazepril, is a non-sulfhydryl angiotensin-converting enzyme inhibitor. Benazepril is converted to benazeprilat by hepatic cleavage of the ester group.

Hydrochlorothiazide USP is a white, or practically white, practically odorless, crystalline powder. It is slightly soluble in water; freely soluble in sodium hydroxide solution, in *n*-butylamine, and in dimethylformamide; sparingly soluble in methanol; and insoluble in ether, in chloroform, and in dilute mineral acids. Hydrochlorothiazide's chemical name is 6-chloro-3,4-dihydro-2*H*-1,2,4-benzothiadiazine-7-sulfonamide 1,1-dioxide; its structural formula is

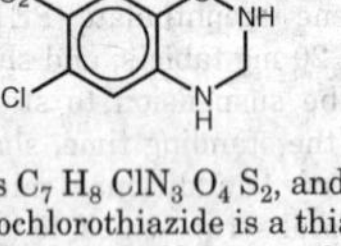

Its empirical formula is $C_7\ H_8\ ClN_3\ O_4\ S_2$, and its molecular weight is 297.73. Hydrochlorothiazide is a thiazide diuretic.

Lotensin HCT is a combination of benazepril hydrochloride and hydrochlorothiazide USP. The tablets are formulated for oral administration with a combination of 5, 10, or 20 mg of benazepril hydrochloride and 6.25, 12.5, or 25 mg of hydrochlorothiazide USP. The inactive ingredients of the tablets are cellulose compounds, crospovidone, hydrogenated castor oil, iron oxides (10/12.5-mg, 20/12.5-mg, and 20/25-mg tablets), lactose, polyethylene glycol, talc, and titanium dioxide.

CLINICAL PHARMACOLOGY

Mechanism of Action

Benazepril and benazeprilat inhibit angiotensin-converting enzyme (ACE) in human subjects and in animals. ACE is a peptidyl dipeptidase that catalyzes the conversion of angiotensin I to the vasoconstrictor substance, angiotensin II. Angiotensin II also stimulates aldosterone secretion by the adrenal cortex.

Inhibition of ACE results in decreased plasma angiotensin II, which leads to decreased vasopressor activity and to decreased aldosterone secretion. The latter decrease may result in a small increase of serum potassium. Hypertensive patients treated with benazepril alone for up to 52 weeks had elevations of serum potassium of up to 0.2 mEq/L. Similar patients treated with benazepril and hydrochlorothiazide for up to 24 weeks had no consistent changes in their serum potassium (see PRECAUTIONS).

Removal of angiotensin II negative feedback on renin secretion leads to increased plasma renin activity. In animal studies, benazepril had no inhibitory effect on the vasopressor response to angiotensin II and did not interfere with the hemodynamic effects of the autonomic neurotransmitters acetylcholine, epinephrine, and norepinephrine.

ACE is identical to kininase, an enzyme that degrades bradykinin. Whether increased levels of bradykinin, a potent vasodepressor peptide, play a role in the therapeutic effects of Lotensin HCT remains to be elucidated.

While the mechanism through which benazepril lowers blood pressure is believed to be primarily suppression of the renin-angiotensin-aldosterone system, benazepril has an antihypertensive effect even in patients with low-renin hypertension.

Hydrochlorothiazide is a thiazide diuretic. Thiazides affect the renal tubular mechanisms of electrolyte reabsorption, directly increasing excretion of sodium and chloride in approximately equivalent amounts. Indirectly, the diuretic action of hydrochlorothiazide reduces plasma volume, with consequent increases in plasma renin activity, increases in aldosterone secretion, increases in urinary potassium loss, and decreases in serum potassium. The renin-aldosterone link is mediated by angiotensin, so coadministration of an ACE inhibitor tends to reverse the potassium loss associated with these diuretics.

The mechanism of the antihypertensive effect of thiazides is unknown.

Pharmacokinetics and Metabolism

Following oral administration of Lotensin HCT, peak plasma concentrations of benazepril are reached within 0.5-1.0 hours. As determined by urinary recovery, the extent of absorption is at least 37%. The absorption of hydrochlorothiazide is somewhat slower (1-2.5 hours) and somewhat more complete (50%-80%). In fasting subjects, the rate and extent of absorption of benazepril and hydrochlorothiazide from Lotensin HCT are not different, respectively, from the rate and extent of absorption of benazepril and hydrochlorothiazide from immediate-release monotherapy formulations.

The absorption of benazepril from Lotensin® tablets is not influenced by the presence of food in the gastrointestinal tract, but possible effects of food upon absorption of either component from Lotensin HCT tablets have not been studied. The reported studies of food effects on hydrochlorothiazide absorption have been inconclusive. The absorption of hydrochlorothiazide is increased by agents that reduce gastrointestinal motility, but it is reported to be reduced by 50% in patients with congestive heart failure.

Cleavage of the ester group (primarily in the liver) converts benazepril to its active metabolite, benazeprilat. Peak plasma concentrations of benazeprilat are reached 1-2 hours after drug intake in the fasting state and 2-4 hours after drug intake in the nonfasting state. The serum protein binding of benazepril is about 96.7% and that of benazeprilat about 95.3%, as measured by equilibrium dialysis; on the basis of in vitro studies, the degree of protein binding should be unaffected by age, hepatic dysfunction, or – over the concentration range of 0.24-23.6 μmol/L – concentration.

Hydrochlorothiazide is not metabolized. Its apparent volume of distribution is 3.6-7.8 L/kg, and its measured plasma protein binding is 67.9%. The drug also accumulates in red blood cells, so that whole blood levels are 1.6-1.8 times those measured in plasma.

In studies of rats given ^{14}C-benazepril, benazepril and its metabolites crossed the blood-brain barrier only to an extremely low extent. Multiple doses of benazepril did not result in accumulation in any tissue except the lung, where, as with other ACE inhibitors in similar studies, there was a slight increase in concentration due to slow elimination in that organ.

Some placental passage occurred when benazepril was administered to pregnant rats. In humans, hydrochlorothiazide crosses the placenta freely, and levels in umbilical-cord blood are similar to those in the maternal circulation.

Benazepril is almost completely metabolized to benazeprilat, which has much greater ACE inhibitory activity than benazepril, and to the glucuronide conjugates of benazepril and benazeprilat. Only trace amounts of an administered dose of benazepril can be recovered unchanged in the urine; about 20% of the dose is excreted as benazeprilat, 4% as benazepril glucuronide, and 8% as benazeprilat glucuronide.

In patients with hepatic dysfunction due to cirrhosis, levels of benazeprilat are essentially unaltered. Similarly, the pharmacokinetics of benazepril and benazeprilat do not appear to be influenced by age.

The kinetics of benazepril are dose-proportional within the dosage range of 5-20 mg. Small deviations from dose proportionality were observed when the broader range of 2-80 mg was studied, possibly due to the saturable binding of the compound to ACE.

The effective half-life of accumulation of benazeprilat following multiple dosing of benazepril hydrochloride is 10-11 hours. Thus, steady-state concentrations of benazeprilat should be reached after 2 or 3 doses of benazepril hydrochloride given once daily.

During chronic administration (28 days) of once-daily doses of benazepril between 5 mg and 20 mg, the kinetics did not change, and there was no significant accumulation. Accumulation ratios based on AUC and urinary recovery of benazeprilat were 1.19 and 1.27, respectively.

When dialysis was started 2 hours after ingestion of 10 mg of benazepril, approximately 6% of benazeprilat was removed in 4 hours of dialysis. The parent compound, benazepril, was not detected in the dialysate.

Benazepril and benazeprilat are cleared predominantly by renal excretion in healthy subjects with normal renal function. Nonrenal (i.e., biliary) excretion accounts for approximately 11%-12% of benazeprilat excretion in healthy subjects. In patients with renal failure, biliary clearance may compensate to an extent for deficient renal clearance.

The disposition of benazepril and benazeprilat in patients with mild-to-moderate renal insufficiency (creatinine clearance > 30 mL/min) is similar to that in patients with normal renal function. In patients with creatinine clearance ≤ 30 mL/min, peak benazeprilat levels and the initial (alpha phase) half-life increase, and time to steady state may be delayed (see DOSAGE AND ADMINISTRATION).

Thiazide diuretics are eliminated by the kidney, with a terminal half-life of 5-15 hours. In a study of patients with impaired renal function (mean creatinine clearance of 19 mL/min), the half-life of hydrochlorothiazide elimination was lengthened to 21 hours.

Pharmacodynamics

Single and multiple doses of 10 mg or more of **benazepril** cause inhibition of plasma ACE activity by at least 80%-90% for at least 24 hours after dosing. For up to 4 hours after a 10-mg dose, pressor responses to exogenous angiotensin I were inhibited by 60%-90%.

Administration of benazepril to patients with mild-to-moderate hypertension results in a reduction of both supine and standing blood pressure to about the same extent, with no compensatory tachycardia.

Symptomatic postural hypotension is infrequent, although it can occur in patients who are salt and/or volume depleted (see WARNINGS, Hypotension).

In single-dose studies, benazepril lowered blood pressure within 1 hour, with peak reductions achieved 2-4 hours after dosing. The antihypertensive effect of a single dose persisted for 24 hours. In multiple-dose studies, once-daily doses of 20-80 mg decreased seated pressure (systolic/diastolic) 24 hours after dosing by about 6-12/4-7 mmHg. The reductions at trough are about 50% of those seen at peak.

Four dose-response studies of benazepril monotherapy using once-daily dosing were conducted in 470 mild-to-moderate hypertensive patients not using diuretics. The minimal effective once-daily dose of benazepril was 10 mg; further falls in blood pressure, especially at morning trough, were seen with higher doses in the studied dosing range (10-80 mg). In studies comparing the same daily dose of benazepril given as a single morning dose or as a twice-daily dose, blood pressure reductions at the time of morning trough blood levels were greater with the divided regimen.

During chronic therapy with benazepril, the maximum reduction in blood pressure with any given dose is generally achieved after 1-2 weeks. The antihypertensive effects of benazepril have continued during therapy for at least 2 years. Abrupt withdrawal of benazepril has not been associated with a rapid increase in blood pressure.

In patients with mild-to-moderate hypertension, total daily doses of Lotensin 20-40 mg were similar in effectiveness to total daily doses of captopril 50-100 mg, hydrochlorothiazide 25-50 mg, nifedipine SR 40-80 mg, and propranolol 80-160 mg.

The antihypertensive effects of benazepril were not appreciably different in patients receiving high- or low-sodium diets.

In hemodynamic studies in dogs, blood pressure reduction was accompanied by a reduction in peripheral arterial resistance, with an increase in cardiac output and renal blood flow and little or no change in heart rate. In normal human volunteers, single doses of benazepril caused an increase in renal blood flow but had no effect on glomerular filtration rate.

In clinical trials of **benazepril/hydrochlorothiazide** using benazepril doses of 5-20 mg and hydrochlorothiazide doses of 6.25-25 mg, the antihypertensive effects were sustained for at least 24 hours, and they increased with increasing dose of either component. Although benazepril monotherapy is somewhat less effective in blacks than in nonblacks, the efficacy of combination therapy appears to be independent of race.

By blocking the renin-angiotensin-aldosterone axis, administration of benazepril tends to reduce the potassium loss associated with the diuretic. In clinical trials of Lotensin HCT, the average change in serum potassium was near zero in subjects who received 5/6.25 mg or 20/12.5 mg, but the average subject who received 10/12.5 mg or 20/25 mg experienced a mild reduction in serum potassium, similar to that experienced by the average subject receiving the same dose of hydrochlorothiazide monotherapy.

INDICATIONS AND USAGE

Lotensin HCT is indicated for the treatment of hypertension.

This fixed combination drug is not indicated for the initial therapy of hypertension (see DOSAGE AND ADMINISTRATION).

In using Lotensin HCT, consideration should be given to the fact that another angiotensin-converting enzyme inhibitor, captopril, has caused agranulocytosis, particularly in patients with renal impairment or collagen-vascular disease. Available data are insufficient to show that benazepril does not have a similar risk (see WARNINGS, Neutropenia/Agranulocytosis).

Black patients receiving ACE inhibitors have been reported to have a higher incidence of angioedema compared to non-blacks.

CONTRAINDICATIONS

Lotensin HCT is contraindicated in patients who are anuric. Lotensin HCT is also contraindicated in patients who are hypersensitive to benazepril, to any other ACE inhibitor, to hydrochlorothiazide, or to other sulfonamide-derived drugs. Hypersensitivity reactions are more likely to occur in patients with a history of allergy or bronchial asthma.

WARNINGS

Anaphylactoid and Possibly Related Reactions

Presumably because angiotensin-converting enzyme inhibitors affect the metabolism of eicosanoids and polypeptides, including endogenous bradykinin, patients receiving ACE inhibitors (including Lotensin HCT) may be subject to a variety of adverse reactions, some of them serious.

Head and Neck Angioedema: Angioedema of the face, extremities, lips, tongue, glottis, and larynx has been reported in patients treated with angiotensin-converting enzyme inhibitors. In U.S. clinical trials, symptoms consistent with angioedema were seen in none of the subjects who received placebo and in about 0.5% of the subjects who received benazepril. Angioedema associated with laryngeal edema can be fatal. If laryngeal stridor or angioedema of the face, tongue, or glottis occurs, treatment with Lotensin HCT should be discontinued and appropriate therapy instituted immediately. *When involvement of the tongue, glottis, or larynx appears likely to cause airway obstruction, appropriate therapy, e.g., subcutaneous epinephrine injection 1:1000 (0.3-0.5 mL) should be promptly administered* (see PRECAUTIONS and ADVERSE REACTIONS).

Intestinal Angioedema: Intestinal angioedema has been reported in patients treated with ACE inhibitors. These patients presented with abdominal pain (with or without nausea or vomiting); in some cases there was no prior history of facial angioedema and C-1 esterase levels were normal. The angioedema was diagnosed by procedures including abdominal CT scan or ultrasound, or at surgery, and symptoms resolved after stopping the ACE inhibitor. Intestinal angioedema should be included in the differential diagnosis of patients on ACE inhibitors presenting with abdominal pain.

Anaphylactoid Reactions During Desensitization: Two patients undergoing desensitizing treatment with hymenoptera venom while receiving ACE inhibitors sustained life-threatening anaphylactoid reactions. In the same patients, these reactions were avoided when ACE inhibitors were temporarily withheld, but they reappeared upon inadvertent rechallenge.

Anaphylactoid Reactions During Membrane Exposure: Anaphylactoid reactions have been reported in patients dialyzed with high-flux membranes and treated concomitantly with an ACE inhibitor. Anaphylactoid reactions have also been reported in patients undergoing low-density lipoprotein apheresis with dextran sulfate absorption.

Hypotension

Lotensin HCT can cause symptomatic hypotension. Like other ACE inhibitors, benazepril has been only rarely associated with hypotension in uncomplicated hypertensive patients. Symptomatic hypotension is most likely to occur in patients who have been volume and/or salt depleted as a result of prolonged diuretic therapy, dietary salt restriction, dialysis, diarrhea, or vomiting. Volume and/or salt depletion should be corrected before initiating therapy with Lotensin HCT.

Lotensin HCT should be used cautiously in patients receiving concomitant therapy with other antihypertensives. The thiazide component of Lotensin HCT may potentiate the action of other antihypertensive drugs, especially ganglionic or peripheral adrenergic-blocking drugs. The antihypertensive effects of the thiazide component may also be enhanced in the postsympathectomy patient.

In patients with congestive heart failure, with or without associated renal insufficiency, ACE inhibitor therapy may cause excessive hypotension, which may be associated with oliguria, azotemia, and (rarely) with acute renal failure and death. In such patients, Lotensin HCT therapy should be started under close medical supervision; they should be followed closely for the first 2 weeks of treatment and whenever the dose of benazepril or diuretic is increased.

If hypotension occurs, the patient should be placed in a supine position, and, if necessary, treated with intravenous infusion of physiological saline. Lotensin HCT treatment usually can be continued following restoration of blood pressure and volume.

Impaired Renal Function

Lotensin HCT should be used with caution in patients with severe renal disease. Thiazides may precipitate azotemia in such patients, and the effects of repeated dosing may be cumulative.

When the renin-angiotensin-aldosterone system is inhibited by benazepril, changes in renal function may be anticipated in susceptible individuals. In patients with **severe congestive heart failure,** whose renal function may depend on the activity of the renin-angiotensin-aldosterone system, treatment with angiotensin-converting enzyme inhibitors (including benazepril) may be associated with oliguria and/or progressive azotemia and (rarely) with acute renal failure and/or death.

In a small study of hypertensive patients with **unilateral or bilateral renal artery stenosis,** treatment with benazepril was associated with increases in blood urea nitrogen and serum creatinine; these increases were reversible upon discontinuation of benazepril therapy, concomitant diuretic therapy, or both. When such patients are treated with Lotensin HCT, renal function should be monitored during the first few weeks of therapy.

Some benazepril-treated hypertensive patients with **no apparent preexisting renal vascular disease** have developed increases in blood urea nitrogen and serum creatinine, usually minor and transient, especially when benazepril has been given concomitantly with a diuretic. Dosage reduction of Lotensin HCT may be required. **Evaluation of the hypertensive patient should always include assessment of renal function** (see DOSAGE AND ADMINISTRATION).

Neutropenia/Agranulocytosis

Another angiotensin-converting enzyme inhibitor, captopril, has been shown to cause agranulocytosis and bone marrow depression, rarely in uncomplicated patients (incidence probably less than once per 10,000 exposures) but more frequently (incidence possibly as great as once per 1000 exposures) in patients with renal impairment, especially those who also have collagen-vascular diseases such as systemic lupus erythematosus or scleroderma. Available data from clinical trials of benazepril are insufficient to show that benazepril does not cause agranulocytosis at similar rates. Monitoring of white blood cell counts should be considered in patients with collagen-vascular disease, especially if the disease is associated with impaired renal function.

Fetal/Neonatal Morbidity and Mortality

ACE inhibitors can cause fetal and neonatal morbidity and death when administered to pregnant women. Several dozen cases have been reported in the world literature. When pregnancy is detected, Lotensin HCT should be discontinued as soon as possible.

The use of ACE inhibitors during the second and third trimesters of pregnancy has been associated with fetal and neonatal injury, including hypotension, neonatal skull hypoplasia, anuria, reversible or irreversible renal failure, and death. Oligohydramnios has also been reported, presumably resulting from decreased fetal renal function; oligohydramnios in this setting has been associated with fetal limb contractures, craniofacial deformation, and hypoplastic lung development. Prematurity, intrauterine growth retardation, and patent ductus arteriosus have also been reported, although it is not clear whether these occurrences were due to the ACE-inhibitor exposure.

These adverse effects do not appear to have resulted from intrauterine ACE- inhibitor exposure that has been limited to the first trimester. Mothers whose embryos and fetuses are exposed to ACE inhibitors only during the first trimester should be so informed. Nonetheless, when patients become pregnant, physicians should make every effort to discontinue the use of benazepril as soon as possible.

Rarely (probably less often than once in every thousand pregnancies), no alternative to ACE inhibitors will be found. In these rare cases, the mothers should be apprised of the potential hazards to their fetuses, and serial ultrasound examinations should be performed to assess the intraamniotic environment.

If oligohydramnios is observed, benazepril should be discontinued unless it is considered life-saving for the mother. Contraction stress testing (CST), a nonstress test (NST), or biophysical profiling (BPP) may be appropriate, depending upon the week of pregnancy. Patients and physicians should be aware, however, that oligohydramnios may not appear until after the fetus has sustained irreversible injury.

Infants with histories of in utero exposure to ACE inhibitors should be closely observed for hypotension, oliguria, and hyperkalemia. If oliguria occurs, attention should be directed toward support of blood pressure and renal perfusion. Exchange transfusion or peritoneal dialysis may be required as means of reversing hypotension and/or substituting for disordered renal function. Benazepril, which crosses the placenta, can theoretically be removed from the neonatal circulation by these means; there are occasional reports of benefit from these maneuvers, but experience is limited.

Intrauterine exposure to thiazide diuretics is associated with fetal or neonatal jaundice, thrombocytopenia, and possibly other adverse reactions that have occurred in adults.

No teratogenic effects were seen when benazepril and hydrochlorothiazide were administered to pregnant rats at a dose ratio of 4:5. On a mg/kg basis, the doses used were up to 167 times the maximum recommended human dose. Similarly, no teratogenic effects were seen when benazepril and hydrochlorothiazide were administered to pregnant mice at total doses up to 160 mg/kg/day, with benazepril:hydrochlorothiazide ratios of 15:1. When hydrochlorothiazide was orally administered without benazepril to pregnant mice and rats during their respective periods of major organogenesis, at doses up to 3000 and 1000 mg/kg/day respectively, there was no evidence of harm to the fetus. Similarly, no teratogenic effects of benazepril were seen in studies of pregnant rats, mice, and rabbits; on a mg/kg basis, the doses used in these studies were 300 times (in rats), 90 times (in mice), and more than 3 times (in rabbits) the maximum recommended human dose.

Hepatic Failure

Rarely, ACE inhibitors have been associated with a syndrome that starts with cholestatic jaundice and progresses to fulminant hepatic necrosis and (sometimes) death. The mechanism of this syndrome is not understood. Patients receiving ACE inhibitors who develop jaundice or marked elevations of hepatic enzymes should discontinue the ACE inhibitor and receive appropriate medical follow-up.

Impaired Hepatic Function

Lotensin HCT should be used with caution in patients with impaired hepatic function or progressive liver disease, since minor alterations of fluid and electrolyte balance may precipitate hepatic coma (see Hepatic Failure, above). In patients with hepatic dysfunction due to cirrhosis, levels of benazeprilat are essentially unaltered. No formal pharmacokinetic studies have been carried out in hypertensive patients with impaired liver function.

Systemic Lupus Erythematosus

Thiazide diuretics have been reported to cause exacerbation or activation of systemic lupus erythematosus.

PRECAUTIONS

General

Derangements of Serum Electrolytes: In clinical trials of benazepril monotherapy, hyperkalemia (serum potassium at least 0.5 mEq/L greater than the upper limit of normal) occurred in approximately 1% of hypertensive patients receiving benazepril. In most cases, these were isolated values which resolved despite continued therapy. Risk factors for the development of hyperkalemia included renal insufficiency, diabetes mellitus, and the concomitant use of potassium-sparing diuretics, potassium supplements, and/or potassium-containing salt substitutes.

Conversely, treatment with thiazide diuretics has been associated with hypokalemia, hyponatremia, and hypochloremic alkalosis. These disturbances have sometimes been manifest as one or more of dryness of mouth, thirst, weakness, lethargy, drowsiness, restlessness, muscle pains or cramps, muscular fatigue, hypotension, oliguria, tachycardia, nausea, and vomiting. Hypokalemia can also sensitize or exaggerate the response of the heart to the toxic effects of digitalis. The risk of hypokalemia is greatest in patients with cirrhosis of the liver, in patients experiencing a brisk diuresis, in patients who are receiving inadequate oral intake of electrolytes, and in patients receiving concomitant therapy with corticosteroids or ACTH.

The opposite effects of benazepril and hydrochlorothiazide on serum potassium will approximately balance each other in many patients, so that no net effect upon serum potassium will be seen. In other patients, one or the other effect may be dominant. Initial and periodic determinations of serum electrolytes to detect possible electrolyte imbalance should be performed at appropriate intervals.

Chloride deficits are generally mild and require specific treatment only under extraordinary circumstances (e.g., in liver disease or renal disease). Dilutional hyponatremia may occur in edematous patients; appropriate therapy is water restriction rather than administration of salt, except in rare instances when the hyponatremia is life-threatening. In actual salt depletion, appropriate replacement is the therapy of choice.

Calcium excretion is decreased by thiazides. In a few patients on prolonged thiazide therapy, pathological changes in the parathyroid gland have been observed, with hypercalcemia and hypophosphatemia. More serious complications of hyperparathyroidism (renal lithiasis, bone resorption, and peptic ulceration) have not been seen.

Thiazides increase the urinary excretion of magnesium, and hypomagnesemia may result.

Other Metabolic Disturbances: Thiazide diuretics tend to reduce glucose tolerance and to raise serum levels of cholesterol, triglycerides, and uric acid. These effects are usually minor, but frank gout or overt diabetes may be precipitated in susceptible patients.

Cough: Presumably due to the inhibition of the degradation of endogenous bradykinin, persistent nonproductive cough has been reported with all ACE inhibitors, always resolving after discontinuation of therapy. ACE inhibitor-induced cough should be considered in the differential diagnosis of cough.

Surgery/Anesthesia: In patients undergoing surgery or during anesthesia with agents that produce hypotension, benazepril will block the angiotensin II formation that could otherwise occur secondary to compensatory renin release. Hypotension that occurs as a result of this mechanism can be corrected by volume expansion.

Information for Patients

Angioedema: Angioedema, including laryngeal edema, can occur at any time with treatment with ACE inhibitors. A patient receiving Lotensin HCT should be told to report immediately any signs or symptoms suggesting angioedema (swelling of face, eyes, lips, or tongue, or difficulty in breathing) and to take no more drug until after consulting with the prescribing physician.

Pregnancy: Female patients of childbearing age should be told about the consequences of second- and third-trimester exposure to ACE inhibitors, and they should also be told that these consequences do not appear to have resulted from intrauterine ACE-inhibitor exposure that has been limited to the first trimester. These patients should be asked to report pregnancies to their physicians as soon as possible.

Symptomatic Hypotension: A patient receiving Lotensin HCT should be cautioned that lightheadedness can occur, especially during the first days of therapy, and that it should be reported to the prescribing physician. The patient should be told that if syncope occurs, Lotensin HCT should be discontinued until the physician has been consulted.

All patients should be cautioned that inadequate fluid intake, excessive perspiration, diarrhea, or vomiting can lead to an excessive fall in blood pressure, with the same consequences of lightheadedness and possible syncope.

Hyperkalemia: A patient receiving Lotensin HCT should be told not to use potassium supplements or salt substitutes containing potassium without consulting the prescribing physician.

Neutropenia: Patients should be told to promptly report any indication of infection (e.g., sore throat, fever), which could be a sign of neutropenia.

Laboratory Tests

The hydrochlorothiazide component of Lotensin HCT may decrease serum PBI levels without signs of thyroid disturbance.

Continued on next page

Lotensin HCT—Cont.

Therapy with Lotensin HCT should be interrupted for a few days before carrying out tests of parathyroid function.

Drug Interactions

Potassium Supplements and Potassium-Sparing Diuretics: As noted above (Derangements of Serum Electrolytes), the net effect of Lotensin HCT may be to elevate a patient's serum potassium, to reduce it, or to leave it unchanged. Potassium-sparing diuretics (spironolactone, amiloride, triamterene, and others) or potassium supplements can increase the risk of hyperkalemia. If concomitant use of such agents is indicated, they should be given with caution, and the patient's serum potassium should be monitored frequently.

Lithium: Increased serum lithium levels and symptoms of lithium toxicity have been reported in patients receiving ACE inhibitors during therapy with lithium. Because renal clearance of lithium is reduced by thiazides, the risk of lithium toxicity is presumably raised further when, as in therapy with Lotensin HCT, a thiazide diuretic is coadministered with the ACE inhibitor. Lotensin HCT and lithium should be coadministered with caution, and frequent monitoring of serum lithium levels is recommended.

Other: Benazepril has been used concomitantly with beta-adrenergic-blocking agents, calcium-blocking agents, cimetidine, diuretics, digoxin, hydralazine, and naproxen without evidence of clinically important adverse interactions. Other ACE inhibitors have had less than additive effects with beta-adrenergic blockers, presumably because drugs of both classes lower blood pressure by inhibiting parts of the renin-angiotensin system.

Interaction studies with warfarin and acenocoumarol have failed to identify any clinically important effects of benazepril on the serum concentrations or clinical effects of these anticoagulants.

Insulin requirements in diabetic patients may be increased, decreased, or unchanged.

Thiazides may decrease arterial responsiveness to norepinephrine, but not enough to preclude effectiveness of the pressor agent for therapeutic use.

Thiazides may increase the responsiveness to tubocurarine.

The diuretic, natriuretic, and antihypertensive effects of thiazide diuretics may be reduced by concurrent administration of nonsteroidal anti-inflammatory agents.

Cholestyramine and colestipol resins: Absorption of hydrochlorothiazide is impaired in the presence of anionic exchange resins. Single doses of either cholestyramine or colestipol resins bind the hydrochlorothiazide and reduce its absorption from the gastrointestinal tract by up to 85% and 43%, respectively.

Carcinogenesis, Mutagenesis, Impairment of Fertility

No evidence of carcinogenicity was found when **benazepril** was given to rats and mice for 104 weeks at doses up to 150 mg/kg/day. On a body-weight basis, this dose is over 100 times the maximum recommended human dose; on a body-surface-area basis, this dose is 18 times (rats) and 9 times (mice) the maximum recommended human dose. No mutagenic activity was detected in the Ames test in bacteria (with or without metabolic activation), in an in vitro test for forward mutations in cultured mammalian cells, or in a nucleus anomaly test. At doses of 50-500 mg/kg/day (38-375 times the maximum recommended human dose on a body-weight basis; 6-61 times the maximum recommended dose on a body-surface-area basis), benazepril had no adverse effect on the reproductive performance of male and female rats.

Under the auspices of the National Toxicology Program, rats and mice received **hydrochlorothiazide** in their feed for two years, at doses up to 600 mg/kg/day in mice and up to 100 mg/kg/day in rats. These studies uncovered no evidence of a carcinogenic potential of hydrochlorothiazide in rats or female mice, but there was equivocal evidence of hepatocarcinogenicity in male mice. Hydrochlorothiazide was not genotoxic in vitro assays using strains TA 98, TA 100, TA 1535, TA 1537, and TA 1538 of *Salmonella typhimurium* (the Ames test); in the Chinese Hamster Ovary (CHO) test for chromosomal aberrations; or in in vivo assays using mouse germinal cell chromosomes, Chinese hamster bone marrow chromosomes, and the *Drosophila* sex-linked recessive lethal trait gene. Positive test results were obtained in the in vitro CHO Sister Chromatid Exchange (clastogenicity) test and in the Mouse Lymphoma Cell (mutagenicity) assays, using concentrations of hydrochlorothiazide of 43-1300 µg/mL. Positive test results were also obtained in the *Aspergillus nidulans* nondisjunction assay, using an unspecified concentration of hydrochlorothiazide.

Hydrochlorothiazide had no adverse effects on the fertility of mice and rats of either sex in studies wherein these species were exposed, via their diets, to doses up to 100 and 4 mg/kg/day, respectively, prior to mating and throughout gestation.

Pregnancy

Pregnancy Categories C (first trimester) and D (second and third trimesters): See WARNINGS, Fetal/Neonatal Morbidity and Mortality.

Nursing Mothers

Minimal amounts of unchanged benazepril and of benazeprilat are excreted into the breast milk of lactating women treated with benazepril, so that a newborn child ingesting nothing but breast milk would receive less than 0.1% of the maternal doses of benazepril and benazeprilat. Thiazides, on the other hand, are definitely excreted into breast milk. Because of the potential for serious adverse reactions in nursing infants from hydrochlorothiazide and the unknown effects of benazepril in infants, a decision should be made whether to discontinue nursing or to discontinue Lotensin HCT, taking into account the importance of the drug to the mother.

Geriatric Use

Of the total number of patients who received Lotensin HCT in U.S. clinical studies of Lotensin HCT, 19% were 65 or older while about 1.5% were 75 or older. Overall differences in effectiveness or safety were not observed between these patients and younger patients, and other reported clinical experience has not identified differences in responses between the elderly and younger patients, but greater sensitivity of some older individuals cannot be ruled out.

Benazepril and benazeprilat are substantially excreted by the kidney. Because elderly patients are more likely to have decreased renal function, care should be taken in dose selection, and it may be useful to monitor renal function.

Pediatric Use

Safety and effectiveness in pediatric patients have not been established.

ADVERSE REACTIONS

Lotensin HCT has been evaluated for safety in over 2500 patients with hypertension; over 500 of these patients were treated for at least 6 months, and over 200 were treated for more than 1 year.

The reported side effects were generally mild and transient, and there was no relationship between side effects and age, sex, race, or duration of therapy. Discontinuation of therapy due to side effects was required in approximately 7% of U.S. patients treated with Lotensin HCT and in 4% of patients treated with placebo.

The most common reasons for discontinuation of therapy with Lotensin HCT in U.S. studies were cough (1.0%; see PRECAUTIONS), "dizziness" (1.0%), headache (0.6%), and fatigue (0.6%).

The side effects considered possibly or probably related to study drug that occurred in U.S. placebo-controlled trials in more than 1% of patients treated with Lotensin HCT are shown in the table below.

Reactions Possibly or Probably Drug Related
Patients in U.S. Placebo-Controlled Studies

	LOTENSIN HCT N=655		Placebo N=235	
	N	%	N	%
"Dizziness"	41	6.3	8	3.4
Fatigue	34	5.2	6	2.6
Postural Dizziness	23	3.5	1	0.4
Headache	20	3.1	10	4.3
Cough	14	2.1	3	1.3
Hypertonia	10	1.5	3	1.3
Vertigo	10	1.5	2	0.9
Nausea	9	1.4	2	0.9
Impotence	8	1.2	0	0.0
Somnolence	8	1.2	1	0.4

Other side effects considered possibly or probably related to study drug that occurred in U.S. placebo-controlled trials in 0.3% to 1.0% of patients treated with Lotensin HCT were the following:

Angioedema: Edema of the lips or face without other manifestations of angioedema (0.3%). See WARNINGS, Angioedema.

Cardiovascular: Hypotension (seen in 0.6% of patients), postural hypotension (0.3%), palpitations, and flushing.

Gastrointestinal: Vomiting, diarrhea, dyspepsia, anorexia, and constipation.

Neurologic and Psychiatric: Insomnia, nervousness, paresthesia, libido decrease, dry mouth, taste perversion, and tinnitus.

Dermatologic: Rash and sweating.

Other: Gout, urinary frequency, arthralgia, myalgia, asthenia, and pain (including chest pain and abdominal pain).

Other adverse experiences reported in 0.3% or more of Lotensin HCT patients in U.S. controlled clinical trials, and rarer events seen in postmarketing experience, were the following; asterisked entries occurred in more than 1% of patients (in some, a causal relationship to Lotensin HCT is uncertain):

Angioedema: Edema of the lips or face without other manifestations of angioedema. See WARNINGS, Angioedema.

Cardiovascular: Syncope, peripheral vascular disorder, and tachycardia.

Body as a Whole: Infection, back pain,* flu syndrome,* fever, chills, and neck pain.

Dermatologic: Photosensitivity and pruritus.

Gastrointestinal: Gastroenteritis, flatulence, and tooth disorder.

Neurologic and Psychiatric: Hypesthesia, abnormal vision, abnormal dreams, and retinal disorder.

Respiratory: Upper respiratory infection,* epistaxis, bronchitis, rhinitis,* sinusitis,* and voice alteration.

Other: Conjunctivitis, arthritis, urinary tract infection, alopecia, and urinary frequency.*

Fetal/Neonatal Morbidity and Mortality: See WARNINGS, Fetal/Neonatal Morbidity and Mortality.

Monotherapy with **benazepril** has been evaluated for safety in over 6000 patients. In clinical trials, the observed adverse reactions to benazepril were similar to those seen in trials of Lotensin HCT. In postmarketing experience with benazepril, there have been rare reports of Stevens-Johnson syndrome, pancreatitis, hemolytic anemia, pemphigus, and thrombocytopenia. Another potentially important adverse experience, eosinophilic pneumonitis, has been attributed to other ACE inhibitors.

Hydrochlorothiazide has been extensively prescribed for many years, but there has not been enough systematic collection of data to support an estimate of the frequency of the observed adverse reactions. Within organ-system groups, the reported reactions are listed here in decreasing order of severity, without regard to frequency.

Cardiovascular: Orthostatic hypotension (may be potentiated by alcohol, barbiturates, or narcotics).

Digestive: Pancreatitis, jaundice (intrahepatic cholestatic) (see WARNINGS), sialadenitis, vomiting, diarrhea, cramping, nausea, gastric irritation, constipation, and anorexia.

Neurologic: Vertigo, lightheadedness, transient blurred vision, headache, paresthesia, xanthopsia, weakness, and restlessness.

Musculoskeletal: Muscle spasm.

Hematologic: Aplastic anemia, agranulocytosis, leukopenia, and thrombocytopenia.

Metabolic: Hyperglycemia, glycosuria, and hyperuricemia.

Hypersensitivity: Necrotizing angiitis, Stevens-Johnson syndrome, respiratory distress (including pneumonitis and pulmonary edema), purpura, urticaria, rash, and photosensitivity.

Clinical Laboratory Test Findings

Serum Electrolytes: See PRECAUTIONS.

Creatinine: Minor reversible increases in serum creatinine were observed in patients with essential hypertension treated with Lotensin HCT. Such increases occurred most frequently in patients with renal artery stenosis (see PRECAUTIONS).

PBI and Tests of Parathyroid Function: See PRECAUTIONS.

Other (Causal Relationships Unknown): Other clinically important changes in standard laboratory tests were rarely associated with Lotensin HCT administration. Elevations in blood urea nitrogen, uric acid, glucose, SGOT, and SGPT (see WARNINGS) have been reported. In the somewhat larger patient population exposed to benazepril monotherapy in U.S. trials, the same abnormalities were reported, together with scattered accounts of hyponatremia, melena, electrocardiographic changes, leukopenia, eosinophilia, and proteinuria.

OVERDOSAGE

No specific information is available on the treatment of overdosage with Lotensin HCT; treatment should be symptomatic and supportive. Therapy with Lotensin HCT should be discontinued, and the patient should be observed. Dehydration, electrolyte imbalance, and hypotension should be treated by established procedures.

Single oral doses of 1 g/kg of benazepril caused reduced activity in mice, and doses of 3 g/kg were associated with significant lethality. Reduction of activity in rats was not seen until they had received doses of 5 g/kg, and doses of 6 g/kg were not lethal. In single-dose studies of hydrochlorothiazide, most rats survived doses up to 2.75 g/kg.

Data from human overdoses of benazepril are scanty, but the most common manifestation of human benazepril overdosage is likely to be hypotension. In human hydrochlorothiazide overdose, the most common signs and symptoms observed have been those of dehydration and electrolyte depletion (hypokalemia, hypochloremia, hyponatremia). If digitalis has also been administered, hypokalemia may accentuate cardiac arrhythmias.

Laboratory determinations of serum levels of benazepril and its metabolites are not widely available, and such determinations have, in any event, no established role in the management of benazepril overdose.

No data are available to suggest physiological maneuvers (e.g., maneuvers to change the pH of the urine) that might accelerate elimination of benazepril and its metabolites. Benazeprilat is only slightly dialyzable, but dialysis might be considered in overdosed patients with severely impaired renal function (see WARNINGS).

Angiotensin II could presumably serve as a specific antagonist-antidote in the setting of benazepril overdose, but angiotensin II is essentially unavailable outside of scattered research facilities. Because the hypotensive effect of benazepril is achieved through vasodilation and effective hypovolemia, it is reasonable to treat benazepril overdose by infusion of normal saline solution.

DOSAGE AND ADMINISTRATION

Benazepril is an effective treatment of hypertension in once-daily doses of 10-80 mg, while hydrochlorothiazide is effective in doses of 12.5-50 mg per day. In clinical trials of benazepril/hydrochlorothiazide combination therapy using benazepril doses of 5-20 mg and hydrochlorothiazide doses of 6.25-25 mg, the antihypertensive effects increased with increasing dose of either component.

The side effects (see WARNINGS) of benazepril are generally rare and apparently independent of dose; those of hydrochlorothiazide are a mixture of dose-dependent phenomena (primarily hypokalemia) and dose-independent phenomena (e.g., pancreatitis), the former much more common than the latter. Therapy with any combination of benazepril and hydrochlorothiazide will be associated with both sets of dose-independent side effects, but regimens in which benazepril is combined with low doses of hydrochlorothiazide produce minimal effects on serum potassium. In clinical trials of Lotensin HCT, the average change in serum potassium was near zero in subjects who received 5/6.25 mg or 20/12.5 mg, but the average subject who received 10/12.5 mg or 20/25 mg experienced a mild reduction in serum potassium, similar to that experienced by the average subject receiving the same dose of hydrochlorothiazide monotherapy.

To minimize dose-independent side effects, it is usually appropriate to begin combination therapy only after a patient has failed to achieve the desired effect with monotherapy.

Dose Titration Guided by Clinical Effect: A patient whose blood pressure is not adequately controlled with benazepril monotherapy may be switched to Lotensin HCT 10/12.5 or Lotensin HCT 20/12.5. Further increases of either or both components could depend on clinical response. The hydrochlorothiazide dose should generally not be increased until 2–3 weeks have elapsed. Patients whose blood pressures are adequately controlled with 25 mg of daily hydrochlorothiazide, but who experience significant potassium loss with this regimen, may achieve similar blood-pressure control without electrolyte disturbance if they are switched to Lotensin HCT 5/6.25.

Replacement Therapy: The combination may be substituted for the titrated individual components.

Use in Renal Impairment: Regimens of therapy with Lotensin HCT need not take account of renal function as long as the patient's creatinine clearance is >30 mL/min/1.73m^2 (serum creatinine roughly ≤3 mg/dL or 265 µmol/L). In patients with more severe renal impairment, loop diuretics are preferred to thiazides, so Lotensin HCT is not recommended (see WARNINGS).

HOW SUPPLIED

Lotensin HCT is available in tablets of four different strengths:

Benazepril	Hydrochlorothiazide	Tablet Color
5 mg	6.25 mg	white
10 mg	12.5 mg	light pink
20 mg	12.5 mg	grayish-violet
20 mg	25 mg	red

Tablets of each strength are supplied in bottles that contain a desiccant and 100 tablets.

The National Drug Codes for the various packages are

Dose	Bottle of 100
5/6.25	NDC 0083-0057-30
10/12.5	NDC 0083-0072-30
20/12.5	NDC 0083-0074-30
20/25	NDC 0083-0075-30

Tablets are oblong and scored, with "Lotensin HCT" on one side and a portion of the NDC code ("57," "72," "74," or "75") on the other.

Storage: Do not store above 30 °C (86 °F). Protect from moisture and light. *Dispense in tight, light-resistant container (USP).*

T2003-43

REV: AUGUST 2003 89001404

NOVARTIS

Manufactured by:
Novartis Pharmaceuticals Corporation
Suffern, New York 10901
Distributed by:
Novartis Pharmaceuticals Corporation
East Hanover, New Jersey 07936

Shown in Product Identification Guide, page 325

LOTREL® ℞

[lō' trĕl]

(amlodipine besylate and benazepril hydrochloride)
Combination Capsules
2.5 mg/10 mg
5 mg/10 mg
5 mg/20 mg
10 mg/20 mg
Rx only

Prescribing Information

The following prescribing information is based on official labeling in effect July 2004.

USE IN PREGNANCY
When used in pregnancy during the second and third trimesters, ACE inhibitors can cause injury and even death to the developing fetus. When pregnancy is detected, Lotrel should be discontinued as soon as possible. *See WARNINGS, Fetal/Neonatal Morbidity and Mortality.*

DESCRIPTION

Benazepril hydrochloride is a white to off-white crystalline powder, soluble (>100 mg/mL) in water, in ethanol, and in methanol. Benazepril hydrochloride's chemical name is 3-[[1-(ethoxycarbonyl)-3-phenyl-(1S)-propyl]amino]-2,3,4,5-tetrahydro-2-oxo-1*H*-1-(3S)-benzazepine-1-acetic acid monohydrochloride; its structural formula is

[structural formula: H, O, N, COCH₂CH₃, CH₂CH₂, H, •HCl, N, CH₂COOH]

Its empirical formula is $C_{24}H_{28}N_2O_5 \bullet HCl$, and its molecular weight is 460.96.

Benazeprilat, the active metabolite of benazepril, is a non-sulfhydryl angiotensin-converting enzyme (ACE) inhibitor. Benazepril is converted to benazeprilat by hepatic cleavage of the ester group.

Amlodipine besylate is a white to pale yellow crystalline powder, slightly soluble in water and sparingly soluble in ethanol. Its chemical name is (R,S)3-ethyl-5-methyl-2-(2-aminoethoxymethyl)-4-(2-chlorophenyl)-1,4-dihydro-6-methyl-3,5-pyridinedicarboxylate benzenesulfonate; its structural formula is

[structural formula: Cl, SO₃H, H₃CO₂C, CO₂CH₂CH₃, H₃C, N, H, CH₂OCH₂CH₂NH₂]

Its empirical formula is $C_{20}H_{25}ClN_2O_5 \bullet C_6H_6O_3S$, and its molecular weight is 567.1.

Amlodipine besylate is the besylate salt of amlodipine, a dihydropyridine calcium channel blocker.

Lotrel is a combination of amlodipine besylate and benazepril hydrochloride. The capsules are formulated in four different strengths for oral administration with a combination of amlodipine besylate equivalent to 2.5 mg, 5 mg or 10 mg of amlodipine, with 10 mg or 20 mg of benazepril hydrochloride providing for the following available combinations: 2.5/10 mg, 5/10 mg, 5/20 mg and 10/20 mg. The inactive ingredients of the capsules are calcium phosphate, cellulose compounds, colloidal silicon dioxide, crospovidone, gelatin, hydrogenated castor oil, iron oxides, lactose, magnesium stearate, polysorbate 80, silicon dioxide, sodium lauryl sulfate, sodium starch (potato) glycolate, starch (corn), talc, and titanium dioxide.

CLINICAL PHARMACOLOGY

Mechanism of Action

Benazepril and benazeprilat inhibit angiotensin-converting enzyme (ACE) in human subjects and in animals. ACE is a peptidyl dipeptidase that catalyzes the conversion of angiotensin I to the vasoconstrictor substance angiotensin II. Angiotensin II also stimulates aldosterone secretion by the adrenal cortex.

Inhibition of ACE results in decreased plasma angiotensin II, which leads to decreased vasopressor activity and to decreased aldosterone secretion. The latter decrease may result in a small increase of serum potassium. Hypertensive patients treated with benazepril and amlodipine for up to 56 weeks had elevations of serum potassium up to 0.2 mEq/L *(see PRECAUTIONS).*

Removal of angiotensin II negative feedback on renin secretion leads to increased plasma renin activity. In animal studies, benazepril had no inhibitory effect on the vasopressor response to angiotensin II and did not interfere with the hemodynamic effects of the autonomic neurotransmitters acetylcholine, epinephrine, and norepinephrine.

ACE is identical to kininase, an enzyme that degrades bradykinin. Whether increased levels of bradykinin, a potent vasodepressor peptide, play a role in the therapeutic effects of Lotrel remains to be elucidated.

While the mechanism through which benazepril lowers blood pressure is believed to be primarily suppression of the renin-angiotensin-aldosterone system, benazepril has an antihypertensive effect even in patients with low-renin hypertension.

Amlodipine is a dihydropyridine calcium antagonist (calcium ion antagonist or slow channel blocker) that inhibits the transmembrane influx of calcium ions into vascular smooth muscle and cardiac muscle. Experimental data suggest that amlodipine binds to both dihydropyridine and non-dihydropyridine binding sites. The contractile processes of cardiac muscle and vascular smooth muscle are dependent upon the movement of extracellular calcium ions into these cells through specific ion channels. Amlodipine inhibits calcium ion influx across cell membranes selectively, with a greater effect on vascular smooth muscle cells than on cardiac muscle cells. Negative inotropic effects can be detected *in vitro* but such effects have not been seen in intact animals at therapeutic doses. Serum calcium concentration is not affected by amlodipine. Within the physiologic pH range, amlodipine is an ionized compound (pKa=8.6), and its kinetic interaction with the calcium channel receptor is characterized by a gradual rate of association and dissociation with the receptor binding site, resulting in a gradual onset of effect.

Amlodipine is a peripheral arterial vasodilator that acts directly on vascular smooth muscle to cause a reduction in peripheral vascular resistance and reduction in blood pressure.

Pharmacokinetics and Metabolism

The rate and extent of absorption of benazepril and amlodipine from Lotrel are not significantly different, respectively, from the rate and extent of absorption of benazepril and amlodipine from individual tablet formulations. Absorption from the individual tablets is not influenced by the presence of food in the gastrointestinal tract; food effects on absorption from Lotrel have not been studied. Following oral administration of Lotrel, peak plasma concentrations of benazepril are reached in 0.5-2 hours. Cleavage of the ester group (primarily in the liver) converts benazepril to its active metabolite, benazeprilat, which reaches peak plasma concentrations in 1.5-4 hours. The extent of absorption of benazepril is at least 37%.

Peak plasma concentrations of amlodipine are reached 6-12 hours after administration of Lotrel; the extent of absorption is 64%-90%.

The apparent volumes of **distribution** of amlodipine and benazeprilat are about 21 L/kg and 0.7 L/kg, respectively. Approximately 93% of circulating amlodipine is bound to plasma proteins, and the bound fraction of benazeprilat is slightly higher. On the basis of *in vitro* studies, benazeprilat's degree of protein binding should be unaffected by age, by hepatic dysfunction, or – over the therapeutic concentration range – by concentration.

Benazeprilat has much greater ACE-inhibitory activity than benazepril, and the **metabolism** of benazepril to benazeprilat is almost complete. Only trace amounts of an administered dose of benazepril can be recovered unchanged in the urine; about 20% of the dose is excreted as benazeprilat, 8% as benazeprilat glucuronide, and 4% as benazepril glucuronide.

Amlodipine is extensively metabolized in the liver, with 10% of the parent compound and 60% of the metabolites excreted in the urine. In patients with hepatic dysfunction, decreased clearance of amlodipine may increase the area-under-the-plasma-concentration curve by 40%-60%, and dosage reduction may be required *(see DOSAGE AND ADMINISTRATION).* In patients with renal impairment, the pharmacokinetics of amlodipine are essentially unaffected.

Benazeprilat's effective **elimination** half-life is 10-11 hours, while that of amlodipine is about 2 days, so steady-state levels of the two components are achieved after about a week of once-daily dosing. The clearance of benazeprilat from the plasma is primarily renal, but biliary excretion accounts for 11%-12% of benazeprilat elimination in normal subjects. In patients with severe renal insufficiency (creatinine clearance less than 30 mL/min), peak benazeprilat levels and the time to steady state may be increased *(see DOSAGE AND ADMINISTRATION).* In patients with hepatic impairment, on the other hand, the pharmacokinetics of benazeprilat are essentially unaffected.

Although the pharmacokinetics of benazepril and benazeprilat are unaffected by **age**, clearance of amlodipine is decreased in the elderly, with resulting increases of 35%-70% in peak plasma levels, elimination half-life, and area-under-the-plasma-concentration curve. Dose adjustment may be required.

Pharmacodynamics

Single and multiple doses of 10 mg or more of **benazepril** cause inhibition of plasma ACE activity by at least 80%-90% for at least 24 hours after dosing. For up to 4 hours after a 10-mg dose, pressor responses to exogenous angiotensin I were inhibited by 60%-90%.

Administration of benazepril to patients with mild-to-moderate hypertension results in a reduction of both supine and standing blood pressure to about the same extent, with no compensatory tachycardia. Symptomatic postural hypotension is infrequent, although it can occur in patients who are salt and/or volume depleted *(see WARNINGS, Hypotension).*

The antihypertensive effects of benazepril were not appreciably different in patients receiving high- or low-sodium diets.

In normal human volunteers, single doses of benazepril caused an increase in renal blood flow but had no effect on glomerular filtration rate.

Following administration of therapeutic doses to patients with hypertension, **amlodipine** produces vasodilation resulting in a reduction of supine and standing blood pressures. These decreases in blood pressure are not accompanied by a significant change in heart rate or plasma catecholamine levels with chronic dosing. Plasma concentrations correlate with effect in both young and elderly patients.

As with other calcium channel blockers, hemodynamic measurements of cardiac function at rest and during exercise (or pacing) in patients with normal ventricular function treated with amlodipine have generally demonstrated a small increase in cardiac index without significant influence on dP/dt or on left ventricular end diastolic pressure or volume. In hemodynamic studies, amlodipine has not been associated with a negative inotropic effect when administered in the therapeutic dose range to intact animals and humans, even when coadministered with beta blockers to humans.

Amlodipine does not change sinoatrial (SA) nodal function or atrioventricular (AV) conduction in intact animals or humans. In clinical studies in which amlodipine was administered in combination with beta blockers to patients with either hypertension or angina, no adverse effects on electrocardiographic parameters were observed.

Continued on next page

Lotrel—Cont.

Over 950 patients received Lotrel once daily in six double-blind, placebo-controlled studies. Lotrel lowered blood pressure within 1 hour, with peak reductions achieved 2-8 hours after dosing. The antihypertensive effect of a single dose persisted for 24 hours.

Once-daily doses of benazepril/amlodipine using benazepril doses of 10-20 mg and amlodipine doses of 2.5-10 mg decreased seated pressure (systolic/diastolic) 24 hours after dosing by about 10-25/6-13 mmHg.

Combination therapy was effective in blacks and nonblacks. Both components contributed to the antihypertensive efficacy in nonblacks, but virtually all of the antihypertensive effect in blacks could be attributed to the amlodipine component. Among nonblack patients in placebo-controlled trials comparing Lotrel to the individual components, the blood pressure lowering effects of the combination were shown to be additive and in some cases synergistic.

During chronic therapy with Lotrel, the maximum reduction in blood pressure with any given dose is generally achieved after 1-2 weeks. The antihypertensive effects of Lotrel have continued during therapy for at least 1 year. Abrupt withdrawal of Lotrel has not been associated with a rapid increase in blood pressure.

INDICATIONS AND USAGE

Lotrel is indicated for the treatment of hypertension.

This fixed combination drug is not indicated for the initial therapy of hypertension ***(see DOSAGE AND ADMINISTRATION).***

In using Lotrel, consideration should be given to the fact that an ACE inhibitor, captopril, has caused agranulocytosis, particularly in patients with renal impairment or collagen-vascular disease. Available data are insufficient to show that benazepril does not have a similar risk *(see WARNINGS, Neutropenia/Agranulocytosis).*

Black patients receiving ACE inhibitors have been reported to have a higher incidence of angioedema compared to nonblacks.

CONTRAINDICATIONS

Lotrel is contraindicated in patients who are hypersensitive to benazepril, to any other ACE inhibitor, or to amlodipine.

WARNINGS

Anaphylactoid and Possibly Related Reactions

Presumably because angiotensin-converting enzyme inhibitors affect the metabolism of eicosanoids and polypeptides, including endogenous bradykinin, patients receiving ACE inhibitors (including Lotrel) may be subject to a variety of adverse reactions, some of them serious. These reactions usually occur after one of the first few doses of the ACE inhibitor, but they sometimes do not appear until after months of therapy.

Head and Neck Angioedema: Angioedema of the face, extremities, lips, tongue, glottis, and larynx has been reported in patients treated with ACE inhibitors. In U.S. clinical trials, symptoms consistent with angioedema were seen in none of the subjects who received placebo and in about 0.5% of the subjects who received benazepril. Angioedema associated with laryngeal edema can be fatal. If laryngeal stridor or angioedema of the face, tongue, or glottis occurs, treatment with Lotrel should be discontinued and appropriate therapy instituted immediately. *When involvement of the tongue, glottis, or larynx appears likely to cause airway obstruction, appropriate therapy, e.g., subcutaneous epinephrine injection 1:1000 (0.3-0.5 mL), should be promptly administered (see ADVERSE REACTIONS).*

Intestinal Angioedema: Intestinal angioedema has been reported in patients treated with ACE inhibitors. These patients presented with abdominal pain (with or without nausea or vomiting); in some cases there was no prior history of facial angioedema and C-1 esterase levels were normal. The angioedema was diagnosed by procedures including abdominal CT scan or ultrasound, or at surgery, and symptoms resolved after stopping the ACE inhibitor. Intestinal angioedema should be included in the differential diagnosis of patients on ACE inhibitors presenting with abdominal pain.

Anaphylactoid Reactions During Desensitization: Two patients undergoing desensitizing treatment with hymenoptera venom while receiving ACE inhibitors sustained life-threatening anaphylactoid reactions. In the same patients, these reactions were avoided when ACE inhibitors were temporarily withheld, but they reappeared upon inadvertent rechallenge.

Anaphylactoid Reactions During Membrane Exposure: Anaphylactoid reactions have been reported in patients dialyzed with high-flux membranes and treated concomitantly with an ACE inhibitor. Anaphylactoid reactions have also been reported in patients undergoing low-density lipoprotein apheresis with dextran sulfate absorption.

Increased Angina and/or Myocardial Infarction: Rarely, patients, particularly those with severe obstructive coronary artery disease, have developed documented increased frequency, duration, and/or severity of angina or acute myocardial infarction on starting calcium channel blocker therapy or at the time of dosage increase. The mechanism of this effect has not been elucidated.

Hypotension

Lotrel can cause symptomatic hypotension. Like other ACE inhibitors, benazepril has been only rarely associated with hypotension in uncomplicated hypertensive patients. Symptomatic hypotension is most likely to occur in patients who have been volume and/or salt depleted as a result of prolonged diuretic therapy, dietary salt restriction, dialysis, diarrhea, or vomiting. Volume and/or salt depletion should be corrected before initiating therapy with Lotrel.

Since the vasodilation induced by amlodipine is gradual in onset, acute hypotension has rarely been reported after oral administration of amlodipine. Nonetheless, caution should be exercised when administering Lotrel as with any other peripheral vasodilator, particularly in patients with severe aortic stenosis.

In patients with congestive heart failure, with or without associated renal insufficiency, ACE inhibitor therapy may cause excessive hypotension, which may be associated with oliguria, azotemia, and (rarely) with acute renal failure and death. In such patients, Lotrel therapy should be started under close medical supervision; they should be followed closely for the first 2 weeks of treatment and whenever the dose of the benazepril component is increased or a diuretic is added or its dose increased.

If hypotension occurs, the patient should be placed in a supine position, and if necessary, treated with intravenous infusion of physiologic saline. Lotrel treatment usually can be continued following restoration of blood pressure and volume.

Neutropenia/Agranulocytosis

Another ACE inhibitor, captopril, has been shown to cause agranulocytosis and bone marrow depression, rarely in uncomplicated patients (incidence probably less than once per 10,000 exposures) but more frequently (incidence possibly as great as once per 1000 exposures) in patients with renal impairment, especially those who also have collagen-vascular diseases such as systemic lupus erythematosus or scleroderma. Available data from clinical trials of benazepril are insufficient to show that benazepril does not cause agranulocytosis at similar rates. Monitoring of white blood cell counts should be considered in patients with collagen-vascular disease, especially if the disease is associated with impaired renal function.

Fetal/Neonatal Morbidity and Mortality

ACE inhibitors can cause fetal and neonatal morbidity and death when administered to pregnant women. Several dozen cases have been reported in the world literature. When pregnancy is detected, Lotrel should be discontinued as soon as possible.

The use of ACE inhibitors during the second and third trimesters of pregnancy has been associated with fetal and neonatal injury, including hypotension, neonatal skull hypoplasia, anuria, reversible or irreversible renal failure, and death. Oligohydramnios has also been reported, presumably resulting from decreased fetal renal function; oligohydramnios in this setting has been associated with fetal limb contractures, craniofacial deformation, and hypoplastic lung development. Prematurity, intrauterine growth retardation, and patent ductus arteriosus have also been reported, although it is not clear whether these occurrences were due to the ACE inhibitor exposure.

These adverse effects do not appear to have resulted from intrauterine ACE inhibitor exposure that has been limited to the first trimester. Mothers whose embryos and fetuses are exposed to ACE inhibitors only during the first trimester should be so informed. Nonetheless, when patients become pregnant, physicians should make every effort to discontinue the use of benazepril as soon as possible.

Rarely (probably less often than once in every thousand pregnancies), no alternative to ACE inhibitors will be found. In these rare cases, the mothers should be apprised of the potential hazards to their fetuses, and serial ultrasound examinations should be performed to assess the intra-amniotic environment.

If oligohydramnios is observed, benazepril should be discontinued unless it is considered life-saving for the mother. Contraction stress testing (CST), a nonstress test (NST), or biophysical profiling (BPP) may be appropriate, depending upon the week of pregnancy. Patients and physicians should be aware, however, that oligohydramnios may not appear until after the fetus has sustained irreversible injury.

Infants with histories of *in utero* exposure to ACE inhibitors should be closely observed for hypotension, oliguria, and hyperkalemia. If oliguria occurs, attention should be directed toward support of blood pressure and renal perfusion. Exchange transfusion or peritoneal dialysis may be required as means of reversing hypotension and/or substituting for disordered renal function. Benazepril, which crosses the placenta, can theoretically be removed from the neonatal circulation by these means; there are occasional reports of benefit from these maneuvers, but experience is limited.

Lotrel has not been adequately studied in pregnant women. When rats received benazepril:amlodipine at doses ranging from 5:2.5 to 50:25 mg/kg/day, dystocia was observed with increasing dose-related incidence at all doses tested. On a mg/m^2 basis, the 2.5 mg/kg/day dose of amlodipine is 3.6 times the amlodipine dose delivered when the maximum recommended dose of Lotrel is given to a 50-kg woman. Similarly, the 5 mg/kg/day dose of benazepril is approximately 2 times the benazepril dose delivered when the maximum recommended dose of Lotrel is given to a 50-kg woman.

No teratogenic effects were seen when benazepril and amlodipine were administered in combination to pregnant rats or rabbits. Rats received dose ratios up to 50:25 mg/kg/day (benazepril:amlodipine) (24 times the maximum recommended human dose on a mg/m^2 basis, assuming a 50-kg woman). Rabbits received doses of up to 1.5:0.75 (benazepril:amlodipine) mg/kg/day; on a mg/m^2 basis, this is 0.97 times the size of a maximum recommended dose of Lotrel given to a 50-kg woman.

Similar results were seen in animal studies involving benazepril alone and amlodipine alone.

Hepatic Failure

Rarely, ACE inhibitors have been associated with a syndrome that starts with cholestatic jaundice and progresses to fulminant hepatic necrosis and (sometimes) death. The mechanism of this syndrome is not understood. Patients receiving ACE inhibitors who develop jaundice or marked elevations of hepatic enzymes should discontinue the ACE inhibitor and receive appropriate medical follow-up.

PRECAUTIONS

General

Impaired Renal Function: Lotrel should be used with caution in patients with severe renal disease.

When the renin-angiotensin-aldosterone system is inhibited by benazepril, changes in renal function may be anticipated in susceptible individuals. In patients with **severe congestive heart failure,** whose renal function may depend on the activity of the renin-angiotensin-aldosterone system, treatment with ACE inhibitors (including benazepril) may be associated with oliguria and/or progressive azotemia and (rarely) with acute renal failure and/or death.

In a small study of hypertensive patients with **unilateral or bilateral renal artery stenosis**, treatment with benazepril was associated with increases in blood urea nitrogen and serum creatinine; these increases were reversible upon discontinuation of benazepril therapy, concomitant diuretic therapy, or both. When such patients are treated with Lotrel, renal function should be monitored during the first few weeks of therapy.

Some benazepril-treated hypertensive patients with **no apparent preexisting renal vascular disease** have developed increases in blood urea nitrogen and serum creatinine, usually minor and transient, especially when benazepril has been given concomitantly with a diuretic. Dosage reduction of Lotrel may be required. **Evaluation of the hypertensive patient should always include assessment of renal function** *(see DOSAGE AND ADMINISTRATION).*

Hyperkalemia: In U.S. placebo-controlled trials of Lotrel, hyperkalemia (serum potassium at least 0.5 mEq/L greater than the upper limit of normal) not present at baseline occurred in approximately 1.5% of hypertensive patients receiving Lotrel. Increases in serum potassium were generally reversible. Risk factors for the development of hyperkalemia include renal insufficiency, diabetes mellitus, and the concomitant use of potassium-sparing diuretics, potassium supplements, and/or potassium-containing salt substitutes.

Patients With Congestive Heart Failure: Although hemodynamic studies and a controlled trial in patients with NYHA Class II-III heart failure have shown that amlodipine did not lead to clinical deterioration as measured by exercise tolerance, left ventricular ejection fraction, and clinical symptomatology, studies have not been performed in patients with NYHA Class IV heart failure. In general, all calcium channel blockers should be used with caution in patients with heart failure.

Patients With Hepatic Failure: In patients with hepatic dysfunction due to cirrhosis, levels of benazeprilat are essentially unaltered. However, since amlodipine is extensively metabolized by the liver and the plasma elimination half-life ($t_{½}$) is 56 hours in patients with impaired hepatic function, caution should be exercised when administering Lotrel to patients with severe hepatic impairment *(see also WARNINGS).*

Cough: Presumably due to the inhibition of the degradation of endogenous bradykinin, persistent nonproductive cough has been reported with all ACE inhibitors, always resolving after discontinuation of therapy. ACE inhibitor-induced cough should be considered in the differential diagnosis of cough.

Surgery/Anesthesia: In patients undergoing surgery or during anesthesia with agents that produce hypotension, benazepril will block the angiotensin II formation that could otherwise occur secondary to compensatory renin release. Hypotension that occurs as a result of this mechanism can be corrected by volume expansion.

Drug Interactions

Diuretics: Patients on diuretics, especially those in whom diuretic therapy was recently instituted, may occasionally experience an excessive reduction of blood pressure after initiation of therapy with Lotrel. The possibility of hypotensive effects with Lotrel can be minimized by either discontinuing the diuretic or increasing the salt intake prior to initiation of treatment with Lotrel.

Potassium Supplements and Potassium-Sparing Diuretics: Benazepril can attenuate potassium loss caused by thiazide diuretics. Potassium-sparing diuretics (spironolactone, amiloride, triamterene, and others) or potassium supplements can increase the risk of hyperkalemia. If concomitant use of such agents is indicated, they should be given with caution, and the patient's serum potassium should be monitored frequently.

Lithium: Increased serum lithium levels and symptoms of lithium toxicity have been reported in patients receiving ACE inhibitors during therapy with lithium. Lotrel and lithium should be coadministered with caution, and frequent monitoring of serum lithium levels is recommended.

Other: Benazepril has been used concomitantly with oral anticoagulants, beta-adrenergic-blocking agents, calcium-blocking agents, cimetidine, diuretics, digoxin, hydralazine, and naproxen without evidence of clinically important adverse interactions.

In clinical trials, amlodipine has been safely administered with thiazide diuretics, beta blockers, ACE inhibitors, long-acting nitrates, sublingual nitroglycerin, digoxin, warfarin, nonsteroidal anti-inflammatory drugs, antibiotics, and oral hypoglycemic drugs.

In vitro data in human plasma indicate that amlodipine has no effect on the protein binding of drugs tested (digoxin, phenytoin, warfarin, and indomethacin). Special studies have indicated that the coadministration of amlodipine with digoxin did not change serum digoxin levels or digoxin renal clearance in normal volunteers; that coadministration with cimetidine did not alter the pharmacokinetics of amlodipine; and that coadministration with warfarin did not change the warfarin-induced prothrombin response time.

Carcinogenesis, Mutagenesis, Impairment of Fertility

No evidence of carcinogenicity was found when **benazepril** was given, via dietary administration, to rats and mice for 104 weeks at doses up to 150 mg/kg/day. On a body-weight basis, this dose is over 100 times the maximum recommended human dose; on a body-surface-area basis, this dose is 18 times (rats) and 9 times (mice) the maximum recommended human dose. No mutagenic activity was detected in the Ames test in bacteria, in an *in vitro* test for forward mutations in cultured mammalian cells, or in a nucleus anomaly test. At doses of 50-500 mg/kg/day (38-375 times the maximum recommended human dose on a body-weight basis; 6-61 times the maximum recommended dose on a body-surface-area basis), benazepril had no adverse effect on the reproductive performance of male and female rats.

Rats and mice treated with amlodipine in the diet for 2 years, at concentrations calculated to provide daily dosage levels of 0.5, 1.25, and 2.5 mg/kg/day, showed no evidence of carcinogenicity. For mice, but not for rats, the highest dose was close to the maximum tolerated dose. On a mg/m^2 basis, this dose given to mice was approximately equal to the maximum recommended clinical dose. On the same basis, the same dose given to rats was approximately twice the maximum recommended clinical dose.

Mutagenicity studies with amlodipine revealed no drug-related effects at either the gene or chromosome levels.

There was no effect on the fertility of rats treated with amlodipine (males for 64 days and females for 14 days prior to mating) at doses up to 10 mg/kg/day (8 times the maximum recommended human dose of 10 mg on a mg/m^2 basis, assuming a 50-kg person).

No adverse effects on fertility occurred when the benazepril:amlodipine combination was given orally to rats of either sex at dose ratios up to 15:7.5 mg/kg/day (benazepril: amlodipine), prior to mating and throughout gestation.

Pregnancy

Pregnancy Categories C (first trimester) and D (second and third trimesters): *See WARNINGS, Fetal/Neonatal Morbidity and Mortality.*

Nursing Mothers

Minimal amounts of unchanged benazepril and of benazeprilat are excreted into the breast milk of lactating women treated with benazepril, so that a newborn child ingesting nothing but breast milk would receive less than 0.1% of the maternal doses of benazepril and benazeprilat.

It is not known whether amlodipine is excreted in human milk. In the absence of this information, it is recommended that nursing be discontinued while Lotrel is administered.

Geriatric Use

Of the total number of patients who received Lotrel in U.S. clinical studies of Lotrel, over 19% were 65 or older while about 2% were 75 or older. Overall differences in effectiveness or safety were not observed between these patients and younger patients. Clinical experience has not identified differences in responses between the elderly and younger patients, but greater sensitivity of some older individuals cannot be ruled out.

Benazepril and benazeprilat are substantially excreted by the kidney. Because elderly patients are more likely to have decreased renal function, care should be taken in dose selection, and it may be useful to monitor renal function.

Amlodipine is extensively metabolized in the liver. In the elderly, clearance of amlodipine is decreased with resulting increases in peak plasma levels, elimination half-life and area-under-the-plasma-concentration curve. Thus a lower starting dose may be required in older patients *(see DOSAGE AND ADMINISTRATION).*

Pediatric Use

Safety and effectiveness in pediatric patients have not been established.

ADVERSE REACTIONS

Lotrel has been evaluated for safety in over 1,850 patients with hypertension; over 500 of these patients were treated for at least 6 months, and over 400 were treated for more than 1 year.

In a pooled analysis of 5 placebo-controlled trials involving Lotrel doses up to 5/20, the reported side effects were generally mild and transient, and there was no relationship between side effects and age, sex, race, or duration of therapy. Discontinuation of therapy due to side effects was required in approximately 4% of patients treated with Lotrel and in 3% of patients treated with placebo.

The most common reasons for discontinuation of therapy with Lotrel in these studies were cough and edema.*

The side effects considered possibly or probably related to study drug that occurred in these trials in more than 1% of patients treated with Lotrel are shown in the table below.

PERCENT INCIDENCE BY SEX OF CERTAIN ADVERSE EVENTS

	Benazepril/Amlodipine		Benazepril		Amlodipine		Placebo	
	Male N=329	Female N=431	Male N=269	Female N=285	Male N=277	Female N=198	Male N=217	Female N=191
Edema	0.6	3.2	0.0	1.8	2.2	9.1	1.4	3.1
Flushing	0.3	0.0	0.0	0.7	0.4	2.0	0.5	0.0
Palpitations	0.3	0.5	0.4	1.4	0.4	2.0	0.5	0.5
Somnolence	0.3	0.0	0.4	0.4	0.4	0.5	0.0	0.0

PERCENT INCIDENCE IN U.S. PLACEBO-CONTROLLED TRIALS

	Benazepril/ Amlodipine N=760	Benazepril N=554	Amlodipine N=475	Placebo N=408
Cough	3.3	1.8	0.4	0.2
Headache	2.2	3.8	2.9	5.6
Dizziness	1.3	1.6	2.3	1.5
Edema*	2.1	0.9	5.1	2.2

*Edema refers to all edema, such as dependent edema, angioedema, facial edema.

The incidence of edema was statistically greater in patients treated with amlodipine monotherapy than in patients treated with the combination. Edema and certain other side effects are associated with amlodipine monotherapy in a dose-dependent manner, and appear to affect women more than men. The addition of benazepril resulted in lower incidences as shown in the following table; the protective effect of benazepril was independent of race and (within the range of doses tested) of dose.

[See first table above]

In a trial (n=386) comparing placebo, Lotrel 5/20, and Lotrel 10/20, edema and dizziness were most commonly reported in the Lotrel 10/20 group.

Other side effects considered possibly or probably related to study drug that occurred in U.S. placebo-controlled trials of patients treated with Lotrel or in postmarketing experience were the following:

Angioedema: Includes edema of the lips or face without other manifestations of angioedema *(see WARNINGS, Angioedema).*

Body as a Whole: Asthenia and fatigue.

CNS: Insomnia, nervousness, anxiety, tremor, and decreased libido.

Dermatologic: Flushing, hot flashes, rash, skin nodule, and dermatitis.

Digestive: Dry mouth, nausea, abdominal pain, constipation, diarrhea, dyspepsia, and esophagitis.

Metabolic and Nutritional: Hypokalemia.

Musculoskeletal: Back pain, musculoskeletal pain, cramps, and muscle cramps.

Respiratory: Pharyngitis.

Urogenital: Sexual problems such as impotence, and polyuria.

Other infrequently reported events were seen in clinical trials (causal relationship unlikely) or in postmarketing experience. These included chest pain, ventricular extrasystole, gout, neuritis, tinnitus, alopecia and upper respiratory tract infection.

Fetal/Neonatal Morbidity and Mortality: *See WARNINGS, Fetal/Neonatal Morbidity and Mortality.*

Monotherapies of benazepril and amlodipine have been evaluated for safety in clinical trials in over 6,000 and 11,000 patients, respectively. The observed adverse reactions to the monotherapies in these trials were similar to those seen in trials of Lotrel. In postmarketing experience with benazepril, there have been rare reports of Stevens-Johnson syndrome, pancreatitis, hemolytic anemia, pemphigus, and thrombocytopenia. Jaundice and hepatic enzyme elevations (mostly consistent with cholestasis) severe enough to require hospitalization have been reported in association with use of amlodipine. Other potentially important adverse experiences attributed to other ACE inhibitors and calcium channel blockers include: eosinophilic pneumonitis (ACE inhibitors) and gynecomastia (CCB's).

Clinical Laboratory Test Findings

Serum Electrolytes: *See PRECAUTIONS.*

Creatinine: Minor reversible increases in serum creatinine were observed in patients with essential hypertension treated with Lotrel. Increases in creatinine are more likely to occur in patients with renal insufficiency or those pretreated with a diuretic and, based on experience with other ACE inhibitors, would be expected to be especially likely in patients with renal artery stenosis *(see PRECAUTIONS, General).*

Other (causal relationships unknown): Clinically important changes in standard laboratory tests were rarely associated with Lotrel administration. Elevations of serum bilirubin and uric acid have been reported as have scattered incidents of elevations of liver enzymes.

OVERDOSAGE

Only a few cases of human overdose with amlodipine have been reported. One patient was asymptomatic after a 250-mg ingestion; another, who combined 70 mg of amlodipine with an unknown large quantity of a benzodiazepine, developed refractory shock and died.

Human overdoses with any combination of amlodipine and benazepril have not been reported. In scattered reports of human overdoses with benazepril and other ACE inhibitors, there are no reports of death.

When mice were given single oral doses of benazepril/amlodipine, mortality was 20% at 50:25 mg/kg, 10% at 100:50 mg/kg, and 100% at 500:250 mg/kg. In rats, mortality was 25% (pooling two studies) at 500:250 mg/kg and 100% at 900:450 mg/kg.

Treatment: To obtain up-to-date information about the treatment of overdose, a good resource is your certified Regional Poison-Control Center. Telephone numbers of certified poison-control centers are listed in the Physicians' Desk Reference** (PDR). In managing overdose, consider the possibilities of multiple-drug overdoses, drug-drug interactions, and unusual drug kinetics in your patient.

The most likely effect of overdose with Lotrel is vasodilation, with consequent hypotension and tachycardia. Simple repletion of central fluid volume (Trendelenburg positioning, infusion of crystalloids) may be sufficient therapy, but pressor agents (norepinephrine or high-dose dopamine) may be required. Overdoses of other dihydropyridine calcium channel blockers are reported to have been treated with calcium chloride and glucagon, but evidence of a dose-response relation has not been seen, and these interventions must be regarded as unproven. With abrupt return of peripheral vascular tone, overdoses of other dihydropyridine calcium channel blockers have sometimes progressed to pulmonary edema, and patients must be monitored for this complication.

Analyses of bodily fluids for concentrations of amlodipine, benazepril, or their metabolites are not widely available. Such analyses are, in any event, not known to be of value in therapy or prognosis.

No data are available to suggest physiologic maneuvers (e.g., maneuvers to change the pH of the urine) that might accelerate elimination of amlodipine, benazepril, or their metabolites. Benazeprilat is only slightly dialyzable; attempted clearance of amlodipine by hemodialysis or hemoperfusion has not been reported, but amlodipine's high protein binding makes it unlikely that these interventions will be of value.

Angiotensin II could presumably serve as a specific antagonist-antidote to benazepril, but angiotensin II is essentially unavailable outside of scattered research laboratories.

DOSAGE AND ADMINISTRATION

Amlodipine is an effective treatment of hypertension in once-daily doses of 2.5-10 mg while benazepril is effective in doses of 10-80 mg. In clinical trials of amlodipine/benazepril combination therapy using amlodipine doses of 2.5-10 mg and benazepril doses of 10-20 mg, the antihypertensive effects increased with increasing dose of amlodipine in all patient groups, and the effects increased with increasing dose of benazepril in nonblack groups. All patient groups benefited from the reduction in amlodipine-induced edema *(see below).*

The hazards *(see WARNINGS)* of benazepril are generally independent of dose; those of amlodipine are a mixture of dose-dependent phenomena (primarily peripheral edema) and dose-independent phenomena, the former much more common than the latter. When benazepril is added to a regimen of amlodipine, the incidence of edema is substantially reduced. Therapy with any combination of amlodipine and benazepril will thus be associated with both sets of dose-independent hazards, but the incidence of edema will generally be less than that seen with similar (or higher) doses of amlodipine monotherapy.

Rarely, the dose-independent hazards of benazepril are serious. To minimize dose-independent hazards, it is usually appropriate to begin therapy with Lotrel only after a patient has either (a) failed to achieve the desired antihypertensive effect with one or the other monotherapy, or (b) demonstrated inability to achieve adequate antihypertensive effect with amlodipine therapy without developing edema.

Dose Titration Guided by Clinical Effect: A patient whose blood pressure is not adequately controlled with amlodipine (or another dihydropyridine) alone or with benazepril (or another ACE inhibitor) alone may be switched to combination therapy with Lotrel. The addition of benazepril to a regimen of amlodipine should not be expected to provide additional antihypertensive effect in African-Americans. However, all patient groups benefit from the reduction in amlodipine-induced edema. Dosage must be guided by clinical response; steady-state levels of benazepril and amlodipine will be reached after approximately 2 and 7 days of dosing, respectively.

In patients whose blood pressures are adequately controlled with amlodipine but who experience unacceptable edema,

Continued on next page

Lotrel—Cont.

combination therapy may achieve similar (or better) blood pressure control without edema. Especially in nonblacks, it may be prudent to minimize the risk of excessive response by reducing the dose of amlodipine as benazepril is added to the regimen.

Replacement Therapy: For convenience, patients receiving amlodipine and benazepril from separate tablets may instead wish to receive capsules of Lotrel containing the same component doses.

Use in Patients With Metabolic Impairments: Regimens of therapy with Lotrel need not take account of renal function as long as the patient's creatinine clearance is >30 mL/min/1.73m^2 (serum creatinine roughly ≤3 mg/dL or 265 µmol/L). In patients with more severe renal impairment, the recommended initial dose of benazepril is 5 mg. Lotrel is not recommended in these patients.

In small, elderly, frail, or hepatically impaired patients, the recommended initial dose of amlodipine, as monotherapy or as a component of combination therapy, is 2.5 mg.

HOW SUPPLIED

Lotrel is available as capsules containing amlodipine besylate equivalent to 2.5 mg, 5 mg or 10 mg of amlodipine, with 10 mg or 20 mg of benazepril hydrochloride providing for the following available combinations: 2.5/10 mg, 5/10 mg, 5/20 mg and 10/20 mg. All four strengths are packaged with a desiccant in bottles of 100 capsules.

Capsules are imprinted with "Lotrel" and a portion of the NDC code.

Dose	Capsule Color/Code	NDC Code Bottle of 100
2.5/10 mg	white with 2 gold bands/2255	NDC 0083-2255-30
5/10 mg	light brown with 2 white bands//2260	NDC 0083-2260-30
5/20 mg	pink with 2 white bands/2265	NDC 0083-2265-30
10/20 mg	purple (amethyst) with 2 white bands/0364	NDC 0078-0364-05

Storage: Store at 25°C (77°F); excursions permitted to 15-30°C (59-86°F).

[See USP controlled room temperature.]

Protect from moisture. Dispense in tight container (USP).

T2004-36

REV: JUNE 2004 Printed in U.S.A. 89008409

Manufactured by:

Novartis Pharmaceuticals Corporation

Suffern, New York 10901

Distributed by:

Novartis Pharmaceuticals Corporation

East Hanover, New Jersey 07936

Shown in Product Identification Guide, page 325

MIACALCIN® ℞

[mī "ă-kal 'sin]

(calcitonin-salmon)

Injection, Synthetic

Rx Only

Prescribing Information

The following prescribing information is based on official labeling in effect July 2003.

DESCRIPTION

Calcitonin is a polypeptide hormone secreted by the parafollicular cells of the thyroid gland in mammals and by the ultimobranchial gland of birds and fish.

Miacalcin® (calcitonin-salmon) Injection, Synthetic is a synthetic polypeptide of 32 amino acids in the same linear sequence that is found in calcitonin of salmon origin. This is shown by the following graphic formula:

```
  ┌────────────────────────────┐
H-Cys-Ser-Asn-Leu-Ser-Thr-Cys-Val-Leu-
  1   2   3   4   5   6   7   8   9

Gly-Lys-Leu-Ser-Gln-Glu-Leu-His-Lys-Leu-
10  11  12  13  14  15  16  17  18  19

Gln-Thr-Tyr-Pro-Arg-Thr-Asn-Thr-Gly-Ser-
20  21  22  23  24  25  26  27  28  29

Gly-Thr-Pro-NH2
30  31  32
```

It is provided in sterile solution for subcutaneous or intramuscular injection. Each milliliter contains; calcitonin-salmon 200 I.U., acetic acid, USP, 2.25 mg; phenol, USP, 5.0 mg; sodium acetate trihydrate, USP, 2.0 mg; sodium chloride, USP, 7.5 mg; water for injection, USP, qs to 1.0 mL. The activity of Miacalcin® (calcitonin-salmon) is stated in International Units based on bioassay in comparison with the International Reference Preparation of calcitonin-salmon for Bioassay, distributed by the National Institute for Biological Standards and Control, Holly Hill, London.

CLINICAL PHARMACOLOGY

Calcitonin acts primarily on bone, but direct renal effects and actions on the gastrointestinal tract are also recognized. Calcitonin-salmon appears to have actions essentially identical to calcitonins of mammalian origin, but its potency per mg is greater and it has a longer duration of action. The actions of calcitonin on bone and its role in normal human bone physiology are still incompletely understood.

Bone—Single injections of calcitonin cause a marked transient inhibition of the ongoing bone resorptive process. With prolonged use, there is a persistent, smaller decrease in the rate of bone resorption. Histologically, this is associated with a decreased number of osteoclasts and an apparent decrease in their resorptive activity. Decreased osteocytic resorption may also be involved. There is some evidence that initially bone formation may be augmented by calcitonin through increased osteoblastic activity. However, calcitonin will probably not induce a long-term increase in bone formation.

Animal studies indicate that endogenous calcitonin, primarily through its action on bone, participates with parathyroid hormone in the homeostatic regulation of blood calcium. Thus, high blood calcium levels cause increased secretion of calcitonin which, in turn, inhibits bone resorption. This reduces the transfer of calcium from bone to blood and tends to return blood calcium to the normal level. The importance of this process in humans has not been determined. In normal adults, who have a relatively low rate of bone resorption, the administration of exogenous calcitonin results in only a slight decrease in serum calcium. In normal children and in patients with generalized Paget's disease, bone resorption is more rapid and decreases in serum calcium are more pronounced in response to calcitonin.

Paget's Disease of Bone (osteitis deformans)—Paget's disease is a disorder of uncertain etiology characterized by abnormal and accelerated bone formation and resorption in one or more bones. In most patients only small areas of bone are involved and the disease is not symptomatic. In a small fraction of patients, however, the abnormal bone may lead to bone pain and bone deformity, cranial and spinal nerve entrapment, or spinal cord compression. The increased vascularity of the abnormal bone may lead to high output congestive heart failure.

Active Paget's disease involving a large mass of bone may increase the urinary hydroxyproline excretion (reflecting breakdown of collagen-containing bone matrix) and serum alkaline phosphatase (reflecting increased bone formation).

Calcitonin-salmon, presumably by an initial blocking effect on bone resorption, causes a decreased rate of bone turnover with a resultant fall in the serum alkaline phosphatase and urinary hydroxyproline excretion in approximately 2/3 of patients treated. These biochemical changes appear to correspond to changes toward more normal bone, as evidenced by a small number of documented examples of: 1) radiologic regression of Pagetic lesions, 2) improvement of impaired auditory nerve and other neurologic function, 3) decreases (measured) in abnormally elevated cardiac output. These improvements occur extremely rarely, if ever, spontaneously (elevated cardiac output may disappear over a period of years when the disease slowly enters a sclerotic phase; in the cases treated with calcitonin, however, the decreases were seen in less than one year.)

Some patients with Paget's disease who have good biochemical and/or symptomatic responses initially, later relapse. Suggested explanations have included the formation of neutralizing antibodies and the development of secondary hyperparathyroidism, but neither suggestion appears to explain adequately the majority of relapses.

Although the parathyroid hormone levels do appear to rise transiently during each hypocalcemic response to calcitonin, most investigators have been unable to demonstrate persistent hypersecretion of parathyroid hormone in patients treated chronically with calcitonin-salmon.

Circulating antibodies to calcitonin after 2–18 months' treatment have been reported in about half of the patients with Paget's disease in whom antibody studies were done, but calcitonin treatment remained effective in many of these cases. Occasionally, patients with high antibody titers are found. These patients usually will have suffered a biochemical relapse of Paget's disease and are unresponsive to the acute hypocalcemic effects of calcitonin.

Hypercalcemia—In clinical trials, calcitonin-salmon has been shown to lower the elevated serum calcium of patients with carcinoma (with or without demonstrated metastases), multiple myeloma or primary hyperparathyroidism (lesser response). Patients with higher values for serum calcium tend to show greater reduction during calcitonin therapy. The decrease in calcium occurs about 2 hours after the first injection and lasts for about 6–8 hours. Calcitonin-salmon given every 12 hours maintained a calcium lowering effect for about 5–8 days, the time period evaluated for most patients during the clinical studies. The average reduction of 8-hour post-injection serum calcium during this period was about 9 percent.

Kidney—Calcitonin increases the excretion of filtered phosphate, calcium, and sodium by decreasing their tubular reabsorption. In some patients, the inhibition of bone resorption by calcitonin is of such magnitude that the consequent reduction of filtered calcium load more than compensates for the decrease in tubular reabsorption of calcium. The result in these patients is a decrease rather than an increase in urinary calcium.

Transient increases in sodium and water excretion may occur after the initial injection of calcitonin. In most patients, these changes return to pretreatment levels with continued therapy.

Gastrointestinal Tract—Increasing evidence indicates that calcitonin has significant actions on the gastrointestinal tract. Short-term administration results in marked transient decreases in the volume and acidity of gastric juice and in the volume and the trypsin and amylase content of pancreatic juice. Whether these effects continue to be elicited after each injection of calcitonin during chronic therapy has not been investigated.

Metabolism—The metabolism of calcitonin-salmon has not yet been studied clinically. Information from animal studies with calcitonin-salmon and from clinical studies with calcitonins of porcine and human origin suggest that calcitonin-salmon is rapidly metabolized by conversion to smaller inactive fragments, primarily in the kidneys, but also in the blood and peripheral tissues. A small amount of unchanged hormone and its inactive metabolites are excreted in the urine.

It appears that calcitonin-salmon cannot cross the placental barrier and its passage to the cerebrospinal fluid or to breast milk has not been determined.

INDICATIONS AND USAGE

Miacalcin® (calcitonin-salmon) Injection, Synthetic is indicated for the treatment of symptomatic Paget's disease of bone, for the treatment of hypercalcemia, and for the treatment of postmenopausal osteoporosis.

Paget's Disease—At the present time, effectiveness has been demonstrated principally in patients with moderate to severe disease characterized by polyostotic involvement with elevated serum alkaline phosphatase and urinary hydroxyproline excretion.

In these patients, the biochemical abnormalities were substantially improved (more than 30% reduction) in about 2/3 of patients studied, and bone pain was improved in a similar fraction. A small number of documented instances of reversal of neurologic deficits has occurred, including improvement in the basilar compression syndrome, and improvement of spinal cord and spinal nerve lesions. At present, there is too little experience to predict the likelihood of improvement of any given neurologic lesion. Hearing loss, the most common neurologic lesion of Paget's disease, is improved infrequently (4 of 29 patients studied audiometrically).

Patients with increased cardiac output due to extensive Paget's disease have had measured decreases in cardiac output while receiving calcitonin. The number of treated patients in this category is still too small to predict how likely such a result will be.

The large majority of patients with localized, especially monostotic disease do not develop symptoms and most patients with mild symptoms can be managed with analgesics. There is no evidence that the prophylactic use of calcitonin is beneficial in asymptomatic patients, although treatment may be considered in exceptional circumstances in which there is extensive involvement of the skull or spinal cord with the possibility of irreversible neurologic damage. In these instances, treatment would be based on the demonstrated effect of calcitonin on Pagetic bone, rather than on clinical studies in the patient population in question.

Hypercalcemia—Miacalcin® (calcitonin-salmon) Injection, Synthetic is indicated for early treatment of hypercalcemic emergencies, along with other appropriate agents, when a rapid decrease in serum calcium is required, until more specific treatment of the underlying disease can be accomplished. It may also be added to existing therapeutic regimens for hypercalcemia such as intravenous fluids and furosemide, oral phosphate or corticosteroids, or other agents.

Postmenopausal Osteoporosis—Miacalcin® (calcitonin-salmon) Injection, Synthetic is indicated for the treatment of postmenopausal osteoporosis in females greater than 5 years postmenopause with low bone mass relative to healthy premenopausal females. Miacalcin® (calcitonin-salmon) Injection should be reserved for patients who refuse or cannot tolerate estrogens or in whom estrogens are contraindicated. Use of Miacalcin® (calcitonin-salmon) Injection is recommended in conjunction with adequate calcium and vitamin D intake to prevent the progressive loss of bone mass. No evidence currently exists to indicate whether or not Miacalcin® (calcitonin-salmon) decreases the risk of vertebral crush fractures or spinal deformity. A recent controlled study, which was discontinued prior to completion because of questions regarding its design and implementation, failed to demonstrate any benefit of salmon calcitonin on fracture rate. No adequate controlled trials have examined the effect of salmon calcitonin injection on vertebral bone mineral density beyond 1 year of treatment. Two placebo-controlled studies with salmon calcitonin have shown an increase in total body calcium at 1 year, followed by a trend to decreasing total body calcium (still above baseline) at 2 years. The minimum effective dose of Miacalcin® (calcitonin-salmon) for prevention of vertebral bone mineral density loss has not been established. It has been suggested that those postmenopausal patients having increased rates of bone turnover may be more likely to respond to antiresorptive agents such as Miacalcin® (calcitonin-salmon).

CONTRAINDICATIONS

Clinical allergy to synthetic calcitonin-salmon.

WARNINGS

Allergic Reactions

Because calcitonin is protein in nature, the possibility of a systemic allergic reaction exists. **Administration of calcitonin-salmon has been reported in a few cases to**

cause serious allergic-type reactions (e.g. bronchospasm, swelling of the tongue or throat, and anaphylactic shock), and in one case, death attributed to anaphylaxis. The usual provisions should be made for the emergency treatment of such a reaction should it occur. Allergic reactions should be differentiated from generalized flushing and hypotension.

For patients with suspected sensitivity to calcitonin, skin testing should be considered prior to treatment utilizing a dilute, sterile solution of Miacalcin® (calcitonin-salmon) Injection, Synthetic. Physicians may wish to refer patients who require skin testing to an allergist. A detailed skin testing protocol is available from the Medical Services Department of Novartis Pharmaceuticals Corporation.

The incidence of osteogenic sarcoma is known to be increased in Paget's disease. Pagetic lesions, with or without therapy, may appear by X-ray to progress markedly, possibly with some loss of definition of periosteal margins. Such lesions should be evaluated carefully to differentiate these from osteogenic sarcoma.

PRECAUTIONS

1. General

The administration of calcitonin possibly could lead to hypocalcemic tetany under special circumstances although no cases have yet been reported. Provisions for parenteral calcium administration should be available during the first several administrations of calcitonin.

2. Laboratory Tests

Periodic examinations of urine sediment of patients on chronic therapy are recommended.

Coarse granular casts and casts containing renal tubular epithelial cells were reported in young adult volunteers at bed rest who were given calcitonin-salmon to study the effect of immobilization on osteoporosis. There was no other evidence of renal abnormality and the urine sediment became normal after calcitonin was stopped. Urine sediment abnormalities have not been reported by other investigators.

3. Instructions for the Patient

Careful instruction in sterile injection technique should be given to the patient, and to other persons who may administer Miacalcin® (calcitonin-salmon) Injection, Synthetic.

4. Carcinogenesis, Mutagenesis, and Impairment of Fertility

An increased incidence of pituitary adenomas has been observed in one-year toxicity studies in Sprague-Dawley rats administered calcitonin-salmon at dosages of 20 and 80 I.U./kg/day and in Fisher 344 rats given 80 I.U./kg/day.

The relevance of these findings to humans is unknown. Calcitonin-salmon was not mutagenic in tests using *Salmonella typhimurium, Escherichia coli,* and Chinese Hamster V79 cells.

5. Pregnancy: Teratogenic Effects

Category C

Calcitonin-salmon has been shown to cause a decrease in fetal birth weights in rabbits when given in doses 14–56 times the dose recommended for human use. Since calcitonin does not cross the placental barrier, this finding may be due to metabolic effects on the pregnant animal. There are no adequate and well-controlled studies in pregnant women. Miacalcin® (calcitonin-salmon) Injection, Synthetic should be used during pregnancy only if the potential benefit justifies the potential risk to the fetus.

6. Nursing Mothers

It is not known whether this drug is excreted in human milk. As a general rule, nursing should not be undertaken while a patient is on this drug since many drugs are excreted in human milk. Calcitonin has been shown to inhibit lactation in animals.

7. Pediatric Use

Disorders of bone in children referred to as juvenile Paget's disease have been reported rarely. The relationship of these disorders to adult Paget's disease has not been established and experience with the use of calcitonin in these disorders is very limited. There is no adequate data to support the use of Miacalcin® (calcitonin-salmon) Injection, Synthetic in children.

ADVERSE REACTIONS

Gastrointestinal System

Nausea with or without vomiting has been noted in about 10% of patients treated with calcitonin. It is most evident when treatment is first initiated and tends to decrease or disappear with continued administration.

Dermatologic/Hypersensitivity

Local inflammatory reactions at the site of subcutaneous or intramuscular injection have been reported in about 10% of patients. Flushing of face or hands occurred in about 2–5% of patients. Skin rashes, nocturia, pruritus of the ear lobes, feverish sensation, pain in the eyes, poor appetite, abdominal pain, edema of feet, and salty taste have been reported in patients treated with calcitonin-salmon. Administration of calcitonin-salmon has been reported in a few cases to cause serious allergic-type reactions (e.g. bronchospasm, swelling of the tongue or throat, and anaphylactic shock), and in one case, death attributed to anaphylaxis *(see WARNINGS).*

OVERDOSAGE

A dose of 1000 I.U. subcutaneously may produce nausea and vomiting as the only adverse effects. Doses of 32 units per kg per day for 1–2 days demonstrate no other adverse effects.

Data on chronic high dose administration are insufficient to judge toxicity.

DOSAGE AND ADMINISTRATION

Paget's Disease—The recommended starting dose of calcitonin-salmon in Paget's disease is 100 I.U. (0.5 mL) per day administered subcutaneously (preferred for outpatient self-administration) or intramuscularly. Drug effect should be monitored by periodic measurement of serum alkaline phosphatase and 24-hour urinary hydroxyproline (if available) and evaluations of symptoms. A decrease toward normal of the biochemical abnormalities is usually seen, if it is going to occur, within the first few months. Bone pain may also decrease during that time. Improvement of neurologic lesions, when it occurs, requires a longer period of treatment, often more than one year.

In many patients, doses of 50 I.U. (0.25 mL) per day or every other day are sufficient to maintain biochemical and clinical improvement. At the present time, however, there are insufficient data to determine whether this reduced dose will have the same effect as the higher dose on forming more normal bone structure. It appears preferable, therefore, to maintain the higher dose in any patient with serious deformity or neurological involvement.

In any patient with a good response initially who later relapses, either clinically or biochemically, the possibility of antibody formation should be explored. The patient may be tested for antibodies by an appropriate specialized test or evaluated for the possibility of antibody formation by critical clinical evaluation.

Patient compliance should also be assessed in the event of relapse.

In patients who relapse, whether because of antibodies or for unexplained reasons, a dosage increase beyond 100 I.U. per day does not usually appear to elicit an improved response.

Hypercalcemia—The recommended starting dose of Miacalcin® (calcitonin-salmon) Injection, Synthetic in hypercalcemia is 4 I.U./kg body weight every 12 hours by subcutaneous or intramuscular injection. If the response to this dose is not satisfactory after one or two days, the dose may be increased to 8 I.U./kg every 12 hours. If the response remains unsatisfactory after two more days, the dose may be further increased to a maximum of 8 I.U./kg every 6 hours.

Postmenopausal Osteoporosis—The minimum effective dose of salmon calcitonin for the prevention of vertebral bone mineral density loss has not been established. Data from a single one-year placebo-controlled study with salmon calcitonin injection suggested that 100 I.U. (subcutaneously or intramuscularly) every other day might be effective in preserving vertebral bone mineral density. Baseline and interval monitoring of biochemical markers of bone resorption/turnover (e.g., fasting AM, second-voided urine hydroxyproline to creatinine ratio) and of bone mineral density may be useful in achieving the minimum effective dose.

Patients should also receive supplemental calcium such as calcium carbonate 1.5 g daily and an adequate vitamin D intake (400 units daily). An adequate diet is also essential. If the volume of Miacalcin® (calcitonin-salmon) Injection, Synthetic to be injected exceeds 2 mL, intramuscular injection is preferable and multiple sites of injection should be used.

Parenteral drug products should be inspected visually for particulate matter and discoloration prior to administration whenever solution and container permit.

HOW SUPPLIED

Miacalcin® (calcitonin-salmon) Injection, Synthetic is available as a sterile solution in individual 2 mL vials containing 200 I.U. per mL (NDC 0078-0149-23).

Store in Refrigerator—Between 2°C-8°C (36°F-46°F).

Manufactured by
Novartis Pharma AG,
Basle, Switzerland for
Novartis Pharmaceuticals Corporation
East Hanover, NJ 07936

T2002-50
REV: JULY 2002 89016801

Shown in Product Identification Guide, page 325

MIACALCIN® ℞

[*mī "ă-kăl-sĭn*]
(calcitonin-salmon)
Nasal Spray
Rx only

Prescribing Information

The following prescribing information is based on official labeling in effect July 2004.

DESCRIPTION

Calcitonin is a polypeptide hormone secreted by the parafollicular cells of the thyroid gland in mammals and by the ultimobranchial gland of birds and fish.

Miacalcin® (calcitonin-salmon) Nasal Spray is a synthetic polypeptide of 32 amino acids in the same linear sequence that is found in calcitonin of salmon origin. This is shown by the following graphic formula:

[See chemical structure at top of next column]

It is provided in a 3.7 mL fill glass bottle as a solution for nasal administration. This is sufficient medication for at least 30 doses.

Active Ingredient: calcitonin-salmon, 2200 I.U. per mL (corresponding to 200 I.U. per 0.09 mL actuation).

H-Cys-Ser-Asn-Leu-Ser-Thr-Cys-Val-Leu-
1 2 3 4 5 6 7 8 9
Gly-Lys-Leu-Ser-Gln-Glu-Leu-His-Lys-Leu-
10 11 12 13 14 15 16 17 18 19
Gln-Thr-Tyr-Pro-Arg-Thr-Asn-Thr-Gly-Ser-
20 21 22 23 24 25 26 27 28 29
Gly-Thr-Pro-NH_2
30 31 32

Inactive Ingredients: sodium chloride, benzalkonium chloride, hydrochloric acid (added as necessary to adjust pH) and purified water.

The activity of Miacalcin® Nasal Spray is stated in International Units based on bioassay in comparison with the International Reference Preparation of calcitonin-salmon for Bioassay, distributed by the National Institute of Biologic Standards and Control, Holly Hill, London.

CLINICAL PHARMACOLOGY

Calcitonin acts primarily on bone, but direct renal effects and actions on the gastrointestinal tract are also recognized. Calcitonin-salmon appears to have actions essentially identical to calcitonins of mammalian origin, but its potency per mg is greater and it has a longer duration of action.

The information below, describing the clinical pharmacology of calcitonin, has been derived from studies with *injectable* calcitonin. The mean bioavailability of Miacalcin® (calcitonin-salmon) Nasal Spray is approximately 3% of that of injectable calcitonin in normal subjects and, therefore, the conclusions concerning the CLINICAL PHARMACOLOGY of this preparation may be different.

The actions of calcitonin on bone and its role in normal human bone physiology are still not completely elucidated, although calcitonin receptors have been discovered in osteoclasts and osteoblasts.

Single injections of calcitonin cause a marked transient inhibition of the ongoing bone resorptive process. With prolonged use, there is a persistent, smaller decrease in the rate of bone resorption. Histologically, this is associated with a decreased number of osteoclasts and an apparent decrease in their resorptive activity. *In vitro* studies have shown that calcitonin-salmon causes inhibition of osteoclast function with loss of the ruffled osteoclast border responsible for resorption of bone. This activity resumes following removal of calcitonin-salmon from the test system. There is some evidence from the *in vitro* studies that bone formation may be augmented by calcitonin through increased osteoblastic activity.

Animal studies indicate that endogenous calcitonin, primarily through its action on bone, participates with parathyroid hormone in the homeostatic regulation of blood calcium. Thus, high blood calcium levels cause increased secretion of calcitonin which, in turn, inhibits bone resorption. This reduces the transfer of calcium from bone to blood and tends to return blood calcium towards the normal level. The importance of this process in humans has not been determined. In normal adults, who have a relatively low rate of bone resorption, the administration of exogenous calcitonin results in only a slight decrease in serum calcium in the limits of the normal range. In normal children and in patients with Paget's disease in whom bone resorption is more rapid, decreases in serum calcium are more pronounced in response to calcitonin.

Bone biopsy and radial bone mass studies at baseline and after 26 months of daily injectable calcitonin indicate that calcitonin therapy results in formation of normal bone.

Postmenopausal Osteoporosis – Osteoporosis is a disease characterized by low bone mass and architectural deterioration of bone tissue leading to enhanced bone fragility and a consequent increase in fracture risk as patients approach or fall below a bone mineral density associated with increased frequency of fracture. The most common type of osteoporosis occurs in postmenopausal females. Osteoporosis is a result of a disproportionate rate of bone resorption compared to bone formation which disrupts the structural integrity of bone, rendering it more susceptible to fracture. The most common sites of these fractures are the vertebrae, hip, and distal forearm (Colles' fractures). Vertebral fractures occur with the highest frequency and are associated with back pain, spinal deformity and a loss of height.

Miacalcin® (calcitonin-salmon) Nasal Spray, given by the intranasal route, has been shown to increase spinal bone mass in postmenopausal women with established osteoporosis but not in early postmenopausal women.

Calcium Homeostasis – In two clinical studies designed to evaluate the pharmacodynamic response to Miacalcin® Nasal Spray, administration of 100-1600 I.U. to healthy volunteers resulted in rapid and sustained small decreases (but still within the normal range) in both total serum calcium and serum ionized calcium. Single doses greater than 400 I.U. did not produce any further biological response to the drug. The development of hypocalcemia has not been reported in studies in healthy volunteers or postmenopausal females.

Kidney – Studies with injectable calcitonin show increases in the excretion of filtered phosphate, calcium, and sodium by decreasing their tubular reabsorption. Comparable studies have not been carried out with Miacalcin® Nasal Spray.

Gastrointestinal Tract – Some evidence from studies with injectable preparations suggest that calcitonin may have sig-

Continued on next page

Miacalcin Nasal Spray—Cont.

nificant actions on the gastrointestinal tract. Short-term administration of injectable calcitonin results in marked transient decreases in the volume and acidity of gastric juice and in the volume and the trypsin and amylase content of pancreatic juice. Whether these effects continue to be elicited after each injection of calcitonin during chronic therapy has not been investigated. These studies have not been conducted with Miacalcin® Nasal Spray.

Pharmacokinetics and Metabolism

The data on bioavailability of Miacalcin® Nasal Spray obtained by various investigators using different methods show great variability. Miacalcin® Nasal Spray is absorbed rapidly by the nasal mucosa. Peak plasma concentrations of drug appear 31-39 minutes after nasal administration compared to 16-25 minutes following parenteral dosing. In normal volunteers approximately 3% (range 0.3%-30.6%) of a nasally administered dose is bioavailable compared to the same dose administered by intramuscular injection. The half-life of elimination of calcitonin-salmon is calculated to be 43 minutes. There is no accumulation of the drug on repeated nasal administration at 10 hour intervals for up to 15 days. Absorption of nasally administered calcitonin has not been studied in postmenopausal women.

INDICATION AND USAGE

Postmenopausal Osteoporosis – Miacalcin® (calcitonin-salmon) Nasal Spray is indicated for the treatment of postmenopausal osteoporosis in females greater than 5 years postmenopause with low bone mass relative to healthy premenopausal females. Miacalcin® Nasal Spray should be reserved for patients who refuse or cannot tolerate estrogens or in whom estrogens are contraindicated. Use of Miacalcin® (calcitonin-salmon) Nasal Spray is recommended in conjunction with an adequate calcium (at least 1000 mg elemental calcium per day) and vitamin D (400 I.U. per day) intake to retard the progressive loss of bone mass. The evidence of efficacy is based on increases in spinal bone mineral density observed in clinical trials.

Two randomized, placebo controlled trials were conducted in 325 postmenopausal females (227 Miacalcin® Nasal Spray treated and 98 placebo treated) with spinal, forearm or femoral bone mineral density (BMD) at least one standard deviation below normal for healthy premenopausal females. These studies conducted over two years demonstrated that 200 I.U. daily of Miacalcin® Nasal Spray increases lumbar vertebral BMD relative to baseline and relative to placebo in osteoporotic females who were greater than 5 years postmenopause. Miacalcin® Nasal Spray produced statistically significant increases in lumbar vertebral BMD compared to placebo as early as six months after initiation of therapy with persistence of this level for up to 2 years of observation.

No effects of Miacalcin® Nasal Spray on cortical bone of the forearm or hip were demonstrated. However, in one study, BMD of the hip showed a statistically significant increase compared with placebo in a region composed of predominantly trabecular bone after one year of treatment changing to a trend at 2 years that was no longer statistically significant.

CONTRAINDICATIONS

Clinical allergy to calcitonin-salmon.

WARNINGS

Allergic Reactions

Because calcitonin is a polypeptide, the possibility of a systemic allergic reaction exists. A few cases of allergic-type reactions have been reported in patients receiving Miacalcin® (calcitonin-salmon) Nasal Spray, including one case of anaphylactic shock, which appears to have been due to the preservative because the patient could tolerate injectable calcitonin-salmon without incident. With injectable calcitonin-salmon there have been a few reports of serious allergic-type reactions (e.g., bronchospasm, swelling of the tongue or throat, anaphylactic shock, and in one case death attributed to anaphylaxis). The usual provisions should be made for the emergency treatment of such a reaction should it occur. Allergic reactions should be differentiated from generalized flushing and hypotension.

For patients with suspected sensitivity to calcitonin, skin testing should be considered prior to treatment utilizing a dilute, sterile solution of Miacalcin® Injection, Synthetic. Physicians may wish to refer patients who require skin testing to an allergist. A detailed skin testing protocol is available from the Medical Services Department of Novartis Pharmaceuticals Corporation.

PRECAUTIONS

1. Drug Interactions

Formal studies designed to evaluate drug interactions with calcitonin-salmon have not been done. No drug interaction studies have been performed with Miacalcin® (calcitonin-salmon) Nasal Spray ingredients.

Currently, no drug interactions with calcitonin-salmon have been observed. The effects of prior use of diphosphonates in postmenopausal osteoporosis patients have not been assessed; however, in patients with Paget's Disease prior diphosphonate use appears to reduce the antiresorptive response to Miacalcin® Nasal Spray.

2. Periodic Nasal Examinations

Periodic nasal examinations with visualization of the nasal mucosa, turbinates, septum and mucosal blood vessel status are recommended.

The development of mucosal alterations or transient nasal conditions occurred in up to 9% of patients who received Miacalcin® Nasal Spray and in up to 12% of patients who received placebo nasal spray in studies in postmenopausal females. The majority of patients (approximately 90%) in whom nasal abnormalities were noted also reported nasally related complaints/symptoms as adverse events. Therefore, a nasal examination should be performed prior to start of treatment with nasal calcitonin and at any time nasal complaints occur.

In all postmenopausal patients treated with Miacalcin® Nasal Spray, the most commonly reported nasal adverse events included rhinitis (12%), epistaxis (3.5%), and sinusitis (2.3%). Smoking was shown not to have any contributory effect on the occurrence of nasal adverse events. One patient (0.3%) treated with Miacalcin® Nasal Spray who was receiving 400 I.U. daily developed a small nasal wound. In clinical trials in another disorder (Paget's Disease), 2.8% of patients developed nasal ulcerations.

If severe ulceration of the nasal mucosa occurs, as indicated by ulcers greater than 1.5 mm in diameter or penetrating below the mucosa, or those associated with heavy bleeding, Miacalcin® Nasal Spray should be discontinued. Although smaller ulcers often heal without withdrawal of Miacalcin® Nasal Spray, medication should be discontinued temporarily until healing occurs.

3. Information for Patients

Careful instructions on pump assembly, priming of the pump and nasal introduction of Miacalcin® Nasal Spray should be given to the patient. Although instructions for patients are supplied with individual bottles, procedures for use should be demonstrated to each patient. Patients should notify their physician if they develop significant nasal irritation.

Patients should be advised of the following:

- Store new, unassembled bottles in the refrigerator between 2°C-8°C (36°F-46°F).
- Protect the product from freezing.
- Before priming the pump and using a new bottle, allow it to reach room temperature.
- Store bottle in use at room temperature between 15°C-30°C (59°F-86°F) in an upright position, for up to 35 days. Each bottle contains at least 30 doses.
- See *DOSAGE AND ADMINISTRATION, Priming (Activation) of Pump* for complete instructions on priming the pump and administering Miacalcin® Nasal Spray. You should keep track of the number of doses used from the bottle.

  After 30 doses, each spray may not deliver the correct amount of medication, even if the bottle is not completely empty.

4. Carcinogenicity, Mutagenicity, and Impairment of Fertility

An increased incidence of non-functioning pituitary adenomas has been observed in one-year toxicity studies in Sprague-Dawley and Fischer 344 Rats administered (subcutaneously) calcitonin-salmon at dosages of 80 I.U. per kilogram per day (16-19 times the recommended human parenteral dose and about 130-160 times the human intranasal dose based on body surface area). The findings suggest that calcitonin-salmon reduced the latency period for development of pituitary adenomas that do not produce hormones, probably through the perturbation of physiologic processes involved in the evolution of this commonly occurring endocrine lesion in the rat. Although administration of calcitonin-salmon reduces the latency period of the development of nonfunctional proliferative lesions in rats, it did not induce the hyperplastic/neoplastic process.

Calcitonin-salmon was tested for mutagenicity using *Salmonella typhimurium* (5 strains) and *Escherichia coli* (2 strains), with and without rat liver metabolic activation, and found to be non-mutagenic. The drug was also not mutagenic in a chromosome aberration test in mammalian V79 cells of the Chinese Hamster *in vitro*.

5. Laboratory Tests

Urine sediment abnormalities have not been reported in ambulatory volunteers treated with Miacalcin® Nasal Spray. Coarse granular casts containing renal tubular epithelial cells were reported in young adult volunteers at bed rest who were given injectable calcitonin-salmon to study the effect of immobilization on osteoporosis. There was no evidence of renal abnormality and the urine sediment became normal after calcitonin was stopped. Periodic examinations of urine sediment should be considered.

6. Pregnancy

Teratogenic Effects

Category C

Calcitonin-salmon has been shown to cause a decrease in fetal birth weights in rabbits when given by injection in doses 8-33 times the parenteral dose and 70-278 times the intranasal dose recommended for human use based on body surface area.

Since calcitonin does not cross the placental barrier, this finding may be due to metabolic effects on the pregnant animal. There are no adequate and well controlled studies in pregnant women with calcitonin-salmon. Miacalcin® Nasal Spray is *not* indicated for use in pregnancy.

7. Nursing Mothers

It is not known whether this drug is excreted in human milk. As a general rule, nursing should not be undertaken while a patient is on this drug since many drugs are excreted in human milk. Calcitonin has been shown to inhibit lactation in animals.

8. Geriatric Use

Clinical trials using Miacalcin® Nasal Spray have included postmenopausal patients up to 77 years of age. No unusual adverse events or increased incidence of common adverse events have been noted in patients over 65 years of age.

9. Pediatric Use

There are no data to support the use of Miacalcin® Nasal Spray in children. Disorders of bone in children referred to as idiopathic juvenile osteoporosis have been reported rarely. The relationship of these disorders to postmenopausal osteoporosis has not been established and experience with the use of calcitonin in these disorders is very limited.

ADVERSE REACTIONS

The incidence of adverse reactions reported in studies involving postmenopausal osteoporotic patients chronically exposed to Miacalcin® (calcitonin-salmon) Nasal Spray (N=341) and to placebo nasal spray (N=131) and reported in greater than 3% of Miacalcin® Nasal Spray treated patients are presented below in the following table. Most adverse reactions were mild to moderate in severity. Nasal adverse events were most common with 70% mild, 25% moderate, and 5% severe in nature (placebo rates were 71% mild, 27% moderate, and 2% severe).

Adverse Reactions Occurring in at Least 3% of Postmenopausal Patients Treated Chronically

Adverse Reaction	Miacalcin® (calcitonin-salmon) Nasal Spray N=341 % of Patients	Placebo N=131 % of Patients
Rhinitis	12.0	6.9
Symptom of Nose†	10.6	16.0
Back Pain	5.0	2.3
Arthralgia	3.8	5.3
Epistaxis	3.5	4.6
Headache	3.2	4.6

†Symptom of nose includes: nasal crusts, dryness, redness or erythema, nasal sores, irritation, itching, thick feeling, soreness, pallor, infection, stenosis, runny/blocked, small wound, bleeding wound, tenderness, uncomfortable feeling and sore across bridge of nose.

In addition, the following adverse events were reported in fewer than 3% of patients during chronic therapy with Miacalcin® Nasal Spray. Adverse events reported in 1%-3% of patients are identified with an asterisk(*). The remainder occurred in less than 1% of patients. Other than flushing, nausea, possible allergic reactions, and possible local irritative effects in the respiratory tract, a relationship to Miacalcin® Nasal Spray has not been established.

Body as a whole – General Disorders: influenza-like symptoms*, fatigue*, periorbital edema, fever

Integumentary: erythematous rash*, skin ulceration, eczema, alopecia, pruritus, increased sweating

Musculoskeletal/Collagen: arthrosis*, myalgia*, arthritis, polymyalgia rheumatica, stiffness

Respiratory/Special Senses: sinusitis*, upper respiratory tract infection*, bronchospasm*, pharyngitis, bronchitis, pneumonia, coughing, dyspnea, taste perversion, parosmia

Cardiovascular: hypertension*, angina pectoris*, tachycardia, palpitation, bundle branch block, myocardial infarction

Gastrointestinal: dyspepsia*, constipation*, abdominal pain*, nausea*, diarrhea*, vomiting, flatulence, increased appetite, gastritis, dry mouth

Liver/Metabolic: cholelithiasis, hepatitis, thirst, weight increase

Endocrine: goiter, hyperthyroidism

Urinary System: cystitis*, pyelonephritis, hematuria, renal calculus

Central and Peripheral Nervous System: dizziness*, paresthesia*, vertigo, migraine, neuralgia, agitation

Hearing/Vestibular: tinnitus, hearing loss, earache

Vision: abnormal lacrimation*, conjunctivitis*, blurred vision, vitreous floater

Vascular: flushing, cerebrovascular accident, thrombophlebitis

Hematologic/Resistance Mechanisms: lymphadenopathy*, infection*, anemia

Psychiatric: depression*, insomnia, anxiety, anorexia

Common adverse reactions associated with the use of injectable calcitonin-salmon occurred less frequently in patients treated with Miacalcin® Nasal Spray than in those patients treated with injectable calcitonin. Nausea, with or without vomiting, which occurred in 1.8% of patients treated with the nasal spray (and 1.5% of those receiving placebo nasal spray) occurs in about 10% of patients who take injectable calcitonin-salmon. Flushing, which occurred in less than 1% of patients treated with the Nasal Spray, occurs in 2%-5% of patients treated with injectable calcitonin-salmon. Although the administered dosages of injectable and nasal spray calcitonin-salmon are comparable (50–100 units daily of injectable versus 200 units daily of nasal spray), the nasal dosage form has a mean bioavailability of about 3% (range

0.3%-30.6%) and therefore provides less drug to the systemic circulation, possibly accounting for the decrease in frequency of adverse reactions.

The collective foreign marketing experience with Miacalcin® Nasal Spray does not show evidence of any notable difference in the incidence profile of reported adverse reactions when compared with that seen in the clinical trials.

OVERDOSAGE

No instances of overdose with Miacalcin® (calcitonin-salmon) Nasal Spray have been reported and no serious adverse reactions have been associated with high doses. There is no known potential for drug abuse for calcitonin-salmon. Single doses of Miacalcin® Nasal Spray up to 1600 I.U., doses up to 800 I.U. per day for three days and chronic administration of doses up to 600 I.U. per day have been studied without serious adverse effects. A dose of 1000 I.U. of Miacalcin® injectable solution given subcutaneously may produce nausea and vomiting. A dose of Miacalcin® injectable solution of 32 I.U. per kg per day for one or two days demonstrated no additional adverse effects.

There have been no reports of hypocalcemic tetany. However, the pharmacologic actions of Miacalcin® Nasal Spray suggest that this could occur in overdose. Therefore, provisions for parenteral administration of calcium should be available for the treatment of overdose.

DOSAGE AND ADMINISTRATION

The recommended dose of Miacalcin® (calcitonin-salmon) Nasal Spray in postmenopausal osteoporotic females is one spray (200 I.U.) per day administered intranasally, alternating nostrils daily.

Drug effect may be monitored by periodic measurements of lumbar vertebral bone mass to document stabilization of bone loss or increases in bone density. Effects of Miacalcin® Nasal Spray on biochemical markers of bone turnover have not been consistently demonstrated in studies in postmenopausal osteoporosis. Therefore, these parameters should not be solely utilized to determine clinical response to Miacalcin® Nasal Spray therapy in these patients.

Priming (Activation) of Pump

Before the first dose and administration, Miacalcin® Nasal Spray should be at room temperature. To prime the pump, the bottle should be held upright and the two white side arms of the pump depressed toward the bottle until a full spray is produced. The pump is primed once the first full spray is emitted. To administer, the nozzle should be carefully placed into the nostril with the head in the upright position, and the pump firmly depressed toward the bottle. The pump should not be primed before each daily dose.

HOW SUPPLIED

Miacalcin® (calcitonin-salmon) Nasal Spray

Available as a metered dose clear solution in 3.7 mL fill clear glass bottle. It is available in a dosage strength of 200 I.U. per activation (0.09 mL per spray). A screw-on pump is provided. The pump, following priming, will deliver 0.09 mL of solution. Miacalcin® Nasal Spray contains 2200 I.U. per mL calcitonin-salmon and is provided in an individual box containing one glass bottle and one screw-on pump .... (NDC 0078-0311-54).

Store and Dispense

Store unopened bottle in refrigerator between 2°C-8°C (36°F-46°F). Protect from freezing.

Store bottle in use at room temperature between 15°C-30°C (59°F-86°F) in an upright position, for up to 35 days. Each bottle contains at least 30 doses.

Manufactured by:
Novartis Pharma S.A.S.
Huningue, France
Distributed by:
Novartis Pharmaceuticals Corp.
East Hanover, New Jersey 07936

T2003-11

REV: APRIL 2003 PRINTED IN U.S.A. 89014604

©Novartis

MYFORTIC®

[mi-for-tic]
(mycophenolic acid*)
delayed-release tablets
***as mycophenolate sodium**
Rx only

Prescribing Information

The following prescribing information is based on official labeling in effect July, 2004.

WARNING

Increased susceptibility to infection and the possible development of lymphoma and other neoplasms may result from immunosuppression. Only physicians experienced in immunosuppressive therapy and management of organ transplant recipients should use Myfortic® (mycophenolic acid). Patients receiving Myfortic should be managed in facilities equipped and staffed with adequate laboratory and supportive medical resources. The physician responsible for maintenance therapy should have complete information requisite for the follow-up of the patient.

Table 1
Mean ± SD Pharmacokinetic Parameters for MPA Following the Oral Administration of Myfortic® to Renal Transplant Patients on Cyclosporine, USP (MODIFIED) Based Immunosuppression

Study Patient	Myfortic® Dosing	n	Dose (mg)	T_{max}* (hr)		C_{max} (µg/mL)	AUC_{0-12hr} (µg*hr/mL)
Adult	Single	24	720	2	(0.8-8)	26.1 ± 12.0	66.5 ± 22.6**
Pediatric***	Single	10	450/m²	2.5	(1.5-24)	36.3 ± 20.9	74.3 ± 22.5**
Adult	Multiple × 6 days, BID	10	720	2	(1.5-3.0)	37.0 ± 13.3	67.9 ± 20.3
Adult	Multiple × 28 days, BID	36	720	2.5	(1.5-8)	31.2 ± 18.1	71.2 ± 26.3
Adult	Chronic, multiple dose, BID						
	2 weeks post-transplant	12	720	1.8	(1.0-5.3)	15.0 ± 10.7	28.6 ± 11.5
	3 months post-transplant	12	720	2	(0.5-2.5)	26.2 ± 12.7	52.3 ± 17.4
	6 months post-transplant	12	720	2	(0-3)	24.1 ± 9.6	57.2 ± 15.3
Adult	Chronic, multiple dose, BID	18	720	1.5	(0-6)	18.9 ± 7.9	57.4 ± 15.0

*median (range), ** $AUC_{0-\infty}$, *** age range of 5-16 years

DESCRIPTION

Myfortic® (mycophenolic acid) delayed-release tablets are an enteric formulation of mycophenolate sodium that delivers the active moiety mycophenolic acid (MPA). Myfortic is an immunosuppressive agent. As the sodium salt, MPA is chemically designated as (E)-6-(4-hydroxy-6-methoxy-7-methyl-3-oxo-1,3-dihydroisobenzofuran-5-yl)-4-methylhex-4-enoic acid sodium salt.

Its empirical formula is $C_{17}H_{19}O_6$ Na. The molecular weight is 342.32 and the structural formula is

Myfortic, as the sodium salt, is a white to off-white, crystalline powder and is highly soluble in aqueous media at physiological pH and practically insoluble in 0.1 N hydrochloric acid.

Myfortic is available for oral use as delayed-release tablets containing either 180 mg or 360 mg of mycophenolic acid. Inactive ingredients include colloidal silicon dioxide, crospovidone, lactose anhydrous, magnesium stearate, povidone (K-30), and starch. The enteric coating of the tablet consists of hypromellose phthalate, titanium dioxide, iron oxide yellow, and indigotine (180 mg) or iron oxide red (360 mg).

CLINICAL PHARMACOLOGY

Mechanism of Action

MPA is an uncompetitive and reversible inhibitor of inosine monophosphate dehydrogenase (IMPDH), and therefore inhibits the *de novo* pathway of guanosine nucleotide synthesis without incorporation to DNA. Because T- and B-lymphocytes are critically dependent for their proliferation on *de novo* synthesis of purines, whereas other cell types can utilize salvage pathways, MPA has potent cytostatic effect on lymphocytes.

Mycophenolate sodium has been shown to prevent the occurrence of acute rejection in rat models of kidney and heart allotransplantation. Mycophenolate sodium also decreases antibody production in mice.

Pharmacokinetics

Absorption

In vitro studies demonstrated that the enteric-coated Myfortic® (mycophenolic acid) tablet does not release MPA under acidic conditions (pH <5) as in the stomach but is highly soluble in neutral pH conditions as in the intestine. Following Myfortic oral administration without food in several pharmacokinetic studies conducted in renal transplant patients, consistent with its enteric-coated formulation, the median delay (T_{lag}) in the rise of MPA concentration ranged between 0.25 and 1.25 hours and the median time to maximum concentration (T_{max}) of MPA ranged between 1.5 and 2.75 hours. In comparison, following the administration of mycophenolate mofetil, the median T_{max} ranged between 0.5 and 1.0 hours. In stable renal transplant patients on cyclosporine, USP (MODIFIED) based immunosuppression, gastrointestinal absorption and absolute bioavailability of MPA following the administration of Myfortic delayed-release tablet was 93% and 72%, respectively. Myfortic pharmacokinetics is dose proportional over the dose range of 360 to 2160 mg.

Distribution

The mean (± SD) volume of distribution at steady state and elimination phase for MPA is 54 (± 25) L and 112 (± 48) L, respectively. MPA is highly protein bound to albumin, >98%. The protein binding of mycophenolic acid glucuronide (MPAG) is 82%. The free MPA concentration may increase under conditions of decreased protein binding (uremia, hepatic failure, and hypoalbuminemia).

Metabolism

MPA is metabolized principally by glucuronyl transferase to glucuronidated metabolites. The phenolic glucuronide of MPA, mycophenolic acid glucuronide (MPAG), is the predominant metabolite of MPA and does not manifest pharmacological activity. The acyl glucuronide is a minor metabolite and has comparable pharmacological activity to MPA. In stable renal transplant patients on cyclosporine, USP (MODIFIED) based immunosuppression, approximately 28% of the oral Myfortic dose was converted to MPAG by pre-systemic metabolism. The AUC ratio of MPA:MPAG:acyl glucuronide is approximately 1:24:0.28 at steady state. The mean clearance of MPA was 140 (± 30) mL/min.

Elimination

The majority of MPA dose administered is eliminated in the urine primarily as MPAG (>60%) and approximately 3% as unchanged MPA following Myfortic administration to stable renal transplant patients. The mean renal clearance of MPAG was 15.5 (± 5.9) mL/min. MPAG is also secreted in the bile and available for deconjugation by gut flora. MPA resulting from the deconjugation may then be reabsorbed and produce a second peak of MPA approximately 6-8 hours after Myfortic dosing. The mean elimination half-life of MPA and MPAG ranged between 8 and 16 hours, and 13 and 17 hours, respectively.

Food Effect

Compared to the fasting state, administration of Myfortic 720 mg with a high fat meal (55 g fat, 1000 calories) had no effect on the systemic exposure (AUC) of MPA. However, there was a 33% decrease in the maximal concentration (C_{max}), a 3.5-hr delay in the T_{lag} (range, -6 to 18 hr), and 5.0-hr delay in the T_{max} (range, -9 to 20 hr) of MPA. To avoid the variability in MPA absorption between doses, Myfortic should be taken on an empty stomach *(see DOSAGE AND ADMINISTRATION and PRECAUTIONS, Information for Patients).*

Pharmacokinetics in Renal Transplant Patients

The mean pharmacokinetic parameters for MPA following the administration of Myfortic in renal transplant patients on cyclosporine, USP (MODIFIED) based immunosuppression are shown in Table 1. Single dose Myfortic pharmacokinetics predicts multiple dose pharmacokinetics. However, in the early post-transplant period, mean MPA AUC and C_{max} were approximately one-half of those measured six months post-transplant.

After near equimolar dosing of Myfortic 720 mg BID and mycophenolate mofetil 1000 mg BID (739 mg as MPA) in both the single and multiple dose cross-over trials, mean systemic MPA exposure (AUC) was similar.

[See table 1 above]

Special Populations

Renal Insufficiency: No specific pharmacokinetic studies in individuals with renal impairment were conducted with Myfortic. However, based on studies of renal impairment with mycophenolate mofetil, MPA exposure is not expected to be appreciably increased over the range of normal to severely-impaired renal function following Myfortic administration. In contrast, MPAG exposure would be increased markedly with decreased renal function; MPAG exposure being approximately 8-fold higher in the setting of anuria. Although dialysis may be used to remove the inactive metabolite MPAG, it would not be expected to remove clinically significant amounts of the active moiety MPA. This is in large part due to the high plasma protein binding of MPA.

Hepatic Insufficiency: No specific pharmacokinetic studies in individuals with hepatic impairment were conducted with Myfortic. In a single dose (mycophenolate mofetil 1000 mg) study of 18 volunteers with alcoholic cirrhosis and 6 healthy volunteers, hepatic MPA glucuronidation processes appeared to be relatively unaffected by hepatic parenchymal disease when the pharmacokinetic parameters of healthy volunteers and alcoholic cirrhosis patients within this study were compared. However, it should be noted that for unexplained reasons, the healthy volunteers in this study had about a 50% lower AUC compared to healthy volunteers in other studies, thus making comparison between volunteers with alcoholic cirrhosis and healthy volunteers difficult. Effects of hepatic disease on this process probably depend on the particular disease. Hepatic disease, such as primary biliary cirrhosis, with other etiologies may show a different effect.

Pediatrics: Limited data are available on the use of Myfortic at a dose of 450 mg/m² body surface area in children. The mean MPA pharmacokinetic parameters for stable pediatric renal transplant patients, 5-16 years, on cyclosporine, USP (MODIFIED) are shown in Table 1. At the same dose administered based on body surface area, the respective mean C_{max} and AUC of MPA determined in children were higher by 33% and 18% than those determined for adults. The clinical impact of the increase in MPA exposure is not known.

Gender: There are no significant gender differences in Myfortic pharmacokinetics.

Elderly: Pharmacokinetics in the elderly have not formally been studied.

Continued on next page

Myfortic—Cont.

CLINICAL STUDIES

The safety and efficacy of Myfortic® (mycophenolic acid) in combination with cyclosporine, USP (MODIFIED) and corticosteroids for the prevention of organ rejection was assessed in two multicenter, randomized, double-blind trials in *de novo* and maintenance renal transplant patients compared to mycophenolate mofetil.

The *de novo* study was conducted in 423 renal transplant patients (ages 18-75 years) in Austria, Canada, Germany, Hungary, Italy, Norway, Spain, UK and USA. Cadaveric donor specimens accounted for 84% of randomized patients. Patients were administered either Myfortic 1.44 g/day or mycophenolate mofetil 2 g/day within 48 hours post-transplant for 12 months in combination with cyclosporine, USP (MODIFIED) and corticosteroids. Forty-one percent of patients received antibody therapy as induction treatment. Treatment failure was defined as the first occurrence of biopsy-proven acute rejection, graft loss, death or loss to follow-up at 6 months. The incidence of treatment failure was similar in Myfortic and mycophenolate mofetil-treated patients at 6 and 12 months (Table 2). The cumulative incidence of graft loss, death and lost to follow-up at 12 months is also given in Table 2.

Table 2
Treatment Failure in *de novo* Renal Transplant Patients (Percent of Patients) at 6- and 12-Months of Treatment when Administered in Combination with Cyclosporine* and Corticosteroids

	Myfortic® 1.44 g/day (n=213)		mycophenolate mofetil 2 g/day (n=210)	
6 Months	n	(%)	n	(%)
Treatment failure#	55	(25.8)	55	(26.2)
Biopsy-proven acute rejection	46	(21.6)	48	(22.9)
Graft loss	7	(3.3)	9	(4.3)
Death	1	(0.5)	2	(1.0)
Lost to follow-up**	3	(1.4)	0	
12 Months	n	(%)	n	(%)
Graft loss or death or lost to follow-up***	20	(9.4)	18	(8.6)
Treatment failure	61	(28.6)	59	(28.1)
Biopsy-proven acute rejection	48	(22.5)	51	(24.3)
Graft loss	9	(4.2)	9	(4.3)
Death	2	(0.9)	5	(2.4)
Lost to follow-up**	5	(2.3)	0	

* USP (MODIFIED)
** Lost to follow-up indicates patients who were lost to follow-up without prior biopsy-proven acute rejection, graft loss or death
*** Lost to follow-up indicates patients who were lost to follow-up without prior graft loss or death (9 Myfortic patients and 4 mycophenolate mofetil patients)
# 95% confidence interval of the difference in treatment failure at 6 months (Myfortic – mycophenolate mofetil) is (-8.7%, 8.0%).

The maintenance study was conducted in 322 renal transplant patients (ages 18-75 years), who were at least 6 months post-transplant receiving 2 g/day mycophenolate mofetil in combination with cyclosporine USP (MODIFIED), with or without corticosteroids for at least two weeks prior to entry in the study. Patients were randomized to Myfortic 1.44 g/day or mycophenolate mofetil 2 g/day for 12 months. The study was conducted in Austria, Belgium, Canada, Germany, Italy, Spain, and USA. Treatment failure was defined as the first occurrence of biopsy-proven acute rejection, graft loss, death, or loss to follow-up at 6 and 12 months. The incidences of treatment failure at 6 and 12 months were similar between Myfortic- and mycophenolate mofetil-treated patients (Table 3). The cumulative incidence of graft loss, death and lost to follow-up at 12 months is also given in Table 3.

Table 3
Treatment Failure in Maintenance Transplant Patients (Percent of Patients) at 6- and 12-Months of Treatment when Administered in Combination with Cyclosporine* and with or without Corticosteroids

	Myfortic® 1.44 g/day (n=159)		mycophenolate mofetil 2 g/day (n=163)	
6 Months	n	(%)	n	(%)
Treatment failure#	7	(4.4)	11	(6.7)
Biopsy-proven acute rejection	2	(1.3)	2	(1.2)
Graft loss	0		1	(0.6)
Death	0		1	(0.6)
Lost to follow-up**	5	(3.1)	7	(4.3)
12 Months	n	(%)	n	(%)
Graft loss or death or lost to follow-up***	10	(6.3)	17	(10.4)
Treatment failure	12	(7.5)	20	(12.3)
Biopsy-proven acute rejection	2	(1.3)	5	(3.1)
Graft loss	0		1	(0.6)
Death	2	(1.3)	4	(2.5)
Lost to follow-up**	8	(5.0)	10	(6.1)

* USP (MODIFIED)
** Lost to follow-up indicates patients who were lost to follow-up without prior biopsy-proven acute rejection, graft loss or death
*** Lost to follow-up indicates patients who were lost to follow-up without prior graft loss or death (8 Myfortic patients and 12 mycophenolate mofetil patients)
# 95% confidence interval of the difference in treatment failure at 6 months (Myfortic – mycophenolate mofetil) is (-7.4%, 2.7%).

The safety and efficacy of Myfortic has not been studied in hepatic or cardiac transplant trials.

INDICATIONS AND USAGE

Myfortic® (mycophenolic acid) delayed-release tablets are indicated for the prophylaxis of organ rejection in patients receiving allogeneic renal transplants, administered in combination with cyclosporine and corticosteroids.

CONTRAINDICATIONS

Myfortic® (mycophenolic acid) is contraindicated in patients with a hypersensitivity to mycophenolate sodium, mycophenolic acid, mycophenolate mofetil, or to any of its excipients.

WARNINGS (see boxed WARNING)

Patients receiving immunosuppressive regimens involving combinations of drugs, including Myfortic® (mycophenolic acid), as part of an immunosuppressive regimen are at increased risk of developing lymphomas and other malignancies, particularly of the skin *(see ADVERSE REACTIONS)*. The risk appears to be related to the intensity and duration of immunosuppression rather than to the use of any specific agent. Oversuppression of the immune system can also increase susceptibility to infection, including opportunistic infections, fatal infections, and sepsis.

Fatal infections can occur in patients receiving immunosuppressive therapy *(see ADVERSE REACTIONS)*.

As usual for patients with increased risk for skin cancer, exposure to sunlight and UV light should be limited by wearing protective clothing and using a sunscreen with a high protection factor.

Myfortic has been administered in combination with the following agents in clinical trials: antithymocyte/lymphocyte immunoglobulin, muromonab-CD3, basiliximab, daclizumab, cyclosporine, and corticosteroids. The efficacy and safety of Myfortic in combination with other immunosuppression agents have not been determined.

The rates for lymphoproliferative disease or lymphoma in Myfortic treated patients were comparable to the mycophenolate mofetil group in the *de novo* and maintenance studies *(see ADVERSE REACTIONS)*.

There are no adequate and well-controlled studies in pregnant women conducted with MPA, Myfortic, or mycophenolate mofetil. Since MPA may cause fetal harm when administered to a pregnant woman, Myfortic should not be used in pregnant women unless the potential benefit justifies the potential risk to the fetus.

Women of childbearing potential should have a negative serum or urine pregnancy test with a sensitivity of at least 50 mIU/mL within 1 week prior to beginning therapy. It is recommended that Myfortic therapy should not be initiated by the physician until a report of a negative pregnancy test has been obtained.

Effective contraception must be used before beginning Myfortic therapy, during therapy, and for 6 weeks following discontinuation of therapy, even where there has been a history of infertility, unless due to hysterectomy. Two reliable forms of contraception must be used simultaneously unless abstinence is the chosen method. If pregnancy does occur during treatment, the physician and patient should discuss the potential risk to the fetus *(see PRECAUTIONS, Pregnancy, and Information for Patients)*.

Patients receiving Myfortic should be monitored for neutropenia *(see PRECAUTIONS, Laboratory Tests)*. The development of neutropenia may be related to Myfortic itself, concomitant medications, viral infections, or some combination of these events. If neutropenia develops (ANC $<1.3\times10^3/\mu L$), dosing with Myfortic should be interrupted or the dose reduced, appropriate diagnostic tests performed, and the patient managed appropriately *(see DOSAGE AND ADMINISTRATION)*.

Patients receiving Myfortic should be instructed to immediately report any evidence of infection, unexpected bruising, bleeding, or any other manifestation of bone marrow suppression.

PRECAUTIONS

General

Gastrointestinal bleeding (requiring hospitalization) has been reported in *de novo* renal transplant patients (1.0%) and maintenance patients (1.3%) treated with Myfortic® (mycophenolic acid) (up to 12 months). Intestinal perforations, gastrointestinal hemorrhage, gastric ulcers and duodenal ulcers have rarely been observed. Most patients receiving Myfortic were also receiving other drugs known to be associated with these complications. Patients with active peptic ulcer disease were excluded from enrollment in studies with Myfortic. Because MPA derivatives have been associated with an increased incidence of digestive system adverse events, including infrequent cases of gastrointestinal tract ulceration, hemorrhage, and perforation, Myfortic should be administered with caution in patients with active serious digestive system disease *(see ADVERSE REACTIONS)*.

Subjects with severe chronic renal impairment (GFR <25 mL/min/1.73 m^2) may present higher plasma MPA and MPAG AUCs relative to subjects with lesser degrees of renal impairment or normal healthy volunteers. No data are available on the safety of long-term exposure to these levels of MPAG.

In the *de novo* study, 18.3% of Myfortic patients versus 16.7% in the mycophenolate mofetil group experienced delayed graft function (DGF). Although patients with DGF experienced a higher incidence of certain adverse events (anemia, leukopenia, and hyperkalemia) than patients without DGF, these events in DGF patients were not more frequent in patients receiving Myfortic compared to mycophenolate mofetil. No dose adjustment is recommended for these patients; however, such patients should be carefully observed *(see CLINICAL PHARMACOLOGY and DOSAGE AND ADMINISTRATION)*.

In view of the significant reduction in the AUC of MPA by cholestyramine when administered with mycophenolate mofetil, caution should be used in the concomitant administration of Myfortic with drugs that interfere with enterohepatic recirculation because of the potential to reduce the efficacy *(see PRECAUTIONS, Drug Interactions)*.

On theoretical grounds, because Myfortic is an IMPDH Inhibitor, it should be avoided in patients with rare hereditary deficiency of hypoxanthine-guanine phosphoribosyl-transferase (HGPRT) such as Lesch-Nyhan and Kelley-Seegmiller syndrome.

During treatment with Myfortic, the use of live attenuated vaccines should be avoided and patients should be advised that vaccinations may be less effective *(see PRECAUTIONS, Drug Interactions, Live Vaccines)*.

Information for Patients

It is recommended that Myfortic be administered on an empty stomach, one hour before or two hours after food intake *(see DOSAGE AND ADMINISTRATION)*.

In order to maintain the integrity of the enteric coating of the tablet, patients should be instructed not to crush, chew, or cut Myfortic tablets and to swallow the tablets whole. Patients should be informed of the need for repeated appropriate laboratory tests while they are receiving Myfortic. Patients should be given complete dosage instructions and informed of the increased risk of lymphoproliferative disease and certain other malignancies.

Women of childbearing potential should be instructed of the potential risks during pregnancy, and that they should use effective contraception before beginning Myfortic therapy, during therapy, and for 6 weeks after Myfortic has been stopped *(see WARNINGS and PRECAUTIONS, Pregnancy)*.

Laboratory Tests

Complete blood count should be performed weekly during the first month, twice monthly for the second and the third month of treatment, then monthly through the first year. If neutropenia develops (ANC $<1.3\times10^3/\mu L$) dosing with Myfortic should be interrupted or the dose reduced, appropriate tests performed, and the patient managed accordingly *(see WARNINGS)*.

Drug Interactions

The following drug interaction studies have been conducted with Myfortic:

Antacids: Absorption of a single dose of Myfortic was decreased when administered to 12 stable renal transplant patients also taking magnesium-aluminum containing antacids (30 mL): the mean C_{max} and $AUC_{(0-t)}$ values for MPA were 25% and 37% lower, respectively, than when Myfortic was administered alone under fasting conditions. It is recommended that Myfortic and antacids not be administered simultaneously.

Cyclosporine: When studied in stable renal transplant patients, cyclosporine, USP (MODIFIED) pharmacokinetics were unaffected by steady state dosing of Myfortic.

The following recommendations are derived from drug interaction studies conducted following the administration of mycophenolate mofetil:

Acyclovir/Ganciclovir: May be taken with Myfortic; however, during the period of treatment, physicians should monitor blood cell counts. Both acyclovir/ganciclovir and MPAG concentrations are increased in the presence of renal impairment, their coexistence may compete for tubular secretion and further increase in the concentrations of the two.

Azathioprine/Mycophenolate Mofetil: Given that azathioprine and mycophenolate mofetil inhibit purine metabolism, it is recommended that Myfortic not be administered concomitantly with azathioprine or mycophenolate mofetil.

Cholestyramine and Drugs that Bind Bile Acids: These drugs interrupt enterohepatic recirculation and reduce MPA exposure when coadministered with mycophenolate mofetil. Therefore, do not administer Myfortic with cholestyramine or other agents that may interfere with enterohepatic recirculation or drugs that may bind bile acids, for example bile acid sequestrates or oral activated charcoal, because of the potential to reduce the efficacy of Myfortic.

Oral Contraceptives: Given the different metabolism of Myfortic and oral contraceptives, no drug interaction between these two classes of drug is expected. However, in a drug-drug interaction study, mean levonorgesterol AUC was decreased by 15% when coadministered with mycophenolate mofetil. Therefore, it is recommended that oral contraceptives are coadministered with Myfortic with caution and additional birth control methods be considered *(see PRECAUTIONS, Pregnancy).*

Live Vaccines: During treatment with Myfortic, the use of live attenuated vaccines should be avoided and patients should be advised that vaccinations may be less effective. Influenza vaccination may be of value. Prescribers should refer to national guidelines for influenza vaccination *(see PRECAUTIONS, General).*

Drugs that alter the gastrointestinal flora may interact with Myfortic by disrupting enterohepatic recirculation. Interference of MPAG hydrolysis may lead to less MPA available for absorption.

Carcinogenesis, Mutagenesis, Impairment of Fertility

In a 104-week oral carcinogenicity study in rats, mycophenolate sodium was not tumorigenic at daily doses up to 9 mg/kg, the highest dose tested. This dose resulted in approximately 0.6-1.2 times the systemic exposure (based upon plasma AUC) observed in renal transplant patients at the recommended dose of 1.44 g/day. Similar results were observed in a parallel study in rats performed with mycophenolate mofetil. In a 104-week oral carcinogenicity study in mice, mycophenolate mofetil was not tumorigenic at a daily dose level as high as 180 mg/kg (which corresponds to 0.6 times the proposed mycophenolate sodium therapeutic dose based upon body surface area).

The genotoxic potential of mycophenolate sodium was determined in five assays. Mycophenolate sodium was genotoxic in the mouse lymphoma/thymidine kinase assay, the micronucleus test in V79 Chinese hamster cells and the *in vivo* mouse micronucleus assay. Mycophenolate sodium was not genotoxic in the bacterial mutation assay (*Salmonella typhimurium* TA 1535, 97a, 98, 100, & 102) or the chromosomal aberration assay in human lymphocytes. Mycophenolate mofetil generated similar genotoxic activity. The genotoxic activity of MPA is probably due to the depletion of the nucleotide pool required for DNA synthesis as a result of the pharmacodynamic mode of action of MPA (inhibition of nucleotide synthesis).

Mycophenolate sodium had no effect on male rat fertility at daily oral doses as high as 18 mg/kg and exhibited no testicular or spermatogenic effects at daily oral doses of 20 mg/kg for 13 weeks (approximately two-fold the therapeutic systemic exposure of MPA). No effects on female fertility were seen up to a daily dose of 20 mg/kg, which was approximately three-fold higher than the recommended therapeutic dose based upon systemic exposure.

Pregnancy Category C

In a teratology study performed with mycophenolate sodium in rats, at a dose as low as 1 mg/kg, malformations in the offspring were observed, including anophthalmia, exencephaly and umbilical hernia. The systemic exposure at this dose represents 0.05 times the clinical exposure at the dose of 1.44 g/day Myfortic. In teratology studies in rabbits, fetal resorptions and malformations occurred from 80 mg/kg/day, in the absence of maternal toxicity (dose levels are equivalent to about 0.8 times the recommended clinical dose, corrected for BSA). There are no relevant qualitative or quantitative differences in the teratogenic potential of mycophenolate sodium and mycophenolate mofetil. There are no adequate and well-controlled studies in pregnant women. Myfortic should be used in pregnant women only if the potential benefit outweighs the potential risk to the fetus.

It is recommended that Myfortic therapy should not be initiated until a negative pregnancy test has been obtained. Patients should be instructed to consult their physician immediately should pregnancy occur.

Effective contraception must be used before beginning Myfortic therapy, during therapy, and for six weeks following discontinuation of therapy *(see WARNINGS).*

Nursing Mothers

It is not known whether MPA is excreted in human milk. Because of the potential for serious adverse reactions in nursing infants from MPA, a decision should be made whether to discontinue the drug or to discontinue nursing while on treatment or within 6 weeks after stopping therapy, taking into account the importance of the drug to the mother.

Pediatric Use

***De novo* Renal Transplant**

The safety and effectiveness of Myfortic in *de novo* pediatric renal transplant patients have not been established.

Stable Renal Transplant

There are no pharmacokinetic data available for pediatric patients <5 years. The safety and effectiveness of Myfortic have been established in the age group 5-16 years in stable pediatric renal transplant patients. Use of Myfortic in this age group is supported by evidence from adequate and well-controlled studies of Myfortic in stable adult renal transplant patients. Limited pharmacokinetic data are available for stable pediatric renal transplant patients in the age group 5-16 years. Pediatric doses for patients with BSA <1.19 m^2 cannot be accurately administered using currently available formulations of Myfortic tablets *(see CLINICAL PHARMACOLOGY, Special Populations, and DOSAGE AND ADMINISTRATION).*

Table 4

Adverse Events (%) in Controlled *de novo* and Maintenance Renal Studies Reported in ≥20% of Patients

	***de novo* Renal Study**		**Maintenance Renal Study**	
	Myfortic® 1.44 g/day (n=213)	**mycophenolate mofetil 2 g/day (n=210)**	**Myfortic® 1.44 g/day (n=159)**	**mycophenolate mofetil 2 g/day (n=163)**
Blood and Lymphatic System Disorders				
Anemia	21.6	21.9	–	–
Leukopenia	19.2	20.5	–	–
Gastrointestinal System Disorders				
Constipation	38.0	39.5	–	–
Nausea	29.1	27.1	24.5	19
Diarrhea	23.5	24.8	21.4	24.5
Vomiting	23.0	20.0	–	–
Dyspepsia	22.5	19.0	–	–
Infections and Infestations				
Urinary Tract Infection	29.1	33.3	–	–
CMV Infection	20.2	18.1	–	–
Nervous System Disorder				
Insomnia	23.5	23.8	–	–
Surgical and Medical Procedure				
Post-operative Pain	23.9	18.6	–	–

Table 5

Viral and Fungal Infections (%) Reported Over 0-12 Months

	***de novo* Renal Study**		**Maintenance Renal Study**	
	Myfortic® 1.44 g/day (n=213)	**mycophenolate mofetil 2 g/day (n=210)**	**Myfortic® 1.44 g/day (n=159)**	**mycophenolate mofetil 2 g/day (n=163)**
	(%)	**(%)**	**(%)**	**(%)**
Any Cytomegalovirus	21.6	20.5	1.9	1.8
–Cytomegalovirus Disease	4.7	4.3	0	0.6
Herpes Simplex	8.0	6.2	1.3	2.5
Herpes Zoster	4.7	3.8	1.9	3.1
Any Fungal Infection	10.8	11.9	2.5	1.8
–Candida NOS	5.6	6.2	0	1.8
–Candida Albicans	2.3	3.8	0.6	0

Geriatric Use

Patients ≥65 years may generally be at increased risk of adverse drug reactions due to immunosuppression. Clinical studies of Myfortic did not include sufficient numbers of subjects aged 65 and over to determine whether they respond differently from younger subjects. Other reported clinical experience has not identified differences in responses between the elderly and younger patients. In general, dose selection for an elderly patient should be cautious, reflecting the greater frequency of decreased hepatic, renal, or cardiac function, and of concomitant disease or other drug therapy.

ADVERSE REACTIONS

The incidence of adverse events for Myfortic® (mycophenolic acid) was determined in randomized, comparative,

active-controlled, double-blind, double-dummy trials in prevention of acute rejection in *de novo* and maintenance kidney transplant patients.

The principal adverse reactions associated with the administration of Myfortic include constipation, nausea, and urinary tract infection in *de novo* patients and nausea, diarrhea and nasopharyngitis in maintenance patients.

Adverse events reported in ≥20% of patients receiving Myfortic or mycophenolate mofetil in the 12-month *de novo* renal study and maintenance renal study, when used in combination with cyclosporine, USP (MODIFIED) and corticosteroids, are listed in Table 4. Adverse event rates were similar between Myfortic and mycophenolate mofetil in both *de novo* and maintenance patients.

[See table 4 above]

Table 5 summarizes the incidence of opportunistic infections in *de novo* and maintenance transplant patients, which were similar in both treatment groups.

[See table 5 above]

The following opportunistic infections occurred rarely in the above controlled trials: aspergillus and cryptococcus.

The incidence of malignancies and lymphoma is consistent with that reported in the literature for this patient population. Lymphoma developed in 2 *de novo* patients (0.9%), (one diagnosed 9 days after treatment initiation) and in 2 maintenance patients (1.3%) (one was AIDS-related), receiving Myfortic with other immunosuppressive agents in the 12-month controlled-clinical trials. Non-melanoma skin carcinoma occurred in 0.9% *de novo* and 1.8% maintenance patients. Other types of malignancy occurred in 0.5% *de novo* and 0.6% maintenance patients.

The following adverse events were reported between 3% to <20% incidence in *de novo* and maintenance patients treated with Myfortic in combination with cyclosporine and corticosteroids are listed in Table 6.

[See table 6 at top of next page]

The following additional adverse reactions have been associated with the exposure to MPA when administered as a sodium salt or as mofetil ester:

Gastrointestinal: Colitis (sometimes caused by CMV), pancreatitis, esophagitis, intestinal perforation, gastrointestinal hemorrhage, gastric ulcers, duodenal ulcers, and ileus *(see PRECAUTIONS).*

Resistance Mechanism Disorders: Serious life-threatening infections such as meningitis and infectious endocarditis have been reported occasionally and there is evidence of a higher frequency of certain types of serious infections such as tuberculosis and atypical mycobacterial infection.

Respiratory: Interstitial lung disorders, including fatal pulmonary fibrosis, have been reported rarely with MPA administration and should be considered in the differential diagnosis of pulmonary symptoms ranging from dyspnea to respiratory failure in post-transplant patients receiving MPA derivatives.

OVERDOSAGE

Signs and Symptoms

There has been no reported experience of acute overdose of Myfortic® (mycophenolic acid) in humans.

Possible signs and symptoms of acute overdose could include the following: hematological abnormalities such as leukopenia and neutropenia, and gastrointestinal symptoms such as abdominal pain, diarrhea, nausea and vomiting, and dyspepsia.

Treatment and Management

General supportive measures and symptomatic treatment should be followed in all cases of overdosage. Although dialysis may be used to remove the inactive metabolite MPAG, it would not be expected to remove clinically significant amounts of the active moiety MPA due to the 98% plasma protein binding of MPA. By interfering with enterohepatic circulation of MPA, activated charcoal or bile acid sequestrants, such as cholestyramine, may reduce the systemic MPA exposure.

DOSAGE AND ADMINISTRATION

The recommended dose of Myfortic® (mycophenolic acid) is 720 mg administered twice daily (1440 mg total daily dose) on an empty stomach, one hour before or two hours after food intake *(see CLINICAL PHARMACOLOGY, Food Effect).*

Myfortic delayed-release tablets and mycophenolate mofetil tablets and capsules should not be used interchangeably without physician supervision because the rate of absorption following the administration of these two products is not equivalent.

Patients are to be instructed that Myfortic tablets should not be crushed, chewed, or cut prior to ingesting. The tablets should be swallowed whole in order to maintain the integrity of the enteric coating.

Continued on next page

Table 6
Adverse Events Reported in 3% to <20% of Patients Treated with Myfortic® in Combination with Cyclosporine* and Corticosteroids

	***de novo* Renal Study**	**Maintenance Renal Study**
Blood and Lymphatic Disorders	Lymphocele, thrombocytopenia	Leukopenia, anemia
Cardiac Disorder	Tachycardia	–
Eye Disorder	Vision blurred	–
Endocrine Disorders	Cushingoid, hirsutism	–
Gastrointestinal Disorder	Abdominal pain upper, flatulence, abdominal distension, sore throat, abdominal pain lower, abdominal pain, gingival hyperplasia, loose stool	Vomiting, dyspepsia, abdominal pain, constipation, gastroesophageal reflux disease, loose stool, flatulence, abdominal pain upper
General Disorders and Administration Site Conditions	Edema, edema lower limb, pyrexia, pain, fatigue, edema peripheral, chest pain	Fatigue, pyrexia, edema, chest pain, peripheral edema
Infections and Infestations	Nasopharyngitis, herpes simplex, upper respiratory tract infection, oral candidiasis, herpes zoster, sinusitis, wound infection, implant infection, pneumonia	Nasopharyngitis, upper respiratory tract infection, urinary tract infection, influenza, sinusitis
Injury, Poisoning, and Procedural Complications	Drug toxicity	Post procedural pain
Investigations	Blood creatinine increased, hemoglobin decrease, blood pressure increased, liver function tests abnormal	Blood creatinine increase, weight increase
Metabolism and Nutrition Disorders	Hypocalcemia, hyperuricemia, hyperlipidemia, hypokalemia, hypophosphatemia, hypercholesterolemia, hyperkalemia, hypomagnesemia, diabetes mellitus, hyperphosphatemia, dehydration, fluid overload, hyperglycemia, hypercalcemia	Dehydration, hypokalemia, hypercholesterolemia
Musculoskeletal and Connective Tissue Disorders	Back pain, arthralgia, pain in limb, muscle cramps, myalgia	Arthralgia, pain in limb, back pain, muscle cramps, peripheral swelling, myalgia
Nervous System Disorders	Tremor, headache, dizziness (excluding vertigo)	Headache, dizziness
Psychiatric Disorders	Anxiety	Insomnia, depression
Renal and Urinary Disorders	Renal tubular necrosis, renal impairment, dysuria, hematuria, hydronephrosis, bladder spasm, urinary retention	–
Respiratory, Thoracic and Mediastinal Disorders	Cough, dyspnea, dyspnea exertional	Cough, dyspnea, pharyngolaryngeal pain, sinus congestion
Skin and Subcutaneous Tissue Disorder	Acne, pruritus	Rash, contusion
Surgical and Medical Procedures	Complications of transplant surgery, post-operative complications, post-operative wound complication	–
Vascular Disorder	Hypertension, hypertension aggravated, hypotension	Hypertension

*USP (MODIFIED)

Myfortic—Cont.

Pediatric: Based on a pharmacokinetic study conducted in stable renal pediatric transplant patients, the recommended dose of Myfortic in stable pediatric patients is 400 mg/m^2 body surface area (BSA) administered twice daily (up to a maximum dose of 720 mg administered twice daily). Patients with a BSA of 1.19 to 1.58 m^2 may be dosed either with three Myfortic 180 mg tablets or one 180 mg tablet plus one 360 mg tablet twice daily (1080 mg daily dose). Patients with a BSA of >1.58 m^2 may be dosed either with four Myfortic 180 mg tablets or two Myfortic 360 mg tablets twice daily (1440 mg daily dose). Pediatric doses for patients with BSA <1.19 m^2 cannot be accurately administered using currently available formulations of Myfortic tablets.

Geriatrics: The maximum recommended dose is 720 mg administered twice daily.

Treatment During Rejection Episodes

Renal transplant rejection does not lead to changes in MPA pharmacokinetics; dosage reduction or interruption of Myfortic is not required.

Patients with Renal Impairment

No dose adjustments are needed in patients experiencing delayed renal graft function post-operatively. Patients with severe chronic renal impairment (GFR <25 mL/min/1.73 m^2 BSA) should be carefully followed for potential adverse reactions due to increase in free MPA and total MPAG concentrations *(see CLINICAL PHARMACOLOGY, Pharmacokinetics, Special Populations).*

Patients with Hepatic Impairment

No dose adjustments are needed for renal transplant patients with hepatic parenchymal disease. However, it is not known whether dosage adjustments are needed for hepatic disease with other etiologies *(see CLINICAL PHARMACOLOGY, Pharmacokinetics).*

HOW SUPPLIED

Myfortic® (mycophenolic acid) delayed-released tablets

360 mg tablet: Pale orange-red film-coated ovaloid tablet with imprint (debossing) "CT" on one side, containing 360 mg mycophenolic acid formulated as a sodium salt.

Bottles of 120 .... NDC 0078-0386-66

180 mg tablet: Lime green film-coated round tablet with bevelled edges and the imprint (debossing) "C" on one side, containing 180 mg mycophenolic acid formulated as a sodium salt.

Bottles of 120 .... NDC 0078-0385-66

Storage

Store at 25°C (77°F); excursions permitted to 15-30°C (59-86°F) [see USP Controlled Room Temperature].

Protect from moisture.

Dispense in a tight container (USP).

Handling

Tablets should not be crushed or cut.

T2004-08
FEBRUARY 2004 Printed in U.S.A. 89022201
Manufactured by:
Novartis Pharma Stein AG
Stein, Switzerland

Distributed by:
Novartis Pharmaceuticals Corporation
East Hanover, New Jersey 07936

Shown in Product Identification Guide, page 325

NEORAL® SOFT GELATIN CAPSULES ℞

[nē ō 'ral]

(cyclosporine capsules, USP) MODIFIED

NEORAL® ORAL SOLUTION

(cyclosporine oral solution, USP) MODIFIED

℞ only

Prescribing Information

The following prescribing information is based on official labeling in effect July 2004.

WARNING

Only physicians experienced in management of systemic immunosuppressive therapy for the indicated disease should prescribe Neoral®. At doses used in solid organ transplantation, only physicians experienced in immunosuppressive therapy and management of organ transplant recipients should prescribe Neoral®. Patients receiving the drug should be managed in facilities equipped and staffed with adequate laboratory and supportive medical resources. The physician responsible for maintenance therapy should have complete information requisite for the follow-up of the patient.

Neoral®, a systemic immunosuppressant, may increase the susceptibility to infection and the development of neoplasia. In kidney, liver, and heart transplant patients Neoral® may be administered with other immunosuppressive agents. Increased susceptibility to infection and the possible development of lymphoma and other neoplasms may result from the increase in the degree of immunosuppression in transplant patients.

Neoral® Soft Gelatin Capsules (cyclosporine capsules, USP) MODIFIED and Neoral® Oral Solution (cyclosporine oral solution, USP) MODIFIED have increased bioavailability in comparison to Sandimmune® Soft Gelatin Capsules (cyclosporine capsules, USP) and Sandimmune® Oral Solution (cyclosporine oral solution, USP). Neoral® and Sandimmune® are not bioequivalent and cannot be used without physician supervision. For a given trough concentration, cyclosporine exposure will be greater with Neoral® than with Sandimmune®. If a patient who is receiving exceptionally high doses of Sandimmune® is converted to Neoral®, particular caution should be exercised. Cyclosporine blood concentrations should be monitored in transplant and rheumatoid arthritis patients taking Neoral® to avoid toxicity due to high concentrations. Dose adjustments should be made in transplant patients to minimize possible organ rejection due to low concentrations. Comparison of blood concentrations in the published literature with blood concentrations obtained using current assays must be done with detailed knowledge of the assay methods employed.

For Psoriasis Patients *(See also Boxed WARNINGS above)*

Psoriasis patients previously treated with PUVA and to a lesser extent, methotrexate or other immunosuppressive agents, UVB, coal tar, or radiation therapy, are at an increased risk of developing skin malignancies when taking Neoral®.

Cyclosporine, the active ingredient in Neoral®, in recommended dosages, can cause systemic hypertension and nephrotoxicity. The risk increases with increasing dose and duration of cyclosporine therapy. Renal dysfunction, including structural kidney damage, is a potential consequence of cyclosporine, and therefore, renal function must be monitored during therapy.

DESCRIPTION

Neoral® is an oral formulation of cyclosporine that immediately forms a microemulsion in an aqueous environment.

Cyclosporine, the active principle in Neoral®, is a cyclic polypeptide immunosuppressant agent consisting of 11 amino acids. It is produced as a metabolite by the fungus species *Beauveria nivea*.

Chemically, cyclosporine is designated as [*R*-[*R**,*R**-(*E*)]]-cyclic-(L-alanyl-D-alanyl-*N*-methyl-L-leucyl-*N*-methyl-L-leucyl-*N*-methyl-L-valyl-3-hydroxy-*N*,4-dimethyl-L-2-amino-6-octenoyl-L-α-amino-butyryl-*N*-methylglycyl-*N*-methyl-L-leucyl-L-valyl-*N*-methyl-L-leucyl).

Neoral® Soft Gelatin Capsules (cyclosporine capsules, USP) MODIFIED are available in 25 mg and 100 mg strengths.

Each 25 mg capsule contains:
cyclosporine .... 25 mg
alcohol, USP dehydrated .... 11.9% v/v (9.5% wt/vol.)

Each 100 mg capsule contains:
cyclosporine .... 100 mg
alcohol, USP dehydrated .... 11.9% v/v (9.5% wt/vol.)

Inactive Ingredients: Corn oil-mono-di-triglycerides, polyoxyl 40 hydrogenated castor oil NF, DL-α-tocopherol USP, gelatin NF, glycerol, iron oxide black, propylene glycol USP, titanium dioxide USP, carmine, and other ingredients.

Neoral® Oral Solution (cyclosporine oral solution, USP) modified is available in 50 mL bottles.

Each mL contains:

cyclosporine .... 100 mg/mL

alcohol, USP dehydrated .... 11.9% v/v (9.5% wt/vol.)

Inactive Ingredients: Corn oil-mono-di-triglycerides, polyoxyl 40 hydrogenated castor oil NF, DL-α-tocopherol USP, propylene glycol USP.

The chemical structure of cyclosporine (also known as cyclosporin A) is:

```
      H3C
         \
          CH
          ||
          HC
            \
             CH2
        H   |
    HO  C  CH-CH3
        |
MeVal-N-CH-C-Abu-MeGly
   |    |   ||      |
 MeLeu CH3  O     MeLeu
   |                |
 MeLeu-D-Ala-Ala-MeLeu-Val
```

$C_{62}H_{111}N_{11}O_{12}$ Mol. Wt. 1202.63

CLINICAL PHARMACOLOGY

Cyclosporine is a potent immunosuppressive agent that in animals prolongs survival of allogeneic transplants involving skin, kidney, liver, heart, pancreas, bone marrow, small intestine, and lung. Cyclosporine has been demonstrated to suppress some humoral immunity and to a greater extent, cell-mediated immune reactions such as allograft rejection, delayed hypersensitivity, experimental allergic encephalomyelitis, Freund's adjuvant arthritis, and graft vs. host disease in many animal species for a variety of organs.

The effectiveness of cyclosporine results from specific and reversible inhibition of immunocompetent lymphocytes in the G_0- and G_1-phase of the cell cycle. T-lymphocytes are preferentially inhibited. The T-helper cell is the main target, although the T-suppressor cell may also be suppressed. Cyclosporine also inhibits lymphokine production and release including interleukin-2.

No effects on phagocytic function (changes in enzyme secretions, chemotactic migration of granulocytes, macrophage migration, carbon clearance *in vivo*) have been detected in animals. Cyclosporine does not cause bone marrow suppression in animal models or man.

Pharmacokinetics: The immunosuppressive activity of cyclosporine is primarily due to parent drug. Following oral administration, absorption of cyclosporine is incomplete. The extent of absorption of cyclosporine is dependent on the individual patient, the patient population, and the formulation. Elimination of cyclosporine is primarily biliary with only 6% of the dose (parent drug and metabolites) excreted in urine. The disposition of cyclosporine from blood is generally biphasic, with a terminal half-life of approximately 8.4 hours (range 5–18 hours). Following intravenous administration, the blood clearance of cyclosporine (assay: HPLC) is approximately 5–7 mL/min/kg in adult recipients of renal or liver allografts. Blood cyclosporine clearance appears to be slightly slower in cardiac transplant patients.

The Neoral® Soft Gelatin Capsules (cyclosporine capsules, USP) MODIFIED and Neoral® Oral Solution (cyclosporine oral solution, USP) MODIFIED are bioequivalent. Neoral® Oral Solution diluted with orange juice or apple juice is bioequivalent to Neoral Oral Solution diluted with water. The effect of milk on the bioavailability of cyclosporine when administered as Neoral Oral Solution has not been evaluated.

The relationship between administered dose and exposure (area under the concentration versus time curve, AUC) is linear within the therapeutic dose range. The intersubject variability (total, %CV) of cyclosporine exposure (AUC) when Neoral® or Sandimmune® is administered ranges from approximately 20% to 50% in renal transplant patients. This intersubject variability contributes to the need for individualization of the dosing regimen for optimal therapy *(see DOSAGE AND ADMINISTRATION)*. Intrasubject variability of AUC in renal transplant recipients (%CV) was 9%–21% for Neoral® and 19%–26% for Sandimmune®. In the same studies, intrasubject variability of trough concentrations (%CV) was 17%–30% for Neoral® and 16%–38% for Sandimmune®.

Absorption: Neoral® has increased bioavailability compared to Sandimmune®. The absolute bioavailability of cyclosporine administered as Sandimmune® is dependent on the patient population, estimated to be less than 10% in liver transplant patients and as great as 89% in some renal transplant patients. The absolute bioavailability of cyclosporine administered as Neoral® has not been determined in adults. In studies of renal transplant, rheumatoid arthritis and psoriasis patients, the mean cyclosporine AUC was approximately 20% to 50% greater and the peak blood cyclosporine concentration (C_{max}) was approximately 40% to 106% greater following administration of Neoral® compared to following administration of Sandimmune®. The dose normalized AUC in *de novo* liver transplant patients administered Neoral® 28 days after transplantation was 50% greater and C_{max} was 90% greater than in those patients administered Sandimmune®. AUC and C_{max} are also increased (Neoral® relative to Sandimmune®) in heart transplant patients, but data are very limited. Although the AUC and C_{max} values are higher on Neoral® relative to Sandimmune®, the pre-dose trough concentrations (dose-normalized) are similar for the two formulations.

Pharmacokinetic Parameters (mean ± SD)

Patient Population	Dose/day[1] (mg/d)	Dose/weight (mg/kg/d)	AUC[2] (ng•hr/mL)	C_{max} (ng/mL)	Trough[3] (ng/mL)	CL/F (mL/min)	CL/F (mL/min/kg)
De novo renal transplant[4] Week 4 (N=37)	597±174	7.95±2.81	8772±2089	1802±428	361±129	593±204	7.8±2.9
Stable renal transplant[4] (N=55)	344±122	4.10±1.58	6035±2194	1333±469	251±116	492±140	5.9±2.1
De novo liver transplant[5] Week 4 (N=18)	458±190	6.89±3.68	7187±2816	1555±740	268±101	577±309	8.6±5.7
De novo rheumatoid arthritis[6] (N=23)	182±55.6	2.37±0.36	2641±877	728±263	96.4±37.7	613±196	8.3±2.8
De novo psoriasis[6] Week 4 (N=18)	189±69.8	2.48±0.65	2324±1048	655±186	74.9±46.7	723±186	10.2±3.9

[1]Total daily dose was divided into two doses administered every 12 hours
[2]AUC was measured over one dosing interval
[3]Trough concentration was measured just prior to the morning Neoral® dose, approximately 12 hours after the previous dose
[4]Assay: TDx specific monoclonal fluorescence polarization immunoassay
[5]Assay: Cyclo-trac specific monoclonal radioimmunoassay
[6]Assay: INCSTAR specific monoclonal radioimmunoassay

Following oral administration of Neoral®, the time to peak blood cyclosporine concentrations (T_{max}) ranged from 1.5–2.0 hours. The administration of food with Neoral® decreases the cyclosporine AUC and C_{max}. A high fat meal (669 kcal, 45 grams fat) consumed within one-half hour before Neoral® administration decreased the AUC by 13% and C_{max} by 33%. The effects of a low fat meal (667 kcal, 15 grams fat) were similar.

The effect of T-tube diversion of bile on the absorption of cyclosporine from Neoral® was investigated in eleven *de novo* liver transplant patients. When the patients were administered Neoral® with and without T-tube diversion of bile, very little difference in absorption was observed, as measured by the change in maximal cyclosporine blood concentrations from pre-dose values with the T-tube closed relative to when it was open: 6.9±41% (range -55% to 68%).

[See table above]

Distribution: Cyclosporine is distributed largely outside the blood volume. The steady state volume of distribution during intravenous dosing has been reported as 3–5 L/kg in solid organ transplant recipients. In blood, the distribution is concentration dependent. Approximately 33%–47% is in plasma, 4%–9% in lymphocytes, 5%–12% in granulocytes, and 41%–58% in erythrocytes. At high concentrations, the binding capacity of leukocytes and erythrocytes becomes saturated. In plasma, approximately 90% is bound to proteins, primarily lipoproteins. Cyclosporine is excreted in human milk. *(See PRECAUTIONS, Nursing Mothers)*

Metabolism: Cyclosporine is extensively metabolized by the cytochrome P-450 3A enzyme system in the liver, and to a lesser degree in the gastrointestinal tract, and the kidney. The metabolism of cyclosporine can be altered by the co-administration of a variety of agents. *(See PRECAUTIONS, Drug Interactions)* At least 25 metabolites have been identified from human bile, feces, blood, and urine. The biological activity of the metabolites and their contributions to toxicity are considerably less than those of the parent compound. The major metabolites (M1, M9, and M4N) result from oxidation at the 1-beta, 9-gamma, and 4-N-demethylated positions, respectively. At steady state following the oral administration of Sandimmune®, the mean AUCs for blood concentrations of M1, M9, and M4N are about 70%, 21%, and 7.5% of the AUC for blood cyclosporine concentrations, respectively. Based on blood concentration data from stable renal transplant patients (13 patients administered Neoral® and Sandimmune® in a crossover study), and bile concentration data from *de novo* liver transplant patients (4 administered Neoral®, 3 administered Sandimmune®), the percentage of dose present as M1, M9, and M4N metabolites is similar when either Neoral® or Sandimmune® is administered.

Excretion: Only 0.1% of a cyclosporine dose is excreted unchanged in the urine. Elimination is primarily biliary with only 6% of the dose (parent drug and metabolites) excreted in the urine. Neither dialysis nor renal failure alter cyclosporine clearance significantly.

Drug Interactions: *(See PRECAUTIONS, Drug Interactions)* When diclofenac or methotrexate was co-administered with cyclosporine in rheumatoid arthritis patients, the AUC of diclofenac and methotrexate, each was significantly increased. *(See PRECAUTIONS, Drug Interactions)* No clinically significant pharmacokinetic interactions occurred between cyclosporine and aspirin, ketoprofen, piroxicam, or indomethacin.

Special Populations: ***Pediatric Population:*** Pharmacokinetic data from pediatric patients administered Neoral® or Sandimmune® are very limited. In 15 renal transplant patients aged 3–16 years, cyclosporine whole blood clearance after IV administration of Sandimmune® was 10.6±3.7 mL/min/kg (assay: Cyclo-trac specific RIA). In a study of 7 renal transplant patients aged 2–16, the cyclosporine clearance ranged from 9.8–15.5 mL/min/kg. In 9 liver transplant patients aged 0.6–5.6 years, clearance was 9.3±5.4 mL/min/kg (assay: HPLC).

In the pediatric population, Neoral® also demonstrates an increased bioavailability as compared to Sandimmune®. In 7 liver *de novo* transplant patients aged 1.4–10 years, the absolute bioavailability of Neoral® was 43% (range 30%–68%) and for Sandimmune® in the same individuals absolute bioavailability was 28% (range 17%–42%).

[See table at top of next page]

Geriatric Population: Comparison of single dose data from both normal elderly volunteers (N=18, mean age 69 years) and elderly rheumatoid arthritis patients (N=16, mean age 68 years) to single dose data in young adult volunteers (N=16, mean age 26 years) showed no significant difference in the pharmacokinetic parameters.

CLINICAL TRIALS

Rheumatoid Arthritis: The effectiveness of Sandimmune® and Neoral® in the treatment of severe rheumatoid arthritis was evaluated in 5 clinical studies involving a total of 728 cyclosporine treated patients and 273 placebo treated patients.

A summary of the results is presented for the "responder" rates per treatment group, with a responder being defined as a patient having *completed* the trial with a 20% improvement in the tender and the swollen joint count and a 20% improvement in 2 of 4 of investigator global, patient global, disability, and erythrocyte sedimentation rates (ESR) for the Studies 651 and 652 and 3 of 5 of investigator global, patient global, disability, visual analog pain, and ESR for Studies 2008, 654 and 302.

Study 651 enrolled 264 patients with active rheumatoid arthritis with at least 20 involved joints, who had failed at least one major RA drug, using a 3:3:2 randomization to one of the following three groups: (1) cyclosporine dosed at 2.5–5 mg/kg/day, (2) methotrexate at 7.5–15 mg/week, or (3) placebo. Treatment duration was 24 weeks. The mean cyclosporine dose at the last visit was 3.1 mg/kg/day. *See Graph below.*

Study 652 enrolled 250 patients with active RA with >6 active painful or tender joints who had failed at least one major RA drug. Patients were randomized using a 3:3:2 randomization to 1 of 3 treatment arms: (1) 1.5–5 mg/kg/day of cyclosporine, (2) 2.5–5 mg/kg/day of cyclosporine, and (3) placebo. Treatment duration was 16 weeks. The mean cyclosporine dose for group 2 at the last visit was 2.92 mg/kg/day. *See Graph below.*

Study 2008 enrolled 144 patients with active RA and >6 active joints who had unsuccessful treatment courses of aspirin and gold or Penicillamine. Patients were randomized to 1 of 2 treatment groups (1) cyclosporine 2.5–5 mg/kg/day with adjustments after the first month to achieve a target trough level and (2) placebo. Treatment duration was 24 weeks. The mean cyclosporine dose at the last visit was 3.63 mg/kg/day. *See Graph below.*

Study 654 enrolled 148 patients who remained with active joint counts of 6 or more despite treatment with maximally tolerated methotrexate doses for at least three months. Patients continued to take their current dose of methotrexate and were randomized to receive, in addition, one of the following medications: (1) cyclosporine 2.5 mg/kg/day with dose increases of 0.5 mg/kg/day at weeks 2 and 4 if there was no evidence of toxicity and further increases of 0.5 mg/kg/day at weeks 8 and 16 if a <30% decrease in active joint count occurred without any significant toxicity; dose decreases could be made at any time for toxicity or (2) placebo. Treatment duration was 24 weeks. The mean cyclosporine dose at the last visit was 2.8 mg/kg/day (range: 1.3–4.1). *See Graph below.*

Study 302 enrolled 299 patients with severe active RA, 99% of whom were unresponsive or intolerant to at least one prior major RA drug. Patients were randomized to 1 of 2 treatment groups (1) Neoral® and (2) cyclosporine, both of which were started at 2.5 mg/kg/day and increased after 4 weeks for inefficacy in increments of 0.5 mg/kg/day to a maximum of 5 mg/kg/day and decreased at any time for

Continued on next page

Neoral—Cont.

toxicity. Treatment duration was 24 weeks. The mean cyclosporine dose at the last visit was 2.91 mg/kg/day (range: 0.72–5.17) for Neoral® and 3.27 mg/kg/day (range: 0.73–5.68) for cyclosporine. *See Graph below.*

[See figure above]

INDICATIONS AND USAGE

Kidney, Liver, and Heart Transplantation: Neoral® is indicated for the prophylaxis of organ rejection in kidney, liver, and heart allogeneic transplants. Neoral® has been used in combination with azathioprine and corticosteroids.

Rheumatoid Arthritis: Neoral® is indicated for the treatment of patients with severe active, rheumatoid arthritis where the disease has not adequately responded to methotrexate. Neoral® can be used in combination with methotrexate in rheumatoid arthritis patients who do not respond adequately to methotrexate alone.

Psoriasis: Neoral® is indicated for the treatment of *adult, nonimmunocompromised* patients with severe (i.e., extensive and/or disabling), recalcitrant, plaque psoriasis who have failed to respond to at least one systemic therapy (e.g., PUVA, retinoids, or methotrexate) or in patients for whom other systemic therapies are contraindicated, or cannot be tolerated.

While rebound rarely occurs, most patients will experience relapse with Neoral® as with other therapies upon cessation of treatment.

CONTRAINDICATIONS

General: Neoral® is contraindicated in patients with a hypersensitivity to cyclosporine or to any of the ingredients of the formulation.

Rheumatoid Arthritis: Rheumatoid arthritis patients with abnormal renal function, uncontrolled hypertension, or malignancies should not receive Neoral®.

Psoriasis: Psoriasis patients who are treated with Neoral® should not receive concomitant PUVA or UVB therapy, methotrexate or other immunosuppressive agents, coal tar or radiation therapy. Psoriasis patients with abnormal renal function, uncontrolled hypertension, or malignancies should not receive Neoral®.

WARNINGS

(See also Boxed WARNING)

All Patients: Cyclosporine, the active ingredient of Neoral® can cause nephrotoxicity and hepatotoxicity. The risk increases with increasing doses of cyclosporine. Renal dysfunction including structural kidney damage is a potential consequence of Neoral® and therefore renal function must be monitored during therapy. **Care should be taken in using cyclosporine with nephrotoxic drugs.** ***(See PRECAUTIONS)***

Patients receiving Neoral® require frequent monitoring of serum creatinine. *(See Special Monitoring under DOSAGE AND ADMINISTRATION)* Elderly patients should be monitored with particular care, since decreases in renal function also occur with age. If patients are not properly monitored and doses are not properly adjusted, cyclosporine therapy can be associated with the occurrence of structural kidney damage and persistent renal dysfunction.

An increase in serum creatinine and BUN may occur during Neoral® therapy and reflect a reduction in the glomerular filtration rate. Impaired renal function at any time requires close monitoring, and frequent dosage adjustment may be indicated. The frequency and severity of serum creatinine elevations increase with dose and duration of cyclosporine therapy. These elevations are likely to become more pronounced without dose reduction or discontinuation.

Because Neoral® is not bioequivalent to Sandimmune®, conversion from Neoral® to Sandimmune® using a 1:1 ratio (mg/kg/day) may result in lower cyclosporine blood concentrations. Conversion from Neoral® to Sandimmune® should be made with increased monitoring to avoid the potential of underdosing.

Kidney, Liver, and Heart Transplant: Cyclosporine, the active ingredient of Neoral®, can cause nephrotoxicity and hepatotoxicity when used in high doses. It is not unusual for serum creatinine and BUN levels to be elevated during cyclosporine therapy. These elevations in renal transplant patients do not necessarily indicate rejection, and each patient must be fully evaluated before dosage adjustment is initiated.

Based on the historical Sandimmune® experience with oral solution, nephrotoxicity associated with cyclosporine had been noted in 25% of cases of renal transplantation, 38% of cases of cardiac transplantation, and 37% of cases of liver transplantation. Mild nephrotoxicity was generally noted 2–3 months after renal transplant and consisted of an arrest in the fall of the pre-operative elevations of BUN and creatinine at a range of 35–45 mg/dl and 2.0–2.5 mg/dl respectively. These elevations were often responsive to cyclosporine dosage reduction.

More overt nephrotoxicity was seen early after transplantation and was characterized by a rapidly rising BUN and creatinine. Since these events are similar to renal rejection episodes, care must be taken to differentiate between them. This form of nephrotoxicity is usually responsive to cyclosporine dosage reduction.

Although specific diagnostic criteria which reliably differentiate renal graft rejection from drug toxicity have not been found, a number of parameters have been significantly associated with one or the other. It should be noted however, that up to 20% of patients may have simultaneous nephrotoxicity and rejection.

Pediatric Pharmacokinetic Parameters (mean ± SD)

Patient Population	Dose/day (mg/d)	Dose/weight (mg/kg/d)	AUC[1] (ng•hr/mL)	C_{max} (ng/mL)	CL/F (mL/min)	CL/F (mL/min/kg)
Stable liver transplant[2]						
Age 2–8, Dosed TID (N=9)	101±25	5.95±1.32	2163±801	629±219	285±94	16.6±4.3
Age 8–15, Dosed BID (N=8)	188±55	4.96±2.09	4272±1462	975±281	378±80	10.2±4.0
Stable liver transplant[3]						
Age 3, Dosed BID (N=1)	120	8.33	5832	1050	171	11.9
Age 8–15, Dosed BID (N=5)	158±55	5.51±1.91	4452±2475	1013±635	328±121	11.0±1.9
Stable renal transplant[3]						
Age 7–15, Dosed BID (N=5)	328±83	7.37±4.11	6922±1988	1827±487	418±143	8.7±2.9

[1]AUC was measured over one dosing interval
[2]Assay: Cyclo-trac specific monoclonal radioimmunoassay
[3]Assay: TDx specific monoclonal fluorescence polarization immunoassay

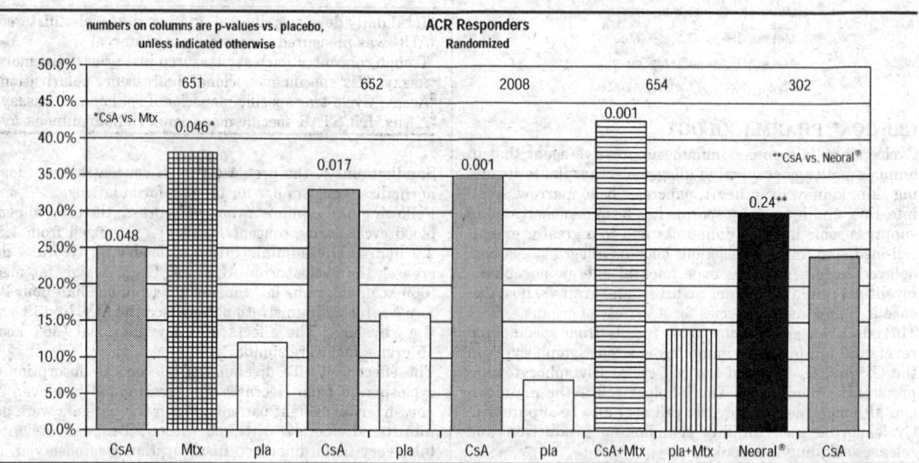

[See table at top of next page]

A form of a cyclosporine-associated nephropathy is characterized by serial deterioration in renal function and morphologic changes in the kidneys. From 5%–15% of transplant recipients who have received cyclosporine will fail to show a reduction in rising serum creatinine despite a decrease or discontinuation of cyclosporine therapy. Renal biopsies from these patients will demonstrate one or several of the following alterations: tubular vacuolization, tubular microcalcifications, peritubular capillary congestion, arteriolopathy, and a striped form of interstitial fibrosis with tubular atrophy. Though none of these morphologic changes is entirely specific, a diagnosis of cyclosporine-associated structural nephrotoxicity requires evidence of these findings.

When considering the development of cyclosporine-associated nephropathy, it is noteworthy that several authors have reported an association between the appearance of interstitial fibrosis and higher cumulative doses or persistently high circulating trough levels of cyclosporine. This is particularly true during the first 6 post-transplant months when the dosage tends to be highest and when, in kidney recipients, the organ appears to be most vulnerable to the toxic effects of cyclosporine. Among other contributing factors to the development of interstitial fibrosis in these patients are prolonged perfusion time, warm ischemia time, as well as episodes of acute toxicity, and acute and chronic rejection. The reversibility of interstitial fibrosis and its correlation to renal function have not yet been determined. Reversibility of arteriolopathy has been reported after stopping cyclosporine or lowering the dosage.

Impaired renal function at any time requires close monitoring, and frequent dosage adjustment may be indicated.

In the event of severe and unremitting rejection, when rescue therapy with pulse steroids and monoclonal antibodies fail to reverse the rejection episode, it may be preferable to switch to alternative immunosuppressive therapy rather than increase the Neoral® dose to excessive levels.

Occasionally patients have developed a syndrome of thrombocytopenia and microangiopathic hemolytic anemia which may result in graft failure. The vasculopathy can occur in the absence of rejection and is accompanied by avid platelet consumption within the graft as demonstrated by Indium 111 labeled platelet studies. Neither the pathogenesis nor the management of this syndrome is clear. Though resolution has occurred after reduction or discontinuation of cyclosporine and 1) administration of streptokinase and heparin or 2) plasmapheresis, this appears to depend upon early detection with Indium 111 labeled platelet scans. *(See ADVERSE REACTIONS)*

Significant hyperkalemia (sometimes associated with hyperchloremic metabolic acidosis) and hyperuricemia have been seen occasionally in individual patients.

Hepatotoxicity associated with cyclosporine use had been noted in 4% of cases of renal transplantation, 7% of cases of cardiac transplantation, and 4% of cases of liver transplantation. This was usually noted during the first month of therapy when high doses of cyclosporine were used and consisted of elevations of hepatic enzymes and bilirubin. The chemistry elevations usually decreased with a reduction in dosage.

As in patients receiving other immunosuppressants, those patients receiving cyclosporine are at increased risk for development of lymphomas and other malignancies, particularly those of the skin. The increased risk appears related to the intensity and duration of immunosuppression rather than to the use of specific agents. Because of the danger of oversuppression of the immune system resulting in increased risk of infection or malignancy, a treatment regimen containing multiple immunosuppressants should be used with caution.

There have been reports of convulsions in adult and pediatric patients receiving cyclosporine, particularly in combination with high dose methylprednisolone.

Encephalopathy has been described both in postmarketing reports and in the literature. Manifestations include impaired consciousness, convulsions, visual disturbances (including blindness), loss of motor function, movement disorders and psychiatric disturbances. In many cases, changes in the white matter have been detected using imaging techniques and pathologic specimens. Predisposing factors such as hypertension, hypomagnesemia, hypocholesterolemia, high-dose corticosteroids, high cyclosporine blood concentrations, and graft-versus-host disease have been noted in many but not all of the reported cases. The changes in most cases have been reversible upon discontinuation of cyclosporine, and in some cases improvement was noted after reduction of dose. It appears that patients receiving liver transplant are more susceptible to encephalopathy than those receiving kidney transplant.

Care should be taken in using cyclosporine with nephrotoxic drugs. *(See PRECAUTIONS)*

Rheumatoid Arthritis: Cyclosporine nephropathy was detected in renal biopsies of 6 out of 60 (10%) rheumatoid arthritis patients after the average treatment duration of 19 months. Only one patient, out of these 6 patients, was treated with a dose ≤4 mg/kg/day. Serum creatinine improved in all but one patient after discontinuation of cyclosporine. The "maximal creatinine increase" appears to be a factor in predicting cyclosporine nephropathy.

There is a potential, as with other immunosuppressive agents, for an increase in the occurrence of malignant lymphomas with cyclosporine. It is not clear whether the risk with cyclosporine is greater than that in rheumatoid arthritis patients or in rheumatoid arthritis patients on cytotoxic treatment for this indication. Five cases of lymphoma were detected: four in a survey of approximately 2,300 patients treated with cyclosporine for rheumatoid arthritis, and another case of lymphoma was reported in a clinical trial. Although other tumors (12 skin cancers, 24 solid tumors of diverse types, and 1 multiple myeloma) were also reported in this survey, epidemiologic analyses did not support a relationship to cyclosporine other than for malignant lymphomas.

Patients should be thoroughly evaluated before and during Neoral® treatment for the development of malignancies. Moreover, use of Neoral® therapy with other immunosuppressive agents may induce an excessive immunosuppression which is known to increase the risk of malignancy.

Psoriasis: *(See also Boxed WARNINGS for Psoriasis)* Since cyclosporine is a potent immunosuppressive agent with a number of potentially serious side effects, the risks and benefits of using Neoral® should be considered before treatment of patients with psoriasis. Cyclosporine, the active ingredient in Neoral®, can cause nephrotoxicity and hypertension *(see PRECAUTIONS)* and the risk increases with increasing dose and duration of therapy. Patients who may be at increased risk such as those with abnormal renal function, uncontrolled hypertension or malignancies, should not receive Neoral®.

Renal dysfunction is a potential consequence of Neoral® therefore renal function must be monitored during therapy. Patients receiving Neoral® require frequent monitoring of serum creatinine. *(See Special Monitoring under DOSAGE AND ADMINISTRATION)* Elderly patients should be monitored with particular care, since decreases in renal function also occur with age. If patients are not properly monitored and doses are not properly adjusted, cyclosporine therapy can cause structural kidney damage and persistent renal dysfunction.

An increase in serum creatinine and BUN may occur during Neoral® therapy and reflects a reduction in the glomerular filtration rate.

Kidney biopsies from 86 psoriasis patients treated for a mean duration of 23 months with 1.2–7.6 mg/kg/day of cyclosporine showed evidence of cyclosporine nephropathy in 18/86 (21%) of the patients. The pathology consisted of renal tubular atrophy and interstitial fibrosis. On repeat biopsy of 13 of these patients maintained on various dosages of cyclosporine for a mean of 2 additional years, the number with cyclosporine induced nephropathy rose to 26/86 (30%). The majority of patients (19/26) were on a dose of ≥5.0 mg/kg/day (the highest recommended dose is 4 mg/kg/day). The patients were also on cyclosporine for greater than 15 months (18/26) and/or had a clinically significant increase in serum creatinine for greater than 1 month (21/26). Creatinine levels returned to normal range in 7 of 11 patients in whom cyclosporine therapy was discontinued.

There is an increased risk for the development of skin and lymphoproliferative malignancies in cyclosporine-treated psoriasis patients. The relative risk of malignancies is comparable to that observed in psoriasis patients treated with other immunosuppressive agents.

Tumors were reported in 32 (2.2%) of 1439 psoriasis patients treated with cyclosporine worldwide from clinical trials. Additional tumors have been reported in 7 patients in cyclosporine postmarketing experience. Skin malignancies were reported in 16 (1.1%) of these patients; all but 2 of them had previously received PUVA therapy. Methotrexate was received by 7 patients. UVB and coal tar had been used by 2 and 3 patients, respectively. Seven patients had either a history of previous skin cancer or a potentially predisposing lesion was present prior to cyclosporine exposure. Of the 16 patients with skin cancer, 11 patients had 18 squamous cell carcinomas and 7 patients had 10 basal cell carcinomas. There were two lymphoproliferative malignancies; one case of non-Hodgkin's lymphoma which required chemotherapy, and one case of mycosis fungoides which regressed spontaneously upon discontinuation of cyclosporine. There were four cases of benign lymphocytic infiltration: 3 regressed spontaneously upon discontinuation of cyclosporine, while the fourth regressed despite continuation of the drug. The remainder of the malignancies, 13 cases (0.9%), involved various organs.

Patients should not be treated concurrently with cyclosporine and PUVA or UVB, other radiation therapy, or other immunosuppressive agents, because of the possibility of excessive immunosuppression and the subsequent risk of malignancies. *(See CONTRAINDICATIONS)* Patients should also be warned to protect themselves appropriately when in the sun, and to avoid excessive sun exposure. Patients should be thoroughly evaluated before and during treatment for the presence of malignancies remembering that malignant lesions may be hidden by psoriatic plaques. Skin lesions not typical of psoriasis should be biopsied before starting treatment. Patients should be treated with Neoral® only after complete resolution of suspicious lesions, and only if there are no other treatment options. *(See Special Monitoring for Psoriasis Patients)*

PRECAUTIONS

General: ***Hypertension:*** Cyclosporine is the active ingredient of Neoral®. Hypertension is a common side effect of cyclosporine therapy which may persist. *(See ADVERSE REACTIONS and DOSAGE AND ADMINISTRATION for monitoring recommendations)* Mild or moderate hypertension is encountered more frequently than severe hypertension and the incidence decreases over time. In recipients of kidney, liver, and heart allografts treated with cyclosporine, antihypertensive therapy may be required. *(See Special Monitoring of Rheumatoid Arthritis and Psoriasis Patients)* However, since cyclosporine may cause hyperkalemia, potassium-sparing diuretics should not be used. While calcium antagonists can be effective agents in treating cyclosporine-associated hypertension, they can interfere with cyclosporine metabolism. *(See Drug Interactions)*

Vaccination: During treatment with cyclosporine, vaccination may be less effective; and the use of live attenuated vaccines should be avoided.

Special Monitoring of Rheumatoid Arthritis Patients: Before initiating treatment, a careful physical examination, including blood pressure measurements (on at least two occasions) and two creatinine levels to estimate baseline

Nephrotoxicity vs. Rejection

Parameter	Nephrotoxicity	Rejection
History	Donor >50 years old or hypotensive Prolonged kidney preservation Prolonged anastomosis time Concomitant nephrotoxic drugs	Anti-donor immune response Retransplant patient
Clinical	Often >6 weeks postop[b] Prolonged initial nonfunction (acute tubular necrosis)	Often <4 weeks postop[b] Fever >37.5°C Weight gain >0.5 kg Graft swelling and tenderness Decrease in daily urine volume >500 mL (or 50%)
Laboratory	CyA serum trough level >200 ng/mL Gradual rise in Cr (<0.15 mg/dl/day)[a] Cr plateau <25% above baseline BUN/Cr ≥20	CyA serum trough level <150 ng/mL Rapid rise in Cr (>0.3 mg/dl/day)[a] Cr >25% above baseline BUN/Cr <20
Biopsy	Arteriolopathy (medial hypertrophy[a], hyalinosis, nodular deposits, intimal thickening, endothelial vacuolization, progressive scarring) Tubular atrophy, isometric vacuolization, isolated calcifications Minimal edema Mild focal infiltrates[c] Diffuse interstitial fibrosis, often striped form	Endovasculitis[c] (proliferation[a], intimal arteritis[b], necrosis, sclerosis) Tubulitis with RBC[b] and WBC[b] casts, some irregular vacuolization Interstitial edema[c] and hemorrhage[b] Diffuse moderate to severe mononuclear infiltrates[d] Glomerulitis (mononuclear cells)[c]
Aspiration Cytology	CyA deposits in tubular and endothelial cells Fine isometric vacuolization of tubular cells	Inflammatory infiltrate with mononuclear phagocytes, macrophages, lymphoblastoid cells, and activated T-cells These strongly express HLA-DR antigens
Urine Cytology	Tubular cells with vacuolization and granularization	Degenerative tubular cells, plasma cells, and lymphocyturia >20% of sediment
Manometry	Intracapsular pressure <40 mm Hg[b]	Intracapsular pressure >40 mm Hg[b]
Ultrasonography	Unchanged graft cross sectional area	Increase in graft cross sectional area AP diameter ≥ Transverse diameter
Magnetic Resonance Imagery	Normal appearance	Loss of distinct corticomedullary junction, swelling image intensity of parachyma approaching that of psoas, loss of hilar fat
Radionuclide Scan	Normal or generally decreased perfusion Decrease in tubular function (^{131}I-hippuran) > decrease in perfusion (^{99m}Tc DTPA)	Patchy arterial flow Decrease in perfusion > decrease in tubular function Increased uptake of Indium 111 labeled platelets or Tc-99m in colloid
Therapy	Responds to decreased cyclosporine	Responds to increased steroids or antilymphocyte globulin

[a]$p < 0.05$, [b]$p < 0.01$, [c]$p < 0.001$, [d]$p < 0.0001$

should be performed. Blood pressure and serum creatinine should be evaluated every 2 weeks during the initial 3 months and then monthly if the patient is stable. It is advisable to monitor serum creatinine and blood pressure always after an increase of the dose of nonsteroidal anti-inflammatory drugs and after initiation of new nonsteroidal anti-inflammatory drug therapy during Neoral® treatment. If co-administered with methotrexate, CBC and liver function tests are recommended to be monitored monthly. *(See also Precautions, General, Hypertension)*

In patients who are receiving cyclosporine, the dose of Neoral® should be decreased by 25%–50% if hypertension occurs. If hypertension persists, the dose of Neoral® should be further reduced or blood pressure should be controlled with antihypertensive agents. In most cases, blood pressure has returned to baseline when cyclosporine was discontinued.

In placebo-controlled trials of rheumatoid arthritis patients, systolic hypertension (defined as an occurrence of two systolic blood pressure readings >140 mmHg) and diastolic hypertension (defined as two diastolic blood pressure readings >90 mmHg) occurred in 33% and 19% of patients treated with cyclosporine, respectively. The corresponding placebo rates were 22% and 8%.

Special Monitoring for Psoriasis Patients: Before initiating treatment, a careful dermatological and physical examination, including blood pressure measurements (on at least two occasions) should be performed. Since Neoral® is an immunosuppressive agent, patients should be evaluated for the presence of occult infection on their first physical examination and for the presence of tumors initially, and throughout treatment with Neoral®. Skin lesions not typical for psoriasis should be biopsied before starting Neoral®. Patients with malignant or premalignant changes of the skin should be treated with Neoral® only after appropriate treatment of such lesions and if no other treatment option exists.

Baseline laboratories should include serum creatinine (on two occasions), BUN, CBC, serum magnesium, potassium, uric acid, and lipids.

The risk of cyclosporine nephropathy is reduced when the starting dose is low (2.5 mg/kg/day), the maximum dose does not exceed 4.0 mg/kg/day, serum creatinine is monitored regularly while cyclosporine is administered, and the dose of Neoral® is decreased when the rise in creatinine is greater than or equal to 25% above the patient's pretreatment level. The increase in creatinine is generally reversible upon timely decrease of the dose of Neoral® or its discontinuation.

Serum creatinine and BUN should be evaluated every 2 weeks during the initial 3 months of therapy and then monthly if the patient is stable. If the serum creatinine is greater than or equal to 25% above the patient's pretreatment level, serum creatinine should be repeated within two weeks. If the change in serum creatinine remains greater than or equal to 25% above baseline, Neoral® should be reduced by 25%–50%. If at **any time** the serum creatinine increases by greater than or equal to 50% above pretreatment level, Neoral® should be reduced by 25%–50%. Neoral® should be discontinued if reversibility (within 25% of baseline) of serum creatinine is not achievable after two dosage modifications. It is advisable to monitor serum creatinine after an increase of the dose of nonsteroidal anti-inflammatory drug and after initiation of new nonsteroidal anti-inflammatory therapy during Neoral® treatment.

Blood pressure should be evaluated every 2 weeks during the initial 3 months of therapy and then monthly if the patient is stable, or more frequently when dosage adjustments are made. Patients without a history of previous hypertension before initiation of treatment with Neoral®, should have the drug reduced by 25%–50% if found to have sustained hypertension. If the patient continues to be hypertensive despite multiple reductions of Neoral®, then Neoral® should be discontinued. For patients with treated hypertension, before the initiation of Neoral® therapy, their medication should be adjusted to control hypertension while on Neoral®. Neoral® should be discontinued if a change in hypertension management is not effective or tolerable.

CBC, uric acid, potassium, lipids, and magnesium should also be monitored every 2 weeks for the first 3 months of therapy, and then monthly if the patient is stable or more frequently when dosage adjustments are made. Neoral® dosage should be reduced by 25%–50% for any abnormality of clinical concern.

In controlled trials of cyclosporine in psoriasis patients, cyclosporine blood concentrations did not correlate well with either improvement or with side effects such as renal dysfunction.

Information for Patients: Patients should be advised that any change of cyclosporine formulation should be made cautiously and only under physician supervision because it may result in the need for a change in dosage.

Patients should be informed of the necessity of repeated laboratory tests while they are receiving cyclosporine. Patients should be advised of the potential risks during pregnancy and informed of the increased risk of neoplasia. Patients should also be informed of the risk of hypertension and renal dysfunction.

Patients should be advised that during treatment with cyclosporine, vaccination may be less effective and the use of live attenuated vaccines should be avoided.

Patients should be given careful dosage instructions. Neoral® Oral Solution (cyclosporine oral solution, USP) MODIFIED should be diluted, preferably with orange or apple juice that is at room temperature. The combination of Neoral® Oral Solution (cyclosporine oral solution, USP) MODIFIED with milk can be unpalatable.

Continued on next page

Neoral—Cont.

Patients should be advised to take Neoral® on a consistent schedule with regard to time of day and relation to meals. Grapefruit and grapefruit juice affect metabolism, increasing blood concentration of cyclosporine, thus should be avoided.

Laboratory Tests: In all patients treated with cyclosporine, renal and liver functions should be assessed repeatedly by measurement of serum creatinine, BUN, serum bilirubin, and liver enzymes. Serum lipids, magnesium, and potassium should also be monitored. Cyclosporine blood concentrations should be routinely monitored in transplant patients *(see DOSAGE AND ADMINISTRATION, Blood Concentration Monitoring in Transplant Patients)*, and periodically monitored in rheumatoid arthritis patients.

Drug Interactions: All of the individual drugs cited below are well substantiated to interact with cyclosporine. In addition, concomitant non-steroidal anti-inflammatory drugs, particularly in the setting of dehydration, may potentiate renal dysfunction.

[See first table at right]

Drugs That Alter Cyclosporine Concentrations: Compounds that decrease cyclosporine absorption such as orlistat should be avoided. Cyclosporine is extensively metabolized by cytochrome P-450 3A. Substances that inhibit this enzyme could decrease metabolism and increase cyclosporine concentrations. Substances that are inducers of cytochrome P-450 activity could increase metabolism and decrease cyclosporine concentrations. Monitoring of circulating cyclosporine concentrations and appropriate Neoral® dosage adjustment are essential when these drugs are used concomitantly. *(See Blood Concentration Monitoring)*

[See second table at right]

The HIV protease inhibitors (e.g., indinavir, nelfinavir, ritonavir, and saquinavir) are known to inhibit cytochrome P-450 3A and thus could potentially increase the concentrations of cyclosporine, however no formal studies of the interaction are available. Care should be exercised when these drugs are administered concomitantly.

Grapefruit and grapefruit juice affect metabolism, increasing blood concentrations of cyclosporine, thus should be avoided.

Drugs/Dietary Supplements That Decrease Cyclosporine Concentrations

Antibiotics	*Anticonvulsants*	*Other Drugs/ Dietary Supplements*
nafcillin	carbamazepine	octreotide
rifampin	phenobarbital	ticlopidine
	phenytoin	orlistat
		St. John's Wort

There have been reports of a serious drug interaction between cyclosporine and the herbal dietary supplement, St. John's Wort. This interaction has been reported to produce a marked reduction in the blood concentrations of cyclosporine, resulting in subtherapeutic levels, rejection of transplanted organs, and graft loss.

Rifabutin is known to increase the metabolism of other drugs metabolized by the cytochrome P-450 system. The interaction between rifabutin and cyclosporine has not been studied. Care should be exercised when these two drugs are administered concomitantly.

Nonsteroidal Anti-inflammatory Drug (NSAID) Interactions: Clinical status and serum creatinine should be closely monitored when cyclosporine is used with nonsteroidal anti-inflammatory agents in rheumatoid arthritis patients. *(See WARNINGS)*

Pharmacodynamic interactions have been reported to occur between cyclosporine and both naproxen and sulindac, in that concomitant use is associated with additive decreases in renal function, as determined by ^{99m}Tc-diethylenetriaminepentaacetic acid (DTPA) and (*p*-aminohippuric acid) PAH clearances. Although concomitant administration of diclofenac does not affect blood levels of cyclosporine, it has been associated with approximate doubling of diclofenac blood levels and occasional reports of reversible decreases in renal function. Consequently, the dose of diclofenac should be in the lower end of the therapeutic range.

Methotrexate Interaction: Preliminary data indicate that when methotrexate and cyclosporine were co-administered to rheumatoid arthritis patients (N=20), methotrexate concentrations (AUCs) were increased approximately 30% and the concentrations (AUCs) of its metabolite, 7-hydroxy methotrexate, were decreased by approximately 80%. The clinical significance of this interaction is not known. Cyclosporine concentrations do not appear to have been altered (N=6).

Other Drug Interactions: Cyclosporine may reduce the clearance of digoxin, colchicine, prednisolone and HMG-CoA inhibitors (statins). Severe digitalis toxicity has been seen within days of starting cyclosporine in several patients taking digoxin. There are also reports on the potential of cyclosporine to enhance the toxic effects of colchicine such as myopathy and neuropathy, especially patients with renal dysfunction. If digoxin or colchicine are used concurrently with cyclosporine, close clinical observation is required in order to enable early detection of toxic manifestations of digoxin or colchicine, followed by reduction of dosage or its withdrawal.

Literature and postmarketing cases of myotoxicity, including muscle pain and weakness, myositis, and rhabdomyolysis, have been reported with concomitant administration of cyclosporine with lovastatin, simvastatin, atorvastatin, pravastatin and, rarely, fluvastatin. When concurrently administered with cyclosporine, the dosage of these statins should be reduced according to label recommendations. Statin therapy needs to be temporarily withheld or discontinued in patients with signs and symptoms myopathy or those with risk factors predisposing to severe renal injury, including renal failure, secondary to rhabdomyolysis.

Cyclosporine should not be used with potassium-sparing diuretics because hyperkalemia can occur.

During treatment with cyclosporine, vaccination may be less effective. The use of live vaccines should be avoided. Frequent gingival hyperplasia with nifedipine, and convulsions with high dose methylprednisolone have been reported.

Psoriasis patients receiving other immunosuppressive agents or radiation therapy (including PUVA and UVB) should not receive concurrent cyclosporine because of the possibility of excessive immunosuppression.

For additional information on Cyclosporine Drug Interactions please contact Novartis Medical Affairs Department at 888-NOW-NOVA [888-669-6682].

Carcinogenesis, Mutagenesis, and Impairment of Fertility: Carcinogenicity studies were carried out in male and female rats and mice. In the 78-week mouse study, evidence of a statistically significant trend was found for lymphomas in females, and the incidence of hepatocellular carcinomas in mid-dose males significantly exceeded the control value. In the 24-month rat study, pancreatic islet cell adenomas significantly exceeded the control rate in the low dose level. Doses used in the mouse and rat studies were 0.01 to 0.16 times the clinical maintenance dose (6 mg/kg). The hepatocellular carcinomas and pancreatic islet cell adenomas were not dose related. Published reports indicate that cotreatment of hairless mice with UV irradiation and cyclosporine or other immunosuppressive agents shorten the time to skin tumor formation compared to UV irradiation alone.

Cyclosporine was not mutagenic in appropriate test systems. Cyclosporine has not been found to be mutagenic/genotoxic in the Ames Test, the V79-HGPRT Test, the micronucleus test in mice and Chinese hamsters, the chromosome-aberration tests in Chinese hamster bone marrow, the mouse dominant lethal assay, and the DNA-repair test in sperm from treated mice. A recent study analyzing sister chromatid exchange (SCE) induction by cyclosporine using human lymphocytes *in vitro* gave indication of a positive effect (i.e., induction of SCE), at high concentrations in this system.

No impairment in fertility was demonstrated in studies in male and female rats.

Widely distributed papillomatosis of the skin was observed after chronic treatment of dogs with cyclosporine at 9 times the human initial psoriasis treatment dose of 2.5 mg/kg, where doses are expressed on a body surface area basis. This papillomatosis showed a spontaneous regression upon discontinuation of cyclosporine.

An increased incidence of malignancy is a recognized complication of immunosuppression in recipients of organ transplants and patients with rheumatoid arthritis and psoriasis. The most common forms of neoplasms are non-Hodgkin's lymphoma and carcinomas of the skin. The risk of malignancies in cyclosporine recipients is higher than in the normal, healthy population but similar to that in patients receiving other immunosuppressive therapies. Reduction or discontinuance of immunosuppression may cause the lesions to regress.

In psoriasis patients on cyclosporine, development of malignancies, especially those of the skin has been reported. *(See WARNINGS)* Skin lesions not typical for psoriasis should be biopsied before starting cyclosporine treatment. Patients with malignant or premalignant changes of the skin should be treated with cyclosporine only after appropriate treatment of such lesions and if no other treatment option exists.

Pregnancy: ***Pregnancy Category C.*** Cyclosporine was not teratogenic in appropriate test systems. Only at dose levels toxic to dams, were adverse effects seen in reproduction studies in rats. Cyclosporine has been shown to be embryo- and fetotoxic in rats and rabbits following oral administration at maternally toxic doses. Fetal toxicity was noted in rats at 0.8 and rabbits at 5.4 times the transplant doses in

Drugs That May Potentiate Renal Dysfunction

Antibiotics	*Antineoplastics*	*Anti-inflammatory Drugs*	*Gastrointestinal Agents*
gentamycin	melphalan	azapropazon	cimetidine
tobramycin		diclofenac	ranitidine
vancomycin	*Antifungals*	naproxen	*Immunosuppressives*
trimethoprim with sulfamethoxazole	amphotericin B	sulindac	tacrolimus
	ketoconazole	colchicine	

Drugs That Increase Cyclosporine Concentrations

Calcium Channel Blockers	*Antifungals*	*Antibiotics*	*Glucocorticoids*	*Other Drugs*	
diltiazem	fluconazole	clarithromycin	methylprednisolone	allopurinol	metoclopramide
nicardipine	itraconazole	erythromycin		bromocriptine	colchicine
verapamil	ketoconazole	quinupristin/ dalfopristin		danazol	amiodarone

		Randomized Kidney Patients		Cyclosporine Patients (Sandimmune®)		
Body System	**Adverse Reactions**	**Sandimmune® (N=227) %**	**Azathioprine (N=228) %**	**Kidney (N=705) %**	**Heart (N=112) %**	**Liver (N=75) %**
Genitourinary	Renal Dysfunction	32	6	25	38	37
Cardiovascular	Hyertension	26	18	13	53	27
	Cramps	4	<1	2	<1	0
Skin	Hirsutism	21	<1	21	28	45
	Acne	6	8	2	2	1
Central Nervous System	Tremor	12	0	21	31	55
	Convulsions	3	1	1	4	5
	Headache	2	<1	2	15	4
Gastrointestinal	Gum Hyperplasia	4	0	9	5	16
	Diarrhea	3	<1	3	4	8
	Nausea/Vomiting	2	<1	4	10	4
	Hepatotoxicity	<1	<1	4	7	4
	Abdominal Discomfort	<1	0	<1	7	0
Autonomic Nervous System	Paresthesia	3	0	1	2	1
	Flushing	<1	0	4	0	4
Hematopoietic	Leukopenia	2	19	<1	6	0
	Lymphoma	<1	0	1	6	1
Respiratory	Sinusitis	<1	0	4	3	7
Miscellaneous	Gynecomastia	<1	0	<1	4	3

Infectious Complications in Historical Randomized Studies in Renal Transplant Patients Using Sandimmune®

Complication	**Cyclosporine Treatment (N=227) % of Complications**	**Azathioprine with Steroids* (N=228) % of Complications**
Septicemia	5.3	4.8
Abscesses	4.4	5.3
Systemic Fungal Infection	2.2	3.9
Local Fungal Infection	7.5	9.6
Cytomegalovirus	4.8	12.3
Other Viral Infections	15.9	18.4
Urinary Tract Infections	21.1	20.2
Wound and Skin Infections	7.0	10.1
Pneumonia	6.2	9.2

*Some patients also received ALG.

humans of 6.0 mg/kg, where dose corrections are based on body surface area. Cyclosporine was embryo- and fetotoxic as indicated by increased pre- and post-natal mortality and reduced fetal weight together with related skeletal retardation.

There are no adequate and well-controlled studies in pregnant women. Neoral® should be used during pregnancy only if the potential benefit justifies the potential risk to the fetus.

The following data represent the reported outcomes of 116 pregnancies in women receiving cyclosporine during pregnancy, 90% of whom were transplant patients, and most of whom received cyclosporine throughout the entire gestational period. The only consistent patterns of abnormality were premature birth (gestational period of 28 to 36 weeks) and low birth weight for gestational age. Sixteen fetal losses occurred. Most of the pregnancies (85 of 100) were complicated by disorders; including, pre-eclampsia, eclampsia, premature labor, abruptio placentae, oligohydramnios, Rh incompatibility, and fetoplacental dysfunction. Pre-term delivery occurred in 47%. Seven malformations were reported in 5 viable infants and in 2 cases of fetal loss. Twenty-eight percent of the infants were small for gestational age. Neonatal complications occurred in 27%. Therefore, the risks and benefits of using Neoral® during pregnancy should be carefully weighed.

Because of the possible disruption of maternal-fetal interaction, the risk/benefit ratio of using Neoral® in psoriasis patients during pregnancy should carefully be weighed with serious consideration for discontinuation of Neoral®.

Nursing Mothers: Since cyclosporine is excreted in human milk, breast-feeding should be avoided.

Pediatric Use: Although no adequate and well-controlled studies have been completed in children, transplant recipients as young as one year of age have received Neoral® with no unusual adverse effects. The safety and efficacy of Neoral® treatment in children with juvenile rheumatoid arthritis or psoriasis below the age of 18 have not been established.

Geriatric Use: In rheumatoid arthritis clinical trials with cyclosporine, 17.5% of patients were age 65 or older. These patients were more likely to develop systolic hypertension on therapy, and more likely to show serum creatinine rises ≥50% above the baseline after 3–4 months of therapy.

Clinical studies of Neoral® in transplant and psoriasis patients did not include a sufficient number of subjects aged 65 and over to determine whether they respond differently from younger subjects. Other reported clinical experiences have not identified differences in response between the elderly and younger patients. In general, dose selection for an elderly patient should be cautious, usually starting at the low end of the dosing range, reflecting the greater frequency of decreased hepatic, renal, or cardiac function, and of concomitant disease or other drug therapy.

ADVERSE REACTIONS

Kidney, Liver, and Heart Transplantation: The principal adverse reactions of cyclosporine therapy are renal dysfunction, tremor, hirsutism, hypertension, and gum hyperplasia.

Hypertension, which is usually mild to moderate, may occur in approximately 50% of patients following renal transplantation and in most cardiac transplant patients.

Glomerular capillary thrombosis has been found in patients treated with cyclosporine and may progress to graft failure. The pathologic changes resembled those seen in the hemolytic-uremic syndrome and included thrombosis of the renal microvasculature, with platelet-fibrin thrombi occluding glomerular capillaries and afferent arterioles, microangiopathic hemolytic anemia, thrombocytopenia, and decreased renal function. Similar findings have been observed when other immunosuppressives have been employed post-transplantation.

Hypomagnesemia has been reported in some, but not all, patients exhibiting convulsions while on cyclosporine therapy. Although magnesium-depletion studies in normal subjects suggest that hypomagnesemia is associated with neurologic disorders, multiple factors, including hypertension, high dose methylprednisolone, hypocholesterolemia, and nephrotoxicity associated with high plasma concentrations of cyclosporine appear to be related to the neurological manifestations of cyclosporine toxicity.

In controlled studies, the nature, severity, and incidence of the adverse events that were observed in 493 transplanted patients treated with Neoral® were comparable with those observed in 208 transplanted patients who received Sandimmune® in these same studies when the dosage of the two drugs was adjusted to achieve the same cyclosporine blood trough concentrations.

Based on the historical experience with Sandimmune®, the following reactions occurred in 3% or greater of 892 patients involved in clinical trials of kidney, heart, and liver transplants.

[See third table on previous page]

Among 705 kidney transplant patients treated with cyclosporine oral solution (Sandimmune®) in clinical trials, the reason for treatment discontinuation was renal toxicity in 5.4%, infection in 0.9%, lack of efficacy in 1.4%, acute tubular necrosis in 1.0%, lymphoproliferative disorders in 0.3%, hypertension in 0.3%, and other reasons in 0.7% of the patients.

The following reactions occurred in 2% or less of Sandimmune®-treated patients: allergic reactions, anemia, anorexia, confusion, conjunctivitis, edema, fever, brittle fingernails, gastritis, hearing loss, hiccups, hyperglycemia, muscle pain, peptic ulcer, thrombocytopenia, tinnitus.

Neoral®/Sandimmune® Rheumatoid Arthritis
Percentage of Patients with Adverse Events ≥3% in any Cyclosporine Treated Group

Body System	Preferred Term	Studies 651+652+2008 Sandimmune®† (N=269)	Study 302 Sandimmune® (N=155)	Study 654 Methotrexate & Sandimmune® (N=74)	Study 654 Methotrexate & Placebo (N=73)	Study 302 Neoral® (N=143)	Studies 651+652+2008 Placebo (N=201)
Autonomic Nervous System Disorders							
	Flushing	2%	2%	3%	0%	5%	2%
Body As A Whole—General Disorders							
	Accidental Trauma	0%	1%	10%	4%	4%	0%
	Edema NOS*	5%	14%	12%	4%	10%	<1%
	Fatigue	6%	3%	8%	12%	3%	7%
	Fever	2%	3%	0%	0%	2%	4%
	Influenza-like symptoms	<1%	6%	1%	0%	3%	2%
	Pain	6%	9%	10%	15%	13%	4%
	Rigors	1%	1%	4%	0%	3%	1%
Cardiovascular Disorders							
	Arrhythmia	2%	5%	5%	6%	2%	1%
	Chest Pain	4%	5%	1%	1%	6%	1%
	Hypertension	8%	26%	16%	12%	25%	2%
Central and Peripheral Nervous System Disorders							
	Dizziness	8%	6%	7%	3%	8%	3%
	Headache	17%	23%	22%	11%	25%	9%
	Migraine	2%	3%	0%	0%	3%	1%
	Paresthesia	8%	7%	8%	4%	11%	1%
	Tremor	8%	7%	7%	3%	13%	4%
Gastrointestinal System Disorders							
	Abdominal Pain	15%	15%	15%	7%	15%	10%
	Anorexia	3%	3%	1%	0%	3%	3%
	Diarrhea	12%	12%	18%	15%	13%	8%
	Dyspepsia	12%	12%	10%	8%	8%	4%
	Flatulence	5%	5%	5%	4%	4%	1%
	Gastrointestinal Disorder NOS*	0%	2%	1%	4%	4%	0%
	Gingivitis	4%	3%	0%	0%	0%	1%
	Gum Hyperplasia	2%	4%	1%	3%	4%	1%
	Nausea	23%	14%	24%	15%	18%	14%
	Rectal Hemorrhage	0%	3%	0%	0%	1%	1%
	Stomatitis	7%	5%	16%	12%	6%	8%
	Vomiting	9%	8%	14%	7%	6%	5%
Hearing and Vestibular Disorders							
	Ear Disorder NOS*	0%	5%	0%	0%	1%	0%
Metabolic and Nutritional Disorders							
	Hypomagnesemia	0%	4%	0%	0%	6%	0%
Musculoskeletal System Disorders							
	Arthropathy	0%	5%	0%	1%	4%	0%
	Leg Cramps/Involuntary Muscle Contractions	2%	11%	11%	3%	12%	1%
Psychiatric Disorders							
	Depression	3%	6%	3%	1%	1%	2%
	Insomnia	4%	1%	1%	0%	3%	2%
Renal							
	Creatinine elevations ≥30%	43%	39%	55%	19%	48%	13%
	Creatinine elevations ≥50%	24%	18%	26%	8%	18%	3%
Reproductive Disorders, Female							
	Leukorrhea	1%	0%	4%	0%	1%	0%
	Menstrual Disorder	3%	2%	1%	0%	1%	1%
Respiratory System Disorders							
	Bronchitis	1%	3%	1%	0%	1%	3%
	Coughing	5%	3%	5%	7%	4%	4%
	Dyspnea	5%	1%	3%	3%	1%	2%
	Infection NOS*	9%	5%	0%	7%	3%	10%
	Pharyngitis	3%	5%	5%	6%	4%	4%
	Pneumonia	1%	0%	4%	0%	1%	1%
	Rhinitis	0%	3%	11%	10%	1%	0%
	Sinusitis	4%	4%	8%	4%	3%	3%
	Upper Respiratory Tract	0%	14%	23%	15%	13%	0%
Skin and Appendages Disorders							
	Alopecia	3%	0%	1%	1%	4%	4%
	Bullous Eruption	1%	0%	4%	1%	1%	1%
	Hypertrichosis	19%	17%	12%	0%	15%	3%
	Rash	7%	12%	10%	7%	8%	10%
	Skin Ulceration	1%	1%	3%	4%	0%	2%
Urinary System Disorders							
	Dysuria	0%	0%	11%	3%	1%	2%
	Micturition Frequency	2%	4%	3%	1%	2%	2%
	NPN, Increased	0%	19%	12%	0%	18%	0%
	Urinary Tract Infection	0%	3%	5%	4%	3%	0%
Vascular (Extracardiac) Disorders							
	Purpura	3%	4%	1%	1%	2%	0%

†Includes patients in 2.5 mg/kg/day dose group only. *NOS = Not Otherwise Specified.

The following reactions occurred rarely: anxiety, chest pain, constipation, depression, hair breaking, hematuria, joint pain, lethargy, mouth sores, myocardial infarction, night sweats, pancreatitis, pruritus, swallowing difficulty, tingling, upper GI bleeding, visual disturbance, weakness, weight loss.

[See fourth table on previous page]

Rheumatoid Arthritis: The principal adverse reactions associated with the use of cyclosporine in rheumatoid arthritis are renal dysfunction *(see WARNINGS)*, hypertension *(see PRECAUTIONS)*, headache, gastrointestinal disturbances, and hirsutism/hypertrichosis.

In rheumatoid arthritis patients treated in clinical trials within the recommended dose range, cyclosporine therapy was discontinued in 5.3% of the patients because of hypertension and in 7% of the patients because of increased creatinine. These changes are usually reversible with timely dose decrease or drug discontinuation. The frequency and severity of serum creatinine elevations increase with dose and duration of cyclosporine therapy. These elevations are likely to become more pronounced without dose reduction or discontinuation.

The following adverse events occurred in controlled clinical trials:

[See table above]

Continued on next page

Neoral—Cont.

In addition, the following adverse events have been reported in 1% to <3% of the rheumatoid arthritis patients in the cyclosporine treatment group in controlled clinical trials.

Autonomic Nervous System: dry mouth, increased sweating;
Body as a Whole: allergy, asthenia, hot flushes, malaise, overdose, procedure NOS*, tumor NOS*, weight decrease, weight increase;
Cardiovascular: abnormal heart sounds, cardiac failure, myocardial infarction, peripheral ischemia;
Central and Peripheral Nervous System: hypoesthesia, neuropathy, vertigo;
Endocrine: goiter;
Gastrointestinal: constipation, dysphagia, enanthema, eructation, esophagitis, gastric ulcer, gastritis, gastroenteritis, gingival bleeding, glossitis, peptic ulcer, salivary gland enlargement, tongue disorder, tooth disorder;
Infection: abscess, bacterial infection, cellulitis, folliculitis, fungal infection, herpes simplex, herpes zoster, renal abscess, moniliasis, tonsillitis, viral infection;
Hematologic: anemia, epistaxis, leukopenia, lymphadenopathy;
Liver and Biliary System: bilirubinemia;
Metabolic and Nutritional: diabetes mellitus, hyperkalemia, hyperuricemia, hypoglycemia;
Musculoskeletal System: arthralgia, bone fracture, bursitis, joint dislocation, myalgia, stiffness, synovial cyst, tendon disorder;
Neoplasms: fibroadenosis, carcinoma;
Psychiatric: anxiety, confusion, decreased libido, emotional lability, impaired concentration, increased libido, nervousness, paroniria, somnolence;
Reproductive (Female): breast pain, uterine hemorrhage;
Respiratory System: abnormal chest sounds, bronchospasm;
Skin and Appendages: abnormal pigmentation, angioedema, dermatitis, dry skin, eczema, nail disorder, pruritus, skin disorder, urticaria;
Special Senses: abnormal vision, cataract, conjunctivitis, deafness, eye pain, taste perversion, tinnitus, vestibular disorder;
Urinary System: abnormal urine, hematuria, increased BUN, micturition urgency, nocturia, polyuria, pyelonephritis, urinary incontinence.

*NOS = Not Otherwise Specified.

Psoriasis: The principal adverse reactions associated with the use of cyclosporine in patients with psoriasis are renal dysfunction, headache, hypertension, hypertriglyceridemia, hirsutism/hypertrichosis, paresthesia or hyperesthesia, influenza-like symptoms, nausea/vomiting, diarrhea, abdominal discomfort, lethargy, and musculoskeletal or joint pain.

In psoriasis patients treated in US controlled clinical studies within the recommended dose range, cyclosporine therapy was discontinued in 1.0% of the patients because of hypertension and in 5.4% of the patients because of increased creatinine. In the majority of cases, these changes were reversible after dose reduction or discontinuation of cyclosporine.

There has been one reported death associated with the use of cyclosporine in psoriasis. A 27-year-old male developed renal deterioration and was continued on cyclosporine. He had progressive renal failure leading to death.

Frequency and severity of serum creatinine increases with dose and duration of cyclosporine therapy. These elevations are likely to become more pronounced and may result in irreversible renal damage without dose reduction or discontinuation.

[See table below]

The following events occurred in 1% to less than 3% of psoriasis patients treated with cyclosporine:

Body as a Whole: fever, flushes, hot flushes; ***Cardiovascular:*** chest pain; ***Central and Peripheral Nervous System:*** appetite increased, insomnia, dizziness, nervousness, vertigo; ***Gastrointestinal:*** abdominal distention, constipation, gingival bleeding; ***Liver and Biliary System:*** hyperbilirubinemia; ***Neoplasms:*** skin malignancies [squamous cell (0.9%) and basal cell (0.4%) carcinomas]; ***Reticuloendothelial:*** platelet, bleeding, and clotting disorders, red blood cell disorder; ***Respiratory:*** infection, viral and other infection; ***Skin and Appendages:*** acne, folliculitis, keratosis, pruritus, rash, dry skin; ***Urinary System:*** micturition frequency; ***Vision:*** abnormal vision.

Mild hypomagnesemia and hyperkalemia may occur but are asymptomatic. Increases in uric acid may occur and attacks of gout have been rarely reported. A minor and dose related hyperbilirubinemia has been observed in the absence of hepatocellular damage. Cyclosporine therapy may be associated with a modest increase of serum triglycerides or cholesterol. Elevations of triglycerides (>750 mg/dL) occur in about 15% of psoriasis patients; elevations of cholesterol (>300 mg/dL) are observed in less than 3% of psoriasis patients. Generally these laboratory abnormalities are reversible upon dose reduction or discontinuation of cyclosporine.

OVERDOSAGE

There is a minimal experience with cyclosporine overdosage. Forced emesis can be of value up to 2 hours after administration of Neoral®. Transient hepatotoxicity and nephrotoxicity may occur which should resolve following drug withdrawal. General supportive measures and symptomatic treatment should be followed in all cases of overdosage. Cyclosporine is not dialyzable to any great extent, nor is it cleared well by charcoal hemoperfusion. The oral dosage at which half of experimental animals are estimated to die is 31 times, 39 times, and >54 times the human maintenance dose for transplant patients (6 mg/kg; corrections based on body surface area) in mice, rats, and rabbits.

DOSAGE AND ADMINISTRATION

Neoral® Soft Gelatin Capsules (cyclosporine capsules, USP) MODIFIED and Neoral® Oral Solution (cyclosporine oral solution, USP) MODIFIED

Neoral® has increased bioavailability in comparison to Sandimmune®. Neoral® and Sandimmune® are not bioequivalent and cannot be used interchangeably without physician supervision.

The daily dose of Neoral® should always be given in two divided doses (BID). It is recommended that Neoral® be administered on a consistent schedule with regard to time of day and relation to meals. Grapefruit and grapefruit juice affect metabolism, increasing blood concentration of cyclosporine, thus should be avoided.

Newly Transplanted Patients: The initial oral dose of Neoral® can be given 4–12 hours prior to transplantation or be given postoperatively. The initial dose of Neoral® varies depending on the transplanted organ and the other immunosuppressive agents included in the immunosuppressive protocol. In newly transplanted patients, the initial oral dose of Neoral® is the same as the initial oral dose of Sandimmune®. Suggested initial doses are available from the results of a 1994 survey of the use of Sandimmune® in US transplant centers. The mean ± SD initial doses were 9±3 mg/kg/day for renal transplant patients (75 centers), 8±4 mg/kg/day for liver transplant patients (30 centers), and 7±3 mg/kg/day for heart transplant patients (24 centers). Total daily doses were divided into two equal daily doses. The Neoral® dose is subsequently adjusted to achieve a pre-defined cyclosporine blood concentration. *(See Blood Concentration Monitoring in Transplant Patients, below)* If cyclosporine trough blood concentrations are used, the target range is the same for Neoral® as for Sandimmune®. Using the same trough concentration target range for Neoral® as for Sandimmune® results in greater cyclosporine exposure when Neoral® is administered. *(See Pharmacokinetics, Absorption)* Dosing should be titrated based on clinical assessments of rejection and tolerability. Lower Neoral® doses may be sufficient as maintenance therapy.

Adjunct therapy with adrenal corticosteroids is recommended initially. Different tapering dosage schedules of prednisone appear to achieve similar results. A representative dosage schedule based on the patient's weight started with 2.0 mg/kg/day for the first 4 days tapered to 1.0 mg/kg/day by 1 week, 0.6 mg/kg/day by 2 weeks, 0.3 mg/kg/day by 1 month, and 0.15 mg/kg/day by 2 months and thereafter as a maintenance dose. Steroid doses may be further tapered on an individualized basis depending on status of patient and function of graft. Adjustments in dosage of prednisone must be made according to the clinical situation.

Conversion from Sandimmune® to Neoral® in Transplant Patients: In transplanted patients who are considered for conversion to Neoral® from Sandimmune®, Neoral® should be started with the same daily dose as was previously used with Sandimmune® (1:1 dose conversion). The Neoral® dose should subsequently be adjusted to attain the preconversion cyclosporine blood trough concentration. Using the same trough concentration target range for Neoral® as for Sandimmune® results in greater cyclosporine exposure when Neoral® is administered. *(See Pharmacokinetics, Absorption)* Patients with suspected poor absorption of Sandimmune® require different dosing strategies. *(See Transplant Patients with Poor Absorption of Sandimmune®, below)* In some patients, the increase in blood trough concentration is more pronounced and may be of clinical significance.

Until the blood trough concentration attains the preconversion value, it is strongly recommended that the cyclosporine blood trough concentration be monitored every 4 to 7 days after conversion to Neoral®. In addition, clinical safety parameters such as serum creatinine and blood pressure should be monitored every two weeks during the first two months after conversion. If the blood trough concentrations are outside the desired range and/or if the clinical safety parameters worsen, the dosage of Neoral® must be adjusted accordingly.

Transplant Patients with Poor Absorption of Sandimmune®: Patients with lower than expected cyclosporine blood trough concentrations in relation to the oral dose of Sandimmune® may have poor or inconsistent absorption of cyclosporine from Sandimmune®. After conversion to Neoral®, patients tend to have higher cyclosporine concentrations. **Due to the increase in bioavailability of cyclosporine following conversion to Neoral®, the cyclosporine blood trough concentration may exceed the target range. Particular caution should be exercised when converting patients to Neoral® at doses greater than 10 mg/kg/day.** The dose of Neoral® should be titrated individually based on cyclosporine trough concentrations, tolerability, and clinical response. In this population the cyclosporine blood trough concentration should be measured more frequently, at least twice a week (daily, if initial dose exceeds 10 mg/kg/day) until the concentration stabilizes within the desired range.

Rheumatoid Arthritis: The initial dose of Neoral® is 2.5 mg/kg/day, taken twice daily as a divided (BID) oral dose. Salicylates, nonsteroidal anti-inflammatory agents, and oral corticosteroids may be continued. *(See WARNINGS and PRECAUTIONS, Drug Interactions)* Onset of action generally occurs between 4 and 8 weeks. If insufficient clinical benefit is seen and tolerability is good (including serum creatinine less than 30% above baseline), the dose may be increased by 0.5–0.75 mg/kg/day after 8 weeks and again after 12 weeks to a maximum of 4 mg/kg/day. If no benefit is seen by 16 weeks of therapy, Neoral® therapy should be discontinued.

Dose decreases by 25%–50% should be made at any time to control adverse events, e.g., hypertension elevations in serum creatinine (30% above patient's pretreatment level) or clinically significant laboratory abnormalities. *(See WARNINGS and PRECAUTIONS)*

If dose reduction is not effective in controlling abnormalities or if the adverse event or abnormality is severe, Neoral® should be discontinued. The same initial dose and dosage range should be used if Neoral® is combined with the rec-

Adverse Events Occurring in 3% or More of Psoriasis Patients in Controlled Clinical Trials

Body System*	Preferred Term	Neoral® (N=182)	Sandimmune® (N=185)
Infection or Potential Infection		24.7%	24.3%
	Influenza-like Symptoms	9.9%	8.1%
	Upper Respiratory Tract Infections	7.7%	11.3%
Cardiovascular System		28.0%	25.4%
	Hypertension**	27.5%	25.4%
Urinary System		24.2%	16.2%
	Increased Creatinine	19.8%	15.7%
Central and Peripheral Nervous System		26.4%	20.5%
	Headache	15.9%	14.0%
	Paresthesia	7.1%	4.8%
Musculoskeletal System		13.2%	8.7%
	Arthralgia	6.0%	1.1%
Body As A Whole–General		29.1%	22.2%
	Pain	4.4%	3.2%
Metabolic and Nutritional		9.3%	9.7%
Reproductive, Female		8.5% (4 of 47 females)	11.5% (6 of 52 females)
Resistance Mechanism		18.7%	21.1%
Skin and Appendages		17.6%	15.1%
	Hypertrichosis	6.6%	5.4%
Respiratory System		5.0%	6.5%
	Bronchospasm, coughing, dyspnea, rhinitis	5.0%	4.9%
Psychiatric		5.0%	3.8%
Gastrointestinal System		19.8%	28.7%
	Abdominal pain	2.7%	6.0%
	Diarrhea	5.0%	5.9%
	Dyspepsia	2.2%	3.2%
	Gum hyperplasia	3.8%	6.0%
	Nausea	5.5%	5.9%
White cell and RES		4.4%	2.7%

*Total percentage of events within the system
**Newly occurring hypertension = SBP≥160 mm Hg and/or DBP≥90 mm Hg

ommended dose of methotrexate. Most patients can be treated with Neoral® doses of 3 mg/kg/day or below when combined with methotrexate doses of up to 15 mg/week. *(See CLINICAL PHARMACOLOGY, Clinical Trials)*
There is limited long-term treatment data. Recurrence of rheumatoid arthritis disease activity is generally apparent within 4 weeks after stopping cyclosporine.
Psoriasis: The initial dose of Neoral® should be 2.5 mg/kg/day. Neoral® should be taken twice daily, as a divided (1.25 mg/kg BID) oral dose. Patients should be kept at that dose for at least 4 weeks, barring adverse events. If significant clinical improvement has not occurred in patients by that time, the patient's dosage should be increased at 2-week intervals. Based on patient response, dose increases of approximately 0.5 mg/kg/day should be made to a maximum of 4.0 mg/kg/day.
Dose decreases by 25%–50% should be made at any time to control adverse events, e.g., hypertension, elevations in serum creatinine (≥25% above the patient's pretreatment level), or clinically significant laboratory abnormalities. If dose reduction is not effective in controlling abnormalities, or if the adverse event or abnormality is severe, Neoral® should be discontinued. *(See Special Monitoring of Psoriasis Patients)*
Patients generally show some improvement in the clinical manifestations of psoriasis in 2 weeks. Satisfactory control and stabilization of the disease may take 12–16 weeks to achieve. Results of a dose-titration clinical trial with Neoral® indicate that an improvement of psoriasis by 75% or more (based on PASI) was achieved in 51% of the patients after 8 weeks and in 79% of the patients after 16 weeks. Treatment should be discontinued if satisfactory response cannot be achieved after 6 weeks at 4 mg/kg/day or the patient's maximum tolerated dose. Once a patient is adequately controlled and appears stable the dose of Neoral® should be lowered, and the patient treated with the lowest dose that maintains an adequate response (this should not necessarily be total clearing of the patient). In clinical trials, cyclosporine doses at the lower end of the recommended dosage range were effective in maintaining a satisfactory response in 60% of the patients. Doses below 2.5 mg/kg/day may also be equally effective.
Upon stopping treatment with cyclosporine, relapse will occur in approximately 6 weeks (50% of the patients) to 16 weeks (75% of the patients). In the majority of patients rebound does not occur after cessation of treatment with cyclosporine. Thirteen cases of transformation of chronic plaque psoriasis to more severe forms of psoriasis have been reported. There were 9 cases of pustular and 4 cases of erythrodermic psoriasis. Long term experience with Neoral® in psoriasis patients is limited and continuous treatment for extended periods greater than one year is not recommended. Alternation with other forms of treatment should be considered in the long term management of patients with this life long disease.
Neoral® Oral Solution (cyclosporine oral solution, USP) MODIFIED–Recommendations for Administration:
To make Neoral® Oral Solution (cyclosporine oral solution, USP) MODIFIED more palatable, it should be diluted with orange or apple juice that is at room temperature. Patients should avoid switching diluents frequently. Grapefruit juice affects metabolism of cyclosporine and should be avoided. The combination of Neoral® solution with milk can be unpalatable. The effect of milk on the bioavailability of cyclosorine when adminstered as Neoral® Oral Solution has not been evaluated.
Take the prescribed amount of Neoral® Oral Solution (cyclosporine oral solution, USP) MODIFIED from the container using the dosing syringe supplied, after removal of the protective cover, and transfer the solution to a glass of orange or apple juice. Stir well and drink at once. Do not allow diluted oral solution to stand before drinking. Use a glass container (not plastic). Rinse the glass with more diluent to ensure that the total dose is consumed. After use, dry the outside of the dosing syringe with a clean towel and replace the protective cover. Do not rinse the dosing syringe with water or other cleaning agents. If the syringe requires cleaning, it must be completely dry before resuming use.
Blood Concentration Monitoring in Transplant Patients:
Transplant centers have found blood concentration of cyclosporine to be an essential component of patient management. Of importance to blood concentration analysis are the type of assay used, the transplanted organ, and other immunosuppressant agents being administered. While no fixed relationship has been established, blood concentration monitoring may assist in the clinical evaluation of rejection and toxicity, dose adjustments, and the assessment of compliance.
Various assays have been used to measure blood concentrations of cyclosporine. Older studies using a nonspecific assay often cited concentrations that were roughly twice those of the specific assays. Therefore, comparison between concentrations in the published literature and an individual patient concentration using current assays must be made with detailed knowledge of the assay methods employed. Current assay results are also not interchangeable and their use should be guided by their approved labeling. A discussion of the different assay methods is contained in *Annals of Clinical Biochemistry* 1994;31:420–446. While several assays and assay matrices are available, there is a consensus that parent-compound-specific assays correlate best with clinical events. Of these, HPLC is the standard reference, but the monoclonal antibody RIAs and the monoclonal antibody FPIA offer sensitivity, reproducibility, and convenience. Most clinicians base their monitoring on trough cyclosporine concentrations. *Applied Pharmacokinetics, Principles of Therapeutic Drug Monitoring* (1992) contains a broad discussion of cyclosporine pharmacokinetics and drug monitoring techniques. Blood concentration monitoring is not a replacement for renal function monitoring or tissue biopsies.

HOW SUPPLIED

Neoral® Soft Gelatin Capsules (cyclosporine capsules, USP) MODIFIED
25 mg
Oval, blue-gray imprinted in red, "Neoral" over "25 mg."
Packages of 30 unit-dose blisters (NDC 0078-0246-15).
100 mg
Oblong, blue-gray imprinted in red, "Neoral" over "100 mg."
Packages of 30 unit-dose blisters (NDC 0078-0248-15).
Store and Dispense: In the original unit-dose container at controlled room temperature 68°–77°F (20°–25°C).
Neoral® Oral Solution (cyclosporine oral solution, USP) MODIFIED: A clear, yellow liquid supplied in 50 mL bottles containing 100 mg/mL (NDC 0078-0274-22).
Store and Dispense: In the original container at controlled room temperature 68°–77°F (20°–25°C). Do not store in the refrigerator. Once opened, the contents must be used within two months. At temperatures below 68°F (20°C) the solution may gel; light flocculation or the formation of a light sediment may also occur. There is no impact on product performance or dosing using the syringe provided. Allow to warm to room temperature 77°F (25°C) to reverse these changes.
Neoral® Soft Gelatin Capsules (cyclosporine capsules, USP) MODIFIED
Manufactured by R.P. Scherer GmbH, EBERBACH/BADEN, GERMANY
Manufactured for Novartis Pharmaceuticals Corporation, East Hanover, NJ 07936
Neoral® Oral Solution (cyclosporine oral solution, USP) MODIFIED
Manufactured by Novartis Pharma S.A.S, F-68330 Huningue, France
Manufactured for Novartis Pharmaceuticals Corporation, East Hanover, NJ 07936
Distributed by:
Novartis Pharmaceuticals Corporation
East Hanover, New Jersey 07936
T2004-19
REV: MARCH 2004 PRINTED IN USA 89005007
©Novartis

Shown in Product Identification Guide, page 325

RITALIN® HYDROCHLORIDE Ⓒ℞

[rit ' ah-lin]
(methylphenidate hydrochloride) tablets USP

RITALIN-SR® Ⓒ℞

(methylphenidate hydrochloride) USP sustained-release tablets
Rx only

Prescribing Information
The following prescribing information is based on official labeling in effect July 2003.

DESCRIPTION

Ritalin hydrochloride, methylphenidate hydrochloride USP, is a mild central nervous system (CNS) stimulant, available as tablets of 5, 10, and 20 mg for oral administration; Ritalin-SR is available as sustained-release tablets of 20 mg for oral administration. Methylphenidate hydrochloride is methyl α-phenyl-2-piperidineacetate hydrochloride, and its structural formula is

COOCH3 | CH—CH · HCl | HN

Methylphenidate hydrochloride USP is a white, odorless, fine crystalline powder. Its solutions are acid to litmus. It is freely soluble in water and in methanol, soluble in alcohol, and slightly soluble in chloroform and in acetone. Its molecular weight is 269.77.
Inactive Ingredients. Ritalin tablets: D&C Yellow No. 10 (5-mg and 20-mg tablets), FD&C Green No. 3 (10-mg tablets), lactose, magnesium stearate, polyethylene glycol, starch (5-mg and 10-mg tablets), sucrose, talc, and tragacanth (20-mg tablets).
Ritalin-SR tablets: Cellulose compounds, cetostearyl alcohol, lactose, magnesium stearate, mineral oil, povidone, titanium dioxide, and zein.

CLINICAL PHARMACOLOGY

Ritalin is a mild central nervous system stimulant.
The mode of action in man is not completely understood, but Ritalin presumably activates the brain stem arousal system and cortex to produce its stimulant effect.
There is neither specific evidence which clearly establishes the mechanism whereby Ritalin produces its mental and behavioral effects in children, nor conclusive evidence regarding how these effects relate to the condition of the central nervous system.
Ritalin in the SR tablets is more slowly but as extensively absorbed as in the regular tablets. Relative bioavailability of the SR tablet compared to the Ritalin tablet, measured by the urinary excretion of Ritalin major metabolite (α-phenyl-2-piperidine acetic acid) was 105% (49%-168%) in children and 101% (85%-152%) in adults. The time to peak rate in children was 4.7 hours (1.3-8.2 hours) for the SR tablets and 1.9 hours (0.3-4.4 hours) for the tablets. An average of 67% of SR tablet dose was excreted in children as compared to 86% in adults.
In a clinical study involving adult subjects who received SR tablets, plasma concentrations of Ritalin's major metabolite appeared to be greater in females than in males. No gender differences were observed for Ritalin plasma concentration in the same subjects.

INDICATIONS

Attention Deficit Disorders, Narcolepsy
Attention Deficit Disorders (previously known as Minimal Brain Dysfunction in Children). Other terms being used to describe the behavioral syndrome below include: Hyperkinetic Child Syndrome, Minimal Brain Damage, Minimal Cerebral Dysfunction, Minor Cerebral Dysfunction.
Ritalin is indicated as an integral part of a total treatment program which typically includes other remedial measures (psychological, educational, social) for a stabilizing effect in children with a behavioral syndrome characterized by the following group of developmentally inappropriate symptoms: moderate-to-severe distractibility, short attention span, hyperactivity, emotional lability, and impulsivity. The diagnosis of this syndrome should not be made with finality when these symptoms are only of comparatively recent origin. Nonlocalizing (soft) neurological signs, learning disability, and abnormal EEG may or may not be present, and a diagnosis of central nervous system dysfunction may or may not be warranted.
Special Diagnostic Considerations
Specific etiology of this syndrome is unknown, and there is no single diagnostic test. Adequate diagnosis requires the use not only of medical but of special psychological, educational, and social resources.
Characteristics commonly reported include: chronic history of short attention span, distractibility, emotional lability, impulsivity, and moderate-to-severe hyperactivity; minor neurological signs and abnormal EEG. Learning may or may not be impaired. The diagnosis must be based upon a complete history and evaluation of the child and not solely on the presence of one or more of these characteristics.
Drug treatment is not indicated for all children with this syndrome. Stimulants are not intended for use in the child who exhibits symptoms secondary to environmental factors and/or primary psychiatric disorders, including psychosis. Appropriate educational placement is essential and psychosocial intervention is generally necessary. When remedial measures alone are insufficient, the decision to prescribe stimulant medication will depend upon the physician's assessment of the chronicity and severity of the child's symptoms.

CONTRAINDICATIONS

Marked anxiety, tension, and agitation are contraindications to Ritalin, since the drug may aggravate these symptoms. Ritalin is contraindicated also in patients known to be hypersensitive to the drug, in patients with glaucoma, and in patients with motor tics or with a family history or diagnosis of Tourette's syndrome.
Ritalin is contraindicated during treatment with monoamine oxidase inhibitors, and also within a minimum of 14 days following discontinuation of a monoamine oxidase inhibitor (hypertensive crises may result).

WARNINGS

Ritalin should not be used in children under six years, since safety and efficacy in this age group have not been established.
Sufficient data on safety and efficacy of long-term use of Ritalin in children are not yet available. Although a causal relationship has not been established, suppression of growth (i.e., weight gain, and/or height) has been reported with the long-term use of stimulants in children. Therefore, patients requiring long-term therapy should be carefully monitored.
Ritalin should not be used for severe depression of either exogenous or endogenous origin. Clinical experience suggests that in psychotic children, administration of Ritalin may exacerbate symptoms of behavior disturbance and thought disorder.
Ritalin should not be used for the prevention or treatment of normal fatigue states.
There is some clinical evidence that Ritalin may lower the convulsive threshold in patients with prior history of seizures, with prior EEG abnormalities in absence of seizures, and, very rarely, in absence of history of seizures and no prior EEG evidence of seizures. Safe concomitant use of anticonvulsants and Ritalin has not been established. In the presence of seizures, the drug should be discontinued.
Use cautiously in patients with hypertension. Blood pressure should be monitored at appropriate intervals in all patients taking Ritalin, especially those with hypertension.
Symptoms of visual disturbances have been encountered in rare cases. Difficulties with accommodation and blurring of vision have been reported.
Drug Interactions
Ritalin may decrease the hypotensive effect of guanethidine. Use cautiously with pressor agents.

Continued on next page

Ritalin/Ritalin-SR—Cont.

Human pharmacologic studies have shown that Ritalin may inhibit the metabolism of coumarin anticoagulants, anticonvulsants (phenobarbital, diphenylhydantoin, primidone), phenylbutazone, and tricyclic drugs (imipramine, clomipramine, desipramine). Downward dosage adjustments of these drugs may be required when given concomitantly with Ritalin.

Serious adverse events have been reported in concomitant use with clonidine, although no causality for the combination has been established. The safety of using methylphenidate in combination with clonidine or other centrally acting alpha-2 agonists has not been systematically evaluated.

Usage in Pregnancy

Adequate animal reproduction studies to establish safe use of Ritalin during pregnancy have not been conducted. However, in a recently conducted study, methylphenidate has been shown to have teratogenic effects in rabbits when given in doses of 200 mg/kg/day, which is approximately 167 times and 78 times the maximum recommended human dose on a mg/kg and a mg/m^2 basis, respectively. In rats, teratogenic effects were not seen when the drug was given in doses of 75 mg/kg/day, which is approximately 62.5 and 13.5 times the maximum recommended human dose on a mg/kg and a mg/m^2 basis, respectively. Therefore, until more information is available, Ritalin should not be prescribed for women of childbearing age unless, in the opinion of the physician, the potential benefits outweigh the possible risks.

Drug Dependence

Ritalin should be given cautiously to emotionally unstable patients, such as those with a history of drug dependence or alcoholism, because such patients may increase dosage on their own initiative.

Chronically abusive use can lead to marked tolerance and psychic dependence with varying degrees of abnormal behavior. Frank psychotic episodes can occur, especially with parenteral abuse. Careful supervision is required during drug withdrawal, since severe depression as well as the effects of chronic overactivity can be unmasked. Long-term follow-up may be required because of the patient's basic personality disturbances.

PRECAUTIONS

Patients with an element of agitation may react adversely; discontinue therapy if necessary.

Periodic CBC, differential, and platelet counts are advised during prolonged therapy.

Drug treatment is not indicated in all cases of this behavioral syndrome and should be considered only in light of the complete history and evaluation of the child. The decision to prescribe Ritalin should depend on the physician's assessment of the chronicity and severity of the child's symptoms and their appropriateness for his/her age. Prescription should not depend solely on the presence of one or more of the behavioral characteristics.

When these symptoms are associated with acute stress reactions, treatment with Ritalin is usually not indicated.

Long-term effects of Ritalin in children have not been well established.

Carcinogenesis/Mutagenesis

In a lifetime carcinogenicity study carried out in B6C3F1 mice, methylphenidate caused an increase in hepatocellular adenomas and, in males only, an increase in hepatoblastomas, at a daily dose of approximately 60 mg/kg/day. This dose is approximately 30 times and 2.5 times the maximum recommended human dose on a mg/kg and mg/m^2 basis, respectively. Hepatoblastoma is a relatively rare rodent malignant tumor type. There was no increase in total malignant hepatic tumors. The mouse strain used is sensitive to the development of hepatic tumors, and the significance of these results to humans is unknown.

Methylphenidate did not cause any increases in tumors in a lifetime carcinogenicity study carried out in F344 rats; the highest dose used was approximately 45 mg/kg/day, which is approximately 22 times and 4 times the maximum recommended human dose on a mg/kg and mg/m^2 basis, respectively.

Methylphenidate was not mutagenic in the in vitro Ames reverse mutation assay or in the in vitro mouse lymphoma cell forward mutation assay. Sister chromatid exchanges and chromosome aberrations were increased, indicative of a weak clastogenic response, in an in vitro assay in cultured Chinese Hamster Ovary (CHO) cells. The genotoxic potential of methylphenidate has not been evaluated in an in vivo assay.

ADVERSE REACTIONS

Nervousness and insomnia are the most common adverse reactions but are usually controlled by reducing dosage and omitting the drug in the afternoon or evening. Other reactions include hypersensitivity (including skin rash, urticaria, fever, arthralgia, exfoliative dermatitis, erythema multiforme with histopathological findings of necrotizing vasculitis, and thrombocytopenic purpura); anorexia; nausea; dizziness; palpitations; headache; dyskinesia; drowsiness; blood pressure and pulse changes, both up and down; tachycardia; angina; cardiac arrhythmia; abdominal pain; weight loss during prolonged therapy. There have been rare reports of Tourette's syndrome. Toxic psychosis has been reported. Although a definite causal relationship has not been established, the following have been reported in patients taking this drug: instances of abnormal liver function, ranging from transaminase elevation to hepatic coma; isolated cases of cerebral arteritis and/or occlusion; leukopenia and/or anemia; transient depressed mood; a few instances of scalp hair loss. Very rare reports of neuroleptic malignant syndrome (NMS) have been received, and, in most of these, patients were concurrently receiving therapies associated with NMS. In a single report, a ten year old boy who had been taking methylphenidate for approximately 18 months experienced an NMS-like event within 45 minutes of ingesting his first dose of venlafaxine. It is uncertain whether this case represented a drug-drug interaction, a response to either drug alone, or some other cause.

In children, loss of appetite, abdominal pain, weight loss during prolonged therapy, insomnia, and tachycardia may occur more frequently; however, any of the other adverse reactions listed above may also occur.

DOSAGE AND ADMINISTRATION

Dosage should be individualized according to the needs and responses of the patient.

Adults

Tablets: Administer in divided doses 2 or 3 times daily, preferably 30 to 45 minutes before meals. Average dosage is 20 to 30 mg daily. Some patients may require 40 to 60 mg daily. In others, 10 to 15 mg daily will be adequate. Patients who are unable to sleep if medication is taken late in the day should take the last dose before 6 p.m.

SR Tablets: Ritalin-SR tablets have a duration of action of approximately 8 hours. Therefore, Ritalin-SR tablets may be used in place of Ritalin tablets when the 8-hour dosage of Ritalin-SR corresponds to the titrated 8-hour dosage of Ritalin. Ritalin-SR tablets must be swallowed whole and never crushed or chewed.

Children (6 years and over)

Ritalin should be initiated in small doses, with gradual weekly increments. Daily dosage above 60 mg is not recommended.

If improvement is not observed after appropriate dosage adjustment over a one-month period, the drug should be discontinued.

Tablets: Start with 5 mg twice daily (before breakfast and lunch) with gradual increments of 5 to 10 mg weekly.

SR Tablets: Ritalin-SR tablets have a duration of action of approximately 8 hours. Therefore, Ritalin-SR tablets may be used in place of Ritalin tablets when the 8-hour dosage of Ritalin-SR corresponds to the titrated 8-hour dosage of Ritalin. Ritalin-SR tablets must be swallowed whole and never crushed or chewed.

If paradoxical aggravation of symptoms or other adverse effects occur, reduce dosage, or, if necessary, discontinue the drug.

Ritalin should be periodically discontinued to assess the child's condition. Improvement may be sustained when the drug is either temporarily or permanently discontinued.

Drug treatment should not and need not be indefinite and usually may be discontinued after puberty.

OVERDOSAGE

Signs and symptoms of acute overdosage, resulting principally from overstimulation of the central nervous system and from excessive sympathomimetic effects, may include the following: vomiting, agitation, tremors, hyperreflexia, muscle twitching, convulsions (may be followed by coma), euphoria, confusion, hallucinations, delirium, sweating, flushing, headache, hyperpyrexia, tachycardia, palpitations, cardiac arrhythmias, hypertension, mydriasis, and dryness of mucous membranes.

Consult with a Certified Poison Control Center regarding treatment for up-to-date guidance and advice.

Treatment consists of appropriate supportive measures. The patient must be protected against self-injury and against external stimuli that would aggravate overstimulation already present. Gastric contents may be evacuated by gastric lavage. In the presence of severe intoxication, use a carefully titrated dosage of a *short-acting* barbiturate before performing gastric lavage. Other measures to detoxify the gut include administration of activated charcoal and a cathartic.

Intensive care must be provided to maintain adequate circulation and respiratory exchange; external cooling procedures may be required for hyperpyrexia.

Efficacy of peritoneal dialysis or extracorporeal hemodialysis for Ritalin overdosage has not been established.

HOW SUPPLIED

Tablets 5 mg — round, yellow (imprinted CIBA 7)

Bottles of 100 .... NDC 0083-0007-30

Tablets 10 mg — round, pale green, scored (imprinted CIBA 3)

Bottles of 100 .... NDC 0083-0003-30

Tablets 20 mg — round, pale yellow, scored (imprinted CIBA 34)

Bottles of 100 .... NDC 0083-0034-30

Do not store above 30°C (86°F). Protect from light.

Dispense in tight, light-resistant container (USP).

SR Tablets 20 mg — round, white, coated (imprinted CIBA 16)

Bottles of 100 .... NDC 0083-0016-30

Note: SR Tablets are color-additive free.

Do not store above 30°C (86°F). Protect from moisture.

Dispense in tight, light-resistant container (USP).

T2001-08

REV: JANUARY 2001 89002403

Novartis Pharmaceuticals Corporation
East Hanover, New Jersey 07936

Shown in Product Identification Guide, page 325

RITALIN LA® Ⓒ℞

[rĭ-tă-lĭn]

(methylphenidate hydrochloride)

extended-release capsules

Rx only

Prescribing Information

The following prescribing information is based on official labeling in effect July 2004.

DESCRIPTION

Methylphenidate hydrochloride is a central nervous system (CNS) stimulant.

Ritalin LA® (methylphenidate hydrochloride) extended-release capsules is an extended-release formulation of methylphenidate with a bi-modal release profile. Ritalin LA® uses the proprietary SODAS™ (Spheroidal Oral Drug Absorption System) technology. Each bead-filled Ritalin LA capsule contains half the dose as immediate-release beads and half as enteric-coated, delayed-release beads, thus providing an immediate release of methylphenidate and a second delayed release of methylphenidate. Ritalin LA 10, 20, 30, and 40 mg capsules provide in a single dose the same amount of methylphenidate as dosages of 5, 10, 15, or 20 mg of Ritalin® tablets given b.i.d.

The active substance in Ritalin LA is methyl α-phenyl-2-piperidineacetate hydrochloride, and its structural formula is

Methylphenidate hydrochloride USP is a white, odorless, fine crystalline powder. Its solutions are acid to litmus. It is freely soluble in water and in methanol, soluble in alcohol, and slightly soluble in chloroform and in acetone. Its molecular weight is 269.77.

Inactive ingredients: ammonio methacrylate copolymer, black iron oxide (10 and 40 mg capsules only), gelatin, methacrylic acid copolymer, polyethylene glycol, red iron oxide (10 and 40 mg capsules only), sugar spheres, talc, titanium dioxide, triethyl citrate, and yellow iron oxide (10, 30, and 40 mg capsules only).

CLINICAL PHARMACOLOGY

Pharmacodynamics

Methylphenidate hydrochloride, the active ingredient in Ritalin LA® (methylphenidate hydrochloride) extended-release capsules, is a central nervous system (CNS) stimulant. The mode of therapeutic action in Attention Deficit Hyperactivity Disorder (ADHD) is not known. Methylphenidate is thought to block the reuptake of norepinephrine and dopamine into the presynaptic neuron and increase the release of these monoamines into the extraneuronal space. Methylphenidate is a racemic mixture comprised of the *d*- and *l-threo* enantiomers. The *d-threo* enantiomer is more pharmacologically active than the *l-threo* enantiomer.

Pharmacokinetics

Absorption

Ritalin LA produces a bi-modal plasma concentration-time profile (i.e., two distinct peaks approximately four hours apart) when orally administered to children diagnosed with ADHD and to healthy adults. The initial rate of absorption for Ritalin LA is similar to that of Ritalin tablets as shown by the similar rate parameters between the two formulations, i.e., initial lag time (T_{lag}), first peak concentration (C_{max1}), and time to the first peak (T_{max1}), which is reached in 1-3 hours. The mean time to the interpeak minimum (T_{minip}), and time to the second peak (T_{max2}) are also similar for Ritalin LA given once daily and Ritalin tablets given in two doses 4 hours apart *(see Figure 1 and Table 1)*, although the ranges observed are greater for Ritalin LA.

Ritalin LA given once daily exhibits a lower second peak concentration (C_{max2}), higher interpeak minimum concentrations (C_{minip}), and less peak and trough fluctuations than Ritalin tablets given in two doses given 4 hours apart. This is due to an earlier onset and more prolonged absorption from the delayed-release beads *(see Figure 1 and Table 1)*. The relative bioavailability of Ritalin LA given once daily is comparable to the same total dose of Ritalin tablets given in two doses 4 hours apart in both children and in adults.

[See figure 1 at top of next column]

[See table 1 at bottom of next page]

Dose Proportionality

After oral administration of Ritalin LA 20 mg and 40 mg capsules to adults there is a slight upward trend in the methylphenidate area under the curve (AUC) and peak plasma concentrations (C_{max1} and C_{max2}).

Distribution

Binding to plasma proteins is low (10%-33%), and the apparent distribution volume at steady state with intravenous administration has been reported to be approximately 6 L/kg.

Figure 1. Mean plasma concentration time-profile of methylphenidate after a single dose of Ritalin® LA 40 mg q.d. and Ritalin® 20 mg given in two doses four hours apart

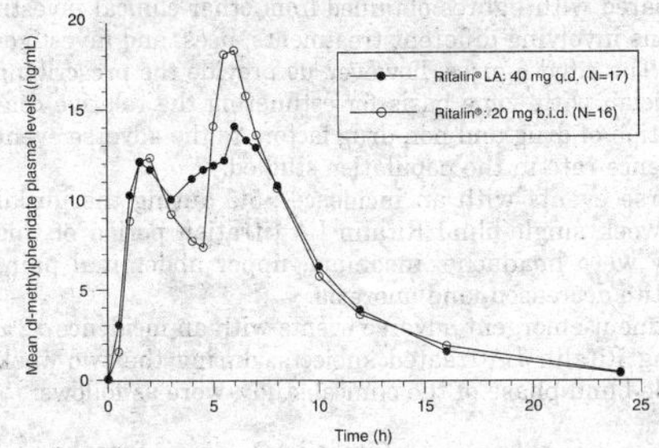

Metabolism

The absolute oral bioavailability of methylphenidate in children has been reported to be about 30% (range 10%-52%), suggesting pronounced presystemic metabolism. Biotransformation of methylphenidate is rapid and extensive leading to the main, de-esterified metabolite α-phenyl-2-piperidine acetic acid (ritalinic acid). Only small amounts of hydroxylated metabolites (e.g., hydroxymethylphenidate and hydroxyritalinic acid) are detectable in plasma. Therapeutic activity is principally due to the parent compound.

Elimination

In studies with Ritalin LA and Ritalin tablets in adults, methylphenidate from Ritalin tablets is eliminated from plasma with an average half-life of about 3.5 hours, (range 1.3-7.7 hours). In children the average half-life is about 2.5 hours, with a range of about 1.5-5.0 hours. The rapid half-life in both children and adults may result in unmeasurable concentrations between the morning and mid-day doses with Ritalin tablets. No accumulation of methylphenidate is expected following multiple once a day oral dosing with Ritalin LA. The half-life of ritalinic acid is about 3-4 hours. After oral administration of an immediate release formulation of methylphenidate, 78%-97% of the dose is excreted in the urine and 1%-3% in the feces in the form of metabolites within 48-96 hours. Only small quantities (<1%) of unchanged methylphenidate appear in the urine. Most of the dose is excreted in the urine as ritalinic acid (60%-86%), the remainder being accounted for by minor metabolites.

Food Effects

Administration times relative to meals and meal composition may need to be individually titrated.

When Ritalin LA was administered with a high fat breakfast to adults, Ritalin LA had a longer lag time until absorption began and variable delays in the time until the first peak concentration, the time until the interpeak minimum, and the time until the second peak. The first peak concentration and the extent of absorption were unchanged after food relative to the fasting state, although the second peak was approximately 25% lower. The effect of a high fat lunch was not examined.

There were no differences in the pharmacokinetics of Ritalin LA when administered with applesauce, compared to administration in the fasting condition. There is no evidence of dose dumping in the presence or absence of food.

For patients unable to swallow the capsule, the contents may be sprinkled on applesauce and administered *(see DOSAGE AND ADMINISTRATION).*

Special Populations

Age: The pharmacokinetics of Ritalin LA was examined in 18 children with ADHD between 7 and 12 years of age. Fifteen of these children were between 10 and 12 years of age. The time until the between peak minimum, and the time until the second peak were delayed and more variable in children compared to adults. After a 20-mg dose of Ritalin LA, concentrations in children were approximately twice the concentrations observed in 18 to 35 year old adults. This higher exposure is almost completely due to the smaller body size and total volume of distribution in children, as apparent clearance normalized to body weight is independent of age.

Gender: There were no apparent gender differences in the pharmacokinetics of methylphenidate between healthy male and female adults when administered Ritalin LA.

Renal Insufficiency: Ritalin LA has not been studied in renally-impaired patients. Renal insufficiency is expected to have minimal effect on the pharmacokinetics of methylphenidate since less than 1% of a radiolabeled dose is excreted in the urine as unchanged compound, and the major metabolite (ritalinic acid), has little or no pharmacologic activity.

Hepatic Insufficiency: Ritalin LA has not been studied in patients with hepatic insufficiency. Hepatic insufficiency is expected to have minimal effect on the pharmacokinetics of methylphenidate since it is metabolized primarily to ritalinic acid by nonmicrosomal hydrolytic esterases that are widely distributed throughout the body.

Clinical Studies

Ritalin LA® (methylphenidate hydrochloride) extended-release capsules was evaluated in a randomized, double-blind, placebo-controlled, parallel group clinical study in which 134 children, ages 6 to 12, with DSM-IV diagnoses of attention deficit hyperactivity disorder (ADHD) received a single morning dose of Ritalin LA in the range of 10-40 mg/day, or placebo, for up to 2 weeks. The doses used were the optimal doses established in a previous individual dose titration phase. In that titration phase, 53 of 164 patients (32%) started on a daily dose of 10 mg and 111 of 164 patients (68%) started on a daily dose of 20 mg or higher. The patient's regular schoolteacher completed the Conners ADHD/DSM-IV Scale for Teachers (CADS-T) at baseline and the end of each week. The CADS-T assesses symptoms of hyperactivity and inattention. The change from baseline of the (CADS-T) scores during the last week of treatment was analyzed as the primary efficacy parameter. Patients treated with Ritalin LA showed a statistically significant improvement in symptom scores from baseline over patients who received placebo. *(See Figure 2.)* This demonstrates that a single morning dose of Ritalin LA exerts a treatment effect in ADHD.

Figure 2. CADS-T total subscale - Mean change from baseline*

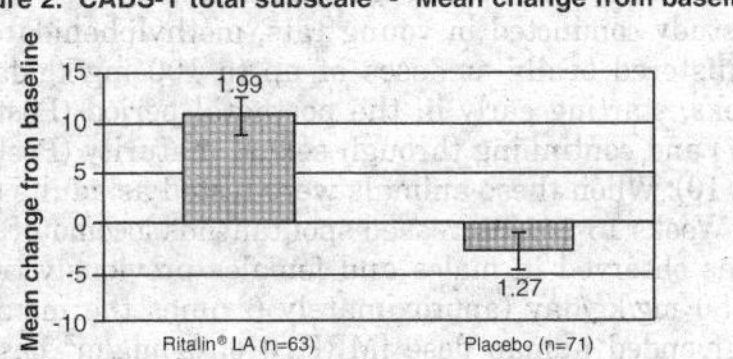

*Error bars represent standard error of the mean

INDICATIONS AND USAGE

Ritalin LA® (methylphenidate hydrochloride) extended-release capsules is indicated for the treatment of Attention Deficit Hyperactivity Disorder (ADHD).

The efficacy of Ritalin LA in the treatment of ADHD was established in one controlled trial of children aged 6 to 12 who met DSM-IV criteria for ADHD *(see CLINICAL PHARMACOLOGY).*

A diagnosis of Attention Deficit Hyperactivity Disorder (ADHD; DSM-IV) implies the presence of hyperactive-impulsive or inattentive symptoms that caused impairment and were present before age 7 years. The symptoms must cause clinically significant impairment, e.g., in social, academic, or occupational functioning, and be present in two or more settings, e.g., school (or work) and at home. The symptoms must not be better accounted for by another mental disorder. For the Inattentive Type, at least six of the following symptoms must have persisted for at least 6 months: lack of attention to details/careless mistakes; lack of sustained attention; poor listener; failure to follow through on tasks; poor organization; avoids tasks requiring sustained mental effort; loses things; easily distracted; forgetful. For the Hyperactive-Impulsive Type, at least six of the following symptoms must have persisted for at least 6 months: fidgeting/squirming; leaving seat; inappropriate running/climbing; difficulty with quiet activities; "on the go;" excessive talking; blurting answers; can't wait turn; intrusive. The Combined Types requires both inattentive and hyperactive-impulsive criteria to be met.

Special Diagnostic Considerations

Specific etiology of this syndrome is unknown, and there is no single diagnostic test. Adequate diagnosis requires the use not only of medical but of special psychological, educational, and social resources. Learning may or may not be impaired. The diagnosis must be based upon a complete history and evaluation of the child and not solely on the presence of the required number of DSM-IV characteristics.

Need for Comprehensive Treatment Program

Ritalin LA is indicated as an integral part of a total treatment program for ADHD that may include other measures (psychological, educational, social) for patients with this syndrome. Drug treatment may not be indicated for all children with this syndrome. Stimulants are not intended for use in the child who exhibits symptoms secondary to environmental factors and/or other primary psychiatric disorders, including psychosis. Appropriate educational placement is essential and psychosocial intervention is often helpful. When remedial measures alone are insufficient, the decision to prescribe stimulant medication will depend upon the physician's assessment of the chronicity and severity of the child's symptoms.

Long-Term Use

The effectiveness of Ritalin LA for long-term use, i.e., for more than 2 weeks, has not been systematically evaluated in controlled trials. Therefore, the physician who elects to use Ritalin LA for extended periods should periodically re-evaluate the long-term usefulness of the drug for the individual patient *(see DOSAGE AND ADMINISTRATION).*

CONTRAINDICATIONS

Agitation

Ritalin LA® (methylphenidate hydrochloride) extended-release capsules is contraindicated in marked anxiety, tension, and agitation, since the drug may aggravate these symptoms.

Hypersensitivity to Methylphenidate

Ritalin LA is contraindicated in patients known to be hypersensitive to methylphenidate or other components of the product.

Glaucoma

Ritalin LA is contraindicated in patients with glaucoma.

Tics

Ritalin LA is contraindicated in patients with motor tics or with a family history or diagnosis of Tourette's syndrome. *(See ADVERSE REACTIONS.)*

Monoamine Oxidase Inhibitors

Ritalin LA is contraindicated during treatment with monoamine oxidase inhibitors, and also within a minimum of 14 days following discontinuation of treatment with a monoamine oxidase inhibitor (hypertensive crises may result).

WARNINGS

Depression

Ritalin LA® (methylphenidate hydrochloride) extended-release capsules should not be used to treat severe depression.

Fatigue

Ritalin LA should not be used for the prevention or treatment of normal fatigue states.

Long-Term Suppression of Growth

Sufficient data on the safety of long-term use of methylphenidate in children are not yet available. Although a causal relationship has not been established, suppression of growth (i.e., weight gain, and/or height) has been reported with the long-term use of stimulants in children. Therefore, patients requiring long-term therapy should be carefully monitored. Patients who are not growing or gaining weight as expected should have their treatment interrupted. In the double-blind placebo-controlled study of Ritalin LA, the mean weight gain was greater for patients receiving placebo (+1.0 kg) than for patients receiving Ritalin LA (+0.1 kg).

Psychosis

Clinical experience suggests that in psychotic patients, administration of methylphenidate may exacerbate symptoms of behavior disturbance and thought disorder.

Seizures

There is some clinical evidence that methylphenidate may lower the convulsive threshold in patients with prior history of seizures, with prior EEG abnormalities in the absence of seizures, and, very rarely, in the absence of history of seizures and no prior EEG evidence of seizures. Safe concomitant use of anticonvulsants and methylphenidate has not been established. In the presence of seizures, Ritalin LA should be discontinued.

Table 1
Mean ± SD and range of pharmacokinetic parameters of methylphenidate after a single dose of Ritalin LA® and Ritalin® given in two doses 4 hours apart

Population	Children		Adult Males	
Formulation	Ritalin®	Ritalin LA®	Ritalin®	Ritalin LA®
Dose	10 mg & 10 mg	20 mg	10 mg & 10 mg	20 mg
N	21	18	9	8
T_{lag} (h)	0.24 ± 0.44	0.28 ± 0.46	1.0 ± 0.5	0.7 ± 0.2
	0-1	0-1	0.7-1.3	0.3-1.0
T_{max1} (h)	1.8 ± 0.6	2.0 ± 0.8	1.9 ± 0.4	2.0 ± 0.9
	1-3	1-3	1.3-2.7	1.3-4.0
C_{max1} (ng/mL)	10.2 ± 4.2	10.3 ± 5.1	4.3 ± 2.3	5.3 ± 0.9
	4.2-20.2	5.5-26.6	1.8-7.5	3.8-6.9
T_{minip} (h)	4.0 ± 0.2	4.5 ± 1.2	3.8 ± 0.4	3.6 ± 0.6
	4-5	2-6	3.3-4.3	2.7-4.3
C_{minip} (ng/mL)	5.8 ± 2.7	6.1 ± 4.1	1.2 ± 1.4	3.0 ± 0.8
	3.1-14.4	2.9-21.0	0.0-3.7	1.7-4.0
T_{max2} (h)	5.6 ± 0.7	6.6 ± 1.5	5.9 ± 0.5	5.5 ± 0.8
	5-8	5-11	5.0-6.5	4.3-6.5
C_{max2} (ng/mL)	15.3 ± 7.0	10.2 ± 5.9	5.3 ± 1.4	6.2 ± 1.6
	6.2-32.8	4.5-31.1	3.6-7.2	3.9-8.3
$AUC_{(0-\infty)}$	102.4 ± 54.6	86.6 ± 64.0[a]	37.8 ± 21.9	45.8 ± 10.0
(ng/mL × h-1)	40.5-261.6	43.3-301.44	14.3-85.3	34.0-61.6
$t_{1/2}$ (h)	2.5 ± 0.8	2.4 ± 0.7[a]	3.5 ± 1.9	3.3 ± 0.4
	1.8-5.3	1.5-4.0	1.3-7.7	3.0-4.2

[a] N = 15

Continued on next page

Ritalin LA—Cont.

Hypertension and other Cardiovascular Conditions
Use cautiously in patients with hypertension. Blood pressure should be monitored at appropriate intervals in patients taking Ritalin LA, especially patients with hypertension. Studies of methylphenidate have shown modest increases of resting pulse and systolic and diastolic blood pressure. Therefore, caution is indicated in treating patients whose underlying medical conditions might be compromised by increases in blood pressure or heart rate, e.g., those with pre-existing hypertension, heart failure, recent myocardial infarction, or hyperthyroidism.

Visual Disturbance
Symptoms of visual disturbances have been encountered in rare cases. Difficulties with accommodation and blurring of vision have been reported with methylphenidate.

Use in Children Under Six Years of Age
Ritalin LA should not be used in children under six years of age, since safety and efficacy in this age group have not been established.

Drug Dependence
Ritalin LA should be given cautiously to patients with a history of drug dependence or alcoholism. Chronic abusive use can lead to marked tolerance and psychological dependence with varying degrees of abnormal behavior. Frank psychotic episodes can occur, especially with parenteral abuse. Careful supervision is required during withdrawal from abusive use, since severe depression may occur. Withdrawal following chronic therapeutic use may unmask symptoms of the underlying disorder that may require follow-up.

PRECAUTIONS

Hematologic Monitoring
Periodic CBC, differential, and platelet counts are advised during prolonged therapy.

Information for Patients
Patient information is provided at the end of this insert. To assure safe and effective use of Ritalin LA® (methylphenidate hydrochloride) extended-release capsules, the patient information should be discussed with patients.

Drug Interactions
Methylphenidate is metabolized primarily by de-esterification (nonmicrosomal hydrolytic esterases) to ritalinic acid and not through oxidative pathways.
The effects of gastrointestinal pH alterations on the absorption of methylphenidate from Ritalin LA have not been studied. Since the modified release characteristics of Ritalin LA are pH dependent, the coadministration of antacids or acid suppressants could alter the release of methylphenidate.
Methylphenidate may decrease the hypotensive effect of guanethidine. Because of possible effects on blood pressure, methylphenidate should be used cautiously with pressor agents.
Human pharmacologic studies have shown that methylphenidate may inhibit the metabolism of coumarin anticoagulants, anticonvulsants (e.g., phenobarbital, phenytoin, primidone), and tricyclic drugs (e.g., imipramine, clomipramine, desipramine). Downward dose adjustment of these drugs may be required when given concomitantly with methylphenidate. It may be necessary to adjust the dosage and monitor plasma drug concentrations (or, in the case of coumarin, coagulation times), when initiating or discontinuing concomitant methylphenidate.
Serious adverse events have been reported in concomitant use of methylphenidatewith clonidine, although no causality for the combination has been established. The safety of using methylphenidate in combination with clonidine or other centrally acting alpha-2-agonists has not been systematically evaluated.

Carcinogenesis/Mutagenesis/Impairment of Fertility
In a lifetime carcinogenicity study carried out in B6C3F1 mice, methylphenidate caused an increase in hepatocellular adenomas and, in males only, an increase in hepatoblastomas, at a daily dose of approximately 60 mg/kg/day. This dose is approximately 30 times and 4 times the maximum recommended human dose on a mg/kg and mg/m^2 basis, respectively. Hepatoblastoma is a relatively rare rodent malignant tumor type. There was no increase in total malignant hepatic tumors. The mouse strain used is sensitive to the development of hepatic tumors, and the significance of these results to humans is unknown.
Methylphenidate did not cause any increases in tumors in a lifetime carcinogenicity study carried out in F344 rats; the highest dose used was approximately 45 mg/kg/day, which is approximately 22 times and 5 times the maximum recommended human dose on a mg/kg and mg/m^2 basis, respectively.
In a 24-week carcinogenicity study in the transgenic mouse strain p53+/-, which is sensitive to genotoxic carcinogens, there was no evidence of carcinogenicity. Male and female mice were fed diets containing the same concentration of methylphenidate as in the lifetime carcinogenicity study; the high-dose groups were exposed to 60-74 mg/kg/day of methylphenidate.
Methylphenidate was not mutagenic in the *in vitro* Ames reverse mutation assay or in the *in vitro* mouse lymphoma cell forward mutation assay. Sister chromatid exchanges and chromosome aberrations were increased, indicative of a weak clastogenic response, in an *in vitro* assay in cultured Chinese Hamster Ovary (CHO) cells. Methylphenidate was negative *in vivo* in males and females in the mouse bone marrow micronucleus assay.
Methylphenidate did not impair fertility in male or female mice that were fed diets containing the drug in an 18-week Continuous Breeding study. The study was conducted at doses up to 160 mg/kg/day, approximately 80-fold and 8-fold the highest recommended dose on a mg/kg and mg/m^2 basis, respectively.

Pregnancy
Pregnancy Category C
In studies conducted in rats and rabbits, methylphenidate was administered orally at doses of up to 75 and 200 mg/kg/day, respectively, during the period of organogenesis. Teratogenic effects (increased incidence of fetal spina bifida) were observed in rabbits at the highest dose, which is approximately 40 times the maximum recommended human dose (MRHD) on a mg/m^2 basis. The no effect level for embryo-fetal development in rabbits was 60 mg/kg/day (11 times the MRHD on a mg/m^2 basis). There was no evidence of specific teratogenic activity in rats, although increased incidences of fetal skeletal variations were seen at the highest dose level (7 times the MRHD on a mg/m^2 basis), which was also maternally toxic. The no effect level for embryo-fetal development in rats was 25 mg/kg/day (2 times the MRHD on a mg/m^2 basis). When methylphenidate was administered to rats throughout pregnancy and lactation at doses of up to 45 mg/kg/day, offspring body weight gain was decreased at the highest dose (4 times the MRHD on a mg/m^2 basis), but no other effects on postnatal development were observed. The no effect level for pre- and postnatal development in rats was 15 mg/kg/day (equal to the MRHD on a mg/m^2 basis).
Adequate and well-controlled studies in pregnant women have not been conducted. Ritalin LA should be used during pregnancy only if the potential benefit justifies the potential risk to the fetus.

Nursing Mothers
It is not known whether methylphenidate is excreted in human milk. Because many drugs are excreted in human milk, caution should be exercised if Ritalin LA is administered to a nursing woman.

Pediatric Use
Long-term effects of methylphenidate in children have not been well established. Ritalin LA should not be used in children under six years of age (*see WARNINGS*).
In a study conducted in young rats, methylphenidate was administered orally at doses of up to 100 mg/kg/day for 9 weeks, starting early in the postnatal period (Postnatal Day 7) and continuing through sexual maturity (Postnatal Week 10). When these animals were tested as adults (Postnatal Weeks 13-14), decreased spontaneous locomotor activity was observed in males and females previously treated with 50 mg/kg/day (approximately 6 times the maximum recommended human dose [MRHD] on a mg/m^2 basis) or greater, and a deficit in the acquisition of a specific learning task was seen in females exposed to the highest dose (12 times the MRHD on a mg/m^2 basis). The no effect level for juvenile neurobehavioral development in rats was 5 mg/kg/day (half the MRHD on a mg/m^2 basis). The clinical significance of the long-term behavioral effects observed in rats is unknown.

ADVERSE REACTIONS

The clinical program for Ritalin LA® (methylphenidate hydrochloride) extended-release capsules consisted of six studies: two controlled clinical studies conducted in children with ADHD aged 6-12 years and four clinical pharmacology studies conducted in healthy adult volunteers. These studies included a total of 256 subjects; 195 children with ADHD and 61 healthy adult volunteers. The subjects received Ritalin LA in doses of 10-40 mg per day. Safety of Ritalin LA was assessed by evaluating frequency and nature of adverse events, routine laboratory tests, vital signs, and body weight.
Adverse events during exposure were obtained primarily by general inquiry and recorded by clinical investigators using terminology of their own choosing. Consequently, it is not possible to provide a meaningful estimate of the proportion of individuals experiencing adverse events without first grouping similar types of events into a smaller number of standardized event categories. In the tables and listings that follow, MEDRA terminology has been used to classify reported adverse events. The stated frequencies of adverse events represent the proportion of individuals who experienced, at least once, a treatment-emergent adverse event of the type listed. An event was considered treatment emergent if it occurred for the first time or worsened while receiving therapy following baseline evaluation.

Adverse Events in a Double-Blind, Placebo-Controlled Clinical Trial with Ritalin LA
Treatment-Emergent Adverse Events
A placebo-controlled, double-blind, parallel-group study was conducted to evaluate the efficacy and safety of Ritalin LA in children with ADHD aged 6-12 years. All subjects received Ritalin LA for up to 4 weeks, and had their dose optimally adjusted, prior to entering the double-blind phase of the trial. In the two-week double-blind treatment phase of this study, patients received either placebo or Ritalin LA at their individually-titrated dose (range 10 mg-40 mg).
The prescriber should be aware that these figures cannot be used to predict the incidence of adverse events in the course of usual medical practice where patient characteristics and other factors differ from those which prevailed in the clinical trials. Similarly, the cited frequencies cannot be compared with figures obtained from other clinical investigations involving different treatments, uses, and investigators. The cited figures, however, do provide the prescribing physician with some basis for estimating the relative contribution of drug and non-drug factors to the adverse event incidence rate in the population studied.
Adverse events with an incidence >5% during the initial four-week single-blind Ritalin LA titration period of this study were headache, insomnia, upper abdominal pain, appetite decreased, and anorexia.
Treatment-emergent adverse events with an incidence >2% among Ritalin LA-treated subjects, during the two-week double-blind phase of the clinical study, were as follows:

Preferred term	Ritalin LA® N=65 N (%)	Placebo N=71 N (%)
Anorexia	2 (3.1)	0 (0.0)
Insomnia	2 (3.1)	0 (0.0)

Adverse Events Associated with Discontinuation of Treatment
In the two-week double-blind treatment phase of a placebo-controlled parallel-group study in children with ADHD, only one Ritalin LA-treated subject (1/65, 1.5%) discontinued due to an adverse event (depression).
In the single-blind titration period of this study, subjects received Ritalin LA for up to 4 weeks. During this period a total of six subjects (6/161, 3.7%) discontinued due to adverse events. The adverse events leading to discontinuation were anger (in 2 patients), hypomania, anxiety, depressed mood, fatigue, migraine and lethargy.

Adverse Events with Other Methylphenidate HCl Dosage Forms
Nervousness and insomnia are the most common adverse reactions reported with other methylphenidate products. In children, loss of appetite, abdominal pain, weight loss during prolonged therapy, insomnia, and tachycardia may occur more frequently; however, any of the other adverse reactions listed below may also occur.
Other reactions include:
Cardiac: angina, arrhythmia, palpitations, pulse increased or decreased, tachycardia
Gastrointestinal: abdominal pain, nausea
Immune: hypersensitivity reactions including skin rash, urticaria, fever, arthralgia, exfoliative dermatitis, erythema multiforme with histopathological findings of necrotizing vasculitis, and thrombocytopenic purpura.
Metabolism/Nutrition: anorexia, weight loss during prolonged therapy
Nervous System: dizziness, drowsiness, dyskinesia, headache, rare reports of Tourette's syndrome, toxic psychosis
Vascular: blood pressure increased or decreased, cerebral arteritis and/or occlusion
Although a definite causal relationship has not been established, the following have been reported in patients taking methylphenidate:
Blood/Lymphatic: leukopenia and/or anemia
Hepatobiliary: abnormal liver function, ranging from transaminase elevation to hepatic coma
Psychiatric: transient depressed mood
Skin/Subcutaneous: scalp hair loss
Very rare reports of neuroleptic malignant syndrome (NMS) have been received, and, in most of these, patients were concurrently receiving therapies associated with NMS. In a single report, a ten-year-old boy who had been taking methylphenidate for approximately 18 months experienced an NMS-like event within 45 minutes of ingesting his first dose of venlafaxine. It is uncertain whether this case represented a drug-drug interaction, a response to either drug alone, or some other cause.

DRUG ABUSE AND DEPENDENCE

Ritalin LA® (methylphenidate hydrochloride) extended-release capsules, like other products containing methylphenidate, is a Schedule II controlled substance. *(See WARNINGS for boxed warning containing drug abuse and dependence information.)*

OVERDOSAGE

Signs and Symptoms
Signs and symptoms of acute overdosage, resulting principally from overstimulation of the central nervous system and from excessive sympathomimetic effects, may include the following: vomiting, agitation, tremors, hyperreflexia, muscle twitching, convulsions (may be followed by coma), euphoria, confusion, hallucinations, delirium, sweating, flushing, headache, hyperpyrexia, tachycardia, palpitations, cardiac arrhythmias, hypertension, mydriasis, and dryness of mucous membranes.

Poison Control Center
Consult with a Certified Poison Control Center regarding treatment for up-to-date guidance and advice.

Recommended Treatment
As with the management of all overdosage, the possibility of multiple drug ingestion should be considered.
When treating overdose, practitioners should bear in mind that there is a prolonged release of methylphenidate from Ritalin LA® (methylphenidate hydrochloride) extended-release capsules.
Treatment consists of appropriate supportive measures. The patient must be protected against self-injury and

against external stimuli that would aggravate overstimulation already present. Gastric contents may be evacuated by gastric lavage as indicated. Before performing gastric lavage, control agitation and seizures if present and protect the airway. Other measures to detoxify the gut include administration of activated charcoal and a cathartic. Intensive care must be provided to maintain adequate circulation and respiratory exchange; external cooling procedures may be required for hyperpyrexia.

Efficacy of peritoneal dialysis or extracorporeal hemodialysis for methylphenidate overdosage has not been established; also, dialysis is considered unlikely to be of benefit due to the large volume of distribution of methylphenidate.

DOSAGE AND ADMINISTRATION

Administration of Dose

Ritalin LA® (methylphenidate hydrochloride) extended-release capsules is for oral administration once daily in the morning. Ritalin LA may be swallowed as whole capsules or alternatively may be administered by sprinkling the capsule contents on a small amount of applesauce *(see specific instructions below)*. Ritalin LA and/or their contents should not be crushed, chewed, or divided.

The capsules may be carefully opened and the beads sprinkled over a spoonful of applesauce. The applesauce should not be warm because it could affect the modified release properties of this formulation. The mixture of drug and applesauce should be consumed immediately in its entirety. The drug and applesauce mixture should not be stored for future use.

Dosing Recommendations

Dosage should be individualized according to the needs and responses of the patients.

Initial Treatment

The recommended starting dose of Ritalin LA is 20 mg once daily. Dosage may be adjusted in weekly 10 mg increments to a maximum of 60 mg/day taken once daily in the morning, depending on tolerability and degree of efficacy observed. Daily dosage above 60 mg is not recommended. When in the judgement of the clinician a lower initial dose is appropriate, patients may begin treatment with Ritalin LA 10 mg.

Patients Currently Receiving Methylphenidate

The recommended dose of Ritalin LA for patients currently taking methylphenidate b.i.d. or sustained release (SR) is provided below.

Previous Methylphenidate Dose	Recommended Ritalin LA® Dose
5 mg methylphenidate b.i.d.	10 mg q.d.
10 mg methylphenidate b.i.d. or 20 mg methylphenidate-SR	20 mg q.d.
15 mg methylphenidate b.i.d.	30 mg q.d.
20 mg methylphenidate b.i.d. or 40 mg of methylphenidate-SR	40 mg q.d.
30 mg methylphenidate b.i.d. or 60 mg methylphenidate-SR	60 mg q.d.

For other methylphenidate regimens, clinical judgment should be used when selecting the starting dose. Ritalin LA dosage may be adjusted at weekly intervals in 10 mg increments.

Daily dosage above 60 mg is not recommended.

Maintenance/Extended Treatment

There is no body of evidence available from controlled trials to indicate how long the patient with ADHD should be treated with Ritalin LA. It is generally agreed, however, that pharmacological treatment of ADHD may be needed for extended periods. Nevertheless, the physician who elects to use Ritalin LA for extended periods in patients with ADHD should periodically re-evaluate the long-term usefulness of the drug for the individual patient with trials off medication to assess the patient's functioning without pharmacotherapy. Improvement may be sustained when the drug is either temporarily or permanently discontinued.

Dose Reduction and Discontinuation

If paradoxical aggravation of symptoms or other adverse events occur, the dosage should be reduced, or, if necessary, the drug should be discontinued. If improvement is not observed after appropriate dosage adjustment over a one-month period, the drug should be discontinued.

HOW SUPPLIED

Ritalin LA capsules 10 mg: white/light brown (imprinted NVR R10)

Bottles of 100 .... NDC 0078-0424-05

Ritalin LA capsules 20 mg: white (imprinted NVR R20)

Bottles of 100 .... NDC 0078-0370-05

Ritalin LA capsules 30 mg: yellow (imprinted NVR R30)

Bottles of 100 .... NDC 0078-0371-05

Ritalin LA capsules 40 mg: light brown (imprinted NVR R40)

Bottles of 100 .... NDC 0078-0372-05

Store at 25°C (77°F), excursions permitted 15°C-30°C (59°F-86°F). [See USP controlled room temperature]

Dispense in tight container (USP).

Ritalin LA® is a trademark of Novartis AG.

SODAS™ is a trademark of Elan Corporation, plc.

This product is covered by US patents including US 5,837,284 and 6,228,398.

REFERENCE

American Psychiatric Association. Diagnosis and Statistical Manual of Mental Disorders. 4th edition. Washington DC: American Psychiatric Association 1994.

REV: APRIL 2004 T2004-34
T2004-35

INFORMATION FOR PATIENTS TAKING RITALIN LA®, OR FOR THEIR PARENTS OR CAREGIVERS

Once Daily

Ritalin LA® Ⓒ

(methylphenidate hydrochloride)

extended-release capsules

This information for patients or their parents or caregivers is about Ritalin LA. Please read this before you start taking Ritalin LA. Also, read the information you get each time you renew your prescription, in case anything has changed. Remember, this information does not take the place of your doctor's instructions. If you have any questions about this information or about Ritalin LA, talk to your doctor or pharmacist.

WHAT IS RITALIN LA?

Ritalin LA is a once-a-day treatment for Attention Deficit Hyperactivity Disorder, or ADHD. Ritalin LA contains the drug methylphenidate (Ritalin®), a central nervous system stimulant that has been used to treat ADHD for more than 30 years. Ritalin is available in several forms including Ritalin LA, an extended-release form of methylphenidate hydrochloride available as 10, 20, 30, and 40 mg extended-release capsules. Ritalin LA is taken by mouth, once each day in the morning, before breakfast.

WHAT IS ATTENTION DEFICIT HYPERACTIVITY DISORDER?

ADHD has three main types of symptoms: inattention, hyperactivity, and impulsiveness. Symptoms of inattention include not paying attention, making careless mistakes, not listening, not finishing tasks, not following directions, and being easily distracted. Symptoms of hyperactivity and impulsiveness include fidgeting, talking excessively, running around at inappropriate times, and interrupting others. Some patients have more symptoms of hyperactivity and impulsiveness while others have more symptoms of inattentiveness. Some patients have all three types of symptoms. Many people have symptoms like these from time to time, but patients with ADHD have these symptoms more than others their age. Symptoms must be present for at least 6 months to be certain of the diagnosis.

HOW DOES RITALIN LA WORK?

When you take a Ritalin LA capsule, half of the beads provide an immediate dose of methylphenidate and the other half provide a delayed second release of the drug to continue to help lessen the symptoms of ADHD during the day. Methylphenidate, the active ingredient in Ritalin LA, helps increase attention and decrease impulsiveness and hyperactivity in patients with ADHD.

BEFORE RITALIN LA TREATMENT

It is very important that ADHD be accurately diagnosed and that the need for medication be carefully assessed. It is important to remember that Ritalin is only part of the overall management of ADHD. Parents, teachers, physicians and other professionals are part of a team that must work together.

Before Ritalin treatment, your doctor should be made aware of any current or past physical or mental problems. Tell your doctor if there is a history of drug or alcohol abuse, depression, psychosis, epilepsy or seizure disorders, high blood pressure, glaucoma, facial tics (involuntary movements), or a family history of Tourette's syndrome.

Both your doctor and your pharmacist should also be informed of all medicines that you are taking, even if these drugs are not taken on a regular basis and are available without prescription. Your doctor will decide whether you can take Ritalin with other medicines. Methylphenidate is known to interact with a number of other drugs. These include medicines to treat depression, such as monoamine oxidase inhibitors; to control seizures; and to thin blood. Sometimes these interactions may require a change in dosage, or occasionally stopping one of the drugs involved.

Tell your doctor if you are pregnant or nursing a baby.

WHO SHOULD NOT TAKE RITALIN LA?

You should NOT take Ritalin LA if:

- You have significant anxiety, tension, or agitation since Ritalin LA may make these conditions worse.
- You are allergic to methylphenidate or any of the other ingredients in Ritalin LA.
- You have glaucoma, an eye disease.
- You have tics or Tourette's syndrome, or a family history of Tourette's syndrome.
- You are taking a monoamine oxidase inhibitor, a type of drug, or have discontinued a monoamine oxidase inhibitor in the last 14 days.

Talk to your doctor if you believe any of these conditions apply to you.

HOW SHOULD I TAKE RITALIN LA?

Take Ritalin LA once each day in the morning.

Take the dose prescribed by your doctor. Your doctor may adjust the amount of drug you take until it is right for you. From time to time, your doctor may interrupt your treatment to check your symptoms while you are not taking the drug.

Ritalin LA capsules may be taken at the same time as food or without food, although food may delay the absorption of Ritalin LA. The Ritalin LA capsule may be swallowed as whole capsules or the capsule may be opened and sprinkled on a small amount of applesauce. The capsule should not be crushed or chewed or its contents divided.

To sprinkle the contents of the capsule, open the capsule carefully and sprinkle the beads over a spoonful of applesauce. The applesauce should not be warm because it could affect the modified release properties of this formulation. The mixture of drug and applesauce should be consumed immediately in its entirety. The drug and applesauce mixture should not be stored for future use.

If you also take antiacids or drugs that suppress stomach acids, you should discuss with your physician or pharmacist how to take these drugs with Ritalin LA.

WHAT ARE THE POSSIBLE SIDE EFFECTS OF RITALIN LA?

The most common side effects of Ritalin LA are:

- Nervousness
- Stomach pain
- Sleeplessness
- Decreased appetite

Other side effects seen with methylphenidate, the active ingredient in Ritalin LA, include nausea, vomiting, dizziness, tics, allergic reactions, increased blood pressure and psychosis (abnormal thinking or hallucinations).

Dependence

Abuse of methylphenidate can lead to dependence. Tell your doctor if you have ever abused or been dependent on alcohol or drugs, or if you are now abusing or dependent on alcohol or drugs.

Blurred Vision

Tell your doctor if you have blurred vision when taking Ritalin LA. This could be a sign of a serious problem.

Slower Growth

Slower growth (weight gain and/or height) has been reported with long-term use of methylphenidate in children. Your doctor will be carefully watching your height and weight. If you are not growing or gaining weight as your doctor expects, your doctor may stop your Ritalin LA treatment.

This is not a complete list of possible side effects. Ask your doctor about other side effects. If you develop any side effect, talk to your doctor.

WHAT MUST I DISCUSS WITH MY DOCTOR BEFORE TAKING RITALIN LA?

Talk to your doctor ***before*** taking RITALIN LA if you:

- Are being treated for depression or have symptoms of depression such as feelings of sadness, worthlessness, and hopelessness.
- Have motion tics (hard-to-control, repeated twitching of any parts of your body) or verbal tics (hard-to-control repeating of sounds or words).
- Have someone in your family with motion tics, verbal tics, or Tourette's syndrome.
- Have abnormal thoughts or visions, hear abnormal sounds, or have been diagnosed with psychosis.
- Have had seizures (convulsions, epilepsy) or abnormal EEGs (electroencephalograms).
- Have high blood pressure.
- Have an abnormal heart rate or rhythm.

Tell your doctor ***immediately*** if you develop any of the above conditions or symptoms while taking Ritalin LA.

CAN I TAKE RITALIN LA WITH OTHER MEDICINES?

Tell your doctor about ***all*** medicines that you are taking or intend to take. Your doctor should decide whether you can take Ritalin LA with other medicines. These include:

- Other medicines that a doctor has prescribed.
- All medicines that you buy yourself without a prescription.
- Any herbal remedies that you may be taking.

Monoamine Oxidase (MAO) Inhibitors

You should not take Ritalin LA with (MAO) inhibitors or within 14 days of stopping a MAO inhibitor.

Starting a New Medicine

While on Ritalin LA, do not start taking a new medicine or herbal remedy before checking with your doctor.

Other Medicines You May Be Taking

Ritalin LA may change the way your body reacts to certain medicines. These include medicines used to treat depression, prevent seizures, or prevent blood clots (commonly called "blood thinners"). Your doctor may need to change your dose of these medicines if you are taking them with Ritalin LA.

Other Important Safety Information

Pregnancy and Nursing

Before taking Ritalin LA, tell your doctor if you are pregnant or plan on becoming pregnant. If you take methylphenidate, it may be in your breast milk. Tell your doctor if you are nursing a baby.

Overdose

Call your doctor ***immediately*** if you take more than the amount of Ritalin LA prescribed by your doctor.

WHAT ELSE SHOULD I KNOW ABOUT RITALIN LA?

Ritalin LA has not been studied in children under 6 years of age.

Ritalin LA may be a part of your overall treatment for ADHD. Your doctor may also recommend that you have counseling or other therapy.

As with all medicines, never share Ritalin LA with anyone else and take only the number of Ritalin LA capsules prescribed by your doctor.

Ritalin LA should be stored in a safe place at room temperature (between 59°F-86°F). Do not store this medicine in

Continued on next page

Ritalin LA—Cont.

hot, damp, or humid places. Keep the container of Ritalin LA in a safe place, away from high-traffic areas where other people could have accidental or unauthorized access to the medication. Keep track of the number of capsules so that you will know if any are missing. Someone who has easy access to Ritalin may be able to give the capsules to others or misuse the medication.

Keep out of the reach of children.

This leaflet summarizes the most important information about Ritalin LA. If you would like more information, talk with your doctor. You can ask your pharmacist or doctor for information about Ritalin LA that is written for health professionals.

You can also call 1-888 NOWNOVA (1-888-669-6682).

T2004-35

T2004-34/T2004-35

REV: APRIL 2004 PRINTED IN U.S.A. 89015703
Manufactured for
Novartis Pharmaceuticals Corporation
East Hanover, New Jersey 07936
By ELAN HOLDINGS INC.
Pharmaceutical Division
Gainesville, GA 30504
©Novartis

Shown in Product Identification Guide, page 325

SANDIMMUNE® SOFT GELATIN CAPSULES ℞

[*săn-dī-mūn*]

(cyclosporine capsules, USP)

SANDIMMUNE® ORAL SOLUTION ℞

(cyclosporine oral solution, USP)

SANDIMMUNE® INJECTION ℞

(cyclosporine injection, USP)

FOR INFUSION ONLY

Rx only

Prescribing Information

The following prescribing information is based on official labeling in effect July 2004.

WARNING

Only physicians experienced in immunosuppressive therapy and management of organ transplant patients should prescribe Sandimmune® (cyclosporine). Patients receiving the drug should be managed in facilities equipped and staffed with adequate laboratory and supportive medical resources. The physician responsible for maintenance therapy should have complete information requisite for the follow-up of the patient.

Sandimmune® (cyclosporine) should be administered with adrenal corticosteroids but not with other immunosuppressive agents. Increased susceptibility to infection and the possible development of lymphoma may result from immunosuppression.

Sandimmune® Soft Gelatin Capsules (cyclosporine capsules, USP) and Sandimmune® Oral Solution (cyclosporine oral solution, USP) have decreased bioavailability in comparison to Neoral® Soft Gelatin Capsules (cyclosporine capsules, USP) MODIFIED and Neoral® Oral Solution (cyclosporine oral solution, USP) MODIFIED.

Sandimmune® and Neoral® are not bioequivalent and cannot be used interchangeably without physician supervision.

The absorption of cyclosporine during chronic administration of Sandimmune® Soft Gelatin Capsules and Oral Solution was found to be erratic. It is recommended that patients taking the soft gelatin capsules or oral solution over a period of time be monitored at repeated intervals for cyclosporine blood levels and subsequent dose adjustments be made in order to avoid toxicity due to high levels and possible organ rejection due to low absorption of cyclosporine. This is of special importance in liver transplants. Numerous assays are being developed to measure blood levels of cyclosporine. Comparison of levels in published literature to patient levels using current assays must be done with detailed knowledge of the assay methods employed. *(See Blood Level Monitoring under DOSAGE AND ADMINISTRATION)*

DESCRIPTION

Cyclosporine, the active principle in Sandimmune® (cyclosporine) is a cyclic polypeptide immunosuppressant agent consisting of 11 amino acids. It is produced as a metabolite by the fungus species *Beauveria nivea*.

Chemically, cyclosporine is designated as [*R*-[*R**,*R**-(E)]]-cyclic (L-alanyl-D-alanyl-*N*-methyl-L-leucyl-*N*-methyl-L-leucyl-*N*-methyl-L-valyl-3-hydroxy-*N*,4-dimethyl-L-2-amino-6-octenoyl-L-α-amino-butyryl-*N*-methylglycyl-*N*-methyl-L-leucyl-L-valyl-*N*-methyl-L-leucyl).

Sandimmune® Soft Gelatin Capsules (cyclosporine capsules, USP) are available in 25 mg and 100 mg strengths.

Each 25 mg capsule contains:
cyclosporine, USP .... 25 mg
alcohol, USP dehydrated .... max 12.7% by volume

Each 100 mg capsule contains:
cyclosporine, USP .... 100 mg
alcohol, USP dehydrated .... max 12.7% by volume

Inactive Ingredients: corn oil, gelatin, glycerol, Labrafil M 2125 CS (polyoxyethylated glycolysed glycerides), red iron oxide (25 mg and 100 mg capsule only), sorbitol, titanium dioxide, and other ingredients.

Sandimmune® Oral Solution (cyclosporine oral solution, USP) is available in 50 mL bottles.

Each mL contains:
cyclosporine, USP .... 100 mg
alcohol, Ph. Helv. .... 12.5% by volume

dissolved in an olive oil, Ph. Helv./Labrafil M 1944 CS (polyoxyethylated oleic glycerides) vehicle which must be further diluted with milk, chocolate milk, or orange juice before oral administration.

Sandimmune® Injection (cyclosporine injection, USP) is available in a 5 mL sterile ampul for I.V. administration.

Each mL contains:
cyclosporine, USP .... 50 mg
*Cremophor® EL (polyoxyethylated castor oil) .... 650 mg
alcohol, Ph. Helv. .... 32.9% by volume
nitrogen .... qs

which must be diluted further with 0.9% Sodium Chloride Injection or 5% Dextrose Injection before use.

The chemical structure of cyclosporine (also known as cyclosporin A) is

```
              H3C
                 \
                  CH
                  ||
                  HC
                    \
                     CH2
                H    |
            HO  |   CH-CH3
               \C/
                |
MeVal-N-CH-C-Abu-MeGly
   |   |     ||        |
MeLeu CH3    O       MeLeu
   |                   |
MeLeu-D-Ala-Ala-MeLeu-Val
```

$C_{62}H_{111}N_{11}O_{12}$ Mol. Wt. 1202.63

CLINICAL PHARMACOLOGY

Sandimmune® (cyclosporine) is a potent immunosuppressive agent which in animals prolongs survival of allogeneic transplants involving skin, heart, kidney, pancreas, bone marrow, small intestine, and lung. Sandimmune® (cyclosporine) has been demonstrated to suppress some humoral immunity and to a greater extent, cell-mediated reactions such as allograft rejection, delayed hypersensitivity, experimental allergic encephalomyelitis, Freund's adjuvant arthritis, and graft vs. host disease in many animal species for a variety of organs.

Successful kidney, liver, and heart allogeneic transplants have been performed in man using Sandimmune® (cyclosporine).

The exact mechanism of action of Sandimmune® (cyclosporine) is not known. Experimental evidence suggests that the effectiveness of cyclosporine is due to specific and reversible inhibition of immunocompetent lymphocytes in the G_0- or G_1-phase of the cell cycle. T-lymphocytes are preferentially inhibited. The T-helper cell is the main target, although the T-suppressor cell may also be suppressed. Sandimmune® (cyclosporine) also inhibits lymphokine production and release including interleukin-2 or T-cell growth factor (TCGF).

No functional effects on phagocytic (changes in enzyme secretions not altered, chemotactic migration of granulocytes, macrophage migration, carbon clearance *in vivo*) or tumor cells (growth rate, metastasis) can be detected in animals. Sandimmune® (cyclosporine) does not cause bone marrow suppression in animal models or man.

The absorption of cyclosporine from the gastrointestinal tract is incomplete and variable. Peak concentrations (C_{max}) in blood and plasma are achieved at about 3.5 hours. C_{max} and area under the plasma or blood concentration/time curve (AUC) increase with the administered dose; for blood the relationship is curvilinear (parabolic) between 0 and 1400 mg. As determined by a specific assay, C_{max} is approximately 1.0 ng/mL/mg of dose for plasma and 2.7-1.4 ng/mL/mg of dose for blood (for low to high doses). Compared to an intravenous infusion, the absolute bioavailability of the oral solution is approximately 30% based upon the results in 2 patients. The bioavailability of Sandimmune® Soft Gelatin Capsules (cyclosporine capsules, USP) is equivalent to Sandimmune® Oral Solution, (cyclosporine oral solution, USP).

Cyclosporine is distributed largely outside the blood volume. In blood the distribution is concentration dependent. Approximately 33%-47% is in plasma, 4%-9% in lymphocytes, 5%-12% in granulocytes, and 41%-58% in erythrocytes. At high concentrations, the uptake by leukocytes and erythrocytes becomes saturated. In plasma, approximately 90% is bound to proteins, primarily lipoproteins.

The disposition of cyclosporine from blood is biphasic with a terminal half-life of approximately 19 hours (range: 10-27 hours). Elimination is primarily biliary with only 6% of the dose excreted in the urine.

Cyclosporine is extensively metabolized but there is no major metabolic pathway. Only 0.1% of the dose is excreted in the urine as unchanged drug. Of 15 metabolites characterized in human urine, 9 have been assigned structures. The major pathways consist of hydroxylation of the Cγ-carbon of 2 of the leucine residues, Cη-carbon hydroxylation, and cyclic ether formation (with oxidation of the double bond) in the side chain of the amino acid 3-hydroxyl-*N*,4-dimethyl-L-2-amino-6-octenoic acid and *N*-demethylation of *N*-methyl leucine residues. Hydrolysis of the cyclic peptide chain or conjugation of the aforementioned metabolites do not appear to be important biotransformation pathways.

INDICATIONS AND USAGE

Sandimmune® (cyclosporine) is indicated for the prophylaxis of organ rejection in kidney, liver, and heart allogeneic transplants. It is always to be used with adrenal corticosteroids. The drug may also be used in the treatment of chronic rejection in patients previously treated with other immunosuppressive agents.

Because of the risk of anaphylaxis, Sandimmune® Injection (cyclosporine injection, USP) should be reserved for patients who are unable to take the soft gelatin capsules or oral solution.

CONTRAINDICATIONS

Sandimmune® Injection (cyclosporine injection, USP) is contraindicated in patients with a hypersensitivity to Sandimmune® (cyclosporine) and/or Cremophor® EL (polyoxyethylated castor oil).

WARNINGS

(See boxed WARNINGs): **Sandimmune® (cyclosporine), when used in high doses, can cause hepatotoxicity and nephrotoxicity.**

It is not unusual for serum creatinine and BUN levels to be elevated during Sandimmune® (cyclosporine) therapy. These elevations in renal transplant patients do not necessarily indicate rejection, and each patient must be fully evaluated before dosage adjustment is initiated.

Nephrotoxicity has been noted in 25% of cases of renal transplantation, 38% of cases of cardiac transplantation, and 37% of cases of liver transplantation. Mild nephrotoxicity was generally noted 2-3 months after transplant and consisted of an arrest in the fall of the preoperative elevations of BUN and creatinine at a range of 35-45 mg/dl and 2.0-2.5 mg/dl respectively. These elevations were often responsive to dosage reduction.

More overt nephrotoxicity was seen early after transplantation and was characterized by a rapidly rising BUN and creatinine. Since these events are similar to rejection episodes care must be taken to differentiate between them. This form of nephrotoxicity is usually responsive to Sandimmune® (cyclosporine) dosage reduction.

Although specific diagnostic criteria which reliably differentiate renal graft rejection from drug toxicity have not been found, a number of parameters have been significantly associated to one or the other. It should be noted however, that up to 20% of patients may have simultaneous nephrotoxicity and rejection.

[See first table at top of next page]

A form of chronic progressive cyclosporine-associated nephrotoxicity is characterized by serial deterioration in renal function and morphologic changes in the kidneys. From 5%-15% of transplant recipients will fail to show a reduction in a rising serum creatinine despite a decrease or discontinuation of cyclosporine therapy. Renal biopsies from these patients will demonstrate an interstitial fibrosis with tubular atrophy. In addition, toxic tubulopathy, peritubular capillary congestion, arteriolopathy, and a striped form of interstitial fibrosis with tubular atrophy may be present. Though none of these morphologic changes is entirely specific, a histologic diagnosis of chronic progressive cyclosporine-associated nephrotoxicity requires evidence of these.

When considering the development of chronic nephrotoxicity it is noteworthy that several authors have reported an association between the appearance of interstitial fibrosis and higher cumulative doses or persistently high circulating trough levels of cyclosporine. This is particularly true during the first 6 posttransplant months when the dosage tends to be highest and when, in kidney recipients, the organ appears to be most vulnerable to the toxic effects of cyclosporine. Among other contributing factors to the development of interstitial fibrosis in these patients must be included, prolonged perfusion time, warm ischemia time, as well as episodes of acute toxicity, and acute and chronic rejection. The reversibility of interstitial fibrosis and its correlation to renal function have not yet been determined.

Impaired renal function at any time requires close monitoring, and frequent dosage adjustment may be indicated. In patients with persistent high elevations of BUN and creatinine who are unresponsive to dosage adjustments, consideration should be given to switching to other immunosuppressive therapy. In the event of severe and unremitting rejection, it is preferable to allow the kidney transplant to be rejected and removed rather than increase the Sandimmune® (cyclosporine) dosage to a very high level in an attempt to reverse the rejection.

Occasionally patients have developed a syndrome of thrombocytopenia and microangiopathic hemolytic anemia which may result in graft failure. The vasculopathy can occur in the absence of rejection and is accompanied by avid platelet consumption within the graft as demonstrated by Indium 111 labeled platelet studies. Neither the pathogenesis nor the management of this syndrome is clear. Though resolution has occurred after reduction or discontinuation of Sandimmune® (cyclosporine) and 1) administration of streptokinase and heparin or 2) plasmapheresis, this appears to depend upon early detection with Indium 111 labeled platelet scans. *(See ADVERSE REACTIONS)*

Significant hyperkalemia (sometimes associated with hyperchloremic metabolic acidosis) and hyperuricemia have been seen occasionally in individual patients.

Hepatotoxicity has been noted in 4% of cases of renal transplantation, 7% of cases of cardiac transplantation, and 4% of cases of liver transplantation. This was usually noted during the first month of therapy when high doses of Sandimmune® (cyclosporine) were used and consisted of elevations of hepatic enzymes and bilirubin. The chemistry elevations usually decreased with a reduction in dosage.

As in patients receiving other immunosuppressants, those patients receiving Sandimmune® (cyclosporine) are at increased risk for development of lymphomas and other malignancies, particularly those of the skin. The increased risk appears related to the intensity and duration of immunosuppression rather than to the use of specific agents. Because of the danger of oversuppression of the immune system, which can also increase susceptibility to infection, Sandimmune® (cyclosporine) should not be administered with other immunosuppressive agents except adrenal corticosteroids. The efficacy and safety of cyclosporine in combination with other immunosuppressive agents have not been determined.

There have been reports of convulsions in adult and pediatric patients receiving cyclosporine, particularly in combination with high dose methylprednisolone.

Encephalopathy has been described both in postmarketing reports and in the literature. Manifestations include impaired consciousness, convulsions, visual disturbances (including blindness), loss of motor function, movement disorders and psychiatric disturbances. In many cases, changes in the white matter have been detected using imaging techniques and pathologic specimens. Predisposing factors such as hypertension, hypomagnesemia, hypocholesterolemia, high-dose corticosteroids, high cyclosporine blood concentrations, and graft-versus-host disease have been noted in many but not all of the reported cases. The changes in most cases have been reversible upon discontinuation of cyclosporine, and in some cases improvement was noted after reduction of dose. It appears that patients receiving liver transplant are more susceptible to encephalopathy than those receiving kidney transplant.

Rarely (approximately 1 in 1000), patients receiving Sandimmune® Injection (cyclosporine injection, USP) have experienced anaphylactic reactions. Although the exact cause of these reactions is unknown, it is believed to be due to the Cremophor® EL (polyoxyethylated castor oil) used as the vehicle for the I.V. formulation. These reactions have consisted of flushing of the face and upper thorax, acute respiratory distress with dyspnea and wheezing, blood pressure changes, and tachycardia. One patient died after respiratory arrest and aspiration pneumonia. In some cases, the reaction subsided after the infusion was stopped.

Patients receiving Sandimmune® Injection (cyclosporine injection, USP) should be under continuous observation for at least the first 30 minutes following the start of the infusion and at frequent intervals thereafter. If anaphylaxis occurs, the infusion should be stopped. An aqueous solution of epinephrine 1:1000 should be available at the bedside as well as a source of oxygen.

Anaphylactic reactions have not been reported with the soft gelatin capsules or oral solution which lack Cremophor® EL (polyoxyethylated castor oil). In fact, patients experiencing anaphylactic reactions have been treated subsequently with the soft gelatin capsules or oral solution without incident.

Care should be taken in using Sandimmune® (cyclosporine) with nephrotoxic drugs. *(See PRECAUTIONS)*

Because Sandimmune® (cyclosporine) is not bioequivalent to Neoral®, conversion from Neoral® to Sandimmune® (cyclosporine) using a 1:1 ratio (mg/kg/day) may result in a lower cyclosporine blood concentration. Conversion from Neoral® to Sandimmune® (cyclosporine) should be made with increased blood concentration monitoring to avoid the potential of underdosing.

Nephrotoxicity vs Rejection

Parameter	Nephrotoxicity	Rejection
History	Donor > 50 years old or hypotensive Prolonged kidney preservation Prolonged anastomosis time Concomitant nephrotoxic drugs	Antidonor immune response Retransplant patient
Clinical	Often > 6 weeks postop[b] Prolonged initial nonfunction (acute tubular necrosis)	Often < 4 weeks postop[b] Fever > 37.5°C Weight gain > 0.5 kg Graft swelling and tenderness Decrease in daily urine volume > 500 mL (or 50%)
Laboratory	CyA serum trough level > 200 ng/mL Gradual rise in Cr (< 0.15 mg/dl/day)[a] Cr plateau < 25% above baseline BUN/Cr ≥ 20	CyA serum trough level < 150 ng/mL Rapid rise in Cr (> 0.3 mg/dl/day)[a] Cr > 25% above baseline BUN/Cr < 20
Biopsy	Arteriolopathy (medial hypertrophy[a], hyalinosis, nodular deposits, intimal thickening, endothelial vacuolization, progressive scarring) Tubular atrophy, isometric vacuolization, isolated calcifications Minimal edema Mild focal infiltrates[c] Diffuse interstitial fibrosis, often striped form	Endovasculitis[c] (proliferation[a], intimal arteritis[b], necrosis, sclerosis) Tubulitis with RBC[b] and WBC[b] casts, some irregular vacuolization Interstitial edema[c] and hemorrhage[b] Diffuse moderate to severe mononuclear infiltrates[d] Glomerulitis (mononuclear cells)[c]
Aspiration Cytology	CyA deposits in tubular and endothelial cells Fine isometric vacuolization of tubular cells	Inflammatory infiltrate with mononuclear phagocytes, macrophages, lymphoblastoid cells, and activated T-cells These strongly express HLA-DR antigens
Urine Cytology	Tubular cells with vacuolization and granularization	Degenerative tubular cells, plasma cells, and lymphocyturia > 20% of sediment
Manometry	Intracapsular pressure < 40 mm Hg[b]	Intracapsular pressure > 40 mm Hg[b]
Ultrasonography	Unchanged graft cross-sectional area	Increase in graft cross-sectional area AP diameter ≥ Transverse diameter
Magnetic Resonance Imagery	Normal appearance	Loss of distinct corticomedullary junction, swelling, image intensity of parachyma approaching that of psoas, loss of hilar fat
Radionuclide Scan	Normal or generally decreased perfusion Decrease in tubular function (^{131} I-hippuran) > decrease in perfusion (^{99}m Tc DTPA)	Patchy arterial flow Decrease in perfusion > decrease in tubular function Increased uptake of Indium 111 labeled platelets or Tc-99m in colloid
Therapy	Responds to decreased Sandimmune® (cyclosporine)	Responds to increased steroids or antilymphocyte globulin

$^{a}p < 0.05$, $^{b}p < 0.01$, $^{c}p < 0.001$, $^{d}p < 0.0001$

Drugs That May Potentiate Renal Dysfunction

Antibiotics	*Antineoplastic*	*Anti-Inflammatory Drugs*	*Gastrointestinal Agents*
gentamicin	melphalan	azapropazon	cimetidine
tobramycin		diclofenac	ranitidine
vancomycin	*Antifungals*	naproxen	
trimethoprim	amphotericin B	sulindac	*Immunosuppressives*
with sulfamethoxazole	ketoconazole	colchicine	tacrolimus

PRECAUTIONS

General

Patients with malabsorption may have difficulty in achieving therapeutic levels with Sandimmune® Soft Gelatin Capsules or Oral Solution.

Hypertension is a common side effect of Sandimmune® (cyclosporine) therapy. *(See ADVERSE REACTIONS)* Mild or moderate hypertension is more frequently encountered than severe hypertension and the incidence decreases over time. Antihypertensive therapy may be required. Control of blood pressure can be accomplished with any of the common antihypertensive agents. However, since cyclosporine may cause hyperkalemia, potassium-sparing diuretics should not be used. While calcium antagonists can be effective agents in treating cyclosporine-associated hypertension, care should be taken since interference with cyclosporine metabolism may require a dosage adjustment. *(See Drug Interactions*

During treatment with Sandimmune® (cyclosporine), vaccination may be less effective; and the use of live attenuated vaccines should be avoided.

Information for Patients

Patients should be advised that any change of cyclosporine formulation should be made cautiously and only under physician supervision because it may result in the need for a change in dosage.

Patients should be informed of the necessity of repeated laboratory tests while they are receiving the drug. They should be given careful dosage instructions, advised of the potential risks during pregnancy, and informed of the increased risk of neoplasia.

Patients using cyclosporine oral solution with its accompanying syringe for dosage measurement should be cautioned not to rinse the syringe either before or after use. Introduction of water into the product by any means will cause variation in dose.

Laboratory Tests

Renal and liver functions should be assessed repeatedly by measurement of BUN, serum creatinine, serum bilirubin, and liver enzymes.

Drug Interactions

All of the individual drugs cited below are well substantiated to interact with cyclosporine. In addition, concomitant non-steroidal anti-inflammatory drugs, particularly in the setting of dehydration, may potentiate renal dysfunction.

[See second table above]

Drugs That Alter Cyclosporine Concentrations: Compounds that decrease cyclosporine absorption such as orlistat should be avoided. Cyclosporine is extensively metabolized by cytochrome P-450 3A. Substances that inhibit this enzyme could decrease metabolism and increase cyclosporine concentrations. Substances that are inducers of cytochrome P-450 activity could increase metabolism and decrease cyclosporine concentrations. Monitoring of circulating cyclosporine concentrations and appropriate Sandimmune® (cyclosporine) dosage adjustment are essential when these drugs are used concomitantly. *(See Blood Concentration Monitoring)*

[See first table at top of next page]

The HIV protease inhibitors (e.g., indinavir, nelfinavir, ritonavir, and saquinavir) are known to inhibit cytochrome P-450 3A and thus could potentially increase the concentrations of cyclosporine, however no formal studies of the interaction are available. Care should be exercised when these drugs are administered concomitantly.

Grapefruit and grapefruit juice affect metabolism, increasing blood concentrations of cyclosporine, thus should be avoided.

[See second table at top of next page]

There have been reports of a serious drug interaction between cyclosporine and the herbal dietary supplement, St. John's Wort. This interaction has been reported to produce a marked reduction in the blood concentrations of cyclosporine, resulting in subtherapeutic levels, rejection of transplanted organs, and graft loss.

Rifabutin is known to increase the metabolism of other drugs metabolized by the cytochrome P-450 system. The interaction between rifabutin and cyclosporine has not been studied. Care should be exercised when these two drugs are administered concomitantly.

Nonsteroidal Anti-inflammatory Drug (NSAID) Interactions: Clinical status and serum creatinine should be closely monitored when cyclosporine is used with nonsteroidal anti-inflammatory agents in rheumatoid arthritis patients. *(See WARNINGS)*

Pharmacodynamic interactions have been reported to occur between cyclosporine and both naproxen and sulindac, in that concomitant use is associated with additive decreases in renal function, as determined by ^{99m}Tc-diethylenetriaminepentaacetic acid (DTPA) and (*p*-aminohippuric acid) PAH clearances. Although concomitant administration of diclofenac does not affect blood levels of cyclosporine, it has been associated with approximate doubling of diclofenac blood levels and occasional reports of reversible decreases in renal function. Consequently, the dose of diclofenac should be in the lower end of the therapeutic range.

Methotrexate Interaction: Preliminary data indicate that when methotrexate and cyclosporine were co-administered to rheumatoid arthritis patients (N=20), methotrexate concentrations (AUCs) were increased approximately 30% and the concentrations (AUCs) of its metabolite, 7-hydroxy methotrexate, were decreased by approximately 80%. The clinical significance of this interaction is not known. Cyclosporine concentrations do not appear to have been altered (N=6).

Other Drug Interactions: Cyclosporine may reduce the clearance of digoxin, colchicine, prednisolone and HMG-CoA reductase inhibitors (statins). Severe digitalis toxicity has been seen within days of starting cyclosporine in several patients taking digoxin. There are also reports on the potential of cyclosporine to enhance the toxic effects of colchicine such as myopathy and neuropathy, especially in patients with renal dysfunction. If digoxin or colchicine are used concurrently with cyclosporine, close clinical observation is required in order to enable early detection of toxic manifestations of digoxin or colchicine, followed by reduction of dosage or its withdrawal.

Literature and postmarketing cases of myotoxicity, including muscle pain and weakness, myositis, and rhabdomyolysis, have been reported with concomitant administration of

Continued on next page

Sandimmune—Cont.

cyclosporine with lovastatin, simvastatin, atorvastatin, pravastatin, and rarely, fluvastatin. When concurrently administered with cyclosporine, the dosage of these statins should be reduced according to label recommendations. Statin therapy needs to be temporarily withheld or discontinued in patients with signs and symptoms of myopathy or those with risk factors predisposing to severe renal injury, including renal failure, secondary to rhabdomyolysis.
Cyclosporine should not be used with potassium-sparing diuretics because hyperkalemia can occur.
During treatment with cyclosporine, vaccination may be less effective. The use of live vaccines should be avoided.
Frequent gingival hyperplasia with nifedipine, and convulsions with high dose methylprednisolone have been reported.
Psoriasis patients receiving other immunosuppressive agents or radiation therapy (including PUVA and UVB) should not receive concurrent cyclosporine because of the possibility of excessive immunosuppression.
For additional information on Cyclosporine Drug Interactions please contact Novartis Medical Affairs Department at 888-NOW-NOVA (888-669-6682).

Carcinogenesis, Mutagenesis, and Impairment of Fertility
Cyclosporine gave no evidence of mutagenic or teratogenic effects in appropriate test systems. Only at dose levels toxic to dams, were adverse effects seen in reproduction studies in rats. *(See Pregnancy)*
Carcinogenicity studies were carried out in male and female rats and mice. In the 78-week mouse study, at doses of 1, 4, and 16 mg/kg/day, evidence of a statistically significant trend was found for lymphocytic lymphomas in females, and the incidence of hepatocellular carcinomas in mid-dose males significantly exceeded the control value. In the 24-month rat study, conducted at 0.5, 2, and 8 mg/kg/day, pancreatic islet cell adenomas significantly exceeded the control rate in the low dose level. The hepatocellular carcinomas and pancreatic islet cell adenomas were not dose related.
No impairment in fertility was demonstrated in studies in male and female rats.
Cyclosporine has not been found mutagenic/genotoxic in the Ames Test, the V79-HGPRT Test, the micronucleus test in mice and Chinese hamsters, the chromosome-aberration tests in Chinese hamster bone marrow, the mouse dominant lethal assay, and the DNA-repair test in sperm from treated mice. A recent study analyzing sister chromatid exchange (SCE) induction by cyclosporine using human lymphocytes *in vitro* gave indication of a positive effect (i.e., induction of SCE), at high concentrations in this system.
An increased incidence of malignancy is a recognized complication of immunosuppression in recipients of organ transplants. The most common forms of neoplasms are non-Hodgkin's lymphoma and carcinomas of the skin. The risk of malignancies in cyclosporine recipients is higher than in the normal, healthy population but similar to that in patients receiving other immunosuppressive therapies. It has been reported that reduction or discontinuance of immunosuppression may cause the lesions to regress.

Pregnancy
Pregnancy Category C. Sandimmune® Oral Solution (cyclosporine oral solution, USP) has been shown to be embryo- and fetotoxic in rats and rabbits when given in doses 2-5 times the human dose. At toxic doses (rats at 30 mg/kg/day and rabbits at 100 mg/kg/day), Sandimmune® Oral Solution (cyclosporine oral solution, USP) was embryo- and fetotoxic as indicated by increased pre- and postnatal mortality and reduced fetal weight together with related skeletal retardations. In the well-tolerated dose range (rats at up to 17 mg/kg/day and rabbits at up to 30 mg/kg/day), Sandimmune® Oral Solution (cyclosporine oral solution, USP) proved to be without any embryolethal or teratogenic effects.
There are no adequate and well-controlled studies in pregnant women. Sandimmune® (cyclosporine) should be used during pregnancy only if the potential benefit justifies the potential risk to the fetus.
The following data represent the reported outcomes of 116 pregnancies in women receiving Sandimmune® (cyclosporine) during pregnancy, 90% of whom were transplant patients, and most of whom received Sandimmune® (cyclosporine) throughout the entire gestational period. Since most of the patients were not prospectively identified, the results are likely to be biased toward negative outcomes. The only consistent patterns of abnormality were premature birth (gestational period of 28 to 36 weeks) and low birth weight for gestational age. It is not possible to separate the effects of Sandimmune® (cyclosporine) on these pregnancies from the effects of the other immunosuppressants, the underlying maternal disorders, or other aspects of the transplantation milieu. Sixteen fetal losses occurred. Most of the pregnancies (85 of 100) were complicated by disorders; including, preeclampsia, eclampsia, premature labor, abruptio placentae, oligohydramnios, Rh incompatibility and fetoplacental dysfunction. Preterm delivery occurred in 47%. Seven malformations were reported in 5 viable infants and in 2 cases of fetal loss. Twenty-eight percent of the infants were small for gestational age. Neonatal complications occurred in 27%. In a report of 23 children followed up to 4 years, postnatal development was said to be normal. More information on cyclosporine use in pregnancy is available from Novartis Pharmaceuticals Corporation.

Drugs That Increase Cyclosporine Concentrations

Calcium Channel Blockers	Antifungals	Antibiotics	Glucocorticoids	Other Drugs
diltiazem	fluconazole	clarithromycin	methylprednisolone	allopurinol
nicardipine	itraconazole	erythromycin		bromocriptine
verapamil	ketoconazole	quinupristin/ dalfopristin		danazol
				metoclopromide
				colchicine
				amiodarone

Drugs/Dietary Supplements That Decrease Cyclosporine Concentrations

Antibiotics	Anticonvulsants	Other Drugs/Dietary Supplements
nafcillin	carbamazepine	octreotide
rifampin	phenobarbital	ticlopidine
	phenytoin	orlistat
		St. John's Wort

Body System/ Adverse Reactions	Randomized Kidney Patients Sandimmune® (N=227) %	Randomized Kidney Patients Azathioprine (N=228) %	All Sandimmune® (cyclosporine) Patients Kidney (N=705) %	All Sandimmune® (cyclosporine) Patients Heart (N=112) %	All Sandimmune® (cyclosporine) Patients Liver (N=75) %
Genitourinary					
Renal Dysfunction	32	6	25	38	37
Cardiovascular					
Hypertension	26	18	13	53	27
Cramps	4	<1	2	<1	0
Skin					
Hirsutism	21	<1	21	28	45
Acne	6	8	2	2	1
Central Nervous System					
Tremor	12	0	21	31	55
Convulsions	3	1	1	4	5
Headache	2	<1	2	15	4
Gastrointestinal					
Gum Hyperplasia	4	0	9	5	16
Diarrhea	3	<1	3	4	8
Nausea/Vomiting	2	<1	4	10	4
Hepatotoxicity	<1	<1	4	7	4
Abdominal Discomfort	<1	0	<1	7	0
Autonomic Nervous System					
Paresthesia	3	0	1	2	1
Flushing	<1	0	4	0	4
Hematopoietic					
Leukopenia	2	19	<1	6	0
Lymphoma	<1	0	1	6	1
Respiratory					
Sinusitis	<1	0	4	3	7
Miscellaneous					
Gynecomastia	<1	0	<1	4	3

Nursing Mothers
Since Sandimmune® (cyclosporine) is excreted in human milk, nursing should be avoided.

Pediatric Use
Although no adequate and well-controlled studies have been conducted in children, patients as young as 6 months of age have received the drug with no unusual adverse effects.

Geriatric Use
Clinical studies of Sandimmune® (cyclosporine) did not include sufficient numbers of subjects aged 65 and over to determine whether they respond differently from younger subjects. Other reported clinical experience has not identified differences in responses between the elderly and younger patients. In general dose selection for an elderly patient should be cautious, usually starting at the low end of the dosing range, reflecting the greater frequency of decreased hepatic, renal, or cardiac function, and of concomitant disease or other drug therapy.

ADVERSE REACTIONS

The principal adverse reactions of Sandimmune® (cyclosporine) therapy are renal dysfunction, tremor, hirsutism, hypertension, and gum hyperplasia.
Hypertension, which is usually mild to moderate, may occur in approximately 50% of patients following renal transplantation and in most cardiac transplant patients.
Glomerular capillary thrombosis has been found in patients treated with cyclosporine and may progress to graft failure. The pathologic changes resemble those seen in the hemolytic-uremic syndrome and include thrombosis of the renal microvasculature, with platelet-fibrin thrombi occluding glomerular capillaries and afferent arterioles, microangiopathic hemolytic anemia, thrombocytopenia, and decreased renal function. Similar findings have been observed when other immunosuppressives have been employed posttransplantation.
Hypomagnesemia has been reported in some, but not all, patients exhibiting convulsions while on cyclosporine therapy. Although magnesium-depletion studies in normal subjects suggest that hypomagnesemia is associated with neurologic disorders, multiple factors, including hypertension, high dose methylprednisolone, hypocholesterolemia, and nephrotoxicity associated with high plasma concentrations of cyclosporine appear to be related to the neurological manifestations of cyclosporine toxicity.
The following reactions occurred in 3% or greater of 892 patients involved in clinical trials of kidney, heart, and liver transplants:
[See third table above]
The following reactions occurred in 2% or less of patients: allergic reactions, anemia, anorexia, confusion, conjunctivitis, edema, fever, brittle fingernails, gastritis, hearing loss, hiccups, hyperglycemia, muscle pain, peptic ulcer, thrombocytopenia, tinnitus.
The following reactions occurred rarely: anxiety, chest pain, constipation, depression, hair breaking, hematuria, joint pain, lethargy, mouth sores, myocardial infarction, night sweats, pancreatitis, pruritus, swallowing difficulty, tingling, upper GI bleeding, visual disturbance, weakness, weight loss.
[See first table at bottom of next page]
[See second table at bottom of next page]
Cremophor® EL (polyoxyethylated castor oil) is known to cause hyperlipemia and electrophoretic abnormalities of lipoproteins. These effects are reversible upon discontinuation of treatment but are usually not a reason to stop treatment.

OVERDOSAGE

There is a minimal experience with overdosage. Because of the slow absorption of Sandimmune® Soft Gelatin Capsules or Oral Solution, forced emesis would be of value up to 2 hours after administration. Transient hepatotoxicity and nephrotoxicity may occur which should resolve following drug withdrawal. General supportive measures and symptomatic treatment should be followed in all cases of overdosage. Sandimmune® (cyclosporine) is not dialyzable to any great extent, nor is it cleared well by charcoal hemoperfusion. The oral LD_{50} is 2329 mg/kg in mice, 1480 mg/kg in rats, and > 1000 mg/kg in rabbits. The I.V. LD_{50} is 148 mg/kg in mice, 104 mg/kg in rats, and 46 mg/kg in rabbits.

DOSAGE AND ADMINISTRATION

Sandimmune® Soft Gelatin Capsules (cyclosporine capsules, USP) and Sandimmune® Oral Solution (cyclosporine oral solution, USP): Sandimmune® Soft Gelatin Capsules (cyclosporine capsules, USP) and Sandimmune® Oral Solution (cyclosporine oral solution, USP) have decreased bioavailability in comparison to Neoral® Soft Gelatin Capsules (cyclosporine capsules, USP) MODIFIED and Neoral® Oral Solution (cyclosporine oral solution, USP) MODIFIED. Sandimmune® and Neoral® are not bioequivalent and cannot be used interchangeably without physician supervision.
The initial oral dose of Sandimmune® (cyclosporine) should be given 4-12 hours prior to transplantation as a single dose of 15 mg/kg. Although a daily single dose of 14-18 mg/kg was used in most clinical trials, few centers continue to use the highest dose, most favoring the lower end of the scale. There is a trend towards use of even lower initial doses for renal transplantation in the ranges of 10-14 mg/kg/day. The initial single daily dose is continued postoperatively for 1-2

weeks and then tapered by 5% per week to a maintenance dose of 5-10 mg/kg/day. Some centers have successfully tapered the maintenance dose to as low as 3 mg/kg/day in selected *renal* transplant patients without an apparent rise in rejection rate.
(See Blood Level Monitoring below)
In pediatric usage, the same dose and dosing regimen may be used as in adults although in several studies children have required and tolerated higher doses than those used in adults.
Adjunct therapy with adrenal corticosteroids is recommended. Different tapering dosage schedules of prednisone appear to achieve similar results. A dosage schedule based on the patient's weight started with 2.0 mg/kg/day for the first 4 days tapered to 1.0 mg/kg/day by 1 week, 0.6 mg/kg/day by 2 weeks, 0.3 mg/kg/day by 1 month, and 0.15 mg/kg/day by 2 months and thereafter as a maintenance dose. Another center started with an initial dose of 200 mg tapered by 40 mg/day until reaching 20 mg/day. After 2 months at this dose, a further reduction to 10 mg/day was made. Adjustments in dosage of prednisone must be made according to the clinical situation.
To make Sandimmune® Oral Solution (cyclosporine oral solution, USP) more palatable, the oral solution may be diluted with milk, chocolate milk, or orange juice preferably at room temperature. Patients should avoid switching diluents frequently. Sandimmune® Soft Gelatin Capsules and Oral Solution should be administered on a consistent schedule with regard to time of day and relation to meals.
Take the prescribed amount of Sandimmune® (cyclosporine) from the container using the dosage syringe supplied after removal of the protective cover, and transfer the solution to a glass of milk, chocolate milk, or orange juice. Stir well and drink at once. Do not allow to stand before drinking. It is best to use a glass container and rinse it with more diluent to ensure that the total dose is taken. After use, replace the dosage syringe in the protective cover. Do not rinse the dosage syringe with water or other cleaning agents either before or after use. If the dosage syringe requires cleaning, it must be completely dry before resuming use. Introduction of water into the product by any means will cause variation in dose.

Sandimmune® Injection (cyclosporine injection, USP)
FOR INFUSION ONLY
Note: Anaphylactic reactions have occurred with Sandimmune® Injection (cyclosporine injection, USP). *(See WARNINGS)*
Patients unable to take Sandimmune® Soft Gelatin Capsules or Oral Solution pre- or postoperatively may be treated with the I.V. concentrate. **Sandimmune® Injection (cyclosporine injection, USP) is administered at 1/3 the oral dose.** The initial dose of Sandimmune® Injection (cyclosporine injection, USP) should be given 4-12 hours prior to transplantation as a single I.V. dose of 5-6 mg/kg/day. This daily single dose is continued postoperatively until the patient can tolerate the soft gelatin capsules or oral solution. Patients should be switched to Sandimmune® Soft Gelatin Capsules or Oral Solution as soon as possible after surgery. In pediatric usage, the same dose and dosing regimen may be used, although higher doses may be required.
Adjunct steroid therapy is to be used. *(See aforementioned)*
Immediately before use, the I.V. concentrate should be diluted 1 mL Sandimmune® Injection (cyclosporine injection, USP) in 20 mL-100 mL 0.9% Sodium Chloride Injection or 5% Dextrose Injection and given in a slow intravenous infusion over approximately 2-6 hours.

Diluted infusion solutions should be discarded after 24 hours.
The Cremophor® EL (polyoxyethylated castor oil) contained in the concentrate for intravenous infusion can cause phthalate stripping from PVC.
Parenteral drug products should be inspected visually for particulate matter and discoloration prior to administration, whenever solution and container permit.

Blood Level Monitoring
Several study centers have found blood level monitoring of cyclosporine useful in patient management. While no fixed relationships have yet been established, in one series of 375 consecutive cadaveric renal transplant recipients, dosage was adjusted to achieve specific whole blood 24-hour trough levels of 100-200 ng/mL as determined by high-pressure liquid chromatography (HPLC).
Of major importance to blood level analysis is the type of assay used. The above levels are specific to the parent cyclosporine molecule and correlate directly to the new monoclonal specific radioimmunoassays (mRIA-sp). Nonspecific assays are also available which detect the parent compound molecule and various of its metabolites. Older studies often cited levels using a nonspecific assay which were roughly twice those of specific assays. Assay results are not interchangeable and their use should be guided by their approved labeling. If plasma specimens are employed, levels will vary with the temperature at the time of separation from whole blood. Plasma levels may range from 1/2-1/5 of whole blood levels. Refer to individual assay labeling for complete instructions. In addition, *Transplantation Proceedings* (June 1990) contains position papers and a broad consensus generated at the Cyclosporine-Therapeutic Drug Monitoring conference that year. Blood level monitoring is not a replacement for renal function monitoring or tissue biopsies.

HOW SUPPLIED

Sandimmune® Soft Gelatin Capsules (cyclosporine capsules, USP)
25 mg: Oblong, pink, branded "⚠, 78/240". Unit dose packages of 30 capsules,
3 blister cards of 10 capsules .... NDC 0078-0240-15
100 mg: Oblong, dusty rose, branded "⚠, 78/241". Unit dose packages of 30 capsules,
3 blister cards of 10 capsules .... NDC 0078-0241-15
Store and Dispense: Store at 25°C (77°F); excursions permitted to 15-30°C (59-86°F) [see USP Controlled Room Temperature].
An odor may be detected upon opening the unit dose container, which will dissipate shortly thereafter. This odor does not affect the quality of the product.

Sandimmune® Oral Solution (cyclosporine oral solution, USP)
Supplied in 50 mL bottles containing 100 mg of cyclosporine per mL .... NDC 0078-0110-22.
A dosage syringe is provided for dispensing.
Store and Dispense: In the original container at temperatures below 30°C (86°F). Do not store in the refrigerator. Protect from freezing. Once opened, the contents must be used within 2 months.

Sandimmune® Injection (cyclosporine injection, USP)
FOR INTRAVENOUS INFUSION
Supplied as a 5 mL sterile ampul containing 50 mg of cyclosporine per mL, in boxes of
10 ampuls .... NDC 0078-0109-01

Store and Dispense: At temperatures below 30°C (86°F) and protected from light.

---

*Cremophor is the registered trademark of BASF Aktiengesellschaft.

Sandimmune® Soft Gelatin Capsules (cyclosporine capsules, USP)
Manufactured by:
R.P. Scherer GmbH, Eberbach/Baden, Germany
Distributed by:
Novartis Pharmaceuticals Corporation
East Hanover, New Jersey 07936

Sandimmune® Oral Solution (cyclosporine oral solution, USP)
Manufactured by:
Novartis Pharma S.A.S.
Huningue, France
Distributed by:
Novartis Pharmaceuticals Corporation
East Hanover, New Jersey 07936

Sandimmune® Injection (cyclosporine injection, USP)
FOR INFUSION ONLY
Manufactured by:
Novartis Pharma Stein AG
Stein, Switzerland
Distributed by:
Novartis Pharmaceuticals Corporation
East Hanover, New Jersey 07936

T2004-40
REV: MAY 2004 PRINTED IN U.S.A. 89016103

Shown in Product Identification Guide, page 325

Renal Transplant Patients In Whom Therapy Was Discontinued

Reason for Discontinuation	Randomized Patients Sandimmune® (N=227) %	Azathioprine (N=228) %	All Sandimmune® Patients (N=705) %
Renal Toxicity	5.7	0	5.4
Infection	0	0.4	0.9
Lack of Efficacy	2.6	0.9	1.4
Acute Tubular Necrosis	2.6	0	1.0
Lymphoma/Lymphoproliferative Disease	0.4	0	0.3
Hypertension	0	0	0.3
Hematological Abnormalities	0	0.4	0
Other	0	0	0.7

Sandimmune® (cyclosporine) was discontinued on a temporary basis and then restarted in 18 additional patients.

Infectious Complications in the Randomized Renal Transplant Patients

Complication	Sandimmune® Treatment (N=227) % of Complications	Standard Treatment* (N=228) % of Complications
Septicemia	5.3	4.8
Abscesses	4.4	5.3
Systemic Fungal Infection	2.2	3.9
Local Fungal Infection	7.5	9.6
Cytomegalovirus	4.8	12.3
Other Viral Infections	15.9	18.4
Urinary Tract Infections	21.1	20.2
Wound and Skin Infections	7.0	10.1
Pneumonia	6.2	9.2

*Some patients also received ALG.

SANDOSTATIN® ℞

[*săn-dō-stă-tĭn*]
(octreotide acetate)
Injection
Rx only

Prescribing Information
The following prescribing information is base on official labeling in effect July 2003.

DESCRIPTION

Sandostatin® (octreotide acetate) Injection, a cyclic octapeptide prepared as a clear sterile solution of octreotide, acetate salt, in a buffered lactic acid solution for administration by deep subcutaneous (intrafat) or intravenous injection. Octreotide acetate, known chemically as L-Cysteinamide, D-phenylalanyl-L-cysteinyl-L-phenylalanyl-D-tryptophyl-L-lysyl-L-threonyl-N-[2-hydroxy-1-(hydroxymethyl)propyl]-, cyclic (2→7)-disulfide; [R-(R*, R*)] acetate salt, is a long-acting octapeptide with pharmacologic actions mimicking those of the natural hormone somatostatin.
Sandostatin® (octreotide acetate) Injection is available as: sterile 1 mL ampuls in 3 strengths, containing 50, 100, or 500 mcg octreotide (as acetate), and sterile 5 mL multi-dose vials in 2 strengths, containing 200 and 1000 mcg/mL of octreotide (as acetate).
Each ampul also contains:
lactic acid, USP .... 3.4 mg
mannitol, USP .... 45 mg
sodium bicarbonate, USP .... qs to pH 4.2 ± 0.3
water for injection, USP .... qs to 1 mL
Each mL of the multi-dose vials also contains:
lactic acid, USP .... 3.4 mg
mannitol, USP .... 45 mg
phenol, USP .... 5.0 mg
sodium bicarbonate, USP .... qs to pH 4.2 ± 0.3
water for injection, USP .... qs to 1 mL
Lactic acid and sodium bicarbonate are added to provide a buffered solution, pH to 4.2 ± 0.3.
The molecular weight of octreotide acetate is 1019.3 (free peptide, $C_{49}H_{66}N_{10}O_{10}S_2$) and its amino acid sequence is:

H-D-Phe-Cys-Phe-D-Trp-Lys-Thr-Cys-Thr-ol,
x CH_3COOH where x = 1.4 to 2.5

CLINICAL PHARMACOLOGY

Sandostatin® (octreotide acetate) exerts pharmacologic actions similar to the natural hormone, somatostatin. It is an even more potent inhibitor of growth hormone, glucagon, and insulin than somatostatin. Like somatostatin, it also suppresses LH response to GnRH, decreases splanchnic blood flow, and inhibits release of serotonin, gastrin, vasoactive intestinal peptide, secretin, motilin, and pancreatic polypeptide.
By virtue of these pharmacological actions, Sandostatin® (octreotide acetate) has been used to treat the symptoms associated with metastatic carcinoid tumors (flushing and diarrhea), and Vasoactive Intestinal Peptide (VIP) secreting adenomas (watery diarrhea).
Sandostatin® (octreotide acetate) substantially reduces growth hormone and/or IGF-I (somatomedin C) levels in patients with acromegaly.
Single doses of Sandostatin® (octreotide acetate) have been shown to inhibit gallbladder contractility and to decrease bile secretion in normal volunteers. In controlled clinical trials the incidence of gallstone or biliary sludge formation was markedly increased (see *WARNINGS*).

Continued on next page

Sandostatin—Cont.

Sandostatin® (octreotide acetate) suppresses secretion of thyroid stimulating hormone (TSH).

Pharmacokinetics

After subcutaneous injection, octreotide is absorbed rapidly and completely from the injection site. Peak concentrations of 5.2 ng/mL (100 mcg dose) were reached 0.4 hours after dosing. Using a specific radioimmunoassay, intravenous and subcutaneous doses were found to be bioequivalent. Peak concentrations and area under the curve values were dose proportional after intravenous single doses up to 200 mcg and subcutaneous single doses up to 500 mcg and after subcutaneous multiple doses up to 500 mcg t.i.d. (1500 mcg/day).

In healthy volunteers the distribution of octreotide from plasma was rapid ($t\alpha\frac{1}{2}$ = 0.2 h), the volume of distribution (Vdss) was estimated to be 13.6 L, and the total body clearance ranged from 7 L/hr to 10 L/hr. In blood, the distribution into the erythrocytes was found to be negligible and about 65% was bound in the plasma in a concentration-independent manner. Binding was mainly to lipoprotein and, to a lesser extent, to albumin.

The elimination of octreotide from plasma had an apparent half-life of 1.7 to 1.9 hours compared with 1-3 minutes with the natural hormone. The duration of action of Sandostatin® (octreotide acetate) is variable but extends up to 12 hours depending upon the type of tumor. About 32% of the dose is excreted unchanged into the urine. In an elderly population, dose adjustments may be necessary due to a significant increase in the half-life (46%) and a significant decrease in the clearance (26%) of the drug.

In patients with acromegaly, the pharmacokinetics differ somewhat from those in healthy volunteers. A mean peak concentration of 2.8 ng/mL (100 mcg dose) was reached in 0.7 hours after subcutaneous dosing. The volume of distribution (Vdss) was estimated to be 21.6 ± 8.5 L and the total body clearance was increased to 18 L/h. The mean percent of the drug bound was 41.2%. The disposition and elimination half-lives were similar to normals.

In patients with renal impairment the elimination of octreotide from plasma was prolonged and total body clearance reduced. In mild renal impairment (Cl_{CR} 40-60 mL/min) octreotide $t_{½}$ was 2.4 hours and total body clearance was 8.8 L/hr, in moderate impairment (Cl_{CR} 10-39 mL/min) $t_{½}$ was 3.0 hours and total body clearance 7.3 L/hr, and in severely renally impaired patients not requiring dialysis (Cl_{CR} <10 mL/min) $t_{½}$ was 3.1 hours and total body clearance was 7.6 L/hr. In patients with severe renal failure requiring dialysis, total body clearance was reduced to about half that found in healthy subjects (from approximately 10 L/hr to 4.5 L/hr).

Patients with liver cirrhosis showed prolonged elimination of drug, with octreotide $t_{½}$ increasing to 3.7 hr and total body clearance decreasing to 5.9 L/hr, whereas patients with fatty liver disease showed $t_{½}$ increased to 3.4 hr and total body clearance of 8.2 L/hr.

INDICATIONS AND USAGE

Acromegaly

Sandostatin® (octreotide acetate) is indicated to reduce blood levels of growth hormone and IGF-I (somatomedin C) in acromegaly patients who have had inadequate response to or cannot be treated with surgical resection, pituitary irradiation, and bromocriptine mesylate at maximally tolerated doses. The goal is to achieve normalization of growth hormone and IGF-I (somatomedin C) levels *(see DOSAGE AND ADMINISTRATION)*. In patients with acromegaly, Sandostatin® (octreotide acetate) reduces growth hormone to within normal ranges in 50% of patients and reduces IGF-I (somatomedin C) to within normal ranges in 50%-60% of patients. Since the effects of pituitary irradiation may not become maximal for several years, adjunctive therapy with Sandostatin® (octreotide acetate) to reduce blood levels of growth hormone and IGF-I (somatomedin C) offers potential benefit before the effects of irradiation are manifested.

Improvement in clinical signs and symptoms or reduction in tumor size or rate of growth were not shown in clinical trials performed with Sandostatin® (octreotide acetate); these trials were not optimally designed to detect such effects.

Carcinoid Tumors

Sandostatin® (octreotide acetate) is indicated for the symptomatic treatment of patients with metastatic carcinoid tumors where it suppresses or inhibits the severe diarrhea and flushing episodes associated with the disease.

Sandostatin® (octreotide acetate) studies were not designed to show an effect on the size, rate of growth or development of metastases.

Vasoactive Intestinal Peptide Tumors (VIPomas)

Sandostatin® (octreotide acetate) is indicated for the treatment of the profuse watery diarrhea associated with VIP secreting tumors. Sandostatin® (octreotide acetate) studies were not designed to show an effect on the size, rate of growth or development of metastases.

CONTRAINDICATIONS

Sensitivity to this drug or any of its components.

WARNINGS

Single doses of Sandostatin® (octreotide acetate) have been shown to inhibit gallbladder contractility and decrease bile secretion in normal volunteers. In clinical trials (primarily patients with acromegaly or psoriasis), the incidence of biliary tract abnormalities was 63% (27% gallstones, 24% sludge without stones, 12% biliary duct dilatation). The incidence of stones or sludge in patients who received Sandostatin® (octreotide acetate) for 12 months or longer was 52%. Less than 2% of patients treated with Sandostatin® (octreotide acetate) for 1 month or less developed gallstones. The incidence of gallstones did not appear related to age, sex or dose. Like patients without gallbladder abnormalities, the majority of patients developing gallbladder abnormalities on ultrasound had gastrointestinal symptoms. The symptoms were not specific for gallbladder disease. A few patients developed acute cholecystitis, ascending cholangitis, biliary obstruction, cholestatic hepatitis, or pancreatitis during Sandostatin® (octreotide acetate) therapy or following its withdrawal. One patient developed ascending cholangitis during Sandostatin® (octreotide acetate) therapy and died.

PRECAUTIONS

General

Sandostatin® (octreotide acetate) alters the balance between the counter-regulatory hormones, insulin, glucagon and growth hormone, which may result in hypoglycemia or hyperglycemia. Sandostatin® (octreotide acetate) also suppresses secretion of thyroid stimulating hormone, which may result in hypothyroidism. Cardiac conduction abnormalities have also occurred during treatment with Sandostatin® (octreotide acetate). However, the incidence of these adverse events during long-term therapy was determined vigorously only in acromegaly patients who, due to their underlying disease and/or the subsequent treatment they receive, are at an increased risk for the development of diabetes mellitus, hypothyroidism, and cardiovascular disease. Although the degree to which these abnormalities are related to Sandostatin® (octreotide acetate) therapy is not clear, new abnormalities of glycemic control, thyroid function and ECG developed during Sandostatin® (octreotide acetate) therapy as described below.

The hypoglycemia or hyperglycemia which occurs during Sandostatin® (octreotide acetate) therapy is usually mild, but may result in overt diabetes mellitus or necessitate dose changes in insulin or other hypoglycemic agents. Hypoglycemia and hyperglycemia occurred on Sandostatin® (octreotide acetate) in 3% and 16% of acromegalic patients, respectively. Severe hyperglycemia, subsequent pneumonia, and death following initiation of Sandostatin® (octreotide acetate) therapy was reported in one patient with no history of hyperglycemia.

In acromegalic patients, 12% developed biochemical hypothyroidism only, 8% developed goiter, and 4% required initiation of thyroid replacement therapy while receiving Sandostatin® (octreotide acetate). Baseline and periodic assessment of thyroid function (TSH, total and/or free T_4) is recommended during chronic therapy.

In acromegalics, bradycardia (<50 bpm) developed in 25%; conduction abnormalities occurred in 10% and arrhythmias occurred in 9% of patients during Sandostatin® (octreotide acetate) therapy. Other EKG changes observed included QT prolongation, axis shifts, early repolarization, low voltage, R/S transition, and early R wave progression. These ECG changes are not uncommon in acromegalic patients. Dose adjustments in drugs such as beta-blockers that have bradycardia effects may be necessary. In one acromegalic patient with severe congestive heart failure, initiation of Sandostatin® (octreotide acetate) therapy resulted in worsening of CHF with improvement when drug was discontinued. Confirmation of a drug effect was obtained with a positive rechallenge.

Several cases of pancreatitis have been reported in patients receiving Sandostatin® (octreotide acetate) therapy.

Sandostatin® (octreotide acetate) may alter absorption of dietary fats in some patients.

In patients with severe renal failure requiring dialysis, the half-life of Sandostatin® (octreotide acetate) may be increased, necessitating adjustment of the maintenance dosage.

Depressed vitamin B_{12} levels and abnormal Schilling's tests have been observed in some patients receiving Sandostatin® (octreotide acetate) therapy, and monitoring of vitamin B_{12} levels is recommended during chronic Sandostatin® (octreotide acetate) therapy.

Information for Patients

Careful instruction in sterile subcutaneous injection technique should be given to the patients and to other persons who may administer Sandostatin® (octreotide acetate) Injection.

Laboratory Tests

Laboratory tests that may be helpful as biochemical markers in determining and following patient response depend on the specific tumor. Based on diagnosis, measurement of the following substances may be useful in monitoring the progress of therapy:

Acromegaly:	Growth Hormone, IGF-I (somatomedin C) Responsiveness to Sandostatin® (octreotide acetate) may be evaluated by determining growth hormone levels at 1-4 hour intervals for 8-12 hours post dose. Alternatively, a single measurement of IGF-I (somatomedin C) level may be made two weeks after drug initiation or dosage change.
Carcinoid:	5-HIAA (urinary 5-hydroxyindole acetic acid), plasma serotonin, plasma Substance P
VIPoma:	VIP (plasma vasoactive intestinal peptide)

Baseline and periodic total and/or free T_4 measurements should be performed during chronic therapy *(see PRECAUTIONS — General)*.

Drug Interactions

Sandostatin® (octreotide acetate) has been associated with alterations in nutrient absorption, so it may have an effect on absorption of orally administered drugs. Concomitant administration of Sandostatin® (octreotide acetate) with cyclosporine may decrease blood levels of cyclosporine and result in transplant rejection.

Patients receiving insulin, oral hypoglycemic agents, beta blockers, calcium channel blockers, or agents to control fluid and electrolyte balance, may require dose adjustments of these therapeutic agents.

Drug Laboratory Test Interactions

No known interference exists with clinical laboratory tests, including amine or peptide determinations.

Carcinogenesis/Mutagenesis/Impairment of Fertility

Studies in laboratory animals have demonstrated no mutagenic potential of Sandostatin® (octreotide acetate).

No carcinogenic potential was demonstrated in mice treated subcutaneously for 85-99 weeks at doses up to 2000 mcg/kg/day (8× the human exposure based on body surface area). In a 116-week subcutaneous study in rats, a 27% and 12% incidence of injection site sarcomas or squamous cell carcinomas was observed in males and females, respectively, at the highest dose level of 1250 mcg/kg/day (10× the human exposure based on body surface area) compared to an incidence of 8%-10% in the vehicle-control groups. The increased incidence of injection site tumors was most probably caused by irritation and the high sensitivity of the rat to repeated subcutaneous injections at the same site. Rotating injection sites would prevent chronic irritation in humans. There have been no reports of injection site tumors in patients treated with Sandostatin® (octreotide acetate) for up to 5 years. There was also a 15% incidence of uterine adenocarcinomas in the 1250 mcg/kg/day females compared to 7% in the saline-control females and 0% in the vehicle-control females. The presence of endometritis coupled with the absence of corpora lutea, the reduction in mammary fibroadenomas, and the presence of uterine dilatation suggest that the uterine tumors were associated with estrogen dominance in the aged female rats which does not occur in humans.

Sandostatin® (octreotide acetate) did not impair fertility in rats at doses up to 1000 mcg/kg/day, which represents 7× the human exposure based on body surface area.

Pregnancy Category B

Reproduction studies have been performed in rats and rabbits at doses up to 16 times the highest human dose based on body surface area and have revealed no evidence of impaired fertility or harm to the fetus due to Sandostatin® (octreotide acetate). There are, however, no adequate and well-controlled studies in pregnant women. Because animal reproduction studies are not always predictive of human response, this drug should be used during pregnancy only if clearly needed.

Nursing Mothers

It is not known whether this drug is excreted in human milk. Because many drugs are excreted in milk, caution should be exercised when Sandostatin® (octreotide acetate) is administered to a nursing woman.

Pediatric Use

Experience with Sandostatin® (octreotide acetate) in the pediatric population is limited. Although formal controlled clinical trials have not been performed to evaluate safety and effectiveness in this age group, there are reports of 49 cases in the literature of neonates and infants with congenital hyperinsulinism [also called familial hyperinsulinism (HI), persistent hyperinsulinemic hypoglycemia of infancy (PHHI), or nesidioblastosis] who have received Sandostatin® as an inhibitor of insulin release. The following efficacy and safety information is derived from these 49 patients.

Sandostatin® has been used to stabilize plasma glucose levels prior to pancreatectomy and to treat recurrent postoperative hypoglycemia. Although most use of octreotide in this setting is short-term, a few reports in the literature have documented longer-term therapy in pediatric patients (2.2-5.5 years). Octreotide is an alternative medical treatment to diazoxide for control of hypoglycemia in this disorder. Of 31 pediatric patients who received Sandostatin® as prescribed for congenital hyperinsulinism and for which long-term follow-up was available, octreotide obviated the need for surgery in 3 patients (10%) and was replaced by diazoxide in 4 patients (13%) due to uncontrolled hypoglycemia. Although the remainder of these patients required surgery, there have been a few reports in the literature of patients who have responded to octreotide after failing treatment with surgery and/or diazoxide. Doses of 3-40 mcg/kg/day have been used. At these doses, the majority of side effects were gastrointestinal: diarrhea, steatorrhea, vomiting, and abdominal distention, each reported in 22%-35% (n = 11-17) of patients. However, they were generally short-lived – with resolution of vomiting and distention in 2-4 days, and diarrhea/steatorrhea, within 2-4 weeks. Steatorrhea was controlled in most patients with pancreatic enzyme supplements. Poor growth was reported in 37% of patients (n = 7) who received Sandostatin® for 1-4.33 years. It was associated with low serum growth hormone and/or IGF-1 levels in 4/6 patients in whom these parameters were measured. Catch-up growth occurred in 3/3 patients who were followed after Sandostatin® was discontinued. Poor weight gain was reported in 32% of patients (n = 6). Tachyphylaxis was reported in 35% (n = 17) of patients. Asymptomatic gallstones with sludge was reported in one infant after one year of therapy and was treated with ursodeoxycholic acid. There has been a single report of an infant with nesidioblastosis who experienced a seizure thought to be independent of Sandostatin® therapy. A single death has been reported in a 16-month-old male with enterocutaneous fistula who developed sudden abdominal pain and increased nasogastric drainage and expired 8 hours after receiving a single 100 mcg subcutaneous dose of Sandostatin®.

ADVERSE REACTIONS

Gallbladder Abnormalities

Gallbladder abnormalities, especially stones and/or biliary sludge, frequently develop in patients on chronic Sandostatin® (octreotide acetate) therapy (*see WARNINGS*).

Cardiac

In acromegalics, sinus bradycardia (<50 bpm) developed in 25%; conduction abnormalities occurred in 10% and arrhythmias developed in 9% of patients during Sandostatin® (octreotide acetate) therapy (*see PRECAUTIONS—General*).

Gastrointestinal

Diarrhea, loose stools, nausea and abdominal discomfort were each seen in 34%-61% of acromegalic patients in U.S. studies although only 2.6% of the patients discontinued therapy due to these symptoms. These symptoms were seen in 5%-10% of patients with other disorders.

The frequency of these symptoms was not dose-related, but diarrhea and abdominal discomfort generally resolved more quickly in patients treated with 300 mcg/day than in those treated with 750 mcg/day. Vomiting, flatulence, abnormal stools, abdominal distention, and constipation were each seen in less than 10% of patients.

Hypo/Hyperglycemia

Hypoglycemia and hyperglycemia occurred in 3% and 16% of acromegalic patients, respectively, but only in about 1.5% of other patients. Symptoms of hypoglycemia were noted in approximately 2% of patients.

Hypothyroidism

In acromegalics, biochemical hypothyroidism alone occurred in 12% while goiter occurred in 6% during Sandostatin® (octreotide acetate) therapy (*see PRECAUTIONS—General*). In patients without acromegaly, hypothyroidism has only been reported in several isolated patients and goiter has not been reported.

Other Adverse Events

Pain on injection was reported in 7.7%, headache in 6% and dizziness in 5%. Pancreatitis was also observed (*see WARNINGS* and *PRECAUTIONS*).

Other Adverse Events 1%-4%

Other events (relationship to drug not established), each observed in 1%-4% of patients, included fatigue, weakness, pruritus, joint pain, backache, urinary tract infection, cold symptoms, flu symptoms, injection site hematoma, bruise, edema, flushing, blurred vision, pollakiuria, fat malabsorption, hair loss, visual disturbance and depression.

Other Adverse Events <1%

Events reported in less than 1% of patients and for which relationship to drug is not established are listed: *Gastrointestinal*: hepatitis, jaundice, increase in liver enzymes, GI bleeding, hemorrhoids, appendicitis, gastric/peptic ulcer, gallbladder polyp; *Integumentary*: rash, cellulitis, petechiae, urticaria, basal cell carcinoma; *Musculoskeletal*: arthritis, joint effusion, muscle pain, Raynaud's phenomenon; *Cardiovascular*: chest pain, shortness of breath, thrombophlebitis, ischemia, congestive heart failure, hypertension, hypertensive reaction, palpitations, orthostatic BP decrease, tachycardia; *CNS*: anxiety, libido decrease, syncope, tremor, seizure, vertigo, Bell's Palsy, paranoia, pituitary apoplexy, increased intraocular pressure, amnesia, hearing loss, neuritis; *Respiratory*: pneumonia, pulmonary nodule, status asthmaticus; *Endocrine*: galactorrhea, hypoadrenalism, diabetes insipidus, gynecomastia, amenorrhea, polymenorrhea, oligomenorrhea, vaginitis; *Urogenital*: nephrolithiasis, hematuria; *Hematologic*: anemia, iron deficiency, epistaxis; *Miscellaneous*: otitis, allergic reaction, increased CK, weight loss.

Evaluation of 20 patients treated for at least 6 months has failed to demonstrate titers of antibodies exceeding background levels. However, antibody titers to Sandostatin® (octreotide acetate) were subsequently reported in three patients and resulted in prolonged duration of drug action in two patients. Anaphylactoid reactions, including anaphylactic shock, have been reported in several patients receiving Sandostatin® (octreotide acetate).

OVERDOSAGE

No frank overdose has occurred in any patient to date. Intravenous bolus doses of 1 mg (1000 mcg) given to healthy volunteers and of 30 mg (30,000 mcg) IV over 20 minutes and of 120 mg (120,000 mcg) IV over 8 hours to research patients have not resulted in serious ill effects.

Up-to-date information about the treatment of overdose can often be obtained from a certified Regional Poison Control Center. Telephone numbers of certified Regional Poison Control Centers are listed in the Physicians' Desk Reference®.*

Mortality occurred in mice and rats given 72 mg/kg and 18 mg/kg IV, respectively.

Drug Abuse and Dependence

There is no indication that Sandostatin® (octreotide acetate) has potential for drug abuse or dependence. Sandostatin® (octreotide acetate) levels in the central nervous system are negligible, even after doses up to 30,000 mcg.

DOSAGE AND ADMINISTRATION

Sandostatin® (octreotide acetate) may be administered subcutaneously or intravenously. Subcutaneous injection is the usual route of administration of Sandostatin® (octreotide acetate) for control of symptoms. Pain with subcutaneous administration may be reduced by using the smallest volume that will deliver the desired dose. Multiple subcutaneous injections at the same site within short periods of time should be avoided. Sites should be rotated in a systematic manner.

Parenteral drug products should be inspected visually for particulate matter and discoloration prior to administration. **Do not use if particulates and/or discoloration are observed.** Proper sterile technique should be used in the preparation of parenteral admixtures to minimize the possibility of microbial contamination. **Sandostatin® (octreotide acetate) is not compatible in Total Parenteral Nutrition (TPN) solutions because of the formation of a glycosyl octreotide conjugate which may decrease the efficacy of the product.**

Sandostatin® (octreotide acetate) is stable in sterile isotonic saline solutions or sterile solutions of dextrose 5% in water for 24 hours. It may be diluted in volumes of 50-200 mL and infused intravenously over 15-30 minutes or administered by IV push over 3 minutes. In emergency situations (e.g.: carcinoid crisis) it may be given by rapid bolus.

The initial dosage is usually 50 mcg administered twice or three times daily. Upward dose titration is frequently required. Dosage information for patients with specific tumors follows.

Acromegaly

Dosage may be initiated at 50 mcg t.i.d. Beginning with this low dose may permit adaptation to adverse gastrointestinal effects for patients who will require higher doses. IGF-I (somatomedin C) levels every 2 weeks can be used to guide titration. Alternatively, multiple growth hormone levels at 0-8 hours after Sandostatin® (octreotide acetate) administration permit more rapid titration of dose. The goal is to achieve growth hormone levels less than 5 ng/mL or IGF-I (somatomedin C) levels less than 1.9 U/mL in males and less than 2.2 U/mL in females. The dose most commonly found to be effective is 100 mcg t.i.d., but some patients require up to 500 mcg t.i.d. for maximum effectiveness. Doses greater than 300 mcg/day seldom result in additional biochemical benefit, and if an increase in dose fails to provide additional benefit, the dose should be reduced. IGF-I (somatomedin C) or growth hormone levels should be reevaluated at 6-month intervals.

Sandostatin® (octreotide acetate) should be withdrawn yearly for approximately 4 weeks from patients who have received irradiation to assess disease activity. If growth hormone or IGF-I (somatomedin C) levels increase and signs and symptoms recur, Sandostatin® (octreotide acetate) therapy may be resumed.

Carcinoid Tumors

The suggested daily dosage of Sandostatin® (octreotide acetate) during the first 2 weeks of therapy ranges from 100-600 mcg/day in 2-4 divided doses (mean daily dosage is 300 mcg). In the clinical studies, the median daily maintenance dosage was approximately 450 mcg, but clinical and biochemical benefits were obtained in some patients with as little as 50 mcg, while others required doses up to 1500 mcg/day. However, experience with doses above 750 mcg/day is limited.

VIPomas

Daily dosages of 200-300 mcg in 2-4 divided doses are recommended during the initial 2 weeks of therapy (range 150-750 mcg) to control symptoms of the disease. On an individual basis, dosage may be adjusted to achieve a therapeutic response, but usually doses above 450 mcg/day are not required.

HOW SUPPLIED

Sandostatin® (octreotide acetate) Injection is available in 1 mL ampuls and 5 mL multi-dose vials as follows:

Ampuls

50 mcg/mL octreotide (as acetate)
Package of 10 ampuls .... (NDC 0078-0180-01)
100 mcg/mL octreotide (as acetate)
Package of 10 ampuls .... (NDC 0078-0181-01)
500 mcg/mL octreotide (as acetate)
Package of 10 ampuls .... (NDC 0078-0182-01)

Multi-Dose Vials

200 mcg/mL octreotide (as acetate)
Box of one .... (NDC 0078-0183-25)
1000 mcg/mL octreotide (as acetate)
Box of one .... (NDC 0078-0184-25)

Storage

For prolonged storage, Sandostatin® (octreotide acetate) ampuls and multi-dose vials should be stored at refrigerated temperatures 2°C-8°C (36°F-46°F) and protected from light. At room temperature, (20°C-30°C or 70°F-86°F), Sandostatin® (octreotide acetate) is stable for 14 days if protected from light. The solution can be allowed to come to room temperature prior to administration. Do not warm artificially. After initial use, multiple-dose vials should be discarded within 14 days. Ampuls should be opened just prior to administration and the unused portion discarded.

*Medical Economics Company, Inc.

T2002-82

REV: OCTOBER 2002 89017902

NOVARTIS

Manufactured by:
Novartis Pharma Stein AG
Schaffhauserstrasse
CH-4332 Stein, Switzerland
Distributed by:
Novartis Pharmaceuticals Corporation
East Hanover, New Jersey 07936
©Novartis

Shown in Product Identification Guide, page 325

SANDOSTATIN LAR® DEPOT ℞

[săn-dō-stă-tĭn]

(octreotide acetate for injectable suspension)

Rx only

Prescribing Information

The following prescribing information is based on official labeling in effect July 2004.

DESCRIPTION

Octreotide is the acetate salt of a cyclic octapeptide. It is a long-acting octapeptide with pharmacologic properties mimicking those of the natural hormone somatostatin. Octreotide is known chemically as L-Cysteinamide, D-phenylalanyl-L-cysteinyl-L-phenylalanyl-D-tryptophyl-L-lysyl-L-threonyl-N-[2-hydroxy-1-(hydroxymethyl) propyl]-, cyclic (2→7)-disulfide; [R-(R*,R*)].

Sandostatin LAR® Depot (octreotide acetate for injectable suspension) is available in a vial containing the sterile drug product, which when mixed with diluent, becomes a suspension that is given as a monthly intragluteal injection. The octreotide is uniformly distributed within the microspheres which are made of a biodegradable glucose star polymer, D,L-lactic and glycolic acids copolymer. Sterile mannitol is added to the microspheres to improve suspendability.

Sandostatin LAR® Depot is available as: sterile 5-mL vials in 3 strengths delivering 10 mg, 20 mg or 30 mg octreotide free peptide. Each vial of Sandostatin LAR® Depot delivers:

[See first table at top of next page]

Each syringe of diluent contains:

carboxymethylcellulose sodium	12.5 mg
mannitol	15.0 mg
water for injection	2.5 mL

The molecular weight of octreotide is 1019.3 (free peptide, $C_{49}H_{66}N_{10}O_{10}S_2$) and its amino acid sequence is:

H-D-Phe-Cys-Phe-D-Trp-Lys-Thr-Cys-Thr-ol•xCH_3COOH
where x = 1.4 to 2.5

CLINICAL PHARMACOLOGY

Sandostatin LAR® Depot (octreotide acetate for injectable suspension) is a long-acting dosage form consisting of microspheres of the biodegradable glucose star polymer, D,L-lactic and glycolic acids copolymer, containing octreotide. It maintains all of the clinical and pharmacological characteristics of the immediate-release dosage form Sandostatin® (octreotide acetate) Injection with the added feature of slow release of octreotide from the site of injection, reducing the need for frequent administration. This slow release occurs as the polymer biodegrades, primarily through hydrolysis. Sandostatin LAR® Depot is designed to be injected intramuscularly (intragluteally) once every four weeks.

Octreotide exerts pharmacologic actions similar to the natural hormone, somatostatin. It is an even more potent inhibitor of growth hormone, glucagon, and insulin than somatostatin. Like somatostatin, it also suppresses LH response to GnRH, decreases splanchnic blood flow, and inhibits release of serotonin, gastrin, vasoactive intestinal peptide, secretin, motilin, and pancreatic polypeptide.

By virtue of these pharmacological actions, octreotide has been used to treat the symptoms associated with metastatic carcinoid tumors (flushing and diarrhea), and Vasoactive Intestinal Peptide (VIP) secreting adenomas (watery diarrhea).

Octreotide substantially reduces and in many cases can normalize growth hormone and/or IGF-1 (somatomedin C) levels in patients with acromegaly.

Single doses of Sandostatin® Injection given subcutaneously have been shown to inhibit gallbladder contractility and to decrease bile secretion in normal volunteers. In controlled clinical trials the incidence of gallstone or biliary sludge formation was markedly increased (*see WARNINGS*).

Octreotide may cause clinically significant suppression of thyroid stimulating hormone (TSH).

Pharmacokinetics

The magnitude and duration of octreotide serum concentrations after an intramuscular injection of the long-acting depot formulation Sandostatin LAR® Depot reflect the release of drug from the microsphere polymer matrix. Drug release is governed by the slow biodegradation of the microspheres in the muscle, but once present in the systemic circulation, octreotide distributes and is eliminated according to its known pharmacokinetic properties which are as follows:

1. Pharmacokinetics of Octreotide Acetate

According to data obtained with the immediate-release formulation, Sandostatin® Injection solution, after subcutaneous injection, octreotide is absorbed rapidly and completely from the injection site. Peak concentrations of 5.2 ng/mL (100 mcg dose) were reached 0.4 hours after dosing. Using a specific radioimmunoassay, intravenous and subcutaneous doses were found to be bioequivalent. Peak concentrations and area-under-the-curve values were dose proportional

Continued on next page

Sandostatin LAR—Cont.

both after subcutaneous or intravenous single doses up to 400 mcg and with multiple doses of 200 mcg t.i.d. (600 mcg/day). Clearance was reduced by about 66% suggesting nonlinear kinetics of the drug at daily doses of 600 mcg/day as compared to 150 mcg/day. The relative decrease in clearance with doses above 600 mcg/day is not defined.

In healthy volunteers the distribution of octreotide from plasma was rapid ($t\alpha_{1/2}$ = 0.2 h), the volume of distribution (Vdss) was estimated to be 13.6 L and the total body clearance was 10 L/h.

In blood, the distribution of octreotide into the erythrocytes was found to be negligible and about 65% was bound in the plasma in a concentration-independent manner. Binding was mainly to lipoprotein and, to a lesser extent, to albumin.

The elimination of octreotide from plasma had an apparent half-life of 1.7 hours, compared with the 1-3 minutes with the natural hormone, somatostatin. The duration of action of subcutaneously administered Sandostatin® Injection solution is variable but extends up to 12 hours depending upon the type of tumor, necessitating multiple daily dosing with this immediate-release dosage form. About 32% of the dose is excreted unchanged into the urine. In an elderly population, dose adjustments may be necessary due to a significant increase in the half-life (46%) and a significant decrease in the clearance (26%) of the drug.

In patients with acromegaly, the pharmacokinetics differ somewhat from those in healthy volunteers. A mean peak concentration of 2.8 ng/mL (100 mcg dose) was reached in 0.7 hours after subcutaneous dosing. The volume of distribution (Vdss) was estimated to be 21.6 ± 8.5 L and the total body clearance was increased to 18 L/h. The mean percent of the drug bound was 41.2%. The disposition and elimination half-lives were similar to normals.

In patients with severe renal failure requiring dialysis, clearance was reduced to about half that found in healthy subjects (from approximately 10 L/h to 4.5 L/h).

The effect of hepatic diseases on the disposition of octreotide is unknown.

2. Pharmacokinetics of Sandostatin LAR® Depot

After a single IM injection of the long-acting depot dosage form Sandostatin LAR® Depot in healthy volunteer subjects, the serum octreotide concentration reached a transient initial peak of about 0.03 ng/mL/mg within 1 hour after administration progressively declining over the following 3 to 5 days to a nadir of <0.01 ng/mL/mg, then slowly increasing and reaching a plateau about two to three weeks post injection. Plateau concentrations were maintained over a period of nearly 2-3 weeks, showing dose proportional peak concentrations of about 0.07 ng/mL/mg. After about 6 weeks post injection, octreotide concentration slowly decreased, to <0.01 ng/mL/mg by weeks 12 to 13, concomitant with the terminal degradation phase of the polymer matrix of the dosage form. The relative bioavailability of the long-acting release Sandostatin LAR® Depot compared to immediate-release Sandostatin® Injection solution given subcutaneously was 60%-63%.

In patients with acromegaly, the octreotide concentrations after single doses of 10 mg, 20 mg and 30 mg Sandostatin LAR® Depot were dose proportional. The transient day 1 peak, amounting to 0.3 ng/mL, 0.8 ng/mL, and 1.3 ng/mL, respectively, was followed by plateau concentrations of 0.5 ng/mL, 1.3 ng/mL, and 2.0 ng/mL, respectively, achieved about 3 weeks post injection. These plateau concentrations were maintained for nearly two weeks.

Following multiple doses of Sandostatin LAR® Depot given every 4 weeks, steady-state octreotide serum concentrations were achieved after the third injection. Concentrations were dose proportional and higher by a factor of approximately 1.6 to 2.0 compared to the concentrations after a single dose. The steady-state octreotide concentrations were 1.2 ng/mL and 2.1 ng/mL, respectively, at trough and 1.6 ng/mL and 2.6 ng/mL, respectively, at peak with 20 mg and 30 mg Sandostatin LAR® Depot given every 4 weeks. No accumulation of octreotide beyond that expected from the overlapping release profiles occurred over a duration of up to 28 monthly injections of Sandostatin LAR® Depot. With the long-acting depot formulation Sandostatin LAR® Depot administered IM every 4 weeks the peak-to-trough variation in octreotide concentrations ranged from 44%-68%, compared to the 163%-209% variation encountered with the daily subcutaneous t.i.d. regimen of Sandostatin® Injection solution.

In patients with carcinoid tumors, the mean octreotide concentrations after 6 doses of 10 mg, 20 mg and 30 mg Sandostatin LAR® Depot administered by IM injection every four weeks were 1.2 ng/mL, 2.5 ng/mL, and 4.2 ng/mL, respectively. Concentrations were dose proportional and steady-state concentrations were reached after two injections of 20 mg and 30 mg and after three injections of 10 mg.

Sandostatin LAR® Depot has not been studied in patients with renal impairment.

Sandostatin LAR® Depot has not been studied in patients with hepatic impairment.

CLINICAL TRIALS

The clinical trials of Sandostatin LAR® Depot (octreotide acetate for injectable suspension) were performed in patients who had been receiving Sandostatin® (octreotide acetate) Injection for a period of weeks to as long as 10 years. The acromegaly studies with Sandostatin LAR® Depot de-

Name of Ingredient	10 mg	20 mg	30 mg
octreotide acetate	11.2 mg*	22.4 mg*	33.6 mg*
D,L-lactic and glycolic acids copolymer	188.8 mg	377.6 mg	566.4 mg
mannitol	41.0 mg	81.9 mg	122.9 mg

*Equivalent to 10/20/30 mg octreotide base.

Table 1
Hormonal Response in Acromegalic Patients Receiving 27 to 28 Injections During[1] Treatment with Sandostatin LAR® Depot

	Sandostatin® Injection S.C.		Sandostatin LAR® Depot	
Mean Hormone Level	**N**	**%**	**N**	**%**
GH <5.0 ng/mL	69/88	78	73/88	83
<2.5 ng/mL	44/88	50	41/88	47
<1.0 ng/mL	6/88	7	10/88	11
IGF-1 normalized	36/88	41	45/88	51
GH <5.0 ng/mL + IGF-1 normalized	36/88	41	45/88	51
<2.5 ng/mL + IGF-1 normalized	30/88	34	37/88	42
<1.0 ng/mL + IGF-1 normalized	5/88	6	10/88	11

[1]Average of monthly levels of GH and IGF-1 over the course of the trials

Table 2
Hormonal Response in Acromegalic Patients Receiving 12 Injections During[1] Treatment with Sandostatin LAR® Depot

	Sandostatin® Injection S.C.		Sandostatin LAR® Depot	
Mean Hormone Level	**N**	**%**	**N**	**%**
GH <5.0 ng/mL	116/122	95	118/122	97
<2.5 ng/mL	84/122	69	80/122	66
<1.0 ng/mL	25/122	21	28/122	23
IGF-1 normalized	82/122	67	82/122	67
GH <5.0 ng/mL + IGF-1 normalized	80/122	66	82/122	67
<2.5 ng/mL + IGF-1 normalized	65/122	53	70/122	57
<1.0 ng/mL + IGF-1 normalized	23/122	19	27/122	22

[1]Average of monthly levels of GH and IGF-1 over the course of the trial

scribed below were performed in patients who achieved GH levels of <10 ng/mL (and, in most cases <5 ng/mL) while on subcutaneous Sandostatin® Injection. However, some patients enrolled were partial responders to subcutaneous Sandostatin® Injection, i.e., GH levels were reduced by >50% on subcutaneous Sandostatin® Injection compared to the untreated state, although not suppressed to <5 ng/mL.

Acromegaly

Sandostatin LAR® Depot was evaluated in three clinical trials in acromegalic patients.

In two of the clinical trials, a total of 101 patients were entered who had, in most cases, achieved a GH level <5 ng/mL on Sandostatin® Injection given in doses of 100 mcg or 200 mcg t.i.d. Most patients were switched to 20 mg or 30 mg doses of Sandostatin LAR® Depot given once every 4 weeks for up to 27 to 28 injections. A few patients received doses of 10 mg and a few required doses of 40 mg. Growth hormone and IGF-1 levels were at least as well controlled with Sandostatin LAR® Depot as they had been on Sandostatin® Injection and this level of control remained for the entire duration of the trials.

A third trial was a 12-month study that enrolled 151 patients who had a GH level <10 ng/mL after treatment with Sandostatin® Injection (most had levels <5 ng/mL). The starting dose of Sandostatin LAR® Depot was 20 mg every 4 weeks for 3 doses. Thereafter, patients received 10 mg, 20 mg or 30 mg every 4 weeks, depending upon the degree of GH suppression. (The recommended regimen for these dosage changes is described under *DOSAGE AND ADMINISTRATION*). Growth hormone and IGF-1 were at least as well controlled on Sandostatin LAR® Depot as they had been on Sandostatin® Injection.

Table 1 summarizes the data on hormonal control (GH and IGF-1) for those patients in the first two clinical trials who received all 27 to 28 injections of Sandostatin LAR® Depot.

[See table 1 above]

For the 88 patients in Table 1, a mean GH level of <2.5 ng/mL was observed in 47% receiving Sandostatin LAR® Depot. Over the course of the trials 42% of patients maintained mean growth hormone levels of <2.5 ng/mL and mean normal IGF-1 levels.

Table 2 summarizes the data on hormonal control (GH and IGF-1) for those patients in the third clinical trial who received all 12 injections of Sandostatin LAR® Depot.

[See table 2 above]

For the 122 patients in Table 2, who received all 12 injections in the third trial, a mean GH level of <2.5 ng/mL was observed in 66% receiving Sandostatin LAR® Depot. Over the course of the trial 57% of patients maintained mean growth hormone levels of <2.5 ng/mL and mean normal IGF-1 levels. In comparing the hormonal response in these trials, note that a higher percentage of patients in the third trial suppressed their mean GH to <5 ng/mL on subcutaneous Sandostatin® Injection, 95%, compared to 78% across the two previous trials.

In all three trials, GH, IGF-1, and clinical symptoms were similarly controlled on Sandostatin LAR® Depot as they had been on Sandostatin® Injection.

Of the 25 patients who completed the trials and were partial responders to Sandostatin® Injection (GH >5.0 ng/mL but reduced by >50% relative to untreated levels), 1 patient (4%) responded to Sandostatin LAR® Depot with a reduction of GH to <2.5 ng/mL and 8 patients (32%) responded with a reduction of GH to <5.0 ng/mL.

Carcinoid Syndrome

A 6-month clinical trial of malignant carcinoid syndrome was performed in 93 patients who had previously been shown to be responsive to Sandostatin® Injection. Sixty-seven patients were randomized at baseline to receive, double-blind, doses of 10 mg, 20 mg or 30 mg Sandostatin LAR® Depot every 28 days and 26 patients continued, unblinded, on their previous Sandostatin® Injection regimen (100-300 mcg t.i.d.).

In any given month after steady-state levels of octreotide were reached, approximately 35%-40% of the patients who received Sandostatin LAR® Depot required supplemental subcutaneous Sandostatin® Injection therapy usually for a few days, to control exacerbation of carcinoid symptoms. In any given month the percentage of patients randomized to subcutaneous Sandostatin® Injection, who required supplemental treatment with an increased dose of Sandostatin® Injection, was similar to the percentage of patients randomized to Sandostatin LAR® Depot. Over the six-month treatment period approximately 50%-70% of patients who completed the trial on Sandostatin LAR® Depot required subcutaneous Sandostatin® Injection supplemental therapy to control exacerbation of carcinoid symptoms although steady-state serum Sandostatin LAR® Depot levels had been reached.

Table 3 presents the average number of daily stools and flushing episodes in malignant carcinoid patients.

[See table 3 at top of next page]

Overall, mean daily stool frequency was as well controlled on Sandostatin LAR® Depot as on Sandostatin® Injection (approximately 2 to 2.5 stools/day).

Mean daily flushing episodes were similar at all doses of Sandostatin LAR® Depot and on Sandostatin® Injection (approximately 0.5 to 1 episode/day).

In a subset of patients with variable severity of disease, median 24 hour urinary 5-HIAA (5-hydroxyindole acetic acid) levels were reduced by 38%-50% in the groups randomized to Sandostatin LAR® Depot.

The reductions are within the range reported in the published literature for patients treated with octreotide (about 10%-50%).

Seventy-eight patients with malignant carcinoid syndrome who had participated in this 6-month trial, subsequently participated in a 12-month extension study in which they received 12 injections of Sandostatin LAR® Depot at 4-week intervals. For those who remained in the extension trial, diarrhea and flushing were as well controlled as during the 6-month trial. Because malignant carcinoid disease is progressive, as expected, a number of deaths (8 patients: 10%) occurred due to disease progression or complications from the underlying disease. An additional 22% of patients prematurely discontinued Sandostatin LAR® Depot due to disease progression or worsening of carcinoid symptoms.

INDICATIONS AND USAGE

Acromegaly

Sandostatin LAR® Depot (octreotide acetate for injectable suspension) is indicated for long-term maintenance therapy in acromegalic patients for whom medical treatment is appropriate and who have been shown to respond to and can tolerate Sandostatin® (octreotide acetate) Injection. The goal of treatment in acromegaly is to reduce GH and IGF-1 levels to normal. Sandostatin LAR® Depot can be used in patients who have had an inadequate response to surgery or in those for whom surgical resection is not an option. It may also be used in patients who have received radiation and have had an inadequate therapeutic response *(see CLINICAL TRIALS and DOSAGE AND ADMINISTRATION).*

Carcinoid Tumors

Sandostatin LAR® Depot is indicated for long-term treatment of the severe diarrhea and flushing episodes associated with metastatic carcinoid tumors in patients in whom initial treatment with Sandostatin® Injection has been shown to be effective and tolerated.

Vasoactive Intestinal Peptide Tumors (VIPomas)

Sandostatin LAR® Depot is indicated for long-term treatment of the profuse watery diarrhea associated with VIP-secreting tumors in patients in whom initial treatment with Sandostatin® Injection has been shown to be effective and tolerated.

In patients with acromegaly, carcinoid syndrome and VIPomas, the effect of Sandostatin® Injection and Sandostatin LAR® Depot on tumor size, rate of growth and development of metastases, has not been determined.

CONTRAINDICATIONS

Sensitivity to this drug or any of its components.

WARNINGS

Adverse events that have been reported in patients receiving Sandostatin® (octreotide acetate) Injection can also be expected in patients receiving Sandostatin LAR® Depot (octreotide acetate for injectable suspension). Incidence figures in the *WARNINGS* and *ADVERSE REACTIONS* sections, below, are those obtained in clinical trials of Sandostatin® Injection and Sandostatin LAR® Depot.

Gallbladder and Related Events

Single doses of Sandostatin® Injection have been shown to inhibit gallbladder contractility and decrease bile secretion in normal volunteers. In clinical trials with Sandostatin® Injection (primarily patients with acromegaly or psoriasis) in patients who had not previously received octreotide, the incidence of biliary tract abnormalities was 63% (27% gallstones, 24% sludge without stones, 12% biliary duct dilatation). The incidence of stones or sludge in patients who received Sandostatin® Injection for 12 months or longer was 52%. The incidence of gallbladder abnormalities did not appear to be related to age, sex or dose but was related to duration of exposure.

In clinical trials 52% of acromegalic patients, most of whom received Sandostatin LAR® Depot for 12 months or longer, developed new biliary abnormalities including gallstones, microlithiasis, sediment, sludge and dilatation. The incidence of new cholelithiasis was 22%, of which 7% were microstones.

In clinical trials 62% of malignant carcinoid patients who received Sandostatin LAR® Depot for up to 18 months developed new biliary abnormalities including gallstones, sludge and dilatation. New gallstones occurred in a total of 24% of patients.

Across all trials, a few patients developed acute cholecystitis, ascending cholangitis, biliary obstruction, cholestatic hepatitis, or pancreatitis during octreotide therapy or following its withdrawal. One patient developed ascending cholangitis during Sandostatin® Injection therapy and died. Despite the high incidence of new gallstones in patients receiving octreotide, 1% of patients developed acute symptoms requiring cholecystectomy.

PRECAUTIONS *(See ADVERSE REACTIONS.)*

General

Growth hormone secreting tumors may sometimes expand and cause serious complications (e.g., visual field defects). Therefore, all patients with these tumors should be carefully monitored.

Octreotide alters the balance between the counter-regulatory hormones, insulin, glucagon and growth hormone, which may result in hypoglycemia or hyperglycemia. Octreotide also suppresses secretion of thyroid stimulating hormone, which may result in hypothyroidism. Cardiac conduction abnormalities have also occurred during treatment with octreotide.

Glucose Metabolism

The hypoglycemia or hyperglycemia which occurs during octreotide therapy is usually mild, but may result in overt diabetes mellitus or necessitate dose changes in insulin or other hypoglycemic agents. Severe hyperglycemia, subsequent pneumonia, and death following initiation of Sandostatin® (octreotide acetate) Injection therapy was reported in one patient with no history of hyperglycemia *(see ADVERSE REACTIONS).*

Table 3
Average No. of Daily Stools and Flushing Episodes in Patients with Malignant Carcinoid Syndrome

Treatment	N	Daily Stools (Average No.) Baseline	Daily Stools (Average No.) Last Visit	Daily Flushing Episodes (Average No.) Baseline	Daily Flushing Episodes (Average No.) Last Visit
Sandostatin® Injection S.C.	26	3.7	2.6	3.0	0.5
Sandostatin LAR® Depot					
10 mg	22	4.6	2.8	3.0	0.9
20 mg	20	4.0	2.1	5.9	0.6
30 mg	24	4.9	2.8	6.1	1.0

In patients with concomitant Type I diabetes mellitus, Sandostatin Injection and Sandostatin LAR® Depot (octreotide acetate for injectable suspension) are likely to affect glucose regulation, and insulin requirements may be reduced. Symptomatic hypoglycemia, which may be severe, has been reported in these patients. In non-diabetics and Type II diabetics with partially intact insulin reserves, Sandostatin Injection or Sandostatin LAR Depot administration may result in decreases in plasma insulin levels and hyperglycemia. It is therefore recommended that glucose tolerance and antidiabetic treatment be periodically monitored during therapy with these drugs.

Thyroid Function

Hypothyroidism has been reported in acromegaly and carcinoid patients receiving octreotide therapy. Baseline and periodic assessment of thyroid function (TSH, total and/or free T_4) is recommended during chronic octreotide therapy *(see ADVERSE REACTIONS).*

Cardiac Function

In both acromegalic and carcinoid syndrome patients, bradycardia, arrhythmias and conduction abnormalities have been reported during octreotide therapy. Other EKG changes were observed such as QT prolongation, axis shifts, early repolarization, low voltage, R/S transition, early R wave progression, and non-specific ST-T wave changes. The relationship of these events to octreotide acetate is not established because many of these patients have underlying cardiac disease *(see PRECAUTIONS).* Dose adjustments in drugs such as beta-blockers that have bradycardia effects may be necessary. In one acromegalic patient with severe congestive heart failure, initiation of Sandostatin® Injection therapy resulted in worsening of CHF with improvement when drug was discontinued. Confirmation of a drug effect was obtained with a positive rechallenge *(see ADVERSE REACTIONS).*

Nutrition

Octreotide may alter absorption of dietary fats in some patients.

Depressed vitamin B_{12} levels and abnormal Schilling's tests have been observed in some patients receiving octreotide therapy, and monitoring of vitamin B_{12} levels is recommended during therapy with Sandostatin LAR® Depot.

Octreotide has been investigated for the reduction of excessive fluid loss from the G.I. tract in patients with conditions producing such a loss. If such patients are receiving total parenteral nutrition (TPN), serum zinc may rise excessively when the fluid loss is reversed. Patients on TPN and octreotide should have periodic monitoring of zinc levels.

Information for Patients

Patients with carcinoid tumors and VIPomas should be advised to adhere closely to their scheduled return visits for reinjection in order to minimize exacerbation of symptoms. Patients with acromegaly should also be urged to adhere to their return visit schedule to help assure steady control of GH and IGF-1 levels.

Laboratory Tests

Laboratory tests that may be helpful as biochemical markers in determining and following patient response depend on the specific tumor. Based on diagnosis, measurement of the following substances may be useful in monitoring the progress of therapy:

Acromegaly: Growth Hormone, IGF-1 (somatomedin C)
Responsiveness to octreotide may be evaluated by determining growth hormone levels at 1-4 hour intervals for 8-12 hours after subcutaneous injection of Sandostatin® Injection (not Sandostatin LAR® Depot). Alternatively, a single measurement of IGF-1 (somatomedin C) level may be made two weeks after initiation of Sandostatin® Injection or dosage change. After patients are switched from Sandostatin® Injection to Sandostatin LAR® Depot, GH and IGF-1 determinations may be made after 3 monthly injections of Sandostatin LAR® Depot. (Steady-state serum levels of octreotide are reached only after a period of 3 months of monthly injections.) Growth hormone can be determined using the mean of 4 assays taken at 1-hour intervals. Somatomedin C can be determined with a single assay. All GH and IGF-1 determinations should be made 4 weeks after the previous Sandostatin LAR® Depot.

Carcinoid: 5-HIAA (urinary 5-hydroxyindole acetic acid), plasma serotonin, plasma Substance P

VIPoma: VIP (plasma vasoactive intestinal peptide)

Baseline and periodic total and/or free T_4 measurements should be performed during chronic therapy *(see PRECAUTIONS—General).*

Drug Interactions

Octreotide has been associated with alterations in nutrient absorption, so it may have an effect on absorption of orally administered drugs. Concomitant administration of octreotide injection with cyclosporine may decrease blood levels of cyclosporine and result in transplant rejection.

Patients receiving insulin, oral hypoglycemic agents, beta-blockers, calcium channel blockers, or agents to control fluid and electrolyte balance, may require dose adjustments of these therapeutic agents.

Concomitant administration of octreotide and bromocriptine increases the availability of bromocriptine. Limited published data indicate that somatostatin analogs might decrease the metabolic clearance of compounds known to be metabolized by cytochrome P450 enzymes, which may be due to the suppression of growth hormones. Since it cannot be excluded that octreotide may have this effect, other drugs mainly metabolized by CYP3A4 and which have a low therapeutic index (e.g., quinidine, terfenadine) should therefore be used with caution.

Drug Laboratory Test Interactions

No known interference exists with clinical laboratory tests, including amine or peptide determinations.

Carcinogenesis/Mutagenesis/Impairment of Fertility

Studies in laboratory animals have demonstrated no mutagenic potential of Sandostatin®. No mutagenic potential of the polymeric carrier in Sandostatin LAR® Depot, D,L-lactic and glycolic acids copolymer, was observed in the Ames mutagenicity test.

No carcinogenic potential was demonstrated in mice treated subcutaneously with octreotide for 85-99 weeks at doses up to 2000 mcg/kg/day (8× the human exposure based on body surface area). In a 116-week subcutaneous study in rats administered octreotide, a 27% and 12% incidence of injection site sarcomas or squamous cell carcinomas was observed in males and females, respectively, at the highest dose level of 1250 mcg/kg/day (10× the human exposure based on body surface area) compared to an incidence of 8%-10% in the vehicle-control groups. The increased incidence of injection site tumors was most probably caused by irritation and the high sensitivity of the rat to repeated subcutaneous injections at the same site. Rotating injection sites would prevent chronic irritation in humans. There have been no reports of injection site tumors in patients treated with Sandostatin® Injection for at least 5 years. There was also a 15% incidence of uterine adenocarcinomas in the 1250 mcg/kg/day females compared to 7% in the saline-control females and 0% in the vehicle-control females. The presence of endometritis coupled with the absence of corpora lutea, the reduction in mammary fibroadenomas, and the presence of uterine dilatation suggest that the uterine tumors were associated with estrogen dominance in the aged female rats which does not occur in humans.

Octreotide did not impair fertility in rats at doses up to 1000 mcg/kg/day, which represents 7× the human exposure based on body surface area.

Pregnancy Category B

Reproduction studies have been performed in rats and rabbits at doses up to 16 times the highest human dose based on body surface area and have revealed no evidence of impaired fertility or harm to the fetus due to octreotide. There are, however, no adequate and well-controlled studies in pregnant women. Because animal reproduction studies are not always predictive of human response, this drug should be used during pregnancy only if clearly needed.

Nursing Mothers

It is not known whether this drug is excreted in human milk. Because many drugs are excreted in milk, caution should be exercised when Sandostatin LAR® Depot is administered to a nursing woman.

Pediatric Use

Sandostatin LAR® Depot has not been studied in pediatric patients.

Experience with Sandostatin® Injection in the pediatric population is limited. Its use has been primarily in patients with congenital hyperinsulinism (also called nesidioblastosis). The youngest patient to receive the drug was 1 month old. At doses of 1-40 mcg/kg body weight/day, the majority of side effects observed were gastrointestinal-steatorrhea, diarrhea, vomiting and abdominal distention. Poor growth has been reported in several patients treated with Sandostatin® Injection for more than 1 year; catch-up growth occurred after Sandostatin® Injection was discontinued. A 16-month-old male with enterocutaneous fistula developed sudden abdominal pain and increased nasogastric drainage and died 8 hours after receiving a single 100 mcg subcutaneous dose of Sandostatin® Injection.

Continued on next page

Sandostatin LAR—Cont.

ADVERSE REACTIONS *(See WARNINGS and PRECAUTIONS.)*

Gallbladder abnormalities, especially stones and/or biliary sludge, frequently develop in patients on chronic octreotide therapy *(see WARNINGS)*. Few patients, however, develop acute symptoms requiring cholecystectomy.

Cardiac

In acromegalics, sinus bradycardia (<50 bpm) developed in 25%; conduction abnormalities occurred in 10% and arrhythmias developed in 9% of patients during Sandostatin® (octreotide acetate) Injection therapy. Electrocardiograms were performed only in carcinoid patients receiving Sandostatin LAR® Depot (octreotide acetate for injectable suspension). In carcinoid syndrome patients sinus bradycardia developed in 19%; conduction abnormalities occurred in 9%, and arrhythmias developed in 3%. The relationship of these events to octreotide acetate is not established because many of these patients have underlying cardiac disease *(see PRECAUTIONS)*.

Gastrointestinal

The most common symptoms are gastrointestinal. The overall incidence of the most frequent of these symptoms in clinical trials of acromegalic patients treated for approximately 1 to 4 years is shown in Table 4.

[See table 4 below]

Only 2.6% of the patients on Sandostatin® Injection in U.S. clinical trials discontinued therapy due to these symptoms. No acromegalic patient receiving Sandostatin LAR® Depot discontinued therapy for a G.I. event.

In patients receiving Sandostatin LAR® Depot the incidence of diarrhea was dose related. Diarrhea, abdominal pain, and nausea developed primarily during the first month of treatment with Sandostatin LAR® Depot. Thereafter, new cases of these events were uncommon. The vast majority of these events were mild-to-moderate in severity.

In rare instances gastrointestinal adverse effects may resemble acute intestinal obstruction, with progressive abdominal distention, severe epigastric pain, abdominal tenderness, and guarding.

Dyspepsia, steatorrhea, discoloration of feces, and tenesmus were reported in 4%-6% of patients.

In a clinical trial of carcinoid syndrome, nausea, abdominal pain, and flatulence were reported in 27%-38% and constipation or vomiting in 15%-21% of patients treated with Sandostatin LAR® Depot. Diarrhea was reported as an adverse event in 14% of patients but since most of the patients had diarrhea as a symptom of carcinoid syndrome, it is difficult to assess the actual incidence of drug-related diarrhea.

Hypo/Hyperglycemia

In acromegaly patients treated with either Sandostatin® Injection or Sandostatin LAR® Depot, hypoglycemia occurred in approximately 2% and hyperglycemia in approximately 15% of patients. In carcinoid patients, hypoglycemia occurred in 4% and hyperglycemia in 27% of patients treated with Sandostatin LAR® Depot *(see PRECAUTIONS)*.

Hypothyroidism

In acromegaly patients receiving Sandostatin® Injection, 12% developed biochemical hypothyroidism, 8% developed goiter, and 4% required initiation of thyroid replacement therapy while receiving Sandostatin® Injection. In acromegalics treated with Sandostatin LAR® Depot hypothyroidism was reported as an adverse event in 2% and goiter in 2%. Two patients receiving Sandostatin LAR® Depot, required initiation of thyroid hormone replacement therapy. In carcinoid patients, hypothyroidism has only been reported in isolated patients and goiter has not been reported *(see PRECAUTIONS)*.

Pain at the Injection Site

Pain on injection, which is generally mild-to-moderate, and short-lived (usually about 1 hour) is dose related, being reported by 2%, 9%, and 11% of acromegalics receiving doses of 10 mg, 20 mg and 30 mg, respectively, of Sandostatin LAR® Depot. In carcinoid patients, where a diary was kept, pain at the injection site was reported by about 20%-25% at a 10-mg dose and about 30%-50% at the 20-mg and 30-mg dose.

Other Adverse Events 16%-20%

Other adverse events (relationship to drug not established) in acromegalic and/or carcinoid syndrome patients receiving Sandostatin LAR® Depot were upper respiratory infection, flu-like symptoms, fatigue, dizziness, headache, malaise, fever, dyspnea, back pain, chest pain, arthropathy.

Other Adverse Events 5%-15%

Other adverse events (relationship to drug not established) occurring in an incidence of 5%-15% in patients receiving Sandostatin LAR® Depot were:

Body As a Whole: asthenia, rigors, allergy
Cardiovascular: hypertension, peripheral edema
Central and Peripheral Nervous System: paresthesia, hypoesthesia
Gastrointestinal: dyspepsia, anorexia, hemorrhoids
Hearing and Vestibular: earache
Heart Rate and Rhythm: palpitations
Hematologic: anemia
Metabolic and Nutritional: dehydration, weight decrease
Musculoskeletal System: myalgia, leg cramps, arthralgia
Psychiatric: depression, anxiety, confusion, insomnia
Resistance Mechanism: viral infection, otitis media
Respiratory System: coughing, pharyngitis, rhinitis, sinusitis
Skin and Appendages: rash, pruritus, increased sweating
Urinary System: urinary tract infection, renal calculus

Other Adverse Events 1%-4%

Other events (relationship to drug not established), each occurring in an incidence of 1%-4% in patients receiving Sandostatin LAR® Depot and reported by at least 2 patients were:

Application Site: injection site inflammation
Body As a Whole: syncope, ascites, hot flushes
Cardiovascular: cardiac failure, angina pectoris, hypertension aggravated
Central and Peripheral Nervous System: vertigo, abnormal gait, neuropathy, neuralgia, tremor, dysphonia, hyperkinesia, hypertonia
Gastrointestinal: rectal bleeding, melena, gastritis, gastroenteritis, colitis, gingivitis, taste perversion, stomatitis, glossitis, dry mouth, dysphagia, steatorrhea, diverticulitis
Hearing and Vestibular: tinnitus
Heart Rate and Rhythm: tachycardia
Liver and Biliary: jaundice
Metabolic and Nutritional: hypokalemia, cachexia, gout, hypoproteinemia
Platelet, Bleeding, Clotting: pulmonary embolism, epistaxis
Psychiatric: amnesia, somnolence, nervousness, hallucinations
Reproductive, Female: menstrual irregularities, breast pain
Reproductive, Male: impotence
Resistance Mechanism: cellulitis, renal abcess, moniliasis, bacterial infection
Respiratory System: bronchitis, pneumonia, pleural effusion
Skin and Appendages: alopecia, urticaria, acne
Urinary System: incontinence, albuminuria
Vascular: cerebral vascular disorder, phlebitis, hematoma
Vision: abnormal vision

Rare Adverse Events

Other events (relationship to drug not established) of potential clinical significance occurring rarely (<1%) in clinical trials of octreotide either as Sandostatin® Injection or Sandostatin LAR® Depot, or reported post-marketing in patients with acromegaly, carcinoid syndrome, or other disorders include:

Body As a Whole: anaphylactoid reactions, including anaphylactic shock, facial edema, generalized edema, abdomen enlarged, malignant hyperpyrexia
Cardiovascular: aneurysm, myocardial infarction, angina pectoris, aggravated, pulmonary hypertension, cardiac arrest, orthostatic hypotension
Central and Peripheral Nervous System: hemiparesis, paresis, convulsions, paranoia, pituitary apoplexy, visual field defect, migraine, aphasia, scotoma, Bell's palsy
Endocrine Disorders: hypoadrenalism, diabetes insipidus, gynecomastia, galactorrhea
Gastrointestinal: G.I. hemorrhage, intestinal obstruction, hepatitis, increase in liver enzymes, fatty liver, peptic/gastric ulcer, gallbladder polyp, appendicitis, pancreatitis
Hearing and Vestibular: deafness
Heart Rate and Rhythm: atrial fibrillation
Hematologic: pancytopenia, thrombocytopenia
Metabolic and Nutritional: renal insufficiency, creatinine increased, CK increased, diabetes mellitus
Musculoskeletal: Raynaud's syndrome, arthritis, joint effusion
Neoplasms: breast carcinoma, basal cell carcinoma
Platelet, Bleeding, and Clotting: arterial thrombosis of the arm
Psychiatric: suicide attempt, libido decrease
Reproductive, Female: lactation, nonpuerperal
Respiratory: pulmonary nodule, status asthmaticus, pneumothorax
Skin and Appendages: cellulitis, petechiae, urticaria
Urinary System: renal failure, hematuria
Vascular: intracranial hemorrhage, retinal vein thrombosis
Vision: glaucoma

Antibodies to Octreotide

Studies to date have shown that antibodies to octreotide develop in up to 25% of patients treated with octreotide acetate. These antibodies do not influence the degree of efficacy response to octreotide; however, in two acromegalic patients who received Sandostatin® Injection, the duration of GH suppression following each injection was about twice as long as in patients without antibodies. It has not been determined whether octreotide antibodies will also prolong the duration of GH suppression in patients being treated with Sandostatin LAR® Depot.

OVERDOSAGE

No frank overdose has occurred in any patient to date. Sandostatin® (octreotide acetate) Injection given in intravenous bolus doses of 1 mg (1000 mcg) to healthy volunteers did not result in serious ill effects, nor did doses of 30 mg (30,000 mcg) given IV over 20 minutes and of 120 mg (120,000 mcg) given IV over 8 hours to research patients. Doses of 2.5 mg (2500 mcg) of Sandostatin® Injection subcutaneously have, however, caused hypoglycemia, flushing, dizziness, and nausea.

Up-to-date information about the treatment of overdose can often be obtained from a certified Regional Poison Control Center. Telephone numbers of certified Regional Poison Control Centers are listed in the *Physicians' Desk Reference®**.

Mortality occurred in mice and rats given 72 mg/kg and 18 mg/kg IV, respectively, of octreotide.

Drug Abuse and Dependence

There is no indication that octreotide has potential for drug abuse or dependence. Octreotide levels in the central nervous system are negligible, even after doses up to 30,000 mcg.

DOSAGE AND ADMINISTRATION

Sandostatin LAR® Depot (octreotide acetate for injectable suspension) must be administered under the supervision of a physician. **Do not directly inject diluent without preparing suspension.** It is important to closely follow the mixing instructions included in the packaging. Sandostatin LAR® Depot must be administered immediately after mixing. Sandostatin LAR® Depot should be administered intragluteally at four-week intervals. Administration of Sandostatin LAR® Depot at intervals greater than 4 weeks is not recommended because there is no adequate information on whether such patients could be satisfactorily controlled. Deltoid injections are to be avoided because of significant discomfort at the injection site when given in that area. **Sandostatin LAR® Depot should never be administered by the IV or S.C. routes.** The following dosage regimens are recommended.

Acromegaly

1. Patients Not Currently Receiving Octreotide Acetate

Patients not currently receiving octreotide acetate should begin therapy with Sandostatin® (octreotide acetate) Injection given subcutaneously in an initial dose of 50 mcg t.i.d. Beginning with this low dose may permit adaptation to adverse gastrointestinal effects for patients who require higher doses. Multiple growth hormone (GH) determinations at 0-8 hours after a subcutaneous Sandostatin® Injection will guide dosage titration. The goal is to attempt to normalize GH and IGF-1 (somatomedin C) levels. Most patients require doses of 100 mcg to 200 mcg t.i.d. for maximum effect but some patients require up to 500 mcg t.i.d. Injection sites should be rotated in a systematic manner to avoid irritation.

Although responsiveness of GH to octreotide acetate can be ascertained quickly, patients should be maintained on Sandostatin® Injection s.c. for at least 2 weeks to determine tolerance to octreotide.

The most common adverse events are gastrointestinal, which usually begin within the first few days of administration and usually subside within 2 to 8 weeks. In clinical trials, <3% of patients discontinued Sandostatin® Injection because of G.I. symptoms.

Patients who are considered to be "responders" to the drug, based on GH and IGF-1 levels, and who tolerate the drug, can then be switched to Sandostatin LAR® Depot in the dosage scheme described under 2, below (Patients Currently Receiving Sandostatin® Injection).

2. Patients Currently Receiving Sandostatin® (octreotide acetate) Injection

Patients currently receiving Sandostatin® Injection can be switched directly to Sandostatin LAR® Depot in a dose of 20 mg given IM intragluteally at 4-week intervals for 3 months. **(Deltoid injections are to be avoided because of significant discomfort at the injection site when given in that area.)** Gluteal injection sites should be alternated to avoid irritation.

At the end of 3 months Sandostatin LAR® Depot dosage may be continued at the same level or increased or decreased based on the following regimen:

GH ≤2.5 ng/mL, IGF-1 normal and clinical symptoms controlled: maintain Sandostatin LAR® Depot dosage at 20 mg every 4 weeks.

Table 4
Number (%) of Acromegalic Patients with Common G.I. Adverse Events

Adverse Event	Sandostatin® Injection S.C. t.i.d. n=114 N	%	Sandostatin LAR® Depot q. 28 days n=261 N	%
Diarrhea	66	(57.9)	95	(36.4)
Abdominal Pain or Discomfort	50	(43.9)	76	(29.1)
Flatulence	15	(13.2)	67	(25.7)
Constipation	10	(8.8)	49	(18.8)
Nausea	34	(29.8)	27	(10.3)
Vomiting	5	(4.4)	17	(6.5)

GH >2.5 ng/mL, IGF-1 elevated, and/or clinical symptoms uncontrolled, increase Sandostatin LAR® Depot dosage to 30 mg every 4 weeks.

GH ≤1 ng/mL, IGF-1 normal and clinical symptoms controlled, reduce Sandostatin LAR® Depot dosage to 10 mg every 4 weeks.

Patients whose GH, IGF-1, and symptoms are not adequately controlled at a dose of 30 mg may have the dose increased to 40 mg every 4 weeks. Doses higher than 40 mg are not recommended.

Administration of Sandostatin LAR® Depot at intervals greater than 4 weeks is not recommended because there is no adequate information on whether such patients could be satisfactorily controlled.

In patients who have received pituitary irradiation, Sandostatin LAR® Depot should be withdrawn yearly for approximately 8 weeks to assess disease activity. If GH or IGF-1 levels increase and signs and symptoms recur, Sandostatin LAR® Depot therapy may be resumed.

3. Special Populations: Renal Failure

In patients with renal failure requiring dialysis, the half-life of octreotide may be increased, necessitating adjustment of the maintenance dosage *(see CLINICAL PHARMACOLOGY and Pharmacokinetics of Octreotide Acetate).*

Carcinoid Tumors and VIPomas

1. Patients Not Currently Receiving Octreotide Acetate

Patients not currently receiving octreotide acetate should begin therapy with Sandostatin® Injection given subcutaneously. The suggested daily dosage for carcinoid tumors during the first 2 weeks of therapy ranges from 100-600 mcg/day in 2-4 divided doses (mean daily dosage is 300 mcg). Some patients may require doses up to 1500 mcg/day. The suggested daily dosage for VIPomas is 200-300 mcg in 2-4 divided doses (range 150-750 mcg); dosage may be adjusted on an individual basis to control symptoms but usually doses above 450 mcg/day are not required.

Sandostatin® Injection should be continued for at least 2 weeks. Thereafter, patients who are considered "responders" to octreotide acetate and who tolerate the drug may be switched to Sandostatin LAR® Depot in the dosage regimen described under 2, below (Patients Currently Receiving Sandostatin® Injection).

2. Patients Currently Receiving Sandostatin® (octreotide acetate) Injection

Patients currently receiving Sandostatin® Injection can be switched to Sandostatin LAR® Depot in a dosage of 20 mg given IM intragluteally at 4-week intervals for 2 months. **Deltoid injections are to be avoided because of significant discomfort at the injection site when given in that area.** Gluteal injection sites should be alternated to avoid irritation. Because of the need for serum octreotide to reach therapeutically effective levels following initial injection of Sandostatin LAR® Depot, carcinoid tumor and VIPoma patients should continue to receive Sandostatin® Injection s.c. for at least 2 weeks in the same dosage they were taking before the switch. Failure to continue subcutaneous injections for this period may result in exacerbation of symptoms. (Some patients may require 3 or 4 weeks of such therapy.)

After two months of a 20-mg dosage of Sandostatin LAR® Depot, dosage may be increased to 30 mg every 4 weeks if symptoms are not adequately controlled. Patients who achieve good control on a 20-mg dose may have their dose lowered to 10 mg for a trial period. If symptoms recur, dosage should then be increased to 20 mg every 4 weeks. Many patients can, however, be satisfactorily maintained at a 10-mg dosage every 4 weeks. A dose of 10 mg is not recommended as a starting dose, however, because therapeutically effective levels of octreotide are reached more rapidly with a 20-mg dose.

Dosages higher than 30 mg are not recommended because there is no information on their usefulness.

Despite good overall control of symptoms, patients with carcinoid tumors and VIPomas often experience periodic exacerbation of symptoms (regardless of whether they are being maintained on Sandostatin® Injection or Sandostatin LAR® Depot). During these periods they may be given Sandostatin® Injection s.c. for a few days at the dosage they were receiving prior to switch to Sandostatin LAR® Depot. When symptoms are again controlled, the Sandostatin® Injection s.c. can be discontinued.

Administration of Sandostatin LAR® Depot at intervals greater than 4 weeks is not recommended because there is no adequate information on whether such patients could be adequately controlled.

3. Special Populations: Renal Failure

In patients with renal failure requiring dialysis, the half-life of octreotide may be increased, necessitating adjustment of the maintenance dosage *(see CLINICAL PHARMACOLOGY and Pharmacokinetics of Octreotide Acetate).*

HOW SUPPLIED

Sandostatin LAR® Depot (octreotide acetate for injectable suspension) is available in single-use kits containing a 5-mL vial of 10 mg, 20 mg or 30 mg strength, a syringe containing 2.5 mL of diluent, two sterile 1 1/2″ 19 gauge needles, and two alcohol wipes. An instruction booklet for the preparation of drug suspension for injection is also included with each kit.

Drug Product Kits

10 mg kit	NDC 0078-0340-61
20 mg kit	NDC 0078-0341-61
30 mg kit	NDC 0078-0342-61
Demonstration kit	NDC 0078-9342-61

Storage

For prolonged storage, Sandostatin LAR® Depot should be stored at refrigerated temperatures between 2°C and 8°C (36°F-46°F) and protected from light until the time of use. Sandostatin LAR® Depot drug product kit should remain at room temperature for 30-60 minutes prior to preparation of the drug suspension. However, after preparation the drug suspension must be administered immediately.

*Trademark of Medical Economics Company, Inc.

REV: APRIL 2004 T2004-23
89018502

Sandostatin LAR® Depot vials are manufactured by:
Biochemie GmbH, Schaftenau, Austria
(Subsidiary of Novartis Pharma AG, Basle, Switzerland)
The diluent syringes are manufactured by:
Solvay Pharmaceuticals B.V.
Olst, The Netherlands
Distributed by:
Novartis Pharmaceuticals Corporation
East Hanover, New Jersey 07936
©Novartis

Shown in Product Identification Guide, page 325

SIMULECT® ℞

[*sĭm ew lĕkt*]
(basiliximab)
For Injection
Rx only

Prescribing Information

The following prescribing information is based on official labeling in effect July 2004.

WARNING

Only physicians experienced in immunosuppression therapy and management of organ transplantation patients should prescribe Simulect® (basiliximab). The physician responsible for Simulect® administration should have complete information requisite for the follow-up of the patient. Patients receiving the drug should be managed in facilities equipped and staffed with adequate laboratory and supportive medical resources.

DESCRIPTION

Simulect® (basiliximab) is a chimeric (murine/human) monoclonal antibody ($IgG_{1\kappa}$), produced by recombinant DNA technology, that functions as an immunosuppressive agent, specifically binding to and blocking the interleukin-2 receptor α-chain (IL-2Rα, also known as CD25 antigen) on the surface of activated T-lymphocytes. Based on the amino acid sequence, the calculated molecular weight of the protein is 144 kilodaltons. It is a glycoprotein obtained from fermentation of an established mouse myeloma cell line genetically engineered to express plasmids containing the human heavy and light chain constant region genes and mouse heavy and light chain variable region genes encoding the RFT5 antibody that binds selectively to the IL-2Rα.

The active ingredient, basiliximab, is water soluble. The drug product, Simulect®, is a sterile lyophilisate which is available in 6 mL colorless glass vials and is available in 10 mg and 20 mg strengths.

Each 10-mg vial contains 10 mg basiliximab, 3.61 mg monobasic potassium phosphate, 0.50 mg disodium hydrogen phosphate (anhydrous), 0.80 mg sodium chloride, 10 mg sucrose, 40 mg mannitol and 20 mg glycine, to be reconstituted in 2.5 mL of Sterile Water for Injection, USP. No preservatives are added.

Each 20-mg vial contains 20 mg basiliximab, 7.21 mg monobasic potassium phosphate, 0.99 mg disodium hydrogen phosphate (anhydrous), 1.61 mg sodium chloride, 20 mg sucrose, 80 mg mannitol and 40 mg glycine, to be reconstituted in 5 mL of Sterile Water for Injection, USP. No preservatives are added.

CLINICAL PHARMACOLOGY

General

Mechanism of Action: Basiliximab functions as an IL-2 receptor antagonist by binding with high affinity ($K_a = 1 \times 10^{10}\ M^{-1}$) to the alpha chain of the high affinity IL-2 receptor complex and inhibiting IL-2 binding. Basiliximab is specifically targeted against IL-2Rα, which is selectively expressed on the surface of activated T-lymphocytes. This specific high affinity binding of Simulect® to IL-2Rα competitively inhibits IL-2-mediated activation of lymphocytes, a critical pathway in the cellular immune response involved in allograft rejection.

While in the circulation, Simulect® impairs the response of the immune system to antigenic challenges. Whether the ability to respond to repeated or ongoing challenges with those antigens returns to normal after Simulect® is cleared is unknown *(see PRECAUTIONS).*

Pharmacokinetics

Adults: Single-dose and multiple-dose pharmacokinetic studies have been conducted in patients undergoing first kidney transplantation. Cumulative doses ranged from 15 mg up to 150 mg. Peak mean ± SD serum concentration following intravenous infusion of 20 mg over 30 minutes is 7.1 ± 5.1 mg/L. There is a dose-proportional increase in C_{max} and AUC up to the highest tested single dose of 60 mg. The volume of distribution at steady state is 8.6 ± 4.1 L. The extent and degree of distribution to various body compartments have not been fully studied. The terminal half-life is 7.2 ± 3.2 days. Total body clearance is 41 ± 19 mL/h. No clinically relevant influence of body weight or gender on distribution volume or clearance has been observed in adult patients. Elimination half-life was not influenced by age (20-69 years), gender or race *(see DOSAGE AND ADMINISTRATION).*

Pediatric: The pharmacokinetics of Simulect® have been assessed in 39 pediatric patients undergoing renal transplantation. In infants and children (1-11 years of age, n=25), the distribution volume and clearance were reduced by about 50% compared to adult renal transplantation patients. The volume of distribution at steady state was 4.8 ± 2.1 L, half-life was 9.5 ± 4.5 days and clearance was 17 ± 6 mL/h. Disposition parameters were not influenced to a clinically relevant extent by age (1-11 years of age), body weight (9-37 kg) or body surface area (0.44-1.20 m^2) in this age group. In adolescents (12-16 years of age, n=14), disposition was similar to that in adult renal transplantation patients. The volume of distribution at steady state was 7.8 ± 5.1 L, half-life was 9.1 ± 3.9 days and clearance was 31 ± 19 mL/h *(see DOSAGE AND ADMINISTRATION).*

Pharmacodynamics

Complete and consistent binding to IL-2Rα in adults is maintained as long as serum Simulect® levels exceed 0.2 µg/mL. As concentrations fall below this threshold, the IL-2Rα sites are no longer fully bound and the number of T-cells expressing unbound IL-2Rα returns to pretherapy values within 1-2 weeks. The relationship between serum concentration and receptor saturation was assessed in 13 pediatric patients and was similar to that characterized in adult renal transplantation patients. *In vitro* studies using human tissues indicate that Simulect® binds only to lymphocytes.

The duration of clinically relevant IL-2 receptor blockade after the recommended course of Simulect® is not known. When basiliximab was added to a regimen of cyclosporine, USP (MODIFIED) and corticosteroids in adult patients, the duration of IL-2Rα saturation was 36 ± 14 days (mean ± SD), similar to that observed in pediatric patients (36 ± 14 days) *(see DOSAGE AND ADMINISTRATION).* When basiliximab was added to a triple therapy regimen consisting of cyclosporine, USP (MODIFIED), corticosteroids, and azathioprine in adults, the duration was 50 ± 20 days and when added to cyclosporine, USP (MODIFIED), corticosteroids, and mycophenolate mofetil in adults, the duration was 59 ± 17 days *(see PRECAUTIONS, Drug Interactions).* No significant changes to circulating lymphocyte numbers or cell phenotypes were observed by flow cytometry.

CLINICAL STUDIES

The safety and efficacy of Simulect® for the prophylaxis of acute organ rejection in adults following cadaveric- or living-donor renal transplantation were assessed in four randomized, double-blind, placebo-controlled clinical studies (1,184 patients). Of these four, two studies (Study 1 [EU/CAN] and Study 2 [US study]) compared two 20-mg doses of Simulect® with placebo, each administered intravenously as an infusion, as part of a standard immunosuppressive regimen comprised of cyclosporine, USP (MODIFIED) and corticosteroids. The other two controlled studies compared two 20-mg doses of Simulect® with placebo, each administered intravenously as a bolus injection, as part of a standard triple-immunosuppressive regimen comprised of cyclosporine, USP (MODIFIED), corticosteroids and either azathioprine or mycophenolate mofetil (Study 3 and Study 4, respectively). The first dose of Simulect® or placebo was administered within 2 hours prior to transplantation surgery (Day 0) and the second dose administered on Day 4 post-transplantation. The regimen of Simulect® was chosen to provide 30-45 days of IL-2Rα saturation.

729 patients were enrolled in the two studies using a dual maintenance immunosuppressive regimen comprised of cyclosporine, USP (MODIFIED) and corticosteroids, of which 363 patients were treated with Simulect® and 358 patients were placebo-treated. Study 1 was conducted at 21 sites in Europe and Canada (EU/CAN Study); Study 2 was conducted at 21 sites in the USA (US Study). Patients 18-75 years of age undergoing first cadaveric (Study 1 and Study 2) or living-donor (Study 2 only) renal transplantation, with ≥1 HLA mismatch, were enrolled.[1,2]

The primary efficacy endpoint in both studies was the incidence of death, graft loss or an episode of acute rejection during the first 6 months post-transplantation. Secondary efficacy endpoints included the primary efficacy variable measured during the first 12 months post-transplantation, the incidence of biopsy-confirmed acute rejection during the first 6 and 12 months post-transplantation, and patient survival and graft survival, each measured at 12 months post-transplantation. Table 1 summarizes the results of these studies. Figure 1 displays the Kaplan-Meier estimates of the percentage of patients by treatment group experiencing the primary efficacy endpoint during the first 12 months post-transplantation for Study 2. Patients in both studies receiving Simulect® experienced a significantly lower incidence of biopsy-confirmed rejection episodes at both 6 and 12 months post-transplantation. There was no difference in the rate of delayed graft function, patient survival, or graft survival between Simulect®-treated patients and placebo-treated patients in either study.

There was no evidence that the clinical benefit of Simulect® was limited to specific subpopulations based on age, gender, race, donor type (cadaveric or living donor allograft) or history of diabetes mellitus.

Continued on next page

Simulect—Cont.

[See table 1 at right]

Figure 1
Kaplan-Meier Estimate of the Percentage of Subjects with Death, Graft Loss or First Rejection Episode (Dual Therapy)

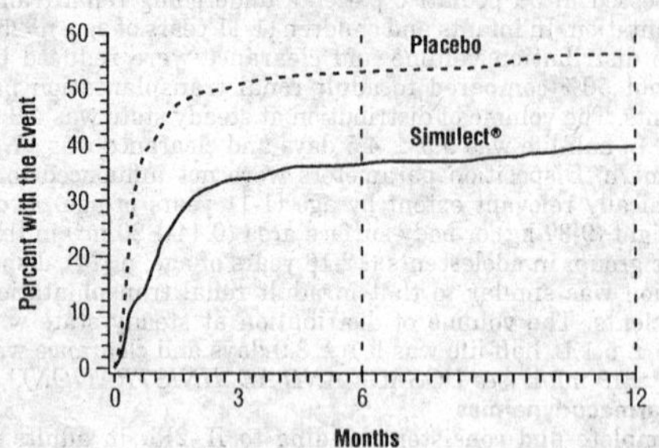

Two double-blind, randomized, placebo-controlled studies (Study 3 and Study 4) assessed the safety and efficacy of Simulect® for the prophylaxis of acute renal transplant rejection in adults when used in combination with a triple immunosuppressive regimen. In Study 3, 340 patients were concomitantly treated with cyclosporine, USP (MODIFIED), corticosteroids and azathioprine (AZA), of which 168 patients were treated with Simulect® and 172 patients were treated with placebo. In Study 4, 123 patients were concomitantly treated with cyclosporine, USP (MODIFIED), corticosteroids and mycophenolate mofetil (MMF), of which 59 patients were treated with Simulect® and 64 patients were treated with placebo. Patients 18-70 years of age undergoing first or second cadaveric or living donor (related or unrelated) renal transplantation were enrolled in both studies. The results of Study 3 are shown in Table 2. These results are consistent with the findings from Study 1 and Study 2.

[See table 2 at right]

In Study 4, the percentage of patients experiencing biopsy-proven acute rejection by 6 months was 15% (9 of 59 patients) in the Simulect® group and 27% (17 of 64 patients) in the placebo group. Although numerically lower, the difference in acute rejection was not significant.

In a multicenter, randomized, double-blind, placebo-controlled trial of Simulect® for the prevention of allograft rejection in liver transplant recipients (n=381) receiving concomitant cyclosporine, USP (MODIFIED) and steroids, the incidence of the combined endpoint of death, graft loss, or first biopsy-confirmed rejection episode at either 6 or 12 months was similar between patients randomized to receive Simulect® and those randomized to receive placebo.

The efficacy of Simulect® for the prophylaxis of acute rejection in recipients of a second renal allograft has not been demonstrated.

Long Term Follow-up

Five-year patient survival and graft survival data were provided by 71% and 58% of the original subjects of Study 1 and Study 2, respectively. Subjects in both studies continued to receive a dual-therapy regimen with cyclosporine, USP (MODIFIED) and corticosteroid. No difference was observed between groups in the 5-year graft survival in either Study 1 (91% Simulect® group, 92% placebo group) or Study 2 (85% Simulect® group, 86% placebo group). In Study 1, patient survival was lower in the Simulect®-treated patients compared to the placebo-treated patients (142/163 [87%] versus 156/164 [95%], respectively). The cause of this difference in survival is unknown. The data do not indicate an increase in malignancy- or infection-related mortality. In Study 2, patient survival in the placebo group (90%) was the same compared to Simulect® group (90%).

INDICATIONS AND USAGE

Simulect® is indicated for the prophylaxis of acute organ rejection in patients receiving renal transplantation when used as part of an immunosuppressive regimen that includes cyclosporine, USP (MODIFIED) and corticosteroids. The efficacy of Simulect® for the prophylaxis of acute rejection in recipients of other solid organ allografts has not been demonstrated.

CONTRAINDICATIONS

Simulect® is contraindicated in patients with known hypersensitivity to basiliximab or any other component of the formulation. *See composition of Simulect® under DESCRIPTION.*

WARNINGS. *See Boxed WARNING.*

General

Simulect® should be administered under qualified medical supervision. Patients should be informed of the potential benefits of therapy and the risks associated with administration of immunosuppressive therapy.

While neither the incidence of lympho-proliferative disorders nor opportunistic infections was higher in Simulect®-treated patients than in placebo-treated patients, patients on immunosuppressive therapy are at increased risk for developing these complications and should be monitored accordingly.

Hypersensitivity

Severe acute (onset within 24 hours) hypersensitivity reactions including anaphylaxis have been observed both on initial exposure to Simulect® and/or following re-exposure after several months. These reactions may include hypotension, tachycardia, cardiac failure, dyspnea, wheezing, bronchospasm, pulmonary edema, respiratory failure, urticaria, rash, pruritus, and/or sneezing. If a severe hypersensitivity reaction occurs, therapy with Simulect® should be permanently discontinued. Medications for the treatment of severe hypersensitivity reactions including anaphylaxis should be available for immediate use. Patients previously administered Simulect® should only be re-exposed to a subsequent course of therapy with extreme caution. The potential risks of such re-administration, specifically those associated with immunosuppression, are not known.

Table 1
Efficacy Parameters (Percentage of Patients)

Dual-therapy Regimen (cyclosporine* and corticosteroids)	Study 1 Placebo (N=185)	Study 1 Simulect® (N=190)	Study 1 p-value	Study 2 Placebo (N=173)	Study 2 Simulect® (N=173)	Study 2 p-value
Primary endpoint						
Death, graft loss or acute rejection episode (0-6 months)	57%	42%	0.003	55%	38%	0.002
Secondary endpoints						
Death, graft loss or acute rejection episode (0-12 months)	60%	46%	0.007	58%	41%	0.001
Biopsy-confirmed rejection episode (0-6 months)	44%	30%	0.007	46%	33%	0.015
Biopsy-confirmed rejection episode (0-12 months)	46%	32%	0.005	49%	35%	0.009
Patient survival (12 months)	97%	95%	0.29	96%	97%	0.56
Patients with functioning graft (12 months)	87%	88%	0.70	93%	95%	0.50

*USP (MODIFIED)

Table 2
Efficacy Parameters (Percentage of Patients)

Study 3: Triple-therapy Regimen (cyclosporine*, corticosteroids, and azathioprine)	Placebo (N=172)	Simulect® (N=168)	p-value
Primary endpoint			
Acute rejection episode (0-6 months)	35%	21%	0.005
Secondary endpoints			
Death, graft loss or acute rejection episode (0-6 months)	40%	26%	0.008
Biopsy-confirmed rejection episode (0-6 months)	29%	18%	0.023
Patient survival (12 months)	97%	98%	1.000
Patients with functioning graft (12 months)	88%	90%	0.599

*USP (MODIFIED)

PRECAUTIONS

General

It is not known whether Simulect® use will have a long-term effect on the ability of the immune system to respond to antigens first encountered during Simulect®-induced immunosuppression.

Immunogenicity

Of renal transplantation patients treated with Simulect® and tested for anti-idiotype antibodies, 4/339 developed an anti-idiotype antibody response, with no deleterious clinical effect upon the patient. In none of these cases was there evidence that the presence of anti-idiotype antibody accelerated Simulect® clearance or decreased the period of receptor saturation. In Study 2, the incidence of human anti-murine antibody (HAMA) in renal transplantation patients treated with Simulect® was 2/138 in patients not exposed to muromonab-CD3 and 4/34 in patients who subsequently received muromonab-CD3. The available clinical data on the use of muromonab-CD3 in patients previously treated with Simulect® suggest that subsequent use of muromonab-CD3 or other murine anti-lymphocytic antibody preparations is not precluded.

These data reflect the percentage of patients whose test results were considered positive for antibodies to Simulect® in an ELISA assay, and are highly dependent on the sensitivity and specificity of the assay. Additionally the observed incidence of antibody positivity in an assay may be influenced by several factors including sample handling, concomitant medications, and underlying disease. For these reasons, comparison of the incidence of antibodies to Simulect® with the incidence of antibodies to other products may be misleading.

Drug Interactions

No dose adjustment is necessary when Simulect® is added to triple-immunosuppression regimens including cyclosporine, corticosteroids, and either azathioprine or mycophenolate mofetil. Three clinical trials have investigated Simulect® use in combination with triple-therapy regimens. Pharmacokinetics were assessed in two of these trials. Total body clearance of Simulect® was reduced by an average 22% and 51% when azathioprine and mycophenolate mofetil, respectively, were added to a regimen consisting of cyclosporine, USP (MODIFIED) and corticosteroids. Nonetheless, the range of individual Simulect® clearance values in the presence of azathioprine (12-57 mL/h) or mycophenolate mofetil (7-54 mL/h) did not extend outside the range observed with dual therapy (10-78 mL/h). The following medications have been administered in clinical trials with Simulect® with no increase in adverse reactions: ATG/ALG, azathioprine, corticosteroids, cyclosporine, mycophenolate mofetil, and muromonab-CD3.

Carcinogenesis/Mutagenesis/Impairment of Fertility

No mutagenic potential of Simulect® was observed in the *in vitro* assays with Salmonella (Ames) and V79 Chinese hamster cells. No long-term or fertility studies in laboratory animals have been performed to evaluate the potential of Simulect® to produce carcinogenicity or fertility impairment, respectively.

Pregnancy Category B

There are no adequate and well-controlled studies in pregnant women. No maternal toxicity, embryotoxicity, or teratogenicity was observed in cynomolgus monkeys 100 days post coitum following dosing with basiliximab during the organogenesis period; blood levels in pregnant monkeys were 13-fold higher than those seen in human patients. Immunotoxicology studies have not been performed in the offspring. Because IgG molecules are known to cross the placental barrier, because the IL-2 receptor may play an important role in development of the immune system, and because animal reproduction studies are not always predictive of human response, Simulect® should only be used in pregnant women when the potential benefit justifies the potential risk to the fetus. Women of childbearing potential should use effective contraception before beginning Simulect® therapy, during therapy, and for 4 months after completion of Simulect® therapy.

Nursing Mothers

It is not known whether Simulect® is excreted in human milk. Because many drugs including human antibodies are excreted in human milk, and because of the potential for adverse reactions, a decision should be made to discontinue nursing or to discontinue the drug, taking into account the importance of the drug to the mother.

Pediatric Use

No randomized, placebo-controlled studies have been completed in pediatric patients. In a safety and pharmacokinetic study, 41 pediatric patients (1-11 years of age [n=27], 12-16 years of age [n=14], median age 8.1 years) were treated with Simulect® via intravenous bolus injection in addition to standard immunosuppressive agents including cyclosporine, USP (MODIFIED), corticosteroids, azathioprine, and mycophenolate mofetil. The acute rejection rate at six months was comparable to that in adults in the triple-therapy trials. The most frequently reported adverse events were hypertension, hypertrichosis, and rhinitis (49% each), urinary tract infections (46%), and fever (39%). Overall, the adverse event profile was consistent with general clinical experience in the pediatric renal transplantation population and with the profile in the controlled adult renal transplantation studies. The available pharmacokinetic data in children and adolescents are described in *CLINICAL PHARMACOLOGY* and *DOSAGE AND ADMINISTRATION.*

It is not known whether the immune response to vaccines, infection, and other antigenic stimuli administered or encountered during Simulect® therapy is impaired or whether such response will remain impaired after Simulect® therapy.

Geriatric Use
Controlled clinical studies of Simulect® have included a small number of patients 65 years and older (Simulect® 28; placebo 32). From the available data comparing Simulect® and placebo-treated patients, the adverse event profile in patients ≥65 years of age is not different from patients <65 years of age and no age-related dosing adjustment is required. Caution must be used in giving immunosuppressive drugs to elderly patients.

ADVERSE REACTIONS

Because clinical trials are conducted under widely varying conditions, adverse reaction rates observed in the clinical trials of a drug cannot be directly compared to rates in the clinical trials of another drug and may not reflect the rates observed in practice. The adverse reaction information from clinical trials does, however, provide a basis for identifying the adverse events that appear to be related to drug use and for approximating rates.
The incidence of adverse events for Simulect® was determined in four randomized, double-blind, placebo-controlled clinical trials for the prevention of renal allograft rejection. Two of the studies (Study 1 and Study 2), used a dual maintenance immunosuppressive regimen comprised of cyclosporine, USP (MODIFIED) and corticosteroids, whereas the other two studies (Study 3 and Study 4) used a triple-immunosuppressive regimen comprised of cyclosporine, USP (MODIFIED), corticosteroids, and either azathioprine or mycophenolate mofetil.
Simulect® did not appear to add to the background of adverse events seen in organ transplantation patients as a consequence of their underlying disease and the concurrent administration of immunosuppressants and other medications. Adverse events were reported by 96% of the patients in the placebo-treated group and 96% of the patients in the Simulect®-treated group. In the four placebo-controlled studies, the pattern of adverse events in 590 patients treated with the recommended dose of Simulect® was similar to that in 594 patients treated with placebo. Simulect® did not increase the incidence of serious adverse events observed compared with placebo.
The most frequently reported adverse events were gastrointestinal disorders, reported in 69% of Simulect®-treated patients and 67% of placebo-treated patients.
The incidence and types of adverse events were similar in Simulect®-treated and placebo-treated patients. The following adverse events occurred in ≥10% of Simulect®-treated patients:
Gastrointestinal System: constipation, nausea, abdominal pain, vomiting, diarrhea, dyspepsia;
Body as a Whole-General: pain, peripheral edema, fever, viral infection;
Metabolic and Nutritional: hyperkalemia, hypokalemia, hyperglycemia, hypercholesterolemia, hypophosphatemia, hyperuricemia;
Urinary System: urinary tract infection;
Respiratory System: dyspnea, upper respiratory tract infection;
Skin and Appendages: surgical wound complications, acne;
Cardiovascular Disorders-General: hypertension;
Central and Peripheral Nervous System: headache, tremor;
Psychiatric: insomnia;
Red Blood Cell: anemia.
The following adverse events, not mentioned above, were reported with an incidence of ≥3% and <10% in pooled analysis of patients treated with Simulect® in the four controlled clinical trials, or in an analysis of the two dual-therapy trials:
Body as a Whole-General: accidental trauma, asthenia, chest pain, increased drug level, infection, face edema, fatigue, dependent edema, generalized edema, leg edema, malaise, rigors, sepsis;
Cardiovascular: abnormal heart sounds, aggravated hypertension, angina pectoris, cardiac failure, chest pain, hypotension;
Endocrine: increased glucocorticoids;
Gastrointestinal: enlarged abdomen, esophagitis, flatulence, gastrointestinal disorder, gastroenteritis, GI hemorrhage, gum hyperplasia, melena, moniliasis, ulcerative stomatitis;
Heart Rate and Rhythm: arrhythmia, atrial fibrillation, tachycardia;
Metabolic and Nutritional: acidosis, dehydration, diabetes mellitus, fluid overload, hypercalcemia, hyperlipemia, hypertriglyceridemia, hypocalcemia, hypoglycemia, hypomagnesemia, hypoproteinemia, weight increase;
Musculoskeletal: arthralgia, arthropathy, back pain, bone fracture, cramps, hernia, myalgia, leg pain;
Nervous System: dizziness, neuropathy, paraesthesia, hypoesthesia;
Platelet and Bleeding: hematoma, hemorrhage, purpura, thrombocytopenia, thrombosis;
Psychiatric: agitation, anxiety, depression;
Red Blood Cell: polycythemia;
Reproductive Disorders, Male: genital edema, impotence;
Respiratory: bronchitis, bronchospasm, abnormal chest sounds, coughing, pharyngitis, pneumonia, pulmonary disorder, pulmonary edema, rhinitis, sinusitis;
Skin and Appendages: cyst, herpes simplex, herpes zoster, hypertrichosis, pruritus, rash, skin disorder, skin ulceration;
Urinary: albuminuria, bladder disorder, dysuria, frequent micturition, hematuria, increased non-protein nitrogen, oliguria, abnormal renal function, renal tubular necrosis, surgery, ureteral disorder, urinary retention;
Vascular Disorders: vascular disorder;
Vision Disorders: cataract, conjunctivitis, abnormal vision;
White Blood Cell: leucopenia. Among these events, leucopenia and hypertriglyceridemia occurred more frequently in the two triple-therapy studies using azathioprine and mycophenolate mofetil than in the dual-therapy studies.

Malignancies
The incidence of malignancies in the controlled clinical trials of renal transplant was not significantly different between groups at 1 year (9/590 Simulect®-treated patients vs. 12/594 placebo-treated patients) or among patients with 5-year follow-up from Studies 1 and 2 (21/295 Simulect®-treated patients vs. 21/291 placebo-treated patients). The incidence of lymphoproliferative disease was not significantly different between groups, and less than 1% in the Simulect®-treated patients.

Infections
The overall incidence of cytomegalovirus infection was similar in Simulect®- and placebo-treated patients (15% vs. 17%) receiving a dual- or triple-immunosuppression regimen. However, in patients receiving a triple-immunosuppression regimen, the incidence of serious cytomegalovirus infection was higher in Simulect®-treated patients compared to placebo-treated patients (11% vs. 5%). The rates of infections, serious infections, and infectious organisms were similar in the Simulect®- and placebo-treatment groups among dual- and triple-therapy treated patients.

Post-Marketing Experience
Severe acute hypersensitivity reactions including anaphylaxis characterized by hypotension, tachycardia, cardiac failure, dyspnea, wheezing, bronchospasm, pulmonary edema, respiratory failure, urticaria, rash, pruritus, and/or sneezing, as well as capillary leak syndrome and cytokine release syndrome, have been reported during post-marketing experience with Simulect®.

OVERDOSAGE

A maximum tolerated dose of Simulect® has not been determined in patients. During the course of clinical studies, Simulect® has been administered to adult renal transplantation patients in single doses of up to 60 mg, or in divided doses over 3-5 days of up to 120 mg, without any associated serious adverse events. There has been one spontaneous report of a pediatric renal transplantation patient who received a single 20-mg dose (2.3 mg/kg) without adverse events.

DOSAGE AND ADMINISTRATION

Simulect® is used as part of an immunosuppressive regimen that includes cyclosporine, USP (MODIFIED) and corticosteroids. Simulect® is for central or peripheral intravenous administration only. Reconstituted Simulect® should be given either as a bolus injection or diluted to a volume of 25 mL (10-mg vial) or 50 mL (20-mg vial) with normal saline or dextrose 5% and administered as an intravenous infusion over 20 to 30 minutes. Bolus administration may be associated with nausea, vomiting and local reactions, including pain.
Simulect® should only be administered once it has been determined that the patient will receive the graft and concomitant immunosuppression. Patients previously administered Simulect® should only be re-exposed to a subsequent course of therapy with extreme caution.
Parenteral drug products should be inspected visually for particulate matter and discoloration before administration. After reconstitution, Simulect® should be a clear-to-opalescent, colorless solution. If particulate matter is present or the solution is colored, do not use.
Care must be taken to assure sterility of the prepared solution because the drug product does not contain any antimicrobial preservatives or bacteriostatic agents.
It is recommended that after reconstitution, the solution should be used immediately. If not used immediately, it can be stored at 2°C to 8°C for 24 hours or at room temperature for 4 hours. Discard the reconstituted solution if not used within 24 hours.
No incompatibility between Simulect® and polyvinyl chloride bags or infusion sets has been observed. No data are available on the compatibility of Simulect® with other intravenous substances. Other drug substances should not be added or infused simultaneously through the same intravenous line.

Adults
In adult patients, the recommended regimen is two doses of 20 mg each. The first 20-mg dose should be given within 2 hours prior to transplantation surgery. The recommended second 20-mg dose should be given 4 days after transplantation. The second dose should be withheld if complications such as severe hypersensitivity reactions to Simulect® or graft loss occur.

Pediatric
In pediatric patients weighing less than 35 kg, the recommended regimen is two doses of 10 mg each. In pediatric patients weighing 35 kg or more, the recommended regimen is two doses of 20 mg each. The first dose should be given within 2 hours prior to transplantation surgery. The recommended second dose should be given 4 days after transplantation. The second dose should be withheld if complications such as severe hypersensitivity reactions to Simulect® or graft loss occur.

Reconstitution of 10 mg Simulect® Vial
To prepare the reconstituted solution, add 2.5 mL of Sterile Water for Injection, USP, using aseptic technique, to the vial containing the Simulect® powder. Shake the vial gently to dissolve the powder.
The reconstituted solution is isotonic and may be given either as a bolus injection or diluted to a volume of 25 mL with normal saline or dextrose 5% for infusion. When mixing the solution, gently invert the bag in order to avoid foaming; DO NOT SHAKE.

Reconstitution of 20 mg Simulect® Vial
To prepare the reconstituted solution, add 5 mL of Sterile Water for Injection, USP, using aseptic technique, to the vial containing the Simulect® powder. Shake the vial gently to dissolve the powder.
The reconstituted solution is isotonic and may be given either as a bolus injection or diluted to a volume of 50 mL with normal saline or dextrose 5% for infusion. When mixing the solution, gently invert the bag in order to avoid foaming; DO NOT SHAKE.

HOW SUPPLIED

Simulect® (basiliximab) is supplied in a single-use glass vial.
Each carton contains one of the following:
1 Simulect® 10 mg vial .... NDC 0078-0393-61
1 Simulect® 20 mg vial .... NDC 0078-0331-84
Store lyophilized Simulect® under refrigerated conditions (2°C to 8°C; 36°F to 46°F).
Do not use beyond the expiration date stamped on the vial.

REFERENCES

1. Kahan, B.D., Rajagopalan P.R. and Hall M., Transplantation, 67, 276-284 (1999).
2. Nashan, B., Moore R., Amlot P., Schmidt A.-G., Abeywickrama K. and Soulillou J.-P., Lancet 350, 1193-1198 (1997).

US License No. 1244
T2003-86
REV: NOVEMBER 2003 89007806
Novartis Pharmaceuticals Corporation
East Hanover, New Jersey 07936

Shown in Product Identification Guide, page 325

STALEVO® 50 ℞
STALEVO® 100
STALEVO® 150

[*stă-lē-vō*]
(carbidopa, levodopa and entacapone)
Tablets
Rx only

Prescribing Information
The following prescribing information is based on official labeling in effect July 2004.

DESCRIPTION

Stalevo® (carbidopa, levodopa and entacapone) is a combination of carbidopa, levodopa and entacapone for the treatment of Parkinson's disease.
Carbidopa, an inhibitor of aromatic amino acid decarboxylation, is a white, crystalline compound, slightly soluble in water, with a molecular weight of 244.3. It is designated chemically as (-)-L-(α-hydrazino-(α-methyl-β-(3,4-dihydroxybenzene) propanoic acid monohydrate. Its empirical formula is $C_{10}H_{14}N_2O_4 \bullet H_2O$, and its structural formula is

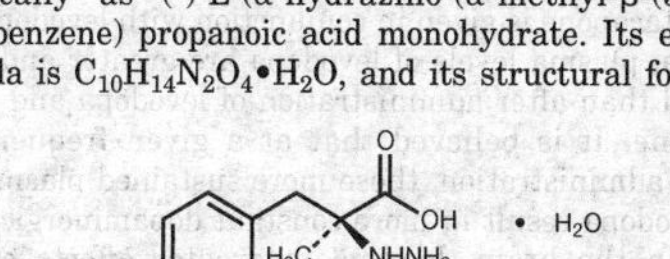

Tablet content is expressed in terms of anhydrous carbidopa, which has a molecular weight of 226.3.
Levodopa, an aromatic amino acid, is a white, crystalline compound, slightly soluble in water, with a molecular weight of 197.2. It is designated chemically as (-)-L-α-amino-β-(3,4-dihydroxybenzene) propanoic acid. Its empirical formula is $C_9H_{11}NO_4$, and its structural formula is

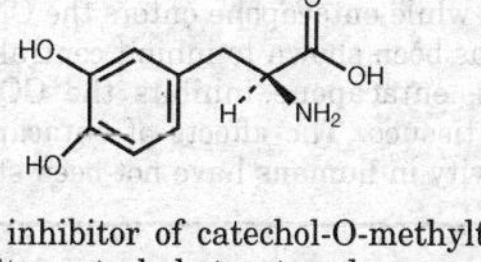

Entacapone, an inhibitor of catechol-O-methyltransferase (COMT), is a nitro-catechol-structured compound with a molecular weight of 305.3. The chemical name of entacapone is (E)-2-cyano-3-(3,4-dihydroxy-5-nitrophenyl)-N,N-diethyl-2-propenamide. Its empirical formula is $C_{14}H_{15}N_3O_5$ and its structural formula is
[See chemical structure at top of next column]
Stalevo® (carbidopa, levodopa and entacapone) is supplied as tablets in three strengths:

Continued on next page

Stalevo—Cont.

Stalevo 50, containing 12.5 mg of carbidopa, 50 mg of levodopa and 200 mg of entacapone;
Stalevo 100, containing 25 mg of carbidopa, 100 mg of levodopa and 200 mg of entacapone;
Stalevo 150, containing 37.5 mg of carbidopa, 150 mg of levodopa and 200 mg of entacapone.

The inactive ingredients of the Stalevo tablet are corn starch, croscarmellose sodium, glycerol 85%, hypromellose, magnesium stearate, mannitol, polysorbate 80, povidone, sucrose, red iron oxide, titanium dioxide, and yellow iron oxide.

CLINICAL PHARMACOLOGY

Parkinson's disease is a progressive, neurodegenerative disorder of the extrapyramidal nervous system affecting the mobility and control of the skeletal muscular system. Its characteristic features include resting tremor, rigidity, and bradykinetic movements.

Mechanism of Action

Levodopa

Current evidence indicates that symptoms of Parkinson's disease are related to depletion of dopamine in the corpus striatum. Administration of dopamine is ineffective in the treatment of Parkinson's disease apparently because it does not cross the blood-brain barrier. However, levodopa, the metabolic precursor of dopamine, does cross the blood-brain barrier, and presumably is converted to dopamine in the brain. This is thought to be the mechanism whereby levodopa relieves symptoms of Parkinson's disease.

Carbidopa

When levodopa is administered orally it is rapidly decarboxylated to dopamine in extracerebral tissues so that only a small portion of a given dose is transported unchanged to the central nervous system. Carbidopa inhibits the decarboxylation of peripheral levodopa, making more levodopa available for transport to the brain. When coadministered with levodopa, carbidopa increases plasma levels of levodopa and reduces the amount of levodopa required to produce a given response by about 75%. Carbidopa prolongs the plasma half-life of levodopa from 50 minutes to 1.5 hours and decreases plasma and urinary dopamine and its major metabolite, homovanillic acid. The T_{max} of levodopa, however, was unaffected by the coadministration.

Entacapone

Entacapone is a selective and reversible inhibitor of catechol-O-methyltransferase (COMT).

In mammals, COMT is distributed throughout various organs with the highest activities in the liver and kidney. COMT also occurs in neuronal tissues, especially in glial cells. COMT catalyzes the transfer of the methyl group of S-adenosyl-L-methionine to the phenolic group of substrates that contain a catechol structure. Physiological substrates of COMT include DOPA, catecholamines (dopamine, norepinephrine, and epinephrine) and their hydroxylated metabolites. The function of COMT is the elimination of biologically active catechols and some other hydroxylated metabolites. When decarboxylation of levodopa is prevented by carbidopa, COMT becomes the major metabolizing enzyme for levodopa, catalyzing its metabolism to 3-methoxy-4-hydroxy-L-phenylalanine (3-OMD).

When entacapone is given in conjunction with levodopa and carbidopa, plasma levels of levodopa are greater and more sustained than after administration of levodopa and carbidopa alone. It is believed that at a given frequency of levodopa administration, these more sustained plasma levels of levodopa result in more constant dopaminergic stimulation in the brain, leading to greater effects on the signs and symptoms of Parkinson's disease. The higher levodopa levels may also lead to increased levodopa adverse effects, sometimes requiring a decrease in the dose of levodopa.

When 200 mg entacapone is coadministered with levodopa/carbidopa, it increases levodopa plasma exposure (AUC) by 35%-40% and prolongs its elimination half-life in Parkinson's disease patients from 1.3 to 2.4 hours. Plasma levels of the major COMT-mediated dopamine metabolite, 3-methoxy-4-hydroxy-L-phenylalanine (3-OMD), are also markedly decreased proportionally with increasing dose of entacapone.

In animals, while entacapone enters the CNS to a minimal extent, it has been shown to inhibit central COMT activity. In humans, entacapone inhibits the COMT enzyme in peripheral tissues. The effects of entacapone on central COMT activity in humans have not been studied.

Pharmacokinetics

The pharmacokinetics of Stalevo® (carbidopa, levodopa and entacapone) tablets have been studied in healthy subjects (age 45-75 years old). Overall, following administration of corresponding doses of levodopa, carbidopa and entacapone as Stalevo or as carbidopa/levodopa product plus Comtan® (entacapone) tablets, the mean plasma concentrations of levodopa, carbidopa, and entacapone are comparable.

Absorption/Distribution:

Both levodopa and entacapone are rapidly absorbed and eliminated, and their distribution volume is moderately small. Carbidopa is absorbed and eliminated slightly more slowly compared with levodopa and entacapone. There are substantial inter- and intra-individual variations in the absorption of levodopa, carbidopa and entacapone, particularly concerning its C_{max}.

The food-effect on the Stalevo tablet has not been evaluated.

Levodopa

The pharmacokinetic properties of levodopa following the administration of single-dose Stalevo® (carbidopa, levodopa and entacapone) tablets are summarized in Table 1.

[See table 1 below]

Since levodopa competes with certain amino acids for transport across the gut wall, the absorption of levodopa may be impaired in some patients on a high protein diet. Meals rich in large neutral amino acids may delay and reduce the absorption of levodopa *(see PRECAUTIONS)*.

Levodopa is bound to plasma protein only to a minor extent (about 10%-30%).

Carbidopa

Following administration of Stalevo as a single dose to healthy male and female subjects, the peak concentration of carbidopa was reached within 2.5 to 3.4 hours on average. The mean C_{max} ranged from about 40 to 125 ng/mL and the mean AUC from 170 to 700 ng•h/mL, with different Stalevo strengths providing 12.5 mg, 25 mg, or 37.5 mg of carbidopa.

Carbidopa is approximately 36% bound to plasma protein.

Entacapone

Following administration of Stalevo as a single dose to healthy male and female subjects, the peak concentration of entacapone in plasma was reached within 1.0 to 1.2 hours on average. The mean C_{max} of entacapone was about 1200 ng/mL and the AUC 1250 to 1450 ng•h/mL after administration of different Stalevo strengths all providing 200 mg of entacapone.

The plasma protein binding of entacapone is 98% over the concentration range of 0.4-50 μg/mL. Entacapone binds mainly to serum albumin.

Metabolism and Elimination:

Levodopa

The elimination half-life of levodopa, the active moiety of antiparkinsonian activity, was 1.7 hours (range 1.1-3.2 hours).

Levodopa is extensively metabolized to various metabolites. Two major pathways are decarboxylation by dopa decarboxylase (DDC) and O-methylation by catechol-O-methyltransferase (COMT).

Carbidopa

The elimination half-life of carbidopa was on average 1.6 to 2 hours (range 0.7-4.0 hours).

Carbidopa is metabolized to two main metabolites (α-methyl-3-methoxy-4-hydroxyphenylpropionic acid and α-methyl-3,4-dihydroxy-phenylpropionic acid). These 2 metabolites are primarily eliminated in the urine unchanged or as glucuronide Unchanged carbidopa accounts for 30% of the total urinary excretion.

Entacapone

The elimination half-life of entacapone was on average 0.8 to 1 hour (0.3-4.5 hours).

Entacapone is almost completely metabolized prior to excretion with only a very small amount (0.2% of dose) found unchanged in urine. The main metabolic pathway is isomerization to the *cis*-isomer, the only active metabolite. Entacapone and the *cis*-isomer are eliminated in the urine as glucuronide conjugates. The glucuronides account for 95% of all urinary metabolites (70% as parent and 25% as *cis*-isomer glucuronides). The glucuronide conjugate of the *cis*-isomer is inactive. After oral administration of a ^{14}C-labeled dose of entacapone, 10% of labeled parent and metabolite is excreted in urine and 90% in feces.

Due to short elimination half-lives, no true accumulation of levodopa or entacapone occurs when they are administered repeatedly.

Special Populations:

Hepatic Impairment:

Stalevo® (carbidopa, levodopa and entacapone)

While there are no studies on the pharmacokinetics of carbidopa and levodopa in patients with hepatic impairment, Stalevo should be administered cautiously to patients with biliary obstruction or hepatic disease since biliary excretion appears to be the major route of excretion of entacapone and hepatic impairment had a significant effect on the pharmacokinetics of entacapone when 200 mg entacapone was administered alone.

Entacapone

Hepatic impairment had a significant effect on the pharmacokinetics of entacapone when 200 mg entacapone was administered alone. A single 200 mg dose of entacapone, without levodopa/dopa decarboxylase inhibitor coadministration, showed approximately two-fold higher AUC and C_{max} values in patients with a history of alcoholism and hepatic impairment (n=10) compared to normal subjects (n=10). All patients had biopsy-proven liver cirrhosis caused by alcohol. According to Child-Pugh grading 7 patients with liver disease had mild hepatic impairment and 3 patients had moderate hepatic impairment. As only about 10% of the entacapone dose is excreted in urine, as parent compound and conjugated glucuronide, biliary excretion appears to be the major route of excretion of this drug. Consequently, Stalevo should be administered with care to patients with biliary obstruction or hepatic disease.

Renal Impairment:

Stalevo® (carbidopa, levodopa and entacapone)

Stalevo should be administered cautiously to patients with severe renal disease. There are no studies on the pharmacokinetics of levodopa and carbidopa in patients with renal impairment.

Entacapone

No important effects of renal function on the pharmacokinetics of entacapone were found. The pharmacokinetics of entacapone have been investigated after a single 200 mg entacapone dose, without levodopa/dopa decarboxylase inhibitor coadministration, in a specific renal impairment study. There were three groups: normal subjects (n=7; creatinine clearance >1.12 mL/sec/1.73 m^2), moderate impairment (n=10; creatinine clearance ranging from 0.60-0.89 mL/sec/1.73 m^2), and severe impairment (n=7; creatinine clearance ranging from 0.20-0.44 mL/sec/1.73 m^2).

Concurrent Diseases:

Stalevo should be administered cautiously to patients with biliary obstruction, hepatic disease, severe cardiovascular or pulmonary disease, bronchial asthma, renal, or endocrine disease.

Elderly:

Stalevo tablets have not been studied in Parkinson's disease patients or in healthy volunteers older than 75 years old.

In the pharmacokinetics studies conducted in healthy volunteers following single dose of carbidopa/levodopa/entacapone (as Stalevo or as separate carbidopa/levodopa and Comtan tablets):

Levodopa

The AUC of levodopa is significantly (on average 10%-20%) higher in elderly (60-75 years) than younger subjects (45-60 years). There is no significant difference in the C_{max} of levodopa between younger (45-60 years) and elderly subjects (60-75 years).

Carbidopa

There is no significant difference in the C_{max} and AUC of carbidopa, between younger (45-60 years) and elderly subjects (60-75 years).

Entacapone

The AUC of entacapone is significantly (on average, 15%) higher in elderly (60-75 years) than younger subjects (45-60 years). There is no significant difference in the C_{max} of entacapone between younger (45-60 years) and elderly subjects (60-75 years).

Gender:

The bioavailability of levodopa is significantly higher in females when given with or without carbidopa and/or entacapone. Following a single dose of carbidopa, levodopa and entacapone together, either as Stalevo or as separate carbidopa/levodopa and Comtan tablets in healthy volunteers (age range 45-74 years):

Levodopa

The plasma exposure (AUC and C_{max}) of levodopa is significantly higher in females than males (on average, 40% for AUC and 30% for C_{max}). These differences are primarily explained by body weight. Other published literature showed significant gender effect (higher concentrations in females) even after correction for body weight.

Carbidopa

There is no gender difference in the pharmacokinetics of carbidopa.

Entacapone

There is no gender difference in the pharmacokinetics of entacapone.

Drug Interactions: See PRECAUTIONS, Drug Interactions.

Clinical Studies

Each Stalevo tablet, provided in three single-dose strengths, contains carbidopa and levodopa in ratio 1:4 and a 200 mg dose of entacapone. The three Stalevo tablet strengths have been shown to be bioequivalent to the corresponding doses of standard-release carbidopa/levodopa 25/100 mg tablets and Comtan 200 mg tablets.

The effectiveness of entacapone as an adjunct to levodopa in the treatment of Parkinson's disease was established in three 24-week multicenter, randomized, double-blind placebo-controlled trials in patients with Parkinson's disease. In two of these trials, the patients' disease was "fluctuating," i.e., was characterized by documented periods of "On" (periods of relatively good functioning) and "Off" (periods of relatively poor functioning), despite optimum levodopa therapy. There was also a withdrawal period fol-

Table 1
Pharmacokinetic Characteristics of Levodopa With Different Tablet Strengths of Stalevo® (mean ± SD)

Tablet Strength	$AUC_{0-\infty}$ (ng·h/mL)	C_{max} (ng/mL)	T_{max} (h)
12.5 - 50 - 200 mg	1040 ± 314	470 ± 154	1.1 ± 0.5
25 - 100 - 200 mg	2910 ± 715	975 ± 247	1.4 ± 0.6
37.5 - 150 - 200 mg	3770 ± 1120	1270 ± 329	1.5 ± 0.9

lowing 6 months of treatment. In the third trial patients were not required to have been experiencing fluctuations. Prior to the controlled part of these trials, patients were stabilized on levodopa for 2-4 weeks.

There is limited experience of using entacapone in patients who do not experience fluctuations.

In the first two studies to be described, patients were randomized to receive placebo or entacapone 200 mg administered concomitantly with each dose of carbidopa-levodopa (up to 10 times daily, but averaging 4-6 doses per day). The formal double-blind portion of both trials was 6 months long. Patients recorded the time spent in the "On" and "Off" states in home diaries periodically throughout the duration of the trial. In one study, conducted in the Nordic countries, the primary outcome measure was the total mean time spent in the "On" state during an 18-hour diary recorded day (6 a.m. to midnight). In the other study, the primary outcome measure was the proportion of awake time spent over 24 hours in the "On" state.

In addition to the primary outcome measure, the amount of time spent in the "Off" state was evaluated, and patients were also evaluated by subparts of the Unified Parkinson's Disease Rating Scale (UPDRS), a frequently used multi-item rating scale intended to assess mentation (Part I), activities of daily living (Part II), motor function (Part III), complications of therapy (Part IV), and disease staging (Part V & VI); an investigator's and patient's global assessment of clinical condition, a 7-point subjective scale designed to assess global functioning in Parkinson's disease; and the change in daily carbidopa-levodopa dose.

In one of the studies, 171 patients were randomized in 16 centers in Finland, Norway, Sweden, and Denmark (Nordic Study), all of whom received concomitant levodopa plus dopa-decarboxylase inhibitor (either carbidopa-levodopa or benserazide-levodopa). In the second trial, 205 patients were randomized in 17 centers in North America (US and Canada); all patients received concomitant carbidopa-levodopa.

The following tables display the results of these two trials:

[See table 2 above]

[See table 3 at top of next page]

Effects on "On" time did not differ by age, sex, weight, disease severity at baseline, levodopa dose and concurrent treatment with dopamine agonists or selegiline.

Withdrawal of Entacapone:

In the North American Study, abrupt withdrawal of entacapone, without alteration of the dose of carbidopa-levodopa, resulted in a significant worsening of fluctuations, compared to placebo. In some cases, symptoms were slightly worse than at baseline, but returned to approximately baseline severity within two weeks following levodopa dose increase on average by 80 mg. In the Nordic Study, similarly, a significant worsening of parkinsonian symptoms was observed after entacapone withdrawal, as assessed two weeks after drug withdrawal.

At this phase, the symptoms were approximately at baseline severity following levodopa dose increase by about 50 mg.

In the third placebo-controlled trial, a total of 301 patients were randomized in 32 centers in Germany and Austria. In this trial, as in the other two trials, entacapone 200 mg was administered with each dose of levodopa/dopa decarboxylase inhibitor (up to 10 times daily) and UPDRS Parts II and III and total daily "On" time were the primary measures of effectiveness. The following results were seen for the primary measures, as well as for some secondary measures:

[See table 4 on next page]

Table 2
Nordic Study

	Baseline	Change from Baseline at Month 6*	p-value vs. placebo
Primary Measure from Home Diary (from an 18-hour Diary Day)			
Hours of Awake Time "On"			
Placebo	9.2	+0.1	—
Entacapone	9.3	+1.5	<0.001
Duration of "On" Time After First AM Dose (Hrs)			
Placebo	2.2	0.0	—
Entacapone	2.1	+0.2	<0.05
Secondary Measures from Home Diary (from an 18-hour Diary Day)			
Hours of Awake Time "Off"			
Placebo	5.3	0.0	—
Entacapone	5.5	-1.3	<0.001
Proportion of Awake Time "On"*(%)**			
Placebo	63.8	+0.6	—
Entacapone	62.7	+9.3	<0.001
Levodopa Total Daily Dose (mg)			
Placebo	705	+14	—
Entacapone	701	-87	<0.001
Frequency of Levodopa Daily Intakes			
Placebo	6.1	+0.1	—
Entacapone	6.2	-0.4	<0.001
Other Secondary Measures			
	Baseline	**Change from Baseline at Month 6**	**p-value vs. placebo**
Investigator's Global (overall) % Improved**			
Placebo	—	28	—
Entacapone	—	56	<0.01
Patient's Global (overall) % Improved**			
Placebo	—	22	—
Entacapone	—	39	N.S.‡
UPDRS Total			
Placebo	37.4	-1.1	—
Entacapone	38.5	-4.8	<0.01
UPDRS Motor			
Placebo	24.6	-0.7	—
Entacapone	25.5	-3.3	<0.05
UPDRS ADL			
Placebo	11.0	-0.4	—
Entacapone	11.2	-1.8	<0.05

* Mean; the month 6 values represent the average of weeks 8, 16, and 24, by protocol-defined outcome measure.
** At least one category change at endpoint.
*** Not an endpoint for this study but primary endpoint in the North American Study.
‡ Not significant.

INDICATIONS

Stalevo® (carbidopa, levodopa and entacapone) is indicated to treat patients with idiopathic Parkinson's disease:

1. To substitute (with equivalent strength of each of the three components) for immediate-release carbidopa/levodopa and entacapone previously administered as individual products.
2. To replace immediate-release carbidopa/levodopa therapy (without entacapone) when patients experience the signs and symptoms of end-of-dose "wearing-off" (only for patients taking a total daily dose of levodopa of 600 mg or less and not experiencing dyskinesias, *see DOSAGE AND ADMINISTRATION*).

CONTRAINDICATIONS

Stalevo® (carbidopa, levodopa and entacapone) tablets are contraindicated in patients who have demonstrated hypersensitivity to any component (carbidopa, levodopa, or entacapone) of the drug or its excipients.

Monoamine oxidase (MAO) and COMT are the two major enzyme systems involved in the metabolism of catecholamines. It is theoretically possible, therefore, that the combination of entacapone and a non-selective MAO inhibitor (e.g., phenelzine and tranylcypromine) would result in inhibition of the majority of the pathways responsible for normal catecholamine metabolism. As with carbidopa-levodopa, nonselective monoamine oxidase (MAO) inhibitors are contraindicated for use with Stalevo. These inhibitors must be discontinued at least two weeks prior to initiating therapy with Stalevo. Stalevo may be administered concomitantly with the manufacturer's recommended dose of MAO inhibitors with selectivity for MAO type B (e.g., selegiline HCl). *(See PRECAUTIONS, Drug Interactions.)*

Stalevo is contraindicated in patients with narrow-angle glaucoma.

Because levodopa may activate malignant melanoma, Stalevo should not be used in patients with suspicious, undiagnosed skin lesions or a history of melanoma.

WARNINGS

The addition of carbidopa to levodopa reduces the peripheral effects (nausea, vomiting) due to decarboxylation of levodopa; however, carbidopa does not decrease the adverse reactions due to the central effects of levodopa. Because carbidopa as well as entacapone permits more levodopa to reach the brain and more dopamine to be formed, certain adverse CNS effects, e.g., dyskinesia (involuntary movements) may occur at lower dosages and sooner with levodopa preparations containing carbidopa and entacapone than with levodopa alone.

The occurrence of dyskinesias may require dosage reduction *(see PRECAUTIONS, Dyskinesia)*.

Stalevo® (carbidopa, levodopa and entacapone) may cause mental disturbances. These reactions are thought to be due to increased brain dopamine following administration of levodopa. All patients should be observed carefully for the development of depression with concomitant suicidal tendencies. Patients with past or current psychoses should be treated with caution.

Stalevo should be administered cautiously to patients with severe cardiovascular or pulmonary disease, bronchial asthma, renal, hepatic or endocrine disease.

As with levodopa, care should be exercised in administering Stalevo to patients with a history of myocardial infarction who have residual atrial, nodal, or ventricular arrhythmias. In such patients, cardiac function should be monitored carefully during the period of initial dosage adjustment, in a facility with provisions for intensive cardiac care.

As with levodopa, treatment with Stalevo may increase the possibility of upper gastrointestinal hemorrhage in patients with a history of peptic ulcer.

Neuroleptic Malignant Syndrome (NMS)

Sporadic cases of a symptom complex resembling NMS have been reported in association with dose reductions or withdrawal of therapy with carbidopa-levodopa. Therefore, patients should be observed carefully when the dosage of Stalevo is reduced abruptly or discontinued, especially if the patient is receiving neuroleptics. NMS is an uncommon but life-threatening syndrome characterized by fever or hyperthermia. Neurological findings, including muscle rigidity, involuntary movements, altered consciousness, mental status changes; other disturbances, such as autonomic dysfunction, tachycardia, tachypnea, sweating, hyper- or hypotension; laboratory findings, such as creatine phosphokinase elevation, leukocytosis, myoglobinuria, and increased serum myoglobin have been reported.

The early diagnosis of this condition is important for the appropriate management of these patients. Considering NMS as a possible diagnosis and ruling out other acute illnesses (e.g., pneumonia, systemic infection, etc.) is essential. This may be especially complex if the clinical presentation includes both serious medical illness and untreated or inadequately treated extrapyramidal signs and symptoms (EPS). Other important considerations in the differential diagnosis include central anticholinergic toxicity, heat stroke, drug fever, and primary central nervous system (CNS) pathology.

The management of NMS should include: 1) intensive symptomatic treatment and medical monitoring and 2) treatment of any concomitant serious medical problems for which specific treatments are available. Dopamine agonists, such as bromocriptine, and muscle relaxants, such as dantrolene, are often used in the treatment of NMS, however, their effectiveness has not been demonstrated in controlled studies.

Drugs Metabolized by Catechol-O-Methyltransferase (COMT)

When a single 400 mg dose of entacapone was given together with intravenous isoprenaline (isoproterenol) and epinephrine without coadministered levodopa/dopa decarboxylase inhibitor, the overall mean maximal changes in heart rate during infusion were about 50% and 80% higher than with placebo, for isoprenaline and epinephrine, respectively.

Therefore, drugs known to be metabolized by COMT, such as isoproterenol, epinephrine, norepinephrine, dopamine, dobutamine, alpha-methyldopa, apomorphine, isoetherine, and bitolterol should be administered with caution in patients receiving entacapone regardless of the route of administration (including inhalation), as their interaction may result in increased heart rates, possibly arrhythmias, and excessive changes in blood pressure.

Ventricular tachycardia was noted in one 32-year-old healthy male volunteer in an interaction study after epinephrine infusion and oral entacapone administration. Treatment with propranolol was required. A causal relationship to entacapone administration appears probable but cannot be attributed with certainty.

Continued on next page

Stalevo—Cont.

PRECAUTIONS

General

As with levodopa, periodic evaluations of hepatic, hematopoietic, cardiovascular, and renal function are recommended during extended therapy.

Patients with chronic wide-angle glaucoma may be treated cautiously with Stalevo® (carbidopa, levodopa and entacapone) provided the intraocular pressure is well controlled and the patient is monitored carefully for changes in intraocular pressure during therapy.

Hypotension/Syncope

In the large controlled trials of entacapone, approximately 1.2% and 0.8% of 200 mg entacapone and placebo patients treated also with levodopa/dopa decarboxylase inhibitor, respectively, reported at least one episode of syncope. Reports of syncope were generally more frequent in patients in both treatment groups who had an episode of documented hypotension (although the episodes of syncope, obtained by history, were themselves not documented with vital sign measurement).

Diarrhea

In clinical trials of entacapone, diarrhea developed in 60 of 603 (10.0%) and 16 of 400 (4.0%) of patients treated with 200 mg of entacapone or placebo in combination with levodopa/dopa decarboxylase inhibitor, respectively. In patients treated with entacapone, diarrhea was generally mild to moderate in severity (8.6%) but was regarded as severe in 1.3%. Diarrhea resulted in withdrawal in 10 of 603 (1.7%) patients, 7 (1.2%) with mild and moderate diarrhea and 3 (0.5%) with severe diarrhea. Diarrhea generally resolved after discontinuation of entacapone. Two patients with diarrhea were hospitalized. Typically, diarrhea presents within 4-12 weeks after entacapone is started, but it may appear as early as the first week and as late as many months after the initiation of treatment.

Hallucinations

Dopaminergic therapy in Parkinson's disease patients has been associated with hallucinations. In clinical trials of entacapone, hallucinations developed in approximately 4.0% of patients treated with 200 mg entacapone or placebo in combination with levodopa/dopa decarboxylase inhibitor. Hallucinations led to drug discontinuation and premature withdrawal from clinical trials in 0.8% and 0% of patients treated with 200 mg entacapone and placebo, respectively. Hallucinations led to hospitalization in 1.0% and 0.3% of patients in the 200 mg entacapone and placebo groups, respectively.

Dyskinesia

Entacapone may potentiate the dopaminergic side effects of levodopa and may therefore cause and/or exacerbate preexisting dyskinesia. Although decreasing the dose of levodopa may ameliorate this side effect, many patients in controlled trials continued to experience frequent dyskinesias despite a reduction in their dose of levodopa. The rates of withdrawal for dyskinesia were 1.5% and 0.8% for 200 mg entacapone and placebo, respectively.

Other Events Reported with Dopaminergic Therapy

The events listed below are rare events known to be associated with the use of drugs that increase dopaminergic activity, although they are most often associated with the use of direct dopamine agonists.

Rhabdomyolysis: Cases of severe rhabdomyolysis have been reported with entacapone when used in combination with levodopa. The complicated nature of these cases makes it impossible to determine what role, if any, entacapone played in their pathogenesis. Severe prolonged motor activity including dyskinesia may account for rhabdomyolysis. One case, however, included fever and alteration of consciousness. It is therefore possible that the rhabdomyolysis may be a result of the syndrome described in Hyperpyrexia and Confusion *(see PRECAUTIONS, Other Events Reported with Dopaminergic Therapy).*

Hyperpyrexia and Confusion: Cases of a symptom complex resembling the neuroleptic malignant syndrome characterized by elevated temperature, muscular rigidity, altered consciousness, and elevated CPK have been reported in association with the rapid dose reduction or withdrawal of other dopaminergic drugs. No cases have been reported following the abrupt withdrawal or dose reduction of entacapone treatment during clinical studies.

Prescribers should exercise caution when discontinuing carbidopa, levodopa and entacapone combination treatment. When considered necessary, withdrawal should proceed slowly. If a decision is made to discontinue treatment with Stalevo, recommendations include monitoring the patient closely and adjusting other dopaminergic treatments as needed. This syndrome should be considered in the differential diagnosis for any patient who develops a high fever or severe rigidity. Tapering entacapone has not been systematically evaluated.

Fibrotic Complications: Cases of retroperitoneal fibrosis, pulmonary infiltrates, pleural effusion, and pleural thickening have been reported in some patients treated with ergot derived dopaminergic agents. These complications may resolve when the drug is discontinued, but complete resolution does not always occur. Although these adverse events are believed to be related to the ergoline structure of these compounds, whether other, nonergot derived drugs (e.g., entacapone, levodopa) that increase dopaminergic activity can cause them is unknown. It should be noted that the expected incidence of fibrotic complications is so low that even if entacapone caused these complications at rates similar to those attributable to other dopaminergic therapies, it is unlikely that it would have been detected in a cohort of the size exposed to entacapone. Four cases of pulmonary fibrosis were reported during clinical development of entacapone; three of these patients were also treated with pergolide and one with bromocriptine. The duration of treatment with entacapone ranged from 7-17 months.

Table 3
North American Study

	Baseline	Change from Baseline at Month 6*	p-value vs. placebo
Primary Measure from Home Diary (for a 24-hour Diary Day)			
Percent of Awake Time "On"			
Placebo	60.8	+2.0	—
Entacapone	60.0	+6.7	<0.05
Secondary Measures from Home Diary (for a 24-hour Diary Day)			
Hours of Awake Time "Off"			
Placebo	6.6	-0.3	—
Entacapone	6.8	-1.2	<0.01
Hours of Awake Time "On"			
Placebo	10.3	+0.4	—
Entacapone	10.2	+1.0	N.S.‡
Levodopa Total Daily Dose (mg)			
Placebo	758	+19	—
Entacapone	804	-93	<0.001
Frequency of Levodopa Daily Intakes			
Placebo	6.0	+0.2	—
Entacapone	6.2	0.0	N.S.‡
Other Secondary Measures			
	Baseline	**Change from Baseline at Month 6**	**p-value vs. placebo**
Investigator's Global (overall) % Improved**			
Placebo	—	21	—
Entacapone	—	34	<0.05
Patient's Global (overall) % Improved**			
Placebo	—	20	—
Entacapone	—	31	<0.05
UPDRS Total***			
Placebo	35.6	+2.8	—
Entacapone	35.1	-0.6	<0.05
UPDRS Motor***			
Placebo	22.6	+1.2	—
Entacapone	22.0	-0.9	<0.05
UPDRS ADL***			
Placebo	11.7	+1.1	—
Entacapone	11.9	0.0	<0.05

* Mean; the month 6 values represent the average of weeks 8, 16, and 24, by protocol-defined outcome measure.
** At least one category change at endpoint.
*** Score change at endpoint similarly to the Nordic Study.
‡ Not significant.

Table 4
German-Austrian Study

	Baseline	Change from Baseline at Month 6	p-value vs. placebo (LOCF)
Primary Measures			
UPDRS ADL*			
Placebo	12.0	+0.5	—
Entacapone	12.4	-0.4	<0.05
UPDRS Motor*			
Placebo	24.1	+0.1	—
Entacapone	24.9	-2.5	<0.05
Hours of Awake Time "On" (Home Diary)**			
Placebo	10.1	+0.5	—
Entacapone	10.2	+1.1	N.S.‡
Other Secondary Measures			
	Baseline	**Change from Baseline at Month 6**	**p-value vs. placebo**
UPDRS Total*			
Placebo	37.7	+0.6	—
Entacapone	39.0	-3.4	<0.05
Percent of Awake Time "On" (Home Diary)**			
Placebo	59.8	+3.5	—
Entacapone	62.0	+6.5	N.S.‡
Hours of Awake Time "Off" (Home Diary)**			
Placebo	6.8	-0.6	—
Entacapone	6.3	-1.2	0.07
Levodopa Total Daily Dose (mg)*			
Placebo	572	+4	—
Entacapone	566	-35	N.S.‡
Frequency of Levodopa Daily Intake*			
Placebo	5.6	+0.2	—
Entacapone	5.4	0.0	<0.01
Global (overall) % Improved***			
Placebo	—	34	—
Entacapone	—	38	N.S.‡

* Total population; score change at endpoint.
** Fluctuating population, with 5-10 doses; score change at endpoint.
*** Total population; at least one category change at endpoint.
‡ Not significant.

Renal Toxicity

In a one-year toxicity study, entacapone (plasma exposure 20 times that in humans receiving the maximum recommended daily dose of 1600 mg) caused an increased incidence of nephrotoxicity in male rats that was characterized by regenerative tubules, thickening of basement membranes, infiltration of mononuclear cells and tubular protein casts. These effects were not associated with changes in clinical chemistry parameters, and there is no established method for monitoring for the possible occurrence of these lesions in humans. Although this toxicity could represent a species-specific effect, there is not yet evidence that this is so.

Hepatic Impairment

Patients with hepatic impairment should be treated with caution. The AUC and C_{max} of entacapone approximately doubled in patients with documented liver disease compared to controls. *(See CLINICAL PHARMACOLOGY, Pharmacokinetics, and DOSAGE AND ADMINISTRATION).*

Biliary Obstruction

Caution should be exercised when administering Stalevo to patients with biliary obstruction, as entacapone is excreted mostly via the bile.

Information for Patients

The patient should be instructed to take Stalevo only as prescribed. The patient should be informed that Stalevo is a standard-release formulation of carbidopa-levodopa combined with entacapone that is designed to begin release of ingredients within 30 minutes after ingestion. It is important that Stalevo be taken at regular intervals according to the schedule outlined by the physician. The patient should be cautioned not to change the prescribed dosage regimen and not to add any additional antiparkinsonian medications, including other carbidopa-levodopa preparations, without first consulting the physician.

Patients should be advised that sometimes a "wearing-off" effect may occur at the end of the dosing interval. The physician should be notified for possible treatment adjustments if such response poses a problem to patient's everyday life.

Patients should be advised that occasionally, dark color (red, brown, or black) may appear in saliva, urine, or sweat after ingestion of Stalevo. Although the color appears to be clinically insignificant, garments may become discolored.

The patient should be advised that a change in diet to foods that are high in protein may delay the absorption of levodopa and may reduce the amount taken up in the circulation. Excessive acidity also delays stomach emptying, thus delaying the absorption of levodopa. Iron salts (such as in multi-vitamin tablets) may also reduce the amount of levodopa available to the body. The above factors may reduce the clinical effectiveness of the levodopa, carbidopa-levodopa and Stalevo therapy.

NOTE: The suggested advice to patients being treated with Stalevo is intended to aid in the safe and effective use of this medication. It is not a disclosure of all possible adverse or intended effects.

Patients should be informed that hallucinations can occur.

Patients should be advised that they may develop postural (orthostatic) hypotension with or without symptoms such as dizziness, nausea, syncope, and sweating. Hypotension may occur more frequently during initial therapy or when total daily levodopa dosage is increased. Accordingly, patients should be cautioned against rising rapidly after sitting or lying down, especially if they have been doing so for prolonged periods, and especially at the initiation of treatment with Stalevo.

Patients should be advised that they should neither drive a car nor operate other complex machinery until they have gained sufficient experience on Stalevo to gauge whether or not it affects their mental and/or motor performance adversely. Because of the possible additive sedative effects, caution should be used when patients are taking other CNS depressants in combination with Stalevo.

Patients should be informed that nausea may occur, especially at the initiation of treatment with Stalevo.

Patients should be advised of the possibility of an increase in dyskinesia.

Carbidopa-levodopa combination and entacapone are known to affect embryo-fetal development in the rabbit and in the rat, respectively. Accordingly, patients should be advised to notify their physicians if they become pregnant or intend to become pregnant during therapy *(see PRECAUTIONS, Pregnancy).*

Carbidopa and entacapone are known to be excreted into maternal milk in rats. Because of the possibility that carbidopa, levodopa and entacapone may be excreted into human maternal milk, patients should be advised to notify their physicians if they intend to breast-feed or are breast-feeding an infant.

Laboratory Tests

Abnormalities in laboratory tests may include elevations of liver function tests such as alkaline phosphatase, SGOT (AST), SGPT (ALT), lactic dehydrogenase, and bilirubin. Abnormalities in blood urea nitrogen and positive Coombs' test have also been reported. Commonly, levels of blood urea nitrogen, creatinine, and uric acid are lower during administration of Stalevo than with levodopa.

Stalevo may cause a false-positive reaction for urinary ketone bodies when a test tape is used for determination of ketonuria. This reaction will not be altered by boiling the urine specimen. False-negative tests may result with the use of glucose-oxidase methods of testing for glucosuria.

Cases of falsely diagnosed pheochromocytoma in patients on carbidopa-levodopa therapy have been reported very rarely. Caution should be exercised when interpreting the plasma and urine levels of catecholamines and their metabolites in patients on carbidopa-levodopa therapy.

Entacapone is a chelator of iron. The impact of entacapone on the body's iron stores is unknown; however, a tendency towards decreasing serum iron concentrations was noted in clinical trials. In a controlled clinical study serum ferritin levels (as marker of iron deficiency and subclinical anemia) were not changed with entacapone compared to placebo after one year of treatment and there was no difference in rates of anemia or decreased hemoglobin levels.

Drug Interactions

Caution should be exercised when the following drugs are administered concomitantly with Stalevo.

Anti-hypertensive agents: Symptomatic postural hypotension has occurred when carbidopa-levodopa was added to the treatment of patients receiving antihypertensive drugs. Therefore, when therapy with Stalevo is started, dosage adjustment of the antihypertensive drug may be required.

MAO inhibitors: For patients receiving nonselective MAO inhibitors, *see CONTRAINDICATIONS*. Concomitant therapy with selegiline and carbidopa-levodopa may be associated with severe orthostatic hypotension not attributable to carbidopa-levodopa alone.

Tricyclic antidepressants: There have been rare reports of adverse reactions, including hypertension and dyskinesia, resulting from the concomitant use of tricyclic antidepressants and carbidopa-levodopa.

Dopamine D2 receptor antagonists (e.g., phenothiazines, butyrophenones, risperidone) and isoniazid: Dopamine D2 receptor antagonists (e.g., phenothiazines, butyrophenones, risperidone) and isoniazid may reduce the therapeutic effects of levodopa.

Phenytoin and papaverine: The beneficial effects of levodopa in Parkinson's disease have been reported to be reversed by phenytoin and papaverine. Patients taking these drugs with carbidopa-levodopa should be carefully observed for loss of therapeutic response.

Iron salts: Iron salts may reduce the bioavailability of levodopa, carbidopa and entacapone. The clinical relevance is unclear.

Metoclopramide: Although metoclopramide may increase the bioavailability of levodopa by increasing gastric emptying, metoclopramide may also adversely affect disease control by its dopamine receptor antagonistic properties.

Drugs known to interfere with biliary excretion, glucuronidation, and intestinal beta-glucuronidase (probenecid, cholestyramine, erythromycin, rifampicin, ampicillin and chloramphenicol): As most entacapone excretion is via the bile, caution should be exercised when drugs known to interfere with biliary excretion, glucuronidation, and intestinal beta-glucuronidase are given concurrently with entacapone. These include probenecid, cholestyramine, and some antibiotics (e.g., erythromycin, rifampicin, ampicillin and chloramphenicol).

Pyridoxine: Stalevo can be given to patients receiving supplemental pyridoxine. Oral coadministration of 10-25 mg of pyridoxine hydrochloride (vitamin B6) with levodopa may reverse the effects of levodopa by increasing the rate of aromatic amino acid decarboxylation. Carbidopa inhibits this action of pyridoxine; therefore, Stalevo can be given to patients receiving supplemental pyridoxine.

Effect of levodopa and carbidopa in Stalevo on the metabolism of other drugs: Inhibition or induction effect of levodopa and carbidopa has not been investigated.

Effect of entacapone in Stalevo on the metabolism of other drugs: Entacapone is unlikely to inhibit the metabolism of other drugs that are metabolized by major P450s including CYP1A2, CYP2A6, CYP2C9, CYP2C19, CYP2D6, CYP2E1 and CYP3A. *In vitro* studies of human CYP enzymes showed that entacapone inhibited the CYP enzymes 1A2, 2A6, 2C9, 2C19, 2D6, 2E1 and 3A only at very high concentrations (IC50 from 200 to over 1000 μM; an oral 200 mg dose achieves a highest level of approximately 5 μM in people); these enzymes would therefore not be expected to be inhibited in clinical use. However, no information is available regarding the induction effect from entacapone.

Drugs that are highly protein bound (such as warfarin, salicylic acid, phenylbutazone, and diazepam):

Levodopa

Levodopa is bound to plasma protein only to a minor extent (about 10%-30%).

Carbidopa

Carbidopa is approximately 36% bound to plasma protein.

Entacapone

Entacapone is highly protein bound (98%). *In vitro* studies have shown no binding displacement between entacapone and other highly bound drugs, such as warfarin, salicylic acid, phenylbutazone, and diazepam.

Hormone Levels

Of the ingredients in Stalevo, levodopa is known to depress prolactin secretion and increase growth hormone levels.

Carcinogenesis

In a two-year bioassay of carbidopa-levodopa, no evidence of carcinogenicity was found in rats receiving doses of approximately two times the maximum daily human dose of carbidopa and four times the maximum daily human dose of levodopa.

Two-year carcinogenicity studies of entacapone were conducted in mice and rats. Rats were treated once daily by oral gavage with entacapone doses of 20, 90, or 400 mg/kg. An increased incidence of renal tubular adenomas and carcinomas was found in male rats treated with the highest dose of entacapone. Plasma exposures (AUC) associated with this dose were approximately 20 times higher than estimated plasma exposures of humans receiving the maximum recommended daily dose of entacapone (MRDD = 1600 mg). Mice were treated once daily by oral gavage with doses of 20, 100 or 600 mg/kg of entacapone (0.05, 0.3, and two times the MRDD for humans on a mg/m^2 basis). Because of a high incidence of premature mortality in mice receiving the highest dose of entacapone, the mouse study is not an adequate assessment of carcinogenicity. Although no treatment related tumors were observed in animals receiving the lower doses, the carcinogenic potential of entacapone has not been fully evaluated. The carcinogenic potential of entacapone administered in combination with carbidopa-levodopa has not been evaluated.

Mutagenesis

Carbidopa was positive in the Ames test in the presence and absence of metabolic activation, was mutagenic in the *in vitro* mouse lymphoma/thymidine kinase assay in the absence of metabolic activation, and was negative in the *in vivo* mouse micronucleus test.

Entacapone was mutagenic and clastogenic in the *in vitro* mouse lymphoma/thymidine kinase assay in the presence and absence of metabolic activation, and was clastogenic in cultured human lymphocytes in the presence of metabolic activation. Entacapone, either alone or in combination with carbidopa-levodopa, was not clastogenic in the *in vivo* mouse micronucleus test or mutagenic in the bacterial reverse mutation assay (Ames test).

Impairment of Fertility

In reproduction studies with carbidopa-levodopa, no effects on fertility were found in rats receiving doses of approximately two times the maximum daily human dose of carbidopa and four times the maximum daily human dose of levodopa.

Entacapone did not impair fertility or general reproductive performance in rats treated with up to 700 mg/kg/day (plasma AUCs 28 times those in humans receiving the MRDD). Delayed mating, but no fertility impairment, was evident in female rats treated with 700 mg/kg/day of entacapone.

Pregnancy

Pregnancy Category C

Carbidopa-levodopa caused both visceral and skeletal malformations in rabbits at all doses and ratios of carbidopa-levodopa tested, which ranged from 10 times/5 times the maximum recommended human dose of carbidopa-levodopa to 20 times/10 times the maximum recommended human dose of carbidopa-levodopa. There was a decrease in the number of live pups delivered by rats receiving approximately two times the maximum recommended human dose of carbidopa and approximately five times the maximum recommended human dose of levodopa during organogenesis. No teratogenic effects were observed in mice receiving up to 20 times the maximum recommended human dose of carbidopa-levodopa.

It has been reported from individual cases that levodopa crosses the human placental barrier, enters the fetus, and is metabolized. Carbidopa concentrations in fetal tissue appeared to be minimal.

In embryo-fetal development studies, entacapone was administered to pregnant animals throughout organogenesis at doses of up to 1000 mg/kg/day in rats and 300 mg/kg/day in rabbits. Increased incidences of fetal variations were evident in litters from rats treated with the highest dose, in the absence of overt signs of maternal toxicity. The maternal plasma drug exposure (AUC) associated with this dose was approximately 34 times the estimated plasma exposure in humans receiving the maximum recommended daily dose (MRDD) of 1600 mg. Increased frequencies of abortions and late/total resorptions and decreased fetal weights were observed in the litters of rabbits treated with maternotoxic doses of 100 mg/kg/day (plasma AUCs 0.4 times those in humans receiving the MRDD) or greater. There was no evidence of teratogenicity in these studies.

However, when entacapone was administered to female rats prior to mating and during early gestation, an increased incidence of fetal eye anomalies (macrophthalmia, microphthalmia, anophthalmia) was observed in the litters of dams treated with doses of 160 mg/kg/day (plasma AUCs seven times those in humans receiving the MRDD) or greater, in the absence of maternotoxicity. Administration of up to 700 mg/kg/day (plasma AUCs 28 times those in humans receiving the MRDD) to female rats during the latter part of gestation and throughout lactation, produced no evidence of developmental impairment in the offspring.

There is no experience from clinical studies regarding the use of Stalevo in pregnant women. Therefore, Stalevo should be used during pregnancy only if the potential benefit justifies the potential risk to the fetus.

Nursing Women

In animal studies, carbidopa and entacapone were excreted into maternal rat milk. It is not known whether entacapone or carbidopa-levodopa are excreted in human milk. Because many drugs are excreted in human milk, caution should be exercised when Stalevo is administered to a nursing woman.

Pediatric Use

Safety and effectiveness in pediatric patients have not been established.

Continued on next page

Stalevo—Cont.

ADVERSE REACTIONS

Carbidopa-levodopa

The most common adverse reactions reported with carbidopa-levodopa have included dyskinesias, such as choreiform, dystonic, and other involuntary movements and nausea.

The following other adverse reactions have been reported with carbidopa-levodopa:

Body as a Whole: Chest pain, asthenia.

Cardiovascular: Cardiac irregularities, hypotension, orthostatic effects including orthostatic hypotension, hypertension, syncope, phlebitis, palpitation.

Gastrointestinal: Dark saliva, gastrointestinal bleeding, development of duodenal ulcer, anorexia, vomiting, diarrhea, constipation, dyspepsia, dry mouth, taste alterations.

Hematologic: Agranulocytosis, hemolytic and non-hemolytic anemia, thrombocytopenia, leukopenia.

Hypersensitivity: Angioedema, urticaria, pruritus, Henoch-Schönlein purpura, bullous lesions (including pemphigus-like reactions).

Musculoskeletal: Back pain, shoulder pain, muscle cramps.

Nervous System/Psychiatric: Psychotic episodes including delusions, hallucinations, and paranoid ideation, neuroleptic malignant syndrome *(see WARNINGS)*, bradykinetic episodes ("on-off" phenomenon), confusion, agitation, dizziness, somnolence, dream abnormalities including nightmares, insomnia, paresthesia, headache, depression with or without development of suicidal tendencies, dementia, increased libido. Convulsions also have occurred; however, a causal relationship with carbidopa-levodopa has not been established.

Respiratory: Dyspnea, upper respiratory infection.

Skin: Rash, increased sweating, alopecia, dark sweat.

Urogenital: Urinary tract infection, urinary frequency, dark urine.

Laboratory Tests: Decreased hemoglobin and hematocrit; abnormalities in alkaline phosphatase, SGOT (AST), SGPT (ALT), lactic dehydrogenase, bilirubin, blood urea nitrogen (BUN), Coombs' test; elevated serum glucose; white blood cells, bacteria, and blood in the urine.

Other adverse reactions that have been reported with levodopa alone and with various carbidopa-levodopa formulations, and may occur with Stalevo® (carbidopa, levodopa and entacapone) are:

Body as a Whole: Abdominal pain and distress, fatigue.

Cardiovascular: Myocardial infarction.

Gastrointestinal: Gastrointestinal pain, dysphagia, sialorrhea, flatulence, bruxism, burning sensation of the tongue, heartburn, hiccups.

Metabolic: Edema, weight gain, weight loss.

Musculoskeletal: Leg pain.

Nervous System/Psychiatric: Ataxia, extrapyramidal disorder, failing, anxiety, gait abnormalities, nervousness, decreased mental acuity, memory impairment, disorientation, euphoria, blepharospasm (which may be taken as an early sign of excess dosage; consideration of dosage reduction may be made at this time), trismus, increased tremor, numbness, muscle twitching, activation of latent Horner's syndrome, peripheral neuropathy.

Respiratory: Pharyngeal pain, cough.

Skin: Malignant melanoma *(see also CONTRAINDICATIONS)*, flushing.

Special Senses: Oculogyric crisis, diplopia, blurred vision, dilated pupils.

Urogenital: Urinary retention, urinary incontinence, priapism.

Miscellaneous: Bizarre breathing patterns, faintness, hoarseness, malaise, hot flashes, sense of stimulation.

Laboratory Tests: Decreased white blood cell count and serum potassium; increased serum creatinine and uric acid; protein and glucose in urine.

Entacapone

The most commonly observed adverse events (>5%) in the double-blind, placebo-controlled trials of entacapone (n=1003) associated with the use of entacapone alone and not seen at an equivalent frequency among the placebo-treated patients were: dyskinesia/hyperkinesia, nausea, urine discoloration, diarrhea, and abdominal pain.

Approximately 14% of the 603 patients given entacapone in the double-blind, placebo-controlled trials discontinued treatment due to adverse events compared to 9% of the 400 patients who received placebo. The most frequent causes of discontinuation in decreasing order are: psychiatric reasons (2% vs. 1%), diarrhea (2% vs. 0%), dyskinesia/hyperkinesia (2% vs. 1%), nausea (2% vs. 1%), abdominal pain (1% vs. 0%), and aggravation of Parkinson's disease symptoms (1% vs. 1%).

Adverse Event Incidence in Controlled Clinical Studies of Entacapone

Table 5 lists treatment emergent adverse events that occurred in at least 1% of patients treated with entacapone participating in the double-blind, placebo-controlled studies and that were numerically more common in the entacapone group, compared to placebo. In these studies, either entacapone or placebo was added to carbidopa-levodopa (or benserazide-levodopa).

[See table 5 below]

The prescriber should be aware that these figures cannot be used to predict the incidence of adverse events in the course of usual medical practice where patient characteristics and other factors differ from those that prevailed in the clinical studies. Similarly, the cited frequencies cannot be compared with figures obtained from other clinical investigations involving different treatments, uses, and investigators. The cited figures do, however, provide the prescriber with some basis for estimating the relative contribution of drug and nondrug factors to the adverse events observed in the population studied.

Effects of Gender and Age on Adverse Reactions

No differences were noted in the rate of adverse events attributable to entacapone alone by age or gender.

DRUG ABUSE AND DEPENDENCE

Controlled substance class: Stalevo® (carbidopa, levodopa and entacapone) is not a controlled substance.

Physical and psychological dependence: Stalevo has not been systematically studied, in animal or humans, for its potential for abuse, tolerance or physical dependence. In premarketing clinical experience, carbidopa-levodopa did not reveal any tendency for a withdrawal syndrome or any drug-seeking behavior. However, there are rare post-marketing reports of abuse and dependence of medications containing levodopa. In general, these reports consist of patients taking increasing doses of medication in order to achieve a euphoric state.

OVERDOSAGE

Management of acute overdosage with Stalevo® (carbidopa, levodopa and entacapone) is the same as management of acute overdosage with levodopa and entacapone. Pyridoxine is not effective in reversing the actions of Stalevo.

Hospitalization is advised, and general supportive measures should be employed, along with immediate gastric lavage and repeated doses of charcoal over time. This may hasten the elimination of entacapone in particular, by decreasing its absorption/reabsorption from the GI tract. Intravenous fluids should be administered judiciously and an adequate airway maintained.

The adequacy of the respiratory, circulatory and renal systems should be carefully monitored and appropriate supportive measures employed. Electrocardiographic monitoring should be instituted and the patient carefully observed for the development of arrhythmias; if required, appropriate antiarrhythmic therapy should be given. The possibility that the patient may have taken other drugs, increasing the risk of drug interactions (especially catechol-structured drugs) should be taken into consideration. To date, no experience has been reported with dialysis; hence, its value in overdosage is not known. Hemodialysis or hemoperfusion is unlikely to reduce entacapone levels due to its high binding to plasma proteins.

There are very few cases of overdosage with levodopa reported in the published literature. Based on the limited available information, the acute symptoms of levodopa/dopa decarboxylase inhibitor overdosage can be expected to arise from dopaminergic overstimulation. Doses of a few grams may result in CNS disturbances, with an increasing likelihood of cardiovascular disturbance (e.g., hypotension, tachycardia) and more severe psychiatric problems at higher doses. An isolated report of rhabdomyolysis and another of transient renal insufficiency suggest that levodopa overdosage may give rise to systemic complications, secondary to dopaminergic overstimulation.

There have been no reported cases of either accidental or intentional overdose with entacapone tablets. However, COMT inhibition by entacapone treatment is dose-dependent. A massive overdose of entacapone may theoretically produce a 100% inhibition of the COMT enzyme in people, thereby preventing the O-methylation of endogenous and exogenous catechols.

The highest single dose of entacapone administered to humans was 800 mg, resulting in a plasma concentration of 14.1 µg/mL. The highest daily dose given to humans was 2400 mg, administered in one study as 400 mg six times daily with carbidopa-levodopa for 14 days in 15 Parkinson's disease patients, and in another study as 800 mg t.i.d. for 7 days in 8 healthy volunteers. At this daily dose, the peak plasma concentrations of entacapone averaged 2.0 µg/mL (at 45 min., compared to 1.0 and 1.2 µg/mL with 200 mg entacapone at 45 min.). Abdominal pain and loose stools were the most commonly observed adverse events during this study. Daily doses as high as 2000 mg entacapone have been administered as 200 mg 10 times daily with carbidopa-levodopa or benserazide-levodopa for at least 1 year in 10 patients, for at least 2 years in 8 patients and for at least 3 years in 7 patients. Overall, however, clinical experience with daily doses above 1600 mg is limited.

The range of lethal plasma concentrations of entacapone based on animal data was 80-130 µg/mL in mice. Respiratory difficulties, ataxia, hypoactivity, and convulsions were observed in mice after high oral (gavage) doses.

DOSAGE AND ADMINISTRATION

Individual tablets should not be fractionated and only one tablet should be administered at each dosing interval.

Generally speaking, Stalevo® (carbidopa, levodopa and entacapone) should be used as a substitute for patients already stabilized on equivalent doses of carbidopa-levodopa and entacapone. However, some patients who have been stabilized on a given dose of carbidopa-levodopa may be treated with Stalevo if a decision has been made to add entacapone *(see below)*.

The optimum daily dosage of Stalevo must be determined by careful titration in each patient. Stalevo tablets are available in three strengths, each in a 1:4 ratio of carbidopa to levodopa and combined with 200 mg of entacapone in a standard-release formulation (Stalevo 50 containing 12.5 mg of carbidopa, 50 mg of levodopa and 200 mg of entacapone; Stalevo 100 containing 25 mg of carbidopa,

Table 5
Summary of Patients with Adverse Events After Start of Trial Drug Administration
At Least 1% in Entacapone Group and >Placebo

SYSTEM ORGAN CLASS Preferred Term	Entacapone (n = 603) % of patients	Placebo (n = 400) % of patients
SKIN AND APPENDAGES DISORDERS		
Sweating Increased	2	1
MUSCULOSKELETAL SYSTEM DISORDERS		
Back Pain	2	1
CENTRAL & PERIPHERAL NERVOUS SYSTEM DISORDERS		
Dyskinesia	25	15
Hyperkinesia	10	5
Hypokinesia	9	8
Dizziness	8	6
SPECIAL SENSES, OTHER DISORDERS		
Taste Perversion	1	0
PSYCHIATRIC DISORDERS		
Anxiety	2	1
Somnolence	2	0
Agitation	1	0
GASTROINTESTINAL SYSTEM DISORDERS		
Nausea	14	8
Diarrhea	10	4
Abdominal Pain	8	4
Constipation	6	4
Vomiting	4	1
Mouth Dry	3	0
Dyspepsia	2	1
Flatulence	2	0
Gastritis	1	0
Gastrointestinal Disorders NOS	1	0
RESPIRATORY SYSTEM DISORDERS		
Dyspnea	3	1
PLATELET, BLEEDING & CLOTTING DISORDERS		
Purpura	2	1
URINARY SYSTEM DISORDERS		
Urine Discoloration	10	0
BODY AS A WHOLE - GENERAL DISORDERS		
Back Pain	4	2
Fatigue	6	4
Asthenia	2	1
RESISTANCE MECHANISM DISORDERS		
Infection Bacterial	1	0

100 mg of levodopa and 200 mg of entacapone; and Stalevo 150 containing 37.5 mg of carbidopa, 150 mg of levodopa and 200 mg of entacapone).

Therapy should be individualized and adjusted according to the desired therapeutic response.

Studies show that peripheral dopa decarboxylase is saturated by carbidopa at approximately 70 mg to 100 mg a day. Patients receiving less than this amount of carbidopa are more likely to experience nausea and vomiting. Experience with total daily dosages of carbidopa greater than 200 mg is limited.

Clinical experience with daily doses above 1600 mg of entacapone is limited. It is recommended that no more than one Stalevo tablet be taken at each dosing administration. Thus the maximum recommended daily dose of Stalevo is eight tablets per day.

How to transfer patients taking carbidopa-levodopa preparations and Comtan® (entacapone) tablets to Stalevo® (carbidopa, levodopa and entacapone) tablets

There is no experience in transferring patients currently treated with formulations of carbidopa-levodopa other than immediate-release carbidopa-levodopa with a 1:4 ratio (controlled-release formulations, or standard-release presentations with a 1:10 ratio of carbidopa-levodopa) and entacapone to Stalevo.

Patients who are currently treated with Comtan 200 mg tablet with each dose of standard-release carbidopa-levodopa, can be directly switched to the corresponding strength of Stalevo containing the same amounts of levodopa and carbidopa. For example, patients receiving one tablet of standard-release carbidopa-levodopa 25/100 mg and one tablet of Comtan 200 mg at each administration can be switched to a single Stalevo 100 tablet (containing 25 mg of carbidopa, 100 mg of levodopa and 200 mg of entacapone).

How to transfer patients not currently treated with Comtan® (entacapone) tablets from carbidopa-levodopa to Stalevo® (carbidopa, levodopa and entacapone) tablets

In patients with Parkinson's disease who experience the signs and symptoms of end-of-dose "wearing-off" on their current standard-release carbidopa-levodopa treatment, clinical experience shows that patients with a history of moderate or severe dyskinesias or taking more than 600 mg of levodopa per day are likely to require a reduction in daily levodopa dose when entacapone is added to their treatment. Since dose adjustment of the individual components is impossible with fixed-dose products, it is recommended that patients first be titrated individually with a carbidopa-levodopa product (ratio 1:4) and an entacapone product, and then transferred to a corresponding dose of Stalevo once the patient's status has stabilized.

In patients who take a total daily levodopa dose up to 600 mg, and who do not have dyskinesias, an attempt can be made to transfer to the corresponding daily dose of Stalevo. Even in these patients, a reduction of carbidopa-levodopa or entacapone may be necessary however, the provider is reminded that this may not be possible with Stalevo. Since entacapone prolongs and enhances the effects of levodopa, therapy should be individualized and adjusted if necessary according to the desired therapeutic response.

Maintenance of Stalevo® Treatment

Therapy should be individualized and adjusted for each patient according to the desired therapeutic response.

When less levodopa is required, the total daily dosage of carbidopa-levodopa should be reduced by either decreasing the strength of Stalevo at each administration or by decreasing the frequency of administration by extending the time between doses.

When more levodopa is required, the next higher strength of Stalevo should be taken and/or the frequency of doses should be increased, up to a maximum of 8 times daily and not to exceed the maximum daily dose recommendations as outlined above.

Addition of Other Antiparkinsonian Medications

Standard drugs for Parkinson's disease may be used concomitantly while Stalevo is being administered, although dosage adjustments may be required.

Interruption of Therapy

Sporadic cases of a symptom complex resembling Neuroleptic Malignant Syndrome (NMS) have been associated with dose reductions and withdrawal of levodopa preparations. Patients should be observed carefully if abrupt reduction or discontinuation of Stalevo is required, especially if the patient is receiving neuroleptics. *(See WARNINGS.)*

If general anesthesia is required, Stalevo may be continued as long as the patient is permitted to take fluids and medication by mouth. If therapy is interrupted temporarily, the patient should be observed for symptoms resembling NMS, and the usual daily dosage may be administered as soon as the patient is able to take oral medication.

Special Populations

Patients with Impaired Hepatic Function

Patients with hepatic impairment should be treated with caution. The AUC and C_{max} of entacapone approximately doubled in patients with documented liver disease, compared to controls. However, these studies were conducted with single-dose entacapone without levodopa/dopa decarboxylase inhibitor coadministration, and therefore the effects of liver disease on the kinetics of chronically administered entacapone have not been evaluated *(see CLINICAL PHARMACOLOGY, Pharmacokinetics of Entacapone)*.

HOW SUPPLIED

Stalevo® (carbidopa, levodopa and entacapone) is supplied as film-coated tablets for oral administration in the following three strengths:

Stalevo 50 film-coated tablets containing 12.5 mg of carbidopa, 50 mg of levodopa and 200 mg of entacapone.

The round, bi-convex shaped tablets are brownish- or greyish-red, unscored, and embossed "LCE 50" on one side.

HDPE bottle of 100 tablets .... NDC 0078-0407-05
HDPE bottle of 250 tablets .... NDC 0078-0407-28

Stalevo 100 film-coated tablets containing 25 mg of carbidopa, 100 mg of levodopa and 200 mg of entacapone.

The oval-shaped tablets are brownish- or greyish-red, unscored, and embossed "LCE 100" on one side.

HDPE bottle of 100 tablets .... NDC 0078-0408-05
HDPE bottle of 250 tablets .... NDC 0078-0408-28

Stalevo 150 film-coated tablets containing 37.5 mg of carbidopa, 150 mg of levodopa and 200 mg of entacapone

The elongated-ellipse shaped tablets are brownish- or greyish-red, unscored, and embossed "LCE 150" on one side.

HDPE bottle of 100 tablets .... NDC 0078-0409-05
HDPE bottle of 250 tablets .... NDC 0078-0409-28

Store at 25°C (77°F); excursions permitted to 15°C-30°C (59°F-86°F).

[see USP Controlled Room Temperature.]

Dispense in tight container (USP).

JANUARY 2004
Printed in U.S.A.
T2004-05
89019602
Manufactured by:
Orion Corporation
ORION PHARMA
Orionintie 1, FIN-02200 Espoo, Finland
Marketed by:
Novartis Pharmaceuticals Corporation
East Hanover, New Jersey 07936

Shown in Product Identification Guide, page 326

STARLIX® ℞

[stăr-līks']
(nateglinide)
tablets
Rx only

Prescribing Information

The following prescribing information is based on official labeling in effect July, 2004.

DESCRIPTION

Starlix® (nateglinide) is an oral antidiabetic agent used in the management of Type 2 diabetes mellitus [also known as non-insulin dependent diabetes mellitus (NIDDM) or adult-onset diabetes]. Starlix, (-)-N-[(trans-4-isopropylcyclohexane)carbonyl]-D-phenylalanine, is structurally unrelated to the oral sulfonylurea insulin secretagogues.

The structural formula is as shown

$C_{19}H_{27}NO_3$
317.43

Nateglinide is a white powder with a molecular weight of 317.43. It is freely soluble in methanol, ethanol, and chloroform, soluble in ether, sparingly soluble in acetonitrile and octanol, and practically insoluble in water. Starlix biconvex tablets contain 60 mg, or 120 mg, of nateglinide for oral administration.

Inactive Ingredients: colloidal silicon dioxide, croscarmellose sodium, hydroxypropyl methylcellulose, iron oxides (red or yellow), lactose monohydrate, magnesium stearate, microcrystalline cellulose, polyethylene glycol, povidone, talc, and titanium dioxide.

CLINICAL PHARMACOLOGY

Mechanism of Action

Nateglinide is an amino-acid derivative that lowers blood glucose levels by stimulating insulin secretion from the pancreas. This action is dependent upon functioning beta-cells in the pancreatic islets. Nateglinide interacts with the ATP-sensitive potassium ($K+_{ATP}$) channel on pancreatic beta-cells. The subsequent depolarization of the beta cell opens the calcium channel, producing calcium influx and insulin secretion. The extent of insulin release is glucose dependent and diminishes at low glucose levels. Nateglinide is highly tissue selective with low affinity for heart and skeletal muscle.

Pharmacokinetics

Absorption

Following oral administration immediately prior to a meal, nateglinide is rapidly absorbed with mean peak plasma drug concentrations (C_{max}) generally occurring within 1 hour (T_{max}) after dosing. When administered to patients with Type 2 diabetes over the dosage range 60 mg to 240 mg three times a day for one week, nateglinide demonstrated linear pharmacokinetics for both AUC (area under the time/plasma concentration curve) and C_{max}. T_{max} was also found to be independent of dose in this patient population. Absolute bioavailability is estimated to be approximately 73%. When given with or after meals, the extent of nateglinide absorption (AUC) remains unaffected. However, there is a delay in the rate of absorption characterized by a decrease in C_{max} and a delay in time to peak plasma concentration (T_{max}). Plasma profiles are characterized by multiple plasma concentration peaks when nateglinide is administered under fasting conditions. This effect is diminished when nateglinide is taken prior to a meal.

Distribution

Based on data following intravenous (IV) administration of nateglinide, the steady-state volume of distribution of nateglinide is estimated to be approximately 10 liters in healthy subjects. Nateglinide is extensively bound (98%) to serum proteins, primarily serum albumin, and to a lesser extent α_1 acid glycoprotein. The extent of serum protein binding is independent of drug concentration over the test range of 0.1-10 µg/mL.

Metabolism

Nateglinide is metabolized by the mixed-function oxidase system prior to elimination. The major routes of metabolism are hydroxylation followed by glucuronide conjugation. The major metabolites are less potent antidiabetic agents than nateglinide. The isoprene minor metabolite possesses potency similar to that of the parent compound nateglinide.

In vitro data demonstrate that nateglinide is predominantly metabolized by cytochrome P450 isoenzymes CYP2C9 (70%) and CYP3A4 (30%).

Excretion

Nateglinide and its metabolites are rapidly and completely eliminated following oral administration. Within 6 hours after dosing, approximately 75% of the administered ^{14}C-nateglinide was recovered in the urine. Eighty-three percent of the ^{14}C-nateglinide was excreted in the urine with an additional 10% eliminated in the feces. Approximately 16% of the ^{14}C-nateglinide was excreted in the urine as parent compound. In all studies of healthy volunteers and patients with Type 2 diabetes, nateglinide plasma concentrations declined rapidly with an average elimination half-life of approximately 1.5 hours. Consistent with this short elimination half-life, there was no apparent accumulation of nateglinide upon multiple dosing of up to 240 mg three times daily for 7 days.

Drug Interactions

In vitro drug metabolism studies indicate that Starlix is predominantly metabolized by the cytochrome P450 isozyme CYP2C9 (70%) and to a lesser extent CYP3A4 (30%). Starlix is a potential inhibitor of the CYP2C9 isoenzyme *in vivo* as indicated by its ability to inhibit the *in vitro* metabolism of tolbutamide. Inhibition of CYP3A4 metabolic reactions was not detected in *in vitro* experiments.

Glyburide: In a randomized, multiple-dose crossover study, patients with Type 2 diabetes were administered 120 mg Starlix three times a day before meals for 1 day in combination with glyburide mg daily. There were no clinically relevant alterations in the pharmacokinetics of either agent.

Metformin: When Starlix 120 mg three times daily before meals was administered in combination with metformin 500 mg three times daily to patients with Type 2 diabetes, there were no clinically relevant changes in the pharmacokinetics of either agent.

Digoxin: When Starlix 120 mg before meals was administered in combination with a single 1-mg dose of digoxin to healthy volunteers, there were no clinically relevant changes in the pharmacokinetics of either agent.

Warfarin: When healthy subjects were administered Starlix mg three times daily before meals for four days in combination with a single dose of warfarin 30 mg on day 2, there were no alterations in the pharmacokinetics of either agent. Prothrombin time was not affected.

Diclofenac: Administration of morning and lunch doses of Starlix 120 mg in combination with single 75-mg dose of diclofenac in healthy volunteers resulted in no significant changes to the pharmacokinetics of either agent.

Special Populations

Geriatric: Age did not influence the pharmacokinetic properties of nateglinide. Therefore, no dose adjustments are necessary for elderly patients.

Gender: No clinically significant differences in nateglinide pharmacokinetics were observed between men and women. Therefore, no dose adjustment based on gender is necessary.

Race: Results of a population pharmacokinetic analysis including subjects of Caucasian, Black, and other ethnic origins suggest that race has little influence on the pharmacokinetics of nateglinide.

Renal Impairment: Compared to healthy matched subjects, patients with Type 2 diabetes and moderate-to-severe renal insufficiency (CrCl 15-50 mL/min) not on dialysis displayed similar apparent clearance, AUC, and C_{max}. Patients with Type 2 diabetes and renal failure on dialysis exhibited reduced overall drug exposure. However, hemodialysis patients also experienced reductions in plasma protein binding compared to the matched healthy volunteers.

Hepatic Impairment: The peak and total exposure of nateglinide in non-diabetic subjects with mild hepatic insufficiency were increased by 30% compared to matched healthy subjects. Starlix® (nateglinide) should be used with caution in patients with chronic liver disease. *(See PRECAUTIONS Hepatic Impairment.)*

Pharmacodynamics

Starlix is rapidly absorbed and stimulates pancreatic insulin secretion within 20 minutes of oral administration. When Starlix is dosed three times daily before meals there

Continued on next page

Starlix—Cont.

is a rapid rise in plasma insulin, with peak levels approximately 1 hour after dosing and a fall to baseline by 4 hours after dosing.

In a double-blind, controlled clinical trial in which Starlix was administered before each of three meals, plasma glucose levels were determined over a 12-hour, daytime period after 7 weeks of treatment. Starlix was administered 10 minutes before meals. The meals were based on standard diabetic weight maintenance menus with the total caloric content based on each subject's height. Starlix produced statistically significant decreases in fasting and postprandial glycemia compared to placebo.

CLINICAL STUDIES

A total of 3,566 patients were randomized in nine double-blind, placebo- or active-controlled studies 8 to 24 weeks in duration to evaluate the safety and efficacy of Starlix® (nateglinide). 3,513 patients had efficacy values beyond baseline. In these studies Starlix was administered up to 30 minutes before each of three main meals daily.

Starlix® Monotherapy Compared to Placebo

In a randomized, double-blind, placebo-controlled, 24-week study, patients with Type 2 diabetes with HbA_{1C} ≥6.8% on diet alone were randomized to receive either Starlix (60 mg or 120 mg three times daily before meals) or placebo. Baseline HbA_{1C} ranged from 7.9% to 8.1% and 77.8% of patients were previously untreated with oral antidiabetic therapy. Patients previously treated with antidiabetic medications were required to discontinue that medication for at least 2 months before randomization. The addition of Starlix before meals resulted in statistically significant reductions in mean HbA_{1C} and mean fasting plasma glucose (FPG) compared to placebo *(see Table 1)*. The reductions in HbA_{1C} and FPG were similar for patients naïve to, and those previously exposed to, antidiabetic medications.

In this study, one episode of severe hypoglycemia (plasma glucose <36 mg/dL) was reported in a patient treated with Starlix 120 mg three times daily before meals. No patients experienced hypoglycemia that required third party assistance. Patients treated with Starlix had statistically significant mean increases in weight compared to placebo *(see Table 1)*.

In another randomized, double-blind, 24-week, active- and placebo-controlled study, patients with Type 2 diabetes were randomized to receive Starlix (120 mg three times daily before meals), metformin 500 mg (three times daily), a combination of Starlix 120 mg (three times daily before meals) and metformin 500 mg (three times daily), or placebo. Baseline HbA_{1C} ranged from 8.3% to 8.4%. Fifty-seven percent of patients were previously untreated with oral antidiabetic therapy. Starlix monotherapy resulted in significant reductions in mean HbA_{1C} and mean FPG compared to placebo that were similar to the results of the study reported above *(see Table 2)*.

[See table 1 above]

Starlix® Monotherapy Compared to Other Oral Antidiabetic Agents

Glyburide

In a 24-week, double-blind, active-controlled trial, patients with Type 2 diabetes who had been on a sulfonylurea for ≥ 3 months and who had a baseline HbA_{1C} ≥6.5% were randomized to receive Starlix (60 mg or 120 mg three times daily before meals) or glyburide 10 mg once daily. Patients randomized to Starlix had significant increases in mean HbA_{1C} and mean FPG at endpoint compared to patients randomized to glyburide.

Metformin

In another randomized, double-blind, 24-week, active- and placebo-controlled study, patients with Type 2 diabetes were randomized to receive Starlix (120 mg three times daily before meals), metformin 500 mg (three times daily), a combination of Starlix 120 mg (three times daily before meals) and metformin 500 mg (three times daily), or placebo. Baseline HbA_{1C} ranged from 8.3% to 8.4%. Fifty-seven percent of patients were previously untreated with oral antidiabetic therapy. The reductions in mean HbA_{1C} and mean FPG at endpoint with metformin monotherapy were significantly greater than the reductions in these variables with Starlix monotherapy *(see Table 2)*. Relative to placebo, Starlix monotherapy was associated with significant increases in mean weight whereas metformin monotherapy was associated with significant decreases in mean weight. Among the subset of patients naïve to antidiabetic therapy, the reductions in mean HbA_{1C} and mean FPG for Starlix monotherapy were similar to those for metformin monotherapy *(see Table 2)*. Among the subset of patients previously treated with other antidiabetic agents, primarily glyburide, HbA_{1C} in the Starlix monotherapy group increased slightly from baseline, whereas HbA_{1C} was reduced in the metformin monotherapy group *(see Table 2)*.

Starlix® Combination Therapy

Metformin

In another randomized, double-blind, 24-week, active- and placebo-controlled study, patients with Type 2 diabetes were randomized to receive Starlix (120 mg three times daily before meals), metformin 500 mg (three times daily), a combination of Starlix 120 mg (three times daily before meals) and metformin 500 mg (three times daily), or placebo. Baseline HbA_{1C} ranged from 8.3% to 8.4%. Fifty-seven percent of patients were previously untreated with oral antidiabetic therapy. Patients previously treated with antidiabetic medications were required to discontinue medication for at least 2 months before randomization. The combination of Starlix and metformin resulted in statistically significantly greater reductions in HbA_{1C} and FPG compared to either Starlix or metformin monotherapy *(see Table 2)*. Starlix, alone or in combination with metformin, significantly reduced the prandial glucose elevation from pre-meal to 2-hours post-meal compared to placebo and metformin alone.

Table 1
Endpoint results for a 24-week, fixed dose study of Starlix® monotherapy

	Placebo	Starlix® 60 mg three times daily before meals	Starlix® 120 mg three times daily before meals
HbA_{1c} (%)	**N=168**	**N=167**	**N=168**
Baseline (mean)	8.0	7.9	8.1
Change from baseline (mean)	+0.2	−0.3	−0.5
Difference from placebo (mean)		−0.5[a]	−0.7[a]
FPG (mg/dL)	**N=172**	**N=171**	**N=169**
Baseline (mean)	167.9	161.0	166.5
Change from baseline (mean)	+9.1	+0.4	−4.5
Difference from placebo (mean)		−8.7[a]	−13.6[a]
Weight (kg)	**N=170**	**N=169**	**N=166**
Baseline (mean)	85.8	83.7	86.3
Change from baseline (mean)	−0.7	+0.3	+0.9
Difference from placebo (mean)		+1.0[a]	+1.6[a]

[a]p-value ≤ 0.004

Table 2
Endpoint results for a 24-week study of Starlix® monotherapy and combination with metformin

	Placebo	Starlix® 120 mg three times daily before meals	Metformin 500 mg three times daily	Starlix® 120 mg before meals plus Metformin*
HbA_{1c} (%)				
All	**N=160**	**N=171**	**N=172**	**N=162**
Baseline (mean)	8.3	8.3	8.4	8.4
Change from baseline (mean)	+0.4	−0.4[bc]	−0.8[c]	−1.5
Difference from placebo		−0.8[a]	−1.2[a]	−1.9[a]
Naïve	**N=98**	**N=99**	**N=98**	**N=81**
Baseline (mean)	8.2	8.1	8.3	8.2
Change from baseline (mean)	+0.3	−0.7[c]	−0.8[c]	−1.6
Difference from placebo		−1.0[a]	−1.1[a]	−1.9[a]
Non-Naïve	**N=62**	**N=72**	**N=74**	**N=81**
Baseline (mean)	8.3	8.5	8.7	8.7
Change from baseline (mean)	+0.6	+0.004[bc]	−0.8[c]	−1.4
Difference from placebo		−0.6[a]	−1.4[a]	−2.0[a]
FPG (mg/dL)				
All	**N=166**	**N=173**	**N=174**	**N=167**
Baseline (mean)	194.0	196.5	196.0	197.7
Change from baseline (mean)	+8.0	−13.1[bc]	−30.0[c]	−44.9
Difference from placebo		−21.1[a]	−38.0[a]	−52.9[a]
Weight (kg)				
All	**N=160**	**N=169**	**N=169**	**N=160**
Baseline (mean)	85.0	85.0	86.0	87.4
Change from baseline (mean)	−0.4	+0.9[bc]	−0.1	+0.2
Difference from placebo		+1.3[a]	+0.3	+0.6

[a]p-value ≤0.05 vs. placebo
[b]p-value ≤0.03 vs. metformin
[c]p-value ≤0.05 vs. combination
*Metformin was administered three times daily

In this study, one episode of severe hypoglycemia (plasma glucose ≤36 mg/dL) was reported in a patient receiving the combination of Starlix and metformin and four episodes of severe hypoglycemia were reported in a single patient in the metformin treatment arm. No patient experienced an episode of hypoglycemia that required third party assistance. Compared to placebo, Starlix monotherapy was associated with a statistically significant increase in weight, while no significant change in weight was observed with combined Starlix and metformin therapy *(see Table 2)*.

In another 24-week, double-blind, placebo-controlled trial, patients with Type 2 diabetes with HbA_{1C} ≥6.8% after treatment with metformin (≥1500 mg daily for ≥1 month) were first entered into a four-week run-in period of metformin monotherapy (2000 mg daily) and then randomized to receive Starlix (60 mg or 120 mg three times daily before meals) or placebo in addition to metformin. Combination therapy with Starlix and metformin was associated with statistically significantly greater reductions in HbA_{1C} compared to metformin monotherapy (−0.4% and −0.6% for Starlix 60 mg and Starlix 120 mg plus metformin, respectively).

[See table 2 above]

Rosiglitazone

A 24-week, double blind multicenter, placebo-controlled trial was performed in patients with Type 2 diabetes not adequately controlled after a therapeutic response to rosiglitazone monotherapy 8 mg daily. The addition of Starlix (120 mg three times per day with meals) was associated with statistically significantly greater reductions in HbA_{1C} compared to rosiglitazone monotherapy. The difference was −0.77% at 24 weeks. The mean change in weight from baseline was about +3 kg for patients treated with Starlix plus rosiglitazone vs about +1 kg for patients treated with placebo plus rosiglitazone.

Glyburide

In a 12-week study of patients with Type 2 diabetes inadequately controlled on glyburide 10 mg once daily, the addition of Starlix (60 mg or 120 mg three times daily before meals) did not produce any additional benefit.

INDICATIONS AND USAGE

Starlix® (nateglinide) is indicated as monotherapy to lower blood glucose in patients with Type 2 diabetes (non-insulin dependent diabetes mellitus, NIDDM) whose hyperglycemia cannot be adequately controlled by diet and physical exercise and who have not been chronically treated with other antidiabetic agents.

Starlix is also indicated for use in combination with metformin or a thiazolidinedione. In patients whose hyperglycemia is inadequately controlled with metformin or after a therapeutic response to a thiazolidinedione, Starlix may be added to, but not substituted for, those drugs.

Patients whose hyperglycemia is not adequately controlled with glyburide or other insulin secretagogues should not be switched to Starlix, nor should Starlix be added to their treatment regimen.

CONTRAINDICATIONS

Starlix® (nateglinide) is contraindicated in patients with:

1. Known hypersensitivity to the drug or its inactive ingredients.
2. Type 1 diabetes.
3. Diabetic ketoacidosis. This condition should be treated with insulin.

PRECAUTIONS

Hypoglycemia: All oral blood glucose lowering drugs that are absorbed systemically are capable of producing hypoglycemia. The frequency of hypoglycemia is related to the severity of the diabetes, the level of glycemic control, and other patient characteristics. Geriatric patients, malnourished patients, and those with adrenal or pituitary insufficiency or severe renal impairment are more susceptible to the glucose lowering effect of these treatments. The risk of hypoglycemia may be increased by strenuous physical exercise, ingestion of alcohol, insufficient caloric intake on an acute or chronic basis, or combinations with other oral antidiabetic agents. Hypoglycemia may be difficult to recognize in patients with autonomic neuropathy and/or those who use beta-blockers. Starlix® (nateglinide) should be administered prior to meals to reduce the risk of hypoglycemia. Patients who skip meals should also skip their scheduled dose of Starlix to reduce the risk of hypoglycemia.

Hepatic Impairment: Starlix should be used with caution in patients with moderate-to-severe liver disease because such patients have not been studied.

Loss of Glycemic Control

Transient loss of glycemic control may occur with fever, infection, trauma, or surgery. Insulin therapy may be needed instead of Starlix therapy at such times. Secondary failure, or reduced effectiveness of Starlix over a period of time, may occur.

Information for Patients

Patients should be informed of the potential risks and benefits of Starlix and of alternative modes of therapy. The risks and management of hypoglycemia should be explained. Patients should be instructed to take Starlix 1 to 30 minutes before ingesting a meal, but to skip their scheduled dose if they skip the meal so that the risk of hypoglycemia will be reduced. Drug interactions should be discussed with patients. Patients should be informed of potential drug-drug interactions with Starlix.

Laboratory Tests

Response to therapies should be periodically assessed with glucose values and HbA_{1C} levels.

Drug Interactions

Nateglinide is highly bound to plasma proteins (98%), mainly albumin. *In vitro* displacement studies with highly protein-bound drugs such as furosemide, propranolol, captopril, nicardipine, pravastatin, glyburide, warfarin, phenytoin, acetylsalicylic acid, tolbutamide, and metformin showed no influence on the extent of nateglinide protein binding. Similarly, nateglinide had no influence on the serum protein binding of propranolol, glyburide, nicardipine, warfarin, phenytoin, acetylsalicylic acid, and tolbutamide *in vitro*. However, prudent evaluation of individual cases is warranted in the clinical setting.

Certain drugs, including nonsteroidal anti-inflammatory agents (NSAIDs), salicylates, monoamine oxidase inhibitors, and non-selective beta-adrenergic-blocking agents may potentiate the hypoglycemic action of Starlix and other oral antidiabetic drugs.

Certain drugs including thiazides, corticosteroids, thyroid products, and sympathomimetics may reduce the hypoglycemic action of Starlix and other oral antidiabetic drugs.

When these drugs are administered or withdrawn from patients receiving Starlix, the patient should be observed closely for changes in glycemic control.

Drug/Food Interactions

The pharmacokinetics of nateglinide were not affected by the composition of a meal (high protein, fat, or carbohydrate). However, peak plasma levels were significantly reduced when Starlix was administered 10 minutes prior to a liquid meal. Starlix did not have any effect on gastric emptying in healthy subjects as assessed by acetaminophen testing.

Carcinogenesis/Mutagenesis/Impairment of Fertility

Carcinogenicity: A two-year carcinogenicity study in Sprague-Dawley rats was performed with oral doses of nateglinide up to 900 mg/kg/day, which produced AUC exposures in male and female rats approximately 30 and 40 times the human therapeutic exposure respectively with a recommended Starlix dose of 120 mg, three times daily before meals. A two-year carcinogenicity study in B6C3F1 mice was performed with oral doses of nateglinide up to 400 mg/kg/day, which produced AUC exposures in male and female mice approximately 10 and 30 times the human therapeutic exposure with a recommended Starlix dose of 120 mg, three times daily before meals. No evidence of a tumorigenic response was found in either rats or mice.

Mutagenesis: Nateglinide was not genotoxic in the *in vitro* Ames test, mouse lymphoma assay, chromosome aberration assay in Chinese hamster lung cells, or in the *in vivo* mouse micronucleus test.

Impairment of Fertility: Fertility was unaffected by administration of nateglinide to rats at doses up to 600 mg/kg (approximately 16 times the human therapeutic exposure with a recommended Starlix dose of 120 mg three times daily before meals).

Pregnancy

Pregnancy Category C

Nateglinide was not teratogenic in rats at doses up to 1000 mg/kg (approximately 60 times the human therapeutic exposure with a recommended Starlix dose of 120 mg, three times daily before meals). In the rabbit, embryonic development was adversely affected and the incidence of gallbladder agenesis or small gallbladder was increased at a dose of 500 mg/kg (approximately 40 times the human therapeutic exposure with a recommended Starlix dose of 120 mg, three times daily before meals). There are no adequate and well-controlled studies in pregnant women. Starlix should not be used during pregnancy.

Labor and Delivery

The effect of Starlix on labor and delivery in humans is not known.

Nursing Mothers

Studies in lactating rats showed that nateglinide is excreted in the milk; the $AUC_{0\text{-}48h}$ ratio in milk to plasma was approximately 1:4. During the peri- and postnatal period body weights were lower in offspring of rats administered nateglinide 1000 mg/kg (approximately 60 times the human therapeutic exposure with a recommended Starlix dose of 120 mg, three times daily before meals). It is not known whether Starlix is excreted in human milk. Because many drugs are excreted in human milk, Starlix should not be administered to a nursing woman.

Pediatric Use

The safety and effectiveness of Starlix in pediatric patients have not been established.

Geriatric Use

No differences were observed in safety or efficacy of Starlix between patients age 65 and over, and those under age 65. However, greater sensitivity of some older individuals to Starlix therapy cannot be ruled out.

ADVERSE REACTIONS

In clinical trials, approximately 2,600 patients with Type 2 diabetes were treated with Starlix® (nateglinide). Of these, approximately 1,335 patients were treated for 6 months or longer and approximately 190 patients for one year or longer.

Hypoglycemia was relatively uncommon in all treatment arms of the clinical trials. Only 0.3% of Starlix patients discontinued due to hypoglycemia. Gastrointestinal symptoms, especially diarrhea and nausea, were no more common in patients using the combination of Starlix and metformin than in patients receiving metformin alone. Likewise, peripheral edema was no more common in patients using the combination of Starlix and rosiglitazone than in patients receiving rosiglitazone alone. The following table lists events that occurred more frequently in Starlix patients than placebo patients in controlled clinical trials.

Common Adverse Events (≥2% in Starlix® patients) in Starlix® Monotherapy Trials (% of patients)

	Placebo N=458	Starlix N=1441
Preferred Term		
Upper Respiratory Infection	8.1	10.5
Back Pain	3.7	4.0
Flu Symptoms	2.6	3.6
Dizziness	2.2	3.6
Arthropathy	2.2	3.3
Diarrhea	3.1	3.2
Accidental Trauma	1.7	2.9
Bronchitis	2.6	2.7
Coughing	2.2	2.4
Hypoglycemia	0.4	2.4

During post-marketing experience, rare cases of hypersensitivity reactions such as rash, itching and urticaria have been reported.

Laboratory Abnormalities

Uric acid: There were increases in mean uric acid levels for patients treated with Starlix alone, Starlix in combination with metformin, metformin alone, and glyburide alone. The respective differences from placebo were 0.29 mg/dL, 0.45 mg/dL, 0.28 mg/dL, and 0.19 mg/dL. The clinical significance of these findings is unknown.

OVERDOSAGE

In a clinical study in patients with Type 2 diabetes, Starlix® (nateglinide) was administered in increasing doses up to 720 mg a day for 7 days and there were no clinically significant adverse events reported. There have been no instances of overdose with Starlix in clinical trials. However, an overdose may result in an exaggerated glucose-lowering effect with the development of hypoglycemic symptoms. Hypoglycemic symptoms without loss of consciousness or neurological findings should be treated with oral glucose and adjustments in dosage and/or meal patterns. Severe hypoglycemic reactions with coma, seizure, or other neurological symptoms should be treated with intravenous glucose. As nateglinide is highly protein bound, dialysis is not an efficient means of removing it from the blood.

DOSAGE AND ADMINISTRATION

Starlix® (nateglinide) should be taken 1 to 30 minutes prior to meals.

Monotherapy and Combination with Metformin or a Thiazolidinedione

The recommended starting and maintenance dose of Starlix, alone or in combination with metformin or a thiazolidinedione, is 120 mg three times daily before meals.

The 60-mg dose of Starlix, either alone or in combination with metformin or a thiazolidinedione, may be used in patients who are near goal HbA_{1C} when treatment is initiated.

Dosage in Geriatric Patients

No special dose adjustments are usually necessary. However, greater sensitivity of some individuals to Starlix therapy cannot be ruled out.

Dosage in Renal and Hepatic Impairment

No dosage adjustment is necessary in patients with mild-to-severe renal insufficiency or in patients with mild hepatic insufficiency. Dosing of patients with moderate-to-severe hepatic dysfunction has not been studied. Therefore, Starlix should be used with caution in patients with moderate-to-severe liver disease *(see PRECAUTIONS, Hepatic Impairment).*

HOW SUPPLIED

Starlix® (nateglinide) tablets

60 mg

Pink, round, beveled edge tablet with "STARLIX" debossed on one side and "60" on the other.

Bottles of 100 .... NDC 0078-0351-05
Bottles of 500 .... NDC 0078-0351-08

120 mg

Yellow, ovaloid tablet with "STARLIX" debossed on one side and "120" on the other.

Bottles of 100 .... NDC 0078-0352-05
Bottles of 500 .... NDC 0078-0352-08

Storage

Store at 25°C (77°F); excursions permitted to 15°C–30°C (59°F-86°F).

Dispense in a tight container, USP.

T2004-03

REV: JANUARY 2004 Printed in U.S.A. 89010106

Manufactured by:
Novartis Pharma Stein AG
Stein, Switzerland

Distributed by:
Novartis Pharmaceuticals Corporation
East Hanover, New Jersey 07936
©Novartis

Shown in Product Identification Guide, page 326

TEGRETOL® ℞

[tĕ-grĕ-tōl]

(carbamazepine USP)

Chewable Tablets of 100 mg – red-speckled, pink
Tablets of 200 mg – pink
Suspension of 100 mg/5 mL

TEGRETOL® -XR ℞

(carbamazepine extended-release tablets)

100 mg, 200 mg, 400 mg

Rx only

Prescribing Information

The following prescribing information is based on official labeling in effect July 2004.

WARNING

APLASTIC ANEMIA AND AGRANULOCYTOSIS HAVE BEEN REPORTED IN ASSOCIATION WITH THE USE OF TEGRETOL. DATA FROM A POPULATION-BASED CASE CONTROL STUDY DEMONSTRATE THAT THE RISK OF DEVELOPING THESE REACTIONS IS 5-8 TIMES GREATER THAN IN THE GENERAL POPULATION. HOWEVER, THE OVERALL RISK OF THESE REACTIONS IN THE UNTREATED GENERAL POPULATION IS LOW, APPROXIMATELY SIX PATIENTS PER ONE MILLION POPULATION PER YEAR FOR AGRANULOCYTOSIS AND TWO PATIENTS PER ONE MILLION POPULATION PER YEAR FOR APLASTIC ANEMIA.

ALTHOUGH REPORTS OF TRANSIENT OR PERSISTENT DECREASED PLATELET OR WHITE BLOOD CELL COUNTS ARE NOT UNCOMMON IN ASSOCIATION WITH THE USE OF TEGRETOL, DATA ARE NOT AVAILABLE TO ESTIMATE ACCURATELY THEIR INCIDENCE OR OUTCOME. HOWEVER, THE VAST MAJORITY OF THE CASES OF LEUKOPENIA HAVE NOT PROGRESSED TO THE MORE SERIOUS CONDITIONS OF APLASTIC ANEMIA OR AGRANULOCYTOSIS.

BECAUSE OF THE VERY LOW INCIDENCE OF AGRANULOCYTOSIS AND APLASTIC ANEMIA, THE VAST MAJORITY OF MINOR HEMATOLOGIC CHANGES OBSERVED IN MONITORING OF PATIENTS ON TEGRETOL ARE UNLIKELY TO SIGNAL THE OCCURRENCE OF EITHER ABNORMALITY. NONETHELESS, COMPLETE PRETREATMENT HEMATOLOGICAL TESTING SHOULD BE OBTAINED AS A BASELINE. IF A PATIENT IN THE COURSE OF TREATMENT EXHIBITS LOW OR DECREASED WHITE BLOOD CELL OR PLATELET COUNTS, THE PATIENT SHOULD BE MONITORED CLOSELY. DISCONTINUATION OF THE DRUG SHOULD BE CONSIDERED IF ANY EVIDENCE OF SIGNIFICANT BONE MARROW DEPRESSION DEVELOPS.

Before prescribing Tegretol, the physician should be thoroughly familiar with the details of this prescribing information, particularly regarding use with other drugs, especially those which accentuate toxicity potential.

DESCRIPTION

Tegretol, carbamazepine USP, is an anticonvulsant and specific analgesic for trigeminal neuralgia, available for oral administration as chewable tablets of 100 mg, tablets of 200 mg, XR tablets of 100, 200, and 400 mg, and as a suspension of 100 mg/5 mL (teaspoon). Its chemical name is

Continued on next page

Tegretol/Tegretol-XR—Cont.

5*H*-dibenz[*b,f*]azepine-5-carboxamide, and its structural formula is

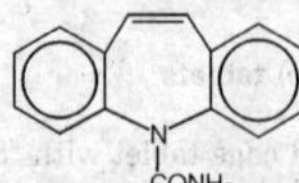

Carbamazepine USP is a white to off-white powder, practically insoluble in water and soluble in alcohol and in acetone. Its molecular weight is 236.27.

Inactive Ingredients Tablets: Colloidal silicon dioxide, D&C Red No. 30 Aluminum Lake (chewable tablets only), FD&C Red No. 40 (200-mg tablets only), flavoring (chewable tablets only), gelatin, glycerin, magnesium stearate, sodium starch glycolate (chewable tablets only), starch, stearic acid, and sucrose (chewable tablets only). Suspension: Citric acid, FD&C Yellow No. 6, flavoring, polymer, potassium sorbate, propylene glycol, purified water, sorbitol, sucrose, and xanthan gum. Tegretol-XR tablets: cellulose compounds, dextrates, iron oxides, magnesium stearate, mannitol, polyethylene glycol, sodium lauryl sulfate, titanium dioxide (200-mg tablets only).

CLINICAL PHARMACOLOGY

In controlled clinical trials, Tegretol has been shown to be effective in the treatment of psychomotor and grand mal seizures, as well as trigeminal neuralgia.

Mechanism of Action

Tegretol has demonstrated anticonvulsant properties in rats and mice with electrically and chemically induced seizures. It appears to act by reducing polysynaptic responses and blocking the post-tetanic potentiation. Tegretol greatly reduces or abolishes pain induced by stimulation of the infraorbital nerve in cats and rats. It depresses thalamic potential and bulbar and polysynaptic reflexes, including the linguomandibular reflex in cats. Tegretol is chemically unrelated to other anticonvulsants or other drugs used to control the pain of trigeminal neuralgia. The mechanism of action remains unknown.

The principal metabolite of Tegretol, carbamazepine-10,11-epoxide, has anticonvulsant activity as demonstrated in several *in vivo* animal models of seizures. Though clinical activity for the epoxide has been postulated, the significance of its activity with respect to the safety and efficacy of Tegretol has not been established.

Pharmacokinetics

In clinical studies, Tegretol suspension, conventional tablets, and XR tablets delivered equivalent amounts of drug to the systemic circulation. However, the suspension was absorbed somewhat faster, and the XR tablet slightly slower, than the conventional tablet. The bioavailability of the XR tablet was 89% compared to suspension. Following a b.i.d. dosage regimen, the suspension provides higher peak levels and lower trough levels than those obtained from the conventional tablet for the same dosage regimen. On the other hand, following a t.i.d. dosage regimen, Tegretol suspension affords steady-state plasma levels comparable to Tegretol tablets given b.i.d. when administered at the same total mg daily dose. Following a b.i.d. dosage regimen, Tegretol-XR tablets afford steady-state plasma levels comparable to conventional Tegretol tablets given q.i.d., when administered at the same total mg daily dose. Tegretol in blood is 76% bound to plasma proteins. Plasma levels of Tegretol are variable and may range from 0.5-25 µg/mL, with no apparent relationship to the daily intake of the drug. Usual adult therapeutic levels are between 4 and 12 µg/mL. In polytherapy, the concentration of Tegretol and concomitant drugs may be increased or decreased during therapy, and drug effects may be altered *(see PRECAUTIONS, Drug Interactions)*. Following chronic oral administration of suspension, plasma levels peak at approximately 1.5 hours compared to 4-5 hours after administration of conventional Tegretol tablets, and 3-12 hours after administration of Tegretol-XR tablets. The CSF/serum ratio is 0.22, similar to the 24% unbound Tegretol in serum. Because Tegretol induces its own metabolism, the half-life is also variable. Autoinduction is completed after 3-5 weeks of a fixed dosing regimen. Initial half-life values range from 25-65 hours, decreasing to 12-17 hours on repeated doses. Tegretol is metabolized in the liver. Cytochrome P450 3A4 was identified as the major isoform responsible for the formation of carbamazepine-10,11-epoxide from Tegretol. After oral administration of ^{14}C-carbamazepine, 72% of the administered radioactivity was found in the urine and 28% in the feces. This urinary radioactivity was composed largely of hydroxylated and conjugated metabolites, with only 3% of unchanged Tegretol.

The pharmacokinetic parameters of Tegretol disposition are similar in children and in adults. However, there is a poor correlation between plasma concentrations of carbamazepine and Tegretol dose in children. Carbamazepine is more rapidly metabolized to carbamazepine-10,11-epoxide (a metabolite shown to be equipotent to carbamazepine as an anticonvulsant in animal screens) in the younger age groups than in adults. In children below the age of 15, there is an inverse relationship between CBZ-E/CBZ ratio and increasing age (in one report from 0.44 in children below the age of 1 year to 0.18 in children between 10-15 years of age).

The effects of race and gender on carbamazepine pharmacokinetics have not been systematically evaluated.

INDICATIONS AND USAGE

Epilepsy

Tegretol is indicated for use as an anticonvulsant drug. Evidence supporting efficacy of Tegretol as an anticonvulsant was derived from active drug-controlled studies that enrolled patients with the following seizure types:

1. Partial seizures with complex symptomatology (psychomotor, temporal lobe). Patients with these seizures appear to show greater improvement than those with other types.
2. Generalized tonic-clonic seizures (grand mal).
3. Mixed seizure patterns which include the above, or other partial or generalized seizures. Absence seizures (petit mal) do not appear to be controlled by Tegretol *(see PRECAUTIONS, General)*.

Trigeminal Neuralgia

Tegretol is indicated in the treatment of the pain associated with true trigeminal neuralgia.

Beneficial results have also been reported in glossopharyngeal neuralgia.

This drug is not a simple analgesic and should not be used for the relief of trivial aches or pains.

CONTRAINDICATIONS

Tegretol should not be used in patients with a history of previous bone marrow depression, acute intermittent porphyria, hypersensitivity to the drug, or known sensitivity to any of the tricyclic compounds, such as amitriptyline, desipramine, imipramine, protriptyline, nortriptyline, etc. Likewise, on theoretical grounds its use with monoamine oxidase inhibitors is not recommended. Before administration of Tegretol, MAO inhibitors should be discontinued for a minimum of 14 days, or longer if the clinical situation permits.

WARNINGS

Patients with a history of adverse hematologic reaction to any drug may be particularly at risk.

Severe dermatologic reactions, including toxic epidermal necrolysis (Lyell's syndrome) and Stevens-Johnson syndrome, have been reported with Tegretol. These reactions have been extremely rare. However, a few fatalities have been reported.

Tegretol has shown mild anticholinergic activity; therefore, patients with increased intraocular pressure should be closely observed during therapy.

Because of the relationship of the drug to other tricyclic compounds, the possibility of activation of a latent psychosis and, in elderly patients, of confusion or agitation should be borne in mind.

As with all antiepileptic drugs, Tegretol should be withdrawn gradually to minimize the potential of increased seizure frequency.

Usage in Pregnancy

Carbamazepine can cause fetal harm when administered to a pregnant woman.

Epidemiological data suggest that there may be an association between the use of carbamazepine during pregnancy and congenital malformations, including spina bifida. There have been reports in association with carbamazepine of other congenital anomalies and developmental disorders (e.g., craniofacial defects, cardiovascular malformations and anomalies involving various body systems). In treating or counseling women of childbearing potential, the prescribing physician will wish to weigh the benefits of therapy against the risks. If this drug is used during pregnancy, or if the patient becomes pregnant while taking this drug, the patient should be apprised of the potential hazard to the fetus.

Retrospective case reviews suggest that, compared with monotherapy, there may be a higher prevalence of teratogenic effects associated with the use of anticonvulsants in combination therapy. Therefore, if therapy is to be continued, monotherapy may be preferable for pregnant women.

In humans, transplacental passage of carbamazepine is rapid (30-60 minutes), and the drug is accumulated in the fetal tissues, with higher levels found in liver and kidney than in brain and lung.

Carbamazepine has been shown to have adverse effects in reproduction studies in rats when given orally in dosages 10-25 times the maximum human daily dosage (MHDD) of 1200 mg on a mg/kg basis or 1.5-4 times the MHDD on a mg/m^2 basis. In rat teratology studies, 2 of 135 offspring showed kinked ribs at 250 mg/kg and 4 of 119 offspring at 650 mg/kg showed other anomalies (cleft palate, 1; talipes, 1; anophthalmos, 2). In reproduction studies in rats, nursing offspring demonstrated a lack of weight gain and an unkempt appearance at a maternal dosage level of 200 mg/kg.

Antiepileptic drugs should not be discontinued abruptly in patients in whom the drug is administered to prevent major seizures because of the strong possibility of precipitating status epilepticus with attendant hypoxia and threat to life. In individual cases where the severity and frequency of the seizure disorder are such that removal of medication does not pose a serious threat to the patient, discontinuation of the drug may be considered prior to and during pregnancy, although it cannot be said with any confidence that even minor seizures do not pose some hazard to the developing embryo or fetus.

Tests to detect defects using currently accepted procedures should be considered a part of routine prenatal care in childbearing women receiving carbamazepine.

There have been a few cases of neonatal seizures and/or respiratory depression associated with maternal Tegretol and other concomitant anticonvulsant drug use. A few cases of neonatal vomiting, diarrhea, and/or decreased feeding have also been reported in association with maternal Tegretol use. These symptoms may represent a neonatal withdrawal syndrome.

PRECAUTIONS

General

Before initiating therapy, a detailed history and physical examination should be made.

Tegretol should be used with caution in patients with a mixed seizure disorder that includes atypical absence seizures, since in these patients Tegretol has been associated with increased frequency of generalized convulsions *(see INDICATIONS AND USAGE)*.

Therapy should be prescribed only after critical benefit-to-risk appraisal in patients with a history of cardiac conduction disturbance; cardiac, hepatic, or renal damage; adverse hematologic or hypersensitivity reaction to other drugs, including reactions to other anticonvulsants; or interrupted courses of therapy with Tegretol.

Hepatic effects, ranging from slight elevations in liver enzymes to rare cases of hepatic failure have been reported *(see ADVERSE REACTIONS and PRECAUTIONS, Laboratory Tests)*. In some cases, hepatic effects may progress despite discontinuation of the drug.

Multi-organ hypersensitivity reactions occurring days to weeks or months after initiating treatment have been reported in rare cases *(see ADVERSE REACTIONS, Other and PRECAUTIONS, Information for Patients)*.

Discontinuation of carbamazepine should be considered if any evidence of hypersensitivity develops.

Hypersensitivity reactions to carbamazepine have been reported in patients who previously experienced this reaction to anticonvulsants including phenytoin and phenobarbital. A history of hypersensitivity reactions should be obtained for a patient and the immediate family members. If positive, caution should be used in prescribing carbamazepine.

Since a given dose of Tegretol suspension will produce higher peak levels than the same dose given as the tablet, it is recommended that patients given the suspension be started on lower doses and increased slowly to avoid unwanted side effects *(see DOSAGE AND ADMINISTRATION)*.

Information for Patients

Patients should be made aware of the early toxic signs and symptoms of a potential hematologic problem, as well as dermatologic, hypersensitivity or hepatic reactions. These symptoms may include, but are not limited to, fever, sore throat, rash, ulcers in the mouth, easy bruising, lymphadenopathy and petechial or purpuric hemorrhage, and in the case of liver reactions, anorexia, nausea/vomiting, or jaundice. The patient should be advised that, because these signs and symptoms may signal a serious reaction, that they must report any occurrence immediately to a physician. In addition, the patient should be advised that these signs and symptoms should be reported even if mild or when occurring after extended use.

Caution should be exercised if alcohol is taken in combination with Tegretol therapy, due to a possible additive sedative effect.

Since dizziness and drowsiness may occur, patients should be cautioned about the hazards of operating machinery or automobiles or engaging in other potentially dangerous tasks.

Laboratory Tests

Complete pretreatment blood counts, including platelets and possibly reticulocytes and serum iron, should be obtained as a baseline. If a patient in the course of treatment exhibits low or decreased white blood cell or platelet counts, the patient should be monitored closely. Discontinuation of the drug should be considered if any evidence of significant bone marrow depression develops.

Baseline and periodic evaluations of liver function, particularly in patients with a history of liver disease, must be performed during treatment with this drug since liver damage may occur *(see PRECAUTIONS, General and ADVERSE REACTIONS)*. Carbamazepine should be discontinued, based on clinical judgment, if indicated by newly occurring or worsening clinical or laboratory evidence of liver dysfunction or hepatic damage, or in the case of active liver disease.

Baseline and periodic eye examinations, including slit-lamp, funduscopy, and tonometry, are recommended since many phenothiazines and related drugs have been shown to cause eye changes.

Baseline and periodic complete urinalysis and BUN determinations are recommended for patients treated with this agent because of observed renal dysfunction.

Monitoring of blood levels *(see CLINICAL PHARMACOLOGY)* has increased the efficacy and safety of anticonvulsants. This monitoring may be particularly useful in cases of dramatic increase in seizure frequency and for verification of compliance. In addition, measurement of drug serum levels may aid in determining the cause of toxicity when more than one medication is being used.

Thyroid function tests have been reported to show decreased values with Tegretol administered alone.

Hyponatremia has been reported in association with Tegretol use, either alone or in combination with other drugs.

Interference with some pregnancy tests has been reported.

Drug Interactions

There has been a report of a patient who passed an orange rubbery precipitate in his stool the day after ingesting Tegretol suspension immediately followed by Thorazine®* solution. Subsequent testing has shown that mixing Tegretol suspension and chlorpromazine solution (both generic and brand name) as well as Tegretol suspension and liquid Mellaril® resulted in the occurrence of this precipitate. Because the extent to which this occurs with other liquid medications is not known, Tegretol suspension should not be administered simultaneously with other liquid medicinal agents or diluents. *(see DOSAGE AND ADMINISTRATION).*

Clinically meaningful drug interactions have occurred with concomitant medications and include, but are not limited to, the following:

Agents That May Affect Tegretol Plasma Levels

CYP 3A4 inhibitors inhibit Tegretol metabolism and can thus increase plasma carbamazepine levels. Drugs that have been shown, or would be expected, to increase plasma carbamazepine levels include

cimetidine, danazol, diltiazem, macrolides, erythromycin, troleandomycin, clarithromycin, fluoxetine, fluvoxamine, nefazodone, loratadine, terfenadine, isoniazid, niacinamide, nicotinamide, propoxyphene, azoles (e.g., ketaconazole, itraconazole, fluconazole), acetazolamide, verapamil, grapefruit juice, protease inhibitors, valproate.*

CYP 3A4 inducers can increase the rate of Tegretol metabolism. Drugs that have been shown, or that would be expected, to decrease plasma carbamazepine levels include

cisplatin, doxorubicin HCl, felbamate,† rifampin, phenobarbital, phenytoin, primidone, methsuximide, theophylline.

*increased levels of the active 10,11-epoxide

†decreased levels of carbamazepine and increased levels of the 10,11-epoxide

Effect of Tegretol on Plasma Levels of Concomitant Agents

Increased levels: clomipramine HCl, phenytoin, primidone

Tegretol induces hepatic CYP activity. Tegretol causes, or would be expected to cause, decreased levels of the following:

acetaminophen, alprazolam, dihydropyridine calcium channel blockers (e.g., felodipine), cyclosporine, corticosteroids (e.g., prednisolone, dexamethasone), clonazepam, clozapine, dicumarol, doxycycline, ethosuximide, haloperidol, itraconazole, lamotrigine, levothyroxine, methadone, methsuximide, midazolam, olanzapine, oral and other hormonal contraceptives, oxcarbazepine, phensuximide, phenytoin, praziquantel, protease inhibitors, risperidone, theophylline, tiagabine, topiramate, tramadol, tricyclic antidepressants (e.g., imipramine, amitriptyline, nortriptyline), valproate, warfarin, ziprasidone, zonisamide.

Concomitant administration of carbamazepine and lithium may increase the risk of neurotoxic side effects.

Alterations of thyroid function have been reported in combination therapy with other anticonvulsant medications.

Concomitant use of Tegretol with hormonal contraceptive products (e.g., oral, and levonorgestrel subdermal implant contraceptives) may render the contraceptives less effective because the plasma concentrations of the hormones may be decreased. Breakthrough bleeding and unintended pregnancies have been reported. Alternative or back-up methods of contraception should be considered.

Carcinogenesis, Mutagenesis, Impairment of Fertility

Carbamazepine, when administered to Sprague-Dawley rats for two years in the diet at doses of 25, 75, and 250 mg/kg/day, resulted in a dose-related increase in the incidence of hepatocellular tumors in females and of benign interstitial cell adenomas in the testes of males.

Carbamazepine must, therefore, be considered to be carcinogenic in Sprague-Dawley rats. Bacterial and mammalian mutagenicity studies using carbamazepine produced negative results. The significance of these findings relative to the use of carbamazepine in humans is, at present, unknown.

Usage in Pregnancy

Pregnancy Category D *(see WARNINGS).*

Labor and Delivery

The effect of Tegretol on human labor and delivery is unknown.

Nursing Mothers

Tegretol and its epoxide metabolite are transferred to breast milk. The ratio of the concentration in breast milk to that in maternal plasma is about 0.4 for Tegretol and about 0.5 for the epoxide. The estimated doses given to the newborn during breast feeding are in the range of 2-5 mg daily for Tegretol and 1-2 mg daily for the epoxide.

Because of the potential for serious adverse reactions in nursing infants from carbamazepine, a decision should be made whether to discontinue nursing or to discontinue the drug, taking into account the importance of the drug to the mother.

Pediatric Use

Substantial evidence of Tegretol's effectiveness for use in the management of children with epilepsy *(see Indications for specific seizure types)* is derived from clinical investigations performed in adults and from studies in several *in vitro* systems which support the conclusion that (1) the pathogenetic mechanisms underlying seizure propagation are essentially identical in adults and children, and (2) the mechanism of action of carbamazepine in treating seizures is essentially identical in adults and children.

Taken as a whole, this information supports a conclusion that the generally accepted therapeutic range of total carbamazepine in plasma (i.e., 4-12 mcg/mL) is the same in children and adults.

The evidence assembled was primarily obtained from short-term use of carbamazepine. The safety of carbamazepine in children has been systematically studied up to 6 months. No longer-term data from clinical trials is available.

Geriatric Use

No systematic studies in geriatric patients have been conducted.

ADVERSE REACTIONS

If adverse reactions are of such severity that the drug must be discontinued, the physician must be aware that abrupt discontinuation of any anticonvulsant drug in a responsive epileptic patient may lead to seizures or even status epilepticus with its life-threatening hazards.

The most severe adverse reactions have been observed in the hemopoietic system *(see boxed WARNING)*, the skin, liver, and the cardiovascular system.

The most frequently observed adverse reactions, particularly during the initial phases of therapy, are dizziness, drowsiness, unsteadiness, nausea, and vomiting. To minimize the possibility of such reactions, therapy should be initiated at the low dosage recommended.

The following additional adverse reactions have been reported:

Hemopoietic System: Aplastic anemia, agranulocytosis, pancytopenia, bone marrow depression, thrombocytopenia, leukopenia, leukocytosis, eosinophilia, acute intermittent porphyria.

Skin: Pruritic and erythematous rashes, urticaria, toxic epidermal necrolysis (Lyell's syndrome) *(see WARNINGS)*, Stevens-Johnson syndrome *(see WARNINGS)*, photosensitivity reactions, alterations in skin pigmentation, exfoliative dermatitis, erythema multiforme and nodosum, purpura, aggravation of disseminated lupus erythematosus, alopecia, and diaphoresis. In certain cases, discontinuation of therapy may be necessary. Isolated cases of hirsutism have been reported, but a causal relationship is not clear.

Cardiovascular System: Congestive heart failure, edema, aggravation of hypertension, hypotension, syncope and collapse, aggravation of coronary artery disease, arrhythmias and AV block, thrombophlebitis, thromboembolism, and adenopathy or lymphadenopathy.

Some of these cardiovascular complications have resulted in fatalities. Myocardial infarction has been associated with other tricyclic compounds.

Liver: Abnormalities in liver function tests, cholestatic and hepatocellular jaundice, hepatitis; very rare cases of hepatic failure.

Pancreatic: Pancreatitis.

Respiratory System: Pulmonary hypersensitivity characterized by fever, dyspnea, pneumonitis, or pneumonia.

Genitourinary System: Urinary frequency, acute urinary retention, oliguria with elevated blood pressure, azotemia, renal failure, and impotence. Albuminuria, glycosuria, elevated BUN, and microscopic deposits in the urine have also been reported.

Testicular atrophy occurred in rats receiving Tegretol orally from 4-52 weeks at dosage levels of 50-400 mg/kg/day. Additionally, rats receiving Tegretol in the diet for 2 years at dosage levels of 25, 75, and 250 mg/kg/day had a dose-related incidence of testicular atrophy and aspermatogenesis. In dogs, it produced a brownish discoloration, presumably a metabolite, in the urinary bladder at dosage levels of 50 mg/kg and higher. Relevance of these findings to humans is unknown.

Nervous System: Dizziness, drowsiness, disturbances of coordination, confusion, headache, fatigue, blurred vision, visual hallucinations, transient diplopia, oculomotor disturbances, nystagmus, speech disturbances, abnormal involuntary movements, peripheral neuritis and paresthesias, depression with agitation, talkativeness, tinnitus, and hyperacusis.

There have been reports of associated paralysis and other symptoms of cerebral arterial insufficiency, but the exact relationship of these reactions to the drug has not been established.

Isolated cases of neuroleptic malignant syndrome have been reported with concomitant use of psychotropic drugs.

Digestive System: Nausea, vomiting, gastric distress and abdominal pain, diarrhea, constipation, anorexia, and dryness of the mouth and pharynx, including glossitis and stomatitis.

Eyes: Scattered punctate cortical lens opacities, as well as conjunctivitis, have been reported. Although a direct causal relationship has not been established, many phenothiazines and related drugs have been shown to cause eye changes.

Musculoskeletal System: Aching joints and muscles, and leg cramps.

Metabolism: Fever and chills. Inappropriate antidiuretic hormone (ADH) secretion syndrome has been reported. Cases of frank water intoxication, with decreased serum sodium (hyponatremia) and confusion, have been reported in association with Tegretol use *(see PRECAUTIONS, Laboratory Tests)*. Decreased levels of plasma calcium have been reported.

Other: Multi-organ hypersensitivity reactions occurring days to weeks or months after initiating treatment have been reported in rare cases. Signs or symptoms may include, but are not limited to, fever, skin rashes, vasculitis, lymphadenopathy, disorders mimicking lymphoma, arthralgia, leukopenia, eosinophilia, hepato-splenomegaly and abnormal liver function tests. These signs and symptoms may occur in various combinations and not necessarily concurrently. Signs and symptoms may initially be mild. Various organs, including but not limited to, liver, skin, immune system, lungs, kidneys, pancreas, myocardium, and colon may be affected *(see PRECAUTIONS, General and PRECAUTIONS, Information for Patients).*

Isolated cases of a lupus erythematosus-like syndrome have been reported. There have been occasional reports of elevated levels of cholesterol, HDL cholesterol, and triglycerides in patients taking anticonvulsants.

A case of aseptic meningitis, accompanied by myoclonus and peripheral eosinophilia, has been reported in a patient taking carbamazepine in combination with other medications. The patient was successfully dechallenged, and the meningitis reappeared upon rechallenge with carbamazepine.

DRUG ABUSE AND DEPENDENCE

No evidence of abuse potential has been associated with Tegretol, nor is there evidence of psychological or physical dependence in humans.

OVERDOSAGE

Acute Toxicity

Lowest known lethal dose: adults, 3.2 g (a 24-year-old woman died of a cardiac arrest and a 24-year-old man died of pneumonia and hypoxic encephalopathy); children, 4 g (a 14-year-old girl died of a cardiac arrest), 1.6 g (a 3-year-old girl died of aspiration pneumonia).

Oral LD_{50} in animals (mg/kg): mice, 1100-3750; rats, 3850-4025; rabbits, 1500-2680; guinea pigs, 920.

Signs and Symptoms

The first signs and symptoms appear after 1-3 hours. Neuromuscular disturbances are the most prominent. Cardiovascular disorders are generally milder, and severe cardiac complications occur only when very high doses (>60 g) have been ingested.

Respiration: Irregular breathing, respiratory depression.

Cardiovascular System: Tachycardia, hypotension or hypertension, shock, conduction disorders.

Nervous System and Muscles: Impairment of consciousness ranging in severity to deep coma. Convulsions, especially in small children. Motor restlessness, muscular twitching, tremor, athetoid movements, opisthotonos, ataxia, drowsiness, dizziness, mydriasis, nystagmus, adiadochokinesia, ballism, psychomotor disturbances, dysmetria. Initial hyperreflexia, followed by hyporeflexia.

Gastrointestinal Tract: Nausea, vomiting.

Kidneys and Bladder: Anuria or oliguria, urinary retention.

Laboratory Findings: Isolated instances of overdosage have included leukocytosis, reduced leukocyte count, glycosuria, and acetonuria. EEG may show dysrhythmias.

Combined Poisoning: When alcohol, tricyclic antidepressants, barbiturates, or hydantoins are taken at the same time, the signs and symptoms of acute poisoning with Tegretol may be aggravated or modified.

Treatment

The prognosis in cases of severe poisoning is critically dependent upon prompt elimination of the drug, which may be achieved by inducing vomiting, irrigating the stomach, and by taking appropriate steps to diminish absorption. If these measures cannot be implemented without risk on the spot, the patient should be transferred at once to a hospital, while ensuring that vital functions are safeguarded. There is no specific antidote.

Elimination of the Drug: Induction of vomiting.

Gastric lavage. Even when more than 4 hours have elapsed following ingestion of the drug, the stomach should be repeatedly irrigated, especially if the patient has also consumed alcohol.

Measures to Reduce Absorption: Activated charcoal, laxatives.

Measures to Accelerate Elimination: Forced diuresis.

Dialysis is indicated only in severe poisoning associated with renal failure. Replacement transfusion is indicated in severe poisoning in small children.

Respiratory Depression: Keep the airways free; resort, if necessary, to endotracheal intubation, artificial respiration, and administration of oxygen.

Hypotension, Shock: Keep the patient's legs raised and administer a plasma expander. If blood pressure fails to rise despite measures taken to increase plasma volume, use of vasoactive substances should be considered.

Convulsions: Diazepam or barbiturates.

Warning: Diazepam or barbiturates may aggravate respiratory depression (especially in children), hypotension, and coma. However, barbiturates should <u>not</u> be used if drugs that inhibit monoamine oxidase have also been taken by the patient either in overdosage or in recent therapy (within 1 week).

Surveillance: Respiration, cardiac function (ECG monitoring), blood pressure, body temperature, pupillary reflexes, and kidney and bladder function should be monitored for several days.

Treatment of Blood Count Abnormalities: If evidence of significant bone marrow depression develops, the following recommendations are suggested: (1) stop the drug, (2) perform daily CBC, platelet, and reticulocyte counts, (3) do a bone marrow aspiration and trephine biopsy immediately and repeat with sufficient frequency to monitor recovery.

Continued on next page

Dosage Information

Indication	Initial Dose			Subsequent Dose			Maximum Daily Dose		
	Tablet*	XR†	Suspension	Tablet*	XR†	Suspension	Tablet*	XR†	Suspension
Epilepsy Under 6 yr	10-20 mg/kg/day b.i.d. or t.i.d.		10-20 mg/kg/day q.i.d.	Increase weekly to achieve optimal clinical response, t.i.d. or q.i.d.		Increase weekly to achieve optimal clinical response, t.i.d. or q.i.d.	35 mg/kg/24 hr *(see DOSAGE AND ADMINISTRATION section above)*		35 mg/kg/24 hr *(see DOSAGE AND ADMINISTRATION section above)*
6-12 yr	100 mg b.i.d. (200 mg/day)	100 mg b.i.d. (200 mg/day)	1/2 tsp q.i.d. (200 mg/day)	Add up to 100 mg/day at weekly intervals, t.i.d. or q.i.d.	Add 100 mg/day at weekly intervals, b.i.d.	Add up to 1 tsp (100 mg)/day at weekly intervals, t.i.d. or q.i.d.	1000 mg/24 hr		
Over 12 yr	200 mg b.i.d. (400 mg/day)	200 mg b.i.d. (400 mg/day)	1 tsp q.i.d. (400 mg/day)	Add up to 200 mg/day at weekly intervals, t.i.d. or q.i.d.	Add up to 200 mg/day at weekly intervals, b.i.d.	Add up to 2 tsp (200 mg)/day at weekly intervals, t.i.d. or q.i.d.	1000 mg/24 hr (12-15 yr) 1200 mg/24 hr (>15 yr) 1600 mg/24 hr (adults, in rare instances)		
Trigeminal Neuralgia	100 mg b.i.d. (200 mg/day)	100 mg b.i.d. (200 mg/day)	1/2 tsp q.i.d. (200 mg/day)	Add up to 200 mg/day in increments of 100 mg every 12 hr	Add up to 200 mg/day in increments of 100 mg every 12 hr	Add up to 2 tsp (200 mg)/day in increments of 50 mg (1/2 tsp) q.i.d.	1200 mg/24 hr		

*Tablet = Chewable or conventional tablets
†XR = Tegretol®-XR extended-release tablets

Tegretol/Tegretol-XR—Cont.

Special periodic studies might be helpful as follows: (1) white cell and platelet antibodies, (2) ^{59}Fe-ferrokinetic studies, (3) peripheral blood cell typing, (4) cytogenetic studies on marrow and peripheral blood, (5) bone marrow culture studies for colony-forming units, (6) hemoglobin electrophoresis for A_2 and F hemoglobin, and (7) serum folic acid and B_{12} levels.

A fully developed aplastic anemia will require appropriate, intensive monitoring and therapy, for which specialized consultation should be sought.

DOSAGE AND ADMINISTRATION *(see table below)*

Tegretol suspension in combination with liquid chlorpromazine or thioridazine results in precipitate formation, and, in the case of chlorpromazine, there has been a report of a patient passing an orange rubbery precipitate in the stool following coadministration of the two drugs. *(see PRECAUTIONS, Drug Interactions)*. Because the extent to which this occurs with other liquid medications is not known, Tegretol suspension should not be administered simultaneously with other liquid medications or diluents.

Monitoring of blood levels has increased the efficacy and safety of anticonvulsants *(see PRECAUTIONS, Laboratory Tests)*. Dosage should be adjusted to the needs of the individual patient. A low initial daily dosage with a gradual increase is advised. As soon as adequate control is achieved, the dosage may be reduced very gradually to the minimum effective level. Medication should be taken with meals.

Since a given dose of Tegretol suspension will produce higher peak levels than the same dose given as the tablet, it is recommended to start with low doses (children 6-12 years: 1/2 teaspoon q.i.d.) and to increase slowly to avoid unwanted side effects.

Conversion of patients from oral Tegretol tablets to Tegretol suspension: Patients should be converted by administering the same number of mg per day in smaller, more frequent doses (i.e., b.i.d. tablets to t.i.d. suspension).

Tegretol-XR is an extended-release formulation for twice-a-day administration. When converting patients from Tegretol conventional tablets to Tegretol-XR, the same total daily mg dose of Tegretol-XR should be administered. **Tegretol-XR tablets must be swallowed whole and never crushed or chewed.** Tegretol-XR tablets should be inspected for chips or cracks. Damaged tablets, or tablets without a release portal, should not be consumed. Tegretol-XR tablet coating is not absorbed and is excreted in the feces; these coatings may be noticeable in the stool.

Epilepsy *(see INDICATIONS AND USAGE)*

Adults and children over 12 years of age - Initial: Either 200 mg b.i.d. for tablets and XR tablets, or 1 teaspoon q.i.d. for suspension (400 mg/day). Increase at weekly intervals by adding up to 200 mg/day using a b.i.d. regimen of Tegretol-XR or a t.i.d. or q.i.d. regimen of the other formulations until the optimal response is obtained. Dosage generally should not exceed 1000 mg daily in children 12-15 years of age, and 1200 mg daily in patients above 15 years of age. Doses up to 1600 mg daily have been used in adults in rare instances.

Maintenance: Adjust dosage to the minimum effective level, usually 800-1200 mg daily.

Children 6-12 years of age - Initial: Either 100 mg b.i.d. for tablets or XR tablets, or 1/2 teaspoon q.i.d. for suspension (200 mg/day). Increase at weekly intervals by adding up to 100 mg/day using a b.i.d. regimen of Tegretol-XR or a t.i.d. or q.i.d. regimen of the other formulations until the optimal response is obtained. Dosage generally should not exceed 1000 mg daily. ***Maintenance:*** Adjust dosage to the minimum effective level, usually 400-800 mg daily.

Children under 6 years of age - Initial: 10-20 mg/kg/day b.i.d. or t.i.d. as tablets, or q.i.d. as suspension. Increase weekly to achieve optimal clinical response administered t.i.d. or q.i.d. ***Maintenance:*** Ordinarily, optimal clinical response is achieved at daily doses below 35 mg/kg. If satisfactory clinical response has not been achieved, plasma levels should be measured to determine whether or not they are in the therapeutic range. No recommendation regarding the safety of carbamazepine for use at doses above 35 mg/kg/24 hours can be made.

Combination Therapy: Tegretol may be used alone or with other anticonvulsants. When added to existing anticonvulsant therapy, the drug should be added gradually while the other anticonvulsants are maintained or gradually decreased, except phenytoin, which may have to be increased *(see PRECAUTIONS, Drug Interactions, and Pregnancy Category D)*.

Trigeminal Neuralgia *(see INDICATIONS AND USAGE)*

Initial: On the first day, either 100 mg b.i.d. for tablets or XR tablets, or 1/2 teaspoon q.i.d. for suspension, for a total daily dose of 200 mg. This daily dose may be increased by up to 200 mg/day using increments of 100 mg every 12 hours for tablets or XR tablets, or 50 mg (1/2 teaspoon) q.i.d. for suspension, only as needed to achieve freedom from pain. Do not exceed 1200 mg daily. ***Maintenance:*** Control of pain can be maintained in most patients with 400-800 mg daily. However, some patients may be maintained on as little as 200 mg daily, while others may require as much as 1200 mg daily. At least once every 3 months throughout the treatment period, attempts should be made to reduce the dose to the minimum effective level or even to discontinue the drug. [See table above]

HOW SUPPLIED

Chewable Tablets 100 mg - round, red-speckled, pink, single-scored (imprinted Tegretol on one side and 52 twice on the scored side)

Bottles of 100 .... NDC 0083-0052-30
Unit Dose (blister pack)
Box of 100 (strips of 10) .... NDC 0083-0052-32

Do not store above 30°C (86°F). *Protect from light and moisture. Dispense in tight, light-resistant container (USP). Meets USP Dissolution Test 1.*

Tablets 200 mg - capsule-shaped, pink, single-scored (imprinted Tegretol on one side and 27 twice on the partially scored side)

Bottles of 100 .... NDC 0083-0027-30
Bottles of 1000 .... NDC 0083-0027-40
Unit Dose (blister pack)
Box of 100 (strips of 10) .... NDC 0083-0027-32

Do not store above 30°C (86°F). *Protect from moisture. Dispense in tight container (USP). Meets USP Dissolution Test 2.*

XR Tablets 100 mg - round, yellow, coated (imprinted T on one side and 100 mg on the other), release portal on one side

Bottles of 100 .... NDC 0083-0061-30

XR Tablets 200 mg - round, pink, coated (imprinted T on one side and 200 mg on the other), release portal on one side

Bottles of 100 .... NDC 0083-0062-30

XR Tablets 400 mg - round, brown, coated (imprinted T on one side and 400 mg on the other), release portal on one side

Bottles of 100 .... NDC 0083-0060-30

Store at controlled room temperature 15°C-30°C (59°F-86°F). *Protect from moisture. Dispense in tight container (USP).*

Suspension 100 mg/5 mL (teaspoon) - yellow-orange, citrus-vanilla flavored

Bottles of 450 mL .... NDC 0083-0019-76

Shake well before using.

Do not store above 30°C (86°F). *Dispense in tight, light-resistant container, (USP).*

*Thorazine® is a registered trademark of GlaxoSmithKline.

Tegretol Chewable Tablets Manufactured by:
Novartis Pharmaceuticals Corporation
East Hanover, New Jersey 07936

Tegretol Tablets Manufactured by:
Novartis Pharmaceuticals Corporation
East Hanover, New Jersey 07936

Tegretol Suspension Manufactured by:
Patheon Inc.
Whitby Operations
Whitby Ontario, Canada
L1N 5Z5

Tegretol-XR Tablets Manufactured by:
Novartis Pharma GmbH
D-79664 Wehr, Germany

Distributed by:
Novartis Pharmaceuticals Corporation
East Hanover, New Jersey 07936

REV: SEPTEMBER 2003 2337-25-03A T2003-70
89007010

Shown in Product Identification Guide, page 326

TRILEPTAL® ℞

[trī-lĕp-tăl]

(oxcarbazepine)

Tablets

Oral Suspension

Rx only

Prescribing Information

The following prescribing information is based on official labeling in effect July 2004,

DESCRIPTION

Trileptal® (oxcarbazepine) is an antiepileptic drug available as 150 mg, 300 mg and 600 mg film-coated tablets for oral administration. Trileptal is also available as a 300 mg/5 mL (60 mg/mL) oral suspension. Oxcarbazepine is 10,11-Dihydro-10-oxo-5*H*-dibenz[b, *f*]azepine-5-carboxamide, and its structural formula is

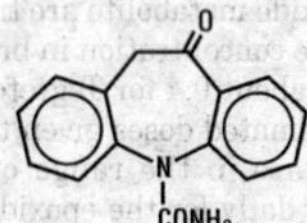

Oxcarbazepine is a white to faintly orange crystalline powder. It is slightly soluble in chloroform, dichloromethane, acetone, and methanol and practically insoluble in ethanol, ether and water. Its molecular weight is 252.27.

Trileptal film-coated tablets contain the following inactive ingredients: colloidal silicon dioxide, crospovidone, hydroxypropyl methylcellulose, magnesium stearate, microcrystalline cellulose, polyethylene glycol, talc and titanium dioxide, yellow iron oxide.

Trileptal oral suspension contains the following inactive ingredients: ascorbic acid; dispersible cellulose; ethanol; macrogol stearate; methyl parahydroxybenzoate; propylene glycol; propyl parahydroxybenzoate; purified water; sodium saccharin; sorbic acid; sorbitol; yellow-plum-lemon aroma.

CLINICAL PHARMACOLOGY

Mechanism of Action

The pharmacological activity of Trileptal® (oxcarbazepine) is primarily exerted through the 10-monohydroxy metabolite (MHD) of oxcarbazepine *(see Metabolism and Excretion subsection)*. The precise mechanism by which oxcarbazepine and MHD exert their antiseizure effect is unknown; however, *in vitro* electrophysiological studies indicate that they produce blockade of voltage-sensitive sodium channels, resulting in stabilization of hyperexcited neural membranes, inhibition of repetitive neuronal firing, and diminution of propagation of synaptic impulses. These actions are thought to be important in the prevention of seizure spread in the intact brain. In addition, increased potassium conductance and modulation of high-voltage activated calcium channels may contribute to the anticonvulsant effects of the drug. No significant interactions of oxcarbazepine or MHD with brain neurotransmitter or modulator receptor sites have been demonstrated.

Pharmacodynamics

Oxcarbazepine and its active metabolite (MHD) exhibit anticonvulsant properties in animal seizure models. They protected rodents against electrically induced tonic extension seizures and, to a lesser degree, chemically induced clonic seizures, and abolished or reduced the frequency of chronically recurring focal seizures in Rhesus monkeys with aluminum implants. No development of tolerance (i.e., attenuation of anticonvulsive activity) was observed in the maximal electroshock test when mice and rats were treated daily for 5 days and 4 weeks, respectively, with oxcarbazepine or MHD.

Pharmacokinetics

Following oral administration of Trileptal tablets, oxcarbazepine is completely absorbed and extensively metabolized to its pharmacologically active 10-monohydroxy metabolite (MHD). The half-life of the parent is about 2 hours, while the half-life of MHD is about 9 hours, so that MHD is responsible for most antiepileptic activity.

Based on MHD concentrations, Trileptal tablets and suspension were shown to have similar bioavailability.

After single dose administration of Trileptal tablets to healthy male volunteers under fasted conditions, the median t_{max} was 4.5 (range 3 to 13) hours. After single dose administration of Trileptal oral suspension to healthy male volunteers under fasted conditions, the median t_{max} was 6 hours.

In a mass balance study in people, only 2% of total radioactivity in plasma was due to unchanged oxcarbazepine, with approximately 70% present as MHD, and the remainder attributable to minor metabolites.

Effect of Food: Food has no effect on the rate and extent of absorption of oxcarbazepine from Trileptal tablets. Although not directly studied, the oral bioavailability of the Trileptal suspension is unlikely to be affected under fed conditions. Therefore, Trileptal tablets and suspension can be taken with or without food.

Steady-state plasma concentrations of MHD are reached within 2-3 days in patients when Trileptal is given twice a day. At steady-state the pharmacokinetics of MHD are linear and show dose proportionality over the dose range of 300 to 2400 mg/day.

Distribution

The apparent volume of distribution of MHD is 49L.

Approximately 40% of MHD is bound to serum proteins, predominantly to albumin. Binding is independent of the serum concentration within the therapeutically relevant range. Oxcarbazepine and MHD do not bind to alpha-1-acid glycoprotein.

Metabolism and Excretion

Oxcarbazepine is rapidly reduced by cytosolic enzymes in the liver to its 10-monohydroxy metabolite, MHD, which is primarily responsible for the pharmacological effect of Trileptal. MHD is metabolized further by conjugation with glucuronic acid. Minor amounts (4% of the dose) are oxidized to the pharmacologically inactive 10,11-dihydroxy metabolite (DHD).

Oxcarbazepine is cleared from the body mostly in the form of metabolites which are predominantly excreted by the kidneys. More than 95% of the dose appears in the urine, with less than 1% as unchanged oxcarbazepine. Fecal excretion accounts for less than 4% of the administered dose. Approximately 80% of the dose is excreted in the urine either as glucuronides of MHD (49%) or as unchanged MHD (27%); the inactive DHD accounts for approximately 3% and conjugates of MHD and oxcarbazepine account for 13% of the dose.

Special Populations

Hepatic Impairment

The pharmacokinetics and metabolism of oxcarbazepine and MHD were evaluated in healthy volunteers and hepatically-impaired subjects after a single 900 mg oral dose. Mild-to-moderate hepatic impairment did not affect the pharmacokinetics of oxcarbazepine and MHD. No dose adjustment for Trileptal is recommended in patients with mild-to-moderate hepatic impairment. The pharmacokinetics of oxcarbazepine and MHD have not been evaluated in severe hepatic impairment.

Renal Impairment

There is a linear correlation between creatinine clearance and the renal clearance of MHD. When Trileptal is administered as a single 300 mg dose in renally impaired patients (creatinine clearance <30 mL/min), the elimination half-life of MHD is prolonged to 19 hours, with a two-fold increase in AUC. Dose adjustment for Trileptal is recommended in these patients *(see PRECAUTIONS and DOSAGE AND ADMINISTRATION sections)*.

Pediatric Use

After a single-dose administration of 5 or 15 mg/kg of Trileptal, the dose-adjusted AUC values of MHD were 30%-40% lower in children below the age of 8 years than in children above 8 years of age. The clearance in children greater than 8 years old approaches that of adults.

Geriatric Use

Following administration of single (300 mg) and multiple (600 mg/day) doses of Trileptal to elderly volunteers (60-82 years of age), the maximum plasma concentrations and AUC values of MHD were 30%-60% higher than in younger volunteers (18-32 years of age). Comparisons of creatinine clearance in young and elderly volunteers indicate that the difference was due to age-related reductions in creatinine clearance.

Gender

No gender related pharmacokinetic differences have been observed in children, adults, or the elderly.

Race

No specific studies have been conducted to assess what effect, if any, race may have on the disposition of oxcarbazepine.

CLINICAL STUDIES

The effectiveness of Trileptal® (oxcarbazepine) as adjunctive and monotherapy for partial seizures in adults and as adjunctive therapy in children aged 4-16 was established in 6 multicenter randomized, double-blind controlled trials. The effectiveness of Trileptal as monotherapy for partial seizures in children aged 4-16 was determined from data obtained in the studies described, as well as by pharmacokinetic/pharmacodynamic considerations.

Trileptal Monotherapy Trials

Four randomized, double-blind, multicenter trials demonstrated the efficacy of Trileptal as monotherapy. Two trials compared Trileptal to placebo and two trials used a randomized withdrawal design to compare a high dose (2400 mg) with a low dose (300 mg) of Trileptal, after substituting Trileptal 2400 mg/day for one or more antiepileptic drugs (AEDs). All doses were administered on a BID schedule.

One placebo-controlled trial was conducted in 102 patients (11-62 years of age) with refractory partial seizures who had completed an inpatient evaluation for epilepsy surgery. Patients had been withdrawn from all AEDs and were required to have 2-10 partial seizures within 48 hours prior to randomization. Patients were randomized to receive either placebo or Trileptal given as 1500 mg/day on Day 1 and 2400 mg/day thereafter for an additional 9 days, or until one of the following three exit criteria occurred: 1) the occurrence of a fourth partial seizure, excluding Day 1, 2) two new-onset secondarily generalized seizures, where such seizures were not seen in the 1-year period prior to randomization, or 3) occurrence of serial seizures or status epilepticus. The primary measure of effectiveness was a between group comparison of the time to meet exit criteria. There was a statistically significant difference in favor of Trileptal *(see Figure 1)*, p=0.0001.

Figure 1: Kaplan-Meier estimates of exit rate by treatment group

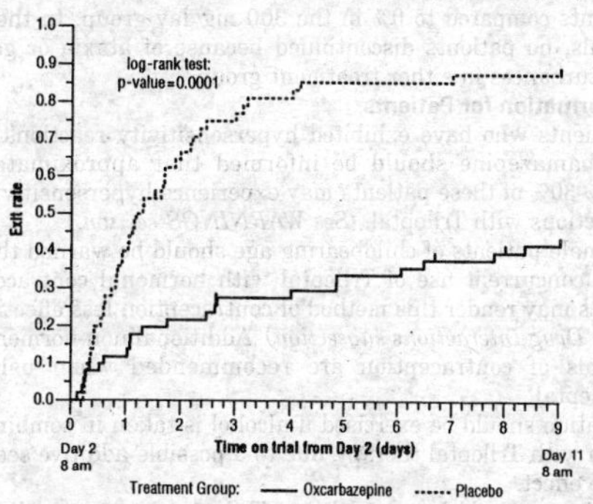

The second placebo-controlled trial was conducted in 67 untreated patients (8-69 years of age) with newly-diagnosed and recent-onset partial seizures. Patients were randomized to placebo or Trileptal, initiated at 300 mg BID and titrated to 1200 mg/day (given as 600 mg BID) in 6 days, followed by maintenance treatment for 84 days. The primary measure of effectiveness was a between group comparison of the time to first seizure. The difference between the two treatments was statistically significant in favor of Trileptal *(see Figure 2)*, p=0.046.

[See figure 2 at top of next column]

A third trial substituted Trileptal monotherapy at 2400 mg/day for carbamazepine in 143 patients (12-65 years of age) whose partial seizures were inadequately controlled on carbamazepine (CBZ) monotherapy at a stable dose of 800 to 1600 mg/day, and maintained this Trileptal dose for 56 days (baseline phase). Patients who were able to tolerate titration of Trileptal to 2400 mg/day during simultaneous carbamazepine withdrawal were randomly assigned to either 300 mg/day of Trileptal or 2400 mg/day Trileptal. Patients were observed for 126 days or until one of the following 4 exit criteria occurred: 1) a doubling of the 28-day seizure

Figure 2: Kaplan-Meier estimates of first seizure event rate by treatment group

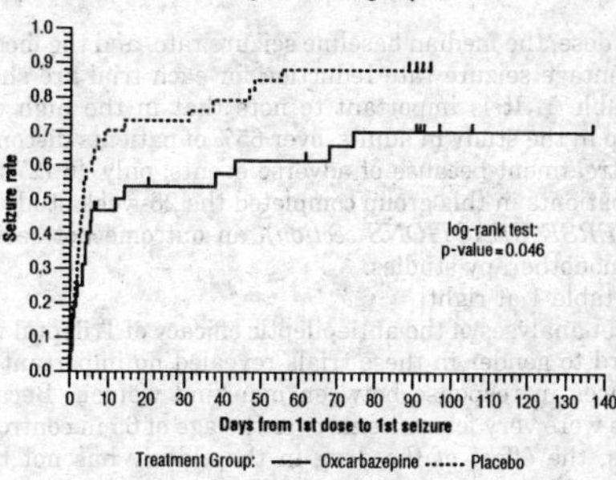

frequency compared to baseline, 2) a two-fold increase in the highest consecutive 2-day seizure frequency during baseline, 3) a single generalized seizure if none had occurred during baseline, or 4) a prolonged generalized seizure. The primary measure of effectiveness was a between group comparison of the time to meet exit criteria. The difference between the curves was statistically significant in favor of the Trileptal 2400 mg/day group *(see Figure 3)*, p=0.0001.

Figure 3: Kaplan-Meier estimates of exit rate by treatment group

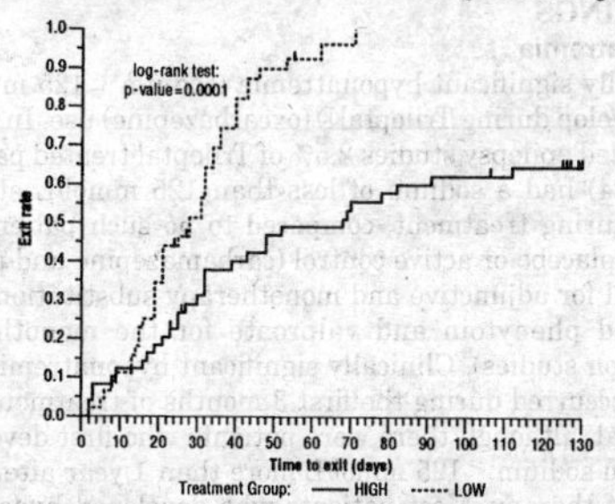

Another monotherapy substitution trial was conducted in 87 patients (11-66 years of age) whose seizures were inadequately controlled on 1 or 2 AEDs. Patients were randomized to either Trileptal 2400 mg/day or 300 mg/day and their standard AED regimen(s) were eliminated over the first 6 weeks of double-blind therapy. Double-blind treatment continued for another 84 days (total double-blind treatment of 126 days) or until one of the 4 exit criteria described for the previous study occurred. The primary measure of effectiveness was a between group comparison of the percentage of patients meeting exit criteria. The results were statistically significant in favor of the Trileptal 2400 mg/day group (14/34; 41.2%) compared to the Trileptal 300 mg/day group (42/45; 93.3%) (p<0.0001). The time to meeting one of the exit criteria was also statistically significant in favor of the Trileptal 2400 mg/day group *(see Figure 4)*, p=0.0001.

Figure 4: Kaplan-Meier estimates of exit rate by treatment group

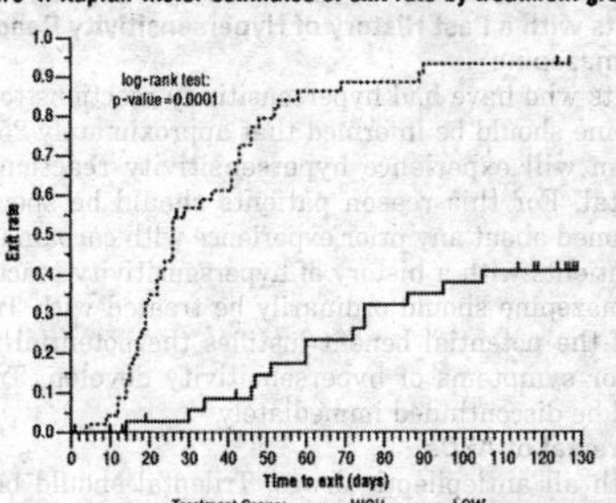

Trileptal Adjunctive Therapy Trials

The effectiveness of Trileptal as an adjunctive therapy for partial seizures was established in two multicenter, randomized, double-blind, placebo-controlled trials, one in 692 patients (15-66 years of age) and one in 264 pediatric patients (3-17 years of age). Patients in these trials were on 1-3 concomitant AEDs. In both of the trials, patients were stabilized on optimum dosages of their concomitant AEDs during an 8-week baseline phase. Patients who experienced at least 8 (minimum of 1-4 per month) partial seizures during the baseline phase were randomly assigned to placebo or to a specific dose of Trileptal in addition to their other AEDs. In these studies, the dose was increased over a 2-week period until either the assigned dose was reached, or intolerance prevented increases. Patients then entered a 14 (pediatrics) or 24 week (adults) maintenance period.

In the adult trial, patients received fixed doses of 600, 1200 or 2400 mg/day. In the pediatric trial, patients received maintenance doses in the range of 30-46 mg/kg/day, depending on baseline weight. The primary measure of effectiveness in both trials was a between group comparison of the percentage change in partial seizure frequency in the double-blind Treatment Phase relative to Baseline Phase. This comparison was statistically significant in favor of Trileptal at all doses tested in both trials (p=0.0001 for all doses for both trials). The number of patients randomized to

Continued on next page

Trileptal—Cont.

each dose, the median baseline seizure rate, and the median percentage seizure rate reduction for each trial are shown in Table 1. It is important to note that in the high dose group in the study in adults, over 65% of patients discontinued treatment because of adverse events; only 46 (27%) of the patients in this group completed the 28-week study *(see ADVERSE REACTIONS section)*, an outcome not seen in the monotherapy studies.

[See table 1 at right]

Subset analyses of the antiepileptic efficacy of Trileptal with regard to gender in these trials revealed no important differences in response between men and women. Because there were very few patients over the age of 65 in controlled trials, the effect of the drug in the elderly has not been adequately assessed.

INDICATIONS AND USAGE

Trileptal® (oxcarbazepine) is indicated for use as monotherapy or adjunctive therapy in the treatment of partial seizures in adults and children ages 4-16 with epilepsy.

CONTRAINDICATIONS

Trileptal® (oxcarbazepine) should not be used in patients with a known hypersensitivity to oxcarbazepine or to any of its components.

WARNINGS

Hyponatremia

Clinically significant hyponatremia (sodium <125 mmol/L) can develop during Trileptal® (oxcarbazepine) use. In the 14 controlled epilepsy studies 2.5% of Trileptal treated patients (38/1524) had a sodium of less than 125 mmol/L at some point during treatment, compared to no such patients assigned placebo or active control (carbamazepine and phenobarbital for adjunctive and monotherapy substitution studies, and phenytoin and valproate for the monotherapy initiation studies). Clinically significant hyponatremia generally occurred during the first 3 months of treatment with Trileptal, although there were patients who first developed a serum sodium <125 mmol/L more than 1 year after initiation of therapy. Most patients who developed hyponatremia were asymptomatic but patients in the clinical trials were frequently monitored and some had their Trileptal dose reduced, discontinued, or had their fluid intake restricted for hyponatremia. Whether or not these maneuvers prevented the occurrence of more severe events is unknown. Cases of symptomatic hyponatremia have been reported during post-marketing use. In clinical trials, patients whose treatment with Trileptal was discontinued due to hyponatremia generally experienced normalization of serum sodium within a few days without additional treatment.

Measurement of serum sodium levels should be considered for patients during maintenance treatment with Trileptal, particularly if the patient is receiving other medications known to decrease serum sodium levels (for example, drugs associated with inappropriate ADH secretion) or if symptoms possibly indicating hyponatremia develop (e.g., nausea, malaise, headache, lethargy, confusion, obtundation, or increase in seizure frequency or severity).

Patients with a Past History of Hypersensitivity Reaction to Carbamazepine

Patients who have had hypersensitivity reactions to carbamazepine should be informed that approximately 25%-30% of them will experience hypersensitivity reactions with Trileptal. For this reason patients should be specifically questioned about any prior experience with carbamazepine, and patients with a history of hypersensitivity reactions to carbamazepine should ordinarily be treated with Trileptal only if the potential benefit justifies the potential risk. If signs or symptoms of hypersensitivity develop, Trileptal should be discontinued immediately.

Withdrawal of AEDs

As with all antiepileptic drugs, Trileptal should be withdrawn gradually to minimize the potential of increased seizure frequency.

PRECAUTIONS

Cognitive/Neuropsychiatric Adverse Events

Use of Trileptal® (oxcarbazepine) has been associated with central nervous system related adverse events. The most significant of these can be classified into three general categories: 1) cognitive symptoms including psychomotor slowing, difficulty with concentration, and speech or language problems, 2) somnolence or fatigue, and 3) coordination abnormalities, including ataxia and gait disturbances.

In one, large, fixed dose study, Trileptal was added to existing AED therapy (up to three concomitant AEDs). By protocol, the dosage of the concomitant AEDs could not be reduced as Trileptal was added, reduction in Trileptal dosage was not allowed if intolerance developed, and patients were discontinued if unable to tolerate their highest target maintenance doses. In this trial, 65% of patients were discontinued because they could not tolerate the 2400 mg/day dose of Trileptal on top of existing AEDs. The adverse events seen in this study were primarily CNS related and the risk for discontinuation was dose related.

In this trial, 7.1% of oxcarbazepine-treated patients and 4% of placebo-treated patients experienced a cognitive adverse event. The risk of discontinuation for these events was about 6.5 times greater on oxcarbazepine than on placebo. In addition, 26% of oxcarbazepine-treated patients and 12% of placebo-treated patients experienced somnolence. The risk of discontinuation for somnolence was about 10 times

Table 1
Summary of percentage change in partial seizure frequency from baseline for placebo-controlled adjunctive therapy trials

Trial	Treatment Group	N	Baseline Median Seizure Rate*	Median % Reduction
1 (pediatrics)	Trileptal	136	12.5	34.8[1]
	Placebo	128	13.1	9.4
2 (adults)	Trileptal 2400 mg/day	174	10.0	49.9[1]
	Trileptal 1200 mg/day	177	9.8	40.2[1]
	Trileptal 600 mg/day	168	9.6	26.4[1]
	Placebo	173	8.6	7.6

[1]p=0.0001; *= # per 28 days

Table 2
Summary of AED Interactions with Trileptal

AED Coadministered	Dose of AED (mg/day)	Trileptal dose (mg/day)	Influence of Trileptal on AED Concentration (Mean change, 90% Confidence Interval)	Influence of AED on MHD Concentration (Mean change, 90% Confidence Interval)
Carbamazepine	400-2000	900	nc[1]	40% decrease [CI: 17% decrease, 57% decrease]
Phenobarbital	100-150	600-1800	14% increase [CI: 2% increase, 24% increase]	25% decrease [CI: 12% decrease, 51% decrease]
Phenytoin	250-500	600-1800 >1200-2400	nc[1,2] up to 40% increase[3] [CI: 12% increase, 60% increase]	30% decrease [CI: 3% decrease, 48% decrease]
Valproic acid	400-2800	600-1800	nc[1]	18% decrease [CI: 13% decrease, 40% decrease]

[1] nc denotes a mean change of less than 10%
[2] Pediatrics
[3] Mean increase in adults at high Trileptal doses

greater on oxcarbazepine than on placebo. Finally, 28.7% of oxcarbazepine-treated patients and 6.4% of placebo-treated patients experienced ataxia or gait disturbances. The risk for discontinuation for these events was about 7 times greater on oxcarbazepine than on placebo.

In a single placebo-controlled monotherapy trial evaluating 2400 mg/day of Trileptal, no patients in either treatment group discontinued double-blind treatment because of cognitive adverse events, somnolence, ataxia, or gait disturbance.

In the two dose-controlled conversion to monotherapy trials comparing 2400 mg/day and 300 mg/day Trileptal, 1.1% of patients in the 2400 mg/day group discontinued double-blind treatment because of somnolence or cognitive adverse events compared to 0% in the 300 mg/day group. In these trials, no patients discontinued because of ataxia or gait disturbances in either treatment group.

Information for Patients

Patients who have exhibited hypersensitivity reactions to carbamazepine should be informed that approximately 25%-30% of these patients may experience hypersensitivity reactions with Trileptal. *(See WARNINGS section.)*

Female patients of childbearing age should be warned that the concurrent use of Trileptal with hormonal contraceptives may render this method of contraception less effective *(see Drug Interactions subsection)*. Additional non-hormonal forms of contraception are recommended when using Trileptal.

Caution should be exercised if alcohol is taken in combination with Trileptal therapy, due to a possible additive sedative effect.

Patients should be advised that Trileptal may cause dizziness and somnolence. Accordingly, patients should be advised not to drive or operate machinery until they have gained sufficient experience on Trileptal to gauge whether it adversely affects their ability to drive or operate machinery.

Laboratory Tests

Serum sodium levels below 125 mmol/L have been observed in patients treated with Trileptal *(see WARNINGS section)*. Experience from clinical trials indicates that serum sodium levels return toward normal when the Trileptal dosage is reduced or discontinued, or when the patient was treated conservatively (e.g., fluid restriction).

Laboratory data from clinical trials suggest that Trileptal use was associated with decreases in T_4, without changes in T_3 or TSH.

Drug Interactions

Oxcarbazepine can inhibit CYP2C19 and induce CYP3A4/5 with potentially important effects on plasma concentrations of other drugs. In addition, several AEDs that are cytochrome P450 inducers can decrease plasma concentrations of oxcarbazepine and MHD.

Oxcarbazepine was evaluated in human liver microsomes to determine its capacity to inhibit the major cytochrome P450 enzymes responsible for the metabolism of other drugs. Results demonstrate that oxcarbazepine and its pharmacologically active 10-monohydroxy metabolite (MHD) have little or no capacity to function as inhibitors for most of the human cytochrome P450 enzymes evaluated (CYP1A2, CYP2A6, CYP2C9, CYP2D6, CYP2E1, CYP4A9 and CYP4A11) with the exception of CYP2C19 and CYP3A4/5. Although inhibition of CYP3A4/5 by oxcarbazepine and MHD did occur at high concentrations, it is not likely to be of clinical significance. The inhibition of CYP2C19 by oxcarbazepine and MHD, however, is clinically relevant *(see below)*.

In vitro, the UDP-glucuronyl transferase level was increased, indicating induction of this enzyme. Increases of 22% with MHD and 47% with oxcarbazepine were observed. As MHD, the predominant plasma substrate, is only a weak inducer of UDP-glucuronyl transferase, it is unlikely to have an effect on drugs that are mainly eliminated by conjugation through UDP-glucuronyl transferase (e.g., valproic acid, lamotrigine).

In addition, oxcarbazepine and MHD induce a subgroup of the cytochrome P450 3A family (CYP3A4 and CYP3A5) responsible for the metabolism of dihydropyridine calcium antagonists and oral contraceptives, resulting in a lower plasma concentration of these drugs.

As binding of MHD to plasma proteins is low (40%), clinically significant interactions with other drugs through competition for protein binding sites are unlikely.

Antiepileptic Drugs

Potential interactions between Trileptal and other AEDs were assessed in clinical studies. The effect of these interactions on mean AUCs and C_{min} are summarized in Table 2.

[See table 2 above]

In vivo, the plasma levels of phenytoin increased by up to 40% when Trileptal was given at doses above 1200 mg/day. Therefore, when using doses of Trileptal greater than 1200 mg/day during adjunctive therapy, a decrease in the dose of phenytoin may be required. The increase of phenobarbital level, however, is small (15%) when given with Trileptal.

Strong inducers of cytochrome P450 enzymes (i.e., carbamazepine, phenytoin and phenobarbital) have been shown to decrease the plasma levels of MHD (29%-40%).

No autoinduction has been observed with Trileptal.

Hormonal Contraceptives

Coadministration of Trileptal with an oral contraceptive has been shown to influence the plasma concentrations of the two hormonal components, ethinylestradiol (EE) and levonorgestrel (LNG). The mean AUC values of EE were decreased by 48% [90% CI: 22-65] in one study and 52% [90% CI: 38-52] in another study. The mean AUC values of LNG were decreased by 32% [90% CI: 20-45] in one study and 52% [90% CI: 42-52] in another study. Therefore, concurrent use of Trileptal with hormonal contraceptives may render these contraceptives less effective *(see Drug Interactions subsection)*. Studies with other oral or implant contraceptives have not been conducted.

Calcium Antagonists

After repeated coadministration of Trileptal, the AUC of felodipine was lowered by 28% [90% CI: 20-33].

Verapamil produced a decrease of 20% [90% CI: 18-27] of the plasma levels of MHD.

Other Drug Interactions

Cimetidine, erythromycin and dextropropoxyphene had no effect on the pharmacokinetics of MHD. Results with warfarin show no evidence of interaction with either single or repeated doses of Trileptal.

Drug/Laboratory Test Interactions

There are no known interactions of Trileptal with commonly used laboratory tests.

Carcinogenesis/Mutagenesis/Impairment of Fertility

In 2-year carcinogenicity studies, oxcarbazepine was administered in the diet at doses of up to 100 mg/kg/day to mice and by gavage at doses of up to 250 mg/kg to rats, and the pharmacologically active 10-hydroxy metabolite (MHD) was administered orally at doses of up to 600 mg/kg/day to rats. In mice, a dose-related increase in the incidence of hepatocellular adenomas was observed at oxcarbazepine doses ≥70 mg/kg/day or approximately 0.1 times the maximum recommended human dose [MRHD] on a mg/m^2 basis. In rats, the incidence of hepatocellular carcinomas was increased in females treated with oxcarbazepine at doses ≥25 mg/kg/day (0.1 times the MRHD on a mg/m^2 basis), and incidences of hepatocellular adenomas and/or carcinomas were increased in males and females treated with MHD at doses of 600 mg/kg/day (2.4 times the MRHD on a mg/m^2 basis) and ≥250 mg/kg/day (equivalent to the MRHD on a mg/m^2 basis), respectively. There was an increase in the incidence of benign testicular interstitial cell tumors in rats at 250 mg oxcarbazepine/kg/day and at ≥250 mg MHD/kg/day, and an increase in the incidence of granular cell tumors in the cervix and vagina in rats at 600 mg MHD/kg/day.

Oxcarbazepine increased mutation frequencies in the Ames test *in vitro* in the absence of metabolic activation in one of five bacterial strains. Both oxcarbazepine and MHD produced increases in chromosomal aberrations and polyploidy in the Chinese hamster ovary assay *in vitro* in the absence of metabolic activation. MHD was negative in the Ames test, and no mutagenic or clastogenic activity was found with either oxcarbazepine or MHD in V79 Chinese hamster cells *in vitro*. Oxcarbazepine and MHD were both negative for clastogenic or aneugenic effects (micronucleus formation) in an *in vivo* rat bone marrow assay.

In a fertility study in which rats were administered MHD (50, 150, or 450 mg/kg) orally prior to and during mating and early gestation, estrous cyclicity was disrupted and numbers of corpora lutea, implantations, and live embryos were reduced in females receiving the highest dose (approximately 2 times the MRHD on a mg/m^2 basis).

Pregnancy Category C

Increased incidences of fetal structural abnormalities and other manifestations of developmental toxicity (embryolethality, growth retardation) were observed in the offspring of animals treated with either oxcarbazepine or its active 10-hydroxy metabolite (MHD) during pregnancy at doses similar to the maximum recommended human dose.

When pregnant rats were given oxcarbazepine (30, 300, or 1000 mg/kg) orally throughout the period of organogenesis, increased incidences of fetal malformations (craniofacial, cardiovascular, and skeletal) and variations were observed at the intermediate and high doses (approximately 1.2 and 4 times, respectively, the maximum recommended human dose [MRHD] on a mg/m^2 basis). Increased embryofetal death and decreased fetal body weights were seen at the high dose. Doses ≥300 mg/kg were also maternally toxic (decreased body weight gain, clinical signs), but there is no evidence to suggest that teratogenicity was secondary to the maternal effects.

In a study in which pregnant rabbits were orally administered MHD (20, 100, or 200 mg/kg) during organogenesis, embryofetal mortality was increased at the highest dose (1.5 times the MRHD on a mg/m^2 basis). This dose produced only minimal maternal toxicity.

In a study in which female rats were dosed orally with oxcarbazepine (25, 50, or 150 mg/kg) during the latter part of gestation and throughout the lactation period, a persistent reduction in body weights and altered behavior (decreased activity) were observed in offspring exposed to the highest dose (0.6 times the MRHD on a mg/m^2 basis). Oral administration of MHD (25, 75, or 250 mg/kg) to rats during gestation and lactation resulted in a persistent reduction in offspring weights at the highest dose (equivalent to the MRHD on a mg/m^2 basis).

There are no adequate and well-controlled clinical studies of Trileptal in pregnant women; however, Trileptal is closely related structurally to carbamazepine, which is considered to be teratogenic in humans. Given this fact, and the results of the animal studies described, it is likely that Trileptal is a human teratogen. Trileptal should be used during pregnancy only if the potential benefit justifies the potential risk to the fetus.

Labor and Delivery

The effect of Trileptal on labor and delivery in humans has not been evaluated.

Nursing Mothers

Oxcarbazepine and its active metabolite (MHD) are excreted in human breast milk. A milk-to-plasma concentration ratio of 0.5 was found for both. Because of the potential for serious adverse reactions to Trileptal in nursing infants, a decision should be made about whether to discontinue nursing or to discontinue the drug in nursing women, taking into account the importance of the drug to the mother.

Table 3
Treatment-Emergent Adverse Event Incidence in a Controlled Clinical Study of Adjunctive Therapy in Adults (Events in at least 2% of patients treated with 2400 mg/day of Trileptal and numerically more frequent than in the placebo group)

	Oxcarbazepine Dosage (mg/day)			
Body System/ Adverse Event	OXC 600 N=163 %	OXC 1200 N=171 %	OXC 2400 N=126 %	Placebo N=166 %
Body as a Whole				
Fatigue	15	12	15	7
Asthenia	6	3	6	5
Edema Legs	2	1	2	1
Weight Increase	1	2	2	1
Feeling Abnormal	0	1	2	0
Cardiovascular System				
Hypotension	0	1	2	0
Digestive System				
Nausea	15	25	29	10
Vomiting	13	25	36	5
Pain Abdominal	10	13	11	5
Diarrhea	5	6	7	6
Dyspepsia	5	5	6	2
Constipation	2	2	6	4
Gastritis	2	1	2	1
Metabolic and Nutritional Disorders				
Hyponatremia	3	1	2	1
Musculoskeletal System				
Muscle Weakness	1	2	2	0
Sprains and Strains	0	2	2	1
Nervous System				
Headache	32	28	26	23
Dizziness	26	32	49	13
Somnolence	20	28	36	12
Ataxia	9	17	31	5
Nystagmus	7	20	26	5
Gait Abnormal	5	10	17	1
Insomnia	4	2	3	1
Tremor	3	8	16	5
Nervousness	2	4	2	1
Agitation	1	1	2	1
Coordination Abnormal	1	3	2	1
EEG Abnormal	0	0	2	0
Speech Disorder	1	1	3	0
Confusion	1	1	2	1
Cranial Injury NOS	1	0	2	1
Dysmetria	1	2	3	0
Thinking Abnormal	0	2	4	0
Respiratory System				
Rhinitis	2	4	5	4
Skin and Appendages				
Acne	1	2	2	0
Special Senses				
Diplopia	14	30	40	5
Vertigo	6	12	15	2
Vision Abnormal	6	14	13	4
Accommodation Abnormal	0	0	2	0

Patients with Renal Impairment

In renally-impaired patients (creatinine clearance <30 mL/min), the elimination half-life of MHD is prolonged with a corresponding increase in AUC *(see CLINICAL PHARMACOLOGY, Pharmacokinetics subsection)*. Trileptal therapy should be initiated at one-half the usual starting dose and increased, if necessary, at a slower than usual rate until the desired clinical response is achieved.

Pediatric Use

Trileptal is indicated for use as adjunctive therapy or monotherapy for partial seizures in patients aged 4-16 years old. Trileptal has been given to about 623 patients between the ages of 3-17 in controlled clinical trials (185 treated as monotherapy) and about 615 patients between the ages of 3-17 in other trials. *(See ADVERSE REACTIONS for a description of the adverse events associated with Trileptal use in this population.)*

Geriatric Use

There were 52 patients over age 65 in controlled clinical trials and 565 patients over the age of 65 in other trials. Following administration of single (300 mg) and multiple (600 mg/day) doses of Trileptal in elderly volunteers (60-82 years of age), the maximum plasma concentrations and AUC values of MHD were 30%-60% higher than in younger volunteers (18-32 years of age). Comparisons of creatinine clearance in young and elderly volunteers indicate that the difference was due to age-related reductions in creatinine clearance.

ADVERSE REACTIONS

Most Common Adverse Events in All Clinical Studies

Adjunctive Therapy/Monotherapy in Adults Previously Treated with other AEDs: The most commonly observed (≥5%) adverse experiences seen in association with Trileptal® (oxcarbazepine) and substantially more frequent than in placebo-treated patients were: Dizziness, somnolence, diplopia, fatigue, nausea, vomiting, ataxia, abnormal vision, abdominal pain, tremor, dyspepsia, abnormal gait.

Approximately 23% of these 1537 adult patients discontinued treatment because of an adverse experience. The adverse experiences most commonly associated with discontinuation were: Dizziness (6.4%), diplopia (5.9%), ataxia (5.2%), vomiting (5.1%), nausea (4.9%), somnolence (3.8%), headache (2.9%), fatigue (2.1%), abnormal vision (2.1%), tremor (1.8%), abnormal gait (1.7%), rash (1.4%), hyponatremia (1.0%).

Monotherapy in Adults not Previously Treated with other AEDs: The most commonly observed (≥5%) adverse experiences seen in association with Trileptal in these patients were similar to those in previously treated patients.

Approximately 9% of these 295 adult patients discontinued treatment because of an adverse experience. The adverse experiences most commonly associated with discontinuation were: Dizziness (1.7%), nausea (1.7%), rash (1.7%), headache (1.4%).

Adjunctive Therapy/Monotherapy in Pediatric Patients Previously Treated with other AEDs: The most commonly observed (≥5%) adverse experiences seen in association with Trileptal in these patients were similar to those seen in adults.

Approximately 11% of these 456 pediatric patients discontinued treatment because of an adverse experience. The adverse experiences most commonly associated with discontinuation were: Somnolence (2.4%), vomiting (2.0%), ataxia (1.8%), diplopia (1.3%), dizziness (1.3%), fatigue (1.1%), nystagmus (1.1%).

Monotherapy in Pediatric Patients not Previously Treated with other AEDs: The most commonly observed (≥5%) adverse experiences seen in association with Trileptal in these patients were similar to those in adults.

Approximately 9.2% of 152 pediatric patients discontinued treatment because of an adverse experience. The adverse experiences most commonly associated (≥1%) with discontinuation were rash (5.3%) and maculopapular rash (1.3%).

Incidence in Controlled Clinical Studies: The prescriber should be aware that the figures in Tables 3, 4, 5 and 6 cannot be used to predict the frequency of adverse experiences in the course of usual medical practice where patient characteristics and other factors may differ from those prevailing during clinical studies. Similarly, the cited frequencies cannot be directly compared with figures obtained from other clinical investigations involving different treatments, uses, or investigators. An inspection of these frequencies,

Continued on next page

Trileptal—Cont.

however, does provide the prescriber with one basis to estimate the relative contribution of drug and nondrug factors to the adverse event incidences in the population studied.

Controlled Clinical Studies of Adjunctive Therapy/Monotherapy in Adults Previously Treated with other AEDs: Table 3 lists treatment-emergent signs and symptoms that occurred in at least 2% of adult patients with epilepsy treated with Trileptal or placebo as adjunctive treatment and were numerically more common in the patients treated with any dose of Trileptal. Table 4 lists treatment-emergent signs and symptoms in patients converted from other AEDs to either high dose Trileptal or low dose (300 mg) Trileptal. Note that in some of these monotherapy studies patients who dropped out during a preliminary tolerability phase are not included in the tables.

[See table 3 at top of previous page]

Table 4
Treatment-Emergent Adverse Event Incidence in Controlled Clinical Studies of Monotherapy in Adults Previously Treated with Other AEDs (Events in at least 2% of patients treated with 2400 mg/day of Trileptal and numerically more frequent than in the low dose control group)

Body System/ Adverse Event	Oxcarbazepine Dosage (mg/day) 2400 N=86 %	300 N=86 %
Body as a Whole		
Fatigue	21	5
Fever	3	0
Allergy	2	0
Edema Generalized	2	1
Pain Chest	2	0
Digestive System		
Nausea	22	7
Vomiting	15	5
Diarrhea	7	5
Dyspepsia	6	1
Anorexia	5	3
Pain Abdominal	5	3
Mouth Dry	3	0
Hemorrhage Rectum	2	0
Toothache	2	1
Hemic and Lymphatic System		
Lymphadenopathy	2	0
Infections and Infestations		
Infection Viral	7	5
Infection	2	0
Metabolic and Nutritional Disorders		
Hyponatremia	5	0
Thirst	2	0
Nervous System		
Headache	31	15
Dizziness	28	8
Somnolence	19	5
Anxiety	7	5
Ataxia	7	1
Confusion	7	0
Nervousness	7	0
Insomnia	6	3
Tremor	6	3
Amnesia	5	1
Convulsions Aggravated	5	2
Emotional Lability	3	2
Hypoesthesia	3	1
Coordination Abnormal	2	1
Nystagmus	2	0
Speech Disorder	2	0
Respiratory System		
Upper Respiratory Tract Infection	10	5
Coughing	5	0
Bronchitis	3	0
Pharyngitis	3	0
Skin and Appendages		
Hot Flushes	2	1
Purpura	2	0
Special Senses		
Vision Abnormal	14	2
Diplopia	12	1
Taste Perversion	5	0
Vertigo	3	0
Earache	2	1
Ear Infection NOS	2	0
Urogenital and Reproductive System		
Urinary Tract Infection	5	1
Micturition Frequency	2	1
Vaginitis	2	0

Controlled Clinical Study of Monotherapy in Adults not Previously Treated with other AEDs: Table 5 lists treatment-emergent signs and symptoms in a controlled clinical study of monotherapy in adults not previously treated with other AEDs that occurred in at least 2% of adult patients with epilepsy treated with Trileptal or placebo and were numerically more common in the patients treated with Trileptal.

Table 5
Treatment-Emergent Adverse Event Incidence in a Controlled Clinical Study of Monotherapy in Adults not Previously Treated with Other AEDs (Events in at least 2% of patients treated with Trileptal and numerically more frequent than in the placebo group)

Body System/ Adverse Event	Oxcarbazepine N=55 %	Placebo N=49 %
Body as a Whole		
Falling Down NOS	4	0
Digestive System		
Nausea	16	12
Diarrhea	7	2
Vomiting	7	6
Constipation	5	0
Dyspepsia	5	4
Musculoskeletal System		
Pain Back	4	2
Nervous System		
Dizziness	22	6
Headache	13	10
Ataxia	5	0
Nervousness	5	2
Amnesia	4	2
Coordination Abnormal	4	2
Tremor	4	0
Respiratory System		
Upper Respiratory Tract Infection	7	0
Epistaxis	4	0
Infection Chest	4	0
Sinusitis	4	2
Skin and Appendages		
Rash	4	2
Special Senses		
Vision Abnormal	4	0

Controlled Clinical Studies of Adjunctive Therapy/Monotherapy in Pediatric Patients Previously Treated with other AEDs: Table 6 lists treatment-emergent signs and symptoms that occurred in at least 2% of pediatric patients with epilepsy treated with Trileptal or placebo as adjunctive treatment and were numerically more common in the patients treated with Trileptal.

Table 6
Treatment-Emergent Adverse Event Incidence in Controlled Clinical Studies of Adjunctive Therapy/ Monotherapy in Pediatric Patients Previously Treated with Other AEDs (Events in at least 2% of patients treated with Trileptal and numerically more frequent than in the placebo group)

Body System/ Adverse Event	Oxcarbazepine N=171 %	Placebo N=139 %
Body as a Whole		
Fatigue	13	9
Allergy	2	0
Asthenia	2	1
Digestive System		
Vomiting	33	14
Nausea	19	5
Constipation	4	1
Dyspepsia	2	0
Nervous System		
Headache	31	19
Somnolence	31	13
Dizziness	28	8
Ataxia	13	4
Nystagmus	9	1
Emotional Lability	8	4
Gait Abnormal	8	3
Tremor	6	4
Speech Disorder	3	1
Concentration Impaired	2	1
Convulsions	2	1
Muscle Contractions Involuntary	2	1
Respiratory System		
Rhinitis	10	9
Pneumonia	2	1
Skin and Appendages		
Bruising	4	2
Sweating Increased	3	0
Special Senses		
Diplopia	17	1
Vision Abnormal	13	1
Vertigo	2	0

Other Events Observed in Association with the Administration of Trileptal

In the paragraphs that follow, the adverse events other than those in the preceding tables or text, that occurred in a total of 565 children and 1574 adults exposed to Trileptal and that are reasonably likely to be related to drug use are presented. Events common in the population, events reflecting chronic illness and events likely to reflect concomitant illness are omitted particularly if minor. They are listed in order of decreasing frequency. Because the reports cite events observed in open label and uncontrolled trials, the role of Trileptal in their causation cannot be reliably determined.

Body as a Whole: Fever, malaise, pain chest precordial, rigors, weight decrease.

Cardiovascular System: Bradycardia, cardiac failure, cerebral hemorrhage, hypertension, hypotension postural, palpitation, syncope, tachycardia.

Digestive System: Appetite increased, blood in stool, cholelithiasis, colitis, duodenal ulcer, dysphagia, enteritis, eructation, esophagitis, flatulence, gastric ulcer, gingival bleeding, gum hyperplasia, hematemesis, hemorrhage rectum, hemorrhoids, hiccup, mouth dry, pain biliary, pain right hypochondrium, retching, sialoadenitis, stomatitis, stomatitis ulcerative.

Hemic and Lymphatic System: Leukopenia, thrombocytopenia.

Laboratory Abnormality: Gamma-GT increased, hyperglycemia, hypocalcemia, hypoglycemia, hypokalemia, liver enzymes elevated, serum transaminase increased.

Musculoskeletal System: Hypertonia muscle.

Nervous System: Aggressive reaction, amnesia, anguish, anxiety, apathy, aphasia, aura, convulsions aggravated, delirium, delusion, depressed level of consciousness, dysphonia, dystonia, emotional lability, euphoria, extrapyramidal disorder, feeling drunk, hemiplegia, hyperkinesia, hyperreflexia, hypoesthesia, hypokinesia, hyporeflexia, hypotonia, hysteria, libido decreased, libido increased, manic reaction, migraine, muscle contractions involuntary, nervousness, neuralgia, oculogyric crisis, panic disorder, paralysis, paroniria, personality disorder, psychosis, ptosis, stupor, tetany.

Respiratory System: Asthma, dyspnea, epistaxis, laryngismus, pleurisy.

Skin and Appendages: Acne, alopecia, angioedema, bruising, dermatitis contact, eczema, facial rash, flushing, folliculitis, heat rash, hot flushes, photosensitivity reaction, pruritus genital, psoriasis, purpura, rash erythematous, rash maculopapular, vitiligo, urticaria.

Special Senses: Accommodation abnormal, cataract, conjunctival hemorrhage, edema eye, hemianopia, mydriasis, otitis externa, photophobia, scotoma, taste perversion, tinnitus, xerophthalmia.

Surgical and Medical Procedures: Procedure dental oral, procedure female reproductive, procedure musculoskeletal, procedure skin.

Urogenital and Reproductive System: Dysuria, hematuria, intermenstrual bleeding, leukorrhea, menorrhagia, micturition frequency, pain renal, pain urinary tract, polyuria, priapism, renal calculus.

Other: Systemic lupus erythematosus.

Post-Marketing and Other Experience

The following adverse events not seen in controlled clinical trials have been observed in named patient programs or post-marketing experience:

Body as a Whole: Multiorgan hypersensitivity disorders characterized by features such as rash, fever, lymphadenopathy, abnormal liver function tests, eosinophilia and arthralgia.

Skin and Appendages: Erythema multiforme, Stevens-Johnson syndrome, toxic epidermal necrolysis.

DRUG ABUSE AND DEPENDENCE

Abuse

The abuse potential of Trileptal® (oxcarbazepine) has not been evaluated in human studies.

Dependence

Intragastric injections of oxcarbazepine to four cynomolgus monkeys demonstrated no signs of physical dependence as measured by the desire to self-administer oxcarbazepine by lever pressing activity.

OVERDOSAGE

Human Overdose Experience

Isolated cases of overdose with Trileptal® (oxcarbazepine) have been reported. The maximum dose taken was approximately 24,000 mg. All patients recovered with symptomatic treatment.

Treatment and Management

There is no specific antidote. Symptomatic and supportive treatment should be administered as appropriate. Removal of the drug by gastric lavage and/or inactivation by administering activated charcoal should be considered.

DOSAGE AND ADMINISTRATION

Trileptal® (oxcarbazepine) is recommended as adjunctive treatment and monotherapy in the treatment of partial seizures in adults and children ages 4-16. All dosing should be given in a twice-a-day (BID) regimen. Trileptal oral suspension and Trileptal film-coated tablets may be interchanged at equal doses.

Trileptal should be kept out of the reach and sight of children.

Before using Trileptal oral suspension, shake the bottle well and prepare the dose immediately afterwards. The prescribed amount of oral suspension should be withdrawn from the bottle using the oral dosing syringe supplied. Trileptal oral suspension can be mixed in a small glass of water just prior to administration or, alternatively, may be swallowed directly from the syringe. After each use, close the bottle and rinse the syringe with warm water and allow it to dry thoroughly.

Trileptal can be taken with or without food *(see CLINICAL PHARMACOLOGY, Pharmacokinetics)*.

Adults

Adjunctive Therapy

Treatment with Trileptal should be initiated with a dose of 600 mg/day, given in a BID regimen. If clinically indicated, the dose may be increased by a maximum of 600 mg/day at approximately weekly intervals; the recommended daily dose is 1200 mg/day. Daily doses above 1200 mg/day show somewhat greater effectiveness in controlled trials, but most patients were not able to tolerate the 2400 mg/day dose, primarily because of CNS effects. It is recommended that the patient be observed closely and plasma levels of the concomitant AEDs be monitored during the period of Trileptal titration, as these plasma levels may be altered, especially at Trileptal doses greater than 1200 mg/day *(see PRECAUTIONS, Drug Interactions subsection)*.

Conversion to Monotherapy

Patients receiving concomitant AEDs may be converted to monotherapy by initiating treatment with Trileptal at 600 mg/day (given in a BID regimen) while simultaneously initiating the reduction of the dose of the concomitant AEDs. The concomitant AEDs should be completely withdrawn over 3-6 weeks, while the maximum dose of Trileptal should be reached in about 2-4 weeks. Trileptal may be increased as clinically indicated by a maximum increment of 600 mg/day at approximately weekly intervals to achieve the recommended daily dose of 2400 mg/day. A daily dose of 1200 mg/day has been shown in one study to be effective in patients in whom monotherapy has been initiated with Trileptal. Patients should be observed closely during this transition phase.

Initiation of Monotherapy

Patients not currently being treated with AEDs may have monotherapy initiated with Trileptal. In these patients, Trileptal should be initiated at a dose of 600 mg/day (given in a BID regimen); the dose should be increased by 300 mg/day every third day to a dose of 1200 mg/day. Controlled trials in these patients examined the effectiveness of a 1200 mg/day dose; a dose of 2400 mg/day has been shown to be effective in patients converted from other AEDs to Trileptal monotherapy *(see above)*.

Pediatric Patients Age 4-16

Adjunctive Therapy

Treatment should be initiated at a daily dose of 8-10 mg/kg generally not to exceed 600 mg/day, given in a BID regimen. The target maintenance dose of Trileptal should be achieved over 2 weeks, and is dependent upon patient weight, according to the following chart:

20-29 kg - 900 mg/day
29.1-39 kg - 1200 mg/day
>39 kg - 1800 mg/day

In the clinical trial, in which the intention was to reach these target doses, the median daily dose was 31 mg/kg with a range of 6-51 mg/kg.

The pharmacokinetics of Trileptal are similar in older children (age >8 yrs) and adults. However, younger children (age <8 yrs) have an increased clearance (by about 30%-40%) compared with older children and adults. In the controlled trial, pediatric patients 8 years old and below received the highest maintenance doses.

Children below 2 years of age have not been studied in controlled clinical trials.

Conversion to Monotherapy

Patients receiving concomitant antiepileptic drugs may be converted to monotherapy by initiating treatment with Trileptal at approximately 8-10 mg/kg/day given in a BID regimen, while simultaneously initiating the reduction of the dose of the concomitant antiepileptic drugs. The concomitant antiepileptic drugs can be completely withdrawn over 3-6 weeks while Trileptal may be increased as clinically indicated by a maximum increment of 10 mg/kg/day at approximately weekly intervals to achieve the recommended daily dose. Patients should be observed closely during this transition phase.

The recommended total daily dose of Trileptal is shown in the table below.

Initiation of Monotherapy

Patients not currently being treated with antiepileptic drugs may have monotherapy initiated with Trileptal. In these patients, Trileptal should be initiated at a dose of 8-10 mg/kg/day given in a BID regimen. The dose should be increased by 5 mg/kg/day every third day to the recommended daily dose shown in the table below.

Table 7
Range of Maintenance Doses of Trileptal for Children by Weight During Monotherapy

Weight in kg	From Dose (mg/day)	To Dose (mg/day)
20	600	900
25	900	1200
30	900	1200
35	900	1500
40	900	1500
45	1200	1500
50	1200	1800
55	1200	1800
60	1200	2100
65	1200	2100
70	1500	2100

Patients with Hepatic Impairment

In general, dose adjustments are not required in patients with mild-to-moderate hepatic impairment *(see CLINICAL PHARMACOLOGY, Pharmacokinetics, Special Populations subsection)*.

Patients with Renal Impairment

In patients with impaired renal function (creatine clearance <30 mL/min) Trileptal therapy should be initiated at one-half the usual starting dose (300 mg/day) and increased slowly to achieve the desired clinical response *(see CLINICAL PHARMACOLOGY, Pharmacokinetics, Special Populations subsection)*.

HOW SUPPLIED

Tablets

150 mg Film-Coated Tablets: yellow, ovaloid, slightly biconvex, scored on both sides. Imprinted with T/D on one side and C/G on the other side.

Bottle of 100 .... NDC 0078-0336-05
Bottle of 1000 .... NDC 0078-0336-09
Unit Dose (blister pack)
Box of 100 (strips of 10) .... NDC 0078-0336-06

300 mg Film-Coated Tablets: yellow, ovaloid, slightly biconvex, scored on both sides. Imprinted with TE/TE on one side and CG/CG on the other side.

Bottle of 100 .... NDC 0078-0337-05
Bottle of 1000 .... NDC 0078-0337-09
Unit Dose (blister pack)
Box of 100 (strips of 10) .... NDC 0078-0337-06

600 mg Film-Coated Tablets: yellow, ovaloid, slightly biconvex, scored on both sides. Imprinted with TF/TF on one side and CG/CG on the other side.

Bottle of 100 .... NDC 0078-0338-05
Bottle of 1000 .... NDC 0078-0338-09
Unit Dose (blister pack)
Box of 100 (strips of 10) .... NDC 0078-0338-06

Store at 25°C (77°F); excursions permitted to 15-30°C (59-86°F) [see USP Controlled Room Temperature]. Dispense in tight container (USP).

Suspension

300 mg/5 mL (60 mg/mL) Oral Suspension: off-white to slightly brown or slightly red suspension. Available in amber glass bottles containing 250 mL of oral suspension. Supplied with a 10 mL dosing syringe and press-in bottle adapter.

Bottle containing 250 mL
of oral suspension .... NDC 0078-0357-52

Store Trileptal® (oxcarbazepine) oral suspension in the original container. Shake well before using.

Use within 7 weeks of first opening the bottle.

Store at 25°C (77°F); excursions permitted to 15-30°C (59-86°F) [see USP Controlled Room Temperature].

T2004-29
REV: MARCH 2004 Printed in U.S.A. 89004905

Tablets Manufactured by:
Novartis Pharmaceuticals Corporation
Suffern, New York 10901
Oral Suspension Manufactured by:
Novartis Pharma S.A.S.
F-68330 Huningue, France
Distributed by:
Novartis Pharmaceuticals Corporation
East Hanover, New Jersey 07936
©Novartis

Shown in Product Identification Guide, page 326

VIVELLE® ℞

[vī-věl]

estradiol transdermal system
Continuous delivery for twice-weekly application
Rx only

Prescribing Information

The following prescribing information is based on official labeling in effect July 2004.

ESTROGENS INCREASE THE RISK OF ENDOMETRIAL CANCER

Close clinical surveillance of all women taking estrogens is important. Adequate diagnostic measures, including endometrial sampling when indicated, should be undertaken to rule out malignancy in all cases of undiagnosed persistent or recurring abnormal vaginal bleeding. There is currently no evidence that the use of "natural" estrogens results in a different endometrial risk profile than synthetic estrogens of equivalent estrogen dose.

CARDIOVASCULAR AND OTHER RISKS

Estrogens with and without progestins should not be used for the prevention of cardiovascular disease.

The Women's Health Initiative (WHI) study reported increased risks of myocardial infarction, stroke, invasive breast cancer, pulmonary emboli, and deep vein thrombosis in postmenopausal women during 5 years of treatment with conjugated equine estrogens (CE 0.625 mg) combined with medroxyprogesterone acetate (MPA 2.5 mg) relative to placebo *(see CLINICAL PHARMACOLOGY, Clinical Studies)*. Other doses of conjugated estrogens with medroxyprogesterone, and other combinations of estrogens and progestins were not studied in the WHI and, in the absence of comparable data, these risks should be assumed to be similar for all estrogens and estrogen-progestin combinations. Because of these risks, estrogens with or without progestins should be prescribed at the lowest effective doses and for the shortest duration consistent with treatment goals and risks for the individual woman.

DESCRIPTION

The Vivelle® (estradiol transdermal system) contains estradiol in a multipolymeric adhesive. The system is designed to release estradiol continuously upon application to intact skin.

Five systems are available to provide nominal *in vivo* delivery of 0.025, 0.0375, 0.05, 0.075, or 0.1 mg of estradiol per day via skin of average permeability. Each corresponding system having an active surface area of 7.25, 11.0, 14.5, 22.0, or 29.0 cm^2 contains 2.17, 3.28, 4.33, 6.57, or 8.66 mg of estradiol USP, respectively. The composition of the systems per unit area is identical.

Estradiol USP is a white, crystalline powder, chemically described as estra-1,3,5(10)-triene-3,17β-diol.

The structural formula is

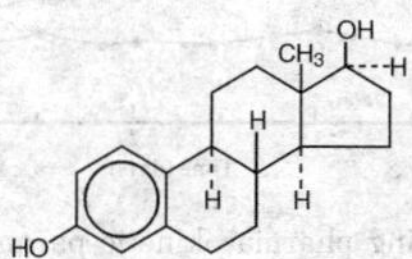

The molecular formula of estradiol is $C_{18}H_{24}O_2$. The molecular weight is 272.39.

The Vivelle system comprises three layers. Proceeding from the visible surface toward the surface attached to the skin, these layers are (1) a translucent flexible film consisting of an ethylene vinyl alcohol copolymer film, a polyurethane film, urethane polymer and epoxy resin, (2) an adhesive formulation containing estradiol USP, acrylic adhesive, polyisobutylene, ethylene vinyl acetate copolymer, 1,3 butylene glycol, styrene-butadiene rubber, oleic acid NF, lecithin, propylene glycol, bentonite NF, mineral oil USP, and dipropylene glycol, and (3) a polyester release liner that is attached to the adhesive surface and must be removed before the system can be used.

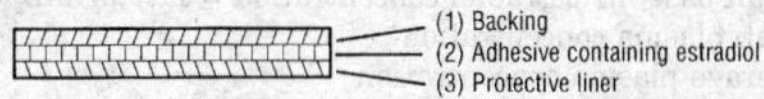

The active component of the system is estradiol. The remaining components of the system are pharmacologically inactive.

CLINICAL PHARMACOLOGY

Endogenous estrogens are largely responsible for the development and maintenance of the female reproductive system and secondary sexual characteristics. Although circulating estrogens exist in a dynamic equilibrium of metabolic interconversions, estradiol is the principal intracellular human estrogen and is substantially more potent than its metabolites, estrone and estriol, at the receptor level.

The primary source of estrogen in normally cycling adult women is the ovarian follicle, which secretes 70 to 500 µg of estradiol daily, depending on the phase of the menstrual cycle. After menopause, most endogenous estrogen is produced by conversion of androstenedione, secreted by the adrenal cortex, to estrone by peripheral tissues. Thus, estrone and the sulfate conjugated form, estrone sulfate, are the most abundant circulating estrogens in postmenopausal women.

Estrogens act through binding to nuclear receptors in estrogen-responsive tissues. To date, two estrogen receptors have been identified. They vary in proportion from tissue to tissue.

Circulating estrogens modulate the pituitary secretion of the gonadotropins, luteinizing hormone (LH) and follicle stimulating hormone (FSH) through a negative feedback mechanism. Estrogens act to reduce the elevated levels of these hormones seen in postmenopausal women.

Pharmacokinetics

Absorption

In a multiple-dose study consisting of three consecutive patch applications of the Vivelle system, which was conducted in 17 healthy, postmenopausal women, blood levels of estradiol and estrone were compared following application of these units to sites on the abdomen and buttocks in a crossover fashion. Patches that deliver nominal estradiol doses of approximately 0.0375 mg/day and 0.1 mg/day were applied to abdominal application sites while the 0.1 mg/day doses were also applied to sites on the buttocks. These systems increased estradiol levels above baseline within 4 hours and maintained respective mean levels of 25 and 79 pg/mL above baseline following application to the abdomen; slightly higher mean levels of 88 pg/mL above baseline were observed following application to the buttocks. At the same time, increases in estrone plasma concentrations averaged about 12 and 50 pg/mL, respectively, following application to the abdomen and 61 pg/mL for the buttocks. While plasma concentrations of estradiol and estrone remained slightly above baseline at 12 hours following removal of the

Continued on next page

Vivelle—Cont.

patches in this study, results from another study show these levels to return to baseline values within 24 hours following removal of the patches.

The figure (see Figure 1) illustrates the mean plasma concentrations of estradiol at steady state during application of these patches at four different dosages.

Figure 1
Steady-State Estradiol Plasma Concentrations for Systems Applied to the Abdomen
Nonbaseline-Corrected Levels

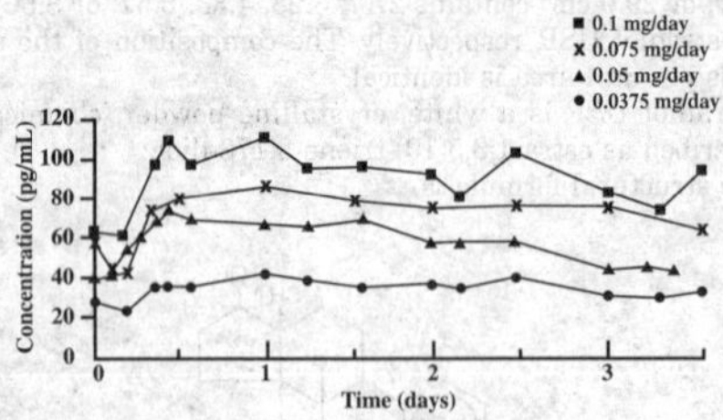

The corresponding pharmacokinetic parameters are summarized in Table 1 below.

Table 1
Steady-State Estradiol Pharmacokinetic Parameters for Systems Applied to the Abdomen (mean ± standard deviation)
Nonbaseline-Corrected Data*

Dosage (mg/day)	C_{max} † (pg/mL)	C_{avg} ‡ (pg/mL)	C_{min} (84 hr)§ (pg/mL)
0.0375	46 ± 16	34 ± 10	30 ± 10
0.05	83 ± 41	57 ± 23#	41 ± 11#
0.075	99 ± 35	72 ± 24	60 ± 24
0.1	133 ± 51	89 ± 38	90 ± 44
0.1¶	145 ± 71	104 ± 52	85 ± 47

* Mean baseline estradiol concentration = 11.7 pg/mL
† Peak plasma concentration
‡ Average plasma concentration
§ Minimum plasma concentration at 84 hr
# Measured over 80 hr
¶ Applied to the buttocks

Distribution

The distribution of exogenous estrogens is similar to that of endogenous estrogens. Estrogens are widely distributed in the body and are generally found in higher concentrations in the sex hormone target organs. Estrogens circulate in the blood largely bound to sex hormone binding globulin (SHBG) and, to a lesser extent, albumin.

Metabolism

Exogenous estrogens are metabolized in the same manner as endogenous estrogens. Circulating estrogens exist in a dynamic equilibrium of metabolic interconversions. These transformations take place mainly in the liver. Estradiol is converted reversibly to estrone, and both can be converted to estriol, which is the major urinary metabolite. Estrogens also undergo enterohepatic recirculation via sulfate and glucuronide conjugation in the liver, biliary secretion of conjugates into the intestine, and hydrolysis in the gut followed by reabsorption. In postmenopausal women, a significant portion of the circulating estrogens exist as sulfate conjugated, especially estrone sulfate, which serves as a circulating reservoir for the formation of more active estrogens.

Excretion

Estradiol, estrone, and estriol are excreted in the urine along with glucuronide and sulfate conjugates. Studies conducted with the Vivelle system show the drug has an apparent mean half-life of 4.4 ± 2.3 hours. After removal of the transdermal systems, serum concentrations of estradiol and estrone returned to baseline levels within 24 hours.

Special Populations

Vivelle was only investigated in postmenopausal women.

Drug Interactions

In vitro and *in vivo* studies have shown that estrogens are metabolized partially by cytochrome P450 3A4 (CYP3A4). Therefore, inducers or inhibitors of CYP3A4 may affect estrogen drug metabolism. Inducers of CYP3A4 such as St. John's Wort preparations (Hypericum perforatum), phenobarbital, carbamazepine and rifampin may reduce plasma concentrations of estrogens, possibly resulting in a decrease in therapeutic effects and/or changes in the uterine bleeding profile. Inhibitors of CYP3A4 such as erythromycin, clarithromycin, ketoconazole, itraconazole, ritonavir and grapefruit juice may increase plasma concentrations of estrogens and may result in side effects.

Adhesion

Data showing the number of systems in controlled studies that required replacement due to inadequate adhesion is not available.

CLINICAL STUDIES

In two controlled clinical trials of 356 subjects, the 0.075 and 0.1 mg doses were superior to placebo in relieving vasomotor symptoms at Week 4, and maintained efficacy through Weeks 8 and 12 of treatment. In this original study, the 0.0375 and 0.05 mg doses, however, did not differ from placebo until approximately Week 6; therefore, an additional 12-week placebo-controlled study in 255 patients was performed to establish the efficacy of the lowest dose of 0.0375 mg. The baseline mean daily number of hot flushes in these 255 patients was 11.5. Results at Weeks 4, 8, and 12 of treatment are shown in the figure below. *(See Figure 2.)*

Figure 2
Mean (SD) Change from Baseline in Mean Daily Number of Flushes for Vivelle 0.0375 mg Versus Placebo in a 12-Week Trial

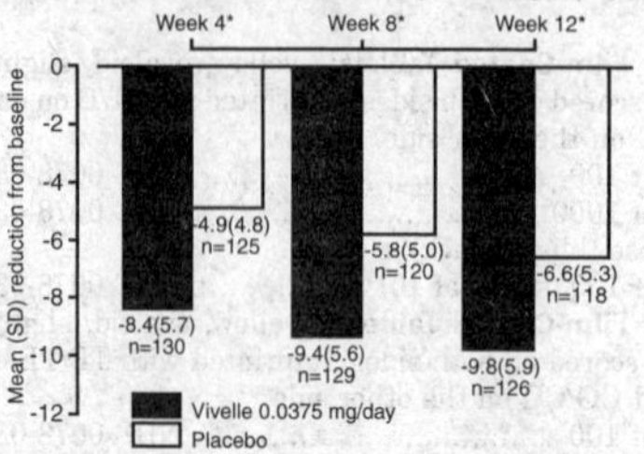

*Indicates statistically significant difference (p<0.05) between Vivelle and placebo

The 0.0375-mg dose was superior to placebo in reducing both the frequency and severity of vasomotor symptoms at Week 4 and maintained efficacy through Weeks 8 and 12 of treatment. The following doses of Vivelle: 0.0375 mg, 0.05 mg, 0.075 mg, and 0.1 mg, are effective for the control of vasomotor symptoms.

Efficacy and safety of the Vivelle system in the prevention of postmenopausal osteoporosis have been studied in a 2-year double-blind, randomized, placebo-controlled, parallel group study. A total of 261 hysterectomized (161) and non-hysterectomized (100), surgically or naturally menopausal women (within 5 years of menopause), with no evidence of osteoporosis (lumbar spine bone mineral density within 2 standard deviations of average peak bone mass, i.e., ≥0.827 g/cm²) were enrolled in this study; 194 patients were randomized to one of the four doses of Vivelle (0.1, 0.05, 0.0375, or 0.025 mg/day) and 67 patients to placebo. Over 2 years, study systems were applied to the buttock or the abdomen twice a week. Non-hysterectomized women received oral medroxyprogesterone acetate (2.5 mg/day) throughout the study.

The study population comprised naturally (82%) or surgically (18%) menopausal, hysterectomized (61%) or non-hysterectomized (39%) women with a mean age of 52.0 years (range 27 to 62 years); the mean duration of menopause was 31.7 months (range 2 to 72 months). Two hundred thirty-two (89%) of randomized subjects (173 on active drug, 59 on placebo) contributed data to the analysis of percent change from baseline in bone mineral density (BMD) of the AP lumbar spine, the primary efficacy variable. Patients were given supplemental dietary calcium (1000 mg elemental calcium/day) but no supplemental vitamin D. There was an increase in BMD of the AP lumbar spine in all Vivelle dose groups; in contrast to this, a decrease in AP lumbar spine BMD was observed in placebo patients. All Vivelle doses were significantly superior to placebo ($p<0.05$) at all time points with the exception of Vivelle 0.05 mg/day at 6 months. The highest dose of Vivelle was superior to the three lower doses. There were no statistically significant differences in pairwise comparisons among the three lower doses.

(See Figure 3.)

Figure 3
Bone Mineral Density - AP Lumbar Spine
Least Squares Means of Percentage Change from Baseline All Randomized Patients with at Least One Post-Baseline Assessment Available with Last Post-Baseline Observation Carried Forward

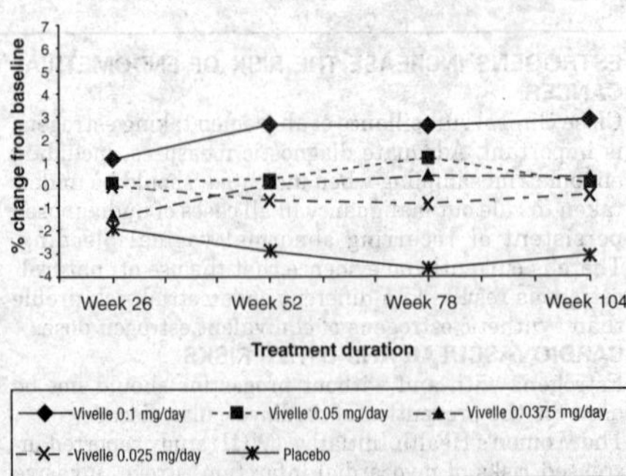

Analysis of percent change from baseline in femoral neck BMD, a secondary efficacy outcome variable, showed qualitatively similar results; all doses of Vivelle were significantly superior to placebo ($p<0.05$) at 24 months. The highest Vivelle dose was superior to placebo at all time points. A mixture of significant and non-significant results were obtained for the lower dose groups at earlier time points. The highest Vivelle dose was superior to the three lower doses, and there were no significant differences among the three lower doses at this skeletal site. *(See Figure 4.)*

Figure 4
Bone Mineral Density - Femoral Neck
Least Squares Means of Percentage Change from Baseline All Randomized Patients with at Least One Post-Baseline Assessment Available with Last Post-Baseline Observation Carried Forward

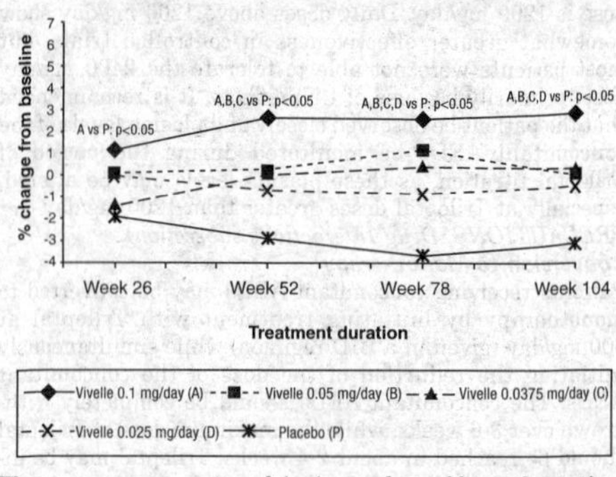

The mean serum osteocalcin (a marker of bone formation) and urinary excretion of cross-link N-telopeptides of type 1 collagen (a marker of bone resorption) decreased numerically in most of the active treatment groups relative to baseline. However, the decreases in both markers were inconsistent across treatment groups and the differences between active treatment groups and placebo were not statistically significant.

Women's Health Initiative Studies

The Women's Health Initiative (WHI) enrolled a total of 27,000 predominantly healthy postmenopausal women to assess the risks and benefits of the use of 0.625 mg conjugated equine estrogens (CE) per day alone and of 0.625 mg conjugated equine estrogens plus 2.5 mg medroxyprogesterone acetate (MPA) per day compared to placebo in the prevention of certain chronic diseases. The primary endpoint was the incidence of coronary heart disease (CHD) (nonfatal myocardial infarction and CHD death), with invasive breast cancer as the primary adverse outcome studied. A "global index" included the earliest occurrence of CHD, invasive breast cancer, stroke, pulmonary embolism (PE), endometrial cancer, colorectal cancer, hip fracture, or death due to other cause. The study did not evaluate the effects of CE or CE/MPA on menopausal symptoms.

The CE-only substudy is continuing and results have not been reported. The CE/MPA substudy was stopped early because, according to the predefined stopping rule, the increased risk of breast cancer and cardiovascular events exceeded the specified benefits included in the "global index." Results of the CE/MPA substudy, which included 16,608 women (average age of 63 years, range 50 to 79, 83.9% White, 6.5% Black, 5.5% Hispanic), after an average follow-up of 5.2 years are presented in Table 2 below.

[See table 2 at bottom of next page]

For those outcomes included in the "global index," absolute excess risks per 10,000 person-years in the group treated with CE/MPA were 7 more CHD events, 8 more strokes, 8 more PEs, and 8 more invasive breast cancers, while absolute risk reductions per 10,000 person-years were 6 fewer colorectal cancers and 5 fewer hip fractures. The absolute excess risk of events included in the "global index" was 19 per 10,000 person-years. There was no difference between the groups in terms of all-cause mortality. *(See BOXED WARNINGS, WARNINGS, and PRECAUTIONS.)*

INDICATIONS AND USAGE

Vivelle is indicated in the following:

1. Treatment of moderate-to-severe vasomotor symptoms associated with the menopause.
2. Treatment of moderate-to-severe symptoms of vulvar and vaginal atrophy associated with the menopause. When prescribing solely for the treatment of symptoms of vulvar and vaginal atrophy, topical vaginal products should be considered.
3. Treatment of hypoestrogenism due to hypogonadism, castration, or primary ovarian failure.
4. Prevention of postmenopausal osteoporosis. When prescribing solely for the prevention of postmenopausal osteoporosis, therapy should only be considered for women at significant risks of osteoporosis and non-estrogen medications should be carefully considered.

   The mainstays for decreasing the risk of postmenopausal osteoporosis are weight-bearing exercise, adequate calcium and vitamin D intake, and when indicated, pharmacologic therapy. Postmenopausal women require an average of 1500 mg/day of elemental calcium. Therefore, when not contraindicated, calcium supplementation may be helpful for women with suboptimal dietary intake. Vitamin D supplementation of 400-800 IU/day may also be required to ensure adequate daily intake in postmenopausal women.

CONTRAINDICATIONS

Estrogens should not be used in individuals with any of the following conditions:

1. Undiagnosed abnormal genital bleeding.
2. Known, suspected or history of cancer of the breast except in appropriately selected patients being treated for metastatic disease.
3. Known or suspected estrogen-dependent neoplasia.
4. Active deep vein thrombosis, pulmonary embolism or a history of these conditions.

5. Active or recent (e.g., within the past year) arterial thromboembolic disease (e.g., stroke, myocardial infarction).
6. Vivelle (estradiol transdermal system) should not be used in patients with known hypersensitivity to its ingredients.
7. Known or suspected pregnancy. There is no indication for Vivelle in pregnancy. There appears to be little or no increased risk of birth defects in women who have used estrogens and progestins from oral contraceptives inadvertently during early pregnancy *(see PRECAUTIONS)*.

WARNINGS

See BOXED WARNINGS.

The use of unopposed estrogens in women who have a uterus is associated with an increased risk of endometrial cancer.

1. **Cardiovascular Disorders**

Estrogen and estrogen/progestin therapy have been associated with an increased risk of cardiovascular events such as myocardial infarction and stroke, as well as venous thrombosis and pulmonary embolism (venous thromboembolism or VTE). Should any of these occur or be suspected, estrogens should be discontinued immediately.

Risk factors for cardiovascular disease (e.g., hypertension, diabetes mellitus, tobacco use, hypercholesterolemia, and obesity) should be managed appropriately.

a. ***Coronary Heart Disease and Stroke.*** In the Women's Health Initiative (WHI) study, an increase in the number of myocardial infarctions and strokes has been observed in women receiving CE alone compared to placebo. These observations are preliminary, and the study is continuing. *(See CLINICAL PHARMACOLOGY, Clinical Studies.)*

In the CE/MPA substudy of WHI an increased risk of coronary heart disease (CHD) events (defined as nonfatal myocardial infarction and CHD death) was observed in women receiving CE/MPA compared to women receiving placebo (37 vs. 30 per 10,000 person-years). The increase in risk was observed in Year 1 and persisted.

In the same substudy of WHI, an increased risk of stroke was observed in women receiving CE/MPA compared to women receiving placebo (29 vs. 21 per 10,000 person-years). The increase in risk was observed after the first year and persisted.

In postmenopausal women with documented heart disease (n = 2,763, average age 66.7 years) a controlled clinical trial of secondary prevention of cardiovascular disease (Heart and Estrogen/Progestin Replacement Study [HERS]) treatment with CE/MPA-0.625 mg/2.5 mg per day demonstrated no cardiovascular benefit. During an average follow-up of 4.1 years, treatment with CE/MPA did not reduce the overall rate of CHD events in postmenopausal women with established coronary heart disease. There were more CHD events in the CE/MPA-treated group than in the placebo group in Year 1, but not during the subsequent years. Two thousand three hundred and twenty-one women from the original HERS trial agreed to participate in an open-label extension of HERS, HERS II. Average follow-up in HERS II was an additional 2.7 years, for a total of 6.8 years overall. Rates of CHD events were comparable among women in the CE/MPA group and the placebo group in HERS, HERS II, and overall.

Large doses of estrogen (5 mg conjugated estrogens per day), comparable to those used to treat cancer of the prostate and breast, have been shown in a large prospective clinical trial in men to increase the risks of nonfatal myocardial infarction, pulmonary embolism, and thrombophlebitis.

b. ***Venous Thromboembolism (VTE).*** In the Women's Health Initiative (WHI) study, an increase in VTE has been observed in women receiving CE compared to placebo. These observations are preliminary, and the study is continuing. *(See CLINICAL PHARMACOLOGY, Clinical Studies.)*

In the CE/MPA substudy of WHI, a 2-fold greater rate of VTE, including deep venous thrombosis and pulmonary embolism, was observed in women receiving CE/MPA compared to women receiving placebo. The rate of VTE was 34 per 10,000 woman-years in the CE/MPA group compared to 16 per 10,000 woman-years in the placebo group. The increase in VTE risk was observed during the first year and persisted.

If feasible, estrogens should be discontinued at least 4 to 6 weeks before surgery of the type associated with an increased risk of thromboembolism, or during periods of prolonged immobilization.

2. **Malignant Neoplasms**

a. ***Endometrial Cancer.*** The use of unopposed estrogens in women with intact uteri has been associated with an increased risk of endometrial cancer. The reported endometrial cancer risk among unopposed estrogen users is about 2- to 12-fold greater than in nonusers and appears dependent on duration of treatment and on estrogen dose. Most studies show no significant increased risk associated with the use of estrogens for less than 1 year. The greatest risk appears associated with prolonged use with increased risks of 15- to 24-fold for five to ten years or more, and this risk has been shown to persist for at least 8 to15 years after estrogen therapy is discontinued.

Clinical surveillance of all women taking estrogen/progestin combinations is important. Adequate diagnostic measures, including endometrial sampling when indicated, should be undertaken to rule out malignancy in all cases of undiagnosed persistent or recurring abnormal vaginal bleeding. There is no evidence that the use of natural estrogens results in a different endometrial risk profile than synthetic estrogens of equivalent estrogen dose. Adding a progestin to estrogen therapy has been shown to reduce the risk of endometrial hyperplasia, which may be a precursor to endometrial cancer.

b. ***Breast Cancer.*** Estrogen and estrogen/progestin therapy in postmenopausal women has been associated with an increased risk of breast cancer. In the CE/MPA substudy of the Women's Health Initiative (WHI) study, a 26% increase of invasive breast cancer (38 vs. 30 per 10,000 woman-years) after an average of 5.2 years of treatment was observed in women receiving CE/MPA compared to women receiving placebo. The increased risk of breast cancer became apparent after 4 years on CE/MPA. The women reporting prior postmenopausal use of estrogen and/or estrogen with progestin had a higher relative risk for breast cancer associated with CE/MPA than those who had never used these hormones. *(See CLINICAL PHARMACOLOGY, Clinical Studies.)*

In the WHI, no increased risk of breast cancer in CE-treated women compared to placebo was reported after an average of 5.2 years of therapy. These data are preliminary and that substudy of WHI is continuing.

Epidemiologic studies have reported an increased risk of breast cancer in association with increasing duration of postmenopausal treatment with estrogens with or without a progestin. This association was reanalyzed in original data from 51 studies that involved various doses and types of estrogens, with and without progestins. In the re-analysis, an increased risk of having breast cancer diagnosed became apparent after about 5 years of continued treatment, and subsided after treatment had been discontinued for 5 years or longer. Some later studies have suggested that postmenopausal treatment with estrogens and progestin increase the risk of breast cancer more than treatment with estrogen alone.

A postmenopausal woman without a uterus who requires estrogen should receive estrogen-alone therapy, and should not be exposed unnecessarily to progestins.

All postmenopausal women should receive yearly breast exams by a health care provider and perform monthly breast self-examinations. In addition, mammography examinations should be scheduled as suggested by providers based on patient age and risk factors.

3. **Gallbladder Disease**

A 2- to 4-fold increase in the risk of gallbladder disease requiring surgery in postmenopausal women receiving estrogens has been reported.

4. **Hypercalcemia**

Administration of estrogen may lead to severe hypercalcemia in patients with breast cancer and bone metastases. If this occurs, the drug should be stopped and appropriate measures taken to reduce the serum calcium level.

5. **Visual Abnormalities**

Retinal vascular thrombosis has been reported in patients receiving estrogens. Discontinue medication pending examination if there is sudden partial or complete loss of vision, or a sudden onset of proptosis, diplopia, or migraine. If examination reveals papilledema or retinal vascular lesions, estrogens should be discontinued.

PRECAUTIONS

General

1. ***Addition of a Progestin When a Woman Has Not Had a Hysterectomy.*** Studies of the addition of a progestin for 10 or more days of a cycle of estrogen administration, or daily with estrogen in a continuous regimen, have reported a lowered incidence of endometrial hyperplasia than would be induced by estrogen treatment alone. Endometrial hyperplasia may be a precursor to endometrial cancer. There are, however, possible risks that may be associated with the use of progestins with estrogens compared to estrogen-alone regimens. These include:
   a. A possible increased risk of breast cancer.
   b. Adverse effects on lipoprotein metabolism (e.g., lowering HDL, raising LDL).
   c. Impairment of glucose tolerance.
2. ***Elevated Blood Pressure.*** In a small number of case reports, substantial increases in blood pressure have been attributed to idiosyncratic reactions to estrogens. In a large, randomized, placebo-controlled clinical trial, a generalized effect of estrogen therapy on blood pressure was not seen. Blood pressure should be monitored at regular intervals with estrogen use.
3. ***Familial Hyperlipoproteinemia.*** In patients with familial defects of lipoprotein metabolism, estrogen therapy may be associated with elevations of plasma triglycerides leading to pancreatitis and other complications.
4. ***Impaired Liver Function.*** Although transdermally administered estrogen therapy avoids first-pass hepatic metabolism, estrogens may be poorly metabolized in patients with impaired liver function. For patients with a history of jaundice associated with past estrogen use or with pregnancy, caution should be exercised and in the case of recurrence, medication should be discontinued.
5. ***Hypothyroidism.*** Estrogen administration leads to increased thyroid-binding globulin (TBG) levels. Patients with normal thyroid function can compensate for the increased TBG by making more thyroid hormone, thus maintaining free T_4 and T_3 serum concentrations in the normal range. Patients dependent on thyroid hormone replacement therapy who are also receiving estrogens may require increased doses of their thyroid replacement therapy. These patients should have their thyroid function monitored in order to maintain their free thyroid hormone levels in an acceptable range.
6. ***Fluid Retention.*** Because estrogens may cause some degree of fluid retention, conditions which might be influenced by this factor, such as asthma, epilepsy, migraine, and cardiac or renal dysfunction, warrant careful observation when estrogens are prescribed.
7. ***Hypocalcemia.*** Estrogens should be used with caution in individuals with severe hypocalcemia.
8. ***Ovarian Cancer.*** Use of estrogen-only products, in particular for 10 or more years, has been associated with an increased risk of ovarian cancer in some epidemiological studies. Other studies did not show a significant association. Data are insufficient to determine whether there is an increased risk with estrogen/progestin combination therapy in postmenopausal women.
9. ***Exacerbation of Endometriosis.*** Endometriosis may be exacerbated with administration of estrogen therapy.
10. ***Exacerbation of Other Conditions.*** Estrogens may cause an exacerbation of asthma, diabetes mellitus, epilepsy, migraine or porphyria and should be used with caution in women with these conditions.

Patient Information

Physicians are advised to discuss the Patient Information leaflet with patients for whom they prescribe Vivelle.

Laboratory Tests

Estrogen administration should be initiated at the lowest dose for the approved indication and then guided by clinical response, rather than by serum hormone levels (e.g., estradiol, FSH).

Table 2
Relative and Absolute Risk Seen in the CE/MPA Substudy of WHI[a]

Event[c]	Relative Risk CE/MPA vs. Placebo at 5.2 Years (95% CI*)	Placebo n=8102	CE/MPA n=8506
		Absolute Risk per 10,000 Person-Years	
CHD Events	1.29 (1.02-1.63)	30	37
Non-Fatal MI	1.32 (1.02-1.72)	23	30
CHD Death	1.18 (0.70-1.97)	6	7
Invasive Breast Cancer[b]	1.26 (1.00-1.59)	30	38
Stroke	1.41 (1.07-1.85)	21	29
Pulmonary Embolism	2.13 (1.39-3.25)	8	16
Colorectal Cancer	0.63 (0.43-0.92)	16	10
Endometrial Cancer	0.83 (0.47-1.47)	6	5
Hip Fracture	0.66 (0.45-0.98)	15	10
Death Due to Causes Other Than the Events Above	0.92 (0.74-1.14)	40	37
Global Index[c]	1.15 (1.03-1.28)	151	170
Deep Vein Thrombosis[d]	2.07 (1.49-2.87)	13	26
Vertebral Fractures[d]	0.66 (0.44-0.98)	15	9
Other Osteoporotic Fractures[d]	0.77 (0.69-0.86)	170	131

[a] Adapted from JAMA, 2002: 288: 321-333
[b] Includes metastatic and non-metastatic breast cancer with the exception of in situ breast cancer
[c] A subset of the events was combined in a "global index," defined as the earliest occurrence of CHD events, invasive breast cancer, stroke, pulmonary embolism, endometrial cancer, colorectal cancer, hip fracture, or death due to other causes
[d] Not included in global index
*Nominal confidence intervals unadjusted for multiple looks and multiple comparisons

Continued on next page

Vivelle—Cont.

Drug/Laboratory Test Interactions

1. Accelerated prothrombin time, partial thromboplastin time, and platelet aggregation time; increased platelet count; increased factors II, VII antigen, VIII antigen, VIII coagulant activity, IX, X, XII, VII-X complex, II-VII-X complex; and beta-thromboglobulin; decreased levels of anti-factor Xa and antithrombin III; decreased antithrombin III activity; increased levels of fibrinogen and fibrinogen activity; increased plasminogen antigen and activity.
2. Increased thyroid-binding globulin (TBG) leading to increased circulating total thyroid hormone, as measured by protein-bound iodine (PBI), T_4 levels (by column or by radioimmunoassay) or T_3 levels by radioimmunoassay. T_3 resin uptake is decreased, reflecting the elevated TBG. Free T_4 and free T_3 concentrations are unaltered. Patients on thyroid replacement therapy may require higher doses of thyroid hormone.
3. Other binding proteins may be elevated in serum, i.e., corticosteroid-binding globulin (CBG), sex hormone-binding globulin (SHBG), leading to increased circulating corticosteroids and sex steroids, respectively. Free or biologically active hormone concentrations are unchanged. Other plasma proteins may be increased (angiotensinogen/renin substrate, alpha-1-antitrypsin, ceruloplasmin).
4. Increased plasma HDL and HDL_2 subfraction concentrations, reduced LDL cholesterol concentration, increased triglycerides levels.
5. Impaired glucose tolerance.
6. Reduced response to metyrapone test.

Carcinogenesis, Mutagenesis, Impairment of Fertility

Long-term, continuous administration of natural and synthetic estrogens in certain animal species increases the frequency of carcinomas of the breast, uterus, cervix, vagina, testis, and liver. *(See BOXED WARNINGS, CONTRAINDICATIONS, and WARNINGS.)*

Pregnancy

Estrogens should not be used during pregnancy. *(See CONTRAINDICATIONS.)*

Nursing Mothers

Estrogen administration to nursing mothers has been shown to decrease the quantity and quality of the milk. Detectable amounts of estrogens have been identified in the milk of mothers receiving this drug. Caution should be exercised when Vivelle is administered to a nursing woman.

Pediatric Use

Estrogen therapy has been used for the induction of puberty in adolescents with some forms of pubertal delay. Safety and effectiveness in pediatric patients have not otherwise been established.

Large and repeated doses of estrogen over an extended time period have been shown to accelerate epiphyseal closure, which could result in short adult stature if treatment is initiated before the completion of physiologic puberty in normally developing children. If estrogen is administered to patients whose bone growth is not complete, periodic monitoring of bone maturation and effects on epiphyseal centers is recommended during estrogen administration.

Estrogen treatment of prepubertal girls also induces premature breast development and vaginal cornification, and may induce vaginal bleeding. *(See INDICATIONS and DOSAGE AND ADMINISTRATION.)*

Geriatric Use

The safety and effectiveness in geriatric patients have not been established.

ADVERSE REACTIONS

See BOXED WARNINGS, WARNINGS and PRECAUTIONS. Because clinical trials are conducted under widely varying conditions, adverse reaction rates observed in the clinical trials of a drug cannot be directly compared to rates in the clinical trials of another drug and may not reflect the rates observed in practice. The adverse reaction information from clinical trials does, however, provide a basis for identifying the adverse events that appear to be related to drug use and for approximating rates.

The following adverse events have been reported with Vivelle therapy:

[See table 3 below]

The following additional adverse reactions have been reported with estrogens:

1. **Genitourinary System.** Changes in vaginal bleeding pattern and abnormal withdrawal bleeding or flow; breakthrough bleeding; spotting; increase in size of uterine leiomyomata; vaginitis, including vaginal candidiasis; change in amount of cervical secretion; changes in cervical ectropion; ovarian cancer; endometrial hyperplasia; endometrial cancer.
2. **Breasts.** Tenderness, enlargement, pain, nipple discharge, galactorrhea; fibrocystic breast changes; breast cancer.
3. **Cardiovascular.** Deep and superficial venous thrombosis; pulmonary embolism; thrombophlebitis; myocardial infarction; stroke; increase in blood pressure.

Table 3

Summary of Most Frequently Reported Adverse Experiences/Medical Events Regardless of Relationship Reported at a Frequency ≥5%

	Vivelle 0.025 mg/day† (N=47) N (%)	Vivelle 0.0375 mg/day† (N=130) N (%)	Vivelle 0.05 mg/day† (N=103) N (%)	Vivelle 0.075 mg/day† (N=46) N (%)	Vivelle 0.1 mg/day† (N=132) N (%)	Placebo (N=157) N (%)
Gastrointestinal Disorders						
Constipation	2 (4.3)	5 (3.8)	4 (3.9)	3 (6.5)	2 (1.5)	4 (2.5)
Dyspepsia	4 (8.5)	12 (9.2)	3 (2.9)	2 (4.3)	0	10 (6.4)
Nausea	2 (4.3)	8 (6.2)	4 (3.9)	0	7 (5.3)	5 (3.2)
General Disorders and Administration Site Conditions*						
Influenza-like Illness	3 (6.4)	6 (4.6)	8 (7.8)	0	3 (2.3)	10 (6.4)
Pain NOS*	0	8 (6.2)	0	2 (4.3)	7 (5.3)	7 (4.5)
Infections and Infestations						
Influenza	4 (8.5)	4 (3.1)	6 (5.8)	0	10 (7.6)	14 (8.9)
Nasopharyngitis	3 (6.4)	16 (12.3)	10 (9.7)	9 (19.6)	11 (8.3)	24 (15.3)
Sinusitis NOS*	4 (8.5)	17 (13.1)	13 (12.6)	3 (6.5)	7 (5.3)	16 (10.2)
Upper Respiratory Tract Infection NOS*	3 (6.4)	8 (6.2)	11 (10.7)	4 (8.7)	6 (4.5)	9 (5.7)
Investigations						
Weight Increased	4 (8.5)	5 (3.8)	2 (1.9)	2 (4.3)	0	3 (1.9)
Musculoskeletal and Connective Tissue Disorders						
Arthralgia	0	11 (8.5)	4 (3.9)	2 (4.3)	5 (3.8)	9 (5.7)
Back Pain	4 (8.5)	10 (7.7)	9 (8.7)	4 (8.7)	14 (10.6)	10 (6.4)
Neck Pain	3 (6.4)	4 (3.1)	4 (3.9)	0	6 (4.5)	2 (1.3)
Pain in Limb	0	10 (7.7)	7 (6.8)	2 (4.3)	6 (4.5)	9 (5.7)
Nervous System Disorders						
Headache NOS*	7 (14.9)	35 (26.9)	32 (31.1)	23 (50.0)	34 (25.8)	37 (23.6)
Sinus Headache	0	12 (9.2)	5 (4.9)	5 (10.9)	2 (1.5)	8 (5.1)
Psychiatric Disorders						
Anxiety NEC**	3 (6.4)	5 (3.8)	0	0	2 (1.5)	4 (2.5)
Depression	5 (10.6)	4 (3.1)	7 (6.8)	0	4 (3.0)	6 (3.8)
Insomnia	3 (6.4)	6 (4.6)	4 (3.9)	2 (4.3)	2 (1.5)	9 (5.7)
Reproductive System and Breast Disorders						
Breast Tenderness	8 (17.0)	10 (7.7)	8 (7.8)	3 (6.5)	17 (12.9)	0
Dysmenorrhea	0	0	0	3 (6.5)	0	0
Intermenstrual Bleeding	3 (6.4)	9 (6.9)	6 (5.8)	0	14 (10.6)	7 (4.5)
Respiratory, Thoracic and Mediastinal Disorders						
Sinus Congestion	0	4 (3.1)	3 (2.9)	3 (6.5)	6 (4.5)	7 (4.5)
Vascular Disorders						
Hot Flushes NOS*	3 (6.4)	0	3 (2.9)	0	0	6 (3.8)
Hypertension NOS*	2 (4.3)	0	3 (2.9)	0	0	2 (1.3)

† Represents milligrams of estradiol delivered daily by each system

* NOS represents not otherwise specified

** NEC represents not elsewhere classified

*** Application site erythema and application site irritation were observed in a small number of patients (3.2% or less of patients across treatment groups)

4. **Gastrointestinal.** Nausea, vomiting; abdominal cramps, bloating; cholestatic jaundice; increased incidence of gall bladder disease; pancreatitis.
5. **Skin.** Chloasma or melasma, which may persist when drug is discontinued; erythema multiforme; erythema nodosum; hemorrhagic eruption; loss of scalp hair; hirsutism; pruritus, rash.
6. **Eyes.** Retinal vascular thrombosis; steepening of corneal curvature; intolerance to contact lenses.
7. **Central Nervous System.** Headache; migraine; dizziness; mental depression; chorea; nervousness; mood disturbances; irritability; exacerbation of epilepsy.
8. **Miscellaneous.** Increase or decrease in weight; reduced carbohydrate tolerance; aggravation of porphyria; edema; arthralgias; leg cramps; changes in libido; anaphylactoid/anaphylactic reactions including urticaria and angioedema; hypocalcemia; exacerbation of asthma; increased triglycerides.

Post-Marketing Adverse Events

Although a causal relationship with Vivelle has not been established, adverse events reported from marketing experience include: isolated reports of anaphylaxis, rare elevated liver function tests, and reports of leg pain.

OVERDOSAGE

Serious ill effects have not been reported following acute ingestion of large doses of estrogen-containing oral contraceptives by young children. Overdosage of estrogen may cause nausea and vomiting, and withdrawal bleeding may occur in females.

DOSAGE AND ADMINISTRATION

The adhesive side of the Vivelle system should be placed on a clean, dry area of the trunk of the body (including the abdomen or buttocks). *The Vivelle system should not be applied to the breasts.* The Vivelle system should be replaced twice weekly. The sites of application must be rotated, with an interval of at least 1 week allowed between applications to a particular site. The area selected should not be oily, damaged, or irritated. The waistline should be avoided, since tight clothing may rub the system off. The system should be applied immediately after opening the pouch and removing the protective liner. The system should be pressed firmly in place with the palm of the hand for about 10 seconds, making sure there is good contact, especially around the edges. In the event that a system should fall off, the same system may be reapplied. If necessary, a new system may be applied. In either case, the original treatment schedule should be continued. If a woman has forgotten to apply a patch, she should apply a new patch as soon as possible. The new patch should be applied on the original treatment schedule. The interruption of treatment in women taking Vivelle might increase the likelihood of breakthrough bleeding, spotting and recurrence of symptoms.

Initiation of Therapy

When estrogen is prescribed for a postmenopausal woman with a uterus, progestin should also be initiated to reduce the risk of endometrial cancer. A woman without a uterus does not need progestin. Use of estrogen alone or in combination with a progestin, should be limited to the shortest duration consistent with treatment goals and risks for the individual woman. Patients should be reevaluated periodically as clinically appropriate (e.g., 3-month to 6-month intervals) to determine whether treatment is still necessary *(see BOXED WARNINGS and WARNINGS)*. For women who have a uterus, adequate diagnostic measures, such as endometrial sampling, when indicated, should be undertaken to rule out malignancy in cases of undiagnosed persistent or recurring abnormal vaginal bleeding.

Patients should be started at the lowest dose. For treatment of moderate-to-severe vasomotor symptoms and vulvar and vaginal atrophy associated with the menopause, start therapy with Vivelle estradiol transdermal system 0.0375 mg/day applied to the skin twice weekly. For the prevention of postmenopausal osteoporosis, the minimum dose that has been shown to be effective is 0.025 mg/day. The dosage may be adjusted as necessary. Reproductive system-associated adverse events were encountered more frequently in the highest dose group (0.1 mg/day) than in other active treatment groups or in placebo-treated patients. In women not currently taking oral estrogens or in women switching from another estradiol transdermal therapy, treatment with the Vivelle estradiol transdermal system may be initiated at once. In women who are currently taking oral estrogens, treatment with the Vivelle estradiol transdermal system should be initiated 1 week after withdrawal of oral hormone therapy, or sooner if menopausal symptoms reappear in less than 1 week.

Therapeutic Regimen

Vivelle may be given continuously in patients who do not have an intact uterus. In those patients with an intact uterus, Vivelle may be given continuously or on a cyclic schedule (e.g., three weeks on drug followed by one week off drug) with a progestin.

HOW SUPPLIED

Vivelle estradiol transdermal system 0.025 mg/day—each 7.25 cm^2 system contains 2.17 mg of estradiol USP for nominal* delivery of 0.025 mg of estradiol per day.

Patient Calendar Pack of 8 systems .... NDC 0078-0348-42

Vivelle estradiol transdermal system 0.0375 mg/day—each 11.0 cm^2 system contains 3.28 mg of estradiol USP for nominal* delivery of 0.0375 mg of estradiol per day.

Patient Calendar Pack of 8 systems .... NDC 0083-2325-08

Vivelle estradiol transdermal system 0.05 mg/day—each 14.5 cm^2 system contains 4.33 mg of estradiol USP for nominal* delivery of 0.05 mg of estradiol per day.
Patient Calendar Pack of 8 systems .... NDC 0083-2326-08
Vivelle estradiol transdermal system 0.075 mg/day—each 22.0 cm^2 system contains 6.57 mg of estradiol USP for nominal* delivery of 0.075 mg of estradiol per day.
Patient Calendar Pack of 8 systems .... NDC 0083-2327-08
Vivelle estradiol transdermal system 0.1 mg/day—each 29.0 cm^2 system contains 8.66 mg of estradiol USP for nominal* delivery of 0.1 mg of estradiol per day.
Patient Calendar Pack of 8 systems .... NDC 0083-2328-08

***See DESCRIPTION**
Do not store above 30°C (86°F). Do not store unpouched. Apply immediately upon removal from the protective pouch.
REV: FEBRUARY 2004 T2004-15

PATIENT INFORMATION

Vivelle® T2004-16
estradiol transdermal system
Rx only

Read this PATIENT INFORMATION before you start taking Vivelle® (estradiol transdermal system) and read all the information that you get each time you refill Vivelle. There may be new information. This information does not take the place of talking to your health care provider about your medical condition or your treatment.
The Vivelle patch that your health care provider has prescribed for you releases small amounts of an estrogen hormone through the skin.
This leaflet describes the risks and benefits of treatment with Vivelle. Vivelle is not for everyone. Talk to your health care provider if you have any questions or concerns about this medication.

What is the most important information I should know about Vivelle?
- Estrogens increase the chances of getting cancer of the uterus.
  Report any unusual vaginal bleeding right away while you are taking estrogens. Vaginal bleeding after menopause may be a warning sign of cancer of the uterus (womb). Your health care provider should check any unusual vaginal bleeding to find out the cause.
- Do not use estrogens with or without progestins to prevent heart disease, heart attacks, or strokes.
  Using estrogens with or without progestins may increase your chances of getting heart attacks, strokes, breast cancer, and blood clots. You and your health care provider should talk regularly about whether you still need treatment with Vivelle.

WHAT IS VIVELLE ?
Vivelle is a patch that contains the estrogen hormone, estradiol. When applied to the skin as directed below, Vivelle releases estrogen through the skin into the bloodstream.
WHAT IS VIVELLE USED FOR?
Vivelle is used after menopause to:
- **Reduce moderate-to-severe hot flashes.**
  Estrogens are hormones made by a woman's ovaries. The ovaries normally stop making estrogens when a woman is between 45 and 55 years old. This drop in body estrogen levels causes the "Change in life" or menopause (the end of monthly menstrual periods). Sometimes, both ovaries are removed during an operation before natural menopause takes place. The sudden drop in estrogen levels causes "surgical menopause."
  When the estrogen levels begin dropping, some women develop very uncomfortable symptoms, such as feelings of warmth in the face, neck, and chest or sudden strong feelings of heat and sweating ("hot flashes" or "hot flushes"). In some women the symptoms are mild, and they will not need estrogens. In other women, symptoms can be more severe. You and your health care provider should talk regularly about whether you still need treatment with Vivelle.
- **Treat moderate-to-severe dryness, itching and burning in or around the vagina.**
  You and your health care provider should talk regularly about whether you still need treatment with Vivelle to control these problems.
- **Treat certain conditions in which a young woman's ovaries do not produce enough estrogens naturally.**
- **Help reduce your chances of getting osteoporosis (thin, weak bones).**
  Osteoporosis from menopause is a thinning of the bones that makes them weaker and easier to break. If you use Vivelle only to prevent osteoporosis from menopause, talk with your health care provider about whether a different treatment or medicine without estrogens might be better for you. You and your health care provider should talk regularly about whether you should continue with Vivelle.
  Weight-bearing exercise, like walking or running, and taking calcium and vitamin D supplements may also lower your chances of getting postmenopausal osteoporosis. It is important to talk about exercise and supplements with your health care provider before starting them.

WHO SHOULD NOT TAKE VIVELLE?
Do not start taking Vivelle if you:
- **Have unusual vaginal bleeding.**
- **Currently have or have had certain cancers.**
  Estrogens may increase the chances of getting certain types of cancers, including cancer of the breast or uterus. If you have or had cancer, talk with your health care provider about whether you should take Vivelle
- **Had a stroke or heart attack in the recent past (for example, in the past year).**
- **Currently have or have had blood clots.**
- **Are allergic to Vivelle or any of its ingredients.**
  See the end of this leaflet for a list of ingredients in Vivelle.
- **Think you may be, or know that you are, pregnant.**

TELL YOUR HEALTH CARE PROVIDER:
- **If you are breastfeeding.**
  The hormone in Vivelle can pass into your milk.
- **About all of your medical problems.**
  Your health care provider may need to check you more carefully if you have certain conditions such as asthma (wheezing), epilepsy (seizures), migraine, endometriosis, or problems with your heart, liver, thyroid, kidneys, or have high calcium levels in your blood.
- **About all the medicines you take,** including prescription and nonprescription medicines, vitamins, and herbal supplements.
  Some medicines may affect how Vivelle works. Vivelle may also affect how other medicines work.
- **If you are going to have surgery or will be on bed rest.**
  You may need to stop taking estrogens.

HOW SHOULD I TAKE VIVELLE?
Estrogens should be used only as long as needed and at the lowest possible dose that works. You and your health care provider should talk regularly (for example every 3 to 6 months) about whether you still need treatment with Vivelle.
How and Where to Apply Vivelle
Each system is individually sealed in a protective pouch. Tear open this pouch at the indentation (do not use scissors) and remove the system.

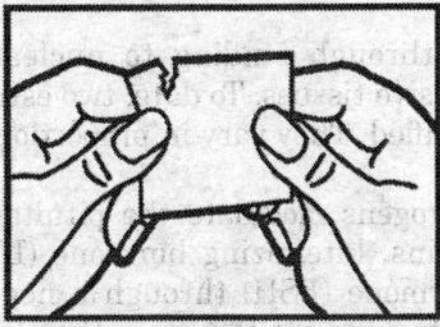

A stiff protective liner covers the adhesive side of the system—the side that will be placed against your skin. This liner must be removed before applying the system. Hold the unit with the protective liner facing you.

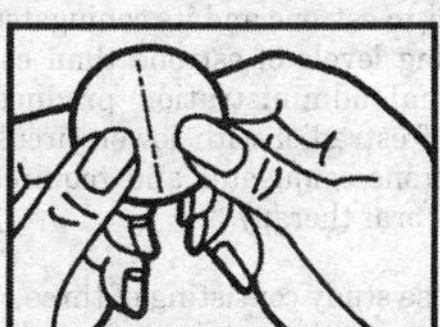

Peel off one side of the protective liner and discard it. Try to avoid touching the sticky side of the system with your fingers.

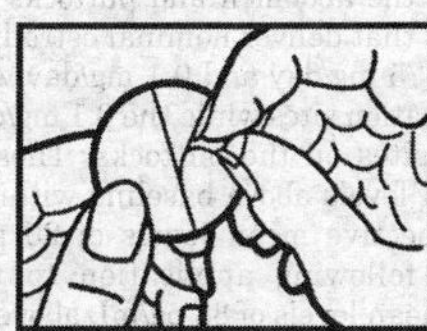

Using the other half of the liner as a handle, apply the sticky side of the system to a dry area of the skin on the trunk of the body (including the abdomen or buttocks). Press the sticky side on the skin and smooth down.

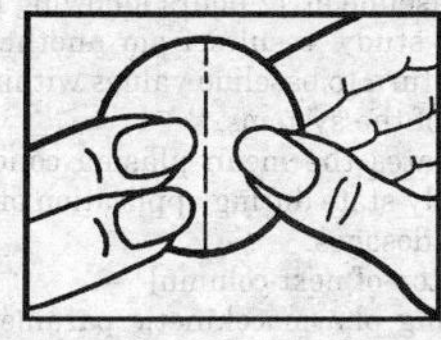

Fold back the remaining side of the system. Grasp the straight edge of the protective liner and pull it off the system.

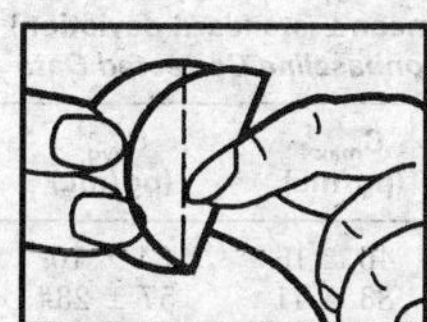

Press the system firmly in place.

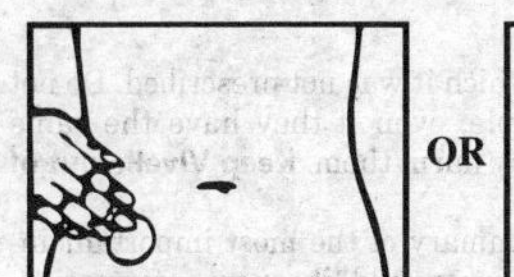

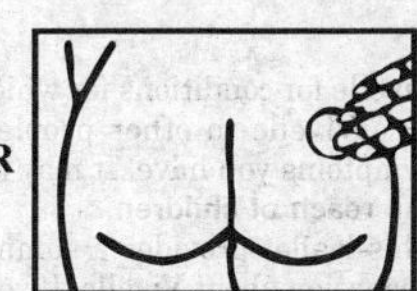

Some women may find that it is more comfortable to wear Vivelle on the buttocks. *Do not apply Vivelle to your breasts.* The sites of application must be rotated, with an interval of at least 1 week allowed between applications to a particular site. The area selected should not be oily, damaged, or irritated. Avoid the waistline, since tight clothing may rub the system off. Apply the system immediately after opening the pouch and removing the protective liner. Press the system firmly in place with the palm of your hand for about 10 seconds, making sure there is good contact, especially around the edges.
The Vivelle system should be worn continuously until it is time to replace it with a new system. You may wish to experiment with different locations when applying a new system, to find ones that are most comfortable for you and where clothing will not rub on the system.
When to Apply Vivelle
The Vivelle system should be replaced twice weekly. Your Vivelle package contains a calendar checklist to help you remember a schedule. Mark the 2-day schedule you plan to follow. Always change the system on the 2 days of the week you have marked.
When changing the system, remove the used Vivelle system and discard it. Any adhesive that might remain on your skin can be easily rubbed off. Then place the new Vivelle system on a different skin site. (The same skin site should not be used again for at least 1 week after removal of the system.)
Please note: Contact with water when you are bathing, swimming, or showering will not affect the system. In the event that a system should fall off, put this same system back on and continue to follow your original treatment schedule. If necessary, you may apply a new system but continue to follow your original schedule.

WHAT ARE THE POSSIBLE SIDE EFFECTS OF ESTROGENS?
Less Common but Serious Side Effects Include:
— Breast Cancer
— Cancer of the Uterus
— Stroke
— Heart Attack
— Blood Clots
— Gallbladder Disease
— Ovarian Cancer
These are Some of the Warning Signs of Serious Side Effects:
— Breast Lumps
— Unusual Vaginal Bleeding
— Dizziness and Faintness
— Changes in Speech
— Severe Headaches
— Chest Pain
— Shortness of Breath
— Pains in Your Legs
— Changes in Vision
— Vomiting
Call your health care provider right away if you get any of these warning signs, or any other unusual symptom that concerns you.
Common Side Effects Include:
— Headache
— Breast Pain
— Irregular Vaginal Bleeding or Spotting
— Stomach/Abdominal Cramps, Bloating
— Nausea and Vomiting
— Hair Loss
Other Side Effects Include:
— High Blood Pressure
— Liver Problems
— High Blood Sugar
— Fluid Retention
— Enlargement of Benign Tumors of the Uterus ("Fibroids")
— Vaginal Yeast Infection
Other side effects of Vivelle may be possible. If you have questions, talk to your health care provider or pharmacist.

WHAT CAN I DO TO LOWER MY CHANCES OF A SERIOUS SIDE EFFECT WITH VIVELLE?
- Talk with your health care provider regularly about whether you should continue taking Vivelle.
- See your health care provider right away if you get vaginal bleeding while taking Vivelle.
- Have a breast exam and mammogram (breast X-ray) every year unless your health care provider tells you something else. If members of your family have had breast cancer or if you have ever had breast lumps or an abnormal mammogram, you may need to have breast exams more often.
- If you have high blood pressure, high cholesterol (fat in the blood), diabetes, are overweight, or if you use tobacco, you may have higher chances for getting heart disease. Ask your health care provider for ways to lower your chances for getting heart disease.

GENERAL INFORMATION ABOUT SAFE AND EFFECTIVE USE OF VIVELLE
Medicines are sometimes prescribed for conditions that are not mentioned in patient information leaflets. Do not take

Continued on next page

Vivelle—Cont.

Vivelle for conditions for which it was not prescribed. Do not give Vivelle to other people, even if they have the same symptoms you have. It may harm them. **Keep Vivelle out of the reach of children.**

This leaflet provides a summary of the most important information about Vivelle. If you would like more information, talk with your health care provider or pharmacist. You can ask for information about Vivelle that is written for health professionals. You can get more information by calling the toll-free number 888-NOW-NOVA (888-669-6682).

WHAT ARE THE INGREDIENTS IN VIVELLE?

The Vivelle system comprises three layers. Proceeding from the visible surface toward the surface attached to the skin, these layers are (1) a translucent flexible film consisting of an ethylene vinyl alcohol copolymer film, a polyurethane film, urethane polymer and epoxy resin, (2) an adhesive formulation containing estradiol USP, acrylic adhesive, polyisobutylene, ethylene vinyl acetate copolymer, 1,3 butylene glycol, styrene-butadiene rubber, oleic acid NF, lecithin, propylene glycol, bentonite NF, mineral oil USP, and dipropylene glycol, and (3) a polyester release liner that is attached to the adhesive surface and must be removed before the system can be used.

The active component of the system is estradiol. The remaining components of the system are pharmacologically inactive.

T2004-16
T2004-15/T2004-16
REV: FEBRUARY 2004 Printed in U.S.A 89008105
101985-2

Distributed by:
Novartis Pharmaceuticals Corporation, East Hanover, New Jersey 07936
©Novartis

Shown in Product Identification Guide, page 326

VIVELLE-DOT® ℞

[*vī-vĕl*]
estradiol transdermal system
Continuous delivery for twice-weekly application
Rx only

Prescribing Information

The following prescribing information is based on official labeling in effect July 2004

ESTROGENS INCREASE THE RISK OF ENDOMETRIAL CANCER.

Close clinical surveillance of all women taking estrogens is important. Adequate diagnostic measures, including endometrial sampling when indicated, should be undertaken to rule out malignancy in all cases of undiagnosed persistent or recurring abnormal vaginal bleeding. There is currently no evidence that the use of "natural" estrogens results in a different endometrial risk profile than synthetic estrogens of equivalent estrogen dose.

CARDIOVASCULAR AND OTHER RISKS

Estrogens with and without progestins should not be used for the prevention of cardiovascular disease.

The Women's Health Initiative (WHI) study reported increased risks of myocardial infarction, stroke, invasive breast cancer, pulmonary emboli, and deep vein thrombosis in postmenopausal women during 5 years of treatment with conjugated equine estrogens (CE 0.625 mg) combined with medroxyprogesterone acetate (MPA 2.5 mg) relative to placebo *(see CLINICAL PHARMACOLOGY, Clinical Studies)*. Other doses of conjugated estrogens with medroxyprogesterone, and other combinations of estrogens and progestins were not studied in the WHI and, in the absence of comparable data, these risks should be assumed to be similar for all estrogens and estrogen-progestin combinations. Because of these risks, estrogens with or without progestins should be prescribed at the lowest effective doses and for the shortest duration consistent with treatment goals and risks for the individual woman.

DESCRIPTION

Vivelle-Dot® (estradiol transdermal system) contains estradiol in a multipolymeric adhesive. The system is designed to release estradiol continuously upon application to intact skin.

Five dosage strengths of Vivelle-Dot are available to provide nominal *in vivo* delivery rates of 0.025, 0.0375, 0.05, 0.075, or 0.1 mg of estradiol per day via the skin. Each corresponding system has an active surface area of 2.5, 3.75, 5.0, 7.5, or 10.0 cm^2 and contains 0.39, 0.585, 0.78, 1.17, or 1.56 mg of estradiol USP, respectively. The composition of the systems per unit area is identical.

Estradiol USP is a white, crystalline powder, chemically described as estra-1,3,5 (10)-triene-3,17β-diol.

The structural formula is
[See chemical structure at top of next column]

The molecular formula of estradiol is $C_{18}H_{24}O_2$. The molecular weight is 272.39.

Vivelle-Dot is comprised of three layers. Proceeding from the visible surface toward the surface attached to the skin, these layers are (1) a translucent polyolefin film (2) an adhesive formulation containing estradiol, acrylic adhesive, silicone adhesive, oleyl alcohol, NF, povidone, USP and dipropylene glycol, and (3) a polyester release liner which is attached to the adhesive surface and must be removed before the system can be used.

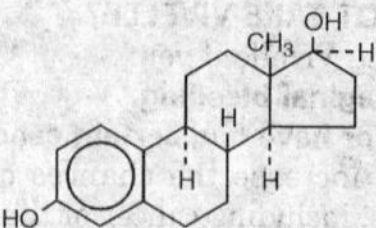

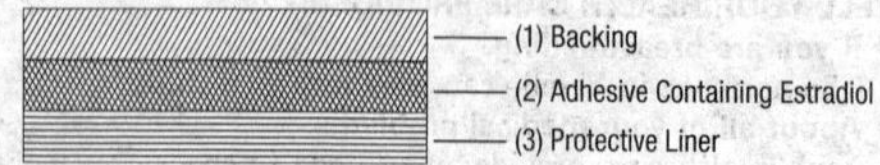

The active component of the system is estradiol. The remaining components of the system are pharmacologically inactive.

CLINICAL PHARMACOLOGY

Endogenous estrogens are largely responsible for the development and maintenance of the female reproductive system and secondary sexual characteristics. Although circulating estrogens exist in a dynamic equilibrium of metabolic interconversions, estradiol is the principal intracellular human estrogen and is substantially more potent than its metabolites, estrone and estriol, at the receptor level.

The primary source of estrogen in normally cycling adult women is the ovarian follicle, which secretes 70 to 500 µg of estradiol daily, depending on the phase of the menstrual cycle. After menopause, most endogenous estrogen is produced by conversion of androstenedione, secreted by the adrenal cortex, to estrone by peripheral tissues. Thus, estrone and the sulfate conjugated form, estrone sulfate, are the most abundant circulating estrogens in postmenopausal women.

Estrogens act through binding to nuclear receptors in estrogen-responsive tissues. To date, two estrogen receptors have been identified. They vary in proportion from tissue to tissue.

Circulating estrogens modulate the pituitary secretion of the gonadotropins, luteinizing hormone (LH) and follicle stimulating hormone (FSH) through a negative feedback mechanism. Estrogens act to reduce the elevated levels of these hormones seen in postmenopausal women.

Pharmacokinetics

The skin metabolizes estradiol only to a small extent. In contrast, orally administered estradiol is rapidly metabolized by the liver to estrone and its conjugates, giving rise to higher circulating levels of estrone than estradiol. Therefore, transdermal administration produces therapeutic plasma levels of estradiol with lower circulating levels of estrone and estrone conjugates and requires smaller total doses than does oral therapy.

Absorption

In a multiple-dose study consisting of three consecutive system applications of the original formulation [Vivelle® (estradiol transdermal system)] which was conducted in 17 healthy, postmenopausal women, blood levels of estradiol and estrone were compared following application of these units to sites on the abdomen and buttocks in a crossover fashion. Systems that deliver nominal estradiol doses of approximately 0.0375 mg/day and 0.1 mg/day were applied to abdominal application sites while the 0.1 mg/day doses were also applied to sites on the buttocks. These systems increased estradiol levels above baseline within 4 hours and maintained respective mean levels of 25 and 79 pg/mL above baseline following application to the abdomen; slightly higher mean levels of 88 pg/mL above baseline were observed following application to the buttocks. At the same time, increases in estrone plasma concentrations averaged about 12 and 50 pg/mL, respectively, following application to the abdomen and 61 pg/mL for the buttocks. While plasma concentrations of estradiol and estrone remained slightly above baseline at 12 hours following removal of the systems in this study, results from another study show these levels to return to baseline values within 24 hours following removal of the systems.

Figure 1 illustrates the mean plasma concentrations of estradiol at steady-state during application of these patches at four different dosages.
[See figure 1 at top of next column]

The corresponding pharmacokinetic parameters are summarized in the table below.

Table 1
Steady-State Estradiol Pharmacokinetic Parameters for Systems Applied to the Abdomen (mean ± standard deviation)
Nonbaseline-Corrected Data*

Dosage (mg/day)	C_{max}[†] (pg/mL)	C_{avg}[‡] (pg/mL)	C_{min} (84 hr)[§] (pg/mL)
0.0375	46 ± 16	34 ± 10	30 ± 10
0.05	83 ± 41	57 ± 23#	41 ± 11#
0.075	99 ± 35	72 ± 24	60 ± 24
0.1	133 ± 51	89 ± 38	90 ± 44
0.1¶	145 ± 71	104 ± 52	85 ± 47

*Mean baseline estradiol concentration = 11.7 pg/mL
†Peak plasma concentration
‡Average plasma concentration
§Minimum plasma concentration at 84 hr
#Measured over 80 hr
¶Applied to the buttocks

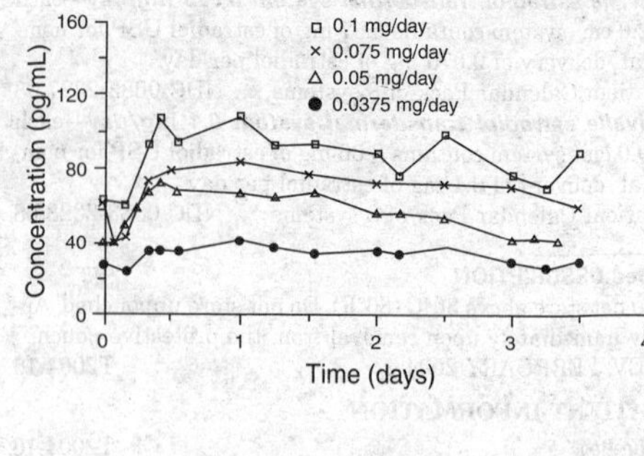

Vivelle-Dot® (estradiol transdermal system), the revised formulation with smaller system sizes, was shown to be bioequivalent to the original formulation, Vivelle® (estradiol transdermal system), used in the clinical trials.

Distribution

No specific investigation of the tissue distribution of estradiol absorbed from Vivelle-Dot in humans has been conducted. The distribution of exogenous estrogens is similar to that of endogenous estrogens. Estrogens are widely distributed in the body and are generally found in higher concentrations in the sex hormone target organs. Estrogens circulate in the blood largely bound to sex hormone binding globulin (SHBG) and, to a lesser extent, albumin.

Metabolism

Exogenous estrogens are metabolized in the same manner as endogenous estrogens. Circulating estrogens exist in a dynamic equilibrium of metabolic interconversions. These transformations take place mainly in the liver. Estradiol is converted reversibly to estrone, and both can be converted to estriol, which is the major urinary metabolite. Estrogens also undergo enterohepatic recirculation via sulfate and glucuronide conjugation in the liver, biliary secretion of conjugates into the intestine, and hydrolysis in the gut followed by reabsorption. In postmenopausal women a significant portion of the circulating estrogens exist as sulfate conjugates, especially estrone sulfate, which serves as a circulating reservoir for the formation of more active estrogens.

Excretion

Estradiol, estrone and estriol are excreted in the urine along with glucuronide and sulfate conjugates. The half-life values calculated after dosing with the Vivelle-Dot ranged from 5.9 to 7.7 hours. After removal of the transdermal systems, serum concentrations of estradiol and estrone returned to baseline levels within 24 hours.

Special Populations

Vivelle-Dot was only investigated in postmenopausal women.

Drug Interactions

In vitro and *in vivo* studies have shown that estrogens are metabolized partially by cytochrome P450 3A4 (CYP3A4). Therefore, inducers or inhibitors of CYP3A4 may affect estrogen drug metabolism. Inducers of CYP3A4 such as St. John's Wort preparations (Hypericum perforatum), phenobarbital, carbamazepine and rifampin may reduce plasma concentrations of estrogens, possibly resulting in a decrease in therapeutic effects and/or changes in the uterine bleeding profile. Inhibitors of CYP3A4 such as erythromycin, clarithromycin, ketoconazole, itraconazole, ritonavir and grapefruit juice may increase plasma concentrations of estrogens and may result in side effects.

Adhesion

Based on combined data from three short-term clinical trials consisting of 471 observations, 85% of Vivelle-Dot adhered completely to the skin over the 3.5-day wear period. Three (3%) of the systems detached and were reapplied or replaced during the 3.5-day wear period. Approximately 80% of the transdermal systems evaluated in these studies were Vivelle-Dot 0.05 mg/day.

CLINICAL STUDIES

Effects on vasomotor symptoms

In a pharmacokinetic study, Vivelle-Dot was shown to be bioequivalent to Vivelle. In two controlled clinical trials with Vivelle, of 356 subjects, the 0.075 and 0.1 mg doses were superior to placebo in relieving vasomotor symptoms at Week 4, and maintained efficacy through Weeks 8 and 12 of treatment. In this original study, the 0.0375 and 0.05 mg doses, however, did not differ from placebo until approximately Week 6, therefore, an additional 12-week placebo-controlled study in 255 patients was performed with Vivelle to establish the efficacy of the lowest dose of 0.0375 mg. The baseline mean daily number of hot flushes in these 255 patients was 11.5. Results at Weeks 4, 8, and 12 of treatment are shown in the figure below. *(See Figure 2.)*

Figure 2
Mean (SD) change from baseline in mean daily number of flushes for Vivelle® 0.375 mg versus Placebo in a 12-week trial.

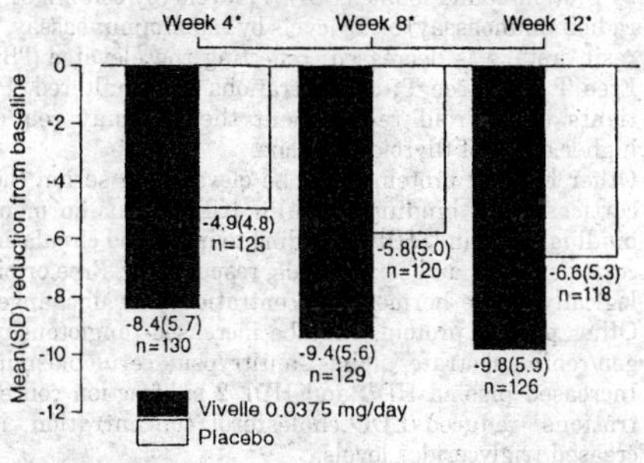

*Indicates statistically significant difference (p<0.05) between Vivelle and placebo

The 0.0375 mg dose was superior to placebo in reducing both the frequency and severity of vasomotor symptoms at Week 4 and maintained efficacy through Weeks 8 and 12 of treatment. All doses of Vivelle (0.0375 mg, 0.05 mg, 0.075 mg, and 0.1 mg) are effective for the control of vasomotor symptoms.

Effects on bone mineral density

Efficacy and safety of Vivelle in the prevention of postmenopausal osteoporosis have been studied in a 2-year double-blind, randomized, placebo-controlled, parallel group study. A total of 261 hysterectomized (161) and non-hysterectomized (100), surgically or naturally menopausal women (within 5 years of menopause), with no evidence of osteoporosis (lumbar spine bone mineral density within 2 standard deviations of average peak bone mass, i.e., $\geq$0.827 g/cm^2) were enrolled in this study; 194 patients were randomized to one of the four doses of Vivelle (0.1, 0.05, 0.0375, or 0.025 mg/day) and 67 patients to placebo. Over 2 years, study systems were applied to the buttock or the abdomen twice a week. Non-hysterectomized women received oral medroxyprogesterone acetate (2.5 mg/day) throughout the study.

The study population comprised naturally (82%) or surgically (18%) menopausal, hysterectomized (61%) or non-hysterectomized (39%) women with a mean age of 52.0 years (range 27 to 62 years); the mean duration of menopause was 31.7 months (range 2 to 72 months). Two hundred thirty-two (89%) of randomized subjects (173 on active drug, 59 on placebo) contributed data to the analysis of percent change from baseline in bone mineral density (BMD) of the AP lumbar spine, the primary efficacy variable. Patients were given supplemental dietary calcium (1000 mg elemental calcium/day) but no supplemental vitamin D. There was an increase in BMD of the AP lumbar spine in all Vivelle dose groups; in contrast to this, a decrease in AP lumbar spine BMD was observed in placebo patients. All Vivelle doses were significantly superior to placebo (p<0.05) at all time points with the exception of Vivelle 0.05 mg/day at 6 months. The highest dose of Vivelle was superior to the three lower doses. There were no statistically significant differences in pairwise comparisons among the three lower doses. *(See Figure 3.)*

Figure 3
Bone Mineral Density - AP Lumbar Spine
Least Squares Means of Percentage Change from Baseline
All Randomized Patients with at Least One Post-Baseline Assessment Available with Last Post-Baseline Observation Carried Forward

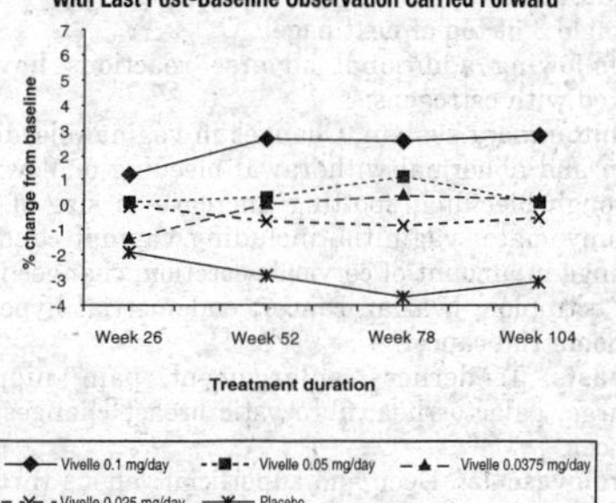

Analysis of percent change from baseline in femoral neck BMD, a secondary efficacy outcome variable, showed qualitatively similar results; all doses of Vivelle were significantly superior to placebo (p<0.05) at 24 months. The highest Vivelle dose was superior to placebo at all time points. A mixture of significant and non-significant results were obtained for the lower dose groups at earlier time points. The highest Vivelle dose was superior to the three lower doses, and there were no significant differences among the three lower doses at this skeletal site. *(See Figure 4.)*

[See figure 4 at top of next column]

The mean serum osteocalcin (a marker of bone formation) and urinary excretion of cross-link N-telopeptides of type 1 collagen (a marker of bone resorption) decreased numerically in most of the active treatment groups relative to baseline. However, the decreases in both markers were inconsistent across treatment groups and the differences between active treatment groups and placebo were not statistically significant.

Table 2
Relative and Absolute Risk Seen in the CE/MPA Substudy of WHI[a]

Event[c]	Relative Risk CE/MPA vs. Placebo at 5.2 Years (95% CI*)	Placebo n=8102	CE/MPA n=8506
		Absolute Risk per 10,000 Person-Years	
CHD events	1.29 (1.02–1.63)	30	37
Non-fatal MI	1.32 (1.02–1.72)	23	30
CHD death	1.18 (0.70–1.97)	6	7
Invasive breast cancer[b]	1.26 (1.00–1.59)	30	38
Stroke	1.41 (1.07–1.85)	21	29
Pulmonary embolism	2.13 (1.39–3.25)	8	16
Colorectal cancer	0.63 (0.43–0.92)	16	10
Endometrial cancer	0.83 (0.47–1.47)	6	5
Hip fracture	0.66 (0.45–0.98)	15	10
Death due to causes other than the events above	0.92 (0.74–1.14)	40	37
Global index[c]	1.15 (1.03–1.28)	151	170
Deep vein thrombosis[d]	2.07 (1.49–2.87)	13	26
Vertebral fractures[d]	0.66 (0.44–0.98)	15	9
Other osteoporotic fractures[d]	0.77 (0.69–0.86)	170	131

[a] Adapted from JAMA, 2002: 288: 321-333
[b] Includes metastatic and non-metastatic breast cancer with the exception of *in situ* breast cancer
[c] A subset of the events was combined in a "global index," defined as the earliest occurrence of CHD events, invasive breast cancer, stroke, pulmonary embolism, endometrial cancer, colorectal cancer, hip fracture, or death due to other causes
[d] Not included in global index
* Nominal confidence intervals unadjusted for multiple looks and multiple comparisons

Figure 4
Bone Mineral Density - Femoral Neck
Least Squares Means of Percentage Change from Baseline
All Randomized Patients with at Least One Post-Baseline Assessment Available with Last Post-Baseline Observation Carried Forward

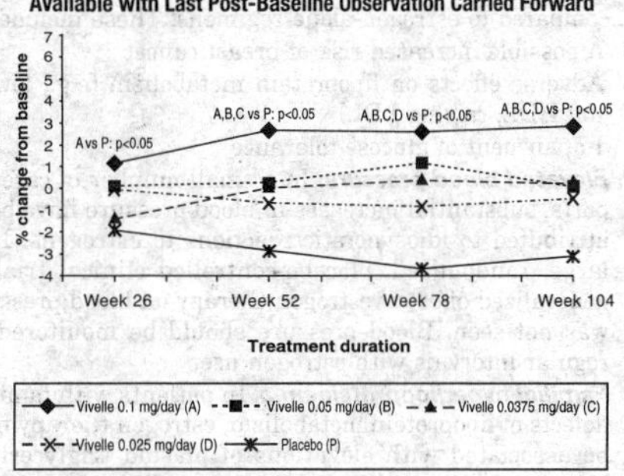

Women's Health Initiative Studies

The Women's Health Initiative (WHI) enrolled a total of 27,000 predominantly healthy postmenopausal women to assess the risks and benefits of the use of 0.625 mg conjugated equine estrogens (CE) per day alone and of 0.625 mg conjugated equine estrogens plus 2.5 mg medroxyprogesterone acetate (MPA) per day compared to placebo in the prevention of certain chronic diseases. The primary endpoint was the incidence of coronary heart disease (CHD) (nonfatal myocardial infarction and CHD death), with invasive breast cancer as the primary adverse outcome studied. A "global index" included the earliest occurrence of CHD, invasive breast cancer, stroke, pulmonary embolism (PE), endometrial cancer, colorectal cancer, hip fracture, or death due to other causes. The study did not evaluate the effects of CE or CE/MPA on menopausal symptoms.

The CE-only substudy is continuing and results have not been reported. The CE/MPA substudy was stopped early because, according to the predefined stopping rule, the increased risk of breast cancer and cardiovascular events exceeded the specified benefits included in the "global index." Results of the CE/MPA substudy, which included 16,608 women (average age of 63 years, range 50 to 79, 83.9% White, 6.5% Black, 5.5% Hispanic), after an average follow-up of 5.2 years are presented in Table 2 below.

[See table 2 above]

For those outcomes included in the "global index" absolute excess risks per 10,000 person-years in the group treated with CE/MPA were 7 more CHD events, 8 more strokes, 8 more PEs, and 8 more invasive breast cancers, while absolute risk reductions per 10,000 person-years were 6 fewer colorectal cancers and 5 fewer hip fractures. The absolute excess risk of events included in the "global index" was 19 per 10,000 person-years. There was no difference between the groups in terms of all-cause mortality. *(See BOXED WARNINGS, WARNINGS, and PRECAUTIONS.)*

INDICATIONS AND USAGE

Vivelle-Dot® (estradiol transdermal system) is indicated in:

1. Treatment of moderate-to-severe vasomotor symptoms associated with the menopause.
2. Treatment of moderate-to-severe symptoms of vulvar and vaginal atrophy associated with the menopause. When prescribing solely for the treatment of symptoms of vulvar and vaginal atrophy, topical vaginal products should be considered.
3. Treatment of hypoestrogenism due to hypogonadism, castration, or primary ovarian failure.
4. Prevention of postmenopausal osteoporosis. When prescribing solely for the prevention of postmenopausal osteoporosis, therapy should only be considered for women at significant risks of osteoporosis and non-estrogen medications should be carefully considered.

The mainstays for decreasing the risk of postmenopausal osteoporosis are weight-bearing exercise, adequate calcium and vitamin D intake, and when indicated, pharmacologic therapy. Postmenopausal women require an average of 1500 mg/day of elemental calcium. Therefore, when not contraindicated, calcium supplementation may be helpful for women with suboptimal dietary intake. Vitamin D supplementation of 400–800 IU/day may also be required to ensure adequate daily intake in postmenopausal women.

CONTRAINDICATIONS

Estrogens should not be used in individuals with any of the following conditions:

1. Undiagnosed abnormal genital bleeding.
2. Known, suspected or history of cancer of the breast except in appropriately selected patients being treated for metastatic disease.
3. Known or suspected estrogen-dependent neoplasia.
4. Active deep vein thrombosis, pulmonary embolism or a history of these conditions.
5. Active or recent (e.g., within the past year) arterial thromboembolic disease (e.g., stroke, myocardial infarction).
6. Vivelle-Dot® (estradiol transdermal system) should not be used in patients with known hypersensitivity to its ingredients.
7. Known or suspected pregnancy. There is no indication for Vivelle-Dot in pregnancy. There appears to be little or no increased risk of birth defects in women who have used estrogens and progestins from oral contraceptives inadvertently during early pregnancy *(see PRECAUTIONS)*.

WARNINGS

See *BOXED WARNINGS*.

The use of unopposed estrogens in women who have a uterus is associated with an increased risk of endometrial cancer.

1. Cardiovascular disorders

Estrogen and estrogen/progestin therapy have been associated with an increased risk of cardiovascular events such as myocardial infarction and stroke, as well as venous thrombosis and pulmonary embolism (venous thromboembolism or VTE). Should any of these occur or be suspected, estrogens should be discontinued immediately.

Risk factors for cardiovascular disease (e.g., hypertension, diabetes mellitus, tobacco use, hypercholesterolemia, and obesity) should be managed appropriately.

a. Coronary heart disease and stroke

In the Women's Health Initiative study (WHI), an increase in the number of myocardial infarctions and strokes has been observed in women receiving CE alone compared to placebo. These observations are preliminary, and the study is continuing. *(See CLINICAL PHARMACOLOGY, Clinical Studies)*.

In the CE/MPA substudy of WHI an increased risk of coronary heart disease (CHD) events (defined as nonfatal myocardial infarction and CHD death) was observed in women receiving CE/MPA compared to women receiving placebo (37 vs 30 per 10,000 person years). The increase in risk was observed in year one and persisted.

In the same substudy of WHI, an increased risk of stroke was observed in women receiving CE/MPA compared to women receiving placebo (29 vs 21 per 10,000 person-years). The increase in risk was observed after the first year and persisted.

In postmenopausal women with documented heart disease (n=2,763, average age 66.7 years) a controlled clinical trial of secondary prevention of cardiovascular disease (Heart and Estrogen/Progestin Replacement Study; HERS) treatment with CE/MPA-0.625 mg/

Continued on next page

Vivelle-Dot—Cont.

2.5 mg per day demonstrated no cardiovascular benefit. During an average follow-up of 4.1 years, treatment with CE/MPA did not reduce the overall rate of CHD events in postmenopausal women with established coronary heart disease. There were more CHD events in the CE/MPA-treated group than in placebo group in year 1, but not during the subsequent years. Two thousand three hundred and twenty one women from the original HERS trial agreed to participate in an open label extension of HERS, HERS II. Average follow-up in HERS II was an additional 2.7 years, for a total of 6.8 years overall. Rates of CHD events were comparable among women in the CE/MPA group and the placebo group in HERS, HERS II, and overall.

Large doses of estrogen (5 mg conjugated estrogens per day), comparable to those used to treat cancer of the prostate and breast, have been shown in a large prospective clinical trial in men to increase the risks of nonfatal myocardial infarction, pulmonary embolism, and thrombophlebitis.

b. Venous thromboembolism (VTE)

In the Women's Health Initiative study (WHI), an increase in VTE has been observed in women receiving CE compared to placebo. These observations are preliminary, and the study is continuing. *(See CLINICAL PHARMACOLOGY, Clinical Studies).*

In the CE/MPA substudy of WHI, a 2-fold greater rate of VTE, including deep venous thrombosis and pulmonary embolism, was observed in women receiving CE/MPA compared to women receiving placebo. The rate of VTE was 34 per 10,000 woman-years in the CE/MPA group compared to 16 per 10,000 woman-years in the placebo group. The increase in VTE risk was observed during the first year and persisted.

If feasible, estrogens should be discontinued at least 4 to 6 weeks before surgery of the type associated with an increased risk of thromboembolism, or during periods of prolonged immobilization.

2. Malignant Neoplasms

a. Endometrial cancer

The use of unopposed estrogens in women with intact uteri has been associated with an increased risk of endometrial cancer. The reported endometrial cancer risk among unopposed estrogen users is about 2- to 12-fold greater than in nonusers and appears dependent on duration of treatment and on estrogen dose. Most studies show no significant increased risk associated with the use of estrogens for less than 1 year. The greatest risk appears associated with prolonged use with increased risks of 15- to 24-fold for five to ten years or more, and this risk has been shown to persist for at least 8 to15 years after estrogen therapy is discontinued.

Clinical surveillance of all women taking estrogen/progestin combinations is important. Adequate diagnostic measures, including endometrial sampling when indicated, should be undertaken to rule out malignancy in all cases of undiagnosed persistent or recurring abnormal vaginal bleeding. There is no evidence that the use of natural estrogens results in a different endometrial risk profile than synthetic estrogens of equivalent estrogen dose. Adding a progestin to estrogen therapy has been shown to reduce the risk of endometrial hyperplasia, which may be a precursor to endometrial cancer.

b. Breast cancer

Estrogen and estrogen/progestin therapy in postmenopausal women has been associated with an increased risk of breast cancer. In the CE/MPA substudy of the Women's Health Initiative study (WHI), a 26% increase of invasive breast cancer (38 vs 30 per 10,000 woman-years) after an average of 5.2 years of treatment was observed in women receiving CE/MPA compared to women receiving placebo. The increased risk of breast cancer became apparent after 4 years on CE/MPA. The women reporting prior postmenopausal use of estrogen and/or estrogen with progestin had a higher relative risk for breast cancer associated with CE/MPA than those who had never used these hormones. *(See CLINICAL PHARMACOLOGY, Clinical Studies.)*

In the WHI, no increased risk of breast cancer in CE-treated women compared to placebo was reported after an average of 5.2 years of therapy. These data are preliminary and that substudy of WHI is continuing.

Epidemiologic studies have reported an increased risk of breast cancer in association with increasing duration of postmenopausal treatment with estrogens with or without a progestin. This association was reanalyzed in original data from 51 studies that involved various doses and types of estrogens, with and without progestins. In the reanalysis, an increased risk of having breast cancer diagnosed became apparent after about 5 years of continued treatment, and subsided after treatment had been discontinued for 5 years or longer. Some later studies have suggested that postmenopausal treatment with estrogens and progestin increase the risk of breast cancer more than treatment with estrogen alone.

A postmenopausal woman without a uterus who requires estrogen should receive estrogen-alone therapy, and should not be exposed unnecessarily to progestins. All postmenopausal women should receive yearly breast exams by a health care provider and perform monthly breast self-examinations. In addition, mammography examinations should be scheduled as suggested by providers based on patient age and risk factors.

3. Gallbladder Disease

A 2- to 4-fold increase in the risk of gallbladder disease requiring surgery in postmenopausal women receiving estrogens has been reported.

4. Hypercalcemia

Administration of estrogen may lead to severe hypercalcemia in patients with breast cancer and bone metastases. If this occurs, the drug should be stopped and appropriate measures taken to reduce the serum calcium level.

5. Visual abnormalities

Retinal vascular thrombosis has been reported in patients receiving estrogens. Discontinue medication pending examination if there is sudden partial or complete loss of vision, or a sudden onset of proptosis, diplopia, or migraine. If examination reveals papilledema or retinal vascular lesions, estrogens should be discontinued.

PRECAUTIONS

A. General

1. Addition of a progestin when a woman has not had a hysterectomy. Studies of the addition of a progestin for 10 or more days of a cycle of estrogen administration, or daily with estrogen in a continuous regimen, have reported a lowered incidence of endometrial hyperplasia than would be induced by estrogen treatment alone. Endometrial hyperplasia may be a precursor to endometrial cancer. There are, however, possible risks that may be associated with the use of progestins with estrogens compared to estrogen-alone regimens. These include:

a. A possible increased risk of breast cancer

b. Adverse effects on lipoprotein metabolism (e.g., lowering HDL, raising LDL)

c. Impairment of glucose tolerance

2. Elevated blood pressure. In a small number of case reports, substantial increases in blood pressure have been attributed to idiosyncratic reactions to estrogens. In a large, randomized, placebo-controlled clinical trial, a generalized effect of estrogen therapy on blood pressure was not seen. Blood pressure should be monitored at regular intervals with estrogen use.

3. Familial hyperlipoproteinemia. In patients with familial defects of lipoprotein metabolism, estrogen therapy may be associated with elevations of plasma triglycerides leading to pancreatitis and other complications.

4. Impaired liver function. Although transdermally administered estrogen therapy avoids first-pass hepatic metabolism, estrogens may be poorly metabolized in patients with impaired liver function. For patients with a history of jaundice associated with past estrogen use or with pregnancy, caution should be exercised and in the case of recurrence, medication should be discontinued.

5. Hypothyroidism. Estrogen administration leads to increased thyroid-binding globulin (TBG) levels. Patients with normal thyroid function can compensate for the increased TBG by making more thyroid hormone, thus maintaining free T_4 and T_3 serum concentrations in the normal range. Patients dependent on thyroid hormone replacement therapy who are also receiving estrogens may require increased doses of their thyroid replacement therapy. These patients should have their thyroid function monitored in order to maintain their free thyroid hormone levels in an acceptable range.

6. Fluid retention. Because estrogens may cause some degree of fluid retention, conditions which might be influenced by this factor, such as asthma, epilepsy, migraine, and cardiac or renal dysfunction, warrant careful observation when estrogens are prescribed.

7. Hypocalcemia. Estrogens should be used with caution in individuals with severe hypocalcemia.

8. Ovarian cancer. Use of estrogen-only products, in particular for ten or more years, has been associated with an increased risk of ovarian cancer in some epidemiological studies. Other studies did not show a significant association. Data are insufficient to determine whether there is an increased risk with estrogen/progestin combination therapy in postmenopausal women.

9. Exacerbation of endometriosis. Endometriosis may be exacerbated with administration of estrogen therapy.

10. Exacerbation of other conditions. Estrogens may cause an exacerbation of asthma, diabetes mellitus, epilepsy, migraine or porphyria and should be used with caution in women with these conditions.

B. Patient Information. Physicians are advised to discuss the **Patient Information** leaflet with patients for whom they prescribe Vivelle-Dot.

C. Laboratory Tests. Estrogen administration should be initiated at the lowest dose for the approved indication and then guided by clinical response, rather than by serum hormone levels (e.g., estradiol, FSH).

D. Drug/Laboratory Test Interactions.

1. Accelerated prothrombin time, partial thromboplastin time, and platelet aggregation time; increased platelet count; increased factors II, VII antigen, VIII antigen, VIII coagulant activity, IX, X, XII, VII-X complex, II-VII-X complex; and beta-thromboglobulin; decreased levels of anti-factor Xa and antithrombin III; decreased antithrombin III activity; increased levels of fibrinogen and fibrinogen activity; increased plasminogen antigen and activity.

2. Increased thyroid-binding globulin (TBG) leading to increased circulating total thyroid hormone, as measured by protein-bound iodine (PBI), T_4 levels (by column or by radioimmunoassay) or T_3 levels by radioimmunoassay. T_3 resin uptake is decreased, reflecting the elevated TBG. Free T_4 and free T_3 concentrations are unaltered. Patients on thyroid replacement therapy may require higher doses of thyroid hormone.

3. Other binding proteins may be elevated in serum (i.e., corticosteroid binding globulin [CBG], sex hormone-binding globulin [SHBG], leading to increased circulating corticosteroids and sex steroids, respectively. Free or biologically active hormone concentrations are unchanged. Other plasma proteins may be increased (angiotensinogen/renin substrate, alpha-1-antitrypsin, ceruloplasmin).

4. Increased plasma HDL and HDL-2 subfraction concentrations, reduced LDL cholesterol concentration, increased triglycerides levels.

5. Impaired glucose tolerance.

6. Reduced response to metyrapone test.

E. Carcinogenesis, Mutagenesis, Impairment of Fertility. Long-term, continuous administration of natural and synthetic estrogens in certain animal species increases the frequency of carcinomas of the breast, uterus, cervix, vagina, testis, and liver. *(See BOXED WARNINGS, CONTRAINDICATIONS, and WARNINGS.)*

F. Pregnancy. Estrogens should not be used during pregnancy. *(See CONTRAINDICATIONS.)*

G. Nursing Mothers. Estrogen administration to nursing mothers has been shown to decrease the quantity and quality of the milk. Detectable amounts of estrogens have been identified in the milk of mothers receiving this drug. Caution should be exercised when Vivelle-Dot is administered to a nursing woman.

H. Pediatric Use. Estrogen therapy has been used for the induction of puberty in adolescents with some forms of pubertal delay. Safety and effectiveness in pediatric patients have not otherwise been established.

Large and repeated doses of estrogen over an extended time period have been shown to accelerate epiphyseal closure, which could result in short adult stature if treatment is initiated before the completion of physiologic puberty in normally developing children. If estrogen is administered to patients whose bone growth is not complete, periodic monitoring of bone maturation and effects on epiphyseal centers is recommended during estrogen administration.

Estrogen treatment of prepubertal girls also induces premature breast development and vaginal cornification, and may induce vaginal bleeding. *(See INDICATIONS and DOSAGE AND ADMINISTRATION.)*

I. Geriatric Use. The safety and effectiveness in geriatric patients have not been established.

ADVERSE REACTIONS

See BOXED WARNINGS, WARNINGS and PRECAUTIONS.

Because clinical trials are conducted under widely varying conditions, adverse reaction rates observed in the clinical trials of a drug cannot be directly compared to rates in the clinical trials of another drug and may not reflect the rates observed in practice. The adverse reaction information from clinical trials does, however, provide a basis for identifying the adverse events that appear to be related to drug use and for approximating rates.

The following adverse events have been reported with Vivelle-Dot therapy:

[See table 3 at top of next page]

The following additional adverse reactions have been reported with estrogens:

1. Genitourinary system. Changes in vaginal bleeding pattern and abnormal withdrawal bleeding or flow; breakthrough bleeding; spotting; increase in size of uterine leiomyomata; vaginitis, including vaginal candidiasis; change in amount of cervical secretion; changes in cervical ectropion; ovarian cancer; endometrial hyperplasia; endometrial cancer.

2. Breasts. Tenderness, enlargement, pain, nipple discharge, galactorrhea; fibrocystic breast changes; breast cancer.

3. Cardiovascular. Deep and superficial venous thrombosis; pulmonary embolism; thrombophlebitis; myocardial infarction; stroke; increase in blood pressure.

4. Gastrointestinal. Nausea, vomiting; abdominal cramps, bloating; cholestatic jaundice; increased incidence of gallbladder disease; pancreatitis.

5. Skin. Chloasma or melasma, which may persist when drug is discontinued; erythema multiforme; erythema nodosum; hemorrhagic eruption; loss of scalp hair; hirsutism; pruritus, rash.

6. Eyes. Retinal vascular thrombosis; steepening of corneal curvature; intolerance to contact lenses.

7. Central nervous system. Headache; migraine; dizziness; mental depression; chorea; nervousness; mood disturbances; irritability; exacerbation of epilepsy.

8. Miscellaneous. Increase or decrease in weight; reduced carbohydrate tolerance; aggravation of porphyria; edema; arthralgias; leg cramps; changes in libido; anaphylactoid/anaphylactic reactions including urticaria and angioedema; hypocalcemia; exacerbation of asthma; increased triglycerides.

OVERDOSAGE

Serious ill effects have not been reported following acute ingestion of large doses of estrogen-containing oral contraceptives by young children. Overdosage of estrogen may cause nausea and vomiting, and withdrawal bleeding may occur in females.

DOSAGE AND ADMINISTRATION

The adhesive side of Vivelle-Dot® (estradiol transdermal system) should be placed on a clean, dry area of the abdomen. *Vivelle-Dot should not be applied to the breasts.* Vivelle-Dot should be replaced twice weekly. The sites of application must be rotated, with an interval of at least 1 week allowed between applications to a particular site. The area selected should not be oily, damaged, or irritated. The waistline should be avoided, since tight clothing may rub the system off. The system should be applied immediately after opening the pouch and removing the protective liner. The system should be pressed firmly in place with the palm of the hand for about 10 seconds, making sure there is good contact, especially around the edges. In the event that a system should fall off the same system may be reapplied. If the same system cannot be reapplied a new system should be applied to another location. In either case, the original treatment schedule should be continued. If a woman has forgotten to apply a patch, she should apply a new patch as soon as possible. The new patch should be applied on the original treatment schedule. The interruption of treatment in women taking Vivelle-Dot might increase the likelihood of breakthrough bleeding, spotting and recurrence of symptoms.

Initiation of Therapy

When estrogen is prescribed for a postmenopausal woman with a uterus, progestin should also be initiated to reduce the risk of endometrial cancer. A woman without a uterus does not need progestin. Use of estrogen alone or in combination with a progestin, should be limited to the shortest duration consistent with treatment goals and risks for the individual woman. Patients should be reevaluated periodically as clinically appropriate (e.g., 3-month to 6-month intervals) to determine whether treatment is still necessary *(See BOXED WARNINGS and WARNINGS).* For women who have a uterus, adequate diagnostic measures, such as endometrial sampling, when indicated, should be undertaken to rule out malignancy in cases of undiagnosed persistent or recurring abnormal vaginal bleeding.

Patients should be started at the lowest dose. For treatment of moderate-to-severe vasomotor symptoms and vulvar and vaginal atrophy associated with the menopause, start therapy with Vivelle-Dot 0.0375 mg/day applied to the skin twice weekly. For the prevention of postmenopausal osteoporosis, the minimum dose that has been shown to be effective is 0.025 mg/day. The dosage may be adjusted as necessary. Reproductive system-associated adverse events were encountered more frequently in the highest dose group (0.1 mg/day) than in other active treatment groups or in placebo-treated patients.

In women not currently taking oral estrogens or in women switching from another estradiol transdermal therapy, treatment with Vivelle-Dot may be initiated at once. In women who are currently taking oral estrogens, treatment with Vivelle-Dot should be initiated 1 week after withdrawal of oral hormone therapy, or sooner if menopausal symptoms reappear in less than 1 week.

Therapeutic Regimen

Vivelle-Dot may be given continuously in patients who do not have an intact uterus. In those patients with an intact uterus, Vivelle-Dot may be given on a cyclic schedule (e.g., three weeks on drug followed by one week off drug).

HOW SUPPLIED

Vivelle-Dot® (estradiol transdermal system), 0.025 mg/day - each 2.5 cm^2 system contains 0.39 mg of estradiol USP for nominal* delivery of 0.025 mg of estradiol per day.

Patient Calendar Pack of
8 Systems .... NDC 0078-0365-42

Carton of 3 Patient Calendar Packs of
8 Systems .... NDC 0078-0365-45

Vivelle-Dot® (estradiol transdermal system), 0.0375 mg/day - each 3.75 cm^2 system contains 0.585 mg of estradiol USP for nominal* delivery of 0.0375 mg of estradiol per day.

Patient Calendar Pack of
8 Systems .... NDC 0078-0343-42

Carton of 3 Patient Calendar Packs
of 8 Systems .... NDC 0078-0343-45

Vivelle-Dot® (estradiol transdermal system), 0.05 mg/day - each 5.0 cm^2 system contains 0.78 mg of estradiol USP for nominal* delivery of 0.05 mg of estradiol per day.

Patient Calendar Pack of
8 Systems .... NDC 0078-0344-42

Carton of 3 Patient Calendar Packs of
8 Systems .... NDC 0078-0344-45

Vivelle-Dot® (estradiol transdermal system), 0.075 mg/day - each 7.5 cm^2 system contains 1.17 mg of estradiol USP for nominal* delivery of 0.075 mg of estradiol per day.

Patient Calendar Pack of
8 Systems .... NDC 0078-0345-42

Carton of 3 Patient Calendar Packs of
8 Systems .... NDC 0078-0345-45

Vivelle-Dot® (estradiol transdermal system), 0.1 mg/day - each 10.0 cm^2 system contains 1.56 mg of estradiol USP for nominal* delivery of 0.1 mg of estradiol per day.

Patient Calendar Pack of
8 Systems .... NDC 0078-0346-42

Table 3
Summary of Most Frequently Reported Adverse Experiences/Medical Events Regardless of Relationship Reported at a Frequency ≥5%

	Vivelle 0.025 mg/day† (N=47) N (%)		Vivelle 0.0375 mg/day† (N=130) N (%)		Vivelle 0.05 mg/day† (N=103) N (%)		Vivelle 0.075 mg/day† (N=46) N (%)		Vivelle 0.1 mg/day† (N=132) N (%)		Placebo (N=157) N (%)	
Gastrointestinal disorders												
Constipation	2	(4.3)	5	(3.8)	4	(3.9)	3	(6.5)	2	(1.5)	4	(2.5)
Dyspepsia	4	(8.5)	12	(9.2)	3	(2.9)	2	(4.3)	0		10	(6.4)
Nausea	2	(4.3)	8	(6.2)	4	(3.9)	0		7	(5.3)	5	(3.2)
General disorders and administration site conditions* **												
Influenza like illness	3	(6.4)	6	(4.6)	8	(7.8)	0		3	(2.3)	10	(6.4)
Pain NOS*	0		8	(6.2)	0		2	(4.3)	7	(5.3)	7	(4.5)
Infections and infestations												
Influenza	4	(8.5)	4	(3.1)	6	(5.8)	0		10	(7.6)	14	(8.9)
Nasopharyngitis	3	(6.4)	16	(12.3)	10	(9.7)	9	(19.6)	11	(8.3)	24	(15.3)
Sinusitis NOS*	4	(8.5)	17	(13.1)	13	(12.6)	3	(6.5)	7	(5.3)	16	(10.2)
Upper respiratory tract infections NOS*	3	(6.4)	8	(6.2)	11	(10.7)	4	(8.7)	6	(4.5)	9	(5.7)
Investigations												
Weight increased	4	(8.5)	5	(3.8)	2	(1.9)	2	(4.3)	0		3	(1.9)
Musculoskeletal and connective tissue disorders												
Arthralgia	0		11	(8.5)	4	(3.9)	2	(4.3)	5	(3.8)	9	(5.7)
Back pain	4	(8.5)	10	(7.7)	9	(8.7)	4	(8.7)	14	(10.6)	10	(6.4)
Neck pain	3	(6.4)	4	(3.1)	4	(3.9)	0		6	(4.5)	2	(1.3)
Pain in limb	0		10	(7.7)	7	(6.8)	2	(4.3)	6	(4.5)	9	(5.7)
Nervous system disorders												
Headache NOS*	7	(14.9)	35	(26.9)	32	(31.1)	23	(50.0)	34	(25.8)	37	(23.6)
Sinus headache	0		12	(9.2)	5	(4.9)	5	(10.9)	2	(1.5)	8	(5.1)
Psychiatric disorders												
Anxiety NEC**	3	(6.4)	5	(3.8)	0		0		2	(1.5)	4	(2.5)
Depression	5	(10.6)	4	(3.1)	7	(6.8)	0		4	(3.0)	6	(3.8)
Insomnia	3	(6.4)	6	(4.6)	4	(3.9)	2	(4.3)	2	(1.5)	9	(5.7)
Reproductive system and breast disorders												
Breast tenderness	8	(17.0)	10	(7.7)	8	(7.8)	3	(6.5)	17	(12.9)	0	
Dysmenorrhea	0		0		0		3	(6.5)	0		0	
Intermenstrual bleeding	3	(6.4)	9	(6.9)	6	(5.8)	0		14	(10.6)	7	(4.5)
Respiratory, thoracic and mediastinal disorders												
Sinus congestion	0		4	(3.1)	3	(2.9)	3	(6.5)	6	(4.5)	7	(4.5)
Vascular disorders												
Hot flushes NOS*	3	(6.4)	0		3	(2.9)	0		0		6	(3.8)
Hypertension NOS*	2	(4.3)	0		3	(2.9)	0		0		2	(1.3)

† Represents milligrams of estradiol delivered daily by each system
* NOS represents not otherwise specified
** NEC represents not elsewhere classified
*** Application site erythema and application site irritation were observed in a small number of patients (3.2% or less of patients across treatment groups)

Carton of 3 Patient Calendar Packs of
8 Systems .... NDC 0078-0346-45

**See DESCRIPTION.*
Store at controlled room temperature at 25°C (77°F).
Do not store unpouched. Apply immediately upon removal from the protective pouch.
REV: FEBRUARY 2004 T2004-17

PATIENT INFORMATION

Vivelle-Dot®
(estradiol transdermal system)

Read this PATIENT INFORMATION before you start taking Vivelle-Dot® (estradiol transdermal system) and read all the information that you get each time you refill Vivelle-Dot. There may be new information. This information does not take the place of talking to your health care provider about your medical condition or your treatment.

The Vivelle-Dot® (estradiol transdermal system) patch that your health care provider has prescribed for you releases small amounts of an estrogen hormone through the skin. This leaflet describes the risks and benefits of treatment with Vivelle-Dot. Vivelle-Dot is not for everyone. Talk to your health care provider if you have any questions or concerns about this medication.

What is the most important information I should know about Vivelle-Dot?

- Estrogens increase the chances of getting cancer of the uterus.
- Report any unusual vaginal bleeding right away while you are taking estrogens. Vaginal bleeding after menopause may be a warning sign of cancer of the uterus (womb). Your health care provider should check any unusual vaginal bleeding to find out the cause.
- Do not use estrogens with or without progestins to prevent heart disease, heart attacks, or strokes.
  Using estrogens with or without progestins may increase your chances of getting heart attacks, strokes, breast cancer, and blood clots. You and your health care provider should talk regularly about whether you still need treatment with Vivelle-Dot.

What is Vivelle-Dot®?

Vivelle-Dot is a patch that contains the estrogen hormone, estradiol. When applied to the skin as directed below, Vivelle-Dot releases estrogen through the skin into the bloodstream.

What is Vivelle-Dot used for?

Vivelle-Dot is used after menopause to:

- **reduce moderate-to-severe hot flashes.**
  Estrogens are hormones made by a woman's ovaries. The ovaries normally stop making estrogens when a woman is between 45 and 55 years old. This drop in body estrogen levels causes the "Change in life" or menopause (the end of monthly menstrual periods). Sometimes, both ovaries are removed during an operation before natural menopause takes place. The sudden drop in estrogen levels causes "surgical menopause."
  When the estrogen levels begin dropping, some women develop very uncomfortable symptoms, such as feelings of warmth in the face, neck, and chest or sudden strong feelings of heat and sweating ("hot flashes" or "hot flushes"). In some women the symptoms are mild, and they will not need estrogens. In other women, symptoms can be more severe. You and your health care provider should talk regularly about whether you still need treatment with Vivelle-Dot.
- **treat moderate-to-severe dryness, itching and burning in or around the vagina.**
  You and your health care provider should talk regularly about whether you still need treatment with Vivelle-Dot to control these problems.
- **treat certain conditions in which a young woman's ovaries do not produce enough estrogens naturally.**
- **help reduce your chances of getting osteoporosis (thin weak bones).**
  Osteoporosis from menopause is a thinning of the bones that makes them weaker and easier to break. If you use Vivelle-Dot only to prevent osteoporosis from menopause, talk with your health care provider about whether a different treatment or medicine without estrogens might be better for you. You and your health care provider should talk regularly about whether you should continue with Vivelle-Dot. Weight-bearing exercise, like walking or running, and taking calcium and vitamin D supplements may also lower your chances of getting postmenopausal osteoporosis. It is important to talk about exercise and supplements with your health care provider before starting them.

Who should not take Vivelle-Dot?

Do not start taking Vivelle-Dot if you:

- **have unusual vaginal bleeding.**
- **currently have or have had certain cancers**
  Estrogens may increase the chances of getting certain types of cancers, including cancer of the breast or uterus.

Continued on next page

Vivelle-Dot—Cont.

If you have or had cancer, talk with your health care provider about whether you should take Vivelle-Dot.

- **had a stroke or heart attack in the recent past (for example in the past year).**
- **currently have or have had blood clots.**
- **are allergic to Vivelle-Dot or any of its ingredients.** See the end of this leaflet for a list of ingredients in Vivelle-Dot.
- **think you may be, or know that you are, pregnant.**

Tell your health care provider:

- **if you are breastfeeding.** The hormone in Vivelle-Dot can pass into your milk.
- **about all of your medical problems:** Your health care provider may need to check you more carefully if you have certain conditions such as asthma (wheezing), epilepsy (seizures), migraine, endometriosis, or problems with your heart, liver, thyroid, kidneys, or have high calcium levels in your blood.
- **about all the medicines you take,** including prescription and nonprescription medicines, vitamins, and herbal supplements. Some medicines may affect how Vivelle-Dot works. Vivelle-Dot may also affect how other medicines work.
- **if you are going to have surgery or will be on bed rest.** You may need to stop taking estrogens.

How should I take Vivelle-Dot?

Estrogens should be used only as long as needed and at the lowest possible dose that works. You and your health care provider should talk regularly (for example every 3 to 6 months) about whether you still need treatment with Vivelle-Dot.

Application Instructions for Vivelle-Dot (estradiol transdermal system)

1. Determine Your Schedule for Your Twice-a-Week Application

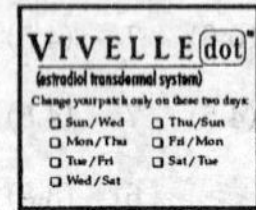

- Decide upon which two days you will change your patch.
- Your Vivelle-Dot® (estradiol transdermal system) individual carton contains a calendar card printed on its inner flap. Mark the two-day schedule you plan to follow on your carton's inner flap.
- BE CONSISTENT.
- If you forget to change your patch on the correct date, apply a new one as soon as you remember.
- No matter what day this happens, stick to the schedule you have marked on the inner flap of your carton (your calendar card).

2. Where to Apply Vivelle-Dot®

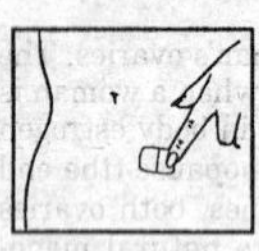

- Apply patch to lower abdomen, below the waistline. Avoid the waistline, since clothing may cause the patch to rub off.
- DO NOT APPLY PATCH TO BREASTS.
- When changing your patch, based on your twice-a-week schedule, apply your new patch to a different site. Do not apply a new patch to that same area for at least one week.

3. Before You Apply Vivelle-Dot®

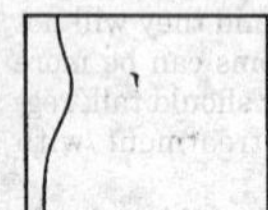

- **Make sure your skin is:**
- Clean (freshly washed), dry and cool.
- Free of any powder, oil, moisturizer or lotion.
- Free of cuts and/or irritations (rashes or other skin problems).

4. How to Apply Vivelle-Dot®

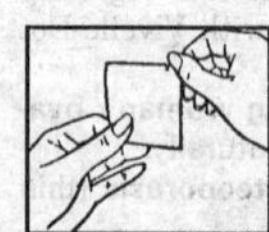

- Each patch is individually sealed in a protective pouch.
- Tear open the pouch at the tear notch (do not use scissors).
- Remove the patch.

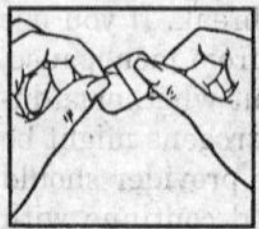

- **Apply the patch immediately after removing from pouch.**
- Holding the patch with the rigid protective liner facing you, remove **half** of the liner, which covers the sticky surface of the patch.

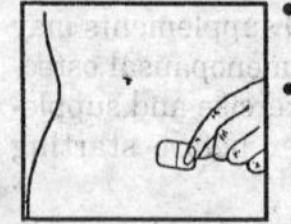

- **AVOID TOUCHING THE STICKY SIDE OF THE PATCH WITH YOUR FINGERS.**
- Using the other half of the rigid protective liner as a handle, apply the sticky side of the patch to the selected area of the abdomen.

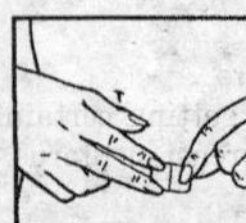

- Press the sticky side of the patch firmly into place.
- Smooth it down.
- While still holding the sticky side down, fold back the other half of the patch.

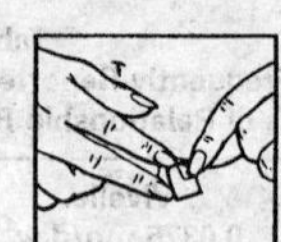

- Grasp an edge of the remaining protective liner and gently pull it off.
- **AVOID TOUCHING THE STICKY SIDE OF THE PATCH WITH YOUR FINGERS.**

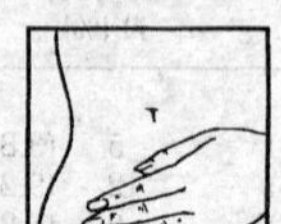

- Press the entire patch firmly into place with the palm of your hand.
- Continue to apply pressure, with the palm of your hand over the patch, for approximately 10 seconds.

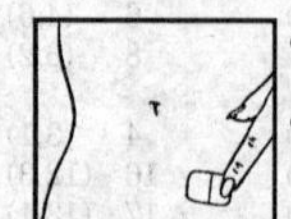

- Make sure that the patch is properly adhered to your skin.
- Go over the edges with your finger to ensure good contact around the patch.

PLEASE NOTE:

- Contact with water while bathing, swimming or showering will not affect the patch.
- In the event that a patch should fall off, **AVOID TOUCHING THE STICKY SIDE WITH YOUR FINGERS.** Put the same patch back on a different site, making sure to press the patch firmly into place for at least 10 seconds.
- Continue to follow your original twice-a-week schedule you have marked on the inner flap of your individual carton (your calendar card).
- If necessary, if the same patch cannot be reapplied, apply a new patch at another location but continue to follow your original schedule.

5. How to Change and Discard Vivelle-Dot®

- When changing the patch, peel off the used patch slowly.
- Fold the used patch in half (sticky sides together) and discard appropriately, in the trash.
- **PLEASE KEEP OUT OF REACH OF CHILDREN.**
- If any adhesive residue remains on your skin after removing the patch, allow the area to dry for 15 minutes. Then, gently rub the area with oil or lotion to remove the adhesive from your skin.
- Keep in mind, **the new patch must be applied to a different area of your abdomen.** This area must be clean, dry, cool and free of powder, oil and/or lotion.

What are the possible side effects of estrogens?

Less common but serious side effects include:

— Breast cancer
— Cancer of the uterus
— Stroke
— Heart attack
— Blood clots
— Gallbladder disease
— Ovarian cancer

These are some of the warning signs of serious side effects:

— Breast lumps
— Unusual vaginal bleeding
— Dizziness and faintness
— Changes in speech
— Severe headaches
— Chest pain
— Shortness of breath
— Pains in your legs
— Changes in vision
— Vomiting

Call your health care provider right away if you get any of these warning signs, or any other unusual symptom that concerns you.

Common side effects include:

— Headache
— Breast pain
— Irregular vaginal bleeding or spotting
— Stomach/abdominal cramps, bloating
— Nausea and vomiting
— Hair loss

Other side effects include:

— High blood pressure
— Liver problems
— High blood sugar
— Fluid retention
— Enlargement of benign tumors of the uterus ("fibroids")
— Vaginal yeast infection

Other side effects of Vivelle-Dot may be possible. If you have questions, talk to your health care provider or pharmacist.

What can I do to lower my chances of a serious side effect with Vivelle-Dot?

- Talk with your health care provider regularly about whether you should continue taking Vivelle-Dot.
- See your health care provider right away if you get vaginal bleeding while taking Vivelle-Dot.
- Have a breast exam and mammogram (breast X-ray) every year unless your health care provider tells you something else. If members of your family have had breast cancer or if you have ever had breast lumps or an abnormal mammogram, you may need to have breast exams more often.
- If you have high blood pressure, high cholesterol (fat in the blood), diabetes, are overweight, or if you use tobacco, you may have higher chances for getting heart disease. Ask your health care provider for ways to lower your chances for getting heart disease.

General information about safe and effective use of Vivelle-Dot

Medicines are sometimes prescribed for conditions that are not mentioned in patient information leaflets. Do not take Vivelle-Dot for conditions for which it was not prescribed. Do not give Vivelle-Dot to other people, even if they have the same symptoms you have. It may harm them. **Keep Vivelle-Dot out of the reach of children.**

This leaflet provides a summary of the most important information about Vivelle-Dot. If you would like more information, talk with your health care provider or pharmacist. You can ask for information about Vivelle-Dot that is written for health professionals. You can get more information by calling the toll free number 888-NOW-NOVA (888-669-6682).

What are the ingredients in Vivelle-Dot?

Vivelle-Dot is comprised of three layers. Proceeding from the visible surface toward the surface attached to the skin, these layers are (1) a translucent polyolefin film (2) an adhesive formulation containing estradiol, acrylic adhesive, silicone adhesive, oleyl alcohol, NF, povidone, USP and dipropylene glycol, and (3) a polyester release liner which is attached to the adhesive surface and must be removed before the system can be used.

The active component of the system is estradiol. The remaining components of the system are pharmacologically inactive.

Other Information

Do not store above 25°C (77°F). Do not store outside of their pouches. Apply immediately upon removal from the protective pouch.

Medicines are sometimes prescribed for conditions that are not mentioned in patient information leaflets. Do not use Vivelle-Dot® (estradiol transdermal system) for conditions for which it was not prescribed.

Do not give Vivelle-Dot to other people, even if they have the same symptoms you have. It may harm them.

Keep this and all drugs out of the reach of children. In case of overdose, remove the system and call your doctor, hospital, or poison control center immediately.

This leaflet summarizes the most important information about Vivelle-Dot. If you would like more information, talk to your health care provider. You can ask for information about Vivelle-Dot that is written for health professionals.

T2004-04
T2004-17/T2004-04

REV: FEBRUARY 2004 Printed in U.S.A 89001006
100922-3
Manufactured by: Noven Pharmaceuticals Inc., Miami, FL 33186
Distributed by: Novartis Pharmaceuticals Corporation, East Hanover, New Jersey 07936

Shown in Product Identification Guide, page 326

VOLTAREN® ℞

[*vōl-tă-rĕn*]
(diclofenac sodium) enteric-coated tablets
Tablets of 25 mg, 50 mg, and 75 mg
Rx only

Prescribing Information

The following prescribing information is based on official labeling in effect July 2003.

DESCRIPTION

Voltaren® (diclofenac sodium enteric-coated tablets), is a benzene-acetic acid derivative. Voltaren is available as Delayed-Release (enteric-coated) Tablets of 25 mg (yellow), 50 mg (light brown), and 75 mg (light pink) for oral administration. The chemical name is 2-[(2,6-dichlorophenyl)amino] benzeneacetic acid, monosodium salt. The molecular weight is 318.14. Its molecular formula is $C_{14}H_{10}Cl_2NNaO_2$, and it has the following structural formula

CH_2COONa
NH
Cl Cl

The inactive ingredients in Voltaren include: hydroxypropyl methylcellulose, iron oxide, lactose, magnesium stearate, methacrylic acid copolymer, microcrystalline cellulose, polyethylene glycol, povidone, propylene glycol, sodium hydroxide, sodium starch glycolate, talc, titanium dioxide, D&C Yellow No. 10 Aluminum Lake (25-mg tablet only), FD&C Blue No. 1 Aluminum Lake (50-mg tablet only).

CLINICAL PHARMACOLOGY

Pharmacodynamics

Voltaren® (diclofenac sodium enteric-coated tablets), is a nonsteroidal anti-inflammatory drug (NSAID) that exhibits anti-inflammatory, analgesic, and antipyretic activities in animal models. The mechanism of action of Voltaren, like that of other NSAIDs, is not completely understood but may be related to prostaglandin synthetase inhibition.

Pharmacokinetics

Absorption

Diclofenac is 100% absorbed after oral administration compared to IV administration as measured by urine recovery.

However, due to first-pass metabolism, only about 50% of the absorbed dose is systemically available (see Table 1). Food has no significant effect on the extent of diclofenac absorption. However, there is usually a delay in the onset of absorption of 1 to 4.5 hours and a reduction in peak plasma levels of < 20%.

Table 1. Pharmacokinetic Parameters for Diclofenac

PK Parameter	Normal Healthy Adults (20-48 yrs.)	
	Mean	Coefficient of Variation (%)
Absolute Bioavailability (%) [N = 7]	55	40
T_{max} (hr) [N = 56]	2.3	69
Oral Clearance (CL/F; mL/min) [N = 56]	582	23
Renal Clearance (% unchanged drug in urine) [N = 7]	<1	—
Apparent Volume of Distribution (V/F; L/kg) [N = 56]	1.4	58
Terminal Half-life (hr) [N = 56]	2.3	48

Distribution
The apparent volume of distribution (V/F) of diclofenac sodium is 1.4 L/kg.
Diclofenac is more than 99% bound to human serum proteins, primarily to albumin. Serum protein binding is constant over the concentration range (0.15-105 μg/mL) achieved with recommended doses.
Diclofenac diffuses into and out of the synovial fluid. Diffusion into the joint occurs when plasma levels are higher than those in the synovial fluid, after which the process reverses and synovial fluid levels are higher than plasma levels. It is not known whether diffusion into the joint plays a role in the effectiveness of diclofenac.
Metabolism
Five diclofenac metabolites have been identified in human plasma and urine. The metabolites include 4′-hydroxy-, 5-hydroxy-, 3′-hydroxy-, 4′,5-dihydroxy- and 3′-hydroxy-4′-methoxy diclofenac. In patients with renal dysfunction, peak concentrations of metabolites 4′-hydroxy- and 5-hydroxy-diclofenac were approximately 50% and 4% of the parent compound after single oral dosing compared to 27% and 1% in normal healthy subjects. However, diclofenac metabolites undergo further glucuronidation and sulfation followed by biliary excretion.
One diclofenac metabolite 4′-hydroxy-diclofenac has very weak pharmacologic activity.
Excretion
Diclofenac is eliminated through metabolism and subsequent urinary and biliary excretion of the glucuronide and the sulfate conjugates of the metabolites. Little or no free unchanged diclofenac is excreted in the urine. Approximately 65% of the dose is excreted in the urine and approximately 35% in the bile as conjugates of unchanged diclofenac plus metabolites. Because renal elimination is not a significant pathway of elimination for unchanged diclofenac, dosing adjustment in patients with mild to moderate renal dysfunction is not necessary. The terminal half-life of unchanged diclofenac is approximately 2 hours.
Special Populations
Pediatric: The pharmacokinetics of Voltaren has not been investigated in pediatric patients.
Race: Pharmacokinetics differences due to race have not been identified.
Hepatic Insufficiency: Hepatic metabolism accounts for almost 100% of Voltaren elimination, so patients with hepatic disease may require reduced doses of Voltaren compared to patients with normal hepatic function.
Renal Insufficiency: Diclofenac pharmacokinetics has been investigated in subjects with renal insufficiency. No differences in the pharmacokinetics of diclofenac have been detected in studies of patients with renal impairment. In patients with renal impairment (inulin clearance 60-90, 30-60, and <30 mL/min; N=6 in each group), AUC values and elimination rate were comparable to those in healthy subjects.

INDICATIONS AND USAGE

Voltaren® (diclofenac sodium enteric-coated tablets), is indicated:
- For relief of signs and symptoms of osteoarthritis
- For relief of signs and symptoms of rheumatoid arthritis
- For acute or long-term use in the relief of signs and symptoms of ankylosing spondylitis

CONTRAINDICATIONS

Voltaren® (diclofenac sodium enteric-coated tablets), is contraindicated in patients with known hypersensitivity to diclofenac. Voltaren should not be given to patients who have experienced asthma, urticaria, or other allergic-type reactions after taking aspirin or other NSAIDs. Severe, rarely fatal, anaphylactic-like reactions to NSAIDs have been reported in such patients (see WARNINGS - Anaphylactoid Reactions, and PRECAUTIONS - Preexisting Asthma).

WARNINGS

Gastrointestinal (GI) Effects - Risk of GI Ulceration, Bleeding, and Perforation:
Serious gastrointestinal toxicity such as inflammation, bleeding, ulceration, and perforation of the stomach, small intestine or large intestine, can occur at any time, with or without warning symptoms, in patients treated with nonsteroidal anti-inflammatory drugs (NSAIDs). Minor upper gastrointestinal problems, such as dyspepsia, are common and may also occur at any time during NSAID therapy. Therefore, physicians and patients should remain alert for ulceration and bleeding even in the absence of previous GI tract symptoms. Patients should be informed about the signs and/or symptoms of serious GI toxicity and the steps to take if they occur. The utility of periodic laboratory monitoring has not been demonstrated, nor has it been adequately assessed. Only one in five patients, who develop a serious upper GI adverse event on NSAID therapy, is symptomatic. It has been demonstrated that upper GI ulcers, gross bleeding or perforation, caused by NSAIDs, appear to occur in approximately 1% of patients treated for 3-6 months, and in about 2%-4% of patients treated for one year. These trends continue thus, increasing the likelihood of developing a serious GI event at some time during the course of therapy. However, even short-term therapy is not without risk.
NSAIDs should be prescribed with extreme caution in those with a prior history of ulcer disease or gastrointestinal bleeding. Most spontaneous reports of fatal GI events are in elderly or debilitated patients and therefore special care should be taken in treating this population. **To minimize the potential risk for an adverse GI event, the lowest effective dose should be used for the shortest possible duration.** For high risk patients, alternate therapies that do not involve NSAIDs should be considered.
Studies have shown that patients with a *prior history of peptic ulcer disease and/or gastrointestinal bleeding* and who use NSAIDs, have a greater than 10-fold risk for developing a GI bleed than patients with neither of these risk factors. In addition to a past history of ulcer disease, pharmacoepidemiological studies have identified several other co-therapies or co-morbid conditions that may increase the risk for GI bleeding such as: treatment with oral corticosteroids, treatment with anticoagulants, longer duration of NSAID therapy, smoking, alcoholism, older age, and poor general health status.
Anaphylactoid Reactions
As with other NSAIDs, anaphylactoid reactions may occur in patients without known prior exposure to Voltaren® (diclofenac sodium enteric-coated tablets). Voltaren should not be given to patients with the aspirin triad. This symptom complex typically occurs in asthmatic patients who experience rhinitis with or without nasal polyps, or who exhibit severe, potentially fatal bronchospasm after taking aspirin or other NSAIDs. (See CONTRAINDICATIONS and PRECAUTIONS - Preexisting Asthma.) Emergency help should be sought in cases where an anaphylactoid reaction occurs.
Advanced Renal Disease
In cases with advanced kidney disease, treatment with Voltaren is not recommended. If NSAID therapy, however, must be initiated, close monitoring of the patient's kidney function is advisable (see PRECAUTIONS - Renal Effects).
Pregnancy
In late pregnancy, as with other NSAIDs, Voltaren should be avoided because it may cause premature closure of the ductus arteriosus.

PRECAUTIONS

General
Voltaren® (diclofenac sodium enteric-coated tablets), cannot be expected to substitute for corticosteroids or to treat corticosteroid insufficiency. Abrupt discontinuation of corticosteroids may lead to disease exacerbation. Patients on prolonged corticosteroid therapy should have their therapy tapered slowly if a decision is made to discontinue corticosteroids.
The pharmacological activity of Voltaren in reducing fever and inflammation may diminish the utility of these diagnostic signs in detecting complications of presumed noninfectious, painful conditions.
Hepatic Effects
Borderline elevations of one or more liver tests may occur in up to 15% of patients taking NSAIDs including Voltaren. These laboratory abnormalities may progress, may remain unchanged, or may be transient with continued therapy. Based on this experience, in patients on chronic treatment with Voltaren, periodic monitoring of transaminases is recommended (see PRECAUTIONS - Laboratory Tests). Notable elevations of ALT or AST (three or more times the upper limit of normal) have been reported in approximately 2%-4% of patients, including marked elevations (eight or more times the upper limit of normal) in about 1% of patients in clinical trials with diclofenac. In addition, rare cases of severe hepatic reactions, including jaundice and fatal fulminant hepatitis, liver necrosis and hepatic failure, some of them with fatal outcomes have been reported.
A patient with symptoms and/or signs suggesting liver dysfunction, or in whom an abnormal liver test has occurred, should be evaluated for evidence of the development of a more severe hepatic reaction while on therapy with Voltaren. If clinical signs and symptoms consistent with liver disease develop, or if systemic manifestations occur (e.g., eosinophilia, rash, etc.), Voltaren should be discontinued.
Renal Effects
Caution should be used when initiating treatment with Voltaren in patients with considerable dehydration. It is advisable to rehydrate patients first and then start therapy with Voltaren. Caution is also recommended in patients with preexisting kidney disease (see WARNINGS - Advanced Renal Disease).
As with other NSAIDs, long-term administration of diclofenac has resulted in renal papillary necrosis and other renal medullary changes. Renal toxicity has also been seen in patients in which renal prostaglandins have a compensatory role in the maintenance of renal perfusion. In these patients, administration of a nonsteroidal anti-inflammatory drug may cause a dose-dependent reduction in prostaglandin formation and, secondarily, in renal blood flow, which may precipitate overt renal decompensation. Patients at greatest risk of this reaction are those with impaired renal function, heart failure, liver dysfunction, those taking diuretics and ACE inhibitors, and the elderly. Discontinuation of nonsteroidal anti-inflammatory drug therapy is usually followed by recovery to the pretreatment state.
Voltaren metabolites are eliminated primarily by the kidneys. The extent to which the metabolites may accumulate in patients with renal failure has not been studied. As with other NSAIDs, metabolites of which are excreted by the kidney, patients with significantly impaired renal function should be more closely monitored.
Hematological Effects
Anemia is sometimes seen in patients receiving NSAIDs, including Voltaren. This may be due to fluid retention, GI loss, or an incompletely described effect upon erythropoiesis. Patients on long-term treatment with NSAIDs, including Voltaren, should have their hemoglobin or hematocrit checked if they exhibit any signs or symptoms of anemia.
All drugs which inhibit the biosynthesis of prostaglandins may interfere to some extent with platelet function and vascular responses to bleeding.
NSAIDs inhibit platelet aggregation and have been shown to prolong bleeding time in some patients. Unlike aspirin, their effect on platelet function is quantitatively less, of shorter duration, and reversible. Voltaren does not generally affect platelet counts, prothrombin time (PT), or partial thromboplastin time (PTT). Patients receiving Voltaren who may be adversely affected by alterations in platelet function, such as those with coagulation disorders or patients receiving anticoagulants, should be carefully monitored.
Fluid Retention and Edema
Fluid retention and edema have been observed in some patients taking NSAIDs. Therefore, as with other NSAIDs, Voltaren should be used with caution in patients with fluid retention, hypertension, or heart failure.
Preexisting Asthma
Patients with asthma may have aspirin-sensitive asthma. The use of aspirin in patients with aspirin-sensitive asthma has been associated with severe bronchospasm which can be fatal. Since cross-reactivity, including bronchospasm, between aspirin and other nonsteroidal anti-inflammatory drugs has been reported in such aspirin-sensitive patients, Voltaren should not be administered to patients with this form of aspirin sensitivity and should be used with caution in all patients with preexisting asthma.
Information for Patients
Voltaren, like other drugs of its class, can cause discomfort and, rarely, more serious side effects, such as gastrointestinal bleeding, which may result in hospitalization and even fatal outcomes. Although serious GI tract ulcerations and bleeding can occur without warning symptoms, patients should be alert for the signs and symptoms of ulcerations and bleeding, and should ask for medical advice when observing any indicative sign or symptoms. Patients should be apprised of the importance of this follow-up (see WARNINGS - Risk of Gastrointestinal Ulceration, Bleeding and Perforation).
Patients should report to their physicians' signs or symptoms of gastrointestinal ulceration or bleeding, skin rash, weight gain, or edema.
Patients should be informed of the warning signs and symptoms of hepatotoxicity (e.g., nausea, fatigue, lethargy, pruritus, jaundice, right upper quadrant tenderness, and "flu-like" symptoms). If these occur, patients should be instructed to stop therapy and seek immediate medical therapy.
Patients should also be instructed to seek immediate emergency help in the case of an anaphylactoid reaction (see WARNINGS).
In late pregnancy, as with other NSAIDs, Voltaren should be avoided because it will cause premature closure of the ductus arteriosus.
Laboratory Tests
Patients on long-term treatment with NSAIDs, should have their CBC and a chemistry profile (including transaminases) checked periodically. If clinical signs and symptoms consistent with liver or renal disease develop, systemic manifestations occur (e.g., eosinophilia, rash, etc.) or if abnormal liver tests persist or worsen, Voltaren should be discontinued.

Continued on next page

Voltaren—Cont.

Drug Interactions

Aspirin: When Voltaren is administered with aspirin, its protein binding is reduced. The clinical significance of this interaction is not known; however, as with other NSAIDs, concomitant administration of diclofenac and aspirin is not generally recommended because of the potential of increased adverse effects.

Methotrexate: NSAIDs have been reported to competitively inhibit methotrexate accumulation in rabbit kidney slices. This may indicate that they could enhance the toxicity of methotrexate. Caution should be used when NSAIDs are administered concomitantly with methotrexate.

Cyclosporine: Voltaren, like other NSAIDs, may affect renal prostaglandins and increase the toxicity of certain drugs. Therefore, concomitant therapy with Voltaren may increase cyclosporine's nephrotoxicity. Caution should be used when Voltaren is administered concomitantly with cyclosporine.

ACE-inhibitors: Reports suggest that NSAIDs may diminish the antihypertensive effect of ACE-inhibitors. This interaction should be given consideration in patients taking NSAIDs concomitantly with ACE-inhibitors.

Furosemide: Clinical studies, as well as post-marketing observations, have shown that Voltaren can reduce the natriuretic effect of furosemide and thiazides in some patients. This response has been attributed to inhibition of renal prostaglandin synthesis. During concomitant therapy with NSAIDs, the patient should be observed closely for signs of renal failure (see PRECAUTIONS - Renal Effects), as well as to assure diuretic efficacy.

Lithium: NSAIDs have produced an elevation of plasma lithium levels and a reduction in renal lithium clearance. The mean minimum lithium concentration increased 15% and the renal clearance was decreased by approximately 20%. These effects have been attributed to inhibition of renal prostaglandin synthesis by the NSAID. Thus, when NSAIDs and lithium are administered concurrently, subjects should be observed carefully for signs of lithium toxicity.

Warfarin: The effects of warfarin and NSAIDs on GI bleeding are synergistic, such that users of both drugs together have a risk of serious GI bleeding higher than users of either drug alone.

Pregnancy

Teratogenic Effects: Pregnancy Category C

Reproductive studies conducted in rats and rabbits have not demonstrated evidence of developmental abnormalities. However, animal reproduction studies are not always predictive of human response. There are no adequate and well-controlled studies in pregnant women.

Nonteratogenic Effects: Because of the known effects of nonsteroidal anti-inflammatory drugs on the fetal cardiovascular system (closure of ductus arteriosus), use during pregnancy (particularly late pregnancy) should be avoided.

Labor and Delivery

In rat studies with NSAIDs, as with other drugs known to inhibit prostaglandin synthesis, an increased incidence of dystocia, delayed parturition, and decreased pup survival occurred. The effects of Voltaren on labor and delivery in pregnant women are unknown.

Nursing Mothers

It is not known whether this drug is excreted in human milk. Because many drugs are excreted in human milk and because of the potential for serious adverse reactions in nursing infants from Voltaren, a decision should be made whether to discontinue nursing or to discontinue the drug, taking into account the importance of the drug to the mother.

Pediatric Use

Safety and effectiveness in pediatric patients have not been established.

Geriatric Use

As with any NSAIDs, caution should be exercised in treating the elderly (65 years and older).

ADVERSE REACTIONS

In patients taking Voltaren® (diclofenac sodium enteric-coated tablets), or other NSAIDs, the most frequently reported adverse experiences occurring in approximately 1%-10% of patients are:

Gastrointestinal experiences including: abdominal pain, constipation, diarrhea, dyspepsia, flatulence, gross bleeding/perforation, heartburn, nausea, GI ulcers (gastric/duodenal) and vomiting.

Abnormal renal function, anemia, dizziness, edema, elevated liver enzymes, headaches, increased bleeding time, pruritus, rashes and tinnitus.

Additional adverse experiences reported occasionally include:

Body as a Whole: fever, infection, sepsis

Cardiovascular System: congestive heart failure, hypertension, tachycardia, syncope

Digestive System: dry mouth, esophagitis, gastric/peptic ulcers, gastritis, gastrointestinal bleeding, glossitis, hematemesis, hepatitis, jaundice

Hemic and Lymphatic System: ecchymosis, eosinophilia, leukopenia, melena, purpura, rectal bleeding, stomatitis, thrombocytopenia

Metabolic and Nutritional: weight changes

Nervous System: anxiety, asthenia, confusion, depression, dream abnormalities, drowsiness, insomnia, malaise, nervousness, paresthesia, somnolence, tremors, vertigo

Respiratory System: asthma, dyspnea

Skin and Appendages: alopecia, photosensitivity, sweating increased

Special Senses: blurred vision

Urogenital System: cystitis, dysuria, hematuria, interstitial nephritis, oliguria/polyuria, proteinuria, renal failure.

Other adverse reactions, which occur rarely are:

Body as a Whole: anaphylactic reactions, appetite changes, death

Cardiovascular System: arrhythmia, hypotension, myocardial infarction, palpitations, vasculitis

Digestive System: colitis, eructation, liver failure, pancreatitis

Hemic and Lymphatic System: agranulocytosis, hemolytic anemia, aplastic anemia, lymphadenopathy, pancytopenia

Metabolic and Nutritional: hyperglycemia

Nervous System: convulsions, coma, hallucinations, meningitis

Respiratory System: respiratory depression, pneumonia

Skin and Appendages: angioedema, toxic epidermal necrolysis, erythema multiforme, exfoliative dermatitis, Stevens-Johnson syndrome, urticaria

Special Senses: conjunctivitis, hearing impairment.

OVERDOSAGE

Symptoms following acute NSAID overdoses are usually limited to lethargy, drowsiness, nausea, vomiting, and epigastric pain, which are generally reversible with supportive care. Gastrointestinal bleeding can occur. Hypertension, acute renal failure, respiratory depression and coma may occur, but are rare. Anaphylactoid reactions have been reported with therapeutic ingestion of NSAIDs, and may occur following an overdose.

Patients should be managed by symptomatic and supportive care following a NSAID overdose. There are no specific antidotes. Emesis and/or activated charcoal (60 to 100 g in adults, 1 to 2 g/kg in children) and/or osmotic cathartic may be indicated in patients seen within 4 hours of ingestion with symptoms or following a large overdose (5 to 10 times the usual dose). Forced diuresis, alkalinization of urine, hemodialysis, or hemoperfusion may not be useful due to high protein binding.

DOSAGE AND ADMINISTRATION

As with other NSAIDs, the lowest dose should be sought for each patient. Therefore, after observing the response to initial therapy with Voltaren® (diclofenac sodium enteric-coated tablets), the dose and frequency should be adjusted to suit an individual patient's needs.

For the relief of osteoarthritis, the recommended dosage is 100-150 mg/day in divided doses (50 mg b.i.d. or t.i.d., or 75 mg b.i.d.).

For the relief of rheumatoid arthritis, the recommended dosage is 150-200 mg/day in divided doses (50 mg t.i.d. or q.i.d., or 75 mg b.i.d.).

For the relief of ankylosing spondylitis, the recommended dosage is 100-125 mg/day, administered as 25 mg q.i.d., with an extra 25-mg dose at bedtime if necessary.

Different formulations of diclofenac [Voltaren® (diclofenac sodium enteric-coated tablets); Voltaren®-XR (diclofenac sodium extended-release tablets); Cataflam® (diclofenac potassium immediate-release tablets)] are not necessarily bioequivalent even if the milligram strength is the same.

HOW SUPPLIED

Voltaren® Tablets

25 mg – yellow, biconvex, triangular-shaped, enteric-coated tablets (imprinted VOLTAREN 25 on one side in black ink)
Bottles of 100 .... NDC 0028-0258-01

50 mg – light brown, biconvex, triangular-shaped, enteric-coated tablets (imprinted VOLTAREN 50 on one side in black ink)
Bottles of 100 .... NDC 0028-0262-01

75 mg – light pink, biconvex, triangular-shaped, enteric-coated tablets (imprinted VOLTAREN 75 on one side in black ink)
Bottles of 100 .... NDC 0028-0264-01

Do not store above 30°C (86°F). Protect from moisture.

Dispense in tight container (USP).

REV: FEBRUARY 2003 T2003-20
89016302

NOVARTIS

Distributed by:
Manufactured by:
Mova Pharmaceuticals Corp.
Caguas, Puerto Rico 00726
Novartis Pharmaceuticals Corp.
East Hanover, NJ 07936

Shown in Product Identification Guide, page 326

VOLTAREN®-XR ℞

[vōl-tă-rĭn]

(diclofenac sodium) extended-release tablets
Tablets of 100 mg
Rx only

Prescribing Information

The following prescribing information is based on official labeling in effect July 2003.

DESCRIPTION

Voltaren®-XR, (diclofenac sodium extended-release tablets), is a benzeneacetic acid derivative. Voltaren-XR is available as Extended-Release Tablets of 100 mg (light pink) for oral administration. The chemical name is 2-[(2,6-dichlorophenyl)amino] benzeneacetic acid, monosodium salt. The molecular weight is 318.14. Its molecular formula is $C_{14}H_{10}Cl_2NNaO_2$, and it has the following structural formula

The inactive ingredients in Voltaren-XR include: cetyl alcohol, hydroxypropyl methylcellulose, iron oxide, magnesium stearate, polyethylene glycol, polysorbate, povidone, silicon dioxide, sucrose, talc, titanium dioxide.

CLINICAL PHARMACOLOGY

Pharmacodynamics

Voltaren®-XR (diclofenac sodium extended-release tablets), is a nonsteroidal anti-inflammatory drug (NSAID) that exhibits anti-inflammatory, analgesic, and antipyretic activities in animal models. The mechanism of action of Voltaren-XR, like that of other NSAIDs, is not completely understood but may be related to prostaglandin synthetase inhibition.

Pharmacokinetics

Absorption

Diclofenac is 100% absorbed after oral administration compared to IV administration as measured by urine recovery. However, due to first-pass metabolism, only about 50% of the absorbed dose is systemically available (see Table 1). When Voltaren-XR is taken with food, there is a delay of 1 to 2 hours in the T_{max} and a two-fold increase in C_{max} values. The extent of absorption of diclofenac, however, is not significantly affected by food intake.

Table 1. Pharmacokinetic Parameters for Diclofenac

PK Parameter	Normal Healthy Adults (18-48 yrs.) Mean	Coefficient of Variation (%)
Absolute Bioavailability (%) [N = 7]	55	40
T_{max} (hr) [N = 12]	5.3	28
Oral Clearance (CL/F; mL/min) [N = 12]	895	56
Renal Clearance (% unchanged drug in urine) [N = 7]	<1	—
Apparent Volume of Distribution (V/F; L/kg) [N = 56]	1.4	58
Terminal Half-life (hr) [N = 56]	2.3	48

Distribution

The apparent volume of distribution (V/F) of diclofenac sodium is 1.4 L/kg. Diclofenac is more than 99% bound to human serum proteins, primarily to albumin. Serum protein binding is constant over the concentration range (0.15-105 g/mL) achieved with recommended doses.

Diclofenac diffuses into and out of the synovial fluid. Diffusion into the joint occurs when plasma levels are higher than those in the synovial fluid, after which the process reverses and synovial fluid levels are higher than plasma levels. It is not known whether diffusion into the joint plays a role in the effectiveness of diclofenac.

Metabolism

Five diclofenac metabolites have been identified in human plasma and urine. The metabolites include 4′-hydroxy-, 5-hydroxy-, 3′-hydroxy-, 4′,5-dihydroxy- and 3′-hydroxy-4′-methoxy diclofenac. In patients with renal dysfunction, peak concentrations of metabolites 4′-hydroxy- and 5-hydroxy-diclofenac were approximately 50% and 4% of the parent compound after single oral dosing compared to 27% and 1% in normal healthy subjects. However, diclofenac metabolites undergo further glucuronidation and sulfation followed by biliary excretion.

One diclofenac metabolite 4′-hydroxy-diclofenac has very weak pharmacologic activity.

Excretion

Diclofenac is eliminated through metabolism and subsequent urinary and biliary excretion of the glucuronide and the sulfate conjugates of the metabolites. Little or no free unchanged diclofenac is excreted in the urine. Approximately 65% of the dose is excreted in the urine and approximately 35% in the bile as conjugates of unchanged diclofenac plus metabolites. Because renal elimination is not a significant pathway of elimination for unchanged diclofenac, dosing adjustment in patients with mild to moderate renal dysfunction is not necessary. The terminal half-life of unchanged diclofenac is approximately 2 hours.

Special Populations

Pediatric: The pharmacokinetics of Voltaren-XR has not been investigated in pediatric patients.

Race: Pharmacokinetics differences due to race have not been identified.

Hepatic Insufficiency: Hepatic metabolism accounts for almost 100% of Voltaren-XR elimination, so patients with hepatic disease may require reduced doses of Voltaren-XR compared to patients with normal hepatic function.

Renal Insufficiency: Diclofenac pharmacokinetics has been investigated in subjects with renal insufficiency. No differences in the pharmacokinetics of diclofenac have been detected in studies of patients with renal impairment. In patients with renal impairment (inulin clearance 60-90, 30-60, and <30 mL/min; N=6 in each group), AUC values and elimination rate were comparable to those in healthy subjects.

INDICATIONS AND USAGE

Voltaren®-XR (diclofenac sodium extended-release tablets) is indicated:

- For relief of signs and symptoms of osteoarthritis
- For relief of signs and symptoms of rheumatoid arthritis

CONTRAINDICATIONS

Voltaren®-XR (diclofenac sodium extended-release tablets) is contraindicated in patients with known hypersensitivity to diclofenac. Voltaren-XR should not be given to patients who have experienced asthma, urticaria, or allergic-type reactions after taking aspirin or other NSAIDs. Severe, rarely fatal, anaphylactic-like reactions to NSAIDs have been reported in such patients (see WARNINGS - Anaphylactoid Reactions, and PRECAUTIONS - Preexisting Asthma).

WARNINGS

Gastrointestinal (GI) Effects - Risk of GI Ulceration, Bleeding, and Perforation:

Serious gastrointestinal toxicity such as inflammation, bleeding, ulceration, and perforation of the stomach, small intestine or large intestine, can occur at any time, with or without warning symptoms, in patients treated with nonsteroidal anti-inflammatory drugs (NSAIDs). Minor upper gastrointestinal problems, such as dyspepsia, are common and may also occur at any time during NSAID therapy. Therefore, physicians and patients should remain alert for ulceration and bleeding even in the absence of previous GI tract symptoms. Patients should be informed about the signs and/or symptoms of serious GI toxicity and the steps to take if they occur. The utility of periodic laboratory monitoring has not been demonstrated, nor has it been adequately assessed. Only one in five patients, who develop a serious upper GI adverse event on NSAID therapy, is symptomatic. It has been demonstrated that upper GI ulcers, gross bleeding or perforation, caused by NSAIDs, appear to occur in approximately 1% of patients treated for 3-6 months, and in about 2%-4% of patients treated for one year. These trends continue thus, increasing the likelihood of developing a serious GI event at some time during the course of therapy. However, even short term therapy is not without risk.

NSAIDs should be prescribed with extreme caution in those with a prior history of ulcer disease or gastrointestinal bleeding. Most spontaneous reports of fatal GI events are in elderly or debilitated patients and therefore special care should be taken in treating this population. **To minimize the potential risk for an adverse GI event, the lowest effective dose should be used for the shortest possible duration.** For high risk patients, alternate therapies that do not involve NSAIDs should be considered.

Studies have shown that patients with *a prior history of peptic ulcer disease and/or gastrointestinal bleeding* and who use NSAIDs, have a greater than 10-fold risk for developing a GI bleed than patients with neither of these risk factors. In addition to a past history of ulcer disease, pharmacoepidemiological studies have identified several other co-therapies or co-morbid conditions that may increase the risk for GI bleeding such as: treatment with oral corticosteroids, treatment with anticoagulants, longer duration of NSAID therapy, smoking, alcoholism, older age, and poor general health status.

Anaphylactoid Reactions

As with other NSAIDs, anaphylactoid reactions may occur in patients without known prior exposure to Voltaren®-XR (diclofenac sodium extended-release tablets). Voltaren-XR should not be given to patients with the aspirin triad. This symptom complex typically occurs in asthmatic patients who experience rhinitis with or without nasal polyps, or who exhibit severe, potentially fatal bronchospasm after taking aspirin or other NSAIDs. (See CONTRAINDICATIONS and PRECAUTIONS - Preexisting Asthma.) Emergency help should be sought in cases where an anaphylactoid reaction occurs.

Advanced Renal Disease

In cases with advanced kidney disease, treatment with Voltaren-XR is not recommended. If NSAID therapy, however, must be initiated, close monitoring of the patient's kidney function is advisable (see PRECAUTIONS - Renal Effects).

Pregnancy

In late pregnancy, as with other NSAIDs, Voltaren-XR should be avoided because it may cause premature closure of the ductus arteriosus.

PRECAUTIONS

General

Voltaren®-XR (diclofenac sodium extended-release tablets) cannot be expected to substitute for corticosteroids or to treat corticosteroid insufficiency. Abrupt discontinuation of corticosteroids may lead to disease exacerbation. Patients on prolonged corticosteroid therapy should have their therapy tapered slowly if a decision is made to discontinue corticosteroids.

The pharmacological activity of Voltaren-XR in reducing fever and inflammation may diminish the utility of these diagnostic signs in detecting complications of presumed noninfectious, painful conditions.

Hepatic Effects

Borderline elevations of one or more liver tests may occur in up to 15% of patients taking NSAIDs including Voltaren-XR. These laboratory abnormalities may progress, may remain unchanged, or may be transient with continuing therapy. Based on this experience, in patients on chronic treatment with Voltaren-XR, periodic monitoring of transaminases is recommended (See PRECAUTIONS - Laboratory Tests). Notable elevations of ALT or AST (three or more times the upper limit of normal) have been reported in approximately 2%-4% of patients, including marked elevations (eight or more times the upper limit of normal) in about 1% of patients in clinical trials with diclofenac. In addition, rare cases of severe hepatic reactions, including jaundice and fatal fulminant hepatitis, liver necrosis and hepatic failure, some of them with fatal outcomes have been reported.

A patient with symptoms and/or signs suggesting liver dysfunction, or in whom an abnormal liver test has occurred, should be evaluated for evidence of the development of a more severe hepatic reaction while on therapy with Voltaren-XR. If clinical signs and symptoms consistent with liver disease develop, or if systemic manifestations occur (e.g., eosinophilia, rash, etc.), Voltaren-XR should be discontinued.

Renal Effects

Caution should be used when initiating treatment with Voltaren-XR in patients with considerable dehydration. It is advisable to rehydrate patients first and then start therapy with Voltaren-XR. Caution is also recommended in patients with pre-existing kidney disease (see WARNINGS - Advanced Renal Disease).

As with other NSAIDs, long-term administration of diclofenac has resulted in renal papillary necrosis and other renal medullary changes. Renal toxicity has also been seen in patients in which renal prostaglandins have a compensatory role in the maintenance of renal perfusion. In these patients, administration of a nonsteroidal anti-inflammatory drug may cause a dose-dependent reduction in prostaglandin formation and, secondarily, in renal blood flow, which may precipitate overt renal decompensation. Patients at greatest risk of this reaction are those with impaired renal function, heart failure, liver dysfunction, those taking diuretics and ACE inhibitors, and the elderly. Discontinuation of non-steroidal anti-inflammatory drug therapy is usually followed by recovery to the pretreatment state.

Voltaren-XR metabolites are eliminated primarily by the kidneys. The extent to which the metabolites may accumulate in patients with renal failure has not been studied. As with other NSAIDs, metabolites of which are excreted by the kidney, patients with significantly impaired renal function should be more closely monitored.

Hematological Effects

Anemia is sometimes seen in patients receiving NSAIDs, including Voltaren-XR. This may be due to fluid retention, GI loss, or an incompletely described effect upon erythropoiesis. Patients on long-term treatment with NSAIDs, including Voltaren-XR, should have their hemoglobin or hematocrit checked if they exhibit any signs or symptoms of anemia.

All drugs which inhibit the biosynthesis of prostaglandins may interfere to some extent with platelet function and vascular responses to bleeding.

NSAIDs inhibit platelet aggregation and have been shown to prolong bleeding time in some patients. Unlike aspirin, their effect on platelet function is quantitatively less, of shorter duration, and reversible. Voltaren-XR does not generally affect platelet counts, prothrombin time (PT), or partial thromboplastin time (PTT). Patients receiving Voltaren-XR who may be adversely affected by alterations in platelet function, such as those with coagulation disorders or patients receiving anticoagulants, should be carefully monitored.

Fluid Retention and Edema

Fluid retention and edema have been observed in some patients taking NSAIDs. Therefore, as with other NSAIDs, Voltaren-XR should be used with caution in patients with fluid retention, hypertension, or heart failure.

Preexisting Asthma

Patients with asthma may have aspirin-sensitive asthma. The use of aspirin in patients with aspirin-sensitive asthma has been associated with severe bronchospasm which can be fatal. Since cross-reactivity, including bronchospasm, between aspirin and other nonsteroidal anti-inflammatory drugs has been reported in such aspirin-sensitive patients, Voltaren-XR should not be administered to patients with this form of aspirin sensitivity and should be used with caution in all patients with preexisting asthma.

Information for Patients

Voltaren-XR, like other drugs of its class, can cause discomfort and, rarely, more serious side effects, such as gastrointestinal bleeding, which may result in hospitalization and even fatal outcomes. Although serious GI tract ulcerations and bleeding can occur without warning symptoms, patients should be alert for the signs and symptoms of ulcerations and bleeding, and should ask for medical advice when observing any indicative sign or symptoms. Patients should be apprised of the importance of this follow-up (see WARNINGS - Risk of Gastrointestinal Ulceration, Bleeding and Perforation).

Patients should report to their physicians' signs or symptoms of gastrointestinal ulceration or bleeding, skin rash, weight gain, or edema.

Patients should be informed of the warning signs and symptoms of hepatotoxicity (e.g., nausea, fatigue, lethargy, pruritus, jaundice, right upper quadrant tenderness, and "flu-like" symptoms). If these occur, patients should be instructed to stop therapy and seek immediate medical therapy.

Patients should also be instructed to seek immediate emergency help in the case of an anaphylactoid reaction (see WARNINGS).

In late pregnancy, as with other NSAIDs, Voltaren-XR should be avoided because it will cause premature closure of the ductus arteriosus.

Laboratory Tests

Patients on long-term treatment with NSAIDs, should have their CBC and a chemistry profile (including transaminases) checked periodically. If clinical signs and symptoms consistent with liver or renal disease develop, systemic manifestations occur (e.g., eosinophilia, rash, etc.) or if abnormal liver tests persist or worsen, Voltaren-XR should be discontinued.

Drug Interactions

Aspirin: When Voltaren-XR is administered with aspirin, its protein binding is reduced. The clinical significance of this interaction is not known; however, as with other NSAIDs, concomitant administration of diclofenac and aspirin is not generally recommended because of the potential of increased adverse effects.

Methotrexate: NSAIDs have been reported to competitively inhibit methotrexate accumulation in rabbit kidney slices. This may indicate that they could enhance the toxicity of methotrexate. Caution should be used when NSAIDs are administered concomitantly with methotrexate.

Cyclosporine: Voltaren-XR, like other NSAIDs, may affect renal prostaglandins and increase the toxicity of certain drugs. Therefore, concomitant therapy with Voltaren-XR may increase cyclosporine's nephrotoxicity. Caution should be used when Voltaren-XR is administered concomitantly with cyclosporine.

ACE-inhibitors: Reports suggest that NSAIDs may diminish the antihypertensive effect of ACE-inhibitors. This interaction should be given consideration in patients taking NSAIDs concomitantly with ACE-inhibitors.

Furosemide: Clinical studies, as well as post marketing observations, have shown that Voltaren-XR can reduce the natriuretic effect of furosemide and thiazides in some patients. This response has been attributed to inhibition of renal prostaglandin synthesis. During concomitant therapy with NSAIDs, the patient should be observed closely for signs of renal failure (see PRE-CAUTIONS - Renal Effects), as well as to assure diuretic efficacy.

Lithium: NSAIDs have produced an elevation of plasma lithium levels and a reduction in renal lithium clearance. The mean minimum lithium concentration increased 15% and the renal clearance was decreased by approximately 20%. These effects have been attributed to inhibition of renal prostaglandin synthesis by the NSAID. Thus, when NSAIDs and lithium are administered concurrently, subjects should be observed carefully for signs of lithium toxicity.

Warfarin: The effects of warfarin and NSAIDs on GI bleeding are synergistic, such that users of both drugs together have a risk of serious GI bleeding higher than users of either drug alone.

Pregnancy

Teratogenic Effects: Pregnancy Category C

Reproductive studies conducted in rats and rabbits have not demonstrated evidence of developmental abnormalities. However, animal reproduction studies are not always predictive of human response. There are no adequate and well-controlled studies in pregnant women.

Nonteratogenic Effects

Because of the known effects of nonsteroidal anti-inflammatory drugs on the fetal cardiovascular system (closure of ductus arteriosus), use during pregnancy (particularly late pregnancy) should be avoided.

Labor and Delivery

In rat studies with NSAIDs, as with other drugs known to inhibit prostaglandin synthesis, an increased incidence of dystocia, delayed parturition, and decreased pup survival occurred. The effects of Voltaren-XR on labor and delivery in pregnant women are unknown.

Nursing Mothers

It is not known whether this drug is excreted in human milk. Because many drugs are excreted in human milk and because of the potential for serious adverse reactions in nursing infants from Voltaren-XR, a decision should be made whether to discontinue nursing or to discontinue the drug, taking into account the importance of the drug to the mother.

Pediatric Use

Safety and effectiveness in pediatric patients have not been established.

Geriatric Use

As with any NSAIDs, caution should be exercised in treating the elderly (65 years and older).

Continued on next page

Voltaren-XR—Cont.

ADVERSE REACTIONS

In patients taking Voltaren®-XR (diclofenac sodium extended-release tablets) or other NSAIDs, the most frequently reported adverse experiences occurring in approximately 1%-10% of patients are:

Gastrointestinal experiences including: abdominal pain, constipation, diarrhea, dyspepsia, flatulence, gross bleeding/perforation, heartburn, nausea, GI ulcers (gastric/duodenal) and vomiting.

Abnormal renal function, anemia, dizziness, edema, elevated liver enzymes, headaches, increased bleeding time, pruritus, rashes and tinnitus.

Additional adverse experiences reported occasionally include:

Body as a Whole: fever, infection, sepsis

Cardiovascular System: congestive heart failure, hypertension, tachycardia, syncope

Digestive System: dry mouth, esophagitis, gastric/peptic ulcers, gastritis, gastrointestinal bleeding, glossitis, hematemesis, hepatitis, jaundice

Hemic and Lymphatic System: ecchymosis, eosinophilia, leukopenia, melena, purpura, rectal bleeding, stomatitis, thrombocytopenia

Metabolic and Nutritional: weight changes

Nervous System: anxiety, asthenia, confusion, depression, dream abnormalities, drowsiness, insomnia, malaise, nervousness, paresthesia, somnolence, tremors, vertigo

Respiratory System: asthma, dyspnea

Skin and Appendages: alopecia, photosensitivity, sweating increased

Special Senses: blurred vision

Urogenital System: cystitis, dysuria, hematuria, interstitial nephritis, oliguria/polyuria, proteinuria, renal failure.

Other adverse reactions, which occur rarely are:

Body as a Whole: anaphylactic reactions, appetite changes, death

Cardiovascular System: arrhythmia, hypotension, myocardial infarction, palpitations, vasculitis

Digestive System: colitis, eructation, liver failure, pancreatitis

Hemic and Lymphatic System: agranulocytosis, hemolytic anemia, aplastic anemia, lymphadenopathy, pancytopenia

Metabolic and Nutritional: hyperglycemia

Nervous System: convulsions, coma, hallucinations, meningitis

Respiratory System: respiratory depression, pneumonia

Skin and Appendages: angioedema, toxic epidermal necrolysis, erythema multiforme, exfoliative dermatitis, Stevens-Johnson syndrome, urticaria

Special Senses: conjunctivitis, hearing impairment.

OVERDOSAGE

Symptoms following acute NSAID overdoses are usually limited to lethargy, drowsiness, nausea, vomiting, and epigastric pain, which are generally reversible with supportive care. Gastrointestinal bleeding can occur. Hypertension, acute renal failure, respiratory depression and coma may occur, but are rare. Anaphylactoid reactions have been reported with therapeutic ingestion of NSAIDs, and may occur following an overdose.

Patients should be managed by symptomatic and supportive care following a NSAID overdose. There are no specific antidotes. Emesis and/or activated charcoal (60 to 100 g in adults, 1 to 2 g/kg in children) and/or osmotic cathartic may be indicated in patients seen within 4 hours of ingestion with symptoms or following a large overdose (5 to 10 times the usual dose). Forced diuresis, alkalinization of urine, hemodialysis, or hemoperfusion may not be useful due to high protein binding.

DOSAGE AND ADMINISTRATION

For the relief of osteoarthritis, the recommended dosage is 100 mg q.d.

For the relief of rheumatoid arthritis, the recommended dosage is 100 mg q.d. In the rare patient where Voltaren®-XR (diclofenac sodium extended-release tablets) 100 mg/day is unsatisfactory, the dose may be increased to 100 mg b.i.d. if the benefits outweigh the clinical risks of increased side effects.

Different formulations of diclofenac [Voltaren (diclofenac sodium enteric-coated tablets); Voltaren-XR (diclofenac sodium extended-release tablets); Cataflam (diclofenac potassium immediate-release tablets)] are not necessarily bioequivalent even if the milligram strength is the same.

HOW SUPPLIED

Voltaren-XR Extended-Release Tablets

100 mg

Light pink, film-coated, round, biconvex with beveled edges (imprinted Voltaren XR on one side and 100 on the other side in black ink)

Bottles of 100 .... NDC 0028-0205-01

Do not store above 30°C (86°F). Protect from moisture.

Dispense in tight container (USP).

REV: OCTOBER 2002 T2002-42 89008903

NOVARTIS

Manufactured by:
Novartis Pharma Stein AG
Stein, Switzerland For
Novartis Pharmaceuticals Corporation
East Hanover, NJ 07936

Shown in Product Identification Guide, page 326

ZELNORM® ℞

[zəl-nōrm]
(tegaserod maleate)
Tablets
Rx only

Prescribing Information

The following prescribing information is based on official labeling in effect August 2004.

DESCRIPTION

Zelnorm® (tegaserod maleate) tablets contain tegaserod as the hydrogen maleate salt. As the maleate salt, tegaserod is chemically designated as 3-(5-methoxy-1H-indol-3-ylmethylene)-N-pentylcarbazimidamide hydrogen maleate. Its empirical formula is $C_{16}H_{23}N_5O \bullet C_4H_4O_4$. The molecular weight is 417.47 and the structural formula is

$\cdot C_4H_4O_4$

Tegaserod as the maleate salt is a white to off-white crystalline powder and is slightly soluble in ethanol and very slightly soluble in water. Each 1.385 mg of tegaserod as the maleate is equivalent to 1 mg of tegaserod. Zelnorm is available for oral use in the following tablet formulations:

- 2-mg and 6-mg tablets (blister packs) containing 2 mg and 6 mg tegaserod, respectively and the following inactive ingredients: crospovidone, glyceryl monostearate, hypromellose, lactose monohydrate, poloxamer 188, and polyethylene glycol 4000.
- 6-mg tablets (bottles) containing 6 mg tegaserod and the following inactive ingredients: crospovidone, glyceryl behenate, hypromellose, lactose monohydrate, and colloidal silicon dioxide.

CLINICAL PHARMACOLOGY

Mechanism of Action

Irritable bowel syndrome with constipation and chronic idiopathic constipation are both lower gastrointestinal dysmotility disorders. Clinical investigations have shown that both motor and sensory functions of the gut appear to be altered in patients suffering from irritable bowel syndrome (IBS), while in patients with chronic idiopathic constipation, reduced intestinal motility is the predominant cause of the condition. Both the enteric nervous system, which acts to integrate and process information in the gut, and 5-hydroxytryptamine (5-HT, serotonin) are thought to represent key elements in the etiology of both IBS and idiopathic constipation. Approximately 95% of serotonin is found throughout the gastrointestinal tract, primarily stored in enterochromaffin cells but also in enteric nerves acting as a neurotransmitter. Serotonin has been shown to be involved in regulating motility, visceral sensitivity and intestinal secretion. Investigations suggest an important role of serotonin Type-4 (5-HT_4) receptors in the maintenance of gastrointestinal functions in humans. 5-HT_4 receptor mRNA has been found throughout the human gastrointestinal tract.

Tegaserod is a 5-HT_4 receptor partial agonist that binds with high affinity at human 5-HT_4 receptors, whereas it has no appreciable affinity for 5-HT_3 or dopamine receptors. It has moderate affinity for 5-HT_1 receptors. Tegaserod, by acting as an agonist at neuronal 5-HT_4 receptors, triggers the release of further neurotransmitters such as calcitonin gene-related peptide from sensory neurons. The activation of 5-HT_4 receptors in the gastrointestinal tract stimulates the peristaltic reflex and intestinal secretion, as well as inhibits visceral sensitivity. *In vivo* studies showed that tegaserod enhanced basal motor activity and normalized impaired motility throughout the gastrointestinal tract. In addition, studies demonstrated that tegaserod moderated visceral sensitivity during colorectal distension in animals.

Pharmacokinetics

Absorption

Peak plasma concentrations are reached approximately 1 hour after oral dosing. The absolute bioavailability of tegaserod when administered to fasting subjects is approximately 10%. The pharmacokinetics are dose proportional over the 2 mg to 12 mg range given twice daily for 5 days. There was no clinically relevant accumulation of tegaserod in plasma when a 6 mg b.i.d. dose was given for 5 days. *(See DOSAGE AND ADMINISTRATION.)*

Food Effects

When the drug is administered with food, the bioavailability of tegaserod is reduced by 40%-65% and C_{max} by approximately 20%-40%. Similar reductions in plasma concentration occur when tegaserod is administered to subjects within 30 minutes prior to a meal, or 2.5 hours after a meal. T_{max} of tegaserod is prolonged from approximately 1 hour to 2 hours when taken following a meal, but decreased to 0.7 hours when taken 30 minutes prior to a meal.

Distribution

Tegaserod is approximately 98% bound to plasma proteins, predominantly alpha-1-acid glycoprotein. Tegaserod exhibits its pronounced distribution into tissues following intravenous dosing with a volume of distribution at steady-state of 368 ± 223 L.

Metabolism

Tegaserod is metabolized mainly via two pathways. The first is a presystemic acid catalyzed hydrolysis in the stomach followed by oxidation and conjugation which produces the main metabolite of tegaserod, 5-methoxyindole-3-carboxylic acid glucuronide. The main metabolite has negligible affinity for 5-HT_4 receptors *in vitro*. In humans, systemic exposure to tegaserod was not altered at neutral gastric pH values. The second metabolic pathway of tegaserod is direct glucuronidation which leads to generation of three isomeric N-glucuronides.

Elimination

The plasma clearance of tegaserod is 77 ± 15 L/h with an estimated terminal half-life ($T_{1/2}$) of 11 ± 5 hours following intravenous dosing. Approximately two-thirds of the orally administered dose of tegaserod is excreted unchanged in the feces, with the remaining one-third excreted in the urine, primarily as the main metabolite.

Sub Populations

Patients: The pharmacokinetics of tegaserod in IBS patients are comparable to those in healthy subjects. The pharmacokinetics of tegaserod in patients with chronic idiopathic constipation have not been studied.

Reduced Renal Function: No change in the pharmacokinetics of tegaserod was observed in subjects with severe renal impairment requiring hemodialysis (creatinine clearance ≤15 mL/min/1.73 m²). C_{max} and AUC of the main pharmacologically inactive metabolite of tegaserod, 5-methoxy-indole-3-carboxylic acid glucuronide, increased 2- and 10-fold respectively, in subjects with severe renal impairment compared to healthy controls. No dosage adjustment is required in patients with mild-to-moderate renal impairment. Tegaserod is not recommended in patients with severe renal impairment.

Reduced Hepatic Function: In subjects with mild hepatic impairment, mean AUC was 31% higher and C_{max} 16% higher compared to subjects with normal hepatic function. No dosage adjustment is required in patients with mild impairment, however, caution is recommended when using tegaserod in this patient population. Tegaserod has not adequately been studied in patients with moderate and severe hepatic impairment, and is therefore not recommended in these patients.

Gender: Gender has no effect on the pharmacokinetics of tegaserod.

Race: Data were inadequate to assess the effect of race on the pharmacokinetics of tegaserod.

Age: In a clinical pharmacology study conducted to assess the pharmacokinetics of tegaserod administered to healthy young (18-40 years) and healthy elderly (65-85 years) subjects, peak plasma concentration and exposure were 22% and 40% greater, respectively, in elderly females than young females but still within the variability seen in tegaserod pharmacokinetics in healthy subjects. Based on an analysis across several pharmacokinetic studies in healthy subjects, there is no age effect on the pharmacokinetics of tegaserod when allowing for body weight as a covariate. Therefore, dose adjustment in elderly patients who have IBS with constipation is not necessary.

CLINICAL STUDIES

IBS with Constipation

Results in Women: In three multicenter, double-blind, placebo-controlled studies, 2,470 women (mean age 43 years [range 17-89 years]; 86% Caucasian, 10% African American) with at least a 3-month history of IBS symptoms prior to the study baseline period that included abdominal pain, bloating and constipation received either Zelnorm® (tegaserod maleate) 6 mg b.i.d. or placebo. In all patients, constipation was characterized by at least two of the following three symptoms each occurring ≥25% of the time over a 3-month period: <3 bowel movements/week, hard or lumpy stools, or straining with a bowel movement. The study design consisted of a 4-week placebo-free baseline period followed by a 12-week double-blind treatment period. Study 1 and 2 evaluated a fixed dose regimen of tegaserod 6 mg b.i.d. while Study 3 utilized a dose-titration design.

Each week of the 4-week placebo-free baseline period and the 12-week double-blind treatment period, patients were asked the question, "Please consider how you felt this past week in regard to your IBS, in particular your overall well-being, and symptoms of abdominal discomfort, pain and altered bowel habit. Compared to the way you usually felt before entering the study, how would you rate your relief of symptoms during the past week?" The response variable consisted of the following 5 categories: completely relieved, considerably relieved, somewhat relieved, unchanged, or worse. Patients were classified as responders within a month if they were considerably or completely relieved for at least two of the four weeks, or if they were at least somewhat relieved for each of the four weeks.

Calculated response rates during month 1 and during month 3 as described above are shown in the table below. The differences in response rates vs. placebo were greater at month 1 than month 3.

[See table at top of next page]

The same efficacy variable (i.e., complete relief, considerable relief, somewhat relief, unchanged, worse) was analyzed on a weekly basis. The proportion of female patients with complete, considerable or somewhat relief at weeks 1, 4, 6, 8 and 12 are shown in the figure below.

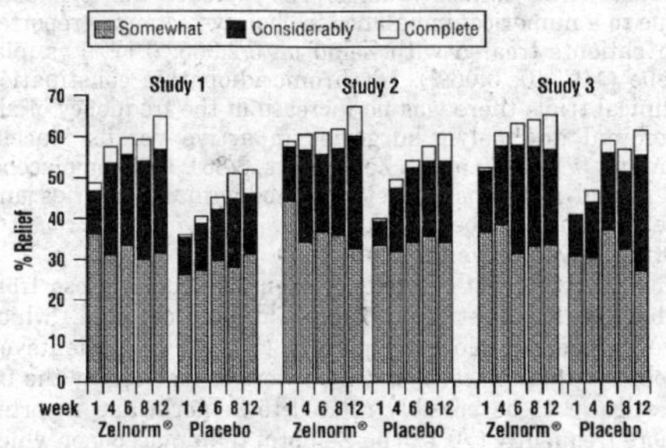

In addition, individual symptoms of abdominal pain/discomfort and bloating were assessed daily using a 6 or 7 point intensity scale. A positive response was defined as at least a 1 point reduction in the scale. During the first four weeks in the fixed dose studies, 8 to 11% more Zelnorm-treated patients than placebo patients were responders for abdominal pain/discomfort. Similarly, 9 to 12% more Zelnorm-treated patients were responders for bloating. Corresponding differences at month 3 were 1 to 10% for abdominal pain/discomfort and 4 to 11% for bloating. Patients on Zelnorm also experienced an increase in median number of stools from 3.8/week at baseline to 6.3/week at month 1 and 6.0/week at month 3, while placebo patients increased from 4.0/week to 5.1/week at month 1 and 5.5/week at month 3.

Results in Men: In two randomized, placebo-controlled, double-blind studies enrolling 288 males, there were no significant differences between placebo and Zelnorm response rates in subgroup analyses by gender.

Chronic Idiopathic Constipation

In two multicenter, double-blind, placebo-controlled studies, 2,612 patients with chronic constipation were randomized to receive either Zelnorm® (tegaserod maleate) 6 mg b.i.d., 2 mg b.i.d., or placebo.

Results in Patients Under Age 65: A total of 2,281 patients were less than 65 years of age. Patients (91% female, mean age 43 [range 18-64], 90% Caucasian, 4.3% African American) had constipation defined as less than 3 complete spontaneous bowel movements [CSBM] per week and at least one of the following symptoms for at least 25% of defecations: straining, hard/very hard stools, incomplete evacuation. A bowel movement was evaluated by the patient as complete if it resulted in a feeling of complete emptying of their bowel. A bowel movement was considered to be spontaneous [SBM] if no laxatives were taken in the preceding 24 hours.The study population consisted of patients with a 6 month or longer history of constipation symptoms (median 12 years). Patients with constipation known to be due to other known colon diseases, pelvic floor dysfunction, metabolic or neurological disturbances, or concomitant medications were excluded.

After a 2-week baseline, patients were randomized to a 12-week double-blind treatment with Zelnorm 6 mg b.i.d., Zelnorm 2 mg b.i.d., or placebo. This treatment period was followed, in Study 1, by an extension period where patients received either 6 mg b.i.d. or 2 mg b.i.d. for an additional 13 months. The drop out rate for lack of efficacy for the additional 13-month period was 19% for 6 mg b.i.d. and 22% for 2 mg b.i.d.. In Study 2, the 12-week treatment period was followed by a 4-week drug-free withdrawal period.

Patients were classified as responders (primary efficacy variable) if they achieved an average increase of at least one CSBM per week during the first four weeks of treatment compared to baseline, and had at least 7 days of exposure in the study.

The response rate for the primary efficacy variable in patients under 65 years of age was higher in the Zelnorm 6 mg b.i.d. group compared to the placebo group for each of the 2 trials ($p < 0.0001$, Table 2). This difference was statistically significant for CSBM changes averaged over the first 4 weeks of treatment and the full 12 weeks of treatment. The results with Zelnorm 2 mg b.i.d. showed significant changes during the first 4 weeks, however, no statistically significant changes were observed over 12 weeks in one study.

Proportion Of Patients Under Age 65 With An Increase Of 1 Or More CSBM For The Two Trials Combined

	Zelnorm® 6 mg b.i.d	Zelnorm® 2 mg b.i.d.	Placebo
Weeks 1–4	43% (337/789)	39% (286/732)	25% (184/737)
Weeks 1–12	45% (355/789)	38% (281/732)	28% (206/737)

Infrequent Defecation

At baseline, the median number of CSBM's per week was zero and the mean number of CSBM's per week was 0.5. Regardless of baseline, Zelnorm significantly increased the number of complete spontaneous bowel movements compared to placebo at each week ($p<0.05$).

[See figure at top of next column]

Zelnorm also significantly increased the number of SBM's compared to placebo at each week ($p<0.05$).

	Month 1			Month 3		
	Proportion of Responders (Females)			Proportion of Responders (Females)		
Study	Zelnorm® 6 mg b.i.d.	Placebo	Difference (95% Confidence Interval)	Zelnorm® 6 mg b.i.d.	Placebo	Difference (95% Confidence Interval)
1	76/244 (31%)	42/240 (17%)	14% (6% to 21%)	95/244 (39%)	66/240 (28%)	11% (3% to 20%)
2	265/767 (35%)	164/752 (22%)	13% (8% to 17%)	334/767 (44%)	292/752 (39%)	5% (0% to 10%)
3	80/233 (34%)	47/234 (20%)	14% (6% to 22%)	100/233 (43%)	88/234 (38%)	5% (-4% to 14%)

Response: ≥2 of 4 weeks complete or considerable relief or 4 of 4 weeks with at least somewhat relief.

Frequency Of Complete Spontaneous Bowel Movement (CSBM) Over 12 Week Treatment And 4 Week Withdrawal Period In Study 2

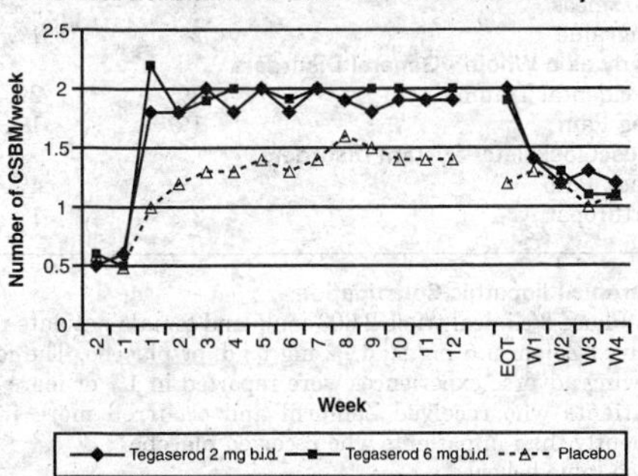

Constipation Symptoms

Patients treated with Zelnorm experienced a statistically significant reduction in the individual symptoms of straining, abdominal distension/bloating, and abdominal discomfort/pain, and a statistically significant improvement in stool consistency and frequency compared to placebo when averaged over the 12 weeks ($p<0.05$). In addition, a global constipation relief score, computed as an average of 4 scores measuring abdominal discomfort/pain, abdominal distension/bloating, bothersomeness of constipation and satisfaction with bowel habits, showed statistically significant improvement for Zelnorm compared to placebo when averaged over the 12 weeks ($p<0.05$).

Results in Patients Age 65 and Over: Subgroup analyses of patients 65 and older (n=331) showed no significant treatment effects for Zelnorm over placebo.

INDICATIONS AND USAGE

IBS with Constipation

Zelnorm® (tegaserod maleate) is indicated for the short-term treatment of women with irritable bowel syndrome (IBS) whose primary bowel symptom is constipation.

The safety and effectiveness of Zelnorm in men with IBS with constipation have not been established.

Chronic Idiopathic Constipation

Zelnorm® (tegaserod maleate) is indicated for the treatment of patients less than 65 years of age with chronic idiopathic constipation. The effectiveness of Zelnorm in patients 65 years or older with chronic idiopathic constipation has not been established *(see Geriatric Use)*.

The efficacy of Zelnorm for the treatment of IBS with constipation or chronic idiopathic constipation has not been studied beyond 12 weeks.

CONTRAINDICATIONS

Zelnorm® (tegaserod maleate) is contraindicated in those patients with:

- severe renal impairment
- moderate or severe hepatic impairment
- a history of bowel obstruction, symptomatic gallbladder disease, suspected sphincter of Oddi dysfunction, or abdominal adhesions
- a known hypersensitivity to the drug or any of its excipients

WARNINGS

Serious consequences of diarrhea, including hypovolemia, hypotension, and syncope have been reported in the clinical studies and during marketed use of Zelnorm® (tegaserod maleate). In some cases, these complications have required hospitalization for rehydration. Zelnorm should be discontinued immediately in patients who develop severe diarrhea, hypotension or syncope. Zelnorm should not be initiated in patients who are currently experiencing or frequently experience diarrhea *(see ADVERSE REACTIONS)*.

PRECAUTIONS

General

Zelnorm® (tegaserod maleate) should be discontinued immediately in patients with new or sudden worsening of abdominal pain.

Ischemic Colitis

Ischemic colitis and other forms of intestinal ischemia have been reported in patients receiving Zelnorm during marketed use of the drug *(see ADVERSE REACTIONS: Post-Marketing Experience)*. In some cases, hospitalization was required. Zelnorm should be discontinued immediately in patients who develop symptoms of ischemic colitis, such as rectal bleeding, bloody diarrhea or new or worsening abdominal pain. Patients experiencing these symptoms should be evaluated promptly and have appropriate diagnostic testing performed. Treatment with Zelnorm should not be resumed in patients who develop findings consistent with ischemic colitis or other forms of intestinal ischemia.

Information for Patients

Patients should take Zelnorm before a meal.

Patients should stop Zelnorm treatment and consult their physician if they experience new or worsening abdominal pain with or without rectal bleeding.

Patients should also be aware of the possible occurrence of diarrhea during therapy. Diarrhea can be a pharmacologic response to Zelnorm. The majority of the Zelnorm patients reporting diarrhea had a single episode. In most cases, diarrhea occurred within the first week of treatment. Typically, diarrhea resolved with continued therapy. Patients should consult their physician if they experience severe diarrhea, or if the diarrhea is accompanied by severe cramping, abdominal pain, or dizziness. Patients should not initiate therapy with Zelnorm if they are currently experiencing or frequently experience diarrhea. *(See ADVERSE REACTIONS.)*

Drug Interactions

In vitro drug-drug interaction data with tegaserod indicated no inhibition of the cytochrome P450 isoenzymes CYP2C8, CYP2C9, CYP2C19, CYP2E1 and CYP3A4, whereas inhibition of CYP1A2 and CYP2D6 could not be excluded. However, *in vivo*, no clinically relevant drug-drug interactions have been observed with dextromethorphan (CYP2D6 prototype substrate), and theophylline (CYP1A2 prototype substrate). There was no effect on the pharmacokinetics of digoxin, oral contraceptives, and warfarin. The main human metabolite of tegaserod hydrogen maleate, 5-methoxyindole-3-carboxylic acid glucuronide, did not inhibit the activity of any of the above cytochrome P450 isoenzymes in *in vitro* tests.

Dextromethorphan: A pharmacokinetic interaction study demonstrated that co-administration of tegaserod and dextromethorphan did not change the pharmacokinetics of either compound to a clinically relevant extent. Dose adjustment of either drug is not necessary when tegaserod is combined with dextromethorphan. Therefore, tegaserod is not expected to alter the pharmacokinetics of drugs metabolized by CYP2D6 (e.g., fluoxetine, omeprazole, captopril).

Theophylline: A pharmacokinetic interaction study demonstrated that co-administration of tegaserod and theophylline did not affect the pharmacokinetics of theophylline. Dose adjustment of theophylline is not necessary when tegaserod is co-administered. Therefore, tegaserod is not expected to alter the pharmacokinetics of drugs metabolized by CYP1A2 (e.g., estradiol, omeprazole).

Digoxin: A pharmacokinetic interaction study with digoxin demonstrated that concomitant administration of tegaserod reduced peak plasma concentration and exposure of digoxin by approximately 15%. This reduction of bioavailability is not considered clinically relevant. When tegaserod is co-administered with digoxin dose adjustment is unlikely to be required.

Warfarin: A pharmacokinetic and pharmacodynamic interaction study with warfarin demonstrated no effect of concomitant administration of tegaserod on warfarin pharmacokinetics and pharmacodynamics. Dose adjustment of warfarin is not necessary when tegaserod is co-administered.

Oral Contraceptives: Co-administration of tegaserod did not affect the steady-state pharmacokinetics of ethinylestradiol and reduced peak concentrations and exposure of levonorgestrel by 8%. Tegaserod is not expected to alter the risk of ovulation in subjects taking oral contraceptives. No alteration in oral contraceptive medication is necessary when tegaserod is co-administered.

Carcinogenesis, Mutagenesis, Impairment of Fertility

Tegaserod was not carcinogenic in rats given oral dietary doses up to 180 mg/kg/day (approximately 93 to 111 times the human exposure at 6 mg b.i.d. based on plasma $AUC_{0\text{-}24\ hr}$) for 110 to 124 weeks.

In mice, dietary administration of tegaserod for 104 weeks produced mucosal hyperplasia and adenocarcinoma of small intestine at 600 mg/kg/day (approximately 83 to 110 times the human exposure at 6 mg b.i.d. based on plasma $AUC_{0\text{-}24\ hr}$). There was no evidence of carcinogenicity at a lower dose of 200 mg/kg/day (approximately 24 to 35 times the human exposure at 6 mg b.i.d. based on plasma $AUC_{0\text{-}24\ hr}$) or 60 mg/kg/day (approximately 3 to 4 times the human exposure at 6 mg b.i.d. based on plasma $AUC_{0\text{-}24\ hr}$).

Continued on next page

Zelnorm—Cont.

Tegaserod was not genotoxic in the *in vitro* Chinese hamster lung fibroblast (CHL/V79) cell chromosomal aberration test, the *in vitro* Chinese hamster lung fibroblast (CHL/V79) cell forward mutation test, the *in vitro* rat hepatocyte unscheduled DNA synthesis (UDS) test or the *in vivo* mouse micronucleus test. The results of Ames test for mutagenicity were equivocal.

Tegaserod at oral doses up to 240 mg/kg/day (approximately 57 times the human exposure at 6 mg b.i.d. based on plasma $AUC_{0-24\ hr}$) in male rats and 150 mg/kg/day (approximately 42 times the human exposure at 6 mg b.i.d. based on plasma $AUC_{0-24\ hr}$) in female rats was found to have no effect on fertility and reproductive performance.

Pregnancy, Teratogenic Effects: Pregnancy Category B

Reproduction studies have been performed in rats at oral doses up to 100 mg/kg/day (approximately 15 times the human exposure at 6 mg b.i.d. based on plasma $AUC_{0-24\ hr}$) and rabbits at oral doses up to 120 mg/kg/day (approximately 51 times the human exposure at 6 mg b.i.d. based on plasma $AUC_{0-24\ hr}$) and have revealed no evidence of impaired fertility or harm to the fetus due to tegaserod. Because animal reproduction studies are not always predictive of human response, this drug should be used during pregnancy only if clearly needed.

Nursing Mothers

Tegaserod and its metabolites are excreted in the milk of lactating rats with a high milk to plasma ratio. It is not known whether tegaserod is excreted in human milk. Many drugs, which are excreted in human milk, have potential for serious adverse reactions in nursing infants. Based on the potential for tumorigenicity shown for tegaserod in the mouse carcinogenicity study, a decision should be made whether to discontinue nursing or to discontinue the drug, taking into account the importance of the drug to the mother.

Pediatric Use

Zelnorm has not been studied in pediatric patients.

Geriatric Use

IBS with Constipation

Of 4,035 patients in Phase 3 clinical studies of Zelnorm, 290 were at least 65 years of age, while 52 were at least 75 years old. No overall differences in safety were observed between these patients and younger patients with regard to adverse events.

No dose adjustment is necessary when administering Zelnorm to patients with IBS with constipation over 65 years old. *(See CLINICAL PHARMACOLOGY.)*

Chronic Idiopathic Constipation

Of 2,612 patients in Phase 3 clinical studies of Zelnorm, 331 were at least 65 years of age. Efficacy in patients 65 years of age or greater showed no significant difference between drug and placebo responses. Patients 65 years of age or greater who received Zelnorm experienced a higher incidence of diarrhea and discontinuations due to diarrhea than patients younger than 65.

ADVERSE REACTIONS

IBS with Constipation

In Phase 3 clinical trials 2,632 female and male patients received Zelnorm® (tegaserod maleate) 6 mg b.i.d. or placebo. The frequency and type of adverse events for females and males were similar. The following adverse experiences were reported in 1% or more of patients who received Zelnorm and occurred more frequently on Zelnorm than placebo:

Adverse Events Occurring in ≥1% of IBS Patients and More Frequently on Zelnorm® (tegaserod maleate) than Placebo

System/Adverse Experience	Zelnorm® 6 mg b.i.d. (n=1,327)	Placebo (n=1,305)
Gastrointestinal System Disorders		
Abdominal Pain	12%	11%
Diarrhea	9%	4%
Nausea	8%	7%
Flatulence	6%	5%
Central and Peripheral Nervous System		
Headache	15%	12%
Dizziness	4%	3%
Migraine	2%	1%
Body as a Whole - General Disorders		
Accidental Trauma	3%	2%
Leg Pain	1%	<1%
Musculoskeletal System Disorders		
Back Pain	5%	4%
Arthropathy	2%	1%

Chronic Idiopathic Constipation

In Phase 3 clinical trials 2,603 male and female patients received Zelnorm 6 mg b.i.d., 2 mg b.i.d. or placebo. The following adverse experiences were reported in 1% or more of patients who received Zelnorm and occurred more frequently than in patients who received placebo.

[See table below]

Zelnorm was not associated with changes in ECG intervals.

Zelnorm-Induced Diarrhea

IBS with Constipation

In the Phase 3 clinical studies, 8.8% of patients receiving Zelnorm reported diarrhea as an adverse experience compared to 3.8% of patients receiving placebo. The majority of the Zelnorm patients reporting diarrhea had a single episode. In most cases, diarrhea occurred within the first week of treatment. Typically, diarrhea resolved with continued therapy. Overall, the discontinuation rate from the studies due to diarrhea was 1.6% among the Zelnorm-treated patients. In clinical studies, a small number of patients (0.04%) experienced clinically significant diarrhea including hospitalization, hypovolemia, hypotension and need for intravenous fluids. Diarrhea can be the pharmacologic response to Zelnorm.

Chronic Idiopathic Constipation

In the two Phase 3 studies, 6.6% of patients treated with Zelnorm 6 mg b.i.d. and 4.2% of patients treated with Zelnorm 2 mg b.i.d. reported diarrhea as an adverse event, versus 3.0% of patients receiving placebo.

The diarrhea episodes experienced by patients treated with tegaserod occurred early after initiation of treatment (median of 5.5 days), were of short duration (median of 2.5 days), and occurred only once in the majority of patients. Typically, diarrhea resolved with continued therapy; only 0.9% of patients treated with Zelnorm 6 mg b.i.d. discontinued the study due to diarrhea (compared to 0.3% in the Zelnorm 2 mg b.i.d. group and 0.2% in the placebo group).

Adverse Events Occurring in ≥1% of Chronic Idiopathic Constipation Patients And More Frequently On Either Dose of Zelnorm® Than Placebo

System/ Adverse Experience	Zelnorm® 6 mg b.i.d. (n=881)	Zelnorm® 2 mg b.i.d. (n=861)	Placebo (n=861)
Gastrointestinal System Disorders			
Diarrhea	7%	4%	3%
Abdominal Pain	5%	6%	5%
Nausea	5%	5%	4%
Abdominal Distension	4%	3%	4%
Abdominal Pain Upper	2%	2%	2%
Vomiting	2%	1%	1%
Central and Peripheral Nervous System			
Dizziness	2%	1%	2%
Insomnia	2%	1%	1%
Headache Aggravated	1%	1%	0%
General Disorders and Administration Site Conditions			
Fatigue	1%	1%	1%
Infections and Infestations			
Upper Respiratory Tract Infection	4%	3%	2%
Sinusitis	3%	3%	2%
Fungal Infection	0%	1%	1%
Musculoskeletal and Connective Tissue Disorders			
Back Pain	3%	2%	3%
Myalgia	1%	1%	1%
Reproductive System and Breast Disorders			
Dysmenorrhea	1%	2%	1%
Respiratory, Thoracic and Mediastinal Disorders			
Pharyngitis	1%	1%	1%
Sinus Congestion	1%	0%	1%
Renal and Urinary Disorders			
Urinary Tract Infection	1%	2%	1%
Skin and Subcutaneous Tissue Disorders			
Rash	1%	1%	0%
Pruritus	0%	1%	0%

Abdominal Surgeries, Including Cholecystectomy

An increase in abdominal surgeries was observed on Zelnorm (9/2,965; 0.3%) vs. placebo (3/1,740; 0.2%) in the Phase 3 IBS clinical studies. The increase was primarily due to a numerical imbalance in cholecystectomies reported in patients treated with Zelnorm (5/2,965; 0.17%) vs. placebo (1/1,740; 0.06%). In chronic idiopathic constipation clinical trials there was no increase in the frequency of abdominal and pelvic surgeries in active versus placebo groups: 9/1,752; 0.5% on Zelnorm vs. 8/861; 0.9% on placebo. A causal relationship between abdominal surgeries and Zelnorm has not been established.

Other Adverse Events

The following list of adverse events includes those from Phase 3 clinical studies (6 mg b.i.d. or 2 mg b.i.d.) which were reported more frequently (>0.2%) in patients on Zelnorm than placebo; or which were considered by the investigator to be possibly related to Zelnorm and reported more frequently (>0.1%) on Zelnorm than placebo; or which lead to discontinuation more frequently (≥0.1% and in more than 1 patient) on Zelnorm than placebo. The list also contains those serious adverse events from all clinical trials in patients treated with either 6 mg b.i.d. or 2 mg b.i.d. Zelnorm which were either considered by the investigator as possibly drug related, or occurred in at least 2 more patients on Zelnorm than on placebo. Although the events reported occurred during treatment with Zelnorm, they were not necessarily caused by it.

Cardiac Disorders: Angina pectoris, supraventricular tachycardia, syncope

Ear and Labyrinth Disorders: Vertigo

Eye Disorders: Visual disturbance

Gastrointestinal Disorders: Hemorrhoids, proctalgia, stomach discomfort, fecal incontinence, irritable bowel syndrome, dyspepsia, gastroesophageal reflux, gastritis

General Disorders and Administration Site Conditions: Chest pain, peripheral edema

Hepatobiliary Disorders: Cholelithiasis

Immune System Disorders: Hypersensitivity reactions

Investigations: Creatinine phosphokinase increased, increased eosinophil count, low neutrophil count

Metabolism and Nutrition Disorders: Increased appetite

Neoplasms Benign, Malignant and Unspecified (including cysts and polyps): Breast carcinoma

Psychiatric Disorders: Depression, sleep disorder, restlessness

Respiratory, Thoracic and Mediastinal Disorders: Dyspnea, pharyngolaryngeal pain

Reproductive System and Breast Disorders: Miscarriage, menorrhagia

Surgical and Medical Procedures: Cholecystectomy

Vascular Disorders: Flushing, hypotension

Post-Marketing Experience

Voluntary reports of adverse events occurring with the use of Zelnorm include the following: ischemic colitis *(see PRECAUTIONS)*, mesenteric ischemia, gangrenous bowel, rectal bleeding, syncope, hypotension, hypovolemia, electrolyte disorders, suspected sphincter of Oddi spasm, bile duct stone, cholecystitis with elevated transaminases, and hypersensitivity reaction including rash, urticaria, pruritus and serious allergic Type I reactions. Because these cases are reported voluntarily from a population of unknown size, estimates of frequency cannot be made. No causal relationship between these events and Zelnorm use has been established.

Post-marketing reports of diarrhea, which can be a pharmacologic response to Zelnorm, have also been received.

OVERDOSAGE

There have been no reports of human overdosage with Zelnorm® (tegaserod maleate). Single oral doses of 120 mg of tegaserod were administered to 3 healthy volunteers in 1 study. All 3 subjects developed diarrhea and headache. Two of these subjects also reported intermittent abdominal pain, and 1 developed orthostatic hypotension. In 28 healthy subjects exposed to doses of tegaserod of 90 to 180 mg/d for several days, adverse events were diarrhea (100%), headache (57%), abdominal pain (18%), flatulence (18%), nausea (7%) and vomiting (7%).

Based on the large distribution volume and high protein binding of tegaserod it is unlikely that tegaserod could be removed by dialysis. In cases of overdosage treat symptomatically and institute supportive measures as appropriate.

DOSAGE AND ADMINISTRATION

IBS with Constipation: The recommended dosage of Zelnorm® (tegaserod maleate) is 6 mg taken twice daily orally before meals for 4-6 weeks. For those women who respond to therapy at 4-6 weeks, an additional 4-6 week course can be considered.

Chronic Idiopathic Constipation: The recommended dosage of Zelnorm is 6 mg taken twice daily orally before meals. Physicians and patients should periodically assess the need for continued therapy.

HOW SUPPLIED

Zelnorm® (tegaserod maleate) is available as whitish to slightly yellowish, marbled, circular flat tablets with a bevelled edge containing 2 mg or 6 mg tegaserod as follows:

2-mg Tablet - white round engraved with "NVR" and "DL"
Unit Dose (blister pack)
Box of 60 (strips of 10) .... NDC 0078-0355-80

6-mg Tablet - white round engraved with "NVR" and "EH"
Unit Dose (blister pack)
Box of 60 (strips of 10) .... NDC 0078-0356-80
Bottle of 60 .... NDC 0078-0426-20

Store at 25°C (77°F); excursions permitted to 15–30°C (59–86°F).
See USP Controlled Room Temperature. Protect from moisture.

T2004-53
T2004-54

Information for the Patient

Zelnorm®
(tegaserod maleate)
Tablets
(pronounced ZEL-norm, te-gas-a-rod mal-ē-ate)
Rx only

Read this information carefully before you start taking Zelnorm® (ZEL-norm). Read the information you get each time you get more Zelnorm. There may be new information. This information does not take the place of talking to your doctor about your medical condition or treatment.

What is the most important information I should know about Zelnorm?

If you get new or worse abdominal (stomach) pain, or blood in your stools, stop taking Zelnorm right away and tell your doctor. Your doctor may need to do tests to find out if you have a serious problem with your bowel that may require special treatment or hospitalization.

Sometimes Zelnorm causes diarrhea. Stop taking Zelnorm and call your doctor right away if you get so much diarrhea that you get lightheaded, dizzy, or faint.

What is Zelnorm?

Zelnorm is a medicine for:

- The short-term treatment of women who have irritable bowel syndrome (IBS) with constipation (not enough or hard bowel movements) as their main bowel problem. Zelnorm does not work for all women who use it. Zelnorm has not been shown to work in men with IBS with constipation.
- The treatment of patients less than 65 years of age with chronic idiopathic constipation. Chronic constipation means constipation lasting over 6 months. Idiopathic constipation means constipation not due to other diseases or drugs. Zelnorm has not been shown to work in patients with chronic idiopathic constipation who are 65 years of age or older.

Zelnorm increases the movement of stools (bowel movement) through the bowels. Zelnorm does not cure IBS with constipation or chronic idiopathic constipation. For those with IBS with constipation who are helped, Zelnorm reduces pain and discomfort in the abdominal area, bloating, and constipation. For those with chronic idiopathic constipation, Zelnorm increases bowel movements, reduces straining, bloating and abdominal discomfort. If you stop taking Zelnorm, your symptoms may return within 1 or 2 weeks.

Who should not take Zelnorm?

You should not start taking Zelnorm if:

- You now have diarrhea or have diarrhea often.
- You have bad kidney or liver disease.
- You have ever had bowel obstruction (intestinal blockage), symptomatic gallbladder disease, or abdominal adhesions causing pain and/or intestinal blockage.
- You are allergic to Zelnorm or any of its ingredients. The active ingredient in Zelnorm is tegaserod maleate. The inactive ingredients are listed at the end of this leaflet.

Zelnorm may not be right for you. Tell your doctor if you:

- Are pregnant or plan to become pregnant. Zelnorm is not recommended for use by pregnant women.
- Are breast-feeding. Do not breast-feed while you are taking Zelnorm. The drug is likely to pass into breast milk.
- Are taking or planning to take any other medicines, including those you can get without a prescription.

How should I take Zelnorm?

- You should take Zelnorm twice a day on an empty stomach shortly before you eat a meal, or as your doctor prescribes it.
- For IBS with Constipation: You should take Zelnorm for 4 to 6 weeks to treat your IBS symptoms. If you feel better, your doctor may prescribe an additional 4 to 6 weeks of Zelnorm.
- For Chronic Idiopathic Constipation: You should talk to your doctor regularly about whether you need to stay on Zelnorm.
- If you miss a dose of Zelnorm, just skip that dose. Do not take two tablets to make up the missed dose. Instead, just wait until the next time you are supposed to take it and then take your normal dose.

What are the possible side effects of Zelnorm?

Headache and diarrhea were the most common side effects seen with Zelnorm.

Diarrhea was an occasional side effect of treatment with Zelnorm. Most people who got diarrhea had it during the first week after starting Zelnorm. Typically, diarrhea went away with continued therapy. If you get bad diarrhea, or if you get diarrhea together with bad cramping, abdominal pain, fainting, or dizziness, tell your doctor. Your doctor may tell you to stop taking Zelnorm or suggest other ways to manage your diarrhea.

There have been rare cases of rectal bleeding and severe abdominal pain in patients treated with Zelnorm. Some of these problems were related to insufficient blood flow to part of the bowel. It is not known if this was related to Zelnorm use.

In studies, a very small number of patients were reported to have abdominal surgery. In IBS with constipation studies there were a few more reports of abdominal surgery in patients taking Zelnorm than in patients taking a sugar pill. Most of these were related to the gallbladder. It is not known if Zelnorm may increase your chance of abdominal surgery. Gallbladder surgery has been reported to occur more often in IBS patients than in the general population. This list is not complete. Your doctor or pharmacist can give you a more complete list of possible side effects. Talk to your doctor about any side effects you may have.

General information about the safe and effective use of Zelnorm

Keep Zelnorm at room temperature. Do not use Zelnorm past the expiration date shown on the package.

Medicines are sometimes prescribed for conditions that are not mentioned in patient information leaflets. Do not use Zelnorm for a condition for which it was not prescribed. Do not give Zelnorm to other people, even if they have the same symptoms that you have. This leaflet summarizes the most important information about Zelnorm. For more information, talk with your doctor. You can ask your doctor or pharmacist for information about Zelnorm that is written for health professionals. You can also contact the company that makes Zelnorm at 1-866-427-6682 or www.zelnorm.com.

Inactive Ingredients: Zelnorm is available for oral use in the following tablet formulations:

- 2-mg and 6-mg tablets (blister packs) containing the following inactive ingredients: crospovidone, glyceryl monostearate, hypromellose, lactose monohydrate, poloxamer 188, and polyethylene glycol 4000.
- 6-mg tablets (bottles) containing the following inactive ingredients: crospovidone, glyceryl behenate, hypromellose, lactose monohydrate, and colloidal silicon dioxide.

T2004-54
T2004-53/T2004-54

REV: AUGUST 2004 PRINTED IN U.S.A. 89015305
Distributed by:
Novartis Pharmaceuticals Corporation
East Hanover, New Jersey 07936

Shown in Product Identification Guide, page 326

ZOMETA® ℞

[zō-mĕ-ta]
(zoledronic acid) Injection
Concentrate for Intravenous Infusion
Rx only

Prescribing Information

The following prescribing information is based on official labeling in effect July 2004.

DESCRIPTION

Zometa® contains zoledronic acid, a bisphosphonic acid which is an inhibitor of osteoclastic bone resorption. Zoledronic acid is designated chemically as (1-Hydroxy-2-imidazol-1-yl-phosphonoethyl) phosphonic acid monohydrate and its structural formula is

[Structural formula: imidazole ring–CH₂–C(OH)(PO₃H₂)₂ • H₂O]

Zoledronic acid is a white crystalline powder. Its molecular formula is $C_5H_{10}N_2O_7P_2 \bullet H_2O$ and its molar mass is 290.1g/Mol. Zoledronic acid is highly soluble in 0.1N sodium hydroxide solution, sparingly soluble in water and 0.1N hydrochloric acid, and practically insoluble in organic solvents. The pH of a 0.7% solution of zoledronic acid in water is approximately 2.0.

Zometa® (zoledronic acid) Injection is available in vials as a sterile liquid concentrate solution for intravenous infusion. Each 5 mL vial contains 4.264 mg of zoledronic acid monohydrate, corresponding to 4 mg zoledronic acid on an anhydrous basis.

Inactive Ingredients: mannitol, USP, as bulking agent, water for injection and sodium citrate, USP, as buffering agent.

CLINICAL PHARMACOLOGY

General

The principal pharmacologic action of zoledronic acid is inhibition of bone resorption. Although the antiresorptive mechanism is not completely understood, several factors are thought to contribute to this action. *In vitro*, zoledronic acid inhibits osteoclastic activity and induces osteoclast apoptosis. Zoledronic acid also blocks the osteoclastic resorption of mineralized bone and cartilage through its binding to bone. Zoledronic acid inhibits the increased osteoclastic activity and skeletal calcium release induced by various stimulatory factors released by tumors.

Pharmacokinetics

Distribution

Single or multiple (q 28 days) 5-minute or 15-minute infusions of 2, 4, 8 or 16 mg Zometa® were given to 64 patients with cancer and bone metastases. The post-infusion decline of zoledronic acid concentrations in plasma was consistent with a triphasic process showing a rapid decrease from peak concentrations at end-of-infusion to <1% of C_{max} 24 hours post infusion with population half-lives of $t_{1/2\alpha}$ 0.24 hours and $t_{1/2\beta}$ 1.87 hours for the early disposition phases of the drug. The terminal elimination phase of zoledronic acid was prolonged, with very low concentrations in plasma between Days 2 and 28 post infusion, and a terminal elimination half-life $t_{1/2\gamma}$ of 146 hours. The area under the plasma concentration versus time curve (AUC_{0-24h}) of zoledronic acid was dose proportional from 2 to 16 mg. The accumulation of zoledronic acid measured over three cycles was low, with mean AUC_{0-24h} ratios for cycles 2 and 3 versus 1 of 1.13 ± 0.30 and 1.16 ± 0.36, respectively.

In vitro and *ex vivo* studies showed low affinity of zoledronic acid for the cellular components of human blood. Binding to human plasma proteins was approximately 22% and was independent of the concentration of zoledronic acid.

Metabolism

Zoledronic acid does not inhibit human P450 enzymes *in vitro*. Zoledronic acid does not undergo biotransformation *in vivo*. In animal studies, <3% of the administered intravenous dose was found in the feces, with the balance either recovered in the urine or taken up by bone, indicating that the drug is eliminated intact via the kidney. Following an intravenous dose of 20 nCi ^{14}C-zoledronic acid in a patient with cancer and bone metastases, only a single radioactive species with chromatographic properties identical to those of parent drug was recovered in urine, which suggests that zoledronic acid is not metabolized.

Excretion

In 64 patients with cancer and bone metastases on average (± s.d.) 39 ± 16% of the administered zoledronic acid dose was recovered in the urine within 24 hours, with only trace amounts of drug found in urine post Day 2. The cumulative percent of drug excreted in the urine over 0-24 hours was independent of dose. The balance of drug not recovered in urine over 0-24 hours, representing drug presumably bound to bone, is slowly released back into the systemic circulation, giving rise to the observed prolonged low plasma concentrations. The 0-24 hour renal clearance of zoledronic acid was 3.7 ± 2.0 L/h.

Zoledronic acid clearance was independent of dose but dependent upon the patient's creatinine clearance. In a study in patients with cancer and bone metastases, increasing the infusion time of a 4-mg dose of zoledronic acid from 5 minutes (n=5) to 15 minutes (n=7) resulted in a 34% decrease in the zoledronic acid concentration at the end of the infusion ([mean ± SD] 403 ± 118 ng/mL vs 264 ± 86 ng/mL) and a 10% increase in the total AUC (378 ± 116 ng × h/mL vs 420 ± 218 ng × h/mL). The difference between the AUC means was not statistically significant.

Special Populations

Pharmacokinetic data in patients with hypercalcemia are not available.

Pediatrics: Pharmacokinetic data in pediatric patients are not available.

Geriatrics: The pharmacokinetics of zoledronic acid were not affected by age in patients with cancer and bone metastases who ranged in age from 38 years to 84 years.

Race: The pharmacokinetics of zoledronic acid were not affected by race in patients with cancer and bone metastases.

Hepatic Insufficiency: No clinical studies were conducted to evaluate the effect of hepatic impairment on the pharmacokinetics of zoledronic acid.

Renal Insufficiency: The pharmacokinetic studies conducted in 64 cancer patients represented typical clinical populations with normal to moderately impaired renal function. Compared to patients with normal renal function (N=37), patients with mild renal impairment (N=15) showed an average increase in plasma AUC of 15%, whereas patients with moderate renal impairment (N=11) showed an average increase in plasma AUC of 43%. Limited pharmacokinetic data are available for Zometa in patients with severe renal impairment (creatinine clearance <30 mL/min). Based on population PK/PD modeling, the risk of renal deterioration appears to increase with AUC, which is doubled at a creatinine clearance of 10 mL/min. Creatinine clearance is calculated by the Cockcroft-Gault formula:

[See table below]

Zometa systemic clearance in individual patients can be calculated from the population clearance of Zometa, CL (L/h)=$6.5(CL_{cr}/90)^{0.4}$. These formulae can be used to predict the Zometa AUC in patients, where CL = Dose/AUC. The average AUC in patients with normal renal function was 0.42 mg*h/L (%CV 33) following a 4-mg dose of Zometa. However, efficacy and safety of adjusted dosing based on these formulae have not been prospectively assessed. *(See WARNINGS.)*

Pharmacodynamics

Hypercalcemia of Malignancy

Clinical studies in patients with hypercalcemia of malignancy (HCM) showed that single-dose infusions of Zometa are associated with decreases in serum calcium and phosphorus and increases in urinary calcium and phosphorus excretion.

Osteoclastic hyperactivity resulting in excessive bone resorption is the underlying pathophysiologic derangement in hypercalcemia of malignancy (HCM, tumor-induced hypercalcemia) and metastatic bone disease. Excessive release of calcium into the blood as bone is resorbed results in polyuria and gastrointestinal disturbances, with progressive dehydration and decreasing glomerular filtration rate. This, in

Continued on next page

$$CrCl = \frac{[140\text{-age (years)}] \times \text{weight (kg)}}{[72 \times \text{serum creatinine (mg/dL)}]} \quad \{\times\ 0.85 \text{ for female patients}\}$$

Zometa—Cont.

turn, results in increased renal resorption of calcium, setting up a cycle of worsening systemic hypercalcemia. Reducing excessive bone resorption and maintaining adequate fluid administration are, therefore, essential to the management of hypercalcemia of malignancy.

Patients who have hypercalcemia of malignancy can generally be divided into two groups according to the pathophysiologic mechanism involved: humoral hypercalcemia and hypercalcemia due to tumor invasion of bone. In humoral hypercalcemia, osteoclasts are activated and bone resorption is stimulated by factors such as parathyroid-hormone-related protein, which are elaborated by the tumor and circulate systemically. Humoral hypercalcemia usually occurs in squamous-cell malignancies of the lung or head and neck or in genitourinary tumors such as renal-cell carcinoma or ovarian cancer. Skeletal metastases may be absent or minimal in these patients.

Extensive invasion of bone by tumor cells can also result in hypercalcemia due to local tumor products that stimulate bone resorption by osteoclasts. Tumors commonly associated with locally mediated hypercalcemia include breast cancer and multiple myeloma.

Total serum calcium levels in patients who have hypercalcemia of malignancy may not reflect the severity of hypercalcemia, since concomitant hypoalbuminemia is commonly present. Ideally, ionized calcium levels should be used to diagnose and follow hypercalcemic conditions; however, these are not commonly or rapidly available in many clinical situations. Therefore, adjustment of the total serum calcium value for differences in albumin levels (corrected serum calcium, CSC) is often used in place of measurement of ionized calcium; several nomograms are in use for this type of calculation *(see DOSAGE AND ADMINISTRATION)*.

Clinical Trials in Hypercalcemia of Malignancy

Two identical multicenter, randomized, double-blind, double-dummy studies of Zometa 4 mg given as a 5-minute intravenous infusion or pamidronate 90 mg given as a 2-hour intravenous infusion were conducted in 185 patients with hypercalcemia of malignancy (HCM). **NOTE: Administration of Zometa 4 mg given as a 5-minute intravenous infusion has been shown to result in an increased risk of renal toxicity, as measured by increases in serum creatinine, which can progress to renal failure. The incidence of renal toxicity and renal failure has been shown to be reduced when Zometa 4 mg is given as a 15-minute intravenous infusion. Zometa should be administered by intravenous infusion over no less than 15 minutes. *(See WARNINGS and DOSAGE AND ADMINISTRATION.)***

The treatment groups in the clinical studies were generally well balanced with regards to age, sex, race, and tumor types. The mean age of the study population was 59 years; 81% were Caucasian, 15% were Black, and 4% were of other races. Sixty percent of the patients were male. The most common tumor types were lung, breast, head and neck, and renal.

In these studies, HCM was defined as a corrected serum calcium (CSC) concentration of ≥12.0 mg/dL (3.00 mmol/L). The primary efficacy variable was the proportion of patients having a complete response, defined as the lowering of the CSC to ≤10.8 mg/dL (2.70 mmol/L) within 10 days after drug infusion.

To assess the effects of Zometa versus those of pamidronate, the two multicenter HCM studies were combined in a preplanned analysis. The results of the primary analysis revealed that the proportion of patients that had normalization of corrected serum calcium by Day 10 were 88% and 70% for Zometa 4 mg and pamidronate 90 mg, respectively (P=0.002). *(See Figure 1.)* **In these studies, no additional benefit was seen for Zometa 8 mg over Zometa 4 mg; however, the risk of renal toxicity of Zometa 8 mg was significantly greater than that seen with Zometa 4 mg.**

Figure 1
Proportion of Complete Responders by Day 10 in Pooled HCM Studies

% Complete Responders
100%
80%
60%
40%
20%
0%
P=0.002
Zometa® 4 mg (n=86)
Pamidronate 90 mg (n=99)

Secondary efficacy variables from the pooled HCM studies included the proportion of patients who had normalization of corrected serum calcium (CSC) by Day 4; the proportion of patients who had normalization of CSC by Day 7; time to relapse of HCM; and duration of complete response. Time to relapse of HCM was defined as the duration (in days) of normalization of serum calcium from study drug infusion until the last CSC value <11.6 mg/dL (<2.90 mmol/L). Patients who did not have a complete response were assigned a time to relapse of 0 days. Duration of complete response was defined as the duration (in days) from the occurrence of a complete response until the last CSC ≤10.8 mg/dL (2.70 mmol/L). The results of these secondary analyses for Zometa 4 mg and pamidronate 90 mg are shown in Table 1.

Table 1
Secondary Efficacy Variables in Pooled HCM Studies

	Zometa® 4 mg		Pamidronate 90 mg	
Complete Response	**N**	**Response Rate**	**N**	**Response Rate**
By Day 4	86	45.3%	99	33.3%
By Day 7	86	82.6%*	99	63.6%
Duration of Response	**N**	**Median Duration (Days)**	**N**	**Median Duration (Days)**
Time to Relapse	86	30*	99	17
Duration of Complete Response	76	32	69	18

*P less than 0.05 vs. pamidronate 90 mg.

Table 2
Overview of Effiency Population for Phase III Studies (Core Phase)

Study No.	No. of Patients	Median Duration (Planned Duration) Zometa® 4 mg	Zometa® Dose	Control	Patient Population
010	1648	12.0 months (13 months)	4 and 8* mg Q3-4 weeks	Pamidronate 90 mg Q3-4 weeks	Multiple myeloma or metastatic breast cancer
039	643	10.5 months (15 months)	4 and 8* mg Q3 weeks	Placebo	Metastatic prostate cancer
011	773	3.8 months (9 months)	4 and 8* mg Q3 weeks	Placebo	Metastatic solid tumor other than breast or prostate cancer

* Patients who were randomized to the 8-mg Zometa group are not included in any of the analyses in this package insert.

Table 3
Solid Tumor Patients by Cancer Type and Treatment Arm

Cancer Type	Zometa® 4 mg N	Placebo N	Cancer Type	Zometa® 4 mg N	Placebo N
NSCLC	124	121	Genitourinary	6	6
Renal	26	19	Malignant Melanoma	5	4
Small Cell Lung	19	22	Hepatobiliary	3	4
Colorectal	19	16	Thyroid	2	4
Unknown	17	14	Other	3	2
Bladder	11	16	Sarcoma	3	3
GI (Other)	10	12	Neuroendocrine/Carcinoid	2	3
Head and Neck	6	4	Mesothelioma	1	0

[See table 1 above]

Clinical Trials in Multiple Myeloma and Bone Metastases of Solid Tumors

Table 2 describes an overview of the efficacy population in three randomized Zometa trials in patients with multiple myeloma and bone metastases of solid tumors. These trials included a pamidronate-controlled study in breast cancer and multiple myeloma, a placebo-controlled study in prostate cancer and a placebo-controlled study in other solid tumors. The prostate cancer study required documentation of previous bone metastases and 3 consecutive rising PSAs while on hormonal therapy. The other placebo-controlled solid tumor study included patients with bone metastases from malignancies other than breast cancer and prostate cancer, listed in Table 3. These trials were comprised of a core phase and an extension phase. In trials 010 and 011, only the core phase was evaluated for efficacy as a high percentage of patients did not choose to participate in the extension phase. In study 039, both the core and extension phases were evaluated for efficacy showing the Zometa advantage during the first 15 months was maintained without decrement or improvement for 24 months. The design of the clinical trials 010, 011, and 039 does not permit assessment of whether more than one year administration of Zometa is beneficial. The optimal duration of Zometa administration is not known.

[See table 2 above]
[See table 3 above]

Patients evaluable for efficacy were treated with Zometa for a median duration of 12.0 months for multiple myeloma and breast cancer, 10.5 months for prostate cancer, and 3.8 months for the other solid tumors. The studies were amended twice because of renal toxicity. The Zometa infusion duration was increased from 5 minutes to 15 minutes. After all patients had been accrued, but while dosing and follow-up continued, patients in the 8-mg Zometa treatment arm were switched to 4 mg. Patients who were randomized to the Zometa 8-mg group are not included in these analyses.

Each study evaluated skeletal-related events (SREs), defined as any of the following: pathologic fracture, radiation therapy to bone, surgery to bone, or spinal cord compression. Change in antineoplastic therapy due to increased pain was a SRE in the prostate cancer study only. Planned analyses included the proportion of patients with a SRE during the study (the primary endpoint) and time to the first SRE. Results for the two Zometa placebo-controlled studies are given in Table 4.

[See table 4 at top of next page]

In the breast cancer and myeloma trial, efficacy was determined by a non-inferiority analysis comparing Zometa to pamidronate 90 mg for the proportion of patients with a SRE. This analysis required an estimation of pamidronate efficacy. Historical data from 1128 patients in three pamidronate placebo-controlled trials demonstrated that pamidronate decreased the proportion of patients with a SRE by 13.1% (95% CI = 7.3%,18.9%). Results of the comparison of treatment with Zometa compared to pamidronate are given in Table 5.

[See table 5 at top of next page]

INDICATIONS AND USAGE

Hypercalcemia of Malignancy

Zometa® (zoledronic acid) Injection is indicated for the treatment of hypercalcemia of malignancy.

Vigorous saline hydration, an integral part of hypercalcemia therapy, should be initiated promptly and an attempt should be made to restore the urine output to about 2 L/day throughout treatment. Mild or asymptomatic hypercalcemia may be treated with conservative measures (i.e., saline hydration, with or without loop diuretics). Patients should be hydrated adequately throughout the treatment, but overhydration, especially in those patients who have cardiac failure, must be avoided. Diuretic therapy should not be employed prior to correction of hypovolemia. The safety and efficacy of Zometa in the treatment of hypercalcemia associated with hyperparathyroidism or with other non-tumor-related conditions has not been established.

Multiple Myeloma and Bone Metastases of Solid Tumors

Zometa is indicated for the treatment of patients with multiple myeloma and patients with documented bone metastases from solid tumors, in conjunction with standard antineoplastic therapy. Prostate cancer should have progressed after treatment with at least one hormonal therapy.

CONTRAINDICATIONS

Zometa® (zoledronic acid) Injection is contraindicated in patients with clinically significant hypersensitivity to zoledronic acid or other bisphosphonates, or any of the excipients in the formulation of Zometa.

WARNINGS

Due to the risk of clinically significant deterioration in renal function, which may progress to renal failure, single doses of Zometa® (zoledronic acid) should not exceed 4 mg and the duration of infusion should be no less than 15 minutes. In the trials and in post-marketing experience, renal deterioration, progression to renal failure and dialysis, have occurred in patients, including those treated with the approved dose of 4 mg infused over 15 minutes. There have been instances of this occurring after the initial Zometa dose.

SAFETY AND PHARMACOKINETIC DATA ARE LIMITED IN PATIENTS WITH SEVERE RENAL IMPAIRMENT AND THE RISK OF RENAL DETERIORATION IS INCREASED *(see ADVERSE EVENTS, Renal Toxicity)*.

- **ZOMETA TREATMENT IS NOT RECOMMENDED IN PATIENTS WITH BONE METASTASES WITH SEVERE RENAL IMPAIRMENT.** In the clinical studies, patients with serum creatinine>265 μmol/L or >3.0 mg/dL were excluded and there were only eight of 564 patients treated with Zometa 4 mg by 15-minute infusion with a baseline creatinine >2 mg/dL. Limited pharmacokinetic data exists in patients with creatinine clearance <30 mL/min *(see CLINI-*

CAL PHARMACOLOGY). Pre-existing renal insufficiency and multiple cycles of Zometa and other bisphosphonates are risk factors for subsequent renal deterioration with Zometa. Risk factors predisposing to renal deterioration, such as dehydration or the use of other nephrotoxic drugs, should be evaluated.

- **ZOMETA TREATMENT IN PATIENTS WITH HYPERCALCEMIA OF MALIGNANCY WITH SEVERE RENAL IMPAIRMENT SHOULD BE CONSIDERED ONLY AFTER EVALUATING THE RISKS AND BENEFITS OF TREATMENT.** In the clinical studies, patients with serum creatinine >400 μmol/L or >4.5 mg/dL were excluded.

Patients who receive Zometa should have serum creatinine assessed prior to each treatment. Patients treated with Zometa for multiple myeloma and bone metastases of solid tumors should have the dose withheld if renal function has deteriorated. *(See DOSAGE AND ADMINISTRATION.)* Patients with hypercalcemia of malignancy with evidence of deterioration in renal function should be appropriately evaluated as to whether the potential benefit of continued treatment with Zometa outweighs the possible risk.

PREGNANCY: ZOMETA SHOULD NOT BE USED DURING PREGNANCY. Zometa may cause fetal harm when administered to a pregnant woman. In reproductive studies in the pregnant rat, subcutaneous doses equivalent to 2.4 or 4.8 times the human systemic exposure (an i.v. dose of 4 mg based on an AUC comparison) resulted in pre- and post-implantation losses, decreases in viable fetuses and fetal skeletal, visceral and external malformations. *(See PRECAUTIONS, Pregnancy Category D.)*

There are no studies in pregnant women using Zometa. If the patient becomes pregnant while taking this drug, the patient should be apprised of the potential harm to the fetus. Women of childbearing potential should be advised to avoid becoming pregnant.

PRECAUTIONS

General

Standard hypercalcemia-related metabolic parameters, such as serum levels of calcium, phosphate, and magnesium, as well as serum creatinine, should be carefully monitored following initiation of therapy with Zometa® (zoledronic acid) Injection. If hypocalcemia, hypophosphatemia, or hypomagnesemia occur, short-term supplemental therapy may be necessary.

Patients with hypercalcemia of malignancy must be adequately rehydrated prior to administration of Zometa. Loop diuretics should not be used until the patient is adequately rehydrated and should be used with caution in combination with Zometa in order to avoid hypocalcemia. Zometa should be used with caution with other nephrotoxic drugs.

Renal Insufficiency: Limited clinical data are available regarding use of Zometa in patients with renal impairment. Zometa is excreted intact primarily via the kidney, and the risk of adverse reactions, in particular renal adverse reactions, may be greater in patients with impaired renal function. Serum creatinine should be monitored in all patients treated with Zometa prior to each dose.

Studies of Zometa in the treatment of hypercalcemia of malignancy excluded patients with serum creatinine ≥400 μmol/L or ≥4.5 mg/dL. Bone metastasis trials excluded patients with serum creatinine >265 μmol/L or >3.0 mg/dL and there were only eight of 564 patients treated with Zometa 4 mg by 15-minute infusion with a baseline serum creatinine >2 mg/dL. No clinical or pharmacokinetics data are available to guide dose selection or to provide guidance on how to safely use Zometa in patients with severe renal impairment. For multiple myeloma and bone metastases of solid tumors, the use of Zometa in patients with severe renal impairment is not recommended. For hypercalcemia of malignancy, Zometa should be used in patients with severe renal impairment only if the expected clinical benefits outweigh the risk of renal failure and after considering other available treatment options. *(See WARNINGS.)* Dose adjustments of Zometa are not necessary in treating patients for hypercalcemia presenting with mild-to-moderate renal impairment prior to initiation of therapy (serum creatinine <400 μmol/L or <4.5 mg/dL).

Patients receiving Zometa for hypercalcemia of malignancy with evidence of deterioration in renal function should be appropriately evaluated and consideration should be given as to whether the potential benefit of continued treatment with Zometa outweighs the possible risk. In patients receiving Zometa for multiple myeloma and bone metastases of solid tumors, who show evidence of deterioration in renal function, Zometa treatment should be withheld until serum creatinine returns to within 10% of baseline. *(See WARNINGS and DOSAGE AND ADMINISTRATION.)*

Hepatic Insufficiency: Only limited clinical data are available for use of Zometa to treat hypercalcemia of malignancy in patients with hepatic insufficiency, and these data are not adequate to provide guidance on dosage selection or how to safely use Zometa in these patients.

Patients with Asthma: While not observed in clinical trials with Zometa, administration of other bisphosphonates has been associated with bronchoconstriction in aspirin-sensitive asthmatic patients. Zometa should be used with caution in patients with aspirin-sensitive asthma.

Laboratory Tests

Serum creatinine should be monitored prior to each dose of Zometa. Serum calcium, electrolytes, phosphate, magnesium, and hematocrit/hemoglobin should also be monitored regularly. *(See WARNINGS, PRECAUTIONS, DOSAGE AND ADMINISTRATION, and ADVERSE REACTIONS.)*

Table 4
Zometa® Compared to Placebo in Patients with Bone Metastases from Prostate Cancer or Other Solid Tumors

	I. Analysis of Proportion of Patients with a SRE[1]				II. Analysis of Time to the First SRE		
Study	Study Arm & Patient Number	Proportion	Difference[2] & 95% CI	P-value	Median (Days)	Hazard Ratio[3] & 95% CI	P-value
Prostate Cancer	Zometa 4 mg (n=214)	33%	-11% (-20%, -1%)	0.02	NR	0.67 (0.49, 0.91)	0.011
	Placebo (n=208)	44%			321		
Solid Tumors	Zometa 4 mg (n=257)	38%	-7% (-15%, 2%)	0.13	230	0.73 (0.55, 0.96)	0.023
	Placebo (n=250)	44%			163		

[1]SRE = Skeletal Related Event
[2]Difference for the proportion of patients with a SRE of Zometa 4 mg versus placebo.
[3]Hazard ratio for the first occurrence of SRE of Zometa 4 mg versus placebo.

Table 5
Zometa® Compared to Pamidronate in Patients with Multiple Myeloma or Bone Metastases from Breast Cancer

	I. Analysis of Proportion of Patients with a SRE[1]				II. Analysis of Time to the First SRE		
Study	Study Arm & Patient Number	Proportion	Difference[2] & 95% CI	P-value	Median (Days)	Hazard Ratio[3] & 95% CI	P-value
Multiple Myeloma & Breast Cancer	Zometa 4 mg (n=561)	44%	-2% (-7.9%, 3.7%)	0.46	373	0.92 (0.77, 1.09)	0.32
	Pamidronate 90 mg (n=555)	46%			363		

[1]SRE = Skeletal Related Event
[2]Difference for the proportion of patients with a SRE of Zometa 4 mg versus pamidronate 90 mg.
[3]Hazard ratio for the first occurrence of SRE of Zometa 4 mg versus pamidronate 90 mg.

Table 6
Grade 3-4 Laboratory Abnormalities for Serum Creatinine, Serum Calcium, Serum Phosphorus, and Serum Magnesium in Two Clinical Trials in Patients with HCM

	Grade 3				Grade 4			
Laboratory Parameter	**Zometa® 4 mg**		**Pamidronate 90 mg**		**Zometa® 4 mg**		**Pamidronate 90 mg**	
	n/N	**(%)**	**n/N**	**(%)**	**n/N**	**(%)**	**n/N**	**(%)**
Serum Creatinine[1]	2/86	(2.3%)	3/100	(3.0%)	0/86	—	1/100	(1.0%)
Hypocalcemia[2]	1/86	(1.2%)	2/100	(2.0%)	0/86	—	0/100	—
Hypophosphatemia[3]	36/70	(51.4%)	27/81	(33.3%)	1/70	(1.4%)	4/81	(4.9%)
Hypomagnesemia[4]	0/71	—	0/84	—	0/71	—	1/84	(1.2%)

[1]Grade 3 (>3× Upper Limit of Normal); Grade 4 (>6× Upper Limit of Normal)
[2]Grade 3 (<7 mg/dL); Grade 4 (<6 mg/dL)
[3]Grade 3 (<2 mg/dL); Grade 4 (<1 mg/dL)
[4]Grade 3 (<0.8 mEq/L); Grade 4 (<0.5 mEq/L)

Drug Interactions

In vitro studies indicate that zoledronic acid is approximately 22% bound to plasma proteins. *In vitro* studies also indicate that zoledronic acid does not inhibit microsomal CYP450 enzymes. *In vivo* studies showed that zoledronic acid is not metabolized, and is excreted into the urine as the intact drug. However, no *in vivo* drug interaction studies have been performed.

Caution is advised when bisphosphonates are administered with aminoglycosides, since these agents may have an additive effect to lower serum calcium level for prolonged periods. This has not been reported in Zometa clinical trials. Caution should also be exercised when Zometa is used in combination with loop diuretics due to an increased risk of hypocalcemia. Caution is indicated when Zometa is used with other potentially nephrotoxic drugs.

In multiple myeloma patients, the risk of renal dysfunction may be increased when Zometa is used in combination with thalidomide.

Carcinogenesis, Mutagenesis, Impairment of Fertility

Carcinogenesis: Standard lifetime carcinogenicity bioassays were conducted in mice and rats. Mice were given oral doses of zoledronic acid of 0.1, 0.5, or 2.0 mg/kg/day. There was an increased incidence of Harderian gland adenomas in males and females in all treatment groups (at doses ≥0.002 times a human intravenous dose of 4 mg, based on a comparison of relative body surface areas). Rats were given oral doses of zoledronic acid of 0.1, 0.5, or 2.0 mg/kg/day. No increased incidence of tumors was observed (at doses ≤0.2 times the human intravenous dose of 4 mg, based on a comparison of relative body surface areas).

Mutagenesis: Zoledronic acid was not genotoxic in the Ames bacterial mutagenicity assay, in the Chinese hamster ovary cell assay, or in the Chinese hamster gene mutation assay, with or without metabolic activation. Zoledronic acid was not genotoxic in the *in vivo* rat micronucleus assay.

Impairment of Fertility: Female rats were given subcutaneous doses of zoledronic acid of 0.01, 0.03, or 0.1 mg/kg/day beginning 15 days before mating and continuing through gestation. Effects observed in the high-dose group (with systemic exposure of 1.2 times the human systemic exposure following an intravenous dose of 4 mg, based on AUC comparison) included inhibition of ovulation and a decrease in the number of pregnant rats. Effects observed in both the mid-dose group (with systemic exposure of 0.2 times the human systemic exposure following an intravenous dose of 4 mg, based on an AUC comparison) and high-dose group included an increase in pre-implantation losses and a decrease in the number of implantations and live fetuses.

Pregnancy Category D *(See WARNINGS.)*

Bisphosphonates are incorporated into the bone matrix, from where they are gradually released over periods of weeks to years. The extent of bisphosphonate incorporation into adult bone, and hence, the amount available for release back into the systemic circulation, is directly related to the total dose and duration of bisphosphonate use. Although there are no data on fetal risk in humans, bisphosphonates do cause fetal harm in animals, and animal data suggest that uptake of bisphosphonates into fetal bone is greater than into maternal bone. Therefore, there is a theoretical risk of fetal harm (e.g., skeletal and other abnormalities) if a woman becomes pregnant after completing a course of bisphosphonate therapy. The impact of variables such as time between cessation of bisphosphonate therapy to conception, the particular bisphosphonate used, and the route of administration (intravenous versus oral) on this risk has not been established.

In female rats given subcutaneous doses of zoledronic acid of 0.01, 0.03, or 0.1 mg/kg/day beginning 15 days before mating and continuing through gestation, the number of stillbirths was increased and survival of neonates was decreased in the mid- and high-dose groups (≥0.2 times the human systemic exposure following an intravenous dose of 4 mg, based on an AUC comparison). Adverse maternal effects were observed in all dose groups (with a systemic exposure of ≥0.07 times the human systemic exposure following an intravenous dose of 4 mg, based on an AUC comparison) and included dystocia and periparturient mortality in pregnant rats allowed to deliver. Maternal mortality may have been related to drug-induced inhibition of skeletal calcium mobilization, resulting in periparturient hypocalcemia. This appears to be a bisphosphonate class effect.

In pregnant rats given a subcutaneous dose of zoledronic acid of 0.1, 0.2, or 0.4 mg/kg/day during gestation, adverse fetal effects were observed in the mid- and high-dose groups (with systemic exposures of 2.4 and 4.8 times, respectively, the human systemic exposure following an intravenous dose

Continued on next page

Zometa—Cont.

of 4 mg, based on an AUC comparison). These adverse effects included increases in pre- and post-implantation losses, decreases in viable fetuses, and fetal skeletal, visceral, and external malformations. Fetal skeletal effects observed in the high-dose group included unossified or incompletely ossified bones, thickened, curved or shortened bones, wavy ribs, and shortened jaw. Other adverse fetal effects observed in the high-dose group included reduced lens, rudimentary cerebellum, reduction or absence of liver lobes, reduction of lung lobes, vessel dilation, cleft palate, and edema. Skeletal variations were also observed in the low-dose group (with systemic exposure of 1.2 times the human systemic exposure following an intravenous dose of 4 mg, based on an AUC comparison). Signs of maternal toxicity were observed in the high-dose group and included reduced body weights and food consumption, indicating that maximal exposure levels were achieved in this study.

In pregnant rabbits given subcutaneous doses of zoledronic acid of 0.01, 0.03, or 0.1 mg/kg/day during gestation (≤0.5 times the human intravenous dose of 4 mg, based on a comparison of relative body surface areas), no adverse fetal effects were observed. Maternal mortality and abortion occurred in all treatment groups (at doses ≥0.05 times the human intravenous dose of 4 mg, based on a comparison of relative body surface areas). Adverse maternal effects were associated with, and may have been caused by, drug-induced hypocalcemia.

Nursing Mothers

It is not known whether Zometa is excreted in human milk. Because many drugs are excreted in human milk, and because Zometa binds to bone long-term, Zometa should not be administered to a nursing woman.

Pediatric Use

The safety and effectiveness of Zometa in pediatric patients have not been established. Because of long-term retention in bone, Zometa should only be used in children if the potential benefit outweighs the potential risk.

Geriatric Use

Clinical studies of Zometa in hypercalcemia of malignancy included 34 patients who were 65 years of age or older. No significant differences in response rate or adverse reactions were seen in geriatric patients receiving Zometa as compared to younger patients. Controlled clinical studies of Zometa in the treatment of multiple myeloma and bone metastases of solid tumors in patients over age 65 revealed similar efficacy and safety in older and younger patients. Because decreased renal function occurs more commonly in the elderly, special care should be taken to monitor renal function.

ADVERSE REACTIONS

Hypercalcemia of Malignancy

Adverse reactions to Zometa® (zoledronic acid) injection are usually mild and transient and similar to those reported for other bisphosphonates. Intravenous administration has been most commonly associated with fever. Occasionally, patients experience a flu-like syndrome consisting of fever, chills, bone pain and/or arthralgias, and myalgias. Gastrointestinal reactions such as nausea and vomiting have been reported following intravenous infusion of Zometa. Local reactions at the infusion site, such as redness or swelling, were observed infrequently. In most cases, no specific treatment is required and the symptoms subside after 24-48 hours.

Rare cases of rash, pruritus, and chest pain have been reported following treatment with Zometa.

As with other bisphosphonates, cases of conjunctivitis and hypomagnesemia have been reported following treatment with Zometa.

Grade 3 and Grade 4 laboratory abnormalities for serum creatinine, serum calcium, serum phosphorus, and serum magnesium observed in two clinical trials of Zometa in patients with HCM are shown in Table 6.

[See table 6 at top of previous page]

Table 7 provides adverse events that were reported by 10% or more of the 189 patients treated with Zometa 4 mg or pamidronate 90 mg from the two controlled multi-center HCM trials. Adverse events are listed regardless of presumed causality to study drug.

Table 8

Percentage of Patients with Adverse Events ≥10% Reported in Three Bone Metastases Clinical Trials By Body System

	Zometa® 4 mg		Pamidronate 90 mg		Placebo	
	n	(%)	n	(%)	n	(%)
Patients Studied						
Total No. of Patients	1031	(100)	556	(100)	455	(100)
Total No. of Patients with any AE	1015	(98)	548	(99)	445	(98)
Blood and Lymphatic						
Anemia	344	(33)	175	(32)	128	(28)
Neutropenia	124	(12)	83	(15)	35	(8)
Thrombocytopenia	102	(10)	53	(10)	20	(4)
Gastrointestinal						
Nausea	476	(46)	266	(48)	171	(38)
Vomiting	333	(32)	183	(33)	122	(27)
Constipation	320	(31)	162	(29)	174	(38)
Diarrhea	249	(24)	162	(29)	83	(18)
Abdominal Pain	143	(14)	81	(15)	48	(11)
Dyspepsia	105	(10)	74	(13)	31	(7)
Stomatitis	86	(8)	65	(12)	14	(3)
Sore Throat	82	(8)	61	(11)	17	(4)
General Disorders and Administration Site						
Fatigue	398	(39)	240	(43)	130	(29)
Pyrexia	328	(32)	172	(31)	89	(20)
Weakness	252	(24)	108	(19)	114	(25)
Edema Lower Limb	215	(21)	126	(23)	84	(19)
Rigors	112	(11)	62	(11)	28	(6)
Infections						
Urinary Tract Infection	124	(12)	50	(9)	41	(9)
Upper Respiratory Tract Infection	101	(10)	82	(15)	30	(7)
Metabolism						
Anorexia	231	(22)	81	(15)	105	(23)
Weight Decreased	164	(16)	50	(9)	61	(13)
Dehydration	145	(14)	60	(11)	59	(13)
Appetite Decreased	130	(13)	48	(9)	45	(10)
Musculoskeletal						
Bone Pain	569	(55)	316	(57)	284	(62)
Myalgia	239	(23)	143	(26)	74	(16)
Arthralgia	216	(21)	131	(24)	73	(16)
Back Pain	156	(15)	106	(19)	40	(9)
Pain in Limb	143	(14)	84	(15)	52	(11)
Neoplasms						
Malignant Neoplasm Aggravated	205	(20)	97	(17)	89	(20)
Nervous						
Headache	191	(19)	149	(27)	50	(11)
Dizziness (excluding vertigo)	180	(18)	91	(16)	58	(13)
Insomnia	166	(16)	111	(20)	73	(16)
Paresthesia	149	(15)	85	(15)	35	(8)
Hypoesthesia	127	(12)	65	(12)	43	(10)
Psychiatric						
Depression	146	(14)	95	(17)	49	(11)
Anxiety	112	(11)	73	(13)	37	(8)
Confusion	74	(7)	39	(7)	47	(10)
Respiratory						
Dyspnea	282	(27)	155	(28)	107	(24)
Cough	224	(22)	129	(23)	65	(14)
Skin						
Alopecia	125	(12)	80	(14)	36	(8)
Dermatitis	114	(11)	74	(13)	38	(8)

Table 7

Percentage of Patients with Adverse Events ≥10% Reported in Hypercalcemia of Malignancy Clinical Trials By Body System

	Zometa® 4 mg		Pamidronate 90 mg	
	n	(%)	n	(%)
Patients Studied				
Total No. of Patients Studied	86	(100)	103	(100)
Total No. of Patients with any AE	81	(94.2)	95	(92.2)
Body as a Whole				
Fever	38	(44.2)	34	(33.0)
Progression of Cancer	14	(16.3)	21	(20.4)
Digestive				
Nausea	25	(29.1)	28	(27.2)
Constipation	23	(26.7)	13	(12.6)
Diarrhea	15	(17.4)	17	(16.5)
Abdominal Pain	14	(16.3)	13	(12.6)
Vomiting	12	(14.0)	17	(16.5)
Anorexia	8	(9.3)	14	(13.6)
Cardiovascular				
Hypotension	9	(10.5)	2	(1.9)
Hemic and Lymphatic System				
Anemia	19	(22.1)	18	(17.5)
Infections				
Moniliasis	10	(11.6)	4	(3.9)
Laboratory Abnormalities				
Hypophosphatemia	11	(12.8)	2	(1.9)
Hypokalemia	10	(11.6)	16	(15.5)
Hypomagnesemia	9	(10.5)	5	(4.9)
Musculoskeletal				
Skeletal Pain	10	(11.6)	10	(9.7)
Nervous				
Insomnia	13	(15.1)	10	(9.7)
Anxiety	12	(14.0)	8	(7.8)
Confusion	11	(12.8)	13	(12.6)
Agitation	11	(12.8)	8	(7.8)
Respiratory				
Dyspnea	19	(22.1)	20	(19.4)
Coughing	10	(11.6)	12	(11.7)
Urogenital				
Urinary Tract Infection	12	(14.0)	15	(14.6)

The following adverse events from the two controlled multicenter HCM trials (n=189) were reported by a greater percentage of patients treated with Zometa 4 mg than with pamidronate 90 mg and occurred with a frequency of greater than or equal to 5% but less than 10%. Adverse events are listed regardless of presumed causality to study drug.

Body as a Whole: asthenia, chest pain, leg edema, mucositis, and metastases; ***Digestive System:*** dysphagia; ***Hemic and Lymphatic System:*** granulocytopenia, thrombocytopenia, and pancytopenia; ***Infection:*** non-specific infection; ***Laboratory Abnormalities:*** hypocalcemia; ***Metabolic and Nutritional:*** dehydration; ***Musculoskeletal:*** arthralgias; ***Nervous System:*** headache, somnolence; ***Respiratory System:*** pleural effusion

NOTE: In the HCM clinical trials, pamidronate 90 mg was given as a 2-hour intravenous infusion. The relative safety of pamidronate 90 mg given as a 2-hour intravenous infusion compared to the same dose given as a 24-hour intravenous infusion has not been adequately studied in controlled clinical trials.

Multiple Myeloma and Bone Metastases of Solid Tumors

The safety analysis includes patients treated in the core and extension phases of the trials. The analysis includes the 2042 patients treated with Zometa 4 mg, pamidronate 90 mg or placebo in the three controlled multicenter Bone Metastases trials, including 969 patients completing the efficacy phase of the trial, and 619 patients that continued in the safety extension phase. Only 347 patients completed the extension phases and were followed two years (or 21 months for the other solid tumor patients). The median duration of exposure for safety analysis for Zometa 4 mg (core plus extension phases) was 12.8 months for breast cancer and multiple myeloma, 10.8 months for prostate cancer, and 4.0 months for other solid tumors.

Table 8 describes adverse events that were reported by ≥10% of patients. Adverse events are listed regardless of presumed causality to study drug.

[See table 8 at left]

Grade 3 and Grade 4 laboratory abnormalities for serum creatinine, serum calcium, serum phosphorus, and serum magnesium observed in three clinical trials of Zometa in patients with Bone Metastases are shown in Tables 9 and 10.

[See table 9 at top of next page]

[See table 10 at top of next page]

Among the less frequently occurring adverse events (<15% of patients), rigors, hypokalemia, influenza-like illness, and hypocalcemia showed a trend for more events with bisphosphonate administration (Zometa 4 mg and pamidronate groups) compared to the placebo group.

Less common adverse events reported more often with Zometa 4 mg than pamidronate included decreased weight, which was reported in 16% of patients in the Zometa 4 mg group compared with 9% in the pamidronate group. Decreased appetite was reported in slightly more patients in the Zometa 4 mg (13%) compared with the pamidronate (9%) and placebo (10%) groups, but the clinical significance of these small differences is not clear.

Renal Toxicity

In the bone metastases trials renal deterioration was defined as an increase of 0.5 mg/dL for patients with normal baseline creatinine (<1.4 mg/dL) or an increase of 1.0 mg/dL for patients with an abnormal baseline creatinine (≥1.4 mg/dL). The following are data on the incidence of renal deterioration in patients receiving Zometa 4 mg over 15 minutes in these trials. *(See Table 11.)*

Table 11
Percentage of Patients with Renal Function Deterioration Who Were Randomized Following the 15-Minute Infusion Amendment

Patient Population/Baseline Creatinine				
Multiple Myeloma and Breast Cancer	**Zometa® 4 mg**		**Pamidronate 90 mg**	
	n/N	**(%)**	**n/N**	**(%)**
Normal	27/246	(11%)	23/246	(9.3%)
Abnormal	2/26	(7.7%)	2/22	(9.1%)
Total	29/272	(10.7%)	25/268	(9.3%)
Solid Tumors	**Zometa® 4 mg**		**Placebo**	
	n/N	**(%)**	**n/N**	**(%)**
Normal	17/154	(11%)	10/143	(7%)
Abnormal	1/11	(9.1%)	1/20	(5%)
Total	18/165	(10.9%)	11/163	(6.7%)
Prostate Cancer	**Zometa® 4 mg**		**Placebo**	
	n/N	**(%)**	**n/N**	**(%)**
Normal	12/82	(14.6%)	8/68	(11.8%)
Abnormal	4/10	(40%)	2/10	(20%)
Total	16/92	(17.4%)	10/78	(12.8%)

The risk of deterioration in renal function appeared to be related to time on study, whether patients were receiving Zometa (4 mg over 15 minutes), placebo, or pamidronate.

Evaluation of serum creatinine is recommended prior to each cycle of therapy with Zometa. In patients receiving Zometa for multiple myeloma and bone metastases of solid tumors, who show evidence of deterioration in renal function, Zometa treatment should be withheld until serum creatinine returns to within 10% of baseline.

In the trials and in post-marketing experience, renal deterioration, progression to renal failure and dialysis have occurred in patients with normal and abnormal baseline renal function, including patients treated with 4 mg infused over a 15-minute period. There have been instances of this occurring after the initial Zometa dose.

Post-Marketing Experience

Cases of osteonecrosis (primarily involving the jaws) have been reported in patients treated with bisphosphonates. The majority of the reported cases are in cancer patients attendant to a dental procedure. Osteonecrosis of the jaws has multiple well documented risk factors including a diagnosis of cancer, concomitant therapies (e.g., chemotherapy, radiotherapy, corticosteroids) and co-morbid conditions (e.g., anemia, coagulopathies, infection, pre-existing oral disease). Although causality cannot be determined, it is prudent to avoid dental surgery as recovery may be prolonged.

OVERDOSAGE

There is no experience of acute overdose with Zometa® (zoledronic acid) Injection. Two patients received Zometa 32 mg over 5 minutes in clinical trials. Neither patient experienced any clinical or laboratory toxicity. Overdosage may cause clinically significant hypocalcemia, hypophosphatemia, and hypomagnesemia. Clinically relevant reductions in serum levels of calcium, phosphorus, and magnesium should be corrected by intravenous administration of calcium gluconate, potassium or sodium phosphate, and magnesium sulfate, respectively.

In an open-label study of zoledronic acid 4 mg in breast-cancer patients, a female patient received a single 48-mg dose of zoledronic acid in error. Two days after the overdose the patient experienced a single episode of hyperthermia (38°C), which resolved after treatment. All other evaluations were normal, and the patient was discharged seven days after the overdose.

A patient with Non-Hodgkin's lymphoma received zoledronic acid 4 mg daily on four successive days for a total dose of 16 mg. The patient developed paresthesia and abnormal liver function tests with increased GGT (nearly 100U/L, each value unknown). The outcome of this case is not known.

In controlled clinical trials, administration of Zometa 4 mg as an intravenous infusion over 5 minutes has been shown to increase the risk of renal toxicity compared to the same dose administered as a 15-minute intravenous infusion. In controlled clinical trials, Zometa 8 mg has been shown to be associated with an increased risk of renal toxicity compared to Zometa 4 mg, even when given as a 15-minute intravenous infusion, and was not associated with added benefit in patients with hypercalcemia of malignancy. **Single doses of Zometa should not exceed 4 mg and the duration of the intravenous infusion should be no less than 15 minutes. *(See WARNINGS.)* In the trials and in post-marketing experience, renal deterioration, progression to renal failure and dialysis, have occurred in patients, including those treated with the approved dose of 4 mg infused over 15 minutes. There have been instances of this occurring after the initial Zometa dose.**

Table 9
Grade 3 Laboratory Abnormalities for Serum Creatinine, Serum Calcium, Serum Phosphorus, and Serum Magnesium in Three Clinical Trials in Patients with Bone Metastases

	Grade 3					
Laboratory Parameter	**Zometa® 4 mg**		**Pamidronate 90 mg**		**Placebo**	
	n/N	**(%)**	**n/N**	**(%)**	**n/N**	**(%)**
Serum Creatinine[1]*	7/529	(1.3%)	4/268	(1.5%)	4/241	(1.7%)
Hypocalcemia[2]	6/973	(0.6%)	4/536	(0.7%)	0/415	—
Hypophosphatemia[3]	115/973	(11.8%)	38/537	(7.1%)	14/415	(3.4%)
Hypermagnesemia[4]	19/971	(2.0%)	2/535	(0.4%)	8/415	(1.9%)
Hypomagnesemia[5]	1/971	(0.1%)	0/535	—	1/415	(0.2%)

[1]Grade 3 (>3× Upper Limit of Normal); Grade 4 (>6× Upper Limit of Normal)
*Serum creatinine data for all patients randomized after the 15-minute infusion amendment
[2]Grade 3 (<7 mg/dL); Grade 4 (<6 mg/dL)
[3]Grade 3 (<2 mg/dL); Grade 4 (<1 mg/dL)
[4]Grade 3 (>3 mEq/L); Grade 4 (>8 mEq/L)
[5]Grade 3 (<0.9 mEq/L); Grade 4 (<0.7 mEq/L)

Table 10
Grade 4 Laboratory Abnormalities for Serum Creatinine, Serum Calcium, Serum Phosphorus, and Serum Magnesium in Three Clinical Trials in Patients with Bone Metastases

	Grade 4					
Laboratory Parameter	**Zometa® 4 mg**		**Pamidronate 90 mg**		**Placebo**	
	n/N	**(%)**	**n/N**	**(%)**	**n/N**	**(%)**
Serum Creatinine[1]*	2/529	(0.4%)	1/268	(0.4%)	0/241	—
Hypocalcemia[2]	7/973	(0.7%)	3/536	(0.6%)	2/415	(0.5%)
Hypophosphatemia[3]	5/973	(0.5%)	0/537	—	1/415	(0.2%)
Hypermagnesemia[4]	0/971	—	0/535	—	2/415	(0.5%)
Hypomagnesemia[5]	2/971	(0.2%)	1/535	(0.2%)	0/415	—

[1]Grade 3 (>3× Upper Limit of Normal); Grade 4 (>6× Upper Limit of Normal)
*Serum creatinine data for all patients randomized after the 15-minute infusion amendment
[2]Grade 3 (<7 mg/dL); Grade 4 (<6 mg/dL)
[3]Grade 3 (<2 mg/dL); Grade 4 (<1 mg/dL)
[4]Grade 3 (>3 mEq/L); Grade 4 (>8 mEq/L)
[5]Grade 3 (<0.9 mEq/L); Grade 4 (<0.7 mEq/L)

DOSAGE AND ADMINISTRATION

Hypercalcemia of Malignancy

Consideration should be given to the severity of, as well as the symptoms of, tumor-induced hypercalcemia when considering use of Zometa® (zoledronic acid) Injection. Vigorous saline hydration alone may be sufficient to treat mild, asymptomatic hypercalcemia.

The maximum recommended dose of Zometa in hypercalcemia of malignancy (albumin-corrected serum calcium* ≥12 mg/dL [3.0 mmol/L]) is 4 mg. The 4-mg dose must be given as a single-dose intravenous infusion over **no less than 15 minutes.**

Patients should be adequately rehydrated prior to administration of Zometa. *(See WARNINGS and PRECAUTIONS.)*

Retreatment with Zometa 4 mg, may be considered if serum calcium does not return to normal or remain normal after initial treatment. It is recommended that a minimum of 7 days elapse before retreatment, to allow for full response to the initial dose. Renal function must be carefully monitored in all patients receiving Zometa and possible deterioration in renal function must be assessed prior to retreatment with Zometa. *(See WARNINGS and PRECAUTIONS.)*

*Albumin-corrected serum calcium (Cca, mg/dL) = Ca + 0.8 (mid-range albumin-measured albumin in mg/dL).

Multiple Myeloma and Metastatic Bone Lesions From Solid Tumors

The recommended dose of Zometa in patients with multiple myeloma and metastatic bone lesions from solid tumors is 4 mg infused over 15 minutes every three or four weeks. The optimal duration of therapy is not known. Treatment of patients with severe renal impairment is not recommended because of lack of safety and efficacy information in this patient population and increased risk of renal toxicity. In the clinical studies, patients with serum creatinine >265 μmol/L or >3.0 mg/dL were excluded. There were only eight of 564 patients treated with Zometa 4 mg by 15-minute infusion who had a baseline serum creatinine >2 mg/dL.

Patients should also be administered an oral calcium supplement of 500 mg and a multiple vitamin containing 400 IU of Vitamin D daily.

Serum creatinine should be measured before each Zometa dose and treatment should be withheld for renal deterioration. In the clinical studies, renal deterioration was defined as follows:

- For patients with normal baseline creatinine, increase of 0.5 mg/dL
- For patients with abnormal baseline creatinine, increase of 1.0 mg/dL

In the clinical studies, Zometa treatment was resumed only when the creatinine returned to within 10% of the baseline value.

Preparation of Solution

Vials of Zometa concentrate for infusion contain overfill allowing for the withdrawal of 5 mL of concentrate (equivalent to 4 mg zoledronic acid). This concentrate should immediately be diluted in 100 mL of sterile 0.9% Sodium Chloride, USP, or 5% Dextrose Injection, USP. Do not store undiluted concentrate in a syringe, to avoid inadvertent injection. The dose must be given as a single intravenous infusion over no less than 15 minutes.

If not used immediately after dilution with infusion media, for microbiological integrity, the solution should be refrigerated at 2°C-8°C (36°F-46°F). The refrigerated solution should then be equilibrated to room temperature prior to administration. The total time between dilution, storage in the refrigerator, and end of administration must not exceed 24 hours.

Zometa must not be mixed with calcium-containing infusion solutions, such as Lactated Ringer's solution, and should be administered as a single intravenous solution in a line separate from all other drugs.

Method of Administration: **Due to the risk of clinically significant deterioration in renal function, which may progress to renal failure, single doses of Zometa should not exceed 4 mg and the duration of infusion should be no less than 15 minutes. *(See WARNINGS.)* In the trials and in post-marketing experience, renal deterioration, progression to renal failure and dialysis, have occurred in patients, including those treated with the approved dose of 4 mg infused over 15 minutes. There have been instances of this occurring after the initial Zometa dose.**

There must be strict adherence to the intravenous administration recommendations for Zometa in order to decrease the risk of deterioration in renal function.

Note: **Parenteral drug products should be inspected visually for particulate matter and discoloration prior to administration, whenever solution and container permit.**

HOW SUPPLIED

Each 5 mL vial contains 4.264 mg zoledronic acid monohydrate, corresponding to 4 mg zoledronic acid on an anhydrous basis, 220 mg of mannitol, USP, water for injection and 24 mg of sodium citrate, USP.

Carton of 1 vial .... NDC 0078-0387-25

Store at 25°C (77°F); excursions permitted to 15°C-30°C (59°F-86°F).

T2004-27

REV: MARCH 2004 Printed in U.S.A.

Manufactured by
Novartis Pharma Stein AG
Stein, Switzerland for
Novartis Pharmaceuticals Corporation
East Hanover, NJ 07936
©Novartis

Shown in Product Identification Guide, page 326

Continued on next page

Novavax, Inc.
508 LAPP ROAD
MALVERN, PA 19355

Direct Inquires to:
Professional Services Department
(888) 466-8282
For Medical Information Contact:
In Emergencies:
(888) 466-8282

AVC™ ℞
(sulfanilamide)
Cream

Prescribing Information as of March 1999

DESCRIPTION

AVC™ is a preparation for vaginal administration for the treatment of *Candida albicans* infections and available in the following forms:

AVC Cream

Each tube contains:
Sulfanilamide 15.0%
in a water-miscible, non-staining base made from lactose, propylene glycol, stearic acid, diglycol stearate, methylparaben, propylparaben, trolamine, and water; buffered with lactic acid to an acid pH of approximately 4.3.

Sulfanilamide is an anti-infective agent. It is *p*-amino-benzenesulfonamide with the chemical structure:

H_2N–[benzene ring]–SO_2NH_2

Sulfanilamide occurs as a white odorless crystalline powder with a slightly bitter taste and sweet aftertaste. It is slightly soluble in water, alcohol, acetone, glycerin, propylene glycol, hydrochloric acid, and solutions of potassium and sodium hydroxide. It is practically insoluble in chloroform, ether, benzene, and petroleum ether.

CLINICAL PHARMACOLOGY

Sulfanilamide has been a useful ingredient of vaginal formulations for about four decades. It blocks certain metabolic processes essential for the growth of susceptible bacteria. In AVC, the sulfanilamide is in a specially compounded base buffered to the pH (about 4.3) of the normal vagina to encourage the presence of the normally occurring Döderlein's bacilli of the vagina.

The use of AVC for the treatment of vulvovaginitis caused by *Candida albicans* is supported by three clinical investigations. The three studies show AVC with sulfanilamide to be significantly more effective ($p \leq 0.01$) than placebo as follows:

In Study I, the ratio of effectiveness was 71% for the AVC with sulfanilamide versus 49% for placebo with 30 days of treatment;

In Study II, the percentages were 48% and 24%, respectively, with 15 days of treatment;

In Study III, the percentages were 66% versus 33%, respectively, with 30 days of treatment.

INDICATIONS AND USAGE

For the treatment of vulvovaginitis caused by *Candida albicans*. (See CLINICAL PHARMACOLOGY.)

CONTRAINDICATIONS

AVC should not be used in patients known to be sensitive to this product or to the sulfonamides.

PRECAUTIONS

General

Because sulfonamides are absorbed from the vaginal mucosa, the usual precautions for oral sulfonamides apply. Patients should be observed for skin rash or evidence of systemic toxicity, and if these develop, the medications should be discontinued.

Deaths associated with administration of oral sulfonamides have reportedly occurred from hypersensitivity reactions, agranulocytosis, aplastic anemia, and other blood dyscrasias. Goiter production, diuresis, and hypoglycemia have reportedly occurred rarely in patients receiving oral sulfonamides. Cross-sensitivity may exist with these agents. Rats appear to be especially susceptible to the goitrogenic effects of sulfonamides, and long-term administration has reportedly produced thyroid malignancies in this species.

Vaginal applicators should be used with caution after the seventh month of pregnancy.

Information For Patients

The doctor should advise the patient that in the event unusual local itching and burning occur, or other unusual symptoms develop, medication should be discontinued and not restarted without further consultation.

Drug Interactions

Drug interactions have not been documented with AVC.

Carcinogenesis, Mutagenesis, Impairment of Fertility

No data are available on long-term potential of AVC for carcinogenicity, mutagenicity, or impairment of fertility in animals or humans.

Pregnancy.

Teratogenic Effects. Pregnancy Category C:

Animal reproductive studies have been conducted with sulfonamides, including sulfanilamide (see below). It is not known whether AVC can cause fetal harm when administered to a pregnant woman or can affect reproductive capacity. AVC should be given to a pregnant woman only if clearly needed.

Sulfonamides, including sulfanilamide, readily pass through the placenta and reach fetal circulation. The concentration in the fetus is from 50–90% of that in the maternal blood and if high enough, can cause toxic effects. The safe use of sulfonamides, including sulfanilamide, in pregnancy has not been established. The teratogenic potential of most sulfonamides has not been thoroughly investigated in either animals or humans. However, a significant increase in the incidence of cleft palate and other bony abnormalities of off-spring has been observed with certain sulfonamides of the short-, intermediate-, and long-acting types (including sulfanilamide) when given to pregnant rats and mice at high oral doses (seven to 25 times the human therapeutic oral dose).

Nursing Mothers

Sulfanilamide should be avoided in nursing mothers because absorbed sulfonamides will appear in maternal milk, and have caused kernicterus in the newborn. Because of the potential for serious adverse reactions in nursing infants from sulfonamides, a decision should be made whether to discontinue nursing or to discontinue the drug.

Pediatric Use

Safety and effectiveness of AVC in pediatric patients have not been established.

ADVERSE REACTIONS

Local sensitivity reactions such as increased discomfort or a burning sensation have occasionally been reported following the use of topical sulfonamides. With the use of AVC Cream, sensitivity reactions (only local) were reported for 0.2% of the investigational patients.

Treatment should be discontinued if either local or systemic manifestations of sulfonamide toxicity or sensitivity occur.

DRUG ABUSE AND DEPENDENCE

Tolerance, abuse, or dependence with AVC have not been reported.

OVERDOSAGE

There have been no reports of accidental overdosage with AVC.

The acute oral LD_{50} of sulfanilamide is 3700–4200 mg/kg in mice.

The minimum human lethal dose of AVC has not been established.

It is not known if AVC is dialyzable.

DOSAGE AND ADMINISTRATION

One applicatorful (about 6 g) once or twice daily. Improvements in symptoms should occur within a few days, but treatment should be continued for a period of 30 days.

Douching with a suitable solution before insertion may be recommended for hygienic purposes.

HOW SUPPLIED

AVC Cream

NDC 66500-103-04 4 oz tube with applicator
Store at room temperature, below 86°F. Protect from cold.
Product darkens with age. Potency is maintained throughout labeled shelf life when stored as directed.
Store at room temperature, below 86°F. Protect from excessive cold and moisture.
Prescribing Information as of July 2003
Manufactured by:
King Pharmaceuticals, Inc.
Bristol, TN 37620
50007637
Distributed by:
Novavax, Inc.
Columbia, MD 21046

ESTRASORB® ℞
[ĕs'trā-sōrb]
(estradiol topical emulsion)
Rx only
Prescribing Information

ESTROGENS INCREASE THE RISK OF ENDOMETRIAL CANCER

Close clinical surveillance of all women taking estrogen is important. Adequate diagnostic measures, including endometrial sampling when indicated, should be undertaken to rule out malignancy in all cases of undiagnosed persistent or recurring abnormal vaginal bleeding. There is no evidence that the use of "natural" estrogens results in a different endometrial risk profile than synthetic estrogens at equivalent estrogenic doses.

CARDIOVASCULAR AND OTHER RISKS

Estrogens with or without progestins should not be used for the prevention of cardiovascular disease.

The Women's Health Initiative (WHI) study reported increased risks of myocardial infarction, stroke, invasive breast cancer, pulmonary emboli, and deep vein thrombosis in postmenopausal women during 5 years of treatment with conjugated equine estrogens (CE 0.625 mg) combined with medroxyprogesterone acetate (MPA 2.5 mg) relative to placebo (see **CLINICAL PHARMACOLOGY, Clinical Studies**). Other doses of conjugated estrogens and medroxyprogesterone acetate, and other combinations of estrogens and progestins were not studies in the WHI and, in the absence of comparable data, these risks should be assumed to be similar. Because of these risks, estrogens with or without progestins should be prescribed at the lowest effective doses and for the shortest duration consistent with treatment goals and risks for the individual woman.

DESCRIPTION

Estrasorb® (estradiol topical emulsion) is designed to deliver estradiol to the blood circulation following topical application of an emulsion. Each gram of Estrasorb contains 2.5 mg of estradiol hemihydrate USP, EP, which is encapsulated using a micellar nanoparticle technology. Estrasorb is packaged in foil pouches containing 1.74 grams of drug product. Daily topical application of the contents of two foil pouches provides systemic delivery of 0.05 mg of estradiol per day.

Estradiol hemihydrate USP, EP (estradiol) is a white, crystalline powder, chemically described as (17β)-estra-1,3,5(10)-triene-3, 17-diol, hemihydrate. The molecular formula of estradiol hemihydrate is $C_{18}H_{24}O_2$, ½ H_2O, and the molecular weight is 281.4 g/mol.

The structural formula is:

[Structural formula of estradiol: OH, CH_3, HO]

The active ingredient in Estrasorb is estradiol. The remaining components (soybean oil, water, polysorbate 80, and ethanol) are pharmacologically inactive.

CLINICAL PHARMACOLOGY

Endogenous estrogens are largely responsible for the development and maintenance of the female reproductive system and secondary sexual characteristics. Although circulating estrogens exist in a dynamic equilibrium of metabolic interconversions, estradiol is the principal intracellular human estrogen and is substantially more potent than its metabolites, estrone and estriol, at the receptor level.

The primary source of estrogen in normally cycling adult women is the ovarian follicle, which secretes 70 to 500 mcg of estradiol daily, depending on the phase of the menstrual cycle. After menopause, most endogenous estrogen is produced by conversion of androstenedione, secreted by the adrenal cortex, to estrone by peripheral tissues. Thus, estrone and its sulfate-conjugated form, estrone sulfate, are the most abundant circulating estrogens in postmenopausal women. Estrogens act through binding to nuclear receptors in estrogen-responsive tissues. To date, two estrogen receptors have been identified. These vary in proportion from tissue to tissue.

Circulating estrogens modulate the pituitary secretion of the gonadotropins, luteinizing hormone (LH) and follicle stimulating hormone (FSH) through a negative feedback mechanism. Estrogens act to reduce the elevated levels of these hormones seen in postmenopausal women.

Pharmacokinetics

Absorption

In a multiple-dose study, 125 patients were treated for 28 days once daily with placebo or 1.15 grams, 2.30 grams, or 3.45 grams of Estrasorb containing 2.5 mg of estradiol per gram. The mean change from baseline in serum estradiol concentrations increased in a dose-dependent manner compared with placebo (Figure 1 below).

Figure 1. Mean serum estradiol concentrations (pg/mL) following topical application of placebo or 1.15 Grams, 2.30 Grams or 3.45 Grams of Estrasorb containing 2.5 mg of estradiol per Gram

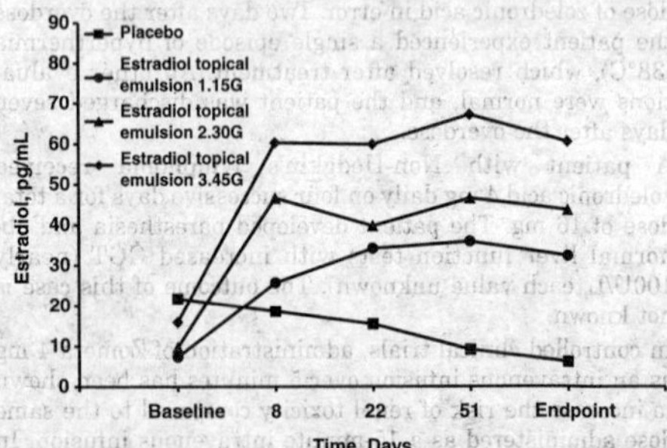

Serum estradiol concentrations were also assessed in a second study involving 200 postmenopausal women, who applied either a 3.45 gram daily dose of Estrasorb (containing 2.5 mg of estradiol per gram; n = 100) or placebo (n = 100) for 12 weeks. Trough estradiol concentrations in the Estrasorb treatment group increased from a mean of 8.9 pg/mL at baseline to 58.6 pg/mL and 70.2 pg/mL at Weeks 2 and 4, respectively (Figure 2). Trough levels of Estrasorb remained at a plateau throughout the rest of the study: 67.3 pg/mL at Week 8 and 63.0 pg/mL at the end of the study.

Figure 2. Mean (SE) Trough Serum Estradiol Concentrations Following Daily Topical Application of 3.45 Grams of Estrasorb Containing 2.5 mg of Estradiol per Gram for 12 weeks.

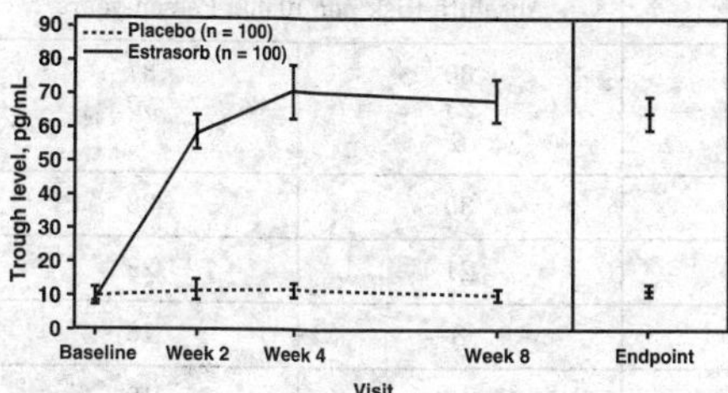

SE = Standard error of the mean.

Application of sunscreen 10 minutes prior to the application of Estrasorb increased the exposure to estradiol by approximately 35%. When sunscreen is applied 25 minutes after the application of Estrasorb, the increase in exposure to estradiol was approximately 15%. (See **PRECAUTIONS**.)

Distribution

No specific investigation of the tissue distribution of estradiol absorbed from Estrasorb in humans has been conducted. The distribution of exogenous estrogens is similar to that of endogenous estrogens. Estrogens are widely distributed in the body and are generally found in higher concentrations in the sex hormone target organs. Estrogens circulate in the blood largely bound to sex hormone binding globulin (SHBG) and albumin.

Metabolism

Exogenous estrogens are metabolized in the same manner as endogenous estrogens. Circulating estrogens exist in a dynamic equilibrium of metabolic interconversions. These transformations take place mainly in the liver. Estradiol is converted reversibly to estrone, and both can be converted to estriol, which is the major urinary metabolite. Estrogens also undergo enterohepatic recirculation via sulfate and glucuronide conjugation in the liver, biliary secretion of conjugates into the intestines, and hydrolysis in the gut followed by reabsorption. In postmenopausal women a significant proportion of the circulating estrogens exists as sulfate conjugates, especially estrone sulfate, which serves as a circulating reservoir for the formation of more active estrogens.

Excretion

Estradiol, estrone, and estriol are excreted in the urine along with glucuronide and sulfate conjugates.

Special Populations

Estrasorb was only investigated in postmenopausal women. Estrasorb has not been studied in patients with hepatic or renal impairment.

Drug Interactions

In vitro and in vivo studies have shown that estrogens are metabolized partially by cytochrome P450 3A4 (CYP3A4). Therefore, inducers or inhibitors of CYP3A4 may affect estrogen drug metabolism. Inducers of CYP3A4 such as St. John's Wort preparations (Hypericum perforatum), phenobarbital, carbamazepine, and rifampin may reduce plasma concentrations of estrogens, possibly resulting in a decrease in therapeutic effects and/or changes in the uterine bleeding profile. Inhibitors of CYP3A4 such as erythromycin, clarithromycin, ketoconazole, itraconazole, ritonavir and grapefruit juice may increase plasma concentrations of estrogens and may result in side effects.

Clinical Studies

Effects on Vasomotor Symptoms

In a 12-week randomized, placebo-controlled clinical trial, a total of 200 postmenopausal women (average age 52 ± 6 years, 79% Caucasian in the Estrasorb treatment group; average age 51.8 ± 6 years, 72% Caucasian in the placebo treatment group) were assigned to receive Estrasorb (3.45 grams containing 2.5 mg of estradiol per gram) or placebo for a 12 weeks duration. Estrasorb was shown to be statistically better than placebo at Weeks 4 and 12 for relief of both the frequency and severity of moderate to severe vasomotor symptoms (p-value <0.001 for Weeks 4 and 12). Frequency results are shown in Table 1. Severity results are shown in Table 2.

[See table 1 above]

[See table 2 above]

Table 1. Mean Number and Mean Change From Baseline in the Number of Moderate to Severe Vasomotor Symptoms Per Day (Intent-To-Treat Population)

Time point	Treatment Group	
	Placebo	Estrasorb
Baseline (observed value)	(N = 100)	(N = 100)
Mean Number of Hot Flushes (SD)	13.63 (5.48)	13.05 (5.78)
Week 4	(N = 97)	(N = 96)
Mean Number of Hot Flushes (SD)	7.46 (6.42)	4.42 (5.60)
Mean Change from Baseline (SD)	−5.97 (4.76)	−8.56 (6.19)
P-value vs. Placebo	NA	<0.001
Week 12	(N = 90)	(N = 90)
Mean Number of Hot Flushes (SD)	5.88 (6.17)	2.00 (3.64)
Mean Change from Baseline (SD)	−7.20 (5.39)	−11.11 (6.84)
P-value vs. Placebo	NA	<0.001

SD = Standard Deviation; NA = Not applicable

Table 2: Mean Change from Baseline in the Severity Score[a] of Hot Flushes Per Day, Intent-to-Treat Population, Most Recent Value Carried Forward

Time point	Treatment Group	
	Placebo	Estrasorb
Baseline (observed value)	(N = 100)	(N = 100)
Mean Severity Score per Day (SD)	2.44 (0.37)	2.36 (0.36)
Week 4	(N = 97)	(N = 96)
Mean Severity Score per Day (SD)	1.99 (0.81)	1.47 (1.03)
Mean Change from Baseline (SD)	−0.45 (0.75)	−0.89 (1.04)
P-value versus Placebo	NA	<0.001
Week 12	(N = 90)	(N = 90)
Mean Severity Score per Day (SD)	1.88 (0.98)	0.92 (1.00)
Mean Change from Baseline (SD)	−0.55 (0.91)	−1.44 (1.04)
P-value vs. Placebo	NA	<0.001

SD = Standard deviation; NA = Not applicable

[a]The severity score per day is determined by calculating the sum of recorded daily severity and dividing this number by the total number of hot flushes on that day.

Potential for estradiol transfer

Estradiol was detected on the skin at 2 and 8 hours post-application. Washing the application area with soap and water 8 hours post-application removed detectable estradiol from the application site.

Upon physical contact of Estrasorb application sites by adult males at 2 and 8 hours post-application over a two-day period in a second study, a mean increase of approximately 25% in serum estradiol concentration was identified. (See **DOSAGE AND ADMINISTRATION**.)

Women's Health Initiative Studies

The Women's Health Initiative (WHI) enrolled a total of 27,000 predominantly healthy postmenopausal women to assess the risks and benefits of either the use of 0.625 mg conjugated equine estrogens (CE) per day alone or the use of 0.625 mg conjugated equine estrogens plus 2.5 mg medroxyprogesterone acetate (MPA) per day compared to placebo in the prevention of certain chronic diseases. The primary endpoint was the incidence of coronary heart disease (CHD) (nonfatal myocardial infarction and CHD death), with invasive breast cancer as the primary adverse outcome studied. A "global index" included the earliest occurrence of CHD, invasive breast cancer, stroke, pulmonary embolism (PE), endometrial cancer, colorectal cancer, hip fracture, or death due to other cause. The study did not evaluate the effects of CE or CE/MPA on menopausal symptoms.

The CE-only substudy is continuing and results have not been reported. The CE/MPA substudy was stopped early because, according to the predefined stopping rule, the increased risk of breast cancer and cardiovascular events exceeded the specified benefits included in the "global index." Results of the CE/MPA substudy, which included 16,608 women (average age of 63 years, range 50 to 79; 83.9% White, 6.5% Black, 5.5% Hispanic), after an average follow-up of 5.2 years are presented in Table 3 below.

[See table 3 at top of next page]

For those outcomes included in the "global index," absolute excess risks per 10,000 person-years in the group treated with CE/MPA were 7 more CHD events, 8 more strokes, 8 more PEs, and 8 more invasive breast cancers, while absolute risk reductions per 10,000 person-years were 6 fewer colorectal cancers and 5 fewer hip fractures. The absolute excess risk of events included in the "global index" was 19 per 10,000 person-years. There was no difference between the groups in terms of all-cause mortality. (See **BOXED WARNINGS, WARNINGS,** and **PRECAUTIONS**.)

INDICATIONS AND USAGE

Estrasorb is indicated for the treatment of moderate to severe vasomotor symptoms associated with menopause.

CONTRAINDICATIONS

Estrogens should not be used in women with any of the following conditions:

1. Undiagnosed abnormal genital bleeding.
2. Known, suspected, or history of cancer of the breast except in appropriately selected patients being treated for metastatic disease.
3. Known or suspected estrogen-dependent neoplasia.
4. Active deep vein thrombosis, pulmonary embolism or history of these conditions.
5. Active or recent (e.g., within the past year) arterial thromboembolic disease (e.g., stroke, myocardial infarction).
6. Liver dysfunction or disease.
7. Estrasorb should not be used in patients with known hypersensitivity to its ingredients.
8. Known or suspected pregnancy. There is no indication for Estrasorb in pregnancy. There appears to be little or no increased risk of birth defects in women who have used estrogens and progestins from oral contraceptives inadvertently during early pregnancy (See PRECAUTIONS.)

WARNINGS

See **BOXED WARNINGS.**

The use of unopposed estrogens in women who have a uterus is associated with an increased risk of endometrial cancer.

1. Cardiovascular disorders.

Estrogen and estrogen/progestin therapy have been associated with an increased risk of cardiovascular events such as myocardial infarction and stroke, as well as venous thrombosis and pulmonary embolism (venous thromboembolism or VTE). Should any of these occur or be suspected, estrogens should be discontinued immediately.

Risk factors for arterial vascular disease (e.g., hypertension, diabetes mellitus, tobacco use, hypercholesterolemia, and obesity) and/or venous thromboembolism (e.g., personal history or family history of VTE, obesity, and systemic lupus erythematosus) should be managed appropriately.

a. *Coronary heart disease and stroke.* In the Women's Health Initiative (WHI) study, an increase in the number of myocardial infarctions and strokes has been observed in women receiving CE compared to placebo. These observations are preliminary, and the study is continuing. (See **CLINICAL PHARMACOLOGY, Clinical Studies.**)

In the CE/MPA substudy of WHI an increased risk of coronary heart disease (CHD) events (defined as non-fatal myocardial infarction and CHD death) was observed in women receiving CE/MPA compared to women receiving placebo (37 vs 30 per 10,000 person-years). The increase in risk was observed after the first year and persisted.

In the same substudy of WHI, an increased risk of stroke was observed in women receiving CE/MPA compared to women receiving placebo (29 vs 21 per 10,000 person-years). The increase in risk was observed after the first year and persisted.

In postmenopausal women with documented heart disease (n = 2,763, average age 66.7 years) a controlled clinical trial of secondary prevention of cardiovascular disease (Heart and Estrogen/Progestin Replacement Study; HERS) treatment with CE/MPA (0.625 mg/2.5 mg per day) demonstrated no cardiovascular benefit. During an average follow-up of 4.1 years, treatment with CE/MPA did not reduce the overall rate of CHD events in postmenopausal women with established coronary heart disease. There were more CHD events in the CE/MPA-treated group than in the placebo group in year 1, but not during the subsequent years. Two thousand three hundred and twenty one women from the original HERS trial agreed to participate in an open label extension of HERS, HERS II. Average follow-up in HERS II was an additional 2.7 years, for a total of 6.8 years overall. Rates of CHD events were comparable among women in the CE/MPA group and the placebo group in HERS, HERS II, and overall.

Continued on next page

Estrasorb—Cont.

Large doses of estrogen (5 mg conjugated estrogens per day), comparable to those used to treat cancer of the prostate and breast, have been shown in a large prospective clinical trial in men to increase the risks of nonfatal myocardial infarction, pulmonary embolism, and thrombophlebitis.

b. *Venous thromboembolism (VTE).* In the Woman's Health Initiative (WHI) study, an increase in VTE has been observed in women receiving CE compared to placebo. These observations are preliminary, and the study is continuing. (See **CLINICAL PHARMACOLOGY, Clinical Studies.**)

In the CE/MPA substudy of WHI, a 2-fold greater rate of VTE, including deep venous thrombosis and pulmonary embolism, was observed in women receiving CE/MPA compared to women receiving placebo. The rate of VTE was 34 per 10,000 person-years in the CE/MPA group compared to 16 per 10,000 person-years in the placebo group. The increase in VTE risk was observed during the first year and persisted.

If feasible, estrogens should be discontinued at least 4 to 6 weeks before surgery of the type associated with an increased risk of thromboembolism, or during periods of prolonged immobilization.

2. Malignant neoplasms.

a. *Endometrial cancer.* The use of unopposed estrogens in women with intact uteri has been associated with an increased risk of endometrial cancer. The reported endometrial cancer risk among unopposed estrogen users is about 2- to 12-fold greater than in nonusers, and appears dependent on duration of treatment and on estrogen dose. Most studies show no significant increased risk associated with the use of estrogens for less than 1 year. The greatest risk appears associated with prolonged use, with increased risks of 15- to 24-fold for use over 5 to 10 years or more, and this risk has been shown to persist at least 8 to 15 years after estrogen therapy is discontinued.

Clinical surveillance of all women taking estrogen/progestin combinations is important. Adequate diagnostic measures, including endometrial sampling when indicated, should be undertaken to rule out malignancy in all cases of undiagnosed persistent or recurring abnormal vaginal bleeding. There is no evidence that the use of natural estrogens results in a different endometrial risk profile than synthetic estrogens of equivalent estrogen dose. Adding a progestin to postmenopausal estrogen therapy has been shown to reduce the risk of endometrial hyperplasia, which may be a precursor to endometrial cancer.

b. *Breast cancer.* Estrogen and estrogen/progestin therapy in postmenopausal women has been associated with an increased risk of breast cancer. In the CE/MPA substudy of the Women's Health Initiative (WHI) study, a 26% increase in invasive breast cancer (38 vs 30 per 10,000 person-years) after an average of 5.2 years of treatment was observed in women receiving CE/MPA compared to women receiving placebo. The increased risk of breast cancer became apparent after 4 years of treatment with CE/MPA. The women reporting prior postmenopausal use of estrogens and/or estrogens with progestin had a higher relative risk for breast cancer associated with CE/MPA than those who had never used these hormones. (See **CLINICAL PHARMACOLOGY, Clinical Studies.**)

In the WHI, no increased risk of breast cancer in CE-treated women compared to placebo was reported after an average of 5.2 years of therapy. These data are preliminary and that substudy of WHI is continuing.

Epidemiologic studies have reported an increased risk of breast cancer in association with increasing duration of postmenopausal treatment with estrogens with or without a progestin. This association was reanalyzed in original data from 51 studies that involved various doses and types of estrogens, with and without progestin. In the reanalysis, an increased risk of having breast cancer diagnosed became apparent after about 5 years of continuous treatment and subsided after treatment had been discontinued for 5 years or longer. Some later studies have suggested that postmenopausal treatment with estrogens and progestin increases the risk of breast cancer more than treatment with estrogen alone.

3. Gallbladder disease. A 2- to 4-fold increase in the risk of gallbladder disease requiring surgery in postmenopausal women receiving estrogens has been reported.

4. Hypercalcemia. Estrogen administration may lead to severe hypercalcemia in patients with breast cancer and bone metastases. If hypercalcemia occurs, the drug should be stopped and appropriate measures taken to reduce the serum calcium level.

5. Visual abnormalities. Retinal vascular thrombosis has been reported in patients receiving estrogens. Discontinue medication pending examination if there is sudden partial or complete loss of vision, or a sudden onset of proptosis, diplopia, or migraine. If examination reveals papilledema or retinal vascular lesions, estrogens should be discontinued.

Table 3. RELATIVE AND ABSOLUTE RISK SEEN IN THE CE/MPA SUBSTUDY OF WHI[a]

Event[c]	Relative Risk Prempro vs Placebo at 5.2 Years (95% CI*)	Placebo n = 8102	CE/MPA n = 8506
		Absolute Risk per 10,000 Person-years	
CHD events	1.29 (1.02–1.63)	30	37
Non-fatal MI	*1.32 (1.02–1.72)*	*23*	*30*
CHD death	*1.18 (0.70–1.97)*	*6*	*7*
Invasive breast cancer[b]	1.26 (1.00–1.59)	30	38
Stroke	1.41 (1.07–1.85)	21	29
Pulmonary embolism	2.13 (1.39–3.25)	8	16
Colorectal cancer	0.63 (0.43–0.92)	16	10
Endometrial cancer	0.83 (0.47–1.47)	6	5
Hip fracture	0.66 (0.45–0.98)	15	10
Death due to causes other than the events above	0.92 (0.74–1.14)	40	37
Global Index[c]	1.15 (1.03–1.28)	151	170
Deep vein thrombosis[d]	2.07 (1.49–2.87)	13	26
Vertebral fractures[d]	0.66 (0.44–0.98)	15	9
Other osteoporotic fractures[d]	0.77 (0.69–0.86)	170	131

a: adapted from JAMA, 2002; 288:321–333
b: includes metastatic and non-metastatic breast cancer with the exception of in situ breast cancer
c: a subset of the events was combined in a "global index", defined as the earliest occurrence of CHD events, invasive breast cancer, stroke, pulmonary embolism, endometrial cancer, colorectal cancer, hip fracture, or death due to other causes
d: not included in Global Index
* nominal confidence intervals unadjusted for multiple looks and multiple comparisons

PRECAUTIONS

A. General

1. *Addition of a progestin when a woman has not had a hysterectomy.* Studies of the addition of a progestin for 10 or more days of a cycle of estrogen administration, or daily with estrogen in a continuous regimen, have reported a lower incidence of endometrial hyperplasia than would be induced by estrogen treatment alone. Endometrial hyperplasia may be a precursor to endometrial cancer. There are, however, possible risks that may be associated with the use of progestins with estrogens compared to estrogen-alone regimens. These include:

a. A possible increased risk of breast cancer.
b. Adverse effects on lipoprotein metabolism (e.g., lowering HDL, raising LDL)
c. Impairment of glucose metabolism.

2. *Elevated blood pressure.* In a small number of case reports, substantial increases in blood pressure have been attributed to idiosyncratic reactions to estrogens. In a large, randomized, placebo-controlled, clinical trial, a generalized effect of estrogen therapy on blood pressure was not seen. Blood pressure should be monitored at regular intervals with estrogen use.

3. *Familial hyperlipoproteinemia.* In patients with familial defects of lipoprotein metabolism, estrogen therapy may be associated with elevations of plasma triglycerides, leading to pancreatitis and other complications.

4. *Impaired liver function.* Although topically administered estrogen therapy avoids first-pass hepatic metabolism, estrogens may be poorly metabolized in patients with impaired liver function. For patient with a history of cholestatic jaundice associated with past estrogen use or with pregnancy, caution should be exercised and in the case of recurrence, medication should be discontinued.

5. *Hypothyroidism.* Estrogen administration leads to increased thyroid-binding globulin (TBG) levels. Patients with normal thyroid function can compensate for the increased TBG by making more thyroid hormone, thus maintaining free T_4 and T_3 serum concentrations in the normal range. Patients dependent on thyroid hormone replacement therapy who are also receiving estrogens may require increased doses of their thyroid replacement therapy. These patients should have their thyroid function monitored in order to maintain their free thyroid hormone levels in an acceptable range.

6. *Fluid retention.* Because estrogens may cause some degree of fluid retention, conditions that might be influenced by this factor, such as a cardiac or renal dysfunction, warrant careful observation when estrogens are prescribed.

7. *Hypocalcemia.* Estrogens should be used with caution in individuals with severe hypocalcemia.

8. *Ovarian cancer.* Use of estrogen-only products, in particular for ten or more years, has been associated with an increased risk of ovarian cancer in some epidemiological studies. Other studies did not show a significant association. Data are insufficient to determine whether there is an increased risk with combined estrogen/progestin therapy in postmenopausal women.

9. *Exacerbation of endometriosis.* Endometriosis may be exacerbated with administration of estrogens.

A few cases of malignant transformation of residual endometrial implants have been reported in women treated post-hysterectomy with estrogen-only therapy. For patients known to have residual endometriosis post-hysterectomy, the addition of progestin should be considered.

10. *Exacerbation of other conditions.* Estrogens may cause an exacerbation of asthma, diabetes mellitus, epilepsy, migraine, porphyria, systemic lupus erythematosus, and hepatic hemangiomas and should be used with caution in patients with these conditions.

11. *Application of sunscreen.* Estrasorb should not be used in close proximity to sunscreen application because estradiol absorption may be increased. (See **CLINICAL PHARMACOLOGY, Pharmacokinetics, *Absorption.***)

B. Patient Information

Physicians are advised to discuss the contents of the PATIENT INFORMATION leaflet with patients for whom they prescribe Estrasorb.

C. Laboratory Tests

Estrogen administration should be initiated at the lowest dose approved for the indication and then guided by clinical rather than by serum hormone levels (e.g., estradiol, FSH).

D. Drug/Laboratory Test Interactions

1. Accelerated prothrombin time, partial thromboplastin time, and platelet aggregation time; increased platelet count; increased factors II, VII antigen, VIII antigen, VIII coagulant activity, IX, X, XII, VII-X complex, II-VII-X complex, and beta-thromboglobulin; decreased levels of antifactor Xa and antithrombin III; decreased antithrombin III activity; increased levels of fibrinogen and fibrinogen activity; increased plasminogen antigen and activity.

2. Increased thyroid-binding globulin (TBG) levels leading to increased circulating total thyroid hormone, as measured by protein-bound iodine (PBI), T_4 levels (by column or by radioimmunoassay) or T_3 levels by radioimmunoassay. T_3 resin uptake is decreased, reflecting the elevated TBG. Free T_4 and free T_3 concentrations are unaltered. Patients on thyroid replacement therapy may require higher doses of thyroid hormone.

3. Other binding proteins may be elevated in serum (i.e., corticosteroid binding globulin, and sex hormone binding globulin), leading to increased circulating corticosteroids and sex steroids, respectively. Free or biologically active hormone concentrations are unchanged. Other plasma proteins may be increased (angiotensinogen/renin substrate, alpha-1-antitrypsin, ceruloplasmin).

4. Increased plasma HDL and HDL_2 cholesterol subfraction concentrations, reduced LDL cholesterol concentration, and increased triglycerides levels.

5. Impaired glucose tolerance.

6. Reduced response to metyrapone test.

E. Carcinogenesis, Mutagenesis, Impairment of Fertility

Long-term continuous administration of natural and synthetic estrogens in certain animal species increases the frequency of carcinomas of the breast, uterus, cervix, vagina, testis, and liver (See **BOXED WARNINGS, CONTRAINDICATIONS,** and **WARNINGS.**)

F. Pregnancy

Estrasorb should not be used during pregnancy. (See **CONTRAINDICATIONS.**)

G. Nursing Mothers

Estrogen administration to nursing mothers has been shown to decrease the quantity and quality of the milk. Detectable amounts of estrogens have been identified in the milk of mothers receiving this drug. Caution should be exercised when Estrasorb is administered to a nursing woman.

H. Pediatric Use

Estrogen therapy has been used for the induction of puberty in adolescents with some forms of pubertal delay. Safety and effectiveness in pediatric patients have not otherwise been established.

Table 4. Number (%) of Patients Reporting ≥ 5% Treatment-Emergent Adverse Events

Body system/ Preferred term	Statistic	Treatment group	
		Placebo (n = 134)	Estrasorb 3.45 grams (n = 139)
Number of subjects with ≥ 1 TEAE	n (%)	82 (61)	95 (68)
Body as a whole	n (%)	40 (30)	49 (35)
Headache	n (%)	17 (13)	12 (9)
Infection	n (%)	10 (7)	16 (12)
Respiratory	n (%)	15 (11)	19 (14)
Sinusitis	n (%)	6 (4)	9 (6)
Skin and appendages	n (%)	7 (5)	15 (11)
Pruritus	n (%)	0	5 (4)
Urogenital	n (%)	20 (15)	44 (32)
Breast pain	n (%)	4 (3)	14 (10)
Endomentrial disorder	n (%)	11 (8)	21 (15)

TEAE = Treatment-emergent adverse event.

I. Geriatric Use
There have not been sufficient numbers of geriatric patients involved in studies utilizing Estrasorb to determine whether those over 65 years of age differ from younger subjects in their response to Estrasorb.

ADVERSE REACTIONS

See **BOXED WARNINGS, WARNINGS,** and **PRECAUTIONS**.
Because clinical trials are conducted under widely varying conditions, adverse reaction rates observed in the clinical trials of a drug cannot be directly compared to rates in the clinical trials of another drug and may not reflect the rates observed in practice. The adverse reaction information from clinical trials does, however, provide a basis for identifying the adverse events that appear to be related to drug use and for approximating rates.
Table 4 summarizes the treatment-emergent adverse events with Estrasorb therapy.
[See table 4 above]
The following adverse reactions have been reported with estrogen therapy:

1. **Genitourinary system.** Changes in vaginal bleeding pattern and abnormal withdrawal bleeding or flow; breakthrough bleeding, spotting; increase in size of uterine leiomyomata; vaginal candidiasis; change in amount of cervical secretion; changes in cervical ectropion; ovarian cancer, endometrial hyperplasia; endometrial cancer.
2. **Breasts.** Tenderness, enlargement, pain, nipple discharge, galactorrhea; fibrocystic breast changes; breast cancer.
3. **Cardiovascular.** Deep and superficial venous thrombosis; pulmonary embolism; thrombophlebitis; myocardial infarction; stroke; increase in blood pressure.
4. **Gastrointestinal.** Nausea, vomiting; abdominal cramps, bloating; cholestatic jaundice; increased incidence of gall bladder disease; pancreatitis.
5. **Skin.** Chloasma or melasma that may persist when drug is discontinued; erythema multiforme; erythema nodosum; hemorrhagic eruption; loss of scalp hair; hirsutism; pruritis, rash.
6. **Eyes.** Retinal vascular thrombosis, steepening of corneal curvature, intolerance to contact lenses.
7. **Central Nervous System.** Headache, migraine, dizziness; mental depression; chorea; nervousness; mood disturbance; anxiety; irritability; insomnia; somnolence; exacerbation of epilepsy.
8. **Miscellaneous.** Increase or decrease in weight; reduced carbohydrate tolerance; aggravation of porphyria; edema; arthralgia; leg cramps; changes in libido; anaphylactoid/anaphylactic reactions; hypocalcemia; exacerbation of asthma; increased triglycerides.

OVERDOSAGE

Serious ill effects have not been reported following acute ingestion of large doses of estrogen-containing products by young children. Overdosage of estrogen may cause nausea and vomiting, and withdrawal bleeding may occur in women.

DOSAGE AND ADMINISTRATION

When estrogen is prescribed for a postmenopausal woman with a uterus, progestin should also be initiated to reduce the risk of endometrial cancer. A woman without a uterus does not need progestin. Use of estrogen, alone or in combination with a progestin, should be with the lowest effective dose and for the shortest duration consistent with treatment goals and risks for the individual women. Patients should be re-evaluated periodically as clinically appropriate (e.g., at 3-month to 6-month intervals) to determine if treatment is still necessary (see **BOXED WARNINGS** and **WARNINGS**). For women with a uterus, adequate diagnostic measures, such as endometrial sampling, when indicated, should be undertaken to rule out malignancy in cases of undiagnosed persistent or recurring abnormal vaginal bleeding.
For the treatment of moderate to severe vasomotor symptoms associated with the menopause, the single approved dose of Estrasorb is 3.48 grams daily. The lowest effective dose of Estrasorb for this indication has not been determined. (See **BOXED WARNINGS** and **WARNINGS**.)

Instructions for daily application of two 1.74-gram foil-laminated pouches

1. Estrasorb should be applied in a comfortable sitting position to clean, dry skin on both legs each morning. Each foil-laminated pouch of Estrasorb should be opened individually.
2. Cut or tear the first foil-laminated pouch at the notches indicated near the top of the pouch.

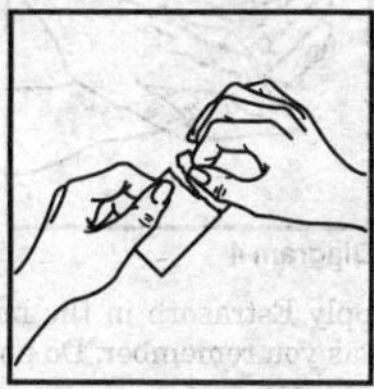

3. Apply the emulsion in the pouch to the top of the left thigh, being careful to push the entire contents from the bottom through the neck of the pouch.

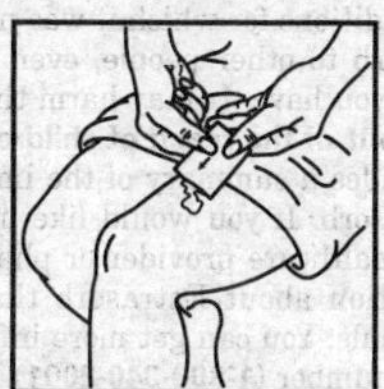

4. Using one hand or both hands rub the emulsion into the entire left thigh and left calf for three minutes until thoroughly absorbed. Rub any excess material remaining on both hands on the buttocks.

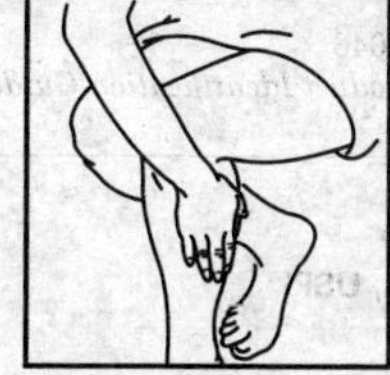

5. Cut or tear the second foil-laminated pouch at the notches indicated near the top of the pouch. Apply the emulsion in the pouch to the top of the right thigh, being careful to push the entire contents from the bottom through the neck of the pouch. Using one hand or both hands rub the emulsion into the entire right thigh and right calf for three minutes until thoroughly absorbed. Rub any excess material remaining on both hands on the buttocks. Estrasorb absorption was not studied on other parts of the body.
6. Allow the application areas to dry completely before covering with clothing to avoid transfer to other individuals.
7. On completion of Estrasorb application, both hands should be washed with soap and water to remove any residual estradiol.

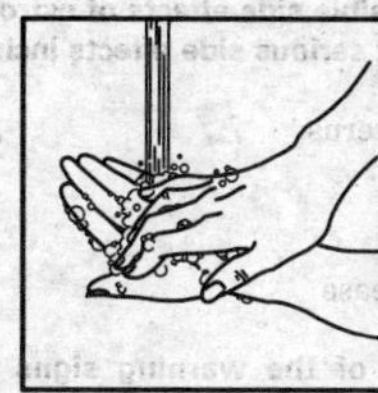

HOW SUPPLIED

Estrasorb (estradiol topical emulsion), nominal 0.05 mg/day:
Estrasorb is packaged in foil-laminated pouches. A daily dose of Estrasorb is two foil-laminated pouches. Each pouch contains 1.74-grams. Each 1.74-gram, foil-laminated pouch contains 4.35 mg of estradiol hemihydrate USP, EP. Each box of Estrasorb contains fourteen 1.74-gram, foil-laminated pouches, packaged in a 1-month supply carton of 56 pouches.
Store at 20–25°C (68–77°F); excursions permitted to 15–30°C (59–86°F) [see USP Controlled Room Temperature]

PATIENT INFORMATION

(Updated October 9, 2003)
Estrasorb®
(estradiol topical emulsion)
Read this PATIENT INFORMATION before you start taking Estrasorb and read what you get each time you refill Estrasorb. There may be new information. This information does not take the place of talking to your healthcare provider about your medical condition or your treatment.

What is the most important information I should know about Estrasorb?

- Estrogens increase the chances of getting cancer of the uterus.

Report any unusual vaginal bleeding right away while you are using Estrasorb. Vaginal bleeding after menopause may be a warning sign of cancer of the uterus (womb). Your healthcare provider should check any unusual vaginal bleeding to find out the cause.

- Do not use estrogens with or without progestins to prevent heart disease, heart attacks, or strokes.

Using estrogens with or without progestins may increase your chances of getting heart attacks, strokes, breast cancer, and blood clots. You and your healthcare provider should talk regularly about whether you still need treatment with estrogens.

What is Estrasorb?
Estrasorb contains an estrogen hormone called estradiol. When applied to the skin as directed below, Estrasorb releases estradiol, which is absorbed through the skin into the bloodstream.
What is Estrasorb used for?
Estrasorb is used after menopause to:

- **reduce moderate to severe hot flashes.**

Estrogens are hormones made by a woman's ovaries. The ovaries normally stop making estrogens when a woman is between 45 to 55 years old. This drop in body estrogen levels causes the "change of life" or menopause (the end of monthly menstrual periods). Sometimes, both ovaries are removed during an operation before natural menopause takes place. The sudden drop in estrogen levels causes "surgical menopause."
When the estrogen levels begin dropping, some women develop very uncomfortable symptoms, such as feelings of warmth in the face, neck, and chest, or sudden strong feelings of heat and sweating ("hot flashes" or "hot flushes"). In some women, the symptoms are mild, and they will not need estrogens. In other women, symptoms can be more severe. You and your healthcare provider should talk regularly about whether you still need treatment with Estrasorb.
Who should not use Estrasorb?
Do not start using Estrasorb if you:

- **have unusual vaginal bleeding**
- **currently have or have had certain cancers**
  Estrogens may increase the chances of getting certain types of cancers, including cancer of the breast or uterus. If you have had cancer, talk with your health care provider about whether you should use Estrasorb.
- **had a stroke or heart attack in the past year**
- **currently have or have had blood clots**
- **are allergic to Estrasorb or any of its ingredients**
  See the end of this leaflet for a list of ingredients in Estrasorb.
- **think you may be pregnant.**

Tell your healthcare provider:

- **if you are breast feeding.** The hormone in Estrasorb can pass into your breast milk.
- **about all of your medical problems.** Your healthcare provider may need to check you more carefully if you have certain conditions, such as asthma (wheezing), epilepsy (seizures), migraine, endometriosis, lupus, problems with your heart, liver, thyroid, kidneys, or have high calcium levels in your blood.
- **if you are going to have surgery or will be on bed rest.** You may need to stop using Estrasorb.

Continued on next page

Estrasorb—Cont.

What are the possible side effects of estrogens?
Less common but serious side effects include:
- Breast cancer
- Cancer of the uterus
- Stroke
- Heart attack
- Blood clots
- Gallbladder disease
- Ovarian cancer

These are some of the warning signs of serious side effects:
- Breast lumps
- Unusual vaginal bleeding
- Dizziness and faintness
- Changes in speech
- Severe headaches
- Chest pain
- Shortness of breath
- Pains in your legs
- Changes in vision
- Vomiting

Call your healthcare provider right away if you get any of these warning signs, or any other unusual symptom that concerns you.

Common side effects include:
- Headache
- Breast pain
- Irregular vaginal bleeding or spotting
- Stomach/abdominal cramps, bloating
- Nausea and vomiting
- Skin irritation, redness, or rash may occur at the site of application
- Hair loss

Other side effects include:
- High blood pressure
- Liver problems
- High blood sugar
- Fluid retention
- Enlargement of benign tumors of the uterus ("fibroids")
- Vaginal yeast infection

These are not all of the possible side effects of Estrasorb. For more information, ask your healthcare provider or pharmacist.

What can I do to lower my chances of getting a serious side effect with Estrasorb?
- Talk with your healthcare provider regularly about whether you should continue using Estrasorb.
- If you have a uterus, talk to your healthcare provider about whether the addition of a progestin is right for you.
- See your healthcare provider right away if you get vaginal bleeding while using Estrasorb.
- Have a breast exam and mammogram (breast X-ray) every year unless your healthcare provider tells you something else. If members of your family have had breast cancer or if you have ever had breast lumps or an abnormal mammogram (breast x-ray examination), you may need to have breast exams more often.
- If you have high blood pressure, high cholesterol (fat in the blood), diabetes, are overweight, or if you use tobacco, you may have higher chances of getting heart disease. Ask your healthcare provider for ways to lower your chances for getting heart disease.

This leaflet provides a summary of the most important information about estrogens. If you want more information, ask your healthcare provider or pharmacist to show you the professional labeling (drug information).

How should I use Estrasorb?
Estrasorb should be used only as long as needed. You and your healthcare provider should talk regularly (for example, every 3 to 6 months) about whether you still need treatment with Estrasorb. Estrasorb is an emulsion that is applied each day to the skin of both thighs and calves. It is not known if Estrasorb will be absorbed as well if applied to other parts of the body. Estrasorb is packaged in foil pouches. A daily dose of Estrasorb is two foil pouches. Do not open the pouches until just before you apply Estrasorb. Apply Estrasorb in the morning. If you shower or take a bath, be sure your skin is dry before using Estrasorb. Do not apply Estrasorb to any skin on your thighs and calves that appears to be red or irritated. Do not apply sunscreen and Estrasorb at the same time because sunscreen may affect the amount of estradiol you absorb.

How to apply Estrasorb
- Estrasorb is best applied when you are sitting comfortably. The skin on both legs should be clean and dry.
- Cut or tear the first pouch across the notches to open it (Diagram 1).

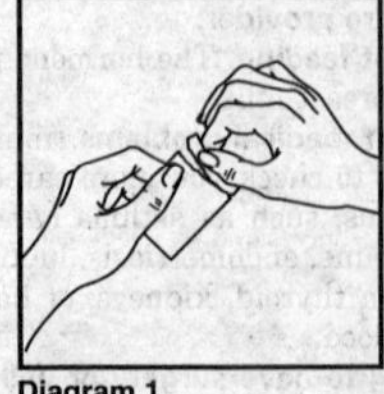

Diagram 1

- Place the pouch flat on top of your left thigh, with the open end facing your knee. Hold the other end with one hand and use the forefinger of your other hand to push all of the contents of the pouch onto your left thigh (Diagram 2).

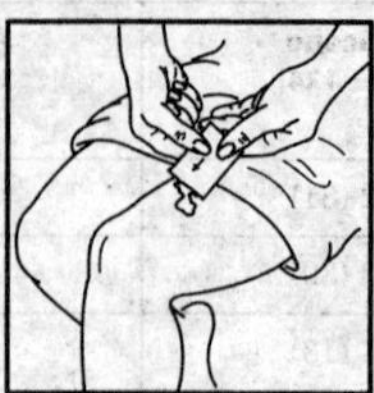

Diagram 2

- With one hand or both hands rub the material into your entire left thigh and left calf for three minutes until thoroughly absorbed (Diagram 3).

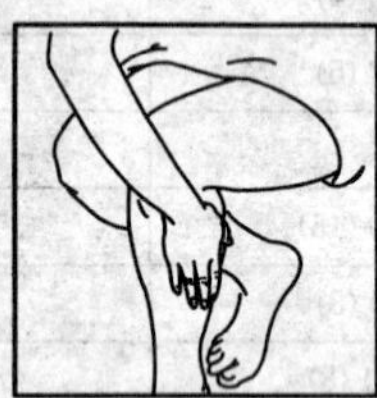

Diagram 3

Rub any excess material remaining on the hands on your buttocks.
- Cut or tear the second pouch across the notches to open it (see Diagram 1). Place the pouch flat on top of your right thigh, with the open end facing your knee. Hold the unopened end with one hand and use the forefinger of your other hand to push all of the contents of the pouch onto your right thigh (see Diagram 2).
- With one hand or both hands rub the material into your entire right thigh and right calf for three minutes until thoroughly absorbed (see Diagram 3). Rub any excess material remaining on the hands on your buttocks.
- To reduce the chances of Estrasorb transfer to other individuals upon contact, allow the application areas to dry completely and cover with clothing.
- Wash your hands with soap and water after you have finished the applications to ensure that any excess material has been removed (Diagram 4).

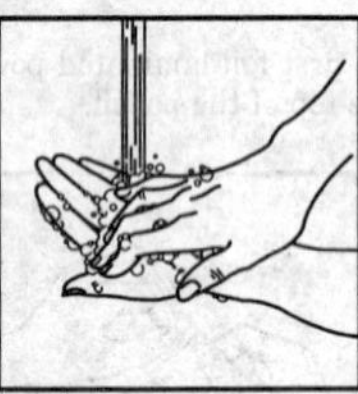

Diagram 4

If you forget to apply Estrasorb in the morning just apply Estrasorb as soon as you remember. Do not apply Estrasorb more than once each day.

General information about the safe and effective use of Estrasorb.
Medicines are sometimes prescribed for conditions that are not mentioned in patient information leaflets. Do not use Estrasorb for conditions for which it was not prescribed. Do not give Estrasorb to other people, even if they have the same symptoms you have. It may harm them.

Keep Estrasorb out of the reach of children.
This leaflet provides a summary of the important information about Estrasorb. If you would like more information, talk with your healthcare provider or pharmacist. You can ask for information about Estrasorb that is written for health professionals. You can get more information by calling the toll free number (**1-800-340-2001**).

What are the ingredients in Estrasorb?
17β-estradiol, Soybean oil, Water, Polysorbate 80, Ethanol

Manufactured by:
Novavax, Inc.
Columbia, MD 21046
Distributed by:
Novavax, Inc.
Columbia, MD 21046

Shown in Product Identification Guide, page 326

GYNODIOL™ ℞
(estradiol tablets, USP)
℞ only

DESCRIPTION
Gynodiol™ (estradiol tablets, USP) is a white, crystalline solid, chemically described as estra-1,3,5(10)-triene-3,17β-diol. It has a molecular formula of $C_{18}H_{24}O_2$ and molecular weight of 272.39. The structural formula is:
[See chemical structure at top of next column]

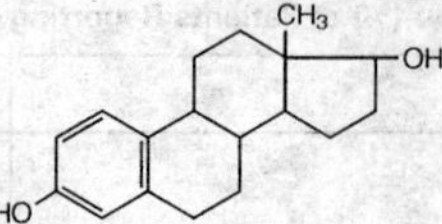

Gynodiol™ (estradiol tablets, USP) for oral administration, contain: 0.5 mg, 1 mg, 1.5 mg, or 2 mg of micronized estradiol per tablet.
Gynodiol™ (estradiol tablets, USP) 0.5 mg contain the following inactive ingredients: lactose monohydrate, croscarmellose sodium, carboxymethylcellulose sodium, pregelatinized starch, magnesium stearate, polysorbate 80, FD&C Blue No. 1 Aluminum Lake, D&C Red No. 27 Aluminum Lake.
Gynodiol™ (estradiol tablets, USP) 1 mg contain the following inactive ingredients: lactose monohydrate, croscarmellose sodium, carboxymethylcellulose sodium, pregelatinized starch, magnesium stearate, polysorbate 80, D&C Red No. 27 Aluminum Lake.
Gynodiol™ (estradiol tablets, USP) 1.5 mg contain the following inactive ingredients: lactose monohydrate, croscarmellose sodium, carboxymethylcellulose sodium, pregelatinized starch, magnesium stearate, polysorbate 80, FD&C Blue No. 1 Aluminum Lake, D&C Yellow No. 10 Aluminum Lake.
Gynodiol™ (estradiol tablets, USP) 2 mg contain the following inactive ingredients: lactose monohydrate, croscarmellose sodium, carboxymethylcellulose sodium, pregelatinized starch, magnesium stearate, FD&C Blue No. 2 Aluminum Lake, polysorbate 80.

HOW SUPPLIED
Gynodiol™ (estradiol tablets, USP) 0.5 mg; round, lavender colored tablet with bisect, debossed with ◇ and 0768. Available in containers of 30 (NDC 66500-768-00), and 100 (NDC 0421-0768-01).
Gynodiol™ (estradiol tablets, USP) 1 mg; round, rose colored tablet with bisect, debossed with ◇ and 1259: Available in containers of 30 (NDC 66500-259-00), and 100 (NDC 66500-259-01).
Gynodiol™ (estradiol tablets, USP) 1.5 mg; round, aqua colored tablet with bisect, debossed with ◇and 0158: Available in containers of 30 (NDC 66500-158-00), and 100 (NDC 66500-158-01).
Gynodiol™ (estradiol tablets, USP) 2 mg; round, blue colored tablet with bisect, debossed with ◇and 0748: Available in containers of 30 (NDC 66500-748-00), and 100 (NDC 0421-0748-01).
Store at controlled room temperature 15°–30°C (59°–86°F).

NOVANATAL™ ℞
[nō' vă-nā-tĕl]
Prenatal Multi-vitamin/Mineral Tablets

DESCRIPTION
NovaNatal™ is a white elliptical film-coated tablet with "102" debossed on one side and scored on the opposite side.
Each tablet contains:

Vitamin D (D_3)	400 IU
Vitamin E (dl-Alpha Tocopheryl Acetate)	30 IU
Vitamin C (Ascorbic Acid)	120 mg
Folic Acid	1 mg
Vitamin B_1 (Thiamine Mononitrate)	3 mg
Vitamin B_2 (Riboflavin)	3 mg
Niacin (Niacinamide)	20 mg
Vitamin B_6 (Pyridoxine HCl)	3 mg
Vitamin B_{12} (Cyanocobalamin)	8 mcg
Calcium (Calcium Carbonate)	200 mg
Iodine (Potassium Iodide)	150 mcg
Zinc (Zinc Oxide)	15 mg
Iron (Carbonyl Iron)	29 mg

INDICATIONS AND USAGE
NovaNatal™ is indicated for use in improving the nutritional status of women throughout pregnancy and in the postnatal period for both lactating and nonlactating mothers. NovaNatal™ is also beneficial in improving the nutritional status of women prior to conception.

CONTRAINDICATIONS
This product is contraindicated in patients with a known hypersensitivity to any of the ingredients.

WARNING
Folic acid alone is improper therapy in the treatment of pernicious anemia and other megaloblasitc anemias where vitamin B_{12} is deficient.

WARNING: Accidental overdose of iron-containing products is a leading cause of fatal poisoning in children under six. Keep this product out of reach of children. In case of accidental overdose, call a doctor or poison control center immediately.

PRECAUTIONS
Folic acid in doses above 0.1mg daily may obscure pernicious anemia in that hematological remission can occur while neurological manifestations remain progressive.

ADVERSE REACTIONS
Allergic sensitization has been reported following both oral and parenteral administration of folic acid.

DOSAGE AND ADMINISTRATION
One tablet daily or as directed by a physician.

HOW SUPPLIED

NovaNatal™ tablets for oral administration are supplied as white elliptical film-coated tablets with "102" debossed on one side and scored on the opposite side in bottles of 90 tablets. NDC 66500-102-01.

Store at controlled room temperature 15°-30° (59°-86°F)

RX only

Manufactured for
Novavax, Inc
Columbia, MD 21046 Rev. 6/03

Novo Nordisk Pharmaceuticals, Inc.

100 COLLEGE ROAD WEST
PRINCETON, NJ 08540

Direct Inquiries to:
Novo Nordisk Pharmaceuticals, Inc.
(800) 727-6500
8:00am - 7:00pm EST M–F
In Emergencies after hours and weekends:
609-987-5800
Novo Nordisk Diabetes Care® Hotline
1-800-727-6500
Norditropin Hotline
1-888-NOVO-HGH
NovoSeven® Hotline
1-877-NOVO-777
Hormone Therapy® Hotline
1-(866) NOVO-FEM
866-668-6336

ACTIVELLA® ℞

estradiol/norethindrone acetate tablets
1 mg estradiol
0.5 mg norethindrone acetate

DESCRIPTION

Activella® is a single tablet containing an estrogen, estradiol (E_2), and a progestin, norethindrone acetate (NETA), for oral administration. Each tablet contains 1 mg estradiol and 0.5 mg norethindrone acetate and the following excipients: lactose monohydrate, starch (corn), copovidone, talc, magnesium stearate, hypromellose and triacetin.

Estradiol (E_2) is a white or almost white crystalline powder. Its chemical name is estra-1, 3, 5 (10)-triene-3, 17β-diol hemihydrate with the empirical formula of $C_{18}H_{24}O_2$, 1/2 H_2O and a molecular weight of 281.4. The structural formula of E_2 is as follows:

OH
HO
Estradiol

Norethindrone acetate (NETA) is a white or yellowish-white crystalline powder. Its chemical name is 17β-acetoxy-19-nor-17α-pregn-4-en-20-yn-3-one with the empirical formula of $C_{22}H_{28}O_3$ and a molecular weight of 340.5. The structural formula of NETA is as follows:

O
Norethindrone Acetate

CLINICAL PHARMACOLOGY

Estrogen drug products act by regulating the transcription of a limited number of genes. Estrogens diffuse through cell membranes and bind to and activate the nuclear estrogen receptor, a DNA-binding protein that is found in estrogen-responsive tissues. The activated estrogen receptor binds to specific DNA sequences, or hormone-response elements, that enhance the transcription of adjacent genes and in turn lead to the observed effects. Estrogen receptors have been identified in tissues of the reproductive tract, breast, pituitary, hypothalamus, liver, and bone in women.

Estrogens are largely responsible for the development and maintenance of the female reproductive system and secondary sexual characteristics. Although circulating estrogens exist in a dynamic equilibrium of metabolic interconversions, estradiol is the principal intracellular human estrogen and is substantially more potent than its metabolites, estrone and estriol, at the receptor level. The primary source of estrogen in normally cycling adult women is the ovarian follicle, which secretes 70 to 500 μg of estradiol daily, depending on the phase of the menstrual cycle. After menopause, most endogenous estrogen is produced by conversion in peripheral tissues of androstenedione which is secreted by the adrenal cortex, to estrone. Thus, estrone and the sulfate conjugated form, estrone sulfate, are the most abundant circulating estrogens in postmenopausal women. Circulating estrogens modulate the pituitary secretion of the gonadotropins, luteinizing hormone (LH), and follicle-stimulating hormone (FSH) through a negative feedback mechanism, and estrogen replacement therapy acts to reduce the elevated levels of these hormones seen in postmenopausal women. Progestin compounds enhance cellular differentiation and generally oppose the actions of estrogens by decreasing estrogen receptor levels, increasing local metabolism of estrogens to less active metabolites, or inducing gene products that blunt cellular responses to estrogen.

Progestins exert their effects in target cells by binding to specific progesterone receptors that interact with progesterone response elements in target genes. Progesterone receptors have been identified in the female reproductive tract, breast, pituitary, hypothalamus, and central nervous system. Progestins produce similar endometrial changes to those of the naturally occurring hormone progesterone.

The use of unopposed estrogen therapy has been associated with an increased risk of endometrial hyperplasia, a possible precursor of endometrial adenocarcinoma. The addition of a progestin, in adequate doses and appropriate duration, to an estrogen replacement regimen reduces the incidence of endometrial hyperplasia, and the attendant risk of carcinoma in women with intact uterus.

PHARMACOKINETICS

ABSORPTION

Estradiol is well absorbed through the gastrointestinal tract. Following oral administration of Activella® (estradiol/norethindrone acetate tablets), peak plasma estradiol concentrations are reached slowly within 5–8 hours. When given orally, estradiol is extensively metabolized (first-pass effect) to estrone sulfate, with smaller amounts of other conjugated and unconjugated estrogens. After oral administration, norethindrone acetate is rapidly absorbed and transformed to norethindrone. It undergoes first-pass metabolism in the liver and other enteric organs, and reaches a peak plasma concentration within 0.5–1.5 hours. The oral bioavailability of estradiol and norethindrone following administration of Activella® when compared to a combination oral solution is 53% and 100%, respectively. The pharmacokinetic parameters of estradiol (E_2). estrone (E_1), and norethindrone (NET) following single oral administration of Activella® in 25 volunteers are summarized in TABLE 1.

TABLE 1
PHARMACOKINETIC PARAMETERS AFTER A SINGLE DOSE OF ACTIVELLA® IN HEALTHY POSTMENOPAUSAL WOMEN

	Activella® (n=25) Mean[c] ± SD
Estradiol [a] (E_2)	
AUC (0–72h)(pg/ml*h)	1053 ± 310
C_{max} (pg/ml)	34.6 ± 10.8
t_{max} (h)	6.8 ± 2.9
$t_{1/2}$ (h) [d]	13.2 ± 4.7
Estrone [a] (E_1)	
AUC (0–72h)(pg/ml*h)	5223 ± 1618
C_{max} (pg/ml)	251.1 ± 91.0
t_{max} (h)	5.7 ± 1.4
$t_{1/2}$ (h) [d]	12.2 ± 4.6
Norethindrone (NET)	
AUC (0–72h)(pg/ml*h)	23681 ± 9023[b]
C_{max} (pg/ml)	5308 ± 1510
t_{max} (h)	1.0 ± 0.0
$t_{1/2}$ (h)	11.4 ± 2.7

AUC = area under the curve,
C_{max} = maximum plasma concentration,
t_{max} = time at maximum plasma concentration,
$t_{1/2}$ = half-life,
SD = standard deviation
[a] baseline unadjusted data; [b] (n=23); [c] arithmetic mean;
[d] baseline adjusted data

Following continuous dosing with once-daily administration of Activella® (estradiol/norethindrone acetate tablets), serum levels of estradiol, estrone, and norethindrone reached steady-state within two weeks with an accumulation of 33–47% above levels following single dose adminstration. Unadjusted circulating levels of E_2, E_1, and NET during Activella® treatment at steady state (dosing at time 0) are provided in Figures 1a and 1b.

[See figure 1a at top of next column]
[See figure 1b at top of next column]

DISTRIBUTION

The distribution of exogenous estrogens is similar to that of endogenous estrogens. Estrogens are widely distributed in the body and are generally found in higher concentrations in the sex hormone target organs. Estradiol circulates in the blood bound to sex-hormone-binding globulin (SHBG) (37%) and to albumin (61%), while only approximately 1–2% is unbound. Norethindrone also binds to a similar extent to SHBG (36%) and to albumin (61%).

METABOLISM AND EXCRETION

Estradiol: Exogenous estrogens are metabolized in the same manner as endogenous estrogens. Circulating estrogens exist in a dynamic equilibrium of metabolic interconversions. These transformations take place mainly in the liver. Estradiol is converted reversibly to estrone, and both can be converted to estriol, which is the major urinary metabolite.

Figure 1a
Levels of Estradiol and Estrone at Steady State during Continuous Dosing with Activella® (n=24)

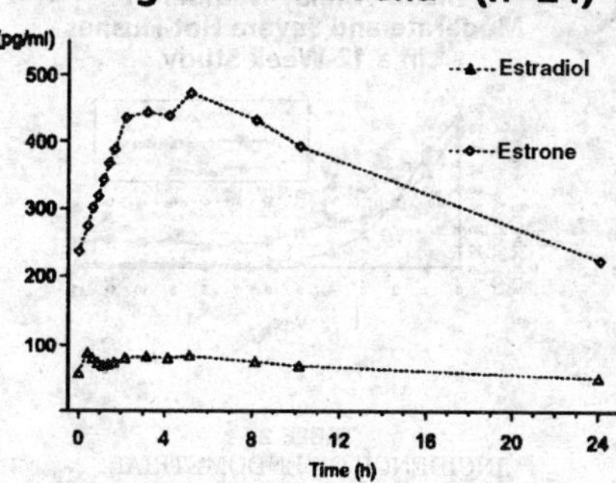

Figure 1b
Levels of Norethindrone at Steady State during Continuous Dosing with Activella® (n=24)

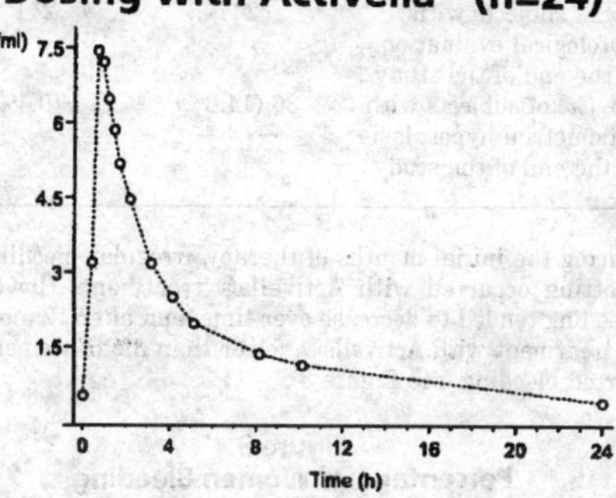

Estrogens also undergo enterohepatic recirculation via sulfate and glucuronide conjugation in the liver, biliary secretion of conjugates into the intestine, and hydrolysis in the gut followed by reabsorption. In postmenopausal women, a significant portion of the circulating estrogens exist as sulfate conjugates, especially estrone sulfate, which serves as a circulating reservoir for the formation of more active estrogens. The half-life of estradiol following single dose administration of Activella® (estradiol/norethindrone acetate tablets) is 12–14 hours.

Norethindrone Acetate: The most important metabolites of norethindrone are isomers of 5α-dihydro-norethindrone and tetrahydro-norethindrone, which are excreted mainly in the urine as sulfate or glucuronide conjugates. The terminal half-life of norethindrone is about 8–11 hours.

DRUG-DRUG INTERACTIONS

Coadministration of estradiol with norethindrone acetate did not elicit any apparent influence on the pharmacokinetics of norethindrone. Similarly, no relevant interaction of norethindrone on the pharmacokinetics of estradiol was found within the NETA dose range investigated in a single dose study.

FOOD-DRUG INTERACTIONS

A single-dose study in 24 healthy postmenopausal women was conducted to investigate any potential impact of administration of Activella® with and without food. Administration of Activella® with food did not modify the bioavailability of estradiol, although increases in AUC_{0-72} of 19% and decreases in C_{max} of 36% for norethindrone were seen.

CLINICAL STUDIES

VASOMOTOR SYMPTOMS

Activella® is effective in reducing the number of moderate-to-severe vasomotor symptoms in postmenopausal women. In a 12-week radomized clinical trial involving 92 subjects, Activella® was compared to 1 mg of estradiol and to placebo. The mean number and intensity of hot flushes were significantly reduced from baseline to week 12 in both the Activella® and the 1 mg estradiol group compared to placebo (see Figure 2).

[See figure 2 at top of next column]

ENDOMETRIAL HYPERPLASIA

Activella® (estradiol/norethindrone acetate tablets) reduced the incidence of estrogen-induced endometrial hyperplasia at 1 year in a randomized, controlled clinical trial. This trial enrolled 1,176 subjects who were randomized to one of 4 arms: 1 mg estradiol unopposed (n=296), 1 mg E_2 + 0.1 mg NETA (n=294), 1 mg E_2 + 0.25 mg NETA (n=291), and Activella® [1 mg E_2 + 0.5 mg NETA] (n=295). At the end of the study, endometrial biopsy results were available for 988 subjects. The results of the 1 mg estradiol unopposed arm compared to Activella® are shown in TABLE 2.

Continued on next page

Activella—Cont.

Figure 2
Mean Weekly Number of Moderate and Severe Hot Flushes in a 12-Week Study

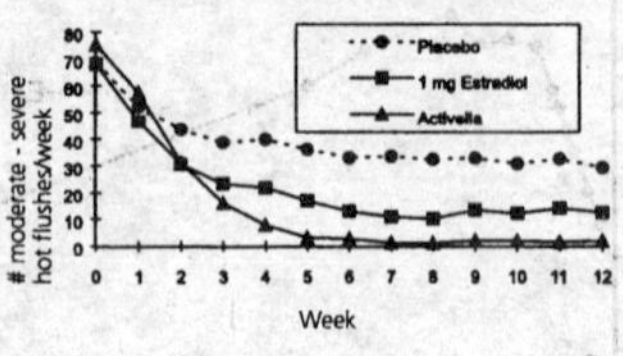

TABLE 2
INCIDENCE OF ENDOMETRIAL HYPERPLASIA WITH UNOPPOSED ESTRADIOL AND ACTIVELLA® IN A 12-MONTH STUDY

	1 mg E_2 (n=296)	Activella® (n=295)
No. of subjects with histological evaluation at the end of the study	247	241
No. (%) of subjects with endometrial hyperplasia at the end of the study	36 (14.6%)	1 (0.4%)

During the initial months of therapy, irregular bleeding or spotting occurred with Activella® treatment. However, bleeding tended to decrease over time, and after 12 months of treatment with Activella®, fewer than 3% of women reported bleeding (see Figure 3).

Figure 3
Percentage of Women Bleeding at Each Month in a 12-Month Study

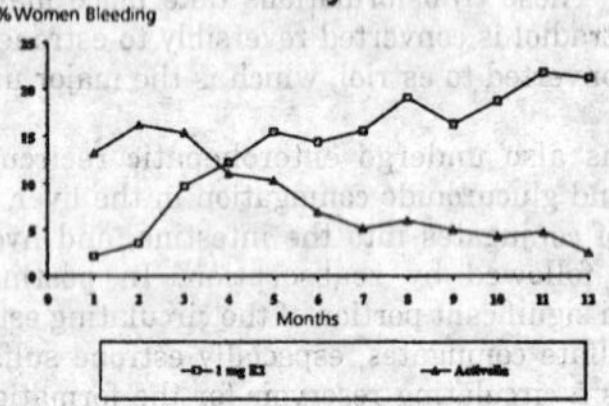

n=number of women
1 mg E2 (3, 6, 9 and 12 months): n=278, 255, 226, 212
Activella® (3, 6, 9 and 12 months): n=273, 246, 238, 232

INFORMATION REGARDING LIPID EFFECTS
A 12-month, placebo-controlled clinical trial in 80 postmenopausal Caucasian women at low risk for cardiovascular disease compared the effects of Activella® to placebo on lipid parameters. These results are shown in TABLE 3.

TABLE 3
PERCENTAGE CHANGE FROM BASELINE IN SELECTED LIPID PARAMETERS WITH ACTIVELLA® IN A 12-MONTH PLACEBO-CONTROLLED STUDY

Lipid Parameter %	Activella® (n=35)	Placebo (n=34)
Total Cholesterol	−10.5%	−0.8%
HDL-C[1]	−12.4%	−6.1%
LDL-C[2]	−10.8%	0.8%
LDL: HDL Ratio	0.1%	9.2%
Triglycerides	2.2%	4.4%

[1] High density lipoprotein-cholesterol
[2] Low density lipoprotein-cholesterol

EFFECT ON BONE MINERAL DENSITY
The results of two randomized, multicenter, calcium-supplemented (500–1000 mg/day), placebo-controlled, 2 year clinical trials have shown that Activella® (estradiol/norethindrone acetate tablets) is effective in preventing bone loss in postmenopausal women. A total of 462 postmenopausal women with intact uteri and baseline BMD values for lumbar spine within 2 standard deviations of the mean in healthy young women were enrolled. In a US trial, 327 postmenopausal women (mean time from menopause 2.5 to 3.1 years) with a mean age of 53 years were randomized to 7 groups (0.25 mg, 0.5 mg, and 1 mg of estradiol alone, 1 mg estradiol with 0.25 mg norethindrone acetate, 1 mg estradiol with 0.5 mg norethindrone acetate, and 2 mg estradiol with 1 mg norethindrone acetate, and placebo. In a European trial, 135 postmenopausal women (mean time from menopause 8.4 to 9.3 years) with a mean age of 58 years were randomized to 1 mg estradiol with 0.25 mg norethindrone acetate, 1 mg estradiol with 0.5 mg norethindrone acetate, and placebo.

TABLE 4
PERCENTAGE CHANGE (MEAN±SEM) IN BONE MINERAL DENSITY (BMD) (Intent to Treat Analysis, Last Observation Carried Forward)

	US Trial		EU Trial	
	Placebo (n=37)	Activella® (n=37)	Placebo (n=40)	Activella® (n=38)
Lumbar spine	−2.1±0.5	3.8±0.5*	−0.9±0.6	5.4±0.8*
Femoral neck	−2.3±0.6	1.8±0.7*	−1.0±0.7	0.7±0.9
Femoral trochanter	−2.0±0.7	3.7±0.7*	0.8±1.1	6.3±1.2*
Ward's triangle	–	–	−1.6±1.3	2.7±1.7
Distal radius	–	–	−0.7±0.5	2.1±0.5*
Total body	–	–	0.4±0.4	3.0±0.5*

US = United States, EU = European
* Significantly (p<0.001) different from placebo

Approximately 58% and 67% of the randomized subjects in the two clinical trials, respectively, completed the two clinical trials. BMD was measured using dual-energy x-ray absorptiometry (DEXA).
A summary of the results comparing Activella® and placebo from the two prevention trials is shown in Table 4.
[See table 4 above]
The overall difference in mean percentage change in BMD at the lumbar spine between Activella® and placebo was 5.9% in the US trial (1000 mg/day calcium) and 6.3% in the European trial (500 mg/day calcium). Activella® also increased BMD at the femoral neck and femoral trochanter compared to placebo. The increase in lumbar spine BMD in the US and European clinical trials is displayed in Figure 4.

FIGURE 4
Percentage Change in Bone Mineral Density (BMD) of the Lumbar Spine (L1-L4) (Intent to Treat Analysis with Last Observation Carried Forward)

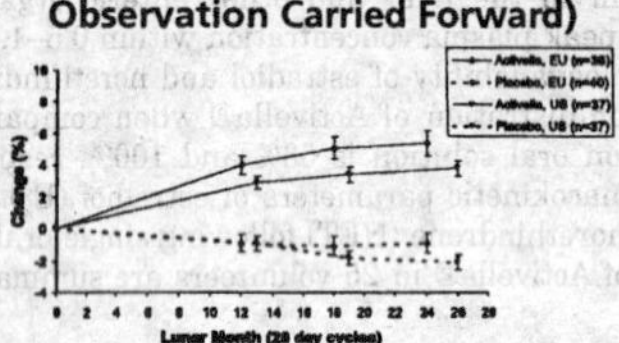

EFFECT ON BONE TURNOVER
Activella® (estradiol/norethindrone acetate tablets) significantly reduced serum and urine markers of bone turnover with a marked decrease in bone resorption makers (e.g., urinary pyridinoline crosslinks Type 1 collagen C-telopeptide, pyridinoline, deoxypyridinoline) and to a lesser extent in bone formation markers (e.g., serum osteocalcin, bone-specific alkaline phosphatase, C-terminal propetide of Type 1 collagen). The suppression of bone turnover markers was evident by 3 months and persisted throughout the 24-month treatment period.

INDICATIONS AND USAGE

Activella® therapy is indicated in women with an intact uterus for the:
1. Treatment of moderate to severe vasomotor symptoms associated with the menopause. There is no adequate evidence that estrogens are effective for nervous symptoms or depression that might occur during menopause and they should not be used to treat these conditions.
2. Treatment of vulvar and vaginal atrophy.
3. Prevention of postmenopausal osteoporosis.
Most prospective studies of efficacy for the osteoporosis prevention indication have been carried out in white postmenopausal women, without stratification by other risk factors, and tend to show a universally beneficial effect on bone. Since estrogen administration is associated with risk, patient selection must be individualized based on the balance of risks and benefits.
Case-control studies have shown an approximately 60-percent reduction in hip and wrist fractures in women whose estrogen replacement was begun within a few years after menopause. Studies also suggest that estrogen reduces the rate of vertebral fractures. When estrogen therapy is discontinued, bone mass declines at a rate comparable to the immediate postmenopausal period. White and Asian women are at higher risk for osteoporosis than black women, and thin women are at a higher risk than heavier women, who generally have higher endogenous estrogen levels. Early menopause is one of the strongest predictors for the development of osteoporosis. Other factors associated with osteoporosis include genetic factors (small build, family history), lifestyle (cigarette smoking, alcohol abuse, sedentary exercise habits) and nutrition (below average body weight and dietary calcium intake).
The mainstays of prevention and management of osteoporosis are weight-bearing exercise, adequate calcium intake, and, when indicated, estrogen. Postmenopausal women absorb dietary calcium less efficiently than premenopausal women and require an average of 1500 mg/day of elemental calcium to remain in neutral calcium balance. The average calcium intake in the USA is 400–600 mg/day. Therefore, when not contraindicated, calcium supplementation may be helpful for women with suboptimal dietary intake.

CONTRAINDICATIONS

Estrogens/progestins combined should not be used in women under any of the following conditions or circumstances.
1. Known or suspected pregnancy, including use for missed abortions or as a diagnostic test for pregnancy. Estrogen or progestin may cause fetal harm when administered to a pregnant woman.
2. Known or suspected breast cancer, or past history of breast cancer associated with the use of estrogens.
3. Known or suspected estrogen-dependent neoplasia, e.g., endometrial cancer.
4. Abnormal genital bleeding unknown etiology.
5. Known or suspected active deep venous thrombosis, thromboembolic disorders or stroke or past history of these conditions associated with estrogen use.
6. Liver dysfunction or disease.
7. Hypersensitivity to any of the components of Activella® (estradiol/norethindrone acetate tablets).

WARNINGS

ALL WARNINGS BELOW PERTAIN TO THE USE OF THIS COMBINATION PRODUCT.
Based on experience with estrogens and/or progestins:
1. Induction of malignant neoplasms
Endometrial cancer. The reported endometrial cancer risk among unopposed estrogen users is about 2- to 12-fold greater than in non-users, and appears dependent on duration of treatment and on estrogen dose. There is no significant increased risk associated with the use of estrogens for less than one year. The greatest risk appears to be associated with prolonged use with increased risks of 15- to 24-fold with five or more years of use. In three studies, persistence of risk was demonstrated for 8 to over 15 years after cessation of estrogen treatment. In one study, a significant decrease in the incidence of endometrial cancer occurred six months after withdrawal. Progestins taken with estrogens have been shown to significantly reduce, but not eliminate, the risk of endometrial cancer associated with estrogen use.
In a large clinical trial, the incidence of endometrial hyperplasia with Activella® was 0.4% (one simple hyperplasia without atypia) compared to 14.6% with 1 mg estradiol unopposed (see CLINICAL STUDIES).
Clinical surveillance of all women taking estrogen/progestin combinations is important. Adequate diagnostic measures, including endometrial sampling when indicated, should be undertaken to rule out malignancy in all cases of undiagnosed persistent or recurring abnormal vaginal bleeding. There is no evidence that "natural" estrogens are more or less hazardous than "synthetic" estrogens at equivalent estrogen doses.
Breast cancer. While the majority of studies have not shown an increased risk of breast cancer in women who have ever used estrogen replacement therapy, some have reported a moderately increased risk (relative risks of 1.3–2.0) in those taking higher doses, or in those taking lower doses for prolonged periods of time, especially in excess of 10 years.
While the effects of added progestins on the risk of breast cancer are also unknown, available epidemiological evidence suggest that progestins do not reduce, and may enhance, the moderately increased breast cancer risk that has been reported with prolonged estrogen replacement therapy.
In a one-year trial among 1,176 women who received either unopposed 1 mg estradiol or a combination of 1 mg estradiol plus one of three different doses of NETA (0.1, 0.25 and 0.5 mg), seven new cases of breast cancer were diagnosed, two of which occurred among the group of 295 Activella® (estradiol/norethindrone acetate tablets) treated women.
Women on hormone replacement therapy should have regular breast examinations and should be instructed in breast self-examination, and women over the age of 40 should have regular mammograms.
2. Congenital lesions with malignant potential. Estrogen therapy during pregnancy is associated with an increased risk of fetal congenital reproductive tract disorders, and possible other birth defects.
Studies of women who received diethylstilbestrol (DES) during pregnancy have shown that female offspring have an increased risk of vaginal adenosis, squamous cell dysplasia of the uterine cervix, and clear cell vaginal cancer later in life; male offspring have an increased risk of urogenital abnormalities and possibly testicular cancer later in life.
Although some of these changes are benign, others are precursors of malignancy.

3. Cardiovascular disease. Large doses of estrogens (5 mg conjugated estrogen per day), comparable to those used to treat cancer of the prostate and breast, have been shown in a large prospective clinical trial in men to increase the risk of nonfatal myocardial infarction, pulmonary embolism, and thrombophlebitis.
These risks cannot necessarily be extrapolated from men to women or from unopposed estrogen to combination estrogen/progestin therapy. However, to avoid the theoretical cardiovascular risk to women caused by high estrogen doses, the dose for estrogen replacement therapy should not exceed the lowest effective dose.
4. Hypercalcemia. Administration of estrogens may lead to severe hypercalcemia in patients with breast cancer and bone metastases. If this occurs, the drugs should be stopped and appropriate measures taken to reduce the serum calcium level.
5. Effects during pregnancy. Use in pregnancy is not recommended.
6. Gallbladder disease. Two studies have reported a 2- to 4-fold increase in the risk of surgically confirmed gallbladder disease in women receiving postmenopausal estrogens. Among the 1,516 women treated in clinical trials with 1 mg estradiol alone or in combination with several doses of NETA, 3 women had surgically confirmed cholelithiasis, none of them on Activella® (estradiol/norethindrone acetate tablets) treatment.
7. Elevated blood pressure. Occasional blood pressure increases during estrogen replacement therapy have been attributed to idiosyncratic reactions to estrogens. More often, blood pressure has remained the same or has dropped. One study showed that postmenopausal estrogen users have higher blood pressure than non-users. Two other studies showed slightly lower blood pressure among estrogen users compared to non-users. Postmenopausal estrogen use does not increase the risk of stroke. Nonetheless, blood pressure should be monitored at regular intervals with estrogen use.
8. Thromboembolic disorders. The physician should be alert to the earliest manifestations of thrombotic disorders (thrombophlebitis, cerebrovascular disorders, pulmonary embolism, and retinal thrombosis). Should any of these occur or be suspected, the drugs should be discontinued immediately. In a one-year study where 295 women were exposed to Activella®, there were two cases of deep vein thromboses reported.
9. Visual abnormalities. Discontinue medication pending examination if there is a sudden partial or complete loss of vision, or a sudden onset of proptosis, diplopia, or migraine. If examinations reveal papilledema or retinal vascular lesions, medication should be withdrawn.

PRECAUTIONS

GENERAL

Based on experience with estrogens and/or progestins:
1. Cardiovascular risk. A causal relationship between estrogen replacement therapy and reduction of cardiovascular disease in postmenopausal women has not been proven. Furthermore, the effect of added progestins on this putative benefit is not yet known.
In recent years, many published studies have suggested that there may be a cause-effect relationship between postmenopausal oral estrogen replacement therapy without added progestins and a decrease in cardiovascular disease in women. Although most of the observational studies that assessed this statistical association have reported a 20% to 50% reduction in coronary heart disease risk and associated mortality in estrogen takers, the following should be considered when interpreting these reports. Because only one of these studies was randomized and it was too small to yield statistically significant results, all relevant studies were subject to selection bias. Thus, the apparently reduced risk of coronary artery disease cannot be attributed with certainty to estrogen replacement therapy. It may instead have been caused by life-style and medical characteristics of the women studied with the result that healthier women were selected for estrogen therapy. In general, treated women were of higher socioeconomic and educational status, more slender, more physically active, more likely to have undergone surgical menopause, and less likely to have diabetes than the untreated women. Although some studies attempted to control for these selection factors, it is common for properly designed randomized trials to fail to confirm benefits suggested by less rigorous study designs. Thus, ongoing and future large-scale randomized trials may fail to confirm this apparent benefit.
Current medical practice often includes the use of concomitant progestin therapy in women with intact uterus. While the effects of added progestins on the risk of ischemic heart disease are not known, all available progestins attenuate at least some of the favorable effects of estrogens on HDL levels, although they maintain the favorable effect of estrogens on LDL levels.
The safety data regarding Activella® (estradiol/norethindrone acetate tablets) were obtained primarily from clinical trials and epidemiologic studies of postmenopausal Caucasian women, who were at generally low risk of cardiovascular disease and higher than average risk for osteoporosis. The safety profile of Activella® derived from these study populations cannot necessarily be extrapolated to other populations of diverse racial and/or demographic composition. When considering prescribing Activella®, physicians are advised to weigh the potential benefits and risks of therapy as applicable to each individual patient.
2. Use in hysterectomized women. Existing data do not support the use of the combination of estrogen and progestin in postmenopausal women without a uterus. Risks that may be associated with the inclusion of progestin in estrogen replacement regimens include deterioration in glucose tolerance, and less favorable effects on lipid metabolism compared to the effects of estrogen alone.
The effects of Activella® on glucose tolerance and lipid metabolism have been studied (see CLINICAL PHARMACOLOGY, Clinical Studies, and PRECAUTIONS, Drug/Laboratory Test Interactions).
3. Physical examination. A complete medical and family history should be taken prior to the initiation of any estrogen/progestin therapy. The pretreatment and periodic physical examinations should include special reference to blood pressure, breasts, abdomen, and pelvic organs, and should include a Papanicolaou smear. As a general rule, estrogen should not be prescribed for longer than one year without another physical examination being performed.
4. Fluid retention. Because estrogens/progestins may cause some degree of fluid retention, conditions that might be influenced by this factor, such as asthma, epilepsy, migraine, and cardiac or renal dysfunction, require careful observation.
5. Uterine bleeding. Certain patients may develop abnormal uterine bleeding. In cases of undiagnosed abnormal uterine bleeding, adequate diagnostic measures are indicated (see WARNINGS).
6. The pathologist should be advised of estrogen/progestin therapy when relevant specimens are submitted.
Based on experience with estrogens:
1. Familial hyperlipoproteinemia. Estrogen therapy may be associated with massive elevations of plasma triglycerides leading to pancreatitis and other complications in patients with familial defects in lipoprotein metabolism.
2. Hypercoagulability. Some studies have shown that women taking estrogen replacement therapy have hypercoagulability primarily related to decreased antithrombin activity. This effect appears dose- and duration-dependent and is less pronounced than that associated with oral contraceptive use. Also, postmenopausal women tend to have changes in levels of coagulation parameters at baseline compared to premenopausal women. Epidemiological studies have suggested that estrogen use is associated with a higher relative risk of developing venous thromboembolism, i.e., deep vein thrombosis or pulmonary embolism. The studies found a 2-3- fold higher risk for estrogen users compared to non-users. There is insufficient information on hypercoagulability in women who have had previous thromboembolic disease. The effects of Activella® (estradiol/norethindrone acetate tablets) (n=40) compared to placebo (n=40) on selected clotting factors were evaluated in a 12-month study with postmenopausal women.
Activella® decreased factor VII, plasminogen activator inhibitor-1, and, to a lesser extent, antithrombin III activity, compared to placebo. Fibrinogen remained unchanged during Activella® treatment in comparison with an increase over time in the placebo group.
3. Mastodynia. Certain patients may develop undesirable manifestations of estrogenic stimulation such as mastodynia. In clinical trials, less than one-fifth of the women treated with Activella® reported breast tenderness or breast pain. The majority of the cases were reported as breast tenderness, primarily during the initial months of the treatment.
Based on experience with progestins:
1. Lipoprotein metabolism. (see CLINICAL STUDIES)
2. Impaired glucose tolerance. Diabetic patients should be carefully observed while receiving estrogen/progestin therapy.
The effects of Activella® on glucose tolerance have been studied (see PRECAUTIONS, Drug/Laboratory Test Interactions).
3. Depression. Patients who have a history of depression should be observed and the drugs discontinued if the depression recurs to a serious degree.

INFORMATION FOR THE PATIENT

See text of Patient Package Insert which appears after the **How Supplied** section.

DRUG/LABORATORY TEST INTERACTIONS

The following interactions have been observed with estrogen therapy, and/or Activella® (estradiol/norethindrone acetate tablets):
1. Activella® decreases factor VII, plasminogen activator inhibitor-1, and, to a lesser extent, antithrombin III activity.
2. Estrogen therapy increases thyroid-binding globulin (TBG) leading to increased circulating total thyroid hormone, as measured by protein-bound iodine (PBI), T_4 levels (by column or by radioimmunoassay) or T_3 levels by radioimmunoassay. T_3 resin uptake is decreased, reflecting the elevated TBG. Free T_4 and free T_3 concentrations are unaltered.
3. Estrogen therapy may elevate other binding proteins in serum i.e., corticosteroid-binding globulin (CBG), sex-hormone-binding globulin (SHBG), leading to increased circulating corticosteroids and sex steroids respectively. Free or biologically active hormone concentrations are unchanged. Other plasma proteins may be increased (angiotensinogen/renin substrate, alpha-1-antitrypsin, ceruloplasmin). In a 12-month clinical trial, SHBG was found to increase with Activella®.
4. Estrogen therapy increases plasma HDL and HDL-2 subfraction concentrations, reduces LDL cholesterol concentration, and increases triglyceride levels. (For effects during Activella® treatment, see CLINICAL PHARMACOLOGY, Clinical Studies).
5. Activella® treatment of healthy postmenopausal women does not decrease glucose tolerance when assessed by an oral glucose tolerance test; the insulin response decreases without any increase in the glucose serum levels. Activella® treatment does not deteriorate insulin sensitivity in healthy postmenopausal women when assessed by an hyperinsulinemic euglycemic clamp.
6. Estrogen therapy reduces response to metyrapone test.
7. Estrogen therapy reduces serum folate concentration.

CARCINOGENESIS, MUTAGENESIS, and IMPAIRMENT OF INFERTILITY

Long-term continuous administration of natural and synthetic estrogens in certain animal species increases the frequency of carcinomas of the breast, uterus, cervix, vagina, testis, and liver. (See CONTRAINDICATIONS and WARNINGS.)

PREGNANCY CATEGORY X:

Estrogens/progestins should not be used during pregnancy. (See CONTRAINDICATIONS and WARNINGS.)

NURSING MOTHERS:

Detectable amounts of estradiol and norethindrone acetate have been identified in the milk of mothers receiving these products and has been reported to decrease the quantity and the quality of the milk.
As a general principle, the administration of any drug to nursing mothers should be done only when clearly necessary since many drugs are excreted in human milk.

Continued on next page

TABLE 5
ALL TREATMENT-EMERGENT ADVERSE EVENTS REGARDLESS OF RELATIONSHIP REPORTED AT A FREQUENCY OF ≥5% WITH ACTIVELLA®

	Endometrial Hyperplasia Study (12-Months)		Vasomotor Symptoms Study (3-Months)		Osteoporosis Study (2 Years)	
	Activella® (n=295)	1 mg E2 (n=296)	Activella® (n=29)	Placebo (n=34)	Activella® (n=47)	Placebo (n=48)
Body as a Whole						
Back Pain	6%	5%	3%	3%	6%	4%
Headache	16%	16%	17%	18%	11%	6%
Digestive System						
Nausea	3%	5%	10%	0%	11%	0%
Gastroenteritis	2%	2%	0%	0%	6%	4%
Nervous System						
Insomnia	6%	4%	3%	3%	0%	8%
Emotional Lability	1%	1%	0%	0%	6%	0%
Respiratory System						
Upper Respiratory Tract Infection	18%	15%	10%	6%	15%	19%
Sinusitis	7%	11%	7%	0%	15%	10%
Metabolic and Nutritional						
Weight increase	0%	0%	0%	0%	9%	6%
Urogenital System						
Breast Pain	24%	10%	21%	0%	17%	8%
Post-Menopausal Bleeding	5%	15%	10%	3%	11%	0%
Uterine Fibroid	5%	4%	0%	0%	4%	8%
Ovarian Cyst	3%	2%	7%	0%	0%	8%
Resistance Mechanism						
Infection Viral	4%	6%	0%	3%	6%	6%
Moniliasis Genital	4%	7%	0%	0%	6%	0%
Secondary Terms						
Injury Accidental	4%	3%	3%	0%	17%*	4%*
Other Events	2%	3%	3%	0%	6%	4%

* including one upper extremity fracture in each group

Activella—Cont.

PEDIATRIC USE:
Safety and effectiveness in pediatric patients have not been established.
GERIATRIC USE:
Clinical studies of Activella® (estradiol/norethindrone acetate tablets) did not include sufficient number of subjects aged 65 and over to determine if they responded differently from younger subjects. Other reported clinical experience has not identified differences in responses between elderly and younger subjects. In general, dose selection for an elderly patient should be cautious, usually starting at the low end of the dosing range, reflecting the greater frequency of decreased hepatic, renal, or cardiac function, and of concomitant disease or other drug therapy.

ADVERSE REACTIONS

(See WARNINGS regarding induction of neoplasia, adverse effects on the fetus, increased incidence of gallbladder disease, elevated blood pressure, thromboembolic disorders, cardiovascular disease, visual abnormalities, and hypercalcemia and PRECAUTIONS regarding cardiovascular disease.)
Adverse events reported by investigators in the Phase 3 studies regardless of causality assessment are shown in TABLE 5.
[See table 5 at top of previous page]
The following adverse reactions have been reported with estrogen and/or progestin therapy:
Genitourinary system: changes in vaginal bleeding pattern and abnormal withdrawal bleeding or flow, breakthrough bleeding, spotting, increase in size of uterine leiomyomata, vaginal candidiasis, changes in amount of cervical secretion, premenstrual-like syndrome, cystitis-like syndrome.
Breasts: tenderness, enlargement.
Gastrointestinal: nausea, vomiting, changes in appetite, cholestatic jaundice, abdominal pain, flatulence, bloating, increased incidence of gallbladder disease.
Skin: chloasma or melasma that may persist when drug is discontinued, erythema multiforme, erythema nodosum, hemorrhagic eruption, loss of scalp hair, hirsutism, itching, skin rash and pruritus.
Cardiovascular: changes in blood pressure, cerebrovascular accidents, deep venous thrombosis and pulmonary embolism.
CNS: headache, migraine, dizziness, depression, chorea, insomnia, nervousness.
Eyes: steepening of corneal curvature, intolerance to contact lenses.
Miscellaneous: increase or decrease in weight, aggravation of porphyria, edema, changes in libido, fatigue, allergic reactions, back pain, arthralgia, myalgia.

OVERDOSAGE

Acute Overdose: Serious ill effects have not been reported following acute ingestion of large doses of estrogen/progestin-containing oral contraceptives by young children. Overdosage may cause nausea and vomiting and withdrawal bleeding may occur in females.

DOSAGE AND ADMINISTRATION

Activella® (estradiol/norethindrone acetate tablets) therapy consists of a single tablet to be taken once daily. For the treatment of moderate to severe vasomotor symptoms associated with the menopause, treatment of vulvar and vaginal atrophy, and the prevention of postmenopausal osteoporosis – Activella® 1 mg E_2 / 0.5 mg NETA daily. The doses of 17beta-estradiol and norethindrone acetate in Activella® may not be the lowest effective dose-combination for the prevention of osteoporosis.
Treated patients with an intact uterus should be monitored closely for signs of endometrial cancer, and appropriate diagnostic measures should be taken to rule out malignancy in the event of persistent or recurring abnormal vaginal bleeding.

HOW SUPPLIED

Activella®, 1 mg estradiol and 0.5 mg norethindrone acetate, is a white, film-coated tablet, engraved with NOVO 288 on one side and the APIS bull on the other. It is round, 6 mm in diameter and bi-convex.
Activella® is supplied as:
28 tablets in a calendar dial pack dispenser NDC 0169-5174-02.
Store in a dry place protected from light. Store at 25°C (77°F); excursions permitted to 15–30°C (59–86°F).
[See USP Controlled Room Temperature]

Rx only
Activella® is a trademark owned by
Novo Nordisk A/S
Revised July 2003
Novo Nordisk Pharmaceuticals, Inc.
Princeton, NJ 08540
1-866-668-6336
www.novonordisk-us.com
Manufactured by
Novo Nordisk AS
2880 Bagsvaerd, Denmark

HUMAN INSULIN DELIVERY SYSTEMS

Novo Nordisk® Pharmaceuticals, Inc. offers durable insulin delivery systems.

DURABLE INSULIN DELIVERY SYSTEMS

The following durable insulin delivery devices, which are sold separately, are available:
1. NovoPen® 3 Insulin Delivery Device
2. NovoPen® Junior
3. NovoPen® 3 PenMate® (optional) for use with NovoPen® Junior or NovoPen® 3
4. Innovo®
5. InDuo®

These devices are used with Novo Nordisk® 3mL PenFill® Cartridges and Novo Fine 30 or NovoFine® 31 Disposable Needles which are sold separately.
For information about obtaining NovoPen® 3 Insulin Delivery Devices for patients, call 1-800-727-6500.
Novolin® PenFill® 1.5 ml, Novolin® Prefilled Syringe (1.5 ml), and NovoPen® 1.5 are no longer marketed by Novo Nordisk®.

DISPOSABLE INSULIN DELIVERY SYSTEMS

The following disposable insulin delivery devices are available:
1. Novolin® InnoLet® human insulin (rDNA origin) disposable prefilled insulin syringe.
2. NovoLog® FlexPen® insulin aspart (rDNA origin) injection in a 3 mL Prefilled syringe, NovoLog Mix 70/30 FlexPen 70% insulin aspart (rDNA origin) protamine suspension and 30% insulin aspart (rDNA origin) injection in a 3 mL Prefilled syringe

These disposable insulin delivery systems are for use with NovoFine® 30 and NovoFine® 31 Disposable Needles which are sold separately.

INNOVO®

[ĭn-ō-vō]

[See figure below]

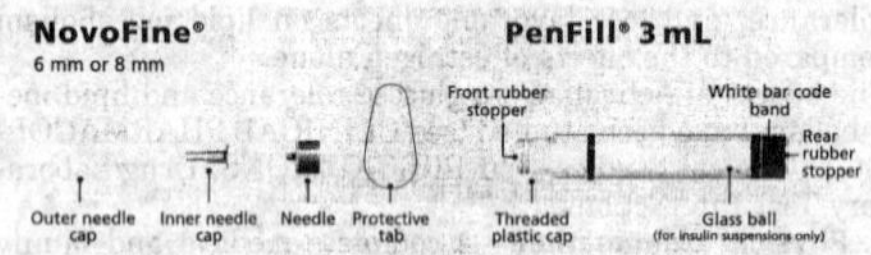

⚠ If Innovo® has been dropped or knocked, you must carry out a function check (see "Function check" section).
Innovo® insulin doser should only be used in combination with products that are compatible and allow Innovo® to function safely and effectively.
PenFill® 3 mL cartridges and NovoFine® needles are designed to be used with Innovo® insulin doser.
Needles and cartridges not included.
Innovo®, PenFill® and NovoFine® are trademarks owned by Novo Nordisk A/S.
Protected by US Patent Nos. 5,957,889; 5,961,496; and 6,045,537. Additional patents pending.
The CE-mark on a medical device indicates that the product conforms with the provisions in the EC Directive for Medical Devices 93/42/EEC. Innovo® fullfils the specification limits for dose accuracy according to ISO 11608 -1 Pen-Injectors for Medical use, Part 1: Requirements and test methods.

Contents

Introduction

Thank you for choosing Innovo®, the insulin doser designed to make insulin therapy easier to live with.
This manual contains instructions for using, storing, and cleaning your Innovo®. Here are some of the unique features Innovo® has to offer:
Easy to carry. Innovo® is short and compact, making it easy to carry in your pocket or purse.
Easy to inject. Innovo® is designed to fit perfectly in your hand, and is ideal for making quick and discreet injections.
Easy to read. The display on Innovo® is large and clear, making it easy to read the dose of insulin dialed and delivered.
Easy to remember. Innovo® has a built-in memory function, displaying your previous dose of insulin and the time passed since your last delivery.
Easy to dial. Innovo® is accurate and can easily be dialed to deliver doses from 1 to 70 units, in steps of 1 unit.
Easy to change dose. The insulin dose can easily be changed without wasting insulin simply by dialing up or down.
Easy to change PenFill®. Innovo® is specially designed for the easy changing of PenFill® 3 mL cartridges and NovoFine® needles with a length of up to 8 mm.
Easy reminders. Innovo® has a battery that lasts for about 5 years from manufacturing date when used at a rate of four daily injections (including the priming air shots). After this time, the display flashes to tell you that Innovo® will expire. Be sure to replace Innovo® within 30 days. The battery cannot be changed. This is to guarantee quality and safety at all times.
Thank you for choosing Innovo®. It is important that you follow the instructions carefully to make insulin therapy as easy to live with as possible.
Please complete and return the Innovo® warranty card.
Customer service and satisfaction are our top priority. If you have any questions about your Innovo®, please call Novo Nordisk Pharmaceuticals, Inc. Our toll free number is 1-800-727-6500.

Getting started

Pull off the cap. Put the cap to one side and keep it. You will need to replace the cap after your injection.

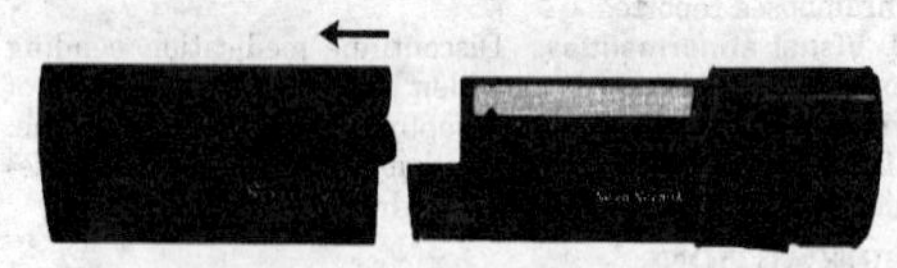

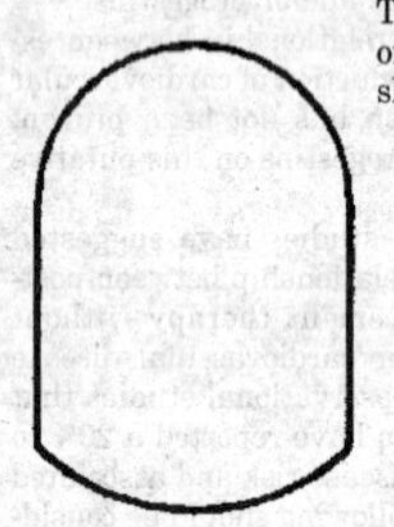

The very first time the cap is pulled off, the display stays blank until the slide is opened.

Make sure that the push button is pressed completely in.
A Otherwise the slide will be locked.
Open the slide in the direction of the arrow shown below.
B

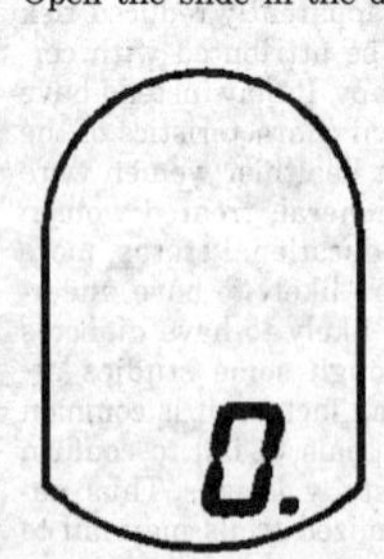

The display now shows 0.

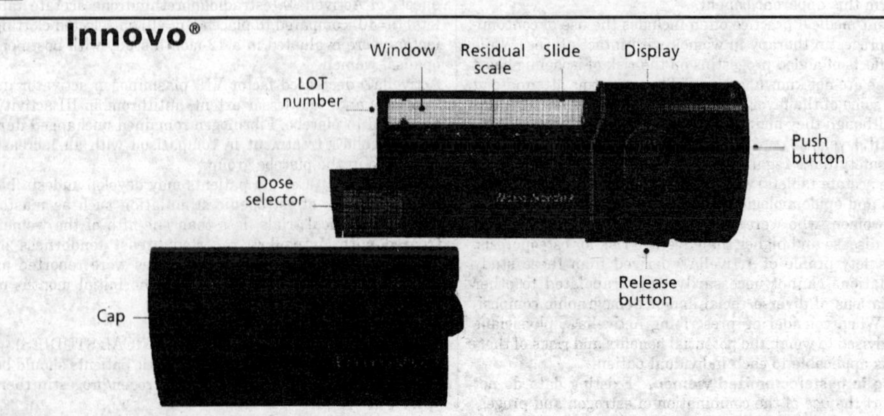

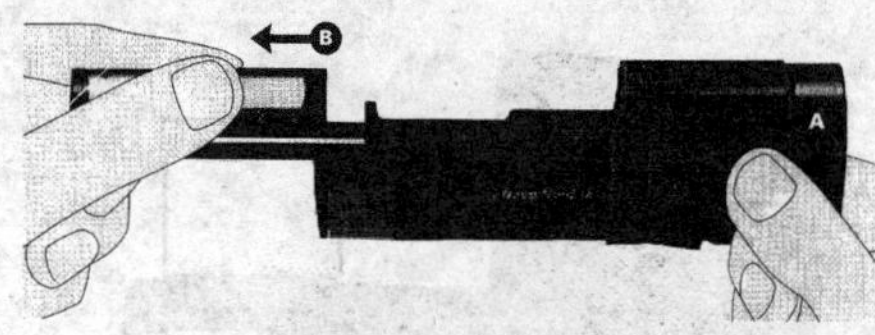

In the PenFill® Information For The Patient you will find instructions on how to:

- check that PenFill® is full and intact. If not, do not use it.
- resuspend the insulin, if PenFill® contains an insulin suspension (cloudy insulin).

Use only a new PenFill® when loading Innovo®. Never load a partially filled PenFill®. Never try to refill a used PenFill®.

Put PenFill® into Innovo® by pushing it slightly backwards as shown. The end with the rear rubber stopper goes in first.

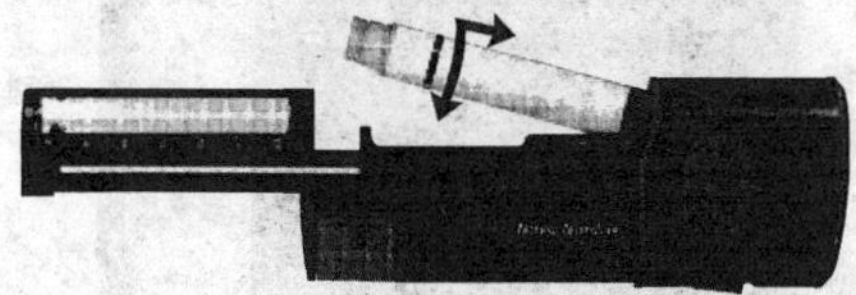

Make sure that the threaded plastic cap fits firmly into place.

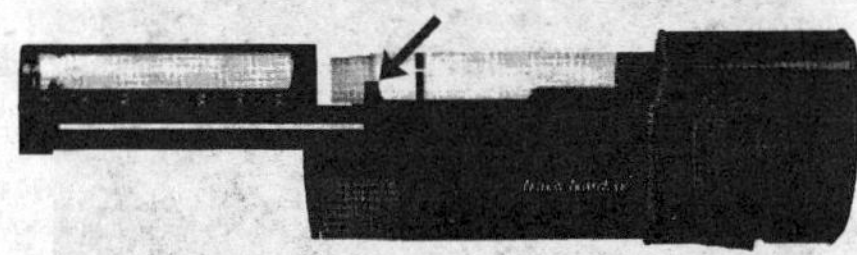

Close the slide completely. The release button is locked until the slide has been closed.
Keep the slide closed until PenFill® is empty.

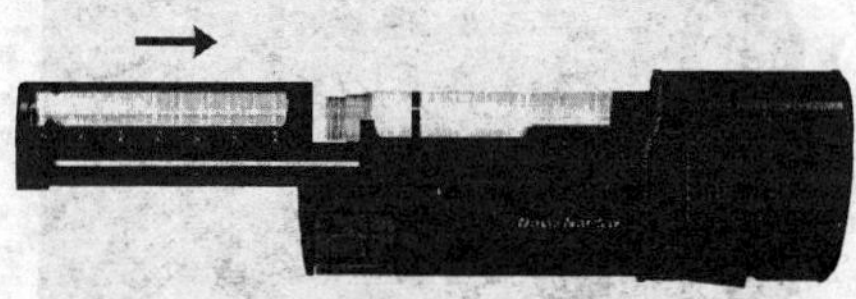

Wipe the front rubber stopper with an alcohol swab.
Never place a NovoFine® needle on your Innovo® until you are ready to prime Innovo® by doing an air shot before giving an injection.
Take the protective tab off a NovoFine® needle and screw the needle tightly onto the threaded plastic cap.
Pull off the outer and inner needle caps. Do not bend or damage the needle before use.
[See first two figures at top of next column]

Priming Innovo® by doing an air shot

⚠Always prime your Innovo® by doing an air shot, to ensure the insulin flow:

- before each injection
- after changing PenFill®
- after changing the needle
- after opening and closing the slide.

It is important that insulin appears at the tip of the needle before you make your injection. Otherwise you will not receive the full insulin dose.

How to prime your Innovo® by doing an air shot

1. Make sure that a needle is mounted, the push button is pressed completely in, and the slide is closed. If the slide is not closed, the release button will be locked.
2. Press the release button **A**. You will see that the push button jumps out.

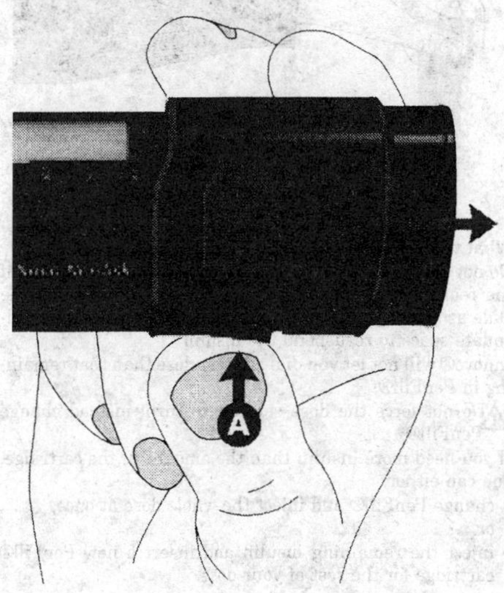

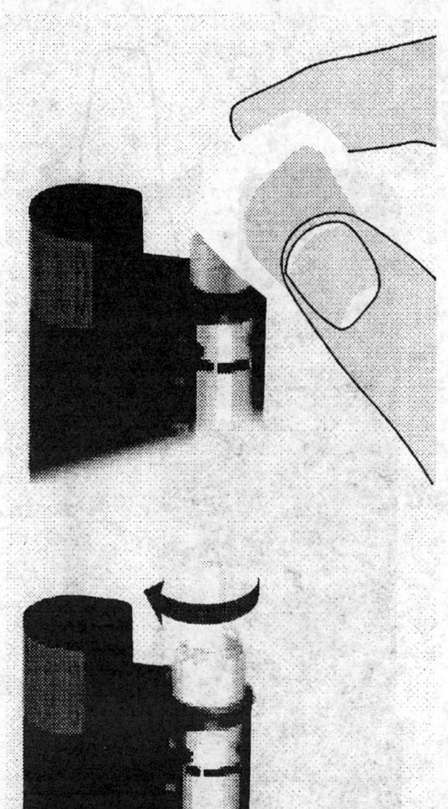

3. Dial 1 unit **B**.

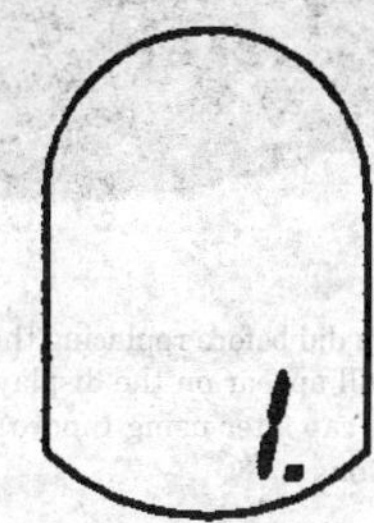

When inserting a new PenFill®, start with 8 units.
After opening and closing the slide you will need to dial a larger number of units, depending on the amount of insulin left in PenFill®.

4. Hold Innovo® with the needle upwards and tap the slide gently with your finger a few times **C**.
5. Press the push button completely in until it locks **D**.
6. A drop of insulin should appear at the needle tip.
7. If not, repeat the priming procedure dialing 1 unit. Repeat until a drop of insulin appears.
[See first figure at top of next column]

Choosing your dose

⚠Make sure that a needle is mounted and that the push button is pressed completely in.

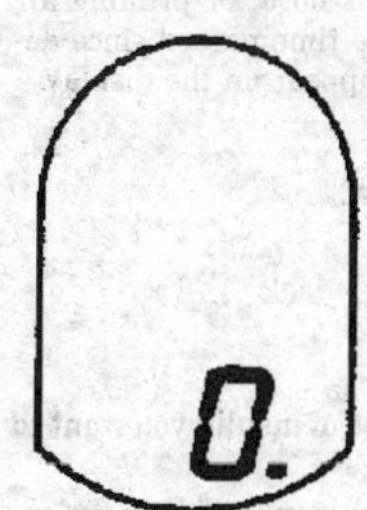

Press the release button **A** and the push button will jump out. The display will show 0.

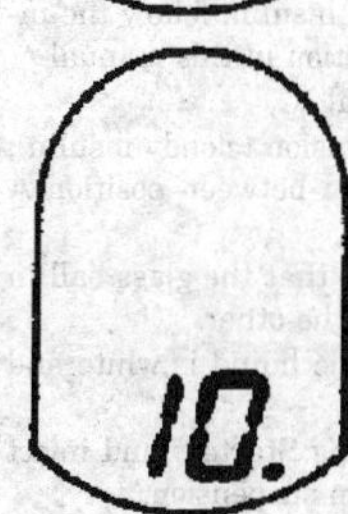

Dial the number of units you need by turning the dose selector at a steady speed **B**. In this example a dose of 10 units has been dialed. The number of units you have dialed is shown in the display. You cannot use the clicks as you dial to determine the dose.

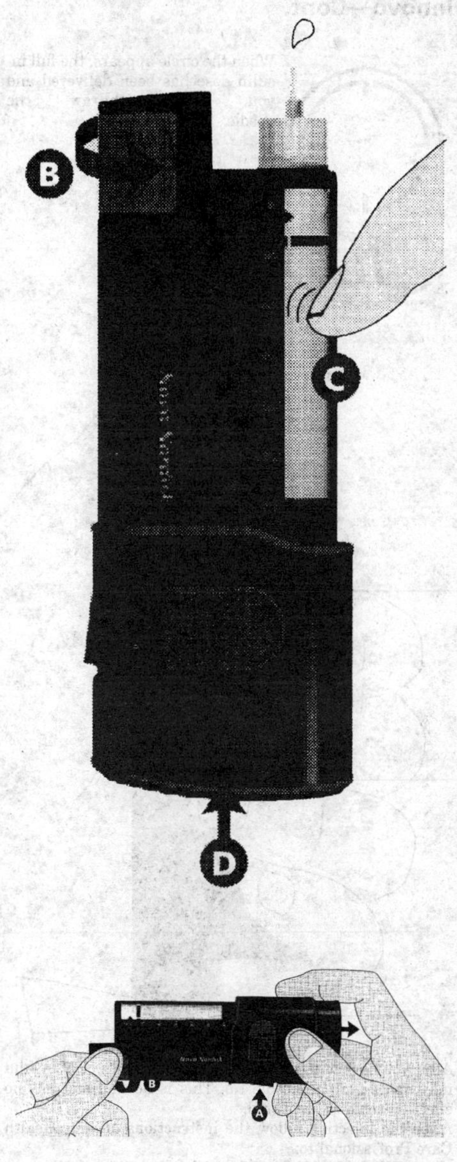

Changing a dose

If you accidentally dial a larger dose than you need, dial back to the correct number of units. The dose dialed can be changed until you press the push button.

Canceling a dose

If you want to cancel a chosen dose, dial back to zero and press the push button completely in. Your last delivered dose (or priming air shot) and the time passed since its delivery will reappear on the display.

Giving the injection

Follow the injection technique recommended by your Health Care Professional.

⚠To inject, press the push button completely in until it locks. You may feel that it becomes a little harder to press the push button towards the end of the injection. This is normal.

⚠Do not change the dose after you have pressed the push button.

With all insulin injection devices the needle should be left under the skin for at least 6 seconds to ensure that the full insulin dose has been delivered. Innovo® helps you to do this by providing a built-in timer.

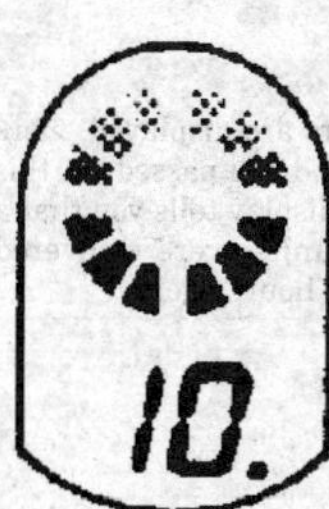

When the push button is pressed completely in, the segments turn on two by two telling you to leave the needle under your skin.

Continued on next page

Innovo—Cont.

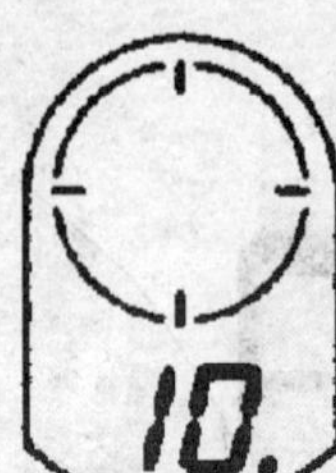

When the circle appears, the full insulin dose has been delivered and you can withdraw the needle.

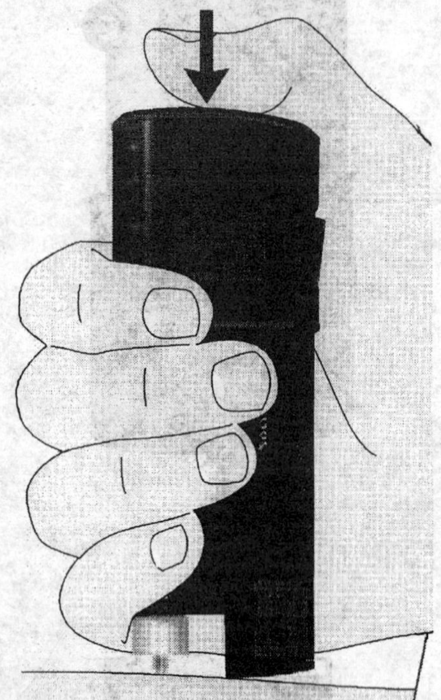

After you have withdrawn the needle, a few drops of insulin may appear at the needle tip. This is normal and has no effect on the dose delivered.

After the injection follow the instructions of your Health Care Professional to:

- carefully replace the outer needle cap on the needle.
- unscrew the needle and discard it properly.

Always replace the cap after using Innovo®.

[See figure at top of next column]

Checking your previous injection

Pull off the cap.

After the display test, your previous dose (or priming air shot) and the time passed since delivery can be seen on the display. Each timer segment represents 1 hour.

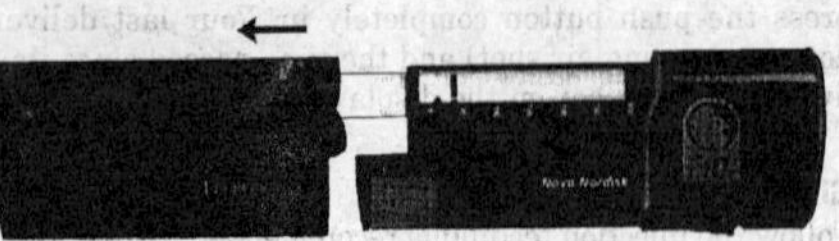

For example, if 4 segments are displayed, more than 4 hours have passed since the previous injection.

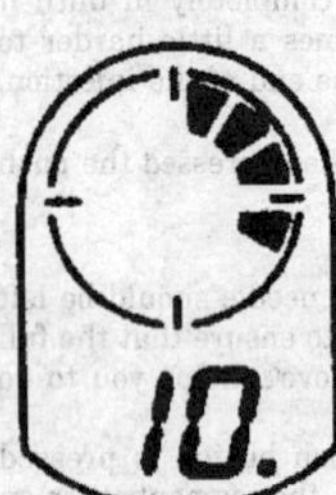

If 12 segments are displayed, more than 12 hours have passed. In this example the display tells you that a dose of 10 units were delivered more than 12 hours ago.

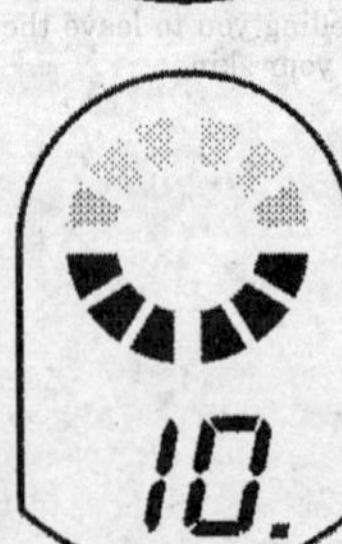

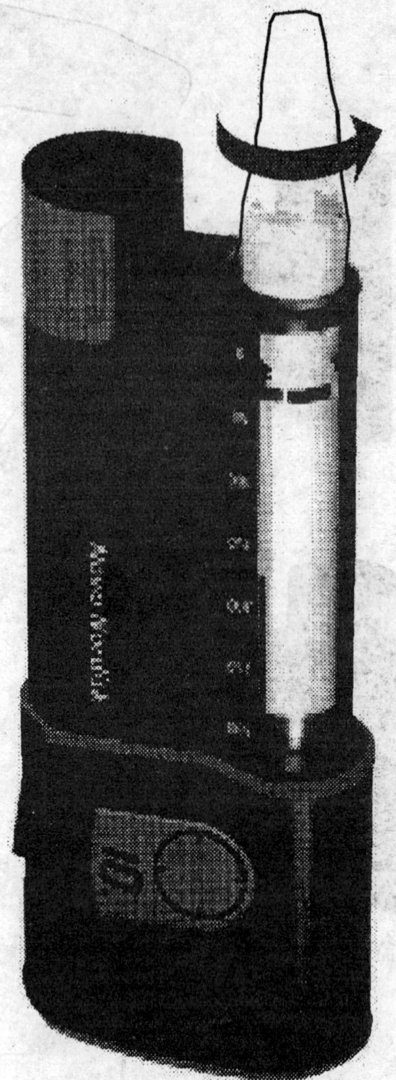

If the last thing you did before replacing the cap was to dial a dose, this dose will appear on the display.

Always replace the cap after using Innovo®.

Subsequent injections

Pull off the cap.

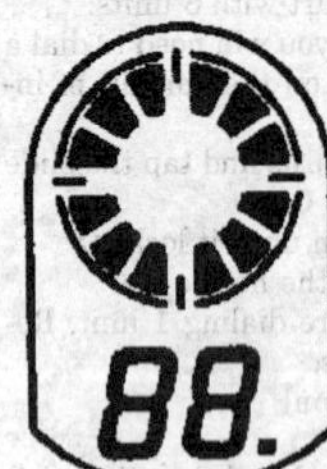

When the cap is pulled off, all the display symbols are turned on telling you that the display is fully functioning.

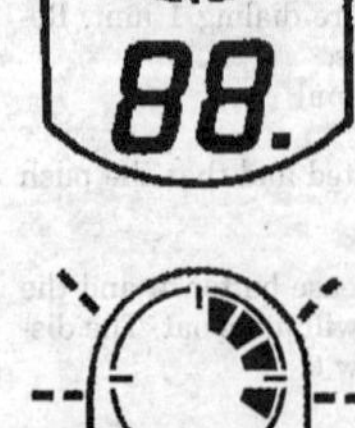

Your previous dose (or priming air shot) and the time passed since delivery then appear on the display.

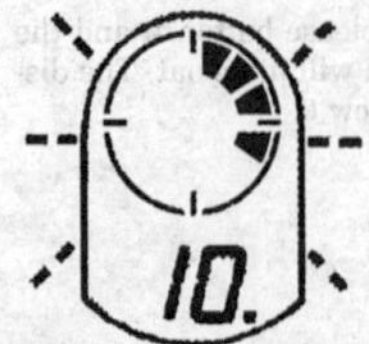

Check that Innovo® contains the type of insulin you want to inject.

If PenFill® contains a soluble (clear) insulin, follow the instructions from "Getting Started" section in this manual.

[See first figure at top of next column]

If Innovo® contains an insulin suspension (cloudy insulin), you must turn Innovo® up and down between position **A** and **B** – as shown in the picture.

The movement must be performed so that the glass ball in the cartridge moves from one end to the other.

Do this at least 10 times, until all the liquid is white and uniformly cloudy.

Then carry on as shown from "Getting Started" and inject shortly after resuspending the insulin suspension.

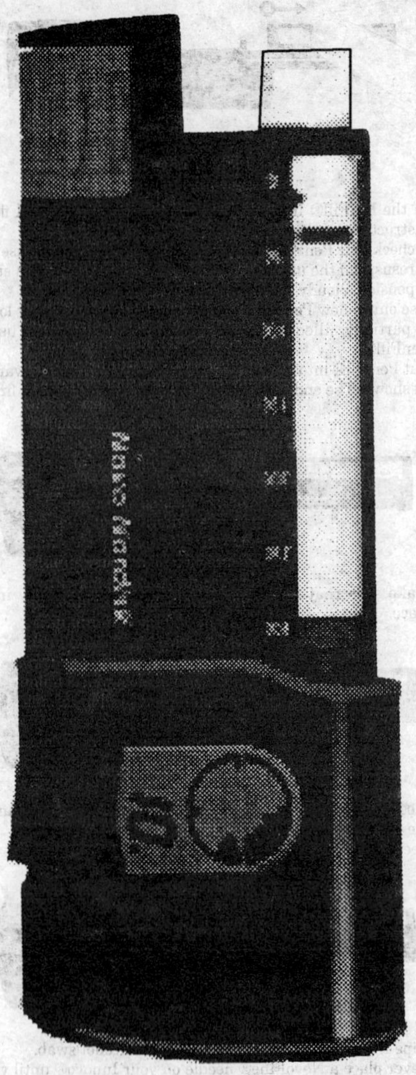

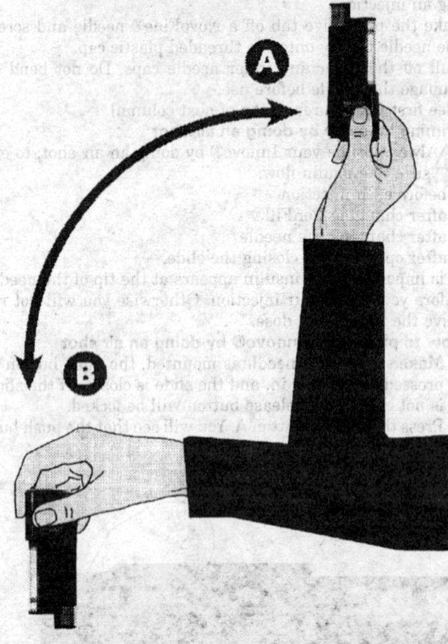

What to do when PenFill® is nearly empty

Do not try to inject an insulin suspension (cloudy insulin) if the rear rubber stopper is below the arrow marks on the slide as shown in the picture. The glass ball must have adequate space to resuspend the insulin.

Innovo® will not let you dial a larger dose than that remaining in PenFill®.

⚠Do not force the dose selector to turn; instead change PenFill®.

If you need more insulin than the amount in the cartridge, you can either:

- change PenFill® and inject the whole dose at once,

  or
- inject the remaining insulin and insert a new PenFill® cartridge for the rest of your dose.

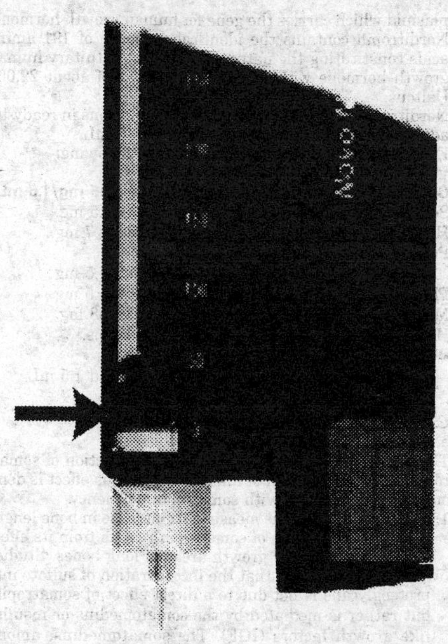

Change PenFill® as described in the "Changing PenFill®" section. Then prime Innovo® by doing an air shot as described in the "Priming Innovo® by doing an air shot" section.

Dial the remaining number of units to complete your dose. Inject, making sure that you have now injected your full dose.

If you have changed PenFill® so your total dose was divided into two doses, note that Innovo® will only remember the second of the two doses given.

Changing PenFill®

- Make sure that the push button is pressed completely in.
- Unscrew the needle.
- Open the slide.
- Take out the used PenFill® cartridge.
- Take a new PenFill® cartridge and continue as described from "Getting Started".

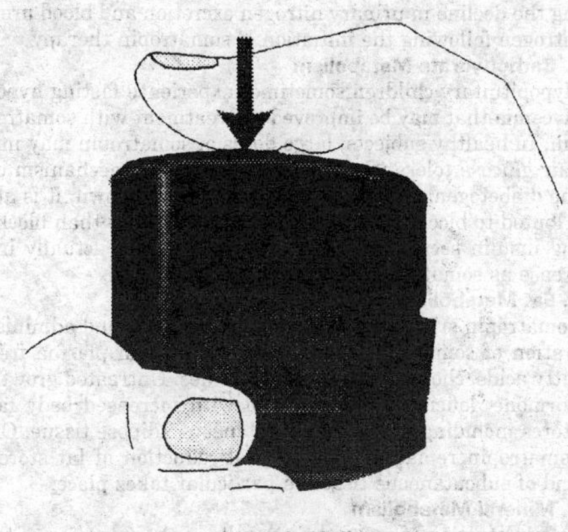

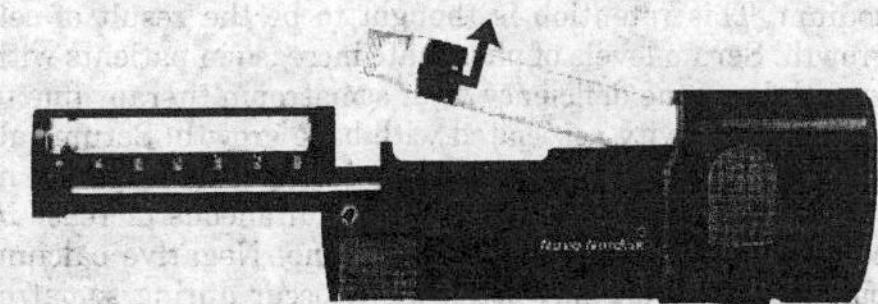

Function check

You should check the functioning of your Innovo®:

- if you think that Innovo® is not working properly
- regularly for your peace of mind (for example once a month or before starting a new box of PenFill® cartridges).

To perform a function check:

1. Screw on a new NovoFine® needle as described on page 9.
2. Prime Innovo® by doing an air shot as described on pages 10–11.
3. Put the outer needle cap over the needle.
4. Dispense 20 units into the outer needle cap.

The insulin should fill the lower part of the outer needle cap. If Innovo® has released too much or too little insulin, repeat the test.

If it happens again, do not use your Innovo®. Contact Novo Nordisk Pharmaceuticals, Inc. at our toll free number (1-800-727-6500), or see the warranty section for further information.

Do not try to repair a faulty Innovo®.

[See figure at top of next column]

What do I do if...?

Here are the answers to some questions you might ask when using your Innovo® insulin doser.

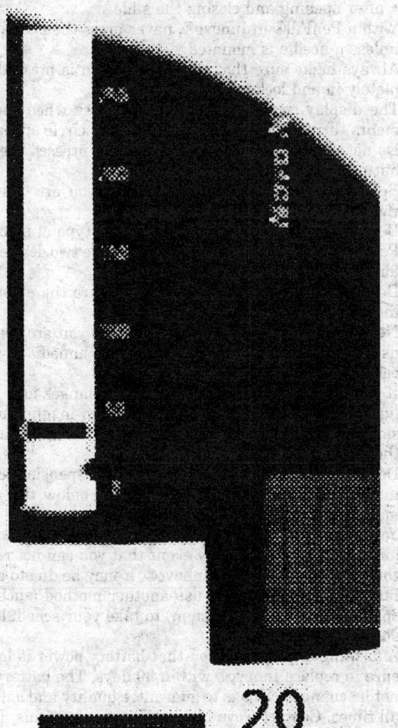

Display

The display does not respond when I turn the dose selector.

Press the release button so that the push button jumps out before a dose can be dialed.

The display shows a minus sign.

The dose selector has been dialed below 0. Dial forward until the display shows the correct number of units.

The display is off.

If the display goes off, press the release button, and the push button will jump out. Press the push button completely in, and the display should reappear.

If the display does not reappear, open and close the slide. Prime Innovo® by doing an air shot as described on page 10.

If the display remains off, Innovo® is not working. Do not use Innovo® but contact Novo Nordisk Pharmaceuticals, Inc. to get a new Innovo®. Our toll free number is 1-800-727-6500.

Priming by doing an air shot

No insulin appears when I try to prime Innovo® by doing an air shot.

The needle may be blocked. Change the needle and prime Innovo® by doing air shots until insulin appears at the needle tip.

Check that the push button is pressed completely in and locked. Open the slide and make sure that PenFill® is inserted correctly. If PenFill® is damaged or empty, change it.

Check that the slide is closed, and prime Innovo® until insulin appears at the needle tip.

No insulin appears when I prime Innovo® and the push button will not go in.

The needle may be blocked. Change the needle and prime Innovo® until insulin appears at the needle tip.

To open the slide, dial back to zero and press the push button completely in until it locks.

Then change PenFill® as described in "Changing PenFill®" section.

Choosing the dose

I cannot release the push button.

Make sure that the slide is closed completely. The release button is locked until the slide is closed.

I want to cancel or change the dialed dose.

Dial back to zero and press the push button completely in. Your last dose and the time passed since delivery will reappear on the display. You can increase, decrease or cancel the dialed dose up until the time you press the push button.

Do not change the dose after you have pressed the push button.

Insulin is delivered when I turn the dose selector.

You have dialed the maximum dose of 70 units and then carried on dialing. If you need to inject a dose of insulin larger than 70 units, you must divide the dose into amounts equal to or less than 70 units.

Injection

The push button blocks during the injection.

Do not try to force the push button in.

The needle may be blocked. Change the needle and prime Innovo® by doing an air shot as described in "Priming Innovo® by doing an air shot" section.

Check if PenFill® is damaged. Dial back to zero and press the push button completely in until it locks. Then open the slide and change PenFill® as described in "Changing PenFill®" section. Prime Innovo® by doing an air shot until insulin appears at the needle tip.

Please observe that part of the insulin dose may have been injected.

If the push button still cannot be pressed completely in, contact Novo Nordisk Pharmaceuticals, Inc. Our toll free number is 1-800-727-6500.

Changing PenFill®

I cannot open the slide.

The needle must be removed. If the push button is out, dial back to zero, and press the push button completely in until it locks. Then open the slide.

If the slide still cannot be opened, contact Novo Nordisk Pharmaceuticals, Inc. Our toll free number is 1-800-727-6500. Do not try to force the slide open.

Function check

I do not think that my Innovo® is working properly.

Carry out the function check described on page 23. Make sure that the lower part of the outer needle cap is filled with 20 units of insulin.

Never use your Innovo® unless you are sure that it is working properly.

How to store and look after your Innovo® insulin doser

Your Innovo® insulin doser is designed to work accurately and safely. It should be handled with care. Avoid situations where your Innovo® insulin doser can be damaged. Always replace the cap after using Innovo®.

Please read the Information For The Patient in the PenFill® pack. This will tell you how to store the cartridges and how long to keep them.

Storage and handling

- Do not expose your Innovo® insulin doser to temperatures below -25°C / -13°F.
- With PenFill® inserted, store Innovo® at room temperature (up to 25°C / 77°F).
- Your Innovo® is tough but can still be damaged. Handle it with care and protect it against direct sunlight, water, dust and dirt.

Cleaning

- Clean off dirt and dust with a dry, soft brush.
- You can clean your Innovo® by wiping it with cotton moistened with ethyl or isopropyl alcohol.
- Do not soak Innovo® in alcohol, wash it or lubricate it. This may damage the mechanism.

Remember

- Do not try to repair a faulty Innovo®.
- Innovo® must only be used according to the instructions in this manual. The manufacturer will not be held responsible for any equipment problems if you have not followed these instructions.
- If you suspect that Innovo® is faulty, contact Novo Nordisk Pharmaceuticals, Inc. Our toll free number is 1-800-727-6500.

Display Information

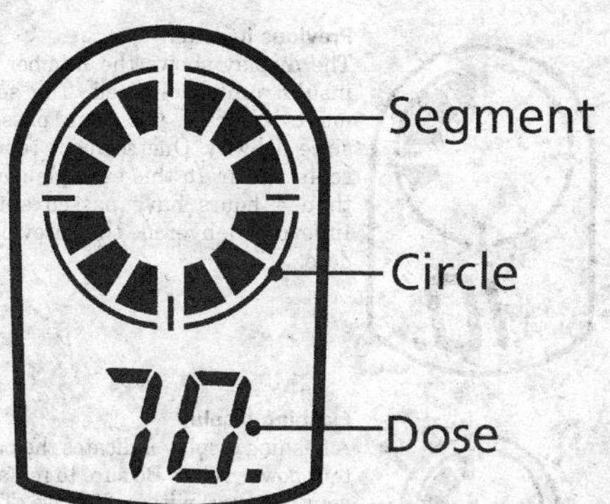

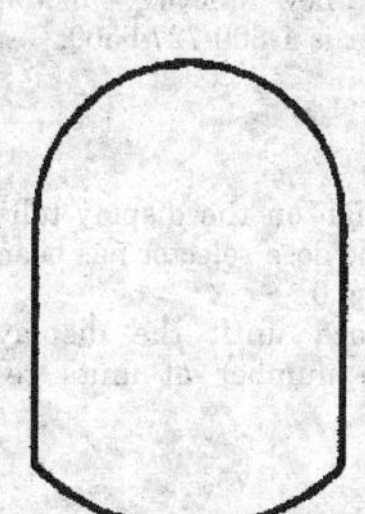

Display is off

The very first time the cap is pulled off, the display stays blank until the slide is opened.

⚠ If the display goes off, press the release button, and the push button will jump out. Press the push button completely in, and the display should reappear. If the display does not reappear, open and close the slide.

Prime Innovo® as described on page 10.

If the display remains off, Innovo® is not working. Do not use Innovo® but contact Novo Nordisk Pharmaceuticals, Inc. to get a new Innovo®. Our toll free number is 1-800-727-6500.

Continued on next page

Innovo—Cont.

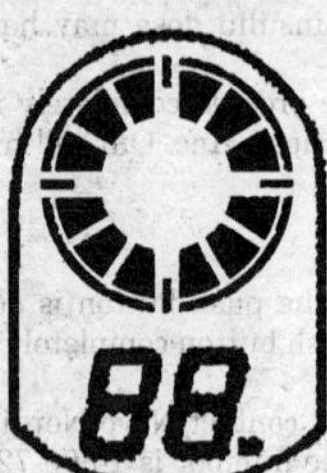

Display test
When the cap is pulled off, all the display symbols are turned on, telling you that the display is fully functional.

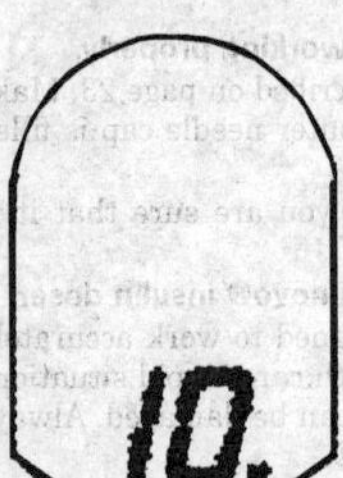

Dialing a dose
The display shows the number of insulin units dialed.

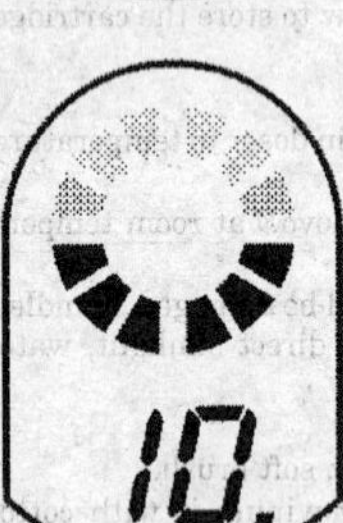

During delivery
The segments turning on two by two tell you to leave the needle under the skin during injection.

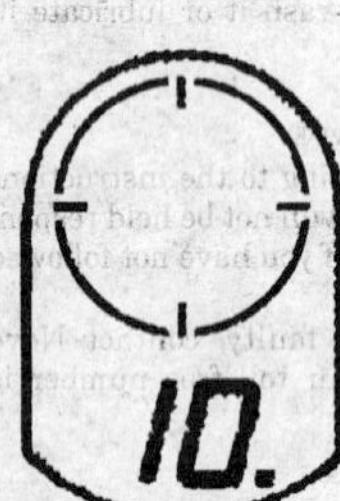

After delivery
The display shows the number of insulin units delivered. The circle confirms that the delivery has been completed.

Previous injection
The display shows the number of insulin units delivered. The segments indicate the time passed since delivery. One segment represents 1 hour. In this example more than 4 hours have passed since Innovo® delivered the previous dose.

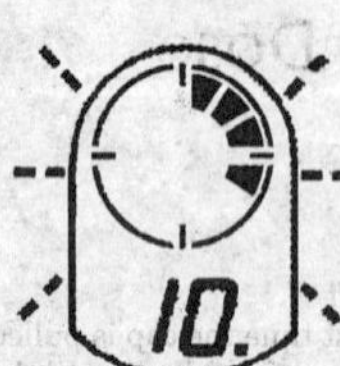

Flashing display
A flashing display indicates the battery power is low. Be sure to replace your Innovo® within 30 days. The battery cannot be changed. Contact Novo Nordisk Pharmaceuticals, Inc. to get a new Innovo®. Our toll free number is 1-800-727-6500.

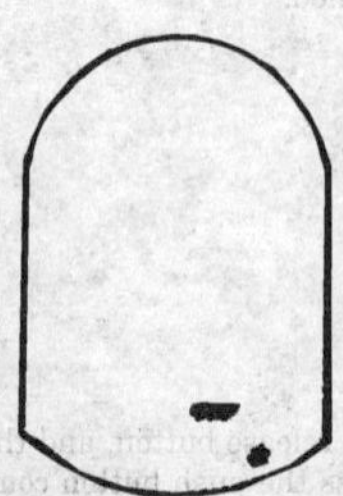

Minus sign
A minus sign on the display tells you that the dose selector has been dialed below 0.
Dial forward until the display shows the number of units required.

⚠Important information

- Always keep a spare insulin delivery system available, in case your Innovo® is lost or damaged.
- Always prime your Innovo® by doing an air shot (as described on pages 10-11) to ensure the insulin flow:
  - before each injection
  - after changing PenFill®
  - after changing the needle
  - after opening and closing the slide
- With a PenFill® in Innovo®, never press the push button unless a needle is mounted.
- Always make sure that the push button is pressed completely in and locks.
- The display confirms completed delivery when the segments turn on two by two and then the circle appears.
- Do not change the dose after you have pressed the push button.
- Before each injection make sure that you are using the right type of insulin.
- If you are treated with more than one type of insulin in PenFill® 3 mL cartridges, you should use two devices, one for each type of insulin.
- Do not use the residual scale to measure the amount of insulin to be injected.
- Never place a needle on Innovo® until you are ready to use it, and take the needle off Innovo® immediately after each injection.
  If you do not remove it, temperature changes may cause liquid to leak out of the needle. With an insulin suspension (cloudy insulin), this may change the concentration of the insulin.
- Do not initiate injection of an insulin suspension (cloudy insulin) if the rear rubber stopper is below the arrow marks on the slide.
- Your Innovo® insulin doser is designed to work accurately and safely. In the unlikely event that you can not release the push button on your Innovo®, it may be due to a malfunction and you should use another method (such as a spare insulin delivery system) to take your scheduled insulin doses.
- A flashing display tells you that battery power is low. Be sure to replace Innovo® within 30 days. The battery cannot be changed. This is to guarantee quality and safety at all times. Contact Novo Nordisk Pharmaceuticals, Inc. to get a new Innovo®. Our toll free number is 1-800-727-6500.
- Innovo® is tough but could still be damaged. So handle it with care, do not drop it and avoid knocking it against hard surfaces. If Innovo® has been dropped or knocked, you must carry out a function check (see page 23).
- Never use your Innovo® unless you are sure that it is working properly.
- Always replace the cap after using Innovo®.
- Do not play with the dose selector or the push button as this can cause Innovo® to wear out.
- Keep Innovo®, PenFill® and NovoFine® out of the reach of children.
- Your Innovo® is for use by you alone. Do not allow anyone else to to use it, even though you attach a new NovoFine® needle for each injection.
- Health Care Professionals, relatives and other carers should follow general precautionary measures for removal and disposal of needles to eliminate the risk of unintended needle penetration.

Warranty Information
Should your Innovo® device be defective in materials or workmanship within three (3) years of purchase, Novo Nordisk Pharmaceuticals, Inc. will replace it at no charge if you mail the defective unit along with a description of the problem and the sales receipt or other proof of purchase to:
Novo Nordisk Pharmaceuticals, Inc. Product Safety 100 College Road West Princeton, New Jersey 08540
No other warranty is made with respect to Innovo®.
This warranty will become invalid and neither Novo Nordisk A/S, Novo Nordisk Pharmaceuticals, Inc., or Bristol-Myers Squibb Co., will assume responsibility in the case of defects or damages arising from:

- The use of Innovo® with products other than PenFill® 3 mL cartridges, NovoFine® single-use disposable needles, or other products specifically recommended by Novo Nordisk.
- The use of Innovo® in a manner other than in strict accordance with the instructions in this booklet or other instructions issued by Novo Nordisk.
- Physical damage to Innovo® caused by neglect, misuse, unauthorized repair, accident, or other breakage.

For assistance or further
information, write to:
Novo Nordisk Pharmaceuticals, Inc.
Customer Relations
100 College Road West
Princeton, NJ 08540
Or call: 1-800-727-6500
Novo Nordisk A/S 2001/2003
Novo Nordisk Pharmaceuticals, Inc.
Princeton, NJ 08540
www.novonordisk-us.com

NORDITROPIN® CARTRIDGES ℞

[nŏrd" ĕ trōp' ĭn]
Somatropin (rDNA origin) injection
5 mg/1.5 mL, 10 mg/1.5 mL or 15 mg/1.5 mL
℞ Only

DESCRIPTION

Norditropin® is the Novo Nordisk A/S registered trademark for somatropin, a polypeptide hormone of recombinant DNA origin. The hormone is synthesized by a special strain of *E. coli* bacteria that has been modified by the addition of a plasmid which carries the gene for human growth hormone. Norditropin contains the identical sequence of 191 amino acids constituting the naturally occurring pituitary human growth hormone with a molecular weight of about 22,000 Daltons.
Norditropin cartridges are supplied as solutions in ready-to-administer cartridges with a volume of 1.5 mL.
Each **Norditropin cartridge** contains the following:

Component	5 mg/1.5 mL	10 mg/1.5 mL	15 mg/1.5 mL
Somatropin	5 mg	10 mg	15 mg
Histidine	1 mg	1 mg	1.7 mg
Poloxamer 188	4.5 mg	4.5 mg	4.5 mg
Phenol	4.5 mg	4.5 mg	4.5 mg
Mannitol	60 mg	60 mg	58 mg
HCl/NaOH	q.s.	q.s.	q.s.
Water for Injection	ad 1.5 mL	ad 1.5 mL	ad 1.5 mL

CLINICAL PHARMACOLOGY

a. Tissue Growth
The primary and most intensively studied action of somatropin is the stimulation of linear growth. This effect is demonstrated in patients with somatropin deficiency.

1. Skeletal growth – the measurable increase in bone length after administration of somatropin results from its effect on the cartilaginous growth areas of long bones. Studies *in vitro* have shown that the incorporation of sulfate into proteoglycans is not due to a direct effect of somatropin, but rather is mediated by the somatomedins or insulin-like growth factors (IGF). The somatomedins, among them somatomedin C, are polypeptide hormones which are synthesized in the liver, kidney, and various other tissue. Somatomedin C is low in the serum of hypopituitary dwarfs and hypophysectomized humans or animals, but its presence can be demonstrated after treatment with somatropin.
2. Cell growth – it has been shown that the total number of skeletal muscle cells is markedly decreased in short stature children lacking endogenous somatropin compared with normal children, and that treatment with somatropin results in an increase in both the number and size of muscle cells.
3. Organ growth – somatropin influences the size of internal organs, and it also increases red cell mass.

b. Protein Metabolism
Linear growth is facilitated in part by increased cellular protein synthesis. This synthesis and growth are reflected by nitrogen retention which can be quantitated by observing the decline in urinary nitrogen excretion and blood urea nitrogen following the initiation of somatropin therapy.

c. Carbohydrate Metabolism
Hypopituitary children sometimes experience fasting hypoglycemia that may be improved by treatment with somatropin. In healthy subjects, large doses of somatropin may impair glucose tolerance. Although the precise mechanism of the diabetogenic effect of somatropin is not known, it is attributed to blocking the action of insulin rather than blocking insulin secretion. Insulin levels in serum actually increase as somatropin levels increase.

d. Fat Metabolism
Somatropin stimulates intracellular lipolysis, and administration of somatropin leads to an increase in plasma free fatty acids, cholesterol, and triglycerides. Untreated growth hormone deficiency is associated with increased body fat stores including increased subcutaneous adipose tissue. On somatropin replacement a general reduction of fat stores and of subcutaneous tissue in particular takes place.

e. Mineral Metabolism
Administration of somatropin results in the retention of total body potassium and phosphorus and to a lesser extent sodium. This retention is thought to be the result of cell growth. Serum levels of phosphate increase in patients with growth hormone deficiency after somatropin therapy due to metabolic activity associated with bone growth. Serum calcium levels are not altered. Although calcium excretion in the urine is increased, there is a simultaneous increase in calcium absorption from the intestine. Negative calcium balance, however, may occasionally occur during somatropin treatment.

f. Connective Tissue Metabolism
Somatropin stimulates the synthesis of chrondroitin sulfate and collagen as well as the urinary excretion of hydroxyproline.

g. Pharmacokinetics
A 180-min IV infusion of Norditropin (33 ng/kg/min) was given to 9 GHD patients. A mean (±SD) hGH steady-state serum level of approximately 23.1 (±15.0) ng/mL was reached at 150 min and a mean clearance rate of approximately 2.3 (±1.8) mL/min/kg or 139 (±105) mL/min for hGH was obtained. Following infusion, serum hGH levels had a biexponential decay with a terminal elimination half-life ($T_{1/2}$) of approximately 21.1 (±5.1) min.
In a study conducted in 18 GHD adult patients, where a SC dose of 0.024 mg/kg or 3 IU/m^2 was given in the thigh, the mean (±SD) C_{max} values of 13.8 (±5.8) and 17.1 (±10.0) ng/mL were obtained for the 4 and 8 mg Norditropin vials, respectively, at approximately 4 to 5 hr. post dose. The mean apparent terminal $T_{1/2}$ values were estimated to be approximately 7 to 10 hr. However, the absolute bioavailability for Norditropin after the SC route of administration is currently not known.
Norditropin cartridge formulation is bioequivalent to Norditropin vial formulation.

INDICATIONS AND USAGE

Norditropin is indicated for the long-term treatment of children who have growth failure due to inadequate secretion of endogenous growth hormone.

CONTRAINDICATIONS

Norditropin should not be used in subjects with closed epiphyses.

Norditropin should not be used in hypopituitary children who have evidence of actively growing intracranial tumors. Therapy with somatropin should be discontinued if there is evidence of recurrent tumor growth.

Norditropin should not be used or should be discontinued when there is any evidence of active malignancy. Anti-malignancy treatment must be complete with evidence of remission prior to the institution of growth hormone therapy.

Norditropin should not be used in any subjects with known hypersensitivity to any of the constituents of the preparation.

Growth hormone should not be initiated to treat patients with acute critical illness due to complications following open heart or abdominal surgery, multiple accidental trauma or to patients having acute respiratory failure. Two placebo-controlled clinical trials in non-growth hormone deficient adult patients (n=522) with these conditions revealed a significant increase in mortality (41.9% vs. 19.3%) among somatropin treated patients (doses 5.3–8 mg/day) compared to those receiving placebo (see WARNINGS).

WARNINGS

Norditropin (somatropin [rDNA origin] injection) cartridges must be used with their corresponding color-coded NordiPen® delivery device. A Norditropin cartridge must not be inserted into a pen with a different color code.

See CONTRAINDICATIONS for information on increased mortality in patients with acute critical illnesses in intensive care units due to complications following open heart or abdominal surgery, multiple accidental trauma or with acute respiratory failure. The safety of continuing growth hormone treatment in patients receiving replacement doses for approved indications who concurrently develop these illnesses has not been established. Therefore, the potential benefit of treatment continuation with growth hormone in patients having acute critical illnesses should be weighed against the potential risk.

PRECAUTIONS

Norditropin should be used only by physicians with experience in the diagnosis and management of patients with growth hormone deficiency.

Patients with growth hormone deficiency secondary to an intracranial lesion should be examined frequently for progression or recurrence of the underlying disease process.

Because growth hormone may induce a state of insulin resistance, patients should be observed for evidence of glucose intolerance.

Concomitant glucocorticoid therapy may inhibit the growth promoting effect of Norditropin. Patients with coexisting ACTH deficiency should have their glucocorticoid replacement dose carefully adjusted to avoid an inhibitory effect on growth.

A state of hypothyroidism may develop during Norditropin treatment. Since untreated hypothyroidism may interfere with the response to Norditropin, patients should have a periodic thyroid function test and should be treated with thyroid hormone when indicated.

Patients with endocrine disorders, including growth hormone deficiency, may develop slipped capital epiphyses more frequently. Any child with the onset of a limp or complaints of hip or knee pain during growth hormone therapy should be evaluated.

Intracranial hypertension (IH) with papilledema, visual changes, headache, nausea and/or vomiting has been reported in a small number of patients treated with growth hormone products. Symptoms usually occurred within the first eight (8) weeks of the initiation of growth hormone therapy. In all reported cases, IH-associated signs and symptoms resolved after termination of therapy or a reduction of the growth hormone dose. Funduscopic examination of patients is recommended at the initiation and periodically during the course of growth hormone therapy.

Progression of scoliosis can occur in children who experience rapid growth. Because growth hormone increases growth rate, patients with a history of scoliosis who are treated with growth hormone should be monitored for progression of scoliosis.

Carcinogenesis, Mutagenesis, Impairment of Fertility: Carcinogenicity, mutagenicity, and fertility studies have not been conducted with Norditropin cartridges.

Pregnancy: Pregnancy Category C. Animal reproduction studies have not been conducted with Norditropin cartridge formulation. It is also not known whether Norditropin can cause fetal harm when administered to a pregnant woman or can affect reproduction capacity. Norditropin should be given to a pregnant woman only if clearly needed.

Nursing Mothers: It is not known whether this drug is excreted in human milk. Because many drugs are excreted in human milk, caution should be exercised when Norditropin is administered to a nursing woman.

ADVERSE REACTIONS

As with all protein drugs, a small percentage of patients may develop antibodies to the protein. Growth hormone antibody with binding capacity lower than 2 mg/L has not been associated with growth attenuation. In some cases, when binding capacity is greater than 2 mg/L, interference with growth response has been observed.

In clinical trials, patients receiving Norditropin for up to 12 months have been tested for induction of antibodies and 0/358 patients developed antibodies with binding capacities above 2 mg/L. Among these patients, 165 had previously been treated with other preparations of growth hormone and 193 were previously untreated naive patients.

Since antibodies to somatropin have the potential to inhibit further linear growth, only patients failing to respond to treatment should be tested for antibodies.

The following adverse events have been reported from clinical studies: headache, localized muscle pain, weakness, mild hyperglycemia and glucosuria.

Leukemia has been reported in a small number of children who have been treated with growth hormone, including growth hormone of pituitary origin and recombinant somatrem and somatropin. On the basis of current evidence, experts cannot conclude that growth hormone therapy is responsible for these occurrences. If there is any risk to an individual patient, it is minimal.

Fluid retention and peripheral edema may occur.

OVERDOSAGE

The maximum dose generally recommended should not be exceeded due to the potential risk of side effects.

DOSAGE AND ADMINISTRATION

The Norditropin dosage and schedule for administration must be individualized for each patient. Generally, subcutaneous administration in the evening, 6–7 times a week, is recommended. It is further recommended to give the injections in the thighs and to vary the injection site on the thigh on a rotating basis. Dosage can be calculated according to body weight.

Generally recommended dosage:

Subcutaneous injection:

0.024–0.034 mg/kg body weight, 6–7 times a week.

Norditropin cartridges must be administered using the NordiPen injection pen. Each cartridge size has a color-coded corresponding pen which is graduated to deliver the appropriate dose based on the concentration of Norditropin in the cartridge.

Norditropin MUST NOT BE INJECTED if the solution is cloudy or contains particulate matter. Use it only if it is clear and colorless.

Measuring the Prescribed Dose:

5 mg/1.5 mL, 10 mg/1.5 mL and 15 mg/1.5 mL Norditropin cartridges

Each cartridge of Norditropin must be inserted into its corresponding NordiPen injection pen. Instructions for delivering the dosage are provided in the NordiPen instruction booklet.

Storage:

Norditropin cartridges must be stored at 2–8°C/36–46°F (refrigerator). Do not freeze. Avoid direct light.

Norditropin cartridges retain their biological potency until the date of expiry indicated on the label. After a Norditropin cartridge has been inserted into the NordiPen injector, it must be stored in the pen in the refrigerator and used within 4 weeks.

HOW SUPPLIED

Norditropin® (somatropin [rDNA origin] injection) 5 mg/1.5 mL, 10 mg/1.5 mL and 15 mg/1.5 mL cartridges:

Norditropin is supplied in 5 mg/1.5 mL, 10 mg/1.5 mL or 15 mg/1.5 mL cartridges which must be administered using the corresponding color-coded NordiPen® injection pen.

Norditropin 5 mg/1.5 mL cartridge (orange) NDC 0169-7768-11

Norditropin 10 mg/1.5 mL cartridge (blue) NDC 0169-7769-11

Norditropin 15 mg/1.5 mL cartridge (green) NDC 0169-7770-11

Date of Issue: December/2002

For information contact:
Novo Nordisk Pharmaceuticals, Inc.
100 College Road West
Princeton, New Jersey 08540, USA
1–888–NOVO-HGH
www.norditropin.com

Manufactured by:
Novo Nordisk A/S
2880 Bagsvaerd, Denmark

HUMAN INSULIN **OTC**

NOVOLIN® 70/30

70% NPH, Human Insulin Isophane Suspension and 30% Regular, Human Insulin Injection (recombinant DNA origin)

100 units/mL

Please read this leaflet carefully.

WARNING

ANY CHANGE OF INSULIN SHOULD BE MADE CAUTIOUSLY AND ONLY UNDER MEDICAL SUPERVISION. CHANGES IN PURITY, STRENGTH, BRAND (MANUFACTURER), TYPE (REGULAR, NPH, LENTE®, ETC.), SPECIES (BEEF, PORK, BEEF-PORK, HUMAN) AND/OR METHOD OF MANUFACTURE (RECOMBINANT DNA VERSUS ANIMAL-SOURCE INSULIN) MAY RESULT IN THE NEED FOR A CHANGE IN DOSAGE.

SPECIAL CARE SHOULD BE TAKEN WHEN THE TRANSFER IS FROM A STANDARD BEEF OR MIXED SPECIES INSULIN TO A PURIFIED PORK OR HUMAN INSULIN. IF A DOSAGE ADJUSTMENT IS NEEDED, IT WILL USUALLY BECOME APPARENT EITHER IN THE FIRST FEW DAYS OR OVER A PERIOD OF SEVERAL WEEKS. ANY CHANGE IN TREATMENT SHOULD BE CAREFULLY MONITORED.

PLEASE READ THE SECTIONS "INSULIN REACTION AND SHOCK" AND "DIABETIC KETOACIDOSIS AND COMA" FOR SYMPTOMS OF HYPOGLYCEMIA (LOW BLOOD GLUCOSE) AND HYPERGLYCEMIA (HIGH BLOOD GLUCOSE).

INSULIN USE IN DIABETES

Your physician has explained that you have diabetes and that your treatment involves injections of insulin or insulin therapy combined with an oral antidiabetic medicine. Insulin is normally produced by the pancreas, a gland that lies behind the stomach. Without insulin, glucose (a simple sugar made from digested food) is trapped in the bloodstream and cannot enter the cells of the body. Some patients who don't make enough of their own insulin, or who cannot use the insulin they do make properly, must take insulin by injection in order to control their blood glucose levels.

Each case of diabetes is different and requires direct and continued medical supervision. Your physician has told you the type, strength and amount of insulin you should use and the time(s) at which you should inject it, and has also discussed with you a diet and exercise schedule. You should contact your physician if you experience any difficulties or if you have questions.

TYPES OF INSULINS

Standard and purified animal insulins as well as human insulins are available. Standard and purified insulins differ in their degree of purification and content of noninsulin material. Standard and purified insulins also vary in species source; they may be of beef, pork, or mixed beef and pork origin. Human insulin is identical in structure to the insulin produced by the human pancreas, and thus differs from animal insulins. Insulins vary in time of action and in strength; see PRODUCT DESCRIPTION and SYRINGES for additional information.

Your physician has prescribed the insulin that is right for you; be sure you have purchased the correct insulin and check it carefully before you use it.

PRODUCT DESCRIPTION

This vial contains **Novolin® 70/30** which is a mixture of 70% NPH, Human Insulin Isophane Suspension (recombinant DNA origin) and 30% Regular, Human Insulin Injection (recombinant DNA origin) USP. The concentration of this product is 100 units of insulin per milliliter. It is a cloudy or milky suspension of human insulin with protamine and zinc. The insulin substance (the cloudy material) settles at the bottom of the vial, therefore, the vial must be gently agitated or rotated so that the contents are uniformly mixed before a dose is withdrawn. **Novolin® 70/30** has an intermediate duration of action. The effect of **Novolin® 70/30** begins approximately $^1/_2$ hour after injection. The effect is maximal between 2 and approximately 12 hours. The full duration of action may last up to 24 hours after injection.

The time course of action of any insulin may vary considerably in different individuals, or at different times in the same individual. Because of this variation, the time periods listed here should be considered as general guidelines only.

This human insulin (recombinant DNA origin) is structurally identical to the insulin produced by the human pancreas. This human insulin is produced by recombinant DNA technology utilizing *Saccharomyces cerevisiae* (bakers' yeast) as the production organism.

STORAGE

Insulin should be stored in a cold place, preferably in a refrigerator, but not in the freezing compartment. **Do not let it freeze.** Keep the insulin vial in its carton so that it will stay clean and protected from light. If refrigeration is not possible, the bottle of insulin which you are currently using can be kept unrefrigerated as long as it is kept as cool as possible and away from heat and sunlight.

Never use **Novolin® 70/30** if the precipitate (the white deposit at the bottom of the vial) has become lumpy or granular in appearance or has formed a deposit of solid particles on the wall of the vial. This insulin should not be used if the liquid in the vial remains clear after the vial has been gently agitated.

Never use insulin after the expiration date which is printed on the vial label and carton.

SYRINGES

Use the Correct Syringe

Doses of insulin are measured in units. Some insulins are available in two strengths: U-100 and U-40. One milliliter (mL) of U-100 contains 100 units of insulin. One milliliter (mL) of U-40 contains 40 units of insulin. Be sure to use the proper syringe for the strength of the insulin prescribed for you. Syringes are clearly marked **"For use with U-100 insulin"** or **"For use with U-40 insulin"**. Low dose U-100 syringes are also available. Failure to use the proper syringe can lead to mistakes in dosage.

Continued on next page

Novolin 70/30—Cont.

Novo Nordisk insulin vials are intended for use with standard insulin syringes. Novo Nordisk has not evaluated the use of these vials with other devices for insulin delivery or with devices intended to aid in giving injections. Consult your doctor and the manufacturer of these devices before use with this product.

Disposable Syringes

Disposable syringes and needles require no sterilization provided the package is intact. They should be used only once and discarded.

Reusable Syringes

Reusable syringes and needles must be sterilized before each use.

1. Boil the syringe parts and needles in a pan of water for at least five minutes. Keep a special pan for this purpose. Heavily chlorinated water should not be used; distilled water is preferable.
   If boiling is not possible, the syringe parts and needles may be sterilized by immersion in 70% ethyl alcohol or 91% isopropyl alcohol for at least five minutes. **Do not use bathing, rubbing or medicated alcohol for sterilization.**
2. Assemble the syringe and fit the needle on the tip of the syringe being careful not to touch the surface of the plunger or needle.
3. Push the plunger in and out several times until the water (or alcohol) has been completely expelled. (The syringe should be thoroughly dried before its use.)

IMPORTANT

Failure to comply with the above and following antiseptic measures may lead to infections at the injection site.

PREPARING THE INJECTION

1. Clean your hands and the injection site with soap and water or with alcohol. Wipe the rubber stopper with an alcohol swab. (Note: Remove the tamper-resistant cap at first use. If the cap has already been removed, do not use this product, return it to your pharmacy.)
2. For insulin suspensions, roll the vial of insulin gently in your hands to mix it. Vigorous shaking immediately before the dose is drawn into the syringe may result in the formation of bubbles or froth which could cause dosage errors.
3. Pull back the plunger until the black tip reaches the marking for the number of units you will inject.
4. Push the needle through the rubber stopper into the vial.
5. Push the plunger all the way in. This inserts air into the bottle.
6. Turn the vial and syringe upside down and slowly pull the plunger back to a few units beyond the correct dose.
7. If there are air bubbles, flick the syringe firmly with your finger to raise the air bubbles to the needle, then slowly push the plunger to the correct unit marking.
8. Lift the vial off the syringe.

GIVING THE INJECTION

1. The following areas are suitable for subcutaneous insulin injection: thighs, upper arms, buttocks, abdomen. Do not change areas without consulting your physician. The actual point of injection should be changed each time; injection sites should be about an inch apart.
2. The injection site should be clean and dry. Pinch up skin area to be injected and hold it firmly.
3. Hold the syringe like a pencil and push the needle quickly and firmly into the pinched-up area.
4. Release the skin and push plunger all the way in to inject insulin beneath the skin. To ensure that all the insulin is injected keep the needle in the skin for several seconds after injection with your finger on the plunger. Do not inject into a muscle unless your physician has advised it. You should never inject insulin into a vein.
5. Remove needle. If slight bleeding occurs, press lightly with a dry cotton swab for a few seconds—**do not rub.**

Note:

The dose should be injected over 2–4 seconds. Preparations of insulin suspensions which are injected slowly may clog the tip of the needle, resulting in an inability to complete the injection. Syringe plugging does not occur when the drug is injected more rapidly. Use the injection technique recommended by your physician.

MIXING INSULIN

Novolin® 70/30 is a premixed insulin containing 70% NPH, Human Insulin Isophane Suspension, recombinant DNA origin (**Novolin® N**) and 30% Regular, Human Insulin Injection, recombinant DNA origin (**Novolin® R**). You should not attempt to change the ratio of this product by adding additional NPH or Regular insulin to this vial. If your physician has prescribed insulin mixed in a proportion other than 70% NPH and 30% Regular, you should use the separate insulin formulations (**Novolin® N** and **Novolin® R**) in the amounts recommended by your physician.

USAGE IN PREGNANCY

It is particularly important to maintain good control of your diabetes during pregnancy and special attention must be paid to your diet, exercise and insulin regimens. If you are pregnant or nursing a baby, consult your physician or nurse educator.

INSULIN REACTION AND SHOCK

Insulin reaction "hypoglycemia" occurs when the blood glucose falls very low. This can happen if you take too much insulin, miss or delay a meal, exercise more than usual or work too hard without eating, or become ill (especially with vomiting or fever). Hypoglycemia can also happen if you combine insulin therapy and other medications that lower blood glucose, such as oral antidiabetic agents or other prescription and over-the-counter drugs. The first symptoms of an insulin reaction usually come on suddenly. They may include a cold sweat, fatigue, nervousness or shakiness, rapid heartbeat, or nausea. Personality change or confusion may also occur. If you drink or eat something right away (a glass of milk or orange juice, or several sugar candies), you can often stop the progression of symptoms. If symptoms persist, call your physician — an insulin reaction can lead to unconsciousness. If a reaction results in loss of consciousness, emergency medical care should be obtained immediately. If you have had repeated reactions or if an insulin reaction has led to a loss of consciousness, contact your physician. Severe hypoglycemia can result in temporary or permanent impairment of brain function and death.

In certain cases, the nature and intensity of the warning symptoms of hypoglycemia may change. A few patients have reported that after being transferred to human insulin, the early warning symptoms of hypoglycemia were less pronounced than they had been with animal-source insulin.

DIABETIC KETOACIDOSIS AND COMA

Diabetic ketoacidosis may develop if your body has too little insulin. The most common causes are acute illness or infection or failure to take enough insulin by injection. If you are ill you should check your urine for ketones. The symptoms of diabetic ketoacidosis usually come on gradually, over a period of hours or days, and include a drowsy feeling, flushed face, thirst and loss of appetite. Notify your physician right away if the urine test is positive for ketones (acetone) or if you have any of these symptoms. Fast, heavy breathing and rapid pulse are more severe symptoms and you should have medical attention right away. Severe, sustained hyperglycemia may result in diabetic coma and death.

ADVERSE REACTIONS

A few people with diabetes develop red, swollen and itchy skin where the insulin has been injected. This is called a "local reaction" and it may occur if the injection is not properly made, if the skin is sensitive to the cleansing solution, or if you are allergic to the insulin being used. If you have a local reaction, tell your physician.

Generalized insulin allergy occurs rarely, but when it does it may cause a serious reaction, including skin rash over the body, shortness of breath, fast pulse, sweating, and a drop in blood pressure. If any of these symptoms develop, you should seek emergency medical care.

If severe allergic reactions to insulin have occurred (i.e., generalized rash, swelling or breathing difficulties) you should be skin-tested with **each** new insulin preparation before it is used.

IMPORTANT NOTES

1. A change in the type, strength, species or purity of insulin could require a dosage adjustment. Any change in insulin should be made under medical supervision.
2. You may have learned how to test your urine or your blood for glucose. It is important to do these tests regularly and to record the results for review with your physician or nurse educator.
3. If you have an acute illness, especially with vomiting or fever, continue taking your insulin. If possible, stay on your regular diet. If you have trouble eating, drink fruit juices, regular soft drinks, or clear soups; if you can, eat small amounts of bland foods. Test your urine for glucose and ketones and, if possible, test your blood glucose. Note the results and contact your physician for possible insulin dose adjustment. If you have severe and prolonged vomiting, seek emergency medical care.
4. You should always carry identification which states that you have diabetes.
5. Always ask your physician or pharmacist before taking any drug.

Always consult your physician if you have any questions about your condition or the use of insulin.

Helpful information for people with diabetes is published by American Diabetes Association, 1660 Duke Street, Alexandria, VA 22314.

For information contact: Novo Nordisk Pharmaceuticals, Inc., Princeton, NJ 08540

Manufactured by Novo Nordisk A/S, DK-2880 Bagsvaerd, Denmark and by Novo Nordisk Pharmaceutical Industries, Inc., 3612 Powhatan Road, Clayton, NC. 27520

Date of issue: February 1999

HOW SUPPLIED

Vials, U-100, 100 units/mL, 10 mL, (List No. 183711) (1's)

Shown in Product Identification Guide, page 326

NOVOLIN® N OTC

NPH, Human Insulin Isophane Suspension (recombinant DNA origin)

100 units/mL

PRODUCT DESCRIPTION

This vial contains **Novolin® N** commonly known as NPH, Human Insulin Isophane Suspension (recombinant DNA origin). The concentration of this product is 100 units of insulin per milliliter. It is a cloudy or milky suspension of human insulin with protamine and zinc. The insulin substance (the cloudy material) settles at the bottom of the vial, therefore, the vial must be gently agitated or rotated so that the contents are uniformly mixed before a dose is withdrawn. **Novolin® N** has an intermediate duration of action. The effect of **Novolin® N** begins approximately $1^1/_2$ hours after injection. The effect is maximal between 4 and 12 hours. The full duration of action may last up to 24 hours after injection. The time course of action of any insulin may vary considerably in different individuals, or at different times in the same individual. Because of this variation, the time periods listed here should be considered as general guidelines only. This human insulin (recombinant DNA origin) is structurally identical to the insulin produced by the human pancreas. This human insulin is produced by recombinant DNA technology utilizing *Saccharomyces cerevisiae* (bakers' yeast) as the production organism.

STORAGE

Insulin should be stored in a cold place, preferably in a refrigerator, but not in the freezing compartment. **Do not let it freeze.** Keep the insulin vial in its carton so that it will stay clean and protected from light. If refrigeration is not possible, the bottle of insulin which you are currently using can be kept unrefrigerated as long as it is kept as cool as possible and away from heat and sunlight.

Never use **Novolin® N** if the precipitate (the white deposit at the bottom of the vial) has become lumpy or granular in appearance or has formed a deposit of solid particles on the wall of the vial. This insulin should not be used if the liquid in the vial remains clear after the vial has been gently agitated.

Never use insulin after the expiration date which is printed on the vial label and carton.

MIXING TWO TYPES OF INSULIN

Different insulins should be mixed only under instruction from a physician. Hypodermic syringes may vary in the amount of space between the bottom line and the needle ("dead space"), so if you are mixing two types of insulin be sure to discuss any change in the model and brand of syringe you are using with your physician or pharmacist. When you are mixing two types of insulin, always draw the Regular (clear) insulin into the syringe first.

SEE NOVOLIN® 70/30 for complete package insert information on Warning: Insulin Use in Diabetes: Types of Insulin: Syringes: Important: Preparing the Injection: Giving the Injection: Usage in Pregnancy: Insulin Reaction and Shock; Diabetic Ketoacidosis and Coma: Adverse Reactions: Important Notes.

HOW SUPPLIED

Vials, U-100, 100 units/mL, 10 mL, (List No. 183411) (1's)

Manufactured by: Novo Nordisk A/S, DK-2880 Bagsvaerd, Denmark and by Novo Nordisk Pharmaceutical Industries, Inc., 3612 Powhatan Road, Clayton, NC. 27520

Date of Issue: February 1999

Shown in Product Identification Guide, page 326

NOVOLIN® R OTC

Regular, Human Insulin Injection (recombinant DNA origin) USP

100 units/mL

PRODUCT DESCRIPTION

This vial contains **Novolin® R**, commonly known as Regular, Human Insulin Injection (recombinant DNA origin). The concentration of this product is 100 units of insulin per milliliter. It is a clear, colorless solution which has a short duration of action. The effect of **Novolin® R** begins approximately $^1/_2$ hour after injection. The effect is maximal between $2^1/_2$ and 5 hours and ends approximately 8 hours after injection. The time course of action of any insulin may vary considerably in different individuals or at different times in the same individual. Because of this variation, the time periods listed here should be considered as general guidelines only.

This human insulin (recombinant DNA origin) is structurally identical to the insulin produced by the human pancreas. This human insulin is produced by recombinant DNA technology utilizing *Saccharomyces cerevisiae* (bakers' yeast) as the production organism.

STORAGE

Insulin should be stored in a cold place, preferably in a refrigerator, but not in the freezing compartment. **Do not let it freeze.** Keep the insulin vial in its carton so that it will stay clean and protected from light. If refrigeration is not possible, the bottle of insulin which you are currently using can be kept unrefrigerated as long as it is kept as cool as possible and away from heat and sunlight.

Never use **Novolin® R** if it becomes viscous (thickened) or cloudy; use it only if it is clear and colorless.

Never use insulin after the expiration date which is printed on the vial label and carton.

MIXING TWO TYPES OF INSULIN—SEE NOVOLIN® N.

IMPORTANT NOTES

1. Due to risk of precipitation in some pump catheters, Novolin® R is not recommended for use in insulin pumps.
2. A change in the type, strength, species or purity of insulin could require a dosage adjustment. Any change in insulin should be made under medical supervision.

3. You may have learned how to test your urine or your blood for glucose. It is important to do these tests regularly and to record the results for review with your physician or nurse educator.
4. If you have an acute illness, especially with vomiting or fever, continue taking your insulin. If possible, stay on your regular diet. If you have trouble eating, drink fruit juices, regular soft drinks, or clear soups; if you can, eat small amounts of bland foods. Test your urine for glucose and ketones and, if possible, test your blood glucose. Note the results and contact your physician for possible insulin dose adjustment. If you have severe and prolonged vomiting, seek emergency medical care.
5. You should always carry identification which states that you have diabetes.
6. Always ask your physician or pharmacist before taking any drug.

Always consult your physician if you have any questions about your condition or the use of insulin.

See Novolin® 70/30 for complete package insert information on Warning: Insulin use in Diabetes: Types of Insulin: Syringes: Important: Preparing the Injection: Giving the Injection: Usage in Pregnancy: Insulin Reaction and Shock: Diabetic Ketoacidosis and Coma: Adverse Reactions.

HOW SUPPLIED

Vials, U-100, 100 units/mL, 10 mL, (List No. 183311) (1's)
Manufactured by: Novo Nordisk A/S, DK 2880 Bagsvaerd, Denmark and by Novo Nordisk Pharmaceutical Industries, Inc., 3612 Powhatan Road, Clayton, NC. 27520
Date of Issue: February 1999

Shown in Product Identification Guide, page 326

NOVOLIN® INNOLET® ℞

[nō-vō-lĭn]
insulin delivery system

Novolin® InnoLet®

[See first graphic at right]

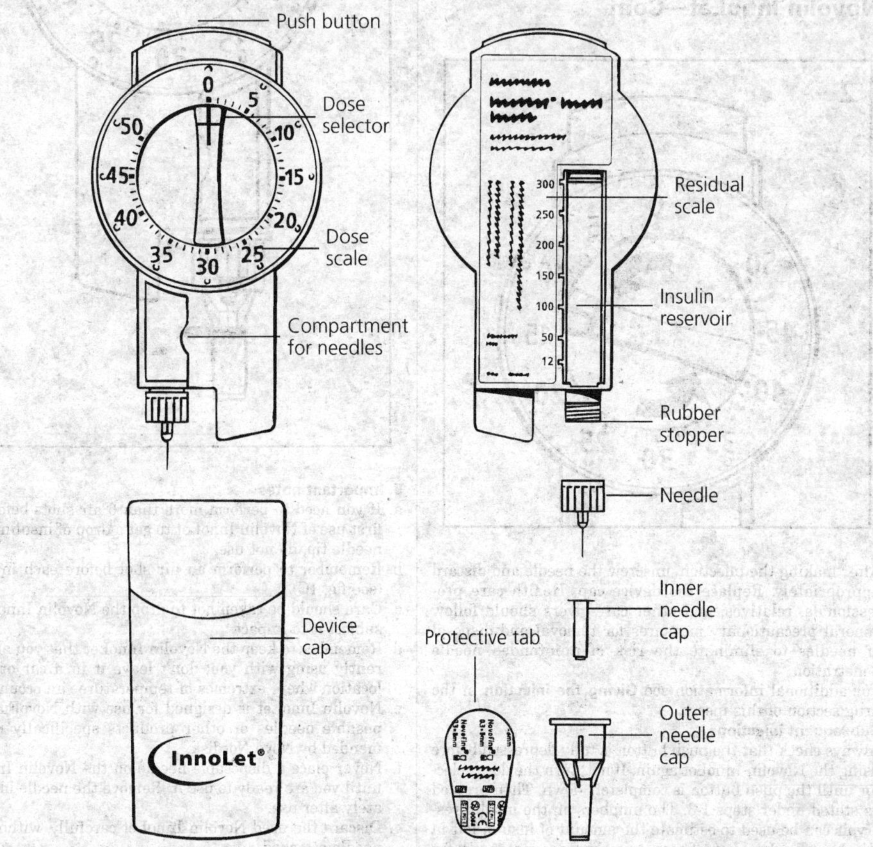

Novolin® InnoLet® directions for use

Novolin® InnoLet® is a disposable dial-a-dose insulin delivery system able to deliver 1-50 units in increments of 1 unit. Novolin InnoLet is designed for use with NovoFine® single-use needles or other products specifically recommended by Novo Nordisk®. Novolin InnoLet is not recommended for the blind or severely visually impaired patients without the assistance of a sighted individual trained in the proper use of this product.

Please read these instructions completely before using this device.

1. Preparing the Novolin® InnoLet®:
Pull off the device cap.

1A. Turn the Novolin InnoLet up and down between positions A and B so the glass ball is moved from one end of the insulin reservoir to the other. Do this at least 10 times, until the liquid appears uniformly white and cloudy.

To ensure even mixing of the remaining insulin there must be at least 12 units of insulin left in the reservoir. If there are less than 12 units left, do not use the Novolin InnoLet. This step is not necessary for Novolin R InnoLet.

Wipe rubber stopper with an alcohol swab.

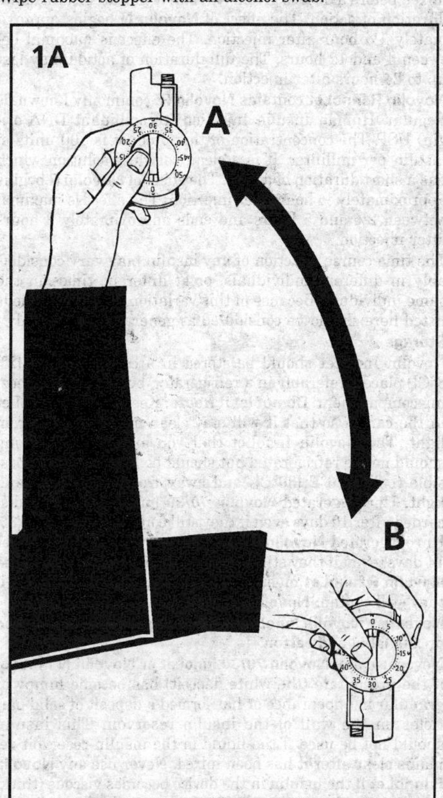

1B. Remove the protective tab from the disposable needle and screw the needle onto the Novolin InnoLet. Never place a disposable needle on your Novolin InnoLet until you are ready to give an injection. Remove the needle immediately after use. If the needle is not removed, some liquid may be expelled from the Novolin InnoLet causing a change in insulin concentration (strength) for Novolin 70/30 InnoLet and Novolin N InnoLet.

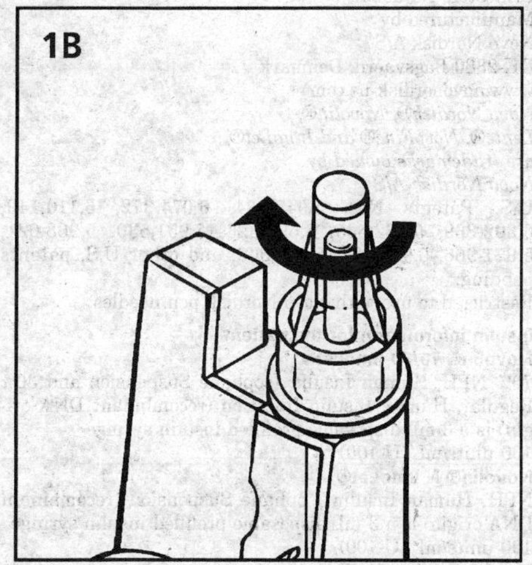

1C. Giving the air shot prior to each injection:
Small amounts of air may collect in the needle and insulin reservoir during normal use. To avoid the injection of air and ensure proper dosing, dial 2 units by turning the dose selector clockwise. Hold the Novolin InnoLet with the needle up and tap the Novolin InnoLet gently with your finger so any air bubbles collect in the top of the reservoir. Remove both the plastic outer and inner needle caps.

With the needle pointing up, press the push button as far as it will go and the dose selector returns to zero. See if a drop of insulin appears at the needle tip (see fig. 1C). If not, repeat the procedure until insulin appears. Before the first use of Novolin InnoLet you may need to perform up to 6 air shots to get a drop of insulin at the needle tip. If you need to make more than 6 air shots, do not use, and return the product to Novo Nordisk. A small air bubble may remain but it will not be injected because the operating mechanism prevents the reservoir from being completely emptied.

[See figure 1C at top of next column]

2. Setting the dose

Always check that the push button is fully depressed and the dose selector is set to zero. Hold the Novolin InnoLet in front of you and dial the dose selector clockwise to set the required dose. Do not put your hand over the push button when dialing the dose. If the button is not allowed to

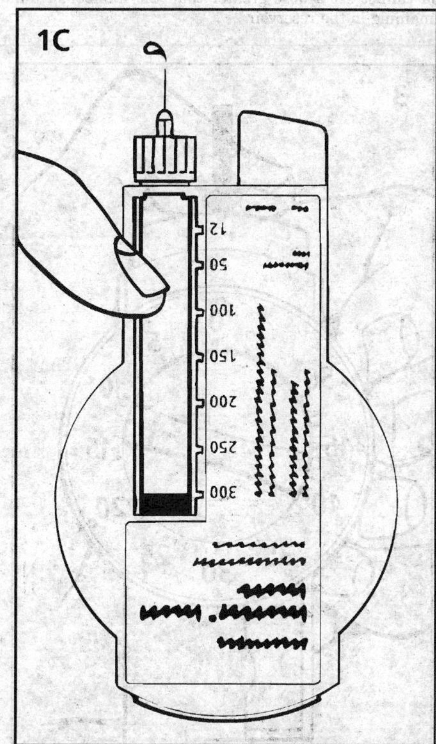

rise freely, insulin will be pushed out of the needle. When setting your dose, you will hear a click for every single unit dialed. Do not rely on this clicking sound as a means of determining your dose. If you have set a wrong dose, simply dial the dose selector forward or backwards until the right number of units has been set.

50 units is the maximum dose.

[See figure 2 at top of next column]

3. Giving the injection

Use the injection technique recommended by your doctor. Check that you have set the proper dose and depress the push button as far as it will go. Make sure not to block the dose selector while injecting as the dose selector must be allowed to return to zero when you press the push button. When depressing the push button you may hear a clicking sound. Do not rely on this clicking sound as a means of confirming delivery of your dose.

Continued on next page

Novolin InnoLet—Cont.

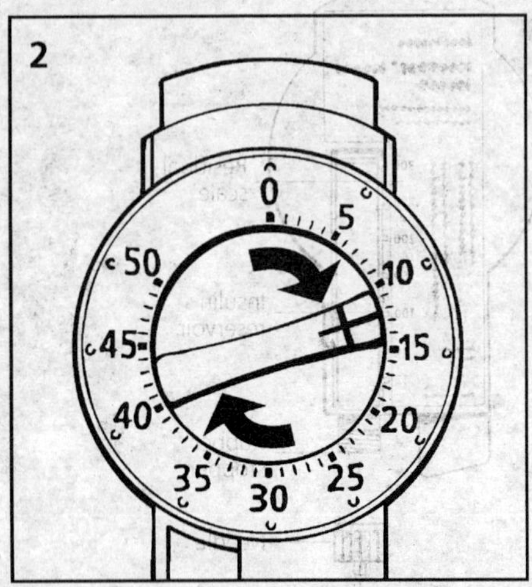

After making the injection, unscrew the needle and discard appropriately. Replace the device cap. Health care professionals, relatives, and other care-givers should follow general precautionary measures for removal and disposal of needles to eliminate the risk of unintended needle penetration.

For additional information see **Giving the injection** in the drug section of this insert.

Subsequent injections

Always check that the push button is fully depressed before using the Novolin InnoLet again. If not, turn the dose selector until the push button is completely down. Then proceed as stated under steps 1-3. The numbers on the insulin reservoir can be used to estimate the amount of insulin left in the Novolin InnoLet. These numbers are not used for measuring the insulin dose.

You cannot set a dose greater than the number of units remaining in the reservoir.

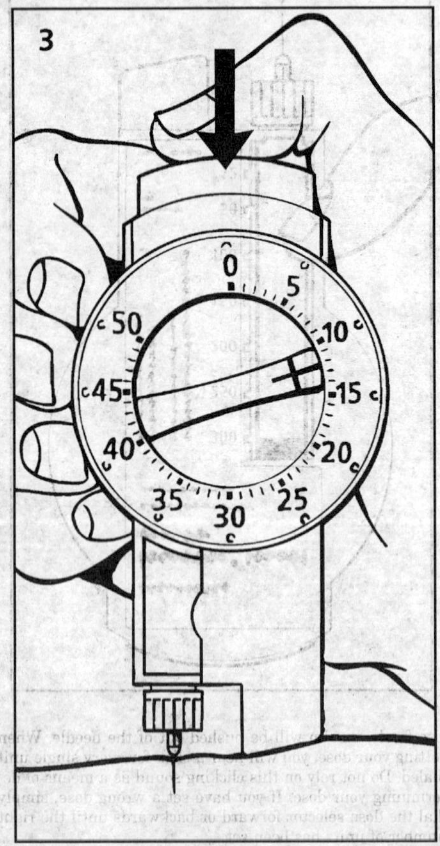

4. Function check

If you think that your Novolin InnoLet is not working properly, follow this procedure:

a. Screw on a new NovoFine needle.
b. Perform air shot as described in section 1C.
c. Put the outer needle cap onto the needle.
d. Dispense 20 units into the needle cap.

[See figure 4 at top of next column]

The insulin will fill the lower part of the cap (as shown in fig. 4). If the Novolin InnoLet has released too much or too little insulin, repeat the test. If it happens again, contact Novo Nordisk and do not use your Novolin InnoLet.

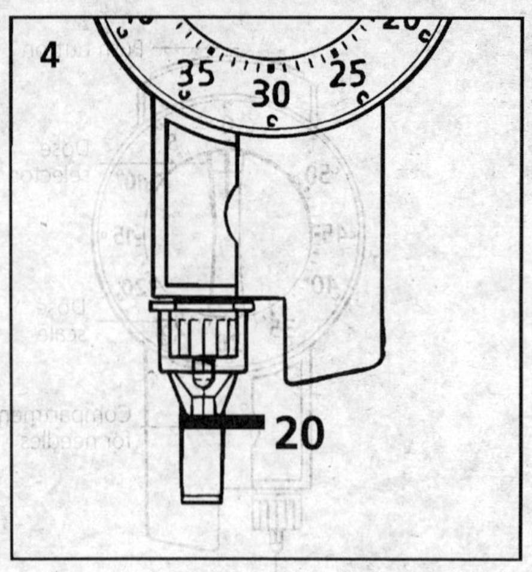

5. Important notes

a. If you need to perform more than 6 air shots before the first use of Novolin InnoLet to get a drop of insulin at the needle tip, do not use.
b. Remember to perform an air shot before each injection (see fig. 1C).
c. Care should be taken not to drop the Novolin InnoLet or subject it to impact.
d. Remember to keep the Novolin InnoLet that you are currently using with you; don't leave it in a car or other location where extremes of temperature can occur.
e. Novolin InnoLet is designed for use with NovoFine disposable needles or other products specifically recommended by Novo Nordisk.
f. Never place a disposable needle on the Novolin InnoLet until you are ready to use it. Remove the needle immediately after use.
g. Discard the used Novolin InnoLet carefully, without the needle attached.
h. Always carry a spare Novolin InnoLet with you in case your Novolin InnoLet is damaged or lost.
i. Novo Nordisk cannot be held responsible for adverse reactions occurring as a consequence of using the insulin delivery system with products that are not recommended by Novo Nordisk.
j. Keep Novolin InnoLet out of the reach of children.

Call 800-727-6500 for additional information.
Novo Nordisk Pharmaceuticals, Inc.
Princeton, NJ 08540
Manufactured by
Novo Nordisk A/S
DK-2880 Bagsvaerd, Denmark
www.novonordisk-us.com
Novo Nordisk®, Novolin®, Lente®, NovoFine® and InnoLet® are trademarks owned by Novo Nordisk A/S
U.S. Patents Nos. 5,947,934, 6,074,372, 6,110,149, 6,302,869, 5,462,535, 5,599,323, 5,951,530, 5,968,021, 5,971,966, 5,980,491, 5,984,906, and other U.S. patents pending.
Restricted to use with Novo Nordisk pen needles.

Insulin information for the patient

Novolin® 70/30 InnoLet®

70% NPH, Human Insulin Isophane Suspension and 30% Regular, Human Insulin Injection (recombinant DNA origin) is a 3 mL disposable prefilled insulin syringe
100 units/mL (U-100)

Novolin® N InnoLet®

NPH, Human Insulin Isophane Suspension (recombinant DNA origin) is a 3 mL disposable prefilled insulin syringe
100 units/mL (U-100)

Novolin® R InnoLet®

Regular, Human Insulin Injection (recombinant DNA origin) USP is a 3mL disposable prefilled insulin syringe
100 units/mL (U-100)

Please read both sides of this insert carefully before using this product.

Novolin® InnoLet® is for single-person use only.

See Important notes section.

WARNING

ANY CHANGE OF INSULIN SHOULD BE MADE CAUTIOUSLY AND ONLY UNDER MEDICAL SUPERVISION. CHANGES IN PURITY, STRENGTH, BRAND (MANUFACTURER), TYPE (REGULAR, NPH, LENTE®, ETC.), SPECIES (BEEF, PORK, BEEF-PORK, HUMAN), AND/OR METHOD OF MANUFACTURE (RECOMBINANT DNA VERSUS ANIMAL-SOURCE INSULIN) MAY RESULT IN THE NEED FOR A CHANGE IN DOSAGE.

SPECIAL CARE SHOULD BE TAKEN WHEN THE TRANSFER IS FROM A STANDARD BEEF OR MIXED SPECIES INSULIN TO A PURIFIED PORK OR HUMAN INSULIN. IF A DOSAGE ADJUSTMENT IS NEEDED, IT WILL USUALLY BECOME APPARENT EITHER IN THE FIRST FEW DAYS OR OVER A PERIOD OF SEVERAL WEEKS. ANY CHANGE IN TREATMENT SHOULD BE CAREFULLY MONITORED.

PLEASE READ THE SECTIONS "INSULIN REACTION AND SHOCK" AND "DIABETIC KETOACIDOSIS AND COMA" FOR SYMPTOMS OF HYPOGLYCEMIA (LOW BLOOD GLUCOSE) AND HYPERGLYCEMIA (HIGH BLOOD GLUCOSE).

Insulin use in diabetes

Your physician has explained that you have diabetes and that your treatment involves injections of insulin or insulin therapy combined with an oral antidiabetic medicine. Insulin is normally produced by the pancreas, a gland that lies behind the stomach. Without insulin, glucose (a simple sugar made from digested food) is trapped in the bloodstream and cannot enter the cells of the body. Some patients who don't make enough of their own insulin, or who cannot use the insulin they do make properly, must take insulin by injection in order to control their blood glucose levels. Each case of diabetes is different and requires direct and continued medical supervision.

Your physician has told you the type, strength and amount of insulin you should use and the time(s) at which you should inject it, and has also discussed with you a diet and exercise schedule. You should contact your physician if you experience any difficulties or if you have questions.

Types of insulins

Standard and purified animal insulins as well as human insulins are available. Standard and purified insulins differ in their degree of purification and content of noninsulin material. Standard and purified insulins also vary in species source; they may be of beef, pork, or mixed beef and pork origin. Human insulin is identical in structure to the insulin produced by the human pancreas, and thus differs from animal insulins. Insulins vary in time of action; see **Product description** for additional information.

Your physician has prescribed the insulin that is right for you; be sure you have purchased the correct insulin and check it carefully before you use it.

Product description

A package contains five (5) Novolin® InnoLet®. Novolin human insulin (recombinant DNA origin) is structurally identical to the insulin produced by the human pancreas. This human insulin is produced by recombinant DNA technology utilizing *Saccharomyces cerevisiae* (bakers' yeast) as the production organism.

Novolin 70/30 InnoLet contains a mixture of 70% NPH, Human Insulin Isophane Suspension and 30% Regular, Human Insulin Injection (recombinant DNA origin). The concentration of this product is 100 units of insulin per milliliter. It is a cloudy or milky suspension of human insulin with protamine and zinc. The insulin substance (the cloudy material) settles at the bottom of the insulin reservoir, therefore, the **Novolin 70/30 InnoLet** must be rotated up and down so that the contents are uniformly mixed before a dose is given. **Novolin 70/30 InnoLet** has an intermediate duration of action. The effect of **Novolin 70/30 InnoLet** begins approximately 1/2 hour after injection. The effect is maximal between 2 and approximately 12 hours. The full duration of action may last up to 24 hours after injection.

Novolin N InnoLet contains **Novolin N**, commonly known as NPH, Human Insulin Isophane Suspension (recombinant DNA origin). The concentration of this product is 100 units of insulin per milliliter. It is a cloudy or milky suspension of human insulin with protamine and zinc. The insulin substance (the cloudy material) settles at the bottom of the insulin reservoir, therefore, the **Novolin N InnoLet** must be rotated up and down so that the contents are uniformly mixed before a dose is given. **Novolin N** has an intermediate duration of action. The effect of **Novolin N** begins approximately 1½ hour after injection. The effect is maximal between 4 and 12 hours. The full duration of action may last up to 24 hours after injection.

Novolin R InnoLet contains **Novolin R**, commonly known as Regular, Human Insulin Injection (recombinant DNA origin) USP. The concentration of this product is 100 units of insulin per milliliter. It is a clear, colorless solution which has a short duration of action. The effect of **Novolin R** begins approximately ½ hour after injection. The effect is maximal between 2½ and 5 hours and ends approximately 8 hours after injection.

The time course of action of any insulin may vary considerably in different individuals, or at different times in the same individual. Because of this variation, the time periods listed here should be considered as general guidance only.

Storage

Novolin InnoLet should be stored in a cold (36°-46°F [2°-8°C]) place, preferably in a refrigerator, but not in the freezing compartment. **Do not let it freeze.** Keep Novolin InnoLet in the carton so that it will stay clean and protected from light. The Novolin InnoLet that you are currently using should not be refrigerated but should be kept as cool as possible (below 86°F [30°C]) and away from direct heat and light. Unrefrigerated **Novolin 70/30 InnoLet** must be discarded after 10 days even if they still contain **Novolin 70/30.** Unrefrigerated **Novolin N InnoLet** must be discarded after 14 days, even if they still contain **Novolin N**. Unrefrigerated **Novolin R InnoLet** must be discarded after 28 days, even if they still contain **Novolin R.**

Never use Novolin InnoLet after the expiration date printed on the label and carton.

Never use any **Novolin 70/30 InnoLet** or **Novolin N InnoLet** if the precipitate (the white deposit) has become lumpy or granular in appearance or has formed a deposit of solid particles on the wall of the insulin reservoir. This insulin should not be used if the liquid in the insulin reservoir remains clear after it has been mixed. Never use any **Novolin R InnoLet** if the insulin in the device becomes viscous (thickened) or cloudy; use it only if it is clear and colorless.

Important

Failure to comply with the following antiseptic measures may lead to infections at the injection site.

— Disposable needles are for single use; they should be used only once and destroyed.

— Clean your hands and the injection site with soap and water or with alcohol.

— Wipe the rubber stopper on the insulin cartridge with an alcohol swab.

Preparing the injection

Never place a single-use disposable needle on your Novolin InnoLet until you are ready to give an injection, and remove the needle immediately after each injection. Follow the directions for use of the Novolin InnoLet in the device section of this insert.

Novolin InnoLet may contain a small amount of air. To prevent an injection of air and make certain insulin is delivered, an air shot must be done before each injection. Directions for performing an air shot are provided in the device section of this insert.

Giving the injection

1. The following areas are suitable for subcutaneous insulin injection: thighs, upper arms, buttocks, abdomen. Do not change areas without consulting your physician. The actual point of injection should be changed each time; injection sites should be about an inch apart.
2. The injection site should be clean and dry. Pinch up skin area to be injected and hold it firmly.
3. Hold the device upright and push the needle quickly and firmly into the pinched-up area. Release the skin and push the push-button all the way in to inject insulin beneath the skin. After the injection, the needle should remain under the skin for at least 6 seconds. Keep the push button fully depressed until the needle is withdrawn from the skin. This will ensure that the full dose has been delivered.
4. Do not inject into a muscle unless your physician has advised it. You should never inject insulin into a vein.
5. Remove the needle. If slight bleeding occurs, press lightly with a dry cotton swab for a few seconds - **do not rub.**

For additional information see **Giving the injection** in the device section of this insert.

Usage in pregnancy

It is particularly important to maintain good control of your diabetes during pregnancy and special attention must be paid to your diet, exercise and insulin regimens. If you are pregnant or nursing a baby, consult your physician or nurse educator.

Insulin reaction and shock

Insulin reaction (hypoglycemia) occurs when the blood glucose falls very low. This can happen if you take too much insulin, miss or delay a meal, exercise more than usual or work too hard without eating, or become ill (especially with vomiting or fever). Hypoglycemia can also happen if you combine insulin therapy and other medications that lower blood glucose, such as oral antidiabetic agents or other prescription and over-the-counter drugs. The first symptoms of an insulin reaction usually come on suddenly. They may include a cold sweat, fatigue, nervousness or shakiness, rapid heartbeat, or nausea. Personality change or confusion may also occur. If you drink or eat something right away (a glass of milk or orange juice, or several sugar candies), you can often stop the progression of symptoms. If symptoms persist, call your physician - an insulin reaction can lead to unconsciousness. If a reaction results in loss of consciousness, emergency medical care should be obtained immediately. If you have had repeated reactions or if an insulin reaction has led to a loss of consciousness, contact your physician. Severe hypoglycemia can result in temporary or permanent impairment of brain function and death.

In certain cases, the nature and intensity of the warning symptoms of hypoglycemia may change. A few patients have reported that after being transferred to human insulin, the early warning symptoms of hypoglycemia were less pronounced than they had been with animal-source insulin.

Diabetic ketoacidosis and coma

Diabetic ketoacidosis may develop if your body has too little insulin. The most common causes are acute illness or infection or failure to take enough insulin by injection. If you are ill you should check your urine for ketones. The symptoms of diabetic ketoacidosis usually come on gradually, over a period of hours or days, and include a drowsy feeling, flushed face, thirst and loss of appetite. Notify your physician right away if the urine test is positive for ketones (acetone) or if you have any of these symptoms. Fast, heavy breathing and rapid pulse are more severe symptoms and you should have medical attention right away. Severe, sustained hyperglycemia may result in diabetic coma and death.

ADVERSE REACTIONS

A few people with diabetes develop red, swollen and itchy skin where the insulin has been injected. This is called a "local reaction" and it may occur if the injection is not properly made, if the skin is sensitive to the cleansing solution, or if you are allergic to the insulin being used. If you have a local reaction, tell your physician.

Generalized insulin allergy occurs rarely, but when it does it may cause a serious reaction, including skin rash over the body, shortness of breath, fast pulse, sweating, and a drop in blood pressure. If any of these symptoms develop, you should seek emergency medical care.

If severe allergic reactions to insulin have occurred (i.e., generalized rash, swelling or breathing difficulties) you should be skin-tested with each new insulin preparation before it is used.

Important notes

1. A change in the type, strength, species or purity of insulin could require a dosage adjustment. Any change in insulin should be made under medical supervision.
2. To avoid possible transmission of disease, Novolin InnoLet is for single-person use only.
3. You may have learned how to test your urine or your blood for glucose. It is important to do these tests regularly and to record the results for review with your physician or nurse educator.
4. If you have an acute illness, especially with vomiting or fever, continue taking your insulin. If possible, stay on your regular diet. If you have trouble eating, drink fruit juices, regular soft drinks, or clear soups; if you can, eat small amounts of bland foods. Test your urine for glucose and ketones and, if possible, test your blood glucose. Note the results and contact your physician for possible insulin dose adjustment. If you have severe and prolonged vomiting, seek emergency medical care.
5. You should always carry identification which states that you have diabetes.
6. Always ask your physician or pharmacist before taking any drug.

Always consult your physician if you have any questions about your condition or the use of insulin.

Helpful information for people with diabetes is published by American Diabetes Association, 1660 Duke Street, Alexandria, VA 22314

Date of Issue: May 2003

Call 800-727-6500 for additional information.

Novo Nordisk
Pharmaceuticals, Inc.
Princeton, NJ 08540
Manufactured by
Novo Nordisk A/S
DK-2880 Bagsvaerd, Denmark
www.novonordisk-us.com

Novo Nordisk®, Novolin®, Lente®, NovoFine® and InnoLet® are trademarks owned by Novo Nordisk A/S

Shown in Product Identification Guide, page 326

HUMAN INSULIN **OTC**

NOVOLIN® 70/30 PenFill®

70% NPH, Human Insulin Isophane Suspension and 30% Regular, Human Insulin Injection (recombinant DNA origin)

3 mL Disposable Cartridge

100 units/ml

NOVOLIN® N PenFill® **OTC**

NPH, Human Insulin Isophane Suspension (recombinant DNA origin)

3 mL Disposable Cartridge

100 units/ml

NOVOLIN® R PenFill® **OTC**

Regular, Human Insulin Injection (recombinant DNA origin)

3 mL Disposable Cartridge

100 units/ml

Please read this leaflet carefully before using this product. Please note the special directions under "PREPARING THE INJECTION".

Novolin® PenFill® cartridges are designed for use with **NovoPen®3, NovoPen®Junior, NovoPen 3 Demi®, InDuo™,** and **Innovo® Insulin Delivery Devices** and **NovoFine®** disposable needles or other products specifically recommended by Novo Nordisk.

PenFill® cartridge is for single-person use only.

See IMPORTANT NOTES section.

WARNING

ANY CHANGE OF INSULIN SHOULD BE MADE CAUTIOUSLY AND ONLY UNDER MEDICAL SUPERVISION. CHANGES IN PURITY, STRENGTH, BRAND (MANUFACTURER), TYPE (REGULAR, NPH, LENTE®, ETC.), SPECIES (BEEF, PORK, BEEF-PORK, HUMAN), AND/OR METHOD OF MANUFACTURE (RECOMBINANT DNA VERSUS ANIMAL-SOURCE INSULIN) MAY RESULT IN THE NEED FOR A CHANGE IN DOSAGE.

SPECIAL CARE SHOULD BE TAKEN WHEN THE TRANSFER IS FROM A STANDARD BEEF OR MIXED SPECIES INSULIN TO A PURIFIED PORK OR HUMAN INSULIN. IF A DOSAGE ADJUSTMENT IS NEEDED, IT WILL USUALLY BECOME APPARENT EITHER IN THE FIRST FEW DAYS OR OVER A PERIOD OF SEVERAL WEEKS. ANY CHANGE IN TREATMENT SHOULD BE CAREFULLY MONITORED.

PLEASE READ THE SECTIONS "INSULIN REACTION AND SHOCK" AND "DIABETIC KETOACIDOSIS AND COMA" FOR SYMPTOMS OF HYPOGLYCEMIA (LOW BLOOD GLUCOSE) AND HYPERGLYCEMIA (HIGH BLOOD GLUCOSE).

INSULIN USE IN DIABETES

Your physician has explained that you have diabetes and that your treatment involves injections of insulin or insulin therapy combined with an oral antidiabetic medicine. Insulin is normally produced by the pancreas, a gland that lies behind the stomach. Without insulin, glucose (a simple sugar made from digested food) is trapped in the bloodstream and cannot enter the cells of the body. Some patients who don't make enough of their own insulin, or who cannot use the insulin they do make properly, must take insulin by injection in order to control their blood glucose levels. Each case of diabetes is different and requires direct and continued medical supervision. Your physician has told you the type, strength and amount of insulin you should use and the time(s) at which you should inject it, and has also discussed with you a diet and exercise schedule. You should contact your physician if you experience any difficulties or if you have questions.

TYPES OF INSULINS

Standard and purified animal insulins as well as human insulins are available. Standard and purified insulins differ in their degree of purification and content of noninsulin material. Standard and purified insulins also vary in species source; they may be of beef, pork, or mixed beef and pork origin. Human insulin is identical in structure to the insulin produced by the human pancreas, and thus differs from animal insulins. Insulins vary in time of action; see PRODUCT DESCRIPTION for additional information.

Your physician has prescribed the insulin that is right for you; be sure you have purchased the correct insulin and check it carefully before you use it.

PRODUCT DESCRIPTION

A package contains five (5) **Novolin® PenFill®** 3mL cartridges.

Novolin® 70/30 PenFill contain **Novolin® 70/30** which is a mixture of 70% NPH, Human Insulin Isophane Suspension and 30% Regular, Human Insulin Injection (recombinant DNA origin). The concentration of this product is 100 units of insulin per milliliter. It is a cloudy or milky suspension of human insulin with protamine and zinc. The insulin substance (the cloudy material) settles at the bottom of the cartridge, therefore, the cartridge must be rotated up and down as described under PREPARING THE INJECTION so that the contents are uniformly mixed before the dose is given. **Novolin® 70/30** has an intermediate duration of action. The effect of **Novolin® 70/30** begins approximately 1/2 hour after injection. The effect is maximal between 2 and approximately 12 hours. The full duration of action may last up to 24 hours after injection.

The time course of action of any insulin may vary considerably in different individuals, or at different times in the same individual. Because of this variation, the time periods listed here should be considered as general guidance only. This human insulin (recombinant DNA origin) is structurally identical to the insulin produced by the human pancreas. This human insulin is produced by recombinant DNA technology utilizing *Saccharomyces cerevisiae* (bakers' yeast) as the production organism.

Novolin® N PenFill® cartridges contain **Novolin® N,** commonly known as NPH, Human Insulin Isophane Suspension (recombinant DNA origin). The concentration of this product is 100 units of insulin per milliliter. It is a cloudy or milky suspension of human insulin with protamine and zinc. The insulin substance (the cloudy material) settles at the bottom of the cartridge; therefore, the cartridge must be rotated up and down as described under PREPARING THE INJECTION so that the contents are uniformly mixed before a dose is given.

Novolin® N has an intermediate duration of action. The effect of **Novolin® N** begins approximately 1½ hours after injection. The effect is maximal between 4 and 12 hours. The full duration of action may last up to 24 hours after injection. The time course of action of any insulin may vary considerably in different individuals, or at different times in the same individual. Because of this variation, the time periods listed here should be considered as general guidance only. This human insulin (recombinant DNA origin) is structurally identical to the insulin produced by the human pancreas. This human insulin is produced by recombinant DNA technology utilizing *Saccharomyces cerevisiae* (bakers' yeast) as the production organism.

Novolin® R PenFill® cartridges contain **Novolin® R,** commonly known as Regular, Human Insulin Injection (recombinant DNA origin). The concentration of this product is 100 units of insulin per milliliter. It is a clear, colorless solution which has a short duration of action. The effect of **Novolin® R** begins approximately ½ hour after injection. The effect is maximal between 2½ and 5 hours and ends approximately 8 hours after injection. The time course of action of any insulin may vary considerably in different individuals, or at different times in the same individual. Because of this variation, the time periods listed here should be considered as general guidance only.

This human insulin (recombinant DNA origin) is structurally identical to the insulin produced by the human pancreas. This human insulin is produced by recombinant DNA technology utilizing *Saccharomyces cerevisiae* (bakers' yeast) as the production organism.

INSULIN DELIVERY SYSTEMS

These Novolin PenFill 3mL cartridges are designed for use with NovoPen® 3, NovoPen® Junior, NovoPen 3 Demi®, InDuo™, and Innovo® Insulin Delivery Devices and NovoFine® disposable needles or other products specifically recommended by Novo Nordisk.

Continued on next page

Novolin PenFill—Cont.

STORAGE

Insulin should be stored in a cold (36°–46°F [2–8°C]) place, preferably in a refrigerator, but not in the freezing compartment. **Do not let it freeze.** Keep **Novolin® 70/30 PenFill®**, **Novolin® N PenFill®** and **Novolin® R PenFill®** cartridges in the carton so that they will stay clean and protected from light. The **Novolin® 70/30 PenFill®**, **Novolin® N PenFIll®** and **Novolin® R PenFill®** cartridges that you are currently using should not be refrigerated but should be kept as cool as possible (below 86°F [30°C]) and away from direct heat and light. **Novolin® N PenFill®** 3.0ml cartridges can be kept unrefrigerated for 14 days, and **Novolin® 70/30 PenFill®** 3.0ml cartridges can be kept unrefrigerated for 10 days. **Novolin® R PenFill®** 3.0ml cartridges can be kept unrefrigerated for 28 days. Unrefrigerated cartridges must be discarded after these time periods, even if they still contain insulin.

Never use insulin after the expiration date which is printed on the label and carton.

Never use any **Novolin® 70/30 PenFill®** or **Novolin® N PenFill®** cartridge if the precipitate (the white deposit), has become lumpy or granular in appearance or has formed a deposit of solid particles on the wall of the cartridge. This insulin should not be used if the liquid in the cartridge remains clear after it has been mixed.

Never use any **Novolin® R PenFill®** cartridge if the insulin becomes viscous (thickened) or cloudy; use it only if it is clear and colorless.

IMPORTANT

Failure to comply with the following antiseptic measures may lead to infections at the injection site.

— Disposable needles are for single use; they should be used only once and destroyed.

— Clean your hands and the injection site with soap and water or with alcohol.

— Wipe the rubber stopper on the insulin cartridge with an alcohol swab.

PREPARING THE INJECTION

Novolin® R PenFill®

Never place a single-use disposable needle on your device until you are ready to give an injection, and remove the needle immediately after each injection. Follow the directions for use in the instruction manual for your insulin delivery device. **Insulin PenFill® cartridges may contain a small amount of air. To prevent an injection of air and make certain insulin is delivered, an air shot must be done before each injection. Directions for performing an air shot are provided in your insulin delivery device instruction manual.**

Novolin® 70/30 PenFill® and **Novolin® N PenFill®**

Never place a single-use disposable needle on your insulin delivery device until you are ready to give an injection, and remove it immediately after each injection. If the needle is not removed, some liquid may be expelled from the cartridge causing a change in the insulin concentration (strength).

The cloudy material in an insulin suspension will settle to the bottom of the cartridge, so the contents must be mixed before injection. These **Novolin® PenFill®** cartridges contain a glass ball to aid mixing.

When using a new cartridge, turn the cartridge up and down between positions A and B—See Figure 1. Do this at least 10 times until the liquid appears uniformly white and cloudy.

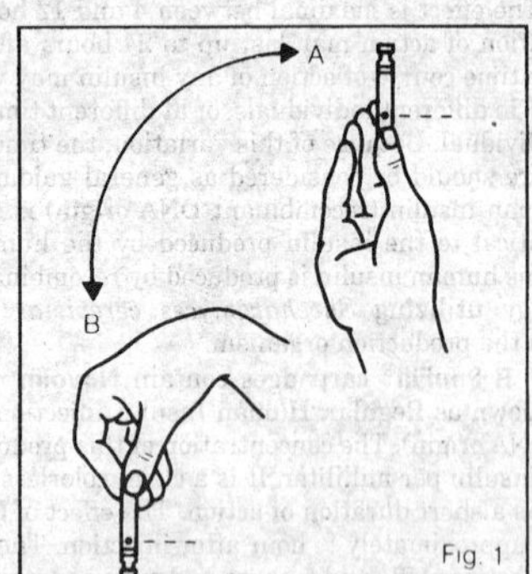

Fig. 1

Assemble your insulin delivery device following the directions in your instruction manual.

For subsequent injections when a cartridge is already in the device, turn the device up and down between positions A and B—See Figure 2. Do this at least 10 times until the liquid appears uniformly white and cloudy. Follow the directions in your insulin delivery device instruction manual.

[See figure 2 at top of next column]

Note: Never initiate a new injection unless there is sufficient insulin in the cartridge to ensure proper mixing (the glass ball needs adequate room for movement to mix the suspension).

Insulin PenFill® cartridges may contain a small amount of air. To prevent an injection of air and make certain insulin is delivered, an air shot must be done before each injection. Directions for performing an air shot are provided in your delivery device instruction manual.

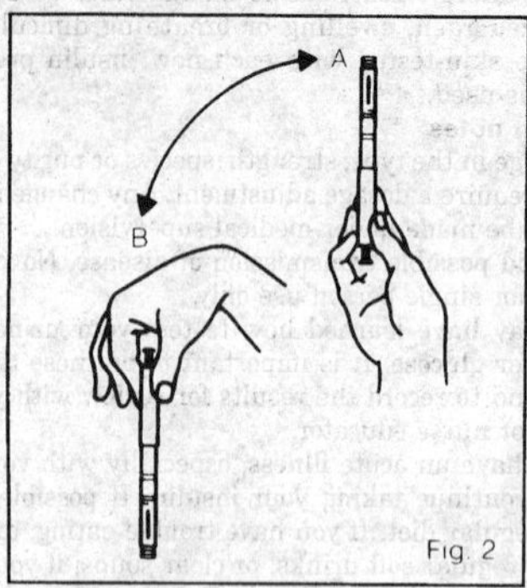

Fig. 2

GIVING THE INJECTION

1. The following areas are suitable for subcutaneous insulin injection: thighs, upper arms, buttocks, abdomen. Do not change areas without consulting your physician. The actual point of injection should be changed each time; injection sites should be about an inch apart.
2. The injection site should be clean and dry. Pinch up skin area to be injected and hold it firmly.
3. Hold the device like a pencil and push the needle quickly and firmly into the pinched-up area.
4. Release the skin and push the push-button all the way in to inject insulin beneath the skin. After the injection, the needle should remain under the skin for at least 6 seconds. Keep the push button fully depressed until the needle is withdrawn from the skin. This will ensure that the full dose has been delivered.
5. Do not inject into a muscle unless your physician has advised it. You should never inject insulin into a vein. Follow the directions for use of your insulin delivery device.
6. Remove the needle. If slight bleeding occurs, press lightly with a dry cotton swab for a few seconds—**do not rub.**

Note: Use the injection technique recommended by your physician.

USAGE IN PREGNANCY

It is particularly important to maintain good control of your diabetes during pregnancy and special attention must be paid to your diet, exercise and insulin regimens. If you are pregnant or nursing a baby, consult your physician or nurse educator.

INSULIN REACTION AND SHOCK

Insulin reaction (hypoglycemia) occurs when the blood glucose falls very low. This can happen if you take too much insulin, miss or delay a meal, exercise more than usual or work too hard without eating, or become ill (especially with vomiting or fever). Hypoglycemia can also happen if you combine insulin therapy and other medications that lower blood glucose, such as oral antidiabetic agents or other prescription and over-the-counter drugs. The first symptoms of an insulin reaction usually come on suddenly. They may include a cold sweat, fatigue, nervousness or shakiness, rapid heartbeat, or nausea. Personality change or confusion may also occur. If you drink or eat something right away (a glass of milk or orange juice, or several sugar candies), you can often stop the progression of symptoms. If symptoms persist, call your physician—an insulin reaction can lead to unconsciousness. If a reaction results in loss of consciousness, emergency medical care should be obtained immediately. If you have had repeated reactions or if an insulin reaction has led to a loss of consciousness, contact your physician. Severe hypoglycemia can result in temporary or permanent impairment of brain function and death.

In certain cases, the nature and intensity of the warning symptoms of hypoglycemia may change. A few patients have reported that after being transferred to human insulin, the early warning symptoms of hypoglycemia were less pronounced than they had been with animal-source insulin.

DIABETIC KETOACIDOSIS AND COMA

Diabetic ketoacidosis may develop if your body has too little insulin. The most common causes are acute illness or infection or failure to take enough insulin by injection. If you are ill you should check your urine for ketones. The symptoms of diabetic ketoacidosis usually come on gradually, over a period of hours or days, and include a drowsy feeling, flushed face, thirst and loss of appetite. Notify your physician right away if the urine test is positive for ketones (acetone) or if you have any of these symptoms. Fast, heavy breathing and rapid pulse are more severe symptoms and you should have medical attention right away. Severe, sustained hyperglycemia may result in diabetic coma and death.

ADVERSE REACTIONS

A few people with diabetes develop red, swollen and itchy skin where the insulin has been injected. This is called a "local reaction" and it may occur if the injection is not properly made, if the skin is sensitive to the cleansing solution, or if you are allergic to the insulin being used. If you have a local reaction, tell your physican.

Generalized insulin allergy occurs rarely, but when it does it may cause a serious reaction, including skin rash over the body, shortness of breath, fast pulse, sweating, and a drop in blood pressure. If any of these symptoms develop, you should seek emergency medical care.

If severe allergic reactions to insulin have occured (i.e., generalized rash, swelling or breathing difficulties) you should be skin-tested with **each** new insulin preparation before it is used.

IMPORTANT NOTES

1. A change in the type, strength, species or purity of insulin could require a dosage adjustment. Any change in insulin should be made under medical supervision.
2. To avoid possible transmission of disease, PenFill® cartridge is for single-person use only.
3. Before use, check that the PenFill® cartridge is intact (e.g. no cracks). Do not use if any damage is seen, or if the part of the rubber piston that you see is wider than the white bar code band.
4. You may have learned how to test your urine or your blood for glucose. It is important to do these tests regularly and to record the results for review with your physician or nurse educator.
5. If you have an acute illness, especially with vomiting or fever, continue taking your insulin. If possible, stay on your regular diet. If you have trouble eating, drink fruit juices, regular soft drinks, or clear soups; if you can, eat small amounts of bland foods. Test your urine for glucose and ketones and, if possible, test your blood glucose. Note the results and contact your physician for possible insulin dose adjustment. If you have severe and prolonged vomiting, seek emergency medical care.
6. You should always carry identification which states that you have diabetes.
7. Always ask your physician or pharmacist before taking any drug.
8. Do not try to refill a PenFill® cartridge.

Always consult your physician if you have any questions about your conditon or the use of insulin.

Helpful information for people with diabetes is published by American Diabetes Association, 1660 Duke Street, Alexandria, VA 22314

Date of issue: July 2002

Protected by U.S. Patent No 6,126,646 and Des. 347,894 and other U.S. Patents Pending, restricted to use with Novo Nordisk insulin delivery devices and Novo Nordisk pen needles.

Novo Nordisk Pharmaceuticals, Inc.
Princeton, NJ 08540
Call 1-800-727-6500 for additional information
(Se habla espanol)
www.novonordisk-us.com

Manufactured by: Novo Nordisk A/S, DK-2880 Bagsvaerd, Denmark and Novo Nordisk Pharmaceutical Industries, Inc., Clayton, NC 27520

HOW SUPPLIED

Novolin® 70/30 PenFill® cartridges, U100, 100 units/mL, 3 mL, (List no. 347718) (5's)

Novolin® N PenFill® cartridges, U100, 100 units/mL, 3 mL, (List no. 347418) (5's)

Novolin® R PenFill® cartridges, U100, 100 units/mL, 3 mL, (List no. 347318) (5's)

NOVOFINE® 30 ℞

Disposable Needle

DESCRIPTION

The self contained disposable needle consists of a protective plastic outer cap, a smooth plastic needle cap and a protective tab. (The needle should not be used if the protective tab is missing or damaged.)

Each **NovoFine® 30** is 30 gauge, one-third ($^1/_3$) inch (8mm) in length and is intended for single use only. Each **NovoFine® 30** is cut to a sharp, low-angle point and coated with silicone for easier penetration.

NovoFine® 30 is for use with all Novo Nordisk® Insulin Delivery Systems.

List# 185250

NovoFine® is a trademark of Novo Nordisk A/S.

NovoFine® 31

Disposable Needle

DESCRIPTION

The self contained disposable needle consists of a protective plastic outer cap, a smooth plastic needle cap and a protective tab. (The needle should not be used if the protective tab is missing or damaged.)

Each **NovoFine® 31** is a 31 gauge, one-fourth (1/4″) inch (6mm) in length and is intended for single use only. Each **NovoFine® 31** is cut to a sharp, low-angle point and coated with silicone for easier penetration.

NovoFine® 31 is for use with all Novo Nordisk® Insulin Delivery Systems.

List 185295

NovoFine® is a trademark of Novo Nordisk A/S.

NOVOLOG® ℞

Insulin aspart (rDNA origin) Injection

DESCRIPTION

NovoLog® (insulin aspart [rDNA origin] injection) is a human insulin analog that is a rapid-acting, parenteral blood glucose-lowering agent.

NovoLog is homologous with regular human insulin with the exception of a single substitution of the amino acid proline by aspartic acid in position B28, and is produced by recombinant DNA technology utilizing *Saccharomyces cerevisiae* (baker's yeast) as the production organism. Insulin aspart has the empirical formula $C_{256}H_{381}N_{65}O_{79}S_6$ and a molecular weight of 5825.8.

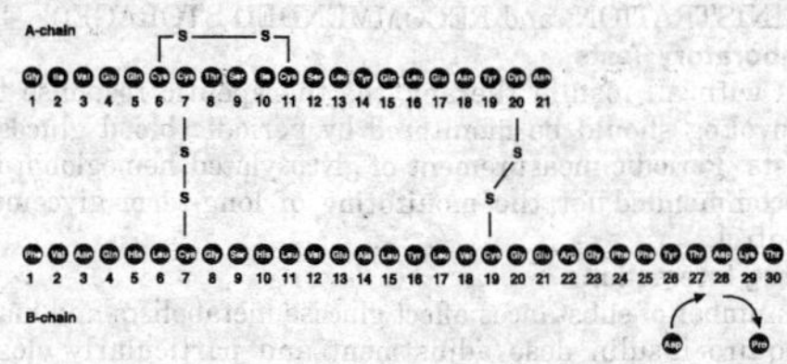

Figure 1. Structural formula of insulin aspart.

NovoLog is a sterile, aqueous, clear, and colorless solution, that contains insulin aspart (B28 asp regular human insulin analog) 100 Units/mL, glycerin 16 mg/mL, phenol 1.50 mg/mL, metacresol 1.72 mg/mL, zinc 19.6 µg/mL, disodium hydrogen phosphate dihydrate 1.25 mg/mL, and sodium chloride 0.58 mg/mL. NovoLog has a pH of 7.2–7.6. Hydrochloric acid 10% and/or sodium hydroxide 10% may be added to adjust pH.

CLINICAL PHARMACOLOGY

Mechanism of Action

The primary activity of NovoLog is the regulation of glucose metabolism. Insulins, including NovoLog, bind to the insulin receptors on muscle and fat cells and lower blood glucose by facilitating the cellular uptake of glucose and simultaneously inhibiting the output of glucose from the liver. In standard biological assays in mice and rabbits, one unit of NovoLog has the same glucose-lowering effect as one unit of regular human insulin. In humans, the effect of NovoLog is more rapid in onset and of shorter duration, compared to regular human insulin, due to its faster absorption after subcutaneous injection (see Figure 2 and Figure 3).

Pharmacokinetics

The single substitution of the amino acid proline with aspartic acid at position B28 in NovoLog reduces the molecule's tendency to form hexamers as observed with regular human insulin. NovoLog is therefore more rapidly absorbed after subcutaneous injection compared to regular human insulin.

Bioavailability and Absorption—NovoLog has a faster absorption, a faster onset of action, and a shorter duration of action than regular human insulin after subcutaneous injection (see Figure 2 and Figure 3). The relative bioavailability of NovoLog compared to regular human insulin indicates that the two insulins are absorbed to a similar extent.

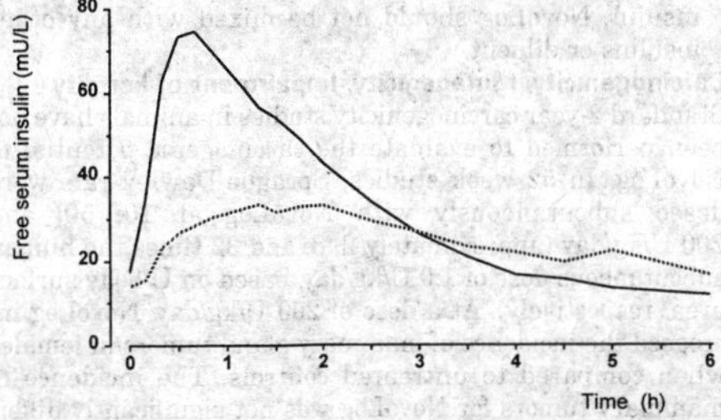

Figure 2. Serial mean serum free insulin concentration collected up to 6 hours following a singel pre-meal dose of NovoLog (solid curve) or regular human insulin (hatched curve) injected immediately before a meal in 22 patients with Type 1 diabetes.

In studies in healthy volunteers (total n=107) and patients with Type 1 diabetes (total n=40), NovoLog consistently reached peak serum concentrations approximately twice as fast as regular human insulin. The median time to maximum concentration in these trials was 40 to 50 minutes for NovoLog versus 80 to 120 minutes for regular human insulin. In a clinical trial in patients with Type 1 diabetes, NovoLog and regular human insulin, both administered subcutaneously at a dose of 0.15 U/kg body weight, reached mean maximum concentrations of 82.1 and 35.9 mU/L, respectively. Pharmacokinetic/pharmacodynamic characteristics of insulin aspart have not been established in patients with Type 2 diabetes.

The intra-individual variability in time to maximum serum insulin concentration for healthy male volunteers was significantly less for NovoLog than for regular human insulin. The clinical significance of this observation has not been established.

In a clinical study in healthy non-obese subjects, the pharmacokinetic differences between NovoLog and regular human insulin described above, were observed independent of the injection site (abdomen, thigh, or upper arm). Differences in pharmacokinetics between NovoLog and regular human insulin are not associated with differences in overall glycemic control

Table 1. Results of two six-month, active-control, open-label trials in patients with Type 1 diabetes (Studies A and B) and one six-month, active-control, open-label trial in patients with Type 2 diabetes (Study C).

Study	Treatment (n)	Mean HbA1c (%)		Hypoglycemia[1] (events/month/ patient)	% of Patients Using Various Numbers of Insulin Injections/Day[2]				
					Rapid-acting			Basal	
		Baseline	Month 6		1–2	3	4–5	1	2
A	NovoLog (n=694) Novolin R (n=346)	8.0 8.0	7.9 8.0	0.06 0.06	3 6	75 75	22 19	54 63	46 37
B	NovoLog (n=573) Novolin R (n=272)	7.9 8.0	7.8 7.9	0.08 0.06	4 4	90 91	6 4	94 93	6 7
C	NovoLog (n=90) Novolin R (n=86)	8.1 7.8	7.7 7.8	0.02 0.01	4 2	93 93	4 5	97 93	4 7

[1] Events requiring intervention from a third party during the last three months of treatment
[2] Percentages are rounded to the nearest whole number

Distribution and Elimination—NovoLog has a low binding to plasma proteins, 0–9%, similar to regular human insulin. After subcutaneous administration in normal male volunteers (n=24), NovoLog was more rapidly eliminated than regular human insulin with an average apparent half-life of 81 minutes compared to 141 minutes for regular human insulin.

Pharmacodynamics

Studies in normal volunteers and patients with diabetes demonstrated that NovoLog has a more rapid onset of action than regular human insulin.

In a 6-hour study in patients with Type 1 diabetes (n=22), the maximum glucose-lowering effect of NovoLog occurred between 1 and 3 hours after subcutaneous injection (see Figure 3).

The duration of action for NovoLog is 3 to 5 hours compared to 5 to 8 hours for regular human insulin. The time course of action of insulin and insulin analogs such as NovoLog may vary considerably in different individuals or within the same individual. The parameters of NovoLog activity (time of onset, peak time and duration) as designated in Figure 3 should be considered only as general guidelines. The rate of insulin absorption and consequently the onset of activity is known to be affected by the site of injection, exercise, and other variables (see PRECAUTIONS, General). Differences in pharmacodynamics between NovoLog and regular human insulin are not associated with differences in overall glycemic control.

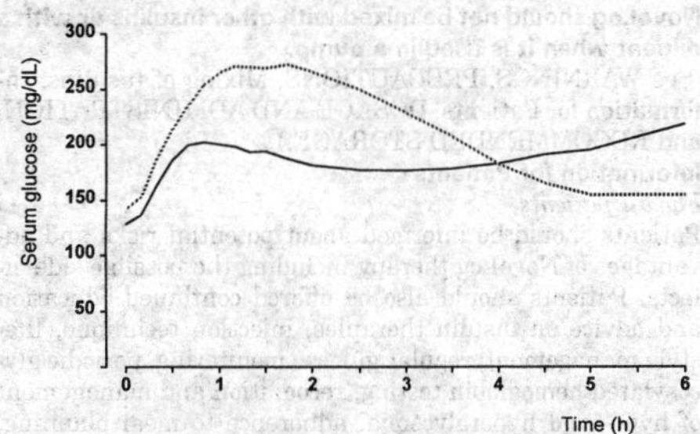

Figure 3. Serial mean serum glucose collected up to 6 hours following a single pre-meal dose of NovoLog (solid curve) or regular human insulin (hatched curve) injected immediately before a meal in 22 patients with Type 1 diabetes.

Special Populations

Children and Adolescents—The pharmacokinetic and pharmacodynamic properties of NovoLog and regular human insulin were evaluated in a single dose study in 18 children (6–12 years, n=9) and adolescents (13–17 years [Tanner grade ≥ 2], n=9) with Type 1 diabetes. The relative differences in pharmacokinetics and pharmacodynamics in children and adolescents with Type 1 diabetes between NovoLog and regular human insulin were similar to those in healthy adult subjects and adults with Type 1 diabetes.

Geriatrics—The effect of age on the pharmacokinetics and pharmacodynamics of NovoLog has not been studied.

Gender—In healthy volunteers, no difference in insulin aspart levels was seen between men and women when body weight differences were taken into account. There was no significant difference in efficacy noted (as assessed by HbA1c) between genders in a trial in patients with Type 1 diabetes.

Obesity—In a study of 23 patients with type 1 diabetes and a wide range of body mass index (BMI, 22—39 kg/m^2), the pharmacokinetic parameters, AUC and Cmax, of NovoLog were generally unaffected by BMI. Clearance of NovoLog was reduced by 28% in patients with BMI >32 compared to patients with BMI <23 when a single dose of 0.1 U/kg NovoLog was administered. However, only 3 patients with BMI <23 were studied.

Ethnic Origin—The effect of ethnic origin on the pharmacokinetics of NovoLog has not been studied.

Renal Impairment—Some studies with human insulin have shown increased circulating levels of insulin in patients with renal failure. A single subcutaneous dose of NovoLog was administered in a study of 18 patients with creatinine clearance values ranging from normal to <30 mL/min and not requiring hemodialysis. No apparent effect of creatinine clearance values on AUC and Cmax of NovoLog was found. However, only 2 patients with severe renal impairment were studied (<30 mL/min). Careful glucose monitoring and dose adjustments of insulin, including NovoLog, may be necessary in patients with renal dysfunction (see PRECAUTIONS, Renal Impairment).

Hepatic Impairment—Some studies with human insulin have shown increased circulating levels of insulin in patients with liver failure. In an open-label, single-dose study of 24 patients with Child-Pugh Scores ranging from 0 (healthy volunteers) to 12 (severe hepatic impairment), no correlation was found between the degree of hepatic failure and any NovoLog pharmacokinetic parameter. Careful glucose monitoring and dose adjustments of insulin, including NovoLog, may be necessary in patients with hepatic dysfunction (see PRECAUTIONS, Hepatic Impairment).

Pregnancy—The effect of pregnancy on the pharmacokinetics and glucodynamics of Novolog has not been studied (see PRECAUTIONS, Pregnancy).

Smoking—The effect of smoking on the pharmacokinetics/ pharmacodynamics of NovoLog has not been studied.

CLINICAL STUDIES

To evaluate the safety and efficacy of NovoLog in patients with Type 1 diabetes, two six-month, open-label, active-control (NovoLog vs. Novolin® R) studies were conducted (see Table 1). NovoLog was administered by subcutaneous injection immediately prior to meals and regular human insulin was administered by subcutaneous injection 30 minutes before meals. NPH insulin was administered as the basal insulin in either single or divided daily doses. Glycemic control (as measured by HbA1c), the rates of hypoglycemia (as determined from the number of events requiring intervention from a third party), and the incidence of ketosis were clinically comparable for the two treatment regimens. The mean total daily doses of insulin were greater (1–3 U/day) in the NovoLog-treated patients compared to patients who received regular human insulin. This difference was primarily due to basal insulin requirements. To achieve the stated levels of glycemic control, some patients required more than three doses of meal-related insulin and/or more than one dose of basal insulin (see Table 1). No serum glucose measurements were obtained in these studies. To evaluate the safety and efficacy of NovoLog in patients with Type 2 diabetes, one six-month, open-label, active-control (NovoLog vs. Novolin R) study was conducted (see Table 1). NovoLog was administered by subcutaneous injection immediately prior to meals and regular human insulin was administered by subcutaneous injection 30 minutes before meals. NPH insulin was administered as the basal insulin in either single or divided daily doses. Glycemic contraol (as measured by HbA1c) and the rates of hypoglycemia (as determined from the number of events requiring intervention from a third party) were clinically comparable for the two treatment regimens. The mean total daily dose of insulin was greater (2 U/day) in the NovoLog-treated patients compared to patients who received regular human insulin. This difference was primarily due to basal insulin requirements. To achieve the stated levels of glycemic control, some patients required more than three doses of meal-related insulin and/or more than one dose of basal insulin (see Table 1).

[See table 1 above]

To evaluate the use of NovoLog by subcutaneous infusion with an external pump, two open-label, parallel design studies (6 weeks [n=29] and 16 weeks [n=118]) compared NovoLog versus Velosulin® (buffered regular human insulin) in patients with Type 1 diabetes. Glycemic control (as measured by HbA1c) and rates of hypoglycemia were comparable. Patients with Type 2 diabetes were also studied in an open-label, parallel design trial (16 weeks [n=127]) using NovoLog by subcutaneous infusion compared to preprandial injection (in conjunction with basal NPH injections). Reductions in HbA1c and rates of hypoglycemia were comparable. (See INDICATIONS AND USAGE, WARNINGS, PRECAUTIONS, Mixing of Insulins, Information for Patients, DOSAGE AND ADMINISTRATION, and RECOMMENDED STORAGE.)

Continued on next page

NovoLog—Cont.

INDICATIONS AND USAGE

NovoLog is indicated for the treatment of adult patients with diabetes mellitus, for the control of hyperglycemia. Because NovoLog has a more rapid onset and a shorter duration of action than human regular insulin, NovoLog given by injection should normally be used in regimens with an intermediate or long-acting insulin. NovoLog may also be infused subcutaneously by external insulin pumps. (See WARNINGS, PRECAUTIONS [especially Usage in Pumps], Information for Patients [especially For Patients Using Pumps], Mixing of Insulins, DOSAGE AND ADMINISTRATION, RECOMMENDED STORAGE.)

CONTRAINDICATIONS

NovoLog is contraindicated during episodes of hypoglycemia and in patients hypersensitive to NovoLog or one of its excipients.

WARNINGS

NovoLog differs from regular human insulin by a more rapid onset and a shorter duration of activity. Because of the fast onset of action, the injection of NovoLog should immediately be followed by a meal. Because of the short duration of action of NovoLog, patients with diabetes also require a longer-acting insulin to maintain adequate glucose control. Glucose monitoring is recommended for all patients with diabetes and is particularly important for patients using external pump infusion therapy.

Hypoglycemia is the most common adverse effect of insulin therapy, including NovoLog.

As with all insulins, the timing of hypoglycemia may differ among various insulin formulations.

Any change of insulin dose should be made cautiously and only under medical supervision. Changes in insulin strength, manufacturer, type (e.g., regular, NPH, analog), species (animal, human), or method of manufacture (rDNA versus animal-source insulin) may result in the need for a change in dosage.

Insulin Pumps: When used in an external insulin pump for subcutaneous infusion, NovoLog should not be diluted or mixed with any other insulin. Physicians and patients should carefully evaluate information on pump use in the NovoLog physician and patient package inserts and in the pump manufacturer's manual (e.g. NovoLog-specific information should be followed for in-use time, frequency of changing infusion sets, or other details specific to NovoLog usage, because NovoLog-specific information may differ from general pump manual instructions). Pump or infusion set malfunctions or insulin degradation can lead to hyperglycemia and ketosis in a short time because of the small subcutaneous depot of insulin. This is especially pertinent for rapid-acting insulin analogs that are more rapidly absorbed through skin and have shorter duration of action. These differences may be particularly relevant when patients are switched from multiple injection therapy or infusion with buffered regular insulin. Prompt identification and correction of the cause of hyperglycemia or ketosis is necessary. Interim therapy with subcutaneous injection may be required. (See PRECAUTIONS, Mixing of Insulins, Information for Patients, DOSAGE AND ADMINISTRATION, and RECOMMENDED STORAGE.)

PRECAUTIONS

General

Hypoglycemia and hypokalemia are among the potential clinical adverse effects associated with the use of all insulins. Because of differences in the action of NovoLog and other insulins, care should be taken in patients in whom such potential side effects might be clinically relevant (e.g., patients who are fasting, have autonomic neuropathy, or are using potassium-lowering drugs or patients taking drugs sensitive to serum potassium level).

Lipodystrophy and hypersensitivity are among other potential clinical adverse effects associated with the use of all insulins.

As with all insulin preparations, the time course of NovoLog action may vary in different individuals or at different times in the same individual and is dependent on site of injection, blood supply, temperature, and physical activity. Adjustment of dosage of any insulin may be necessary if patients change their physical activity or their usual meal plan. Insulin requirements may be altered during illness, emotional disturbances, or other stresses.

Hypoglycemia—As with all insulin preparations, hypoglycemic reactions may be associated with the administration of NovoLog. Rapid changes in serum glucose levels may induce symptoms of hypoglycemia in persons with diabetes, regardless of the glucose value. Early warning symptoms of hypoglycemia may be different or less pronounced under certain conditions, such as long duration of diabetes, diabetic nerve disease, use of medications such as beta-blockers, or intensified diabetes control (see PRECAUTIONS, Drug Interactions). Such situations may result in severe hypoglycemia (and, possibly, loss of consciousness) prior to patients' awareness of hypoglycemia.

Renal Impairment—As with other insulins, the dose requirements for NovoLog may be reduced in patients with renal impairment (see CLINICAL PHARMACOLOGY, Pharmacokinetics).

Hepatic Impairment—As with other insulins, the dose requirements for NovoLog may be reduced in patients with hepatic impairment (see CLINICAL PHARMACOLOGY, Pharmacokinetics).

Allergy—Local Allergy—As with other insulin therapy, patients may experience redness, swelling, or itching at the site of injection. These minor reactions usually resolve in a few days to a few weeks, but in some occasions, may require discontinuation of NovoLog. In some instances, these reactions may be related to factors other than insulin, such as irritants in a skin cleansing agent or poor injection technique.

Systemic Allergy—Less common, but potentially more serious, is generalized allergy to insulin, which may cause rash (including pruritus) over the whole body, shortness of breath, wheezing, reduction in blood pressure, rapid pulse, or sweating. Severe cases of generalized allergy, including anaphylactic reaction, may be life threatening.

Localized reactions and generalized myalgias have been reported with the use of cresol as an injectable excipient.

In controlled clinical trials using injection therapy, allergic reactions were reported in 3 of 735 patients (0.4%) who received regular human insulin and 10 of 1394 patients (0.7%) who received NovoLog. During these and other trials, 3 of 2341 patients treated with NovoLog were discontinued due to allergic reactions.

Antibody Production—Increases in levels of anti-insulin antibodies that react with both human insulin and insulin aspart have been observed in patients treated with NovoLog. The number of patients treated with insulin aspart experiencing these increases is greater than the number among those treated with human regular insulin. Data from a 12-month controlled trial in patients with Type 1 diabetes suggest that the increase in these antibodies is transient. The differences in antibody levels between the human regular insulin and insulin aspart treatment groups observed at 3 and 6 months were no longer evident at 12 months. The clinical significance of these antibodies is not known. They do not appear to cause deterioration in HbAlc or to necessitate increases in insulin dose.

Pregnancy and Lactation

Female patients should be advised to tell their physician if they intend to become, or if they become pregnant. Information is not available on the use of NovoLog during pregnancy or lactation.

Usage in Pumps

NovoLog is recommended for use in Disetronic H-TRON® plus V100 with Disetronic 3.15 plastic cartridges and Classic or Tender infusion sets; MiniMed Models 505, 506, or 507 with MiniMed 3 mL syringes and Polyfin® or Sof-set® infusion sets.

In-vitro studies have shown that pump malfunction, loss of cresol, and insulin degradation, may occur with the use of NovoLog for more than two days at 37°C (98.6°F) in infusion sets and reservoirs. NovoLog in clinical use should not be exposed to temperatures greater than 37°C (98.6°F).

NovoLog should not be mixed with other insulins or with a diluent when it is used in a pump.

(See WARNINGS, PRECAUTIONS, Mixing of Insulins, Information for Patients, DOSAGE AND ADMINISTRATION, and RECOMMENDED STORAGE.)

Information for Patients

For all patients

Patients should be informed about potential risks and advantages of NovoLog therapy including the possible side effects. Patients should also be offered continued education and advice on insulin therapies, injection technique, lifestyle management, regular glucose monitoring, periodic glycosylated hemoglobin testing, recognition and management of hypo- and hyperglycemia, adherence to meal planning, complications of insulin therapy, timing of dose, instruction for use of injection or subcutaneous infusion devices, devices, and proper storage of insulin.

Patients should be informed that frequent, patient-performed blood glucose measurements are needed to achieve optimal glycemic control and avoid both hyper- and hypoglycemia. Female patients should be advised to discuss with their physician if they intend to, or if they become, pregnant because information is not available on the use of NovoLog during pregnancy or lactation (see PRECAUTIONS, Pregnancy).

For patients using pumps

Patients using external pump infusion therapy should be trained in intensive insulin therapy with multiple injections and in the function of their pump and pump accessories. NovoLog is recommended for use with Disetronic H-TRON plus V100 with Disetronic 3.15 plastic cartridges and Classic or Tender infusion sets; MiniMed Models 505, 506, and 507 with MiniMed 3 mL syringes and Polyfin or Sof-set infusion sets. The use of NovoLog in quick-release infusion sets and cartridge adapters has not been assessed.

To avoid insulin degradation, infusion set occlusion, and loss of the preservative (cresol), the infusion sets (reservoir syringe, tubing, and catheter) and the NovoLog® in the reservoir should be replaced, and a new infusion site selected every 48 hours or less. Insulin exposed to temperatures higher than 37°C (98.6°F) should be discarded. The temperature of the insulin may exceed ambient temperature when the pump housing, cover, tubing, or sport case is exposed to sunlight or radiant heat. Infusion sites that are erythematous, pruritic, or thickened should be reported to medical personnel, and a new site selected because continued infusion may increase the skin reaction and/or alter the absorption of NovoLog.

Pump or infusion set malfunctions or insulin degradation can lead to hyperglycemia and ketosis in a short time because of the small subcutaneous depot of insulin. This is especially pertinent for rapid-acting insulin analogs that are more rapidly absorbed through skin and have shorter duration of action.

These differences are particularly relevant when patients are switched from infused buffered regular insulin or multiple injection therapy. Prompt identification and correction of the cause of hyperglycemia or ketosis is necessary. Problems include pump malfunction, infusion set occlusion, leakage, disconnection or kinking, and degraded insulin. Less commonly, hypoglycemia from pump malfunction may occur. If these problems cannot be promptly corrected, patients should resume therapy with subcutaneous insulin injection and contact their physician. (See WARNINGS, PRECAUTIONS, Mixing of Insulins, DOSAGE AND ADMINISTRATION, and RECOMMENDED STORAGE.)

Laboratory Tests

As with all insulin therapy, the therapeutic response to NovoLog should be monitored by periodic blood glucose tests. Periodic measurement of glycosylated hemoglobin is recommended for the monitoring of long-term glycemic control.

Drug Interactions

A number of substances affect glucose metabolism and may require insulin dose adjustment and particularly close monitoring.

- The following are examples of substances that may increase the blood-glucose-lowering effect and susceptibility to hypoglycemia: oral antidiabetic products, ACE inhibitors, disopyramide, fibrates, fluoxetine, monoamine oxidase (MAO) inhibitors, propoxyphene, salicylates, somatostatin analog (e.g., octreotide), sulfonamide antibiotics.
- The following are examples of substances that may reduce the blood-glucose-lowering effect: corticosteroids, niacin, danazol, diuretics, sympathomimetic agents (e.g., epinephrine, salbutamol, terbutaline), isoniazid, phenothiazine derivatives, somatropin, thyroid hormones, estrogens, progestogens (e.g., in oral contaceptives).
- Beta-blockers, clonidine, lithium salts, and alcohol may either potentiate or weaken the blood-glucose-lowering effect of insulin. Pentamidine may cause hypoglycemia, which may sometimes be followed by hyperglycemia.
- In addition, under the influence of sympatholytic medicinal products such as beta-blockers, clonidine, guanethidine, and reserpine, the signs of hypoglycemia may be reduced or absent (see CLINICAL PHARMACOLOGY).

Mixing of Insulins

- A clinical study in healthy male volunteers (n=24) demonstrated that mixing NovoLog with NPH human insulin immediately before injection produced some attenuation in the peak concentration of NovoLog, but that the time to peak and the total bioavailability of NovoLog were not significantly affected. If NovoLog is mixed with NPH human insulin, NovoLog should be drawn into the syringe first. The injection should be made immediately after mixing. Because there are no data on the compatibility of NovoLog and crystalline zinc insulin preparations, NovoLog should not be mixed with these preparations.
- The effects of mixing NovoLog with insulins of animal source or insulin preparations produced by other manufacturers have not been studied (see WARNINGS).
- Mixtures should not be administered intravenously.
- When used in external subcutaneous infusion pumps for insulin, NovoLog should not be mixed with any other insulins or diluent.

Carcinogenicity, Mutagenicity, Impairment of Fertility

Standard 2-year carcinogenicity studies in animals have not been performed to evaluate the carcinogenic potential of NovoLog. In 52 week studies, Sprague-Dawley rats were dosed subcutaneously with NovoLog at 10, 50, and 200 U/kg/day (approximately 2, 8, and 32 times the human subcutaneous dose of 1.0 U/kg/day, based on U/body surface area, respectively). At a dose of 200 U/kg/day, NovoLog increased the incidence of mammary gland tumors in females when compared to untreated controls. The incidence of mammary tumors for NovoLog was not significantly different than for regular human insulin. The relevance of these findings to humans is not known. NovoLog was not genotoxic in the following tests: Ames test, mouse lymphoma cell forward gene mutation test, human peripheral blood lymphocyte chromosome aberration test, *in vivo* micronucleus test in mice, and in *ex vivo* UDS test in rat liver hepatocytes. In fertility studies in male and female rats, at subcutaneous doses up to 200 U/kg/day (approximately 32 times the human subcutaneous dose, based on U/body surface area), no direct adverse effects on male and female fertility, or general reproductive performance of animals was observed.

Pregnancy—Teratogenic Effects—Pregnancy Category C

There are no adequate well-controlled clinical studies of the use of NovoLog in pregnant women. NovoLog should be used during pregnancy only if the potential benefit justifies the potential risk to the fetus.

It is essential for patients with diabetes or history of gestational diabetes to maintain good metabolic control before conception and throughout pregnancy. Insulin requirements may decrease during the first trimester, generally increase during the second and third trimesters, and rapidly decline after delivery. Careful monitoring of glucose control is essential in such patients.

Subcutaneous reproduction and teratology studies have been performed with NovoLog and regular human insulin in rats and rabbits. In these studies, NovoLog was given to female rats before mating, during mating, and throughout pregnancy, and to rabbits during organogenesis. The effects of NovoLog did not differ from those observed with subcutaneous regular human insulin. NovoLog, like human insulin, caused pre- and post-implantation losses and visceral/skeletal abnormalities in rats at a dose of 200 U/kg/day (approximately 32 times the human subcutaneous dose of 1.0 U/kg/day, based on U/body surface area) and in rabbits at a dose of 10 U/kg/day (approximately three times the human subcutaneous dose of 1.0 U/kg/day, based on U/body surface area). The effects are probably secondary to maternal hypoglycemia at high doses. No significant effects were observed in rats at a dose of 50 U/kg/day and rabbits at a dose of 3 U/kg/day. These doses are approximately 8 times the human subcutaneous dose of 1.0 U/kg/day for rats and equal to the human subcutaneous dose of 1.0 U/kg/day for rabbits, based on U/body surface area.

Nursing Mothers

It is unknown whether insulin aspart is excreted in human milk. Many drugs, including human insulin, are excreted in human milk. For this reason, caution should be exercised when NovoLog is administered to a nursing mother.

Pediatric Use

Safety and effectiveness of NovoLog in children have not been studied.

Geriatric Use

Of the total number of patients (n=1,375) treated with NovoLog in 3 human insulin-controlled clinical studies, 2.6% (n=36) were 65 years of age or over. Half of these patients had Type 1 diabetes (18/1285) and half had Type 2 (18/90) diabetes. The HbA1c response to NovoLog, as compared to human insulin, did not differ by age, particularly in patients with Type 2 diabetes. Additional studies in larger populations of patients 65 years of age or over are needed to permit conclusions regarding the safety of NovoLog in elderly compared to younger patients. Pharmacokinetic/pharmacodynamic studies to assess the effect of age on the onset of NovoLog action have not been performed.

ADVERSE REACTIONS

Clinical trials comparing NovoLog with regular human insulin did not demonstrate a difference in frequency of adverse events between the two treatments.

Adverse events commonly associated with human insulin therapy include the following:

Body as a Whole—*Allergic reactions* (see PRECAUTIONS, Allergy).

Skin and Appendages—*Injection site reaction, lipodystrophy, pruritus, rash* (see PRECAUTIONS, Allergy, Information for Patients, Usage in Pumps).

Other—*Hypoglycemia* Hyperglycemia and Ketosis (see WARNINGS and PRECAUTIONS).

In controlled clinical trials, small, but persistent elevations in alkaline phosphatase result were observed in some patients treated with NovoLog. The clinical significance of this finding is unknown.

OVERDOSAGE

Hypoglycemia may occur as a result of an excess of insulin relative to food intake, energy expenditure, or both. Mild episodes of hypoglycemia usually can be treated with oral glucose. Adjustments in drug dosage, meal patterns, or exercise, may be needed. More severe episodes with coma, seizure, or neurologic impairment may be treated with intramuscular/subcutaneous glucagon or concentrated intravenous glucose. Sustained carbohydrate intake and observation may be necessary because hypoglycemia may recur after apparent clinical recovery.

DOSAGE AND ADMINISTRATION

NovoLog should generally be given immediately before a meal (start of meal within 5–10 minutes after injection) because of its fast onset of action. The dosage of NovoLog should be individualized and determined, based on the physician's advice, in accordance with the needs of the patient. The total daily individual insulin requirement is usually between 0.5–1.0 U/kg/day. When used in a meal-related subcutaneous injection treatment regimen, 50–70% of total insulin requirements may be provided by NovoLog and the remainder provided by an intermediate-acting or long-acting insulin. When used in external insulin infusion pumps, the initial programming of the pump is based on the total daily insulin dose of the previous regimen. Although there is significant interpatient variability, approximately 50% of the total dose is given as meal-related boluses of NovoLog and the remainder as basal infusion. Because of NovoLog's comparatively rapid onset and short duration of glucose lowering activity, some patients may require more basal insulin and more total insulin to prevent pre-meal hyperglycemia when using NovoLog than when using human regular insulin. Additional basal insulin injections, or higher basal rates in external subcutaneous infusion pumps may be necessary.

Infusion sets and the insulin in the infusion sets must be changed every 48 hours or sooner to assure the activity of NovoLog and proper pump function.

(See WARNINGS, PRECAUTIONS, Information for Patients.)

NovoLog should be administered by subcutaneous injection in the abdominal wall, the thigh, or the upper arm, or by continuous subcutaneous infusion in the abdominal wall. Injection sites and infusion sites should be rotated within the same region. As with all insulins, the duration of action will vary according to the dose, injection site, blood flow, temperature, and level of physical activity.

Parenteral drug products should be inspected visually for particulate matter and discoloration prior to administration, whenever solution and container permit. Never use any NovoLog® if it has become viscous (thickened) or cloudy; use it only if it is clear and colorless. NovoLog should not be used after the printed expiration date.

HOW SUPPLIED

NovoLog is available in the following package sizes: each presentation containing 100 Units of insulin aspart per mL (U-100).

10 mL vials	NDC 0169-7501-11
3 mL PenFill cartridges*	NDC 0169-3303-12
3 mL NovoLog FlexPen® Prefilled syringe	NDC 0169-6339-10

*NovoLog PenFill cartridges are for use with NovoFine® disposable needles and the following 3 mL PenFill cartridge compatible delivery devices: NovoPen® 3, NovoPen Junior, Innovo®, and InDuo®.

NovoLog FlexPen Prefilled syringes are for use with NovoFine disposable needles.

RECOMMENDED STORAGE

NovoLog in unopened vials, cartridges, and NovoLog FlexPen Prefilled syringes should be stored between 2° and 8°C (36° to 46°F). *Do not freeze.* **Do not use NovoLog® if it has been frozen or exposed to temperatures that exceed 37°C (98.6°F).** After a cartridges or vials has been punctured, it may be kept at temperatures below 30°C (86°F) for up to 28 days, but should not be exposed to excessive heat or sunlight. Opened vials may be refrigerated. Cartridges should not be refrigerated after insertion into the NovoPen 3. Infusion sets (resevoirs, tubing, and catheters) and the NovoLog in the resevoir should be discarded after no more than 48 hours of use or after exposed to temperatures that exceed 37°C (98.6°F).

Rx only

Date of Issue: March 19, 2004

Manufactured For
Novo Nordisk
Pharmaceuticals, Inc.
Princeton, New Jersey 08540
By Novo Nordisk A/S
2880 Bagsvaerd, Denmark
www.novonordisk-us.com

NovoLog®, Novolin®, Velosulin®, PenFill®, FlexPen®, NovoFine®, NovoPen®, and Innovo® are trademarks of Novo Nordisk A/S

H-TRON® is a trademark of Disetronic Medical Systems, Inc.

Polyfin® and Sof-set® are trademarks of Medtronic Minimed, Inc.

In Duo® is a trademark of LifeScan, Inc., a Johnson & Johnson Company.

Information For The Patient
NovoLog® (Insulin aspart [rDNA origin] Injection)
3 mL PenFill® Disposable Cartridge (300 units per cartridge)
10 mL Vial (1000 units per vial)
100 units/mL (U-100)

- What is the most important information I should know about NovoLog?
  - For all NovoLog users
  - For pump users
- What is NovoLog?
- Who should not use NovoLog?
- What should I know about using insulin?
- What should I know about using NovoLog?
- What should I avoid when using NovoLog?
- What are the possible side effects of NovoLog?
- How should I store NovoLog?
- General advice
- Injection and pump infusion instructions
  - How should I inject NovoLog?
  - Using Vials
  - Using Cartridges
  - How should I infuse NovoLog with an external subcutaneous insulin infusion pump?
  - How should I mix insulin?

Read this information carefully before you begin treatment. Read the information you get whenever you get more medicine. There may be new information. This information does not take the place of talking with your doctor about your medical condition or your treatment. If you have any questions about NovoLog (NO-voe-log), ask your doctor. Only your doctor can determine if NovoLog is right for you.

What is the most important information I should know about NovoLog?

For all NovoLog Users

- NovoLog (NO-voe-log) is different from regular human insulin and buffered regular human insulin (Velosulin). It works faster (rapid onset of action) and will not work as long (shorter duration of action) as regular human insulin or buffered regular human insulin (Velosulin).
- Because the onset of action is fast, you should eat a meal 5–10 minutes after a NovoLog injection or NovoLog bolus infusion dose given by an external pump. (A bolus is a large dose.) Eating right after the dose will reduce the risk of low blood sugar (hypoglycemia).
- The shorter duration of NovoLog's action means that you may need to use an intermediate or longer-acting insulin (basal insulin) or higher basal rates of NovoLog insulin infusion in the pump. This will give the best glucose control and will help you avoid hyperglycemia (high blood sugar) and ketoacidosis (too much acid [low pH] in your body).
- Glucose monitoring is recommended for all patients who use insulin.

If you use NovoLog by injection, you may need to increase some or all of the following:

- your total dose of insulin
- your dose of intermediate or long-acting insulin (for example, NPH)
- the number of injections of basal insulin

If you infuse NovoLog into the skin (subcutaneous tissue) by pump, you may need to increase some or all of the following:

- your total insulin dose
- the basal infusion dose
- the proportion of total insulin given as a basal infusion

Age and exposure to heat affect the stability of NovoLog and its preservative. Also, NovoLog does not work well after it has been frozen. Therefore, do not use old insulin or insulin that has been exposed to temperature extremes. Hyperglycemia may be a sign that the insulin is no longer working and needs to be replaced.

Do not mix NovoLog:

- with any other insulins when used in a pump
- with Lantus® (insulin glargine [rDNA origin] injection) when used with injections by syringe
  (You may, however, mix NovoLog with NPH when used with injections by syringe.
  See: How should I mix insulins?)

For Pumps Users

- Glucose monitoring is very important for patients using external pumps subcutaneous infusion therapy. You should be aware that pump or infusion set malfunctions that result in inadequate insulin infusion can quickly lead to hyperglycemia and ketosis. Accordingly, problems with the infusion pump, the flow of insulin, or the quality of the insulin should be identified and corrected as quickly as possible. There is only a small amount of insulin infused into the skin with a pump. The faster absorption through the skin of rapid-acting insulin analogs and shorter duration of action may give you less time to identify and correct the problem than with buffered regular insulin.
- Therefore, you should dose with insulin from a new vial of NovoLog if unexplained hyperglycemia or pump alarms do not respond to all of the following:
  - a repeat dose (injection or bolus) of NovoLog
  - a change in the infusion set, including the NovoLog in the reservoir
  - a change in the infusion site

  If these measures do not work, you may need to resume skin (subcutaneous) injections with syringes or insulin pens. Continue to monitor your glucose and ketones. If problems continue, you must contact your doctor.
- When NovoLog is used in an external subcutaneous insulin infusion pump, you should use only recommended pumps and infusion sets (insulin reservoirs, tubing, catheters). The infusion set, reservoir insulin, and infusion site should be changed:
  - at intervals of 48 hours or less
  - with unexpected hyperglycemia or ketosis
  - when alarms sound, as specified by your MiniMed or Disetronic pump manual
  - if the insulin or pump has been exposed to temperatures over 98.6°F (37°C), as it might be in a sauna with long showers, or on a hot day
  - if the insulin or pump could have absorbed radiant heat, for example from sunlight, that would heat the insulin to over 98.6°F (37°C). Dark colored pump cases or sport covers can increase this type of heat. The location where the pump is worn may also affect the temperature

Patients who develop "pump bumps" (skin reactions at the infusion site) may need to change infusion sites more often.

For your safety, read the section "What are the possible side effects of NovoLog?" to review the symptoms of low blood sugar (hypoglycemia) and high blood sugar (hyperglycemia).

What is NovoLog?

NovoLog is a clear, colorless, sterile solution for injection or infusion under the skin (subcutaneously). NovoLog is a human-made form of insulin to lower your blood sugar faster than human regular insulin. Because the insulin is human-made by recombinant DNA technology (rDNA) and is chemically different from the insulin made by the human body, it is called an insulin analog. The active ingredient in NovoLog is insulin aspart. The concentration of insulin aspart is 100 units per milliliter, or U100. NovoLog also contains: glycerin, phenol, metacresol, zinc, disodium hydrogen phosphate dihydrate, and sodium chloride. Hydrochloric acid and/or sodium hydroxide may be added to adjust the pH. These ingredients help to preserve or stabilize NovoLog insulin. The pH (balance between acid and alkaline conditions) is important to the stability of NovoLog. Increases in temperature can affect the stability of NovoLog, so it may not work well.

Who should not use NovoLog?

Do not use NovoLog if:

- your blood sugar (glucose) is too low (hypoglycemia)
- you do not plan to eat right after your injection or infusion
- you are allergic to insulin aspart or any of the ingredients contained in NovoLog (check with your doctor if you are not sure)

The effects of NovoLog on an unborn child or on a nursing baby are unknown. Therefore, tell your doctor if you plan to become pregnant or breast feed, or if you become pregnant. You may need to use another medicine.

Continued on next page

NovoLog—Cont.

Tell your doctor about all medicines and supplements that you are using. Some medicines, including non-prescription medicines and dietary supplements, may affect your diabetes.

What should I know about using insulin?

- Make any change of insulin cautiously and only under medical supervision. Changes in the strength, manufacturer, type (for example: Regular, NPH, Lente®), species (beef, pork, beef-pork, human) or method of manufacture (recombinant [rDNA] or animal source insulin) may cause a need for a change in the timing or dose of the new insulin.
- Glucose monitoring will help you and your health care provider adjust dosages.
- Always carry a quick source of sugar, such as candy or glucose tablets, to treat low blood sugars (hypoglycemia).
- Always carry identification that states that you have diabetes.

What should I know about using NovoLog?

See the end of this Patient Information for instructions for using NovoLog in injections and pumps.

- NovoLog starts working 10–20 minutes after injection or infusion. The greatest blood sugar lowering effect is between 1 and 3 hours after injection or infusion. This blood sugar lowering lasts for 3 to 5 hours. (The time periods are only general guidelines)
- Because the onset of action is rapid, you should eat a meal within 5–10 minutes after a NovoLog injection or a NovoLog bolus dose from an external pump to avoid low blood sugar (hypoglycemia).
- The shorter duration of NovoLog's action means that you may need to use an intermediate or longer-acting insulin (basal insulin) or higher basal rates of NovoLog insulin infusion in the pump. This will help you avoid hyperglycemia and ketoacidosis.
- Do not inject or infuse in skin that has become reddened or bumpy or thickened after infusion or injection. Insulin absorption in these areas may not be the same as that in normal skin, and may change the onset and duration of insulin action.
- Use NovoLog only if it appears clear and colorless. Do not use NovoLog if it appears cloudy, thickened, or colored, or if it contains solid particles.

What should I avoid while using NovoLog?

- Drinking alcohol may lead to hypoglycemia.
- Do not miss meals after injections of NovoLog or bolus infusions of NovoLog.

What are the possible side effects of NovoLog?

Insulins can cause hypoglycemia (low blood sugar), hyperglycemia (high blood sugar), allergy, and skin reactions.

Hypoglycemia (insulin reaction). This is the most common side effect. It occurs when there is a conflict between the amount of carbohydrates (source of glucose) from your food, the amount of glucose used by your body, and the amount and timing of insulin dosing. Therefore, **hypoglycemia can occur with:**

- **The wrong insulin dose.** This can happen with any of the following:
  - too much insulin is injected
  - the bolus dose of insulin infusion is set too high
  - the basal infusion dose is set too high
  - the pump does not work right, delivering too much insulin
- **Medicines that directly lower glucose or increase sensitivity to insulin.** This can happen with oral (taken by mouth) antidiabetes drugs, sulfa antibiotics (for infections), ACE inhibitors (for blood pressure and heart failure), salicylates, including aspirin and NSAIDS (for pain), some antidepressants, and with other medicines.
- **Medical conditions that limit the body's glucose reserve, lengthen the time insulin stays in the body, or that increase sensitivity to insulin.** These conditions include diseases of the adrenal glands, the pituitary, the thyroid gland, the liver, and the kidney.
- **Not enough carbohydrate (sugar or starch) intake.** This can happen if:
  - a meal or snack is missed or delayed
  - you have vomiting or diarrhea that decreases the amount of glucose absorbed by your body
  - alcohol interferes with carbohydrate metabolism
- **Too much glucose use by the body.** This can happen from:
  - too much exercise
  - higher than normal metabolism rates due to fever or an overactive thyroid

Hypoglycemia can be mild or severe. Its onset may be rapid. Patients with very good (tight) glucose control, patients with diabetic neuropathy (nerve problems), or patients using some Beta-blockers (used for high blood pressure and heart conditions) may have few warning symptoms before severe hypoglycemia develops. Hypoglycemia may reduce your ability to drive a car or use mechanical equipment without risk of injury to yourself or others. Severe hypoglycemia can cause temporary or permanent harm to your heart or brain. **It may cause unconsciousness, seizures, or death.** Symptoms of hypoglycemia include:

- anxiety, irritability, restlessness, trouble concentrating, personality changes, mood changes, or other abnormal behavior
- tingling in your hands, feet, lips, or tongue
- dizziness, light-headedness, or drowsiness
- nightmares or trouble sleeping
- headache
- blurred vision or slurred speech
- palpitations (rapid heart beat)
- sweating
- tremor (shaking) or unsteady gait (walking)

Mild to moderate hypoglycemia can be treated by eating or drinking carbohydrates (milk, orange juice, sugar candies, or glucose tablets). More severe or continuing hypoglycemia may require the help of another person or emergency medical personnel. Patients who are unable to take sugar by mouth or who are unconscious may need treatment with a glucagon injection or glucose given intravenously (in the vein).

Talk with your doctor about severe, continuing, or frequent hypoglycemia, and hypoglycemia for which you had few warning symptoms.

Hyperglycemia (high blood sugar) is another common side effect. It also occurs when there is a conflict between the amount of carbohydrates (source of glucose) from your food, the amount of glucose used by your body, and the amount and timing of insulin dosing. Therefore, **hyperglycemia can occur with:**

- **The wrong insulin dose.** This can happen from any of the following:
  - too little or no insulin is injected
  - the bolus dose of insulin infusion is set too low
  - the basal infusion dose is set too low
  - the pump or catheter system does not work right, delivering too little insulin
  - the insulin's ability to lower glucose is changed by incorrect storage (freezing, excessive heat), or usage after the expiration date
- **Medicines that directly increase glucose or decrease sensitivity to insulin.** This can happen, for example, with thiazide water pills (used for blood pressure), corticosteroids, birth control pills, and protease inhibitors (used for AIDS).
- **Medical conditions that increase the body's production of glucose or decrease sensitivity to insulin.** These medical conditions include fevers, infections, heart attacks, and stress.
- **Too much carbohydrate intake.** This can happen if you
  - eat larger meals
  - eat more often
  - increase the proportion of carbohydrate in your meals

Hyperglycemia can be mild or severe. It can **progress to diabetic acidosis (DKA) (ketoacidosis) or very high glucose levels (hyperosmolar coma) and result in unconsciousness and death.** Although diabetic acidosis occurs most often in patients with Type 1 diabetes, it can occur in patients with Type 2 diabetes who become severely ill. Urine or blood tests will show acetone, ketones, and high level of glucose.

Hyperosmolar coma occurs most often in patients with Type 2 diabetes. Urine and blood tests will show very high levels of glucose.

Glucose monitoring is very important for patients using external pump infusion therapy. You should be aware that pump or infusion set malfunctions that result in inadequate insulin infusion can quickly lead to hyperglycemia and ketosis. Accordingly, problems with the infusion pump, the flow of insulin, or the quality of the insulin should be identified and corrected as quickly as possible. The faster absorption of rapid-acting insulin analogs through the skin and shorter duration of action may give you less time to identify and correct the problem.

Because some patients experience few symptoms of hyperglycemia and ketosis, it is important to monitor your glucose several times a day. Symptoms of hyperglycemia include:

- confusion or drowsiness
- fruity smelling breath
- rapid, deep breathing
- increased thirst
- decreased appetite, nausea, or vomiting
- abdominal (stomach area) pain
- rapid heart rate
- increased urination and dehydration (too little fluid in your body)

Mild hyperglycemia can be treated by extra doses of insulin and drinking fluids (rehydration). Patients using pumps should check pump function and replace the insulin in the reservoir-syringe, as well as change the tubing and catheter and the infusion site. **Patients using pumps may need to resume insulin injections with syringes or injection pens.** Glucose and acetone-ketone levels should be monitored more often until they return to normal. **More severe or continuing hyperglycemia requires prompt evaluation and treatment by your health care provider.**

Allergy can be serious. Generalized allergy is an uncommon, but possibly life-threatening, reaction to insulin products. Symptoms include:

- itchy rash over the entire body
- shortness of breath or wheezing
- confusion
- low blood pressure
- rapid heart beat
- sweating

If you think you are having a generalized allergic reaction, get emergency medical help right away.

Allergic reactions at the injection site (itching, redness, hardness, or swelling) are more common than generalized allergy. They may need several days or weeks to clear up. Pump patients with site reactions may need to change their infusion sites more often than every 48 hours. Patients should avoid injection or infusion of insulin into skin areas that have reactions. Tell your doctor about such reactions, because they can become more severe, or they change the absorption of insulin.

Lipodystrophy is a common change in the fat below the injection site. These changes include loss of fat (depressions in the skin called lipoatrophy) or thickening of the tissue under the skin (lipohypertrophy). Pump patients with lipodystrophy may need to change their infusion sites more often than every 48 hours. Patients should avoid injection or infusion of insulin into skin areas that have these reactions. Tell your doctor about such reactions because they can become more severe, or they may change the absorption of insulin.

How should I store NovoLog?

- **NovoLog can be damaged by high temperatures.** Therefore, be sure to protect it from high air temperatures, heat from the sun, saunas, long showers, and other heat sources. This is especially important if you use a pump or an insulin pen, because you carry these devices with you and they may be exposed to different temperatures as you go about your daily activities. **Throw NovoLog away if it has been in temperatures greater than 98.6°F (37°C).**
- **Unopened NovoLog** should be stored in a refrigerator but not in the freezer and protected from light. Even if it has been refrigerated and protected from sunlight and unopened, it should not be used after the expiration date on the label and the carton. Unopened vials and cartridges can be stored unrefrigerated at temperatures below 86°F (30°C) and protected from light for up to 28 days.
- **Punctured vials and cartridges** can be stored unrefrigerated at temperatures below 86°F (30°C) and protected from light for up to 28 days. Punctured vials may be stored in the refrigerator. Cartridges inserted into their NovoPen® 3 device should not be stored in the refrigerator.
- **The NovoLog in the pump reservoir and the complete infusion set** (reservoir, tubing, catheter-needle) should be replaced **at least every 48 hours.** Replacement should be more often than every 48 hours if you have hyperglycemia, the pump alarm sounds, or the insulin flow is blocked (occlusion).
- Never use NovoLog if it has been stored improperly.

General advice

This leaflet summarizes the most important information about NovoLog. If you would like more information, talk with your doctor. You can ask your pharmacist or doctor for information about NovoLog that is written for health professionals.

Injection and pump infusion instructions

- NovoLog comes in 10 mL (milliliter) vials or in 3 mL cartridges. NovoLog can be withdrawn from vials with syringes for injection or for insertion into the reservoirs of external subcutaneous infusion pumps (Disetronic H-TRON® plus V100 or MiniMed Models 505, 506, or 507).
- Doses of insulin are measured in units. NovoLog is available as a U-100 insulin. One milliliter (mL) of U-100 contains 100 units of insulin aspart (1 mL=1 cc). Only U-100 type syringes should be used for injection to ensure proper dosing.
- Disposable syringes and needles are sterile if the package is sealed. They should be used only once and throw away properly, to protect others from harm.
- NovoLog PenFill® cartridges are for use with NovoFine® disposable needles and the following 3 mL PenFill® compatible delivery devices: NovoPen® 3, NovoPen® Junior, Innovo® and InDuo™. Never share needles.

How should I inject NovoLog?

Using Vials

1. The vial and the insulin should be inspected. The insulin should be clear and colorless. The tamper-resistant cap should be in place to be removed by you. If the cap had been removed before your first use of the vial, or if the insulin is cloudy or colored, you should return the vial to the pharmacy. Do not use it.
2. Both the injection site and your hands should be cleaned with soap and water or with alcohol. The injection site should be dry before you inject.
3. The rubber stopper should be wiped with an alcohol wipe.
4. The plunger of the syringe should be pulled back until the black tip is at the level for the number of units to be injected.
5. Insert the neeedle of the syringe through the rubber stopper of the vial. Push in the syringe plunger completely to put air into the vial.
6. Turn the vial upside-down with the needle-syringe still attached, and pull the plunger back a few units past the correct dose.
7. Remove any air bubbles by flicking the syringe and squirting air bubbles out the needle. Continue pushing the plunger until you have the correct dose.
8. Lift the vial off the syringe.
9. Inject NovoLog into the subcutaneous (under the skin) tissue (not into muscle or blood vessels) in the abdomen, thighs, upper arms, or buttocks. Pinch the skin fold between your fingers and push the needle straight into the pinched skin. Because insulin absorption and activity can be affected by the site you choose, you should discuss the injection site with your doctor.

10. Release the pinched skin and push the plunger in completely. Keep the needle in the skin for a few seconds before withdrawing the syringe.
11. Press the injection site for a few seconds to reduce bleeding. Do not rub.
12. To avoid needle sticks, throw away the syringe and needle without recapping. Discuss sterile technique and proper disposal of your used insulin supplies with your doctor.

Using Cartridges

1. The cartridge and the insulin should be inspected. The insulin should be clear and colorless. The tamper-resistant foil should be in place to be removed by you. If the foil had been punctured or removed before your first use of the cartridge or if the insulin is cloudy or colored, you should return the cartridge to the pharmacy. Do not use it.
2. Both the injection site and your hands should be cleaned with soap and water or with alcohol. The injection site should be dry before you inject. Do not use skin that is reddened, itchy, or thickened as an infusion site.
3. Insert a 3 mL cartridge in the pen-device barrel. Attach a new needle to the end of the cartridge and turn the pen device upside-down so that any air bubbles can be eliminated by flicking the pen device and squirting air bubbles out the needle. (This should eliminate extra air for all future doses from that cartridge. However, the needle will need to be changed for each dose.)
4. Set the dose to be delivered by twisting the top of the pen-device until the correct number appears in the window.
5. Inject NovoLog into the subcutaneous (under the skin) tissue (not into muscle or blood vessels) in the abdomen, thighs, upper arms, or buttocks. Pinch the skin fold between your fingers and push the needle straight into the pinched skin. Because insulin absorption and activity can be affected by the site you choose, you should discuss the injections site with your doctor.
6. Release the pinched skin. Inject the dose by pressing the flat plunger button on the top of the pen-device. Keep the needle in the skin for a few seconds before withdrawing the pen-device.
7. Press the injection site for a few seconds to reduce bleeding. Do not rub.
8. Throw away the disposable needle without recapping to avoid needle sticks. Discuss sterile technique and proper disposal of your used insulin supplies with your doctor.

How should I infuse NovoLog with an external subcutaneous insulin infusion pump?

NovLog is recommended for use with the Disetronic H-Tron plus V100 and MiniMed 505, 506, and 507 pumps. The Disetronic 3.15 plastic cartridge and Tenders or Classic tubing can be used with the Disetronic pump. The MiniMed 3 mL syringe and Polyfin® or Sof-set® tubing can be used in the MiniMed pumps. The use of NovoLog in quick-release infusion sets and cartridge adapters has not been assessed.

1. Inspect your insulin as you would for an injection. The insulin should be clear and colorless and without particles. The tamper-resistant cap should be in place to be removed by you. If the cap had been removed before your first use of the vial or if the insulin is cloudy or colored, you should return the vial to the pharmacy. Do not use it.
2. Both the infusion site and your hands should be cleaned with soap and water or with alcohol. The infusion site should be dry before you insert the catheter-needle and tubing. Do not use skin that is reddened, itchy, bumpy or thickened as an infusion site because the onset and duration of NovoLog action may not be the same as that in normal skin.
3. Fill the reservoir-syringe with 2 days worth of NovoLog plus about 25 extra units to prime the pump and fill up the dead space of the infusion tubing.
4. Remove air bubbles from the reservoir according to the pump manufacturers' instructions.
5. Attach the infusion set to the reservoir. Make sure the connection is tight. Prime the infusion set until you see a drop of insulin coming out of the infusion needle-catheter. Flick the tubing to remove air bubbles. Follow the pump manufacturers' instructions for additional priming.
6. Prime the needle-catheter and insert the infusion set into the skin according to the pump manufacturer.
7. Program the pump for mealtime NovoLog boluses and NovoLog basal insulin infusion according to instructions from your doctor and the manufacturer of your pump equipment.
8. Change the infusion site, the insulin reservoir, the tubing, the catheter-needle, and the insulin every 48 hours or less, even if you have not used all of the insulin. This will help ensure that NovoLog and the pump works well. (See "What is the most important information I should know about NovoLog?")
9. Change the infusion site, the insulin reservoir, the tubing, the catheter-needle, and the insulin if you experience a pump alarm, catheter blockage, hyperglycemia, or if your pump insulin has been exposed to heat greater than 98.6°F (37°C). (See "What is the most important information I should know about NovoLog?") Hyperglycemia identified with glucose monitoring may be the first indication of a problem with the pump, infusion set, or NovoLog. Hyperglycemia in the absence of an alarm still requires you to investigate because pump alarms are designed to detect back-pressure and occlusion. The alarms may not detect all the changes to NovoLog that could result in hyperglycemia. You may need to resume subcutaneous insulin injections if the cause of the problem cannot be promptly identified or fixed. (See "Hyperglycemia" under "What are the possible side effects of NovoLog?") Remember that long stretches of tubing increase the risk of kinking and expose the insulin in the tubing to more variations in temperature.

These instructions give you specific information for use of NovoLog in external subcutaneous infusion pumps, but are not a substitute for pump education.

How should I mix insulins?

NovoLog should be mixed only when syringe injections are used. NovoLog can be mixed with NPH human insulin immediately before use. The NovoLog should be drawn into the syringe before the NPH. Mixing with other insulins has not been studied. **NovoLog should not be mixed with Lantus® (insulin glargine [rDNA origin] injection). Mixed insulins should NEVER be used in a pump or for intravenous infusion.**

1. Add together the doses of NPH and NovoLog. The total dose will determine the final volume in the syringe after drawing up both insulins into the syringe.
2. Roll the NPH vial between your hands until the liquid is equally cloudy throughout.
3. Draw into the syringe the same amount of air as the NPH dose. Inject this air into the NPH vial and then remove the needle without withdrawing or touching any of the NPH insulin. (Transferring NPH to the NovoLog vial will contaminate the NovoLog vial and may change how quickly it works.)
4. Draw into the syringe the same amount of air as the NovoLog dose. Inject this air into the NovoLog vial. With the needle in place, turn the vial upside-down and withdraw the correct dose of NovoLog. The tip of the needle must be in the NovoLog to get the full dose and not an air dose.
5. Insert the needle into the NPH vial. Turn the NPH vial upside down with the syringe-needle still in it. Withdraw the correct dose of NPH.
6. Inject immediately to reduce changes in how quickly the insulin works.

Helpful information for people with diabetes is published by the American Diabetes Association, 1660 Duke Street, Alexandria, VA 22314

For information contact:
Novo Nordisk Pharmaceuticals Inc.,
100 College Road West
Princeton, New Jersey 08540
1-800-727-6500
www.novonordisk-us.com

Manufactured by
Novo Nordisk A/S
2880 Bagsvaerd, Denmark

License under U.S. Patent No. 5,618,913 and Des. 347,894

NovoLog®, PenFill®, NovoPen®, Innovo®, NovoFine®, and Lente® are trademarks of Novo Nordisk A/S.
Lantus® is a trademark of Aventis Pharmaceuticals Inc.
Polyfin® and Sofset® are trademarks of Medtronic MiniMed, Inc.
H-TRON® is a trademark of Disetronic Medical Systems, Inc.
InDuo™ is trademark of LifeScan, Inc., a Johnson & Johnson company.

Date of Issue: May 15, 2002

Shown in Product Identification Guide, page 326

NOVOLOG® MIX 70/30 ℞

[nō'vō-lŏg]

70% insulin aspart protamine suspension and 30% insulin aspart injection, (rDNA origin)

DESCRIPTION

NovoLog Mix 70/30 (70% insulin aspart protamine suspension and 30% insulin aspart injection, [rDNA origin]) is a human insulin analog suspension containing 70% insulin aspart protamine crystals and 30% soluble insulin aspart. NovoLog Mix 70/30 is a blood glucose-lowering agent with a rapid onset and an intermediate duration of action. Insulin aspart is homologous with regular human insulin with the exception of a single substitution of the amino acid proline by aspartic acid in position B28, and is produced by recombinant DNA technology utilizing *Saccharomyces cerevisiae* (baker's yeast) as the production organism. Insulin aspart (NovoLog®) has the empirical formula $C_{256}H_{381}N_{65}O_{79}S_6$ and a molecular weight of 5825.8 Da.

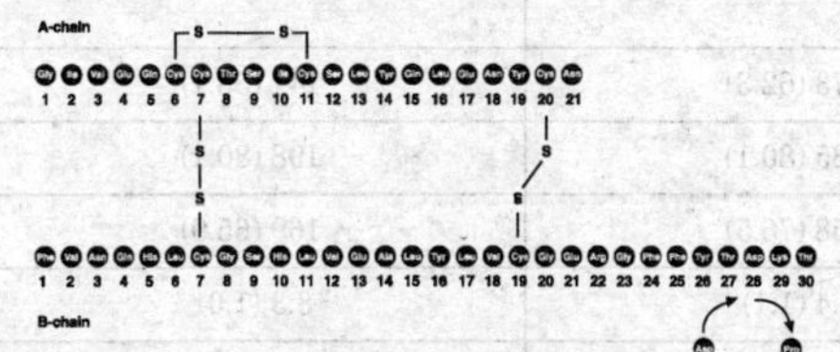

Figure 1. Structural formula of insulin aspart

NovoLog Mix 70/30 is a uniform, white, sterile suspension that contains insulin aspart (B28 asp regular human insulin analog) 100 Units/mL, mannitol 36.4 mg/mL, phenol 1.50 mg/mL, metacresol 1.72 mg/mL, zinc 19.6 μg/mL, disodium hydrogen phosphate dihydrate 1.25 mg/mL, sodium chloride 0.58 mg/mL, and protamine sulfate 0.33 mg/mL. NovoLog Mix 70/30 has a pH of 7.20-7.44. Hydrochloric acid or sodium hydroxide may be added to adjust pH.

CLINICAL PHARMACOLOGY

Mechanism of action

The primary activity of NovoLog Mix 70/30 is the regulation of glucose metabolism. Insulins, including NovoLog Mix 70/30, exert their specific action through binding to insulin receptors. Insulin binding activates mechanisms to lower blood glucose by facilitating cellular uptake of glucose into skeletal muscle and fat, simultaneously inhibiting the output of glucose from the liver.

In standard biological assays in mice and rabbits, one unit of NovoLog has the same glucose-lowering effect as one unit of regular human insulin. However, the effect of NovoLog Mix 70/30 is more rapid in onset compared to Novolin® (human insulin) 70/30 due to its faster absorption after subcutaneous injection.

Pharmacokinetics

Bioavailability and Absorption-

The single substitution of the amino acid proline with aspartic acid at position B28 in insulin aspart (NovoLog) reduces the molecule's tendency to form hexamers as observed with regular human insulin. The rapid absorption characteristics of NovoLog are maintained by NovoLog Mix 70/30. The insulin aspart in the soluble component of NovoLog Mix 70/30 is absorbed more rapidly from the subcutaneous layer than regular human insulin. The remaining 70% is in crystalline form as insulin aspart protamine which has a prolonged absorption profile after subcutaneous injection.

The relative bioavailability of NovoLog Mix 70/30 compared to NovoLog and Novolin 70/30 indicates that they are absorbed to similar degrees. In euglycemic clamp studies in healthy volunteers (n=23) after dosing with 0.2 U/kg of NovoLog Mix 70/30, a mean maximum serum concentration (C_{max}) of 23.4 ± 5.3 mU/L was reached after 60 minutes. The mean half-life (t1/2) of NovoLog Mix 70/30 was about 8 to 9 hours. Serum insulin levels returned to baseline 15 to 18 hours after a subcutaneous dose. Similar data were seen in a separate euglycemic clamp study in healthy volunteers (n=24) after dosing with 0.3 U/kg of NovoLog Mix 70/30. A C_{max} of 61.3 ± 20.1 mU/L was reached after 85 minutes. Serum insulin levels returned to baseline 12 hours after a subcutaneous dose.

The C_{max} and the area under the insulin concentration-time curve (AUC) after administration of NovoLog Mix 70/30 differed by approximately 20% from those after administration of NovoLog Mix 50/50 (investigational drug, not marketed.) and Novolin 70/30 (see Fig. 2 and 3 for pharmacokinetic profiles).

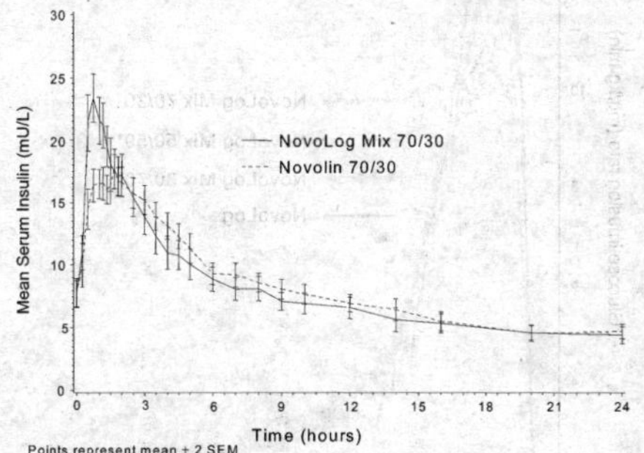

Figure 2. Pharmacokinetic Profiles of NovoLog Mix 70/30 and Novolin® 70/30

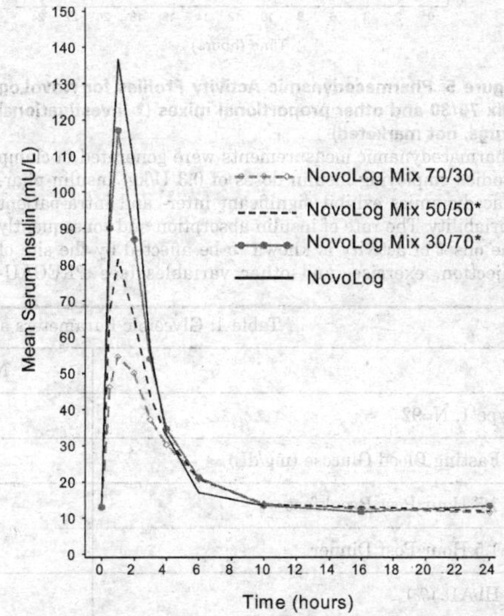

Figure 3. Pharmacokinetic profiles for Novolog Mix 70/30 and other proportional mixes (*investigational drugs, not marketed).

Pharmacokinetic measurements were generated in clamp studies employing insulin doses of 0.3 U/kg. Insulin kinetics exhibit significant inter- and intra-patient variability. The rate of insulin absorption and consequently the onset of ac-

Continued on next page

NovoLog Mix 70/30—Cont.

tivity is known to be affected by the site of injection, exercise, and other variables (see PRECAUTIONS, General). Differences in pharmacokinetics between NovoLog Mix 70/30 and products to which it has been compared are not associated with differences in overall glycemic control.
Distribution and Elimination— NovoLog has a low binding to plasma proteins, 0 to 9%, similar to regular human insulin. After subcutaneous administration in normal male volunteers (n=24), NovoLog was more rapidly eliminated than regular human insulin with an average apparent half-life of 81 minutes compared to 141 minutes for regular human insulin.

Pharmacodynamics

The two euglycemic clamp studies described above assessed glucose utilization after dosing of healthy volunteers. NovoLog Mix 70/30 has a more rapid onset of action than regular human insulin in studies of normal volunteers and patients with diabetes. The peak pharmacodynamic effect of NovoLog Mix 70/30 occurs between 1 and 4 hours after injection. The duration of action may be as long as 24 hours (see Figures 4 and 5).

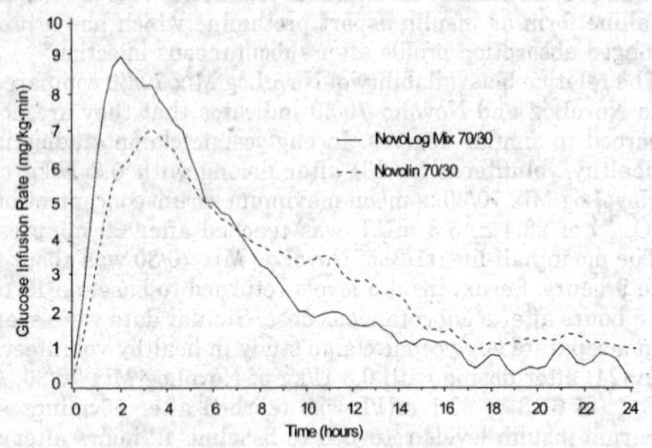

Figure 4. Pharmacodynamic Activity Profile of NovoLog Mix 70/30 and Novolin 70/30 in healthy subjects

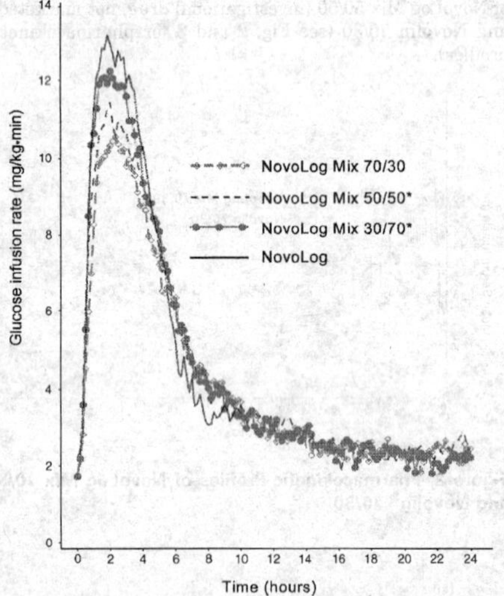

Figure 5. Pharmacodynamic Activity Profiles for NovoLog Mix 70/30 and other proportional mixes (* investigational drugs, not marketed)

Pharmacodynamic measurements were generated in clamp studies employing insulin doses of 0.3 U/kg. Insulin pharmacodynamics exhibit significant inter- and intra-patient variability. The rate of insulin absorption and consequently the onset of activity is known to be affected by the site of injection, exercise, and other variables (see PRECAUTIONS, General). Differences in pharmacodynamics between NovoLog Mix 70/30 and products to which it has been compared are not associated with differences in overall glycemic control.

Special populations

Children and adolescents—The pharmacokinetic and pharmacodynamic properties of NovoLog Mix 70/30 have not been assessed in children and adolescents less than 18 years of age.
Geriatrics—The effect of age on the pharmacokinetics and pharmacodynamics of NovoLog Mix 70/30 has not been studied.
Gender—The effect of gender on the pharmacokinetics and pharmacodynamics of NovoLog Mix 70/30 has not been studied.
Obesity—The effect of obesity and/or subcutaneous fat thickness on the pharmacokinetics and pharmacodynamics of NovoLog Mix 70/30 has not been studied but data on the rapid acting component (NovoLog) show no significant effect.
Ethnic origin—The effect of ethnic origin on the pharmacokinetics and pharmacodynamics of NovoLog Mix 70/30 has not been studied.
Renal impairment—The effect of renal function on the pharmacokinetics and pharmacodynamics of NovoLog Mix 70/30 has not been studied but data on the rapid acting component (NovoLog) show no significant effect. Some studies with human insulin have shown increased circulating levels of insulin in patients with renal failure. Careful glucose monitoring and dose adjustments of insulin, including NovoLog Mix 70/30, may be necessary in patients with renal dysfunction (see PRECAUTIONS, Renal Impairment).
Hepatic impairment—The effect of hepatic impairment on the pharmacokinetics and pharmacodynamics of NovoLog Mix 70/30 has not been studied but data on the rapid-acting component (NovoLog) show no significant effect. Some studies with human insulin have shown increased circulating levels of insulin in patients with liver failure. Careful glucose monitoring and dose adjustments of insulin, including NovoLog Mix 70/30, may be necessary in patients with hepatic dysfunction (see PRECAUTIONS, Hepatic Impairment).
Pregnancy—The effect of pregnancy on the pharmacokinetics and pharmacodynamics of NovoLog Mix 70/30 has not been studied (see PRECAUTIONS, Pregnancy).
Smoking—The effect of smoking on the pharmacokinetics and pharmacodynamics of NovoLog Mix 70/30 has not been studied.

CLINICAL STUDIES

In a three-month, open-label trial, patients with Type 1 (n=146) or Type 2 (n=178) diabetes were treated BID (before breakfast and before supper) with NovoLog Mix 70/30 or Novolin 70/30. The small changes in HbA1c were comparable across the treatment groups (see Table 1).
[See table 1 below]
The significance, with respect to the long-term clinical sequelae of diabetes, of the differences in postprandial hyperglycemia between treatment groups has not been established.
Specific anti-insulin antibodies as well as cross-reacting anti-insulin antibodies were monitored in the 3-month, open-label comparator trial as well as in a long-term extension trial (see PRECAUTIONS, Allergy).

INDICATIONS AND USAGE

NovoLog Mix 70/30 is indicated for the treatment of patients with diabetes mellitus for the control of hyperglycemia.

CONTRAINDICATIONS

NovoLog Mix 70/30 is contraindicated during episodes of hypoglycemia and in patients hypersensitive to NovoLog Mix 70/30 or one of its excipients.

WARNINGS

Because NovoLog Mix 70/30 has peak pharmacodynamic activity one hour after injection, it should be administered with meals.
NovoLog Mix 70/30 should not be administered intravenously.
NovoLog Mix 70/30 is not to be used in insulin infusion pumps.
NovoLog Mix 70/30 should not be mixed with any other insulin product.
Hypoglycemia is the most common adverse effect of insulin therapy, including NovoLog Mix 70/30. As with all insulins, the timing of hypoglycemia may differ among various insulin formulations.
Glucose monitoring is recommended for all patients with diabetes.
Any change of insulin dose should be made cautiously and only under medical supervision. Changes in insulin strength, manufacturer, type (e.g., regular, NPH, analog), species (animal, human), or method of manufacture (rDNA versus animal-source insulin) may result in the need for a change in dosage.

PRECAUTIONS

General

Hypoglycemia and hypokalemia are among the potential clinical adverse effects associated with the use of all insulins. Because of differences in the action of NovoLog Mix 70/30 and other insulins, care should be taken in patients in whom such potential side effects might be clinically relevant (e.g., patients who are fasting, have autonomic neuropathy, or are using potassium-lowering drugs or patients taking drugs sensitive to serum potassium level).
Fixed ratio insulins are typically dosed on a twice daily basis, i.e., before breakfast and supper, with each dose intended to cover two meals or a meal and snack (see DOSAGE AND ADMINISTRATION). Because there is diurnal variation in insulin resistance and endogenous insulin secretion, variability in the time and content of meals, and variability in the time and extent of exercise, fixed ratio insulin mixtures may not provide optimal glycemic control for all patients. The dose of insulin required to provide adequate glycemic control for one of the meals may result in hyper- or hypoglycemia for the other meal. The pharmacodynamic profile may also be inadequate for patients (e.g. pregnant women) who require more frequent meals.
Adjustments in insulin dose or insulin type may be needed during illness, emotional stress, and other physiologic stress in addition to changes in meals and exercise.
The pharmacokinetic and pharmacodynamic profiles of all insulins may be altered by the site used for injection and the degree of vascularization of the site. Smoking, temperature, and exercise contribute to variations in blood flow and insulin absorption. These and other factors contribute to inter- and intra-patient variability.
Lipodystrophy and hypersensitivity are among other potential clinical adverse effects associated with the use of all insulins.
Hypoglycemia—As with all insulin preparations, hypoglycemic reactions may be associated with the administration of NovoLog Mix 70/30. Rapid changes in serum glucose concentrations may induce symptoms of hypoglycemia in persons with diabetes, regardless of the glucose value. Early warning symptoms of hypoglycemia may be different or less pronounced under certain conditions, such as long duration of diabetes, diabetic nerve disease, use of medications such as beta-blockers, or intensified diabetes control.
Renal Impairment—Clinical or pharmacology studies with NovoLog Mix 70/30 in diabetic patients with various degrees of renal impairment have not been conducted. As with other insulins, the requirements for NovoLog Mix 70/30 may be reduced in patients with renal impairment.
Hepatic Impairment—Clinical or pharmacology studies with NovoLog Mix 70/30 in diabetic patients with various degrees of hepatic impairment have not been conducted. As with other insulins, the requirements for NovoLog Mix 70/30 may be reduced in patients with hepatic impairment.
Allergy—
Local Reactions—Erythema, swelling, and pruritus at the injection site have been observed with NovoLog Mix 70/30 as with other insulin therapy. Reactions may be related to the insulin molecule, other components in the insulin preparation including protamine and cresol, components in skin cleansing agents, or injection techniques.
Systemic Reactions—Less common, but potentially more serious, is generalized allergy to insulin, which may cause rash (including pruritus) over the whole body, shortness of breath, wheezing, reduction in blood pressure, rapid pulse, or sweating. Severe cases of generalized allergy, including anaphylactic reaction, may be life threatening. Localized reactions and generalized myalgias have been reported with the use of cresol as an injectable excipient.
Antibody production—Specific anti-insulin antibodies as well as cross-reacting anti-insulin antibodies were monitored in the 3-month, open-label comparator trial as well as in a long-term extension trial. Changes in cross-reactive antibodies were more common after NovoLog Mix 70/30 than with Novolin 70/30 but these changes did not correlate with change in HbA1c or increase in insulin dose. The clinical significance of these antibodies has not been established. Antibodies did not increase further after long-term exposure (>6 months) to NovoLog Mix 70/30.
Information for patients—
Patients should be informed about potential risks and advantages of NovoLog Mix 70/30 therapy including the possible side effects. Patients should also be offered continued education and advice on insulin therapies, injection technique, life-style management, regular glucose monitoring, periodic glycosylated hemoglobin testing, recognition and management of hypo- and hyperglycemia, adherence to

Table 1: Glycemic Parameters at the End of Treatment [Mean (SD)]

	NovoLog Mix 70/30	Novolin 70/30
Type 1, N=92		
Fasting Blood Glucose (mg/dL)	173 (62.3)	141 (58.7)
1.5 Hour Post Breakfast	185 (80.1)	198 (80.1)
1.5 Hour Post Dinner	158 (76.5)	169 (65.9)
HbA1c (%)	8.4 (1.1)	8.3 (1.0)
Type 2, N=169		
Fasting Blood Glucose (mg/dL)	151 (39.2)	151 (67.6)
1.5 Hour Post Breakfast	180 (64.1)	198 (80.1)
1.5 Hour Post Dinner	166 (49.8)	189 (49.8)
HbA1c (%)	7.9 (1.0)	8.1 (1.1)

meal planning, complications of insulin therapy, timing of dose, instruction for use of injection devices, and proper storage of insulin.
Female patients should be advised to discuss with their physician if they intend to, or if they become, pregnant because information is not available on the use of NovoLog Mix 70/30 during pregnancy or lactation (see PRECAUTIONS, Pregnancy).
Laboratory Tests—The therapeutic response to NovoLog Mix 70/30 should be assessed by measurement of serum or blood glucose and glycosylated hemoglobin.
Drug Interactions A number of substances affect glucose metabolism and may require insulin dose adjustment and particularly close monitoring. The following are examples of substances that may increase the blood-glucose-lowering effect and susceptibility to hypoglycemia: oral antidiabetic products, ACE inhibitors, disopyramide, fibrates, fluoxetine, monoamine oxidase (MAO) inhibitors, propoxyphene, salicylates, somatostatin analog (e.g. octreotide), sulfonamide antibiotics.
The following are examples of substances that may reduce the blood-glucose-lowering effect: corticosteroids, niacin, danazol, diuretics, sympathomimetic agents (e.g., epinephrine, salbutamol, terbutaline), isoniazid, phenothiazine derivatives, somatropin, thyroid hormones, estrogens, progestogens (e.g., in oral contraceptives).
Beta-blockers, clonidine, lithium salts, and alcohol may either potentiate or weaken the blood-glucose- lowering effect of insulin.
Pentamidine may cause hypoglycemia, which may sometimes be followed by hyperglycemia.
In addition, under the influence of sympatholytic medical products such as beta-blockers, clonidine, guanethidine, and reserpine, the signs of hypoglycemia may be reduced or absent (see CLINICAL PHARMACOLOGY).

Mixing of insulins
NovoLog Mix 70/30 should not be mixed with any other insulin product.

Carcinogenicity, Mutagenicity, Impairment of Fertility
Standard 2-year carcinogenicity studies in animals have not been performed to evaluate the carcinogenic potential of NovoLog Mix 70/30. In 52-week studies, Sprague-Dawley rats were dosed subcutaneously with NovoLog, the rapid-acting component of NovoLog Mix 70/30, at 10, 50, and 200 U/kg/day (approximately 2, 8, and 32 times the human subcutaneous dose of 1.0 U/kg/day, based on U/body surface area, respectively). At a dose of 200 U/kg/day, NovoLog increased the incidence of mammary gland tumors in females when compared to untreated controls. The incidence of mammary tumors for NovoLog was not significantly different than for regular human insulin. The relevance of these findings to humans is not known. NovoLog was not genotoxic in the following tests: Ames test, mouse lymphoma cell forward gene mutation test, human peripheral blood lymphocyte chromosome aberration test, in vivo micronucleus test in mice, and in ex vivo UDS test in rat liver hepatocytes. In fertility studies in male and female rats, NovoLog at subcutaneous doses up to 200 U/kg/day (approximately 32 times the human subcutaneous dose, based on U/body surface area) had no direct adverse effects on male and female fertility, or on general reproductive performance of animals.

Pregnancy—Teratogenic Effects—Pregnancy Category C
Animal reproduction studies have not been conducted with NovoLog Mix 70/30. However, reproductive toxicology and teratology studies have been performed with NovoLog (the rapid-acting component of NovoLog Mix 70/30) and regular human insulin in rats and rabbits. In these studies, NovoLog was given to female rats before mating, during mating, and throughout pregnancy, and to rabbits during organogenesis. The effects of NovoLog did not differ from those observed with subcutaneous regular human insulin. NovoLog, like human insulin, caused pre- and post-implantation losses and visceral/skeletal abnormalities in rats at a dose of 200 U/kg/day (approximately 32-times the human subcutaneous dose of 1.0 U/kg/day, based on U/body surface area), and in rabbits at a dose of 10 U/kg/day (approximately three times the human subcutaneous dose of 1.0 U/kg/day, based on U/body surface area). The effects are probably secondary to maternal hypoglycemia at high doses. No significant effects were observed in rats at a dose of 50 U/kg/day and rabbits at a dose of 3 U/kg/day.
These doses are approximately 8 times the human subcutaneous dose of 1.0 U/kg/day for rats and equal to the human subcutaneous dose of 1.0 U/kg/day for rabbits based on U/body surface area.
It is not known whether NovoLog Mix 70/30 can cause fetal harm when administered to a pregnant woman or can affect reproductive capacity. There are no adequate and well-controlled studies of the use of NovoLog Mix 70/30 or NovoLogâ in pregnant women. NovoLog Mix 70/30 should be used during pregnancy only if the potential benefit justifies the potential risk to the fetus.
Nursing mothers—It is unknown whether NovoLog Mix 70/30 is excreted in human milk as is human insulin. There are no adequate and well-controlled studies of the use of NovoLog Mix 70/30 or NovoLog in lactating women.
Pediatric Use—Safety and effectiveness of NovoLog Mix 70/30 in children have not been established.
Geriatric Use—Clinical studies of NovoLog Mix 70/30 did not include sufficient numbers of patients aged 65 and over to determine whether they respond differently than younger patients. In general, dose selection for an elderly patient should be cautious, usually starting at the low end of the dosing range reflecting the greater frequency of decreased hepatic, renal, or cardiac function, and of concomitant disease or other drug therapy in this population.

Table 2. Summary of pharmacodynamic properties of insulin products (pooled cross-study comparison) and recommended interval between dosing and meal initiation

Insulin Products	*Dose (U/kg) Used in Study*	*Recommended interval between dosing an meal initiation (minutes)**	*Time of Peak Activity (hours after dosing) (mean±SD)*	Percent of Total Activity Occurring in the First 4 hours *(mean, range)*
NovoLog	0.3	10–20	2.2±0.98	65%±11%
Novolin R	0.2	30	3.3	60%±16%
Novolin 50/50	0.5	30	4.0±0.6	54%±12%
NovoLog Mix 70/30	0.3	10–20	2.4±0.80	45%±22%
Novolin 70/30	0.3	30	4.2±0.39	25%±5%
Novolin N	0.3	n/a	8.0±5.3	21%±11%

*Applicable only to Novolin R and NovoLog alone or as components of insulin mixes.

ADVERSE REACTIONS
Clinical trials comparing NovoLog Mix 70/30 with Novolin 70/30 did not demonstrate a difference in frequency of adverse events between the two treatments.
Adverse events commonly associated with human insulin therapy include the following:
Body as whole: *Allergic reactions* (see PRECAUTIONS, Allergy).
Skin and Appendages: *Local injection site reactions or rash or pruritus, as with other insulin therapies, occurred in 7% of all patients on NovoLog Mix 70/30 and 5% on Novolin 70/30. Rash led to withdrawal of therapy in <1% of patients on either drug* (see PRECAUTIONS, Allergy).
Hypoglycemia: see WARNINGS and PRECAUTIONS.
Other: Small elevations in alkaline phosphatase were observed in patients treated in NovoLog controlled clinical trials. There have been no clinical consequences of these laboratory findings.

OVERDOSAGE
Hypoglycemia may occur as a result of an excess of insulin relative to food intake, energy expenditure, or both. Mild episodes of hypoglycemia usually can be treated with oral glucose. Adjustments in drug dosage, meal patterns, or exercise, may be needed. More severe episodes with coma, seizure, or neurologic impairment may be treated with intramuscular/subcutaneous glucagon or concentrated intravenous glucose. Sustained carbohydrate intake and observation may be necessary because hypoglycemia may recur after apparent clinical recovery.

DOSAGE AND ADMINISTRATION
General
Fixed ratio insulins are typically dosed on a twice daily basis, i.e. before breakfast and supper, with each dose intended to cover two meals or a meal and snack. NovoLog Mix 70/30 is intended only for subcutaneous injection (into the abdominal wall, thigh, or upper arm). NovoLog Mix 70/30 should not be administered intravenously. The absorption rate of NovoLog Mix 70/30 from the subcutaneous tissue allows dosing within 15 minutes of meal initiation.
Dose regimens of NovoLog Mix 70/30 will vary among patients and should be determined by the health care professional familiar with the patient's metabolic needs, eating habits, and other lifestyle variables. As with all insulins, the duration of action may vary according to the dose, injection site, blood flow, temperature, and level of physical activity and conditioning.
[See table 2 above]

Administration using PenFill® Cartridges for 3 mL PenFill cartridge compatible delivery devices, NovoLog Mix 70/30 FlexPen Prefilled syringes, or vials:
PenFill Cartridges for 3 mL PenFill cartridge compatible delivery devices*: NovoLog Mix 70/30 PenFill suspension should be visually inspected and resuspended immediately before use. The resuspended NovoLog Mix 70/30 must appear uniformly white and cloudy. Before inserting the cartridge into the insulin delivery system, roll the cartridge between your palms 10 times. Thereafter, turn the cartridge upside down so that the glass ball moves from one end of the cartridge to the other. Do this at least 10 times. The rolling and turning procedure must be repeated until the suspension appears uniformly white and cloudy. Inject immediately. Before each subsequent injection, turn the 3 mL PenFill cartridge compatible delivery devices* upside down so that the glass ball moves from one end of the cartridge to the other. Repeat this 10 times until the suspension appears uniformly white and cloudy. Inject immediately. **After use, needles on the insulin pen delivery devices should not be recapped. Used syringes, needles, or lancets should be placed in sharps containers (such as red biohazard containers), hard plastic containers (such as detergent bottles), or metal containers (such as an empty coffee can). Such containers should be sealed and disposed of properly.**

* NovoLog Mix 70/30 PenFill cartridges are for use with the following 3 mL PenFill cartridge compatible delivery devices: NovoPen® 3, Innovo®, and InDuo®.

Disposable NovoLog Mix 70/30 FlexPen® Prefilled Syringes:
NovoLog Mix 70/30 suspension should be visually inspected and resuspended immediately before use. The resuspended NovoLog Mix 70/30 must appear uniformly white and cloudy. Before use, roll the disposable NovoLog Mix 70/30 FlexPen prefilled syringe between your palms 10 times. Thereafter, turn the disposable NovoLog Mix 70/30 FlexPen prefilled syringe upside down so that the glass ball moves from one end of the reservoir to the other. Do this at least 10 times. The rolling and turning procedure must be repeated until the suspension appears uniformly white and cloudy. Inject immediately. Before each subsequent injection, turn the disposable NovoLog Mix 70/30 FlexPen Prefilled syringe upside down so that the glass ball moves from one end of the reservoir to the other at least 10 times and until the suspension appears uniformly white and cloudy. Inject immediately. **After use, needles on the disposable NovoLog Mix 70/30 FlexPen prefilled syringes should not be recapped. Used syringes, needles, or lancets should be placed in sharps containers (such as red biohazard containers), hard plastic containers (such as detergent bottles), or metal containers (such as an empty coffee can). Such containers should be sealed and disposed of properly.**
Vial: NovoLog Mix 70/30 vial must be resuspended immediately before use. Roll the vial gently 10 times in your hand to mix it. The resuspended NovoLog Mix 70/30 must appear uniformly white and cloudy.

HOW SUPPLIED
NovoLog Mix 70/30 is available in the following package sizes: each presentation contains 100 Units of insulin aspart per mL (U-100).

10 mL vials	NDC 0169-3685-12
3 mL PenFill cartridges*	NDC 0169-3682-13
3 mL NovoLog Mix 70/30 FlexPen Prefilled Syringe	NDC 0169-3696-19

*NovoLog Mix 70/30 PenFill cartridges are for use with the following 3 mL PenFill cartridge compatible delivery devices: NovoPen 3, Innovo, and InDuo.

RECOMMENDED STORAGE
NovoLog Mix 70/30 should be stored between 2°C and 8°C (36° F to 46°F). *Do not freeze.* **Do not use NovoLog Mix 70/30 if it has been frozen.**
Vials:
The vials should be stored in a refrigerator, not in a freezer. If refrigeration is not possible, the bottle in use can be kept unrefrigerated at room temperature below 30° C (86°F) for up to 28 days, as long as it is kept as cool as possible and away from direct heat and light.
Unpunctured vials can be used until the expiration date printed on the label if they are stored in a refrigerator. Keep unused vials in the carton so they will stay clean and protected from light.
PenFill cartridges or NovoLog Mix 70/30 FlexPen Prefilled syringes:
Once a cartridge or a NovoLog Mix 70/30 FlexPen prefilled syringe is punctured, it may be used for up to 14 days if it is kept at room temperature below 30°C (86°F). Cartridges or NovoLog Mix 70/30 FlexPen prefilled syringes in use must NOT be stored in the refrigerator. Keep all PenFill cartridges and disposable NovoLog Mix 70/30 FlexPen Prefilled syringes away from direct heat and sunlight. Unpunctured PenFill cartridges and NovoLog Mix 70/30 FlexPen Prefilled syringes can be used until the expiration date printed on the label if they are stored in a refrigerator. Keep unused PenFill cartridges and NovoLog Mix 70/30 FlexPen Prefilled syringes in the carton so they will stay clean and protected from light.
Rx Only.
Date of issue: November 18, 2002
Novo Nordisk®, NovoLog®, FlexPen®, Innovo®, Novolin®, NovoPen®, PenFill® and NovoFine® are trademarks owned by Novo Nordisk® A/S. In Duo® is a trademark of LifeScan, Inc., a Johnson and Johnson company.

License under U.S. Patent No. 5,618,913 and Des. 347,894.
Manufactured by:
Novo Nordisk A/S
2880 Bagsvaerd, Denmark

Continued on next page

NovoLog Mix 70/30—Cont.

Manufactured for:
Novo Nordisk Pharmaceuticals, Inc.
Princeton, NJ 08540
www.novonordisk-us.com

Patient Information for 10 mL vials and 3 mL PenFill cartridges (100 Units/mL, U-100)

NovoLog® Mix 70/30
70% insulin aspart protamine
suspension and 30% insulin aspart
injection, (rDNA origin)

What is the most important information I should know about NovoLog Mix 70/30?

WARNINGS

THIS NOVO NORDISK® HUMAN INSULIN ANALOG MIXTURE IS DIFFERENT FROM OTHER INSULIN MIXTURES BECAUSE IT HAS A RAPID ONSET OF ACTION. THE RAPID ONSET OF ACTION MEANS THAT YOU SHOULD TAKE YOUR DOSE OF NOVOLOG MIX 70/30 (70% INSULIN ASPART [rDNA ORIGIN] PROTAMINE SUSPENSION AND 30% INSULIN ASPART [rDNA ORIGIN] INJECTION) WITHIN 15 MINUTES OF A MEAL.
ANY CHANGE OF INSULIN SHOULD BE MADE CAUTIOUSLY AND ONLY UNDER MEDICAL SUPERVISION. CHANGES IN STRENGTH, MANUFACTURER, TYPE (E.G., REGULAR, NPH, ANALOG), SPECIES (BEEF, PORK, BEEF-PORK, HUMAN), OR METHOD OF MANUFACTURE (rDNA VERSUS ANIMAL-SOURCE INSULIN) MAY RESULT IN THE NEED FOR A CHANGE IN THE TIMING OR DOSAGE OF NOVOLOG MIX 70/30.
PATIENTS TAKING NOVOLOG MIX 70/30 MAY REQUIRE A CHANGE IN DOSAGE FROM THAT USED WITH OTHER INSULINS. IF AN ADJUSTMENT IS NEEDED, IT MAY OCCUR WITH THE FIRST DOSE OR DURING THE FIRST SEVERAL WEEKS OR MONTHS.

What is NovoLog Mix 70/30?

NovoLog Mix 70/30 (NO-voe-log-MIX-SEV-en-tee-THIR-tee) is a mixed insulin analog similar to human insulin mixes used to treat diabetes. The active ingredient in NovoLog Mix 70/30 is insulin aspart, which is made through biotechnology. Another ingredient, protamine, is used to slow the absorption of the insulin analog by your body.

NovoLog Mix 70/30 comes in:

- 10 mL vials (small bottles) for use with a syringe
- 3 mL PenFill® cartridges for use with 3 mL PenFill cartridge compatible delivery devices*
- 3 mL Novolog Mix 70/30 FlexPen Prefilled syringe

*3 mL PenFill cartridge compatible delivery devices: NovoPen® 3, Innovo®, and InDuo®.

Who should not take NovoLog Mix 70/30?

Do not take NovoLog Mix 70/30 if:

- Your blood sugar is too low (hypoglycemia).
- You are allergic to NovoLog Mix 70/30 or any of its ingredients. Check with your doctor or pharmacist if you want information about the ingredients
- You are not planning to eat within 15 minutes of your injection

Tell your doctor if:

- **You have liver or kidney problems.** Your dose may need to be changed.
- **You are pregnant or planning to become pregnant.** It is not known whether NovoLog Mix 70/30 can cause any harm to the baby if it is taken during pregnancy.
- **You are breast-feeding or planning to breast-feed.** It is not known whether NovoLog Mix 70/30 is passed through in human milk as is human insulin. Many drugs, including human insulin, are present in human milk, and may affect the baby.
- **You take any other medicines,** including prescription and non-prescription medicines and herbal supplements. Your NovoLog Mix 70/30 needs may change if you take other medicines. Be sure to mention if you take the following:
- oral hypoglycemic medicines (medicines you take by mouth to treat non insulin-dependent [Type 2] diabetes)
- monoamine oxidase (MAO) inhibitors (used to treat depression)
- beta-blocking agents (used to treat certain heart conditions or high blood pressure)
- angiotensin converting enzyme (ACE) inhibitors (used to treat certain heart conditions or high blood pressure)
- salicylates, including aspirin (used to relieve pain or lower fever)
- anabolic steroids and glucocorticoids
- oral contraceptives (used for birth control)
- diuretics such as thiazides (used to treat high blood pressure or swelling [edema])
- thyroid hormones (used to treat thyroid gland problems)
- danazol (used to treat endometriosis)
- octeotide (used to treat gigantism or other rare endocrine tumors)
- sulfa antibiotics (used to treat infections)

How should I take NovoLog Mix 70/30?

- Follow your doctor's instructions about monitoring your blood sugar.
- Before injecting, make sure that you have the correct type and strength of insulin. Carefully follow the instructions on how to use your insulin syringe or pen
- Inject your NovoLog Mix 70/30 fifteen-minutes or less before a meal.
- Inject NovoLog Mix 70/30 under your skin (subcutaneously). Never inject it into a vein.
- The effect of an injected insulin dose may occur faster if the insulin is injected into your abdomen (stomach area). However, you may also inject under the skin or your thigh, or upper arm.
- Change (rotate) injection sites within the same body area.
- Measure your blood sugar level as directed by your doctor.
- Carefully follow the instructions given by your doctor about the type of insulin you are using, its dose, and time of its injection. Any change in insulin should be made cautiously and only with your doctor's guidance. Your insulin needs may change due to a number of factors, such as illness, stress, medicines, or changes in diet or exercise routines. Follow your doctor's instructions to make these changes in your dose regimen.
- Clean your hands and the injection site with soap and water or with alcohol before you start the injection process.

See the end of this patient information for instructions about preparing and giving the injection.

What should I do during illness?

Even if you have a short term (acute) illness, especially with vomiting or fever, continue taking your insulin. If possible, stay on your regular diet. If you have trouble eating, drink fruit juices, regular soft drinks, or clear soups. If you can, eat small amounts of bland foods. Test your urine for glucose and ketones and, if possible, test your blood glucose. Note the results and contact your health care provider for possible insulin dose adjustment. If you have severe and continued vomiting, get emergency medical care.

What should I avoid while taking NovoLog Mix 70/30?

Alcohol, including beer and wine, may increase and lengthen the risk of hypoglycemia (too low blood sugar) when you take NovoLog Mix 70/30. Be careful when you drive a car or operate machinery. Your ability to concentrate or react may be reduced if you have hypoglycemia. Ask your doctor if you should drive if you have:

- frequent hypoglycemia
- reduced or absent warning signs of hypoglycemia

What are the possible side effects of NovoLog Mix 70/30?

Common side effects include blood sugar that is too low (hypoglycemia).

Hypglycemia (too little glucose in the blood) is one of the most frequent problems experienced by insulin users. It can be brought about by:

1. Missing or delaying meals.
2. Taking too much insulin
3. Exercising or working more than usual
4. An infection or illness (especially with diarrhea or vomiting)
5. A change in the body's need for insulin
6. Diseases of the adrenal, pituitary, or thyroid gland, or kidney or liver disease that is getting worse
7. Interactions with other drugs that lower blood glucose, such as oral (taken by mouth) antidiabetic medicines, salicylates (for example, aspirin), sulfa antibiotics, and certain antidepressants
8. Drinking of alcohol

What are symptoms of **mild to moderate** hypoglycemia:

- Sweating
- Dizziness
- Palpitation (fast heart beat)
- Tremor (shakiness)
- Hunger
- Restlessness
- Tingling in the hands, feet, lips, or tongue
- Lightheadedness
- Trouble concentrating
- Headache
- Drowsiness
- Sleep problems
- Anxiety
- Blurred vision
- Slurred speech
- Depressed mood
- Irritability
- Abnormal behavior
- Unsteady movement
- Personality change

What are symptoms of **severe** hypoglycemia:

- Disorientation
- Unconsciousness
- Seizures (convulsions)
- Death

If you develop serious hypoglycemic reactions, get medical help right away.

Without recognition of early warning symptoms, you may not be able to take steps to avoid more serious hypoglycemia. Be alert for all of the various types of symptoms that may indicate hypoglycemia. Patients who experience hypoglycemia without early warning symptoms should monitor their blood glucose frequently, especially prior to activities such as driving. If the blood glucose is below your normal fasting glucose, you should consider eating or drinking sugar-containing foods to treat your hypoglycemia. Mild to moderate hypoglycemia may be treated by eating foods or drinks that contain sugar. Patients should always carry a quick source of sugar, such as candy mints or glucose tablets. More severe hypoglycemia may require the assistance of another person. Patients who are unable to take sugar orally or who are unconscious require an injection of glucagon or should be treated with intravenous administration of glucose at a medical facility. You should learn to recognize your own symptoms of hypoglycemia. If you are uncertain about these symptoms, you should monitor your blood glucose frequently to help you learn to recognize the symptoms that you experience with hypoglycemia. If you have frequent episodes of hypoglycemia or experience difficulty in recognizing the symptoms, you should consult your doctor to discuss possible changes in therapy, meal plans, and/or exercise programs to help you avoid hypoglycemia.

Common side effects include blood sugar that is too high (hyperglycemia) and diabetic ketoacidosis.

Hyperglycemia (too much glucose in the blood) may develop if your body has too little insulin. Hyperglycemia can be brought about by any of the following:

1. Not taking your insulin or taking less than the doctor has prescribed
2. Eating much more than your meal plan suggests
3. Developing a fever, infection, or being under stress

In patients with type 1 or insulin-dependent diabetes, long-lasting hyperglycemia can cause diabetic ketoacidosis (DKA). The first symptoms of DKA usually come on slowly, over a period of hours or days, and include feeling drowsy, flushed face, thirst, loss of appetite, and fruity odor on the breath. With DKA, urine tests show large amounts of glucose and ketones. Heavy breathing and a rapid pulse are more severe symptoms. If uncorrected, long-lasting hyperglycemia or DKA can lead to nausea, vomiting, stomach pains, dehydration, loss of consciousness, or even death. Therefore, it is important that you obtain medical help right away.

Other possible side effects include the following:

- **Serious allergic reaction.**
  Get medical help right away if you develop a rash over your whole body, have trouble breathing, a fast heartbeat, or sweating. These are signs of a dangerous allergic reaction (systemic allergic reaction). These reactions are not common.
- **Reaction at the injection site** (local allergic reaction). You may get redness, swelling and itching at the injection site. If you have serious or continuing reactions, you may need to stop using NovoLog Mix 70/30 and use another insulin. Do not inject insulin into skin sites with these reactions. No type of insulin should be injected into skin sites with these reactions.
- **Skin thickens or pits at the injection site,** especially if the injection site is not rotated (changed).
- **Vision changes** that may require evaluation by an ophthalmologist (medical doctors specializing in eye disease) or changes in your eyeglasses or contact lens prescription.
- **Fluid retention or swelling of your hands and feet.**
- **Low potassium in your blood** (hypokalemia)

There are other possible side effects from NovoLog Mix 70/30. Ask your doctor or pharmacist for further information. Tell your doctor or pharmacist if you have any other unwanted effects that you believe are caused by this insulin.

How should I store NovoLog Mix 70/30?

- **Unused insulin:**
  Store insulin in a refrigerator (36°F to 46°F; 2°C to 8°C), but not in the freezer. Do not use NovoLog Mix 70/30 if it has been frozen. Keep unused PenFill® cartridges and vials in the carton so they will stay clean and protected from light.
- **After starting to use the insulin:**
  Do not refrigerate disposable PenFill cartridges in use (the rubber stopper has been punctured). However, keep them as cool as possible (below 30°C [86°F]). The vials should be stored in a refrigerator, not in a freezer. If refrigeration is not possible, the bottle that you are currently using can be kept unrefrigerated at room temperature (below 30°C [86°F]) up to 28 days, as long as it is kept as cool as possible. Keep all disposable PenFill cartridges away from direct heat and sunlight.
- **Throw away unrefrigerated disposable NovoLog Mix 70/30 PenFill cartridges after 14 days, even if they still contain insulin. Throw away unrefrigerated vials after 28 days, even if they still contain insulin.**

General information about NovoLog Mix 70/30

Use NovoLog Mix 70/30 only to treat your diabetes.

Do not give it to any other person. Ask your doctor or pharmacist about any concerns you have. They can answer your questions and give you written information about NovoLog Mix 70/30 written for health care professionals.

How should I prepare and deliver the injection using different delivery devices?

Using the 10 mL vial:

1. At your first use, remove the tamper-resistant cap of the vial. If the cap has already been removed, do not use this vial and return it to your pharmacy.
2. Wipe the rubber stopper with an alcohol swab.
3. Roll the vial gently 10 times in your hands to mix it. Do not shake it vigorously.
   Vigorous shaking right before the dose is drawn into the syringe may cause bubbles or froth, which could cause dosage errors.
   The insulin should be used only if it uniformly appears white and cloudy.
4. Pull back the plunger until the black tip reaches the marking for the number of units you will inject.
5. Push the needle through the rubber stopper into the vial.
6. Push the plunger all the way in. This inserts air into the vial.
7. Turn the vial and syringe upside down together and slowly pull the plunger back to a few units beyond the correct dose.
8. If there are air bubbles in the syringe, tap the syringe gently with your finger to raise the air bubbles to the needle. Then slowly push the plunger to the correct unit marking.

9. Lift the vial off the syringe.
10. Inject right away. If there is a delay after you rolled the vial, you will have to roll it again to remix the insulin. (See injection instructions "How should I inject NovoLog Mix 70/30 with a syringe?")
11. After the injection, remove the needle **without recapping** and dispose of it in a puncture-resistant container. Used syringes, needles, or lancets should be placed in sharps containers (such as red biohazard containers), hard plastic containers (such as detergent bottles), or metal containers (such as an empty coffee can). Such containers should be sealed and disposed of properly.

Using the NovoLog Mix 70/30 3 mL PenFill cartridge in 3 mL PenFill cartridge compatible delivery devices* (*see 3 mL PenFill cartridge compatible delivery devices section):

1. Read the instruction manuals for the 3 mL PenFill cartridge compatible delivery devices* before the device is used.
2. For PenFill cartridge:
   Before inserting the PenFill cartridge in the 3 mL PenFill cartridge compatible delivery devices* for the first time, roll the cartridge between your palms 10 times. Then turn the PenFill cartridge up and down between positions **a** and **b** (see Diagram 1) so the glass ball moves from one end of the cartridge to the other. Do this at least 10 times. The procedure must be repeated until the insulin appears uniformly white and cloudy. Insert the PenFill cartridge into the 3 mL PenFill cartridge compatible delivery devices* and inject right away.
   Diagram #1

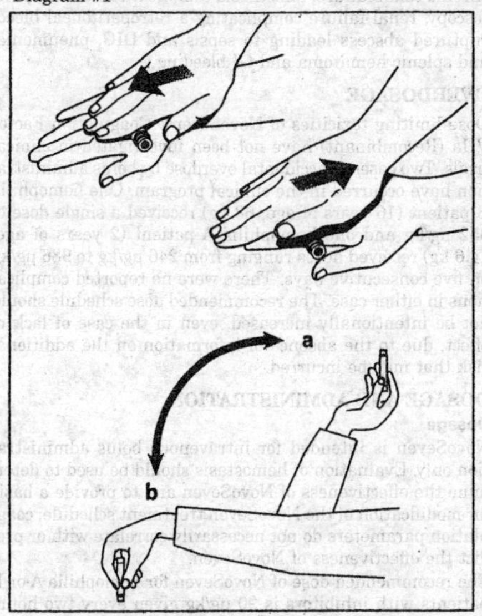

3. Place the needle onto the 3 mL PenFill cartridge compatible delivery devices* immediately before use.
4. Airshots/priming should be done prior to each injection. Directions for performing an airshot or priming are provided in your insulin delivery device instruction manual.
5. Inject the insulin right away. If there is a delay after you mix the insulin and the injection, you will have to mix the insulin again before injecting the insulin. (See "How should I inject NovoLog Mix 70/30 with 3 mL PenFill cartridge compatible devices*?" below.)
6. After the injection, remove the needle **without recapping** and dispose of it in a puncture-resistant container. Used syringes, needles, or lancets should be placed in sharps containers (such as red biohazard containers), hard plastic containers (such as detergent bottles), or metal containers (such as an empty coffee can). Such containers should be sealed and disposed of properly.

After the first use of PenFill® cartridge:

1. If the PenFill cartridge is already in the 3 mL PenFill cartridge compatible delivery devices*, it should be turned upside down between positions **a** and **b** (see Diagram 1), so that the glass ball moves from one end of the PenFill cartridge to the other. Do this until the insulin appears uniformly white and cloudy.
2. Airshots/priming should be done prior to each injection. Directions for performing an airshot or priming are provided in your insulin delivery device instruction manual.
3. Inject right away. If there is a delay between mixing of the insulin and the injection, the insulin will need to be mixed again. (See "How should I inject NovoLog Mix 70/30 with 3 mL PenFill cartridge compatible devices*?" below.)
4. After the injection, remove the needle **without recapping** and dispose of it in a puncture-resistant container. Used syringes, needles, or lancets should be placed in sharps containers (such as red biohazard containers), hard plastic containers (such as detergent bottles), or metal containers (such as an empty coffee can). Such containers should be sealed and disposed of properly.

How should I Inject NovoLog Mix 70/30 insulin with 3 mL PenFill cartridge compatible delivery devices*?

1. Pinch your skin between two fingers, push the needle into the skinfold, and push the plunger to inject the insulin under your skin. The needle should be perpendicular to the skin. This means the needle will be straight in.
2. Keep the needle under your skin for at least 6 seconds to make sure you have injected all the insulin.
3. If blood appears after you pull the needle from your skin, press the injection site slightly with a finger. Do not rub the area.

***3 mL PenFill cartridge compatible delivery devices**
NovoPen 3, Innovo, InDuo
Helpful information for people with diabetes is published by the American Diabetes Association,
1660 Duke Street, Alexandria, VA 22314.
Date of Issue: November 18, 2002
For information about NovoLog® Mix 70/30 contact:
Novo Nordisk Pharmaceuticals, Inc.
100 College Road West
Princeton, New Jersey 08540
1-800-727-6500
www.novonordisk-us.com
Manufactured by
Novo Nordisk A/S
DK-2880 Bagsvaerd, Denmark
Novo Nordisk®, NovoLog®, FlexPen®, Innovo®, Novolin®, NovoPen®, PenFill®, and NovoFine® are trademarks owned by Novo Nordisk A/S.
InDuo™ is a trademark of LifeScan, Inc., a Johnson & Johnson company.
License under U.S. Patent No. 5,618,913 and Des. 347,894

Shown in Product Identification Guide, page 326

NOVOSEVEN® ℞

Coagulation Factor VIIa (Recombinant)
For Intravenous Use Only
℞ Only

DESCRIPTION

NovoSeven® is recombinant human coagulation Factor VIIa (rFVIIa), intended for promoting hemostasis by activating the extrinsic pathway of the coagulation cascade.[1] NovoSeven is a vitamin K-dependent glycoprotein consisting of 406 amino acid residues (MW 50 K Dalton). NovoSeven is structurally similar to human plasma-derived Factor VIIa.

The gene for human Factor VII is cloned and expressed in baby hamster kidney cells (BHK cells). Recombinant FVII is secreted into the culture media (containing newborn calf serum) in its single-chain form and then proteolytically converted by autocatalysis to the active two-chain form, rFVIIa, during a chromatographic purification process. The purification process has been demonstrated to remove exogenous viruses (MuLV, SV40, Pox virus, Reovirus, BEV, IBR virus). No human serum or other proteins are used in the production or formulation of NovoSeven.

NovoSeven is supplied as a sterile, white lyophilized powder of rFVIIa in single-use vials.

Each vial of lyophilized drug contains the following:
[See table below]

After reconstitution with the appropriate volume of **Sterile Water for Injection, USP (not supplied)**, each vial contains approximately 0.6 mg/mL NovoSeven (corresponding to 600 µg/mL). The reconstituted vials have a pH of approximately 5.5 in sodium chloride (3 mg/mL), calcium chloride dihydrate (1.5 mg/mL), glycylglycine (1.3 mg/mL), polysorbate 80 (0.1 mg/mL), and mannitol (30 mg/mL).

The reconstituted product is a clear colorless solution which contains no preservatives. NovoSeven contains trace amounts of proteins derived from the manufacturing and purification processes such as mouse IgG (maximum of 1.2 ng/mg), bovine IgG (maximum of 30 ng/mg), and protein from BHK-cells and media (maximum of 19 ng/mg).

CLINICAL PHARMACOLOGY

Pharmacodynamics

NovoSeven is recombinant Factor VIIa and, when complexed with tissue factor can activate coagulation Factor X to Factor Xa, as well as coagulation Factor IX to Factor IXa. Factor Xa, in complex with other factors, then converts prothrombin to thrombin, which leads to the formation of a hemostatic plug by converting fibrinogen to fibrin and thereby inducing local hemostasis.

Pharmacokinetics

Single-dose pharmacokinetics of NovoSeven (17.5, 35, and 70 µg/kg) exhibited dose-porportional behavior in 15 subjects with hemophilia A or B.[2] Factor VII clotting activities were measured in plasma drawn prior to and during a 24-hour period after NovoSeven administration. The median apparent volume of distribution at steady state was 103 mL/kg (range 78–139). Median clearance was 33 mL/kg/hr (range 27–49). The median residence time was 3.0 hours (range 2.4–3.3), and the $t_{1/2}$ was 2.3 hours (range 1.7–2.7). The median *in vivo* plasma recovery was 44% (30–71%).

CLINICAL STUDIES

No direct comparisons to other coagulation products have been conducted, therefore no conclusions regarding the comparative safety or efficacy can be made.

Open Protocol Use

The largest number of patients who received NovoSeven during the investigational phase of product development were in an open protocol study[3,4,5] that began enrollment in 1988, shortly after the completion of the pharmacokinetic study. These patients included persons with hemophilia types A or B (with or without inhibitors), persons with acquired inhibitors to Factor VIII or Factor IX, and a few FVII deficient patients. The clinical situations were diverse and included muscle/joint bleeds, mucocutaneous bleeds, surgical prophylaxis, intracerebral bleeds, and other emergent situations. Dose schedules were suggested by Novo Nordisk, but they were subject to the option of the investigator. Clinical outcomes were not reported in a standardized manner. Therefore, the clinical data from the Open Protocol is problematic for the evaluation of the safety and efficacy of the product by statistical methods. The following two cases describe the extremes of the clinical outcomes that were observed under the Open Protocol:

Case #1: A one-year-old hemophilia B patient had both an inhibitor to Factor IX and would experience severe anaphylactic reactions to any product containing Factor IX. His life threatening hypersensitivity reaction to Factor IX precluded the use of other coagulation products and NovoSeven was requested under the compassionate use program because it contained Factor VIIa and no other coagulation factors. Between the child's ages of one to three, he was successfully treated with NovoSeven for 23 spontaneous joint, muscle, and oral bleeds. NovoSeven was administered by intravenous bolus dosing at 90 µg/kg every two hours. Hemostasis was achieved each time within one to eight days therapy, without reported sequelae. Adverse events were infrequent, minor, and considered unrelated to NovoSeven treatment.

Case #2: A 36-year-old hemophilia A patient with long standing inhibitors experienced pain between his shoulder-blades (DAY 0); he treated himself at home for three days with an activated Prothrombin Complex Concentrate (aPCC). From DAY 16-DAY 18, the patient treated himself at home with another aPCC. On DAY 18, he awoke with paraparesis of the lower extremities and was hospitalized. A large epidural hematoma (C6 to T12) was seen on MRI. The following day (DAY 19), the patient began treatment with NovoSeven, 90 µg/kg every 2 (and later every 3) hours (DAY 19–36). Neurologic and symptomatic improvement was observed. On DAY 29, the NovoSeven dose interval was increased to every four hours. On DAY 31, the patient experienced a massive upper gastrointestinal bleed secondary to stress ulcers (likely dexamethasone induced). He was hypotensive for over two hours, and by the next day, he was requiring large volumes of fluid support and developed abdominal pain. A laparotomy on DAY 32 revealed necrotic large bowel which required resection. Intraoperative and post operative hemostasis was satisfactory on NovoSeven and there was no evidence of thrombosis of the larger mesenteric vessels either at surgery or in the pathologic specimen. On the fourth day post-op (DAY 36), NovoSeven investigational supplies were depleted, and the patient began receiving an aPCC (72 U/kg every 6 hours) and four units of packed red cells per day. During aPCC therapy, bleeding increased; there was coffee ground emesis in the naso-gastric tube. After two days (DAY 38), additional NovoSeven was provided, but the patient was then experiencing severe adult respiratory distress syndrome (ARDS). Within 24 hours of resuming NovoSeven treatment (DAY 40), the patient's life support was voluntarily removed. An autopsy noted the history of bleeding ulcer, ischemic colon, thrombocytopenia, diffuse hemorrhage, lung changes consistent with ARDS, history of epidural hemorrhage, arthropathy, and generalized edema. His stomach had no signs of the ulcers seen the week before on endoscopy indicating healing. On gross neuropathologic exam, his epidural hematoma had resolved.

Dosing Study

A double-blind, randomized comparison trial[6] of two dose levels of NovoSeven in the treatment of joint, muscle and mucocutaneous hemorrhages was conducted in hemophilia A and B patients with and without inhibitors. Patients received NovoSeven as soon as they could be evaluated in the treatment centers (4 to 18 hours after experiencing a bleed). Thirty-five patients were treated at the 35 µg/kg dose (59 joint, 15 muscle and 5 mucocutaneous bleeding episodes) and 43 patients were treated at the 70 µg/kg dose (85 joint and 14 muscle bleeding episodes).

Dosing was to be repeated at 2.5 hour intervals but ranged up to four hours for some patients. Efficacy was assessed at

Continued on next page

Contents	1.2 mg (60 KIU) Vial	2.4 mg (120 KIU) Vial	4.8 mg (240 KIU) Vial
rFVIIa	1200 µg	2400 µg	4800 µg
sodium chloride*	5.84 mg	11.68 mg	23.36 mg
calcium chloride dihydrate*	2.94 mg	5.88 mg	11.76 mg
glycylglycine	2.64 mg	5.28 mg	10.56 mg
polysorbate 80	0.14 mg	0.28 mg	0.56 mg
mannitol	60.0 mg	120.0 mg	240.0 mg

*per mg of rFVIIa: 0.44 mEq sodium, 0.06 mEq calcium

NovoSeven—Cont.

12±2 hours or at end of treatment, whichever occurred first. Based on a subjective evaluation by the investigator, the respective efficacy rates for the 35 and 70 μg/kg groups were: excellent 59% and 60%, effective 12% and 11%, and partially effective 17% and 20%. The average number of injections required to achieve hemostasis was 2.8 and 3.2 for the 35 and 70 μg/kg groups, respectively.

One patient in the 35 μg/kg group and three in the 70 μg/kg group experienced serious adverse events that were not considered related to NovoSeven. Two unrelated deaths occurred; one patient died of AIDS and the other of intracranial hemorrhage secondary to trauma.

INDICATIONS AND USAGE

NovoSeven is indicated for the treatment of bleeding episodes in hemophilia A or B patients with inhibitors to Factor VIII or Factor IX. NovoSeven should be administered to patients only under the supervision of a physician experienced in the treatment of hemophilia.

CONTRAINDICATIONS

NovoSeven® Coagulation Factor VIIa (Recombinant) should not be administered to patients with known hypersensitivity to NovoSeven or any of the components of NovoSeven. NovoSeven is contraindicated in patients with known hypersensitivity to mouse, hamster, or bovine proteins.

WARNINGS

The extent of the risk of thrombotic adverse events after treatment with NovoSeven is not known, but is considered to be low. Patients with disseminated intravascular coagulation (DIC), advanced atherosclerotic disease, crush injury, or septicemia may have an increased risk of developing thrombotic events due to circulating TF or predisposing coagulopathy. (See **ADVERSE REACTIONS**)

Additional data on the adverse event profile in general and regarding the frequency of thrombotic events in particular is being collected through a postmarket surveillance program. The Hemophilia Research Society (HRS) Registry surveillance program is designed to collect data on all uses of NovoSeven to expand the base of experience regarding the use of NovoSeven. All prescribers can obtain information regarding contribution of patient data to this program by calling 1-877-362-7355.

PRECAUTIONS

General

Patients who receive NovoSeven should be monitored if they develop signs or symptoms of activation of the coagulation system or thrombosis. When there is laboratory confirmation of intravascular coagulation or presence of clinical thrombosis, the rFVIIa dosage should be reduced or the treatment stopped, depending on the patient's symptoms.

Due to limited clinical studies which clearly address the effect of post-hemostatic dosing, precautions should be exercised when NovoSeven is used for prolonged dosing. (See **DOSAGE AND ADMINISTRATION**)

Information for Patients

Patients receiving NovoSeven should be informed of the benefits and risks associated with treatment. Patients should be warned about the early signs of hypersensitivity reactions, including hives, urticaria, tightness of the chest, wheezing, hypotension, and anaphylaxis.

Laboratory Tests

Laboratory coagulation parameters may be used as an adjunct to the clinical evaluation of hemostasis in monitoring the effectiveness and treatment schedule of NovoSeven although these parameters have shown no direct correlation to achieving hemostasis. Assays of prothrombin time (PT), activated partial thromboplastin time (aPTT), and plasma FVII clotting activity (FVII:C), may give different results with different reagents. Treatment with NovoSeven has been shown to produce the following characteristics:

PT: As shown below, in patients with hemophilia A/B with inhibitors, the PT shortened to about a 7-second plateau at a FVII:C level of approximately 5 U/mL. For FVII:C levels > 5 U/mL, there is no further change in PT.

[See figure at top of next column]

aPTT: While administration of NovoSeven shortens the prolonged aPTT in hemophilia A/B patients with inhibitors, normalization has usually not been observed in doses shown to induce clinical improvement. Data indicate that clinical improvement was associated with a shortening of aPTT of 15 to 20 seconds.

FVIIa:C: FVIIa:C levels were measured two hours after NovoSeven administration of 35 μg/kg and 90 μg/kg following two days of dosing at two hour intervals. Average steady state levels were 11 and 28 U/mL for the two dose levels, respectively.

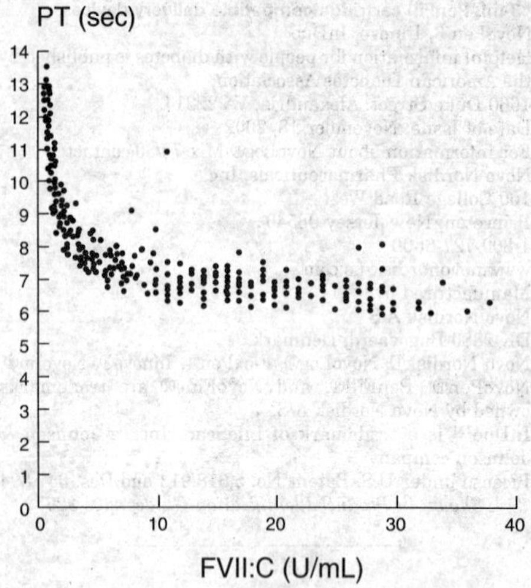

Drug Interactions

The risk of a potential interaction between NovoSeven and coagulation factor concentrates has not been adequately evaluated in preclinical or clinical studies. Simultaneous use of activated prothrombin complex concentrates or prothrombin complex concentrates should be avoided.

Although the specific drug interaction was not studied in a clinical trial, there have been more than 50 episodes of concomitant use of antifibrinolytic therapies (*i.e.*, tranexamic acid, aminocaproic acid) and NovoSeven.

NovoSeven should not be mixed with infusion solutions until clinical data are available to direct this use.

Carcinogenesis, Mutagenesis, Impairment of Fertility

Two mutagenicity studies have given no indication of carcinogenic potential for NovoSeven. The clastogenic activity of NovoSeven was evaluated in both *in vitro* studies (*i.e.*, cultured human lymphocytes) and *in vivo* studies (*i.e.*, mouse micronucleus test). Neither of these studies indicated clastogenic activity of NovoSeven. Other gene mutation studies have not been performed with NovoSeven (*e.g.*, Ames test). No chronic carcinogenicity studies have been performed with NovoSeven.

A reproductive study in male and female rats at dose levels up to 3.0 mg/kg/day had no effect on mating performance, fertility, or litter characteristics.

Pregnancy

Pregnancy Category C. Treatment of rats and rabbits with NovoSeven® in reproduction studies has been associated with mortality at doses up to 6 mg/kg and 5 mg/kg. At 6 mg/kg in rats, the abortion rate was 0 out of 25 litters; in rabbits at 5 mg/kg, the abortion rate was 2 out of 25 litters. Twenty-three out of 25 female rats given 6 mg/kg of NovoSeven gave birth successfully, however, two of the 23 litters died during the early period of lactation. No evidence of teratogenicity was observed after dosing with NovoSeven. There are no adequate and well-controlled studies in pregnant women. NovoSeven should be used during pregnancy only if the potential benefit justifies the potential risk to the fetus. The patients in whom NovoSeven is indicated are male.

Labor and Delivery

NovoSeven was administered to a FVII deficient patient (25 years of age, 66 kg) during a vaginal delivery (36 μg/kg) and during a tubal ligation (90 μg/kg). No adverse reactions were reported during labor, vaginal delivery, or the tubal ligation.

Nursing Mothers

It is not known whether NovoSeven is excreted in human milk. Because many drugs are excreted in human milk, and because of the potential for serious adverse reactions in nursing infants, a decision should be made whether to discontinue nursing or to discontinue the drug, taking into account the importance of the drug to the mother.

Pediatric Use

The safety and effectiveness of NovoSeven was not determined to be different in various age groups, from infants to adolescents (0 to 16 years of age). Clinical trials were conducted with dosing determined according to body weight and not according to age.

Geriatric Use

Clinical studies in hemophilia did not enroll geriatric patients.

ADVERSE REACTIONS

NovoSeven has been generally well tolerated in clinical studies in 298 patients with hemophilia A or B with inhibitors treated for 1,939 bleeding episodes. The table below lists adverse events that were reported in ≥2% of NovoSeven patients and were considered to be at least possibly related or of unknown relationship to NovoSeven administration.

[See table below]

Body System Event	# of episodes reported (n=1,939 treatments)	# of unique patients (n=298 patients)
Body as a whole		
Fever	16	13
Platelets, Bleeding, and Clotting		
Hemorrhage NOS	15	8
Fibrinogen plasma decreased	10	5
Skin and Musculoskeletal		
Hemarthrosis	14	8
Cardiovascular		
Hypertension	9	6

Events which were reported in 1% of patients and were considered to be at least possibly or of unknown relationship to NovoSeven administration were: allergic reaction, arthrosis, bradycardia, coagulation disorder, DIC, edema, fibrinolysis increased, headache, hypotension, injection site reaction, pain, pneumonia, prothrombin decreased, pruritus, purpura, rash, renal function abnormal, therapeutic response decreased, and vomiting.

In the 298 hemophilia patients, thrombosis was reported in two patients.

Serious adverse events that were probably or possibly related, or where the relationship to NovoSeven was not specified occurred in 14 of the 298 patients (4.7%). Six of these 14 patients died of the following conditions: worsening of chronic renal failure, anesthesia complications during proctoscopy, renal failure complicating a retroperitoneal bleed, ruptured abscess leading to sepsis and DIC, pneumonia, and splenic hematoma and GI bleeding.

OVERDOSAGE

Dose limiting toxicities of NovoSeven® Coagulation Factor VIIa (Recombinant) have not been investigated in clinical trials. Two cases of accidental overdose by bolus administration have occurred in the clinical program. One hemophilia B patient (16 years of age, 68 kg) received a single dose of 352 μg/kg and one hemophilia A patient (2 years of age, 14.6 kg) received doses ranging from 246 μg/kg to 986 μg/kg on five consecutive days. There were no reported complications in either case. The recommended dose schedule should not be intentionally increased, even in the case of lack of effect, due to the absence of information on the additional risk that may be incurred.

DOSAGE AND ADMINISTRATION

Dosage

NovoSeven is intended for intravenous bolus administration only. Evaluation of hemostasis should be used to determine the effectiveness of NovoSeven and to provide a basis for modification of the NovoSeven treatment schedule; coagulation parameters do not necessarily correlate with or predict the effectiveness of NovoSeven.

The recommended dose of NovoSeven for hemophilia A or B patients with inhibitors is 90 μg/kg given every two hours until hemostasis is achieved, or until the treatment has been judged to be inadequate. Doses between 35 and 120 μg/kg have been used successfully in clinical trials, and both the dose and administration interval may be adjusted based on the severity of the bleeding and degree of hemostasis achieved.[7] The minimal effective dose has not been established. For patients treated for joint or muscle bleeds, a decision on outcome was reached for a majority of patients within eight doses although more doses were required for severe bleeds. A majority of patients who reported adverse experiences received more than twelve doses.

Post-Hemostatic Dosing: The appropriate duration of post-hemostatic dosing has not been studied. For severe bleeds, dosing should continue at 3–6 hour intervals after hemostasis is achieved, to maintain the hemostatic plug. The biological and clinical effects of prolonged elevated levels of Factor VIIa have not been studied; therefore, the duration of post-hemostatic dosing should be minimized, and patients should be appropriately monitored by a physician experienced in the treatment of hemophilia during this time period.

Reconstitution

Reconstitution should be performed using the following procedures:

1. Always use aseptic technique.
2. Bring NovoSeven (white, lyophilized powder) and the specified volume of Sterile Water for Injection, USP, (diluent) to room temperature, but not above 37°C (98.6°F). The specified volume of diluent corresponding to the amount of NovoSeven is as follows.
   1.2 mg (1200 μg) vial + 2.2 mL **Sterile Water for Injection, USP**
   2.4 mg (2400 μg) vial + 4.3 mL **Sterile Water for Injection, USP**
   4.8 mg (4800 μg) vial + 8.5 mL **Sterile Water for Injection, USP**
   After reconstitution with the specified volume of diluent, each vial contains approximately 0.6 mg/mL NovoSeven (600 μg/mL).
3. Remove caps from the NovoSeven vials to expose the central portion of the rubber stopper. Cleanse the rubber stoppers with an alcohol swab and allow to dry prior to use.
4. Draw back the plunger of a sterile syringe (attached to sterile needle) and admit air into the syringe.

5. Insert the needle of the syringe into the sterile water for injection vial. Inject air into the vial and withdraw the quantity required for reconstitution.
6. Insert the syringe needle containing the diluent into the NovoSeven vial through the center of the rubber stopper, aiming the needle against the side so that the stream of liquid runs down the vial wall (the NovoSeven vial does not contain a vacuum). **Do not inject the diluent directly on the NovoSeven powder.**
7. Gently swirl the vial until all the material is dissolved. The reconstituted solution is a clear, colorless solution which may be used up to 3 hours after reconstitution.

Administration

Administration should take place within 3 hours after reconstitution. Any unused solution should be discarded. Do not store reconstituted NovoSeven in syringes. NovoSeven is intended for intravenous bolus injection only and should not be mixed with infusion solutions. As with all parenteral drug products, reconstituted NovoSeven should be inspected visually for particulate matter and discoloration prior to administration. Do not use if particulate matter or discoloration is observed. Administration should be performed using the following procedures:

1. Always use aseptic technique.
2. Draw back the plunger of a sterile syringe (attached to sterile needle) and admit air into the syringe.
3. Insert needle into the vial of reconstituted NovoSeven. Inject air into the vial and then withdraw the appropriate amount of reconstituted NovoSeven into the syringe.
4. Remove and discard the needle from the syringe; attach a suitable intravenous injection needle and administer as a slow bolus injection over 2 to 5 minutes, depending on the dose administered.
5. Discard any unused reconstituted NovoSeven after 3 hours.

HOW SUPPLIED

NovoSeven® Coagulation Factor VIIa (Recombinant) is supplied as a white, lyophilized powder in single-use vials, one vial per carton. The vials are made of Class I, Type I, hydrolytic, neutral, white glass, closed with a latex-free, bromobutyl rubber stopper, and sealed with an aluminum cap. The vials are equipped with a snap-off polypropylene cap. The amount of rFVIIa in milligrams and in micrograms is stated on the label as follows:

1.2 mg per vial (1200 µg/vial) NDC 0169-7060-01
2.4 mg per vial (2400 µg/vial) NDC 0169-7061-01
4.8 mg per vial (4800 µg/vial) NDC 0169-7062-01

Storage

Prior to reconstitution, keep refrigerated (2–8°C /36–46°F). Avoid exposure to direct sunlight. Do not use past the expiration date.

After reconstitution, NovoSeven may be stored either at room temperature or refrigerated for up to 3 hours. Do not freeze reconstituted NovoSeven or store it in syringes.

REFERENCES

1. Roberts, H.R.: Thoughts on the mechanism of action of FVIIa, 2nd Symposium on New Aspects of Hemophilia Treatment, Copenhagen, Denmark, 1991, pgs. 153–156.
2. Lindley, C.M., et al.: Pharmacokinetics and pharmacodynamics of recombinant Factor VIIa, Clinical Pharmacology & Therapeutics, Vol. 55, No. 6, June 1994, pgs. 638–648.
3. Lusher, J., et al.: Clinical experience with recombinant Factor VIIa, Blood Coagulation and Fibrinolysis 1998, 9:119–128.
4. Bech, M. R.: Recombinant Factor VIIa in Joint and Muscle Bleeding Episodes, Haemostasis 1996;26(suppl 1): 135–138.
5. Lusher, J.M.: Recombinant Factor VIIa (NovoSeven®) in the Treatment of Internal Bleeding in Patients with Factor VIII and IX Inhibitors, Haemostasis 1996; 26(suppl 1):124–130.
6. Lusher, J.M., et al.: A randomized, double-blind comparison of two dosage levels of recombinant factor VIIa in the treatment of joint, muscle and mucocutaneous haemorrhages in persons with hemophilia A and B, with and without inhibitor, Haemophilia 1988, 4:790–798.
7. Hedner, U.: Dosing and Monitoring NovoSeven® Treatment, Haemostasis 1996;26(suppl 1):102–108.

Date of issue: February/2003
License Number: 1261

U.S. Patent Nos. 4,382,083; 4,479,938; 4,784,950, 5,180,583 and 6,310,183
For Information contact:
Novo Nordisk Pharmaceuticals, Inc.
100 College Road West
Princeton, NJ 08540, USA
1-877-NOVO-777
www.novoseven-us.com
Manufactured by:
Novo Nordisk A/S
2880 Bagsvaerd, Denmark

PRANDIN® ℞
(repaglinide) Tablets
(0.5, 1, and 2 mg)

DESCRIPTION

PRANDIN® (repaglinide) is an oral blood glucose-lowering drug of the meglitinide class used in the management of type 2 diabetes mellitus (also known as non-insulin dependent diabetes mellitus or NIDDM). Repaglinide, S(+) 2-ethoxy-4(2((3-methyl-1-(2-(1-piperidinyl) phenyl)-butyl) amino)-2-oxoethyl) benzoic acid, is chemically unrelated to the oral sulfonylurea insulin secretagogues.

The structural formula is as shown below:

Repaglinide is a white to off-white powder with molecular formula $C_{27}H_{36}N_2O_4$ and a molecular weight of 452.6. PRANDIN tablets contain 0.5 mg, 1 mg, or 2 mg of repaglinide. In addition each tablet contains the following inactive ingredients: calcium hydrogen phosphate (anhydrous), microcrystalline cellulose, maize starch, polacrilin potassium, povidone, glycerol (85%), magnesium stearate, meglumine, and poloxamer. The 1 mg and 2 mg tablets contain iron oxides (yellow and red, respectively) as coloring agents.

CLINICAL PHARMACOLOGY

Mechanism of Action

Repaglinide lowers blood glucose levels by stimulating the release of insulin from the pancreas. This action is dependent upon functioning beta (β) cells in the pancreatic islets. Insulin release is glucose-dependent and diminishes at low glucose concentrations.

Repaglinide closes ATP-dependent potassium channels in the β-cell membrane by binding at characterizable sites. This potassium channel blockade depolarizes the β-cell, which leads to an opening of calcium channels. The resulting increased calcium influx induces insulin secretion. The ion channel mechanism is highly tissue selective with low affinity for heart and skeletal muscle.

Pharmacokinetics

Absorption: After oral administration, repaglinide is rapidly and completely absorbed from the gastrointestinal tract. After single and multiple oral doses in healthy subjects or in patients, peak plasma drug levels (C_{max}) occur within 1 hour (T_{max}). Repaglinide is rapidly eliminated from the blood stream with a half-life of approximately 1 hour. The mean absolute bioavailability is 56%. When repaglinide was given with food, the mean T_{max} was not changed, but the mean C_{max} and AUC (area under the time/plasma concentration curve) were decreased 20% and 12.4%, respectively.

Distribution: After intravenous (IV) dosing in healthy subjects, the volume of distribution at steady state (V_{ss}) was 31 L, and the total body clearance (CL) was 38 L/h. Protein binding and binding to human serum albumin was greater than 98%.

Metabolism: Repaglinide is completely metabolized by oxidative biotransformation and direct conjugation with glucuronic acid after either an IV or oral dose. The major metabolites are an oxidized dicarboxylic acid (M2), the aromatic amine (M1), and the acyl glucuronide (M7). The cytochrome P-450 enzyme system, specifically 3A4, has been shown to be involved in the N-dealkylation of repaglinide to M2 and the further oxidation to M1. Metabolites do not contribute to the glucose-lowering effect of repaglinide.

Excretion: Within 96 hours after dosing with ^{14}C-repaglinide as a single, oral dose, approximately 90% of the radiolabel was recovered in the feces and approximately 8% in the urine. Only 0.1% of the dose is cleared in the urine as parent compound. The major metabolite (M2) accounted for 60% of the administered dose. Less than 2% of parent drug was recovered in feces.

Pharmacokinetic parameters: The pharmacokinetic parameters of repaglinide obtained from a single-dose, crossover study in healthy subjects and from a multiple-dose, parallel, dose-proportionality (0.5, 1, 2 and 4 mg) study in patients with type 2 diabetes are summarized in the following table:

Parameter	Patient with type 2 diabetes[a]
Dose 0.5 mg 1 mg 2 mg 4 mg	$AUC_{0-24\ hr}$ Mean ±SD (ng/mL*hr): 68.9 ± 154.4 125.8 ± 129.8 152.4 ± 89.6 447.4 ± 211.3
Dose 0.5 mg 1 mg 2 mg 4 mg	$C_{max\ 0-5\ hr}$ Mean ±SD (ng/mL): 9.8 ± 10.2 18.3 ± 9.1 26.0 ± 13.0 65.8 ± 30.1
Dose 0.5–4 mg	$T_{max\ 0-5\ hr}$ Means (SD) 1.0–1.4 (0.3–0.5) hr
Dose 0.5–4 mg	$T_{1/2}$ Means (Ind Range) 1.0–1.4 (0.4–8.0) hr

Parameter	Healthy Subjects
CL based on i.v.	38± 16 L/hr
V_{ss} based on i.v.	31± 12 L
AbsBio	56± 9%

a: dosed preprandially with three meals
CL = total body clearance
V_{ss} = volume of distribution at steady state
AbsBio = absolute bioavailability

These data indicate that repaglinide did not accumulate in serum. Clearance of oral repaglinide did not change over the 0.5–4 mg dose range, indicating a linear relationship between dose and plasma drug levels.

Variability of exposure: Repaglinide AUC after multiple doses of 0.25 to 4 mg with each meal varies over a wide range. The intra-individual and inter-individual coefficients of variation were 36% and 69%, respectively. AUC over the therapeutic dose range included 69 to 1005 ng/mL*hr, but AUC exposure up to 5417 ng/mL*hr was reached in dose escalation studies without apparent adverse consequences.

Special populations:

Geriatric. Healthy volunteers were treated with a regimen of 2 mg taken before each of 3 meals. There were no significant differences in repaglinide pharmacokinetics between the group of patients <65 years of age and a comparably sized group of patients ≥65 years of age. (See **PRECAUTIONS, Geriatric Use**)

Pediatric. No studies have been performed in pediatric patients.

Gender. A comparison of pharmacokinetics in males and females showed the AUC over the 0.5 mg to 4 mg dose range to be 15% to 70% higher in females with type 2 diabetes. This difference was not reflected in the frequency of hypoglycemic episodes (male: 16%; female: 17%) or other adverse events. With respect to gender, no change in general dosage recommendation is indicated since dosage for each patient should be individualized to achieve optimal clinical response.

Race. No pharmacokinetic studies to assess the effects of race have been performed, but in a U.S. 1-year study in patients with type 2 diabetes, the blood glucose-lowering effect was comparable between Caucasians (n=297) and African-Americans (n=33). In a U.S. dose-response study, there was no apparent difference in exposure (AUC) between Caucasians (n=74) and Hispanics (n=33).

Drug-Drug Interactions:

Drug interaction studies performed in healthy volunteers show that PRANDIN had no clinically relevant effect on the pharmacokinetic properties of digoxin, theophylline, or warfarin. Co-administration of cimetidine with PRANDIN did not significantly alter the absorption and disposition of repaglinide.

Additionally, the following drugs were studied in healthy volunteers with co-administration of PRANDIN. Listed below are the results:

Gemfibrozil and Itraconazole: Co-administration of gemfibrozil (600 mg) and a single dose of 0.25 mg PRANDIN (after 3 days of twice-daily 600 mg gemfibrozil) resulted in an 8.1-fold higher repaglinide AUC and prolonged repaglinide half-life from 1.3 to 3.7 hr. Co-administration with itraconazole and a single dose of 0.25 mg PRANDIN (on the third day of a regimen of 200 mg initial dose, twice-daily 100 mg itraconazole) resulted in a 1.4-fold higher repaglinide AUC. Co-administration of both gemfibrozil and itraconazole with PRANDIN resulted in a 19-fold higher repaglinide AUC and prolonged repaglinide half-life to 6.1 hr. Plasma repaglinide concentration at 7 h increased 28.6-fold with gemfibrozil co-administration and 70.4-fold with the gemfibrozil-itraconazole combination (see **PRECAUTIONS, Drug-Drug Interactions**).

Ketoconazole: Co-administration of 200 mg ketoconazole and a single dose of 2 mg PRANDIN (after 4 days of once daily ketoconazole 200 mg) resulted in a 15% and 16% increase in repaglinide AUC and C_{max}, respectively. The increases were from 20.2 ng/mL to 23.5 ng/mL for C_{max} and from 38.9 ng/mL *hr to 44.9 ng/mL *hr for AUC.

Rifampin: Co-administration of 600 mg rifampin and a single dose of 4 mg PRANDIN (after 6 days of once daily rifampin 600 mg) resulted in a 32% and 26% decrease in repaglinide AUC and C_{max}, respectively. The decreases were from 40.4 ng/mL to 29.7 ng/mL for C_{max} and from 56.8 ng/mL *hr to 38.7 ng/mL *hr for AUC.

Levonorgestrel & Ethinyl Estradiol:

Co-administration of a combination tablet of 0.15 mg levonorgestrel and 0.03 mg ethinyl estradiol administered once daily for 21 days with 2 mg PRANDIN administered three times daily (days 1–4) and a single dose on Day 5 resulted in 20% increases in repaglinide, levonorgestrel, and ethinyl estradiol C_{max}. The increase in repaglinide C_{max} was from 40.5 ng/mL to 47.4 ng/mL. Ethinyl estradiol AUC parameters were increased by 20%, while repaglinide and levonorgestrel AUC values remained unchanged.

Simvastatin: Co-administration of 20 mg simvastatin and a single dose of 2 mg PRANDIN (after 4 days of once daily simvastatin 20 mg and three times daily PRANDIN 2 mg) resulted in a 26% increase in repaglinide C_{max} from 23.6 ng/mL to 29.7 ng/mL. AUC was unchanged.

Continued on next page

Prandin—Cont.

Nifedipine: Co-administration of 10 mg nifedipine with a single dose of 2 mg PRANDIN (after 4 days of three times daily nifedipine 10 mg and three times daily PRANDIN 2 mg) resulted in unchanged AUC and C_{max} values for both drugs.

Clarithromycin: Co-administration of 250 mg clarithromycin and a single dose of 0.25 mg PRANDIN (after 4 days of twice daily clarithromycin 250 mg) resulted in a 40% and 67% increase in repaglinide AUC and C_{max}, respectively. The increase in AUC was from 5.3 ng/mL *hr. to 7.5 ng/mL *hr and the increase in C_{max} was from 4.4 ng/mL to 7.3 ng/mL.

Renal insufficiency. Single-dose and steady-state pharmacokinetics of repaglinide were compared between patients with type 2 diabetes and normal renal function (CrCl > 80 mL/min), mild to moderate renal function impairment (CrCl = 40–80 mL/min), and severe renal function impairment (CrCl = 20–40 mL/min). Both AUC and C_{max} of repaglinide were similar in patients with normal and mild to moderately impaired renal function (mean values 56.7 ng/mL*hr vs 57.2 ng/mL*hr and 37.5 ng/mL vs 37.7 ng/mL, respectively). Patients with severely reduced renal function had elevated mean AUC and C_{max} values (98.0 ng/mL*hr and 50.7 ng/mL, respectively), but this study showed only a weak correlation between repaglinide levels and creatinine clearance. Initial dose adjustment does not appear to be necessary for patients with mild to moderate renal dysfunction. **However, patients with type 2 diabetes who have *severe* renal function impairment should initiate PRANDIN therapy with the 0.5 mg dose—subsequently, patients should be carefully titrated. Studies were not conducted in patients with creatinine clearances below 20 mL/min or patients with renal failure requiring hemodialysis.**

Hepatic insufficiency. A single-dose, open-label study was conducted in 12 healthy subjects and 12 patients with chronic liver disease (CLD) classified by Child-Pugh scale and caffeine clearance. Patients with moderate to severe impairment of liver function had higher and more prolonged serum concentrations of both total and unbound repaglinide than healthy subjects ($AUC_{healthy}$: 91.6 ng/mL*hr; $AUC_{CLD\ patients}$: 368.9 ng/mL*hr; $C_{max,\ healthy}$: 46.7 ng/mL; $C_{max,\ CLD\ patients}$: 105.4 ng/mL). AUC was statistically correlated with caffeine clearance. No difference in glucose profiles was observed across patient groups. Patients with impaired liver function may be exposed to higher concentrations of repaglinide and its associated metabolites than would patients with normal liver function receiving usual doses. Therefore, **PRANDIN should be used cautiously in patients with impaired liver function. Longer intervals between dose adjustments should be utilized to allow full assessment of response.**

Clinical Trials

A four-week, double-blind, placebo-controlled dose-response trial was conducted in 138 patients with type 2 diabetes using doses ranging from 0.25 to 4 mg taken with each of three meals. PRANDIN therapy resulted in dose-proportional glucose-lowering over the full dose range. Plasma insulin levels increased after meals and reverted toward baseline before the next meal. Most of the fasting blood glucose-lowering effect was demonstrated within 1–2 weeks.

In a double-blind, placebo-controlled, 3-month dose titration study, PRANDIN or placebo doses for each patient were increased weekly from 0.25 mg through 0.5, 1, and 2 mg, to a maximum of 4 mg, until a fasting plasma glucose (FPG) level <160 mg/dL was achieved or the maximum dose reached. The dose that achieved the targeted control or the maximum dose was continued to end of study. FPG and 2-hour post-prandial glucose (PPG) increased in patients receiving placebo and decreased in patients treated with repaglinide. Differences between the repaglinide- and placebo-treated groups were -61 mg/dL (FPG) and -104 mg/dL (PPG). The between-group change in HbA_{1c}, which reflects long-term glycemic control, was 1.7% units.

[See table below]

Another double-blind, placebo-controlled trial was carried out in 362 patients treated for 24 weeks. The efficacy of 1 and 4 mg preprandial doses was demonstrated by lowering of fasting blood glucose and by HbA_{1c} at the end of the study. HbA_{1c} for the PRANDIN-treated groups (1 and 4 mg groups combined) at the end of the study was decreased compared to the placebo-treated group in previously naïve patients and in patients previously treated with oral hypoglycemic agents by 2.1% units and 1.7% units, respectively. In this fixed-dose trial, patients who were naïve to oral hypoglycemic agent therapy and patients in relatively good glycemic control at baseline (HbA_{1c} below 8%) showed greater blood glucose-lowering including a higher frequency of hypoglycemia. Patients who were previously treated and who had baseline HbA_{1c} ≥8% reported hypoglycemia at the same rate as patients randomized to placebo. There was no average gain in body weight when patients previously treated with oral hypoglycemic agents were switched to PRANDIN. The average weight gain in patients treated with PRANDIN and not previously treated with sulfonylurea drugs was 3.3%.

The dosing of PRANDIN relative to meal-related insulin release was studied in three trials including 58 patients. Glycemic control was maintained during a period in which the meal and dosing pattern was varied (2, 3, or 4 meals per day; before meals × 2, 3 or 4) compared with a period of 3 regular meals and 3 doses per day (before meals × 3). It was also shown that PRANDIN can be administered at the start of a meal, 15 minutes before, or 30 minutes before the meal with the same blood glucose lowering effect.

PRANDIN was compared to other insulin secretagogues in 1-year controlled trials to demonstrate comparability of efficacy and safety. Hypoglycemia was reported in 16% of 1228 PRANDIN patients, 20% of 417 glyburide patients, and 19% of 81 glipizide patients. Of PRANDIN-treated patients with symptomatic hypoglycemia, none developed coma or required hospitalization.

PRANDIN was studied in combination with metformin in 83 patients not satisfactorily controlled on exercise, diet, and metformin alone. PRANDIN dosage was titrated for 4 to 8 weeks, followed by a 3-month maintenance period. Combination therapy with PRANDIN and metformin resulted in significantly greater improvement in glycemic control as compared to repaglinide or metformin monotherapy. HbA_{1c} was improved by 1% unit and FPG decreased by an additional 35 mg/dL. In this study where metformin dosage was kept constant, the combination therapy of PRANDIN and metformin showed dose-sparing effects with respect to PRANDIN. The greater efficacy response of the combination group was achieved at a lower daily repaglinide dosage than in the PRANDIN monotherapy group (see Table).

PRANDIN and Metformin Therapy: Mean Changes from Baseline in Glycemic Parameters and Weight After 4 to 5 Months of Treatment[1]

	PRANDIN	Combination	Metformin
N	28	27	27
Median Final Dose (mg/day)	12	6 (PRANDIN) 1500 (metformin)	1500
HbA_{1c} (% units)	−0.38	−1.41*	−0.33
FPG (mg/dL)	8.8	−39.2*	−4.5
Weight (kg)	3.0	2.4#	−0.90

1: based on intent-to-treat analysis
*: p<0.05, for pairwise comparisons with PRANDIN and metformin.
#: p<0.05, for pairwise comparison with metformin.

A combination therapy regimen of PRANDIN and pioglitazone was compared to monotherapy with either agent alone in a 24-week trial that enrolled 246 patients previously treated with sulfonylurea or metformin monotherapy (HbA_{1c} > 7.0%). Numbers of patients treated were: PRANDIN (N = 61), pioglitazone (N = 62), combination (N = 123). PRANDIN dosage was titrated during the first 12 weeks, followed by a 12-week maintenance period. Combination therapy resulted in significantly greater improvement in glycemic control as compared to monotherapy (figure below). The changes from baseline for completers in FPG (mg/dL) and HbA_{1c} (%), respectively were: −39.8 and −0.1 for PRANDIN, −35.3 and −0.1 for pioglitazone and −92.4 and −1.9 for the combination. In this study where pioglitazone dosage was kept constant, the combination therapy group showed dose-sparing effects with respect to PRANDIN (see figure legend). The greater efficacy response of the combination group was achieved at a lower daily repaglinide dosage than in the PRANDIN monotherapy group. Mean weight increases associated with combination, PRANDIN and pioglitazone therapy were 5.5 kg, 0.3 kg, and 2.0 kg respectively.

HbA_{1c} Values from PRANDIN / Pioglitazone Combination Study

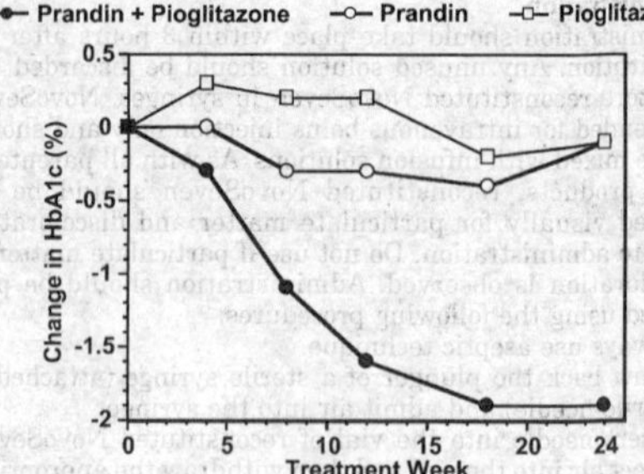

HbA_{1c} values by study week for patients who completed study (combination, N = 101; PRANDIN, N = 35, pioglitazone, N = 26).

Subjects with FPG above 270 mg/dL were withdrawn from the study.

Pioglitazone dose: fixed at 30 mg/day; PRANDIN median final dose: 6 mg/day for combination and 10 mg/day for monotherapy.

A combination therapy regimen of PRANDIN and rosiglitazone was compared to monotherapy with either agent alone in a 24-week trial that enrolled 252 patients previously treated with sulfonylurea or metformin (HbA_{1c} > 7.0%). Combination therapy resulted in significantly greater improvement in glycemic control as compared to monotherapy (table below). The glycemic effects of the combination therapy were dose-sparing with respect to both total daily PRANDIN dosage and total daily rosiglitazone dosage (see table legend). A greater efficacy response of the combination therapy group was achieved with half the median daily dose of PRANDIN and rosiglitazone, as compared to the respective monotherapy groups. Mean weight change associated with combination therapy was greater than that of PRANDIN monotherapy.

Mean Changes from Baseline in Glycemic Parameters and Weight in a 24-Week PRANDIN/ Rosiglitazone Combination Study[1]

	PRANDIN	Combination	Rosiglitazone
N	63	127	62
HbA_{1c} (%)			
Baseline	9.3	9.1	9.0
Change by 24 weeks	−0.17	−1.43*	−0.56
FPG (mg/dL)			
Baseline	269	257	252
Change by 24 weeks	−54	−94*	−67
Change in Weight (kg)	+1.3	+4.5#	+3.3

1: based on intent-to-treat analysis
*: p-value ≤ 0.001 for comparison to either monotherapy
#: p-value < 0.001 for comparison to PRANDIN
Final median doses: rosiglitazone - 4 mg/day for combination and 8 mg/day for monotherapy; PRANDIN - 6 mg/day for combination and 12 mg/day for monotherapy

PRANDIN vs. Placebo Treatment: Mean FPG, PPG, and HbA_{1c} Changes from baseline after 3 months of treatment:

	FPG	(mg/dL)	PPG	(mg/dL)	HbA_{1c}	(%)
	PL	R	PL	R	PL	R
Baseline	215.3	220.2	245.2	261.7	8.1	8.5
Change from baseline (at last visit)	30.3	-31.0*	56.5	-47.6*	1.1	-0.6*

FPG = fasting plasma glucose
PPG = post-prandial glucose
PL = placebo (N=33)
R = repaglinide (N=66)
* p<0.05 for between group difference

INDICATIONS AND USAGE

PRANDIN is indicated as an adjunct to diet and exercise to lower the blood glucose in patients with type 2 diabetes mellitus (NIDDM) whose hyperglycemia cannot be controlled satisfactorily by diet and exercise alone.

PRANDIN is also indicated for combination therapy use (with metformin or thiazolidinediones) to lower blood glucose in patients whose hyperglycemia cannot be controlled by diet and exercise plus monotherapy with any of the following agents: metformin, sulfonylureas, repaglinide, or thiazolidinediones. If glucose control has not been achieved after a suitable trial of combination therapy, consideration should be given to discontinuing these drugs and using insulin. Judgments should be based on regular clinical and laboratory evaluations.

In initiating treatment for patients with type 2 diabetes, diet and exercise should be emphasized as the primary form of treatment. Caloric restriction, weight loss, and exercise are essential in the obese diabetic patient. Proper dietary management and exercise alone may be effective in controlling the blood glucose and symptoms of hyperglycemia. In addition to regular physical activity, cardiovascular risk factors should be identified and corrective measures taken where possible.

If this treatment program fails to reduce symptoms and/or blood glucose, the use of an oral blood glucose-lowering agent or insulin should be considered. Use of PRANDIN must be viewed by both the physician and patient as a treatment in addition to diet, and not as a substitute for diet or as a convenient mechanism for avoiding dietary restraint. Furthermore, loss of blood glucose control on diet alone may be transient, thus requiring only short-term administration of PRANDIN.

During maintenance programs, PRANDIN should be discontinued if satisfactory lowering of blood glucose is no longer achieved. Judgments should be based on regular clinical and laboratory evaluations.

In considering the use of PRANDIN or other antidiabetic therapies, it should be recognized that blood glucose control in type 2 diabetes has not been definitely established to be effective in preventing the long-term cardiovascular complications of diabetes. However, in patients with Type 1 diabetes, the Diabetes Control and Complications Trial (DCCT) demonstrated that improved glycemic control, as reflected by HbA_{1c} and fasting glucose levels, was associated with a reduction in the diabetic complications retinopathy, neuropathy, and nephropathy.

CONTRAINDICATIONS

PRANDIN is contraindicated in patients with:

1. Diabetic ketoacidosis, with or without coma. This condition should be treated with insulin.
2. Type 1 diabetes.
3. Known hypersensitivity to the drug or its inactive ingredients.

PRECAUTIONS

General: Hypoglycemia: All oral blood glucose-lowering drugs are capable of producing hypoglycemia. Proper patient selection, dosage, and instructions to the patients are important to avoid hypoglycemic episodes. Hepatic insufficiency may cause elevated repaglinide blood levels and may diminish gluconeogenic capacity, both of which increase the risk of serious hypoglycemia. Elderly, debilitated, or malnourished patients, and those with adrenal, pituitary, hepatic or severe renal insufficiency may be particularly susceptible to the hypoglycemic action of glucose-lowering drugs.

Hypoglycemia may be difficult to recognize in the elderly and in people taking beta-adrenergic blocking drugs. Hypoglycemia is more likely to occur when caloric intake is deficient, after severe or prolonged exercise, when alcohol is ingested, or when more than one glucose-lowering drug is used.

The frequency of hypoglycemia is greater in patients with type 2 diabetes who have not been previously treated with oral blood glucose-lowering drugs (naïve) or whose HbA_{1c} is less than 8%. PRANDIN should be administered with meals to lessen the risk of hypoglycemia.

Loss of control of blood glucose: When a patient stabilized on any diabetic regimen is exposed to stress such as fever, trauma, infection, or surgery, a loss of glycemic control may occur. At such times, it may be necessary to discontinue PRANDIN and administer insulin. The effectiveness of any hypoglycemic drug in lowering blood glucose to a desired level decreases in many patients over a period of time, which may be due to progression of the severity of diabetes or to diminished responsiveness to the drug. This phenomenon is known as secondary failure, to distinguish it from primary failure in which the drug is ineffective in an individual patient when the drug is first given. Adequate adjustment of dose and adherence to diet should be assessed before classifying a patient as a secondary failure.

Information for Patients

Patients should be informed of the potential risks and advantages of PRANDIN and of alternative modes of therapy. They should also be informed about the importance of adherence to dietary instructions, of a regular exercise program, and of regular testing of blood glucose and HbA_{1c}. The risks of hypoglycemia, its symptoms and treatment, and conditions that predispose to its development and concomitant administration of other glucose-lowering drugs should be explained to patients and responsible family members. Primary and secondary failure should also be explained.

Patients should be instructed to take PRANDIN before meals (2, 3, or 4 times a day preprandially). Doses are usually taken within 15 minutes of the meal but time may vary from immediately preceding the meal to as long as 30 minutes before the meal. **Patients who skip a meal (or add an extra meal) should be instructed to skip (or add) a dose for that meal.**

Laboratory Tests

Response to all diabetic therapies should be monitored by periodic measurements of fasting blood glucose and glycosylated hemoglobin levels with a goal of decreasing these levels towards the normal range. During dose adjustment, fasting glucose can be used to determine the therapeutic response. Thereafter, both glucose and glycosylated hemoglobin should be monitored. Glycosylated hemoglobin may be especially useful for evaluating long-term glycemic control. Postprandial glucose level testing may be clinically helpful in patients whose pre-meal blood glucose levels are satisfactory but whose overall glycemic control (HbA_{1c}) is inadequate.

Commonly Reported Adverse Events (% of Patients)*

EVENT	PRANDIN N = 352	PLACEBO N = 108	PRANDIN N = 1228	SU N = 498
	Placebo controlled studies		Active controlled studies	
Metabolic				
Hypoglycemia	31**	7	16	20
Respiratory				
URI	16	8	10	10
Sinusitis	6	2	3	4
Rhinitis	3	3	7	8
Bronchitis	2	1	6	7
Gastrointestinal				
Nausea	5	5	3	2
Diarrhea	5	2	4	6
Constipation	3	2	2	3
Vomiting	3	3	2	1
Dyspepsia	2	2	4	2
Musculoskeletal				
Arthralgia	6	3	3	4
Back Pain	5	4	6	7
Other				
Headache	11	10	9	8
Paresthesia	3	3	2	1
Chest pain	3	1	2	1
Urinary tract infection	2	1	3	3
Tooth disorder	2	0	<1	<1
Allergy	2	0	1	<1

*: Events ≥ 2% for the PRANDIN group in the placebo-controlled studies and ≥ events in the placebo group
: See trial description in **CLINICAL PHARMACOLOGY, Clinical Trials

Drug-Drug Interactions

In vitro data indicate that repaglinide metabolism may be inhibited by antifungal agents like ketoconazole and miconazole, and antibacterial agents like erythromycin (cytochrome P-450 enzyme system 3A4 inhibitors). Drugs that induce the cytochrome P-450 enzyme system 3A4 may increase repaglinide metabolism; such drugs include rifampin, barbiturates, and carbamezepine. See **CLINICAL PHARMACOLOGY** section, **Drug-Drug Interactions.**

In vivo data from a study that evaluated the co-administration of a cytochrome P–450 enzyme inhibitor, clarithromycin, with PRANDIN resulted in a clinically significant increase in repaglinide plasma levels. This increase in repaglinide plasma levels may necessitate a PRANDIN dose adjustment. See **CLINICAL PHARMACOLOGY** section, **Drug-Drug Interactions.**

In vivo data from a study that evaluated the co-administration of gemfibrozil with PRANDIN in healthy subjects resulted in a significant increase in repaglinide blood levels. **Patients taking PRANDIN should not start taking gemfibrozil; patients taking gemfibrozil should not start taking PRANDIN. Concomitant use may result in enhanced and prolonged blood glucose-lowering effects of repaglinide. Caution should be used in patients already on PRANDIN and gemfibrozil - blood glucose levels should be monitored and PRANDIN dose adjustment may be needed. Rare post-marketing events of serious hypoglycemia have been reported in patients taking PRANDIN and gemfibrozil together. Gemfibrozil and itraconazole had a synergistic metabolic inhibitory effect on PRANDIN. Therefore, patients taking PRANDIN and gemfibrozil should not take itraconazole.** See **CLINICAL PHARMACOLOGY** section, **Drug-Drug Interactions.**

The hypoglycemic action of oral blood glucose-lowering agents may be potentiated by certain drugs including nonsteroidal anti-inflammatory agents and other drugs that are highly protein bound, salicylates, sulfonamides, chloramphenicol, coumarins, probenecid, monoamine oxidase inhibitors, and beta adrenergic blocking agents. When such drugs are administered to a patient receiving oral blood glucose-lowering agents, the patient should be observed closely for hypoglycemia. When such drugs are withdrawn from a patient receiving oral blood glucose-lowering agents, the patient should be observed closely for loss of glycemic control. Certain drugs tend to produce hyperglycemia and may lead to loss of glycemic control. These drugs include the thiazides and other diuretics, corticosteroids, phenothiazines, thyroid products, estrogens, oral contraceptives, phenytoin, nicotinic acid, sympathomimetics, calcium channel blocking drugs, and isoniazid. When these drugs are administered to a patient receiving oral blood glucose-lowering agents, the patient should be observed for loss of glycemic control. When these drugs are withdrawn from a patient receiving oral blood glucose-lowering agents, the patient should be observed closely for hypoglycemia.

Carcinogenesis, Mutagenesis, and Impairment of Fertility

Long-term carcinogenicity studies were performed for 104 weeks at doses up to and including 120 mg/kg body weight/day (rats) and 500 mg/kg body weight/day (mice) or approximately 60 and 125 times clinical exposure, respectively, on a mg/m^2 basis. No evidence of carcinogenicity was found in mice or female rats. In male rats, there was an increased incidence of benign adenomas of the thyroid and liver. The relevance of these findings to humans is unclear. The no-effect doses for these observations in male rats were 30 mg/kg body weight/day for thyroid tumors and 60 mg/kg body weight/day for liver tumors, which are over 15 and 30 times, respectively, clinical exposure on a mg/m^2 basis.

Repaglinide was non-genotoxic in a battery of *in vivo* and *in vitro* studies: Bacterial mutagenesis (Ames test), *in vitro* forward cell mutation assay in V79 cells (HGPRT), *in vitro* chromosomal aberration assay in human lymphocytes, unscheduled and replicating DNA synthesis in rat liver, and *in vivo* mouse and rat micronucleus tests.

Fertility of male and female rats was unaffected by repaglinide administration at doses up to 80 mg/kg body weight/day (females) and 300 mg/kg body weight/day (males); over 40 times clinical exposure on a mg/m^2 basis.

Pregnancy

Pregnancy category C

Teratogenic Effects: Safety in pregnant women has not been established. Repaglinide was not teratogenic in rats or rabbits at doses 40 times (rats) and approximately 0.8 times (rabbit) clinical exposure (on a mg/m^2 basis) throughout pregnancy. Because animal reproduction studies are not always predictive of human response, PRANDIN should be used during pregnancy only if it is clearly needed.

Because recent information suggests that abnormal blood glucose levels during pregnancy are associated with a higher incidence of congenital abnormalities, many experts recommend that insulin be used during pregnancy to maintain blood glucose levels as close to normal as possible.

Nonteratogenic Effects: Offspring of rat dams exposed to repaglinide at 15 times clinical exposure on a mg/m^2 basis during days 17 to 22 of gestation and during lactation developed nonteratogenic skeletal deformities consisting of shortening, thickening, and bending of the humerus during the postnatal period. This effect was not seen at doses up to 2.5 times clinical exposure (on a mg/m^2 basis) on days 1 to 22 of pregnancy or at higher doses given during days 1 to 16 of pregnancy. Relevant human exposure has not occurred to date and therefore the safety of PRANDIN administration throughout pregnancy or lactation cannot be established.

Nursing Mothers

In rat reproduction studies, measurable levels of repaglinide were detected in the breast milk of the dams and lowered blood glucose levels were observed in the pups. Cross fostering studies indicated that skeletal changes (see **Nonteratogenic Effects**) could be induced in control pups nursed by treated dams, although this occurred to a lesser degree than those pups treated *in utero*. Although it is not known whether repaglinide is excreted in human milk some oral agents are known to be excreted by this route. Because the potential for hypoglycemia in nursing infants may exist, and because of the effects on nursing animals, a decision should be made as to whether PRANDIN should be discontinued in nursing mothers, or if mothers should discontinue nursing. If PRANDIN is discontinued and if diet alone is inadequate for controlling blood glucose, insulin therapy should be considered.

Pediatric Use

No studies have been performed in pediatric patients.

Geriatric Use

In repaglinide clinical studies of 24 weeks or greater duration, 415 patients were over 65 years of age. In one-year,

Continued on next page

Prandin—Cont.

active-controlled trials, no differences were seen in effectiveness or adverse events between these subjects and those less than 65 other than the expected age-related increase in cardiovascular events observed for PRANDIN and comparator drugs. There was no increase in frequency or severity of hypoglycemia in older subjects. Other reported clinical experience has not identified differences in responses between the elderly and younger patients, but greater sensitivity of some older individuals to PRANDIN therapy cannot be ruled out.

ADVERSE REACTIONS

Hypoglycemia: See **PRECAUTIONS** and **OVERDOSAGE** sections.

PRANDIN has been administered to 2931 individuals during clinical trials. Approximately 1500 of these individuals with type 2 diabetes have been treated for at least 3 months, 1000 for at least 6 months, and 800 for at least 1 year. The majority of these individuals (1228) received PRANDIN in one of five 1-year, active-controlled trials. The comparator drugs in these 1-year trials were oral sulfonylurea drugs (SU) including glyburide and glipizide. Over one year, 13% of PRANDIN patients were discontinued due to adverse events, as were 14% of SU patients. The most common adverse events leading to withdrawal were hyperglycemia, hypoglycemia, and related symptoms (see **PRECAUTIONS**). Mild or moderate hypoglycemia occurred in 16% of PRANDIN patients, 20% of glyburide patients, and 19% of glipizide patients.

The table below lists common adverse events for PRANDIN patients compared to both placebo (in trials 12 to 24 weeks duration) and to glyburide and glipizide in one year trials. The adverse event profile of PRANDIN was generally comparable to that for sulfonylurea drugs (SU).

[See table at top of previous page]

Cardiovascular events also occur commonly in patients with type 2 diabetes. In one-year comparator trials, the incidence of individual events was not greater than 1% except for chest pain (1.8%) and angina (1.8%). The individual incidence of other cardiovascular events (hypertension, abnormal EKG, myocardial infarction, arrhythmias, and palpitations) was ≤1% and not different for PRANDIN and the comparator drugs.

The incidence of serious cardiovascular adverse events added together, including ischemia, was slightly higher for repaglinide (4%) than for sulfonylurea drugs (3%) in controlled comparator clinical trials. In 1-year controlled trials, PRANDIN treatment was not associated with excess mortality rates compared to rates observed with other oral hypoglycemic agent therapies.

Summary of Serious Cardiovascular Events (% of total patients with events)

	PRANDIN	SU*
Total Exposed	1228	498
Serious CV Events	4%	3%
Cardiac Ischemic Events	2%	2%
Deaths due to CV Events	0.5%	0.4%

* glyburide and glipizide

Infrequent adverse events (<1% of patients)

Less common adverse clinical or laboratory events observed in clinical trials included elevated liver enzymes, thrombocytopenia, leukopenia, and anaphylactoid reactions (one patient).

Combination therapy with thiazolidinediones

During 24-week treatment clinical trials of PRANDIN-rosiglitazone or PRANDIN-pioglitazone combination therapy (a total of 250 patients in combination therapy), hypoglycemia (blood glucose < 50 mg/dL) occurred in 7% of combination therapy patients in comparison to 7% for PRANDIN monotherapy, and 2% for thiazolidinedione monotherapy.

Peripheral edema was reported in 12 out of 250 PRANDIN-thiazolidinedione combination therapy patients and 3 out of 124 thiazolidinedione monotherapy patients, with no cases reported in these trials for PRANDIN monotherapy. When corrected for dropout rates of the treatment groups, the percentage of patients having events of peripheral edema per 24 weeks of treatment were 5% for PRANDIN-thiazolidinedione combination therapy, and 4% for thiazolidinedione monotherapy. There were reports in 2 of 250 patients (0.8%) treated with PRANDIN-thiazolidinedione therapy of episodes of edema with congestive heart failure. Both patients had a prior history of coronary artery disease and recovered after treatment with diuretic agents. No comparable cases in the monotherapy treatment groups were reported.

Mean change in weight from baseline was +4.9 kg for PRANDIN-thiazolidinedione therapy. There were no patients on PRANDIN-thiazolidinedione combination therapy who had elevations of liver transaminases (defined as 3 times the upper limit of normal levels).

Although no causal relationship has been established, postmarketing experience includes reports of the following rare adverse events: alopecia, hemolytic anemia, pancreatitis, Stevens-Johnson Syndrome, and severe hepatic dysfunction.

OVERDOSAGE

In a clinical trial, patients received increasing doses of PRANDIN up to 80 mg a day for 14 days. There were few adverse effects other than those associated with the intended effect of lowering blood glucose. Hypoglycemia did not occur when meals were given with these high doses. Hypoglycemic symptoms without loss of consciousness or neurologic findings should be treated aggressively with oral glucose and adjustments in drug dosage and/or meal patterns. Close monitoring may continue until the physician is assured that the patient is out of danger. Patients should be closely monitored for a minimum of 24 to 48 hours, since hypoglycemia may recur after apparent clinical recovery. There is no evidence that repaglinide is dialyzable using hemodialysis.

Severe hypoglycemic reactions with coma, seizure, or other neurological impairment occur infrequently, but constitute medical emergencies requiring immediate hospitalization. If hypoglycemic coma is diagnosed or suspected, the patient should be given a rapid intravenous injection of concentrated (50%) glucose solution. This should be followed by a continuous infusion of more dilute (10%) glucose solution at a rate that will maintain the blood glucose at a level above 100 mg/dL.

DOSAGE AND ADMINISTRATION

There is no fixed dosage regimen for the management of type 2 diabetes with PRANDIN.

The patient's blood glucose should be monitored periodically to determine the minimum effective dose for the patient; to detect primary failure, i.e., inadequate lowering of blood glucose at the maximum recommended dose of medication; and to detect secondary failure, i.e., loss of an adequate blood glucose-lowering response after an initial period of effectiveness. Glycosylated hemoglobin levels are of value in monitoring the patient's longer term response to therapy.

Short-term administration of PRANDIN may be sufficient during periods of transient loss of control in patients usually well controlled on diet.

PRANDIN doses are usually taken within 15 minutes of the meal but time may vary from immediately preceding the meal to as long as 30 minutes before the meal.

Starting Dose

For patients not previously treated or whose HbA_{1c} is <8%, the starting dose should be 0.5 mg with each meal. For patients previously treated with blood glucose-lowering drugs and whose HbA_{1c} is ≥ 8%, the initial dose is 1 or 2 mg with each meal preprandially (see previous paragraph).

Dose Adjustment

Dosing adjustments should be determined by blood glucose response, usually fasting blood glucose. Postprandial glucose levels testing may be clinically helpful in patients whose pre-meal blood glucose levels are satisfactory but whose overall glycemic control (HbA_{1c}) is inadequate. The preprandial dose should be doubled up to 4 mg with each meal until satisfactory blood glucose response is achieved. At least one week should elapse to assess response after each dose adjustment.

The recommended dose range is 0.5 mg to 4 mg taken with meals. PRANDIN may be dosed preprandially 2, 3, or 4 times a day in response to changes in the patient's meal pattern. The maximum recommended daily dose is 16 mg.

Patient Management

Long-term efficacy should be monitored by measurement of HbA_{1c} levels approximately every 3 months. Failure to follow an appropriate dosage regimen may precipitate hypoglycemia or hyperglycemia. Patients who do not adhere to their prescribed dietary and drug regimen are more prone to exhibit unsatisfactory response to therapy including hypoglycemia. When hypoglycemia occurs in patients taking a combination of PRANDIN and a thiazolidinedione or PRANDIN and metformin, the dose of PRANDIN should be reduced.

Patients Receiving Other Oral Hypoglycemic Agents

When PRANDIN is used to replace therapy with other oral hypoglycemic agents, PRANDIN may be started on the day after the final dose is given. Patients should then be observed carefully for hypoglycemia due to potential overlapping of drug effects. When transferred from longer half-life sulfonylurea agents (e.g., chlorpropamide) to repaglinide, close monitoring may be indicated for up to one week or longer.

Combination Therapy

If PRANDIN monotherapy does not result in adequate glycemic control, metformin or a thiazolidinedione may be added. If metformin or thiazolidinedione monotherapy does not provide adequate control, PRANDIN may be added. The starting dose and dose adjustments for PRANDIN combination therapy is the same as for PRANDIN monotherapy. The dose of each drug should be carefully adjusted to determine the minimal dose required to achieve the desired pharmacologic effect. Failure to do so could result in an increase in the incidence of hypoglycemic episodes. Appropriate monitoring of FPG and HbA_{1c} measurements should be used to ensure that the patient is not subjected to excessive drug exposure or increased probability of secondary drug failure.

HOW SUPPLIED

PRANDIN (repaglinide) tablets are supplied as unscored, biconvex tablets available in 0.5 mg (white), 1 mg (yellow) and 2 mg (peach) strengths. Tablets are embossed with the Novo Nordisk (Apis) bull symbol and colored to indicate strength.

0.5 mg tablets (white)	Bottles of 100	NDC 00169-0081-81
	Bottles of 500	NDC 00169-0081-82
	Bottles of 1000	NDC 00169-0081-83
1 mg tablets (yellow)	Bottles of 100	NDC 00169-0082-81
	Bottles of 500	NDC 00169-0082-82
	Bottles of 1000	NDC 00169-0082-83
2 mg tablets (peach)	Bottles of 100	NDC 00169-0084-81
	Bottles of 500	NDC 00169-0084-82
	Bottles of 1000	NDC 00169-0084-83

Do not store above 25°C (77°F).
Protect from moisture.
Keep bottles tightly closed.
Dispense in tight containers with safety closures.
Licensed under US Patent Nos. RE37,035, 5,312,924 and 6,143,769

PRANDIN® is a registered trademark of Novo Nordisk A/S.

Manufactured in Germany for
Novo Nordisk
Pharmaceuticals, Inc.
Princeton, NJ 08540
1-800-727-6500
www.novonordisk-us.com

Shown in Product Identification Guide, page 326

VAGIFEM® ℞

[văg ə′ fĕm]

(estradiol vaginal tablets)
25µg
PHYSICIAN PACKAGE INSERT

ESTROGENS HAVE BEEN REPORTED TO INCREASE THE RISK OF ENDOMETRIAL CARCINOMA.

Three independent, case controlled studies have reported an increased risk of endometrial cancer in postmenopausal women exposed to exogenous estrogens for more than one year. This risk was independent of the other known risk factors for endometrial cancer. These studies are further supported by the finding that incident rates of endometrial cancer have increased sharply since 1969 in eight different areas of the United States with population-based cancer-reporting systems, an increase which may be related to the rapidly expanding use of estrogens during the last decade.

The three case-controlled studies reported that the risk of endometrial cancer in estrogen users was about 4.5 to 13.9 times greater than in nonusers. The risk appears to depend on both duration of treatment and on estrogen dose. In view of these findings, when estrogens are used for the treatment of menopausal symptoms, the lowest dose that will control symptoms should be utilized and medication should be discontinued as soon as possible. When prolonged treatment is medically indicated, the patient should be reassessed, on at least a semi-annual basis, to determine the need for continued therapy.

Close clinical surveillance of all women taking estrogens is important. In all cases of undiagnosed persistent or reoccurring abnormal vaginal bleeding, adequate diagnostic measures should be undertaken to rule out malignancy.

There is no evidence at present that "natural" estrogens are more or less hazardous than "synthetic" estrogens at equi-estrogenic doses.

DESCRIPTION

VAGIFEM® (estradiol vaginal tablets) are small, white, film-coated tablets containing 25.8µg of estradiol hemihydrate equivalent to 25µg of estradiol.

Each tablet contains the following inactive ingredients: hypromellose, lactose monohydrate, maize starch and magnesium stearate. The film coating contains hypromellose and polyethylene glycol. Each white tablet is 6 mm in diameter and is placed in a disposable applicator.

Each tablet-filled applicator is packaged separately in a blister pack. 17β-estradiol hemihydrate is a white, almost white or colorless crystalline solid, chemically described as estra-1,3,5 (10)-triene-3, 17 diol.

The chemical formula is $C_{18}H_{24}O_2 \cdot {}^1/_2\, H_2O$ with a molecular weight of 281.4.

The structural formula is:

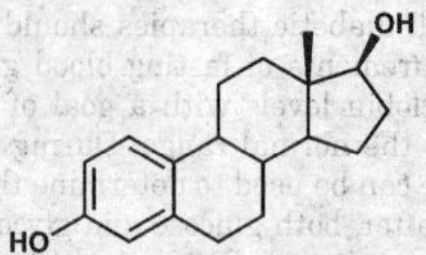

CLINICAL PHARMACOLOGY

In vivo estrogens diffuse through cell membranes, distribute throughout the cell, bind to and activate the estrogen receptors, thereby eliciting their biological effects. Estrogen receptors have been identified in tissue of the reproductive tract, breast, pituitary, hypothalamus, liver and bone of women. The estrogen contained in VAGIFEM, 17 β-estradiol is chemically and biologically identical to the endogenous human 17 β-estradiol and is, therefore, classified as a human estrogen.

Estrogens regulate growth, differentiation and functioning of many different tissues within and outside of the reproductive system. Estrogens are intricately involved with other hormones, especially progesterone, and during the ovulatory phase of the menstrual cycle cause proliferation of the endometrium. Most of the activity of estrogens appear to be exerted via estrogen receptors in target cells of tissues of the woman's reproductive tract: breast, pituitary, hypothalamus, brain, liver, and bone.

The steroid-receptor complex is bound to the cell's DNA and induces synthesis of specific proteins.

Maturation of the vaginal epithelium is dependent on estrogen as it increases the number of superficial and intermediate cells as compared with basal cells. Estrogen keeps the pH of the vagina at approximately 4.5 which enhances normal bacterial flora, predominately, *Lactobacillus döderlein*.

Pharmacokinetics

Absorption

Estrogen drug products are well absorbed through the skin, mucous membranes, and the gastrointestinal (GI) tract. The vaginal delivery of estrogens circumvents first-pass metabolism.

A single-center, randomized, double-blind comparison study conducted in the U.S. showed that vaginal application of VAGIFEM® over a 12-week course demonstrated a mean C_{max} of estradiol of 50 pg/mL and that there was no significant accumulation of estradiol as measured by the AUC_{0-24} (See Table 1 below).

Table 1:
MEAN (±STANDARD DEVIATION) PHARMACOKINETIC PARAMETERS FOR ESTRADIOL
(Uncorrected for base line)

	Timepoint Day 1	Day 14	Day 84
PK Parameter:			
AUC (pg.hr/mL)	538 (±265)	567 (±246)	563 (±341)
C_{max} (pg/mL)	51 (±34)	47 (±21)	49 (±27)

Distribution

Circulating, unbound estrogens are known to modulate pharmacological response. Estrogens circulate in the blood bound to sex-hormone binding globulin (SHBG) and albumin. A dynamic equilibrium exists between the conjugated and the unconjugated forms of estradiol and estrone, which undergo rapid interconversion.

Metabolism

Exogenously-delivered or endogenously-derived estrogens are primarily metabolized in the liver to estrone and estriol, which are also found in the systemic circulation. VAGIFEM intravaginal administration avoids first-pass metabolism that occurs with oral estrogens.

The levels of E_1 seen during 12 weeks of VAGIFEM administration do not show any accumulation of E_1, and the observed values are within the postmenopausal range. See Table 2 below.

Table 2:
MEAN (±STANDARD DEVIATION) PHARMACOKINETIC PARAMETERS FOR ESTRONE
(Uncorrected for base line)

	Timepoint Day 1	Day 14	Day 84
E1:			
AUC (pg.hr/mL)	649 (±230)	744 (±267)	681 (±271)
C_{max} (pg/mL)	35 (±12)	39 (±13)	35 (±12)

Excretion

Estrogen metabolites are primarily excreted in the urine as glucoronides and sulfates.

Drug-Drug Interactions

No formal drug-drug interaction studies have been done with VAGIFEM.

CLINICAL STUDIES

A placebo-controlled comparison study was done in the U.S., in which 230 patients were randomized to receive either placebo, VAGIFEM, or 10μg estradiol vaginal tablets.

Patients inserted one tablet intravaginally each day for 14 days, then one tablet twice weekly for the remaining 10 weeks. All patients were assessed for vaginal symptoms. VAGIFEM® was superior to placebo in the relief of symptoms of the dryness, soreness, and irritation associated with atrophic vaginitis. This change of symptoms was seen at Week 7 and was maintained throughout to Week 12. (See Figure 1)

An open, controlled comparison study was done in Canada in which 159 patients were randomized to receive either VAGIFEM or the conjugated estrogen vaginal cream, comparator drug. Two (2) grams (~ 1.25 mg conjugated estrogens) of the comparator drug, which is the highest approved dose, was given daily for 3 weeks, withheld for 1 week, then repeated cyclically (3 weeks on, 1 week off) for up to 24 weeks; VAGIFEM was administered daily for 2 weeks, then twice weekly for the remaining 22 weeks. Of all patients entering into treatment phase of the study 10% of patients discontinued their treatment in the VAGIFEM group and 32% discontinued their treatment in the comparator group. In this study, patients were assessed for relief of symptoms. VAGIFEM 25μg was not less effective than the approved comparator product at the 2.0 gm dose in the relief of symptoms.

Symptoms of dryness, soreness, and irritation were rated as 0 = none, 1 = mild, 2 = moderate and 3 = severe. The average severity score of the three symptoms over time for the placebo controlled and comparator studies are shown in the following figures:

Figure 1
(Placebo controlled)

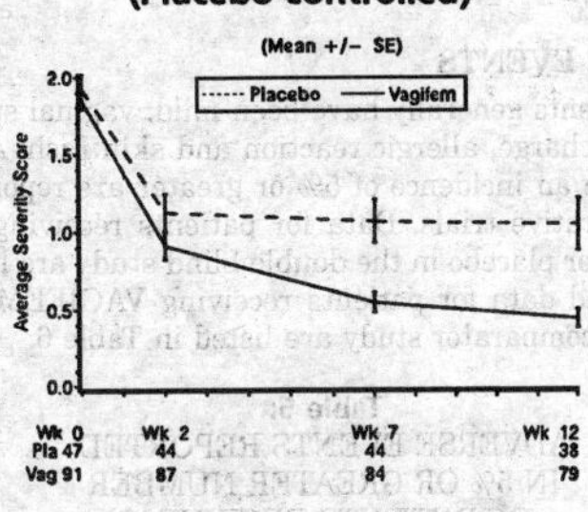

Figure 2
(Comparator)

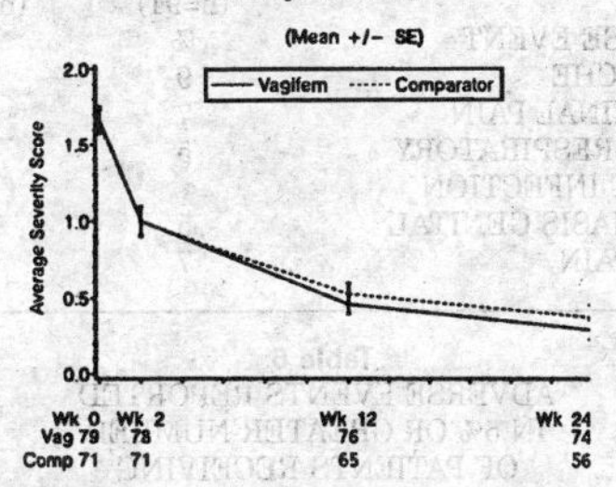

The endometrium was evaluated at the end of each study by endometrial biopsy. See Tables 3 & 4 below.

Table 3:
ENDOMETRIAL BIOPSY RESULTS COMPARING VAGIFEM WITH PLACEBO OVER 12 WEEKS OF TREATMENT
(US Trial)

	VAGIFEM	Placebo
Total Number of Patients enrolled	91	47
Patients with uterus (non-hysterectomized)	48	24
Total Biopsies	32	21
Atrophic Endometrium	27 (84%)	18 (86%)
Weakly Proliferative	0 (0%)	0 (0%)
Proliferative	1 (3%)	0 (0%)
Simple Hyperplasia	1 (3%)	0 (0%)
Complex Hyperplasia	0 (0%)	0 (0%)
Insufficient Tissue	3 (9%)	3 (14%)

Table 4:
ENDOMETRIAL BIOPSY RESULTS COMPARING VAGIFEM TO COMPARATOR GIVEN OVER 24 WEEKS

	VAGIFEM	Comparator
Total Number of Patients enrolled	80	79
Patients with uterus (non-hysterectomized)	80	79
Total Biopsies	49	49
Atrophic Endometrium	34 (68%)	15 (30%)
Weakly Proliferative	0 (0%)	4 (8%)
Proliferative	1 (2%)	7 (14%)
Simple Hyperplasia	0 (0%)	1 (2%)
Complex Hyperplasia	0 (0%)	1 (2%)
Insufficient Tissue	14 (28%)	21 (42%)

INDICATIONS AND USE

VAGIFEM® is indicated for the treatment of atrophic vaginitis.

CONTRAINDICATIONS

The use of VAGIFEM is contraindicated in women who exhibit one or more of the following:

1. Known or suspected breast carcinoma.
2. Known or suspected estrogen-dependent neoplasia; e.g. endometrial carcinoma.
3. Abnormal genital bleeding of unknown etiology.
4. Known or suspected pregnancy. (See PRECAUTIONS)
5. Porphyria.
6. Hypersensitivity to any VAGIFEM constituents.
7. Active thrombophlebitis or thromboembolic disorders.
8. A past history of thrombophlebitis, thrombosis, or thromboembolic disorders associated with previous estrogen use (except when used in treatment of breast malignancy).

WARNINGS

1. *Induction of malignant neoplasms.* Long-term, continuous administration of natural and synthetic estrogens in certain animal species increases the frequency of carcinomas of the breast, cervix, vagina, and liver. There are now reports that estrogens increase risk of carcinoma of the endometrium in humans (See Boxed Warning).

At the present time there is no satisfactory evidence that estrogens given to postmenopausal women increase the risk of cancer of the breast, although a recent long-term follow-up of a single physician's practice has raised this possibility. Because of the animal data, there is a need for caution in prescribing estrogens for women with a strong family history of breast cancer or who have breast nodules, fibrocystic disease, or abnormal mammograms.

2. *Gallbladder disease.* A recent study has reported a 2- to 3-fold increase in the risk of surgically confirmed gallbladder disease in women receiving postmenopausal estrogens, similar to the 2-fold increase previously noted in users of oral contraceptives.

3. *Effects similar to those caused by estrogen-progestogen oral contraceptives.* There are several serious adverse effects of oral contraceptives, most of which have not, up to now, been documented as consequences of postmenopausal estrogen therapy. This may reflect the comparatively low doses of estrogens used in postmenopausal women. It would be expected that the larger doses of estrogen used to treat prostatic or breast cancer are more likely to result in these adverse effects, and, in fact, it has been shown that there is an increased risk of thrombosis in men receiving estrogens for prostatic cancer.

a. *Thromboembolic disease.* It is now well established that users of oral contraceptives have an increased risk of various thromboembolic and thrombotic vascular diseases, such as thrombophlebitis, pulmonary embolism, stroke, and myocardial infarction. Cases of retinal thrombosis, mesenteric thrombosis, and optic neuritis have been reported in oral-contraceptive users. There is evidence that the risk of several of these adverse reactions is related to the dose of the drug. An increased risk of postsurgery thromboembolic complications has also been reported in users of oral contraceptives. If feasible, estrogen should be discontinued at least 4 weeks before surgery of the type associated with an increased risk of thromboembolism, or during periods of prolonged immobilization.

While an increased rate of thromboembolism and thrombotic disease in postmenopausal users of estrogens has not been found, this does not rule out the possibility that such an increase may be present, or that subgroups of women who have underlying risk factors, or who are receiving large doses of estrogens, may have increased risk. Therefore, estrogens should not be used (except in treatment of malignancy) in a person with a history of such disorders in association with estrogen use. They should be used with caution in patients with cerebral vascular or coronary artery disease and only for those in whom estrogens are clearly needed.

Large doses of estrogens (5 mg conjugated estrogens per day), comparable to those used to treat cancer of the prostate and breast, have been shown in a large prospective clinical trial in men, to increase the risk of nonfatal myocardial infarction, pulmonary embolism, and thrombophlebitis. When estrogen doses of this size are used, any of the thromboembolic and thrombotic adverse effects associated with oral contraceptive use should be considered a clear risk.

b. *Hepatic adenoma.* Benign hepatic adenomas appear to be associated with the oral contraceptives.

Although benign, and rare, these may rupture and may cause death through intra-abdominal hemorrhage. Such lesions have not yet been reported in association with other estrogen or progestogen preparations but should be considered in estrogen users having abdominal pain and tenderness, abdominal mass, or hypovolemic shock.

Hepatocellular carcinoma has also been reported in women taking estrogen-containing oral contraceptives. The relationship of this malignancy to these drugs is not known at this time.

c. *Elevated blood pressure.* Women using oral contraceptives sometimes experience increased blood pressure which, in most cases, returns to normal on discontinuing the drug. There is now a report that this may occur with the use of estrogens in the menopause and blood pressure should be monitored with estrogen use, especially if high doses are used.

d. *Glucose tolerance.* A worsening of glucose tolerance has been observed in a significant percentage of patients on estrogen-containing oral contraceptives. For this reason, diabetic patients should be carefully observed while using estrogens.

4. *Hypercalcemia.* Administration of estrogens may lead to severe hypercalcemia in patients with breast cancer and

Continued on next page

Vagifem—Cont.

bone metastases. If this occurs, the drug should be stopped and appropriate measures taken to reduce the serum calcium level.

5. *Rare Event:* Trauma induced by the VAGIFEM® applicator may occur, especially in patients with severely atrophic vaginal mucosa.

PRECAUTIONS

A. General Precautions.

1. A complete medical and family history should be taken prior to the initiation of any estrogen therapy.
The pretreatment and periodic physical examinations should include special references to blood pressure, breast, abdomen, and pelvic organs, and should include a Papanicolaou smear. As a general rule, estrogens should not be prescribed for longer than one year without another physical exam being performed.
2. Fluid retention—Because estrogens may cause some degree of fluid retention, conditions which might be influenced by this factor, such as asthma, epilepsy, migraine, and cardiac and renal dysfunction, require careful observation.
3. Familial Hyperlipoproteinemia—Estrogen therapy may be associated with massive elevations of plasma triglycerides leading to pancreatitis and other complications in patients with familial defects of lipoprotein metabolism.
4. Certain patients may develop undesirable manifestations of excessive estrogenic stimulation, such as abnormal or excessive uterine bleeding, mastodynia, etc.
5. Prolonged administration of unopposed estrogen therapy has been reported to increase the risk of endometrial hyperplasia in some patients.
6. Preexisting uterine leiomyomata may increase in size during estrogen use.
7. The pathologist should be advised of estrogen therapy when relevant specimens are submitted.
8. Patients with a history of jaundice during pregnancy have an increased risk of recurrence of jaundice while receiving estrogen-containing oral contraceptive therapy. If jaundice develops in any patient receiving estrogen, the medication should be discontinued while the cause is investigated.
9. Estrogens may be poorly metabolized in patients with impaired liver function and should be administered with caution in such patients.
10. Because estrogens influence the metabolism of calcium and phosphorus, they should be used with caution in patients with metabolic bone diseases that are associated with hypercalcemia or in patients with renal insufficiency.
11. Because of the effects of estrogens on epiphyseal closure, they should be used judiciously in young patients in whom bone growth is not yet complete.
12. Insertion of the VAGIFEM® applicator—Patients with severly atrophic vaginal mucosa should be instructed to exercise care during insertion of the applicator. After gynecological surgery, any vaginal applicator should be used with caution and only if clearly indicated.
13. Vaginal infection—Vaginal infection is generally more common in postmenopausal women due to the lack of normal flora seen in fertile women, especially lactobacilla; hence the subsequent higher pH. Vaginal infections should be treated with appropriate antimicrobial therapy before initiation of VAGIFEM therapy.

B. Information for the Patient

See text of patient Package Insert which appears above.

C. Drug/Laboratory Test Interactions

Certain endocrine and liver function tests may be affected by estrogen-containing oral contraceptives. The following similar changes may be expected with larger doses of estrogens:

a. Increased prothrombin and factors VII, VIII, IX, and X, decreased antithrombin III; increased norepinephrine induced platelet aggregability.
b. Increased thyroid binding globulin (TBG) leading to increased circulating total thyroid hormone, as measured by PBI, T_4 by column, or T_4 by radioimmunoassay. Free T_4 resin uptake is decreased, reflecting the elevated TBG, free T_4 concentration is unaltered.
c. Impaired glucose tolerance.
d. Reduced response to metyrapone test.
e. Reduced serum folate concentration.
f. Increased serum triglyceride and phospholipid concentration.

D. Carcinogenesis, Mutagenesis and Impairment of Fertility

Long term continuous administration of natural and synthetic estrogens in certain animal species increases the frequency of carcinomas of the breast, uterus, vagina and liver. (See CONTRAINDICATIONS AND WARNINGS)

E. Pregnancy Category X

Estrogens are not indicated for use during pregnancy or the immediate postpartum period. Estrogens are ineffective for the prevention or treatment of threatened or habitual abortion. Treatment with diethylstilbesterol (DES) during pregnancy has been associated with an increased risk of congenital defects and cancer in the reproductive organs of the fetus, and possibly other birth defects. The use of DES during pregnancy has also been associated with a subsequent increased risk of breast cancer in the mothers.

F. Nursing Mothers

As a general principle, administration of any drug to nursing mothers should be done only when clearly necessary since many drugs are excreted in human milk. In addition, estrogen administration to nursing mothers has been shown to decrease the quantity and quality of the milk. Estrogens are not indicated for the prevention of postpartum breast engorgement.

G. Pediatric Use

Safety and effectiveness in pediatric patients have not been established.

H. Geriatric Use

Clinical studies of VAGIFEM® did not include sufficient numbers of subjects aged 65 and over to determine whether they respond differently from younger subjects. Other reported clinical experience has not identified differences in responses between the elderly and younger patients. In general, dose selection for an elderly patient should be cautious, usually starting at the low end of the dosing range, reflecting the greater frequency of decreased hepatic, renal, or cardiac function, and of concomitant disease or other drug therapy.

ADVERSE EVENTS

Adverse events generally have been mild: vaginal spotting, vaginal discharge, allergic reaction and skin rash. Adverse events with an incidence of 5% or greater are reported for two comparative trials. Data for patients receiving either VAGIFEM or placebo in the double blind study are listed in Table 5, and data for patients receiving VAGIFEM in the open label comparator study are listed in Table 6.

Table 5:
ADVERSE EVENTS REPORTED IN 5% OR GREATER NUMBER OF PATIENTS RECEIVING VAGIFEM® IN THE PLACEBO CONTROLLED TRIAL.

	VAGIFEM	Placebo
	(n=91)	(n=47)
ADVERSE EVENT	%	%
HEADACHE	9	6
ABDOMINAL PAIN	7	4
UPPER RESPIRATORY TRACT INFECTION	5	4
MONILIASIS GENITAL	5	2
BACK PAIN	7	6

Table 6:
ADVERSE EVENTS REPORTED IN 5% OR GREATER NUMBER OF PATIENTS RECEIVING VAGIFEM® IN THE OPEN LABEL STUDY.

	VAGIFEM
	(n=80)
ADVERSE EVENT	%
PRURITUS GENITAL	6
HEADACHE	10
UPPER RESPIRATORY TRACT INFECTION	11

Other adverse events that occurred in 3–5% of VAGIFEM subjects included: allergy, bronchitis, dyspepsia, haematuria, hot flashes, insomnia, pain, sinusitis, vaginal discomfort, vaginitis. A causal relationship to VAGIFEM has not been established.

OVERDOSAGE

Numerous reports of ingestion of large doses of estrogen containing oral contraceptives by young children indicate that acute serious ill effects do not occur. Overdosage with estrogens may cause nausea, and withdrawal bleeding may occur in females.

DOSAGE AND ADMINISTRATION

VAGIFEM is gently inserted into the vagina as far as it can comfortably go without force, using the supplied applicator.

- Initial dose: One (1) VAGIFEM tablet, inserted vaginally, once daily for two (2) weeks. It is advisable to have the patient administer treatment at the same time each day.
- Maintenance dose: One (1) VAGIFEM tablet, inserted vaginally, twice weekly.

The need to continue therapy should be assessed by the physician with the patient. Attempts to discontinue or taper medication should be made at three to six month intervals.

HOW SUPPLIED

Each VAGIFEM® (estradiol vaginal tablets), 25µg is contained in a disposable, single-use applicator, packaged in a blister pack. Cartons contain 8 or 18 applicators with inset tablets.

8 applicators: NDC 0169-5173-03
18 applicators: NDC 0169-5173-04

STORAGE: Store at 25°C (77°F); excursions permitted to 15°C–30°C (59°F–86°F). [See USP Controlled Room Temperature.]

Rx only

Vagifem® is a trademark owned by Novo Nordisk AS
Revised July 2003
Novo Nordisk Pharmaceuticals, Inc.
Princeton, NJ 08540
1-888-824-4336
www.novonordisk-us.com

Manufactured by
Novo Nordisk AS
2880 Bagsværd, Denmark

INFORMATION FOR PATIENTS

Introduction

This leaflet describes when and how to use VAGIFEM® (estradiol vaginal tablets) and the risks and benefits of estrogen treatment. Please read this information carefully before starting treatment.

Estrogens have important benefits but also some risks. You must decide, with your doctor or health care provider, whether the risks to you of estrogen use are acceptable because of their benefits. If you use estrogens, check with your health care provider to be sure you are using the dose that is appropriate for you, and that you don't use them longer than necessary. How long you need to use estrogens should be decided by you and your health care provider. Estrogens are hormones made by the ovaries of normal women. Between ages 45 and 55, the ovaries normally stop making estrogens. This leads to a drop in body estrogen levels which causes the "change of life" or menopause (the end of monthly menstrual periods). If both ovaries are removed during an operation before natural menopause takes place, the sudden drop in estrogen levels causes "surgical menopause."

When the estrogen levels begin dropping, some women develop very uncomfortable symptoms, such as feeling of warmth in the face, neck, and chest, or sudden intense episodes of heat and sweating ("hot flashes" or "hot flushes"). Using estrogen drugs can help the body adjust to lower estrogen levels and reduce these symptoms. Most women have only mild menopausal symptoms or none at all and may not need to use estrogen drugs. VAGIFEM DOES NOT PROVIDE ENOUGH ESTROGEN TO REDUCE THESE SYMPTOMS.

The declining estrogen levels associated with advancing age after menopause may also result in thinning and drying of the tissue in the vagina and urinary tract (urogenital atrophy). Vaginal symptoms of this condition include dryness in the vagina (atrophic vaginitis), genital itching and burning, and pain with intercourse. Urinary symptoms may include urinary urgency and pain on urination. Small amounts of estrogens delivered directly to the local tissue can be used to help reduce these symptoms.

Use of VAGIFEM®

(estradiol vaginal tablets)

VAGIFEM is a local estrogen therapy designed to relieve vaginal symptoms, a major component of the urogenital symptoms found in post-menopausal estrogen deficiency. VAGIFEM® (estradiol vaginal tablets) exerts its effect locally in the lower urogenital tract, particularly the vagina, and has not been associated with significant effects in other estrogen-sensitive organs or tissues of the body. Consequently, VAGIFEM provides relief of local symptoms of menopause only.

Description

VAGIFEM® (estradiol vaginal tablets) contains 25µg (micrograms) of estrogen (estradiol). VAGIFEM releases estradiol into the vagina. A gel layer forms when the tablet comes in contact with the vagina. The estradiol is released from this gel layer. See Figure 1.

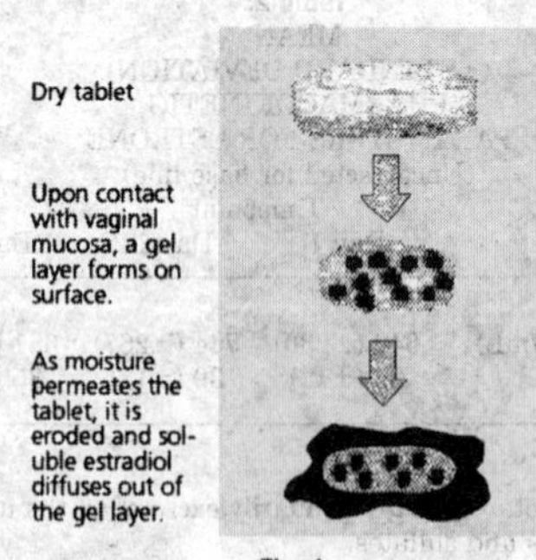
Dry tablet
Upon contact with vaginal mucosa, a gel layer forms on surface.
As moisture permeates the tablet, it is eroded and soluble estradiol diffuses out of the gel layer.

Fig. 1

Dosage

One (1) VAGIFEM tablet inserted vaginally once daily for the first two (2) weeks. Then one (1) tablet twice weekly. (See table below).

Administration Regimen

Days:	1	2	3	4	5	6	7
Week 1 1 Vagifem tablet everyday	/	/	/	/	/	/	/
Week 2 1 Vagifem tablet everyday	/	/	/	/	/	/	/
Week 3 and Thereafter 1 Vagifem tablet twice weekly			/			/	

Directions for use of VAGIFEM®:

Step 1: Tear off a single applicator.

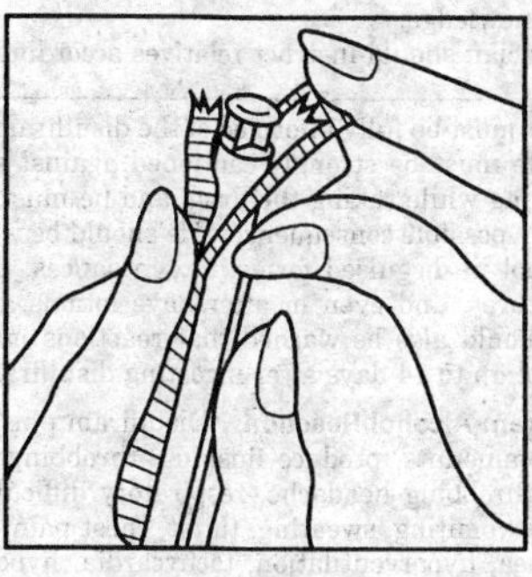

Fig.2

Step 2: Separate the plastic wrap and remove the applicator from the plastic wrap. See Figure 2.

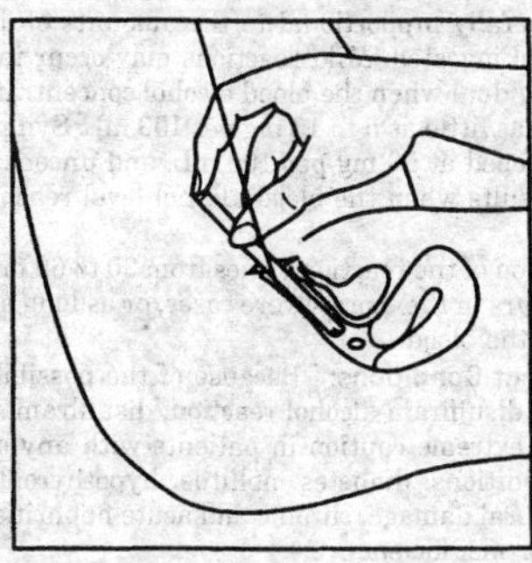

Fig.3

Step 3: First select the best position for vaginal insertion of VAGIFEM® (estradiol vaginal tablets) that is most comfortable for you. See suggested reclining Figure 3 or standing Figure 4 position illustrated below:

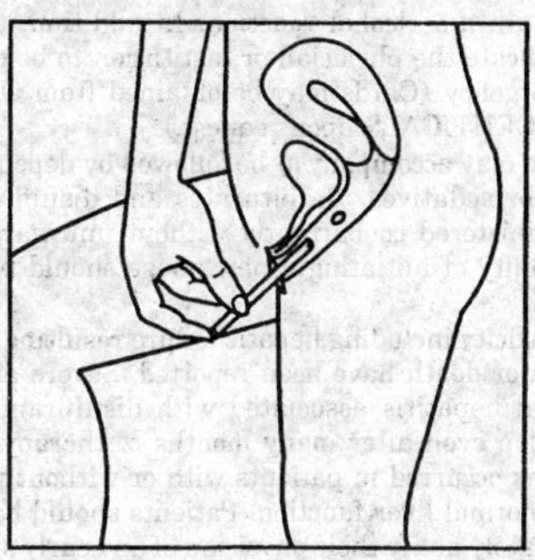

Fig.4

Step 4: The applicator should be held so that the finger of one hand can press the applicator plunger. See Figure 5.

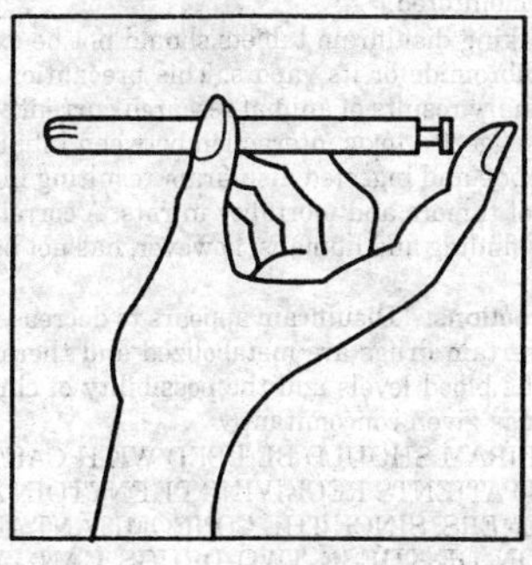

Fig.5

Step 5: The other hand should be used to guide the applicator gently and comfortably through the vaginal opening (see Figures 3 and 4 above). If the tablet has come out of the applicator prior to insertion, do not attempt to replace it. Use a fresh tablet-filled applicator.

Step 6: The applicator should be inserted (without forcing) as far as comfortably possible, or until half of the applicator is inside your vagina, whichever is less.

Step 7: Once the tablet-filled applicator has been inserted, gently press the plunger until a click is heard and the plunger is fully depressed. This will eject the tablet inside your vagina where it will dissolve slowly over several hours.

Step 8: After depressing the plunger, gently remove the applicator and dispose of it the same way you would a plastic tampon applicator. The applicator is of no further use and should be discarded properly. Insertion may be done at any time of the day. It is advisable to use the same time daily for all applications of VAGIFEM® (estradiol vaginal tablets). If you have any questions, please consult your health care provider or pharmacist.

Who Should Not Use VAGIFEM®

(estradiol vaginal tablets)

VAGIFEM should not be used:

During pregnancy—Women who are definitely postmenopausal cannot become pregnant. Women who believe they are postmenopausal because their menstrual cycles have recently stopped should confirm that they are not pregnant before using any form of estrogen-containing drug. Using estrogens while pregnant may cause the unborn child to have birth defects. Estrogens do not prevent miscarriage.

In the presence of unusual vaginal bleeding which has not been evaluated by a health care provider. Unusual vaginal bleeding after menopause can be a warning sign of cancer of the uterus. Estrogens may increase the risk of cancer of the uterus in women who have had their menopause ("change of life"). If you use any estrogen-containing drug, it is important to visit your health care provider regularly and report any unusual vaginal bleeding right away. Your health care provider should evaluate any unusual vaginal bleeding to find out the cause.

If there is a history of certain types of cancer—Estrogens may increase the risk of certain types of cancer, usually uterine or breast. VAGIFEM has not been associated with an increased risk of uterine cancer. Although there are reports of increased risk of breast cancer in women on hormone replacement therapy, VAGIFEM is administered locally and is not expected to pose an increased risk.

After childbirth or when breast-feeding a baby—VAGIFEM should not be used to try to stop the breasts from filling with milk after a baby is born. Women who are breast-feeding should avoid using any drugs because many drugs pass through to the baby in the milk. While nursing a baby, drugs should only be taken on the advice of your healthcare giver.

Possible Risks from Treatment with Estrogens

The following risk factors apply to estrogens in general:

Cancer of the uterus—Estrogens increase the risk of developing a condition (endometrial hyperplasia) that may lead to cancer of the lining of the uterus (endometrial cancer). The risk of endometrial cancer is greater in estrogen users than nonusers. Studies have shown that this increased risk depends on estrogen dose, duration of treatment, and treatment regimen.

Using progestin therapy together with estrogen therapy may reduce the higher risk of uterine cancer related to estrogen use.

If the uterus has been removed (total hysterectomy), there is no danger of developing cancer of the uterus.

Cancer of the breast—Most studies have not shown a higher risk of breast cancer in women who have ever used estrogens. However, some studies have reported that breast cancer developed more often (up to twice the usual rate) in women who used estrogens for long periods of time (especially more than 10 years) or who used higher doses for shorter time periods. VAGIFEM® (estradiol vaginal tablets) is not expected to increase this risk since it is a low dose, applied topically in the vagina, is minimally absorbed into the systemic circulation and is used for relatively short periods of time. Regular breast examinations by a health professional and monthly self-examination are recommended for all women.

Gallbladder disease and abnormal blood clotting—Gallbladder disease and abnormal blood clotting are risk factors associated with medium to high doses of estrogen. Most studies of low-dose estrogen usage by women do not show an increased risk of these complications, and to date there have not been complications with VAGIFEM (estradiol vaginal tablets) treatment.

Side Effects

Few side effects have been reported: vaginal spotting, vaginal discharge, allergic reaction and skin rash.

Estrogens in General

In addition to the risks listed above, the following side effects have been reported with estrogen use:

Nausea and vomiting, breast tenderness or enlargement, enlargement of benign tumors ("fibroids") of the uterus, retention of excess fluid.

Estrogen may worsen some conditions, such as asthma, epilepsy, migraine, heart disease, or kidney disease. Spotty darkening of the skin, particularly on the face.

If you use estrogens, you may reduce your risks by doing these things: See your health care provider regularly. While you are using estrogens, it is important to visit your health care provider at least annually for a check-up. If you develop vaginal bleeding while taking estrogens, call your health care provider; you may need further evaluation. If members of your family have had breast cancer or if you have ever had breast lumps or an abnormal mammogram (breast X-ray), you may need to have more frequent breast examinations. Reassess your need for estrogens. You and your health care provider should reevaluate whether or not you still need estrogens at least every six months.

Be alert for warning signs. If any of these warning signals (or any other unusual symptoms) happen while you are using estrogens, call your health care provider immediately: Abnormal bleeding from the vagina (possible uterine cancer); pains in the calves or chest, sudden shortness of breath, or coughing blood (possible clot in the legs, heart, or lungs); severe headache or vomiting, dizziness, faintness, changes in vision or speech, weakness or numbness of an arm or leg (possible clot in the brain or eye); breast lumps (possible breast cancer; ask your health care provider to show you how to examine your breasts monthly); yellowing of skin or eyes (possible liver problem); pain, swelling, or tenderness in the abdomen (possible gallbladder problem).

1. Estrogens increase the risk of developing a condition called endometrial hyperplasia that may lead to cancer of the lining of the uterus. Progestin, another hormone drug, is usually prescribed with higher-dose estrogen preparations in order to lower the risk of developing endometrial hyperplasia. Progestins are not usually needed for women using VAGIFEM® (estradiol vaginal tablets) alone.
2. Vaginal infection is generally more common in postmenopausal women. Vaginal infections should be treated by your health care provider with the appropriate antimicrobial therapy before initiation of VAGIFEM. If a vaginal infection develops during use of VAGIFEM, it may be continued while the infection is being treated. See your health care provider if you have vaginal discomfort or suspect you have a vaginal infection.
3. Your health care provider has prescribed this drug for you and you alone. Do not give the drug to anyone else.
4. Keep this and all drugs out of the reach of children.
5. This leaflet provides a summary of important information about VAGIFEM. If you want more information, ask your health care provider or pharmacist to show you the professional labeling. The professional labeling is also published in a book called the "Physicians' Desk Reference" which is available in book stores and public libraries. Generic drugs carry virtually the same labeling information as their brand name versions.

HOW SUPPLIED

Each VAGIFEM® (estradiol vaginal tablets), 25μg is contained in a disposable, single-use applicator, packaged in a blister pack. Cartons contain 8 or 18 applicators with inset tablets.

8 applicators: NDC 0169-5173-03

18 applicators: NDC 0169-5173-04

STORAGE: Store at 25°C (77°F); excursions permitted to 15°C–30°C (59°F–86°F). [See USP Controlled Room Temperature.]

Rx only

Vagifem® is a trademark owned
by Novo Nordisk A/S
Revised July 2003
Novo Nordisk Pharmaceuticals, Inc.
Princeton, NJ 08540
1-888-824-4336
www.novonordisk-us.com
Manufactured by
Novo Nordisk A/S
2880 Bagsværd, Denmark

Novogyne Pharmaceuticals

A joint venture between

NOVARTIS PHARMACEUTICALS CORPORATION
EAST HANOVER, NEW JERSEY 07936
and
NOVEN PHARMACEUTICALS, INC.
MIAMI, FLORIDA 33186

For Information Contact:

Customer Response Department
(888) NOW-NOVARTIS (888-669-6682)

Product information for **Vivelle®** (estradiol transdermal system), **Vivelle-Dot®** (estradiol transdermal system) and CombiPatch® (estradiol/norethindrone acetate transdermal system) are referenced under the distributor, NOVARTIS PHARMACEUTICALS CORPORATION.

NOTICE

Before prescribing or administering
any product described in
PHYSICIANS' DESK REFERENCE
check the **PDR Supplements**
for revised information.

Obiken Japan Applied Microbiology Research Institute Ltd.

326 OTOGURO TAMAHO-CHO
NAKAKOMA-GUN, YAMANASHI, 409-3812,
JAPAN

For Direct Inquiries contact:
TEL: 81-55-240-3511
FAX: 81-55-240-3512
E-MAIL: info@oubiken.co.jp or sale@oubiken.co.jp
URL: http://www.oubiken.co.jp

ABPC® (Agaricus Blazei Practical Compound) OTC

ABPC® is the processed food, which is mycelia of Agaricus blazei mushroom treated by digestive enzyme and is applied as dietary supplement.

***PRODUCT DESCRIPTION**

Agaricus blazei Murrill H-1, which we have originally isolated from wild Agaricus blazei mushroom, is used to produce ABPC® (Enzyme digested Agaricus blazei mushroom mycelium processed food).
ABPC® is prepared from mycelium of Agaricus blazei mushroom cultured in the fermentor that we have originally designed. Mycelia processed by enzyme.
After completion of enzyme treatment, the product are freeze-dried and powdered.
It is essential for keeping the quality of product consistently from lots to lots that mycelium is cultured by fermentor.
The amount of β-D-glucan of the mycellia by this method (ca 30% (wt/wt)) is more than that of Agaricus blazei fruit body (ca 8% (wt/wt)).
Agaricus blazei mushroom has been used habitually in Brazil and other South American countries for the sake of health.
ABPC® is one of the best processed foods for the sake of health, because it protects us from physiological imbalance due to irregular habits and aging, or enhances immune system.
We, OBIKEN has obtained the U. S. patent concerning with the mycelium culturing method. U. S. patent number: USP6465218 registered October 15, 2002 and have been assessed, registered ISO9001:2000 for design/development and manufacturing ABPC® in March 14, 2003.

CLINICAL DATA

The first publication as regarding clinical test of ABPC® was the treatment report at 35th Conference of Japan Society of Clinical Oncology in 1997, where Dr. Yukie NIWA (Tosashimizu Hospital, Tosashimizu-city, Kochi), Dr. Jiro ITAMI (Shibata Hospital) presented the cases of high survival rate of breast cancer, stomach cancer and spleen cancer among 1,260 patients. The test have been conducted at the hospitals including Kanazawa Medical University, University of Yamanashi Faculty of Medical, Juntendo University School of Medicine, Akiyama Neurosurgery Hospital and Sano Surgical Hospital.

***RECOMMENDED DOSAGE**

ABPC® is the dietary supplement which is produced by culturing mycelium of Agaricus blazei mushroom in fermentor. It enhances immune system and one of the best processed food for keeping good health.
As a dietary supplement, ABPC® should be taken 1 to 2 sticks per day, usually with water or lukewarm water, or could be taken by chewing. It may be used before or after meal. Store at room temperature in the dark.

Ingredients: The content of ABPC® per stick (contain 1.00 gr) is as followings.

1) ABPC powder freeze-dried
:68% (Wt/Wt)
2) Lactose
:20% (Wt/Wt)
3) Calcium from egg shell
:10% (Wt/Wt)
4) Lipid
:2% (Wt/Wt)
5) Energy : 345Kcal/100gr

ADVERSE REACTIONS

Since we have released ABPC® in Japan 7 years ago, no adverse reaction have been reported. The acute toxicity test with mice[1),2),3)] proved satety of ABPC®.

References;
1) Test report dated December 4, 1997 conducted by The Japan Food Analysis Center
2) Test report dated June 14, 2002 conducted by Japan Applied Microbiology Research Institute Ltd.
3) Test report dated June 26, 2002 conducted by The Japan Food Analysis Center

WARNING

Women who are pregnant or in a period of lactation and infant should better avoid to take. Although no sign of adverse reaction observed in taking a large amount, it is better not to exceed 5 times of daily dosage.

HOW SUPPLIED

The box contains 90 sticks (Total amount 90 gr). Each stick contains 1.0 gr granule of ABPC®.
However, We can also supply in the shape of tablet.

*These statements have not been evaluated by the Food And Drug Administration. This products are not intended to diagnose, treat, cure OR prevent any disease.

Shown in Product Identification Guide, page 327

Odyssey Pharmaceuticals, Inc.

72 EAGLE ROCK AVENUE
EAST HANOVER, NJ 07936

Direct Inquiries to:
(877) 427-9068

ANTABUSE® TABLETS ℞
(Disulfiram Tablets, USP)
IN ALCOHOLISM
℞ only

> **WARNING:**
> Disulfiram should *never* be administered to a patient when he is in a state of alcohol intoxication, or without his full knowledge.
> The physician should instruct relatives accordingly.

DESCRIPTION

Disulfiram is an alcohol antagonist drug.
CHEMICAL NAME:
bis(diethylthiocarbamoyl) disulfide.
STRUCTURAL FORMULA:

$$(C_2H_5)_2N\overset{S}{\overset{\|}{C}}-S-S-\overset{S}{\overset{\|}{C}}N(C_2H_5)_2$$

$C_{10}H_{20}N_2S_4$ M.W. 296.54

Disulfiram occurs as a white to off-white, odorless, and almost tasteless powder, soluble in water to the extent of about 20 mg in 100 mL, and in alcohol to the extent of about 3.8 g in 100 mL.
Each tablet for oral administration contains 250 mg or 500 mg disulfiram, USP. Tablets also contain colloidal silicon dioxide, anhydrous lactose, magnesium stearate, microcrystalline cellulose, sodium starch glycolate, and stearic acid.

CLINICAL PHARMACOLOGY

Disulfiram produces a sensitivity to alcohol which results in a highly unpleasant reaction when the patient under treatment ingests even small amounts of alcohol.
Disulfiram blocks the oxidation of alcohol at the acetaldehyde stage. During alcohol metabolism following disulfiram intake, the concentration of acetaldehyde occurring in the blood may be 5 to 10 times higher than that found during metabolism of the same amount of alcohol alone.
Accumulation of acetaldehyde in the blood produces a complex of highly unpleasant symptoms referred to hereinafter as the disulfiram-alcohol reaction. This reaction, which is proportional to the dosage of both disulfiram and alcohol, will persist as long as alcohol is being metabolized. Disulfiram does not appear to influence the rate of alcohol elimination from the body.
Disulfiram is absorbed slowly from the gastrointestinal tract and is eliminated slowly from the body. One (or even two) weeks after a patient has taken his last dose of disulfiram, ingestion of alcohol may produce unpleasant symptoms.
Prolonged administration of disulfiram does not produce tolerance; the longer a patient remains on therapy, the more exquisitely sensitive he becomes to alcohol.

INDICATIONS AND USAGE

Disulfiram is an aid in the management of selected chronic alcohol patients who *want* to remain in a state of enforced sobriety so that supportive and psychotherapeutic treatment may be applied to best advantage.
Disulfiram is not a cure for alcoholism. When used alone, without proper motivation and supportive therapy, it is unlikely that it will have any substantive effect on the drinking pattern of the chronic alcoholic.

CONTRAINDICATIONS

Patients who are receiving or have recently received metronidazole, paraldehyde, alcohol, or alcohol-containing preparations, e.g., cough syrups, tonics and the like, should not be given disulfiram.
Disulfiram is contraindicated in the presence of severe myocardial disease or coronary occlusion, psychoses, and hypersensitivity to disulfiram or to other thiuram derivatives used in pesticides and rubber vulcanization.

WARNINGS

> Disulfiram should *never* be administered to a patient when he is in a state of alcohol intoxication, or without his full knowledge.
> The physician should instruct relatives accordingly.

The patient must be fully informed of the disulfiram-alcohol reaction. He must be strongly cautioned against surreptitious drinking while taking the drug, and he must be fully aware of the possible consequences. He should be warned to avoid alcohol in disguised forms, i.e., in sauces, vinegars, cough mixtures, and even in aftershave lotions and back rubs. He should also be warned that reactions may occur with alcohol up to 14 days after ingesting disulfiram.

The Disulfiram-Alcohol Reaction: Disulfiram plus alcohol, even small amounts, produce flushing, throbbing in head and neck, throbbing headache, respiratory difficulty, nausea, copious vomiting, sweating, thirst, chest pain, palpitation, dyspnea, hyperventilation, tachycardia, hypotension, syncope, marked uneasiness, weakness, vertigo, blurred vision, and confusion. In severe reactions there may be respiratory depression, cardiovascular collapse, arrhythmias, myocardial infarction, acute congestive heart failure, unconsciousness, convulsions, and death.
The intensity of the reaction varies with each individual, but is generally proportional to the amounts of disulfiram and alcohol ingested. Mild reactions may occur in the sensitive individual when the blood alcohol concentration is increased to as little as 5 to 10 mg per 100 mL. Symptoms are fully developed at 50 mg per 100 mL, and unconsciousness usually results when the blood alcohol level reaches 125 to 150 mg.
The duration of the reaction varies from 30 to 60 minutes, to several hours in the more severe cases, or as long as there is alcohol in the blood.

Concomitant Conditions: Because of the possibility of an accidental disulfiram-alcohol reaction, disulfiram should be used with extreme caution in patients with any of the following conditions: diabetes mellitus, hypothyroidism, epilepsy, cerebral damage, chronic and acute nephritis, hepatic cirrhosis or insufficiency.

PRECAUTIONS

Patients with a history of rubber contact dermatitis should be evaluated for hypersensitivity to thiuram derivatives before receiving disulfiram (see **CONTRAINDICATIONS**).
It is suggested that every patient under treatment carry an *Identification Card* stating that he is receiving disulfiram and describing the symptoms most likely to occur as a result of the disulfiram-alcohol reaction. In addition, this card should indicate the physician or institution to be contacted in an emergency. (Cards may be obtained from ODYSSEY PHARMACEUTICALS upon request.)
Alcoholism may accompany or be followed by dependence on narcotics or sedatives. Barbiturates and disulfiram have been administered concurrently without untoward effects; the possibility of initiating a new abuse should be considered.
Hepatic toxicity including hepatic failure resulting in transplantation or death have been reported. Severe and sometimes fatal hepatitis associated with disulfiram therapy may develop even after many months of therapy. Hepatic toxicity has occurred in patients with or without prior history of abnormal liver function. Patients should be advised to immediately notify their physician of any early symptoms of hepatitis, such as fatigue, weakness, malaise, anorexia, nausea, vomiting, jaundice, or dark urine.
Baseline and follow-up liver function tests (10–14 days) are suggested to detect any hepatic dysfunction that may result with disulfiram therapy. In addition, a complete blood count and serum chemistries, including liver function tests, should be monitored.
Patients taking disulfiram tablets should not be exposed to ethylene dibromide or its vapors. This precaution is based on preliminary results of animal research currently in progress that suggest a toxic interaction between inhaled ethylene dibromide and ingested disulfiram resulting in a higher incidence of tumors and mortality in rats. A correlation between this finding and humans, however, has not been demonstrated.

Drug Interactions: Disulfiram appears to decrease the rate at which certain drugs are metabolized and therefore may increase the blood levels and the possibility of clinical toxicity of drugs given concomitantly.

DISULFIRAM SHOULD BE USED WITH CAUTION IN THOSE PATIENTS RECEIVING PHENYTOIN AND ITS CONGENERS, SINCE THE CONCOMITANT ADMINISTRATION OF THESE TWO DRUGS CAN LEAD TO PHENYTOIN INTOXICATION. PRIOR TO ADMINISTERING DISULFIRAM TO A PATIENT ON PHENYTOIN THERAPY, A BASELINE PHENYTOIN SERUM LEVEL SHOULD BE OBTAINED. SUBSEQUENT TO INITIATION OF DISULFIRAM THERAPY, SERUM LEVELS OF PHENYTOIN SHOULD BE DETERMINED ON DIFFERENT DAYS FOR EVIDENCE OF AN INCREASE OR FOR A CONTINUING RISE IN LEVELS. INCREASED PHENYTOIN LEVELS SHOULD BE TREATED WITH APPROPRIATE DOSAGE ADJUSTMENT.

It may be necessary to adjust the dosage of oral anticoagulants upon beginning or stopping disulfiram, since disulfiram may prolong prothrombin time.

Patients taking isoniazid when disulfiram is given should be observed for the appearance of unsteady gait or marked changes in mental status, the disulfiram should be discontinued if such signs appear.

In rats, simultaneous ingestion of disulfiram and nitrite in the diet for 78 weeks has been reported to cause tumors, and it has been suggested that disulfiram may react with nitrites in the rat stomach to form a nitrosamine, which is tumorigenic. Disulfiram alone in the rat's diet did not lead to such tumors. The relevance of this finding to humans is not known at this time.

Usage in Pregnancy: The safe use of this drug in pregnancy has not been established. Therefore, disulfiram should be used during pregnancy only when, in the judgement of the physician, the probable benefits outweigh the possible risks.

Pediatric Use: Safety and effectiveness in pediatric patients have not been established.

Nursing Mothers: It is not known whether this drug is excreted in human milk. Since many drugs are so excreted, disulfiram should not be given to nursing mothers.

Geriatric Use: A determination has not been made whether controlled clinical studies of disulfiram included sufficient numbers of subjects aged 65 and over to define a difference in response from younger subjects. Other reported clinical experience has not identified differences in responses between the elderly and younger patients. In general, dose selection for an elderly patient should be cautious, usually starting at the low end of the dosing range, reflecting the greater frequency of decreased hepatic, renal or cardiac function, and of concomitant disease or other drug therapy.

ADVERSE REACTIONS

(See **CONTRAINDICATIONS**, **WARNINGS**, and **PRECAUTIONS**.)

OPTIC NEURITIS, PERIPHERAL NEURITIS, POLYNEURITIS, AND PERIPHERAL NEUROPATHY MAY OCCUR FOLLOWING ADMINISTRATION OF DISULFIRAM.

Multiple cases of hepatitis, including both cholestatic and fulminant hepatitis, as well as hepatic failure resulting in transplantation or death, have been reported with administration of disulfiram.

Occasional skin eruptions are, as a rule, readily controlled by concomitant administration of an antihistaminic drug.

In a small number of patients, a transient mild drowsiness, fatigability, impotence, headache, acneform eruptions, allergic dermatitis, or a metallic or garlic-like aftertaste may be experienced during the first two weeks of therapy. These complaints usually disappear spontaneously with the continuation of therapy, or with reduced dosage.

Psychotic reactions have been noted, attributable in most cases to high dosage, combined toxicity (with metronidazole or isoniazid), or to the unmasking of underlying psychoses in patients stressed by the withdrawal of alcohol.

OVERDOSAGE

No specific information is available on the treatment of overdosage with disulfiram. It is recommended that the physician contact the local Poison Control Center.

DOSAGE AND ADMINISTRATION

Disulfiram should never be administered until the patient has abstained from alcohol for at least 12 hours.

Initial Dosage Schedule: In the first phase of treatment, a *maximum* of 500 mg daily is given in a single dose for one to two weeks. Although usually taken in the morning, disulfiram may be taken on retiring by patients who experience a sedative effect. Alternatively, to minimize, or eliminate, the sedative effect, dosage may be adjusted downward.

Maintenance Regimen: The average maintenance dose is 250 mg daily (range, 125 to 500 mg), it should not exceed 500 mg daily.

Note: Occasionally patients, while seemingly on adequate maintenance doses of disulfiram, report that they are able to drink alcoholic beverages with impunity and without any symptomatology. All appearances to the contrary, such patients must be presumed to be disposing of their tablets in some manner without actually taking them. Until such patients have been observed reliably taking their daily disulfiram tablets (preferably crushed and well mixed with liquid), it cannot be concluded that disulfiram is ineffective.

Duration of Therapy: The daily, uninterrupted administration of disulfiram must be continued until the patient is fully recovered socially and a basis for permanent self-control is established. Depending on the individual patient, maintenance therapy may be required for months or even years.

Trial with Alcohol: During early experience with disulfiram, it was thought advisable for each patient to have at least one supervised alcohol-drug reaction. More recently, the test reaction has been largely abandoned. Furthermore, such a test reaction should never be administered to a patient over 50 years of age. A clear, detailed and convincing description of the reaction is felt to be sufficient in most cases.

However, where a test reaction is deemed necessary, the suggested procedure is as follows:

After the first one to two weeks' therapy with 500 mg daily, a drink of 15 mL (1/2 oz) of 100 proof whiskey, or equivalent, is taken slowly. This test dose of alcoholic beverage may be repeated once only, so that the total dose does not exceed 30 mL (1 oz) of whiskey. Once a reaction develops, no more alcohol should be consumed. Such tests should be carried out only when the patient is hospitalized, or comparable supervision and facilities, including oxygen, are available.

Management of Disulfiram-Alcohol Reaction: In severe reactions, whether caused by an excessive test dose or by the patient's unsupervised ingestion of alcohol, supportive measures to restore blood pressure and treat shock should be instituted. Other recommendations include: oxygen, carbogen (95% oxygen and 5% carbon dioxide), vitamin C intravenously in massive doses (1 g) and ephedrine sulfate. Antihistamines have also been used intravenously. Potassium levels should be monitored, particularly in patients on digitalis, since hypokalemia has been reported.

HOW SUPPLIED

Disulfiram Tablets, USP:

250 mg—White, round, unscored tablets in bottles of 100 and 1000.
Debossed: OP 706

500 mg—White, round, scored tablets in bottles of 50, 100 and 500.
Debossed: OP 707 on one side and scored on the other side.

Dispense in a tight, light-resistant container as defined in the USP.

Store at 20°–25°C (68°–77°F). [See USP Controlled Room Temperature].

Distributed by Odyssey Pharmaceuticals, Inc., East Hanover, New Jersey 07936

Manufactured by PLIVA®, Inc., East Hanover, NJ 07936

Rev. 12/03

Shown in Product Identification Guide, page 327

CUSTODIOL® ℞

Bretschneider HTK Solution
For Kidney, Liver and Heart Preservation

DESCRIPTION

Composition

1,000 ml CUSTODIOL® contain:

[See table below]

Physical Properties

pH 7.02–7.20 at 25°C (pH 7.4–7.45 at 4°C)

Osmolality: 310 mosmol/kg

Caution: Federal law restricts sale of this device to or on the order of a physician or licensed practitioner.

INDICATIONS FOR USE

CUSTODIOL® HTK Solution is indicated for perfusion and flushing of donor kidneys, liver, and heart prior to removal from the donor or immediately after removal from the donor. The solution is left in the organ vasculature during hypothermic storage and transportation (not for continuous perfusion) to the recipient.

WARNINGS AND PRECAUTIONS

Warning: Perfusion of the kidney, liver and/or heart should be carried out with a maximum hydrostatic pressure of 120 mm Hg.

Warning: CUSTODIOL® is not indicated for intravenous or intraarterial administration. It is indicated only for selective perfusion of the kidney, liver and heart and for cooling of the surface areas, i.e., for the preservation of the donor organ during the transport from donor to recipient. CUSTODIOL® may not be used for systemic infusion.

Warning: CUSTODIOL® is not indicated for continuous perfusion.

Warning: Keep out of reach of children.

Caution: The product must be used before the expiration date stated on the package.

Caution: The product must be stored according to the recommendations prior to use.

ADVERSE EVENTS

No side effects have been encountered that could be attributed to this product.

Interactions with other Medical Products

Interactions with such therapeutic agents as glycosides, diuretics, nitrates, antihypertensives, beta blockers and calcium antagonists, which are used perioperatively, have not been reported.

OVERDOSES (Symptoms, Countermeasures)

In the case of entry of the HTK solution into the general circulation, the resultant change in the concentration of sodium and calcium is very slight. After checking sodium and calcium levels in the extracorporeal circulation both of these electrolytes should be replaced if necessary.

INSTRUCTIONS FOR USE (Recommendations)

Required Equipment:

- Perfusion apparatus with a Y-piece for bottle or bags
- Perfusion cannula tube 2.5 to 3 mm
- Tube clamp
- Perfusion stand with a height setting of up to 200 cm with tape measure.
- Cooling Equipment (5 to 8° C) for use in cardiac surgery
- Perfusion tube with an internal diameter of 6 mm
- Transport Container with sterile pouch for transport of the cooled organ from donor to recipient.

Filtration of CUSTODIOL® is not necessary or recommended.

Tolerance of Ischemia by the Kidney

The kidney may be stored with ice cold CUSTODIOL® solution at about 2 to 4°C with a period of (cold) ischemia of up to 48 hours. Warm ischemia time, that is to say the average time period required for the completion of anastomosis of the vessels, is usually 30 minutes. Taking this time as a basis, the organ recovers completely with optimal immediate function within 24 hours.

Tolerance of Ischemia by the Liver

The liver may be stored with ice cold CUSTODIOL® solution at about 2 to 4°C with a period of (cold) ischemia of up to 15 hours. Warm ischemia time, that is to say the average time period required for the completion of anastomosis of the vessels, is usually 30 minutes. Taking this time as a basis, the organ recovers completely with optimal immediate function within 24 hours.

Tolerance of Ischemia by the Heart

The Heart may be stored with ice cold CUSTODIOL® solution at about 2 to 4°C with a period of (cold) ischemia of up to 4 hours. Warm ischemia time, that is to say the average time period required for the completion of anastomosis of the vessels, is usually 30 minutes.

Introduction of Renal Perfusion

Following successful laparotomy, the kidney is prepared by ligature of the capsular vessels. The perfusion catheter for selective kidney perfusion is fixed in the renal artery using a tourniquet. Cold perfusion (2–4°C) is performed under hydrostatic pressure (maximum of 120 mmHg). Within the first minute of perfusion, the renal vein is incised and clamped off adjacent to the vena cava. The escaping perfusate is removed from the abdominal cavity. After approximately 10 minutes of perfusion, the kidney is resected before transplantation.

Introduction of Hepatic Perfusion

The donor should be heparinised appropriately, and the aorta or the iliac bifurcation and the portal vein will be exposed. The perfusion tubing should be of the largest possible diameter and the cannulae should have an internal bore of at least 5 mm. Because of the low viscosity of the solution, perfusion is performed under hydrostatic pressure only (maximum of 120 mmHg). Perfusion of the portal vein can be performed by cannulating the superior or inferior mesenteric vein and advancing the catheter up to the origin of the portal vein. After performing cannulation, clamping off the aorta and opening the vena cava, bubble-free perfusion is begun via both lines simultaneously. As a general rule, 8–12 liters of HTK at 2–4°C should be perfused (about 300 ml per kg of body weight) and this will require about 10 minutes.

Should the center decide to use the so-called aorto-single flush technique, the total amount of the preservation solution needed is perfused only via the aortal line. Once again, a pressurized infusion is not necessary or recommended. A Y-perfusion system is recommended in addition to perfusion tubing of the largest possible caliber and perfusion cannulae with an internal bore of at least Charrière 15 (5 mm). The time required for perfusion is extended by about 5 minutes. At the implant site, the back-table preparation includes the reperfusion of approximately 500 ml cold HTK solution. The perfusion is stopped when the anastomoses of the inferior vena cava are completed at the end of the second warm ischemia time. It is permissible, in view of the flow properties and low potassium concentration of the HTK solution, to perform flushing of the organ or testing for leaks in the anastomoses with HTK solution itself, if necessary. Alternatively, any standard flushing solution may be used. Simultaneous reperfusion via the artery and the portal vein are preferable, though primary reperfusion through the portal vein alone is acceptable.

Introduction of Cardiac Perfusion

The inactivation of the heart renders it susceptible to overstretching. Decompression of the left ventricle must therefore be performed at the commencement of cardioplegia. For adult hearts the following recommendation is appropriate: The solution, cooled to 5°C–8°C, is perfused into the coronary arteries by hydrostatic pressure of 100 mmHg (equivalent to initial height of perfusion bottle above level of heart

Continued on next page

0.8766 g	Sodium chloride	=	15.0	mmol/l
0.6710 g	Potassium chloride	=	9.0	mmol/l
0.1842 g	Potassium hydrogen 2-Ketoglutarate	=	1.0	mmol/l
0.8132 g	Magnesium chloride • 6 H_2O	=	4.0	mmol/l
3.7733 g	Histidine • HCl • H_2O	=	18.0	mmol/l
27.9289 g	Histidine	=	180.0	mmol/l
0.4085 g	Tryptophan	=	2.0	mmol/l
5.4651 g	Mannitol	=	30.0	mmol/l
0.0022 g	Calcium chloride - $2H_2O$	=	0.015	mmol/l

in sterile Water for injection

Anion: Cl^- 50 mval

Custodiol HTK—Cont.

= 140 cm). After cardiac arrest has ensued (within the first minute after starting perfusion) the perfusion bottle should be lowered to about 50–70 cm above the level of the heart, equivalent to 40–50 mmHg. In patients with pronounced coronary stenosis, a higher perfusion pressure (about 50 mmHg) will be necessary for a somewhat longer time. The overall perfusion time should be 6–8 minutes, so as to ensure homogeneous equilibration. Even for small hearts, a perfusion rate of 1 ml/min/gram-estimated-heart-weight at a perfusion pressure of 40–50 mmHg and a perfusion time of 6–8 min should be enough to ensure equilibration. The heart may then be excised. The heart should tolerate a cold ischemic time of up to four hours.

Transport of a Donor Organ

The transport of a donor organ to the recipient utilizes a sterile pouch accommodating the size of the organ in an ice cold CUSTODIOL® solution. The organ must be completely covered by the solution. The pouch is sealed with adhesive tape and is placed into a second container which is also filled with CUSTODIOL® solution in order to prevent a breakdown of insulation and cooling by trapped air. The double-bagged organ is placed into a sterile plastic container and closed with a secure lid. The plastic bag is then placed into a transport container packed with ice for transport. Information about the donor, copies of the laboratory results and blood samples from the donor are also included. The transport of the donor organ in CUSTODIOL® solution must be accomplished as quickly as possible.

CLINICAL EXPERIENCE

Kidney Transplant Trials

A major multi-center prospective randomized clinical trial has been carried out in Europe comparing three perfusion and preservation solutions for use in kidney transplants[1]. The three solutions were the CUSTODIOL® HTK solution, the Belzer UW solution, and the Euro-Collins (EC) solution. Forty-seven centers participated and followed a strict protocol. Over a thousand kidneys were included in the study. In the HTK-UW study, there were 342 donors and 611 transplants (the UW group had 168 donors and 297 transplants, the HTK group had 174 donors and 314 transplants). In the HTK-EC study, there were 317 donors and 569 transplants (the EC group had 155 donors and 277 transplants, the HTK group had 162 donors and 292 transplants).

This study directly compared kidney survival in the HTK group with the UW group, and also with the EC solution, and showed that for kidney transplants, the HTK solution performs as well overall as the UW solution, and significantly better than EC solution for initial nonfunction. The average cold ischemia time in the HTK-UW study was 25.8 hours in the HTK group and 25.5 hours in the UW group. In the HTK-EC group, the average cold ischemia time was 24.1 hours in the HTK group and 24.2 hours in the EC group. The overall kidney survival rates from the 47-center study for HTK versus UW, and HTK versus EC, at four time points were:

	HTK	UW	HTK	EC
1 Month	91%	91%	85%	86%
12 Months	83%	82%	80%	74%
24 Months	77%	74%	76%	71%
36 Months	74%	68%	70%	67%

Delayed graft function that required two or more dialysis sessions during the first week was 20% (107/544) in the pooled HTK groups, 25% (66/266) for the UW group, and 32% (85/268) for the EC group. Initial nonfunction (INF) occurred in 33% of the kidneys in both HTK and UW groups, and in the other study, INF occurred in 29% of the HTK group and 43% of the EC group.

[1]de Boer J, De Meester J, Smits JMA, Doxiadis IIN, Groenewoud AF, Persijn GG (1999). Eurotransplant randomized multicenter study comparing kidney graft preservation with HTK, UW, and EC. *Transplantation* in press, publication about December 1999

Liver Transplant Trials

Several clinical studies have been reported that examined the performance of CUSTODIOL® HTK Solution in liver transplants. These studies have collected data on survival rates and other outcome measures. The primary evidence for effectiveness has come from a four-center prospective clinical study carried out under the auspices of the Eurotransplant organization of Leiden, The Netherlands. The four centers were located at Essen, Innsbruck, Gottingen, and Vienna. The results from this and other studies are discussed below.

Gubernatis summarized the experience at the Medizinische Hochschule Hanover, Clinic for Abdominal and Transplantation Surgery, for livers preserved in UW solution and in HTK solution. This was a retrospective study of transplants conducted at Hanover between 1988 and 1996. During this period there were 515 liver transplants using the UW solution and 232 using HTK solution. These transplants were carried out in 416 patients using UW and 197 using HTK (some were re-transplants). The survival curves for all patients out to five years were essentially indistinguishable and certainly not significantly different statistically. An update on the Hanover experience through 1999 showed that 461 livers had been preserved with HTK solution and 607 with UW solution. Prof. Gubernatis reiterated his earlier conclusion that the two solutions were equivalent in their ability to preserve the liver for transplant.

A randomized prospective study was organized under the direction of Prof. J. Erhard at Essen, comparing 30 livers preserved with HTK Solution with 30 livers preserved with UW solution. There were two cases of initial nonfunction (INF) in the UW group and one case of INF in the HTK group. Graft survival at 3 months was 87% in the HTK group and 80% in the UW group ($p = 0.21$). Patient survival at 30 months was 77% in the HTK group and 74% in the UW group.

A multi-center prospective clinical study was carried out in Europe to evaluate the performance of the HTK solution in liver transplants.[2] Four transplant centers participated. 228 livers were included in the study (205 were initial transplants, 23 were re-transplants). This trial took place during 1996-1999 under the auspices of Eurotransplant. The four transplant centers participating were: Innsbruck Transplant Center; Vienna Transplant Center; University Clinic, Essen; and University Hospital, Göttingen. The (patient) survival rate at one year observed in this study was 82.5%. The following table shows the patient survival at different times in the direct comparison study at Essen, the four-center prospective study, and the Hanover retrospective study. These data show that the patient survival rates for HTK-preserved livers are similar to those for UW-preserved livers.

[2]Pokorny H, Grünberger T, Rockenschaub S, Windhager T, Rosensting A, Lange R, et al (2000). Preservation of the liver with HTK--a multicenter experience. Poster presented at International Congress of the Transplant Society, Rome, Italy.

[See table below]

	HTK-Ess	UW-Ess	HTK (4-Ctr)	HTK-Han	UW-Han
1 Month	87%*	80%*			
3 Months			82.5%		
12 Months				71%	72%
30 Months	77%	74%		69%	67%

* Graft survival

Heart Transplant Trials

Several clinical studies have been reported that examined the performance of CUSTODIOL® HTK Solution in heart transplants. These studies have collected data on survival rates and other outcome measures.

At the Bad Oeynhausen transplant center, during the period 1989–2002, 1233 hearts were preserved with the HTK Solution. 19 hearts were preserved with other solutions. The data reported here represent the entire experience of the center, with no cases excluded. The following table summarizes the experience at Bad Oeynhausen:

The Bad Oeynhausen Experience in Cardiac Transplantation

	HTK Solution	Other Solutions*
Number of Subjects	1233	19
Age of Donor		
Median	33.8	36.2
Minimum	0	16
Maximum	72	65
Donor Cause of Death		
Traumatic Bleeding	501	6
Spontaneous Bleeding	491	9
Hypoxia	97	2
Gun Shot Wound	33	1
Domino	1	1
Cerebral Ischemia	43	
Brain Tumor	31	
Intoxication	18	
Other	18	
Cold Ischemia Time		
Median	194.6	213.1
Standard Deviation	42.3	43.1
Minimum	68	108
Maximum	340	289
Recipient Gender		
Male	1014 (82.2 %)	17 (89.5 %)
Female	219 (17.8 %)	2 (10.5 %)
Recipient Age		
Median	50.4	53.9
Standard Deviation	17.0	13.3
Maximum	77.9	66.4
Minimum	0	15.5
Recipient Diagnosis		
Cardiomyopathy	625	8
Coronary Artery Disease	479	9
Valve Disease	65	1
Congenital Disease	37	
Retransplant	21	1
Acute Myocarditis	2	
Other Diseases	4	
Causes of Death Post-TX		
Graft Rejection	52	1
MOF	25	
Graft Vasculopathy	3	
Acute Bleeding	1	
Infection	49	2
Acute left ventricular failure	11	
Right Ventricular Failure	13	
Neurological Complications	13	2
Pulmonary Complications	3	
Abdominal Complications	6	
Perioperative Complications	8	
Primary Graft Failure	23 (1.9%)	0
Deaths in First Year	248 (21%)	7 (37%)
Deaths in First Three Months	184 (16%)	5 (27%)

*The other solutions included UW, Roe, Ringer's lactate, normal saline, Plasmalyte A, Plegisol, Carmichael's, and Stanford.

Wieselthaler et al[3]. reported a randomized prospective study conducted at the University of Vienna comparing CUSTODIOL® solution to Celsior, another cardiac cold storage solution. 48 patients were randomized to either the CUSTODIOL® group or the Celsior group. Following are the results from this study:

[3]Wieselthaler GM, Chevtchik O, Konetschny, Moldi R, Milinger E, Mares P, Griessmacher A, Grimm M. Wolner E, Laufer G (1999). Improved graft function using a new myocardial preservation solution. Preliminary data a randonmized prospective study. *Transplantation Proceedings*, 31: 2067–2070

	HTK	Celsior
Number of Subjects	24	24
Perioperative Graft Failure	2/24 (8.3%)	2/24 (8.3%)
Patient Survival at 30 Days	22/24 (91.7%)	23/24 (95.8%)
Graft Survival at 30 Days	22/25 (88.0%)	23/25 (92.0%)
Spontaneous Stable Cardiac Rhythm Immediately after Opening Aortic Cross-Clamp	9/24 (37.5%)	19/24 (79.2)%
Cold Ischemia Time (Min)		
Mean	199	183
Standard Deviation	54	43
Minimum	96	165
Maximum	290	282
Donor Age (Yrs)		
Mean	38	38
Standard Deviation	12	11
Recipient Age (Yrs)		
Mean	55	57
Standard Deviation	9	11
Donor Heart Dysfunction	7/24	2/24
Causes of First Graft Failure		
Infection		1
Acute Graft Failure	2	1
Deaths in Retransplanted Patients	1/1	0/1

Adverse Events Observed in the Clinical Studies

Kidney Studies

There were no unexpected adverse events in these clinical studies. The adverse events that occurred were expected because of the nature of transplantation. None are believed to be affected by any of the solutions.

Kidney failure rates in the first 48 hours were comparable in all groups: UW-15/297 and HTK-18/314; EC-15/277 and HTK-13/272.

In the HTK-UW kidney study, acute rejection episodes occurred in 99/314 (32%) in the HTK group and 105/297 (35%) in the UW group. In the HTK-EC study, acute rejection episodes occurred in 99/292 (34%) in the HTK group and 108/277 (39%) in the EC group.

Liver Studies

There were no unexpected adverse events in these clinical studies. The adverse events that occurred were expected because of the nature of transplantation.

In the multi-center trial, primary disfunction rate (PDF) was 10.3%, with a primary non-function rate (PNF) of 3.6%. Bile duct complications were seen in 19% of transplants. This compares with data from Eurotransplant on the UW solution: PDR of 15.2% and PNR of 7.8%.

Heart Studies

There were no unexpected adverse events in these clinical studies. The adverse events that occurred were expected because of the nature of heart transplantation.

In the Bad Oeynhausen experience, the primary dysfunction rate (PNF) was 1.9%.

HOW SUPPLIED

Bottles of	500 ml
Bottles of	1000 ml
Bags of	2000 ml
Bags of	5000 ml

Store at +2°C to +15°C (35°F–59°F) and protect from light.

Registration #: K 992209
#: K 020924
#: K 032794

Distributed by
Odyssey Pharmaceuticals, Inc.
East Hanover, NJ 07936
Manufactured by
DR. FRANZ KÖHLER CHEMIE GMBH
P.O. Box 1117, D-64659 Alsbach-Hähnlein, Germany
P08-0725 / 10500216 Iss. 5/04

NYSTATIN VAGINAL TABLETS, USP ℞
100,000 Units

DESCRIPTION

Nystatin is an antimycotic polyene antibiotic obtained from *Streptomyces noursei.*

Nystatin Vaginal Tablets, USP are available as oval-shaped compressed tablets for intravaginal administration, each containing 100,000 units Nystatin, USP. Inactive ingredients include corn starch, ethylcellulose, anhydrous lactose, microcrystalline cellulose, polyethylene glycol and stearic acid.

CLINICAL PHARMACOLOGY

Nystatin is both fungistatic and fungicidal *in vitro* against a wide variety of yeasts and yeast-like fungi. Nystatin acts by binding to sterols in the cell membrane of sensitive fungi with a resultant change in membrane permeability allowing leakage of intracellular components. Nystatin exhibits no appreciable activity against bacteria, protozoa, trichomonads or viruses.

Nystatin is not absorbed from intact skin or mucous membranes.

INDICATIONS AND USAGE

Nystatin Vaginal Tablets, USP are effective for the local treatment of vulvovaginal candidiasis (moniliasis). The diagnosis should be confirmed, prior to therapy, by KOH smears and/or cultures. Other pathogens commonly associated with vulvovaginitis (Trichomonas and *Haemophilus vaginalis*) do not respond to nystatin and should be ruled out by appropriate laboratory methods.

CONTRAINDICATIONS

This preparation is contraindicated in patients with a history of hypersensitivity to any of its components.

PRECAUTIONS

General: Discontinue treatment if sensitization or irritation is reported during use.

Information for Patients: The patient should be informed of symptoms of sensitization or irritation and told to report them promptly.

The patient should be warned against interruption or discontinuation of medication even during menstruation and even though symptomatic relief may occur within a few days.

The patient should be advised that adjunctive measures such as therapeutic douches are unnecessary and sometimes inadvisable, but cleansing douches may be used by nonpregnant women, if desired, for esthetic purposes.

Laboratory Tests: If there is a lack of response to Nystatin Vaginal Tablets, USP, appropriate microbiological studies should be repeated to confirm the diagnosis and rule out other pathogens before instituting another course of antimycotic therapy (see **INDICATIONS AND USAGE**).

Carcinogenesis, Mutagenesis, Impairment of Fertility: Long-term studies in animals have not been performed to evaluate carcinogenic potential, mutagenesis, or whether this medication effects fertility in females.

Pregnancy: *Teratogenic Effects: Pregnancy Category A.* There have been no reports that use of Nystatin Vaginal Tablets by pregnant women increases the risk of fetal abnormalities or affects later growth, development and functional maturation of the child. Nevertheless, because the possibility of harm cannot be ruled out, Nystatin Vaginal Tablets should be used during pregnancy only if the physician considers it essential to the welfare of the patient.

Animal reproduction studies have not been conducted with nystatin vaginal tablets.

Pediatric Use: Safety and effectiveness in pediatric patients have not been established.

ADVERSE REACTIONS

Nystatin is virtually nontoxic and nonsensitizing and is well tolerated by all age groups, even on prolonged administration. Rarely, irritation or sensitization may occur (see **PRECAUTIONS**).

DOSAGE AND ADMINISTRATION

The usual dosage is one tablet (100,000 units nystatin) daily for two weeks. The tablets should be deposited high in the vagina by means of the applicator. "Instructions for the Patient" are enclosed in each package.

HOW SUPPLIED: Nystatin Vaginal Tablets, USP:

Pale yellow mottled oval-shaped, flat façe, beveled tablet (Debossed ODYSSEY on one side and 705 on the other) are available in packages of 15 individually foil wrapped tablets, with applicator and "Instructions for the Patient".

Store at controlled room temperature 15°–30°C (59°–86°F).

Distributed by Odyssey Pharmaceuticals, Inc.
East Hanover, NJ 07936
Manufactured by PLIVA®, Inc.
East Hanover, NJ 07936
Iss. 3/03

Shown in Product Identification Guide, page 327

SANCTURA™ ℞
[sánk-tur-ă]
(trospium chloride)
20 mg Tablets

PRESCRIBING INFORMATION

DESCRIPTION

Sanctura™ (trospium chloride) is a quaternary ammonium compound with the chemical name of spiro[8-azoniabicyclo[3,2,1]octane-8,1′-pyrrolidinium]-3-[(hydroxydiphenyl-acetyl)-oxy]chloride(1α, 3β, 5β)-(9CI). The empirical formula of trospium chloride is $C_{25}H_{30}ClNO_3$; and its molecular weight is 427.97. The structural formula of trospium chloride is represented below:

Trospium chloride is a fine, colorless to slightly yellow, crystalline solid. The compound's solubility in water is approximately 1 g/2 mL.

Each Sanctura tablet contains 20 mg of trospium chloride and is to be given orally. Each tablet also contains the following inactive ingredients: sucrose, wheat starch, microcrystalline cellulose, talc, lactose monohydrate, calcium carbonate, titanium dioxide, stearic acid, croscarmellose sodium, povidone, polyethylene glycol 8000, colloidal silicon dioxide, ferric oxide, carboxymethylcellulose sodium, white wax, magnesium stearate, and carnauba wax.

CLINICAL PHARMACOLOGY

Sanctura is an antispasmodic, antimuscarinic agent.

Trospium chloride antagonizes the effect of acetylcholine on muscarinic receptors in cholinergically innervated organs. Its parasympatholytic action reduces the tonus of smooth muscle in the bladder. Receptor assays showed that trospium chloride has negligible affinity for nicotinic receptors as compared to muscarinic receptors at concentrations obtained from therapeutic doses.

Pharmacodynamics

Placebo-controlled studies employing urodynamic variables were conducted in patients with conditions characterized by involuntary detrusor contractions. The results demonstrate that Sanctura increases maximum cystometric bladder capacity and volume at first detrusor contraction.

Pharmacokinetics

Absorption: After oral administration, less than 10% of the dose is absorbed. Mean absolute bioavailability of a 20 mg dose is 9.6% (range: 4.0-16.1%). Peak plasma concentrations (C_{max}) occur between 5 to 6 hours post-dose. Mean C_{max} increases greater than dose-proportionally; a 3-fold and 4-fold increase in C_{max} was observed for dose increases from 20 mg to 40 mg and from 20 mg to 60 mg, respectively. AUC exhibits dose linearity for single doses up to 60 mg. Sanctura exhibits diurnal variability in exposure with a decrease in C_{max} and AUC of up to 59% and 33%, respectively, for evening relative to morning doses.

Effect of Food: Administration with a high fat meal resulted in reduced absorption, with AUC and C_{max} values 70-80% lower than those obtained when Sanctura was administered while fasting. Therefore, it is recommended that Sanctura should be taken at least one hour prior to meals or on an empty stomach. (See DOSAGE AND ADMINISTRATION and PRECAUTIONS: Information for Patients).

Distribution: Protein binding ranged from 50 to 85% when therapeutic concentration levels (0.5 - 50 ng/mL) were incubated with human serum *in vitro*.

The ^{3}H-trospium chloride ratio of plasma to whole blood was 1.6:1. This ratio indicates that the majority of ^{3}H-trospium chloride is distributed in plasma. The apparent volume of distribution for a 20 mg oral dose is 395 (± 140) liters.

Metabolism: The metabolic pathway of trospium in humans has not been fully defined. Of the 10% of the dose absorbed, metabolites account for approximately 40% of the excreted dose following oral administration. The major metabolic pathway is hypothesized as ester hydrolysis with subsequent conjugation of benzylic acid to form azoniaspironortropanol with glucuronic acid. Cytochrome P450 is not expected to contribute significantly to the elimination of trospium. *In vitro* data from human liver microsomes investigating the inhibitory effect of trospium on seven cytochrome P450 isoenzyme substrates (CYP1A2, 2A6, 2C9, 2C19, 2D6, 2E1, and 3A4) suggest a lack of inhibition at clinically relevant concentrations of trospium.

Excretion: The plasma half-life for Sanctura following oral administration is approximately 20 hours. After administration of oral ^{14}C-trospium chloride, the majority of the dose (85.2%) was recovered in feces and a smaller amount (5.8% of the dose) was recovered in urine; 60% of the radioactivity excreted in urine was unchanged trospium.

The mean renal clearance for trospium (29.07 L/hour) is 4-fold higher than average glomerular filtration rate, indicating that active tubular secretion is a major route of elimination for trospium. There may be competition for elimination with other compounds that are also renally eliminated (See PRECAUTIONS: Drug Interactions).

A summary of mean (± standard deviation) pharmacokinetic parameters for a single 20 mg dose of Sanctura is provided in Table 1.

Table 1. Mean (± SD) Pharmacokinetic Parameter Estimates for a Single 20 mg Sanctura Dose in Healthy Volunteers.

C_{max} (ng/mL)	$AUC_{0-\infty}$ (ng/mL•hr)	T_{max} (hr)	$t_{½}$ (hr)
3.5 ± 4.0	36.4 ± 21.8	5.3 ± 1.2	18.3 ± 3.2

The mean plasma concentration-time (+ SD) profile for Sanctura is shown in Figure 1.

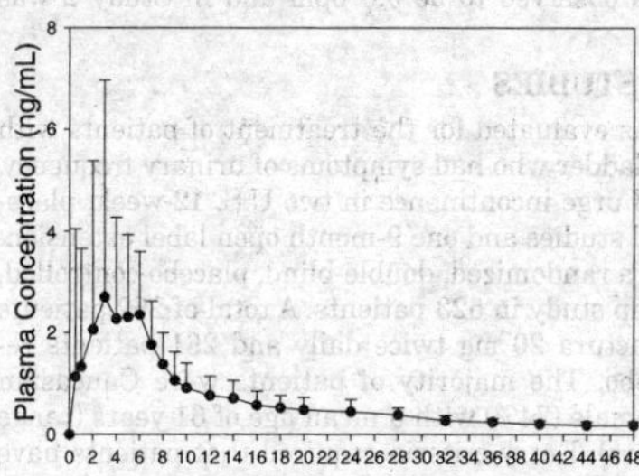

Figure 1. Mean (+ SD) Concentration-Time Profile for a Single 20 mg Oral Dose of Sanctura in Healthy Volunteers.

Pharmacokinetics in Special Populations

Age: Age did not appear to significantly affect the pharmacokinetics of Sanctura, however, increased anticholinergic side effects unrelated to drug exposure were observed in patients ≥75 years of age. (See PRECAUTIONS: Geriatric Use and DOSAGE AND ADMINISTRATION).

Pediatric: The pharmacokinetics of Sanctura were not evaluated in pediatric patients.

Gender: Studies comparing the pharmacokinetics in different genders had conflicting results. When a single 40 mg Sanctura dose was administered to 16 elderly subjects, exposure was 45% lower in elderly females compared to elderly males. When 20 mg Sanctura was dosed BID for 4 days to 6 elderly males and 6 elderly females (60 to 75 years), AUC and C_{max} were 26% and 68% higher, respectively, in females without hormone replacement therapy than in males.

Race: Pharmacokinetic differences due to race have not been studied.

Renal Insufficiency: Severe renal impairment significantly altered the disposition of Sanctura. A 4.5-fold and 2 fold increase in mean $AUC_{0-\infty}$ and C_{max}, respectively, and the appearance of an additional elimination phase with a long half-life (~33 hr) was detected in patients with severe renal insufficiency (CLcr < 30 mL/min) compared with healthy, nearly age-matched subjects. The different pharmacokinetic behavior of Sanctura in patients with severe renal insufficiency necessitates adjustment of dosage frequency. The pharmacokinetics of Sanctura have not been studied in people with moderate or mild renal impairment (CLcr ranging from 30-80 mL/min).(See PRECAUTIONS: General and DOSAGE AND ADMINISTRATION).

Continued on next page

Sanctura—Cont.

Hepatic Insufficiency: There is no information regarding the effect of severe hepatic impairment on exposure to Sanctura. Maximum trospium concentration (C_{max}) increased 12% and 63% in subjects with mild and moderate hepatic impairment, respectively, compared to healthy subjects. Mean area under the plasma concentration-time curve (AUC) was similar. Caution should be used when administering Sanctura to patients with moderate and severe hepatic dysfunction. (See PRECAUTIONS: General).

Drug-Drug Interactions
No *in vivo* drug-drug interaction studies have been performed to assess the effect of concomitant medications on the pharmacokinetics of Sanctura or to assess the effect of Sanctura on the pharmacokinetics of other drugs. Sanctura is metabolized by esterases and excreted by the kidneys by a combination of tubular secretion and glomerular filtration. Based on *in vitro* data, no clinically relevant interactions with the metabolism of trospium are expected. However, drugs which are actively secreted may interact with trospium by competing for renal tubular secretion. (See PRECAUTIONS: Drug Interactions).

Electrophysiology
The effect of 20 mg BID and up to 100 mg BID Sanctura on QT interval was evaluated in a single-blind, randomized, placebo and active (moxifloxacin 400 mg QD) controlled 5 day parallel trial in 170 male and female healthy volunteer subjects aged 18 to 45 years. The QT interval was measured over a 24 hour period at steady state. The 100 mg BID dose of Sanctura was chosen because this achieves the C_{max} expected in severe renal impairment. Sanctura was not associated with an increase in individual corrected (QTcI) or Fridericia corrected (QTcF) QT interval at any time during steady state measurement, while moxifloxacin was associated with a 6.4 msec increase in QTcF.
In this study, asymptomatic, non-specific T wave inversions were observed more often in subjects receiving Sanctura than in subjects receiving moxifloxacin or placebo following five days of treatment. This finding was not observed during routine safety monitoring in 2 other placebo-controlled clinical trials in 591 Sanctura-treated overactive bladder patients (See CLINICAL STUDIES). The clinical significance of T wave inversion in this study is unknown. Sanctura is associated with an increase in heart rate that correlates with increasing plasma concentrations. In the study described above, Sanctura demonstrated a mean increase in heart rate compared to placebo of 9.1 bpm for the 20 mg dose and of 18.0 bpm for the 100 mg dose. In the two U.S. placebo-controlled trials in patients with overactive bladder, the mean increase in heart rate compared to placebo in Study 1 was observed to be 3.0 bpm and in Study 2 was 4.0 bpm.

CLINICAL STUDIES

Sanctura was evaluated for the treatment of patients with overactive bladder who had symptoms of urinary frequency, urgency, and urge incontinence in two U.S. 12-week, placebo-controlled studies and one 9-month open label extension.
Study 1 was a randomized, double-blind, placebo-controlled, parallel-group study in 523 patients. A total of 262 patients received Sanctura 20 mg twice daily and 261 patients received placebo. The majority of patients were Caucasian (85%) and female (74%) with a mean age of 61 years (range 21 to 90 years). Entry criteria required that patients have urge or mixed incontinence (with a predominance of urge), urge incontinence episodes of at least 7 per week, and greater than 70 micturitions per week. The patient's medical history and urinary diary during the treatment-free baseline confirmed the diagnosis. Reductions in urinary frequency, urge incontinence episodes and urinary void volume for placebo and Sanctura treatment groups are summarized in Table 2 and Figures 2 and 3.
[See table 2 above]

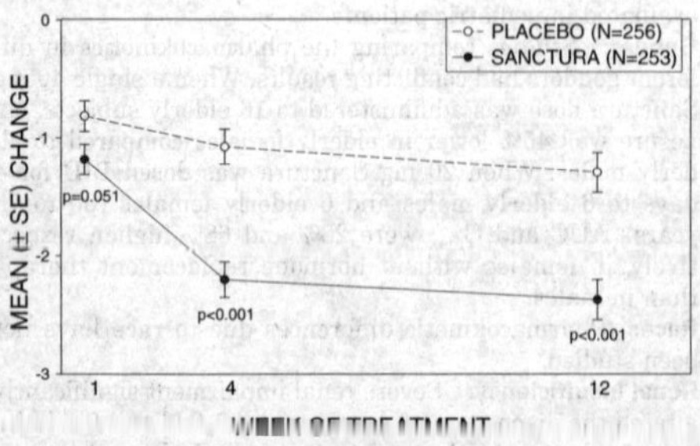

Figure 2 - Mean Change from Baseline in Urinary Frequency/24 Hours, by Visit: Study 1

[See figure 3 at top of next column]
Study 2 was nearly identical in design to Study 1. A total of 329 patients received Sanctura 20 mg twice daily and 329 patients received placebo. The majority of patients were Caucasian (88%) and female (82%) with a mean age of 61 years (range 19 to 94 years). Entry criteria were identical to Study 1. Reductions in urinary frequency, urge incontinence episodes, and urinary void volume for placebo and Sanctura treatment groups are summarized in Table 3 and Figures 4 and 5.

Table 2. Mean (SE) change from baseline to end of treatment (Week 12 or last observation carried forward) for urinary frequency, urge incontinence episodes, and void volume in Study 1.

Efficacy endpoint	Placebo N=256	Sanctura N=253	P-value
Urinary frequency/24 hours[a, *]			
Mean baseline	12.9	12.7	
Mean change from baseline	-1.3 (0.2)	-2.4 (0.2)	<0.001
Urge incontinence episodes/week[b, *]			
Mean baseline	30.1	27.3	
Mean change from baseline	-13.9 (1.2)	-15.4 (1.1)	0.012
Urinary void volume/toilet void (mL)[a, c]			
Mean baseline	156.6	155.1	
Mean change from baseline	7.7 (3.1)	32.1 (3.1)	<0.001

[a] Treatment differences assessed by analysis of variance for ITT:LOCF data set.
[b] Treatment differences assessed by ranked analysis of variance for ITT:LOCF data set.
[c] Placebo N=253, Sanctura N=248.
* Denotes co-primary endpoint
ITT=intent-to-treat, LOCF=last observation carried forward.

Table 3. Mean (SE) change from baseline to end of treatment (Week 12 or last observation carried forward) for urinary frequency, urge incontinence episodes, and void volume in Study 2.

Efficacy endpoint	Placebo N=325	Sanctura N=323	P-value
Urinary frequency/24 hours[a, *]			
Mean baseline	13.2	12.9	
Mean change from baseline	-1.8 (0.2)	-2.7 (0.2)	<0.001
Urge incontinence episodes/week[b]			
Mean baseline	27.3	26.9	
Mean change from baseline	-12.1 (1.0)	-16.1 (1.0)	<0.001
Urinary void volume/toilet void (mL)[a, c]			
Mean baseline	154.6	154.8	
Mean change from baseline	9.4 (2.8)	35.6 (2.8)	<0.001

[a] Treatment differences assessed by analysis of variance for ITT:LOCF data set.
[b] Treatment differences assessed by ranked analysis of variance for ITT:LOCF data set.
[c] Placebo N=320, Sanctura N=319.
* Denotes primary endpoint
ITT=intent-to-treat, LOCF=last observation carried forward.

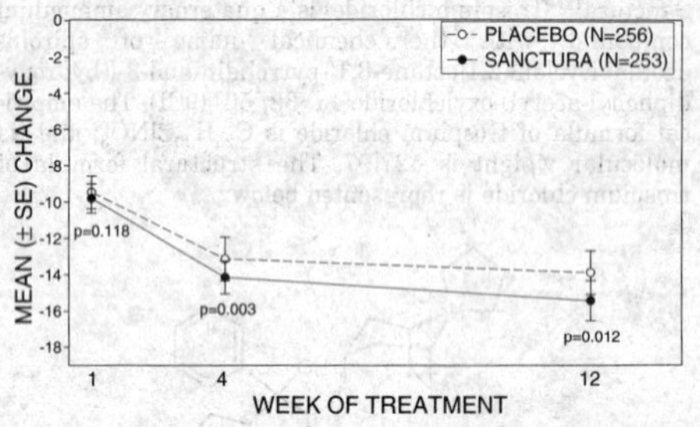

Figure 3 - Mean Change from Baseline in Urge Incontinence/Week, by Visit: Study 1

[See table 3 above]

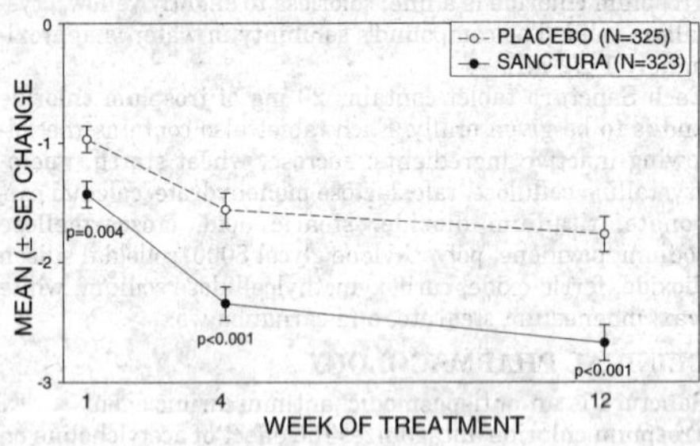

Figure 4 - Mean Change from Baseline in Urinary Frequency/24 Hours, by Visit: Study 2

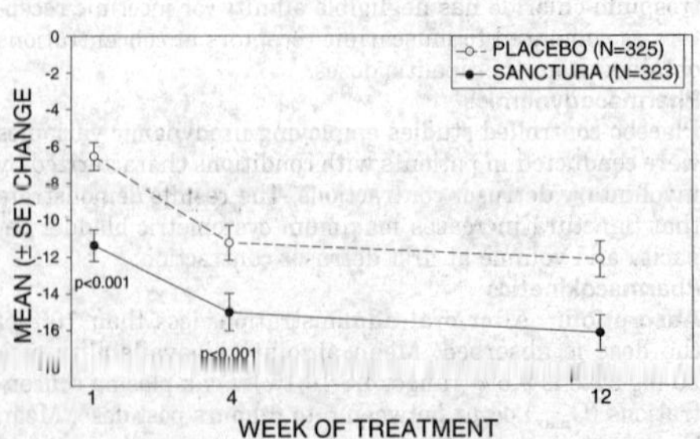

Figure 5 - Mean Change from Baseline in Urge Incontinence/Week, by Visit: Study 2

INDICATIONS AND USAGE

Sanctura is indicated for the treatment of overactive bladder with symptoms of urge urinary incontinence, urgency, and urinary frequency.

CONTRAINDICATIONS

Sanctura is contraindicated in patients with urinary retention, gastric retention, or uncontrolled narrow-angle glaucoma and in patients who are at risk for these conditions. Sanctura is also contraindicated in patients who have demonstrated hypersensitivity to the drug or its ingredients.

PRECAUTIONS

General
Risk of Urinary Retention: Sanctura should be administered with caution to patients with clinically significant bladder outflow obstruction because of the risk of urinary retention.
Decreased Gastrointestinal Motility: Sanctura should be administered with caution to patients with gastrointestinal obstructive disorders because of the risk of gastric retention (See CONTRAINDICATIONS). Sanctura, like other anticholinergic drugs, may decrease gastrointestinal motility and should be used with caution in patients with conditions such as ulcerative colitis, intestinal atony and myasthenia gravis.
Controlled Narrow-angle Glaucoma: In patients being treated for narrow-angle glaucoma, Sanctura should only be used if the potential benefits outweigh the risks and in that circumstance only with careful monitoring.
Patients with Renal Insufficiency: Dose modification is recommended in patients with severe renal insufficiency (CLcr < 30mL/min). In such patients, Sanctura should be administered as 20 mg once a day at bedtime (See DOSAGE AND ADMINISTRATION).
Patients with Hepatic Impairment: Caution should be used when administering Sanctura in patients with moderate or severe hepatic dysfunction (See CLINICAL PHARMACOLOGY: Pharmacokinetics in Special Populations).
Information for Patients
Patients should be informed that anticholinergic agents, such as Sanctura, may produce clinically significant adverse effects related to anticholinergic pharmacological activity. For example, heat prostration (fever and heat stroke due to decreased sweating) can occur when anticholinergics such as Sanctura are used in a hot environment. Because anticholinergics such as Sanctura may also produce dizziness or blurred vision, patients should be advised to exercise caution. Patients should be informed that alcohol may enhance the drowsiness caused by anticholinergic agents.
Sanctura should be taken 1 hour prior to meals or on an empty stomach. If a dose is skipped, patients are advised to take their next dose 1 hour prior to their next meal.
Drug Interactions
The concomitant use of Sanctura with other anticholinergic agents that produce dry mouth, constipation, and other anticholinergic pharmacological effects may increase the frequency and/or severity of such effects. Anticholinergic agents may potentially alter the absorption of some concomitantly administered drugs due to anticholinergic effects on gastrointestinal motility.
Drugs Eliminated by Active Tubular Secretion: Although studies to assess drug-drug interactions with Sanctura have not been conducted, Sanctura has the potential for pharmacokinetic interactions with other drugs that are eliminated by active tubular secretion (e.g. digoxin, procainamide, pancuronium, morphine, vancomycin, metformin and tenofovir). Coadministration of Sanctura with drugs that are eliminated by active renal tubular secretion may increase

the serum concentration of Sanctura and/or the coadministered drug due to competition for this elimination pathway. Careful patient monitoring is recommended in patients receiving such drugs (See CLINICAL PHARMACOLOGY: Excretion, and CLINICAL PHARMACOLOGY: Drug-Drug Interactions).

Drug-Laboratory-Test Interactions

Interactions between Sanctura and laboratory tests have not been studied.

Carcinogenesis, Mutagenesis, Impairment of Fertility

Carcinogenicity studies with trospium chloride were conducted in mice and rats. A 78-week carcinogenicity study in mice and a 104-week carcinogenicity study in rats were conducted at doses of 2, 20, and 200 mg/kg/day. No evidence of a carcinogenic effect was found in either mice or rats. The 200 mg/kg/day dose in the mouse and rat represents approximately 25 and 60 times, respectively, the human dose based on body surface area. At 200 mg/kg/day in the mouse and rat after 4 weeks the AUC was 34 and 753 ng•h/mL, respectively. The exposure in the rat is 8.6-fold higher than the AUC following 40 mg daily exposure in healthy young or elderly subjects (88 ng•h/mL).

Trospium chloride was not mutagenic in tests for detection of gene mutations in bacteria (Ames test) and mammalian cells (L5178Y mouse lymphoma and CHO cells) or in vivo in the rat micronucleus test.

No evidence of impaired fertility was observed in rats administered doses up to 200 mg/kg/day (about 10 multiples of the expected clinical exposure via AUC).

Pregnancy: Teratogenic Effects

Pregnancy Category C: Trospium chloride has been shown to cause maternal toxicity in rats and a decrease in fetal survival in rats administered approximately 10 times the expected clinical exposure (AUC). The no effect levels for maternal and fetal toxicity were approximately equivalent to the expected clinical exposure in rats, and about 5-6 times the expected clinical exposure in rabbits. No malformations or developmental delays were observed. There are no adequate and well controlled studies in pregnant women. Sanctura should be used during pregnancy only if the potential benefit justifies the potential risk to the fetus.

Nursing Mothers

Trospium chloride (2 mg/kg PO and 50 µg/kg IV) was excreted, to a limited extent (<1%), into the milk of lactating rats. The activity observed in the milk was primarily from the parent compound. It is not known whether this drug is excreted in human milk. Because many drugs are excreted in human milk, caution should be exercised when Sanctura is administered to a nursing woman. Sanctura should be used during lactation only if the potential benefit justifies the potential risk to the newborn.

Pediatric Use

The safety and effectiveness of Sanctura in pediatric patients have not been established.

Geriatric Use

Of the 591 patients with overactive bladder who received treatment with Sanctura in the two U.S., placebo-controlled, efficacy and safety studies, 249 patients (42%) were 65 years of age and older. Eighty-eight Sanctura-treated patients (15%) were ≥ 75 years of age.

In these 2 studies, the incidence of commonly reported anticholinergic adverse events in patients treated with Sanctura (including dry mouth, constipation, dyspepsia, UTI, and urinary retention) was higher in patients 75 years of age and older as compared to younger patients. This effect may be related to an enhanced sensitivity to anticholinergic agents in this patient population (See CLINICAL PHARMACOLOGY: Pharmacokinetics in Special Populations and DOSAGE AND ADMINISTRATION). Therefore, based upon tolerability, the dose frequency of Sanctura may be reduced to 20 mg once daily in patients 75 years of age and older.

ADVERSE REACTIONS

The safety of Sanctura was evaluated in Phase 2 and 3 controlled clinical trials in a total of 2975 patients, who were treated with Sanctura (N=1673), placebo (N=1056) or active control medications (N=246). Of this total, 1181 patients participated in two, twelve-week, Phase 3, U.S., efficacy and safety studies and a 9-month open-label extension. Of this total, 591 patients received Sanctura 20 mg twice daily. In all controlled trials combined, 232 and 208 patients received treatment with Sanctura for at least 24 and 52 weeks, respectively.

In all placebo-controlled trials combined, the incidence of serious adverse events was 2.9% among patients receiving Sanctura 20 mg BID and 1.5% among patients receiving placebo. Of these, 0.2% and 0.3% were judged to be at least possibly related to treatment with Sanctura or placebo, respectively, by the investigator.

Table 4 lists treatment emergent adverse events from the combined 12-week U.S. safety and efficacy trials that were judged to be at least possibly related to treatment with Sanctura by the investigator, were reported by at least 1% of patients, and were reported more frequently in the Sanctura group than in the placebo group.

The 2 most common adverse events reported by patients receiving Sanctura 20 mg BID were dry mouth and constipation. The single most frequently reported adverse event for Sanctura, dry mouth, occurred in 20.1% of Sanctura treated patients and 5.8% of patients receiving placebo. In the two Phase 3 U.S. studies, dry mouth led to discontinuation in 1.9% of patients treated with Sanctura 20 mg BID. For the patients who reported dry mouth, most had their first occurrence of the event within the first month of treatment.

Table 4. Incidence (%) of adverse events judged at least possibly related to treatment with Sanctura, reported in ≥ 1% of all patients treated with Sanctura and more frequent with Sanctura (20 mg BID) than placebo in Studies 1 and 2 combined.

Adverse Event	Placebo (N=590)	Sanctura 20 mg BID (N=591)
Gastrointestinal disorders		
Dry mouth	34 (5.8)	119 (20.1)
Constipation	27 (4.6)	57 (9.6)
Abdominal pain upper	7 (1.2)	9 (1.5)
Constipation aggravated	5 (0.8)	8 (1.4)
Dyspepsia	2 (0.3)	7 (1.2)
Flatulence	5 (0.8)	7 (1.2)
Nervous system disorders		
Headache	12 (2.0)	25 (4.2)
General Disorders		
Fatigue	8 (1.4)	11 (1.9)
Renal and Urinary Disorders	8 (1.4)	11 (1.9)
Urinary retention	2 (0.3)	7 (1.2)
Eye Disorders		
Dry eyes NOS	2 (0.3)	7 (1.2)

Abbreviations: BID=twice daily, NOS=not otherwise specified.

Other adverse events from the Phase 3, U.S., placebo-controlled trials judged possibly related to treatment with Sanctura by the investigator, occurring in ≥0.5% of Sanctura-treated patients, and more common with Sanctura than placebo are: tachycardia NOS, vision blurred, abdominal distension, vomiting NOS, dysgeusia, dry throat, and dry skin.

During controlled clinical studies, one event of angioneurotic edema was reported.

Postmarketing Surveillance

Additional spontaneous adverse events, regardless of relationship to drug, reported from marketing experience with trospium chloride include: gastritis, palpitations, supraventricular tachycardia, chest pain, Stevens-Johnson syndrome, anaphylactic reaction, syncope, rhabdomyolysis, vision abnormal, hallucinations and delirium, and "hypertensive crisis".

OVERDOSAGE

Management of Overdosage

Overdosage with Sanctura may result in severe anticholinergic effects. Treatment should be provided according to symptoms and supportive. In the event of overdosage, ECG monitoring is recommended.

A 7-month-old baby experienced tachycardia and mydriasis after administration of a single dose of trospium 10 mg given by a sibling. The baby's weight was reported as 5 kg. Following admission into the hospital and about 1 hour after ingestion of the trospium, medicinal charcoal was administered for detoxification. While hospitalized, the baby experienced mydriasis and tachycardia up to 230 beats/minute. Therapeutic intervention was not deemed necessary. The baby was discharged as completely recovered the following day.

DOSAGE AND ADMINISTRATION

The recommended dose is 20 mg twice daily. Sanctura should be dosed at least one hour before meals or given on an empty stomach.

Dosage modification is recommended in the following patient populations:

For patients with severe renal impairment (CLcr < 30 mL/min), the recommended dose is 20 mg once daily at bedtime (See PRECAUTIONS: General).

In geriatric patients ≥ 75 years of age, dose may be titrated down to 20 mg once daily based upon tolerability (See PRECAUTIONS: Geriatric Use).

HOW SUPPLIED

Sanctura™ tablets 20 mg (brownish yellow, biconvex, glossy coated tablets printed with black ink) are supplied as follows:

60 count HDPE bottle- NDC 65473-980-04
500 count HDPE bottle- NDC 65473-980-02
14 count blister (PVC/Paper backed foil) - NDC 65473-980-70
14 count blister (PVC-Aclar/Paper backed foil) - NDC 65473-980-71

Store at controlled room temperature 20° to 25°C (68° to 77°F) (see USP).

Rx only

Manufactured for:
Odyssey Pharmaceuticals, Inc.
East Hanover, NJ 07936 USA
and
Indevus Pharmaceuticals, Inc.
Lexington, MA 02421 USA
Manufactured by:
Madaus AG
Troisdorf, Germany
Address Medical Inquiries to:
www.SANCTURA.com or (877)-427-9068

SURMONTIL® ℞

(trimipramine maleate)
℞ only

DESCRIPTION

Surmontil (trimipramine maleate) is 5-(3-dimethylamino-2-methylpropyl)-10,11-dihydro-5H-dibenz (b,f) azepine acid maleate (racemic form).

$\cdot C_4H_4O_4$

CH_2—*CH(CH_3)—CH_2—N(CH_3)$_2$

Molecular Formula: $C_{20}H_{26}N_2 \cdot C_4H_4O_4$
Molecular Weight: 410.5

Surmontil capsules contain trimipramine maleate equivalent to 25 mg, 50 mg, or 100 mg of trimipramine as the base. The inactive ingredients present are FD&C Blue 1, gelatin, lactose, magnesium stearate, and titanium dioxide. The 25 mg dosage strength also contains D&C Yellow 10 and FD&C Yellow 6; the 50 mg dosage strength also contains D&C Red 28, FD&C Red 40, and FD&C Yellow 6.

Trimipramine maleate is prepared as a racemic mixture which can be resolved into levorotatory and dextrorotatory isomers. The asymmetric center responsible for optical isomerism is marked in the formula by an asterisk. Trimipramine maleate is an almost odorless, white or slightly cream-colored, crystalline substance, melting at 140°–144° C. It is very slightly soluble in ether and water, is slightly soluble in ethyl alcohol and acetone, and freely soluble in chloroform and methanol at 20° C.

CLINICAL PHARMACOLOGY

Surmontil is an antidepressant with an anxiety-reducing sedative component to its action. The mode of action of Surmontil on the central nervous system is not known. However, unlike amphetamine-type compounds it does not act primarily by stimulation of the central nervous system. It does not act by inhibition of the monoamine oxidase system.

The single-dose pharmacokinetics of trimipramine were evaluated in a comparative study of 24 elderly subjects and 24 younger subjects; no clinically relevant differences were demonstrated based on age or gender.

INDICATIONS AND USAGE

Surmontil is indicated for the relief of symptoms of depression. Endogenous depression is more likely to be alleviated than other depressive states. In studies with neurotic outpatients, the drug appeared to be equivalent to amitriptyline in the less-depressed patients but somewhat less effective than amitriptyline in the more severely depressed patients. In hospitalized depressed patients, trimipramine and imipramine were equally effective in relieving depression.

CONTRAINDICATIONS

Surmontil is contraindicated in cases of known hypersensitivity to the drug. The possibility of cross-sensitivity to other dibenzazepine compounds should be kept in mind. Surmontil should not be given in conjunction with drugs of the monoamine oxidase inhibitor class (e.g., tranylcypromine, isocarboxazid or phenelzine sulfate). The concomitant use of monoamine oxidase inhibitors (MAOI) and tricyclic compounds similar to Surmontil has caused severe hyperpyretic reactions, convulsive crises, and death in some patients. At least two weeks should elapse after cessation of therapy with MAOI before instituting therapy with Surmontil. Initial dosage should be low and increased gradually with caution and careful observation of the patient. The drug is contraindicated during the acute recovery period after a myocardial infarction.

WARNINGS

General Consideration for Use

Extreme caution should be used when this drug is given to patients with any evidence of cardiovascular disease because of the possibility of conduction defects, arrhythmias, myocardial infarction, strokes, and tachycardia.

Caution is advised in patients with increased intraocular pressure, history of urinary retention, or history of narrow-angle glaucoma because of the drug's anticholinergic properties; hyperthyroid patients or those on thyroid medication because of the possibility of cardiovascular toxicity; patients with a history of seizure disorder, because this drug has been shown to lower the seizure threshold; patients receiving guanethidine or similar agents, since Surmontil (trimipramine maleate) may block the pharmacologic effects of these drugs.

Since the drug may impair the mental and/or physical abilities required for the performance of potentially hazardous tasks, such as operating an automobile or machinery, the patient should be cautioned accordingly.

PRECAUTIONS

General

The possibility of suicide is inherent in any severely depressed patient and persists until a significant remission occurs. When a patient with a serious suicidal potential is not hospitalized, the prescription should be for the smallest amount feasible.

Continued on next page

Surmontil—Cont.

In schizophrenic patients activation of the psychosis may occur and require reduction of dosage or the addition of a major tranquilizer to the therapeutic regime.
Manic or hypomanic episodes may occur in some patients, in particular those with cyclic-type disorders. In some cases therapy with Surmontil must be discontinued until the episode is relieved, after which therapy may be reinstituted at lower dosages if still required.
Concurrent administration of Surmontil and electroshock therapy may increase the hazards of therapy. Such treatment should be limited to those patients for whom it is essential. When possible, discontinue the drug for several days prior to elective surgery.
Surmontil should be used with caution in patients with impaired liver function.
Chronic animal studies showed occasional occurrence of hepatic congestion, fatty infiltration, or increased serum liver enzymes at the highest dose of 60 mg/kg/day.
Both elevation and lowering of blood sugar have been reported with tricyclic antidepressants.

Drug Interactions

Cimetidine

There is evidence that cimetidine inhibits the elimination of tricyclic antidepressants. Downward adjustment of Surmontil dosage may be required if cimetidine therapy is initiated; upward adjustment if cimetidine therapy is discontinued.

Alcohol

Patients should be warned that the concomitant use of alcoholic beverages may be associated with exaggerated effects.

Catecholamines/Anticholinergics

It has been reported that tricyclic antidepressants can potentiate the effects of catecholamines. Similarly, atropine-like effects may be more pronounced in patients receiving anticholinergic therapy. Therefore, particular care should be exercised when it is necessary to administer tricyclic antidepressants with sympathomimetic amines, local decongestants, local anesthetics containing epinephrine, atropine or drugs with an anticholinergic effect. In resistant cases of depression in adults, a dose of 2.5 mg/kg/day may have to be exceeded. If a higher dose is needed, ECG monitoring should be maintained during the initiation of therapy and at appropriate intervals during stabilization of dose.

Drugs Metabolized by P450 2D6

The biochemical activity of the drug metabolizing isozyme cytochrome P450 2D6 (debrisoquin hydroxylase) is reduced in a subset of the caucasian population (about 7–10% of caucasians are so called "poor metabolizers"); reliable estimates of the prevalence of reduced P450 2D6 isozyme activity among Asian, African, and other populations are not yet available. Poor metabolizers have higher than expected plasma concentrations of tricyclic antidepressants (TCAs) when given usual doses. Depending on the fraction of drug metabolized by P450 2D6, the increase in plasma concentration may be small, or quite large (8 fold increase in plasma AUC of the TCA).
In addition, certain drugs inhibit the activity of the isozyme and make normal metabolizers resemble poor metabolizers. An individual who is stable on a given dose of TCA may become abruptly toxic when given one of these inhibiting drugs as concomitant therapy. The drugs that inhibit cytochrome P450 2D6 include some that are not metabolized by the enzyme (quinidine; cimetidine) and many that are substrates for P450 2D6 (many other antidepressants, phenothiazines, and the Type 1C antiarrhythmics propafenone and flecainide). While all the selective serotonin reuptake inhibitors (SSRIs), e.g., fluoxetine, sertraline, and paroxetine, inhibit P450 2D6, they may vary in the extent of inhibition. The extent to which SSRI TCA interactions may pose clinical problems will depend on the degree of inhibition and the pharmacokinetics of the SSRI involved. Nevertheless, caution is indicated in the co-administration of TCAs with any of the SSRIs and also in switching from one class to the other. Of particular importance, sufficient time must elapse before initiating TCA treatment in a patient being withdrawn from fluoxetine, given the long half-life of the parent and active metabolite (at least 5 weeks may be necessary).
Concomitant use of tricyclic antidepressants with drugs that can inhibit cytochrome P450 2D6 may require lower doses than usually prescribed for either the tricyclic antidepressant or the other drug. Furthermore, whenever one of these other drugs is withdrawn from co-therapy, an increased dose of tricyclic antidepressant may be required. It is desirable to monitor TCA plasma levels whenever a TCA is going to be co-administered with another drug known to be an inhibitor of P450 2D6.

Carcinogenesis, Mutagenesis, Impairment of Fertility

Semen studies in man (four schizophrenics and nine normal volunteers) revealed no significant changes in sperm morphology. It is recognized that drugs having a parasympathetic effect, including tricyclic antidepressants, may alter the ejaculatory response.
Chronic animal studies showed occasional evidence of degeneration of seminiferous tubules at the highest dose of 60 mg/kg/day.

Pregnancy

Teratogenic Effects—Pregnancy Category C

Surmontil has shown evidence of embryotoxicity and/or increased incidence of major anomalies in rats or rabbits at doses 20 times the human dose. There are no adequate and well-controlled studies in pregnant women. Surmontil should be used during pregnancy only if the potential benefit justifies the potential risk to the fetus.

Pediatric Use

This drug is not recommended for use in children, since safety and effectiveness in the pediatric age group have not been established.

Geriatric Use

Clinical studies of Surmontil® (trimipramine maleate) were not adequate to determine whether subjects aged 65 and over respond differently from younger subjects.
The pharmacokinetics of trimipramine were not substantially altered in the elderly (see **CLINICAL PHARMACOLOGY**).
Surmontil is known to be substantially excreted by the kidney. Clinical circumstances, some of which may be more common in the elderly, such as hepatic or renal impairment, should be considered (see **PRECAUTIONS—General**).
Greater sensitivity (e.g., confusional states, sedation) of some older individuals cannot be ruled out (see **ADVERSE REACTIONS**). In general, dose selection for an elderly patient should be cautious, usually starting at a lower dose (see **DOSAGE AND ADMINISTRATION**).

ADVERSE REACTIONS

Note: The pharmacological similarities among the tricyclic antidepressants require that each of the reactions be considered when Surmontil is administered. Some of the adverse reactions included in this listing have not in fact been reported with Surmontil.

Cardiovascular

Hypotension, hypertension, tachycardia, palpitation, myocardial infarction, arrhythmias, heart block, stroke.

Psychiatric

Confusional states (especially the elderly) with hallucinations, disorientation, delusions; anxiety, restlessness, agitation; insomnia and nightmares; hypomania; exacerbation of psychosis.

Neurological

Numbness, tingling, paresthesias of extremities; incoordination, ataxia, tremors; peripheral neuropathy; extrapyramidal symptoms; seizures, alterations in EEG patterns; tinnitus; syndrome of inappropriate ADH (antidiuretic hormone) secretion.

Anticholinergic

Dry mouth and, rarely, associated sublingual adenitis; blurred vision, disturbances of accommodation, mydriasis, constipation, paralytic ileus; urinary retention, delayed micturition, dilation of the urinary tract.

Allergic

Skin rash, petechiae, urticaria, itching, photosensitization, edema of face and tongue.

Hematologic

Bone-marrow depression including agranulocytosis, eosinophilia; purpura; thrombocytopenia. Leukocyte and differential counts should be performed in any patient who develops fever and sore throat during therapy; the drug should be discontinued if there is evidence of pathological neutrophil depression.

Gastrointestinal

Nausea and vomiting, anorexia, epigastric distress, diarrhea, peculiar taste, stomatitis, abdominal cramps, black tongue.

Endocrine

Gynecomastia in the male; breast enlargement and galactorrhea in the female; increased or decreased libido, impotence; testicular swelling; elevation or depression of blood-sugar levels.

Other

Jaundice (simulating obstructive); altered liver function; weight gain or loss; perspiration; flushing; urinary frequency; drowsiness, dizziness, weakness, and fatigue; headache; parotid swelling; alopecia.

Withdrawal Symptoms

Though not indicative of addiction, abrupt cessation of treatment after prolonged therapy may produce nausea, headache, and malaise.

DOSAGE AND ADMINISTRATION

Dosage should be initiated at a low level and increased gradually, noting carefully the clinical response and any evidence of intolerance.
Lower dosages are recommended for elderly patients and adolescents. Lower dosages are also recommended for outpatients as compared to hospitalized patients who will be under close supervision. It is not possible to prescribe a single dosage schedule of Surmontil that will be therapeutically effective in all patients. The physical psychodynamic factors contributing to depressive symptomatology are very complex; spontaneous remissions or exacerbations of depressive symptoms may occur with or without drug therapy. Consequently, the recommended dosage regimens are furnished as a guide which may be modified by factors such as the age of the patient, chronicity and severity of the disease, medical condition of the patient, and degree of psychotherapeutic support.
Most antidepressant drugs have a lag period of ten days to four weeks before a therapeutic response is noted. Increasing the dose will not shorten this period but rather increase the incidence of adverse reactions.

Usual Adult Dose

Outpatients and Office Patients—Initially, 75 mg/day in divided doses, increased to 150 mg/day. Dosages over 200 mg/day are not recommended. Maintenance therapy is in the range of 50 to 150 mg/day. For convenient therapy and to facilitate patient compliance, the total dosage requirement may be given at bedtime.
Hospitalized Patients—Initially, 100 mg/day in divided doses. This may be increased gradually in a few days to 200 mg/day, depending upon individual response and tolerance. If improvement does not occur in 2 to 3 weeks, the dose may be increased to the maximum recommended dose of 250 to 300 mg/day.
Adolescent and Geriatric Patients—Initially, a dose of 50 mg/day is recommended, with gradual increments up to 100 mg/day, depending upon patient response and tolerance.
Maintenance—Following remission, maintenance medication may be required for a longer period of time, at the lowest dose that will maintain remission. Maintenance therapy is preferably administered as a single dose at bedtime. To minimize relapse, maintenance therapy should be continued for about three months.

OVERDOSAGE*

Deaths may occur from overdosage with this class of drugs. Multiple drug ingestion (including alcohol) is common in deliberate tricyclic antidepressant overdose. As the management is complex and changing, it is recommended that the physician contact a poison control center for current information on treatment. Signs and symptoms of toxicity develop rapidly after tricyclic antidepressant overdose, therefore, hospital monitoring is required as soon as possible.

Manifestations

Critical manifestations of overdose include: cardiac dysrhythmias, severe hypotension, convulsions, and CNS depression, including coma. Changes in the electrocardiogram, particularly in QRS axis or width, are clinically significant indicators of tricyclic antidepressant toxicity.
Other signs of overdose may include: confusion, disturbed concentration, transient visual hallucinations, dilated pupils, agitation, hyperactive reflexes, stupor, drowsiness, muscle rigidity, vomiting, hypothermia, hyperpyrexia, or any of the symptoms listed under **ADVERSE REACTIONS**.

Management

General

Obtain an ECG and immediately initiate cardiac monitoring. Protect the patient's airway, establish an intravenous line and initiate gastric decontamination. A minimum of six hours of observation with cardiac monitoring and observation for signs of CNS or respiratory depression, hypotension, cardiac dysrhythmias and/or conduction blocks, and seizures is necessary. If signs of toxicity occur at any time during this period, extended monitoring is required. There are case reports of patients succumbing to fatal dysrhythmias late after overdose; these patients had clinical evidence of significant poisoning prior to death and most received inadequate gastrointestinal decontamination. Plasma drug levels may not reflect the severity of the poisoning. Therefore, monitoring of plasma drug levels alone should not guide management of the patient.

Gastrointestinal Decontamination

All patients suspected of tricyclic antidepressant overdose should receive gastrointestinal decontamination. This should include large volume gastric lavage followed by activated charcoal. If consciousness is impaired, the airway should be secured prior to lavage. Emesis is contraindicated.

Cardiovascular

A maximal limb-lead QRS duration of ≥ 0.10 seconds has been associated with an increased incidence of seizures. A QRS duration of ≥ 0.16 seconds has been associated with an increased incidence of ventricular dysrhythmias. Intravenous sodium bicarbonate should be used to maintain the serum pH in the range of 7.45 to 7.55. If the pH response is inadequate, hyperventilation may also be used. Concomitant use of hyperventilation and sodium bicarbonate should be done with extreme caution, with frequent pH monitoring. A pH > 7.60 or a $pCO_2 < 20$ mm Hg is undesirable. Dysrhythmias unresponsive to sodium bicarbonate therapy/hyperventilation may respond to lidocaine, bretylium or phenytoin. Type 1A and 1C antiarrhythmics are generally contraindicated (e.g., quinidine, disopyramide, and procainamide).
In rare instances, hemoperfusion may be beneficial in acute refractory cardiovascular instability in patients with acute toxicity. However, hemodialysis, peritoneal dialysis, exchange transfusions, and forced diuresis generally have been reported as ineffective in tricyclic antidepressant poisoning.

CNS

In patients with CNS depression, early intubation is advised because of the potential for abrupt deterioration. Seizures should be controlled with benzodiazepines, or if these are ineffective, other anticonvulsants (e.g., phenobarbital, phenytoin). Physostigmine is not recommended except to treat life-threatening symptoms that have been unresponsive to other therapies, and then only in consultation with a poison control center.

Psychiatric Follow-up

Since overdosage is often deliberate, patients may attempt suicide by other means during the recovery phase. Psychiatric referral may be appropriate.

Pediatric Management

The principles of management of child and adult overdosages are similar. It is strongly recommended that the physician contact the local poison control center for specific pediatric treatment.

*Poisindex® Toxicologic Management. Topic: Antidepressants, Tricyclic Micromedex Inc. Vol. 85.

HOW SUPPLIED

Surmontil® (trimipramine maleate) Capsules

25 mg — Opaque blue and yellow capsule in bottles of 100.
Printed OP and 718

50 mg — Opaque blue and orange capsule in bottles of 100.
Printed OP and 719

100 mg — Opaque blue and white capsule in bottles of 100.
Printed OP and 720

Store at room temperature, approximately 25°C (77°F).
Keep bottles tightly closed.
Dispense in a tight container.

Manufactured for Odyssey Pharmaceuticals, Inc.
East Hanover, NJ 07936
By Wyeth Laboratories
A Wyeth-Ayerst Co.
Guayama, Puerto Rico 00784
P08-0718 **CI 7476-2** Rev. 10/01

Shown in Product Identification Guide, page 327

URECHOLINE® ℞

[ū-rĕch-ō-līn]

Bethanechol Chloride, USP

5-mg, 10-mg, 25-mg, and 50-mg scored tablets

DESCRIPTION

Bethanechol chloride, a cholinergic agent, is a synthetic ester which is structurally and pharmacologically related to acetylcholine.

It is designated chemically as 2-[(aminocarbonyl)oxy]-*N, N, N*-trimethyl-1-propanaminium chloride. Its molecular formula is $C_7H_{17}ClN_2O_2$ and its structural formula is:

$$\left[\begin{array}{l} CH_3CHCH_2N^+(CH_3)_3 \\ \quad | \\ \quad OCONH_2 \end{array} \right] Cl^-$$

It is a white, hygroscopic crystalline powder having a slight amine-like odor, freely soluble in water, and has a molecular weight of 196.68.

Each tablet for oral administration contains 5 mg, 10 mg, 25 mg or 50 mg bethanechol chloride, USP. Tablets also contain the following inactive ingredients: anhydrous lactose, colloidal silicon dioxide, magnesium stearate, microcrystalline cellulose, sodium starch glycolate, and (25 mg and 50 mg) D&C Yellow #10 and FD&C Yellow #6.

CLINICAL PHARMACOLOGY

Bethanechol chloride acts principally by producing the effects of stimulation of the parasympathetic nervous system. It increases the tone of the detrusor urinae muscle, usually producing a contraction sufficiently strong to initiate micturition and empty the bladder. It stimulates gastric motility, increases gastric tone and often restores impaired rhythmic peristalsis.

Stimulation of the parasympathetic nervous system releases acetylcholine at the nerve endings. When spontaneous stimulation is reduced and therapeutic intervention is required, acetylcholine can be given, but it is rapidly hydrolyzed by cholinesterase and its effects are transient. Bethanechol chloride is not destroyed by cholinesterase and its effects are more prolonged than those of acetylcholine.

Effects on the GI and urinary tracts sometimes appear within 30 minutes after oral administration of bethanechol chloride, but more often 60 to 90 minutes are required to reach maximum effectiveness. Following oral administration, the usual duration of action of bethanechol is one hour, although large doses (300 to 400 mg) have been reported to produce effects for up to six hours. Subcutaneous injection produces a more intense action on bladder muscle than does oral administration of the drug.

Because of the selective action of bethanechol, nicotinic symptoms of cholinergic stimulation are usually absent or minimal when orally or subcutaneously administered in therapeutic doses, while muscarinic effects are prominent. Muscarinic effects usually occur within 5 to 15 minutes after subcutaneous injection, reach a maximum in 15 to 30 minutes, and disappear within two hours. Doses that stimulate micturition and defecation and increase peristalsis do not ordinarily stimulate ganglia or voluntary muscles. Therapeutic test doses in normal human subjects have little effect on heart rate, blood pressure or peripheral circulation.

Bethanechol chloride does not cross the blood-brain barrier because of its charged quaternary amine moiety. The metabolic rate and mode of excretion of the drug have not been elucidated.

A clinical study (Diokno, A.C.; Lapides, J.; *Urol* 10: 23–24, July 1977) was conducted on the relative effectiveness of oral and subcutaneous doses of bethanechol chloride on the stretch response of bladder muscle in patients with urinary retention. Results showed that 5 mg of the drug given subcutaneously stimulated a response that was more rapid in onset and of larger magnitude than an oral dose of 50 mg, 100 mg, or 200 mg. All the oral doses, however, had a longer duration of effect than the subcutaneous dose. Although the 50 mg oral dose caused little change in intravesical pressure in this study, this dose has been found in other studies to be clinically effective in the rehabilitation of patients with decompensated bladders.

INDICATIONS AND USAGE

Bethanechol chloride is indicated for the treatment of acute postoperative and postpartum nonobstructive (functional) urinary retention and for neurogenic atony of the urinary bladder with retention.

CONTRAINDICATIONS

Hypersensitivity to bethanechol chloride tablets, hyperthyroidism, peptic ulcer, latent or active bronchial asthma, pronounced bradycardia or hypotension, vasomotor instability, coronary artery disease, epilepsy and parkinsonism.

Bethanechol chloride should not be employed when the strength or integrity of the gastrointestinal or bladder wall is in question, or in the presence of mechanical obstruction; when increased muscular activity of the gastrointestinal tract or urinary bladder might prove harmful, as following recent urinary bladder surgery, gastrointestinal resection and anastomosis, or when there is possible gastrointestinal obstruction; in bladder neck obstruction, spastic gastrointestinal disturbances, acute inflammatory lesions of the gastrointestinal tract, or peritonitis; or in marked vagotonia.

PRECAUTIONS

General: In urinary retention, if the sphincter fails to relax as bethanechol contracts the bladder, urine may be forced up the ureter into the kidney pelvis. If there is bacteriuria, this may cause reflux infection.

Information for Patients: Bethanechol chloride tablets should preferably be taken one hour before or two hours after meals to avoid nausea or vomiting. Dizziness, lightheadedness or fainting may occur, especially when getting up from a lying or sitting position.

Drug Interactions: Special care is required if this drug is given to patients receiving ganglion blocking compounds because a critical fall in blood pressure may occur. Usually, severe abdominal symptoms appear before there is such a fall in the blood pressure.

Carcinogenesis, Mutagenesis, Impairment of Fertility: Long-term studies in animals have not been performed to evaluate the effects upon fertility, mutagenic or carcinogenic potential of bethanechol chloride.

Pregnancy: ***Teratogenic Effects:*** Pregnancy Category C. Animal reproduction studies have not been conducted with bethanechol chloride. It is also not known whether bethanechol chloride can cause fetal harm when administered to a pregnant woman or can affect reproduction capacity. Bethanechol chloride should be given to a pregnant woman only if clearly needed.

Nursing Mothers: It is not known whether this drug is secreted in human milk. Because many drugs are secreted in human milk and because of the potential for serious adverse reactions from bethanechol chloride in nursing infants, a decision should be made whether to discontinue nursing or to discontinue the drug, taking into account the importance of the drug to the mother.

Pediatric Use: Safety and effectiveness in pediatric patients have not been established.

ADVERSE REACTIONS

Adverse reactions are rare following oral administration of bethanechol, but are more common following subcutaneous injection. Adverse reactions are more likely to occur when dosage is increased.

The following adverse reactions have been observed: *Body as a Whole:* malaise; *Digestive:* abdominal cramps or discomfort, colicky pain, nausea and belching, diarrhea, borborygmi, salivation; *Renal:* urinary urgency; *Nervous System:* headache; *Cardiovascular:* a fall in blood pressure with reflex tachycardia, vasomotor response; *Skin:* flushing producing a feeling of warmth, sensation of heat about the face, sweating; *Respiratory:* bronchial constriction, asthmatic attacks; *Special Senses:* lacrimation, miosis.

Causal Relationship Unknown: The following adverse reactions have been reported, and a causal relationship to therapy with bethanechol has not been established: *Body as a Whole:* malaise; *Nervous System:* seizures.

OVERDOSAGE

Early signs of overdosage are abdominal discomfort, salivation, flushing of the skin ("hot feeling"), sweating, nausea, and vomiting.

Atropine Sulfate is a specific antidote. The recommended dose for adults is 0.6 mg. Repeat doses can be given every two hours, according to clinical response. The recommended dosage in infants and children up to 12 years of age is 0.01 mg/kg (to a maximum single dose of 0.4 mg) repeated every two hours as needed until the desired effect is obtained or adverse effects of atropine preclude further usage. Subcutaneous injection of atropine is preferred except in emergencies when the intravenous route may be employed.

The oral LD_{50} of bethanechol chloride is 1510 mg/kg in the mouse.

DOSAGE AND ADMINISTRATION

Dosage must be individualized, depending on the type and severity of the condition to be treated.

Preferably give the drug when the stomach is empty. If taken soon after eating, nausea and vomiting may occur.

The usual adult oral dose ranges from 10 to 50 mg three or four times a day. The minimum effective dose is determined by giving 5 to 10 mg initially and repeating the same amount at hourly intervals until satisfactory response occurs, or until a maximum of 50 mg has been given. The effects of the drug sometimes appear within 30 minutes and are usually maximal within 60 to 90 minutes. The drug effects persist for about one hour.

If necessary, the effects of the drug can be abolished promptly by atropine (see **OVERDOSAGE**).

HOW SUPPLIED

Urecholine® Tablets

5 mg—White, round, scored tablets in bottles of 100. Debossed OP 697

10 mg—White, round, scored tablets in bottles of 100. Debossed OP 703

25 mg—Yellow, round, scored tablets in bottles of 100. Debossed OP 704

50 mg—Yellow round, scored tablets in bottles of 100. Debossed OP 700

Dispense in a tight container as defined in the USP.

Store at controlled room temperature 15°–30°C (59°–86°F).

Distributed by Odyssey Pharmaceuticals, Inc.,
East Hanover, New Jersey 07936
Manufactured by PLIVA®, Inc,
East Hanover, NJ 07936

Iss. 1/03

Shown in Product Identification Guide, page 327

VIVACTIL® ℞

[vī văc tĭl]

(Protriptyline HCl, USP) 5 mg and 10 mg Tablets

DESCRIPTION

Protriptyline HCl is *N*-methyl-5*H*-dibenzo[*a,d*]-cycloheptene-5-propanamine hydrochloride. Its molecular formula is $C_{19}H_{21}N{\bullet}HCl$ and its structural formula is:

H CH₂CH₂CH₂NHCH₃ • HCl

Protriptyline HCl, a dibenzocycloheptene derivative, has a molecular weight of 299.84. It is a white to yellowish powder that is freely soluble in water and soluble in dilute HCl.

Protriptyline HCl is supplied as 5 mg or 10 mg film-coated tablets. Inactive ingredients are anhydrous lactose, carnauba wax, corn starch, dibasic calcium phosphate, hydroxypropyl cellulose, hydroxypropyl methylcellulose, magnesium stearate, microcrystalline cellulose, polyethylene glycol, polysorbate 80, propylene glycol, sodium starch glycolate, titanium dioxide, and the 5 mg tablets contain FD&C Yellow #6 and FD&C Red #40; the 10 mg tablets contain D&C Yellow #10 and D&C Red #30.

CLINICAL PHARMACOLOGY

Protriptyline hydrochloride is an antidepressant agent. The mechanism of its antidepressant action in man is not known. It is not a monoamine oxidase inhibitor, and it does not act primarily by stimulation of the central nervous system.

Protriptyline has been found in some studies to have a more rapid onset of action than imipramine or amitriptyline. The initial clinical effect may occur within one week. Sedative and tranquilizing properties are lacking. The rate of excretion is slow.

INDICATIONS AND USAGE

Protriptyline hydrochloride tablets are indicated for the treatment of symptoms of mental depression in patients who are under close medical supervision. Its activating properties make it particularly suitable for withdrawn and anergic patients.

CONTRAINDICATIONS

Protriptyline hydrochloride tablets are contraindicated in patients who have shown prior hypersensitivity to it.

It should not be given concomitantly with a monoamine oxidase inhibiting compound. Hyperpyretic crises, severe convulsions, and deaths have occurred in patients receiving tricyclic antidepressant and monoamine oxidase inhibiting drugs simultaneously. When it is desired to substitute protriptyline for a monoamine oxidase inhibitor, a minimum of 14 days should be allowed to elapse after the latter is discontinued. Protriptyline should then be initiated cautiously with gradual increase in dosage until optimum response is achieved.

Protriptyline is contraindicated in patients taking cisapride because of the possibility of adverse cardiac interactions including prolongation of the QT interval, cardiac arrhythmias and conduction system disturbances.

This drug should not be used during the acute recovery phase following myocardial infarction.

WARNINGS

Protriptyline may block the antihypertensive effect of guanethidine or similarly acting compounds.

Protriptyline should be used with caution in patients with a history of seizures, and, because of its autonomic activity, in patients with a tendency to urinary retention, or increased intraocular tension.

Tachycardia and postural hypotension may occur more frequently with protriptyline than with other antidepressant drugs. Protriptyline should be used with caution in elderly

Continued on next page

Vivactil—Cont.

patients and patients with cardiovascular disorders; such patients should be observed closely because of the tendency of the drug to produce tachycardia, hypotension, arrhythmias, and prolongation of the conduction time. Myocardial infarction and stroke have occurred with drugs of this class. On rare occasions, hyperthyroid patients or those receiving thyroid medication may develop arrhythmias when this drug is given.
In patients who may use alcohol excessively, it should be borne in mind that the potentiation may increase the danger inherent in any suicide attempt or overdosage.
Pediatric Use: The safety and effectiveness of protriptyline in pediatric patients have not been established.
Usage in Pregnancy: Safe use in pregnancy and lactation has not been established; therefore, use in pregnant women, nursing mothers or women who may become pregnant requires that possible benefits be weighed against possible hazards to mother and child.
In mice, rats, and rabbits, doses about ten times greater than the recommended human doses had no apparent adverse effects on reproduction.

PRECAUTIONS

General—When protriptyline HCl is used to treat the depressive component of schizophrenia, psychotic symptoms may be aggravated. Likewise, in manic-depressive psychosis, depressed patients may experience a shift toward the manic phase if they are treated with an antidepressant drug. Paranoid delusions, with or without associated hostility, may be exaggerated. In any of these circumstances, it may be advisable to reduce the dose of protriptyline or to use a major tranquilizing drug concurrently.
Symptoms, such as anxiety or agitation, may be aggravated in overactive or agitated patients.
The possibility of suicide in depressed patients remains during treatment and until significant remission occurs. This type of patient should not have access to large quantities of the drug.
Concurrent administration of protriptyline and electroshock therapy may increase the hazards of therapy. Such treatment should be limited to patients for whom it is essential.
Discontinue the drug several days before elective surgery, if possible.
Both elevation and lowering of blood sugar levels have been reported.
Information for Patients: While on therapy with protriptyline, patients should be advised as to the possible impairment of mental and/or physical abilities required for performance of hazardous tasks, such as operating machinery or driving a motor vehicle.
Drug Interactions: When protriptyline is given with anticholinergic agents or sympathomimetic drugs, including epinephrine combined with local anesthetics, close supervision and careful adjustment of dosages are required.
Hyperpyrexia has been reported when tricyclic antidepressants are administered with anticholinergic agents or with neuroleptic drugs, particularly during hot weather.
Cimetidine is reported to reduce hepatic metabolism of certain tricyclic antidepressants, thereby delaying elimination and increasing steady-state concentrations of these drugs. Clinically significant effects have been reported with the tricyclic antidepressants when used concomitantly with cimetidine. Increases in plasma levels of tricyclic antidepressants, and in the frequency and severity of side-effects, particularly anticholinergic, have been reported when cimetidine was added to the drug regimen. Discontinuation of cimetidine in well-controlled patients receiving tricyclic antidepressants and cimetidine may decrease the plasma levels and efficacy of the antidepressants.
Tricyclic antidepressants may enhance the seizure risk in patients taking ULTRAM (tramadol hydrochloride).
Protriptyline may enhance the response to alcohol and the effects of barbiturates and other CNS depressants.
Drugs Metabolized by Cytochrome P450 2D6: The biochemical activity of the drug metabolizing isozyme cytochrome P450 2D6 (debrisoquine hydroxylase) is reduced in a subset of the Caucasian population (about 7% to 10% of Caucasians are so called "poor metabolizers"); reliable estimates of the prevalence of reduced P450 2D6 isozyme activity among Asian, African, and other populations are not yet available. Poor metabolizers have higher than expected plasma concentrations of tricyclic antidepressants (TCAs) when given usual doses. Depending on the fraction of drug metabolized by P450 2D6, the increase in plasma concentration may be small or quite large (8 fold increase in plasma AUC of the TCA).
In addition, certain drugs inhibit the activity of this isozyme and make normal metabolizers resemble poor metabolizers. An individual who is stable on a given dose of TCA may become abruptly toxic when given one of these inhibiting drugs as concomitant therapy. The drugs that inhibit cytochrome P450 2D6 include some that are not metabolized by the enzyme (quinidine; cimetidine) and many that are substrates for P450 2D6 (many other antidepressants, phenothiazines, and the Type 1C anti-arrhythmics, propafenone and flecainide). While all the selective serotonin reuptake inhibitors (SSRIs), e.g., fluoxetine, sertraline, and paroxetine, inhibit P450 2D6, they may vary in the extent of inhibition. The extent to which SSRI-TCA interactions may pose clinical problems will depend on the degree of inhibition and the pharmacokinetics of the SSRI involved. Nevertheless, caution is indicated in the coadministration of TCAs with any of the SSRIs and also in switching from one class to the other. Of particular importance, sufficient time must elapse before initiating TCA treatment in a patient being withdrawn from fluoxetine, given the long half-life of the parent and active metabolite (at least 5 weeks may be necessary).
Concomitant use of tricyclic antidepressants with drugs that can inhibit cytochrome P450 2D6 may require lower doses than usually prescribed for either the tricyclic antidepressant or the other drug. Furthermore, whenever one of these other drugs is withdrawn from co-therapy, an increased dose of tricyclic antidepressant may be required. It is desirable to monitor TCA plasma levels whenever a TCA is going to be coadministered with another drug known to be an inhibitor of P450 2D6.
Pediatric Use: The safety and effectiveness of protriptyline in pediatric patients have not been established.
Geriatric Use: Clinical studies of protriptyline did not include sufficient numbers of subjects aged 65 and over to determine whether they respond differently from younger subjects. Other reported clinical experience has not identified differences in responses between the elderly and younger patients. In general, dose selection for an elderly patient should be cautious, usually starting at the low end of the dosing range, reflecting the greater frequency of decreased hepatic, renal, or cardiac function, and of concomitant disease or other drug therapy. (see WARNINGS, DOSAGE AND ADMINISTRATION, and ADVERSE REACTIONS.)

ADVERSE REACTIONS

Within each category the following adverse reactions are listed in order of decreasing severity. Included in the listing are a few adverse reactions which have not been reported with this specific drug. However, the pharmacological similarities among the tricyclic antidepressant drugs require that each of the reactions be considered when protriptyline is administered. Protriptyline is more likely to aggravate agitation and anxiety and produce cardiovascular reactions such as tachycardia and hypotension.
Cardiovascular: Myocardial infarction; stroke; heart block; arrhythmias; hypotension, particularly orthostatic hypotension; hypertension; tachycardia; palpitation.
Psychiatric: Confusional states (especially in the elderly) with hallucinations, disorientation, delusions, anxiety, restlessness, agitation; hypomania; exacerbation of psychosis; insomnia, panic, and nightmares.
Neurological: Seizures; incoordination; ataxia; tremors; peripheral neuropathy; numbness, tingling, and paresthesias of extremities; extrapyramidal symptoms; drowsiness; dizziness; weakness and fatigue; headache; syndrome of inappropriate ADH (antidiuretic hormone) secretion; tinnitus; alteration in EEG patterns.
Anticholinergic: Paralytic ileus; hyperpyrexia; urinary retention, delayed micturition, dilatation of the urinary tract; constipation; blurred vision, disturbance of accommodation, increased intraocular pressure, mydriasis; dry mouth and rarely associated sublingual adenitis.
Allergic: Drug fever; petechiae, skin rash, urticaria, itching, photosensitization (avoid excessive exposure to sunlight); edema (general, or of face and tongue).
Hematologic: Agranulocytosis; bone marrow depression; leukopenia; thrombocytopenia; purpura; eosinophilia.
Gastrointestinal: Nausea and vomiting; anorexia; epigastric distress; diarrhea; peculiar taste; stomatitis; abdominal cramps; black tongue.
Endocrine: Impotence, increased or decreased libido; gynecomastia in the male; breast enlargement and galactorrhea in the female; testicular swelling; elevation or depression of blood sugar levels.
Other: Jaundice (simulating obstructive); altered liver function; parotid swelling; alopecia; flushing; weight gain or loss; urinary frequency, nocturia; perspiration.
Withdrawal Symptoms: Though not indicative of addiction, abrupt cessation of treatment after prolonged therapy may produce nausea, headache, and malaise.

OVERDOSAGE

Deaths may occur from overdosage with this class of drugs. Multiple drug ingestion (including alcohol) is common in deliberate tricyclic antidepressant overdose. As management of overdose is complex and changing, it is recommended that the physician contact a poison control center for current information on treatment. Signs and symptoms of toxicity develop rapidly after tricyclic antidepressant overdose, therefore, hospital monitoring is required as soon as possible.
MANIFESTATIONS Critical manifestations of overdosage include: cardiac dysrhythmias, severe hypotension, convulsions, and CNS depression, including coma. Changes in the electrocardiogram, particularly in QRS axis or width, are clinically significant indicators of tricyclic antidepressant toxicity.
Other signs of overdose may include: confusion, disturbed concentration, transient visual hallucinations, dilated pupils, agitation, hyperactive reflexes, stupor, drowsiness, muscle rigidity, vomiting, hypothermia, hyperpyrexia, or any of the symptoms listed under **ADVERSE REACTIONS**.
MANAGEMENT
General Obtain an ECG and immediately initiate cardiac monitoring. Protect the patient's airway, establish an intravenous line and initiate gastric decontamination. A minimum of six hours of observation with cardiac monitoring and observation for signs of CNS or respiratory depression, hypotension, cardiac dysrhythmias and/or conduction blocks, and seizures is necessary. If signs of toxicity occur at any time during this period, extended monitoring is required. There are case reports of patients succumbing to fatal dysrhythmias late after overdose. These patients had clinical evidence of significant poisoning prior to death and most received inadequate gastrointestinal decontamination. Monitoring of plasma drug levels should not guide management of the patient.
Gastrointestinal Decontamination All patients suspected of a tricyclic antidepressant overdose should receive gastrointestinal decontamination. This should include large volume gastric lavage followed by activated charcoal. If consciousness is impaired, the airway should be secured prior to lavage. Emesis is contraindicated.
Cardiovascular A maximal limb-lead QRS duration of ≥0.10 seconds may be the best indication of the severity of the overdose. Intravenous sodium bicarbonate should be used to maintain the serum pH in the range of 7.45 to 7.55. If the pH response is inadequate, hyperventilation may also be used. Concomitant use of hyperventilation and sodium bicarbonate should be done with extreme caution, with frequent pH monitoring. A pH >7.60 or a pCO2 <20 mmHg is undesirable. Dysrhythmias unresponsive to sodium bicarbonate therapy/hyperventilation may respond to lidocaine, bretylium or phenytoin. Type 1A and 1C antiarrhythmics are generally contraindicated (e.g., quinidine, disopyramide, and procainamide).
In rare instances, hemoperfusion may be beneficial in acute refractory cardiovascular instability in patients with acute toxicity. However, hemodialysis, peritoneal dialysis, exchange transfusions, and forced diuresis generally have been reported as ineffective in tricyclic antidepressant poisoning.
CNS In patients with CNS depression, early intubation is advised because of the potential for abrupt deterioration. Seizures should be controlled with benzodiazepines or, if these are ineffective, other anticonvulsants (e.g., phenobarbital, phenytoin). Physostigmine is not recommended except to treat life-threatening symptoms that have been unresponsive to other therapies, and then only in close consultation with a poison control center.
PSYCHIATRIC FOLLOW-UP Since overdosage is often deliberate, patients may attempt suicide by other means during the recovery phase. Psychiatric referral may be appropriate.
PEDIATRIC MANAGEMENT The principles of management of child and adult overdosages are similar. It is strongly recommended that the physician contact the local poison control center for specific pediatric treatment.

DOSAGE AND ADMINISTRATION

Dosage should be initiated at a low level and increased gradually, noting carefully the clinical response and any evidence of intolerance.
Usual Adult Dosage—Fifteen to 40 mg a day divided into 3 or 4 doses. If necessary, dosage may be increased to 60 mg a day. Dosages above this amount are not recommended. Increases should be made in the morning dose.
Adolescent and Elderly Patients—In general, lower dosages are recommended for these patients. Five mg 3 times a day may be given initially, and increased gradually if necessary. In elderly patients, the cardiovascular system must be monitored closely if the daily dose exceeds 20 mg.
When satisfactory improvement has been reached, dosage should be reduced to the smallest amount that will maintain relief of symptoms.
Minor adverse reactions require reduction in dosage. Major adverse reactions or evidence of hypersensitivity require prompt discontinuation of the drug.
The safety and effectiveness of protriptyline in pediatric patients have not been established.

HOW SUPPLIED

Vivactil® Tablets:
5 mg - Orange, oval, film-coated tablets in bottles of 100. Debossed OP 701
10 mg - Yellow, oval, film-coated tablets in bottles of 100. Debossed OP 702
Dispense in a tight container as defined in the USP.
Store at controlled room temperature 15°–30°C (59°–86°F). [see USP].

METABOLISM

Metabolic studies indicate that protriptyline is well absorbed from the gastrointestinal tract and is rapidly sequestered in tissues. Relatively low plasma levels are found after administration, and only a small amount of unchanged drug is excreted in the urine of dogs and rabbits. Preliminary studies indicate that demethylation of the secondary amine moiety occurs to a significant extent, and that metabolic transformation probably takes place in the liver. It penetrates the brain rapidly in mice and rats, and moreover that which is present in the brain is almost all unchanged drug.
Studies on the disposition of radioactive protriptyline in human test subjects showed significant plasma levels within 2 hours, peaking at 8 to 12 hours, then declining gradually. Urinary excretion studies in the same subjects showed significant amounts of radioactivity in 2 hours. The rate of excretion was slow. Cumulative urinary excretion during 16 days accounted for approximately 50% of the drug. The fecal route of excretion did not seem to be important.

Distributed by Odyssey Pharmaceuticals, Inc.,
East Hanover, New Jersey 07936
Manufactured by PLIVA®, Inc.
East Hanover, NJ 07936
Iss. 1/03
Shown in Product Identification Guide, page 327

VOSPIRE ER™ ℞
[*vō'spēr*]
(Albuterol Sulfate)
Extended-Release Tablets

DESCRIPTION

Albuterol extended-release tablets contain albuterol sulfate, the racemic form of albuterol and a relatively selective beta$_2$-adrenergic bronchodilator, in an extended-release formulation. Albuterol sulfate has the chemical name (±) α_1-[(*tert*-butylamino)methyl]-4-hydroxy-*m*-xylene-α, α'-diol sulfate (2:1) (salt), and the following structural formula:

[HOCH$_2$, HO–(ring)–CHCH$_2$NHC(CH$_3$)$_3$ (OH)]$_2$ •H$_2$SO$_4$

Albuterol sulfate has a molecular weight of 576.7, and the molecular formula is $(C_{13}H_{21}NO_3)_2 \bullet H_2SO_4$. Albuterol sulfate is a white crystalline powder, soluble in water and slightly soluble in ethanol.

The World Health Organization recommended name for albuterol base is salbutamol.

Each tablet for oral administration contains 4 mg or 8 mg of albuterol as 4.8 mg or 9.6 mg, respectively, of albuterol sulfate in a cellulosic material that serves as a diffusion-release membrane. In addition each tablet contains the following inactive ingredients: Calcium sulfate, carnauba wax, ethylcellulose, ferric oxide black, hypromellose, ink-thinner XI, lactose monohydrate, magnesium stearate, polyethylene glycol, propylene glycol, shellac, stearic acid, titanium dioxide, triacetin, D&C Yellow #10, (4 mg only) and FD&C Blue #1 (4 mg only).

CLINICAL PHARMACOLOGY

In vitro studies and *in vivo* pharmacologic studies have demonstrated that albuterol has a preferential effect on beta$_2$-adrenergic receptors compared with isoproterenol. While it is recognized that beta$_2$-adrenergic receptors are the predominant receptors in bronchial smooth muscle, data indicates that there is a population of beta$_2$-receptors in the human heart existing in a concentration between 10% and 50%. The precise function of these receptors has not been established. (See Warnings).

The pharmacologic effects of beta-adrenergic agonist drugs, including albuterol, are at least in part attributable to stimulation through beta-adrenergic receptors on intracellular adenyl cyclase, the enzyme that catalyzes the conversion of adenosine triphosphate (ATP) to cyclic-3', 5'-adenosine monophosphate (cyclic AMP). Increased cyclic AMP levels are associated with relaxation of bronchial smooth muscle and inhibition of release of mediators of immediate hypersensitivity from cells, especially from mast cells.

Albuterol has been shown in most controlled clinical trials to have more effect on the respiratory tract, in the form of bronchial smooth muscle relaxation, than isoproterenol at comparable doses while producing fewer cardiovascular effects.

Albuterol is longer acting than isoproterenol in most patients by any route of administration because it is not a substrate for the cellular uptake processes for catecholamines nor for catechol-O-methyl transferase.

Preclinical: Intravenous studies in rats with albuterol sulfate have demonstrated that albuterol crosses the blood-brain barrier and reaches brain concentrations amounting to approximately 5.0% of the plasma concentrations. In structures outside the blood-brain barrier (pineal and pituitary glands), albuterol concentrations were found to be 100 times those in the whole brain.

Studies in laboratory animals (minipigs, rodents, and dogs) have demonstrated the occurrence of cardiac arrhythmias and sudden death (with histologic evidence of myocardial necrosis) when beta-agonists and methylxanthines were administered concurrently. The clinical significance of these findings is unknown.

Pharmacokinetics and Disposition: In a single-dose study comparing one 8 mg albuterol extended-release tablet with two 4 mg immediate-release albuterol tablets, USP in 17 normal adult volunteers, the extent of availability of albuterol extended-release tablets was shown to be about 80% of albuterol tablets, USP with or without food. In addition, lower mean peak plasma concentration and longer time to reach the peak level were observed with albuterol extended-release tablets as compared with albuterol tablets, USP. The single-dose study results also showed that food decreases the rate of absorption of albuterol from albuterol extended-release tablets without altering the extent of bioavailability. In addition, the study indicated that food causes a more gradual increase in the fraction of the available dose absorbed from the extended-release formulation as compared with the fasting condition.

Mean Values at Steady State

	C_{max} (ng/mL)	C_{min} (ng/mL)	T_{max} (h)	$T_{1/2}$ (h)	AUC (ng-h/mL)
Albuterol Extended-Release Tablets	13.7	8.1	6.0	9.3	134
Albuterol Tablets, USP	13.9	8.1	2.6	7.2	132

In another single-dose study in adults, 8 mg and 4 mg albuterol extended-release tablets were shown to deliver dose-proportional plasma concentrations in the fasting state. Definitive studies for the effect of food on 4 mg albuterol extended-release tablets have not been conducted. However, since food lowers the rate of absorption of 8 mg albuterol extended-release tablets, it is expected that food reduces the rate of absorption of 4 mg albuterol extended-release tablets also.

Albuterol extended-release tablets have been formulated to provide duration of action of up to 12 hours. In an 8-day, multiple-dose, crossover study, 15 normal adult male volunteers were given 8 mg albuterol extended-release tablets every 12 hours or 4 mg albuterol tablets, USP every 6 hours. Each dose of albuterol extended-release tablets and the corresponding doses of albuterol tablets, USP were administered in the postprandial state. Steady-state plasma concentrations were reached within 2 days for both formulations. Fluctuations (C_{max}-C_{min}/$C_{average}$) in plasma concentrations were similar for albuterol extended-release tablets administered at 12-hour intervals and albuterol tablets, USP administered every 6 hours. In addition, the relative bioavailability of albuterol extended-release tablets was approximately 100% of the immediate-release tablet at steady state. A summary of these results is shown in the following table:

[See table above]

The mean plasma albuterol concentration versus time data at steady state after the administration of albuterol extended-release tablets 8 mg every 12 hours are displayed in the following graph:

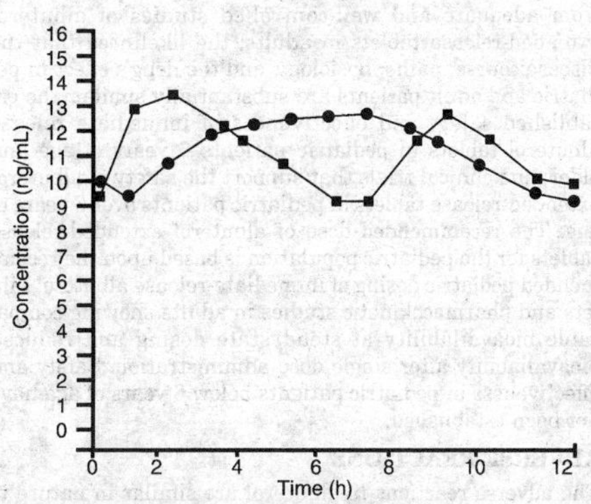

Pharmacokinetic studies of 4- and 8-mg albuterol extended-release tablets have not been conducted in pediatric patients. Bioavailability of 4- and 8-mg albuterol extended-release tablets in pediatric patients relative to 2- and 4-mg immediate release albuterol has been extrapolated from adult studies showing comparability at steady-state dosing and reduced bioavailability after single dose administration.

INDICATIONS AND USAGE

Albuterol extended-release tablets are indicated for the relief of bronchospasm in adults and children 6 years of age and older with reversible obstructive airway disease.

CONTRAINDICATIONS

Albuterol extended-release tablets are contraindicated in patients with a history of hypersensitivity to albuterol or any of its components.

WARNINGS

Immediate hypersensitivity reactions may occur after administration of albuterol, as demonstrated by rare cases of urticaria, angioedema, rash, bronchospasm, and oropharyngeal edema.

Cardiovascular Effects: Albuterol extended-release tablets, like all other beta-adrenergic agonists, can produce a clinically significant cardiovascular effect in some patients, as measured by pulse rate, blood pressure, and/or symptoms. Although such effects are uncommon after administration of albuterol extended-release tablets at recommended doses, if they occur, the drug may need to be discontinued. In addition, beta-agonists have been reported to produce electrocardiogram (ECG) changes, such as flattening of the T wave, prolongation of the QTc interval, and ST segment depression. The clinical significance of these findings is unknown. Therefore, albuterol extended-release tablets, like all sympathomimetic amines, should be used with caution in patients with cardiovascular disorders, especially coronary insufficiency, cardiac arrhythmias, and hypertension.

Deterioration of Asthma: Asthma may deteriorate acutely over a period of hours or chronically over several days or longer. If the patient needs more doses of albuterol extended-release tablets than usual, this may be a marker of destabilization of asthma and requires reevaluation of the patient and the treatment regimen, giving special consideration to the possible need for anti-inflammatory treatment; e.g., corticosteroids.

Use of Anti-Inflammatory Agents: The use of beta adrenergic agonist bronchodilators alone may not be adequate to control asthma in many patients. Early consideration should be given to adding anti-inflammatory agents; e.g., corticosteroids.

Paradoxical Bronchospasm: Albuterol extended-release tablets can produce paradoxical bronchospasm, which may be life threatening. If paradoxical bronchospasm occurs, albuterol extended-release tablets should be discontinued immediately and alternative therapy instituted.

Rarely, erythema multiforme and Stevens-Johnson syndrome have been associated with the administration of oral albuterol in children.

PRECAUTIONS

General: Albuterol, as with all sympathomimetic amines, should be used with caution in patients with cardiovascular disorders, especially coronary insufficiency, cardiac arrhythmias, and hypertension; in patients with convulsive disorders, hyperthyroidism, or diabetes mellitus; and in patients who are unusually responsive to sympathomimetic amines. Clinically significant changes in systolic and diastolic blood pressure have been seen and could be expected to occur in some patients after use of any beta-adrenergic bronchodilator.

In controlled clinical trials in adults, patients treated with albuterol extended-release tablets had increases in selected serum chemistry values and decreases in selected hematologic values. Increases in SGPT were more frequent among patients treated with albuterol extended-release tablets (12 of 247 patients, 4.9%) than among the theophylline (6 of 188 patients, 3.2%) and placebo (1 of 138 patients, 0.7%) groups. Increases in serum glucose concentration were also more frequent among patients treated with albuterol extended-release tablets (23 of 234 patients, 9.8%) than among theophylline (11 of 173 patients, 6.45%) and placebo (3 of 129 patients, 2.3%) groups. Increases in SGOT were also more frequent among patients treated with albuterol extended-release tablets (10 of 248 patients, 4%) and theophylline (5 of 193, 2.6%) than among patients treated with placebo. Decreases in white blood cell counts were more frequent in patients treated with albuterol extended-release tablets (10 of 247 patients, 4%) compared with patients receiving theophylline (2 of 185 patients, 1.1%) and patients receiving placebo (1 of 141 patients, 0.7%). Decreases in hemoglobin and hematocrit were more frequent in patients receiving albuterol extended-release tablets (16 of 228 patients, 7.0%, and 17 of 230 patients, 7.4%, respectively) than in patients receiving theophylline (5 of 171 patients, 2.9%, and 9 of 173 patients, 5.2%, respectively) and patients receiving placebo (5 of 129 patients, 3.9%, and 3 of 132 patients, 2.3%, respectively). The clinical significance of these results is unknown.

Large doses of intravenous albuterol have been reported to aggravate pre-existing diabetes mellitus and ketoacidosis. As with other beta-agonists, albuterol may produce significant hypokalemia in some patients, possibly through intracellular shunting, which has the potential to produce adverse cardiovascular effects. The decrease is usually transient, not requiring supplementation.

Information for Patients:

Albuterol extended-release tablets must be swallowed whole with the aid of liquids. DO NOT CHEW OR CRUSH THESE TABLETS.

The action of albuterol extended-release tablets should last up to 12 hours or longer. Albuterol extended-release tablets should not be used more frequently than recommended. Do not increase the dose or frequency of albuterol extended-release tablets without consulting your physician. If you find that treatment with albuterol extended-release tablets becomes less effective for symptomatic relief, your symptoms become worse, and/or you need to use the product more frequently than usual, you should seek medical attention immediately. While you are using albuterol extended-release tablets, other inhaled drugs and asthma medications should be taken only as directed by your physician. Common adverse effects include palpitations, chest pain, rapid heart rate, tremor or nervousness. If you are pregnant or nursing, contact your physician about use of albuterol extended-release tablets. Effective and safe use of albuterol extended-release tablets includes an understanding of the way that it should be administered.

Drug Interactions: The concomitant use of albuterol extended-release tablets and other oral sympathomimetic

Continued on next page

Vospire ER—Cont.

agents is not recommended since such combined use may lead to deleterious cardiovascular effects. This recommendation does not preclude the judicious use of an aerosol bronchodilator of the adrenergic stimulant type in patients receiving albuterol extended-release tablets. Such concomitant use, however, should be individualized and not given on a routine basis. If regular coadministration is required, then alternative therapy should be considered.

Monoamine Oxidase Inhibitors or Tricyclic Antidepressants: Albuterol should be administered with extreme caution to patients being treated with monoamine oxidase inhibitors or tricyclic antidepressants, or within 2 weeks of discontinuation of such agents, because the action of albuterol on the vascular system may be potentiated.

Beta Blockers: Beta-adrenergic receptor blocking agents not only block the pulmonary effect of beta-agonists, such as albuterol extended-release tablets, but may produce severe bronchospasm in asthmatic patients. Therefore, patients with asthma should not normally be treated with beta-blockers. However, under certain circumstances, e.g., as prophylaxis after myocardial infarction, there may be no acceptable alternatives to the use of beta-adrenergic blocking agents in patients with asthma. In this setting, cardioselective beta-blockers could be considered, although they should be administered with caution.

Diuretics: The ECG changes and/or hypokalemia that may result from the administration of non potassium-sparing diuretics (such as loop or thiazide diuretics) can be acutely worsened by beta-agonists, especially when the recommended dose of the beta-agonist is exceeded. Although the clinical significance of these effects is not known, caution is advised in the coadministration of beta-agonists with non potassium-sparing diuretics.

Digoxin: Mean decreases of 16% to 22% in serum digoxin levels were demonstrated after single dose intravenous and oral administration of albuterol, respectively, to normal volunteers who had received digoxin for 10 days. The clinical significance of these findings for patients with obstructive airway disease who are receiving albuterol and digoxin on a chronic basis is unclear. Nevertheless, it would be prudent to carefully evaluate the serum digoxin levels in patients who are currently receiving digoxin and albuterol.

Carcinogenesis, Mutagenesis, Impairment of Fertility: In a 2-year study in Sprague-Dawley rats, albuterol sulfate caused a significant dose-related increase in the incidence of benign leiomyomas of the mesovarium at dietary doses of 2.0, 10, and 50 mg/kg, (approximately 1/2, 3, and 15 times, respectively, the maximum recommended daily oral dose for adults on a mg/m^2 basis, or, approximately 2/5, 2, and 10 times, respectively, the maximum recommended daily oral dose for children on a mg/m^2 basis). In another study this effect was blocked by the coadministration of propranolol, a non-selective beta-adrenergic antagonist. In an 18 month study in CD-1 mice, albuterol sulfate showed no evidence of tumorigenicity at dietary doses of up to 500 mg/kg (approximately 65 times the maximum recommended daily oral dose for adults on a mg/m^2 basis, or, approximately 50 times the maximum recommended daily oral dose for children on a mg/m^2 basis). In a 22 month study in the Golden hamster, albuterol sulfate showed no evidence of tumorigenicity at dietary doses of 50 mg/kg, (approximately 7 times the maximum recommended daily oral dose for adults and children on a mg/m^2 basis).

Albuterol sulfate was not mutagenic in the Ames test with or without metabolic activation using tester strains *S. typhimurium* TA 1537, TA 1538, and TA98 or *E. coli* WP2, WP2uvrA, and WP67. No forward mutation was seen in yeast strain *S. cerevisiae* S9 nor any mitotic gene conversion in yeast strain *S. cerevisiae* JD1 with or without metabolic activation. Fluctuation assays in *S. typhimurium* TA98 and *E. coli* WP2, both with metabolic activation, were negative. Albuterol sulfate was not clastogenic in a human peripheral lymphocyte assay or in an AH1 strain mouse micronucleus assay at intraperitoneal doses of up to 200 mg/kg.

Reproduction studies in rats demonstrated no evidence of impaired fertility at oral doses up to 50 mg/kg, (approximately 15 times the maximum recommended daily oral dose for adults on a mg/m^2 basis).

Pregnancy: Teratogenic Effects: Pregnancy Category C: Albuterol Sulfate has been shown to be teratogenic in mice. A study in CD-1 mice at subcutaneous (SC) doses of 0.025, 0.25, and 2.5 mg/kg, (approximately 3/1000, 3/100, and 3/10 times the maximum recommended daily oral dose for adults on a mg/m^2 basis), showed cleft palate formation in 5 of 111 (4.5%) fetuses at 0.25 mg/kg and in 10 of 108 (9.3%) fetuses at 2.5 mg/kg. The drug did not induce cleft palate formation at the lowest dose, 0.025 mg/kg. Cleft palate also occurred in 22 of 72 (30.5%) fetuses of females treated with 2.5 mg/kg, of isoproterenol (positive control) subcutaneously (approximately 3/10 times the maximum recommended daily oral dose for adults on a mg/m^2 basis). A reproduction study in Stride Dutch rabbits revealed cranioschisis in 7/19 fetuses (37%) when albuterol sulfate was administered orally at a 50 mg/kg dose, (approximately 25 times the maximum recommended daily oral dose for adults on a mg/m^2 basis).

There are no adequate and well-controlled studies in pregnant women. Albuterol should be used during pregnancy only if the potential benefit justifies the potential risk to the fetus.

During worldwide marketing experience, various congenital anomalies, including cleft palate and limb defects, have been rarely reported in the offspring of patients being treated with albuterol. Some of the mothers were taking multiple medications during their pregnancies. No consistent pattern of defects can be discerned, and a relationship between albuterol use and congenital anomalies has not been established.

Labor and Delivery: Because of the potential for beta-agonist interference with uterine contractility, use of albuterol extended-release tablets for relief of bronchospasm during labor should be restricted to those patients in whom the benefits clearly outweigh the risks.

Tocolysis: Albuterol has not been approved for the management of pre-term labor. The benefit:risk ratio when albuterol is administered for tocolysis has not been established. Serious adverse reactions, including pulmonary edema, have been reported during or following treatment of premature labor with beta$_2$-agonists, including albuterol.

Nursing Mothers: It is not known whether albuterol is excreted in human milk. Because of the potential for tumorigenicity shown for albuterol in animal studies, a decision should be made whether to discontinue nursing or to discontinue the drug, taking into account the importance of the drug to the mother.

Pediatric Use: The safety and effectiveness of albuterol extended-release tablets have been established in pediatric patients 6 years of age or older. Use of albuterol extended-release tablets in these age groups is supported by evidence from adequate and well-controlled studies of albuterol extended-release tablets in adults; the likelihood that the disease course, pathophysiology, and the drug's effect in pediatric and adult patients are substantially similar; the established safety and effectiveness of immediate release albuterol tablets in pediatric patients 6 years of age and older; and clinical trials that support the safety of albuterol extended-release tablets in pediatric patients over 6 years of age. The recommended dose of albuterol extended-release tablets for the pediatric population is based upon the recommended pediatric dosing of immediate-release albuterol tablets and pharmacokinetic studies in adults showing comparable bioavailability at steadystate dosing and reduced bioavailability after single dose administration. Safety and effectiveness in pediatric patients below 6 years of age have not been established.

ADVERSE REACTIONS

The adverse reactions to albuterol are similar in nature to reactions to other sympathomimetic agents. The most frequent adverse reactions to albuterol are nervousness, tremor, headache, tachycardia, and palpitations. Less frequent adverse reactions are muscle cramps, insomnia, nausea, weakness, dizziness, drowsiness, flushing, restlessness, irritability, chest discomfort, and difficulty in micturition.

Rare cases of urticaria, angioedema, rash, bronchospasm, and oropharyngeal edema have been reported after the use of albuterol.

In addition, albuterol, like other sympathomimetic agents, can cause adverse reactions such as hypertension, angina, vomiting, vertigo, central nervous system stimulation, unusual taste, and drying or irritation of the oropharynx.

In controlled clinical trials of adult patients conducted in the United States, the following incidence of adverse events was reported:

[See table below]

A trend was observed among patients treated with albuterol extended-release tablets toward increasing frequency of muscle cramps with increasing patient age (12-20 years, 1.2%; 21-30 years, 2.6%; 31-40 years, 6.9%; 41-50 years, 6.9%), compared with no such events in the placebo group. Also observed was an increasing frequency of tremor with increasing patient age (12-20 years, 29.4%; 21-30 years, 29.9%; 31-40 years, 27.6%; 41-50 years, 37.9%), compared to 2.9% or less in the placebo group.

The reactions are generally transient in nature, and it is usually not necessary to discontinue treatment with albuterol extended-release tablets.

OVERDOSAGE

The expected symptoms with overdosage are those of excessive beta-adrenergic stimulation and/or occurrence or exaggeration of any of the symptoms listed under ADVERSE REACTIONS; e.g., seizures, angina, hypertension or hypotension, tachycardia with rates up to 200 beats per minute, arrhythmias, nervousness, headache, tremor, dry mouth, palpitation, nausea, dizziness, fatigue, malaise, and insomnia. Hypokalemia may also occur. As with all sympathomimetic aerosol medications, cardiac arrest and even death may be associated with abuse of albuterol extended-release tablets.

Treatment consists of discontinuation of albuterol extended-release tablets together with appropriate symptomatic therapy. The judicious use of a cardioselective beta-receptor blocker may be considered, bearing in mind that such medication can produce bronchospasm. There is insufficient evidence to determine if dialysis is beneficial for overdosage of albuterol extended-release tablets.

The oral median lethal dose of albuterol sulfate in mice is greater than 2000 mg/kg, (approximately 250 times the maximum recommended daily oral dose for adults on a mg/m^2 basis, or, approximately 200 times the maximum recommended daily oral dose for children on a mg/m^2 basis). In mature rats, the subcutaneous median lethal dose of albuterol sulfate is approximately 450 mg/kg (approximately 110 times the maximum recommended daily oral dose for adults on a mg/m^2 basis, or, approximately 90 times the maximum recommended daily oral dose for children on a mg/m^2 basis). In small young rats, the subcutaneous median lethal dose is approximately 2000 mg/kg, (approximately 500 times the maximum recommended daily oral dose for adults on a mg/m^2 basis, or, approximately 400 times the maximum recommended daily oral dose for children on a mg/m^2 basis).

DOSAGE AND ADMINISTRATION

The following dosages of albuterol extended-release tablets are expressed in terms of albuterol base:

Usual Dosage:

Adults and Children over 12 years of age: The usual recommended dosage for adults and pediatric patients over 12 years of age is 8 mg every 12 hours. In some patients, 4 mg every 12 hours may be sufficient.

Children 6 to 12 years of age: The usual recommended dosage for children 6 through 12 years of age is 4 mg every 12 hours.

Dosage adjustment in Adults and Children over 12 years of age: In unusual circumstances, such as adults of low body weight, it may be desirable to use a starting dosage of 4 mg every 12 hours and progress to 8 mg every 12 hours according to response.

If control of reversible airway obstruction is not achieved with the recommended doses in patients on otherwise optimized asthma therapy, the doses may be cautiously increased stepwise under the control of the supervising physician to a maximum dose of 32 mg per day in divided doses (i.e., every 12 hours).

Dosage adjustment in Children 6 to 12 years of age: If control of reversible airway obstruction is not achieved with the recommended doses in patients on otherwise optimized asthma therapy, the doses may be cautiously increased stepwise under the control of the supervising physician to a maximum dose of 24 mg per day in divided doses (i.e., every 12 hours).

Switching from oral albuterol, USP products: Patients currently maintained on albuterol tablets, USP or albuterol sulfate syrup can be switched to albuterol extended-release tablets. For example, the administration of one 4 mg albuterol extended-release tablet every 12 hours is comparable to one 2 mg albuterol tablet, USP every 6 hours. Multiples of this regimen up to the maximum recommended daily dose also apply.

Albuterol extended-release tablets must be swallowed whole with the aid of liquids. **DO NOT CHEW OR CRUSH THESE TABLETS.**

HOW SUPPLIED

Albuterol Extended-Release Tablets, equivalent to 4 mg and 8 mg of Albuterol:

4 mg – Green, round, coated tablets in bottles of 100. Printed V on one side and 4 on the other side in black ink.

8 mg – White, round, coated tablets in bottles of 100. Printed V on one side and 8 on the other side in black ink.

Dispense in a well-closed, light-resistant container as defined in the USP. Replace cap securely after each opening. **Store at 20°–25°C (68°–77°F) [See USP Controlled Room Temperature].**

Distributed by Odyssey Pharmaceuticals, Inc.
East Hanover, New Jersey 07936
Manufactured by:
PLIVA, Inc.
East Hanover, NJ 07936
2/04

Shown in Product Identification Guide, page 327

Event	Albuterol Extended-Release Tablets (n=330)	Theophylline (n=197)	Other Beta-agonists (n=20)	Placebo (n=178)
Tremor	24.2%	6.1%	35.0%	1.1%
Headache	18.8%	26.9%	35.0%	20.8%
Nervousness	8.5%	5.1%	10.0%	2.8%
Nausea/Vomiting	4.2%	19.8%	5.0%	3.9%
Tachycardia	2.7%	0.5%	5.0%	0%
Muscle Cramps	2.7%	0.5%	5.0%	0.6%
Palpitations	2.4%	0.5%	0%	1.1%
Insomnia	2.4%	6.1%	0%	1.7%
Dizziness	1.5%	2.0%	0%	5.1%
Somnolence	0.3%	1.0%	0%	0.6%

Organon USA, Inc.
56 LIVINGSTON AVE.
ROSELAND, NJ 07068

Direct Inquiries to:
(973) 325-4500

Currently available products are listed below. For complete product line information and price lists, direct inquiries to Organon Inc. Customer Service. For specific product information, contact Organon Inc. Medical Services Department.

NUVARING® ℞

[*nū'vă-ring*]
(etonogestrel/ethinyl estradiol vaginal ring)

delivers 0.120 mg/0.015 mg per day

Patients should be counseled that this product does not protect against HIV infection (AIDS) and other sexually transmitted diseases.

FOR VAGINAL USE ONLY

DESCRIPTION

NuvaRing® (etonogestrel/ethinyl estradiol vaginal ring) is a non-biodegradable, flexible, transparent, colorless to almost colorless, combination contraceptive vaginal ring containing two active components, a progestin, etonogestrel (13-ethyl-17-hydroxy-11-methylene-18,19-dinor-17α-pregn-4-en-20-yn-3-one) and an estrogen, ethinyl estradiol (19-nor-17α-pregna-1,3,5(10)-trien-20-yne-3, 17-diol). When placed in the vagina, each ring releases on average 0.120 mg/day of etonogestrel and 0.015 mg/day of ethinyl estradiol over a three-week period of use. NuvaRing® is made of ethylene vinylacetate copolymers (28% and 9% vinyl acetate) and magnesium stearate and contains 11.7 mg etonogestrel and 2.7 mg ethinyl estradiol. NuvaRing® has an outer diameter of 54 mm and a cross-sectional diameter of 4 mm. The molecular weights for etonogestrel and ethinyl estradiol are 324.46 and 296.40, respectively. The structural formulas are as follows:

ETONOGESTREL $C_{22}H_{28}O_2$ — ETHINYL ESTRADIOL $C_{20}H_{24}O_2$

CLINICAL PHARMACOLOGY

Combination hormonal contraceptives act by suppression of gonadotropins. Although the primary effect of this action is inhibition of ovulation, other alterations include changes in the cervical mucus (which increase the difficulty of sperm entry into the uterus) and the endometrium (which reduce the likelihood of implantation).
Receptor binding studies, as well as studies in animals, have shown that etonogestrel, the biologically active metabolite of desogestrel, combines high progestational activity with low intrinsic androgenicity. The relevance of this later finding in humans is unknown.

Pharmacokinetics

Absorption

Etonogestrel: Etonogestrel released by NuvaRing® is rapidly absorbed. Bioavailability of etonogestrel after vaginal administration is approximately 100%. The serum etonogestrel and ethinyl estradiol concentrations (pg/mL) observed during three weeks of NuvaRing® use are summarized in Table I.

Ethinyl estradiol: Ethinyl estradiol released by NuvaRing® is rapidly absorbed. Bioavailability of ethinyl estradiol after vaginal administration is approximately 55.6%, which is comparable to that with oral administration of ethinyl estradiol. The serum ethinyl estradiol concentrations observed during three weeks of NuvaRing® use are summarized in Table I.

[See table I above]

The pharmacokinetic profile of etonogestrel and ethinyl estradiol during use of NuvaRing® is shown in Figure 1.

[See figure 1 at top of next column]

The pharmacokinetic parameters of etonogestrel and ethinyl estradiol were determined during one cycle of NuvaRing® use in 16 healthy female subjects and are summarized in Table II.

[See table II above]

Distribution

Etonogestrel: Etonogestrel is approximately 32% bound to sex hormone binding globulin (SHBG) and approximately 66% bound to albumin in blood.

Ethinyl estradiol: Ethinyl estradiol is highly but not specifically bound to serum albumin (approximately 98.5%) and induces an increase in the serum concentrations of SHBG.

Metabolism

In vitro data shows that both etonogestrel and ethinyl estradiol are metabolized in liver microsomes by the cyto-

TABLE I: MEAN (SD) SERUM ETONOGESTREL AND ETHINYL ESTRADIOL CONCENTRATIONS (n=16).

	1 week	2 weeks	3 weeks
Etonogestrel (pg/mL)	1578 (408)	1476 (362)	1374 (328)
Ethinyl-estradiol (pg/mL)	19.1 (4.5)	18.3 (4.3)	17.6 (4.3)

TABLE II: MEAN (SD) PHARMACOKINETIC PARAMETERS OF NuvaRing® (n=16).

Hormone	C_{max} pg/mL	T_{max} hr	$t_{1/2}$ hr	CL L/hr
Etonogestrel	1716 (445)	200.3 (69.6)	29.3 (6.1)	3.4 (0.8)
Ethinyl Estradiol	34.7 (17.5)	59.3 (67.5)	44.7 (28.8)	34.8 (11.6)

C_{max} - maximum serum drug concentration
T_{max} - time at which maximum serum drug concentration occurs
$t_{1/2}$ - elimination half-life, calculated by $0.693/K_{elim}$
CL - apparent clearance

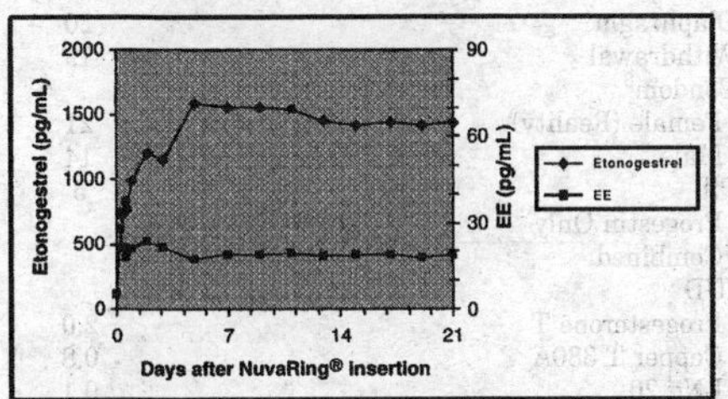

Figure 1. Mean serum concentration-time profile of etonogestrel and ethinyl estradiol during three weeks of NuvaRing® use.

chrome P450 3A4 isoenzyme. Ethinyl estradiol is primarily metabolized by aromatic hydroxylation, but a wide variety of hydroxylated and methylated metabolites are formed. These are present as free metabolites and as sulfate and glucuronide conjugates. The hydroxylated ethinyl estradiol metabolites have weak estrogenic activity. The biological activity of etonogestrel metabolites is unknown.

Excretion

Etonogestrel and ethinyl estradiol are primarily eliminated in urine, bile and feces.

Special Populations

Race

No formal studies were conducted to evaluate the effect of race on the pharmacokinetics of NuvaRing® (etonogestrel/ethinyl estradiol vaginal ring).

Hepatic Insufficiency

No formal studies were conducted to evaluate the effect of hepatic disease on the pharmacokinetics, safety, and efficacy of NuvaRing®. However, steroid hormones may be poorly metabolized in patients with impaired liver function (see PRECAUTIONS).

Renal Insufficiency

No formal studies were conducted to evaluate the effect of renal disease on the pharmacokinetics, safety, and efficacy of NuvaRing®.

Drug. Drug Interactions

Interactions between contraceptive steroids and other drugs have been reported in the literature (see PRECAUTIONS).
The pharmacokinetics of NuvaRing® were evaluated in one cycle in 24 healthy female subjects randomized to a single-dose vaginal administration on Day 8 of 100 mg of a nonoxynol-9 spermicide gel or a 1200 mg miconazole nitrate antimycotic capsule. In this study, it was determined that the vaginally-administered, oil-based miconazole nitrate capsule increased the serum concentrations of etonogestrel and ethinyl estradiol by approximately 17% and 16%, respectively. The clinical significance of these findings is unknown; however, the contraceptive effectiveness of NuvaRing® is not expected to change. It was determined that the single dose of 100 mg vaginally-administered, water-based nonoxynol-9 gel did not affect the serum concentrations of etonogestrel or ethinyl estradiol. The effects of chronic administration of either of these products with NuvaRing® are unknown.

INDICATIONS AND USAGE

NuvaRing® is indicated for the prevention of pregnancy in women who elect to use this product as a method of contraception. Like oral contraceptives, NuvaRing® is highly effective if used as recommended in this label.
In two large clinical trials of 13 cycles of NuvaRing® use, pregnancy rates were between one and two per 100 women-years of use. Table III lists the pregnancy rates for users of various contraceptive methods.

[See table III at top of next page]

CONTRAINDICATIONS

NuvaRing® should not be used in women who currently have the following conditions:

- Thrombophlebitis or thromboembolic disorders
- A past history of deep vein thrombophlebitis or thromboembolic disorders
- Cerebral vascular or coronary artery disease (current or history)
- Valvular heart disease with complications
- Severe hypertension
- Diabetes with vascular involvement
- Headaches with focal neurological symptoms
- Major surgery with prolonged immobilization
- Known or suspected carcinoma of the breast or personal history of breast cancer
- Carcinoma of the endometrium or other known or suspected estrogen-dependent neoplasia
- Undiagnosed abnormal genital bleeding
- Cholestatic jaundice of pregnancy or jaundice with prior hormonal contraceptive use
- Hepatic tumors (benign or malignant), active liver disease
- Known or suspected pregnancy
- Heavy smoking (≥15 cigarettes per day) and over age 35
- Hypersensitivity to any of the components of NuvaRing®

WARNINGS

Cigarette smoking increases the risk of serious cardiovascular side effects from combination oral contraceptive use. The risk increases with age and with heavy smoking (15 or more cigarettes per day) and is quite marked in women over 35 years of age. Women who use combination hormonal contraceptives, including NuvaRing®, should be strongly advised not to smoke.

NuvaRing® and other contraceptives that contain both an estrogen and a progestin are called combination hormonal contraceptives. There is no epidemiologic data available to determine whether safety and efficacy with the vaginal route of administration of combination hormonal contraceptives would be different than the oral route. Practitioners prescribing NuvaRing® should be familiar with the following information relating to these risks.
The use of oral contraceptives is associated with increased risks of several serious conditions including myocardial infarction, thromboembolism, stroke, hepatic neoplasia, and gallbladder disease, although the risk of serious morbidity or mortality is very small in healthy women without underlying risk factors. The risk of morbidity and mortality increases signficantly in the presence of other underlying risk factors such as hypertension, hyperlipidemias, obesity, and diabetes.
The information contained in this package insert is principally based on studies carried out in patients who used oral contraceptives with formulations of higher doses of estrogens and progestogens than those in common use today. The effect of long-term use of oral contraceptives with lower doses of both estrogens and progestogens remains to be determined.
Throughout this labeling, epidemiologic studies reported are of two types: retrospective or case control studies and prospective or cohort studies. Case control studies provide a measure of the relative risk of a disease, namely, a *ratio* of the incidence of a disease among oral contraceptive users to that among non-users. The relative risk does not provide information on the actual clinical occurrence of a disease. Cohort studies provide a measure of attributable risk, which is the *difference* in the incidence of disease between oral contraceptive users and non-users. The attributable risk does provide information about the actual occurrence of a disease in the population. For further information, the reader is referred to a text on epidemiologic methods.

1. THROMBOEMBOLIC DISORDERS AND OTHER VASCULAR PROBLEMS

a. Thromboembolism

An increased risk of thromboembolic and thrombotic disease associated with the use of oral contraceptives is well established. Case control studies have found the relative risk of users compared to non-users to be 3 for the first episode of superficial venous thrombosis, 4 to 11 for deep vein thrombosis or pulmonary embolism, and 1.5 to 6 for women with predisposing conditions for venous thromboembolic disease. Cohort studies have shown the relative risk to be somewhat lower, about 3 for new cases and about 4.5 for new cases requiring hospitalization. The risk of thrombo-

Continued on next page

NuvaRing—Cont.

embolic disease associated with oral contraceptives is not related to length of use and disappears after pill use is stopped.

Several epidemiology studies indicate that third generation oral contraceptives, including those containing desogestrel (etonogestrel, the progestin in NuvaRing®, is the biologically active metabolite of desogestrel), are associated with a higher risk of venous thromboembolism than certain second generation oral contraceptives. In general, these studies indicate an approximate two-fold increased risk, which corresponds to an additional one to two cases of venous thromboembolism per 10,000 women-years of use. However, data from additional studies have not shown this two-fold increase in risk. It is unknown if NuvaRing® has a different risk of venous thromboembolism than second generation oral contraceptives.

A two- to four-fold increase in relative risk of postoperative thromboembolic complications has been reported with the use of oral contraceptives. The relative risk of venous thrombosis in women who have predisposing conditions is twice that of women without such medical conditions. If feasible, combination hormonal contraceptives, including NuvaRing®, should be discontinued at least four weeks prior to and for two weeks after elective surgery of a type associated with an increase in risk of thromboembolism and during and following prolonged immobilization. Since the immediate postpartum period is also associated with an increased risk of thromboembolism, combination hormonal contraceptives, such as NuvaRing®, should be started no earlier than four weeks after delivery in women who elect not to breast feed.

The clinician should be alert to the earliest manifestations of thrombotic disorders (thrombophlebitis, pulmonary embolism, cerebrovascular disorders, and retinal thrombosis). Should any of these occur or be suspected, NuvaRing® should be discontinued immediately.

b. Myocardial infarction

An increased risk of myocardial infarction has been attributed to oral contraceptive use. This risk is primarily in smokers or women with other underlying risk factors for coronary artery disease such as hypertension, hypercholesterolemia, morbid obesity, and diabetes. The relative risk of heart attack for current combination oral contraceptive users has been estimated to be 2 to 6. The risk is very low in women under the age of 30.

Smoking in combination with oral contraceptive use has been shown to contribute substantially to the incidence of myocardial infarction in women in their mid-thirties or older with smoking accounting for the majority of excess cases. Mortality rates associated with circulatory disease have been shown to increase substantially in smokers, over the age of 35 and nonsmokers over the age of 40 among women who use oral contraceptives (see Table IV).

[See table IV at right]

Oral contraceptives may compound the effects of well-known risk factors, such as hypertension, diabetes, hyperlipidemias, age, and obesity. In particular, some progestogens are known to decrease HDL cholesterol and cause glucose intolerance, while estrogens may create a state of hyperinsulinism. Oral contraceptives have been shown to increase blood pressure among users (see WARNINGS). Similar effects on risk factors have been associated with an increased risk of heart disease. NuvaRing® must be used with caution in women with cardiovascular disease risk factors.

c. Cerebrovascular diseases

Oral contraceptives have been shown to increase both the relative and attributable risks of cerebrovascular events (thrombotic and hemorrhagic strokes), although, in general, the risk is greatest among older (>35 years), hypertensive women who also smoke. Hypertension was found to be a risk factor for both users and non-users, for both types of strokes, while smoking interacted to increase the risk for hemorrhagic strokes.

In a large study, the relative risk of thrombotic strokes has been shown to range from 3 for normotensive users to 14 for users with severe hypertension. The relative risk of hemorrhagic stroke is reported to be 1.2 for non-smokers who used oral contraceptives, 2.6 for smokers who did not use oral contraceptives, 7.6 for smokers who used oral contraceptives, 1.8 for normotensive users and 25.7 for users with severe hypertension. The attributable risk is also greater in older women.

d. Dose-related risk of vascular disease from oral contraceptives

A positive association has been observed between the amount of estrogen and progestogen in oral contraceptives and the risk of vascular disease. A decline in serum high-density lipoproteins (HDL) has been reported with many progestational agents. A decline in serum high-density lipoproteins has been associated with an increased incidence of ischemic heart disease. Because estrogens increase HDL cholesterol, the net effect of an oral contraceptive depends on a balance achieved between doses of estrogen and progestogen and the nature and absolute amount of progestogens used in the contraceptives. The activity and amount of both hormones should be considered in the choice of a hormonal contraceptive.

e. Persistence of risk of vascular disease

There are two studies that have shown persistence of risk of vascular disease for ever-users of oral contraceptives. In a study in the United States, the risk of developing myocardial infarction after discontinuing oral contraceptives persists for at least nine years for women 40–49 years old who had used oral contraceptives for five or more years, but this increased risk was not demonstrated in other age groups. In another study in Great Britain, the risk of developing cerebrovascular disease persisted for at least six years after discontinuation of oral contraceptives, although excess risk was very small. However, both studies were performed with oral contraceptive formulations containing 50 micrograms or more of estrogen.

It is unknown whether NuvaRing® is distinct from combination oral contraceptives with regard to the occurrence of venous or arterial thrombosis.

2. **ESTIMATES OF MORTALITY FROM CONTRACEPTIVE USE**

One study gathered data from a variety of sources that have estimated the mortality rate associated with different methods of contraception at different ages (Table V). These estimates include the combined risk of death associated with contraceptive methods plus the risk attributable to pregnancy in the event of method failure. Each method of contraception has its specific benefits and risks. The study concluded that with the exception of oral contraceptive users age 35 and older who smoke and age 40 and older who did not smoke, mortality associated with all methods of birth control is low and below that associated with childbirth.

TABLE III: PERCENTAGE OF WOMEN EXPERIENCING AN UNINTENDED PREGNANCY DURING THE FIRST YEAR OF TYPICAL USE AND THE FIRST YEAR OF PERFECT USE OF CONTRACEPTION AND THE PERCENTAGE CONTINUING USE AT THE END OF THE FIRST YEAR: UNITED STATES.

	% of Women Experiencing an Unintended Pregnancy within the First Year of Use		% of Women Continuing Use at One Year[3]
Method (1)	**Typical Use[1] (2)**	**Perfect Use[2] (3)**	**(4)**
Chance[4]	85	85	
Spermicides[5]	26	6	40
Periodic abstinence	25		63
Calendar		9	
Ovulation Method		3	
Sympto-Thermal[6]		2	
Post-Ovulation		1	
Cap[7]			
Parous Women	40	26	42
Nulliparous Women	20	9	56
Sponge			
Parous Women	40	20	42
Nulliparous Women	20	9	56
Diaphragm[7]	20	6	56
Withdrawal	19	4	
Condom[8]			
Female (Reality)	21	5	56
Male	14	3	61
Pill	5		71
Progestin Only		0.5	
Combined		0.1	
IUD			
Progesterone T	2.0	1.5	81
Copper T 380A	0.8	0.6	78
LNg 20	0.1	0.1	81
Depo-Provera	0.3	0.3	70
Norplant and Norplant-2	0.05	0.05	88
Female sterilization	0.5	0.5	100
Male sterilization	0.15	0.10	100

Emergency Contraceptive Pills: Treatment initiated within 72 hours after unprotected intercourse reduces the risk of pregnancy by at least 75%.[9]

Lactation Amenorrhea Method: LAM is a highly effective, temporary method of contraception.[10]

Adapted from Hatcher et al., Contraceptive Technology, 17th Revised Edition. New York, NY: Irvington Publishers, 1998.

[1] Among *typical* couples who initiate use of a method (not necessarily for the first time), the percentage who experience an accidental pregnancy during the first year if they do not stop use for any other reason.

[2] Among couples who initiate use of a method (not necessarily for the first time) and who use it *perfectly* (both consistently and correctly), the percentage who experience an accidental pregnancy during the first year if they do not stop use for any other reason.

[3] Among couples attempting to avoid pregnancy, the percentage who continue to use a method for one year.

[4] The percents becoming pregnant in columns (2) and (3) are based on data from populations where contraception is not used and from women who cease using contraception in order to become pregnant. Among such populations, about 89% become pregnant within one year. This estimate was lowered slightly (to 85%) to represent the percent who would become pregnant within one year among women now relying on reversible methods of contraception if they abandoned contraception altogether.

[5] Foams, creams, gels, vaginal suppositories, and vaginal film.

[6] Cervical mucus (ovulation) method supplemented by calendar in the pre-ovulatory and basal body temperature in the post-ovulatory phases.

[7] With spermicidal cream or jelly.

[8] Without spermicides.

[9] The treatment schedule is one dose within 72 hours after unprotected intercourse, and a second dose 12 hours after the first dose. The FDA has declared the following brands of oral contraceptives to be safe and effective for emergency contraception. Ovral (one dose is two white pills), Alesse (one dose is five pink pills), Nordette or Levlen (one dose is four yellow pills).

[10] However, to maintain effective protection against pregnancy, another method of contraception must be used as soon as menstruation resumes, the frequency or duration of breastfeeds is reduced, bottle feeds are introduced, or the baby reaches six months of age.

TABLE IV: CIRCULATORY DISEASE MORTALITY RATES PER 100,000 WOMAN-YEARS BY AGE, SMOKING STATUS, AND COMBINATION ORAL CONTRACEPTIVE USE.

AGE	EVER-USERS NON-SMOKERS	EVER-USERS SMOKERS	CONTROLS NON-SMOKERS	CONTROLS SMOKERS
15–24	0.0	10.5	0.0	0.0
25–34	4.4	14.2	2.7	4.2
35–44	21.5	63.4	6.4	15.2
45+	52.4	206.7	11.4	27.9

(Adapted from P.M. Layde and V. Beral, Lancet, 1981;1:541–546.)

The observation of a possible increase in risk of mortality with age for oral contraceptive users is based on data gathered in the 1970's, but not reported until 1983. However, current clinical practice involves the use of lower estrogen-dose formulations combined with careful consideration of risk factors.

Because of these changes in practice and, also, because of some limited new data which suggest that the risk of cardiovascular disease with the use of oral contraceptives may now be less than previously observed, the Fertility and Maternal Health Drugs Advisory Committee was asked to review the topic in 1989. The Committee concluded that although cardiovascular disease risks may be increased with oral contraceptive use after age 40 in healthy non-smoking women (even with the newer low-dose formulations), there are also greater potential health risks associated with pregnancy in older women and with the alternative surgical and medical procedures which may be necessary if such women do not have access to effective and acceptable means of contraception. Therefore, the Committee recommended that the benefits of low-dose oral contraceptive use by healthy non-smoking women over 40 may outweigh the possible risks. Although the data are mainly obtained with oral contraceptives, this is likely to apply to NuvaRing® as well. Women of all ages who take hormonal contraceptives, should take the lowest possible dose formulation that is effective and meets the needs of the individual patient.

[See table V above]

TABLE V: ANNUAL NUMBER OF BIRTH-RELATED OR METHOD-RELATED DEATHS ASSOCIATED WITH CONTROL OF FERTILITY PER 100,000 NON-STERILE WOMEN, BY FERTILITY CONTROL METHOD ACCORDING TO AGE.

Method of control and outcome	15–19	20–24	25–29	30–34	35–39	40–44
No fertility control methods*	7.0	7.4	9.1	14.8	25.7	28.2
Oral contraceptives non-smoker**	0.3	0.5	0.9	1.9	13.8	31.6
Oral contraceptives smoker**	2.2	3.4	6.6	13.5	51.1	117.2
IUD**	0.8	0.8	1.0	1.0	1.4	1.4
Condom*	1.1	1.6	0.7	0.2	0.3	0.4
Diaphragm/spermicide*	1.9	1.2	1.2	1.3	2.2	2.8
Periodic abstinence*	2.5	1.6	1.6	1.7	2.9	3.6

* Deaths are birth related
** Deaths are method related

Adapted from H.W. Ory, *Family Planning Perspectives* 1983;15:50–56.

3. **CARCINOMA OF THE REPRODUCTIVE ORGANS AND BREASTS**

Numerous epidemiologic studies have been performed on the incidence of breast, endometrial, ovarian, and cervical cancer in women using combination oral contraceptives.

The risk of having breast cancer diagnosed may be slightly increased among current and recent users of combination oral contraceptives. However, this excess risk appears to decrease over time after COC discontinuation and by 10 years after cessation the increased risk disappears. Some studies report an increased risk with duration of use while other studies do not and no consistent relationships have been found with dose or type of steroid. Some studies have found a small increase in risk for women who first use COCs before age 20. Most studies show a similar pattern of risk with COC use regardless of a woman's reproductive history or her family breast cancer history.

In addition, breast cancers diagnosed in current or ever oral contraceptive users may be less clinically advanced than in never-users.

Women who currently have or have had breast cancer should not use hormonal contraceptives because breast cancer is usually a hormonally sensitive tumor.

Some studies suggest that combination oral contraceptive use has been associated with an increase in the risk of cervical intraepithelial neoplasia in some populations of women. However, there continues to be controversy about the extent to which such findings may be due to differences in sexual behavior and other factors.

In spite of many studies of the relationship between oral contraceptive use and breast and cervical cancers, a cause-and-effect relationship has not been established. It is unknown whether NuvaRing® is distinct from oral contraceptives with regard to the above statements.

4. **HEPATIC NEOPLASIA**

Benign hepatic adenomas are associated with oral contraceptive use, although the incidence of benign tumors is rare in the United States. Indirect calculations have estimated the attributable risk to be in the range of 3.3 cases per 100,000 for users, a risk that increases after four or more years of use. Rupture of rare, benign, hepatic adenomas may cause death through intra-abdominal hemorrhage.

Studies from Britain have shown an increased risk of developing hepatocellular carcinoma in long term (>8 years) oral contraceptive users. However, these cancers are extremely rare in the US and the attributable risk (the excess incidence) of liver cancers in oral contraceptive users approaches less than one per million users. It is unknown whether NuvaRing® is distinct from oral contraceptives in this regard.

5. **OCULAR LESIONS**

There have been clinical case reports of retinal thrombosis associated with the use of oral contraceptives. NuvaRing® should be discontinued if there is unexplained partial or complete loss of vision, onset of proptosis or diplopia, papilledema, or retinal vascular lesions. Appropriate diagnostic and therapeutic measures should be undertaken immediately.

6. **HORMONAL CONTRACEPTIVE USE BEFORE OR DURING EARLY PREGNANCY**

Hormonal contraceptives should not be used during pregnancy.

Extensive epidemiologic studies have revealed no increased risk of birth defects in women who have used oral contraceptives prior to pregnancy. Studies also do not suggest a teratogenic effect, particularly in so far as cardiac anomalies and limb reduction defects are concerned, when oral contraceptives are taken inadvertently during early pregnancy.

Combination hormonal contraceptives, such as NuvaRing®, should not be used to induce withdrawal bleeding as a test for pregnancy. NuvaRing® should not be used during pregnancy to treat threatened or habitual abortion. It is recommended that for any patient who has not adhered to the prescribed regimen for use of NuvaRing® and has missed a menstrual period or who has missed two consecutive periods, pregnancy should be ruled out.

7. **GALLBLADDER DISEASE**

Combination hormonal contraceptives, such as NuvaRing®, may worsen existing gallbladder disease and may accelerate the development of this disease in previously asymptomatic women. Women with a history of combination hormonal contraceptive-related cholestasis are more likely to have the condition recur with subsequent combination hormonal contraceptive use.

8. **CARBOHYDRATE AND LIPID METABOLIC EFFECTS**

Hormonal contraceptives have been shown to cause a decrease in glucose tolerance in some users. However, in the non-diabetic woman, combination hormonal contraceptives appear to have no effect on fasting blood glucose. Prediabetic and diabetic women should be carefully observed while taking combination hormonal contraceptives, such as NuvaRing®. In a clinical study involving 37 NuvaRing®-treated subjects, glucose tolerance tests showed no clinically significant changes in serum glucose levels from baseline to cycle six.

A small proportion of women will have persistent hypertriglyceridemia while using oral contraceptives. Changes in serum triglycerides and lipoprotein levels have been reported in combination hormonal contraceptive users.

9. **ELEVATED BLOOD PRESSURE**

An increase in blood pressure has been reported in women taking oral contraceptives and this increase is more likely in older oral contraceptive users and with continued use. Data from the Royal College of General Practitioners and subsequent randomized trials have shown that the incidence of hypertension increases with increasing concentrations of progestogens.

Women with a history of hypertension or hypertension-related diseases, or renal disease should be encouraged to use another method of contraception. If these women elect to use NuvaRing®, they should be monitored closely and if significant elevation of blood pressure occurs, NuvaRing® should be discontinued. For most women, elevated blood pressure will return to normal after stopping hormonal contraceptives, and there is no difference in the occurrence of hypertension between former and never-users.

10. **HEADACHE**

The onset or exacerbation of migraine or development of headache with a new pattern which is recurrent, persistent, or severe requires discontinuation of NuvaRing® and evaluation of the cause.

11. **BLEEDING IRREGULARITIES**

Bleeding Patterns

Breakthrough bleeding and spotting are sometimes encountered in women using NuvaRing®. If abnormal bleeding while using NuvaRing® persists or is severe, appropriate investigation should be instituted to rule out the possibility of organic pathology or pregnancy, and appropriate treatment should be instituted when necessary. In the event of amenorrhea, pregnancy should be ruled out.

Bleeding patterns were evaluated in two large clinical studies. During cycles 1 through 13, breakthrough bleeding/spotting occurred in 7.2 to 11.7% of cycles in a study of 1177 US and Canadian subjects, and in 2.6 to 6.4% of cycles in a second study of 1145 European and Israeli subjects. Absence of withdrawal bleeding occurred in 2.3 to 3.8% of cycles in the US and Canadian trial subjects and in 0.6 to 2.1% of cycles in the European and Israeli trials subjects. Bleeding patterns for individual women over multiple cycles were not evaluated.

Some women may encounter amenorrhea or oligomenorrhea after discontinuing use of NuvaRing®, especially when such a condition was pre-existent.

12. **ECTOPIC PREGNANCY**

Ectopic as well as intrauterine pregnancy may occur in contraceptive failures.

PRECAUTIONS

1. **GENERAL**

Patients should be counseled that this product does not protect against HIV infection (AIDS) and other sexually transmitted diseases.

2. **PHYSICAL EXAMINATION AND FOLLOW-UP**

It is good medical practice for women using NuvaRing®, as for all women, to have an annual medical evaluation including physical examination and relevant laboratory tests. The physical examination should include special reference to blood pressure, breasts, abdomen, pelvic organs and vagina (including cervical cytology). In case of undiagnosed, persistent or recurrent abnormal vaginal bleeding, appropriate measures should be conducted to rule out malignancy. Women with a family history of breast cancer or who have breast nodules should be monitored with particular care.

3. **LIPID DISORDERS**

Women who are being treated for hyperlipidemias should be followed closely if they elect to use NuvaRing®. Some progestogens may elevate LDL levels and may render the control of hyperlipidemias more difficult.

4. **LIVER FUNCTION**

If jaundice develops in any woman using NuvaRing®, product use should be discontinued. The hormones in NuvaRing® may be poorly metabolized in patients with impaired liver function.

5. **FLUID RETENTION**

Steroid hormones like those in NuvaRing®, may cause some degree of fluid retention. NuvaRing® should be prescribed with caution, and only with careful monitoring, in patients with conditions which might be aggravated by fluid retention.

6. **EMOTIONAL DISORDERS**

Women who become significantly depressed while using combination hormonal contraceptives, such as NuvaRing®, should stop the medication and use another method of contraception in an attempt to determine whether the symptom is drug related. Women with a history of depression should be carefully observed and NuvaRing® discontinued if significant depression occurs.

7. **CONTACT LENSES**

Contact lens wearers who develop visual changes or changes in lens tolerance should be assessed by an ophthalmologist.

8. **DRUG INTERACTIONS**

Changes in Contraceptive Effectiveness Associated with Co-Administration of Other Drugs

Contraceptive effectiveness may be reduced when hormonal contraceptives are co-administered with some antibiotics, antifungals, anticonvulsants, and other drugs that increase metabolism of contraceptive steroids. This could result in unintended pregnancy or breakthrough bleeding. Examples include barbiturates, griseofulvin, rifampin, phenylbutazone, phenytoin, carbamazepine, felbamate, oxcarbazepine, topiramate and possibly with ampicillin and tetracyclines. Women may need to use an additional contraceptive method when taking medications which may make hormonal contraceptives less effective.

Several of the anti-HIV protease inhibitors have been studied with co-administration of oral combination hormonal contraceptives; significant changes (increase and decrease) in the mean AUC of the estrogen and progestin have been noted in some cases. The efficacy and safety of oral contraceptive products may be affected; it is unknown whether this applies to NuvaRing®. Healthcare providers should refer to the label of the individual anti-HIV protease inhibitors for further drug-drug interaction information.

Herbal products containing St. John's Wort (hypericum perforatum) may induce hepatic enzymes (cytochrome P450) and p-glycoprotein transporter and may reduce the effectiveness of contraceptive steroids. This may also result in breakthrough bleeding.

Increase in Plasma Hormone Levels Associated with Co-Administered Drugs

Co-administration of atorvastatin and certain oral contraceptives containing ethinyl estradiol increase AUC values for ethinyl estradiol by approximately 20%. Ascorbic acid and acetaminophen may increase plasma ethinyl estradiol levels, possibly by inhibition of conjugation. CYP 3A4 inhibitors such as itraconazole or ketoconazole may increase plasma hormone levels.

Changes in Plasma Levels of Co-Administered Drugs

Combination hormonal contraceptives containing some synthetic estrogens (e.g., ethinyl estradiol) may inhibit

Continued on next page

NuvaRing—Cont.

the metabolism of other compounds. Increased plasma concentrations of cyclosporine, prednisolone, and theophylline have been reported with concomitant administration of oral contraceptives. In addition, oral contraceptives may induce the conjugation of other compounds. Decreased plasma concentrations of acetaminophen and increased clearance of temazepam, salicylic acid, morphine and clofibric acid have been noted when these drugs were administered with oral contraceptives.

9. INTERACTIONS WITH LABORATORY TESTS

Certain endocrine and liver function tests and blood components may be affected by combined hormonal contraceptives:

a Increased prothrombin and factors VII, VIII, IX and X; decreased antithrombin 3, increased norepinephrine-induced platelet aggregability.
b. Increased thyroid binding globulin (TBG) leading to increased circulating total thyroid hormone, as measured by protein-bound iodine (PBI), T4 by column or by radioimmunoassay. Free T3 resin uptake is decreased, reflecting the elevated TBG; free T4 concentration is unaltered.
c. Other binding proteins may be elevated in serum.
d. Sex hormone-binding globulins are increased and result in elevated levels of total circulating sex steroids; however, free or biologically active levels either decrease or remain unchanged.
e. Triglycerides may be increased and levels of various other lipids and lipoproteins may be affected.
f. Glucose tolerance may be decreased.
g. Serum folate levels may be depressed by oral contraceptive therapy. This may be of clinical significance if a woman becomes pregnant shortly after discontinuing NuvaRing®.

10. CARCINOGENESIS, MUTAGENESIS, IMPAIRMENT OF FERTILITY

In a 24-month carcinogenicity study in rats with subdermal implants releasing 10 and 20 µg etonogestrel per day (approximately 0.3 and 0.6 times the systemic steady state exposure of women using NuvaRing®), no drug-related carcinogenic potential was observed. Etonogestrel was not genotoxic in the *in-vitro* Ames/Salmonella reverse mutation assay, the chromosomal aberration assay in Chinese hamster ovary cells or in the *in-vivo* mouse micronucleus test. Fertility returned after withdrawal from treatment. See WARNINGS.

11. PREGNANCY

Pregnancy Category X (see CONTRAINDICATIONS and WARNINGS).

Teratology studies have been performed in rats and rabbits using the oral route of administration at doses up to 130 and 260 times, respectively, the human NuvaRing® dose (based on body surface area) and have revealed no evidence of harm to the fetus due to etonogestrel.

12. NURSING MOTHERS

The effects of NuvaRing® in nursing mothers have not been evaluated and are unknown. Small amounts of contraceptive steroids have been identified in the milk of nursing mothers and a few adverse effects on the child have been reported, including jaundice and breast enlargement. In addition, contraceptive steroids given in the postpartum period may interfere with lactation by decreasing the quantity and quality of breast milk. Long-term follow-up of children whose mothers used combination hormonal contraceptives while breast feeding has shown no deleterious effects on infants. However, women who are breast feeding should be advised not to use NuvaRing® but to use other forms of contraception until the child is weaned.

13. PEDIATRIC USE

Safety and efficacy of NuvaRing® have been established in women of reproductive age. Safety and efficacy are expected to be the same for postpubertal adolescents under the age of 16 and for users 16 years and older. Use of this product before menarche is not indicated.

14. GERIATRIC USE

This product has not been studied in women over 65 years of age and is not indicated in this population.

15. VAGINAL USE

NuvaRing® may not be suitable for women with conditions that make the vagina more susceptible to vaginal irritation or ulceration. Some women are aware of the ring at random times during the 21 days of use or during intercourse. During intercourse some sexual partners may feel NuvaRing® in the vagina. However, clinical studies revealed that 90% of couples did not find this to be a problem.

If NuvaRing® has been removed or expelled during the three-week use period, it should be rinsed with cool to lukewarm (not hot) water and re-inserted as soon as possible, but at the latest within three hours of removal or expulsion. If NuvaRing® is lost, a new vaginal ring should be inserted and the regimen should be continued without alteration. If the ring has been out of the vagina for more than three hours, contraceptive effectiveness may be reduced and an additional method of contraception, such as male condoms or spermicide, **must** be used until the ring has been used continuously for seven days. NuvaRing® may interfere with the correct placement and position of a diaphragm. A diaphragm is therefore not recommended as a back-up method with NuvaRing® use.

16. EXPULSION

NuvaRing® can be accidentally expelled, for example, when it has not been inserted properly, or while removing a tampon, moving the bowels, straining, or with severe constipation. If this occurs, the vaginal ring can be rinsed with cool to lukewarm (not hot) water and reinserted promptly (see VAGINAL USE above and INFORMATION FOR THE PATIENT, DOSAGE AND ADMINISTRATION). If NuvaRing® is lost, a new vaginal ring should be inserted and the regimen should be continued without alteration. If the ring has been out of the vagina for more than three hours, contraceptive effectiveness may be reduced and an additional method of contraception, such as male condoms or spermicide, **MUST** be used until NuvaRing® has been used **continuously for seven days.** Vaginal stenosis, cervical prolapse, rectoceles, and cystoceles are conditions that under some circumstances may make expulsion more likely to occur.

INFORMATION FOR THE PATIENT

The patient should be instructed regarding the proper use of NuvaRing® (see Patient Information printed below).

ADVERSE REACTIONS

The most common adverse events reported by 5 to 14% of women using NuvaRing® in clinical trials (n=2501) were the following: vaginitis, headache, upper respiratory tract infection, leukorrhea, sinusitis, weight gain, and nausea.

The most frequent system-organ class adverse events leading to discontinuation in 1 to 2.5% of women using NuvaRing® in the trials included the following: device related events (foreign body sensation, coital problems, device expulsion), vaginal symptoms (discomfort/vaginitis/leukorrhea), headache, emotional lability, and weight gain.

Listed below are adverse reactions that have been associated with the use of combination hormonal contraceptives. These are also likely to apply to combination vaginal hormonal contraceptives, such as NuvaRing®.

An increased risk of the following serious adverse reactions has been associated with the use of combination hormonal contraceptives (see CONTRAINDICATIONS and WARNINGS):

- Thrombophlebitis and venous thrombosis with or without embolism
- Arterial thromboembolism
- Pulmonary embolism
- Myocardial infarction
- Cerebral hemorrhage
- Cerebral thrombosis
- Hypertension
- Gallbladder disease
- Hepatic adenomas or benign liver tumors

There is evidence of an association between the following conditions and the use of combination hormonal contraceptives:

- Mesenteric thrombosis
- Retinal thrombosis

The following additional adverse reactions have been reported in users of combination hormonal contraceptives and are believed to be drug-related:

- Nausea
- Vomiting
- Gastrointestinal symptoms (such as abdominal cramps and bloating)
- Breakthrough bleeding
- Spotting
- Change in menstrual flow
- Amenorrhea
- Temporary infertility after discontinuation of treatment
- Edema
- Melasma which may persist
- Breast changes: tenderness, enlargement, secretion
- Change in weight (increase or decrease)
- Change in cervical erosion and secretion
- Diminution in lactation when given immediately postpartum
- Cholestatic jaundice
- Migraine
- Rash (allergic)
- Mental depression
- Reduced tolerance to carbohydrates
- Vaginal candidiasis
- Change in corneal curvature (steepening)
- Intolerance to contact lenses

The following additional adverse reactions have been reported in users of combination hormonal contraceptives and a causal association has been neither confirmed nor refuted:

- Pre-menstrual syndrome
- Cataracts
- Changes in appetite
- Cystitis-like syndrome
- Headache
- Nervousness
- Dizziness
- Hirsutism
- Loss of scalp hair
- Erythema multiforme
- Erythema nodosum
- Hemorrhagic eruption
- Vaginitis
- Porphyria
- Impaired renal function
- Hemolytic uremic syndrome
- Acne
- Changes in libido
- Colitis
- Budd-Chiari Syndrome

OVERDOSAGE

Overdosage of combination hormonal contraceptives may cause nausea, vomiting, vaginal bleeding, or other menstrual irregularities. Given the nature and design of NuvaRing® it is unlikely that overdosage will occur. If NuvaRing® is broken, it does not release a higher dose of hormones. Serious ill effects have not been reported following acute ingestion of large doses of oral contraceptives by young children. There are no antidotes and further treatment should be symptomatic.

DOSAGE AND ADMINISTRATION

To achieve maximum contraceptive effectiveness, NuvaRing® must be used as directed (see When to Start NuvaRing® below). One NuvaRing® is inserted in the vagina by the woman herself. **The ring is to remain in place continuously for three weeks.** It is removed for a one-week break, during which a withdrawal bleed usually occurs. A new ring is inserted one week after the last ring was removed.

The user can choose the insertion position that is most comfortable to her, for example, standing with one leg up, squatting, or lying down. The ring is to be compressed and inserted into the vagina. The exact position of NuvaRing® inside the vagina is not critical for its function. The vaginal ring must be inserted on the appropriate day and left in place for three consecutive weeks. This means that the ring is removed three weeks later on the same day of the week as it was inserted and at about the same time. NuvaRing® can be removed by hooking the index finger under the forward rim or by grasping the rim between the index and middle finger and pulling it out. The used ring should be placed in the sachet (foil pouch) and discarded in a waste receptacle out of the reach of children and pets (do not flush in toilet). After a one-week break, during which a withdrawal bleed usually occurs, a new ring is inserted on the same day of the week as it was inserted in the previous cycle. The withdrawal bleed usually starts on day 2–3 after removal of the ring and may not have finished before the next ring is inserted. In order to maintain contraceptive effectiveness, the new ring must be inserted one week after the previous one was removed even if menstrual bleeding has not finished.

When to Start NuvaRing®

IMPORTANT: The possibility of ovulation and conception prior to the first use of NuvaRing® should be considered.

No preceding hormonal contraceptive use in the past month

Counting the first day of menstruation as "Day 1," NuvaRing® should be inserted on or prior to Day 5 of the cycle, even if the patient has not finished bleeding. During the first cycle, an additional method of contraception, such as male condoms or spermicides, is recommended until after the first seven days of continuous ring use.

Switching from a combination oral contraceptive

NuvaRing® may be inserted anytime within seven days after the last combined (estrogen plus progestin) oral contraceptive tablet and no later than the day that a new cycle of pills would have been started. No back-up method is needed.

Switching from a progestin-only method

There are several types of progestin-only methods. Women should insert the first NuvaRing® as follows:

- Any day of the month when switching from a progestin-only pill; do not skip any days between the last pill and the first day of NuvaRing® use
- On the same day as contraceptive implant removal
- On the same day as removal of a progestin-containing IUD, or
- On the day when the next contraceptive injection would be due

In all of these cases, the patient should be advised to use an additional method of contraception, such as male condoms or spermicide, for the first seven days after insertion of the ring.

Following complete first trimester abortion

The patient may start using NuvaRing® within the first five days following a complete first trimester abortion and does not need to use an additional method of contraception. If use of NuvaRing® is not started within five days following a first trimester abortion, the patient should follow the instructions for "No preceding hormonal contraceptive use in the past month." In the meantime she should be advised to use a non-hormonal contraceptive method.

Following delivery or second trimester abortion

The use of NuvaRing® for contraception may be initiated four weeks postpartum in women who elect not to breast feed. Women who are breast feeding should be advised not to use NuvaRing® but to use other forms of contraception until the child is weaned. NuvaRing® use may be initiated four weeks after a second trimester abortion. When NuvaRing® is used postpartum or postabortion, the increased risk of thromboembolic disease must be considered. (See CONTRAINDICATIONS and WARNINGS concerning thromboembolic disease. See PRECAUTIONS for "Nursing Mothers".) If the patient begins using NuvaRing® postpartum, and has not yet had a period, the possibility of ovulation and conception occurring prior to initiation of NuvaRing® should be considered, and she should be instructed to use an additional method of contraception, such as male condoms or spermicide, for the first seven days.

Deviations from the Recommended Regimen

To prevent loss of contraceptive efficacy patients should not deviate from the recommended regimen.

Inadvertent removal, expulsion, or prolonged ring-free interval

If NuvaRing® has been out of the vagina during the three-week use period, it can be rinsed with cool to lukewarm (not hot) water and should be **re-inserted as soon as possible,** at the latest within three hours. If the ring has been out of the vagina for more than three hours, contraceptive effectiveness may be reduced and an additional method of contraception, such as male condoms or spermicide, **MUST** be used until NuvaRing® has been used **continuously for seven days.**

If the ring-free interval has been extended beyond one week, the possibility of pregnancy should be considered, and an additional method of contraception, such as male condoms or spermicide, **MUST** be used until NuvaRing® has been used **continuously for seven days.**

Prolonged Use of NuvaRing®

If NuvaRing® has been left in place for up to one extra week (i.e., up to four weeks total), it should be removed and the patient should insert a new ring after the one-week ring-free interval. The mean serum etonogestrel concentration during the fourth week of continuous use of NuvaRing® was 1272 ± 311 pg/mL compared to a mean concentration range of 1578 ± 408 to 1374 ± 328 pg/mL during weeks one to three. The mean serum ethinyl estradiol concentration during the fourth week of continuous use of NuvaRing® was 16.8 ± 4.6 pg/mL compared to a mean concentration range of 19.1 ± 4.5 to 17.6 ± 4.3 pg/mL during weeks one to three. If NuvaRing® has been left in place for longer than four weeks, pregnancy should be ruled out, and an additional method of contraception, such as male condoms or spermicide, **MUST** be used until a new NuvaRing® has been used **continuously for seven days.**

In the event of a missed menstrual period

1. If the patient has not adhered to the prescribed regimen (NuvaRing® has been out of the vagina for more than three hours or the preceding ring-free interval was extended beyond one week) the possibility of pregnancy should be considered at the time of the first missed period and NuvaRing® use should be discontinued if pregnancy is confirmed.
2. If the patient has adhered to the prescribed regimen and misses two consecutive periods, pregnancy should be ruled out.
3. If the patient has retained one NuvaRing® for longer than four weeks, pregnancy should be ruled out.

HOW SUPPLIED

Each NuvaRing® (etonogestrel/ethinyl estradiol vaginal ring) is individually packaged in a reclosable aluminum laminate sachet consisting of three layers, from outside to inside: polyester, aluminum foil, and low-density polyethylene. The ring should be replaced in this reclosable sachet after use for convenient disposal.

Box of 3 sachets	NDC 0052-0273-03
Box of 1 sachet	NDC 0052-0273-01

Storage

Prior to dispensing to the user, store refrigerated 2–8°C (36–46°F). After dispensing to the user, NuvaRing® can be stored for up to 4 months at 25°C (77°F); excursions permitted to 15–30°C (59–86°F) [see USP Controlled Room Temperature]. Avoid storing NuvaRing® in direct sunlight or at temperatures above 30°C (86°F). For the Dispenser: When NuvaRing® is dispensed to the user, place an expiration date on the label. The date should not exceed either 4 months from the date of dispensing or the expiration date, whichever comes first.

℞ only

REFERENCES FURNISHED UPON REQUEST

PATIENT INFORMATION

NuvaRing® (etonogestrel/ethinyl estradiol vaginal ring)

℞ only

Read this leaflet carefully before you use NuvaRing® so that you understand the benefits and risks of using this form of birth control. The leaflet gives you information about the possible serious side effects of NuvaRing®. This leaflet will also tell you how to use NuvaRing® properly so that it will give you the best possible protection against pregnancy. Read the information you get whenever you get a new prescription or refill, because there may be new information. This information does not take the place of talking with your healthcare provider.

What is NuvaRing®?

NuvaRing® (NEW-vah-ring) is a flexible combined contraceptive vaginal ring. It is used to prevent pregnancy. **It does not protect against HIV infection (AIDS) and other sexually transmitted diseases (STD's) such as chlamydia, genital herpes, genital warts, gonorrhea, hepatitis B, and syphilis.** NuvaRing® contains a combination of a progestin and estrogen, two kinds of female hormones. You insert the ring in your vagina and leave it there for three weeks. You then remove it for a one-week ring-free period. After the ring is inserted, it releases a continuous low dose of hormones into your body.

Contraceptives that contain both an estrogen and a progestin are called combination hormonal contraceptives. Most studies on combination contraceptives have used oral (taken by mouth) contraceptives. NuvaRing® may have the same risks that have been found for combination oral contraceptives. This leaflet will tell you about risks of taking combination oral contraceptives that may also apply to NuvaRing® users. In addition it will tell you how to use NuvaRing® properly so that it willl give you the best possible protection against pregnancy.

Who should not use NuvaRing®?

Cigarette smoking increases the risk of serious cardiovascular side effects when you use combination oral contraceptives. This risk increases even more if you are over age 35 and if you smoke 15 or more cigarettes a day. Women who use combination hormonal contraceptives, including NuvaRing®, are strongly advised not to smoke.

Do not use **NuvaRing®** if you have any of the following conditions:

- pregnancy or suspected pregnancy
- blood clots in your legs (thrombosis), lungs (pulmonary embolism), or eyes now or in the past
- chest pain (angina pectoris)
- heart attack or stroke
- severe high blood pressure
- diabetes with complications of the kidneys, eyes, nerves, or blood vessels
- headaches with neurological symptoms
- known or suspected breast cancer or cancer of the lining of the uterus, cervix, or vagina (now or in the past)
- unexplained vaginal bleeding
- yellowing of the whites of the eyes or of the skin (jaundice) during pregnancy or during past use of oral contraceptives (birth control pills)
- liver tumors or active liver disease
- disease of the heart valves with complications
- need for a long period of bedrest following major surgery
- an allergic reaction to any of the components of NuvaRing®

Tell your healthcare provider if you have ever had any of the conditions just listed. Your healthcare provider can suggest another method of birth control.

Talk with your healthcare provider about when to start NuvaRing® if you are recovering from the birth of a child or a second trimester miscarriage or abortion or if you are breast feeding.

In addition, talk to your healthcare provider about using NuvaRing® if you have any of the following conditions. Women with any of these conditions should be checked often by their doctor or healthcare provider if they choose to use NuvaRing®.

- a family history of breast cancer
- breast nodules, fibrocystic disease, an abnormal breast x-ray, or abnormal mammogram
- diabetes
- high blood pressure
- high cholesterol or triglycerides
- headaches or epilepsy
- mental depression
- gallbladder or kidney disease
- major surgery (You may need to stop using NuvaRing® for a while to reduce your chance of getting blood clots.)
- any condition that makes the vagina get irritated easily
- prolapsed (dropped) uterus, dropped bladder (cystocele), or rectal prolapse (rectocele)
- severe constipation

How should I use NuvaRing®?

For the best protection from pregnancy, use NuvaRing® exactly as directed. Insert one NuvaRing® in the vagina and **keep it in place for three weeks in a row.** Remove it for a one-week break and then insert a new ring. During the one-week break, you will usually have your menstrual period. Your healthcare provider should examine you at least once a year to see if there are any signs of side effects of NuvaRing® use.

When should I start NuvaRing®?

Follow the instructions in one of the sections below to find out when to start using NuvaRing®.

If you **did not** use a hormonal contraceptive in the past month

Counting the first day of your menstrual period as "Day 1," insert your first NuvaRing® between Day 1 and Day 5 of the cycle, but at the latest on Day 5, even if you have not finished bleeding. During this first cycle, use an extra method of birth control, such as male condoms or spermicide, for the first seven days of ring use.

If you are switching from a combination oral contraceptive (birth control pill containing both progestin and estrogen)

Insert NuvaRing® anytime during the first seven days after the last combined (estrogen and progestin) oral contraceptive tablet and no later than the day when you would have started a new pill cycle. No extra birth control method is needed.

If you are switching from a progestin-only contraceptive (mini-pill, implant, injection, or IUD)

- When switching from a mini-pill, start using NuvaRing® on any day of the month. Do not skip days between your last pill and first day of NuvaRing® use.
- When switching from an implant, start using NuvaRing® on the same day you have your implant removed.
- When switching from an injectable contraceptive, start using NuvaRing® on the day when your next injection is due.
- When switching from a progestin-containing IUD, start using NuvaRing® on the same day you have your IUD removed.

When you are switching from a progestin-only contraceptive, use an extra method of birth control, such as male condoms or spermicide, for the first seven days after inserting NuvaRing®.

Following first trimester abortion or miscarriage

If you start using NuvaRing® within five days after a complete first trimester abortion or miscarriage, you do not need to use an extra method of contraception.

If NuvaRing® is not started within five days after a first trimester abortion or miscarriage, begin NuvaRing® at the time of your next menstrual period. Counting the first day of your menstrual period as "Day 1," insert NuvaRing® on or before Day 5 of the cycle, even if you have not finished bleeding. During this first cycle, use an extra method of birth control, such as male condoms or spermicide, for the first seven days of ring use.

How do I insert NuvaRing®?

1. Each NuvaRing® comes in a reclosable foil pouch. After washing and drying your hands, remove NuvaRing® from its foil pouch. Keep the foil pouch for proper disposal of the ring after use. Choose the position that is most comfortable for you. For example, lying down, squatting, or standing with one leg up (Figures 1a, 1b, and 1c, respectively).

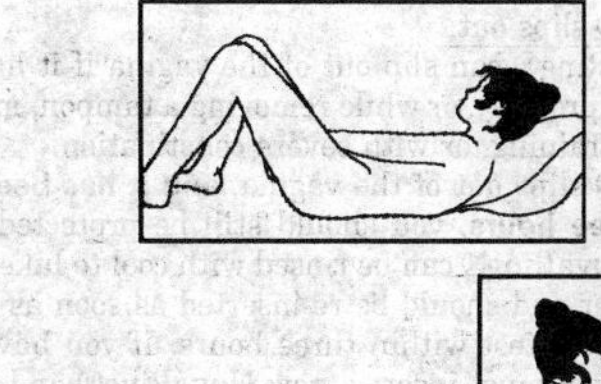

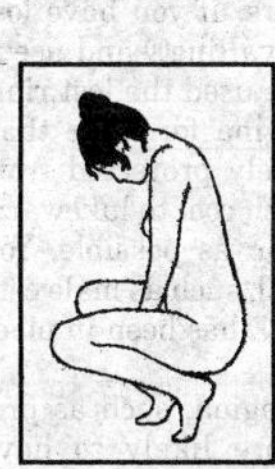

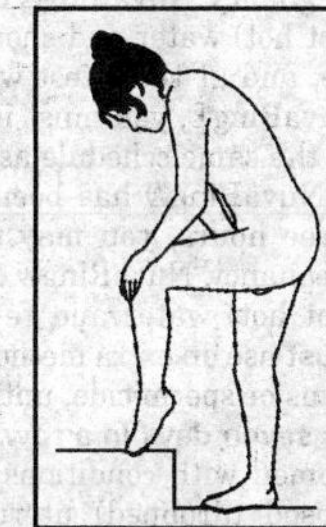

Figures 1a, 1b, 1c. Positions for NuvaRing® insertion.

2. Hold NuvaRing® between your thumb and index finger (Figure 2a) and press the opposites sides of the ring together (Figure 2b).

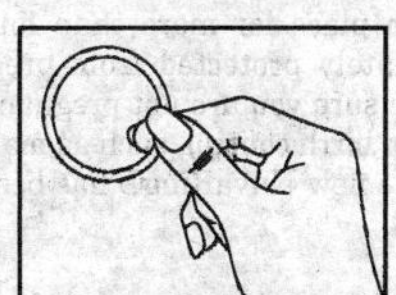

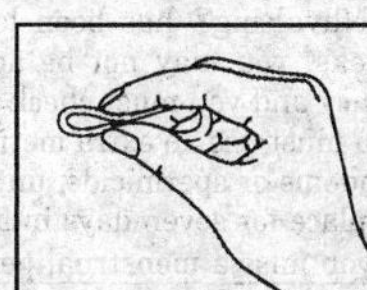

Figures 2a and 2b. Holding NuvaRing® and pressing the sides together.

3. Gently push the folded ring into your vagina (Figures 3a, 3b, and 3c). The exact position of NuvaRing® in the vagina is not important for it to work.

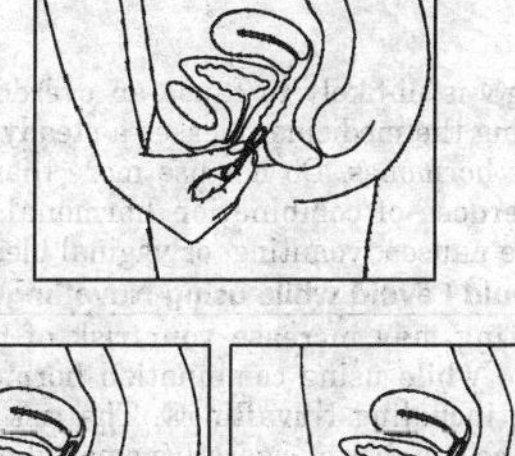

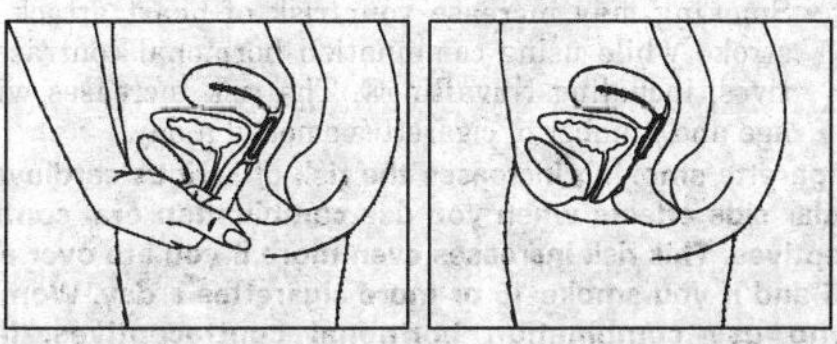

Figures 3a, 3b, and 3c. Inserting NuvaRing®.

Although some women may be aware of NuvaRing® in the vagina, most women do not feel it once it is in place. If you feel discomfort, NuvaRing® if probably not inserted back far

Continued on next page

NuvaRing—Cont.

enough in the vagina. Use your finger to gently push NuvaRing® further into your vagina. **There is no danger of NuvaRing® being pushed too far up in the vagina or getting lost.** NuvaRing® can be inserted only as far as the end of the vagina, where the cervix (the narrow, lower end of the uterus) will block NuvaRing® from going any further.

4. Once inserted, keep NuvaRing® in place for three weeks in a row.

How do I remove NuvaRing®?

1. Remove the ring three weeks after insertion on the same day of the week as it was inserted, at about the same time. For example, when NuvaRing® is inserted on a Sunday at about 10:00 PM, the ring should be removed on the Sunday three weeks later at about 10:00 PM. You can remove NuvaRing® by hooking the index finger under the forward rim or by holding the rim between the index and middle finger and pulling it out.
2. Place the used ring in the foil pouch and properly dispose of it in a waste receptacle out of the reach of children and pets. Do not throw it in the toilet. Your menstrual period will usually start two to three days after the ring is removed and may not have finished before the next ring is inserted. **To continue to have pregnancy protection, you must insert the new ring one week after the last one was removed, even if your menstrual period has not stopped.**

When do I insert a new ring?

After a one-week ring-free break, insert a new ring on the same day of the week as it was inserted in the last cycle. For example, if NuvaRing® was inserted on a Sunday at about 10:00 PM, after the one-week break you should insert a new ring on a Sunday at about 10:00 PM.

If NuvaRing® slips out:

Rarely, NuvaRing® can slip out of the vagina if it has not been inserted properly, or while removing a tampon, moving the bowels, straining, or with severe constipation.

If NuvaRing® slips out of the vagina, **and it has been out less than three hours,** you should still be protected from pregnancy. NuvaRing® can be rinsed with cool to lukewarm (not hot) water and should be re-inserted as soon as possible, and at the latest within three hours. If you have lost NuvaRing®, you must insert a new NuvaRing® and use it on the same schedule as you would have used the lost ring.

If NuvaRing® has been out of the vagina for more than three hours, you may not be adequately protected from pregnancy. NuvaRing® can be rinsed with cool to lukewarm (not hot) water and re-inserted as soon as possible. You **must** use an extra method of birth control, such as male condoms or spermicide, until the NuvaRing® has been in place for **seven days in a row.**

Women with conditions affecting the vagina, such as prolapsed (dropped) uterus, may be more likely to have NuvaRing® slip out of the vagina. If NuvaRing® slips out repeatedly, you should consult with your healthcare provider.

If NuvaRing® is in your vagina too long:

If NuvaRing® has been left in your vagina for an extra week or less (four weeks total or less), remove it and insert a new ring after a one-week ring-free break.

If NuvaRing® has been left in place for more than four weeks, you may not be adequately protected from pregnancy and you must check to be sure you are not pregnant. You must use an extra method of birth control, such as male condoms or spermicide, until the new NuvaRing® has been in place for seven days in a row.

If you miss a menstrual period:

You must check to be sure that you are not pregnant if:

1. you miss a period and NuvaRing® was out of the vagina for more than three hours during the three weeks of ring use
2. you miss a period and you had waited longer than one week to insert a new ring
3. you have followed the instructions and you miss two periods in a row
4. you have left NuvaRing® in place for longer than four weeks

Overdose

NuvaRing® is unlikely to cause an overdose because the ring holding the medicine releases a steady amount of contraceptive hormones. Do not use more than one ring at a time. Overdose of combination hormonal contraceptives may cause nausea, vomiting, or vaginal bleeding.

What should I avoid while using NuvaRing®?

- Smoking may increase your risk of heart attack or stroke while using combination hormonal contraceptives, including NuvaRing®. The risk increases with age and number of cigarettes smoked a day.

Cigarette smoking increases the risk of serious cardiovascular side effects when you use combination oral contraceptives. This risk increases even more if you are over age 35 and if you smoke 15 or more cigarettes a day. Women who use combination hormonal contraceptives, like NuvaRing®, are strongly advised not to smoke.

Do not breast feed while using NuvaRing®. Some of the medicine may pass through the milk to the baby and could cause yellowing of the skin (jaundice) and breast enlargement. NuvaRing® could also decrease the amount and quality of your breast milk.

The hormones in NuvaRing® can interact with many other medicines and herbal supplements. Tell your healthcare provider about any medicines you are taking, including prescription medicines, over-the-counter medicines, herbal remedies, and vitamins.

The blood levels of the hormones released by NuvaRing® were increased when women used an oil-based vaginal medication (miconazole nitrate) for a yeast infection while NuvaRing® was in place. The pregnancy protection of NuvaRing® is not likely to be changed by use of these products. The blood levels of the hormones released by NuvaRing® were not changed when women used vaginal, water-based spermicides (nonoxynol or N-9 products) along with NuvaRing®.

While using NuvaRing®, you should not rely upon a diaphragm when you need a back-up method of birth control because NuvaRing® may interfere with the correct placement and position of a diaphragm.

If you are scheduled for any laboratory tests, tell your doctor or healthcare provider you are using NuvaRing®. Contraceptive hormones may change certain blood tests results.

What are the possible risks and side effects of NuvaRing®?

- **Blood clots**
  The hormones in NuvaRing® may cause changes in your blood clotting system which may allow your blood to clot more easily. If blood clots form in your legs, they can travel to the lungs and cause a sudden blockage of a vessel carrying blood to the lungs. Rarely, clots occur in the blood vessels of the eye and may cause blindness, double vision, or other vision problems. The risk of getting blood clots may be greater with the type of progestin in NuvaRing® than with some other progestins in certain low-dose birth control pills. It is unknown if the risk of blood clots is different with NuvaRing® use than with the use of certain birth control pills.
- **Heart attacks and strokes**
  Hormonal contraceptives may increase your risk of strokes (blockage of blood flow to the brain) or heart attacks (blockage of blood flow to the heart). Any of these conditions can cause death or serious disability. Smoking greatly increases the risk of having heart attacks and strokes. Furthermore, smoking and the use of combination hormonal contraceptives, like NuvaRing®, greatly increases the chances of developing and dying of heart disease. If you use combination hormonal contraceptives, including NuvaRing®, you should not smoke.
- **High blood pressure and heart disease**
  Combination hormonal contraceptives, including NuvaRing®, can worsen conditions like high blood pressure, diabetes, and problems with cholesterol and triglycerides.
- **Cancer of the breast**
  Various studies give conflicting reports on the relationship between breast cancer and hormone contraceptive use. Combination hormonal contraceptives, including NuvaRing®, may slightly increase your chance of having breast cancer diagnosed. After you stop using hormonal contraceptives, the chance of having breast cancer diagnosed begins to go back down. You should have regular breast examinations by a healthcare provider and examine your own breasts monthly. Tell your healthcare provider if you have a family history of breast cancer or if you have had breast nodules or an abnormal mammogram.
- **Gallbladder disease**
  Combination hormonal contraceptive users may have a higher chance of having gallbladder disease.
- **Liver tumors**
  In rare cases, combination hormonal contraceptives, like NuvaRing®, can cause non-cancerous (benign) but dangerous liver tumors. These benign liver tumors can break and cause fatal internal bleeding. In addition, it is possible that women who use combination hormonal contraceptives, like NuvaRing®, have a higher chance of getting liver cancer. However, liver cancers are extremely rare.

The common side effects reported by NuvaRing® users are:

- vaginal infections and irritation
- vaginal discharge (leukorrhea)
- headache
- weight gain
- nausea

In addition to the risks and side effects listed above, users of combination hormonal contraceptives have reported the following side effects:

- vomiting
- change in appetite
- abdominal cramps and bloating
- breast tenderness or enlargement
- irregular vaginal bleeding or spotting
- changes in menstrual cycle
- temporary infertility after treatment
- fluid retention (edema)
- spotty darkening of the skin, particularly on the face
- rash
- weight changes
- depression
- intolerance to contact lenses

Call your healthcare provider right away if you get any of the symptoms listed below. They may be signs of a serious problem:

- sharp chest pain, coughing blood, or sudden shortness of breath (possible clot in the lung)
- pain in the calf (back of lower leg; possible clot in the leg)
- crushing chest pain or heaviness in the chest (possible heart attack)
- sudden severe headache or vomiting, dizziness or fainting, problems with vision or speech, weakness, or numbness in an arm or leg (possible stroke)
- sudden partial or complete loss of vision (possible clot in the eye)
- yellowing of the skin or whites of the eyes (jaundice), especially with fever, tiredness, loss of appetite, dark colored urine, or light colored bowel movements (possible liver problems)
- severe pain, swelling or tenderness in the abdomen (gallbladder or liver problems)
- breast lumps (possible breast cancer or benign breast disease)
- irregular vaginal bleeding or spotting that happens in more than one menstrual cycle or lasts for more than a few days
- swelling (edema) of your fingers or ankles
- difficulty in sleeping, weakness, lack of energy, fatigue, or a change in mood (possible severe depression)

How effective is NuvaRing®?

If NuvaRing® is used according to the directions, your chance of getting pregnant is about 1 to 2% a year. This means that, for every 100 women who use NuvaRing® for a year, about one or two will become pregnant. Your chance of getting pregnant increases if NuvaRing® is not used exactly according to the directions.

By comparison, the chances of getting pregnant in the first year of typical use (not always following directions exactly) of other methods of birth control are as follows:

No birth control method:	85%
Spermicides alone:	26%
Periodic abstinence methods (calendar, ovulation, thermometer):	25%
Withdrawal:	19%
Cervical Cap with spermicides:	20 to 40%
Vaginal sponge:	20 to 40%
Diaphragm with spermicides:	20%
Condom alone (male):	14%
Condom alone (female):	21%
Oral contraceptives:	5%
IUD:	less than 1 to 2%
Implants:	less than 1%
Injection:	less than 1%
Sterilization:	less than 1%

Other information

- Place the used ring in the reclosable foil pouch and properly dispose of it in a waste receptacle out of the reach of children and pets.
- Store NuvaRing® at room temperature, 25°C (77°F). Temperatures can be from 59–86°F (15–30°C). Avoid direct sunlight or storing above 86°F (30°C).

Medicines are sometimes prescribed for conditions that are not mentioned in patient information leaflets. Do not use NuvaRing® for a condition for which it was not prescribed. Do not give NuvaRing® to anyone else who may want to use it.

This leaflet summarizes the most important information about NuvaRing®. If you would like more information, talk with your healthcare provider. You can ask your pharmacist or healthcare provider for information about NuvaRing® that is written for health professionals.

ORGANON
Manufactured for Organon USA Inc.
West Orange, NJ 07052
by N.V. Organon, Oss, The Netherlands
©2001 Organon USA Inc. 5310192 10/03 20

Shown in Product Identification Guide, page 327

REMERON® ℞
(mirtazapine) Tablets

HOW SUPPLIED

REMERON® (mirtazapine) Tablets are supplied as:

15 mg Tablets — oval, scored, yellow, coated, with "Organon" debossed on one side and "$\frac{TZ}{3}$" on the other side.
Bottles of 30 NDC 0052-0105-30

30 mg Tablets — oval, scored, red-brown, coated, with "Organon" debossed on one side and "$\frac{TZ}{5}$" on the other side.
Bottles of 30 NDC 0052-0107-30

45 mg Tablets — oval, white, coated, with "Organon" debossed on one side and "$\frac{TZ}{7}$" on the other side.
Bottles of 30 NDC 0052-0109-30

Storage

Store at 25°C (77°F); excursions permitted to 15–30°C (59–86°F) [see USP Controlled Room Temperature]. Protect from light and moisture.

℞ only

Organon
Manufactured for Organon Inc., West Orange, NJ 07052
by N.V. Organon, Oss, The Netherlands
5310179 5/02 17

REMERONSolTab® ℞
[rĕ'mər-ŏn-sŏl-tăb]
(mirtazapine)
Orally Disintegrating Tablets
Once-A-Day

HOW SUPPLIED
REMERONSolTab® (mirtazapine) Orally Disintegrating Tablets are supplied as:
15 mg Tablets — round, white with "TZ/1" debossed on one side.
Box of 30 5 × 6 Unit Dose Blisters NDC 0052-0106-30
Long Term Care Carton
Box of 30 5 × 6 Unit Dose Blisters NDC 0052-0106-93
30 mg Tablets — round, white with "TZ/2" debossed on one side.
Box of 30 5 × 6 Unit Dose Blisters NDC 0052-0108-30
Long Term Care Carton
Box of 30 5 × 6 Unit Dose Blisters NDC 0052-0108-93
45 mg Tablets — round, white with "TZ/4" debossed on one side.
Box of 30 5 × 6 Unit Dose Blisters NDC 0052-0110-30
Storage
Store at 25°C (77°F); excursions permitted to 15–30°C (59–86°F) [see USP Controlled Room Temperature]. Protect from light and moisture. Use immediately upon opening individual tablet blister.
Rx only
Organon
Manufactured for Organon Inc., West Orange, NJ 07052
by CIMA Labs Inc., Eden Prairie, MN 55344
5310216 6/02 16
Shown in Product Identification Guide, page 327

TICE® BCG ℞
[tīs]
BCG LIVE
(FOR INTRAVESICAL USE)

WARNING
TICE® BCG contains live, attenuated mycobacteria. Because of the potential risk for transmission, it should be prepared, handled, and disposed of as a biohazard material (see PRECAUTIONS and DOSAGE AND ADMINISTRATION).
BCG infections have been reported in health care workers, primarily from exposures resulting from accidental needle sticks or skin lacerations during the preparation of BCG for administration. Nosocomial infections have been reported in patients receiving parenteral drugs that were prepared in areas in which BCG was reconstituted. BCG is capable of dissemination when administered by the intravesical route, and serious infections, including fatal infections, have been reported in patients receiving intravesical BCG (see WARNINGS PRECAUTIONS, and ADVERSE REACTIONS).

HOW SUPPLIED
TICE® BCG is supplied in a box of one vial of TICE® BCG. Each vial contains 1 to 8 × 10^8 CFU, which is equivalent to approximately 50 mg (wet weight), as lyophilized (freeze-dried) powder, NDC 0052-0602-02.
STORAGE
The intact vials of TICE® BCG should be stored refrigerated, at 2–8°C (36–46°F).
This agent contains live bacteria and should be protected from **direct** sunlight. The product should not be used after the expiration date printed on the label.
Rx Only
Manufactured for: Organon, Inc.
West Orange, NJ 07052
Manufactured by: Organon Teknika Corporation
100 Rodolphe Street
Building 1300
Durham, NC 27712
U.S. License No. 956
TICE® is a registered trademark owned by the University of Illinois and licensed to Organon Teknika Corporation.
RM129.3 July 2002
Shown in Product Identification Guide, page 327

ZEMURON® ℞
[zĕmū-rŏn]
(rocuronium bromide) Injection

THIS DRUG SHOULD BE ADMINISTERED BY ADEQUATELY-TRAINED INDIVIDUALS FAMILIAR WITH ITS ACTIONS, CHARACTERISTICS, AND HAZARDS.

DESCRIPTION
ZEMURON® (rocuronium bromide) Injection is a nondepolarizing neuromuscular blocking agent with a rapid to intermediate onset depending on dose and intermediate duration. Rocuronium bromide is chemically designated as 1-[17β-(acetyloxy)-3α-hydroxy-2β-(4-morpholinyl)-5α-androstan-16β-yl]-1-(2-propenyl)pyrrolidinium bromide.

TABLE 1: Percent of Excellent or Good Intubating Conditions and Median (Range) Time to Completion of Intubation in Patients with Intubation Initiated at 60 to 70 Seconds

ZEMURON® Dose (mg/kg) Administered over 5 sec	Percent of Patients With Excellent or Good Intubating Conditions	Time to Completion of Intubation (min)
Adults* 18 to 64 yrs		
0.45 (n=43)	86%	1.6 (1.0–7.0)
0.6 (n=51)	96%	1.6 (1.0–3.2)
Infants 3 mo to 1 yr		
0.6 (n=18)	100%	1.0 (1.0–1.5)
Pediatric 1 to 12 yrs		
0.6 (n=12)	100%	1.0 (0.5–2.3)

* Excludes patients undergoing cesarean section
Excellent intubating conditions = jaw relaxed, vocal cords apart and immobile, no diaphragmatic movement
Good intubating conditions = same as excellent but with some diaphragmatic movement

TABLE 2: Median (Range) Time to Onset and Clinical Duration Following Initial (Intubating) Dose During Opioid/Nitrous Oxide/Oxygen Anesthesia (Adults) and Halothane Anesthesia (Pediatric Patients)

ZEMURON® Dose (mg/kg) Administered over 5 sec	Time to ≥80% Block (min)	Time to Maximum Block (min)	Clinical Duration (min)
Adults 18 to 64 yrs			
0.45 (n=50)	1.3 (0.8–6.2)	3.0 (1.3–8.2)	22 (12–31)
0.6 (n=142)	1.0 (0.4–6.0)	1.8 (0.6–13.0)	31 (15–85)
0.9 (n=20)	1.1 (0.3–3.8)	1.4 (0.8–6.2)	58 (27–111)
1.2 (n=18)	0.7 (0.4–1.7)	1.0 (0.6–4.7)	67 (38–160)
Geriatric ≥65 yrs			
0.6 (n=31)	2.3 (1.0–8.3)	3.7 (1.3–11.3)	46 (22–73)
0.9 (n=5)	2.0 (1.0–3.0)	2.5 (1.2–5.0)	62 (49–75)
1.2 (n=7)	1.0 (0.8–3.5)	1.3 (1.2–4.7)	94 (64–138)
Infants 3 mo to 1 yr			
0.6 (n=17)	—	0.8 (0.3–3.0)	41 (24–68)
0.8 (n=9)	—	0.7 (0.5–0.8)	40 (27–70)
Pediatric 1 to 12 yrs			
0.6 (n=27)	0.8 (0.4–2.0)	1.0 (0.5–3.3)	26 (17–39)
0.8 (n=18)	—	0.5 (0.3–1.0)	30 (17–56)

n = the number of patients who had time to maximum block recorded
Clinical duration = time until return to 25% of control T_1. Patients receiving doses of 0.45 mg/kg who achieved less than 90% block (16% of these patients) had about 12 to 15 minutes to 25% recovery.

The structural formula is:

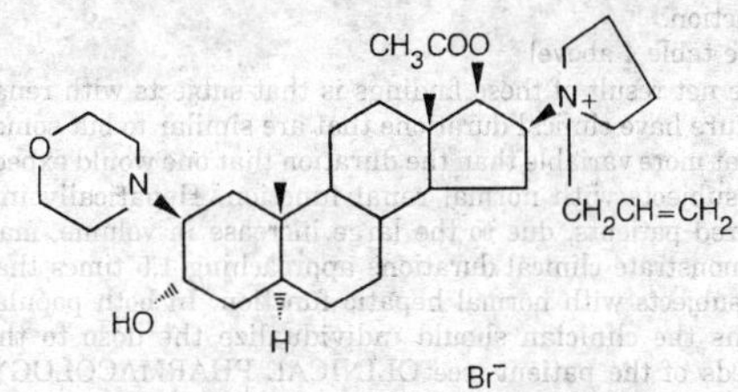

The chemical formula is $C_{32}H_{53}BrN_2O_4$ with a molecular weight of 609.70. The partition coefficient of rocuronium bromide in n-octanol/water is 0.5 at 20°C.
ZEMURON® is supplied as a sterile, nonpyrogenic, isotonic solution that is clear, colorless to yellow/orange, for intravenous injection only. Each mL contains 10 mg rocuronium bromide and 2 mg sodium acetate. The aqueous solution is adjusted to isotonicity with sodium chloride and to a pH of 4 with acetic acid and/or sodium hydroxide.

CLINICAL PHARMACOLOGY
ZEMURON® (rocuronium bromide) Injection is a nondepolarizing neuromuscular blocking agent with a rapid to intermediate onset depending on dose and intermediate duration. It acts by competing for cholinergic receptors at the motor end-plate. This action is antagonized by acetylcholinesterase inhibitors, such as neostigmine and edrophonium.
Pharmacodynamics
The ED_{95} (dose required to produce 95% suppression of the first [T_1] mechanomyographic [MMG] response of the adductor pollicis muscle [thumb] to indirect supramaximal train-of-four stimulation of the ulnar nerve) during opioid/nitrous oxide/oxygen anesthesia is approximately 0.3 mg/kg. Patient variability around the ED_{95} dose suggests that 50% of patients will exhibit T_1 depression of 91 to 97%.
Table 1 presents intubating conditions in patients with intubation initiated at 60 to 70 seconds.
[See table 1 above]
Table 2 presents the time to onset and clinical duration for the initial dose of ZEMURON® (rocuronium bromide) Injection under opioid/nitrous oxide/oxygen anesthesia in adults and geriatric patients, and under halothane anesthesia in pediatric patients.
[See table 2 above]
The time to ≥80% block and clinical duration as a function of dose are presented in Figures 1 and 2.
[See figure 1 at top of next column]

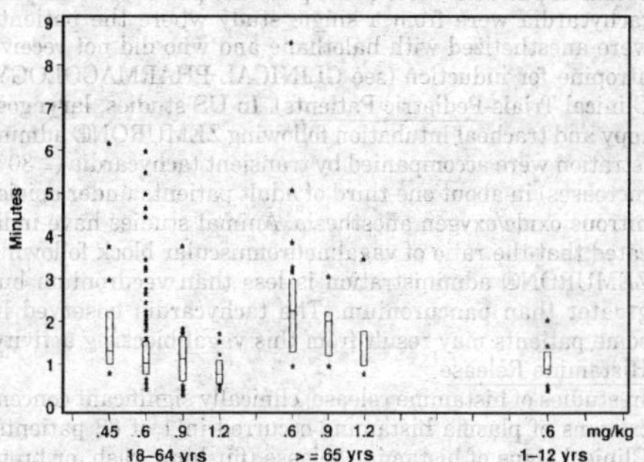

FIGURE 1: Time to ≥80% Block *vs.* Initial Dose of ZEMURON® by Age Group (Median, 25th and 75th percentile, and individual values)

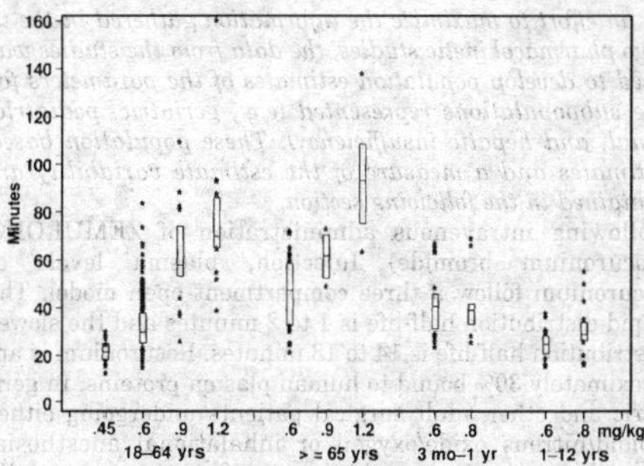

FIGURE 2: Duration of Clinical Effect *vs.* Initial Dose of ZEMURON® by Age Group (Median, 25th and 75th percentile, and individual values)

The clinical durations for the first five maintenance doses, in patients receiving five or more maintenance doses are represented in Figure 3 (see DOSAGE AND ADMINISTRATION-Maintenance Dosing).
[See figure 3 at top of next column]
Once spontaneous recovery has reached 25% of control T_1, the neuromuscular block produced by ZEMURON® is readily reversed with anticholinesterase agents, e.g., edrophonium or neostigmine.
The median spontaneous recovery from 25 to 75% T_1 was 13 minutes in adult patients. When neuromuscular block was reversed in 36 adults at a T_1 of 22 to 27%, recovery to a T_1 of 89 (50–132)% and T_4/T_1 of 69 (38–92)% was achieved within 5 minutes. Only five of 320 adults reversed received an ad-

Continued on next page

Zemuron—Cont.

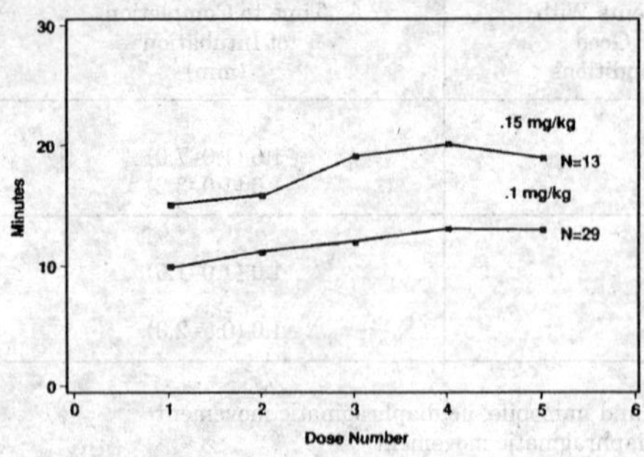

FIGURE 3: Duration of Clinical Effect *vs.* Number of ZEMURON® Maintenance Doses, by Dose

ditional dose of reversal agent. The median (range) dose of neostigmine was 0.04 (0.01–0.09) mg/kg and the median (range) dose of edrophonium was 0.5 (0.3–1.0) mg/kg.
In geriatric patients (n=51) reversed with neostigmine, the median T_4/T_1 increased from 40 to 88% in 5 minutes.
Pediatric patients (n=27) who received 0.5 mg/kg edrophonium had increases in the median T_4/T_1 from 37% at reversal to 93% after 2 minutes. Pediatric patients (n=58) who received 1 mg/kg edrophonium had increases in the median T_4/T_1 from 72% at reversal to 100% after 2 minutes. Infants (n=10) who were reversed with 0.03 mg/kg neostigmine recovered from 25 to 75% T_1 within 4 minutes.
There were no reports of less than satisfactory clinical recovery of neuromuscular function.
The neuromuscular blocking action of ZEMURON® may be enhanced in the presence of potent inhalation anesthetics (see PRECAUTIONS-Inhalation Anesthetics).

Hemodynamics

There were no dose-related effects on the incidence of changes from baseline (≥30%) in mean arterial blood pressure (MAP) or heart rate associated with ZEMURON® administration over the dose range of 0.12 to 1.2 mg/kg ($4 \times ED_{95}$) within 5 minutes after ZEMURON® administration and prior to intubation. Increases or decreases in MAP were observed in 2 to 5% of geriatric and other adult patients, and in about 1% of pediatric patients. Heart rate changes (≥30%) occurred in 0 to 2% of geriatric and other adult patients. Tachycardia (≥30%) occurred in 12 of 127 pediatric patients. Most of the pediatric patients developing tachycardia were from a single study where the patients were anesthetized with halothane and who did not receive atropine for induction (see CLINICAL PHARMACOLOGY-Clinical Trials-Pediatric Patients). In US studies, laryngoscopy and tracheal intubation following ZEMURON® administration were accompanied by transient tachycardia (≥30% increases) in about one-third of adult patients under opioid/nitrous oxide/oxygen anesthesia. Animal studies have indicated that the ratio of vagal:neuromuscular block following ZEMURON® administration is less than vecuronium but greater than pancuronium. The tachycardia observed in some patients may result from this vagal blocking activity.

Histamine Release

In studies of histamine release, clinically significant concentrations of plasma histamine occurred in 1 of 88 patients. Clinical signs of histamine release (flushing, rash, or bronchospasm) associated with the administration of ZEMURON® were assessed in clinical trials and reported in 9 of 1137 (0.8%) patients.

Pharmacokinetics

In an effort to maximize the information gathered in the in vivo pharmacokinetic studies, the data from the studies was used to develop population estimates of the parameters for the subpopulations represented (e.g., geriatric, pediatric, renal, and hepatic insufficiency). These population based estimates and a measure of the estimate variability are contained in the following section.

Following intravenous administration of ZEMURON® (rocuronium bromide) Injection, plasma levels of rocuronium follow a three compartment open model. The rapid distribution half-life is 1 to 2 minutes and the slower distribution half-life is 14 to 18 minutes. Rocuronium is approximately 30% bound to human plasma proteins. In geriatric and other adult surgical patients undergoing either opioid/nitrous oxide/oxygen or inhalational anesthesia, the observed pharmacokinetic profile was essentially unchanged.
[See table 3 above]
In general, studies with normal adult subjects did not reveal any differences in the pharmacokinetics of rocuronium due to gender.
Studies of distribution, metabolism, and excretion in cats and dogs indicate that rocuronium is eliminated primarily by the liver. The rocuronium analog 17-desacetyl-rocuronium, a metabolite, has been rarely observed in the plasma or urine of humans administered single doses of 0.5 to 1 mg/kg with or without a subsequent infusion (for up to 12 hr) of rocuronium. In the cat, 17-desacetyl-rocuronium has approximately one-twentieth the neuromuscular blocking potency of rocuronium. The effects of renal failure and hepatic disease on the pharmacokinetics and pharmacodynamics of rocuronium in humans are consistent with these findings.
In general, patients undergoing cadaver kidney transplant have a small reduction in clearance which is offset pharmacokinetically by a corresponding increase in volume, such that the net effect is an unchanged plasma half-life. Patients with demonstrated liver cirrhosis have a marked increase in their volume of distribution resulting in a plasma half-life approximately twice that of patients with normal hepatic function. Table 4 shows pharmacokinetic parameters in subjects with either impaired renal or hepatic function.
[See table 4 above]
The net result of these findings is that subjects with renal failure have clinical durations that are similar to but somewhat more variable than the duration that one would expect in subjects with normal renal function. Hepatically impaired patients, due to the large increase in volume, may demonstrate clinical durations approaching 1.5 times that of subjects with normal hepatic function. In both populations the clinician should individualize the dose to the needs of the patient (see CLINICAL PHARMACOLOGY-Individualization of Dosage).
Tissue redistribution accounts for most (about 80%) of the initial amount of rocuronium administered. As tissue compartments fill with continued dosing (4 to 8 hours), less drug is redistributed away from the site of action and, for an infusion-only dose, the rate to maintain neuromuscular blockade falls to about 20% of the initial infusion rate. The use of a loading dose and a smaller infusion rate reduces the need for adjustment of dose.

TABLE 3: Mean (SD) Pharmacokinetic Parameters in Adults (n=22; ages 27 to 58 yrs) and Geriatric (n=20; ≥65 yrs) During Opioid/Nitrous Oxide/Oxygen Anesthesia

PK Parameters	Adults (Ages 27 to 58 yrs)	Geriatrics (≥65 yrs)
Clearance (L/kg/hr)	0.25 (0.08)	0.21 (0.06)
Volume of Distribution at Steady State (L/kg)	0.25 (0.04)	0.22 (0.03)
$t_{1/2}$ β Elimination (hr)	1.4 (0.4)	1.5 (0.4)

TABLE 4: Mean (SD) Pharmacokinetic Parameters in Adults with Normal Renal and Hepatic Function (n=10, ages 23 to 65), Renal Transplant Patients (n=10, ages 21 to 45) and Hepatic Dysfunction Patients (n=9, ages 31 to 67) During Isoflurane Anesthesia

PK Parameters	Normal Renal and Hepatic Function	Renal Transplant Patients	Hepatic Dysfunction Patients
Clearance (L/kg/hr)	0.16 (0.05)*	0.13 (0.04)	0.13 (0.06)
Volume of Distribution at Steady State (L/kg)	0.26 (0.03)	0.34 (0.11)	0.53 (0.14)
$t_{1/2}$ β Elimination (hr)	2.4 (0.8)*	2.4 (1.1)	4.3 (2.6)

* Differences in the calculated $t_{1/2}$ β and CI between this study and the study in young adults *vs.* geriatrics (≥65 years) is related to the different sample populations and anesthetic techniques.

TABLE 5: Mean (SD) Pharmacokinetic Parameters of Rocuronium in Pediatric Patients (ages 3 to <12 mos, n=6; 1 to <3 yrs, n=5; 3 to <8 yrs, n=7) During Halothane Anesthesia

	Patient Age Range		
PK Parameters	3 to <12 mos	1 to <3 yrs	3 to <8 yrs
Clearance (L/kg/hr)	0.35 (0.08)	0.32 (0.07)	0.44 (0.16)
Volume of Distribution at Steady State (L/kg)	0.30 (0.04)	0.26 (0.06)	0.21 (0.03)
$t_{1/2}$ β Elimination (hr)	1.3 (0.5)	1.1 (0.7)	0.8 (0.3)

Special Populations

Pediatrics

The clinical duration of effects of ZEMURON® (rocuronium bromide) Injection did not vary with age in patients 4 months to 8 years of age. The terminal half-life and other pharmacokinetic parameters of rocuronium in these pediatric patients are presented in Table 5.
[See table 5 above]

Clinical Trials

In US clinical trials, a total of 1137 patients received ZEMURON® (rocuronium bromide) Injection, including 176 pediatric, 140 geriatric, 55 obstetric, and 766 other adults. Most patients (90%) were ASA physical status I or II, about 9% were ASA III, and 10 patients (undergoing coronary artery bypass grafting or valvular surgery) were ASA IV. In European clinical trials, a total of 1394 patients received ZEMURON®, including 52 pediatric, 128 geriatric (≥65 years) and 1214 other adults.

Adult Patients

Intubation using doses of ZEMURON® 0.6 to 0.85 mg/kg was evaluated in 203 adults in 11 clinical trials. Excellent to good intubating conditions were generally achieved within 2 minutes and maximum block occurred within 3 minutes in most patients. Doses within this range provide clinical relaxation for a median (range) time of 33 (14–85) minutes under opioid/nitrous oxide/oxygen anesthesia. Larger doses (0.9 and 1.2 mg/kg) were evaluated in two trials with 19 and 16 patients under opioid/nitrous oxide/oxygen anesthesia and provided 58 (27–111) and 67 (38–160) minutes of clinical relaxation, respectively.

Cardiovascular Disease

In one clinical trial, 10 patients with clinically significant cardiovascular disease undergoing coronary artery bypass graft received an initial dose of 0.6 mg/kg ZEMURON®. Neuromuscular block was maintained during surgery with bolus maintenance doses of 0.3 mg/kg. Following induction, continuous 8 mcg/kg/min infusion of ZEMURON® produced relaxation sufficient to support mechanical ventilation for 6 to 12 hours in the surgical intensive care unit (SICU) while the patients were recovering from surgery. Hypertension and tachycardia were reported in some patients but these occurrences were less frequent in patients receiving beta or calcium channel blocking drugs. In 7 of these 10 patients, ZEMURON® was associated with transient increases (≥30%) in pulmonary vascular resistance. In another clinical trial of 17 patients undergoing abdominal aortic surgery, transient increases (≥30%) in pulmonary vascular resistance were observed in 4 of 17 patients receiving ZEMURON® 0.6 or 0.9 mg/kg.

Rapid Sequence Intubation

Intubating conditions were assessed in 230 patients in six clinical trials where anesthesia was induced with either thiopental (3 to 6 mg/kg) or propofol (1.5 to 2.5 mg/kg) in combination with either fentanyl (2 to 5 mcg/kg) or alfentanil (1 mg). Most of the patients also received a premedication such as midazolam or temazepam. Most patients had intubation attempted within 60 to 90 seconds of administration of ZEMURON® 0.6 mg/kg or succinylcholine 1 to 1.5 mg/kg. Excellent or good intubating conditions were achieved in 119/120 (99% [95% confidence interval 95–99.9%]) patients receiving ZEMURON® and in 108/110 (98% [94–99.8%]) patients receiving succinylcholine. The duration of action of ZEMURON® 0.6 mg/kg is longer than succinylcholine and at this dose is approximately equivalent to the duration of other intermediate acting neuromuscular blocking drugs.

Geriatric Patients

ZEMURON® was evaluated in 55 geriatric patients (ages 65 to 80 years) in six clinical trials. Doses of 0.6 mg/kg provided excellent to good intubating conditions in a median (range) time of 2.3 (1–8) minutes. Recovery times from 25 to 75% after these doses were not prolonged in geriatric patients compared to other adult patients.

Pediatric Patients

ZEMURON® 0.6 or 0.8 mg/kg was evaluated for intubation in 75 pediatric patients (n=28; age 3 to 12 months, n=47; age 1 to 12 years) in three trials using halothane (1 to 5%) nitrous oxide (60 to 70%) in oxygen. Of the pediatric patients anesthetized with halothane who did not receive atropine for induction, about 80% experienced a transient increase (≥30%) in heart rate after intubation. One of the 19 infants anesthetized with halothane and fentanyl who received atropine for induction experienced this magnitude of change.

Obese Patients

ZEMURON® was dosed according to actual body weight (ABW) in most clinical trials. The administration of ZEMURON® in the 47 of 330 (14%) patients who were at least 30% or more above their ideal body weight (IBW) was not associated with clinically significant differences in the onset, duration, recovery, or reversal of ZEMURON®-induced neuromuscular block.

In one clinical trial in obese patients, ZEMURON® 0.6 mg/kg was dosed according to ABW (n=12) or IBW (n=11). Obese patients dosed according to IBW had a longer time to maximum block, a shorter median (range) clinical duration of 25 (14–29) minutes, and did not achieve intubating conditions comparable to those dosed based on ABW. These results support the recommendation that obese patients be dosed based on actual body weight.

Obstetric Patients

ZEMURON® 0.6 mg/kg was administered with thiopental, 3 to 4 mg/kg (n=13) or 4 to 6 mg/kg (n=42), for rapid sequence induction of anesthesia for Cesarean section. No neonate had APGAR scores <7 at 5 minutes. The umbilical venous plasma concentrations were 18% of maternal concentrations at delivery. Intubating conditions were poor or inadequate in 5 of 13 women receiving 3 to 4 mg/kg thiopental when intubation was attempted 60 seconds after drug injection. Therefore, ZEMURON® is not recommended for rapid sequence induction in Cesarean section patients.

Individualization of Dosage

DOSES OF ZEMURON® (rocuronium bromide) INJECTION SHOULD BE INDIVIDUALIZED AND A PERIPHERAL NERVE STIMULATOR SHOULD BE USED TO MEASURE NEUROMUSCULAR FUNCTION DURING ZEMURON® ADMINISTRATION IN ORDER TO MONITOR DRUG EFFECT, DETERMINE THE NEED FOR ADDITIONAL DOSES, AND CONFIRM RECOVERY FROM NEUROMUSCULAR BLOCK.

Based on the known actions of ZEMURON®, the following factors should be considered when administering ZEMURON®:

Renal or Hepatic Impairment

No differences from patients with normal hepatic and kidney function were observed for onset time at a dose of 0.6 mg/kg ZEMURON®. When compared to patients with normal renal and hepatic function, the mean clinical duration is similar in patients with end-stage renal disease undergoing renal transplant, and is about 1.5 times longer in patients with hepatic disease. Patients with renal failure may have a greater variation in duration of effect (see CLINICAL PHARMACOLOGY-Pharmacokinetics and PRECAUTIONS-Hepatic Disease and PRECAUTIONS-Renal Failure).

Reduced Plasma Cholinesterase Activity

No differences from patients with normal plasma cholinesterase activity are expected since rocuronium metabolism does not depend on plasma cholinesterase.

Drugs or Conditions Causing Potentiation of, or Resistance to, Neuromuscular Block

The neuromuscular blocking action of ZEMURON® is potentiated by isoflurane and enflurane anesthesia. Potentiation is minimal when administration of the recommended dose of ZEMURON® occurs prior to the administration of these potent inhalation agents. The median clinical duration of a dose of 0.57 to 0.85 mg/kg was 34, 38, and 42 minutes under opioid/nitrous oxide/oxygen, enflurane and isoflurane maintenance anesthesia, respectively. During 1 to 2 hours of infusion, the infusion rate of ZEMURON® required to maintain about 95% block was decreased by as much as 40% under enflurane and isoflurane anesthesia (see PRECAUTIONS-Inhalation Anesthetics).

When ZEMURON® is administered to patients chronically receiving anticonvulsant agents such as carbamazepine or phenytoin, shorter durations of neuromuscular block may occur and infusion rates may be higher due to the development of resistance to nondepolarizing muscle relaxants (see PRECAUTIONS-Anticonvulsants).

Pulmonary Hypertension

ZEMURON may be associated with increased pulmonary vascular resistance, so caution is appropriate in patients with pulmonary hypertension or valvular heart disease (see CLINICAL PHARMACOLOGY-Clinical Trials).

Obesity

In obese patients, the initial dose of ZEMURON® 0.6 mg/kg should be based upon the patient's actual body weight (see CLINICAL PHARMACOLOGY-Clinical Trials-Obese Patients).

Based on the known actions of other nondepolarizing neuromuscular blocking agents, the following additional factors should be considered when administering ZEMURON®:

Drugs or Conditions Causing Potentiation of, or Resistance to, Neuromuscular Block

Resistance to nondepolarizing agents, consistent with upregulation of skeletal muscle acetylcholine receptors, is associated with burns, disuse atrophy, denervation, and direct muscle trauma. Receptor up-regulation may also contribute to the resistance to nondepolarizing muscle relaxants which sometimes develops in patients with cerebral palsy, patients chronically receiving anticonvulsant agents such as carbamazepine or phenytoin or with chronic exposure to nondepolarizing agents (see PRECAUTIONS).

Other nondepolarizing neuromuscular blocking agents have been found to exhibit profound neuromuscular blocking effects in cachectic or debilitated patients, patients with neuromuscular diseases, and patients with carcinomatosis. In these or other patients in whom potentiation of neuromuscular block or difficulty with reversal may be anticipated, a decrease from the recommended initial dose should be considered.

Certain antibiotics, magnesium salts, lithium, local anesthetics, procainamide, and quinidine have been shown to increase the duration of neuromuscular block and decrease infusion requirements of other neuromuscular blocking agents. In patients in whom potentiation of neuromuscular block may be anticipated, a decrease from the recommended initial dose should be considered (see PRECAUTIONS-Antibiotics and PRECAUTIONS-Other).

Severe acid-base and/or electrolyte abnormalities may potentiate or cause resistance to the neuromuscular blocking action of ZEMURON® (see PRECAUTIONS-Other). No data are available in such patients and no dosing recommendations can be made.

Burns

Patients with burns are known to develop resistance to nondepolarizing neuromuscular blocking agents, probably due to upregulation of post-synaptic skeletal muscle cholinergic receptors (see CLINICAL PHARMACOLOGY-Individualization of Dosage).

INDICATIONS AND USAGE

ZEMURON® (rocuronium bromide) Injection is a nondepolarizing neuromuscular blocking agent with a rapid to intermediate onset depending on dose and intermediate duration and is indicated for inpatients and outpatients as an adjunct to general anesthesia to facilitate both rapid sequence and routine tracheal intubation, and to provide skeletal muscle relaxation during surgery or mechanical ventilation.

CONTRAINDICATIONS

ZEMURON® (rocuronium bromide) Injection is contraindicated in patients known to have hypersensitivity to rocuronium bromide.

WARNINGS

ZEMURON® (rocuronium bromide) INJECTION SHOULD BE ADMINISTERED IN CAREFULLY ADJUSTED DOSAGES BY OR UNDER THE SUPERVISION OF EXPERIENCED CLINICIANS WHO ARE FAMILIAR WITH THE DRUG'S ACTIONS AND THE POSSIBLE COMPLICATIONS OF ITS USE. THE DRUG SHOULD NOT BE ADMINISTERED UNLESS FACILITIES FOR INTUBATION, ARTIFICIAL RESPIRATION, OXYGEN THERAPY, AND AN ANTAGONIST ARE IMMEDIATELY AVAILABLE. IT IS RECOMMENDED THAT CLINICIANS ADMINISTERING NEUROMUSCULAR BLOCKING AGENTS SUCH AS ZEMURON® EMPLOY A PERIPHERAL NERVE STIMULATOR TO MONITOR DRUG RESPONSE, NEED FOR ADDITIONAL RELAXANT, AND ADEQUACY OF SPONTANEOUS RECOVERY OR ANTAGONISM.

ZEMURON® HAS NO KNOWN EFFECT ON CONSCIOUSNESS, PAIN THRESHOLD, OR CEREBRATION. THEREFORE, ITS ADMINISTRATION MUST BE ACCOMPANIED BY ADEQUATE ANESTHESIA OR SEDATION.

In patients with myasthenia gravis or myasthenic (Eaton-Lambert) syndrome, small doses of nondepolarizing neuromuscular blocking agents may have profound effects. In such patients, a peripheral nerve stimulator and use of a small test dose may be of value in monitoring the response to administration of muscle relaxants.

ZEMURON®, which has an acid pH, should not be mixed with alkaline solutions (e.g., barbiturate solutions) in the same syringe or administered simultaneously during intravenous infusion through the same needle.

Anaphylaxis

Although rare, severe anaphylactic reactions to neuromuscular blocking agents, including ZEMURON® (rocuronium bromide) Injection, have been reported. These reactions have, in some cases, been life threatening. Due to the potential severity of these reactions, the necessary precautions, such as the immediate availability of appropriate emergency treatment, should be taken.

Special precautions should be taken in patients who have had previous anaphylactic reactions to other neuromuscular blocking agents, since allergic cross-reactivity has been reported in this class of drugs.

PRECAUTIONS

Long-term Use in ICU

ZEMURON® (rocuronium bromide) Injection has not been studied for long-term use in the ICU. As with other nondepolarizing neuromuscular blocking drugs, apparent tolerance to ZEMURON® may develop rarely during chronic administration in the ICU. While the mechanism for development of this resistance is not known, receptor upregulation may be a contributing factor. It is STRONGLY RECOMMENDED THAT NEUROMUSCULAR TRANSMISSION BE MONITORED CONTINUOUSLY DURING ADMINISTRATION AND RECOVERY WITH THE HELP OF A NERVE STIMULATOR. ADDITIONAL DOSES OF ZEMURON® OR ANY OTHER NEUROMUSCULAR BLOCKING AGENT SHOULD NOT BE GIVEN UNTIL THERE IS A DEFINITE RESPONSE (ONE TWITCH OF THE TRAIN-OF-FOUR) TO NERVE STIMULATION. Prolonged paralysis and/or skeletal muscle weakness may be noted during initial attempts to wean from the ventilator patients who have chronically received neuromuscular blocking drugs in the ICU. Therefore, ZEMURON® should only be used in this setting if, in the opinion of the prescribing physician, the specific advantages of the drug outweigh the risk.

Labor and Delivery

The use of ZEMURON® (rocuronium bromide) Injection in Cesarean section has been studied in a limited number of patients. ZEMURON® is not recommended for rapid sequence induction in Cesarean section patients (see CLINICAL PHARMACOLOGY-Clinical Trials).

Hepatic Disease

Since ZEMURON® (rocuronium bromide) Injection is primarily excreted by the liver, it should be used with caution in patients with clinically significant hepatic disease. ZEMURON® 0.6 mg/kg has been studied in a limited number of patients (n=9) with clinically significant hepatic disease under steady-state isoflurane anesthesia. After ZEMURON® 0.6 mg/kg, the median (range) clinical duration of 60 (35–166) minutes was moderately prolonged compared to 42 minutes in patients with normal hepatic function. The median recovery time of 53 minutes was also prolonged in patients with cirrhosis compared to 20 minutes in patients with normal hepatic function. Four of eight patients with cirrhosis, who received ZEMURON® 0.6 mg/kg under opioid/nitrous oxide/oxygen anesthesia, did not achieve complete block. These findings are consistent with the increase in volume of distribution at steady state observed in patients with significant hepatic disease (see CLINICAL PHARMACOLOGY-Pharmacokinetics). If used for rapid sequence induction in patients with ascites, an increased initial dosage may be necessary to assure complete block. Duration will be prolonged in these cases. The use of doses higher than 0.6 mg/kg has not been studied.

Renal Failure

Due to the limited role of the kidney in the excretion of ZEMURON® (rocuronium bromide) Injection, usual dosing guidelines should be adequate. ZEMURON® 0.6 mg/kg has been evaluated in three single center trials (n=30, ages 19 to 61 years) in patients undergoing renal transplant surgery, or shunt procedures in preparation for dialysis. After ZEMURON® 0.6 mg/kg, the time to maximum block was about 1 to 2 minutes and was not different from patients without renal dysfunction. The mean (SD) clinical duration of 54 (22) minutes was not considered prolonged compared to 46 (12) minutes in normal patients; however, there was substantial variation (range, 22–90 minutes). The spontaneous recovery rate from 25 to 75% of control in renal dysfunction patients of 27 (11) minutes was similar to 28 (20) minutes in normal patients (see CLINICAL PHARMACOLOGY-Pharmacokinetics).

Anaphylaxis

There have been rare reports of severe anaphylactic reactions to ZEMURON® (rocuronium bromide) Injection, including some that have been life threatening. Clinicians should be prepared for the possibility of these reactions and take the necessary precautions, including the immediate availability of emergency treatment (see WARNINGS).

Malignant Hyperthermia (MH)

In an animal study in MH-susceptible swine, the administration of ZEMURON® (rocuronium bromide) Injection did not appear to trigger malignant hyperthermia. ZEMURON® has not been studied in MH-susceptible patients. Because ZEMURON® is always used with other agents, and the occurrence of malignant hyperthermia during anesthesia is possible even in the absence of known triggering agents, clinicians should be familiar with early signs, confirmatory diagnosis and treatment of malignant hyperthermia prior to the start of any anesthetic.

Altered Circulation Time

Conditions associated with slower circulation time, e.g., cardiovascular disease or advanced age, may be associated with a delay in onset time. Because higher doses of ZEMURON® (rocuronium bromide) Injection produce a longer duration of action, the initial dosage should usually not be increased in these patients to reduce onset time; instead, when feasible, more time should be allowed for the drug to achieve onset of effect.

Drug Interactions

The use of ZEMURON® (rocuronium bromide) Injection before succinylcholine, for the purpose of attenuating some of the side effects of succinylcholine, has not been studied.

If ZEMURON® is administered following administration of succinylcholine, it should not be given until recovery from succinylcholine has been observed. The median duration of action of ZEMURON® 0.6 mg/kg administered after a 1 mg/kg dose of succinylcholine when T_1 returned to 75% of control was 36 minutes (range 14–57, n=12) *vs.* 28 minutes (17–51, n=12) without succinylcholine.

There are no controlled studies documenting the use of ZEMURON® before or after other nondepolarizing muscle relaxants. Interactions have been observed when other nondepolarizing muscle relaxants have been administered in succession.

Inhalation Anesthetics

Use of inhalation anesthetics has been shown to enhance the activity of other neuromuscular blocking agents, enflurane > isoflurane > halothane.

Isoflurane and enflurane may also prolong the duration of action of initial and maintenance doses of ZEMURON® and decrease the average infusion requirement of ZEMURON® by 40% compared to opioid/nitrous oxide/oxygen anesthesia. No definite interaction between ZEMURON® and halothane has been demonstrated. In one study, use of enflurane in 10 patients resulted in a 20% increase in mean clinical duration of the initial intubating dose, and a 37% increase in the duration of subsequent maintenance doses, when compared in the same study to 10 patients under opioid/nitrous oxide/oxygen anesthesia. The clinical duration of in-

Continued on next page

Zemuron—Cont.

itial doses of ZEMURON® of 0.57 to 0.85 mg/kg under enflurane or isoflurane anesthesia, as used clinically, was increased by 11% and 23%, respectively. The duration of maintenance doses was affected to a greater extent, increasing by 30 to 50% under either enflurane or isoflurane anesthesia. Potentiation by these agents is also observed with respect to the infusion rates of ZEMURON® required to maintain approximately 95% neuromuscular block. Under isoflurane and enflurane anesthesia, the infusion rates are decreased by approximately 40% compared to opioid/nitrous oxide/oxygen anesthesia. The median spontaneous recovery time (from 25 to 75% of control T_1) is not affected by halothane, but is prolonged by enflurane (15% longer) and isoflurane (62% longer). Reversal-induced recovery of ZEMURON® neuromuscular block is minimally affected by anesthetic technique.

Intravenous Anesthetics

The use of propofol for induction and maintenance of anesthesia does not alter the clinical duration or recovery characteristics following recommended doses of ZEMURON®.

Anticonvulsants

In 2 of 4 patients receiving chronic anticonvulsant therapy, apparent resistance to the effects of ZEMURON® was observed in the form of diminished magnitude of neuromuscular block, or shortened clinical duration. As with other nondepolarizing neuromuscular blocking drugs, if ZEMURON® is administered to patients chronically receiving anticonvulsant agents such as carbamazepine or phenytoin, shorter durations of neuromuscular block may occur and infusion rates may be higher due to the development of resistance to nondepolarizing muscle relaxants. While the mechanism for development of this resistance is not known, receptor upregulation may be a contributing factor (see CLINICAL PHARMACOLOGY-Individualization of Dosage).

Antibiotics

Drugs which may enhance the neuromuscular blocking action of nondepolarizing agents such as ZEMURON® include certain antibiotics (e.g., aminoglycosides; vancomycin; tetracyclines; bacitracin; polymyxins; colistin; and sodium colistimethate). If these antibiotics are used in conjunction with ZEMURON®, prolongation of neuromuscular block should be considered a possibility.

Other

Experience concerning injection of quinidine during recovery from use of other muscle relaxants suggests that recurrent paralysis may occur. This possibility must also be considered for ZEMURON®.

ZEMURON®-induced neuromuscular blockade was modified by alkalosis and acidosis in experimental pigs. Both respiratory and metabolic acidosis prolonged the recovery time. The potency of ZEMURON® was significantly enhanced in metabolic acidosis and alkalosis, but was reduced in respiratory alkalosis. In addition, experience with other drugs has suggested that acute (e.g., diarrhea) or chronic (e.g., adrenocortical insufficiency) electrolyte imbalance may alter neuromuscular blockade. Since electrolyte imbalance and acid-base imbalance are usually mixed, either enhancement or inhibition may occur. Magnesium salts, administered for the management of toxemia of pregnancy, may enhance neuromuscular blockade.

A local tolerance study in rabbits demonstrated that ZEMURON® was well tolerated following intravenous, intra-arterial and perivenous administration with only a slight irritation of surrounding tissues observed after perivenous administration. In humans, if extravasation occurs, it may be associated with signs or symptoms of local irritation; the injection or infusion should be terminated immediately and restarted in another vein (see DOSAGE AND ADMINISTRATION).

Drug/Laboratory Test Interactions

None known.

Carcinogenesis, Mutagenesis, Impairment of Fertility

Studies in animals have not been performed to evaluate carcinogenic potential or impairment of fertility. Mutagenicity studies (Ames test, analysis of chromosomal aberrations in mammalian cells, and micronucleus test) conducted with ZEMURON® (rocuronium bromide) Injection did not suggest mutagenic potential.

Pregnancy

Pregnancy Category C

Developmental toxicology studies have been performed in pregnant, conscious, nonventilated rabbits and rats. Inhibition of neuromuscular function was the endpoint for high-dose selection. The maximum tolerated dose served as the high-dose and was administered intravenously three times a day to rats (0.3 mg/kg, 15 to 30% of human intubation dose of 0.6 to 1.2 mg/kg based on the body surface unit of mg/m^2) from day 6 to 17 and to rabbits (0.02 mg/kg, 25% human dose) from day 6 to 18 of pregnancy. High-dose treatment caused acute symptoms of respiratory dysfunction due to the pharmacological activity of the drug. Teratogenicity was not observed in these animal species. The incidence of late embryonic death was increased at the high-dose in rats most likely due to oxygen deficiency. Therefore, this finding probably has no relevance for humans because immediate mechanical ventilation of the intubated patient will effectively prevent embryo-fetal hypoxia. However, there are no adequate and well-controlled studies in pregnant women. ZEMURON® (rocuronium bromide) Injection should be used during pregnancy only if the potential benefit justifies the potential risk to the fetus.

TABLE 6: Infusion Rates Using ZEMURON® Injection (0.5 mg/mL)*

Patient Weight		Drug Delivery Rate (mcg/kg/min)									
(kg)	(lbs)	4	5	6	7	8	9	10	12	14	16
		Infusion Delivery Rate (mL/hr)									
10	22	4.8	6.0	7.2	8.4	9.6	10.8	12.0	14.4	16.8	19.2
15	33	7.2	9.0	10.8	12.6	14.4	16.2	18.0	21.6	25.2	28.8
20	44	9.6	12.0	14.4	16.8	19.2	21.6	24.0	28.8	33.6	38.4
25	55	12.0	15.0	18.0	21.0	24.0	27.0	30.0	36.0	42.0	48.0
35	77	16.8	21.0	25.2	29.4	33.6	37.8	42.0	50.4	58.8	67.2
50	110	24.0	30.0	36.0	42.0	48.0	54.0	60.0	72.0	84.0	96.0
60	132	28.8	36.0	43.2	50.4	57.6	64.8	72.0	86.4	100.8	115.2
70	154	33.6	42.0	50.4	58.8	67.2	75.6	84.0	100.8	117.6	134.4
80	176	38.4	48.0	57.6	67.2	76.8	86.4	96.0	115.2	134.4	153.6
90	198	43.2	54.0	64.8	75.6	86.4	97.2	108.0	129.6	151.2	172.8
100	220	48.0	60.0	72.0	84.0	96.0	108.0	120.0	144.0	168.0	192.0

Pediatric Use

The use of ZEMURON® (rocuronium bromide) Injection in pediatric patients less than 3 months of age and greater than 14 years of age has not been studied. See Pharmacodynamics subsection of CLINICAL PHARMACOLOGY and Use in Pediatrics subsection of DOSAGE AND ADMINISTRATION for clinical experience and recommendations for use in pediatric patients 3 months to 14 years of age.

Geriatric Use

ZEMURON® (rocuronium bromide) Injection was administered to 140 geriatric patients (≥65 years) in US clinical trials and 128 geriatric patients in European clinical trials. The observed pharmacokinetic profile for geriatric patients (n=20) was similar to that for other adult surgical patients (see CLINICAL PHARMACOLOGY). Onset time and duration of action were slightly longer for geriatric patients (n=43) in clinical trials. For clinical experiences and recommendations for use in geriatric patients, see Pharmacodynamics and Clinical Trials subsections of CLINICAL PHARMACOLOGY and Use in Geriatrics subsection of DOSAGE AND ADMINISTRATION.

ADVERSE REACTIONS

Clinical studies in the US (n=1137) and Europe (n=1394) totaled 2531 patients. Prolonged neuromuscular block is associated with neuromuscular blockers as a class. Prolonged neuromuscular block (166 minutes) occurred after 0.6 mg/kg ZEMURON® (rocuronium bromide) Injection in an obese 67 year-old female with hepatic dysfunction who had received gentamicin before surgery. The patients exposed in the US clinical studies provide the basis for calculation of adverse reaction rates. The following adverse experiences were reported in patients administered ZEMURON® (all events judged by investigators during the clinical trials to have a possible causal relationship):

Adverse experiences in greater than 1% of patients: — NONE

Adverse experiences in less than 1% of patients Probably Related or Relationship Unknown:

Cardiovascular:	arrhythmia, abnormal electrocardiogram, tachycardia
Digestive:	nausea, vomiting
Respiratory:	asthma (bronchospasm, wheezing, or rhonchi), hiccup
Skin and Appendages:	rash, injection site edema, pruritus

In the European studies, the most commonly reported adverse experiences were transient hypotension (2%) and hypertension (2%); it is in greater frequency than the US studies (0.1% and 0.1%). Changes in heart rate and blood pressure were defined differently from the US studies in which changes in cardiovascular parameters were not considered as adverse events unless judged by the investigator as unexpected, clinically significant, or thought to be histamine related.

In clinical practice, there have been reports, primarily from European sources, of severe allergic reactions (anaphylactic and anaphylactoid reactions and shock) with ZEMURON®, including some that have been life threatening and rarely fatal (see WARNINGS and PRECAUTIONS).

OVERDOSAGE

No cases of significant accidental or intentional overdose with ZEMURON® (rocuronium bromide) Injection have been reported. Overdosage with neuromuscular blocking agents may result in neuromuscular block beyond the time needed for surgery and anesthesia. The primary treatment is maintenance of a patent airway and controlled ventilation until recovery of normal neuromuscular function is assured. Once evidence of recovery from neuromuscular block is observed, further recovery may be facilitated by administration of an anticholinesterase agent (e.g., neostigmine, edrophonium) in conjunction with an appropriate anticholinergic agent (see Antagonism of Neuromuscular Blockade).

Antagonism of Neuromuscular Blockade

ANTAGONISTS (SUCH AS NEOSTIGMINE) SHOULD NOT BE ADMINISTERED PRIOR TO THE DEMONSTRATION OF SOME SPONTANEOUS RECOVERY FROM NEUROMUSCULAR BLOCKADE. THE USE OF A NERVE STIMULATOR TO DOCUMENT RECOVERY AND ANTAGONISM OF NEUROMUSCULAR BLOCKADE IS RECOMMENDED.

Patients should be evaluated for adequate clinical evidence of antagonism, e.g., 5 second head lift, adequate phonation, ventilation, and upper airway maintenance. Ventilation must be supported until no longer required.

Antagonism may be delayed in the presence of debilitation, carcinomatosis, and concomitant use of certain broad spectrum antibiotics, or anesthetic agents and other drugs which enhance neuromuscular blockade or separately cause respiratory depression. Under such circumstances the management is the same as that of prolonged neuromuscular blockade.

DOSAGE AND ADMINISTRATION

ZEMURON® (rocuronium bromide) INJECTION IS FOR INTRAVENOUS USE ONLY. THIS DRUG SHOULD BE ADMINISTERED BY OR UNDER THE SUPERVISION OF EXPERIENCED CLINICIANS FAMILIAR WITH THE USE OF NEUROMUSCULAR BLOCKING AGENTS. INDIVIDUALIZATION OF DOSAGE SHOULD BE CONSIDERED IN EACH CASE (see CLINICAL PHARMACOLOGY-Individualization of Dosage).

The dosage information which follows is derived from studies based upon units of drug per unit of body weight. It is intended to serve as an initial guide to clinicians familiar with other neuromuscular blocking agents to acquire experience with ZEMURON®. The monitoring of twitch response is recommended to evaluate recovery from ZEMURON® and decrease the hazards of overdosage if additional doses are administered (see CLINICAL PHARMACOLOGY-Pharmacodynamics and DOSAGE AND ADMINISTRATION-Maintenance Dosing).

It is recommended that clinicians administering neuromuscular blocking agents such as ZEMURON® employ a peripheral nerve stimulator to monitor drug response, determine the need for additional relaxant and adequacy of spontaneous recovery or antagonism.

Rapid Sequence Intubation

In appropriately premedicated and adequately anesthetized patients, ZEMURON® (rocuronium bromide) Injection 0.6 to 1.2 mg/kg will provide excellent or good intubating conditions in most patients in less than 2 minutes (see CLINICAL PHARMACOLOGY-Clinical Trials).

Dose for Tracheal Intubation

The recommended initial dose regardless of anesthetic technique is 0.6 mg/kg. Neuromuscular block sufficient for intubation (≥80% block) is attained in a median (range) time of 1 (0.4–6) minute(s) and most patients have intubation completed within 2 minutes. Maximum blockade is achieved in most patients in less than 3 minutes. This dose may be expected to provide 31 (15–85) minutes of clinical relaxation under opioid/nitrous oxide/oxygen anesthesia. Under halothane, isoflurane, and enflurane anesthesia, some extension of the period of clinical relaxation should be expected (see PRECAUTIONS-Inhalation Anesthetics).

A lower dose of ZEMURON® (rocuronium bromide) Injection (0.45 mg/kg) may be used. Neuromuscular block sufficient for intubation (≥80% block) is attained in a median (range) time of 1.3 (0.8–6.2) minute(s) and most patients have intubation completed within 2 minutes. Maximum blockade is achieved in most patients in less than 4 minutes. This dose may be expected to provide 22 (12–31) minutes of clinical relaxation under opioid/nitrous oxide/

oxygen anesthesia. Patients receiving this low dose of 0.45 mg/kg who achieve less than 90% block (about 16% of these patients) may have a more rapid time to 25% recovery, 12 to 15 minutes.

Should there be reason for the selection of a larger bolus dose in individual patients, initial doses of 0.9 or 1.2 mg/kg can be administered during surgery under opioid/nitrous oxide/oxygen anesthesia without adverse effects to the cardiovascular system. These doses will provide ≥80% block in most patients in less than 2 minutes, with maximum blockade occurring in most patients in less than 3 minutes. Doses of 0.9 and 1.2 mg/kg may be expected to provide 58 (27–111) and 67 (38–160) minutes, respectively, of clinical relaxation under opioid/nitrous oxide/oxygen anesthesia.

Maintenance Dosing

Maintenance doses of 0.1, 0.15, and 0.2 mg/kg ZEMURON® (rocuronium bromide) Injection, administered at 25% recovery of control T_1 (defined as 3 twitches of train-of-four), provide a median (range) of 12 (2–31), 17 (6–50) and 24 (7–69) minutes of clinical duration under opioid/nitrous oxide/oxygen anesthesia (see CLINICAL PHARMACOLOGY-Pharmacodynamics). In all cases, dosing should be guided based on the clinical duration following initial dose or prior maintenance dose and not administered until recovery of neuromuscular function is evident. A clinically insignificant cumulation of effect with repetitive maintenance dosing has been observed (see CLINICAL PHARMACOLOGY-Pharmacodynamics).

Use by Continuous Infusion

Infusion at an initial rate of 10 to 12 mcg/kg/min of ZEMURON® (rocuronium bromide) Injection should be initiated only after early evidence of spontaneous recovery from an intubating dose. Due to rapid redistribution (see CLINICAL PHARMACOLOGY-Pharmacokinetics) and the associated rapid spontaneous recovery, initiation of the infusion after substantial return of neuromuscular function (more than 10% of control T_1), may necessitate additional bolus doses to maintain adequate block for surgery.

Upon reaching the desired level of neuromuscular block, the infusion of ZEMURON® must be individualized for each patient. The rate of administration should be adjusted according to the patient's twitch response as monitored with the use of a peripheral nerve stimulator. In clinical trials, infusion rates have ranged from 4 to 16 mcg/kg/min.

Inhalation anesthetics, particularly enflurane and isoflurane, may enhance the neuromuscular blocking action of nondepolarizing muscle relaxants. In the presence of steady-state concentrations of enflurane or isoflurane, it may be necessary to reduce the rate of infusion by 30 to 50%, at 45 to 60 minutes after the intubating dose.

Spontaneous recovery and reversal of neuromuscular blockade following discontinuation of ZEMURON® infusion may be expected to proceed at rates comparable to that following comparable total doses administered by repetitive bolus injections (see CLINICAL PHARMACOLOGY-Pharmacodynamics).

Infusion solutions of ZEMURON® can be prepared by mixing ZEMURON® with an appropriate infusion solution such as 5% glucose in water or lactated Ringers (see DOSAGE AND ADMINISTRATION-Compatibility). These infusion solutions should be used within 24 hours of mixing. Unused portions of infusion solutions should be discarded.

Infusion rates of ZEMURON® can be individualized for each patient using the following tables as guidelines:

[See table 6 at top of previous page]
[See table 7 above]
[See table 8 at right]

Infusion solutions should be used within 24 hours of mixing. Unused portions of infusion solutions should be discarded.

Use in Pediatrics

Initial doses of 0.6 mg/kg in pediatric patients under halothane anesthesia produce excellent to good intubating conditions within 1 minute. The median (range) time to maximum block was 1 (0.5–3.3) minute(s). This dose will provide a median (range) time of clinical relaxation of 41 (24–68) minutes in 3 month to 1 year-old infants and 27 (17–41) minutes in 1 to 12 year-old pediatric patients. Maintenance doses of 0.075 to 0.125 mg/kg, administered upon return of T_1 to 25% of control, provide clinical relaxation for 7 to 10 minutes.

Spontaneous recovery proceeds at approximately the same rate in infants (3 months to 1 year) as in adults, but is more rapid in pediatric patients (1 to 12 years) than adults (see CLINICAL PHARMACOLOGY-Pharmacodynamics). A continuous infusion of ZEMURON® (rocuronium bromide) Injection initiated at a rate of 12 mcg/kg/min upon return of T_1 to 10% of control (one twitch present in the train-of-four), may also be used to maintain neuromuscular blockade in pediatric patients. The infusion of ZEMURON® must be individualized for each patient. The rate of administration should be adjusted according to the patient's twitch response as monitored with the use of a peripheral nerve stimulator. Spontaneous recovery and reversal of neuromuscular blockade following discontinuation of ZEMURON® infusion may be expected to proceed at rates comparable to that following similar total exposure to single bolus doses (see CLINICAL PHARMACOLOGY-Pharmacodynamics).

Use in Obese Patients

An analysis across all US controlled clinical studies indicates that the pharmacodynamics of ZEMURON® (rocuronium bromide) Injection are not different between obese and non-obese patients when dosed based upon their actual body weight.

TABLE 7: Infusion Rates Using ZEMURON® Injection (1 mg/mL)**

Patient Weight		Drug Delivery Rate (mcg/kg/min)									
(kg)	(lbs)	4	5	6	7	8	9	10	12	14	16
		Infusion Delivery Rate (mL/hr)									
10	22	2.4	3.0	3.6	4.2	4.8	5.4	6.0	7.2	8.4	9.6
15	33	3.6	4.5	5.4	6.3	7.2	8.1	9.0	10.8	12.6	14.4
20	44	4.8	6.0	7.2	8.4	9.6	10.8	12.0	14.4	16.8	19.2
25	55	6.0	7.5	9.0	10.5	12.0	13.5	15.0	18.0	21.0	24.0
35	77	8.4	10.5	12.6	14.7	16.8	18.9	21.0	25.2	29.4	33.6
50	110	12.0	15.0	18.0	21.0	24.0	27.0	30.0	36.0	42.0	48.0
60	132	14.4	18.0	21.6	25.2	28.8	32.4	36.0	43.2	50.4	57.6
70	154	16.8	21.0	25.2	29.4	33.6	37.8	42.0	50.4	58.8	67.2
80	176	19.2	24.0	28.8	33.6	38.4	43.2	48.0	57.6	67.2	76.8
90	198	21.6	27.0	32.4	37.8	43.2	48.6	54.0	64.8	75.6	86.4
100	220	24.0	30.0	36.0	42.0	48.0	54.0	60.0	72.0	84.0	96.0

TABLE 8: Infusion Rates Using ZEMURON® Injection (5 mg/mL)***

Patient Weight		Drug Delivery Rate (mcg/kg/min)									
(kg)	(lbs)	4	5	6	7	8	9	10	12	14	16
		Infusion Delivery Rate (mL/hr)									
10	22	0.5	0.6	0.7	0.8	1.0	1.1	1.2	1.4	1.7	1.9
15	33	0.7	0.9	1.1	1.3	1.4	1.6	1.8	2.2	2.5	2.9
20	44	1.0	1.2	1.4	1.7	1.9	2.2	2.4	2.9	3.4	3.8
25	55	1.2	1.5	1.8	2.1	2.4	2.7	3.0	3.6	4.2	4.8
35	77	1.7	2.1	2.5	2.9	3.4	3.8	4.2	5.0	5.9	6.7
50	110	2.4	3.0	3.6	4.2	4.8	5.4	6.0	7.2	8.4	9.6
60	132	2.9	3.6	4.3	5.0	5.8	6.5	7.2	8.6	10.1	11.5
70	154	3.4	4.2	5.0	5.9	6.7	7.6	8.4	10.1	11.8	13.4
80	176	3.8	4.8	5.8	6.7	7.7	8.6	9.6	11.5	13.4	15.4
90	198	4.3	5.4	6.5	7.6	8.6	9.7	10.8	13.0	15.1	17.3
100	220	4.8	6.0	7.2	8.4	9.6	10.8	12.0	14.4	16.8	19.2

* 50 mg ZEMURON® in 100 mL solution
** 100 mg ZEMURON® in 100 mL solution
** 500 mg ZEMURON® in 100 mL solution

Use in Geriatrics

Geriatric patients (≥65 years) exhibited a slightly prolonged median (range) clinical duration of 46 (22–73), 62 (49–75), and 94 (64–138) minutes under opioid/nitrous oxide/oxygen anesthesia following doses of 0.6, 0.9, and 1.2 mg/kg, respectively. Maintenance doses of 0.1 and 0.15 mg/kg ZEMURON® (rocuronium bromide) Injection, administered at 25% recovery of T_1, provide approximately 13 and 33 minutes of clinical duration under opioid/nitrous oxide/oxygen anesthesia. The median (range) rate of spontaneous recovery of T_1 from 25 to 75% in geriatric patients is 17 (7–56) minutes which is not different from that in other adults (see CLINICAL PHARMACOLOGY-Pharmacokinetics and CLINICAL PHARMACOLOGY-Pharmacodynamics).

Compatibility

Diluent Compatibility

ZEMURON® (rocuronium bromide) Injection is compatible in solution with:

0.9% NaCl solution	sterile water for injection
5% glucose in water	lactated Ringers
5% glucose in saline	

ZEMURON® is compatible in the above solutions at concentrations up to 5 mg/mL for 24 hours at room temperature in plastic bags, glass bottles, and plastic syringe pumps.

Drug Admixture Incompatibility

ZEMURON® is physically incompatible when mixed with the following drugs:

amphotericin	hydrocortisone sodium succinate
amoxicillin	insulin
azathioprine	intralipid
cefazolin	ketorolac
cloxacillin	lorazepam
dexamethasone	methohexital
diazepam	methylprednisolone
erythromycin	thiopental
famotidine	trimethoprim
furosemide	vancomycin

Parenteral drug products should be inspected visually for particulate matter and clarity prior to administration whenever solution and container permit. Do not use solution if particulate matter is present.

Safety and Handling

There is no specific work exposure limit for ZEMURON® (rocuronium bromide) Injection. In case of eye contact, flush with water for at least 10 minutes.

HOW SUPPLIED

ZEMURON® (rocuronium bromide) Injection is available in the following:

ZEMURON® 5 mL multiple dose vials containing 50 mg rocuronium bromide injection (10 mg/mL)
Box of 10 NDC 0052-0450-15

ZEMURON® 10 mL multiple dose vials containing 100 mg rocuronium bromide injection (10 mg/mL)
Box of 10 NDC 0052-0450-16

The packaging of this product contains **no** natural rubber (latex).

Storage

ZEMURON® (rocuronium bromide) Injection should be stored in a refrigerator, 2–8°C (36–46°F). DO NOT FREEZE. Upon removal from refrigeration to room temperature storage conditions (25°C/77°F), use ZEMURON® within 60 days. Use opened vials of ZEMURON® within 30 days.

℞ only

ORGANON
Manufactured for Organon USA Inc.
West Orange, NJ 07052
by Baxter Pharmaceutical Solutions LLC
Bloomington, IN 47403
5310153-01 2/04 04

Shown in Product Identification Guide, page 327

Ortho Biotech Products, L.P.
430 ROUTE 22 EAST
P.O. BOX 6914
BRIDGEWATER, NJ 08807-0914

Direct Inquiries to:
(800) 325-7504
Prompt #1, Customer Service
Prompt #2, Medical Information
FAX: (908) 526-9230

LEUSTATIN® ℞
[lew' stăt-ĭn]
(cladribine)
Injection
For Intravenous Infusion Only

> **WARNING**
> LEUSTATIN (cladribine) Injection should be administered under the supervision of a qualified physician experienced in the use of antineoplastic therapy. Suppression of bone marrow function should be anticipated. This is usually reversible and appears to be dose dependent. Serious neurological toxicity (including irreversible paraparesis and quadraparesis) has been repor ted in patients who received LEUSTATIN Injection by continuous infusion at high doses (4 to 9 times the recommended dose for Hairy Cell Leukemia). Neurologic toxicity appears to demonstrate a dose relationship; however, severe neurological toxicity has been reported rarely following treatment with standard cladribine dosing regimens.
> Acute nephrotoxicity has been observed with high doses of LEUSTATIN (4 to 9 times the recommended dose for Hairy Cell Leukemia), especially when given concomitantly with other nephrotoxic agents/therapies.

DESCRIPTION

LEUSTATIN (cladribine) Injection (also commonly known as 2-chloro-2′-deoxy-β-D-adenosine) is a synthetic antineoplastic agent for continuous intravenous infusion. It is a clear, colorless, sterile, preservative-free, isotonic solution. LEUSTATIN Injection is available in single-use vials containing 10 mg (1 mg/mL) of cladribine, a chlorinated purine nucleoside analog. Each milliliter of LEUSTATIN Injection contains 1 mg of the active ingredient and 9 mg (0.15 mEq) of sodium chloride as an inactive ingredient. The solution has a pH range of 5.5 to 8.0. Phosphoric acid and/or dibasic sodium phosphate may have been added to adjust the pH to 6.3±0.3.

The chemical name for cladribine is 2-chloro-6-amino-9-(2-deoxy-β-D-erythropento-furanosyl) purine and the structure is represented below:

cladribine

MW 285.7

CLINICAL PHARMACOLOGY

Cellular Resistance and Sensitivity:

The selective toxicity of 2-chloro-2′-deoxy-β-D-adenosine towards certain normal and malignant lymphocyte and monocyte populations is based on the relative activities of deoxycytidine kinase and deoxynucleotidase. Cladribine passively crosses the cell membrane. In cells with a high ratio of deoxycytidine kinase to deoxynucleotidase, it is phosphorylated by deoxycytidine kinase to 2-chloro-2′-deoxy-β-D-adenosine monophosphate (2-CdAMP). Since 2-chloro-2′-deoxy-β-D-adenosine is resistant to deamination by adenosine deaminase and there is little deoxynucleotide deaminase in lymphocytes and monocytes, 2-CdAMP accumulates intracellularly and is subsequently converted into the active triphosphate deoxynucleotide, 2-chloro-2′-deoxy-β-D-adenosine triphosphate (2-CdATP). It is postulated that cells with high deoxycytidine kinase and low deoxynucleotidase activities will be selectively killed by 2-chloro-2′-deoxy-β-D-adenosine as toxic deoxynucleotides accumulate intracellularly.

Cells containing high concentrations of deoxynucleotides are unable to properly repair single-strand DNA breaks. The broken ends of DNA activate the enzyme poly (ADP-ribose) polymerase resulting in NAD and ATP depletion and disruption of cellular metabolism. There is evidence, also, that 2-CdATP is incorporated into the DNA of dividing cells, resulting in impairment of DNA synthesis. Thus, 2-chloro-2′-deoxy-β-D-adenosine can be distinguished from other chemotherapeutic agents affecting purine metabolism in that it is cytotoxic to both actively dividing and quiescent lymphocytes and monocytes, inhibiting both DNA synthesis and repair.

PHARMACOKINETICS

In a clinical investigation, 17 patients with Hairy Cell Leukemia and normal renal function were treated for 7 days with the recommended treatment regimen of LEUSTATIN Injection (0.09 mg/kg/day) by continuous intravenous infusion. The mean steady-state serum concentration was estimated to be 5.7 ng/mL with an estimated systemic clearance of 663.5 mL/h/kg when LEUSTATIN was given by continuous infusion over 7 days. In Hairy Cell Leukemia patients, there does not appear to be a relationship between serum concentrations and ultimate clinical outcome.

In another study, 8 patients with hematologic malignancies received a two (2) hour infusion of LEUSTATIN® Injection (0.12 mg/kg). The mean end-of-infusion plasma LEUSTATIN concentration was 48±19 ng/mL. For 5 of these patients, the disappearance of LEUSTATIN could be described by either a biphasic or triphasic decline. For these patients with normal renal function, the mean terminal half-life was 5.4 hours. Mean values for clearance and steady-state volume of distribution were 978±422 mL/h/kg and 4.5±2.8 L/kg, respectively.

Cladribine plasma concentration after intravenous administration declines multi-exponentially with an average half-life of 6.7±2.5 hours. In general, the apparent volume of distribution of cladribine is approximately 9 L/kg, indicating an extensive distribution in body tissues.

Cladribine penetrates into cerebrospinal fluid. One report indicates that concentrations are approximately 25% of those in plasma.

LEUSTATIN is bound approximately 20% to plasma proteins.

Except for some understanding of the mechanism of cellular toxicity, no other information is available on the metabolism of LEUSTATIN in humans. An average of 18% of the administered dose has been reported to be excreted in urine of patients with solid tumors during a 5-day continuous intravenous infusion of 3.5-8.1 mg/m^2/day of LEUSTATIN. The effect of renal and hepatic impairment on the elimination of cladribine has not been investigated in humans.

CLINICAL STUDIES

Two single-center open label studies of LEUSTATIN (cladribine) have been conducted in patients with Hairy Cell Leukemia with evidence of active disease requiring therapy. In the study conducted at the Scripps Clinic and Research Foundation (Study A), 89 patients were treated with a single course of LEUSTATIN Injection given by continuous intravenous infusion for 7 days at a dose of 0.09 mg/kg/day. In the study conducted at the M.D. Anderson Cancer Center (Study B), 35 patients were treated with a 7-day continuous intravenous infusion of LEUSTATIN Injection at a comparable dose of 3.6 mg/m^2/day. A complete response (CR) required clearing of the peripheral blood and bone marrow of hairy cells and recovery of the hemoglobin to 12 g/dL, platelet count to 100 × 10^9/L, and absolute neutrophil count to 1500 × 10^6/L. A good partial response (GPR) required the same hematologic parameters as a complete response, and that fewer than 5% hairy cells remain in the bone marrow. A par tial response (PR) required that hairy cells in the bone marrow be decreased by at least 50% from baseline and the same response for hematologic parameters as for complete response. A pathologic relapse was defined as an increase in bone marrow hairy cells to 25% of pretreatment levels. A clinical relapse was defined as the recurrence of cytopenias, specifically, decreases in hemoglobin ≥ 2 g/dL, ANC ≥ 25% or platelet counts ≥ 50,000. Patients who met the criteria for a complete response but subsequently were found to have evidence of bone marrow hairy cells (< 25% of pretreatment levels) were reclassified as partial responses and were not considered to be complete responses with relapse.

Among patients evaluable for efficacy (N=106), using the hematologic and bone marrow response criteria described above, the complete response rates in patients treated with LEUSTATIN Injection were 65% and 68% for Study A and Study B, respectively, yielding a combined complete response rate of 66%. Overall response rates (i.e., Complete plus Good Partial plus Partial Responses) were 89% and 86% in Study A and Study B, respectively, for a combined overall response rate of 88% in evaluable patients treated with LEUSTATIN Injection.

Using an intent-to-treat analysis (N=123) and further requiring no evidence of splenomegaly as a criterion for CR (i.e., no palpable spleen on physical examination and ≤ 13 cm on CT scan), the complete response rates for Study A and Study B were 54% and 53%, respectively, giving a combined CR rate of 54%. The overall response rates (CR + GPR + PR) were 90% and 85%, for Studies A and B, respectively, yielding a combined overall response rate of 89%.

RESPONSE RATES TO LEUSTATIN TREATMENT IN PATIENTS WITH HAIRY CELL LEUKEMIA

	CR	Overall
Evaluable Patients N=106	66%	88%
Intent-to-treat Population N=123	54%	89%

In these studies, 60% of the patients had not received prior chemotherapy for Hairy Cell Leukemia or had undergone splenectomy as the only prior treatment and were receiving LEUSTATIN as a first-line treatment. The remaining 40% of the patients received LEUSTATIN as a second-line treatment, having been treated previously with other agents, including α-interferon and/or deoxycoformycin. The overall response rate for patients without prior chemotherapy was 92%, compared with 84% for previously treated patients. LEUSTATIN is active in previously treated patients; however, retrospective analysis suggests that the overall response rate is decreased in patients previously treated with splenectomy or deoxycoformycin and in patients refractory to α-interferon.

OVERALL RESPONSE RATES (CR+GPR+PR) TO LEUSTATIN TREATMENT IN PATIENTS WITH HAIRY CELL LEUKEMIA

	OVERALL RESPONSE (N=123)	NR + RELAPSE
No Prior Chemotherapy	68/74 92%	6 + 4 14%
Any Prior Chemotherapy	41/49 84%	8 + 3 22%
Previous Splenectomy	32/41* 78%	9 + 1 24%
Previous Interferon	40/48 83%	8 + 3 23%
Interferon Refractory	6/11* 55%	5 + 2 64%
Previous Deoxycoformycin	3/6* 50%	3 +1 66%

NR = No Response
* $P < 0.05$

After a reversible decline, normalization of peripheral blood counts (Hemoglobin >12.0 g/dL, Platelets >100 × 10^9/L, Absolute Neutrophil Count (ANC) >1500 × 10^6/L) was achieved by 92% of evaluable patients. The median time to normalization of peripheral counts was 9 weeks from the start of treatment (Range: 2 to 72). The median time to normalization of Platelet Count was 2 weeks, the median time to normalization of ANC was 5 weeks and the median time to normalization of Hemoglobin was 8 weeks. With normalization of Platelet Count and Hemoglobin, requirements for platelet and RBC transfusions were abolished after Months 1 and 2, respectively, in those patients with complete response. Platelet recovery may be delayed in a minority of patients with severe baseline thrombocytopenia. Corresponding to normalization of ANC, a trend toward a reduced incidence of infection was seen after the third month, when compared to the months immediately preceding LEUSTATIN therapy (see also WARNINGS, PRECAUTIONS and ADVERSE REACTIONS).

LEUSTATIN TREATMENT IN PATIENTS WITH HAIRY CELL LEUKEMIA TIME TO NORMALIZATION OF PERIPHERAL BLOOD COUNTS

Parameter	Median Time to Normalization of Count*
Platelet Count	2 weeks
Absolute Neutrophil Count	5 weeks
Hemoglobin	8 weeks
ANC, Hemoglobin and Platelet Count	9 weeks

*Day 1 = First day of infusion

For patients achieving a complete response, the median time to response (i.e., absence of hairy cells in bone marrow and peripheral blood together with normalization of peripheral blood parameters), measured from treatment start, was approximately 4 months. Since bone marrow aspiration and biopsy were frequently not performed at the time of peripheral blood normalization, the median time to complete response may actually be shorter than that which was recorded. At the time of data cut-off, the median duration of complete response was greater than 8 months and ranged to 25+ months. Among 93 responding patients, seven had shown evidence of disease progression at the time of the data cut-off. In four of these patients, disease was limited to the bone marrow without peripheral blood abnormalities (pathologic progression), while in three patients there were also peripheral blood abnormalities (clinical progression). Seven patients who did not respond to a first course of LEUSTATIN received a second course of therapy. In the five patients who had adequate follow-up, additional courses did not appear to improve their overall response.

INDICATIONS FOR USE

LEUSTATIN Injection is indicated for the treatment of active Hairy Cell Leukemia as defined by clinically significant anemia, neutropenia, thrombocytopenia or disease-related symptoms.

CONTRAINDICATIONS

LEUSTATIN Injection is contraindicated in those patients who are hypersensitive to this drug or any of its components.

WARNINGS

Severe bone marrow suppression, including neutropenia, anemia and thrombocytopenia, has been commonly observed in patients treated with LEUSTATIN, especially at high doses. At initiation of treatment, most patients in the clinical studies had hematologic impairment as a manifestation of active Hairy Cell Leukemia. Following treatment with LEUSTATIN, further hematologic impairment occurred before recovery of peripheral blood counts began. During the first two weeks after treatment initiation, mean Platelet Count, ANC, and Hemoglobin concentration declined and subsequently increased with normalization of mean counts by Day 12, Week 5 and Week 8, respectively. The myelosuppressive effects of LEUSTATIN were most notable during the first month following treatment. Forty-four percent (44%) of patients received transfusions with RBCs and 14% received transfusions with platelets during Month 1. Careful hematologic monitoring, especially during the first 4 to 8 weeks after treatment with LEUSTATIN Injection, is recommended (see PRECAUTIONS).

Fever (T ≥ 100°F) was associated with the use of LEUSTATIN in approximately two-thirds of patients (131/196) in the first month of therapy. Virtually all of these patients were treated empirically with parenteral antibiotics. Overall, 47% (93/196) of all patients had fever in the setting of neutropenia (ANC ≤ 1000), including 62 patients (32%) with severe neutropenia (i.e., ANC ≤ 500).

In a Phase I investigational study using LEUSTATIN in high doses (4 to 9 times the recommended dose for Hairy Cell Leukemia) as part of a bone marrow transplant conditioning regimen, which also included high dose cyclophosphamide and total body irradiation, acute nephrotoxicity and delayed onset neurotoxicity were observed. Thirty-one (31) poor-risk patients with drug-resistant acute leukemia in relapse (29 cases) or non-Hodgkins Lymphoma (2 cases) received LEUSTATIN for 7 to 14 days prior to bone marrow transplantation. During infusion, 8 patients experienced gastrointestinal symptoms. While the bone marrow was initially cleared of all hematopoietic elements, including tumor cells, leukemia eventually recurred in all treated patients. Within 7 to 13 days after starting treatment with LEUSTATIN, 6 patients (19%) developed manifestations of renal dysfunction (e.g., acidosis, anuria, elevated serum creatinine, etc.) and 5 required dialysis. Several of these patients were also being treated with other medications having known nephrotoxic potential. Renal dysfunction was reversible in 2 of these patients. In the 4 patients whose renal function had not recovered at the time of death, autopsies were performed; in 2 of these, evidence of tubular damage was noted. Eleven (11) patients (35%) experienced delayed onset neurologic toxicity. In the majority, this was characterized by progressive irreversible motor weakness (paraparesis/ quadriparesis) of the upper and/or lower extremities, first noted 35 to 84 days after starting high dose therapy with LEUSTATIN. Non-invasive testing (electromyography and nerve conduction studies) was consistent with demyelinating disease. Severe neurologic toxicity has also been noted with high doses of another drug in this class.

Axonal peripheral polyneuropathy was observed in a dose escalation study at the highest dose levels (approximately 4 times the recommended dose for Hairy Cell Leukemia) in patients not receiving cyclophosphamide or total body irradiation. Severe neurological toxicity has been reported rarely following treatment with standard cladribine dosing regimens.

In patients with Hairy Cell Leukemia treated with the recommended treatment regimen (0.09 mg/kg/day for 7 consecutive days), there have been no reports of nephrologic toxicities.

Of the 196 Hairy Cell Leukemia patients entered in the two trials, there were 8 deaths following treatment. Of these, 6 were of infectious etiology, including 3 pneumonias, and 2 occurred in the first month following LEUSTATIN therapy. Of the 8 deaths, 6 occurred in previously treated patients who were refractory to α-interferon.

Benzyl alcohol is a constituent of the recommended diluent for the 7-day infusion solution. Benzyl alcohol has been reported to be associated with a fatal "Gasping Syndrome" in premature infants (see DOSAGE AND ADMINISTRATION).

Pregnancy Category D: LEUSTATIN Injection should not be given during pregnancy.

Cladribine is teratogenic in mice and rabbits and consequently has the potential to cause fetal harm when administered to a pregnant woman. A significant increase in fetal variations was observed in mice receiving 1.5 mg/kg/day (4.5 mg/m^2) and increased resorptions, reduced litter size and increased fetal malformations were observed when mice received 3.0 mg/kg/day (9 mg/m^2). Fetal death and malformations were observed in rabbits that received 3.0 mg/kg/day (33.0 mg/m^2). No fetal effects were seen in mice at 0.5 mg/kg/day (1.5 mg/m^2) or in rabbits at 1.0 mg/kg/day (11.0 mg/m^2).

Although there is no evidence of teratogenicity in humans due to LEUSTATIN, other drugs which inhibit DNA synthesis (e.g., methotrexate and aminopterin) have been reported to be teratogenic in humans. LEUSTATIN has been shown to be embryotoxic in mice when given at doses equivalent to the recommended dose.

There are no adequate and well controlled studies in pregnant women. If LEUSTATIN is used during pregnancy, or if the patient becomes pregnant while taking this drug, the patient should be apprised of the potential hazard to the fetus. Women of childbearing age should be advised to avoid becoming pregnant.

PRECAUTIONS

General: LEUSTATIN Injection is a potent antineoplastic agent with potentially significant toxic side effects. It should be administered only under the supervision of a physician experienced with the use of cancer chemotherapeutic agents. Patients undergoing therapy should be closely observed for signs of hematologic and non-hematologic toxicity. Periodic assessment of peripheral blood counts, particularly during the first 4 to 8 weeks post-treatment, is recommended to detect the development of anemia, neutropenia and thrombocytopenia and for early detection of any potential sequelae (e.g., infection or bleeding). As with other potent chemotherapeutic agents, monitoring of renal and hepatic function is also recommended, especially in patients with underlying kidney or liver dysfunction (see WARNINGS and ADVERSE REACTIONS).

Fever was a frequently observed side effect during the first month on study. Since the majority of fevers occurred in neutropenic patients, patients should be closely monitored during the first month of treatment and empiric antibiotics should be initiated as clinically indicated. Although 69% of patients developed fevers, less than 1/3 of febrile events were associated with documented infection. Given the known myelosuppressive effects of LEUSTATIN, practitioners should carefully evaluate the risks and benefits of administering this drug to patients with active infections (see WARNINGS and ADVERSE REACTIONS).

There are inadequate data on dosing of patients with renal or hepatic insufficiency. Development of acute renal insufficiency in some patients receiving high doses of LEUSTATIN has been described. Until more information is available, caution is advised when administering the drug to patients with known or suspected renal or hepatic insufficiency (see WARNINGS).

Rare cases of tumor lysis syndrome have been reported in patients treated with cladribine with other hematologic malignancies having a high tumor burden.

LEUSTATIN Injection must be diluted in designated intravenous solutions prior to administration (see DOSAGE AND ADMINISTRATION).

Laboratory Tests: During and following treatment, the patient's hematologic profile should be monitored regularly to determine the degree of hematopoietic suppression. In the clinical studies, following reversible declines in all cell counts, the mean Platelet Count reached 100 × 10^9/L by Day 12, the mean Absolute Neutrophil Count reached 1500 × 10^6/L by Week 5 and the mean Hemoglobin reached 12 g/dL by Week 8. After peripheral counts have normalized, bone marrow aspiration and biopsy should be performed to confirm response to treatment with LEUSTATIN. Febrile events should be investigated with appropriate laboratory and radiologic studies. Periodic assessment of renal function and hepatic function should be performed as clinically indicated.

Drug Interactions: There are no known drug interactions with LEUSTATIN Injection. Caution should be exercised if LEUSTATIN Injection is administered before, after, or in conjunction with other drugs known to cause immunosuppression or myelosuppression (see WARNINGS).

Carcinogenesis: No animal carcinogenicity studies have been conducted with cladribine. However, its carcinogenic potential cannot be excluded based on demonstrated genotoxicity of cladribine.

Mutagenesis: As expected for compounds in this class, the actions of cladribine yield DNA damage. In mammalian cells in culture, cladribine caused the accumulation of DNA strand breaks. Cladribine was also incorporated into DNA of human lymphoblastic leukemia cells. Cladribine was not mutagenic *in vitro* (Ames and Chinese hamster ovary cell gene mutation tests) and did not induce unscheduled DNA synthesis in primary rat hepatocyte cultures. However, cladribine was clastogenic both *in vitro* (chromosome aberrations in Chinese hamster ovary cells) and *in vivo* (mouse bone marrow micronucleus test).

Impairment of Fertility: When administered intravenously to Cynomolgus monkeys, cladribine has been shown to cause suppression of rapidly generating cells, including testicular cells. The effect on human fertility is unknown.

Pregnancy: Pregnancy Category D: (see WARNINGS).

Nursing Mothers: It is not known whether this drug is excreted in human milk. Because many drugs are excreted in human milk and because of the potential for serious adverse reactions in nursing infants from cladribine, a decision should be made whether to discontinue nursing or discontinue the drug, taking into account the importance of the drug for the mother.

Pediatric Use: Safety and effectiveness in pediatric patients have not been established. In a Phase I study involving patients 1-21 years old with relapsed acute leukemia, LEUSTATIN was given by continuous intravenous infusion in doses ranging from 3 to 10.7 mg/m^2/day for 5 days (one-half to twice the dose recommended in Hairy Cell Leukemia). In this study, the dose-limiting toxicity was severe myelosuppression with profound neutropenia and thrombocytopenia. At the highest dose (10.7 mg/m^2/day), 3 of 7 patients developed irreversible myelosuppression and fatal systemic bacterial or fungal infections. No unique toxicities were noted in this study[1] (see WARNINGS and ADVERSE REACTIONS).

Geriatric Use: Clinical studies of LEUSTATIN did not include sufficient numbers of subjects aged 65 and over to determine whether they respond differently from younger subjects. Other reported clinical experience has not identified differences in responses between the elderly and younger patients. In general, dose selection for an elderly patient should be cautious, reflecting the greater frequency of decreased hepatic, renal, or cardiac function, and of concomitant disease or other drug therapy in elderly patients.

ADVERSE REACTIONS

Safety data are based on 196 patients with Hairy Cell Leukemia: the original cohort of 124 patients plus an additional 72 patients enrolled at the same two centers after the original enrollment cutoff. In Month 1 of the Hairy Cell Leukemia clinical trials, severe neutropenia was noted in 70% of patients, fever in 69%, and infection was documented in 28%. Other adverse experiences reported frequently during the first 14 days after initiating treatment included: fatigue (45%), nausea (28%), rash (27%), headache (22%) and injection site reactions (19%). Most non-hematologic adverse experiences were mild to moderate in severity.

Myelosuppression was frequently observed during the first month after starting treatment. Neutropenia (ANC < 500 × 10^6/L) was noted in 70% of patients, compared with 26% in whom it was present initially. Severe anemia (Hemoglobin < 8.5 g/dL) developed in 37% of patients, compared with 10% initially and thrombocytopenia (Platelets < 20 × 10^9/L) developed in 12% of patients, compared to 4% in whom it was noted initially.

During the first month, 54 of 196 patients (28%) exhibited documented evidence of infection. Serious infections (e.g., septicemia, pneumonia) were reported in 6% of all patients; the remainder were mild or moderate. Several deaths were attributable to infection and/or complications related to the underlying disease. During the second month, the overall rate of documented infection was 6%; these infections were mild to moderate and no severe systemic infections were seen. After the third month, the monthly incidence of infection was either less than or equal to that of the months immediately preceding LEUSTATIN therapy.

During the first month, 11% of patients experienced severe fever (i.e., ≥104°F). Documented infections were noted in fewer than one-third of febrile episodes. Of the 196 patients studied, 19 were noted to have a documented infection in the month prior to treatment. In the month following treatment, there were 54 episodes of documented infection: 23 (42%) were bacterial, 11 (20%) were viral and 11 (20%) were fungal. Seven (7) of 8 documented episodes of herpes zoster occurred during the month following treatment. Fourteen (14) of 16 episodes of documented fungal infections occurred in the first two months following treatment. Virtually all of these patients were treated empirically with antibiotics (see WARNINGS and PRECAUTIONS).

Analysis of lymphocyte subsets indicates that treatment with cladribine is associated with prolonged depression of the CD4 counts. Prior to treatment, the mean CD4 count was 766/µL. The mean CD4 count nadir, which occurred 4 to 6 months following treatment, was 272/µL. Fifteen (15) months after treatment, mean CD4 counts remained below 500/µL. CD8 counts behaved similarly, though increasing counts were observed after 9 months. The clinical significance of the prolonged CD4 lymphopenia is unclear.

Another event of unknown clinical significance includes the observation of prolonged bone marrow hypocellularity. Bone marrow cellularity of < 35% was noted after 4 months in 42 of 124 patients (34%) treated in the two pivotal trials. This hypocellularity was noted as late as day 1010. It is not known whether the hypocellularity is the result of disease related marrow fibrosis or if it is the result of cladribine toxicity. There was no apparent clinical effect on the peripheral blood counts.

The vast majority of rashes were mild and occurred in patients who were receiving or had recently been treated with other medications (e.g., allopurinol or antibiotics) known to cause rash.

Most episodes of nausea were mild, not accompanied by vomiting, and did not require treatment with antiemetics. In patients requiring antiemetics, nausea was easily controlled, most frequently with chlorpromazine.

Adverse reactions reported during the first 2 weeks following treatment initiation (regardless of relationship to drug) by > 5% of patients included:

Body as a Whole: fever (69%), fatigue (45%), chills (9%), asthenia (9%), diaphoresis (9%), malaise (7%), trunk pain (6%)

Gastrointestinal: nausea (28%), decreased appetite (17%), vomiting (13%), diarrhea (10%), constipation (9%), abdominal pain (6%)

Hemic / Lymphatic: purpura (10%), petechiae (8%), epistaxis (5%)

Nervous System: headache (22%), dizziness (9%), insomnia (7%)

Cardiovascular System: edema (6%), tachycardia (6%)

Respiratory System: abnormal breath sounds (11%), cough (10%), abnormal chest sounds (9%), shortness of breath (7%)

Skin / Subcutaneous Tissue: rash (27%), injection site reactions (19%), pruritis (6%), pain (6%), erythema (6%)

Musculoskeletal System: myalgia (7%), arthralgia (5%)

Adverse experiences related to intravenous administration included: injection site reactions (9%) (i.e., redness, swell-

Continued on next page

Leustatin—Cont.

ing, pain), thrombosis (2%), phlebitis (2%) and a broken catheter (1%). These appear to be related to the infusion procedure and/or indwelling catheter, rather than the medication or the vehicle.
From Day 15 to the last follow-up visit, the only events reported by > 5% of patients were: fatigue (11%), rash (10%), headache (7%), cough (7%), and malaise (5%).
For a description of adverse reactions associated with use of high doses in non-Hairy Cell Leukemia patients, see WARNINGS.
The following additional adverse events have been reported since the drug became commercially available. These adverse events have been reported primarily in patients who received multiple courses of LEUSTATIN Injection:
Hematologic: bone marrow suppression with prolonged pancytopenia, including some reports of aplastic anemia; hemolytic anemia, which was reported in patients with lymphoid malignancies, occurring within the first few weeks following treatment.
Hepatic: reversible, generally mild increases in bilirubin and transaminases.
Nervous System: Neurological toxicity; however, severe neurotoxicity has been reported rarely following treatment with standard cladribine dosing regimens.
Respiratory System: pulmonary interstitial infiltrates; in most cases, an infectious etiology was identified.
Skin/Subcutaneous: urticaria, hypereosinophilia. In isolated cases Stevens-Johnson and toxic epidermal necrolysis have been reported in patients who were receiving or had recently been treated with other medications (e.g., allopurinol or antibiotics) known to cause these syndromes.
Opportunistic infections have occurred in the acute phase of treatment due to the immunosuppression mediated by LEUSTATIN Injection.

OVERDOSAGE

High doses of LEUSTATIN have been associated with: irreversible neurologic toxicity (paraparesis/quadriparesis), acute nephrotoxicity, and severe bone marrow suppression resulting in neutropenia, anemia and thrombocytopenia (see WARNINGS). There is no known specific antidote to overdosage. Treatment of overdosage consists of discontinuation of LEUSTATIN, careful observation and appropriate supportive measures. It is not known whether the drug can be removed from the circulation by dialysis or hemofiltration.

DOSAGE AND ADMINISTRATION

Usual Dose:
The recommended dose and schedule of LEUSTATIN Injection for active Hairy Cell Leukemia is as a single course given by continuous infusion for 7 consecutive days at a dose of 0.09 mg/kg/day. Deviations from this dosage regimen are not advised. If the patient does not respond to the initial course of LEUSTATIN Injection for Hairy Cell Leukemia, it is unlikely that they will benefit from additional courses. Physicians should consider delaying or discontinuing the drug if neurotoxicity or renal toxicity occurs (see WARNINGS).
Specific risk factors predisposing to increased toxicity from LEUSTATIN have not been defined. In view of the known toxicities of agents of this class, it would be prudent to proceed carefully in patients with known or suspected renal insufficiency or severe bone marrow impairment of any etiology. Patients should be monitored closely for hematologic and non-hematologic toxicity (see WARNINGS and PRECAUTIONS).
Preparation and Administration of Intravenous Solutions:
LEUSTATIN Injection must be diluted with the designated diluent prior to administration. Since the drug product does not contain any anti-microbial preservative or bacteriostatic agent, **aseptic technique and proper environmental precautions must be observed in preparation of LEUSTATIN Injection solutions.**
To prepare a single daily dose: Add the calculated dose (0.09 mg/kg or 0.09 mL/kg) of LEUSTATIN Injection to an infusion bag containing 500 mL of 0.9% Sodium Chloride Injection, USP. Infuse continuously over 24 hours. Repeat daily for a total of 7 consecutive days. **The use of 5% dextrose as a diluent is not recommended because of increased degradation of cladribine.** Admixtures of LEUSTATIN Injection are chemically and physically stable for at least 24 hours at room temperature under normal room fluorescent light in Baxter Viaflex®† PVC infusion containers. **Since limited compatability data are available, adherence to the recommended diluents and infusion systems is advised.**

	Dose of LEUSTATIN Injection	Recommended Diluent	Quantity of Diluent
24-hour infusion method	1 (day) × 0.09 mg/kg	0.9% Sodium Chloride Injection, USP	500 mL

To prepare a 7-day infusion: The 7-day infusion solution should only be prepared with Bacteriostatic 0.9% Sodium Chloride Injection, USP (0.9% benzyl alcohol preserved). In order to minimize the risk of microbial contamination, both LEUSTATIN Injection and the diluent should be passed through a sterile 0.22μ disposable hydrophilic syringe filter as each solution is being introduced into the infusion reservoir. First add the calculated dose of LEUSTATIN Injection (7 days × 0.09 mg/kg or mL/kg) to the infusion reservoir through the sterile filter. Then add a calculated amount of Bacteriostatic 0.9% Sodium Chloride Injection, USP (0.9% benzyl alcohol preserved) also through the filter to bring the total volume of the solution to 100 mL. After completing solution preparation, clamp off the line, disconnect and discard the filter. Aseptically aspirate air bubbles from the reservoir as necessary using the syringe and a dry second sterile filter or a sterile vent filter assembly. Reclamp the line and discard the syringe and filter assembly. Infuse continuously over 7 days. Solutions prepared with Bacteriostatic Sodium Chloride Injection for individuals weighing more than 85 kg may have reduced preservative effectiveness due to greater dilution of the benzyl alcohol preservative. Admixtures for the 7-day infusion have demonstrated acceptable chemical and physical stability for at least 7 days in the SIMS Deltec MEDICATION CASSETTE™ Reservoir ‡.

	Dose of LEUSTATIN Injection	Recommended Diluent	Quantity of Diluent
7-day infusion method (use sterile 0.22μ filter when preparing infusion solution)	7 (days) × 0.09 mg/kg	Bacteriostatic 0.9% Sodium Chloride Injection, USP (0.9% benzyl alcohol)	q.s. to 100 mL

Since limited compatibility data are available, adherence to the recommended diluents and infusion systems is advised. Solutions containing LEUSTATIN Injection should not be mixed with other intravenous drugs or additives or infused simultaneously via a common intravenous line, since compatibility testing has not been performed. Preparations containing benzyl alcohol should not be used in neonates (see WARNINGS).
Care must be taken to assure the sterility of prepared solutions. Once diluted, solutions of LEUSTATIN Injection should be administered promptly or stored in the refrigerator (2° to 8°C) for no more than 8 hours prior to start of administration. Vials of LEUSTATIN Injection are for single-use only. Any unused portion should be discarded in an appropriate manner (see Handling and Disposal).
Parenteral drug products should be inspected visually for particulate matter and discoloration prior to administration, whenever solution and container permit. A precipitate may occur dur ing the exposure of LEUSTATIN Injection to low temperatures; it may be resolubilized by allowing the solution to warm naturally to room temperature and by shaking vigorously. **DO NOT HEAT OR MICROWAVE.**
Chemical Stability of Vials:
When stored in refrigerated conditions between 2° to 8°C (36° to 46°F) protected from light, unopened vials of LEUSTATIN Injection are stable until the expiration date indicated on the package. Freezing does not adversely affect the solution. If freezing occurs, thaw naturally to room temperature. DO NOT heat or microwave. Once thawed, the vial of LEUSTATIN Injection is stable until expiry if refrigerated. DO NOT refreeze. Once diluted, solutions containing LEUSTATIN Injection should be administered promptly or stored in the refrigerator (2° to 8°C) for no more than 8 hours prior to administration.
Handling and Disposal:
The potential hazards associated with cytotoxic agents are well established and proper precautions should be taken when handling, preparing, and administering LEUSTATIN Injection. The use of disposable gloves and protective garments is recommended. If LEUSTATIN Injection contacts the skin or mucous membranes, wash the involved surface immediately with copious amounts of water. Several guidelines on this subject have been published.[2–8] There is no general agreement that all of the procedures recommended in the guidelines are necessary or appropriate. Refer to your Institution's guidelines and all applicable state/local regulations for disposal of cytotoxic waste.

HOW SUPPLIED

LEUSTATIN Injection is supplied as a sterile, preservative-free, isotonic solution containing 10mg (1mg/mL) of cladribine as 10 mL filled into a single-use clear flint glass 20 mL vial. LEUSTATIN Injection is supplied in 10 mL (1 mg/mL) single-use vials (NDC 59676-201-01) available in a treatment set (case) of seven vials.
Store refrigerated 2° to 8°C (36° to 46°F). Protect from light during storage.

References:

1. Santana VM, Mirro J, Harwood FC, et al: A phase I clinical trial of 2-Chloro-deoxyadenosine in pediatric patients with acute leukemia. *J. Clin. Onc.*, **9**: 416 (1991).
2. Recommendations for the Safe Handling of Parenteral Antineoplastic Drugs. NIH Publication No. 83-2621. For sale by the Superintendent of Documents, U. S. Government Printing Office, Washington, D. C. 20402.
3. AMA Council Report. Guidelines for Handling Parenteral Antineoplastics, *JAMA*, March 15 (1985).
4. National Study Commission on Cytotoxic Exposure–Recommendations for Handling Cytotoxic Agents. Available from Louis P. Jeffrey, Sc.D., Chairman, National Study Commission on Cytotoxic Exposure, Massachusetts College of Pharmacy and Allied Health Sciences, 179 Longwood Avenue, Boston, Massachusetts 02115.
5. Clinical Oncological Society of Australia: Guidelines and Recommendations for Safe Handling of Antineoplastic Agents, *Med. J. Australia* **1**:425 (1983).
6. Jones RB, et al. Safe Handling of Chemotherapeutic Agents: A Report from the Mount Sinai Medical Center. Ca—*A Cancer Journal for Clinicians*, Sept/Oct. 258-263 (1983).
7. American Society of Hospital Pharmacists Technical Assistance Bulletin on Handling Cytotoxic Drugs in Hospitals. *Am. J. Hosp. Pharm.*, **42**:131 (1985).
8. OSHA Work-Practice Guidelines for Personnel Dealing with Cytotoxic (antineoplastic) Drugs. *Am. J. Hosp. Pharm.*, **43**:1193 (1986).

CAUTION: Rx ONLY

† Viaflex® containers, manufactured by Baxter Healthcare Corporation—Code No. 2B8013 (tested in 1991)
‡ MEDICATION CASSETTE™ Reservoir, manufactured by SIMS Deltec, Inc.—Reorder No. 602100A (tested in 1991)

ORTHO BIOTECH PRODUCTS, L.P.
Raritan, New Jersey 08869
ORTHO BIOTECH
©OBPLP 2000 Printed in U.S.A. G38-10-940-9
Revised May 2003

ORTHOCLONE OKT®3 STERILE SOLUTION ℞
(muromonab-CD3)
For Intravenous Use Only

WARNING:
Only physicians experienced in immunosuppressive therapy and management of solid organ transplant patients should use ORTHOCLONE OKT3 (muromonab-CD3). Patients treated with ORTHOCLONE OKT3 must be managed in a facility equipped and staffed for cardiopulmonary resuscitation and where the patient can be closely monitored for an appropriate period based on his or her health status.
Anaphylactic and anaphylactoid reactions may occur following administration of any dose or course of ORTHOCLONE OKT3. In addition, serious, occasionally life-threatening or lethal, systemic, cardiovascular, and central nervous system reactions have been reported following administration of ORTHOCLONE OKT3. These have included: pulmonary edema, especially in patients with volume overload; shock, cardiovascular collapse, cardiac or respiratory arrest, seizures, coma, cerebral edema, cerebral herniation, blindness, and paralysis. Fluid status should be carefully monitored prior to and during ORTHOCLONE OKT3 administration. Pretreatment with methylprednisolone is recommended to minimize symptoms of Cytokine Release Syndrome. (See: WARNINGS: Cytokine Release Syndrome, Central Nervous System Events, Anaphylactic Reactions; DOSAGE AND ADMINISTRATION.)

DESCRIPTION

ORTHOCLONE OKT3 (muromonab-CD3) Sterile Solution is a murine monoclonal antibody to the CD3 antigen of human T cells which functions as an immunosuppressant. It is for intravenous use only. The antibody is a biochemically purified IgG_{2a} immunoglobulin with a heavy chain of approximately 50,000 daltons and a light chain of approximately 25,000 daltons. It is directed to a glycoprotein with a molecular weight of 20,000 in the human T cell surface which is essential for T cell functions. Because it is a monoclonal antibody preparation, ORTHOCLONE OKT3 Sterile Solution is a homogeneous, reproducible antibody product with consistent, measurable reactivity to human T cells.
Each 5 mL ampule of ORTHOCLONE OKT3 Sterile Solution contains 5 mg (1 mg/mL) of muromonab-CD3 in a clear colorless solution which may contain a few fine translucent protein particles. Each ampule contains a buffered solution (pH 7.0 ± 0.5) of monobasic sodium phosphate (2.25 mg), dibasic sodium phosphate (9.0 mg), sodium chloride (43 mg), and polysorbate 80 (1.0 mg) in water for injection.
The proper name, muromonab-CD3, is derived from the descriptive term murine monoclonal antibody. The CD3 designation identifies the specificity of the antibody as the Cell Differentiation (CD) cluster 3 defined by the First International Workshop on Human Leukocyte Differentiation Antigens.

CLINICAL PHARMACOLOGY

ORTHOCLONE OKT3 reverses graft rejection, probably by blocking the function of T cells which play a major role in acute allograft rejection. ORTHOCLONE OKT3 reacts with and blocks the function of a 20,000 dalton molecule (CD3) in the membrane of human T cells that has been associated *in vitro* with the antigen recognition structure of T cells and is essential for signal transduction. In *in vitro* cytolytic assays, ORTHOCLONE OKT3 blocks both the generation and function of effector cells. Binding of ORTHOCLONE OKT3 to T lymphocytes results in early activation of T cells, which leads to cytokine release, followed by blocking T cell functions. After termination of ORTHOCLONE OKT3 therapy, T cell function usually returns to normal within one week. *In vivo*, ORTHOCLONE OKT3 reacts with most peripheral blood T cells and T cells in body tissues, but has not been found to react with other hematopoietic elements or other tissues of the body.

A rapid and concomitant decrease in the number of circulating CD3 positive cells, including those that are CD2, CD4, or CD8 positive has been observed in patients studied within minutes after the administration of ORTHOCLONE OKT3. This decrease in the number of CD3 positive T cells results from the specific interaction between ORTHOCLONE OKT3 and the CD3 antigen on the surface of all T lymphocytes. T cell activation results in the release of numerous cytokines/lymphokines, which are felt to be responsible for many of the acute clinical manifestations seen following ORTHOCLONE OKT3 administration. (See: WARNINGS: Cytokine Release Syndrome, Central Nervous System Events.)

While CD3 positive cells are not detectable between days two and seven, increasing numbers of circulating CD2, CD4, and CD8 positive cells have been observed. The presence of these CD2, CD4, and CD8 positive cells has not been shown to affect reversal of rejection. After termination of ORTHOCLONE OKT3 therapy, CD3 positive cells reappear rapidly and reach pre-treatment levels within a week. In some patients however, increasing numbers of CD3 positive cells have been observed prior to termination of ORTHOCLONE OKT3 therapy. This reappearance of CD3 positive cells has been attributed to the development of neutralizing antibodies to ORTHOCLONE OKT3, which in turn block its ability to bind to the CD3 antigen on T lymphocytes. (See: PRECAUTIONS: Sensitization.)

Pediatric patients are known to have higher CD3 lymphocyte counts than adults. Pediatric patients receiving ORTHOCLONE OKT®3 therapy often require progressively higher doses of ORTHOCLONE OKT3 to achieve depletion of CD3 positive cells (<25 cells/mm^3) and ensure therapeutic ORTHOCLONE OKT3 serum concentrations (>800 ng/mL). (See: DOSAGE AND ADMINISTRATION; PRECAUTIONS: Laboratory Tests.)

Serum levels of ORTHOCLONE OKT3 are measurable using an enzyme-linked immunosorbent assay (ELISA). During the initial clinical trials in renal allograft rejection, in patients treated with 5 mg per day for 14 days, mean serum trough levels of the drug rose over the first three days and then averaged 900 ng/mL on days 3 to 14. Serum concentrations measured daily during treatment with ORTHOCLONE OKT3 in renal, hepatic, and cardiac allograft recipients revealed that pediatric patients less than 10 years of age have higher levels than patients 10-50 years of age. Subsequent clinical experience has demonstrated that serum levels greater than or equal to 800 ng/mL of ORTHOCLONE OKT3 blocks the function of cytotoxic T cells *in vitro* and *in vivo*. Reduced T cell clearance or low plasma ORTHOCLONE OKT3 levels provide a basis for adjusting ORTHOCLONE OKT3 dosage or for discontinuing therapy. (See: WARNINGS: Anaphylactic Reactions; PRECAUTIONS: Laboratory Tests; ADVERSE EVENTS: Hypersensitivity Reactions; DOSAGE AND ADMINISTRATION.)

Following administration of ORTHOCLONE OKT3 *in vivo*, leukocytes have been observed in cerebrospinal and peritoneal fluids. The mechanism for this effect is not completely understood, but probably is related to cytokines altering membrane permeability, rather than an active inflammatory process. (See: WARNINGS: Cytokine Release Syndrome, Central Nervous System Events.)

CLINICAL STUDIES

Acute Renal Rejection:

In a controlled randomized clinical trial, ORTHOCLONE OKT3 was compared with conventional high-dose steroid therapy in reversing acute renal allograft rejection. In this trial, 122 evaluable patients undergoing acute rejection of cadaveric renal transplants were treated either with ORTHOCLONE OKT3 daily for a mean of 14 days, with concomitant lowering of the dosage of azathioprine and maintenance steroids (62 patients), or with conventional high-dose steroids (60 patients). ORTHOCLONE OKT3 reversed 94% of the rejections compared to a 75% reversal rate obtained with conventional high-dose steroid treatment (p=0.006). The one year Kaplan-Meier (actuarial) estimates of graft survival rates for these patients who had acute rejection were 62% and 45% for ORTHOCLONE OKT3 and steroid-treated patients, respectively (p=0.04). At two years the rates were 56% and 42%, respectively (p=0.06).

One- and two-year patient survivals were not significantly different between the two groups, being 85% and 75% for ORTHOCLONE OKT3 treated patients and 90% and 85% for steroid-treated patients.

In additional open clinical trials, the observed rate of reversal of acute renal allograft rejection was 92% (n=126) for ORTHOCLONE OKT3 therapy. ORTHOCLONE OKT3 was also effective in reversing acute renal allograft rejections in 65% (n=225) of cases where steroids and lymphocyte immune globulin preparations were contraindicated or were not successful.

The effectiveness of ORTHOCLONE OKT3 for prophylaxis of renal allograft rejection has not been established.

Acute Cardiac or Hepatic Allograft Rejection:

ORTHOCLONE OKT3 was studied for use in reversing acute cardiac and hepatic allograft rejection in patients who are unresponsive to high-doses of steroids. The rate of reversal in acute cardiac allograft rejection was 90% (n=61) and was 83% for hepatic allograft rejection (n=124) in patients unresponsive to treatment with steroids.

Controlled randomized trials have not been conducted to evaluate the effectiveness of ORTHOCLONE OKT3 compared to conventional therapy as first line treatment for acute cardiac and hepatic allograft rejection.

INDICATIONS AND USAGE

ORTHOCLONE OKT3 is indicated for the treatment of acute allograft rejection in renal transplant patients.

ORTHOCLONE OKT3 is indicated for the treatment of steroid-resistant acute allograft rejection in cardiac and hepatic transplant patients.

The dosage of other immunosuppressive agents used in conjunction with ORTHOCLONE OKT3 should be reduced to the lowest level compatible with an effective therapeutic response. (See: WARNINGS and ADVERSE EVENTS: Infections, Neoplasia; DOSAGE AND ADMINISTRATION.)

CONTRAINDICATIONS

ORTHOCLONE OKT3 should not be given to patients who:

- are hypersensitive to this or any other product of murine origin;
- have anti-mouse antibody titers ≥1:1000;
- are in (uncompensated) heart failure or in fluid overload, as evidenced by chest X-ray or a greater than 3 percent weight gain within the week prior to planned ORTHOCLONE OKT3 administration;
- have uncontrolled hypertension;
- have a history of seizures, or are predisposed to seizures;
- are determined or suspected to be pregnant, or who are breast-feeding. (See: PRECAUTIONS: Pregnancy, Nursing Mothers.)

WARNINGS

SEE BOXED WARNING

Cytokine Release Syndrome

Most patients develop an acute clinical syndrome [i.e., Cytokine Release Syndrome (CRS)] that has been attributed to the release of cytokines by activated lymphocytes or monocytes and is temporally associated with the administration of the first few doses of ORTHOCLONE OKT®3 (particularly, the first two to three doses). This clinical syndrome has ranged from a more frequently reported mild, self-limited, "flu-like" illness to a less frequently reported severe, life-threatening shock-like reaction, which may include serious cardiovascular and central nervous system manifestations. The syndrome typically begins approximately 30 to 60 minutes after administration of a dose of ORTHOCLONE OKT3 (but may occur later) and may persist for several hours. The frequency and severity of this symptom complex is usually greatest with the first dose. With each successive dose of ORTHOCLONE OKT3, both the frequency and severity of the Cytokine Release Syndrome tends to diminish. Increasing the amount of ORTHOCLONE OKT3 or resuming treatment after a hiatus may result in a reappearance of the CRS.

Common clinical manifestations of CRS may include: high fever (often spiking, up to 107°F), chills/rigors, headache, tremor, nausea/vomiting, diarrhea, abdominal pain, malaise, muscle/joint aches and pains, and generalized weakness. Less frequently reported adverse experiences include: minor dermatologic reactions (e.g., rash, pruritus, etc.) and a spectrum of often serious, occasionally fatal, cardiorespiratory and central nervous system adverse experiences.

Cardiorespiratory findings may include: dyspnea, shortness of breath, bronchospasm/wheezing, tachypnea, respiratory arrest/failure/distress, cardiovascular collapse, cardiac arrest, angina/myocardial infarction, chest pain/tightness, tachycardia (including ventricular), hypertension, hemodynamic instability, hypotension including profound shock, heart failure, pulmonary edema (cardiogenic and non-cardiogenic), adult respiratory distress syndrome, hypoxemia, apnea, and arrhythmias. (See: BOXED WARNING; PRECAUTIONS; ADVERSE EVENTS.)

In the initial studies of renal allograft rejection, potentially fatal, severe pulmonary edema occurred in 5% of the initial 107 patients. Fluid overload was present before treatment in all of these cases. It occurred in none of the subsequent 311 patients treated with first-dose volume/weight restrictions. In subsequent trials and in post-marketing experience, severe pulmonary edema has occurred in patients who appeared to be euvolemic. The pathogenesis of pulmonary edema may involve all or some of the following: volume overload; increased pulmonary vascular permeability; and/or reduced left ventricular compliance/contractility.

During the first 1 to 3 days of ORTHOCLONE OKT3 therapy, some patients have experienced an acute and transient decline in the glomerular filtration rate (GFR) and diminished urine output with a resulting increase in the level of serum creatinine. Massive release of cytokines appears to lead to reversible renal functional impairment and/or delayed renal allograft function. Similarly, transient elevations in hepatic transaminases have been reported following administration of the first few doses of ORTHOCLONE OKT3.

Patients at risk for more serious complications of CRS may include those with the following conditions: unstable angina; recent myocardial infarction or symptomatic ischemic heart disease; heart failure of any etiology; pulmonary edema of any etiology; any form of chronic obstructive pulmonary disease; intravascular volume overload or depletion of any etiology (e.g., excessive dialysis, recent intensive diuresis, blood loss, etc.); cerebrovascular disease; patients with advanced symptomatic vascular disease or neuropathy; a history of seizures; and septic shock. Efforts should be made to correct or stabilize background conditions prior to the initiation of therapy. (See: PRECAUTIONS.)

Prior to administration of ORTHOCLONE OKT3, the patient's volume (fluid) status and a chest X-ray should be assessed to rule out volume overload, uncontrolled hypertension, or uncompensated heart failure. Patients should not weigh >3% above their minimum weight during the week prior to injection.

The Cytokine Release Syndrome is associated with increased serum levels of cytokines (e.g., TNF-α, IL-2, IL-6, IFN-γ) that peak between 1 and 4 hours following administration of ORTHOCLONE OKT3. The serum levels of cytokines and the manifestations of CRS may be reduced by pretreatment with 8 mg/kg of methylprednisolone (i.e., high-dose steroids), given 1 to 4 hours prior to administration of the first dose of ORTHOCLONE OKT3, and by closely following recommendations for dosage and treatment duration. (See: DOSAGE AND ADMINISTRATION.) It is not known if corticosteroid pretreatment decreases organ damage and sequelae associated with CRS. For example, increased intracranial pressure and cerebral herniation have occurred despite pretreatment with currently recommended doses and schedules of methyprednisolone.

If any of the more serious presentations of the Cytokine Release Syndrome occur, intensive treatment including oxygen, intravenous fluids, corticosteroids, pressor amines, antihistamines, intubation, etc., may be required.

Central Nervous System Events

Seizures, encephalopathy, cerebral edema, aseptic meningitis, and headache have been reported, even following the first dose, during therapy with ORTHOCLONE OKT®3. Seizures, some accompanied by loss of consciousness or cardiorespiratory arrest, or death, have occurred independently or in conjunction with any of the neurologic syndromes described below.

A few cases of fatal cerebral herniations subsequent to cerebral edema have been reported. All patients, particularly pediatric patients, must be carefully evaluated for fluid retention and hypertension before the initiation of ORTHOCLONE OKT3 therapy. Close monitoring for neurologic symptoms must be performed during the first twenty-four (24) hours following each of the first few doses of ORTHOCLONE OKT3 injection.

Patients should be closely monitored for convulsions and manifestations of encephalopathy, including: impaired cognition, confusion, obtundation, altered mental status, disorientation, auditory/visual hallucinations, psychosis (delirium, paranoia), mood changes (e.g., mania, agitation, combativeness, etc.), diffuse hypotonus, hyperreflexia, myoclonus, tremor, asterixis, involuntary movements, major motor seizures, lethargy/stupor/coma, and diffuse weakness. Approximately one-third of patients with a diagnosis of encephalopathy may have had coexisting aseptic meningitis syndrome.

Signs and symptoms of the aseptic meningitis syndrome described in association with the use of ORTHOCLONE OKT3 have included: fever, headache, meningismus (stiff neck), and photophobia. Diagnosis is confirmed by cerebrospinal fluid (CSF) analysis demonstrating leukocytosis with pleocytosis, elevated protein and normal or decreased glucose, with negative viral, bacterial, and fungal cultures. The possibility of infection should be evaluated in any immunosuppressed transplant patient with clinical findings suggesting meningitis. Approximately one-third of the patients with a diagnosis of aseptic meningitis had coexisting signs and symptoms of encephalopathy. Most patients with the aseptic meningitis syndrome had a benign course and recovered without any permanent sequelae during therapy or subsequent to its completion or discontinuation. However, because meningitis is a frequent infection encountered in pediatric allograft recipients, and the immunosuppression associated with transplantation increases the risk of opportunistic infection, pediatric patients with signs or symptoms suggestive of meningeal irritation while receiving ORTHOCLONE OKT3 should have lumbar punctures performed to rule out an infectious etiology. (See: PRECAUTIONS: Pediatric Use.)

Signs or symptoms of encephalopathy, meningitis, seizures, and cerebral edema, with or without headache, typically have been reversible. Headache, aseptic meningitis, seizures, and less severe forms of encephalopathy resolved in most patients despite continued treatment with ORTHOCLONE OKT3. However, some events resulted in permanent neurologic impairment.

The following additional central nervous system events have each been reported: irreversible blindness, impaired vision, quadri- or paraparesis/plegia, cerebrovascular accident (hemiparesis/plegia), aphasia, transient ischemic attack, subarachnoid hemorrhage, palsy of the VI cranial nerve, hearing decrease, and deafness.

Patients who may be at greater risk for CNS adverse experiences include those: with known or suspected CNS disorders (e.g., history of seizure disorder, etc.); with cerebrovascular disease (small or large vessel); with conditions having associated neurologic problems (e.g., head trauma, uremia,

Continued on next page

Orthoclone OKT3—Cont.

infection, fluid and electrolyte disturbance, etc.); with underlying vascular diseases; or who are receiving a medication concomitantly that may, by itself, affect the central nervous system. (See: WARNINGS, PRECAUTIONS and ADVERSE EVENTS: Cytokine Release Syndrome.)

Anaphylactic Reactions

Serious and occasionally fatal, immediate (usually within 10 minutes) hypersensitivity (anaphylactic) reactions have been reported in patients treated with ORTHOCLONE OKT3. **Manifestations of anaphylaxis may appear similar to manifestations of the Cytokine Release Syndrome (described above). It may be impossible to determine the mechanism responsible for any systemic reaction(s).** Reactions attributed to hypersensitivity have been reported less frequently than those attributed to cytokine release. Acute hypersensitivity reactions may be characterized by: cardiovascular collapse, cardiorespiratory arrest, loss of consciousness, hypotension/shock, tachycardia, tingling, angioedema (including laryngeal, pharyngeal, or facial edema), airway obstruction, bronchospasm, dyspnea, urticaria, and pruritus.

Serious allergic events, including anaphylactic or anaphylactoid reactions, have been reported in patients re-exposed to ORTHOCLONE OKT3 subsequent to their initial course of therapy. Pretreatment with antihistamines and/or steroids may not reliably prevent anaphylaxis in this setting. Possible allergic hazards of retreatment should be weighed against expected therapeutic benefits and alternatives. If a patient is retreated with ORTHOCLONE OKT3, it is particularly important that epinephrine and other emergency life-support equipment should be immediately available.

If hypersensitivity is suspected, discontinue the drug immediately; do not resume therapy or re-expose the patient to ORTHOCLONE OKT3. Serious acute hypersensitivity reactions may require emergency treatment with 0.3 mL to 0.5 mL aqueous epinephrine (1:1000 dilution) subcutaneously and other resuscitative measures including oxygen, intravenous fluids, antihistamines, corticosteroids, pressor amines, and airway management, as clinically indicated. (See: PRECAUTIONS: Cytokine Release Syndrome vs. Anaphylactic Reactions; ADVERSE EVENTS: Hypersensitivity Reactions.)

Consequences of Immunosuppression

Serious and sometimes fatal infections and neoplasias have been reported in association with all immunosuppressive therapies, including those regimens containing ORTHOCLONE OKT®3.

Infections: ORTHOCLONE OKT3 is usually added to immunosuppressive therapeutic regimens, thereby augmenting the degree of immunosuppression. This increase in the total amount of immunosuppression may alter the spectrum of infections observed and increase the risk, the severity, and the morbidity of infectious complications. During the first month post-transplant, patients are at greatest risk for the following infections: (1) those present prior to transplant, perhaps exacerbated by post-transplant immunosuppression; (2) infection conveyed by the donor organ; and (3) the usual post-operative urinary tract, intravenous line related, wound, or pulmonary infections due to bacterial pathogens. (See: ADVERSE EVENTS: Infections.)

Approximately one to six months post-transplant, patients are at risk for viral infections [e.g., cytomegalovirus (CMV), Epstein-Barr virus (EBV), herpes simplex virus (HSV), etc.] which produce serious systemic disease and which also increase the overall state of immunosuppression.

Reactivation (1 to 4 months post-transplant) of EBV and CMV has been reported. When administration of an anti-lymphocyte antibody, including ORTHOCLONE OKT3, is followed by an immunosuppressive regimen including cyclosporine, there is an increased risk of reactivating CMV and impaired ability to limit its proliferation, resulting in symptomatic and disseminated disease. EBV infection, either primary or reactivated, may play an important role in the development of post-transplant lymphoproliferative disorders. (See: WARNINGS and ADVERSE EVENTS: Neoplasia.)

In the pediatric transplant population, viral infections often include pathogens uncommon in adults, such as varicella zoster virus (VZV), adenovirus, and respiratory syncytial virus (RSV). A large proportion of pediatric patients have not been infected with the herpes viruses prior to transplantation and, therefore, are susceptible to developing primary infections from the grafted organ and/or blood products.

Anti-infective prophylaxis may reduce the morbidity associated with certain potential pathogens and should be considered for pediatric and other high-risk patients. Judicious use of immunosuppressive drugs, including type, dosage, and duration, may limit the risk and seriousness of some opportunistic infections. It is also possible to reduce the risk of serious CMV or EBV infection by avoiding transplantation of a CMV-seropositive (donor) and/or EBV-seropositive (donor) organ into a seronegative patient.

Neoplasia: As a result of depressed cell-mediated immunity from immunosuppressive agents, organ transplant patients have an increased risk of developing malignancies. This risk is evidenced almost exclusively by the occurrence of lymphoproliferative disorders, squamous cell carcinomas of the skin and lip, and sarcomas. In immunosuppressed patients, T cell cytotoxicity is impaired allowing for transformation and proliferation of EBV-infected B lymphocytes. Transformed B lymphocytes are thought to initiate oncogenesis, which ultimately culminates in the development of most post-transplant lymphoproliferative disorders. Patients, especially pediatric patients, with primary EBV infection may be at a higher risk for the development of EBV-associated lymphoproliferative disorders. Data support an association between the development of lymphoproliferative disorders at the time of active EBV infection and ORTHOCLONE OKT3 administration in pediatric liver allograft recipients. (See: ADVERSE EVENTS Infections, Neoplasia.)

Following the initiation of ORTHOCLONE OKT3 therapy, patients should be continuously monitored for evidence of lymphoproliferative disorders through physical examination and histological evaluation of any suspect lymphoid tissue. Close surveillance is advised, since early detection with subsequent reduction of total immunosuppression may result in regression of some of these lymphoproliferative disorders. Since the potential for the development of lymphoproliferative disorders is related to the duration and extent (intensity) of total immunosuppression, physicians are advised: to adhere to the recommended dosage and duration of ORTHOCLONE OKT3 therapy; to limit the number of courses of ORTHOCLONE OKT3 and other anti- T lymphocyte antibody preparations administered within a short period of time; and, if appropriate, to reduce the dosage(s) of immunosuppressive drugs used concomitantly to the lowest level compatible with an effective therapeutic response. (See: DOSAGE AND ADMINISTRATION.)

A recent study examined the incidence of non-Hodgkin's lymphoma (NHL) among 45,000 kidney transplant recipients and over 7,500 heart transplant recipients. This study suggested that all transplant patients, regardless of the immunosuppressive regimen employed, are at increased risk of NHL over the general population. The relative risk was highest among those receiving the most aggressive regimens.

The long-term risk of neoplastic events in patients being treated with ORTHOCLONE OKT3 has not been determined.

PRECAUTIONS

General

When using combinations of immunosuppressive agents, the dose of each agent, including ORTHOCLONE OKT®3, should be reduced to the lowest level compatible with an effective therapeutic response so as to reduce the potential for and severity of infections and malignant transformations.

Fever: If the temperature of the patient exceeds 37.8°C (100°F), it should be lowered by antipyretics before administration of each dose of ORTHOCLONE OKT3. The possibility of infection should be evaluated.

Severe Cytokine Release Syndrome Versus Anaphylactic Reactions: **It may not be possible to distinguish between an acute hypersensitivity reaction (e.g., anaphylaxis, angioedema, etc.) and the Cytokine Release Syndrome. Potentially serious signs and symptoms having an immediate onset (usually within 10 minutes) following administration of ORTHOCLONE OKT3 are probably due to acute hypersensitivity. If hypersensitivity is suspected, discontinue the drug immediately; do not resume therapy or re-expose the patient to ORTHOCLONE OKT3.** Clinical manifestations beginning approximately 30 to 60 minutes (or later) following administration of ORTHOCLONE OKT3 are more likely cytokine-mediated. (See: WARNINGS: Cytokine Release Syndrome Anaphylactic Reactions.)

Central Nervous System Events: Since some seizures (and other serious central nervous system events) following ORTHOCLONE OKT3 administration have been life-threatening, anti-seizure precautions (e.g., an airway ready for use, if needed) should be taken. (See: WARNINGS and ADVERSE EVENTS: Central Nervous System Events.)

Infection / Viral-Induced Lymphoproliferative Disorders: If infection or a viral induced lymphoproliferative disorder occurs, culture or biopsy as soon as possible, promptly institute appropriate anti-infective therapy, and (if possible) reduce/discontinue immunosuppressive therapy. (See: WARNINGS, ADVERSE EVENTS.)

Low Protein-Binding Filter: Use a low protein-binding 0.2 or 0.22 micrometer (μm) filter to prepare the injections. (See: ADMINISTRATION INSTRUCTIONS.)

Sensitization: ORTHOCLONE OKT3 is a mouse (immunoglobulin) protein that can induce human anti-mouse antibody production (i.e., sensitization) in some patients following exposure; a titer ≥1:1000 is a contraindication for use. (See: WARNINGS, ADVERSE EVENTS.)

In the initial clinical trials using low doses of prednisone and azathioprine during ORTHOCLONE OKT3 therapy for renal allograft rejection, antibodies to ORTHOCLONE OKT3 were observed with an incidence of 21% (n=43) for IgM, 86% (n=43) for IgG and 29% (n=35) for IgE. The mean time of appearance of IgG antibodies was 20 ± 2 days (mean ± SD). Early IgG antibodies appeared towards the end of the second week of treatment in 3% (n=86) of the patients.

Subsequent clinical experience has shown that the dose, duration, and type of immunosuppressive medications used in combination with ORTHOCLONE OKT3 may affect both the incidence and magnitude of the host antibody response. Furthermore, immunosuppressive agents used concomitantly with ORTHOCLONE OKT3 (i.e., steroids, azathioprine, prednisone, or cyclosporine) have altered the time course of anti-mouse antibody development and the specificity of the antibodies formed (i.e., idiotypic, isotypic, allotypic).

Thrombosis: As with other immunosuppressive therapies, arterial, venous, and capillary thromboses of allografts and other vascular beds (e.g., heart, lungs, brain, bowel, etc.) have been reported in patients treated with ORTHOCLONE OKT3. In addition, microangiopathic changes (e.g., platelet microthrombi) in the renal allograft associated in some patients with microangiopathic hemolytic anemia have been reported. This was observed in 5 of 93 (5%) patients receiving doses above the recommended dose. The relationship to dose remains uncertain; however, the relative risk appears to be greater with doses above the recommended dose. Patients with a history of thrombosis or underlying vascular disease should be given ORTHOCLONE OKT3 only when the potential benefits clearly outweigh the increased risks of therapy.

Information for Patients:

Patients should be advised:

- of the signs and symptoms associated with the Cytokine Release Syndrome and the potentially serious nature of this syndrome (e.g., systemic, cardiovascular, central nervous system events).
- to seek medical attention for skin rash, urticaria, rapid heart beat, respiratory distress, dysphagia, or any swelling suggesting an allergic reaction or angioedema.
- that ORTHOCLONE OKT3 may impair mental alertness and coordination and may effect the ability to operate an automobile or machinery.
- of other risks associated with the use of ORTHOCLONE OKT3. (See: BOXED WARNING; WARNINGS; PRECAUTIONS; ADVERSE EVENTS.)

Laboratory Tests: The following tests should be monitored prior to and during ORTHOCLONE OKT®3 therapy:

- Renal: BUN, serum creatinine, etc.;
- Hepatic: transaminases, alkaline phosphatase, bilirubin;
- Hematopoietic: WBCs and differential, platelet count, etc.;
- Chest X-ray within 24 hours before initiating ORTHOCLONE OKT3 treatment to rule out heart failure or fluid overload.
- Blood Tests: Periodic assessment of organ system functions (renal, hepatic, and hematopoietic) should be performed.

During therapy with ORTHOCLONE OKT3: In adults, periodic monitoring to ensure plasma ORTHOCLONE OKT3 levels (≥800 ng/mL) or T cell clearance (CD3 positive T cells <25 cells/mm^3) is recommended. In pediatric patients, <u>both</u> plasma ORTHOCLONE OKT3 levels (≥800 ng/mL) <u>and</u> T cell clearance (CD3 positive T cells <25 cells/mm^3) should be monitored daily. (See: CLINICAL PHARMACOLOGY.)

Carcinogenesis: Long-term studies have not been performed in laboratory animals to evaluate the carcinogenic potential of ORTHOCLONE OKT3; however, neoplasia has been reported in patients receiving this product. (See: WARNINGS and ADVERSE EVENTS: Neoplasia.)

Pregnancy Category C: Animal reproductive studies have not been conducted with ORTHOCLONE OKT3. It is also not known whether ORTHOCLONE OKT3 can cause fetal harm when administered to a pregnant woman or can affect reproduction capacity. However, ORTHOCLONE OKT3 is an IgG antibody and may cross the human placenta. The effect on the fetus of the release of cytokines and/or immunosuppression after treatment with ORTHOCLONE OKT3 is not known. ORTHOCLONE OKT3 should be given to a pregnant woman only if clearly needed. If this drug is used during pregnancy, or the patient becomes pregnant while taking this drug, the patient should be apprised of the potential hazard to the fetus. (See: CONTRAINDICATIONS, WARNINGS, and ADVERSE EVENTS.)

Nursing Mothers: It is not known whether ORTHOCLONE OKT3 is excreted in human milk. Because many drugs are excreted in human milk and because of the potential for serious adverse events/oncogenesis shown for ORTHOCLONE OKT3 in human studies, a decision should be made to discontinue nursing or to discontinue the drug, taking into account the importance of the drug to the mother. (See: CONTRAINDICATIONS.)

Pediatric Use: Safety and effectiveness have been established in infants (1 mo. up to 2 yr.); children (2 yr. up to 12 yr.); and adolescents (12 yr. up to 16 yr.). Use of ORTHOCLONE OKT3 in these age groups is supported by clinical studies that included adults and pediatric patients. In those studies, the safety and efficacy of ORTHOCLONE OKT3 in pediatric patients receiving renal or hepatic transplants was similar to that in the overall cohort. There were insufficient data to compare the safety and efficacy of ORTHOCLONE OKT3 in pediatric patients in a study of patients receiving cardiac transplants. Additional pharmacokinetic, pharmacodynamic, and clinical studies in infants, children, and adolescents have been reported in published literature.

Pediatric patients are known to have higher CD3 lymphocyte counts than adults; therefore, progressively higher doses of ORTHOCLONE OKT3 are often required to achieve therapeutic levels of lymphocyte clearance. (See: DOSAGE AND ADMINISTRATION.)

<u>Specific Safety Concerns in Pediatric Patients</u>

Deaths Due to Cerebral Herniation:

The postmarketing data base indicates that pediatric patients may be at increased risk of developing cerebral edema with or without herniation compared to adults. In the period between 1986 and 1996, twenty-five cases (6 in pediatric patients) of cerebral edema were identified with subsequent cerebral herniation and death in five cases (4 in pediatric patients). Herniation in the pediatric patients and one 19 year old subject occurred within a few hours to one day after the first dose (2.5 or 5 mg) of ORTHOCLONE OKT3 administered in the investigational setting for prophylaxis of renal allograft rejection. All pediatric patients and especially those receiving a renal allograft must be carefully evaluated for fluid retention and hypertension before the initiation of ORTHOCLONE OKT3 therapy. (See: WARNINGS: Cytokine Release Syndrome; DOSAGE AND ADMINISTRATION: General.) Patients should be closely monitored for neurologic symptoms during the first twenty four (24) hours following each of the first few doses of ORTHOCLONE OKT3 injection.

Other Serious Central Nervous System Adverse Events:
Other significant neurologic complications reported in pediatric transplant recipients receiving ORTHOCLONE OKT3 include status epilepticus, cerebral edema, diffuse encephalopathy, cerebritis, seizures, cortical dysfunction, and intracranial hemorrhage. Permanent neurologic impairments (e.g., blindness, deafness, paralysis) have been reported rarely. Because meningitis is a frequent infection encountered in pediatric allograft recipients, and the immunosuppression associated with transplantation increases the risk of opportunistic infection, patients with meningeal irritation following treatment with ORTHOCLONE OKT3 therapy should be evaluated with lumbar puncture as early as possible to rule out an infectious etiology.

Viral Infection:
The overall incidence of infections appeared to be similar in pediatric patients compared to the overall population studied. In the pediatric population, viral infections often include pathogens uncommon in adults, such as varicella zoster virus (VZV), adenovirus, enterovirus, parainfluenza virus, and respiratory syncytial virus (RSV). In addition, many viral diseases often manifest differently in pediatric patients than they do in adults. Because a large proportion of pediatric patients have not been infected by herpes viruses (e.g., EBV, HSV, CMV) prior to transplantation they may be more susceptible to acquiring primary infections from the grafted organ and/or blood products when immunosuppressed. Antiviral prophylactic therapy may be particularly useful in these high risk pediatric patients. (See: ADVERSE EVENTS: Infections.)

Neoplasia:
Patients with primary EBV infection may be at higher risk for the development of EBV-associated lymphoproliferative disorders. There are data to support an association between the development of lymphoproliferative disorders at the time of active EBV infection and ORTHOCLONE OKT®3 administration in pediatric liver allograft recipients. Antiviral prophylactic therapy may be particularly useful in these high risk pediatric patients.

Gastrointestinal Fluid Losses:
Parenteral hydration may be required for gastrointestinal fluid loss secondary to diarrhea and/or vomiting resulting from the "Cytokine Release Syndrome".

Thrombosis:
Pediatric patients may be at an increased risk of thrombosis. Pediatric patients weighing less than 15 kg are at high-risk for hepatic artery thrombosis. Thrombosis has been reported in pediatric transplant recipients treated with ORTHOCLONE OKT3. A number of factors, including surgical technique, the presence of a hypercoaguable state, and the absence of prior dialysis experience may be relevant to the pathophysiology of the increased risk of thrombosis. (See: BOXED WARNING; WARNINGS; PRECAUTIONS; ADVERSE EVENTS; DOSAGE AND ADMINISTRATION.)

ADVERSE EVENTS

Cytokine Release Syndrome
In controlled clinical trials for treatment of acute renal allograft rejection, patients treated with ORTHOCLONE OKT3 plus concomitant low-dose immunosuppressive therapy (primarily azathioprine and corticosteroids) were observed to have an increased incidence of adverse experiences during the first two days of treatment, as compared with the group of patients receiving azathioprine and high-dose steroid therapy. During this period the majority of patients experienced pyrexia (90%), of which 19% were 40.0°C (104°F) or above, and chills (59%). In addition, other adverse experiences occurring in 8% or more of the patients during the first two days of ORTHOCLONE OKT3 therapy included: dyspnea (21%), nausea (19%), vomiting (19%), chest pain (14%), diarrhea (14%), tremor (13%), wheezing (13%), headache (11%), tachycardia (10%), rigor (8%), and hypertension (8%). A similar spectrum of clinical manifestations has been observed in open clinical studies and in post-marketing experience involving patients treated with ORTHOCLONE OKT3 for rejection following renal, cardiac, and hepatic transplantation.
Additional serious and occasionally fatal cardiorespiratory manifestations have been reported following any of the first few doses. (See: WARNINGS: Cytokine Release Syndrome ADVERSE EVENTS: Cardiovascular, Respiratory.)
In the acute renal allograft rejection trials, potentially fatal pulmonary edema had been reported following the first two doses in less than 2% of the patients treated with ORTHOCLONE OKT3. Pulmonary edema was usually associated with fluid overload. However, post-marketing experience revealed that pulmonary edema has occurred in patients who appeared to be euvolemic, presumably as a consequence of cytokine-mediated increased vascular permeability ("leaky capillaries") and/or reduced myocardial contractility/compliance (i.e., left ventricular dysfunction). (See: WARNINGS: Cytokine Release Syndrome DOSAGE AND ADMINISTRATION.)

Infections
In the controlled randomized renal allograft rejection trial conducted before cyclosporine was marketed, the most common infections during the first 45 days of ORTHOCLONE OKT3 therapy were due to herpes simplex virus (27%) and cytomegalovirus (19%). Other severe and life-threatening infections were *Staphylococcus epidermidis* (5%), *Pneumocystis carinii* (3%), *Legionella* (2%), *Cryptococcus* (2%), *Serratia* (2%) and gram-negative bacteria (2%). The incidence of infections was similar in patients treated with ORTHOCLONE OKT3 and in patients treated with high-dose steroids.
In a clinical trial of acute hepatic allograft rejection, refractory to conventional treatment, the most common infections reported in patients treated with ORTHOCLONE OKT3 during the first 45 days of the study were cytomegalovirus (16% of patients, of which 43% of infections were severe), fungal infections (15% of patients, of which 30% were severe), and herpes simplex virus (8% of patients, of which 10% were severe). Other severe and life-threatening infections were gram-positive infections (9% of patients), gram-negative infections (8% of patients), viral infections (2% of patients), and *Legionella* (1% of patients). In another trial studying the use of ORTHOCLONE OKT®3 in patients with hepatic allografts, the incidence of fungal infections was 34% and infections with the herpes simplex virus was 31%.
In a clinical trial studying the use of ORTHOCLONE OKT3 in patients with acute cardiac rejection refractory to conventional treatment, the most common infections in the ORTHOCLONE OKT3 group reported during the first 45 days of the study were herpes simplex virus (5% of patients, of which 20% were severe), fungal infections (4% of patients, of which 75% were severe), and cytomegalovirus (3% of patients, of which 33% were severe). No other severe or life-threatening infections were reported during this period.
In a retrospective analysis of pediatric patients treated for acute hepatic rejection, the most common infections reported in patients treated with ORTHOCLONE OKT3 therapy were due to bacterial infections (47%), fungal infections (21%), cytomegalovirus (19%), herpes simplex virus (15%), adenovirus (8%), and Epstein-Barr virus (8%). The overall rates of viral, fungal, and bacterial infections were similar in patients treated with ORTHOCLONE OKT3 (n=53) and in patients whose rejection was treated with steroids alone (n=27). In another study of 149 pediatric liver allograft patients where 59 episodes of steroid-resistant rejection were treated with ORTHOCLONE OKT3, the incidence of invasive cytomegalovirus infection was higher in patients receiving ORTHOCLONE OKT3 than in those receiving steroids alone.
Clinically significant infections (e.g., pneumonia, sepsis, etc.) due to the following pathogens have been reported:

Bacterial: *Clostridium* species (including *perfringens*), *Corynebacterium*, Enterococcus, *Enterobacter aerogenes*, *Escherichia coli*, *Klebsiella* species, *Lactobacillus*, *Legionella*, *Listeria monocytogenes*, *Mycobacteria* species, *Nocardia asteroides*, *Proteus* species, *Providencia* species, *Pseudomonas aeruginosa*, *Serratia* species, *Staphylococcus* species, *Streptococcus* species, *Yersinia enterocolitica*, and other gram-negative bacteria.
*Fungal:** *Aspergillus*, *Candida*, *Cryptococcus*, *Dermatophytes*.
Protozoa: *Pneumocystis carinii*, *Toxoplasma gondii*.
Viral: cytomegalovirus* (CMV), Epstein-Barr virus* (EBV), herpes simplex virus* (HSV), hepatitis viruses, varicella zoster virus (VZV), adenovirus, enterovirus, respiratory syncytial virus (RSV), parainfluenza virus.

As a consequence of being a potent immunosuppressive, the incidence and severity of infections with designated(*) pathogens, especially the herpes family of viruses, may be increased. (See: WARNINGS: Infections.)

Neoplasia
In patients treated with ORTHOCLONE OKT3, post-transplant lymphoproliferative disorders have ranged from lymphadenopathy or benign polyclonal B cell hyperplasias to malignant and often fatal monoclonal B cell lymphomas. In post-marketing experience, approximately one-third of the lymphoproliferations reported were benign and two-thirds were malignant. Lymphoma types included: B cell, large cell, polyclonal, non-Hodgkin's, lymphocytic, T cell, Burkitt's. The majority were not histologically classified. Malignant lymphomas appear to develop early after transplantation, the majority within the first four months post-treatment. Many of these have been rapidly progressive. Some were fulminant, involving the allografted organ and were widely disseminated at the time of diagnosis. Carcinomas of the skin included: basal cell, squamous cell, sarcoma, melanoma, and keratoacanthoma. Other neoplasms infrequently reported include: multiple myeloma, leukemia, carcinoma of the breast, adenocarcinoma, cholangiocarcinoma, and recurrences of pre-existing hepatoma and renal cell carcinoma. (See: WARNINGS: Neoplasia.)

Hypersensitivity Reactions
Reported adverse reactions resulting from the formation of antibodies to ORTHOCLONE OKT3 have included antigen-antibody (immune complex) mediated syndromes and IgE-mediated reactions. Hypersensitivity reactions have ranged from a mild, self-limited rash or pruritus to severe, life-threatening anaphylactic reactions/shock or angioedema (including: swelling of lips, eyelids, laryngeal spasm and airway obstruction with hypoxia). (See: WARNINGS: Anaphylactic Reactions.)
Other hypersensitivity reactions have included: ineffectiveness of treatment, serum sickness, arthritis, allergic interstitial nephritis, immune complex deposition resulting in glomerulonephritis, vasculitis (including temporal and retinal), and eosinophilia.

Adverse Reactions by Body System
Adverse events reported in greater than or equal to 1% of clinical trial patients treated with ORTHOCLONE OKT3 (n=393) are shown in Table 1:

Table 1: Adverse Events Reported in Clinical Trials (≥1% incidence, n=393)

Body System	Incidence (%)
Autonomic Nervous System Disorders	
Diaphoresis	7
Vasodilation	7
Body as a Whole, General Disorders	
Anorexia	4
Asthenia	10
Chills	43
Fatigue	9
Lethargy	6
Malaise	5
Pain, trunk	6
Pyrexia	77
Cardiovascular Disorders, General	
Arrhythmia	4
Bradycardia	4
Hypertension	19
Hypotension	25
Pain, chest	9
Tachycardia	26
Vascular Occlusion	2
Central & Peripheral Nervous System Disorders	
Convulsions	1
Dizziness	6
Headache	28
Meningitis	1
Tremor	14
Gastrointestinal System Disorders	
Diarrhea	37
Nausea	32
Pain, abdominal	6
Pain, GI	7
Vomiting	25
Hematopoietic Disorders	
Anemia	2
Leukocytosis	1
Thrombocytopenia	2
Metabolic and Nutritional Disorders	
Edema	12
Musculoskeletal System Disorders	
Arthralgia	7
Myalgia	1
Psychiatric Disorders	
Confusion	6
Depression	3
Nervousness	5
Somnolence	2
Renal Disorders	
Renal Dysfunction	3
Respiratory System Disorders	
Abnormal Chest Sound	10
Dyspnea	16
Hyperventilation	7
Hypoxia	1
Pneumonia	1
Pulmonary Edema	2
Respiratory Congestion	4
Wheezing	6
Skin and Appendages Disorders	
Pruritus	7
Rash	14
Rash Erythematous	2
Special Senses	
Photophobia	1
Tinnitus	1
White Cell and Reticuloendothelial System Disorders	
Leukopenia	7

Selected Adverse Events Reported In Clinical Trials (< 1% incidence, n=393):
Cardiovascular Disorders, General: Angina, Cardiac Arrest, Fluctuation in Blood Pressure, Heart Failure, Myocardial Infarction, Shock, Thrombosis.
Central and Peripheral Nervous System Disorders: Coma, Encephalopathy, Epilepsy, Hypotonia.
Gastrointestinal Disorders: Gastrointestinal Hemorrhage.
Hemapoietic Disorders: Coagulation Disorder, Lymphadenopathy, Lymphopenia.
Hepatobiliary: Hepatitis, SGOT Increased, SGPT Increased.
Psychiatric Disorders: Hallucinations, Mood Changes, Paranoia, Psychosis.
Renal Disorders: Anuria, Oliguria.
Respiratory System Disorders: Apnea, Pneumonitis.

Continued on next page

Orthoclone OKT3—Cont.

Special Senses: Conjunctivitis, Hearing Decrease.

Worldwide Postmarketing Experience - Body Systems/ Events Listed Alphabetically:

Body as a Whole, General Disorders: Fever (including spiking temperatures as high as 107°F), Flu-like Syndrome.

Cardiovascular Disorders: Cardiovascular Collapse, Hemodynamic Instability, Left Ventricular Dysfunction.

Central and Peripheral Nervous System Disorders: Agitation, Aphasia, Asterixis, Cerebritis, Cerebral Edema, Cerebral Herniation, Cerebrovascular Accident, CNS Infection, CNS Malignancy, Cranial Nerve VI Palsy, Encephalitis, Hyperreflexia, Involuntary Movements, Intracranial Hemorrhage, Impaired Cognition, Myoclonus, Obnubilation, Paresis/plegia including quadriparesis/plegia, Status Epilepticus, Stupor, Transient Ischemic Attack, Vertigo.

In a post-marketing survey involving 214 renal transplant patients, the incidence of aseptic meningitis syndrome was 6%. Fever (89%), headache (44%), neck stiffness (14%), and photophobia (10%) were the most commonly reported symptoms; a combination of these four symptoms occurred in 5% of patients.

Between 1987 and 1992, 75 post-marketing reports have described seizures, averaging about 12 per year, and including 23 fatalities. More than two-thirds of these reports (53) were of domestic spontaneous origin, and their age and sex distributions were broad. Post-licensure reports generally provide insufficient data to allow accurate estimation of risk or of incidence.

Gastrointestinal Disorders: Bowel Infarction.

Hematopoietic Disorders: Aplastic anemia, Arterial, Venous and Capillary Thrombosis of allografts and other vascular beds e.g., heart, lung, brain and bowel etc., Disseminated Intravascular Coagulation, Microangiopathic Changes (e.g., platelet microthrombi), Microangiopathic Hemolytic Anemia, Neutropenia, Pancytopenia.

Hepatobiliary: Hepatitis or Hepato/splenomegaly, usually secondary to viral infection or lymphoma.

Musculoskeletal Disorders: Arthritis, Stiffness/Aches/ Pains.

Renal Disorders: Azotemia, Abnormal Urinary Cytology including exfoliation of damaged lymphocytes, collecting duct cells and cellular casts, Delayed Graft Function, Renal Insufficiency/Renal Failure, usually transient and reversible and occasionally in association with Cytokine Release Syndrome.

Respiratory System Disorders: Adult Respiratory Distress Syndrome, Respiratory Arrest, Respiratory Failure.

Skin and Appendages: Erythema, Flushing, Stevens-Johnson Syndrome, Urticaria.

Special Senses: Blindness, Blurred Vision, Deafness, Diplopia, Otitis Media, Nasal and Ear Stuffiness, Papilledema.

OVERDOSAGE

Symptoms of overdosage with ORTHOCLONE OKT®3 may include hyperthermia, severe chills, myalgia, vomiting, diarrhea, edema, oliguria, pulmonary edema, and acute renal failure. A high incidence (5%) of microangiopathic hemolytic anemia/HUS syndrome in patients receiving 10 mg per day of ORTHOCLONE OKT3 was also reported. In the event of acute overdosage with ORTHOCLONE OKT3, the patient should be carefully observed and given symptomatic and supportive treatment.

DOSAGE AND ADMINISTRATION

Adults

The recommended dose of ORTHOCLONE OKT3 for the treatment of acute renal, steroid-resistant cardiac, or steroid-resistant hepatic allograft rejection is 5 mg per day in a single (bolus) intravenous injection in less than one minute for 10 to 14 days. For acute renal rejection, treatment should begin upon diagnosis. For steroid-resistant cardiac or hepatic allograft rejection, treatment should begin when the treating physician deems a rejection has not been reversed by an adequate course of corticosteroid therapy. (See: CLINICAL PHARMACOLOGY; PRECAUTIONS: Sensitization, Laboratory Tests.)

Pediatric Patients

The initial recommended dose is 2.5 mg per day in pediatric patients weighing less than or equal to 30 kg and 5 mg per day in pediatric patients weighing greater than 30 kg in a single (bolus) intravenous injection in less than one minute for 10 to 14 days. Daily increases in ORTHOCLONE OKT3 doses (i.e., 2.5 mg increments) may be required to achieve depletion of CD3 positive cells (<25 cells/mm^3) and ensure therapeutic ORTHOCLONE OKT3 serum concentrations (> 800 ng/mL). Pediatric patients may require augmentation of the ORTHOCLONE OKT3 dose. For acute renal rejection, treatment should begin upon diagnosis. For steroid-resistant cardiac or hepatic allograft rejection, treatment should begin when the treating physician deems a rejection has not been reversed by an adequate course of corticosteroid therapy. (See: CLINICAL PHARMACOLOGY; PRECAUTIONS; Laboratory Tests; Pediatric Use.)

General

For the first few doses, patients should be monitored in a facility equipped and staffed for cardiopulmonary resuscitation (CPR). Patients receiving subsequent doses of ORTHOCLONE OKT3, should also be monitored in a facility equipped and staffed for CPR. Vital signs should be monitored frequently. Patients receiving ORTHOCLONE OKT3 should also be carefully monitored for signs and symptoms of Cytokine Release Syndrome, particularly after the first few doses but also after a treatment hiatus with resumption of therapy. The patient's temperature should be lowered to <37.8°C (100°F) before the administration of any dose of ORTHOCLONE OKT3.

Prior to administration of ORTHOCLONE OKT3, the patient's volume status should be assessed carefully. It is imperative, especially prior to the first few doses, that there be no clinical evidence of volume overload, uncontrolled hypertension, or uncompensated heart failure. Patients should have a clear chest X-ray and should not weigh more than 3% above their minimum weight during the week prior to injection.

To decrease the incidence and severity of Cytokine Release Syndrome, associated with the first dose of ORTHOCLONE OKT3, it is strongly recommended that methylprednisolone sodium succinate 8.0 mg/kg be administered intravenously 1 to 4 hours prior to the initial dose of ORTHOCLONE OKT3. Acetaminophen and antihistamines given concomitantly with ORTHOCLONE OKT3 may also help to reduce some early reactions. (See: WARNINGS and ADVERSE EVENTS: Cytokine Release Syndrome.)

When using concomitant immunosuppressive drugs, the dose of each should be reduced to the lowest level compatible with an effective therapeutic response in order to reduce the potential for malignancy and infections. Maintenance immunosuppression should be resumed approximately three days prior to the cessation of ORTHOCLONE OKT®3 therapy. (See: WARNINGS and ADVERSE EVENTS: Infection, Neoplasia.)

Reduced T cell clearance or low plasma ORTHOCLONE OKT3 levels provide a basis for adjusting ORTHOCLONE OKT3 dosage or for discontinuing therapy. (See: WARNINGS: Anaphylactic Reactions; PRECAUTIONS: Laboratory Tests; ADVERSE EVENTS: Hypersensitivity Reactions.)

ADMINISTRATION INSTRUCTIONS

1. Before administration, ORTHOCLONE OKT3 should be inspected for particulate matter and discoloration. Because ORTHOCLONE OKT3 is a protein solution, it may develop fine translucent particles (shown not to affect potency).
2. No bacteriostatic agent is present in this product. Adherence to aseptic technique is advised. Once the ampule is opened, use immediately and discard the unused portion.
3. Prepare ORTHOCLONE OKT3 for injection by drawing solution into a syringe through a low protein-binding 0.2 or 0.22 micrometer (µm) filter. Detach filter and attach a new needle for a single intravenous (bolus) injection.
4. Because no data is available on compatibility of ORTHOCLONE OKT3 with other intravenous substances or additives, other medications/substances should not be added or infused simultaneously through the same intravenous line. If the same intravenous line is used for sequential infusion of several different drugs, the line should be flushed with saline before and after injection of ORTHOCLONE OKT3.
5. Administer ORTHOCLONE OKT3 as a single intravenous (bolus) injection in less than one minute. Do **not** administer by intravenous infusion or in conjunction with other drug solutions.

HOW SUPPLIED

ORTHOCLONE OKT3 is supplied as a sterile solution in packages of 5 ampules (NDC 59676-101-01). Each 5 mL ampule contains 5 mg of muromonab-CD3.

Storage: Store in a refrigerator at 2° to 8°C (36° to 46°F). DO NOT FREEZE OR SHAKE.

REFERENCES

1. Adair JC, Woodley SL, O'Connell JB, et al. Aseptic Meningitis following Cardiac Transplantation: Clinical Characteristics and Relationship to Immunosuppressive Regimen. Neurology 41:249–252, 1991.
2. Chatenoud L, Legendre C, Ferran C, *et al.* Corticosteroid Inhibition of the OKT3 - Induced Cytokine-Related Syndrome - Dosage and Kinetics Prerequisites. Transplantation 51:334–338, 1991.
3. Cockfield SM, Preiksaitis J, Harvey E, Jones C, Herbert D, Keown P, and Halloran PF, *et al.* Is Sequential Use of ALG and OKT3 in Renal Transplants Associated with an Increased Incidence of Fulminant Post Transplant Lymphoproliferative Disorders? Transplant. Proc. 23: 1106–1107, 1991.
4. Ettenger RB, Marik J, Rosenthal JT, *et al.* OKT3 for Rejection Reversal in Pediatric Renal Transplantation. Clin. Transplantation 2:180–184, 1988.
5. Gaston RS, Deierhoi MH, Patterson T, *et al.* OKT3 First-Dose Reaction: Association with T Cell Subsets and Cytokine Release. Kid. International 39:141–148, 1991.
6. Goldman M, Abramowicz D, DePauw L, *et al.* OKT3-Induced Cytokine Released Attenuation by High-Dose Methylprednisolone. Lancet 2:802–803, 1989.
7. Ortho Multicenter Transplant Study Group. A Randomized Clinical Trial of OKT3 Monoclonal Antibody for Acute Rejection of Cadaveric Renal Transplants. N. Engl. J. Med. 313:337–342, 1985.
8. Penn I. The Changing Patterns of Posttransplant Malignancies. Transplant. Proc. 23:1101–1103,1991.
9. Rubin RH and Tolkoff-Rubin NE. The Impact of Infection on the Outcome of Transplantation. Transplant. Proc. 23:2068–2074, 1991.
10. Schroeder TJ, Ryckman FC, Hurtubise PE, *et al.* Immunological Monitoring During and Following OKT3 Therapy in Children. Clin. Transplantation 5:191–196, 1991.
11. Goldstein G, Fuccello AJ, Norman DJ, *et al.* OKT3 Monoclonal Antibody Plasma Levels During Therapy and the Subsequent Development of Host Antibodies to OKT3. Transplantation 42:507–511, 1986.
12. Schroeder TJ, Michael AT, First MR, *et al.* Variations in Serum OKT3 Concentration Based Upon Age, Sex, Transplanted Organ, Treatment Regimen, and Anti-OKT3 Status. Therapeutic Drug Monitoring 16:361–367, 1994.
13. First MR, Schroeder TJ, Hurtubise PE, *et al.* Immune Monitoring During Retreatment with OKT3. Transplan. Proc. 21:1753–1754, 1989.

ORTHO BIOTECH PRODUCTS, L.P.
Raritan, New Jersey 08869
U.S.A. ORTHO BIOTECH
 631-10-191-4
Revised January 2003

ORTHOVISC® ℞
High Molecular Weight Hyaluronan

CAUTION

Federal law restricts this device to sale by or on the order of a physician (or properly licensed practitioner).

DESCRIPTION

ORTHOVISC® is a sterile, non-pyrogenic, clear, viscoelastic solution of hyaluronan contained in a single-use syringe. ORTHOVISC® consists of high molecular weight (1.0-2.9 million daltons), ultra-pure natural hyaluronan dissolved in physiological saline. Hyaluronan is a natural complex sugar of the glycosaminoglycan family. The hyaluronan is extracted from rooster combs.

INDICATIONS

ORTHOVISC® is indicated in the treatment of pain in osteoarthritis (OA) of the knee in patients who have failed to respond adequately to conservative non-pharmacologic therapy and to simple analgesics, e.g. acetaminophen.

CONTRAINDICATIONS

- Do not administer to patients with known hypersensitivity (allergy) to hyaluronate preparations.
- Do not administer to patients with known allergies to avian or avian-derived products (including eggs, feathers, or poultry).
- Do not inject ORTHOVISC® in the knees of patients with infections or skin diseases in the area of the injection site or joint.

WARNINGS

- Do not concomitantly use disinfectants containing quarternary ammonium salts for skin preparation as hyaluronic acid can precipitate in their presence.
- Transient increases in inflammation in the injected knee following ORTHOVISC® injection have been reported in some patients with inflammatory osteoarthritis.

PRECAUTIONS

General

- Strict aseptic injection technique should be used during the application of ORTHOVISC®.
- The safety and effectiveness of the use of ORTHOVISC® in joints other than the knee have not been demonstrated.
- The effectiveness of a single treatment cycle of less than 3 injections has not been established. Pain relief may not be seen until after the third injection.
- The safety and effectiveness has not been established for more than one course of treatment.
- STERILE CONTENTS. The pre-filled syringe is intended for single use only. The contents of the syringe should be used immediately after opening. Discard any unused ORTHOVISC®. Do not resterilize.
- Do not use ORTHOVISC® if the package has been opened or damaged.
- Store ORTHOVISC® in its original package at room temperature (below 77°F/25°C). DO NOT FREEZE.
- Remove joint effusion, if present, before injecting ORTHOVISC®.
- Only medical professionals trained in accepted injection techniques for delivering agents into the knee joint should inject ORTHOVISC® for the indicated use.

Information for Patients

- Transient pain or swelling may occur after the intraarticular (IA) injection.
- As with any invasive joint procedure, it is recommended that patients avoid strenuous activity or prolonged (i.e., more than one hour) weight-bearing activities such as running or tennis within 48 hours following the intra-articular injection.

Use in Specific Populations

- **Pregnancy:** The safety and effectiveness of the use of ORTHOVISC® in pregnant women has not been tested.
- **Nursing Mothers:** It is not known if ORTHOVISC® is excreted in human milk. The safety and effectiveness of the use of the product in lactating women has not been tested.
- **Children:** The safety and effectiveness of the use of ORTHOVISC® in children has not been tested.

ADVERSE EVENTS

ORTHOVISC® was investigated in 3 randomized, controlled clinical studies conducted in the U.S. An integrated safety analysis was conducted, pooling the ORTHOVISC® groups from the 3 studies and pooling the control groups, which were either intraarticular saline injections or arthrocentesis. In the integrated analysis, there were 562 patients in the groups treated with ORTHOVISC® (434 receiving 3 injections and 128 receiving 4 injections), 296 in the group treated with physiological saline, and 123 in the group treated with arthrocentesis.

Adverse events occurring at >5% of the overall integrated population included: arthralgia (12.6% in the ORTHOVISC® group, 17.2% in the saline group, and 0.8% in the arthrocentesis group); back pain (6.9% in the ORTHOVISC® group, 12.2% in the saline group, 2 and 4.9% in the arthrocentesis group); and headache NOS (12.1% in the ORTHOVISC® group, 16.6% in the saline group, and 17.9% in the arthrocentesis group). Injection site adverse events (including erythema, edema, pain and reaction NOS) occurred at rates of 0.4%, 0.9%, 2.5% and 0.2%, respectively, in the ORTHOVISC® group, compared to 0.0%, 0.3%, 2.0%, and 0.7% in the saline group and 0.0%, 0.0%, 0.8% and 0.8% in the arthrocentesis group.

Local adverse events reported on a by-patient basis for the combined ITT populations of the three studies are presented in Table 1.

[See table 1 above]

Table 1
Local individual adverse events reported on a by-patient basis for the combined ITT populations of the three studies.

Adverse Event	ORTHOVISC N = 562		Saline N = 296		Arthrocentesis N = 123	
Any Adverse Event	349	(62.1%)	204	(68.9%)	65	(52.8%)
Injection site erythema	2	(0.4%)	0	(0%)	0	(0%)
Injection site edema	5	(0.9%)	1	(0.3%)	0	(0%)
Injection site pain	14	(2.5%)	6	(2.0%)	1	(0.8%)
Injection site reaction NOS[1]	1	(0.2%)	2	(0.7%)	1	(0.8%)
Pain NOS[1]	14	(2.5%)	11	(3.7%)	1	(0.8%)
Arthralgia	71	(12.6%)	51	(17.2%)	1	(0.8%)
Arthritis NOS[1]	4	(0.7%)	5	(1.7%)	0	(0%)
Arthropathy NOS[1]	5	(0.9%)	3	(1.0%)	0	(0%)
Baker's cyst	2	(0.4%)	2	(0.7%)	0	(0%)
Bursitis	6	(1.1%)	6	(2.0%)	2	(1.6%)
Joint disorder NOS[1]	2	(0.4%)	0	(0%)	0	(0%)
Joint effusion	2	(0.4%)	1	(0.3%)	1	(0.8%)
Joint stiffness	3	(0.5%)	2	(0.7%)	0	(0%)
Joint swelling	4	(0.7%)	2	(0.7%)	1	(0.8%)
Localized osteoarthritis	5	(0.9%)	1	(0.3%)	1	(0.8%)
Aggravated osteoarthritis	2	(0.4%)	0	(0%)	1	(0.8%)
Knee arthroplasty	3	(0.5%)	2	(0.7%)	0	(0%)

Notes: [1]NOS = Not otherwise specified.

CLINICAL STUDIES

The effectiveness of ORTHOVISC® for the treatment of osteoarthritis of the knee was evaluated in three main studies; two randomized, controlled, double-blind multicenter studies (OAK9501 and OAK2001) that involved unilateral treatment, and one study (OAK9801) that involved bilateral treatment. Because bilateral treatment confounded the assessment of effectiveness of the OAK9801 study, the effectiveness data are summarized for the OAK9501 and OAK2001 studies. Safety data for all three studies are reported in "Adverse Events."

Study Design/Analysis

The objective of the randomized studies was to assess the effectiveness of ORTHOVISC® for the treatment of joint pain of patients with idiopathic osteoarthritis of the knee. The OAK9501 study randomized patients to 3 weekly injections of either ORTHOVISC® (O3) or saline. The OAK2001 study randomized patients to one of three treatments: 4 ORTHOVISC® injections (O4), 3 ORTHOVISC® injections + 1 arthrocentesis (O3A1) procedure, or 4 arthrocentesis (A4) procedures. Follow-up occurred at weeks 7/8, 11/12, 15/16 and 21/22, with final follow-up at week 27/28. When each study was analyzed individually, the primary analyses for each study did not show statistical significance. A combined analysis was additionally performed. The combined data consisted of data obtained from a subgroup of patients from each of the studies (the "ITT Subgroup" from OAK9501 and the "Evaluable Subgroup" from OAK2001) who had Kellgren-Lawrence radiographic grades of II or III at baseline and WOMAC pain in the contralateral knee of <175mm (out of 500) and is referred to as the effectiveness subgroup population. For the effectiveness subgroup population, the primary effectiveness analysis performed was to determine the proportion of patients achieving a 20% improvement from baseline in the WOMAC Pain Score in conjunction with a minimum absolute improvement of 50 mm from baseline in the WOMAC Pain Score, and a 40% and 50% improvement from baseline in WOMAC Pain Score at four assessment points between Weeks 7/8 to 21/22 for the index knee.

Study Population

OAK9501 included 226 patients at 10 centers, and OAK2001 involved 373 patients at 24 centers. Within the individual studies, baseline and demographic variables were similar among groups. Table 2 below summarizes the baseline and patient demographic characteristics for the combined effectiveness subgroup.

[See table 2 above]

Table 2
Baseline and patient demographics summary—effectiveness subgroup.[1]

Characteristic	O3 N = 83	Saline × 3 N = 81	O4 N = 104	O3A1 N = 90	A4 N = 100
No. (%) female	51 (61.4%)	49 (60.5%)	46 (44.2%)	59 (65.5%)	50 (50.0%)
Mean ±SD age (years)	65 ± 8	68 ± 9	59 ± 9	59 ± 9	59 ± 8
Mean ±SD BMI (kg/m^2)	32 ± 7	30 ± 6	29 ± 4	30 ± 4	30 ± 4
Mean ±SD WOMAC Pain (0-500mm) Study Knee	274 ± 65	268 ± 70	288 ± 60	290 ± 50	293 ± 59
Mean ±SD WOMAC Pain (0-500mm) Contralateral	83 ± 57	87 ± 54	69 ± 47	70 ± 47	68 ± 48
Mean ±SD Investigator Global (0-100mm)	53 ± 19	51 ± 19	59 ± 14	58 ± 14	58 ± 15
Mean ±SD Patient Global (0-100mm)	56 ± 20	53 ± 22	67 ± 15	62 ± 17	64 ± 15

Notes: [1]Patients with Kellgren-Lawrence radiographic grades of II or III at baseline and WOMAC pain in the contralateral knee of <175mm (out of 500).

Combined Study Results

In the combined analysis of OAK9501 and OAK2001, two subgroup populations (representing patients with baseline Kellgren-Lawrence grade II or III radiographic findings and contralateral knee pain <175 mm on the WOMAC Pain Score) were analyzed together, comprising 5 treatment groups (4 ORTHOVISC® injections [O4], 3 ORTHOVISC® injections followed by 1 arthrocentesis [O3A1], 3 ORTHOVISC® injections [O3], 4 arthrocentesis procedures [A4] and 3 saline injections [Saline]). For the GEE analyses, the O3A1 and O3 groups were also pooled to form a sixth group [O3A1/O3].

The primary effectiveness analysis was performed to determine the proportion of patients achieving a 20% improvement from baseline in WOMAC Pain Score in conjunction with a minimum absolute improvement of 50 mm from baseline in the WOMAC Pain Score, and a 40% and 50% improvement from baseline in WOMAC Pain Score at four assessment points between Weeks 8 to 22 for the index knee. A significantly larger proportion of O4 patients achieved 40% and 50% improvements from baseline in WOMAC Pain Score compared to both A4 and Saline over 7-22 weeks (based on GEE analysis). Similarly, a significantly larger proportion of O3 and O3A1/O3 patients achieved 40% and 50% improvements from baseline in WOMAC Pain Score than Saline patients (based on GEE analysis) (Table 3). Table 4 presents the mean number of patients from the effectiveness subgroup over the four follow-up visits that achieved improvement over weeks 8 through 22.

Table 3
GEE Results (P-Values) for the Effectiveness Subgroups for the Primary Endpoints

Endpoint	O4 vs. A4	O4 vs. Saline	O3 vs. Saline
20% improvement from baseline and 50 mm absolute improvement in WOMAC Pain	0.0738	0.1116	0.0789
40% improvement in WOMAC Pain Score from baseline	**0.0094***	**0.0015***	**0.0166***
50% improvement in WOMAC Pain Score from baseline	**0.0360***	**0.0015***	**0.0274***

O4 4 weekly ORTHOVISC® injections—OAK2001 Study
O3 3 weekly ORTHOVISC® injections—OAK9501 Study
A4 4 control [arthrocentesis only] procedures—OAK2001 Study
Saline 3 control [saline injection] procedures—OAK9501 Study
* Statistically significant

[See table 4 at top of next page]

O4 4 weekly ORTHOVISC® injections—OAK2001 Study
O3A1 3 weekly ORTHOVISC® injections + 1 control [arthrocentesis only] procedure—OAK2001 Study
O3 3 weekly ORTHOVISC® injections—OAK9501 Study
A4 4 control [arthrocentesis only] procedures—OAK2001 Study
Saline 3 control [saline injection] procedures—OAK9501 Study

Summary

In summary, with respect to patients achieving ≥40% and ≥50% improvement compared to baseline, the four injection ORTHOVISC® regimen demonstrated effectiveness compared to both Saline and Arthrocentesis control procedures, and the three-weekly injection regimen demonstrated effectiveness compared to Saline in the indicated patient population.

DETAILED DEVICE DESCRIPTION

Hyaluronan is a high molecular weight polysaccharide composed of repeating disaccharide units of sodium glucuronate and N-acetylglucosamine.

Each syringe contains the following in a 2 ml dose sterile-filled into a syringe:

Hyaluronan	30 mg
Sodium Chloride	18 mg
Water for Injection	q.s. up to 2.0 ml

ORTHOVISC® does not contain any synthetic additives.

Continued on next page

Table 4
Summary of mean number patients achieving primary individual patient success criteria—effectiveness subgroups from OAK9501 and OAK2001—over weeks 8 through 22 (4 visits).

	O4 N = 104	O3A1 N = 90	A4 N = 100	O3 N = 83	Saline × 3 N = 81
Mean No. (%) patients achieving ≥20% improvement from baseline and absolute improvement of 50 mm in WOMAC Pain	77.5 (74.5%)	58.3 (64.7%)	64.5 (64.5%)	59.3 (71.4%)	50.8 (62.7%)
Mean No. (%) patients achieving ≥40% improvement from baseline	68.0 (65.4%)	47.0 (52.2%)	48.8 (48.8%)	45.8 (55.1%)	34.3 (42.3%)
Mean No. (%) patients achieving ≥50% improvement from baseline	59.3 (57.0%)	40.5 (45.0%)	43.5 (43.5%)	38.5 (46.4%)	28.3 (34.9%)

Orthovisc—Cont.

HOW SUPPLIED

ORTHOVISC® is supplied as a sterile-filled solution, in a single-use syringe, sealed in a sterile pouch inside a carton. The product is presented as a sterile, non-pyrogenic solution in a 2 ml syringe. Each syringe is labeled "ORTHOVISC®" for ready identification. A rubber cap is provided on the syringe tip to prevent leakage and protect sterility of the product.

DIRECTIONS FOR USE

ORTHOVISC® is injected into the knee joint in a series of intra-articular injections one week apart for a total of three or four injections. Standard intra-articular injection site preparation, aseptic technique and precautions should be used.

- After removal of the protective rubber cap on the tip of the syringe, securely attach a small gauge needle (18-21 gauge) to the tip.
- Inject ORTHOVISC® into the knee joint using proper injection technique.
- Inject the full contents of the syringe into one knee only.
- If treatment is bilateral, a separate syringe should be used for each knee.

ORTHOVISC® is a registered trademark of Anika Therapeutics, Inc.
Manufactured by:
Anika Therapeutics, Inc.
236 West Cummings Park
Woburn, Massachusetts USA 01801
Distributed by:
ORTHO BIOTECH
Ortho Biotech Products, L.P.
Raritan, NJ 08869-0670 USA
AML 530-220 01/04 Product Code 59676-360-01

Patient Information

ORTHOVISC® High Molecular Weight Hyaluronan

What is ORTHOVISC®?
ORTHOVISC® is a viscous (thick) sterile mixture made from highly purified hyaluronan from rooster combs. Hyaluronan is a natural chemical found in the body. High amounts of hyaluronan are found in the joint tissues and in the fluid that fills the joints. The body's own hyaluronan acts like a lubricant and a shock absorber in the joint. It is needed for the joint to work properly. When you have osteoarthritis, there may not be enough natural hyaluronan in the joint, and the quality of that hyaluronan may be poorer than normal. ORTHOVISC® is given in a shot (injection) directly into the knee joint.

What is ORTHOVISC® used for?
ORTHOVISC® is used to relieve knee pain due to osteoarthritis. It is used for patients who do not get adequate pain relief from simple pain relievers like acetaminophen or from exercise and physical therapy.

What are the benefits of ORTHOVISC®?
Clinical trials conducted in the U.S. have shown that ORTHOVISC® provides pain relief to patients who have not been able to find pain relief with simple pain medication or exercise compared to saline placebo injections.

What other treatments are available for osteoarthritis?
If you have pain due to osteoarthritis of the knee, there are things you can do that do not involve ORTHOVISC® injections. These include:

Non-drug treatments:
- Avoiding activities that cause pain in your knee
- Exercise
- Physical therapy
- Removal of excess fluid from the knee

Drug therapy:
- Pain medication such as acetaminophen and narcotics
- Drugs that reduce inflammation, such as aspirin and other "nonsteroidal anti-inflammatory" agents (NSAIDs) (such as ibuprofen and naproxen)
- Corticosteroids that are injected directly into the knee joint

Are there any reasons why you should not take ORTHOVISC®?
- You should not take this product if you are allergic to hyaluronate products.
- You should not take this product if you are allergic to products from birds (poultry, feathers, eggs, etc.). If you are injected with ORTHOVISC® and are allergic to bird products, you could develop an allergic reaction to the injections.
- You should not have an injection into the knee if you have infections or skin diseases around the injection site.

Things you should know about ORTHOVISC®
- ORTHOVISC® should be injected by a qualified physician.
- Tell your physician if you are allergic to products from birds, such as feathers, eggs and poultry. If you are allergic to bird products and you have ORTHOVISC® injections, you may have a severe reaction and even die from the injection.
- For 48 hours after you receive the injection, you should avoid activities such as jogging, tennis, heavy lifting or standing on your feet for a long time (more than one hour).
- The safety and effectiveness of ORTHOVISC® in joints other than the knee has not been demonstrated in U.S. studies.
- The safety and effectiveness of ORTHOVISC® has not been shown in pregnant or nursing women. You should tell your doctor if you are pregnant or nursing.
- The safety and effectiveness of ORTHOVISC® has not been shown in children.
- The safety and effectiveness has not been established for more than one course of treatment.

Possible complications
- Side effects are sometimes seen when ORTHOVISC® is injected into the knee joint. These can include: pain, swelling, heat, rash, itching, bruising and/or redness. You may also feel achy. These reactions are generally mild and do not last long.
- If any of these symptoms or signs appear after you are given ORTHOVISC® or if you have any other problems, you should call your doctor.

How is ORTHOVISC® given?
Your doctor will inject ORTHOVISC® (30 mg/2 mL) into your knee once a week, for a total of 3 or 4 injections.

Distributed by:
ORTHO BIOTECH
Ortho Biotech Products, L.P.
Raritan, NJ 08869
Manufactured by:
Anika Therapeutics, Inc.
236 West Cummings Park
Woburn, MA 01890
AML 530-220 01/04 PI
Distributed By:
ORTHO BIOTECH
Ortho Biotech Products, L.P. Bridgewater, NJ 08807-0914 USA
©Ortho Biotech Products, L.P. 2004 ORTHOVISC® is a registered trademark of Anika Therapeutics, Inc.
Printed in U.S.A 2/04 08VSC1001
Manufactured By:
Anika Therapeutics, Inc. Woburn, MA 01801 USA

Shown in Product Identification Guide, page 327

PROCRIT® ℞

[*prō-krit*]
(Epoetin alfa)
FOR INJECTION

DESCRIPTION

Erythropoietin is a glycoprotein which stimulates red blood cell production. It is produced in the kidney and stimulates the division and differentiation of committed erythroid progenitors in the bone marrow. PROCRIT® (Epoetin alfa), a 165 amino acid glycoprotein manufactured by recombinant DNA technology, has the same biological effects as endogenous erythropoietin.[1] It has a molecular weight of 30,400 daltons and is produced by mammalian cells into which the human erythropoietin gene has been introduced. The product contains the identical amino acid sequence of isolated natural erythropoietin.

PROCRIT® is formulated as a sterile, colorless liquid in an isotonic sodium chloride/sodium citrate buffered solution or a sodium chloride/sodium phosphate buffered solution for intravenous (IV) or subcutaneous (SC) administration.

Single-dose, Preservative-free Vial: Each 1 mL of solution contains 2000, 3000, 4000 or 10,000 Units of Epoetin alfa, 2.5 mg Albumin (Human), 5.8 mg sodium citrate, 5.8 mg sodium chloride, and 0.06 mg citric acid in Water for Injection, USP (pH 6.9 ± 0.3). This formulation contains no preservative.

Single-dose, Preservative-free Vial: 1 mL (40,000 Units/mL). Each 1 mL of solution contains 40,000 Units of Epoetin alfa, 2.5 mg Albumin (Human), 1.2 mg sodium phosphate monobasic monohydrate, 1.8 mg sodium phosphate dibasic anhydrate, 0.7 mg sodium citrate, 5.8 mg sodium chloride, and 6.8 mcg citric acid in Water for Injection, USP (pH 6.9 ± 0.3). This formulation contains no preservative.

Multidose, Preserved Vial: 2 mL (20,000 Units, 10,000 Units/mL). Each 1 mL of solution contains 10,000 Units of Epoetin alfa, 2.5 mg Albumin (Human), 1.3 mg sodium citrate, 8.2 mg sodium chloride, 0.11 mg citric acid, and 1% benzyl alcohol as preservative in Water for Injection, USP (pH 6.1 ± 0.3).

Multidose, Preserved Vial: 1 mL (20,000 Units/mL). Each 1 mL of solution contains 20,000 Units of Epoetin alfa, 2.5 mg Albumin (Human), 1.3 mg sodium citrate, 8.2 mg sodium chloride, 0.11 mg citric acid, and 1% benzyl alcohol as preservative in Water for Injection, USP (pH 6.1 ± 0.3).

CLINICAL PHARMACOLOGY

Chronic Renal Failure Patients

Endogenous production of erythropoietin is normally regulated by the level of tissue oxygenation. Hypoxia and anemia generally increase the production of erythropoietin, which in turn stimulates erythropoiesis.[2] In normal subjects, plasma erythropoietin levels range from 0.01 to 0.03 Units/mL and increase up to 100- to 1000-fold during hypoxia or anemia.[2] In contrast, in patients with chronic renal failure (CRF), production of erythropoietin is impaired, and this erythropoietin deficiency is the primary cause of their anemia.[3,4]

Chronic renal failure is the clinical situation in which there is a progressive and usually irreversible decline in kidney function. Such patients may manifest the sequelae of renal dysfunction, including anemia, but do not necessarily require regular dialysis. Patients with end-stage renal disease (ESRD) are those patients with CRF who require regular dialysis or kidney transplantation for survival.

PROCRIT® has been shown to stimulate erythropoiesis in anemic patients with CRF, including both patients on dialysis and those who do not require regular dialysis.[4–13] The first evidence of a response to the three times weekly (TIW) administration of PROCRIT® is an increase in the reticulocyte count within 10 days, followed by increases in the red cell count, hemoglobin, and hematocrit, usually within 2 to 6 weeks.[4,5] Because of the length of time required for erythropoiesis – several days for erythroid progenitors to mature and be released into the circulation – a clinically significant increase in hematocrit is usually not observed in less than 2 weeks and may require up to 6 weeks in some patients. Once the hematocrit reaches the suggested target range (30% to 36%), that level can be sustained by PROCRIT® therapy in the absence of iron deficiency and concurrent illnesses.

The rate of hematocrit increase varies between patients and is dependent upon the dose of PROCRIT®, within a therapeutic range of approximately 50 to 300 Units/kg TIW.[4] A greater biologic response is not observed at doses exceeding 300 Units/kg TIW.[6] Other factors affecting the rate and extent of response include availability of iron stores, the baseline hematocrit, and the presence of concurrent medical problems.

Zidovudine-treated HIV-infected Patients

Responsiveness to PROCRIT® in HIV-infected patients is dependent upon the endogenous serum erythropoietin level prior to treatment. Patients with endogenous serum erythropoietin levels ≤ 500 mUnits/mL, and who are receiving a dose of zidovudine ≤ 4200 mg/week, may respond to PROCRIT® therapy. Patients with endogenous serum erythropoietin levels > 500 mUnits/mL do not appear to respond to PROCRIT® therapy. In a series of four clinical trials involving 255 patients, 60% to 80% of HIV-infected patients treated with zidovudine had endogenous serum erythropoietin levels ≤ 500 mUnits/mL.

Response to PROCRIT® in zidovudine-treated HIV-infected patients is manifested by reduced transfusion requirements and increased hematocrit.

Cancer Patients on Chemotherapy

A series of clinical trials enrolled 131 anemic cancer patients who received PROCRIT® TIW and who were receiving cyclic cisplatin- or non cisplatin-containing chemotherapy. Endogenous baseline serum erythropoietin levels varied among patients in these trials with approximately 75% (n = 83/110) having endogenous serum erythropoietin levels ≤ 132 mUnits/mL, and approximately 4% (n = 4/110) of patients having endogenous serum erythropoietin levels > 500 mUnits/mL. In general, patients with lower baseline serum erythropoietin levels responded more vigorously to PROCRIT® than patients with higher baseline erythropoietin levels. Although no specific serum erythropoietin level can be stipulated above which patients would be unlikely to respond to PROCRIT® therapy, treatment of patients with grossly elevated serum erythropoietin levels (eg, > 200 mUnits/mL) is not recommended.

Pharmacokinetics

In adult and pediatric patients with CRF, the elimination half-life of plasma erythropoietin after intravenously administered PROCRIT® ranges from 4 to 13 hours.[14-16] The half-life is approximately 20% longer in CRF patients than that in healthy subjects. After SC administration, peak plasma levels are achieved within 5 to 24 hours. The half-life is similar between adult patients with serum creatinine level greater than 3 and not on dialysis and those maintained on dialysis.

The pharmacokinetic profile of PROCRIT® in children and adolescents appears to be similar to that of adults. Limited data are available in neonates.[17]

The pharmacokinetics PROCRIT® have not been studied in HIV-infected patients.

A pharmacokinetic study comparing 150 Units/kg SC TIW to 40,000 Units SC weekly dosing regimen was conducted for 4 weeks in healthy subjects (n = 12) and for 6 weeks in anemic cancer patients (n = 32) receiving cyclic chemotherapy. There was no accumulation of serum erythropoietin after the 2 dosing regimens during the study period. The 40,000 Units weekly regimen had a higher C_{max} (3- to 7-fold), longer T_{max} (2- to 3-fold), higher AUC_{0-168h} (2- to 3-fold) of erythropoietin and lower clearance (50%) than the 150 Units/kg TIW regimen. In anemic cancer patients, the average $t_{1/2}$ was similar (40 hours with range of 16 to 67 hours) after both dosing regimens. After the 150 Units/kg TIW dosing, the values of T_{max} and clearance are similar (13.3 ± 12.4 vs. 14.2 ± 6.7 hours, and 20.2 ± 15.9 vs. 23.6 ± 9.5 mL/h/kg) between Week 1 when patients were receiving chemotherapy (n = 14) and Week 3 when patients were not receiving chemotherapy (n = 4). Differences were observed after the 40,000 Units weekly dosing with longer T_{max} (38 ± 18 hours) and lower clearance (9.2 ± 4.7 mL/h/kg) during Week 1 when patients were receiving chemotherapy (n = 18) compared with those (22 ± 4.5 hours, 13.9 ± 7.6 mL/h/kg) during Week 3 when patients were not receiving chemotherapy (n = 7).

The bioequivalence between the 10,000 Units/mL citrate-buffered Epoetin alfa formulation and the 40,000 Units/mL phosphate-buffered Epoetin alfa formulation has been demonstrated after SC administration of single 750 Units/kg doses to healthy subjects.

INDICATIONS AND USAGE

Treatment of Anemia of Chronic Renal Failure Patients

PROCRIT® is indicated for the treatment of anemia associated with CRF, including patients on dialysis (ESRD) and patients not on dialysis. PROCRIT® is indicated to elevate or maintain the red blood cell level (as manifested by the hematocrit or hemoglobin determinations) and to decrease the need for transfusions in these patients.

Non-dialysis patients with symptomatic anemia considered for therapy should have a hemoglobin less than 10 g/dL.

PROCRIT® is not intended for patients who require immediate correction of severe anemia. PROCRIT® may obviate the need for maintenance transfusions but is not a substitute for emergency transfusion.

Prior to initiation of therapy, the patient's iron stores should be evaluated. Transferrin saturation should be at least 20% and ferritin at least 100 ng/mL. Blood pressure should be adequately controlled prior to initiation of PROCRIT® therapy, and must be closely monitored and controlled during therapy.

PROCRIT® should be administered under the guidance of a qualified physician (see DOSAGE AND ADMINISTRATION).

Treatment of Anemia in Zidovudine-treated HIV-infected Patients

PROCRIT® is indicated for the treatment of anemia related to therapy with zidovudine in HIV-infected patients. PROCRIT® is indicated to elevate or maintain the red blood cell level (as manifested by the hematocrit or hemoglobin determinations) and to decrease the need for transfusions in these patients. PROCRIT® is not indicated for the treatment of anemia in HIV-infected patients due to other factors such as iron or folate deficiencies, hemolysis, or gastrointestinal bleeding, which should be managed appropriately.

PROCRIT®, at a dose of 100 Units/kg TIW, is effective in decreasing the transfusion requirement and increasing the red blood cell level of anemic, HIV-infected patients treated with zidovudine, when the endogenous serum erythropoietin level is ≤ 500 mUnits/mL and when patients are receiving a dose of zidovudine ≤ 4200 mg/week.

Treatment of Anemia in Cancer Patients on Chemotherapy

PROCRIT® is indicated for the treatment of anemia in patients with non-myeloid malignancies where anemia is due to the effect of concomitantly administered chemotherapy. PROCRIT® is indicated to decrease the need for transfusions in patients who will be receiving concomitant chemotherapy for a minimum of 2 months. PROCRIT® is not indicated for the treatment of anemia in cancer patients due to other factors such as iron or folate deficiencies, hemolysis, or gastrointestinal bleeding, which should be managed appropriately.

Reduction of Allogeneic Blood Transfusion in Surgery Patients

PROCRIT® is indicated for the treatment of anemic patients (hemoglobin > 10 to ≤ 13 g/dL) scheduled to undergo elective, noncardiac, nonvascular surgery to reduce the need for allogeneic blood transfusions.[18-20] PROCRIT® is indicated for patients at high risk for perioperative transfusions with significant, anticipated blood loss. PROCRIT® is not indicated for anemic patients who are willing to donate autologous blood. The safety of the perioperative use of PROCRIT® has been studied only in patients who are receiving anticoagulant prophylaxis.

Proportion of Patients Transfused During Chemotherapy (Efficacy Population[a])

Chemotherapy Regimen	On Study[b]		During Months 2 and 3[c]	
	PROCRIT®	Placebo	PROCRIT®	Placebo
Regimens without cisplatin	44% (15/34)	44% (16/36)	21% (6/29)	33% (11/33)
Regimens containing cisplatin	50% (14/28)	63% (19/30)	23% (5/22)[d]	56% (14/25)
Combined	47% (29/62)	53% (35/66)	22% (11/51)[d]	43% (25/58)

[a] Limited to patients remaining on study at least 15 days (1 patient excluded from PROCRIT®, 2 patients excluded from placebo).
[b] Includes all transfusions from day 1 through the end of study.
[c] Limited to patients remaining on study beyond week 6 and includes only transfusions during weeks 5–12.
[d] Unadjusted 2-sided $p < 0.05$.

CLINICAL EXPERIENCE: RESPONSE TO PROCRIT®

Chronic Renal Failure Patients

Response to PROCRIT® was consistent across all studies. In the presence of adequate iron stores (see IRON EVALUATION), the time to reach the target hematocrit is a function of the baseline hematocrit and the rate of hematocrit rise.

The rate of increase in hematocrit is dependent upon the dose of PROCRIT® administered and individual patient variation. In clinical trials at starting doses of 50 to 150 Units/kg TIW, adult patients responded with an average rate of hematocrit rise of:

Starting Dose (TIW IV)	Hematocrit Increase Points/Day	Points/2 Weeks
50 Units/kg	0.11	1.5
100 Units/kg	0.18	2.5
150 Units/kg	0.25	3.5

Over this dose range, approximately 95% of all patients responded with a clinically significant increase in hematocrit, and by the end of approximately 2 months of therapy virtually all patients were transfusion-independent. Changes in the quality of life of adult patients treated with PROCRIT® were assessed as part of a phase 3 clinical trial.[5,8] Once the target hematocrit (32% to 38%) was achieved, statistically significant improvements were demonstrated for most quality of life parameters measured, including energy and activity level, functional ability, sleep and eating behavior, health status, satisfaction with health, sex life, well-being, psychological effect, life satisfaction, and happiness. Patients also reported improvement in their disease symptoms. They showed a statistically significant increase in exercise capacity (VO_2 max), energy, and strength with a significant reduction in aching, dizziness, anxiety, shortness of breath, muscle weakness, and leg cramps.[8,21]

Adult Patients on Dialysis: Thirteen clinical studies were conducted, involving IV administration to a total of 1010 anemic patients on dialysis for 986 patient-years of PROCRIT® therapy. In the three largest of these clinical trials, the median maintenance dose necessary to maintain the hematocrit between 30% to 36% was approximately 75 Units/kg TIW. In the US multicenter phase 3 study, approximately 65% of the patients required doses of 100 Units/kg TIW, or less, to maintain their hematocrit at approximately 35%. Almost 10% of patients required a dose of 25 Units/kg, or less, and approximately 10% required a dose of more than 200 Units/kg TIW to maintain their hematocrit at this level.

A multicenter unit dose study was also conducted in 119 patients receiving peritoneal dialysis who self-administered PROCRIT® subcutaneously for approximately 109 patient-years of experience. Patients responded to PROCRIT® administered SC in a manner similar to patients receiving IV administration.[22]

Pediatric Patients on Dialysis: One hundred twenty-eight children from 2 months to 19 years of age with CRF requiring dialysis were enrolled in 4 clinical studies of PROCRIT®. The largest study was a placebo-controlled, randomized trial in 113 children with anemia (hematocrit ≤ 27%) undergoing peritoneal dialysis or hemodialysis. The initial dose of PROCRIT® was 50 Units/kg IV or SC TIW. The dose of study drug was titrated to achieve either a hematocrit of 30% to 36% or an absolute increase in hematocrit of 6 percentage points over baseline.

At the end of the initial 12 weeks, a statistically significant rise in mean hematocrit (9.4% vs 0.9%) was observed only in the PROCRIT® arm. The proportion of children achieving a hematocrit of 30%, or an increase in hematocrit of 6 percentage points over baseline, at any time during the first 12 weeks was higher in the PROCRIT® arm (96% vs 58%). Within 12 weeks of initiating PROCRIT® therapy, 92.3% of the pediatric patients were transfusion-independent as compared to 65.4% who received placebo. Among patients who received 36 weeks of PROCRIT®, hemodialysis patients required a higher median maintenance dose (167 Units/kg/week [n = 28] vs 76 Units/kg/week [n = 36]) and took longer to achieve a hematocrit of 30% to 36% (median time to response 69 days vs 32 days) than patients undergoing peritoneal dialysis.

Patients With CRF Not Requiring Dialysis

Four clinical trials were conducted in patients with CRF not on dialysis involving 181 patients treated with PROCRIT® for approximately 67 patient-years of experience. These patients responded to PROCRIT® therapy in a manner similar to that observed in patients on dialysis. Patients with CRF not on dialysis demonstrated a dose-dependent and sustained increase in hematocrit when PROCRIT® was administered by either an IV or SC route, with similar rates of rise of hematocrit when PROCRIT® was administered by either route. Moreover, PROCRIT® doses of 75 to 150 Units/kg per week have been shown to maintain hematocrits of 36% to 38% for up to 6 months. Correcting the anemia of progressive renal failure will allow patients to remain active even though their renal function continues to decrease.[23-24]

Zidovudine-treated HIV-infected Patients

PROCRIT® has been studied in four placebo-controlled trials enrolling 297 anemic (hematocrit < 30%) HIV-infected (AIDS) patients receiving concomitant therapy with zidovudine (all patients were treated with Epoetin alfa manufactured by Amgen Inc). In the subgroup of patients (89/125 PROCRIT® and 88/130 placebo) with prestudy endogenous serum erythropoietin levels ≤ 500 mUnits/mL, PROCRIT® reduced the mean cumulative number of units of blood transfused per patient by approximately 40% as compared to the placebo group.[25] Among those patients who required transfusions at baseline, 43% of patients treated with PROCRIT® versus 18% of placebo-treated patients were transfusion-independent during the second and third months of therapy. PROCRIT® therapy also resulted in significant increases in hematocrit in comparison to placebo. When examining the results according to the weekly dose of zidovudine received during month 3 of therapy, there was a statistically significant ($p < 0.003$) reduction in transfusion requirements in patients treated with PROCRIT® (n = 51) compared to placebo treated patients (n = 54) whose mean weekly zidovudine dose was ≤ 4200 mg/week.[25]

Approximately 17% of the patients with endogenous serum erythropoietin levels ≤ 500 mUnits/mL receiving PROCRIT® in doses from 100 to 200 Units/kg TIW achieved a hematocrit of 38% without administration of transfusions or significant reduction in zidovudine dose. In the subgroup of patients whose prestudy endogenous serum erythropoietin levels were > 500 mUnits/mL, PROCRIT® therapy did not reduce transfusion requirements or increase hematocrit, compared to the corresponding responses in placebo-treated patients.

In a 6 month open-label PROCRIT® study, patients responded with decreased transfusion requirements and sustained increases in hematocrit and hemoglobin with doses of PROCRIT® up to 300 Units/kg TIW.[25-27]

Responsiveness to PROCRIT® therapy may be blunted by intercurrent infectious/inflammatory episodes and by an increase in zidovudine dosage. Consequently, the dose of PROCRIT® must be titrated based on these factors to maintain the desired erythropoietic response.

Cancer Patients on Chemotherapy

Three-Times Weekly (TIW) Dosing

PROCRIT® administered TIW has been studied in a series of six placebo-controlled, double-blind trials that enrolled 131 anemic cancer patients receiving PROCRIT® or matching placebo. Across all studies, 72 patients were treated with concomitant non cisplatin-containing chemotherapy regimens and 59 patients were treated with concomitant cisplatin-containing chemotherapy regimens. Patients were randomized to PROCRIT® 150 Units/kg or placebo subcutaneously TIW for 12 weeks in each study.

The results of the pooled data from these six studies are shown in the table below. Because of the length of time required for erythropoiesis and red cell maturation, the efficacy of PROCRIT® (reduction in proportion of patients requiring transfusions) is not manifested until 2 to 6 weeks after initiation of PROCRIT®.

[See first table above]

Intensity of chemotherapy in the above trials was not directly assessed, however the degree and timing of neutropenia was comparable across all trials. Available evidence suggests that patients with lymphoid and solid cancers respond similarly to PROCRIT® therapy, and that patients with or without tumor infiltration of the bone marrow respond similarly to PROCRIT® therapy.

Continued on next page

Procrit—Cont.

Weekly (QW) Dosing

PROCRIT® was also studied in a placebo-controlled, double-blind trial utilizing weekly dosing in a total of 344 anemic cancer patients. In this trial, 61 (35 placebo arm and 26 in the PROCRIT® arm) patients were treated with concomitant cisplatin containing regimens and 283 patients received concomitant chemotherapy regimens that did not contain cisplatinum. Patients were randomized to PROCRIT® 40,000 Units weekly (n = 174) or placebo (n = 170) SC for a planned treatment period of 16 weeks. If hemoglobin had not increased by > 1 g/dL, after 4 weeks of therapy or the patient received RBC transfusion during the first 4 weeks of therapy, study drug was increased to 60,000 Units weekly. Forty-three percent of patients in the Epoetin alfa group required an increase in PROCRIT® dose to 60,000 Units weekly.[25]

Results demonstrated that PROCRIT® therapy reduced the proportion of patients transfused in day 29 through week 16 of the study as compared to placebo. Twenty-five patients (14%) in the PROCRIT® group received transfusions compared to 48 patients (28%) in the placebo group (p = 0.0010) between day 29 and week 16 or the last day on study.

Comparable intensity of chemotherapy for patients enrolled in the two study arms was suggested by similarities in mean dose and frequency of administration for the 10 most commonly administered chemotherapy agents, and similarity in the incidence of changes in chemotherapy during the trial in the two arms.

Surgery Patients

PROCRIT® has been studied in a placebo-controlled, double-blind trial enrolling 316 patients scheduled for major, elective orthopedic hip or knee surgery who were expected to require ≥ 2 units of blood and who were not able or willing to participate in an autologous blood donation program. Based on previous studies which demonstrated that pretreatment hemoglobin is a predictor of risk of receiving transfusion,[20,28] patients were stratified into one of three groups based on their pretreatment hemoglobin [≤ 10 (n = 2), > 10 to ≤ 13 (n = 96), and > 13 to ≤ 15 g/dL (n = 218)] and then randomly assigned to receive 300 Units/kg PROCRIT®, 100 Units/kg PROCRIT® or placebo by SC injection for 10 days before surgery, on the day of surgery, and for 4 days after surgery.[18] All patients received oral iron and a low-dose post-operative warfarin regimen.[18]

Treatment with PROCRIT® 300 Units/kg significantly (p = 0.024) reduced the risk of allogeneic transfusion in patients with a pretreatment hemoglobin of > 10 to ≤ 13 g/dL; 5/31 (16%) of PROCRIT® 300 Units/kg, 6/26 (23%) of PROCRIT® 100 Units/kg, and 13/29 (45%) of placebo-treated patients were transfused.[18] There was no significant difference in the number of patients transfused between PROCRIT® (9% 300 Units/kg, 6% 100 Units/kg) and placebo (13%) in the > 13 to ≤ 15 g/dL hemoglobin stratum. There were too few patients in the ≤ 10 g/dL group to determine if PROCRIT® is useful in this hemoglobin strata. In the > 10 to ≤ 13 g/dL pretreatment stratum, the mean number of units transfused per PROCRIT®-treated patient (0.45 units blood for 300 Units/kg, 0.42 units blood for 100 Units/kg) was less than the mean transfused per placebo-treated patient (1.14 units) (overall p = 0.028). In addition, mean hemoglobin, hematocrit, and reticulocyte counts increased significantly during the presurgery period in patients treated with PROCRIT®.[18]

PROCRIT® was also studied in an open-label, parallel-group trial enrolling 145 subjects with a pretreatment hemoglobin level of ≥ 10 to ≤ 13 g/dL who were scheduled for major orthopedic hip or knee surgery and who were not participating in an autologous program.[19] Subjects were randomly assigned to receive one of two SC dosing regimens of PROCRIT® (600 Units/kg once weekly for 3 weeks prior to surgery and on the day of surgery or 300 Units/kg once daily for 10 days prior to surgery, on the day of surgery and for 4 days after surgery). All subjects received oral iron and appropriate pharmacologic anticoagulation therapy.

From pretreatment to presurgery, the mean increase in hemoglobin in 600 Units/kg weekly group (1.44 g/dL) was greater than observed in the 300 Units/kg daily group.[19] The mean increase in absolute reticulocyte count was smaller in the weekly group ($0.11 \times 10^6/mm^3$) compared to the daily group ($0.17 \times 10^6/mm^3$). Mean hemoglobin levels were similar for the two treatment groups throughout the post-surgical period.

The erythropoietic response observed in both treatment groups resulted in similar transfusion rates [11/69 (16%) in the 600 Units/kg weekly group and 14/71 (20%) in the 300 Units/kg daily group].[19] The mean number of units transfused per subject was approximately 0.3 units in both treatment groups.

CONTRAINDICATIONS

PROCRIT® is contraindicated in patients with:

1. Uncontrolled hypertension.
2. Known hypersensitivity to mammalian cell-derived products.
3. Known hypersensitivity to Albumin (Human).

WARNINGS

Pediatric Use

The multidose preserved formulation contains benzyl alcohol. Benzyl alcohol has been reported to be associated with an increased incidence of neurological and other complications in premature infants which are sometimes fatal.

Thrombotic Events and Increased Mortality

A randomized, prospective trial of 1265 hemodialysis patients with clinically evident cardiac disease (ischemic heart disease or congestive heart failure) was conducted in which patients were assigned to PROCRIT® treatment targeted to a maintenance hematocrit of either 42 ± 3% or 30 ± 3%.[42] Increased mortality was observed in 634 patients randomized to a target hematocrit of 42% [221 deaths (35% mortality)] compared to 631 patients targeted to remain at a hematocrit of 30% [185 deaths (29% mortality)]. The reason for increased mortality observed in these studies is unknown, however, the incidence of non-fatal myocardial infarctions (3.1% vs 2.3%), vascular access thromboses (39% vs 29%), and all other thrombotic events (22% vs 18%) were also higher in the group randomized to achieve a hematocrit of 42%.

Increased mortality was also observed in a randomized placebo-controlled study of PROCRIT® in adult patients who did not have CRF who were undergoing coronary artery bypass surgery (7 deaths in 126 patients randomized to PROCRIT® versus no deaths among 56 patients receiving placebo). Four of these deaths occurred during the period of study drug administration and all four deaths were associated with thrombotic events. While the extent of the population affected is unknown, in patients at risk for thrombosis, the anticipated benefits of PROCRIT® treatment should be weighed against the potential for increased risks associated with therapy.

In a randomized, prospective trial conducted with another Epoetin alfa product, in 939 women with metastatic carcinoma of the breast who were receiving chemotherapy, patients were assigned to receive either Epoetin alfa or placebo for up to a year, in a weekly schedule, with the primary goal of showing improved survival and improved quality of life in the Epoetin alfa treatment arm.[25] This study utilized a treatment strategy designed to maintain hemoglobin levels of 12 to 14 g/dL (hematocrit 36 to 42%). Increased mortality in the first 4 months after randomization was observed among 469 patients who received the erythropoietin product [41 deaths (8.7% mortality)] compared to 470 patients who received placebo [16 deaths (3.4% mortality)]. In the first four months of the study, the incidence of fatal thrombotic vascular events (1.1% vs 0.2%) and death attributed to disease progression (6.0% vs 2.8%) were both higher in the group randomized to receive Epoetin alfa as compared to placebo. Based on Kaplan-Meier estimates, the proportion of subjects surviving at 12 months after randomization was lower in the Epoetin alfa group than in the placebo group (70% vs 76%), p = 0.012, log rank. However, due to insufficient monitoring and data collection, reliable comparisons cannot be made concerning the effect of Epoetin alfa on overall time to disease progression, progression-free survival, and overall survival.

Pure Red Cell Aplasia

Pure red cell aplasia (PRCA), in association with neutralizing antibodies to native erythropoietin, has been observed in patients treated with recombinant erythropoietins. PRCA has been reported in a limited number of patients exposed to PROCRIT®. This has been reported predominantly in patients with CRF. Any patient with loss of response to PROCRIT® should be evaluated for the etiology of loss of effect (see PRECAUTIONS: LACK OR LOSS OF RESPONSE). PROCRIT® should be discontinued in any patient with evidence of PRCA and the patient evaluated for the presence of binding and neutralizing antibodies to PROCRIT®, native erythropoietin, and any other recombinant erythropoietin administered to the patient. Amgen/Ortho Biotech Products, L.P. should be contacted to assist in this evaluation. In patients with PRCA secondary to neutralizing antibodies to erythropoietin, PROCRIT® should not be administered and such patients should not be switched to another product as anti-erythropoietin antibodies cross-react with other erythropoietins (see ADVERSE REACTIONS).

Albumin (Human)

PROCRIT® contains albumin, a derivative of human blood. Based on effective donor screening and product manufacturing processes, it carries an extremely remote risk for transmission of viral diseases. A theoretical risk for transmission of Creutzfeldt-Jakob disease (CJD) also is considered extremely remote. No cases of transmission of viral diseases or CJD have ever been identified for albumin.

Chronic Renal Failure Patients

Hypertension: Patients with uncontrolled hypertension should not be treated with PROCRIT®; blood pressure should be controlled adequately before initiation of therapy. Up to 80% of patients with CRF have a history of hypertension.[29] Although there does not appear to be any direct pressor effects of PROCRIT®, blood pressure may rise during PROCRIT® therapy. During the early phase of treatment when the hematocrit is increasing, approximately 25% of patients on dialysis may require initiation of, or increases in, antihypertensive therapy. Hypertensive encephalopathy and seizures have been observed in patients with CRF treated with PROCRIT®.

Special care should be taken to closely monitor and aggressively control blood pressure in patients treated with PROCRIT®. Patients should be advised as to the importance of compliance with antihypertensive therapy and dietary restrictions. If blood pressure is difficult to control by initiation of appropriate measures, the hemoglobin may be reduced by decreasing or withholding the dose of PROCRIT®. A clinically significant decrease in hemoglobin may not be observed for several weeks.

It is recommended that the dose of PROCRIT® be decreased if the hemoglobin increase exceeds 1 g/dL in any 2-week period, because of the possible association of excessive rate of rise of hemoglobin with an exacerbation of hypertension. In CRF patients on hemodialysis with clinically evident ischemic heart disease or congestive heart failure, the hemoglobin should be managed carefully, not to exceed 12 g/dL (see THROMBOTIC EVENTS).

Seizures: Seizures have occurred in patients with CRF participating in PROCRIT® clinical trials.

In adult patients on dialysis, there was a higher incidence of seizures during the first 90 days of therapy (occurring in approximately 2.5% of patients) as compared with later timepoints.

Given the potential for an increased risk of seizures during the first 90 days of therapy, blood pressure and the presence of premonitory neurologic symptoms should be monitored closely. Patients should be cautioned to avoid potentially hazardous activities such as driving or operating heavy machinery during this period.

While the relationship between seizures and the rate of rise of hemoglobin is uncertain, it is recommended that the dose of PROCRIT® be decreased if the hemoglobin increase exceeds 1 g/dL in any 2-week period.

Thrombotic Events: During hemodialysis, patients treated with PROCRIT® may require increased anticoagulation with heparin to prevent clotting of the artificial kidney (see ADVERSE REACTIONS for more information about thrombotic events).

Other thrombotic events (eg, myocardial infarction, cerebrovascular accident, transient ischemic attack) have occurred in clinical trials at an annualized rate of less than 0.04 events per patient year of PROCRIT® therapy. These trials were conducted in adult patients with CRF (whether on dialysis or not) in whom the target hematocrit was 32% to 40%. However, the risk of thrombotic events, including vascular access thrombosis, was significantly increased in adult patients with ischemic heart disease or congestive heart failure receiving PROCRIT® therapy with the goal of reaching a normal hematocrit (42%) as compared to a target hematocrit of 30%. Patients with pre-existing cardiovascular disease should be monitored closely.

Zidovudine-treated HIV-infected Patients

In contrast to CRF patients, PROCRIT® therapy has not been linked to exacerbation of hypertension, seizures, and thrombotic events in HIV-infected patients.

PRECAUTIONS

The parenteral administration of any biologic product should be attended by appropriate precautions in case allergic or other untoward reactions occur (see CONTRAINDICATIONS). In clinical trials, while transient rashes were occasionally observed concurrently with PROCRIT® therapy, no serious allergic or anaphylactic reactions were reported (see ADVERSE REACTIONS for more information regarding allergic reactions).

The safety and efficacy of PROCRIT® therapy have not been established in patients with a known history of a seizure disorder or underlying hematologic disease (eg, sickle cell anemia, myelodysplastic syndromes, or hypercoagulable disorders).

In some female patients, menses have resumed following PROCRIT® therapy; the possibility of pregnancy should be discussed and the need for contraception evaluated.

Hematology

Exacerbation of porphyria has been observed rarely in patients with CRF treated with PROCRIT®. However, PROCRIT® has not caused increased urinary excretion of porphyrin metabolites in normal volunteers, even in the presence of a rapid erythropoietic response. Nevertheless, PROCRIT® should be used with caution in patients with known porphyria.

In preclinical studies in dogs and rats, but not in monkeys, PROCRIT® therapy was associated with subclinical bone marrow fibrosis. Bone marrow fibrosis is a known complication of CRF in humans and may be related to secondary hyperparathyroidism or unknown factors. The incidence of bone marrow fibrosis was not increased in a study of adult patients on dialysis who were treated with PROCRIT® for 12 to 19 months, compared to the incidence of bone marrow fibrosis in a matched group of patients who had not been treated with PROCRIT®.

Hemoglobin in CRF patients should be measured twice a week; zidovudine-treated HIV-infected and cancer patients should have hemoglobin measured once a week until hemoglobin has been stabilized, and measured periodically thereafter.

Lack or Loss of Response

If the patient fails to respond or to maintain a response to doses within the recommended dosing range, the following etiologies should be considered and evaluated:

1. Iron deficiency: Virtually all patients will eventually require supplemental iron therapy (see IRON EVALUATION).
2. Underlying infectious, inflammatory, or malignant processes.
3. Occult blood loss.
4. Underlying hematologic diseases (ie, thalassemia, refractory anemia, or other myelodysplastic disorders).
5. Vitamin deficiencies: Folic acid or vitamin B12.
6. Hemolysis.
7. Aluminum intoxication.
8. Osteitis fibrosa cystica.

9. Pure Red Cell Aplasia (PRCA):In the absence of another etiology, the patient should be evaluated for evidence of PRCA and sera should be tested for the presence of antibodies to recombinant erythropoietins.

Iron Evaluation

During PROCRIT® therapy, absolute or functional iron deficiency may develop. Functional iron deficiency, with normal ferritin levels but low transferrin saturation, is presumably due to the inability to mobilize iron stores rapidly enough to support increased erythropoiesis. Transferrin saturation should be at least 20% and ferritin should be at least 100 ng/mL.

Prior to and during PROCRIT® therapy, the patient's iron status, including transferrin saturation (serum iron divided by iron binding capacity) and serum ferritin, should be evaluated. Virtually all patients will eventually require supplemental iron to increase or maintain transferrin saturation to levels which will adequately support erythropoiesis stimulated by PROCRIT®. All surgery patients being treated with PROCRIT® should receive adequate iron supplementation throughout the course of therapy in order to support erythropoiesis and avoid depletion of iron stores.

Drug Interactions

No evidence of interaction of PROCRIT® with other drugs was observed in the course of clinical trials.

Carcinogenesis, Mutagenesis, and Impairment of Fertility

Carcinogenic potential of PROCRIT® has not been evaluated. PROCRIT® does not induce bacterial gene mutation (Ames Test), chromosomal aberrations in mammalian cells, micronuclei in mice, or gene mutation at the HGPRT locus. In female rats treated IV with PROCRIT®, there was a trend for slightly increased fetal wastage at doses of 100 and 500 Units/kg.

Pregnancy Category C

PROCRIT® has been shown to have adverse effects in rats when given in doses 5 times the human dose. There are no adequate and well-controlled studies in pregnant women. PROCRIT® should be used during pregnancy only if potential benefit justifies the potential risk to the fetus.

In studies in female rats, there were decreases in body weight gain, delays in appearance of abdominal hair, delayed eyelid opening, delayed ossification, and decreases in the number of caudal vertebrae in the F1 fetuses of the 500 Units/kg group. In female rats treated IV, there was a trend for slightly increased fetal wastage at doses of 100 and 500 Units/kg. PROCRIT® has not shown any adverse effect at doses as high as 500 Units/kg in pregnant rabbits (from day 6 to 18 of gestation).

Nursing Mothers

Postnatal observations of the live offspring (F1 generation) of female rats treated with PROCRIT® during gestation and lactation revealed no effect of PROCRIT® at doses of up to 500 Units/kg. There were, however, decreases in body weight gain, delays in appearance of abdominal hair, eyelid opening, and decreases in the number of caudal vertebrae in the F1 fetuses of the 500 Units/kg group. There were no PROCRIT®-related effects on the F2 generation fetuses.

It is not known whether PROCRIT® is excreted in human milk. Because many drugs are excreted in human milk, caution should be exercised when PROCRIT® is administered to a nursing woman.

Pediatric Use

See WARNINGS: PEDIATRIC USE.

Pediatric Patients on Dialysis: PROCRIT® is indicated in infants (1 month to 2 years), children (2 years to 12 years), and adolescents (12 years to 16 years) for the treatment of anemia associated with CRF requiring dialysis. Safety and effectiveness in pediatric patients less than 1 month old have not been established (see CLINICAL EXPERIENCE: CHRONIC RENAL FAILURE, *PEDIATRIC PATIENTS ON DIALYSIS*). The safety data from these studies show that there is no increased risk to pediatric CRF patients on dialysis when compared to the safety profile of PROCRIT® in adult CRF patients (see ADVERSE REACTIONS and WARNINGS). Published literature[30–33] provides supportive evidence of the safety and effectiveness of PROCRIT® in pediatric CRF patients on dialysis.

Pediatric Patients Not Requiring Dialysis: Published literature[33,34] has reported the use of PROCRIT® in 133 pediatric patients with anemia associated with CRF not requiring dialysis, ages 3 months to 20 years, treated with 50 to 250 Units/kg SC or IV, QW to TIW. Dose-dependent increases in hemoglobin and hematocrit were observed with reductions in transfusion requirements.

Pediatric HIV-infected Patients: Published literature[35,36] has reported the use of PROCRIT® in 20 zidovudine-treated anemic HIV-infected pediatric patients ages 8 months to 17 years, treated with 50 to 400 Units/kg SC or IV, 2 to 3 times per week. Increases in hemoglobin levels and in reticulocyte counts, and decreases in or elimination of blood transfusions were observed.

Pediatric Cancer Patients on Chemotherapy: Published literature[37,38] has reported the use of PROCRIT® in approximately 64 anemic pediatric cancer patients ages 6 months to 18 years, treated with 25 to 300 Units/kg SC or IV, 3 to 7 times per week. Increases in hemoglobin and decreases in transfusion requirements were noted.

Chronic Renal Failure Patients

Patients with CRF Not Requiring Dialysis

Blood pressure and hemoglobin should be monitored no less frequently than for patients maintained on dialysis. Renal function and fluid and electrolyte balance should be closely monitored, as an improved sense of well-being may obscure the need to initiate dialysis in some patients.

Hematology

Sufficient time should be allowed to determine a patient's responsiveness to a dosage of PROCRIT® before adjusting the dose. Because of the time required for erythropoiesis and the red cell half-life, an interval of 2 to 6 weeks may occur between the time of a dose adjustment (initiation, increase, decrease, or discontinuation) and a significant change in hemoglobin.

In order to avoid reaching the suggested target hemoglobin too rapidly, or exceeding the suggested target range (hemoglobin of 10 g/dL to 12 g/dL), the guidelines for dose and frequency of dose adjustments (see DOSAGE AND ADMINISTRATION) should be followed.

For patients who respond to PROCRIT® with a rapid increase in hemoglobin (eg, more than 1 g/dL in any 2-week period), the dose of PROCRIT® should be reduced because of the possible association of excessive rate of rise of hemoglobin with an exacerbation of hypertension.

The elevated bleeding time characteristic of CRF decreases toward normal after correction of anemia in adult patients treated with PROCRIT®. Reduction of bleeding time also occurs after correction of anemia by transfusion.

Laboratory Monitoring

The hemoglobin should be determined twice a week until it has stabilized in the suggested target range and the maintenance dose has been established. After any dose adjustment, the hemoglobin should also be determined twice weekly for at least 2 to 6 weeks until it has been determined that the hemoglobin has stabilized in response to the dose change. The hemoglobin should then be monitored at regular intervals.

A complete blood count with differential and platelet count should be performed regularly. During clinical trials, modest increases were seen in platelets and white blood cell counts. While these changes were statistically significant, they were not clinically significant and the values remained within normal ranges.

In patients with CRF, serum chemistry values (including blood urea nitrogen [BUN], uric acid, creatinine, phosphorus, and potassium) should be monitored regularly. During clinical trials in adult patients on dialysis, modest increases were seen in BUN, creatinine, phosphorus, and potassium. In some adult patients with CRF not on dialysis treated with PROCRIT®, modest increases in serum uric acid and phosphorus were observed. While changes were statistically significant, the values remained within the ranges normally seen in patients with CRF.

Diet

As the hemoglobin increases and patients experience an improved sense of well-being and quality of life, the importance of compliance with dietary and dialysis prescriptions should be reinforced. In particular, hyperkalemia is not uncommon in patients with CRF. In US studies in patients on dialysis, hyperkalemia has occurred at an annualized rate of approximately 0.11 episodes per patient-year of PROCRIT® therapy, often in association with poor compliance to medication, diet, and/or dialysis.

Dialysis Management

Therapy with PROCRIT® results in an increase in hematocrit and a decrease in plasma volume which could affect dialysis efficiency. In studies to date, the resulting increase in hematocrit did not appear to adversely affect dialyzer function[9,10] or the efficiency of high flux hemodialysis.[11] During hemodialysis, patients treated with PROCRIT® may require increased anticoagulation with heparin to prevent clotting of the artificial kidney.

Patients who are marginally dialyzed may require adjustments in their dialysis prescription. As with all patients on dialysis, the serum chemistry values (including BUN, creatinine, phosphorus, and potassium) in patients treated with PROCRIT® should be monitored regularly to assure the adequacy of the dialysis prescription.

Information for Patients

In those situations in which the physician determines that a home dialysis patient can safely and effectively self-administer PROCRIT®, the patient should be instructed as to the proper dosage and administration. Home dialysis patients should be referred to the full "Information For Home Dialysis Patients" insert; it is not a disclosure of all possible effects. Patients should be informed of the signs and symptoms of allergic drug reaction and advised of appropriate actions. If home use is prescribed for a home dialysis patient, the patient should be thoroughly instructed in the importance of proper disposal and cautioned against the reuse of needles, syringes, or drug product. A puncture-resistant container for the disposal of used syringes and needles should be available to the patient. The full container should be disposed of according to the directions provided by the physician.

Renal Function

In adult patients with CRF not on dialysis, renal function and fluid and electrolyte balance should be closely monitored, as an improved sense of well-being may obscure the need to initiate dialysis in some patients. In patients with CRF not on dialysis, placebo-controlled studies of progression of renal dysfunction over periods of greater than 1 year have not been completed. In shorter term trials in adult patients with CRF not on dialysis, changes in creatinine and creatinine clearance were not significantly different in patients treated with PROCRIT® compared with placebo-treated patients. Analysis of the slope of 1/serum creatinine versus time plots in these patients indicates no significant change in the slope after the initiation of PROCRIT® therapy.

Zidovudine-treated HIV-infected Patients

Hypertension

Exacerbation of hypertension has not been observed in zidovudine-treated HIV-infected patients treated with PROCRIT®. However, PROCRIT® should be withheld in these patients if pre-existing hypertension is uncontrolled, and should not be started until blood pressure is controlled. In double-blind studies, a single seizure has been experienced by a patient treated with PROCRIT®.[25]

Cancer Patients on Chemotherapy

Hypertension

Hypertension, associated with a significant increase in hemoglobin, has been noted rarely in patients treated with PROCRIT®. Nevertheless, blood pressure in patients treated with PROCRIT® should be monitored carefully, particularly in patients with an underlying history of hypertension or cardiovascular disease.

Seizures

In double-blind, placebo-controlled trials, 3.2% (n = 2/63) of patients treated with PROCRIT® TIW and 2.9% (n = 2/68) of placebo-treated patients had seizures. Seizures in 1.6% (n = 1/63) of patients treated with PROCRIT® TIW occurred in the context of a significant increase in blood pressure and hematocrit from baseline values. However, both patients treated with PROCRIT® also had underlying CNS pathology which may have been related to seizure activity.

In a placebo-controlled, double-blind trial utilizing weekly dosing with PROCRIT®, 1.2% (n = 2/168) of safety-evaluable patients treated with PROCRIT® and 1% (n = 1/165) of placebo-treated patients had seizures. Seizures in the patients treated with weekly PROCRIT® occurred in the context of a significant increase in hemoglobin from baseline values however significant increases in blood pressure were not seen. These patients may have had other CNS pathology.

Thrombotic Events

In double-blind, placebo-controlled trials, 3.2% (n = 2/63) of patients treated with PROCRIT® TIW and 11.8% (n = 8/68) of placebo-treated patients had thrombotic events (eg, pulmonary embolism, cerebrovascular accident) (See WARNINGS; THROMBOTIC EVENTS AND INCREASED MORTALITY).

In a placebo-controlled, double-blind trial utilizing weekly dosing with PROCRIT®, 6.0% (n = 10/168) of safety-evaluable patients treated with PROCRIT® and 3.6% (n = 6/165) (p = 0.444) of placebo-treated patients had clinically significant thrombotic events (deep vein thrombosis requiring anticoagulant therapy, embolic event including pulmonary embolism, myocardial infarction, cerebral ischemia, left ventricular failure and thrombotic microangiopathy). A definitive relationship between the rate of hemoglobin increase and the occurrence of clinically significant thrombotic events could not be evaluated due to the limited schedule of hemoglobin measurements in this study.

Tumor Growth Factor Potential

PROCRIT® is a growth factor that primarily stimulates red cell production. Erythropoietin receptors are also found to be present on the surface of some malignant cell lines and tumor biopsy specimens. However, it is not known if these receptors are functional. A randomized, placebo-controlled trial was conducted in 224 chemotherapy-naive, non-anemic patients with small cell lung cancer receiving cisplatin-based combination chemotherapy, to investigate whether the concurrent use of PROCRIT® stimulated tumor growth as assessed by impact on overall response rate. Patients were randomized to receive PROCRIT® 150 Units/kg or placebo subcutaneously TIW during chemotherapy. The overall response rates, after 3 cycles of treatment, were 72% and 67%, in the PROCRIT® and placebo arms, respectively. Complete response rates (17% vs. 14%) and median overall survival (10.5 mos vs. 10.4 mos) were similar in the PROCRIT® and placebo arms.[25]

Two additional studies explored effect on survival and/or progression of administrations of other exogenous erythropoietin with higher hemoglobin targets.

In a randomized, placebo-controlled study using another Epoetin alfa product, conducted in 939 women with metastatic breast cancer, study drug dosing was titrated to attempt to maintain hemoglobin levels between 12 and 14 g/dL. At four months, death attributed to disease progression was higher (6% vs 3%) in women receiving Epoetin alfa. Overall mortality was significantly higher at 12 months in the Epoetin alfa arm (See WARNINGS; THROMBOTIC EVENTS AND INCREASED MORTALITY).

In a randomized, placebo-controlled study using Epoetin beta, conducted in 351 patients with head and neck cancer, study drug was administered with the aim of achieving a hemoglobin level of 14 g/dL in women and 15 g/dL in men. Locoregional progression-free survival was significantly shorter (median PFS: 406 days Epoetin beta vs 745 days placebo, p = 0.04) in patients receiving Epoetin beta.[43]

There is insufficient information to establish whether use of Epoetin products, including PROCRIT®, have an adverse effect on time to tumor progression or progression-free survival.

These trials permitted or required dosing to achieve hemoglobin of greater than 12 g/dL. Until further information is available, the recommended target hemoglobin should not exceed 12 g/dL in men or women.

Surgery Patients

Thrombotic/Vascular Events

In perioperative clinical trials with orthopedic patients, the overall incidence of thrombotic/vascular events was similar

Continued on next page

Procrit—Cont.

in Epoetin alfa and placebo-treated patients who had a pretreatment hemoglobin of > 10 to ≤ 13 g/dL. In patients with a hemoglobin of > 13 g/dL treated with 300 Units/kg of Epoetin alfa, the possibility that PROCRIT® treatment may be associated with an increased risk of postoperative thrombotic/vascular events cannot be excluded.[18–20,28]

In one study in which Epoetin alfa was administered in the perioperative period to patients undergoing coronary artery bypass graft surgery, there were 7 deaths in the group treated with Epoetin alfa (n = 126) and no deaths in the placebo-treated group (n = 56). Among the 7 deaths in the patients treated with Epoetin alfa, 4 were at the time of therapy (between study day 2 and 8). The 4 deaths at the time of therapy (3%) were associated with thrombotic/vascular events. A causative role of Epoetin alfa cannot be excluded (see WARNINGS).

Hypertension

Blood pressure may rise in the perioperative period in patients being treated with PROCRIT®. Therefore, blood pressure should be monitored carefully.

ADVERSE REACTIONS

Immunogenicity

As with all therapeutic proteins, there is the potential for immunogenicity. The observed incidence of antibody positivity in an assay may be influenced by several factors including assay methodology, sample handling, timing of sample collection, concomitant medications, and underlying disease. For these reasons, comparison of the incidence of antibodies to PROCRIT® with the incidence of antibodies to other products may be misleading.

A few cases of PRCA associated with antibodies with neutralizing activity have been reported in patients receiving PROCRIT® (see WARNINGS: PURE RED CELL APLASIA). These cases were observed in patients treated by either SC or IV routes of administration and occurred predominantly in CRF patients.

Chronic Renal Failure Patients

PROCRIT® is generally well-tolerated. The adverse events reported are frequent sequelae of CRF and are not necessarily attributable to PROCRIT® therapy. In double-blind, placebo-controlled studies involving over 300 patients with CRF, the events reported in greater than 5% of patients treated with PROCRIT® during the blinded phase were:

	Percent of Patients Reporting Event	
Event	**Patients Treated With PROCRIT® (n = 200)**	**Placebo-treated Patients (n = 135)**
Hypertension	24%	19%
Headache	16%	12%
Arthralgias	11%	6%
Nausea	11%	9%
Edema	9%	10%
Fatigue	9%	14%
Diarrhea	9%	6%
Vomiting	8%	5%
Chest Pain	7%	9%
Skin Reaction (Administration Site)	7%	12%
Asthenia	7%	12%
Dizziness	7%	13%
Clotted Access	7%	2%

Significant adverse events of concern in patients with CRF treated in double-blind, placebo-controlled trials occurred in the following percent of patients during the blinded phase of the studies:

Seizure	1.1%	1.1%
CVA/TIA	0.4%	0.6%
MI	0.4%	1.1%
Death	0	1.7%

In the US PROCRIT® studies in adult patients on dialysis (over 567 patients), the incidence (number of events per patient-year) of the most frequently reported adverse events were: hypertension (0.75), headache (0.40), tachycardia (0.31), nausea/vomiting (0.26), clotted vascular access (0.25), shortness of breath (0.14), hyperkalemia (0.11), and diarrhea (0.11). Other reported events occurred at a rate of less than 0.10 events per patient per year.

Events reported to have occurred within several hours of administration of PROCRIT® were rare, mild, and transient, and included injection site stinging in dialysis patients and flu-like symptoms such as arthralgias and myalgias.

In all studies analyzed to date, PROCRIT® administration was generally well-tolerated, irrespective of the route of administration.

Pediatric CRF Patients: In pediatric patients with CRF on dialysis, the pattern of most adverse events was similar to that found in adults. Additional adverse events reported during the double-blind phase in > 10% of pediatric patients in either treatment group were: abdominal pain, dialysis access complications including access infections and peritonitis in those receiving peritoneal dialysis, fever, upper respiratory infection, cough, pharyngitis, and constipation. The rates are similar between the treatment groups for each event.

Hypertension: Increases in blood pressure have been reported in clinical trials, often during the first 90 days of therapy. On occasion, hypertensive encephalopathy and seizures have been observed in patients with CRF treated with PROCRIT®. When data from all patients in the US phase 3 multicenter trial were analyzed, there was an apparent trend of more reports of hypertensive adverse events in patients on dialysis with a faster rate of rise of hematocrit (greater than 4 hematocrit points in any 2-week period). However, in a double-blind, placebo-controlled trial, hypertensive adverse events were not reported at an increased rate in the group treated with PROCRIT® (150 Units/kg TIW) relative to the placebo group.

Seizures: There have been 47 seizures in 1010 patients on dialysis treated with PROCRIT® in clinical trials, with an exposure of 986 patient-years for a rate of approximately 0.048 events per patient-year. However, there appeared to be a higher rate of seizures during the first 90 days of therapy (occurring in approximately 2.5% of patients) when compared to subsequent 90-day periods. The baseline incidence of seizures in the untreated dialysis population is difficult to determine; it appears to be in the range of 5% to 10% per patient-year.[39–41]

Thrombotic Events: In clinical trials where the maintenance hematocrit was 35 ± 3% on PROCRIT®, clotting of the vascular access (A-V shunt) has occurred at an annualized rate of about 0.25 events per patient-year, and other thrombotic events (eg, myocardial infarction, cerebral vascular accident, transient ischemic attack, and pulmonary embolism) occurred at a rate of 0.04 events per patient-year. In a separate study of 1111 untreated dialysis patients, clotting of the vascular access occurred at a rate of 0.50 events per patient-year. However, in CRF patients on hemodialysis who also had clinically evident ischemic heart disease or congestive heart failure, the risk of A-V shunt thrombosis was higher (39% vs 29%, $p < 0.001$), and myocardial infarction, vascular ischemic events, and venous thrombosis were increased, in patients targeted to a hematocrit of 42 ± 3% compared to those maintained at 30 ± 3% (see WARNINGS).

In patients treated with commercial PROCRIT®, there have been rare reports of serious or unusual thrombo-embolic events including migratory thrombophlebitis, microvascular thrombosis, pulmonary embolus, and thrombosis of the retinal artery, and temporal and renal veins. A causal relationship has not been established.

Allergic Reactions: There have been no reports of serious allergic reactions or anaphylaxis associated with PROCRIT® administration during clinical trials. Skin rashes and urticaria have been observed rarely and when reported have generally been mild and transient in nature. There have been rare reports of potentially serious allergic reactions including urticaria with associated respiratory symptoms or circumoral edema, or urticaria alone. Most reactions occurred in situations where a causal relationship could not be established. Symptoms recurred with rechallenge in a few instances, suggesting that allergic reactivity may occasionally be associated with PROCRIT® therapy. If an anaphylactoid reaction occurs, PROCRIT® should be immediately discontinued and appropriate therapy initiated.

Zidovudine-treated HIV-infected Patients

Adverse events reported in clinical trials with PROCRIT® in zidovudine-treated HIV-infected patients were consistent with the progression of HIV infection. In double-blind, placebo-controlled studies of 3 months duration involving approximately 300 zidovudine-treated HIV-infected patients, adverse events with an incidence of ≥ 10% in either patients treated with PROCRIT® or placebo-treated patients were:

	Percent of Patients Reporting Event	
Event	**Patients Treated With PROCRIT® (n = 144)**	**Placebo-treated Patients (n = 153)**
Pyrexia	38%	29%
Fatigue	25%	31%
Headache	19%	14%
Cough	18%	14%
Diarrhea	16%	18%
Rash	16%	8%
Congestion, Respiratory	15%	10%
Nausea	15%	12%
Shortness of Breath	14%	13%
Asthenia	11%	14%
Skin Reaction, (Medication Site)	10%	7%
Dizziness	9%	10%

In the 297 patients studied, PROCRIT® was not associated with significant increases in opportunistic infections or mortality.[25] In 71 patients from this group treated with PROCRIT® at 150 Units/kg TIW, serum p24 antigen levels did not appear to increase.[27] Preliminary data showed no enhancement of HIV replication in infected cell lines *in vitro*.[25]

Peripheral white blood cell and platelet counts are unchanged following PROCRIT® therapy.

Allergic Reactions: Two zidovudine-treated HIV-infected patients had urticarial reactions within 48 hours of their first exposure to study medication. One patient was treated with PROCRIT® and one was treated with placebo (PROCRIT® vehicle alone). Both patients had positive immediate skin tests against their study medication with a negative saline control. The basis for this apparent pre-existing hypersensitivity to components of the PROCRIT® formulation is unknown, but may be related to HIV-induced immunosuppression or prior exposure to blood products.

Seizures: In double-blind and open-label trials of PROCRIT® in zidovudine-treated HIV-infected patients, 10 patients have experienced seizures.[25] In general, these seizures appear to be related to underlying pathology such as meningitis or cerebral neoplasms, not PROCRIT® therapy.

Cancer Patients on Chemotherapy

Adverse experiences reported in clinical trials with PROCRIT® administered TIW in cancer patients were consistent with the underlying disease state. In double-blind, placebo-controlled studies of up to 3 months duration involving 131 cancer patients, adverse events with an incidence > 10% in either patients treated with PROCRIT® or placebo-treated patients were as indicated below:

	Percent of Patients Reporting Event	
Event	**Patients Treated With PROCRIT® (n = 63)**	**Placebo-treated Patients (n = 68)**
Pyrexia	29%	19%
Diarrhea	21%*	7%
Nausea	17%*	32%
Vomiting	17%	15%
Edema	17%*	1%
Asthenia	13%	16%
Fatigue	13%	15%
Shortness of Breath	13%	9%
Paresthesia	11%	6%
Upper Respiratory Infection	11%	4%
Dizziness	5%	12%
Trunk Pain	3%*	16%

* Statistically significant

Although some statistically significant differences between patients treated with PROCRIT® and placebo-treated patients were noted, the overall safety profile of PROCRIT® appeared to be consistent with the disease process of advanced cancer. During double-blind and subsequent open-label therapy in which patients (n = 72 for total exposure to PROCRIT®) were treated for up to 32 weeks with doses as high as 927 Units/kg, the adverse experience profile of PROCRIT® was consistent with the progression of advanced cancer.

Three hundred thirty-three (333) cancer patients enrolled in a placebo-controlled, double-blind trial utilizing Weekly dosing with PROCRIT® for up to 4 months were evaluable for adverse events. The incidence of adverse events was similar in both treatment and placebo arms.

Surgery Patients

Adverse events with an incidence of ≥ 10% are shown in the following table:

[See table at top of next page]

Thrombotic/Vascular Events: In three double-blind, placebo-controlled orthopedic surgery studies, the rate of deep venous thrombosis (DVT) was similar among Epoetin alfa and placebo-treated patients in the recommended population of patients with a pretreatment hemoglobin of > 10 to ≤ 13 g/dL.[18,19,28] However, in 2 of 3 orthopedic surgery studies the overall rate (all pretreatment hemoglobin groups combined) of DVTs detected by postoperative ultrasonography and/or surveillance venography was higher in the group treated with Epoetin alfa than in the placebo-treated group (11% vs 6%). This finding was attributable to the difference in DVT rates observed in the subgroup of patients with pretreatment hemoglobin > 13 g/dL. However, the incidence of DVTs was within the range of that reported in the literature for orthopedic surgery patients.

In the orthopedic surgery study of patients with pretreatment hemoglobin of > 10 to ≤ 13 g/dL which compared two dosing regimens (600 Units/kg weekly × 4 and 300 Units/kg daily × 15), 4 subjects in the 600 Units/kg weekly PROCRIT® group (5%) and no subjects in the 300 Units/kg daily group had a thrombotic vascular event during the study period.[19]

In a study examining the use of Epoetin alfa in 182 patients scheduled for coronary artery bypass graft surgery, 23% of patients treated with Epoetin alfa and 29% treated with placebo experienced thrombotic/vascular events. There were 4 deaths among the Epoetin alfa-treated patients that were associated with a thrombotic/vascular event. A causative role of Epoetin alfa cannot be excluded (see WARNINGS).

OVERDOSAGE

The maximum amount of PROCRIT® that can be safely administered in single or multiple doses has not been determined. Doses of up to 1500 Units/kg TIW for 3 to 4 weeks have been administered to adults without any direct toxic effects of PROCRIT® itself.[6] Therapy with PROCRIT® can result in polycythemia if the hemoglobin is not carefully monitored and the dose appropriately adjusted. If the suggested target range is exceeded, PROCRIT® may be temporarily withheld until the hemoglobin returns to the suggested target range; PROCRIT® therapy may then be resumed using a lower dose (see DOSAGE AND ADMINISTRATION). If polycythemia is of concern, phlebotomy may be indicated to decrease the hemoglobin.

DOSAGE AND ADMINISTRATION

Chronic Renal Failure Patients

The recommended range for the starting dose of PROCRIT® is 50 to 100 Units/kg TIW for adult patients. The recommended starting dose for pediatric CRF patients on dialysis is 50 Units/kg TIW. The dose of PROCRIT® should be reduced as the hemoglobin approaches 12 g/dL or increases by more than 1 g/dL in any 2-week period. The dosage of PROCRIT® must be individualized to maintain the hemoglobin within the suggested target range. At the physician's discretion, the suggested target hemoglobin range may be expanded to achieve maximal patient benefit.

PROCRIT® may be given either as an IV or SC injection. In patients on hemodialysis, PROCRIT® usually has been administered as an IV bolus TIW. While the administration of PROCRIT® is independent of the dialysis procedure, PROCRIT® may be administered into the venous line at the end of the dialysis procedure to obviate the need for additional venous access. In adult patients with CRF not on dialysis, PROCRIT® may be given either as an IV or SC injection.

Patients who have been judged competent by their physicians to self-administer PROCRIT® without medical or other supervision may give themselves either an IV or SC injection. The table below provides general therapeutic guidelines for patients with CRF:

Starting Dose:	
Adults	50 to 100 Units/kg TIW; IV or SC
Pediatric Patients	50 Units/kg TIW; IV or SC
Reduce Dose When:	1. Hgb approaches 12 g/dL or, 2. Hgb increases > 1 g/dL in any 2-week period
Increase Dose If:	Hgb does not increase by 2 g/dL after 8 weeks of therapy, and hgb is below suggested target range
Maintenance Dose:	Individually titrate
Suggested Target Hgb Range:	10 g/dL to 12 g/dL

During therapy, hematological parameters should be monitored regularly (see LABORATORY MONITORING).

Pretherapy Iron Evaluation: Prior to and during PROCRIT® therapy, the patient's iron stores, including transferrin saturation (serum iron divided by iron binding capacity) and serum ferritin, should be evaluated. Transferrin saturation should be at least 20%, and ferritin should be at least 100 ng/mL. Virtually all patients will eventually require supplemental iron to increase or maintain transferrin saturation to levels that will adequately support erythropoiesis stimulated by PROCRIT®.

Dose Adjustment: The dose should be adjusted for each patient to achieve and maintain a target hemoglobin not to exceed 12 g/dL.

Increases in dose should not be made more frequently than once a month. If the hemoglobin is increasing and approaching 12 g/dL, the dose should be reduced by approximately 25%. If the hemoglobin continues to increase, dose should be temporarily withheld until the hemoglobin begins to decrease, at which point therapy should be reinitiated at a dose approximately 25% below the previous dose. If the hemoglobin increases by more than 1 g/dL in a 2-week period, the dose should be decreased by approximately 25%.

If the increase in the hemoglobin is less than 1 g/dL over 4 weeks and iron stores are adequate (see PRECAUTIONS: LABORATORY MONITORING), the dose of PROCRIT® may be increased by approximately 25% of the previous dose. Further increases may be made at 4-week intervals until the specified hemoglobin is obtained.

Maintenance Dose: The maintenance dose must be individualized for each patient on dialysis. In the US phase 3 multicenter trial in patients on hemodialysis, the median maintenance dose was 75 Units/kg TIW, with a range from 12.5 to 525 Units/kg TIW. Almost 10% of the patients required a dose of 25 Units/kg, or less, and approximately 10% of the patients required more than 200 Units/kg TIW to maintain their hematocrit in the suggested target range. In pediatric hemodialysis and peritoneal dialysis patients, the median maintenance dose was 167 Units/kg/week (49 to 447 Units/kg per week) and 76 Units/kg per week (24 to 323 Units/kg/week) administered in divided doses (TIW or BIW), respectively to achieve the target range of 30% to 36%.

If the hemoglobin remains below, or falls below, the suggested target range, iron stores should be re-evaluated. If the transferrin saturation is less than 20%, supplemental iron should be administered. If the transferrin saturation is greater than 20%, the dose of PROCRIT® may be increased. Such dose increases should not be made more frequently than once a month, unless clinically indicated, as the response time of the hemoglobin to a dose increase can be 2 to 6 weeks. Hemoglobin should be measured twice weekly for 2 to 6 weeks following dose increases. In adult patients with CRF not on dialysis, the maintenance dose must also be individualized. PROCRIT® doses of 75 to 150 Units/kg/week have been shown to maintain hematocrits of 36% to 38% for up to 6 months.

Event	Percent of Patients Reporting Event: Patients Treated With PROCRIT® 300 U/kg (n = 112)[a]	Patients Treated With PROCRIT 100 U/kg (n = 101)[a]	Placebo-treated Patients (n = 103)[a]	Patients Treated With PROCRIT 600 U/kg (n = 73)[b]	Patients Treated With PROCRIT 300 U/kg (n = 72)[b]
Pyrexia	51%	50%	60%	47%	42%
Nausea	48%	43%	45%	45%	58%
Constipation	43%	42%	43%	51%	53%
Skin Reaction (Medication Site)	25%	19%	22%	26%	29%
Vomiting	22%	12%	14%	21%	29%
Skin Pain	18%	18%	17%	5%	4%
Pruritus	16%	16%	14%	14%	22%
Insomnia	13%	16%	13%	21%	18%
Headache	13%	11%	9%	10%	19%
Dizziness	12%	9%	12%	11%	21%
Urinary Tract Infection	12%	3%	11%	11%	8%
Hypertension	10%	11%	10%	5%	10%
Diarrhea	10%	7%	12%	10%	6%
Deep Venous Thrombosis	10%	3%	5%	0%	0%
Dyspepsia	9%	11%	6%	7%	8%
Anxiety	7%	2%	11%	11%	4%
Edema	6%	11%	8%	11%	7%

[a] Study including patients undergoing orthopedic surgery treated with PROCRIT® or placebo for 15 days

[b] Study including patients undergoing orthopedic surgery treated with PROCRIT® 600 Units/kg weekly × 4 or 300 Units/kg daily ×15

[c] Determined by clinical symptoms

Lack or Loss of Response: Over 95% of patients with CRF responded with clinically significant increases in hematocrit, and virtually all patients were transfusion-independent within approximately 2 months of initiation of PROCRIT® therapy.

If a patient fails to respond or maintain a response, other etiologies should be considered and evaluated as clinically indicated (see PRECAUTIONS: LACK OR LOSS OF RESPONSE).

Zidovudine-treated HIV-infected Patients

Prior to beginning PROCRIT®, it is recommended that the endogenous serum erythropoietin level be determined (prior to transfusion). Available evidence suggests that patients receiving zidovudine with endogenous serum erythropoietin levels > 500 mUnits/mL are unlikely to respond to therapy with PROCRIT®.

Starting Dose: For adult patients with serum erythropoietin levels ≤ 500 mUnits/mL who are receiving a dose of zidovudine ≤ 4200 mg/week, the recommended starting dose of PROCRIT® is 100 Units/kg as an IV or SC injection TIW for 8 weeks. For pediatric patients, see PRECAUTIONS: PEDIATRIC USE.

Increase Dose: During the dose adjustment phase of therapy, the hemoglobin should be monitored weekly. If the response is not satisfactory in terms of reducing transfusion requirements or increasing hemoglobin after 8 weeks of therapy, the dose of PROCRIT® can be increased by 50 to 100 Units/kg TIW. Response should be evaluated every 4 to 8 weeks thereafter and the dose adjusted accordingly by 50 to 100 Units/kg increments TIW. If patients have not responded satisfactorily to a PROCRIT® dose of 300 Units/kg TIW, it is unlikely that they will respond to higher doses of PROCRIT®.

Maintenance Dose: After attainment of the desired response (ie, reduced transfusion requirements or increased hemoglobin), the dose of PROCRIT® should be titrated to maintain the response based on factors such as variations in zidovudine dose and the presence of intercurrent infectious or inflammatory episodes. If the hemoglobin exceeds 13 g/dL, the dose should be discontinued until the hemoglobin drops to 12 g/dL. The dose should be reduced by 25% when treatment is resumed and then titrated to maintain the desired hemoglobin.

Cancer Patients on Chemotherapy

Although no specific serum erythropoietin level can be stipulated above which patients would be unlikely to respond to PROCRIT® therapy, treatment of patients with grossly elevated serum erythropoietin levels (eg, > 200 mUnits/mL) is not recommended. The hemoglobin should be monitored on a weekly basis in patients receiving PROCRIT® therapy until hemoglobin becomes stable. The dose of PROCRIT® should be titrated to maintain the desired hemoglobin.

Two PROCRIT® dosing regimens may be used in adults; 150 Units/kg SC TIW or 40,000 Units SC Weekly. For pediatric patients, see PRECAUTIONS: PEDIATRIC USE.

TIW Dosing	
Starting Dose:	
Adults	150 Units/kg SC TIW
Pediatric Patients	See PRECAUTIONS: PEDIATRIC USE
Reduce Dose by 25% when:	1. Hgb approaches 12 g/dL or, 2. Hgb increases > 1 g/dL in any 2-week period
Withhold Dose if:	Hgb exceeds 13 g/dL, until the hemoglobin fall to 12 g/dL, and restart dose at 25% below the previous dose
Increase Dose to 300 Units/kg TIW if:	response is not satisfactory [no reduction in transfusion requirements or rise in hemoglobin] after 8 weeks
Suggested Target Hgb Range:	10 g/dL to 12 g/dL

During therapy, hematological parameters should be monitored regularly (see PRECAUTIONS: LABORATORY MONITORING).

Weekly Dosing

- The starting dose in adults is 40,000 Units SC Weekly. If after 4 weeks of therapy, the hemoglobin has not increased by ≥ 1 g/dL, in the absence of RBC transfusion, the PROCRIT® dose should be increased to 60,000 Units Weekly.
- If patients have not responded satisfactorily to a PROCRIT® dose of 60,000 Units Weekly after 4 weeks, it is unlikely that they will respond to higher doses of PROCRIT®.
- PROCRIT® should be withheld if the hemoglobin exceeds 13 g/dL and reinitiated with a 25% dose reduction when the hemoglobin is less than 12 g/dL.
- If PROCRIT® treatment produces a very rapid hemoglobin response (e.g., an increase of more than 1 g/dL in any 2-week period), the dose of PROCRIT® should be reduced by 25%.

Surgery Patients

Prior to initiating treatment with PROCRIT® a hemoglobin should be obtained to establish that it is > 10 to ≤ 13 g/dL.[18] The recommended dose of PROCRIT® is 300 Units/kg/day subcutaneously for 10 days before surgery, on the day of surgery, and for 4 days after surgery.

An alternate dose schedule is 600 Units/kg PROCRIT® subcutaneously in once weekly doses (21, 14 and 7 days before surgery) plus a fourth dose on day of surgery.[19]

All patients should receive adequate iron supplementation. Iron supplementation should be initiated no later than the beginning of treatment with PROCRIT® and should continue throughout the course of therapy.

PREPARATION AND ADMINISTRATION OF PROCRIT®

1. Do not shake. It is not necessary to shake PROCRIT®. Prolonged vigorous shaking may denature any glycoprotein, rendering it biologically inactive.
2. Parenteral drug products should be inspected visually for particulate matter and discoloration prior to administration. Do not use any vials exhibiting particulate matter or discoloration.
3. Using aseptic techniques, attach a sterile needle to a sterile syringe. Remove the flip top from the vial containing PROCRIT®, and wipe the septum with a disinfectant. Insert the needle into the vial, and withdraw into the syringe an appropriate volume of solution.
4. **Single-dose:** 1 mL vial contains no preservative. Use one dose per vial; do not re-enter vial. Discard unused portions.
   Multidose: 1 mL and 2 mL vials contain preservative. Store at 2° to 8°C after initial entry and between doses. Discard 21 days after initial entry.
5. Do not dilute or administer in conjunction with other drug solutions. However, at the time of SC administration, preservative-free PROCRIT® from single-use vials may be admixed in a syringe with bacteriostatic 0.9% sodium chloride injection, USP, with benzyl alcohol 0.9% (bacteriostatic saline) at a 1:1 ratio using aseptic technique. The benzyl alcohol in the bacteriostatic saline acts as a local anesthetic which may ameliorate SC injection

Continued on next page

Procrit—Cont.

site discomfort. Admixing is not necessary when using the multidose vials of PROCRIT® containing benzyl alcohol.

HOW SUPPLIED

PROCRIT®, containing Epoetin alfa, is available in vials containing color coded labels and caps.

1 mL **Single-Dose, Preservative-free** Solution

Each dosage form is supplied in the following packages:

Cartons containing six (6) **single-dose** vials:
- 2000 Units/mL (NDC 59676-302-01) (Purple)
- 3000 Units/mL (NDC 59676-303-01) (Magenta)
- 4000 Units/mL (NDC 59676-304-01) (Green)
- 10,000 Units/mL (NDC 59676-310-01) (Red)

Cartons containing four (4) **single-dose** vials:
- 40,000 Units/mL (NDC 59676-340-01) (Orange)

Trays containing twenty-five (25) **single-dose** vials:
- 2000 Units/mL (NDC 59676-302-02) (Purple)
- 3000 Units/mL (NDC 59676-303-02) (Magenta)
- 4000 Units/mL (NDC 59676-304-02) (Green)
- 10,000 Units/mL (NDC 59676-310-02) (Red)

2 mL **Multidose, Preserved** Solution

Cartons containing six (6) **multidose** vials:
- 10,000 Units/mL (NDC 59676-312-01) (Blue)

1 mL **Multidose, Preserved** Solution

Cartons containing six (6) **multidose** vials:
- 20,000 Units/mL (NDC 59676-320-01) (Lime)

STORAGE

Store at 2° to 8° C (36° to 46° F). Do not freeze or shake.

REFERENCES

1. Egrie JC, Strickland TW, Lane J, et al. Characterization and Biological Effects of Recombinant Human Erythropoietin. *Immunobiol.* 1986;72:213–224. 2. Graber SE, Krantz SB. Erythropoietin and the Control of Red Cell Production. *Ann Rev Med.* 1978;29:51–66. 3. Eschbach JW, Adamson JW. Anemia of End-Stage Renal Disease (ESRD). *Kidney Intl.* 1985;28:1–5. 4. Eschbach JW, Egrie JC, Downing MR, et al. Correction of the Anemia of End-Stage Renal Disease with Recombinant Human Erythropoietin. *NEJM.* 1987;316:73–78. 5. Eschbach JW, Abdulhadi MH, Browne JK, et al. Recombinant Human Erythropoietin in Anemic Patients with End-Stage Renal Disease. *Ann Intern Med.* 1989;111:992–1000. 6. Eschbach JW, Egrie JC, Downing MR, et al. The Use of Recombinant Human Erythropoietin (r-HuEPO): Effect in End-Stage Renal Disease (ESRD). In: Friedman, Beyer, DeSanto, Giordano, eds. *Prevention Of Chronic Uremia.* Philadelphia, PA: Field and Wood Inc. 1989;148–155. 7. Egrie JC, Eschbach JW, McGuire T, Adamson JW. Pharmacokinetics of Recombinant Human Erythropoietin (r-HuEPO) Administered to Hemodialysis (HD) Patients. *Kidney Intl.* 1988;33:262. 8. Evans RW, Rader B, Manninen DL, et al. The Quality of Life of Hemodialysis Recipients Treated with Recombinant Human Erythropoietin. *JAMA.* 1990;263:825–830. 9. Paganini E, Garcia J, Ellis P, et al. Clinical Sequelae of Correction of Anemia with Recombinant Human Erythropoietin (r-HuEPO); Urea Kinetics, Dialyzer Function and Reuse. *Am J Kid Dis.* 1988;11:16. 10. Delano BG, Lundin AP, Golansky R, et al. Dialyzer Urea and Creatinine Clearances Not Significantly Changed in r-HuEPO Treated Maintenance Hemodialysis (MD) Patients. *Kidney Intl.* 1988;33: 219. 11. Stivelman J, Van Wyck D, and Ogden D. Use of Recombinant Erythropoietin (r-HuEPO) with High Flux Dialysis (HFD) Does Not Worsen Azotemia or Shorten Access Survival. *Kidney Intl.* 1988;33:239. 12. Lim VS, DeGowin RL, Zavala D, et al. Recombinant Human Erythropoietin Treatment in Pre-Dialysis Patients: A Double-Blind Placebo Controlled Trial. *Ann Int Med.* 1989;110:108–114. 13. Stone WJ, Graber SE, Krantz SB, et al. Treatment of the Anemia of Pre-Dialysis Patients with Recombinant Human Erythropoietin: A Randomized, Placebo-Controlled Trial. *Am J Med Sci.* 1988;296:171–179. 14. Braun A, Ding R, Seidel C, Fies T, Kurtz A, Scharer K. Pharmacokinetics of recombinant human erythropoietin applied subcutaneously to children with chronic renal failure. *Pediatr Nephrol* 1993;7:61–64. 15. Geva P, Sherwood JB. Pharmacokinetics of recombinant human erythropoietin (rHuEPO) in pediatric patients on chronic cycling peritoneal dialysis (CCPD). *Blood.* 1991;78 (Suppl 1):91a. 16. Jabs K, Grant JR, Harmon W, et al. Pharmacokinetics of Epoetin alfa (rHuEPO) in pediatric hemodialysis (HD) patients. *J Am Soc Nephrol.* 1991;2:380. 17. Kling PJ, Widness JA, Guillery EN, Veng-Pedersen P, Peters C, DeAlarcon PA. Pharmacokinetics and pharmacodynamics of erythropoietin during therapy in an infant with renal failure. *J Pediatr.* 1992;121:822–825. 18. de Andrade JR and Jove M. Baseline Hemoglobin as a Predictor of Risk of Transfusion and Response to Epoetin alfa in Orthopedic Surgery Patients. *Am. J. of Orthoped.* 1996;25 (8): 533–542. 19. Goldberg MA and McCutchen JW. A Safety and Efficacy Comparison Study of Two Dosing Regimens of Epoetin alfa in Patients Undergoing Major Orthopedic Surgery. *Am. J. of Orthoped.* 1996;25 (8): 544–552. 20. Faris PM and Ritter MA. The Effects of Recombinant Human Erythropoietin on Perioperative Transfusion Requirements in Patients Having a Major Orthopedic Operation. *J. Bone and Joint Surgery.* 1996;78–A:62–72. 21. Lundin AP, Akerman MJH, Chesler RM, et al. Exercise in Hemodialysis Patients after Treatment with Recombinant Human Erythropoietin. *Nephron.* 1991;58:315–319. 22. Amgen Inc., data on file. 23. Eschbach JW, Kelly MR, Haley NR, et al. Treatment of the Anemia of Progressive Renal Failure with Recombinant Human Erythropoietin. *NEJM.* 1989;321:158–163. 24. The US Recombinant Human Erythropoietin Predialysis Study Group. Double-Blind, Placebo-Controlled Study of the Therapeutic Use of Recombinant Human Erythropoietin for Anemia Associated with Chronic Renal Failure in Predialysis Patients. *Am J Kid Dis.* 1991;18:50–59. 25. Ortho Biologics, Inc., data on file. 26. Danna RP, Rudnick SA, Abels RI. Erythropoietin Therapy for the Anemia Associated with AIDS and AIDS Therapy and Cancer. In: MB Garnick, ed. *Erythropoietin in Clinical Applications — An International Perspective.* New York, NY:Marcel Dekker. 1990;301–324. 27. Fischl M, Galpin JE, Levine JD, et al. Recombinant Human Erythropoietin for Patients with AIDS Treated with Zidovudine. *NEJM.* 1990;322:1488–1493. 28. Laupacis A. Effectiveness of Perioperative Recombinant Human Erythropoietin in Elective Hip Replacement. *Lancet.* 1993;341: 1228–1232. 29. Kerr DN. Chronic Renal Failure. In: Beeson PB, McDermott W, Wyngaarden JB, eds, *Cecil Textbook of Medicine.* Philadelphia, PA: W.B. Saunders; 1979;1351–1367. 30. Campos A, Garin EH. Therapy of renal anemia in children and adolescents with recombinant human erythropoietin (rHuEPO). *Clin Pediatr* (Phila). 1992;31:94–99. 31. Montini G, Zacchello G, Baraldi E, et al. Benefits and risks of anemia correction with recombinant human erythropoietin in children maintained by hemodialysis. *J Pediatr.* 1990;117:556–560. 32. Offner G, Hoyer PF, Latta K, Winkler L, Brodehl J, Scigalla P. One year's experience with recombinant erythropoietin in children undergoing continuous ambulatory or cycling peritoneal dialysis. *Pediatr Nephrol.* 1990;4:498–500. 33. Muller-Wiefel DE, Scigalla P. Specific problems of renal anemia in childhood. *Contrib Nephrol.* 1988;66:71–84. 34. Scharer K, Klare B, Dressel P, Gretz N. Treatment of renal anemia by subcutaneous erythropoietin in children with preterminal chronic renal failure. *Acta Paediatr.* 1993;82:953–958. 35. Mueller BU, Jacobsen RN, Jarosinski P, et al. Erythropoietin for zidovudine-associated anemia in children with HIV infection. *Pediatr AIDS and HIV Infect: Fetus to Adolesc.* 1994;5:169–173. 36. Zuccotti GV, Plebani A, Biasucci G, et al. Granulocyte-colony stimulating factor and erythropoietin therapy in children with human immunodeficiency virus infection. *J Int Med Res.* 1996;24:115–121. 37. Beck MN, Beck D. Recombinant erythropoietin in acute chemotherapy-induced anemia of children with cancer. *Med Pediatr Oncol.* 1995;25:17–21. 38. Bennetts G, Bertolone S, Bray G, Dinndorf P, Feusner J, Cairo M. Erythropoietin reduces volumes of red cell transfusions required in some subsets of children with acute lymphocytic leukemia. *Blood.* 1995;86:853a. 39. Raskin NH, Fishman RA. Neurologic Disorders in Renal Failure (First of Two Parts). *NEJM.* 1976;294:143–148. 40. Raskin NH and Fishman RA. Neurologic Disorders in Renal Failure (Second of Two Parts). *NEJM.* 1976;294:204–210. 41. Messing RO, Simon RP. Seizures as a Manifestation of Systemic Disease. *Neurologic Clinics.* 1986;4:563–584. 42. Besarab A, Bolton WK, Browne JK, et al. The effects of normal as compared with low hematocrit values in patients with cardiac disease who are receiving hemodialysis and epoetin. *NEJM.* 1998;339:584–90. 43. Henke, M, Laszig, R, Rübe, C, et al. Erythropoietin to treat head and neck cancer patients with anaemia undergoing radiotherapy: randomized, double-blind, placebo-controlled trial. *The Lancet.* 2003;362: 1255–1260.

Manufactured by:
Amgen Inc.
One Amgen Center Drive
Thousand Oaks, CA 91320-1799
Distributed by:
Ortho Biotech Products, L.P.
Raritan, New Jersey 08869-0670
ORTHO BIOTECH
Revised June 2004

638-10-979-3
Printed in U. S. A.

PROCRIT®
EPOETIN ALFA

INFORMATION FOR HOME DIALYSIS PATIENTS

What is PROCRIT® and how does it work?

PROCRIT® is a copy of human erythropoietin, a hormone produced primarily by healthy kidneys. PROCRIT® replaces the erythropoietin that the failed kidneys can no longer produce, and signals the bone marrow to make the oxygen-carrying red blood cells once again. PROCRIT® is produced in mammalian cells that have been genetically altered by the addition of a gene of the natural substance erythropoietin.

How should I take PROCRIT®?

In those situations where your doctor has determined that you, as a home dialysis patient, can self-administer PROCRIT®, you will receive instruction on how much PROCRIT® to use, how to inject it, how often you should inject it, and how you should dispose of the unused portions of each vial. You will be instructed to monitor your blood pressure carefully every day and to report any changes outside of the guidelines that your doctor has given you. When the number of red blood cells increases, your blood pressure can also increase, so your doctor may prescribe some new or additional blood pressure medication. Be sure to follow your doctor's orders. You may also be instructed to have certain laboratory tests, such as additional hematocrit or iron level measurements, done more frequently.You may be asked to report these tests to your doctor or dialysis center. Also, your doctor may prescribe additional iron for you to take. Be sure to comply with your doctor's orders. Continue to check your access, as your doctor or nurse has shown you, to make sure it is working. Be sure to let your health care professional know right away if there is a problem.

Allergy to PROCRIT®

Patients occasionally experience redness, swelling, or itching at the site of injection of PROCRIT®. This may indicate an allergy to the components of PROCRIT®, or it may indicate a local reaction. If you have a local reaction, consult your doctor. A potentially more serious reaction would be a generalized allergy to PROCRIT®, which could cause a rash over the whole body, shortness of breath, wheezing, reduction in blood pressure, fast pulse, or sweating. Severe cases of generalized allergy may be life-threatening. If you think you are having a generalized allergic reaction, stop taking PROCRIT® and notify a doctor or emergency medical personnel immediately.

How will I know if PROCRIT® is working?

The effectiveness of PROCRIT® is measured by the increase in hematocrit (the amount of red blood cells in the blood) that results from PROCRIT® therapy. The rise in hematocrit is not immediate. It usually takes about 2 to 6 weeks before the hematocrit starts to rise. The amount of time it takes, and the dose of PROCRIT® that is needed to make the hematocrit increase, varies from patient to patient.

What is the most important information I should know about PROCRIT® and CHRONIC RENAL FAILURE?

PROCRIT® has been prescribed for you by your doctor because you:

1. Have anemia due to your kidney disease.
2. Are able to dialyze at home.
3. Have been determined to be able to administer PROCRIT® without direct medical or other supervision.

A lack of energy or feeling of tiredness is the major symptom of anemia. Additional symptoms include shortness of breath, chest pain, and feeling cold all the time. The reason for these symptoms is that there is a lack of red blood cells. Red blood cells carry oxygen, which is important for all of the body's functions. When there are fewer red blood cells, the body does not get all the oxygen it needs.

Kidneys remove toxins from the blood; they also measure the amount of oxygen in the blood. If there is not enough oxygen, the kidneys will produce a hormone called erythropoietin. Erythropoietin is released into the bloodstream and travels to the bone marrow where red blood cells are made. Erythropoietin signals the bone marrow to make more oxygen-carrying red blood cells.

As the kidneys fail, they stop cleansing toxins from your blood. They also make less erythropoietin than they should. Therefore, the bone marrow does not receive a strong-enough signal to make the oxygen-carrying red blood cells. Fewer red blood cells are produced so the muscles, brain, and other parts of the body do not get the oxygen they need to function properly.

Most patients treated with PROCRIT® no longer need blood transfusions. However, certain medical conditions, or unexpected blood loss, may result in the need for a transfusion.

What do I need to know if I am giving myself PROCRIT® injections?

When you receive your PROCRIT® from the dialysis center, doctor's office or home dialysis supplier, always check to see that:

1. The name PROCRIT® appears on the carton and vial label.
2. You will be able to use PROCRIT® before the expiration date stamped on the package.

The PROCRIT® solution in the vial should always be clear and colorless. Do not use PROCRIT® if the contents of the vial appear discolored or cloudy, or if the vial appears to contain lumps, flakes, or particles. In addition, if the vial has been shaken vigorously, the solution may appear to be frothy and should not be used. Therefore, care should be taken not to shake the PROCRIT® vial vigorously before use. Unless you have been prescribed Multidose PROCRIT® (1 mL or 2 mL vials with a big "M" on the label, each containing a total of 20,000 Units of PROCRIT®), vials of PROCRIT® are for single use. Any unused portion of a vial should not be used. However, Multidose PROCRIT® may be used to inject multiple doses as prescribed by your doctor, and may be stored in the refrigerator (but not the freezing compartment) between doses for up to 21 days, and can be used for multiple doses. Follow your doctor's or dialysis center's instructions on what to do with the used vials.

How should I store PROCRIT®?

PROCRIT® should be stored in the refrigerator, but not in the freezing compartment. Do not let the vial freeze and do not leave it in direct sunlight. Do not use a vial of PROCRIT® that has been frozen or after the expiration date that is stamped on the label. If you have any questions about the safety of a vial of PROCRIT® that has been subjected to temperature extremes, be sure to check with your dialysis unit staff.

Always use the correct syringe.

Your doctor has instructed you on how to give yourself the correct dosage of PROCRIT®. This dosage will usually be measured in Units per milliliter or cc's. It is important to use a syringe that is marked in tenths of milliliters (for example, 0.2 mL or cc). Failure to use the proper syringe can lead to a mistake in dosage, and you may receive too much or too little PROCRIT®. Too little PROCRIT® may not be effective in increasing your hematocrit, and too much PROCRIT® may lead to a hematocrit that is too high. Only use disposable syringes and needles as they do not require sterilization; they should be used once and disposed of as instructed by your doctor.

IMPORTANT: TO HELP AVOID CONTAMINATION AND POSSIBLE INFECTION, FOLLOW THESE INSTRUCTIONS EXACTLY.

PREPARING THE DOSE

1. Wash your hands thoroughly with soap and water before preparing the medication.
2. Check the date on the PROCRIT® vial to be sure that the drug has not expired.

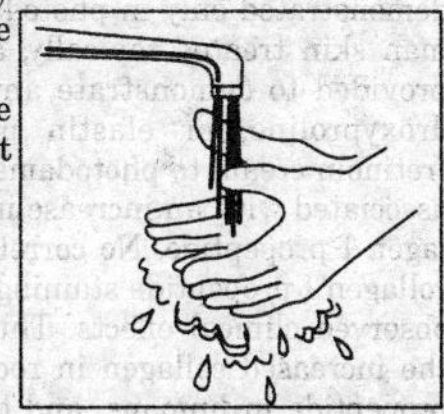

3. Remove the vial of PROCRIT® from the refrigerator and allow it to reach room temperature. Unless you are using a Multidose vial, each PROCRIT® vial is designed to be used only once. It is not necessary to shake PROCRIT®. Prolonged vigorous shaking may damage the product. Assemble the other supplies you will need for your injection.

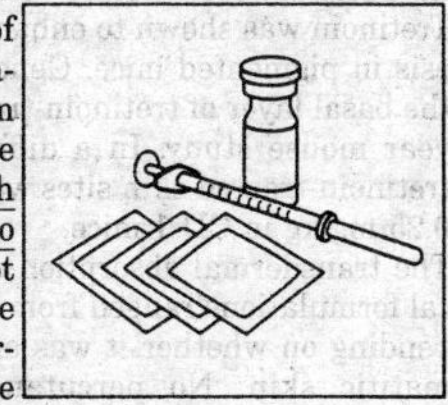

4. Hemodialysis patients should wipe off the venous port of the hemodialysis tubing with an antiseptic swab. Peritoneal dialysis patients should cleanse the skin with an antiseptic swab where the injection is to be made.

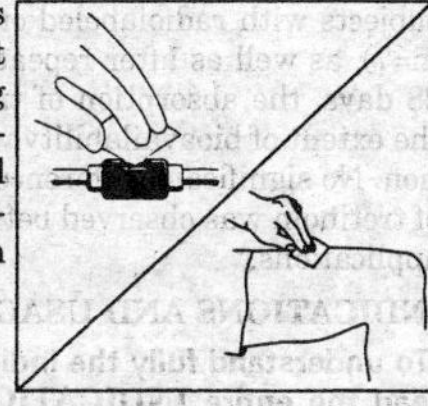

5. Flip off the red protective cap but do not remove the gray rubber stopper. Wipe the top of the gray rubber stopper with an antiseptic swab.

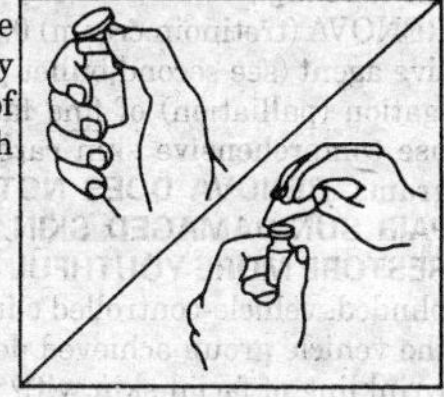

6. Using a syringe and needle designed for subcutaneous injection, draw air into the syringe by pulling back on the plunger. The amount of air should be equal to your PROCRIT® dose.
7. Carefully remove the needle cover. Put the needle through the gray rubber stopper of the PROCRIT® vial.

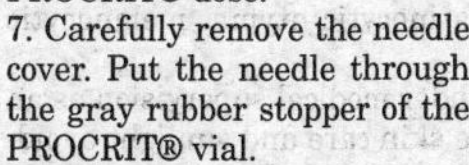

8. Push the plunger in to discharge air into the vial. The air injected into the vial will allow PROCRIT® to be easily withdrawn into the syringe.
9. Turn the vial and syringe upside down in one hand. Be sure the tip of the needle is in the PROCRIT® solution. Your other hand will be free to move the plunger. Draw back on the plunger slowly to draw the correct dose of PROCRIT® into the syringe.
10. Check for air bubbles. The air is harmless, but too large an air bubble will reduce the PROCRIT® dose. To remove air bubbles, gently tap the syringe to move the air bubbles to the top of the syringe, then use the plunger to push the solution and the air back into the vial. Then re-measure your correct dose of PROCRIT®.

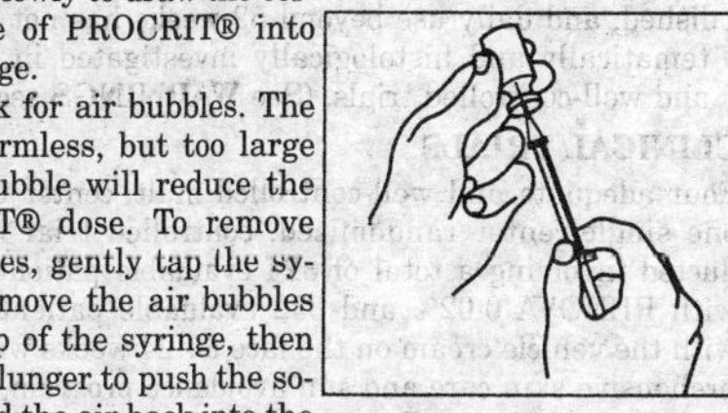

11. Double check your dose. Remove the needle from the vial. Do not lay the syringe down or allow the needle to touch anything.

INJECTING THE DOSE

Patients on home hemodialysis using the intravenous injection route:

1. Insert the needle of the syringe into the previously cleansed venous port and inject the PROCRIT®.
2. Remove the syringe and dispose of the whole unit. Use the disposable syringe only once. Dispose of syringes and needles as directed by your doctor, by following these simple steps:

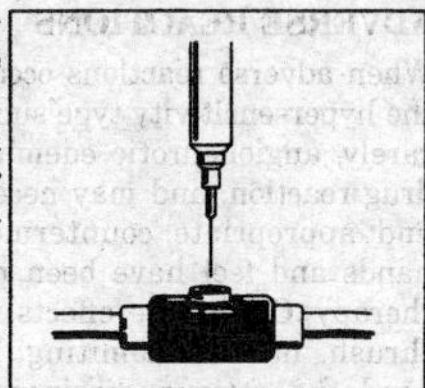

— Place all used needles and syringes in a hard plastic container with a screw-on-cap, or a metal container with a plastic lid, such as a coffee can properly labeled as to content. If a metal container is used, cut a small hole in the plastic lid and tape the lid to the metal container. If a hard-plastic container is used, always screw the cap on tightly after each use. When the container is full, tape around the cap or lid, and dispose of according to your doctor's instructions.
— Do not use glass or clear plastic containers, or any container that will be recycled or returned to a store.
— Always store the container out of the reach of children.
— Please check with your doctor, nurse, or pharmacist for other suggestions. There may be special state and local laws that they will discuss with you.

Patients on home peritoneal dialysis or home hemodialysis using the subcutaneous route:

1. With one hand, stabilize the previously cleansed skin by spreading it or by pinching up a large area with your free hand.
2. Hold the syringe with the other hand, as you would a pencil. Double check that the correct amount of PROCRIT® is in the syringe. Insert the needle straight into the skin (90 degree angle). Pull the plunger back slightly. If blood comes into the syringe, do not inject PROCRIT®, as the needle has entered a blood vessel; withdraw the syringe and inject at a different site. Inject the PROCRIT® by pushing the plunger all the way down.

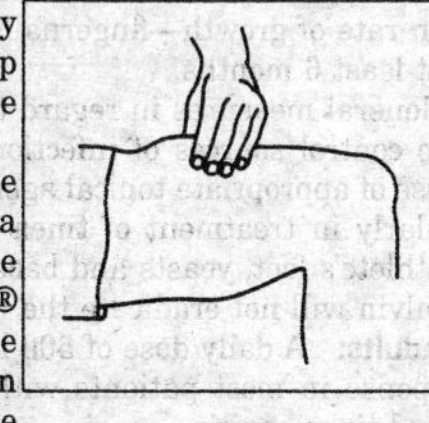

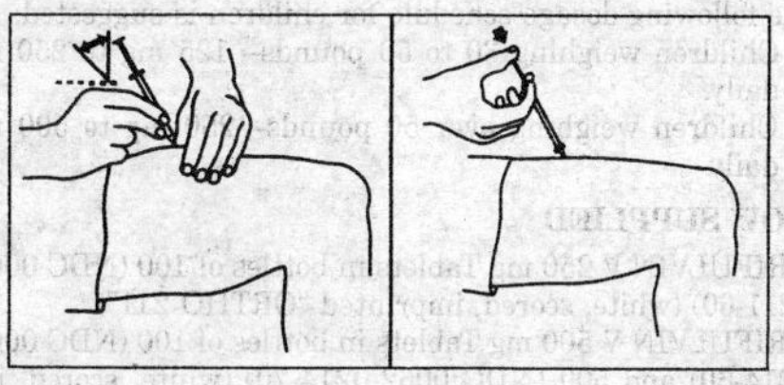

3. Hold an antiseptic swab near the needle and pull the needle straight out of the skin. Press the antiseptic swab over the injection site for several seconds.
4. Use the disposable syringe only once. Dispose of syringes and needles as directed by your doctor, by following these simple steps:
— Place all used needles and syringes in a hard plastic container with a screw-on-cap, or a metal container with a plastic lid, such as a coffee can properly labeled as to content. If a metal container is used, cut a small hole in the plastic lid and tape the lid to the metal container. If a hard-plastic container is used, always screw the cap on tightly after each use. When the container is full, tape around the cap or lid, and dispose of according to your doctor's instructions.
— Do not use glass or clear plastic containers, or any container that will be recycled or returned to a store.
— Always store the container out of the reach of children.
— Please check with your doctor, nurse, or pharmacist for other suggestions. There may be special state and local laws that they will discuss with you.
5. Always change the site for each injection as directed. Occasionally a problem may develop at the injection site. If you notice a lump, swelling, or bruising that doesn't go away, contact your doctor. You may wish to record the site just used so that you can keep track.

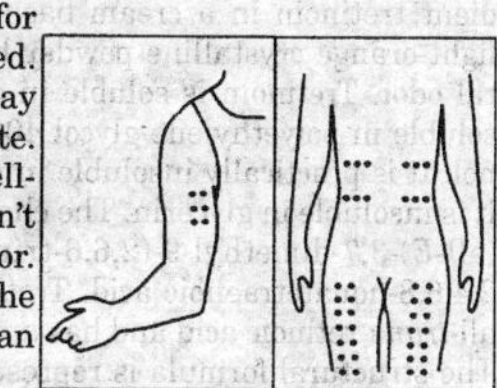

USAGE IN PREGNANCY

If you are pregnant or nursing a baby, consult your doctor before using PROCRIT®.

IMPORTANT NOTES

Since you are a home dialysis patient and your doctor allows you to self-administer PROCRIT®, please note the following:

1. Always follow the instructions of your doctor concerning the dosage and administration of PROCRIT®. Do not change the dose or instructions for administration of PROCRIT® without consulting your doctor.
2. Your doctor will tell you what to do if you miss a dose of PROCRIT®. Always keep a spare syringe and needle on hand.
3. Always consult your doctor if you notice anything unusual about your condition or your use of PROCRIT®.

Manufactured by:
Amgen Inc.
One Amgen Center Drive
Thousand Oaks, CA 91320-1799
Distributed by:
Ortho Biotech Products, L.P.
Raritan, New Jersey 08869-0670
ORTHO BIOTECH

Printed in U.S.A.
Revised June 2004
638-10-979-3

Shown in Product Identification Guide, page 327

SPORANOX® ℞
[*spə 'ah-näks"*]
(itraconazole) Injection

For full prescribing information, see listing under JANSSEN PHARMACEUTICA PRODUCTS, L.P.

Shown in Product Identification Guide, page 327

SPORANOX® ℞
[*spə 'ah-näks"*]
(itraconazole) Oral Solution

For full prescribing information, see listing under JANSSEN PHARMACEUTICA PRODUCTS, L.P.

Shown in Product Identification Guide, page 327

OrthoNeutrogena Division of Ortho-McNeil Pharmaceuticals, Inc.

5760 WEST 96th STREET
LOS ANGELES, CA 90045

For Medical Information Contact:
Dermatological Medical Information
(800) 426-7762

GRIFULVIN V ® ℞
[*gri 'fulvən*]
(griseofulvin tablets) microsize and (griseofulvin oral suspension) microsize Suspension and Tablets

DESCRIPTION

Griseofulvin is an antibiotic derived from a species of *Penicillium.* Each GRIFULVIN V Tablet contains either 250 mg or 500 mg of griseofulvin microsize, and also contains calcium stearate, colloidal silicon dioxide, starch, and wheat gluten. Additionally, the 250 mg tablet also contains dibasic calcium phosphate. Each 5 mL of GRIFULVIN V Suspension contains 125 mg of griseofulvin microsize and also contains alcohol 0.2%, docusate sodium, FD&C Red No. 40, FD&C Yellow No. 6, flavors, magnesium aluminium silicate, menthol, methylparaben, propylene glycol, propylparaben, saccharin sodium, simethicone emulsion, sodium alginate, sucrose, and purified water.

CLINICAL PHARMACOLOGY

GRIFULVIN V (griseofulvin microsize) acts systemically to inhibit the growth of *Trichophyton, Microsporum* and *Epidermophyton* genera of fungi. Fungistatic amounts are deposited in the keratin, which is gradually exfoliated and replaced by noninfected tissue.

Griseofulvin absorption from the gastrointestinal tract varies considerably among individuals, mainly because of insolubility of the drug in aqueous media of the upper G.I. tract. The peak serum level found in fasting adults given 0.5 g occurs at about four hours and ranges between 0.5 and 2.0 mcg/mL.

It should be noted that some individuals are consistently "poor absorbers" and tend to attain lower blood levels at all times. This may explain unsatisfactory therapeutic results in some patients. Better blood levels can probably be attained in most patients if the tablets are administered after a meal with a high fat content.

INDICATIONS AND USAGE

Major indications for GRIFULVIN V are:

Tinea capitis (ringworm of the scalp)
Tinea corporis (ringworm of the body)
Tinea pedis (athlete's foot)
Tinea unguium (onychomycosis; ringworm of the nails)
Tinea cruris (ringworm of the thigh)
Tinea barbae (barber's itch)

GRIFULVIN V inhibits the growth of those genera of fungi that commonly cause ringworm infections of the hair, skin, and nails, such as:

Trichophyton rubrum
Trichophyton tonsurans
Trichophyton mentagrophytes
Trichophyton interdigitalis
Trichophyton verrucosum
Trichophyton sulphureum

Continued on next page

Grifulvin V—Cont.

Trichophyton schoenleini
Microsporum audouini
Microsporum canis
Microsporum gypseum
Epidermophyton floccosum
Trichophyton megnini
Trichophyton gallinae
Trichophyton crateriform

Note: Prior to therapy, the type of fungi responsible for the infection should be identified. The use of the drug is not justified in minor or trivial infections which will respond to topical antifungal agents alone.

It is *not* effective in:
Bacterial infections
Candidiasis (Moniliasis)
Histoplasmosis
Actinomycosis
Sporotrichosis
Chromoblastomycosis
Coccidioidomycosis
North American Blastomycosis
Cryptococcosis (Torulosis)
Tinea versicolor
Nocardiosis

CONTRAINDICATIONS

This drug is contraindicated in patients with porphyria, hepatocellular failure, and in individuals with a history of hypersensitivity to griseofulvin.
Two cases of conjoined twins have been reported in patients taking griseofulvin during the first trimester of pregnancy. Griseofulvin should not be prescribed to pregnant patients.

WARNINGS

Prophylactic Usage: Safety and efficacy of prophylactic use of this drug have not been established.
Chronic feeding of griseofulvin, at levels ranging from 0.5-2.5% of the diet, resulted in the development of liver tumors in several strains of mice, particularly in males. Smaller particle sizes result in an enhanced effect. Lower oral dosage levels have not been tested. Subcutaneous administration of relatively small doses of griseofulvin once a week during the first three weeks of life has also been reported to induce hepatomata in mice. Although studies in other animal species have not yielded evidence of tumorigenicity, these studies were not of adequate design to form a basis for conclusions in this regard.
In subacute toxicity studies, orally administered griseofulvin produced hepatocellular necrosis in mice, but this has not been seen in other species. Disturbances in porphyrin metabolism have been reported in griseofulvin-treated laboratory animals. Griseofulvin has been reported to have a colchicine-like effect on mitosis and cocarcinogenicity with methylcholanthrene in cutaneous tumor induction in laboratory animals.
Reports of animal studies in the Soviet literature state that a griseofulvin preparation was found to be embryotoxic and teratogenic on oral administration to pregnant Wistar rats. Rat reproduction studies done in the United States and Great Britain were inconclusive in this regard. Pups with abnormalities have been reported in the litters of a few bitches treated with griseofulvin. Because the potential for adverse effects on the human fetus cannot be ruled out, additional contraceptive precautions should be taken during treatment with griseofulvin and for a month after termination of treatment. GRIFULVIN V should not be prescribed to women intending to become pregnant within one month following cessation of therapy.
Suppression of spermatogenesis has been reported to occur in rats but investigation in man failed to confirm this. Griseofulvin interferes with chromosomal distribution during cell division, causing aneuploidy in plant and mammalian cells. These effects have been demonstrated *in vitro* at concentrations that may be achieved in the serum with the recommended therapeutic dosage.
Since griseofulvin has demonstrated harmful effects *in vitro* on the genotype in bacteria, plants, and fungi, males should wait at least six months after completing griseofulvin therapy before fathering a child.

PRECAUTIONS

Patients on prolonged therapy with any potent medication should be under close observation. Periodic monitoring of organ system function, including renal, hepatic and hemopoietic, should be done.
Since griseofulvin is derived from species of penicillin, the possibility of cross sensitivity with penicillin exists; however, known penicillin-sensitive patients have been treated without difficulty.
Since a photosensitivity reaction is occasionally associated with griseofulvin therapy, patients should be warned to avoid exposure to intense natural or artificial sunlight. Should a photosensitivity reaction occur, lupus erythematosus may be aggravated.
Drug Interactions: Patients on warfarin-type anticoagulant therapy may require dosage adjustment of the anticoagulant during and after griseofulvin therapy. Concomitant use of barbiturates usually depresses griseofulvin activity and may necessitate raising the dosage.
The concomitant administration of griseofulvin has been reported to reduce the efficacy of oral contraceptives and to increase the incidence of breakthrough bleeding.

ADVERSE REACTIONS

When adverse reactions occur, they are most commonly of the hypersensitivity type such as skin rashes, urticaria and rarely, angioneurotic edema or erythema multiforme-like drug reaction, and may necessitate withdrawal of therapy and appropriate countermeasures. Paresthesias of the hands and feet have been reported rarely after extended therapy. Other side effects reported occasionally are oral thrush, nausea, vomiting, epigastric distress, diarrhea, headache, fatigue, dizziness, insomnia, mental confusion and impairment of performance of routine activities.
Proteinuria and leukopenia have been reported rarely. Administration of the drug should be discontinued if granulocytopenia occurs.
When rare, serious reactions occur with griseofulvin, they are usually associated with high dosages, long periods of therapy, or both.

DOSAGE AND ADMINISTRATION

Accurate diagnosis of the infecting organism is essential. Identification should be made either by direct microscopic examination of a mounting of infected tissue in a solution of potassium hydroxide or by culture on an appropriate medium.
Medication must be continued until the infecting organism is completely eradicated as indicated by appropriate clinical or laboratory examination. Representative treatment periods are tinea capitis, 4 to 6 weeks; tinea corporis, 2 to 4 weeks; tinea pedis, 4 to 8 weeks; tinea unguium—depending on rate of growth—fingernails, at least 4 months; toenails, at least 6 months.
General measures in regard to hygiene should be observed to control sources of infection or reinfection. Concomitant use of appropriate topical agents is usually required, particularly in treatment of tinea pedis since in some forms of athlete's foot, yeasts and bacteria may be involved. Griseofulvin will not eradicate the bacterial or monilial infection.
Adults: A daily dose of 500 mg. will give a satisfactory response in most patients with tinea corporis, tinea cruris, and tinea capitis.
For those fungus infections more difficult to eradicate such as tinea pedis and tinea unguium, a daily dose of 1.0 g is recommended.
Children: Approximately 5 mg per pound of body weight per day is an effective dose for most children. On this basis the following dosage schedule for children is suggested:
Children weighing 30 to 50 pounds—125 mg to 250 mg daily.
Children weighing over 50 pounds—250 mg to 500 mg daily.

HOW SUPPLIED

GRIFULVIN V 250 mg Tablets in bottles of 100 (NDC 0062-0211-60) (white, scored, imprinted "ORTHO 211").
GRIFULVIN V 500 mg Tablets in bottles of 100 (NDC 0062-0214-60) and 500 (NDC 0062-0214-70) (white, scored, imprinted "ORTHO 214").
Dispense GRIFULVIN V Tablets in a tight container as defined in the USP.
GRIFULVIN V Suspension 125 mg per 5 mL in bottles of 4 fl oz (120mL) (NDC 0062-0206-04).
Dispense GRIFULVIN V Suspension in a tight, light-resistant container as defined in the USP.
STORE AT ROOM TEMPERATURE
Revised January 1997
631-10-560-2
Shown in Product Identification Guide, page 327

RENOVA® ℞

(tretinoin cream) 0.02%
FOR TOPICAL USE ON THE FACE. NOT FOR OPHTHALMIC, ORAL, OR INTRAVAGINAL USE.

DESCRIPTION

RENOVA (tretinoin cream) 0.02% contains the active ingredient tretinoin in a cream base. Tretinoin is a yellow- to light-orange crystalline powder having a characteristic floral odor. Tretinoin is soluble in dimethylsulfoxide, slightly soluble in polyethylene glycol 400, octanol, and 100% ethanol. It is practically insoluble in water and mineral oil, and it is insoluble in glycerin. The chemical name for tretinoin is (all-*E*)-3,7-dimethyl-9-(2,6,6-trimethyl-1-cyclonexen-1-yl)-2,4,6,8-nonatetraenoic acid. Tretinoin is also referred to as all-*trans*-retinoic acid and has a molecular weight of 300.44. The structural formula is represented below.

TRETINOIN

Tretinoin is available as RENOVA at a concentration of 0.02% w/w in an oil-in-water emulsion formulation consisting of benzyl alcohol, butylated hydroxytoluene, caprylic/capric triglyceride, cetyl alcohol, edetate disodium, fragrance, methylparaben, propylparaben, purified water, stearic acid, stearyl alcohol, steareth 2, steareth 20, and xanthan gum.

CLINICAL PHARMACOLOGY

Tretinoin is an endogenous retinoid metabolite of Vitamin A that binds to intracellular receptors in the cytosol and nucleus, but cutaneous levels of tretinoin in excess of physiologic concentrations occur following application of a tretinoin-containing topical drug product. Although tretinoin activates three members of the retinoic acid (RAR) nuclear receptors (RARα, RARβ, and RARγ) which may act to modify gene expression, subsequent protein synthesis, and epithelial cell growth and differentiation, it has not been established whether the clinical effects of tretinoin are mediated through activation of retinoic acid receptors, other mechanisms such as irritation, or both.
The effect of tretinoin on skin with chronic photodamage has not been evaluated in animal studies. When hairless albino mice were treated topically with tretinoin shortly after a period of UVB irradiation, new collagen formation was demonstrated only in photodamaged skin. However, in human skin treated topically, adequate data have not been provided to demonstrate any increase in desmosine, hydroxyproline, or elastin mRNA. Application of 0.1% tretinoin cream to photodamaged human forearm skin was associated with an increase in antibody staining for procollagen I propeptide. No correlation was made between procollagen I propeptide staining with collagen I levels or with observed clinical effects. Thus, the relationships between the increased collagen in rodents, increased procollagen I propeptide in humans, and the clinical effects of tretinoin have not yet been clearly defined.
Tretinoin was shown to enhance UV-stimulated melanogenesis in pigmented mice. Generalized amyloid deposition in the basal layer of tretinoin-treated skin was noted in a two-year mouse study. In a different study, hyalinization at tretinoin-treated skin sites was noted at doses beginning at 0.25 mg/kg in CD-1 mice.
The transdermal absorption of tretinoin from various topical formulations ranged from 1% to 31% of applied dose, depending on whether it was applied to healthy skin or dermatitic skin. No percutaneous absorption study was conducted with RENOVA 0.02% in human volunteers. When percutaneous absorption of the oil-in-water emulsion formulation at 0.05% concentration was assessed in healthy male subjects with radiolabeled cream after a single application (n=7), as well as after repeated daily applications (n=7) for 28 days, the absorption of tretinoin was less than 2% and the extent of bioavailability was less after repeated application. No significant difference in endogenous concentrations of tretinoin was observed between single and repeated daily applications.

INDICATIONS AND USAGE

(To understand fully the indication for this product, please read the entire INDICATIONS AND USAGE section of the labeling.)
RENOVA (tretinoin cream) 0.02% is indicated as an adjunctive agent (see second bullet point below) for use in the mitigation (palliation) of fine facial wrinkles in patients who use comprehensive skin care and sunlight avoidance programs. **RENOVA DOES NOT ELIMINATE WRINKLES, REPAIR SUN-DAMAGED SKIN, REVERSE PHOTOAGING, or RESTORE MORE YOUTHFUL or YOUNGER SKIN.** In double-blinded, vehicle-controlled clinical studies, many patients in the vehicle group achieved desired palliative effects on fine wrinkling of facial skin with the use of comprehensive skin care and sunlight avoidance programs including sunscreens, protective clothing, and non-prescription emollient creams.

- RENOVA 0.02% has NOT DEMONSTRATED A MITIGATING EFFECT on significant signs of chronic sunlight exposure such as coarse or deep wrinkling, tactile roughness, mottled hyperpigmentation, lentigines, telangiectasia, skin laxity, keratinocytic atypia, melanocytic atypia, or dermal elastosis
- RENOVA should be used under medical supervision as an adjunct to a comprehensive skin care and sunlight avoidance program that includes the use of effective sunscreens (minimum SPF of 15) and protective clothing.
- Patients with visible actinic keratoses and patients with a history of skin cancer were excluded from clinical trials of RENOVA 0.02%. Thus the effectiveness and safety of RENOVA 0.02% in these populations are not known at this time.
- Neither the safety nor the effectiveness of RENOVA for the prevention or treatment of actinic keratoses or skin neoplasms has been established.
- Neither the safety nor the efficacy of using RENOVA 0.02% daily for greater than 52 weeks has been established, and daily use beyond 52 weeks has not been systematically and histologically investigated in adequate and well-controlled trials. (See **WARNINGS** section.)

CLINICAL TRIALS

Four adequate and well-controlled multi-center trials and one single-center randomized, controlled trial were conducted involving a total of 324 evaluable patients treated with RENOVA 0.02% and 332 evaluable patients treated with the vehicle cream on the face for 24 weeks with a comprehensive skin care and sun avoidance program, to assess the effects on fine and coarse wrinkling, mottled hyperpigmentation, tactile skin roughness, and laxity. Patients were evaluated at baseline on a 10 unit scale and changes from that baseline rating were categorized as follows:

Worsening:	Increase of 1 unit or more.
No improvement:	No change.
Minimal improvement:	Reduction of 1 unit.
Mild improvement:	Reduction of 2 units.
Moderate improvement:	Reduction of 3 units or more.

In these trials, the fine and coarse wrinkling, mottled hyperpigmentation, tactile roughness, and laxity of the facial skin were thought to be caused by multiple factors which included intrinsic aging or environmental factors, such as chronic sunlight exposure.
Two of the five trials provided adequate demonstration of efficacy for mitigation of fine facial wrinkling. No two of the five trials adequately demonstrated efficacy for mitigation of coarse wrinkling, mottled hyperpigmentation, tactile skin roughness, and laxity. Data for fine wrinkling (the indication for which RENOVA 0.02% demonstrated efficacy) from all five trials (four studies in lightly pigmented subjects with Fitzpatrick Skin Types I-III and one study in darkly pigmented subjects with Fitzpatrick Skin Types IV-VI) is provided below:

FINE WRINKLING IN LIGHTLY PIGMENTED SUBJECTS

	Subjects using RENOVA 0.02% + CSP* (N=279)	Vehicle + CSP* (N=280)
Worsened	1%	3%
No Change	40%	58%
Minimal Improvement	35%	27%
Mild Improvement	15%	9%
Moderate Improvement	10%	3%

A single-center study (N = 107) in darkly pigmented, mostly African-American, subjects with Fitzpatrick Skin Types IV-VI demonstrated minimal or mild improvement in fine facial wrinkling in 43% of patients using Vehicle + CSP* compared to 29% of subjects using RENOVA 0.02% + CSP*. Although fewer darkly pigmented subjects improved with RENOVA 0.02% than with vehicle, these findings may reflect the small size of this study.

*CSP = Comprehensive skin protection and sunlight avoidance programs including use of sunscreens, protective clothing, and non-prescription emollient creams.

Self-assessment of fine wrinkles after 24 weeks of treatment with either RENOVA 0.02% or Vehicle from the four studies in lightly pigmented patients showed the following:

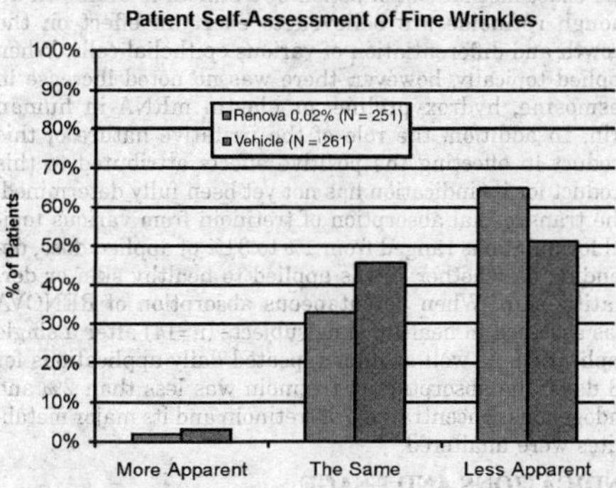

No studies have been conducted comparing the facial irritation or efficacy of RENOVA 0.02% to RENOVA 0.05% (older marketed formulation).
Patients may lose some of the mitigating effects of RENOVA 0.02% after 12 weeks of discontinuation of RENOVA 0.02% from their comprehensive skin care and sunlight avoidance program.

CONTRAINDICATIONS

This drug is contraindicated in individuals with a history of sensitivity reactions to any of its components. It should be discontinued if hypersensitivity to any of its ingredients is noted.

WARNINGS

- RENOVA 0.02% is a dermal irritant, and the results of continued irritation of the skin for greater than 52 weeks in chronic use with RENOVA are not known. There is evidence of atypical changes in melanocytes and keratinocytes and of increased dermal elastosis in some patients treated with RENOVA 0.05% for longer than 48 weeks. The significance of these findings and their relevance for RENOVA 0.02% are unknown.
- RENOVA should not be administered if the patient is also taking drugs known to be photosensitizers (e.g., thiazides, tetracyclines, fluoroquinolones, phenothiazines, sulfonamides) because of the possibility of augmented phototoxicity.

Exposure to sunlight (including sunlamps) should be avoided or minimized during use of RENOVA because of heightened sunburn susceptibility. Patients should be warned to use sunscreens (minimum SPF of 15) and protective clothing when using RENOVA. Patients with sunburn should be advised not to use RENOVA until fully recovered. Patients who may have considerable sun exposure, e.g., due to their occupation, and those patients with inherent sensitivity to sunlight should exercise caution when using RENOVA and follow the precautions outlined in the Patient Package Insert.
RENOVA should be kept out of the eyes, mouth, angles of the nose, and mucous membranes. Topical use may cause severe local erythema, pruritus, burning, stinging, and peeling at the site of application. If the degree of local irritation warrants, patients should be directed to use less medication, decrease the frequency of application, discontinue use temporarily, or discontinue use altogether and consider additional appropriate therapy.
Tretinoin has been reported to cause severe irritation on eczematous skin and should be used only with caution in patients with this condition.
Application of larger amounts of medication than recommended has not been shown to lead to more rapid or better results, and marked redness, peeling, or discomfort may occur.

PRECAUTIONS

General: RENOVA should be used only as an adjunct to a comprehensive skin care and sunlight avoidance program. (See **INDICATIONS AND USAGE** section.)
If a drug sensitivity, chemical irritation, or a systemic adverse reaction develops, use of RENOVA should be discontinued.
Weather extremes, such as wind or cold, may be more irritating to patients using tretinoin-containing products.
Information for Patients: RENOVA 0.02% is to be used as described below unless otherwise directed by your physician:

1. It is for use on the face.
2. Avoid contact with the eyes, ears, nostrils, angles of the nose, and mouth. RENOVA may cause severe redness, itching, burning, stinging, and peeling if used on these areas.
3. In the evening, gently wash your face with a mild soap. Pat skin dry and wait 20–30 minutes before applying RENOVA. Apply only a small pearl-sized (about ¼ inch or 5 millimeter diameter) amount of RENOVA to your face at one time. This should be enough to cover the entire affected area lightly.
4. Do not wash your face for at least one hour after applying RENOVA.
5. For best results, you are advised not to apply another skin care product or cosmetic for at least one hour after applying RENOVA.
6. In the morning, apply a moisturizing sunscreen, SPF 15 or greater.
7. RENOVA is a serious medication. Do not use RENOVA if you are pregnant or attempting to become pregnant. If you become pregnant while using RENOVA, please contact your physician immediately.
8. Avoid sunlight and other medicines that may increase your sensitivity to sunlight.
9. RENOVA does not remove wrinkles or repair sun-damaged skin.

Please refer to the Patient Package Insert for additional patient information.
Drug Interactions: Concomitant topical medications, medicated or abrasive soaps, shampoos, cleansers, cosmetics with a strong drying effect, products with high concentrations of alcohol, astringents, spices or lime, permanent wave solutions, electrolysis, hair depilatories or waxes, and products that may irritate the skin should be used with caution in patients being treated with RENOVA because they may increase irritation with RENOVA.
RENOVA should not be administered if the patient is also taking drugs known to be photosensitizers (e.g., thiazides, tetracyclines, fluoroquinolones, phenothiazines, sulfonamides) because of the possibility of augmented phototoxicity.
Carcinogenesis, Mutagenesis, Impairment of Fertility: In a 91-week dermal study in which CD-1 mice were administered 0.017% and 0.035% formulations of tretinoin, cutaneous squamous cell carcinomas and papillomas in the treatment area were observed in some female mice. These concentrations are near the tretinoin concentration of this clinical formulation (0.02%). A dose-related incidence of liver tumors in male mice was observed at those same doses. The maximum systemic doses associated with the 0.017% and 0.035% formulations are 0.5 and 1.0 mg/kg/day. These doses are 10 and 20 times the maximum human systemic dose, when adjusted for total body surface area. The biological significance of these findings is not clear because they occurred at doses that exceeded the dermal maximally tolerated dose (MTD) of tretinoin and because they were within the background natural occurrence rate for these tumors in this strain of mice. There was no evidence of carcinogenic potential when 0.025 mg/kg/day of tretinoin was administered topically to mice (0.5 times the maximum human systemic dose, adjusted for total body surface area). For purposes of comparisons of the animal exposure to systemic human exposure, the maximum human systemic dose is defined as 1 gram of 0.02% RENOVA applied daily to a 50 kg person (0.004 mg tretinoin/kg body weight).
Studies in hairless albino mice suggest that concurrent exposure to tretinoin may enhance the tumorigenic potential of carcinogenic doses of UVB and UVA light from a solar simulator. This effect has been confirmed in a later study in pigmented mice, and dark pigmentation did not overcome the enhancement of photocarcinogenesis by 0.05% tretinoin. Although the significance of these studies to humans is not clear, patients should minimize exposure to sunlight or artificial ultraviolet irradiation sources.
The mutagenic potential of tretinoin was evaluated in the Ames assay and in the *in vivo* mouse micronucleus assay, both of which were negative.
In dermal Segment I fertility studies in rats, slight (not statistically significant) decreases in sperm count and motility were seen at 0.5 mg/kg/day (20 times the maximum human systemic dose adjusted for total body surface area), and slight (not statistically significant) increases in the number and percent of nonviable embryos in females treated with 0.25 mg/kg/day (10 times the maximum human systemic dose adjusted for total body surface area) and above were observed. A dermal Segment III study with RENOVA has not been performed in any species. In oral Segment I and Segment III studies in rats with tretinoin, decreased survival of neonates and growth retardation were observed at doses in excess of 2 mg/kg/day (83 times the human topical dose adjusted for total body surface area).
Pregnancy:
Teratogenic effects: Pregnancy Category C.
ORAL tretinoin has been shown to be teratogenic in rats, mice, rabbits, hamsters, and subhuman primates. It was teratogenic and fetotoxic in Wistar rats when given orally or topically in doses greater than 1 mg/kg/day (42 times the maximum human systemic dose normalized for total body surface area). However, variations in teratogenic doses among various strains of rats have been reported. In the cynomolgus monkey, which, metabolically, is closer to humans for tretinoin than the other species examined, fetal malformations were reported at doses of 10 mg/kg/day or greater, but none were observed at 5 mg/kg/day (417 times the maximum human systemic dose adjusted for total body surface area), although increased skeletal variations were observed at all doses. A dose-related increase in embryolethality and abortion was reported. Similar results have also been reported in pigtail macaques.
TOPICAL tretinoin in animal teratogenicity tests has generated equivocal results. There is evidence for teratogenicity (shortened or kinked tail) of topical tretinoin in Wistar rats at doses greater than 1 mg/kg/day (42 times the maximum human systemic dose adjusted for total body surface area). Anomalies (humerus: short 13%, bent 6%, os parietal incompletely ossified 14%) have also been reported when 10 mg/kg/day was dermally applied.
There are other reports in New Zealand White rabbits administered doses of greater than 0.2 mg/kg/day (17 times the maximum human systemic dose adjusted for total body surface area) of an increased incidence of domed head and hydrocephaly, typical of retinoid-induced fetal malformations in this species.
In contrast, several well-controlled animal studies have shown that dermally applied tretinoin may be fetotoxic, but not overtly teratogenic, in rats and rabbits at doses of 1.0 and 0.5 mg/kg/day, respectively (42 times the maximum human systemic dose adjusted for total body surface area in both species).
With widespread use of any drug, a small number of birth defect reports associated temporally with the administration of the drug would be expected by chance alone. Thirty human cases of temporally-associated congenital malformations have been reported during two decades of clinical use of another formulation of topical tretinoin (Retin-A). Although no definite pattern of teratogenicity and no causal association has been established from these cases, 5 of the reports describe the rare birth defect category holoprosencephaly (defects associated with incomplete midline development of the forebrain). The significance of these spontaneous reports in terms of risk to the fetus is not known.
Non-teratogenic effects:
Dermal tretinoin has been shown to be fetotoxic in rabbits when administered 0.5 mg/kg/day (42 times the maximum human systemic dose normalized for total body surface area). Oral tretinoin has been shown to be fetotoxic, resulting in skeletal variations and increased intrauterine death, in rats when administered 2.5 mg/kg/day (104 times the maximum human systemic dose adjusted for total body surface area).
There are, however, no adequate and well-controlled studies in pregnant women. RENOVA should not be used during pregnancy.
Nursing Mothers: It is not known whether this drug is excreted in human milk. Since many drugs are excreted in human milk, mitigation of fine facial wrinkles with RENOVA 0.02% may be postponed in nursing mothers until after completion of the nursing period.
Pediatric Use: Safety and effectiveness in patients less than 18 years of age have not been established.
Geriatric Use: In clinical studies with RENOVA 0.02%, patients aged 65 to 71 did not demonstrate a significant difference for improvement in fine wrinkling when compared to patients under the age of 65. Patients aged 65 and over may demonstrate slightly more irritation, although the differences were not statistically significant in the clinical studies for RENOVA 0.02%. Safety and effectiveness of RENOVA 0.02% in individuals older than 71 years of age have not been established.

ADVERSE REACTIONS

(See **WARNINGS** and **PRECAUTIONS** sections.)
In double-blind, vehicle-controlled studies involving 339 patients who applied RENOVA 0.02% to their faces, adverse

Continued on next page

Renova 0.02%—Cont.

reactions associated with the use of RENOVA were limited primarily to the skin. Almost all patients reported one or more local reactions such as peeling, dry skin, burning, stinging, erythema, and pruritus. In 32% of all study patients, skin irritation was reported that was severe, led to temporary discontinuation of RENOVA 0.02%, or led to use of a mild topical corticosteroid. About 7% of patients using RENOVA 0.02%, compared to less than 1% of the control patients, had sufficiently severe local irritation to warrant short-term use of mild topical corticosteroids to alleviate local irritation. About 4% of patients had to discontinue use of RENOVA because of adverse reactions.

Approximately 2% of spontaneous post-marketing adverse event reporting for RENOVA 0.05% were for skin hypo- or hyperpigmentation. Other spontaneously reported adverse events for RENOVA 0.05% predominantly appear to be local reactions similar to those seen in clinical trials.

OVERDOSAGE

Application of larger amounts of medication than recommended has not been shown to lead to more rapid or better results, and marked redness, peeling, or discomfort may occur. Oral ingestion of the drug may lead to the same side effects as those associated with excessive oral intake of Vitamin A.

DOSAGE AND ADMINISTRATION

- Do NOT use RENOVA if the patient is pregnant or is attempting to become pregnant or is at high risk of pregnancy,
- Do NOT use RENOVA if the patient is sunburned or if the patient has eczema or other chronic skin conditions of the face,
- Do NOT use RENOVA if the patient is inherently sensitive to sunlight,
- Do NOT use RENOVA if the patient is also taking drug(s) known to be photosensitizers (e.g., thiazides, tetracyclines, fluoroquinolones, phenothiazines, sulfonamides) because of the possibility of augmented phototoxicity.

Patients require detailed instruction to obtain maximal benefits and to understand all the precautions necessary to use this product with greatest safety. The physician should review the Patient Package Insert.

RENOVA should be applied to the face once a day in the evening, using only enough to cover the entire affected area lightly. Patients should gently wash their faces with a mild soap, pat the skin dry, and wait 20 to 30 minutes before applying RENOVA. The patient should apply a small pearl-sized (about ¼ inch or 5 millimeter diameter) amount of cream to cover the entire affected area lightly. Caution should be taken when applying the cream to avoid the eyes, ears, nostrils, and mouth.

Application of RENOVA may cause a transitory feeling of warmth or slight stinging.

Mitigation (palliation) of fine facial wrinkling may occur gradually over the course of therapy. Up to six months of therapy may be required before the effects are seen.

With discontinuation of RENOVA therapy, some patients may lose the mitigating effects of RENOVA on fine facial wrinkles. **The safety and effectiveness of using RENOVA 0.02% daily for greater than 52 weeks have not been established.**

Application of larger amounts of medication than recommended may not lead to more rapid or better results, and marked redness, peeling, or discomfort may occur.

Patients treated with RENOVA may use cosmetics but the areas to be treated should be cleansed before the medication is applied. (See **PRECAUTIONS** section.)

HOW SUPPLIED

RENOVA® (tretinoin cream), 0.02% is available in tubes containing 40 grams (NDC 0062-0187-02).

Storage: Store at 25° (77°F), excursions permitted to 15–30°C (59°–86°F).

QUESTIONS: Physicians and Pharmacists can call 1-800-426-7762, from 8:30 a.m. to 4:30 p.m. Eastern Time, Monday through Friday.

Rx only.

RENOVA

(reh-NO-vah)

Generic Name: Tretinoin Cream (0.02%)

Use only on the Face

Read this leaflet carefully before you start to use your medicine. Read the information you get every time you get more medicine. There may be new information about the drug. This leaflet does not take the place of talks with your doctor. It is important for you to talk with your doctor about how to use RENOVA for the best results and how to reduce side effects.

What is the Most Important Information about RENOVA?

RENOVA is a serious medicine. **Do not use RENOVA if you are pregnant or attempting to become pregnant.** If you become pregnant while using RENOVA, please contact your doctor immediately.

Avoid sunlight and other medicines that may increase your sensitivity to sunlight (See "Who should **not** use RENOVA?").

RENOVA 0.02% does not remove wrinkles or repair sun-damaged skin. (See "What is RENOVA?" for more details.)

What is RENOVA?

RENOVA 0.02% is a prescription medicine that may reduce fine facial wrinkles. It is for patients who are using a total skin care and sunlight avoidance program. RENOVA does not remove wrinkles or repair sun-damaged skin. RENOVA does not work for everyone who uses it. It may work better for some patients than for others.

RENOVA should be used only under the guidance of your doctor as part of a sunlight avoidance and total skin care program. This program should include avoiding sunlight as much as possible, using clothing to protect you from sunlight, using sunscreens with a minimum SPF of 15, and using face creams that add moisture to the skin.

When you use RENOVA, you will not see improvement right away. Generally, you may notice some effects in 3 to 4 months. If RENOVA treatment is stopped, the improvement may gradually disappear.

The use of RENOVA 0.02% in patients for more than 52 weeks has not been studied. Therefore, it is not known if RENOVA 0.02% is safe or works if used longer than 52 weeks. In a study in people with medium to dark skin color, RENOVA 0.02% has not demonstrated a benefit over a sunlight avoidance program and total skin care. RENOVA 0.02% has not been studied in people with visible actinic keratoses or in people with a history of skin cancer.

Who should not use RENOVA?

Do not use RENOVA if:

- you are pregnant or plan to become pregnant. If you become pregnant while using RENOVA, please contact your doctor immediately.
- you are sunburned or your skin is irritated
- you are highly sensitive to sunlight
- you are allergic to any of the ingredients in RENOVA. The active ingredient is tretinoin. Ask your doctor or pharmacist about the inactive ingredients.

RENOVA can cause increased skin irritation and increased chance of sunburn.

Tell your doctor if you have any skin condition. RENOVA may not be right for you.

Because RENOVA may make your skin more likely to burn from sunlight, tell your doctor if you are using other medicines that increase sensitivity to sunlight. You should not use RENOVA with such medicines. These include, but are not limited to:

- thiazides (to treat high blood pressure)
- tetracyclines, fluoroquinolones, sulfonamides (to treat infection)
- phenothiazines (to treat serious emotional problems)

If you are taking any prescription or non-prescription medicines, check with your doctor to make sure you can use RENOVA with them.

We do not know if RENOVA is passed to infants through breast milk. Therefore, tell your doctor if you are breast feeding.

How should I use RENOVA?

Use RENOVA as part of a total skin care and sun avoidance program. Follow your doctors instructions on how to use RENOVA. RENOVA is usually applied to the face once a day in the evening, following the 3 steps listed below:

1. Gently wash your face with a mild soap.
2. Pat the skin dry and wait 20–30 minutes before applying RENOVA.
3. Apply only a small pearl-sized amount (about ¼ inch or 5 mm diameter) of RENOVA to the face at one time. It should be enough to cover your affected area lightly.

Be especially careful when applying RENOVA to avoid your eyes, ears, nostrils, angles of the nose, and mouth. RENOVA may cause severe redness, itching, burning, stinging, and peeling if used on these areas.

Using too much RENOVA may increase discomfort and skin redness and peeling.

You may use cosmetics one hour after applying RENOVA. If you do, be sure to clean your face before applying RENOVA again. Skin moisturizers should be used at least every morning to protect the treated areas from dryness.

Use sunscreen and wear protective clothing to protect the treated areas from sunlight. If you sunburn easily, or if you spend a lot of time exposed to sunlight, be especially careful to protect your skin.

What should I avoid while using RENOVA?

RENOVA can make your treated skin more sensitive to sunlight. Therefore, keep out of the sunlight as much as possible and do not use sunlamps. Avoid as much as possible products that can increase skin irritation, such as:

- other skin medicines
- medicated or abrasive (rough) soaps
- permanent wave solutions
- chemical hair removers or waxes
- electrolysis
- products with alcohol, spices, astringents, or lime
- cleansers, shampoos, or cosmetics with a strong drying effect
- other products that may irritate your skin

What are the possible side effects of RENOVA?

You may feel brief warmth or stinging on your skin after you use RENOVA. Most patients report peeling, dry skin, burning, stinging, itching, and redness,. These are usually mild to moderate and occur early in treatment. Contact your doctor if the side effects are a problem.

General advice about prescription medicines

Medicines are sometimes prescribed for conditions that are not mentioned in patient information leaflets. Only use RENOVA to treat the condition that your doctor has prescribed it for. Do not give RENOVA to other people. It may harm them.

This leaflet summarizes the most important information about RENOVA. If you would like more information, talk with your doctor. You can ask your pharmacist or doctor for information about RENOVA that is written for health professionals.

ORTHO DERMATOLOGICAL

Ortho Dermatological
Division of Ortho-McNeil
Pharmaceutical, Inc.
Skillman, New Jersey 08558

 Issued September 2000 Printed in USA

U.S. Patents 4,603,146 and 4,877,805 653-10-856-1

Shown in Product Identification Guide, page 327

RENOVA® ℞

[*rē' nōvă*]

(TRETINOIN EMOLLIENT CREAM)
0.05%
FOR TOPICAL USE ON THE FACE ONLY

Prescribing Information

DESCRIPTION

RENOVA (tretinoin emollient cream) 0.05% contains the active ingredient tretinoin (a retinoid) in an emollient cream base. Tretinoin is a yellow to light orange crystalline powder having a characteristic floral odor. Tretinoin is soluble in dimethylsulfoxide, slightly soluble in polyethylene glycol 400, octanol, and 100% ethanol. It is practically insoluble in water and mineral oil, and it is insoluble in glycerin. The chemical name for tretinoin is (all-E)-3,7-dimethyl-9-(2,6,6-trimethyl-1-cyclonexen-1-yl)-2,4,6,8-nonatetraenoic acid. Tretinoin is also referred to as all-*trans*-retinoic acid and has a molecular weight of 300.44. The structural formula is represented below.

TRETINOIN

Tretinoin is available as RENOVA at a concentration of 0.05% w/w in a water in oil emulsion formulation consisting of light mineral oil, NF; sorbitol solution, USP; hydroxyoctacosanyl hydroxystearate; methoxy PEG-22/dodecyl glycol copolymer; PEG-45/dodecyl glycol copolymer; stearoxytrimethylsilane and stearyl alcohol; dimethicone 50 cs; methylparaben, NF; edetate disodium, USP; quaternium-15; butylated hydroxytoluene, NF; citric acid monohydrate, USP; fragrance; and purified water, USP.

CLINICAL PHARMACOLOGY

The exact mechanism of action of tretinoin is unknown although retinoids are believed to exert an effect on the growth and differentiation of various epithelial cells. When applied topically, however, there was no noted increase in desmosine, hydroxyproline, or elastin mRNA in human skin. In addition, the role of the irritative nature of this product in effecting the positive effects attributed to this product for its indication has not yet been fully determined.

The transdermal absorption of tretinoin from various topical formulations ranged from 1% to 31% of applied dose, depending on whether it was applied to healthy skin or dermatitic skin. When percutaneous absorption of RENOVA was assessed in healthy male subjects (n=14) after a single application, as well as after repeated daily applications for 28 days, the absorption of tretinoin was less than 2% and endogenous concentrations of tretinoin and its major metabolites were unaltered.

INDICATIONS AND USAGE

(To understand fully the indication for this product, please read the entire INDICATIONS AND USAGE section of the labeling.)

RENOVA (tretinoin emollient cream) 0.05% is indicated as an adjunctive agent (see second bullet point below) for use in the mitigation (palliation) of fine wrinkles, mottled hyperpigmentation, and tactile roughness of facial skin in patients who do not achieve such palliation using comprehensive skin care and sun avoidance programs alone (see bullet point 3 for populations in which effectiveness has not been established). **RENOVA DOES NOT ELIMINATE WRINKLES, REPAIR SUN DAMAGED SKIN, REVERSE PHOTO-AGING, or RESTORE A MORE YOUTHFUL or YOUNGER DERMAL HISTOLOGIC PATTERN.** Many patients achieve desired palliative effects on fine wrinkling, mottled hyperpigmentation, and tactile roughness of facial skin with the use of comprehensive skin care and sun avoidance programs including sunscreens, protective clothing, and emollient creams **NOT** containing tretinoin.

- RENOVA has demonstrated NO MITIGATING EFFECT on significant signs of chronic sun exposure such as coarse or deep wrinkling, skin yellowing, lentigines, telangiectasia, skin laxity, keratinocytic atypia, melanocytic atypia, or dermal elastosis.
- RENOVA should only be used under medical supervision as an adjunct to a comprehensive skin care and sun avoidance program that includes the use of effective sunscreens (minimum SPF of 15) and protective clothing when desired results on fine wrinkles, mottled hyperpigmentation, and roughness of facial skin have not been achieved with a comprehensive skin care and sun avoidance program alone.
- The effectiveness of RENOVA in the mitigation of fine wrinkles, mottled hyperpigmentation, and tactile rough-

ness of facial skin has not been established in people greater than 50 years of age OR in people with moderately to heavily pigmented skin. In addition, patients with visible actinic keratoses and patients with a history of skin cancer were excluded from clinical trials of RENOVA. Thus the effectiveness and safety of RENOVA in these populations are not known at this time.

- Neither the safety nor the effectiveness of RENOVA for the prevention or treatment of actinic keratoses or skin neoplasms has been established.
- Neither the safety nor the efficacy of using RENOVA daily for greater than 48 weeks has been established, and daily use beyond 48 weeks has not been systematically and histologically investigated in adequate and well-controlled trials. (See **WARNINGS** section.)

CLINICAL TRIALS DATA

Two adequate and well-controlled trials were conducted involving a total of 161 evaluable patients (under 50 years of age) treated with RENOVA and 154 evaluable patients treated with the vehicle emollient cream on the face for 24 weeks as an adjunct to a comprehensive skin care and sun avoidance program, to assess the effects on fine wrinkling, mottled hyperpigmentation, and tactile skin roughness. Patients were evaluated at baseline on a 10 point scale and changes from that baseline rating were categorized as follows:

No Improvement:	No change or an increase of 1 unit or more.
Minimal Improvement:	Reduction of 1 unit.
Moderate Improvement:	Reduction of 2 units or more.

In these trials, the fine wrinkles, mottled hyperpigmentation, and tactile roughness of the facial skin were thought to be caused by multiple factors which included intrinsic aging or environmental factors, such as chronic sun exposure.

The results of these assessments are as follows:

[See table above]

Most of the improvement in these signs was noted during the first 24 weeks of therapy. Thereafter, therapy primarily maintained the improvement realized during the first 24 weeks.

A majority of patients will lose most mitigating effects of RENOVA on fine wrinkles, mottled hyperpigmentation, and tactile roughness of facial skin with discontinuation of a comprehensive skin care and sun avoidance program including RENOVA; however, the safety and effectiveness of using RENOVA daily for greater than 48 weeks have not been established.

CONTRAINDICATIONS

This drug is contraindicated in individuals with a history of sensitivity reactions to any of its components. It should be discontinued if hypersensitivity to any of its ingredients is noted.

WARNINGS

- RENOVA is a dermal irritant, and the results of continued irritation of the skin for greater than 48 weeks in chronic, long term use are not known. There is evidence of atypical changes in melanocytes and keratinocytes, and of increased dermal elastosis in some patients treated with RENOVA for longer than 48 weeks. The significance of these findings is unknown.
- Safety and effectiveness of RENOVA in individuals with moderately or heavily pigmented skin have not been established.
- RENOVA should not be administered if the patient is also taking drugs known to be photosensitizers (e.g., thiazides, tetracyclines, fluoroquinolones, phenothiazines, sulfonamides) because of the possibility of augmented phototoxicity.

Because of heightened burning susceptibility, exposure to sunlight (including sunlamps) should be avoided or minimized during use of RENOVA. Patients must be warned to use sunscreens (minimum SPF of 15) and protective clothing when using RENOVA. Patients with sunburn should be advised not to use RENOVA until fully recovered. Patients who may have considerable sun exposure due to their occupation and those patients with inherent sensitivity to sunlight should exercise particular caution when using RENOVA and assure that the precautions outlined in the Patient Package Insert are observed.

RENOVA should be kept out of the eyes, mouth, angles of the nose, and mucous membranes. Topical use may cause severe local erythema, pruritus, burning, stinging, and peeling at the site of application. If the degree of local irritation warrants, patients should be directed to use less medication, decrease the frequency of application, discontinue use temporarily, or discontinue use altogether.

Tretinoin has been reported to cause severe irritation on eczematous skin and should be used only with utmost caution in patients with this condition.

Application of larger amounts of medication than recommended will not lead to more rapid or better results, and marked redness, peeling, or discomfort may occur.

PRECAUTIONS

General: RENOVA should only be used as an adjunct to a comprehensive skin care and sun avoidance program. (See **INDICATIONS AND USAGE** section.)

If a drug sensitivity, chemical irritation, or a systemic adverse reaction develops, use of RENOVA should be discontinued.

Weather extremes, such as wind or cold, may be more irritating to patients using RENOVA.

FINE WRINKLING

	NO IMPROVEMENT	MINIMAL IMPROVEMENT	MODERATE IMPROVEMENT
RENOVA +CSP*	36%	40%	24%
Vehicle + CSP	62%	30%	8%

MOTTLED HYPERPIGMENTATION

	NO IMPROVEMENT	MINIMAL IMPROVEMENT	MODERATE IMPROVEMENT
RENOVA +CSP	35%	27%	38%
Vehicle + CSP	53%	21%	27%

TACTILE SKIN ROUGHNESS

	NO IMPROVEMENT	MINIMAL IMPROVEMENT	MODERATE IMPROVEMENT
RENOVA +CSP	49%	35%	16%
Vehicle + CSP	67%	23%	10%

* CSP = Comprehensive skin protection and sun avoidance programs including use of sunscreens, protective clothing, and emollient cream.

Information for Patients: See Patient Package Insert.

Drug Interactions: Concomitant topical medications, medicated or abrasive soaps, shampoos, cleansers, cosmetics with a strong drying effect, products with high concentrations of alcohol, astringents, spices or lime, permanent wave solutions, electrolysis, hair depilatories or waxes, and products that may irritate the skin should be used with caution in patients being treated with RENOVA because they may increase irritation with RENOVA.

RENOVA should not be administered if the patient is also taking drugs known to be photosensitizers (e.g., thiazides, tetracyclines, fluoroquinolones, phenothiazines, sulfonamides) because of the possibility of augmented phototoxicity.

Carcinogenesis, Mutagenesis, Impairment of Fertility: In a life-time dermal study in CD-1 mice, at 100 and 200 times the average recommended human topical clinical dose, a few skin tumors in the female mice and liver tumors in male mice were observed. The biological significance of these findings is not clear because they occurred at doses that exceeded the dermal maximally tolerated dose (MTD) of tretinoin and because they were within the background natural occurrence rate for these tumors in this strain of mice. There was no evidence of carcinogenic potential when tretinoin was administered topically at a dose 5 times the average recommended human topical clinical dose. For purposes of comparisons of the animal exposure to human exposure, the "recommended human topical clinical dose" is defined as 500 mg of 0.05% RENOVA applied daily to a 50 kg person.

In a chronic, two-year bioassay of Vitamin A acid in mice performed by Tsubura and Yamamoto, generalized amyloid deposition was reported in all groups in the basal layer of the Vitamin A treated skin. In CD-1 mice, a similar study reported hyalinization at the treated skin sites and the incidence of this finding was 0/50, 3/50, 3/50, and 2/50 in male mice and 1/50, 0/50, 4/50, and 2/50 in female mice from the vehicle control, 0.25 mg/kg, 0.5 mg/kg, and 1 mg/kg groups, respectively.

Studies in hairless albino mice suggest that tretinoin may enhance the tumorigenic potential of carcinogenic doses of UVB and UVA light from a solar simulator. In other studies, when lightly pigmented hairless mice treated with tretinoin were exposed to carcinogenic doses of UVB light, the incidence and rate of development of skin tumors were either reduced or no effect was seen. Due to significantly different experimental conditions, no strict comparison of these disparate data is possible at this time. Although the significance of these studies to humans is not clear, patients should minimize exposure to sun.

The mutagenic potential of tretinoin was evaluated in the Ames assay and in the in vivo mouse micronucleus assay, both of which were negative.

Dermal Segment I and III studies with RENOVA have not been performed in any species. In oral Segment I and Segment III studies in rats with tretinoin, decreased survival of neonates and growth retardation were observed at doses in excess of 2 mg/kg/day (>400 times the average recommended human topical clinical dose).

Pregnancy:

Teratogenic effects: Pregnancy Category C.

ORAL tretinoin has been shown to be teratogenic in rats, mice, rabbits, hamsters, and subhuman primates. It was teratogenic and fetotoxic in rats when given orally in doses 1000 times the average recommended human topical clinical dose. However, variations in teratogenic doses among various strains of rats have been reported. In the cynomolgus monkey, which, metabolically, is closer to humans for tretinoin than the other species examined, fetal malformations were reported at doses of 10 mg/kg/day or greater, but none were observed at 5 mg/kg/day (1000 times the average recommended human topical clinical dose), although increased skeletal variations were observed at all doses. A dose-related increased embryolethality and abortion was reported. Similar results have also been reported in pigtail macaques.

TOPICAL tretinoin in animal teratogenicity tests has generated equivocal results. There is evidence for teratogenicity (shortened or kinked tail) of topical tretinoin in Wistar rats at doses greater than 1 mg/kg/day (200 times the recommended human topical clinical dose). Anomalies (humerus: short 13%, bent 6%, os parietal incompletely ossified 14%) have also been reported when 10 mg/kg/day was dermally applied.

There are other reports in New Zealand White rabbits with doses of approximately 80 times the recommended human topical clinical dose of an increased incidence of domed head and hydrocephaly, typical of retinoid-induced fetal malformations in this species.

In contrast, several well-controlled animal studies have shown that dermally applied tretinoin was not teratogenic at doses of 100 and 200 times the recommended human topical clinical dose, in rats and rabbits, respectively.

With widespread use of any drug, a small number of birth defect reports associated temporally with the administration of the drug would be expected by chance alone. Thirty cases of temporally-associated congenital malformations have been reported during two decades of clinical use of another formulation of topical tretinoin (Retin-A). Although no definite pattern of teratogenicity and no causal association has been established from these cases, 5 of the reports describe the rare birth defect category holoprosencephaly (defects associated with incomplete midline development of the forebrain). The significance of these spontaneous reports in terms of risk to the fetus is not known.

Non-teratogenic effects:

Dermal tretinoin has been shown to be fetotoxic in rabbits when administered in doses 100 times the recommended topical human clinical dose. Oral tretinoin has been shown to be fetotoxic in rats when administered in doses 500 times the recommended topical human clinical dose.

There are, however, no adequate and well-controlled studies in pregnant women. RENOVA should not be used during pregnancy.

Nursing Mothers: It is not known whether this drug is excreted in human milk. Because many drugs are excreted in human milk, caution should be exercised when RENOVA is administered to a nursing woman.

Pediatric Use: Safety and effectiveness in patients less than 18 years of age have not been established.

Geriatric Use: Safety and effectiveness in individuals older than 50 years of age have not been established.

ADVERSE REACTIONS

(See **WARNINGS** and **PRECAUTIONS** sections.)

In double-blind, vehicle-controlled studies involving 179 patients who applied RENOVA to their face, adverse reactions associated with the use of RENOVA were limited primarily to the skin. During these trials, 4% of patients had to discontinue use of RENOVA because of adverse reactions. These discontinuations were due to skin irritation or related cutaneous adverse reactions.

Local reactions such as peeling, dry skin, burning, stinging, erythema, and pruritus were reported by almost all subjects during therapy with RENOVA. These signs and symptoms were usually of mild to moderate severity and generally occurred early in therapy. In most patients the dryness, peeling, and redness recurred after an initial (24 week) decline.

Continued on next page

Renova 0.05%—Cont.

OVERDOSAGE

Application of larger amounts of medication than recommended will not lead to more rapid or better results, and marked redness, peeling, or discomfort may occur. Oral ingestion of the drug may lead to the same side effects as those associated with excessive oral intake of Vitamin A.

DOSAGE AND ADMINISTRATION

- Do NOT use RENOVA if the patient is pregnant or is attempting to become pregnant or is at high risk of pregnancy,
- Do NOT use RENOVA if the patient is sunburned or if the patient has eczema or other chronic skin condition(s),
- Do NOT use RENOVA if the patient is inherently sensitive to sunlight,
- Do NOT use RENOVA if the patient is also taking drugs known to be photosensitizers (e.g., thiazides, tetracyclines, fluoroquinolones, phenothiazines, sulfonamides) because of the possibility of augmented phototoxicity.

Patients require detailed instruction to obtain maximal benefits and to understand all the precautions necessary to use this product with greatest safety. The physician should review the Patient Package Insert.

RENOVA should be applied to the face once a day before retiring using only enough to cover the entire affected area lightly. Patients should gently wash their face with a mild soap, pat the skin dry, and wait 20 to 30 minutes before applying RENOVA. The patient should apply a pea-sized amount of cream to cover the entire face lightly. Special caution should be taken when applying the cream to avoid the eyes, ears, nostrils, and mouth.

Application of RENOVA may cause a transitory feeling of warmth or slight stinging.

Mitigation (palliation) of facial fine wrinkling, mottled hyperpigmentation and tactile roughness may occur gradually over the course of therapy. Up to six months of therapy may be required before the effects are seen. Most of the improvement noted with RENOVA is seen during the first 24 weeks of therapy. Thereafter, therapy primarily maintains the improvement realized during the first 24 weeks.

With discontinuation of RENOVA therapy, a majority of patients will lose most mitigating effects of RENOVA on fine wrinkles, mottled hyperpigmentation, and tactile roughness of facial skin; **however, the safety and effectiveness of using RENOVA daily for greater than 48 weeks have not been established.**

Application of larger amounts of medication than recommended will not lead to more rapid or better results, and marked redness, peeling, or discomfort may occur.

Patients treated with RENOVA may use cosmetics but the areas to be treated should be cleansed thoroughly before the medication is applied. (See **PRECAUTIONS** section.)

HOW SUPPLIED

RENOVA is available in these sizes:

NDC 0062-0185-00 20 gram tube
NDC 0062-0185-05 40 gram tube
NDC 0062-0185-03 60 gram tube

Storage: Store between 15° and 25°C (59° and 77°F). DO NOT FREEZE.

QUESTIONS: Physicians and Pharmacists can call 1-800-426-7762, from 8:30 a.m. to 4:30 p.m. Eastern Time, Monday through Friday.

Rx only.

DERMATOLOGICAL DIVISION
ORTHO PHARMACEUTICAL CORPORATION
Raritan, New Jersey 08869

© OPC 1991 Revised February 1998 653-10-870-7
U.S. Patents 4,603,146, 4,423,041 and 4,877,805

Shown in Product Identification Guide, page 327

RETIN-A MICRO® ℞

[ret-in-A My-Kroe]

(tretinoin gel) microsphere
0.1%/0.04%

FOR TOPICAL USE ONLY. NOT FOR OPHTHALMIC, ORAL, OR INTRAVAGINAL USE.

DESCRIPTION

Retin-A Micro (tretinoin gel) microsphere, 0.1% and 0.04%, is a formulation containing 0.1% or 0.04%, by weight, tretinoin for topical treatment of acne vulgaris. This formulation uses patented methyl methacrylate/glycol dimethacrylate crosspolymer porous microspheres (MICROSPONGE® System) to enable inclusion of the active ingredient, tretinoin, in an aqueous gel. Other components of this formulation are purified water, carbomer 974P (0.04% formulation), carbomer 934P (0.1% formulation), glycerin, disodium EDTA, propylene glycol, sorbic acid, PPG-20 methyl glucose ether distearate, cyclomethicone and dimethicone copolyol, benzyl alcohol, trolamine, and butylated hydroxytoluene.

Chemically, tretinoin is all-*trans*-retinoic acid, also known as (all-*E*)-3,7-dimethyl-9-(2,6,6-trimethyl-1-cyclohexen-1-yl)-2,4,6,8-nonatetraenoic acid. It is a member of the retinoid family of compounds, and a metabolite of naturally occurring Vitamin A. Tretinoin has a molecular weight of 300.44. Tretinoin has the following structure:

H_3C CH_3 CH_3 CH_3 COOH CH_3

CLINICAL PHARMACOLOGY

Tretinoin is a retinoid metabolite of Vitamin A that binds to intracellular receptors in the cytosol and nucleus, but cutaneous levels of tretinoin in excess of physiologic concentrations occur following application of a tretinoin-containing topical drug product.

Although tretinoin activates three members of the retinoid acid (RAR) nuclear receptors (RARα, RARβ, and RARγ) which may act to modify gene expression, subsequent protein synthesis, and epithelial cell growth and differentiation, it has not been established whether the clinical effects of tretinoin are mediated through activation of retinoic acid receptors, other mechanisms, or both.

Mode of Action: Although the exact mode of action of tretinoin is unknown, current evidence suggests that the effectiveness of tretinoin in acne is due primarily to its ability to modify abnormal follicular keratinization. Comedones form in follicles with an excess of keratinized epithelial cells. Tretinoin promotes detachment of cornified cells and the enhanced shedding of corneocytes from the follicle. By increasing the mitotic activity of follicular epithelia, tretinoin also increases the turnover rate of thin, loosely-adherent corneocytes. Through these actions, the comedo contents are extruded and the formation of the microcomedo, the precursor lesion of acne vulgaris, is reduced.

Additionally, tretinoin acts by modulating the proliferation and differentiation of epidermal cells. These effects are mediated by tretinoin's interaction with a family of nuclear retinoic acid receptors. Activation of these nuclear receptors causes changes in gene expression. The exact mechanisms whereby tretinoin-induced changes in gene expression regulate skin function are not understood.

Pharmacokinetics: Tretinoin is a metabolite of Vitamin A metabolism in man. Percutaneous absorption, as determined by the cumulative excretion of radiolabeled drug into urine and feces, was assessed in 44 healthy men and women. Estimates of *in vivo* bioavailability, mean (SD)%, following both single and multiple daily applications, for a period of 28 days with the 0.1% gel, were 0.82 (0.11)% and 1.41 (0.54)%, respectively. The plasma concentrations of tretinoin and its metabolites, 13-*cis*-retinoic acid, all-*trans*-4-oxo-retinoic acid, and 13-*cis*-4-oxo-retinoic acid, generally ranged from 1 to 3 ng/mL and were essentially unaltered after either single or multiple daily applications of Retin-A Micro (tretinoin gel) microsphere, 0.1%, relative to baseline levels. Clinical pharmacokinetic studies have not been performed with Retin-A Micro (tretinoin gel) microsphere, 0.04%.

INDICATIONS AND USAGE

Retin-A Micro (tretinoin gel) microsphere, 0.1% and 0.04%, is indicated for topical application in the treatment of acne vulgaris. The safety and efficacy of the use of this product in the treatment of other disorders have not been established.

CLINICAL STUDIES

Retin-A Micro (tretinoin gel) microsphere, 0.1%: In two vehicle-controlled studies, Retin-A Micro (tretinoin gel) microsphere 0.1%, applied once daily was significantly more effective than vehicle in reducing the severity of acne lesion counts. The mean reductions in lesion counts from baseline after treatment for 12 weeks are shown in the following table:

Mean Percent Reduction In Lesion Counts
Retin-A Micro (tretinoin gel) microsphere, 0.1%

	Retin-A Micro (tretinoin gel) microsphere, 0.1%		Vehicle gel	
	Study #1 72 pts	Study #2 71 pts	Study #1 72 pts	Study #2 67 pts
Non-inflammatory lesion counts	49%	32%	22%	3%
Inflammatory lesion counts	37%	29%	18%	24%
Total lesion counts	45%	32%	23%	16%

[See first table above]

Retin-A Micro (tretinoin gel) microsphere, 0.1%, was also significantly superior to the vehicle in the investigator's global evaluation of the clinical response. In Study #1, thirty-five percent (35%) of patients using Retin-A Micro (tretinoin gel) microsphere, 0.1%, achieved an excellent result, as compared to eleven percent (11%) of patients on the vehicle control. In Study #2, twenty-eight percent (28%) of patients using Retin-A Micro (tretinoin gel) microsphere, 0.1%, achieved an excellent result, as compared to nine percent (9%) of the patients on the vehicle control.

Retin-A Micro (tretinoin gel) microsphere, 0.04%: In two vehicle-controlled clinical studies, Retin-A Micro (tretinoin gel) microsphere, 0.04%, applied once daily was more effective ($p < 0.05$) than vehicle in reducing the acne lesion counts. The mean reductions in lesion counts from baseline after treatment for 12 weeks are shown in the following table:

Mean Percent Reduction In Lesion Counts
Retin-A Micro (tretinoin gel) microsphere, 0.04%

	Retin-A Micro (tretinoin gel) microsphere, 0.04%		Vehicle gel	
	Study #1 108 pts	Study #2 111 pts	Study #1 110 pts	Study #2 103 pts
Non-inflammatory lesion counts	37%	29%	−2%*	14%
Inflammatory lesion counts	44%	41%	13%	30%
Total lesion counts	40%	35%	8%	20%

*–That is, a mean percent increase of 2%

[See second table above]

Retin-A Micro (tretinoin gel) microsphere, 0.04%, was also superior ($p < 0.05$) to the vehicle in the investigator's global evaluation of the clinical response. In Study #1, fourteen percent (14%) of patients using Retin-A Micro (tretinoin gel) microsphere, 0.04%, achieved an excellent result compared to five percent (5%) of patients on vehicle control. In Study #2, nineteen percent (19%) of patients using Retin-A Micro (tretinoin gel) microsphere, 0.04%, achieved an excellent result compared to nine percent (9%) of patients on vehicle control.

No studies were conducted comparing the efficacy of Retin-A Micro 0.04% to Retin-A Micro 0.1%. There is no evidence that Retin-A Micro 0.1% is more efficacious than Retin-A Micro 0.04% or that Retin-A Micro 0.04% is safer than Retin-A Micro 0.1%.

CONTRAINDICATIONS

This drug is contraindicated in individuals with a history of sensitivity reactions to any of its components. It should be discontinued if hypersensitivity to any of its ingredients is noted.

PRECAUTIONS

General:

- The skin of certain individuals may become excessively dry, red, swollen, or blistered. If the degree of irritation warrants, patients should be directed to temporarily reduce the amount or frequency of application of the medication, discontinue use temporarily, or discontinue use all together. Efficacy at reduced frequencies of application has not been established. If a reaction suggesting sensitivity occurs, use of the medication should be discontinued. Excessive skin dryness may also be experienced; if so, use of an appropriate emollient during the day may be helpful.
- Unprotected exposure to sunlight, including sunlamps, should be minimized during the use of Retin-A Micro (tretinoin gel) microsphere, 0.1% and 0.04%, and patients with sunburn should be advised not to use the product until fully recovered because of heightened susceptibility to sunlight as a result of the use of tretinoin. Patients who may be required to have considerable sun exposure due to occupation and those with inherent sensitivity to the sun

should exercise particular caution. Use of sunscreen products (SPF 15) and protective clothing over treated areas are recommended when exposure cannot be avoided.

- Weather extremes, such as wind or cold, also may be irritating to patients under treatment with tretinoin.
- Retin-A Micro (tretinoin gel) microsphere, 0.1% and 0.04%, should be kept away from the eyes, the mouth, paranasal creases of the nose, and mucous membranes.
- Tretinoin has been reported to cause severe irritation on eczematous skin and should be used with utmost caution in patients with this condition.

Information for Patients: See Patient Information leaflet.

Drug Interactions: Concomitant topical medication, medicated or abrasive soaps and cleansers, products that have a strong drying effect, products with high concentrations of alcohol, astringents, or spices should be used with caution because of possible interaction with tretinoin. Avoid contact with the peel of limes. Particular caution should be exercised with the concomitant use of topical over-the-counter acne preparations containing benzoyl peroxide, sulfur, resorcinol, or salicylic acid with Retin-A Micro (tretinoin gel) microsphere, 0.1% and 0.04%. It also is advisable to allow the effects of such preparations to subside before use of Retin-A Micro (tretinoin gel) microsphere, 0.1% and 0.04%, is begun.

Carcinogenesis, Mutagenesis, Impairment of Fertility: In a 91-week dermal study in which CD-1 mice were administered 0.017% and 0.035% formulations of tretinoin, cutaneous squamous cell carcinomas and papillomas in the treatment area were observed in some female mice. These concentrations are near the tretinoin concentration of these clinical formulations (0.04% and 0.1%). A dose-related incidence of liver tumors in male mice was observed at those same doses. The maximum systemic doses associated with the administered 0.017% and 0.035% formulations are 0.5 and 1.0 mg/kg/day, respectively. These doses are two and four times the maximum human systemic dose applied topically, when normalized for total body surface area. The biological significance of these findings is not clear because they occurred at doses that exceeded the dermal maximally tolerated dose (MTD) of tretinoin and because they were within the background natural occurrence rate for these tumors in this strain of mice. There was no evidence of carcinogenic potential when 0.025 mg/kg/day of tretinoin was administered topically to mice (0.1 times the maximum human systemic dose, normalized for total body surface area). For purposes of comparisons of the animal exposure to systemic human exposure, the maximum human systemic dose applied topically is defined as 1 gram of Retin-A Micro (tretinoin gel) microsphere, 0.1%, applied daily to a 50 kg person (0.02 mg tretinoin/kg body weight).

Dermal carcinogenicity testing has not been performed with Retin-A Micro (tretinoin gel) microsphere, 0.04% or 0.1%.

Studies in hairless albino mice suggest that concurrent exposure to tretinoin may enhance the tumorigenic potential of carcinogenic doses of UVB and UVA light from a solar simulator. This effect has been confirmed in a later study in pigmented mice, and dark pigmentation did not overcome the enhancement of photocarcinogenesis by 0.05% tretinoin. Although the significance of these studies to humans is not clear, patients should minimize exposure to sunlight or artificial ultraviolet irradiation sources.

The mutagenic potential of tretinoin was evaluated in the Ames assay and in the *in vivo* mouse micronucleus assay, both of which were negative.

The components of the microspheres have shown potential for genetic toxicity and teratogenesis. EGDMA, a component of the excipient acrylates copolymer, was positive for induction of structural chromosomal aberrations in the *in vitro* chromosomal aberration assay in mammalian cells in the absence of metabolic activation, and negative for genetic toxicity in the Ames assay, the HGPRT forward mutation assay, and the mouse micronucleus assay.

In dermal Segment I fertility studies of another tretinoin formulation in rats, slight (not statistically significant) decreases in sperm count and motility were seen at 0.5 mg/kg/day (4 times the maximum human systemic dose applied topically, and normalized for total body surface area), and slight (not statistically significant) increases in the number and percent of nonviable embryos in females treated with 0.25 mg/kg/day (2 times the maximum human systemic dose applied topically and normalized for total body surface area) and above were observed. In oral Segment I and Segment III studies in rats with tretinoin, decreased survival of neonates and growth retardation were observed at doses in excess of 2 mg/kg/day (17 times the human topical dose normalized for total body surface area).

Dermal fertility and perinatal development studies with Retin-A Micro (tretinoin gel) microsphere, 0.1% or 0.04%, have not been performed in any species.

Pregnancy: Teratogenic Effects: Pregnancy Category C.

In a study of pregnant rats treated with topical application of Retin-A Micro (tretinoin gel) microsphere, 0.1%, at doses of 0.5 to 1 mg/kg/day on gestation days 6-15 (4 to 8 times the maximum human systemic dose of tretinoin normalized for total body surface area after topical administration of Retin-A Micro (tretinoin gel) microsphere, 0.1%) some alterations were seen in vertebrae and ribs of offspring. In another study, pregnant New Zealand white rabbits were treated with Retin-A Micro (tretinoin gel) microsphere, 0.1%, at doses of 0.2, 0.5, and 1.0 mg/kg/day, administered topically for 24 hours a day while wearing Elizabethan collars to prevent ingestion of the drug. There appeared to be increased incidences of certain alterations, including domed head and hydrocephaly, typical of retinoid-induced fetal malformations in this species, at 0.5 and 1.0 mg/kg/day. Similar malformations were not observed at 0.2 mg/kg/day, 3 times the maximum human systemic dose of tretinoin after topical administration of Retin-A Micro (tretinoin gel) microsphere, 0.1%, normalized for total body surface area. In a repeat study of the highest topical dose (1.0 mg/kg/day) in pregnant rabbits, these effects were not seen, but a few alterations that may be associated with tretinoin exposure were seen. Other pregnant rabbits exposed topically for six hours to 0.5 or 0.1 mg/kg/day tretinoin while restrained in stocks to prevent ingestion, did not show any teratogenic effects at doses up to 17 times (1.0 mg/kg/day) the maximum human systemic dose after topical administration of Retin-A Micro (tretinoin gel) microsphere, 0.1%, adjusted for total body surface area, but fetal resorptions were increased at 0.5 mg/kg. In addition, topical tretinoin in non Retin-A Micro (tretinoin gel) microsphere formulations was not teratogenic in rats and rabbits when given in doses of 42 and 27 times the maximum human systemic dose after topical administration of Retin-A Micro (tretinoin gel) microsphere, 0.1%, normalized for total body surface area, respectively, (assuming a 50 kg adult applied a daily dose of 1.0 g of 0.1% gel topically). At these topical doses, however, delayed ossification of several bones occurred in rabbits. In rats, a dose-dependent increase of supernumerary ribs was observed.

Oral tretinoin has been shown to be teratogenic in rats, mice, rabbits, hamsters, and subhuman primates. Tretinoin was teratogenic in Wistar rats when given orally or topically in doses greater than 1 mg/kg/day (8 times the maximum human systemic dose normalized for total body surface area). However, variations in teratogenic doses among various strains of rats have been reported. In the cynomolgus monkey, which metabolically is more similar to humans than other species in its handling of tretinoin, fetal malformations were reported for doses of 10 mg/kg/day or greater, but none were observed at 5 mg/kg/day (83 times the maximum human systemic dose normalized for total body surface area), although increased skeletal variations were observed at all doses. Dose-related increases in embryolethality and abortion also were reported. Similar results have also been reported in pigtail macaques.

Topical tretinoin in animal teratogenicity tests has generated equivocal results. There is evidence for teratogenicity (shortened or kinked tail) of topical tretinoin in Wistar rats at doses greater than 1 mg/kg/day (8 times the maximum human systemic dose normalized for total body surface area). Anomalies (humerus: short 13%, bent 6%, os parietal incompletely ossified 14%) have also been reported when 10 mg/kg/day was topically applied. Supernumerary ribs have been a consistent finding in rats when dams were treated topically or orally with retinoids.

There are no adequate and well-controlled studies in pregnant women. Retin-A Micro should be used during pregnancy only if the potential benefit justifies the potential risk to the fetus.

With widespread use of any drug, a small number of birth defect reports associated temporally with the administration of the drug would be expected by chance alone. Thirty human cases of temporally associated congenital malformations have been reported during two decades of clinical use of Retin-A. Although no definite pattern of teratogenicity and no causal association has been established from these cases, five of the reports describe the rare birth defect category holoprosencephaly (defects associated with incomplete midline development of the forebrain). The significance of these spontaneous reports in terms of risk to the fetus is not known.

Non-Teratogenic Effects: Topical tretinoin has been shown to be fetotoxic in rabbits when administered 0.5 mg/kg/day (8 times the maximum human systemic dose applied topically and normalized for total body surface area), resulting in fetal resorptions and variations in ossification. Oral tretinoin has been shown to be fetotoxic, resulting in skeletal variations and increased intrauterine death in rats when administered 2.5 mg/kg/day (21 times the maximum human systemic dose applied topically and normalized for total body surface area).

There are, however no adequate and well-controlled studies in pregnant women.

Animal Toxicity Studies: In male mice treated topically with Retin-A Micro (tretinoin gel) microsphere, 0.1%, at 0.5, 2.0, or 5.0 mg/kg/day tretinoin (2, 8, or 21 times the maximum human systemic dose after topical administration of Retin-A Micro (tretinoin gel) microsphere, 0.1%, normalized for total body surface area) for 90 days, a reduction in testicular weight, but with no pathological changes were observed at the two highest doses. Similarly, in female mice there was a reduction in ovarian weights, but without any underlying pathological changes, at 5.0 mg/kg/day (21 times the maximum human dose). In this study there was a dose-related increase in the plasma concentration of tretinoin 4 hours after the first dose. A separate toxicokinetic study in mice indicates that systemic exposure is greater after topical application to unrestrained animals than to restrained animals, suggesting that the systemic toxicity observed is probably related to ingestion. Male and female dogs treated with Retin-A Micro (tretinoin gel) microsphere, 0.1%, at 0.2, 0.5, or 1.0 mg/kg/day tretinoin (5, 12, or 25 times the maximum human systemic dose after topical administration of Retin-A Micro (tretinoin gel) microsphere, 0.1%, normalized for total body surface area, respectively) for 90 days showed no evidence of reduced testicular or ovarian weights or pathological changes.

Nursing Mothers: It is not known whether this drug is excreted in human milk. Because many drugs are excreted in human milk, caution should be exercised when Retin-A Micro (tretinoin gel) microsphere, 0.1% or 0.04%, is administered to a nursing woman.

Pediatric Use: Safety and effectiveness in children below the age of 12 have not been established.

Geriatric Use: Safety and effectiveness in a geriatric population have not been established. Clinical studies of Retin-A Micro did not include sufficient numbers of subjects aged 65 and over to determine whether they respond differently from younger subjects.

ADVERSE REACTIONS

Irritation Potential:

Acne clinical trial results: In separate clinical trials for each concentration, acne patients treated with Retin-A Micro (tretinoin gel) microsphere, 0.1% or 0.04%, analysis over the twelve week period showed that cutaneous irritation scores for erythema, peeling, dryness, burning/stinging, or itching peaked during the initial two weeks of therapy, decreasing thereafter.

Approximately half of the patients treated with Retin-A Micro, 0.04% had cutaneous irritation at Week 2. Of those patients who did experience cutaneous side effects, most had signs or symptoms that were mild in severity (severity was ranked on a 4-point ordinal scale: 0=none, 1=mild, 2=moderate, and 3=severe). Less than 10% of patients experienced moderate cutaneous irritation and there was no severe irritation at Week 2.

In studies on Retin-A Micro (tretinoin gel) microsphere, 0.04%, throughout the treatment period the majority of patients experienced some degree of irritation (mild, moderate, or severe) with 1% (2/225) of patients having scores indicative of a severe irritation rating; and 1.3% (3/225) of patients treated with Retin-A Micro (tretinoin gel) microsphere, 0.04%, discontinued treatment due to irritation, which included dryness in one patient and peeling and urticaria in another.

In studies on Retin-A Micro (tretinoin gel) microsphere, 0.1%, no more than 3% of patients had cutaneous irritation scores indicative of a severe irritation rating; although, 6% (14/224) of patients treated with Retin-A Micro (tretinoin gel) microsphere, 0.1% discontinued treatment due to irritation. Of these 14 patients, four had severe irritation after 3 to 5 days of treatment, with blistering in one patient.

Results in studies of subjects without acne: In a half-face comparison trial conducted for up to 14 days in women with sensitive skin, but without acne, Retin-A Micro (tretinoin gel) microsphere, 0.1% was statistically less irritating than tretinoin cream, 0.1%. In addition, a cumulative 21 day irritation evaluation in subjects with normal skin showed that Retin-A Micro (tretinoin gel) microsphere, 0.1%, had a lower irritation profile than tretinoin cream, 0.1%. The clinical significance of these irritation studies for patients with acne is not established. Comparable effectiveness of Retin-A Micro (tretinoin gel) microsphere, 0.1% and tretinoin cream, 0.1%, has not been established. The lower irritancy of Retin-A Micro (tretinoin gel) microsphere, 0.1% in subjects without acne may be attributable to the properties of its vehicle. The contribution to decreased irritancy by the MICROSPONGE® System has not been established. No irritation studies have been performed to compare Retin-A Micro (tretinoin gel) microsphere, 0.04%, with either Retin-A Micro (tretinoin gel) microsphere, 0.1%, or tretinoin cream, 0.1%.

The skin of certain sensitive individuals may become excessively red, edematous, blistered, or crusted. If these effects occur, the medication should either be discontinued until the integrity of the skin is restored, or the medication should be adjusted to a level the patient can tolerate. However, efficacy has not been established for lower dosing frequencies (see **DOSAGE AND ADMINISTRATION** Section).

True contact allergy to topical tretinoin is rarely encountered. Temporary hyper- or hypopigmentation has been reported with repeated application of tretinoin. Some individuals have been reported to have heightened susceptibility to sunlight while under treatment with tretinoin.

OVERDOSAGE

Retin-A Micro (tretinoin gel) microsphere, 0.1% and 0.04%, is intended for topical use only. If medication is applied excessively, no more rapid or better results will be obtained and marked redness, peeling, or discomfort may occur. Oral ingestion of large amounts of the drug may lead to the same side effects as those associated with excessive oral intake of Vitamin A.

DOSAGE AND ADMINISTRATION

Retin-A Micro (tretinoin gel) microsphere, 0.1% and 0.04%, should be applied once a day, in the evening, to the skin where acne lesions appear, using enough to cover the entire affected area lightly. Application of excessive amounts of gel may result in "caking" of the gel, and will not provide incremental efficacy.

A transitory feeling of warmth or slight stinging may be noted on application. In cases where it has been necessary to temporarily discontinue therapy or to reduce the frequency of application, therapy may be resumed or the frequency of application increased as the patient becomes able to tolerate the treatment. Frequency of application should be closely monitored by careful observation of the clinical

Continued on next page

Retin-A Micro—Cont.

therapeutic response and skin tolerance. Efficacy has not been established for less than once daily dosing frequencies. During the early weeks of therapy, an apparent exacerbation of inflammatory lesions may occur. If tolerated, this should not be considered a reason to discontinue therapy. Therapeutic results may be noticed after two weeks, but more than seven weeks of therapy are required before consistent beneficial effects are observed.
Patients treated with Retin-A Micro (tretinoin gel) microsphere, 0.1% and 0.04%, may use cosmetics, but the areas to be treated should be cleansed thoroughly before the medication is applied.

HOW SUPPLIED

Retin-A Micro® (tretinoin gel) microsphere, 0.1% is supplied as:
20g (NDC 0062-0190-02) and 45g (NDC 0062-0190-03) tubes.
Retin-A Micro® (tretinoin gel) microsphere, 0.04% is supplied as:
20g (NDC 0062-0204-02) and 45g (NDC 0062-0204-03) tubes.
Storage Conditions: Store at 15°–25°C (59°–77°F).
Rx only.
Patent Nos.: 4,690,825; 5,145,675 & 5,955,109
ORTHO DERMATOLOGICAL
Division of Ortho-McNeil Pharmaceutical, Inc.
Skillman, New Jersey 08558
643-11-706-2
643-10-706-2

Retin-A Micro® is a registered trademark of Ortho-McNeil Pharmaceutical, Inc.
MICROSPONGE® is a registered trademark of Enhanced Derm Technologies Inc.
Redwood City, CA
Shown in Product Identification Guide, page 327

SPECTAZOLE® ℞

[*spĕk-tră-zōl*]
(econazole nitrate 1%)
Cream
For Topical Use Only

Prescribing Information

DESCRIPTION

SPECTAZOLE Cream contains the antifungal agent, econazole nitrate 1%, in a water-miscible base consisting of pegoxol 7 stearate, peglicol 5 oleate, mineral oil, benzoic acid, butylated hydroxyanisole, and purified water. The white to off-white soft cream is for topical use only.
Chemically, econazole nitrate is 1-[2-{(4-chloro-phenyl) methoxy}-2-(2,4-dichlorophenyl)ethyl]-1H-imidazole mononitrate. Its structure is as follows:

[Structure: imidazole–CH2-CH-O-CH2–(4-chlorophenyl), with 2,4-dichlorophenyl; ·HNO3]

CLINICAL PHARMACOLOGY

After topical application to the skin of normal subjects, systemic absorption of econazole nitrate is extremely low. Although most of the applied drug remains on the skin surface, drug concentrations were found in the stratum corneum which, by far, exceeded the minimum inhibitory concentration for dermatophytes. Inhibitory concentrations were achieved in the epidermis and as deep as the middle region of the dermis. Less than 1% of the applied dose was recovered in the urine and feces.
Microbiology: Econazole nitrate has been shown to be active against most strains of the following microorganisms, both *in vitro* and in clinical infections as described in the INDICATIONS AND USAGE section.

Dermatophytes	**Yeasts**
Epidermophyton floccosum	*Candida albicans*
Microsporum audouini	*Malassezia furfur*
Microsporum canis	
Microsporum gypseum	
Trichophyton mentagrophytes	
Trichophyton rubrum	
Trichophyton tonsurans	

Econazole nitrate exhibits broad-spectrum antifungal activity against the following organisms *in vitro,* **but the clinical significance of these data is unknown.**

Dermatophytes	**Yeasts**
Trichophyton verrucosum	*Candida guillermondii*
	Candida parapsilosis
	Candida tropicalis

INDICATIONS AND USAGE

SPECTAZOLE Cream is indicated for topical application in the treatment of tinea pedis, tinea cruris, and tinea corporis caused by *Trichophyton rubrum, Trichophyton mentagrophytes, Trichophyton tonsurans, Microsporum canis, Microsporum audouini, Microsporum gypseum,* and *Epidermophyton floccosum,* in the treatment of cutaneous candidiasis, and in the treatment of tinea versicolor.

CONTRAINDICATIONS

SPECTAZOLE Cream is contraindicated in individuals who have shown hypersensitivity to any of its ingredients.

WARNINGS

SPECTAZOLE is not for ophthalmic use.

PRECAUTIONS

General: If a reaction suggesting sensitivity or chemical irritation should occur, use of the medication should be discontinued.
For external use only. Avoid introduction of SPECTAZOLE Cream into the eyes.
Carcinogenicity Studies: Long-term animal studies to determine carcinogenic potential have not been performed.
Fertility (Reproduction): Oral administration of econazole nitrate in rats has been reported to produce prolonged gestation. Intravaginal administration in humans has not shown prolonged gestation or other adverse reproductive effects attributable to econazole nitrate therapy.
Pregnancy: Pregnancy Category C. Econazole nitrate has not been shown to be teratogenic when administered orally to mice, rabbits or rats. Fetotoxic or embryotoxic effects were observed in Segment I oral studies with rats receiving 10 to 40 times the human dermal dose. Similar effects were observed in Segment II or Segment III studies with mice, rabbits and/or rats receiving oral doses 80 or 40 times the human dermal dose.
Econazole nitrate should be used in the first trimester of pregnancy only when the physician considers it essential to the welfare of the patient. The drug should be used during the second and third trimesters of pregnancy only if clearly needed.
Nursing Mothers: It is not known whether econazole nitrate is excreted in human milk. Following oral administration of econazole nitrate to lactating rats, econazole and/or metabolites were excreted in milk and were found in nursing pups. Also, in lactating rats receiving large oral doses (40 or 80 times the human dermal dose), there was a reduction in post partum viability of pups and survival to weaning; however, at these high doses, maternal toxicity was present and may have been a contributing factor. Caution should be exercised when econazole nitrate is administered to a nursing woman.

ADVERSE REACTIONS

During clinical trials, approximately 3% of patients treated with econazole nitrate 1% cream reported side effects thought possibly to be due to the drug, consisting mainly of burning, itching, stinging, and erythema. One case of pruritic rash has also been reported.

OVERDOSE

Overdosage of econazole nitrate in humans has not been reported to date. In mice, rats, guinea pigs and dogs, the oral LD 50 values were found to be 462, 668, 272, and >160 mg/kg, respectively.

DOSAGE AND ADMINISTRATION

Sufficient SPECTAZOLE Cream should be applied to cover affected areas once daily in patients with tinea pedis, tinea cruris, tinea corporis, and tinea versicolor, and twice daily (morning and evening) in patients with cutaneous candidiasis.
Early relief of symptoms is experienced by the majority of patients and clinical improvement may be seen fairly soon after treatment is begun; however, candidal infections and tinea cruris and corporis should be treated for two weeks and tinea pedis for one month in order to reduce the possibility of recurrence. If a patient shows no clinical improvement after the treatment period, the diagnosis should be redetermined. Patients with tinea versicolor usually exhibit clinical and mycological clearing after two weeks of treatment.

HOW SUPPLIED

SPECTAZOLE (econazole nitrate 1%) Cream is supplied in tubes of 15 grams (NDC 0062-5460-02), 30 grams (NDC 0062-5460-01), and 85 grams (NDC 0062-5460-03).
Store SPECTAZOLE Cream below 86°F.
Ortho Dermatological, Division of
Ortho-McNeil Pharmaceutical, Inc.
Skillman, New Jersey 08558
©OMP 2001 Revised January 2001 631-11-331-1
Shown in Product Identification Guide, page 327

For information on over-the-counter drugs,
consult **PDR For Nonprescription Drugs and Dietary Supplements.**

Ortho-Clinical Diagnostics

A Johnson & Johnson Company
1001 U.S. HWY 202
RARITAN, NEW JERSEY 08869-0606

Direct Inquiries to:
Customer Service
(800) 828-6316

Rh_o(D) Immune Globulin (Human)
RhoGAM® ℞
Ultra-Filtered (300 μg)
MICRhoGAM®
Ultra-Filtered (50 μg)
Rx Only
For Intramuscular Injection Only
Preservative-free, latex-free delivery system

DESCRIPTION

RhoGAM® and MICRhoGAM® Rh_o(D) Immune Globulin (Human) are sterile solutions containing IgG anti-D (anti-Rh) for use in preventing Rh immunization. They are manufactured from human plasma containing anti-D. A single dose of RhoGAM contains sufficient anti-D (approximately 300 μg)* to suppress the immune response to 15 mL (or less) of Rh-positive red blood cells.[2,3] A single dose of MICRhoGAM contains sufficient anti-D (approximately 50 μg)* to suppress the immune response to 2.5 mL (or less) of Rh-positive red blood cells. The anti-D dose is measured by comparison to the RhoGAM in-house reference standard, the potency of which is established relative to the International Reference Preparation 68/419.
All donors are carefully screened by history and laboratory testing to reduce the risk of transmitting blood-borne pathogens from infected donors. Fractionation of the plasma is performed by a modification of the cold alcohol procedure that has been shown to significantly lower viral titers.[4] Following fractionation, an additional viral-clearance filtration step is incorporated into the manufacturing process. This filtration step removes viruses via a size-exclusion mechanism utilizing a patented Viresolve† 180 ultrafiltration membrane with defined pore-size distribution of 12–18 nanometers. The ultrafiltration step utilizes tangential flow filtration to permit filtration of IgG while effectively retarding enveloped and non-enveloped viruses above the pore-size distribution cutoff. The filter is inert to the product. Non-enveloped viruses are known to be resistant to chemical and physical inactivation.[5,6] Laboratory spiking studies have shown that the cumulative viral removal capability of the RhoGAM/MICRhoGAM manufacturing process exceeds 13 logs for human immunodeficiency virus (HIV). Clearance of model viruses for hepatitis C virus (HCV), hepatitis B virus (HBV) and parvovirus B19 (a non-enveloped virus) exceeds 11 logs.[4] The donor selection process, the fractionation process and the Viresolve ultrafiltration step are designed to increase product safety by reducing the risk of transmission of enveloped and non-enveloped viruses. Rh_o(D) Immune Globulin (Human) intended for intramuscular use and prepared by cold alcohol fractionation has not been reported to transmit hepatitis or other infectious diseases.[7]
The safety of Rh_o(D) Immune Globulin (Human) has been further shown in an empirical study of viral marker rates in female blood donors in the United States.[8] This study revealed that Rh-negative donors, of whom an estimated 55–60% had received Rh_o(D) Immune Globulin (Human) for pregnancy-related indications, had prevalence and incidence viral marker rates similar to those of Rh-positive female donors who had not received Rh_o(D) Immune Globulin (Human). Even after the fractionation and virus-filtration steps, there remains a risk of contracting blood-borne pathogens from a plasma-derived product.
The final product contains approximately 5 ± 1% gamma globulin, 2.9 mg/mL sodium chloride, 0.01% polysorbate 80 and 15 mg/mL glycine. Small amounts of IgA, typically less than 15 μg per dose, are present.[9] The pH range is 6.20–6.55. The product contains no preservative and utilizes a latex-free delivery system.

*The anti-D content of RhoGAM/MICRhoGAM is expressed as μg per dose. It can be expressed as International Units (IU) per dose. The conversion factor is 1 μg = 5 IU.[1]
†Viresolve is a trademark of Millipore Corporation.

CLINICAL PHARMACOLOGY

Mechanism of Action

RhoGAM® and MICRhoGAM® act by suppressing the immune response of Rh-negative individuals to Rh-positive red blood cells. The mechanism of action is unknown. RhoGAM, MICRhoGAM and other Rh_o(D) Immune Globulin (Human) products are not effective in altering the course or consequences of Rh immunization once it has occurred.

Obstetrical Use

The Rh-negative obstetrical patient may be exposed to red blood cells from her Rh-positive fetus during the normal course of pregnancy or after obstetrical procedures or abdominal trauma. Clinical studies have proven that the incidence of Rh immunization as a result of pregnancy was reduced to 1–2% from 12–13% when RhoGAM was given within 72 hours following delivery.[10,11] Antepartum administration of Rh immune globulin at 28 weeks, as well as within 72 hours of delivery, has been shown to reduce the Rh immunization rate to about 0.1–0.2%.[12,13]

Clinical studies demonstrated that administration of MICRhoGAM within three hours following abortion was 100% effective in preventing Rh immunization.[14]

Use after Rh Incompatible Transfusion

An Rh-negative individual transfused with one unit of Rh-positive red blood cells has about an 80% likelihood of producing anti-D.[3] However, Rh immunization can occur after exposure to < 1 mL of Rh-positive red blood cells. Protection from Rh immunization is accomplished by administering the appropriate dose of RhoGAM or MICRhoGAM, which is ≥ 20 µg per mL of Rh-positive red blood cells, within 72 hours of transfusion of incompatible red cells.[2,15] (See **DOSAGE AND ADMINISTRATION** section.)

Pharmacokinetic Properties

Pharmacokinetic studies after intramuscular injection were performed on eight Rh-negative subjects.[16] Six subjects received a single dose (300 µg) of RhoGAM, while two subjects received four doses (1200 µg). Plasma anti-D levels were monitored for four months using a validated method with sensitivity of approximately 1 ng/mL. The parameters measured and/or calculated included the following:

Cmax = maximum plasma concentration obtained (ng/mL)
Tmax = time to attain Cmax (days)
T1/2 = elimination half-life (days)
Vd = volume of distribution (liters)

Mean Pharmacokinetic Parameters for RhoGAM

Parameter	Single Dose (n = 6)	Four Doses (n = 2)	Dose Ratio (1/4)
Cmax	37.1	146.3	0.253
Tmax	5	5	0.999
T1/2	24.2	27.0	0.933
Vd	8.59	8.16	1.053

INDICATIONS AND USAGE

Pregnancy and Other Obstetrical Conditions in Rh-Negative Women, Unless the Father or Baby are Conclusively Rh Negative

- Pregnancy/delivery of an Rh-positive baby irrespective of the ABO groups of the mother and baby
- Abortion/threatened abortion at any stage of gestation
- Ectopic pregnancy
- Antepartum fetal-maternal hemorrhage (suspected or proven) resulting from antepartum hemorrhage (e.g., placenta previa), amniocentesis, chorionic villus sampling, percutaneous umbilical blood sampling, other obstetrical manipulative procedure (e.g., version) or abdominal trauma
- Transfusion of Rh incompatible blood or blood products

Transfusion

- Prevention of Rh immunization in any Rh-negative person after incompatible transfusion of Rh-positive blood or blood products (e.g., red cells, platelet concentrates, granulocyte concentrates)

CONTRAINDICATIONS

Individuals known to have had an anaphylactic or severe systemic reaction to human globulin should not receive RhoGAM®, MICRhoGAM® or any other $Rh_o(D)$ Immune Globulin (Human).

WARNINGS

RhoGAM® and MICRhoGAM® are made from human plasma. Because these products are made from human blood, they may carry a risk of transmitting infectious agents, e.g., viruses, and, theoretically, the Creutzfeldt-Jakob disease (CJD) agent. The risk that such products will transmit an infectious agent has been reduced by screening plasma donors for prior exposure to certain viruses, by testing for the presence of certain current virus infections and by removing certain viruses during the manufacturing process. Following fractionation, an additional viral-clearance filtration step is incorporated into the manufacturing process. This filtration step removes viruses via a size-exclusion mechanism utilizing a patented Viresolve 180 ultrafiltration membrane with a defined pore-size distribution of 12–18 nanometers. The filter is inert to the product. This virus removal process has been shown in laboratory spiking studies to reduce the levels of some viruses ranging from 18–200 nanometers in size, including enveloped viruses as well as non-enveloped viruses.[4] All of the above steps are designed to increase product safety by reducing the risk of transmission of lipid-enveloped and non-lipid-enveloped viruses. Despite these measures, such products can still potentially transmit disease. There is also the possibility that unknown infectious agents may be present in such products. ALL infections thought by a physician possibly to have been transmitted by these products should be reported by the physician or other healthcare provider in the United States to Ortho-Clinical Diagnostics, Inc. at 1-800-421-3311. Outside the United States, the company distributing these products should be contacted. The physician should discuss the risks and benefits of these products with the patient. RhoGAM and MICRhoGAM are manufactured and distributed by Ortho-Clinical Diagnostics, Inc., Raritan, NJ 08869.

PRECAUTIONS

For intramuscular use only. Do not inject RhoGAM® or MICRhoGAM® intravenously. In the case of postpartum use, the product is intended for maternal administration. Do not inject the newborn infant.

Patients should be observed for at least 20 minutes after administration.

Allergic responses to RhoGAM or MICRhoGAM may occur. Patients should be informed of the early signs of hypersensitivity reactions, including hives, generalized urticaria, tightness of the chest, wheezing, hypotension and anaphylaxis. The treatment depends upon the nature and severity of the reaction.

RhoGAM and MICRhoGAM contain a small quantity of IgA (less than 15 µg per dose).[9] Although high doses of intravenous immunoglobulin containing IgA at levels of 270–720 µg/mL have been given without incident during treatment of patients with high-titered antibodies to IgA,[17] the attending physician must weigh the benefit against the potential risks of hypersensitivity reactions.

The presence of passively acquired anti-D in the maternal serum may cause a positive antibody screening test. This does not preclude further antepartum or postpartum prophylaxis.

Some babies born of women given $Rh_o(D)$ Immune Globulin (Human) antepartum have weakly positive direct antiglobulin (Coombs) tests at birth.

Fetal-maternal hemorrhage may cause false blood typing results in the mother. Late in pregnancy or following delivery, there may be sufficient fetal Rh-positive red blood cells in the circulation of the Rh-negative mother to cause a positive antiglobulin test for weak D (D^u). When there is any doubt as to the patient's Rh type, RhoGAM or MICRhoGAM should be administered.

Pregnancy Category C

Animal reproduction studies have not been conducted with RhoGAM or MICRhoGAM. The available evidence suggests that $Rh_o(D)$ Immune Globulin (Human) does not harm the fetus or affect future pregnancies or the reproduction capacity of the maternal recipient.[18,19]

ADVERSE REACTIONS

Adverse experience (AE) complaints related to RhoGAM® Ultra-Filtered and MICRhoGAM® Ultra-Filtered are received at a rate of approximately one complaint per 60,000 doses distributed for use.[20] These AE complaints are split between reports of anti-D formation despite RhoGAM or MICRhoGAM administration and reports of local reactions at the site of administration.

Local AE reactions include swelling, induration, redness and mild pain at the site of injection, and a small number of patients have noted a slight elevation in temperature. Rarely, these reactions have been treated with antihistamines or corticosteroids. Systemic reactions to RhoGAM or MICRhoGAM are extremely rare. There have been no reported fatalities due to anaphylaxis or any other cause related to RhoGAM or MICRhoGAM administration.

As with any $Rh_o(D)$ Immune Globulin (Human), administration to patients who have received Rh-positive red blood cells may result in signs and symptoms of a hemolytic reaction, including fever, back pain, nausea and vomiting, hypo- or hypertension, hemoglobinuria/emia, elevated bilirubin and creatinine and decreased haptoglobin.

DOSAGE AND ADMINISTRATION

For intramuscular use only. Do not inject RhoGAM® or MICRhoGAM® intravenously. In the case of postpartum use, the product is intended for maternal administration. Do not inject the newborn infant.

Parenteral drug products should be inspected visually for particulate matter and discoloration prior to administration.

A single dose (approximately 50 µg)* is contained in each prefilled syringe of MICRhoGAM. This dose will suppress the immune response to 2.5 mL of Rh-positive red blood cells. MICRhoGAM is therefore indicated within 72 hours after termination of pregnancy up to and including 12 weeks' gestation. At or beyond 13 weeks' gestation, RhoGAM should be administered instead of MICRhoGAM.

A single dose (approximately 300 µg)* is contained in each prefilled syringe of RhoGAM. This is the usual dose for the indications associated with pregnancy unless there is clinical or laboratory evidence of a fetal-maternal hemorrhage (FMH) in excess of 15 mL of Rh-positive red blood cells. RhoGAM should be administered within 72 hours of known or suspected exposure to Rh-positive red blood cells. The indications and recommended dosage for RhoGAM and MICRhoGAM are summarized in the following table.

Indications and Recommended Dosage

Indication	Indicated Dose[a] (approximately)
Postpartum (if the newborn is Rh-positive)	300 µg[b]
Antepartum: Prophylaxis at 26 to 28 weeks' gestation[c]	300 µg
Antepartum: Amniocentesis, chorionic villus sampling (CVS) and percutaneous umbilical blood sampling (PUBS)	300 µg
Antepartum: Abdominal trauma or obstetrical manipulation	300 µg
Antepartum: Ectopic pregnancy[d]	300 µg
Antepartum: Abortion or threatened abortion at any stage of gestation with continuation of pregnancy[d]	300 µg
Transfusion of Rh-incompatible blood or blood products[d]	300 µg

[a] Additional doses of RhoGAM are indicated when the patient has been exposed to > 15 mL of Rh-positive red blood cells. This may be determined by use of qualitative or quantitative tests for FMH (see below).

[b] See **DESCRIPTION** section.

[c] If antepartum prophylaxis is indicated, it is essential that the mother receive a postpartum dose if the infant is Rh-positive.

[d] If abortion or termination of pregnancy occurs up to and including 12 weeks' gestation, or less than 2.5 mL of Rh-incompatible red blood cells were administered, a single dose of MICRhoGAM $Rh_o(D)$ Immune Globulin (Human) (approximately 50 µg)* may be used instead of RhoGAM.

If RhoGAM is administered for one of the above indications early in pregnancy (before 26 to 28 weeks), there is an obligation to maintain a level of passively acquired anti-D by administration of RhoGAM at 12-week intervals. RhoGAM should be administered within 72 hours of delivery or exposure to Rh-positive red blood cells. There is little information concerning the effectiveness of Rh Immune Globulin when given beyond this 72-hour period. In one study, Rh Immune Globulin provided protection against Rh immunization in about 50% of subjects when given 13 days after exposure to Rh-positive cells.[21] If delivery occurs within three weeks after the last antepartum dose, the postpartum dose may be withheld, but a test for FMH should be performed to determine if exposure to > 15 mL of red cells has occurred.[22]

Multiple doses of RhoGAM are required if an FMH exceeds 15 mL, an event that is possible but unlikely prior to the third trimester of pregnancy and is most likely at delivery. Patients known or suspected to be at increased risk of FMH should be tested for FMH by qualitative or quantitative methods.[23] In efficacy studies, RhoGAM was shown to suppress Rh immunization in all subjects when given at a dose of ≥ 20 µg per mL of Rh-positive red blood cells.[3] Thus, a single dose of RhoGAM will suppress the immune response after exposure to ≤ 15 mL of Rh-positive red blood cells. However, in clinical practice, laboratory methods used to determine the amount of exposure (volume of transfusion or FMH) to Rh-positive red blood cells are imprecise.[24,25] Therefore, administration of more than 20 µg of RhoGAM per mL of Rh-positive red blood cells should be considered whenever a large FMH or red cell exposure is suspected or documented.[25]

When multiple doses are required, consult your pharmacy for pooling directions. Multiple doses may be administered at the same time or at spaced intervals, as long as the total dose is administered within three days of exposure.

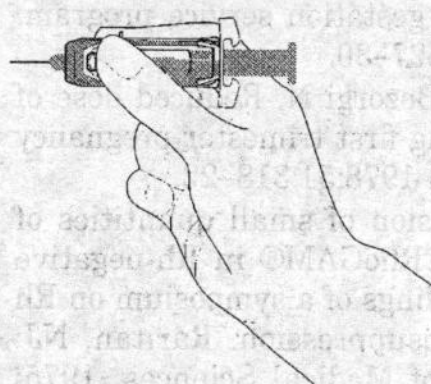

Administer injection.
Administer injection per standard protocol.
Note: When administering an intramuscular injection, place fingers in contact with syringe barrel through windows in shield to prevent possible premature activation of safety guard.

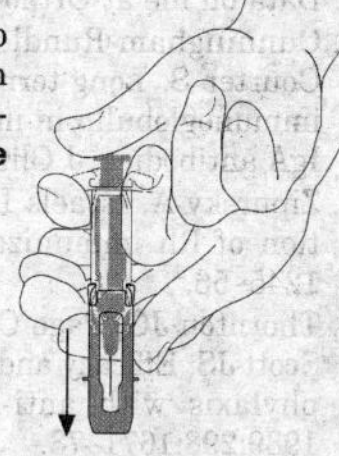

Slide safety guard over needle.
After injection, use free hand to slide safety guard over needle. An audible "click" indicates proper activation. **Keep hands behind needle at all times.**

Overdosage

Patients who receive RhoGAM or MICRhoGAM for Rh-incompatible transfusion should be monitored by clinical and laboratory means due to the risk of a hemolytic reaction.

HOW SUPPLIED

RhoGAM® is available in packages containing:

- 5 prefilled single-dose syringes of RhoGAM (Product Code 780710) NDC 0562-7807-06
- 5 package inserts
- 5 control forms
- 5 patient identification cards

and

- 25 prefilled single-dose syringes of RhoGAM (Product Code 780715) NDC 0562-7807-26
- 25 package inserts
- 25 control forms
- 25 patient identification cards

MICRhoGAM® is available in packages containing:

- 5 prefilled single-dose syringes of MICRhoGAM (Product Code 780810) NDC 0562-7808-06
- 5 package inserts
- 5 control forms

Continued on next page

Rho(D)/RhoGAM/MICRhoGAM—Cont.

- 5 patient identification cards

and

- 25 prefilled single-dose syringes of MICRhoGAM (Product Code 780815) NDC 0562-7808-26
- 25 package inserts
- 25 control forms
- 25 patient identification cards

STORAGE

Store at 2 to 8°C. Do not store frozen.

REFERENCES

1. Gunson HH, Bowell PJ, Kirkwood TBL. Collaborative study to recalibrate the International Reference Preparation of anti-D immunoglobulin. J Clin Pathol 1980;33: 249–53.
2. Pollack W, Ascari WQ, Kochesky RJ, O'Connor RR, Ho TY, Tripodi D. Studies on Rh prophylaxis. I. Relationship between doses of anti-Rh and size of antigenic stimulus. Transfusion 1971;11:333–39.
3. Pollack W, Ascari WQ, Crispen JF, O'Connor RR, Ho TY. Studies on Rh prophylaxis. II. Rh immune prophylaxis after transfusion with Rh-positive blood. Transfusion 1971;11:340–44.
4. Data on file at Ortho-Clinical Diagnostics, Inc.
5. Prowse C, Ludlam CA, Yap PL. Human parvovirus B19 and blood products. Vox Sang 1997;72:1–10.
6. Mannucci PM, Gdovin S, Gringeri A, Colombo M, Mele A, Schinaia N, Ciavarella N, Emerson SU, Purcell RH. Transmission of hepatitis A to patients with hemophilia by Factor VIII concentrates treated with organic solvent and detergent to inactivate viruses. Ann Intern Med 1994;120:1–7.
7. Tabor E. The epidemiology of virus transmission by plasma derivatives: clinical studies verifying the lack of transmission of hepatitis B and C viruses and HIV type 1. Transfusion 1999;39:1160–68.
8. Watanabe KK, Busch MP, Schreiber GB, Zuck TF. Evaluation of the safety of Rh Immunoglobulin by monitoring viral markers among Rh-negative female blood donors. Vox Sang 2000;8:1–6.
9. Data on file at Ortho-Clinical Diagnostics, Inc.
10. Pollack W, Gorman JG, Freda VJ, Ascari WQ, Allen AE, Baker WJ. Results of clinical trials of RhoGAM in women. Transfusion 1968;8:151–53.
11. Freda VJ, Gorman JG, Pollack W, Bowe E. Prevention of Rh hemolytic disease—ten years' clinical experience with Rh immune globulin. New Engl J Med 1975; 292: 1014–16.
12. Bowman JM, Chown B, Lewis M, Pollock JM. Rh isoimmunization during pregnancy: antenatal prophylaxis. Can Med Assoc J 1978;118:623–27.
13. Bowman JM, Pollock JM. Antenatal prophylaxis of Rh isoimmunization: 28-weeks' gestation service program. Can Med Assoc J 1978;118:627–30.
14. Stewart FH, Burnhill MS, Bozorgi N. Reduced dose of Rh immunoglobulin following first trimester pregnancy termination. Obstet Gynecol 1978;51:318–22.
15. Crispen J. Immunosuppression of small quantities of Rh-positive blood with MICRhoGAM® in Rh-negative male volunteers. In: Proceedings of a symposium on Rh antibody mediated immunosuppression. Raritan, NJ: Ortho Research Institute of Medical Sciences, 1975: 51–54.
16. Data on file at Ortho-Clinical Diagnostics, Inc.
17. Cunningham-Rundles C, Zhuo Z, Mankarious S, Courter S. Long-term use of IgA-depleted intravenous immunoglobulin in immunodeficient subjects with anti-IgA antibodies. J Clin Immunol 1993;13:272–78.
18. Zipursky A, Israels LG. The pathogenesis and prevention of Rh immunization. Can Med Assoc J 1967;97: 1245–56.
19. Thornton JG, Page C, Foote G, Arthur GR, Tovey LAD, Scott JS. Efficacy and long term effects of antenatal prophylaxis with anti-D immunoglobulin. Brit Med J 1989;298:1671–73.
20. Data on file at Ortho-Clinical Diagnostics, Inc.
21. Samson D, Mollison PL. Effect on primary Rh immunization of delayed administration of anti-Rh. Immunol 1975;28:349–57.
22. Garratty G, ed. Hemolytic disease of the newborn. Arlington, VA: American Association of Blood Banks, 1984: 78.
23. Urbaniak SJ. Statement from the Consensus Conference on Anti-D Prophylaxis, The Royal College of Physicians of Edinburgh & The Royal College of Obstetricians and Gynaecologists, UK. Vox Sang 1998;74: 127–28.
24. Bayliss KM, Kueck DD, Johnson ST, Fueger JT, McFadden PW, Mikulski D, Gottschall JL. Detecting fetomaternal hemorrhage: a comparison of five methods. Transfusion 1991;31:303–7.
25. Kumpel BM. Quantification of anti-D and fetomaternal hemorrhage by flow cytometry (editorial). Transfusion 2000;40:6–9.

ORTHO-CLINICAL DIAGNOSTICS, INC.
A Johnson & Johnson Company
Raritan, New Jersey 08869
U.S. License 1236
U.S. Patent 3,449,314

Ortho-McNeil Pharmaceutical

RARITAN, NJ 08869-0602

www.ortho-mcneil.com
For Medical Information Contact:
(800) 682-6532
In Emergencies:
(908) 218-7325
For Patient Education Materials Contact:
877-323-2200
For Customer Service (Sales and Ordering):
800-631-5273

To obtain Prescribing Information on the following products, please call 1-877-323-2200:

BICITRA
DITROPAN
HALDOL Tablets/Concentrate/Injection
MODICON Tablets
MYCELEX TROCHE
ORTHO Diaphragm Kits
ORTHO-NOVUM 1/50 Tablets
ORTHO-NOVUM Tablets
PANCREASE
PANCREASE MT
PARAFON FORTE DSC
POLYCITRA-K
TERAZOL 7 Vaginal Cream
TERAZOL 3 Vaginal Cream
TERAZOL 3 Vaginal Suppositories
TESTODERM
TESTODERM With Adhesive
TOLECTIN 200/400/600
TYLOX Capsules
URISPAS
VASCOR Tablets

AXERT® ℞

[aks'ərt]

(almotriptan malate) Tablets

Prescribing Information

DESCRIPTION

AXERT Tablets contain almotriptan malate, a selective 5-hydroxytryptamine$_{1B/1D}$ (5-HT$_{1B/1D}$) receptor agonist. Almotriptan malate is chemically designated as 1-[[[3-[2-(Dimethylamino)ethyl]- 1H-indol-5-yl]methyl]sulfonyl]pyrrolidine (±)-hydroxybutanedioate (1:1), and its structural formula is:

[structural formula: pyrrolidine N–SO₂–CH₂ on indole, CH₂CH₂–N(CH₃)–CH₃ · HOOC–CH₂–CH(OH)–COOH]

Its empirical formula is $C_{17}H_{25}N_3O_2S{\cdot}C_4H_6O_5$, representing a molecular weight of 469.56. Almotriptan is a white to slightly yellow crystalline powder that is soluble in water. AXERT Tablets for oral administration contain almotriptan malate equivalent to 6.25 or 12.5 mg of almotriptan. Each compressed tablet contains the following inactive ingredients: mannitol, cellulose, povidone, sodium starch glycolate, sodium stearyl fumarate, titanium dioxide, hydroxypropyl methylcellulose, polyethylene glycol, propylene glycol, iron oxide (6.25 mg only), FD&C Blue No. 2 (12.5 mg only), and carnauba wax.

CLINICAL PHARMACOLOGY

Mechanism of Action: Almotriptan binds with high affinity to 5-HT$_{1D}$, 5-HT$_{1B}$, and 5-HT$_{1F}$ receptors. Almotriptan has weak affinity for 5-HT$_{1A}$ and 5-HT$_7$ receptors, but has no significant affinity or pharmacological activity at 5-HT$_2$, 5-HT$_3$, 5-HT$_4$, 5-HT$_6$; alpha or beta adrenergic; adenosine (A$_1$, A$_2$); angiotensin (AT$_1$, AT$_2$); dopamine (D$_1$, D$_2$); endothelin (ET$_A$, ET$_B$); or tachykinin (NK$_1$, NK$_2$, NK$_3$) binding sites.

Current theories on the etiology of migraine headache suggest that symptoms are due to local cranial vasodilatation and/or to the release of vasoactive and pro-inflammatory peptides from sensory nerve endings in an activated trigeminal system. The therapeutic activity of almotriptan in migraine can most likely be attributed to agonist effects at 5-HT$_{1B/1D}$ receptors on the extracerebral, intracranial blood vessels that become dilated during a migraine attack, and on nerve terminals in the trigeminal system. Activation of these receptors results in cranial vessel constriction, inhibition of neuropeptide release, and reduced transmission in trigeminal pain pathways.

Pharmacokinetics

General: Almotriptan is well absorbed after oral administration (absolute bioavailability about 70%) with peak plasma levels 1 to 3 hours after administration; food does not affect pharmacokinetics. Almotriptan has a mean half-life of 3 to 4 hours. It is eliminated primarily by renal excretion (about 75% of the oral dose). Almotriptan is minimally protein bound (approximately 35%) and the mean apparent volume of distribution is approximately 180 to 200 liters.

Metabolism and Excretion: Almotriptan is metabolized by one minor and two major pathways. Monoamine oxidase (MAO)-mediated oxidative deamination (approximately 27% of the dose), and cytochrome P450-mediated oxidation (approximately 12% of the dose) are the major routes of metabolism, while flavin monooxygenase is the minor route. MAO-A is responsible for the formation of the indoleacetic acid metabolite, whereas cytochrome P450 (3A4 and 2D6) catalyzes the hydroxylation of the pyrrolidine ring to an intermediate that is further oxidized by aldehyde dehydrogenase to the gamma-aminobutyric acid derivative. Both metabolites are inactive.

Approximately 40% of an administered dose is excreted unchanged in urine. Renal clearance exceeds the glomerular filtration rate by approximately 3-fold, indicating an active mechanism. Approximately 13% of the administered dose is excreted via feces, both unchanged and metabolized.

Special Populations

Geriatric: Renal and total clearance, and amount of drug excreted in the urine were lower in elderly healthy volunteers (age 65 to 76 years) than in younger healthy volunteers (age 19 to 34 years), resulting in longer terminal half-life (3.7 h vs. 3.2 h) and a 25% higher area under the plasma concentration-time curve in the elderly subjects. The differences, however, do not appear to be clinically significant.

Pediatric: The pharmacokinetics of almotriptan in pediatric patients have not been evaluated.

Gender: No significant gender differences have been observed in pharmacokinetic parameters.

Race: No significant differences have been observed in pharmacokinetic parameters between Caucasian and African-American volunteers.

Hepatic impairment: The pharmacokinetics of almotriptan have not been assessed in this population. Based on the known mechanisms of clearance of almotriptan, the maximum decrease expected in almotriptan clearance due to hepatic impairment would be 60% (see DOSAGE AND ADMINISTRATION).

Renal impairment: The clearance of almotriptan was approximately 65% lower in patients with severe renal impairment (Cl/F=19.8 L/h; creatinine clearance between 10 and 30 mL/min) and approximately 40% lower in patients with moderate renal impairment (Cl/F=34.2 L/h; creatinine clearance between 31 and 71 mL/min) than in healthy volunteers (Cl/F=57 L/h). Maximal plasma concentrations of almotriptan increased by approximately 80% in these patients (see DOSAGE AND ADMINISTRATION).

Drug Interactions (see also PRECAUTIONS, Drug Interactions)

All drug interaction studies were performed in healthy volunteers using a single 12.5 mg dose of almotriptan and multiple doses of the other drug.

Monoamine oxidase inhibitors: Coadministration of almotriptan and moclobemide (150 mg bid for 8 days) resulted in a 27% decrease in almotriptan clearance.

Propranolol: Coadministration of almotriptan and propranolol (80 mg bid for 7 days) resulted in no significant changes in the pharmacokinetics of almotriptan.

Selective serotonin reuptake inhibitors: Coadministration of almotriptan and fluoxetine (60 mg daily for 8 days), a potent inhibitor of CYP4502D6, had no effect on almotriptan clearance, but maximal concentrations of almotriptan were increased 18%. This difference is not clinically significant.

Verapamil: Coadministration of almotriptan and verapamil (120 mg sustained release tablets bid for 7 days), an inhibitor of CYP4503A4, resulted in a 20% increase in the area under the plasma concentration-time curve, and in a 24% increase in maximal plasma concentrations of almotriptan. Neither of these changes is clinically significant.

Ketoconazole and other potent CYP3A4 inhibitors: Coadministration of almotriptan and the potent CYP3A4 inhibitor ketoconazole (400 mg qd for 3 days) resulted in an approximately 60% increase in the area under the plasma concentration-time curve and maximal plasma concentrations of almotriptan. Although the interaction between almotriptan and other potent CYP3A4 inhibitors (eg, itraconazole, ritonavir, and erythromycin) has not been studied, increased exposures to almotriptan may be expected when almotriptan is used concomitantly with these medications.

CLINICAL STUDIES

The efficacy of AXERT Tablets was established in 3 multicenter, randomized, double-blind, placebo-controlled European trials. Patients enrolled in these studies were primarily female (86%) and Caucasian (more than 98%), with a mean age of 41 years (range of 18 to 72). Patients were instructed to treat a moderate to severe migraine headache. Two hours after taking one dose of study medication, patients evaluated their headache pain. If the pain had not decreased in severity to mild or to no pain, the patient was allowed to take an escape medication. If the pain had decreased to mild or to no pain at 2 hours but subsequently increased in severity between 2 and 24 hours, it was considered a relapse and the patient was instructed to take a second dose of study medication. Associated symptoms of nausea, vomiting, photophobia, and phonophobia were also evaluated.

In these studies, the percentage of patients achieving a response (mild or no pain) 2 hours after treatment was significantly greater in patients who received either AXERT 6.25 mg or 12.5 mg, compared with those who received placebo. A higher percentage of patients reported pain relief after treatment with the 12.5 mg dose than with the 6.25 mg dose. Doses greater than 12.5 mg did not lead to significantly better response. These results are summarized in Table 1.

Table 1. Response Rates 2 Hours Following Treatment of Initial Headache

	Placebo	AXERT 6.25 mg	AXERT 12.5 mg
Study 1	33.8% (N=80)	55.4%* (N=166)	58.5%† (N=164)
Study 2	40.0% (N=95)	—	57.1%‡ (N=175)
Study 3	33.0% (N=176)	55.6%† (N=360)	64.9%† (N=370)

*p value 0.002 in comparison with placebo
†p value <0.001 in comparison with placebo
‡p value 0.008 in comparison with placebo

These results cannot be validly compared with results of anti-migraine treatments in other studies. Because studies are conducted at different times, with different samples of patients, by different investigators, employing different criteria and/or different interpretations of the same criteria, under different conditions (dose, dosing regimen, etc.), quantitative estimates of treatment responses and the timing of response may be expected to vary considerably from study to study.

The estimated probability of achieving pain relief within 2 hours following initial treatment with AXERT is shown in Figure 1.

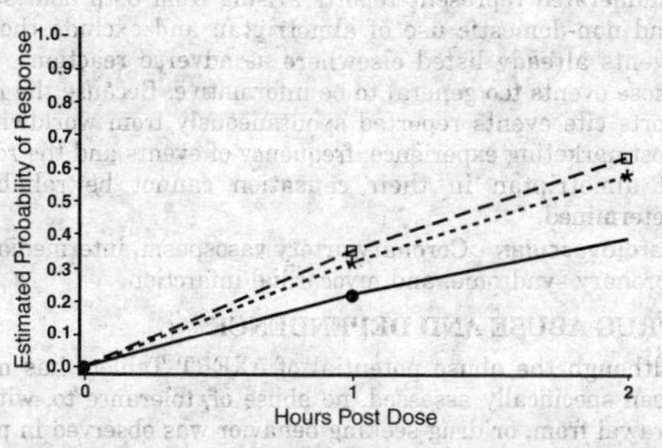

Figure 1. Estimated Probability of Achieving an Initial Headache Response (mild or no pain) in 2 Hours.

This Kaplan-Meier plot is based on data obtained in the three placebo-controlled clinical trials that provided evidence of efficacy (Studies 1, 2, and 3). Patients not achieving pain relief by 2 hours were censored at 2 hours.

For patients with migraine-associated photophobia, phonophobia, nausea, and vomiting at baseline, there was a decreased incidence of these symptoms following administration of AXERT compared with placebo.

Two to 24 hours following the initial dose of study medication, patients were allowed to take an escape medication or a second dose of study medication for pain response. The estimated probability of patients taking escape medication or a second dose of study medication over the 24 hours following the initial dose of study medication is shown in Figure 2.

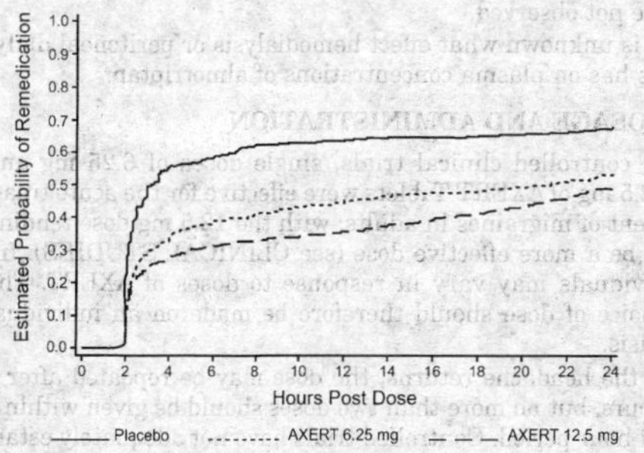

Figure 2. Estimated Probability of Patients Taking Escape Medication or a Second Dose of Study Medication Over the 24 Hours Following the Initial Dose of Study Treatment

This Kaplan-Meier plot is based on data obtained in the three placebo-controlled trials that provided evidence of efficacy (Studies 1, 2, and 3). Patients not using additional treatment were censored at 24 hours. Remedication was not allowed within 2 hours after the initial dose of AXERT.

The efficacy of AXERT was unaffected by the presence of aura; by gender, weight, or age of the patient; or by concomitant use of common migraine prophylactic drugs (eg, beta-blockers, calcium channel blockers, tricyclic antidepressants), or oral contraceptives. There were insufficient data to assess the effect of race on efficacy.

INDICATIONS AND USAGE

AXERT Tablets are indicated for the acute treatment of migraine with or without aura in adults.

AXERT is not intended for the prophylactic therapy of migraine or for use in the management of hemiplegic or basilar migraine (see CONTRAINDICATIONS). Safety and effectiveness of AXERT have not been established for cluster headache, which is present in an older, predominantly male population.

CONTRAINDICATIONS

AXERT Tablets should not be given to patients with ischemic heart disease (angina pectoris, history of myocardial infarction, or documented silent ischemia), or to patients who have symptoms or findings consistent with ischemic heart disease, coronary artery vasospasm, including Prinzmetal's variant angina, or other significant underlying cardiovascular disease (see WARNINGS).

Because AXERT may increase blood pressure, it should not be given to patients with uncontrolled hypertension (see WARNINGS).

AXERT should not be administered within 24 hours of treatment with another $5\text{-}HT_1$ agonist, or an ergotamine-containing or ergot-type medication like dihydroergotamine or methysergide.

AXERT should not be given to patients with hemiplegic or basilar migraine.

AXERT is contraindicated in patients who are hypersensitive to almotriptan or any of its ingredients.

WARNINGS

AXERT Tablets should only be used where a clear diagnosis of migraine has been established.

Risk of Myocardial Ischemia and/or Infarction and Other Adverse Cardiac Events: Because of the potential of this class of compounds ($5\text{-}HT_{1B/1D}$ agonists) to cause coronary vasospasm, AXERT should not be given to patients with documented ischemic or vasospastic coronary artery disease (see CONTRAINDICATIONS). It is strongly recommended that $5\text{-}HT_1$ agonists (including AXERT) not be given to patients in whom unrecognized coronary artery disease (CAD) is predicted by the presence of risk factors (eg, hypertension, hypercholesterolemia, smoker, obesity, diabetes, strong family history of CAD, female with surgical or physiological menopause, or male over 40 years of age) unless a cardiovascular evaluation provides satisfactory clinical evidence that the patient is reasonably free of coronary artery and ischemic myocardial disease or other significant underlying cardiovascular disease. The sensitivity of cardiac diagnostic procedures to detect cardiovascular diseases or predisposition to coronary artery vasospasm is modest at best. If, during the cardiovascular evaluation, the patient's medical history, electrocardiogram (ECG), or other investigations reveal findings indicative of, or consistent with, coronary artery vasospasm or myocardial ischemia, AXERT should not be administered (see CONTRAINDICATIONS).

For patients with risk factors predictive of CAD, who are determined to have a satisfactory cardiovascular evaluation, it is strongly recommended that administration of the first dose of AXERT take place in the setting of a physician's office or similar medically staffed and equipped facility, unless the patient has previously received almotriptan. Because cardiac ischemia can occur in the absence of clinical symptoms, consideration should be given to obtaining an ECG during the interval immediately following the first use of AXERT in a patient with risk factors.

It is recommended that patients who are intermittent long-term users of AXERT and who have or acquire risk factors predictive of CAD, as described above, undergo periodic interval cardiovascular evaluation as they continue to use AXERT.

The systematic approach described above is intended to reduce the likelihood that patients with unrecognized cardiovascular disease will be inadvertently exposed to AXERT.

Cardiac Events and Fatalities Associated with $5\text{-}HT_1$ Agonists: Serious adverse cardiac events, including acute myocardial infarction, have been reported within a few hours following administration of almotriptan. Life-threatening disturbances of cardiac rhythm, and death have been reported within a few hours following the administration of other $5\text{-}HT_1$ agonists. Considering the extent of use of $5\text{-}HT_1$ agonists in patients with migraine, the incidence of these events is extremely low.

AXERT can cause coronary vasospasm; at least one of these events occurred in a patient with no cardiac history and with documented absence of coronary artery disease. Because of the close proximity of the events to use of AXERT, a causal relationship cannot be excluded.

Premarketing experience with almotriptan: Among the 3865 subjects/patients who received AXERT in premarketing clinical trials, one patient was hospitalized for observation after a scheduled ECG was found to be abnormal (negative T-waves on the left leads) 48 hours after taking a single 6.25 mg dose of almotriptan. The patient, a 48-year-old female, had previously taken 3 other doses for earlier migraine attacks. Myocardial enzymes at the time of the abnormal ECG were normal. The patient was diagnosed as having had myocardial ischemia, and it was also found that she had a family history of coronary disease. An ECG performed 2 days later was normal, as was a follow-up coronary angiography. The patient recovered without incident.

Postmarketing experience with almotriptan: Serious cardiovascular events have been reported in association with the use of AXERT. The uncontrolled nature of postmarketing surveillance, however, makes it impossible to definitively determine the proportion of the reported cases that were actually caused by almotriptan or to reliably assess causation in individual cases.

Cerebrovascular Events and Fatalities with $5\text{-}HT_1$ Agonists: Cerebral hemorrhage, subarachnoid hemorrhage, stroke, and other cerebrovascular events have been reported in patients treated with other $5\text{-}HT_1$ agonists, and some have resulted in fatalities. In a number of cases, it appears possible that the cerebrovascular events were primary, the agonist having been administered in the incorrect belief that the symptoms experienced were a consequence of migraine, when they were not. It should be noted that patients with migraine may be at increased risk of certain cerebrovascular events (eg, stroke, hemorrhage, transient ischemic attack).

Other Vasospasm-Related Events: $5\text{-}HT_1$ agonists may cause vasospastic reactions other than coronary artery vasospasm. Both peripheral vascular ischemia and colonic ischemia with abdominal pain and bloody diarrhea have been reported with $5\text{-}HT_1$ agonists.

Increases in Blood Pressure: Significant elevations in systemic blood pressure, including hypertensive crisis, have been reported on rare occasions in patients with and without a history of hypertension treated with other $5\text{-}HT_1$ agonists. AXERT is contraindicated in patients with uncontrolled hypertension (see CONTRAINDICATIONS). In volunteers, small increases in mean systolic and diastolic blood pressure relative to placebo were seen over the first 4 hours after administration of 12.5 mg of almotriptan (0.21 and 1.35 mm Hg, respectively). The effect of almotriptan on blood pressure was also assessed in patients with hypertension controlled by medication. In this population, mean increases in systolic and diastolic blood pressure relative to placebo over the first 4 hours after administration of 12.5 mg of almotriptan were 4.87 and 0.26 mm Hg, respectively. The slight increases in blood pressure in both volunteers and controlled hypertensive patients were not considered clinically significant.

An 18% increase in mean pulmonary artery pressure was seen following dosing with another $5\text{-}HT_1$ agonist in a study evaluating subjects undergoing cardiac catheterization.

PRECAUTIONS

General: As with other $5\text{-}HT_{1B/1D}$ agonists, sensations of tightness, pain, pressure, and heaviness in the precordium, throat, neck, and jaw have been reported after treatment with AXERT Tablets. These events have not been associated with arrhythmias or ischemic ECG changes in clinical trials. Because drugs in this class, including almotriptan, may cause coronary artery vasospasm, patients who experience signs or symptoms suggestive of angina following dosing should be evaluated for the presence of CAD or a predisposition to Prinzmetal's variant angina before receiving additional doses of medication, and should be monitored electrocardiographically if dosing is resumed and similar symptoms recur. Similarly, patients who experience other symptoms or signs suggestive of decreased arterial flow, such as ischemic bowel syndrome or Raynaud's syndrome following the use of any $5\text{-}HT_1$ agonist are candidates for further evaluation (see WARNINGS).

AXERT should also be administered with caution to patients with diseases that may alter the absorption, metabolism, or excretion of drugs, such as those with impaired hepatic or renal function (see CLINICAL PHARMACOLOGY, Special Populations).

For a given attack, if a patient does not respond to the first dose of AXERT, the diagnosis of migraine headache should be reconsidered before the administration of a second dose.

Binding to Melanin-Containing Tissues: When pigmented rats were given a single oral dose of 5 mg/kg of radiolabeled almotriptan, the elimination half-life of radioactivity from the eye was 22 days. This finding suggests that almotriptan and/or its metabolites may bind to the melanin of the eye. Because almotriptan could accumulate in melanin-rich tissues over time, there is the possibility that it could cause toxicity in these tissues over extended use. However, no adverse retinal effects related to treatment with almotriptan were noted in a 52-week toxicity study in dogs given up to 12.5 mg/kg/day (resulting in systemic exposure [plasma AUC] to parent drug approximately 20 times that in humans receiving the maximum recommended daily dose of 25 mg). Although no systematic monitoring of ophthalmologic function was undertaken in clinical trials, and no specific recommendations for ophthalmologic monitoring are offered, prescribers should be aware of the possibility of long-term ophthalmologic effects.

Corneal Opacities: Three male dogs (out of a total of 14 treated) in a 52-week toxicity study of oral almotriptan, developed slight corneal opacities that were noted after 51, but not after 25, weeks of treatment. The doses at which this occurred were 2, 5, and 12.5 mg/kg/day. The opacity reversed in the affected dog at 12.5 mg/kg/day after a 4-week drug-free period. Systemic exposure (plasma AUC) to parent drug at 2 mg/kg/day was approximately 2.5 times the exposure in humans receiving the maximum recommended daily dose of 25 mg. A no-effect dose was not established.

Information for Patients: See PATIENT INFORMATION at the end of this labeling for the text of the separate leaflet provided for patients.

Laboratory Tests: No specific laboratory tests are recommended for monitoring patients.

Continued on next page

Axert—Cont.

Drug Interactions (see also CLINICAL PHARMACOLOGY, Drug Interactions)
Ergot-containing drugs: These drugs have been reported to cause prolonged vasospastic reactions. Because there is a theoretical basis that these effects may be additive, use of ergotamine-containing or ergot-type medications (like dihydroergotamine or methysergide) and AXERT within 24 hours of each other should be avoided (see CONTRAINDICATIONS).
Monoamine oxidase inhibitors: Coadministration of moclobemide resulted in a 27% decrease in almotriptan clearance and an increase in C_{max} of approximately 6%. No dose adjustment is necessary.
Other 5-HT$_{1B/1D}$ agonists: Concomitant use of other 5-HT$_{1B/1D}$ agonists within 24 hours of treatment with AXERT is contraindicated (see CONTRAINDICATIONS).
Propranolol: The pharmacokinetics of almotriptan were not affected by coadministration of propranolol.
Selective serotonin reuptake inhibitors (SSRIs): SSRIs (eg, fluoxetine, fluvoxamine, paroxetine, sertraline) have been rarely reported to cause weakness, hyperreflexia, and incoordination when coadministered with 5-HT$_1$ agonists. If concomitant treatment with AXERT and an SSRI is clinically warranted, appropriate observation of the patient is advised.
Verapamil: Coadministration of almotriptan and verapamil resulted in a 24% increase in plasma concentrations of almotriptan. No dose adjustment is necessary.
Ketoconazole and other potent CYP3A4 inhibitors: Coadministration of almotriptan and the potent CYP3A4 inhibitor ketoconazole (400 mg qd for 3 days) resulted in an approximately 60% increase in the area under the plasma concentration-time curve and maximal plasma concentrations of almotriptan. Although the interaction between almotriptan and other potent CYP3A4 inhibitors (eg, itraconazole, ritonavir, and erythromycin) has not been studied, increased exposures to almotriptan may be expected when almotriptan is used concomitantly with these medications.
Drug/Laboratory Test Interactions: AXERT is not known to interfere with commonly employed clinical laboratory tests.
Carcinogenesis, Mutagenesis, Impairment of Fertility
Carcinogenesis: The carcinogenic potential of almotriptan was evaluated by oral gavage for up to 103 weeks in mice at doses up to 250 mg/kg/day and in rats for up to 104 weeks at doses up to 75 mg/kg/day. These doses were associated with plasma exposures (AUC) to parent drug that were approximately 40 and 78 times, in mice and rats respectively, the plasma AUC observed in humans receiving the maximum recommended daily dose (MRDD) of 25 mg. Because of high mortality rates in both studies, which reached statistical significance in high dose female mice, all female rats, all male mice, and high dose female mice were terminated between weeks 96 and 98. There was no increase in tumors related to almotriptan administration.
Mutagenesis: Almotriptan was not mutagenic, with or without metabolic activation, in two *in vitro* gene mutation assays, the Ames test and the thymidine locus mouse lymphoma assay. Almotriptan was not clastogenic in an *in vivo* mouse micronucleus assay. Almotriptan produced an equivocal weakly positive response in *in vitro* cytogenetics assays in human lymphocytes.
Impairment of fertility: When female rats received almotriptan by oral gavage prior to and during mating and up to implantation at doses of 25, 100, and 400 mg/kg/day, prolongation of the estrous cycle was observed at a dose of 100 mg/kg/day (40 times the maximum recommended daily dose [MRDD] of 25 mg on a mg/m^2 basis). No effects on fertility were noted in female rats at 25 mg/kg/day (approximately 10 times the MRDD on a mg/m^2 basis).
Pregnancy: Pregnancy Category C: When almotriptan was administered by oral gavage to pregnant rats throughout the period of organogenesis at doses of 125, 250, 500, and 1000 mg/kg/day, an increase in embryolethality was seen at the highest dose (maternal exposure, based on plasma AUC of parent drug, was approximately 958 times the human exposure at the maximum recommended daily dose [MRDD] of 25 mg). Increased incidences of fetal skeletal variations (decreased ossification) were noted at doses greater than 125 mg/kg/day (maternal exposure 80 times human exposure at MRDD). Similar studies in rabbits conducted with almotriptan at doses of 5, 20, and 60 mg/kg/day demonstrated increases in embryolethality at the high dose (50 times the MRDD on a mg/m^2 basis). When almotriptan was administered to rats throughout the periods of gestation and lactation at doses of 25, 100, and 400 mg/kg/day, gestation length was increased and litter size and offspring body weight were decreased at the high dose (160 times the MRDD on a mg/m^2 basis). The decrease in pup weight persisted throughout lactation. The no-observed-effect level in this study was 100 mg/kg/day (40 times the MRDD on a mg/m^2 basis).
There are no adequate and well-controlled studies in pregnant women; therefore AXERT should be used during pregnancy only if the potential benefit justifies the potential risk to the fetus.
Nursing Mothers: It is not known whether almotriptan is excreted in human milk. Because many drugs are excreted in human milk, caution should be exercised when AXERT is administered to a nursing woman. Lactating rats dosed with almotriptan had milk levels equivalent to maternal plasma levels at 0.5 hours and 7 times higher than plasma levels at 6 hours after dosing.
Pediatric Use: Safety and effectiveness of AXERT in pediatric patients have not been established; therefore, AXERT is not recommended for use in patients under 18 years of age.
Postmarketing experience with other triptans include a limited number of reports that describe pediatric patients who have experienced clinically serious adverse events that are similar in nature to those reported rarely in adults. The long-term safety of almotriptan in pediatric patients has not been studied.
Geriatric Use: Clinical studies of AXERT did not include sufficient numbers of subjects aged 65 and over to determine whether they respond differently from younger subjects. Clearance of almotriptan was lower in elderly volunteers than in younger individuals but there were no observed differences in the safety and tolerability between the two populations (see CLINICAL PHARMACOLOGY, Special Populations). In general, dose selection for an elderly patient should be cautious, usually starting at the low end of the dosing range, reflecting the greater frequency of decreased hepatic, renal or cardiac function, and of concomitant disease or other drug therapy. The recommended dose of AXERT for elderly patients with normal renal function for their age is the same as that recommended for younger adults.

ADVERSE REACTIONS

Serious cardiac events, including myocardial infarction and coronary artery vasospasm, have occurred following the use of AXERT Tablets. These events are extremely rare and have been reported in patients with risk factors predictive of CAD. Events reported in association with drugs in this class have included coronary artery vasospasm, transient myocardial ischemia, myocardial infarction, ventricular tachycardia, and ventricular fibrillation (see CONTRAINDICATIONS, WARNINGS and PRECAUTIONS).
Incidence in Controlled Clinical Trials: Adverse events were assessed in controlled clinical trials that included 1840 patients who received one or two doses of AXERT and 386 patients who received placebo.
The most common adverse events during treatment with AXERT were nausea, somnolence, headache, paresthesia, and dry mouth. In long-term open-label studies where patients were allowed to treat multiple attacks for up to one year, 5% (63 out of 1347 patients) withdrew due to adverse experiences.
Table 2 lists the adverse events that occurred in at least 1% of the patients treated with AXERT, and at an incidence greater than in patients treated with placebo, regardless of drug relationship. These events reflect experience gained under closely monitored conditions of clinical trials in a highly selected patient population. In actual clinical practice or in other clinical trials, these frequency estimates may not apply, as the conditions of use, reporting behavior, and the kinds of patients treated may differ.

Table 2. Incidence of Adverse Events in Controlled Clinical Trials (Reported in at Least 1% of Patients Treated with AXERT, and at an Incidence Greater than Placebo)

Adverse Event	Percent of Patients Reporting the Event		
	AXERT 6.25 mg (n=527)	AXERT 12.5 mg (n=1313)	Placebo (n=386)
Digestive			
Nausea	1	2	1
Dry Mouth	1	1	0.5
Nervous			
Paresthesia	1	1	0.5

AXERT is generally well tolerated. Most adverse events were mild in intensity and were transient, and did not lead to long-lasting effects. The incidence of adverse events in controlled clinical trials was not affected by gender, weight, age, presence of aura, or use of prophylactic medications or oral contraceptives. There were insufficient data to assess the effect of race on the incidence of adverse events.
Other Events: In this section, the frequencies of less commonly reported adverse events are presented. However, the role of AXERT in their causation cannot be reliably determined. Furthermore, variability associated with adverse event reporting, the terminology used to describe adverse events, etc., limit the value of the quantitative frequency estimates provided. Event frequencies are calculated as the number of patients who used AXERT in controlled clinical trials and reported an event, divided by the total number of patients exposed to AXERT in these studies. All reported events are included, except the ones already listed in the previous table, those unlikely to be drug-related, and those poorly characterized. Events are further classified within body system categories and enumerated in order of decreasing frequency using the following definitions: frequent adverse events are those occurring in at least 1/100 patients; infrequent adverse events are those occurring in 1/100 to 1/1000 patients; and rare adverse events are those occurring in fewer than 1/1000 patients.
Body: Frequent was headache. Infrequent were abdominal cramp or pain, asthenia, chills, back pain, chest pain, neck pain, fatigue, and rigid neck. Rare were fever and photosensitivity reaction.
Cardiovascular: Infrequent were vasodilation, palpitations, and tachycardia. Rare were hypertension and syncope.
Digestive: Infrequent were diarrhea, vomiting, and dyspepsia. Rare were colitis, gastritis, gastroenteritis, esophageal reflux, increased thirst, and increased salivation.
Metabolic: Infrequent were hyperglycemia and increased serum creatine phosphokinase. Rare were increased gamma glutamyl transpeptidase and hypercholesteremia.
Musculoskeletal: Infrequent were myalgia and muscular weakness. Rare were arthralgia, arthritis, and myopathy.
Nervous: Frequent were dizziness and somnolence. Infrequent were tremor, vertigo, anxiety, hypesthesia, restlessness, CNS stimulation, insomnia, and shakiness. Rare were change in dreams, impaired concentration, abnormal coordination, depressive symptoms, euphoria, hyperreflexia, hypertonia, nervousness, neuropathy, nightmares, and nystagmus.
Respiratory: Infrequent were pharyngitis, rhinitis, dyspnea, laryngismus, sinusitis, bronchitis, and epistaxis. Rare were hyperventilation, laryngitis, and sneezing.
Skin: Infrequent were diaphoresis, dermatitis, erythema, pruritus, and rash.
Special Senses: Infrequent were ear pain, conjunctivitis, eye irritation, hyperacusis, and taste alteration. Rare were diplopia, dry eyes, eye pain, otitis media, parosmia, scotoma, and tinnitus.
Urogenital: Infrequent was dysmenorrhea.
Postmarketing Experience: The following section enumerates potentially important adverse events that have occurred in clinical practice and that have been reported spontaneously to various surveillance systems. The events enumerated represent reports arising from both domestic and non-domestic use of almotriptan and exclude those events already listed elsewhere as adverse reactions, or those events too general to be informative. Because the reports cite events reported spontaneously from worldwide postmarketing experience, frequency of events and the role of almotriptan in their causation cannot be reliably determined.
Cardiovascular: Coronary artery vasospasm, intermediate coronary syndrome, and myocardial infarction.

DRUG ABUSE AND DEPENDENCE

Although the abuse potential of AXERT Tablets has not been specifically assessed, no abuse of, tolerance to, withdrawal from, or drug-seeking behavior was observed in patients who received AXERT in clinical trials or their extensions. The 5-HT$_{1B/1D}$ agonists, as a class, have not been associated with drug abuse.

OVERDOSAGE

Patients and volunteers receiving single oral doses of 100 to 150 mg of almotriptan did not experience significant adverse events. Six additional normal volunteers received single oral doses of 200 mg without serious adverse events. During clinical trials with AXERT Tablets, one patient ingested 62.5 mg in a 5 hour period and another patient ingested 100 mg in a 38 hour period. Neither patient experienced adverse reactions.
Based on the pharmacology of 5-HT agonists, hypertension or other more serious cardiovascular symptoms could occur after overdosage. Gastrointestinal decontamination (ie, gastric lavage followed by activated charcoal) should be considered in patients suspected of an overdose with AXERT. Clinical and electrocardiographic monitoring should be continued for at least 20 hours, even if clinical symptoms are not observed.
It is unknown what effect hemodialysis or peritoneal dialysis has on plasma concentrations of almotriptan.

DOSAGE AND ADMINISTRATION

In controlled clinical trials, single doses of 6.25 mg and 12.5 mg of AXERT Tablets were effective for the acute treatment of migraines in adults, with the 12.5 mg dose tending to be a more effective dose (see CLINICAL STUDIES). Individuals may vary in response to doses of AXERT. The choice of dose should therefore be made on an individual basis.
If the headache returns, the dose may be repeated after 2 hours, but no more than two doses should be given within a 24 hour period. Controlled trials have not adequately established the effectiveness of a second dose if the initial dose is ineffective.
The safety of treating an average of more than four headaches in a 30 day period has not been established.
Hepatic impairment: The pharmacokinetics of almotriptan have not been assessed in this population. The maximum decrease expected in the clearance of almotriptan due to hepatic impairment is 60%. Therefore, the maximum daily dose should not exceed 12.5 mg over a 24 hour period, and a starting dose of 6.25 mg should be used (see CLINICAL PHARMACOLOGY, Pharmacokinetics).
Renal impairment: In patients with severe renal impairment, the clearance of almotriptan was decreased. Therefore, the maximum daily dose should not exceed 12.5 mg over a 24 hour period, and a starting dose of 6.25 mg should be used (see CLINICAL PHARMACOLOGY, Pharmacokinetics).

HOW SUPPLIED

AXERT Tablets are available as follows:

6.25 mg: white, circular, biconvex tablet, printed in red with the code 2080.

Unit Dose (aluminum blister pack)
6 tablets NDC 0062-2080-06

12.5 mg: white, circular, biconvex tablet, printed in blue with a stylized A.

Unit Dose (aluminum blister pack)
6 tablets NDC 0062-2085-06

Store at 25°C (77°F); excursions permitted to 15°-30°C (59°-86°F) [see USP Controlled Room Temperature].

℞ only

US Patent No. 5,565,447

PATIENT INFORMATION

Patient information about
AXERT® Tablets
Generic name: almotriptan malate

Please read this information before you start taking AXERT Tablets. Also, read this leaflet each time you renew your prescription, just in case anything has changed. Remember, this leaflet does not take the place of careful discussions with your doctor. You and your doctor should discuss AXERT when you start taking your medication and at regular checkups.

What is AXERT and what is it used for?

AXERT is a medication used to treat migraine attacks in adults. AXERT is a member of a class of drugs called selective serotonin receptor agonists.

Use AXERT only for a migraine attack. Do not use AXERT to treat headaches that might be caused by other conditions. Tell your doctor about your symptoms. Your doctor will decide if you have migraine.

There is more information about migraine at the end of this leaflet.

Who should not take AXERT?*

Do not take AXERT if you
- have ever had heart disease.
- have uncontrolled high blood pressure.
- have hemiplegic or basilar migraine. If you are not sure, ask your doctor.
- have taken another serotonin receptor agonist in the last 24 hours. These include naratriptan (AMERGE®), rizatriptan (MAXALT®), sumatriptan (IMITREX®), or zolmitriptan (ZOMIG®).
- have taken ergotamine-type medicines in the last 24 hours. These include ergotamine (BELLERGAL-S®, CAFERGOT®, ERGOMAR®, WIGRAINE®), dihydroergotamine (D.H.E. 45®), or methysergide (SANSERT®).
- had an allergic reaction to AXERT or any of its ingredients. The active ingredient is almotriptan malate. Ask your doctor or pharmacist about inactive ingredients.

Tell your doctor if you take
- monoamine oxidase (MAO) inhibitors, such as phenelzine sulfate (NARDIL®) or tranylcypromine sulfate (PARNATE®) for depression or another condition, or if it has been less than two weeks since you stopped taking a MAO inhibitor.
- ketoconazole (NIZORAL®), itraconazole (SPORANOX®), ritonavir (NORVIR®), or erythromycin (EMYCIN®), or if it has been less than one week since you stopped taking one of these drugs.

These medicines may affect how AXERT works, or AXERT may affect how these medicines work.

To help your doctor decide if AXERT is right for you or if you need to be checked while taking AXERT, tell your doctor about any
- past or present medical problems.
- past or present high blood pressure, chest pain, shortness of breath, or heart disease.
- liver or kidney problems.
- risk factors for heart disease, such as:
  - — high blood pressure
  - — diabetes
  - — high cholesterol
  - — overweight
  - — smoking
  - — family members with heart disease
  - — you are past menopause
  - — you are a male over 40 years old.
- plans to become pregnant, or if you are pregnant, might be pregnant, or do not use effective birth control.
- plans to breast-feed, or if you are already breast-feeding.
- medicines you take or plan to take, including prescription and non-prescription medicines and herbal supplements. Be sure to include medicines you normally take for a migraine.

How should I take AXERT?
- When you have a migraine headache, take your medicine as directed by your doctor.
- If your headache comes back after your first dose, you may take a second dose 2 hours or more after the first dose. If your pain continues after the first dose, do not take a second dose without first checking with your doctor.
- Do not take more than two AXERT Tablets in a 24 hour period.
- If you take too much medicine, contact your doctor, hospital emergency department, or poison control center right away.

What should I avoid while taking AXERT?

Check with your doctor before you take any new medicines, including prescription and non-prescription medicines and supplements. There are some medicines that you should not take during the period 24 hours before and 24 hours after taking AXERT. Some of them are listed in the section "Who should not take AXERT?"

What are the possible side effects of AXERT?

AXERT is generally well tolerated. The side effects are usually mild and do not last long. The following is **not** a complete list of side effects. Ask your doctor to tell you about the other side effects.

The **most common** side effects are
- Nausea
- Sleepiness
- Tingling or burning feeling (paresthesia)
- Headache
- Dry mouth.

If you experience sleepiness, you should evaluate your ability to perform complex tasks such as driving or operating heavy machinery.

Tell your doctor about any other symptoms that you develop while taking AXERT. If the symptoms continue or worsen, get medical help right away. Also, tell your doctor if you develop a rash or itching after taking AXERT. You may be allergic to the medicine.

In very rare cases, patients taking this class of medicines experience serious heart problems, stroke, or increased blood pressure. Extremely rarely, patients have died. Therefore, tell your doctor right away if you feel tightness, pain, pressure or heaviness in your chest, throat, neck, or jaw after taking AXERT. Do not take AXERT again until your doctor has checked you.

What is migraine and how does it differ from other headaches?

Migraine is an intense, throbbing, typically one-sided headache. It often includes nausea, vomiting, sensitivity to light, and sensitivity to sound. The pain and symptoms from a migraine headache may be worse than the pain and symptoms of a common headache.

Some people have visual symptoms before the headache, such as flashing lights or wavy lines, called an aura.

Migraine attacks typically last for hours or, rarely, for more than a day. They can return often. The strength and frequency of migraine attacks may vary.

Based on your symptoms, your doctor will decide whether you have migraine.

Migraine headaches tend to occur in members of the same family. Both men and women get migraine, but it is more common in women.

What may trigger a migraine attack?

Certain things may trigger migraine attacks in some people. Some of these triggers are
- Certain foods or drinks, such as cheese, chocolate, citrus fruit (oranges, grapefruit, lemons, lime, and others), caffeine, and alcohol
- Stress
- Change in behavior, such as too much or too little sleep, missing a meal, or a change in diet
- Hormone changes in women, such as during monthly menstrual periods.

You may be able to prevent migraine attacks or make them come less often if you understand what triggers your attacks. Keeping a headache diary may help you identify and monitor the possible triggers that cause your migraine. Once you identify the triggers, you and your doctor can change your lifestyle to avoid those triggers.

How does AXERT work during a migraine attack?

Treatment with AXERT
- reduces swelling of blood vessels surrounding the brain. This swelling is associated with the headache pain of a migraine attack.
- blocks the release of substances from nerve endings that cause more pain and other symptoms of migraine.
- interrupts the sending of specific pain signals to your brain.

It is thought that each of these actions contributes to relief of your symptoms by AXERT.

How should I store AXERT?

Keep your medicine in a safe place where children cannot reach it. It may be harmful to children. Store your medicine away from heat, light, or moisture, at a controlled room temperature. If your medicine has expired, throw it away as instructed. If your doctor decides to stop your treatment, do not keep any leftover medicine unless your doctor tells you to do so. Throw away your medicine as instructed. Be sure that discarded tablets are out of the reach of children.

General advice about prescription medicines

Medicines are sometimes prescribed for conditions that are not mentioned in patient information leaflets. Do not use AXERT for a condition for which it was not prescribed. Do not give AXERT to other people, even if they have the same symptoms you have. People may be harmed if they take medicines that have not been prescribed for them.

This leaflet provides a summary of information about AXERT. If you have any questions or concerns about either AXERT or migraines, talk to your doctor. In addition, talk to your pharmacist or other health care provider.

* The brands listed are the trademarks of their respective owners and are not trademarks of Ortho-McNeil Pharmaceutical, Inc.

ORTHO-McNEIL

Mfd. for: Ortho-McNeil Pharmaceutical, Inc.
Raritan, NJ 08869

Mfd. by: Shire US Manufacturing Inc.
Owings Mills, MD 21117, USA

Licensed from: Almirall Prodesfarma

Issued: May 2003 818 426 003
692270
635-10-626-1

Shown in Product Identification Guide, page 328

DITROPAN XL® ℞
[*dī-trō-păn*]
(oxybutynin chloride)
Extended Release Tablets

Prescribing Information

DESCRIPTION

DITROPAN XL® (oxybutynin chloride) Extended Release Tablets DITROPAN XL® (oxybutynin chloride) is an antispasmodic, anticholinergic agent. Each DITROPAN XL Extended Release Tablet contains 5 mg, 10 mg, or 15 mg of oxybutynin chloride USP, formulated as a once-a-day controlled-release tablet for oral administration. Oxybutynin chloride is administered as a racemate of R- and S-enantiomers.

Chemically, oxybutynin chloride is d,l (racemic) 4-diethylamino-2-butynyl phenylcyclohexylglycolate hydrochloride. The empirical formula of oxybutynin chloride is $C_{22}H_{31}NO_3$ • HCl.

Its structural formula is:

C_6H_5–C(C$_6H_{11}$)(OH)–C(=O)–O–CH$_2$–C≡C–CH$_2$–N(C$_2$H$_5$)$_2$ • HCl

Oxybutynin chloride is a white crystalline solid with a molecular weight of 393.9. It is readily soluble in water and acids, but relatively insoluble in alkalis.

DITROPAN XL also contains the following inert ingredients: cellulose acetate, hypromellose, lactose, magnesium stearate, polyethylene glycol, polyethylene oxide, synthetic iron oxides, titanium dioxide, polysorbate 80, sodium chloride, and butylated hydroxytoluene.

System Components and Performance

DITROPAN XL uses osmotic pressure to deliver oxybutynin chloride at a controlled rate over approximately 24 hours. The system, which resembles a conventional tablet in appearance, comprises an osmotically active bilayer core surrounded by a semipermeable membrane. The bilayer core is composed of a drug layer containing the drug and excipients, and a push layer containing osmotically active components. There is a precision-laser drilled orifice in the semipermeable membrane on the drug-layer side of the tablet. In an aqueous environment, such as the gastrointestinal tract, water permeates through the membrane into the tablet core, causing the drug to go into suspension and the push layer to expand. This expansion pushes the suspended drug out through the orifice. The semipermeable membrane controls the rate at which water permeates into the tablet core, which in turn controls the rate of drug delivery. The controlled rate of drug delivery into the gastrointestinal lumen is thus independent of pH or gastrointestinal motility. The function of DITROPAN XL depends on the existence of an osmotic gradient between the contents of the bilayer core and the fluid in the gastrointestinal tract. Since the osmotic gradient remains constant, drug delivery remains essentially constant. The biologically inert components of the tablet remain intact during gastrointestinal transit and are eliminated in the feces as an insoluble shell.

CLINICAL PHARMACOLOGY

Oxybutynin chloride exerts a direct antispasmodic effect on smooth muscle and inhibits the muscarinic action of acetylcholine on smooth muscle. Oxybutynin chloride exhibits only one-fifth of the anticholinergic activity of atropine on the rabbit detrusor muscle, but four to ten times the antispasmodic activity. No blocking effects occur at skeletal neuromuscular junctions or autonomic ganglia (antinicotinic effects).

Oxybutynin chloride relaxes bladder smooth muscle. In patients with conditions characterized by involuntary bladder contractions, cystometric studies have demonstrated that oxybutynin increases bladder (vesical) capacity, diminishes the frequency of uninhibited contractions of the detrusor muscle, and delays the initial desire to void. Oxybutynin thus decreases urgency and the frequency of both incontinent episodes and voluntary urination.

Antimuscarinic activity resides predominantly in the R-isomer. A metabolite, desethyloxybutynin, has pharmacological activity similar to that of oxybutynin in *in vitro* studies.

Pharmacokinetics

Absorption

Following the first dose of DITROPAN XL® (oxybutynin chloride), oxybutynin plasma concentrations rise for 4 to 6 hours; thereafter steady concentrations are maintained for up to 24 hours, minimizing fluctuations between peak and trough concentrations associated with oxybutynin.

The relative bioavailabilities of R- and S-oxybutynin from DITROPAN XL are 156% and 187%, respectively, compared

Continued on next page

Ditropan XL—Cont.

with oxybutynin. The mean pharmacokinetic parameters for R- and S-oxybutynin are summarized in Table 1. The plasma concentration-time profiles for R- and S-oxybutynin are similar in shape; Figure 1 shows the profile for R-oxybutynin.

Table 1: Mean (SD) R- and S-Oxybutynin Pharmacokinetic Parameters Following a Single Dose of DITROPAN XL 10 mg (n=43)

Parameters (units)	R-Oxybutynin		S-Oxybutynin	
C_{max} (ng/mL)	1.0	(0.6)	1.8	(1.0)
T_{max} (h)	12.7	(5.4)	11.8	(5.3)
$t_{1/2}$ (h)	13.2	(6.2)	12.4	(6.1)
$AUC_{(0-48)}$ (ng•h/mL)	18.4	(10.3)	34.2	(16.9)
AUC_{inf} (ng•h/mL)	21.3	(12.2)	39.5	(21.2)

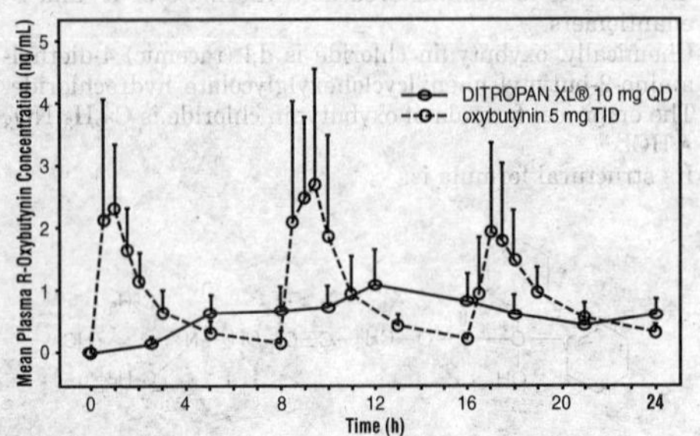

Figure 1. *Mean R-oxybutynin plasma concentrations following a single dose of DITROPAN XL 10mg and oxybutynin 5 mg administered every 8 hours (n=23 for each treatment).*

Steady-state oxybutynin plasma concentrations are achieved by Day 3 of repeated DITROPAN XL dosing, with no observed drug accumulation or change in oxybutynin and desethyloxybutynin pharmacokinetic parameters.

DITROPAN XL steady-state pharmacokinetics was studied in 19 children aged 5-15 years with detrusor overactivity associated with a neurological condition (e.g. spina bifida). The children were on DITROPAN XL total daily dose ranging from 5 to 20 mg (0.10 to 0.77 mg/kg). Sparse sampling technique was used to obtain serum samples. When all available data are normalized to an equivalent of 5 mg per day Ditropan XL, the mean pharmacokinetic parameters derived for R- and S-oxybutynin and R- and S-desethyloxybutynin are summarized in Table 2. The plasma-time concentration profiles for R- and S-oxybutynin are similar in shape; Figure 2 shows the profile for R-oxybutynin when all available data are normalized to an equivalent of 5 mg per day.

[See table 2 above]

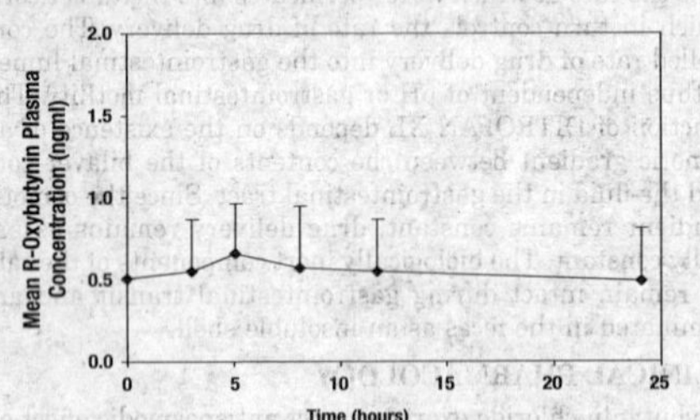

***Figure 2.** Mean steady-state (±SD) R-oxybutynin plasma concentrations following administration of 5 to 20 mg DITROPAN XL once daily in children aged 5-15. Plot represents all available data normalized to an equivalent of DITROPAN XL 5 mg once daily.*

Food Effects

The rate and extent of absorption and metabolism of oxybutynin are similar under fed and fasted conditions.

Distribution

Plasma concentrations of oxybutynin decline biexponentially following intravenous or oral administration. The volume of distribution is 193 L after intravenous administration of 5 mg oxybutynin chloride.

Metabolism

Oxybutynin is metabolized primarily by the cytochrome P450 enzyme systems, particularly CYP3A4 found mostly in the liver and gut wall. Its metabolic products include phenylcyclohexylglycolic acid, which is pharmacologically inactive, and desethyloxybutynin, which is pharmacologically active. Following DITROPAN XL administration, plasma concentrations of R- and S-desethyloxybutynin are 73% and 92%, respectively, of concentrations observed with oxybutynin.

Excretion

Oxybutynin is extensively metabolized by the liver, with less than 0.1% of the administered dose excreted unchanged in the urine. Also, less than 0.1% of the administered dose is excreted as the metabolite desethyloxybutynin.

Table 2
Mean ± SD R- and S-Oxybutynin and R- and S-Desethyloxybutynin Pharmacokinetic Parameters in Children Aged 5-15 Following Administration of 5 to 20 mg DITROPAN XL Once Daily (n=19)
All Available Data Normalized to an Equivalent of DITROPAN XL 5 mg Once Daily

	R-Oxybutynin	S-Oxybutynin	R-Desethyloxybutynin	S-Desethyloxybutynin
C_{max} (ng/mL)	0.7 ± 0.4	1.3 ± 0.8	7.8 ± 3.7	4.2 ± 2.3
T_{max} (hr)	5.0	5.0	5.0	5.0
AUC (ng.hr/mL)	12.8 ± 7.0	23.7 ± 14.4	125.1 ± 66.7	73.6 ± 47.7

Dose Proportionality

Pharmacokinetic parameters of oxybutynin and desethyloxybutynin (C_{max} and AUC) following administration of 5-20 mg of DITROPAN XL are dose proportional.

Special Populations

Geriatric: The pharmacokinetics of DITROPAN XL were similar in all patients studied (up to 78 years of age).

Pediatric: The pharmacokinetics of DITROPAN XL were evaluated in 19 children aged 5-15 years with detrusor overactivity associated with a neurological condition (e.g., spina bifida). The pharmacokinetics of DITROPAN XL in these pediatric patients were consistent with those reported for adults (see Tables 1 and 2, and Figures 1 and 2 above).

Gender: There are no significant differences in the pharmacokinetics of oxybutynin in healthy male and female volunteers following administration of DITROPAN XL.

Race: Available data suggest that there are no significant differences in the pharmacokinetics of oxybutynin based on race in healthy volunteers following administration of DITROPAN XL.

Renal Insufficiency: There is no experience with the use of DITROPAN XL in patients with renal insufficiency.

Hepatic Insufficiency: There is no experience with the use of DITROPAN XL in patients with hepatic insufficiency.

Drug-Drug Interactions: See **PRECAUTIONS:** Drug Interactions.

Clinical Studies

DITROPAN XL was evaluated for the treatment of patients with overactive bladder with symptoms of urge urinary incontinence, urgency, and frequency in three controlled studies and one open label study. The majority of patients were Caucasian (89.0%) and female (91.9%) with a mean age of 59 years (range, 18 to 98 years). Entry criteria required that patients have urge or mixed incontinence (with a predominance of urge) as evidenced by ≥ 6 urge incontinence episodes per week and ≥ 10 micturitions per day. Study 1 was a forced dose escalation design, whereas the other studies used a dose adjustment design in which each patient's final dose was adjusted to a balance between improvement of incontinence symptoms and tolerability of side effects. Controlled studies included patients known to be responsive to oxybutynin or other anticholinergic medications, and these patients were maintained on a final dose for up to 2 weeks. The efficacy results for the three controlled trials are presented in the following tables and figures.

Number of Urge Urinary Incontinence Episodes Per Week

Study 1	n	DITROPAN XL®	n	Placebo
Mean Baseline	34	15.9	16	20.9
Mean (SD) Change from Baseline†	34	-15.8 (8.9)	16	-7.6 (8.6)
95% Confidence Interval for Difference (DITROPAN XL® - Placebo)		(-13.6, -2.8)*		

*The difference between DITROPAN XL® and placebo was statistically significant.

†Covariate adjusted mean with missing observations set to baseline values

[See first figure at top of next column]

Number of Urge Urinary Incontinence Episodes Per Week (continued)

Study 2	n	DITROPAN XL®	n	oxybutynin
Mean Baseline	53	27.6	52	23.0
Mean (SD) Change from Baseline†	53	-17.6 (11.9)	52	-19.4 (11.9)
95% Confidence Interval for Difference (DITROPAN XL® - oxybutynin)		(-2.8, 6.5)*		

†Covariate adjusted mean with missing observations set to baseline values

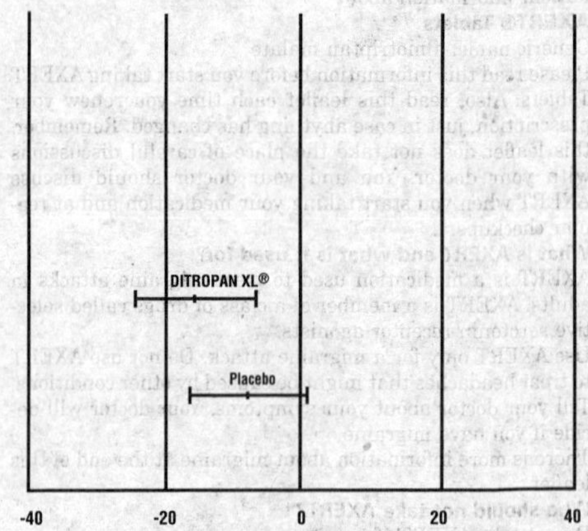

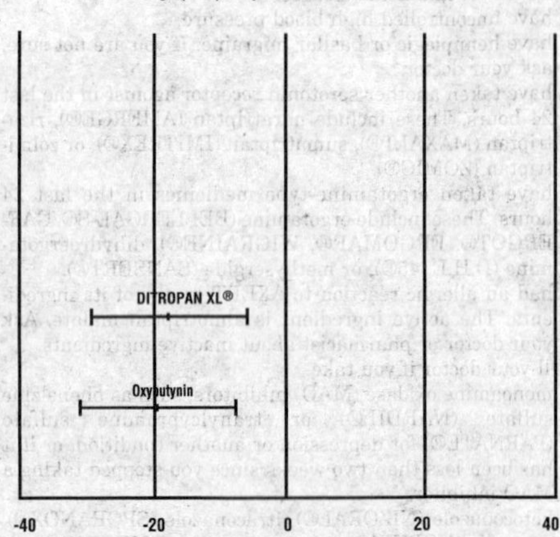

Study 3	n	DITROPAN XL®	n	oxybutynin
Mean Baseline	111	18.9	115	19.5
Mean (SD) Change from Baseline†	111	-14.5 (8.7)	115	-13.8 (8.6)
95% Confidence Interval for Difference (DITROPAN XL® - oxybutynin)		(-3.0, 1.6)**		

**The difference between DITROPAN XL® and oxybutynin fulfilled the criteria for comparable efficacy.

† Covariate adjusted mean with missing observations set to baseline values

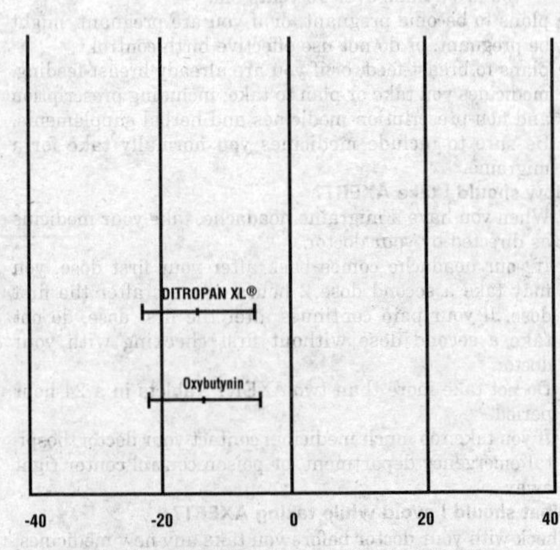

INDICATIONS AND USAGE

DITROPAN XL® (oxybutynin chloride) is a once-daily controlled-release tablet indicated for the treatment of overactive bladder with symptoms of urge urinary incontinence, urgency, and frequency.

DITROPAN XL is also indicated in the treatment of pediatric patients aged 6 years and older with symptoms of detrusor overactivity associated with a neurological condition (e.g., spina bifida).

CONTRAINDICATIONS

DITROPAN XL® (oxybutynin chloride) is contraindicated in patients with urinary retention, gastric retention and other severe decreased gastrointestinal motility conditions, uncontrolled narrow-angle glaucoma and in patients who are at risk for these conditions.

DITROPAN XL is also contraindicated in patients who have demonstrated hypersensitivity to the drug substance or other components of the product.

PRECAUTIONS

General

DITROPAN XL® (oxybutynin chloride) should be used with caution in patients with hepatic or renal impairment and in patients with myasthenia gravis due to the risk of symptom aggravation.

Urinary Retention

DITROPAN XL should be administered with caution to patients with clinically significant bladder outflow obstruction because of the risk of urinary retention (see **CONTRAINDICATIONS**).

Gastrointestinal Disorders

DITROPAN XL should be administered with caution to patients with gastrointestinal obstructive disorders because of the risk of gastric retention (see **CONTRAINDICATIONS**).

DITROPAN XL, like other anticholinergic drugs, may decrease gastrointestinal motility and should be used with caution in patients with conditions such as ulcerative colitis and intestinal atony.

DITROPAN XL should be used with caution in patients who have gastro-esophageal reflux and/or who are concurrently taking drugs (such as bisphosphonates) that can cause or exacerbate esophagitis.

As with any other nondeformable material, caution should be used when administering DITROPAN XL to patients with preexisting severe gastrointestinal narrowing (pathologic or iatrogenic). There have been rare reports of obstructive symptoms in patients with known strictures in association with the ingestion of other drugs in nondeformable controlled-release formulations.

Information for Patients

Patients should be informed that heat prostration (fever and heat stroke due to decreased sweating) can occur when anticholinergics such as oxybutynin chloride are administered in the presence of high environmental temperature.

Because anticholinergic agents such as oxybutynin may produce drowsiness (somnolence) or blurred vision, patients should be advised to exercise caution.

Patients should be informed that alcohol may enhance the drowsiness caused by anticholinergic agents such as oxybutynin.

Patients should be informed that DITROPAN XL should be swallowed whole with the aid of liquids. Patients should not chew, divide, or crush tablets. The medication is contained within a nonabsorbable shell designed to release the drug at a controlled rate. The tablet shell is eliminated from the body; patients should not be concerned if they occasionally notice in their stool something that looks like a tablet.

Drug Interactions

The concomitant use of oxybutynin with other anticholinergic drugs or with other agents which produce dry mouth, constipation, somnolence (drowsiness), and/or other anticholinergic-like effects may increase the frequency and/or severity of such effects.

Anticholinergic agents may potentially alter the absorption of some concomitantly administered drugs due to anticholinergic effects on gastrointestinal motility. This may be of concern for drugs with a narrow therapeutic index.

Mean oxybutynin chloride plasma concentrations were approximately 2 fold higher when DITROPAN XL was administered with ketoconazole, a potent CYP3A4 inhibitor. Other inhibitors of the cytochrome P450 3A4 enzyme system, such as antimycotic agents (e.g., itraconazole and miconazole) or macrolide antibiotics (e.g., erythromycin and clarithromycin), may alter oxybutynin mean pharmacokinetic parameters (i.e., C_{max} and AUC). The clinical relevance of such potential interactions is not known. Caution should be used when such drugs are co-administered.

Carcinogenesis, Mutagenesis, Impairment of Fertility

A 24-month study in rats at dosages of oxybutynin chloride of 20, 80, and 160 mg/kg/day showed no evidence of carcinogenicity. These doses are approximately 6, 25, and 50 times the maximum human exposure, based on surface area.

Oxybutynin chloride showed no increase of mutagenic activity when tested in *Schizosaccharomyces pompholiciformis, Saccharomyces cerevisiae,* and *Salmonella typhimurium* test systems.

Reproduction studies with oxybutynin chloride in the mouse, rat, hamster, and rabbit showed no definite evidence of impaired fertility.

Pregnancy: Teratogenic Effects

Pregnancy Category B

Reproduction studies with oxybutynin chloride in the mouse, rat, hamster, and rabbit showed no definite evidence of impaired fertility or harm to the animal fetus. The safety of DITROPAN XL administration to women who are or who may become pregnant has not been established. Therefore, DITROPAN XL should not be given to pregnant women unless, in the judgment of the physician, the probable clinical benefits outweigh the possible hazards.

Nursing Mothers

It is not known whether oxybutynin is excreted in human milk. Because many drugs are excreted in human milk, caution should be exercised when DITROPAN XL is administered to a nursing woman.

Pediatric Use

The safety and efficacy of DITROPAN XL were studied in 60 children in a 24-week, open-label trial. Patients were aged 6-15 years, all had symptoms of detrusor overactivity in association with a neurological condition (e.g., spina bifida), all used clean intermittent catheterization, and all were current users of oxybutynin chloride. Study results demonstrated that administration of DITROPAN XL 5 to 20 mg/day was associated with an increase from baseline in mean urine volume per catheterization from 108 mL to 136 mL, an increase from baseline in mean urine volume after morning awakening from 148 mL to 189 mL, and an increase from baseline in the mean percentage of catheterizations without a leaking episode from 34% to 51%.

Urodynamic results were consistent with clinical results. Administration of DITROPAN XL resulted in an increase from baseline in mean maximum cystometric capacity from 185 mL to 254 mL, a decrease from baseline in mean detrusor pressure at maximum cystometric capacity from 44 cm H_2O to 33 cm H_2O, and a reduction in the percentage of patients demonstrating uninhibited detrusor contractions (of at least 15 cm H_2O) from 60% to 28%.

DITROPAN XL is not recommended in pediatric patients who can not swallow the tablet whole without chewing, dividing, or crushing, or in children under the age of 6 (see **DOSAGE AND ADMINISTRATION**).

Geriatric Use

The rate and severity of anticholinergic effects reported by patients less than 65 years old and those 65 years and older were similar (see **CLINICAL PHARMACOLOGY, Pharmacokinetics, *Special Populations:*** *Gender*).

ADVERSE REACTIONS

Adverse Events with DITROPAN XL

The safety and efficacy of DITROPAN XL® (oxybutynin chloride) was evaluated in a total of 580 participants who received DITROPAN XL in clinical trials (429 patients, 151 healthy volunteers). These participants were treated with 5-30 mg/day for up to 4.5 months. Safety information is provided for 429 patients from three controlled clinical studies and one open label study (Table 3). The adverse events are reported regardless of causality.

Table 3
Incidence (%) of Adverse Events Reported by ≥5% of Patients Using DITROPAN XL (5-30 mg/day)

Body System	Adverse Event	DITROPAN XL® 5-30 mg/day (n=429)
General	headache	9.8
	asthenia	6.8
	pain	6.8
Digestive	dry mouth	60.8
	constipation	13.1
	diarrhea	9.1
	nausea	8.9
	dyspepsia	6.8
Nervous	somnolence	11.9
	dizziness	6.3
Respiratory	rhinitis	5.6
Special senses	blurred vision	7.7
	dry eyes	6.1
Urogenital	urinary tract infection	5.1

The most common adverse events reported by patients receiving 5-30 mg/day DITROPAN XL were the expected side effects of anticholinergic agents. The incidence of dry mouth was dose-related.

The discontinuation rate for all adverse events was 6.8%. The most frequent adverse event causing early discontinuation of study medication was nausea (1.9%), while discontinuation due to dry mouth was 1.2%.

In addition, the following adverse events were reported by 2 to <5% of patients using DITROPAN XL (5-30 mg/day) in all studies. *General:* abdominal pain, dry nasal and sinus mucous membranes, accidental injury, back pain, flu syndrome; *Cardiovascular:* hypertension, palpitation, vasodilatation; *Digestive:* flatulence, gastroesophageal reflux; *Musculoskeletal:* arthritis; *Nervous:* insomnia, nervousness, confusion; *Respiratory:* upper respiratory tract infection, cough, sinusitis, bronchitis, pharyngitis; *Skin:* dry skin, rash; *Urogenital:* impaired urination (hesitancy), increased post void residual volume, urinary retention, cystitis.

Additional rare adverse events reported from worldwide post-marketing experience with DITROPAN XL include: peripheral edema, cardiac arrhythmia, tachycardia, hallucinations, convulsions, and impotence.

Additional adverse events reported with some other oxybutynin chloride formulations include: cycloplegia, mydriasis, and suppression of lactation.

OVERDOSAGE

The continuous release of oxybutynin from DITROPAN XL® (oxybutynin chloride) should be considered in the treatment of overdosage. Patients should be monitored for at least 24 hours. Treatment should be symptomatic and supportive. Activated charcoal as well as a cathartic may be administered.

Overdosage with oxybutynin chloride has been associated with anticholinergic effects including central nervous system excitation, flushing, fever, dehydration, cardiac arrhythmia, vomiting, and urinary retention.

Ingestion of 100 mg oxybutynin chloride in association with alcohol has been reported in a 13-year-old boy who experienced memory loss, and a 34-year-old woman who developed stupor, followed by disorientation and agitation on awakening, dilated pupils, dry skin, cardiac arrhythmia, and retention of urine. Both patients fully recovered with symptomatic treatment.

DOSAGE AND ADMINISTRATION

DITROPAN XL® (oxybutynin chloride) must be swallowed whole with the aid of liquids, and must not be chewed, divided, or crushed.

DITROPAN XL may be administered with or without food.

Adults: The recommended starting dose of DITROPAN XL is 5 mg once daily. Dosage may be adjusted in 5-mg increments to achieve a balance of efficacy and tolerability (up to a maximum of 30 mg/day). In general, dosage adjustment may proceed at approximately weekly intervals.

Pediatric patients aged 6 years of age and older: The recommended starting dose of DITROPAN XL is 5 mg once daily. Dosage may be adjusted in 5-mg increments to achieve a balance of efficacy and tolerability (up to a maximum of 20 mg/day).

HOW SUPPLIED

DITROPAN XL® (oxybutynin chloride) Extended Release Tablets are available in three dosage strengths, 5 mg (pale yellow), 10 mg (pink), and 15 mg (gray) and are imprinted with "5 XL", "10 XL", or "15 XL". DITROPAN XL Extended Release Tablets are supplied in bottles of 100 tablets.

5 mg	100 count bottle	NDC 17314-8500-1
10 mg	100 count bottle	NDC 17314-8501-1
15 mg	100 count bottle	NDC 17314-8502-1

Storage

Store at 25°C (77°F); excursions permitted to 15-30°C (59-86°F) [see USP Controlled Room Temperature]. Protect from moisture and humidity.

Rx only

For more information call 1-888-395-1232 or visit www.DITROPANXL.com

Manufactured by ALZA Corporation, Mountain View, CA 94043

An ALZA OROS®
Technology Product

DITROPAN XL® and OROS® are registered trademarks of ALZA Corporation.

Distributed and Marketed by Ortho-McNeil Pharmaceutical, Inc., Raritan, NJ 08869

ORTHO-McNEIL

631-10-800-1 Revised June 2003

Shown in Product Identification Guide, page 328

ELMIRON® -100 MG ℞
(pentosan polysulfate sodium) Capsules

Prescribing Information

DESCRIPTION

Pentosan polysulfate sodium is a semi-synthetically produced heparin-like macromolecular carbohydrate derivative which chemically and structurally resembles glycosaminoglycans. It is a white odorless powder, slightly hygroscopic and soluble in water to 50% at pH 6. it has a molecular weight of 4000 to 6000 Dalton with the following structural formula:

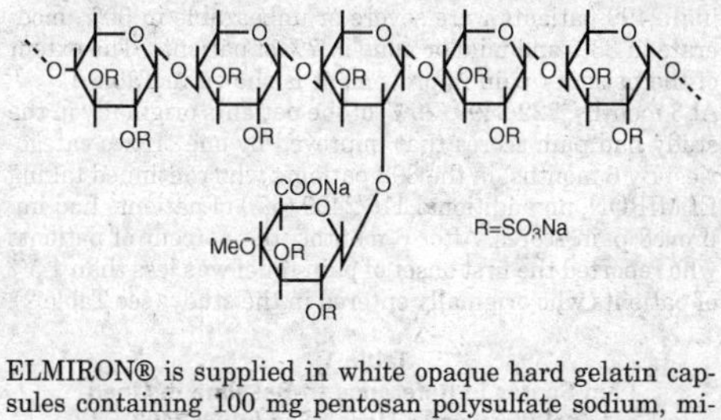

ELMIRON® is supplied in white opaque hard gelatin capsules containing 100 mg pentosan polysulfate sodium, microcrystalline cellulose, and magnesium stearate. It is formulated for oral use.

CLINICAL PHARMACOLOGY

GENERAL: Pentosan polysulfate sodium is a low molecular weight heparin-like compound. It has anticoagulant and

Continued on next page

Elmiron—Cont.

fibrinolytic effects. The mechanism of action of pentosan polysulfate sodium in interstitial cystitis is not known.

PHARMACOKINETICS

Absorption: In preliminary clinical studies with different doses of radio labeled pentosan polysulfate sodium, absorption was approximately 3% of the administered dose (n=3).

Distribution: Preclinical studies with parenterally administered radio labeled pentosan polysulfate sodium showed distribution to the uroepithelium of the genitourinary tract with lesser amounts found in the liver, spleen, lung, skin, periosteum, and bone marrow. Erythrocyte penetration is low in animals.

Metabolism: Preliminary literature studies of metabolism in 5 healthy volunteers with radio labeled drug suggest that 68% of the dose, at about 1 hour after IV administration, undergoes partial desulfation in the liver and spleen. In another study of 3 healthy volunteers, partial depolymerization occurs in the kidney. Both the desulfation and depolymerization can be saturated with continued dosing.

Excretion: In preliminary clinical studies in 8 healthy male volunteers, the elimination half-life of pentosan polysulfate sodium had a mean value at 24 hours after IV injection of 40 mg.

The elimination half-life in urine following orally administered radio labeled pentosan polysulfate sodium was determined to be 4.8 hours for the unchanged drug.

In preliminary human studies in 3 healthy male volunteers, after single doses of radio labeled drug, urinary excretion averaged 3.5% of the administered dose. After multiple doses of pentosan polysulfate sodium, urine excretion of radioactivity averaged 11% of the administered dose.

Further analyses of the urinary fraction obtained after repeated dosing showed that about 3% of the dose may be unchanged pentosan polysulfate sodium.

Special Populations: Dose adjustments in geriatric patients and in patients with hepatic or renal impairment were not studied.

PHARMACODYNAMICS

The mechanism by which pentosan polysulfate sodium achieves its effects in patients is unknown. In preliminary clinical models, pentosan polysulfate sodium adhered to the bladder wall mucosal membrane. The drug may act as a buffer to control cell permeability preventing irritating solutes in the urine from reaching the cells.

Food effects: The effect of food on absorption of pentosan polysulfate sodium is not known. In clinical trials, ELMIRON was administered with water 1 hour before or 2 hours after meals.

Drug-Drug Interactions: Not studied.

CLINICAL TRIALS

ELMIRON was evaluated in two clinical trials for the relief of pain in patients with chronic interstitial cystitis (IC). All patients met the NIH definition of IC based upon the results of cystoscopy, cytology, and biopsy. One blinded, randomized, placebo controlled study evaluated 151 patients (145 women, 5 men, 1 unknown) with a mean age of 44 years (range 18 to 81). Approximately equal numbers of patients received either placebo or ELMIRON 100 mg three times a day for 3 months. Clinical improvement in bladder pain was based upon the patient's own assessment. In this study, 28/74 (38%) of patients who received ELMIRON and 13/74 (18%) of patients who received placebo, showed greater than 50% improvement in bladder pain (p=0.005).

A second clinical trial, the physician's usage study, was a prospectively designed retrospective analysis of 2499 patients who received ELMIRON 300 mg a day without blinding. Of the 2499 patients, 2220 were women, 254 were men, and 25 were of unknown sex. The patients had a mean age of 47 years and 23% were over 60 years of age. By 3 months, 1307 (52%) of the patients had dropped out or were ineligible for analysis, overall, 1192 (48%) received ELMIRON for 3 months; 892 (36%) received ELMIRON for 6 months; and 598 (24%) received ELMIRON for one year.

Patients had unblinded evaluations every 3 months for the patient's rating of overall change in pain in comparison to baseline and for the difference calculated in "pain/discomfort" scores. At baseline, pain/discomfort scores for the original 2499 patients were severe or unbearable in 60%, moderate in 33% and mild or none in 7% of patients. The extent of the patients' pain improvement is shown in Table 1.

At 3 months, 722/2499 (29%) of the patients originally in the study had pain scores that improved by one or two categories. By 6 months, in the 892 patients who continued taking ELMIRON, an additional 116/2499 (5%) of patients had improved pain scores. After 6 months, the percent of patients who reported the first onset of pain relief was less than 1.5% of patients who originally entered in the study (see Table 2).

Table 1:
Pain Scores in Reference to Baseline in Open Label Physician's Usage Study (N=2499)[1]

Efficacy Parameter	3 months[2]	6 months[2]
Patient Rating of Overall Change in Pain (Recollection of difference between current pain and baseline pain)[3]	N=1161 Median=3 Mean=3.44 CI: (3.37, 3.51)	N=724 Median=4 Mean=3.91 CI: (3.83, 3.99)
Change in Pain/ Discomfort Score (Calculated difference in scores at the time point and baseline)[4]	N=1440 Median=1 Mean=0.51 CI: (0.45, 0.57)	N=904 Median=1 Mean=0.66 CI: (0.61, 0.71)

[1] Trial not designed to detect onset of pain relief.
[2] CI=95% confidence interval.
[3] 6-point-scale: 1 = worse, 2 = no better, 3 = slightly improved, 4 = moderately improved, 5 = greatly improved, 6=symptom gone.
[4] 3-point scale: 1=none or mild, 2=moderate, 3=severe or unbearable.

Table 2:
Number (%) of Patients with New Relief of Pain/Discomfort[1] in the Open-Label Physician's Usage Study (N=2499)

	at 3 months[2] (n=1192)	at 6 months[3] (n=892)
Considering only the patients who continued treatment	722/1192 (61%)	116/892 (13%)
Considering all the patients originally enrolled in the study	722/2499 (29%)	116/2499 (5%)

[1] First-time improvement in pain/discomfort score by 1 or 2 categories.
[2] Number (%) of patients with improvement of pain/discomfort score at 3 months when compared to baseline.
[3] Number (%) of patients without pain/ discomfort improvement at 3 months who had improvement at 6 months.

INDICATIONS AND USAGE

ELMIRON (pentosan polysulfate sodium) is indicated for the relief of bladder pain or discomfort associated with interstitial cystitis.

CONTRAINDICATIONS

ELMIRON (pentosan polysulfate sodium) is contraindicated in patients with known hypersensitivity to the drug, structurally related compounds, or excipients.

WARNINGS

None.

PRECAUTIONS

GENERAL

ELMIRON (pentosan polysulfate sodium) is a weak anticoagulant (1/15 the activity of heparin). Bleeding complications of ecchymosis, epistaxis, and gum hemorrhage have been reported (see **ADVERSE REACTIONS**). Patients undergoing invasive procedures or having sign/symptoms of underlying coagulopathy or other increased risk of bleeding (due to other therapies such as coumarin anticoagulants, heparin, t-PA, streptokinase, or high dose aspirin) should be evaluated for hemorrhage. Patients with diseases such as aneurysms, thrombocytopenia, hemophilia, gastrointestinal ulcerations, polyps, or diverticula should be carefully evaluated before starting ELMIRON.

A similar product that was given subcutaneously, sublingually, or intramuscularly (and not initially metabolized by the liver) is associated with delayed immunoallergic thrombocytopenia with symptoms of thrombosis and hemorrhage. Caution should be exercised when using ELMIRON in patients who have a history of heparin induced thrombocytopenia.

Hepatic Insufficiency: Pentosan polysulfate sodium is desulfated by both the liver and the spleen. The extent to which hepatic insufficiency or splenic disorders may increase the bioavailability of the parent or active metabolites of pentosan polysulfate sodium is not known. Caution should be exercised when using ELMIRON in these patients.

Mildly (<2.5 × normal) elevated transaminase, alkaline phosphatase, γ-glutamyl transpeptidase, and lactic dehydrogenase occurred in 1.2% of patients. The increases usually appeared 3 to 12 months after the start of ELMIRON therapy, and were not associated with jaundice or other clinical signs or symptoms. These abnormalities are usually transient, may remain essentially unchanged, or may rarely progress with continued use. Increases in PTT and PT (<1% for both) or thrombocytopenia (0.2%) were noted.

Alopecia is associated with pentosan polysulfate and with heparin products. In clinical trials of ELMIRON, alopecia could begin within the first 4 weeks of treatment. Ninety-seven percent (97%) of the cases of alopecia reported were alopecia areata, limited to a single area on the scalp.

INFORMATION FOR PATIENTS

Patients should take the drug as prescribed, in the dosage prescribed, and no more frequently than prescribed. Patients should be reminded that ELMIRON has a weak anticoagulant effect. This effect may increase bleeding times.

LABORATORY TEST FINDINGS

Pentosan polysulfate sodium did not affect prothrombin time (PT) or partial thromboplastin time (PPT) up to 1200 mg per day in 24 healthy male subjects treated for 8 days. Pentosan polysulfate sodium also inhibits the generation of factor Xa plasma and inhibits thrombin-induced platelet aggregation in human platelet rich plasma ex vivo. (SEE **PRECAUTIONS**—Hepatic Insufficiency Section for additional information).

CARCINOGENICITY, MUTAGENESIS, IMPAIRMENT OF FERTILITY

Long term studies in animals have not been performed to evaluate the carcinogenic potential of ELMIRON. Pentosan polysulfate sodium was not clastogenic or mutagenic when tested in the mouse micronucleus test or the Ames test (*S. typhimurium*). The effect of pentosan polysulfate sodium on spermatogenesis has not been investigated.

PREGNANCY CATEGORY B

Reproduction studies have been performed in mice and rats with intravenous daily doses of 15 mg/kg, and in rabbits with 7.5 mg/kg. These doses are 0.42 and 0.14 times the daily oral human doses of ELMIRON when normalized to body surface area. These studies did not reveal evidence of impaired fertility or harm to the fetus from ELMIRON. Direct in vitro bathing of cultured mouse embryos with pentosan polysulfate sodium (PPS) at a concentration of 1 mg/mL may cause reversible limb bud abnormalities. Adequate and well controlled studies have not been performed in pregnant women. Because animal studies are not always predictive of human response, this drug should be used in pregnancy only if clearly needed.

NURSING MOTHERS

It is not known whether this drug is excreted in human milk. Because many drugs are excreted in human milk, caution should be exercised when ELMIRON is administered to a nursing woman.

PEDIATRIC USE

Safety and effectiveness in pediatric patients below the age of 16 years have not been established.

ADVERSE REACTIONS

ELMIRON was evaluated in clinical trials in a total of 2627 patients (2343 women, 262 men, 22 unknown) with a mean age of 47 [range 18 to 88 with 581 (22%) over 60 years of age]. Of the 2627 patients, 128 patients were in a 3 month trial and the remaining 2499 patients were in a long term, unblinded trial.

Deaths occurred in 6/2627 (0.2%) patients who received the drug over a period of 3 to 75 months. The deaths appear to be related to other concurrent illnesses or procedures, except in one patient for whom the cause was not known.

Serious adverse events occurred in 33/2627 (1.3%) patients. Two patients had severe abdominal pain or diarrhea and dehydration that required hospitalization. Because there was not a control group of patients with interstitial cystitis who were concurrently evaluated, it is difficult to determine which events are associated with ELMIRON and which events are associated with concurrent illness, medicine, or other factors.

Adverse Experience In Placebo-Controlled Clinical Trials of ELMIRON® 100 mg Three Times a Day for 3 Months

Body System/ Adverse Experience		Elmiron n=128	Placebo n=130
CNS	Overall Number of Patients*	3	5
	Insomnia	1	0
	Headache	1	3
	Severe Emotional Lability/Depression	2	1
	Nystagmus/Dizziness	1	1
	Hyperkinesia	1	1
GI	Overall Number of Patients*	7	7
	Nausea	3	3
	Diarrhea	3	6
	Dyspepsia	1	0
	Jaundice	0	1
	Vomiting	0	2
Skin/Allergic	Overall Number of Patients*	2	4
	Rash	0	2
	Pruritus	0	2
	Lacrimation	1	1
	Rhinitis	1	1
	Increased Sweating	1	0
Other	Overall Number of Patients*	1	3

Amenorrhea	0	1
Arthralgia	0	1
Vaginitis	1	1
Total Events	17	27
Total Number of Patients Reporting Adverse Events	13	19

* Within a body system, the individual events do not sum to equal overall number of patients because a patient may have more than one event.

The adverse events described below were reported in an unblinded clinical trial of 2499 interstitial cystitis patients treated with ELMIRON. Of the original 2499 patients, 1192 (48%) received ELMIRON for 3 months; 892 (36%) received ELMIRON for 6 months; and 598 (24%) received ELMIRON for one year, 355 (14%) received ELMIRON for 2 years, and 145 (6%) for 4 years.

FREQUENCY (1 to 4%): Alopecia (4%), diarrhea (4%), nausea (4%), headache (3%), rash (3%), dyspepsia (2%), abdominal pain (2%), liver function abnormalities (1%), dizziness (1%).

FREQUENCY (≤1%): *Digestive:* Vomiting, mouth ulcer, colitis, esophagitis, gastritis, flatulence, constipation, anorexia, gum hemorrhage.

Hematologic: Anemia, ecchymosis, increased prothrombin time, increased partial thromboplastin time, leukopenia, thrombocytopenia.

Hypersensitive Reactions: Allergic reaction, photosensitivity.

Respiratory System: Pharyngitis, rhinitis, epistaxis, dyspnea.

Skin and Appendages: Pruritis, urticaria.

Special Senses: Conjunctivitis, tinnitus, optic neuritis, amblyopia, retinal hemorrhage.

OVERDOSAGE

Overdose has not been reported. Based upon the pharmacodynamics of the drug, toxicity is likely to be reflected as anticoagulation, bleeding, thrombocytopenia, liver function abnormalities, and gastric distress. (See **CLINICAL PHARMACOLOGY** and **PRECAUTIONS** sections). In the event of acute overdosage, the patient should be given gastric lavage if possible, carefully observed and given symptomatic and supportive treatment.

DOSAGE AND ADMINISTRATION

The recommended dose of ELMIRON is 300 mg/day taken as one 100 mg capsule orally three times daily. The capsules should be taken with water at least 1 hour before meals or 2 hours after meals.

Patients receiving ELMIRON should be reassessed after 3 months. If improvement has not occurred and if limiting adverse events are not present, ELMIRON may be continued for another 3 months.

The clinical value and risks of continued treatment in patients whose pain has not improved by 6 months is not known.

HOW SUPPLIED

ELMIRON® is supplied in white opaque hard gelatin capsules imprinted "BNP7600" containing 100 mg pentosan polysulfate sodium. Supplied in bottles of 100 capsules.
NDC NUMBER 17314-9300-1

STORAGE

Store at controlled room temperature 15°–30°C (59°–86°F).

Rx only

ELMIRON® is a Registered Trademark of IVAX Research, Inc. under license to ORTHO-McNEIL PHARMACEUTICAL, INC.

ORTHO-McNEIL
ORTHO-McNEIL PHARMACEUTICAL, INC.
Raritan, New Jersey, 08869
633-20-506-1
Manufactured by:
IVAX Pharmaceuticals, Inc.
Miami, FL 33137-3227
Distributed by
ORTHO-McNEIL PHARMACEUTICAL, INC.
Raritan, New Jersey, 08869-4043
I493001
0802ISS
Patent #5,180,715

Patient Information

Medication Guide

Questions and Answers About
ELMIRON®
(Generic name = pentosan polysulfate sodium) Capsules

What is the most important information I should know about ELMIRON?

ELMIRON (pronounced EL ma ron) is used to treat the pain or discomfort of interstitial cystitis (IC).

You must take ELMIRON as prescribed by your doctor in the dosage prescribed but no more frequently than prescribed.

ELMIRON is a weak anticoagulant (blood thinner) which may increase bleeding.

Call your doctor if you will be undergoing surgery or will begin taking anticoagulant therapy such as Coumadin®, heparin, high doses of aspirin, or anti-inflammatory drugs such as ibuprofen.

What is ELMIRON?

ELMIRON is used to treat the pain or discomfort of interstitial cystitis (IC). It is not known exactly how ELMIRON works, but it is not a pain medication, like aspirin or acetaminophen and therefore must be taken continuously for relief as prescribed.

Who should not take ELMIRON?

- Patients undergoing surgery should speak with their doctor about when to discontinue ELMIRON prior to surgery.
- ELMIRON should be used during pregnancy only if clearly needed.

What does your doctor need to know?

- If you are taking anticoagulant therapy such as Coumadin®, heparin, high doses of aspirin, or anti-inflammatory drugs such as ibuprofen.
- If you are pregnant.
- If you have any liver problems.

How should I take ELMIRON?

You should take 1 capsule of ELMIRON by mouth three times a day, with water at least 1 hour before meals or 2 hours after meals. Each capsule contains 100 mg of ELMIRON.

What should I avoid while taking ELMIRON?

High doses of aspirin or anti-inflammatory drugs such as ibuprofen.

What are the most common side effects of ELMIRON?

The most common side effects are hair loss, diarrhea, nausea, headache, rash, upset stomach, abnormal liver function tests, dizziness and bruising.

Call your doctor if these side effects persist or are bothersome.

If you suspect that someone may have taken more than the prescribed dose of this medicine, contact your local poison control center or emergency room immediately. This medication was prescribed for your particular condition. Do not use it for another condition or give the drug to others.

This leaflet provides a summary of information about ELMIRON. Medicines are sometimes prescribed for uses other than those listed in a Medication Guide. If you have any questions or concerns, or want more information about ELMIRON, contact your doctor or pharmacist. Your pharmacist also has a longer leaflet about ELMIRON that is written for health professionals that you can ask to read.

ELMIRON® is a Registered Trademark of IVAX Research, Inc. under license to ORTHO-McNEIL PHARMACEUTICAL, INC.

ORTHO-McNEIL
ORTHO-McNEIL PHARMACEUTICAL, INC.
Raritan, New Jersey, 08869
633-20-506-1P
Manufactured by:
IVAX Pharmaceuticals, Inc.
Miami, FL 33137-3227
Distributed by
ORTHO-McNEIL PHARMACEUTICAL, INC.
Raritan, New Jersey, 08869-4043
I493001
0802ISS
Patent #5,180,715

Shown in Product Identification Guide, page 328

FLOXIN® TABLETS ℞

(ofloxacin tablets)
[flŏx- ĭn]

DESCRIPTION

FLOXIN® (ofloxacin tablets) Tablets is a synthetic broad-spectrum antimicrobial agent for oral administration. Chemically, ofloxacin, a fluorinated carboxyquinolone, is the racemate, (±)-9-fluoro-2,3-dihydro-3-methyl-10-(4-methyl-1-piperazinyl)-7-oxo-7H-pyrido[1,2,3-de]-1,4-benzoxazine-6-carboxylic acid. The chemical structure is:

Its empirical formula is $C_{18}H_{20}FN_3O_4$, and its molecular weight is 361.4. Ofloxacin is an off-white to pale yellow crystalline powder. The molecule exists as a zwitterion at the pH conditions in the small intestine. The relative solubility characteristics of ofloxacin at room temperature, as defined by USP nomenclature, indicate that ofloxacin is considered to be *soluble* in aqueous solutions with pH between 2 and 5. It is *sparingly* to *slightly soluble* in aqueous solutions with pH 7 (solubility falls to 4 mg/mL) and *freely soluble* in aqueous solutions with pH above 9. Ofloxacin has the potential to form stable coordination compounds with many metal ions. This *in vitro* chelation potential has the following formation order: $Fe^{+3} > Al^{+3} > Cu^{+2} > Ni^{+2} > Pb^{+2} > Zn^{+2} > Mg^{+2} > Ca^{+2} > Ba^{+2}$.

FLOXIN Tablets contain the following inactive ingredients: anhydrous lactose, corn starch, hydroxypropyl cellulose, hydroxypropyl methylcellulose, magnesium stearate, polyethylene glycol, polysorbate 80, sodium starch glycolate, titanium dioxide and may also contain synthetic yellow iron oxide.

CLINICAL PHARMACOLOGY

Following oral administration, the bioavailability of ofloxacin in the tablet formulation is approximately 98%. Maximum serum concentrations are achieved one to two hours after an oral dose. Absorption of ofloxacin after single or multiple doses of 200 to 400 mg is predictable, and the amount of drug absorbed increases proportionately with the dose. Ofloxacin has biphasic elimination. Following multiple oral doses at steady-state administration, the half-lives are approximately 4–5 hours and 20–25 hours. However, the longer half-life represents less than 5% of the total AUC. Accumulation at steady-state can be estimated using a half-life of 9 hours. The total clearance and volume of distribution are approximately similar after single or multiple doses. Elimination is mainly by renal excretion. The following are mean peak serum concentrations in healthy 70–80 kg male volunteers after single oral doses of 200, 300, or 400 mg of ofloxacin or after multiple oral doses of 400 mg. [See table below]

Steady-state concentrations were attained after four oral doses, and the area under the curve (AUC) was approximately 40% higher than the AUC after single doses. Therefore, after multiple-dose administration of 200 mg and 300 mg doses, peak serum levels of 2.2 µg/mL and 3.6 µg/mL, respectively, are predicted at steady-state.

In vitro, approximately 32% of the drug in plasma is protein bound.

The single dose and steady-state plasma profiles of ofloxacin injection were comparable in extent of exposure (AUC) to those of ofloxacin tablets when the injectable and tablet formulations of ofloxacin were administered in equal doses (mg/mg) to the same group of subjects. The mean steady-state $AUC_{(0-12)}$ attained after the intravenous administration of 400 mg over 60 min was 43.5 µg•h/mL; the mean steady-state $AUC_{(0-12)}$ attained after the oral administration of 400 mg was 41.2 µg•h/mL (two one-sided t-test, 90% confidence interval was 103–109).

(See following chart.)

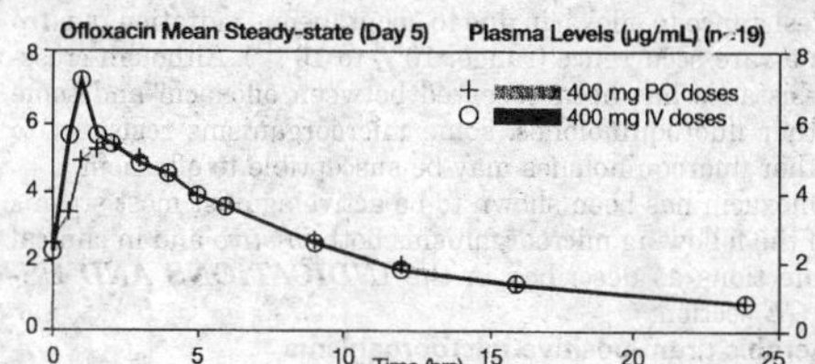

Between 0 and 6 h following the administration of a single 200 mg oral dose of ofloxacin to 12 healthy volunteers, the average urine ofloxacin concentration was approximately 220 µg/mL. Between 12 and 24 hours after administration, the average urine ofloxacin level was approximately 34 µg/mL.

Following oral administration of recommended therapeutic doses, ofloxacin has been detected in blister fluid, cervix, lung tissue, ovary, prostatic fluid, prostatic tissue, skin, and sputum. The mean concentration of ofloxacin in each of these various body fluids and tissues after one or more doses was 0.8 to 1.5 times the concurrent plasma level. Inadequate data are presently available on the distribution or levels of ofloxacin in the cerebrospinal fluid or brain tissue.

Ofloxacin has a pyridobenzoxazine ring that appears to decrease the extent of parent compound metabolism. Between 65% and 80% of an administered oral dose of ofloxacin is excreted unchanged via the kidneys within 48 hours of dosing. Studies indicate that less than 5% of an administered dose is recovered in the urine as the desmethyl or N-oxide metabolites. Four to eight percent of an ofloxacin dose is excreted in the feces. This indicates a small degree of biliary excretion of ofloxacin.

The administration of FLOXIN with food does not affect the C_{max} and AUC_∞ of the drug, but T_{max} is prolonged.

Clearance of ofloxacin is reduced in patients with impaired renal function (creatinine clearance rate ≤ 50 mL/min), and dosage adjustment is necessary. (See ***PRECAUTIONS: General*** and ***DOSAGE AND ADMINISTRATION.***)

Continued on next page

Oral Dose	Serum Concentration 2 hours after admin. (µg/mL)	Area Under the Curve ($AUC_{(0-\infty)}$) (µg·h/mL)
200 mg single dose	1.5	14.1
300 mg single dose	2.4	21.2
400 mg single dose	2.9	31.4
400 mg steady-state	4.6	61.0

Floxin—Cont.

Following oral administration to healthy elderly subjects (65–81 years of age), maximum plasma concentrations are usually achieved one to two hours after single and multiple twice-daily doses, indicating that the rate of oral absorption is unaffected by age or gender. Mean peak plasma concentrations in elderly subjects were 9–21% higher than those observed in younger subjects. Gender differences in the pharmacokinetic properties of elderly subjects have been observed. Peak plasma concentrations were 114% and 54% higher in elderly females compared to elderly males following single and multiple twice-daily doses. [This interpretation was based on study results collected from two separate studies.] Plasma concentrations increase dose-dependently with the increase in doses after single oral dose and at steady state. No differences were observed in the volume of distribution values between elderly and younger subjects. As in younger subjects, elimination is mainly by renal excretion as unchanged drug in elderly subjects, although less drug is recovered from renal excretion in elderly subjects. Consistent with younger subjects, less than 5% of an administered dose was recovered in the urine as the desmethyl and N-oxide metabolites in the elderly. A longer plasma half-life of approximately 6.4 to 7.4 hours was observed in elderly subjects, compared with 4 to 5 hours for young subjects. Slower elimination of ofloxacin is observed in elderly subjects as compared with younger subjects which may be attributable to the reduced renal function and renal clearance observed in the elderly subjects. Because ofloxacin is known to be substantially excreted by the kidney, and elderly patients are more likely to have decreased renal function, dosage adjustment is necessary for elderly patients with impaired renal function as recommended for all patients. (See ***PRECAUTIONS: General*** and ***DOSAGE AND ADMINISTRATION.***)

Microbiology

Ofloxacin is a quinolone antimicrobial agent. The mechanism of action of ofloxacin and other fluoroquinolone antimicrobials involves inhibition of bacterial topoisomerase IV and DNA gyrase (both of which are type II topoisomerases), enzymes required for DNA replication, transcription, repair and recombination.

Ofloxacin has *in vitro* activity against a wide range of gram-negative and gram-positive microorganisms. Ofloxacin is often bactericidal at concentrations equal to or slightly greater than inhibitory concentrations.

Fluoroquinolones, including ofloxacin, differ in chemical structure and mode of action from aminoglycosides, macrolides and β-lactam antibiotics, including penicillins. Fluoroquinolones may, therefore, be active against bacteria resistant to these antimicrobials.

Resistance to ofloxacin due to spontaneous mutation *in vitro* is a rare occurrence (range: 10^{-9} to 10^{-11}). Although cross-resistance has been observed between ofloxacin and some other fluoroquinolones, some microorganisms resistant to other fluoroquinolones may be susceptible to ofloxacin.

Ofloxacin has been shown to be active against most strains of the following microorganisms both *in vitro* and in clinical infections as described in the ***INDICATIONS AND USAGE*** section:

Aerobic gram-positive microorganisms
Staphylococcus aureus (methicillin-susceptible strains)
Streptococcus pneumoniae (penicillin-susceptible strains)
Streptococcus pyogenes

Aerobic gram-negative microorganisms
Citrobacter (diversus) koseri
Enterobacter aerogenes
Escherichia coli
Haemophilus influenzae
Klebsiella pneumoniae
Neisseria gonorrhoeae
Proteus mirabilis
Pseudomonas aeruginosa

As with other drugs in this class, some strains of *Pseudomonas aeruginosa* may develop resistance fairly rapidly during treatment with ofloxacin.

Other microorganisms
Chlamydia trachomatis

The following *in vitro* data are available, **but their clinical significance is unknown.**

Ofloxacin exhibits *in vitro* minimum inhibitory concentrations (MIC values) of 2 μg/mL or less against most (≥ 90%) strains of the following microorganisms; however, the safety and effectiveness of ofloxacin in treating clinical infections due to these microorganisms have not been established in adequate and well-controlled trials:

Aerobic gram-positive microorganisms
Staphylococcus epidermidis (methicillin-susceptible strains)
Staphylococcus saprophyticus
Streptococcus pneumoniae (penicillin-resistant strains)

Aerobic gram-negative microorganisms
Acinetobacter calcoaceticus
Bordetella pertussis
Citrobacter freundii
Enterobacter cloacae
Haemophilus ducreyi
Klebsiella oxytoca
Moraxella catarrhalis
Morganella morganii
Proteus vulgaris
Providencia rettgeri
Providencia stuartii
Serratia marcescens

Anaerobic microorganisms
Clostridium perfringens

Other microorganisms
Chlamydia pneumoniae
Gardnerella vaginalis
Legionella pneumophila
Mycoplasma hominis
Mycoplasma pneumoniae
Ureaplasma urealyticum

Ofloxacin is not active against Treponema pallidum. (See ***WARNINGS.***)

Many strains of other streptococcal species, *Enterococcus* species, and anaerobes are resistant to ofloxacin.

Susceptibility Tests

Dilution techniques: Quantitative methods are used to determine antimicrobial minimum inhibitory concentrations (MIC values). These MIC values provide estimates of the susceptibility of bacteria to antimicrobial compounds. The MIC values should be determined using a standardized procedure. Standardized procedures are based on a dilution method[1] (broth or agar) or equivalent with standardized inoculum concentrations and standardized concentrations of ofloxacin powder. The MIC values should be interpreted according to the following criteria:

For testing aerobic microorganisms other than *Haemophilus influenzae*, *Neisseria gonorrhoeae*, and *Streptococcus pneumoniae*:

MIC (μg/mL)	Interpretation
≤2	Susceptible (S)
4	Intermediate (I)
≥8	Resistant (R)

For testing *Haemophilus influenzae*:[a]

MIC (μg/mL)	Interpretation
≤2.0	Susceptible (S)

[a] This interpretive standard is applicable only to broth microdilution susceptibility tests with *Haemophilus influenzae* using *Haemophilus* Test Medium[1].

The current absence of data on resistant strains precludes defining any results other than "Susceptible." Strains yielding MIC results suggestive of a "nonsusceptible" category should be submitted to a reference laboratory for further testing.

For testing *Neisseria gonorrhoeae*:[b]

MIC (μg/mL)	Interpretation
≤0.25	Susceptible (S)
0.5–1	Intermediate (I)
≥2	Resistant (R)

[b] These interpretive standards are applicable only to agar dilution tests using GC agar base and 1% defined growth supplement incubated in 5% CO_2.

For testing *Streptococcus* species including *Streptococcus pneumoniae*:[c]

MIC (μg/mL)	Interpretation
≤2	Susceptible (S)
4	Intermediate (I)
≥8	Resistant (R)

[c] These interpretive standards are applicable only to broth microdilution susceptibility tests using cation-adjusted Mueller-Hinton broth with 2–5% lysed horse blood.

A report of "Susceptible" indicates that the pathogen is likely to be inhibited if the antimicrobial compound in the blood reaches the concentrations usually achievable. A report of "Intermediate" indicates that the result should be considered equivocal, and, if the microorganism is not fully susceptible to alternative, clinically feasible drugs, the test should be repeated. This category implies possible clinical applicability in body sites where the drug is physiologically concentrated or in situations where high dosage of drug can be used. This category also provides a buffer zone which prevents small uncontrolled technical factors from causing major discrepancies in interpretation. A report of "Resistant" indicates that the pathogen is not likely to be inhibited if the antimicrobial compound in the blood reaches the concentrations usually achievable; other therapy should be selected.

Standardized susceptibility test procedures require the use of laboratory control microorganisms to control the technical aspects of the laboratory procedures. Standard ofloxacin powder should provide the following MIC values:

[See table below]

Microorganism		MIC (μg/mL)
Escherichia coli	ATCC 25922	0.015–0.12
Haemophilus influenzae	ATCC 49247[d]	0.016–0.06
Neisseria gonorrhoeae	ATCC 49226[e]	0.004–0.016
Pseudomonas aeruginosa	ATCC 27853	1–8
Staphylococcus aureus	ATCC 29213	0.12–1
Streptococcus pneumoniae	ATCC 49619[f]	1–4

[d] This quality control range is applicable only to *H. influenzae* ATCC 49247 tested by a microdilution procedure using *Haemophilus* Test Medium (HTM)[1].

[e] This quality control range is applicable only to *N. gonorrhoeae* ATCC 49226 tested by an agar dilution procedure using GC agar base with 1% defined growth supplement incubated in 5% CO_2.

[f] This quality control range is applicable only to *S. pneumoniae* ATCC 49619 tested by a microdilution procedure using cation-adjusted Mueller-Hinton broth with 2–5% lysed horse blood.

Diffusion techniques: Quantitative methods that require measurement of zone diameters also provide reproducible estimates of the susceptibility of bacteria to antimicrobial compounds. One such standardized procedure[2] requires the use of standardized inoculum concentrations. This procedure uses paper disks impregnated with 5-μg ofloxacin to test the susceptibility of microorganisms to ofloxacin.

Reports from the laboratory providing results of the standard single-disk susceptibility test with a 5-μg ofloxacin disk should be interpreted according to the following criteria:

For testing aerobic microorganisms other than *Haemophilus influenzae*, *Neisseria gonorrhoeae*, and *Streptococcus pneumoniae*:

Zone Diameter (mm)	Interpretation
≥16	Susceptible (S)
13–16	Intermediate (I)
≤12	Resistant (R)

For testing *Haemophilus influenzae*:[g]

Zone Diameter (mm)	Interpretation
≥16	Susceptible (S)

[g] This zone diameter standard is applicable only to disk diffusion tests with *Haemophilus influenzae* using *Haemophilus* Test Medium (HTM)[2] incubated in 5% CO_2.

The current absence of data on resistant strains precludes defining any results other than "Susceptible." Strains yielding zone diameter results suggestive of a "nonsusceptible" category should be submitted to a reference laboratory for further testing.

For testing *Neisseria gonorrhoea*:[h]

Zone Diameter (mm)	Interpretation
≥31	Susceptible (S)
25–30	Intermediate (I)
≤24	Resistant (R)

[h] These zone diameter standards are applicable only to disk diffusion tests using GC agar base and 1% defined growth supplement incubated in 5% CO_2.

For testing *Streptococcus* species including *Streptococcus pneumoniae*:[i]

Zone Diameter (mm)	Interpretation
≥16	Susceptible (S)
13–15	Intermediate (I)
≤12	Resistant (R)

[i] These zone diameter standards are applicable only to disk diffusion tests performed using Mueller-Hinton agar supplemented with 5% defibrinated sheep blood and incubated in 5% CO_2.

Interpretation should be as stated above for results using dilution techniques. Interpretation involves correlation of the diameter obtained in the disk test with the MIC for ofloxacin.

As with standardized dilution techniques, diffusion methods require the use of laboratory control microorganisms that are used to control the technical aspects of the laboratory procedures. For the diffusion technique, the 5-μg ofloxacin disk should provide the following zone diameters in these laboratory quality control strains:

[See table at top of next page]

INDICATIONS AND USAGE

FLOXIN (ofloxacin tablets) Tablets are indicated for the treatment of adults with mild to moderate infections (unless otherwise indicated) caused by susceptible strains of the designated microorganisms in the infections listed below. Please see ***DOSAGE AND ADMINISTRATION*** for specific recommendations.

Acute bacterial exacerbations of chronic bronchitis due to *Haemophilus influenzae* or *Streptococcus pneumoniae*.

Community-acquired Pneumonia due to *Haemophilus influenzae* or *Streptococcus pneumoniae*.

Uncomplicated skin and skin structure infections due to *Staphylococcus aureus, Streptococcus pyogenes*, or *Proteus mirabilis*.

Acute, uncomplicated urethral and cervical gonorrhea due to *Neisseria gonorrhoeae*. (See ***WARNINGS.***)

Nongonococcal urethritis and cervicitis due to *Chlamydia trachomatis*. (See ***WARNINGS.***)

Mixed infections of the urethra and cervix due to *Chlamydia trachomatis* and *Neisseria gonorrhoeae*. (See ***WARNINGS.***)

Acute pelvic inflammatory disease (including severe infection) due to *Chlamydia trachomatis* and/or *Neisseria gonorrhoeae*. (See ***WARNINGS.***)

NOTE: If anaerobic microorganisms are suspected of contributing to the infection, appropriate therapy for anaerobic pathogens should be administered.

Uncomplicated cystitis due to *Citrobacter diversus, Enterobacter aerogenes, Escherichia coli, Klebsiella pneumoniae, Proteus mirabilis*, or *Pseudomonas aeruginosa*.

Complicated urinary tract infections due to *Escherichia coli, Klebsiella pneumoniae, Proteus mirabilis, Citrobacter diversus**, or *Pseudomonas aeruginosa**.

Prostatitis due to *Escherichia coli*.

* = Although treatment of infections due to this organism in this organ system demonstrated a clinically significant outcome, efficacy was studied in fewer than 10 patients.

Appropriate culture and susceptibility tests should be performed before treatment in order to isolate and identify organisms causing the infection and to determine their susceptibility to ofloxacin. Therapy with ofloxacin may be initiated before results of these tests are known; once results become available, appropriate therapy should be continued.

As with other drugs in this class, some strains of *Pseudomonas aeruginosa* may develop resistance fairly rapidly during treatment with ofloxacin. Culture and susceptibility testing performed periodically during therapy will provide information not only on the therapeutic effect of the antimicrobial agent but also on the possible emergence of bacterial resistance.

CONTRAINDICATIONS

FLOXIN (ofloxacin) is contraindicated in persons with a history of hypersensitivity associated with the use of ofloxacin or any member of the quinolone group of antimicrobial agents.

WARNINGS

THE SAFETY AND EFFICACY OF OFLOXACIN IN PEDIATRIC PATIENTS AND ADOLESCENTS (UNDER THE AGE OF 18 YEARS), PREGNANT WOMEN, AND LACTATING WOMEN HAVE NOT BEEN ESTABLISHED. (See PRECAUTIONS: Pediatric Use, Pregnancy, and Nursing Mothers subsections.)

In the immature rat, the oral administration of ofloxacin at 5 to 16 times the recommended maximum human dose based on mg/kg or 1–3 times based on mg/m^2 increased the incidence and severity of osteochondrosis. The lesions did not regress after 13 weeks of drug withdrawal. Other quinolones also produce similar erosions in the weight-bearing joints and other signs of arthropathy in immature animals of various species. (See ***ANIMAL PHARMACOLOGY.***)

Convulsions, increased intracranial pressure, and toxic psychosis have been reported in patients receiving quinolones, including ofloxacin. Quinolones, including ofloxacin, may also cause central nervous system stimulation which may lead to: tremors, restlessness/agitation, nervousness/anxiety, lightheadedness, confusion, hallucinations, paranoia and depression, nightmares, insomnia, and rarely suicidal thoughts or acts. These reactions may occur following the first dose. If these reactions occur in patients receiving ofloxacin, the drug should be discontinued and appropriate measures instituted. Insomnia may be more common with ofloxacin than some other products in the quinolone class. As with all quinolones, ofloxacin should be used with caution in patients with a known or suspected CNS disorder that may predispose to seizures or lower the seizure threshold (e.g., severe cerebral arteriosclerosis, epilepsy) or in the presence of other risk factors that may predispose to seizures or lower the seizure threshold (e.g., certain drug therapy, renal dysfunction). (See ***PRECAUTIONS: General, Information for Patients, Drug Interactions*** and ***ADVERSE REACTIONS.***)

Serious and occasionally fatal hypersensitivity (anaphylactic/anaphylactoid) reactions have been reported in patients receiving therapy with quinolones, including ofloxacin. These reactions often occur following the first dose. Some reactions were accompanied by cardiovascular collapse, hypotension/shock, seizure, loss of consciousness, tingling, angioedema (including tongue, laryngeal, throat or facial edema/swelling), airway obstruction (including bronchospasm, shortness of breath and acute respiratory distress), dyspnea, urticaria/hives, itching, and other serious skin reactions. A few patients had a history of hypersensitivity reactions. The drug should be discontinued immediately at the first appearance of a skin rash or any other sign of hypersensitivity. Serious acute hypersensitivity reactions may require treatment with epinephrine and other resuscitative measures, including oxygen, intravenous fluids, antihistamines, corticosteroids, pressor amines, and airway management, as clinically indicated. (See ***PRECAUTIONS*** and ***ADVERSE REACTIONS.***)

Microorganism		Zone Diameter (mm)
Escherichia coli	ATCC 25922	29–33
Haemophilus influenzae	ATCC 49247[j]	31–40
Neisseria gonorrhoeae	ATCC 49226[k]	43–51
Pseudomonas aeruginosa	ATCC 27853	17–21
Staphylococcus aureus	ATCC 25923	24–28
Streptococcus pneumoniae	ATCC 49619[l]	16–21

[j] This quality control range is applicable only to *H. influenzae* ATCC 49247 tested by a disk diffusion procedure using *Haemophilus* Test Medium (HTM)[2] incubated in 5% CO_2.

[k] This quality control range is applicable only to *N. gonorrhoeae* ATCC 49226 tested by a disk diffusion procedure using GC agar base with 1% defined growth supplement incubated in 5% CO_2.

[l] This quality control range is applicable only to *S. pneumoniae* ATCC 49619 tested by a disk diffusion procedure using Mueller-Hinton agar supplemented with 5% defibrinated sheep blood and incubated in 5% CO_2.

Serious and sometimes fatal events, some due to hypersensitivity, and some due to uncertain etiology, have been reported in patients receiving therapy with quinolones, including ofloxacin. These events may be severe and generally occur following the administration of multiple doses. Clinical manifestations may include one or more of the following: fever, rash or severe dermatologic reactions (e.g., toxic epidermal necrolysis, Stevens-Johnson Syndrome); vasculitis; arthralgia; myalgia; serum sickness; allergic pneumonitis; interstitial nephritis; acute renal insufficiency/failure; hepatitis; jaundice; acute hepatic necrosis/failure; anemia, including hemolytic and aplastic; thrombocytopenia, including thrombotic thrombocytopenic purpura; leukopenia; agranulocytosis; pancytopenia; and/or other hematologic abnormalities. The drug should be discontinued immediately at the first appearance of a skin rash or any other sign of hypersensitivity and supportive measures instituted. (See ***PRECAUTIONS: Information for Patients*** and ***ADVERSE REACTIONS.***)

Pseudomembranous colitis has been reported with nearly all antibacterial agents, including ofloxacin, and may range in severity from mild to life-threatening. Therefore, it is important to consider this diagnosis in patients who present with diarrhea subsequent to the administration of any antibacterial agents.

Treatment with antibacterial agents alters the normal flora of the colon and may permit overgrowth of clostridia. Studies indicate a toxin produced by *Clostridium difficile* is one primary cause of "antibiotic-associated colitis".

After the diagnosis of pseudomembranous colitis has been established, therapeutic measures should be initiated. Mild cases of pseudomembranous colitis usually respond to drug discontinuation alone. In moderate to severe cases, consideration should be given to management with fluids and electrolytes, protein supplementation, and treatment with an antibacterial drug clinically effective against *C. difficile* colitis. (See ***ADVERSE REACTIONS.***)

Ruptures of the shoulder, hand, and Achilles tendons that required surgical repair or resulted in prolonged disability have been reported with ofloxacin and other quinolones. Ofloxacin should be discontinued if the patient experiences pain, inflammation, or rupture of a tendon. Patients should rest and refrain from exercise until the diagnosis of tendinitis or tendon rupture has been confidently excluded. Tendon rupture can occur at any time during or after therapy with ofloxacin.

Ofloxacin has not been shown to be effective in the treatment of syphilis. Antimicrobial agents used in high doses for short periods of time to treat gonorrhea may mask or delay the symptoms of incubating syphilis. All patients with gonorrhea should have a serologic test for syphilis at the time of diagnosis. Patients treated with ofloxacin for gonorrhea should have a follow-up serologic test for syphilis after three months and, if positive, treatment with an appropriate antimicrobial should be instituted.

PRECAUTIONS

General:

Adequate hydration of patients receiving ofloxacin should be maintained to prevent the formation of a highly concentrated urine.

Administer ofloxacin with caution in the presence of renal or hepatic insufficiency/impairment. In patients with known or suspected renal or hepatic insufficiency/impairment, careful clinical observation and appropriate laboratory studies should be performed prior to and during therapy since elimination of ofloxacin may be reduced. In patients with impaired renal function (creatinine clearance ≤ 50 mg/mL), alteration of the dosage regimen is necessary. (See ***CLINICAL PHARMACOLOGY*** and ***DOSAGE AND ADMINISTRATION.***)

Moderate to severe phototoxicity reactions have been observed in patients exposed to direct sunlight while receiving some drugs in this class, including ofloxacin. Excessive sunlight should be avoided. Therapy should be discontinued if phototoxicity (e.g., a skin eruption) occurs.

As with other quinolones, ofloxacin should be used with caution in any patient with a known or suspected CNS disorder that may predispose to seizures or lower the seizure threshold (e.g., severe cerebral arteriosclerosis, epilepsy) or in the presence of other risk factors that may predispose to seizures or lower the seizure threshold (e.g., certain drug therapy, renal dysfunction). (See ***WARNINGS*** and ***Drug Interactions.***)

A possible interaction between oral hypoglycemic drugs (e.g., glyburide/glibenclamide) or with insulin and fluoroquinolone antimicrobial agents have been reported resulting in a potentiation of the hypoglycemic action of these drugs. The mechanism for this interaction is not known. If a hypoglycemic reaction occurs in a patient being treated with ofloxacin, discontinue ofloxacin immediately and consult a physician. (See ***Drug Interactions*** and ***ADVERSE REACTIONS.***)

As with any potent drug, periodic assessment of organ system functions, including renal, hepatic, and hematopoietic, is advisable during prolonged therapy. (See ***WARNINGS*** and ***ADVERSE REACTIONS.***)

Information for Patients:

Patients should be advised:

- to drink fluids liberally;
- that mineral supplements, vitamins with iron or minerals, calcium-, aluminum-, or magnesium-based antacids, sucralfate or Videx®, (Didanosine), chewable/buffered tablets or the pediatric powder for oral solution should not be taken within the two-hour period before or within the two-hour period after taking ofloxacin (See ***Drug Interactions***);
- that ofloxacin can be taken without regard to meals;
- that ofloxacin may cause neurologic adverse effects (e.g., dizziness, lightheadedness) and that patients should know how they react to ofloxacin before they operate an automobile or machinery or engage in activities requiring mental alertness and coordination (See ***WARNINGS*** and ***ADVERSE REACTIONS***);
- to discontinue treatment and inform their physician if they experience pain, inflammation, or rupture of a tendon, and to rest and refrain from exercise until the diagnosis of tendinitis or tendon rupture has been confidently excluded;
- that ofloxacin may be associated with hypersensitivity reactions, even following the first dose, to discontinue the drug at the first sign of a skin rash, hives or other skin reactions, a rapid heartbeat, difficulty in swallowing or breathing, any swelling suggesting angioedema (e.g., swelling of the lips, tongue, face; tightness of the throat, hoarseness), or any other symptom of an allergic reaction (See ***WARNINGS*** and ***ADVERSE REACTIONS***);
- to avoid excessive sunlight or artificial ultraviolet light while receiving ofloxacin and to discontinue therapy if phototoxicity (e.g., skin eruption) occurs;
- that if they are diabetic and are being treated with insulin or an oral hypoglycemic drug, to discontinue ofloxacin immediately if a hypoglycemic reaction occurs and consult a physician (See ***PRECAUTIONS: General*** and ***Drug Interactions***);
- that convulsions have been reported in patients taking quinolones, including ofloxacin, and to notify their physician before taking this drug if there is a history of this condition.

Drug Interactions:

Antacids, Sucralfate, Metal Cations, Multivitamins: Quinolones form chelates with alkaline earth and transition metal cations. Administration of quinolones with antacids containing calcium, magnesium, or aluminum, with sucralfate, with divalent or trivalent cations such as iron, or with multivitamins containing zinc or with Videx®, (Didanosine), chewable/buffered tablets or the pediatric powder for oral solution may substantially interfere with the absorption of quinolones resulting in systemic levels considerably lower than desired. These agents should not be taken within the two-hour period before or within the two-hour period after ofloxacin administration. (See ***DOSAGE AND ADMINISTRATION.***)

Caffeine: Interactions between ofloxacin and caffeine have not been detected.

Cimetidine: Cimetidine has demonstrated interference with the elimination of some quinolones. This interference has resulted in significant increases in half-life and AUC of some quinolones. The potential for interaction between ofloxacin and cimetidine has not been studied.

Cyclosporine: Elevated serum levels of cyclosporine have been reported with concomitant use of cyclosporine with some other quinolones. The potential for interaction between ofloxacin and cyclosporine has not been studied.

Drugs metabolized by Cytochrome P450 enzymes: Most quinolone antimicrobial drugs inhibit cytochrome P450 enzyme activity. This may result in a prolonged half-life for some drugs that are also metabolized by this system (e.g., cyclosporine, theophylline/methylxanthines, warfarin) when coadministered with quinolones. The extent of this inhibition varies among different quinolones. (See other ***Drug Interactions.***)

Non-steroidal anti-inflammatory drugs: The concomitant administration of a non-steroidal anti-inflammatory drug

Continued on next page

Floxin—Cont.

with a quinolone, including ofloxacin, may increase the risk of CNS stimulation and convulsive seizures. (See ***WARNINGS*** and ***PRECAUTIONS*: General.**)

Probenecid: The concomitant use of probenecid with certain other quinolones has been reported to affect renal tubular secretion. The effect of probenecid on the elimination of ofloxacin has not been studied.

Theophylline: Steady-state theophylline levels may increase when ofloxacin and theophylline are administered concurrently. As with other quinolones, concomitant administration of ofloxacin may prolong the half-life of theophylline, elevate serum theophylline levels, and increase the risk of theophylline-related adverse reactions. Theophylline levels should be closely monitored and theophylline dosage adjustments made, if appropriate, when ofloxacin is co-administered. Adverse reactions (including seizures) may occur with or without an elevation in the serum theophylline level. (See ***WARNINGS*** and ***PRECAUTIONS*: General.**)

Warfarin: Some quinolones have been reported to enhance the effects of the oral anticoagulant warfarin or its derivatives. Therefore, if a quinolone antimicrobial is administered concomitantly with warfarin or its derivatives, the prothrombin time or other suitable coagulation test should be closely monitored.

Antidiabetic agents (e.g., insulin, glyburide/glibenclamide): Since disturbances of blood glucose, including hyperglycemia and hypoglycemia, have been reported in patients treated concurrently with quinolones and an antidiabetic agent, careful monitoring of blood glucose is recommended when these agents are used concomitantly. (See ***PRECAUTIONS*: General** and **Information for Patients.**)

Carcinogenesis, Mutagenesis, Impairment of Fertility:

Long-term studies to determine the carcinogenic potential of ofloxacin have not been conducted.

Ofloxacin was not mutagenic in the Ames bacterial test, *in vitro* and *in vivo* cytogenetic assay, sister chromatid exchange (Chinese Hamster and Human Cell Lines), unscheduled DNA Repair (UDS) using human fibroblasts, dominant lethal assays, or mouse micronucleus assay. Ofloxacin was positive in the UDS test using rat hepatocytes and Mouse Lymphoma Assay.

Pregnancy: Teratogenic Effects. Pregnancy Category C.

Ofloxacin has not been shown to have any teratogenic effects at oral doses as high as 810 mg/kg/day (11 times the recommended maximum human dose based on mg/m^2 or 50 times based on mg/kg) and 160 mg/kg/day (4 times the recommended maximum human dose based on mg/m^2 or 10 times based on mg/kg) when administered to pregnant rats and rabbits, respectively. Additional studies in rats with oral doses up to 360 mg/kg/day (5 times the recommended maximum human dose based on mg/m^2 or 23 times based on mg/kg) demonstrated no adverse effect on late fetal development, labor, delivery, lactation, neonatal viability, or growth of the newborn. Doses equivalent to 50 and 10 times the recommended maximum human dose of ofloxacin (based on mg/kg) were fetotoxic (i.e., decreased fetal body weight and increased fetal mortality) in rats and rabbits, respectively. Minor skeletal variations were reported in rats receiving doses of 810 mg/kg/ day, which is more than 10 times higher than the recommended maximum human dose based on mg/m^2.

There are, however, no adequate and well-controlled studies in pregnant women. Ofloxacin should be used during pregnancy only if the potential benefit justifies the potential risk to the fetus. (See ***WARNINGS.***)

Nursing Mothers:

In lactating females, a single oral 200-mg dose of ofloxacin resulted in concentrations of ofloxacin in milk that were similar to those found in plasma. Because of the potential for serious adverse reactions from ofloxacin in nursing infants, a decision should be made whether to discontinue nursing or to discontinue the drug, taking into account the importance of the drug to the mother. (See ***WARNINGS*** and ***ADVERSE REACTIONS.***)

Pediatric Use:

Safety and effectiveness in pediatric patients and adolescents below the age of 18 years have not been established. Ofloxacin causes arthropathy (arthrosis) and osteochondrosis in juvenile animals of several species. (See ***WARNINGS.***)

Geriatric Use:

In phase 2/3 clinical trials with ofloxacin, 688 patients (14.2%) were ≥ 65 years of age. Of these, 436 patients (9.0%) were between the ages of 65 and 74 and 252 patients (5.2%) were 75 years or older. There was no apparent difference in the frequency or severity of adverse reactions in elderly adults compared with younger adults. The pharmacokinetic properties of ofloxacin in elderly subjects are similar to those in younger subjects. Drug absorption appears to be unaffected by age. Dosage adjustment is necessary for elderly patients with impaired renal function (creatinine clearance rate ≤ 50 mL/min) due to reduced clearance of ofloxacin. In comparative studies, the frequency and severity of most drug-related nervous system events in patients ≥ 65 years of age were comparable for ofloxacin and control drugs. The only differences identified were an increase in reports of insomnia (3.9% vs 1.5%) and headache (4.7% vs 1.8%) with ofloxacin. It is important to note that these geriatric safety data are extracted from 44 comparative studies where the adverse reaction information from 20 different controls (other antibiotics or placebo) were pooled for comparison with ofloxacin. The clinical significance of such a comparison is not clear. (See ***CLINICAL PHARMACOLOGY*** and ***DOSAGE AND ADMINISTRATION.***)

ADVERSE REACTIONS

The following is a compilation of the data for ofloxacin based on clinical experience with both the oral and intravenous formulations. The incidence of drug-related adverse reactions in patients during Phase 2 and 3 clinical trials was 11%. Among patients receiving multiple-dose therapy, 4% discontinued ofloxacin due to adverse experiences.

In clinical trials, the following events were considered likely to be drug-related in patients receiving multiple doses of ofloxacin:

nausea 3%, insomnia 3%, headache 1%, dizziness 1%, diarrhea 1%, vomiting 1%, rash 1%, pruritus 1%, external genital pruritus in women 1%, vaginitis 1%, dysgeusia 1%.

In clinical trials, the most frequently reported adverse events, regardless of relationship to drug, were:

nausea 10%, headache 9%, insomnia 7%, external genital pruritus in women 6%, dizziness 5%, vaginitis 5%, diarrhea 4%, vomiting 4%.

In clinical trials, the following events, regardless of relationship to drug, occurred in 1 to 3% of patients:

Abdominal pain and cramps, chest pain, decreased appetite, dry mouth, dysgeusia, fatigue, flatulence, gastrointestinal distress, nervousness, pharyngitis, pruritus, fever, rash, sleep disorders, somnolence, trunk pain, vaginal discharge, visual disturbances, and constipation.

Additional events, occurring in clinical trials at a rate of less than 1%, regardless of relationship to drug, were:

Body as a whole:	asthenia, chills, malaise, extremity pain, pain, epistaxis
Cardiovascular System:	cardiac arrest, edema, hypertension, hypotension, palpitations, vasodilation
Gastrointestinal System:	dyspepsia
Genital/Reproductive System:	burning, irritation, pain and rash of the female genitalia; dysmenorrhea; menorrhagia; metrorrhagia
Musculoskeletal System:	arthralgia, myalgia
Nervous System:	seizures, anxiety, cognitive change, depression, dream abnormality, euphoria, hallucinations, paresthesia, syncope, vertigo, tremor, confusion
Nutritional/Metabolic:	thirst, weight loss
Respiratory System:	respiratory arrest, cough, rhinorrhea
Skin/Hypersensitivity:	angioedema, diaphoresis, urticaria, vasculitis
Special Senses:	decreased hearing acuity, tinnitus, photophobia
Urinary System:	dysuria, urinary frequency, urinary retention

The following laboratory abnormalities appeared in ≥ 1.0% of patients receiving multiple doses of ofloxacin. It is not known whether these abnormalities were caused by the drug or the underlying conditions being treated.

Hematopoietic:	anemia, leukopenia, leukocytosis, neutropenia, neutrophilia, increased band forms, lymphocytopenia, eosinophilia, lymphocytosis, thrombocytopenia, thrombocytosis, elevated ESR
Hepatic:	elevated: alkaline phosphatase, AST (SGOT), ALT (SGPT)
Serum chemistry:	hyperglycemia, hypoglycemia, elevated creatinine, elevated BUN
Urinary:	glucosuria, proteinuria, alkalinuria, hyposthenuria, hematuria, pyuria

Post-Marketing Adverse Events:

Additional adverse events, regardless of relationship to drug, reported from worldwide marketing experience with quinolones, including ofloxacin:

Clinical:

Cardiovascular System:	cerebral thrombosis, pulmonary edema, tachycardia, hypotension/shock, syncope
Endocrine/Metabolic:	hyper- or hypoglycemia, especially in diabetic patients on insulin or oral hypoglycemic agents (See ***PRECAUTIONS*: General** and **Drug Interactions.**)
Gastrointestinal System:	hepatic dysfunction including: hepatic necrosis, jaundice (cholestatic or hepatocellular), hepatitis; intestinal perforation; pseudomembranous colitis (the onset of pseudomembranous colitis symptoms may occur during or after antimicrobial treatment), GI hemorrhage; hiccough, painful oral mucosa, pyrosis (See ***WARNINGS.***)
Genital/Reproductive System:	vaginal candidiasis
Hematopoietic:	anemia, including hemolytic and aplastic; hemorrhage, pancytopenia, agranulocytosis, leukopenia, reversible bone marrow depression, thrombocytopenia, thrombotic thrombocytopenic purpura, petechiae, ecchymosis/bruising (See ***WARNINGS.***)
Musculoskeletal:	tendinitis/rupture; weakness; rhabdomyolysis
Nervous System:	nightmares; suicidal thoughts or acts, disorientation, psychotic reactions, paranoia; phobia, agitation, restlessness, aggressiveness/hostility, manic reaction, emotional lability; peripheral neuropathy, ataxia, incoordination; possible exacerbation of: myasthenia gravis and extrapyramidal disorders; dysphasia, lightheadedness (See ***WARNINGS*** and ***PRECAUTIONS.***)
Respiratory System:	dyspnea, bronchospasm, allergic pneumonitis, stridor (See ***WARNINGS.***)
Skin/Hypersensitivity:	anaphylactic (-toid) reactions/shock; purpura, serum sickness, erythema multiforme/Stevens-Johnson Syndrome, erythema nodosum, exfoliative dermatitis, hyperpigmentation, toxic epidermal necrolysis, conjunctivitis, photosensitivity, vesiculobullous eruption (See ***WARNINGS*** and ***PRECAUTIONS.***)
Special Senses:	diplopia, nystagmus, blurred vision, disturbances of: taste, smell, hearing and equilibrium, usually reversible following discontinuation
Urinary System:	anuria, polyuria, renal calculi, renal failure, interstitial nephritis, hematuria (See ***WARNINGS*** and ***PRECAUTIONS.***)

Laboratory:

Hematopoietic:	prolongation of prothrombin time
Serum chemistry:	acidosis, elevation of: serum triglycerides, serum cholesterol, serum potassium, liver function tests including: GGTP, LDH, bilirubin
Urinary:	albuminuria, candiduria

In clinical trials using multiple-dose therapy, ophthalmologic abnormalities, including cataracts and multiple punctate lenticular opacities, have been noted in patients undergoing treatment with other quinolones. The relationship of the drugs to these events is not presently established.

CRYSTALLURIA and CYLINDRURIA HAVE BEEN REPORTED with other quinolones.

OVERDOSAGE

Information on overdosage with ofloxacin is limited. One incident of accidental overdosage has been reported. In this case, an adult female received 3 grams of ofloxacin intravenously over 45 minutes. A blood sample obtained 15 minutes after the completion of the infusion revealed an ofloxacin level of 39.3 µg/mL. In 7 h, the level had fallen to 16.2 µg/mL, and by 24 h to 2.7 µg/mL. During the infusion, the patient developed drowsiness, nausea, dizziness, hot and cold flushes, subjective facial swelling and numbness, slurring of speech, and mild to moderate disorientation. All complaints except the dizziness subsided within 1 h after discontinuation of the infusion. The dizziness, most bothersome while standing, resolved in approximately 9 h. Laboratory testing reportedly revealed no clinically significant changes in routine parameters in this patient.

In the event of an acute overdose, the stomach should be emptied. The patient should be observed and appropriate hydration maintained. Ofloxacin is not efficiently removed by hemodialysis or peritoneal dialysis.

DOSAGE AND ADMINISTRATION

The usual dose of FLOXIN (ofloxacin tablets) Tablets is 200 mg to 400 mg orally every 12 h as described in the following dosing chart. These recommendations apply to patients with normal renal function (i.e., creatinine clearance > 50 mL/min). For patients with altered renal function (i.e., creatinine clearance ≤ 50 mL/min), see the ***Patients with Impaired Renal Function*** subsection.

[See first table at top of next page]

Antacids containing calcium, magnesium, or aluminum; sucralfate; divalent or trivalent cations such as iron; or multivitamins containing zinc; or Videx®, (Didanosine), chewable/buffered tablets or the pediatric powder for oral solution should not be taken within the two-hour period before or within the two-hour period after taking ofloxacin. (See ***PRECAUTIONS.***)

Patients with Impaired Renal Function:

Dosage should be adjusted for patients with a creatinine clearance ≤ 50 mL/min.

Patients with Normal Renal Function:

Infection†	Unit Dose	Frequency	Duration	Daily Dose
Acute Bacterial Exacerbation of Chronic Bronchitis	400 mg	q12h	10 days	800 mg
Comm. Acquired Pneumonia	400 mg	q12h	10 days	800 mg
Uncomplicated Skin and Skin Structure Infections	400 mg	q12h	10 days	800 mg
Acute, Uncomplicated Urethral and Cervical Gonorrhea	400 mg	single dose	1 day	400 mg
Nongonococcal Cervicitis/Urethritis due to *C. trachomatis*	300 mg	q12h	7 days	600 mg
Mixed Infection of the urethra and cervix due to *C. trachomatis* and *N. gonorrhoeae*	300 mg	q12h	7 days	600 mg
Acute Pelvic Inflammatory Disease	400 mg	q12h	10–14 days	800 mg
Uncomplicated Cystitis due to *E. coli* or *K. pneumoniae*	200 mg	q12h	3 days	400 mg
Uncomplicated Cystitis due to other approved pathogens	200 mg	q12h	7 days	400 mg
Complicated UTI's	200 mg	q12h	10 days	400 mg
Prostatitis due to *E. coli*	300 mg	q12h	6 weeks	600 mg

† DUE TO THE DESIGNATED PATHOGENS (See ***INDICATIONS AND USAGE.***)

Creatinine Clearance	Maintenance Dose	Frequency
20–50 mL/min	the usual recommended unit dose	q24h
< 20 mL/min	½ the usual recommended unit dose	q24h

After a normal initial dose, dosage should be adjusted as follows:
[See second table above]
When only the serum creatinine is known, the following formula may be used to estimate creatinine clearance.

Men: Creatinine clearance (mL/min) =

$$\frac{\text{Weight (kg)} \times (140 - \text{age})}{72 \times \text{serum creatinine (mg/dL)}}$$

Women: 0.85 × the value calculated for men.

The serum creatinine should represent a steady-state of renal function.

Patients with Cirrhosis:
The excretion of ofloxacin may be reduced in patients with severe liver function disorders (e.g., cirrhosis with or without ascites). A maximum dose of 400 mg of ofloxacin per day should therefore not be exceeded.

HOW SUPPLIED

FLOXIN (ofloxacin tablets) Tablets are supplied as 200 mg light yellow, 300 mg white, and 400 mg pale gold film-coated tablets. Each tablet is distinguished by "FLOXIN" and the appropriate strength. FLOXIN Tablets are packaged in bottles and in unit-dose blister strips in the following configurations:

200 mg tablets—UROPAK unit-dose/6 tablets (NDC 0062-1540-09)
200 mg tablets—bottles of 50 (NDC 0062-1540-02)
200 mg tablets—unit-dose/100 tablets (NDC 0062-1540-05)
300 mg tablets—bottles of 50 (NDC 0062-1541-02)
300 mg tablets—unit-dose/100 tablets (NDC 0062-1541-05)
400 mg tablets—bottles of 100 (NDC 0062-1542-01)
400 mg tablets—unit-dose/100 tablets (NDC 0062-1542-05)

FLOXIN Tablets should be stored in well-closed containers. Store below 86°F (30°C).

Also Available:
Ofloxacin is also available for intravenous administration in the following configurations:

FLOXIN (ofloxacin injection) I.V. IN SINGLE-USE VIALS (10 mL) containing a concentrated solution with the equivalent of 400 mg of ofloxacin.

FLOXIN (ofloxacin injection) I.V. PRE-MIXED IN FLEXIBLE CONTAINERS (50 mL and 100 mL) containing a dilute solution with the equivalent of 200 mg or 400 mg of ofloxacin, respectively, in 5% Dextrose (D_5W).

ANIMAL PHARMACOLOGY

Ofloxacin, as well as other drugs of the quinolone class, has been shown to cause arthropathies (arthrosis) in immature dogs and rats. In addition, these drugs are associated with an increased incidence of osteochondrosis in rats as compared to the incidence observed in vehicle-treated rats. (See ***WARNINGS.***) There is no evidence of arthropathies in fully mature dogs at intravenous doses up to 3 times the recommended maximum human dose (on a mg/m^2 basis or 5 times based on mg/kg basis), for a one-week exposure period.

Long-term, high-dose systemic use of other quinolones in experimental animals has caused lenticular opacities; however, this finding was not observed in any animal studies with ofloxacin.

Reduced serum globulin and protein levels were observed in animals treated with other quinolones. In one ofloxacin study, minor decreases in serum globulin and protein levels were noted in female cynomolgus monkeys dosed orally with 40 mg/kg ofloxacin daily for one year. These changes, however, were considered to be within normal limits for monkeys.

Crystalluria and ocular toxicity were not observed in any animals treated with ofloxacin.

FLOXIN® is a trademark of ORTHO-McNEIL PHARMACEUTICAL, INC.
U.S. Patent No. 4,382,892

REFERENCES

1. National Committee for Clinical Laboratory Standards. Methods for Dilution Antimicrobial Susceptibility Tests for Bacteria That Grow Aerobically—Fourth Edition. Approved Standard NCCLS Document M7-A4, Vol. 17, No. 2, NCCLS, Wayne, PA, January, 1997.
2. National Committee for Clinical Laboratory Standards. Performance Standards for Antimicrobial Disk Susceptibility Tests—Sixth Edition. Approved Standard NCCLS Document M2-A6, Vol. 17, No. 1, NCCLS, Wayne, PA, January, 1997.

ORTHO-McNEIL
PHARMACEUTICAL, INC.
Raritan, New Jersey 08869
© OMP 1998 Revised February 2000 7516001

HALDOL® Decanoate 50
(haloperidol) ℞

HALDOL® Decanoate 100
(haloperidol) ℞
[hal 'dawl dek "ah-nō 'ōt]
For IM Injection Only

Prescribing Information

DESCRIPTION

Haloperidol decanoate is the decanoate ester of the butyrophenone, HALDOL (haloperidol). It has a markedly extended duration of effect. It is available in sesame oil in sterile form for intramuscular (IM) injection. The structural formula of haloperidol decanoate, 4-(4-chlorophenyl)-1-[4-(4-fluorophenyl)-4-oxobutyl]-4 piperidinyl decanoate, is:

Haloperidol decanoate is almost insoluble in water (0.01 mg/mL), but is soluble in most organic solvents.

Each mL of HALDOL Decanoate 50 for IM injection contains 50 mg haloperidol (present as haloperidol decanoate 70.52 mg) in a sesame oil vehicle, with 1.2% (w/v) benzyl alcohol as a preservative.

Each mL of HALDOL Decanoate 100 for IM injection contains 100 mg haloperidol (present as haloperidol decanoate 141.04 mg) in a sesame oil vehicle, with 1.2% (w/v) benzyl alcohol as a preservative.

CLINICAL PHARMACOLOGY

HALDOL Decanoate 50 and HALDOL Decanoate 100 are the long-acting forms of HALDOL (haloperidol). The basic effects of haloperidol decanoate are no different from those of HALDOL with the exception of duration of action. Haloperidol blocks the effects of dopamine and increases its turnover rate; however, the precise mechanism of action is unknown.

Administration of haloperidol decanoate in sesame oil results in slow and sustained release of haloperidol. The plasma concentrations of haloperidol gradually rise, reaching a peak at about 6 days after the injection, and falling thereafter, with an apparent half-life of about 3 weeks. Steady state plasma concentrations are achieved after the third or fourth dose. The relationship between dose of haloperidol decanoate and plasma haloperidol concentration is roughly linear for doses below 450 mg. It should be noted, however, that the pharmacokinetics of haloperidol decanoate following intramuscular injections can be quite variable between subjects.

INDICATIONS AND USAGE

HALDOL Decanoate 50 and HALDOL Decanoate 100 are indicated for the treatment of schizophrenic patients who require prolonged parenteral antipsychotic therapy.

CONTRAINDICATIONS

Since the pharmacologic and clinical actions of HALDOL Decanoate 50 and HALDOL Decanoate 100 are attributed to HALDOL (haloperidol) as the active medication, Contraindications, Warnings, and additional information are those of HALDOL, modified only to reflect the prolonged action.

HALDOL is contraindicated in severe toxic central nervous system depression or comatose states from any cause and in individuals who are hypersensitive to this drug or have Parkinson's disease.

WARNINGS

Tardive Dyskinesia—A syndrome consisting of potentially irreversible, involuntary, dyskinetic movements may develop in patients treated with antipsychotic drugs. Although the prevalence of the syndrome appears to be highest among the elderly, especially elderly women, it is impossible to rely upon prevalence estimates to predict, at the inception of antipsychotic treatment, which patients are likely to develop the syndrome. Whether antipsychotic drug products differ in their potential to cause tardive dyskinesia is unknown.

Both the risk of developing tardive dyskinesia and the likelihood that it will become irreversible are believed to increase as the duration of treatment and the total cumulative dose of antipsychotic drugs administered to the patient increase. However, the syndrome can develop, although much less commonly, after relatively brief treatment periods at low doses.

There is no known treatment for established cases of tardive dyskinesia, although the syndrome may remit, partially or completely, if antipsychotic treatment is withdrawn. Antipsychotic treatment, itself, however, may suppress (or partially suppress) the signs and symptoms of the syndrome and thereby may possibly mask the underlying process. The effect that symptomatic suppression has upon the long-term course of the syndrome is unknown.

Given these considerations, antipsychotic drugs should be prescribed in a manner that is most likely to minimize the occurrence of tardive dyskinesia. Chronic antipsychotic treatment should generally be reserved for patients who suffer from a chronic illness that 1) is known to respond to antipsychotic drugs, and 2) for whom alternative, equally effective, but potentially less harmful treatments are **not** available or appropriate. In patients who do require chronic treatment, the smallest dose and the shortest duration of treatment producing a satisfactory clinical response should be sought. The need for continued treatment should be reassessed periodically.

If signs and symptoms of tardive dyskinesia appear in a patient on antipsychotics, drug discontinuation should be considered. However, some patients may require treatment despite the presence of the syndrome. (For further information about the description of tardive dyskinesia and its clinical detection, please refer to ADVERSE REACTIONS.)

Neuroleptic Malignant Syndrome (NMS)—A potentially fatal symptom complex sometimes referred to as Neuroleptic Malignant Syndrome (NMS) has been reported in association with antipsychotic drugs. Clinical manifestations of NMS are hyperpyrexia, muscle rigidity, altered mental status (including catatonic signs) and evidence of autonomic instability (irregular pulse or blood pressure, tachycardia, diaphoresis, and cardiac dysrhythmias). Additional signs may include elevated creatine phosphokinase, myoglobinuria (rhabdomyolysis) and acute renal failure.

The diagnostic evaluation of patients with this syndrome is complicated. In arriving at a diagnosis, it is important to identify cases where the clinical presentation includes both serious medical illness (e.g., pneumonia, systemic infection, etc.) and untreated or inadequately treated extrapyramidal signs and symptoms (EPS). Other important considerations in the differential diagnosis include central anticholinergic toxicity, heat stroke, drug fever and primary central nervous system (CNS) pathology.

The management of NMS should include 1) immediate discontinuation of antipsychotic drugs and other drugs not essential to concurrent therapy, 2) intensive symptomatic treatment and medical monitoring, and 3) treatment of any concomitant serious medical problems for which specific treatments are available. There is no general agreement about specific pharmacological treatment regimens for uncomplicated NMS.

If a patient requires antipsychotic drug treatment after recovery from NMS, the potential reintroduction of drug therapy should be carefully considered. The patient should be carefully monitored, since recurrences of NMS have been reported.

Hyperpyrexia and heat stroke, not associated with the above symptom complex, have also been reported with HALDOL.

General—A number of cases of bronchopneumonia, some fatal, have followed the use of antipsychotic drugs, including HALDOL (haloperidol). It has been postulated that lethargy and decreased sensation of thirst due to central inhibition may lead to dehydration, hemoconcentration and reduced pulmonary ventilation. Therefore, if the above signs and symptoms appear, especially in the elderly, the physician should institute remedial therapy promptly.

Although not reported with HALDOL, decreased serum cholesterol and/or cutaneous and ocular changes have been reported in patients receiving chemically-related drugs.

PRECAUTIONS

HALDOL Decanoate 50 and HALDOL Decanoate 100 should be administered cautiously to patients:

— with severe cardiovascular disorders, because of the possibility of transient hypotension and/or precipitation of anginal pain. Should hypotension occur and a vasopressor be required, epinephrine should not be used since HALDOL (haloperidol) may block its vasopressor activ-

Continued on next page

Haldol Decanoate—Cont.

ity, and paradoxical further lowering of the blood pressure may occur. Instead, metaraminol, phenylephrine or norepinephrine should be used.

— receiving anticonvulsant medications, with a history of seizures, or with EEG abnormalities, because HALDOL may lower the convulsive threshold. If indicated, adequate anticonvulsant therapy should be concomitantly maintained.
— with known allergies, or with a history of allergic reactions to drugs.
— receiving anticoagulants, since an isolated instance of interference occurred with the effects of one anticoagulant (phenindione).

If concomitant antiparkinson medication is required, it may have to be continued after HALDOL Decanoate 50 or HALDOL Decanoate 100 is discontinued because of the prolonged action of haloperidol decanoate. If both drugs are discontinued simultaneously, extrapyramidal symptoms may occur. The physician should keep in mind the possible increase in intraocular pressure when anticholinergic drugs, including antiparkinson agents, are administered concomitantly with haloperidol decanoate.

In patients with thyrotoxicosis who are also receiving antipsychotic medication, including haloperidol decanoate, severe neurotoxicity (rigidity, inability to walk or talk) may occur.

When HALDOL is used to control mania in bipolar disorders, there may be a rapid mood swing to depression.

Information for Patients

Haloperidol decanoate may impair the mental and/or physical abilities required for the performance of hazardous tasks such as operating machinery or driving a motor vehicle. The ambulatory patient should be warned accordingly. The use of alcohol with this drug should be avoided due to possible additive effects and hypotension.

Drug Interactions

An encephalopathic syndrome (characterized by weakness, lethargy, fever, tremulousness and confusion, extrapyramidal symptoms, leukocytosis, elevated serum enzymes, BUN, and FBS) followed by irreversible brain damage has occurred in a few patients treated with lithium plus HALDOL. A causal relationship between these events and the concomitant administration of lithium and HALDOL has not been established; however, patients receiving such combined therapy should be monitored closely for early evidence of neurological toxicity and treatment discontinued promptly if such signs appear.

As with other antipsychotic agents, it should be noted that HALDOL may be capable of potentiating CNS depressants such as anesthetics, opiates, and alcohol.

In a study of 12 schizophrenic patients coadministered oral haloperidol and rifampin, plasma haloperidol levels were decreased by a mean of 70% and mean scores on the Brief Psychiatric Rating Scale were increased from baseline. In 5 other schizophrenic patients treated with oral haloperidol and rifampin, discontinuation of rifampin produced a mean 3.3-fold increase in haloperidol concentrations. Thus, careful monitoring of clinical status is warranted when rifampin is administered or discontinued in haloperidol-treated patients.

Carcinogenesis, Mutagenesis, and Impairment of Fertility

No mutagenic potential of haloperidol decanoate was found in the Ames Salmonella microsomal activation assay. Negative or inconsistent positive findings have been obtained in *in vitro* and *in vivo* studies of effects of short-acting haloperidol on chromosome structure and number. The available cytogenetic evidence is considered too inconsistent to be conclusive at this time.

Carcinogenicity studies using oral haloperidol were conducted in Wistar rats (dosed at up to 5 mg/kg daily for 24 months) and in Albino Swiss mice (dosed at up to 5 mg/kg daily for 18 months). In the rat study survival was less than optimal in all dose groups, reducing the number of rats at risk for developing tumors. However, although a relatively greater number of rats survived to the end of the study in high-dose male and female groups, these animals did not have a greater incidence of tumors than control animals. Therefore, although not optimal, this study does suggest the absence of a haloperidol related increase in the incidence of neoplasia in rats at doses up to 20 times the usual daily human dose for chronic or resistant patients.

In female mice at 5 and 20 times the highest initial daily dose for chronic or resistant patients, there was a statistically significant increase in mammary gland neoplasia and total tumor incidence; at 20 times the same daily dose there was a statistically significant increase in pituitary gland neoplasia. In male mice, no statistically significant differences in incidences of total tumors or specific tumor types were noted.

Antipsychotic drugs elevate prolactin levels; the elevation persists during chronic administration. Tissue culture experiments indicate that approximately one-third of human breast cancers are prolactin dependent *in vitro*, a factor of potential importance if the prescription of these drugs is contemplated in a patient with a previously detected breast cancer. Although disturbances such as galactorrhea, amenorrhea, gynecomastia, and impotence have been reported, the clinical significance of elevated serum prolactin levels is unknown for most patients.

An increase in mammary neoplasms has been found in rodents after chronic administration of antipsychotic drugs.

HALDOL DECANOATE DOSING RECOMMENDATIONS

Patients	1st Month	Monthly Maintenance
Stabilized on low daily oral doses (up to 10 mg/day) Elderly or Debilitated	10–15 × Daily Oral Dose	10–15 × Previous Daily Oral Dose
High dose Risk of relapse Tolerant to oral haloperidol	20 × Daily Oral Dose	10–15 × Previous Daily Oral Dose

Neither clinical studies nor epidemiologic studies conducted to date, however, have shown an association between chronic administration of these drugs and mammary tumorigenesis; the available evidence is considered too limited to be conclusive at this time.

Usage in Pregnancy

Pregnancy Category C. Rodents given up to 3 times the usual maximum human dose of haloperidol decanoate showed an increase in incidence of resorption, fetal mortality, and pup mortality. No fetal abnormalities were observed.

Cleft palate has been observed in mice given oral haloperidol at 15 times the usual maximum human dose. Cleft palate in mice appears to be a nonspecific response to stress or nutritional imbalance as well as to a variety of drugs, and there is no evidence to relate this phenomenon to predictable human risk for most of these agents.

There are no adequate and well-controlled studies in pregnant women. There are reports, however, of cases of limb malformations observed following maternal use of HALDOL along with other drugs which have suspected teratogenic potential during the first trimester of pregnancy. Causal relationships were not established with these cases. Since such experience does not exclude the possibility of fetal damage due to HALDOL, haloperidol decanoate should be used during pregnancy or in women likely to become pregnant only if the benefit clearly justifies a potential risk to the fetus.

Nursing Mothers

Since haloperidol is excreted in human breast milk, infants should not be nursed during drug treatment with haloperidol decanoate.

Pediatric Use

Safety and effectiveness of haloperidol decanoate in children have not been established.

Geriatric Use

Clinical studies of haloperidol did not include sufficient numbers of subjects aged 65 and over to determine whether they respond differently from younger subjects. Other reported clinical experience has not consistently identified differences in responses between the elderly and younger patients. However, the prevalence of tardive dyskinesia appears to be highest among the elderly, especially elderly women (see WARNINGS, Tardive dyskinesia). Also, the pharmacokinetics of haloperidol in geriatric patients generally warrants the use of lower doses (see DOSAGE AND ADMINISTRATION).

ADVERSE REACTIONS

Adverse reactions following the administration of HALDOL Decanoate 50 or HALDOL Decanoate 100 are those of HALDOL (haloperidol). Since vast experience has accumulated with HALDOL, the adverse reactions are reported for that compound as well as for haloperidol decanoate. As with all injectable medications, local tissue reactions have been reported with haloperidol decanoate.

CNS Effects:

Extrapyramidal Symptoms (EPS)—EPS during the administration of HALDOL (haloperidol) have been reported frequently, often during the first few days of treatment. EPS can be categorized generally as Parkinson-like symptoms, akathisia, or dystonia (including opisthotonos and oculogyric crisis). While all can occur at relatively low doses, they occur more frequently and with greater severity at higher doses. The symptoms may be controlled with dose reductions or administration of antiparkinson drugs such as benztropine mesylate USP or trihexyphenidyl hydrochloride USP. It should be noted that persistent EPS have been reported; the drug may have to be discontinued in such cases.

Withdrawal Emergent Neurological Signs—Generally, patients receiving short-term therapy experience no problems with abrupt discontinuation of antipsychotic drugs. However, some patients on maintenance treatment experience transient dyskinetic signs after abrupt withdrawal. In certain of these cases the dyskinetic movements are indistinguishable from the syndrome described below under "Tardive Dyskinesia" except for duration. Although the long-acting properties of haloperidol decanoate provide gradual withdrawal, it is not known whether gradual withdrawal of antipsychotic drugs will reduce the rate of occurrence of withdrawal emergent neurological signs.

Tardive Dyskinesia—As with all antipsychotic agents HALDOL has been associated with persistent dyskinesias. Tardive dyskinesia, a syndrome consisting of potentially irreversible, involuntary, dyskinetic movements, may appear in some patients on long-term therapy with haloperidol decanoate or may occur after drug therapy has been discontinued. The risk appears to be greater in elderly patients on high-dose therapy, especially females. The symptoms are persistent and in some patients appear irreversible. The syndrome is characterized by rhythmical involuntary movements of tongue, face, mouth or jaw (e.g., protrusion of tongue, puffing of cheeks, puckering of mouth, chewing movements). Sometimes these may be accompanied by involuntary movements of extremities and the trunk.

There is no known effective treatment for tardive dyskinesia; antiparkinson agents usually do not alleviate the symptoms of this syndrome. It is suggested that all antipsychotic agents be discontinued if these symptoms appear. Should it be necessary to reinstitute treatment, or increase the dosage of the agent, or switch to a different antipsychotic agent, this syndrome may be masked.

It has been reported that fine vermicular movement of the tongue may be an early sign of tardive dyskinesia and if the medication is stopped at that time the full syndrome may not develop.

Tardive Dystonia—Tardive dystonia, not associated with the above syndrome, has also been reported. Tardive dystonia is characterized by delayed onset of choreic or dystonic movements, is often persistent, and has the potential of becoming irreversible.

Other CNS effects—Insomnia, restlessness, anxiety, euphoria, agitation, drowsiness, depression, lethargy, headache, confusion, vertigo, grand mal seizures, exacerbation of psychotic symptoms including hallucinations, and catatonic-like behavioral states which may be responsive to drug withdrawal and/or treatment with anticholinergic drugs.

Body as a Whole: Neuroleptic malignant syndrome (NMS), hyperpyrexia and heat stroke have been reported with HALDOL. (See WARNINGS for further information concerning NMS.)

Cardiovascular Effects: Tachycardia, hypotension, hypertension and ECG changes including prolongation of the Q-T interval and ECG pattern changes compatible with the polymorphous configuration of torsade de pointes.

Hematologic Effects: Reports have appeared citing the occurrence of mild and usually transient leukopenia and leukocytosis, minimal decreases in red blood cell counts, anemia, or a tendency toward lymphomonocytosis. Agranulocytosis has rarely been reported to have occurred with the use of HALDOL, and then only in association with other medication.

Liver Effects: Impaired liver function and/or jaundice have been reported.

Dermatologic Reactions: Maculopapular and acneiform skin reactions and isolated cases of photosensitivity and loss of hair.

Endocrine Disorders: Lactation, breast engorgement, mastalgia, menstrual irregularities, gynecomastia, impotence, increased libido, hyperglycemia, hypoglycemia and hyponatremia.

Gastrointestinal Effects: Anorexia, constipation, diarrhea, hypersalivation, dyspepsia, nausea and vomiting.

Autonomic Reactions: Dry mouth, blurred vision, urinary retention, diaphoresis and priapism.

Respiratory Effects: Laryngospasm, bronchospasm and increased depth of respiration.

Special Senses: Cataracts, retinopathy and visual disturbances.

Other: Cases of sudden and unexpected death have been reported in association with the administration of HALDOL. The nature of the evidence makes it impossible to determine definitively what role, if any, HALDOL played in the outcome of the reported cases. The possibility that HALDOL caused death cannot, of course, be excluded, but it is to be kept in mind that sudden and unexpected death may occur in psychotic patients when they go untreated or when they are treated with other antipsychotic drugs.

Postmarketing Events: Hyperammonemia has been reported in a 5½ year old child with citrullinemia, an inherited disorder of ammonia excretion, following treatment with HALDOL.

OVERDOSAGE

While overdosage is less likely to occur with a parenteral than with an oral medication, information pertaining to HALDOL (haloperidol) is presented, modified only to reflect the extended duration of action of haloperidol decanoate.

Manifestations—In general, the symptoms of overdosage would be an exaggeration of known pharmacologic effects and adverse reactions, the most prominent of which would be: 1) severe extrapyramidal reactions, 2) hypotension, or 3) sedation. The patient would appear comatose with respiratory depression and hypotension which could be severe enough to produce a shock-like state. The extrapyramidal reactions would be manifested by muscular weakness or rigidity and a generalized or localized tremor, as demonstrated by the akinetic or agitans types, respectively. With accidental overdosage, hypertension rather than hypotension occurred in a two-year old child. The risk of ECG changes associated with torsade de pointes should be considered.

(For further information regarding torsade de pointes, please refer to ADVERSE REACTIONS.)

Treatment—Since there is no specific antidote, treatment is primarily supportive. A patent airway must be established by use of an oropharyngeal airway or endotracheal tube or, in prolonged cases of coma, by tracheostomy. Respiratory depression may be counteracted by artificial respiration and mechanical respirators. Hypotension and circulatory collapse may be counteracted by use of intravenous fluids, plasma, or concentrated albumin, and vasopressor agents such as metaraminol, phenylephrine and norepinephrine. Epinephrine should not be used. In case of severe extrapyramidal reactions, antiparkinson medication should be administered, and should be continued for several weeks, and then withdrawn gradually as extrapyramidal symptoms may emerge. ECG and vital signs should be monitored especially for signs of Q-T prolongation or dysrhythmias and monitoring should continue until the ECG is normal. Severe arrhythmias should be treated with appropriate anti-arrhythmic measures.

DOSAGE AND ADMINISTRATION

HALDOL Decanoate 50 and HALDOL Decanoate 100 should be administered by deep intramuscular injection. A 21 gauge needle is recommended. The maximum volume per injection site should not exceed 3 mL. DO NOT ADMINISTER INTRAVENOUSLY.

Parenteral drug products should be inspected visually for particulate matter and discoloration prior to administration, whenever solution and container permit.

HALDOL Decanoate 50 and HALDOL Decanoate 100 are intended for use in schizophrenic patients who require prolonged parenteral antipsychotic therapy. These patients should be previously stabilized on antipsychotic medication before considering a conversion to haloperidol decanoate. Furthermore, it is recommended that patients being considered for haloperidol decanoate therapy have been treated with, and tolerate well, short-acting HALDOL (haloperidol) in order to reduce the possibility of an unexpected adverse sensitivity to haloperidol. Close clinical supervision is required during the initial period of dose adjustment in order to minimize the risk of overdosage or reappearance of psychotic symptoms before the next injection. During dose adjustment or episodes of exacerbation of symptoms of schizophrenia, haloperidol decanoate therapy can be supplemented with short-acting forms of haloperidol.

The dose of HALDOL Decanoate 50 or HALDOL Decanoate 100 should be expressed in terms of its haloperidol content. The starting dose of haloperidol decanoate should be based on the patient's age, clinical history, physical condition, and response to previous antipsychotic therapy. The preferred approach to determining the minimum effective dose is to begin with lower initial doses and to adjust the dose upward as needed. For patients previously maintained on low doses of antipsychotics (e.g. up to the equivalent of 10 mg/day oral haloperidol), it is recommended that the initial dose of haloperidol decanoate be 10–15 times the previous daily dose in oral haloperidol equivalents; limited clinical experience suggests that lower initial doses may be adequate.

Initial Therapy

Conversion from oral haloperidol to haloperidol decanoate can be achieved by using an initial dose of haloperidol decanoate that is 10 to 20 times the previous daily dose in oral haloperidol equivalents.

In patients who are elderly, debilitated, or stable on low doses of oral haloperidol (e.g. up to the equivalent of 10 mg/day oral haloperidol), a range of 10 to 15 times the previous daily dose in oral haloperidol equivalents is appropriate for initial conversion.

In patients previously maintained on higher doses of antipsychotics for whom a low dose approach risks recurrence of psychiatric decompensation and in patients whose long-term use of haloperidol has resulted in a tolerance to the drug, 20 times the previous daily dose in oral haloperidol equivalents should be considered for initial conversion, with downward titration on succeeding injections.

The initial dose of haloperidol decanoate should not exceed 100 mg regardless of previous antipsychotic dose requirements. If, therefore, conversion requires more than 100 mg of haloperidol decanoate as an initial dose, that dose should be administered in two injections, i.e. a maximum of 100 mg initially followed by the balance in 3 to 7 days.

Maintenance Therapy

The maintenance dosage of haloperidol decanoate must be individualized with titration upward or downward based on therapeutic response. The usual maintenance range is 10 to 15 times the previous daily dose in oral haloperidol equivalents dependent on the clinical response of the patient.

[See table at top of previous page]

Close clinical supervision is required during initiation and stabilization of haloperidol decanoate therapy.

Haloperidol decanoate is usually administered monthly or every 4 weeks. However, variation in patient response may dictate a need for adjustment of the dosing interval as well as the dose (See CLINICAL PHARMACOLOGY).

Clinical experience with haloperidol decanoate at doses greater than 450 mg per month has been limited.

HOW SUPPLIED

HALDOL® (haloperidol) Decanoate 50 for IM injection, 50 mg haloperidol as 70.5 mg per mL haloperidol decanoate—NDC 0045-0253, 10 × 1 mL ampuls, 3 × 1 mL ampuls and 5 mL multiple dose vials.

HALDOL® (haloperidol) Decanoate 100 for IM injection, 100 mg haloperidol as 141.04 mg per mL haloperidol decanoate—NDC 0045-0254, 5 × 1 mL ampuls and 5 mL multiple dose vials.

Store at controlled room temperature (15°–30° C, 59°–86° F). Do not refrigerate or freeze.

Protect from light.

ORTHO-McNEIL
OMP DIVISION
ORTHO-McNEIL
PHARMACEUTICAL, INC.
Raritan, New Jersey 08869 Revised September 2001
643-94-253-5

Shown in Product Identification Guide, page 328

LEVAQUIN® ℞
[*lĕvă-kwĭn*]
(levofloxacin) Tablets
LEVAQUIN®
(levofloxacin) Injection
LEVAQUIN®
(levofloxacin in 5% dextrose) Injection

Prescribing Information

To reduce the development of drug-resistant bacteria and maintain the effectiveness of LEVAQUIN® (levofloxacin) and other antibacterial drugs, LEVAQUIN should be used only to treat or prevent infections that are proven or strongly suspected to be caused by bacteria.

DESCRIPTION

LEVAQUIN® is a synthetic broad spectrum antibacterial agent for oral and intravenous administration. Chemically, levofloxacin, a chiral fluorinated carboxyquinolone, is the pure (-)-(S)-enantiomer of the racemic drug substance ofloxacin. The chemical name is (-)-(S)-9-fluoro-2,3-dihydro-3-methyl-10-(4-methyl-1-piperazinyl)-7-oxo-7H-pyrido[1,2,3-de]-1,4-benzoxazine-6-carboxylic acid hemihydrate.

The chemical structure is:

[Chemical structure: F, COOH, N, O, H_3C, CH_3, H, $\cdot ½H_2O$]

Its empirical formula is $C_{18}H_{20}FN_3O_4 \bullet ½ H_2O$ and its molecular weight is 370.38. Levofloxacin is a light yellowish-white to yellow-white crystal or crystalline powder. The molecule exists as a zwitterion at the pH conditions in the small intestine.

The data demonstrate that from pH 0.6 to 5.8, the solubility of levofloxacin is essentially constant (approximately 100 mg/mL). Levofloxacin is considered *soluble to freely soluble* in this pH range, as defined by USP nomenclature. Above pH 5.8, the solubility increases rapidly to its maximum at pH 6.7 (272 mg/mL) and is considered *freely soluble* in this range. Above pH 6.7, the solubility decreases and reaches a minimum value (about 50 mg/mL) at a pH of approximately 6.9.

Levofloxacin has the potential to form stable coordination compounds with many metal ions. This in vitro chelation potential has the following formation order: $Al^{+3}>Cu^{+2}>Zn^{+2}>Mg^{+2}>Ca^{+2}$.

LEVAQUIN Tablets are available as film-coated tablets and contain the following inactive ingredients:

250 mg (as expressed in the anhydrous form): hypromellose, crospovidone, microcrystalline cellulose, magnesium stearate, polyethylene glycol, titanium dioxide, polysorbate 80 and synthetic red iron oxide.

500 mg (as expressed in the anhydrous form): hypromellose, crospovidone, microcrystalline cellulose, magnesium stearate, polyethylene glycol, titanium dioxide, polysorbate 80 and synthetic red and yellow iron oxides.

750 mg (as expressed in the anhydrous form): hypromellose, crospovidone, microcrystalline cellulose, magnesium stearate, polyethylene glycol, titanium dioxide, polysorbate 80.

LEVAQUIN Injection in Single-Use Vials is a sterile, preservative-free aqueous solution of levofloxacin with pH ranging from 3.8 to 5.8. LEVAQUIN Injection in Premix Flexible Containers is a sterile, preservative-free aqueous solution of levofloxacin with pH ranging from 3.8 to 5.8. The appearance of LEVAQUIN Injection may range from a clear yellow to a greenish-yellow solution. This does not adversely affect product potency.

LEVAQUIN Injection in Single-Use Vials contains levofloxacin in Water for Injection. LEVAQUIN Injection in Premix Flexible Containers is a dilute, non-pyrogenic, nearly isotonic premixed solution that contains levofloxacin in 5% Dextrose (D_5W). Solutions of hydrochloric acid and sodium hydroxide may have been added to adjust the pH.

The flexible container is fabricated from a specially formulated non-plasticized, thermoplastic copolyester (CR3). The amount of water that can permeate from the container into the overwrap is insufficient to affect the solution significantly. Solutions in contact with the flexible container can leach out certain of the container's chemical components in very small amounts within the expiration period. The suitability of the container material has been confirmed by tests in animals according to USP biological tests for plastic containers.

CLINICAL PHARMACOLOGY

The mean ±SD pharmacokinetic parameters of levofloxacin determined under single and steady-state conditions following oral (p.o.) or intravenous (i.v.) doses of levofloxacin are summarized in Table 1.

Absorption

Levofloxacin is rapidly and essentially completely absorbed after oral administration. Peak plasma concentrations are usually attained one to two hours after oral dosing. The absolute bioavailability of a 500 mg tablet and a 750 mg tablet of levofloxacin are both approximately 99%, demonstrating complete oral absorption of levofloxacin. Following a single intravenous dose of levofloxacin to healthy volunteers, the mean ±SD peak plasma concentration attained was 6.2 ±1.0 µg/mL after a 500 mg dose infused over 60 minutes and 11.5 ±4.0 µg/mL after a 750 mg dose infused over 90 minutes.

Levofloxacin pharmacokinetics are linear and predictable after single and multiple oral or i.v. dosing regimens. Steady-state conditions are reached within 48 hours following a 500 mg or 750 mg once-daily dosage regimen. The mean ±SD peak and trough plasma concentrations attained following multiple once-daily oral dosage regimens were approximately 5.7 ±1.4 and 0.5 ±0.2 µg/mL after the 500 mg doses, and 8.6 ±1.9 and 1.1 ±0.4 µg/mL after the 750 mg doses, respectively. The mean ±SD peak and trough plasma concentrations attained following multiple once-daily i.v. regimens were approximately 6.4 ±0.8 and 0.6 ±0.2 µg/mL after the 500 mg doses, and 12.1 ±4.1 and 1.3 ±0.71 µg/mL after the 750 mg doses, respectively.

Oral administration of a 500-mg LEVAQUIN tablet with food slightly prolongs the time to peak concentration by approximately 1 hour and slightly decreases the peak concentration by approximately 14%. Therefore, levofloxacin tablets can be administered without regard to food.

The plasma concentration profile of levofloxacin after i.v. administration is similar and comparable in extent of exposure (AUC) to that observed for levofloxacin tablets when equal doses (mg/mg) are administered. Therefore, the oral and i.v. routes of administration can be considered interchangeable. (See following chart.)

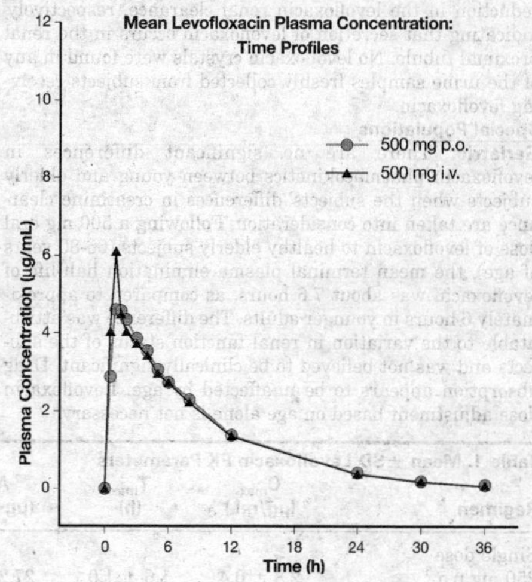

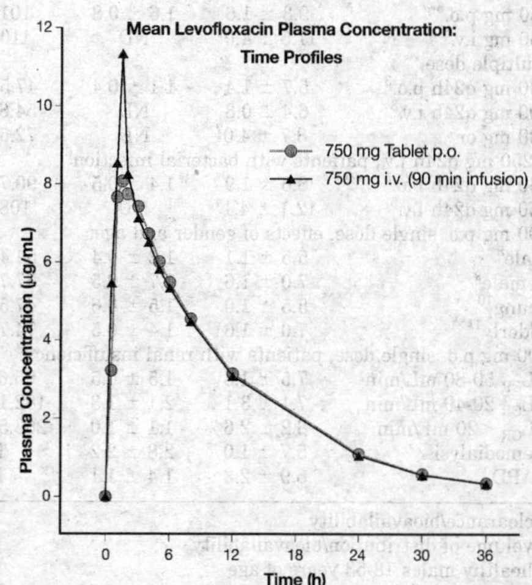

Distribution

The mean volume of distribution of levofloxacin generally ranges from 74 to 112 L after single and multiple 500 mg or 750 mg doses, indicating widespread distribution into body tissues. Levofloxacin reaches its peak levels in skin tissues and in blister fluid of healthy subjects at approximately 3 hours after dosing. The skin tissue biopsy to plasma AUC ratio is approximately 2 and the blister fluid to plasma AUC

Continued on next page

Levaquin—Cont.

ratio is approximately 1 following multiple once-daily oral administration of 750 mg and 500 mg levofloxacin, respectively, to healthy subjects. Levofloxacin also penetrates well into lung tissues. Lung tissue concentrations were generally 2- to 5- fold higher than plasma concentrations and ranged from approximately 2.4 to 11.3 µg/g over a 24-hour period after a single 500 mg oral dose.

In vitro, over a clinically relevant range (1 to 10 µg/mL) of serum/plasma levofloxacin concentrations, levofloxacin is approximately 24 to 38% bound to serum proteins across all species studied, as determined by the equilibrium dialysis method. Levofloxacin is mainly bound to serum albumin in humans. Levofloxacin binding to serum proteins is independent of the drug concentration.

Metabolism

Levofloxacin is stereochemically stable in plasma and urine and does not invert metabolically to its enantiomer, D-ofloxacin. Levofloxacin undergoes limited metabolism in humans and is primarily excreted as unchanged drug in the urine. Following oral administration, approximately 87% of an administered dose was recovered as unchanged drug in urine within 48 hours, whereas less than 4% of the dose was recovered in feces in 72 hours. Less than 5% of an administered dose was recovered in the urine as the desmethyl and N-oxide metabolites, the only metabolites identified in humans. These metabolites have little relevant pharmacological activity.

Excretion

Levofloxacin is excreted largely as unchanged drug in the urine. The mean terminal plasma elimination half-life of levofloxacin ranges from approximately 6 to 8 hours following single or multiple doses of levofloxacin given orally or intravenously. The mean apparent total body clearance and renal clearance range from approximately 144 to 226 mL/min and 96 to 142 mL/min, respectively. Renal clearance in excess of the glomerular filtration rate suggests that tubular secretion of levofloxacin occurs in addition to its glomerular filtration. Concomitant administration of either cimetidine or probenecid results in approximately 24% and 35% reduction in the levofloxacin renal clearance, respectively, indicating that secretion of levofloxacin occurs in the renal proximal tubule. No levofloxacin crystals were found in any of the urine samples freshly collected from subjects receiving levofloxacin.

Special Populations

Geriatric: There are no significant differences in levofloxacin pharmacokinetics between young and elderly subjects when the subjects' differences in creatinine clearance are taken into consideration. Following a 500 mg oral dose of levofloxacin to healthy elderly subjects (66-80 years of age), the mean terminal plasma elimination half-life of levofloxacin was about 7.6 hours, as compared to approximately 6 hours in younger adults. The difference was attributable to the variation in renal function status of the subjects and was not believed to be clinically significant. Drug absorption appears to be unaffected by age. Levofloxacin dose adjustment based on age alone is not necessary.

Pediatric: The pharmacokinetics of levofloxacin in pediatric subjects have not been studied.

Gender: There are no significant differences in levofloxacin pharmacokinetics between male and female subjects when subjects' differences in creatinine clearance are taken into consideration. Following a 500 mg oral dose of levofloxacin to healthy male subjects, the mean terminal plasma elimination half-life of levofloxacin was about 7.5 hours, as compared to approximately 6.1 hours in female subjects. This difference was attributable to the variation in renal function status of the male and female subjects and was not believed to be clinically significant. Drug absorption appears to be unaffected by the gender of the subjects. Dose adjustment based on gender alone is not necessary.

Race: The effect of race on levofloxacin pharmacokinetics was examined through a covariate analysis performed on data from 72 subjects: 48 white and 24 non-white. The apparent total body clearance and apparent volume of distribution were not affected by the race of the subjects.

Renal insufficiency: Clearance of levofloxacin is substantially reduced and plasma elimination half-life is substantially prolonged in patients with impaired renal function (creatinine clearance <50 mL/min), requiring dosage adjustment in such patients to avoid accumulation. Neither hemodialysis nor continuous ambulatory peritoneal dialysis (CAPD) is effective in removal of levofloxacin from the body, indicating that supplemental doses of levofloxacin are not required following hemodialysis or CAPD. (See **PRECAUTIONS: General** and **DOSAGE AND ADMINISTRATION.**)

Hepatic insufficiency: Pharmacokinetic studies in hepatically impaired patients have not been conducted. Due to the limited extent of levofloxacin metabolism, the pharmacokinetics of levofloxacin are not expected to be affected by hepatic impairment.

Bacterial infection: The pharmacokinetics of levofloxacin in patients with serious community-acquired bacterial infections are comparable to those observed in healthy subjects.

Drug-drug interactions: The potential for pharmacokinetic drug interactions between levofloxacin and theophylline, warfarin, cyclosporine, digoxin, probenecid, cimetidine, sucralfate, and antacids has been evaluated. (See **PRECAUTIONS: Drug Interactions.**)

[See table 1 below]

MICROBIOLOGY

Levofloxacin is the L-isomer of the racemate, ofloxacin, a quinolone antimicrobial agent. The antibacterial activity of ofloxacin resides primarily in the L-isomer. The mechanism of action of levofloxacin and other fluoroquinolone antimicrobials involves inhibition of bacterial topoisomerase IV and DNA gyrase (both of which are type II topoisomerases), enzymes required for DNA replication, transcription, repair and recombination.

Levofloxacin has in vitro activity against a wide range of gram-negative and gram-positive microorganisms. Levofloxacin is often bactericidal at concentrations equal to or slightly greater than inhibitory concentrations.

Table 1. Mean ±SD Levofloxacin PK Parameters

Regimen	C_{max} (µg/mL)	T_{max} (h)	AUC (µg·h/mL)	CL/F[1] (mL/min)	Vd/F[2] (L)	$t_{1/2}$ (h)	CL_R (mL/min)
Single dose							
250 mg p.o.[3]	2.8 ± 0.4	1.6 ± 1.0	27.2 ± 3.9	156 ± 20	ND	7.3 ± 0.9	142 ± 21
500 mg p.o.[3]*	5.1 ± 0.8	1.3 ± 0.6	47.9 ± 6.8	178 ± 28	ND	6.3 ± 0.6	103 ± 30
500 mg i.v.[3]	6.2 ± 1.0	1.0 ± 0.1	48.3 ± 5.4	175 ± 20	90 ± 11	6.4 ± 0.7	112 ± 25
750 mg p.o.[5]*	9.3 ± 1.6	1.6 ± 0.8	101 ± 20	129 ± 24	83 ± 17	7.5 ± 0.9	ND
750 mg i.v.[5]	11.5 ± 4.0[4]	ND	110 ± 40	126 ± 39	75 ± 13	7.5 ± 1.6	ND
Multiple dose							
500 mg q24h p.o.[3]	5.7 ± 1.4	1.1 ± 0.4	47.5 ± 6.7	175 ± 25	102 ± 22	7.6 ± 1.6	116 ± 31
500 mg q24h i.v.[3]	6.4 ± 0.8	ND	54.6 ± 11.1	158 ± 29	91 ± 12	7.0 ± 0.8	99 ± 28
500 mg or 250 mg q24h i.v., patients with bacterial infection[6]	8.7 ± 4.0[7]	ND	72.5 ± 51.2[7]	154 ± 72	111 ± 58	ND	ND
750 mg q24h p.o.[5]	8.6 ± 1.9	1.4 ± 0.5	90.7 ± 17.6	143 ± 29	100 ± 16	8.8 ± 1.5	116 ± 28
750 mg q24h i.v.[5]	12.1 ± 4.1[4]	ND	108 ± 34	126 ± 37	80 ± 27	7.9 ± 1.9	ND
500 mg p.o. single dose, effects of gender and age:							
Male[8]	5.5 ± 1.1	1.2 ± 0.4	54.4 ± 18.9	166 ± 44	89 ± 13	7.5 ± 2.1	126 ± 38
Female[9]	7.0 ± 1.6	1.7 ± 0.5	67.7 ± 24.2	136 ± 44	62 ± 16	6.1 ± 0.8	106 ± 40
Young[10]	5.5 ± 1.0	1.5 ± 0.6	47.5 ± 9.8	182 ± 35	83 ± 18	6.0 ± 0.9	140 ± 33
Elderly[11]	7.0 ± 1.6	1.4 ± 0.5	74.7 ± 23.3	121 ± 33	67 ± 19	7.6 ± 2.0	91 ± 29
500 mg p.o. single dose, patients with renal insufficiency:							
CL_{CR} 50-80 mL/min	7.5 ± 1.8	1.5 ± 0.5	95.6 ± 11.8	88 ± 10	ND	9.1 ± 0.9	57 ± 8
CL_{CR} 20-49 mL/min	7.1 ± 3.1	2.1 ± 1.3	182.1 ± 62.6	51 ± 19	ND	27 ± 10	26 ± 13
CL_{CR} <20 mL/min	8.2 ± 2.6	1.1 ± 1.0	263.5 ± 72.5	33 ± 8	ND	35 ± 5	13 ± 3
Hemodialysis	5.7 ± 1.0	2.8 ± 2.2	ND	ND	ND	76 ± 42	ND
CAPD	6.9 ± 2.3	1.4 ± 1.1	ND	ND	ND	51 ± 24	ND

[1] clearance/bioavailability
[2] volume of distribution/bioavailability
[3] healthy males 18-53 years of age
[4] 60 min infusion for 250 mg and 500 mg doses, 90 min infusion for 750 mg dose
[5] healthy male and female subjects 18-54 years of age
[6] 500 mg q48h for patients with moderate renal impairment (CL_{CR} 20-50 mL/min) and infections of the respiratory tract or skin
[7] dose-normalized values (to 500 mg dose), estimated by population pharmacokinetic modeling
[8] healthy males 22-75 years of age
[9] healthy females 18-80 years of age
[10] young healthy male and female subjects 18-36 years of age
[11] healthy elderly male and female subjects 66-80 years of age
* Absolute bioavailability; F = 0.99 ± 0.08 from a 500-mg tablet and F=0.99 ± 0.06 from a 750-mg tablet; ND = not determined.

Fluoroquinolones, including levofloxacin, differ in chemical structure and mode of action from aminoglycosides, macrolides and β-lactam antibiotics, including penicillins. Fluoroquinolones may, therefore, be active against bacteria resistant to these antimicrobials.

Resistance to levofloxacin due to spontaneous mutation in vitro is a rare occurrence (range: 10^{-9} to 10^{-10}). Although cross-resistance has been observed between levofloxacin and some other fluoroquinolones, some microorganisms resistant to other fluoroquinolones may be susceptible to levofloxacin.

Levofloxacin has been shown to be active against most strains of the following microorganisms both in vitro and in clinical infections as described in the **INDICATIONS AND USAGE** section:

Aerobic gram-positive microorganisms

Enterococcus faecalis (many strains are only moderately susceptible)
Staphylococcus aureus (methicillin-susceptible strains)
Staphylococcus epidermidis (methicillin-susceptible strains)
Staphylococcus saprophyticus
Streptococcus pneumoniae (including penicillin-resistant strains*)
Streptococcus pyogenes

*Note: penicillin-resistant *S. pneumoniae* are those strains with a penicillin MIC value of ≥2 µg/mL

Aerobic gram-negative microorganisms

Enterobacter cloacae
Escherichia coli
Haemophilus influenzae
Haemophilus parainfluenzae
Klebsiella pneumoniae
Legionella pneumophila
Moraxella catarrhalis
Proteus mirabilis
Pseudomonas aeruginosa
Serratia marcescens

As with other drugs in this class, some strains of *Pseudomonas aeruginosa* may develop resistance fairly rapidly during treatment with levofloxacin.

Other microorganisms

Chlamydia pneumoniae
Mycoplasma pneumoniae

The following in vitro data are available, **but their clinical significance is unknown.**

Levofloxacin exhibits in vitro minimum inhibitory concentrations (MIC values) of 2 µg/mL or less against most (≥90%) strains of the following microorganisms; however, the safety and effectiveness of levofloxacin in treating clinical infections due to these microorganisms have not been established in adequate and well-controlled trials.

Aerobic gram-positive microorganisms

Staphylococcus haemolyticus
Streptococcus (Group C/F)
Streptococcus (Group G)
Streptococcus agalactiae
Streptococcus milleri
Viridans group streptococci

Aerobic gram-negative microorganisms

Acinetobacter baumannii
Acinetobacter lwoffii
Bordetella pertussis
Citrobacter (diversus) koseri
Citrobacter freundii
Enterobacter aerogenes
Enterobacter sakazakii
Klebsiella oxytoca
Morganella morganii
Pantoea (Enterobacter) agglomerans
Proteus vulgaris
Providencia rettgeri
Providencia stuartii
Pseudomonas fluorescens

Anaerobic gram-positive microorganisms

Clostridium perfringens

Susceptibility Tests

Susceptibility testing for levofloxacin should be performed, as it is the optimal predictor of activity.

Dilution techniques: Quantitative methods are used to determine antimicrobial minimal inhibitory concentrations (MIC values). These MIC values provide estimates of the susceptibility of bacteria to antimicrobial compounds. The MIC values should be determined using a standardized procedure. Standardized procedures are based on a dilution method[1] (broth or agar) or equivalent with standardized inoculum concentrations and standardized concentrations of levofloxacin powder. The MIC values should be interpreted according to the following criteria:

For testing *Enterobacteriaceae*, Enterococci, *Staphylococcus* species, and *Pseudomonas aeruginosa:*

MIC (µg/mL)	Interpretation
≤2	Susceptible (S)
4	Intermediate (I)
≥8	Resistant (R)

For testing *Haemophilus influenzae* and *Haemophilus parainfluenzae:*[a]

MIC (µg/mL)	Interpretation
≤2	Susceptible (S)

[a] These interpretive standards are applicable only to broth microdilution susceptibility testing with *Haemophilus influ-*

enzae and *Haemophilus parainfluenzae* using Haemophilus Test Medium.[1]
The current absence of data on resistant strains precludes defining any categories other than "Susceptible." Strains yielding MIC results suggestive of a "nonsusceptible" category should be submitted to a reference laboratory for further testing.

For testing *Streptococcus* spp. including *S. pneumoniae*:[b]

MIC (µg/mL)	Interpretation
≤2	Susceptible (S)
4	Intermediate (I)
≥8	Resistant (R)

[b] These interpretive standards are applicable only to broth microdilution susceptibility tests using cation-adjusted Mueller-Hinton broth with 2-5% lysed horse blood.

A report of "Susceptible" indicates that the pathogen is likely to be inhibited if the antimicrobial compound in the blood reaches the concentrations usually achievable. A report of "Intermediate" indicates that the result should be considered equivocal, and, if the microorganism is not fully susceptible to alternative, clinically feasible drugs, the test should be repeated. This category implies possible clinical applicability in body sites where the drug is physiologically concentrated or in situations where a high dosage of drug can be used. This category also provides a buffer zone which prevents small uncontrolled technical factors from causing major discrepancies in interpretation. A report of "Resistant" indicates that the pathogen is not likely to be inhibited if the antimicrobial compound in the blood reaches the concentrations usually achievable; other therapy should be selected.
Standardized susceptibility test procedures require the use of laboratory control microorganisms to control the technical aspects of the laboratory procedures. Standard levofloxacin powder should give the following MIC values:

Microorganism		MIC (µg/mL)
Enterococcus faecalis	ATCC 29212	0.25-2
Escherichia coli	ATCC 25922	0.008-0.06
Escherichia coli	ATCC 35218	0.015-0.06
Haemophilus influenzae	ATCC 49247[c]	0.008-0.03
Pseudomonas aeruginosa	ATCC 27853	0.5-4
Staphylococcus aureus	ATCC 29213	0.06-0.5
Streptococcus pneumoniae	ATCC 49619[d]	0.5-2

[c] This quality control range is applicable to only *H. influenzae* ATCC 49247 tested by a broth microdilution procedure using Haemophilus Test Medium (HTM).[1]
[d] This quality control range is applicable to only *S. pneumoniae* ATCC 49619 tested by a broth microdilution procedure using cation-adjusted Mueller-Hinton broth with 2-5% lysed horse blood.

Diffusion techniques: Quantitative methods that require measurement of zone diameters also provide reproducible estimates of the susceptibility of bacteria to antimicrobial compounds. One such standardized procedure[2] requires the use of standardized inoculum concentrations. This procedure uses paper disks impregnated with 5-µg levofloxacin to test the susceptibility of microorganisms to levofloxacin.
Reports from the laboratory providing results of the standard single-disk susceptibility test with a 5-µg levofloxacin disk should be interpreted according to the following criteria:
For testing *Enterobacteriaceae*, Enterococci, *Staphylococcus* species, and *Pseudomonas aeruginosa*:

Zone diameter (mm)	Interpretation
≥17	Susceptible (S)
14-16	Intermediate (I)
≤13	Resistant (R)

For *Haemophilus influenzae* and *Haemophilus parainfluenzae*:[e]

Zone diameter (mm)	Interpretation
≥17	Susceptible (S)

[e] These interpretive standards are applicable only to disk diffusion susceptibility testing with *Haemophilus influenzae* and *Haemophilus parainfluenzae* using Haemophilus Test Medium.[2]

The current absence of data on resistant strains precludes defining any categories other than "Susceptible." Strains yielding zone diameter results suggestive of a "nonsusceptible" category should be submitted to a reference laboratory for further testing.

For *Streptococcus* spp. including *S. pneumoniae*:[f]

Zone diameter (mm)	Interpretation
≥17	Susceptible (S)
14-16	Intermediate (I)
≤13	Resistant (R)

[f] These zone diameter standards for *Streptococcus* spp. including *S. pneumoniae* apply only to tests performed using Mueller-Hinton agar supplemented with 5% sheep blood and incubated in 5% CO_2.

Interpretation should be as stated above for results using dilution techniques. Interpretation involves correlation of the diameter obtained in the disk test with the MIC for levofloxacin.
As with standardized dilution techniques, diffusion methods require the use of laboratory control microorganisms to control the technical aspects of the laboratory procedures. For the diffusion technique, the 5-µg levofloxacin disk should provide the following zone diameters in these laboratory test quality control strains:

Microorganism		Zone Diameter (mm)
Escherichia coli	ATCC 25922	29-37
Haemophilus influenzae	ATCC 49247[g]	32-40
Pseudomonas aeruginosa	ATCC 27853	19-26
Staphylococcus aureus	ATCC 25923	25-30
Streptococcus pneumoniae	ATCC 49619[h]	20-25

[g] This quality control range is applicable to only *H. influenzae* ATCC 49247 tested by a disk diffusion procedure using Haemophilus Test Medium (HTM).[2]
[h] This quality control range is applicable to only *S. pneumoniae* ATCC 49619 tested by a disk diffusion procedure using Mueller-Hinton agar supplemented with 5% sheep blood and incubated in 5% CO_2.

INDICATIONS AND USAGE

To reduce the development of drug-resistant bacteria and maintain the effectiveness of LEVAQUIN® (levofloxacin) and other antibacterial drugs, LEVAQUIN should be used only to treat or prevent infections that are proven or strongly suspected to be caused by susceptible bacteria. When culture and susceptibility information are available, they should be considered in selecting or modifying antibacterial therapy. In the absence of such data, local epidemiology and susceptibility patterns may contribute to the empiric selection of therapy.
LEVAQUIN Tablets/Injection are indicated for the treatment of adults (≥18 years of age) with mild, moderate, and severe infections caused by susceptible strains of the designated microorganisms in the conditions listed below. LEVAQUIN Injection is indicated when intravenous administration offers a route of administration advantageous to the patient (e.g., patient cannot tolerate an oral dosage form). Please see **DOSAGE AND ADMINISTRATION** for specific recommendations.
Acute maxillary sinusitis due to *Streptococcus pneumoniae, Haemophilus influenzae*, or *Moraxella catarrhalis.*
Acute bacterial exacerbation of chronic bronchitis due to *Staphylococcus aureus, Streptococcus pneumoniae, Haemophilus influenzae, Haemophilus parainfluenzae*, or *Moraxella catarrhalis.*
Nosocomial pneumonia due to methicillin-susceptible *Staphylococcus aureus, Pseudomonas aeruginosa, Serratia marcescens, Escherichia coli, Klebsiella pneumoniae, Haemophilus influenzae*, or *Streptococcus pneumoniae.* Adjunctive therapy should be used as clinically indicated. Where *Pseudomonas aeruginosa* is a documented or presumptive pathogen, combination therapy with an anti-pseudomonal β-lactam is recommended. (See **CLINICAL STUDIES.**)
Community-acquired pneumonia due to *Staphylococcus aureus, Streptococcus pneumoniae* (including penicillin-resistant strains, MIC value for penicillin ≥2 µg/mL), *Haemophilus influenzae, Haemophilus parainfluenzae, Klebsiella pneumoniae, Moraxella catarrhalis, Chlamydia pneumoniae, Legionella pneumophila*, or *Mycoplasma pneumoniae.* (See **CLINICAL STUDIES.**)
Complicated skin and skin structure infections due to methicillin-susceptible *Staphylococcus aureus, Enterococcus faecalis, Streptococcus pyogenes*, or *Proteus mirabilis.*
Uncomplicated skin and skin structure infections (mild to moderate) including abscesses, cellulitis, furuncles, impetigo, pyoderma, wound infections, due to *Staphylococcus aureus* or *Streptococcus pyogenes.*
Chronic bacterial prostatitis due to *Escherichia coli, Enterococcus faecalis*, or *Staphylococcus epidermidis.*
Complicated urinary tract infections (mild to moderate) due to *Enterococcus faecalis, Enterobacter cloacae, Escherichia coli, Klebsiella pneumoniae, Proteus mirabilis*, or *Pseudomonas aeruginosa.*
Acute pyelonephritis (mild to moderate) caused by *Escherichia coli.*
Uncomplicated urinary tract infections (mild to moderate) due to *Escherichia coli, Klebsiella pneumoniae*, or *Staphylococcus saprophyticus.*
Appropriate culture and susceptibility tests should be performed before treatment in order to isolate and identify organisms causing the infection and to determine their susceptibility to levofloxacin. Therapy with levofloxacin may be initiated before results of these tests are known; once results become available, appropriate therapy should be selected.
As with other drugs in this class, some strains of *Pseudomonas aeruginosa* may develop resistance fairly rapidly during treatment with levofloxacin. Culture and susceptibility testing performed periodically during therapy will provide information about the continued susceptibility of the pathogens to the antimicrobial agent and also the possible emergence of bacterial resistance.

CONTRAINDICATIONS

Levofloxacin is contraindicated in persons with a history of hypersensitivity to levofloxacin, quinolone antimicrobial agents, or any other components of this product.

WARNINGS

THE SAFETY AND EFFICACY OF LEVOFLOXACIN IN PEDIATRIC PATIENTS, ADOLESCENTS (UNDER THE AGE OF 18 YEARS), PREGNANT WOMEN, AND NURSING WOMEN HAVE NOT BEEN ESTABLISHED. (See **PRECAUTIONS: Pediatric Use, Pregnancy,** and **Nursing Mothers** subsections.)
In immature rats and dogs, the oral and intravenous administration of levofloxacin increased the incidence and severity of osteochondrosis. Other fluoroquinolones also produce similar erosions in the weight bearing joints and other signs of arthropathy in immature animals of various species. (See **ANIMAL PHARMACOLOGY.**)
Convulsions and toxic psychoses have been reported in patients receiving quinolones, including levofloxacin. Quinolones may also cause increased intracranial pressure and central nervous system stimulation which may lead to tremors, restlessness, anxiety, lightheadedness, confusion, hallucinations, paranoia, depression, nightmares, insomnia, and, rarely, suicidal thoughts or acts. These reactions may occur following the first dose. If these reactions occur in patients receiving levofloxacin, the drug should be discontinued and appropriate measures instituted. As with other quinolones, levofloxacin should be used with caution in patients with a known or suspected CNS disorder that may predispose to seizures or lower the seizure threshold (e.g., severe cerebral arteriosclerosis, epilepsy) or in the presence of other risk factors that may predispose to seizures or lower the seizure threshold (e.g., certain drug therapy, renal dysfunction.) (See **PRECAUTIONS: General, Information for Patients, Drug Interactions** and **ADVERSE REACTIONS.**)
Serious and occasionally fatal hypersensitivity and/or anaphylactic reactions have been reported in patients receiving therapy with quinolones, including levofloxacin. These reactions often occur following the first dose. Some reactions have been accompanied by cardiovascular collapse, hypotension/shock, seizure, loss of consciousness, tingling, angioedema (including tongue, laryngeal, throat, or facial edema/swelling), airway obstruction (including bronchospasm, shortness of breath, and acute respiratory distress), dyspnea, urticaria, itching, and other serious skin reactions. Levofloxacin should be discontinued immediately at the first appearance of a skin rash or any other sign of hypersensitivity. Serious acute hypersensitivity reactions may require treatment with epinephrine and other resuscitative measures, including oxygen, intravenous fluids, antihistamines, corticosteroids, pressor amines, and airway management, as clinically indicated. (See **PRECAUTIONS** and **ADVERSE REACTIONS.**)
Serious and sometimes fatal events, some due to hypersensitivity, and some due to uncertain etiology, have been reported rarely in patients receiving therapy with quinolones, including levofloxacin. These events may be severe and generally occur following the administration of multiple doses. Clinical manifestations may include one or more of the following: fever, rash or severe dermatologic reactions (e.g., toxic epidermal necrolysis, Stevens-Johnson Syndrome); vasculitis; arthralgia; myalgia; serum sickness; allergic pneumonitis; interstitial nephritis; acute renal insufficiency or failure; hepatitis; jaundice; acute hepatic necrosis or failure; anemia, including hemolytic and aplastic; thrombocytopenia, including thrombotic thrombocytopenic purpura; leukopenia; agranulocytosis; pancytopenia; and/or other hematologic abnormalities. The drug should be discontinued immediately at the first appearance of a skin rash or any other sign of hypersensitivity and supportive measures instituted. (See **PRECAUTIONS: Information for Patients** and **ADVERSE REACTIONS.**)
Pseudomembranous colitis has been reported with nearly all antibacterial agents, including levofloxacin, and may range in severity from mild to life-threatening. Therefore, it is important to consider this diagnosis in patients who present with diarrhea subsequent to the administration of any antibacterial agent.
Treatment with antibacterial agents alters the normal flora of the colon and may permit overgrowth of clostridia. Studies indicate that a toxin produced by *Clostridium difficile* is one primary cause of "antibiotic-associated colitis."
After the diagnosis of pseudomembranous colitis has been established, therapeutic measures should be initiated. Mild cases of pseudomembranous colitis usually respond to drug discontinuation alone. In moderate to severe cases, consideration should be given to management with fluids and electrolytes, protein supplementation, and treatment with an antibacterial drug clinically effective against *C. difficile* colitis. (See **ADVERSE REACTIONS.**)
Ruptures of the shoulder, hand, or Achilles tendons that required surgical repair or resulted in prolonged disability have been reported in patients receiving quinolones, including levofloxacin. Post-marketing surveillance reports indicate that this risk may be increased in patients receiving concomitant corticosteroids, especially in the elderly. Levofloxacin should be discontinued if the patient experiences pain, inflammation, or rupture of a tendon. Patients should rest and refrain from exercise until the diagnosis of tendinitis or tendon rupture has been confidently excluded. Tendon rupture can occur during or after therapy with quinolones, including levofloxacin.

Continued on next page

Levaquin—Cont.

Body as a Whole – General Disorders:	Ascites, allergic reaction, asthenia, drug level increase, edema, enlarged abdomen, fever, headache, hot flashes, influenza-like symptoms, leg pain, malaise, rigors, substernal chest pain, syncope, multiple organ failure, changed temperature sensation, withdrawal syndrome
Cardiovascular Disorders, General:	Cardiac failure, hypertension, hypertension aggravated hypotension, postural hypotension
Central and Peripheral Nervous System Disorders:	Convulsions (seizures), dysphonia, hyperesthesia, hyperkinesia, hypertonia, hypoesthesia, involuntary muscle contractions, migraine, paresthesia, paralysis, speech disorder, stupor, tremor, vertigo, encephalopathy, abnormal gait, leg cramps, intracranial hypertension, ataxia
Gastro-Intestinal System Disorders:	Dry mouth, dysphagia, esophagitis, gastritis, gastroenteritis, gastroesophageal reflux, G.I. hemorrhage, glossitis, hemorrhoids, intestinal obstruction, pancreatitis, tongue edema, melena, stomatitis
Hearing and Vestibular Disorders:	Earache, tinnitus
Heart Rate and Rhythm Disorders:	Arrhythmia, arrhythmia ventricular, atrial fibrillation, bradycardia, cardiac arrest, ventricular fibrillation, heart block, palpitation, supraventricular tachycardia, ventricular tachycardia, tachycardia
Liver and Biliary System Disorders:	Abnormal hepatic function, cholecystitis, cholelithiasis, elevated bilirubin, hepatic enzymes increased, hepatic failure, jaundice
Metabolic and Nutritional Disorders:	Hypomagnesemia, thirst, dehydration, electrolyte abnormality, fluid overload, gout, hyperglycemia, hyperkalemia, hypernatremia, hypoglycemia, hypokalemia, hyponatremia, hypophosphatemia, nonprotein nitrogen increase, weight decrease
Musculo-Skeletal System Disorders:	Arthralgia, arthritis, arthrosis, myalgia, osteomyelitis, skeletal pain, synovitis, tendonitis, tendon disorder
Myo, Endo, Pericardial and Valve Disorders:	Angina pectoris, endocarditis, myocardial infarction
Neoplasms:	Carcinoma, thrombocythemia
Other Special Senses Disorders:	Parosmia, taste perversion
Platelet, Bleeding and Clotting Disorders:	Hematoma, epistaxis, prothrombin decreased, pulmonary embolism, purpura, thrombocytopenia
Psychiatric Disorders:	Abnormal dreaming, agitation, anorexia, confusion, depression, hallucination, impotence, nervousness, paroniria, sleep disorder, somnolence
Red Blood Cell Disorders:	Anemia
Reproductive Disorders:	Dysmenorrhea, leukorrhea
Resistance Mechanism Disorders:	Abscess, bacterial infection, fungal infection, herpes simplex, moniliasis, otitis media, sepsis, viral infection
Respiratory System Disorders:	Airways obstruction, aspiration, asthma, bronchitis, bronchospasm, chronic obstructive airway disease, coughing, hemoptysis, epistaxis, hypoxia, laryngitis, pharyngitis, pleural effusion, pleurisy, pneumonitis, pneumonia, pneumothorax, pulmonary collapse, pulmonary edema, respiratory depression, respiratory insufficiency, upper respiratory tract infection
Skin and Appendages Disorders:	Alopecia, bullous eruption, dry skin, eczema, genital pruritus, increased sweating, rash, skin exfoliation, skin ulceration, urticaria
Urinary System Disorders:	Abnormal renal function, acute renal failure, dysuria, hematuria, oliguria, urinary incontinence, urinary retention, urinary tract infection
Vascular (Extracardiac) Disorders:	Flushing, gangrene, phlebitis, purpura, thrombophlebitis (deep)
Vision Disorders:	Abnormal vision, eye pain, conjunctivitis
White Cell and RES Disorders:	Agranulocytosis, granulocytopenia, leukocytosis, lymphadenopathy

PRECAUTIONS

General

Prescribing LEVAQUIN in the absence of a proven or strongly suspected bacterial infection or a prophylactic indication is unlikely to provide benefit to the patient and increases the risk of the development of drug-resistant bacteria.

Because a rapid or bolus intravenous injection may result in hypotension, LEVOFLOXACIN INJECTION SHOULD ONLY BE ADMINISTERED BY SLOW INTRAVENOUS INFUSION OVER A PERIOD OF 60 OR 90 MINUTES DEPENDING ON THE DOSAGE. (See **DOSAGE AND ADMINISTRATION**.)

Although levofloxacin is more soluble than other quinolones, adequate hydration of patients receiving levofloxacin should be maintained to prevent the formation of a highly concentrated urine.

Administer levofloxacin with caution in the presence of renal insufficiency. Careful clinical observation and appropriate laboratory studies should be performed prior to and during therapy since elimination of levofloxacin may be reduced. In patients with impaired renal function (creatinine clearance <50 mL/min), adjustment of the dosage regimen is necessary to avoid the accumulation of levofloxacin due to decreased clearance. (See **CLINICAL PHARMACOLOGY** and **DOSAGE AND ADMINISTRATION**.)

Moderate to severe phototoxicity reactions have been observed in patients exposed to direct sunlight while receiving drugs in this class. Excessive exposure to sunlight should be avoided. However, in clinical trials with levofloxacin, phototoxicity has been observed in less than 0.1% of patients. Therapy should be discontinued if phototoxicity (e.g., a skin eruption) occurs.

As with other quinolones, levofloxacin should be used with caution in any patient with a known or suspected CNS disorder that may predispose to seizures or lower the seizure threshold (e.g., severe cerebral arteriosclerosis, epilepsy) or in the presence of other risk factors that may predispose to seizures or lower the seizure threshold (e.g., certain drug therapy, renal dysfunction). (See **WARNINGS** and **Drug Interactions**.)

As with other quinolones, disturbances of blood glucose, including symptomatic hyper- and hypoglycemia, have been reported, usually in diabetic patients receiving concomitant treatment with an oral hypoglycemic agent (e.g., glyburide/glibenclamide) or with insulin. In these patients, careful monitoring of blood glucose is recommended. If a hypoglycemic reaction occurs in a patient being treated with levofloxacin, levofloxacin should be discontinued immediately and appropriate therapy should be initiated immediately. (See **Drug Interactions** and **ADVERSE REACTIONS**.)

Some quinolones, including levofloxacin, have been associated with prolongation of the QT interval on the electrocardiogram and infrequent cases of arrhythmia. During postmarketing surveillance, rare cases of torsades de pointes have been reported in patients taking levofloxacin. These reports generally involved patients with concurrent medical conditions or concomitant medications that may have been contributory. The risk of arrhythmias may be reduced by avoiding concurrent use with other drugs that prolong the QT interval including class Ia or class III antiarrhythmic agents; in addition, use of levofloxacin in the presence of risk factors for torsades de pointes such as hypokalemia, significant bradycardia, and cardiomyopathy should be avoided.

As with any potent antimicrobial drug, periodic assessment of organ system functions, including renal, hepatic, and hematopoietic, is advisable during therapy. (See **WARNINGS** and **ADVERSE REACTIONS**.)

Information for Patients

Patients should be advised:

- Patients should be counseled that antibacterial drugs including LEVAQUIN® (levofloxacin) should only be used to treat bacterial infections. They do not treat viral infections (e.g., the common cold). When LEVAQUIN is prescribed to treat a bacterial infection, patients should be told that although it is common to feel better early in the course of therapy, the medication should be taken exactly as directed. Skipping doses or not completing the full course of therapy may (1) decrease the effectiveness of the immediate treatment and (2) increase the likelihood that bacteria will develop resistance and will not be treatable by LEVAQUIN or other antibacterial drugs in the future.
- to drink fluids liberally;
- that antacids containing magnesium, or aluminum, as well as sucralfate, metal cations such as iron, and multivitamin preparations with zinc or Videx® (didanosine) should be taken at least two hours before or two hours after oral levofloxacin administration. (See **Drug Interactions**);
- that oral levofloxacin can be taken without regard to meals;
- that levofloxacin may cause neurologic adverse effects (e.g., dizziness, lightheadedness) and that patients should know how they react to levofloxacin before they operate an automobile or machinery or engage in other activities requiring mental alertness and coordination. (See **WARNINGS** and **ADVERSE REACTIONS**);
- to discontinue treatment and inform their physician if they experience pain, inflammation, or rupture of a tendon, and to rest and refrain from exercise until the diagnosis of tendinitis or tendon rupture has been confidently excluded;
- that levofloxacin may be associated with hypersensitivity reactions, even following the first dose, and to discontinue the drug at the first sign of a skin rash, hives or other skin reactions, a rapid heartbeat, difficulty in swallowing or breathing, any swelling suggesting angioedema (e.g., swelling of the lips, tongue, face, tightness of the throat, hoarseness), or other symptoms of an allergic reaction. (See **WARNINGS** and **ADVERSE REACTIONS**);
- to avoid excessive sunlight or artificial ultraviolet light while receiving levofloxacin and to discontinue therapy if phototoxicity (i.e., skin eruption) occurs;
- that if they are diabetic and are being treated with insulin or an oral hypoglycemic agent and a hypoglycemic reaction occurs, they should discontinue levofloxacin and consult a physician. (See **PRECAUTIONS: General** and **Drug Interactions**.);
- that concurrent administration of warfarin and levofloxacin has been associated with increases of the International Normalized Ratio (INR) or prothrombin time and clinical episodes of bleeding. Patients should notify their physician if they are taking warfarin.
- that convulsions have been reported in patients taking quinolones, including levofloxacin, and to notify their physician before taking this drug if there is a history of this condition.

Drug Interactions

Antacids, Sucralfate, Metal Cations, Multivitamins

LEVAQUIN Tablets: While the chelation by divalent cations is less marked than with other quinolones, concurrent administration of LEVAQUIN Tablets with antacids containing magnesium, or aluminum, as well as sucralfate, metal cations such as iron, and multivitamin preparations with zinc may interfere with the gastrointestinal absorption of levofloxacin, resulting in systemic levels considerably lower than desired. Tablets with antacids containing magnesium, aluminum, as well as sucralfate, metal cations such as iron, and multivitamins preparations with zinc or Videx® (didanosine) may substantially interfere with the gastrointestinal absorption of levofloxacin, resulting in systemic levels considerably lower than desired. These agents should be taken at least two hours before or two hours after levofloxacin administration.

LEVAQUIN Injection: There are no data concerning an interaction of **intravenous** quinolones with **oral** antacids, sucralfate, multivitamins, Videx® (didanosine), or metal cations. However, no quinolone should be co-administered with any solution containing multivalent cations, e.g., magnesium, through the same intravenous line. (See **DOSAGE AND ADMINISTRATION**.)

Theophylline: No significant effect of levofloxacin on the plasma concentrations, AUC, and other disposition parameters for theophylline was detected in a clinical study involving 14 healthy volunteers. Similarly, no apparent effect of theophylline on levofloxacin absorption and disposition was observed. However, concomitant administration of other quinolones with theophylline has resulted in prolonged elimination half-life, elevated serum theophylline levels, and a subsequent increase in the risk of theophylline-related adverse reactions in the patient population. Therefore, theophylline levels should be closely monitored and appropriate dosage adjustments made when levofloxacin is co-administered. Adverse reactions, including seizures, may occur with or without an elevation in serum theophylline levels. (See **WARNINGS** and **PRECAUTIONS: General**.)

Warfarin: No significant effect of levofloxacin on the peak plasma concentrations, AUC, and other disposition parameters for R- and S-warfarin was detected in a clinical study involving healthy volunteers. Similarly, no apparent effect of warfarin on levofloxacin absorption and disposition was observed. There have been reports during the post-marketing experience in patients that levofloxacin enhances the effects of warfarin. Elevations of the prothrombin time in the setting of concurrent warfarin and levofloxacin use have been associated with episodes of bleeding. Prothrombin time, International Normalized Ratio (INR), or other suitable anticoagulation tests should be closely monitored if levofloxacin is administered concomitantly with warfarin. Patients should also be monitored for evidence of bleeding.

Cyclosporine: No significant effect of levofloxacin on the peak plasma concentrations, AUC, and other disposition parameters for cyclosporine was detected in a clinical study involving healthy volunteers. However, elevated serum levels of cyclosporine have been reported in the patient population when co-administered with some other quinolones. Levofloxacin C_{max} and k_e were slightly lower while T_{max} and $t_{1/2}$ were slightly longer in the presence of cyclosporine than those observed in other studies without concomitant medication. The differences, however, are not considered to be clinically significant. Therefore, no dosage adjustment is required for levofloxacin or cyclosporine when administered concomitantly.

Digoxin: No significant effect of levofloxacin on the peak plasma concentrations, AUC, and other disposition parameters for digoxin was detected in a clinical study involving healthy volunteers. Levofloxacin absorption and disposition kinetics were similar in the presence or absence of digoxin. Therefore, no dosage adjustment for levofloxacin or digoxin is required when administered concomitantly.

Probenecid and Cimetidine: No significant effect of probenecid or cimetidine on the rate and extent of levofloxacin absorption was observed in a clinical study involving healthy volunteers. The AUC and $t_{1/2}$ of levofloxacin were 27-38% and 30% higher, respectively, while CL/F and CL_R were 21-35% lower during concomitant treatment with probenecid or cimetidine compared to levofloxacin alone. Although these differences were statistically significant, the changes were not high enough to warrant dosage adjustment for levofloxacin when probenecid or cimetidine is co-administered.

Non-steroidal anti-inflammatory drugs: The concomitant administration of a non-steroidal anti-inflammatory drug with a quinolone, including levofloxacin, may increase the risk of CNS stimulation and convulsive seizures. (See **WARNINGS** and **PRECAUTIONS: General.**)

Antidiabetic agents: Disturbances of blood glucose, including hyperglycemia and hypoglycemia, have been reported in patients treated concomitantly with quinolones and an antidiabetic agent. Therefore, careful monitoring of blood glucose is recommended when these agents are co-administered.

Carcinogenesis, Mutagenesis, Impairment of Fertility

In a lifetime bioassay in rats, levofloxacin exhibited no carcinogenic potential following daily dietary administration for 2 years; the highest dose (100 mg/kg/day) was 1.4 times the highest recommended human dose (750 mg) based upon relative body surface area. Levofloxacin did not shorten the time to tumor development of UV-induced skin tumors in hairless albino (Skh-1) mice at any levofloxacin dose level and was therefore not photo-carcinogenic under conditions of this study. Dermal levofloxacin concentrations in the hairless mice ranged from 25 to 42 µg/g at the highest levofloxacin dose level (300 mg/kg/day) used in the photo-carcinogenicity study. By comparison, dermal levofloxacin concentrations in human subjects receiving 750 mg of levofloxacin averaged approximately 11.8 µg/g at C_{max}.

Levofloxacin was not mutagenic in the following assays: Ames bacterial mutation assay *(S. typhimurium* and *E. coli)*, CHO/HGPRT forward mutation assay, mouse micronucleus test, mouse dominant lethal test, rat unscheduled DNA synthesis assay, and the mouse sister chromatid exchange assay. It was positive in the in vitro chromosomal aberration (CHL cell line) and sister chromatid exchange (CHL/IU cell line) assays.

Levofloxacin caused no impairment of fertility or reproductive performance in rats at oral doses as high as 360 mg/kg/day, corresponding to 4.2 times the highest recommended human dose based upon relative body surface area and intravenous doses as high as 100 mg/kg/day, corresponding to 1.2 times the highest recommended human dose based upon relative body surface area.

Pregnancy: Teratogenic Effects. Pregnancy Category C.

Levofloxacin was not teratogenic in rats at oral doses as high as 810 mg/kg/day which corresponds to 9.4 times the highest recommended human dose based upon relative body surface area, or at intravenous doses as high as 160 mg/kg/day corresponding to 1.9 times the highest recommended human dose based upon relative body surface area. The oral dose of 810 mg/kg/day to rats caused decreased fetal body weight and increased fetal mortality. No teratogenicity was observed when rabbits were dosed orally as high as 50 mg/kg/day which corresponds to 1.1 times the highest recommended human dose based upon relative body surface area, or when dosed intravenously as high as 25 mg/kg/day, corresponding to 0.5 times the highest recommended human dose based upon relative body surface area.

There are, however, no adequate and well-controlled studies in pregnant women. Levofloxacin should be used during pregnancy only if the potential benefit justifies the potential risk to the fetus. (See **WARNINGS.**)

Nursing Mothers

Levofloxacin has not been measured in human milk. Based upon data from ofloxacin, it can be presumed that levofloxacin will be excreted in human milk. Because of the potential for serious adverse reactions from levofloxacin in nursing infants, a decision should be made whether to discontinue nursing or to discontinue the drug, taking into account the importance of the drug to the mother.

Pediatric Use

Safety and effectiveness in pediatric patients and adolescents below the age of 18 years have not been established. Quinolones, including levofloxacin, cause arthropathy and osteochondrosis in juvenile animals of several species. (See **WARNINGS.**)

Geriatric Use

In phase 3 clinical trials, 1,190 levofloxacin-treated patients (25%) were ≧65 years of age. Of these, 675 patients (14%) were between the ages of 65 and 74 and 515 patients (11%) were 75 years or older. No overall differences in safety or effectiveness were observed between these subjects and younger subjects, and other reported clinical experience has not identified differences in responses between the elderly and younger patients, but greater sensitivity of some older individuals cannot be ruled out.

The pharmacokinetic properties of levofloxacin in younger adults and elderly adults do not differ significantly when creatinine clearance is taken into consideration. However since the drug is known to be substantially excreted by the kidney, the risk of toxic reactions to this drug may be greater in patients with impaired renal function. Because

Patients with Normal Renal Function

Infection*	Unit Dose	Freq.	Duration**	Daily Dose
Comm. Acquired Pneumonia	500 mg	q24h	7-14 days	500 mg
Comm. Acquired Pneumonia	750 mg***	q24h	5 days	750 mg
Nosocomial Pneumonia	750 mg	q24h	7-14 days	750 mg
Complicated SSSI	750 mg	q24h	7-14 days	750 mg
Acute Bacterial Exacerbation of Chronic Bronchitis	500 mg	q24h	7 days	500 mg
Acute Maxillary Sinusitis	500 mg	q24h	10-14 days	500 mg
Uncomplicated SSSI	500 mg	q24h	7-10 days	500 mg
Chronic Bacterial Prostatitis	500 mg	q24h	28 days	500 mg
Complicated UTI	250 mg	q24h	10 days	250 mg
Acute pyelonephritis	250 mg	q24h	10 days	250 mg
Uncomplicated UTI	250 mg	q24h	3 days	250 mg

* **DUE TO THE DESIGNATED PATHOGENS** (See **INDICATIONS AND USAGE.**)

** Sequential therapy (intravenous to oral) may be instituted at the discretion of the physician.

*** Efficacy of this alternative regimen has only been documented for infections caused by penicillin-susceptible *Streptococcus pneumoniae, Haemophilius influenzae, Haemophilus parainfluenzae, Mycoplasma pneumoniae* and *Chlamydia pneumoniae.*

Patients with Impaired Renal Function

Renal Status	Initial Dose	Subsequent Dose
Acute Bacterial Exacerbation of Chronic Bronchitis/Comm. Acquired Pneumonia/Acute Maxillary Sinusitis/ Uncomplicated SSSI/Chronic Bacterial Prostatitis		
CL_{CR} from 50 to 80 mL/min	No dosage adjustment required	
CL_{CR} from 20 to 49 mL/min	500 mg	250 mg q24h
CL_{CR} from 10 to 19 mL/min	500 mg	250 mg q48h
Hemodialysis	500 mg	250 mg q48h
CAPD	500 mg	250 mg q48h
Complicated SSSI/Nosocomial Pneumonia/Comm. Acquired Pneumonia		
CL_{CR} from 50 to 80 mL/min	No dosage adjustment required	
CL_{CR} from 20 to 49 mL/min	750 mg	750 mg q48h
CL_{CR} from 10 to 19 mL/min	750 mg	500 mg q48h
Hemodialysis	750 mg	500 mg q48h
CAPD	750 mg	500 mg q48h
Complicated UTI/Acute Pyelonephritis		
CL_{CR} ≥20 mL/min	No dosage adjustment required	
CL_{CR} from 10 to 19 mL/min	250 mg	250 mg q48h
Uncomplicated UTI	No dosage adjustment required	

CL_{CR}=creatinine clearances
CAPD=chronic ambulatory peritoneal dialysis

elderly patients are more likely to have decreased renal function, care should be taken in dose selection, and it may be useful to monitor renal function.

ADVERSE REACTIONS

The incidence of drug-related adverse reactions in patients during Phase 3 clinical trials conducted in North America was 6.2%. Among patients receiving levofloxacin therapy, 4.3% discontinued levofloxacin therapy due to adverse experiences. The overall incidence, type and distribution of adverse events was similar in patients receiving levofloxacin doses of 750 mg once daily compared to patients receiving doses from 250 mg once daily to 500 mg twice daily.

In clinical trials, the following events were considered likely to be drug-related in patients receiving levofloxacin:
nausea 1.2%, diarrhea 1.0%, vaginitis 0.6%, insomnia 0.4%, abdominal pain 0.4%, flatulence 0.3%, pruritus 0.3%, dizziness 0.3%, rash 0.3%, dyspepsia 0.2%, genital moniliasis 0.2%, moniliasis 0.2%, taste perversion 0.2%, vomiting 0.2%, injection site pain 0.2%, injection site reaction 0.2%, injection site inflammation 0.1%, constipation 0.1%, fungal infection 0.1%, genital pruritis 0.1%, headache 0.1%, nervousness 0.1%, rash erythematous 0.1%, urticaria 0.1% anorexia 0.1%, somnolence 0.1%, agitation 0.1%, rash maculopapular 0.1%, tremor 0.1%, condition aggravated 0.1%, allergic reaction 0.1%.

In clinical trials, the following events occurred in >3% of patients, regardless of drug relationship:
nausea 7.1%, headache 6.2%, diarrhea 5.5%, insomnia 5.1%, constipation 3.5%.

In clinical trials, the following events occurred in 1 to 3% of patients, regardless of drug relationship:
abdominal pain 2.7%,dizziness 2.5%, vomiting 2.5%, dyspepsia 2.3%, vaginitis 1.7%, rash 1.6%, chest pain 1.4%, pruritus 1.3%, sinusitis 1.3%, dyspnea 1.4%, fatigue 1.4%, flatulence 1.2%, pain 1.6%, back pain 1.2%, rhinitis 1.2%, anxiety 1.2%, pharyngitis 1.2%.

In clinical trials, the following events, of potential medical importance, occurred at a rate of 0.1% to 0.9%, regardless of drug relationship:
[See table at top of previous page]

In clinical trials using multiple-dose therapy, ophthalmologic abnormalities, including cataracts and multiple punctate lenticular opacities, have been noted in patients undergoing treatment with other quinolones. The relationship of the drugs to these events is not presently established.

Crystalluria and cylindruria have been reported with other quinolones.

The following markedly abnormal laboratory values appeared in >2% of patients receiving levofloxacin. It is not known whether these abnormalities were caused by the drug or the underlying condition being treated.

Blood Chemistry: decreased glucose (2.2%)
Hematology: decreased lymphocytes (2.2%)

Post-Marketing Adverse Reactions

Additional adverse events reported from worldwide post-marketing experience with levofloxacin include:
allergic pneumonitis, anaphylactic shock, anaphylactoid reaction, dysphonia, abnormal EEG, encephalopathy, eosinophilia, erythema multiforme, hemolytic anemia, multi-system organ failure, increased International Normalized Ratio (INR)/prothrombin time, Stevens-Johnson Syndrome, tendon rupture, torsades de pointes, vasodilation.

OVERDOSAGE

Levofloxacin exhibits a low potential for acute toxicity. Mice, rats, dogs and monkeys exhibited the following clinical signs after receiving a single high dose of levofloxacin: ataxia, ptosis, decreased locomotor activity, dyspnea, prostration, tremors, and convulsions. Doses in excess of 1500 mg/kg orally and 250 mg/kg i.v. produced significant mortality in rodents. In the event of an acute overdosage, the stomach should be emptied. The patient should be observed and appropriate hydration maintained. Levofloxacin is not efficiently removed by hemodialysis or peritoneal dialysis.

DOSAGE AND ADMINISTRATION

LEVAQUIN Injection should only be administered by intravenous infusion. It is not for intramuscular, intrathecal, intraperitoneal, or subcutaneous administration.

CAUTION: RAPID OR BOLUS INTRAVENOUS INFUSION MUST BE AVOIDED. Levofloxacin Injection should be infused intravenously slowly over a period of not less than 60 or 90 minutes, depending on the dosage. (See **PRECAUTIONS.**)

Single-use vials require dilution prior to administration. (See **PREPARATION FOR ADMINISTRATION.**)

The usual dose of LEVAQUIN Tablets or Injection is 250 mg or 500 mg administered orally or by slow infusion over 60 minutes every 24 hours or 750 mg administered orally or by slow infusion over 90 minutes every 24 hours, as indicated by infection and described in the following dosing chart. These recommendations apply to patients with normal renal function (i.e., creatinine clearance > 80 mL/min). For patients with altered renal function see the **Patients with Impaired Renal Function** subsection. Oral doses should be administered at least two hours before or two hours after antacids containing magnesium, aluminum, as well as sucralfate, metal cations such as iron, and multivitamin preparations with zinc or Videx® (didanosine), chewable/buffered tablets or the pediatric powder for oral solution.

[See first table above]
[See second table above]

When only the serum creatinine is known, the following formula may be used to estimate creatinine clearance.

$$\text{Men: Creatinine Clearance (mL/min)} = \frac{\text{Weight (kg)} \times (140 - \text{age})}{72 \times \text{serum creatinine (mg/dL)}}$$

Women: 0.85 × the value calculated for men.

The serum creatinine should represent a steady state of renal function.

Preparation of Levofloxacin Injection for Administration

LEVAQUIN Injection in Single-Use Vials: LEVAQUIN Injection is supplied in single-use vials containing a concentrated levofloxacin solution with the equivalent of 500 mg (20 mL vial) and 750 mg (30 mL vial) of levofloxacin in Water for Injection, USP. The 20 mL and 30 mL vials each

Continued on next page

Levaquin—Cont.

contain 25 mg of levofloxacin/mL. **THESE LEVAQUIN INJECTION SINGLE-USE VIALS MUST BE FURTHER DILUTED WITH AN APPROPRIATE SOLUTION PRIOR TO INTRAVENOUS ADMINISTRATION.** (See **COMPATIBLE INTRAVENOUS SOLUTIONS.**) The concentration of the resulting diluted solution should be 5 mg/mL prior to administration.

This intravenous drug product should be inspected visually for particulate matter prior to administration.

This intravenous drug product should be inspected visually for particulate matter prior to administration. Samples containing visible particles should be discarded.

Since no preservative or bacteriostatic agent is present in this product, aseptic technique must be used in preparation of the final intravenous solution. **Since the vials are for single-use only, any unused portion remaining in the vial should be discarded. When used to prepare two 250 mg doses from the 20 mL vial containing 500 mg of levofloxacin, the full content of the vial should be withdrawn at once using a single-entry procedure, and a second dose should be prepared and stored for subsequent use.** (See **Stability of LEVAQUIN Injection Following Dilution.**)

Since only limited data are available on the compatibility of levofloxacin intravenous injection with other intravenous substances, **additives or other medications should not be added to LEVAQUIN Injection in single-use vials or infused simultaneously through the same intravenous line.** If the same intravenous line is used for sequential infusion of several different drugs, the line should be flushed before and after infusion of LEVAQUIN Injection with an infusion solution compatible with LEVAQUIN Injection and with any other drug(s) administered via this common line.

Prepare the desired dosage of levofloxacin according to the following chart:

[See first table above]

For example, to prepare a 500 mg dose using the 20 mL vial (25 mg/mL), withdraw 20 mL and dilute with a compatible intravenous solution to a total volume of 100 mL.

Compatible Intravenous Solutions: Any of the following intravenous solutions may be used to prepare a 5 mg/mL levofloxacin solution with the approximate pH values:

Intravenous Fluids	Final pH of LEVAQUIN Solution
0.9% Sodium Chloride Injection, USP	4.71
5% Dextrose Injection, USP	4.58
5% Dextrose/0.9% NaCl Injection	4.62
5% Dextrose in Lactated Ringers	4.92
Plasma-Lyte® 56/5% Dextrose Injection	5.03
5% Dextrose, 0.45% Sodium Chloride, and 0.15% Potassium Chloride Injection	4.61
Sodium Lactate Injection (M/6)	5.54

LEVAQUIN Injection Premix in Single-Use Flexible Containers: LEVAQUIN Injection is also supplied in flexible containers containing a premixed, ready-to-use levofloxacin solution in D_5W for single-use. The fill volume is either 50 or 100 mL for the 100 mL flexible container or 150 mL for the 150 mL container. **NO FURTHER DILUTION OF THESE PREPARATIONS ARE NECESSARY. Consequently each 50 mL, 100 mL, and 150 mL premix flexible container already contains a dilute solution with the equivalent of 250 mg, 500 mg, and 750 mg of levofloxacin, respectively (5 mg/mL) in 5% Dextrose (D_5W).**

This parenteral drug product should be inspected visually for particulate matter prior to administration. Samples containing visible particles should be discarded.

Since the premix flexible containers are for single-use only, any unused portion should be discarded.

Since only limited data are available on the compatibility of levofloxacin intravenous injection with other intravenous substances, **additives or other medications should not be added to LEVAQUIN Injection in flexible containers or infused simultaneously through the same intravenous line.** If the same intravenous line is used for sequential infusion of several different drugs, the line should be flushed before and after infusion of LEVAQUIN Injection with an infusion solution compatible with LEVAQUIN Injection and with any other drug(s) administered via this common line.

Instructions for the Use of LEVAQUIN Injection Premix in Flexible Containers

To open:

1. Tear outer wrap at the notch and remove solution container.
2. Check the container for minute leaks by squeezing the inner bag firmly. If leaks are found, or if the seal is not intact, discard the solution, as the sterility may be compromised.
3. Do not use if the solution is cloudy or a precipitate is present.
4. Use sterile equipment.
5. **WARNING: Do not use flexible containers in series connections.** Such use could result in air embolism due to residual air being drawn from the primary container before administration of the fluid from the secondary container is complete.

Desired Dosage Strength	From Appropriate Vial, Withdraw Volume	Volume of Diluent	Infusion Time
250 mg	10 mL (20 mL Vial)	40 mL	60 min
500 mg	20 mL (20 mL Vial)	80 mL	60 min
750 mg	30 mL (30 mL Vial)	120 mL	90 min

Pathogen	N	Levofloxacin No. (%) of Patients Microbiologic/Clinical Outcomes	N	Imipenem/Cilastatin No. (%) of Patients Microbiologic/Clinical Outcomes
MSSA[a]	21	14 (66.7)/13 (61.9)	19	13 (68.4)/15 (78.9)
P. aeruginosa[b]	17	10 (58.8)/11 (64.7)	17	5 (29.4)/ 7 (41.2)
S. marcescens	11	9 (81.8)/ 7 (63.6)	7	2 (28.6)/ 3 (42.9)
E. coli	12	10 (83.3)/ 7 (58.3)	11	7 (63.6)/ 8 (72.7)
K. pneumoniae[c]	11	9 (81.8)/ 5 (45.5)	7	6 (85.7)/ 3 (42.9)
H. influenzae	16	13 (81.3)/10 (62.5)	15	14 (93.3)/11 (73.3)
S. pneumoniae	4	3 (75.0)/ 3 (75.0)	7	5 (71.4)/ 4 (57.1)

[a]Methicillin-susceptible *S. aureus*
[b]See above text for use of combination therapy.
[c]The observed differences in rates for the clinical and microbiological outcomes may reflect other factors that were not accounted for in the study.

Preparation for administration:
1. Close flow control clamp of administration set.
2. Remove cover from port at bottom of container.
3. Insert piercing pin of administration set into port with a twisting motion until the pin is firmly seated. **NOTE: See full directions on administration set carton.**
4. Suspend container from hanger.
5. Squeeze and release drip chamber to establish proper fluid level in chamber during infusion of LEVAQUIN Injection in Premix Flexible Containers.
6. Open flow control clamp to expel air from set. Close clamp.
7. Regulate rate of administration with flow control clamp.

Stability of LEVAQUIN Injection as Supplied

When stored under recommended conditions, LEVAQUIN Injection, as supplied in 20 mL and 30 mL vials, or 100 mL and 150 mL flexible containers, is stable through the expiration date printed on the label.

Stability of LEVAQUIN Injection Following Dilution

LEVAQUIN Injection, when diluted in a compatible intravenous fluid to a concentration of 5 mg/mL, is stable for 72 hours when stored at or below 25°C (77°F) and for 14 days when stored under refrigeration at 5°C (41°F) in plastic intravenous containers. Solutions that are diluted in a compatible intravenous solution and frozen in glass bottles or plastic intravenous containers are stable for 6 months when stored at -20°C (-4°F). **THAW FROZEN SOLUTIONS AT ROOM TEMPERATURE 25°C (77°F) OR IN A REFRIGERATOR 8°C (46°F). DO NOT FORCE THAW BY MICROWAVE IRRADIATION OR WATER BATH IMMERSION. DO NOT REFREEZE AFTER INITIAL THAWING.**

HOW SUPPLIED

LEVAQUIN Tablets

LEVAQUIN (levofloxacin) Tablets are supplied as 250, 500, and 750 mg capsule-shaped, coated tablets. LEVAQUIN Tablets are packaged in bottles and in unit-dose blister strips in the following configurations:

250 mg tablets are terra cotta pink and are imprinted: "LEVAQUIN" on one side and "250" on the other side.
 bottles of 50 (NDC 0045-1520-50)
 unit-dose/100 tablets (NDC 0045-1520-10)

500 mg tablets are peach and are imprinted: "LEVAQUIN" on one side and "500" on the other side.
 bottles of 50 (NDC 0045-1525-50)
 unit-dose/100 tablets (NDC 0045-1525-10)

750 mg tablets are white and are imprinted: "LEVAQUIN" one side and "750" the other side.
 bottles of 20 (NDC 0045-1530-20)
 unit-dose/100 tablets (NDC 0045-1530-10)
 LEVA-Pak 5 tablets (NDC 0045-1530-05)

LEVAQUIN Tablets should be stored at 15° to 30°C (59° to 86°F) in well-closed containers.

LEVAQUIN Tablets are manufactured for OMP DIVISION, ORTHO-McNEIL PHARMACEUTICAL, INC. by Janssen Ortho LLC, Gurabo, Puerto Rico 00778.

LEVAQUIN Injection

Single-Use Vials: LEVAQUIN (levofloxacin) Injection is supplied in single-use vials. Each vial contains a concentrated solution with the equivalent of 500 mg of levofloxacin in 20 mL vials and 750 mg of levofloxacin in 30 mL vials.
25 mg/mL, 20 mL vials (NDC 0045-0069-51)
25 mg/mL, 30 mL vials (NDC 0045-0065-55)

LEVAQUIN Injection in Single-Use Vials should be stored at controlled room temperature and protected from light.

LEVAQUIN Injection in Single-Use Vials is manufactured for OMP DIVISION, ORTHO-McNEIL PHARMACEUTICAL, INC. by OMJ Pharmaceuticals, Inc., San German, Puerto Rico 00683.

Premix in Flexible Containers: LEVAQUIN (levofloxacin in 5% dextrose) Injection is supplied as a single-use, premixed solution in flexible containers. Each bag contains a dilute solution with the equivalent of 250, 500, or 750 mg of levofloxacin, respectively, in 5% Dextrose (D_5W).
5 mg/mL (250 mg), 50 mL flexible container (NDC 0045-0067-01)
5 mg/mL (500 mg), 100 mL flexible container (NDC 0045-0068-01)
5 mg/mL (750 mg), 150 mL flexible container (NDC 0045-0066-01)

LEVAQUIN Injection Premix in Flexible Containers should be stored at or below 25°C (77°F); however, brief exposure up to 40°C (104°F) does not adversely affect the product. Avoid excessive heat and protect from freezing and light.

LEVAQUIN Injection Premix in Flexible Containers is manufactured for OMP DIVISION, ORTHO-McNEIL PHARMACEUTICAL, INC. by ABBOTT Laboratories, North Chicago, IL 60064.

CLINICAL STUDIES

Nosocomial Pneumonia

Adult patients with clinically and radiologically documented nosocomial pneumonia were enrolled in a multicenter, randomized, open-label study comparing intravenous levofloxacin (750 mg once daily) followed by oral levofloxacin (750 mg once daily) for a total of 7-15 days to intravenous imipenem/cilastatin (500-1000 mg q6-8 hours daily) followed by oral ciprofloxacin (750 mg q12 hours daily) for a total of 7-15 days. Levofloxacin-treated patients received an average of 7 days of intravenous therapy (range: 1-16 days); comparator-treated patients received an average of 8 days of intravenous therapy (range: 1-19 days).

Overall, in the clinically and microbiologically evaluable population, adjunctive therapy was empirically initiated at study entry in 56 of 93 (60.2%) patients in the levofloxacin arm and 53 of 94 (56.4%) patients in the comparator arm. The average duration of adjunctive therapy was 7 days in the levofloxacin arm and 7 days in the comparator. In clinically and microbiologically evaluable patients with documented *Pseudomonas aeruginosa* infection, 15 of 17 (88.2%) received ceftazidime (N=11) or piperacillin/tazobactam (N=4) in the levofloxacin arm and 16 of 17 (94.1%) received an aminoglycoside in the comparator arm. Overall, in clinically and microbiologically evaluable patients, vancomycin was added to the treatment regimen of 37 of 93 (39.8%) patients in the levofloxacin arm and 28 of 94 (29.8%) patients in the comparator arm for suspected methicillin-resistant *S. aureus* infection.

Clinical success rates in clinically and microbiologically evaluable patients at the posttherapy visit (primary study endpoint assessed on day 3-15 after completing therapy) were 58.1% for levofloxacin and 60.6% for comparator. The 95% CI for the difference of response rates (levofloxacin minus comparator) was [-17.2, 12.0]. The microbiological eradication rates at the posttherapy visit were 66.7% for levofloxacin and 60.6% for comparator. The 95% CI for the difference of eradication rates (levofloxacin minus comparator) was [-8.3, 20.3]. Clinical success and microbiological eradication rates by pathogen were as follows:

[See second table above]

Community-Acquired Bacterial Pneumonia

7 to 14 Day Treatment Regimen

Adult inpatients and outpatients with a diagnosis of community-acquired bacterial pneumonia were evaluated in two pivotal clinical studies. In the first study, 590 patients were enrolled in a prospective, multi-center, unblinded randomized trial comparing levofloxacin 500 mg once daily orally or intravenously for 7 to 14 days to ceftriaxone 1 to 2 grams intravenously once or in equally divided doses twice daily followed by cefuroxime axetil 500 mg orally twice daily for a total of 7 to 14 days. Patients assigned to treatment with the control regimen were allowed to receive erythromycin (or doxycycline if intolerant of erythromycin) if an infection due to atypical pathogens was suspected or proven. Clinical and microbiologic evaluations were performed during treatment, 5 to 7 days posttherapy, and 3 to 4 weeks posttherapy. Clinical success (cure plus improvement) with levofloxacin at 5 to 7 days posttherapy, the primary efficacy variable in this study, was superior (95%) to the control group (83%). The 95% CI for the difference of response rates (levofloxacin minus comparator) was [-6, 19]. In the second study, 264 patients were enrolled in a prospective, multi-center, non-comparative trial of 500 mg levofloxacin administered orally or intravenously once daily for 7 to 14 days. Clinical success for clinically evaluable patients was 93%. For both studies, the clinical success rate in patients with atypical pneumonia due to *Chlamydia pneumoniae, Mycoplasma pneumoniae*, and *Legionella pneumophila* were 96%, 96%, and 70%, respectively. Microbiologic eradication rates across both studies were as follows:

Pathogen	No. Pathogens	Microbiologic Eradication Rate (%)
H. influenzae	55	98
S. pneumoniae	83	95
S. aureus	17	88
M. catarrhalis	18	94
H. parainfluenzae	19	95
K. pneumoniae	10	100.0

Additional studies were initiated to evaluate the utility of LEVAQUIN in community-acquired pneumonia due to *S. pneumoniae*, with particular interest in penicillin-resistant strains (MIC value for penicillin ≥2 μg/mL). In addition to the studies previously discussed, inpatients and outpatients with mild to severe community-acquired pneumonia were evaluated in six additional clinical studies; one double-blind study, two open label randomized studies, and three open label non-comparative studies. The total number of clinically evaluable patients with *S. pneumoniae* across all 8 studies was 250 for levofloxacin and 41 for comparators. The clinical success rate (cured or improved) among the 250 levofloxacin-treated patients with *S. pneumoniae* was 245/250 (98%). The clinical success rate among the 41 comparator-treated patients with *S. pneumoniae* was 39/41 (95%).

Across these 8 studies, 18 levofloxacin-treated and 4 non-quinolone comparator-treated patients with community-acquired pneumonia due to penicillin-resistant *S. pneumoniae* (MIC value for penicillin ≥2 μg/mL) were identified. Of the 18 levofloxacin-treated patients, 15 were evaluable following the completion of therapy. Fifteen out of the 15 evaluable levofloxacin-treated patients with community-acquired pneumonia due to penicillin-resistant *S. pneumoniae* achieved clinical success (cure or improvement). Of these 15 patients, 6 were bacteremic and 5 were classified as having severe disease. Of the 4 comparator-treated patients with community-acquired pneumonia due to penicillin-resistant *S. pneumoniae,* 3 were evaluable for clinical efficacy. Three out of the 3 evaluable comparator-treated patients achieved clinical success. All three of the comparator-treated patients were bacteremic and had disease classified as severe.

Community-Acquired Bacterial Pneumonia

5-Day Treatment Regimen

To evaluate the safety and efficacy of higher dose and shorter course of levofloxacin, 528 outpatient and hospitalized adults with clinically and radiologically determined mild to severe community-acquired pneumonia were evaluated in a double-blind, randomized, prospective, multicenter study comparing levofloxacin 750 mg, i.v. or p.o., q.d. for five days or levofloxacin 500 mg i.v. or p.o., q.d. for 10 days.

Clinical success rates (cure plus improvement) in the clinically evaluable population were 90.9% in the levofloxacin 750mg group and 91.1% in the levofloxacin 500 mg group. The 95% CI for the difference of response rates (levofloxacin 750 minus levofloxacin 500) was [-5.9, 5.4]. In the clinically evaluable population (31-38 days after enrollment) pneumonia was observed in 7 out of 151 patients in the levofloxacin 750 mg group and 2 out of 147 patients in the levofloxacin 500 mg group. Given the small numbers observed, the significance of this finding can not be determined statistically. The microbiological efficacy of the 5-day regimen was documented for infections listed in the table below.

	Eradication rate
Penicillin susceptible *S. pneumoniae*	19/20
Haemophilus influenzae	12/12
Haemophilus parainfluenzae	10/10
Mycoplasma pneumoniae	26/27
Chlamydia pneumoniae	13/15

Complicated Skin and Skin Structure Infections

Three hundred ninety-nine patients were enrolled in an open-label, randomized, comparative study for complicated skin and skin structure infections. The patients were randomized to receive either levofloxacin 750 mg QD (IV followed by oral), or an approved comparator for a median of 10 ± 4.7 days. As is expected in complicated skin and skin structure infections, surgical procedures were performed in the levofloxacin and comparator groups. Surgery (incision and drainage or debridement) was performed on 45% of the levofloxacin treated patients and 44% of the comparator treated patients, either shortly before or during antibiotic treatment and formed an integral part of therapy for this indication.

Among those who could be evaluated clinically 2-5 days after completion of study drug, overall success rates (improved or cured) were 116/138 (84.1%) for patients treated with levofloxacin and 106/132 (80.3%) for patients treated with the comparator.

Success rates varied with the type of diagnosis ranging from 68% in patients with infected ulcers to 90% in patients with infected wounds and abscesses. These rates were equivalent to those seen with comparator drugs.

Chronic Bacterial Prostatitis

Adult patients with a clinical diagnosis of prostatitis and microbiological culture results from urine sample collected after prostatic massage (VB_3) or expressed prostatic secretion (EPS) specimens obtained via the Meares-Stamey procedure were enrolled in a multicenter, randomized, double-blind study comparing oral levofloxacin 500 mg, once daily for a total of 28 days to oral ciprofloxacin 500 mg, twice daily for a total of 28 days. The primary efficacy endpoint was microbiologic efficacy in microbiologically evaluable patients. A total of 136 and 125 microbiologically evaluable patients were enrolled in the levofloxacin and ciprofloxacin groups, respectively. The microbiologic eradication rate by patient infection at 5-18 days after completion of therapy was 75.0% in the levofloxacin group and 76.8% in the ciprofloxacin group (95% CI [-12.58, 8.98] for levofloxacin minus ciprofloxacin). The overall eradication rates for pathogens of interest are presented below:

Pathogen	Levofloxacin (N=136) N	Levofloxacin (N=136) Eradication	Ciprofloxacin (N=125) N	Ciprofloxacin (N=125) Eradication
E. coli	15	14 (93.3%)	11	9 (81.8%)
E. faecalis	54	39 (72.2%)	44	33 (75.0%)
**S. epidermidis*	11	9 (81.8%)	14	11 (78.6%)

*Eradication rates shown are for patients who had a sole pathogen only; mixed cultures were excluded.

Eradication rates for *S. epidermidis* when found with other co-pathogens are consistent with rates seen in pure isolates. Clinical success (cure + improvement with no need for further antibiotic therapy) rates in microbiologically evaluable population 5-18 days after completion of therapy were 75.0% for levofloxacin-treated patients and 72.8% for ciprofloxacin-treated patients (95% CI [-8.87, 13.27] for levofloxacin minus ciprofloxacin). Clinical long-term success (24-45 days after completion of therapy) rates were 66.7% for the levofloxacin-treated patients and 76.9% for the ciprofloxacin-treated patients (95% CI [-23.40, 2.89] for levofloxacin minus ciprofloxacin).

ANIMAL PHARMACOLOGY

Levofloxacin and other quinolones have been shown to cause arthropathy in immature animals of most species tested. (See **WARNINGS**.) In immature dogs (4-5 months old), oral doses of 10 mg/kg/day for 7 days and intravenous doses of 4 mg/kg/day for 14 days of levofloxacin resulted in arthropathic lesions. Administration at oral doses of 300 mg/kg/day for 7 days and intravenous doses of 60 mg/kg/day for 4 weeks produced arthropathy in juvenile rats.

When tested in a mouse ear swelling bioassay, levofloxacin exhibited phototoxicity similar in magnitude to ofloxacin, but less phototoxicity than other quinolones.

While crystalluria has been observed in some intravenous rat studies, urinary crystals are not formed in the bladder, being present only after micturition and are not associated with nephrotoxicity.

In mice, the CNS stimulatory effect of quinolones is enhanced by concomitant administration of non-steroidal anti-inflammatory drugs.

In dogs, levofloxacin administered at 6 mg/kg or higher by rapid intravenous injection produced hypotensive effects. These effects were considered to be related to histamine release.

In vitro and in vivo studies in animals indicate that levofloxacin is neither an enzyme inducer or inhibitor in the human therapeutic plasma concentration range; therefore, no drug metabolizing enzyme-related interactions with other drugs or agents are anticipated.

REFERENCES

1. National Committee for Clinical Laboratory Standards. Methods for Dilution Antimicrobial Susceptibility Tests for Bacteria That Grow Aerobically Sixth Edition. Approved Standard NCCLS Document M7-A6, Vol. 23, No. 2, NCCLS, Wayne, PA, January, 2003.
2. National Committee for Clinical Laboratory Standards. Performance Standards for Antimicrobial Disk Susceptibility Tests Eighth Edition. Approved Standard NCCLS Document M2-A8, Vol. 23, No. 1, NCCLS, Wayne, PA, January, 2003.

Patient Information About: LEVAQUIN®

(levofloxacin) Tablets

250 mg Tablets, 500 mg Tablets, and 750 mg Tablets

This leaflet contains important information about LEVAQUIN® (levofloxacin), and should be read completely before you begin treatment. This leaflet does not take the place of discussions with your doctor or health care professional about your medical condition or your treatment. This leaflet does not list all benefits and risks of LEVAQUIN® The medicine described here can be prescribed only by a licensed health care professional. If you have any questions about LEVAQUIN® talk to your health care professional. Only your health care professional can determine if LEVAQUIN® is right for you.

What is LEVAQUIN®?

LEVAQUIN® is a quinolone antibiotic used to treat lung, sinus, skin, and urinary tract infections caused by certain germs called bacteria. LEVAQUIN® kills many of the types of bacteria that can infect the lungs, sinuses, skin, and urinary tract and has been shown in a large number of clinical trials to be safe and effective for the treatment of bacterial infections.

Sometimes viruses rather than bacteria may infect the lungs and sinuses (for example the common cold). LEVAQUIN®, like other antibiotics, does not kill viruses.

You should contact your health care professional if you think that your condition is not improving while taking LEVAQUIN®. LEVAQUIN® Tablets are terra cotta pink for the 250 mg tablet, peach colored for the 500 mg tablet, or white for the 750 mg tablet.

How and when should I take LEVAQUIN®?

LEVAQUIN® should be taken once a day for 3, 5, 7, 10, 14 or 28 days depending on your prescription. It should be swallowed and may be taken with or without food. Try to take the tablet at the same time each day and drink fluids liberally.

You may begin to feel better quickly; however, in order to make sure that all bacteria are killed, you should complete the full course of medication. Do not take more than the prescribed dose of LEVAQUIN® even if you missed a dose by mistake. You should not take a double dose.

Who should not take LEVAQUIN®?

You should not take LEVAQUIN® if you have ever had a severe allergic reaction to any of the group of antibiotics known as "quinolones" such as ciprofloxacin. Serious and occasionally fatal allergic reactions have been reported in patients receiving therapy with quinolones, including LEVAQUIN®.

If you are pregnant or are planning to become pregnant while taking LEVAQUIN®, talk to your health care professional before taking this medication. LEVAQUIN® is not recommended for use during pregnancy or nursing, as the effects on the unborn child or nursing infant are unknown. LEVAQUIN® is not recommended for children.

What are possible side effects of LEVAQUIN®?

LEVAQUIN® is generally well tolerated. The most common side effects caused by LEVAQUIN®, which are usually mild, include nausea, diarrhea, itching, abdominal pain, dizziness, flatulence, rash and vaginitis in women.

You should be careful about driving or operating machinery until you are sure LEVAQUIN® is not causing dizziness.

Allergic reactions have been reported in patients receiving quinolones including LEVAQUIN®, even after just one dose. If you develop hives, skin rash or other symptoms of an allergic reaction, you should stop taking this medication and call your health care professional.

Ruptures of shoulder, hand, or Achilles tendons have been reported in patients receiving quinolones, including LEVAQUIN®. If you develop pain, swelling, or rupture of a tendon you should stop taking LEVAQUIN® and contact your health care professional.

Some quinolone antibiotics have been associated with the development of phototoxicity ("sunburns" and "blistering sunburns") following exposure to sunlight or other sources of ultraviolet light such as artificial ultraviolet light used in tanning salons. LEVAQUIN® has been infrequently associated with phototoxicity. You should avoid excessive exposure to sunlight or artificial ultraviolet light while you are taking LEVAQUIN®.

If you have diabetes and you develop a hypoglycemic reaction while on LEVAQUIN®, you should stop taking LEVAQUIN® and call your health care professional.

Convulsions have been reported in patients receiving quinolone antibiotics including LEVAQUIN®. If you have experienced convulsions in the past, be sure to let your physician know that you have a history of convulsions.

Quinolones, including LEVAQUIN®, may also cause central nervous system stimulation which may lead to tremors, restlessness, anxiety, lightheadedness, confusion, hallucinations, paranoia, depression, nightmares, insomnia, and rarely, suicidal thoughts or acts.

If you notice any side effects not mentioned in this leaflet or you have concerns about the side effects you are experiencing, please inform your health care professional.

For more complete information regarding levofloxacin, please refer to the full prescribing information, which may be obtained from your health care professional, pharmacist, or the Physicians Desk Reference (PDR).

What about other medicines I am taking?

Taking warfarin (Coumadin®) and LEVAQUIN® together can further predispose you to the development of bleeding problems. If you take warfarin, be sure to tell your health care professional.

Many antacids and multivitamins may interfere with the absorption of LEVAQUIN® and may prevent it from working properly. You should take LEVAQUIN® either 2 hours before or 2 hours after taking these products.

It is important to let your health care professional know all of the medicines you are using.

Other information

Take your dose of LEVAQUIN® once a day.

Complete the course of medication even if you are feeling better.

Keep this medication out of the reach of children.

This information does not take the place of discussions with your doctor or health care professional about your medical condition or your treatment.

ORTHO-McNEIL

OMP DIVISION

ORTHO-McNEIL PHARMACEUTICAL, INC.

Raritan, New Jersey, USA 08869

U.S. Patent No. 5,053,407.

 Revised February 2004 7518209

Shown in Product Identification Guide, page 328

Continued on next page

ORTHO-CEPT® ℞

[ɔr-thō-sĕpt]

(desogestrel and ethinyl estradiol) Tablets

Prescribing Information

Patients should be counseled that this product does not protect against HIV infection (AIDS) and other sexually transmitted diseases.

DESCRIPTION

ORTHO-CEPT Tablets provide an oral contraceptive regimen of 21 light orange round tablets each containing 0.15 mg desogestrel (13-ethyl-11-methylene-18, 19-dinor-17 alpha-pregn-4-en- 20-yn-17-ol) and 0.03 mg ethinyl estradiol (19-nor-17 alpha-pregna-1,3,5 (10)-trien-20-yne-3, 17, diol). Inactive ingredients include vitamin E, corn starch, povidone, stearic acid, colloidal silicone dioxide, lactose, hypromellose, polyethylene glycol, titanium dioxide, talc and ferric oxide. Each green tablet contains the following inactive ingredients: lactose, pregelatinized starch, magnesium stearate, FD&C Blue No. 1 Aluminum Lake, ferric oxide, hypromellose, polyethylene glycol, titanium dioxide and talc.

desogestrel ethinyl estradiol

CLINICAL PHARMACOLOGY

Pharmacodynamics

Combination oral contraceptives act by suppression of gonadotropins. Although the primary mechanism of this action is inhibition of ovulation, other alterations include changes in the cervical mucus, which increase the difficulty of sperm entry into the uterus, and changes in the endometrium which reduce the likelihood of implantation.

Receptor binding studies, as well as studies in animals, have shown that 3-keto-desogestrel, the biologically active metabolite of desogestrel, combines high progestational activity with minimal intrinsic androgenicity.[91,92] The relevance of this latter finding in humans is unknown.

Pharmacokinetics

Desogestrel is rapidly and almost completely absorbed and converted into 3-keto-desogestrel, its biologically active metabolite. Following oral administration, the relative bioavailability of desogestrel, as measured by serum levels of 3-keto-desogestrel, is approximately 84%.

In the third cycle of use after a single dose of ORTHO-CEPT, maximum concentrations of 3-keto-desogestrel of 2,805 ± 1,203 pg/mL (mean ± SD) are reached at 1.4 ± 0.8 hours. The area under the curve ($AUC_{0-\infty}$) is 33,858 ± 11,043 pg/mL•hr after a single dose. At steady state, attained from at least day 19 onwards, maximum concentrations of 5,840 ± 1,667 pg/mL are reached at 1.4 ± 0.9 hours. The minimum plasma levels of 3-keto-desogestrel at steady state are 1,400 ± 560 pg/mL. The AUC_{0-24} at steady state is 52,299 ± 17,878 pg/mL•hr. The mean $AUC_{0-\infty}$ for 3-keto-desogestrel at single dose is significantly lower than the mean AUC_{0-24} at steady state. This indicates that the kinetics of 3-keto-desogestrel are non-linear due to an increase in binding of 3-keto-desogestrel to sex hormone-binding globulin in the cycle, attributed to increased sex hormone-binding globulin levels which are induced by the daily administration of ethinyl estradiol. Sex hormone-binding globulin levels increased significantly in the third treatment cycle from day 1 (150 ± 64 nmol/L) to day 21 (230 ± 59 nmol/L).

The elimination half-life for 3-keto-desogestrel is approximately 38 ± 20 hours at steady state. In addition to 3-keto-desogestrel, other phase I metabolites are 3α-OH-desogestrel, 3β-OH-desogestrel, and 3α-OH-5α-H-desogestrel. These other metabolites are not known to have any pharmacologic effects, and are further converted in part by conjugation (phase II metabolism) into polar metabolites, mainly sulfates and glucuronides.

Ethinyl estradiol is rapidly and almost completely absorbed. In the third cycle of use after a single dose of ORTHO-CEPT, the relative bioavailability is approximately 83%.

In the third cycle of use after a single dose of ORTHO-CEPT, maximum concentrations of ethinyl estradiol of 95 ± 34 pg/mL are reached at 1.5 ± 0.8 hours. The $AUC_{0-\infty}$ is 1,471 ± 268 pg/mL•hr after a single dose. At steady state, attained from at least day 19 onwards, maximum ethinyl estradiol concentrations of 141 ± 48 pg/mL are reached at about 1.4 ± 0.7 hours. The minimum serum levels of ethinyl estradiol at steady state are 24 ± 8.3 pg/mL. The AUC_{0-24}, at steady state is 1,117 ± 302 pg/mL•hr. The mean $AUC_{0-\infty}$ for ethinyl estradiol following a single dose during treatment cycle 3 does not significantly differ from the mean AUC_{0-24} at steady state. This finding indicates linear kinetics for ethinyl estradiol.

The elimination half-life is 26 ± 6.8 hours at steady state. Ethinyl estradiol is subject to a significant degree of presystemic conjugation (phase II metabolism). Ethinyl estradiol escaping gut wall conjugation undergoes phase I metabolism and hepatic conjugation (phase II metabolism). Major phase I metabolites are 2-OH-ethinyl estradiol and 2-methoxy-ethinyl estradiol. Sulfate and glucuronide conjugates of both ethinyl estradiol and phase I metabolites, which are excreted in bile, can undergo enterohepatic circulation.

INDICATIONS AND USAGE

ORTHO-CEPT Tablets are indicated for the prevention of pregnancy in women who elect to use oral contraceptives as a method of contraception.

Oral contraceptives are highly effective. Table I lists the typical accidental pregnancy rates for users of combination oral contraceptives and other methods of contraception. The efficacy of these contraceptive methods, except sterilization, the IUD, and the Norplant System depends upon the reliability with which they are used. Correct and consistent use of these methods can result in lower failure rates.

In a clinical trial with ORTHO-CEPT, 1,195 subjects completed 11,656 cycles and a total of 10 pregnancies were reported. This represents an overall user-efficacy (typical user-efficacy) pregnancy rate of 1.12 per 100 women-years. This rate includes patients who did not take the drug correctly.

[See table I at left]

ORTHO-CEPT has not been studied for and is not indicated for use in emergency contraception.

CONTRAINDICATIONS

Oral contraceptives should not be used in women who currently have the following conditions:

- Thrombophlebitis or thromboembolic disorders
- A past history of deep vein thrombophlebitis or thromboembolic disorders
- Cerebral vascular or coronary artery disease (current or history)
- Valvular heart disease with complications
- Severe hypertension
- Diabetes with vascular involvement
- Headaches with focal neurological symptoms
- Major surgery with prolonged immobilization
- Known or suspected carcinoma of the breast or personal history of breast cancer
- Carcinoma of the endometrium or other known or suspected estrogen-dependent neoplasia
- Undiagnosed abnormal genital bleeding
- Cholestatic jaundice of pregnancy or jaundice with prior pill use
- Acute or chronic hepatocellular disease with abnormal liver function
- Hepatic adenomas or carcinomas
- Known or suspected pregnancy
- Hypersensitivity to any component of this product

WARNINGS

Cigarette smoking increases the risk of serious cardiovascular side effects from oral contraceptive use. This risk increases with age and with heavy smoking (15 or more cigarettes per day) and is quite marked in women over 35 years of age. Women who use oral contraceptives should be strongly advised not to smoke.

The use of oral contraceptives is associated with increased risks of several serious conditions including myocardial infarction, thromboembolism, stroke, hepatic neoplasia, and gallbladder disease, although the risk of serious morbidity or mortality is very small in healthy women without underlying risk factors. The risk of morbidity and mortality in-

TABLE I: PERCENTAGE OF WOMEN EXPERIENCING AN UNINTENDED PREGNANCY DURING THE FIRST YEAR OF TYPICAL USE AND THE FIRST YEAR OF PERFECT USE OF CONTRACEPTION AND THE PERCENTAGE CONTINUING USE AT THE END OF THE FIRST YEAR, UNITED STATES.

	% of Women Experiencing an Unintended Pregnancy within the First Year of Use		% of Women Continuing Use at One Year[3]
Method (1)	Typical Use[1] (2)	Perfect Use[2] (3)	(4)
Chance[4]	85	85	
Spermicides[5]	26	6	40
Periodic abstinence	25		63
Calendar		9	
Ovulation Method		3	
Sympto-Thermal[6]		2	
Post-Ovulation		1	
Withdrawal	19	4	
Cap[7]			
Parous Women	40	26	42
Nulliparous Women	20	9	56
Sponge			
Parous Women	40	20	42
Nulliparous Women	20	9	56
Diaphragm[7]	20	6	56
Condom[8]			
Female (Reality)	21	5	56
Male	14	3	61
Pill	5		71
Progestin Only		0.5	
Combined		0.1	
IUD			
Progesterone T	2.0	1.5	81
Copper T 380A	0.8	0.6	78
LNg 20	0.1	0.1	81
Depo-Provera	0.3	0.3	70
Norplant and Norplant-2	0.05	0.05	88
Female Sterilization	0.5	0.5	100
Male Sterilization	0.15	0.10	100

Emergency Contraceptive Pills: Treatment initiated within 72 hours after unprotected intercourse reduces the risk of pregnancy by at least 75%.[9]

Lactation Amenorrhea Method: LAM is a highly effective, temporary method of contraception.[10]

Source: Trussell J. Contraceptive efficacy in Hatcher RA, Trussell J, Stewart F, Cates W, Stewart GK, Kowel D, Guest F, Contraceptive Technology: Seventeenth Revised Edition. New York, NY; Irvington Publishers, 1998.

1 Among *typical* couples who initiate use of a method (not necessarily for the first time), the percentage who experience an accidental pregnancy during the first year if they do not stop use for any other reason.

2 Among couples who initiate use of a method (not necessarily for the first time) and who use it *perfectly* (both consistently and correctly), the percentage who experience an accidental pregnancy during the first year if they do not stop use for any other reason.

3 Among couples attempting to avoid pregnancy, the percentage who continue to use a method for one year.

4 The percents becoming pregnant in columns (2) and (3) are based on data from populations where contraception is not used and from women who cease using contraception in order to become pregnant. Among such populations, about 89% become pregnant within one year. This estimate was lowered slightly (to 85%) to represent the percent who would become pregnant within one year among women now relying on reversible methods of contraception if they abandoned contraception altogether.

5 Foams, creams, gels, vaginal suppositories, and vaginal film.

6 Cervical mucus (ovulation) method supplemented by calendar in the pre-ovulatory and basal body temperature in the post-ovulatory phases.

7 With spermicidal cream or jelly.

8 Without spermicides.

9 The treatment schedule is one dose within 72 hours after unprotected intercourse, and a second dose 12 hours after the first dose. The FDA has declared the following brands of oral contraceptives to be safe and effective for emergency contraception: Ovral® (1 dose is 2 white pills), Alesse® (1 dose is 5 pink pills), Nordette® or Levlen® (1 dose is 4 yellow pills).

10 However, to maintain effective protection against pregnancy, another method or contraception must be used as soon as menstruation resumes, the frequency of duration of breastfeeds is reduced, bottle feeds are introduced, or the baby reaches 6 months of age.

creases significantly in the presence of other underlying risk factors such as hypertension, hyperlipidemias, obesity and diabetes.

Practitioners prescribing oral contraceptives should be familiar with the following information relating to these risks.

The information contained in this package insert is principally based on studies carried out in patients who used oral contraceptives with formulations of higher doses of estrogens and progestogens than those in common use today. The effect of long term use of the oral contraceptives with formulations of lower doses of both estrogens and progestogens remains to be determined.

Throughout this labeling, epidemiological studies reported are of two types: retrospective or case control studies and prospective or cohort studies. Case control studies provide a measure of the relative risk of a disease, namely, a *ratio* of the incidence of a disease among oral contraceptive users to that among nonusers. The relative risk does not provide information on the actual clinical occurrence of a disease. Cohort studies provide a measure of attributable risk, which is the *difference* in the incidence of disease between oral contraceptive users and nonusers. The attributable risk does provide information about the actual occurrence of a disease in the population (Adapted from refs. 2 and 3 with the author's permission). For further information, the reader is referred to a text on epidemiological methods.

1. THROMBOEMBOLIC DISORDERS AND OTHER VASCULAR PROBLEMS

a. Thromboembolism

An increased risk of thromboembolic and thrombotic disease associated with the use of oral contraceptives is well established. Case control studies have found the relative risk of users compared to non-users to be 3 for the first episode of superficial venous thrombosis, 4 to 11 for deep vein thrombosis or pulmonary embolism, and 1.5 to 6 for women with predisposing conditions for venous thromboembolic disease.[2, 3, 19-24] Cohort studies have shown the relative risk to be somewhat lower, about 3 for new cases and about 4.5 for new cases requiring hospitalization.[25] The risk of thromboembolic disease associated with oral contraceptives is not related to length of use and disappears after pill use is stopped.[2]

Several epidemiologic studies indicate that third generation oral contraceptives, including those containing desogestrel, are associated with a higher risk of venous thromboembolism than certain second generation oral contraceptives. In general, these studies indicate an approximate 2-fold increased risk, which corresponds to an additional 1-2 cases of venous thromboembolism per 10,000 women-years of use. However, data from additional studies have not shown this 2-fold increase in risk.

A two- to four-fold increase in relative risk of post-operative thromboembolic complications has been reported with the use of oral contraceptives.[9] The relative risk of venous thrombosis in women who have predisposing conditions is twice that of women without such medical conditions.[26] If feasible, oral contraceptives should be discontinued at least four weeks prior to and for two weeks after elective surgery of a type associated with an increase in risk of thromboembolism and during and following prolonged immobilization. Since the immediate postpartum period is also associated with an increased risk of thromboembolism, oral contraceptives should be started no earlier than four weeks after delivery in women who elect not to breast feed.

b. Myocardial infarction

An increased risk of myocardial infarction has been attributed to oral contraceptive use. This risk is primarily in smokers or women with other underlying risk factors for coronary artery disease such as hypertension, hypercholesterolemia, morbid obesity, and diabetes. The relative risk of heart attack for current oral contraceptive users has been estimated to be two to six.[4-10] The risk is very low in women under the age of 30.

Smoking in combination with oral contraceptive use has been shown to contribute substantially to the incidence of myocardial infarctions in women in their mid-thirties or older with smoking accounting for the majority of excess cases.[11] Mortality rates associated with circulatory disease have been shown to increase substantially in smokers, especially in those 35 years of age and older and in nonsmokers over the age of 40 among women who use oral contraceptives. (See Table II)

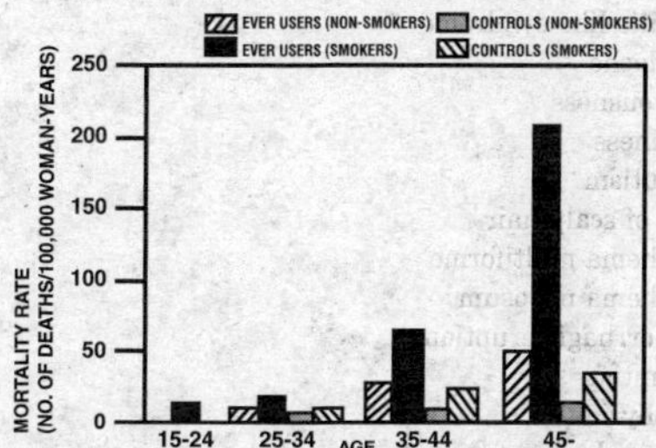

TABLE II. (Adapted from P.M. Layde and V. Beral, ref #12.)

Oral contraceptives may compound the effects of well-known risk factors, such as hypertension, diabetes, hyperlipidemias, age and obesity.[13] In particular, some progestogens are known to decrease HDL cholesterol and cause glucose intolerance, while estrogens may create a state of hyperinsulinism.[14-18] Oral contraceptives have been shown to increase blood pressure among users (see section 9 in WARNINGS). Similar effects on risk factors have been associated with an increased risk of heart disease. Oral contraceptives must be used with caution in women with cardiovascular disease risk factors.

There is some evidence that the risk of myocardial infarction associated with oral contraceptives is lower when the progestogen has minimal androgenic activity than when the activity is greater. Receptor binding and animal studies have shown that desogestrel or its active metabolite has minimal androgenic activity (see CLINICAL PHARMACOLOGY), although these findings have not been confirmed in adequate and well-controlled clinical trials.

c. Cerebrovascular diseases

Oral contraceptives have been shown to increase both the relative and attributable risks of cerebrovascular events (thrombotic and hemorrhagic strokes), although, in general, the risk is greatest among older (> 35 years), hypertensive women who also smoke. Hypertension was found to be a risk factor for both users and nonusers, for both types of strokes, and smoking interacted to increase the risk of stroke.[27-29]

In a large study, the relative risk of thrombotic strokes has been shown to range from 3 for normotensive users to 14 for users with severe hypertension.[30] The relative risk of hemorrhagic stroke is reported to be 1.2 for non-smokers who used oral contraceptives, 2.6 for smokers who did not use oral contraceptives, 7.6 for smokers who used oral contraceptives, 1.8 for normotensive users and 25.7 for users with severe hypertension.[30] The attributable risk is also greater in older women.[3]

d. Dose-related risk of vascular disease from oral contraceptives

A positive association has been observed between the amount of estrogen and progestogen in oral contraceptives and the risk of vascular disease.[31-33] A decline in serum high density lipoproteins (HDL) has been reported with many progestational agents.[14-16] A decline in serum high density lipoproteins has been associated with an increased incidence of ischemic heart disease. Because estrogens increase HDL cholesterol, the net effect of an oral contraceptive depends on a balance achieved between doses of estrogen and progestogen and the nature and absolute amount of progestogens used in the contraceptives. The amount of both hormones should be considered in the choice of an oral contraceptive.

Minimizing exposure to estrogen and progestogen is in keeping with good principles of therapeutics. For any particular estrogen/progestogen combination, the dosage regimen prescribed should be one which contains the least amount of estrogen and progestogen that is compatible with a low failure rate and the needs of the individual patient. New acceptors of oral contraceptive agents should be started on preparations containing the lowest estrogen content which is judged appropriate for the individual patient.

e. Persistence of risk of vascular disease

There are two studies which have shown persistence of risk of vascular disease for ever-users of oral contraceptives. In a study in the United States, the risk of developing myocardial infarction after discontinuing oral contraceptives persists for at least 9 years for women 40-49 years old who had used oral contraceptives for five or more years, but this increased risk was not demonstrated in other age groups.[8] In another study in Great Britain, the risk of developing cerebrovascular disease persisted for at least 6 years after discontinuation of oral contraceptives, although excess risk was very small.[34] However, both studies were performed with oral contraceptive formulations containing 0.050 mg or higher of estrogens.

2. ESTIMATES OF MORTALITY FROM CONTRACEPTIVE USE

One study gathered data from a variety of sources which have estimated the mortality rate associated with different methods of contraception at different ages (Table III). These estimates include the combined risk of death associated with contraceptive methods plus the risk attributable to pregnancy in the event of method failure. Each method of contraception has its specific benefits and risks. The study concluded that with the exception of oral contraceptive users 35 and older who smoke and 40 and older who do not smoke, mortality associated with all methods of birth control is low and below that associated with childbirth.

TABLE III: ANNUAL NUMBER OF BIRTH-RELATED OR METHOD-RELATED DEATHS ASSOCIATED WITH CONTROL OF FERTILITY PER 100,000 NONSTERILE WOMEN, BY FERTILITY CONTROL METHOD ACCORDING TO AGE

Method of control and outcome	15-19	20-24	25-29	30-34	35-39	40-44
No fertility control methods*	7.0	7.4	9.1	14.8	25.7	28.2
Oral contraceptives non-smoker**	0.3	0.5	0.9	1.9	13.8	31.6
Oral contraceptives smoker**	2.2	3.4	6.6	13.5	51.1	117.2
IUD**	0.8	0.8	1.0	1.0	1.4	1.4
Condom*	1.1	1.6	0.7	0.2	0.3	0.4
Diaphragm/spermicide*	1.9	1.2	1.2	1.3	2.2	2.8
Periodic abstinence*	2.5	1.6	1.6	1.7	2.9	3.6

*Deaths are birth-related
**Deaths are method-related

Adapted from H.W. Ory, ref. #35.

The observation of an increase in risk of mortality with age for oral contraceptive users is based on data gathered in the 1970's.[35] Current clinical recommendation involves the use of lower estrogen dose formulations and a careful consideration of risk factors. In 1989, the Fertility and Maternal Health Drugs Advisory Committee was asked to review the use of oral contraceptives in women 40 years of age and over. The Committee concluded that although cardiovascular disease risk may be increased with oral contraceptive use after age 40 in healthy non-smoking women (even with the newer low-dose formulations), there are also greater potential health risks associated with pregnancy in older women and with the alternative surgical and medical procedures which may be necessary if such women do not have access to effective and acceptable means of contraception. The Committee recommended that the benefits of low-dose oral contraceptive use by healthy non-smoking women over 40 may outweigh the possible risks.

Of course, older women, as all women who take oral contraceptives, should take an oral contraceptive which contains the least amount of estrogen and progestogen that is compatible with a low failure rate and individual patient needs. [See table III above]

3. CARCINOMA OF THE REPRODUCTIVE ORGANS AND BREASTS

Numerous epidemiological studies have been performed on the incidence of breast, endometrial, ovarian, and cervical cancer in women using oral contraceptives.

The risk of having breast cancer diagnosed may be slightly increased among current and recent users of combination oral contraceptives. However, this excess risk appears to decrease over time after discontinuation of combination oral contraceptives and by 10 years after cessation the increased risk disappears. Some studies report an increased risk with duration of use while other studies do not and no consistent relationships have been found with dose or type of steroid. Some studies have found a small increase in risk for women who first use combination oral contraceptives before age 20. Most studies show a similar pattern of risk with combination oral contraceptives regardless of a woman's reproductive history or her family breast cancer history.

Breast cancers diagnosed in current or previous oral contraceptive users tend to be less clinically advanced than in nonusers.

Women who currently have or have had breast cancer should not use oral contraceptives because breast cancer is usually a hormonally-sensitive tumor.

Some studies suggest that oral contraceptive use has been associated with an increase in the risk of cervical intraepithelial neoplasia in some populations of women.[45-48] However, there continues to be controversy about the extent to which such findings may be due to differences in sexual behavior and other factors.

In spite of many studies of the relationship between oral contraceptive use and breast and cervical cancers, a cause-and-effect relationship has not been established.

4. HEPATIC NEOPLASIA

Benign hepatic adenomas are associated with oral contraceptive use, although the incidence of benign tumors is rare in the United States. Indirect calculations have estimated the attributable risk to be in the range of 3.3 cases/100,000 for users, a risk that increases after four or more years of use especially with oral contraceptives of higher dose.[49] Rupture of benign, hepatic adenomas may cause death through intra-abdominal hemorrhage.[50,51]

Studies from Britain have shown an increased risk of developing hepatocellular carcinoma in long-term (>8 years) oral contraceptive users. However, these cancers are extremely rare in the U.S. and the attributable risk (the excess incidence) of liver cancers in oral contraceptive users approaches less than one per million users.

5. OCULAR LESIONS

There have been clinical case reports of retinal thrombosis associated with the use of oral contraceptives. Oral contraceptives should be discontinued if there is unexplained partial or complete loss of vision; onset of proptosis or diplopia;

Continued on next page

Ortho-Cept—Cont.

papilledema; or retinal vascular lesions. Appropriate diagnostic and therapeutic measures should be undertaken immediately.

6. ORAL CONTRACEPTIVE USE BEFORE OR DURING EARLY PREGNANCY

Extensive epidemiological studies have revealed no increased risk of birth defects in women who have used oral contraceptives prior to pregnancy.[56–57] The majority of recent studies also do not indicate a teratogenic effect, particularly in so far as cardiac anomalies and limb reduction defects are concerned,[55,56,58,59] when oral contraceptives are taken inadvertently during early pregnancy.

The administration of oral contraceptives to induce withdrawal bleeding should not be used as a test for pregnancy. Oral contraceptives should not be used during pregnancy to treat threatened or habitual abortion.

It is recommended that for any patient who has missed two consecutive periods, pregnancy should be ruled out. If the patient has not adhered to the prescribed schedule, the possibility of pregnancy should be considered at the time of the first missed period. Oral contraceptive use should be discontinued if pregnancy is confirmed.

7. GALLBLADDER DISEASE

Earlier studies have reported an increased lifetime relative risk of gallbladder surgery in users of oral contraceptives and estrogens.[60,61] More recent studies, however, have shown that the relative risk of developing gallbladder disease among oral contraceptive users may be minimal.[62-64] The recent findings of minimal risk may be related to the use of oral contraceptive formulations containing lower hormonal doses of estrogens and progestogens.

8. CARBOHYDRATE AND LIPID METABOLIC EFFECTS

Oral contraceptives have been shown to cause a decrease in glucose tolerance in a significant percentage of users.[17] This effect has been shown to be directly related to estrogen dose.[65] In general, progestogens increase insulin secretion and create insulin resistance, this effect varying with different progestational agents.[17,66] In the nondiabetic woman, oral contraceptives appear to have no effect on fasting blood glucose.[67] Because of these demonstrated effects, prediabetic and diabetic women should be carefully monitored while taking oral contraceptives.

A small proportion of women will have persistent hypertriglyceridemia while on the pill. As discussed earlier (see WARNINGS 1.a. and 1.d.), changes in serum triglycerides and lipoprotein levels have been reported in oral contraceptive users.

9. ELEVATED BLOOD PRESSURE

Women with significant hypertension should not be started on hormonal contraception.[98] An increase in blood pressure has been reported in women taking oral contraceptives[68] and this increase is more likely in older oral contraceptive users[69] and with extended duration of use.[61] Data from the Royal College of General Practitioners[12] and subsequent randomized trials have shown that the incidence of hypertension increases with increasing progestational activity and concentrations of progestogens.

Women with a history of hypertension or hypertension-related diseases, or renal disease[70] should be encouraged to use another method of contraception. If women elect to use oral contraceptives, they should be monitored closely and if significant elevation of blood pressure occurs, oral contraceptives should be discontinued. For most women, elevated blood pressure will return to normal after stopping oral contraceptives,[69] and there is no difference in the occurrence of hypertension among former and never users.[68,70,71]

10. HEADACHE

The onset or exacerbation of migraine or development of headache with a new pattern which is recurrent, persistent or severe requires discontinuation of oral contraceptives and evaluation of the cause.

11. BLEEDING IRREGULARITIES

Breakthrough bleeding and spotting are sometimes encountered in patients on oral contraceptives, especially during the first three months of use. Nonhormonal causes should be considered and adequate diagnostic measures taken to rule out malignancy or pregnancy in the event of breakthrough bleeding, as in the case of any abnormal vaginal bleeding. If pathology has been excluded, time or a change to another formulation may solve the problem. In the event of amenorrhea, pregnancy should be ruled out.

Some women may encounter post-pill amenorrhea or oligomenorrhea, especially when such a condition was preexistent.

12. ECTOPIC PREGNANCY

Ectopic as well as intrauterine pregnancy may occur in contraceptive failures.

PRECAUTIONS

1. GENERAL

Patients should be counseled that this product does not protect against HIV infection (AIDS) and other sexually transmitted diseases.

2. PHYSICAL EXAMINATION AND FOLLOW UP

It is good medical practice for all women to have annual history and physical examinations, including women using oral contraceptives. The physical examination, however, may be deferred until after initiation of oral contraceptives if requested by the woman and judged appropriate by the clinician. The physical examination should include special reference to blood pressure, breasts, abdomen and pelvic organs, including cervical cytology, and relevant laboratory tests. In case of undiagnosed, persistent or recurrent abnormal vaginal bleeding, appropriate measures should be conducted to rule out malignancy. Women with a strong family history of breast cancer or who have breast nodules should be monitored with particular care.

3. LIPID DISORDERS

Women who are being treated for hyperlipidemias should be followed closely if they elect to use oral contraceptives. Some progestogens may elevate LDL levels and may render the control of hyperlipidemias more difficult.

4. LIVER FUNCTION

If jaundice develops in any woman receiving oral contraceptives, the medication should be discontinued. Steroid hormones may be poorly metabolized in patients with impaired liver function.

5. FLUID RETENTION

Oral contraceptives may cause some degree of fluid retention. They should be prescribed with caution, and only with careful monitoring, in patients with conditions which might be aggravated by fluid retention.

6. EMOTIONAL DISORDERS

Women with a history of depression should be carefully observed and the drug discontinued if depression recurs to a serious degree.

7. CONTACT LENSES

Contact lens wearers who develop visual changes or changes in lens tolerance should be assessed by an ophthalmologist.

8. DRUG INTERACTIONS

Changes in contraceptive effectiveness associated with co-administration of other products:

Contraceptive effectiveness may be reduced when hormonal contraceptives are coadministered with antibiotics, anticonvulsants, and other drugs that increase the metabolism of contraceptive steroids. This could result in unintended pregnancy or breakthrough bleeding. Examples include rifampin, barbiturates, phenylbutazone, phenytoin, carbamazepine, felbamate, oxcarbazepine, topiramate, and griseofulvin. Several cases of contraceptive failure and breakthrough bleeding have been reported in the literature with concomitant administration of antibiotics such as ampicillin and tetracyclines. However, clinical pharmacology studies investigating drug interaction between combined oral contraceptives and these antibiotics have reported inconsistent results.

Several of the anti-HIV protease inhibitors have been studied with co-administration of oral combination hormonal contraceptives; significant changes (increase and decrease) in the plasma levels of the estrogen and progestin have been noted in some cases. The safety and efficacy of oral contraceptive products may be affected with co-administration of anti-HIV protease inhibitors. Healthcare professionals should refer to the label of the individual anti-HIV protease inhibitors for further drug-drug interaction information.

Herbal products containing St. John's Wort (hypericum perforatum) may induce hepatic enzymes (cytochrome P450) and p-glycoprotein transporter and may reduce the effectiveness of contraceptive steroids. This may also result in breakthrough bleeding.

Increase in plasma levels associated with co-administered drugs:

Co-administration of atorvastatin and certain oral contraceptives containing ethinyl estradiol increase AUC values for ethinyl estradiol by approximately 20%. Ascorbic acid and acetaminophen may increase plasma ethinyl estradiol levels, possibly by inhibition of conjugation. CYP 3A4 inhibitors such as itraconazole or ketoconazole may increase plasma hormone levels.

Changes in plasma levels of co-administered drugs:

Combination hormonal contraceptives containing some synthetic estrogens (e.g., ethinyl estradiol) may inhibit the metabolism of other compounds. Increased plasma concentrations of cyclosporin, prednisolone, and theophylline have been reported with concomitant administration of oral contraceptives. Decreased plasma concentrations of acetaminophen and increased clearance of temazepam, salicylic acid, morphine and clofibric acid, due to induction of conjugation, have been noted when these drugs were administered with oral contraceptives.

9. INTERACTIONS WITH LABORATORY TESTS

Certain endocrine and liver function tests and blood components may be affected by oral contraceptives:

a. Increased prothrombin and factors VII, VIII, IX, and X; decreased antithrombin 3; increased norepinephrine-induced platelet aggregability.
b. Increased thyroid binding globulin (TBG) leading to increased circulating total thyroid hormone, as measured by protein-bound iodine (PBI), T4 by column or by radioimmunoassay. Free T3 resin uptake is decreased, reflecting the elevated TBG; free T4 concentration is unaltered.
c. Other binding proteins may be elevated in serum.
d. Sex hormone binding globulins are increased and result in elevated levels of total circulating sex steroids however, free or biologically active levels either decrease or remain unchanged.
e. Triglycerides may be increased and levels of various other lipids and lipoproteins may be affected.
f. Glucose tolerance may be decreased.
g. Serum folate levels may be depressed by oral contraceptive therapy. This may be of clinical significance if a woman becomes pregnant shortly after discontinuing oral contraceptives.

10. CARCINOGENESIS

See WARNINGS section.

11. PREGNANCY

Pregnancy Category X. See CONTRAINDICATIONS and WARNINGS sections.

12. NURSING MOTHERS

Small amounts of oral contraceptive steroids have been identified in the milk of nursing mothers and a few adverse effects on the child have been reported, including jaundice and breast enlargement. In addition, oral contraceptives given in the postpartum period may interfere with lactation by decreasing the quantity and quality of breast milk. If possible, the nursing mother should be advised not to use oral contraceptives but to use other forms of contraception until she has completely weaned her child.

13. PEDIATRIC USE

Safety and efficacy of ORTHO-CEPT Tablets have been established in women of reproductive age. Safety and efficacy are expected to be the same for postpubertal adolescents under the age of 16 and for users 16 years and older. Use of this product before menarche is not indicated.

14. GERIATRIC USE

This product has not been studied in women over 65 years of age and is not indicated in this population.

INFORMATION FOR THE PATIENT

See Patient Labeling Printed Below

ADVERSE REACTIONS

An increased risk of the following serious adverse reactions has been associated with the use of oral contraceptives (see WARNINGS section).

- Thrombophlebitis and venous thrombosis with or without embolism
- Arterial thromboembolism
- Pulmonary embolism
- Myocardial infarction
- Cerebral hemorrhage
- Cerebral thrombosis
- Hypertension
- Gallbladder disease
- Hepatic adenomas or benign liver tumors

There is evidence of an association between the following conditions and the use of oral contraceptives:

- Mesenteric thrombosis
- Retinal thrombosis

The following adverse reactions have been reported in patients receiving oral contraceptives and are believed to be drug-related:

- Nausea
- Vomiting
- Gastrointestinal symptoms (such as abdominal cramps and bloating)
- Breakthrough bleeding
- Spotting
- Change in menstrual flow
- Amenorrhea
- Temporary infertility after discontinuation of treatment
- Edema
- Melasma which may persist
- Breast changes: tenderness, enlargement, secretion
- Change in weight (increase or decrease)
- Change in cervical erosion and secretion
- Diminution in lactation when given immediately postpartum
- Cholestatic jaundice
- Migraine
- Rash (allergic)
- Mental depression
- Reduced tolerance to carbohydrates
- Vaginal candidiasis
- Change in corneal curvature (steepening)
- Intolerance to contact lenses

The following adverse reactions have been reported in users of oral contraceptives and a casual association has been neither confirmed nor refuted:

- Pre-menstrual syndrome
- Cataracts
- Changes in appetite
- Cystitis-like syndrome
- Headache
- Nervousness
- Dizziness
- Hirsutism
- Loss of scalp hair
- Erythema multiforme
- Erythema nodosum
- Hemorrhagic eruption
- Vaginitis
- Porphyria
- Impaired renal function
- Hemolytic uremic syndrome
- Acne
- Changes in libido
- Colitis
- Budd-Chiari Syndrome

OVERDOSAGE

Serious ill effects have not been reported following acute ingestion of large doses of oral contraceptives by young children. Overdosage may cause nausea, and withdrawal bleeding may occur in females.

NON-CONTRACEPTIVE HEALTH BENEFITS

The following non-contraceptive health benefits related to the use of oral contraceptives are supported by epidemiological studies which largely utilized oral contraceptive formulations containing estrogen doses exceeding 0.035 mg of ethinyl estradiol or 0.05 mg of mestranol.[73-78]

Effects on menses:

- increased menstrual cycle regularity
- decreased blood loss and decreased incidence of iron deficiency anemia
- decreased incidence of dysmenorrhea

Effects related to inhibition of ovulation:

- decreased incidence of functional ovarian cysts
- decreased incidence of ectopic pregnancies

Effects from long-term use:

- decreased incidence of fibroadenomas and fibrocystic disease of the breast
- decreased incidence of acute pelvic inflammatory disease
- decreased incidence of endometrial cancer
- decreased incidence of ovarian cancer

DOSAGE AND ADMINISTRATION

To achieve maximum contraceptive effectiveness, ORTHO-CEPT must be taken exactly as directed and at intervals not exceeding 24 hours. ORTHO-CEPT is available in the DIALPAK® Tablet Dispenser which is preset for a Sunday Start. Day 1 Start is also provided.

Day 1 Start

The dosage of ORTHO-CEPT for the initial cycle of therapy is one light orange "active" tablet administered daily from the 1st day through the 21st day of the menstrual cycle, counting the first day of menstrual flow as "Day 1." Tablets are taken without interruption as follows: One light orange "active" tablet daily for 21 days, then one green "reminder" tablet daily for 7 days. After 28 tablets have been taken, a new course is started and a light orange "active" tablet is taken the next day.

The use of ORTHO-CEPT for contraception may be initiated 4 weeks postpartum in women who elect not to breast feed. When the tablets are administered during the postpartum period, the increased risk of thromboembolic disease associated with the postpartum period must be considered. (See CONTRAINDICATIONS and WARNINGS concerning thromboembolic disease. See also PRECAUTIONS for "Nursing Mothers".) If the patient starts on ORTHO-CEPT postpartum, and has not yet had a period, she should be instructed to use another method of contraception until a light orange "active" tablet has been taken daily for 7 days. The possibility of ovulation and conception prior to initiation of medication should be considered. If the patient misses one (1) light orange "active" tablet in Weeks 1, 2, or 3, the tablet should be taken as soon as she remembers. If the patient misses two (2) light orange "active" tablets in Week 1 or Week 2, the patient should take two (2) light orange "active" tablets the day she remembers and two (2) light orange "active" tablets the next day; and then continue taking one (1) light orange "active" tablet a day until she finishes the pack. The patient should be instructed to use a back-up method of birth control such as condoms or spermicide if she has sex in the seven (7) days after missing pills. If the patient misses two (2) light orange "active" tablets in the third week or misses three (3) or more light orange "active" tablets in a row, the patient should throw out the rest of the pack and start a new pack that same day. The patient should be instructed to use a back-up method of birth control if she has sex in the seven (7) days after missing pills.

Sunday Start

When taking ORTHO-CEPT, the first light orange "active" tablet should be taken on the first Sunday after menstruation begins. If period begins on Sunday, the first light orange "active" tablet is taken on that day. If switching directly from another oral contraceptive, the first light orange "active" tablet should be taken on the first Sunday after the last ACTIVE tablet of the previous product. Tablets are taken without interruption as follows: One light orange "active" tablet daily for 21 days, then one green "reminder" tablet daily for 7 days. After 28 tablets have been taken, a new course is started and a light orange "active" tablet is taken the next day (Sunday). When initiating a Sunday start regimen, another method of contraception should be used until after the first 7 consecutive days of administration.

The use of ORTHO-CEPT for contraception may be initiated 4 weeks postpartum. When the tablets are administered during the postpartum period, the increased risk of thromboembolic disease associated with the postpartum period must be considered. (See CONTRAINDICATIONS and WARNINGS concerning thromboembolic disease. See also PRECAUTIONS for "Nursing Mothers".) If the patient starts on ORTHO-CEPT postpartum, and has not yet had a period, she should be instructed to use another method of contraception until a light orange "active" tablet has been taken daily for 7 days. The possibility of ovulation and conception prior to initiation of medication should be considered. If the patient misses one (1) light orange "active" tablet in Weeks 1, 2, or 3, the light orange "active" tablet should be taken as soon as she remembers. If the patient misses two (2) light orange "active" tablets in Week 1 or Week 2, the patient should take two (2) light orange "active" tablets the day she remembers and two (2) light orange "active" tablets the next day; and then continue taking one (1) light orange "active" tablet a day until she finishes the pack. The patient should be instructed to use a back-up method of birth control such as condoms or spermicide if she has sex in the seven (7) days after missing pills. If the patient misses two (2) light orange "active" tablets in the third week or misses three (3) or more light orange "active" tablets in a row, the patient should continue taking one light orange "active" tablet every day until Sunday. On Sunday the patient should throw out the rest of the pack and start a new pack that same day. The patient should be instructed to use a back-up method of birth control if she has sex in the seven (7) days after missing pills.

ADDITIONAL INSTRUCTIONS FOR ALL DOSING REGIMENS

Breakthrough bleeding, spotting, and amenorrhea are frequent reasons for patients discontinuing oral contraceptives. In breakthrough bleeding, as in all cases of irregular bleeding from the vagina, nonfunctional causes should be borne in mind. In undiagnosed persistent or recurrent abnormal bleeding from the vagina, adequate diagnostic measures are indicated to rule out pregnancy or malignancy. If pathology has been excluded, time or a change to another formulation may solve the problem. Changing to an oral contraceptive with a higher estrogen content, while potentially useful in minimizing menstrual irregularity, should be done only if necessary since this may increase the risk of thromboembolic disease.

Use of oral contraceptives in the event of a missed menstrual period:

1. If the patient has not adhered to the prescribed schedule, the possibility of pregnancy should be considered at the time of the first missed period and oral contraceptive use should be discontinued if pregnancy is confirmed.
2. If the patient has adhered to the prescribed regimen and misses two consecutive periods, pregnancy should be ruled out.

HOW SUPPLIED

ORTHO-CEPT Tablets are available in a DIALPAK® Tablet Dispenser (NDC 0062-1796-15) containing 28 tablets, as follows: 21 light orange, round, convex, beveled edged, coated tablets imprinted "ORTHO" on one side and "D 150" on the other side containing 0.15 mg desogestrel together with 0.03 mg ethinyl estradiol, and 7 green, round, convex, beveled edged, coated tablets imprinted "ORTHO P" on both sides containing inert ingredients.

STORAGE: Store at 25°C (77°F); excursions permitted to 15°-30°C (59°-86°F).

Rx only

REFERENCES

1. Trussell J. Contraceptive efficacy. In Hatcher RA, Trussell J, Stewart F, Cates W, Stewart GK, Kowal D, Guest F. Contraceptive Technology: Seventeenth Revised Edition. New York NY: Irvington Publishers, 1998, in press. **2.** Stadel BV. Oral contraceptives and cardiovascular disease. (Pt.1). N Engl J Med 1981; 305:612-618. **3.** Stadel BV. Oral contraceptives and cardiovascular disease. (Pt. 2). N Engl J Med 1981; 305:672-677. **4.** Adam SA, Thorogood M. Oral contraception and myocardial infarction revisited: the effects of new preparations and prescribing patterns. Br J Obstet and Gynecol 1981; 88:838-845. **5.** Mann JI, Inman WH. Oral contraceptives and death from myocardial infarction. Br Med J 1975; 2 (5965):245-248. **6.** Mann JI, Vessey MP, Thorogood M, Doll R. Myocardial infarction in young women with special reference to oral contraceptive practice. Br Med J 1975; 2(5956):241-245. **7.** Royal College of General Practitioners' Oral Contraception Study: Further analyses of mortality in oral contraceptive users. Lancet 1981;1:541-546. **8.** Slone D, Shapiro S, Kaufman DW, Rosenberg L, Miettinen OS, Stolley PD. Risk of myocardial infarction in relation to current and discontinued use of oral contraceptives. N Engl J Med 1981; 305:420-424. **9.** Vessey MP. Female hormones and vascular disease—an epidemiological overview. Br J Fam Plann 1980; 6 (Supplement):1-12. **10.** Russell-Briefel RG, Ezzati TM, Fulwood R, Perlman JA, Murphy RS. Cardiovascular risk status and oral contraceptive use, United States, 1976-80. Prevent Med 1986; 15:352-362. **11.** Goldbaum GM, Kendrick JS, Hogelin GC, Gentry EM. The relative impact of smoking and oral contraceptive use on women in the United States. JAMA 1987; 258:1339-1342. **12.** Layde PM, Beral V. Further analyses of mortality in oral contraceptive users: Royal College of General Practitioners' Oral Contraception Study. (Table 5) Lancet 1981; 1:541-546. **13.** Knopp RH. Arteriosclerosis risk: the roles of oral contraceptives and postmenopausal estrogens. J Reprod Med 1986; 31(9) (Supplement):913-921. **14.** Krauss RM, Roy S, Mishell DR, Casagrande J, Pike MC. Effects of two low-dose oral contraceptives on serum lipids and lipoproteins: Differential changes in high-density lipoproteins subclasses. Am J Obstet 1983; 145:446-452. **15.** Wahl P, Walden C, Knopp R, Hoover J, Wallace R, Heiss G, Rifkind B. Effect of estrogen/progestin potency on lipid/lipoprotein cholesterol. N Engl J Med 1983; 308:862-867. **16.** Wynn V, Niththyananthan R. The effect of progestin in combined oral contraceptives on serum lipids with special reference to high-density lipoproteins. Am J Obstet Gynecol 1982; 142:766-771. **17.** Wynn V, Godsland I. Effects of oral contraceptives and carbohydrate metabolism. J Reprod Med 1986; 31(9) (Supplement):892-897. **18.** LaRosa JC. Atherosclerotic risk factors in cardiovascular disease. J Reprod Med 1986;31 (9) (Supplement): 906-912. **19.** Inman WH, Vessey MP. Investigation of death from pulmonary, coronary, and cerebral thrombosis and embolism in women of child-bearing age. Br Med J 1968; 2 (5599):193-199. **20.** Maguire MG, Tonascia J, Sartwell PE, Stolley PD, Tockman MS. Increased risk of thrombosis due to oral contraceptives: a further report. Am J Epidemiol 1979; 110 (2):188-195. **21.** Petitti DB, Wingerd J, Pellegrin F, Ramacharan S. Risk of vascular disease in women: smoking, oral contraceptives, noncontraceptive estrogens, and other factors. JAMA 1979; 242:1150-1154. **22.** Vessey MP, Doll R. Investigation of relation between use of oral contraceptives and throm-boembolic disease. Br Med J 1968; 2 (5599):199-205. **23.** Vessey MP, Doll R. Investigation of relation between use of oral contraceptives and thromboembolic disease. A further report. Br Med J 1969; 2 (5658):651-657. **24.** Porter JB, Hunter JR, Danielson DA, Jick H, Stergachis A. Oral contraceptives and non-fatal vascular disease-recent experience. Obstet Gynecol 1982; 59 (3):299-302. **25.** Vessey M, Doll R, Peto R, Johnson B, Wiggins P. A long-term follow-up study of women using different methods of contraception: an interim report. J Biosocial Sci 1976; 8:375-427. **26.** Royal College of General Practitioners: Oral contraceptives, venous thrombosis, and varicose veins. J Royal Coll Gen Pract 1978; 28:393-399. **27.** Collaborative Group for the Study of Stroke in Young Women: Oral contraception and increased risk of cerebral ischemia or thrombosis. N Engl J Med 1973; 288:871-878. **28.** Petitti DB, Wingerd J. Use of oral contraceptives, cigarette smoking, and risk of subarachnoid hemorrhage. Lancet 1978; 2:234-236. **29.** Inman WH. Oral contraceptives and fatal subarachnoid hemorrhage. Br Med J 1979; 2 (6203):1468-70. **30.** Collaborative Group for the study of Stroke in Young Women: Oral contraceptives and stroke in young women: associated risk factors. JAMA 1975; 231:718-722. **31.** Inman WH, Vessey MP, Westerholm B, Engelund A. Thromboembolic disease and the steroidal content of oral contraceptives. A report to the Committee on Safety of Drugs. Br Med J 1970; 2:203-209. **32.** Meade TW, Greenberg G, Thompson SG. Progestogens and cardiovascular reactions associated with oral contraceptives and a comparison of the safety of 50- and 35-mcg oestrogen preparations. Br Med J 1980; 280 (6224):1157-1161. **33.** Kay CR. Progestogens and arterial disease-evidence from the Royal College of General Practitioners' Study. Am J Obstet Gynecol 1982; 142:762-765. **34.** Royal College of General Practitioners: Incidence of arterial disease among oral contraceptive users. J Royal Coll Gen Pract 1983; 33:75-82. **35.** Ory HW. Mortality associated with fertility and fertility control: 1983. Family Planning Perspectives 1983; 15:50-56. **36.** The Cancer and Steroid Hormone Study of the Centers for Disease Control and the National Institute of Child Health and Human Development: Oral contraceptive use and the risk of breast cancer. N Engl J Med 1986; 315:405-411. **37.** Pike MC, Henderson BE, Krailo MD, Duke A, Roy S. Breast cancer risk in young women and use of oral contraceptives: possible modifying effect of formulation and age at use. Lancet 1983; 2:926-929. **38.** Paul C, Skegg DG, Spears GFS, Kaldor JM. Oral contraceptives and breast cancer: A national study. Br Med J 1986; 293: 723-725. **39.** Miller DR, Rosenberg L, Kaufman DW, Schottenfeld D, Stolley PD, Shapiro S. Breast cancer risk in relation to early oral contraceptive use. Obstet Gynecol 1986; 68:863-868. **40.** Olsson H, Olsson ML, Moller TR, Ranstam J, Holm P. Oral contraceptive use and breast cancer in young women in Sweden (letter). Lancet 1985; 1(8431):748-749. **41.** McPherson K, Vessey M, Neil A, Doll R, Jones L, Roberts M. Early contraceptive use and breast cancer: Results of another case-control study. Br J Cancer 1987; 56: 653-660. **42.** Huggins GR, Zucker PF. Oral contraceptives and neoplasia: 1987 update. Fertil Steril 1987; 47:733-761. **43.** McPherson K, Drife JO. The pill and breast cancer: why the uncertainty? Br Med J 1986; 293:709-710. **44.** Shapiro S. Oral contraceptives—time to take stock. N Engl J Med 1987; 315:450-451. **45.** Ory H, Naib Z, Conger SB, Hatcher RA, Tyler CW. Contraceptive choice and prevalence of cervical dysplasia and carcinoma in situ. Am J Obstet Gynecol 1976;124:573-577. **46.** Vessey MP, Lawless M, McPherson K, Yeates D. Neoplasia of the cervix uteri and contraception: a possible adverse effect of the pill. Lancet 1983; 2:930. **47.** Brinton LA, Huggins GR, Lehman HF, Malli K, Savitz DA, Trapido E, Rosenthal J, Hoover R. Long term use of oral contraceptives and risk of invasive cervical cancer. Int J Cancer 1986; 38:339-344. **48.** WHO Collaborative Study of Neoplasia and Steroid Contraceptives: Invasive cervical cancer and combined oral contraceptives. Br Med J 1985; 290:961-965. **49.** Rooks JB, Ory HW, Ishak KG, Strauss LT, Greenspan JR, Hill AP, Tyler CW. Epidemiology of hepatocellular adenoma: the role of oral contraceptive use. JAMA 1979; 242:644-648. **50.** Bein NN, Goldsmith HS. Recurrent massive hemorrhage from benign hepatic tumors secondary to oral contraceptives. Br J Surg 1977; 64:433-435. **51.** Klatskin G. Hepatic tumors: possible relationship to use of oral contraceptives. Gastroenterology 1977; 73:386-394. **52.** Henderson BE, Preston-Martin S, Edmondson HA, Peters RL, Pike MC. Hepatocellular carcinoma and oral contraceptives. Br J Cancer 1983; 48:437-440. **53.** Neuberger J, Forman D, Doll R, Williams R. Oral contraceptives and hepatocellular carcinoma. Br Med J 1986; 292:1355-1357. **54.** Forman D, Vincent TJ, Doll R. Cancer of the liver and oral contraceptives. Br Med J 1986; 292:1357-1361. **55.** Harlap S, Eldor J. Births following oral contraceptive failures. Obstet Gynecol 1980; 55:447-452. **56.** Savolainen E, Saksela E, Saxen L. Teratogenic hazards of oral contraceptives analyzed in a national malformation register. Am J Obstet

Continued on next page

Ortho-Cept—Cont.

Gynecol 1981; 140:521-524. **57.** Janerich DT, Piper JM, Glebatis DM. Oral contraceptives and birth defects. Am J Epidemiol 1980; 112:73-79. **58.** Ferencz C, Matanoski GM, Wilson PD, Rubin JD, Neill CA, Gutberlet R. Maternal hormone therapy and congenital heart disease. Teratology 1980; 21:225-239. **59.** Rothman KJ, Fyler DC, Goldbatt A, Kreidberg MB. Exogenous hormones and other drug exposures of children with congenital heart disease. Am J Epidemiol 1979; 109:433-439. **60.** Boston Collaborative Drug Surveillance Program: Oral contraceptives and venous thromboembolic disease, surgically confirmed gall-bladder disease, and breast tumors. Lancet 1973; 1:1399-1404. **61.** Royal College of General Practitioners: Oral contraceptives and health. New York, Pittman, 1974. **62.** Layde PM, Vessey MP, Yeates D. Risk of gall bladder disease: a cohort study of young women attending family planning clinics. J Epidemiol Community Health 1982; 36:274-278. **63.** Rome Group for the Epidemiology and Prevention of Cholelithiasis (GREPCO): Prevalence of gallstone disease in an Italian adult female population. Am J Epidemiol 1984; 119:796-805. **64.** Strom BL, Tamragouri RT, Morse ML, Lazar EL, West SL, Stolley PD, Jones JK. Oral contraceptives and other risk factors for gall bladder disease. Clin Pharmacol Ther 1986; 39:335-341. **65.** Wynn V, Adams PW, Godsland IF, Melrose J, Niththyananthan R, Oakley NW, Seedj A. Comparison of effects of different combined oral contraceptive formulations on carbohydrate and lipid metabolism. Lancet 1979; 1:1045-1049. **66.** Wynn V. Effect of progesterone and progestins on carbohydrate metabolism. In Progesterone and Progestin. Edited by Bardin CW, Milgrom E, Mauvis-Jarvis P. New York, Raven Press, 1983; pp. 395-410. **67.** Perlman JA, Roussell-Briefel RG, Ezzati TM, Lieberknecht G. Oral glucose tolerance and the potency of oral contraceptive progestogens. J Chronic Dis 1985; 38:857-864. **68.** Royal College of General Practitioners' Oral Contraception Study: Effect on hypertension and benign breast disease of progestogen component in combined oral contraceptives. Lancet 1977; 1:624. **69.** Fisch IR, Frank J. Oral contraceptives and blood pressure. JAMA 1977; 237:2499-2503. **70.** Laragh AJ. Oral contraceptive induced hypertension - nine years later. Am J Obstet Gynecol 1976; 126:141-147. **71.** Ramcharan S, Peritz E, Pellegrin FA, Williams WT. Incidence of hypertension in the Walnut Creek Contraceptive Drug Study cohort. In Pharmacology of Steroid Contraceptive Drugs. Garattini S, Berendes HW. Eds. New York, Raven Press, 1977; pp. 277-288. (Monographs of the Mario Negri Institute for Pharmacological Research, Milan). **72.** Stockley I. Interactions with oral contraceptives. J Pharm 1976; 216:140-143. **73.** The Cancer and Steroid Hormone Study of the Centers for Disease Control and the National Institute of Child Health and Human Development: Oral contraceptive use and the risk of ovarian cancer. JAMA 1983; 249:1596-1599. **74.** The Cancer and Steroid Hormone Study of the Centers for Disease Control and the National Institute of Child Health and Human Development: Combination oral contraceptive use and the risk of endometrial cancer. JAMA 1987; 257:796-800. **75.** Ory HW. Functional ovarian cysts and oral contraceptives: negative association confirmed surgically. JAMA 1974; 228:68-69. **76.** Ory HW, Cole P, Macmahon B, Hoover R. Oral contraceptives and reduced risk of benign breast disease. N Engl J Med 1976; 294:419-422. **77.** Ory HW. The noncontraceptive health benefits from oral contraceptive use. Fam Plann Perspect 1982; 14:182-184. **78.** Ory HW, Forrest JD, Lincoln R. Making Choices: Evaluating the health risks and benefits of birth control methods. New York, The Alan Guttmacher Institute, 1983; p.1. **79.** Schlesselman J, Stadel BV, Murray P, Lai S. Breast Cancer in relation to early use of oral contraceptives 1988; 259: 1828-1833. **80.** Hennekens CH, Speizer FE, Lipnick RJ, Rosner B, Bain C, Belanger C, Stampfer MJ, Willett W, Peto R. A case-controlled study of oral contraceptive use and breast cancer. JNCI 1984;72:39-42. **81.** LaVecchia C, Decarli A, Fasoli M, Franceschi S, Gentile A, Negri E, Parazzini F, Tognoni G. Oral contraceptives and cancers of the breast and of the female genital tract. Interim results from a case-control study. Br J Cancer 1986; 54:311-317. **82.** Meirik O, Lund E, Adami H, Bergstrom R, Christoffersen T, Bergsjo P. Oral contraceptive use in breast cancer in young women. A Joint National Case-control study in Sweden and Norway. Lancet 1986; 11:650-654. **83.** Kay CR, Hannaford PC. Breast cancer and the pill—A further report from the Royal College of General Practitioners' oral contraception study. Br J Cancer 1988; 58:675-680. **84.** Stadel BV, Lai S, Schlesselman JJ, Murray P. Oral contraceptives and premenopausal breast cancer in nulliparous women. Contraception 1988; 38:287-299. **85.** Miller DR, Rosenberg L, Kaufman DW, Stolley P, Warshauer ME, Shapiro S. Breast cancer before age 45 and oral contraceptive use: New Findings. Am J Epidemiol 1989; 129:269-280. **86.** The UK National Case-Control Study Group, Oral contraceptive use and breast cancer risk in young women. Lancet 1989; 1:973-982. **87.** Schlesselman JJ. Cancer of the breast and reproductive tract in relation to use of oral contraceptives. Contraception 1989; 40:1-38. **88.** Vessey MP, McPherson K, Villard-Mackintosh L, Yeates D. Oral contraceptives and breast cancer: latest findings in a large cohort study. Br J Cancer 1989; 59:613-617. **89.** Jick SS, Walker AM, Stergachis A, Jick H. Oral contraceptives and breast cancer. Br J Cancer 1989; 59:618-621.**90.** Godsland, I et al. The effects of different formulations of oral contraceptive agents on lipid and carbohydrate metabolism. N Engl J Med 1990; 323:1375-81. **91.** Kloosterboer, HJ et al. Selectivity in progesterone and androgen receptor binding of progestogens used in oral contraception. Contraception 1988; 38:325-32. **92.** Van der Vies, J and de Visser, J. Endocrinological studies with desogestrel. Arzneim Forsch/ Drug Res, 1983; 33(I),2:231-6. **93.** Data on file, Organon Inc. **94.** Fotherby, K. Oral contraceptives, lipids and cardiovascular diseases. Contraception 1985; Vol. 31; 4:367-94. **95.** Lawrence, DM et al. Reduced sex hormone binding globulin and derived free testosterone levels in women with severe acne. Clinical Endocrinology 1981; 15:87-91. **96.** Collaborative Group on Hormonal Factors in Breast Cancer. Breast cancer and hormonal contraceptives: collaborative reanalysis of individual data on 53 297 women with breast cancer and 100 239 women without breast cancer from 54 epidemiological studies. Lancet 1996; 347:1713-1727. **97.** Palmer JR, Rosenberg L, Kaufman DW, Warshauer ME, Stooley P, Shapiro S. Oral Contraceptive Use and Liver Cancer. Am J Epidemiol 1989; 130:878-882. **98.** Improving access to quality care in family planning: Medical eligibility criteria for contraceptive use. Geneva, WHO, Family and Reproductive Health, 1996.

BRIEF SUMMARY PATIENT PACKAGE INSERT

ORTHO-CEPT (desogestrel and ethinyl estradiol) Tablets

This product (like all oral contraceptives) is intended to prevent pregnancy. It does not protect against HIV infection (AIDS) and other sexually transmitted diseases.

Oral contraceptives, also known as "birth control pills" or "the pill," are taken to prevent pregnancy, and when taken correctly without missing any pills, have a failure rate of approximately 1% per year. The typical failure rate is approximately 5% per year when women who miss pills are included. For most women, oral contraceptives are also free of serious or unpleasant side effects. However, forgetting to take pills considerably increases the chances of pregnancy.

For the majority of women, oral contraceptives can be taken safely. But there are some women who are at high risk of developing certain serious diseases that can be life-threatening or may cause temporary or permanent disability. The risks associated with taking oral contraceptives increase significantly if you:

- smoke
- have high blood pressure, diabetes, high cholesterol
- have or have had clotting disorders, heart attack, stroke, angina pectoris, cancer of the breast or sex organs, jaundice or malignant or benign liver tumors

Although cardiovascular disease risks may be increased with oral contraceptive use after age 40 in healthy, non-smoking women (even with the newer low-dose formulations), there are also greater potential health risks associated with pregnancy in older women.

You should not take the pill if you suspect you are pregnant or have unexplained vaginal bleeding.

Cigarette smoking increases the risk of serious cardiovascular side effects from oral contraceptive use. This risk increases with age and with heavy smoking (15 or more cigarettes per day) and is quite marked in women over 35 years of age. Women who use oral contraceptives are strongly advised not to smoke.

Most side effects of the pill are not serious. The most common such effects are nausea, vomiting, bleeding between menstrual periods, weight gain, breast tenderness, headache, and difficulty wearing contact lenses. These side effects, especially nausea and vomiting, may subside within the first three months of use.

The serious side effects of the pill occur very infrequently, especially if you are in good health and are young. However, you should know that the following medical conditions have been associated with or made worse by the pill:

1. Blood clots in the legs (thrombophlebitis) or lungs (pulmonary embolism), stoppage or rupture of a blood vessel in the brain (stroke), blockage of blood vessels in the heart (heart attack or angina pectoris) or other organs of the body. As mentioned above, smoking increases the risk of heart attacks and strokes, and subsequent serious medical consequences.
2. In rare cases, oral contraceptives can cause benign but dangerous liver tumors. These benign liver tumors can rupture and cause fatal internal bleeding. In addition, some studies report an increased risk of developing liver cancer. However, liver cancers are rare.
3. High blood pressure, although blood pressure usually returns to normal when the pill is stopped.

The symptoms associated with these serious side effects are discussed in the detailed patient labeling given to you with your supply of pills. Notify your healthcare professional if you notice any unusual physical disturbances while taking the pill. In addition, drugs such as rifampin, as well as some anticonvulsants and some antibiotics and herbal preparations containing St. John's Wort (hypericum perforation) may decrease oral contraceptive effectiveness.

Various studies give conflicting reports on the relationship between breast cancer and oral contraceptive use. Oral contraceptive use may slightly increase your chance of having breast cancer diagnosed, particularly after using hormonal contraceptives at a younger age. After you stop using hormonal contraceptives, the chances of having breast cancer diagnosed begin to go back down. You should have regular breast examinations by a healthcare professional and examine your own breasts monthly. Tell your healthcare professional if you have a family history of breast cancer or if you have had breast nodules or an abnormal mammogram. Women who currently have or have had breast cancer should not use oral contraceptives because breast cancer is usually a hormone-sensitive tumor.

Some studies have found an increase in the incidence of cancer of the cervix in women who use oral contraceptives. However, this finding may be related to factors other than the use of oral contraceptives. There is insufficient evidence to rule out the possibility that the pill may cause such cancers.

Taking the pill provides some important non-contraceptive benefits. These include less painful menstruation, less menstrual blood loss and anemia, fewer pelvic infections, and fewer cancers of the ovary and the lining of the uterus.

Be sure to discuss any medical condition you may have with your healthcare professional. Your healthcare professional will take a medical and family history before prescribing oral contraceptives and will examine you. The physical examination may be delayed to another time if you request it and the healthcare professional believes that it is a good medical practice to postpone it. You should be reexamined at least once a year while taking oral contraceptives. The detailed patient information labeling gives you further information which you should read and discuss with your healthcare professional.

This product (like all oral contraceptives) is intended to prevent pregnancy. It does not protect against transmission of HIV (AIDS) and other sexually transmitted diseases such as chlamydia, genital herpes, genital warts, gonorrhea, hepatitis B, and syphilis.

HOW TO TAKE THE PILL

IMPORTANT POINTS TO REMEMBER

BEFORE YOU START TAKING YOUR PILLS:

1. BE SURE TO READ THESE DIRECTIONS:
Before you start taking your pills.
Anytime you are not sure what to do.
2. THE RIGHT WAY TO TAKE THE PILL IS TO TAKE ONE PILL EVERY DAY AT THE SAME TIME.
If you miss pills you could get pregnant. This includes starting the pack late.
The more pills you miss, the more likely you are to get pregnant.
3. MANY WOMEN HAVE SPOTTING OR LIGHT BLEEDING, OR MAY FEEL SICK TO THEIR STOMACH DURING THE FIRST 1-3 PACKS OF PILLS. If you feel sick to your stomach, do not stop taking the pill. The problem will usually go away. If it doesn't go away, check with your healthcare professional.
4. MISSING PILLS CAN ALSO CAUSE SPOTTING OR LIGHT BLEEDING, even when you make up these missed pills.
On the days you take 2 pills to make up for missed pills, you could also feel a little sick to your stomach.
5. IF YOU HAVE VOMITING OR DIARRHEA, or IF YOU TAKE SOME MEDICINES, including some antibiotics, your pills may not work as well.
Use a back-up method (such as condoms or spermicides) until you check with your healthcare professional.
6. IF YOU HAVE TROUBLE REMEMBERING TO TAKE THE PILL, talk to your healthcare professional about how to make pill-taking easier or about using another method of birth control.
7. IF YOU HAVE ANY QUESTIONS OR ARE UNSURE ABOUT THE INFORMATION IN THIS LEAFLET, call your healthcare professional.

BEFORE YOU START TAKING YOUR PILLS

1. DECIDE WHAT TIME OF DAY YOU WANT TO TAKE YOUR PILL.
It is important to take it at about the same time every day.
2. LOOK AT YOUR PILL PACK:
The pill pack has 21 light orange "active" pills (with hormones) to take for 3 weeks, followed by 1 week of green "reminder" pills (without hormones).
3. ALSO FIND:
1) where on the pack to start taking pills,
2) in what order to take the pills.
3) check picture of pill pack and additional instructions for using this package below.
4. BE SURE YOU HAVE READY AT ALL TIMES:
ANOTHER KIND OF BIRTH CONTROL (such as condoms or spermicides) to use as a back-up method in case you miss pills.
AN EXTRA, FULL PILL PACK.

WHEN TO START THE FIRST PACK OF PILLS

You have a choice of which day to start taking your first pack of pills. ORTHO-CEPT is available in the DIALPAK® Tablet Dispenser which is preset for a Sunday Start. Day 1 Start is also provided. Decide with your healthcare professional which is the best day for you. Pick a time of day which will be easy to remember.

DAY 1 START:

1. Take the first light orange "active" pill of the first pack during the first 24 hours of your period.
2. You will not need to use a back-up method of birth control, since you are starting the pill at the beginning of your period.

SUNDAY START:

1. Take the first light orange "active" pill of the first pack on the Sunday after your period starts, even if you are still bleeding. If your period begins on Sunday, start the pack that same day.
2. Use another method of birth control such as condoms or spermicide as a back-up method if you have sex anytime from the Sunday you start your first pack until the next Sunday (7 days).

WHAT TO DO DURING THE MONTH

1. TAKE ONE PILL AT THE SAME TIME EVERY DAY UNTIL THE PACK IS EMPTY.

Do not skip pills even if you are spotting or bleeding between monthly periods or feel sick to your stomach (nausea).

Do not skip pills even if you do not have sex very often.

2. WHEN YOU FINISH A PACK OR SWITCH YOUR BRAND OF PILLS:

Start the next pack on the day after your last green "reminder" pill. Do not wait any days between packs.

WHAT TO DO IF YOU MISS PILLS

If you **MISS 1** light orange "active" pill:

1. Take it as soon as you remember. Take the next pill at your regular time. This means you may take 2 pills in 1 day.
2. You do not need to use a back-up birth control method if you have sex.

If you **MISS 2** light orange "active" pills in a row in **WEEK 1 OR WEEK 2** of your pack:

1. Take 2 pills on the day you remember and 2 pills the next day.
2. Then take 1 pill a day until you finish the pack.
3. You COULD BECOME PREGNANT if you have sex in the 7 days after you miss pills. You MUST use another birth control method (such as condoms or spermicides) as a back-up method for those 7 days.

If you **MISS 2** light orange "active" pills in a row in **THE 3RD WEEK**:

1. **If you are a Day 1 Starter:**
THROW OUT the rest of the pill pack and start a new pack that same day.
If you are a Sunday Starter:
Keep taking 1 pill every day until Sunday. On Sunday, THROW OUT the rest of the pack and start a new pack of pills that same day.
2. You may not have your period this month but this is expected. However, if you miss your period 2 months in a row, call your healthcare professional because you might be pregnant.
3. You COULD BECOME PREGNANT if you have sex in the 7 days after you miss pills. You MUST use another birth control method (such as condoms or spermicides) as a back-up method for those 7 days.

If you **MISS 3 OR MORE** light orange "active" pills in a row (during the first 3 weeks):

1. **If you are a Day 1 Starter:**
THROW OUT the rest of the pill pack and start a new pack that same day.
If you are a Sunday Starter:
Keep taking 1 pill every day until Sunday. On Sunday, THROW OUT the rest of the pack and start a new pack of pills that same day.
2. You may not have your period this month but this is expected. However, if you miss your period 2 months in a row, call your healthcare professional because you might be pregnant.
3. You COULD BECOME PREGNANT if you have sex in the 7 days after you miss pills. You MUST use another birth control method (such as condoms or spermicides) as a back-up method for those 7 days.

A REMINDER:

If you forget any of the 7 green "reminder" pills in Week 4:
THROW AWAY the pills you missed.
Keep taking 1 pill each day until the pack is empty.
You do not need a back-up method.

FINALLY, IF YOU ARE STILL NOT SURE WHAT TO DO ABOUT THE PILLS YOU HAVE MISSED:

Use a BACK-UP METHOD anytime you have sex.

KEEP TAKING ONE LIGHT ORANGE "ACTIVE" PILL EACH DAY until you can reach your healthcare professional.

INSTRUCTIONS FOR USE

DIALPAK® TABLET DISPENSER

1. The DIALPAK comes to you set up for Sunday Start. If your healthcare professional has instructed you to start pill-taking on the first SUNDAY after your menstrual period has begun, or has instructed you to start pill-taking on the first day of your menstrual period and that day is SUNDAY, go to the directions in Number 3.
2. If you are to start pill-taking on a day other than SUNDAY, the enclosed calendar label has been provided and will be placed over the calendar printed on the plastic in the center of the DIALPAK. To put label in place, identify your correct starting day, locate that day on the label, line that day up with the pill to which the word START and the black Day Arrow are pointing, remove the label from the backing and press the label over the printed calendar on the center plastic.
3. When the compact is open with the cover at top, the pills should be arranged as they are in the picture. If not, turn the ribbed outer ring until the pills are positioned correctly.

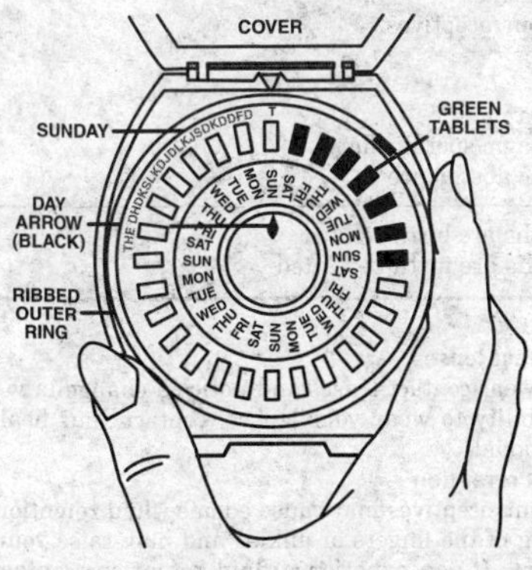

4. The first light orange "active" pill you will take is indicated by START and lines up with the black Day Arrow in the center of the DIALPAK. If not, see the directions in Number 3.
5. Push down on the first light orange "active" pill with your thumb or forefinger. The pill will come out through a hole in the back of the package.
6. The next day, turn the DIAL to the right using the ribbed outer ring to the next light orange "active" pill and your second light orange "active" pill is ready to be taken.
7. After you have taken all 21 light orange "active" pills, take one green "reminder" pill daily for 7 days. During this time your period should begin.
8. After you have taken all the pills, start a new pack of pills even if your period is not yet over.

STORAGE: Store at 25°C (77°F); excursions permitted to 15°-30°C (59°-86°F).

DETAILED PATIENT LABELING

This product (like all oral contraceptives) is intended to prevent pregnancy. It does not protect against HIV infection (AIDS) and other sexually transmitted diseases.

<u>PLEASE NOTE:</u> **This labeling is revised from time to time as important new medical information becomes available. Therefore, please review this labeling carefully.**

The following oral contraceptive product contains a combination of a progestogen and estrogen, the two kinds of female hormones:

ORTHO-CEPT® (desogestrel and ethinyl estradiol) Tablets

Each light orange tablet contains 0.15 mg desogestrel and 0.03 mg ethinyl estradiol. Each green tablet contains inert ingredients.

INTRODUCTION

Any woman who considers using oral contraceptives (the birth control pill or the pill) should understand the benefits and risks of using this form of birth control. This patient labeling will give you much of the information you will need to make this decision and will also help you determine if you are at risk of developing any of the serious side effects of the pill. It will tell you how to use the pill properly so that it will be as effective as possible. However, this labeling is not a replacement for a careful discussion between you and your healthcare professional. You should discuss the information provided in this labeling with him or her, both when you first start taking the pill and during your revisits. You should also follow your healthcare professional's advice with regard to regular check-ups while you are on the pill.

EFFECTIVENESS OF ORAL CONTRACEPTIVES

Oral contraceptives or "birth control pills" or "the pill" are used to prevent pregnancy and are more effective than most other non-surgical methods of birth control. When they are taken correctly without missing any pills, the chance of becoming pregnant is approximately 1% (1 pregnancy per 100 women per year of use). Typical failure rates, including women who do not always take the pills exactly as directed, are approximately 5% per year. The chance of becoming pregnant increases with each missed pill during a menstrual cycle.

In comparison, typical failure rates for other non-surgical methods of birth control during the first year of use are as follows:

Implant: < 1%
Injection: < 1%
IUD: 1 to 2%
Diaphragm with spermicides: 20%
Spermicides alone: 26%
Vaginal sponge: 20 to 40%
Female sterilization: < 1%
Male sterilization: < 1%
Cervical Cap with spermicides: 20 to 40%
Condom alone (male): 14%
Condom alone (female): 21%
Periodic abstinence: 25%
Withdrawal: 19%
No methods: 85%

WHO SHOULD NOT TAKE ORAL CONTRACEPTIVES

Cigarette smoking increases the risk of serious cardiovascular side effects from oral contraceptive use. This risk increases with age and with heavy smoking (15 or more cigarettes per day) and is quite marked in women over 35 years of age. Women who use oral contraceptives are strongly advised not to smoke.

Some women should not use the pill. For example, you should not take the pill if you have any of the following conditions:

- A history of heart attack or stroke
- Blood clots in the legs (thrombophlebitis), lungs (pulmonary embolism), or eyes
- A history of blood clots in the deep veins of your legs
- Chest pain (angina pectoris)
- Known or suspected breast cancer or cancer of the lining of the uterus, cervix or vagina
- Unexplained vaginal bleeding (until a diagnosis is reached by your healthcare professional)
- Yellowing of the whites of the eyes or of the skin (jaundice) during pregnancy or during previous use of the pill
- Liver tumor (benign or cancerous)
- Known or suspected pregnancy
- If you plan to have surgery with prolonged bedrest

Tell your healthcare professional if you have ever had any of these conditions. Your healthcare professional can recommend another method of birth control.

OTHER CONSIDERATIONS BEFORE TAKING ORAL CONTRACEPTIVES

Tell your healthcare professional if you have or have had:

- Breast nodules, fibrocystic disease of the breast, an abnormal breast x-ray or mammogram
- Diabetes
- Elevated cholesterol or triglycerides
- High blood pressure
- Migraine or other headaches or epilepsy
- Mental depression
- Gallbladder, liver, heart or kidney disease
- History of scanty or irregular menstrual periods

Women with any of these conditions should be checked often by their healthcare professional if they choose to use oral contraceptives.

Also, be sure to inform your healthcare professional if you smoke or are on any medications.

RISKS OF TAKING ORAL CONTRACEPTIVES

1. Risk of developing blood clots

Blood clots and blockage of blood vessels are one of the most serious side effects of taking oral contraceptives and can cause death or serious disability. In particular, a clot in the legs can cause thrombophlebitis and a clot that travels to the lungs can cause a sudden blocking of the vessel carrying blood to the lungs. The risks of these side effects may be greater with desogestrel-containing oral contraceptives, such as ORTHO-CEPT, than with certain other low-dose pills. Rarely, clots occur in the blood vessels of the eye and may cause blindness, double vision, or impaired vision.

If you take oral contraceptives and need elective surgery, need to stay in bed for a prolonged illness or injury or have recently delivered a baby, you may be at risk of developing blood clots. You should consult your healthcare professional about stopping oral contraceptives three to four weeks before surgery and not taking oral contraceptives for two weeks after surgery or during bedrest. You should also not take oral contraceptives soon after delivery of a baby. It is advisable to wait for at least four weeks after delivery if you are not breast feeding. If you are breast feeding, you should wait until you have weaned your child before using the pill. (See also the section on Breast Feeding in General Precautions.)

The risk of circulatory disease in oral contraceptive users may be higher in users of high dose pills. The risk of venous thromboembolic disease associated with oral contraceptives does not increase with length of use and disappears after pill use is stopped. The risk of abnormal blood clotting increases with age in both users and nonusers of oral contraceptives, but the increased risk from the oral contraceptive appears to be present at all ages. For women aged 20 to 44 it is estimated that about 1 in 2,000 using oral contraceptives will be hospitalized each year because of abnormal clotting. Among nonusers in the same age group, about 1 in 20,000 would be hospitalized each year. For oral contraceptive users in general, it has been estimated that in women between the ages of 15 and 34 the risk of death due to a circulatory disorder is about 1 in 12,000 per year, whereas for nonusers the rate is about 1 in 50,000 per year. In the age group 35 to 44, the risk is estimated to be about 1 in 2,500 per year for oral contraceptive users and about 1 in 10,000 per year for nonusers.

2. Heart attacks and strokes

Oral contraceptives may increase the tendency to develop strokes (stoppage or rupture of blood vessels in the brain) and angina pectoris and heart attacks (blockage of blood vessels in the heart). Any of these conditions can cause death or serious disability.

Smoking greatly increases the possibility of suffering heart attacks and strokes. Furthermore, smoking and the use of oral contraceptives greatly increase the chances of developing and dying of heart disease.

3. Gallbladder disease

Oral contraceptive users probably have a greater risk than nonusers of having gallbladder disease, although this risk

Continued on next page

Ortho-Cept—Cont.

may be related to pills containing high doses of estrogens.

4. Liver tumors

In rare cases, oral contraceptives can cause benign but dangerous liver tumors. These benign liver tumors can rupture and cause fatal internal bleeding. In addition, some studies report an increased risk of developing liver cancer. However, liver cancers are rare.

5. Cancer of the reproductive organs and breasts

Various studies give conflicting reports on the relationship between breast cancer and oral contraceptive use. Oral contraceptive use may slightly increase your chance of having breast cancer diagnosed, particularly after using hormonal contraceptives at a younger age. After you stop using hormonal contraceptives, the chances of having breast cancer diagnosed begin to go back down. You should have regular breast examinations by a healthcare professional and examine your own breasts monthly. Tell your healthcare professional if you have a family history of breast cancer or if you have had breast nodules or an abnormal mammogram. Women who currently have or have had breast cancer should not use oral contraceptives because breast cancer is usually a hormone-sensitive tumor.

Some studies have found an increase in the incidence of cancer of the cervix in women who use oral contraceptives. However, this finding may be related to factors other than the use of oral contraceptives. There is insufficient evidence to rule out the possibility that pills may cause such cancers.

ESTIMATED RISK OF DEATH FROM A BIRTH CONTROL METHOD OR PREGNANCY

All methods of birth control and pregnancy are associated with a risk of developing certain diseases which may lead to disability or death. An estimate of the number of deaths associated with different methods of birth control and pregnancy has been calculated and is shown in the following table.

ANNUAL NUMBER OF BIRTH-RELATED OR METHOD-RELATED DEATHS ASSOCIATED WITH CONTROL OF FERTILITY PER 100,000 NONSTERILE WOMEN, BY FERTILITY CONTROL METHOD ACCORDING TO AGE

Method of control and outcome	15-19	20-24	25-29	30-34	35-39	40-44
No fertility control methods*	7.0	7.4	9.1	14.8	25.7	28.2
Oral contraceptives non-smoker**	0.3	0.5	0.9	1.9	13.8	31.6
Oral contraceptives smoker**	2.2	3.4	6.6	13.5	51.1	117.2
IUD**	0.8	0.8	1.0	1.0	1.4	1.4
Condom*	1.1	1.6	0.7	0.2	0.3	0.4
Diaphragm/spermicide*	1.9	1.2	1.2	1.3	2.2	2.8
Periodic abstinence*	2.5	1.6	1.6	1.7	2.9	3.6

*Deaths are birth-related
**Deaths are method-related

[See table above]

In the above table, the risk of death from any birth control method is less than the risk of childbirth, except for oral contraceptive users over the age of 35 who smoke and pill users over the age of 40 even if they do not smoke. It can be seen in the table that for women aged 15 to 39, the risk of death was highest with pregnancy (7–26 deaths per 100,000 women, depending on age). Among pill users who do not smoke, the risk of death is always lower than that associated with pregnancy for any age group, although over the age of 40, the risk increases to 32 deaths per 100,000 women, compared to 28 associated with pregnancy at that age. However, for pill users who smoke and are over the age of 35, the estimated number of deaths exceeds those for other methods of birth control. If a woman is over the age of 40 and smokes, her estimated risk of death is four times higher (117/100,000 women) than the estimated risk associated with pregnancy (28/100,000 women) in that age group.

The suggestion that women over 40 who do not smoke should not take oral contraceptives is based on information from older, higher-dose pills. An Advisory Committee of the FDA discussed this issue in 1989 and recommended that the benefits of low-dose oral contraceptive use by healthy, non-smoking women over 40 years of age may outweigh the possible risks. Older women, as all women, who take oral contraceptives, should take an oral contraceptive which contains the least amount of estrogen and progestogen that is compatible with the individual patient needs.

WARNING SIGNALS

If any of these adverse effects occur while you are taking oral contraceptives, call your healthcare professional immediately:

- Sharp chest pain, coughing of blood, or sudden shortness of breath (indicating a possible clot in the lung)
- Pain in the calf (indicating a possible clot in the leg)
- Crushing chest pain or heaviness in the chest (indicating a possible heart attack)
- Sudden severe headache or vomiting, dizziness or fainting, disturbances of vision or speech, weakness, or numbness in an arm or leg (indicating a possible stroke)
- Sudden partial or complete loss of vision (indicating a possible clot in the eye)
- Breast lumps (indicating possible breast cancer or fibrocystic disease of the breast; ask your healthcare professional to show you how to examine your breasts)
- Severe pain or tenderness in the stomach area (indicating a possibly ruptured liver tumor)
- Difficulty in sleeping, weakness, lack of energy, fatigue, or change in mood (possibly indicating severe depression)
- Jaundice or a yellowing of the skin or eyeballs, accompanied frequently by fever, fatigue, loss of appetite, dark colored urine, or light colored bowel movements (indicating possible liver problems)

SIDE EFFECTS OF ORAL CONTRACEPTIVES

1. Vaginal bleeding

Irregular vaginal bleeding or spotting may occur while you are taking the pills. Irregular bleeding may vary from slight staining between menstrual periods to breakthrough bleeding which is a flow much like a regular period. Irregular bleeding occurs most often during the first few months of oral contraceptive use, but may also occur after you have been taking the pill for some time. Such bleeding may be temporary and usually does not indicate any serious problems. It is important to continue taking your pills on schedule. If the bleeding occurs in more than one cycle or lasts for more than a few days, talk to your healthcare professional.

2. Contact lenses

If you wear contact lenses and notice a change in vision or an inability to wear your lenses, contact your healthcare professional.

3. Fluid retention

Oral contraceptives may cause edema (fluid retention) with swelling of the fingers or ankles and may raise your blood pressure. If you experience fluid retention, contact your healthcare professional.

4. Melasma

A spotty darkening of the skin is possible, particularly of the face, which may persist.

5. Other side effects

Other side effects may include nausea and vomiting, change in appetite, headache, nervousness, depression, dizziness, loss of scalp hair, rash, and vaginal infections.

If any of these side effects bother you, call your healthcare professional.

GENERAL PRECAUTIONS

1. Missed periods and use of oral contraceptives before or during early pregnancy

There may be times when you may not menstruate regularly after you have completed taking a cycle of pills. If you have taken your pills regularly and miss one menstrual period, continue taking your pills for the next cycle but be sure to inform your healthcare professional before doing so. If you have not taken the pills daily as instructed and missed a menstrual period, you may be pregnant. If you missed two consecutive menstrual periods, you may be pregnant. Check with your healthcare professional immediately to determine whether you are pregnant. Stop taking oral contraceptives if pregnancy is confirmed.

There is no conclusive evidence that oral contraceptive use is associated with an increase in birth defects, when taken inadvertently during early pregnancy. Previously, a few studies had reported that oral contraceptives might be associated with birth defects, but these findings have not been seen in more recent studies. Nevertheless, oral contraceptives should not be used during pregnancy. You should check with your healthcare professional about risks to your unborn child of any medication taken during pregnancy.

2. While breast feeding

If you are breast feeding, consult your healthcare professional before starting oral contraceptives. Some of the drug will be passed on to the child in the milk. A few adverse effects on the child have been reported, including yellowing of the skin (jaundice) and breast enlargement. In addition, oral contraceptives may decrease the amount and quality of your milk. If possible, do not use oral contraceptives while breast feeding. You should use another method of contraception since breast feeding provides only partial protection from becoming pregnant and this partial protection decreases significantly as you breast feed for longer periods of time. You should consider starting oral contraceptives only after you have weaned your child completely.

3. Laboratory tests

If you are scheduled for any laboratory tests, tell your healthcare professional you are taking birth control pills. Certain blood tests may be affected by birth control pills.

4. Drug interactions

Certain drugs may interact with birth control pills to make them less effective in preventing pregnancy or cause an increase in breakthrough bleeding. Such drugs include rifampin; drugs used for epilepsy such as barbiturates (for example, phenobarbital); topiramate (TOPAMAX®), carbamazepine (Tegretol® is one brand of this drug), phenytoin (Dilantin® is one brand of this drug); phenylbutazone (Butazolidin® is one brand); certain drugs used in the treatment of HIV or AIDS; and possibly certain antibiotics. Pregnancies and breakthrough bleeding have been reported by women who used some form of the herbal supplement St. John's Wort while using combined hormonal contraceptives. You may need to use additional contraception when you take other products which can make oral contraceptives less effective. Be sure to tell your healthcare professional if you are taking or start taking any medications while taking birth control pills.

5. Sexually transmitted diseases

This product (like all oral contraceptives) is intended to prevent pregnancy. It does not protect against transmission of HIV (AIDS) and other sexually transmitted diseases such as chlamydia, genital herpes, genital warts, gonorrhea, hepatitis B, and syphilis.

HOW TO TAKE THE PILL

IMPORTANT POINTS TO REMEMBER

BEFORE YOU START TAKING YOUR PILLS:

1. BE SURE TO READ THESE DIRECTIONS:
Before you start taking your pills.
Anytime you are not sure what to do.
2. THE RIGHT WAY TO TAKE THE PILL IS TO TAKE ONE PILL EVERY DAY AT THE SAME TIME.
If you miss pills you could get pregnant. This includes starting the pack late.
The more pills you miss, the more likely you are to get pregnant.
3. MANY WOMEN HAVE SPOTTING OR LIGHT BLEEDING, OR MAY FEEL SICK TO THEIR STOMACH DURING THE FIRST 1-3 PACKS OF PILLS. If you feel sick to your stomach, do not stop taking the pill. The problem will usually go away. If it doesn't go away, check with your healthcare professional.
4. MISSING PILLS CAN ALSO CAUSE SPOTTING OR LIGHT BLEEDING, even when you make up these missed pills.
On the days you take 2 pills to make up for missed pills, you could also feel a little sick to your stomach.
5. IF YOU HAVE VOMITING OR DIARRHEA, or IF YOU TAKE SOME MEDICINES, including some antibiotics, your pills may not work as well.
Use a back-up method (such as condoms or spermicides) until you check with your healthcare professional.
6. IF YOU HAVE TROUBLE REMEMBERING TO TAKE THE PILL, talk to your healthcare professional about how to make pill-taking easier or about using another method of birth control.
7. IF YOU HAVE ANY QUESTIONS OR ARE UNSURE ABOUT THE INFORMATION IN THIS LEAFLET, call your healthcare professional.

BEFORE YOU START TAKING YOUR PILLS

1. DECIDE WHAT TIME OF DAY YOU WANT TO TAKE YOUR PILL.
It is important to take it at about the same time every day.
2. LOOK AT YOUR PILL PACK:
The pill pack has 21 light orange "active" pills (with hormones) to take for 3 weeks, followed by 1 week of green "reminder" pills (without hormones).
3. ALSO FIND:
1) where on the pack to start taking pills,
2) in what order to take the pills.
CHECK PICTURE OF PILL PACK AND ADDITIONAL INSTRUCTIONS FOR USING THIS PACKAGE IN THE BRIEF SUMMARY PATIENT PACKAGE INSERT.
4. BE SURE YOU HAVE READY AT ALL TIMES:
ANOTHER KIND OF BIRTH CONTROL (such as condoms or spermicides) to use as a back-up method in case you miss pills.
AN EXTRA, FULL PILL PACK.

WHEN TO START THE FIRST PACK OF PILLS

You have a choice of which day to start taking your first pack of pills. ORTHO-CEPT is available in the DIALPAK® Tablet Dispenser which is preset for a Sunday Start. Day 1 Start is also provided. Decide with your healthcare professional which is the best day for you. Pick a time of day which will be easy to remember.

DAY 1 START:

1. Take the first light orange "active" pill of the first pack during the first 24 hours of your period.
2. You will not need to use a back-up method of birth control, since you are starting the pill at the beginning of your period.

SUNDAY START:

1. Take the first light orange "active" pill of the first pack on the Sunday after your period starts, even if you are still bleeding. If your period begins on Sunday, start the pack that same day.
2. Use another method of birth control such as condoms or spermicides as a back-up method if you have sex anytime from the Sunday you start your first pack until the next Sunday (7 days).

WHAT TO DO DURING THE MONTH

1. TAKE ONE PILL AT THE SAME TIME EVERY DAY UNTIL THE PACK IS EMPTY.

Do not skip pills even if you are spotting or bleeding between monthly periods or feel sick to your stomach (nausea).

Do not skip pills even if you do not have sex very often.

2. WHEN YOU FINISH A PACK OR SWITCH YOUR BRAND OF PILLS:

Start the next pack on the day after your last green "reminder" pill. Do not wait any days between packs.

WHAT TO DO IF YOU MISS PILLS

If you **MISS 1** light orange "active" pill:

1. Take it as soon as you remember. Take the next pill at your regular time. This means you may take 2 pills in 1 day.
2. You do not need to use a back-up birth control method if you have sex.

If you **MISS 2** light orange "active" pills in a row in **WEEK 1 OR WEEK 2** of your pack:

1. Take 2 pills on the day you remember and 2 pills the next day.
2. Then take 1 pill a day until you finish the pack.
3. You COULD BECOME PREGNANT if you have sex in the 7 days after you miss pills. You MUST use another birth control method (such as condoms or spermicides) as a back-up method for those 7 days.

If you **MISS 2** light orange "active" pills in a row in **THE 3RD WEEK**:

1. **If you are a Day 1 Starter:**
THROW OUT the rest of the pill pack and start a new pack that same day.
If you are a Sunday Starter:
Keep taking 1 pill every day until Sunday. On Sunday, THROW OUT the rest of the pack and start a new pack of pills that same day.
2. You may not have your period this month but this is expected. However, if you miss your period 2 months in a row, call your healthcare professional because you might be pregnant.
3. You COULD BECOME PREGNANT if you have sex in the 7 days after you miss pills. You MUST use another birth control method (such as condoms or spermicides) as a back-up method for those 7 days.

If you **MISS 3 OR MORE** light orange "active" pills in a row (during the first 3 weeks):

1. **If you are a Day 1 Starter:**
THROW OUT the rest of the pill pack and start a new pack that same day.
If you are a Sunday Starter:
Keep taking 1 pill every day until Sunday. On Sunday, THROW OUT the rest of the pack and start a new pack of pills that same day.
2. You may not have your period this month but this is expected. However, if you miss your period 2 months in a row, call your healthcare professional because you might be pregnant.
3. You COULD BECOME PREGNANT if you have sex in the 7 days after you miss pills. You MUST use another birth control method (such as condoms or spermicides) as a back-up method for those 7 days.

A REMINDER:

If you forget any of the 7 green "reminder" pills in Week 4:
THROW AWAY the pills you missed.
Keep taking 1 pill each day until the pack is empty.
You do not need a back-up method.

FINALLY, IF YOU ARE STILL NOT SURE WHAT TO DO ABOUT THE PILLS YOU HAVE MISSED:

Use a BACK-UP METHOD anytime you have sex.
KEEP TAKING ONE LIGHT ORANGE "ACTIVE" PILL EACH DAY until you can reach your healthcare professional.

PREGNANCY DUE TO PILL FAILURE

When taken correctly without missing any pills, oral contraceptives are highly effective; however the typical failure rate of large numbers of pill users is 5% per year when women who miss pills are included. If failure does occur, the risk to the fetus is minimal.

PREGNANCY AFTER STOPPING THE PILL

There may be some delay in becoming pregnant after you stop using oral contraceptives, especially if you had irregular menstrual cycles before you used oral contraceptives. It may be advisable to postpone conception until you begin menstruating regularly once you have stopped taking the pill and desire pregnancy.

There does not appear to be any increase in birth defects in newborn babies when pregnancy occurs soon after stopping the pill.

OVERDOSAGE

Serious ill effects have not been reported following ingestion of large doses of oral contraceptives by young children. Overdosage may cause nausea and withdrawal bleeding in females. In case of overdosage, contact your healthcare professional.

OTHER INFORMATION

Your healthcare professional will take a medical and family history before prescribing oral contraceptives and will examine you. The physical examination may be delayed to another time if you request it and the healthcare professional believes that it is a good medical practice to postpone it. You should be reexamined at least once a year. Be sure to inform your healthcare professional if there is a family history of any of the conditions listed previously in this leaflet. Be sure to keep all appointments with your healthcare professional because this is a time to determine if there are early signs of side effects of oral contraceptive use.

Do not use the drug for any condition other than the one for which it was prescribed. This drug has been prescribed specifically for you; do not give it to others who may want birth control pills.

HEALTH BENEFITS FROM ORAL CONTRACEPTIVES

In addition to preventing pregnancy, use of combination oral contraceptives may provide certain benefits. They are:

- menstrual cycles may become more regular
- blood flow during menstruation may be lighter and less iron may be lost. Therefore, anemia due to iron deficiency is less likely to occur.
- pain or other symptoms during menstruation may be encountered less frequently.
- ectopic (tubal) pregnancy may occur less frequently.
- noncancerous cysts or lumps in the breast may occur less frequently.
- acute pelvic inflammatory disease may occur less frequently.
- oral contraceptive use may provide some protection against developing two forms of cancer: cancer of the ovaries and cancer of the lining of the uterus.

If you want more information about birth control pills, ask your healthcare professional. They have a more technical leaflet called the Professional Labeling, which you may wish to read. The professional labeling is also published in a book entitled *Physicians' Desk Reference*, available in many book stores and public libraries.

STORAGE: Store at 25°C (77°F); excursions permitted to 15°-30°C (59°-86°F).

Packaged and Distributed by
ORTHO-McNEIL PHARMACEUTICAL, INC.
Raritan, New Jersey 08869
Jointly Manufactured by
ORTHO-McNEIL PHARMACEUTICAL, INC.
Raritan, New Jersey 08869 and
DIOSYNTH bv
Oss, The Netherlands
ORTHO-MCNEIL
© OMP 1998 REVISED JANUARY 2004 10031900
Shown in Product Identification Guide, page 328

ORTHO EVRA® ℞

[ōr'-thō 'ev'-rā]
(NORELGESTROMIN / ETHINYL ESTRADIOL TRANSDERMAL SYSTEM)

Prescribing Information

Patients should be counseled that this product does not protect against HIV infection (AIDS) and other sexually transmitted diseases.

℞ only

DESCRIPTION

ORTHO EVRA® is a combination transdermal contraceptive patch with a contact surface area of 20 cm^2. It contains 6.00 mg norelgestromin and 0.75 mg ethinyl estradiol (EE), and releases 150 micrograms of norelgestromin and 20 micrograms of EE to the bloodstream per 24 hours.

ORTHO EVRA® is a thin, matrix-type transdermal contraceptive patch consisting of three layers. The backing layer is composed of a beige flexible film consisting of a low-density pigmented polyethylene outer layer and a polyester inner layer. It provides structural support and protects the middle adhesive layer from the environment. The middle layer contains polyisobutylene/polybutene adhesive, crospovidone, non-woven polyester fabric and lauryl lactate as inactive components. The active components in this layer are the hormones, norelgestromin and ethinyl estradiol. The third layer is the release liner, which protects the adhesive layer during storage and is removed just prior to application. It is a transparent polyethylene terephthalate (PET) film with a polydimethylsiloxane coating on the side that is in contact with the middle adhesive layer.

The outside of the backing layer is heat-stamped "ORTHO EVRA® 150/20."

The structural formulas of the components are:

norelgestromin ethinyl estradiol

Molecular weight, norelgestromin: 327.47
Molecular weight, ethinyl estradiol: 296.41
Chemical name for norelgestromin: 18, 19-dinorpregn-4-en-20-yn-3-one, 13-ethyl- 17-hydroxy-, 3-oxime, (17α)
Chemical name for ethinyl estradiol: 19-Norpregna-1, 3, 5 (10)-trien-20-yne-3, 17-diol, (17α)

CLINICAL PHARMACOLOGY

Pharmacodynamics

Norelgestromin is the active progestin largely responsible for the progestational activity that occurs in women following application of ORTHO EVRA®. Norelgestromin is also the primary active metabolite produced following oral administration of norgestimate (NGM), the progestin component of the oral contraceptive products ORTHO-CYCLEN® and ORTHO TRI-CYCLEN®.

Combination oral contraceptives act by suppression of gonadotropins. Although the primary mechanism of this action is inhibition of ovulation, other alterations include changes in the cervical mucus (which increase the difficulty of sperm entry into the uterus) and the endometrium (which reduce the likelihood of implantation).

Receptor and human sex hormone-binding globulin (SHBG) binding studies, as well as studies in animals and humans, have shown that both norgestimate and norelgestromin exhibit high progestational activity with minimal intrinsic androgenicity[90–93]. Transdermally-administered norelgestromin, in combination with ethinyl estradiol, does not counteract the estrogen-induced increases in SHBG, resulting in lower levels of free testosterone in serum compared to baseline.

Pharmacokinetic studies with ORTHO EVRA® demonstrated consistent elimination kinetics for norelgestromin and EE with half-life values of approximately 28 hours and 17 hours, respectively. One clinical trial assessed the return of hypothalamic-pituitary-ovarian axis function post-therapy and found that FSH, LH, and Estradiol mean values, though suppressed during therapy, returned to near baseline values during the 6 weeks post therapy.

Pharmacokinetics

Absorption

Following application of ORTHO EVRA®, both norelgestromin and EE rapidly appear in the serum, reach a plateau by approximately 48 hours, and are maintained at an approximate steady-state throughout the wear period. C^{SS} concentrations for norelgestromin and EE during one week of patch wear are approximately 0.6–0.8 ng/ml and 40–50 pg/ml, respectively, and are generally consistent from all studies and application sites. These C^{SS} concentrations are within the reference ranges for norelgestromin (0.6 to 1.2 ng/ml) and EE (25 to 75 pg/ml) established based upon the C_{ave} concentrations observed with subjects taking ORTHO-CYCLEN®.

Daily absorption of norelgestromin and EE from ORTHO EVRA® was determined by comparison to an intravenous infusion of norelgestromin and EE. The results indicated that the average dose of norelgestromin and EE absorbed into the systemic circulation is 150 mcg/day and 20 mcg/day, respectively.

The absorption of norelgestromin and EE following application of ORTHO EVRA® to the abdomen, buttock, upper outer arm and upper torso (excluding breast) was evaluated in a cross-over design study. The results of this study indicated that C^{SS} and AUC for the buttock, upper arm and torso for each analyte were equivalent. While C^{SS} values for the abdomen were within reference ranges for EE 35 mcg/NGM 250 mcg oral contraceptive users, exposure to the drugs was lower and strict bioequivalence requirements for AUC were not met in this study. However, in a separate parallel group multiple application pharmacokinetic study, C^{SS} and AUC for the buttock and abdomen were not statistically different. Therefore, all four sites may be considered therapeutically equivalent.

The absorption of norelgestromin and EE following application of ORTHO EVRA® was studied under conditions encountered in a health club (sauna, whirlpool and treadmill) and in a cold water bath. The results indicated that for norelgestromin there were no significant treatment effects on C^{SS} or AUC when compared to normal wear. For EE, slight increases were observed due to sauna, whirlpool and treadmill, however, the C^{SS} values following these treatments were within the reference range. There was no significant effect of cold water on these parameters.

In multiple dose studies, C^{SS} and AUC for norelgestromin and EE were found to increase slightly over time when compared to Week 1 of Cycle 1. In a three-cycle study, these pharmacokinetic parameters reached steady-state conditions during all three weeks of Cycle 3. (See Table 1, Figures 1 and 2).

[See table 1 at top of next page]

Figure 1: Mean Norelgestromin Serum Concentrations (ng/mL) in Healthy Female Volunteers Following Application of ORTHO EVRA® on the Buttock for Three Consecutive Cycles (Dotted horizontal lines indicate the reference range. Dotted vertical arrow indicates time of patch removal.)

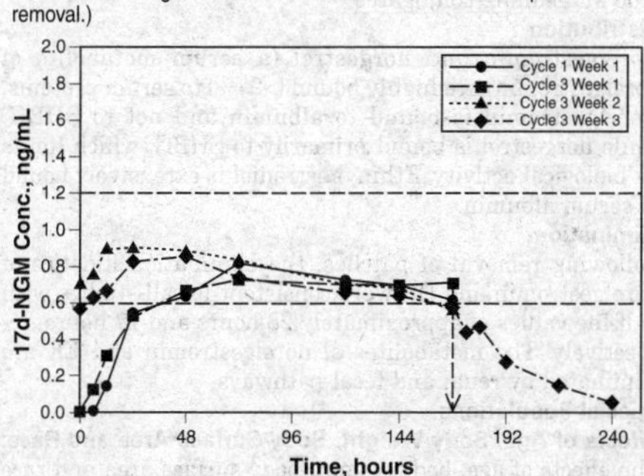

Continued on next page

Ortho Evra—Cont.

Figure 2: Mean Ethinyl Estradiol Serum Concentrations (pg/mL) in Healthy Female Volunteers Following Application of ORTHO EVRA® on the Buttock for Three Consecutive Cycles (Dotted horizontal lines indicate the reference range. Dotted vertical arrows indicates time of patch removal.)

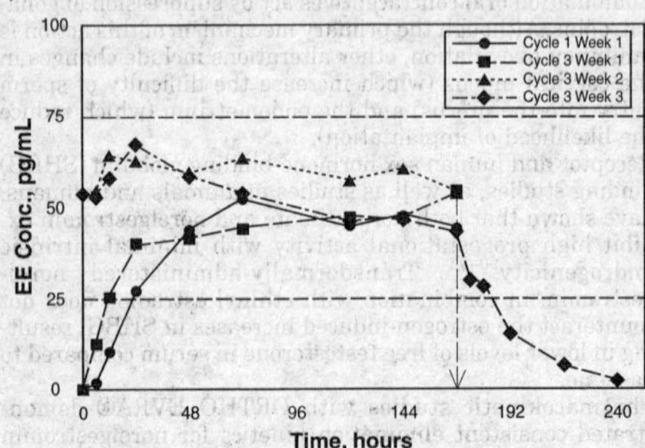

Results from a study of consecutive ORTHO EVRA® wear for 7 days and 10 days indicated that serum concentrations of norelgestromin and EE dropped slightly during the first 6 hours after the patch replacement, still stayed within the reference range and recovered within 12 hours. Target C^{ss} of norelgestromin and EE were maintained during 2 days of extended wear of ORTHO EVRA®.

Figure 3: Mean (SD) Norelgestromin Serum Concentrations (ng/mL) Following Application of ORTHO EVRA® to the Abdomen for 7 Days and 10 Days (Dotted horizontal lines indicate the reference range. Solid vertical arrows indicate actual time of patch removal. Dotted vertical arrows indicates theoretical time of patch removal under normal use.)

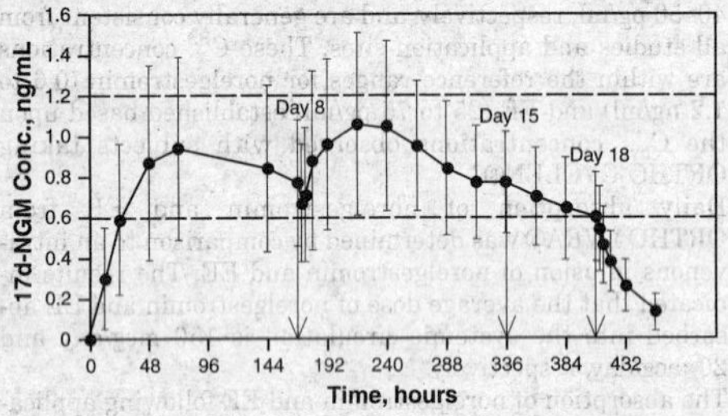

Figure 4: Mean (SD) EE Serum Concentrations (pg/mL) Following Application of ORTHO EVRA® to Abdomen for 7 Days and 10 Days (Dotted horizontal lines indicate the reference range. Solid vertical arrows indicate actual time of patch removal. Dotted vertical arrows indicates theoretical time of patch removal under normal use.)

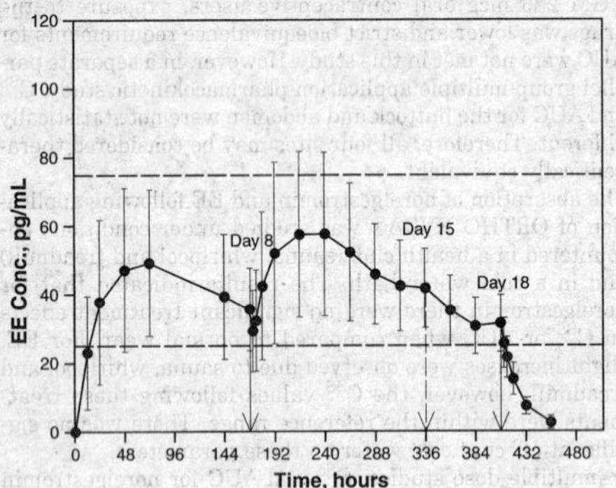

Metabolism

Since ORTHO EVRA® is applied transdermally, first-pass metabolism (via the gastrointestinal tract and/or liver) of norelgestromin and EE that would be expected with oral administration is avoided. Hepatic metabolism of norelgestromin occurs and metabolites include norgestrel, which is highly bound to SHBG, and various hydroxylated and conjugated metabolites. Ethinyl estradiol is also metabolized to various hydroxylated products and their glucuronide and sulfate conjugates.

Distribution

Norelgestromin and norgestrel (a serum metabolite of norelgestromin) are highly bound (>97%) to serum proteins. Norelgestromin is bound to albumin and not to SHBG, while norgestrel is bound primarily to SHBG, which limits its biological activity. Ethinyl estradiol is extensively bound to serum albumin.

Elimination

Following removal of patches, the elimination kinetics of norelgestromin and EE were consistent for all studies with half-life values of approximately 28 hours and 17 hours, respectively. The metabolites of norelgestromin and EE are eliminated by renal and fecal pathways.

Special Populations

Effects of Age, Body Weight, Body Surface Area and Race: The effects of age, body weight, body surface area and race on the pharmacokinetics of norelgestromin and EE were evaluated in 230 healthy women from nine pharmacokinetic

Table 1: Mean (SD) Pharmacokinetic Parameters of Norelgestromin and EE Following 3 Consecutive Cycles of ORTHO EVRA® Wear on the Buttock

Analyte	Parameter	Cycle 1 Week 1	Cycle 3 Week 1	Cycle 3 Week 2	Cycle 3 Week 3
Norelgestromin	C^{ss} [a]	0.70 (0.28)	0.70 (0.29)	0.80 (0.23)	0.70 (0.32)
	AUC_{0-168} [b]	107 (44.2)	105 (45.5)	132 (57.1)	120 (52.8)
	t ½[c]	nc	nc	nc	32.1 (12.9)
EE	C^{ss} [d]	46.4 (17.9)	47.6 (17.3)	59.0 (25.1)	49.6 (27.0)
	AUC_{0-168} [e]	6796 (2673)	7160 (2893)	10054 (4205)	8840 (5176)
	t ½[c]	nc	nc	nc	21.0 (9.07)

[a]ng/mL
[b]ng·h/mL
[c]h
[d]pg/mL
[e]pg·h/mL
nc = not calculated

studies of single 7-day applications of ORTHO EVRA®. For both norelgestromin and EE, increasing age, body weight and body surface area each were associated with slight decreases in C^{ss} and AUC values. However, only a small fraction (10–25%) of the overall variability in the pharmacokinetics of norelgestromin and EE following application of ORTHO EVRA® may be associated with any or all of the above demographic parameters. There was no significant effect of race with respect to Caucasians, Hispanics and Blacks.

Renal and Hepatic Impairment

No formal studies were conducted with ORTHO EVRA® to evaluate the pharmacokinetics, safety, and efficacy in women with renal or hepatic impairment. Steroid hormones may be poorly metabolized in patients with impaired liver function (see PRECAUTIONS).

Drug Interactions

The metabolism of hormonal contraceptives may be influenced by various drugs. Of potential clinical importance are drugs that cause the induction of enzymes that are responsible for the degradation of estrogens and progestins, and drugs that interrupt entero-hepatic recirculation of estrogen (e.g. certain antibiotics)[72].

The proposed mechanism of interaction of antibiotics is different from that of liver enzyme-inducing drugs. Literature suggests possible interactions with the concomitant use of hormonal contraceptives and ampicillin or tetracycline. In a pharmacokinetic drug interaction study, oral administration of tetracycline HCl, 500 mg q.i.d. for 3 days prior to and 7 days during wear of ORTHO EVRA® did not significantly affect the pharmacokinetics of norelgestromin or EE.

The major target for enzyme inducers is the hepatic microsomal estrogen-2-hydroxylase (cytochrome P450 3A4)[99]. See also PRECAUTIONS, Drug Interactions.

Patch Adhesion

In the clinical trials with ORTHO EVRA®, approximately 2% of the cumulative number of patches completely detached. The proportion of subjects with at least 1 patch that completely detached ranged from 2% to 6%, with a reduction from Cycle 1 (6%) to Cycle 13 (2%). For instructions on how to manage detachment of patches, refer to the DOSAGE AND ADMINISTRATION section.

INDICATIONS AND USAGE

ORTHO EVRA® is indicated for the prevention of pregnancy.

Like oral contraceptives, ORTHO EVRA® is highly effective if used as recommended in this label.

In 3 large clinical trials in North America, Europe and South Africa, 3,330 women (ages 18–45) completed 22,155 cycles of ORTHO EVRA® use, pregnancy rates were approximately 1 per 100 women-years of ORTHO EVRA® use. The racial distribution was 91% Caucasian, 4.9% Black, 1.6% Asian, and 2.4% Other.

With respect to weight, 5 of the 15 pregnancies reported with ORTHO EVRA® use were among women with a baseline body weight ≥198 lbs. (90kg), which constituted <3% of the study population. The greater proportion of pregnancies among women at or above 198 lbs. was statistically significant and suggests that ORTHO EVRA® may be less effective in these women.

Health Care Professionals who consider ORTHO EVRA® for women at or above 198 lbs. should discuss the patient's individual needs in choosing the most appropriate contraceptive option.

Table 2 lists the accidental pregnancy rates for users of various methods of contraception. The efficacy of these contraceptive methods, except sterilization, IUD, and Norplant depends upon the reliability with which they are used. Correct and consistent use of methods can result in lower failure rates.

[See table 2 at top of next page]

ORTHO EVRA® has not been studied for and is not indicated for use in emergency contraception.

CONTRAINDICATIONS

ORTHO EVRA® should not be used in women who currently have the following conditions:

- Thrombophlebitis, thromboembolic disorders
- A past history of deep vein thrombophlebitis or thromboembolic disorders
- Cerebrovascular or coronary artery disease (current or past history)
- Valvular heart disease with complications[103]
- Severe hypertension[103]
- Diabetes with vascular involvement[103]
- Headaches with focal neurological symptoms
- Major surgery with prolonged immobilization
- Known or suspected carcinoma of the breast or personal history of breast cancer
- Carcinoma of the endometrium or other known or suspected estrogen-dependent neoplasia
- Undiagnosed abnormal genital bleeding
- Cholestatic jaundice of pregnancy or jaundice with prior hormonal contraceptive use
- Acute or chronic hepatocellular disease with abnormal liver function[103]
- Hepatic adenomas or carcinomas
- Known or suspected pregnancy
- Hypersensitivity to any component of this product

WARNINGS

Cigarette smoking increases the risk of serious cardiovascular side effects from hormonal contraceptive use. This risk increases with age and with heavy smoking (15 or more cigarettes per day) and is quite marked in women over 35 years of age. Women who use hormonal contraceptives, including ORTHO EVRA®, should be strongly advised not to smoke.

ORTHO EVRA® and other contraceptives that contain both an estrogen and a progestin are called combination hormonal contraceptives. There is no epidemiologic data available to determine whether safety and efficacy with the transdermal route of administration would be different than the oral route. Practitioners prescribing ORTHO EVRA® should be familiar with the following information relating to risks.

The use of combination hormonal contraceptives is associated with increased risks of several serious conditions including myocardial infarction, thromboembolism, stroke, hepatic neoplasia, and gallbladder disease, although the risk of serious morbidity or mortality is very small in healthy women without underlying risk factors. The risk of morbidity and mortality increases significantly in the presence of other underlying risk factors such as hypertension, hyperlipidemias, obesity and diabetes.

The information contained in this package insert is principally based on studies carried out in women who used combination oral contraceptives with higher formulations of estrogens and progestins than those in common use today. The effect of long-term use of combination hormonal contraceptives with lower doses of both estrogen and progestin administered by any route remains to be determined.

Throughout this labeling, epidemiological studies reported are of two types: retrospective or case control studies and prospective or cohort studies. Case control studies provide a measure of the relative risk of a disease, namely, a ratio of the incidence of a disease among oral contraceptive users to that among nonusers. The relative risk does not provide information on the actual clinical occurrence of a disease. Cohort studies provide a measure of attributable risk, which is the *difference* in the incidence of disease between hormonal contraceptive users and nonusers. The attributable risk does provide information about the actual occurrence of a disease in the population (adapted from refs. 2 and 3 with the author's permission). For further information, the reader is referred to a text on epidemiological methods.

1. Thromboembolic Disorders And Other Vascular Problems

a. Thromboembolism

An increased risk of thromboembolic and thrombotic disease associated with the use of hormonal contraceptives is well established. Case control studies have found the relative risk of users compared to nonusers to be 3 for the first episode of superficial venous thrombosis, 4 to 11 for deep vein thrombosis or pulmonary embolism, and 1.5 to 6 for women with predisposing conditions for venous thromboembolic disease[2,3,19–24]. Cohort studies have shown the relative risk to be somewhat lower, about 3 for new cases and about 4.5 for new cases requiring hospitalization[25]. The risk of thromboembolic disease associated with hormonal contraceptives is not related to length of use and disappears after hormonal contraceptive use is stopped[2]. A two- to four-fold increase in relative risk of post-operative thromboembolic complications has been reported with the use of hormonal contraceptives[9,26]. The relative risk of venous thrombosis in women who have predisposing conditions is twice that of women without such medical conditions[9,26]. If feasible, hormonal contraceptives should be discontinued at least four weeks prior to and for two weeks after elective surgery of a type associated with an increase in risk of thromboembolism and during and following prolonged immobilization. Since the immediate postpartum period is also associated with an increased risk of thromboembolism, hormonal contraceptives should be started no earlier than four weeks after delivery in women who elect not to breast-feed.

In the large clinical trials (N= 3,330 with 1,704 women-years of exposure), one case of non-fatal pulmonary embolism occurred during ORTHO EVRA® use, and one case of post-operative non-fatal pulmonary embolism was reported following ORTHO EVRA® use. It is unknown if the risk of venous thromboembolism with ORTHO EVRA® use is different than with use of combination oral contraceptives.

As with any combination hormonal contraceptives, the clinician should be alert to the earliest manifestations of thrombotic disorders (thrombophlebitis, pulmonary embolism, cerebrovascular disorders, and retinal thrombosis). Should any of these occur or be suspected, ORTHO EVRA® should be discontinued immediately.

b. Myocardial Infarction

An increased risk of myocardial infarction has been attributed to hormonal contraceptive use. This risk is primarily in smokers or women with other underlying risk factors for coronary artery disease such as hypertension, hypercholesterolemia, morbid obesity, and diabetes. The relative risk of heart attack for current hormonal contraceptive users has been estimated to be two to six[4–10] compared to non-users. The risk is very low under the age of 30.

Smoking in combination with oral contraceptive use has been shown to contribute substantially to the incidence of myocardial infarctions in women in their mid-thirties or older with smoking accounting for the majority of excess cases[11]. Mortality rates associated with circulatory disease have been shown to increase substantially in smokers, especially in those 35 years of age and older among women who use oral contraceptives. (See Figure 5)

Figure 5: Circulatory Disease Mortality Rates Per 100,000 Woman- Years by Age, Smoking Status and Oral Contraceptive Use

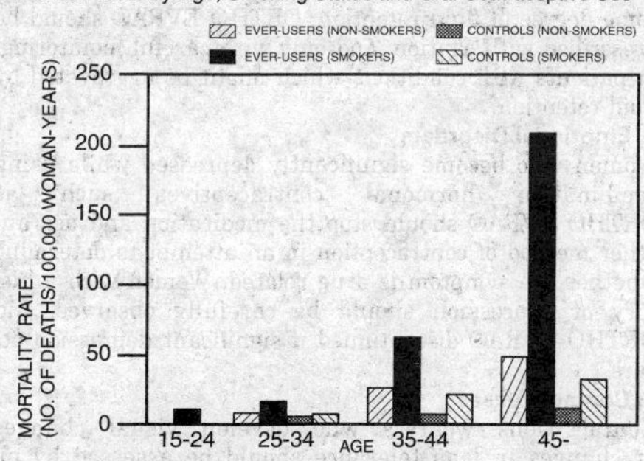

Hormonal contraceptives may compound the effects of well-known risk factors, such as hypertension, diabetes, hyperlipidemias, age and obesity[13]. In particular, some progestins are known to decrease HDL cholesterol and cause glucose intolerance, while estrogens may create a state of hyperinsulinism[14–18]. Hormonal contraceptives have been shown to increase blood pressure among some users (see Section 9 in WARNINGS). Similar effects on risk factors have been associated with an increased risk of heart disease. Hormonal contraceptives, including ORTHO EVRA®, must be used with caution in women with cardiovascular disease risk factors.

Norgestimate and norelgestromin have minimal androgenic activity (see CLINICAL PHARMACOLOGY). There is some evidence that the risk of myocardial infarction associated with hormonal contraceptives is lower when the progestin has minimal androgenic activity than when the activity is greater[97].

c. Cerebrovascular diseases

Hormonal contraceptives have been shown to increase both the relative and attributable risks of cerebrovascular events (thrombotic and hemorrhagic strokes), although, in general, the risk is greatest among older (>35 years), hypertensive women who also smoke. Hypertension was found to be a risk factor for both users and nonusers, for both types of strokes, and smoking interacted to increase the risk of stroke[27–29].

In a large study, the relative risk of thrombotic strokes has been shown to range from 3 for normotensive users to 14 for users with severe hypertension[30]. The relative risk of hemorrhagic stroke is reported to be 1.2 for non-smokers who used hormonal contraceptives, 2.6 for smokers who did not use hormonal contraceptives, 7.6 for smokers who used hormonal contraceptives, 1.8 for normotensive users and 25.7 for users with severe hypertension[30]. The attributable risk is also greater in older women[3].

Table 2: Percentage of Women Experiencing an Unintended Pregnancy During the First Year of Typical Use and the First Year of Perfect Use of Contraception and the Percentage Continuing Use at the End of the First Year. United States.

Method (1)	% of Women Experiencing an Unintended Pregnancy within the First Year of Use: Typical Use[1] (2)	Perfect Use[2] (3)	% of Women Continuing Use at One Year[3] (4)
Chance[4]	85	85	
Spermicides[5]	26	6	40
Periodic abstinence	25		63
Calendar		9	
Ovulation Method		3	
Sympto-Thermal[6]		2	
Post-Ovulation		1	
Cap[7]			
Parous Women	40	26	42
Nulliparous Women	20	9	56
Sponge			
Parous Women	40	20	42
Nulliparous Women	20	9	56
Diaphragm[7]	20	6	56
Withdrawal	19	4	
Condom[8]			
Female (Reality)	21	5	56
Male	14	3	61
Pill	5		71
Progestin Only		0.5	
Combined		0.1	
IUD			
Progesterone T	2.0	1.5	81
Copper T380A	0.8	0.6	78
LNg 20	0.1	0.1	81
Depo-Provera	0.3	0.3	70
Norplant and Norplant-2	0.05	0.05	88
Female Sterilization	0.5	0.5	100
Male Sterilization	0.15	0.10	100

Hatcher et al, 1998, Ref. # 1.

Emergency Contraceptive Pills: Treatment initiated within 72 hours after unprotected intercourse reduces the risk of pregnancy by at least 75%.[9]

Lactational Amenorrhea Method: LAM is highly effective, *temporary* method of contraception.[10]

Source: Trussell J, Contraceptive efficacy. In Hatcher RA, Trussell J, Stewart F, Cates W, Stewart GK, Kowal D, Guest F, Contraceptive Technology: Seventeenth Revised Edition. New York NY: Irvington Publishers, 1998.

[1] Among *typical* couples who initiate use of a method (not necessarily for the first time), the percentage who experience an accidental pregnancy during the first year if they do not stop use for any other reason.

[2] Among couples who initiate use of a method (not necessarily for the first time) and who use it *perfectly* (both consistently and correctly), the percentage who experience an accidental pregnancy during the first year if they do not stop use for any other reason.

[3] Among couples attempting to avoid pregnancy, the percentage who continue to use a method for one year.

[4] The percents becoming pregnant in columns (2) and (3) are based on data from populations where contraception is not used and from women who cease using contraception in order to become pregnant. Among such populations, about 89% become pregnant within one year. This estimate was lowered slightly (to 85%) to represent the percent who would become pregnant within one year among women now relying on reversible methods of contraception if they abandoned contraception altogether.

[5] Foams, creams, gels, vaginal suppositories, and vaginal film.

[6] Cervical mucus (ovulation) method supplemented by calendar in the pre-ovulatory and basal body temperature in the post-ovulatory phases.

[7] With spermicidal cream or jelly.

[8] Without spermicides.

[9] The treatment schedule is one dose within 72 hours after unprotected intercourse, and a second dose 12 hours after the first dose. The Food and Drug Administration has declared the following brands of oral contraceptives to be safe and effective for emergency contraception: Ovral (1 dose is 2 white pills), Alesse (1 dose is 5 pink pills), Nordette or Levlen (1 dose is 2 light-orange pills), Lo/Ovral (1 dose is 4 white pills), Triphasil or Tri-Levlen (1 dose is 4 yellow pills).

[10] However, to maintain effective protection against pregnancy, another method of contraception must be used as soon as menstruation resumes, the frequency or duration of breastfeeds is reduced, bottle feeds are introduced, or the baby reaches six months of age.

d. Dose-related risk of vascular disease from hormonal contraceptives

A positive association has been observed between the amount of estrogen and progestin in hormonal contraceptives and the risk of vascular disease[31–33]. A decline in serum high-density lipoproteins (HDL) has been reported with many progestational agents[14–16]. A decline in serum high-density lipoproteins has been associated with an increased incidence of ischemic heart disease. Because estrogens increase HDL cholesterol, the net effect of a hormonal contraceptive depends on a balance achieved between doses of estrogen and progestin and the activity of the progestin used in the contraceptives. The activity and amount of both hormones should be considered in the choice of a hormonal contraceptive.

e. Persistence of risk of vascular disease

There are two studies that have shown persistence of risk of vascular disease for ever-users of combination hormonal contraceptives. In a study in the United States, the risk of developing myocardial infarction after discontinuing combination hormonal contraceptives persists for at least 9 years for women 40–49 years who had used combination hormonal contraceptives for five or more years, but this increased risk was not demonstrated in other age groups[8]. In another study in Great Britain, the risk of developing cerebrovascular disease persisted for at least 6 years after discontinuation of combination hormonal contraceptives, although excess risk was very small[34]. However, both studies were performed with combination hormonal contraceptive formulations containing 50 micrograms or higher of estrogens.

It is unknown whether ORTHO EVRA® is distinct from other combination hormonal contraceptives with regard to the occurrence of venous and arterial thrombosis.

2. Estimates Of Mortality From Combination Hormonal Contraceptive Use

One study gathered data from a variety of sources that have estimated the mortality rate associated with different methods of contraception at different ages (Table 3). These estimates include the combined risk of death associated with contraceptive methods plus the risk attributable to pregnancy in the event of method failure. Each method of contraception has its specific benefits and risks. The study concluded that with the exception of combination oral contraceptive users 35 and older who smoke, and 40 and older who do not smoke, mortality associated with all methods of birth control is low and below that associated with childbirth.

The observation of a possible increase in risk of mortality with age for combination oral contraceptive users is based on data gathered in the 1970's but not reported until 1983[35]. Current clinical recommendation involves the use of lower estrogen dose formulations and a careful consideration of risk factors. In 1989, the Fertility and Maternal Health Drugs Advisory Committee was asked to review the use of combination hormonal contraceptives in women 40 years of age and over. The Committee concluded that although car-

Continued on next page

Ortho Evra—Cont.

diovascular disease risks may be increased with combination hormonal contraceptive use after age 40 in healthy non-smoking women (even with the newer low-dose formulations), there are also greater potential health risks associated with pregnancy in older women and with the alternative surgical and medical procedures that may be necessary if such women do not have access to effective and acceptable means of contraception. The Committee recommended that the benefits of low-dose combination hormonal contraceptive use by healthy non-smoking women over 40 may outweigh the possible risks[36,37].

Although the data are mainly obtained with oral contraceptives, this is likely to apply to ORTHO EVRA® as well. Women of all ages who use combination hormonal contraceptives, should use the lowest possible dose formulation that is effective and meets the individual patient needs.

[See table 3 below]

3. Carcinoma Of The Reproductive Organs And Breasts

Numerous epidemiological studies give conflicting reports on the relationship between breast cancer and COC use. The risk of having breast cancer diagnosed may be slightly increased among current and recent users of combination oral contraceptives. However, this excess risk appears to decrease over time after COC discontinuation and by 10 years after cessation the increased risk disappears. Some studies report an increased risk with duration of use while other studies do not and no consistent relationships have been found with dose or type of steroid. Some studies have found a small increase in risk for women who first use COCs before age 20. Most studies show a similar pattern of risk with COC use regardless of a woman's reproductive history or her family breast cancer history.

In addition, breast cancers diagnosed in current or ever oral contraceptive users may be less clinically advanced than in never-users.

Women who currently have or have had breast cancer should not use hormonal contraceptives because breast cancer is usually a hormonally sensitive tumor.

Some studies suggest that combination oral contraceptive use has been associated with an increase in the risk of cervical intraepithelial neoplasia in some populations of women[45–48]. However, there continues to be controversy about the extent to which such findings may be due to differences in sexual behavior and other factors.

In spite of many studies of the relationship between oral contraceptive use and breast and cervical cancers, a cause-and-effect relationship has not been established. It is not known whether ORTHO EVRA® is distinct from oral contraceptives with regard to the above statements.

4. Hepatic Neoplasia

Benign hepatic adenomas are associated with hormonal contraceptive use, although the incidence of benign tumors is rare in the United States. Indirect calculations have estimated the attributable risk to be in the range of 3.3 cases/100,000 for users, a risk that increases after four or more years of use, especially with hormonal contraceptives containing 50 micrograms or more of estrogen[49]. Rupture of benign, hepatic adenomas may cause death through intra-abdominal hemorrhage[50,51].

Studies from Britain and the US have shown an increased risk of developing hepatocellular carcinoma in long term ($\geq$ 8 years)[52–54,96] oral contraceptive users. However, these cancers are extremely rare in the U.S. and the attributable risk (the excess incidence) of liver cancers in oral contraceptive users approaches less than one per million users. It is unknown whether ORTHO EVRA® is distinct from oral contraceptives in this regard.

5. Ocular Lesions

There have been clinical case reports of retinal thrombosis associated with the use of hormonal contraceptives. ORTHO EVRA® should be discontinued if there is unexplained partial or complete loss of vision; onset of proptosis or diplopia; papilledema; or retinal vascular lesions. Appropriate diagnostic and therapeutic measures should be undertaken immediately.

6. Hormonal Contraceptive Use Before Or During Early Pregnancy

Extensive epidemiological studies have revealed no increased risk of birth defects in women who have used oral contraceptives prior to pregnancy[56,57]. Studies also do not indicate a teratogenic effect, particularly in so far as cardiac anomalies and limb reduction defects are concerned[55,56,58,59], when oral contraceptives are taken inadvertently during early pregnancy.

Combination hormonal contraceptives such as ORTHO EVRA® should not be used to induce withdrawal bleeding as a test for pregnancy. ORTHO EVRA® should not be used during pregnancy to treat threatened or habitual abortion. It is recommended that for any patient who has missed two consecutive periods, pregnancy should be ruled out. If the patient has not adhered to the prescribed schedule for the use of ORTHO EVRA® the possibility of pregnancy should be considered at the time of the first missed period. Hormonal contraceptive use should be discontinued if pregnancy is confirmed.

7. Gallbladder Disease

Earlier studies have reported an increased lifetime relative risk of gallbladder surgery in users of hormonal contraceptives and estrogens[60,61]. More recent studies, however, have shown that the relative risk of developing gallbladder disease among hormonal contraceptive users may be minimal[62–64]. The recent findings of minimal risk may be related to the use of hormonal contraceptive formulations containing lower hormonal doses of estrogens and progestins.

Combination hormonal contraceptives such as ORTHO EVRA® may worsen existing gallbladder disease and may accelerate the development of this disease in previously asymptomatic women. Women with a history of combination hormonal contraceptive-related cholestasis are more likely to have the condition recur with subsequent combination hormonal contraceptive use.

8. Carbohydrate And Lipid Metabolic Effects

Hormonal contraceptives have been shown to cause a decrease in glucose tolerance in some users[17]. However, in the non-diabetic woman, combination hormonal contraceptives appear to have no effect on fasting blood glucose[67]. Prediabetic and diabetic women in particular should be carefully monitored while taking combination hormonal contraceptives such as ORTHO EVRA®.

In clinical trials with oral contraceptives containing ethinyl estradiol and norgestimate there were no clinically significant changes in fasting blood glucose levels. There were no clinically significant changes in glucose levels over 24 cycles of use. Moreover, glucose tolerance tests showed no clinically significant changes from baseline to cycles 3, 12 and 24. In a 6-cycle clinical trial with ORTHO EVRA® there were no clinically significant changes in fasting blood glucose from baseline to end of treatment.

A small proportion of women will have persistent hypertriglyceridemia while taking hormonal contraceptives. As discussed earlier (see WARNINGS 1a and 1d), changes in serum triglycerides and lipoprotein levels have been reported in hormonal contraceptive users.

9. Elevated Blood Pressure

Women with significant hypertension should not be started on hormonal contraception[103]. Women with a history of hypertension or hypertension-related diseases, or renal disease[70] should be encouraged to use another method of contraception. If women elect to use ORTHO EVRA®, they should be monitored closely and if a clinically significant elevation of blood pressure occurs, ORTHO EVRA® should be discontinued. For most women, elevated blood pressure will return to normal after stopping hormonal contraceptives, and there is no difference in the occurrence of hypertension between former and never users[68–71].

An increase in blood pressure has been reported in women taking hormonal contraceptives[68] and this increase is more likely in older hormonal contraceptive users[69] and with extended duration of use[61]. Data from the Royal College of General Practitioners[12] and subsequent randomized trials have shown that the incidence of hypertension increases with increasing progestational activity.

10. Headache

The onset or exacerbation of migraine headache or the development of headache with a new pattern that is recurrent, persistent or severe requires discontinuation of ORTHO EVRA® and evaluation of the cause.

11. Bleeding Irregularities

Breakthrough bleeding and spotting are sometimes encountered in women using ORTHO EVRA®. Non-hormonal causes should be considered and adequate diagnostic measures taken to rule out malignancy, other pathology, or pregnancy in the event of breakthrough bleeding, as in the case of any abnormal vaginal bleeding. If pathology has been excluded, time or a change to another contraceptive product may resolve the bleeding. In the event of amenorrhea, pregnancy should be ruled out before initiating use of ORTHO EVRA®.

Some women may encounter amenorrhea or oligomenorrhea after discontinuation of hormonal contraceptive use, especially when such a condition was pre-existent.

<u>Bleeding Patterns:</u>

In the clinical trials most women started their withdrawal bleeding on the fourth day of the drug-free interval, and the median duration of withdrawal bleeding was 5 to 6 days. On average 26% of women per cycle had 7 or more total days of bleeding and/or spotting (this includes both withdrawal flow and breakthrough bleeding and/or spotting).

12. Ectopic Pregnancy

Ectopic as well as intrauterine pregnancy may occur in contraceptive failures.

Table 3. Annual Number of Birth-Related or Method-Related Deaths Associated With Control of Fertility Per 100,000 Non-Sterile Women, by Fertility Control Method According to Age

Method of control and outcome	15–19	20–24	25–29	30–34	35–39	40–44
No fertility control methods*	7.0	7.4	9.1	14.8	25.7	28.2
Oral contraceptives, non-smoker**	0.3	0.5	0.9	1.9	13.8	31.6
Oral contraceptives, smoker**	2.2	3.4	6.6	13.5	51.1	117.2
IUD**	0.8	0.8	1.0	1.0	1.4	1.4
Condom*	1.1	1.6	0.7	0.2	0.3	0.4
Diaphragm/spermicide*	1.9	1.2	1.2	1.3	2.2	2.8
Periodic abstinence*	2.5	1.6	1.6	1.7	2.9	3.6

*Deaths are birth-related
**Deaths are method-related
Adapted from H.W. Ory, ref. # 35.

PRECAUTIONS

Women should be counseled that ORTHO EVRA® does not protect against HIV infection (AIDS) and other sexually transmitted infections.

1. Body Weight ≥198 lbs. (90 kg)

Results of clinical trials suggest that ORTHO EVRA® may be less effective in women with body weight ≥198 lbs. (90 kg) than in women with lower body weights.

2. Physical Examination And Follow-Up

It is good medical practice for women using ORTHO EVRA®, as for all women, to have annual medical evaluation and physical examinations. The physical examination, however, may be deferred until after initiation of hormonal contraceptives if requested by the woman and judged appropriate by the clinician. The physical examination should include special reference to blood pressure, breasts, abdomen and pelvic organs, including cervical cytology, and relevant laboratory tests. In case of undiagnosed, persistent or recurrent abnormal vaginal bleeding, appropriate measures should be conducted to rule out malignancy or other pathology. Women with a strong family history of breast cancer or who have breast nodules should be monitored with particular care.

3. Lipid Disorders

Women who are being treated for hyperlipidemias should be followed closely if they elect to use ORTHO EVRA®. Some progestins may elevate LDL levels and may render the control of hyperlipidemias more difficult.

4. Liver Function

If jaundice develops in any woman using ORTHO EVRA®, the medication should be discontinued. The hormones in ORTHO EVRA® may be poorly metabolized in patients with impaired liver function.

5. Fluid Retention

Steroid hormones like those in ORTHO EVRA® may cause some degree of fluid retention. ORTHO EVRA® should be prescribed with caution, and only with careful monitoring, in patients with conditions which might be aggravated by fluid retention.

6. Emotional Disorders

Women who become significantly depressed while using combination hormonal contraceptives such as ORTHO EVRA® should stop the medication and use another method of contraception in an attempt to determine whether the symptom is drug related. Women with a history of depression should be carefully observed and ORTHO EVRA® discontinued if significant depression occurs.

7. Contact Lenses

Contact lens wearers who develop visual changes or changes in lens tolerance should be assessed by an ophthalmologist.

8. Drug Interactions

<u>Changes in Contraceptive Effectiveness Associated with Co-Administration of Other Drugs:</u>

Contraceptive effectiveness may be reduced when hormonal contraceptives are co-administered with some antibiotics, antifungals, anticonvulsants, and other drugs that increase metabolism of contraceptive steroids. This could result in unintended pregnancy or breakthrough bleeding. Examples include barbiturates, griseofulvin, rifampin, phenylbutazone, phenytoin, carbamazepine, felbamate, oxcarbazepine, topiramate and possibly with ampicillin.

The proposed mechanism of interaction of antibiotics is different from that of liver enzyme-inducing drugs. Literature suggests possible interactions with the concomitant use of hormonal contraceptives and ampicillin or tetracycline. In a pharmacokinetic drug interaction study, oral administration of tetracycline HCl, 500 mg q.i.d. for 3 days prior to and 7 days during wear of ORTHO EVRA® did not significantly affect the pharmacokinetics of norelgestromin or EE.

Several of the anti-HIV protease inhibitors have been studied with co-administration of oral combination hormonal contraceptives; significant changes (increase and decrease) in the mean AUC of the estrogen and progestin have been noted in some cases. The efficacy and safety of oral contraceptive products may be affected; it is unknown whether this applies to ORTHO EVRA®. Healthcare professionals should refer to the label of the individual anti-HIV protease inhibitors for further drug-drug interaction information.

Herbal products containing St. John's Wort (hypericum perforatum) may induce hepatic enzymes (cytochrome P450) and p-glycoprotein transporter and may reduce the effectiveness of contraceptive steroids. This may also result in breakthrough bleeding.

Increase in Plasma Hormone Levels Associated with Co-Administered Drugs:
Co-administration of atorvastatin and certain oral contraceptives containing ethinyl estradiol increase AUC values for ethinyl estradiol by approximately 20%. Ascorbic acid and acetaminophen may increase plasma ethinyl estradiol levels, possibly by inhibition of conjugation. CYP 3A4 inhibitors such as itraconazole or ketoconazole may increase plasma hormone levels.
Changes in Plasma Levels of Co-Administered Drugs:
Combination hormonal contraceptives containing some synthetic estrogens (e.g., ethinyl estradiol) may inhibit the metabolism of other compounds. Increased plasma concentrations of cyclosporine, prednisolone, and theophylline have been reported with concomitant administration of oral contraceptives. In addition, oral contraceptives may induce the conjugation of other compounds. Decreased plasma concentrations of acetaminophen and increased clearance of temazepam, salicylic acid, morphine and clofibric acid have been noted when these drugs were administered with oral contraceptives.
Although norelgestromin and its metabolites inhibit a variety of P450 enzymes in human liver microsomes, the clinical consequence of such an interaction on the levels of other concomitant medications is likely to be insignificant. Under the recommended dosing regimen, the in vivo concentrations of norelgestromin and its metabolites, even at the peak serum levels, are relatively low compared to the inhibitory constant (Ki) (based on results of *in vitro* studies).
Health care professionals are advised to also refer to prescribing information of co-administered drugs for recommendations regarding management of concomitant therapy.

9. Interactions With Laboratory Tests
Certain endocrine and liver function tests and blood components may be affected by hormonal contraceptives:
a. Increased prothrombin and factors VII, VIII, IX, and X; decreased antithrombin 3; increased norepinephrine-induced platelet aggregability.
b. Increased thyroid binding globulin (TBG) leading to increased circulating total thyroid hormone, as measured by protein-bound iodine (PBI), T4 by column or by radioimmunoassay. Free T3 resin uptake is decreased, reflecting the elevated TBG, free T4 concentration is unaltered.
c. Other binding proteins may be elevated in serum.
d. Sex hormone binding globulins are increased and result in elevated levels of total circulating endogenous sex steroids and corticoids; however, free or biologically active levels either decrease or remain unchanged.
e. Triglycerides may be increased and levels of various other lipids and lipoproteins may be affected.
f. Glucose tolerance may be decreased.
g. Serum folate levels may be depressed by hormonal contraceptive therapy. This may be of clinical significance if a woman becomes pregnant shortly after discontinuing ORTHO EVRA®.

10. Carcinogenesis
No carcinogenicity studies were conducted with norelgestromin. However, bridging PK studies were conducted using doses of NGM/EE which were used previously in the 2-year rat carcinogenicity study and 10-year monkey toxicity study to support the approval of ORTHO-CYCLEN® and ORTHO TRI-CYCLEN® under NDAs 19-653 and 19-697, respectively. The PK studies demonstrated that rats and monkeys were exposed to 16 and 8 times the human exposure, respectively, with the proposed ORTHO EVRA® transdermal contraceptive system.
Norelgestromin was tested in in-vitro mutagenicity assays (bacterial plate incorporation mutation assay, CHO/HGPRT mutation assay, chromosomal aberration assay using cultured human peripheral lymphocytes) and in one in-vivo test (rat micronucleus assay) and found to have no genotoxic potential.
See WARNINGS Section.

11. Pregnancy
Pregnancy Category X. See CONTRAINDICATIONS and WARNINGS Sections.
Norelgestromin was tested for its reproductive toxicity in a rabbit developmental toxicity study by the SC route of administration. Doses of 0, 1, 2, 4 and 6 mg/kg body weight, which gave systemic exposure of approximately 25 to 125 times the human exposure with ORTHO EVRA®, were administered daily on gestation days 7–19. Malformations reported were paw hyperflexion at 4 and 6 mg/kg and paw hyperextension and cleft palate at 6 mg/kg.

12. Nursing Mothers
The effects of ORTHO EVRA® in nursing mothers have not been evaluated and are unknown. Small amounts of combination hormonal contraceptive steroids have been identified in the milk of nursing mothers and a few adverse effects on the child have been reported, including jaundice and breast enlargement. In addition, combination hormonal contraceptives given in the postpartum period may interfere with lactation by decreasing the quantity and quality of breast milk. Long-term follow-up of infants whose mothers used combination hormonal contraceptives while breast feeding has shown no deleterious effects. However, the nursing mother should be advised not to use ORTHO EVRA® but to use other forms of contraception until she has completely weaned her child.

13. Pediatric Use
Safety and efficacy of ORTHO EVRA® have been established in women of reproductive age. Safety and efficacy are expected to be the same for post-pubertal adolescents under the age of 16 and for users 16 years and older. Use of this product before menarche is not indicated.

14. Geriatric Use
This product has not been studied in women over 65 years of age and is not indicated in this population.

15. Sexually Transmitted Diseases
Patients should be counseled that this product does not protect against HIV infection (AIDS) and other sexually transmitted diseases.

16. Patch Adhesion
Experience with more than 70,000 ORTHO EVRA® patches worn for contraception for 6–13 cycles showed that 4.7% of patches were replaced because they either fell off (1.8%) or were partly detached (2.9%). Similarly, in a small study of patch wear under conditions of physical exertion and variable temperature and humidity, less than 2% of patches were replaced for complete or partial detachment.
If the ORTHO EVRA® patch becomes partially or completely detached and remains detached, insufficient drug delivery occurs. A patch should not be re-applied if it is no longer sticky, if it has become stuck to itself or another surface, if it has other material stuck to it, or if it has become loose or fallen off before. If a patch cannot be re-applied, a new patch should be applied immediately. Supplemental adhesives or wraps should not be used to hold the ORTHO EVRA® patch in place.
If a patch is partially or completely detached for more than one day (24 hours or more) OR if the woman is not sure how long the patch has been detached, she may not be protected from pregnancy. She should stop the current contraceptive cycle and start a new cycle immediately by applying a new patch. Back-up contraception, such as condoms, spermicide, or diaphragm, must be used for the first week of the new cycle.

INFORMATION FOR THE PATIENT
See Patient Labeling printed below.

ADVERSE REACTIONS

The most common adverse events reported by 9 to 22% of women using ORTHO EVRA® in clinical trials (N= 3,330) were the following, in order of decreasing incidence: breast symptoms, headache, application site reaction, nausea, upper respiratory infection, menstrual cramps, and abdominal pain.
The most frequent adverse events leading to discontinuation in 1 to 2.4% of women using ORTHO EVRA® in the trials included the following: nausea and/or vomiting, application site reaction, breast symptoms, headache, and emotional lability.
Listed below are adverse events that have been associated with the use of combination hormonal contraceptives. These are also likely to apply to combination transdermal hormonal contraceptives such as ORTHO EVRA®.
An increased risk of the following serious adverse reactions has been associated with the use of combination hormonal contraceptives (see WARNINGS Section).

- Thrombophlebitis and venous thrombosis with or without embolism
- Arterial thromboembolism
- Pulmonary embolism
- Myocardial infarction
- Cerebral hemorrhage
- Cerebral thrombosis
- Hypertension
- Gallbladder disease
- Hepatic adenomas or benign liver tumors

There is evidence of an association between the following conditions and the use of combination hormonal contraceptives:

- Mesenteric thrombosis
- Retinal thrombosis

The following adverse reactions have been reported in users of combination hormonal contraceptives and are believed to be drug-related:

- Nausea
- Vomiting
- Gastrointestinal symptoms (such as abdominal cramps and bloating)
- Breakthrough bleeding
- Spotting
- Change in menstrual flow
- Amenorrhea
- Temporary infertility after discontinuation of treatment
- Edema
- Melasma which may persist
- Breast changes: tenderness, enlargement, secretion
- Change in weight (increase or decrease)
- Change in cervical erosion and secretion
- Diminution in lactation when given immediately postpartum
- Cholestatic jaundice
- Migraine
- Rash (allergic)
- Mental depression
- Reduced tolerance to carbohydrates
- Vaginal candidiasis
- Change in corneal curvature (steepening)
- Intolerance to contact lenses

The following adverse reactions have been reported in users of combination hormonal contraceptives and a cause and effect association has been neither confirmed nor refuted:

- Pre-menstrual syndrome
- Cataracts
- Changes in appetite
- Cystitis-like syndrome
- Headache
- Nervousness
- Dizziness
- Hirsutism
- Loss of scalp hair
- Erythema multiforme
- Erythema nodosum
- Hemorrhagic eruption
- Vaginitis
- Porphyria
- Impaired renal function
- Hemolytic uremic syndrome
- Acne
- Changes in libido
- Colitis
- Budd-Chiari Syndrome

OVERDOSAGE

Serious ill effects have not been reported following accidental ingestion of large doses of hormonal contraceptives. Overdosage may cause nausea and vomiting, and withdrawal bleeding may occur in females. Given the nature and design of the ORTHO EVRA® patch, it is unlikely that overdosage will occur. Serious ill effects have not been reported following acute ingestion of large doses of oral contraceptives by young children. In case of suspected overdose, all ORTHO EVRA® patches should be removed and symptomatic treatment given.

DOSAGE AND ADMINISTRATION

To achieve maximum contraceptive effectiveness, ORTHO EVRA® must be used exactly as directed.
Complete instructions to facilitate patient counseling on proper system usage may be found in the Detailed Patient Labeling.
Transdermal Contraceptive System Overview
This system uses a 28-day (four-week) cycle. A new patch is applied each week for three weeks (21 total days). Week Four is patch-free. Withdrawal bleeding is expected during this time.
Every new patch should be applied on the same day of the week. This day is known as the "Patch Change Day." For example, if the first patch is applied on a Monday, all subsequent patches should be applied on a Monday. Only one patch should be worn at a time.
On the day after Week Four ends a new four-week cycle is started by applying a new patch. Under no circumstances should there be more than a seven-day patch-free interval between dosing cycles.

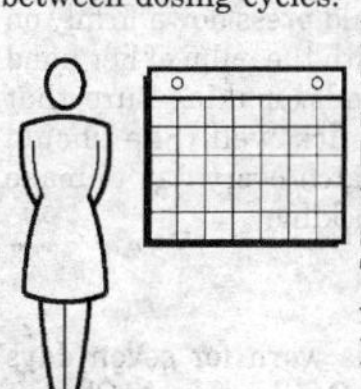

If the woman is starting ORTHO EVRA® for the **first time**, she should **wait until the day she begins her menstrual period**. Either a First Day start or Sunday start may be chosen (see below). The day she applies her first patch will be Day 1. Her "Patch Change Day" will be on this day every week.

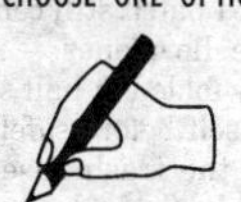

- for **First Day Start**: the patient should apply her first patch during the first 24 hours of her menstrual period.

If therapy starts after Day 1 of the menstrual cycle, a non-hormonal back-up contraceptive (such as condoms, spermicide, or diaphragm) should be used concurrently for the first 7 consecutive days of the first treatment cycle.
OR

- for **Sunday Start**: the woman should apply her first patch on the first Sunday after her menstrual period starts. She must use back-up contraception for the first week of her first cycle.

If the menstrual period begins on a Sunday, the first patch should be applied on that day, and no back-up contraception is needed.
Where to apply the patch. The patch should be applied to clean, dry, intact healthy skin on the buttock, abdomen, upper outer arm or upper torso, in a place where it won't be rubbed by tight clothing. ORTHO EVRA® should not be placed on skin that is red, irritated or cut, nor should it be placed on the breasts.
To prevent interference with the adhesive properties of ORTHO EVRA®, no make-up, creams, lotions, powders or other topical products should be applied to the skin area where the ORTHO EVRA® patch is or will be placed.

Continued on next page

Ortho Evra—Cont.

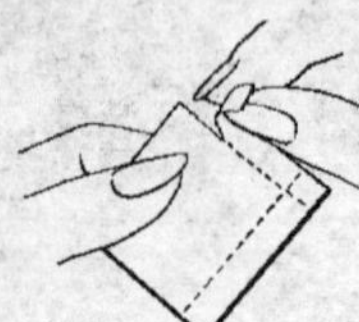

Application of the ORTHO EVRA® patch

The foil pouch is opened by tearing it along the edge using the fingers.

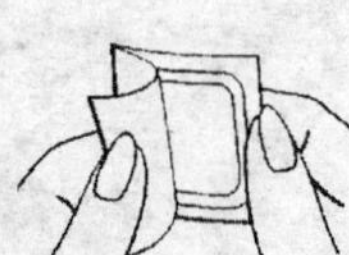

The foil pouch should be peeled apart and open flat.

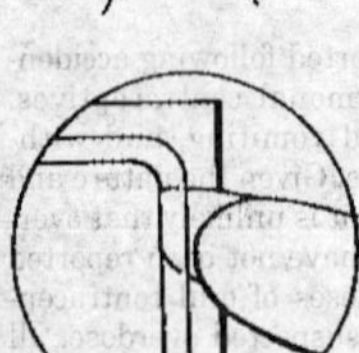

A corner of the patch is grasped firmly and it is gently removed from the foil pouch.

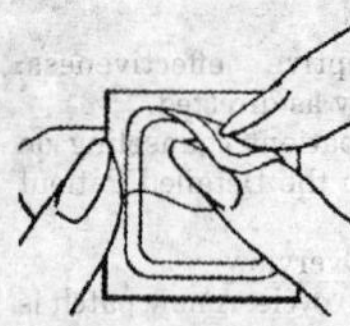

The woman should be instructed to use her fingernail, to lift one corner of the patch and peel the patch **and** the plastic liner off the foil liner. **Sometimes patches can stick to the inside of the pouch – the woman should be careful not to accidentally remove the clear liner as she removes the patch.**

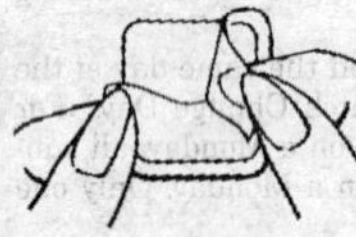

Half of the clear protective liner is to be peeled away. (The woman should avoid touching the sticky surface of the patch).

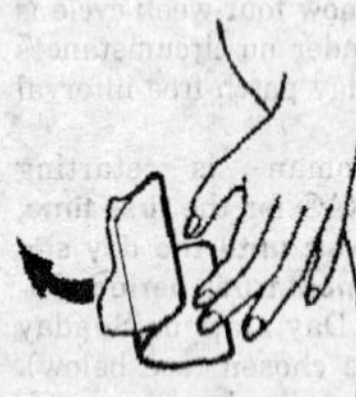

The sticky surface of the patch is applied to the skin and the other half of the liner is removed. The woman should press down firmly on the patch with the palm of her hand for 10 seconds, making sure that the edges stick well. She should check her patch every day to make sure it is sticking.

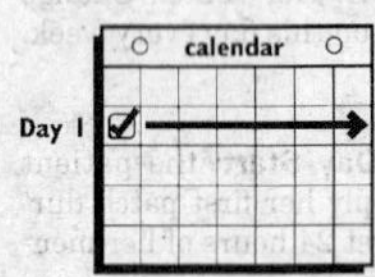

The patch is worn for seven days (one week). On the "Patch Change Day", Day 8, the used patch is removed and a new one is applied immediately. The used patch still contains some active hormones – it should be carefully folded in half so that it sticks to itself before safely disposing of it in the trash. Used patches should not be flushed down the toilet.

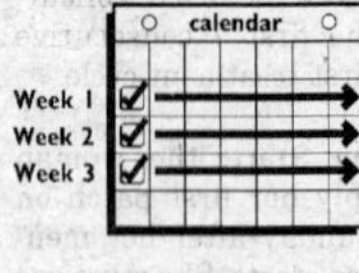

A new patch is applied for Week Two (on Day 8) and again for Week Three (on Day 15), on the usual "Patch Change Day". Patch changes may occur at any time on the Change Day. Each new ORTHO EVRA® patch should be applied to a new spot on the skin to help avoid irritation, although they may be kept within the same anatomic area.

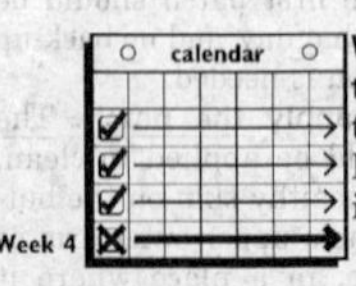

Week Four is patch-free (Day 22 through Day 28), thus completing the four-week contraceptive cycle. Bleeding is expected to begin during this time.

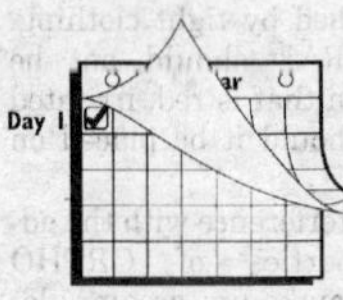

The next four-week cycle is started by applying a new patch on the usual "Patch Change Day," the day after Day 28, no matter when the menstrual period begins or ends.

Under no circumstances should there be more than a seven-day patch-free interval between patch cycles.

If the ORTHO EVRA® patch becomes partially or completely detached and remains detached, insufficient drug delivery occurs.

If a patch is partially or completely detached:

- **for less than one day** (up to 24 hours), the woman should try to reapply it to the same place or replace it with a new patch immediately. No back-up contraception is needed. The woman's "Patch Change Day" will remain the same.
- **for more than one day** (24 hours or more) **OR if the woman is not sure how long the patch has been detached,** SHE MAY NOT BE PROTECTED FROM PREGNANCY. She should stop the current contraceptive cycle and start a new cycle immediately by applying a new patch. There is now a new "Day 1" and a new "Patch Change Day." Back-up contraception, such as condoms, spermicide, or diaphragm, must be used for the first week of the new cycle.

A patch should not be re-applied if it is no longer sticky, if it has become stuck to itself or another surface, if it has other material stuck to it or if it has previously become loose or fallen off. If a patch cannot be re-applied, a new patch should be applied immediately. Supplemental adhesives or wraps should not be used to hold the ORTHO EVRA® patch in place.

If the woman forgets to change her patch...

- **at the start of any patch cycle** (Week One /Day 1): SHE MAY NOT BE PROTECTED FROM PREGNANCY. She should apply the first patch of her new cycle as soon as she remembers. There is now a new "Patch Change Day" and a new "Day 1." The woman must use back-up contraception, such as condoms, spermicide, or diaphragm, for the first week of the new cycle.
- **in the middle of the patch cycle (Week Two/Day 8 or Week Three/Day 15),**
  - — for **one or two days** (up to 48 hours), she should apply a new patch immediately. The next patch should be applied on the usual "Patch Change Day." No back-up contraception is needed. (See Figures 3 and 4 in the Clinical Pharmacology section.)
  - — for **more than two days** (48 hours or more), SHE MAY NOT BE PROTECTED FROM PREGNANCY. She should stop the current contraceptive cycle and start a new four-week cycle immediately by putting on a new patch. There is now a new "Patch Change Day" and a new "Day 1." The woman must use back-up contraception for one week.
- **at the end of the patch cycle (Week Four/Day 22),** Week Four (Day 22): If the woman forgets to remove her patch, she should take it off as soon as she remembers. The next cycle should be started on the usual "Patch Change Day," which is the day after Day 28. No back-up contraception is needed.

Under no circumstances should there be more than a seven-day patch-free interval between cycles. If there are more than seven patch-free days, THE WOMAN MAY NOT BE PROTECTED FROM PREGNANCY and back-up contraception, such as condoms, spermicide, or diaphragm, must be used for seven days. As with combined oral contraceptives, the risk of ovulation increases with each day beyond the recommended drug-free period. If coital exposure has occurred during such an extended patch-free interval, the possibility of fertilization should be considered.

Change Day Adjustment

If the woman wishes to change her Patch Change Day she should complete her current cycle, removing the third ORTHO EVRA® patch on the correct day. During the patch-free week, she may select an earlier Patch Day Change by applying a new ORTHO EVRA® patch on the desired day. In no case should there be more than 7 consecutive patch-free days.

Switching from an Oral Contraceptive

Treatment with ORTHO EVRA® should begin on the first day of withdrawal bleeding. If there is no withdrawal bleeding within 5 days of the last active (hormone-containing) tablet, pregnancy must be ruled out. If therapy starts later than the first day of withdrawal bleeding, a non-hormonal contraceptive should be used concurrently for 7 days. If more than 7 days elapse after taking the last active oral contraceptive tablet, the possibility of ovulation and conception should be considered.

Use after Childbirth

Women who elect not to breast-feed should start contraceptive therapy with ORTHO EVRA® no sooner than 4 weeks after childbirth. If a woman begins using ORTHO EVRA® postpartum, and has not yet had a period, the possibility of ovulation and conception occurring prior to use of ORTHO EVRA® should be considered, and she should be instructed to use an additional method of contraception, such as condoms, spermicide, or diaphragm, for the first seven days. (See *Precautions: Nursing Mothers, and Warnings: Thromboembolic and Other Vascular Problems.*)

Use after Abortion or Miscarriage[106]

After an abortion or miscarriage that occurs in the first trimester, ORTHO EVRA® may be started immediately. An additional method of contraception is not needed if ORTHO EVRA® is started immediately. If use of ORTHO EVRA® is not started within 5 days following a first trimester abortion, the woman should follow the instructions for a woman starting ORTHO EVRA® for the first time. In the meantime she should be advised to use a non-hormonal contraceptive method. Ovulation may occur within 10 days of an abortion or miscarriage.

ORTHO EVRA® should be started no earlier than 4 weeks after a second trimester abortion or miscarriage. When ORTHO EVRA® is used postpartum or postabortion, the increased risk of thromboembolic disease must be considered. (See CONTRAINDICATIONS and WARNINGS concerning thromboembolic disease. See PRECAUTIONS for "Nursing Mothers".)

Breakthrough Bleeding or Spotting

In the event of breakthrough bleeding or spotting (bleeding that occurs on the days that ORTHO EVRA® is worn), treatment should be continued. If breakthrough bleeding persists longer than a few cycles, a cause other than ORTHO EVRA® should be considered.

In the event of no withdrawal bleeding (bleeding that should occur during the patch-free week), treatment should be resumed on the next scheduled Change Day. If ORTHO EVRA® has been used correctly, the absence of withdrawal bleeding is not necessarily an indication of pregnancy. Nevertheless, the possibility of pregnancy should be considered, especially if absence of withdrawal bleeding occurs in 2 consecutive cycles. ORTHO EVRA® should be discontinued if pregnancy is confirmed.

In Case of Vomiting or Diarrhea

Given the nature of transdermal application, dose delivery should be unaffected by vomiting.

In Case of Skin Irritation

If patch use results in uncomfortable irritation, the patch may be removed and a new patch may be applied to a different location until the next Change Day. Only one patch should be worn at a time.

ADDITIONAL INSTRUCTIONS FOR DOSING

Breakthrough bleeding, spotting, and amenorrhea are frequent reasons for patients discontinuing hormonal contraceptives. In case of breakthrough bleeding, as in all cases of irregular bleeding from the vagina, nonfunctional causes should considered. In case of undiagnosed persistent or recurrent abnormal bleeding from the vagina, adequate diagnostic measures are indicated to rule out pregnancy or malignancy. If pathology has been excluded, time or a change to another method of contraception may solve the problem.

Use of hormonal contraceptives in the event of a missed menstrual period:

1. If the woman has not adhered to the prescribed schedule, the possibility of pregnancy should be considered at the time of the first missed period. Hormonal contraceptive use should be discontinued if pregnancy is confirmed.
2. If the woman has adhered to the prescribed regimen and misses one period, she should continue using her contraceptive patches.
3. If the woman has adhered to the prescribed regimen and misses two consecutive periods, pregnancy should be ruled out. ORTHO EVRA® use should be discontinued if pregnancy is confirmed.

HOW SUPPLIED

Each beige ORTHO EVRA® patch contains 6.0 mg norelgestromin and 0.75 mg EE, and releases 150 micrograms of norelgestromin and 20 micrograms of EE to the bloodstream per 24 hours. Each patch surface is heat stamped with ORTHO EVRA® 150/20. Each patch is packaged in a protective pouch.

ORTHO EVRA® is available in folding cartons of 1 cycle each (NDC # 0062-1920-15); each cycle contains 3 patches. ORTHO EVRA® is also available in folding cartons containing a single patch (NDC # 0062-1920-01), intended for use as a replacement in the event that a patch is inadvertently lost or destroyed.

Special Precautions for Storage and Disposal

Store at 25°C (77°F); excursions permitted to 15–30°C (59–86°F).

Store patches in their protective pouches. Apply immediately upon removal from the protective pouch.

Do not store in the refrigerator or freezer.

Used patches still contain some active hormones. Each patch should be carefully folded in half so that it sticks to itself before safely disposing of it in the trash. Used patches should not be flushed down the toilet.

REFERENCES

1. Trussel J. Contraceptive efficacy. In Hatcher RA, Trussel J, Stewart F, Cates W, Stewart GK, Kowal D, Guest F. *Contraceptive Technology: Seventeenth Revised Edition.* New York NY: Irvington Publishers, 1998. **2.** Stadel BV. Oral contraceptives and cardiovascular disease. (Pt.1). N Engl J Med 1981; 305:612-618. **3.** Stadel BV. Oral contraceptives and cardiovascular disease. (Pt.2). N Engl J Med 1981; 305:672–677. **4.** Adam SA, Thorogood M. Oral contraception and myocardial infarction revisited: the effects of new preparations and prescribing patterns. Br J Obstet Gynaecol 1981; 88: 838–845. **5.** Mann JI, Inman WH. Oral contraceptives and death from myocardial infarction. Br Med J 1975; 2(5965): 245–248. **6.** Mann JI, Vessey MP, Thorogood M, Doll R. Myocardial infarction in young women with special reference to oral contraceptive practice. Br Med J 1975; 2(5956):241–245. **7.** Royal College of General Practitioners' Oral Contraception Study: Further analyses of mortality in oral contraceptive users. Lancet 1981; 1:541–546. **8.** Slone D, Shapiro S, Kaufman DW, Rosenberg L, Miettinen OS, Stolley PD. Risk of myocardial infarction in relation to current and discontinued use of oral contraceptives. N Engl J Med 1981; 305:420–424. **9.** Vessey MP. Female hormones and vascular disease-an epidemiological overview. Br J Fam Plann 1980; 6 (Supplement): 1–12. **10.** Russell-Briefel RG, Ezzati TM, Fulwood R, Perlman JA, Murphy RS. Cardiovascular risk status and oral contraceptive use, United States, 1976–80. Prevent Med 1986; 15:352–362. **11.** Goldbaum GM, Kendrick JS, Hogelin GC, Gentry EM. The relative impact of smoking and oral contraceptive use on women in the United States. JAMA 1987; 258:1339–1342. **12.** Layde PM, Beral V. Further analyses of mortality in oral contraceptive users; Royal College of General Practitioners' Oral Contraception

Study. (Table 5) Lancet 1981; 1:541–546. **13.** Knopp RH. Arteriosclerosis risk: the roles of oral contraceptives and postmenopausal estrogens. J Reprod Med 1986; 31(9) (Supplement):913–921. **14.** Krauss RM, Roy S, Mishell DR, Casagrande J, Pike MC. Effects of two low-dose oral contraceptives on serum lipids and lipoproteins: Differential changes in high-density lipoproteins subclasses. Am J Obstet 1983; 145:446–452. **15.** Wahl P, Walden C, Knopp R, Hoover J, Wallace R, Heiss G, Rifkind B. Effect of estrogen/progestin potency on lipid/lipoprotein cholesterol. N Engl J Med 1983; 308:862–867. **16.** Wynn V, Niththyananthan R. The effect of progestin in combined oral contraceptives on serum lipids with special reference to high density lipoproteins. Am J Obstet Gynecol 1982;142:766–771. **17.** Wynn V, Godsland I. Effects of oral contraceptives on carbohydrate metabolism. J Reprod Med 1986;31(9)(Supplement):892–897. **18.** LaRosa JC. Atherosclerotic risk factors in cardiovascular disease. J Reprod Med 1986;31(9)(Supplement): 906–912. **19.** Inman WH, Vessey MP. Investigation of death from pulmonary, coronary, and cerebral thrombosis and embolism in women of child-bearing age. Br Med J 1968;2(5599):193–199. **20.** Maguire MG, Tonascia J, Sartwell PE, Stolley PD, Tockman MS. Increased risk of thrombosis due to oral contraceptives: a further report. Am J Epidemiol 1979;110(2):188–195. **21.** Petitti DB, Wingerd J, Pellegrin F, Ramacharan S. Risk of vascular disease in women: smoking, oral contraceptives, noncontraceptive estrogens, and other factors. JAMA 1979;242:1150–1154. **22.** Vessey MP, Doll R. Investigation of relation between use of oral contraceptives and thromboembolic disease. Br Med J 1968;2(5599):199–205. **23.** Vessey MP, Doll R. Investigation of relation between use of oral contraceptives and thromboembolic disease. A further report. Br Med J 1969; 2(5658): 651–657. **24.** Porter JB, Hunter JR, Danielson DA, Jick H, Stergachis A. Oral contraceptives and non-fatal vascular disease-recent experience. Obstet Gynecol 1982;59(3):299–302. **25.** Vessey M, Doll R, Peto R, Johnson B, Wiggins P. A long-term follow-up study of women using different methods of contraception: an interim report. J Biosocial Sci 1976;8: 375–427. **26.** Royal College of General Practitioners: Oral Contraceptives, venous thrombosis, and varicose veins. J Royal Coll Gen Pract 1978; 28:393–399. **27.** Collaborative Group for the Study of Stroke in Young Women: Oral contraception and increased risk of cerebral ischemia or thrombosis. N Engl J Med 1973;288:871–878. **28.** Petitti DB, Wingerd J. Use of oral contraceptives, cigarette smoking, and risk of subarachnoid hemorrhage. Lancet 1978;2:234–236.**29.** Inman WH. Oral contraceptives and fatal subarachnoid hemorrhage. Br Med J 1979:2(6203):1468–1470.**30.** Collaborative Group for the Study of Stroke in Young Women: Oral Contraceptives and stroke in young women: associated risk factors. JAMA 1975; 231:718–722. **31.** Inman WH, Vessey MP, Westerholm B, Engelund A. Thromboembolic disease and the steroidal content of oral contraceptives. A report to the Committee on Safety of Drugs. Br Med J 1970;2:203-209. **32.** Meade TW, Greenberg G, Thompson SG. Progestogens and cardiovascular reactions associated with oral contraceptives and a comparison of the safety of 50- and 35-mcg oestrogen preparations. Br Med J 1980;280(6224):1157–1161. **33.** Kay CR. Progestogens and arterial disease-evidence from the Royal College of General Practitioners' Study. Am J Obstet Gynecol 1982;142:762–765. **34.** Royal College of General Practitioners: Incidence of arterial disease among oral contraceptive users. J Royal Coll Gen Pract 1983;33:75–82. **35.** Ory HW. Mortality associated with fertility and fertility control: 1983. Family Planning Perspectives 1983;15:50–56. **36.** The Cancer and Steroid Hormone Study of the Centers for Disease Control and the National Institute of Child Health and Human Development: Oral contraceptive use and the risk of breast cancer. N Engl J Med 1986;315:405–411. **37.** Pike MC, Henderson BE, Krailo MD, Duke A, Roy S. Breast cancer in young women and use of oral contraceptives: possible modifying effect of formulation and age at use. Lancet 1983;2:926–929. **38.** Paul C, Skegg DG, Spears GFS, Kaldor JM. Oral contraceptives and breast cancer: A national study. Br Med J 1986; 293:723–725. **39.** Miller DR, Rosenberg L, Kaufman DW, Schottenfeld D, Stolley PD, Shapiro S. Breast cancer risk in relation to early oral contraceptive use. Obstet Gynecol 1986;68:863–868. **40.** Olson H, Olson KL, Moller TR, Ranstam J, Holm P. Oral contraceptive use and breast cancer in young women in Sweden (letter). Lancet 1985; 2:748–749. **41.** McPherson K, Vessey M, Neil A, Doll R, Jones L, Roberts M. Early contraceptive use and breast cancer: Results of another case-control study. Br J Cancer 1987; 56:653–660. **42.** Huggins GR, Zucker PF. Oral contraceptives and neoplasia; 1987 update. Fertil Steril 1987; 47:733–761. **43.** McPherson K, Drife JO. The pill and breast cancer: why the uncertainty? Br Med J 1986; 293:709–710. **44.** Shapiro S. Oral contraceptives-time to take stock. N Engl J Med 1987; 315: 450–451. **45.** Ory H, Naib Z, Conger SB, Hatcher RA, Tyler CW. Contraceptive choice and prevalence of cervical dysplasia and carcinoma in situ. Am J Obstet Gynecol 1976; 124: 573–577. **46.** Vessey MP, Lawless M, McPherson K, Yeates D. Neoplasia of the cervix uteri and contraception: a possible adverse effect of the pill. Lancet 1983; 2:930. **47.** Brinton LA, Huggins GR, Lehman HF, Malli K, Savitz DA, Trapido E, Rosenthal J, Hoover R. Long term use of oral contraceptives and risk of invasive cervical cancer. Int J Cancer 1986; 38:339–344. **48.** WHO Collaborative Study of Neoplasia and Steroid Contraceptives: Invasive cervical cancer and combined oral contraceptives. Br Med J 1985; 290:961–965. **49.** Rooks JB, Ory HW, Ishak KG, Strauss LT, Greenspan JR, Hill AP, Tyler CW. Epidemiology of hepatocellular adenoma: the role of oral contraceptive use. JAMA 1979; 242:644–648. **50.** Bein NN, Goldsmith HS. Recurrent massive hemorrhage from benign hepatic tumors secondary to oral contraceptives. Br J Surg 1977; 64:433–435. **51.** Klatskin G. Hepatic tumors: possible relationship to use of oral contraceptives. Gastroenterology 1977; 73:386–394. **52.** Henderson BE, Preston-Martin S, Edmondson HA, Peters RL, Pike MC. Hepatocellular carcinoma and oral contraceptives. Br J Cancer 1983;48:437–440. **53.** Neuberger J, Forman D, Doll R, Williams R. Oral contraceptives and hepatocellular carcinoma. Br Med J 1986; 292:1355–1357. **54.** Forman D, Vincent TJ, Doll R. Cancer of the liver and oral contraceptives. Br Med J 1986; 292:1357–1361. **55.** Harlap S, Eldor J. Births following oral contraceptive failures. Obstet Gynecol 1980; 55:447–452. **56.** Savolainen E, Saksela E, Saxen L. Teratogenic hazards of oral contraceptives analyzed in a national malformation register. Am J Obstet Gynecol 1981: 140:521–524. **57.** Janerich DT, Piper JM, Glebatis DM. Oral contraceptives and birth defects. Am J Epidemiol 1980; 112:73–79. **58.** Ferencz C, Matanoski GM, Wilson PD, Rubin JD, Neill CA, Gutberlet R. Maternal hormone therapy and congenital heart disease. Teratology 1980; 21:225–239. **59.** Rothman KJ, Fyler DC, Goldblatt A, Kreidberg MB. Exogenous hormones and other drug exposures of children with congenital heart disease. Am J Epidemiol 1979; 109:433-439. **60.** Boston Collaborative Drug Surveillance Program: Oral contraceptives and venous thromboembolic disease, surgically confirmed gallbladder disease, and breast tumors. Lancet 1973; 1:1399–1404. **61.** Royal College of General Practitioners: Oral contraceptives and health. New York, Pittman 1974. **62.** Layde PM, Vessey MP, Yeates D. Risk of gallbladder disease: a cohort study of young women attending family planning clinics. J Epidemiol Community Health 1982; 36:274–278. **63.** Rome Group for Epidemiology and Prevention of Cholelithiasis (GREPCO): Prevalence of gallstone disease in an Italian adult female population. Am J Epidemiol 1984; 119:796–805. **64.** Strom BL, Tamragouri RT, Morse ML, Lazar EL, West SL, Stolley PD, Jones JK. Oral contraceptives and other risk factors for gallbladder disease. Clin Pharmacol Ther 1986; 39:335–341. **65.** Wynn V, Adams PW, Godsland IF, Melrose J, Niththyananthan R, Oakley NW, Seedj A. Comparison of effects of different combined oral contraceptive formulations on carbohydrate and lipid metabolism. Lancet 1979; 1:1045–1049. **66.** Wynn V. Effect of progesterone and progestins on carbohydrate metabolism. In: Progesterone and Progestin. Bardin CW, Milgrom E, Mauvis-Jarvis P. eds. New York, Raven Press 1983; pp. 395–410. **67.** Perlman JA, Roussell-Briefel RG, Ezzati TM, Lieberknecht G. Oral glucose tolerance and the potency of oral contraceptive progestogens. J Chronic Dis 1985;38:857–864. **68.** Royal College of General Practitioners' Oral Contraception Study: Effect on hypertension and benign breast disease of progestogen component in combined oral contraceptives. Lancet 1977; 1:624. **69.** Fisch IR, Frank J. Oral contraceptives and blood pressure. JAMA 1977; 237:2499–2503. **70.** Laragh AJ. Oral contraceptive induced hypertension-nine years later. Am J Obstet Gynecol 1976; 126:141–147. **71.** Ramcharan S, Peritz E, Pellegrin FA, Williams WT. Incidence of hypertension in the Walnut Creek Contraceptive Drug Study cohort: In: Pharmacology of steroid contraceptive drugs. Garattini S, Berendes HW. Eds. New York, Raven Press, 1977; pp. 277–288, (Monographs of the Mario Negri Institute for Pharmacological Research Milan.) **72.** Stockley I. Interactions with oral contraceptives. J Pharm 1976;216:140–143. **73.** The Cancer and Steroid Hormone Study of the Centers for Disease Control and the National Institute of Child Health and Human Development: Oral contraceptive use and the risk of ovarian cancer. JAMA 1983; 249:1596–1599. **74.** The Cancer and Steroid Hormone Study of the Centers for Disease Control and the National Institute of Child Health and Human Development: Combination oral contraceptive use and the risk of endometrial cancer. JAMA 1987; 257:796–800. **75.** Ory HW. Functional ovarian cysts and oral contraceptives: negative association confirmed surgically. JAMA 1974; 228:68–69. **76.** Ory HW, Cole P, MacMahon B, Hoover R. Oral contraceptives and reduced risk of benign breast disease. N Engl J Med 1976; 294:419–422. **77.** Ory HW. The noncontraceptive health benefits from oral contraceptive use. Fam Plann Perspect 1982; 14:182–184. **78.** Ory HW, Forrest JD, Lincoln R. Making choices: Evaluating the health risks and benefits of birth control methods. New York, The Alan Guttmacher Institute, 1983; p.1. **79.** Schlesselman J, Stadel BV, Murray P, Lai S. Breast cancer in relation to early use of oral contraceptives. JAMA 1988; 259:1828–1833. **80.** Hennekens CH, Speizer FE, Lipnick RJ, Rosner B, Bain C, Belanger C, Stampfer MJ, Willett W, Peto R. A case-control study of oral contraceptive use and breast cancer. JNCI 1984; 72:39–42. **81.** LaVecchia C, Decarli A, Fasoli M, Franceschi S, Gentile A, Negri E, Parazzini F, Tognoni G. Oral contraceptives and cancers of the breast and of the female genital tract. Interim results from a case-control study. Br J Cancer 1986; 54:311–317. **82.** Meirik O, Lund E, Adami H, Bergstrom R, Christoffersen T, Bergsjo P. Oral contraceptive use and breast cancer in young women. A Joint National Case-control study in Sweden and Norway. Lancet 1986; 11:650–654. **83.** Kay CR, Hannaford PC. Breast cancer and the pill-A further report from the Royal College of General Practitioners' oral contraception study. Br J Cancer 1988;58:675–680. **84.** Stadel BV, Lai S, Schlesselman JJ, Murray P. Oral contraceptives and premenopausal breast cancer in nulliparous women. Contraception 1988; 38:287–299. **85.** Miller DR, Rosenberg L, Kaufman DW, Stolley P, Warshauer ME, Shapiro S. Breast cancer before age 45 and oral contraceptive use: New Findings. Am J Epidemiol 1989; 129:269–280. **86.** The UK National Case-Control Study Group, Oral contraceptive use and breast cancer risk in young women. Lancet 1989; 1:973–982. **87.** Schlesselman JJ. Cancer of the breast and reproductive tract in relation to use of oral contraceptives. Contraception 1989; 40:1–38. **88.** Vessey MP, McPherson K, Villard-Mackintosh L, Yeates D. Oral contraceptives and breast cancer: latest findings in a large cohort study. Br J Cancer 1989; 59:613–617. **89.** Jick SS, Walker AM, Stergachis A, Jick H. Oral contraceptives and breast cancer. Br J Cancer 1989; 59:618–621. **90.** Anderson FD, Selectivity and minimal androgenicity of norgestimate in monophasic and triphasic oral contraceptives. Acta Obstet Gynecol Scand 1992; 156 (Supplement):15–21. **91.** Chapdelaine A, Desmaris J-L, Derman RJ. Clinical evidence of minimal androgenic activity of norgestimate. Int J Fertil 1989; 34(51):347–352. **92.** Phillips A, Demarest K, Hahn DW, Wong F, McGuire JL. Progestational and androgenic receptor binding affinities and in vivo activities of norgestimate and other progestins. Contraception 1989; 41(4):399–409. **93.** Phillips A, Hahn DW, Klimek S, McGuire JL. A comparison of the potencies and activities of progestogens used in contraceptives. Contraception 1987; 36(2):181–192. **94.** Janaud A, Rouffy J, Upmalis D, Dain M-P. A comparison study of lipid and androgen metabolism with triphasic oral contraceptive formulations containing norgestimate or levonorgestrel Acta Obstet Gynecol Scand 1992; 156 (Supplement):34–38. **95.** Collaborative Group on Hormonal Factors in Breast Cancer. Breast cancer and hormonal contraceptives: collaborative reanalysis of individual data on 53 297 women with breast cancer and 100 239 women without breast cancer from 54 epidemiological studies. Lancet 1996; 347:1713–1727. **96.** Palmer JR, Rosenberg L, Kaufman DW, Warshauer ME, Stolley P, Shapiro S. Oral Contraceptive Use and Liver Cancer. Am J Epidemiol 1989;130:878–882. **97.** Lewis M, Spitzer WO, Heinemann LAJ, MacRae KD, Bruppacher R, Thorogood M on behalf of Transnational Research Group on Oral Contraceptives and Health of Young Women. Third generation oral contraceptives and risk of myocardial infarction: an international case-control study. Br Med J, 1996;312:88–90. **98.** Vessey MP, Smith MA, Yeates D. Return of fertility after discontinuation of oral contraceptives: influence of age and parity. Brit J Fam Plan; 1986; 11:120–124. **99.** Back DJ, Orme M.L'E. Pharmacokinetic drug interactions with oral contraceptives. Clin Pharmacokinet 1990; 18:472–484. **100.** Rosenfeld WE, Doose DR, Walker SA, Nayak RK. Effect of topiramate on the pharmacokinetics of an oral contraceptive containing norethindrone and ethinyl estradiol in patients with epilepsy. Epilepsia 1997 Mar;38(3):317–323. **101.** Shenfield GM. Oral Contraceptives. Are drug interaction of clinical significance? Drug Saf 1993 Jul;9(1):21–37. **102.** Ouellet D, Hsu A, Qian J, Locke CS, Eason CJ, Cavanaugh JH, Leonard JM, Granneman GR. Effect of ritonavir on the pharmacokinetics of ethinyl oestradiol in healthy female volunteers. Br J Clin Pharmacol 1998;46(2):111–116. **103.** Improving access to quality care in family planning: Medical eligibility criteria for contraceptive use. Geneva, WHO, Family and Reproductive Health, 1996 (WHO/FRH/FPP/96.9). **104.** Skolnick JL, Stoler BS, Katz DG, Anderson WH. Rifampicin, oral contraceptives and pregnancy. J Am Med Assoc 1976;236–1382. **105.** Henney JE. Risk of drug interactions with St. John's Wort. JAMA 2000;283(13). **106.** Lahteenmaki P et al, Coagulation factors in women using oral contraceptives or intrauterine devices immediately after abortion. American Journal of Obstetrics and Gynecology, (1981); 141: 175–179.

DETAILED PATIENT LABELING

ORTHO EVRA®
(norelgestromin/ethinyl estradiol transdermal system)
℞ only

This product is intended to prevent pregnancy. It does not protect against HIV (AIDS) or other sexually transmitted diseases.

DESCRIPTION

The contraceptive patch ORTHO EVRA® is a thin, beige, plastic patch that sticks to the skin. The sticky part of the patch contains the hormones norelgestromin and ethinyl estradiol, which are absorbed continuously through the skin and into the bloodstream. Each patch is sealed in a pouch that protects it until you are ready to wear it.

INTRODUCTION

Any woman who considers using the contraceptive patch ORTHO EVRA® should understand the benefits and risks of using this form of birth control. This leaflet will give you much of the information you will need to make this decision and will also help you determine if you are at risk of developing any serious side effects. It will tell you how to use the contraceptive patch properly so that it will be as effective as possible. However, this leaflet is not a replacement for a careful discussion between you and your health care professional. You should discuss the information provided in this leaflet with him or her, both when you first start using the contraceptive patch ORTHO EVRA® and during your revisits. You should also follow your health care professional's advice with regard to regular check-ups while you are using the contraceptive patch.

EFFECTIVENESS OF HORMONAL CONTRACEPTIVE METHODS

Hormonal contraceptives, including ORTHO EVRA®, are used to prevent pregnancy and are more effective than most

Continued on next page

Ortho Evra—Cont.

other non-surgical methods of birth control. When ORTHO EVRA® is used correctly, the chance of becoming pregnant is approximately 1% (1 pregnancy per 100 women per year of use when used correctly), which is comparable to that of the pill. The chance of becoming pregnant increases with incorrect use.

Clinical trials suggested that ORTHO EVRA® may be less effective in women weighing more than 198 lbs. (90 kg). If you weigh more than 198 lbs. (90 kg) you should talk to your health care professional about which method of birth control may be best for you.

Typical failure rates for other methods of birth control during the first year of use are as follows:
Implant: <1%
Injection: <1%
IUD: <1–2%
Diaphragm with spermicides: 20%
Spermicides alone: 26%
Female sterilization: <1%
Male sterilization: <1%
Cervical Cap with spermicide: 20 to 40%
Condom alone (male): 14%
Condom alone (female): 21%
Periodic abstinence: 25%
No birth control method: 85%
Withdrawal: 19%

WHO SHOULD NOT USE ORTHO EVRA®

Hormonal contraceptives include birth control pills, injectables, implants, the vaginal ring, and the contraceptive patch. The following information is derived primarily from studies of birth control pills. The contraceptive patch is expected to be associated with similar risks:

Cigarette smoking increases the risk of serious cardiovascular side effects from hormonal contraceptive use. This risk increases with age and with heavy smoking (15 or more cigarettes per day) and is quite marked in women over 35 years of age. Women who use hormonal contraceptives, including ORTHO EVRA®, should be strongly advised not to smoke.

Some women should not use the ORTHO EVRA® contraceptive patch. For example, you should not use ORTHO EVRA® if you are pregnant or think you may be pregnant. You should also not use ORTHO EVRA® if you have any of the following conditions:

- A history of heart attack or stroke
- Blood clots in the legs (thrombophlebitis), lungs (pulmonary embolism), or eyes
- A history of blood clots in the deep veins of your legs
- Chest pain (angina pectoris)
- Known or suspected breast cancer or cancer of the lining of the uterus, cervix or vagina.
- Unexplained vaginal bleeding (until your doctor reaches a diagnosis)
- Hepatitis or yellowing of the whites of your eyes or of the skin (jaundice) during pregnancy or during previous use of hormonal contraceptives such as ORTHO EVRA®, NORPLANT, or the birth control pill
- Liver tumor (benign or cancerous)
- Known or suspected pregnancy
- Severe high blood pressure
- Diabetes with complications of the kidneys, eyes, nerves, or blood vessels
- Headaches with neurological symptoms
- Use of oral contraceptives (birth control pills)
- Disease of heart valves with complications
- Need for a prolonged period of bed rest following major surgery
- An allergic reaction to any of the components of ORTHO EVRA®

Tell your health care professional if you have ever had any of these conditions. Your health care professional can recommend a non-hormonal method of birth control.

OTHER CONSIDERATIONS BEFORE USING ORTHO EVRA®

Talk to your health care professional about using ORTHO EVRA® if

- you smoke
- you are recovering from the birth of a baby
- you are recovering from a second trimester miscarriage or abortion
- you are breast feeding
- you weigh 198 pounds or more
- you are taking any other medications

Also, tell your health care professional if you have or have had:

- Breast nodules, fibrocystic disease of the breast, an abnormal breast x-ray or mammogram
- A family history of breast cancer
- Diabetes
- Elevated cholesterol or triglycerides
- High blood pressure
- Migraine or other headaches or epilepsy
- Depression
- Gallbladder disease
- Liver disease
- Heart disease
- Kidney disease
- Scanty or irregular menstrual periods

If you have any of these conditions you should be checked often by your health care professional if you use the contraceptive patch.

RISKS OF USING HORMONAL CONTRACEPTIVES, INCLUDING ORTHO EVRA®

The following information is derived primarily from studies of birth control pills. Since ORTHO EVRA® contains hormones similar to those found in birth control pills, it is expected to be associated with similar risks:

1. Risk of developing blood clots

Blood clots and blockage of blood vessels that can cause death or serious disability are some of the most serious side effects of using hormonal contraceptives, including the ORTHO EVRA® contraceptive patch. In particular, a clot in the legs can cause thrombophlebitis, and a clot that travels to the lungs can cause sudden blocking of the vessel carrying blood to the lungs. Rarely, clots occur in the blood vessels of the eye and may cause blindness, double vision, or impaired vision.

If you use ORTHO EVRA® and need elective surgery, need to stay in bed for a prolonged illness or injury or have recently delivered a baby, you may be at risk of developing blood clots. You should consult your doctor about stopping ORTHO EVRA® four weeks before surgery and not using it for two weeks after surgery or during bed rest. You should also not use ORTHO EVRA® soon after delivery of a baby. It is advisable to wait for at least four weeks after delivery if you are not breast-feeding. If you are breast-feeding, you should wait until you have weaned your child before using ORTHO EVRA®. (See also the section on Breast Feeding in General Precautions.)

2. Heart attacks and strokes

Hormonal contraceptives, including ORTHO EVRA®, may increase the risk of developing strokes (blockage or rupture of blood vessels in the brain) and angina pectoris and heart attacks (blockage of blood vessels in the heart). Any of these conditions can cause death or serious disability.

Smoking and the use of hormonal contraceptives including ORTHO EVRA® greatly increase the chances of developing and dying of heart disease. Smoking also greatly increases the possibility of suffering heart attacks and strokes.

3. Gallbladder disease

Women who use hormonal contraceptives, including ORTHO EVRA®, probably have a greater risk than nonusers of having gallbladder disease.

4. Liver tumors

In rare cases, combination oral contraceptives can cause benign but dangerous liver tumors. Since ORTHO EVRA® contains hormones similar to those in birth control pills, this association may also exist with ORTHO EVRA®. These benign liver tumors can rupture and cause fatal internal bleeding. In addition, some studies report an increased risk of developing liver cancer. However, liver cancers are rare.

5. Cancer of the reproductive organs and breasts

Various studies give conflicting reports on the relationship between breast cancer and hormonal contraceptive use. Combination hormonal contraceptives, including ORTHO EVRA®, may slightly increase your chance of having breast cancer diagnosed, particularly after using hormonal contraceptives at a younger age. After you stop using hormonal contraceptives, the chances of having breast cancer diagnosed begin to go back down. You should have regular breast examinations by a health care professional and examine your own breasts monthly. Tell your health care professional if you have a family history of breast cancer or if you have had breast nodules or an abnormal mammogram.

Women who currently have or have had breast cancer should not use oral contraceptives because breast cancer is usually a hormone-sensitive tumor.

Some studies have found an increase in the incidence of cancer of the cervix in women who use oral contraceptives, although this finding may be related to factors other than the use of oral contraceptives. However, there is insufficient evidence to rule out the possibility that oral contraceptives may cause such cancers.

ESTIMATED RISK OF DEATH FROM A BIRTH CONTROL METHOD OR PREGNANCY

All methods of birth control and pregnancy are associated with a risk of developing certain diseases that may lead to disability or death. An estimate of the number of deaths associated with different methods of birth control and pregnancy has been calculated and is shown in the following table.

ORTHO EVRA® is expected to be associated with similar risks as oral contraceptives:

[See table below]

In the above table, the risk of death from any birth control method is less than the risk of childbirth, except for oral contraceptive users over the age of 35 who smoke and pill users over the age of 40 even if they do not smoke. It can be seen in the table that for women aged 15 to 39, the risk of death was highest with pregnancy (7–26 deaths per 100,000 women, depending on age). Among pill users who do not smoke, the risk of death is always lower than that associated with pregnancy for any age group, although over the age of 40, the risk increases to 32 deaths per 100,000 women, compared to 28 associated with pregnancy at that age. However, for pill users who smoke and are over the age of 35, the estimated number of deaths exceeds those for other methods of birth control. If a woman is over the age of 40 and smokes, her estimated risk of death is four times higher (117/100,000 women) than the estimated risk associated with pregnancy (28/100,000 women) in that age group.

In 1989 an Advisory Committee of the FDA concluded that the benefits of low-dose hormonal contraceptive use by healthy, non-smoking women over 40 years of age may outweigh the possible risks.

WARNING SIGNALS

If any of these adverse effects occur while you are using ORTHO EVRA®, call your doctor immediately:

- Sharp chest pain, coughing of blood, or sudden shortness of breath (indicating a possible clot in the lung)
- Pain in the calf (indicating a possible clot in the leg)
- Crushing chest pain or tightness in the chest (indicating a possible heart attack)
- Sudden severe headache or vomiting, dizziness or fainting, disturbances of vision or speech, weakness, or numbness in an arm or leg (indicating a possible stroke)
- Sudden partial or complete loss of vision (indicating a possible clot in the eye)
- Breast lumps (indicating possible breast cancer or fibrocystic disease of the breast; ask your doctor or health care professional to show you how to examine your breasts)
- Severe pain or tenderness in the stomach area (indicating a possibly ruptured liver tumor)
- Severe problems with sleeping, weakness, lack of energy, fatigue, or change in mood (possibly indicating severe depression)
- Jaundice or a yellowing of the skin or eyeballs accompanied frequently by fever, fatigue, loss of appetite, dark colored urine, or light colored bowel movements (indicating possible liver problems)

SIDE EFFECTS OF ORTHO EVRA®

1. Skin irritation

Skin irritation, redness or rash may occur at the site of application. If this occurs, the patch may be removed and a new patch may be applied to a new location until the next Change Day. Single replacement patches are available from pharmacies.

2. Vaginal bleeding

Irregular vaginal bleeding or spotting may occur while you are using ORTHO EVRA®. Irregular bleeding may vary from slight staining between menstrual periods to breakthrough bleeding which is a flow much like a regular period. Irregular bleeding may occur during the first few months of contraceptive patch use but may also occur after you have been using the contraceptive patch for some time. Such bleeding may be temporary and usually does not indicate any serious problems. It is important to continue using your contraceptive patches on schedule. If the bleeding occurs in more than a few cycles or lasts for more than a few days, talk to your health care professional.

3. Problems wearing contact lenses

If you wear contact lenses and notice a change in vision or an inability to wear your lenses, contact your health care professional.

4. Fluid retention or raised blood pressure

Hormonal contraceptives, including the contraceptive patch, may cause edema (fluid retention) with swelling of the fingers or ankles and may raise your blood pressure. If you experience fluid retention, contact your health care professional.

Annual Number of Birth-Related or Method-Related Deaths Associated With Control of Fertility Per 100,000 Nonsterile Women by Fertility Control Method According to Age

Method of control and outcome	15–19	20–24	25–29	30–34	35–39	40–44
No fertility control methods*	7.0	7.4	9.1	14.8	25.7	28.2
Oral contraceptives, non-smoker**	0.3	0.5	0.9	1.9	13.8	31.6
Oral contraceptives, smoker**	2.2	3.4	6.6	13.5	51.1	117.2
IUD**	0.8	0.8	1.0	1.0	11.4	1.4
Condom*	1.1	1.6	0.7	0.2	0.3	0.4
Diaphragm/spermicide*	1.9	1.2	1.2	1.3	2.2	2.8
Periodic abstinence*	2.5	1.6	1.6	1.7	2.9	3.6

*Deaths are birth-related
**Deaths are method-related
Adapted from H.W. Ory, ref. # 35.

5. Melasma
A spotty darkening of the skin is possible, particularly of the face. This may persist after use of hormonal contraceptives is discontinued.

6. Other side effects
The most common side effects of ORTHO EVRA® include nausea and vomiting, breast symptoms, headache, menstrual cramps, and abdominal pain. In addition, change in appetite, nervousness, depression, dizziness, loss of scalp hair, rash, and vaginal infections may occur.

GENERAL PRECAUTIONS

1. Weight > 198 lbs. (90 kg)
Clinical trials suggest that ORTHO EVRA® may be less effective in women weighing more than 198 lbs. (90 kg) compared with its effectiveness in women with lower body weights. If you weigh more than 198 lbs. (90 kg) you should talk to your health care professional about which method of birth control may be best for you.

2. Missed periods and use of ORTHO EVRA® before or during early pregnancy
There may be times when you may not menstruate regularly during your patch-free week. If you have used ORTHO EVRA® correctly and miss one menstrual period, continue using your contraceptive patches for the next cycle but be sure to inform your health care professional before doing so. If you have not used ORTHO EVRA® as instructed and missed a menstrual period, or if you missed two menstrual periods in a row, you could be pregnant. Check with your health care professional immediately to determine whether you are pregnant. Stop using ORTHO EVRA® if you are pregnant.
There is no conclusive evidence that hormonal contraceptive use causes birth defects when taken accidentally during early pregnancy. Previously, a few studies had reported that oral contraceptives might be associated with birth defects, but these findings have not been seen in more recent studies. Nevertheless, hormonal contraceptives, including ORTHO EVRA®, should not be used during pregnancy. You should check with your health care professional about risks to your unborn child from any medication taken during pregnancy.

3. While breast-feeding
If you are breast-feeding, consult your health care professional before starting ORTHO EVRA®. Hormonal contraceptives are passed on to the child in the milk. A few adverse effects on the child have been reported, including yellowing of the skin (jaundice) and breast enlargement. In addition, combination hormonal contraceptives may decrease the amount and quality of your milk. If possible, do not use combination hormonal contraceptives such as ORTHO EVRA® while breast-feeding. You should use a barrier method of contraception since breast-feeding provides only partial protection from becoming pregnant and this partial protection decreases significantly as you breast-feed for longer periods of time. You should consider starting ORTHO EVRA® only after you have weaned your child completely.

4. Laboratory tests
If you are scheduled for any laboratory tests, tell your doctor you are using ORTHO EVRA® since certain blood tests may be affected by hormonal contraceptives.

5. Drug interactions
Certain drugs may interact with hormonal contraceptives, including ORTHO EVRA®, to make them less effective in preventing pregnancy or cause an increase in breakthrough bleeding. Such drugs include rifampin, drugs used for epilepsy such as barbiturates (for example, phenobarbital), anticonvulsants such as topiramate (TOPAMAX), carbamazepine (Tegretol is one brand of this drug), phenytoin (Dilantin is one brand of this drug), phenylbutazone (Butazolidin is one brand), certain drugs used in the treatment of HIV or AIDS, and possibly certain antibiotics. Tetracycline has been shown not to interact with ORTHO EVRA®. Pregnancies and breakthrough bleeding have been reported by users of combined hormonal contraceptives who also used some form of St. John's Wort.
As with all prescription products, you should notify your health care professional of any other medications you are taking. You may need to use a barrier contraceptive when you take drugs that can make ORTHO EVRA® less effective.

6. Sexually transmitted diseases
ORTHO EVRA® is intended to prevent pregnancy. It does not protect against HIV (AIDS) or other sexually transmitted diseases such as chlamydia, genital herpes, genital warts, gonorrhea, hepatitis B, and syphilis.

HOW TO USE ORTHO EVRA®

Instructions for Use

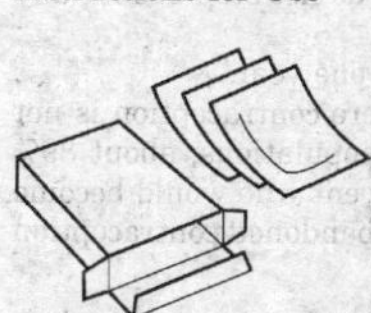

ORTHO EVRA® keeps you from becoming pregnant by transferring hormones to your body through your skin. The patch must stick securely to your skin in order for it to work properly.
This method uses a 28 day (four week) cycle. You should apply a new patch each week for three weeks (21 total days). You should not apply a patch during the fourth week. Your menstrual period should start during this patch-free week.
Every new patch should be applied on the same day of the week. This day will be your 'Patch Change Day.' *For example, if you apply your first patch on a Monday, all of your patches should be applied on a Monday.* You should wear only one patch at a time.
On the day after week four ends, you should begin a new four week cycle by applying a new patch.
Save these instructions.

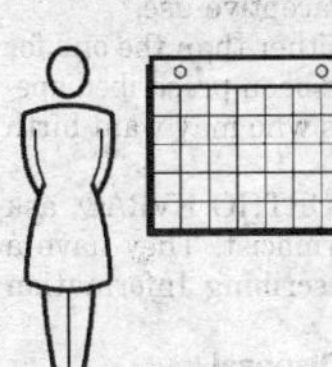

1
If this is the **first time** you are using ORTHO EVRA®, **wait until the day you get your menstrual period.** *The day you apply your first patch will be Day 1. Your 'Patch Change Day' will be on this day every week.*

CHOOSE ONE OPTION:

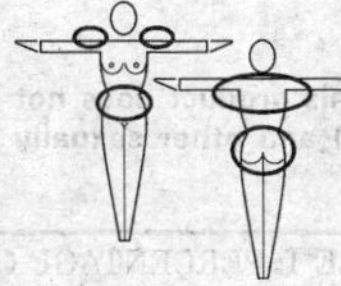

☐ First Day Start
or
☐ Sunday Start

2
You may choose a first day start or Sunday start
- *for **First Day** start:* apply your first patch during the first 24 hours of your menstrual period.

OR
- for ***Sunday** start:* apply your first patch on the first Sunday after your menstrual period starts. *You must use back-up contraception, such as a condom, spermicide, or diaphragm for the first week of your first cycle.*
- *The day you apply your first patch will be Day 1. Your 'Patch Change Day' will be on this day every week.*

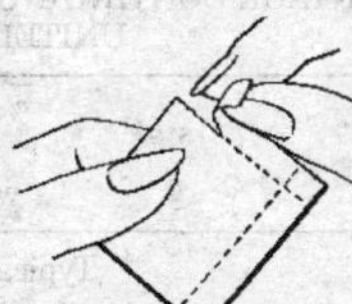

3
Choose a place on your body to put the patch. Put the patch on your buttock, abdomen, upper outer arm or upper torso, in a place where it won't be rubbed by tight clothing. *Never put the patch on your breasts. To avoid irritation, apply each new patch to a different place on your skin.*

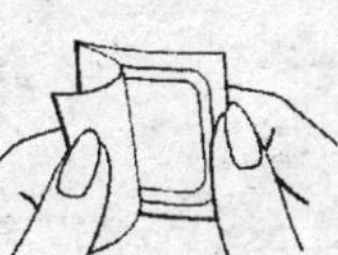

4
Open the foil pouch by tearing it along the top edge <u>and</u> one side edge.

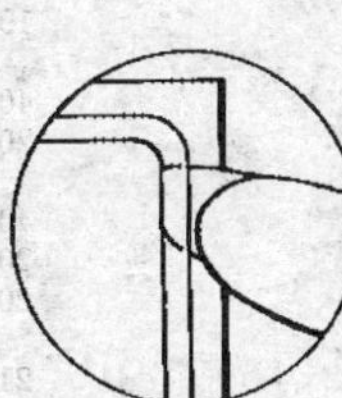

Peel the foil pouch apart and open it flat.

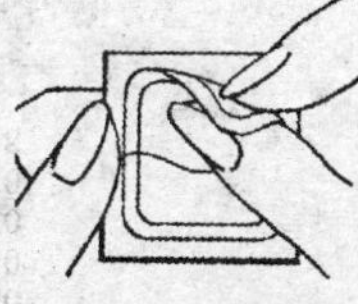

5
You will see that the patch is covered by a layer of clear plastic. It is important to remove the patch **and** the plastic together from the foil pouch.
Using your fingernail, lift one corner of the patch and peel the patch **and** the plastic off the foil liner.

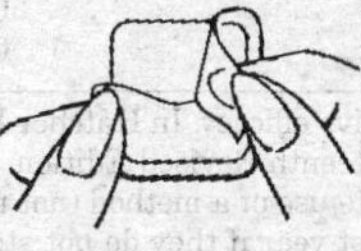

Sometimes patches can stick to the inside of the pouch – be careful not to accidentally remove the clear liner as you remove the patch.

6
Peel away half of the clear plastic and **be careful** not to touch the exposed sticky surface of the patch **with your fingers.**

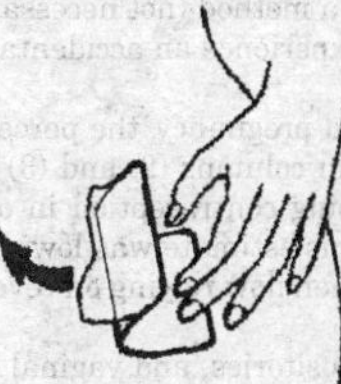

7
Apply the sticky side of the patch to the skin you've cleaned and dried, then remove the other half of the clear plastic.
Press firmly on the patch with the palm of your hand for 10 seconds, making sure the edges stick well. Run your finger around the edge of the patch to make sure it is sticking properly.
Check your patch every day to make sure all the edges are sticking.

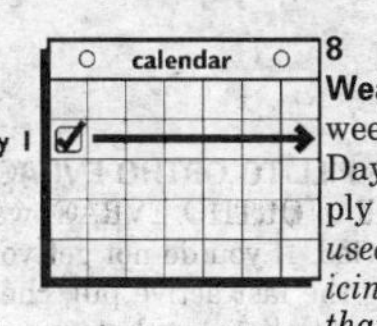

8
Wear the patch for seven days (one week). On your 'Patch Change Day,' Day 8, remove the used patch. Apply a new patch immediately. *The used patch still contains some medicine – carefully fold it in half so that it sticks to itself before safely disposing of it in the trash. Used patches should not be flushed down the toilet.*

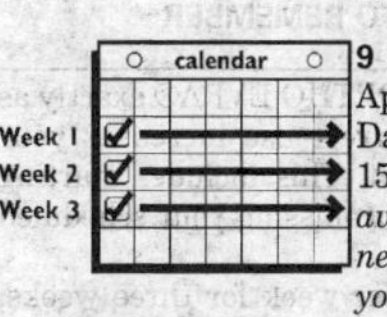

9
Apply a new patch for week two (on Day 8) and for week three (on Day 15), on your 'Patch Change Day.' *To avoid irritation, do not apply the new patch to the same exact place on your skin.*

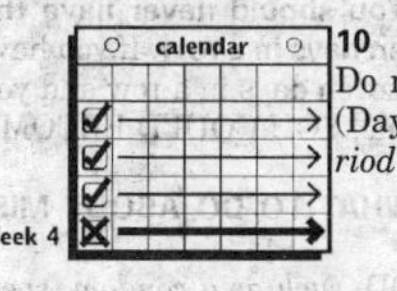

10
Do not wear a patch on week four (Day 22 through Day 28). *Your period should start during this week.*

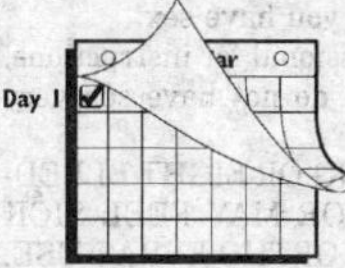

11
Begin your next four week cycle by applying a new patch on your normal 'Patch Change Day,' the day after Day 28 – *no matter when your period begins or ends.*

If your patch has become loose or has fallen off...
- **for less than one day**, try to re-apply it or apply a new patch immediately. No back-up contraception is needed. *Your 'Patch Change Day' will remain the same.*
- **for more than one day OR if you are not sure for how long**, YOU MAY BECOME PREGNANT – **Start a new four week cycle immediately** by putting on a new patch. *You now have a new Day 1 and a new 'Patch Change Day.' You must use back-up contraception, such as a condom, spermicide, or diaphragm for the first week of your new cycle.*
- do not try to re-apply a patch if it's no longer sticky, if it has become stuck to itself or another surface, if it has other material stuck to it or if it has previously become loose or fallen off. No tapes or wraps should be used to keep the patch in place. If you cannot re-apply a patch, apply a new patch immediately.

If you forget to change your patch...
- **at the start of any patch cycle,**
  Week one (Day 1): If you forget to apply your patch, YOU COULD BECOME PREGNANT – *you must use back-up contraception for one week.* Apply the first patch of your new cycle as soon as you remember. *You now have a new 'Patch Change Day' and new Day 1.*
- **in the middle of your patch cycle,**
  Week two or week three: If you forget to change your patch for **one or two days**, apply a new patch as soon as you remember. Apply your next patch on your normal 'Patch Change Day.' No back-up contraception is needed.
  Week two or week three: If you forget to change your patch for **more than two days**, YOU COULD BECOME PREGNANT – **start a new four week cycle as soon as you remember by putting on a new patch.** *You now have a different 'Patch Change Day' and a new Day 1. You must use back-up contraception for the first week of your new cycle.*
- **at the end of your patch cycle,**
  Week four: If you forget to remove your patch, take it off as soon as you remember. Start your next cycle on your normal 'Patch Change Day,' the day after Day 28. No back-up contraception is needed.
- **at the start of your next patch cycle,**
  Day 1 (week one): If you forget to apply your patch, YOU COULD BECOME PREGNANT – apply the first patch of your new cycle as soon as you remember. *You now have a new 'Patch Change Day' and new Day 1. You must use back-up contraception for the first week of your new cycle.*
- ***you should never have the patch off for more than seven days.***

Other information...
- Always apply your patch to clean, dry skin. Avoid skin that is red, irritated or cut. Do not use creams, oils, powder or makeup on your skin where you will put a patch or near a patch you are wearing. It may cause the patch to become loose.
- If patch use results in uncomfortable irritation, the patch may be removed and a new patch may be applied to a new location until the next Change Day. Only one patch should be worn at a time.
- Some medicines may change the way ORTHO EVRA® works. If you are taking any medication, you must talk to your health care professional BEFORE you use the patch. *You may need to use back-up contraception.*
- Store at 25°C (77°F).
- Single replacement patches are available through your pharmacist.
- For further information log on to **www.orthoevra.com** or call toll free **1 877 EVRA 888**

Continued on next page

Ortho Evra—Cont.

WHEN YOU SWITCH FROM THE PILL TO ORTHO EVRA®:
If you are switching from the pill to ORTHO EVRA®, wait until you get your menstrual period. If you do not get your period within five days of taking the last active pill, check with your health care professional to be sure that you are not pregnant.

IMPORTANT POINTS TO REMEMBER

1. IT IS IMPORTANT TO USE ORTHO EVRA® exactly as directed in this leaflet. Incorrect use increases your chances of becoming pregnant. This includes starting your contraceptive cycle late or missing your scheduled CHANGE DAYS.
2. You should wear one patch per week for three weeks, followed by one week off. **You should never have the patch off for more than seven days in a row.** If you have the patch off for more than seven days in a row and you have had sex during this time, YOU COULD BECOME PREGNANT.
3. **IF YOU ARE NOT SURE WHAT TO DO ABOUT MISTAKES WITH PATCH USE:**
   - Use a BACK-UP METHOD, *such as a condom, spermicide, or diaphragm* anytime you have sex.
   - Contact your health care professional for instructions.
4. Do not skip patches even if you do not have sex very often.
5. SOME WOMEN HAVE SPOTTING OR LIGHT BLEEDING, BREAST TENDERNESS OR MAY FEEL SICK TO THEIR STOMACH DURING ORTHO EVRA® USE. If these symptoms occur, do not stop using the contraceptive patch. The problem will usually go away. If it doesn't go away, check with your health care professional.
6. MISTAKES IN USING YOUR PATCHES CAN ALSO CAUSE SPOTTING OR LIGHT BLEEDING.
7. If you miss TWO PERIODS IN A ROW contact your health care professional because you might be pregnant.
8. The amount of drug you get from the ORTHO EVRA® patch should not be affected by VOMITING OR DIARRHEA.
9. IF YOU TAKE CERTAIN MEDICINES, ORTHO EVRA® may not work as well. Use a non-hormonal back-up method (such as condoms, spermicide, or diaphragm) until you check with your health care professional.
10. IF YOU WANT TO MOVE YOUR PATCH CHANGE DAY to a different day of the week, finish your current cycle, removing your third ORTHO EVRA® patch on the correct day. **During week four,** the "patch-free week" (Day 22 through Day 28), you may choose an earlier Patch Change Day by applying a new patch on the day you prefer. You now have a new Day 1 and a new Patch Change Day. **You should never have the patch off for more than seven days in a row.**
11. BE SURE YOU HAVE READY AT ALL TIMES:
    - A NON-HORMONAL BIRTH CONTROL method (such as condoms, spermicide, or diaphragm) to use as a back-up in case of dosing errors.
12. IF YOU HAVE TROUBLE REMEMBERING TO CHANGE YOUR CONTRACEPTIVE PATCH, talk to your health care professional about how to make patch-changing easier or about using another method of birth control.
13. Single replacement patches are available through your pharmacist.
14. For Patch replacement, see "How to use ORTHO EVRA®" section.

IF YOU HAVE ANY QUESTIONS OR ARE UNSURE ABOUT THE INFORMATION IN THIS LEAFLET, call your health care professional.

PREGNANCY DUE TO ORTHO EVRA® FAILURE
The incidence of pregnancy from hormonal contraceptive failure is approximately one percent (i.e., one pregnancy per 100 women per year) if used correctly. The chance of becoming pregnant increases with incorrect use. If contraceptive patch failure does occur, the risk to the fetus is minimal.

PREGNANCY AFTER STOPPING ORTHO EVRA®
There may be some delay in becoming pregnant after you stop using ORTHO EVRA®, especially if you had irregular menstrual cycles before you used hormonal contraceptives. It may be best to postpone conception until you begin menstruation regularly once you have stopped using ORTHO EVRA® and want to become pregnant.
There does not appear to be any increase in birth defects in newborn babies when pregnancy occurs soon after stopping hormonal contraceptives.

OVERDOSAGE
ORTHO EVRA® is unlikely to cause an overdose because the patch releases a steady amount of the hormones. Do not use more than one patch at a time. Serious ill effects have not been reported when large doses of oral contraceptives were accidentally taken by young children. Overdosage may cause nausea and vomiting. Vaginal bleeding may occur in females. In case of overdosage, contact your health care professional or pharmacist.

OTHER INFORMATION
Your health care professional will take a medical and family history before prescribing ORTHO EVRA® and will examine you. The physical examination may be delayed to another time if you request it and the health care professional believes that it is a good medical practice to postpone it. You should be reexamined at least once a year. Be sure to inform your health care professional if there is a family history of any of the conditions listed previously in this leaflet. Be sure to keep all appointments with your health care professional, because this is a time to determine if there are early signs of side effects of hormonal contraceptive use.
Do not use the drug for any condition other than the one for which it was prescribed. This drug has been prescribed specifically for you; do not give it to others who may want birth control.
If you want more information about ORTHO EVRA®, ask your health care professional or pharmacist. They have a more technical leaflet called the Prescribing Information that you may wish to read.

Special Precautions for Storage and Disposal
Store at room temperature.
Store patches in their protective pouches. Apply to the skin immediately upon removal from the protective pouch.
Do not store in the refrigerator or freezer.
Used patches still contain some active hormones. Fold each patch in half so that it sticks to itself before safely disposing of it in the trash. Used patches should not be flushed down the toilet.

ORTHO-McNEIL
ORTHO-McNEIL PHARMACEUTICAL, INC.
Raritan, New Jersey 08869
© OMP 2001 Revised: May 2003 631-10-662-2
Shown in Product Identification Guide, page 328

ORTHO MICRONOR® ℞
[ōr'-thō' mīc-rō-nōr]
(norethindrone)
Tablets

Prescribing Information
Patients should be counseled that this product does not protect against HIV infection (AIDS) and other sexually transmitted diseases.

DESCRIPTION
ORTHO MICRONOR® 28 Day Regimen
Each tablet contains 0.35 mg norethindrone. Inactive ingredients include D&C Green No. 5, D&C Yellow No. 10, lactose, magnesium stearate, povidone and starch.

OH
CH_3
···C≡CH
norethindrone

CLINICAL PHARMACOLOGY
1. MODE OF ACTION
ORTHO MICRONOR progestin-only oral contraceptives prevent conception by suppressing ovulation in approximately half of users, thickening the cervical mucus to inhibit sperm penetration, lowering the midcycle LH and FSH peaks, slowing the movement of the ovum through the fallopian tubes, and altering the endometrium.
2. PHARMACOKINETICS
Serum progestin levels peak about two hours after oral administration, followed by rapid distribution and elimination. By 24 hours after drug ingestion, serum levels are near baseline, making efficacy dependent upon rigid adherence to the dosing schedule. There are large variations in serum levels among individual users. Progestin-only administration results in lower steady-state serum progestin levels and a shorter elimination half-life than concomitant administration with estrogens.

INDICATIONS AND USAGE
1. Indications
Progestin-only oral contraceptives are indicated for the prevention of pregnancy.
2. Efficacy
If used perfectly, the first-year failure rate for progestin-only oral contraceptives is 0.5%. However, the typical failure rate is estimated to be closer to 5%, due to late or omitted pills. Table 1 lists the pregnancy rates for users of all major methods of contraception.
[See table 1 below]

TABLE 1: PERCENTAGE OF WOMEN EXPERIENCING AN UNINTENDED PREGNANCY DURING THE FIRST YEAR OF TYPICAL USE AND THE FIRST YEAR OF PERFECT USE OF CONTRACEPTION AND THE PERCENTAGE CONTINUING USE AT THE END OF THE FIRST YEAR. UNITED STATES.

	% of Women Experiencing an Unintended Pregnancy within the First Year of Use		% of Women Continuing Use at One Year[3]
Method (1)	Typical Use[1] (2)	Perfect Use[2] (3)	(4)
Chance[4]	85	85	
Spermicides[5]	26	6	40
Periodic abstinence	25		63
Calendar		9	
Ovulation Method		3	
Sympto-Thermal[6]		2	
Post-Ovulation		1	
Withdrawal	19	4	
Cap[7]			
Parous Women	40	26	42
Nulliparous Women	20	9	56
Sponge			
Parous Women	40	20	42
Nulliparous Women	20	9	56
Diaphragm[7]	20	6	56
Condom[8]			
Female (Reality)	21	5	56
Male	14	3	61
Pill	5		71
Progestin Only		0.5	
Combined		0.1	
IUD			
Progesterone T	2.0	1.5	81
Copper T380A	0.8	0.6	78
LNg 20	0.1	0.1	81
Depo-Provera	0.3	0.3	70
Norplant and Norplant-2	0.05	0.05	88
Female Sterilization	0.5	0.5	100
Male Sterilization	0.15	0.10	100

Adapted from Trussel J. Contraceptive efficacy. In Hatcher RA, Trussel J, Stewart F, Cates W, Stewart GK, Kowal D, Guest F, Contraceptive Technology: Seventeenth Revised Edition. New York NY: Irvington Publishers, 1998, in press.
1. Among *typical* couples who initiate use of a method (not necessarily for the first time), the percentage who experience an accidental pregnancy during the first year if they do not stop use for any other reason.
2. Among couples who initiate use of a method (not necessarily for the first time) and who use it *perfectly* (both consistently and correctly), the percentage who experience an accidental pregnancy during the first year if they do not stop use for any other reason.
3. Among couples attempting to avoid pregnancy, the percentage who continue to use a method for one year.
4. The percents becoming pregnant in columns (2) and (3) are based on data from populations where contraception is not used and from women who cease using contraception in order to become pregnant. Among such populations, about 89% become pregnant within one year. This estimate was lowered slightly (to 85%) to represent the percent who would become pregnant within one year among women now relying on reversible methods of contraception if they abandoned contraception altogether.
5. Foams, creams, gels, vaginal suppositories, and vaginal film.
6. Cervical mucus (ovulation) method supplemented by calendar in the pre-ovulatory and basal body temperature in the post-ovulatory phases.
7. With spermicidal cream or jelly.
8. Without spermicides.

CONTRAINDICATIONS

Progestin-only oral contraceptives (POPs) should not be used by women who currently have the following conditions:

- Known or suspected pregnancy
- Known or suspected carcinoma of the breast
- Undiagnosed abnormal genital bleeding
- Hypersensitivity to any component of this product
- Benign or malignant liver tumors
- Acute liver disease

WARNINGS

Cigarette smoking increases the risk of serious cardiovascular disease. Women who use oral contraceptives should be strongly advised not to smoke.

ORTHO MICRONOR does not contain estrogen and, therefore, this insert does not discuss the serious health risks that have been associated with the estrogen component of combined oral contraceptives (COCs). The health care provider is referred to the prescribing information of combined oral contraceptives for a discussion of those risks. The relationship between progestin-only oral contraceptives and these risks is not fully defined. The physician should remain alert to the earliest manifestation of symptoms of any serious disease and discontinue oral contraceptive therapy when appropriate.

1. Ectopic Pregnancy

The incidence of ectopic pregnancies for progestin-only oral contraceptive users is 5 per 1000 woman-years. Up to 10% of pregnancies reported in clinical studies of progestin-only oral contraceptive users are extrauterine. Although symptoms of ectopic pregnancy should be watched for, a history of ectopic pregnancy need not be considered a contraindication to use of this contraceptive method. Health providers should be alert to the possibility of an ectopic pregnancy in women who become pregnant or complain of lower abdominal pain while on progestin-only oral contraceptives.

2. Delayed Follicular Atresia/Ovarian Cysts

If follicular development occurs, atresia of the follicle is sometimes delayed and the follicle may continue to grow beyond the size it would attain in a normal cycle. Generally these enlarged follicles disappear spontaneously. Often they are asymptomatic; in some cases they are associated with mild abdominal pain. Rarely they may twist or rupture, requiring surgical intervention.

3. Irregular Genital Bleeding

Irregular menstrual patterns are common among women using progestin-only oral contraceptives. If genital bleeding is suggestive of infection, malignancy or other abnormal conditions, such nonpharmacologic causes should be ruled out. If prolonged amenorrhea occurs, the possibility of pregnancy should be evaluated.

4. Carcinoma of the Breast and Reproductive Organs

Some epidemiological studies of oral contraceptive users have reported an increased relative risk of developing breast cancer, particularly at a younger age and apparently related to duration of use. These studies have predominantly involved combined oral contraceptives and there is insufficient data to determine whether the use of POPs similarly increases the risk.

A meta-analysis of 54 studies found a small increase in the frequency of having breast cancer diagnosed for women who were currently using combined oral contraceptives or had used them within the past ten years. This increase in the frequency of breast cancer diagnosis, within ten years of stopping use, was generally accounted for by cancers localized to the breast. There was no increase in the frequency of having breast cancer diagnosed ten or more years after cessation of use.

Women with breast cancer should not use oral contraceptives because the role of female hormones in breast cancer has not been fully determined.

Some studies suggest that oral contraceptive use has been associated with an increase in the risk of cervical intraepithelial neoplasia in some populations of women. However, there continues to be controversy about the extent to which such findings may be due to differences in sexual behavior and other factors. There is insufficient data to determine whether the use of POPs increases the risk of developing cervical intraepithelial neoplasia.

5. Hepatic Neoplasia

Benign hepatic adenomas are associated with combined oral contraceptive use, although the incidence of benign tumors is rare in the United States. Rupture of benign, hepatic adenomas may cause death through intraabdominal hemorrhage.

Studies have shown an increased risk of developing hepatocellular carcinoma in combined oral contraceptive users. However, these cancers are rare in the U.S. There is insufficient data to determine whether POPs increase the risk of developing hepatic neoplasia.

PRECAUTIONS

1. General

Patients should be counseled that this product does not protect against HIV infection (AIDS) and other sexually transmitted diseases.

2. Physical Examination and Follow up

It is considered good medical practice for sexually active women using oral contraceptives to have annual history and physical examinations. The physical examination may be deferred until after initiation of oral contraceptives if requested by the woman and judged appropriate by the clinician.

TABLE 2: PERCENTAGE OF WOMEN EXPERIENCING AN UNINTENDED PREGNANCY DURING THE FIRST YEAR OF TYPICAL USE AND THE FIRST YEAR OF PERFECT USE OF CONTRACEPTION AND THE PERCENTAGE CONTINUING USE AT THE END OF THE FIRST YEAR. UNITED STATES.

	% of Women Experiencing an Unintended Pregnancy within the First Year of Use		% of Women Continuing Use at One Year[3]
Method (1)	Typical Use[1] (2)	Perfect Use[2] (3)	(4)
Chance[4]	85	85	
Spermicides[5]	26	6	40
Periodic abstinence	25		63
Calendar		9	
Ovulation Method		3	
Sympto-Thermal[6]		2	
Post-Ovulation		1	
Withdrawal	19	4	
Cap[7]			
Parous Women	40	26	42
Nulliparous Women	20	9	56
Sponge			
Parous Women	40	20	42
Nulliparous Women	20	9	56
Diaphragm[7]	20	6	56
Condom[8]			
Female (Reality)	21	5	56
Male	14	3	61
Pill	5		71
Progestin Only		0.5	
Combined		0.1	
IUD			
Progesterone T	2.0	1.5	81
Copper T380A	0.8	0.6	78
LNg 20	0.1	0.1	81
Depo-Provera	0.3	0.3	70
Norplant and Norplant-2	0.05	0.05	88
Female Sterilization	0.5	0.5	100
Male Sterilization	0.15	0.10	100

Adapted from Trussel J. Contraceptive efficacy. In Hatcher RA, Trussel J, Stewart F, Cates W, Stewart GK, Kowal D, Guest F, Contraceptive Technology: Seventeenth Revised Edition. New York NY: Irvington Publishers, 1998, in press.

1. Among *typical* couples who initiate use of a method (not necessarily for the first time), the percentage who experience an accidental pregnancy during the first year if they do not stop use for any other reason.
2. Among couples who initiate use of a method (not necessarily for the first time) and who use it *perfectly* (both consistently and correctly), the percentage who experience an accidental pregnancy during the first year if they do not stop use for any other reason.
3. Among couples attempting to avoid pregnancy, the percentage who continue to use a method for one year.
4. The percents becoming pregnant in columns (2) and (3) are based on data from populations where contraception is not used and from women who cease using contraception in order to become pregnant. Among such populations, about 89% become pregnant within one year. This estimate was lowered slightly (to 85%) to represent the percent who would become pregnant within one year among women now relying on reversible methods of contraception if they abandoned contraception altogether.
5. Foams, creams, gels, vaginal suppositories, and vaginal film.
6. Cervical mucus (ovulation) method supplemented by calendar in the pre-ovulatory and basal body temperature in the post-ovulatory phases.
7. With spermicidal cream or jelly.
8. Without spermicides.

3. Carbohydrate and Lipid Metabolism

Some users may experience slight deterioration in glucose tolerance, with increases in plasma insulin but women with diabetes mellitus who use progestin-only oral contraceptives do not generally experience changes in their insulin requirements. Nonetheless, prediabetic and diabetic women in particular should be carefully monitored while taking POPs.

Lipid metabolism is occasionally affected in that HDL, HDL2, and apolipoprotein A-I and A-II may be decreased; hepatic lipase may be increased. There is usually no effect on total cholesterol, HDL_3, LDL, or VLDL.

4. Drug Interactions

The effectiveness of progestin-only pills is reduced by hepatic enzyme-inducing drugs such as the anticonvulsants phenytoin, carbamazepine, and barbiturates, and the antituberculosis drug rifampin. No significant interaction has been found with broad-spectrum antibiotics.

5. Interactions with Laboratory Tests

The following endocrine tests may be affected by progestin-only oral contraceptive use:

- Sex hormone-binding globulin (SHBG) concentrations may be decreased.
- Thyroxine concentrations may be decreased, due to a decrease in thyroid binding globulin (TBG).

6. Carcinogenesis

See WARNINGS section.

7. Pregnancy

Many studies have found no effects on fetal development associated with long-term use of contraceptive doses of oral progestins. The few studies of infant growth and development that have been conducted have not demonstrated significant adverse effects. It is nonetheless prudent to rule out suspected pregnancy before initiating any hormonal contraceptive use.

8. Nursing Mothers

No adverse effects have been found on breastfeeding performance or on the health, growth or development of the infant. Small amounts of progestin pass into the breast milk, resulting in steroid levels in infant plasma of 1–6% of the levels of maternal plasma.

9. Pediatric Use

Safety and efficacy of ORTHO MICRONOR Tablets have been established in women of reproductive age. Safety and efficacy are expected to be the same for postpubertal adolescents under the age of 16 and for users 16 years and older. Use of this product before menarche is not indicated.

10. Fertility Following Discontinuation

The limited available data indicate a rapid return of normal ovulation and fertility following discontinuation of progestin-only oral contraceptives.

11. Headache

The onset or exacerbation of migraine or development of severe headache with focal neurological symptoms which is recurrent or persistent requires discontinuation of progestin-only contraceptives and evaluation of the cause.

INFORMATION FOR THE PATIENT

1. See Detailed Patient Labeling for detailed information.
2. Counseling issues

The following points should be discussed with prospective users before prescribing progestin-only oral contraceptives:

- The necessity of taking pills at the same time every day, including throughout all bleeding episodes.
- The need to use a backup method such as condoms and spermicides for the next 48 hours whenever a progestin-only oral contraceptive is taken 3 or more hours late.
- The potential side effects of progestin-only oral contraceptives, particularly menstrual irregularities.
- The need to inform the clinician of prolonged episodes of bleeding, amenorrhea or severe abdominal pain.
- The importance of using a barrier method in addition to progestin-only oral contraceptives if a woman is at risk of contracting or transmitting STDs/HIV.

ADVERSE REACTIONS

Adverse reactions reported with the use of POPs include:

- Menstrual irregularity is the most frequently reported side effect.

Continued on next page

Ortho Micronor—Cont.

- Frequent and irregular bleeding are common, while long duration of bleeding episodes and amenorrhea are less likely.
- Headache, breast tenderness, nausea, and dizziness are increased among progestin-only oral contraceptive users in some studies.
- Androgenic side effects such as acne, hirsutism, and weight gain occur rarely.

OVERDOSAGE

There have been no reports of serious ill effects from overdosage, including ingestion by children.

DOSAGE AND ADMINISTRATION

To achieve maximum contraceptive effectiveness, ORTHO MICRONOR must be taken exactly as directed. One tablet is taken every day, at the same time. Administration is continuous, with no interruption between pill packs. See Detailed Patient Labeling for detailed instruction.

HOW SUPPLIED

ORTHO MICRONOR Tablets are available in a DIALPAK® Tablet Dispenser
(NDC 0062-1411-16) containing 28 green tablets (0.35 mg norethindrone).
STORAGE: Store at 25°C (77°F); excursions permitted to 15°–30°C (59–86°F).

REFERENCE

McCann M, and Potter L. Progestin-Only Oral Contraceptives: A Comprehensive Review. Contraception, 50:60 (Suppl. 1), December 1994.

DETAILED PATIENT LABELING

ORTHO MICRONOR® (norethindrone) **Tablets**

This product (like all oral contraceptives) is used to prevent pregnancy. It does not protect against HIV infection (AIDS) or other sexually transmitted diseases.

DESCRIPTION

ORTHO MICRONOR® 28 Day Regimen

Each tablet contains 0.35 mg norethindrone. Inactive ingredients include D&C Green No. 5, D&C Yellow No. 10, lactose, magnesium stearate, povidone and starch.

INTRODUCTION

This leaflet is about birth control pills that contain one hormone, a progestin. Please read this leaflet before you begin to take your pills. It is meant to be used along with talking with your doctor or clinic.

Progestin-only pills are often called "POPs" or "the mini-pill." POPs have less progestin than the combined birth control pill (or "the pill") which contains both an estrogen and a progestin.

HOW EFFECTIVE ARE POPs?

About 1 in 200 POP users will get pregnant in the first year if they all take POPs perfectly (that is, on time, every day). About 1 in 20 "typical" POP users (including women who are late taking pills or miss pills) gets pregnant in the first year of use. Table 2 will help you compare the efficacy of different methods.

[See table 2 at top of previous page]

HOW DO POPs WORK?

POPs can prevent pregnancy in different ways including:

- They make the cervical mucus at the entrance to the womb (the uterus) too thick for the sperm to get through to the egg.
- They prevent ovulation (release of the egg from the ovary) in about half of the cycles.
- They also affect other hormones, the fallopian tubes and the lining of the uterus.

YOU SHOULD NOT TAKE POPs

- If there is any chance you may be pregnant.
- If you have breast cancer.
- If you have bleeding between your periods that has not been diagnosed.
- If you are taking certain drugs for epilepsy (seizures) or for TB. (See "Using POPs with Other Medicines" below.)
- If you are hypersensitive, or allergic, to any component of this product.
- If you have liver tumors, either benign or cancerous.
- If you have acute liver disease.

RISKS OF TAKING POPs

Cigarette smoking greatly increases the possibility of suffering heart attacks and strokes. Women who use oral contraceptives are strongly advised not to smoke.

WARNING: If you have sudden or severe pain in your lower abdomen or stomach area, you may have an ectopic pregnancy or an ovarian cyst. If this happens, you should contact your doctor or clinic immediately.

Ectopic Pregnancy

An ectopic pregnancy is a pregnancy outside the womb. Because POPs protect against pregnancy, the chance of having a pregnancy outside the womb is very low. If you do get pregnant while taking POPs, you have a slightly higher chance that the pregnancy will be ectopic than do users of some other birth control methods.

Ovarian Cysts

These cysts are small sacs of fluid in the ovary. They are more common among POP users than among users of most other birth control methods. They usually disappear without treatment and rarely cause problems.

Cancer of the Reproductive Organs and Breasts

Some studies in women who use combined oral contraceptives that contain both estrogen and a progestin have reported an increase in the risk of developing breast cancer, particularly at a younger age and apparently related to duration of use. There is insufficient data to determine whether the use of POPs similarly increases this risk.

A meta-analysis of 54 studies found a small increase in the frequency of having breast cancer diagnosed for women who were currently using combined oral contraceptives or had used them within the past ten years. This increase in the frequency of breast cancer diagnosis, within ten years of stopping use, was generally accounted for by cancers localized to the breast. There was no increase in the frequency of having breast cancer diagnosed ten or more years after cessation of use.

Some studies have found an increase in the incidence of cancer of the cervix in women who use oral contraceptives. However, this finding may be related to factors other than the use of oral contraceptives and there is insufficient data to determine whether the use of POPs increases the risk of developing cancer of the cervix.

Liver Tumors

In rare cases, combined oral contraceptives can cause benign but dangerous liver tumors. These benign liver tumors can rupture and cause fatal internal bleeding. In addition, some studies report an increased risk of developing liver cancer among women who use combined oral contraceptives. However, liver cancers are rare. There is insufficient data to determine whether POPs increase the risk of liver tumors.

Diabetic Women

Diabetic women taking POPs do not generally require changes in the amount of insulin they are taking. However, your physician may monitor you more closely under these conditions.

SEXUALLY TRANSMITTED DISEASES (STDs)

WARNING: POPs do not protect against getting or giving someone HIV (AIDS) or any other STD, such as chlamydia, gonorrhea, genital warts or herpes.

SIDE EFFECTS

Irregular Bleeding:

The most common side effect of POPs is a change in menstrual bleeding. Your periods may be either early or late, and you may have some spotting between periods. Taking pills late or missing pills can result in some spotting or bleeding.

Other Side Effects:

Less common side effects include headaches, tender breasts, nausea and dizziness. Weight gain, acne and extra hair on your face and body have been reported, but are rare.

If you are concerned about any of these side effects, check with your doctor or clinic.

USING POPs WITH OTHER MEDICINES

Before taking a POP, inform your health care provider of any other medication, including over-the-counter medicine, that you may be taking.

These medicines can make POPs less effective:

Medicines for seizures such as:

- Phenytoin (Dilantin)
- Carbamazepine (Tegretol)
- Phenobarbital

Medicine for TB:

- Rifampin (Rifampicin)

Before you begin taking any new medicines be sure your doctor or clinic knows you are taking a progestin-only birth control pill.

HOW TO TAKE POPs

IMPORTANT POINTS TO REMEMBER

- POPs must be taken at the same time every day, so choose a time and then take the pill at that same time every day. Every time you take a pill late, and especially if you miss a pill, you are more likely to get pregnant.
- Start the next pack the day after the last pack is finished. There is no break between packs. Always have your next pack of pills ready.
- You may have some menstrual spotting between periods. Do not stop taking your pills if this happens.
- If you vomit soon after taking a pill, use a backup method (such as a condom and/or a spermicide) for 48 hours.
- If you want to stop taking POPs, you can do so at any time, but, if you remain sexually active and don't wish to become pregnant, be certain to use another birth control method.
- If you are not sure about how to take POPs, ask your doctor or clinic.

STARTING POPs

- It's best to take your first POP on the first day of your menstrual period.
- If you decide to take your first POP on another day, use a backup method (such as a condom and/or a spermicide) every time you have sex during the next 48 hours.
- If you have had a miscarriage or an abortion, you can start POPs the next day.

IF YOU ARE LATE OR MISS TAKING YOUR POPs

- If you are more than 3 hours late or you miss one or more POPs:
  1) **TAKE** a missed pill as soon as you remember that you missed it,
  2) **THEN** go back to taking POPs at your regular time,
  3) **BUT** be sure to use a backup method (such as a condom and/or a spermcide) every time you have sex for the next 48 hours.
- If you are not sure what to do about the pills you have missed, keep taking POPs and use a backup method until you can talk to your doctor or clinic.

IF YOU ARE BREASTFEEDING

- If you are fully breastfeeding (not giving your baby any food or formula), you may start your pills 6 weeks after delivery.
- If you are partially breastfeeding (giving your baby some food or formula), you should start taking pills by 3 weeks after delivery.

IF YOU ARE SWITCHING PILLS

- If you are switching from the combined pills to POPs, take the first POP the day after you finish the last active combined pill. Do not take any of the 7 inactive pills from the combined pill pack. You should know that many women have irregular periods after switching to POPs, but this is normal and to be expected.
- If you are switching from POPs to the combined pills, take the first active combined pill on the first day of your period, even if your POPs pack is not finished.
- If you switch to another brand of POPs, start the new brand anytime.
- If you are breastfeeding, you can switch to another method of birth control at any time, except do not switch to the combined pills until you stop breastfeeding or at least until 6 months after delivery.

PREGNANCY WHILE ON THE PILL

If you think you are pregnant, contact your physician. Even though research has shown that POPs do not cause harm to the unborn baby, it is always best not to take any drugs or medicines that you don't need when you are pregnant.

You should get a pregnancy test:

- If your period is late and you took one or more pills late or missed taking them and had sex without a backup method.
- Anytime it has been more than 45 days since the beginning of your last period.

WILL POPs AFFECT YOUR ABILITY TO GET PREGNANT LATER?

If you want to become pregnant, simply stop taking POPs. POPs will not delay your ability to get pregnant.

BREASTFEEDING

If you are breastfeeding, POPs will not affect the quality or amount of your breastmilk or the health of your nursing baby.

OVERDOSE

No serious problems have been reported when many pills were taken by accident, even by a small child, so there is usually no reason to treat an overdose.

OTHER QUESTIONS OR CONCERNS

If you have any questions or concerns, check with your doctor or clinic. You can also ask for the more detailed "Professional Labeling" written for doctors and other health care providers.

HOW TO STORE YOUR POPs

Store at 25°C (77°F); excursions permitted to 15°–30°C (59°–86°F).

ORTHO-McNEIL
PHARMACEUTICAL, INC.
Raritan, New Jersey 08869
©OMP 1998 REVISED JANUARY 2002 635-50-894-2

Shown in Product Identification Guide, page 328

ORTHO TRI-CYCLEN® TABLETS ℞
ORTHO-CYCLEN® TABLETS

(norgestimate/ethinyl estradiol)

Prescribing Information

Patients should be counseled that this product does not protect against HIV infection (AIDS) and other sexually transmitted diseases.

DESCRIPTION

Each of the following products is a combination oral contraceptive containing the progestational compound norgestimate and the estrogenic compound ethinyl estradiol.

ORTHO TRI-CYCLEN □ 28 Tablets.

Each white tablet contains 0.180 mg of the progestational compound, norgestimate (18,19-Dinor-17-pregn-4-en-20-yn-3-one,17-(acetyloxy)-13-ethyl-,oxime,(17α)-(+)-) and 0.035 mg of the estrogenic compound, ethinyl estradiol (19-nor-17α-pregna,1,3,5(10)-trien-20-yne-3,17-diol). Inactive ingredients include lactose, magnesium stearate, and pregelatinized starch.

Each light blue tablet contains 0.215 mg of the progestational compound norgestimate (18,19-Dinor-17-pregn-4-en-

20-yn-3-one,17-(acetyloxy)-13-ethyl-,oxime,(17α)-(+)-) and 0.035 mg of the estrogenic compound, ethinyl estradiol (19-nor-17α-pregna,1,3,5(10)-trien-20-yne-3,17-diol). Inactive ingredients include FD&C Blue No. 2 Aluminum Lake, lactose, magnesium stearate, and pregelatinized starch.
Each blue tablet contains 0.250 mg of the progestational compound norgestimate (18,19-Dinor-17-pregn-4-en-20-yn-3-one,17-(acetyloxy)-13-ethyl-,oxime,(17α)-(+)-) and 0.035 mg of the estrogenic compound, ethinyl estradiol (19-nor-17α-pregna,1,3,5(10)-trien-20-yne-3,17-diol). Inactive ingredients include FD&C Blue No. 2 Aluminum Lake, lactose, magnesium stearate, and pregelatinized starch.
Each green tablet contains only inert ingredients, as follows: D&C Yellow No. 10 Aluminum Lake, FD&C Blue No. 2 Aluminum Lake, lactose, magnesium stearate, microcrystalline cellulose and pregelatinized starch.
ORTHO-CYCLEN ☐ 28 Tablets.
Each blue tablet contains 0.250 mg of the progestational compound norgestimate (18,19-Dinor-17-pregn-4-en-20-yn-3-one,17-(acetyloxy)-13-ethyl-,oxime,(17α)-(+)-) and 0.035 mg of the estrogenic compound, ethinyl estradiol (19-nor-17α-pregna,1,3,5(10)-trien-20-yne-3,17-diol). Inactive ingredients include FD&C Blue No. 2 Aluminum Lake, lactose, magnesium stearate, and pregelatinized starch.
Each green tablet contains only inert ingredients, as follows: D&C Yellow No. 10 Aluminum Lake, FD&C Blue No. 2 Aluminum Lake, lactose, magnesium stearate, microcrystalline cellulose and pregelatinized starch.

Norgestimate

Ethinyl Estradiol

CLINICAL PHARMACOLOGY

ORAL CONTRACEPTION

Combination oral contraceptives act by suppression of gonadotropins. Although the primary mechanism of this action is inhibition of ovulation, other alterations include changes in the cervical mucus (which increase the difficulty of sperm entry into the uterus) and the endometrium (which reduce the likelihood of implantation).
Receptor binding studies, as well as studies in animals and humans, have shown that norgestimate and 17-deacetyl norgestimate, the major serum metabolite, combine high progestational activity with minimal intrinsic androgenicity.[90–93] Norgestimate, in combination with ethinyl estradiol, does not counteract the estrogen-induced increases in sex hormone binding globulin (SHBG), resulting in lower serum testosterone.[90,91,94]

ACNE

Acne is a skin condition with a multifactorial etiology. The combination of ethinyl estradiol and norgestimate may increase sex hormone binding globulin (SHBG) and decrease free testosterone resulting in a decrease in the severity of facial acne in otherwise healthy women with this skin condition.
Norgestimate and ethinyl estradiol are well absorbed following oral administration of ORTHO-CYCLEN and ORTHO TRI-CYCLEN. On the average, peak serum concentrations of norgestimate and ethinyl estradiol are observed within two hours (0.5–2.0 hr for norgestimate and 0.75–3.0 hr for ethinyl estradiol) after administration followed by a rapid decline due to distribution and elimination. Although norgestimate serum concentrations following single or multiple dosing were generally below assay detection within 5 hours, a major norgestimate serum metabolite, 17-deacetyl norgestimate, (which exhibits a serum half-life ranging from 12 to 30 hours) appears rapidly in serum with concentrations greatly exceeding that of norgestimate. The 17-deacetylated metabolite is pharmacologically active and the pharmacologic profile is similar to that of norgestimate. The elimination half-life of ethinyl estradiol ranged from approximately 6 to 14 hours.
Both norgestimate and ethinyl estradiol are extensively metabolized and eliminated by renal and fecal pathways. Following administration of ^{14}C-norgestimate, 47% (45–49%) and 37% (16–49%) of the administered radioactivity was eliminated in the urine and feces, respectively. Unchanged norgestimate was not detected in the urine. In addition to 17-deacetyl norgestimate, a number of metabolites of norgestimate have been identified in human urine following administration of radiolabeled norgestimate. These include 18,19-Dinor-17-pregn-4-en-20-yn-3-one,17-hydroxy-13-ethyl,(17α)-(-);18,19-Dinor-5β-17-pregnan-20-yn,3α,17β-dihydroxy-13-ethyl,(17α), various hydroxylated metabolites and conjugates of these metabolites. Ethinyl estradiol is metabolized to various hydroxylated products and their glucuronide and sulfate conjugates.

TABLE I: PERCENTAGE OF WOMEN EXPERIENCING AN UNINTENDED PREGNANCY DURING THE FIRST YEAR OF TYPICAL USE AND THE FIRST YEAR OF PERFECT USE OF CONTRACEPTION AND THE PERCENTAGE CONTINUING USE AT THE END OF THE FIRST YEAR, UNITED STATES.

	% of Women Experiencing an Unintended Pregnancy within the First Year of Use		% of Women Continuing Use at One Year[3]
Method (1)	Typical Use[1] (2)	Perfect Use[2] (3)	(4)
Chance[4]	85	85	
Spermicides[5]	26	6	40
Periodic abstinence	25		63
Calendar		9	
Ovulation Method		3	
Sympto-Thermal[6]		2	
Post-Ovulation		1	
Withdrawal	19	4	
Cap[7]			
Parous Women	40	26	42
Nulliparous Women	20	9	56
Sponge			
Parous Women	40	20	42
Nulliparous Women	20	9	56
Diaphragm[7]	20	6	56
Condom[8]			
Female (Reality)	21	5	56
Male	14	3	61
Pill	5		71
Progestin Only		0.5	
Combined		0.1	
IUD			
Progesterone T	2.0	1.5	81
Copper T380A	0.8	0.6	78
LNg 20	0.1	0.1	81
Depo-Provera	0.3	0.3	70
Norplant and Norplant-2	0.05	0.05	88
Female Sterilization	0.5	0.5	100
Male Sterilization	0.15	0.10	100

Adapted from Hatcher et al., 1998 Ref. #1.
[1]Among *typical* couples who initiate use of a method (not necessarily for the first time), the percentage who experience an accidental pregnancy during the first year if they do not stop use for any other reason.
[2]Among couples who initiate use of a method (not necessarily for the first time) and who use it *perfectly* (both consistently and correctly), the percentage who experience an accidental pregnancy during the first year if they do not stop use for any other reason.
[3]Among couples attempting to avoid pregnancy, the percentage who continue to use a method for one year.
[4]The percents becoming pregnant in columns (2) and (3) are based on data from populations where contraception is not used and from women who cease using contraception in order to become pregnant. Among such populations, about 89% become pregnant within one year. This estimate was lowered slightly (to 85%) to represent the percent who would become pregnant within one year among women now relying on reversible methods of contraception if they abandoned contraception altogether.
[5]Foams, creams, gels, vaginal suppositories, and vaginal film.
[6]Cervical mucus (ovulation) method supplemented by calendar in the pre-ovulatory and basal body temperature in the post-ovulatory phases.
[7]With spermicidal cream or jelly.
[8]Without spermicides.

INDICATIONS AND USAGE

ORTHO-CYCLEN and ORTHO TRI-CYCLEN Tablets are indicated for the prevention of pregnancy in women who elect to use oral contraceptives as a method of contraception.
ORTHO TRI-CYCLEN is indicated for the treatment of moderate acne vulgaris in females, ≥ 15 years of age, who have no known contraindications to oral contraceptive therapy, desire contraception, have achieved menarche and are unresponsive to topical anti-acne medications.
Oral contraceptives are highly effective. Table I lists the typical accidental pregnancy rates for users of combination oral contraceptives and other methods of contraception. The efficacy of these contraceptive methods, except sterilization, depends upon the reliability with which they are used. Correct and consistent use of methods can result in lower failure rates.
[See table I above]
In clinical trials with ORTHO-CYCLEN, 1,651 subjects completed 24,272 cycles and a total of 18 pregnancies were reported. This represents an overall use-efficacy (typical user efficacy) pregnancy rate of 0.96 per 100 women-years. This rate includes patients who did not take the drug correctly.
In four clinical trials with ORTHO TRI-CYCLEN, the use-efficacy pregnancy rate ranged from 0.68 to 1.47 per 100 women-years. In total, 4,756 subjects completed 45,244 cycles and a total of 42 pregnancies were reported. This represents an overall use-efficacy rate of 1.21 per 100 women-years. One of these 4 studies was a randomized comparative clinical trial in which 4,633 subjects completed 22,312 cycles. Of the 2,312 patients on ORTHO TRI-CYCLEN, 8 pregnancies were reported. This represents an overall use-efficacy pregnancy rate of 0.94 per 100 women-years.
In two double-blind, placebo-controlled, six month, multicenter clinical trials, ORTHO TRI-CYCLEN showed a statistically significant decrease in inflammatory lesion count and total lesion count (Table II). The adverse reaction profile of ORTHO TRI-CYCLEN from these two controlled clinical trials is consistent with what has been noted from previous studies involving ORTHO TRI-CYCLEN and are the known risks associated with oral contraceptives.

TABLE II: Acne Vulgaris Indication
Combined Results: Two Multicenter, Placebo-Controlled Trials
Primary Efficacy Variables: Evaluable-for-Efficacy Population

	ORTHO TRI-CYCLEN®	Placebo
	N = 163	N = 161
Mean Age at Enrollment	27.3 years	28.0
Inflammatory Lesions – Mean Percent Reduction	56.6	36.6
Total Lesions – Mean Percent Reduction	49.6	30.3

CONTRAINDICATIONS

Oral contraceptives should not be used in women who currently have the following conditions:

- Thrombophlebitis or thromboembolic disorders
- A past history of deep vein thrombophlebitis or thromboembolic disorders
- Cerebral vascular or coronary artery disease
- Migraine with focal aura
- Known or suspected carcinoma of the breast
- Carcinoma of the endometrium or other known or suspected estrogen dependent neoplasia
- Undiagnosed abnormal genital bleeding
- Cholestatic jaundice of pregnancy or jaundice with prior pill use
- Acute or chronic hepatocellular disease with abnormal liver function
- Hepatic adenomas or carcinomas
- Known or suspected pregnancy
- Hypersensitivity to any component of this product

Continued on next page

Ortho Tri-Cyclen—Cont.

WARNINGS

Cigarette smoking increases the risk of serious cardiovascular side effects from oral contraceptive use. This risk increases with age and with heavy smoking (15 or more cigarettes per day) and is quite marked in women over 35 years of age. Women who use oral contraceptives should be strongly advised not to smoke.

The use of oral contraceptives is associated with increased risks of several serious conditions including myocardial infarction, thromboembolism, stroke, hepatic neoplasia, and gallbladder disease, although the risk of serious morbidity or mortality is very small in healthy women without underlying risk factors. The risk of morbidity and mortality increases significantly in the presence of other underlying risk factors such as hypertension, hyperlipidemias, obesity and diabetes.

Practitioners prescribing oral contraceptives should be familiar with the following information relating to these risks.

The information contained in this package insert is principally based on studies carried out in patients who used oral contraceptives with higher formulations of estrogens and progestogens than those in common use today. The effect of long-term use of the oral contraceptives with lower formulations of both estrogens and progestogens remains to be determined.

Throughout this labeling, epidemiological studies reported are of two types: retrospective or case control studies and prospective or cohort studies. Case control studies provide a measure of the relative risk of a disease, namely, a *ratio* of the incidence of a disease among oral contraceptive users to that among nonusers. The relative risk does not provide information on the actual clinical occurrence of a disease. Cohort studies provide a measure of attributable risk, which is the *difference* in the incidence of disease between oral contraceptive users and nonusers. The attributable risk does provide information about the actual occurrence of a disease in the population (adapted from refs. 2 and 3 with the author's permission). For further information, the reader is referred to a text on epidemiological methods.

1. THROMBOEMBOLIC DISORDERS AND OTHER VASCULAR PROBLEMS

a. Myocardial Infarction

An increased risk of myocardial infarction has been attributed to oral contraceptive use. This risk is primarily in smokers or women with other underlying risk factors for coronary artery disease such as hypertension, hypercholesterolemia, morbid obesity, and diabetes. The relative risk of heart attack for current oral contraceptive users has been estimated to be two to six.[4–10] The risk is very low under the age of 30.

Smoking in combination with oral contraceptive use has been shown to contribute substantially to the incidence of myocardial infarctions in women in their mid-thirties or older with smoking accounting for the majority of excess cases.[11] Mortality rates associated with circulatory disease have been shown to increase substantially in smokers, especially in those 35 years of age and older among women who use oral contraceptives.

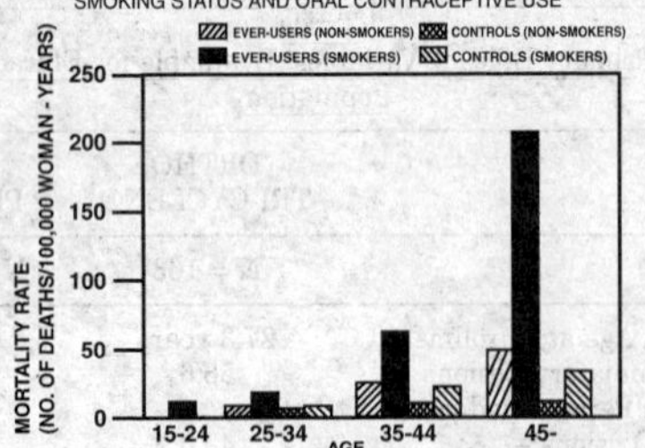

TABLE III. (Adapted from P.M. Layde and V. Beral, ref. #12.)

Oral contraceptives may compound the effects of well-known risk factors, such as hypertension, diabetes, hyperlipidemias, age and obesity.[13] In particular, some progestogens are known to decrease HDL cholesterol and cause glucose intolerance, while estrogens may create a state of hyperinsulinism.[14–18] Oral contraceptives have been shown to increase blood pressure among users (see Section 9 in WARNINGS). Similar effects on risk factors have been associated with an increased risk of heart disease. Oral contraceptives must be used with caution in women with cardiovascular disease risk factors.

Norgestimate has minimal androgenic activity (see CLINICAL PHARMACOLOGY), and there is some evidence that the risk of myocardial infarction associated with oral contraceptives is lower when the progestogen has minimal androgenic activity than when the activity is greater [97].

b. Thromboembolism

An increased risk of thromboembolic and thrombotic disease associated with the use of oral contraceptives is well established. Case control studies have found the relative risk of users compared to nonusers to be 3 for the first episode of superficial venous thrombosis, 4 to 11 for deep vein thrombosis or pulmonary embolism, and 1.5 to 6 for women with predisposing conditions for venous thromboembolic disease.[2,3,19–24] Cohort studies have shown the relative risk to be somewhat lower, about 3 for new cases and about 4.5 for new cases requiring hospitalization.[25] The risk of thromboembolic disease associated with oral contraceptives is not related to length of use and disappears after pill use is stopped.[2]

A two- to four-fold increase in relative risk of post-operative thromboembolic complications has been reported with the use of oral contraceptives.[9] The relative risk of venous thrombosis in women who have predisposing conditions is twice that of women without such medical conditions.[26] If feasible, oral contraceptives should be discontinued at least four weeks prior to and for two weeks after elective surgery of a type associated with an increase in risk of thromboembolism and during and following prolonged immobilization. Since the immediate postpartum period is also associated with an increased risk of thromboembolism, oral contraceptives should be started no earlier than four weeks after delivery in women who elect not to breast feed. After an induced or spontaneous abortion that occurs at or after 20 weeks gestation, hormonal contraceptives may be started either on Day 21 post-abortion or on the first day of the first spontaneous menstruation, whichever comes first [98].

c. Cerebrovascular diseases

Oral contraceptives have been shown to increase both the relative and attributable risks of cerebrovascular events (thrombotic and hemorrhagic strokes), although, in general, the risk is greatest among older (>35 years), hypertensive women who also smoke. Hypertension was found to be a risk factor for both users and nonusers, for both types of strokes, and smoking interacted to increase the risk of stroke.[27–29]

In a large study, the relative risk of thrombotic strokes has been shown to range from 3 for normotensive users to 14 for users with severe hypertension.[30] The relative risk of hemorrhagic stroke is reported to be 1.2 for non-smokers who used oral contraceptives, 2.6 for smokers who did not use oral contraceptives, 7.6 for smokers who used oral contraceptives, 1.8 for normotensive users and 25.7 for users with severe hypertension.[30] The attributable risk is also greater in older women.[3]

d. Dose-related risk of vascular disease from oral contraceptives

A positive association has been observed between the amount of estrogen and progestogen in oral contraceptives and the risk of vascular disease.[31–33] A decline in serum high density lipoproteins (HDL) has been reported with many progestational agents.[14–16] A decline in serum high density lipoproteins has been associated with an increased incidence of ischemic heart disease. Because estrogens increase HDL cholesterol, the net effect of an oral contraceptive depends on a balance achieved between doses of estrogen and progestogen and the activity of the progestogen used in the contraceptives. The activity and amount of both hormones should be considered in the choice of an oral contraceptive.

Minimizing exposure to estrogen and progestogen is in keeping with good principles of therapeutics. For any particular estrogen/progestogen combination, the dosage regimen prescribed should be one which contains the least amount of estrogen and progestogen that is compatible with a low failure rate and the needs of the individual patient. New acceptors of oral contraceptive agents should be started on preparations containing 0.035 mg or less of estrogen.

e. Persistence of risk of vascular disease

There are two studies which have shown persistence of risk of vascular disease for ever-users of oral contraceptives. In a study in the United States, the risk of developing myocardial infarction after discontinuing oral contraceptives persists for at least 9 years for women 40–49 years who had used oral contraceptives for five or more years, but this increased risk was not demonstrated in other age groups.[8] In another study in Great Britain, the risk of developing cerebrovascular disease persisted for at least 6 years after discontinuation of oral contraceptives, although excess risk was very small.[34] However, both studies were performed with oral contraceptive formulations containing 50 micrograms or higher of estrogens.

2. ESTIMATES OF MORTALITY FROM CONTRACEPTIVE USE

One study gathered data from a variety of sources which have estimated the mortality rate associated with different methods of contraception at different ages (Table IV). These estimates include the combined risk of death associated with contraceptive methods plus the risk attributable to pregnancy in the event of method failure. Each method of contraception has its specific benefits and risks. The study concluded that with the exception of oral contraceptive users 35 and older who smoke, and 40 and older who do not smoke, mortality associated with all methods of birth control is low and below that associated with childbirth. The observation of an increase in risk of mortality with age for oral contraceptive users is based on data gathered in the 1970's.[35] Current clinical recommendation involves the use of lower estrogen dose formulations and a careful consideration of risk factors. In 1989, the Fertility and Maternal Health Drugs Advisory Committee was asked to review the use of oral contraceptives in women 40 years of age and over. The Committee concluded that although cardiovascular disease risks may be increased with oral contraceptive use after age 40 in healthy non-smoking women (even with the newer low-dose formulations), there are also greater potential health risks associated with pregnancy in older women and with the alternative surgical and medical procedures which may be necessary if such women do not have access to effective and acceptable means of contraception. The Committee recommended that the benefits of low-dose oral contraceptive use by healthy non-smoking women over 40 may outweigh the possible risks.

Of course, older women, as all women, who take oral contraceptives, should take an oral contraceptive which contains the least amount of estrogen and progestogen that is compatible with a low failure rate and individual patient needs.

[See table IV below]

3. CARCINOMA OF THE REPRODUCTIVE ORGANS AND BREASTS

Numerous epidemiological studies have been performed on the incidence of breast, endometrial, ovarian, and cervical cancer in women using oral contraceptives. While there are conflicting reports, most studies suggest that use of oral contraceptives is not associated with an overall increase in the risk of developing breast cancer. Some studies have reported an increased relative risk of developing breast cancer, particularly at a younger age. This increased relative risk has been reported to be related to duration of use.[36–44,79–89]

A meta-analysis of 54 studies found a small increase in the frequency of having breast cancer diagnosed for women who were currently using combined oral contraceptives or had used them within the past ten years. This increase in the frequency of breast cancer diagnosis, within ten years of stopping use, was generally accounted for by cancers localized to the breast. There was no increase in the frequency of having breast cancer diagnosed ten or more years after cessation of use.[95]

Some studies suggest that oral contraceptive use has been associated with an increase in the risk of cervical intraepithelial neoplasia in some populations of women.[45–48] However, there continues to be controversy about the extent to which such findings may be due to differences in sexual behavior and other factors.

4. HEPATIC NEOPLASIA

Benign hepatic adenomas are associated with oral contraceptive use, although the incidence of benign tumors is rare in the United States. Indirect calculations have estimated the attributable risk to be in the range of 3.3 cases/100,000 for users, a risk that increases after four or more years of use especially with oral contraceptives of higher dose.[49] Rupture of benign, hepatic adenomas may cause death through intra-abdominal hemorrhage.[50,51]

Studies have shown an increased risk of developing hepatocellular carcinoma[52–54,96] in oral contraceptive users. However, these cancers are rare in the U.S.

5. OCULAR LESIONS

There have been clinical case reports of retinal thrombosis associated with the use of oral contraceptives. Oral contraceptives should be discontinued if there is unexplained partial or complete loss of vision; onset of proptosis or diplopia; papilledema; or retinal vascular lesions. Appropriate diagnostic and therapeutic measures should be undertaken immediately.

TABLE IV: ANNUAL NUMBER OF BIRTH-RELATED OR METHOD-RELATED DEATHS ASSOCIATED WITH CONTROL OF FERTILITY PER 100,000 NON-STERILE WOMEN, BY FERTILITY CONTROL METHOD ACCORDING TO AGE

Method of control and outcome	15-19	20-24	25-29	30-34	35-39	40-44
No fertility control methods*	7.0	7.4	9.1	14.8	25.7	28.2
Oral contraceptives non-smoker**	0.3	0.5	0.9	1.9	13.8	31.6
Oral contraceptives smoker**	2.2	3.4	6.6	13.5	51.1	117.2
IUD**	0.8	0.8	1.0	1.0	1.4	1.4
Condom*	1.1	1.6	0.7	0.2	0.3	0.4
Diaphragm/spermicide*	1.9	1.2	1.2	1.3	2.2	2.8
Periodic abstinence*	2.5	1.6	1.6	1.7	2.9	3.6

*Deaths are birth-related
**Deaths are method-related

Adapted from H.W. Ory, ref. #35.

6. ORAL CONTRACEPTIVE USE BEFORE OR DURING EARLY PREGNANCY

Extensive epidemiological studies have revealed no increased risk of birth defects in women who have used oral contraceptives prior to pregnancy.[56,57] The majority of recent studies also do not indicate a teratogenic effect, particularly in so far as cardiac anomalies and limb reduction defects are concerned,[55,56,58,59] when taken inadvertently during early pregnancy.

The administration of oral contraceptives to induce withdrawal bleeding should not be used as a test for pregnancy. Oral contraceptives should not be used during pregnancy to treat threatened or habitual abortion.

It is recommended that for any patient who has missed two consecutive periods, pregnancy should be ruled out before continuing oral contraceptive use. If the patient has not adhered to the prescribed schedule, the possibility of pregnancy should be considered at the time of the first missed period. Oral contraceptive use should be discontinued until pregnancy is ruled out.

7. GALLBLADDER DISEASE

Earlier studies have reported an increased lifetime relative risk of gallbladder surgery in users of oral contraceptives and estrogens.[60,61] More recent studies, however, have shown that the relative risk of developing gallbladder disease among oral contraceptive users may be minimal.[62–64] The recent findings of minimal risk may be related to the use of oral contraceptive formulations containing lower hormonal doses of estrogens and progestogens.

8. CARBOHYDRATE AND LIPID METABOLIC EFFECTS

Oral contraceptives have been shown to cause a decrease in glucose tolerance in a significant percentage of users.[17] This effect has been shown to be directly related to estrogen dose.[65] Progestogens increase insulin secretion and create insulin resistance, this effect varying with different progestational agents.[17,66] However, in the non-diabetic woman, oral contraceptives appear to have no effect on fasting blood glucose.[67] Because of these demonstrated effects, prediabetic and diabetic women in particular should be carefully monitored while taking oral contraceptives.

A small proportion of women will have persistent hypertriglyceridemia while on the pill. As discussed earlier (see WARNINGS 1a and 1d), changes in serum triglycerides and lipoprotein levels have been reported in oral contraceptive users.

In clinical studies with ORTHO-CYCLEN there were no clinically significant changes in fasting blood glucose levels. No statistically significant changes in mean fasting blood glucose levels were observed over 24 cycles of use. Glucose tolerance tests showed minimal, clinically insignificant changes from baseline to cycles 3, 12, and 24.

In clinical studies with ORTHO TRI-CYCLEN there were no clinically significant changes in fasting blood glucose levels. Minimal statistically significant changes were noted in glucose levels over 24 cycles of use. Glucose tolerance tests showed no clinically significant changes from baseline to cycles 3, 12, and 24.

9. ELEVATED BLOOD PRESSURE

Women with significant hypertension should not be started on hormonal contraception.[98] An increase in blood pressure has been reported in women taking oral contraceptives[68] and this increase is more likely in older oral contraceptive users[69] and with extended duration of use.[61] Data from the Royal College of General Practitioners[12] and subsequent randomized trials have shown that the incidence of hypertension increases with increasing progestational activity.

Women with a history of hypertension or hypertension-related diseases, or renal disease[70] should be encouraged to use another method of contraception. If women elect to use oral contraceptives, they should be monitored closely and if significant elevation of blood pressure occurs, oral contraceptives should be discontinued. For most women, elevated blood pressure will return to normal after stopping oral contraceptives, and there is no difference in the occurrence of hypertension between former and never users.[68–71] It should be noted that in two separate large clinical trials (N = 633 and N = 911), no statistically significant changes in mean blood pressure were observed with ORTHO-CYCLEN.

10. HEADACHE

The onset or exacerbation of migraine or development of headache with a new pattern which is recurrent, persistent or severe requires discontinuation of oral contraceptives and evaluation of the cause.

11. BLEEDING IRREGULARITIES

Breakthrough bleeding and spotting are sometimes encountered in patients on oral contraceptives, especially during the first three months of use. Non-hormonal causes should be considered and adequate diagnostic measures taken to rule out malignancy or pregnancy in the event of breakthrough bleeding, as in the case of any abnormal vaginal bleeding. If pathology has been excluded, time or a change to another formulation may solve the problem. In the event of amenorrhea, pregnancy should be ruled out.

Some women may encounter post-pill amenorrhea or oligomenorrhea, especially when such a condition was preexistent.

12. ECTOPIC PREGNANCY

Ectopic as well as intrauterine pregnancy may occur in contraceptive failures.

PRECAUTIONS

1. PHYSICAL EXAMINATION AND FOLLOW UP

It is good medical practice for all women to have annual history and physical examinations, including women using oral contraceptives. The physical examination, however, may be deferred until after initiation of oral contraceptives if requested by the woman and judged appropriate by the clinician. The physical examination should include special reference to blood pressure, breasts, abdomen and pelvic organs, including cervical cytology, and relevant laboratory tests. In case of undiagnosed, persistent or recurrent abnormal vaginal bleeding, appropriate measures should be conducted to rule out malignancy. Women with a strong family history of breast cancer or who have breast nodules should be monitored with particular care.

2. LIPID DISORDERS

Women who are being treated for hyperlipidemias should be followed closely if they elect to use oral contraceptives. Some progestogens may elevate LDL levels and may render the control of hyperlipidemias more difficult.

3. LIVER FUNCTION

If jaundice develops in any woman receiving such drugs, the medication should be discontinued. Steroid hormones may be poorly metabolized in patients with impaired liver function.

4. FLUID RETENTION

Oral contraceptives may cause some degree of fluid retention. They should be prescribed with caution, and only with careful monitoring, in patients with conditions which might be aggravated by fluid retention.

5. EMOTIONAL DISORDERS

Women with a history of depression should be carefully observed and the drug discontinued if depression recurs to a serious degree.

6. CONTACT LENSES

Contact lens wearers who develop visual changes or changes in lens tolerance should be assessed by an ophthalmologist.

7. DRUG INTERACTIONS

Reduced efficacy and increased incidence of breakthrough bleeding and menstrual irregularities have been associated with concomitant use of rifampin. A similar association, though less marked, has been suggested with barbiturates, phenylbutazone, phenytoin sodium, carbamazepine, griseofulvin, topiramate, and possibly with ampicillin and tetracyclines.[72] A possible interaction has been suggested with hormonal contraceptives and the herbal supplement St. Johns Wort based on some reports of oral contraceptive users experiencing breakthrough bleeding shortly after starting St. Johns Wort. Pregnancies have been reported by users of combined hormonal contraceptives who also used some form of St. Johns Wort. Healthcare prescribers are advised to consult the package inserts of medication administered concomitantly with oral contraceptives.

8. INTERACTIONS WITH LABORATORY TESTS

Certain endocrine and liver function tests and blood components may be affected by oral contraceptives:

a. Increased prothrombin and factors VII, VIII, IX, and X; decreased antithrombin 3; increased norepinephrine-induced platelet aggregability.

b. Increased thyroid binding globulin (TBG) leading to increased circulating total thyroid hormone, as measured by protein-bound iodine (PBI), T4 by column or by radioimmunoassay. Free T3 resin uptake is decreased, reflecting the elevated TBG, free T4 concentration is unaltered.

c. Other binding proteins may be elevated in serum.

d. Sex hormone binding globulins are increased and result in elevated levels of total circulating sex steroids; however, free or biologically active levels either decrease or remain unchanged.

e. High-density lipoprotein (HDL-C) and total cholesterol (Total-C) may be increased, low-density lipoprotein (LDL-C) may be increased or decreased, while LDL-C/HDL-C ratio may be decreased and triglycerides may be unchanged.

f. Glucose tolerance may be decreased.

g. Serum folate levels may be depressed by oral contraceptive therapy. This may be of clinical significance if a woman becomes pregnant shortly after discontinuing oral contraceptives.

9. CARCINOGENESIS

See WARNINGS Section.

10. PREGNANCY

Pregnancy Category X. See CONTRAINDICATIONS and WARNINGS Sections.

11. NURSING MOTHERS

Small amounts of oral contraceptive steroids have been identified in the milk of nursing mothers and a few adverse effects on the child have been reported, including jaundice and breast enlargement. In addition, combination oral contraceptives given in the postpartum period may interfere with lactation by decreasing the quantity and quality of breast milk. If possible, the nursing mother should be advised not to use combination oral contraceptives but to use other forms of contraception until she has completely weaned her child.

12. PEDIATRIC USE

Safety and efficacy of ORTHO-CYCLEN Tablets and ORTHO TRI-CYCLEN Tablets have been established in women of reproductive age. Safety and efficacy are expected to be the same for postpubertal adolescents under the age of 16 and for users 16 years and older. Use of this product before menarche is not indicated.

13. SEXUALLY TRANSMITTED DISEASES

Patients should be counseled that this product does not protect against HIV infection (AIDS) and other sexually transmitted diseases.

INFORMATION FOR THE PATIENT

See Patient Labeling printed below.

ADVERSE REACTIONS

An increased risk of the following serious adverse reactions has been associated with the use of oral contraceptives (See WARNINGS Section).

- Thrombophlebitis and venous thrombosis with or without embolism
- Arterial thromboembolism
- Pulmonary embolism
- Myocardial infarction
- Cerebral hemorrhage
- Cerebral thrombosis
- Hypertension
- Gallbladder disease
- Hepatic adenomas or benign liver tumors

The following adverse reactions have been reported in patients receiving oral contraceptives and are believed to be drug-related:

- Nausea
- Vomiting
- Gastrointestinal symptoms (such as abdominal cramps and bloating)
- Breakthrough bleeding
- Spotting
- Change in menstrual flow
- Amenorrhea
- Temporary infertility after discontinuation of treatment
- Edema
- Melasma which may persist
- Breast changes: tenderness, enlargement, secretion
- Change in weight (increase or decrease)
- Change in cervical erosion and secretion
- Diminution in lactation when given immediately postpartum
- Cholestatic jaundice
- Migraine
- Rash (allergic)
- Mental depression
- Reduced tolerance to carbohydrates
- Vaginal candidiasis
- Change in corneal curvature (steepening)
- Intolerance to contact lenses

The following adverse reactions have been reported in users of oral contraceptives and the association has been neither confirmed nor refuted:

- Pre-menstrual syndrome
- Cataracts
- Changes in appetite
- Cystitis-like syndrome
- Headache
- Nervousness
- Dizziness
- Hirsutism
- Loss of scalp hair
- Erythema multiforme
- Erythema nodosum
- Hemorrhagic eruption
- Vaginitis
- Porphyria
- Impaired renal function
- Hemolytic uremic syndrome
- Acne
- Changes in libido
- Colitis
- Budd-Chiari Syndrome

OVERDOSAGE

Serious ill effects have not been reported following acute ingestion of large doses of oral contraceptives by young children. Overdosage may cause nausea and withdrawal bleeding may occur in females.

NON-CONTRACEPTIVE HEALTH BENEFITS

The following non-contraceptive health benefits related to the use of combination oral contraceptives are supported by epidemiological studies which largely utilized oral contraceptive formulations containing estrogen doses exceeding 0.035 mg of ethinyl estradiol or 0.05 mg mestranol.[73–78]

Effects on menses:

- increased menstrual cycle regularity
- decreased blood loss and decreased incidence of iron deficiency anemia
- decreased incidence of dysmenorrhea

Effects related to inhibition of ovulation:

- decreased incidence of functional ovarian cysts
- decreased incidence of ectopic pregnancies

Other effects:

- decreased incidence of fibroadenomas and fibrocystic disease of the breast
- decreased incidence of acute pelvic inflammatory disease
- decreased incidence of endometrial cancer
- decreased incidence of ovarian cancer

DOSAGE AND ADMINISTRATION

ORAL CONTRACEPTION

To achieve maximum contraceptive effectiveness, ORTHO TRI-CYCLEN Tablets and ORTHO-CYCLEN Tablets must be taken exactly as directed and at intervals not exceeding 24 hours. ORTHO TRI-CYCLEN and ORTHO-CYCLEN are available in the DIALPAK® Tablet Dispenser which is preset for a Sunday Start. Day 1 Start is also provided.

28-Day Regimen (Sunday Start)

When taking ORTHO TRI-CYCLEN □ 28 and ORTHO-CYCLEN □ 28 the first tablet should be taken on the first Sunday after menstruation begins. If period begins on Sun-

Continued on next page

Ortho Tri-Cyclen—Cont.

day, the first tablet should be taken that day. Take one active tablet daily for 21 days followed by one green tablet daily for 7 days. After 28 tablets have been taken, a new course is started the next day (Sunday). For the first cycle of a Sunday Start regimen, another method of contraception should be used until after the first 7 consecutive days of administration.

If the patient misses one (1) active tablet in Weeks 1, 2, or 3, the tablet should be taken as soon as she remembers. If the patient misses two (2) active tablets in Week 1 or Week 2, the patient should take two (2) tablets the day she remembers and two (2) tablets the next day; and then continue taking one (1) tablet a day until she finishes the pack. The patient should be instructed to use a back-up method of birth control if she has sex in the seven (7) days after missing pills. If the patient misses two (2) active tablets in the third week or misses three (3) or more active tablets in a row, the patient should continue taking one tablet every day until Sunday. On Sunday the patient should throw out the rest of the pack and start a new pack that same day. The patient should be instructed to use a back-up method of birth control if she has sex in the seven (7) days after missing pills.

Complete instructions to facilitate patient counseling on proper pill usage may be found in the Detailed Patient Labeling ("How to Take the Pill" section).

28-Day Regimen (Day 1 Start)

The dosage of ORTHO TRI-CYCLEN □ 28 and ORTHO-CYCLEN □ 28, for the initial cycle of therapy is one active tablet administered daily from the 1st day through the 21st day of the menstrual cycle, counting the first day of menstrual flow as "Day 1" followed by one green tablet daily for 7 days. Tablets are taken without interruption for 28 days. After 28 tablets have been taken, a new course is started the next day.

If the patient misses one (1) active tablet in Weeks 1, 2, or 3, the tablet should be taken as soon as she remembers. If the patient misses two (2) active tablets in Week 1 or Week 2, the patient should take two (2) tablets the day she remembers and two (2) tablets the next day; and then continue taking one (1) tablet a day until she finishes the pack. The patient should be instructed to use a back-up method of birth control if she has sex in the seven (7) days after missing pills. If the patient misses two (2) active tablets in the third week or misses three (3) or more active tablets in a row, the patient should throw out the rest of the pack and start a new pack that same day. The patient should be instructed to use a back-up method of birth control if she has sex in the seven (7) days after missing pills.

Complete instructions to facilitate patient counseling on proper pill usage may be found in the Detailed Patient Labeling ("How to Take the Pill" section).

The use of ORTHO TRI-CYCLEN and ORTHO-CYCLEN for contraception may be initiated 4 weeks postpartum in women who elect not to breast feed. When the tablets are administered during the postpartum period, the increased risk of thromboembolic disease associated with the postpartum period must be considered. (See CONTRAINDICATIONS and WARNINGS concerning thromboembolic disease. See also PRECAUTIONS for "Nursing Mothers.") The possibility of ovulation and conception prior to initiation of medication should be considered.

(See Discussion of Dose-Related Risk of Vascular Disease from Oral Contraceptives.)

ADDITIONAL INSTRUCTIONS FOR ALL DOSING REGIMENS

Breakthrough bleeding, spotting, and amenorrhea are frequent reasons for patients discontinuing oral contraceptives. In breakthrough bleeding, as in all cases of irregular bleeding from the vagina, nonfunctional causes should be borne in mind. In undiagnosed persistent or recurrent abnormal bleeding from the vagina, adequate diagnostic measures are indicated to rule out pregnancy or malignancy. If pathology has been excluded, time or a change to another formulation may solve the problem. Changing to an oral contraceptive with a higher estrogen content, while potentially useful in minimizing menstrual irregularity, should be done only if necessary since this may increase the risk of thromboembolic disease.

Use of oral contraceptives in the event of a missed menstrual period:

1. If the patient has not adhered to the prescribed schedule, the possibility of pregnancy should be considered at the time of the first missed period and oral contraceptive use should be discontinued and a non-hormonal method should be used until pregnancy is ruled out.
2. If the patient has adhered to the prescribed regimen and misses two consecutive periods, pregnancy should be ruled out before continuing oral contraceptive use.

ACNE

The timing of initiation of dosing with ORTHO TRI-CYCLEN for acne should follow the guidelines for use of ORTHO TRI-CYCLEN as an oral contraceptive. **Consult the DOSAGE AND ADMINISTRATION section for oral contraceptives.** The dosage regimen for ORTHO TRI-CYCLEN for treatment of facial acne, as available in a DIALPAK® Tablet Dispenser, utilizes a 21-day active and a 7-day placebo schedule. Take one active tablet daily for 21 days followed by one green tablet for 7 days. After 28 tablets have been taken, a new course is started the next day.

HOW SUPPLIED

ORTHO TRI-CYCLEN □ 28 Tablets are available in a DIALPAK® Tablet Dispenser (NDC 0062-1903-15) containing 28 tablets. Each white tablet contains 0.180 mg of the progestational compound, norgestimate, together with 0.035 mg of the estrogenic compound, ethinyl estradiol. Each light blue tablet contains 0.215 mg of the progestational compound, norgestimate, together with 0.035 mg of the estrogenic compound, ethinyl estradiol. Each blue tablet contains 0.250 mg of the progestational compound, norgestimate, together with 0.035 mg of the estrogenic compound, ethinyl estradiol. Each green tablet contains inert ingredients.

The white tablets are unscored, with "Ortho" and "180" debossed on each side; the light blue tablets are unscored with "Ortho" and "215" debossed on each side; the blue tablets are unscored with "Ortho" and "250" debossed on each side.

ORTHO TRI-CYCLEN □ 28 Tablets are available for clinic usage in a VERIDATE® Tablet Dispenser (unfilled) and VERIDATE Refills (NDC 0062-1903-20).

ORTHO-CYCLEN □ 28 Tablets are available in a DIALPAK® Tablet Dispenser (NDC 0062-1901-15) containing 28 tablets tablets as follows: 21 blue tablets and 7 green tablets. Each blue tablet contains 0.250 mg of the progestational compound, norgestimate, together with 0.035 mg of the estrogenic compound, ethinyl estradiol which are unscored with "Ortho" and "250" debossed on each side. Each green green tablets contains inert ingredients.

ORTHO-CYCLEN □ 28 Tablets are available for clinic usage in a VERIDATE® Tablet Dispenser (unfilled) and VERIDATE Refills (NDC 0062-1901-20).

℞ only

REFERENCES

1. Trussel J. Contraceptive efficacy. In Hatcher RA, Trussel J, Stewart F, Cates W, Stewart GK, Kowal D, Guest F, Contraceptive Technology: Seventeenth Revised Edition. New York NY: Irvington Publishers, 1998, in press. **2.** Stadel BV, Oral contraceptives and cardiovascular disease. (Pt. 1). N Engl J Med 1981; 305:612–618. **3.** Stadel BV, Oral contraceptives and cardiovascular disease. (Pt. 2). N Engl J Med 1981; 305:672–677. **4.** Adam SA, Thorogood M. Oral contraception and myocardial infarction revisited: the effects of new preparations and prescribing patterns. Br J Obstet Gynaecol 1981; 88:838–845. **5.** Mann JI, Inman WH. Oral contraceptives and death from myocardial infarction. Br Med J 1975; 2(5965):245–248. **6.** Mann JI, Vessey MP, Thorogood M, Doll R. Myocardial infarction in young women with special reference to oral contraceptive practice. Br Med J 1975; 2(5956):241–245. **7.** Royal College of General Practitioners' Oral Contraception Study: further analyses of mortality in oral contraceptive users. Lancet 1981; 1:541–546. **8.** Slone D, Shapiro S, Kaufman DW, Rosenberg L, Miettinen OS, Stolley PD. Risk of myocardial infarction in relation to current and discontinued use of oral contraceptives. N Engl J Med 1981; 305:420–424. **9.** Vessey MP. Female hormones and vascular disease—an epidemiological overview. Br J Fam Plann 1980; 6 (Supplement): 1–12. **10.** Russell-Briefel RG, Ezzati TM, Fulwood R, Perlman JA, Murphy RS. Cardiovascular risk status and oral contraceptive use, United States, 1976-80. Prevent Med 1986; 15:352–362. **11.** Goldbaum GM, Kendrick JS, Hogelin GC, Gentry EM. The relative impact of smoking and oral contraceptive use on women in the United States. JAMA 1987; 258:1339–1342. **12.** Layde PM, Beral V. Further analyses of mortality in oral contraceptive users: Royal College of General Practitioners' Oral Contraception Study. (Table 5) Lancet 1981; 1:541–546. **13.** Knopp RH. Arteriosclerosis risk: the roles of oral contraceptives and postmenopausal estrogens. J Reprod Med 1986; 31(9)(Supplement): 913–921. **14.** Krauss RM, Roy S, Mishell DR, Casagrande J, Pike MC. Effects of two low-dose oral contraceptives on serum lipids and lipoproteins: Differential changes in high-density lipoproteins subclasses. Am J Obstet 1983; 145:446–452. **15.** Wahl P, Walden C, Knopp R, Hoover J, Wallace R, Heiss G, Rifkind B. Effect of estrogen/progestin potency on lipid/lipoprotein cholesterol. N Engl J Med 1983; 308:862–867. **16.** Wynn V, Niththyananthan R. The effect of progestin in combined oral contraceptives on serum lipids with special reference to high density lipoproteins. Am J Obstet Gynecol 1982; 142:766–771. **17.** Wynn V, Godsland I. Effects of oral contraceptives on carbohydrate metabolism. J Reprod Med 1986; 31(9)(Supplement):892–897. **18.** LaRosa JC. Atherosclerotic risk factors in cardiovascular disease. J Reprod Med 1986; 31(9)(Supplement): 906–912. **19.** Inman WH, Vessey MP. Investigation of death from pulmonary, coronary, and cerebral thrombosis and embolism in women of child-bearing age. Br Med J 1968; 2(5599):193–199. **20.** Maguire MG, Tonascia J, Sartwell PE, Stolley PD, Tockman MS. Increased risk of thrombosis due to oral contraceptives: a further report. Am J Epidemiol 1979; 110(2):188–195. **21.** Petitti DB, Wingerd J, Pellegrin F, Ramacharan S. Risk of vascular disease in women: smoking, oral contraceptives, noncontraceptive estrogens, and other factors. JAMA 1979; 242:1150–1154. **22.** Vessey MP, Doll R. Investigation of relation between use of oral contraceptives and thromboembolic disease. Br Med J 1968; 2(5599):199–205. **23.** Vessey MP, Doll R. Investigation of relation between use of oral contraceptives and thromboembolic disease. A further report. Br Med J 1969; 2(5658):651–657. **24.** Porter JB, Hunter JR, Danielson DA, Jick H, Stergachis A. Oral contraceptives and non-fatal vascular disease—recent experience. Obstet Gynecol 1982; 59(3): 299–302. **25.** Vessey M, Doll R, Peto R, Johnson B, Wiggins P. A long-term follow-up study of women using different methods of contraception: an interim report. J Biosocial Sci 1976; 8:375–427. **26.** Royal College of General Practitioners: Oral Contraceptives, venous thrombosis, and varicose veins. J Royal Coll Gen Pract 1978; 28:393–399. **27.** Collaborative Group for the Study of Stroke in Young Women: Oral contraception and increased risk of cerebral ischemia or thrombosis. N Engl J Med 1973; 288:871–878. **28.** Petitti DB, Wingerd J. Use of oral contraceptives, cigarette smoking, and risk of subarachnoid hemorrhage. Lancet 1978; 2:234–236. **29.** Inman WH. Oral contraceptives and fatal subarachnoid hemorrhage. Br Med J 1979; 2(6203):1468–1470. **30.** Collaborative Group for the Study of Stroke in Young Women: Oral Contraceptives and stroke in young women: associated risk factors. JAMA 1975; 231:718–722. **31.** Inman WH, Vessey MP, Westerholm B, Engelund A. Thromboembolic disease and the steroidal content of oral contraceptives. A report to the Committee on Safety of Drugs. Br Med J 1970; 2:203–209. **32.** Meade TW, Greenberg G, Thompson SG. Progestogens and cardiovascular reactions associated with oral contraceptives and a comparison of the safety of 50- and 35-mcg oestrogen preparations. Br Med J 1980; 280(6224):1157–1161. **33.** Kay CR. Progestogens and arterial disease—evidence from the Royal College of General Practitioners' Study. Am J Obstet Gynecol 1982; 142:762–765. **34.** Royal College of General Practitioners: Incidence of arterial disease among oral contraceptive users. J Royal Coll Gen Pract 1983; 33:75–82. **35.** Ory HW. Mortality associated with fertility and fertility control: 1983. Family Planning Perspectives 1983; 15:50–56. **36.** The Cancer and Steroid Hormone Study of the Centers for Disease Control and the National Institute of Child Health and Human Development: Oral contraceptive use and the risk of breast cancer. N Engl J Med 1986; 315:405–411. **37.** Pike MC, Henderson BE, Krailo MD, Duke A, Roy S. Breast cancer in young women and use of oral contraceptives: possible modifying effect of formulation and age at use. Lancet 1983; 2:926–929. **38.** Paul C, Skegg DG, Spears GFS, Kaldor JM. Oral contraceptives and breast cancer: A national study. Br Med J 1986; 293:723–725. **39.** Miller DR, Rosenberg L, Kaufman DW, Schottenfeld D, Stolley PD, Shapiro S. Breast cancer risk in relation to early oral contraceptive use. Obstet Gynecol 1986; 68:863–868. **40.** Olsson H, Olsson ML, Moller TR, Ranstam J, Holm P. Oral contraceptive use and breast cancer in young women in Sweden (letter). Lancet 1985; 1(8431):748–749. **41.** McPherson K, Vessey M, Neil A, Doll R, Jones L, Roberts M. Early contraceptive use and breast cancer: Results of another case-control study. Br J Cancer 1987; 56:653–660. **42.** Huggins GR, Zucker PF. Oral contraceptives and neoplasia: 1987 update. Fertil Steril 1987; 47: 733–761. **43.** McPherson K, Drife JO. The pill and breast cancer: why the uncertainty? Br Med J 1986; 293:709–710. **44.** Shapiro S. Oral contraceptives—time to take stock. N Engl J Med 1987; 315:450–451. **45.** Ory H, Naib Z, Conger SB, Hatcher RA, Tyler CW. Contraceptive choice and prevalence of cervical dysplasia and carcinoma in situ. Am J Obstet Gynecol 1976; 124:573–577. **46.** Vessey MP, Lawless M, McPherson K, Yeates D. Neoplasia of the cervix uteri and contraception: a possible adverse effect of the pill. Lancet 1983; 2:930. **47.** Brinton LA, Huggins GR, Lehman HF, Malli K, Savitz DA, Trapido E, Rosenthal J, Hoover R. Long term use of oral contraceptives and risk of invasive cervical cancer. Int J Cancer 1986; 38:339–344. **48.** WHO Collaborative Study of Neoplasia and Steroid Contraceptives: Invasive cervical cancer and combined oral contraceptives. Br Med J 1985; 290:961–965. **49.** Rooks JB, Ory HW, Ishak KG, Strauss LT, Greenspan JR, Hill AP, Tyler CW. Epidemiology of hepatocellular adenoma: the role of oral contraceptive use. JAMA 1979; 242:644–648. **50.** Bein NN, Goldsmith HS. Recurrent massive hemorrhage from benign hepatic tumors secondary to oral contraceptives. Br J Surg 1977; 64:433–435. **51.** Klatskin G. Hepatic tumors: possible relationship to use of oral contraceptives. Gastroenterology 1977; 73: 386–394. **52.** Henderson BE, Preston-Martin S, Edmondson HA, Peters RL, Pike MC. Hepatocellular carcinoma and oral contraceptives. Br J Cancer 1983; 48:437–440. **53.** Neuberger J, Forman D, Doll R, Williams R. Oral contraceptives and hepatocellular carcinoma. Br Med J 1986; 292:1355–1357. **54.** Forman D, Vincent TJ, Doll R. Cancer of the liver and oral contraceptives. Br Med J 1986; 292:1357–1361. **55.** Harlap S, Eldor J. Births following oral contraceptive failures. Obstet Gynecol 1980; 55:447–452. **56.** Savolainen E, Saksela E, Saxen L. Teratogenic hazards of oral contraceptives analyzed in a national malformation register. Am J Obstet Gynecol 1981; 140:521–524. **57.** Janerich DT, Piper JM, Glebatis DM. Oral contraceptives and birth defects. Am J Epidemiol 1980; 112:73–79. **58.** Ferencz C, Matanoski GM, Wilson PD, Rubin JD, Neill CA, Gutberlet R. Maternal hormone therapy and congenital heart disease. Teratology 1980; 21:225–239. **59.** Rothman KJ, Fyler DC, Goldblatt A, Kreidberg MB. Exogenous hormones and other drug exposures of children with congenital heart disease. Am J Epidemiol 1979; 109:433–439. **60.** Boston Collaborative Drug Surveillance Program: Oral contraceptives and venous thromboembolic disease, surgically confirmed gallbladder disease, and breast tumors. Lancet 1973; 1:1399–1404. **61.** Royal College of General Practitioners: Oral contraceptives and health. New York, Pittman 1974. **62.** Layde PM, Vessey MP, Yeates D. Risk of gallbladder disease: a cohort study of young women attending family planning clinics. J Epidemiol Community Health 1982; 36:274–278. **63.** Rome Group for Epidemiology and Prevention of Cholelithiasis (GREPCO): Prevalence of gallstone disease in an Italian adult female population. Am J Epidemiol 1984; 119:796–

805. **64.** Storm BL, Tamragouri RT, Morse ML, Lazar EL, West SL, Stolley PD, Jones JK. Oral contraceptives and other risk factors for gallbladder disease. Clin Pharmacol Ther 1986; 39:335–341. **65.** Wynn V, Adams PW, Godsland IF, Melrose J, Niththyananthan R, Oakley NW, Seedj A. Comparison of effects of different combined oral contraceptive formulations on carbohydrate and lipid metabolism. Lancet 1979; 1:1045–1049. **66.** Wynn V. Effect of progesterone and progestins on carbohydrate metabolism. In: Progesterone and Progestin. Bardin CW, Milgrom E, Mauvis-Jarvis P. eds. New York, Raven Press 1983; pp. 395–410. **67.** Perlman JA, Roussell-Briefel RG, Ezzati TM, Lieberknecht G. Oral glucose tolerance and the potency of oral contraceptive progestogens. J Chronic Dis 1985; 38:857–864. **68.** Royal College of General Practitioners' Oral Contraception Study: Effect on hypertension and benign breast disease of progestogen component in combined oral contraceptives. Lancet 1977; 1:624. **69.** Fisch IR, Frank J. Oral contraceptives and blood pressure. JAMA 1977; 237:2499–2503. **70.** Laragh AJ. Oral contraceptive induced hypertension—nine years later. Am J Obstet Gynecol 1976; 126:141–147. **71.** Ramcharan S, Peritz E, Pellegrin FA, Williams WT. Incidence of hypertension in the Walnut Creek Contraceptive Drug Study cohort: In: Pharmacology of steroid contraceptive drugs. Garattini S, Berendes HW. eds. New York, Raven Press, 1977; pp. 277–288, (Monographs of the Mario Negri Institute for Pharmacological Research Milan.) **72.** Stockley I. Interactions with oral contraceptives. J Pharm 1976; 216: 140–143. **73.** The Cancer and Steroid Hormone Study of the Centers for Disease Control and the National Institute of Child Health and Human Development: Oral contraceptive use and the risk of ovarian cancer. JAMA 1983; 249:1596–1599. **74.** The Cancer and Steroid Hormone Study of the Centers for Disease Control and the National Institute of Child Health and Human Development: Combination oral contraceptive use and the risk of endometrial cancer. JAMA 1987; 257:796–800. **75.** Ory HW. Functional ovarian cysts and oral contraceptives: negative association confirmed surgically. JAMA 1974; 228:68–69. **76.** Ory HW, Cole P, MacMahon B, Hoover R. Oral contraceptives and reduced risk of benign breast disease. N Engl J Med 1976; 294:419–422. **77.** Ory HW. The noncontraceptive health benefits from oral contraceptive use. Fam Plann Perspect 1982; 14:182–184. **78.** Ory HW, Forrest JD, Lincoln R. Making choices: evaluating the health risks and benefits of birth control methods. New York, The Alan Guttmacher Institute, 1983; p. 1. **79.** Schlesselman J, Stadel BV, Murray P, Lai S. Breast cancer in relation to early use of oral contraceptives. JAMA 1988; 259:1828–1833. **80.** Hennekens CH, Speizer FE, Lipnick RJ, Rosner B, Bain C, Belanger C, Stampfer MJ, Willett W, Peto R. A case-control study of oral contraceptive use and breast cancer. JNCI 1984; 72:39–42. **81.** LaVecchia C, Decarli A, Fasoli M, Franceschi S, Gentile A, Negri E, Parazzini F, Tognoni G. Oral contraceptives and cancers of the breast and of the female genital tract. Interim results from a case-control study. Br J Cancer 1986; 54:311–317. **82.** Meirik O, Lund E, Adami H, Bergstrom R, Christoffersen T, Bergsjo P. Oral contraceptive use and breast cancer in young women. A Joint National Case-control study in Sweden and Norway. Lancet 1986; 11:650–654. **83.** Kay CR, Hannaford PC. Breast cancer and the pill—A further report from the Royal College of General Practitioners' oral contraception study. Br J Cancer 1988; 58:675–680. **84.** Stadel BV, Lai S, Schlesselman JJ, Murray P. Oral contraceptives and premenopausal breast cancer in nulliparous women. Contraception 1988; 38:287–299. **85.** Miller DR, Rosenberg L, Kaufman DW, Stolley P, Warshauer ME, Shapiro S. Breast cancer before age 45 and oral contraceptive use: New findings. Am J Epidemiol 1989; 129:269–280. **86.** The UK National Case-Control Study Group, Oral contraceptive use and breast cancer risk in young women. Lancet 1989; 1:973–982. **87.** Schlesselman JJ. Cancer of the breast and reproductive tract in relation to use of oral contraceptives. Contraception 1989; 40:1–38. **88.** Vessey MP, McPherson K, Villard-Mackintosh L, Yeates D. Oral contraceptives and breast cancer: latest findings in a large cohort study. Br J Cancer 1989; 59:613–617. **89.** Jick SS, Walker AM, Stergachis A, Jick H. Oral contraceptives and breast cancer. Br J Cancer 1989; 59:618–621. **90.** Anderson FD. Selectivity and minimal androgenicity of norgestimate in monophasic and triphasic oral contraceptives. Acta Obstet Gynecol Scand 1992; 156 (Supplement):15–21. **91.** Chapdelaine A, Desmaris J-L, Derman RJ. Clinical evidence of minimal androgenic activity of norgestimate. Int J Fertil 1989; 34(51):347–352. **92.** Phillips A, Demarest K, Hahn DW, Wong F, McGuire JL. Progestational and androgenic receptor binding affinities and in vivo activities of norgestimate and other progestins. Contraception 1989; 41(4):399–409. **93.** Phillips A, Hahn DW, Klimek S, McGuire JL. A comparison of the potencies and activities of progestogens used in contraceptives. Contraception 1987; 36(2):181–192. **94.** Janaud A, Rouffy J, Upmalis D, Dain M-P. A comparison study of lipid and androgen metabolism with triphasic oral contraceptive formulations containing norgestimate or levonorgestrel. Acta Obstet Gynecol Scand 1992; 156 (Supplement):34–38. **95.** Collaborative Group on Hormonal Factors in Breast Cancer. Breast cancer and hormonal contraceptives: collaborative reanalysis of individual data on 53 297 women with breast cancer and 100 239 women without breast cancer from 54 epidemiological studies. Lancet 1996; 347:1713–1727. **96.** Palmer JR, Rosenberg L, Kaufman DW, Warshauer ME, Stolley P, Shapiro S. Oral Contraceptive Use and Liver Cancer. Am J Epidemiol 1989; 130:878–882. **97.** Lewis M, Spitzer WO, Heinemann LAJ, MacRae KD, Bruppacher R, Thorogood M, on behalf of Transnational Research Group on Oral Contraceptives and Health of Young Women. Third generation oral contraceptives and risk of myocardial infarction: an international case-control study. Br Med J 1996;312:88–90. **98.** Improving access to quality care in family planning: Medical eligibility criteria for contraceptive use. Geneva, WHO, Family and Reproductive Health, 1996.

BRIEF SUMMARY PATIENT PACKAGE INSERT

Oral contraceptives, also known as "birth control pills" or "the pill," are taken to prevent pregnancy. ORTHO TRI-CYCLEN may also be taken to treat moderate acne in females who are able to use the pill. When taken correctly to prevent pregnancy, oral contraceptives have a failure rate of less than 1% per year when used without missing any pills. The typical failure rate of large numbers of pill users is 5% per year when women who miss pills are included. For most women oral contraceptives are also free of serious or unpleasant side effects. However, forgetting to take pills considerably increases the chances of pregnancy.

For the majority of women, oral contraceptives can be taken safely. But there are some women who are at high risk of developing certain serious diseases that can be fatal or may cause temporary or permanent disability. The risks associated with taking oral contraceptives increase significantly if you:

- smoke
- have high blood pressure, diabetes, high cholesterol
- have or have had clotting disorders, heart attack, stroke, angina pectoris, cancer of the breast or sex organs, jaundice or malignant or benign liver tumors.

Although cardiovascular disease risks may be increased with oral contraceptive use after age 40 in healthy, non-smoking women (even with the newer low-dose formulations), there are also greater potential health risks associated with pregnancy in older women.

You should not take the pill if you suspect you are pregnant or have unexplained vaginal bleeding.

Cigarette smoking increases the risk of serious cardiovascular side effects from oral contraceptive use. This risk increases with age and with heavy smoking (15 or more cigarettes per day) and is quite marked in women over 35 years of age. Women who use oral contraceptives are strongly advised not to smoke.

Most side effects of the pill are not serious. The most common such effects are nausea, vomiting, bleeding between menstrual periods, weight gain, breast tenderness, and difficulty wearing contact lenses. These side effects, especially nausea and vomiting, may subside within the first three months of use.

The serious side effects of the pill occur very infrequently, especially if you are in good health and are young. However, you should know that the following medical conditions have been associated with or made worse by the pill:

1. Blood clots in the legs (thrombophlebitis), lungs (pulmonary embolism), stoppage or rupture of a blood vessel in the brain (stroke), blockage of blood vessels in the heart (heart attack or angina pectoris) or other organs of the body. As mentioned above, smoking increases the risk of heart attacks and strokes and subsequent serious medical consequences.

2. In rare cases, oral contraceptives can cause benign but dangerous liver tumors. These benign liver tumors can rupture and cause fatal internal bleeding. In addition, some studies report an increased risk of developing liver cancer. However, liver cancers are rare.

3. High blood pressure, although blood pressure usually returns to normal when the pill is stopped.

The symptoms associated with these serious side effects are discussed in the detailed leaflet given to you with your supply of pills. Notify your doctor or health care provider if you notice any unusual physical disturbances while taking the pill. In addition, drugs such as rifampin, as well as some anticonvulsants and some antibiotics may decrease oral contraceptive effectiveness.

There is conflict among studies regarding breast cancer and oral contraceptive use. Some studies have reported an increase in the risk of developing breast cancer, particularly at a younger age. This increased risk appears to be related to duration of use. The majority of studies have found no overall increase in the risk of developing breast cancer. Some studies have found an increase in the incidence of cancer of the cervix in women who use oral contraceptives. However, this finding may be related to factors other than the use of oral contraceptives. There is insufficient evidence to rule out the possibility pills may cause such cancers.

Taking the combination pill provides some important non-contraceptive benefits. These include less painful menstruation, less menstrual blood loss and anemia, fewer pelvic infections, and fewer cancers of the ovary and the lining of the uterus.

Be sure to discuss any medical condition you may have with your health care provider. Your health care provider will take a medical and family history before prescribing oral contraceptives and will examine you. The physical examination may be delayed to another time if you request it and the health care provider believes that it is a good medical practice to postpone it. You should be reexamined at least once a year while taking oral contraceptives. Your pharmacist should have given you the detailed patient information labeling which gives you further information which you should read and discuss with your health care provider.

ORTHO-CYCLEN and ORTHO TRI-CYCLEN (like all oral contraceptives) are intended to prevent pregnancy. ORTHO TRI-CYCLEN is also used to treat moderate acne in females who are able to take oral contraceptives. Oral contraceptives do not protect against transmission of HIV (AIDS) and other sexually transmitted diseases such as chlamydia, genital herpes, genital warts, gonorrhea, hepatitis B, and syphilis.

DETAILED PATIENT LABELING

PLEASE NOTE: This labeling is revised from time to time as important new medical information becomes available. Therefore, please review this labeling carefully.

ORTHO TRI-CYCLEN □ 28 Day Regimen

Each white tablet contains 0.180 mg norgestimate and 0.035 mg ethinyl estradiol. Each light blue tablet contains 0.215 mg norgestimate and 0.035 mg ethinyl estradiol. Each blue tablet contains 0.250 mg norgestimate and 0.035 mg ethinyl estradiol. Each green tablet contains inert ingredients.

ORTHO-CYCLEN □ 28 Day Regimen

Each blue tablet contains 0.250 mg norgestimate and 0.035 mg ethinyl estradiol. Each green tablet contains inert ingredients.

INTRODUCTION

Any woman who considers using oral contraceptives (the birth control pill or the pill) should understand the benefits and risks of using this form of birth control. This patient labeling will give you much of the information you will need to make this decision and will also help you determine if you are at risk of developing any of the serious side effects of the pill. It will tell you how to use the pill properly so that it will be as effective as possible. However, this labeling is not a replacement for a careful discussion between you and your health care provider. You should discuss the information provided in this labeling with him or her, both when you first start taking the pill and during your revisits. You should also follow your health care providers advice with regard to regular check-ups while you are on the pill.

EFFECTIVENESS OF ORAL CONTRACEPTIVES FOR CONTRACEPTION

Oral contraceptives or "birth control pills" or "the pill" are used to prevent pregnancy and are more effective than other non-surgical methods of birth control. When they are taken correctly, the chance of becoming pregnant is less than 1% (1 pregnancy per 100 women per year of use) when used perfectly, without missing any pills. Typical failure rates are actually 5% per year. The chance of becoming pregnant increases with each missed pill during a menstrual cycle.

In comparison, typical failure rates for other non-surgical methods of birth control during the first year of use are as follows:

Implant: <1%
Injection: <1%
IUD: 1 to 2%
Diaphragm with spermicides: 20%
Spermicides alone: 26%
Vaginal sponge: 20 to 40%
Female sterilization: <1%
Male sterilization: <1%
Cervical Cap with spermicides: 20 to 40%
Condom alone (male): 14%
Condom alone (female): 21%
Periodic abstinence: 25%
Withdrawal: 19%
No methods: 85%

WHO SHOULD NOT TAKE ORAL CONTRACEPTIVES

Cigarette smoking increases the risk of serious cardiovascular side effects from oral contraceptive use. This risk increases with age and with heavy smoking (15 or more cigarettes per day) and is quite marked in women over 35 years of age. Women who use oral contraceptives are strongly advised not to smoke.

Some women should not use the pill. For example, you should not take the pill if you are pregnant or think you may be pregnant. You should also not use the pill if you have any of the following conditions:

- A history of heart attack or stroke
- Blood clots in the legs (thrombophlebitis), lungs (pulmonary embolism), or eyes
- A history of blood clots in the deep veins of your legs
- Chest pain (angina pectoris)
- Known or suspected breast cancer or cancer of the lining of the uterus, cervix or vagina
- Unexplained vaginal bleeding (until a diagnosis is reached by your doctor)
- Yellowing of the whites of the eyes or of the skin (jaundice) during pregnancy or during previous use of the pill
- Liver tumor (benign or cancerous)
- Known or suspected pregnancy

Tell your health care provider if you have ever had any of these conditions. Your health care provider can recommend a safer method of birth control.

Continued on next page

Ortho Tri-Cyclen—Cont.

OTHER CONSIDERATIONS BEFORE TAKING ORAL CONTRACEPTIVES

Tell your health care provider if you have or have had:

- Breast nodules, fibrocystic disease of the breast, an abnormal breast x-ray or mammogram
- Diabetes
- Elevated cholesterol or triglycerides
- High blood pressure
- Migraine or other headaches or epilepsy
- Mental depression
- Gallbladder, liver, heart or kidney disease
- History of scanty or irregular menstrual periods

Women with any of these conditions should be checked often by their health care provider if they choose to use oral contraceptives.

Also, be sure to inform your doctor or health care provider if you smoke or are on any medications.

RISKS OF TAKING ORAL CONTRACEPTIVES

1. Risk of developing blood clots

Blood clots and blockage of blood vessels are one of the most serious side effects of taking oral contraceptives and can cause death or serious disability. In particular, a clot in the legs can cause thrombophlebitis and a clot that travels to the lungs can cause a sudden blocking of the vessel carrying blood to the lungs. Rarely, clots occur in the blood vessels of the eye and may cause blindness, double vision, or impaired vision.

If you take oral contraceptives and need elective surgery, need to stay in bed for a prolonged illness or injury or have recently delivered a baby, you may be at risk of developing blood clots. You should consult your doctor about stopping oral contraceptives four weeks before surgery and not taking oral contraceptives for two weeks after surgery or during bed rest. You should also not take oral contraceptives soon after delivery of a baby. It is advisable to wait for at least four weeks after delivery if you are not breast feeding or four weeks after a second trimester abortion. If you are breast feeding, you should wait until you have weaned your child before using the pill. (See also the section on Breast Feeding in General Precautions.)

The risk of circulatory disease in oral contraceptive users may be higher in users of high-dose pills and may be greater with longer duration of oral contraceptive use. In addition, some of these increased risks may continue for a number of years after stopping oral contraceptives. The risk of abnormal blood clotting increases with age in both users and nonusers of oral contraceptives, but the increased risk from the oral contraceptive appears to be present at all ages. For women aged 20 to 44 it is estimated that about 1 in 2,000 using oral contraceptives will be hospitalized each year because of abnormal clotting. Among nonusers in the same age group, about 1 in 20,000 would be hospitalized each year. For oral contraceptive users in general, it has been estimated that in women between the ages of 15 and 34 the risk of death due to a circulatory disorder is about 1 in 12,000 per year, whereas for nonusers the rate is about 1 in 50,000 per year. In the age group 35 to 44, the risk is estimated to be about 1 in 2,500 per year for oral contraceptive users and about 1 in 10,000 per year for nonusers.

2. Heart attacks and strokes

Oral contraceptives may increase the tendency to develop strokes (stoppage or rupture of blood vessels in the brain) and angina pectoris and heart attacks (blockage of blood vessels in the heart). Any of these conditions can cause death or serious disability.

Smoking greatly increases the possibility of suffering heart attacks and strokes. Furthermore, smoking and the use of oral contraceptives greatly increase the chances of developing and dying of heart disease.

3. Gallbladder disease

Oral contraceptive users probably have a greater risk than nonusers of having gallbladder disease, although this risk may be related to pills containing high doses of estrogens.

4. Liver tumors

In rare cases, oral contraceptives can cause benign but dangerous liver tumors. These benign liver tumors can rupture and cause fatal internal bleeding. In addition, some studies report an increased risk of developing liver cancer. However, liver cancers are rare.

5. Cancer of the reproductive organs and breasts

There is conflict among studies regarding breast cancer and oral contraceptive use. Some studies have reported an increase in the risk of developing breast cancer, particularly at a younger age. This increased risk appears to be related to duration of use. The majority of studies have found no overall increase in the risk of developing breast cancer.

A meta-analysis of 54 studies found a small increase in the frequency of having breast cancer diagnosed for women who were currently using combined oral contraceptives or had used them within the past ten years. This increase in the frequency of breast cancer diagnosis, within ten years of stopping use, was generally accounted for by cancers localized to the breast. There was no increase in the frequency of having breast cancer diagnosed ten or more years after cessation of use.

Some studies have found an increase in the incidence of cancer of the cervix in women who use oral contraceptives. However, this finding may be related to factors other than the use of oral contraceptives. There is insufficient evidence to rule out the possibility that pills may cause such cancers.

ESTIMATED RISK OF DEATH FROM A BIRTH CONTROL METHOD OR PREGNANCY

All methods of birth control and pregnancy are associated with a risk of developing certain diseases which may lead to disability or death. An estimate of the number of deaths associated with different methods of birth control and pregnancy has been calculated and is shown in the following table.

[See table below]

In the above table, the risk of death from any birth control method is less than the risk of childbirth, except for oral contraceptive users over the age of 35 who smoke and pill users over the age of 40 even if they do not smoke. It can be seen in the table that for women aged 15 to 39, the risk of death was highest with pregnancy (7–26 deaths per 100,000 women, depending on age). Among pill users who do not smoke, the risk of death was always lower than that associated with pregnancy for any age group, although over the age of 40, the risk increases to 32 deaths per 100,000 women, compared to 28 associated with pregnancy at that age. However, for pill users who smoke and are over the age of 35, the estimated number of deaths exceeds those for other methods of birth control. If a woman is over the age of 40 and smokes, her estimated risk of death is four times higher (117/100,000 women) than the estimated risk associated with pregnancy (28/100,000 women) in that age group.

The suggestion that women over 40 who do not smoke should not take oral contraceptives is based on information from older, higher-dose pills. An Advisory Committee of the FDA discussed this issue in 1989 and recommended that the benefits of low-dose oral contraceptive use by healthy, non-smoking women over 40 years of age may outweigh the possible risks.

WARNING SIGNALS

If any of these adverse effects occur while you are taking oral contraceptives, call your doctor immediately:

- Sharp chest pain, coughing of blood, or sudden shortness of breath (indicating a possible clot in the lung)
- Pain in the calf (indicating a possible clot in the leg)
- Crushing chest pain or heaviness in the chest (indicating a possible heart attack)
- Sudden severe headache or vomiting, dizziness or fainting, disturbances of vision or speech, weakness, or numbness in an arm or leg (indicating a possible stroke)
- Sudden partial or complete loss of vision (indicating a possible clot in the eye)
- Breast lumps (indicating possible breast cancer or fibrocystic disease of the breast; ask your doctor or health care provider to show you how to examine your breasts)
- Severe pain or tenderness in the stomach area (indicating a possibly ruptured liver tumor)
- Difficulty in sleeping, weakness, lack of energy, fatigue, or change in mood (possibly indicating severe depression)
- Jaundice or a yellowing of the skin or eyeballs, accompanied frequently by fever, fatigue, loss of appetite, dark colored urine, or light colored bowel movements (indicating possible liver problems)

ANNUAL NUMBER OF BIRTH-RELATED OR METHOD-RELATED DEATHS ASSOCIATED WITH CONTROL OF FERTILITY PER 100,000 NON-STERILE WOMEN, BY FERTILITY CONTROL METHOD ACCORDING TO AGE

Method of control and outcome	15-19	20-24	25-29	30-34	35-39	40-44
No fertility control methods*	7.0	7.4	9.1	14.8	25.7	28.2
Oral contraceptives non-smoker**	0.3	0.5	0.9	1.9	13.8	31.6
Oral contraceptives smoker**	2.2	3.4	6.6	13.5	51.1	117.2
IUD**	0.8	0.8	1.0	1.0	1.4	1.4
Condom*	1.1	1.6	0.7	0.2	0.3	0.4
Diaphragm/spermicide*	1.9	1.2	1.2	1.3	2.2	2.8
Periodic abstinence*	2.5	1.6	1.6	1.7	2.9	3.6

*Deaths are birth-related
**Deaths are method-related

Adapted from H.W. Ory, ref. #35.

SIDE EFFECTS OF ORAL CONTRACEPTIVES

1. Vaginal bleeding

Irregular vaginal bleeding or spotting may occur while you are taking the pills. Irregular bleeding may vary from slight staining between menstrual periods to breakthrough bleeding which is a flow much like a regular period. Irregular bleeding occurs most often during the first few months of oral contraceptive use, but may also occur after you have been taking the pill for some time. Such bleeding may be temporary and usually does not indicate any serious problems. It is important to continue taking your pills on schedule. If the bleeding occurs in more than one cycle or lasts for more than a few days, talk to your doctor or health care provider.

2. Contact lenses

If you wear contact lenses and notice a change in vision or an inability to wear your lenses, contact your doctor or health care provider.

3. Fluid retention

Oral contraceptives may cause edema (fluid retention) with swelling of the fingers or ankles and may raise your blood pressure. If you experience fluid retention, contact your doctor or health care provider.

4. Melasma

A spotty darkening of the skin is possible, particularly of the face, which may persist.

5. Other side effects

Other side effects may include nausea and vomiting, change in appetite, headache, nervousness, depression, dizziness, loss of scalp hair, rash, and vaginal infections.

If any of these side effects bother you, call your doctor or health care provider.

GENERAL PRECAUTIONS

1. Missed periods and use of oral contraceptives before or during early pregnancy

There may be times when you may not menstruate regularly after you have completed taking a cycle of pills. If you have taken your pills regularly and miss one menstrual period, continue taking your pills for the next cycle but be sure to inform your health care provider before doing so. If you have not taken the pills daily as instructed and missed a menstrual period, you may be pregnant. If you missed two consecutive menstrual periods, you may be pregnant. Check with your health care provider immediately to determine whether you are pregnant. Do not continue to take oral contraceptives until you are sure you are not pregnant, but continue to use another method of contraception.

There is no conclusive evidence that oral contraceptive use is associated with an increase in birth defects, when taken inadvertently during early pregnancy. Previously, a few studies had reported that oral contraceptives might be associated with birth defects, but these findings have not been seen in more recent studies. Nevertheless, oral contraceptives or any other drugs should not be used during pregnancy unless clearly necessary and prescribed by your doctor. You should check with your doctor about risks to your unborn child of any medication taken during pregnancy.

2. While breast feeding

If you are breast feeding, consult your doctor before starting oral contraceptives. Some of the drug will be passed on to the child in the milk. A few adverse effects on the child have been reported, including yellowing of the skin (jaundice) and breast enlargement. In addition, combination oral contraceptives may decrease the amount and quality of your milk. If possible, do not use combination oral contraceptives while breast feeding. You should use another method of contraception since breast feeding provides only partial protection from becoming pregnant and this partial protection decreases significantly as you breast feed for longer periods of time. You should consider starting combination oral contraceptives only after you have weaned your child completely.

3. Laboratory tests

If you are scheduled for any laboratory tests, tell your doctor you are taking birth control pills. Certain blood tests may be affected by birth control pills.

4. Drug interactions

Certain drugs may interact with birth control pills to make them less effective in preventing pregnancy or cause an increase in breakthrough bleeding. Such drugs include rifampin, drugs used for epilepsy such as barbiturates (for example, phenobarbital), anticonvulsants such as topiramate (TOPAMAX), carbamazepine (Tegretol is one brand of this drug), phenytoin (Dilantin is one brand of this drug), phenylbutazone (Butazolidin is one brand), certain drugs used in the treatment of HIV or AIDS, and possibly certain antibiotics. You may need to use additional contraception when you take drugs which can make oral contraceptives less effective. A possible interaction has been suggested with hormonal contraceptives and the herbal supplement St. Johns Wort based on some reports of oral contraceptive users experiencing breakthrough bleeding shortly after starting St. Johns Wort. Pregnancies have been reported by users of combined hormonal contraceptives who also used some form of St. Johns Wort.

5. Sexually transmitted diseases

ORTHO-CYCLEN and ORTHO TRI-CYCLEN (like all oral contraceptives) are intended to prevent pregnancy. ORTHO TRI-CYCLEN is also used to treat moderate acne in females who are able to take oral contraceptives. Oral contraceptives do not protect against transmission of HIV (AIDS) and other sexually transmitted diseases such as chlamydia, genital herpes, genital warts, gonorrhea, hepatitis B, and syphilis.

HOW TO TAKE THE PILL

IMPORTANT POINTS TO REMEMBER

BEFORE YOU START TAKING YOUR PILLS:
1. BE SURE TO READ THESE DIRECTIONS:
Before you start taking your pills.
Anytime you are not sure what to do.
2. THE RIGHT WAY TO TAKE THE PILL IS TO TAKE ONE PILL EVERY DAY AT THE SAME TIME.
If you miss pills you could get pregnant. This includes starting the pack late. The more pills you miss, the more likely you are to get pregnant.
3. MANY WOMEN HAVE SPOTTING OR LIGHT BLEEDING, OR MAY FEEL SICK TO THEIR STOMACH DURING THE FIRST 1-3 PACKS OF PILLS. If you feel sick to your stomach, do not stop taking the pill. The problem will usually go away. If it doesn't go away, check with your doctor or clinic.
4. MISSING PILLS CAN ALSO CAUSE SPOTTING OR LIGHT BLEEDING, even when you make up these missed pills.
On the days you take 2 pills to make up for missed pills, you could also feel a little sick to your stomach.
5. IF YOU HAVE VOMITING OR DIARRHEA, for any reason, or IF YOU TAKE SOME MEDICINES, including some antibiotics, your pills may not work as well. Use a back-up method (such as condoms, foam, or sponge) until you check with your doctor or clinic.
6. IF YOU HAVE TROUBLE REMEMBERING TO TAKE THE PILL, talk to your doctor or clinic about how to make pill-taking easier or about using another method of birth control.
7. IF YOU HAVE ANY QUESTIONS OR ARE UNSURE ABOUT THE INFORMATION IN THIS LEAFLET, call your doctor or clinic.

BEFORE YOU START TAKING YOUR PILLS

1. DECIDE WHAT TIME OF DAY YOU WANT TO TAKE YOUR PILL.
It is important to take it at about the same time every day.
2. LOOK AT YOUR PILL PACK TO SEE IF IT HAS 28 PILLS:
The 28-pill pack has 21 "active" pills (with hormones) to take for 3 weeks. This is followed by 1 week of reminder green pills (without hormones).
ORTHO TRI-CYCLEN: There are 7 white "active" pills, 7 light blue "active" pills, and 7 blue "active" pills.
ORTHO-CYCLEN: There are 21 blue "active" pills.
3. ALSO FIND:
1) where on the pack to start taking pills,
2) in what order to take the pills.
CHECK PICTURE OF PILL PACK AND ADDITIONAL INSTRUCTIONS FOR USING THIS PACKAGE IN THE BRIEF SUMMARY PATIENT PACKAGE INSERT.
4. BE SURE YOU HAVE READY AT ALL TIMES:
ANOTHER KIND OF BIRTH CONTROL (such as condoms, foam, or sponge) to use as a back-up method in case you miss pills.
AN EXTRA, FULL PILL PACK.

WHEN TO START THE FIRST PACK OF PILLS

You have a choice of which day to start taking your first pack of pills. ORTHO TRI-CYCLEN and ORTHO- CYCLEN are available in the DIALPAK® Tablet Dispenser which is preset for a Sunday Start. Day 1 Start is also provided. Decide with your doctor or clinic which is the best day for you. Pick a time of day which will be easy to remember.

SUNDAY START:
ORTHO TRI-CYCLEN: Take the first "active" white pill of the first pack on the Sunday after your period starts, even if you are still bleeding. If your period begins on Sunday, start the pack that same day.
ORTHO-CYCLEN: Take the first "active" blue pill of the first pack on the Sunday after your period starts, even if you are still bleeding. If your period begins on Sunday, start the pack that same day.
Use another method of birth control as a back-up method if you have sex anytime from the Sunday you start your first pack until the next Sunday (7 days). Condoms, foam, or the sponge are good back-up methods of birth control.

DAY 1 START:
ORTHO TRI-CYCLEN: Take the first "active" white pill of the first pack during the first 24 hours of your period.
ORTHO-CYCLEN: Take the first "active" blue pill of the first pack during the first 24 hours of your period.
You will not need to use a back-up method of birth control, since you are starting the pill at the beginning of your period.

WHAT TO DO DURING THE MONTH

1. TAKE ONE PILL AT THE SAME TIME EVERY DAY UNTIL THE PACK IS EMPTY.
Do not skip pills even if you are spotting or bleeding between monthly periods or feel sick to your stomach (nausea).
Do not skip pills even if you do not have sex very often.

2. WHEN YOU FINISH A PACK OR SWITCH YOUR BRAND OF PILLS:
Start the next pack on the day after your last "reminder" pill. Do not wait any days between packs.

WHAT TO DO IF YOU MISS PILLS

ORTHO TRI-CYCLEN:
If you **MISS 1** white, light blue, or blue "active" pill:
1. Take it as soon as you remember. Take the next pill at your regular time. This means you may take 2 pills in 1 day.
2. You do not need to use a back-up birth control method if you have sex.
If you **MISS 2** white or light blue "active" pills in a row in **WEEK 1 OR WEEK 2** of your pack:
1. Take 2 pills on the day you remember and 2 pills the next day.
2. Then take 1 pill a day until you finish the pack.
3. You MAY BECOME PREGNANT if you have sex in the 7 days after you miss pills. You MUST use another birth control method (such as condoms, foam, or sponge) as a back-up method for those 7 days.
If you **MISS 2** blue "active" pills in a row in **THE 3RD WEEK**:
1. **If you are a Sunday Starter:**
Keep taking 1 pill every day until Sunday. On Sunday, THROW OUT the rest of the pack and start a new pack of pills that same day.
If you are a Day 1 Starter:
THROW OUT the rest of the pill pack and start a new pack that same day.
2. You may not have your period this month but this is expected. However, if you miss your period 2 months in a row, call your doctor or clinic because you might be pregnant.
3. You MAY BECOME PREGNANT if you have sex in the 7 days after you miss pills. You MUST use another birth control method (such as condoms, foam, or sponge) as a back-up method for those 7 days.
If you **MISS 3 OR MORE** white, light blue, or blue "active" pills in a row (during the first 3 weeks):
1. **If you are a Sunday Starter:**
Keep taking 1 pill every day until Sunday. On Sunday, THROW OUT the rest of the pack and start a new pack of pills that same day.
If you are a Day 1 Starter:
THROW OUT the rest of the pill pack and start a new pack that same day.
2. You may not have your period this month but this is expected. However, if you miss your period 2 months in a row, call your doctor or clinic because you might be pregnant.
3. You MAY BECOME PREGNANT if you have sex in the 7 days after you miss pills. You MUST use another birth control method (such as condoms, foam, or sponge) as a back-up method for those 7 days.

ORTHO-CYCLEN:
If you **MISS 1** blue "active" pill:
1. Take it as soon as you remember. Take the next pill at your regular time. This means you may take 2 pills in 1 day.
2. You do not need to use a back-up birth control method if you have sex.
If you **MISS 2** blue "active" pills in a row in **WEEK 1 OR WEEK 2** of your pack:
1. Take 2 pills on the day you remember and 2 pills the next day.
2. Then take 1 pill a day until you finish the pack.
3. You MAY BECOME PREGNANT if you have sex in the 7 days after you miss pills. You MUST use another birth control method (such as condoms, foam, or sponge) as a back-up method for those 7 days.
If you **MISS 2** blue "active" pills in a row in **THE 3RD WEEK**:
1. **If you are a Sunday Starter:**
Keep taking 1 pill every day until Sunday. On Sunday, THROW OUT the rest of the pack and start a new pack of pills that same day.
If you are a Day 1 Starter:
THROW OUT the rest of the pill pack and start a new pack that same day.
2. You may not have your period this month but this is expected. However, if you miss your period 2 months in a row, call your doctor or clinic because you might be pregnant.
3. You MAY BECOME PREGNANT if you have sex in the 7 days after you miss pills. You MUST use another birth control method (such as condoms, foam, or sponge) as a back-up method for those 7 days.
If you **MISS 3 OR MORE** blue "active" pills in a row (during the first 3 weeks):
1. **If you are a Sunday Starter:**
Keep taking 1 pill every day until Sunday. On Sunday, THROW OUT the rest of the pack and start a new pack of pills that same day.
If you are a Day 1 Starter:
THROW OUT the rest of the pill pack and start a new pack that same day.
2. You may not have your period this month but this is expected. However, if you miss your period 2 months in a row, call your doctor or clinic because you might be pregnant.
3. You MAY BECOME PREGNANT if you have sex in the 7 days after you miss pills. You MUST use another birth control method (such as condoms, foam, or sponge) as a back-up method for those 7 days.

A REMINDER FOR THOSE ON 28-DAY PACKS:
If you forget any of the 7 green "reminder" pills in Week 4:
THROW AWAY the pills you missed.
Keep taking 1 pill each day until the pack is empty.
You do not need a back-up method.

FINALLY, IF YOU ARE STILL NOT SURE WHAT TO DO ABOUT THE PILLS YOU HAVE MISSED:
Use a BACK-UP METHOD anytime you have sex.
KEEP TAKING ONE "ACTIVE" PILL EACH DAY until you can reach your doctor or clinic.

PREGNANCY DUE TO PILL FAILURE
The incidence of pill failure resulting in pregnancy is approximately one percent (i.e., one pregnancy per 100 women per year) if taken every day as directed, but more typical failure rates are 5%. If failure does occur, the risk to the fetus is minimal.

PREGNANCY AFTER STOPPING THE PILL
There may be some delay in becoming pregnant after you stop using oral contraceptives, especially if you had irregular menstrual cycles before you used oral contraceptives. It may be advisable to postpone conception until you begin menstruating regularly once you have stopped taking the pill and desire pregnancy.
There does not appear to be any increase in birth defects in newborn babies when pregnancy occurs soon after stopping the pill.

OVERDOSAGE
Serious ill effects have not been reported following ingestion of large doses of oral contraceptives by young children. Overdosage may cause nausea and withdrawal bleeding in females. In case of overdosage, contact your health care provider or pharmacist.

OTHER INFORMATION
Your health care provider will take a medical and family history before prescribing oral contraceptives and will examine you. The physical examination may be delayed to another time if you request it and the health care provider believes that it is a good medical practice to postpone it. You should be reexamined at least once a year. Be sure to inform your health care provider if there is a family history of any of the conditions listed previously in this leaflet. Be sure to keep all appointments with your health care provider, because this is a time to determine if there are early signs of side effects of oral contraceptive use.
Do not use the drug for any condition other than the one for which it was prescribed. This drug has been prescribed specifically for you; do not give it to others who may want birth control pills.

HEALTH BENEFITS FROM ORAL CONTRACEPTIVES
In addition to preventing pregnancy, use of combination oral contraceptives may provide certain benefits. They are:
- menstrual cycles may become more regular
- blood flow during menstruation may be lighter and less iron may be lost. Therefore, anemia due to iron deficiency is less likely to occur.
- pain or other symptoms during menstruation may be encountered less frequently
- ectopic (tubal) pregnancy may occur less frequently
- noncancerous cysts or lumps in the breast may occur less frequently
- acute pelvic inflammatory disease may occur less frequently
- oral contraceptive use may provide some protection against developing two forms of cancer: cancer of the ovaries and cancer of the lining of the uterus.

If you want more information about birth control pills, ask your doctor/health care provider or pharmacist. They have a more technical leaflet called the Professional Labeling, which you may wish to read. The professional labeling is also published in a book entitled *Physicians Desk Reference*, available in many book stores and public libraries.
ORTHO-McNEIL PHARMACEUTICAL, INC.
Raritan, New Jersey 08869
 REVISED MARCH 2001 635-50-900-7
Shown in Product Identification Guide, page 328

ORTHO TRI-CYCLEN® LO TABLETS ℞
(norgestimate/ethinyl estradiol)

Prescribing Information

Patients should be counseled that this product does not protect against HIV infection (AIDS) and other sexually transmitted diseases.

DESCRIPTION
ORTHO TRI-CYCLEN® Lo Tablets is a combination oral contraceptive containing the progestational compound norgestimate and the estrogenic compound ethinyl estradiol.
ORTHO TRI-CYCLEN® Lo
28 Tablets
Each white tablet contains 0.180 mg of the progestational compound, norgestimate (+)-13-Ethyl-17-hydroxy-18, 19-dinor-17α-pregn-4-en-20-yn-3-one oxime acetate (ester) and 0.025 mg of the estrogenic compound, ethinyl estradiol (19-nor-17α-pregna,1,3,5(10)-trien-20-yne-3,17-diol). Inactive ingredients include lactose, magnesium stearate, croscarmellose sodium, microcrystalline cellulose, carnauba wax, hydroxypropylmethylcellulose, polyethylene glycol, titanium dioxide, and purified water.
Each light blue tablet contains 0.215 mg of the progestational compound norgestimate (+)-13-Ethyl-17-hydroxy-18, 19-dinor-17α-pregn-4-en-20-yn-3-one oxime acetate (ester) and 0.025 mg of the estrogenic compound, ethinyl estradiol (19-nor-17α-pregna,1,3,5(10)-trien-20-yne-3,17-diol). Inactive ingredients include FD & C Blue No. 2 Aluminum Lake, lactose, magnesium stearate, croscarmellose sodium, micro-

Continued on next page

Ortho Tri-Cyclen Lo—Cont.

crystalline cellulose, carnauba wax, hydroxypropylmethylcellulose, polyethylene glycol, titanium dioxide, and purified water.
Each dark blue tablet contains 0.250 mg of the progestational compound norgestimate (+)-13-Ethyl-17-hydroxy-18, 19-dinor-17α-pregn-4-en-20-yn-3-one oxime acetate (ester) and 0.025 mg of the estrogenic compound, ethinyl estradiol (19-nor-17α-pregna,1,3,5(10)-trien-20-yne-3,17-diol). Inactive ingredients include FD & C Blue No. 2 Aluminum Lake, lactose, magnesium stearate, croscarmellose sodium, microcrystalline cellulose, polysorbate 80, carnauba wax, hydroxypropylmethylcellulose, polyethylene glycol, titanium dioxide, and purified water.
Each green tablet contains only inert ingredients, as follows: FD & C Blue No. 1 Aluminum Lake, lactose, magnesium stearate, pregelatinized starch, ferric oxide, hydroxypropylmethylcellulose, polyethylene glycol, titanium dioxide, talc and purified water.

Norgestimate Ethinyl Estradiol

CLINICAL PHARMACOLOGY

Oral Contraception

Combination oral contraceptives act by suppression of gonadotropins. Although the primary mechanism of this action is inhibition of ovulation, other alterations include changes in the cervical mucus (which increase the difficulty of sperm entry into the uterus) and the endometrium (which reduce the likelihood of implantation).
Receptor binding studies, as well as studies in animals and humans, have shown that norgestimate and 17-deacetyl norgestimate, the major serum metabolite, combine high progestational activity with minimal intrinsic androgenicity.[90–93] Norgestimate, in combination with ethinyl estradiol, does not counteract the estrogen-induced increases in sex hormone binding globulin (SHBG), resulting in lower serum testosterone.[90,91,94]

PHARMACOKINETICS

Absorption

Norgestimate (NGM) and ethinyl estradiol (EE) are rapidly absorbed following oral administration. Norgestimate is rapidly and completely metabolized by first-pass (intestinal and/or hepatic) mechanisms to norelgestromin (NGMN) and norgestrel (NG), which are the major active metabolites of norgestimate. Mean pharmacokinetic parameters for NGMN, NG and EE during three cycles of administration of ORTHO TRI-CYCLEN® Lo are summarized in Table 1. These results indicate that: (1) Peak serum concentrations of NGMN and EE were generally reached by 2 hours after dosing; (2) Accumulation following multiple dosing of the 180 µg NGM / 25 µg dose is approximately 1.5 to 2 fold for NGMN and approximately 1.5 fold for EE compared with single dose administration, in agreement with that predicted based on linear kinetics of NGMN and EE; (3) The kinetics of NGMN are dose proportional following NGM doses of 180 to 250 µg; (4) Steady-state conditions for NGMN following each NGM dose and for EE were achieved during the three cycle study; (5) Non-linear accumulation (4.5–14.5 fold) of norgestrel was observed as a result of high affinity binding to SHBG, which limits its biological activity.[100] The effect of food on the pharmacokinetics of ORTHO TRI-CYCLEN® Lo has not been studied.
Table 1 provides a summary of norelgestromin, norgestrel and ethinyl estradiol pharmacokinetic parameters.
[See table 1 above]

Distribution

Norelgestromin and norgestrel (a serum metabolite of norelgestromin) are highly bound (>97%) to serum proteins. Norelgestromin is bound to albumin and not to SHBG, while norgestrel is bound primarily to SHBG. Ethinyl estradiol is extensively bound (> 97%) to serum albumin.

Metabolism

Norgestimate is extensively metabolized by first-pass mechanisms in the gastrointestinal tract and/or liver. Norgestimate's primary active metabolite is norelgestromin. Subsequent hepatic metabolism of norelgestromin occurs and metabolites include norgestrel, which is also active and various hydroxylated and conjugated metabolites. Ethinyl estradiol is also metabolized to various hydroxylated products and their glucuronide and sulfate conjugates.

Excretion

Following 3 cycles of administration of ORTHO TRI-CYCLEN® Lo, the mean (± SD) elimination half-life values, at steady-state, for norelgestromin, norgestrel and ethinyl estradiol were 28.1 (± 10.6) hours, 36.4 (±10.2) hours and 17.7 (± 4.4) hours, respectively (Table 1). The metabolites of norelgestromin and ethinyl estradiol are eliminated by renal and fecal pathways.

Special Populations

Effects of Body Weight, Body Surface Area, and Age

The effects of body weight, body surface area, age and race on the pharmacokinetics of norelgestromin, norgestrel and ethinyl estradiol were evaluated in 79 healthy women using

Table 1: Mean (SD) Pharmacokinetic Parameters of ORTHO TRI-CYCLEN® Lo During a Three Cycle Study

Analyte[1]	Cycle	Day	C_{max}	t_{max} (h)	AUC_{0-24h}	$t_{1/2}$ (h)
NGMN[(2–4)]	1	1	0.91 (0.27)	1.8 (1.0)	5.86 (1.54)	NC
	3	7	1.42 (0.43)	1.8 (0.7)	11.3 (3.2)	NC
		14	1.57 (0.39)	1.8 (0.7)	13.9 (3.7)	NC
		21	1.82 (0.54)	1.5 (0.7)	16.1 (4.8)	28.1 (10.6)
NG[(2–4)]	1	1	0.32 (0.14)	2.0 (1.1)	2.44 (2.04)	NC
	3	7	1.64 (0.89)	1.9 (0.9)	27.9 (18.1)	NC
		14	2.11 (1.13)	4.0 (6.3)	40.7 (24.8)	NC
		21	2.79 (1.42)	1.7 (1.2)	49.9 (27.6)	36.4 (10.2)
EE[(2,3,5)]	1	1	55.6 (18.1)	1.7 (0.5)	421 (118)	NC
	3	7	91.1 (36.7)	1.3 (0.3)	782 (329)	NC
		14	96.9 (38.5)	1.3 (0.3)	796 (273)	NC
		21	95.9 (38.9)	1.3 (0.6)	771 (303)	17.7 (4.4)

[1] NGMN = Norelgestromin, NG = norgestrel, EE = ethinyl estradiol
[2] C_{max} = peak serum concentration, t_{max} = time to reach peak serum concentration, AUC_{0-24h} = area under serum concentration vs time curve from 0 to 24 hours, $t_{1/2}$ = elimination half-life.
[3] units for all analytes; h = hours
[4] units for NGMN and NG – C_{max} = ng/mL, AUC_{0-24h} = h.ng/mL
[5] units for EE only – C_{max} = pg/mL, AUC_{0-24h} = h.pg/mL
NC = not calculated

Table 2: Percentage Of Women Experiencing An Unintended Pregnancy During The First Year Of Typical Use And The First Year Of Perfect Use Of Contraception And The Percentage Continuing Use At The End Of The First Year. United States.

Method (1)	% of Women Experiencing an Unintended Pregnancy Within the First Year of Use: Typical Use[1] (2)	Perfect Use[2] (3)	% of Women Continuing Use at One Year[3] (4)
Chance[4]	85	85	
Spermicides[5]	26	6	40
Periodic abstinence	25		63
Calendar		9	
Ovulation Method		3	
Sympto-Thermal[6]		2	
Post-Ovulation		1	
Withdrawal	19	4	
Cap[7]			
Parous Women	40	26	42
Nulliparous Women	20	9	56
Sponge			
Parous Women	40	20	42
Nulliparous Women	20	9	56
Diaphragm[7]	20	6	56
Condom[8]			
Female (Reality)	21	5	56
Male	14	3	61
Pill	5		71
Progestin Only		0.5	
Combined		0.1	
IUD			
Progesterone T	2.0	1.5	81
Copper T380A	0.8	0.6	78
LNg 20	0.1	0.1	81
Depo-Provera	0.3	0.3	70
Norplant and Norplant-2	0.05	0.05	88
Female Sterilization	0.5	0.5	100
Male Sterilization	0.15	0.10	100

Emergency Contraceptives Pills: Treatment initiated within 72 hours after unprotected intercourse reduces the risk of pregnancy by at least 75%.[9]
Lactation Amenorrhea Method: LAM is a highly effective, temporary method of contraception.[10]
Source: Trussell J. Contraceptive efficacy. In Hatcher RA, Trussell J, Stewart F, Cates W, Stewart GK, Kowel D, Guest F, Contraceptive Technology: Seventeenth Revised Edition. New York NY: Irvington Publishers, 1998.
[1] Among *typical* couples who initiate use of a method (not necessarily for the first time), the percentage who experience an accidental pregnancy during the first year if they do not stop use for any other reason.
[2] Among couples who initiate use of a method (not necessarily for the first time) and who use it *perfectly* (both consistently and correctly), the percentage who experience an accidental pregnancy during the first year if they do not stop use for any other reason.
[3] Among couples attempting to avoid pregnancy, the percentage who continue to use a method for one year.
[4] The percents becoming pregnant in columns (2) and (3) are based on data from populations where contraception is not used and from women who cease using contraception in order to become pregnant. Among such populations, about 89% become pregnant within one year. This estimate was lowered slightly (to 85%) to represent the percent who would become pregnant within one year among women now relying on reversible methods of contraception if they abandoned contraception altogether.
[5] Foams, creams, gels, vaginal suppositories, and vaginal film.
[6] Cervical mucus (ovulation) method supplemented by calendar in the pre-ovulatory and basal body temperature in the post-ovulatory phases.
[7] With spermicidal cream or jelly.
[8] Without spermicides.
[9] The treatment schedule is one dose within 72 hours after unprotected intercourse, and a second dose 12 hours after the first dose. The FDA has declared the following brands of oral contraceptives to be safe and effective for emergency contraception: Ovral (1 dose is 2 white pills), Alesse (1 dose is 5 pink pills), Nordette or Levlen (1 dose is 4 yellow pills).
[10] However, to maintain effective protection against pregnancy, another method of contraception must be used as soon as menstruation resumes, the frequency or duration of breastfeeds is reduced, bottle feeds are introduced, or the baby reaches 6 months of age.

pooled data following single dose administration of NGM 180 or 250 µg/EE 25 µg tablets in four pharmacokinetic studies. Increasing body weight and body surface area were each associated with decreases in C_{max} and AUC_{0-24h} values for norelgestromin and ethinyl estradiol and increases in CL/F (oral clearance) for ethinyl estradiol. Increasing body weight by 10 kg is predicted to reduce the following parameters: NGMN C_{max} by 9% and AUC_{0-24h} by 19%, norgestrel C_{max} by 12% and AUC_{0-24h} by 46%, EE C_{max} by 13% and AUC_{0-24h} by 12%. These changes were statistically significant. Increasing age was associated with slight decreases (6% with increasing age by 5 years) in C_{max} and AUC_{0-24h} for norelgestromin and were statistically significant, but there was no significant effect for norgestrel or ethinyl estradiol. Only a small to moderate fraction (5–40%) of the overall variability in the pharmacokinetics of norelgestromin and ethinyl estradiol following ORTHO TRI-CYCLEN® Lo Tablets may be explained by any or all of the above demographic parameters.

In clinical studies involving 1673 subjects with a mean weight of 141 pounds, there was no association between pregnancy and weight.

Renal and Hepatic Impairment

No studies with ORTHO TRI-CYCLEN® Lo have been conducted in women with renal or hepatic impairment.

Drug-Drug Interactions

Although norelgestromin and its metabolites inhibit a variety of P450 enzymes in human liver microsomes, under the recommended dosing regimen, the in vivo concentrations of norelgestromin and its metabolites, even at the peak serum levels, are relatively low compared to the inhibitory constant (K_i).

Interactions between oral contraceptives and other drugs have been reported in the literature. No formal drug-drug interaction studies were conducted with ORTHO TRI-CYCLEN® Lo (see PRECAUTIONS).

INDICATIONS AND USAGE

ORTHO TRI-CYCLEN® Lo Tablets are indicated for the prevention of pregnancy in women who elect to use oral contraceptives as a method of contraception.

In an active controlled clinical trial 1,673 subjects completed 11,003 cycles of ORTHO TRI-CYCLEN® Lo use and a total of 20 pregnancies were reported in ORTHO TRI-CYCLEN® Lo users[99]. This represents an overall use-efficacy (typical user efficacy) pregnancy rate of 2.36 per 100 women-years of use.

Oral contraceptives are highly effective for pregnancy prevention. Table 2 lists the typical accidental pregnancy rates for users of combination oral contraceptives and other methods of contraception. The efficacy of these contraceptive methods, except sterilization, the IUD, and the Norplant system, depends upon the reliability with which they are used. Correct and consistent use of methods can result in lower failure rates.

[See table 2 at top of previous page]

ORTHO TRI-CYCLEN® Lo has not been studied for and is not indicated for use in emergency contraception.

CONTRAINDICATIONS

Oral contraceptives should not be used in women who have any of the following conditions:

- Thrombophlebitis or thromboembolic disorders
- A past history of deep vein thrombophlebitis or thromboembolic disorders
- Cerebral vascular or coronary artery disease (current or history)
- Valvular heart disease with complications
- Severe hypertension
- Diabetes with vascular involvement
- Headaches with focal neurological symptoms
- Major surgery with prolonged immobilization
- Known or suspected carcinoma of the breast or personal history of breast cancer
- Carcinoma of the endometrium or other known or suspected estrogen-dependent neoplasia
- Undiagnosed abnormal genital bleeding
- Cholestatic jaundice of pregnancy or jaundice with prior pill use
- Hepatic adenomas or carcinomas
- Known or suspected pregnancy
- Hypersensitivity to any component of this product

WARNINGS

Cigarette smoking increases the risk of serious cardiovascular side effects from oral contraceptive use. This risk increases with age and with heavy smoking (15 or more cigarettes per day) and is quite marked in women over 35 years of age. Women who use oral contraceptives should be strongly advised not to smoke.

The use of oral contraceptives is associated with increased risks of several serious conditions including myocardial infarction, thromboembolism, stroke, hepatic neoplasia, and gallbladder disease, although the risk of serious morbidity or mortality is very small in healthy women without underlying risk factors. The risk of morbidity and mortality increases significantly in the presence of other underlying risk factors such as hypertension, hyperlipidemias, obesity and diabetes.

Practitioners prescribing oral contraceptives should be familiar with the following information relating to these risks.

The information contained in this package insert is principally based on studies carried out in patients who used oral contraceptives with higher formulations of estrogens and progestogens than those in common use today. The effect of long-term use of the oral contraceptives with lower formulations of both estrogens and progestogens remains to be determined.

Throughout this labeling, epidemiological studies reported are of two types: retrospective or case control studies and prospective or cohort studies. Case control studies provide a measure of the relative risk of a disease, namely, a ratio of the incidence of a disease among oral contraceptive users to that among nonusers. The relative risk does not provide information on the actual clinical occurrence of a disease. Cohort studies provide a measure of attributable risk, which is the difference in the incidence of disease between oral contraceptive users and nonusers. The attributable risk does provide information about the actual occurrence of a disease in the population (adapted from refs. 2 and 3 with the author's permission). For further information, the reader is referred to a text on epidemiological methods.

1. Thromboembolic Disorders and Other Vascular Problems

a. Myocardial Infarction

An increased risk of myocardial infarction has been attributed to oral contraceptive use. This risk is primarily in smokers or women with other underlying risk factors for coronary artery disease such as hypertension, hypercholesterolemia, morbid obesity, and diabetes. The relative risk of heart attack for current oral contraceptive users has been estimated to be two to six.[4–10] The risk is very low under the age of 30.

Smoking in combination with oral contraceptive use has been shown to contribute substantially to the incidence of myocardial infarctions in women in their mid-thirties or older with smoking accounting for the majority of excess cases.[11] Mortality rates associated with circulatory disease have been shown to increase substantially in smokers, especially in those 35 years of age and older and in nonsmokers over the age of 40 among women who use oral contraceptives.

Figure 1: Circulatory Disease Mortality Rates Per 100,000 Women-Years By Age, Smoking Status And Oral Contraceptive Use

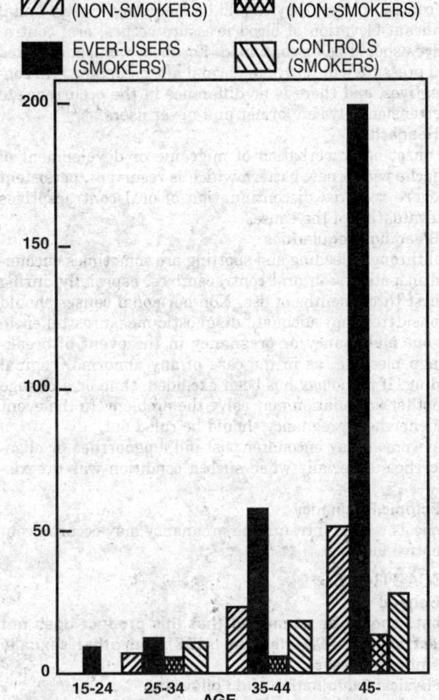

FIGURE 1. Adapted from P.M. Layde and V. Beral, Ref. #12.

Oral contraceptives may compound the effects of well-known risk factors, such as hypertension, diabetes, hyperlipidemias, age and obesity.[13] In particular, some progestogens are known to decrease HDL cholesterol and cause glucose intolerance, while estrogens may create a state of hyperinsulinism.[14–18] Oral contraceptives have been shown to increase blood pressure among users (see section 9 in WARNINGS). Similar effects on risk factors have been associated with an increased risk of heart disease. Oral contraceptives must be used with caution in women with cardiovascular disease risk factors.

Norgestimate has minimal androgenic activity (see CLINICAL PHARMACOLOGY), and there is some evidence that the risk of myocardial infarction associated with oral contraceptives is lower when the progestogen has minimal androgenic activity than when the activity is greater.[97]

b. Thromboembolism

An increased risk of thromboembolic and thrombotic disease associated with the use of oral contraceptives is well established. Case control studies have found the relative risk of users compared to nonusers to be 3 for the first episode of superficial venous thrombosis, 4 to 11 for deep vein thrombosis or pulmonary embolism, and 1.5 to 6 for women with predisposing conditions for venous thromboembolic disease.[2,3,19–24] Cohort studies have shown the relative risk to be somewhat lower, about 3 for new cases and about 4.5 for new cases requiring hospitalization.[25] The risk of thromboembolic disease associated with oral contraceptives is not related to length of use and disappears after pill use is stopped.[2]

A two- to four-fold increase in relative risk of post-operative thromboembolic complications has been reported with the use of oral contraceptives.[9] The relative risk of venous thrombosis in women who have predisposing conditions is twice that of women without such medical conditions.[26] If feasible, oral contraceptives should be discontinued at least four weeks prior to and for two weeks after elective surgery of a type associated with an increase in risk of thromboembolism and during and following prolonged immobilization. Since the immediate postpartum period is also associated with an increased risk of thromboembolism, oral contraceptives should be started no earlier than four weeks after delivery in women who elect not to breast feed.

c. Cerebrovascular diseases

Oral contraceptives have been shown to increase both the relative and attributable risks of cerebrovascular events (thrombotic and hemorrhagic strokes), although, in general, the risk is greatest among older (>35 years), hypertensive women who also smoke. Hypertension was found to be a risk factor for both users and nonusers, for both types of strokes, and smoking interacted to increase the risk of hemorrhagic stroke.[27–29]

In a large study, the relative risk of thrombotic strokes has been shown to range from 3 for normotensive users to 14 for users with severe hypertension.[30] The relative risk of hemorrhagic stroke is reported to be 1.2 for non-smokers who used oral contraceptives, 2.6 for smokers who did not use oral contraceptives, 7.6 for smokers who used oral contraceptives, 1.8 for normotensive users and 25.7 for users with severe hypertension.[30] The attributable risk is also greater in older women.[3]

d. Dose-related risk of vascular disease from oral contraceptives

A positive association has been observed between the amount of estrogen and progestogen in oral contraceptives and the risk of vascular disease.[31–33] A decline in serum high density lipoproteins (HDL) has been reported with many progestational agents.[14–16] A decline in serum high density lipoproteins has been associated with an increased incidence of ischemic heart disease. Because estrogens increase HDL cholesterol, the net effect of an oral contraceptive depends on a balance achieved between doses of estrogen and progestogen and the activity of the progestogen used in the contraceptives. The activity and amount of both hormones should be considered in the choice of an oral contraceptive.

Minimizing exposure to estrogen and progestogen is in keeping with good principles of therapeutics. For any particular estrogen/progestogen combination, the dosage regimen prescribed should be one which contains the least amount of estrogen and progestogen that is compatible with a low failure rate and the needs of the individual patient. New acceptors of oral contraceptive agents should be started on preparations containing the lowest estrogen content which is judged appropriate for an individual patient.

e. Persistence of risk of vascular disease

There are two studies which have shown persistence of risk of vascular disease for ever-users of oral contraceptives. In a study in the United States, the risk of developing myocardial infarction after discontinuing oral contraceptives persists for at least 9 years for women 40–49 years who had used oral contraceptives for five or more years, but this increased risk was not demonstrated in other age groups.[8] In another study in Great Britain, the risk of developing cerebrovascular disease persisted for at least 6 years after discontinuation of oral contraceptives, although excess risk was very small.[34] However, both studies were performed with oral contraceptive formulations containing 50 micrograms or higher of estrogens.

2. Estimates of Mortality from Contraceptive Use

One study gathered data from a variety of sources which have estimated the mortality rate associated with different methods of contraception at different ages (Table 3). These estimates include the combined risk of death associated with contraceptive methods plus the risk attributable to pregnancy in the event of method failure. Each method of contraception has its specific benefits and risks. The study concluded that with the exception of oral contraceptive users 35 and older who smoke, and 40 and older who do not smoke, mortality associated with all methods of birth control is low and below that associated with childbirth. The observation of an increase in risk of mortality with age for oral contraceptive users is based on data gathered in the 1970's.[35] Current clinical recommendation involves the use of lower estrogen dose formulations and a careful consideration of risk factors. In 1989, the Fertility and Maternal Health Drugs Advisory Committee was asked to review the use of oral contraceptives in women 40 years of age and over.

The Committee concluded that although cardiovascular disease risks may be increased with oral contraceptive use after age 40 in healthy non-smoking women (even with the newer low-dose formulations), there are also greater potential health risks associated with pregnancy in older women and with the alternative surgical and medical procedures which may be necessary if such women do not have access to effective and acceptable means of contraception. The Committee recommended that the benefits of low-dose oral contraceptive use by healthy non-smoking women over 40 may outweigh the possible risks.

Of course, older women, as all women, who take oral contraceptives, should take an oral contraceptive which contains the least amount of estrogen and progestogen that is compatible with a low failure rate and individual patient needs.

[See table 3 at top of next page]

3. Carcinoma of the Reproductive Organs and Breasts

Numerous epidemiological studies have been performed on the incidence of breast, endometrial, ovarian, and cervical cancer in women using oral contraceptives.

Continued on next page

Ortho Tri-Cyclen Lo—Cont.

The risk of having breast cancer diagnosed may be slightly increased among current and recent users of combination oral contraceptives. However, this excess risk appears to decrease over time after discontinuation of combination oral contraceptives and by 10 years after cessation the increased risk disappears. Some studies report an increased risk with duration of use while other studies do not and no consistent relationships have been found with dose or type of steroid. Some studies have found a small increase in risk for women who first use combination oral contraceptives before age 20. Most studies show a similar pattern of risk with combination oral contraceptive use regardless of a woman's reproductive history or her family breast cancer history.

Breast cancers diagnosed in current or previous oral contraceptive users tend to be less clinically advanced than in nonusers.

Women who currently have or have had breast cancer should not use oral contraceptives because breast cancer is usually a hormonally-sensitive tumor.

Some studies suggest that oral contraceptive use has been associated with an increase in the risk of cervical intraepithelial neoplasia in some populations of women.[45–48] However, there continues to be controversy about the extent to which such findings may be due to differences in sexual behavior and other factors.

In spite of many studies of the relationship between oral contraceptive use and breast and cervical cancers, a cause-and-effect relationship has not been established.

4. Hepatic Neoplasia

Benign hepatic adenomas are associated with oral contraceptive use, although the incidence of benign tumors is rare in the United States. Indirect calculations have estimated the attributable risk to be in the range of 3.3 cases/100,000 for users, a risk that increases after four or more years of use especially with oral contraceptives of higher dose.[49] Rupture of benign, hepatic adenomas may cause death through intra-abdominal hemorrhage.[50,51]

Studies from Britain have shown an increased risk of developing hepatocellular carcinoma in long-term (>8 years) oral contraceptive users. However, these cancers are extremely rare in the U.S. and the attributable risk (the excess incidence) of liver cancers in oral contraceptive users approaches less than one per million users.

5. Ocular Lesions

There have been clinical case reports of retinal thrombosis associated with the use of oral contraceptives. Oral contraceptives should be discontinued if there is unexplained partial or complete loss of vision; onset of proptosis or diplopia; papilledema; or retinal vascular lesions. Appropriate diagnostic and therapeutic measures should be undertaken immediately.

6. Oral Contraceptive Use Before or During Early Pregnancy

Extensive epidemiological studies have revealed no increased risk of birth defects in women who have used oral contraceptives prior to pregnancy.[56,57] The majority of recent studies also do not indicate a teratogenic effect, particularly in so far as cardiac anomalies and limb reduction defects are concerned,[55,56,58,59] when taken inadvertently during early pregnancy.

The administration of oral contraceptives to induce withdrawal bleeding should not be used as a test for pregnancy. Oral contraceptives should not be used during pregnancy to treat threatened or habitual abortion.

It is recommended that for any patient who has missed two consecutive periods, pregnancy should be ruled out. If the patient has not adhered to the prescribed schedule, the possibility of pregnancy should be considered at the time of the first missed period. Oral contraceptive use should be discontinued if pregnancy is confirmed.

7. Gallbladder Disease

Earlier studies have reported an increased lifetime relative risk of gallbladder surgery in users of oral contraceptives and estrogens.[60,61] More recent studies, however, have shown that the relative risk of developing gallbladder disease among oral contraceptive users may be minimal.[62–64] The recent findings of minimal risk may be related to the use of oral contraceptive formulations containing lower hormonal doses of estrogens and progestogens.

8. Carbohydrate and Lipid Metabolic Effects

Oral contraceptives have been shown to cause a decrease in glucose tolerance in a significant percentage of users.[17] This effect has been shown to be directly related to estrogen dose.[65] Progestogens increase insulin secretion and create insulin resistance, this effect varying with different progestational agents.[17,66] However, in the non-diabetic woman, oral contraceptives appear to have no effect on fasting blood glucose.[67] Because of these demonstrated effects, prediabetic and diabetic women in particular should be carefully monitored while taking oral contraceptives.

A small proportion of women will have persistent hypertriglyceridemia while on the pill. As discussed earlier (see WARNINGS 1a and 1d), changes in serum triglycerides and lipoprotein levels have been reported in oral contraceptive users.

9. Elevated Blood Pressure

Women with significant hypertension should not be started on hormonal contraception.[98] An increase in blood pressure has been reported in women taking oral contraceptives[68] and this increase is more likely in older oral contraceptive users[69] and with extended duration of use.[61] Data from the

Table 3: Annual Number of Birth-Related or Method-Related Deaths Associated with Control of Fertility Per 100,000 Nonsterile Women, By Fertility-Control Method and According to Age

Method of control and outcome	15–19	20–24	25–29	30–34	35–39	40–44
No fertility-control methods*	7.0	7.4	9.1	14.8	25.7	28.2
Oral contraceptives nonsmoker**	0.3	0.5	0.9	1.9	13.8	31.6
Oral contraceptives smoker**	2.2	3.4	6.6	13.5	51.1	117.2
IUD**	0.8	0.8	1.0	1.0	1.4	1.4
Condom*	1.1	1.6	0.7	0.2	0.3	0.4
Diaphragm/spermicide*	1.9	1.2	1.2	1.3	2.2	2.8
Periodic abstinence*	2.5	1.6	1.6	1.7	2.9	3.6

* Deaths are birth-related
**Deaths are method-related
Adapted from H.W. Ory, Family Planning Perspectives, Ref. #35.

Royal College of General Practitioners[12] and subsequent randomized trials have shown that the incidence of hypertension increases with increasing progestational activity and concentrations of progestogens.

Women with a history of hypertension or hypertension-related diseases, or renal disease[70] should be encouraged to use another method of contraception. If women elect to use oral contraceptives, they should be monitored closely and if significant elevation of blood pressure occurs, oral contraceptives should be discontinued. For most women, elevated blood pressure will return to normal after stopping oral contraceptives, and there is no difference in the occurrence of hypertension between former and never users.[68–71]

10. Headache

The onset or exacerbation of migraine or development of headache with a new pattern which is recurrent, persistent or severe requires discontinuation of oral contraceptives and evaluation of the cause.

11. Bleeding Irregularities

Breakthrough bleeding and spotting are sometimes encountered in patients on oral contraceptives, especially during the first three months of use. Non-hormonal causes should be considered and adequate diagnostic measures taken to rule out malignancy or pregnancy in the event of breakthrough bleeding, as in the case of any abnormal vaginal bleeding. If pathology has been excluded, time or a change to another formulation may solve the problem. In the event of amenorrhea, pregnancy should be ruled out.

Some women may encounter post-pill amenorrhea or oligomenorrhea, especially when such a condition was preexistent.

12. Ectopic Pregnancy

Ectopic as well as intrauterine pregnancy may occur in contraceptive failures.

PRECAUTIONS

1. General

Patients should be counseled that this product does not protect against HIV infection (AIDS) and other sexually transmitted diseases.

2. Physical Examination and Follow-Up

It is good medical practice for all women to have annual history and physical examinations, including women using oral contraceptives. The physical examination, however, may be deferred until after initiation of oral contraceptives if requested by the woman and judged appropriate by the clinician. The physical examination should include special reference to blood pressure, breasts, abdomen and pelvic organs, including cervical cytology, and relevant laboratory tests. In case of undiagnosed, persistent or recurrent abnormal vaginal bleeding, appropriate measures should be conducted to rule out malignancy. Women with a strong family history of breast cancer or who have breast nodules should be monitored with particular care.

3. Lipid Disorders

Women who are being treated for hyperlipidemias should be followed closely if they elect to use oral contraceptives. Some progestogens may elevate LDL levels and may render the control of hyperlipidemias more difficult.

4. Liver Function

If jaundice develops in any woman receiving oral contraceptives, the medication should be discontinued. Steroid hormones may be poorly metabolized in patients with impaired liver function.

5. Fluid Retention

Oral contraceptives may cause some degree of fluid retention. They should be prescribed with caution, and only with careful monitoring, in patients with conditions which might be aggravated by fluid retention.

6. Emotional Disorders

Women with a history of depression should be carefully observed and the drug discontinued if depression recurs to a serious degree.

7. Contact Lenses

Contact lens wearers who develop visual changes or changes in lens tolerance should be assessed by an ophthalmologist.

8. Drug Interactions

Changes in contraceptive effectiveness associated with co-administration of other products:

Contraceptive effectiveness may be reduced when hormonal contraceptives are coadministered with antibiotics, anticonvulsants, and other drugs that increase the metabolism of contraceptive steroids. This could result in unintended pregnancy or breakthrough bleeding. Examples include rifampin, barbiturates, phenylbutazone, phenytoin, carbamazepine, felbamate, oxcarbazepine, topiramate, and griseofulvin. Several cases of contraceptive failure and breakthrough bleeding have been reported in the literature with concomitant administration of antibiotics such as ampicillin and tetracyclines. However, clinical pharmacology studies investigating drug interaction between combined oral contraceptives and these antibiotics have reported inconsistent results.

Several of the anti-HIV protease inhibitors have been studied with co-administration of oral combination hormonal contraceptives; significant changes (increase and decrease) in the plasma levels of the estrogen and progestin have been noted in some cases. The safety and efficacy of oral contraceptive products may be affected with coadministration of anti-HIV protease inhibitors. Health care providers should refer to the label of the individual anti-HIV protease inhibitors for further drug-drug interaction information.

Herbal products containing St. John's Wort (hypericum perforatum) may induce hepatic enzymes (cytochrome P450) and p-glycoprotein transporter and may reduce the effectiveness of contraceptive steroids. This may also result in breakthrough bleeding.

Increase in plasma ethinyl estradiol levels associated with co-administered drugs:

Co-administration of atorvastatin and certain oral contraceptives containing ethinyl estradiol increase AUC values for ethinyl estradiol by approximately 20%. Ascorbic acid and acetaminophen may increase plasma ethinyl estradiol levels, possibly by inhibition of conjugation. CYP 3A4 inhibitors such as itraconazole or ketoconazole may increase plasma hormone levels.

Changes in plasma levels of co-administered drugs:

Combination hormonal contraceptives containing some synthetic estrogens (e.g., ethinyl estradiol) may inhibit the metabolism of other compounds. Increased plasma concentrations of cyclosporin, prednisolone, and theophylline have been reported with concomitant administration of oral contraceptives. Decreased plasma concentrations of acetaminophen and increased clearance of temazepam, salicylic acid, morphine and clofibric acid, due to induction of conjugation, have been noted when drugs were administered with oral contraceptives.

9. Interactions with Laboratory Tests

Certain endocrine and liver function tests and blood components may be affected by oral contraceptives:

a. Increased prothrombin and factors VII, VIII, IX, and X; decreased antithrombin 3; increased norepinephrine-induced platelet aggregability.

b. Increased thyroid binding globulin (TBG) leading to increased circulating total thyroid hormone, as measured by protein-bound iodine (PBI), T4 by column or by radioimmunoassay. Free T3 resin uptake is decreased, reflecting the elevated TBG, free T4 concentration is unaltered.

c. Other binding proteins may be elevated in serum.

d. Sex hormone binding globulins are increased and result in elevated levels of total circulating sex steroids; however, free or biologically active levels either decrease or remain unchanged.

e. Triglycerides may be increased and levels of various other lipids and lipoproteins may be affected.

f. Glucose tolerance may be decreased.

g. Serum folate levels may be depressed by oral contraceptive therapy. This may be of clinical significance if a woman becomes pregnant shortly after discontinuing oral contraceptives.

10. Carcinogenesis

See WARNINGS section.

11. Pregnancy

Pregnancy Category X. See CONTRAINDICATIONS and WARNINGS sections.

12. Nursing Mothers

Small amounts of oral contraceptive steroids have been identified in the milk of nursing mothers and a few adverse effects on the child have been reported, including jaundice and breast enlargement. In addition, oral contraceptives given in the postpartum period may interfere with lactation by decreasing the quantity and quality of breast milk. If possible, the nursing mother should be advised not to use combination oral contraceptives but to use other forms of contraception until she has completely weaned her child.

13. Pediatric Use

Safety and efficacy of ORTHO TRI-CYCLEN® Lo Tablets have been established in women of reproductive age. Safety and efficacy are expected to be the same for postpubertal adolescents under the age of 16 and for users 16 years and older. Use of this product before menarche is not indicated.

14. Geriatric Use

This product has not been studied in women over 65 years of age and is not indicated in this population.

INFORMATION FOR THE PATIENT

See Patient Labeling printed below.

ADVERSE REACTIONS

An increased risk of the following serious adverse reactions has been associated with the use of oral contraceptives (see WARNINGS section).

- Thrombophlebitis and venous thrombosis with or without embolism
- Arterial thromboembolism
- Pulmonary embolism
- Myocardial infarction
- Cerebral hemorrhage
- Cerebral thrombosis
- Hypertension
- Gallbladder disease
- Hepatic adenomas or benign liver tumors

There is evidence of an association between the following conditions and the use of oral contraceptives:

- Mesenteric thrombosis
- Retinal thrombosis

The following adverse reactions have been reported in patients receiving oral contraceptives and are believed to be drug-related:

- Nausea
- Vomiting
- Gastrointestinal symptoms (such as abdominal cramps and bloating)
- Breakthrough bleeding
- Spotting
- Change in menstrual flow
- Amenorrhea
- Temporary infertility after discontinuation of treatment
- Edema
- Melasma which may persist
- Breast changes: tenderness, enlargement, secretion
- Change in weight (increase or decrease)
- Change in cervical erosion and secretion
- Diminution in lactation when given immediately postpartum
- Cholestatic jaundice
- Migraine
- Rash (allergic)
- Mental depression
- Reduced tolerance to carbohydrates
- Vaginal candidiasis
- Change in corneal curvature (steepening)
- Intolerance to contact lenses

The following adverse reactions have been reported in users of oral contraceptives and the association has been neither confirmed nor refuted:

- Pre-menstrual syndrome
- Cataracts
- Changes in appetite
- Cystitis-like syndrome
- Headache
- Nervousness
- Dizziness
- Hirsutism
- Loss of scalp hair
- Erythema multiforme
- Erythema nodosum
- Hemorrhagic eruption
- Vaginitis
- Porphyria
- Impaired renal function
- Hemolytic uremic syndrome
- Acne
- Changes in libido
- Colitis
- Budd-Chiari Syndrome

OVERDOSAGE

Serious ill effects have not been reported following acute ingestion of large doses of oral contraceptives by young children. Overdosage may cause nausea and withdrawal bleeding may occur in females.

NON-CONTRACEPTIVE HEALTH BENEFITS

The following non-contraceptive health benefits related to the use of combination oral contraceptives are supported by epidemiological studies which largely utilized oral contraceptive formulations containing estrogen doses exceeding 0.035 mg of ethinyl estradiol or 0.05 mg mestranol.[73–78]

Effects on menses:

- increased menstrual cycle regularity
- decreased blood loss and decreased incidence of iron deficiency anemia
- decreased incidence of dysmenorrhea

Effects related to inhibition of ovulation:

- decreased incidence of functional ovarian cysts
- decreased incidence of ectopic pregnancies

Other effects:

- decreased incidence of fibroadenomas and fibrocystic disease of the breast
- decreased incidence of acute pelvic inflammatory disease
- decreased incidence of endometrial cancer
- decreased incidence of ovarian cancer

DOSAGE AND ADMINISTRATION

Oral Contraception

To achieve maximum contraceptive effectiveness, ORTHO TRI-CYCLEN® Lo Tablets must be taken exactly as directed and at intervals not exceeding 24 hours. The possibility of ovulation and conception prior to initiation of medication should be considered. ORTHO TRI-CYCLEN® Lo is available in the DIALPAK® Tablet Dispenser which is preset for a Sunday Start. Day 1 Start is also provided.

Sunday Start

When taking ORTHO TRI-CYCLEN® Lo the first tablet should be taken on the first Sunday after menstruation begins. If the menstrual period begins on Sunday, the first tablet should be taken that day. Take one white, light blue or dark blue active tablet daily for 21 days followed by one green placebo tablet daily for 7 days. After 28 tablets have been taken, a new course is started the next day (Sunday). For the first cycle of a Sunday Start regimen, another method of contraception should be used until after the first 7 consecutive days of administration.

If the patient misses one (1) active tablet in Weeks 1, 2, or 3, the tablet should be taken as soon as she remembers. If the patient misses two (2) active tablets in Week 1 or Week 2, the patient should take two (2) tablets the day she remembers and two (2) tablets the next day; and then continue taking one (1) tablet a day until she finishes the pack. The patient should be instructed to use a back-up method of birth control if she has sex in the seven (7) days after missing pills. If the patient misses two (2) active tablets in the third week or misses three (3) or more active tablets in a row, the patient should continue taking one tablet every day until Sunday. On Sunday the patient should throw out the rest of the pack and start a new pack that same day. The patient should be instructed to use a back-up method of birth control if she has sex in the seven (7) days after missing pills. Complete instructions to facilitate patient counseling on proper pill usage may be found in the Detailed Patient Labeling ("How to Take the Pill" section).

Day 1 Start

The dosage of ORTHO TRI-CYCLEN® Lo for the initial cycle of therapy is one white, light blue or dark blue active tablet administered daily from the 1st day through the 21st day of the menstrual cycle, counting the first day of menstrual flow as "Day 1" followed by one green placebo tablet daily for 7 days. Tablets are taken without interruption for 28 days. After 28 tablets have been taken, a new course is started the next day.

If the patient misses one (1) active tablet in Weeks 1, 2, or 3, the tablet should be taken as soon as she remembers. If the patient misses two (2) active tablets in Week 1 or Week 2, the patient should take two (2) tablets the day she remembers and two (2) tablets the next day; and then continue taking one (1) tablet a day until she finishes the pack. The patient should be instructed to use a back-up method of birth control if she has sex in the seven (7) days after missing pills. If the patient misses two (2) active tablets in the third week or misses three (3) or more active tablets in a row, the patient should throw out the rest of the pack and start a new pack that same day. The patient should be instructed to use a back-up method of birth control if she has sex in the seven (7) days after missing pills.

Complete instructions to facilitate patient counseling on proper pill usage may be found in the Detailed Patient Labeling ("How to Take the Pill" section).

When switching from another oral contraceptive, ORTHO TRI-CYCLEN® Lo should be started on the same day that a new pack of the previous oral contraceptive would have been started.

The use of ORTHO TRI-CYCLEN® Lo for contraception may be initiated 4 weeks postpartum in women who elect not to breast feed. When the tablets are administered during the postpartum period, the increased risk of thromboembolic disease associated with the postpartum period must be considered. (See CONTRAINDICATIONS and WARNINGS concerning thromboembolic disease. See also PRECAUTIONS for "Nursing Mothers.") The possibility of ovulation and conception prior to initiation of medication should be considered.

(See Discussion of Dose-Related Risk of Vascular Disease from Oral Contraceptives.)

ADDITIONAL INSTRUCTIONS FOR ALL DOSING REGIMENS

Breakthrough bleeding, spotting, and amenorrhea are frequent reasons for patients discontinuing oral contraceptives. In breakthrough bleeding, as in all cases of irregular bleeding from the vagina, nonfunctional causes should be borne in mind. In undiagnosed persistent or recurrent abnormal bleeding from the vagina, adequate diagnostic measures are indicated to rule out pregnancy or malignancy. If pathology has been excluded, time or a change to another formulation may solve the problem. Changing to an oral contraceptive with a higher estrogen content, while potentially useful in minimizing menstrual irregularity, should be done only if necessary since this may increase the risk of thromboembolic disease.

Use of oral contraceptives in the event of a missed menstrual period:

1. If the patient has not adhered to the prescribed schedule, the possibility of pregnancy should be considered at the time of the first missed period and oral contraceptive use should be discontinued if pregnancy is confirmed.
2. If the patient has adhered to the prescribed regimen and misses two consecutive periods, pregnancy should be ruled out before continuing oral contraceptive use.

HOW SUPPLIED

ORTHO TRI-CYCLEN® Lo Tablets are available in a DIALPAK® Tablet Dispenser (NDC 0062-1251-15) containing 28 tablets. Each of the 7 white tablets contains 0.180 mg of the progestational compound, norgestimate, together with 0.025 mg of the estrogenic compound, ethinyl estradiol. Each of the 7 light blue tablets contains 0.215 mg of the progestational compound, norgestimate, together with 0.025 mg of the estrogenic compound, ethinyl estradiol. Each of the 7 dark blue tablets contains 0.250 mg of the progestational compound, norgestimate, together with 0.025 mg of the estrogenic compound, ethinyl estradiol. Each of the 7 green tablets contains inert ingredients.

The white tablets are unscored, with "O-M" and "180" debossed on each side; the light blue tablets are unscored with "O-M" and "215" debossed on each side; the dark blue tablets are unscored with "O-M" and "250" debossed on each side.

ORTHO TRI-CYCLEN® Lo Tablets are available for clinic usage in a VERIDATE® Tablet Dispenser (unfilled) and VERIDATE Refills (NDC 0062-1251-20).

Protect from light.

℞ only

REFERENCES

1. Trussell J. Contraceptive efficacy. In Hatcher RA, Trussell J, Stewart F, Cates W, Stewart GK, Kowal D, Guest F, *Contraceptive Technology: Seventeenth Revised Edition.* New York NY: Irvington Publishers, 1998. **2.** Stadel BV, Oral contraceptives and cardiovascular disease. (Pt.1). N Engl J Med 1981; 305:612–618. **3.** Stadel BV, Oral contraceptives and cardiovascular disease. (Pt.2). N Engl J Med 1981; 305:672–677. **4.** Adam SA, Thorogood M. Oral contraception and myocardial infarction revisited: the effects of new preparations and prescribing patterns. Br J Obstet Gynaecol 1981; 88: 838–845. **5.** Mann Jl, Inman WH. Oral contraceptives and death from myocardial infarction. Br Med J 1975; 2(5965): 245–248. **6.** Mann Jl, Vessey MP, Thorogood M, Doll R. Myocardial infarction in young women with special reference to oral contraceptive practice. Br Med J 1975; 2(5956):241–245. **7.** Royal College of General Practitioners' Oral Contraception Study: Further analyses of mortality in oral contraceptive users. Lancet 1981; 1:541–546. **8.** Slone D, Shapiro S, Kaufman DW, Rosenberg L, Miettinen OS, Stolley PD. Risk of myocardial infarction in relation to current and discontinued use of oral contraceptives. N Engl J Med 1981: 305:420–424. **9.** Vessey MP. Female hormones and vascular disease–an epidemiological overview. Br J Fam Plann 1980; 6(Supplement): 1–12. **10.** Russell-Briefel RG, Ezzati TM, Fulwood R, Perlman JA, Murphy RS. Cardiovascular risk status and oral contraceptive use, United States, 1976–80. Prevent Med 1986; 15:352–362. **11.** Goldbaum GM, Kendrick JS, Hogelin GC, Gentry EM. The relative impact of smoking and oral contraceptive use on women in the United States. JAMA 1987; 258:1339–1342. **12.** Layde PM, Beral V. Further analyses of mortality in oral contraceptive users; Royal College of General Practitioners' Oral Contraception Study. (Table 5) Lancet 1981; 1:541–546. **13.** Knopp RH. Arteriosclerosis risk: the roles of oral contraceptives and postmenopausal estrogens. J Reprod Med 1986; 31(9) (Supplement):913–921. **14.** Krauss RM, Roy S, Mishell DR, Casagrande J, Pike MC. Effects of two low-dose oral contraceptives on serum lipids and lipoproteins: Differential changes in high-density lipoproteins subclasses. Am J Obstet 1983; 145:446–452. **15.** Wahl P, Walden C, Knopp R, Hoover J, Wallace R, Heiss G, Rifkind B. Effect of estrogen/progestin potency on lipid/lipoprotein cholesterol. N Engl J Med 1983; 308:862–867. **16.** Wynn V, Niththyananthan R. The effect of progestin in combined oral contraceptives on serum lipids with special reference to high density lipoproteins. Am J Obstet Gynecol 1982;142:766–771. **17.** Wynn V, Godsland I. Effects of oral contraceptives on carbohydrate metabolism. J Reprod Med 1986;31(9)(Supplement):892–897. **18.** LaRosa JC. Atherosclerotic risk factors in cardiovascular disease. J Reprod Med 1986;31(9)(Supplement): 906–912. **19.** Inman WH, Vessey MP. Investigation of death from pulmonary, coronary, and cerebral thrombosis and embolism in women of child-bearing age. Br Med J 1968;2(5599):193–199. **20.** Maguire MG, Tonascia J, Sartwell PE, Stolley PD, Tockman MS. Increased risk of thrombosis due to oral contraceptives: a further report. Am J Epidemiol 1979;110(2):188–195. **21.** Petitti DB, Wingerd J, Pellegrin F, Ramacharan S. Risk of vascular disease in women: smoking, oral contraceptives, noncontraceptive estrogens, and other factors. JAMA 1979;242:1150–1154. **22.** Vessey MP, Doll R, Investigation of relation between use of oral contraceptives and thromboembolic disease. Br Med J 1968;2(5599):199–205. **23.** Vessey MP, Doll R. Investigation of relation between use of oral contraceptives and thromboembolic disease. A further report. Br Med J 1969; 2(5658): 651–657. **24.** Porter JB, Hunter JR, Danielson DA, Jick H, Stergachis A. Oral contraceptives and non-fatal vascular disease–recent experience. Obstet Gynecol 1982;59(3):299–

Continued on next page

Ortho Tri-Cyclen Lo—Cont.

302. **25.** Vessey M, Doll R, Peto R, Johnson B, Wiggins P. A long-term follow-up study of women using different methods of contraception: an interim report. J Biosocial Sci 1976;8: 375–427. **26.** Royal College of General Practitioners: Oral Contraceptives, venous thrombosis, and varicose veins. J Royal Coll Gen Pract 1978; 28:393–399. **27.** Collaborative Group for the Study of Stroke in Young Women: Oral contraception and increased risk of cerebral ischemia or thrombosis. N Engl J Med 1973;288:871–878. **28.** Petitti DB, Wingerd J. Use of oral contraceptives, cigarette smoking, and risk of subarachnoid hemorrhage. Lancet 1978;2:234–236. **29.** Inman WH. Oral contraceptives and fatal subarachnoid hemorrhage. Br Med J 1979:2(6203):1468–1470. **30.** Collaborative Group for the Study of Stroke in Young Women: Oral Contraceptives and stroke in young women: associated risk factors. JAMA 1975; 231:718–722. **31.** Inman WH, Vessey MP, Westerholm B, Engelund A. Thromboembolic disease and the steroidal content of oral contraceptives. A report to the Committee on Safety of Drugs. Br Med J 1970;2:203–209. **32.** Meade TW, Greenberg G, Thompson SG. Progestogens and cardiovascular reactions associated with oral contraceptives and a comparison of the safety of 50- and 35-mcg oestrogen preparations. Br Med J 1980;280(6224):1157–1161. **33.** Kay CR. Progestogens and arterial disease–evidence from the Royal College of General Practitioners' Study. Am J Obstet Gynecol 1982;142:762–765. **34.** Royal College of General Practitioners: Incidence of arterial disease among oral contraceptive users. J Royal Coll Gen Pract 1983;33:75–82. **35.** Ory HW. Mortality associated with fertility and fertility control: 1983. Family Planning Perspectives 1983;15:50–56. **36.** The Cancer and Steroid Hormone Study of the Centers for Disease Control and the National Institute of Child Health and Human Development: Oral contraceptive use and the risk of breast cancer. N Engl J Med 1986;315:405–411. **37.** Pike MC, Henderson BE, Krailo MD, Duke A, Roy S. Breast cancer in young women and use of oral contraceptives: possible modifying effect of formulation and age at use. Lancet 1983;2:926–929. **38.** Paul C, Skegg DG, Spears GFS, Kaldor JM. Oral contraceptives and breast cancer: A national study. Br Med J 1986; 293:723–725. **39.** Miller DR, Rosenberg L, Kaufman DW, Schottenfeld D, Stolley PD, Shapiro S. Breast cancer risk in relation to early oral contraceptive use. Obstet Gynecol 1986;68:863–868. **40.** Olsson H, Olsson ML, Moller TR, Ranstam J, Holm P. Oral contraceptive use and breast cancer in young women in Sweden (letter). Lancet 1985; 1(8431):748–749. **41.** McPherson K, Vessey M, Neil A, Doll R, Jones L, Roberts M. Early contraceptive use and breast cancer: Results of another case-control study. Br J Cancer 1987; 56:653–660. **42.** Huggins GR, Zucker PF. Oral contraceptives and neoplasia; 1987 update. Fertil Steril 1987; 47:733–761. **43.** McPherson K, Drife JO. The pill and breast cancer: why the uncertainty? Br Med J 1986; 293: 709–710. **44.** Shapiro S. Oral contraceptives–time to take stock. N Engl J Med 1987; 315:450–451. **45.** Ory H, Naib Z, Conger SB, Hatcher RA, Tyler CW. Contraceptive choice and prevalence of cervical dysplasia and carcinoma in situ. Am J Obstet Gynecol 1976; 124:573–577. **46.** Vessey MP, Lawless M, McPherson K, Yeates D. Neoplasia of the cervix uteri and contraception: a possible adverse effect of the pill. Lancet 1983; 2:930. **47.** Brinton LA, Huggins GR, Lehman HF, Malli K, Savitz DA, Trapido E, Rosenthal J, Hoover R. Long term use of oral contraceptives and risk of invasive cervical cancer. Int J Cancer 1986; 38:339–344. **48.** WHO Collaborative Study of Neoplasia and Steroid Contraceptives: Invasive cervical cancer and combined oral contraceptives. Br Med J 1985; 290:961–965. **49.** Rooks JB, Ory HW, Ishak KG, Strauss LT, Greenspan JR, Hill AP, Tyler CW. Epidemiology of hepatocellular adenoma: the role of oral contraceptive use. JAMA 1979; 242:644–648. **50.** Bein NN, Goldsmith HS. Recurrent massive hemorrhage from benign hepatic tumors secondary to oral contraceptives. Br J Surg 1977; 64:433–435. **51.** Klatskin G. Hepatic tumors: possible relationship to use of oral contraceptives. Gastroenterology 1977; 73:386–394. **52.** Henderson BE, Preston-Martin S, Edmondson HA, Peters RL, Pike MC. Hepatocellular carcinoma and oral contraceptives. Br J Cancer 1983;48:437–440. **53.** Neuberger J, Forman D, Doll R, Williams R. Oral contraceptives and hepatocellular carcinoma. Br Med J 1986; 292:1355–1357. **54.** Forman D, Vincent TJ, Doll R, Cancer of the liver and oral contraceptives. Br Med J 1986; 292:1357–1361. **55.** Harlap S, Eldor J. Births following oral contraceptive failures. Obstet Gynecol 1980; 55:447–452. **56.** Savolainen E, Saksela E, Saxen L. Teratogenic hazards of oral contraceptives analyzed in a national malformation register. Am J Obstet Gynecol 1981: 140:521–524. **57.** Janerich DT, Piper JM, Glebatis DM. Oral contraceptives and birth defects. Am J Epidemiol 1980; 112:73–79. **58.** Ferencz C, Matanoski GM, Wilson PD, Rubin JD, Neill CA, Gutberlet R. Maternal hormone therapy and congenital heart disease. Teratology 1980; 21:225–239. **59.** Rothman KJ, Fyler DC, Goldblatt A, Kreidberg MB. Exogenous hormones and other drug exposures of children with congenital heart disease. Am J Epidemiol 1979; 109:433–439. **60.** Boston Collaborative Drug Surveillance Program: Oral contraceptives and venous thromboembolic disease, surgically confirmed gallbladder disease, and breast tumors. Lancet 1973; 1:1399–1404. **61.** Royal College of General Practitioners: Oral contraceptives and health. New York, Pittman 1974. **62.** Layde PM, Vessey MP, Yeates D. Risk of gallbladder disease: a cohort study of young women attending family planning clinics. J Epidemiol Community Health 1982; 36:274–278. **63.** Rome Group for Epidemiology and Prevention of Cholelithiasis (GREPCO): Prevalence of gallstone disease in an Italian adult female population. Am J Epidemiol 1984; 119:796–805. **64.** Storm BL, Tamragouri RT, Morse ML, Lazar EL, West SL, Stolley PD, Jones JK. Oral contraceptives and other risk factors for gallbladder disease. Clin Pharmacol Ther 1986; 39:335–341. **65.** Wynn V, Adams PW, Godsland IF, Melrose J, Niththyananthan R, Oakley NW, Seedj A. Comparison of effects of different combined oral contraceptive formulations on carbohydrate and lipid metabolism. Lancet 1979; 1:1045–1049. **66.** Wynn V. Effect of progesterone and progestins on carbohydrate metabolism. In: Progesterone and Progestin. Bardin CW, Milgrom E, Mauvis-Jarvis P. eds. New York, Raven Press 1983; pp. 395–410. **67.** Perlman JA, Roussell-Briefel RG, Ezzati TM, Lieberknecht G. Oral glucose tolerance and the potency of oral contraceptive progestogens. J Chronic Dis 1985;38:857–864. **68.** Royal College of General Practitioners' Oral Contraception Study: Effect on hypertension and benign breast disease of progestogen component in combined oral contraceptives. Lancet 1977; 1:624. **69.** Fisch IR, Frank J. Oral contraceptives and blood pressure. JAMA 1977; 237:2499–2503. **70.** Laragh AJ. Oral contraceptive induced hypertension–nine years later. Am J Obstet Gynecol 1976; 126:141–147. **71.** Ramcharan S, Peritz E, Pellegrin FA, Williams WT. Incidence of hypertension in the Walnut Creek Contraceptive Drug Study cohort: In: Pharmacology of steroid contraceptive drugs. Garattini S, Berendes HW. Eds. New York, Raven Press, 1977; pp. 277–288, (Monographs of the Mario Negri Institute for Pharmacological Research Milan.) **72.** Stockley I. Interactions with oral contraceptives. J Pharm 1976;216:140–143. **73.** The Cancer and Steroid Hormone Study of the Centers for Disease Control and the National Institute of Child Health and Human Development: Oral contraceptive use and the risk of ovarian cancer. JAMA 1983; 249:1596–1599. **74.** The Cancer and Steroid Hormone Study of the Centers for Disease Control and the National Institute of Child Health and Human Development: Combination oral contraceptive use and the risk of endometrial cancer. JAMA 1987; 257:796–800. **75.** Ory HW. Functional ovarian cysts and oral contraceptives: negative association confirmed surgically. JAMA 1974; 228:68–69. **76.** Ory HW, Cole P, MacMahon B, Hoover R. Oral contraceptives and reduced risk of benign breast disease. N Engl J Med 1976; 294:419–422. **77.** Ory HW. The noncontraceptive health benefits from oral contraceptive use. Fam Plann Perspect 1982; 14:182–184. **78.** Ory HW, Forrest JD, Lincoln R. Making choices: Evaluating the health risks and benefits of birth control methods. New York, The Alan Guttmacher Institute, 1983; p.1. **79.** Schlesselman J, Stadel BV, Murray P, Lai S. Breast cancer in relation to early use of oral contraceptives. JAMA 1988; 259:1828–1833. **80.** Hennekens CH, Speizer FE, Lipnick RJ, Rosner B, Bain C, Belanger C, Stampfer MJ, Willett W, Peto R. A case-control study of oral contraceptive use and breast cancer. JNCI 1984; 72:39–42. **81.** LaVecchia C, Decarli A, Fasoli M, Franceschi S, Gentile A, Negri E, Parazzini F, Tognoni G. Oral contraceptives and cancers of the breast and of the female genital tract. Interim results from a case-control study. Br J Cancer 1986; 54:311–317. **82.** Meirik O, Lund E, Adami H, Bergstrom R, Christoffersen T, Bergsjo P. Oral contraceptive use and breast cancer in young women. A Joint National Case-control study in Sweden and Norway. Lancet 1986; 11:650–654. **83.** Kay CR, Hannaford PC. Breast cancer and the pill–A further report from the Royal College of General Practitioners' oral contraception study. Br J Cancer 1988;58:675–680. **84.** Stadel BV, Lai S, Schlesselman JJ, Murray P. Oral contraceptives and premenopausal breast cancer in nulliparous women. Contraception 1988; 38:287–299. **85.** Miller DR, Rosenberg L, Kaufman DW, Stolley P, Warshauer ME, Shapiro S. Breast cancer before age 45 and oral contraceptive use: New Findings. Am J Epidemiol 1989; 129:269–280. **86.** The UK National Case-Control Study Group, Oral contraceptive use and breast cancer risk in young women. Lancet 1989; 1:973–982. **87.** Schlesselman JJ. Cancer of the breast and reproductive tract in relation to use of oral contraceptives. Contraception 1989; 40:1–38. **88.** Vessey MP, McPherson K, Villard-Mackintosh L, Yeates D. Oral contraceptives and breast cancer: latest findings in a large cohort study. Br J Cancer 1989; 59:613–617. **89.** Jick SS, Walker AM, Stergachis A, Jick H. Oral contraceptives and breast cancer. Br J Cancer 1989; 59:618–621. **90.** Anderson FD, Selectivity and minimal androgenicity of norgestimate in monophasic and triphasic oral contraceptives. Acta Obstet Gynecol Scand 1992; 156 (Supplement):15–21. **91.** Chapdelaine A, Desmaris J-L, Derman RJ. Clinical evidence of minimal androgenic activity of norgestimate. Int J Fertil 1989; 34(51):347–352. **92.** Phillips A, Demarest K, Hahn DW, Wong F, McGuire JL. Progestational and androgenic receptor binding affinities and in vivo activities of norgestimate and other progestins. Contraception 1989; 41(4):399–409. **93.** Phillips A, Hahn DW, Klimek S, McGuire JL. A comparison of the potencies and activities of progestogens used in contraceptives. Contraception 1987; 36(2):181–192. **94.** Janaud A, Rouffy J, Upmalis D, Dain M-P. A comparison study of lipid and androgen metabolism with triphasic oral contraceptive formulations containing norgestimate or levonorgestrel. Acta Obstet Gynecol Scand 1992; 156 (Supplement):34–38. **95.** Collaborative Group on Hormonal Factors in Breast Cancer. Breast cancer and hormonal contraceptives: collaborative reanalysis of individual data on 53,297 women with breast cancer and 100,239 women without breast cancer from 54 epidemiological studies. Lancet 1996; 347:1713–1727. **96.** Palmer JR, Rosenberg L, Kaufman DW, Warshauer ME, Stolley P, Shapiro S. Oral Contraceptive Use and Liver Cancer. Am J Epidemiol 1989;130:878–882. **97.** Lewis M, Spitzer WO, Heinemann LAJ, MacRae KD, Bruppacher R, Thorogood M on behalf of Transnational Research Group on Oral Contraceptives and Health of Young Women. Third generation oral contraceptives and risk of myocardial infarction: an international case-control study. Br Med J, 1996;312:88–90. **98.** Improving access to quality care in family planning: Medical eligibility criteria for contraceptive use. Geneva, WHO, Family and Reproductive Health, 1996. **99.** Hampton RM, Short M, Bieber E, et al. Comparison of a novel norgestimate/ethinyl estradiol oral contraceptive (Ortho Tri-Cyclen Lo) with the oral contraceptive Loestrin Fe 1/20. Contraception 2001;63:289–295. **100.** Sitteri PK, Murai JT, Hammond GL, Nisker JA, Raymoure WJ, Huhn RW. The serum transport of steroid hormones. Rec Prog Horm Res 1982;38:457–510.

BRIEF SUMMARY PATIENT PACKAGE INSERT

Oral contraceptives, also known as "birth control pills" or "the pill," are taken to prevent pregnancy. When taken correctly without missing any pills, oral contraceptives are highly effective; however the typical failure rate of large numbers of pill users is 5% per year when women who miss pills are included. Forgetting to take pills considerably increases the chances of pregnancy. For most women oral contraceptives are also free of serious or unpleasant side effects.

For the majority of women, oral contraceptives can be taken safely. But there are some women who are at high risk of developing certain serious diseases that can be fatal or may cause temporary or permanent disability. The risks associated with taking oral contraceptives increase significantly if you:

- smoke
- have high blood pressure, diabetes, high cholesterol
- have or have had clotting disorders, heart attack, stroke, angina pectoris, cancer of the breast or sex organs, jaundice or malignant or benign liver tumors

Although cardiovascular disease risks may be increased with oral contraceptive use after age 40 in healthy, nonsmoking women (even with the newer low-dose formulations), there are also greater potential health risks associated with pregnancy in older women.

You should not take the pill if you suspect you are pregnant or have unexplained vaginal bleeding.

Cigarette smoking increases the risk of serious cardiovascular side effects from oral contraceptive use. This risk increases with age and with heavy smoking (15 or more cigarettes per day) and is quite marked in women over 35 years of age. Women who use oral contraceptives are strongly advised not to smoke.

Most side effects of the pill are not serious. The most common such effects are nausea, vomiting, bleeding between menstrual periods, weight gain, breast tenderness, and difficulty wearing contact lenses. These side effects, especially nausea and vomiting, may subside within the first three months of use.

The serious side effects of the pill occur very infrequently, especially if you are in good health and are young. However, you should know that the following medical conditions have been associated with or made worse by the pill:

1. Blood clots in the legs (thrombophlebitis), lungs (pulmonary embolism), stoppage or rupture of a blood vessel in the brain (stroke), blockage of blood vessels in the heart (heart attack or angina pectoris) or other organs of the body. As mentioned above, smoking increases the risk of heart attacks and strokes and subsequent serious medical consequences.
2. In rare cases, oral contraceptives can cause benign but dangerous liver tumors. These benign liver tumors can rupture and cause fatal internal bleeding. In addition, some studies report an increased risk of developing liver cancer. However, liver cancers are rare.
3. High blood pressure, although blood pressure usually returns to normal when the pill is stopped.

The symptoms associated with these serious side effects are discussed in the detailed leaflet given to you with your supply of pills. Notify your doctor or health care professional if you notice any unusual physical disturbances while taking the pill. In addition, drugs such as rifampin, as well as some anti-convulsants and some antibiotics, and herbal preparations containing St. John's Wort (hypericum perforatum) may decrease oral contraceptive effectiveness.

Various studies give conflicting reports on the relationship between breast cancer and oral contraceptive use. Oral contraceptive use may slightly increase your chance of having breast cancer diagnosed, particularly after using hormonal contraceptives at a younger age. After you stop using hormonal contraceptives, the chances of having breast cancer diagnosed begin to go back down. You should have regular breast examinations by a health care professional and examine your own breasts monthly. Tell your health care provider if you have a family history of breast cancer or if you have had breast nodules or an abnormal mammogram. Women who currently have or have had breast cancer should not use oral contraceptives because breast cancer is usually a hormone-sensitive tumor.

Some studies have found an increase in the incidence of cancer of the cervix in women who use oral contraceptives.

However, this finding may be related to factors other than the use of oral contraceptives. There is insufficient evidence to rule out the possibility that the pill may cause such cancers.

Taking the combination pill provides some important noncontraceptive benefits. These include less painful menstruation, less menstrual blood loss and anemia, fewer pelvic infections, and fewer cancers of the ovary and the lining of the uterus.

Be sure to discuss any medical condition you may have with your health care professional. Your health care professional will take a medical and family history before prescribing oral contraceptives and will examine you. The physical examination may be delayed to another time if you request it and the health care professional believes that it is a good medical practice to postpone it. You should be reexamined at least once a year while taking oral contraceptives. Your pharmacist should have given you the detailed patient information labeling which gives you further information which you should read and discuss with your health care professional.

ORTHO TRI-CYCLEN® Lo (like all oral contraceptives) is intended to prevent pregnancy. Oral contraceptives do not protect against transmission of HIV (AIDS) and other sexually transmitted diseases such as chlamydia, genital herpes, genital warts, gonorrhea, hepatitis B, and syphilis.

HOW TO TAKE THE PILL

IMPORTANT POINTS TO REMEMBER

BEFORE YOU START TAKING YOUR PILLS:

1. BE SURE TO READ THESE DIRECTIONS:
Before you start taking your pills.
Anytime you are not sure what to do.

2. THE RIGHT WAY TO TAKE THE PILL IS TO TAKE ONE PILL EVERY DAY AT THE SAME TIME.
If you miss pills you could get pregnant. This includes starting the pack late.
The more pills you miss, the more likely you are to get pregnant.

3. MANY WOMEN HAVE SPOTTING OR LIGHT BLEEDING, OR MAY FEEL SICK TO THEIR STOMACH DURING THE FIRST 1–3 PACKS OF PILLS. If you feel sick to your stomach, do not stop taking the pill. The problem will usually go away. If it doesn't go away, check with your health care professional.

4. MISSING PILLS CAN ALSO CAUSE SPOTTING OR LIGHT BLEEDING, even when you make up these missed pills.
On the days you take 2 pills to make up for missed pills, you could also feel a little sick to your stomach.

5. IF YOU HAVE VOMITING OR DIARRHEA, or IF YOU TAKE SOME MEDICINES, including some antibiotics, your pills may not work as well.
Use a back-up method (such as condoms or spermicides) until you check with your health care professional.

6. IF YOU HAVE TROUBLE REMEMBERING TO TAKE THE PILL, talk to your health care professional about how to make pill-taking easier or about using another method of birth control.

7. IF YOU HAVE ANY QUESTIONS OR ARE UNSURE ABOUT THE INFORMATION IN THIS LEAFLET, call your health care professional.

BEFORE YOU START TAKING YOUR PILLS

1. DECIDE WHAT TIME OF DAY YOU WANT TO TAKE YOUR PILL.
It is important to take it at about the same time every day.

2. The 28-pill pack has 21 white, light blue, and dark blue "active" pills (with hormones) to take for 3 weeks. This is followed by 1 week of "reminder" green pills (without hormones).

3. ALSO FIND:
   1) where on the pack to start taking pills,
   2) in what order to take the pills.

CHECK PICTURE OF PILL PACK AND ADDITIONAL INSTRUCTIONS FOR USING THIS PACKAGE IN THE BRIEF SUMMARY PATIENT PACKAGE INSERT.

4. BE SURE YOU HAVE READY AT ALL TIMES:
ANOTHER KIND OF BIRTH CONTROL (such as condoms or spermicide) to use as a back-up method in case you miss pills.
AN EXTRA, FULL PILL PACK.

WHEN TO START THE FIRST PACK OF PILLS

You have a choice of which day to start taking your first pack of pills. ORTHO TRI-CYCLEN® Lo is available in the DIALPAK® Tablet Dispenser which is preset for a Sunday Start. Day 1 Start is also provided. Decide with your health care professional which is the best day for you. Pick a time of day which will be easy to remember.

SUNDAY START:
Take the first "active" white pill of the first pack on the Sunday after your period starts, even if you are still bleeding. If your period begins on Sunday, start the pack that same day. Use another method of birth control (such as condoms or spermicide) as a back-up method if you have sex anytime from the Sunday you start your first pack until the next Sunday (7 days).

DAY 1 START:
Take the first "active" white pill of the first pack during the first 24 hours of your period.
You will not need to use a back-up method of birth control, since you are starting the pill at the beginning of your period.

WHAT TO DO DURING THE MONTH

1. Take One Pill At The Same Time Every Day Until The Pack Is Empty
Do not skip pills even if you are spotting or bleeding between monthly periods or feel sick to your stomach (nausea).
Do not skip pills even if you do not have sex very often.

2. When You Finish A Pack Or Switch Your Brand Of Pills
Start the next pack on the day after your last "reminder" pill. Do not wait any days between packs.

WHAT TO DO IF YOU MISS PILLS

If you **MISS 1** white, light blue or dark blue "active" pill:
1. Take it as soon as you remember. Take the next pill at your regular time. This means you may take 2 pills in 1 day.
2. You do not need to use a back-up birth control method if you have sex.

If you **MISS 2** white or light blue "active" pills in a row in **WEEK 1 OR WEEK 2** of your pack:
1. Take 2 pills on the day you remember and 2 pills the next day.
2. Then take 1 pill a day until you finish the pack.
3. You COULD BECOME PREGNANT if you have sex in the 7 days after you miss pills. You MUST use another birth control method (such as condoms or spermicide) as a back-up method for those 7 days.

If you **MISS 2** dark blue "active" pills in a row in **THE 3RD WEEK:**
1. **If you are a Sunday Starter:**
Keep taking 1 pill every day until Sunday. On Sunday, THROW OUT the rest of the pack and start a new pack of pills that same day.
If you are a Day 1 Starter:
THROW OUT the rest of the pill pack and start a new pack that same day.
2. You may not have your period this month but this is expected. However, if you miss your period 2 months in a row, call your health care professional because you might be pregnant.
3. You COULD BECOME PREGNANT if you have sex in the 7 days after you miss pills. You MUST use another birth control method (such as condoms or spermicide) as a back-up method for those 7 days.

If you **MISS 3 OR MORE** white, light blue or dark blue "active" pills in a row (during the first 3 weeks):
1. **If you are a Sunday Starter:**
Keep taking 1 pill every day until Sunday. On Sunday, THROW OUT the rest of the pack and start a new pack of pills that same day.
If you are a Day 1 Starter:
THROW OUT the rest of the pill pack and start a new pack that same day.
2. You may not have your period this month but this is expected. However, if you miss your period 2 months in a row, call your health care professional because you might be pregnant.
3. You COULD BECOME PREGNANT if you have sex in the 7 days after you miss pills. You MUST use another birth control method (such as condoms or spermicide) as a back-up method for those 7 days.

If you forget any of the 7 green "reminder" pills in Week 4:
THROW AWAY the pills you missed.
Keep taking 1 pill each day until the pack is empty.
You do not need a back-up method.

FINALLY, IF YOU ARE STILL NOT SURE WHAT TO DO ABOUT THE PILLS YOU HAVE MISSED:
Use a BACK-UP METHOD anytime you have sex.
KEEP TAKING ONE "ACTIVE" PILL EACH DAY until you can reach your health care professional.

INSTRUCTIONS FOR USING YOUR DIALPAK® TABLET DISPENSER

Please Read Me!

☐ Sunday Start or ☐ Day 1 Start

There are two ways to start taking birth control pills: Sunday Start or Day 1 Start.Your health care provider will tell you which to use.

Save these instructions.

1

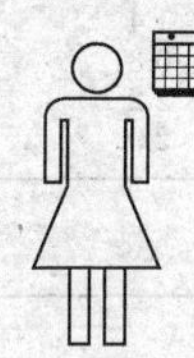

If this is the first time you are taking birth control pills, or if you have not taken birth control pills for 10 days or more, your first step is to **wait until the first day you get your menstrual period.** Then, follow these instructions for either Sunday Start or Day 1 Start.

2

☐ Sunday Start
☐ Day 1 Start

When you get your period:
• You will use a **Sunday Start** if your doctor told you to take your first pill on a Sunday. Take pill "1" on the Sunday after your period starts.
If your period starts on a Sunday, take pill "1" that day.
• You will use a **Day 1 Start** if your doctor told you to take pill "1" on the first day of your period.

3

Dialpak
arrow
dial

SET THE DAY:
☐**Sunday Start:** the arrow on your *empty* Dialpak should point to SU (Sunday).
☐**Day 1 Start:** turn the dial on your *empty* Dialpak until the arrow points to the first day of your period (if your period starts on Tuesday, the arrow will point to TU).

4

refill
snap!
"V"shape

Insert the new refill by lining up the "V" shape on the refill with the "V" shape at the top of your Dialpak. Snap the refill in place. You are ready to take pill "1." You should always begin your pill cycle with pill "1," as shown on the inner part of the refill ring.

5

Remove pill "1" by pushing down on the pill. The pill will come out through a hole in the back of the Dialpak.

6

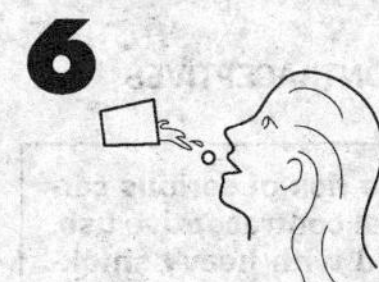

Swallow the pill. You will take one pill each day. If you use a Sunday Start and you are taking the pill for the FIRST TIME, YOU MUST USE A BACK-UP METHOD OF BIRTH CONTROL FOR THE FIRST 7 DAYS. If you use a Day 1 Start, you are protected from becoming pregnant as soon as you take your first pill.

7

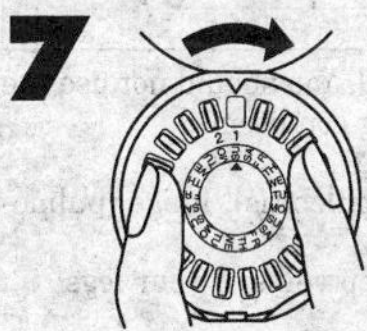

Wait 24 hours to take your next pill. To take pill "2," **turn the dial on your Dialpak** to the next day. Continue to take one pill each day until all the pills have been taken.

8

Take your pill at the same time every day. It is important to take the correct pill each day and not miss any pills. To help you remember, take your pill at the same time as another daily activity, like turning off your alarm clock or brushing your teeth.

9

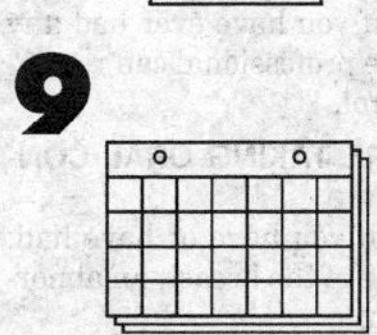

When your refill is empty, keep your Dialpak case. You will start a new refill on the day after pill "28."

10

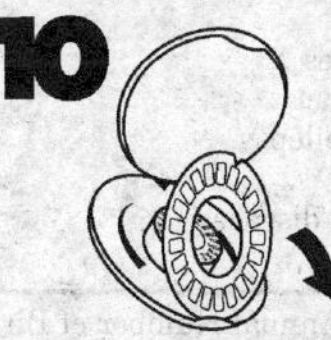

Turn the dial to the pill "1" position to remove the empty refill and insert a new refill. THE FIRST PILL IN EVERY REFILL WILL ALWAYS BE TAKEN ON THE SAME DAY OF THE WEEK, NO MATTER WHEN YOUR NEXT PERIOD STARTS.

DETAILED PATIENT LABELING

PLEASE NOTE: This labeling is revised from time to time as important new medical information becomes available. Therefore, please review this labeling carefully.

ORTHO TRI-CYCLEN® Lo-28 Day Regimen

Each white tablet contains 0.180 mg norgestimate and 0.025 mg ethinyl estradiol.

Each light blue tablet contains 0.215 mg norgestimate and 0.025 mg ethinyl estradiol.

Each dark blue tablet contains 0.250 mg norgestimate and 0.025 mg ethinyl estradiol.

Each green tablet contains inert ingredients.

INTRODUCTION

Any woman who considers using oral contraceptives (the birth control pill or the pill) should understand the benefits and risks of using this form of birth control. This patient labeling will give you much of the information you will need

Continued on next page

Ortho Tri-Cyclen Lo—Cont.

to make this decision and will also help you determine if you are at risk of developing any of the serious side effects of the pill. It will tell you how to use the pill properly so that it will be as effective as possible. However, this labeling is not a replacement for a careful discussion between you and your health care professional. You should discuss the information provided in this labeling with him or her, both when you first start taking the pill and during your revisits. You should also follow your health care professional's advice with regard to regular check-ups while you are on the pill.

EFFECTIVENESS OF ORAL CONTRACEPTIVES FOR CONTRACEPTION

Oral contraceptives or "birth control pills" or "the pill" are used to prevent pregnancy and are more effective than most other non-surgical methods of birth control. When taken correctly without missing any pills, oral contraceptives are highly effective; however, typical failure rates are 5% per year. The chance of becoming pregnant increases with each missed pill during a menstrual cycle.

In comparison, typical failure rates for other non-surgical methods of birth control during the first year of use are as follows:

Implant: <1%
Injection: <1%
IUD: 1 to 2%
Diaphragm with spermicides: 20%
Spermicides alone: 26%
Vaginal sponge: 20 to 40%
Female sterilization: <1%
Male sterilization: <1%
Cervical Cap with spermicide: 20 to 40%
Condom alone (male): 14%
Condom alone (female): 21%
Periodic abstinence: 25%
No methods: 85%
Withdrawal: 19%

WHO SHOULD NOT TAKE ORAL CONTRACEPTIVES

Cigarette smoking increases the risk of serious cardiovascular side effects from oral contraceptive use. This risk increases with age and with heavy smoking (15 or more cigarettes per day) and is quite marked in women over 35 years of age. Women who use oral contraceptives are strongly advised not to smoke.

Some women should not use the pill. You should not use the pill if you have any of the following conditions:

- A history of heart attack or stroke
- Blood clots in the legs (thrombophlebitis), lungs (pulmonary embolism), or eyes
- A history of blood clots in the deep veins of your legs
- Chest pain (angina pectoris)
- Known or suspected breast cancer or cancer of the lining of the uterus, cervix or vagina
- Unexplained vaginal bleeding (until a diagnosis is reached by your doctor)
- Yellowing of the whites of the eyes or of the skin (jaundice) during pregnancy or during previous use of the pill
- Liver tumor (benign or cancerous)
- Known or suspected pregnancy
- If you plan to have surgery with prolonged bedrest

Tell your health care professional if you have ever had any of these conditions. Your health care professional can recommend a safer method of birth control.

OTHER CONSIDERATIONS BEFORE TAKING ORAL CONTRACEPTIVES

Tell your health care professional if you have or have had:

- Breast nodules, fibrocystic disease of the breast, an abnormal breast x-ray or mammogram
- Diabetes
- Elevated cholesterol or triglycerides
- High blood pressure
- Migraine or other headaches or epilepsy
- Mental depression
- Gallbladder, liver, heart or kidney disease
- History of scanty or irregular menstrual periods

Women with any of these conditions should be checked often by their health care professional if they choose to use oral contraceptives.

Also, be sure to inform your health care professional if you smoke or are on any medications.

RISKS OF TAKING ORAL CONTRACEPTIVES

1. Risk of Developing Blood Clots

Blood clots and blockage of blood vessels are one of the most serious side effects of taking oral contraceptives and can cause death or serious disability. In particular, a clot in the legs can cause thrombophlebitis and a clot that travels to the lungs can cause a sudden blocking of the vessel carrying blood to the lungs. Rarely, clots occur in the blood vessels of the eye and may cause blindness, double vision, or impaired vision.

If you take oral contraceptives and need elective surgery, need to stay in bed for a prolonged illness or injury or have recently delivered a baby, you may be at risk of developing blood clots. You should consult your healthcare professional about stopping oral contraceptives four weeks before surgery and not taking oral contraceptives for two weeks after surgery or during bed rest. You should also not take oral contraceptives soon after delivery of a baby. It is advisable to wait for at least four weeks after delivery if you are not breast feeding. If you are breast feeding, you should wait until you have weaned your child before using the pill. (See also the section on Breast Feeding in General Precautions.)

The risk of circulatory disease in oral contraceptive users may be higher in users of high-dose pills and may be greater with longer duration of oral contraceptive use. In addition, some of these increased risks may continue for a number of years after stopping oral contraceptives. The risk of abnormal blood clotting increases with age in both users and nonusers of oral contraceptives, but the increased risk from the oral contraceptive appears to be present at all ages. For women aged 20 to 44 it is estimated that about 1 in 2,000 using oral contraceptives will be hospitalized each year because of abnormal clotting. Among nonusers in the same age group, about 1 in 20,000 would be hospitalized each year. For oral contraceptive users in general, it has been estimated that in women between the ages of 15 and 34 the risk of death due to a circulatory disorder is about 1 in 12,000 per year, whereas for nonusers the rate is about 1 in 50,000 per year. In the age group 35 to 44, the risk is estimated to be about 1 in 2,500 per year for oral contraceptive users and about 1 in 10,000 per year for nonusers.

2. Heart Attacks and Strokes

Oral contraceptives may increase the tendency to develop strokes (stoppage or rupture of blood vessels in the brain) and angina pectoris and heart attacks (blockage of blood vessels in the heart). Any of these conditions can cause death or serious disability.

Smoking greatly increases the possibility of suffering heart attacks and strokes. Furthermore, smoking and the use of oral contraceptives greatly increase the chances of developing and dying of heart disease.

3. Gallbladder Disease

Oral contraceptive users probably have a greater risk than nonusers of having gallbladder disease, although this risk may be related to pills containing high doses of estrogens.

4. Liver Tumors

In rare cases, oral contraceptives can cause benign but dangerous liver tumors. These benign liver tumors can rupture and cause fatal internal bleeding. In addition, some studies report an increased risk of developing liver cancer. However, liver cancers are rare.

5. Cancer of the Reproductive Organs and Breasts

Various studies give conflicting reports on the relationship between breast cancer and oral contraceptive use. Oral contraceptive use may slightly increase your chance of having breast cancer diagnosed, particularly after using hormonal contraceptives at a younger age. After you stop using hormonal contraceptives, the chances of having breast cancer diagnosed begin to go back down. You should have regular breast examinations by a health care professional and examine your own breasts monthly. Tell your health care professional if you have a family history of breast cancer or if you have had breast nodules or an abnormal mammogram. Women who currently have or have had breast cancer should not use oral contraceptives because breast cancer is usually a hormone-sensitive tumor.

Some studies have found an increase in the incidence of cancer of the cervix in women who use oral contraceptives. However, this finding may be related to factors other than the use of oral contraceptives. There is insufficient evidence to rule out the possibility that the pill may cause such cancers.

ESTIMATED RISK OF DEATH FROM A BIRTH CONTROL METHOD OR PREGNANCY

All methods of birth control and pregnancy are associated with a risk of developing certain diseases which may lead to disability or death. An estimate of the number of deaths associated with different methods of birth control and pregnancy has been calculated and is shown in the following table.

[See table 4 below]

Table 4: Annual Number of Birth-Related or Method-Related Deaths Associated with Control of Fertility Per 100,000 Nonsterile Women, By Fertility-Control Method and According to Age

Method of control and outcome	15–19	20–24	25–29	30–34	35–39	40–44
No fertility-control methods*	7.0	7.4	9.1	14.8	25.7	28.2
Oral contraceptives nonsmoker**	[illegible]	[illegible]	[illegible]	[illegible]	[illegible]	[illegible]
Oral contraceptives smoker**	2.2	3.4	6.6	13.5	51.1	117.2
IUD**	0.8	0.8	1.0	1.0	1.4	1.4
Condom*	1.1	1.6	0.7	0.2	0.3	0.4
Diaphragm/spermicide*	1.9	1.2	1.2	1.3	2.2	2.8
Periodic abstinence*	2.5	1.6	1.6	1.7	2.9	3.6

* Deaths are birth-related
**Deaths are method-related

Adapted from H.W. Ory, Family Planning Perspectives, Ref. #35.

In the above table, the risk of death from any birth control method is less than the risk of childbirth, except for oral contraceptive users over the age of 35 who smoke and pill users over the age of 40 even if they do not smoke. It can be seen in the table that for women aged 15 to 39, the risk of death was highest with pregnancy (7–26 deaths per 100,000 women, depending on age). Among pill users who do not smoke, the risk of death was always lower than that associated with pregnancy for any age group, although over the age of 40, the risk increases to 32 deaths per 100,000 women, compared to 28 associated with pregnancy at that age. However, for pill users who smoke and are over the age of 35, the estimated number of deaths exceeds those for other methods of birth control. If a woman is over the age of 40 and smokes, her estimated risk of death is four times higher (117/100,000 women) than the estimated risk associated with pregnancy (28/100,000 women) in that age group.

The suggestion that women over 40 who do not smoke should not take oral contraceptives is based on information from older, higher-dose pills. An Advisory Committee of the FDA discussed this issue in 1989 and recommended that the benefits of low-dose oral contraceptive use by healthy, non-smoking women over 40 years of age may outweigh the possible risks. Older women, as all women, who take oral contraceptives, should take an oral contraceptive which contains the least amount of estrogen and progestogen that is compatible with the individual patient needs.

WARNING SIGNALS

If any of these adverse effects occur while you are taking oral contraceptives, call your doctor immediately:

- Sharp chest pain, coughing of blood, or sudden shortness of breath (indicating a possible clot in the lung)
- Pain in the calf (indicating a possible clot in the leg)
- Crushing chest pain or heaviness in the chest (indicating a possible heart attack)
- Sudden severe headache or vomiting, dizziness or fainting, disturbances of vision or speech, weakness, or numbness in an arm or leg (indicating a possible stroke)
- Sudden partial or complete loss of vision (indicating a possible clot in the eye)
- Breast lumps (indicating possible breast cancer or fibrocystic disease of the breast; ask your doctor or health care professional to show you how to examine your breasts)
- Severe pain or tenderness in the stomach area (indicating a possibly ruptured liver tumor)
- Difficulty in sleeping, weakness, lack of energy, fatigue, or change in mood (possibly indicating severe depression)
- Jaundice or a yellowing of the skin or eyeballs, accompanied frequently by fever, fatigue, loss of appetite, dark colored urine, or light colored bowel movements (indicating possible liver problems)

SIDE EFFECTS OF ORAL CONTRACEPTIVES

1. Vaginal Bleeding

Irregular vaginal bleeding or spotting may occur while you are taking the pills. Irregular bleeding may vary from slight staining between menstrual periods to breakthrough bleeding which is a flow much like a regular period. Irregular bleeding occurs most often during the first few months of oral contraceptive use, but may also occur after you have been taking the pill for some time. Such bleeding may be temporary and usually does not indicate any serious problems. It is important to continue taking your pills on schedule. If the bleeding occurs in more than one cycle or lasts for more than a few days, talk to your health care professional.

2. Contact Lenses

If you wear contact lenses and notice a change in vision or an inability to wear your lenses, contact your health care professional.

3. Fluid Retention

Oral contraceptives may cause edema (fluid retention) with swelling of the fingers or ankles and may raise your blood pressure. If you experience fluid retention, contact your health care professional.

4. Melasma

A spotty darkening of the skin is possible, particularly of the face, which may persist.

5. Other Side Effects

Other side effects may include nausea and vomiting, change in appetite, headache, nervousness, depression, dizziness, loss of scalp hair, rash, and vaginal infections.

If any of these side effects bother you, call your health care professional.

GENERAL PRECAUTIONS

1. Missed Periods and Use of Oral Contraceptives Before or During Early Pregnancy

There may be times when you may not menstruate regularly after you have completed taking a cycle of pills. If you have taken your pills regularly and miss one menstrual period, continue taking your pills for the next cycle but be sure to inform your health care professional. If you have not taken the pills daily as instructed and missed a menstrual period, you may be pregnant. If you missed two consecutive menstrual periods, you may be pregnant. Check with your health care professional immediately to determine whether you are pregnant. Stop taking oral contraceptives if pregnancy is confirmed.

There is no conclusive evidence that oral contraceptive use is associated with an increase in birth defects, when taken inadvertently during early pregnancy. Previously, a few studies had reported that oral contraceptives might be associated with birth defects, but these findings have not been seen in more recent studies. Nevertheless, oral contraceptives should not be used during pregnancy. You should check with your healthcare provider about risks to your unborn child of any medication taken during pregnancy.

2. While Breast-Feeding

If you are breast-feeding, consult your healthcare professional before starting oral contraceptives. Some of the drug will be passed on to the child in the milk. A few adverse effects on the child have been reported, including yellowing of the skin (jaundice) and breast enlargement. In addition, oral contraceptives may decrease the amount and quality of your milk. If possible, do not use oral contraceptives while breast-feeding. You should use another method of contraception since breast feeding provides only partial protection from becoming pregnant and this partial protection decreases significantly as you breast feed for longer periods of time. You should consider starting oral contraceptives only after you have weaned your child completely.

3. Laboratory Tests

If you are scheduled for any laboratory tests, tell your healthcare professional you are taking birth control pills. Certain blood tests may be affected by birth control pills.

4. Drug Interactions

Certain drugs may interact with birth control pills to make them less effective in preventing pregnancy or cause an increase in breakthrough bleeding. Such drugs include rifampin, drugs used for epilepsy such as barbiturates (for example, phenobarbital), topiramate (TOPAMAX), carbamazepine (Tegretol is one brand of this drug), or phenytoin (Dilantin is one brand of this drug); phenylbutazone (Butazolidin is one brand); certain drugs used in the treatment of HIV or AIDS; and possibly certain antibiotics. Pregnancies and breakthrough bleeding have been reported by women who also used some form of the herbal supplement St. John's Wort while using combined hormonal contraceptives. You may need to use additional contraception when you take other products which can make oral contraceptives less effective. Be sure to tell your healthcare provider if you are taking or start taking any medications while taking birth control pills.

5. Sexually Transmitted Diseases

ORTHO TRI-CYCLEN® Lo (like all oral contraceptives) is intended to prevent pregnancy. Oral contraceptives do not protect against transmission of HIV (AIDS) and other sexually transmitted diseases such as chlamydia, genital herpes, genital warts, gonorrhea, hepatitis B, and syphilis.

HOW TO TAKE THE PILL

IMPORTANT POINTS TO REMEMBER

BEFORE YOU START TAKING YOUR PILLS:

1. BE SURE TO READ THESE DIRECTIONS:
Before you start taking your pills.
Anytime you are not sure what to do.

2. THE RIGHT WAY TO TAKE THE PILL IS TO TAKE ONE PILL EVERY DAY AT THE SAME TIME.
If you miss pills you could get pregnant. This includes starting the pack late.
The more pills you miss, the more likely you are to get pregnant.

3. MANY WOMEN HAVE SPOTTING OR LIGHT BLEEDING, OR MAY FEEL SICK TO THEIR STOMACH DURING THE FIRST 1–3 PACKS OF PILLS. If you feel sick to your stomach, do not stop taking the pill. The problem will usually go away. If it doesn't go away, check with your health care professional.

4. MISSING PILLS CAN ALSO CAUSE SPOTTING OR LIGHT BLEEDING, even when you make up these missed pills.
On the days you take 2 pills to make up for missed pills, you could also feel a little sick to your stomach.

5. IF YOU HAVE VOMITING OR DIARRHEA, or IF YOU TAKE SOME MEDICINES, including some antibiotics, your pills may not work as well.
Use a back-up method (such as condoms or spermicides) until you check with your health care professional.

6. IF YOU HAVE TROUBLE REMEMBERING TO TAKE THE PILL, talk to your health care professional about how to make pill-taking easier or about using another method of birth control.

7. IF YOU HAVE ANY QUESTIONS OR ARE UNSURE ABOUT THE INFORMATION IN THIS LEAFLET, call your health care professional.

BEFORE YOU START TAKING YOUR PILLS

1. DECIDE WHAT TIME OF DAY YOU WANT TO TAKE YOUR PILL.
It is important to take it at about the same time every day.

2. The pack has 21 white, light blue, and dark blue "active" pills (with hormones) to take for 3 weeks. This is followed by 1 week of "reminder" green pills (without hormones).

3. ALSO FIND:
 1) where on the pack to start taking pills,
 2) in what order to take the pills.
CHECK PICTURE OF PILL PACK AND ADDITIONAL INSTRUCTIONS FOR USING THIS PACKAGE IN THE BRIEF SUMMARY PATIENT PACKAGE INSERT.

4. BE SURE YOU HAVE READY AT ALL TIMES:
ANOTHER KIND OF BIRTH CONTROL (such as condoms or spermicide) to use as a back-up method in case you miss pills.
AN EXTRA, FULL PILL PACK.

WHEN TO START THE FIRST PACK OF PILLS

You have a choice of which day to start taking your first pack of pills. ORTHO TRI-CYCLEN® Lo is available in the DIALPAK® Tablet Dispenser which is preset for a Sunday Start. Day 1 Start is also provided. Decide with your health care professional which is the best day for you. Pick a time of day which will be easy to remember.

SUNDAY START:

Take the first "active" white pill of the first pack on the Sunday after your period starts, even if you are still bleeding. If your period begins on Sunday, start the pack that same day. Use another method of birth control (such as condoms or spermicide) as a back-up method if you have sex anytime from the Sunday you start your first pack until the next Sunday (7 days).

DAY 1 START:

Take the first "active" white pill of the first pack during the first 24 hours of your period.
You will not need to use a back-up method of birth control, since you are starting the pill at the beginning of your period.

WHAT TO DO DURING THE MONTH

1. Take One Pill At The Same Time Every Day Until The Pack Is Empty

Do not skip pills even if you are spotting or bleeding between monthly periods or feel sick to your stomach (nausea).
Do not skip pills even if you do not have sex very often.

2. When You Finish A Pack Or Switch Your Brand Of Pills

Start the next pack on the day after your last "reminder" pill. Do not wait any days between packs.

WHAT TO DO IF YOU MISS PILLS

If you **MISS 1** white, light blue or dark blue "active" pill:
1. Take it as soon as you remember. Take the next pill at your regular time. This means you may take 2 pills in 1 day.
2. You do not need to use a back-up birth control method if you have sex.

If you **MISS 2** white or light blue "active" pills in a row in **WEEK 1 OR WEEK 2** of your pack:
1. Take 2 pills on the day you remember and 2 pills the next day.
2. Then take 1 pill a day until you finish the pack.
3. You COULD BECOME PREGNANT if you have sex in the 7 days after you miss pills. You MUST use another birth control method (such as condoms or spermicide) as a back-up method for those 7 days.

If you **MISS 2** dark blue "active" pills in a row in **THE 3RD WEEK:**

1. If you are a Sunday Starter:
Keep taking 1 pill every day until Sunday. On Sunday, THROW OUT the rest of the pack and start a new pack of pills that same day.
If you are a Day 1 Starter:
THROW OUT the rest of the pill pack and start a new pack that same day.
2. You may not have your period this month but this is expected. However, if you miss your period 2 months in a row, call your health care professional because you might be pregnant.
3. You COULD BECOME PREGNANT if you have sex in the 7 days after you miss pills. You MUST use another birth control method (such as condoms or spermicide) as a back-up method for those 7 days.

If you **MISS 3 OR MORE** white, light blue or dark blue "active" pills in a row (during the first 3 weeks):

1. If you are a Sunday Starter:
Keep taking 1 pill every day until Sunday. On Sunday, THROW OUT the rest of the pack and start a new pack of pills that same day.
If you are a Day 1 Starter:
THROW OUT the rest of the pill pack and start a new pack that same day.
2. You may not have your period this month but this is expected. However, if you miss your period 2 months in a row, call your health care professional because you might be pregnant.
3. You COULD BECOME PREGNANT if you have sex in the 7 days after you miss pills. You MUST use another birth control method (such as condoms or spermicide) as a back-up method for those 7 days.

If you forget any of the 7 green "reminder" pills in Week 4: THROW AWAY the pills you missed.
Keep taking 1 pill each day until the pack is empty.
You do not need a back-up method.

FINALLY, IF YOU ARE STILL NOT SURE WHAT TO DO ABOUT THE PILLS YOU HAVE MISSED:

Use a BACK-UP METHOD anytime you have sex.
KEEP TAKING ONE "ACTIVE" PILL EACH DAY until you can reach your health care provider.

PREGNANCY DUE TO PILL FAILURE

When taken correctly without missing any pills, oral contraceptives are highly effective; however the typical failure rate of large numbers of pill users is 5% per year when women who miss pills are included. If failure does occur, the risk to the fetus is minimal.

PREGNANCY AFTER STOPPING THE PILL

There may be some delay in becoming pregnant after you stop using oral contraceptives, especially if you had irregular menstrual cycles before you used oral contraceptives. It may be advisable to postpone conception until you begin menstruating regularly once you have stopped taking the pill and desire pregnancy.

There does not appear to be any increase in birth defects in newborn babies when pregnancy occurs soon after stopping the pill.

OVERDOSAGE

Serious ill effects have not been reported following ingestion of large doses of oral contraceptives by young children. Overdosage may cause nausea and withdrawal bleeding in females. In cases of overdosage, contact your health care professional or pharmacist.

OTHER INFORMATION

Your health care professional will take a medical and family history before prescribing oral contraceptives and will examine you. The physical examination may be delayed to another time if you request it and the health care professional believes that it is a good medical practice to postpone it. You should be reexamined at least once a year. Be sure to inform your health care professional if there is a family history of any of the conditions listed previously in this leaflet. Be sure to keep all appointments with your health care professional, because this is a time to determine if there are early signs of side effects of oral contraceptive use.

Do not use the drug for any condition other than the one for which it was prescribed. This drug has been prescribed specifically for you; do not give it to others who may want birth control pills.

HEALTH BENEFITS FROM ORAL CONTRACEPTIVES

In addition to preventing pregnancy, use of combination oral contraceptives may provide certain benefits. They are:

- menstrual cycles may become more regular
- blood flow during menstruation may be lighter and less iron may be lost. Therefore, anemia due to iron deficiency is less likely to occur.
- pain or other symptoms during menstruation may be encountered less frequently
- ectopic (tubal) pregnancy may occur less frequently
- noncancerous cysts or lumps in the breast may occur less frequently
- acute pelvic inflammatory disease may occur less frequently
- oral contraceptive use may provide some protection against developing two forms of cancer: cancer of the ovaries and cancer of the lining of the uterus

If you want more information about birth control pills, ask your doctor/health care professional or pharmacist. They have a more technical leaflet called the Professional Labeling, which you may wish to read. The professional labeling is also published in a book entitled *Physicians' Desk Reference*, available in many bookstores and public libraries.

ORTHO-McNEIL PHARMACEUTICAL, INC.
Raritan, New Jersey 08869
© OMP 2002 Issued August 2002 635-50-951-1

Shown in Product Identification Guide, page 328

TOPAMAX® ℞

[*tō-pă-măks*]
(topiramate)
Tablets

TOPAMAX® ℞

(topiramate capsules)
Sprinkle Capsules

Prescribing Information

DESCRIPTION

Topiramate is a sulfamate-substituted monosaccharide that is intended for use as an antiepileptic drug. TOPAMAX® (topiramate) Tablets are available as 25 mg, 50 mg, 100 mg, and 200 mg round tablets for oral administration. TOPAMAX® (topiramate capsules) Sprinkle Capsules are available as 15 mg and 25 mg sprinkle capsules for oral administration as whole capsules or opened and sprinkled onto soft food.

Continued on next page

Topamax—Cont.

Topiramate is a white crystalline powder with a bitter taste. Topiramate is most soluble in alkaline solutions containing sodium hydroxide or sodium phosphate and having a pH of 9 to 10. It is freely soluble in acetone, chloroform, dimethylsulfoxide, and ethanol. The solubility in water is 9.8 mg/mL. Its saturated solution has a pH of 6.3. Topiramate has the molecular formula $C_{12}H_{21}NO_8S$ and a molecular weight of 339.37. Topiramate is designated chemically as 2,3:4,5-Di-*O*-isopropylidene-β-D-fructopyranose sulfamate and has the following structural formula:

TOPAMAX® (topiramate) Tablets contain the following inactive ingredients: lactose monohydrate, pregelatinized starch, microcrystalline cellulose, sodium starch glycolate, magnesium stearate, purified water, carnauba wax, hypromellose, titanium dioxide, polyethylene glycol, synthetic iron oxide (100 and 200 mg tablets) and polysorbate 80.

TOPAMAX® (topiramate capsules) Sprinkle Capsules contain topiramate coated beads in a hard gelatin capsule. The inactive ingredients are: sugar spheres (sucrose and starch), povidone, cellulose acetate, gelatin, silicone dioxide, sodium lauryl sulfate, titanium dioxide, and black pharmaceutical ink.

CLINICAL PHARMACOLOGY

Mechanism of Action:

The precise mechanism by which topiramate exerts its antiseizure effect is unknown; however, preclinical studies have revealed four properties that may contribute to topiramate's antiepileptic efficacy. Electrophysiological and biochemical evidence suggests that topiramate, at pharmacologically relevant concentrations, blocks voltage-dependent sodium channels, augments the activity of the neurotransmitter gamma-aminobutyrate at some subtypes of the GABA-A receptor, antagonizes the kainate subtype of the glutamate receptor, and inhibits the carbonic anhydrase enzyme, particularly isozymes II and IV.

Pharmacodynamics:

Topiramate has anticonvulsant activity in rat and mouse maximal electroshock seizure (MES) tests. Topiramate is only weakly effective in blocking clonic seizures induced by the $GABA_A$ receptor antagonist, pentylenetetrazole. Topiramate is also effective in rodent models of epilepsy, which include tonic and absence-like seizures in the spontaneous epileptic rat (SER) and tonic and clonic seizures induced in rats by kindling of the amygdala or by global ischemia.

Pharmacokinetics:

The sprinkle formulation is bioequivalent to the immediate release tablet formulation and, therefore, may be substituted as a therapeutic equivalent.

Absorption of topiramate is rapid, with peak plasma concentrations occurring at approximately 2 hours following a 400 mg oral dose. The relative bioavailability of topiramate from the tablet formulation is about 80% compared to a solution. The bioavailability of topiramate is not affected by food.

The pharmacokinetics of topiramate are linear with dose proportional increases in plasma concentration over the dose range studied (200 to 800 mg/day). The mean plasma elimination half-life is 21 hours after single or multiple doses. Steady state is thus reached in about 4 days in patients with normal renal function. Topiramate is 13-17% bound to human plasma proteins over the concentration range of 1-250 µg/mL.

Metabolism and Excretion:

Topiramate is not extensively metabolized and is primarily eliminated unchanged in the urine (approximately 70% of an administered dose). Six metabolites have been identified in humans, none of which constitutes more than 5% of an administered dose. The metabolites are formed via hydroxylation, hydrolysis, and glucuronidation. There is evidence of renal tubular reabsorption of topiramate. In rats, given probenecid to inhibit tubular reabsorption, along with topiramate, a significant increase in renal clearance of topiramate was observed. This interaction has not been evaluated in humans. Overall, oral plasma clearance (CL/F) is approximately 20 to 30 mL/min in humans following oral administration.

Pharmacokinetic Interactions (see also Drug Interactions):

Antiepileptic Drugs

Potential interactions between topiramate and standard AEDs were assessed in controlled clinical pharmacokinetic studies in patients with epilepsy. The effect of these interactions on mean plasma AUCs are summarized under **PRECAUTIONS (Table 3).**

Special Populations:

Renal Impairment:

The clearance of topiramate was reduced by 42% in moderately renally impaired (creatinine clearance 30-69 mL/min/1.73m^2) and by 54% in severely renally impaired subjects (creatinine clearance <30 mL/min/1.73m^2) compared to normal renal function subjects (creatinine clearance >70 mL/min/1.73m^2). Since topiramate is presumed to undergo significant tubular reabsorption, it is uncertain whether this experience can be generalized to all situations of renal impairment. It is conceivable that some forms of renal disease could differentially affect glomerular filtration rate and tubular reabsorption resulting in a clearance of topiramate not predicted by creatinine clearance. In general, however, use of one-half the usual starting and maintenance dose is recommended in patients with moderate or severe renal impairment (see **PRECAUTIONS: General** and **DOSAGE AND ADMINISTRATION**).

Hemodialysis:

Topiramate is cleared by hemodialysis. Using a high efficiency, counterflow, single pass-dialysate hemodialysis procedure, topiramate dialysis clearance was 120 mL/min with blood flow through the dialyzer at 400 mL/min. This high clearance (compared to 20-30 mL/min total oral clearance in healthy adults) will remove a clinically significant amount of topiramate from the patient over the hemodialysis treatment period. Therefore, a supplemental dose may be required (see **DOSAGE AND ADMINISTRATION**).

Hepatic Impairment:

In hepatically impaired subjects, the clearance of topiramate may be decreased; the mechanism underlying the decrease is not well understood.

Age, Gender, and Race:

The pharmacokinetics of topiramate in elderly subjects (65-85 years of age, N=16) were evaluated in a controlled clinical study. The elderly subject population had reduced renal function [creatinine clearance (-20%)] compared to young adults. Following a single oral 100 mg dose, maximum plasma concentration for elderly and young adults was achieved at approximately 1-2 hours. Reflecting the primary renal elimination of topiramate, topiramate plasma and renal clearance were reduced 21% and 19%, respectively, in elderly subjects, compared to young adults. Similarly, topiramate half-life was longer (13%) in the elderly. Reduced topiramate clearance resulted in slightly higher maximum plasma concentration (23%) and AUC (25%) in elderly subjects than observed in young adults. Topiramate clearance is decreased in the elderly only to the extent that renal function is reduced. As recommended for all patients, dosage adjustment may be indicated in the elderly patient when impaired renal function (creatinine clearance rate ≤70 mL/min/1.73 m^2) is evident. It may be useful to monitor renal function in the elderly patient (see **Special Populations: Renal Impairment, PRECAUTIONS: General** and **DOSAGE AND ADMINISTRATION**).

Clearance of topiramate in adults was not affected by gender or race.

Pediatric Pharmacokinetics:

Pharmacokinetics of topiramate were evaluated in patients ages 4 to 17 years receiving one or two other antiepileptic drugs. Pharmacokinetic profiles were obtained after one week at doses of 1, 3, and 9 mg/kg/day. Clearance was independent of dose.

Pediatric patients have a 50% higher clearance and consequently shorter elimination half-life than adults. Consequently, the plasma concentration for the same mg/kg dose may be lower in pediatric patients compared to adults. As in adults, hepatic enzyme-inducing antiepileptic drugs decrease the steady state plasma concentrations of topiramate.

CLINICAL STUDIES

The results of controlled clinical trials established the efficacy of TOPAMAX® (topiramate) Tablets and TOPAMAX® (topiramate capsules) Sprinkle Capsules as adjunctive therapy in adults and pediatric patients ages 2-16 years with partial onset seizures or primary generalized tonic-clonic seizures, and in patients 2 years of age and older with seizures associated with Lennox-Gastaut syndrome.

The studies described in the following sections were conducted using TOPAMAX® (topiramate) Tablets.

Controlled Trials in Patients With Partial Onset Seizures

Adults With Partial Onset Seizures

The effectiveness of topiramate as an adjunctive treatment for adults with partial onset seizures was established in six multicenter, randomized, double-blind, placebo-controlled trials, two comparing several dosages of topiramate and placebo and four comparing a single dosage with placebo, in patients with a history of partial onset seizures, with or without secondarily generalized seizures.

Patients in these studies were permitted a maximum of two antiepileptic drugs (AEDs) in addition to TOPAMAX® Tablets or placebo. In each study, patients were stabilized on optimum dosages of their concomitant AEDs during the baseline phase lasting between 4 and 12 weeks. Patients who experienced a prespecified minimum number of partial onset seizures, with or without secondary generalization, during the baseline phase (12 seizures for 12-week baseline, 8 for 8-week baseline, or 3 for 4-week baseline) were randomly assigned to placebo or a specified dose of TOPAMAX® Tablets in addition to their other AEDs.

Following randomization, patients began the double-blind phase of treatment. In five of the six studies, patients received active drug beginning at 100 mg per day; the dose was then increased by 100 mg or 200 mg/day increments weekly or every other week until the assigned dose was reached, unless intolerance prevented increases. In the sixth study (119), the 25 or 50 mg/day initial doses of topiramate were followed by respective weekly increments of 25 or 50 mg/day until the target dose of 200 mg/day was reached. After titration, patients entered a 4, 8, or 12-week stabilization period. The numbers of patients randomized to each dose, and the actual mean and median doses in the stabilization period are shown in Table 1.

Pediatric Patients Ages 2-16 Years With Partial Onset Seizures

The effectiveness of topiramate as an adjunctive treatment for pediatric patients ages 2 -16 years with partial onset seizures was established in a multicenter, randomized, double-blind, placebo-controlled trial, comparing topiramate and placebo in patients with a history of partial onset seizures, with or without secondarily generalized seizures.

Patients in this study were permitted a maximum of two antiepileptic drugs (AEDs) in addition to TOPAMAX® Tablets or placebo. In this study, patients were stabilized on optimum dosages of their concomitant AEDs during an 8-week baseline phase. Patients who experienced at least six partial onset seizures, with or without secondarily generalized seizures, during the baseline phase were randomly assigned to placebo or TOPAMAX® Tablets in addition to their other AEDs.

Following randomization, patients began the double-blind phase of treatment. Patients received active drug beginning at 25 or 50 mg per day; the dose was then increased by 25 mg to 150 mg/day increments every other week until the assigned dosage of 125, 175, 225, or 400 mg/day based on patients' weight to approximate a dosage of 6 mg/kg per day was reached, unless intolerance prevented increases. After titration, patients entered an 8-week stabilization period.

Controlled Trials in Patients With Primary Generalized Tonic-Clonic Seizures

The effectiveness of topiramate as an adjunctive treatment for primary generalized tonic-clonic seizures in patients 2 years old and older was established in a multicenter, randomized, double-blind, placebo-controlled trial, comparing a single dosage of topiramate and placebo.

Patients in this study were permitted a maximum of two antiepileptic drugs (AEDs) in addition to TOPAMAX® or placebo. Patients were stabilized on optimum dosages of their concomitant AEDs during an 8-week baseline phase. Patients who experienced at least three primary generalized tonic-clonic seizures during the baseline phase were randomly assigned to placebo or TOPAMAX® in addition to their other AEDs.

Following randomization, patients began the double-blind phase of treatment. Patients received active drug beginning at 50 mg per day for four weeks; the dose was then increased by 50 mg to 150 mg/day increments every other week until the assigned dose of 175, 225, or 400 mg/day based on patients' body weight to approximate a dosage of 6 mg/kg per day was reached, unless intolerance prevented increases. After titration, patients entered a 12-week stabilization period.

Controlled Trial in Patients With Lennox-Gastaut Syndrome

The effectiveness of topiramate as an adjunctive treatment for seizures associated with Lennox-Gastaut syndrome was established in a multicenter, randomized, double-blind, placebo-controlled trial comparing a single dosage of topiramate with placebo in patients 2 years of age and older.

Patients in this study were permitted a maximum of two antiepileptic drugs (AEDs) in addition to TOPAMAX® or placebo. Patients who were experiencing at least 60 seizures per month before study entry were stabilized on optimum dosages of their concomitant AEDs during a four week baseline phase. Following baseline, patients were randomly assigned to placebo or TOPAMAX® in addition to their other AEDs. Active drug was titrated beginning at 1 mg/kg per day for a week; the dose was then increased to 3 mg/kg per day for one week then to 6 mg/kg per day. After titration, patients entered an 8-week stabilization period. The primary measures of effectiveness were the percent reduction in drop attacks and a parental global rating of seizure severity.

[See table 1 at top of next page]

In all add-on trials, the reduction in seizure rate from baseline during the entire double-blind phase was measured. The median percent reductions in seizure rates and the responder rates (fraction of patients with at least a 50% reduction) by treatment group for each study are shown below in Table 2. As described above, a global improvement in seizure severity was also assessed in the Lennox-Gastaut trial.

[See table 2 at top of next page]

Subset analyses of the antiepileptic efficacy of TOPAMAX® Tablets in these studies showed no differences as a function of gender, race, age, baseline seizure rate, or concomitant AED.

INDICATIONS AND USAGE

TOPAMAX® (topiramate) Tablets and TOPAMAX® (topiramate capsules) Sprinkle Capsules are indicated as adjunctive therapy for adults and pediatric patients ages [illegible] 16 years with partial [illegible] alized tonic-clonic seizures, and in patients 2 years of age and older with seizures associated with Lennox-Gastaut syndrome.

CONTRAINDICATIONS

TOPAMAX® is contraindicated in patients with a history of hypersensitivity to any component of this product.

WARNINGS

Metabolic Acidosis

Hyperchloremic, non-anion gap, metabolic acidosis (i.e., decreased serum bicarbonate below the normal reference range in the absence of chronic respiratory alkalosis) is associated with topiramate treatment. This metabolic acidosis is caused by renal bicarbonate loss due to the inhibitory effect of topiramate on carbonic anhydrase. Such electrolyte imbalance has been observed with the use of topiramate in placebo-controlled clinical trials and in the post-marketing period. Generally, topiramate-induced metabolic acidosis occurs early in treatment although cases can occur at any time during treatment. Bicarbonate decrements are usually mild-moderate (average decrease of 4 mEq/L at daily doses of 400 mg in adults and at approximately 6 mg/kg/day in pediatric patients); rarely, patients can experience severe decrements to values below 10 mEq/L. Conditions or therapies that predispose to acidosis (such as renal disease, severe respiratory disorders, status epilepticus, diarrhea, surgery, ketogenic diet, or drugs) may be additive to the bicarbonate lowering effects of topiramate.

In adults, the incidence of persistent treatment-emergent decreases in serum bicarbonate (levels of <20 mEq/L at two consecutive visits or at the final visit) in controlled clinical trials for adjunctive treatment of epilepsy was 32% for 400 mg/day, and 1% for placebo. Metabolic acidosis has been observed at doses as low as 50 mg/day. The incidence of a markedly abnormally low serum bicarbonate (i.e., absolute value <17 mEq/L and >5 mEq/L decrease from pretreatment) in these trials was 3% for 400 mg/day, and 0% for placebo. Serum bicarbonate levels have not been systematically evaluated at daily doses greater than 400 mg/day.

In pediatric patients (<16 years of age), the incidence of persistent treatment-emergent decreases in serum bicarbonate in placebo-controlled trials for adjunctive treatment of Lennox-Gastaut syndrome or refractory partial onset seizures was 67% for TOPAMAX (at approximately 6 mg/kg/day), and 10% for placebo. The incidence of a markedly abnormally low serum bicarbonate (i.e., absolute value <17 mEq/L and >5 mEq/L decrease from pretreatment) in these trials was 11% for TOPAMAX and 0% for placebo. Cases of moderately severe metabolic acidosis have been reported in patients as young as 5 months old, especially at daily doses above 5 mg/kg/day.

Although not approved for the prophylaxis of migraine, the incidence of persistent treatment-emergent decreases in serum bicarbonate in placebo-controlled trials for adults for prophylaxis of migraine was 44% for 200 mg/day, 39% for 100 mg/day, 23% for 50 mg/day, and 7% for placebo. The incidence of a markedly abnormally low serum bicarbonate (i.e., absolute value <17 mEq/L and >5 mEq/L decrease from pretreatment) in these trials was 11% for 200 mg/day, 9% for 100 mg/day, 2% for 50 mg/day, and <1% for placebo.

Some manifestations of acute or chronic metabolic acidosis may include hyperventilation, nonspecific symptoms such as fatigue and anorexia, or more severe sequelae including cardiac arrhythmias or stupor. Chronic, untreated metabolic acidosis may increase the risk for nephrolithiasis or nephrocalcinosis, and may also result in osteomalacia (referred to as rickets in pediatric patients) and/or osteoporosis with an increased risk for fractures. Chronic metabolic acidosis in pediatric patients may also reduce growth rates. A reduction in growth rate may eventually decrease the maximal height achieved. The effect of topiramate on growth and bone-related sequelae has not been systematically investigated.

Measurement of baseline and periodic serum bicarbonate during topiramate treatment is recommended. If metabolic acidosis develops and persists, consideration should be given to reducing the dose or discontinuing topiramate (using dose tapering). If the decision is made to continue patients on topiramate in the face of persistent acidosis, alkali treatment should be considered.

Acute Myopia and Secondary Angle Closure Glaucoma

A syndrome consisting of acute myopia associated with secondary angle closure glaucoma has been reported in patients receiving TOPAMAX®. Symptoms include acute onset of decreased visual acuity and/or ocular pain. Opthalmologic findings can include myopia, anterior chamber shallowing, ocular hyperemia (redness) and increased intraocular pressure. Mydriasis may or may not be present. This syndrome may be associated with supraciliary effusion resulting in anterior displacement of the lens and iris, with secondary angle closure glaucoma. Symptoms typically occur within 1 month of initiating TOPAMAX® therapy. In contrast to primary narrow angle glaucoma, which is rare under 40 years of age, secondary angle closure glaucoma associated with topiramate has been reported in pediatric patients as well as adults. The primary treatment to reverse symptoms is discontinuation of TOPAMAX® as rapidly as possible, according to the judgement of the treating physician. Other measures, in conjunction with discontinuation of TOPAMAX®, may be helpful.

Elevated intraocular pressure of any etiology, if left untreated, can lead to serious sequelae including permanent vision loss.

Oligohidrosis and Hyperthermia

Oligohidrosis (decreased sweating), infrequently resulting in hospitalization, has been reported in association with TOPAMAX® use. Decreased sweating and an elevation in body temperature above normal characterized these cases. Some of the cases were reported after exposure to elevated environmental temperatures.

The majority of the reports have been in children. Patients, especially pediatric patients, treated with TOPAMAX® should be monitored closely for evidence of decreased sweating and increased body temperature, especially in hot weather. Caution should be used when TOPAMAX® is prescribed with other drugs that predispose patients to heat-related disorders; these drugs include, but are not limited to, other carbonic anhydrase inhibitors and drugs with anticholinergic activity.

Withdrawal of AEDs

Antiepileptic drugs, including TOPAMAX®, should be withdrawn gradually to minimize the potential of increased seizure frequency.

Cognitive/Neuropsychiatric Adverse Events

Adults

Adverse events most often associated with the use of TOPAMAX® were central nervous system related. In adults, the most significant of these can be classified into three general categories: 1) psychomotor slowing, difficulty with concentration, and speech or language problems, in particular, word-finding difficulties 2) somnolence or fatigue and 3) mood disturbances including irritability and depression. Reports of psychomotor slowing, speech and language problems, and difficulty with concentration and attention were common in adults. Although in some cases these events were mild to moderate, they at times led to withdrawal from treatment. The incidence of psychomotor slowing is only marginally dose-related, but both language problems and difficulty with concentration or attention clearly increased in frequency with increasing dosage in the five double-blind trials [see **ADVERSE REACTIONS, Table 6**]. Somnolence and fatigue were the most frequently reported adverse events during clinical trials with TOPAMAX®. These events were generally mild to moderate and occurred early in therapy. While the incidence of somnolence does not appear to be dose-related, that of fatigue increases at dosages above 400 mg/day.

In the double blind phases of clinical trials with topiramate in approved and investigational indications, suicide attempts occurred at a rate of 3/1000 patient years (13 events/3999 patient years) on topiramate versus 0 (0 events/1430 patient years) on placebo. One completed suicide was reported in a bipolar disorder trial in a patient on topiramate. Additional nonspecific CNS effects occasionally observed with topiramate as add-on therapy include dizziness or imbalance, confusion, and memory problems.

Pediatric Patients

In double-blind clinical studies, the incidences of cognitive/neuropsychiatric adverse events in pediatric patients were generally lower than previously observed in adults. These events included psychomotor slowing, difficulty with concentration/attention, speech disorders/related speech problems and language problems. The most frequently reported

Continued on next page

Table 1: Topiramate Dose Summary During the Stabilization Periods of Each of Five Double-Blind, Placebo-Controlled, Add-On Trials in Adults with Partial Onset Seizures[b]

			Target Topiramate Dosage (mg/day)				
Protocol	Stabilization Dose	Placebo[a]	200	400	600	800	1,000
YD	N	42	42	40	41	—	—
	Mean Dose	5.9	200	390	556	—	—
	Median Dose	6.0	200	400	600	—	—
YE	N	44	—	—	40	45	40
	Mean Dose	9.7	—	—	544	739	796
	Median Dose	10.0	—	—	600	800	1,000
Y1	N	23	—	19	—	—	—
	Mean Dose	3.8	—	395	—	—	—
	Median Dose	4.0	—	400	—	—	—
Y2	N	30	—	—	28	—	—
	Mean Dose	5.7	—	—	522	—	—
	Median Dose	6.0	—	—	600	—	—
Y3	N	28	—	—	—	25	—
	Mean Dose	7.9	—	—	—	568	—
	Median Dose	8.0	—	—	—	600	—
119	N	90	157	—	—	—	—
	Mean Dose	8	200	—	—	—	—
	Median Dose	8	200	—	—	—	—

[a] Placebo dosages are given as the number of tablets. Placebo target dosages were as follows: Protocol Y1, 4 tablets/day; Protocols YD and Y2, 6 tablets/day; Protocol Y3 and 119, 8 tablets/day; Protocol YE, 10 tablets/day.

[b] Dose-response studies were not conducted for other indications or pediatric partial onset seizures.

Table 2: Efficacy Results in Double-Blind, Placebo-Controlled, Add-On Trials

			Target Topiramate Dosage (mg/day)					
Protocol	Efficacy Results	Placebo	200	400	600	800	1,000	≈6 mg/kg/day*
Partial Onset Seizures								
Studies in Adults								
YD	N	45	45	45	46	—	—	—
	Median % Reduction	11.6	27.2[a]	47.5[b]	44.7[c]	—	—	—
	% Responders	18	24	44[d]	46[d]	—	—	—
YE	N	47	—	—	48	48	47	—
	Median % Reduction	1.7	—	—	40.8[c]	41.0[c]	36.0[c]	—
	% Responders	9	—	—	40[c]	41[c]	36[d]	—
Y1	N	24	—	23	—	—	—	—
	Median % Reduction	1.1	—	40.7[e]	—	—	—	—
	% Responders	8	—	35[d]	—	—	—	—
Y2	N	30	—	—	30	—	—	—
	Median % Reduction	−12.2	—	—	46.4[f]	—	—	—
	% Responders	10	—	—	47[c]	—	—	—
Y3	N	28	—	—	—	28	—	—
	Median % Reduction	−20.6	—	—	—	24.3[c]	—	—
	% Responders	0	—	—	—	43[c]	—	—
119	N	91	168	—	—	—	—	—
	Median % Reduction	20.0	44.2[c]	—	—	—	—	—
	% Responders	24	45[c]	—	—	—	—	—
Studies in Pediatric Patients								
YP	N	45	—	—	—	—	—	41
	Median % Reduction	10.5	—	—	—	—	—	33.1[d]
	% Responders	20	—	—	—	—	—	39
Primary Generalized Tonic-Clonic[h]								
YTC	N	40	—	—	—	—	—	39
	Median % Reduction	9.0	—	—	—	—	—	56.7[d]
	% Responders	20	—	—	—	—	—	56[c]
Lennox-Gastaut Syndrome[i]								
YL	N	49	—	—	—	—	—	46
	Median % Reduction	–5.1	—	—	—	—	—	14.8[d]
	% Responders	14	—	—	—	—	—	28[g]
	Improvement in Seizure Severity[j]	28	—	—	—	—	—	52[d]

Comparisons with placebo: [a]p=0.080; [b]p≤0.010; [c]p≤0.001; [d]p≤0.050; [e]p=0.065; [f]p≤0.005; [g]p=0.071; [h]Median % reduction and % responders are reported for PGTC Seizures; [i]Median % reduction and % responders for drop attacks, i.e., tonic or atonic seizures; [j]Percent of subjects who were minimally, much, or very much improved from baseline

* For Protocols YP and YTC, protocol-specified target dosages (<9.3 mg/kg/day) were assigned based on subject's weight to approximate a dosage of 6 mg/kg per day; these dosages corresponded to mg/day dosages of 125, 175, 225, and 400 mg/day.

Topamax—Cont.

neuropsychiatric events in this population were somnolence and fatigue. No patients discontinued treatment due to adverse events in double-blind trials.

Sudden Unexplained Death in Epilepsy (SUDEP)

During the course of premarketing development of TOPAMAX® (topiramate) Tablets, 10 sudden and unexplained deaths were recorded among a cohort of treated patients (2,796 subject years of exposure). This represents an incidence of 0.0035 deaths per patient year. Although this rate exceeds that expected in a healthy population matched for age and sex, it is within the range of estimates for the incidence of sudden unexplained deaths in patients with epilepsy not receiving TOPAMAX® (ranging from 0.0005 for the general population of patients with epilepsy, to 0.003 for a clinical trial population similar to that in the TOPAMAX® program, to 0.005 for patients with refractory epilepsy).

PRECAUTIONS

General:

Kidney Stones

A total of 32/2,086 (1.5%) of adults exposed to topiramate during its development reported the occurrence of kidney stones, an incidence about 2-4 times greater than expected in a similar, untreated population. As in the general population, the incidence of stone formation among topiramate treated patients was higher in men. Kidney stones have also been reported in pediatric patients.

An explanation for the association of TOPAMAX® and kidney stones may lie in the fact that topiramate is a carbonic anhydrase inhibitor. Carbonic anhydrase inhibitors, e.g., acetazolamide or dichlorphenamide, promote stone formation by reducing urinary citrate excretion and by increasing urinary pH. The concomitant use of TOPAMAX® with other carbonic anhydrase inhibitors or potentially in patients on a ketogenic diet may create a physiological environment that increases the risk of kidney stone formation, and should therefore be avoided.

Increased fluid intake increases the urinary output, lowering the concentration of substances involved in stone formation. Hydration is recommended to reduce new stone formation.

Paresthesia

Paresthesia, an effect associated with the use of other carbonic anhydrase inhibitors, appears to be a common effect of TOPAMAX®.

Adjustment of Dose in Renal Failure

The major route of elimination of unchanged topiramate and its metabolites is via the kidney. Dosage adjustment may be required in patients with reduced renal function (see **DOSAGE AND ADMINISTRATION**).

Decreased Hepatic Function

In hepatically impaired patients, topiramate should be administered with caution as the clearance of topiramate may be decreased.

Information for Patients

Patients taking TOPAMAX® should be told to seek immediate medical attention if they experience blurred vision or periorbital pain.

Patients, especially pediatric patients, treated with TOPAMAX® should be monitored closely for evidence of decreased sweating and increased body temperature, especially in hot weather.

Patients, particularly those with predisposing factors, should be instructed to maintain an adequate fluid intake in order to minimize the risk of renal stone formation [see **PRECAUTIONS: General**, for support regarding hydration as a preventative measure].

Patients should be warned about the potential for somnolence, dizziness, confusion, and difficulty concentrating and advised not to drive or operate machinery until they have gained sufficient experience on topiramate to gauge whether it adversely affects their mental and/or motor performance.

Additional food intake may be considered if the patient is losing weight while on this medication.

Please refer to the end of the product labeling for important information on how to take TOPAMAX® (topiramate capsules) Sprinkle Capsules.

Laboratory Tests:

Measurement of baseline and periodic serum bicarbonate during topiramate treatment is recommended (see **WARNINGS**).

Drug Interactions:

Antiepileptic Drugs

Potential interactions between topiramate and standard AEDs were assessed in controlled clinical pharmacokinetic studies in patients with epilepsy. The effects of these interactions on mean plasma AUCs are summarized in the following table:

In Table 3, the second column (AED concentration) describes what happens to the concentration of the AED listed in the first column when topiramate is added.

The third column (topiramate concentration) describes how the coadministration of a drug listed in the first column modifies the concentration of topiramate in experimental settings when TOPAMAX® was given alone.

[See table 3 above]

Other Drug Interactions

Digoxin: In a single-dose study, serum digoxin AUC was decreased by 12% with concomitant TOPAMAX® administration. The clinical relevance of this observation has not been established.

Table 3: Summary of AED Interactions with TOPAMAX®

AED Co-administered	AED Concentration	Topiramate Concentration
Phenytoin	NC or 25% increase[a]	48% decrease
Carbamazepine (CBZ)	NC	40% decrease
CBZ epoxide[b]	NC	NE
Valproic acid	11% decrease	14% decrease
Phenobarbital	NC	NE
Primidone	NC	NE

a = Plasma concentration increased 25% in some patients, generally those on a b.i.d. dosing regimen of phenytoin.
b = is not administered but is an active metabolite of carbamazepine.
NC = Less than 10% change in plasma concentration.
AED = Antiepileptic drug.
NE = Not Evaluated.

Table 4: Incidence of Treatment-Emergent Adverse Events in Placebo-Controlled, Add-On Trials in Adults[a,b] Where Rate Was > 1% in Any Topiramate Group and Greater Than the Rate in Placebo-Treated Patients

		TOPAMAX® Dosage (mg/day)	
Body System/ Adverse Event[c]	Placebo (N=291)	200-400 (N=183)	600-1,000 (N=414)
Body as a Whole – General Disorders			
Fatigue	13	15	30
Asthenia	1	6	3
Back Pain	4	5	3
Chest Pain	3	4	2
Influenza-Like Symptoms	2	3	4
Leg Pain	2	2	4
Hot Flushes	1	2	1
Allergy	1	2	3
Edema	1	2	1
Body Odor	0	1	0
Rigors	0	1	<1
Central & Peripheral Nervous System Disorders			
Dizziness	15	25	32
Ataxia	7	16	14
Speech Disorders/Related Speech Problems	2	13	11
Paresthesia	4	11	19
Nystagmus	7	10	11
Tremor	6	9	9
Language Problems	1	6	10
Coordination Abnormal	2	4	4
Hypoaesthesia	1	2	1
Gait Abnormal	1	3	2
Muscle Contractions Involuntary	1	2	2
Stupor	0	2	1
Vertigo	1	1	2
Gastro-Intestinal System Disorders			
Nausea	8	10	12
Dyspepsia	6	7	6
Abdominal Pain	4	6	7
Constipation	2	4	3
Gastroenteritis	1	2	1
Dry Mouth	1	2	4
Gingivitis	<1	1	1
GI Disorder	<1	1	0
Hearing and Vestibular Disorders			
Hearing Decreased	1	2	1
Metabolic and Nutritional Disorders			
Weight Decrease	3	9	13
Muscle-Skeletal System Disorders			
Myalgia	1	2	2
Skeletal Pain	0	1	0
Platelet, Bleeding & Clotting Disorders			
Epistaxis	1	2	1
Psychiatric Disorders			
Somnolence	12	29	28
Nervousness	6	16	19
Psychomotor Slowing	2	13	21
Difficulty with Memory	3	12	14
Anorexia	4	10	12
Confusion	5	11	14
Depression	5	5	13
Difficulty with Concentration/Attention	2	6	14
Mood Problems	2	4	9
Agitation	2	3	3
Aggressive Reaction	2	3	3
Emotional Lability	1	3	3
Cognitive Problems	1	3	3
Libido Decreased	1	2	<1
Apathy	1	1	3
Depersonalization	1	1	2

(Table continued on next page)

CNS Depressants: Concomitant administration of TOPAMAX® and alcohol or other CNS depressant drugs has not been evaluated in clinical studies. Because of the potential of topiramate to cause CNS depression, as well as other cognitive and/or neuropsychiatric adverse events, topiramate should be used with extreme caution if used in combination with alcohol and other CNS depressants.

Oral Contraceptives: In a pharmacokinetic interaction study in healthy volunteers with a concomitantly administered combination oral contraceptive product containing 1 mg norethindrone (NET) plus 35 mcg ethinyl estradiol (EE), TOPAMAX® given in the absence of other medications at doses of 50 to 200 mg/day was not associated with statistically significant changes in mean exposure (AUC) to either component of the oral contraceptive. In another study, exposure to EE was statistically significantly decreased at doses of 200, 400, and 800 mg/day (18%, 21%, and 30%, respectively) when given as adjunctive therapy in patients taking valproic acid. In both studies, TOPAMAX® (50 mg/day to 800 mg/day) did not significantly affect exposure to NET. Although there was a dose dependent decrease in EE exposure for doses between 200-800 mg/day, there was no significant dose dependent change in EE exposure for doses of 50-200 mg/day. The clinical significance of the changes observed is not known. The possibility of decreased contraceptive efficacy and increased breakthrough bleeding should be

Table 4 (cont.): Incidence of Treatment-Emergent Adverse Events in Placebo-Controlled, Add-On Trials in Adults[a,b] Where Rate Was > 1% in Any Topiramate Group and Greater Than the Rate in Placebo-Treated Patients

		TOPAMAX® Dosage (mg/day)	
Body System/ Adverse Event[c]	Placebo (N=291)	200-400 (N=183)	600-1,000 (N=414)
Reproductive Disorders, Female			
Breast Pain	2	4	0
Amenorrhea	1	2	2
Menorrhagia	0	2	1
Menstrual Disorder	1	2	1
Reproductive Disorders, Male			
Prostatic Disorder	<1	2	0
Resistance Mechanism Disorders			
Infection	1	2	1
Infection Viral	1	2	<1
Moniliasis	<1	1	0
Respiratory System Disorders			
Pharyngitis	2	6	3
Rhinitis	6	7	6
Sinusitis	4	5	6
Dyspnea	1	1	2
Skin and Appendages Disorders			
Skin Disorder	<1	2	1
Sweating Increased	<1	1	<1
Rash Erythematous	<1	1	<1
Special Sense Other, Disorders			
Taste Perversion	0	2	4
Urinary System Disorders			
Hematuria	1	2	<1
Urinary Tract Infection	1	2	3
Micturition Frequency	1	1	2
Urinary Incontinence	<1	2	1
Urine Abnormal	0	1	<1
Vision Disorders			
Vision Abnormal	2	13	10
Diplopia	5	10	10
White Cell and RES Disorders			
Leukopenia	1	2	1

[a] Patients in these add-on trials were receiving 1 to 2 concomitant antiepileptic drugs in addition to TOPAMAX® or placebo.
[b] Values represent the percentage of patients reporting a given adverse event. Patients may have reported more than one adverse event during the study and can be included in more than one adverse event category.
[c] Adverse events reported by at least 1% of patients in the TOPAMAX® 200-400 mg/day group and more common than in the placebo group are listed in this table.

Table 5: Incidence of Treatment-Emergent Adverse Events in Study 119[a,b] Where Rate Was ≥ 2% in the Topiramate Group and Greater Than the Rate in Placebo-Treated Patients

		TOPAMAX® Dosage (mg/day)
Body System/ Adverse Event[c]	Placebo (N=92)	200 (N=171)
Body as a Whole – General Disorders		
Fatigue	4	9
Chest Pain	1	2
Cardiovascular Disorders, General		
Hypertension	0	2
Central & Peripheral Nervous System Disorders		
Paresthesia	2	9
Dizziness	4	7
Tremor	2	3
Hypoasthesia	0	2
Leg Cramps	0	2
Language Problems	0	2
Gastro-Intestinal System Disorders		
Abdominal Pain	3	5
Constipation	0	4
Diarrhea	1	2
Dyspepsia	0	2
Dry Mouth	0	2
Hearing and Vestibular Disorders		
Tinnitus	0	2
Metabolic and Nutritional Disorders		
Weight Decrease	4	8
Psychiatric Disorders		
Somnolence	9	15
Anorexia	7	9
Nervousness	2	9
Difficulty with Concentration/Attention	0	5
Insomnia	3	4
Difficulty with Memory	1	2
Aggressive Reaction	0	2
Respiratory System Disorders		
Rhinitis	0	4
Urinary System Disorders		
Cystitis	0	2
Vision Disorders		
Diplopia	0	2
Vision Abnormal	0	2

[a] Patients in these add-on trials were receiving 1 to 2 concomitant antiepileptic drugs in addition to TOPAMAX® or placebo.
[b] Values represent the percentage of patients reporting a given adverse event. Patients may have reported more than one adverse event during the study and can be included in more than one adverse event category.
[c] Adverse events reported by at least 2% of patients in the TOPAMAX® 200 mg/kg group and more common than in the placebo group are listed in this table.

considered in patients taking combination oral contraceptive products with TOPAMAX®. Patients taking estrogen containing contraceptives should be asked to report any change in their bleeding patterns. Contraceptive efficacy can be decreased even in the absence of breakthrough bleeding.

Metformin: A drug-drug interaction study conducted in healthy volunteers evaluated the steady-state pharmacokinetics of metformin and topiramate in plasma when metformin was given alone and when metformin and topiramate were given simultaneously. The results of this study indicated that metformin mean C_{max} and mean AUC_{0-12h} increased by 18% and 25%, respectively, while mean CL/F decreased 20% when metformin was co-administered with topiramate. Topiramate did not affect metformin t_{max}. The clinical significance of the effect of topiramate on metformin pharmacokinetics is unclear. Oral plasma clearance of topiramate appears to be reduced when administered with metformin. The extent of change in the clearance is unknown. The clinical significance of the effect of metformin on topiramate pharmacokinetics is unclear. When TOPAMAX® is added or withdrawn in patients on metformin therapy, careful attention should be given to the routine monitoring for adequate control of their diabetic disease state.

Others: Concomitant use of TOPAMAX®,a weak carbonic anhydrase inhibitor, with other carbonic anhydrase inhibitors, e.g., acetazolamide or dichlorphenamide, may create a physiological environment that increases the risk of renal stone formation, and should therefore be avoided.

Drug/Laboratory Test Interactions: There are no known interactions of topiramate with commonly used laboratory tests.

Carcinogenesis, Mutagenesis, Impairment of Fertility:
An increase in urinary bladder tumors was observed in mice given topiramate (20, 75, and 300 mg/kg) in the diet for 21 months. The elevated bladder tumor incidence, which was statistically significant in males and females receiving 300 mg/kg, was primarily due to the increased occurrence of a smooth muscle tumor considered histomorphologically unique to mice. Plasma exposures in mice receiving 300 mg/kg were approximately 0.5 to 1 times steady-state exposures measured in patients receiving topiramate monotherapy at the recommended human dose (RHD) of 400 mg, and 1.5 to 2 times steady-state topiramate exposures in patients receiving 400 mg of topiramate plus phenytoin. The relevance of this finding to human carcinogenic risk is uncertain. No evidence of carcinogenicity was seen in rats following oral administration of topiramate for 2 years at doses up to 120 mg/kg (approximately 3 times the RHD on a mg/m^2 basis).

Topiramate did not demonstrate genotoxic potential when tested in a battery of *in vitro* and *in vivo* assays. Topiramate was not mutagenic in the Ames test or the *in vitro* mouse lymphoma assay; it did not increase unscheduled DNA synthesis in rat hepatocytes *in vitro*; and it did not increase chromosomal aberrations in human lymphocytes *in vitro* or in rat bone marrow *in vivo*.

No adverse effects on male or female fertility were observed in rats at doses up to 100 mg/kg (2.5 times the RHD on a mg/m^2 basis).

Pregnancy: Pregnancy Category C.
Topiramate has demonstrated selective developmental toxicity, including teratogenicity, in experimental animal studies. When oral doses of 20, 100, or 500 mg/kg were administered to pregnant mice during the period of organogenesis, the incidence of fetal malformations (primarily craniofacial defects) was increased at all doses. The low dose is approximately 0.2 times the recommended human dose (RHD= 400 mg/day) on a mg/m^2 basis. Fetal body weights and skeletal ossification were reduced at 500 mg/kg in conjunction with decreased maternal body weight gain.

In rat studies (oral doses of 20, 100, and 500 mg/kg or 0.2, 2.5, 30, and 400 mg/kg), the frequency of limb malformations (ectrodactyly, micromelia, and amelia) was increased among the offspring of dams treated with 400 mg/kg (10 times the RHD on a mg/m^2 basis) or greater during the organogenesis period of pregnancy. Embryotoxicity (reduced fetal body weights, increased incidence of structural variations) was observed at doses as low as 20 mg/kg (0.5 times the RHD on a mg/m^2 basis). Clinical signs of maternal toxicity were seen at 400 mg/kg and above, and maternal body weight gain was reduced during treatment with 100 mg/kg or greater.

In rabbit studies (20, 60, and 180 mg/kg or 10, 35, and 120 mg/kg orally during organogenesis), embryo/fetal mortality was increased at 35 mg/kg (2 times the RHD on a mg/m^2 basis) or greater, and teratogenic effects (primarily rib and vertebral malformations) were observed at 120 mg/kg (6 times the RHD on a mg/m^2 basis). Evidence of maternal toxicity (decreased body weight gain, clinical signs, and/or mortality) was seen at 35 mg/kg and above.

When female rats were treated during the latter part of gestation and throughout lactation (0.2, 4, 20, and 100 mg/kg or 2, 20, and 200 mg/kg), offspring exhibited decreased viability and delayed physical development at 200 mg/kg (5 times the RHD on a mg/m^2 basis) and reductions in pre- and/or postweaning body weight gain at 2 mg/kg (0.05 times the RHD on a mg/m^2 basis) and above. Maternal toxicity (decreased body weight gain, clinical signs) was evident at 100 mg/kg or greater.

In a rat embryo/fetal development study with a postnatal component (0.2, 2.5, 30, or 400 mg/kg during organogenesis; noted above), pups exhibited delayed physical development at 400 mg/kg (10 times the RHD on a mg/m^2 basis) and persistent reductions in body weight gain at 30 mg/kg (1 times the RHD on a mg/m^2 basis) and higher.

There are no studies using TOPAMAX® in pregnant women. TOPAMAX® should be used during pregnancy only if the potential benefit outweighs the potential risk to the fetus.

Continued on next page

Topamax—Cont.

In post-marketing experience, cases of hypospadias have been reported in male infants exposed in utero to topiramate, with or without other anticonvulsants; however, a causal relationship with topiramate has not been established.

Labor and Delivery:
In studies of rats where dams were allowed to deliver pups naturally, no drug-related effects on gestation length or parturition were observed at dosage levels up to 200 mg/kg/day. The effect of TOPAMAX® on labor and delivery in humans is unknown.

Nursing Mothers:
Topiramate is excreted in the milk of lactating rats. The excretion of topiramate in human milk has not been evaluated in controlled studies. Limited observations in patients suggest an extensive secretion of topiramate into breast milk. Since many drugs are excreted in human milk, and because the potential for serious adverse reactions in nursing infants to TOPAMAX® is unknown, the potential benefit to the mother should be weighed against the potential risk to the infant when considering recommendations regarding nursing.

Pediatric Use:
Safety and effectiveness in patients below the age of 2 years have not been established. Topiramate is associated with metabolic acidosis. Chronic untreated metabolic acidosis in pediatric patients may cause osteomalacia (rickets) and may reduce growth rates. A reduction in growth rate may eventually decrease the maximal height achieved. The effect of topiramate on growth and bone-related sequelae has not been systematically investigated (see **WARNINGS**).

Geriatric Use:
In clinical trials, 3% of patients were over 60. No age related difference in effectiveness or adverse effects were evident. However, clinical studies of topiramate did not include sufficient numbers of subjects aged 65 and over to determine whether they respond differently than younger subjects. Dosage adjustment may be necessary for elderly with impaired renal function (creatinine clearance rate ≤70 mL/min/1.73 m^2) due to reduced clearance of topiramate (see **CLINICAL PHARMACOLOGY** and **DOSAGE AND ADMINISTRATION**).

Race and Gender Effects:
Evaluation of effectiveness and safety in clinical trials has shown no race or gender related effects.

ADVERSE REACTIONS

The data described in the following section were obtained using TOPAMAX® (topiramate) Tablets.

The most commonly observed adverse events associated with the use of topiramate at dosages of 200 to 400 mg/day in controlled trials in adults with partial onset seizures, primary generalized tonic-clonic seizures, or Lennox-Gastaut syndrome, that were seen at greater frequency in topiramate-treated patients and did not appear to be dose-related were: somnolence, dizziness, ataxia, speech disorders and related speech problems, psychomotor slowing, abnormal vision, difficulty with memory, paresthesia and diplopia [see Table 4]. The most common dose-related adverse events at dosages of 200 to 1,000 mg/day were: fatigue, nervousness, difficulty with concentration or attention, confusion, depression, anorexia, language problems, anxiety, mood problems, and weight decrease [see Table 6].

Adverse events associated with the use of topiramate at dosages of 5 to 9 mg/kg/day in controlled trials in pediatric patients with partial onset seizures, primary generalized tonic-clonic seizures, or Lennox-Gastaut syndrome, that were seen at greater frequency in topiramate-treated patients were: fatigue, somnolence, anorexia, nervousness, difficulty with concentration/attention, difficulty with memory, aggressive reaction, and weight decrease [see Table 7].

In controlled clinical trials in adults, 11% of patients receiving topiramate 200 to 400 mg/day as adjunctive therapy discontinued due to adverse events. This rate appeared to increase at dosages above 400 mg/day. Adverse events associated with discontinuing therapy included somnolence, dizziness, anxiety, difficulty with concentration or attention, fatigue, and paresthesia and increased at dosages above 400 mg/day. None of the pediatric patients who received topiramate adjunctive therapy at 5 to 9 mg/kg/day in controlled clinical trials discontinued due to adverse events.

Approximately 28% of the 1,757 adults with epilepsy who received topiramate at dosages of 200 to 1,600 mg/day in clinical studies discontinued treatment because of adverse events; an individual patient could have reported more than one adverse event. These adverse events were: psychomotor slowing (4.0%), difficulty with memory (3.2%), fatigue (3.2%), confusion (3.1%), somnolence (3.2%), difficulty with concentration/attention (2.9%), anorexia (2.7%), depression (2.6%), dizziness (2.5%), weight decrease (2.5%), nervousness (2.3%), ataxia (2.1%), and paresthesia (2.0%). Approximately 11% of the 310 pediatric patients who received topiramate at dosages up to 30 mg/kg/day discontinued due to adverse events. Adverse events associated with discontinuing therapy included aggravated convulsions (2.3%), difficulty with concentration/attention (1.6%), language problems (1.3%), personality disorder (1.3%), and somnolence (1.3%).

Incidence in Controlled Clinical Trials – Add-On Therapy – Partial Onset Seizures, Primary Generalized Tonic-Clonic Seizures, and Lennox-Gastaut Syndrome

Table 4 lists treatment-emergent adverse events that occurred in at least 1% of adults treated with 200 to 400 mg/day topiramate in controlled trials that were numerically more common at this dose than in the patients treated with placebo. In general, most patients who experienced adverse events during the first eight weeks of these trials no longer experienced them by their last visit. Table 7 lists treatment-emergent adverse events that occurred in at least 1% of pediatric patients treated with 5 to 9 mg/kg topiramate in controlled trials that were numerically more common than in patients treated with placebo.

The prescriber should be aware that these data were obtained when TOPAMAX® was added to concurrent antiepileptic drug therapy and cannot be used to predict the frequency of adverse events in the course of usual medical practice where patient characteristics and other factors may differ from those prevailing during clinical studies. Similarly, the cited frequencies cannot be directly compared with data obtained from other clinical investigations involving different treatments, uses, or investigators. Inspection of these frequencies, however, does provide the prescribing physician with a basis to estimate the relative contribution of drug and non-drug factors to the adverse event incidences in the population studied.

[See table 4 on pages 2544 and 2545]

Incidence in Study 119 – Add-On Therapy – Adults with Partial Onset Seizures

Study 119 was a randomized, double-blind, placebo-controlled, parallel group study with 3 treatment arms: 1) placebo; 2) topiramate 200 mg/day with a 25 mg/day starting dose, increased by 25 mg/day each week for 8 weeks until the 200 mg/day maintenance dose was reached; and 3) topiramate 200 mg/day with a 50 mg/day starting dose, increased by 50 mg/day each week for 4 weeks until the 200 mg/day maintenance dose was reached. All patients were maintained on concomitant carbamazepine with or without another concomitant antiepileptic drug.

The incidence of adverse events did not differ significantly between the 2 topiramate regimens. The cited frequencies of adverse events cannot be directly compared with data obtained in other studies using different patients with different titration rates and taking different combinations of concomitant medications.

[See table 5 on previous page]
[See table 6 below]
[See table 7 at top of next page]

Other Adverse Events Observed

Other events that occurred in more than 1% of adults treated with 200 to 400 mg of topiramate in placebo-controlled trials but with equal or greater frequency in the placebo group were: headache, injury, anxiety, rash, pain, convulsions aggravated, coughing, fever, diarrhea, vomiting, muscle weakness, insomnia, personality disorder, dysmenorrhea, upper respiratory tract infection, and eye pain.

Other Adverse Events Observed During All Clinical Trials

Topiramate, initiated as adjunctive therapy, has been administered to 1,927 adults and 313 pediatric patients with epilepsy during all clinical studies. During these studies, all adverse events were recorded by the clinical investigators using terminology of their own choosing. To provide a meaningful estimate of the proportion of individuals having adverse events, similar types of events were grouped into a smaller number of standardized categories using modified WHOART dictionary terminology. The frequencies presented represent the proportion of patients who experienced an event of the type cited on at least one occasion while receiving topiramate. Reported events are included except those already listed in the previous table or text, those too general to be informative, and those not reasonably associated with the use of the drug.

Events are classified within body system categories and enumerated in order of decreasing frequency using the following definitions: *frequent* occurring in at least 1/100 patients; *infrequent* occurring in 1/100 to 1/1000 patients; *rare* occurring in fewer than 1/1000 patients.

Autonomic Nervous System Disorders: *Infrequent:* vasodilation.

Body as a Whole: *Infrequent:* syncope, abdomen enlarged. *Rare:* alcohol intolerance.

Cardiovascular Disorders, General: *Infrequent:* hypotension, postural hypotension.

Central & Peripheral Nervous System Disorders: *Frequent:* hypertonia. *Infrequent:* neuropathy, apraxia, hyperaesthesia, dyskinesia, dysphonia, scotoma, ptosis, dystonia, visual field defect, encephalopathy, EEG abnormal. *Rare:* upper motor neuron lesion, cerebellar syndrome, tongue paralysis.

Gastrointestinal System Disorders: *Frequent:* diarrhea, vomiting. *Infrequent:* hemorrhoids, stomatitis, melena, gastritis, tongue edema, esophagitis.

Heart Rate and Rhythm Disorders: *Infrequent:* AV block.

Liver and Biliary System Disorders: *Infrequent:* SGPT increased, SGOT increased, gamma-GT increased.

Metabolic and Nutritional Disorders: *Frequent:* dehydration. *Infrequent:* hypokalemia, alkaline phosphatase increased, hypocalcemia, hyperlipemia, acidosis, hyperglycemia, xerophthalmia. *Rare:* hyperchloremia, diabetes mellitus, hypernatremia, hyponatremia, hypocholesterolemia, hypophosphatemia, creatinine increased.

Musculoskeletal System Disorders: *Frequent:* arthralgia. *Infrequent:* arthrosis.

Myo-, Endo-, Pericardial & Valve Disorders: *Infrequent:* angina pectoris.

Neoplasms: *Infrequent:* thrombocythemia. *Rare:* polycythemia.

Platelet, Bleeding, and Clotting Disorders: *Infrequent:* gingival bleeding. *Rare:* pulmonary embolism.

Psychiatric Disorders: *Frequent:* impotence, hallucination, euphoria, psychosis, suicide attempt. *Infrequent:* paranoid reaction, delusion, paranoia, delirium, abnormal dreaming, neurosis. *Rare:* libido increased, manic reaction.

Red Blood Cell Disorders: *Frequent:* anemia. *Rare:* marrow depression, pancytopenia.

Reproductive Disorders, Male: *Infrequent:* ejaculation disorder, breast discharge.

Skin and Appendages Disorders: *Frequent:* acne. *Infrequent:* urticaria, photosensitivity reaction, abnormal hair texture. *Rare:* chloasma.

Special Senses Other, Disorders: *Infrequent:* taste loss, parosmia.

Urinary System Disorders: *Frequent:* dysuria, renal calculus. *Infrequent:* urinary retention, face edema, renal pain, albuminuria, polyuria, oliguria.

Vascular (Extracardiac) Disorders: *Infrequent:* flushing, deep vein thrombosis, phlebitis. *Rare:* vasospasm.

Vision Disorders: *Frequent:* conjunctivitis. *Infrequent:* abnormal accommodation, photophobia, strabismus. *Rare:* mydriasis, iritis.

White Cell and Reticuloendothelial System Disorders: *Infrequent:* lymphadenopathy, eosinophilia, lymphopenia, granulocytopenia. *Rare:* lymphocytosis.

Postmarketing and Other Experience

In addition to the adverse experiences reported during clinical testing of TOPAMAX®, the following adverse experiences have been reported worldwide in patients receiving topiramate post-approval. These adverse experiences have not been listed above and data are insufficient to support an estimate of their incidence or to establish causation. The listing is alphabetized: bullous skin reactions (including erythema multiforme, Stevens-Johnson syndrome, toxic epidermal necrolysis), hepatic failure (including fatalities), hepatitis, pancreatitis, pemphigus, and renal tubular acidosis.

DRUG ABUSE AND DEPENDENCE

The abuse and dependence potential of TOPAMAX® has not been evaluated in human studies.

OVERDOSAGE

Overdoses of TOPAMAX® have been reported. Signs and symptoms included convulsions, drowsiness, speech disturbance, blurred vision, diplopia, mentation impaired, lethargy, abnormal coordination, stupor, hypotension, abdominal pain, agitation, dizziness and depression. The clinical consequences were not severe in most cases, but deaths have been reported after poly-drug overdoses involving TOPAMAX®.

Topiramate overdose has resulted in severe metabolic acidosis (see **WARNINGS**).

A patient who ingested a dose between 96 and 110 g topiramate was admitted to hospital with coma lasting 20-24 hours followed by full recovery after 3 to 4 days.

In acute TOPAMAX® overdose, if the ingestion is recent, the stomach should be emptied immediately by lavage or by induction of emesis. Activated charcoal has been shown to adsorb topiramate *in vitro*. Treatment should be appropriately supportive. Hemodialysis is an effective means of removing topiramate from the body.

Table 6: Incidence (%) of Dose-Related Adverse Events From Placebo-Controlled, Add-On Trials in Adults with Partial Onset Seizures[a]

		TOPAMAX® Dosage (mg/day)		
Adverse Event	Placebo (N=216)	200 (N=45)	400 (N=68)	600-1,000 (N=414)
Fatigue	13	11	12	30
Nervousness	7	13	18	19
Difficulty with Concentration/Attention	1	7	9	14
Confusion	4	9	10	14
Depression	6	9	7	13
Anorexia	4	4	6	12
Language problems	<1	2	9	10
Anxiety	6	2	3	10
Mood problems	2	0	6	9
Weight decrease	3	4	9	13

[a] Dose-response studies were not conducted for other adult indications or for pediatric indications.

DOSAGE AND ADMINISTRATION

TOPAMAX® has been shown to be effective in adults and pediatric patients ages 2-16 years with partial onset seizures or primary generalized tonic-clonic seizures, and in patients 2 years of age and older with seizures associated with Lennox-Gastaut syndrome. In the controlled add-on trials, no correlation has been demonstrated between trough plasma concentrations of topiramate and clinical efficacy. No evidence of tolerance has been demonstrated in humans. Doses above 400 mg/day (600, 800, or 1,000 mg/day) have not been shown to improve responses in dose-response studies in adults with partial onset seizures.

It is not necessary to monitor topiramate plasma concentrations to optimize TOPAMAX® therapy. On occasion, the addition of TOPAMAX® to phenytoin may require an adjustment of the dose of phenytoin to achieve optimal clinical outcome. Addition or withdrawal of phenytoin and/or carbamazepine during adjunctive therapy with TOPAMAX® may require adjustment of the dose of TOPAMAX®. Because of the bitter taste, tablets should not be broken.

TOPAMAX® can be taken without regard to meals.

Adults (17 Years of Age and Over)

The recommended total daily dose of TOPAMAX® as adjunctive therapy in adults with partial seizures is 200-400 mg/day in two divided doses, and 400 mg/day in two divided doses as adjunctive treatment in adults with primary generalized tonic-clonic seizures. It is recommended that therapy be initiated at 25 - 50 mg/day followed by titration to an effective dose in increments of 25 - 50 mg/week. Titrating in increments of 25 mg/week may delay the time to reach an effective dose. Daily doses above 1,600 mg have not been studied.

In the study of primary generalized tonic-clonic seizures the initial titration rate was slower than in previous studies; the assigned dose was reached at the end of 8 weeks (see **CLINICAL STUDIES, Controlled Trials in Patients With Primary Generalized Tonic-Clonic Seizures**).

Pediatric Patients (Ages 2-16 Years) - Partial Seizures, Primary Generalized Tonic-Clonic Seizures, or Lennox-Gastaut Syndrome

The recommended total daily dose of TOPAMAX® (topiramate) as adjunctive therapy for patients with partial seizures, primary generalized tonic-clonic seizures, or seizures associated with Lennox-Gastaut syndrome is approximately 5 to 9 mg/kg/day in two divided doses. Titration should begin at 25 mg (or less, based on a range of 1 to 3 mg/kg/day) nightly for the first week. The dosage should then be increased at 1- or 2-week intervals by increments of 1 to 3 mg/kg/day (administered in two divided doses), to achieve optimal clinical response. Dose titration should be guided by clinical outcome.

In the study of primary generalized tonic-clonic seizures the initial titration rate was slower than in previous studies; the assigned dose of 6 mg/kg/day was reached at the end of 8 weeks (see **CLINICAL STUDIES, Controlled Trials in Patients With Primary Generalized Tonic-Clonic Seizures**).

Administration of TOPAMAX® Sprinkle Capsules

TOPAMAX® (topiramate capsules) Sprinkle Capsules may be swallowed whole or may be administered by carefully opening the capsule and sprinkling the entire contents on a small amount (teaspoon) of soft food. This drug/food mixture should be swallowed immediately and not chewed. It should not be stored for future use.

Patients with Renal Impairment:

In renally impaired subjects (creatinine clearance less than 70 mL/min/1.73m^2), one half of the usual adult dose is recommended. Such patients will require a longer time to reach steady-state at each dose.

Geriatric Patients (Ages 65 Years and Over):

Dosage adjustment may be indicated in the elderly patient when impaired renal function (creatinine clearance rate ≤70 mL/min/1.73 m^2) is evident (see **DOSAGE AND ADMINISTRATION: Patients with Renal Impairment** and **CLINICAL PHARMACOLOGY: Special Populations: Age, Gender, and Race**).

Patients Undergoing Hemodialysis:

Topiramate is cleared by hemodialysis at a rate that is 4 to 6 times greater than a normal individual. Accordingly, a prolonged period of dialysis may cause topiramate concentration to fall below that required to maintain an anti-seizure effect. To avoid rapid drops in topiramate plasma concentration during hemodialysis, a supplemental dose of topiramate may be required. The actual adjustment should take into account 1) the duration of dialysis period, 2) the clearance rate of the dialysis system being used, and 3) the effective renal clearance of topiramate in the patient being dialyzed.

Patients with Hepatic Disease:

In hepatically impaired patients topiramate plasma concentrations may be increased. The mechanism is not well understood.

Table 7: Incidence (%) of Treatment-Emergent Adverse Events in Placebo-Controlled, Add-On Trials in Pediatric Patients Ages 2–16 Years[a,b] (Events That Occurred in at Least 1% of Topiramate-Treated Patients and Occurred More Frequently in Topiramate-Treated Than Placebo-Treated Patients)

Body System/ Adverse Event	Placebo (N=101)	Topiramate (N=98)
Body as a Whole – General Disorders		
Fatigue	5	16
Injury	13	14
Allergic Reaction	1	2
Back Pain	0	1
Pallor	0	1
Cardiovascular Disorders, General		
Hypertension	0	1
Central & Peripheral Nervous System Disorders		
Gait Abnormal	5	8
Ataxia	2	6
Hyperkinesia	4	5
Dizziness	2	4
Speech Disorders/Related Speech Problems	2	4
Hyporeflexia	0	2
Convulsions Grand Mal	0	1
Fecal Incontinence	0	1
Paresthesia	0	1
Gastro-Intestinal System Disorders		
Nausea	5	6
Saliva Increased	4	6
Constipation	4	5
Gastroenteritis	2	3
Dysphagia	0	1
Flatulence	0	1
Gastroesophageal Reflux	0	1
Glossitis	0	1
Gum Hyperplasia	0	1
Heart Rate and Rhythm Disorders		
Bradycardia	0	1
Metabolic and Nutritional Disorders		
Weight Decrease	1	9
Thirst	1	2
Hypoglycemia	0	1
Weight Increase	0	1
Platelet, Bleeding, & Clotting Disorders		
Purpura	4	8
Epistaxis	1	4
Hematoma	0	1
Prothrombin Increased	0	1
Thrombocytopenia	0	1
Psychiatric Disorders		
Somnolence	16	26
Anorexia	15	24
Nervousness	7	14
Personality Disorder (Behavior Problems)	9	11
Difficulty with Concentration/Attention	2	10
Aggressive Reaction	4	9
Insomnia	7	8
Difficulty with Memory NOS	0	5
Confusion	3	4
Psychomotor Slowing	2	3
Appetite Increased	0	1
Neurosis	0	1
Reproductive Disorders, Female		
Leukorrhoea	0	2
Resistance Mechanism Disorders		
Infection Viral	3	7
Respiratory System Disorders		
Pneumonia	1	5
Respiratory Disorder	0	1
Skin and Appendages Disorders		
Skin Disorder	2	3
Alopecia	1	2
Dermatitis	0	2
Hypertrichosis	1	2
Rash Erythematous	0	2
Eczema	0	1
Seborrhoea	0	1
Skin Discoloration	0	1
Urinary System Disorders		
Urinary Incontinence	2	4
Nocturia	0	1
Vision Disorders		
Eye Abnormality	1	2
Vision Abnormal	1	2
Diplopia	0	1
Lacrimation Abnormal	0	1
Myopia	0	1
White Cell and RES Disorders		
Leukopenia	0	2

[a] Patients in these add-on trials were receiving 1 to 2 concomitant antiepileptic drugs in addition to TOPAMAX® or placebo.
[b] Values represent the percentage of patients reporting a given adverse event. Patients may have reported more than one adverse event during the study and can be included in more than one adverse event category.

HOW SUPPLIED

TOPAMAX® (topiramate) Tablets is available as debossed, coated, round tablets in the following strengths and colors:

25 mg white (coded "TOP" on one side; "25" on the other)

50 mg light-yellow (coded "TOPAMAX" on one side; "50" on the other)

100 mg yellow (coded "TOPAMAX" on one side; "100" on the other)

200 mg salmon (coded "TOPAMAX" on one side; "200" on the other)

They are supplied as follows:

25 mg tablets - bottles of 60 count with desiccant (NDC 0045-0639-65)

50 mg tablets – bottles of 60 count with desiccant (NDC 0045-0640-65)

100 mg tablets – bottles of 60 count with desiccant (NDC 0045-0641-65)

200 mg tablets – bottles of 60 count with desiccant (NDC 0045-0642-65)

TOPAMAX® (topiramate capsules) Sprinkle Capsules contain small, white to off white spheres. The gelatin capsules are white and clear.

They are marked as follows:

15 mg capsule with "TOP" and "15 mg" on the side

25 mg capsule with "TOP" and "25 mg" on the side

The capsules are supplied as follows:

15 mg capsules – bottles of 60 (NDC 0045-0647-65)

25 mg capsules – bottles of 60 (NDC 0045-0645-65)

TOPAMAX® (topiramate) Tablets should be stored in tightly-closed containers at controlled room temperature, (59 to 86°F, 15 to 30°C). Protect from moisture.

TOPAMAX® (topiramate capsules) Sprinkle Capsules should be stored in tightly-closed containers at or below 25°C (77°F). Protect from moisture.

Continued on next page

Topamax—Cont.

TOPAMAX® (topiramate) and TOPAMAX® (topiramate capsules) are trademarks of Ortho-McNeil Pharmaceutical.

HOW TO TAKE

TOPAMAX® (topiramate capsules) SPRINKLE CAPSULES

A Guide for Patients and Their Caregivers

Your doctor has given you a prescription for TOPAMAX® (topiramate capsules) Sprinkle Capsules. Here are your instructions for taking this medication. Please read these instructions prior to use.

To Take With Food

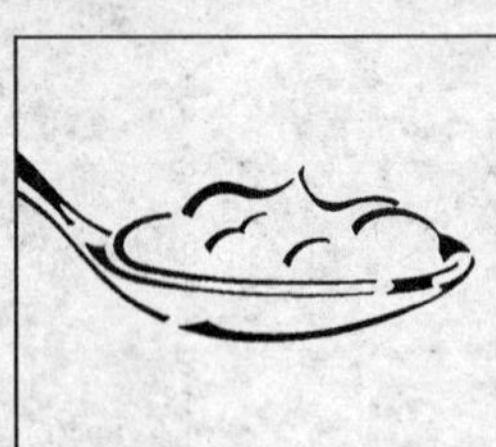

You may sprinkle the contents of TOPAMAX® Sprinkle Capsules on a small amount (teaspoon) of soft food, such as applesauce, custard, ice cream, oatmeal, pudding, or yogurt.

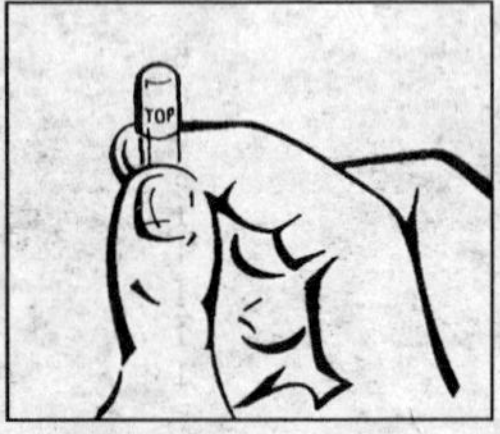

Hold the capsule upright so that you can read the word "TOP."

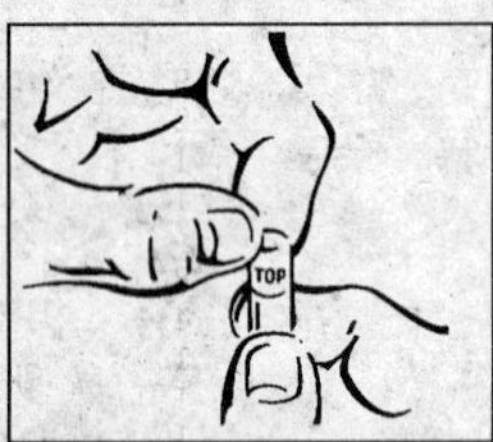

Carefully twist off the clear portion of the capsule. You may find it best to do this over the small portion of the food onto which you will be pouring the sprinkles.

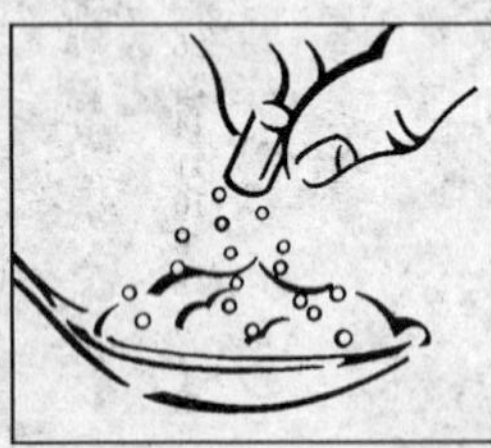

Sprinkle all of the capsule's contents onto a spoonful of soft food, taking care to see that the entire prescribed dosage is sprinkled onto the food.

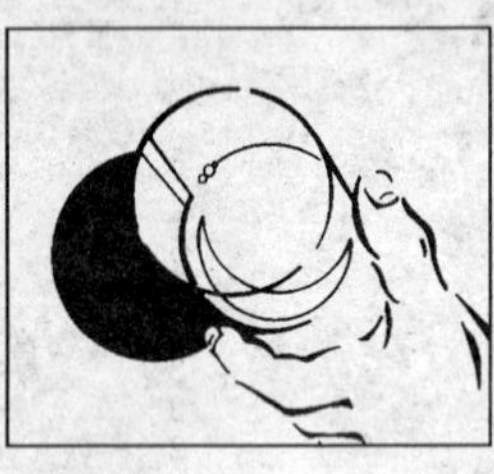

Be sure the patient swallows the entire spoonful of the sprinkle/food mixture immediately. Chewing should be avoided. It may be helpful to have the patient drink fluids immediately in order to make sure all of the mixture is swallowed.

IMPORTANT: Never store any sprinkle/food mixture for use at a later time.

To Take Without Food

TOPAMAX® Sprinkle Capsules may also be swallowed as whole capsules.

For more information about TOPAMAX® Sprinkle Capsules, ask your doctor or pharmacist.

ORTHO-McNEIL
OMP DIVISION
ORTHO-McNEIL PHARMACEUTICAL, INC.
Raritan, NJ 08869

 Revision Date June 2004 7517110

Shown in Product Identification Guide, page 328

TYLENOL® WITH CODEINE ℞

[ti 'len-awl co' dēn]

tablets Ⓒ III

(acetaminophen and codeine phosphate tablets)

elixir Ⓒ V

(acetaminophen and codeine phosphate oral solution USP)

Analgesic For Oral Use

Prescribing Information

DESCRIPTION

Each tablet contains:

No. 3 Codeine Phosphate	30 mg
Acetaminophen	300 mg
No. 4 Codeine Phosphate	60 mg
Acetaminophen	300 mg

Each 5 mL of elixir contains:

Codeine Phosphate	12 mg
Acetaminophen	120 mg

Alcohol 7%

Inactive ingredients: tablets—powdered cellulose, magnesium stearate, sodium metabisulfite†, pregelatinized starch, starch (corn); elixir—alcohol, citric acid, propylene glycol, sodium benzoate, saccharin sodium, sucrose, natural and artificial flavors, FD&C Yellow No. 6.

Acetaminophen, 4′-hydroxyacetanilide, is a non-opiate, non-salicylate analgesic and antipyretic which occurs as a white, odorless, crystalline powder, possessing a slightly bitter taste. Its structure is as follows:

$C_8H_9NO_2$ M.W. 151.16

Codeine is an alkaloid, obtained from opium or prepared from morphine by methylation. Codeine phosphate occurs as fine, white, needle-shaped crystals, or white, crystalline powder. It is affected by light. Its chemical name is: 7,8-didehydro- 4,5α-epoxy-3-methoxy-17-methylmorphinan-6α-ol phosphate (1:1) (salt) hemihydrate. Its structure is as follows:

$C_{18}H_{21}NO_3.H_3PO_4.\ ^1/_2H_2O$ M.W. 406.37

†See WARNINGS

CLINICAL PHARMACOLOGY

TYLENOL with Codeine (acetaminophen and codeine phosphate tablets and oral solution USP) combine the analgesic effects of a centrally acting analgesic, codeine, with a peripherally acting analgesic, acetaminophen. Both ingredients are well absorbed orally. The plasma elimination half-life ranges from 1 to 4 hours for acetaminophen, and from 2.5 to 3 hours for codeine.

Codeine retains at least one-half of its analgesic activity when administered orally. A reduced first-pass metabolism of codeine by the liver accounts for the greater oral efficacy of codeine when compared to most other morphine-like narcotics. Following absorption, codeine is metabolized by the liver and metabolic products are excreted in the urine. Approximately 10 percent of the administered codeine is demethylated to morphine, which may account for its analgesic activity.

Acetaminophen is distributed throughout most fluids of the body, and is metabolized primarily in the liver. Little unchanged drug is excreted in the urine, but most metabolic products appear in the urine within 24 hours.

INDICATIONS AND USAGE

TYLENOL with Codeine tablets (acetaminophen and codeine phosphate tablets) are indicated for the relief of mild to moderately severe pain.

TYLENOL with Codeine elixir (acetaminophen and codeine phosphate oral solution USP) is indicated for the relief of mild to moderate pain.

CONTRAINDICATIONS

TYLENOL with Codeine tablets or elixir (acetaminophen and codeine phosphate tablets and oral solution USP) should not be administered to patients who have previously exhibited hypersensitivity to any component.

WARNINGS

TYLENOL with Codeine tablets (acetaminophen and codeine phosphate tablets) contain sodium metabisulfite, a sulfite that may cause allergic-type reactions including anaphylactic symptoms and life-threatening or less severe asthmatic episodes in certain susceptible people. The overall prevalence of sulfite sensitivity in the general population is unknown and probably low. Sulfite sensitivity is seen more frequently in asthmatic than in nonasthmatic people.

PRECAUTIONS

General

Head Injury and Increased Intracranial Pressure: The respiratory depressant effects of narcotics and their capacity to elevate cerebrospinal fluid pressure may be markedly exaggerated in the presence of head injury, other intracranial lesions or a pre-existing increase in intracranial pressure. Furthermore, narcotics produce adverse reactions which may obscure the clinical course of patients with head injuries.

Acute Abdominal Conditions: The administration of this product or other narcotics may obscure the diagnosis or clinical course of patients with acute abdominal conditions.

Special Risk Patients: This drug should be given with caution to certain patients such as the elderly or debilitated, and those with severe impairment of hepatic or renal function, hypothyroidism, Addison's disease, and prostatic hypertrophy or urethral stricture.

Information for Patients

Codeine may impair the mental and/or physical abilities required for the performance of potentially hazardous tasks such as driving a car or operating machinery. The patient using this drug should be cautioned accordingly.

The patient should understand the single-dose and 24 hour dose limits, and the time interval between doses.

Drug Interactions

Patients receiving other narcotic analgesics, antipsychotics, antianxiety agents, or other CNS depressants (including alcohol) concomitantly with this drug may exhibit an additive CNS depression. When such combined therapy is contemplated, the dose of one or both agents should be reduced.

The concurrent use of anticholinergics with codeine may produce paralytic ileus.

Carcinogenesis, Mutagenesis, Impairment of Fertility

No long-term studies in animals have been performed with acetaminophen or codeine to determine carcinogenic potential or effects on fertility.

Acetaminophen and codeine have been found to have no mutagenic potential using the Ames Salmonella-Microsomal Activation test, the Basc test on Drosophila germ cells, and the Micronucleus test on mouse bone marrow.

Pregnancy

Teratogenic Effects: Pregnancy Category C.

Codeine: A study in rats and rabbits reported no teratogenic effect of codeine administered during the period of organogenesis in doses ranging from 5 to 120 mg/kg. In the rat, doses at the 120 mg/kg level, in the toxic range for the adult animal, were associated with an increase in embryo resorption at the time of implantation. In another study a single 100 mg/kg dose of codeine administered to pregnant mice reportedly resulted in delayed ossification in the offspring. There are no studies in humans, and the significance of these findings to humans, if any, is not known.

TYLENOL with Codeine (acetaminophen and codeine phosphate tablets and oral solution USP) should be used during pregnancy only if the potential benefit justifies the potential risk to the fetus.

Nonteratogenic Effects:

Dependence has been reported in newborns whose mothers took opiates regularly during pregnancy. Withdrawal signs include irritability, excessive crying, tremors, hyperreflexia, fever, vomiting, and diarrhea. These signs usually appear during the first few days of life.

Labor and Delivery

Narcotic analgesics cross the placental barrier. The closer to delivery and the larger the dose used, the greater the possibility of respiratory depression in the newborn. Narcotic analgesics should be avoided during labor if delivery of a premature infant is anticipated. If the mother has received narcotic analgesics during labor, newborn infants should be observed closely for signs of respiratory depression. Resuscitation may be required (see OVERDOSAGE). The effect of codeine, if any, on the later growth, development, and functional maturation of the child is unknown.

Nursing Mothers

Some studies, but not others, have reported detectable amounts of codeine in breast milk. The levels are probably not clinically significant after usual therapeutic dosage. The possibility of clinically important amounts being excreted in breast milk in individuals abusing codeine should be considered.

Pediatric Use

Safe dosage of TYLENOL with Codeine elixir (acetaminophen and codeine phosphate oral solution USP) has not been established in children below the age of three years.

ADVERSE REACTIONS

The most frequently observed adverse reactions include lightheadedness, dizziness, sedation, shortness of breath, nausea and vomiting. These effects seem to be more prominent in ambulatory than in non-ambulatory patients, and some of these adverse reactions may be alleviated if the patient lies down. Other adverse reactions include allergic reactions, euphoria, dysphoria, constipation, abdominal pain and pruritus.

At higher doses, codeine has most of the disadvantages of morphine including respiratory depression.

DRUG ABUSE AND DEPENDENCE

TYLENOL with Codeine tablets (acetaminophen and codeine phosphate tablets) are a Schedule III controlled substance.

TYLENOL with Codeine elixir (acetaminophen and codeine phosphate oral solution USP) is a Schedule V controlled substance.

Codeine can produce drug dependence of the morphine type and, therefore, has the potential for being abused. Psychic dependence, physical dependence and tolerance may develop upon repeated administration of this drug, and it should be prescribed and administered with the same degree of caution appropriate to the use of other oral narcotic-containing medications.

OVERDOSAGE

Acetaminophen

Signs and Symptoms: In acute acetaminophen overdosage, dose-dependent, potentially fatal hepatic necrosis is the most serious adverse effect. Renal tubular necrosis, hypoglycemic coma and thrombocytopenia may also occur.

In adults, hepatic toxicity has rarely been reported with acute overdoses of less than 10 grams and fatalities with less than 15 grams. Importantly, young children seem to be more resistant than adults to the hepatotoxic effect of an acetaminophen overdose. Despite this, the measures outlined below should be initiated in any adult or child suspected of having ingested an acetaminophen overdose.

Early symptoms following a potentially hepatotoxic overdose may include: nausea, vomiting, diaphoresis and general malaise. Clinical and laboratory evidence of hepatic toxicity may not be apparent until 48 to 72 hours post-ingestion.

Treatment: The stomach should be emptied promptly by lavage or by induction of emesis with syrup of ipecac. Patients' estimates of the quantity of a drug ingested are notoriously unreliable. Therefore, if an acetaminophen overdose is suspected, a serum acetaminophen assay should be obtained as early as possible, but no sooner than four hours following ingestion. Liver function studies should be obtained initially and repeated at 24-hour intervals.

The antidote, N-acetylcysteine, should be administered as early as possible, preferably within 16 hours of the overdose ingestion for optimal results, but in any case, within 24 hours. Following recovery, there are no residual, structural or functional hepatic abnormalities.

Codeine

Signs and Symptoms: Serious overdose with codeine is characterized by respiratory depression (a decrease in respiratory rate and/or tidal volume, Cheyne-Stokes respiration, cyanosis), extreme somnolence progressing to stupor or coma, skeletal muscle flaccidity, cold and clammy skin, and sometimes bradycardia and hypotension. In severe overdosage, apnea, circulatory collapse, cardiac arrest and death may occur.

Treatment: Primary attention should be given to the reestablishment of adequate respiratory exchange through provision of a patent airway and the institution of assisted or controlled ventilation. The narcotic antagonist naloxone is a specific antidote against respiratory depression which may result from overdosage or unusual sensitivity to narcotics, including codeine. Therefore, an appropriate dose of naloxone hydrochloride (see package insert) should be administered, preferably by the intravenous route, and simultaneously with efforts at respiratory resuscitation. Since the duration of action of codeine may exceed that of the antagonist, the patient should be kept under continued surveillance and repeated doses of the antagonist should be administered as needed to maintain adequate respiration.

An antagonist should not be administered in the absence of clinically significant respiratory or cardiovascular depression. Oxygen, intravenous fluids, vasopressors and other supportive measures should be employed as indicated.

Gastric emptying may be useful in removing unabsorbed drug.

DOSAGE AND ADMINISTRATION

Dosage should be adjusted according to severity of pain and response of the patient.

It should be kept in mind, however, that tolerance to codeine can develop with continued use and that the incidence of untoward effects is dose related. Adult doses of codeine higher than 60 mg fail to give commensurate relief of pain but merely prolong analgesia and are associated with an appreciably increased incidence of undesirable side effects. Equivalently high doses in children would have similar effects.

The usual adult dosage for tablets is:

	Single Doses (Range)	Maximum 24 Hour Dose
Codeine Phosphate	15mg–60mg	360mg
Acetaminophen	300mg–1000mg	4000mg

Doses may be repeated up to every 4 hours.

The prescriber must determine the number of tablets per dose, and the maximum number of tablets per 24 hours, based upon the above dosage guidance. This information should be conveyed in the prescription.

For children, the dose of codeine phosphate is 0.5 mg/kg.

TYLENOL with Codeine elixir (acetaminophen and codeine phosphate oral solution USP) contains 120 mg of acetaminophen and 12 mg of codeine phosphate/5 mL and is given orally.

The usual doses are:

Children: *(7 to 12 years):* 10 mL (2 teaspoonfuls) 3 or 4 times daily.
(3 to 6 years): 5 mL (1 teaspoonful) 3 or 4 times daily.
(under 3 years): safe dosage has not been established.

Adults: 15 mL (1 tablespoonful) every 4 hours as needed.

HOW SUPPLIED

TYLENOL with Codeine tablets (acetaminophen and codeine phosphate tablets): (round, white, imprinted "McNEIL," "TYLENOL CODEINE" and either "3" or "4"): No. 3—NDC 0045-0513-60 bottles of 100, NDC 0045-0513-70 bottles of 500, NDC 0045-0513-80 bottles of 1000, NDC 0045-0513-72 unit dose (20 × 25); No. 4—NDC 0045-0515-60 bottles of 100, NDC 0045-0515-70 bottles of 500.

TYLENOL with Codeine elixir (acetaminophen and codeine phosphate oral solution USP) contains 120 mg acetaminophen and 12 mg codeine phosphate/5 mL (colored amber, cherry flavored) — NDC 0045-0508-16, bottles of 1 pint.

Store TYLENOL with Codeine tablets at controlled room temperature (15–30°C, 59–86°F).

Store TYLENOL with Codeine elixir at controlled room temperature (15–30°C, 59–86°F). Protect from light. Do not refrigerate. Do not freeze.

Dispense in tight, light-resistant container as defined in the official compendium.

OMP DIVISION
ORTHO-MCNEIL
PHARMACEUTICAL, INC.
RARITAN, NEW JERSEY 08869

633-10-057-3 Revised July 2000

Shown in Product Identification Guide, page 328

ULTRACET™ ℞

[ŭl'tră-sĕt]

(tramadol hydrochloride/acetaminophen tablets)

Prescribing Information

DESCRIPTION

ULTRACET™ (37.5 mg tramadol hydrochloride/325 mg acetaminophen tablets) combines two analgesics, tramadol and acetaminophen.

The chemical name for tramadol hydrochloride is (+)*cis*-2-[(dimethylamino)methyl]-1-(3-methoxyphenyl) cyclohexanol hydrochloride. Its structural formula is:

The molecular weight of tramadol hydrochloride is 299.84. Tramadol hydrochloride is a white, bitter, crystalline and odorless powder.

The chemical name for acetaminophen is *N*-acetyl-*p*-aminophenol. Its structural formula is:

The molecular weight of acetaminophen is 151.17. Acetaminophen is an analgesic and antipyretic agent which occurs as a white, odorless, crystalline powder, possessing a slightly bitter taste.

ULTRACET Tablets contain 37.5 mg tramadol hydrochloride and 325 mg acetaminophen and are light yellow in color. Inactive ingredients in the tablet are powdered cellulose, pregelatinized starch, sodium starch glycolate, starch, purified water, magnesium stearate, OPADRY® Light Yellow, and carnauba wax.

CLINICAL PHARMACOLOGY

The following information is based on studies of tramadol alone or acetaminophen alone, except where otherwise noted:

Pharmacodynamics

Tramadol is a centrally acting synthetic opioid analgesic. Although its mode of action is not completely understood, from animal tests, at least two complementary mechanisms appear applicable: binding of parent and M1 metabolite to μ-opioid receptors and weak inhibition of reuptake of norepinephrine and serotonin.

Opioid activity is due to both low affinity binding of the parent compound and higher affinity binding of the O-demethylated metabolite M1 to μ-opioid receptors. In animal models, M1 is up to 6 times more potent than tramadol in producing analgesia and 200 times more potent in μ-opioid binding. Tramadol-induced analgesia is only partially antagonized by the opiate antagonist naloxone in several animal tests.

The relative contribution of both tramadol and M1 to human analgesia is dependent upon the plasma concentrations of each compound (see CLINICAL PHARMACOLOGY, Pharmacokinetics).

Tramadol has been shown to inhibit reuptake of norepinephrine and serotonin in vitro, as have some other opioid analgesics. These mechanisms may contribute independently to the overall analgesic profile of tramadol.

Apart from analgesia, tramadol administration may produce a constellation of symptoms (including dizziness, somnolence, nausea, constipation, sweating and pruritus) similar to that of other opioids.

Acetaminophen

Acetaminophen is a non-opiate, non-salicylate analgesic.

Pharmacokinetics

Tramadol is administered as a racemate and both the [−] and [+] forms of both tramadol and M1 are detected in the circulation. The pharmacokinetics of plasma tramadol and acetaminophen following oral administration of one ULTRACET tablet are shown in Table 1. Tramadol has a slower absorption and longer half-life when compared to acetaminophen.

[See table 1 below]

A single dose pharmacokinetic study of ULTRACET in volunteers showed no drug interactions between tramadol and acetaminophen. Upon multiple oral dosing to steady state, however, the bioavailability of tramadol and metabolite M1 was lower for the combination tablets compared to tramadol administered alone. The decrease in AUC was 14% for (+)-tramadol, 10.4% for (−)-tramadol, 11.9% for (+)-M1 and 24.2% for (−)-M1. The cause of this reduced bioavailability is not clear. Following single or multiple dose administration of ULTRACET, no significant change in acetaminophen pharmacokinetics was observed when compared to acetaminophen given alone.

Absorption:

The absolute bioavailability of tramadol from ULTRACET tablets has not been determined. Tramadol hydrochloride has a mean absolute bioavailability of approximately 75% following administration of a single 100 mg oral dose of ULTRAM® tablets. The mean peak plasma concentration of racemic tramadol and M1 after administration of two ULTRACET tablets occurs at approximately two and three hours, respectively, post-dose.

Peak plasma concentrations of acetaminophen occur within one hour and are not affected by co-administration with tramadol. Oral absorption of acetaminophen following administration of ULTRACET occurs primarily in the small intestine.

Food Effects:

When ULTRACET was administered with food, the time to peak plasma concentration was delayed for approximately 35 minutes for tramadol and almost one hour for acetaminophen. However, peak plasma concentration or the extent of absorption of either tramadol or acetaminophen were not affected. The clinical significance of this difference is unknown.

Distribution:

The volume of distribution of tramadol was 2.6 and 2.9 L/kg in male and female subjects, respectively, following a 100 mg intravenous dose. The binding of tramadol to human plasma proteins is approximately 20% and binding also appears to be independent of concentration up to 10 μg/mL. Saturation of plasma protein binding occurs only at concentrations outside the clinically relevant range.

Acetaminophen appears to be widely distributed throughout most body tissues except fat. Its apparent volume of distribution is about 0.9 L/kg. A relative small portion (~20%) of acetaminophen is bound to plasma protein.

Metabolism:

Following oral administration, tramadol is extensively metabolized by a number of pathways, including CYP2D6 and CYP3A4, as well as by conjugation of parent and metabolites. Approximately 30% of the dose is excreted in the urine as unchanged drug, whereas 60% of the dose is excreted as metabolites. The major metabolic pathways appear to be *N*- and *O*-demethylation and glucuronidation or sulfation in the liver. Metabolite M1 (*O*-desmethyltramadol) is pharmacologically active in animal models. Formation of M1 is dependent on CYP2D6 and as such is subject to inhibition, which may affect the therapeutic response (see PRECAUTIONS, Drug Interactions).

Approximately 7% of the population has reduced activity of the CYP2D6 isoenzyme of cytochrome P450. These individuals are "poor metabolizers" of debrisoquine, dextromethorphan, tricyclic antidepressants, among other drugs. Based on a population PK analysis of Phase 1 studies in healthy

Continued on next page

Table 1: Summary of Mean (±SD) Pharmacokinetic Parameters of the (+)- and (−) Enantiomers of Tramadol and M1 and Acetaminophen Following A Single Oral Dose Of One Tramadol/Acetaminophen Combination Tablet (37.5 mg/325 mg) in Volunteers

Parameter[a]	(+)-Tramadol	(−)-Tramadol	(+)-M1	(−)-M1	acetaminophen
C_{max} (ng/mL)	64.3 (9.3)	55.5 (8.1)	10.9 (5.7)	12.8 (4.2)	4.2 (0.8)
t_{max} (h)	1.8 (0.6)	1.8 (0.7)	2.1 (0.7)	2.2 (0.7)	0.9 (0.7)
CL/F (mL/min)	588 (226)	736 (244)	— —	— —	365 (84)
$t_{1/2}$ (h)	5.1 (1.4)	4.7 (1.2)	7.8 (3.0)	6.2 (1.6)	2.5 (0.6)

[a]For acetaminophen, C_{max} was measured as μg/mL.

Ultracet—Cont.

subjects, concentrations of tramadol were approximately 20% higher in "poor metabolizers" versus extensive metabolizers, while M1 concentrations were 40% lower. In vitro drug interaction studies in human liver microsomes indicates that inhibitors of CYP2D6 such as fluoxetine and its metabolite norfluoxetine, amitriptyline and quinidine inhibit the metabolism of tramadol to various degrees. The full pharmacological impact of these alterations in terms of either efficacy or safety is unknown. Concomitant use of SEROTONIN re-uptake INHIBITORS and MAO INHIBITORS may enhance the risk of adverse events, including seizure (see WARNINGS) and serotonin syndrome.

Acetaminophen is primarily metabolized in the liver by first-order kinetics and involves three principal separate pathways:

a) conjugation with glucuronide;

b) conjugation with sulfate; and

c) oxidation via the cytochrome, P450-dependent, mixed-function oxidase enzyme pathway to form a reactive intermediate metabolite, which conjugates with glutathione and is then further metabolized to form cysteine and mercapturic acid conjugates. The principal cytochrome P450 isoenzyme involved appears to be CYP2E1, with CYP1A2 and CYP3A4 as additional pathways.

In adults, the majority of acetaminophen is conjugated with glucuronic acid and, to a lesser extent, with sulfate. These glucuronide-, sulfate-, and glutathione-derived metabolites lack biologic activity. In premature infants, newborns, and young infants, the sulfate conjugate predominates.

Elimination:

Tramadol is eliminated primarily through metabolism by the liver and the metabolites are eliminated primarily by the kidneys. The plasma elimination half-lives of racemic tramadol and M1 are approximately 5–6 and 7 hours, respectively, after administration of ULTRACET. The apparent plasma elimination half-life of racemic tramadol increased to 7–9 hours upon multiple dosing of ULTRACET. The half-life of acetaminophen is about 2 to 3 hours in adults. It is somewhat shorter in children and somewhat longer in neonates and in cirrhotic patients. Acetaminophen is eliminated from the body primarily by formation of glucuronide and sulfate conjugates in a dose-dependent manner. Less than 9% of acetaminophen is excreted unchanged in the urine.

Special Populations

Renal:

The pharmacokinetics of ULTRACET in patients with renal impairment have not been studied. Based on studies using tramadol alone, excretion of tramadol and metabolite M1 is reduced in patients with creatinine clearance of less than 30 mL/min, adjustment of dosing regimen in this patient population is recommended. (See DOSAGE AND ADMINISTRATION.) The total amount of tramadol and M1 removed during a 4-hour dialysis period is less than 7% of the administered dose based on studies using tramadol alone.

Hepatic:

The pharmacokinetics and tolerability of ULTRACET in patients with impaired hepatic function has not been studied. Since tramadol and acetaminophen are both extensively metabolized by the liver, the use of ULTRACET in patients with hepatic impairment is not recommended (see PRECAUTIONS and DOSAGE AND ADMINISTRATION).

Geriatric:

A population pharmacokinetic analysis of data obtained from a clinical trial in patients with chronic pain treated with ULTRACET which included 55 patients between 65 and 75 years of age and 19 patients over 75 years of age, showed no significant changes in pharmacokinetics of tramadol and acetaminophen in elderly patients with normal renal and hepatic function (see PRECAUTIONS, Geriatric Use).

Gender:

Tramadol clearance was 20% higher in female subjects compared to males on four phase I studies of ULTRACET in 50 male and 34 female healthy subjects. The clinical significance of this difference is unknown.

Pediatric:

Pharmacokinetics of ULTRACET Tablets have not been studied in pediatric patients below 16 years of age.

Clinical Studies

Single Dose Studies for Treatment of Acute Pain

In pivotal single-dose studies in acute pain, two tablets of ULTRACET administered to patients with pain following oral surgical procedures provided greater relief than placebo or either of the individual components given at the same dose. The onset of pain relief after ULTRACET was faster than tramadol alone. Onset of analgesia occurred in less than one hour. The duration of pain relief after ULTRACET was longer than acetaminophen alone. Analgesia was generally comparable to that of the comparator, ibuprofen.

INDICATIONS AND USAGE

ULTRACET is indicated for the short-term (five days or less) management of acute pain.

CONTRAINDICATIONS

ULTRACET should not be administered to patients who have previously demonstrated hypersensitivity to tramadol, acetaminophen, any other component of this product or opioids. ULTRACET is contraindicated in any situation where opioids are contraindicated, including acute intoxication with any of the following: alcohol, hypnotics, narcotics, centrally acting analgesics, opioids or psychotropic drugs. ULTRACET may worsen central nervous system and respiratory depression in these patients.

WARNINGS

Seizure Risk

Seizures have been reported in patients receiving tramadol within the recommended dosage range. Spontaneous post-marketing reports indicate that seizure risk is increased with doses of tramadol above the recommended range. Concomitant use of tramadol increases the seizure risk in patients taking:

- **Selective serotonin reuptake inhibitors (SSRI antidepressants or anoretics),**
- **Tricyclic antidepressants (TCAs), and other tricyclic compounds (e.g., cyclobenzaprine, promethazine, etc.), or**
- **Other opioids.**

Administration of tramadol may enhance the seizure risk in patients taking:

- **MAO inhibitors (see also WARNINGS—Use with MAO Inhibitors),**
- **Neuroleptics, or**
- **Other drugs that reduce the seizure threshold.**

Risk of convulsions may also increase in patients with epilepsy, those with a history of seizures, or in patients with a recognized risk for seizure (such as head trauma, metabolic disorders, alcohol and drug withdrawal, CNS infections). In tramadol overdose, naloxone administration may increase the risk of seizure.

Anaphylactoid Reactions

Serious and rarely fatal anaphylactoid reactions have been reported in patients receiving therapy with tramadol. When these events do occur it is often following the first dose. Other reported allergic reactions include pruritus, hives, bronchospasm, angioedema, toxic epidermal necrolysis and Stevens-Johnson syndrome. Patients with a history of anaphylactoid reactions to codeine and other opioids may be at increased risk and therefore should not receive ULTRACET (see CONTRAINDICATIONS).

Respiratory Depression

Administer ULTRACET cautiously in patients at risk for respiratory depression. In these patients, alternative non-opioid analgesics should be considered. When large doses of tramadol are administered with anesthetic medications or alcohol, respiratory depression may result. Respiratory depression should be treated as an overdose. If naloxone is to be administered, use cautiously because it may precipitate seizures (see WARNINGS, Seizure Risk and OVERDOSAGE).

Interaction With Central Nervous System (CNS) Depressants

ULTRACET should be used with caution and in reduced dosages when administered to patients receiving CNS depressants such as alcohol, opioids, anesthetic agents, narcotics, phenothiazines, tranquilizers or sedative hypnotics. Tramadol increases the risk of CNS and respiratory depression in these patients.

Increased Intracranial Pressure or Head Trauma

ULTRACET should be used with caution in patients with increased intracranial pressure or head injury. The respiratory depressant effects of opioids include carbon dioxide retention and secondary elevation of cerebrospinal fluid pressure and may be markedly exaggerated in these patients. Additionally, pupillary changes (miosis) from tramadol may obscure the existence, extent, or course of intracranial pathology. Clinicians should also maintain a high index of suspicion for adverse drug reaction when evaluating altered mental status in these patients if they are receiving ULTRACET (see Respiratory Depression).

Use in Ambulatory Patients

Tramadol may impair the mental and or physical abilities required for the performance of potentially hazardous tasks such as driving a car or operating machinery. The patient using this drug should be cautioned accordingly.

Use With MAO Inhibitors and Serotonin Re-uptake Inhibitors

Use ULTRACET with great caution in patients taking monoamine oxidase inhibitors. Animal studies have shown increased deaths with combined administration of MAO inhibitors and tramadol. Concomitant use of tramadol with MAO inhibitors or SSRI's increases the risk of adverse events, including seizure and serotonin syndrome.

Use With Alcohol

ULTRACET should not be used concomitantly with alcohol consumption. The use of ULTRACET in patients with liver disease is not recommended.

Use With Other Acetaminophen-containing Products

Due to the potential for acetaminophen hepatotoxicity at doses higher than the recommended dose, ULTRACET should not be used concomitantly with other acetaminophen-containing products.

Withdrawal

Withdrawal symptoms may occur if ULTRACET is discontinued abruptly. (See DRUG ABUSE AND DEPENDENCE.) These symptoms may include: anxiety, sweating, insomnia, rigors, pain, nausea, tremors, diarrhea, upper respiratory symptoms, piloerection, and rarely hallucinations. Clinical experience suggests that withdrawal symptoms may be relieved by tapering the medication.

Physical Dependence and Abuse

Tramadol may induce psychic and physical dependence of the morphine-type (μ-opioid). (See DRUG ABUSE AND DEPENDENCE.) Tramadol should not be used in opioid-dependent patients. Tramadol has been shown to reinitiate physical dependence in some patients that have been previously dependent on other opioids. Dependence and abuse, including drug-seeking behavior and taking illicit actions to obtain the drug are not limited to those patients with prior history of opioid dependence.

Risk of Overdosage

Serious potential consequences of overdosage with tramadol are central nervous system depression, respiratory depression and death. In treating an overdose, primary attention should be given to maintaining adequate ventilation along with general supportive treatment. (See OVERDOSAGE.)

Serious potential consequences of overdosage with acetaminophen are hepatic (centrilobular) necrosis, leading to hepatic failure and death. Emergency help should be sought immediately and treatment initiated immediately if overdose is suspected, even if symptoms are not apparent.

PRECAUTIONS

General

The recommended dose of ULTRACET should not be exceeded.

Do not co-administer ULTRACET with other tramadol or acetaminophen-containing products. (See WARNINGS, Use With Other Acetaminophen-containing Products and Risk of Overdosage.)

Pediatric Use

The safety and effectiveness of ULTRACET has not been studied in the pediatric population.

Geriatric Use

In general, dose selection for an elderly patient should be cautious, reflecting the greater frequency of decreased hepatic, renal, or cardiac function; of concomitant disease and multiple drug therapy.

Acute Abdominal Conditions

The administration of ULTRACET may complicate the clinical assessment of patients with acute abdominal conditions.

Use in Renal Disease

ULTRACET has not been studied in patients with impaired renal function. Experience with tramadol suggest that impaired renal function results in a decreased rate and extent of excretion of tramadol and its active metabolite, M1. In patients with creatinine clearances of less than 30 mL/min, it is recommended that the dosing interval of ULTRACET be increased not to exceed 2 tablets every 12 hours.

Use in Hepatic Disease

ULTRACET has not been studied in patients with impaired hepatic function. The use of ULTRACET in patients with hepatic impairment is not recommended (see WARNINGS, Use With Alcohol).

Information for Patients

- ULTRACET may impair mental or physical abilities required for the performance of potentially hazardous tasks such as driving a car or operating machinery.
- ULTRACET should not be taken with alcohol containing beverages.
- The patient should be instructed not to take ULTRACET in combination with other tramadol or acetaminophen-containing products, including over-the-counter preparations.
- ULTRACET should be used with caution when taking medications such as tranquilizers, hypnotics or other opiate containing analgesics.
- The patient should be instructed to inform the physician if they are pregnant, think they might become pregnant, or are trying to become pregnant (see PRECAUTIONS, Labor and Delivery).
- The patient should understand the single-dose and 24-hour dose limit and the time interval between doses, since exceeding these recommendations can result in respiratory depression, seizures, hepatic toxicity and death.

Drug Interactions

In vitro studies indicate that tramadol is unlikely to inhibit the CYP3A4-mediated metabolism of other drugs when tramadol is administered concomitantly at therapeutic doses. Tramadol does not appear to induce its own metabolism in humans, since observed maximal plasma concentrations after multiple oral doses are higher than expected based on single-dose data. Tramadol is a mild inducer of selected drug metabolism pathways measured in animals.

Use With Carbamazepine

Patients taking **carbamazepine** may have a significantly reduced analgesic effect of tramadol. Because carbamazepine increases tramadol metabolism and because of the seizure risk associated with tramadol, concomitant administration of ULTRACET and carbamazepine is not recommended.

Use With Quinidine

Tramadol is metabolized to M1 by CYP2D6. **Quinidine** is a selective inhibitor of that isoenzyme; so that concomitant administration of quinidine and tramadol results in increased concentrations of tramadol and reduced concentrations of M1. The clinical consequences of these findings are unknown. In vitro drug interaction studies in human liver microsomes indicate that tramadol has no effect on quinidine metabolism.

Use With Inhibitors of CYP2D6

In vitro drug interaction studies in human liver microsomes indicate that concomitant administration with inhibitors of CYP2D6 such as fluoxetine, paroxetine, and amitriptyline could result in some inhibition of the metabolism of tramadol.

Use With Cimetidine
Concomitant administration of ULTRACET and **cimetidine** has not been studied. Concomitant administration of tramadol and cimetidine does not result in clinically significant changes in tramadol pharmacokinetics. Therefore, no alteration of the ULTRACET dosage regimen is recommended.
Use With MAO Inhibitors
Interactions with **MAO Inhibitors,** due to interference with detoxification mechanisms, have been reported for some centrally acting drugs (see WARNINGS, Use With MAO Inhibitors).
Use With Digoxin
Post-marketing surveillance of tramadol has revealed rare reports of **digoxin** toxicity.
Use With Warfarin Like Compounds
Post-marketing surveillance of both tramadol and acetaminophen individual products have revealed rare alterations of warfarin effect, including elevation of prothrombin times.
While such changes have been generally of limited clinical significance for the individual products, periodic evaluation of prothrombin time should be performed when ULTRACET and warfarin-like compounds are administered concurrently.
Carcinogenesis, Mutagenesis, Impairment of Fertility
There are no animal or laboratory studies on the combination product (tramadol and acetaminophen) to evaluate carcinogenesis, mutagenesis, or impairment of fertility.
A slight but statistically significant increase in two common murine tumors, pulmonary and hepatic, was observed in a mouse carcinogenicity study, particularly in aged mice. Mice were dosed orally up to 30 mg/kg (90 mg/m^2 or 0.5 times the maximum daily human tramadol dosage of 185 mg/m^2) for approximately two years, although the study was not done with the Maximum Tolerated Dose. This finding is not believed to suggest risk in humans. No such finding occurred in rat carcinogenicity study (dosing orally up to 30 mg/kg, 180 mg/m^2, or 1 time the maximum daily human tramadol dosage).
Tramadol was not mutagenic in the following assays: Ames *Salmonella* microsomal activation test, CHO/HPRT mammalian cell assay, mouse lymphoma assay (in the absence of metabolic activation), dominant lethal mutation tests in mice, chromosome aberration test in Chinese hamsters, and bone marrow micronucleus tests in mice and Chinese hamsters. Weakly mutagenic results occurred in the presence of metabolic activation in the mouse lymphoma assay and micronucleus test in rats. Overall, the weight of evidence from these tests indicates that tramadol does not pose a genotoxic risk to humans.
No effects on fertility were observed for tramadol at oral dose levels up to 50 mg/kg (350 mg/m^2) in male rats and 75 mg/kg (450 mg/m^2) in female rats. These dosages are 1.6 and 2.4 times the maximum daily human tramadol dosage of 185 mg/m^2.
Pregnancy
Teratogenic Effects: *Pregnancy Category C*
No drug-related teratogenic effects were observed in the progeny of rats treated orally with tramadol and acetaminophen. The tramadol/acetaminophen combination product was shown to be embryotoxic and fetotoxic in rats at a maternally toxic dose, 50/434 mg/kg tramadol/acetaminophen (300/2604 mg/m^2 or 1.6 times the maximum daily human tramadol/acetaminophen dosage of 185/1591 mg/m^2), but was not teratogenic at this dose level. Embryo and fetal toxicity consisted of decreased fetal weights and increased supernumerary ribs.
Non-teratogenic effects:
Tramadol alone was evaluated in peri- and post-natal studies in rats. Progeny of dams receiving oral (gavage) dose levels of 50 mg/kg (300 mg/m^2 or 1.6 times the maximum daily human tramadol dosage) or greater had decreased weights, and pup survival was decreased early in lactation at 80 mg/kg (480 mg/m^2 or 2.6 times the maximum daily human tramadol dosage).
There are no adequate and well-controlled studies in pregnant women. ULTRACET should be used during pregnancy only if the potential benefit justifies the potential risk to the fetus. Neonatal seizures, neonatal withdrawal syndrome, fetal death and still birth have been reported with tramadol hydrochloride during post-marketing.
Labor and Delivery
ULTRACET should not be used in pregnant women prior to or during labor unless the potential benefits outweigh the risks. Safe use in pregnancy has not been established. Chronic use during pregnancy may lead to physical dependence and post-partum withdrawal symptoms in the newborn. (See DRUG ABUSE AND DEPENDENCE.) Tramadol has been shown to cross the placenta. The mean ratio of serum tramadol in the umbilical veins compared to maternal veins was 0.83 for 40 women given tramadol during labor.
The effect of ULTRACET, if any, on the later growth, development, and functional maturation of the child is unknown.
Nursing Mothers
ULTRACET is not recommended for obstetrical preoperative medication or for post-delivery analgesia in nursing mothers because its safety in infants and newborns has not been studied.
Following a single IV 100 mg dose of tramadol, the cumulative excretion in breast milk within 16 hours post-dose was 100 µg of tramadol (0.1% of the maternal dose) and 27 µg of M1.

ADVERSE REACTIONS

Table 2 reports the incidence rate of treatment-emergent adverse events over five days of ULTRACET use in clinical trials (subjects took an average of at least 6 tablets per day).

Table 2: Incidence of Treatment-Emergent Adverse Events (≥2.0%)

Body System Preferred Term	ULTRACET (N=142) %
Gastrointestinal System	
Constipation	6
Diarrhea	3
Nausea	3
Dry Mouth	2
Psychiatric Disorders	
Somnolence	6
Anorexia	3
Insomnia	2
Central & Peripheral Nervous System	
Dizziness	3
Skin and Appendages	
Sweating Increased	4
Pruritus	2
Reproductive Disorders, Male*	
Prostatic Disorder	2

*Number of males = 62

Incidence at least 1%, causal relationship at least possible or greater: the following lists adverse reactions that occurred with an incidence of at least 1% in single-dose or repeated-dose clinical trials of ULTRACET.
Body as a Whole—Asthenia, fatigue, hot flushes
Central and Peripheral Nervous System—Dizziness, headache, tremor
Gastrointestinal System—Abdominal pain, constipation, diarrhea, dyspepsia, flatulence, dry mouth, nausea, vomiting
Psychiatric Disorders—Anorexia, anxiety, confusion, euphoria, insomnia, nervousness, somnolence
Skin and Appendages—Pruritus, rash, increased sweating.
Selected Adverse events occurring at less than 1%: the following lists clinically relevant adverse reactions that occurred with an incidence of less than 1% in ULTRACET clinical trials.
Body as a Whole—Chest pain, rigors, syncope, withdrawal syndrome
Cardiovascular Disorders—Hypertension, aggravated hypertension, hypotension
Central and Peripheral Nervous System—Ataxia, convulsions, hypertonia, migraine, aggravated migraine, involuntary muscle contractions, paraesthesia, stupor, vertigo
Gastrointestinal System—Dysphagia, melena, tongue edema
Hearing and Vestibular Disorders—Tinnitus
Heart Rate and Rhythm Disorders—Arrhythmia, palpitation, tachycardia
Liver and Biliary System—Hepatic function abnormal
Metabolic and Nutritional Disorders—Weight decrease
Psychiatric Disorders—Amnesia, depersonalization, depression, drug abuse, emotional lability, hallucination, impotence, paroniria, abnormal thinking
Red Blood Cell Disorders—Anemia
Respiratory System—Dyspnea
Urinary System—Albuminuria, micturition disorder, oliguria, urinary retention
Vision Disorders—Abnormal vision
Other clinically significant adverse experiences previously reported with tramadol hydrochloride.
Other events which have been reported with the use of tramadol products and for which a causal association has not been determined include: vasodilation, orthostatic hypotension, myocardial ischemia, pulmonary edema, allergic reactions (including anaphylaxis and urticaria, Stevens-Johnson syndrome/TENS), cognitive dysfunction, difficulty concentrating, depression, suicidal tendency, hepatitis liver failure and gastrointestinal bleeding. Reported laboratory abnormalities included elevated creatinine and liver function tests. Serotonin syndrome (whose symptoms may include mental status change, hyperreflexia, fever, shivering, tremor, agitation, diaphoresis, seizures and coma) has been reported with tramadol when used concomitantly with other serotonergic agents such as SSRIs and MAOIs.
Other clinically significant adverse experiences previously reported with acetaminophen.
Allergic reactions (primarily skin rash) or reports of hypersensitivity secondary to acetaminophen are rare and generally controlled by discontinuation of the drug and, when necessary, symptomatic treatment.

DRUG ABUSE AND DEPENDENCE

Tramadol may induce psychic and physical dependence of the morphine-type (µ-opioid). (See WARNINGS.) Dependence and abuse, including drug-seeking behavior and taking illicit actions to obtain the drug are not limited to those patients with a prior history of opioid dependence. The risk in patients with substance abuse has been observed to be higher. Tramadol is associated with craving and tolerance development. Withdrawal symptoms may occur if tramadol is discontinued abruptly. These symptoms may include: anxiety, sweating, insomnia, rigors, pain, nausea, tremors, diarrhea, upper respiratory symptoms, piloerection, and rarely hallucinations. Clinical experience suggests that withdrawal symptoms may be relieved by reinstitution of opioid therapy followed by a gradual, tapered dose reduction of the medication combined with symptomatic support.

OVERDOSAGE

ULTRACET is a combination product. The clinical presentation of overdose may include the signs and symptoms of tramadol toxicity, acetaminophen toxicity or both. The initial symptoms of tramadol overdosage may include respiratory depression and or seizures. The initial symptoms seen within the first 24 hours following an acetaminophen overdose are: anorexia, nausea, vomiting, malaise, pallor and diaphoresis.
Tramadol
Serious potential consequences of overdosage are respiratory depression, lethargy, coma, seizure, cardiac arrest and death. (See WARNINGS.) Fatalities have been reported in post marketing in association with both intentional and unintentional overdose with tramadol.
Acetaminophen
Serious potential consequences of overdosage with acetaminophen are hepatic centrilobular necrosis, leading to hepatic failure and death. Renal tubular necrosis, hypoglycemia and coagulation defects also may occur. Early symptoms following a potentially hepatotoxic overdose may include: nausea, vomiting, diaphoresis and general malaise. Clinical and laboratory evidence of hepatic toxicity may not be apparent until 48 to 72 hours post ingestion.
Treatment of Overdose
A single or multiple overdose with ULTRACET may be a potentially lethal polydrug overdose, and consultation with a regional poison control center is recommended.
In treating an overdose of ULTRACET, primary attention should be given to maintaining adequate ventilation along with general supportive treatment. While naloxone will reverse some, but not all, symptoms caused by overdosage with tramadol, the risk of seizures is also increased with naloxone administration. In animals, convulsions following the administration of toxic doses of tramadol could be suppressed with barbiturates or benzodiazepines but were increased with naloxone. Naloxone administration did not change the lethality of an overdose in mice. Based on experience with tramadol, hemodialysis is not expected to be helpful in an overdose because it removes less than 7% of the administered dose in a 4-hour dialysis period.
Standard recommendations should be followed for the treatment of acetaminophen overdose.

DOSAGE AND ADMINISTRATION

For the short-term (five days or less) management of acute pain, the recommended dose of ULTRACET is 2 tablets every 4 to 6 hours as needed for pain relief up to a maximum of 8 tablets per day.
Individualization of Dose
In patients with creatinine clearances of less than 30 mL/min, it is recommended that the dosing interval of ULTRACET be increased not to exceed 2 tablets every 12 hours. Dose selection for an elderly patient should be cautious, in view of the potential for greater sensitivity to adverse events.

HOW SUPPLIED

ULTRACET (37.5 mg tramadol hydrochloride/325 mg acetaminophen) Tablets (light yellow, film-coated capsule-shaped tablet) debossed "O–M" on one side and "650" on the other are available as follows:
20's: NDC 0045 0650 50 (Bottles of 20 tablets)
100's: NDC 0045 0650 60 (Bottles of 100 tablets)
500's: NDC 0045 0650 70 (Bottles of 500 tablets)
HUD 100's: NDC 0045 0650 10 (Packages of 100 unit doses in blister packs, 10 cards of 10 tablets each)
Dispense in a tight container. Store at 25°C (77°F); excursions permitted to 15 – 30°C (59 – 86°F).
ORTHO-McNEIL
OMP DIVISION
ORTHO-McNEIL PHARMACEUTICAL, INC.
Raritan, New Jersey 08869
U.S. Patent 5,336,691 635-11-231-1
 Issued August 2001 7517200
Shown in Product Identification Guide, page 328

ULTRAM® ℞
(tramadol hydrochloride tablets)

Prescribing Information

DESCRIPTION

ULTRAM® (tramadol hydrochloride tablets) is a centrally acting analgesic. The chemical name for tramadol hydrochloride is (±)*cis*-2-[(dimethylamino)methyl]-1-(3-methoxyphenyl) cyclohexanol hydrochloride. Its structural formula is:
[See chemical structure at top of next column]
The molecular weight of tramadol hydrochloride is 299.8. Tramadol hydrochloride is a white, bitter, crystalline and odorless powder. It is readily soluble in water and ethanol and has a pKa of 9.41. The n-octanol/water log partition coefficient (logP) is 1.35 at pH 7. ULTRAM tablets contain 50 mg of tramadol hydrochloride and are white in color. In-

Continued on next page

Ultram—Cont.

active ingredients in the tablet are corn starch, hydroxypropyl methylcellulose, lactose, magnesium stearate, microcrystalline cellulose, polyethylene glycol, polysorbate 80, sodium starch glycolate, titanium dioxide and wax.

CLINICAL PHARMACOLOGY

Pharmacodynamics

ULTRAM is a centrally acting synthetic opioid analgesic. Although its mode of action is not completely understood, from animal tests, at least two complementary mechanisms appear applicable: binding of parent and M1 metabolite to μ-opioid receptors and weak inhibition of reuptake of norepinephrine and serotonin.

Opioid activity is due to both low affinity binding of the parent compound and higher affinity binding of the O-demethylated metabolite M1 to μ-opioid receptors. In animal models, M1 is up to 6 times more potent than tramadol in producing analgesia and 200 times more potent in μ-opioid binding. Tramadol-induced analgesia is only partially antagonized by the opiate antagonist naloxone in several animal tests. The relative contribution of both tramadol and M1 to human analgesia is dependent upon the plasma concentrations of each compound (see CLINICAL PHARMACOLOGY, Pharmacokinetics).

Tramadol has been shown to inhibit reuptake of norepinephrine and serotonin *in vitro*, as have some other opioid analgesics. These mechanisms may contribute independently to the overall analgesic profile of ULTRAM. Analgesia in humans begins approximately within one hour after administration and reaches a peak in approximately two to three hours.

Apart from analgesia, ULTRAM administration may produce a constellation of symptoms (including dizziness, somnolence, nausea, constipation, sweating and pruritus) similar to that of other opioids. In contrast to morphine, tramadol has not been shown to cause histamine release. At therapeutic doses, ULTRAM has no effect on heart rate, left-ventricular function or cardiac index. Orthostatic hypotension has been observed.

Pharmacokinetics

The analgesic activity of ULTRAM is due to both parent drug and the M1 metabolite (see CLINICAL PHARMACOLOGY, Pharmacodynamics). Tramadol is administered as a racemate and both the [−] and [+] forms of both tramadol and M1 are detected in the circulation. Tramadol is well absorbed orally with an absolute bioavailability of 75%. Tramadol has a volume of distribution of approximately 2.7L/kg and is only 20% bound to plasma proteins. Tramadol is extensively metabolized by a number of pathways, including CYP2D6 and CYP3A4, as well as by conjugation of parent and metabolites. One metabolite, M1, is pharmacologically active in animal models. The formation of M1 is dependent upon CYP2D6 and as such is subject to inhibition, which may affect the therapeutic response (see PRECAUTIONS, Drug Interactions). Tramadol and its metabolites are excreted primarily in the urine with observed plasma half-lives of 6.3 and 7.4 hours for tramadol and M1, respectively. Linear pharmacokinetics have been observed following multiple doses of 50 and 100 mg to steady-state.

Absorption:

Racemic tramadol is rapidly and almost completely absorbed after oral administration. The mean absolute bioavailability of a 100 mg oral dose is approximately 75%. The mean peak plasma concentration of racemic tramadol and M1 occurs at two and three hours, respectively, after administration in healthy adults. In general, both enantiomers of tramadol and M1 follow a parallel time course in the body following single and multiple doses although small differences (~ 10%) exist in the absolute amount of each enantiomer present.

Steady-state plasma concentrations of both tramadol and M1 are achieved within two days with q.i.d. dosing. There is no evidence of self-induction (see Figure 1 and Table 1 below).

Figure 1: Mean Tramadol and M1 Plasma Concentration Profiles after a Single 100 mg Oral Dose and after Twenty-Nine 100 mg Oral Doses of Tramadol HCl given q.i.d.

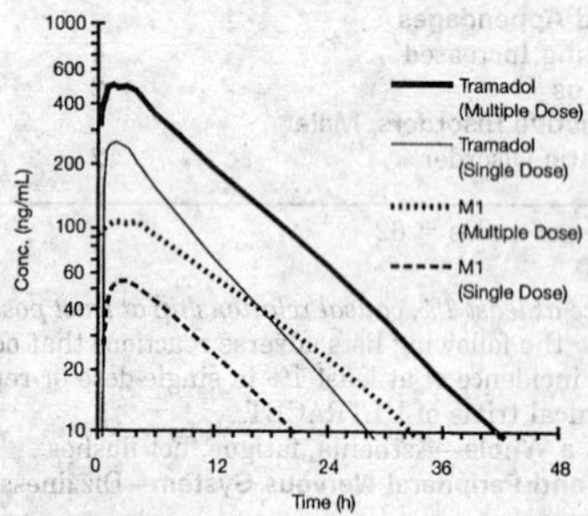

[See table 1 below]

Food Effects: Oral administration of ULTRAM with food does not significantly affect its rate or extent of absorption, therefore, ULTRAM can be administered without regard to food.

Distribution:

The volume of distribution of tramadol was 2.6 and 2.9 liters/kg in male and female subjects, respectively, following a 100 mg intravenous dose. The binding of tramadol to human plasma proteins is approximately 20% and binding also appears to be independent of concentration up to 10 μg/mL. Saturation of plasma protein binding occurs only at concentrations outside the clinically relevant range.

Metabolism:

Tramadol is extensively metabolized after oral administration. Approximately 30% of the dose is excreted in the urine as unchanged drug, whereas 60% of the dose is excreted as metabolites. The remainder is excreted either as unidentified or as unextractable metabolites. The major metabolic pathways appear to be *N*- and *O*- demethylation and glucuronidation or sulfation in the liver. One metabolite (*O*-desmethyltramadol, denoted M1) is pharmacologically active in animal models. Formation of M1 is dependent on CYP2D6 and as such is subject to inhibition, which may affect the therapeutic response (see PRECAUTIONS, Drug Interactions).

Approximately 7% of the population has reduced activity of the CYP2D6 isoenzyme of cytochrome P-450. These individuals are "poor metabolizers" of debrisoquine, dextromethorphan, tricyclic antidepressants, among other drugs. Based on a population PK analysis of Phase I studies in healthy subjects, concentrations of tramadol were approximately 20% higher in "poor metabolizers" versus "extensive metabolizers," while M1 concentrations were 40% lower. Concomitant therapy with inhibitors of CYP2D6 such as fluoxetine, paroxetine and quinidine could result in significant drug interactions. In vitro drug interaction studies in human liver microsomes indicate that inhibitors of CYP2D6 such as fluoxetine and its metabolite norfluoxetine, amitriptyline and quinidine inhibit the metabolism of tramadol to various degrees, suggesting that concomitant administration of these compounds could result in increases in tramadol concentrations and decreased concentrations of M1. The full pharmacological impact of these alterations in terms of either efficacy or safety is unknown. Concomitant use of SEROTONIN re-uptake INHIBITORS and MAO INHIBITORS may enhance the risk of adverse events, including seizure (see WARNINGS) and serotonin syndrome.

Elimination:

Tramadol is eliminated primarily through metabolism by the liver and the metabolites are eliminated primarily by the kidneys. The mean terminal plasma elimination half-lives of racemic tramadol and racemic M1 are 6.3 ± 1.4 and 7.4 ± 1.4 hours, respectively. The plasma elimination half-life of racemic tramadol increased from approximately six hours to seven hours upon multiple dosing.

Special Populations

Renal:

Impaired renal function results in a decreased rate and extent of excretion of tramadol and its active metabolite, M1. In patients with creatinine clearances of less than 30 mL/min, adjustment of the dosing regimen is recommended (see DOSAGE AND ADMINISTRATION). The total amount of tramadol and M1 removed during a 4-hour dialysis period is less than 7% of the administered dose.

Hepatic:

Metabolism of tramadol and M1 is reduced in patients with advanced cirrhosis of the liver, resulting in both a larger area under the concentration time curve for tramadol and longer tramadol and M1 elimination half-lives (13 hrs. for tramadol and 19 hrs. for M1). In cirrhotic patients, adjustment of the dosing regimen is recommended (see DOSAGE AND ADMINISTRATION).

Geriatric:

Healthy elderly subjects aged 65 to 75 years have plasma tramadol concentrations and elimination half-lives comparable to those observed in healthy subjects less than 65 years of age. In subjects over 75 years, maximum serum concentrations are elevated (208 vs. 162 ng/mL) and the elimination half-life is prolonged (7 vs. 6 hours) compared to subjects 65 to 75 years of age. Adjustment of the daily dose is recommended for patients older than 75 years (see DOSAGE AND ADMINISTRATION).

Gender:

The absolute bioavailability of tramadol was 73% in males and 79% in females. The plasma clearance was 6.4 mL/min/kg in males and 5.7 mL/min/kg in females following a 100 mg IV dose of tramadol. Following a single oral dose, and after adjusting for body weight, females had a 12% higher peak tramadol concentration and a 35% higher area under the concentration-time curve compared to males. The clinical significance of this difference is unknown.

Clinical Studies

ULTRAM has been given in single oral doses of 50, 75 and 100 mg to patients with pain following surgical procedures and pain following oral surgery (extraction of impacted molars).

In single-dose models of pain following oral surgery, pain relief was demonstrated in some patients at doses of 50 mg and 75 mg. A dose of 100 mg ULTRAM tended to provide analgesia superior to codeine sulfate 60 mg, but it was not as effective as the combination of aspirin 650 mg with codeine phosphate 60 mg.

ULTRAM has been studied in three long-term controlled trials involving a total of 820 patients, with 530 patients receiving ULTRAM. Patients with a variety of chronic painful conditions were studied in double-blind trials of one to three months duration. Average daily doses of approximately 250 mg of ULTRAM in divided doses were generally comparable to five doses of acetaminophen 300 mg with codeine phosphate 30 mg (TYLENOL® with Codeine #3) daily, five doses of aspirin 325 mg with codeine phosphate 30 mg daily, or two to three doses of acetaminophen 500 mg with oxycodone hydrochloride 5 mg (TYLOX®) daily.

Titration Trials

In a randomized, blinded clinical study with 129 to 132 patients per group, a 10-day titration to a daily ULTRAM dose of 200 mg (50 mg q.i.d.), attained in 50 mg increments every 3 days, was found to result in fewer discontinuations due to dizziness or vertigo than titration over only 4 days or no titration. In a second study with 54 to 59 patients per group, patients who had nausea or vomiting when titrated over 4 days were randomized to re-initiate ULTRAM therapy using slower titration rates.

A 16-day titration schedule, starting with 25 mg qAM and using additional doses in 25 mg increments every third day to 100 mg/day (25 mg q.i.d.), followed by 50 mg increments in the total daily dose every third day to 200 mg/day (50 mg q.i.d.), resulted in fewer discontinuations due to nausea or vomiting and fewer discontinuations due to any cause than did a 10-day titration schedule.

Table 1
Mean (%CV) Pharmacokinetic Parameters for Racemic Tramadol and M1 Metabolite

Population/ Dosage Regimen[a]	Parent Drug/ Metabolite	Peak Conc. (ng/mL)	Time to Peak (hrs)	Clearance/F[b] (mL/min/Kg)	$t_{1/2}$ (hrs)
Healthy Adults, 100 mg qid, MD p.o.	Tramadol	592 (30)	2.3 (61)	5.90 (25)	6.7 (15)
	M1	110 (29)	2.4 (46)	c	7.0 (14)
Healthy Adults, 100 mg SD p.o.	Tramadol	308 (25)	1.6 (63)	8.50 (31)	5.6 (20)
	M1	55.0 (36)	3.0 (51)	c	6.7 (16)
Geriatric, (>75 yrs) 50 mg SD p.o.	Tramadol	208 (31)	2.1 (19)	6.89 (25)	7.0 (23)
	M1	d	d	c	d
Hepatic Impaired, 50 mg SD p.o.	Tramadol	217 (11)	1.9 (16)	4.23 (56)	13.3 (11)
	M1	19.4 (12)	9.8 (20)	c	18.5 (15)
Renal Impaired, CL_{cr} 10-30 mL/min 100 mg SD i.v.	Tramadol	c	c	4.23 (54)	10.6 (31)
	M1	c	c	c	11.5 (40)
Renal Impaired, CL_{cr}<5 mL/min 100 mg SD i.v.	Tramadol	c	c	3.73 (17)	11.0 (29)
	M1	c	c	c	16.9 (18)

a SD = Single dose, MD = Multiple dose, p.o. = Oral administration, i.v. = Intravenous administration, q.i.d. = Four times daily
b F represents the oral bioavailability of tramadol
c Not applicable
d Not measured

Figure 2:

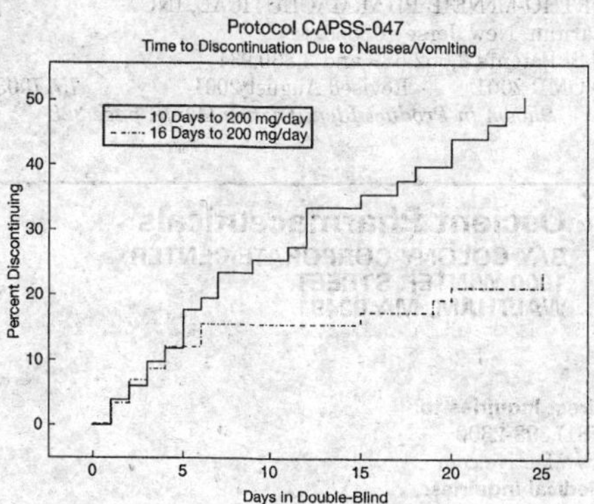

INDICATIONS AND USAGE

ULTRAM is indicated for the management of moderate to moderately severe pain in adults.

CONTRAINDICATIONS

ULTRAM should not be administered to patients who have previously demonstrated hypersensitivity to tramadol, any other component of this product or opioids. ULTRAM is contraindicated in any situation where opioids are contraindicated, including acute intoxication with any of the following: alcohol, hypnotics, narcotics, centrally acting analgesics, opioids or psychotropic drugs. ULTRAM may worsen central nervous system and respiratory depression in these patients.

WARNINGS

Seizure Risk

Seizures have been reported in patients receiving ULTRAM within the recommended dosage range. Spontaneous post-marketing reports indicate that seizure risk is increased with doses of ULTRAM above the recommended range. Concomitant use of ULTRAM increases the seizure risk in patients taking:

- **Selective serotonin reuptake inhibitors (SSRI antidepressants or anorectics),**
- **Tricyclic antidepressants (TCAs), and other tricyclic compounds (e.g., cyclobenzaprine, promethazine, etc.), or**
- **Other opioids.**

Administration of ULTRAM may enhance the seizure risk in patients taking:

- **MAO inhibitors (see also WARNINGS – Use with MAO Inhibitors),**
- **Neuroleptics, or**
- **Other drugs that reduce the seizure threshold.**

Risk of convulsions may also increase in patients with epilepsy, those with a history of seizures, or in patients with a recognized risk for seizure (such as head trauma, metabolic disorders, alcohol and drug withdrawal, CNS infections). In ULTRAM overdose, naloxone administration may increase the risk of seizure.

Anaphylactoid Reactions

Serious and rarely fatal anaphylactoid reactions have been reported in patients receiving therapy with ULTRAM. When these events do occur it is often following the first dose. Other reported allergic reactions include pruritus, hives, bronchospasm, angioedema, toxic epidermal necrolysis and Stevens-Johnson syndrome. Patients with a history of anaphylactoid reactions to codeine and other opioids may be at increased risk and therefore should not receive ULTRAM (see CONTRAINDICATIONS).

Respiratory Depression

Administer ULTRAM cautiously in patients at risk for respiratory depression. In these patients alternative non-opioid analgesics should be considered. When large doses of ULTRAM are administered with anesthetic medications or alcohol, respiratory depression may result. Respiratory depression should be treated as an overdose. If naloxone is to be administered, use cautiously because it may precipitate seizures (see WARNINGS, Seizure Risk and OVERDOSAGE).

Interaction With Central Nervous System (CNS) Depressants

ULTRAM should be used with caution and in reduced dosages when administered to patients receiving CNS depressants such as alcohol, opioids, anesthetic agents, narcotics, phenothiazines, tranquilizers or sedative hypnotics. ULTRAM increases the risk of CNS and respiratory depression in these patients.

Increased Intracranial Pressure or Head Trauma

ULTRAM should be used with caution in patients with increased intracranial pressure or head injury. The respiratory depressant effects of opioids include carbon dioxide retention and secondary elevation of cerebrospinal fluid pressure, and may be markedly exaggerated in these patients. Additionally, pupillary changes (miosis) from tramadol may obscure the existence, extent, or course of intracranial pathology. Clinicians should also maintain a high index of suspicion for adverse drug reaction when evaluating altered mental status in these patients if they are receiving ULTRAM. (See Respiratory Depression.)

Use in Ambulatory Patients

ULTRAM may impair the mental and or physical abilities required for the performance of potentially hazardous tasks such as driving a car or operating machinery. The patient using this drug should be cautioned accordingly.

Use With MAO Inhibitors and Serotonin Re-uptake Inhibitors

Use ULTRAM with great caution in patients taking monoamine oxidase inhibitors. Animal studies have shown increased deaths with combined administration. Concomitant use of ULTRAM with MAO inhibitors or SSRI's increases the risk of adverse events, including seizure and serotonin syndrome.

Withdrawal

Withdrawal symptoms may occur if ULTRAM is discontinued abruptly. (See DRUG ABUSE AND DEPENDENCE.) These symptoms may include: anxiety, sweating, insomnia, rigors, pain, nausea, tremors, diarrhea, upper respiratory symptoms, piloerection, and rarely hallucinations. Clinical experience suggests that withdrawal symptoms may be relieved by tapering the medication.

Physical Dependence and Abuse

ULTRAM may induce psychic and physical dependence of the morphine-type (μ-opioid) (see DRUG ABUSE AND DEPENDENCE). ULTRAM should not be used in opioid-dependent patients. ULTRAM has been shown to reinitiate physical dependence in some patients that have been previously dependent on other opioids. Dependence and abuse, including drug-seeking behavior and taking illicit actions to obtain the drug, are not limited to those patients with prior history of opioid dependence.

Risk of Overdosage

Serious potential consequences of overdosage with ULTRAM (tramadol hydrochloride tablets) are central nervous system depression, respiratory depression and death. In treating an overdose, primary attention should be given to maintaining adequate ventilation along with general supportive treatment (see OVERDOSAGE).

PRECAUTIONS

Acute Abdominal Conditions

The administration of ULTRAM may complicate the clinical assessment of patients with acute abdominal conditions.

Use in Renal and Hepatic Disease

Impaired renal function results in a decreased rate and extent of excretion of tramadol and its active metabolite, M1. In patients with creatinine clearances of less than 30 mL/min, dosing reduction is recommended (see DOSAGE AND ADMINISTRATION). Metabolism of tramadol and M1 is reduced in patients with advanced cirrhosis of the liver. In cirrhotic patients, dosing reduction is recommended (see DOSAGE AND ADMINISTRATION).

With the prolonged half-life in these conditions, achievement of steady-state is delayed, so that it may take several days for elevated plasma concentrations to develop.

Information for Patients

- ULTRAM may impair mental or physical abilities required for the performance of potentially hazardous tasks such as driving a car or operating machinery.
- ULTRAM should not be taken with alcohol containing beverages.
- ULTRAM should be used with caution when taking medications such as tranquilizers, hypnotics or other opiate containing analgesics.
- The patient should be instructed to inform the physician if they are pregnant, think they might become pregnant, or are trying to become pregnant (see PRECAUTIONS, Labor and Delivery).
- The patient should understand the single-dose and 24-hour dose limit and the time interval between doses, since exceeding these recommendations can result in respiratory depression, seizures and death.

Drug Interactions

In vitro studies indicate that tramadol is unlikely to inhibit the CYP3A4-mediated metabolism of other drugs when tramadol is administered concomitantly at therapeutic doses. Tramadol does not appear to induce its own metabolism in humans, since observed maximal plasma concentrations after multiple oral doses are higher than expected based on single-dose data. Tramadol is a mild inducer of selected drug metabolism pathways measured in animals.

Use With Carbamazepine

Patients taking **carbamazepine** may have a significantly reduced analgesic effect of ULTRAM. Because carbamazepine increases tramadol metabolism and because of the seizure risk associated with tramadol, concomitant administration of ULTRAM and carbamazepine is not recommended.

Use With Quinidine

Tramadol is metabolized to M1 by CYP2D6. **Quinidine** is a selective inhibitor of that isoenzyme, so that concomitant administration of quinidine and ULTRAM results in increased concentrations of tramadol and reduced concentrations of M1. The clinical consequences of these findings are unknown. In vitro drug interaction studies in human liver microsomes indicate that tramadol has no effect on quinidine metabolism.

Use With Inhibitors of CYP2D6

In vitro drug interaction studies in human liver microsomes indicate that concomitant administration with inhibitors of CYP2D6 such as fluoxetine, paroxetine, and amitriptyline could result in some inhibition of the metabolism of tramadol.

Use With Cimetidine

Concomitant administration of ULTRAM with **cimetidine** does not result in clinically significant changes in tramadol pharmacokinetics. Therefore, no alteration of the ULTRAM dosage regimen is recommended.

Use With MAO Inhibitors

Interactions with **MAO Inhibitors**, due to interference with detoxification mechanisms, have been reported for some centrally acting drugs (see WARNINGS, Use With MAO Inhibitors).

Use With Digoxin and Warfarin

Post-marketing surveillance has revealed rare reports of digoxin toxicity and alteration of warfarin effect, including elevation of prothrombin times.

Carcinogenesis, Mutagenesis, Impairment of Fertility

A slight, but statistically significant, increase in two common murine tumors, pulmonary and hepatic, was observed in a mouse carcinogenicity study, particularly in aged mice. Mice were dosed orally up to 30 mg/kg (90 mg/m^2 or 0.36 times the maximum daily human dosage of 246 mg/m^2) for approximately two years, although the study was not done with the Maximum Tolerated Dose. This finding is not believed to suggest risk in humans. No such finding occurred in a rat carcinogenicity study (dosing orally up to 30 mg/kg, 180 mg/m^2, or 0.73 times the maximum daily human dosage).

Tramadol was not mutagenic in the following assays: Ames *Salmonella* microsomal activation test, CHO/HPRT mammalian cell assay, mouse lymphoma assay (in the absence of metabolic activation), dominant lethal mutation tests in mice, chromosome aberration test in Chinese hamsters, and bone marrow micronucleus tests in mice and Chinese hamsters. Weakly mutagenic results occurred in the presence of metabolic activation in the mouse lymphoma assay and micronucleus test in rats. Overall, the weight of evidence from these tests indicates that tramadol does not pose a genotoxic risk to humans.

No effects on fertility were observed for tramadol at oral dose levels up to 50 mg/kg (300 mg/m^2) in male rats and 75 mg/kg (450 mg/m^2) in female rats. These dosages are 1.2 and 1.8 times the maximum daily human dosage of 246 mg/m^2, respectively.

Pregnancy, Teratogenic Effects: *Pregnancy Catogery C*

Tramadol has been shown to be embryotoxic and fetotoxic in mice, (120 mg/kg or 360 mg/m^2), rats ($\geq$25 mg/kg or 150 mg/m^2) and rabbits ($\geq$75 mg/kg or 900 mg/m^2) at maternally toxic dosages, but was not teratogenic at these dose levels. These dosages on a mg/m^2 basis are 1.4, $\geq$0.6, and $\geq$3.6 times the maximum daily human dosage (246 mg/m^2) for mouse, rat and rabbit, respectively.

No drug-related teratogenic effects were observed in progeny of mice (up to 140 mg/kg or 420 mg/m^2), rats (up to 80 mg/kg or 480 mg/m^2) or rabbits (up to 300 mg/kg or 3600 mg/m^2) treated with tramadol by various routes. Embryo and fetal toxicity consisted primarily of decreased fetal weights, skeletal ossification and increased supernumerary ribs at maternally toxic dose levels. Transient delays in developmental or behavioral parameters were also seen in pups from rat dams allowed to deliver. Embryo and fetal lethality were reported only in one rabbit study at 300 mg/kg (3600 mg/m^2), a dose that would cause extreme maternal toxicity in the rabbit. The dosages listed for mouse, rat and rabbit are 1.7, 1.9 and 14.6 times the maximum daily human dosage (246 mg/m^2), respectively.

Non-teratogenic Effects

Tramadol was evaluated in peri- and post-natal studies in rats. Progeny of dams receiving oral (gavage) dose levels of 50 mg/kg (300 mg/m^2 or 1.2 times the maximum daily human tramadol dosage) or greater had decreased weights, and pup survival was decreased early in lactation at 80 mg/kg (480 mg/m^2 or 1.9 and higher the maximum daily human dose).

There are no adequate and well-controlled studies in pregnant women. ULTRAM should be used during pregnancy only if the potential benefit justifies the potential risk to the fetus. Neonatal seizures, neonatal withdrawal syndrome, fetal death and still birth have been reported during post-marketing.

Labor and Delivery

ULTRAM should not be used in pregnant women prior to or during labor unless the potential benefits outweigh the risks. Safe use in pregnancy has not been established. Chronic use during pregnancy may lead to physical dependence and post-partum withdrawal symptoms in the newborn (see DRUG ABUSE AND DEPENDENCE). Tramadol has been shown to cross the placenta. The mean ratio of serum tramadol in the umbilical veins compared to maternal veins was 0.83 for 40 women given tramadol during labor.

The effect of ULTRAM, if any, on the later growth, development, and functional maturation of the child is unknown.

Nursing Mothers

ULTRAM is not recommended for obstetrical preoperative medication or for post-delivery analgesia in nursing mothers because its safety in infants and newborns has not been studied. Following a single IV 100 mg dose of tramadol, the cumulative excretion in breast milk within 16 hours post-dose was 100 μg of tramadol (0.1% of the maternal dose) and 27 μg of M1.

Pediatric Use

The safety and efficacy of ULTRAM in patients under 16 years of age have not been established. The use of ULTRAM in the pediatric population is not recommended.

Continued on next page

Ultram—Cont.

Geriatric Use

In general, dose selection for an elderly patient should be cautious, usually starting at the low end of the dosing range, reflecting the greater frequency of decreased hepatic, renal or cardiac function and of concomitant disease or other drug therapy. In patients over 75 years of age, daily doses in excess of 300 mg are not recommended (see CLINICAL PHARMACOLOGY and DOSAGE AND ADMINISTRATION).

A total of 455 elderly (65 years of age or older) subjects were exposed to ULTRAM in controlled clinical trials. Of those, 145 subjects were 75 years of age and older.

In studies including geriatric patients, treatment-limiting adverse events were higher in subjects over 75 years of age compared to those under 65 years of age. Specifically, 30% of those over 75 years of age had gastrointestinal treatment-limiting adverse events compared to 17% of those under 65 years of age. Constipation resulted in discontinuation of treatment in 10% of those over 75.

ADVERSE REACTIONS

ULTRAM was administered to 550 patients during the double-blind or open-label extension periods in U.S. studies of chronic nonmalignant pain. Of these patients, 375 were 65 years old or older. Table 2 reports the cumulative incidence rate of adverse reactions by 7, 30 and 90 days for the most frequent reactions (5% or more by 7 days). The most frequently reported events were in the central nervous system and gastrointestinal system. Although the reactions listed in the table are felt to be probably related to ULTRAM administration, the reported rates also include some events that may have been due to underlying disease or concomitant medication. The overall incidence rates of adverse experiences in these trials were similar for ULTRAM and the active control groups, TYLENOL® with Codeine #3 (acetaminophen 300 mg with codeine phosphate 30 mg), and aspirin 325 mg with codeine phosphate 30 mg, however, the rates of withdrawals due to adverse events appeared to be higher in the ULTRAM groups.

Table 2: Cumulative Incidence of Adverse Reactions for ULTRAM in Chronic Trials of Nonmalignant Pain (N = 427)

	Up to 7 Days	Up to 30 Days	Up to 90 Days
Diziness/Vertigo	26%	31%	33%
Nausea	24%	34%	40%
Constipation	24%	38%	46%
Headache	18%	26%	32%
Somnolence	16%	23%	25%
Vomiting	9%	13%	17%
Pruritus	8%	10%	11%
"CNS Stimulation"[1]	7%	11%	14%
Asthenia	6%	11%	12%
Sweating	6%	7%	9%
Dyspepsia	5%	9%	13%
Dry Mouth	5%	9%	10%
Diarrhea	5%	6%	10%

[1]"CNS Stimulation" is a composite of nervousness, anxiety, agitation, tremor, spasticity, euphoria, emotional lability and hallucinations.

Incidence 1% to less than 5%, possibly causally related: the following lists adverse reactions that occurred with an incidence of 1% to less than 5% in clinical trials, and for which the possibility of a causal relationship with ULTRAM exists.

Body as a Whole: Malaise.
Cardiovascular: Vasodilation.
Central Nervous System: Anxiety, Confusion, Coordination disturbance, Euphoria, Miosis, Nervousness, Sleep disorder.
Gastrointestinal: Abdominal pain, Anorexia, Flatulence.
Musculoskeletal: Hypertonia.
Skin: Rash.
Special Senses: Visual disturbance.
Urogenital: Menopausal symptoms, Urinary frequency, Urinary retention.

Incidence less than 1%, possibly causally related: the following lists adverse reactions that occurred with an incidence of less than 1% in clinical trials and/or reported in post-marketing experience.

Body as a Whole: Accidental injury, Allergic reaction, Anaphylaxis, Death, Suicidal tendency, Weight loss, Serotonin syndrome (mental status change, hyperreflexia, fever, shivering, tremor, agitation, diaphoresis, seizures and coma).
Cardiovascular: Orthostatic hypotension, Syncope, Tachycardia.
Central Nervous System: Abnormal gait, Amnesia, Cognitive dysfunction, Depression, Difficulty in concentration, Hallucinations, Paresthesia, Seizure (see WARNINGS), Tremor.
Respiratory: Dyspnea.
Skin: Stevens-Johnson syndrome/Toxic epidermal necrolysis, Urticaria, Vesicles.
Special Senses: Dysgeusia.
Urogenital: Dysuria, Menstrual disorder.

Other adverse experiences, causal relationship unknown: A variety of other adverse events were reported infrequently in patients taking ULTRAM during clinical trials and/or reported in post-marketing experience. A causal relationship between ULTRAM and these events has not been determined. However, the most significant events are listed below as alerting information to the physician.

Cardiovascular: Abnormal ECG, Hypertension, Hypotension, Myocardial ischemia, Palpitations, Pulmonary edema, Pulmonary embolism.
Central Nervous System: Migraine, Speech disorders.
Gastrointestinal: Gastrointestinal bleeding, Hepatitis, Stomatitis, Liver failure.
Laboratory Abnormalities: Creatinine increase, Elevated liver enzymes, Hemoglobin decrease, Proteinuria.
Sensory: Cataracts, Deafness, Tinnitus.

DRUG ABUSE AND DEPENDENCE

ULTRAM may induce psychic and physical dependence of the morphine-type (μ-opioid). (See WARNINGS.) Dependence and abuse, including drug-seeking behavior and taking illicit actions to obtain the drug are not limited to those patients with prior history of opioid dependence. The risk in patients with substance abuse has been observed to be higher. ULTRAM is associated with craving and tolerance development. Withdrawal symptoms may occur if ULTRAM is discontinued abruptly. These symptoms may include: anxiety, sweating, insomnia, rigors, pain, nausea, tremors, diarrhea, upper respiratory symptoms, piloerection, and rarely hallucinations. Clinical experience suggests that withdrawal symptoms may be relieved by reinstitution of opioid therapy followed by a gradual, tapered dose reduction of the medication combined with symptomatic support.

OVERDOSAGE

Serious potential consequences of overdosage are respiratory depression, lethargy, coma, seizure, cardiac arrest and death. (See WARNINGS.) Fatalities have been reported in post marketing in association with both intentional and unintentional overdose with ULTRAM. In treating an overdose, primary attention should be given to maintaining adequate ventilation along with general supportive treatment. While naloxone will reverse some, but not all, symptoms caused by overdosage with ULTRAM, the risk of seizures is also increased with naloxone administration. In animals convulsions following the administration of toxic doses of tramadol could be suppressed with barbiturates or benzodiazepines but were increased with naloxone. Naloxone administration did not change the lethality of an overdose in mice. Hemodialysis is not expected to be helpful in an overdose because it removes less than 7% of the administered dose in a 4-hour dialysis period.

DOSAGE AND ADMINISTRATION

Adults (17 years of age and over)

For patients with moderate to moderately severe chronic pain not requiring rapid onset of analgesic effect, the tolerability of ULTRAM can be improved by initiating therapy with the following titration regimen: ULTRAM should be started at 25 mg/day qAM and titrated in 25 mg increments as separate doses every 3 days to reach 100 mg/day (25 mg q.i.d.). Thereafter the total daily dose may be increased by 50 mg as tolerated every 3 days to reach 200 mg/day (50 mg q.i.d.). After titration, ULTRAM 50 to 100 mg can be administered as needed for pain relief every 4 to 6 hours **not to exceed 400 mg/day.**

For the subset of patients for whom rapid onset of analgesic effect is required and for whom the benefits outweigh the risk of discontinuation due to adverse events associated with higher initial doses, ULTRAM 50 mg to 100 mg can be administered as needed for pain relief every four to six hours, **not to exceed 400 mg per day.**

Individualization of Dose

Good pain management practice dictates that the dose be individualized according to patient need using the lowest beneficial dose. Studies with tramadol in adults have shown that starting at the lowest possible dose and titrating upward will result in fewer discontinuations and increased tolerability.

- In all patients with **creatinine clearance less than 30 mL/min,** it is recommended that the dosing interval of ULTRAM be increased to 12 hours, with a maximum daily dose of 200 mg. Since only 7% of an administered dose is removed by hemodialysis, **dialysis patients** can receive their regular dose on the day of dialysis.
- The recommended dose for adult patients with **cirrhosis** is 50 mg every 12 hours.
- In general, dose selection for an elderly patient over 65 years old should be cautious, usually starting at the low end of the dosing range, reflecting the greater frequency of decreased hepatic, renal or cardiac function and of concomitant disease or other drug therapy. For elderly patients **over 75 years old,** total dose should not exceed 300 mg/day.

HOW SUPPLIED

ULTRAM (tramadol hydrochloride tablets) Tablets – 50 mg (white, scored, film-coated capsule-shaped tablet) debossed "ULTRAM" on one side and "06 59" on the other side.
100's – NDC 0045-0659-60 bottles of 100 tablets
500's – NDC 0045-0659-70 bottles of 500 tablets
Packages of 100 unit doses in blister packs –
NDC 0045-0659-10 (10 cards of 10 tablets each).
Dispense in a tight container. Store at 25°C (77°F); excursions permitted to 15-30°C (59-89°F).

ORTHO-McNEIL
OMP DIVISION
ORTHO-McNEIL PHARMACEUTICAL, INC.
Raritan, New Jersey 08869
U.S. Patents 3,652,589 and 3,830,934
 Revised August 2001 7517003
Shown in Product Identification Guide, page 328

Oscient Pharmaceuticals

BAY COLONY CORPORATE CENTER
1000 WINTER STREET
WALTHAM, MA 02451

Direct Inquiries to:
(781) 398-2300
www.factive.com
Medical Inquiries:
(866) 4FACTIV
(866) 432-2848

FACTIVE® ℞

[fāk-tēv]
(gemifloxacin mesylate)
Tablets

PRESCRIBING INFORMATION

To reduce the development of drug-resistant bacteria and maintain the effectiveness of FACTIVE and other antibacterial drugs, FACTIVE should be used only to treat infections that are proven or strongly suspected to be caused by bacteria.

DESCRIPTION

FACTIVE (gemifloxacin mesylate) is a synthetic broad-spectrum antibacterial agent for oral administration. Gemifloxacin, a compound related to the fluoroquinolone class of antibiotics, is available as the mesylate salt in the sesquihydrate form. Chemically, gemifloxacin is (*R,S*)-7-[(4Z)-3-(aminomethyl)-4-(methoxyimino)-1-pyrrolidinyl]- 1-cyclopropyl-6-fluoro-1,4-dihydro-4-oxo-1,8-naphthyridine-3-carboxylic acid.

The mesylate salt is a white to light brown solid with a molecular weight of 485.49. Gemifloxacin is considered freely soluble at neutral pH (350 μg/mL at 37°C, pH 7.0). Its empirical formula is $C_{18}H_{20}FN_5O_4 \bullet CH_4O_3S$ and its chemical structure is:

Each white to off-white, oval, film-coated FACTIVE tablet has breaklines and GE 320 debossed on both faces and contains gemifloxacin mesylate equivalent to 320 mg gemifloxacin. The inactive ingredients are crospovidone, hydroxypropyl methylcellulose, magnesium stearate, microcrystalline cellulose, polyethylene glycol, povidone, and titanium dioxide.

CLINICAL PHARMACOLOGY

Pharmacokinetics

The pharmacokinetics of gemifloxacin are approximately linear over the dose range from 40 mg to 640 mg. There was minimal accumulation of gemifloxacin following multiple oral doses up to 640 mg a day for 7 days (mean accumulation <20%). Following repeat oral administration of 320 mg gemifloxacin once daily, steady-state is achieved by the third day of dosing.

Absorption and Bioavailability

Gemifloxacin, given as an oral tablet, is rapidly absorbed from the gastrointestinal tract. Peak plasma concentrations of gemifloxacin were observed between 0.5 and 2 hours following oral tablet administration and the absolute bioavailability of the 320 mg tablet averaged approximately 71% (95% CI 60%-84%). Following repeat oral doses of 320 mg to healthy subjects, the mean ± SD maximal gemifloxacin plasma concentrations (Cmax) and systemic drug exposure (AUC(0–24)) were 1.61 ± 0.51 μg/mL (range 0.70-2.62 μg/mL) and 9.93 ± 3.07 μg•hr/mL (range 4.71-20.1 μg•hr/mL), respectively. In patients with respiratory and urinary tract infections (n=1123), similar estimates of systemic drug exposure were determined using a population pharmacokinetics analysis (geometric mean AUC(0–24), 8.36 μg•hr/mL; range 3.2-47.7 μg•hr/mL.

The pharmacokinetics of gemifloxacin were not significantly altered when a 320 mg dose was administered with a high-fat meal. Therefore FACTIVE tablets may be administered without regard to meals.

Distribution

In vitro binding of gemifloxacin to plasma proteins in healthy subjects is approximately 60 to 70% and is concentration independent. After repeated doses, the in vivo plasma protein binding in healthy elderly and young subjects ranged from 55% to 73% and was unaffected by age. Renal impairment does not significantly affect the protein binding of gemifloxacin. The blood-to-plasma concentration ratio of gemifloxacin was 1.2:1. The geometric mean for Vdss/F is 4.18 L/kg (range, 1.66–12.12 L/kg).

Gemifloxacin is widely distributed throughout the body after oral administration. Concentrations of gemifloxacin in bronchoalveolar lavage fluid exceed those in the plasma. Gemifloxacin penetrates well into lung tissue and fluids. After five daily doses of 320 mg gemifloxacin, concentrations in plasma, bronchoalveolar macrophages, epithelial lining fluid and bronchial mucosa at approximately 2 hours were as in Table 1:

Table 1. Gemifloxacin Concentrations in Plasma and Tissues (320 mg Oral Dosing)

Tissue	Concentration (mean ± SD)	Ratio compared with plasma (mean ± SD)
Plasma	1.40 (0.442) μg/mL	–
Bronchoalveolar Macrophages	107 (77) μg/g	90.5 (106.3)
Epithelial Lining Fluid	2.69 (1.96) μg/mL	1.99 (1.32)
Bronchial Mucosa	9.52 (5.15) μg/g	7.21 (4.03)

Metabolism

Gemifloxacin is metabolized to a limited extent by the liver. The unchanged compound is the predominant drug-related component detected in plasma (approximately 65%) up to 4 hours after dosing. All metabolites formed are minor (<10% of the administered oral dose); the principal ones are N-acetyl gemifloxacin, the E-isomer of gemifloxacin and the carbamyl glucuronide of gemifloxacin. Cytochrome P450 enzymes do not play an important role in gemifloxacin metabolism, and the metabolic activity of these enzymes is not significantly inhibited by gemifloxacin.

Excretion

Gemifloxacin and its metabolites are excreted via dual routes of excretion. Following oral administration of gemifloxacin to healthy subjects, a mean (±SD) of 61± 9.5% of the dose was excreted in the feces and 36± 9.3% in the urine as unchanged drug and metabolites. The mean (±SD) renal clearance following repeat doses of 320 mg was approximately 11.6 ± 3.9 L/hr (range 4.6-17.6 L/hr), which indicates active secretion is involved in the renal excretion of gemifloxacin. The mean (±SD) plasma elimination half-life at steady state following 320 mg to healthy subjects was approximately 7 ± 2 hours (range 4-12 hours).

Special Populations

Pediatric: The pharmacokinetics of gemifloxacin in pediatric subjects have not been studied.

Geriatric: In adult subjects, the pharmacokinetics of gemifloxacin are not affected by age.

Gender: There are no significant differences between gemifloxacin pharmacokinetics in males and females when differences in body weight are taken into account. Population pharmacokinetic studies indicated that following administration of 320 mg gemifloxacin, AUC values were approximately 10% higher in healthy female patients compared to males. Males and females had mean AUC values of 7.98 μg•h/mL (range, 3.21–42.71 μg•h/mL) and 8.80 μg•h/mL (range, 3.33–47.73 μg•h/mL), respectively. No gemifloxacin dosage adjustment based on gender is necessary.

Hepatic Insufficiency: The pharmacokinetics following a single 320 mg dose of gemifloxacin were studied in patients with mild (Child-Pugh Class A) to moderate (Child-Pugh Class B) liver disease. There was a mean increase in AUC (0-inf) of 34% and a mean increase in Cmax of 25% in these patients with hepatic impairment compared to healthy volunteers.

The pharmacokinetics of a single 320 mg dose of gemifloxacin were also studied in patients with severe hepatic impairment (Child-Pugh Class C). There was a mean increase in AUC (0-inf) of 45% and a mean increase in Cmax of 41% in these subjects with hepatic impairment compared to healthy volunteers.

These average pharmacokinetic increases are not considered to be clinically significant. There was no significant change in plasma elimination half-life in the mild, moderate or severe hepatic impairment patients. No dosage adjustment is recommended in patients with mild (Child-Pugh Class A), moderate (Child-Pugh Class B) or severe (Child-Pugh Class C) hepatic impairment. (See **DOSAGE AND ADMINISTRATION**.)

Renal Insufficiency: Results from population pharmacokinetic and clinical pharmacology studies with repeated 320 mg doses indicate the clearance of gemifloxacin is reduced and the plasma elimination is prolonged, leading to an average increase in AUC values of approximately 70% in patients with renal insufficiency. In the pharmacokinetic studies, gemifloxacin Cmax was not significantly altered in subjects with renal insufficiency. Dose adjustment in patients with creatinine clearance >40 mL/min is not required. Modification of the dosage is recommended for patients with creatinine clearance ≤40 mL/min. (See **DOSAGE AND ADMINISTRATION**.)

Hemodialysis removes approximately 20 to 30% of an oral dose of gemifloxacin from plasma.

Photosensitivity Potential: In a study of the skin response to ultraviolet and visible radiation conducted in 40 healthy volunteers, the minimum erythematous dose (MED) was assessed following administration of either gemifloxacin 160 mg once daily, gemifloxacin 320 mg once daily, ciprofloxacin 500 mg b.i.d., or placebo for 7 days. At 5 of the 6 wavelengths tested (295–430 nm), the photosensitivity potential of gemifloxacin was not statistically different from placebo. At 365 nm (UVA region), gemifloxacin showed a photosensitivity potential similar to that of ciprofloxacin 500 mg b.i.d. and the photosensitivity potentials for both drugs were statistically greater than that of placebo. Photosensitivity reactions were reported rarely in clinical trials with gemifloxacin (0.039%). (See **ADVERSE REACTIONS**.)

Drug-Drug Interactions

Antacids/Di- and Trivalent Cations: The systemic availability of gemifloxacin is significantly reduced when an aluminum-and magnesium- containing antacid is concomitantly administered (AUC decreased 85%; Cmax decreased 87%). Administration of an aluminum- and magnesium-containing antacid or ferrous sulfate (325 mg) at 3 hours before or at 2 hours after gemifloxacin did not significantly alter the systemic availability of gemifloxacin. Therefore, aluminum- and/or magnesium- containing antacids, ferrous sulfate (iron), multivitamin preparations containing zinc or other metal cations, or Videx® (didanosine) chewable/buffered tablets or the pediatric powder for oral solution should not be taken within 3 hours before or 2 hours after taking FACTIVE tablets.

Calcium carbonate (1000 mg) given either 2 hr before or 2 hr after gemifloxacin administration showed no notable reduction in gemifloxacin systemic availability. Calcium carbonate administered simultaneously with gemifloxacin resulted in a small, not clinically significant, decrease in gemifloxacin exposure [AUC (0-inf) decreased 21% and Cmax decreased].

Sucralfate: When sucralfate (2 g) was administered 3 hours prior to gemifloxacin, the oral bioavailability of gemifloxacin was significantly reduced (53% decrease in AUC; 69% decrease in Cmax). When sucralfate (2 g) was administered 2 hours after gemifloxacin, the oral bioavailability of gemifloxacin was not significantly affected; therefore FACTIVE should be taken at least 2 hours before sucralfate. (See **PRECAUTIONS**.)

In Vitro Metabolism: Results of in vitro inhibition studies indicate that hepatic cytochrome P450 (CYP450) enzymes do not play an important role in gemifloxacin metabolism. Therefore gemifloxacin should not cause significant in vivo pharmacokinetic interactions with other drugs that are metabolized by CYP450 enzymes.

Theophylline: Gemifloxacin 320 mg at steady-state did not affect the repeat dose pharmacokinetics of theophylline (300 to 400 mg b.i.d. to healthy male subjects).

Digoxin: Gemifloxacin 320 mg at steady-state did not affect the repeat dose pharmacokinetics of digoxin (0.25 mg once daily to healthy elderly subjects).

Oral Contraceptives: The effect of an oral estrogen/progesterone contraceptive product (once daily for 21 days) on the pharmacokinetics of gemifloxacin (320 mg once daily for 6 days) in healthy female subjects indicates that concomitant administration caused an average reduction in gemifloxacin AUC and Cmax of 19% and 12%. These changes are not considered clinically significant. Gemifloxacin 320 mg at steady-state did not affect the repeat dose pharmacokinetics of an ethinylestradiol/levonorgestrol oral contraceptive product (30 μg/150 μg once daily for 21 days to healthy female subjects).

Cimetidine: Co-administration of a single dose of 320 mg gemifloxacin with cimetidine 400 mg four times daily for 7 days resulted in slight average increases in gemifloxacin AUC(0-inf) and Cmax of 10% and 6%, respectively. These increases are not considered clinically significant.

Omeprazole: Co-administration of a single dose of 320 mg gemifloxacin with omeprazole 40 mg once daily for 4 days resulted in slight average increases in gemifloxacin AUC(0-inf) and Cmax of 10% and 11%, respectively. These increases are not considered clinically significant.

Warfarin: Administration of repeated doses of gemifloxacin (320 mg once daily for 7 days) to healthy subjects on stable warfarin therapy had no significant effect on warfarin-induced anticoagulant activity (i.e., International Normalized Ratios for Prothrombin Time). (See **PRECAUTIONS: Drug Interactions**.)

Probenecid: Administration of a single dose of 320 mg gemifloxacin to healthy subjects who also received repeat doses of probenecid (total dose = 4.5 g) reduced the mean renal clearance of gemifloxacin by approximately 50%, resulting in a mean increase of 45% in gemifloxacin AUC(0-inf) and a prolongation of mean half-life by 1.6 hours. Mean gemifloxacin Cmax increased 8%.

Microbiology

Gemifloxacin has in vitro activity against a wide range of Gram-negative and Gram-positive microorganisms. Gemifloxacin is bactericidal with minimum bactericidal concentrations (MBCs) generally within one dilution of the minimum inhibitory concentrations (MICs). Gemifloxacin acts by inhibiting DNA synthesis through the inhibition of both DNA gyrase and topoisomerase IV (TOPO IV), which are essential for bacterial growth. *Streptococcus pneumoniae* showing mutations in both DNA gyrase and TOPO IV (double mutants) are resistant to most fluoroquinolones. Gemifloxacin has the ability to inhibit both enzyme systems at therapeutically relevant drug levels in *S. pneumoniae* (dual targeting), and has MIC values that are still in the susceptible range for some of these double mutants.

The mechanism of action of quinolones, including gemifloxacin, is different from that of macrolides, beta-lactams, aminoglycosides, or tetracyclines; therefore, microorganisms resistant to these classes of drugs may be susceptible to gemifloxacin and other quinolones. There is no known cross-resistance between gemifloxacin and the above mentioned classes of antimicrobials.

The main mechanism of fluoroquinolone resistance is due to mutations in DNA gyrase and/or TOPO IV. Resistance to gemifloxacin develops slowly via multistep mutations and efflux in a manner similar to other fluoroquinolones. The frequency of spontaneous mutation is low (10^{-7} to $<10^{-10}$). Although cross-resistance has been observed between gemifloxacin and other fluoroquinolones, some microorganisms resistant to other fluoroquinolones may be susceptible to gemifloxacin.

Gemifloxacin has been shown to be active against most strains of the following microorganisms, both in vitro and in clinical infections as described in the **INDICATIONS AND USAGE** section.

Aerobic gram-positive microorganisms

Streptococcus pneumoniae (including multi-drug resistant strains [MDRSP])*.

*MDRSP, Multi-drug resistant *Streptococcus pneumoniae* includes isolates previously known as PRSP (penicillin-resistant *Streptococcus pneumoniae*), and are strains resistant to two or more of the following antibiotics: penicillin, 2nd generation cephalosporins, e.g., cefuroxime, macrolides, tetracyclines and trimethoprim/sulfamethoxazole.

Aerobic gram-negative microorganisms

Haemophilus influenzae

Haemophilus parainfluenzae

Klebsiella pneumoniae (many strains are only moderately susceptible)

Moraxella catarrhalis

Other microorganisms

Chlamydia pneumoniae

Mycoplasma pneumoniae

The following data are available, **but their clinical significance is unknown**.

Gemifloxacin exhibits in vitro minimal inhibitory concentrations (MICs) of 0.25 μg/mL or less against most (≥90%) strains of the following microorganisms; however, the safety and effectiveness of gemifloxacin in treating clinical infections due to these microorganisms has not been established in adequate and well-controlled clinical trials:

Aerobic gram-positive microorganisms

Staphylococcus aureus (methicillin-susceptible strains only)

Streptococcus pyogenes

Aerobic gram-negative microorganisms

Acinetobacter lwoffii

Klebsiella oxytoca

Legionella pneumophila

Proteus vulgaris

Susceptibility Tests

Dilution techniques: Quantitative methods are used to determine antimicrobial minimum inhibitory concentrations (MICs). These MICs provide estimates of the susceptibility of bacteria to antimicrobial compounds. The MICs should be determined using a standardized procedure. Standardized procedures are based on a dilution method[1] (broth or agar) or equivalent with standardized inoculum concentrations and standardized concentrations of gemifloxacin powder. The MICs should be interpreted according to the following criteria:

For testing *Enterobacteriaceae:*

MIC (μg/mL)	Interpretation
≤0.25	Susceptible (S)
0.5	Intermediate (I)
≥1.0	Resistant (R)

For testing *Haemophilus influenzae* and *Haemophilus parainfluenzae*[a]:

MIC (μg/mL)	Interpretation
≤0.12	Susceptible (S)

[a] This interpretive standard is applicable only to broth microdilution susceptibility testing with *Haemophilus influenzae* and *Haemophilus parainfluenzae* using *Haemophilus* Test Medium (HTM)[1].

The current absence of data on resistant strains precludes defining any results other than "Susceptible". Strains yielding MIC results suggestive of a "nonsusceptible" category should be submitted to a reference laboratory for further testing.

For testing *Streptococcus pneumoniae*[b]:

MIC (μg/mL)	Interpretation
≤0.12	Susceptible (S)
0.25	Intermediate (I)
≥0.5	Resistant (R)

Continued on next page

Factive—Cont.

[b] These interpretive standards are applicable only to broth microdilution susceptibility tests using cation–adjusted Muller-Hinton broth with 2-5% lysed horse blood.

A report of "Susceptible" indicates that the pathogen is likely to be inhibited if the antimicrobial compound in the blood reaches the concentration usually achievable. A report of "Intermediate" indicates that the result should be considered equivocal, and if the microorganism is not fully susceptible to alternative, clinically feasible drugs, the test should be repeated. This category implies possible clinical applicability in body sites where the drug is physiologically concentrated or in situations where high dosage of drug can be used. This category also provides a buffer zone, which prevents small uncontrolled technical factors from causing major discrepancies in interpretation. A report of "Resistant" indicates that the pathogen is not likely to be inhibited if the antimicrobial compound in the blood reaches the concentration usually achievable; other therapy should be selected.
Standardized susceptibility test procedures require the use of laboratory control microorganisms to control the technical aspects of the laboratory procedures. Standard gemifloxacin powder should provide the following MIC values:
[See first table above]

Diffusion Techniques: Quantitative methods that require measurement of zone diameters also provide reproducible estimates of the susceptibility of bacteria to antimicrobial compounds. One such standardized procedure[2] requires the use of standardized inoculum concentrations. This procedure uses paper disks impregnated with 5µg gemifloxacin to test the susceptibility of microorganisms to gemifloxacin.
Reports from the laboratory providing results of the standard single-disk susceptibility test with a 5µg gemifloxacin disk should be interpreted according to the following criteria:
For testing *Enterobacteriaceae:*

Zone Diameter (mm)	Interpretation
≥20	Susceptible (S)
16-19	Intermediate (I)
≤15	Resistant (R)

For testing *Haemophilus influenzae* and *Haemophilus parainfluenzae*[e]:

Zone Diameter (mm)	Interpretation
≥18	Susceptible (S)

[e] This interpretive standard is applicable only to disk diffusion susceptibility testing with *Haemophilus influenzae* and *Haemophilus parainfluenzae* using *Haemophilus* Test Medium (HTM).[2]

The current absence of data on resistant strains precludes defining any results other than "Susceptible". Strains yielding zone diameter results suggestive of a "nonsusceptible" category should be submitted to a reference laboratory for further testing.
For testing *Streptococcus pneumoniae*[f]:

Zone Diameter (mm)	Interpretation
≥23	Susceptible (S)
20-22	Intermediate (I)
≤19	Resistant (R)

[f] These zone diameter standards apply only to tests performed using Mueller-Hinton agar supplemented with 5% defibrinated sheep blood incubated in 5% CO_2.

Interpretation should be as stated above for results using dilution techniques. Interpretation involves correlation of the diameter obtained in the disk test with the MIC for gemifloxacin.
As with standardized dilution techniques, diffusion methods require the use of laboratory control microorganisms that are used to control the technical aspects of the laboratory procedures. For the diffusion technique, the 5µg gemifloxacin disk should provide the following zone diameters in these laboratory quality control strains:
[See second table above]

INDICATIONS AND USAGE

FACTIVE is indicated for the treatment of infections caused by susceptible strains of the designated microorganisms in the conditions listed below. (See **DOSAGE AND ADMINISTRATION** and **CLINICAL STUDIES.**)

Acute bacterial exacerbation of chronic bronchitis caused by *Streptococcus pneumoniae, Haemophilus influenzae, Haemophilus parainfluenzae,* or *Moraxella catarrhalis.*

Community-acquired pneumonia (of mild to moderate severity) caused by *Streptococcus pneumoniae* (including multi-drug resistant strains [MDRSP])*, *Haemophilus influenzae, Moraxella catarrhalis, Mycoplasma pneumoniae, Chlamydia pneumoniae, or Klebsiella pneumoniae* **.

*MDRSP, Multi-drug resistant *Streptococcus pneumoniae* includes isolates previously known as PRSP (penicillin-resistant *Streptococcus pneumoniae*), and are strains resistant to two or more of the following antibiotics: penicillin, 2nd generation cephalosporins, e.g. cefuroxime, macrolides, tetracyclines and trimethoprim/sulfamethoxazole.
**In the clinical trials, there were 13 subjects with *Klebsiella pneumoniae,* primarily from non-comparative studies.

Microorganism		MIC Range (µg/mL)
Enterococcus faecalis	ATCC 29212	0.016-0.12
Escherichia coli	ATCC 25922	0.004-0.016
Haemophilus influenzae	ATCC 49247[c]	0.002-0.008
Streptococcus pneumoniae	ATCC 49619[d]	0.008-0.03

[c] This quality control range is applicable to only *H. influenzae* ATCC 49247 tested by a broth microdilution procedure using Haemophilus Test Medium (HTM)[1].
[d] This quality control range is applicable to only *S. pneumoniae* ATCC 49619 tested by a broth microdilution procedure using cation-adjusted Mueller-Hinton broth with 2-5% lysed horse blood.

Microorganism		Zone Diameter (mm)
Escherichia coli	ATCC 25922	29-36
Haemophilus influenzae	ATCC 49247[g]	30-37
Streptococcus pneumoniae	ATCC 49619[h]	28-34

[g] This quality control range is applicable to only *H. influenzae* ATCC 49247 tested by a disk diffusion procedure using *Haemophilus* Test Medium (HTM)[2].
[h] This quality control range is applicable to only *S. pneumoniae* ATCC 49619 tested by a disk diffusion procedure using Mueller-Hinton agar supplemented with 5% defibrinated sheep blood and incubated in 5% CO_2.

Ten subjects had mild disease, 2 had moderate disease, and 1 had severe disease. There were two clinical failures in subjects with mild disease (one subject with bacteriologic recurrence).
To reduce the development of drug-resistant bacteria and maintain the effectiveness of FACTIVE and other antibacterial drugs, FACTIVE should be used only to treat infections that are proven or strongly suspected to be caused by susceptible bacteria. When culture and susceptibility information are available, they should be considered in selecting or modifying antibacterial therapy. In the absence of such data, local epidemiology and susceptibility patterns may contribute to the empiric selection of therapy.

CONTRAINDICATIONS

Gemifloxacin is contraindicated in patients with a history of hypersensitivity to gemifloxacin, fluoroquinolone antibiotic agents, or any of the product components.

WARNINGS

THE SAFETY AND EFFECTIVENESS OF FACTIVE IN CHILDREN, ADOLESCENTS (LESS THAN 18 YEARS OF AGE), PREGNANT WOMEN, AND LACTATING WOMEN HAVE NOT BEEN ESTABLISHED. (See PRECAUTIONS: Pediatric Use, Pregnancy and Nursing Mothers subsections.)

QT Effects: **GEMIFLOXACIN MAY PROLONG THE QT INTERVAL IN SOME PATIENTS. GEMIFLOXACIN SHOULD BE AVOIDED IN PATIENTS WITH A HISTORY OF PROLONGATION OF THE QTc INTERVAL, PATIENTS WITH UNCORRECTED ELECTROLYTE DISORDERS (HYPOKALEMIA OR HYPOMAGNESEMIA), AND PATIENTS RECEIVING CLASS IA (E.G., QUINIDINE, PROCAINAMIDE) OR CLASS III (E.G., AMIODARONE, SOTALOL) ANTIARRHYTHMIC AGENTS.**
Pharmacokinetic studies between gemifloxacin and drugs that prolong the QTc interval such as erythromycin, antipsychotics, and tricyclic antidepressants have not been performed. Gemifloxacin should be used with caution when given concurrently with these drugs, as well as in patients with ongoing proarrhythmic conditions, such as clinically significant bradycardia or acute myocardial ischemia. No cardiovascular morbidity or mortality attributable to QTc prolongation occurred with gemifloxacin treatment in over 6775 patients, including 653 patients concurrently receiving drugs known to prolong the QTc interval and 5 patients with hypokalemia.
The likelihood of QTc prolongation may increase with increasing dose of the drug; therefore, the recommended dose should not be exceeded especially in patients with renal or hepatic impairment where the Cmax and AUC are slightly higher. QTc prolongation may lead to an increased risk for ventricular arrhythmias including torsades de pointes. The maximal change in the QTc interval occurs approximately 5-10 hours following oral administration of gemifloxacin.

Hypersensitivity Reactions: Serious and occasionally fatal hypersensitivity and/or anaphylactic reactions have been reported in patients receiving fluoroquinolone therapy. These reactions may occur following the first dose. Some reactions have been accompanied by cardiovascular collapse, hypotension/shock, seizure, loss of consciousness, tingling, angioedema (including tongue, laryngeal, throat or facial edema/swelling), airway obstruction (including bronchospasm, shortness of breath and acute respiratory distress), dyspnea, urticaria, itching and other serious skin reactions. Gemifloxacin should be discontinued immediately at the appearance of any sign of an immediate type I hypersensitivity skin rash or any other manifestation of a hypersensitivity reaction; the need for continued fluoroquinolone therapy should be evaluated. As with other drugs, serious acute hypersensitivity reactions may require treatment with epinephrine and other resuscitative measures, including oxygen, intravenous fluids, antihistamines, corticosteroids, pressor amines and airway management as clinically indicated. (See **PRECAUTIONS** and **ADVERSE REACTIONS.**)
Serious and occasionally fatal events, some due to hypersensitivity and/or some of uncertain etiology, have been reported in patients receiving fluoroquinolones. These events may be severe and generally occur following the administration of multiple doses. Clinical manifestations usually include new onset fever and one or more of the following: rash or severe dermatologic reactions (e.g., toxic epidermal necrolysis, Stevens-Johnson Syndrome); vasculitis, arthralgia, myalgia, serum sickness; allergic pneumonitis, interstitial nephritis; acute renal insufficiency or failure; hepatitis, jaundice, acute hepatic necrosis or failure; anemia, including hemolytic and aplastic; thrombocytopenia, including thrombotic thrombocytopenic purpura; leukopenia; agranulocytosis; pancytopenia; and/or other hematologic abnormalities.

Tendon and Cartilage Effects: Fluoroquinolones as a class have been shown to cause arthropathy and osteochondrosis in immature rats and dogs. The relevance of these findings to humans is unknown. Tendonitis and rupture of the shoulder, hand, and Achilles tendons that required surgical repair or resulted in prolonged disability have been reported in patients receiving fluoroquinolones. Gemifloxacin should be discontinued if the patient experiences pain, inflammation, or rupture of a tendon. Patients should rest and refrain from exercise until the diagnosis of tendonitis or tendon rupture has been confidently excluded. Tendon rupture can occur either during or after treatment. Elderly patients, athletes, and patients taking corticosteroids are more prone to tendonitis.

CNS Effects: In clinical studies with gemifloxacin, Central nervous system (CNS) effects have been reported infrequently. As with other fluoroquinolones, gemifloxacin should be used with caution in patients with CNS diseases such as epilepsy or patients predisposed to convulsions. Although not seen in gemifloxacin clinical trials, convulsions, increased intracranial pressure, and toxic psychosis have been reported in patients receiving other fluoroquinolones. CNS stimulation which may lead to tremors, restlessness, anxiety, lightheadedness, confusion, hallucinations, paranoia, depression, insomnia, and rarely suicidal thoughts or acts may also be caused by other fluoroquinolones. If these reactions occur in patients receiving gemifloxacin, the drug should be discontinued and appropriate measures instituted.

Antibiotic Associated Colitis: Pseudomembranous colitis has been reported with nearly all antibacterial agents, including gemifloxacin, and may range in severity from mild to life-threatening. Therefore, it is important to consider this diagnosis in patients who present with diarrhea subsequent to the administration of any antibacterial agent.
Treatment with antibacterial agents alters the normal flora of the colon and may permit overgrowth of clostridia. Studies indicate that a toxin produced by *Clostridium difficile* is the primary cause of "antibiotic-associated colitis."
After the diagnosis of pseudomembranous colitis has been established, therapeutic measures should be initiated. Mild cases of pseudomembranous colitis usually respond to drug discontinuation alone. In moderate to severe cases, consideration should be given to management with fluids and electrolytes, protein supplementation, and treatment with an antibacterial drug clinically effective against *Clostridium difficile* colitis. (See **ADVERSE REACTIONS.**)

PRECAUTIONS

General: Prescribing FACTIVE in the absence of a proven or strongly suspected bacterial infection is unlikely to provide benefit to the patient and increases the risk of the development of drug-resistant bacteria.

Rash: In clinical studies, the overall rate of drug-related rash was 2.8%. The most common form of rash associated with gemifloxacin was described as maculopapular and mild to moderate in severity; 0.3% was described as urticarial in appearance. Rash usually appeared 8 to 10 days after start of therapy; 60% of the rashes resolved within 7 days, and 80% resolved within 14 days. Approximately 10% of those patients developing rash had a rash described as of severe intensity. Histology was evaluated in a clinical pharmacology study and was consistent with an uncomplicated exanthematous skin reaction and showed no evidence of phototoxicity, vasculitis, or necrosis. There were no documented cases in the clinical trials of more serious skin reactions known to be associated with significant morbidity or mortality.
Rash was more commonly observed in patients <40 years of age, especially females and post-menopausal females taking hormone replacement therapy. The incidence of rash also

correlated with longer treatment duration (>7 days). Prolonging duration of therapy beyond 7 days causes the incidence of rash to increase significantly in all subgroups except men over the age of 40 (see Table 2). Gemifloxacin therapy should be discontinued in patients developing a rash while on treatment (see **ADVERSE REACTIONS** and **CLINICAL STUDIES**).

[See table 2 at right]

Photosensitivity reactions have been reported very rarely in clinical trials with FACTIVE. (See **CLINICAL PHARMACOLOGY**.) However, as with all drugs of this class, it is recommended that patients avoid unnecessary exposure to strong sunlight or artificial UV rays (e.g., sunlamps, solariums), and should be advised of the appropriate use of broad spectrum sun block if in bright sunlight. Treatment should be discontinued if a photosensitivity reaction is suspected.

Hepatic Effects: Liver enzyme elevations (increased ALT and/or AST) occurred at similar rates in patients receiving gemifloxacin 320 mg daily relative to comparator antimicrobial agents (ciprofloxacin, levofloxacin, clarithromycin/cefuroxime axetil, amoxicillin/clavulanate potassium, and ofloxacin). In patients who received gemifloxacin at doses of 480 mg per day or greater there was an increased incidence of elevations in liver enzymes. (See **ADVERSE REACTIONS**.)

There were no clinical symptoms associated with these liver enzyme elevations. The liver enzyme elevations resolved following cessation of therapy. The recommended dose of gemifloxacin 320 mg daily should not be exceeded and the recommended length of therapy should not be exceeded. (See **DOSAGE AND ADMINISTRATION**.)

Alteration of the dosage regimen is necessary for patients with impairment of renal function (creatinine clearance ≤40 mL/min). (See **DOSAGE AND ADMINISTRATION**.)

Adequate hydration of patients receiving gemifloxacin should be maintained to prevent the formation of a highly concentrated urine.

Information for Patients

Patients should be counseled:

- that antibacterial drugs including FACTIVE should only be used to treat bacterial infections. They do not treat viral infections (e.g. the common cold). When FACTIVE is prescribed to treat a bacterial infection, patients should be told that although it is common to feel better early in the course of therapy, the medication should be taken exactly as directed. Skipping doses or not completing the full course of therapy may (1) decrease the effectiveness of the immediate treatment and (2) increase the likelihood that bacteria will develop resistance and will not be treatable by FACTIVE or other antibacterial drugs in the future;
- that FACTIVE has been associated with rash. Patients should discontinue drug and call their healthcare provider if they develop a rash;
- that FACTIVE may be associated with hypersensitivity reactions, including anaphylactic reactions, even following a single dose; patients should immediately discontinue the drug at the sign of a rash or other allergic reaction and seek medical care;
- that FACTIVE may produce changes in the electrocardiogram (QTc interval prolongation);
- that FACTIVE should be avoided in patients receiving Class IA (e.g., quinidine, procainamide) or Class III (e.g., amiodarone, sotalol) antiarrhythmic agents;
- that FACTIVE should be used with caution in patients receiving drugs that may affect the QTc interval such as erythromycin, antipsychotics, and tricyclic antidepressants;
- to inform their physician of any personal or family history of QTc prolongation or proarrhythmic conditions such as recent hypokalemia, significant bradycardia, or recent myocardial ischemia;
- to inform their physician of any other medications when taken concurrently with FACTIVE, including over-the-counter medications and dietary supplements;
- to contact their physician if they experience palpitations or fainting spells while taking FACTIVE;
- that FACTIVE may be taken with or without meals;
- to drink fluids liberally;
- not to take antacids containing magnesium and/or aluminum or products containing ferrous sulfate (iron), multivitamin preparations containing zinc or other metal cations, or Videx® (didanosine) chewable/buffered tablets or the pediatric powder for oral solution within 3 hours before or 2 hours after taking FACTIVE tablets;
- that FACTIVE should be taken at least 2 hours before sucralfate;
- that phototoxicity has been reported with certain quinolones. The potential for FACTIVE to cause phototoxicity was low (3/7659) at the recommended dose in clinical studies. In keeping with good clinical practice, avoid excessive sunlight or artificial ultraviolet light (e.g. tanning beds). If a sunburn-like reaction or skin eruption occurs, contact your physician; (See **CLINICAL PHARMACOLOGY: Photosensitivity Potential**);
- that FACTIVE may cause dizziness; if this occurs, patients should not operate an automobile or machinery or engage in activities requiring mental alertness or coordination;
- that they should discontinue FACTIVE therapy and inform their physician if they feel pain, tenderness or rupture of a tendon. Patients should rest and avoid exercise until the diagnosis of tendonitis or tendon rupture has been excluded;

Table 2. Rash Incidence in FACTIVE Treated Patients from the Clinical Studies Population* by Gender, Age, and Duration of Therapy

Gender & Age (yr) Category	Duration of Gemifloxacin Therapy			
	5 days	7 days	10 days**	14 days**
Female < 40	5/242 (2.1%)	39/324 (12.0%)	20/131 (15.3%)	7/31 (22.6%)
Female ≥ 40	19/1210 (1.6%)	30/695 (4.3%)	19/308 (6.2%)	10/126 (7.9%)
Male < 40	4/218 (1.8%)	20/318 (6.3%)	7/74 (9.5%)	3/39 (7.7%)
Male ≥ 40	9/1321 (0.7%)	23/776 (3.0%)	9/345 (2.6%)	3/116 (2.6%)
Totals	37/2991 (1.2%)	112/2113 (5.3%)	55/858 (6.4%)	23/312 (7.4%)

*includes patients from studies of community-acquired pneumonia, acute bacterial exacerbation of chronic bronchitis, and other indications.
exceeds the recommended duration of therapy (see **DOSAGE AND ADMINISTRATION)

- that convulsions have been reported in patients receiving quinolones; and they should notify their physician before taking this drug if there is a history of this condition.

Drug Interactions: Administration of repeat doses of FACTIVE had no effect on the repeat dose pharmacokinetics of theophylline, digoxin or an ethinylestradiol/levonorgestrol oral contraceptive product in healthy subjects. (See **CLINICAL PHARMACOLOGY: Drug-Drug Interactions.**)

Concomitant administration of FACTIVE and calcium carbonate, cimetidine, omeprazole, or an estrogen/progesterone oral contraceptive produced minor changes in the pharmacokinetics of gemifloxacin, which were considered to be without clinical significance. (See **CLINICAL PHARMACOLOGY**.)

Concomitant administration of FACTIVE with probenecid resulted in a 45% increase in systemic exposure to gemifloxacin. (See **CLINICAL PHARMACOLOGY**.)

FACTIVE had no significant effect on the anticoagulant effect of warfarin in healthy subjects on stable warfarin therapy. However, because some quinolones have been reported to enhance the anticoagulant effects of warfarin or its derivatives in patients, the prothrombin time or other suitable coagulation test should be closely monitored if a quinolone antimicrobial is administered concomitantly with warfarin or its derivatives.

Quinolones form chelates with alkaline earth and transition metals. The absorption of oral gemifloxacin is significantly reduced by the concomitant administration of an antacid containing aluminum and magnesium. Magnesium- and/or aluminum-containing antacids, products containing ferrous sulfate (iron), multivitamin preparations containing zinc or other metal cations, or Videx® (didanosine) chewable/buffered tablets or the pediatric powder for oral solution should not be taken within 3 hours before or 2 hours after FACTIVE. Sucralfate should not be taken within 2 hours of FACTIVE. (See **CLINICAL PHARMACOLOGY**.)

Carcinogenesis, Mutagenesis, Impairment of Fertility

Carcinogenesis: Long term studies in animals to determine the carcinogenic potential of gemifloxacin have not been conducted.

Photocarcinogenesis: Gemifloxacin did not shorten the time to development of UVR-induced skin tumors in hairless albino (Skh-1) mice; thus, it was not photocarcinogenic in this model. These mice received oral gemifloxacin and concurrent irradiation with simulated sunlight 5 days per week for 40 weeks followed by a 12-week treatment-free observation period. The daily dose of UV radiation used in this study was approximately 1/3 of the minimal dose of UV radiation that would induce erythema in Caucasian humans. The median time to the development of skin tumors in the hairless mice was similar in the vehicle control group (36 weeks) and those given up to 100 mg/kg gemifloxacin daily (39 weeks). Following repeat doses of 100 mg/kg gemifloxacin per day, the mice had skin gemifloxacin concentrations of approximately 7.4 µg/g. Plasma levels following this dose were approximately 1.4 µg/mL in the mice around the time of irradiation. There are no data on gemifloxacin skin levels in humans, but the mouse plasma gemifloxacin levels are in the expected range of human plasma Cmax levels (0.7-2.6 µg/mL, with an overall mean of about 1.6 µg/mL) following multiple 320 mg oral doses.

Mutagenesis: Gemifloxacin was not mutagenic in 4 bacterial strains (TA 98, TA 100, TA 1535, TA 1537) used in an Ames *Salmonella* reversion assay. It did not induce micronuclei in the bone marrow of mice following intraperitoneal doses of up to 40 mg/kg and it did not induce unscheduled DNA synthesis in hepatocytes from rats which received oral doses of up to 1600 mg/kg. Gemifloxacin was clastogenic in vitro in the mouse lymphoma and human lymphocyte chromosome aberration assays. It was clastogenic *in vivo* in the rat micronucleus assay at oral and intravenous dose levels (≥800 mg/kg and ≥40 mg/kg, respectively) that produced bone marrow toxicity. Fluoroquinolone clastogenicity is apparently due to inhibition of mammalian topoisomerase activity which has threshold implications.

Impairment of Fertility: Gemifloxacin did not affect the fertility of male or female rats at AUC levels following oral administration (216 and 600 mg/kg/day) that were approximately 3- to 4-fold higher than the AUC levels at the clinically recommended dose.

Pregnancy: Teratogenic Effects. Pregnancy Category C. Gemifloxacin treatment during organogenesis caused fetal growth retardation in mice (oral dosing at 450 mg/kg/day), rats (oral dosing at 600 mg/kg/day) and rabbits (IV dosing at 40 mg/kg/day) at AUC levels which were 2-, 4- and 3-fold those in women given oral doses of 320 mg. In rats, this growth retardation appeared to be reversible in a pre- and postnatal development study (mice and rabbits were not studied for the reversibility of this effect). Treatment of pregnant rats at 8-fold clinical exposure (based upon AUC comparisons) caused fetal brain and ocular malformations in the presence of maternal toxicity. The overall no-effect exposure level in pregnant animals was approximately 0.8 to 3-fold clinical exposure.

The safety of gemifloxacin in pregnant women has not been established. Gemifloxacin should not be used in pregnant women unless the potential benefit to the mother outweighs the risk to the fetus. There are no adequate and well-controlled studies in pregnant women.

Nursing Mothers: Gemifloxacin is excreted in the breast milk of rats. There is no information on excretion of gemifloxacin into human milk. Therefore, gemifloxacin should not be used in lactating women unless the potential benefit to the mother outweighs the risk.

Pediatric Use: Safety and effectiveness in children and adolescents less than 18 years of age have not been established. Fluoroquinolones, including gemifloxacin, cause arthropathy and osteochondrosis in immature animals. (See **WARNINGS**.)

Geriatric Use: Of the total number of subjects in clinical studies of gemifloxacin, 30% (2064) were 65 and over, while 12% (779) were 75 and over. No overall difference in effectiveness was observed between these subjects and younger subjects; the adverse event rates for this group was similar to or lower than that for younger subjects with the exception that the incidence of rash was lower in geriatric patients compared to patients less than 40 years of age.

ADVERSE REACTIONS

In clinical studies, 6775 patients received daily oral doses of 320 mg gemifloxacin. In addition, 1797 healthy volunteers and 81 patients with renal or hepatic impairment received single or repeat doses of gemifloxacin in clinical pharmacology studies. The majority of adverse reactions experienced by patients in clinical trials were considered to be of mild to moderate severity.

Gemifloxacin was discontinued because of an adverse event (possibly or probably related) in 2.2% of patients, primarily due to rash (0.9%), nausea (0.3%), diarrhea (0.3%), urticaria (0.3%) and vomiting (0.2%). Comparator antibiotics were discontinued because of an adverse event at an overall comparable rate of 2.1%, primarily due to diarrhea (0.5%), nausea (0.3%), vomiting (0.3%) and rash (0.3%).

Drug-related adverse events, classified as possibly or probably related with a frequency of ≥1% for patients receiving 320 mg of gemifloxacin versus comparator drug (beta-lactam antibiotics, macrolides or other fluoroquinolones) are as follows: diarrhea 3.6% vs. 4.6%; rash 2.8% vs. 0.6%; nausea 2.7% vs. 3.2%; headache 1.2% vs. 1.5%; abdominal pain 0.9% vs. 1.1%; vomiting 0.9% vs. 1.1%; dizziness 0.8% vs. 1.5%; and taste perversion 0.3% vs. 1.9%.

Gemifloxacin appears to have a low potential for photosensitivity. In clinical trials, treatment-related photosensitivity occurred in only 0.039% (3/7659) of patients.

Additional drug-related adverse events (possibly or probably related) in >0.1% to 1% of patients who received 320 mg of gemifloxacin were: abdominal pain, anorexia, arthralgia, constipation, dermatitis, dizziness, dry mouth, dyspepsia, fatigue, flatulence, fungal infection, gastritis, genital moniliasis, hyperglycemia, insomnia, leukopenia, moniliasis, pruritus, somnolence, taste perversion, thrombocythemia, urticaria, vaginitis, and vomiting.

Other adverse events reported from clinical trials which have potential clinical significance and which were considered to have a suspected relationship to the drug, that occurred in ≤0.1% of patients were: abnormal urine, anemia, asthenia, back pain, bilirubinemia, dyspnea, eczema, eosinophilia, flushing, gastroenteritis, granulocytopenia, hot flashes, increased GGT, leg cramps, myalgia, nervousness, non-specified gastrointestinal disorder, pain, pharyngitis, pneumonia, thrombocytopenia, tremor, vertigo, and vision abnormality.

In clinical trials of acute bacterial exacerbation of chronic bronchitis (ABECB) and community acquired pneumonia (CAP), the incidences of rash were as follows (Table 3):

[See table 3 at top of next page]

(see **PRECAUTIONS**)

Laboratory Changes: The percentages of patients who received multiple doses of gemifloxacin and had a laboratory

Continued on next page

Table 3. Incidence of Rash by Clinical Indication in Patients Treated with Gemifloxacin

	ABECB (5 days) N = 2284		CAP (7 days) N = 643	
	n/N	%	n/N	%
Totals	27/2284	1.2	26/643	4.0
Females, < 40 years	NA*		8/88	9.1
Females, ≥ 40 years	16/1040	1.5	5/214	2.3
Males, < 40 years	NA*		5/101	5.0
Males, ≥ 40 years	11/1203	0.9	8/240	3.3

* insufficient number of patients in this category for a meaningful analysis

Men: Creatinine Clearance (mL/min) = $\frac{\text{Weight (kg)} \times (140 - \text{age})}{72 \times \text{serum creatinine (mg/dL)}}$

Women: 0.85 × the value calculated for men

Factive—Cont.

abnormality are listed below. It is not known whether these abnormalities were related to gemifloxacin or an underlying condition.

Clinical Chemistry: increased ALT (1.5%), increased AST (1.1%), increased creatine phosphokinase (0.6%), increased potassium (0.5%), decreased sodium (0.3%), increased gammaglutamyl transferase (0.5%), increased alkaline phosphatase (0.3%), increased total bilirubin (0.3%), increased blood urea nitrogen (0.3%), decreased calcium (0.2%), decreased albumin (0.3%), increased serum creatinine (0.2%), decreased total protein (0.1%) and increased calcium (<0.1%). CPK elevations were noted infrequently: 0.8% in gemifloxacin patients vs. 0.4% in the comparator patients.

Hematology: increased platelets (0.9%), decreased neutrophils (0.5%), increased neutrophils (0.5%), decreased hematocrit (0.3%), decreased hemoglobin (0.2%), decreased platelets (0.2%), decreased red blood cells (0.1%), increased hematocrit (0.1%), increased hemoglobin (0.1%), and increased red blood cells (0.1%).

In clinical studies, approximately 7% of the gemifloxacin treated patients had elevated ALT values immediately prior to entry into the study. Of these patients, approximately 10% showed a further elevation of their ALT at the on-therapy visit and 5% showed a further elevation at the end of therapy visit. None of these patients demonstrated evidence of hepatocellular jaundice. For the pooled comparators, approximately 6% of patients had elevated ALT values immediately prior to entry into the study. Of these patients, approximately 7% showed a further elevation of their ALT at the on-therapy visit and 4% showed a further elevation at the end of therapy visit.

In a clinical trial where 638 patients received either a single 640 mg dose of gemifloxacin or 250 mg bid of ciprofloxacin for 3 days, there was an increased incidence of ALT elevations in the gemifloxacin arm (3.9%) vs. the comparator arm (1.0%). In this study, two patients experienced ALT elevations of 8 to 10 times the upper limit of normal. These elevations were asymptomatic and reversible.

OVERDOSAGE

Any signs or symptoms of overdosage should be treated symptomatically. No specific antidote is known. In the event of acute oral overdosage, the stomach should be emptied by inducing vomiting or by gastric lavage; the patient should be carefully observed and treated symptomatically with appropriate hydration maintained. Hemodialysis removes approximately 20 to 30% of an oral dose of gemifloxacin from plasma.

Mortality occurred at oral gemifloxacin doses of 1600 mg/kg in rats and 320 mg/kg in mice. The minimum lethal intravenous doses in these species were 160 and 80 mg/kg, respectively. Toxic signs after administration of a single high oral dose (400 mg/kg) of gemifloxacin to rodents included ataxia, lethargy, piloerection, tremor, and clonic convulsions.

DOSAGE AND ADMINISTRATION

FACTIVE can be taken with or without food and should be swallowed whole with a liberal amount of liquid. The recommended dose of FACTIVE is 320 mg daily, according to the following table (Table 4).

Table 4. Recommended Dosage Regimen of FACTIVE

INDICATION	DOSE	DURATION
Acute bacterial exacerbation of chronic bronchitis	Over 320 mg tablet daily	5 days
Community-acquired pneumonia (of mild to moderate severity)	One 320 mg tablet daily	7 days

The recommended dose and duration of FACTIVE should not be exceeded (see Table 2).

Renally Impaired Patients: Dose adjustment in patients with creatinine clearance >40 mL/min is not required. Modification of the dosage is recommended for patients with creatinine clearance ≤40 mL/min. Table 5 provides dosage guidelines for use in patients with renal impairment:

Table 5. Recommended Doses for Patients with Renal Impairment

Creatinine Clearance (mL/min)	Dose
>40	See Usual Dosage
≤40	160 mg q24h

Patients requiring routine hemodialysis or continuous ambulatory peritoneal dialysis (CAPD) should receive 160 mg q24h.

When only the serum creatinine concentration is known, the following formula may be used to estimate creatinine clearance.

[See second table above]

Use in Hepatically Impaired Patients: No dosage adjustment is recommended in patients with mild (Child-Pugh Class A), moderate (Child-Pugh Class B) or severe (Child-Pugh Class C) hepatic impairment.

Use in Elderly: No dosage adjustment is recommended.

HOW SUPPLIED

FACTIVE (gemifloxacin mesylate) is available as white to off-white, oval, film-coated tablets with breaklines and GE 320 debossed on both faces. Each tablet contains gemifloxacin mesylate equivalent to 320 mg of gemifloxacin.

320 mg Unit of Use (CR*) 5's	NDC 67707-320-05
320 mg Unit of Use (CR*) 7's	NDC 67707-320-07
320 mg Hospital Pack (NCR**) 30's	NDC 67707-320-30

*Child Resistant ** Not Child Resistant

STORAGE

Store at 25°C (77°F); excursions permitted to 15°-30°C (59°-86°F) [see USP Controlled Room Temperature]. Protect from light.

ANIMAL PHARMACOLOGY

Quinolones have been shown to cause arthropathy in immature animals. Degeneration of articular cartilage occurred in juvenile dogs given at least 192 mg/kg/day gemifloxacin in a 28-day study (producing about 6 times the systemic exposure at the clinical dose), but not in mature dogs. There was no damage to the articular surfaces of joints in immature rats given repeated doses of up to 800 mg/kg/day.

Some quinolones have been reported to have proconvulsant properties that are potentiated by the concomitant administration of non-steroidal anti-inflammatory drugs (NSAIDs). Gemifloxacin alone had effects in tests of behavior or CNS interaction typically at doses of at least 160 mg/kg. No convulsions occurred in mice given the active metabolite of the NSAID, fenbufen, followed by 80 mg/kg gemifloxacin.

Dogs given 192 mg/kg/day (about 6 times the systemic exposure at the clinical dose) for 28 days, or 24 mg/kg/day (approximately equivalent to the systemic exposure at the clinical dose) for 13 weeks showed reversible increases in plasma ALT activities and local periportal liver changes associated with blockage of small bile ducts by crystals containing gemifloxacin.

Quinolones have been associated with prolongation of the electrocardiographic QT interval in dogs. Gemifloxacin produced no effect on the QT interval in dogs dosed orally to provide about 4 times human therapeutic plasma concentrations at Cmax, and transient prolongation after intravenous administration at more than 4 times human plasma levels at Cmax. Gemifloxacin exhibited weak activity in the cardiac I_{Kr} (hERG) channel inhibition assay, having an IC_{50} of approximately 270 μM.

Gemifloxacin, like many other quinolones, tends to crystallize at the alkaline pH of rodent urine, resulting in a nephropathy in rats that is reversible on drug withdrawal (oral no-effect dose 24 mg/kg/day).

Gemifloxacin was weakly phototoxic to hairless mice given a single 200 mg/kg oral dose and exposed to UVA radiation, however, no evidence of phototoxicity was observed at 100 mg/kg/day dosed orally for 13 weeks in a standard hairless mouse model, using simulated sunlight.

CLINICAL STUDIES

Acute Bacterial Exacerbation of Chronic Bronchitis (ABECB)

FACTIVE (320 mg once daily for 5 days) was evaluated for the treatment of acute bacterial exacerbation of chronic bronchitis in three pivotal double-blind, randomized, actively-controlled clinical trials (studies 068, 070, and 212). The primary efficacy parameter in these studies was the clinical response at follow-up (day 13 to 24). The results of the clinical response at follow-up for the principal ABECB studies demonstrate that FACTIVE 320 mg PO once daily for 5 days was at least as good as the comparators given for 7 days. The results are shown in Table 6 below.

Table 6. Clinical Response at Follow-Up (Test of Cure): Pivotal ABECB Studies

Drug Regimen	Success Rate % (n/N)	Treatment Difference (95% CI)
Study 068		
FACTIVE 320 mg × 5 days	86.0 (239/278)	1.2 (-4.7, 7.0)
Clarithromycin 500 mg bid × 7 days	84.8 (240/283)	
Study 070		
FACTIVE 320 mg × 5 days	93.6 (247/264)	
Amoxicillin/ clavulanate 500 mg/125 mg tid × 7 days	93.2 (248/266)	0.4 (-3.9, 4.6)
Study 212		
FACTIVE 320 mg × 5 days	88.2 (134/152)	3.1 (-4.7, 10.7)
Levofloxacin 500 mg × 7 days	85.1 (126/148)	

Community Acquired Pneumonia (CAP)

The clinical program to evaluate the efficacy of gemifloxacin in the treatment of community acquired pneumonia in adults consisted of three double-blind, randomized, actively-controlled clinical studies (studies 011, 012, and 049) and one open, actively-controlled study (study 185). In addition, two uncontrolled studies (studies 061 and 287) were conducted. Three of the studies, pivotal study 011 and the uncontrolled studies, had a fixed 7-day duration of treatment for FACTIVE. Pivotal study 011 compared a 7-day course of FACTIVE with a 10-day treatment course of amoxicillin/clavulanate (1g/125 mg tid) and clinical success rates were similar between treatment arms. The results of comparative studies 049, 185, and 012 were supportive although treatment duration could have been 7 to 14 days. The results of the clinical studies with a fixed 7-day duration of gemifloxacin are shown in Table 7:

Table 7. Clinical Response at Follow-Up (Test of Cure): CAP Studies with a Fixed 7 Day Duration of Treatment

Drug Regimen	Success Rate % (n/N)	Treatment Difference (95% CI)*
Study 011		
FACTIVE 320 mg × 7 days	88.7 % (102/115)	
Amoxicillin/ clavulanate 500 mg/125 mg tid × 10 days	87.6% (99/113)	1.1 (-7.3, 9.5)
Study 061		
FACTIVE 320 mg × 7 days	91.7% (154/168)	(86.1, 95.2)
Study 287		
FACTIVE 320 mg × 7 days	89.8% (132/147)	(84.9, 94.7)

* For uncontrolled studies, the 95% CI around the success rate is shown

The combined bacterial eradication rates for patients treated with a fixed 7-day treatment regimen of FACTIVE are shown in Table 8:

Table 8. Bacterial Eradication by Pathogen for Patients Treated with FACTIVE in Studies with a Fixed 7-day Duration of Treatment

Pathogen	n/N	%
S. pneumoniae	68/77	88.3
M. pneumoniae	21/22	95.5
H. influenzae	30/35	85.7
C. pneumoniae	13/14	92.9
*K. pneumoniae**	11/13	84.6
M. catarrhalis	10/10	100

* Subjects with *Klebsiella pneumoniae* included in this table were from non-comparative studies 061 and 287. 10 of these subjects had mild disease, 2 had moderate disease, and 1 had severe disease. Both failures were in subjects with mild disease (one of these had a bacteriologic recurrence).

FACTIVE was also effective in the treatment of CAP due to multi-drug resistant *Streptococcus pneumoniae* (MDRSP*). Of 22 patients with MDRSP treated for 7 days, 19 (86.5%) achieved clinical and bacteriological success at follow-up. The clinical and bacteriological success for the 22 patients with 22 MDRSP isolates are shown in Table 9.

*MDRSP: Multi-drug resistant *Streptococcus pneumoniae* includes isolates previously known as PRSP (penicillin-resistant *Streptococcus pneumoniae*), and are strains resistant to two or more of the following antibiotics: penicillin, 2nd generation cephalosporins, e.g., cefuroxime, macrolides, tetracyclines and trimethoprim/sulfamethoxazole.

Table 9. Clinical and Bacteriological Success for 22 Patients Treated with FACTIVE in Studies with a 7-day Duration of Treatment for MDRSP

Screening Susceptibility	Clinical Success		Bacteriological Success	
	n/N[a]	%	n/N[b]	%
Penicillin-resistant	11/11	100	11/11	100
2nd generation cephalosporin-resistant	14/14	100	14/14	100
Macrolide-resistant[c]	16/19	84.2	16/19	84.2
Trimethoprim/ sulfamethoxazole-resistant	16/16	100	16/16	100
Tetracycline-resistant	13/16	81.3	13/16	81.3

a) n = the number of patients successfully treated; N = number of patients with MDRSP (from a total of 22 patients)
b) n = the number of bacteriological isolates successfully treated; N = number of isolates studied (from a total of 22 isolates)
c) Macrolide antibiotics tested include clarithromycin and erythromycin

Cutaneous Manifestations (Rash)
In clinical trials of 6,775 patients, the incidence of rash was higher in patients receiving gemifloxacin than in those receiving comparator drugs (see **PRECAUTIONS** and **ADVERSE REACTIONS**). Rash was more commonly observed in patients <40 years of age, especially females and post-menopausal females taking hormone replacement therapy. The incidence of rash also correlated with longer treatment duration (>7 days). (See Table 2.)
To further characterize gemifloxacin-associated rash, a clinical pharmacology study was conducted. The study enrolled 1,011 healthy female volunteers less than 40 years of age. Subjects were randomized to receive either FACTIVE 320 mg po daily or ciprofloxacin 500 mg po twice daily for 10 days. The objective of the study was to assess the characteristics of rash. The majority of rashes in subjects receiving FACTIVE were maculopapular and of mild to moderate severity; 7% of the rashes were reported as severe, and severity appeared to correlate with the extent of the rash. In 68% of the subjects reporting a severe rash and approximately 25% of all those reporting rash, >60% of the body surface area was involved; the characteristics of the rash were otherwise indistinguishable from those subjects reporting a mild rash. The histopathology was consistent with the clinical observation of uncomplicated exanthematous morbilliform eruption. There were no documented cases of hypersensitivity syndrome or findings suggestive of angioedema or other serious cutaneous reactions.
The majority of rash events (81.9%) occurred on days 8 through 10 day of the planned 10 day course of gemifloxacin; 2.7% of rash events occurred within one day of the start of dosing. The median duration of rash was 6 days. The rash resolved without treatment in the majority of subjects. Approximately 19% received antihistamines and 5% received steroids, although the therapeutic benefit of these therapies is uncertain.
In the second part of this study after a 4 to 6 week wash out period, subjects developing a rash on gemifloxacin were treated with ciprofloxacin or placebo; 5.9% developed rash when treated with ciprofloxacin and 2.0% developed rash when treated with placebo. The characteristics of rash in subjects receiving ciprofloxacin following gemifloxacin were similar to those described in subjects who only received ciprofloxacin. The cross sensitization rate to other fluoroquinolones was not evaluated in this clinical study. There was no evidence of sub-clinical sensitization to gemifloxacin (i.e. subjects who had not developed a rash to gemifloxacin in the first part of the study were not at higher risk of developing a rash to gemifloxacin with a second exposure).
There was no relationship between the incidence of rash and systemic exposure (Cmax and AUC) to either gemifloxacin or its major metabolite, N-acetyl gemifloxacin.

REFERENCES

1. National Committee for Clinical Laboratory Standards. Methods for Dilution Antimicrobial Susceptibility Tests for Bacteria that Grow Aerobically—Sixth Edition. Approved Standard NCCLS Document M7-A6, Vol. 23, No. 2, NCCLS, Wayne, PA, January 2003. **2.** National Committee for Clinical Laboratory Standards. Performance Standards for Antimicrobial Disk Susceptibility Tests—Eighth Edition. Approved Standard NCCLS Document A2-A8, Vol. 23, No. 1, NCCLS Wayne, PA, January 2003.

DATE OF REVISION FEBRUARY 2004

Rx only
OSCIENT PHARMACEUTICALS
Waltham, MA 02453-8443 USA
Licensed from LG Life Sciences, Ltd. Seoul, Korea
02-23-04-1

Patient Information
FACTIVE®
(gemifloxacin mesylate) Tablets

This leaflet summarizes the most important information about FACTIVE. Read the Patient Information that comes with FACTIVE each time you get a new prescription. There may be new information. This leaflet does not list all benefits and risks of treatment and does not take the place of talking with your healthcare provider about your condition or your treatment. FACTIVE can only be prescribed by a healthcare professional. If you would like more information, talk with your healthcare provider or pharmacist.

What is FACTIVE?
FACTIVE is an antibiotic. It is used to treat adults 18 years or older with bronchitis or pneumonia (lung infections) caused by certain bacteria (germs).
Sometimes, other germs called viruses infect the lungs. The common cold is a virus. FACTIVE, like other antibiotics, does not treat viruses.
FACTIVE tablets are white to off white and imprinted with GE 320 on both sides.

Who should not take FACTIVE?
- **Do not take FACTIVE if you are allergic to any of the ingredients in FACTIVE or to any antibiotic called a "quinolone".** If you develop hives, difficulty breathing, or other symptoms of a severe allergic reaction, seek emergency treatment right away. If you develop a skin rash, stop taking FACTIVE and call your healthcare professional. The ingredients in FACTIVE are listed at the end of this leaflet. Ask your healthcare provider or pharmacist if you need a list of quinolones.

FACTIVE may not be right for you. Tell your healthcare provider if you:
- are pregnant, planning to become pregnant, or are breast feeding. The effects of FACTIVE on unborn children and nursing infants are unknown;
- or any family members have a rare heart condition known as congenital prolongation of the QTc interval;
- have low potassium or magnesium levels;
- have a slow heart beat called bradycardia;
- have had a recent heart attack;
- have a history of convulsions;
- have kidney problems.

FACTIVE has not been studied in children under the age of 18. Quinolones may cause joint problems (arthropathy) in children.
Tell your healthcare provider about all the medicines you take including prescription and nonprescription medicines, vitamins, and dietary supplements. **Be sure to tell your healthcare provider if you take:**
- medicines for your heart rhythm called "antiarrhythmics"
- erythromycin
- medicines for your mental health called "antipsychotics" or "tricyclic antidepressants"
- medicines called "corticosteroids", taken by mouth or by injection
- medicines called diuretics such as furosemide and hydrochlorothiazide.

How should I take FACTIVE?
- Take 1 FACTIVE tablet a day for 5 or 7 days, exactly as prescribed.
- Take FACTIVE at the same time each day.
- FACTIVE can be taken with or without food.
- Swallow the FACTIVE tablet whole, and drink plenty of fluids with it. Do not chew the FACTIVE tablet.
- If you miss a dose of FACTIVE, take it as soon as you remember. **Do not take more than 1 dose of FACTIVE in a day.**
- To make sure all bacteria are killed, take all the medicine that was prescribed for you even if you begin to feel better.
- Call your healthcare provider if your condition does not improve while taking FACTIVE.

Do not take the following medicines within 3 hours before FACTIVE or 2 hours after FACTIVE. They may interfere with the absorption of FACTIVE and may prevent it from working properly:
- antacids that contain magnesium or aluminum
- ferrous sulfate (iron)
- multivitamin that contains zinc or other metals
- Videx® (didanosine)

FACTIVE should be taken at least 2 hours before sucralfate.

What are possible side effects of FACTIVE?
FACTIVE is generally well tolerated. The most common side effects with FACTIVE include diarrhea, rash, nausea, headache, vomiting, stomach pain, dizziness, and a change in the way things taste in your mouth. If you get a rash while taking FACTIVE, stop FACTIVE, and call your healthcare provider right away. Do not drive or operate heavy machinery until you know how FACTIVE affects you. FACTIVE can make you dizzy.
FACTIVE and other quinolone antibiotics may cause the following serious side effects:
- a rare heart problem known as prolongation of the QTc interval. This condition can cause an abnormal heartbeat and result in sudden death. You should call your healthcare provider right away if you have any symptoms of prolongation of the QTc interval including heart palpitations (a change in the way your heart beats) or fainting spells;
- central nervous system problems including body shakes (tremors), restless feeling, lightheaded feelings, confusion, and hallucinations (seeing or hearing things that are not there);
- tendon problems including tendonitis or rupture ("tears") of a tendon. If you experience pain, swelling, or rupture of a tendon, stop taking FACTIVE and call your healthcare professional;
- phototoxicity. This can make your skin sunburn easier. Do not use a sunlamp or tanning bed while taking FACTIVE. Use a sunscreen and wear protective clothing if you must be out in the sun.

These are not all the side effects you may experience with FACTIVE. If you get any side effects that concern you, call your healthcare provider.
General information about the safe and effective use of FACTIVE:
Medicines are sometimes prescribed for conditions other than those described in patient information leaflets. Do not use FACTIVE for a condition for which it was not prescribed. Do not give FACTIVE to other people, even if they have the same symptoms that you have. It may harm them.
Keep FACTIVE and all medicines out of the reach of children.

What are the ingredients in FACTIVE?
Active ingredient: gemifloxacin
Inactive Ingredients: crospovidone, hydroxypropyl methycellulose, magnesium stearate, microcrystalline cellulose, polyethylene glycol, povidone, titanium dioxide.

Shown in Product Identification Guide, page 328

Otsuka America Pharmaceutical, Inc.

2440 RESEARCH BLVD
ROCKVILLE, MD 20850

For Direct Inquiries Contact:
Medical Affairs
Otsuka America Pharmaceutical, Inc.
1-800-441-6763
fax 301-721-7284
To request routine or emergency Medical Information, or to report an adverse experience, please call: 1-800-438-9927

ABILIFY® ℞
[ă-bĭl-ĭ-fī]
(aripiprazole) Tablets
Rx only

DESCRIPTION
ABILIFY® (aripiprazole) is a psychotropic drug that is available as tablets for oral administration. Aripiprazole is 7-[4-[4-(2,3-dichlorophenyl)-1-piperazinyl]butoxy]-3,4-dihydrocarbostyril. The empirical formula is $C_{23}H_{27}Cl_2N_3O_2$ and its molecular weight is 448.38. The chemical structure is:

Cl Cl N N-CH₂CH₂CH₂CH₂O N H O

ABILIFY tablets are available in 5-mg, 10-mg, 15-mg, 20-mg, and 30-mg strengths. Inactive ingredients include lactose monohydrate, cornstarch, microcrystalline cellulose, hydroxypropyl cellulose, and magnesium stearate. Colorants include ferric oxide (yellow or red) and FD&C Blue No. 2 Aluminum Lake.

Continued on next page

Abilify—Cont.

CLINICAL PHARMACOLOGY

Pharmacodynamics

Aripiprazole exhibits high affinity for dopamine D_2 and D_3, serotonin 5-HT_{1A} and 5-HT_{2A} receptors (K_i values of 0.34, 0.8, 1.7, and 3.4 nM, respectively), moderate affinity for dopamine D_4, serotonin 5-HT_{2C} and 5-HT_7, alpha$_1$-adrenergic and histamine H_1 receptors (K_i values of 44, 15, 39, 57, and 61 nM, respectively), and moderate affinity for the serotonin reuptake site (K_i=98 nM). Aripiprazole has no appreciable affinity for cholinergic muscarinic receptors (IC_{50} >1000 nM). Aripiprazole functions as a partial agonist at the dopamine D_2 and the serotonin 5-HT_{1A} receptors, and as an antagonist at serotonin 5-HT_{2A} receptor.

The mechanism of action of aripiprazole, as with other drugs having efficacy in schizophrenia, is unknown. However, it has been proposed that the efficacy of aripiprazole is mediated through a combination of partial agonist activity at D_2 and 5-HT_{1A} receptors and antagonist activity at 5-HT_{2A} receptors. Actions at receptors other than D_2, 5-HT_{1A}, and 5-HT_{2A} may explain some of the other clinical effects of aripiprazole, e.g., the orthostatic hypotension observed with aripiprazole may be explained by its antagonist activity at adrenergic alpha$_1$ receptors.

Pharmacokinetics

ABILIFY activity is presumably primarily due to the parent drug, aripiprazole, and to a lesser extent, to its major metabolite, dehydro-aripiprazole, which has been shown to have affinities for D_2 receptors similar to the parent drug and represents 40% of the parent drug exposure in plasma. The mean elimination half-lives are about 75 hours and 94 hours for aripiprazole and dehydro-aripiprazole, respectively. Steady-state concentrations are attained within 14 days of dosing for both active moieties. Aripiprazole accumulation is predictable from single-dose pharmacokinetics. At steady state, the pharmacokinetics of aripiprazole are dose-proportional. Elimination of aripiprazole is mainly through hepatic metabolism involving two P450 isozymes, CYP2D6 and CYP3A4.

Absorption

Aripiprazole is well absorbed, with peak plasma concentrations occurring within 3 to 5 hours; the absolute oral bioavailability of the tablet formulation is 87%. ABILIFY can be administered with or without food. Administration of a 15-mg ABILIFY tablet with a standard high-fat meal did not significantly affect the C_{max} or AUC of aripiprazole or its active metabolite, dehydro-aripiprazole, but delayed T_{max} by 3 hours for aripiprazole and 12 hours for dehydro-aripiprazole.

Distribution

The steady-state volume of distribution of aripiprazole following intravenous administration is high (404 L or 4.9 L/kg), indicating extensive extravascular distribution. At therapeutic concentrations, aripiprazole and its major metabolite are greater than 99% bound to serum proteins, primarily to albumin. In healthy human volunteers administered 0.5 to 30 mg/day aripiprazole for 14 days, there was dose-dependent D_2-receptor occupancy indicating brain penetration of aripiprazole in humans.

Metabolism and Elimination

Aripiprazole is metabolized primarily by three biotransformation pathways: dehydrogenation, hydroxylation, and N-dealkylation. Based on *in vitro* studies, CYP3A4 and CYP2D6 enzymes are responsible for dehydrogenation and hydroxylation of aripiprazole, and N-dealkylation is catalyzed by CYP3A4. Aripiprazole is the predominant drug moiety in the systemic circulation. At steady state, dehydro-aripiprazole, the active metabolite, represents about 40% of aripiprazole AUC in plasma.

Approximately 8% of Caucasians lack the capacity to metabolize CYP2D6 substrates and are classified as poor metabolizers (PM), whereas the rest are extensive metabolizers (EM). PMs have about an 80% increase in aripiprazole exposure and about a 30% decrease in exposure to the active metabolite compared to EMs, resulting in about a 60% higher exposure to the total active moieties from a given dose of aripiprazole compared to EMs. Coadministration of ABILIFY with known inhibitors of CYP2D6, like quinidine in EMs, results in a 112% increase in aripiprazole plasma exposure, and dosing adjustment is needed (see **PRECAUTIONS: Drug-Drug Interactions**). The mean elimination half-lives are about 75 hours and 146 hours for aripiprazole in EMs and PMs, respectively. Aripiprazole does not inhibit or induce the CYP2D6 pathway.

Following a single oral dose of [^{14}C]-labeled aripiprazole, approximately 25% and 55% of the administered radioactivity was recovered in the urine and feces, respectively. Less than 1% of unchanged aripiprazole was excreted in the urine and approximately 18% of the oral dose was recovered unchanged in the feces.

Special Populations

In general, no dosage adjustment for ABILIFY (aripiprazole) is required on the basis of a patient's age, gender, race, smoking status, hepatic function, or renal function (see **DOSAGE AND ADMINISTRATION: Dosage in Special Populations**). The pharmacokinetics of aripiprazole in special populations are described below.

Hepatic Impairment

In a single-dose study (15 mg of aripiprazole) in subjects with varying degrees of liver cirrhosis (Child-Pugh Classes A, B, and C) the AUC of aripiprazole, compared to healthy subjects, increased 31% in mild HI, increased 8% in moderate HI, and decreased 20% in severe HI. None of these differences would require dose adjustment.

Renal Impairment

In patients with severe renal impairment (creatinine clearance <30 mL/min), C_{max} of aripiprazole (given in a single dose of 15 mg) and dehydro-aripiprazole increased by 36% and 53%, respectively, but AUC was 15% lower for aripiprazole and 7% higher for dehydro-aripiprazole. Renal excretion of both unchanged aripiprazole and dehydro-aripiprazole is less than 1% of the dose. No dosage adjustment is required in subjects with renal impairment.

Elderly

In formal single-dose pharmacokinetic studies (with aripiprazole given in a single dose of 15 mg), aripiprazole clearance was 20% lower in elderly (≥65 years) subjects compared to younger adult subjects (18 to 64 years). There was no detectable age effect, however, in the population pharmacokinetic analysis in schizophrenia patients. Also, the pharmacokinetics of aripiprazole after multiple doses in elderly patients appeared similar to that observed in young, healthy subjects. No dosage adjustment is recommended for elderly patients (see **PRECAUTIONS: Geriatric Use**).

Gender

C_{max} and AUC of aripiprazole and its active metabolite, dehydro-aripiprazole, are 30 to 40% higher in women than in men, and correspondingly, the apparent oral clearance of aripiprazole is lower in women. These differences, however, are largely explained by differences in body weight (25%) between men and women. No dosage adjustment is recommended based on gender.

Race

Although no specific pharmacokinetic study was conducted to investigate the effects of race on the disposition of aripiprazole, population pharmacokinetic evaluation revealed no evidence of clinically significant race-related differences in the pharmacokinetics of aripiprazole. No dosage adjustment is recommended based on race.

Smoking

Based on studies utilizing human liver enzymes *in vitro*, aripiprazole is not a substrate for CYP1A2 and also does not undergo direct glucuronidation. Smoking should, therefore, not have an effect on the pharmacokinetics of aripiprazole. Consistent with these *in vitro* results, population pharmacokinetic evaluation did not reveal any significant pharmacokinetic differences between smokers and nonsmokers. No dosage adjustment is recommended based on smoking status.

Drug-Drug Interactions

Potential for Other Drugs to Affect ABILIFY

Aripiprazole is not a substrate of CYP1A1, CYP1A2, CYP2A6, CYP2B6, CYP2C8, CYP2C9, CYP2C19, or CYP2E1 enzymes. Aripiprazole also does not undergo direct glucuronidation. This suggests that an interaction of aripiprazole with inhibitors or inducers of these enzymes, or other factors, like smoking, is unlikely.

Both CYP3A4 and CYP2D6 are responsible for aripiprazole metabolism. Agents that induce CYP3A4 (e.g., carbamazepine) could cause an increase in aripiprazole clearance and lower blood levels. Inhibitors of CYP3A4 (e.g., ketoconazole) or CYP2D6 (e.g., quinidine, fluoxetine, or paroxetine) can inhibit aripiprazole elimination and cause increased blood levels.

Potential for ABILIFY to Affect Other Drugs

Aripiprazole is unlikely to cause clinically important pharmacokinetic interactions with drugs metabolized by cytochrome P450 enzymes. In *in vivo* studies, 10- to 30-mg/day doses of aripiprazole had no significant effect on metabolism by CYP2D6 (dextromethorphan), CYP2C9 (warfarin), CYP2C19 (omeprazole, warfarin), and CYP3A4 (dextromethorphan) substrates. Additionally, aripiprazole and dehydro-aripiprazole did not show potential for altering CYP1A2-mediated metabolism *in vitro* (see **PRECAUTIONS: Drug-Drug Interactions**).

Aripiprazole had no clinically important interactions with the following drugs:

Famotidine: Coadministration of aripiprazole (given in a single dose of 15 mg) with a 40-mg single dose of the H_2 antagonist famotidine, a potent gastric acid blocker, decreased the solubility of aripiprazole and, hence, its rate of absorption, reducing by 37% and 21% the C_{max} of aripiprazole and dehydro-aripiprazole, respectively, and by 13% and 15%, respectively, the extent of absorption (AUC). No dosage adjustment of aripiprazole is required when administered concomitantly with famotidine.

Valproate: When valproate (500-1500 mg/day) and aripiprazole (30 mg/day) were coadministered at steady state, the C_{max} and AUC of aripiprazole were decreased by 25%. No dosage adjustment of aripiprazole is required when administered concomitantly with valproate.

Lithium: A pharmacokinetic interaction of aripiprazole with lithium is unlikely because lithium is not bound to plasma proteins, is not metabolized, and is almost entirely excreted unchanged in urine. Coadministration of therapeutic doses of lithium (1200-1800 mg/day) for 21 days with aripiprazole (30 mg/day) did not result in clinically significant changes in the pharmacokinetics of aripiprazole or its active metabolite, dehydro-aripiprazole (C_{max} and AUC increased by less than 20%). No dosage adjustment of aripiprazole is required when administered concomitantly with lithium.

Dextromethorphan: Aripiprazole at doses of 10 to 30 mg per day for 14 days had no effect on dextromethorphan's O-dealkylation to its major metabolite, dextrorphan, a pathway known to be dependent on CYP2D6 activity. Aripiprazole also had no effect on dextromethorphan's N-demethylation to its metabolite 3-methyoxymorphan, a pathway known to be dependent on CYP3A4 activity. No dosage adjustment of dextromethorphan is required when administered concomitantly with aripiprazole.

Warfarin: Aripiprazole 10 mg per day for 14 days had no effect on the pharmacokinetics of R- and S-warfarin or on the pharmacodynamic end point of International Normalized Ratio, indicating the lack of a clinically relevant effect of aripiprazole on CYP2C9 and CYP2C19 metabolism or the binding of highly protein-bound warfarin. No dosage adjustment of warfarin is required when administered concomitantly with aripiprazole.

Omeprazole: Aripiprazole 10 mg per day for 15 days had no effect on the pharmacokinetics of a single 20-mg dose of omeprazole, a CYP2C19 substrate, in healthy subjects. No dosage adjustment of omeprazole is required when administered concomitantly with aripiprazole.

Clinical Studies

The efficacy of ABILIFY (aripiprazole) in the treatment of schizophrenia was evaluated in four short-term (4- and 6-week), placebo-controlled trials of acutely relapsed inpatients who predominantly met DSM-III/IV criteria for schizophrenia. Three of the four trials were able to distinguish aripiprazole from placebo, but one study, the smallest, did not. Three of these studies also included an active control group consisting of either risperidone (one trial) or haloperidol (two trials), but they were not designed to allow for a comparison of ABILIFY and the active comparators.

In the three positive trials for ABILIFY, four primary measures were used for assessing psychiatric signs and symptoms. The Positive and Negative Syndrome Scale (PANSS) is a multi-item inventory of general psychopathology used to evaluate the effects of drug treatment in schizophrenia. The PANSS positive subscale is a subset of items in the PANSS that rates seven positive symptoms of schizophrenia (delusions, conceptual disorganization, hallucinatory behavior, excitement, grandiosity, suspiciousness/persecution, and hostility). The PANSS negative subscale is a subset of items in the PANSS that rates seven negative symptoms of schizophrenia (blunted affect, emotional withdrawal, poor rapport, passive apathetic withdrawal, difficulty in abstract thinking, lack of spontaneity/flow of conversation, stereotyped thinking). The Clinical Global Impression (CGI) assessment reflects the impression of a skilled observer, fully familiar with the manifestations of schizophrenia, about the overall clinical state of the patient.

In a 4-week trial (n=414) comparing two fixed doses of ABILIFY (15 or 30 mg/day) and haloperidol (10 mg/day) to placebo, both doses of ABILIFY were superior to placebo in the PANSS total score, PANSS positive subscale, and CGI-severity score. In addition, the 15-mg dose was superior to placebo in the PANSS negative subscale.

In a 4-week trial (n=404) comparing two fixed doses of ABILIFY (20 or 30 mg/day) and risperidone (6 mg/day) to placebo, both doses of ABILIFY were superior to placebo in the PANSS total score, PANSS positive subscale, PANSS negative subscale, and CGI-severity score.

In a 6-week trial (n=420) comparing three fixed doses of ABILIFY (10, 15, or 20 mg/day) to placebo, all three doses of ABILIFY were superior to placebo in the PANSS total score, PANSS positive subscale, and the PANSS negative subscale.

In a fourth study, a 4-week trial (n=103) comparing ABILIFY in a range of 5 to 30 mg/day or haloperidol 5 to 20 mg/day to placebo, haloperidol was superior to placebo, in the Brief Psychiatric Rating Scale (BPRS), a multi-item inventory of general psychopathology traditionally used to evaluate the effects of drug treatment in psychosis, and in a responder analysis based on the CGI-severity score, the primary outcomes for that trial. ABILIFY was only significantly different compared to placebo in a responder analysis based on the CGI-severity score.

Thus, the efficacy of 15-mg, 20-mg, and 30-mg daily doses was established in two studies for each dose, whereas the efficacy of the 10-mg dose was established in one study. There was no evidence in any study that the higher dose groups offered any advantage over the lowest dose group.

An examination of population subgroups did not reveal any clear evidence of differential responsiveness on the basis of age, gender, or race.

A longer-term trial enrolled 310 inpatients or outpatients meeting DSM-IV criteria for schizophrenia who were, by history, symptomatically stable on other antipsychotic medications for periods of 3 months or longer. These patients were discontinued from their antipsychotic medications and randomized to ABILIFY 15 mg or placebo for up to 26 weeks of observation for relapse. Relapse during the double-blind phase was defined as CGI-Improvement score of ≥5 (minimally worse), scores ≥5 (moderately severe) on the hostility or uncooperativeness items of the PANSS, or ≥20% increase in the PANSS total score. Patients receiving ABILIFY 15 mg experienced a significantly longer time to relapse over the subsequent 26 weeks compared to those receiving placebo.

INDICATIONS AND USAGE

ABILIFY is indicated for the treatment of schizophrenia. The efficacy of ABILIFY in the treatment of schizophrenia was established in short-term (4- and 6-week) controlled trials of schizophrenic inpatients (see **CLINICAL PHARMACOLOGY: Clinical Studies**).

The efficacy of ABILIFY in maintaining stability in patients with schizophrenia who had been symptomatically stable on other antipsychotic medications for periods of 3 months or longer, were discontinued from those other medications, and were then administered ABILIFY 15 mg/day and observed for relapse during a period of up to 26 weeks was demonstrated in a placebo-controlled trial (see **CLINICAL PHARMACOLOGY: Clinical Studies**). The physician who elects to use ABILIFY for extended periods should periodically re-evaluate the long-term usefulness of the drug for the individual patient (see **DOSAGE AND ADMINISTRATION**).

CONTRAINDICATIONS

ABILIFY is contraindicated in patients with a known hypersensitivity to the product.

WARNINGS

Neuroleptic Malignant Syndrome (NMS)

A potentially fatal symptom complex sometimes referred to as Neuroleptic Malignant Syndrome (NMS) has been reported in association with administration of antipsychotic drugs, including aripiprazole. Two possible cases of NMS occurred during aripiprazole treatment in the premarketing worldwide clinical database. Clinical manifestations of NMS are hyperpyrexia, muscle rigidity, altered mental status, and evidence of autonomic instability (irregular pulse or blood pressure, tachycardia, diaphoresis, and cardiac dysrhythmia). Additional signs may include elevated creatine phosphokinase, myoglobinuria (rhabdomyolysis), and acute renal failure.

The diagnostic evaluation of patients with this syndrome is complicated. In arriving at a diagnosis, it is important to exclude cases where the clinical presentation includes both serious medical illness (e.g., pneumonia, systemic infection, etc) and untreated or inadequately treated extrapyramidal signs and symptoms (EPS). Other important considerations in the differential diagnosis include central anticholinergic toxicity, heat stroke, drug fever, and primary central nervous system pathology.

The management of NMS should include: 1) immediate discontinuation of antipsychotic drugs and other drugs not essential to concurrent therapy; 2) intensive symptomatic treatment and medical monitoring; and 3) treatment of any concomitant serious medical problems for which specific treatments are available. There is no general agreement about specific pharmacological treatment regimens for uncomplicated NMS.

If a patient requires antipsychotic drug treatment after recovery from NMS, the potential reintroduction of drug therapy should be carefully considered. The patient should be carefully monitored, since recurrences of NMS have been reported.

Tardive Dyskinesia

A syndrome of potentially irreversible, involuntary, dyskinetic movements may develop in patients treated with antipsychotic drugs. Although the prevalence of the syndrome appears to be highest among the elderly, especially elderly women, it is impossible to rely upon prevalence estimates to predict, at the inception of antipsychotic treatment, which patients are likely to develop the syndrome. Whether antipsychotic drug products differ in their potential to cause tardive dyskinesia is unknown.

The risk of developing tardive dyskinesia and the likelihood that it will become irreversible are believed to increase as the duration of treatment and the total cumulative dose of antipsychotic drugs administered to the patient increase. However, the syndrome can develop, although much less commonly, after relatively brief treatment periods at low doses.

There is no known treatment for established cases of tardive dyskinesia, although the syndrome may remit, partially or completely, if antipsychotic treatment is withdrawn. Antipsychotic treatment, itself, however, may suppress (or partially suppress) the signs and symptoms of the syndrome and, thereby, may possibly mask the underlying process. The effect that symptomatic suppression has upon the long-term course of the syndrome is unknown.

Given these considerations, ABILIFY (aripiprazole) should be prescribed in a manner that is most likely to minimize the occurrence of tardive dyskinesia. Chronic antipsychotic treatment should generally be reserved for patients who suffer from a chronic illness that (1) is known to respond to antipsychotic drugs, and (2) for whom alternative, equally effective, but potentially less harmful treatments are not available or appropriate. In patients who do require chronic treatment, the smallest dose and the shortest duration of treatment producing a satisfactory clinical response should be sought. The need for continued treatment should be reassessed periodically.

If signs and symptoms of tardive dyskinesia appear in a patient on ABILIFY, drug discontinuation should be considered. However, some patients may require treatment with ABILIFY despite the presence of the syndrome.

Hyperglycemia and Diabetes Mellitus

Hyperglycemia, in some cases extreme and associated with ketoacidosis or hyperosmolar coma or death, has been reported in patients treated with atypical antipsychotics. There have been few reports of hyperglycemia in patients treated with ABILIFY. Although fewer patients have been treated with ABILIFY, it is not known if this more limited experience is the sole reason for the paucity of such reports. Assessment of the relationship between atypical antipsychotic use and glucose abnormalities is complicated by the possibility of an increased background risk of diabetes mellitus in patients with schizophrenia and the increasing incidence of diabetes mellitus in the general population. Given these confounders, the relationship between atypical antipsychotic use and hyperglycemia-related adverse events is not completely understood. However, epidemiological studies which did not include ABILIFY suggest an increased risk of treatment-emergent hyperglycemia-related adverse events in patients treated with the atypical antipsychotics included in these studies. Because ABILIFY was not marketed at the time these studies were performed, it is not known if ABILIFY is associated with this increased risk. Precise risk estimates for hyperglycemia-related adverse events in patients treated with atypical antipsychotics are not available.

Patients with an established diagnosis of diabetes mellitus who are started on atypical antipsychotics should be monitored regularly for worsening of glucose control. Patients with risk factors for diabetes mellitus (e.g., obesity, family history of diabetes) who are starting treatment with atypical antipsychotics should undergo fasting blood glucose testing at the beginning of treatment and periodically during treatment. Any patient treated with atypical antipsychotics should be monitored for symptoms of hyperglycemia including polydipsia, polyuria, polyphagia, and weakness. Patients who develop symptoms of hyperglycemia during treatment with atypical antipsychotics should undergo fasting blood glucose testing. In some cases, hyperglycemia has resolved when the atypical antipsychotic was discontinued; however, some patients required continuation of anti-diabetic treatment despite discontinuation of the suspect drug.

PRECAUTIONS

General

Orthostatic Hypotension

Aripiprazole may be associated with orthostatic hypotension, perhaps due to its α_1-adrenergic receptor antagonism. The incidence of orthostatic hypotension associated events from five short-term, placebo-controlled trials in schizophrenia (n=926) on ABILIFY included: orthostatic hypotension (placebo 1%, aripiprazole 1.9%); orthostatic lightheadedness (placebo 1%, aripiprazole 0.9%), and syncope (placebo 1%, aripiprazole 0.6%). The incidence of a significant orthostatic change in blood pressure (defined as a decrease of at least 30 mmHg in systolic blood pressure when changing from a supine to standing position) for aripiprazole was not statistically different from placebo (14% among aripiprazole-treated patients and 12% among placebo-treated patients).

Aripiprazole should be used with caution in patients with known cardiovascular disease (history of myocardial infarction or ischemic heart disease, heart failure or conduction abnormalities), cerebrovascular disease, or conditions which would predispose patients to hypotension (dehydration, hypovolemia, and treatment with antihypertensive medications).

Seizure

Seizures occurred in 0.1% (1/926) of aripiprazole-treated patients in short-term, placebo-controlled trials. As with other antipsychotic drugs, aripiprazole should be used cautiously in patients with a history of seizures or with conditions that lower the seizure threshold, e.g., Alzheimer's dementia. Conditions that lower the seizure threshold may be more prevalent in a population of 65 years or older.

Potential for Cognitive and Motor Impairment

In short-term, placebo-controlled trials, somnolence was reported in 11% of patients on ABILIFY (aripiprazole) compared to 8% of patients on placebo; somnolence led to discontinuation in 0.1% (1/926) of patients on ABILIFY (aripiprazole) in short-term, placebo-controlled trials. Despite the relatively modest increased incidence of somnolence compared to placebo, ABILIFY, like other antipsychotics, may have the potential to impair judgment, thinking, or motor skills. Patients should be cautioned about operating hazardous machinery, including automobiles, until they are reasonably certain that therapy with ABILIFY does not affect them adversely.

Body Temperature Regulation

Disruption of the body's ability to reduce core body temperature has been attributed to antipsychotic agents. Appropriate care is advised when prescribing aripiprazole for patients who will be experiencing conditions which may contribute to an elevation in core body temperature, e.g., exercising strenuously, exposure to extreme heat, receiving concomitant medication with anticholinergic activity, or being subject to dehydration.

Dysphagia

Esophageal dysmotility and aspiration have been associated with antipsychotic drug use. Aspiration pneumonia is a common cause of morbidity and mortality in elderly patients, in particular those with advanced Alzheimer's dementia. Aripiprazole and other antipsychotic drugs should be used cautiously in patients at risk for aspiration pneumonia (see **PRECAUTIONS:** *Use in Patients with Concomitant Illness*).

Suicide

The possibility of a suicide attempt is inherent in psychotic illnesses, and close supervision of high-risk patients should accompany drug therapy. Prescriptions for ABILIFY should be written for the smallest quantity of tablets consistent with good patient management in order to reduce the risk of overdose.

Use in Patients with Concomitant Illness

Safety Experience in Elderly Patients with Psychosis Associated with Alzheimer's Disease: In a flexible dose (2 to 15 mg/day), 10-week, placebo-controlled study of aripiprazole in elderly patients (mean age: 81.5 years; range: 56 to 95 years) with psychosis associated with Alzheimer's dementia, 4 of 105 patients (3.8%) who received ABILIFY died compared to no deaths among 102 patients who received placebo during or within 30 days after termination of the double-blind portion of the study. Three of the patients (age 92, 91, and 87 years) died following the discontinuation of ABILIFY in the double-blind phase of the study (causes of death were pneumonia, heart failure, and shock). The fourth patient (age 78 years) died following hip surgery while in the double-blind portion of the study. The treatment-emergent adverse events that were reported at an incidence of ≥5% and having a greater incidence than placebo in this study were accidental injury, somnolence, and bronchitis. Eight percent of the ABILIFY-treated patients reported somnolence compared to one percent of placebo patients. In a small pilot, open-label, ascending-dose cohort study (n=30) in elderly patients with dementia, ABILIFY was associated in a dose-related fashion with somnolence.

The safety and efficacy of ABILIFY in the treatment of patients with psychosis associated with dementia have not been established. If the prescriber elects to treat such patients with ABILIFY, vigilance should be exercised, particularly for the emergence of difficulty swallowing or excessive somnolence, which could predispose to accidental injury or aspiration.

Clinical experience with ABILIFY in patients with certain concomitant systemic illnesses (see **CLINICAL PHARMACOLOGY: Special Populations:** *Renal Impairment* and *Hepatic Impairment*) is limited.

ABILIFY has not been evaluated or used to any appreciable extent in patients with a recent history of myocardial infarction or unstable heart disease. Patients with these diagnoses were excluded from premarketing clinical studies.

Information for Patients

Physicians are advised to discuss the following issues with patients for whom they prescribe ABILIFY:

Interference with Cognitive and Motor Performance

Because aripiprazole may have the potential to impair judgment, thinking, or motor skills, patients should be cautioned about operating hazardous machinery, including automobiles, until they are reasonably certain that aripiprazole therapy does not affect them adversely.

Pregnancy

Patients should be advised to notify their physician if they become pregnant or intend to become pregnant during therapy with ABILIFY.

Nursing

Patients should be advised not to breast-feed an infant if they are taking ABILIFY.

Concomitant Medication

Patients should be advised to inform their physicians if they are taking, or plan to take, any prescription or over-the-counter drugs, since there is a potential for interactions.

Alcohol

Patients should be advised to avoid alcohol while taking ABILIFY.

Heat Exposure and Dehydration

Patients should be advised regarding appropriate care in avoiding overheating and dehydration.

Drug-Drug Interactions

Given the primary CNS effects of aripiprazole, caution should be used when ABILIFY is taken in combination with other centrally acting drugs and alcohol. Due to its α_1-adrenergic receptor antagonism, aripiprazole has the potential to enhance the effect of certain antihypertensive agents.

Potential for Other Drugs to Affect ABILIFY (aripiprazole)

Aripiprazole is not a substrate of CYP1A1, CYP1A2, CYP2A6, CYP2B6, CYP2C8, CYP2C9, CYP2C19, or CYP2E1 enzymes. Aripiprazole also does not undergo direct glucuronidation. This suggests that an interaction of aripiprazole with inhibitors or inducers of these enzymes, or other factors, like smoking, is unlikely.

Both CYP3A4 and CYP2D6 are responsible for aripiprazole metabolism. Agents that induce CYP3A4 (e.g., carbamazepine) could cause an increase in aripiprazole clearance and lower blood levels. Inhibitors of CYP3A4 (e.g., ketoconazole) or CYP2D6 (e.g., quinidine, fluoxetine, or paroxetine) can inhibit aripiprazole elimination and cause increased blood levels.

Ketoconazole: Coadministration of ketoconazole (200 mg/day for 14 days) with a 15-mg single dose of aripiprazole increased the AUC of aripiprazole and its active metabolite by 63% and 77%, respectively. The effect of a higher ketoconazole dose (400 mg/day) has not been studied. When concomitant administration of ketoconazole with aripiprazole occurs, aripiprazole dose should be reduced to one-half of its normal dose. Other strong inhibitors of CYP3A4 (itraconazole) would be expected to have similar effects and need similar dose reductions; weaker inhibitors (erythromycin, grapefruit juice) have not been studied. When the CYP3A4 inhibitor is withdrawn from the combination therapy, aripiprazole dose should then be increased.

Quinidine: Coadministration of a 10-mg single dose of aripiprazole with quinidine (166 mg/day for 13 days), a potent inhibitor of CYP2D6, increased the AUC of aripiprazole by 112% but decreased the AUC of its active metabolite, dehydro-aripiprazole, by 35%. Aripiprazole dose should be reduced to one-half of its normal dose when concomitant ad-

Continued on next page

Abilify—Cont.

ministration of quinidine with aripiprazole occurs. Other significant inhibitors of CYP2D6, such as fluoxetine or paroxetine, would be expected to have similar effects and, therefore, should be accompanied by similar dose reductions. When the CYP2D6 inhibitor is withdrawn from the combination therapy, aripiprazole dose should then be increased.

Carbamazepine: Coadministration of carbamazepine (200 mg BID), a potent CYP3A4 inducer, with aripiprazole (30 mg QD) resulted in an approximate 70% decrease in C_{max} and AUC values of both aripiprazole and its active metabolite, dehydro-aripiprazole. When carbamazepine is added to aripiprazole therapy, aripiprazole dose should be doubled. Additional dose increases should be based on clinical evaluation. When carbamazepine is withdrawn from the combination therapy, aripiprazole dose should then be reduced.

No clinically significant effect of famotidine, valproate, or lithium was seen on the pharmacokinetics of aripiprazole (see **CLINICAL PHARMACOLOGY: Drug-Drug Interactions**).

Potential for ABILIFY to Affect Other Drugs

Aripiprazole is unlikely to cause clinically important pharmacokinetic interactions with drugs metabolized by cytochrome P450 enzymes. In *in vivo* studies, 10- to 30-mg/day doses of aripiprazole had no significant effect on metabolism by CYP2D6 (dextromethorphan), CYP2C9 (warfarin), CYP2C19 (omeprazole, warfarin), and CYP3A4 (dextromethorphan) substrates. Additionally, aripiprazole and dehydro-aripiprazole did not show potential for altering CYP1A2-mediated metabolism *in vitro* (see **CLINICAL PHARMACOLOGY: Drug-Drug Interactions**).

Alcohol: There was no significant difference between aripiprazole coadministered with ethanol and placebo coadministered with ethanol on performance of gross motor skills or stimulus response in healthy subjects. As with most psychoactive medications, patients should be advised to avoid alcohol while taking ABILIFY.

Carcinogenesis, Mutagenesis, Impairment of Fertility

Carcinogenesis

Lifetime carcinogenicity studies were conducted in ICR mice and in Sprague-Dawley (SD) and F344 rats. Aripiprazole was administered for 2 years in the diet at doses of 1, 3, 10, and 30 mg/kg/day to ICR mice and 1, 3, and 10 mg/kg/day to F344 rats (0.2 to 5 and 0.3 to 3 times the maximum recommended human dose [MRHD] based on mg/m^2, respectively). In addition, SD rats were dosed orally for 2 years at 10, 20, 40, and 60 mg/kg/day (3 to 19 times the MRHD based on mg/m^2). Aripiprazole did not induce tumors in male mice or rats. In female mice, the incidences of pituitary gland adenomas and mammary gland adenocarcinomas and adenoacanthomas were increased at dietary doses of 3 to 30 mg/kg/day (0.1 to 0.9 times human exposure at MRHD based on AUC and 0.5 to 5 times the MRHD based on mg/m^2). In female rats, the incidence of mammary gland fibroadenomas was increased at a dietary dose of 10 mg/kg/day (0.1 times human exposure at MRHD based on AUC and 3 times the MRHD based on mg/m^2); and the incidences of adrenocortical carcinomas and combined adrenocortical adenomas/carcinomas were increased at an oral dose of 60 mg/kg/day (14 times human exposure at MRHD based on AUC and 19 times the MRHD based on mg/m^2).

Proliferative changes in the pituitary and mammary gland of rodents have been observed following chronic administration of other antipsychotic agents and are considered prolactin-mediated. Serum prolactin was not measured in the aripiprazole carcinogenicity studies. However, increases in serum prolactin levels were observed in female mice in a 13-week dietary study at the doses associated with mammary gland and pituitary tumors. Serum prolactin was not increased in female rats in 4- and 13-week dietary studies at the dose associated with mammary gland tumors. The relevance for human risk of the findings of prolactin-mediated endocrine tumors in rodents is unknown.

Mutagenesis

The mutagenic potential of aripiprazole was tested in the *in vitro* bacterial reverse-mutation assay, the *in vitro* bacterial DNA repair assay, the *in vitro* forward gene mutation assay in mouse lymphoma cells, the *in vitro* chromosomal aberration assay in Chinese hamster lung (CHL) cells, the *in vivo* micronucleus assay in mice, and the unscheduled DNA synthesis assay in rats. Aripiprazole and a metabolite (2,3-DCPP) were clastogenic in the *in vitro* chromosomal aberration assay in CHL cells with and without metabolic activation. The metabolite, 2,3-DCPP, produced increases in numerical aberrations in the *in vitro* assay in CHL cells in the absence of metabolic activation. A positive response was obtained in the *in vivo* micronucleus assay in mice, however, the response was shown to be due to a mechanism not considered relevant to humans.

Impairment of Fertility

Female rats were treated with oral doses of 2, 6, and 20 mg/kg/day (0.6, 2, and 6 times the maximum recommended human dose [MRHD] on a mg/m^2 basis) of aripiprazole from 2 weeks prior to mating through day 7 of gestation. Estrus cycle irregularities and increased corpora lutea were seen at all doses, but no impairment of fertility was seen. Increased pre-implantation loss was seen at 6 and 20 mg/kg, and decreased fetal weight was seen at 20 mg/kg.

Male rats were treated with oral doses of 20, 40, and 60 mg/kg/day (6, 13, and 19 times the MRHD on a mg/m^2 basis) of aripiprazole from 9 weeks prior to mating through mating. Disturbances in spermatogenesis were seen at 60 mg/kg, and prostate atrophy was seen at 40 and 60 mg/kg, but no impairment of fertility was seen.

Pregnancy

Pregnancy Category C

In animal studies, aripiprazole demonstrated developmental toxicity, including possible teratogenic effects in rats and rabbits.

Pregnant rats were treated with oral doses of 3, 10, and 30 mg/kg/day (1, 3, and 10 times the maximum recommended human dose [MRHD] on a mg/m^2 basis) of aripiprazole during the period of organogenesis. Gestation was slightly prolonged at 30 mg/kg. Treatment caused a slight delay in fetal development, as evidenced by decreased fetal weight (30 mg/kg), undescended testes (30 mg/kg), and delayed skeletal ossification (10 and 30 mg/kg). There were no adverse effects on embryofetal or pup survival. Delivered offspring had decreased bodyweights (10 and 30 mg/kg), and increased incidences of hepatodiaphragmatic nodules and diaphragmatic hernia at 30 mg/kg (the other dose groups were not examined for these findings). (A low incidence of diaphragmatic hernia was also seen in the fetuses exposed to 30 mg/kg.) Postnatally, delayed vaginal opening was seen at 10 and 30 mg/kg and impaired reproductive performance (decreased fertility rate, corpora lutea, implants, and live fetuses, and increased post-implantation loss, likely mediated through effects on female offspring) was seen at 30 mg/kg. Some maternal toxicity was seen at 30 mg/kg, however, there was no evidence to suggest that these developmental effects were secondary to maternal toxicity.

Pregnant rabbits were treated with oral doses of 10, 30, and 100 mg/kg/day (2, 3, and 11 times human exposure at MRHD based on AUC and 6, 19, and 65 times the MRHD based on mg/m^2) of aripiprazole during the period of organogenesis. Decreased maternal food consumption and increased abortions were seen at 100 mg/kg. Treatment caused increased fetal mortality (100 mg/kg), decreased fetal weight (30 and 100 mg/kg), increased incidence of skeletal abnormality (fused sternebrae at 30 and 100 mg/kg) and minor skeletal variations (100 mg/kg).

In a study in which rats were treated with oral doses of 3, 10, and 30 mg/kg/day (1, 3, and 10 times the MRHD on a mg/m^2 basis) of aripiprazole perinatally and postnatally (from day 17 of gestation through day 21 postpartum), slight maternal toxicity and slightly prolonged gestation were seen at 30 mg/kg. An increase in stillbirths, and decreases in pup weight (persisting into adulthood) and survival, were seen at this dose.

There are no adequate and well-controlled studies in pregnant women. It is not known whether aripiprazole can cause fetal harm when administered to a pregnant woman or can affect reproductive capacity. Aripiprazole should be used during pregnancy only if the potential benefit outweighs the potential risk to the fetus.

Labor and Delivery

The effect of aripiprazole on labor and delivery in humans is unknown.

Nursing Mothers

Aripiprazole was excreted in milk of rats during lactation. It is not known whether aripiprazole or its metabolites are excreted in human milk. It is recommended that women receiving aripiprazole should not breast-feed.

Pediatric Use

Safety and effectiveness in pediatric and adolescent patients have not been established.

Geriatric Use

Of the 5592 patients treated with aripiprazole in premarketing clinical trials, 659 (12%) were ≥65 years old and 525 (9%) were ≥75 years old. The majority (91%) of the 659 patients were diagnosed with dementia of the Alzheimer's type.

Placebo-controlled studies of aripiprazole in schizophrenia did not include sufficient numbers of subjects aged 65 and over to determine whether they respond differently from younger subjects. There was no effect of age on the pharmacokinetics of a single 15-mg dose of aripiprazole. Aripiprazole clearance was decreased by 20% in elderly subjects (≥65 years) compared to younger adult subjects (18 to 64 years), but there was no detectable effect of age in the population pharmacokinetic analysis in schizophrenia patients.

Studies of elderly patients with psychosis associated with Alzheimer's disease, have suggested that there may be a different tolerability profile in this population compared to younger patients with schizophrenia (see **PRECAUTIONS:** *Use in Patients with Concomitant Illness*). The safety and efficacy of ABILIFY (aripiprazole) in the treatment of patients with psychosis associated with Alzheimer's disease has not been established. If the prescriber elects to treat such patients with ABILIFY, vigilance should be exercised.

ADVERSE REACTIONS

Aripiprazole has been evaluated for safety in 5592 patients who participated in multiple-dose, premarketing trials in schizophrenia, bipolar mania, and dementia of the Alzheimer's type, and who had approximately 3639 patient-years of exposure. A total of 1887 aripiprazole-treated patients were treated for at least 180 days and 1251 aripiprazole-treated patients had at least 1 year of exposure.

The conditions and duration of treatment with aripiprazole included (in overlapping categories) double-blind, comparative and noncomparative open-label studies, inpatient and outpatient studies, fixed- and flexible-dose studies, and short- and longer-term exposure.

Adverse events during exposure were obtained by collecting volunteered adverse events, as well as results of physical examinations, vital signs, weights, laboratory analyses, and ECG. Adverse experiences were recorded by clinical investigators using terminology of their own choosing. In the tables and tabulations that follow, modified COSTART dictionary terminology has been used initially to classify reported adverse events into a smaller number of standardized event categories, in order to provide a meaningful estimate of the proportion of individuals experiencing adverse events.

The stated frequencies of adverse events represent the proportion of individuals who experienced at least once, a treatment-emergent adverse event of the type listed. An event was considered treatment emergent if it occurred for the first time or worsened while receiving therapy following baseline evaluation. There was no attempt to use investigator causality assessments; ie, all reported events are included.

The prescriber should be aware that the figures in the tables and tabulations cannot be used to predict the incidence of side effects in the course of usual medical practice where patient characteristics and other factors differ from those that prevailed in the clinical trials. Similarly, the cited frequencies cannot be compared with figures obtained from other clinical investigations involving different treatment, uses, and investigators. The cited figures, however, do provide the prescribing physician with some basis for estimating the relative contribution of drug and nondrug factors to the adverse event incidence in the population studied.

Adverse Findings Observed in Short-Term, Placebo-Controlled Trials of Patients with Schizophrenia

The following findings are based on a pool of five placebo-controlled trials (four 4-week and one 6-week) in which aripiprazole was administered in doses ranging from 2 to 30 mg/day.

Adverse Events Associated with Discontinuation of Treatment in Short-Term, Placebo-Controlled Trials

Overall, there was no difference in the incidence of discontinuation due to adverse events between aripiprazole-treated (7%) and placebo-treated (9%) patients. The types of adverse events that led to discontinuation were similar between the aripiprazole and placebo-treated patients.

Adverse Events Occurring at an Incidence of 2% or More Among Aripiprazole-Treated Patients and Greater than Placebo in Short-Term Placebo-Controlled Trials

Table 1 enumerates the incidence, rounded to the nearest percent, of treatment-emergent adverse events that occurred during acute therapy (up to 6 weeks), including only those events that occurred in 2% or more of patients treated with aripiprazole (doses ≥2 mg/day) and for which the incidence in patients treated with aripiprazole was greater than the incidence in patients treated with placebo.

Table 1: Treatment-Emergent Adverse Events in Short-Term, Placebo-Controlled Trials

Body System / Adverse Event	Percentage of Patients Reporting Event[a] Aripiprazole (n=926)	Placebo (n=413)
Body as a Whole		
Headache	32	25
Asthenia	7	5
Fever	2	1
Digestive System		
Nausea	14	10
Vomiting	12	7
Constipation	10	8
Nervous System		
Anxiety	25	24
Insomnia	24	19
Lightheadedness	11	7
Somnolence	11	8
Akathisia	10	7
Tremor	3	2
Respiratory System		
Rhinitis	4	3
Coughing	3	2
Skin and Appendages		
Rash	6	5
Special Senses		
Blurred vision	3	1

[a] Events reported by at least 2% of patients treated with aripiprazole, except the following events, which had an incidence equal to or less than placebo: abdominal pain, accidental injury, back pain, dental pain, dyspepsia, diarrhea, dry mouth, myalgia, agitation, psychosis, extrapyramidal syndrome, hypertonia, pharyngitis, upper respiratory tract infection, dysmenorrhea, vaginitis.

An examination of population subgroups did not reveal any clear evidence of differential adverse event incidence on the basis of age, gender, or race.

Dose-Related Adverse Events

Dose response relationships for the incidence of treatment-emergent adverse events were evaluated from four trials comparing various fixed doses (2, 10, 15, 20, and 30 mg/day) of aripiprazole to placebo. This analysis, stratified by study, indicated that the only adverse event to have a possible dose response relationship, and then most prominent only with 30 mg, was somnolence (placebo, 7.7%; 15 mg, 8.7%; 20 mg, 7.5%; 30 mg, 15.3%).

Extrapyramidal Symptoms

In the short-term, placebo-controlled trials, the incidence of reported EPS for aripiprazole-treated patients was 6% vs. 6% for placebo. Objectively collected data from those trials on the Simpson Angus Rating Scale (for EPS), the Barnes Akathisia Scale (for akathisia), and the Assessments of Involuntary Movement Scales (for dyskinesias) also did not show a difference between aripiprazole and placebo, with the exception of the Barnes Akathisia Scale (aripiprazole, 0.08; placebo, -0.05).

Similarly, in a long-term (26-week), placebo-controlled trial, objectively collected data on the Simpson Angus Rating Scale (for EPS), the Barnes Akathisia Scale (for akathisia), and the Assessments of Involuntary Movement Scales (for dyskinesias) did not show a difference between aripiprazole and placebo,

Laboratory Test Abnormalities

A between group comparison for 4- to 6-week placebo-controlled trials revealed no medically important differences between the aripiprazole and placebo groups in the proportions of patients experiencing potentially clinically significant changes in routine serum chemistry, hematology, or urinalysis parameters. Similarly, there were no aripiprazole/placebo differences in the incidence of discontinuations for changes in serum chemistry, hematology, or urinalysis.

In a long-term (26-week), placebo-controlled trial there were no medically important differences between the aripiprazole and placebo patients in the mean change from baseline in prolactin, fasting glucose, triglyceride, HDL, LDL, and total cholesterol measurements.

Weight Gain

In short-term trials, there was a slight difference in mean weight gain between aripiprazole and placebo patients (+0.7 kg vs. -0.05 kg, respectively), and also a difference in the proportion of patients meeting a weight gain criterion of ≥7% of body weight [aripiprazole (8%) compared to placebo (3%)].

Table 2 provides the weight change results from a long-term (26-week), placebo-controlled study of aripiprazole, both mean change from baseline and proportions of patients meeting a weight gain criterion of ≥7% of body weight relative to baseline, categorized by BMI at baseline:

[See table 2 above]

Table Table 3 provides the weight change results from a long-term (52-week), study of aripiprazole, both mean change from baseline and proportions of patients meeting a weight gain criterion of ≥7% of body weight relative to baseline, categorized by BMI at baseline:

Table 2: Weight Change Results Categorized by BMI at Baseline: Placebo-Controlled Study in Schizophrenia, Safety Sample

	BMI <23		BMI 23-27		BMI >27	
	Placebo	Aripiprazole	Placebo	Aripiprazole	Placebo	Aripiprazole
Mean change from baseline (kg)	–0.5	–0.5	–0.6	–1.3	–1.5	–2.1
% with ≥7% increase BW	3.7%	6.8%	4.2%	5.1%	4.1%	5.7%

Table 3: Weight Change Results Categorized by BMI at Baseline

	BMI <23	BMI 23-27	BMI >27
Mean change from baseline (kg)	2.6	1.4	–1.2
% with ≥7% increase BW	30%	19%	8%

ECG Changes

Between group comparisons for pooled, placebo-controlled-trials revealed no significant differences between aripiprazole and placebo in the proportion of patients experiencing potentially important changes in ECG parameters; in fact, within the dose range of 10 to 30 mg/day, aripiprazole tended to slightly shorten the QT_c interval. Aripiprazole was associated with a median increase in heart rate of 4 beats per minute compared to a 1 beat per minute increase among placebo patients.

Additional Findings Observed in Clinical Trials

Adverse Events in a Long-Term, Double-Blind, Placebo-Controlled Trial

The adverse events reported in a 26-week, double-blind trial comparing ABILIFY (aripiprazole) and placebo were generally consistent with those reported in the short-term, placebo-controlled trials, except for a higher incidence of tremor [9% (13/153) for ABILIFY vs. 1% (2/153) for placebo]. In this study, the majority of the cases of tremor were of mild intensity (9/13 mild and 4/13 moderate), occurred early in therapy (9/13 ≤49 days), and were of limited duration (9/13 ≤10 days). Tremor infrequently led to discontinuation (<1%) of ABILIFY. In addition, in a long-term (52-week), active-controlled study, the incidence of tremor for ABILIFY was 4% (34/859).

Other Adverse Events Observed During the Premarketing Evaluation of Aripiprazole

Following is a list of modified COSTART terms that reflect treatment-emergent adverse events as defined in the introduction to the **ADVERSE REACTIONS** section reported by patients treated with aripiprazole at multiple doses ≥2 mg/day during any phase of a trial within the database of 5592 patients. All reported events are included except those already listed in Table 1, or other parts of the **ADVERSE REACTIONS** section, those considered in the **WARNINGS** or **PRECAUTIONS**, those event terms which were so general as to be uninformative, events reported with an incidence of <0.05% and which did not have a substantial probability of being acutely life-threatening, events that are otherwise common as background events, and events considered unlikely to be drug related. It is important to emphasize that, although the events reported occurred during treatment with aripiprazole, they were not necessarily caused by it.

Events are further categorized by body system and listed in order of decreasing frequency according to the following definitions: frequent adverse events are those occurring in at least 1/100 patients (only those not already listed in the tabulated results from placebo-controlled trials appear in this listing); infrequent adverse events are those occurring in 1/100 to 1/1000 patients; rare events are those occurring in fewer than 1/1000 patients.

Body as a Whole: *Frequent* – flu syndrome, peripheral edema, chest pain, neck pain, neck rigidy; *Infrequent* – pelvic pain, suicide attempt, face edema, malaise, photosensitivity, arm rigidity, jaw pain, chills, bloating, jaw tightness, enlarged abdomen, chest tightness; *Rare* – throat pain, back tightness, head heaviness, moniliasis, throat tightness, leg rigidity, neck tightness, Mendelson's syndrome, heat stroke.

Cardiovascular System: *Frequent* – hypertension, tachycardia, hypotension, bradycardia; *Infrequent* – palpitation, hemorrhage, myocardial infarction, prolonged QT interval, cardiac arrest, atrial fibrillation, heart failure, AV block, myocardial ischemia, phlebitis, deep vein thrombosis, angina pectoris, extrasystoles; *Rare* – vasovagal reaction, cardiomegaly, atrial flutter, thrombophlebitis.

Digestive System: *Frequent* – anorexia, nausea and vomiting; *Infrequent* – increased appetite, gastroenteritis, dysphagia, flatulence, gastritis, tooth caries, gingivitis, hemorrhoids, gastroesophageal reflux, gastrointestinal hemorrhage, periodontal abscess, tongue edema, fecal incontinence, colitis, rectal hemorrhage, stomatitis, mouth ulcer, cholecystitis, fecal impaction, oral moniliasis, cholelithiasis, eructation, intestinal obstruction, peptic ulcer; *Rare* – esophagitis, gum hemorrhage, glossitis, hematemesis, melena, duodenal ulcer, cheilitis, hepatitis, hepatomegaly, pancreatitis, intestinal perforation.

Endocrine System: *Infrequent* – hypothyroidism; *Rare* – goiter, hyperthyroidism.

Hemic/Lymphatic System: *Frequent* – ecchymosis, anemia; *Infrequent* – hypochromic anemia, leukopenia, leukocytosis, lymphadenopathy, thrombocytopenia; *Rare* – eosinophilia, thrombocythemia, macrocytic anemia.

Metabolic and Nutritional Disorders: *Frequent* – weight loss, creatine phosphokinase increased; *Infrequent* – dehydration, edema, hypercholesteremia, hyperglycemia, hypokalemia, diabetes mellitus, SGPT increased, hyperlipemia, hypoglycemia, thirst, BUN increased, hyponatremia, SGOT increased, alkaline phosphatase increased, iron deficiency anemia, creatinine increased, bilirubinemia, lactic dehydrogenase increased, obesity; *Rare* – hyperkalemia, gout, hypernatremia, cyanosis, hyperuricemia, hypoglycemic reaction.

Musculoskeletal System: *Frequent* – muscle cramp; *Infrequent* – arthralgia, bone pain, myasthenia, arthritis, arthrosis, muscle weakness, spasm, bursitis; *Rare* – rhabdomyolysis, tendonitis, tenosynovitis, rheumatoid arthritis, myopathy.

Nervous System: *Frequent* – depression, nervousness, increased salivation, hostility, suicidal thought, manic reaction, abnormal gait, confusion, cogwheel rigidity; *Infrequent* – dystonia, twitch, impaired concentration, paresthesia, vasodilation, hypesthesia, extremity tremor, impotence, bradykinesia, decreased libido, panic attack, apathy, dyskinesia, hypersomnia, vertigo, dysarthria, tardive dyskinesia, ataxia, impaired memory, stupor, increased libido, amnesia, cerebrovascular accident, hyperactivity, depersonalization, hypokinesia, restless leg, myoclonus, dysphoria, neuropathy, increased reflexes, slowed thinking, hyperkinesia, hyperesthesia, hypotonia, oculogyric crisis; *Rare* – delirium, euphoria, buccoglossal syndrome, akinesia, blunted affect, decreased consciousness, incoordination, cerebral ischemia, decreased reflexes, obsessive thought, intracranial hemorrhage.

Respiratory System: *Frequent* – dyspnea, pneumonia; *Infrequent* – asthma, epistaxis, hiccup, laryngitis; *Rare* – hemoptysis, aspiration pneumonia, increased sputum, dry nasal passages, pulmonary edema, pulmonary embolism, hypoxia, respiratory failure, apnea.

Skin and Appendages: *Frequent* – dry skin, pruritis, sweating, skin ulcer; *Infrequent* – acne, vesiculobullous rash, eczema, alopecia, psoriasis, seborrhea; *Rare* – maculopapular rash, exfoliative dermatitis, urticaria.

Special Senses: *Frequent* – conjunctivitus, ear pain; *Infrequent* – dry eye, eye pain, tinnitus, otitis media, cataract, altered taste, blepharitis; *Rare* – increased lacrimation, frequent blinking, otitis externa, amblyopia, deafness, diplopia, eye hemorrhage, photophobia.

Urogenital System: *Frequent* – urinary incontinence; *Infrequent* – cystitis, urinary frequency, leukorrhea, urinary retention, hematuria, dysuria, amenorrhea, abnormal ejaculation, vaginal hemorrhage, vaginal moniliasis, kidney failure, uterus hemorrhage, menorrhagia, albuminuria, kidney calculus, nocturia, polyuria, urinary urgency; *Rare* – breast pain, cervicitis, female lactation, anorgasmy, urinary burning, glycosuria, gynecomastia, urolithiasis, priapism.

Other Events Observed During the Postmarketing Evaluation of Aripiprazole

Voluntary reports of adverse events in patients taking aripiprazole that have been received since market introduction and not listed above that may have no causal relationship with the drug include rare occurrences of allergic reaction (e.g., anaphylactic reaction, angioedema, laryngospasm, pruritis, or urticaria).

DRUG ABUSE AND DEPENDENCE

Controlled Substance

ABILIFY (aripiprazole) is not a controlled substance.

Abuse and Dependence

Aripiprazole has not been systematically studied in humans for its potential for abuse, tolerance, or physical dependence. In physical dependence studies in monkeys, withdrawal symptoms were observed upon abrupt cessation of dosing. While the clinical trials did not reveal any tendency for any drug-seeking behavior, these observations were not systematic and it is not possible to predict on the basis of this limited experience the extent to which a CNS-active drug will be misused, diverted, and/or abused once marketed. Consequently, patients should be evaluated carefully for a history of drug abuse, and such patients should be observed closely for signs of ABILIFY (aripiprazole) misuse or abuse (e.g., development of tolerance, increases in dose, drug-seeking behavior).

OVERDOSAGE

Human Experience

In clinical studies, accidental or intentional acute overdosage of aripiprazole was identified in patients with estimated doses up to 1080 mg with no fatalities. The reported signs and symptoms observed with aripiprazole overdose included nausea, vomiting, asthenia, diarrhea, and somnolence. In the patients who were evaluated in hospital settings, there were no reported observations indicating clinically significant adverse change in vital signs, laboratory assessments, or ECG.

During postmarketing experience, the reported signs and symptoms observed in adult patients who overdosed with aripiprazole alone at doses up to 450 mg included tachycardia. In addition, reports of accidental overdose with aripiprazole (up to 195 mg) in children have been received. The potentially medically serious signs and symptoms reported include extrapyramidal symptoms and transient loss of consciousness with recovery.

Management of Overdosage

No specific information is available on the treatment of overdose with aripiprazole. An electrocardiogram should be obtained in case of overdosage and, if QT_c interval prolongation is present, cardiac monitoring should be instituted. Otherwise, management of overdose should concentrate on supportive therapy, maintaining an adequate airway, oxygenation and ventilation, and management of symptoms. Close medical supervision and monitoring should continue until the patient recovers.

Charcoal: In the event of an overdose of ABILIFY (aripiprazole), an early charcoal administration may be useful in partially preventing the absorption of aripiprazole. Administration of 50 g of activated charcoal, one hour after a single 15-mg oral dose of aripiprazole, decreased the mean AUC and C_{max} of aripiprazole by 50%.

Hemodialysis: Although there is no information on the effect of hemodialysis in treating an overdose with aripiprazole, hemodialysis is unlikely to be useful in overdose management since aripiprazole is highly bound to plasma proteins.

DOSAGE AND ADMINISTRATION

Usual Dose

The recommended starting and target dose for ABILIFY is 10 or 15 mg/day administered on a once-a-day schedule without regard to meals. ABILIFY has been systematically evaluated and shown to be effective in a dose range of 10 to 30 mg/day; however, doses higher than 10 or 15 mg/day, the lowest doses in these trials, were not more effective than 10 or 15 mg/day. Dosage increases should not be made before 2 weeks, the time needed to achieve steady state.

Dosage in Special Populations

Dosage adjustments are not routinely indicated on the basis of age, gender, race, or renal or hepatic impairment status (see **CLINICAL PHARMACOLOGY: Special Populations**).

Dosage adjustment for patients taking aripiprazole concomitantly with potential CYP3A4 inhibitors: When concomitant administration of ketoconazole with aripiprazole oc-

Continued on next page

Abilify—Cont.

curs, aripiprazole dose should be reduced to one-half of the usual dose. When the CYP3A4 inhibitor is withdrawn from the combination therapy, aripiprazole dose should then be increased.

Dosage adjustment for patients taking aripiprazole concomitantly with potential CYP2D6 inhibitors: When concomitant administration of potential CYP2D6 inhibitors such as quinidine, fluoxetine, or paroxetine with aripiprazole occurs, aripiprazole dose should be reduced at least to one-half of its normal dose. When the CYP2D6 inhibitor is withdrawn from the combination therapy, aripiprazole dose should then be increased.

Dosage adjustment for patients taking potential CYP3A4 inducers: When a potential CYP3A4 inducer such as carbamazepine is added to aripiprazole therapy, the aripiprazole dose should be doubled (to 20 to 30 mg). Additional dose increases should be based on clinical evaluation. When carbamazepine is withdrawn from the combination therapy, the aripiprazole dose should be reduced to 10 to 15 mg.

Maintenance Therapy

While there is no body of evidence available to answer the question of how long a patient treated with aripiprazole should remain on it, systematic evaluation of patients with schizophrenia who had been symptomatically stable on other antipsychotic medications for periods of 3 months or longer, were discontinued from those medications, and were then administered ABILIFY 15 mg/day and observed for relapse during a period of up to 26 weeks, demonstrated a benefit of such maintenance treatment (see **CLINICAL PHARMACOLOGY: Clinical Studies**). Patients should be periodically reassessed to determine the need for maintenance treatment.

Switching from Other Antipsychotics

There are no systematically collected data to specifically address switching patients with schizophrenia from other antipsychotics to ABILIFY or concerning concomitant administration with other antipsychotics. While immediate discontinuation of the previous antipsychotic treatment may be acceptable for some patients with schizophrenia, more gradual discontinuation may be most appropriate for others. In all cases, the period of overlapping antipsychotic administration should be minimized.

ANIMAL TOXICOLOGY

Aripiprazole produced retinal degeneration in albino rats in a 26-week chronic toxicity study at a dose of 60 mg/kg and in a 2-year carcinogenicity study at doses of 40 and 60 mg/kg. The 40- and 60-mg/kg doses represent 13 and 19 times the maximum recommended human dose (MRHD) based on mg/m^2 and 7 to 14 times human exposure at MRHD based on AUC. Evaluation of the retinas of albino mice and monkeys did not reveal evidence of retinal degeneration. Additional studies to further evaluate the mechanism have not been performed. The relevance of this finding to human risk is unknown.

HOW SUPPLIED

ABILIFY® (aripiprazole) Tablets are available in the following strengths and packages.

The 5-mg ABILIFY tablets are blue, modified rectangular tablets, debossed on one side with "A-007" and "5".

Bottles of 30	NDC 59148-007-13
Blister of 100	NDC 59148-007-35

The 10-mg ABILIFY tablets are pink, modified rectangular tablets, debossed on one side with "A-008" and "10".

Bottles of 30	NDC 59148-008-13
Blister of 100	NDC 59148-008-35

The 15-mg ABILIFY tablets are yellow, round tablets, debossed on one side with "A-009" and "15".

Bottles of 30	NDC 59148-009-13
Blister of 100	NDC 59148-009-35

The 20-mg ABILIFY tablets are white, round tablets, debossed on one side with "A-010" and "20".

Bottles of 30	NDC 59148-010-13
Blister of 100	NDC 59148-010-35

The 30-mg ABILIFY tablets are pink, round tablets, debossed on one side with "A-011" and "30".

Bottles of 30	NDC 59148-011-13
Blister of 100	NDC 59148-011-35

Storage

Store at 25° C (77° F); excursions permitted to 15-30° C (59-86° F) [see USP Controlled Room Temperature].

Marketed by Otsuka America Pharmaceutical, Inc, Rockville, MD 20850 USA
and Bristol-Myers Squibb Co, Princeton, NJ 08543 USA

Manufactured and Distributed by Bristol-Myers Squibb Co, Princeton, NJ 08543 USA
U.S. Patent Nos. 4,734,416 and 5,006,528

Bristol-Myers Squibb Company **Otsuka America**
Princeton, NJ 08543 U.S.A. **Pharmaceutical, Inc.**
D6-B0001-05-04 Revised: May 2004
1152082A3 AP4114A/06-04

Shown in Product Identification Guide, page 328

PLETAL® ℞
[PLAY-tal]
(cilostazol) (sil-OS-tah-zol)
Tablets

CONTRAINDICATION

Cilostazol and several of its metabolites are inhibitors of phosphodiesterase III. Several drugs with this pharmacologic effect have caused decreased survival compared to placebo in patients with class III-IV congestive heart failure. PLETAL is contraindicated in patients with congestive heart failure of any severity.

DESCRIPTION

PLETAL (cilostazol) is a quinolinone derivative that inhibits cellular phosphodiesterase (more specific for phosphodiesterase III). The empirical formula of cilostazol is $C_{20}H_{27}N_5O_2$, and its molecular weight is 369.46. Cilostazol is 6-[4-(1-cyclohexyl-1*H*-tetrazol-5-yl)butoxy]-3,4-dihydro-2(1*H*)-quinolinone, CAS-73963-72-1.

The structural formula is:

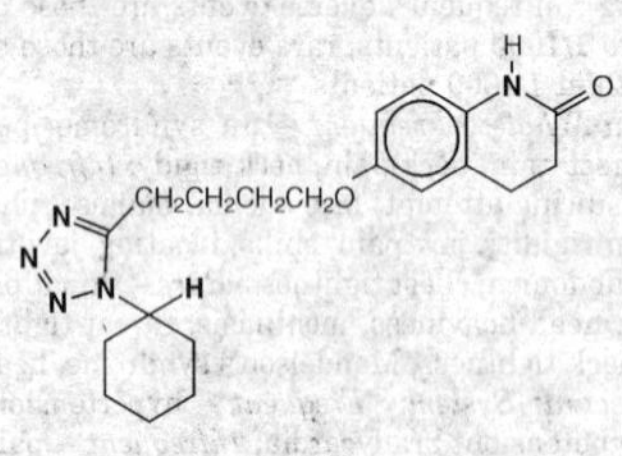

Cilostazol occurs as white to off-white crystals or as a crystalline powder that is slightly soluble in methanol and ethanol, and is practically insoluble in water, 0.1 N HCl, and 0.1 N NaOH.

PLETAL (cilostazol) tablets for oral administration are available in 50 mg triangular and 100 mg round, white debossed tablets. Each tablet, in addition to the active ingredient, contains the following inactive ingredients: carboxymethylcellulose calcium, corn starch, hydroxypropyl methylcellulose 2910, magnesium stearate, and microcrystalline cellulose.

CLINICAL PHARMACOLOGY

Mechanism of Action:

The mechanism of the effects of PLETAL on the symptoms of intermittent claudication is not fully understood. PLETAL and several of its metabolites are cyclic AMP (cAMP) phosphodiesterase III inhibitors (PDE III inhibitors), inhibiting phosphodiesterase activity and suppressing cAMP degradation with a resultant increase in cAMP in platelets and blood vessels, leading to inhibition of platelet aggregation and vasodilation, respectively.

PLETAL reversibly inhibits platelet aggregation induced by a variety of stimuli, including thrombin, ADP, collagen, arachidonic acid, epinephrine, and shear stress. Effects on circulating plasma lipids have been examined in patients taking PLETAL. After 12 weeks, as compared to placebo, PLETAL 100 mg b.i.d. produced a reduction in triglycerides of 29.3 mg/dL (15%) and an increase in HDL-cholesterol of 4.0 mg/dL ($\cong$ 10%).

Cardiovascular Effects:

Cilostazol affects both vascular beds and cardiovascular function. It produces non-homogeneous dilation of vascular beds, with greater dilation in femoral beds than in vertebral, carotid or superior mesenteric arteries. Renal arteries were not responsive to the effects of cilostazol.

In dogs or cynomolgous monkeys, cilostazol increased heart rate, myocardial contractile force, and coronary blood flow as well as ventricular automaticity, as would be expected for a PDE III inhibitor. Left ventricular contractility was increased at doses required to inhibit platelet aggregation. A-V conduction was accelerated. In humans, heart rate increased in a dose-proportional manner by a mean of 5.1 and 7.4 beats per minute in patients treated with 50 and 100 mg b.i.d., respectively. In 264 patients evaluated with Holter monitors, numerically more cilostazol-treated patients had increases in ventricular premature beats and non-sustained ventricular tachycardia events than did placebo-treated patients; the increases were not dose-related.

Pharmacokinetics:

PLETAL is absorbed after oral administration. A high fat meal increases absorption, with an approximately 90% increase in C_{max} and a 25% increase in AUC. Absolute bioavailability is not known. Cilostazol is extensively metabolized by hepatic cytochrome P-450 enzymes, mainly 3A4, and, to a lesser extent, 2C19, with metabolites largely excreted in urine. Two metabolites are active, with one metabolite appearing to account for at least 50% of the pharmacologic (PDE III inhibition) activity after administration of PLETAL. Pharmacokinetics are approximately dose proportional. Cilostazol and its active metabolites have apparent elimination half-lives of about 11-13 hours. Cilostazol and its active metabolites accumulate about 2-fold with chronic administration and reach steady state blood levels within a few days. The pharmacokinetics of cilostazol and its two major active metabolites were similar in healthy normal subjects and patients with intermittent claudication due to peripheral arterial disease (PAD).

The mean ± SEM plasma concentration-time profile at steady state after multiple dosing of PLETAL 100 mg b.i.d. is shown below:

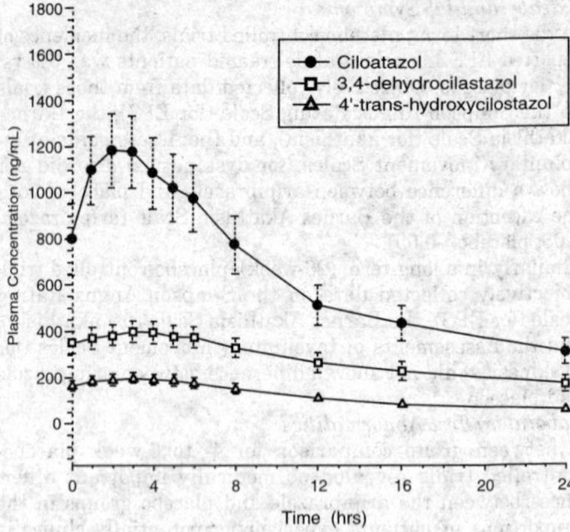

Distribution:

Plasma Protein and Erythrocyte Binding:

Cilostazol is 95-98% protein bound, predominantly to albumin. The mean percent binding for 3,4-dehydro-cilostazol is 97.4% and for 4′-trans-hydroxy-cilostazol is 66%. Mild hepatic impairment did not affect protein binding. The free fraction of cilostazol was 27% higher in subjects with renal impairment than in normal volunteers. The displacement of cilostazol from plasma proteins by erythromycin, quinidine, warfarin, and omeprazole was not clinically significant.

Metabolism and Excretion:

Cilostazol is eliminated predominately by metabolism and subsequent urinary excretion of metabolites. Based on *in vitro* studies, the primary isoenzymes involved in cilostazol's metabolism are CYP3A4 and, to a lesser extent, CYP2C19. The enzyme responsible for metabolism of 3,4-dehydro-cilostazol, the most active of the metabolites, is unknown. Following oral administration of 100 mg radiolabeled cilostazol, 56% of the total analytes in plasma was cilostazol, 15% was 3,4-dehydro-cilostazol (4-7 times as active as cilostazol), and 4% was 4′-trans-hydroxy-cilostazol (one fifth as active as cilostazol). The primary route of elimination was via the urine (74%), with the remainder excreted in feces (20%). No measurable amount of unchanged cilostazol was excreted in the urine, and less than 2% of the dose was excreted as 3,4-dehydro-cilostazol. About 30% of the dose was excreted in urine as 4′-trans-hydroxy-cilostazol. The remainder was excreted as other metabolites, none of which exceeded 5%. There was no evidence of induction of hepatic microenzymes.

Special Populations:

Age and Gender:

The total and unbound oral clearances, adjusted for body weight, of cilostazol and its metabolites were not significantly different with respect to age and/or gender across a 50-to-80-year-old age range.

Smokers:

Population pharmacokinetic analysis suggests that smoking decreased cilostazol exposure by about 20%.

Hepatic Impairment:

The pharmacokinetics of cilostazol and its metabolites were similar in subjects with mild hepatic disease as compared to healthy subjects.

Patients with moderate or severe hepatic impairment have not been studied.

Renal Impairment:

The total pharmacologic activity of cilostazol and its metabolites was similar in subjects with mild to moderate renal impairment and in normal subjects. Severe renal impairment increases metabolite levels and alters protein binding of the parent and metabolites. The expected pharmacologic activity, however, based on plasma concentrations and relative PDE III inhibiting potency of parent drug and metabolites, appeared little changed. Patients on dialysis have not been studied, but, it is unlikely that cilostazol can be removed efficiently by dialysis because of its high protein binding (95-98%).

Pharmacokinetic and Pharmacodynamic Drug-Drug Interactions:

Cilostazol could have pharmacodynamic interactions with other inhibitors of platelet function and pharmacokinetic interactions because of effects of other drugs on its metabolism by CYP3A4 or CYP2C19. A reduced dose of PLETAL should be considered when taken concomitantly with CYP3A4 or CYP2C19 inhibitors. Cilostazol does not appear to inhibit CYP3A4 (see *Pharmacokinetic and Pharmacodynamic Drug-Drug Interactions*, Lovastatin).

Aspirin:

Short-term (≤4 days) coadministration of aspirin with PLETAL increased the inhibition of ADP-induced *ex vivo* platelet aggregation by 22%-37% when compared to either aspirin or PLETAL alone. Short-term (≤4 days) coadministration of aspirin with PLETAL increased the inhibition of arachidonic acid-induced *ex vivo* platelet aggregation by 20% compared to PLETAL alone and by 48% compared to aspirin alone. However, short-term coadministration of aspirin with PLETAL had no clinically significant impact on PT, aPTT, or bleeding time compared to aspirin alone. Effects of long-term coadministration in the general population are unknown. In eight randomized, placebo-controlled, double-blind clinical trials, aspirin was coadministered with cilostazol to 201 patients. The most frequent doses and mean durations of aspirin therapy were 75-81 mg daily for 137 days (107 patients) and 325 mg daily for 54 days (85 patients). There was no apparent increase in incidence of hemorrhagic adverse effects in patients taking cilostazol and aspirin compared to patients taking placebo and equivalent doses of aspirin.

Warfarin:

The cytochrome P-450 isoenzymes involved in the metabolism of R-warfarin are CYP3A4, CYP1A2, and CYP2C19, and in the metabolism of S-warfarin, CYP2C9. Cilostazol did not inhibit either the metabolism or the pharmacologic effects (PT, aPTT, bleeding time, or platelet aggregation) of R- and S-warfarin after a single 25-mg dose of warfarin. The effect of concomitant multiple dosing of warfarin and PLETAL on the pharmacokinetics and pharmacodynamics of both drugs is unknown.

Clopidogrel:

Multiple doses of clopidogrel do not significantly increase steady state plasma concentrations of cilostazol.

Inhibitors of CYP3A4:

Strong Inhibitors of CYP3A4: A priming dose of ketoconazole 400 mg (a strong inhibitor of CYP3A4), was given one day prior to coadministration of single doses of ketoconazole 400 mg and cilostazol 100 mg. This regimen increased cilostazol C_{max} by 94% and AUC by 117%. Other strong inhibitors of CYP3A4, such as itraconazole, fluconazole, miconazole, fluvoxamine, fluoxetine, nefazodone, and sertraline, would be expected to have a similar effect (see DOSAGE AND ADMINISTRATION).

Moderate Inhibitors of CYP3A4

1. *Erythromycin and other macrolide antibiotics:* Erythromycin is a moderately strong inhibitor of CYP3A4. Coadministration of erythromycin 500 mg q 8h with a single dose of cilostazol 100 mg increased cilostazol C_{max} by 47% and AUC by 73%. Inhibition of cilostazol metabolism by erythromycin increased the AUC of 4′-trans-hydroxy-cilostazol by 141%. Other macrolide antibiotics (e.g., clarithromycin), but not all (e.g., azithromycin), would be expected to have a similar effect (see DOSAGE AND ADMINISTRATION).
2. *Diltiazem:* Diltiazem 180 mg decreased the clearance of cilostazol by ~30%. Cilostazol C_{max} increased ~30% and AUC increased ~40% (see DOSAGE AND ADMINISTRATION).
3. *Grapefruit Juice:* Grapefruit juice increased the C_{max} of cilostazol by ~50%, but had no effect on AUC.

Inhibitors of CYP2C19:

Omeprazole: Coadministration of omeprazole did not significantly affect the metabolism of cilostazol, but the systemic exposure to 3,4-dehydro-cilostazol was increased by 69%, probably the result of omeprazole's potent inhibition of CYP2C19 (see DOSAGE AND ADMINISTRATION).

Quinidine:

Concomitant administration of quinidine with a single dose of cilostazol 100 mg did not alter cilostazol pharmacokinetics.

Lovastatin:

The concomitant administration of lovastatin with cilostazol decreases cilostazol $C_{ss,max}$ and AUC_{τ} by 15%. There is also a decrease, although nonsignificant, in cilostazol metabolite concentrations. Coadministration of cilostazol with lovastatin increases lovastatin and β-hydroxi lovastatin AUC approximately 70%. This is most likely clinically insignificant.

CLINICAL EFFICACY

The ability of PLETAL to improve walking distance in patients with stable intermittent claudication was studied in eight large, randomized, placebo-controlled, double-blind trials of 12 to 24 weeks' duration using dosages of 50 mg b.i.d. (n=303), 100 mg b.i.d. (n=998), and placebo (n=973). Efficacy was determined primarily by the change in maximal walking distance from baseline (compared to change on placebo) on one of several standardized exercise treadmill tests.

Compared to patients treated with placebo, patients treated with PLETAL 50 or 100 mg b.i.d. experienced statistically significant improvements in walking distances both for the distance before the onset of claudication pain and the distance before exercise-limiting symptoms supervened (maximal walking distance). The effect of PLETAL on walking distance was seen as early as the first on-therapy observation point of two or four weeks.

The following figure depicts the percent mean improvement in maximal walking distance, at study end for each of the eight studies.

[See figure at top of next column]

Across the eight clinical trials, the range of improvement in maximal walking distance in patients treated with PLETAL 100 mg b.i.d., expressed as the percent mean change from baseline, was 28% to 100%.

The corresponding changes in the placebo group were −10% to 41%.

The Walking Impairment Questionnaire, which was administered in six of the eight clinical trials, assesses the impact of a therapeutic intervention on walking ability. In a pooled analysis of the six trials, patients treated with either PLETAL 100 mg b.i.d. or 50 mg b.i.d. reported improvements in their walking speed and walking distance as compared to placebo. Improvements in walking performance were seen in the various subpopulations evaluated, including those defined by gender, smoking status, diabetes mel-

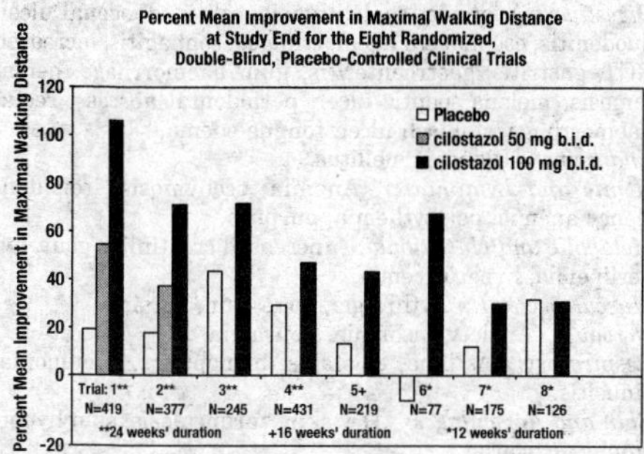

litus, duration of peripheral artery disease, age, and concomitant use of beta blockers or calcium channel blockers. PLETAL has not been studied in patients with rapidly progressing claudication or in patients with leg pain at rest, ischemic leg ulcers, or gangrene. Its long-term effects on limb preservation and hospitalization have not been evaluated. No reliable estimate of its effect on survival is available (see PRECAUTIONS).

INDICATIONS AND USAGE

PLETAL is indicated for the reduction of symptoms of intermittent claudication, as indicated by an increased walking distance.

CONTRAINDICATIONS

Cilostazol and several of its metabolites are inhibitors of phosphodiesterase III. Several drugs with this pharmacologic effect have caused decreased survival compared to placebo in patients with class III-IV congestive heart failure. PLETAL is contraindicated in patients with congestive heart failure of any severity.

PLETAL is contraindicated in patients with haemostatic disorders or active pathologic bleeding, such as bleeding peptic ulcer and intracranial bleeding. PLETAL inhibits platelet aggregation in a reversible manner.

PLETAL is contraindicated in patients with known or suspected hypersensitivity to any of its components.

PRECAUTIONS

PLETAL is contraindicated in patients with congestive heart failure. In patients without congestive heart failure, the long-term effects of PDE III inhibitors (including PLETAL) are unknown. Patients in the 3-6 month placebo-controlled trials of PLETAL were relatively stable (no recent myocardial infarction or strokes, no rest pain or other signs of rapidly progressing disease) and only 19 patients died (0.7% in the placebo group and 0.8% in the group on PLETAL). The calculated relative risk of death of 1.2 has a wide 95% confidence limit (0.5-3.1). There are no data as to longer-term risk or risk in patients with more severe underlying heart disease.

Hematologic adverse reactions: Rare cases have been reported of thrombocytopenia or leukopenia progressing to agranulocytosis when cilostazol was not immediately discontinued. The agranulocytosis, however, was reversible on discontinuation of cilostazol.

Use with Clopidogrel.

There is limited information with respect to the efficacy or safety of the concurrent use of cilostazol and clopidogrel, a platelet-aggregation inhibiting drug indicated for use in patients with peripheral arterial disease. Coadministration significantly increased AUC of dehydro-cilostazol metabolite by 24%. Although it cannot be determined whether there was an additive effect on bleeding times during concomitant administration with cilostazol and clopidgrel, caution should be advised for checking bleeding times during coadministration.

Information for Patients:

Please refer to the patient package insert.

Patients should be advised:

- to read the patient package insert for PLETAL carefully before starting therapy and to reread it each time therapy is renewed in case the information has changed.
- to take PLETAL at least one-half hour before or two hours after food.
- that the beneficial effects of PLETAL on the symptoms of intermittent claudication may not be immediate. Although the patient may experience benefit in 2 to 4 weeks after initiation of therapy, treatment for up to 12 weeks may be required before a beneficial effect is experienced.
- about the uncertainty concerning cardiovascular risk in long-term use or in patients with severe underlying heart disease, as described under PRECAUTIONS.

Hepatic Impairment:

Patients with moderate or severe hepatic impairment have not been studied in clinical trials.

Special caution should be advised when PLETAL is used in patients with severe hepatic impairment.

Renal Impairment:

Patients on dialysis have not been studied, but, it is unlikely that cilostazol can be removed efficiently by dialysis because of its high protein binding (95-98%).

Special caution should be advised when PLETAL is used in patients with severe renal impairment: creatinine clearance < 25 ml/min.

Drug Interactions:

Since PLETAL is extensively metabolized by cytochrome P-450 isoenzymes, caution should be exercised when PLETAL is coadministered with inhibitors of CYP3A4 such as ketoconazole and erythromycin or inhibitors of CYP2C19 such as omeprazole. Pharmacokinetic studies have demonstrated that omeprazole and erythromycin significantly increased the systemic exposure of cilostazol and/or its major metabolites. Population pharmacokinetic studies showed higher concentrations of cilostazol among patients concurrently treated with diltiazem, an inhibitor of CYP3A4 (see CLINICAL PHARMACOLOGY, *Pharmacokinetic and Pharmacodynamic Drug-Drug Interactions*). PLETAL does not, however, appear to cause increased blood levels of drugs metabolized by CYP3A4, as it had no effect on lovastatin, a drug with metabolism very sensitive to CYP3A4 inhibition.

Use with other antiplatelet agents: PLETAL inhibits platelet aggregation but in a reversible manner. Caution is advised in patients at risk of bleeding from surgery or pathologic processes. Platelet aggregability returns to normal within 96 hours of stopping PLETAL. Caution is advised in patients receiving both PLETAL and any other antiplatelet agent, or in patients with thrombocytopenia.

Cardiovascular Toxicity:

Repeated oral administration of cilostazol to dogs (30 or more mg/kg/day for 52 weeks, 150 or more mg/kg/day for 13 weeks, and 450 mg/kg/day for 2 weeks), produced cardiovascular lesions that included endocardial haemorrhage, hemosiderin deposition and fibrosis in the left ventricle, haemorrhage in the right atrial wall, haemorrhage and necrosis of the smooth muscle in the wall of the coronary artery, intimal thickening of the coronary artery, and coronary arteritis and periarteritis. At the lowest dose associated with cardiovascular lesions in the 52-week study, systemic exposure (AUC) to unbound cilostazol was less than that seen in humans at the maximum recommended human dose (MRHD) of 100 mg b.i.d. Similar lesions have been reported in dogs following the administration of other positive inotropic agents (including PDE III inhibitors) and/or vasodilating agents. No cardiovascular lesions were seen in rats following 5 or 13 weeks of administration of cilostazol at doses up to 1500 mg/kg/day. At this dose, systemic exposures (AUCs) to unbound cilostazol were only about 1.5 and 5 times (male and female rats, respectively) the exposure seen in humans at the MRHD. Cardiovascular lesions were also not seen in rats following 52 weeks of administration of cilostazol at doses up to 150 mg/kg/day. At this dose, systemic exposures (AUCs) to unbound cilostazol were about 0.5 and 5 times (male and female rats, respectively) the exposure in humans at the MRHD. In female rats, cilostazol AUCs were similar at 150 and 1500 mg/kg/day. Cardiovascular lesions were also not observed in monkeys after oral administration of cilostazol for 13 weeks at doses up to 1800 mg/kg/day. While this dose of cilostazol produced pharmacologic effects in monkeys, plasma cilostazol levels were less than those seen in humans given the MRHD, and those seen in dogs given doses associated with cardiovascular lesions.

Carcinogenesis, Mutagenesis, Impairment of Fertility:

Dietary administration of cilostazol to male and female rats and mice for up to 104 weeks, at doses up to 500 mg/kg/day in rats and 1000 mg/kg/day in mice, revealed no evidence of carcinogenic potential. The maximum doses administered in both rat and mouse studies were, on a systemic exposure basis, less than the human exposure at the MRHD of the drug. Cilostazol tested negative in bacterial gene mutation, bacterial DNA repair, mammalian cell gene mutation, and mouse *in vivo* bone marrow chromosomal aberration assays. It was, however, associated with a significant increase in chromosomal aberrations in the *in vitro* Chinese Hamster Ovary Cell assay.

Cilostazol did not affect fertility or mating performance of male and female rats at doses as high as 1000 mg/kg/day. At this dose, systemic exposures (AUCs) to unbound cilostazol were less than 1.5 times in males, and about 5 times in females, the exposure in humans at the MRHD.

Pregnancy:

Pregnancy Category C: In a rat developmental toxicity study, oral administration of 1000 mg cilostazol/kg/day was associated with decreased fetal weights, and increased incidences of cardiovascular, renal, and skeletal anomalies (ventricular septal, aortic arch and subclavian artery abnormalities, renal pelvic dilation, 14th rib, and retarded ossification). At this dose, systemic exposure to unbound cilostazol in nonpregnant rats was about 5 times the exposure in humans given the MRHD. Increased incidences of ventricular septal defect and retarded ossification were also noted at 150 mg/kg/day (5 times the MRHD on a systemic exposure basis). In a rabbit developmental toxicity study, an increased incidence of retardation of ossification of the sternum was seen at doses as low as 150 mg/kg/day. In nonpregnant rabbits given 150 mg/kg/day, exposure to unbound cilostazol was considerably lower than that seen in humans given the MRHD, and exposure to 3,4-dehydro-cilostazol was barely detectable.

When cilostazol was administered to rats during late pregnancy and lactation, an increased incidence of stillborn and decreased birth weights of offspring was seen at doses of 150 mg/kg/day (5 times the MRHD on a systemic exposure basis).

There are no adequate and well-controlled studies in pregnant women.

Nursing Mothers:

Transfer of cilostazol into milk has been reported in experimental animals (rats). Because of the potential risk to nursing infants, a decision should be made to discontinue nursing or to discontinue PLETAL.

Continued on next page

Pletal—Cont.

Pediatric Use:
The safety and effectiveness of PLETAL in pediatric patients have not been established.
Geriatric Use:
Of the total number of subjects (n = 2274) in clinical studies of PLETAL, 56 percent were 65-years-old and over, while 16 percent were 75-years-old and over. No overall differences in safety or effectiveness were observed between these subjects and younger subjects, and other reported clinical experience has not identified differences in responses between the elderly and younger patients, but greater sensitivity of some older individuals cannot be ruled out. Pharmacokinetic studies have not disclosed any age-related effects on the absorption, distribution, metabolism, and elimination of cilostazol and its metabolites.

ADVERSE REACTIONS

Adverse events were assessed in eight placebo-controlled clinical trials involving 2274 patients exposed to either 50 or 100 mg b.i.d. PLETAL (n=1301) or placebo (n=973), with a median treatment duration of 127 days for patients on PLETAL and 134 days for patients on placebo.
The only adverse event resulting in discontinuation of therapy in ≥ 3% of patients treated with PLETAL 50 or 100 mg b.i.d. was headache, which occurred with an incidence of 1.3%, 3.5%, and 0.3% in patients treated with PLETAL 50 mg b.i.d., 100 mg b.i.d, or placebo, respectively. Other frequent causes of discontinuation included palpitation and diarrhea, both 1.1% for cilostazol (all doses) versus 0.1% for placebo.
The most commonly reported adverse events, occurring in ≥ 2% of patients treated with PLETAL 50 or 100 mg b.i.d., are shown in the table (to the right).
Other events seen with an incidence of ≥ 2%, but occurring in the placebo group at least as frequently as in the 100 mg b.i.d. group were: asthenia, hypertension, vomiting, leg cramps, hypesthesia, paresthesia, dyspnea, rash, hematuria, urinary tract infection, flu syndrome, angina pectoris, arthritis, and bronchitis.
[See table at bottom of page 2445]
Less frequent adverse events (<2%) that were experienced by patients exposed to PLETAL 50 mg b.i.d. or 100 mg b.i.d. in the eight controlled clinical trials and that occurred at a frequency in the 100 mg b.i.d. group greater than in the placebo group, regardless of suspected drug relationship, are listed below.
Body as a whole: Chills, face edema, fever, generalized edema, malaise, neck rigidity, pelvic pain, retroperitoneal haemorrhage.
Cardiovascular: Atrial fibrillation, atrial flutter, cerebral infarct, cerebral ischemia, congestive heart failure, heart arrest, haemorrhage, hypotension, myocardial infarction, myocardial ischemia, nodal arrhythmia, postural hypotension, supraventricular tachycardia, syncope, varicose vein, vasodilation, ventricular extrasystoles, ventricular tachycardia.
Digestive: Anorexia, cholelithiasis, colitis, duodenal ulcer, duodenitis, esophageal haemorrhage, esophagitis, increased GGT, gastritis, gastroenteritis, gum haemorrhage, hematemesis, melena, peptic ulcer, periodontal abscess, rectal haemorrhage, stomach ulcer, tongue edema.
Endocrine: Diabetes mellitus.
Hemic and Lymphatic: Anemia, ecchymosis, iron deficiency anemia, polycythemia, purpura.
Metabolic and Nutritional: Increased creatinine, gout, hyperlipemia, hyperuricemia.
Musculoskeletal: Arthralgia, bone pain, bursitis.
Nervous: Anxiety, insomnia, neuralgia.
Respiratory: Asthma, epistaxis, hemoptysis, pneumonia, sinusitis.
Skin and Appendages: Dry skin, furunculosis, skin hypertrophy, urticaria.
Special Senses: Amblyopia, blindness, conjunctivitis, diplopia, ear pain, eye haemorrhage, retinal haemorrhage, tinnitus.
Urogenital: Albuminuria, cystitis, urinary frequency, vaginal haemorrhage, vaginitis.

Post-Marketing Experience
The following adverse drug reactions (ADRs) to PLETAL have been reported worldwide since launch of PLETAL in the US. Although the exact rate cannot be calculated, the frequency of these ADRs can be estimated as: very rare (<1/10,000: <0.01%)

- Blood and lymphatic system disorders

Very rare: agranulocytosis, granulocytopenia, thrombocytopenia, leukopenia, bleeding tendency

- Cardiac disorders
  Very rare: Torsades de Pointes, QTc prolongation *(Very rare cases of torsades de pointes and QTc prolongation occurred in patients with cardiac disorders, e.g. complete atrioventricular block, cardiac failure and bradyarrythmia, when treated with cilostazol. Cilostazol was used "off label" due to its positive chronotropic action.)*
- Gastrointestinal disorders
  Very rare: gastrointestinal haemorrhage
- General disorders and administration site conditions
  Very rare: pain, chest pain, hot flushes
- Hepatobiliary disorders
  Very rare: hepatic dysfunction/abnormal liver function tests, jaundice
- Injury, poisoning and procedural complications
  Very rare: extradural haematoma and subdural haematoma
- Investigations
  Very rare: blood glucose increased, blood uric acid increased, platelet count decreased, white blood cell count decreased, increase in BUN (blood urea increased)
- Nervous system disorders
  Very rare: intracranial haemorrhage, cerebral haemorrhage, cerebrovascular accident
- Respiratory, thoracic and mediastinal disorders
  Very rare: pulmonary haemorrhage, interstitial pneumonia
- Skin and subcutaneous tissue disorders
  Very rare: haemorrhage subcutaneous, pruritus, skin eruptions including Stevens Johnson syndrome, skin drug eruption (dermatitis medicamentosa)
- Vascular disorders
  Very rare: subacute thrombosis (These cases of subacute thrombosis occurred in patients treated with aspirin and "off label" use of cilostazol for prevention of thrombotic complication after coronary stenting.)

OVERDOSAGE

Information on acute overdosage with PLETAL in humans is limited. The signs and symptoms of an acute overdose can be anticipated to be those of excessive pharmacologic effect: severe headache, diarrhea, hypotension, tachycardia, and possibly cardiac arrhythmias. The patient should be carefully observed and given supportive treatment. Since cilostazol is highly protein-bound, it is unlikely that it can be efficiently removed by hemodialysis or peritoneal dialysis. The oral LD_{50} of cilostazol is >5.0 g/kg in mice and rats and >2.0 g/kg in dogs.

DOSAGE AND ADMINISTRATION

The recommended dosage of PLETAL is 100 mg b.i.d. taken at least half an hour before or two hours after breakfast and dinner. A dose of 50 mg b.i.d. should be considered during coadministration of such inhibitors of CYP3A4 as ketoconazole, itraconazole, erythromycin and diltiazem, and during coadministration of such inhibitors of CYP2C19 as omeprazole.
Patients may respond as early as 2 to 4 weeks after the initiation of therapy, but treatment for up to 12 weeks may be needed before a beneficial effect is experienced.
Discontinuation of Therapy: The available data suggest that the dosage of PLETAL can be reduced or discontinued without rebound (i.e., platelet hyperaggregability).

HOW SUPPLIED

PLETAL is supplied as 50 mg and 100 mg tablets. The 50 mg tablets are white, triangular, debossed with PLETAL 50, and provided in bottles of 60 tablets (NDC #59148-003-16), and hospital unit dose packs of 100 tablets (NDC #59148-003-35). The 100 mg tablets are white, round, debossed with PLETAL 100, and provided in bottles of 60 tablets (NDC #59148-002-16), and hospital unit dose packs of 100 tablets (NDC #59148-002-35).
Rx ONLY.
STORAGE
Store PLETAL tablets at 25°C (77°F); excursions permitted to 15-30°C (59-86°F) [See USP Controlled Room Temperature].
Manufactured for
OTSUKA AMERICA PHARMACEUTICAL, INC.
Rockville, MD 20850
Manufactured by
OTSUKA PHARMACEUTICAL CO., LTD.
Tokushima 771-0192, Japan
1101/05-04
U.S. Patent No. 4,277,479
Shown in Product Identification Guide, page 328

Most Commonly Reported AEs (Incidence ≥2%) in Patients on PLETAL (PLT) 50 mg b.i.d. or 100 mg b.i.d. and Occurring at a Rate in the 100 mg b.i.d. Group Higher Than in Patients on Placebo

Adverse Events (AEs) by Body System	PLT 50 mg b.i.d. (N=303) %	PLT 100 mg b.i.d. (N=998) %	Placebo (N=973) %
BODY AS A WHOLE			
Abdominal pain	4	5	3
Back pain	6	7	6
Headache	27	34	14
Infection	14	10	8
CARDIOVASCULAR			
Palpitation	5	10	1
Tachycardia	4	4	1
DIGESTIVE			
Abnormal stools	12	15	4
Diarrhea	12	19	7
Dyspepsia	6	6	4
Flatulence	2	3	2
Nausea	6	7	6
METABOLIC & NUTRITIONAL			
Peripheral edema	9	7	4
MUSCULO-SKELETAL			
Myalgia	2	3	2
NERVOUS			
Dizziness	9	10	6
Vertigo	3	1	1
RESPIRATORY			
Cough increased	3	4	3
Pharyngitis	7	10	7
Rhinitis	12	7	5

Ovation Pharmaceuticals, Inc.

FOUR PARKWAY NORTH
DEERFIELD, IL 60015

Direct Inquiries to:
Phone: 847.282.1000
Fax: 847.282.1001
Email: info@ovationpharma.com

CHEMET® ℞
[kĕm' ĕt]
(succimer)

DESCRIPTION

CHEMET (succimer) is an orally active, heavy metal chelating agent. The chemical name for succimer is *meso* 2, 3-dimercaptosuccinic acid (DMSA). Its empirical formula is $C_4H_6O_4S_2$ and molecular weight is 182.2. The *meso*-structural formula is:

COOH
|
H-C-SH
|
H-C-SH
|
COOH

Succimer is a white crystalline powder with an unpleasant, characteristic mercaptan odor and taste.
Each CHEMET opaque white capsule for oral administration, contains beads coated with 100 mg of succimer and is imprinted black with CHEMET 100. Inactive ingredients in medicated beads are: povidone, sodium starch glycolate, starch and sucrose. Inactive ingredients in capsule are: gelatin, iron oxide, titanium dioxide and other ingredients.

CLINICAL PHARMACOLOGY

Succimer is a lead chelator; it forms water soluble chelates and, consequently, increases the urinary excretion of lead.

Preclinical Toxicology: In an ongoing six month chronic oral toxicity study in dogs, thrombocytopenia was observed in animals receiving succimer at 80 or 140 mg/kg/day after three months of dosing. Preliminary gross pathology findings in the affected dogs included ecchymoses in a number of organs. No depressed platelet counts were observed in dogs receiving succimer at 10 mg/kg/day for three months. Platelets were not enumerated in previous oral toxicity studies up to 28 days. In those studies, daily doses of succimer up to 200 mg/kg/day did not produce any significant overt toxicity in rats and dogs. However, six and twenty-eight day oral toxicity studies in dogs have shown that doses of 300 mg/kg/day or higher were toxic and lethal to some dogs. Kidney and gastrointestinal tract were the major target organs for succimer toxicity. Toxicity was manifested by anorexia, emesis, mucoid and/or bloody diarrhea, increased blood urea nitrogen concentration, increased SGPT, SGOT and alkaline phosphatase levels, renal tubular necrosis, purulent nephritis and severe gastrointestinal bleeding and ulceration. Deaths were due to renal failure.

Pharmacokinetics: In a study performed in healthy adult volunteers, after a single dose of ^{14}C-succimer at 16, 32, or 48 mg/kg, absorption was rapid but variable with peak blood radioactivity levels between one and two hours. On average, 49% of the radiolabeled dose was excreted: 39% in the feces, 9% in the urine and 1% as carbon dioxide from the lungs. Since fecal excretion probably represented nonabsorbed drug, most of the absorbed drug was excreted by the kidneys. The apparent elimination half-life of the radiolabeled material in the blood was about two days.

In other studies of healthy adult volunteers receiving a single oral dose of 10 mg/kg, the chemical analysis of succimer and its metabolites in the urine showed that succimer was rapidly and extensively metabolized. Approximately 25% of the administered dose was excreted in the urine with the peak blood level and urinary excretion occurring between two and four hours. Of the total amount of drug eliminated in the urine, approximately 90% was eliminated in altered form as mixed succimer-cysteine disulfides; the remaining 10% was eliminated unchanged. The majority of mixed disulfides consisted of succimer in disulfide linkages with two molecules of L-cysteine, the remaining disulfides contained one L-cysteine per succimer molecule.

Pharmacodynamics: Dose ranging studies were performed in 18 men with blood lead levels of 44-96 µg/dL. Three groups of 6 patients received either 10.0, 6.7 or 3.3 mg/kg succimer orally every 8 hours for 5 days. After five days the mean blood levels of the three groups decreased 72.5%, 58.3% and 35.5% respectively. The mean urinary lead excretions in the initial 24 hours were 28.6, 18.6 and 12.3 times the pretreatment 24 hour urinary lead excretion. As the chelatable pool was reduced during therapy, urinary lead output decreased. A mean of 19 mg of lead was excreted during a five-day course of 30 mg/kg/day succimer. Clinical symptoms, such as headache and colic, and biochemical indices of lead toxicity also improved. Decrease in urinary excretion of d-aminolevulinic acid (ALA) and coproporphyrin paralleled the improvement in erythrocyte d-aminolevulinic acid dehydratase (ALA-D). Three control patients with lead poisoning of similar severity received $CaNa_2EDTA$ intravenously at a dose of 50 mg/kg/day for five days. The mean blood lead level decreased 47.4% and the mean urinary lead excretion was 21 mg in the control patients.

Effect on Essential Minerals: In the above studies succimer had no significant effect on the urinary elimination of iron, calcium or magnesium. Zinc excretion doubled during treatment. The effect of succimer on the excretion of essential minerals was small compared to that of $CaNa_2EDTA$, which can induce more than a ten-fold increase in urinary excretion of zinc and doubling of copper and iron excretion.

Efficacy: A dose ranging study was performed in 15 pediatric patients aged 2 to 7 years with blood lead levels of 30-49 µg/dL and positive $CaNa_2EDTA$ lead mobilization tests. Each group of five patients received 350, 233 or 116 mg/m^2 succimer every 8 hours for 5 days. These doses corresponded to 10, 6.7 and 3.3 mg/kg. Six control patients received 1000 mg/m^2/day $CaNa_2EDTA$ intravenously for 5 days. Following therapy, the mean blood lead levels decreased 78, 63 and 42% respectively in the three groups treated with succimer. The response of the 350 mg/m^2 every 8 hours (10 mg/kg q 8 hr) group was significantly better than that of the other succimer treated groups as well as that of the control group, whose mean blood lead level fell 48%. No adverse reactions or changes in essential mineral excretion were reported in the succimer treated groups. In the $CaNa_2EDTA$ treated group, the cumulative amount of urinary lead excreted was slightly but significantly greater than in the succimer group. After $CaNa_2EDTA$, the urinary excretion of copper, zinc, iron and calcium were significantly increased.

As with other chelators, both adults and pediatric patients experienced a rebound in blood lead levels after discontinuation of CHEMET. In these studies, after treatment with a dose of 350 mg/m^2 (10 mg/kg) every 8 hours for five days, the mean lead level rebounded and plateaued at 60-85% of pretreatment levels two weeks after therapy. The rebound plateau was somewhat higher with lower doses of succimer and with intravenous $CaNa_2EDTA$.

In an attempt to control rebound of blood lead levels, 19 pediatric patients, ages 1-7 years, with blood lead levels of 42-67 µg/dL, were treated with 350 mg/m^2 succimer every 8 hours for five days and then divided into three groups. One group was followed for two weeks with no further therapy, the second group was treated for two weeks with 350 mg/m^2 daily, and the third with 350 mg/m^2 every 12 hours. After the initial 5 days of therapy, the mean blood lead level in all subjects declined 61%. While the untreated group and the group treated with 350 mg/m^2 daily experienced rebound during the ensuing two weeks, the group who received the 350 mg/m^2 every 12 hours experienced no such rebound during the treatment period and less rebound following cessation of therapy.

In another study, ten pediatric patients, ages 21 to 72 months, with blood lead levels of 30-57 µg/dL were treated with succimer 350 mg/m^2 every eight hours for five days followed by an additional 19-22 days of therapy at a dose of 350 mg/m^2 every 12 hours. The mean blood lead levels decreased and remained stable at under 15 µg/dL during the extended dosing period.

In addition to the controlled studies, approximately 250 patients with lead poisoning have been treated with succimer either orally or parenterally in open U.S. and foreign studies with similar results reported. Succimer has been used for the treatment of lead poisoning in one patient with sickle cell anemia and in five patients with glucose-6-phosphodehydrogenase (G6PD) deficiency without adverse reactions.

Lead Encephalopathy: Three adults with lead encephalopathy have been reported in the literature to have improved with succimer therapy. However, data are not available regarding the use of succimer for the treatment of this rare and sometimes fatal complication of lead poisoning in pediatric patients.

Other Heavy Metal Poisoning: No controlled clinical studies have been conducted with succimer in poisoning with other heavy metals. A limited number of patients have received succimer for mercury or arsenic poisoning. These patients showed increased urinary excretion of the heavy metal and varying degrees of symptomatic improvement.

INDICATIONS AND USAGE

CHEMET is indicated for the treatment of lead poisoning in pediatric patients with blood lead levels above 45 µg/dL. CHEMET is not indicated for prophylaxis of lead poisoning in a lead-containing environment; the use of CHEMET should always be accompanied by identification and removal of the source of the lead exposure.

CONTRAINDICATIONS

CHEMET should not be administered to patients with a history of allergy to the drug.

WARNINGS

Keep out of reach of pediatric patients. CHEMET is not a substitute for effective abatement of lead exposure.

Mild to moderate neutropenia has been observed in some patients receiving succimer. While a causal relationship to succimer has not been definitely established, neutropenia has been reported with other drugs in the same chemical class. A complete blood count with white blood cell differential and direct platelet counts should be obtained prior to and weekly during treatment with succimer. Therapy should either be withheld or discontinued if the absolute neutrophil count (ANC) is below 1200/µL and the patient followed closely to document recovery of the ANC to above 1500/µL or to the patient's baseline neutrophil count. There is limited experience with reexposure in patients who have developed neutropenia. Therefore, such patients should be rechallenged only if the benefit of succimer therapy clearly outweighs the potential risk of another episode of neutropenia and then only with careful patient monitoring.

Patients treated with succimer should be instructed to promptly report any signs of infection. If infection is suspected, the above laboratory tests should be conducted immediately.

PRECAUTIONS

The extent of clinical experience with CHEMET is limited. Therefore, patients should be carefully observed during treatment.

General: Elevated blood lead levels and associated symptoms may return rapidly after discontinuation of CHEMET because of redistribution of lead from bone stores to soft tissues and blood. After therapy, patients should be monitored for rebound of blood lead levels, by measuring blood lead levels at least once weekly until stable. However, the severity of lead intoxication (as measured by the initial blood lead level and the rate and degree of rebound of blood lead) should be used as a guide for more frequent blood lead monitoring.

All patients undergoing treatment should be adequately hydrated. Caution should be exercised in using CHEMET therapy in patients with compromised renal function. Limited data suggests that CHEMET is dialyzable, but that the lead chelates are not.

Transient mild elevations of serum transaminases have been observed in 6-10% of patients during the course of succimer therapy. Serum transaminases should be monitored before the start of therapy and at least weekly during therapy. Patients with a history of liver disease should be monitored closely. No data are available regarding the metabolism of succimer in patients with liver disease.

Clinical experience with repeated courses is limited. The safety of uninterrupted dosing longer than three weeks has not been established and it is not recommended.

The possibility of allergic or other mucocutaneous reactions to the drug must be borne in mind on readministration (as well as during initial courses). Patients requiring repeated courses of CHEMET should be monitored during each treatment course. One patient experienced recurrent mucocutaneous vesicular eruptions of increasing severity affecting the oral mucosa, the external urethral meatus and the perianal area on the third, fourth and fifth courses of the drug. The reaction resolved between courses and upon discontinuation of therapy.

Information for Patients: Patients should be instructed to maintain adequate fluid intake. If rash occurs, patients should consult their physician. Patients should be instructed to promptly report any indication of infection, which may be a sign of neutropenia (see WARNINGS and ADVERSE REACTIONS).

In young pediatric patients unable to swallow capsules, the contents of the capsule can be administered in a small amount of food (see DOSAGE AND ADMINISTRATION).

Drug Interaction: CHEMET is not known to interact with other drugs including iron supplements; interactions have not been systematically studied. Concomitant administration of CHEMET with other chelation therapy, such as $CaNa_2EDTA$ is not recommended.

Drug/Laboratory Tests Interaction: Succimer may interfere with serum and urinary laboratory tests. *In vitro* studies have shown succimer to cause false positive results for ketones in urine using nitroprusside reagents such as Ketostix® and falsely decreased measurements of serum uric acid and CPK.

Carcinogenesis, Mutagenesis and Impairment of Fertility: CHEMET has not been tested for carcinogenic potential in long-term animal studies. CHEMET has not been tested in animals for its effect on fertility and reproductive performance in males and females. It was not mutagenic in the Ames bacterial assay and in the mammalian cell forward gene mutation assay.

Pregnancy: *Teratogenic Effects—Pregnancy Category C.* CHEMET has been shown to be teratogenic and fetotoxic in pregnant mice when given subcutaneously in a dose range of 410 to 1640 mg/kg/day during the period of organogenesis. There are no adequate and well controlled studies in pregnant women. CHEMET should be used during pregnancy only if the potential benefit justifies the potential risk to the fetus.

Nursing Mothers: It is not known whether this drug is excreted in human milk. Because many drugs and heavy metals are excreted in human milk, nursing mothers requiring CHEMET therapy should be discouraged from nursing their infants.

Pediatric Use: Refer to the INDICATIONS and DOSAGE AND ADMINISTRATION sections. Safety and efficacy in pediatric patients less than 12 months of age have not been established.

ADVERSE REACTIONS

Clinical experience with CHEMET has been limited. Consequently, the full spectrum and incidence of adverse reactions including the possibility of hypersensitivity or idiosyncratic reactions have not been determined. The most common events attributable to succimer, i.e., gastrointestinal symptoms or increases in serum transaminases, have been observed in about 10% of patients (see PRECAUTIONS). Rashes, some necessitating discontinuation of therapy, have been reported in about 4% of patients. If rash occurs, other causes (e.g. measles) should be considered before ascribing the reaction to succimer. Rechallenge with succimer may be considered if lead levels are high enough to warrant retreatment. One allergic mucocutaneous reaction has been reported on repeated administration of the drug (see PRECAUTIONS). Mild to moderate neutropenia has been observed in some patients receiving succimer (see WARNINGS). Table I presents adverse events reported with the administration of succimer for the treatment of lead and other heavy metal intoxication.

TABLE I
INCIDENCE OF ADVERSE EVENTS IN DOMESTIC STUDIES REGARDLESS OF ATTRIBUTION OR SUCCIMER DOSAGE

	Pediatric Patients (191)		Adults (134)	
	%	(n)	%	(n)
Digestive:	12.0	23	20.9	28
Nausea, vomiting, diarrhea, appetite loss, hemorroidal symptoms, loose stools, metallic taste in mouth.				
Body as a Whole:	5.2	10	15.7	21
Back pain, abdominal cramps, stomach pains, head pain, rib pain, chills, flank pain, fever, flu-like symtpoms, heavy head/tired, head cold, headache, moniliasis.				
Metabolic:	4.2	8	10.4	14
Elevated SGPT, SGOT, alkaline phosphatase, elevated serum cholesterol.				
Nervous:	1.0	2	12.7	17
Drowsiness, dizziness, sensorimotor neuropathy, sleepiness, paresthesia.				
Skin and Appendages:	2.6	5	11.2	15
Papular rash, herpetic rash, rash, mucocutaneous eruptions, pruritus.				
Special Senses:	1.0	2	3.7	5
Cloudy film in eye, ears plugged, otitis media, eyes watery.				
Respiratory:	3.7	7	0.7	1
Throat sore, rhinorrhea, nasal congestion, cough				
Urogenital:	0.0	–	3.7	5
Decreased urination, voiding difficulty, proteinuria increased.				

Continued on next page

Chemet—Cont.

Cardiovascular:	0.0	–	1.8	2
Arrhythmia.				
Heme/Lymphatic:	0.5*	1	1.5*	2
Mild to moderate neutropenia.				
Increased platelet count, intermittent eosinophilia.				
Musculoskeletal:	0.0	–	3.0	4
Kneecap pain, leg pains.				

*Does not include neutropenia—see WARNINGS.

OVERDOSAGE

Doses of 2300 mg/kg in the rat and 2400 mg/kg in the mouse produced ataxia, convulsions, labored respiration and frequently death. No case of overdosage has been reported in humans. Limited data indicate that succimer is dialyzable. In case of acute overdosage, induction of vomiting or gastric lavage followed by administration of an activated charcoal slurry and appropriate supportive therapy are recommended.

DOSAGE AND ADMINISTRATION

Start dosage at 10 mg/kg or 350 mg/m^2 every eight hours for five days. Initiation of therapy at higher doses is not recommended. (See Table II for Dosing chart and number of capsules.) Reduce frequency of administration to 10 mg/kg or 350 mg/m^2 every 12 hours (two-thirds of initial daily dosage) for an additional two weeks of therapy. A course of treatment lasts 19 days. Repeated courses may be necessary if indicated by weekly monitoring of blood lead concentration. A minimum of two weeks between courses is recommended unless blood lead levels indicate the need for more prompt treatment.

TABLE II
CHEMET (SUCCIMER) PEDIATRIC DOSING CHART

LBS	KG	DOSE(MG)*	Number of CAPSULES*
18-35	8-15	100	1
36-55	16-23	200	2
56-75	24-34	300	3
76-100	35-44	400	4
>100	>45	500	5

*To be administered every 8 hours for 5 days, followed by dosing every 12 hours for 14 days.

In young pediatric patients who cannot swallow capsules, CHEMET can be administered by separating the capsule and sprinkling the medicated beads on a small amount of soft food or putting them in a spoon and following with fruit drink.

Identification of the source of lead in the pediatric patient's environment and its abatement are critical to a successful therapy outcome. Chelation therapy is not a substitute for preventing further exposure to lead and should not be used to permit continued exposure to lead.

Patients who have received $CaNa_2EDTA$ with or without BAL may use CHEMET for subsequent treatment after an interval of four weeks. Data on the concomitant use of CHEMET with $CaNa_2EDTA$ with or without BAL are not available, and such use is not recommended.

HOW SUPPLIED

100 mg capsules in bottle of 100 (NDC 67386-201-11)
Store between 15° C and 25° C and avoid excessive heat.
PC3201C
Rev. 7/2003

Distributed by
OVATION
Pharmaceuticals, Inc.
Deerfield, IL 60015, U.S.A.

Shown in Product Identification Guide, page 328

DESOXYN® Ⓒ℞
[dĕ-sŏks-ĭn]
(methamphetamine hydrochloride)
TABLETS, USP **No. 102**

METHAMPHETAMINE HAS A HIGH POTENTIAL FOR ABUSE. IT SHOULD THUS BE TRIED ONLY IN WEIGHT REDUCTION PROGRAMS FOR PATIENTS IN WHOM ALTERNATIVE THERAPY HAS BEEN INEFFECTIVE. ADMINISTRATION OF METHAMPHETAMINE FOR PROLONGED PERIODS OF TIME IN OBESITY MAY LEAD TO DRUG DEPENDENCE AND MUST BE AVOIDED. PARTICULAR ATTENTION SHOULD BE PAID TO THE POSSIBILITY OF SUBJECTS OBTAINING METHAMPHETAMINE FOR NON-THERAPEUTIC USE OR DISTRIBUTION TO OTHERS, AND THE DRUG SHOULD BE PRESCRIBED OR DISPENSED SPARINGLY.

DESCRIPTION

DESOXYN (methamphetamine hydrochloride tablets, USP), chemically known as (S)-N, α-dimethylbenzeneethanamine hydrochloride, is a member of the amphetamine group of sympathomimetic amines. It has the following structural formula:

$$\left[C_6H_5{-}CH_2{-}\underset{\displaystyle CH_3}{\underset{|}{CH}}{-}\overset{+}{N}H_2CH_3 \right] Cl^-$$

DESOXYN tablets contain 5 mg of methamphetamine hydrochloride for oral administration.

Inactive Ingredients:

Corn starch, lactose, sodium paraminobenzoate, stearic acid and talc.

CLINICAL PHARMACOLOGY

Methamphetamine is a sympathomimetic amine with CNS stimulant activity. Peripheral actions include elevation of systolic and diastolic blood pressures and weak bronchodilator and respiratory stimulant action. Drugs of this class used in obesity are commonly known as "anorectics" or "anorexigenics". It has not been established, however, that the action of such drugs in treating obesity is primarily one of appetite suppression. Other central nervous system actions, or metabolic effects, may be involved, for example.

Adult obese subjects instructed in dietary management and treated with "anorectic" drugs, lose more weight on the average than those treated with placebo and diet, as determined in relatively short-term clinical trials.

The magnitude of increased weight loss of drug-treated patients over placebo-treated patients is only a fraction of a pound a week. The rate of weight loss is greatest in the first weeks of therapy for both drug and placebo subjects and tends to decrease in succeeding weeks. The origins of the increased weight loss due to the various possible drug effects are not established. The amount of weight loss associated with the use of an "anorectic" drug varies from trial to trial, and the increased weight loss appears to be related in part to variables other than the drug prescribed, such as the physician-investigator, the population treated, and the diet prescribed. Studies do not permit conclusions as to the relative importance of the drug and non-drug factors on weight loss.

The natural history of obesity is measured in years, whereas the studies cited are restricted to a few weeks duration; thus, the total impact of drug-induced weight loss over that of diet alone must be considered clinically limited.

The mechanism of action involved in producing the beneficial behavioral changes seen in hyperkinetic children receiving methamphetamine is unknown.

In humans, methamphetamine is rapidly absorbed from the gastrointestinal tract. The primary site of metabolism is in the liver by aromatic hydroxylation, N-dealkylation and deamination. At least seven metabolites have been identified in the urine. The biological half-life has been reported in the range of 4 to 5 hours. Excretion occurs primarily in the urine and is dependent on urine pH. Alkaline urine will significantly increase the drug half-life. Approximately 62% of an oral dose is eliminated in the urine within the first 24 hours with about one-third as intact drug and the remainder as metabolites.

INDICATIONS AND USAGE

Attention Deficit Disorder with Hyperactivity—DESOXYN tablets are indicated as an integral part of a total treatment program which typically includes other remedial measures (psychological, educational, social) for a stabilizing effect in children over 6 years of age with a behavioral syndrome characterized by the following group of developmentally inappropriate symptoms: moderate to severe distractibility, short attention span, hyperactivity, emotional lability, and impulsivity. The diagnosis of this syndrome should not be made with finality when these symptoms are only of comparatively recent origin. Nonlocalizing (soft) neurological signs, learning disability, and abnormal EEG may or may not be present, and a diagnosis of central nervous system dysfunction may or may not be warranted.

Exogenous Obesity—as a short-term (i.e., a few weeks) adjunct in a regimen of weight reduction based on caloric restriction, for patients in whom obesity is refractory to alternative therapy, e.g., repeated diets, group programs, and other drugs. The limited usefulness of DESOXYN tablets (see **CLINICAL PHARMACOLOGY**) should be weighed against possible risks inherent in use of the drug, such as those described below.

CONTRAINDICATIONS

DESOXYN tablets are contraindicated during or within 14 days following the administration of monoamine oxidase inhibitors; hypertensive crisis may result. It is also contraindicated in patients with glaucoma, advanced arteriosclerosis, symptomatic cardiovascular disease, moderate to severe hypertension, hyperthyroidism or known hypersensitivity or idiosyncrasy to sympathomimetic amines. Methamphetamine should not be given to patients who are in an agitated state or who have a history of drug abuse.

WARNINGS

Tolerance to the anorectic effect usually develops within a few weeks. When this occurs, the recommended dose should not be exceeded in an attempt to increase the effect; rather, the drug should be discontinued (see **DRUG ABUSE AND DEPENDENCE**).

Decrements in the predicted growth (i.e., weight gain and/or height) rate have been reported with the long-term use of stimulants in children. Therefore, patients requiring long-term therapy should be carefully monitored.

Usage in Nursing Mothers: Amphetamines are excreted in human milk. Mothers taking amphetamines should be advised to refrain from nursing.

PRECAUTIONS

General:

DESOXYN tablets should be used with caution in patients with even mild hypertension.

Methamphetamine should not be used to combat fatigue or to replace rest in normal persons.

Prescribing and dispensing of methamphetamine should be limited to the smallest amount that is feasible at one time in order to minimize the possibility of overdosage.

Information for Patients:

The patient should be informed that methamphetamine may impair the ability to engage in potentially hazardous activities, such as, operating machinery or driving a motor vehicle.

The patient should be cautioned not to increase dosage, except on advice of the physician.

Drug Interactions:

Insulin requirements in diabetes mellitus may be altered in association with the use of methamphetamine and the concomitant dietary regimen.

Methamphetamine may decrease the hypotensive effect of *guanethidine*.

DESOXYN should not be used concurrently with *monoamine oxidase inhibitors* (see **CONTRAINDICATIONS**).

Concurrent administration of *tricyclic antidepressants* and indirect-acting sympathomimetic amines such as the amphetamines, should be closely supervised and dosage carefully adjusted.

Phenothiazines are reported in the literature to antagonize the CNS stimulant action of the amphetamines.

Drug/Laboratory Test Interactions:

Literature reports suggest that amphetamines may be associated with significant elevation of plasma corticosteroids. This should be considered if determination of plasma corticosteroid levels is desired in a person receiving amphetamines.

Carcinogenesis, Mutagenesis, Impairment of Fertility:

Data are not available on long-term potential for carcinogenicity, mutagenicity, or impairment of fertility.

Pregnancy:

Teratogenic effects: Pregnancy Category C. Methamphetamine has been shown to have teratogenic and embryocidal effects in mammals given high multiples of the human dose. There are no adequate and well-controlled studies in pregnant women. DESOXYN tablets should not be used during pregnancy unless the potential benefit justifies the potential risk to the fetus.

Nonteratogenic effects: Infants born to mothers dependent on amphetamines have an increased risk of premature delivery and low birth weight. Also, these infants may experience symptoms of withdrawal as demonstrated by dysphoria, including agitation and significant lassitude.

Nursing Mothers:

See **WARNINGS**.

Pediatric Use:

Safety and effectiveness for use as an anorectic agent in children below the age of 12 years have not been established.

Long-term effects of methamphetamine in children have not been established (see **WARNINGS**).

Drug treatment is not indicated in all cases of the behavioral syndrome characterized by moderate to severe distractibility, short attention span, hyperactivity, emotional lability and impulsivity. It should be considered only in light of the complete history and evaluation of the child. The decision to prescribe DESOXYN tablets should depend on the physician's assessment of the chronicity and severity of the child's symptoms and their appropriateness for his/her age. Prescription should not depend solely on the presence of one or more of the behavioral characteristics.

When these symptoms are associated with acute stress reactions, treatment with DESOXYN tablets is usually not indicated.

Clinical experience suggests that in psychotic children, administration of DESOXYN tablets may exacerbate symptoms of behavior disturbance and thought disorder.

Amphetamines have been reported to exacerbate motor and phonic tics and Tourette's syndrome. Therefore, clinical evaluation for tics and Tourette's syndrome in children and their families should precede use of stimulant medications.

ADVERSE REACTIONS

The following are adverse reactions in decreasing order of severity within each category that have been reported:

Cardiovascular: Elevation of blood pressure, tachycardia and palpitation.

Central Nervous System: Psychotic episodes have been rarely reported at recommended doses. Dizziness, dysphoria, overstimulation, euphoria, insomnia, tremor, restlessness and headache. Exacerbation of motor and phonic tics and Tourette's syndrome.

Gastrointestinal: Diarrhea, constipation, dryness of mouth, unpleasant taste and other gastrointestinal disturbances.

Hypersensitivity: Urticaria.

Endocrine: Impotence and changes in libido.

Miscellaneous: Suppression of growth has been reported with the long-term use of stimulants in children (see **WARNINGS**).

DRUG ABUSE AND DEPENDENCE

Controlled Substance: DESOXYN tablets are subject to control under DEA schedule II.

Abuse: Methamphetamine has been extensively abused. Tolerance, extreme psychological dependence, and severe social disability have occurred. There are reports of patients who have increased the dosage to many times that recommended. Abrupt cessation following prolonged high dosage administration results in extreme fatigue and mental depression; changes are also noted on the sleep EEG. Manifestations of chronic intoxication with methamphetamine include severe dermatoses, marked insomnia, irritability, hyperactivity, and personality changes. The most severe manifestation of chronic intoxication is psychosis often clinically indistinguishable from schizophrenia.

OVERDOSAGE

Manifestations of acute overdosage with methamphetamine include restlessness, tremor, hyperreflexia, rapid respiration, confusion, assaultiveness, hallucinations, panic states, hyperpyrexia, and rhabdomyolysis. Fatigue and depression usually follow the central stimulation. Cardiovascular effects include arrhythmias, hypertension or hypotension, and circulatory collapse. Gastrointestinal symptoms include nausea, vomiting, diarrhea, and abdominal cramps. Fatal poisoning usually terminates in convulsions and coma.

Consult with a Certified Poison Control Center regarding treatment for up to date guidance and advice. Management of acute methamphetamine intoxication is largely symptomatic and includes gastric evacuation, administration of activated charcoal, and sedation. Experience with hemodialysis or peritoneal dialysis is inadequate to permit recommendations in this regard.

Acidification of urine increases methamphetamine excretion, but is believed to increase risk of acute renal failure if myoglobinuria is present. Intravenous phentolamine (Regitine®) has been suggested for possible acute, severe hypertension, if this complicates methamphetamine overdosage. Usually a gradual drop in blood pressure will result when sufficient sedation has been achieved. Chlorpromazine has been reported to be useful in decreasing CNS stimulation and sympathomimetic effects.

DOSAGE AND ADMINISTRATION

DESOXYN tablets are given orally.

Methamphetamine should be administered at the lowest effective dosage, and dosage should be individually adjusted. Late evening medication should be avoided because of the resulting insomnia.

Attention Deficit Disorder with Hyperactivity: For treatment of children 6 years or older with a behavioral syndrome characterized by moderate to severe distractibility, short attention span, hyperactivity, emotional lability and impulsivity: an initial dose of 5 mg DESOXYN once or twice a day is recommended. Daily dosage may be raised in increments of 5 mg at weekly intervals until an optimum clinical response is achieved. The usual effective dose is 20 to 25 mg daily. The total daily dose may be given in two divided doses daily. Where possible, drug administration should be interrupted occasionally to determine if there is a recurrence of behavioral symptoms sufficient to require continued therapy.

For Obesity: One 5 mg tablet should be taken one-half hour before each meal. Treatment should not exceed a few weeks in duration. Methamphetamine is not recommended for use as an anorectic agent in children under 12 years of age.

HOW SUPPLIED

DESOXYN (methamphetamine hydrochloride tablets, USP) is supplied as white tablets imprinted with the letters OV on one side and the number 12 on the opposite side, containing 5 mg methamphetamine hydrochloride in bottles of 100 (**NDC** 67386-102-01).

Recommended Storage: Store below 86°F (30°C).

Revised: May, 2003

Manufactured by:
Abbott Laboratories,
North Chicago, IL 60064, U.S.A.
Distributed by:
OVATION PHARMACEUTICALS, INC.
Deerfield, IL 60015, U.S.A.

Shown in Product Identification Guide, page 328

MEBARAL® Ⓒ℞

[mĕ' bă-rəl]

Brand of MEPHOBARBITAL TABLETS, USP

DESCRIPTION

Mephobarbital, 5-Ethyl-1-methyl-5-phenylbarbituric acid, is a barbiturate with sedative, hypnotic, and anticonvulsant properties. It occurs as a white, nearly odorless, tasteless powder and is slightly soluble in water and in alcohol.

MEBARAL is available as tablets for oral administration.

The structural formula is:

[See chemical structure at top of next column]

Inactive Ingredients: Lactose, Starch, Stearic Acid, Talc.

CLINICAL PHARMACOLOGY

Barbiturates are capable of producing all levels of CNS mood alteration from excitation to mild sedation, to hypnosis, and deep coma. Overdosage can produce death. In high enough therapeutic doses, barbiturates induce anesthesia.

Barbiturates depress the sensory cortex, decrease motor activity, alter cerebellar function, and produce drowsiness, sedation, and hypnosis.

Barbiturates are respiratory depressants. The degree of respiratory depression is dependent upon dose. With hypnotic doses, respiratory depression produced by barbiturates is similar to that which occurs during physiologic sleep with slight decrease in blood pressure and heart rate.

Studies in laboratory animals have shown that barbiturates cause reduction in the tone and contractility of the uterus, ureters, and urinary bladder. However, concentrations of the drugs required to produce this effect in humans are not reached with sedative-hypnotic doses.

Barbiturates do not impair normal hepatic function, but have been shown to induce liver microsomal enzymes, thus increasing and/or altering the metabolism of barbiturates and other drugs. (See PRECAUTIONS-Drug Interactions.)

MEBARAL exerts a strong sedative and anticonvulsant action but has a relatively mild hypnotic effect. It reduces the incidence of epileptic seizures in grand mal and petit mal. MEBARAL usually causes little or no drowsiness or lassitude. Hence, when it is used as a sedative or anticonvulsant, patients usually become more calm, more cheerful, and better adjusted to their surroundings without clouding of mental faculties. MEBARAL is reported to produce less sedation than does phenobarbital.

Barbiturates are weak acids that are absorbed and rapidly distributed to all tissues and fluids with high concentrations in the brain, liver, and kidneys. Lipid solubility of the barbiturates is the dominant factor in their distribution within the body. Barbiturates are bound to plasma and tissue proteins to a varying degree with the degree of binding increasing directly as a function of lipid solubility.

Approximately 50% of an oral dose of mephobarbital is absorbed from the gastrointestinal tract. Therapeutic plasma concentrations for mephobarbital have not been established nor has the half-life been determined. Following oral administration, the onset of action of the drug is 30 to 60 minutes and the duration of action is 10 to 16 hours. The primary route of mephobarbital metabolism is N-demethylation by the microsomal enzymes of the liver to form phenobarbital. Phenobarbital may be excreted in the urine unchanged or further metabolized to *p*-hydroxyphenobarbital and excreted in the urine as glucuronide or sulfate conjugates. About 75% of a single oral dose of mephobarbital is converted to phenobarbital in 24 hours.

Therefore, chronic administration of mephobarbital may lead to an accumulation of phenobarbital (not mephobarbital) in plasma. It has not been determined whether mephobarbital or phenobarbital is the active agent during long-time mephobarbital therapy.

INDICATIONS AND USAGE

MEBARAL is indicated for use as a sedative for the relief of anxiety, tension, and apprehension, and as an anticonvulsant for the treatment of grand mal and petit mal epilepsy.

CONTRAINDICATIONS

Hypersensitivity to any barbiturate. Manifest or latent porphyria.

WARNINGS

Habit Forming

Barbiturates may be habit forming. Tolerance, psychological, and physical dependence may occur with continued use. (See DRUG ABUSE AND DEPENDENCE and CLINICAL PHARMACOLOGY.) Patients who have psychological dependence on barbiturates may increase the dosage or decrease the dosage interval without consulting a physician and may subsequently develop a physical dependence on barbiturates. To minimize the possibility of overdosage or the development of dependence, the prescribing and dispensing of sedative-hypnotic barbiturates should be limited to the amount required for the interval until the next appointment. Abrupt cessation after prolonged use in the dependent person may result in withdrawal symptoms, including delirium, convulsions, and possibly death. Barbiturates should be withdrawn gradually from any patient known to be taking excessive dosage over long periods of time. (See DRUG ABUSE AND DEPENDENCE.)

Acute or Chronic Pain

Caution should be exercised when barbiturates are administered to patients with acute or chronic pain, because paradoxical excitement could be induced or important symptoms could be masked. However, the use of barbiturates as sedatives in the postoperative surgical period and as adjuncts to cancer chemotherapy is well established.

Use in Pregnancy

Barbiturates can cause fetal damage when administered to a pregnant woman. Retrospective, case-controlled studies have suggested a connection between the maternal consumption of barbiturates and a higher than expected incidence of fetal abnormalities. Following oral or parenteral administration, barbiturates readily cross the placental barrier and are distributed throughout fetal tissues with highest concentrations found in the placenta, fetal liver, and brain. Fetal blood levels approach maternal blood levels following parenteral administration.

Withdrawal symptoms occur in infants born to mothers who receive barbiturates throughout the last trimester of pregnancy. (See DRUG ABUSE AND DEPENDENCE.) If this drug is used during pregnancy, or if the patient becomes pregnant while taking this drug, the patient should be apprised of the potential hazard to the fetus.

Synergistic Effects

The concomitant use of alcohol or other CNS depressants may produce additive CNS depressant effects.

PRECAUTIONS

General

Barbiturates may be habit forming. Tolerance and psychological and physical dependence may occur with continuing use. (See DRUG ABUSE AND DEPENDENCE.) Barbiturates should be administered with caution, if at all, to patients who are mentally depressed, have suicidal tendencies, or a history of drug abuse.

Elderly or debilitated patients may react to barbiturates with marked excitement, depression, and confusion. In some persons, barbiturates repeatedly produce excitement rather than depression.

In patients with hepatic damage, barbiturates should be administered with caution and initially in reduced doses. Barbiturates should not be administered to patients showing the premonitory signs of hepatic coma.

Status epilepticus may result from the abrupt discontinuation of MEBARAL, even when administered in small daily doses in the treatment of epilepsy.

Caution and careful adjustment of dosage are required when MEBARAL is used in patients with impaired renal, cardiac or respiratory function, and in patients with myasthenia gravis and myxedema. The least quantity feasible should be prescribed or dispensed at any one time in order to minimize the possibility of acute or chronic overdosage.

Vitamin D Deficiency: MEBARAL may increase vitamin D requirements, possibly by increasing vitamin D metabolism via enzyme induction. Rarely, rickets and osteomalacia have been reported following prolonged use of barbiturates.

Vitamin K: Bleeding in the early neonatal period due to coagulation defects may follow exposure to anticonvulsant drugs *in utero*; therefore, vitamin K should be given to the mother before delivery or to the child at birth.

Information for the Patient

Practitioners should give the following information and instructions to patients receiving barbiturates.

1. The use of barbiturates carries with it an associated risk of psychological and/or physical dependence. The patient should be warned against increasing the dose of the drug without consulting a physician.
2. Barbiturates may impair mental and/or physical abilities required for the performance of potentially hazardous tasks (e.g., driving, operating machinery, etc.).
3. Alcohol should not be consumed while taking barbiturates. Concurrent use of the barbiturates with other CNS depressants (e.g., alcohol, narcotics, tranquilizers, and antihistamines) may result in additional CNS depressant effects.

Laboratory Tests

Prolonged therapy with barbiturates should be accompanied by periodic laboratory evaluation of organ systems, including hematopoietic, renal, and hepatic systems. (See PRECAUTIONS [General] and ADVERSE REACTIONS.)

Drug Interactions

Most reports of clinically significant drug interactions occurring with the barbiturates have involved phenobarbital. However, the application of these data to other barbiturates appears valid and warrants serial blood level determinations of the relevant drugs when there are multiple therapies.

1. *Anticoagulants.* Phenobarbital lowers the plasma levels of dicumarol (name previously used: bishydroxycoumarin) and causes a decrease in anticoagulant activity as measured by the prothrombin time. Barbiturates can induce hepatic microsomal enzymes resulting in increased metabolism and decreased anticoagulant response of oral anticoagulants (e.g., warfarin, acenocoumarol, dicumarol, and phenprocoumon). Patients stabilized on anticoagulant therapy may require dosage adjustments if barbiturates are added to or withdrawn from their dosage regimen.
2. *Corticosteroids.* Barbiturates appear to enhance the metabolism of exogenous corticosteroids probably through the induction of hepatic microsomal enzymes. Patients stabilized on corticosteroid therapy may require dosage adjustments if barbiturates are added to or withdrawn from their dosage regimen.
3. *Griseofulvin.* Phenobarbital appears to interfere with the absorption of orally administered griseofulvin, thus decreasing its blood level. The effect of the resultant decreased blood levels of griseofulvin on therapeutic response has not been established. However, it would be preferable to avoid concomitant administration of these drugs.

Continued on next page

Mebaral—Cont.

4. *Doxycycline.* Phenobarbital has been shown to shorten the half-life of doxycycline for as long as 2 weeks after barbiturate therapy is discontinued.
   This mechanism is probably through the induction of hepatic microsomal enzymes that metabolize the antibiotic. If phenobarbital and doxycycline are administered concurrently, the clinical response to doxycycline should be monitored closely.
5. *Phenytoin, Sodium Valproate, Valproic Acid.* The effect of barbiturates on the metabolism of phenytoin appears to be variable. Some investigators report an accelerating effect, while others report no effect. Because the effect of barbiturates on the metabolism of phenytoin is not predictable, phenytoin and barbiturate blood levels should be monitored more frequently if these drugs are given concurrently. Sodium valproate and valproic acid appear to decrease barbiturate metabolism; therefore, barbiturate blood levels should be monitored and appropriate dosage adjustments made as indicated.
6. *Central Nervous System Depressants.* The concomitant use of other central nervous system depressants, including other sedatives or hypnotics, antihistamines, tranquilizers, or alcohol, may produce additive depressant effects.
7. *Monoamine Oxidase Inhibitors (MAOI).* MAOI prolong the effects of barbiturates probably because metabolism of the barbiturate is inhibited.
8. *Estradiol, Estrone, Progesterone, and other Steroidal Hormones.* Pretreatment with or concurrent administration of phenobarbital may decrease the effect of estradiol by increasing its metabolism. There have been reports of patients treated with antiepileptic drugs (e.g., phenobarbital) who become pregnant while taking oral contraceptives. An alternate contraceptive method might be suggested to women taking phenobarbital.

Carcinogenesis

Animal Data. Phenobarbital sodium is carcinogenic in mice and rats after lifetime administration. In mice, it produced benign and malignant liver cell tumors. In rats, benign liver cell tumors were observed very late in life. Phenobarbital is the major metabolite of MEBARAL.

Human Data. In a 29-year epidemiological study of 9,136 patients who were treated on an anticonvulsant protocol which included phenobarbital, results indicated a higher than normal incidence of hepatic carcinoma. Previously, some of these patients were treated with thorotrast, a drug which is known to produce hepatic carcinomas. Thus, this study did not provide sufficient evidence that phenobarbital sodium is carcinogenic in humans. Phenobarbital is the major metabolite of MEBARAL.

A retrospective study of 84 children with brain tumors matched to 73 normal controls and 78 cancer controls (malignant disease other than brain tumors) suggested an association between exposure to barbiturates prenatally and an increased incidence of brain tumors.

Pregnancy

Teratogenic Effects. Pregnancy Category D-See WARNINGS-Use in Pregnancy.

Nonteratogenic Effects. Reports of infants suffering from long-term barbiturate exposure *in utero* included the acute withdrawal syndrome of seizures and hyperirritability from birth to a delayed onset of up to 14 days. (See DRUG ABUSE AND DEPENDENCE.)

Labor and Delivery. Hypnotic doses of these barbiturates do not appear to significantly impair uterine activity during labor. Full anesthetic doses of barbiturates decrease the force and frequency of uterine contractions. Administration of sedative-hypnotic barbiturates to the mother during labor may result in respiratory depression in the newborn. Premature infants are particularly susceptible to the depressant effects of barbiturates. If barbiturates are used during labor and delivery, resuscitation equipment should be available.

Data are currently not available to evaluate the effect of these barbiturates when forceps delivery or other intervention is necessary. Also, data are not available to determine the effect of these barbiturates on the later growth, development, and functional maturation of the child.

Nursing Mothers. Caution should be exercised when a barbiturate is administered to a nursing woman since small amounts of barbiturates are excreted in the milk.

ADVERSE REACTIONS

The following adverse reactions and their incidence were compiled from surveillance of thousands of hospitalized patients. Because such patients may be less aware of certain of the milder adverse effects of barbiturates, the incidence of these reactions may be somewhat higher in fully ambulatory patients.

More than 1 in 100 Patients. The most common adverse reactions estimated to occur at a rate of 1 to 3 patients per 100 is:

Nervous System: Somnolence.

Less than 1 in 100 Patients. Adverse reactions estimated to occur at a rate of less than 1 in 100 patients listed below, grouped by organ system, and by decreasing order of occurrence are:

Nervous System: Agitation, confusion, hyperkinesia, ataxia, CNS depression, nightmares, nervousness, psychiatric disturbance, hallucinations, insomnia, anxiety, dizziness, thinking abnormality.

Respiratory System: Hypoventilation, apnea.

Cardiovascular System: Bradycardia, hypotension, syncope.

Digestive System: Nausea, vomiting, constipation.

Other Reported Reactions: Headache, hypersensitivity reactions (angioedema, skin rashes, exfoliative dermatitis), fever, liver damage, megaloblastic anemia following chronic phenobarbital use.

DRUG ABUSE AND DEPENDENCE

Mephobarbital is a controlled substance in Narcotic Schedule IV. Barbiturates may be habit forming. Tolerance, psychological dependence, and physical dependence may occur especially following prolonged use of high doses of barbiturates. As tolerance to barbiturates develops, the amount needed to maintain the same level of intoxication increases; tolerance to a fatal dosage, however, does not increase more than two-fold. As this occurs, the margin between an intoxicating dosage and fatal dosage becomes smaller.

Symptoms of acute intoxication with barbiturates include unsteady gait, slurred speech, and sustained nystagmus. Mental signs of chronic intoxication include confusion, poor judgment, irritability, insomnia, and somatic complaints.

Symptoms of barbiturate dependence are similar to those of chronic alcoholism. If an individual appears to be intoxicated with alcohol to a degree that is radically disproportionate to the amount of alcohol in his or her blood the use of barbiturates should be suspected. The lethal dose of a barbiturate is far less if alcohol is also ingested.

The symptoms of barbiturate withdrawal can be severe and may cause death. Minor withdrawal symptoms may appear 8 to 12 hours after the last dose of a barbiturate. These symptoms usually appear in the following order: anxiety, muscle twitching, tremor of hands and fingers, progressive weakness, dizziness, distortion in visual perception, nausea, vomiting, insomnia, and orthostatic hypotension. Major withdrawal symptoms (convulsions and delirium) may occur within 16 hours and last up to 5 days after abrupt cessation of these drugs. Intensity of withdrawal symptoms gradually declines over a period of approximately 15 days. Individuals susceptible to a barbiturate abuse and dependence include alcoholics and opiate abusers, as well as other sedative-hypnotic and amphetamine abusers.

Drug dependence to barbiturates arises from repeated administration of a barbiturate or agent with barbiturate-like effect on a continuous basis, generally in amounts exceeding therapeutic dose levels. The characteristics of drug dependence to barbiturates include: (a) a strong desire or need to continue taking the drug; (b) a tendency to increase the dose; (c) a psychic dependence on the effects of the drug related to subjective and individual appreciation of those effects; and (d) a physical dependence on the effects of the drug requiring its presence for maintenance of homeostasis and resulting in a definite, characteristic, and self-limited abstinence syndrome when the drug is withdrawn.

Treatment of barbiturate dependence consists of cautious and gradual withdrawal of the drug. Barbiturate-dependent patients can be withdrawn by using a number of different withdrawal regimens. In all cases withdrawal takes an extended period of time. One method involves substituting a 30 mg dose of phenobarbital for each 100 mg to 200 mg dose of barbiturate that the patient has been taking. The total daily amount of phenobarbital is then administered in 3 to 4 divided doses, not to exceed 600 mg daily. Should signs of withdrawal occur on the first day of treatment, a loading dose of 100 mg to 200 mg of phenobarbital may be administered IM in addition to the oral dose. After stabilization on phenobarbital, the total daily dose is decreased by 30 mg a day as long as withdrawal is proceeding smoothly. A modification of this regimen involves initiating treatment at the patient's regular dosage level and decreasing the daily dosage by 10% if tolerated by the patient.

Infants physically dependent on barbiturates may be given phenobarbital 3 mg/kg/day to 10 mg/kg/day. After withdrawal symptoms (hyperactivity, disturbed sleep, tremors, hyperreflexia) are relieved, the dosage of phenobarbital should be gradually decreased and completely withdrawn over a 2-week period.

OVERDOSAGE

The toxic dose of barbiturates varies considerably. In general, an oral dose of 1 g of most barbiturates produces serious poisoning in an adult. Death commonly occurs after 2 g to 10 g of ingested barbiturate. Barbiturate intoxication may be confused with alcoholism, bromide intoxication, and with various neurological disorders.

Acute overdosage with barbiturates is manifested by CNS and respiratory depression which may progress to Cheyne-Stokes respiration, areflexia, constriction of the pupils to a slight degree (though in severe poisoning they may show paralytic dilation), oliguria, tachycardia, hypotension, lowered body temperature, and coma. Typical shock syndrome (apnea, circulatory collapse, respiratory arrest, and death) may occur.

In extreme overdose, all electrical activity in the brain may cease, in which case a "flat" EEG normally equated with clinical death cannot be accepted. This effect is fully reversible unless hypoxic damage occurs. Consideration should be given to the possibility of barbiturate intoxication even in situations that appear to involve trauma.

Complications such as pneumonia, pulmonary edema, cardiac arrhythmias, congestive heart failure, and renal failure may occur. Uremia may increase CNS sensitivity to barbiturates if renal function is impaired. Differential diagnosis should include hypoglycemia, head trauma, cerebrovascular accidents, convulsive states, and diabetic coma.

Treatment of overdosage is mainly supportive and consists of the following:

1. Maintenance of an adequate airway, with assisted respiration and oxygen administration as necessary.
2. Monitoring of vital signs and fluid balance.
3. If the patient is conscious and has not lost the gag reflex, emesis may be induced with ipecac. Care should be taken to prevent pulmonary aspiration of vomitus. After completion of vomiting, 30 g activated charcoal in a glass of water may be administered.
4. If emesis is contraindicated, gastric lavage may be performed with a cuffed endotracheal tube in place with the patient in the face down position. Activated charcoal may be left in the emptied stomach and a saline cathartic administered.
5. Fluid therapy and other standard treatment for shock, if needed.
6. If renal function is normal, forced diuresis may aid in the elimination of the barbiturate. Alkalinization of the urine increases renal excretion of some barbiturates, including mephobarbital (which is metabolized to phenobarbital).
7. Although not recommended as a routine procedure, hemodialysis may be used in severe barbiturate intoxications or if the patient is anuric or in shock.
8. Patient should be rolled from side to side every 30 minutes.
9. Antibiotics should be given if pneumonia is suspected.
10. Appropriate nursing care to prevent hypostatic pneumonia, decubiti aspiration, and other complications of patients with altered states of consciousness.

DOSAGE AND ADMINISTRATION

Epilepsy: Average dose for adults: 400 mg to 600 mg (6 grains to 9 grains) daily; children under 5 years: 16 mg to 32 mg (1/4 grain to 1/2 grain) three or four times daily; children over 5 years: 32 mg to 64 mg (1/2 grain to 1 grain) three or four times daily. MEBARAL is best taken at bedtime if seizures generally occur at night, and during the day if attacks are diurnal.

Treatment should be started with a small dose which is gradually increased over four or five days until the optimum dosage is determined. If the patient has been taking some other antiepileptic drug, it should be tapered off as the doses of MEBARAL are increased, to guard against the temporary marked attacks that may occur when any treatment for epilepsy is changed abruptly. Similarly, when the dose is lowered to a maintenance level or to be discontinued, the amount should be reduced gradually over four or five days.

Special Patient Population: Dosage should be reduced in the elderly or debilitated because these patients may be more sensitive to barbiturates. Dosage should be reduced for patients with impaired renal function or hepatic disease.

Combination with Other Drugs: MEBARAL may be used in combination with phenobarbital, either in the form of alternating courses or concurrently. When the two drugs are used at the same time, the dose should be about one-half the amount of each used alone. The average daily dose for an adult is from 50 mg to 100 mg (3/4 grain to 1 1/2 grains) of phenobarbital and from 200 mg to 300 mg (3 grains to 4 1/2 grains) of MEBARAL.

MEBARAL may also be used with phenytoin sodium; in some cases, combined therapy appears to give better results than either agent used alone, since phenytoin sodium is particularly effective for the psychomotor types of seizure but relatively ineffective for petit mal. When the drugs are employed concurrently, a reduced dose of phenytoin sodium is advisable, but the full dose of MEBARAL may be given. Satisfactory results have been obtained with an average daily dose of 230 mg (3 1/2 grains) of phenytoin sodium plus about 600 mg (9 grains) of MEBARAL.

Sedation: Adults: 32 mg to 100 mg (1/2 grain to 1 1/2 grains)–optimum dose, 50 mg (3/4 grain)–three to four times daily. Children: 16 mg to 32 mg (1/4 grain to 1/2 grain) three to four times daily.

HOW SUPPLIED

Tablets—white, round, convex and the 32 mg and 50 mg tablets are scored.

32 mg (1/2 grain), bottles of 250
(NDC 67386-801-02).
50 mg (3/4 grain), bottles of 250
(NDC 67386-802-02).
100 mg (1 1/2 grains), bottles of 250
(NDC 67386-803-02).

Store at room temperature up to 25° C (77° F).

Distributed by
OVATION Pharmaceuticals, Inc.
Deerfield, IL 60015, USA
Printed in USA Revised July 2003

Shown in Product Identification Guide, page 328

NEMBUTAL® ℂ ℞
SODIUM SOLUTION
(pentobarbital sodium injection, USP)
℞ only **No. 501**
Vials
DO NOT USE IF MATERIAL HAS PRECIPITATED

DESCRIPTION

The barbiturates are nonselective central nervous system depressants which are primarily used as sedative hypnotics and also anticonvulsants in subhypnotic doses. The barbiturates and their sodium salts are subject to control under the Federal Controlled Substances Act (See "Drug Abuse and Dependence" section).

The sodium salts of amobarbital, pentobarbital, phenobarbital, and secobarbital are available as sterile parenteral solutions.

Barbiturates are substituted pyrimidine derivatives in which the basic structure common to these drugs is barbituric acid, a substance which has no central nervous system (CNS) activity. CNS activity is obtained by substituting alkyl, alkenyl, or aryl groups on the pyrimidine ring.

NEMBUTAL Sodium Solution (pentobarbital sodium injection) is a sterile solution for intravenous or intramuscular injection. Each mL contains pentobarbital sodium 50 mg, in a vehicle of propylene glycol, 40%, alcohol, 10% and water for injection, to volume. The pH is adjusted to approximately 9.5 with hydrochloric acid and/or sodium hydroxide.

NEMBUTAL Sodium is a short-acting barbiturate, chemically designated as sodium 5-ethyl-5-(1-methylbutyl) barbiturate. The structural formula for pentobarbital sodium is:

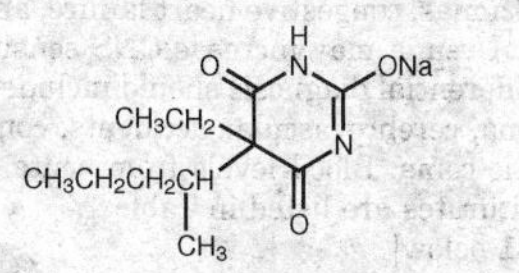

The sodium salt occurs as a white, slightly bitter powder which is freely soluble in water and alcohol but practically insoluble in benzene and ether.

CLINICAL PHARMACOLOGY

Barbiturates are capable of producing all levels of CNS mood alteration from excitation to mild sedation, to hypnosis, and deep coma. Overdosage can produce death. In high enough therapeutic doses, barbiturates induce anesthesia.

Barbiturates depress the sensory cortex, decrease motor activity, alter cerebellar function, and produce drowsiness, sedation, and hypnosis.

Barbiturate-induced sleep differs from physiological sleep. Sleep laboratory studies have demonstrated that barbiturates reduce the amount of time spent in the rapid eye movement (REM) phase of sleep or dreaming stage. Also, Stages III and IV sleep are decreased. Following abrupt cessation of barbiturates used regularly, patients may experience markedly increased dreaming, nightmares, and/or insomnia. Therefore, withdrawal of a single therapeutic dose over 5 or 6 days has been recommended to lessen the REM rebound and disturbed sleep which contribute to drug withdrawal syndrome (for example, decrease the dose from 3 to 2 doses a day for 1 week).

In studies, secobarbital sodium and pentobarbital sodium have been found to lose most of their effectiveness for both inducing and maintaining sleep by the end of 2 weeks of continued drug administration at fixed doses. The short-, intermediate-, and, to a lesser degree, long-acting barbiturates have been widely prescribed for treating insomnia. Although the clinical literature abounds with claims that the short-acting barbiturates are superior for producing sleep while the intermediate-acting compounds are more effective in maintaining sleep, controlled studies have failed to demonstrate these differential effects. Therefore, as sleep medications, the barbiturates are of limited value beyond short-term use.

Barbiturates have little analgesic action at subanesthetic doses. Rather, in subanesthetic doses these drugs may increase the reaction to painful stimuli. All barbiturates exhibit anticonvulsant activity in anesthetic doses. However, of the drugs in this class, only phenobarbital, mephobarbital, and metharbital have been clinically demonstrated to be effective as oral anticonvulsants in subhypnotic doses.

Barbiturates are respiratory depressants. The degree of respiratory depression is dependent upon dose. With hypnotic doses, respiratory depression produced by barbiturates is similar to that which occurs during physiologic sleep with slight decrease in blood pressure and heart rate.

Studies in laboratory animals have shown that barbiturates cause reduction in the tone and contractility of the uterus, ureters, and urinary bladder. However, concentrations of the drugs required to produce this effect in humans are not reached with sedative-hypnotic doses.

Barbiturates do not impair normal hepatic function, but have been shown to induce liver microsomal enzymes, thus increasing and/or altering the metabolism of barbiturates and other drugs. (See "Precautions—*Drug Interactions*" section).

Pharmacokinetics:
Barbiturates are absorbed in varying degrees following oral, rectal, or parenteral administration. The salts are more rapidly absorbed than are the acids.

The onset of action for oral or rectal administration varies from 20 to 60 minutes. For IM administration, the onset of action is slightly faster. Following IV administration, the onset of action ranges from almost immediately for pentobarbital sodium to 5 minutes for phenobarbital sodium. Maximal CNS depression may not occur until 15 minutes or more after IV administration for phenobarbital sodium.

Duration of action, which is related to the rate at which the barbiturates are redistributed throughout the body, varies among persons and in the same person from time to time.

No studies have demonstrated that the different routes of administration are equivalent with respect to bioavailability.

Barbiturates are weak acids that are absorbed and rapidly distributed to all tissues and fluids with high concentrations in the brain, liver, and kidneys. Lipid solubility of the barbiturates is the dominant factor in their distribution within the body. The more lipid soluble the barbiturate, the more rapidly it penetrates all tissues of the body. Barbiturates are bound to plasma and tissue proteins to a varying degree with the degree of binding increasing directly as a function of lipid solubility.

Phenobarbital has the lowest lipid solubility, lowest plasma binding, lowest brain protein binding, the longest delay in onset of activity, and the longest duration of action. At the opposite extreme is secobarbital which has the highest lipid solubility, plasma protein binding, brain protein binding, the shortest delay in onset of activity, and the shortest duration of action. Butabarbital is classified as an intermediate barbiturate.

The plasma half-life for pentobarbital in adults is 15 to 50 hours and appears to be dose dependent.

Barbiturates are metabolized primarily by the hepatic microsomal enzyme system, and the metabolic products are excreted in the urine, and less commonly, in the feces. Approximately 25 to 50 percent of a dose of aprobarbital or phenobarbital is eliminated unchanged in the urine, whereas the amount of other barbiturates excreted unchanged in the urine is negligible. The excretion of unmetabolized barbiturate is one feature that distinguishes the long-acting category from those belonging to other categories which are almost entirely metabolized. The inactive metabolites of the barbiturates are excreted as conjugates of glucuronic acid.

INDICATIONS AND USAGE

Parenteral:
a. Sedatives.
b. Hypnotics, for the short-term treatment of insomnia, since they appear to lose their effectiveness for sleep induction and sleep maintenance after 2 weeks (See "Clinical Pharmacology" section).
c. Preanesthetics.
d. Anticonvulsant, in anesthetic doses, in the emergency control of certain acute convulsive episodes, e.g., those associated with status epilepticus, cholera, eclampsia, meningitis, tetanus, and toxic reactions to strychnine or local anesthetics.

CONTRAINDICATIONS

Barbiturates are contraindicated in patients with known barbiturate sensitivity. Barbiturates are also contraindicated in patients with a history of manifest or latent porphyria.

WARNINGS

1. *Habit forming:* Barbiturates may be habit forming. Tolerance, psychological and physical dependence may occur with continued use. (See "Drug Abuse and Dependence" and "Pharmacokinetics" sections). Patients who have psychological dependence on barbiturates may increase the dosage or decrease the dosage interval without consulting a physician and may subsequently develop a physical dependence on barbiturates. To minimize the possibility of overdosage or the development of dependence, the prescribing and dispensing of sedative-hypnotic barbiturates should be limited to the amount required for the interval until the next appointment. Abrupt cessation after prolonged use in the dependent person may result in withdrawal symptoms, including delirium, convulsions, and possibly death. Barbiturates should be withdrawn gradually from any patient known to be taking excessive dosage over long periods of time. (See "Drug Abuse and Dependence" section).
2. *IV administration:* Too rapid administration may cause respiratory depression, apnea, laryngospasm, or vasodilation with fall in blood pressure.
3. *Acute or chronic pain:* Caution should be exercised when barbiturates are administered to patients with acute or chronic pain, because paradoxical excitement could be induced or important symptoms could be masked. However, the use of barbiturates as sedatives in the postoperative surgical period and as adjuncts to cancer chemotherapy is well established.
4. *Use in pregnancy:* Barbiturates can cause fetal damage when administered to a pregnant woman. Retrospective, case-controlled studies have suggested a connection between the maternal consumption of barbiturates and a higher than expected incidence of fetal abnormalities. Following oral or parenteral administration, barbiturates readily cross the placental barrier and are distributed throughout fetal tissues with highest concentrations found in the placenta, fetal liver, and brain. Fetal blood levels approach maternal blood levels following parenteral administration.
   Withdrawal symptoms occur in infants born to mothers who receive barbiturates throughout the last trimester of pregnancy. (See "Drug Abuse and Dependence" section). If this drug is used during pregnancy, or if the patient becomes pregnant while taking this drug, the patient should be apprised of the potential hazard to the fetus.
5. *Synergistic effects:* The concomitant use of alcohol or other CNS depressants may produce additive CNS depressant effects.

PRECAUTIONS

General:
Barbiturates may be habit forming. Tolerance and psychological and physical dependence may occur with continuing use. (See "Drug Abuse and Dependence" section). Barbiturates should be administered with caution, if at all, to patients who are mentally depressed, have suicidal tendencies, or a history of drug abuse.

Elderly or debilitated patients may react to barbiturates with marked excitement, depression, and confusion. In some persons, barbiturates repeatedly produce excitement rather than depression.

In patients with hepatic damage, barbiturates should be administered with caution and initially in reduced doses. Barbiturates should not be administered to patients showing the premonitory signs of hepatic coma.

Parenteral solutions of barbiturates are highly alkaline. Therefore, extreme care should be taken to avoid perivascular extravasation or intra-arterial injection. Extravascular injection may cause local tissue damage with subsequent necrosis; consequences of intra-arterial injection may vary from transient pain to gangrene of the limb. Any complaint of pain in the limb warrants stopping the injection.

Information for the patient:
Practitioners should give the following information and instructions to patients receiving barbiturates.
1. The use of barbiturates carries with it an associated risk of psychological and/or physical dependence. The patient should be warned against increasing the dose of the drug without consulting a physician.
2. Barbiturates may impair mental and/or physical abilities required for the performance of potentially hazardous tasks (e.g., driving, operating machinery, etc.).
3. Alcohol should not be consumed while taking barbiturates. Concurrent use of the barbiturates with other CNS depressants (e.g., alcohol, narcotics, tranquilizers, and antihistamines) may result in additional CNS depressant effects.

Laboratory tests:
Prolonged therapy with barbiturates should be accompanied by periodic laboratory evaluation of organ systems, including hematopoietic, renal, and hepatic systems. (See "Precautions-*General*" and "Adverse Reactions" sections).

Drug interactions:
Most reports of clinically significant drug interactions occurring with the barbiturates have involved phenobarbital. However, the application of these data to other barbiturates appears valid and warrants serial blood level determinations of the relevant drugs when there are multiple therapies.
1. *Anticoagulants:* Phenobarbital lowers the plasma levels of dicumarol (name previously used: bishydroxycoumarin) and causes a decrease in anticoagulant activity as measured by the prothrombin time. Barbiturates can induce hepatic microsomal enzymes resulting in increased metabolism and decreased anticoagulant response of oral anticoagulants (e.g., warfarin, acenocoumarol, dicumarol, and phenprocoumon). Patients stabilized on anticoagulant therapy may require dosage adjustments if barbiturates are added to or withdrawn from their dosage regimen.
2. *Corticosteroids:* Barbiturates appear to enhance the metabolism of exogenous corticosteroids probably through the induction of hepatic microsomal enzymes. Patients stabilized on corticosteroid therapy may require dosage adjustments if barbiturates are added to or withdrawn from their dosage regimen.
3. *Griseofulvin:* Phenobarbital appears to interfere with the absorption of orally administered griseofulvin, thus decreasing its blood level. The effect of the resultant decreased blood levels of griseofulvin on therapeutic response has not been established. However, it would be preferable to avoid concomitant administration of these drugs.
4. *Doxycycline:* Phenobarbital has been shown to shorten the half-life of doxycycline for as long as 2 weeks after barbiturate therapy is discontinued.
   This mechanism is probably through the induction of hepatic microsomal enzymes that metabolize the antibiotic. If phenobarbital and doxycycline are administered concurrently, the clinical response to doxycycline should be monitored closely.
5. *Phenytoin, sodium valproate, valproic acid:* The effect of barbiturates on the metabolism of phenytoin appears to be variable. Some investigators report an accelerating effect, while others report no effect. Because the effect of barbiturates on the metabolism of phenytoin is not predictable, phenytoin and barbiturate blood levels should be monitored more frequently if these drugs are given concurrently. Sodium valproate and valproic acid appear to decrease barbiturate metabolism; therefore, barbiturate blood levels should be monitored and appropriate dosage adjustments made as indicated.

Continued on next page

Nembutal—Cont.

6. *Central nervous system depressants:* The concomitant use of other central nervous system depressants, including other sedatives or hypnotics, antihistamines, tranquilizers, or alcohol, may produce additive depressant effects.
7. *Monoamine oxidase inhibitors (MAOI):* MAOI prolong the effects of barbiturates probably because metabolism of the barbiturate is inhibited.
8. *Estradiol, estrone, progesterone and other steroidal hormones:* Pretreatment with or concurrent administration of phenobarbital may decrease the effect of estradiol by increasing its metabolism. There have been reports of patients treated with antiepileptic drugs (e.g., phenobarbital) who became pregnant while taking oral contraceptives. An alternate contraceptive method might be suggested to women taking phenobarbital.

Carcinogenesis:
1. *Animal data.* Phenobarbital sodium is carcinogenic in mice and rats after lifetime administration. In mice, it produced benign and malignant liver cell tumors. In rats, benign liver cell tumors were observed very late in life.
2. *Human data.* In a 29-year epidemiological study of 9,136 patients who were treated on an anticonvulsant protocol that included phenobarbital, results indicated a higher than normal incidence of hepatic carcinoma. Previously, some of these patients were treated with thorotrast, a drug that is known to produce hepatic carcinomas. Thus, this study did not provide sufficient evidence that phenobarbital sodium is carcinogenic in humans.

Data from one retrospective study of 235 children in which the types of barbiturates are not identified suggested an association between exposure to barbiturates prenatally and an increased incidence of brain tumor. (Gold, E., et al., "Increased Risk of Brain Tumors in Children Exposed to Barbiturates," Journal of National Cancer Institute, 61:1031-1034, 1978).

Pregnancy:
1. *Teratogenic effects.* Pregnancy Category D—See "Warnings—Use in Pregnancy" section.
2. *Nonteratogenic effects.* Reports of infants suffering from long-term barbiturate exposure in utero included the acute withdrawal syndrome of seizures and hyperirritability from birth to a delayed onset of up to 14 days. (See "Drug Abuse and Dependence" section).

Labor and delivery:
Hypnotic doses of these barbiturates do not appear to significantly impair uterine activity during labor. Full anesthetic doses of barbiturates decrease the force and frequency of uterine contractions. Administration of sedative-hypnotic barbiturates to the mother during labor may result in respiratory depression in the newborn. Premature infants are particularly susceptible to the depressant effects of barbiturates. If barbiturates are used during labor and delivery, resuscitation equipment should be available.
Data are currently not available to evaluate the effect of these barbiturates when forceps delivery or other intervention is necessary. Also, data are not available to determine the effect of these barbiturates on the later growth, development, and functional maturation of the child.

Nursing mothers:
Caution should be exercised when a barbiturate is administered to a nursing woman since small amounts of barbiturates are excreted in the milk.

ADVERSE REACTIONS

The following adverse reactions and their incidence were compiled from surveillance of thousands of hospitalized patients. Because such patients may be less aware of certain of the milder adverse effects of barbiturates, the incidence of these reactions may be somewhat higher in fully ambulatory patients.
More than 1 in 100 patients. The most common adverse reaction estimated to occur at a rate of 1 to 3 patients per 100 is: *Nervous System:* Somnolence.
Less than 1 in 100 patients. Adverse reactions estimated to occur at a rate of less than 1 in 100 patients listed below, grouped by organ system, and by decreasing order of occurrence are:
Nervous system: Agitation, confusion, hyperkinesia, ataxia, CNS depression, nightmares, nervousness, psychiatric disturbance, hallucinations, insomnia, anxiety, dizziness, thinking abnormality.
Respiratory system: Hypoventilation, apnea.
Cardiovascular system: Bradycardia, hypotension, syncope.
Digestive system: Nausea, vomiting, constipation.
Other reported reactions: Headache, injection site reactions, hypersensitivity reactions (angioedema, skin rashes, exfoliative dermatitis), fever, liver damage, megaloblastic anemia following chronic phenobarbital use.

DRUG ABUSE AND DEPENDENCE

Pentobarbital sodium injection is subject to control by the Federal Controlled Substances Act under DEA schedule II.
Barbiturates may be habit forming. Tolerance, psychological dependence, and physical dependence may occur especially following prolonged use of high doses of barbiturates. Daily administration in excess of 400 milligrams (mg) of pentobarbital or secobarbital for approximately 90 days is likely to produce some degree of physical dependence. A dosage of from 600 to 800 mg taken for at least 35 days is sufficient to produce withdrawal seizures. The average daily dose for the barbiturate addict is usually about 1.5 grams. As tolerance to barbiturates develops, the amount needed to maintain the same level of intoxication increases; tolerance to a fatal dosage, however, does not increase more than two-fold. As this occurs, the margin between an intoxicating dosage and fatal dosage becomes smaller.
Symptoms of acute intoxication with barbiturates include unsteady gait, slurred speech, and sustained nystagmus. Mental signs of chronic intoxication include confusion, poor judgment, irritability, insomnia, and somatic complaints.
Symptoms of barbiturate dependence are similar to those of chronic alcoholism. If an individual appears to be intoxicated with alcohol to a degree that is radically disproportionate to the amount of alcohol in his or her blood the use of barbiturates should be suspected. The lethal dose of a barbiturate is far less if alcohol is also ingested.
The symptoms of barbiturate withdrawal can be severe and may cause death. Minor withdrawal symptoms may appear 8 to 12 hours after the last dose of a barbiturate. These symptoms usually appear in the following order: anxiety, muscle twitching, tremor of hands and fingers, progressive weakness, dizziness, distortion in visual perception, nausea, vomiting, insomnia, and orthostatic hypotension. Major withdrawal symptoms (convulsions and delirium) may occur within 16 hours and last up to 5 days after abrupt cessation of these drugs. Intensity of withdrawal symptoms gradually declines over a period of approximately 15 days. Individuals susceptible to barbiturate abuse and dependence include alcoholics and opiate abusers, as well as other sedative-hypnotic and amphetamine abusers.
Drug dependence to barbiturates arises from repeated administration of a barbiturate or agent with barbiturate-like effect on a continuous basis, generally in amounts exceeding therapeutic dose levels. The characteristics of drug dependence to barbiturates include: (a) a strong desire or need to continue taking the drug; (b) a tendency to increase the dose; (c) a psychic dependence on the effects of the drug related to subjective and individual appreciation of those effects; and (d) a physical dependence on the effects of the drug requiring its presence for maintenance of homeostasis and resulting in a definite, characteristic, and self-limited abstinence syndrome when the drug is withdrawn.
Treatment of barbiturate dependence consists of cautious and gradual withdrawal of the drug. Barbiturate-dependent patients can be withdrawn by using a number of different withdrawal regimens. In all cases withdrawal takes an extended period of time. One method involves substituting a 30 mg dose of phenobarbital for each 100 to 200 mg dose of barbiturate that the patient has been taking. The total daily amount of phenobarbital is then administered in 3 to 4 divided doses, not to exceed 600 mg daily. Should signs of withdrawal occur on the first day of treatment, a loading dose of 100 to 200 mg of phenobarbital may be administered IM in addition to the oral dose. After stabilization on phenobarbital, the total daily dose is decreased by 30 mg a day as long as withdrawal is proceeding smoothly. A modification of this regimen involves initiating treatment at the patient's regular dosage level and decreasing the daily dosage by 10 percent if tolerated by the patient.
Infants physically dependent on barbiturates may be given phenobarbital 3 to 10 mg/kg/day. After withdrawal symptoms (hyperactivity, disturbed sleep, tremors, hyperreflexia) are relieved, the dosage of phenobarbital should be gradually decreased and completely withdrawn over a 2-week period.

OVERDOSAGE

The toxic dose of barbiturates varies considerably. In general, an oral dose of 1 gram of most barbiturates produces serious poisoning in an adult. Death commonly occurs after 2 to 10 grams of ingested barbiturate. Barbiturate intoxication may be confused with alcoholism, bromide intoxication, and with various neurological disorders.
Acute overdosage with barbiturates is manifested by CNS and respiratory depression which may progress to Cheyne-Stokes respiration, areflexia, constriction of the pupils to a slight degree (though in severe poisoning they may show paralytic dilation), oliguria, tachycardia, hypotension, lowered body temperature, and coma. Typical shock syndrome (apnea, circulatory collapse, respiratory arrest, and death) may occur.
In extreme overdose, all electrical activity in the brain may cease, in which case a "flat" EEG normally equated with clinical death cannot be accepted. This effect is fully reversible unless hypoxic damage occurs. Consideration should be given to the possibility of barbiturate intoxication even in situations that appear to involve trauma.
Complications such as pneumonia, pulmonary edema, cardiac arrhythmias, congestive heart failure, and renal failure may occur. Uremia may increase CNS sensitivity to barbiturates. Differential diagnosis should include hypoglycemia, head trauma, cerebrovascular accidents, convulsive states, and diabetic coma. Blood levels from acute overdosage for some barbiturates are listed in Table 1.
[See table 1 below]
Treatment of overdosage is mainly supportive and consists of the following:
1. Maintenance of an adequate airway, with assisted respiration and oxygen administration as necessary.
2. Monitoring of vital signs and fluid balance.
3. Fluid therapy and other standard treatment for shock, if needed.
4. If renal function is normal, forced diuresis may aid in the elimination of the barbiturate. Alkalinization of the urine increases renal excretion of some barbiturates, especially phenobarbital, also aprobarbital and mephobarbital (which is metabolized to phenobarbital).
5. Although not recommended as a routine procedure, hemodialysis may be used in severe barbiturate intoxications or if the patient is anuric or in shock.
6. Patient should be rolled from side to side every 30 minutes.
7. Antibiotics should be given if pneumonia is suspected.
8. Appropriate nursing care to prevent hypostatic pneumonia, decubiti, aspiration, and other complications of patients with altered states of consciousness.

DOSAGE AND ADMINISTRATION

Dosages of barbiturates must be individualized with full knowledge of their particular characteristics and recommended rate of administration. Factors of consideration are the patient's age, weight, and condition. Parenteral routes should be used only when oral administration is impossible or impractical.
Intramuscular Administration: IM injection of the sodium salts of barbiturates should be made deeply into a large muscle, and a volume of 5 mL should not be exceeded at any one site because of possible tissue irritation. After IM injection of a hypnotic dose, the patient's vital signs should be monitored. The usual adult dosage of NEMBUTAL Sodium Solution is 150 to 200 mg as a single IM injection; the recommended pediatric dosage ranges from 2 to 6 mg/kg as a single IM injection not to exceed 100 mg.
Intravenous Administration: NEMBUTAL Sodium Solution should not be admixed with any other medication or solution. IV injection is restricted to conditions in which other routes are not feasible, either because the patient is unconscious (as in cerebral hemorrhage, eclampsia, or status epilepticus), or because the patient resists (as in delirium), or because prompt action is imperative. Slow IV injection is essential, and patients should be carefully observed during administration. This requires that blood pressure, respiration, and cardiac function be maintained, vital signs be recorded, and equipment for resuscitation and artificial ventilation be available. The rate of IV injection should not exceed 50 mg/min for pentobarbital sodium.
There is no average intravenous dose of NEMBUTAL Sodium Solution (pentobarbital sodium injection) that can be relied on to produce similar effects in different patients. The possibility of overdose and respiratory depression is remote when the drug is injected slowly in fractional doses.
A commonly used initial dose for the 70 kg adult is 100 mg. Proportional reduction in dosage should be made for pediatric or debilitated patients. At least one minute is necessary to determine the full effect of intravenous pentobarbital. If necessary, additional small increments of the drug may be given up to a total of from 200 to 500 mg for normal adults.
Anticonvulsant use: In convulsive states, dosage of NEMBUTAL Sodium Solution should be kept to a minimum to avoid compounding the depression which may follow con-

Table 1.— *Concentration of Barbiturate in the Blood Versus Degree of CNS Depression*

		Blood barbiturate level in ppm (μg/mL)				
Barbiturate	Onset/ duration	Degree of depression in nontolerant persons*				
		1	2	3	4	5
Pentobarbital	Fast/short	≤2	0.5 to 3	10 to 15	12 to 25	15 to 40
Secobarbital	Fast/short	≤2	0.5 to 5	10 to 15	15 to 25	15 to 40
Amobarbital	Intermediate/ intermediate	≤3	2 to 10	30 to 40	30 to 60	40 to 80
Butabarbital	Intermediate/ intermediate	≤5	3 to 25	40 to 60	50 to 80	60 to 100
Phenobarbital	Slow/long	≤10	5 to 40	50 to 80	70 to 120	100 to 200

*Categories of degree of depression in nontolerant persons:
1. Under the influence and appreciably impaired for purposes of driving a motor vehicle or performing tasks requiring alertness and unimpaired judgment and reaction time.
2. Sedated, therapeutic range, calm, relaxed, and easily aroused.
3. Comatose, difficult to arouse, significant depression of respiration.
4. Compatible with death in aged or ill persons or in presence of obstructed airway, other toxic agents, or exposure to cold.
5. Usual lethal level, the upper end of the range includes those who received some supportive treatment.

vulsions. The injection must be made slowly with due regard to the time required for the drug to penetrate the blood-brain barrier.

Special patient population: Dosage should be reduced in the elderly or debilitated because these patients may be more sensitive to barbiturates. Dosage should be reduced for patients with impaired renal function or hepatic disease.

Inspection: Parenteral drug products should be inspected visually for particulate matter and discoloration prior to administration, whenever solution containers permit. Solutions for injection showing evidence of precipitation should not be used.

HOW SUPPLIED

NEMBUTAL Sodium Solution (pentobarbital sodium injection, USP) is available in the following sizes: 20-mL multiple-dose vial, 1 g per vial (**NDC** 67386-501-52); and 50-mL multiple-dose vial, 2.5 g per vial (**NDC** 67386-501-55).

Each mL contains:

Pentobarbital Sodium, derivative of barbituric acid	50 mg
Propylene glycol	40% v/v
Alcohol	10%
Water for Injection	qs

(pH adjusted to approximately 9.5 with hydrochloric acid and/or sodium hydroxide.)

Vial stoppers are latex free.

Exposure of pharmaceutical products to heat should be minimized. Avoid excessive heat. Protect from freezing. It is recommended that the product be stored at room temperature, 86°F (30°C); however, brief exposure up to 104°F (40°C) does not adversely affect the product.

Revised: July, 2003

Manufactured by Abbott Laboratories,
North Chicago, Illinois 60064 U.S.A.
Distributed by
OVATION PHARMACEUTICALS, INC.
Deerfield, Illinois, U.S.A. 60015

Shown in Product Identification Guide, page 329

PEGANONE® 250 mg ℞

[pĕg-ă-nōn]
ETHOTOIN TABLETS, USP
℞ Only **No. 601**

DESCRIPTION

PEGANONE (ethotoin tablets, USP) is an oral antiepileptic of the hydantoin series and is chemically identified as 3-ethyl-5-phenyl-2,4-imidazolidinedione. It is represented by the following structural formula:

PEGANONE tablets are available in a dosage strength of 250 mg.

Inactive Ingredients

Acacia, lactose, sodium carboxymethylcellulose, stearic acid and talc.

CLINICAL PHARMACOLOGY

PEGANONE (ethotoin tablets, USP) exerts an antiepileptic effect without causing general central nervous system depression. The mechanism of action is probably very similar to that of phenytoin. The latter drug appears to stabilize rather than to raise the normal seizure threshold, and to prevent the spread of seizure activity rather than to abolish the primary focus of seizure discharges.

Ethotoin is fairly rapidly absorbed; the extent of oral absorption is not known. The drug exhibits saturable metabolism with respect to the formation of N-deethyl and p-hydroxyl-ethotoin, the major metabolites. Where plasma concentrations are below about 8 µg/mL, the elimination half-life of ethotoin is in the range of 3 to 9 hours. A study comparing single doses of 500 mg, 1000 mg, and 1500 mg of PEGANONE (ethotoin tablets, USP) demonstrated that ethotoin, and to a lesser extent 5-phenylhydantoin, a major metabolite, exhibits substantial nonlinear kinetics. The degree of nonlinearity with multiple dosing may be increased over that seen after a single dose, given the likelihood of plasma accumulation based on a reported elimination half-life of 6 to 9 hours and a dosing interval of 4 to 6 hours. Experience suggests that therapeutic plasma concentrations fall in the range of 15 to 50 µg/mL; however, this range is not as extensively documented as those quoted for other antiepileptics.

In laboratory animals, the drug was found effective against electroshock convulsions, and to a lesser extent, against complex partial (psychomotor) and pentylenetetrazol-induced seizures. In mice, the duration of antiepileptic activity was prolonged by hepatic injury but not by bilateral nephrectomy; the drug is apparently biotransformed by the liver.

INDICATIONS AND USAGE

PEGANONE (ethotoin tablets, USP) is indicated for the control of tonic-clonic (grand mal) and complex partial (psychomotor) seizures.

CONTRAINDICATIONS

PEGANONE (ethotoin tablets, USP) is contraindicated in patients with hepatic abnormalities or hematologic disorders.

WARNINGS

PEGANONE (ETHOTOIN TABLETS, USP) CAN CAUSE FETAL HARM WHEN ADMINISTERED TO A PREGNANT WOMAN. THERE ARE MULTIPLE REPORTS IN THE CLINICAL LITERATURE WHICH INDICATE THAT THE USE OF ANTIEPILEPTIC DRUGS DURING PREGNANCY RESULTS IN AN INCREASED INCIDENCE OF BIRTH DEFECTS IN THE OFFSPRING. ALTHOUGH DATA ARE MORE EXTENSIVE WITH RESPECT TO PHENYTOIN AND PHENOBARBITAL, REPORTS INDICATE A POSSIBLE SIMILAR ASSOCIATION WITH THE USE OF OTHER ANTIEPILEPTIC DRUGS. THEREFORE, ANTIEPILEPTIC DRUGS SHOULD BE ADMINISTERED TO WOMEN OF CHILD-BEARING POTENTIAL ONLY IF THEY ARE CLEARLY SHOWN TO BE ESSENTIAL IN THE MANAGEMENT OF THEIR SEIZURES.

ANTIEPILEPTIC DRUGS SHOULD NOT BE DISCONTINUED IN PATIENTS IN WHOM THE DRUG IS ADMINISTERED TO PREVENT MAJOR SEIZURES BECAUSE OF THE STRONG POSSIBILITY OF PRECIPITATING STATUS EPILEPTICUS WITH ATTENDANT HYPOXIA AND RISK TO BOTH MOTHER AND THE UNBORN CHILD. CONSIDERATION SHOULD, HOWEVER, BE GIVEN TO DISCONTINUATION OF ANTIEPILEPTICS PRIOR TO AND DURING PREGNANCY WHEN THE NATURE, FREQUENCY AND SEVERITY OF THE SEIZURES DO NOT POSE A SERIOUS THREAT TO THE PATIENT. IT IS NOT, HOWEVER, KNOWN WHETHER EVEN MINOR SEIZURES CONSTITUTE SOME RISK TO THE DEVELOPING EMBRYO OR FETUS.

REPORTS HAVE SUGGESTED THAT THE MATERNAL INGESTION OF ANTIEPILEPTIC DRUGS, PARTICULARLY BARBITURATES, IS ASSOCIATED WITH A NEONATAL COAGULATION DEFECT THAT MAY CAUSE BLEEDING DURING THE EARLY (USUALLY WITHIN 24 HOURS OF BIRTH) NEONATAL PERIOD. THE POSSIBILITY OF THE OCCURRENCE OF THIS DEFECT WITH THE USE OF PEGANONE SHOULD BE KEPT IN MIND. THE DEFECT IS CHARACTERIZED BY DECREASED LEVELS OF VITAMIN K-DEPENDENT CLOTTING FACTORS, AND PROLONGATION OF EITHER THE PROTHROMBIN TIME OR THE PARTIAL THROMBOPLASTIN TIME, OR BOTH. IT HAS BEEN SUGGESTED THAT VITAMIN K BE GIVEN PROPHYLACTICALLY TO THE MOTHER ONE MONTH PRIOR TO AND DURING DELIVERY, AND THE INFANT, INTRAVENOUSLY, IMMEDIATELY AFTER BIRTH.

IF PEGANONE IS USED DURING PREGNANCY, OR IF THE PATIENT BECOMES PREGNANT WHILE TAKING THIS DRUG, THE PATIENT SHOULD BE APPRISED OF THE POTENTIAL HAZARD TO THE FETUS.

PRECAUTIONS

General:

Blood dyscrasias have been reported in patients receiving PEGANONE. Although the etiologic role of PEGANONE has not been definitely established, physicians should be alert for general malaise, sore throat and other symptoms indicative of possible blood dyscrasia.

There is some evidence suggesting that hydantoin-like compounds may interfere with folic acid metabolism, precipitating a megaloblastic anemia. If this should occur during gestation, folic acid therapy should be considered.

Information for Patients:

Patients should be advised to report immediately such signs and symptoms as sore throat, fever, malaise, easy bruising, petechiae, epistaxis, skin rash or others that may be indicative of an infection or bleeding tendency.

Laboratory Tests:

Liver function tests should be performed if clinical evidence suggests the possibility of hepatic dysfunction. Signs of liver damage are indication for withdrawal of the drug.

It is recommended that blood counts and urinalyses be performed when therapy is begun and at monthly intervals for several months thereafter. As in patients receiving other hydantoin compounds and other antiepileptic drugs, blood dyscrasias have been reported in patients receiving PEGANONE (ethotoin tablets, USP). Marked depression of the blood count is indication for withdrawal of the drug.

Drug Interactions:

PEGANONE used in combination with other drugs known to adversely affect the hematopoietic system should be avoided if possible.

A two-way interaction between the hydantoin antiepileptic, phenytoin, and the coumarin anticoagulants has been suggested. Presumably, phenytoin acts as a stimulator of coumarin metabolism and has been reported to cause decreased serum levels of the coumarin anticoagulants and increased prothrombin-proconvertin concentrations. Conversely, the coumarin anticoagulants have been reported to increase the serum levels and prolong the serum half-life of phenytoin by inhibiting its metabolism. Although there is no documentation of such, a similar interaction between ethotoin and the coumarin anticoagulants may occur. Caution is therefore advised when administering PEGANONE to patients receiving coumarin anticoagulants.

Carcinogenesis, Mutagenesis, Impairment of Fertility:

No data are available on long-term potential for carcinogenicity in animals or humans.

Pregnancy:

Pregnancy Category D. See "Warnings" section.

Nonteratogenic Effects:

Reports have suggested that the maternal ingestion of antiepileptic drugs, particularly barbiturates, is associated with a neonatal coagulation defect that may cause bleeding during the early (usually within 24 hours of birth) neonatal period. The possibility of the occurrence of this defect with the use of PEGANONE should be kept in mind. See "**WARNINGS**" section.

Nursing Mothers:

Ethotoin is excreted in breast milk. Because of the potential for serious adverse reactions in nursing infants from ethotoin, a decision should be made whether to discontinue nursing or to discontinue the drug, taking into account the importance of the drug to the mother.

ADVERSE REACTIONS

Adverse reactions associated with PEGANONE, in decreasing order of severity, are:

Isolated cases of lymphadenopathy and systemic lupus erythematosus have been reported in patients taking hydantoin compounds, and lymphadenopathy has occurred with PEGANONE. Withdrawal of therapy has resulted in remission of the clinical and pathological findings. Therefore, if a lymphoma-like syndrome develops, the drug should be withdrawn and the patient should be closely observed for regression of signs and symptoms before treatment is resumed.

Ataxia and gum hypertrophy have occurred only rarely—usually only in patients receiving an additional hydantoin derivative. It is of interest to note that ataxia and gum hypertrophy have subsided in patients receiving other hydantoins when PEGANONE (ethotoin tablets, USP) was given as a substitute antiepileptic.

Occasionally, vomiting or nausea after ingestion of PEGANONE has been reported, but if the drug is administered after meals, the incidence of gastric distress is reduced. Other side effects have included chest pain, nystagmus, diplopia, fever, dizziness, diarrhea, headache, insomnia, fatigue, numbness, skin rash, and Stevens-Johnson syndrome.

OVERDOSAGE

Symptoms of acute overdosage include drowsiness, visual disturbance, nausea and ataxia. Coma is possible at very high dosage.

Treatment should be begun by inducing emesis; gastric lavage may be considered as an alternative. General supportive measures will be necessary. A careful evaluation of blood-forming organs should be made following recovery.

DOSAGE AND ADMINISTRATION

PEGANONE (ethotoin tablets, USP) is administered orally in 4 to 6 divided doses daily. The drug should be taken after food, and doses should be spaced as evenly as practicable. Initial dosage should be conservative. For adults, the initial daily dose should be 1 g or less, with subsequent gradual dosage increases over a period of several days. The optimum dosage must be determined on the basis of individual response. The usual adult maintenance dose is 2 to 3 g daily. Less than 2 g daily has been found ineffective in most adults.

Pediatric dosage depends upon the age and weight of the patient. The initial dose should not exceed 750 mg daily. The usual maintenance dose in children ranges from 500 mg to 1 g daily, although occasionally 2 or (rarely) 3 g daily may be necessary.

If a patient is receiving another antiepileptic drug, it should not be discontinued when PEGANONE therapy is begun. The dosage of the other drug should be reduced gradually as that of PEGANONE is increased. PEGANONE may eventually replace the other drug or the optimal dosage of both antiepileptics may be established.

In tonic-clonic (grand mal) seizures, use of the drug with phenobarbital may be beneficial.

HOW SUPPLIED

PEGANONE (ethotoin tablets, USP) 250 mg grooved, white tablets bearing the letters OV on one side and the number 61 on the other and are supplied in bottles of 100 (**NDC** 67386-601-01).

Recommended storage: Store below 77°F (25°C).

Dispense in a tight light-resistant container, as defined in the USP, with a child-resistant cap.

Revised: October, 2003

Distributed by:
OVATION PHARMACEUTICALS, INC.
Deerfield, IL 60015, U.S.A.

Rev. October, 2003

Shown in Product Identification Guide, page 329

PANHEMATIN® ℞

[păn-hē′ma-tin]
(HEMIN FOR INJECTION)
For I.V. Use Only

PANHEMATIN (hemin for injection) should only be used by physicians experienced in the management of porphyrias in hospitals where the recommended clinical and laboratory diagnostic and monitoring techniques are available.

Continued on next page

Panhematin—Cont.

PANHEMATIN therapy should be considered after an appropriate period of alternate therapy (i.e., 400 g glucose/day for 1 to 2 days). (See "WARNINGS", "PRECAUTIONS" and "DOSAGE AND ADMINISTRATION" sections.)

DESCRIPTION

PANHEMATIN (hemin for injection) is an enzyme inhibitor derived from processed red blood cells. Hemin for injection was known previously as hematin. The term hematin has been used to describe the chemical reaction product of hemin and sodium carbonate solution. Hemin is an iron containing metalloporphyrin. Chemically hemin is represented as chloro [7,12-diethenyl-3,8,13,17-tetramethyl-21H,23H-porphine-2,18-dipropanoato(2-)-N^{21},N^{22},N^{23},N^{24}] iron. The structural formula for hemin is:

CH_3 $CH = CH_2$ $CH_2 = CH$ Cl CH_3 N Fe N CH_3 $CH_2CH_2CO_2H$ CH_3 $CH_2CH_2CO_2H$

PANHEMATIN is a sterile, lyophilized powder suitable for intravenous administration after reconstitution. Each dispensing vial of PANHEMATIN contains the equivalent of 313 mg hemin, 215 mg sodium carbonate and 300 mg of sorbitol. The pH may have been adjusted with hydrochloric acid; the product contains no preservatives. When mixed as directed with Sterile Water for Injection, USP, each 43 mL provides the equivalent of approximately 301 mg hematin (7 mg/mL).

CLINICAL PHARMACOLOGY

Heme acts to limit the hepatic and/or marrow synthesis of porphyrin. This action is likely due to the inhibition of δ-aminolevulinic acid synthetase, the enzyme which limits the rate of the porphyrin/heme biosynthetic pathway. The exact mechanism by which hematin produces symptomatic improvement in patients with acute episodes of the hepatic porphyrias has not been elucidated.[1,9]

Following intravenous administration of hematin in non-jaundiced human patients, an increase in fecal urobilinogen can be observed which is roughly proportional to the amount of hematin administered. This suggests an entero-hepatic pathway as at least one route of elimination. Bilirubin metabolites are also excreted in the urine following hematin injections.[2]

PANHEMATIN (hemin for injection) therapy for the acute porphyrias is not curative. After discontinuation of PANHEMATIN treatment, symptoms generally return although in some cases remission is prolonged. Some neurological symptoms have improved weeks to months after therapy although little or no response was noted at the time of treatment.

Other aspects of human pharmacokinetics have not been defined.

INDICATIONS AND USAGE

PANHEMATIN (hemin for injection) is indicated for the amelioration of recurrent attacks of acute intermittent porphyria temporally related to the menstrual cycle in susceptible women.

Manifestations such as pain, hypertension, tachycardia, abnormal mental status and mild to progressive neurologic signs may be controlled in selected patients with this disorder.

Similar findings have been reported in other patients with acute intermittent porphyria, porphyria variegata and hereditary coproporphyria. PANHEMATIN is not indicated in porphyria cutanea tarda.

CONTRAINDICATIONS

Hemin for injection is contraindicated in patients with known hypersensitivity to this drug.

WARNINGS

PANHEMATIN (hemin for injection) is made from human blood. Products made from human blood may contain infectious agents, such as viruses, that can cause disease. The risk that such products will transmit an infectious agent has been reduced by screening blood donors for prior exposure to certain viruses, by testing for the presence of certain current virus infections, and by inactivating certain viruses. Despite these measures, such products can still potentially transmit disease. There is also the possibility that unknown infectious agents may be present in such products. ALL infections thought by a physician possibly to have been transmitted by this product should be reported by the physician or other healthcare provider to Abbott Laboratories, (800) 633-9110. The physician should discuss the risks and benefits of this product with the patient.

Because this product is made from human blood, it may carry a risk of transmitting infectious agents, e.g., viruses, and theoretically, the Creutzfeldt-Jakob disease (CJD) agent.

PANHEMATIN therapy is intended to limit the rate of porphyria/heme biosynthesis possibly by inhibiting the enzyme δ-aminolevulinic acid synthetase. For this reason, drugs such as estrogens, barbituric acid derivatives and steroid metabolites which increase the activity of δ-aminolevulinic acid synthetase should be avoided.

Also, because PANHEMATIN has exhibited transient, mild anticoagulant effects during clinical studies, concurrent anticoagulant therapy should be avoided.[9] The extent and duration of the hypocoagulable state induced by PANHEMATIN has not been established.

PRECAUTIONS

General:

Clinical benefit from PANHEMATIN depends on prompt administration. Attacks of porphyria may progress to a point where irreversible neuronal damage has occurred. PANHEMATIN therapy is intended to prevent an attack from reaching the critical stage of neuronal degeneration. PANHEMATIN is not effective in repairing neuronal damage.[9]

Recommended dosage guidelines should be strictly followed. Reversible renal shutdown has been observed in a case where an excessive hematin dose (12.2 mg/kg) was administered in a single infusion. Oliguria and increased nitrogen retention occurred although the patient remained asymptomatic.[4] No worsening of renal function has been seen with administration of recommended dosages of hematin.[9]

A large arm vein or a central venous catheter should be utilized for the administration of hemin for injection to avoid the possibility of phlebitis.

Since reconstituted PANHEMATIN is not transparent, any undissolved particulate matter is difficult to see when inspected visually. Therefore, terminal filtration through a sterile 0.45 micron or smaller filter is recommended.

Tests for Diagnosis and Monitoring of Therapy:

Before PANHEMATIN therapy is begun, the presence of acute porphyria must be diagnosed using the following criteria:[9]

a. Presence of clinical symptoms.

b. Positive Watson-Schwartz or Hoesch test. (A negative Watson-Schwartz or Hoesch test indicates a porphyric attack is highly unlikely. When in doubt quantitative measures of δ-aminolevulinic acid and porphobilinogen in serum or urine may aid in diagnosis.)

Urinary concentrations of the following compounds may be *monitored* during PANHEMATIN therapy. Drug effect will be demonstrated by a decrease in one or more of the following compounds:[3–6]

ALA–δ-aminolevulinic acid
UPG–uroporphyrinogen
PBG–porphobilinogen
coproporphyrin

Carcinogenesis, Mutagenesis, Impairment of Fertility:

No data are available on potential for carcinogenicity, mutagenicity or impairment of fertility in animals or humans.

Pregnancy:

Teratogenic effects: Pregnancy Category C. Animal reproduction studies have not been conducted with hematin. It is also not known whether hematin can cause fetal harm when administered to a pregnant woman or can affect reproduction capacity. For this reason hemin for injection should not be given to a pregnant woman unless the expected benefits are sufficiently important to the health and welfare of the patient to outweigh the unknown hazard to the fetus.

Nursing Mothers:

It is not known whether this drug is excreted in human milk. Because many drugs are excreted in human milk, caution should be exercised when hemin for injection is administered to a nursing woman.

Pediatric Use:

Safety and effectiveness in pediatric patients under 16 years of age have not been established.

ADVERSE REACTIONS

Reversible renal shutdown has occurred with administration of excessive doses (See "PRECAUTIONS" section).

Phlebitis with or without leucocytosis and with or without mild pyrexia has occurred after administration of hematin through small arm veins.

There have been post-marketing and literature reports of thrombocytopenia and coagulaopathy (including prolonged prothrombin time and prolonged partial thromboplastin time) in patients receiving PANHEMATIN. The initial literature report[8] described coagulopathy occurring in a patient receiving hematin therapy. This patient exhibited prolonged prothrombin time and partial thromboplastin time, thrombocytopenia, mild hypofibrogenemia, mild elevation of fibrin split products, and a 10% fall in hematocrit.

OVERDOSAGE

Reversible renal shutdown has been observed in a case where an excessive hematin dose (12.2 mg/kg) was administered in a single infusion. Treatment of this case consisted of ethacrynic acid and mannitol.[7]

DOSAGE AND ADMINISTRATION

Before administering hemin for injection, an appropriate period of alternate therapy (i.e., 400 g glucose/day for 1 to 2 days) must be considered. If improvement is unsatisfactory for the treatment of acute attacks of porphyria, an intravenous infusion of PANHEMATIN containing a dose of 1 to 4 mg/kg/day of hematin should be given over a period of 10 to 15 minutes for 3 to 14 days based on the clinical signs. In more severe cases this dose may be repeated no earlier than every 12 hours. No more than 6 mg/kg of hematin should be given in any 24-hour period.

After reconstitution each mL of PANHEMATIN contains the equivalent of approximately 7 mg of hematin. The drug may be administered directly from the vial.

Dosage Calculation Table

1 mg hematin equivalent = 0.14 mL PANHEMATIN
2 mg hematin equivalent = 0.28 mL PANHEMATIN
3 mg hematin equivalent = 0.42 mL PANHEMATIN
4 mg hematin equivalent = 0.56 mL PANHEMATIN

Since reconstituted PANHEMATIN is not transparent, any undissolved particulate matter is difficult to see when inspected visually. Therefore, terminal filtration through a sterile 0.45 micron or smaller filter is recommended.

Preparation of Solution:

Reconstitute PANHEMATIN by aseptically adding 43 mL of Sterile Water for Injection, USP, to the dispensing vial. Immediately after adding diluent, the product should be shaken well for a period of 2 to 3 minutes to aid dissolution.

NOTE: Because PANHEMATIN contains no preservative and because PANHEMATIN undergoes rapid chemical decomposition in solution, it should not be reconstituted until immediately before use. After the first withdrawal from the vial, any solution remaining must be discarded.

No drug or chemical agent should be added to a PANHEMATIN fluid admixture unless its effect on the chemical and physical stability has first been determined.

HOW SUPPLIED

PANHEMATIN (hemin for injection) is supplied as a sterile, lyophilized black powder in single dose dispensing vials (**NDC** 0074-2000-43). When mixed as directed with Sterile Water for Injection, USP, each 43 mL provides the equivalent of approximately 301 mg hematin (7 mg/mL). Store lyophilized powder in refrigerator (2-8°C) until time of use.

REFERENCES

1. Bickers, D., Treatment of the Porphyrias: Mechanisms of Action, *J Invest Dermatol* 77(1):107-113, 1981.
2. Watson, C. J., Hematin and Porphyria, editorial, *N Engl J Med* 293(12):605-607, September 18, 1975.
3. Lamon, J. M., Hematin Therapy for Acute Porphyria, *Medicine* 58(3):252-269, 1979.
4. Dhar, G. J., et al., Effects of Hematin in Hepatic Porphyria, *Ann Intern Med* 83:20-30, 1975.
5. Watson, C. J., et al., Use of Hematin in the Acute Attack of the "Inducible" Hepatic Porphyrias, *Adv Intern Med* 23:265-286, 1978.
6. McColl, K. E., et al., Treatment with Haematin in Acute Hepatic Porphyria, *Q J Med*, New Series L (198):161-174, Spring, 1981.
7. Dhar, G. J., et al., Transitory Renal Failure Following Rapid Administration of a Relatively Large Amount of Hematin in a Patient with Acute Intermittent Porphyria in Clinical Remission, *Acta Med Scand* 203:437-443, 1978.
8. Morris, D. L., et al., Coagulopathy Associated with Hematin Treatment for Acute Intermittent Prophyria, *Ann Intern Med* 95:700-701, 1981.
9. Pierach, C. A., Hematin Therapy for the Porphyric Attack, *Semin Liver Dis* 2(2):125-131, May, 1982.

Revised: August, 2000
ABBOTT LABORATORIES
NORTH CHICAGO, IL 60064, U.S.A.
(No. 2000)
58-6276-R7

Shown in Product Identification Guide, page 329

TRANXENE® T-TAB® TABLETS ©IV ℞

[trănks-ēne]

(clorazepate dipotassium) (Nos. 4389, 4390, 4391)

TRANXENE®-SD &

TRANXENE®-SD HALF STRENGTH

(clorazepate dipotassium) (Nos. 2997, 2699)

SINGLE DOSE TABLETS

DESCRIPTION

Chemically, TRANXENE is a benzodiazepine. The empirical formula is $C_{16}H_{11}ClK_2N_2O_4$; the molecular weight is 408.92; and the structural formula may be represented as follows:

H O N–C CH–CO_2 K • KOH Cl C=N

The compound occurs as a fine, light yellow, practically odorless powder. It is insoluble in the common organic solvents, but very soluble in water. Aqueous solutions are unstable, clear, light yellow, and alkaline.

TRANXENE T-TAB tablets contain either 3.75 mg, 7.5 mg or 15 mg of clorazepate dipotassium for oral administration. TRANXENE-SD and TRANXENE-SD HALF STRENGTH tablets contain 22.5 mg and 11.25 mg of clorazepate dipotassium respectively. TRANXENE-SD and TRANXENE-SD HALF STRENGTH tablets gradually release clorazepate and are designed for once-a-day administration in patients already stabilized on TRANXENE T-TAB tablets.

Inactive ingredients for TRANXENE T-TAB® Tablets: Colloidal silicon dioxide, FD&C Blue No. 2 (3.75 mg only), FD&C Yellow No. 6 (7.5 mg only), FD&C Red No. 3 (15 mg only), magnesium oxide, magnesium stearate, microcrystalline cellulose, potassium carbonate, potassium chloride, and talc. Inactive ingredients for TRANXENE-SD and TRANXENE-SD HALF STRENGTH Tablets: Castor oil wax, FD&C Blue No. 2 (SD Half Strength, 11.25 mg only), iron oxide (SD, 22.5 mg only), lactose, magnesium oxide, magnesium stearate, potassium carbonate, potassium chloride, and talc.

CLINICAL PHARMACOLOGY

Pharmacologically, clorazepate dipotassium has the characteristics of the benzodiazepines. It has depressant effects on the central nervous system. The primary metabolite, nordiazepam, quickly appears in the blood stream. The serum half-life is about 2 days. The drug is metabolized in the liver and excreted primarily in the urine.

Studies in healthy men have shown that clorazepate dipotassium has depressant effects on the central nervous system. Prolonged administration of single daily doses as high as 120 mg was without toxic effects. Abrupt cessation of high doses was followed in some patients by nervousness, insomnia, irritability, diarrhea, muscle aches, or memory impairment.

Since orally administered clorazepate dipotassium is rapidly decarboxylated to form nordiazepam, there is essentially no circulating parent drug. Nordiazepam, the primary metabolite, quickly appears in the blood and is eliminated from the plasma with an apparent half-life of about 40 to 50 hours. Plasma levels of nordiazepam increase proportionally with TRANXENE dose and show moderate accumulation with repeated administration. The protein binding of nordiazepam in plasma is high (97-98%).

Within 10 days after oral administration of a 15 mg (50µCi) dose of ^{14}C-TRANXENE to two volunteers, 62-67% of the radioactivity was excreted in the urine and 15-19% was eliminated in the feces. Both subjects were still excreting measurable amounts of radioactivity in the urine (about 1% of the ^{14}C-dose) on day ten.

Nordiazepam is further metabolized by hydroxylation. The major urinary metabolite is conjugated oxazepam (3-hydroxynordiazepam), and smaller amounts of conjugated p-hydroxynordiazepam and nordiazepam are also found in the urine.

INDICATIONS AND USAGE

TRANXENE is indicated for the management of anxiety disorders or for the short-term relief of the symptoms of anxiety. Anxiety or tension associated with the stress of everyday life usually does not require treatment with an anxiolytic.

TRANXENE tablets are indicated as adjunctive therapy in the management of partial seizures.

The effectiveness of TRANXENE tablets in long-term management of anxiety, that is, more than 4 months, has not been assessed by systematic clinical studies. Long-term studies in epileptic patients, however, have shown continued therapeutic activity. The physician should reassess periodically the usefulness of the drug for the individual patient.

TRANXENE tablets are indicated for the symptomatic relief of acute alcohol withdrawal.

CONTRAINDICATIONS

TRANXENE tablets are contraindicated in patients with a known hypersensitivity to the drug and in those with acute narrow angle glaucoma.

WARNINGS

TRANXENE tablets are not recommended for use in depressive neuroses or in psychotic reactions.

Patients taking TRANXENE tablets should be cautioned against engaging in hazardous occupations requiring mental alertness, such as operating dangerous machinery including motor vehicles.

Since TRANXENE has a central nervous system depressant effect, patients should be advised against the simultaneous use of other CNS-depressant drugs, and cautioned that the effects of alcohol may be increased.

Because of the lack of sufficient clinical experience, TRANXENE tablets are not recommended for use in patients less than 9 years of age.

Physical and Psychological Dependence:

Withdrawal symptoms (similar in character to those noted with barbiturates and alcohol) have occurred following abrupt discontinuance of clorazepate. Withdrawal symptoms associated with the abrupt discontinuation of benzodiazepines have included convulsions, delirium, tremor, abdominal and muscle cramps, vomiting, sweating, nervousness, insomnia, irritability, diarrhea, and memory impairment. The more severe withdrawal symptoms have usually been limited to those patients who had received excessive doses over an extended period of time. Generally milder withdrawal symptoms have been reported following abrupt discontinuance of benzodiazepines taken continuously at therapeutic levels for several months. Consequently, after extended therapy, abrupt discontinuation of clorazepate should generally be avoided and a gradual dosage tapering schedule followed.

Caution should be observed in patients who are considered to have a psychological potential for drug dependence.

Evidence of drug dependence has been observed in dogs and rabbits which was characterized by convulsive seizures when the drug was abruptly withdrawn or the dose was reduced; the syndrome in dogs could be abolished by administration of clorazepate.

Usage in Pregnancy:

An increased risk of congenital malformations associated with the use of minor tranquilizers (chlordiazepoxide, diazepam, and meprobamate) during the first trimester of pregnancy has been suggested in several studies. Clorazepate dipotassium, a benzodiazepine derivative, has not been studied adequately to determine whether it, too, may be associated with an increased risk of fetal abnormality. Because use of these drugs is rarely a matter of urgency, their use during this period should almost always be avoided. The possibility that a woman of childbearing potential may be pregnant at the time of institution of therapy should be considered. Patients should be advised that if they become pregnant during therapy or intend to become pregnant they should communicate with their physician about the desirability of discontinuing the drug.

Usage during Lactation:

TRANXENE tablets should not be given to nursing mothers since it has been reported that nordiazepam is excreted in human breast milk.

PRECAUTIONS

In those patients in which a degree of depression accompanies the anxiety, suicidal tendencies may be present and protective measures may be required. The least amount of drug that is feasible should be available to the patient.

Patients taking TRANXENE tablets for prolonged periods should have blood counts and liver function tests periodically. The usual precautions in treating patients with impaired renal or hepatic function should also be observed.

In elderly or debilitated patients, the initial dose should be small, and increments should be made gradually, in accordance with the response of the patient, to preclude ataxia or excessive sedation.

Information for Patients:

To assure the safe and effective use of benzodiazepines, patients should be informed that, since benzodiazepines may produce psychological and physical dependence, it is essential that they consult with their physician before either increasing the dose or abruptly discontinuing this drug.

Pediatric Use:

See **WARNINGS**.

Geriatric Use:

Clinical studies of TRANXENE were not adequate to determine whether subjects aged 65 and over respond differently than younger subjects. Elderly or debilitated patients may be especially sensitive to the effects of all benzodiazepines, including TRANXENE. In general, elderly or debilitated patients should be started on lower doses of Tranxene and observed closely, reflecting the greater frequency of decreased hepatic, renal, or cardiac function, and concomitant disease or other drug therapy. Dose adjustments should also be made slowly, and with more caution in this patient population (see **PRECAUTIONS** and **DOSAGE AND ADMINISTRATION**).

ADVERSE REACTIONS

The side effect most frequently reported was drowsiness. Less commonly reported (in descending order of occurrence) were: dizziness, various gastrointestinal complaints, nervousness, blurred vision, dry mouth, headache, and mental confusion. Other side effects included insomnia, transient skin rashes, fatigue, ataxia, genitourinary complaints, irritability, diplopia, depression, tremor, and slurred speech.

There have been reports of abnormal liver and kidney function tests and of decrease in hematocrit.

Decrease in systolic blood pressure has been observed.

DOSAGE AND ADMINISTRATION

For the symptomatic relief of anxiety:

TRANXENE T-TAB® tablets are administered orally in divided doses. The usual daily dose is 30 mg. The dose should be adjusted gradually within the range of 15 to 60 mg daily in accordance with the response of the patient. In elderly or debilitated patients it is advisable to initiate treatment at a daily dose of 7.5 to 15 mg.

TRANXENE tablets may also be administered in a single dose daily at bedtime; the recommended initial dose is 15 mg. After the initial dose, the response of the patient may require adjustment of subsequent dosage. Lower doses may be indicated in the elderly patient. Drowsiness may occur at the initiation of treatment and with dosage increment.

TRANXENE-SD (22.5 mg) tablets may be administered as a single dose every 24 hours. This tablet is intended as an alternate dosage form for the convenience of patients stabilized on a dose of 7.5 mg tablets three times a day. TRANXENE-SD tablets should not be used to initiate therapy.

TRANXENE-SD HALF STRENGTH (11.25 mg) tablets may be administered as a single dose every 24 hours. This tablet is intended as an alternate dosage form for the convenience of patients stabilized on a dose of 3.75 mg tablets three times a day. TRANXENE-SD HALF STRENGTH should not be used to initiate therapy.

For the symptomatic relief of acute alcohol withdrawal:

The following dosage schedule is recommended:

1st 24 hours (Day 1)	30 mg initially; followed by 30 to 60 mg in divided doses
2nd 24 hours (Day 2)	45 to 90 mg in divided doses
3rd 24 hours (Day 3)	22.5 to 45 mg in divided doses
Day 4	15 to 30 mg in divided doses

Thereafter, gradually reduce the daily dose to 7.5 to 15 mg. Discontinue drug therapy as soon as patient's condition is stable.

The maximum recommended total daily dose is 90 mg. Avoid excessive reductions in the total amount of drug administered on successive days.

As an Adjunct to Antiepileptic Drugs:

In order to minimize drowsiness, the recommended initial dosages and dosage increments should not be exceeded.

Adults: The maximum recommended initial dose in patients over 12 years old is 7.5 mg three times a day. Dosage should be increased by no more than 7.5 mg every week and should not exceed 90 mg/day.

Children (9–12 years): The maximum recommended initial dose is 7.5 mg two times a day. Dosage should be increased by no more than 7.5 mg every week and should not exceed 60 mg/day.

DRUG INTERACTIONS

If TRANXENE is to be combined with other drugs acting on the central nervous system, careful consideration should be given to the pharmacology of the agents to be employed. Animal experience indicates that clorazepate dipotassium prolongs the sleeping time after hexobarbital or after ethyl alcohol, increases the inhibitory effects of chlorpromazine, but does not exhibit monoamine oxidase inhibition. Clinical studies have shown increased sedation with concurrent hypnotic medications. The actions of the benzodiazepines may be potentiated by barbiturates, narcotics, phenothiazines, monoamine oxidase inhibitors or other antidepressants.

If TRANXENE tablets are used to treat anxiety associated with somatic disease states, careful attention must be paid to possible drug interaction with concomitant medication.

In bioavailability studies with normal subjects, the concurrent administration of antacids at therapeutic levels did not significantly influence the bioavailability of TRANXENE tablets.

OVERDOSAGE

Overdosage is usually manifested by varying degrees of CNS depression ranging from slight sedation to coma. As in the management of overdosage with any drug, it should be borne in mind that multiple agents may have been taken.

The treatment of overdosage should consist of the general measures employed in the management of overdosage of any CNS depressant. Gastric evacuation either by the induction of emesis, lavage, or both, should be performed immediately. General supportive care, including frequent monitoring of the vital signs and close observation of the patient, is indicated. Hypotension, though rarely reported, may occur with large overdoses. In such cases the use of agents such as Levophed® Bitartrate (norepinephrine bitartrate injection, USP) or Aramine® Injection (metaraminol bitartrate injection, USP) should be considered.

While reports indicate that individuals have survived overdoses of clorazepate dipotassium as high as 450 to 675 mg, these doses are not necessarily an accurate indication of the amount of drug absorbed since the time interval between ingestion and the institution of treatment was not always known. Sedation in varying degrees was the most common physiological manifestation of clorazepate dipotassium overdosage. Deep coma when it occurred was usually associated with the ingestion of other drugs in addition to clorazepate dipotassium.

Flumazenil, a specific benzodiazepine receptor antagonist, is indicated for the complete or partial reversal of the sedative effects of benzodiazepines and may be used in situations when an overdose with a benzodiazepine is known or suspected. Prior to the administration of flumazenil, necessary measures should be instituted to secure airway, ventilation, and intravenous access. Flumazenil is intended as an adjunct to, not as a substitute for, proper management of benzodiazepine overdose. Patients treated with flumazenil should be monitored for resedation, respiratory depression, and other residual benzodiazepine effects for an appropriate period after treatment. **The prescriber should be aware of a risk of seizure in association with flumazenil treatment, particularly in long-term benzodiazepine users and in cyclic antidepressant overdose.** The complete flumazenil package insert including CONTRAINDICATIONS, WARNINGS, and PRECAUTIONS should be consulted prior to use.

ANIMAL PHARMACOLOGY AND TOXICOLOGY

Studies in rats and monkeys have shown a substantial difference between doses producing tranquilizing, sedative and toxic effects. In rats, conditioned avoidance response was inhibited at an oral dose of 10 mg/kg; sedation was induced at 32 mg/kg; the LD_{50} was 1320 mg/kg. In monkeys aggressive behavior was reduced at an oral dose of 0.25 mg/kg; sedation (ataxia) was induced at 7.5 mg/kg; the LD_{50} could not be determined because of the emetic effect of large doses, but the LD_{50} exceeds 1600 mg/kg.

Continued on next page

Tranxene—Cont.

Twenty-four dogs were given clorazepate dipotassium orally in a 22-month toxicity study; doses up to 75 mg/kg were given. Drug-related changes occurred in the liver; weight was increased and cholestasis with minimal hepatocellular damage was found, but lobular architecture remained well preserved.
Eighteen rhesus monkeys were given oral doses of clorazepate dipotassium from 3 to 36 mg/kg daily for 52 weeks. All treated animals remained similar to control animals. Although total leucocyte count remained within normal limits it tended to fall in the female animals on the highest doses. Examination of all organs revealed no alterations attributable to clorazepate dipotassium. There was no damage to liver function or structure.
Reproduction Studies:
Standard fertility, reproduction, and teratology studies were conducted in rats and rabbits. Oral doses in rats up to 150 mg/kg and in rabbits up to 15 mg/kg produced no abnormalities in the fetuses. TRANXENE did not alter the fertility indices or reproductive capacity of adult animals. As expected, the sedative effect of high doses interfered with care of the young by their mothers (see *Usage in Pregnancy*).

HOW SUPPLIED

TRANXENE® 3.75 mg scored T-TAB tablets are supplied as blue-colored tablets bearing the letters OV, the distinctive T shape and a two-digit designation, 31:
Bottles of 100 .... (**NDC** 67386-301-01).

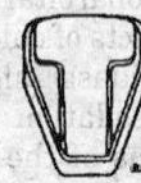
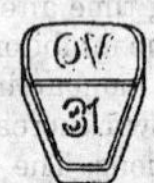

7.5 mg scored T-TAB tablets are supplied as peach-colored tablets bearing the letters OV, the distinctive T shape and a two-digit designation, 32:
Bottles of 100 .... (**NDC** 67386-302-01).
Bottles of 500 .... (**NDC** 67386-302-05).

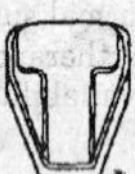
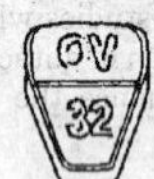

15 mg scored T-TAB tablets are supplied as lavender-colored tablets bearing the letters OV, the distinctive T shape and a two-digit designation, 33:
Bottles of 100 .... (**NDC** 67386-303-01).

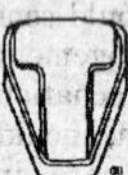
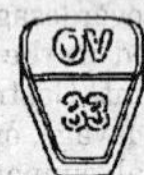

TRANXENE®-SD 22.5 mg single dose tablets are supplied as tan-colored tablets bearing the letters OV and a two-digit designation, 45:
Bottles of 100 .... (**NDC** 67386-405-01).
TRANXENE®-SD HALF STRENGTH 11.25 mg single dose tablets are supplied as blue-colored tablets bearing the letters OV and a two-digit designation, 44:
Bottles of 100 .... (**NDC** 67386-404-01).
Recommended storage: Protect from moisture. Keep bottle tightly closed. Store below 77°F (25°C). Dispense in a USP tight, light-resistant container.
T-TAB, tablet appearance and shape are registered trademarks of Ovation Pharmaceuticals.
U.S. Design Pat. No. D-300,879
®Registered Trademark of
Ovation Pharmaceuticals, Inc.
Revised: December, 2002
Manufactured by Abbott Laboratories,
North Chicago, IL 60064 for:
OVATION PHARMACEUTICALS, INC.
Deerfield, IL 60015
Shown in Product Identification Guide, page 329

NOTICE
Before prescribing or administering
any product described in
PHYSICIANS' DESK REFERENCE
check the **PDR Supplements**
for revised information.

Paddock Laboratories, Inc.

3940 QUEBEC AVENUE NORTH
MINNEAPOLIS, MN 55427

Direct Inquiries to:
(800) 328-5113

For Medical Information Contact:
Regulatory Affairs Department
(800) 328-5113

ACTIDOSE® with SORBITOL OTC

[*act 'ĭ -dose*]
(Activated Charcoal with Sorbitol Suspension)

DESCRIPTION

Actidose with Sorbitol is supplied in bottles and tubes. Each 120 mL package contains 25 grams of activated charcoal in suspension and 48 grams of sorbitol. Each 240 mL package contains 50 grams of activated charcoal in suspension and 96 grams of sorbitol. Each milliliter contains 208 mg (0.208 gram) activated in charcoal and 400 mg (0.4 gram) sorbitol.

HOW SUPPLIED

25 g unit-of-use bottle NDC 0574-0120-04
50 g unit-of-use bottle NDC 0574-0120-08
25 g unit-of-use tube NDC 0574-0120-74
50 g unit-of-use tube NDC 0574-0120-76

ACTIDOSE®-AQUA OTC

[*act 'ĭ 'dose a-qua*]
(Activated Charcoal Suspension)

DESCRIPTION

Actidose-Aqua is supplied in bottles and tubes. Each 72 mL package contains 15 grams of activated charcoal in suspension, each 120 mL package contains 25 grams of activated charcoal in suspension and each 240 mL package contains 50 grams of activated charcoal in suspension. Each milliliter contains 208 mg (0.208 gram) activated charcoal.

HOW SUPPLIED

25 g unit-of-use bottle NDC 0574-0121-04
50 g unit-of-use bottle NDC 0574-0121-08
15 g unit-of-use tube NDC 0574-0121-25
25 g unit-of-use tube NDC 0574-0121-74
50 g unit-of-use tube NDC 0574-0121-76

COLOCORT® ℞

[*cō-lō-cŏrt*]
Hydrocortisone Rectal Suspension, USP
(Retention)
100 mg/60 mL
Disposable Unit for Rectal Use Only

DESCRIPTION

Hydrocortisone is a white to practically white, odorless, crystalline powder, very slightly soluble in water.
Hydrocortisone rectal suspension is a convenient disposable single-dose enema designed for ease of self-administration.
Each disposable unit (60 mL) for rectal administration contains: Hydrocortisone, 100 mg in an aqueous solution containing carbomer 934P, polysorbate 80, purified water, sodium hydroxide and methylparaben, 0.18% as a preservative.

HOW SUPPLIED

Colocort®, Hydrocortisone Rectal Suspension, USP, (Retention) 100 mg/60 mL, is supplied as disposable single-dose bottles with lubricated rectal applicator tips, in boxes of seven × 60 mL (NDC 0574-2020-07) and boxes of one × 60 mL (NDC 0574-2020-01).
Store at controlled room temperature, 15°–30°C (59°–86°F).
Rx only
2124148 (08-01)

EZ-Char® Pellets OTC

(Activated Charcoal USP)

DESCRIPTION

EZ-Char is a pelletized form of activated charcoal designed to be mixed with water and used as a poison adsorbent in poisoning emergencies.

HOW SUPPLIED

25 gram bottle NDC 0574-0122-25
2200353 (07-01)

GLUTOSE 15™ OTC
GLUTOSE 45™

(Oral Glucose Gel)

DESCRIPTION

Glutose gel is a lemon-flavored, dye-free oral glucose gel for treatment of insulin reaction or hypoglycemia. Glutose gel contains Dextrose (d-glucose) USP 40%.

HOW SUPPLIED

Glutose 15: 3 x 15g unit-of-use tubes per package NDC 0574-0069-30
Glutose 45: 1 x 45g multi-use tube per package NDC 0574-0069-45
132931 (07-97)

KIONEX™ POWDER ℞

[*ky-onĕx*]
Sodium Polystyrene
Sulfonate, USP

Cation-Exchange Resin

DESCRIPTION

Kionex™ brand of sodium polystyrene sulfonate is a benzene, diethenyl-, polymer with ethenylbenzene, sulfonated, sodium salt.
The drug is a light brown to brown finely ground, powdered form of sodium polystyrene sulfonate, a cation-exchange resin prepared in the sodium phase with an *in vitro* exchange capacity of approximately 3.1 mEq (*in vivo* approximately 1 mEq) of potassium per gram. The sodium content is approximately 100 mg (4.1 mEq) per gram of the drug. It can be administered orally or in an enema.

HOW SUPPLIED

Store at controlled room temperature 15–30°C (59–86°F).
Kionex should not be heated for to do so may alter the exchange properties of the resin.
Dispense in a tight, light-resistant container as defined in the USP.
Kionex™ (Sodium Polystyrene Sulfonate, USP) is available as a powder in containers of:
1 Pound (454 grams) NDC 0574-2004-16
Rx only 2124142 (04-93)

LAClotion™ 12%* ℞

(ammonium lactate) Lotion

For topical use only. Not for ophthalmic use.

DESCRIPTION

*LAClotion™, (ammonium lactate) lotion specially formulates 12% lactic acid neutralized with ammonium hydroxide, as ammonium lactate to provide a lotion pH of 4.5–5.5. LAClotion also contains light mineral oil, glyceryl stearate, PEG-100 stearate, propylene glycol, polyoxyl 40 stearate, glycerin, magnesium aluminum silicate, laureth-4, cetyl alcohol, methyl and propyl parabens, methylcellulose, and water.

INDICATIONS AND USAGE

LAClotion is indicated for the treatment of dry, scaly skin (xerosis) and ichthyosis vulgaris and for temporary relief of itching associated with these conditions.

DOSAGE AND ADMINISTRATION

Shake well. Apply to the affected areas and rub thoroughly. Use twice daily or as directed by a physician.

HOW SUPPLIED

225 g (NDC 0574-2021-08) plastic bottle and
400 g (NDC 0574-2021-16) plastic bottle.
Rx only 2200236 (01-02)

NYSTOP® ℞

Nystatin Topical
Powder USP
For topical use only.
Not for ophthalmic use.

DESCRIPTION

Nystatin is a polyene antifungal antibiotic obtained from *Streptomyces nursei*.
Nystatin Topical Powder USP is for dermatologic use.
Nystatin Topical Powder USP contains 100,000 USP nystatin units per gram dispersed in talc.

INDICATIONS AND USAGE

Nystatin Topical Powder is indicated in the treatment of cutaneous or mucocutaneous mycotic infections caused by *Candida albicans* and other susceptible *Candida* species.

This preparation is not indicated for systemic, oral, intravaginal or ophthalmic use.

DOSAGE AND ADMINISTRATION

Very moist lesions are best treated with the topical dusting powder.

Adults and Pediatric Patients (Neonates and Older):

Apply to candidal lesions two or three times daily until healing is complete. For fungal infection of the feet caused by *Candida* species, the powder should be dusted on the feet, as well as, in all foot wear.

HOW SUPPLIED

Nystop® Nystatin Topical Powder USP is supplied as 100,000 units nystatin per gram in 15 g, 30 g and 60 g plastic squeeze bottles.

(NDC 0574-2008-15) (NDC 0574-2008-30) (NDC 0574-2008-02)

STORAGE

Store at controlled room temperature 15°–30°C (59°–86°F); avoid excessive heat (40°C; 104°F).

Rx only 2200790 (05-03)

PADDOCK NYSTATIN™ NYSTATIN, USP ℞

For Extemporaneous Preparation of Oral Suspension

DESCRIPTION

Nystatin USP is an antifungal antibiotic obtained from *Streptomyces noursei*.

Nystatin USP is a ready-to-use, non-sterile powder for oral administration which contains no excipients or preservatives. It is available in containers of 50 million, 150 million, 500 million and 2 billion units. Each mg contains a minimum of 5,000 units.

HOW SUPPLIED

Product Code (NDC)	Size (units)	Approx. Weight (grams)
0574-0404-05	50 million	8.3 – 10
0574-0404-15	150 million	25 – 30
0574-0404-50	500 million	83 – 100
0574-0404-02	2 billion	333 – 400

Storage: Store in a refrigerator. 2°–8°C (36°–46°F). Protect from light.

Rx only 2124070 (10-01)

PODOCON-25® ℞

(25% podophyllin in benzoin tincture)

DESCRIPTION

Podocon-25® is composed of Podophyllin (Podophyllum Resin, American) 25% in Benzoin Tincture.

Podophyllin is a cytotoxic agent that has been used topically in the treatment of genital warts. It arrests mitosis in metaphase, an effect it shares with other cytotoxic agents such as the vinca alkaloids. The active agent is podophyllotoxin, whose concentration varies with the type of podophyllin used; the American source normally containing one-fourth the amount of podophyllotoxin as the Indian source.

NOTE: PODOCON-25 IS TO BE APPLIED ONLY BY A PHYSICIAN. IT IS NOT TO BE DISPENSED TO THE PATIENT.

HOW SUPPLIED

Podocon-25 is available in 15-mL bottles with tapered tip applicator attached inside cap. **NDC 0574-0601-15**

Store at room temperature 15°–30° C (59°–86° F) in tight, light-resistant containers.

Rx only

124075 (06-98)

PODOFILOX ℞

Topical Solution 0.5%

DESCRIPTION

Podofilox Topical Solution is an antimitotic drug which can be chemically synthesized or purified from the plant families *Coniferae* and *Berberidaceae* (e.g. species of *Juniperus* and *Podophyllum*). Podofilox Topical Solution 0.5% is formulated for topical administration. Each milliliter of solution contains 5 mg of podofilox, in a vehicle containing lactic acid and sodium lactate in alcohol 95%, USP.

HOW SUPPLIED

3.5 mL Podofilox Topical Solution 0.5% is supplied as a clear liquid in amber glass bottles with child-resistant screw caps. NDC 0574-0611-05. Store at controlled room temperature between 15° and 30°C (59° and 86°F). **Avoid excessive heat. Do not freeze.**

Rx only 124159 (04-01)

Product	Product Identification FRONT/BACK
Acebutolol HCl Capsules 200 mg	G AC 200*
Acebutolol HCl Capsules 400 mg	G AC 400*
Acyclovir Capsules 200 mg	G 0034*
Acyclovir Tablets 400 mg	G 0036
Acyclovir Tablets 800 mg	G / 0037
Akineton Tablets 2 mg	11 (BISECT)
Allopurinol Tablets 100 mg	0524 0405 (BISECT)
Allopurinol Tablets 300 mg	0524 0410 (BISECT)
Amiloride HCl Tablets 5 mg	par 117
Amiodarone HCl Tablets 200 mg	AM 200 G (BISECT)
Atenolol Tablets 25 mg	G/25
Atenolol Tablets 50 mg	G / A/50
Atenolol Tablets 100 mg	G / A/100
Benztropine Mesylate Tablets 0.5 mg	par 164 (BISECT)
Benztropine Mesylate Tablets 1 mg	par 165 (BISECT)
Benztropine Mesylate Tablets 2 mg	par 166 (BISECT)
busPIRone HCl Tablets 5 mg	par 707 / 5 (BISECT)
busPIRone HCl Tablets 7.5 mg	par 725 / 7.5 (BISECT)
busPIRone HCl Tablets 10 mg	par 708 / 10 (BISECT)
busPIRone HCl Tablets 15 mg	par 721 / 5 5 5 (TRISECT AND BISECT)
Capoten Tablets 12.5 mg	CAPOTEN 12.5 (PARTIAL BISECT)
Capoten Tablets 25 mg	CAPOTEN 25 (QUADRISECT)
Capoten Tablets 50 mg	CAPOTEN 50 (BISECT)
Capoten Tablets 100 mg	CAPOTEN 100 (BISECT)
Capozide Tablets 25 mg/ 15 mg	CAPOZIDE 25/15 (QUADRISECT)
Capozide Tablets 25 mg/ 25 mg	CAPOZIDE 25/25 (QUADRISECT)
Capozide Tablets 50 mg/ 15 mg	CAPOZIDE 50/15 (BISECT)
Capozide Tablets 50 mg/ 25 mg	CAPOZIDE 50/25 (BISECT)
Captopril Tablets 12.5 mg	E121 / (BISECT)
Captopril Tablets 25 mg	E122 / (QUADRISECT)
Captopril Tablets 50 mg	E123 / (BISECT)
Captopril Tablets 100 mg	E124 / (BISECT)
Carisoprodol and Aspirin Tablets 200 mg/325 mg	par 246
Chlordiazepoxide Hydrochloride Capsules 5 mg	Par / 958*
Chlordiazepoxide Hydrochloride Capsules 10 mg	Par / 959*
Chlordiazepoxide Hydrochloride Capsules 25 mg	Par / 960*
Clomiphene Citrate Tablets 50 mg	par 701 (BISECT)
Cyproheptadine HCl Tablets 4 mg	par 043 (BISECT)
Dexamethasone Tablets 0.25 mg	par 083 (BISECT)
Dexamethasone Tablets 0.5 mg	par 084 (BISECT)
Dexamethasone Tablets 0.75 mg	par 085 (BISECT)
Dexamethasone Tablets 1.5 mg	par 086 (BISECT)
Dexamethasone Tablets 4 mg	par 087 (BISECT)
Dexamethasone Tablets 6 mg	par 129 (BISECT)
Diphenoxylate HCl and Atropine Sulfate Tablets 2.5 mg/0.025 mg	P 771
Doxazosin Mesylate Tablets 1 mg	DX1 / G
Doxazosin Mesylate Tablets 2 mg	DX 2 / G (BISECT)
Doxazosin Mesylate Tablets 4 mg	DX 4 / G (BISECT)
Doxazosin Mesylate Tablets 8 mg	DX 8 / G (BISECT)
Doxepin HCl Capsules 10 mg	par 217 / par 217*
Doxepin HCl Capsules 25 mg	par 218 / par 218*
Doxepin HCl Capsules 50 mg	par 219 / par 219*
Doxepin HCl Capsules 75 mg	par 220 / par 220*
Doxepin HCl Capsules 100 mg	par 221 / par 221*
Doxepin HCl Capsules 150 mg	par 222 / par 222*
Doxycycline Capsules 50 mg	par 726 / par 726*
Doxycycline Capsules 100 mg	par 727 / par 727*
Enalapril Maleate Tablets 2.5 mg	EN 2.5 / G (BISECT)
Enalapril Maleate Tablets 5.0 mg	EN 5 / G (BISECT)
Enalapril Maleate Tablets 10 mg	EN 10 / G (BISECT)
Enalapril Maleate Tablets 20 mg	EN 20 / G
Enalapril Maleate and Hydrochlorothiazide Tablets 5 mg/ 12.5 mg	C 133
Enalapril Maleate and Hydrochlorothiazide Tablets 10 mg/ 25 mg	C 134
Etodolac Tablets 500 mg	ET 500 / G
Famotidine Tablets 20 mg	C 119
Famotidine Tablets 40 mg	C 120
Flecainide Acetate Tablets 50 mg	FC 50 / G
Flecainide Acetate Tablets 100 mg	FC 100 / G (BISECT)
Flecainide Acetate Tablets 150 mg	FC 150 / G (BISECT)
Fluoxetine HCl Tablets 10 mg	FL 10 / G (BISECT)
Fluoxetine HCl Tablets 20 mg	FL 20 / G (BISECT)
Fluoxetine Capsules 10 mg	G FL 10*
Fluoxetine Capsules 20 mg	FLUOXETINE 20 mg R148*
Fluoxetine Capsules 40 mg	FLUOXETINE 40 mg R149*
Fluoxetine Oral Solution	N/A
Fluphenazine HCl Tablets 1 mg	par 061
Fluphenazine HCl Tablets 2.5 mg	par 062
Fluphenazine HCl Tablets 5 mg	par 076
Fluphenazine HCl Tablets 10 mg	par 064
Glyburide and Metformin HCl Tablets 1.25 mg/250 mg	biconvex 6057
Glyburide and Metformin HCl Tablets 2.5 mg/500 mg	biconvex 6058
Glyburide and Metformin HCl Tablets 5 mg/500 mg	biconvex 6059
Guanfacine Tablets 1 mg	GU 1 / G
Guanfacine Tablets 2 mg	GU 2 / G
HydrALAzine HCl Tablets 10 mg	par 029
HydrALAzine HCl Tablets 25 mg	par 027
HydrALAzine HCl Tablets 50 mg	par 028
HydrALAzine HCl Tablets 100 mg	par 121
Hydra-Zide (Hydralazine HCl and Hydrochlorothiazide) Capsules 25 mg/25 mg	par 143 / par 143*
Hydra-Zide (Hydralazine HCl and Hydrochlorothiazide) Capsules 50 mg/50 mg	par 144 / par 144*

(Table continued on next page)

Par Pharmaceutical, Inc.

ONE RAM RIDGE ROAD
SPRING VALLEY, NY 10977

Direct Inquiries to:
Customer Representative
(800) 828-9393

The following is a listing of products currently available from Par Pharmaceutical, Inc.

[See table on previous page and above]

Parkedale Pharmaceuticals

Please see King Pharmaceuticals, Inc.

Parke-Davis

A Division of Warner-Lambert Company LLC
A Pfizer Company
235 E 42ND STREET
NEW YORK, NY 10017-5755

For updates to the product information listed below, please check the Pfizer Web site: http://www.pfizer.com, or call (800) 438-1985. For complete product listing, please see the Manufacturers' Index.

For Medical Information, Contact:
(800) 438-1985
24 hours a day, seven days a week.

Distribution:
1855 Shelby Oaks Drive North
Memphis, TN 38134
(901) 387-5200
Customer Service:
(800) 533-4535

PARCODE®
(Parke-Davis Accurate Recognition Code)

Code Number	Product Name
001-006	*Unassigned*
007	**Dilantin® Infatabs®** Each tablet contains 50 mg phenytoin, USP.
008-143	*Unassigned*
145-154	*Unassigned*
155	**Lipitor® Tablets** Each tablet contains atorvastatin calcium equivalent to 10 mg atorvastatin.
156	**Lipitor® Tablets** Each tablet contains atorvastatin calcium equivalent to 20 mg atorvastatin.
157	**Lipitor® Tablets** Each tablet contains atorvastatin calcium equivalent to 40 mg atorvastatin.
158	**Lipitor® Tablets** Each tablet contains atorvastatin calcium equivalent to 80 mg atorvastatin.
159-219	*Unassigned*
220	**Accuretic™ Tablets** Each tablet contains 20 mg quinapril and 12.5 mg hydrochlorothiazide.
221	*Unassigned*
222	**Accuretic™ Tablets** Each tablet contains 10 mg quinapril and 12.5 mg hydrochlorothiazide.
223	**Accuretic™ Tablets** Each tablet contains 20 mg quinapril and 25 mg hydrochlorothiazide.
224-236	*Unassigned*
238-269	*Unassigned*
271-361	*Unassigned*
363-364	*Unassigned*
366-400	*Unassigned*
401	**Neurontin® Tablets** Each tablet contains 800 mg gabapentin.
402-415	*Unassigned*
417-424	*Unassigned*
428-512	*Unassigned*

(cont.)

Product	Product Identification FRONT/BACK
Hydra-Zide (Hydralazine HCl and Hydrochlorothiazide) Capsules 100 mg/50 mg	par 145 / par 145*
Hydroxyurea Capsules 500 mg	724 par*
Ibuprofen Tablets 400 mg	IBU 400
Ibuprofen Tablets 600 mg	IBU 600
Ibuprofen Tablets 800 mg	IBU 800
Imipramine HCl Tablets 10 mg	par / 54
Imipramine HCl Tablets 25 mg	par / 55
Imipramine HCl Tablets 50 mg	par / 56
Indapamide Tablets 1.25 mg	IE 1.25 / G
Indapamide Tablets 2.5 mg	IE 2.5 / G
Isosorbide Dinitrate Tablets 5 mg	par 020 (BISECT)
Isosorbide Dinitrate Tablets 10 mg	par 021 (BISECT)
Isosorbide Dinitrate Tablets 20 mg	par 022 (BISECT)
Isosorbide Dinitrate Tablets 30 mg	par 009 (BISECT)
Lisinopril Tablets 2.5 mg	556/par
Lisinopril Tablets 5 mg	557/par
Lisinopril Tablets 10 mg	558/par
Lisinopril Tablets 20 mg	559/par
Lisinopril Tablets 30 mg	635/par
Lisinopril Tablets 40 mg	560/par
Lovastatin Tablets 10 mg	LV 10 / G
Lovastatin Tablets 20 mg	LV 20 / G
Lovastatin Tablets 40 mg	LV 40 / G
Meclizine HCl Tablets 12.5 mg	par / 034
Meclizine HCl Tablets 25 mg	par / 035
Megestrol Acetate Tablets 20 mg	par 289 (BISECT)
Megestrol Acetate Tablets 40 mg	par 290 (BISECT)
Megestrol Acetate Oral Suspension 40 mg/mL	NA
Mercaptopurine Tablets 50 mg	P02
Metaproterenol Sulfate Tablets 10 mg	par 258 (BISECT)
Metaproterenol Sulfate Tablets 20 mg	par 259 (BISECT)
Metformin Tablets 500 mg	MF 1 / G
Metformin Tablets 850 mg	MF 2 / G
Metformin Tablets 1000 mg	MF 3 / G (BISECT)
Methimazole Tablets 5 mg	EM 5 (BISECT)
Methimazole Tablets 10 mg	EM 10 (BISECT)
Methimazole Tablets 20 mg	EM 20 (BISECT)
Minoxidil Tablets 2.5 mg	par 256 / MINOXIDIL 2 ½ (BISECT)
Minoxidil Tablets 10 mg	par 257 / MINOXIDIL 10 (BISECT)
Mirtazapine Tablets 15 mg	MR/15 / G
Mirtazapine Tablets 30 mg	MR/30 / G
Mirtazapine Tablets 45 mg	MR/45 / G
Nefazodone Hydrochloride Tablets 50 mg	DRL 50/1
Nefazodone Hydrochloride Tablets 100 mg	DRL 100/2
Nefazodone Hydrochloride Tablets 150 mg	DRL 150/3
Nefazodone Hydrochloride Tablets 200 mg	DRL 200/4
Nefazodone Hydrochloride Tablets 250 mg	DRL 250/5
Nicardipine HCl Capsules 20 mg	G 0041*
Nicardipine HCl Capsules 30 mg	G 0042*
Nizatidine Capsules 150 mg	G NZ 150*
Nizatidine Capsules 300 mg	G NZ 300*
Ofloxacin Tablets 200 mg	par 200 / 682
Ofloxacin Tablets 300 mg	par 300 / 683
Ofloxacin Tablets 400 mg	par 400 / 684
Orphengesic (Orphenadrine Citrate/Aspirin/Caffeine) Tablets 25 mg/385 mg/30 mg	par 472
Orphengesic Forte (Orphenadrine Citrate/Aspirin/Caffeine) Tablets 50 mg/770 mg/60 mg	par 473 (BISECT)
Oxaprozin Tablets 600 mg	00 53 / G (BISECT)
Paroxetine Hydrochloride Tablets 10 mg	par 876
Paroxetine Hydrochloride Tablets 20 mg	par 877
Paroxetine Hydrochloride Tablets 30 mg	par 878
Paroxetine Hydrochloride Tablets 40 mg	par 879
Prochlorperazine Maleate Tablets 5 mg	TL 113 (BISECT)
Prochlorperazine Maleate Tablets 10 mg	TL 115 (BISECT)
Questran (cholestyramine oral suspension) Powder 4 g	NA
Questran Light (cholestyramine oral suspension) Powder 4 g	NA
Ranitidine Tablets 150 mg	par 544
Ranitidine Tablets 300 mg	par 545
Ranitidine HCl Capsules 150 mg	CD 129*
Ranitidine HCl Capsules 300 mg	CD 130*
Ribasphere™ (Ribavirin Capsules) 200 mg	riba 200
Selegiline HCl Tablets 5 mg	SE 5 / G
Sotalol HCl Tablets 80 mg	S 80 / G (BISECT)
Sotalol HCl Tablets 120 mg	S 120 / G (BISECT)
Sotalol HCl Tablets 160 mg	S 160 / G (BISECT)
Sotalol HCl Tablets 240 mg	S 240 / G (BISECT)
SSD (1% Silver Sulfadiazine) Cream	NA
SSD AF (1% Silver Sulfadiazine) Cream	NA
Sumycin (tetracycline HCl) Tablets 250 mg	663
Sumycin (tetracycline HCl) Tablets 500 mg	603
Sumycin (tetracycline HCl) Syrup 125 mg/ 5 mL	NA
Ticlopidine HCl Tablets 250 mg	T250 / G
Tizanidine HCl Tablets 2 mg	R179 (BISECT)
Tizanidine HCl Tablets 4 mg	R180 (QUADRISECT)
Torsemide Tablets 5 mg	par 651/5 (Bisect)
Torsemide Tablets 10 mg	par 652/10 (Bisect)
Torsemide Tablets 20 mg	par 653/20 (Bisect)
Torsemide Tablets 100 mg	par 654/100 (Bisect)
Tramadol Hydrochloride Tablets 50 mg	TL/50 / G
Triazolam Tablets 0.125 mg	TR 125 / G
Triazolam Tablets 0.25 mg	TR 250 / G (BISECT)
ZORprin Tablets 800 mg	57

* body/cap of capsule

513	**Neurontin® Tablets** Each tablet contains 600 mg gabapentin.
514-524	*Unassigned*
526	*Unassigned*
527	**Accupril® Tablets** Each tablet contains quinapril hydrochloride equivalent to 5 mg quinapril.
528-529	*Unassigned*
530	**Accupril® Tablets** Each tablet contains quinapril hydrochloride equivalent to 10 mg quinapril.
531	*Unassigned*
532	**Accupril® Tablets** Each tablet contains quinapril hydrochloride equivalent to 20 mg quinapril.
533-534	*Unassigned*
535	**Accupril® Tablets** Each tablet contains quinapril hydrochloride equivalent to 40 mg quinapril.
536	*Unassigned*
538-554	*Unassigned*
556-621	*Unassigned*
622	**Ferrous Fumarate Tablets** Each tablet contains 75 mg ferrous fumarate.
623-736	*Unassigned*
738-802	*Unassigned*
803	**Neurontin® Capsules** Each capsule contains 100 mg gabapentin.
804	*Unassigned*
805	**Neurontin® Capsules** Each capsule contains 300 mg gabapentin.
806	**Neurontin® Capsules** Each capsule contains 400 mg gabapentin.
807-914	*Unassigned*
917-999	*Unassigned*

ACCUPRIL® ℞

[*ă'kew-prĭl*]

(Quinapril Hydrochloride Tablets)

USE IN PREGNANCY
When used in pregnancy during the second and third trimesters, ACE inhibitors can cause injury and even death to the developing fetus. When pregnancy is detected, ACCUPRIL should be discontinued as soon as possible. See WARNINGS, Fetal/Neonatal Morbidity and Mortality.

DESCRIPTION

ACCUPRIL® (quinapril hydrochloride) is the hydrochloride salt of quinapril, the ethyl ester of a non-sulfhydryl, angiotensin-converting enzyme (ACE) inhibitor, quinaprilat.

Quinapril hydrochloride is chemically described as [3S-[2[R*(R*)], 3R*]]-2-[2-[[1-(ethoxycarbonyl)-3-phenylpropyl] amino]-1-oxopropyl]-1,2,3,4-tetrahydro-3-isoquinolinecarboxylic acid, monohydrochloride. Its empirical formula is $C_{25}H_{30}N_2O_5$ •HCl and its structural formula is:

M.W.=474.98

Quinapril hydrochloride is a white to off-white amorphous powder that is freely soluble in aqueous solvents.

ACCUPRIL tablets contain 5 mg, 10 mg, 20 mg, or 40 mg of quinapril for oral administration. Each tablet also contains candelilla wax, crospovidone, gelatin, lactose, magnesium carbonate, magnesium stearate, synthetic red iron oxide, and titanium dioxide.

CLINICAL PHARMACOLOGY

Mechanism of Action: Quinapril is deesterified to the principal metabolite, quinaprilat, which is an inhibitor of ACE activity in human subjects and animals. ACE is a peptidyl dipeptidase that catalyzes the conversion of angiotensin I to the vasoconstrictor, angiotensin II. The effect of quinapril in hypertension and in congestive heart failure (CHF) appears to result primarily from the inhibition of circulating and tissue ACE activity, thereby reducing angiotensin II formation. Quinapril inhibits the elevation in blood pressure caused by intravenously administered angiotensin I, but has no effect on the pressor response to angiotensin II, norepinephrine or epinephrine. Angiotensin II also stimulates the secretion of aldosterone from the adrenal cortex, thereby facilitating renal sodium and fluid reabsorption. Reduced aldosterone secretion by quinapril may result in a small increase in serum potassium. In controlled hypertension trials, treatment with ACCUPRIL alone resulted in mean increases in potassium of 0.07 mmol/L (see PRECAUTIONS). Removal of angiotensin II negative feedback on renin secretion leads to increased plasma renin activity (PRA).

While the principal mechanism of antihypertensive effect is thought to be through the renin-angiotensin-aldosterone system, quinapril exerts antihypertensive actions even in patients with low renin hypertension. ACCUPRIL was an effective antihypertensive in all races studied, although it was somewhat less effective in blacks (usually a predominantly low renin group) than in nonblacks. ACE is identical to kininase II, an enzyme that degrades bradykinin, a potent peptide vasodilator; whether increased levels of bradykinin play a role in the therapeutic effect of quinapril remains to be elucidated.

Pharmacokinetics and Metabolism: Following oral administration, peak plasma quinapril concentrations are observed within one hour. Based on recovery of quinapril and its metabolites in urine, the extent of absorption is at least 60%. The rate and extent of quinapril absorption are diminished moderately (approximately 25-30%) when ACCUPRIL tablets are administered during a high-fat meal. Following absorption, quinapril is deesterified to its major active metabolite, quinaprilat (about 38% of oral dose), and to other minor inactive metabolites. Following multiple oral dosing of ACCUPRIL, there is an effective accumulation half-life of quinaprilat of approximately 3 hours, and peak plasma quinaprilat concentrations are observed approximately 2 hours post-dose. Quinaprilat is eliminated primarily by renal excretion, up to 96% of an IV dose, and has an elimination half-life in plasma of approximately 2 hours and a prolonged terminal phase with a half-life of 25 hours. The pharmacokinetics of quinapril and quinaprilat are linear over a single-dose range of 5-80 mg doses and 40-160 mg in multiple daily doses. Approximately 97% of either quinapril or quinaprilat circulating in plasma is bound to proteins.

In patients with renal insufficiency, the elimination half-life of quinaprilat increases as creatinine clearance decreases. There is a linear correlation between plasma quinaprilat clearance and creatinine clearance. In patients with end-stage renal disease, chronic hemodialysis or continuous ambulatory peritoneal dialysis has little effect on the elimination of quinapril and quinaprilat. Elimination of quinaprilat may be reduced in elderly patients (≥65 years) and in those with heart failure; this reduction is attributable to decrease in renal function (see DOSAGE AND ADMINISTRATION). Quinaprilat concentrations are reduced in patients with alcoholic cirrhosis due to impaired deesterification of quinapril. Studies in rats indicate that quinapril and its metabolites do not cross the blood-brain barrier.

Pharmacodynamics and Clinical Effects

Hypertension: Single doses of 20 mg of ACCUPRIL provide over 80% inhibition of plasma ACE for 24 hours. Inhibition of the pressor response to angiotensin I is shorter-lived, with a 20 mg dose giving 75% inhibition for about 4 hours, 50% inhibition for about 8 hours, and 20% inhibition at 24 hours. With chronic dosing, however, there is substantial inhibition of angiotensin II levels at 24 hours by doses of 20-80 mg.

Administration of 10 to 80 mg of ACCUPRIL to patients with mild to severe hypertension results in a reduction of sitting and standing blood pressure to about the same extent with minimal effect on heart rate. Symptomatic postural hypotension is infrequent although it can occur in patients who are salt- and/or volume-depleted (see WARNINGS). Antihypertensive activity commences within 1 hour with peak effects usually achieved by 2 to 4 hours after dosing. During chronic therapy, most of the blood pressure lowering effect of a given dose is obtained in 1-2 weeks. In multiple-dose studies, 10-80 mg per day in single or divided doses lowered systolic and diastolic blood pressure throughout the dosing interval, with a trough effect of about 5-11/3-7 mm Hg. The trough effect represents about 50% of the peak effect. While the dose-response relationship is relatively flat, doses of 40-80 mg were somewhat more effective at trough than 10-20 mg, and twice daily dosing tended to give a somewhat lower trough blood pressure than once daily dosing with the same total dose. The antihypertensive effect of ACCUPRIL continues during long-term therapy, with no evidence of loss of effectiveness.

Hemodynamic assessments in patients with hypertension indicate that blood pressure reduction produced by quinapril is accompanied by a reduction in total peripheral resistance and renal vascular resistance with little or no change in heart rate, cardiac index, renal blood flow, glomerular filtration rate, or filtration fraction.

Use of ACCUPRIL with a thiazide diuretic gives a blood-pressure lowering effect greater than that seen with either agent alone.

In patients with hypertension, ACCUPRIL 10-40 mg was similar in effectiveness to captopril, enalapril, propranolol, and thiazide diuretics.

Therapeutic effects appear to be the same for elderly (≥65 years of age) and younger adult patients given the same daily dosages, with no increase in adverse events in elderly patients.

Heart Failure: In a placebo-controlled trial involving patients with congestive heart failure treated with digitalis and diuretics, parenteral quinaprilat, the active metabolite of quinapril, reduced pulmonary capillary wedge pressure and systemic vascular resistance and increased cardiac output/index. Similar favorable hemodynamic effects were seen with oral quinapril in baseline-controlled trials, and such effects appeared to be maintained during chronic oral quinapril therapy. Quinapril reduced renal hepatic vascular resistance and increased renal and hepatic blood flow with glomerular filtration rate remaining unchanged.

A significant dose response relationship for improvement in maximal exercise tolerance has been observed with ACCUPRIL therapy. Beneficial effects on the severity of heart failure as measured by New York Heart Association (NYHA) classification and Quality of Life and on symptoms of dyspnea, fatigue, and edema were evident after 6 months in a double-blind, placebo-controlled study. Favorable effects were maintained for up to two years of open label therapy. The effects of quinapril on long-term mortality in heart failure have not been evaluated.

INDICATIONS AND USAGE

Hypertension

ACCUPRIL is indicated for the treatment of hypertension. It may be used alone or in combination with thiazide diuretics.

Heart Failure

ACCUPRIL is indicated in the management of heart failure as adjunctive therapy when added to conventional therapy including diuretics and/or digitalis.

In using ACCUPRIL, consideration should be given to the fact that another angiotensin-converting enzyme inhibitor, captopril, has caused agranulocytosis, particularly in patients with renal impairment or collagen vascular disease. Available data are insufficient to show that ACCUPRIL does not have a similar risk (see WARNINGS).

Angioedema in black patients: Black patients receiving ACE inhibitor monotherapy have been reported to have a higher incidence of angioedema compared to non-blacks. It should also be noted that in controlled clinical trials ACE inhibitors have an effect on blood pressure that is less in black patients than in non-blacks.

CONTRAINDICATIONS

ACCUPRIL is contraindicated in patients who are hypersensitive to this product and in patients with a history of angioedema related to previous treatment with an ACE inhibitor.

WARNINGS

Anaphylactoid and Possibly Related Reactions

Presumably because angiotensin-converting inhibitors affect the metabolism of eicosanoids and polypeptides, including endogenous bradykinin, patients receiving ACE inhibitors (including **ACCUPRIL**) may be subject to a variety of adverse reactions, some of them serious.

Head and Neck Angioedema: Angioedema of the face, extremities, lips, tongue, glottis, and larynx has been reported in patients treated with ACE inhibitors and has been seen in 0.1% of patients receiving ACCUPRIL.

In two similarly sized U.S. postmarketing trials that, combined, enrolled over 3,000 black patients and over 19,000 non-blacks, angioedema was reported in 0.30% and 0.55% of blacks (in study 1 and 2 respectively) and 0.39% and 0.17% of non-blacks.

Angioedema associated with laryngeal edema can be fatal. If laryngeal stridor or angioedema of the face, tongue, or glottis occurs, treatment with ACCUPRIL should be discontinued immediately, the patient treated in accordance with accepted medical care, and carefully observed until the swelling disappears. In instances where swelling is confined to the face and lips, the condition generally resolves without treatment; antihistamines may be useful in relieving symptoms. **Where there is involvement of the tongue, glottis, or larynx likely to cause airway obstruction, emergency therapy including, but not limited to, subcutaneous epinephrine solution 1:1000 (0.3 to 0.5 mL) should be promptly administered** (see ADVERSE REACTIONS).

Intestinal Angioedema: Intestinal angioedema has been reported in patients treated with ACE inhibitors. These patients presented with abdominal pain (with or without nausea or vomiting); in some cases there was no prior history of facial angioedema and C-1 esterase levels were normal. The angioedema was diagnosed by procedures including abdominal CT scan or ultrasound, or at surgery, and symptoms resolved after stopping the ACE inhibitor. Intestinal angioedema should be included in the differential diagnosis of patients on ACE inhibitors presenting with abdominal pain.

Patients with a history of angioedema: Patients with a history of angioedema unrelated to ACE inhibitor therapy may be at increased risk of angioedema while receiving an ACE inhibitor (see also CONTRAINDICATIONS).

Anaphylactoid reactions during desensitization: Two patients undergoing desensitizing treatment with hymenoptera venom while receiving ACE inhibitors sustained life-threatening anaphylactoid reactions. In the same patients, these reactions were avoided when ACE inhibitors were temporarily withheld, but they reappeared upon inadvertent rechallenge.

Anaphylactoid reactions during membrane exposure: Anaphylactoid reactions have been reported in patients dialyzed with high-flux membranes and treated concomitantly with an ACE inhibitor. Anaphylactoid reactions have also been reported in patients undergoing low-density lipoprotein apheresis with dextran sulfate absorption.

Hepatic Failure: Rarely, ACE inhibitors have been associated with a syndrome that starts with cholestatic jaundice

Continued on next page

Accupril—Cont.

and progresses to fulminant hepatic necrosis and (sometimes) death. The mechanism of this syndrome is not understood. Patients receiving ACE inhibitors who develop jaundice or marked elevations of hepatic enzymes should discontinue the ACE inhibitor and receive appropriate medical follow-up.

Hypotension: Excessive hypotension is rare in patients with uncomplicated hypertension treated with ACCUPRIL alone. Patients with heart failure given ACCUPRIL commonly have some reduction in blood pressure, but discontinuation of therapy because of continuing symptomatic hypotension usually is not necessary when dosing instructions are followed. Caution should be observed when initiating therapy in patients with heart failure (see DOSAGE AND ADMINISTRATION). In controlled studies, syncope was observed in 0.4% of patients (N=3203); this incidence was similar to that observed for captopril (1%) and enalapril (0.8%).

Patients at risk of excessive hypotension, sometimes associated with oliguria and/or progressive azotemia, and rarely with acute renal failure and/or death, include patients with the following conditions or characteristics: heart failure, hyponatremia, high dose diuretic therapy, recent intensive diuresis or increase in diuretic dose, renal dialysis, or severe volume and/or salt depletion of any etiology. It may be advisable to eliminate the diuretic (except in patients with heart failure), reduce the diuretic dose or cautiously increase salt intake (except in patients with heart failure) before initiating therapy with ACCUPRIL in patients at risk for excessive hypotension who are able to tolerate such adjustments.

In patients at risk of excessive hypotension, therapy with ACCUPRIL should be started under close medical supervision. Such patients should be followed closely for the first two weeks of treatment and whenever the dose of ACCUPRIL and/or diuretic is increased. Similar considerations may apply to patients with ischemic heart or cerebrovascular disease in whom an excessive fall in blood pressure could result in a myocardial infarction or a cerebrovascular accident.

If excessive hypotension occurs, the patient should be placed in the supine position and, if necessary, receive an intravenous infusion of normal saline. A transient hypotensive response is not a contraindication to further doses of ACCUPRIL, which usually can be given without difficulty once the blood pressure has stabilized. If symptomatic hypotension develops, a dose reduction or discontinuation of ACCUPRIL or concomitant diuretic may be necessary.

Neutropenia/Agranulocytosis: Another ACE inhibitor, captopril, has been shown to cause agranulocytosis and bone marrow depression rarely in patients with uncomplicated hypertension, but more frequently in patients with renal impairment, especially if they also have a collagen vascular disease, such as systemic lupus erythematosus or scleroderma. Agranulocytosis did occur during ACCUPRIL treatment in one patient with a history of neutropenia during previous captopril therapy. Available data from clinical trials of ACCUPRIL are insufficient to show that, in patients without prior reactions to other ACE inhibitors, ACCUPRIL does not cause agranulocytosis at similar rates. As with other ACE inhibitors, periodic monitoring of white blood cell counts in patients with collagen vascular disease and/or renal disease should be considered.

Fetal/Neonatal Morbidity and Mortality: ACE inhibitors can cause fetal and neonatal morbidity and death when administered to pregnant women. Several dozen cases have been reported in the world literature. When pregnancy is detected, ACE inhibitors should be discontinued as soon as possible.

The use of ACE inhibitors during the second and third trimesters of pregnancy has been associated with fetal and neonatal injury, including hypotension, neonatal skull hypoplasia, anuria, reversible or irreversible renal failure, and death. Oligohydramnios has also been reported, presumably resulting from decreased fetal renal function; oligohydramnios in this setting has been associated with fetal limb contractures, craniofacial deformation, and hypoplastic lung development. Prematurity, intrauterine growth retardation, and patent ductus arteriosus have also been reported, although it is not clear whether these occurrences were due to the ACE inhibitor exposure.

These adverse effects do not appear to have resulted from intrauterine ACE inhibitor exposure that has been limited to the first trimester. Mothers whose embryos and fetuses are exposed to ACE inhibitors only during the first trimester should be so informed. Nonetheless, when patients become pregnant, physicians should make every effort to discontinue the use of ACCUPRIL as soon as possible.

Rarely (probably less often than once in every thousand pregnancies), no alternative to ACE inhibitors will be found. In these rare cases, the mothers should be apprised of the potential hazards to their fetuses, and serial ultrasound examinations should be performed to assess the intraamniotic environment.

If oligohydramnios is observed, ACCUPRIL should be discontinued unless it is considered life-saving for the mother. Contraction stress testing (CST), a non-stress test (NST), or biophysical profiling (BPP) may be appropriate, depending upon the week of pregnancy. Patients and physicians should be aware, however, that oligohydramnios may not appear until after the fetus has sustained irreversible injury.

Infants with histories of *in utero* exposure to ACE inhibitors should be closely observed for hypotension, oliguria, and hyperkalemia. If oliguria occurs, attention should be directed toward support of blood pressure and renal perfusion. Exchange transfusion or dialysis may be required as a means of reversing hypotension and/or substituting for disordered renal function. Removal of ACCUPRIL, which crosses the placenta, from the neonatal circulation is not significantly accelerated by these means.

No teratogenic effects of ACCUPRIL were seen in studies of pregnant rats and rabbits. On a mg/kg basis, the doses used were up to 180 times (in rats) and one time (in rabbits) the maximum recommended human dose.

PRECAUTIONS

General

Impaired renal function: As a consequence of inhibiting the renin-angiotensin-aldosterone system, changes in renal function may be anticipated in susceptible individuals. In patients with severe heart failure whose renal function may depend on the activity of the renin-angiotensin-aldosterone system, treatment with ACE inhibitors, including ACCUPRIL, may be associated with oliguria and/or progressive azotemia and rarely acute renal failure and/or death.

In clinical studies in hypertensive patients with unilateral or bilateral renal artery stenosis, increases in blood urea nitrogen and serum creatinine have been observed in some patients following ACE inhibitor therapy. These increases were almost always reversible upon discontinuation of the ACE inhibitor and/or diuretic therapy. In such patients, renal function should be monitored during the first few weeks of therapy.

Some patients with hypertension or heart failure with no apparent preexisting renal vascular disease have developed increases in blood urea and serum creatinine, usually minor and transient, especially when ACCUPRIL has been given concomitantly with a diuretic. This is more likely to occur in patients with preexisting renal impairment. Dosage reduction and/or discontinuation of any diuretic and/or ACCUPRIL may be required.

Evaluation of patients with hypertension or heart failure should always include assessment of renal function (see DOSAGE AND ADMINISTRATION).

Hyperkalemia and potassium-sparing diuretics: In clinical trials, hyperkalemia (serum potassium ≥5.8 mmol/L) occurred in approximately 2% of patients receiving ACCUPRIL. In most cases, elevated serum potassium levels were isolated values which resolved despite continued therapy. Less than 0.1% of patients discontinued therapy due to hyperkalemia. Risk factors for the development of hyperkalemia include renal insufficiency, diabetes mellitus, and the concomitant use of potassium-sparing diuretics, potassium supplements, and/or potassium-containing salt substitutes, which should be used cautiously, if at all, with ACCUPRIL (see PRECAUTIONS, Drug Interactions).

Cough: Presumably due to the inhibition of the degradation of endogenous bradykinin, persistent non-productive cough has been reported with all ACE inhibitors, always resolving after discontinuation of therapy. ACE inhibitor-induced cough should be considered in the differential diagnosis of cough.

Surgery/anesthesia: In patients undergoing major surgery or during anesthesia with agents that produce hypotension, ACCUPRIL will block angiotensin II formation secondary to compensatory renin release. If hypotension occurs and is considered to be due to this mechanism, it can be corrected by volume expansion.

Information for Patients

Pregnancy: Female patients of childbearing age should be told about the consequences of second- and third-trimester exposure to ACE inhibitors, and they should also be told that these consequences do not appear to have resulted from intrauterine ACE-inhibitor exposure that has been limited to the first trimester. These patients should be asked to report pregnancies to their physicians as soon as possible.

Angioedema: Angioedema, including laryngeal edema can occur with treatment with ACE inhibitors, especially following the first dose. Patients should be so advised and told to report immediately any signs or symptoms suggesting angioedema (swelling of face, extremities, eyes, lips, tongue, difficulty in swallowing or breathing) and to stop taking the drug until they have consulted with their physician (see WARNINGS).

Symptomatic hypotension: Patients should be cautioned that lightheadedness can occur, especially during the first few days of ACCUPRIL therapy, and that it should be reported to a physician. If actual syncope occurs, patients should be told to not take the drug until they have consulted with their physician (see WARNINGS).

All patients should be cautioned that inadequate fluid intake or excessive perspiration, diarrhea, or vomiting can lead to an excessive fall in blood pressure because of reduction in fluid volume, with the same consequences of lightheadedness and possible syncope.

Patients planning to undergo any surgery and/or anesthesia should be told to inform their physician that they are taking an ACE inhibitor.

Hyperkalemia: Patients should be told not to use potassium supplements or salt substitutes containing potassium without consulting their physician (see PRECAUTIONS).

Neutropenia: Patients should be told to report promptly any indication of infection (eg, sore throat, fever) which could be a sign of neutropenia.

NOTE: As with many other drugs, certain advice to patients being treated with ACCUPRIL is warranted. This information is intended to aid in the safe and effective use of this medication. It is not a disclosure of all possible adverse or intended effects.

Drug Interactions

Concomitant diuretic therapy: As with other ACE inhibitors, patients on diuretics, especially those on recently instituted diuretic therapy, may occasionally experience an excessive reduction of blood pressure after initiation of therapy with ACCUPRIL. The possibility of hypotensive effects with ACCUPRIL may be minimized by either discontinuing the diuretic or cautiously increasing salt intake prior to initiation of treatment with ACCUPRIL. If it is not possible to discontinue the diuretic, the starting dose of quinapril should be reduced (see DOSAGE AND ADMINISTRATION).

Agents increasing serum potassium: Quinapril can attenuate potassium loss caused by thiazide diuretics and increase serum potassium when used alone. If concomitant therapy of ACCUPRIL with potassium-sparing diuretics (eg, spironolactone, triamterene, or amiloride), potassium supplements, or potassium-containing salt substitutes is indicated, they should be used with caution along with appropriate monitoring of serum potassium (see PRECAUTIONS).

Tetracycline and other drugs that interact with magnesium: Simultaneous administration of tetracycline with ACCUPRIL reduced the absorption of tetracycline by approximately 28% to 37%, possibly due to the high magnesium content in ACCUPRIL tablets. This interaction should be considered if coprescribing ACCUPRIL and tetracycline or other drugs that interact with magnesium.

Lithium: Increased serum lithium levels and symptoms of lithium toxicity have been reported in patients receiving concomitant lithium and ACE inhibitor therapy. These drugs should be coadministered with caution and frequent monitoring of serum lithium levels is recommended. If a diuretic is also used, it may increase the risk of lithium toxicity.

Other agents: Drug interaction studies of ACCUPRIL with other agents showed:

- Multiple dose therapy with propranolol or cimetidine has no effect on the pharmacokinetics of single doses of ACCUPRIL.
- The anticoagulant effect of a single dose of warfarin (measured by prothrombin time) was not significantly changed by quinapril coadministration twice-daily.
- ACCUPRIL treatment did not affect the pharmacokinetics of digoxin.
- No pharmacokinetic interaction was observed when single doses of ACCUPRIL and hydrochlorothiazide were administered concomitantly.
- Co-administration of multiple 10 mg doses of atorvastatin with 80 mg of ACCUPRIL resulted in no significant change in the steady-state pharmacokinetic parameters of atorvastatin.

Carcinogenesis, Mutagenesis, Impairment of Fertility

Quinapril hydrochloride was not carcinogenic in mice or rats when given in doses up to 75 or 100 mg/kg/day (50 to 60 times the maximum human daily dose, respectively, on an mg/kg basis and 3.8 to 10 times the maximum human daily dose when based on an mg/m^2 basis) for 104 weeks. Female rats given the highest dose level had an increased incidence of mesenteric lymph node hemangiomas and skin/subcutaneous lipomas. Neither quinapril nor quinaprilat were mutagenic in the Ames bacterial assay with or without metabolic activation. Quinapril was also negative in the following genetic toxicology studies: *in vitro* mammalian cell point mutation, sister chromatid exchange in cultured mammalian cells, micronucleus test with mice, *in vitro* chromosome aberration with V79 cultured lung cells, and in an *in vivo* cytogenetic study with rat bone marrow. There were no adverse effects on fertility or reproduction in rats at doses up to 100 mg/kg/day (60 and 10 times the maximum daily human dose when based on mg/kg and mg/m^2, respectively).

Pregnancy

Pregnancy Categories C (first trimester) and D (second and third trimesters): See WARNINGS, Fetal/Neonatal Morbidity and Mortality.

Nursing Mothers

Because ACCUPRIL is secreted in human milk, caution should be exercised when this drug is administered to a nursing woman.

Pediatric Use

The safety and effectiveness of ACCUPRIL in pediatric patients have not been established.

Geriatric Use

Clinical studies of ACCUPRIL did not include sufficient numbers of subjects aged 65 and over to determine whether they respond differently from younger subjects. Other reported clinical experience has not identified differences in responses between the elderly and younger patients. In general, dose selection for an elderly patient should be cautious, usually starting at the low end of the dosing range, reflecting the greater frequency of decreased hepatic, renal or cardiac function, and of concomitant disease or other drug therapy.

This drug is known to be substantially excreted by the kidney, and the risk of toxic reactions to this drug may be greater in patients with impaired renal function. Because

elderly patients are more likely to have decreased renal function, care should be taken in dose selection, and it may be useful to monitor renal function.
Elderly patients exhibited increased area under the plasma concentration time curve and peak levels for quinaprilat compared to values observed in younger patients; this appeared to relate to decreased renal function rather than to age itself.

ADVERSE REACTIONS

Hypertension
ACCUPRIL has been evaluated for safety in 4960 subjects and patients. Of these, 3203 patients, including 655 elderly patients, participated in controlled clinical trials. ACCUPRIL has been evaluated for long-term safety in over 1400 patients treated for 1 year or more.
Adverse experiences were usually mild and transient.
In placebo-controlled trials, discontinuation of therapy because of adverse events was required in 4.7% of patients with hypertension.
Adverse experiences probably or possibly related to therapy or of unknown relationship to therapy occurring in 1% or more of the 1563 patients in placebo-controlled hypertension trials who were treated with ACCUPRIL are shown below.

Adverse Events in Placebo-Controlled Trials

	Accupril (N=1563) Incidence (Discontinuance)	Placebo (N=579) Incidence (Discontinuance)
Headache	5.6 (0.7)	10.9 (0.7)
Dizziness	3.9 (0.8)	2.6 (0.2)
Fatigue	2.6 (0.3)	1.0
Coughing	2.0 (0.5)	0.0
Nausea and/or Vomiting	1.4 (0.3)	1.9 (0.2)
Abdominal Pain	1.0 (0.2)	0.7

Heart Failure
ACCUPRIL has been evaluated for safety in 1222 ACCUPRIL treated patients. Of these, 632 patients participated in controlled clinical trials. In placebo-controlled trials, discontinuation of therapy because of adverse events was required in 6.8% of patients with congestive heart failure.
Adverse experiences probably or possibly related or of unknown relationship to therapy occurring in 1% or more of the 585 patients in placebo-controlled congestive heart failure trials who were treated with ACCUPRIL are shown below.

	Accupril (N=585) Incidence (Discontinuance)	Placebo (N=295) Incidence (Discontinuance)
Dizziness	7.7 (0.7)	5.1 (1.0)
Coughing	4.3 (0.3)	1.4
Fatigue	2.6 (0.2)	1.4
Nausea and/or Vomiting	2.4 (0.2)	0.7
Chest Pain	2.4	1.0
Hypotension	2.9 (0.5)	1.0
Dyspnea	1.9 (0.2)	2.0
Diarrhea	1.7	1.0
Headache	1.7	1.0 (0.3)
Myalgia	1.5	2.0
Rash	1.4 (0.2)	1.0
Back Pain	1.2	0.3

See PRECAUTIONS, Cough.
Hypertension and/or Heart Failure
Clinical adverse experiences probably, possibly, or definitely related, or of uncertain relationship to therapy occurring in 0.5% to 1.0% (except as noted) of the patients with CHF or hypertension treated with ACCUPRIL (with or without concomitant diuretic) in controlled or uncontrolled trials (N=4847) and less frequent, clinically significant events seen in clinical trials or post-marketing experience (the rarer events are in italics) include (listed by body system):
General: back pain, malaise, viral infections, *anaphylactoid reaction.*
Cardiovascular: palpitation, vasodilation, tachycardia, *heart failure, hyperkalemia, myocardial infarction, cerebrovascular accident, hypertensive crisis, angina pectoris, orthostatic hypotension, cardiac rhythm disturbances, cardiogenic shock*
Hematology: *hemolytic anemia*
Gastrointestinal: flatulence, dry mouth or throat, constipation, *gastrointestinal hemorrhage, pancreatitis, abnormal liver function tests, dyspepsia*
Nervous/Psychiatric: somnolence, vertigo, syncope, nervousness, depression, insomnia, paresthesia
Integumentary: alopecia, increased sweating, pemphigus, pruritus, *exfoliative dermatitis, photosensitivity reaction, dermatopolymyositis*
Urogenital: urinary tract infection, impotence, *acute renal failure, worsening renal failure*
Respiratory: *eosinophilic pneumonitis*
Other: amblyopia, edema, arthralgia, pharyngitis, *agranulocytosis, hepatitis, thrombocytopenia*
Fetal/Neonatal Morbidity and Mortality
See WARNINGS, Fetal/Neonatal Morbidity and Mortality.
Angioedema
Angioedema has been reported in patients receiving ACCUPRIL (0.1%). Angioedema associated with laryngeal edema may be fatal. If angioedema of the face, extremities, lips, tongue, glottis, and/or larynx occurs, treatment with ACCUPRIL should be discontinued and appropriate therapy instituted immediately. (See WARNINGS.)
Clinical Laboratory Test Findings
Hematology: (See WARNINGS)
Hyperkalemia: (See PRECAUTIONS)
Creatinine and Blood Urea Nitrogen: Increases (>1.25 times the upper limit of normal) in serum creatinine and blood urea nitrogen were observed in 2% and 2%, respectively, of all patients treated with ACCUPRIL alone. Increases are more likely to occur in patients receiving concomitant diuretic therapy than in those on ACCUPRIL alone. These increases often remit on continued therapy. In controlled studies of heart failure, increases in blood urea nitrogen and serum creatinine were observed in 11% and 8%, respectively, of patients treated with ACCUPRIL; most often these patients were receiving diuretics with or without digitalis.

OVERDOSAGE

Doses of 1440 to 4280 mg/kg of quinapril cause significant lethality in mice and rats.
No specific information is available on the treatment of overdosage with quinapril. The most likely clinical manifestation would be symptoms attributable to severe hypotension.
Laboratory determinations of serum levels of quinapril and its metabolites are not widely available, and such determinations have, in any event, no established role in the management of quinapril overdose.
No data are available to suggest physiological maneuvers (eg, maneuvers to change pH of the urine) that might accelerate elimination of quinapril and its metabolites.
Hemodialysis and peritoneal dialysis have little effect on the elimination of quinapril and quinaprilat. Angiotensin II could presumably serve as a specific antagonist-antidote in the setting of quinapril overdose, but angiotensin II is essentially unavailable outside of scattered research facilities. Because the hypotensive effect of quinapril is achieved through vasodilation and effective hypovolemia, it is reasonable to treat quinapril overdose by infusion of normal saline solution.

DOSAGE AND ADMINISTRATION

Hypertension
Monotherapy: The recommended initial dosage of ACCUPRIL in patients not on diuretics is 10 or 20 mg once daily. Dosage should be adjusted according to blood pressure response measured at peak (2-6 hours after dosing) and trough (predosing). Generally, dosage adjustments should be made at intervals of at least 2 weeks. Most patients have required dosages of 20, 40, or 80 mg/day, given as a single dose or in two equally divided doses. In some patients treated once daily, the antihypertensive effect may diminish toward the end of the dosing interval. In such patients an increase in dosage or twice daily administration may be warranted. In general, doses of 40-80 mg and divided doses give a somewhat greater effect at the end of the dosing interval.
Concomitant Diuretics: If blood pressure is not adequately controlled with ACCUPRIL monotherapy, a diuretic may be added. In patients who are currently being treated with a diuretic, symptomatic hypotension occasionally can occur following the initial dose of ACCUPRIL. To reduce the likelihood of hypotension, the diuretic should, if possible, be discontinued 2 to 3 days prior to beginning therapy with ACCUPRIL (see WARNINGS). Then, if blood pressure is not controlled with ACCUPRIL alone, diuretic therapy should be resumed.
If the diuretic cannot be discontinued, an initial dose of 5 mg ACCUPRIL should be used with careful medical supervision for several hours and until blood pressure has stabilized.
The dosage should subsequently be titrated (as described above) to the optimal response (see WARNINGS, PRECAUTIONS, and Drug Interactions).
Renal Impairment: Kinetic data indicate that the apparent elimination half-life of quinaprilat increases as creatinine clearance decreases. Recommended starting doses, based on clinical and pharmacokinetic data from patients with renal impairment, are as follows:

Creatinine Clearance	Maximum Recommended Initial Dose
>60 mL/min	10 mg
30-60 mL/min	5 mg
10-30 mL/min	2.5 mg
<10 mL/min	Insufficient data for dosage recommendation

Patients should subsequently have their dosage titrated (as described above) to the optimal response.
Elderly (≥65 years): The recommended initial dosage of ACCUPRIL in elderly patients is 10 mg given once daily followed by titration (as described above) to the optimal response.
Heart Failure
ACCUPRIL is indicated as adjunctive therapy when added to conventional therapy including diuretics and/or digitalis. The recommended starting dose is 5 mg twice daily. This dose may improve symptoms of heart failure, but increases in exercise duration have generally required higher doses. Therefore, if the initial dosage of ACCUPRIL is well tolerated, patients should then be titrated at weekly intervals until an effective dose, usually 20 to 40 mg daily given in two equally divided doses, is reached or undesirable hypotension, orthostatis, or azotemia (see WARNINGS) prohibit reaching this dose.
Following the initial dose of ACCUPRIL, the patient should be observed under medical supervision for at least two hours for the presence of hypotension or orthostatis and, if present, until blood pressure stabilizes. The appearance of hypotension, orthostatis, or azotemia early in dose titration should not preclude further careful dose titration. Consideration should be given to reducing the dose of concomitant diuretics.
DOSE ADJUSTMENTS IN PATIENTS WITH HEART FAILURE AND RENAL IMPAIRMENT OR HYPONATREMIA
Pharmacokinetic data indicate that quinapril elimination is dependent on level of renal function. In patients with heart failure and renal impairment, the recommended initial dose of ACCUPRIL is 5 mg in patients with a creatinine clearance above 30 mL/min and 2.5 mg in patients with a creatinine clearance of 10 to 30 mL/min. There is insufficient data for dosage recommendation in patients with a creatinine clearance less than 10 mL/min (see DOSAGE AND ADMINISTRATION, Heart Failure WARNINGS, and PRECAUTIONS, Drug Interactions).
If the initial dose is well tolerated, ACCUPRIL may be administered the following day as a twice daily regimen. In the absence of excessive hypotension or significant deterioration of renal function, the dose may be increased at weekly intervals based on clinical and hemodynamic response.

HOW SUPPLIED

ACCUPRIL tablets are supplied as follows:
5-mg tablets: brown, film-coated, elliptical scored tablets, coded "PD 527" on one side and "5" on the other.
N0071-0527-23 bottles of 90 tablets
N0071-0527-40 10 × 10 unit dose blisters
10-mg tablets: brown, film-coated, triangular tablets, coded "PD 530" on one side and "10" on the other.
N0071-0530-23 bottles of 90 tablets
N0071-0530-40 10 × 10 unit dose blisters
20-mg tablets: brown, film-coated, round tablets, coded "PD 532" on one side and "20" on the other.
N0071-0532-23 bottles of 90 tablets
N0071-0532-40 10 × 10 unit dose blisters
40-mg tablets: brown, film-coated, elliptical tablets, coded "PD 535" on one side and "40" on the other.
N0071-0535-23 bottles of 90 tablets
Dispense in well-closed containers as defined in the USP.
Storage: Store at controlled room temperature 15°-30°C (59°-86°F).
Protect from light.
Rx only

Revised February 2003
Manufactured by:
Pfizer Pharmaceuticals, Ltd.
Vega Baja, PR 00694
Distributed by:
Parke-Davis
Division of Pfizer Inc, NY, NY 10017
69-5825-00-2
Shown in Product Identification Guide, page 329

ACCURETIC™ ℞

[*ă' kew-rĕ' tĭk*]
(quinapril HCl/hydrochlorothiazide) Tablets

USE IN PREGNANCY
When used in pregnancy during the second and third trimesters, ACE inhibitors can cause injury and even death to the developing fetus. When pregnancy is detected, ACCURETIC should be discontinued as soon as possible. See **WARNINGS: Fetal/Neonatal Morbidity and Mortality.**

DESCRIPTION

ACCURETIC is a fixed-combination tablet that combines an angiotensin-converting enzyme (ACE) inhibitor, quinapril hydrochloride, and a thiazide diuretic, hydrochlorothiazide. Quinapril hydrochloride is chemically described as [3S-[2[R*(R*)], 3R*]]-2-[2-[[1-(ethoxycarbonyl)-3-phenylpropyl] amino]-1-oxopropyl]-1,2,3,4-tetrahydro-3-isoquinolinecarboxylic acid, monohydrochloride. Its empirical formula is $C_{25}H_{30}N_2O_5 \cdot HCl$ and its structural formula is:
[See chemical structure at top of next column]
Quinapril hydrochloride is a white to off-white amorphous powder that is freely soluble in aqueous solvents.

Continued on next page

Accuretic—Cont.

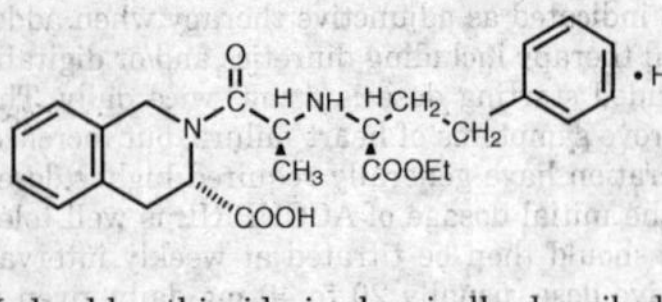

• HCl

M.W. = 474.98

Hydrochlorothiazide is chemically described as: 6-Chloro-3,4-dihydro-2H-1,2,4-benzothiadiazine-7-sulfonamide 1,1-dioxide. Its empirical formula is $C_7H_8ClN_3O_4S_2$ and its structural formula is:

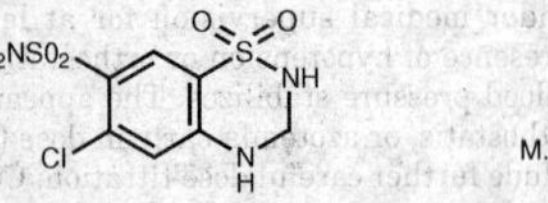

M.W. = 297.72

Hydrochlorothiazide is a white to off-white, crystalline powder which is slightly soluble in water but freely soluble in sodium hydroxide solution.

ACCURETIC is available for oral use as fixed combination tablets in three strengths of quinapril with hydrochlorothiazide: 10 mg with 12.5 mg (ACCURETIC 10/12.5), 20 mg with 12.5 mg (ACCURETIC 20/12.5), and 20 mg with 25 mg (ACCURETIC 20/25). Inactive ingredients: candelilla wax, crospovidone, hydroxypropyl cellulose, hypromellose, iron oxide red, iron oxide yellow, lactose, magnesium carbonate, magnesium stearate, polyethylene glycol, povidone, and titanium dioxide.

CLINICAL PHARMACOLOGY

Mechanism of Action: The principal metabolite of quinapril, quinaprilat, is an inhibitor of ACE activity in human subjects and animals. ACE is peptidyl dipeptidase that catalyzes the conversion of angiotensin I to the vasoconstrictor, angiotensin II. The effect of quinapril in hypertension appears to result primarily from the inhibition of circulating and tissue ACE activity, thereby reducing angiotensin II formation. Quinapril inhibits the elevation in blood pressure caused by intravenously administered angiotensin I, but has no effect on the pressor response to angiotensin II, norepinephrine, or epinephrine. Angiotensin II also stimulates the secretion of aldosterone from the adrenal cortex, thereby facilitating renal sodium and fluid reabsorption. Reduced aldosterone secretion by quinapril may result in a small increase in serum potassium. In controlled hypertension trials, treatment with quinapril alone resulted in mean increases in potassium of 0.07 mmol/L (see **PRECAUTIONS**). Removal of angiotensin II negative feedback on renin secretion leads to increased plasma renin activity (PRA).

While the principal mechanism of antihypertensive effect is thought to be through the renin-angiotensin-aldosterone system, quinapril exerts antihypertensive actions even in patients with low renin hypertension. Quinapril was an effective antihypertensive in all races studied, although it was somewhat less effective in blacks (usually a predominantly low renin group) than in non-blacks. ACE is identical to kininase II, an enzyme that degrades bradykinin, a potent peptide vasodilator; whether increased levels of bradykinin play a role in the therapeutic effect of quinapril remains to be elucidated.

Hydrochlorothiazide is a thiazide diuretic. Thiazides affect the renal tubular mechanisms of electrolyte reabsorption, directly increasing excretion of sodium and chloride in approximately equivalent amounts. Indirectly, the diuretic action of hydrochlorothiazide reduces plasma volume, with consequent increases in plasma renin activity, increases in aldosterone secretion, increases in urinary potassium loss, and decreases in serum potassium. The renin-aldosterone link is mediated by angiotensin, so coadministration of an ACE inhibitor tends to reverse the potassium loss associated with these diuretics.

The mechanism of the antihypertensive effect of thiazides is unknown.

Pharmacokinetics and Metabolism: The rate and extent of absorption of quinapril and hydrochlorothiazide from ACCURETIC tablets are not different, respectively, from the rate and extent of absorption of quinapril and hydrochlorothiazide from immediate-release monotherapy formulations, either administered concurrently or separately. Following oral administration of Accupril (quinapril monotherapy) tablets, peak plasma quinapril concentrations are observed within 1 hour. Based on recovery of quinapril and its metabolites in urine, the extent of absorption is at least 60%. The absorption of hydrochlorothiazide is somewhat slower (1 to 2.5 hours) and more complete (50% to 80%).

The rate of quinapril absorption was reduced by 14% when ACCURETIC tablets were administered with a high-fat meal as compared to fasting, while the extent of absorption was not affected. The rate of hydrochlorothiazide absorption was reduced by 12% when ACCURETIC tablets were administered with a high-fat meal, while the extent of absorption was not significantly affected. Therefore, ACCURETIC may be administered without regard to food.

Following absorption, quinapril is deesterified to its major active metabolite, quinaprilat (about 38% of oral dose), and to other minor inactive metabolites. Following multiple oral dosing of quinapril, there is an effective accumulation half-life of quinaprilat of approximately 3 hours, and peak plasma quinaprilat concentrations are observed approximately 2 hours postdose. Approximately 97% of either quinapril or quinaprilat circulating in plasma is bound to proteins. Hydrochlorothiazide is not metabolized. Its apparent volume of distribution is 3.6 to 7.8 L/kg, consistent with measured plasma protein binding of 67.9%. The drug also accumulates in red blood cells, so that whole blood levels are 1.6 to 1.8 times those measured in plasma.

Some placental passage occurred when quinapril was administered to pregnant rats. Studies in rats indicate that quinapril and its metabolites do not cross the blood-brain barrier. Hydrochlorothiazide crosses the placenta freely but not the blood-brain barrier.

Quinaprilat is eliminated primarily by renal excretion, up to 96% of an IV dose, and has an elimination half-life in plasma of approximately 2 hours and a prolonged terminal phase with a half-life of 25 hours. Hydrochlorothiazide is excreted unchanged by the kidney. When plasma levels have been followed for at least 24 hours, the plasma half-life has been observed to vary between 4 to 15 hours. At least 61% of the oral dose is eliminated unchanged within 24 hours.

In patients with renal insufficiency, the elimination half-life of quinaprilat increases as creatinine clearance decreases. There is a linear correlation between plasma quinaprilat clearance and creatinine clearance. In patients with end-stage renal disease, chronic hemodialysis or continuous ambulatory peritoneal dialysis have little effect on the elimination of quinapril and quinaprilat. Elimination of quinaprilat is reduced in elderly patients (≥65 years) and in those with heart failure; this reduction is attributable to decrease in renal function (see **DOSAGE AND ADMINISTRATION**). Quinaprilat concentrations are reduced in patients with alcoholic cirrhosis due to impaired deesterification of quinapril. In a study of patients with impaired renal function (mean creatinine clearance of 19 mL/min), the half-life of hydrochlorothiazide elimination was lengthened to 21 hours.

The pharmacokinetics of quinapril and quinaprilat are linear over a single-dose range of 5- to 80-mg doses and 40- to 160-mg in multiple daily doses.

Pharmacodynamics and Clinical Effects: Single doses of 20 mg of quinapril provide over 80% inhibition of plasma ACE for 24 hours. Inhibition of the pressor response to angiotensin I is shorter-lived, with a 20-mg dose giving 75% inhibition for about 4 hours, 50% inhibition for about 8 hours, and 20% inhibition at 24 hours. With chronic dosing, however, there is substantial inhibition of angiotensin II levels at 24 hours by doses of 20 to 80 mg.

Administration of 10 to 80 mg of quinapril to patients with mild to severe hypertension results in a reduction of sitting and standing blood pressure to about the same extent with minimal effect on heart rate. Symptomatic postural hypotension is infrequent, although it can occur in patients who are salt- and/or volume-depleted (see **WARNINGS**).

Antihypertensive activity commences within 1 hour with peak effects usually achieved by 2 to 4 hours after dosing. During chronic therapy, most of the blood pressure lowering effect of a given dose is obtained in 1 to 2 weeks. In multiple-dose studies, 10 to 80 mg per day in single or divided doses lowered systolic and diastolic blood pressure throughout the dosing interval, with a trough effect of about 5 to 11/3 to 7 mm Hg. The trough effect represents about 50% of the peak effect.

While the dose-response relationship is relatively flat, doses of 40 to 80 mg were somewhat more effective at trough than 10 to 20 mg, and twice-daily dosing tended to give a somewhat lower trough blood pressure than once-daily dosing with the same total dose. The antihypertensive effect of quinapril continues during long-term therapy, with no evidence of loss of effectiveness.

Hemodynamic assessments in patients with hypertension indicate that blood pressure reduction produced by quinapril is accompanied by a reduction in total peripheral resistance and renal vascular resistance with little or no change in heart rate, cardiac index, renal blood flow, glomerular filtration rate, or filtration fraction.

Therapeutic effects of quinapril appear to be the same for elderly (≥65 years of age) and younger adult patients given the same daily dosages, with no increase in adverse events in elderly patients. In patients with hypertension, quinapril 10 to 40 mg was similar in effectiveness to captopril, enalapril, propranolol, and thiazide diuretics.

After oral administration of hydrochlorothiazide, diuresis begins within 2 hours, peaks in about 4 hours, and lasts about 6 to 12 hours. Use of quinapril with a thiazide diuretic gives blood pressure lowering effect greater than that seen with either agent alone. In clinical trials of quinapril/hydrochlorothiazide using quinapril doses of 2.5 to 40 mg and hydrochlorothiazide doses of 6.25 to 25 mg, the antihypertensive effects were sustained for at least 24 hours, and increased with increasing dose of either component. Although quinapril monotherapy is somewhat less effective in blacks than in non-blacks, the efficacy of combination therapy appears to be independent of race. By blocking the renin-angiotensin-aldosterone axis, administration of quinapril tends to reduce the potassium loss associated with the diuretic. In clinical trials of ACCURETIC, the average change in serum potassium was near zero when 2.5 to 40 mg of quinapril was combined with hydrochlorothiazide 6.25 mg, and the average subject who received 10 to 20/12.5 to 25 mg experienced a milder reduction in serum potassium than that experienced by the average subject receiving the same dose of hydrochlorothiazide monotherapy.

INDICATIONS AND USAGE

ACCURETIC is indicated for the treatment of hypertension. This fixed combination is not indicated for the initial therapy of hypertension (see **DOSAGE AND ADMINISTRATION**).

In using ACCURETIC, consideration should be given to the fact that another angiotensin-converting enzyme inhibitor, captopril, has caused agranulocytosis, particularly in patients with renal impairment or collagen-vascular disease. Available data are insufficient to show that quinapril does not have a similar risk (see **WARNINGS: Neutropenia/Agranulocytosis**).

Angioedema in Black Patients: Black patients receiving ACE inhibitor monotherapy have been reported to have a higher incidence of angioedema compared to non-blacks. It should also be noted that in controlled clinical trials, ACE inhibitors have an effect on blood pressure that is less in black patients than in non-blacks.

CONTRAINDICATIONS

ACCURETIC is contraindicated in patients who are hypersensitive to quinapril or hydrochlorothiazide and in patients with a history of angioedema related to previous treatment with an ACE inhibitor.

Because of the hydrochlorothiazide components, this product is contraindicated in patients with anuria or hypersensitivity to other sulfonamide-derived drugs.

WARNINGS

Anaphylactoid and Possibly Related Reactions: Presumably because angiotensin converting inhibitors affect the metabolism of eicosanoids and polypeptides, including endogenous bradykinin, patients receiving ACE inhibitors (including quinapril) may be subject to a variety of adverse reactions, some of them serious.

Head and Neck Angioedema: Angioedema of the face, extremities, lips, tongue, glottis, and larynx has been reported in patients treated with ACE inhibitors and has been seen in 0.1% of patients receiving quinapril. In two similarly sized US postmarketing quinapril trials that, combined, enrolled over 3,000 black patients and over 19,000 non-blacks, angioedema was reported in 0.30% and 0.55% of blacks (in Study 1 and 2, respectively) and 0.39% and 0.17% of non-blacks. Angioedema associated with laryngeal edema can be fatal. If laryngeal stridor or angioedema of the face, tongue, or glottis occurs, treatment with ACCURETIC should be discontinued immediately, the patient treated in accordance with accepted medical care, and carefully observed until the swelling disappears. In instances where swelling is confined to the face and lips, the condition generally resolves without treatment; antihistamines may be useful in relieving symptoms. **Where there is involvement of the tongue, glottis, or larynx likely to cause airway obstruction, emergency therapy including, but not limited to, subcutaneous epinephrine solution 1:1000 (0.3 to 0.5 mL) should be promptly administered** (see **PRECAUTIONS** and **ADVERSE REACTIONS**).

Intestinal Angioedema: Intestinal angioedema has been reported in patients treated with ACE inhibitors. These patients presented with abdominal pain (with or without nausea or vomiting); in some cases there was no prior history of facial angioedema and C-1 esterase levels were normal. The angioedema was diagnosed by procedures including abdominal CT scan or ultrasound, or at surgery, and symptoms resolved after stopping the ACE inhibitor. Intestinal angioedema should be included in the differential diagnosis of patients on ACE inhibitors presenting with abdominal pain.

Patients With a History of Angioedema: Patients with a history of angioedema unrelated to ACE inhibitor therapy may be at increased risk of angioedema while receiving an ACE inhibitor (see also **CONTRAINDICATIONS**).

Anaphylactoid Reactions During Desensitization: Two patients undergoing desensitizing treatment with Hymenoptera venom while receiving ACE inhibitors sustained life-threatening anaphylactoid reactions. In the same patients, these reactions were avoided when ACE inhibitors were temporarily withheld, but they reappeared upon inadvertent challenge.

Anaphylactoid Reactions During Membrane Exposure: Anaphylactoid reactions have been reported in patients dialyzed with high-flux membranes and treated concomitantly with an ACE inhibitor. Anaphylactoid reactions have also been reported in patients undergoing low-density lipoprotein apheresis with dextran sulfate absorption.

Hepatic Failure: Rarely, ACE inhibitors have been associated with a syndrome that starts with cholestatic jaundice and progresses to fulminant hepatic necrosis and (sometimes) death. The mechanism of this syndrome is not understood. Patients receiving ACE inhibitors who develop jaundice or marked elevations of hepatic enzymes should discontinue the ACE inhibitor and receive appropriate medical follow-up.

Hypotension: ACCURETIC can cause symptomatic hypotension, probably not more frequently than either monotherapy. It was reported in 1.2% of 1,571 patients receiving ACCURETIC during clinical trials. Like other ACE inhibitors, quinapril has been only rarely associated with hypotension in uncomplicated hypertensive patients.

Symptomatic hypotension sometimes associated with oliguria and/or progressive azotemia, and rarely acute renal failure and/or death, include patients with the following conditions or characteristics: heart failure, hyponatremia, high dose diuretic therapy, recent intensive diuresis or increase in diuretic dose, renal dialysis or severe volume and/or salt depletion of any etiology. Volume and/or salt depletion should be corrected before initiating therapy with ACCURETIC.

ACCURETIC should be used cautiously in patients receiving concomitant therapy with other antihypertensives. The thiazide component of ACCURETIC may potentiate the action of other antihypertensive drugs, especially ganglionic or peripheral adrenergic-blocking drugs. The antihypertensive effects of the thiazide component may also be enhanced in the postsympathectomy patients.

In patients at risk of excessive hypotension, therapy with ACCURETIC should be started under close medical supervision. Such patients should be followed closely for the first 2 weeks of treatment and whenever the dosage of quinapril or diuretic is increased. Similar considerations may apply to patients with ischemic heart or cerebrovascular disease in whom an excessive fall in blood pressure could result in myocardial infarction or cerebrovascular accident.

If excessive hypotension occurs, the patient should be placed in a supine position and, if necessary, treated with intravenous infusion of normal saline. ACCURETIC treatment usually can be continued following restoration of blood pressure and volume. If symptomatic hypotension develops, a dose reduction or discontinuation of ACCURETIC may be necessary.

Impaired Renal Function: ACCURETIC should be used with caution in patients with severe renal disease. Thiazides may precipitate azotemia in such patients, and the effects of repeated dosing may be cumulative.

When the renin-angiotensin-aldosterone system is inhibited by quinapril, changes in renal function may be anticipated in susceptible individuals. In patients with severe congestive heart failure, whose renal function may depend on the activity of the renin-angiotensin-aldosterone system, treatment with angiotensin-converting enzyme inhibitors (including quinapril) may be associated with oliguria and/or progressive azotemia and (rarely) with acute renal failure and/or death.

In clinical studies in hypertensive patients with unilateral renal artery stenosis, treatment with ACE inhibitors was associated with increases in blood urea nitrogen and serum creatinine; these increases were reversible upon discontinuation of ACE inhibitor, concomitant diuretic, or both. When such patients are treated with ACCURETIC, renal function should be monitored during the first few weeks of therapy.

Some quinapril-treated hypertensive patients with no apparent preexisting renal vascular diseases have developed increases in blood urea nitrogen and serum creatinine, usually minor and transient, especially when quinapril has been given concomitantly with a diuretic. This is more likely to occur in patients with pre-existing renal impairment. Dosage reduction of ACCURETIC may be required. **Evaluation of the hypertensive patients should also include assessment of the renal function.** (see **DOSAGE AND ADMINISTRATION**).

Neutropenia/Agranulocytosis: Another ACE inhibitor, captopril, has been shown to cause agranulocytosis and bone marrow depression rarely in patients with uncomplicated hypertension, but more frequently in patients with renal impairment, especially if they also have a collagen vascular disease, such as systemic lupus erythematosus or scleroderma. Agranulocytosis did occur during quinapril treatment in one patient with a history of neutropenia during previous captopril therapy. Available data from clinical trials of quinapril are insufficient to show that, in patients without prior reactions to other ACE inhibitors, quinapril does not cause agranulocytosis at similar rates. As with other ACE inhibitors, periodic monitoring of white blood cell counts in patients with collagen vascular disease and/or renal disease should be considered.

Fetal/Neonatal Morbidity and Mortality: ACE inhibitors can cause fetal and neonatal morbidity and death when administered to pregnant women. Several dozen cases have been reported in the world literature. When pregnancy is detected, ACCURETIC should be discontinued as soon as possible.

The use of ACE inhibitors during the second and third trimesters of pregnancy has been associated with fetal and neonatal injury, including hypotension, neonatal skull hypoplasia, anuria, reversible or irreversible renal failure, and death. Oligohydramnios has also been reported, presumably resulting from decreased fetal renal function; oligohydramnios in this setting has been associated with fetal limb contractures, craniofacial deformation, and hypoplastic lung development. Prematurity, intrauterine growth retardation, and patent ductus arteriosus have also been reported, although it is not clear whether these occurrences were due to the ACE inhibitor exposure.

These adverse effects do not appear to have resulted from intrauterine ACE inhibitor exposure that has been limited to the first trimester. Mothers whose embryos and fetuses are exposed to ACE inhibitors only during the first trimester should be so informed. Nonetheless, when patients become pregnant, physicians should make every effort to discontinue the use of quinapril as soon as possible.

Rarely (probably less often than once in every thousand pregnancies), no alternative ACE inhibitors will be found. In these rare cases, the mothers should be apprised of the potential hazards to their fetuses, and serial ultrasound examinations should be performed to assess the intraamniotic environment.

If oligohydramnios is observed, quinapril should be discontinued unless it is considered life-saving for the mother. Contraction stress testing (CST), a nonstress test (NST), or biophysical profiling (BPP) may be appropriate, depending upon the week of pregnancy. Patients and physicians should be aware, however, that oligohydramnios may not appear until after the fetus has sustained irreversible injury.

Infants with histories of *in utero* exposure to ACE inhibitors should be closely observed for hypotension, oliguria, and hyperkalemia. If oliguria occurs, attention should be directed toward support of blood pressure and renal perfusion. Exchange transfusion or peritoneal dialysis may be required as a means of reversing hypotension and/or substituting for disordered renal function. Removal of quinapril, which crosses the placenta, from the neonatal circulation is not significantly accelerated by these means.

Intrauterine exposure to thiazide diuretics is associated with fetal or neonatal jaundice, thrombocytopenia, and possibly other adverse reactions that occurred in adults.

No teratogenic effects of quinapril were seen in studies of pregnant rats and rabbits. On a mg/kg basis, the doses used were up to 180 times (in rats) and one time (in rabbits) the maximum recommended human dose. No teratogenic effects of ACCURETIC were seen in studies of pregnant rats and rabbits. On a mg/kg (quinapril/hydrochlorothiazide) basis, the doses used were up to 188/94 times (in rats) and 0.6/0.3 times (in rabbits) the maximum recommended human dose.

Impaired Hepatic Function: ACCURETIC should be used with caution in patients with impaired hepatic function or progressive liver disease, since minor alterations of fluid and electrolyte balance may precipitate hepatic coma. Also, since the metabolism of quinapril to quinaprilat is normally dependent upon hepatic esterases, patients with impaired liver function could develop markedly elevated plasma levels of quinapril. No normal pharmacokinetic studies have been carried out in hypertensive patients with impaired liver function.

Systemic Lupus Erythematosus: Thiazide diuretics have been reported to cause exacerbation or activation of systemic lupus erythematosus.

PRECAUTIONS

General

Derangements of Serum Electrolytes: In clinical trials, hyperkalemia (serum potassium $\geq$5.8 mmol/L) occurred in approximately 2% of patients receiving quinapril. In most cases, elevated serum potassium levels were isolated values which resolved despite continued therapy. Less than 0.1% of patients discontinued therapy due to hyperkalemia. Risk factors for the development of hyperkalemia include renal insufficiency, diabetes mellitus, and the concomitant use of potassium-sparing diuretics, potassium supplements, and/or potassium-containing salt substitutes.

Treatment with thiazide diuretics has been associated with hypokalemia, hyponatremia, and hypochloremic alkalosis. These disturbances have sometimes been manifest as one or more of dryness of mouth, thirst, weakness, lethargy, drowsiness, restlessness, muscle pains or cramps, muscular fatigue, hypotension, oliguria, tachycardia, nausea, and vomiting. Hypokalemia can also sensitize or exaggerate the response of the heart to the toxic effects of digitalis. The risk of hypokalemia is greatest in patients with cirrhosis of the liver, in patients experiencing a brisk diuresis, in patients who are receiving inadequate oral intake of electrolytes, and in patients receiving concomitant therapy with corticosteroids or ACTH.

The opposite effects of quinapril and hydrochlorothiazide on serum potassium will approximately balance each other in many patients, so that no net effect upon serum potassium will be seen. In other patients, one or the other effect may be dominant. Initial and periodic determinations of serum electrolytes to detect possible electrolyte imbalance should be performed at appropriate intervals.

Chloride deficits secondary to thiazide therapy are generally mild and require specific treatment only under extraordinary circumstances (eg, in liver disease or renal disease). Dilutional hyponatremia may occur in edematous patients in hot weather; appropriate therapy is water restriction rather than administration of salt, except in rare instances when the hyponatremia is life threatening. In actual salt depletion, appropriate replacement is the therapy of choice.

Calcium excretion is decreased by thiazides. In a few patients on prolonged thiazide therapy, pathological changes in the parathyroid gland have been observed, with hypercalcemia and hypophosphatemia. More serious complications of hyperparathyroidism (renal lithiasis, bone resorption, and peptic ulceration) have not been seen.

Thiazides increase the urinary excretion of magnesium, and hypomagnesemia may result.

Other Metabolic Disturbances: Thiazide diuretics tend to reduce glucose tolerance and to raise serum levels of cholesterol, triglycerides, and uric acid. These effects are usually minor, but frank gout or overt diabetes may be precipitated in susceptible patients.

Cough: Presumably due to the inhibition of the degradation of endogenous bradykinin, persistent nonproductive cough has been reported with all ACE inhibitors, resolving after discontinuation of therapy. ACE inhibitor-induced cough should be considered in the differential diagnosis of cough.

Surgery/Anesthesia: In patients undergoing surgery or during anesthesia with agents that produce hypotension, quinapril will block the angiotensin II formation that could otherwise occur secondary to compensatory renin release. Hypotension that occurs as a result of this mechanism can be corrected by volume expansion.

Information for Patients

Angioedema: Angioedema, including laryngeal edema, can occur with treatment with ACE inhibitors, especially following the first dose. Patients receiving ACCURETIC should be told to report immediately any signs or symptoms suggesting angioedema (swelling of face, eyes, lips, or tongue, or difficulty in breathing) and to take no more drug until after consulting with the prescribing physician.

Pregnancy: Female patients of childbearing age should be told about the consequences of second- and third-trimester exposure to ACE inhibitors, and they should also be told that these consequences do not appear to have resulted from intrauterine ACE-inhibitor exposure that has been limited to the first trimester. These patients should be asked to report pregnancies to their physicians as soon as possible.

Symptomatic Hypotension: A patient receiving ACCURETIC should be cautioned that lightheadedness can occur, especially during the first days of therapy, and that it should be reported to the prescribing physician. The patient should be told that if syncope occurs, ACCURETIC should be discontinued until the physician has been consulted.

All patients should be cautioned that inadequate fluid intake, excessive perspiration, diarrhea, or vomiting can lead to an excessive fall in blood pressure because of reduction in fluid volume, with the same consequences of lightheadedness and possible syncope.

Patients planning to undergo major surgery and/ or general or spinal anesthesia should be told to inform their physicians that they are taking an ACE inhibitor.

Hyperkalemia: A patient receiving ACCURETIC should be told not to use potassium supplements or salt substitutes containing potassium without consulting the prescribing physician.

Neutropenia: Patients should be told to promptly report any indication of infection (eg, sore throat, fever) which could be a sign of neutropenia.

NOTE: As with many other drugs, certain advice to patients being treated with quinapril is warranted. This information is intended to aid in the safe and effective use of this medication. It is not a disclosure of all possible adverse or intended effects.

Laboratory Tests

The hydrochlorothiazide component of ACCURETIC may decrease serum PBI levels without signs of thyroid disturbance.

Therapy with ACCURETIC should be interrupted for a few days before carrying out tests of parathyroid function.

Drug Interactions

Potassium Supplements and Potassium-Sparing Diuretics: As noted above ("Derangements of Serum Electrolytes"), the net effect of ACCURETIC may be to elevate a patient's serum potassium, to reduce it, or to leave it unchanged. Potassium-sparing diuretics (spironolactone, amiloride, triamterene, and others) or potassium supplements can increase the risk of hyperkalemia. If concomitant use of such agents is indicated, they should be given with caution, and the patient's serum potassium should be monitored frequently.

Lithium: Increased serum lithium levels and symptoms of lithium toxicity have been reported in patients receiving ACE inhibitors during therapy with lithium. Because renal clearance of lithium is reduced by thiazides, the risk of lithium toxicity is presumably raised further when, as in therapy with ACCURETIC, a thiazide diuretic is coadministered with the ACE inhibitor. ACCURETIC and lithium should be coadministered with caution, and frequent monitoring of serum lithium levels is recommended.

Tetracycline and Other Drugs That Interact with Magnesium: Simultaneous administration of tetracycline with quinapril reduced the absorption of tetracycline by approximately 28% to 37%, possibly due to the high magnesium content in quinapril tablets. This interaction should be considered if coprescribing quinapril and tetracycline or other drugs that interact with magnesium.

Other Agents:

Drug interaction studies of quinapril and other agents showed:

- Multiple dose therapy with propranolol or cimetidine has no effect on the pharmacokinetics of single doses of quinapril.
- The anticoagulant effect of a single dose of warfarin (measured by prothrombin time) was not significantly changed by quinapril coadministration twice daily.
- Quinapril treatment did not affect the pharmacokinetics of digoxin.
- No pharmacokinetic interaction was observed when single doses of quinapril and hydrochlorothiazide were administered concomitantly.

When administered concurrently, the following drugs may interact with thiazide diuretics.

- Alcohol, Barbiturates, or Narcotics—potentiation of orthostatic hypotension may occur.
- Antidiabetic Drugs (oral hypoglycemic agents and insulin)—dosage adjustments of the antidiabetic drug may be required.
- Cholestyramine and Colestipol Resin—absorption of hydrochlorothiazide is impaired in the presence of anionic exchange resins. Single doses of either cholestyramine or colestipol resins bind the hydrochlorothiazide and reduce its absorption from the gastrointestinal tract by up to 85% and 43%, respectively.

Continued on next page

Accuretic—Cont.

- Corticosteroids, ACTH—intensified electrolyte depletion, particularly hypokalemia.
- Pressor Amines (eg, norepinephrine)—possible decreased response to pressor amines, but not sufficient to preclude their therapeutic use.
- Skeletal Muscle Relaxants, Nondepolarizing (eg, tubocurarine)—possible increased responsiveness to the muscle relaxant.
- Nonsteroidal Antiinflammatory Drugs—the diuretic, natriuretic, and antihypertensive effects of thiazide diuretics may be reduced by concurrent administration of nonsteroidal antiinflammatory agents.

Carcinogenesis, Mutagenesis, Impairment of Fertility
Carcinogenicity, mutagenicity, and fertility studies have not been conducted in animals with ACCURETIC.
Quinapril hydrochloride was not carcinogenic in mice or rats when given in doses up to 75 or 100 mg/kg/day (50 or 60 times the maximum human daily dose, respectively, on a mg/kg basis and 3.8 or 10 times the maximum human daily dose on a mg/m^2 basis) for 104 weeks. Female rats given the highest dose level had an increased incidence of mesenteric lymph node hemangiomas and skin/subcutaneous lipomas. Neither quinapril nor quinaprilat were mutagenic in the Ames bacterial assay with or without metabolic activation. Quinapril was also negative in the following genetic toxicology studies: *in vitro* mammalian cell point mutation, sister chromatid exchange in cultured mammalian cells, micronucleus test with mice, *in vitro* chromosome aberration with V79 cultured lung cells, and in an *in vivo* cytogenetic study with rat bone marrow. There were no adverse effects on fertility or reproduction in rats at doses up to 100 mg/kg/day (60 and 10 times the maximum daily human dose when based on mg/kg and mg/m^2, respectively).
Under the auspices of the National Toxicology Program, rats and mice received hydrochlorothiazide in their feed for 2 years, at doses up to 600 mg/kg/day in mice and up to 100 mg/kg/day in rats. These studies uncovered no evidence of a carcinogenic potential of hydrochlorothiazide in rats or female mice, but there was "equivocal" evidence of hepatocarcinogenicity in male mice. Hydrochlorothiazide was not genotoxic in *in vitro* assays using strains TA 98, TA 100, TA 1535, TA 1537, and TA 1538 of *Salmonella typhimurium* (the Ames test); in the Chinese hamster ovary (CHO) test for chromosomal aberrations; or *in vivo* assays using mouse germinal cell chromosomes, Chinese hamster bone marrow chromosomes, and the *Drosophila* sex-linked recessive lethal trait gene. Positive test results were obtained in the *in vitro* CHO sister chromatid exchange (clastogenicity) test and in the mouse lymphoma cell (mutagenicity) assays, using concentrations of hydrochlorothiazide of 43 to 1300 µg/mL. Positive test results were also obtained in the *Aspergillus nidulans* nondisjunction assay, using an unspecified concentration of hydrochlorothiazide.
Hydrochlorothiazide had no adverse effects on the fertility of mice and rats of either sex in studies wherein these species were exposed, via their diets, to doses of up to 100 and 4 mg/kg/day, respectively, prior to mating and throughout gestation.

Pregnancy
Pregnancy Categories C (first trimester) and D (second and third trimesters): See WARNINGS: Fetal/Neonatal Morbidity and Mortality.

Nursing Mothers
Because quinapril and hydrochlorothiazide are secreted in human milk, caution should be exercised when ACCURETIC is administered to a nursing woman.
Because of the potential for serious adverse reactions in nursing infants from hydrochlorothiazide and the unknown effects of quinapril in infants, a decision should be made whether to discontinue nursing or to discontinue ACCURETIC, taking into account the importance of the drug to the mother.

Geriatric Use
Clinical studies of quinapril HCl/hydrochlorothiazide did not include sufficient numbers of subjects aged 65 and over to determine whether they respond differently from younger subjects. Other reported clinical experience has not identified differences in responses between the elderly and younger patients. In general, dose selection for an elderly patient should be cautious, usually starting at the low end of the dosing range, reflecting the greater frequency of decreased hepatic, renal, or cardiac function, and of concomitant disease or other drug therapy.

Pediatric Use
Safety and effectiveness of ACCURETIC in children have not been established.

ADVERSE REACTIONS

ACCURETIC has been evaluated for safety in 1571 patients in controlled and uncontrolled studies. Of these, 498 were given quinapril plus hydrochlorothiazide for at least 1 year, with 153 patients extending combination therapy for over 2 years. In clinical trials with ACCURETIC, no adverse experience specific to the combination has been observed. Adverse experiences that have occurred have been limited to those that have been previously reported with quinapril or hydrochlorothiazide.
Adverse experiences were usually mild and transient, and there was no relationship between side effects and age, sex, race, or duration of therapy. Discontinuation of therapy because of adverse effects was required in 2.1% in patients in

	Percent of Patients in Controlled Trials	
	Quinapril/HCTZ N = 943	Placebo N = 100
Headache	6.7	30.0
Dizziness	4.8	4.0
Coughing	3.2	2.0
Fatigue	2.9	3.0
Myalgia	2.4	5.0
Viral Infection	1.9	4.0
Rhinitis	2.0	3.0
Nausea and/or Vomiting	1.8	6.0
Abdominal Pain	1.7	4.0
Back Pain	1.5	2.0
Diarrhea	1.4	1.0
Upper Respiratory Infection	1.3	4.0
Insomnia	1.2	2.0
Somnolence	1.2	0.0
Bronchitis	1.2	1.0
Dyspepsia	1.2	2.0
Asthenia	1.1	1.0
Pharyngitis	1.1	2.0
Vasodilatation	1.0	1.0
Vertigo	1.0	2.0
Chest Pain	1.0	2.0

BODY AS A WHOLE:	Asthenia, Malaise
CARDIOVASCULAR:	Palpitation, Tachycardia, *Heart Failure, Hyperkalemia, Myocardial Infarction, Cerebrovascular Accident, Hypertensive Crisis, Angina Pectoris, Orthostatic Hypotension, Cardiac Rhythm Disturbance*
GASTROINTESTINAL:	Mouth or Throat Dry, *Gastrointestinal Hemorrhage, Pancreatitis, Abnormal Liver Function Tests*
NERVOUS/PSYCHIATRIC:	Nervousness, Vertigo, *Paresthesia*
RESPIRATORY:	Sinusitis, Dyspnea
INTEGUMENTARY:	Pruritus, Sweating Increased, *Erythema Multiforme, Exfoliative Dermatitis, Photosensitivity Reaction, Alopecia, Pemphigus*
UROGENITAL SYSTEM:	*Acute Renal Failure, Impotence*
OTHER:	*Agranulocytosis, Thrombocytopenia, Arthralgia*
Angioedema:	Angioedema has been reported in 0.1% of patients receiving quinapril (0.1%) (see **WARNINGS**).
Fetal/Neonatal Morbidity and Mortality:	See **WARNINGS:** Fetal/Neonatal Morbidity and Mortality

BODY AS A WHOLE:	Weakness.
CARDIOVASCULAR:	Orthostatic hypotension (may be potentiated by alcohol, barbiturates, or narcotics).
DIGESTIVE:	Pancreatitis, jaundice (intrahepatic cholestatic), sialadenitis, vomiting, diarrhea, cramping, nausea, gastric irritation, constipation, and anorexia.
NEUROLOGIC:	Vertigo, lightheadedness, transient blurred vision, headache, paresthesia, xanthopsia, weakness, and restlessness.
MUSCULOSKELETAL:	Muscle spasm.
HEMATOLOGIC:	Aplastic anemia, agranulocytosis, leukopenia, thrombocytopenia, and hemolytic anemia.
RENAL:	Renal failure, renal dysfunction, interstitial nephritis (see **WARNINGS**).
METABOLIC:	Hyperglycemia, glycosuria, and hyperuricemia.
HYPERSENSITIVITY:	Necrotizing angiitis, Stevens-Johnson syndrome, respiratory distress (including pneumonitis and pulmonary edema), purpura, urticaria, rash, and photosensitivity.

controlled studies. The most common reasons for discontinuation of therapy with ACCURETIC were cough (1.0%; see **PRECAUTIONS**) and headache (0.7%).
Adverse experiences probably or possibly related to therapy or of unknown relationship to therapy occurring in 1% or more of the 943 patients treated with quinapril plus hydrochlorothiazide in controlled trials are shown below.
[See first table above]
Clinical adverse experiences probably, possibly, or definitely related or of uncertain relationship to therapy occurring in ≥0.5% to <1.0% (except as noted) of the patients treated with quinapril/HCTZ in controlled and uncontrolled trials (N=1571) and less frequent, clinically significant events seen in clinical trials or postmarketing experience (the rarer events are in italics) include (listed by body system):
[See second table above]

Postmarketing Experience
The following serious nonfatal adverse events, regardless of their relationship to quinapril and HCTZ combination tablets, have been reported during extensive postmarketing experience:
BODY AS A WHOLE: Shock, accidental injury, neoplasm, cellulitis, ascites, generalized edema, hernia and anaphylactoid reaction.
CARDIOVASCULAR SYSTEM: Bradycardia, cor pulmonale, vasculitis, and deep thrombosis.
DIGESTIVE SYSTEM: Gastrointestinal carcinoma, cholestatic jaundice, hepatitis, esophagitis, vomiting, and diarrhea.
HEMIC SYSTEM: Anemia.
METABOLIC AND NUTRITIONAL DISORDERS: Weight loss.
MUSCULOSKELETAL SYSTEM: Myopathy, myositis, and arthritis.
NERVOUS SYSTEM: Paralysis, hemiplegia, speech disorder, abnormal gait, meningism, and amnesia.
RESPIRATORY SYSTEM: Pneumonia, asthma, respiratory infiltration, and lung disorder.
SKIN AND APPENDAGES: Urticaria, macropapular rash, and petechiases.
SPECIAL SENSES: Abnormal vision.
UROGENITAL SYSTEM: Kidney function abnormal, albuminuria, pyuria, hematuria, and nephrosis.
Quinapril monotherapy has been evaluated for safety in 4960 patients. In clinical trials adverse events which occurred with quinapril were also seen with ACCURETIC. In addition, the following were reported for quinapril at an incidence >0.5%: depression, back pain, constipation, syncope, and amblyopia.
Hydrochlorothiazide has been extensively prescribed for many years, but there has not been enough systematic collection of data to support an estimate of the frequency of the observed adverse reactions. Within organ-system groups, the reported reactions are listed here in decreasing order of severity, without regard to frequency.
[See third table above]

Clinical Laboratory Test Findings
Serum Electrolytes: See **PRECAUTIONS**.
Creatinine, Blood Urea Nitrogen: Increases (>1.25 times the upper limit of normal) in serum creatinine and blood urea nitrogen were observed in 3% and 4%, respectively, of patients treated with ACCURETIC. Most increases were minor and reversible, which can occur in patients with essential hypertension but most frequently in patients with renal artery stenosis (see **PRECAUTIONS**).
PBI and Tests of Parathyroid Function: See **PRECAUTIONS**.
Hematology: See **WARNINGS**.
Other (causal relationships unknown): Other clinically important changes in standard laboratory tests were rarely associated with ACCURETIC administration. Elevations in uric acid, glucose, magnesium, cholesterol, triglyceride, and calcium (see **PRECAUTIONS**) have been reported.

OVERDOSAGE

No specific information is available on the treatment of overdosage with ACCURETIC or quinapril monotherapy; treatment should be symptomatic and supportive. Therapy with ACCURETIC should be discontinued, and the patient should be observed. Dehydration, electrolyte imbalance, and hypotension should be treated by established procedures.
The oral median lethal dose of quinapril/hydrochlorothiazide in combination ranges from 1063/664 to 4640/2896 mg/kg in mice and rats. Doses of 1440 to 4280 mg/kg of quinapril cause significant lethality in mice and rats. In single-dose studies of hydrochlorothiazide, most rats survived doses up to 2.75 g/kg.
Data from human overdoses of ACE inhibitors are scanty; the most likely manifestation of human quinapril overdosage is hypotension. In human hydrochlorothiazide overdose, the most common signs and symptoms observed have been

those of dehydration and electrolyte depletion (hypokalemia, hypochloremia, hyponatremia). If digitalis has also been administered, hypokalemia may accentuate cardiac arrhythmias.
Laboratory determinations of serum levels of quinapril and its metabolites are not widely available, and such determinations have, in any event, no established role in the management of quinapril overdose.
No data are available to suggest physiological maneuvers (eg, maneuvers to change the pH of the urine) that might accelerate elimination of quinapril and its metabolites. Hemodialysis and peritoneal dialysis have little effect on the elimination of quinapril and quinaprilat.
Angiotensin II could presumably serve as a specific antagonist-antidote in the setting of quinapril overdose, but angiotensin II is essentially unavailable outside of scattered research facilities. Because the hypotensive effect of quinapril is achieved through vasodilation and effective hypovolemia, it is reasonable to treat quinapril overdose by infusion of normal saline solution.

DOSAGE AND ADMINISTRATION

As individual monotherapy, quinapril is an effective treatment of hypertension in once-daily doses of 10 to 80 mg and hydrochlorothiazide is effective in doses of 12.5 to 50 mg. In clinical trials of quinapril/hydrochlorothiazide combination therapy using quinapril doses of 2.5 to 40 mg and hydrochlorothiazide doses of 6.25 to 25 mg, the antihypertensive effects increased with increasing dose of either component.
The side effects (see **WARNINGS**) of quinapril are generally rare and apparently independent of dose; those of hydrochlorothiazide are a mixture of dose-dependent phenomena (primarily hypokalemia) and dose-independent phenomena (eg, pancreatitis), the former much more common than the latter. Therapy with any combination of quinapril and hydrochlorothiazide will be associated with both sets of dose-independent side effects, but regimens that combine low doses of hydrochlorothiazide with quinapril produce minimal effects on serum potassium. In clinical trials of ACCURETIC, the average change in serum potassium was near zero in subjects who received HCTZ 6.25 mg in the combination, and the average subject who received 10 to 40/12.5 to 25 mg experienced a milder reduction in serum potassium than that experienced by the average subject receiving the same dose of hydrochlorothiazide monotherapy.
To minimize dose-independent side effects, it is usually appropriate to begin combination therapy only after a patient has failed to achieve the desired effect with monotherapy.

Therapy Guided by Clinical Effect

Patients whose blood pressures are not adequately controlled with quinapril monotherapy may instead be given ACCURETIC 10/12.5 or 20/12.5. Further increases of either or both components could depend on clinical response. The hydrochlorothiazide dose should generally not be increased until 2 to 3 weeks have elapsed. Patients whose blood pressures are adequately controlled with 25 mg of daily hydrochlorothiazide, but who experience significant potassium loss with this regimen, may achieve blood pressure control with less electrolyte disturbance if they are switched to ACCURETIC 10/12.5 or 20/12.5.

Replacement Therapy

For convenience, patients who are adequately treated with 20 mg of quinapril and 25 mg of hydrochlorothiazide and experience no significant electrolyte disturbances may instead wish to receive ACCURETIC 20/25.

Use in Renal Impairment

Regimens of therapy with ACCURETIC need not take account of renal function as long as the patient's creatinine clearance is >30 mL/min/1.73 m^2 (serum creatinine roughly ≤3 mg/dL or 265 μmol/L). In patients with more severe renal impairment, loop diuretics are preferred to thiazides. Therefore, ACCURETIC is not recommended for use in these patients.

HOW SUPPLIED

ACCURETIC is available in tablets of three different strengths:
10/12.5 tablets: pink, scored elliptical, biconvex, film-coated tablets coded "PD 222" on one side. Each tablet contains 10 mg of quinapril and 12.5 mg of hydrochlorothiazide.
N0071-0222-23: 90 tablet bottles
20/12.5 tablets: pink, scored triangular, film-coated tablets coded "PD 220" on one side. Each tablet contains 20 mg of quinapril and 12.5 mg of hydrochlorothiazide.
N0071-0220-23: 90 tablet bottles
20/25 tablets: pink, round, biconvex, film-coated tablets coded "PD 223" on one side. Each tablet contains 20 mg of quinapril and 25 mg of hydrochlorothiazide.
N0071-0223-23: 90 tablet bottles
Dispense in tight containers as defined in the USP.
Store at Controlled Room Temperature 20°-25°C (68°-77°F) [see USP].
Rx only
69-5822-00-2
Manufactured by:
Pfizer Pharmaceuticals, Ltd
Vega Baja, PR 00694
MADE IN GERMANY
Distributed by:
PARKE-DAVIS
Division of Pfizer Inc
NY, NY 10017

Revised August 2003
Shown in Product Identification Guide, page 329

LIPITOR® ℞
[lĭ′pĭ-tōr]
(Atorvastatin Calcium)
Tablets

DESCRIPTION

Lipitor® (atorvastatin calcium) is a synthetic lipid-lowering agent. Atorvastatin is an inhibitor of 3-hydroxy-3-methylglutaryl-coenzyme A (HMG-CoA) reductase. This enzyme catalyzes the conversion of HMG-CoA to mevalonate, an early and rate-limiting step in cholesterol biosynthesis.
Atorvastatin calcium is [R-(R*, R*)]-2-(4-fluorophenyl)-β, δ-dihydroxy-5-(1-methylethyl)-3-phenyl-4-[(phenylamino)carbonyl]-1H-pyrrole-1-heptanoic acid, calcium salt (2:1) trihydrate. The empirical formula of atorvastatin calcium is $(C_{33}H_{34}FN_2O_5)_2Ca \cdot 3H_2O$ and its molecular weight is 1209.42. Its structural formula is:

Atorvastatin calcium is a white to off-white crystalline powder that is insoluble in aqueous solutions of pH 4 and below. Atorvastatin calcium is very slightly soluble in distilled water, pH 7.4 phosphate buffer, and acetonitrile, slightly soluble in ethanol, and freely soluble in methanol.
Lipitor tablets for oral administration contain 10, 20, 40 or 80 mg atorvastatin and the following inactive ingredients: calcium carbonate, USP; candelilla wax, FCC; croscarmellose sodium, NF; hydroxypropyl cellulose, NF; lactose monohydrate, NF; magnesium stearate, NF; microcrystalline cellulose, NF; Opadry White YS-1-7040 (hypromellose, polyethylene glycol, talc, titanium dioxide); polysorbate 80, NF; simethicone emulsion.

CLINICAL PHARMACOLOGY

Mechanism of Action

Atorvastatin is a selective, competitive inhibitor of HMG-CoA reductase, the rate-limiting enzyme that converts 3-hydroxy-3-methylglutaryl-coenzyme A to mevalonate, a precursor of sterols, including cholesterol. Cholesterol and triglycerides circulate in the bloodstream as part of lipoprotein complexes. With ultracentrifugation, these complexes separate into HDL (high-density lipoprotein), IDL (intermediate-density lipoprotein), LDL (low-density lipoprotein), and VLDL (very-low-density lipoprotein) fractions. Triglycerides (TG) and cholesterol in the liver are incorporated into VLDL and released into the plasma for delivery to peripheral tissues. LDL is formed from VLDL and is catabolized primarily through the high-affinity LDL receptor. Clinical and pathologic studies show that elevated plasma levels of total cholesterol (total-C), LDL-cholesterol (LDL-C), and apolipoprotein B (apo B) promote human atherosclerosis and are risk factors for developing cardiovascular disease, while increased levels of HDL-C are associated with a decreased cardiovascular risk.
In animal models, Lipitor lowers plasma cholesterol and lipoprotein levels by inhibiting HMG-CoA reductase and cholesterol synthesis in the liver and by increasing the number of hepatic LDL receptors on the cell-surface to enhance uptake and catabolism of LDL; Lipitor also reduces LDL production and the number of LDL particles. Lipitor reduces LDL-C in some patients with homozygous familial hypercholesterolemia (FH), a population that rarely responds to other lipid-lowering medication(s).
A variety of clinical studies have demonstrated that elevated levels of total-C, LDL-C, and apo B (a membrane complex for LDL-C) promote human atherosclerosis. Similarly, decreased levels of HDL-C (and its transport complex, apo A) are associated with the development of atherosclerosis. Epidemiologic investigations have established that cardiovascular morbidity and mortality vary directly with the level of total-C and LDL-C, and inversely with the level of HDL-C.
Lipitor reduces total-C, LDL-C, and apo B in patients with homozygous and heterozygous FH, nonfamilial forms of hypercholesterolemia, and mixed dyslipidemia. Lipitor also reduces VLDL-C and TG and produces variable increases in HDL-C and apolipoprotein A-1. Lipitor reduces total-C, LDL-C, VLDL-C, apo B, TG, and non-HDL-C, and increases HDL-C in patients with isolated hypertriglyceridemia. Lipitor reduces intermediate density lipoprotein cholesterol (IDL-C) in patients with dysbetalipoproteinemia.
Like LDL, cholesterol-enriched triglyceride-rich lipoproteins, including VLDL, intermediate density lipoprotein (IDL), and remnants, can also promote atherosclerosis. Elevated plasma triglycerides are frequently found in a triad with low HDL-C levels and small LDL particles, as well as in association with non-lipid metabolic risk factors for coronary heart disease. As such, total plasma TG has not consistently been shown to be an independent risk factor for CHD. Furthermore, the independent effect of raising HDL or lowering TG on the risk of coronary and cardiovascular morbidity and mortality has not been determined.

Pharmacodynamics

Atorvastatin as well as some of its metabolites are pharmacologically active in humans. The liver is the primary site of action and the principal site of cholesterol synthesis and LDL clearance. Drug dosage rather than systemic drug concentration correlates better with LDL-C reduction. Individualization of drug dosage should be based on therapeutic response (see DOSAGE AND ADMINISTRATION).

Pharmacokinetics and Drug Metabolism

Absorption: Atorvastatin is rapidly absorbed after oral administration; maximum plasma concentrations occur within 1 to 2 hours. Extent of absorption increases in proportion to atorvastatin dose. The absolute bioavailability of atorvastatin (parent drug) is approximately 14% and the systemic availability of HMG-CoA reductase inhibitory activity is approximately 30%. The low systemic availability is attributed to presystemic clearance in gastrointestinal mucosa and/or hepatic first-pass metabolism. Although food decreases the rate and extent of drug absorption by approximately 25% and 9%, respectively, as assessed by Cmax and AUC, LDL-C reduction is similar whether atorvastatin is given with or without food. Plasma atorvastatin concentrations are lower (approximately 30% for Cmax and AUC) following evening drug administration compared with morning. However, LDL-C reduction is the same regardless of the time of day of drug administration (see DOSAGE AND ADMINISTRATION).
Distribution: Mean volume of distribution of atorvastatin is approximately 381 liters. Atorvastatin is ≥98% bound to plasma proteins. A blood/plasma ratio of approximately 0.25 indicates poor drug penetration into red blood cells. Based on observations in rats, atorvastatin is likely to be secreted in human milk (see CONTRAINDICATIONS, Pregnancy and Lactation, and PRECAUTIONS, Nursing Mothers).
Metabolism: Atorvastatin is extensively metabolized to ortho- and parahydroxylated derivatives and various beta-oxidation products. *In vitro* inhibition of HMG-CoA reductase by ortho- and parahydroxylated metabolites is equivalent to that of atorvastatin. Approximately 70% of circulating inhibitory activity for HMG-CoA reductase is attributed to active metabolites. *In vitro* studies suggest the importance of atorvastatin metabolism by cytochrome P450 3A4, consistent with increased plasma concentrations of atorvastatin in humans following coadministration with erythromycin, a known inhibitor of this isozyme (see PRECAUTIONS, Drug Interactions). In animals, the ortho-hydroxy metabolite undergoes further glucuronidation.
Excretion: Atorvastatin and its metabolites are eliminated primarily in bile following hepatic and/or extra-hepatic metabolism; however, the drug does not appear to undergo enterohepatic recirculation. Mean plasma elimination half-life of atorvastatin in humans is approximately 14 hours, but the half-life of inhibitory activity for HMG-CoA reductase is 20 to 30 hours due to the contribution of active metabolites. Less than 2% of a dose of atorvastatin is recovered in urine following oral administration.

Special Populations

Geriatric: Plasma concentrations of atorvastatin are higher (approximately 40% for Cmax and 30% for AUC) in healthy elderly subjects (age ≥65 years) than in young adults. Clinical data suggest a greater degree of LDL-lowering at any dose of drug in the elderly patient population compared to younger adults (see PRECAUTIONS section; Geriatric Use subsection).
Pediatric: Pharmacokinetic data in the pediatric population are not available.
Gender: Plasma concentrations of atorvastatin in women differ from those in men (approximately 20% higher for Cmax and 10% lower for AUC); however, there is no clinically significant difference in LDL-C reduction with Lipitor between men and women.
Renal Insufficiency: Renal disease has no influence on the plasma concentrations or LDL-C reduction of atorvastatin; thus, dose adjustment in patients with renal dysfunction is not necessary (see DOSAGE AND ADMINISTRATION).
Hemodialysis: While studies have not been conducted in patients with end-stage renal disease, hemodialysis is not expected to significantly enhance clearance of atorvastatin since the drug is extensively bound to plasma proteins.
Hepatic Insufficiency: In patients with chronic alcoholic liver disease, plasma concentrations of atorvastatin are markedly increased. Cmax and AUC are each 4-fold greater in patients with Childs-Pugh A disease. Cmax and AUC are approximately 16-fold and 11-fold increased, respectively, in patients with Childs-Pugh B disease (see CONTRAINDICATIONS).

Clinical Studies

Prevention of Cardiovascular Disease

In the Anglo-Scandinavian Cardiac Outcomes Trial (ASCOT), the effect of LIPITOR (atorvastatin calcium) on fatal and non-fatal coronary heart disease was assessed in 10,305 hypertensive patients 40-80 years of age (mean of 63 years), without a previous myocardial infarction and with TC levels ≤251 mg/dl (6.5 mmol/l). Additionally all patients had at least 3 of the following cardiovascular risk factors: male gender (81.1%), age >55 years (84.5%), smoking (33.2%), diabetes (24.3%), history of CHD in a first-degree relative (26%), TC:HDL >6 (14.3%), peripheral vascular disease (5.1%), left ventricular hypertrophy (14.4%), prior cerebrovascular event (9.8%), specific ECG abnormality (14.3%), proteinuria/albuminuria (62.4%)]. In this double-

Continued on next page

Lipitor—Cont.

blind, placebo-controlled study patients were treated with anti-hypertensive therapy (Goal BP <140/90 mm Hg for non-diabetic patients, <130/80 mm Hg for diabetic patients) and allocated to either LIPITOR 10 mg daily (n=5168) or placebo (n=5137), using a covariate adaptive method which took into account the distribution of fourteen baseline characteristics of patients already enrolled and minimized the imbalance of those characteristics across the groups. Patients were followed for a median duration of 3.3 years.

The effect of 10 mg/day of LIPITOR on lipid levels was similar to that seen in previous clinical trials.

LIPITOR significantly reduced the rate of coronary events [either fatal coronary heart disease (46 events in the placebo group vs 40 events in the LIPITOR group) or nonfatal MI (108 events in the placebo group vs 60 events in the LIPITOR group)] with a relative risk reduction of 36% [(based on incidences of 1.9% for LIPITOR vs 3.0% for placebo), p=0.0005 (see Figure 1)]. The risk reduction was consistent regardless of age, smoking status, obesity or presence of renal dysfunction. The effect of LIPITOR was seen regardless of baseline LDL levels. Due to the small number of events, results for women were inconclusive.

Figure 1: Effect of LIPITOR 10 mg/day on Cumulative Incidence of Nonfatal Myocardial Infarction or Coronary Heart Disease Death (in ASCOT-LLA)

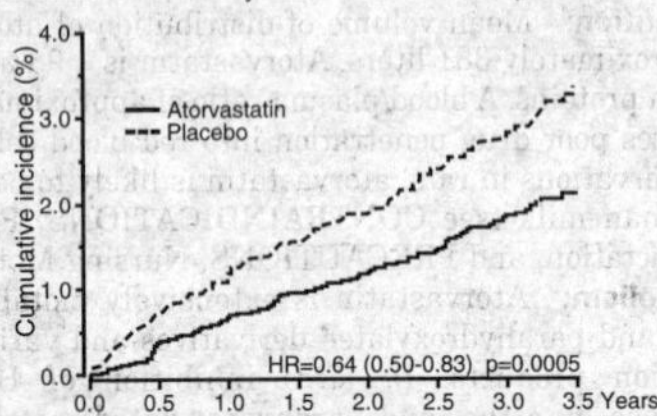

LIPITOR also significantly decreased the relative risk for revascularization procedures by 42%. Although the reduction of fatal and non-fatal strokes did not reach a pre-defined significance level (p = 0.01), a favorable trend was observed with a 26% relative risk reduction (incidences of 1.7% for LIPITOR and 2.3% for placebo). There was no significant difference between the treatment groups for death due to cardiovascular causes (p=0.51) or noncardiovascular causes (p=0.17).

Hypercholesterolemia (Heterozygous Familial and Nonfamilial) and Mixed Dyslipidemia (*Fredrickson* Types IIa and IIb)

Lipitor reduces total-C, LDL-C, VLDL-C, apo B, and TG, and increases HDL-C in patients with hypercholesterolemia and mixed dyslipidemia. Therapeutic response is seen within 2 weeks, and maximum response is usually achieved within 4 weeks and maintained during chronic therapy.

Lipitor is effective in a wide variety of patient populations with hypercholesterolemia, with and without hypertriglyceridemia, in men and women, and in the elderly. Experience in pediatric patients has been limited to patients with homozygous FH. In two multicenter, placebo-controlled, dose-response studies in patients with hypercholesterolemia, Lipitor given as a single dose over 6 weeks significantly reduced total-C, LDL-C, apo B, and TG (Pooled results are provided in Table 1).

[See table 1 above]

In patients with *Fredrickson* Types IIa and IIb hyperlipoproteinemia pooled from 24 controlled trials, the median (25th and 75th percentile) percent changes from baseline in HDL-C for atorvastatin 10, 20, 40, and 80 mg were 6.4 (-1.4, 14), 8.7 (0, 17), 7.8 (0, 16), and 5.1 (-2.7, 15), respectively. Additionally, analysis of the pooled data demonstrated consistent and significant decreases in total-C, LDL-C, TG, total-C/HDL-C, and LDL-C/HDL-C.

In three multicenter, double-blind studies in patients with hypercholesterolemia, Lipitor was compared to other HMG-CoA reductase inhibitors. After randomization, patients were treated for 16 weeks with either Lipitor 10 mg per day or a fixed dose of the comparative agent (Table 2).

[See table 2 above]

The impact on clinical outcomes of the differences in lipid-altering effects between treatments shown in Table 2 is not known. Table 2 does not contain data comparing the effects of atorvastatin 10 mg and higher doses of lovastatin, pravastatin, and simvastatin. The drugs compared in the studies summarized in the table are not necessarily interchangeable.

Hypertriglyceridemia (*Fredrickson* Type IV)

The response to Lipitor in 64 patients with isolated hypertriglyceridemia treated across several clinical trials is shown in the table below. For the atorvastatin-treated patients, median (min, max) baseline TG level was 565 (267-1502).

[See table 3 above]

Dysbetalipoproteinemia (*Fredrickson* Type III)

The results of an open-label crossover study of 16 patients (genotypes: 14 apo E2/E2 and 2 apo E3/E2) with dysbetalipoproteinemia (*Fredrickson* Type III) are shown in the table below.

[See table 4 above]

Homozygous Familial Hypercholesterolemia

In a study without a concurrent control group, 29 patients ages 6 to 37 years with homozygous FH received maximum daily doses of 20 to 80 mg of Lipitor. The mean LDL-C reduction in this study was 18%. Twenty-five patients with a reduction in LDL-C had a mean response of 20% (range of 7% to 53%, median of 24%); the remaining 4 patients had 7% to 24% increases in LDL-C. Five of the 29 patients had absent LDL-receptor function. Of these, 2 patients also had a portacaval shunt and had no significant reduction in LDL-C. The remaining 3 receptor-negative patients had a mean LDL-C reduction of 22%.

Heterozygous Familial Hypercholesterolemia in Pediatric Patients

In a double-blind, placebo-controlled study followed by an open-label phase, 187 boys and postmenarchal girls 10-17 years of age (mean age 14.1 years) with heterozygous familial hypercholesterolemia (FH) or severe hypercholesterolemia were randomized to Lipitor (n=140) or placebo (n=47) for 26 weeks and then all received Lipitor for 26 weeks. Inclusion in the study required 1) a baseline LDL-C level ≥ 190 mg/dL or 2) a baseline LDL-C ≥ 160 mg/dL and positive family history of FH or documented premature cardiovascular disease in a first- or second-degree relative. The mean baseline LDL-C value was 218.6 mg/dL (range: 138.5-385.0 mg/dL) in the Lipitor group compared to 230.0 mg/dL (range: 160.0-324.5 mg/dL) in the placebo group. The dosage of Lipitor (once daily) was 10 mg for the first 4 weeks and up-titrated to 20 mg if the LDL-C level was > 130 mg/dL. The number of Lipitor-treated patients who required up-titration to 20 mg after Week 4 during the double-blind phase was 80 (57.1%).

Lipitor significantly decreased plasma levels of total-C, LDL-C, triglycerides, and apolipoprotein B during the 26 week double-blind phase (see Table 5).

[See table 5 above]

The mean achieved LDL-C value was 130.7 mg/dL (range: 70.0-242.0 mg/dL) in the Lipitor group compared to

TABLE 1. Dose-Response in Patients With Primary Hypercholesterolemia (Adjusted Mean % Change From Baseline)[a]

Dose	N	TC	LDL-C	Apo B	TG	HDL-C	Non-HDL-C/ HDL-C
Placebo	21	4	4	3	10	-3	7
10	22	-29	-39	-32	-19	6	-34
20	20	-33	-43	-35	-26	9	-41
40	21	-37	-50	-42	-29	6	-45
80	23	-45	-60	-50	-37	5	-53

[a]Results are pooled from 2 dose-response studies.

TABLE 2. Mean Percent Change From Baseline at End Point (Double-Blind, Randomized, Active-Controlled Trials)

Treatment (Daily Dose)	N	Total-C	LDL-C	Apo B	TG	HDL-C	Non-HDL-C/ HDL-C
Study 1							
Atorvastatin 10 mg	707	-27[a]	-36[a]	-28[a]	-17[a]	+7	-37[a]
Lovastatin 20 mg	191	-19	-27	-20	-6	+7	-28
95% CI for Diff[1]		-9.2, -6.5	-10.7, -7.1	-10.0, -6.5	-15.2, -7.1	-1.7, 2.0	-11.1, -7.1
Study 2							
Atorvastatin 10 mg	222	-25[b]	-35[b]	-27[b]	-17[b]	+6	-36[b]
Pravastatin 20 mg	77	-17	-23	-17	-9	+8	-28
95% CI for Diff[1]		-10.8, -6.1	-14.5, -8.2	-13.4, -7.4	-14.1, -0.7	-4.9, 1.6	-11.5, -4.1
Study 3							
Atorvastatin 10 mg	132	-29[c]	-37[c]	-34[c]	-23[c]	+7	-39[c]
Simvastatin 10 mg	45	-24	-30	-30	-15	+7	-33
95% CI for Diff[1]		-8.7, -2.7	-10.1, -2.6	-8.0, -1.1	-15.1, -0.7	-4.3, 3.9	-9.6, -1.9

[1] A negative value for the 95% CI for the difference between treatments favors atorvastatin for all except HDL-C, for which a positive value favors atorvastatin. If the range does not include 0, this indicates a statistically significant difference.
[a] Significantly different from lovastatin, ANCOVA, p ≤0.05
[b] Significantly different from pravastatin, ANCOVA, p ≤0.05
[c] Significantly different from simvastatin, ANCOVA, p ≤0.05

TABLE 3. Combined Patients With Isolated Elevated TG: Median (min, max) Percent Changes From Baseline

	Placebo (N=12)	Atorvastatin 10 mg (N=37)	Atorvastatin 20 mg (N=13)	Atorvastatin 80 mg (N=14)
Triglycerides	-12.4 (-36.6, 82.7)	-41.0 (-76.2, 49.4)	-38.7 (-62.7, 29.5)	-51.8 (-82.8, 41.3)
Total-C	-2.3 (-15.5, 24.4)	-28.2 (-44.9, -6.8)	-34.9 (-49.6, -15.2)	-44.4 (-63.5, -3.8)
LDL-C	3.6 (-31.3, 31.6)	-26.5 (-57.7, 9.8)	-30.4 (-53.9, 0.3)	-40.5 (-60.6, -13.8)
HDL-C	3.8 (-18.6, 13.4)	13.8 (-9.7, 61.5)	11.0 (-3.2, 25.2)	7.5 (-10.8, 37.2)
VLDL-C	-1.0 (-31.9, 53.2)	-48.8 (-85.8, 57.3)	-44.6 (-62.2, -10.8)	-62.0 (-88.2, 37.6)
non-HDL-C	-2.8 (-17.6, 30.0)	-33.0 (-52.1, -13.3)	-42.7 (-53.7, -17.4)	-51.5 (-72.9, -4.3)

TABLE 4. Open-Label Crossover Study of 16 Patients With Dysbetalipoproteinemia (*Fredrickson* Type III)

	Median (min, max) at Baseline (mg/dL)	Median % Change (min, max) Atorvastatin 10 mg	Median % Change (min, max) Atorvastatin 80 mg
Total-C	442 (225, 1320)	-37 (-85, 17)	-58 (-90, -31)
Triglycerides	678 (273, 5990)	-39 (-92, -8)	-53 (-95, -30)
IDL-C + VLDL-C	215 (111, 613)	-32 (-76, 9)	-63 (-90, -8)
non-HDL-C	411 (218, 1272)	-43 (-87, -19)	-64 (-92, -36)

TABLE 5
Lipid-altering Effects of Lipitor in Adolescent Boys and Girls with Heterozygous Familial Hypercholesterolemia or Severe Hypercholesterolemia (Mean Percent Change from Baseline at Endpoint in Intention-to-Treat Population)

DOSAGE	N	Total-C	LDL-C	HDL-C	TG	Apolipoprotein B
Placebo	47	-1.5	-0.4	-1.9	1.0	0.7
Lipitor	140	-31.4	-39.6	2.8	-12.0	-34.0

228.5 mg/dL (range: 152.0-385.0 mg/dL) in the placebo group during the 26 week double-blind phase.

The safety and efficacy of doses above 20 mg have not been studied in controlled trials in children. The long-term efficacy of Lipitor therapy in childhood to reduce morbidity and mortality in adulthood has not been established.

INDICATIONS AND USAGE

Prevention of Cardiovascular Disease

In adult patients without clinically evident coronary heart disease, but with multiple risk factors for coronary heart disease such as age ≥ 55 years, smoking, hypertension, low HDL-C, or a family history of early coronary heart disease, Lipitor is indicated to:

- Reduce the risk of myocardial infarction
- Reduce the risk for revascularization procedures and angina

Hypercholesterolemia

Lipitor is indicated:

1. as an adjunct to diet to reduce elevated total-C, LDL-C, apo B, and TG levels and to increase HDL-C in patients with primary hypercholesterolemia (heterozygous familial and nonfamilial) and mixed dyslipidemia (*Fredrickson* Types IIa and IIb);
2. as an adjunct to diet for the treatment of patients with elevated serum TG levels (*Fredrickson* Type IV);
3. for the treatment of patients with primary dysbetalipoproteinemia (*Fredrickson* Type III) who do not respond adequately to diet;
4. to reduce total-C and LDL-C in patients with homozygous familial hypercholesterolemia as an adjunct to other lipid-lowering treatments (eg, LDL apheresis) or if such treatments are unavailable;
5. as an adjunct to diet to reduce total-C, LDL-C, and apo B levels in boys and postmenarchal girls, 10 to 17 years of age, with heterozygous familial hypercholesterolemia if after an adequate trial of diet therapy the following findings are present:
   a. LDL-C remains ≥ 190 mg/dL or
   b. LDL-C remains ≥ 160 mg/dL and:
      - there is a positive family history of premature cardiovascular disease or
      - two or more other CVD risk factors are present in the pediatric patient

Therapy with lipid-altering agents should be a component of multiple-risk-factor intervention in individuals at increased risk for atherosclerotic vascular disease due to hypercholesterolemia. Lipid-altering agents should be used in addition to a diet restricted in saturated fat and cholesterol only when the response to diet and other nonpharmacological measures has been inadequate (see *National Cholesterol Education Program (NCEP) Guidelines*, summarized in Table 6).

[See table 6 above]

After the LDL-C goal has been achieved, if the TG is still ≥200 mg/dL, non HDL-C (total-C minus HDL-C) becomes a secondary target of therapy. Non-HDL-C goals are set 30 mg/dL higher than LDL-C goals for each risk category.

Prior to initiating therapy with Lipitor, secondary causes for hypercholesterolemia (eg, poorly controlled diabetes mellitus, hypothyroidism, nephrotic syndrome, dysproteinemias, obstructive liver disease, other drug therapy, and alcoholism) should be excluded, and a lipid profile performed to measure total-C, LDL-C, HDL-C, and TG. For patients with TG <400 mg/dL (<4.5 mmol/L), LDL-C can be estimated using the following equation: LDL-C = total-C - (0.20 × [TG] + HDL-C). For TG levels >400 mg/dL (>4.5 mmol/L), this equation is less accurate and LDL-C concentrations should be determined by ultracentrifugation.

Lipitor has not been studied in conditions where the major lipoprotein abnormality is elevation of chylomicrons (*Fredrickson* Types I and V).

The NCEP classification of cholesterol levels in pediatric patients with a familial history of hypercholesterolemia or premature cardiovascular disease is summarized below:

Category	Total-C (mg/dL)	LDL-C (mg/dL)
Acceptable	<170	<110
Borderline	170-199	110-129
High	≥200	≥130

CONTRAINDICATIONS

Active liver disease or unexplained persistent elevations of serum transaminases.

Hypersensitivity to any component of this medication.

Pregnancy and Lactation

Atherosclerosis is a chronic process and discontinuation of lipid-lowering drugs during pregnancy should have little impact on the outcome of long-term therapy of primary hypercholesterolemia. Cholesterol and other products of cholesterol biosynthesis are essential components for fetal development (including synthesis of steroids and cell membranes). Since HMG-CoA reductase inhibitors decrease cholesterol synthesis and possibly the synthesis of other biologically active substances derived from cholesterol, they may cause fetal harm when administered to pregnant women. Therefore, HMG-CoA reductase inhibitors are contraindicated during pregnancy and in nursing mothers. ATORVASTATIN SHOULD BE ADMINISTERED TO WOMEN OF CHILDBEARING AGE ONLY WHEN SUCH PATIENTS ARE HIGHLY UNLIKELY TO CONCEIVE AND HAVE BEEN INFORMED OF THE POTENTIAL

TABLE 6. NCEP Treatment Guidelines: LDL-C Goals and Cutpoints for Therapeutic Lifestyle Changes and Drug Therapy in Different Risk Categories

Risk Category	LDL Goal (mg/dL)	LDL Level at Which to Initiate Therapeutic Lifestyle Changes (mg/dL)	LDL Level at Which to Consider Drug Therapy (mg/dL)
CHD[a] or CHD risk equivalents (10-year risk >20%)	<100	≥100	≥130 (100-129: drug optional)[b]
2+ Risk Factors (10-year risk ≤20%)	<130	≥130	10-year risk 10%-20%: ≥130 10-year risk <10%: ≥160
0-1 Risk factor[c]	<160	≥160	≥190 (160-189: LDL-lowering drug optional)

[a] CHD, coronary heart disease

[b] Some authorities recommend use of LDL-lowering drugs in this category if an LDL-C level of <100 mg/dL cannot be achieved by therapeutic lifestyle changes. Others prefer use of drugs that primarily modify triglycerides and HDL-C, e.g., nicotinic acid or fibrate. Clinical judgement also may call for deferring drug therapy in this subcategory.

[c] Almost all people with 0-1 risk factor have 10-year risk <10%; thus, 10-year risk assessment in people with 0-1 risk factor is not necessary.

HAZARDS. If the patient becomes pregnant while taking this drug, therapy should be discontinued and the patient apprised of the potential hazard to the fetus.

WARNINGS

Liver Dysfunction

HMG-CoA reductase inhibitors, like some other lipid-lowering therapies, have been associated with biochemical abnormalities of liver function. **Persistent elevations (>3 times the upper limit of normal [ULN] occurring on 2 or more occasions) in serum transaminases occurred in 0.7% of patients who received atorvastatin in clinical trials. The incidence of these abnormalities was 0.2%, 0.2%, 0.6%, and 2.3% for 10, 20, 40, and 80 mg, respectively.**

One patient in clinical trials developed jaundice. Increases in liver function tests (LFT) in other patients were not associated with jaundice or other clinical signs or symptoms. Upon dose reduction, drug interruption, or discontinuation, transaminase levels returned to or near pretreatment levels without sequelae. Eighteen of 30 patients with persistent LFT elevations continued treatment with a reduced dose of atorvastatin.

It is recommended that liver function tests be performed prior to and at 12 weeks following both the initiation of therapy and any elevation of dose, and periodically (eg, semiannually) thereafter. Liver enzyme changes generally occur in the first 3 months of treatment with atorvastatin. Patients who develop increased transaminase levels should be monitored until the abnormalities resolve. Should an increase in ALT or AST of >3 times ULN persist, reduction of dose or withdrawal of atorvastatin is recommended.

Atorvastatin should be used with caution in patients who consume substantial quantities of alcohol and/or have a history of liver disease. Active liver disease or unexplained persistent transaminase elevations are contraindications to the use of atorvastatin (see CONTRAINDICATIONS).

Skeletal Muscle

Rare cases of rhabdomyolysis with acute renal failure secondary to myoglobinuria have been reported with atorvastatin and with other drugs in this class.

Uncomplicated myalgia has been reported in atorvastatin-treated patients (see ADVERSE REACTIONS). Myopathy, defined as muscle aches or muscle weakness in conjunction with increases in creatine phosphokinase (CPK) values >10 times ULN, should be considered in any patient with diffuse myalgias, muscle tenderness or weakness, and/or marked elevation of CPK. Patients should be advised to report promptly unexplained muscle pain, tenderness or weakness, particularly if accompanied by malaise or fever. Atorvastatin therapy should be discontinued if markedly elevated CPK levels occur or myopathy is diagnosed or suspected.

The risk of myopathy during treatment with drugs in this class is increased with concurrent administration of cyclosporine, fibric acid derivatives, erythromycin, niacin, or azole antifungals. Physicians considering combined therapy with atorvastatin and fibric acid derivatives, erythromycin, immunosuppressive drugs, azole antifungals, or lipid-lowering doses of niacin should carefully weigh the potential benefits and risks and should carefully monitor patients for any signs or symptoms of muscle pain, tenderness, or weakness, particularly during the initial months of therapy and during any periods of upward dosage titration of either drug. Periodic creatine phosphokinase (CPK) determinations may be considered in such situations, but there is no assurance that such monitoring will prevent the occurrence of severe myopathy.

Atorvastatin therapy should be temporarily withheld or discontinued in any patient with an acute, serious condition suggestive of a myopathy or having a risk factor predisposing to the development of renal failure secondary to rhabdomyolysis (eg, severe acute infection, hypotension, major surgery, trauma, severe metabolic, endocrine and electrolyte disorders, and uncontrolled seizures).

PRECAUTIONS

General

Before instituting therapy with atorvastatin, an attempt should be made to control hypercholesterolemia with appropriate diet, exercise, and weight reduction in obese patients, and to treat other underlying medical problems (see INDICATIONS AND USAGE).

Information for Patients

Patients should be advised to report promptly unexplained muscle pain, tenderness, or weakness, particularly if accompanied by malaise or fever.

Drug Interactions

The risk of myopathy during treatment with drugs of this class is increased with concurrent administration of cyclosporine, fibric acid derivatives, niacin (nicotinic acid), erythromycin, azole antifungals (see WARNINGS, Skeletal Muscle).

Antacid: When atorvastatin and Maalox® TC suspension were coadministered, plasma concentrations of atorvastatin decreased approximately 35%. However, LDL-C reduction was not altered.

Antipyrine: Because atorvastatin does not affect the pharmacokinetics of antipyrine, interactions with other drugs metabolized via the same cytochrome isozymes are not expected.

Colestipol: Plasma concentrations of atorvastatin decreased approximately 25% when colestipol and atorvastatin were coadministered. However, LDL-C reduction was greater when atorvastatin and colestipol were coadministered than when either drug was given alone.

Cimetidine: Atorvastatin plasma concentrations and LDL-C reduction were not altered by coadministration of cimetidine.

Digoxin: When multiple doses of atorvastatin and digoxin were coadministered, steady-state plasma digoxin concentrations increased by approximately 20%. Patients taking digoxin should be monitored appropriately.

Erythromycin: In healthy individuals, plasma concentrations of atorvastatin increased approximately 40% with coadministration of atorvastatin and erythromycin, a known inhibitor of cytochrome P450 3A4 (see WARNINGS, Skeletal Muscle).

Oral Contraceptives: Coadministration of atorvastatin and an oral contraceptive increased AUC values for norethindrone and ethinyl estradiol by approximately 30% and 20%. These increases should be considered when selecting an oral contraceptive for a woman taking atorvastatin.

Warfarin: Atorvastatin had no clinically significant effect on prothrombin time when administered to patients receiving chronic warfarin treatment.

Endocrine Function

HMG-CoA reductase inhibitors interfere with cholesterol synthesis and theoretically might blunt adrenal and/or gonadal steroid production. Clinical studies have shown that atorvastatin does not reduce basal plasma cortisol concentration or impair adrenal reserve. The effects of HMG-CoA reductase inhibitors on male fertility have not been studied in adequate numbers of patients. The effects, if any, on the pituitary-gonadal axis in premenopausal women are unknown. Caution should be exercised if an HMG-CoA reductase inhibitor is administered concomitantly with drugs that may decrease the levels or activity of endogenous steroid hormones, such as ketoconazole, spironolactone, and cimetidine.

CNS Toxicity

Brain hemorrhage was seen in a female dog treated for 3 months at 120 mg/kg/day. Brain hemorrhage and optic nerve vacuolation were seen in another female dog that was sacrificed in moribund condition after 11 weeks of escalating doses up to 280 mg/kg/day. The 120 mg/kg dose resulted in a systemic exposure approximately 16 times the human plasma area-under-the-curve (AUC, 0-24 hours) based on the maximum human dose of 80 mg/day. A single tonic convulsion was seen in each of 2 male dogs (one treated at 10 mg/kg/day and one at 120 mg/kg/day) in a 2-year study. No CNS lesions have been observed in mice after chronic treatment for up to 2 years at doses up to 400 mg/kg/day or in rats at doses up to 100 mg/kg/day. These doses were 6 to 11 times (mouse) and 8 to 16 times (rat) the human AUC (0-24) based on the maximum recommended human dose of 80 mg/day.

Continued on next page

Lipitor—Cont.

CNS vascular lesions, characterized by perivascular hemorrhages, edema, and mononuclear cell infiltration of perivascular spaces, have been observed in dogs treated with other members of this class. A chemically similar drug in this class produced optic nerve degeneration (Wallerian degeneration of retinogeniculate fibers) in clinically normal dogs in a dose-dependent fashion at a dose that produced plasma drug levels about 30 times higher than the mean drug level in humans taking the highest recommended dose.

Carcinogenesis, Mutagenesis, Impairment of Fertility

In a 2-year carcinogenicity study in rats at dose levels of 10, 30, and 100 mg/kg/day, 2 rare tumors were found in muscle in high-dose females: in one, there was a rhabdomyosarcoma and, in another, there was a fibrosarcoma. This dose represents a plasma AUC (0-24) value of approximately 16 times the mean human plasma drug exposure after an 80 mg oral dose.

A 2-year carcinogenicity study in mice given 100, 200, or 400 mg/kg/day resulted in a significant increase in liver adenomas in high-dose males and liver carcinomas in high-dose females. These findings occurred at plasma AUC (0-24) values of approximately 6 times the mean human plasma drug exposure after an 80 mg oral dose.

In vitro, atorvastatin was not mutagenic or clastogenic in the following tests with and without metabolic activation: the Ames test with *Salmonella typhimurium* and *Escherichia coli,* the HGPRT forward mutation assay in Chinese hamster lung cells, and the chromosomal aberration assay in Chinese hamster lung cells. Atorvastatin was negative in the *in vivo* mouse micronucleus test.

Studies in rats performed at doses up to 175 mg/kg (15 times the human exposure) produced no changes in fertility. There was aplasia and aspermia in the epididymis of 2 of 10 rats treated with 100 mg/kg/day of atorvastatin for 3 months (16 times the human AUC at the 80 mg dose); testis weights were significantly lower at 30 and 100 mg/kg and epididymal weight was lower at 100 mg/kg. Male rats given 100 mg/kg/day for 11 weeks prior to mating had decreased sperm motility, spermatid head concentration, and increased abnormal sperm. Atorvastatin caused no adverse effects on semen parameters, or reproductive organ histopathology in dogs given doses of 10, 40, or 120 mg/kg for two years.

Pregnancy

Pregnancy Category X

See CONTRAINDICATIONS

Safety in pregnant women has not been established. Atorvastatin crosses the rat placenta and reaches a level in fetal liver equivalent to that of maternal plasma. Atorvastatin was not teratogenic in rats at doses up to 300 mg/kg/day or in rabbits at doses up to 100 mg/kg/day. These doses resulted in multiples of about 30 times (rat) or 20 times (rabbit) the human exposure based on surface area (mg/m^2).

In a study in rats given 20, 100, or 225 mg/kg/day, from gestation day 7 through to lactation day 21 (weaning), there was decreased pup survival at birth, neonate, weaning, and maturity in pups of mothers dosed with 225 mg/kg/day. Body weight was decreased on days 4 and 21 in pups of mothers dosed at 100 mg/kg/day; pup body weight was decreased at birth and at days 4, 21, and 91 at 225 mg/kg/day. Pup development was delayed (rotorod performance at 100 mg/kg/day and acoustic startle at 225 mg/kg/day; pinnae detachment and eye opening at 225 mg/kg/day). These doses correspond to 6 times (100 mg/kg) and 22 times (225 mg/kg) the human AUC at 80 mg/day. Rare reports of congenital anomalies have been received following intrauterine exposure to HMG-CoA reductase inhibitors. There has been one report of severe congenital bony deformity, tracheo-esophageal fistula, and anal atresia (VATER association) in a baby born to a woman who took lovastatin with dextroamphetamine sulfate during the first trimester of pregnancy. Lipitor should be administered to women of child-bearing potential only when such patients are highly unlikely to conceive and have been informed of the potential hazards. If the woman becomes pregnant while taking Lipitor, it should be discontinued and the patient advised again as to the potential hazards to the fetus.

Nursing Mothers

Nursing rat pups had plasma and liver drug levels of 50% and 40%, respectively, of that in their mother's milk. Because of the potential for adverse reactions in nursing infants, women taking Lipitor should not breast-feed (see CONTRAINDICATIONS).

Pediatric Use

Safety and effectiveness in patients 10-17 years of age with heterozygous familial hypercholesterolemia have been evaluated in a controlled clinical trial of 6 months duration in adolescent boys and postmenarchal girls. Patients treated with Lipitor had an adverse experience profile generally similar to that of patients treated with placebo, the most common adverse experiences observed in both groups, regardless of causality assessment, were infections. **Doses greater than 20 mg have not been studied in this patient population.** In this limited controlled study, there was no detectable effect on growth or sexual maturation in boys or on menstrual cycle length in girls (see CLINICAL PHARMACOLOGY, Clinical Studies section; ADVERSE REACTIONS, Pediatric Patients (ages 10-17 years); and DOSAGE AND ADMINISTRATION, Heterozygous Familial Hypercholesterolemia in Pediatric Patients (10-17 years of age). Adolescent females should be counseled on appropriate contraceptive methods while on Lipitor therapy (see CONTRAINDICATIONS and PRECAUTIONS, Pregnancy). **Lipitor has not been studied in controlled clinical trials involving pre-pubertal patients or patients younger than 10 years of age.**

Clinical efficacy with doses up to 80 mg/day for 1 year have been evaluated in an uncontrolled study of patients with homozygous FH including 8 pediatric patients (see CLINICAL PHARMACOLOGY, Clinical Studies: Homozygous Familial Hypercholesterolemia).

Geriatric Use

The safety and efficacy of atorvastatin (10-80 mg) in the geriatric population (≥65 years of age) was evaluated in the ACCESS study. In this 54-week open-label trial 1,958 patients initiated therapy with atorvastatin 10 mg. Of these, 835 were elderly (≥65 years) and 1,123 were non-elderly. The mean change in LDL-C from baseline after 6 weeks of treatment with atorvastatin 10 mg was –38.2% in the elderly patients versus –34.6% in the non-elderly group.

The rates of discontinuation due to adverse events were similar between the two age groups. There were no differences in clinically relevant laboratory abnormalities between the age groups.

ADVERSE REACTIONS

Lipitor is generally well-tolerated. Adverse reactions have usually been mild and transient. In controlled clinical studies of 2502 patients, <2% of patients were discontinued due to adverse experiences attributable to atorvastatin. The most frequent adverse events thought to be related to atorvastatin were constipation, flatulence, dyspepsia, and abdominal pain.

Clinical Adverse Experiences

Adverse experiences reported in ≥2% of patients in placebo-controlled clinical studies of atorvastatin, regardless of causality assessment, are shown in Table 7.

[See table 7 below]

Anglo-Scandinavian Cardiac Outcomes Trial (ASCOT)

In ASCOT (see CLINICAL PHARMACOLOGY, *Clinical Studies)* involving 10,305 participants treated with Lipitor 10 mg daily (n=5,168) or placebo (n=5,137), the safety and tolerability profile of the group treated with Lipitor was comparable to that of the group treated with placebo during a median of 3.3 years of follow-up.

The following adverse events were reported, regardless of causality assessment in patients treated with atorvastatin in clinical trials. The events in italics occurred in ≥2% of patients and the events in plain type occurred in <2% of patients.

Body as a Whole: *Chest pain,* face edema, fever, neck rigidity, malaise, photosensitivity reaction, generalized edema.

Digestive System: *Nausea,* gastroenteritis, liver function tests abnormal, colitis, vomiting, gastritis, dry mouth, rectal hemorrhage, esophagitis, eructation, glossitis, mouth ulceration, anorexia, increased appetite, stomatitis, biliary pain, cheilitis, duodenal ulcer, dysphagia, enteritis, melena, gum hemorrhage, stomach ulcer, tenesmus, ulcerative stomatitis, hepatitis, pancreatitis, cholestatic jaundice.

Respiratory System: *Bronchitis, rhinitis,* pneumonia, dyspnea, asthma, epistaxis.

Nervous System: *Insomnia, dizziness,* paresthesia, somnolence, amnesia, abnormal dreams, libido decreased, emotional lability, incoordination, peripheral neuropathy, torticollis, facial paralysis, hyperkinesia, depression, hypesthesia, hypertonia.

Musculoskeletal System: *Arthritis,* leg cramps, bursitis, tenosynovitis, myasthenia, tendinous contracture, myositis.

Skin and Appendages: Pruritus, contact dermatitis, alopecia, dry skin, sweating, acne, urticaria, eczema, seborrhea, skin ulcer.

Urogenital System: *Urinary tract infection,* urinary frequency, cystitis, hematuria, impotence, dysuria, kidney calculus, nocturia, epididymitis, fibrocystic breast, vaginal hemorrhage, albuminuria, breast enlargement, metrorrhagia, nephritis, urinary incontinence, urinary retention, urinary urgency, abnormal ejaculation, uterine hemorrhage.

Special Senses: Amblyopia, tinnitus, dry eyes, refraction disorder, eye hemorrhage, deafness, glaucoma, parosmia, taste loss, taste perversion.

Cardiovascular System: Palpitation, vasodilatation, syncope, migraine, postural hypotension, phlebitis, arrhythmia, angina pectoris, hypertension.

Metabolic and Nutritional Disorders: *Peripheral edema,* hyperglycemia, creatine phosphokinase increased, gout, weight gain, hypoglycemia.

Hemic and Lymphatic System: Ecchymosis, anemia, lymphadenopathy, thrombocytopenia, petechia.

Postintroduction Reports

Adverse events associated with Lipitor therapy reported since market introduction, that are not listed above, regardless of causality assessment, include the following: anaphylaxis, angioneurotic edema, bullous rashes (including erythema multiforme, Stevens-Johnson syndrome, and toxic epidermal necrolysis), and rhabdomyolysis.

Pediatric Patients (ages 10-17 years)

In a 26-week controlled study in boys and postmenarchal girls (n=140), the safety and tolerability profile of Lipitor 10 to 20 mg daily was generally similar to that of placebo (see CLINICAL PHARMACOLOGY, Clinical Studies section and PRECAUTIONS, Pediatric Use).

OVERDOSAGE

There is no specific treatment for atorvastatin overdosage. In the event of an overdose, the patient should be treated symptomatically, and supportive measures instituted as required. Due to extensive drug binding to plasma proteins, hemodialysis is not expected to significantly enhance atorvastatin clearance.

DOSAGE AND ADMINISTRATION

The patient should be placed on a standard cholesterol-lowering diet before receiving Lipitor and should continue on this diet during treatment with Lipitor.

Hypercholesterolemia (Heterozygous Familial and Nonfamilial) and Mixed Dyslipidemia (*Fredrickson* Types IIa and IIb)

The recommended starting dose of Lipitor is 10 or 20 mg once daily. Patients who require a large reduction in LDL-C (more than 45%) may be started at 40 mg once daily. The dosage range of Lipitor is 10 to 80 mg once daily. Lipitor can be administered as a single dose at any time of the day, with or without food. The starting dose and maintenance doses of Lipitor should be individualized according to patient characteristics such as goal of therapy and response (see *NCEP Guidelines,* summarized in Table 5). After initiation and/or upon titration of Lipitor, lipid levels should be analyzed within 2 to 4 weeks and dosage adjusted accordingly.

Since the goal of treatment is to lower LDL-C, the NCEP recommends that LDL-C levels be used to initiate and assess treatment response. Only if LDL-C levels are not available, should total-C be used to monitor therapy.

Heterozygous Familial Hypercholesterolemia in Pediatric Patients (10-17 years of age)

The recommended starting dose of Lipitor is 10 mg/day; the maximum recommended dose is 20 mg/day (doses greater than 20 mg have not been studied in this patient population). Doses should be individualized according to the recommended goal of therapy (see NCEP Pediatric Panel Guidelines[1], CLINICAL PHARMACOLOGY, and INDICATIONS AND USAGE). Adjustments should be made at intervals of 4 weeks or more.

[1] National Cholesterol Education Program (NCEP): Highlights of the Report of the Expert Panel on Blood Cholesterol Levels in Children Adolescents, *Pediatrics.* 89(3):495-501. 1992.

Homozygous Familial Hypercholesterolemia

The dosage of Lipitor in patients with homozygous FH is 10 to 80 mg daily. Lipitor should be used as an adjunct to other lipid-lowering treatments (eg, LDL apheresis) in these patients or if such treatments are unavailable.

TABLE 7. Adverse Events in Placebo-Controlled Studies (% of Patients)

BODY SYSTEM/ Adverse Event	Placebo N = 270	Atorvastatin 10 mg N = 863	Atorvastatin 20 mg N = 36	Atorvastatin 40 mg N = 79	Atorvastatin 80 mg N = 94
BODY AS A WHOLE					
Infection	10.0	10.3	2.8	10.1	7.4
Headache	7.0	5.4	16.7	2.5	6.4
Accidental Injury	3.7	4.2	0.0	1.3	3.2
Flu Syndrome	1.9	2.2	0.0	2.5	3.2
Abdominal Pain	0.7	2.8	0.0	3.8	2.1
Back Pain	3.0	2.8	0.0	3.8	1.1
Allergic Reaction	2.6	0.9	2.8	1.3	0.0
Asthenia	1.9	2.2	0.0	3.8	0.0
DIGESTIVE SYSTEM					
Constipation	1.8	2.1	0.0	2.5	1.1
Diarrhea	1.5	2.7	0.0	3.8	5.3
Dyspepsia	4.1	2.3	2.8	1.3	2.1
Flatulence	3.3	2.1	2.8	1.3	1.1
RESPIRATORY SYSTEM					
Sinusitis	2.6	2.8	0.0	2.5	6.4
Pharyngitis	1.5	2.5	0.0	1.3	2.1
SKIN AND APPENDAGES					
Rash	0.7	3.9	2.8	3.8	1.1
MUSCULOSKELETAL SYSTEM					
Arthralgia	1.5	2.0	0.0	5.1	0.0
Myalgia	1.1	3.2	5.6	1.3	0.0

Concomitant Therapy
Atorvastatin may be used in combination with a bile acid binding resin for additive effect. The combination of HMG-CoA reductase inhibitors and fibrates should generally be avoided (see WARNINGS, Skeletal Muscle, and PRECAUTIONS, Drug Interactions for other drug-drug interactions).
Dosage in Patients With Renal Insufficiency
Renal disease does not affect the plasma concentrations nor LDL-C reduction of atorvastatin; thus, dosage adjustment in patients with renal dysfunction is not necessary (see CLINICAL PHARMACOLOGY, Pharmacokinetics).

HOW SUPPLIED

Lipitor is supplied as white, elliptical, film-coated tablets of atorvastatin calcium containing 10, 20, 40 and 80 mg atorvastatin.
10 mg tablets: coded "PD 155" on one side and "10" on the other.
NDC 0071-0155-23 bottles of 90
NDC 0071-0155-34 bottles of 5000
NDC 0071-0155-40 10 × 10 unit dose blisters
20 mg tablets: coded "PD 156" on one side and "20" on the other.
NDC 0071-0156-23 bottles of 90
NDC 0071-0156-40 10 × 10 unit dose blisters
NDC 0071-0156-94 bottles of 5000
40 mg tablets: coded "PD 157" on one side and "40" on the other.
NDC 0071-0157-23 bottles of 90
NDC 0071-0157-73 bottles of 500
80 mg tablets: coded "PD 158" on one side and "80" on the other.
NDC 0071-0158-23 bottles of 90
NDC 0071-0158-73 bottles of 500
Storage
Store at controlled room temperature 20-25°C (68-77°F) [see USP].
Rx Only

Manufactured by:
Pfizer Ireland Pharmaceuticals
Dublin, Ireland
Distributed by:
Pfizer Parke-Davis
Division of Pfizer Inc, NY, NY 10017
LAB-0021-7.0 Revised July 2004
Shown in Product Identification Guide, page 329

NEURONTIN® ℞
[nər-ŏn-tĭn]
(gabapentin) Capsules

NEURONTIN®
(gabapentin) Tablets

NEURONTIN®
(gabapentin) Oral Solution

DESCRIPTION

Neurontin® (gabapentin) Capsules, Neurontin® (gabapentin) Tablets, and Neurontin® (gabapentin) Oral Solution are supplied as imprinted hard shell capsules containing 100 mg, 300 mg, and 400 mg of gabapentin, elliptical film-coated tablets containing 600 mg and 800 mg of gabapentin or an oral solution containing 250 mg/5 mL of gabapentin.
The inactive ingredients for the capsules are lactose, cornstarch, and talc. The 100 mg capsule shell contains gelatin and titanium dioxide. The 300 mg capsule shell contains gelatin, titanium dioxide, and yellow iron oxide. The 400 mg capsule shell contains gelatin, red iron oxide, titanium dioxide, and yellow iron oxide. The imprinting ink contains FD&C Blue No. 2 and titanium dioxide.
The inactive ingredients for the tablets are poloxamer 407, copolyvidonum, cornstarch, magnesium stearate, hydroxypropyl cellulose, talc, candelilla wax and purified water.
The inactive ingredients for the oral solution are glycerin, xylitol, purified water and artificial cool strawberry anise flavor.
Gabapentin is described as 1-(aminomethyl)cyclohexaneacetic acid with a molecular formula of $C_9H_{17}NO_2$ and a molecular weight of 171.24. The structural formula of gabapentin is:

CH_2NH_2
CH_2CO_2H

Gabapentin is a white to off-white crystalline solid with a pK_{a1} of 3.7 and a pK_{a2} of 10.7. It is freely soluble in water and both basic and acidic aqueous solutions. The log of the partition coefficient (n-octanol/0.05M phosphate buffer) at pH 7.4 is –1.25.

CLINICAL PHARMACOLOGY

Mechanism of Action
The mechanism by which gabapentin exerts its analgesic action is unknown, but in animal models of analgesia, gabapentin prevents allodynia (pain-related behavior in response to a normally innocuous stimulus) and hyperalgesia (exaggerated response to painful stimuli). In particular, gabapentin prevents pain-related responses in several models of neuropathic pain in rats or mice (e.g. spinal nerve ligation models, streptozocin-induced diabetes model, spinal cord injury model, acute herpes zoster infection model). Gabapentin also decreases pain-related responses after peripheral inflammation (carrageenan footpad test, late phase of formalin test). Gabapentin did not alter immediate pain-related behaviors (rat tail flick test, formalin footpad acute phase, acetic acid abdominal constriction test, footpad heat irradiation test). The relevance of these models to human pain is not known.
The mechanism by which gabapentin exerts its anticonvulsant action is unknown, but in animal test systems designed to detect anticonvulsant activity, gabapentin prevents seizures as do other marketed anticonvulsants. Gabapentin exhibits antiseizure activity in mice and rats in both the maximal electroshock and pentylenetetrazole seizure models and other preclinical models (e.g., strains with genetic epilepsy, etc.). The relevance of these models to human epilepsy is not known.
Gabapentin is structurally related to the neurotransmitter GABA (gamma-aminobutyric acid) but it does not modify $GABA_A$ or $GABA_B$ radioligand binding, it is not converted metabolically into GABA or a GABA agonist, and it is not an inhibitor of GABA uptake or degradation. Gabapentin was tested in radioligand binding assays at concentrations up to 100 μM and did not exhibit affinity for a number of other common receptor sites, including benzodiazepine, glutamate, N-methyl-D-aspartate (NMDA), quisqualate, kainate, strychnine-insensitive or strychnine-sensitive glycine, alpha 1, alpha 2, or beta adrenergic, adenosine A1 or A2, cholinergic muscarinic or nicotinic, dopamine D1 or D2, histamine H1, serotonin S1 or S2, opiate mu, delta or kappa, cannabinoid 1, voltage-sensitive calcium channel sites labeled with nitrendipine or diltiazem, or at voltage-sensitive sodium channel sites labeled with batrachotoxinin A 20-alpha-benzoate. Furthermore, gabapentin did not alter the cellular uptake of dopamine, noradrenaline, or serotonin.
In vitro studies with radiolabeled gabapentin have revealed a gabapentin binding site in areas of rat brain including neocortex and hippocampus. A high-affinity binding protein in animal brain tissue has been identified as an auxiliary subunit of voltage-activated calcium channels. However, functional correlates of gabapentin binding, if any, remain to be elucidated.
Pharmacokinetics and Drug Metabolism
All pharmacological actions following gabapentin administration are due to the activity of the parent compound; gabapentin is not appreciably metabolized in humans.
Oral Bioavailability: Gabapentin bioavailability is not dose proportional; i.e., as dose is increased, bioavailability decreases. Bioavailability of gabapentin is approximately 60%, 47%, 34%, 33%, and 27% following 900, 1200, 2400, 3600, and 4800 mg/day given in 3 divided doses, respectively. Food has only a slight effect on the rate and extent of absorption of gabapentin (14% increase in AUC and C_{max}).
Distribution: Less than 3% of gabapentin circulates bound to plasma protein. The apparent volume of distribution of gabapentin after 150 mg intravenous administration is 58±6 L (Mean±SD). In patients with epilepsy, steady-state predose (C_{min}) concentrations of gabapentin in cerebrospinal fluid were approximately 20% of the corresponding plasma concentrations.
Elimination: Gabapentin is eliminated from the systemic circulation by renal excretion as unchanged drug. Gabapentin is not appreciably metabolized in humans.
Gabapentin elimination half-life is 5 to 7 hours and is unaltered by dose or following multiple dosing. Gabapentin elimination rate constant, plasma clearance, and renal clearance are directly proportional to creatinine clearance (see Special Populations: Patients With Renal Insufficiency, below). In elderly patients, and in patients with impaired renal function, gabapentin plasma clearance is reduced. Gabapentin can be removed from plasma by hemodialysis.
Dosage adjustment in patients with compromised renal function or undergoing hemodialysis is recommended (see DOSAGE AND ADMINISTRATION, Table 5).
Special Populations: *Adult Patients With Renal Insufficiency:* Subjects (N=60) with renal insufficiency (mean creatinine clearance ranging from 13-114 mL/min) were administered single 400 mg oral doses of gabapentin. The mean gabapentin half-life ranged from about 6.5 hours (patients with creatinine clearance >60 mL/min) to 52 hours (creatinine clearance <30 mL/min) and gabapentin renal clearance from about 90 mL/min (>60 mL/min group) to about 10 mL/min (<30 mL/min). Mean plasma clearance (CL/F) decreased from approximately 190 mL/min to 20 mL/min.

TABLE 1. Controlled PHN Studies: Duration, Dosages, and Number of Patients

Study	Study Duration	Gabapentin (mg/day)[a] Target Dose	Patients Receiving Gabapentin	Patients Receiving Placebo
1	8 weeks	3600	113	116
2	7 weeks	1800, 2400	223	111
		Total	336	227

[a] Given in 3 divided doses (TID)

Dosage adjustment in adult patients with compromised renal function is necessary (see DOSAGE AND ADMINISTRATION). Pediatric patients with renal insufficiency have not been studied.
Hemodialysis: In a study in anuric adult subjects (N=11), the apparent elimination half-life of gabapentin on nondialysis days was about 132 hours; during dialysis the apparent half-life of gabapentin was reduced to 3.8 hours. Hemodialysis thus has a significant effect on gabapentin elimination in anuric subjects.
Dosage adjustment in patients undergoing hemodialysis is necessary (see DOSAGE AND ADMINISTRATION).
Hepatic Disease: Because gabapentin is not metabolized, no study was performed in patients with hepatic impairment.
Age: The effect of age was studied in subjects 20-80 years of age. Apparent oral clearance (CL/F) of gabapentin decreased as age increased, from about 225 mL/min in those under 30 years of age to about 125 mL/min in those over 70 years of age. Renal clearance (CLr) and CLr adjusted for body surface area also declined with age; however, the decline in the renal clearance of gabapentin with age can largely be explained by the decline in renal function. Reduction of gabapentin dose may be required in patients who have age related compromised renal function. (See PRECAUTIONS, Geriatric Use, and DOSAGE AND ADMINISTRATION.)
Pediatric: Gabapentin pharmacokinetics were determined in 48 pediatric subjects between the ages of 1 month and 12 years following a dose of approximately 10 mg/kg. Peak plasma concentrations were similar across the entire age group and occurred 2 to 3 hours postdose. In general, pediatric subjects between 1 month and <5 years of age achieved approximately 30% lower exposure (AUC) than that observed in those 5 years of age and older. Accordingly, oral clearance normalized per body weight was higher in the younger children. Apparent oral clearance of gabapentin was directly proportional to creatinine clearance. Gabapentin elimination half-life averaged 4.7 hours and was similar across the age groups studied.
A population pharmacokinetic analysis was performed in 253 pediatric subjects between 1 month and 13 years of age. Patients received 10 to 65 mg/kg/day given TID. Apparent oral clearance (CL/F) was directly proportional to creatinine clearance and this relationship was similar following a single dose and at steady state. Higher oral clearance values were observed in children <5 years of age compared to those observed in children 5 years of age and older, when normalized per body weight. The clearance was highly variable in infants <1 year of age. The normalized CL/F values observed in pediatric patients 5 years of age and older were consistent with values observed in adults after a single dose. The oral volume of distribution normalized per body weight was constant across the age range.
These pharmacokinetic data indicate that the effective daily dose in pediatric patients with epilepsy ages 3 and 4 years should be 40 mg/kg/day to achieve average plasma concentrations similar to those achieved in patients 5 years of age and older receiving gabapentin at 30 mg/kg/day (see DOSAGE AND ADMINISTRATION).
Gender: Although no formal study has been conducted to compare the pharmacokinetics of gabapentin in men and women, it appears that the pharmacokinetic parameters for males and females are similar and there are no significant gender differences.
Race: Pharmacokinetic differences due to race have not been studied. Because gabapentin is primarily renally excreted and there are no important racial differences in creatinine clearance, pharmacokinetic differences due to race are not expected.
Clinical Studies
Postherpetic Neuralgia
Neurontin® was evaluated for the management of postherpetic neuralgia (PHN) in 2 randomized, double-blind, placebo-controlled, multicenter studies; N=563 patients in the intent-to-treat (ITT) population (Table 1). Patients were enrolled if they continued to have pain for more than 3 months after healing of the herpes zoster skin rash.
[See table 1 above]
Each study included a 1-week baseline during which patients were screened for eligibility and a 7- or 8-week double-blind phase (3 or 4 weeks of titration and 4 weeks of fixed dose). Patients initiated treatment with titration to a maximum of 900 mg/day gabapentin over 3 days. Dosages were then to be titrated in 600 to 1200 mg/day increments at 3- to 7-day intervals to target dose over 3 to 4 weeks. In

Continued on next page

Neurontin—Cont.

Study 1, patients were continued on lower doses if not able to achieve the target dose. During baseline and treatment, patients recorded their pain in a daily diary using an 11-point numeric pain rating scale ranging from 0 (no pain) to 10 (worst possible pain). A mean pain score during baseline of at least 4 was required for randomization (baseline mean pain score for Studies 1 and 2 combined was 6.4). Analyses were conducted using the ITT population (all randomized patients who received at least one dose of study medication). Both studies showed significant differences from placebo at all doses tested.

A significant reduction in weekly mean pain scores was seen by Week 1 in both studies, and significant differences were maintained to the end of treatment. Comparable treatment effects were observed in all active treatment arms. Pharmacokinetic/pharmacodynamic modeling provided confirmatory evidence of efficacy across all doses. Figures 1 and 2 show these changes for Studies 1 and 2.

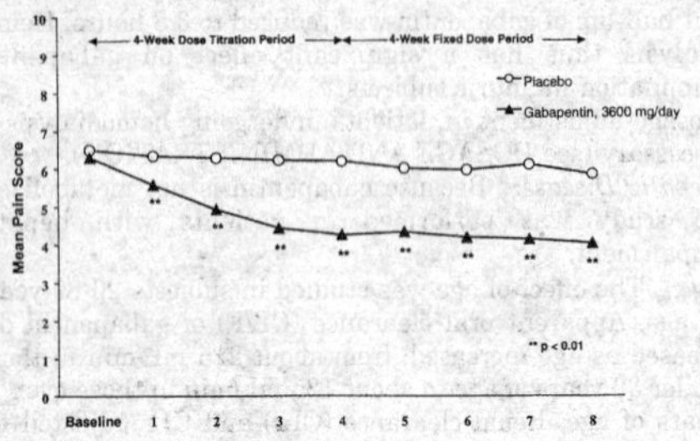

Figure 1. Weekly Mean Pain Scores (Observed Cases in ITT Population): Study 1

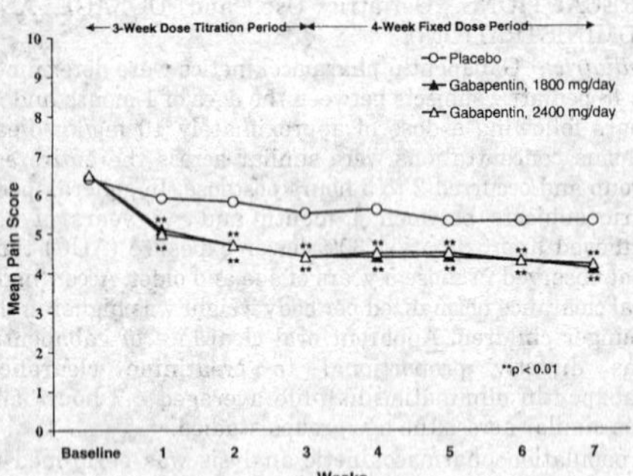

Figure 2. Weekly Mean Pain Scores (Observed Cases in ITT Population): Study 2

The proportion of responders (those patients reporting at least 50% improvement in endpoint pain score compared with baseline) was calculated for each study (Figure 3).

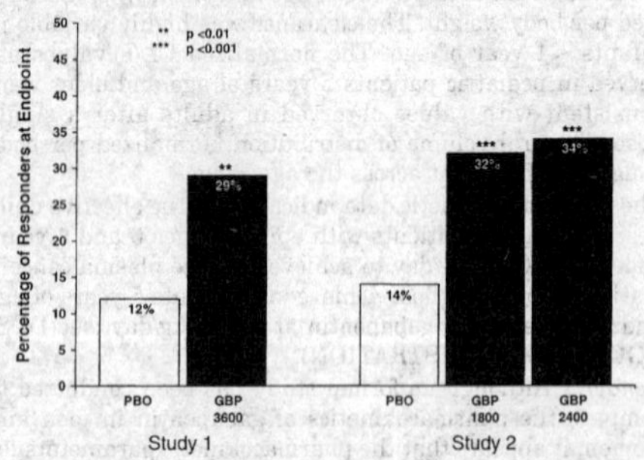

Figure 3. Proportion of Responders (patients with ≥50% reduction in pain score) at Endpoint: Controlled PHN Studies

Epilepsy

The effectiveness of Neurontin® as adjunctive therapy (added to other antiepileptic drugs) was established in multicenter placebo-controlled, double-blind, parallel-group clinical trials in adult and pediatric patients (3 years and older) with refractory partial seizures.

Evidence of effectiveness was obtained in three trials conducted in 705 patients (age 12 years and above) and one trial conducted in 247 pediatric patients (3 to 12 years of age). The patients enrolled had a history of at least 4 partial seizures per month in spite of receiving one or more antiepileptic drugs at therapeutic levels and were observed on their established antiepileptic drug regimen during a 12-week baseline period (6 weeks in the study of pediatric patients). In patients continuing to have at least 2 (or 4 in some studies) seizures per month, Neurontin® or placebo was then added on to the existing therapy during a 12-week treatment period. Effectiveness was assessed primarily on the basis of the percent of patients with a 50% or greater reduction in seizure frequency from baseline to treatment (the "responder rate") and a derived measure called response ratio, a measure of change defined as (T - B)/(T + B), where B is the patient's baseline seizure frequency and T is the patient's seizure frequency during treatment. Response ratio is distributed within the range -1 to +1. A zero value indicates no change while complete elimination of seizures would give a value of -1; increased seizure rates would give positive values. A response ratio of -0.33 corresponds to a 50% reduction in seizure frequency. The results given below are for all partial seizures in the intent-to-treat (all patients who received any doses of treatment) population in each study, unless otherwise indicated.

One study compared Neurontin® 1200 mg/day divided TID with placebo. Responder rate was 23% (14/61) in the Neurontin® group and 9% (6/66) in the placebo group; the difference between groups was statistically significant. Response ratio was also better in the Neurontin® group (-0.199) than in the placebo group (-0.044), a difference that also achieved statistical significance.

A second study compared primarily 1200 mg/day divided TID Neurontin® (N=101) with placebo (N=98). Additional smaller Neurontin® dosage groups (600 mg/day, N=53; 1800 mg/day, N=54) were also studied for information regarding dose response. Responder rate was higher in the Neurontin® 1200 mg/day group (16%) than in the placebo group (8%), but the difference was not statistically significant. The responder rate at 600 mg (17%) was also not significantly higher than in the placebo, but the responder rate in the 1800 mg group (26%) was statistically significantly superior to the placebo rate. Response ratio was better in the Neurontin® 1200 mg/day group (-0.103) than in the placebo group (-0.022); but this difference was also not statistically significant (p = 0.224). A better response was seen in the Neurontin® 600 mg/day group (-0.105) and 1800 mg/day group (-0.222) than in the 1200 mg/day group, with the 1800 mg/day group achieving statistical significance compared to the placebo group.

A third study compared Neurontin® 900 mg/day divided TID (N=111) and placebo (N=109). An additional Neurontin® 1200 mg/day dosage group (N=52) provided dose-response data. A statistically significant difference in responder rate was seen in the Neurontin® 900 mg/day group (22%) compared to that in the placebo group (10%). Response ratio was also statistically significantly superior in the Neurontin® 900 mg/day group (-0.119) compared to that in the placebo group (-0.027), as was response ratio in 1200 mg/day Neurontin® (-0.184) compared to placebo.

Analyses were also performed in each study to examine the effect of Neurontin® on preventing secondarily generalized tonic-clonic seizures. Patients who experienced a secondarily generalized tonic-clonic seizure in either the baseline or in the treatment period in all three placebo-controlled studies were included in these analyses. There were several response ratio comparisons that showed a statistically significant advantage for Neurontin® compared to placebo and favorable trends for almost all comparisons.

Analysis of responder rate using combined data from all three studies and all doses (N=162, Neurontin®; N=89, placebo) also showed a significant advantage for Neurontin® over placebo in reducing the frequency of secondarily generalized tonic-clonic seizures.

In two of the three controlled studies, more than one dose of Neurontin® was used. Within each study the results did not show a consistently increased response to dose. However, looking across studies, a trend toward increasing efficacy with increasing dose is evident (see Figure 4).

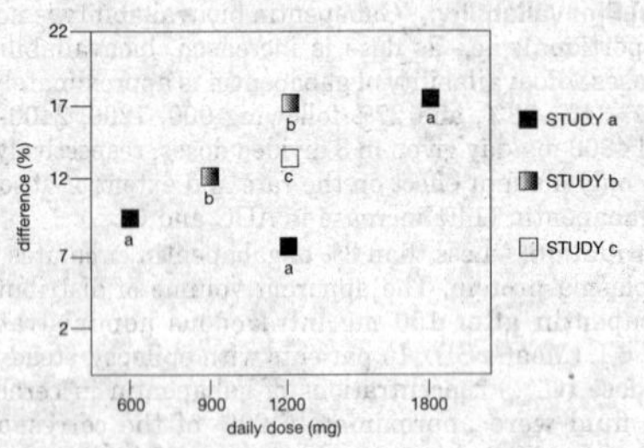

FIGURE 4. Responder Rate in Patients Receiving Neurontin® Expressed as a Difference from Placebo by Dose and Study: Adjunctive Therapy Studies in Patients ≥12 Years of Age with Partial Seizures

In the figure, treatment effect magnitude, measured on the Y axis in terms of the difference in the proportion of gabapentin and placebo assigned patients attaining a 50% or greater reduction in seizure frequency from baseline, is plotted against the daily dose of gabapentin administered (X axis).

Although no formal analysis by gender has been performed, estimates of response (Response Ratio) derived from clinical trials (398 men, 307 women) indicate no important gender differences exist. There was no consistent pattern indicating that age had any effect on the response to Neurontin®. There were insufficient numbers of patients of races other than Caucasian to permit a comparison of efficacy among racial groups.

A fourth study in pediatric patients age 3 to 12 years compared 25 – 35 mg/kg/day Neurontin® (N=118) with placebo (N=127). For all partial seizures in the intent-to-treat population, the response ratio was statistically significantly better for the Neurontin® group (-0.146) than for the placebo group (-0.079). For the same population, the responder rate for Neurontin® (21%) was not significantly different from placebo (18%).

A study in pediatric patients age 1 month to 3 years compared 40 mg/kg/day Neurontin® (N=38) with placebo (N=38) in patients who were receiving at least one marketed antiepileptic drug and had at least one partial seizure during the screening period (within 2 weeks prior to baseline). Patients had up to 48 hours of baseline and up to 72 hours of double-blind video EEG monitoring to record and count the occurrence of seizures. There were no statistically significant differences between treatments in either the response ratio or responder rate.

INDICATIONS AND USAGE

Postherpetic Neuralgia

Neurontin® (gabapentin) is indicated for the management of postherpetic neuralgia in adults.

Epilepsy

Neurontin® (gabapentin) is indicated as adjunctive therapy in the treatment of partial seizures with and without secondary generalization in patients over 12 years of age with epilepsy. Neurontin is also indicated as adjunctive therapy in the treatment of partial seizures in pediatric patients age 3 – 12 years.

CONTRAINDICATIONS

Neurontin® is contraindicated in patients who have demonstrated hypersensitivity to the drug or its ingredients.

WARNINGS

Neuropsychiatric Adverse Events—Pediatric Patients 3-12 years of age

Gabapentin use in pediatric patients with epilepsy 3–12 years of age is associated with the occurrence of central nervous system related adverse events. The most significant of these can be classified into the following categories: 1) emotional lability (primarily behavioral problems), 2) hostility, including aggressive behaviors, 3) thought disorder, including concentration problems and change in school performance, and 4) hyperkinesia (primarily restlessness and hyperactivity). Among the gabapentin-treated patients, most of the events were mild to moderate in intensity.

In controlled trials in pediatric patients 3–12 years of age the incidence of these adverse events was: emotional lability 6% (gabapentin-treated patients) vs 1.3% (placebo-treated patients); hostility 5.2% vs 1.3%; hyperkinesia 4.7% vs 2.9%; and thought disorder 1.7% vs 0%. One of these events, a report of hostility, was considered serious. Discontinuation of gabapentin treatment occurred in 1.3% of patients reporting emotional lability and hyperkinesia and 0.9% of gabapentin-treated patients reporting hostility and thought disorder. One placebo-treated patient (0.4%) withdrew due to emotional lability.

Withdrawal Precipitated Seizure, Status Epilepticus

Antiepileptic drugs should not be abruptly discontinued because of the possibility of increasing seizure frequency.

In the placebo-controlled studies in patients >12 years of age, the incidence of status epilepticus in patients receiving Neurontin® was 0.6% (3 of 543) versus 0.5% in patients receiving placebo (2 of 378). Among the 2074 patients >12 years of age treated with Neurontin® across all studies (controlled and uncontrolled) 31 (1.5%) had status epilepticus. Of these, 14 patients had no prior history of status epilepticus either before treatment or while on other medications. Because adequate historical data are not available, it is impossible to say whether or not treatment with Neurontin® is associated with a higher or lower rate of status epilepticus than would be expected to occur in a similar population not treated with Neurontin®.

Tumorigenic Potential

In standard preclinical *in vivo* lifetime carcinogenicity studies, an unexpectedly high incidence of pancreatic acinar adenocarcinomas was identified in male, but not female, rats. (See PRECAUTIONS: Carcinogenesis, Mutagenesis, Impairment of Fertility.) The clinical significance of this finding is unknown. Clinical experience during gabapentin's premarketing development provides no direct means to assess its potential for inducing tumors in humans.

In clinical studies in adjunctive therapy in epilepsy comprising 2085 patient-years of exposure in patients >12 years of age, new tumors were reported in 10 patients (2 breast, 3 brain, 2 lung, 1 adrenal, 1 non-Hodgkin's lymphoma, 1 endometrial carcinoma *in situ*), and preexisting tumors worsened in 11 patients (9 brain, 1 breast, 1 prostate) during or up to 2 years following discontinuation of Neurontin®. Without knowledge of the background incidence and recurrence in a similar population not treated with Neurontin®, it is impossible to know whether the incidence seen in this cohort is or is not affected by treatment.

Sudden and Unexplained Death in Patients With Epilepsy

During the course of premarketing development of Neurontin® 8 sudden and unexplained deaths were recorded among a cohort of 2203 patients treated (2103 patient-years of exposure).

Some of these could represent seizure-related deaths in which the seizure was not observed, e.g., at night. This represents an incidence of 0.0038 deaths per patient-year. Although this rate exceeds that expected in a healthy population matched for age and sex, it is within the range of estimates for the incidence of sudden unexplained deaths in patients with epilepsy not receiving Neurontin® (ranging from 0.0005 for the general population of epileptics to 0.003 for a clinical trial population similar to that in the Neurontin® program, to 0.005 for patients with refractory epilepsy). Consequently, whether these figures are reassuring or raise further concern depends on comparability of the populations reported upon to the Neurontin® cohort and the accuracy of the estimates provided.

PRECAUTIONS

Information for Patients

Patients should be instructed to take Neurontin® only as prescribed.

Patients should be advised that Neurontin® may cause dizziness, somnolence and other symptoms and signs of CNS depression. Accordingly, they should be advised neither to drive a car nor to operate other complex machinery until they have gained sufficient experience on Neurontin® to gauge whether or not it affects their mental and/or motor performance adversely.

Patients who require concomitant treatment with morphine may experience increases in gabapentin concentrations. Patients should be carefully observed for signs of CNS depression, such as somnolence, and the dose of Neurontin® or morphine should be reduced appropriately (see Drug Interactions).

Laboratory Tests

Clinical trials data do not indicate that routine monitoring of clinical laboratory parameters is necessary for the safe use of Neurontin®. The value of monitoring gabapentin blood concentrations has not been established. Neurontin® may be used in combination with other antiepileptic drugs without concern for alteration of the blood concentrations of gabapentin or of other antiepileptic drugs.

Drug Interactions

In vitro studies were conducted to investigate the potential of gabapentin to inhibit the major cytochrome P450 enzymes (CYP1A2, CYP2A6, CYP2C9, CYP2C19, CYP2D6, CYP2E1, and CYP3A4) that mediate drug and xenobiotic metabolism using isoform selective marker substrates and human liver microsomal preparations. Only at the highest concentration tested (171 µg/mL; 1 mM) was a slight degree of inhibition (14%-30%) of isoform CYP2A6 observed. No inhibition of any of the other isoforms tested was observed at gabapentin concentrations up to 171 µg/mL (approximately 15 times the C_{max} at 3600 mg/day).

Gabapentin is not appreciably metabolized nor does it interfere with the metabolism of commonly coadministered antiepileptic drugs.

The drug interaction data described in this section were obtained from studies involving healthy adults and adult patients with epilepsy.

Phenytoin: In a single (400 mg) and multiple dose (400 mg TID) study of Neurontin® in epileptic patients (N=8) maintained on phenytoin monotherapy for at least 2 months, gabapentin had no effect on the steady-state trough plasma concentrations of phenytoin and phenytoin had no effect on gabapentin pharmacokinetics.

Carbamazepine: Steady-state trough plasma carbamazepine and carbamazepine 10, 11 epoxide concentrations were not affected by concomitant gabapentin (400 mg TID; N=12) administration. Likewise, gabapentin pharmacokinetics were unaltered by carbamazepine administration.

Valproic Acid: The mean steady-state trough serum valproic acid concentrations prior to and during concomitant gabapentin administration (400 mg TID; N=17) were not different and neither were gabapentin pharmacokinetic parameters affected by valproic acid.

Phenobarbital: Estimates of steady-state pharmacokinetic parameters for phenobarbital or gabapentin (300 mg TID; N=12) are identical whether the drugs are administered alone or together.

Naproxen: Coadministration (N=18) of naproxen sodium capsules (250 mg) with Neurontin® (125 mg) appears to increase the amount of gabapentin absorbed by 12% to 15%. Gabapentin had no effect on naproxen pharmacokinetic parameters. These doses are lower than the therapeutic doses for both drugs. The magnitude of interaction within the recommended dose ranges of either drug is not known.

Hydrocodone: Coadministration of Neurontin® (125 to 500 mg; N=48) decreases hydrocodone (10 mg; N=50) C_{max} and AUC values in a dose-dependent manner relative to administration of hydrocodone alone; C_{max} and AUC values are 3% to 4% lower, respectively, after administration of 125 mg Neurontin® and 21% to 22% lower, respectively, after administration of 500 mg Neurontin®. The mechanism for this interaction is unknown. Hydrocodone increases gabapentin AUC values by 14%. The magnitude of interaction at other doses is not known.

Morphine: A literature article reported that when a 60-mg controlled-release morphine capsule was administered 2 hours prior to a 600-mg Neurontin® capsule (N=12), mean gabapentin AUC increased by 44% compared to gabapentin administered without morphine (see PRECAUTIONS). Morphine pharmacokinetic parameter values were not affected by administration of Neurontin® 2 hours after morphine. The magnitude of interaction at other doses is not known.

Cimetidine: In the presence of cimetidine at 300 mg QID (N=12) the mean apparent oral clearance of gabapentin fell by 14% and creatinine clearance fell by 10%. Thus cimetidine appeared to alter the renal excretion of both gabapentin and creatinine, an endogenous marker of renal function. This small decrease in excretion of gabapentin by cimetidine is not expected to be of clinical importance. The effect of gabapentin on cimetidine was not evaluated.

Oral Contraceptive: Based on AUC and half-life, multiple-dose pharmacokinetic profiles of norethindrone and ethinyl estradiol following administration of tablets containing 2.5 mg of norethindrone acetate and 50 mcg of ethinyl estradiol were similar with and without coadministration of gabapentin (400 mg TID; N=13). The Cmax of norethindrone was 13% higher when it was coadministered with gabapentin; this interaction is not expected to be of clinical importance.

Antacid (Maalox®): Maalox reduced the bioavailability of gabapentin (N=16) by about 20%. This decrease in bioavailability was about 5% when gabapentin was administered 2 hours after Maalox. It is recommended that gabapentin be taken at least 2 hours following Maalox administration.

Effect of Probenecid: Probenecid is a blocker of renal tubular secretion. Gabapentin pharmacokinetic parameters without and with probenecid were comparable. This indicates that gabapentin does not undergo renal tubular secretion by the pathway that is blocked by probenecid.

Drug/Laboratory Tests Interactions

Because false positive readings were reported with the Ames N-Multistix SG® dipstick test for urinary protein when gabapentin was added to other antiepileptic drugs, the more specific sulfosalicylic acid precipitation procedure is recommended to determine the presence of urine protein.

Carcinogenesis, Mutagenesis, Impairment of Fertility

Gabapentin was given in the diet to mice at 200, 600, and 2000 mg/kg/day and to rats at 250, 1000, and 2000 mg/kg/day for 2 years. A statistically significant increase in the incidence of pancreatic acinar cell adenomas and carcinomas was found in male rats receiving the high dose; the no-effect dose for the occurrence of carcinomas was 1000 mg/kg/day. Peak plasma concentrations of gabapentin in rats receiving the high dose of 2000 mg/kg were 10 times higher than plasma concentrations in humans receiving 3600 mg per day, and in rats receiving 1000 mg/kg/day peak plasma concentrations were 6.5 times higher than in humans receiving 3600 mg/day. The pancreatic acinar cell carcinomas did not affect survival, did not metastasize and were not locally invasive. The relevance of this finding to carcinogenic risk in humans is unclear.

Studies designed to investigate the mechanism of gabapentin-induced pancreatic carcinogenesis in rats indicate that gabapentin stimulates DNA synthesis in rat pancreatic acinar cells *in vitro* and, thus, may be acting as a tumor promoter by enhancing mitogenic activity. It is not known whether gabapentin has the ability to increase cell proliferation in other cell types or in other species, including humans.

Gabapentin did not demonstrate mutagenic or genotoxic potential in three *in vitro* and four *in vivo* assays. It was negative in the Ames test and the *in vitro* HGPRT forward mutation assay in Chinese hamster lung cells; it did not produce significant increases in chromosomal aberrations in the *in vitro* Chinese hamster lung cell assay; it was negative in the *in vivo* chromosomal aberration assay and in the *in vivo* micronucleus test in Chinese hamster bone marrow; it was negative in the *in vivo* mouse micronucleus assay; and it did not induce unscheduled DNA synthesis in hepatocytes from rats given gabapentin.

No adverse effects on fertility or reproduction were observed in rats at doses up to 2000 mg/kg (approximately 5 times the maximum recommended human dose on a mg/m^2 basis).

Pregnancy

Pregnancy Category C: Gabapentin has been shown to be fetotoxic in rodents, causing delayed ossification of several bones in the skull, vertebrae, forelimbs, and hindlimbs. These effects occurred when pregnant mice received oral doses of 1000 or 3000 mg/kg/day during the period of organogenesis, or approximately 1 to 4 times the maximum dose of 3600 mg/day given to epileptic patients on a mg/m^2 basis. The no-effect level was 500 mg/kg/day or approximately ½ of the human dose on a mg/m^2 basis.

When rats were dosed prior to and during mating, and throughout gestation, pups from all dose groups (500, 1000 and 2000 mg/kg/day) were affected. These doses are equivalent to less than approximately 1 to 5 times the maximum human dose on a mg/m^2 basis. There was an increased incidence of hydroureter and/or hydronephrosis in rats in a study of fertility and general reproductive performance at 2000 mg/kg/day with no effect at 1000 mg/kg/day, in a teratology study at 1500 mg/kg/day with no effect at 300 mg/kg/day, and in a perinatal and postnatal study at all doses studied (500, 1000 and 2000 mg/kg/day). The doses at which the effects occurred are approximately 1 to 5 times the maximum human dose of 3600 mg/day on a mg/m^2 basis; the no-effect doses were approximately 3 times (Fertility and General Reproductive Performance study) and approximately equal to (Teratogenicity study) the maximum human dose on a mg/m^2 basis. Other than hydroureter and hydronephrosis, the etiologies of which are unclear, the incidence of malformations was not increased compared to controls in offspring of mice, rats, or rabbits given doses up to 50 times (mice), 30 times (rats), and 25 times (rabbits) the human daily dose on a mg/kg basis, or 4 times (mice), 5 times (rats), or 8 times (rabbits) the human daily dose on a mg/m^2 basis.

In a teratology study in rabbits, an increased incidence of postimplantation fetal loss occurred in dams exposed to 60, 300, and 1500 mg/kg/day, or less than approximately ¼ to 8 times the maximum human dose on a mg/m^2 basis. There are no adequate and well-controlled studies in pregnant women. This drug should be used during pregnancy only if the potential benefit justifies the potential risk to the fetus.

Use in Nursing Mothers

Gabapentin is secreted into human milk following oral administration. A nursed infant could be exposed to a maximum dose of approximately 1 mg/kg/day of gabapentin. Because the effect on the nursing infant is unknown, Neurontin® should be used in women who are nursing only if the benefits clearly outweigh the risks.

Pediatric Use

Safety and effectiveness of Neurontin® (gabapentin) in the management of postherpetic neuralgia in pediatric patients have not been established.

Effectiveness as adjunctive therapy in the treatment of partial seizures in pediatric patients below the age of 3 years has not been established (see CLINICAL PHARMACOLOGY, Clinical Studies).

Geriatric Use

The total number of patients treated with Neurontin® in controlled clinical trials in patients with postherpetic neuralgia was 336, of which 102 (30%) were 65 to 74 years of age, and 168 (50%) were 75 years of age and older. There was a larger treatment effect in patients 75 years of age and older compared with younger patients who received the same dosage. Since gabapentin is almost exclusively eliminated by renal excretion, the larger treatment effect observed in patients ≥75 years may be a consequence of increased gabapentin exposure for a given dose that results from an age-related decrease in renal function. However, other factors cannot be excluded. The types and incidence of adverse events were similar across age groups except for peripheral edema and ataxia, which tended to increase in incidence with age.

Clinical studies of Neurontin® in epilepsy did not include sufficient numbers of subjects aged 65 and over to determine whether they responded differently from younger subjects. Other reported clinical experience has not identified differences in responses between the elderly and younger patients. In general, dose selection for an elderly patient should be cautious, usually starting at the low end of the dosing range, reflecting the greater frequency of decreased hepatic, renal, or cardiac function, and of concomitant disease or other drug therapy.

This drug is known to be substantially excreted by the kidney, and the risk of toxic reactions to this drug may be greater in patients with impaired renal function. Because elderly patients are more likely to have decreased renal function, care should be taken in dose selection, and dose should be adjusted based on creatinine clearance values in these patients (see CLINICAL PHARMACOLOGY, ADVERSE REACTIONS, and DOSAGE AND ADMINISTRATION sections).

ADVERSE REACTIONS

Postherpetic Neuralgia

The most commonly observed adverse events associated with the use of Neurontin® in adults, not seen at an equivalent frequency among placebo-treated patients, were dizziness, somnolence, and peripheral edema.

In the 2 controlled studies in postherpetic neuralgia, 16% of the 336 patients who received Neurontin® and 9% of the 227 patients who received placebo discontinued treatment because of an adverse event. The adverse events that most frequently led to withdrawal in Neurontin®-treated patients were dizziness, somnolence, and nausea.

Incidence in Controlled Clinical Trials

Table 2 lists treatment-emergent signs and symptoms that occurred in at least 1% of Neurontin®-treated patients with postherpetic neuralgia participating in placebo-controlled trials and that were numerically more frequent in the Neurontin® group than in the placebo group. Adverse events were usually mild to moderate in intensity.

TABLE 2. Treatment-Emergent Adverse Event Incidence in Controlled Trials in Postherpetic Neuralgia (Events in at least 1% of Neurontin®-Treated Patients and Numerically More Frequent Than in the Placebo Group)

Body System/ Preferred Term	Neurontin® N=336 %	Placebo N=227 %
Body as a Whole		
Asthenia	5.7	4.8
Infection	5.1	3.5
Headache	3.3	3.1
Accidental injury	3.3	1.3
Abdominal pain	2.7	2.6
Digestive System		
Diarrhea	5.7	3.1
Dry mouth	4.8	1.3
Constipation	3.9	1.8
Nausea	3.9	3.1
Vomiting	3.3	1.8
Flatulence	2.1	1.8
Metabolic and Nutritional Disorders		
Peripheral edema	8.3	2.2
Weight gain	1.8	0.0
Hyperglycemia	1.2	0.4
Nervous System		
Dizziness	28.0	7.5
Somnolence	21.4	5.3
Ataxia	3.3	0.0
Thinking abnormal	2.7	0.0
Abnormal gait	1.5	0.0
Incoordination	1.5	0.0
Amnesia	1.2	0.9

Continued on next page

Neurontin—Cont.

Hypesthesia	1.2	0.9
Respiratory System		
Pharyngitis	1.2	0.4
Skin and Appendages		
Rash	1.2	0.9
Special Senses		
Amblyopia[a]	2.7	0.9
Conjunctivitis	1.2	0.0
Diplopia	1.2	0.0
Otitis media	1.2	0.0

[a] Reported as blurred vision

Other events in more than 1% of patients but equally or more frequent in the placebo group included pain, tremor, neuralgia, back pain, dyspepsia, dyspnea, and flu syndrome. There were no clinically important differences between men and women in the types and incidence of adverse events. Because there were few patients whose race was reported as other than white, there are insufficient data to support a statement regarding the distribution of adverse events by race.

Epilepsy

The most commonly observed adverse events associated with the use of Neurontin® in combination with other antiepileptic drugs in patients >12 years of age, not seen at an equivalent frequency among placebo-treated patients, were somnolence, dizziness, ataxia, fatigue, and nystagmus. The most commonly observed adverse events reported with the use of Neurontin® in combination with other antiepileptic drugs in pediatric patients 3 to 12 years of age, not seen at an equal frequency among placebo-treated patients, were viral infection, fever, nausea and/or vomiting, somnolence, and hostility (see WARNINGS, Neuropsychiatric Adverse Events).

Approximately 7% of the 2074 patients >12 years of age and approximately 7% of the 449 pediatric patients 3 to 12 years of age who received Neurontin® in premarketing clinical trials discontinued treatment because of an adverse event. The adverse events most commonly associated with withdrawal in patients >12 years of age were somnolence (1.2%), ataxia (0.8%), fatigue (0.6%), nausea and/or vomiting (0.6%), and dizziness (0.6%). The adverse events most commonly associated with withdrawal in pediatric patients were emotional lability (1.6%), hostility (1.3%), and hyperkinesia (1.1%).

Incidence in Controlled Clinical Trials

Table 3 lists treatment-emergent signs and symptoms that occurred in at least 1% of Neurontin®-treated patients >12 years of age with epilepsy participating in placebo-controlled trials and were numerically more common in the Neurontin® group. In these studies, either Neurontin® or placebo was added to the patient's current antiepileptic drug therapy. Adverse events were usually mild to moderate in intensity.

The prescriber should be aware that these figures, obtained when Neurontin® was added to concurrent antiepileptic drug therapy, cannot be used to predict the frequency of adverse events in the course of usual medical practice where patient characteristics and other factors may differ from those prevailing during clinical studies. Similarly, the cited frequencies cannot be directly compared with figures obtained from other clinical investigations involving different treatments, uses, or investigators. An inspection of these frequencies, however, does provide the prescribing physician with one basis to estimate the relative contribution of drug and nondrug factors to the adverse event incidences in the population studied.

TABLE 3. Treatment-Emergent Adverse Event Incidence in Controlled Add-On Trials In Patients >12 years of age (Events in at least 1% of Neurontin® patients and numerically more frequent than in the placebo group)

Body System/ Adverse Event	Neurontin®[a] N=543 %	Placebo[a] N=378 %
Body As A Whole		
Fatigue	11.0	5.0
Weight Increase	2.9	1.6
Back Pain	1.8	0.5
Peripheral Edema	1.7	0.5
Cardiovascular		
Vasodilatation	1.1	0.3
Digestive System		
Dyspepsia	2.2	0.5
Mouth or Throat Dry	1.7	0.5
Constipation	1.5	0.8
Dental Abnormalities	1.5	0.3
Increased Appetite	1.1	0.8
Hematologic and Lymphatic Systems		
Leukopenia	1.1	0.5
Musculoskeletal System		
Myalgia	2.0	1.9
Fracture	1.1	0.8
Nervous System		
Somnolence	19.3	8.7
Dizziness	17.1	6.9
Ataxia	12.5	5.6
Nystagmus	8.3	4.0
Tremor	6.8	3.2
Nervousness	2.4	1.9
Dysarthria	2.4	0.5
Amnesia	2.2	0.0
Depression	1.8	1.1
Thinking Abnormal	1.7	1.3
Twitching	1.3	0.5
Coordination Abnormal	1.1	0.3
Respiratory System		
Rhinitis	4.1	3.7
Pharyngitis	2.8	1.6
Coughing	1.8	1.3
Skin and Appendages		
Abrasion	1.3	0.0
Pruritus	1.3	0.5
Urogenital System		
Impotence	1.5	1.1
Special Senses		
Diplopia	5.9	1.9
Amblyopia[b]	4.2	1.1
Laboratory Deviations		
WBC Decreased	1.1	0.5

[a] Plus background antiepileptic drug therapy
[b] Amblyopia was often described as blurred vision.

Other events in more than 1% of patients >12 years of age but equally or more frequent in the placebo group included: headache, viral infection, fever, nausea and/or vomiting, abdominal pain, diarrhea, convulsions, confusion, insomnia, emotional lability, rash, acne.

Among the treatment-emergent adverse events occurring at an incidence of at least 10% of Neurontin®-treated patients, somnolence and ataxia appeared to exhibit a positive dose-response relationship.

The overall incidence of adverse events and the types of adverse events seen were similar among men and women treated with Neurontin®. The incidence of adverse events increased slightly with increasing age in patients treated with either Neurontin® or placebo. Because only 3% of patients (28/921) in placebo-controlled studies were identified as nonwhite (black or other), there are insufficient data to support a statement regarding the distribution of adverse events by race.

Table 4 lists treatment-emergent signs and symptoms that occurred in at least 2% of Neurontin®-treated patients age 3 to 12 years of age with epilepsy participating in placebo-controlled trials and were numerically more common in the Neurontin® group. Adverse events were usually mild to moderate in intensity.

TABLE 4. Treatment-Emergent Adverse Event Incidence in Pediatric Patients Age 3 to 12 Years in a Controlled Add-On Trial (Events in at least 2% of Neurontin® patients and numerically more frequent than in the placebo group)

Body System/ Adverse Event	Neurontin®[a] N=119 %	Placebo[a] N=128 %
Body As A Whole		
Viral Infection	10.9	3.1
Fever	10.1	3.1
Weight Increase	3.4	0.8
Fatigue	3.4	1.6
Digestive System		
Nausea and/or Vomiting	8.4	7.0
Nervous System		
Somnolence	8.4	4.7
Hostility	7.6	2.3
Emotional Lability	4.2	1.6
Dizziness	2.5	1.6
Hyperkinesia	2.5	0.8
Respiratory System		
Bronchitis	3.4	0.8
Respiratory Infection	2.5	0.8

[a] Plus background antiepileptic drug therapy

Other events in more than 2% of pediatric patients 3 to 12 years of age but equally or more frequent in the placebo group included: pharyngitis, upper respiratory infection, headache, rhinitis, convulsions, diarrhea, anorexia, coughing, and otitis media.

Other Adverse Events Observed During All Clinical Trials Clinical Trials in Adults and Adolescents (Except Clinical Trials in Neuropathic Pain)

Neurontin® has been administered to 2074 patients >12 years of age during all adjunctive therapy clinical trials (except clinical trials in patients with neuropathic pain), only some of which were placebo-controlled. During these trials, all adverse events were recorded by the clinical investigators using terminology of their own choosing. To provide a meaningful estimate of the proportion of individuals having adverse events, similar types of events were grouped into a smaller number of standardized categories using modified COSTART dictionary terminology. These categories are used in the listing below. The frequencies presented represent the proportion of the 2074 patients >12 years of age exposed to Neurontin® who experienced an event of the type cited on at least one occasion while receiving Neurontin®. All reported events are included except those already listed in Table 3, those too general to be informative, and those not reasonably associated with the use of the drug.

Events are further classified within body system categories and enumerated in order of decreasing frequency using the following definitions: frequent adverse events are defined as those occurring in at least 1/100 patients; infrequent adverse events are those occurring in 1/100 to 1/1000 patients; rare events are those occurring in fewer than 1/1000 patients.

Body As A Whole: *Frequent:* asthenia, malaise, face edema; *Infrequent:* allergy, generalized edema, weight decrease, chill; *Rare:* strange feelings, lassitude, alcohol intolerance, hangover effect.

Cardiovascular System: *Frequent:* hypertension; *Infrequent:* hypotension, angina pectoris, peripheral vascular disorder, palpitation, tachycardia, migraine, murmur; *Rare:* atrial fibrillation, heart failure, thrombophlebitis, deep thrombophlebitis, myocardial infarction, cerebrovascular accident, pulmonary thrombosis, ventricular extrasystoles, bradycardia, premature atrial contraction, pericardial rub, heart block, pulmonary embolus, hyperlipidemia, hypercholesterolemia, pericardial effusion, pericarditis.

Digestive System: *Frequent:* anorexia, flatulence, gingivitis; *Infrequent:* glossitis, gum hemorrhage, thirst, stomatitis, increased salivation, gastroenteritis, hemorrhoids, bloody stools, fecal incontinence, hepatomegaly; *Rare:* dysphagia, eructation, pancreatitis, peptic ulcer, colitis, blisters in mouth, tooth discolor, perlèche, salivary gland enlarged, lip hemorrhage, esophagitis, hiatal hernia, hematemesis, proctitis, irritable bowel syndrome, rectal hemorrhage, esophageal spasm.

Endocrine System: *Rare:* hyperthyroid, hypothyroid, goiter, hypoestrogen, ovarian failure, epididymitis, swollen testicle, cushingoid appearance.

Hematologic and Lymphatic System: *Frequent:* purpura most often described as bruises resulting from physical trauma; *Infrequent:* anemia, thrombocytopenia, lymphadenopathy; *Rare:* WBC count increased, lymphocytosis, non-Hodgkin's lymphoma, bleeding time increased.

Musculoskeletal System: *Frequent:* arthralgia; *Infrequent:* tendinitis, arthritis, joint stiffness, joint swelling, positive Romberg test; *Rare:* costochondritis, osteoporosis, bursitis, contracture.

Nervous System: *Frequent:* vertigo, hyperkinesia, paresthesia, decreased or absent reflexes, increased reflexes, anxiety, hostility; *Infrequent:* CNS tumors, syncope, dreaming abnormal, aphasia, hypesthesia, intracranial hemorrhage, hypotonia, dysesthesia, paresis, dystonia, hemiplegia, facial paralysis, stupor, cerebellar dysfunction, positive Babinski sign, decreased position sense, subdural hematoma, apathy, hallucination, decrease or loss of libido, agitation, paranoia, depersonalization, euphoria, feeling high, doped-up sensation, suicidal, psychosis; *Rare:* choreoathetosis, orofacial dyskinesia, encephalopathy, nerve palsy, personality disorder, increased libido, subdued temperament, apraxia, fine motor control disorder, meningismus, local myoclonus, hyperesthesia, hypokinesia, mania, neurosis, hysteria, antisocial reaction, suicide gesture.

Respiratory System: *Frequent:* pneumonia; *Infrequent:* epistaxis, dyspnea, apnea; *Rare:* mucositis, aspiration pneumonia, hyperventilation, hiccup, laryngitis, nasal obstruction, snoring, bronchospasm, hypoventilation, lung edema.

Dermatological: *Infrequent:* alopecia, eczema, dry skin, increased sweating, urticaria, hirsutism, seborrhea, cyst, herpes simplex; *Rare:* herpes zoster, skin discolor, skin papules, photosensitive reaction, leg ulcer, scalp seborrhea, psoriasis, desquamation, maceration, skin nodules, subcutaneous nodule, melanosis, skin necrosis, local swelling.

Urogenital System: *Infrequent:* hematuria, dysuria, urination frequency, cystitis, urinary retention, urinary incontinence, vaginal hemorrhage, amenorrhea, dysmenorrhea, menorrhagia, breast cancer, unable to climax, ejaculation abnormal; *Rare:* kidney pain, leukorrhea, pruritus genital, renal stone, acute renal failure, anuria, glycosuria, nephrosis, nocturia, pyuria, urination urgency, vaginal pain, breast pain, testicle pain.

Special Senses: *Frequent:* abnormal vision; *Infrequent:* cataract, conjunctivitis, eyes dry, eye pain, visual field defect, photophobia, bilateral or unilateral ptosis, eye hemorrhage, hordeolum, hearing loss, earache, tinnitus, inner ear infection, otitis, taste loss, unusual taste, eye twitching, ear fullness; *Rare:* eye itching, abnormal accommodation, perforated ear drum, sensitivity to noise, eye focusing problem, watery eyes, retinopathy, glaucoma, iritis, corneal disorders, lacrimal dysfunction, degenerative eye changes, blindness, retinal degeneration, miosis, chorioretinitis, strabismus, eustachian tube dysfunction, labyrinthitis, otitis externa, odd smell.

Clinical trials in Pediatric Patients With Epilepsy

Adverse events occurring during epilepsy clinical trials in 449 pediatric patients 3 to 12 years of age treated with gabapentin that were not reported in adjunctive trials in adults are:

Body as a Whole: dehydration, infectious mononucleosis
Digestive System: hepatitis
Hemic and Lymphatic System: coagulation defect
Nervous System: aura disappeared, occipital neuralgia
Psychobiologic Function: sleepwalking
Respiratory System: pseudocroup, hoarseness

Clinical Trials in Adults With Neuropathic Pain of Various Etiologies

Safety information was obtained in 1173 patients during double-blind and open-label clinical trials including neuropathic pain conditions for which efficacy has not been demonstrated. Adverse events reported by investigators were grouped into standardized categories using modified COSTART IV terminology. Listed below are all reported events except those already listed in Table 2 and those not reasonably associated with the use of the drug.

Events are further classified within body system categories and enumerated in order of decreasing frequency using the following definitions: frequent adverse events are defined as those occurring in at least 1/100 patients; infrequent adverse events are those occurring in 1/100 to 1/1000 patients; rare events are those occurring in fewer than 1/1000 patients.

Body as a Whole: *Infrequent:* chest pain, cellulitis, malaise, neck pain, face edema, allergic reaction, abscess, chills, chills and fever, mucous membrane disorder; *Rare:* body odor, cyst, fever, hernia, abnormal BUN value, lump in neck, pelvic pain, sepsis, viral infection.

Cardiovascular System: *Infrequent:* hypertension, syncope, palpitation, migraine, hypotension, peripheral vascular disorder, cardiovascular disorder, cerebrovascular accident, congestive heart failure, myocardial infarction, vasodilatation; *Rare:* angina pectoris, heart failure, increased capillary fragility, phlebitis, thrombophlebitis, varicose vein.

Digestive System: *Infrequent:* gastroenteritis, increased appetite, gastrointestinal disorder, oral moniliasis, gastritis, tongue disorder, thirst, tooth disorder, abnormal stools, anorexia, liver function tests abnormal, periodontal abscess; *Rare:* cholecystitis, cholelithiasis, duodenal ulcer, fecal incontinence, gamma glutamyl transpeptidase increased, gingivitis, intestinal obstruction, intestinal ulcer, melena, mouth ulceration, rectal disorder, rectal hemorrhage, stomatitis.

Endocrine System: *Infrequent:* diabetes mellitus.

Hemic and Lymphatic System: *Infrequent:* ecchymosis, anemia; *Rare:* lymphadenopathy, lymphoma-like reaction, prothrombin decreased.

Metabolic and Nutritional: *Infrequent:* edema, gout, hypoglycemia, weight loss; *Rare:* alkaline phosphatase increased, diabetic ketoacidosis, lactic dehydrogenase increased.

Musculoskeletal: *Infrequent:* arthritis, arthralgia, myalgia, arthrosis, leg cramps, myasthenia; *Rare:* shin bone pain, joint disorder, tendon disorder.

Nervous System: *Frequent:* confusion, depression; *Infrequent:* vertigo, nervousness, paresthesia, insomnia, neuropathy, libido decreased, anxiety, depersonalization, reflexes decreased, speech disorder, abnormal dreams, dysarthria, emotional lability, nystagmus, stupor, circumoral paresthesia, euphoria, hyperesthesia, hypokinesia; *Rare:* agitation, hypertonia, libido increased, movement disorder, myoclonus, vestibular disorder.

Respiratory System: *Infrequent:* cough increased, bronchitis, rhinitis, sinusitis, pneumonia, asthma, lung disorder, epistaxis; *Rare:* hemoptysis, voice alteration.

Skin and Appendages: *Infrequent:* pruritus, skin ulcer, dry skin, herpes zoster, skin disorder, fungal dermatitis, furunculosis, herpes simplex, psoriasis, sweating, urticaria, vesiculobullous rash; *Rare:* acne, hair disorder, maculopapular rash, nail disorder, skin carcinoma, skin discoloration, skin hypertrophy.

Special Senses: *Infrequent:* abnormal vision, ear pain, eye disorder, taste perversion, deafness; *Rare:* conjunctival hyperemia, diabetic retinopathy, eye pain, fundi with microhemorrhage, retinal vein thrombosis, taste loss.

Urogenital System: *Infrequent:* urinary tract infection, dysuria, impotence, urinary incontinence, vaginal moniliasis, breast pain, menstrual disorder, polyuria, urinary retention; *Rare:* cystitis, ejaculation abnormal, swollen penis, gynecomastia, nocturia, pyelonephritis, swollen scrotum, urinary frequency, urinary urgency, urine abnormality.

Postmarketing and Other Experience

In addition to the adverse experiences reported during clinical testing of Neurontin®, the following adverse experiences have been reported in patients receiving marketed Neurontin®. These adverse experiences have not been listed above and data are insufficient to support an estimate of their incidence or to establish causation. The listing is alphabetized: angioedema, blood glucose fluctuation, erythema multiforme, elevated liver function tests, fever, hyponatremia, jaundice, movement disorder such as dyskinesia, Stevens-Johnson syndrome.

Adverse events following the abrupt discontinuation of gabapentin have also been reported. The most frequently reported events were anxiety, insomnia, nausea, pain and sweating.

DRUG ABUSE AND DEPENDENCE

The abuse and dependence potential of Neurontin® has not been evaluated in human studies.

OVERDOSAGE

A lethal dose of gabapentin was not identified in mice and rats receiving single oral doses as high as 8000 mg/kg. Signs of acute toxicity in animals included ataxia, labored breathing, ptosis, sedation, hypoactivity, or excitation.

Acute oral overdoses of Neurontin® up to 49 grams have been reported. In these cases, double vision, slurred speech, drowsiness, lethargy and diarrhea were observed. All patients recovered with supportive care.

TABLE 5. Neurontin® Dosage Based on Renal Function

Renal Function Creatinine Clearance (mL/min)	Total Daily Dose Range (mg/day)	Dose Regimen (mg)				
≥60	900-3600	300 TID	400 TID	600 TID	800 TID	1200 TID
>30-59	400-1400	200 BID	300 BID	400 BID	500 BID	700 BID
>15-29	200-700	200 QD	300 QD	400 QD	500 QD	700 QD
15[a]	100-300	100 QD	125 QD	150 QD	200 QD	300 QD
		Post-Hemodialysis Supplemental Dose (mg)[b]				
Hemodialysis		125[b]	150[b]	200[b]	250[b]	350[b]

[a] For patients with creatinine clearance <15 mL/min, reduce daily dose in proportion to creatinine clearance (e.g., patients with a creatinine clearance of 7.5 mL/min should receive one-half the daily dose that patients with a creatinine clearance of 15 mL/min receive).

[b] Patients on hemodialysis should receive maintenance doses based on estimates of creatinine clearance as indicated in the upper portion of the table and a supplemental post-hemodialysis dose administered after each 4 hours of hemodialysis as indicated in the lower portion of the table.

Gabapentin can be removed by hemodialysis. Although hemodialysis has not been performed in the few overdose cases reported, it may be indicated by the patient's clinical state or in patients with significant renal impairment.

DOSAGE AND ADMINISTRATION

Neurontin® is given orally with or without food. Patients should be informed that, should they break the scored 600 or 800 mg tablet in order to administer a half-tablet, they should take the unused half-tablet as the next dose. Half-tablets not used within several days of breaking the scored tablet should be discarded.

If Neurontin® dose is reduced, discontinued or substituted with an alternative medication, this should be done gradually over a minimum of 1 week.

Postherpetic Neuralgia

In adults with postherpetic neuralgia, Neurontin® therapy may be initiated as a single 300-mg dose on Day 1, 600 mg/day on Day 2 (divided BID), and 900 mg/day on Day 3 (divided TID). The dose can subsequently be titrated up as needed for pain relief to a daily dose of 1800 mg (divided TID). In clinical studies, efficacy was demonstrated over a range of doses from 1800 mg/day to 3600 mg/day with comparable effects across the dose range. Additional benefit of using doses greater than 1800 mg/day was not demonstrated.

Epilepsy

Neurontin® is recommended for add-on therapy in patients 3 years of age and older. Effectiveness in pediatric patients below the age of 3 years has not been established.

Patients >12 years of age: The effective dose of Neurontin® is 900 to 1800 mg/day and given in divided doses (three times a day) using 300 or 400 mg capsules, or 600 or 800 mg tablets. The starting dose is 300 mg three times a day. If necessary, the dose may be increased using 300 or 400 mg capsules, or 600 or 800 mg tablets three times a day up to 1800 mg/day. Dosages up to 2400 mg/day have been well tolerated in long-term clinical studies. Doses of 3600 mg/day have also been administered to a small number of patients for a relatively short duration, and have been well tolerated. The maximum time between doses in the TID schedule should not exceed 12 hours.

Pediatric Patients Age 3–12 years: The starting dose should range from 10-15 mg/kg/day in 3 divided doses, and the effective dose reached by upward titration over a period of approximately 3 days. The effective dose of Neurontin® in patients 5 years of age and older is 25–35 mg/kg/day and given in divided doses (three times a day). The effective dose in pediatric patients ages 3 and 4 years is 40 mg/kg/day and given in divided doses (three times a day) (see CLINICAL PHARMACOLOGY, Pediatrics). Neurontin® may be administered as the oral solution, capsule, or tablet, or using combinations of these formulations. Dosages up to 50 mg/kg/day have been well-tolerated in a long-term clinical study. The maximum time interval between doses should not exceed 12 hours.

It is not necessary to monitor gabapentin plasma concentrations to optimize Neurontin® therapy. Further, because there are no significant pharmacokinetic interactions among Neurontin® and other commonly used antiepileptic drugs, the addition of Neurontin® does not alter the plasma levels of these drugs appreciably.

If Neurontin® is discontinued and/or an alternate anticonvulsant medication is added to the therapy, this should be done gradually over a minimum of 1 week.

Dosage in Renal Impairment

Creatinine clearance is difficult to measure in outpatients. In patients with stable renal function, creatinine clearance (C_{Cr}) can be reasonably well estimated using the equation of Cockroft and Gault:

for females $C_{Cr}=(0.85)(140\text{-age})(\text{weight})/[(72)(S_{Cr})]$

for males $C_{Cr}=(140\text{-age})(\text{weight})/[(72)(S_{Cr})]$

where age is in years, weight is in kilograms and S_{Cr} is serum creatinine in mg/dL.

Dosage adjustment in patients ≥12 years of age with compromised renal function or undergoing hemodialysis is recommended as follows (see dosing recommendations above for effective doses in each indication).

[See table 5 above]

The use of Neurontin® in patients <12 years of age with compromised renal function has not been studied.

Dosage in Elderly

Because elderly patients are more likely to have decreased renal function, care should be taken in dose selection, and dose should be adjusted based on creatinine clearance values in these patients.

HOW SUPPLIED

Neurontin® (gabapentin) capsules, tablets and oral solution are supplied as follows:

100 mg capsules;
White hard gelatin capsules printed with "PD" on one side and "Neurontin®/100 mg" on the other; available in:
Bottles of 100: N 0071-0803-24
Unit dose 50's: N 0071-0803-40

300 mg capsules;
Yellow hard gelatin capsules printed with "PD" on one side and "Neurontin®/300 mg" on the other; available in:
Bottles of 100: N 0071-0805-24
Unit dose 50's: N 0071-0805-40

400 mg capsules;
Orange hard gelatin capsules printed with "PD" on one side and "Neurontin®/400 mg" on the other; available in:
Bottles of 100: N 0071-0806-24
Unit dose 50's: N 0071-0806-40

600 mg tablets;
White elliptical film-coated scored tablets debossed with "NT" and "16" on one side; available in:
Bottles of 100: N 0071-0513-24

800 mg tablets;
White elliptical film-coated scored tablets debossed with "NT" and "26" on one side; available in:
Bottles of 100: N 0071-0401-24

250 mg/5 mL oral solution;
Clear colorless to slightly yellow solution; each 5 mL of oral solution contains 250 mg of gabapentin; available in:
Bottles containing 470 mL: N0071-2012-23

Storage (Capsules)

Store at 25°C (77°F); excursions permitted to 15° - 30°C (59° - 86°F) [see USP Controlled Room Temperature].

Storage (Tablets)

Store at 25°C (77°F); excursions permitted to 15° - 30°C (59° - 86°F) [see USP Controlled Room Temperature].

Storage (Oral Solution)

Store refrigerated, 2°-8°C (36°-46°F)

Rx only

Revised May 2004

Capsules and Tablets:
Manufactured by:
Pfizer Pharmaceuticals, Ltd.
Vega Baja, PR 00694

Oral Solution:
Manufactured for:
Pfizer Pharmaceuticals, Ltd.
Vega Baja, PR 00694

Distributed by:
Parke-Davis
Division of Pfizer Inc, NY, NY 10017

LAB-0106-6

Shown in Product Identification Guide, page 329

PBM Pharmaceuticals, Inc.

**204 NORTH MAIN STREET
GORDONSVILLE, VA 22942**

Direct Inquiries to:
Customer Service
866-366-6282
Fax 302-266-7556

ANIMI-3™ ℞
[ă-nĭ-mĭ 3]

Each Capsule contains:

Folic Acid	1 mg
Vitamin B6	12.5 mg
Vitamin B12	500 mcg
Omega-3 Acids	500 mg
-Docosahexaenoic Acid (DHA)	350 mg
-Eicosapentaenoic Acid (EPA)	35 mg

Rx Only

DESCRIPTION

Animi-3™ Capsules are intended for oral administration. Each Capsule Contains: 1 mg Folic Acid USP, 12.5 mg Vitamin B-6 USP, 500 mcg Vitamin B-12 USP and Pharmaceutical Grade Omega-3 Fish Oil providing 500 mg Omega-3 Acids; including 350 mg Docosahexaenoic Acid (DHA) and 35 mg Eicosapentaenoic Acid (EPA).

Also Contains: Yellow Beeswax NF, Sunflower Oil FCC, Bleached Lecithin NF, Pyridoxine Hydrochloride USP, Cyanocobalamin USP, Ascorbic Acid USP, Mixed Tocopherols NF, Ascorbyl Palmitate NF and a soft shell capsule (which contains; Gelatin USP, Glycerin NF, Titanium Dioxide USP, FD&C Red 40 and USP Purified Water).

HOW SUPPLIED

Animi-3™ supplied as red opaque oblong Capsules. Each Capsule is imprinted with "PBM 540" in black opacode.

Animi-3™ Capsules are available in bottles of 60 capsules (NDC 66213-540-60).

PBM Pharmaceuticals, Inc.
Gordonsville, VA 22942
Rev. 0504

DONNATAL EXTENTABS® ℞
Rev. 06/04
Rx Only

DESCRIPTION

Each Donnatal Extentabs® tablet contains:

Phenobarbital, USP ($^3/_4$ gr.)	48.6 mg
Hyoscyamine Sulfate, USP	0.3111 mg
Atropine Sulfate, USP	0.0582 mg
Scopolamine Hydrobromide, USP	0.0195 mg

Each Donnatal Extentabs® tablet contains the equivalent of three Donnatal® tablets. Extentabs are designed to release the ingredients gradually to provide effects for up to twelve (12) hours.

In addition, each tablet contains the following inactive ingredients: Anhydrous Lactose, Calcium Sulfate Granular, Colloidal Silicon Dioxide, Dibasic Calcium Phosphate, Lactose Monohydrate, Magnesium Stearate, and Stearic Acid. Film Coating and Polishing Solution contains: D&C Yellow #10 Aluminum Lake, FD&C Blue #1 Aluminum Lake, Hydroxypropyl Methylcellulose, Polydextrose, Polyethylene Glycol, Titanium Dioxide, and Triacetin. The printing ink contains Titanium Dioxide.

HOW SUPPLIED

Donnatal Extentabs® Tablets are supplied as: film coated green, round, compressed tablets printed "P421" in black ink.

Bottles of 100 tablets
Bottles of 500 tablets

Store at controlled room temperature 20°–25°C (68°–77°F). Protect from light and moisture.

Dispense in a well-closed, light-resistant container as defined in the USP using a child-resistant closure.

Also available: Donnatal® Tablets in bottles of 100 and 1000 tablets and Donnatal® Elixir in 4 fl oz bottles and 1 pint bottles.

PBM Pharmaceuticals, Inc.
Gordonsville, VA 22942

For information on over-the-counter drugs, consult **PDR For Nonprescription Drugs and Dietary Supplements.**

Pedinol Pharmacal Inc.

**30 BANFI PLAZA NORTH
FARMINGDALE, NY 11735**

Direct Inquiries to:
Director of Professional Services
(631) 293-9500
E-Mail:
INFO@Pedinol.com

CASTELLANI PAINT Modified OTC
CASTELLANI PAINT Modified–Colorless OTC

DESCRIPTION

Castellani Paint Modified is a first aid antiseptic and drying agent. Care should be taken to avoid spilling. Guard against staining as Castellani Paint Modified will stain skin and clothing.

HOW SUPPLIED

Bottle Size	1 oz. (29.57 mL)	1 pt. (453.6 mL)
Color	NDC 0884-2893-01	NDC 0884-2893-16
Colorless	NDC 0884-2993-01	NDC 0884-2993-16

Store at controlled room temperature 15°–30°C (59°–86°F)

FORMALYDE-10® SPRAY ℞

DESCRIPTION

Formalyde-10 Spray is a topical solution containing Formaldehyde 10% to safeguard against offensive odor and dry excessive moisture of the feet. Drying agent for pre & post-surgical removal of warts where dryness is required.

HOW SUPPLIED

Available in 2 oz. (59.14 mL) plastic spray bottle.
NDC 0884-4789-02
Store at controlled room temperature 15°–30°C (59°–86°F)

FUNGOID® TINCTURE OTC
(miconazole nitrate 2% USP)
For external use only. Not for ophthalmic use.

DESCRIPTION

FUNGOID TINCTURE (miconazole nitrate 2%) cures athlete's foot (tinea pedis) and ringworm (tinea corporis). FUNGOID TINCTURE can be used for the treatment of superficial skin infections caused by yeast (Candida albicans).

HOW SUPPLIED

FUNGOID TINCTURE is supplied in a 1 oz. (29.57 mL) bottle with brush applicator (NDC 0884-0293-01) and a 0.25 oz. (7.39 mL) bottle with brush applicator (NDC 0884-0293-25). Store at controlled room temperature 15°–30° C (59°–86° F).

Gris-PEG® ℞
(griseofulvin ultramicrosize)
Tablets, USP
125 mg; 250 mg

DESCRIPTION

Gris-PEG® Tablets contain ultramicrosize crystals of griseofulvin, an antibiotic derived from a species of *Penicillium.*

Each Gris-PEG® contains:

Active Ingredient: griseofulvin ultramicrosize .... 125 mg
Inactive Ingredients: colloidal silicon dioxide, lactose, magnesium stearate; methylcellulose; methylparaben; polyethylene glycol 400 and 8000, polyvinylpyrrolidone, and titanium dioxide.

or

Active Ingredient: griseofulvin ultramicrosize .... 250 mg
Inactive Ingredients: colloidal silicon dioxide; magnesium stearate; methylcellulose; methylparaben; polyethylene glycol 400 and 8000; povidone, sodium lauryl sulfate; and titanium dioxide.

ACTION

Microbiology – Griseofulvin in fungistatic with *in vitro* activity against various species of *Microsporum, Epidermophyton* and *Trichophyton.* It has no effect on bacteria or other genera of fungi.

Human Pharmacology – Following oral administration, griseofulvin is deposited in the keratin precursor cells and has a greater affinity for diseased tissue. The drug is tightly bound to the new keratin which becomes highly resistant to fungal invasions.

The efficiency of gastrointestinal absorption of ultramicrocrystalline griseofulvin is approximately one and one-half times that of the conventional microsize griseofulvin. This factor permits the oral intake of two-thirds as much ultramicrocrystalline griseofulvin as the microsize form. However, there is currently no evidence that this lower dose confers any significant clinical differences with regard to safety and/or efficacy.

INDICATIONS

Gris-PEG® (griseofulvin ultramicrosize) is indicated for the treatment of the following ringworm infections; tinea corporis (ringworm of the body), tinea pedis (athlete's foot), tinea cruris (ringworm of the groin and thigh), tinea barbae (barber's itch), tinea capitis (ringworm of the scalp), and tinea unguium (onychomycosis, ringworm of the nails), when caused by one or more of the following genera of fungi: *Trichophyton rubrum, Trichophyton tonsurans, Trichophyton mentagrophytes, Trichophyton interdigitalis, Trichophyton verrucosum, Trichophyton megnini, Trichophyton gallinae, Trichophyton crateriform, Trichophyton sulphureum, Trichophyton schoenleini, Microsporum audouini, Microsporum canis, Microsporum gypseum* and *Epidermophyton floccosum.* Note: Prior to therapy, the type of fungi responsible for the infection should be identified. The use of the drug is not justified in minor or trivial infections which will respond to topical agents alone. Griseofulvin in *not* effective in the following: bacterial infections, candidiasis (moniliasis), histoplasmosis, actinomycosis, sporotrichosis, chromoblastomycosis, coccidioidomycosis, North American blastomycosis, cryptococcosis (torulosis), tinea versicolor and nocardiosis.

CONTRAINDICATIONS

Two cases of conjoined twins have been reported since 1977 in patients taking griseofulvin during the first trimester of pregnancy. Griseofulvin should not be prescribed to pregnant patients. If the patient becomes pregnant while taking this drug, the patient should be apprised of the potential hazard to the fetus. This drug is contraindicated in patients with porphyria or hepatocellular failure and in individuals with a history of hypersensitivity to griseofulvin.

WARNINGS

Prophylactic Usage – Safety and efficacy of griseofulvin for prophylaxis of fungal infections have not been established.

Animal Toxicology – Chronic feeding of griseofulvin, at levels ranging from 0.5%–2.5% of the diet resulted in the development of liver tumors in several strains of mice, particularly in males. Smaller particle sizes result in an enhanced effect. Lower oral dosage levels have not been tested. Subcutaneous administration of relatively small doses of griseofulvin once a week during the first three weeks of life has also been reported to induce hepatomata in mice. Thyroid tumors, mostly adenomas but some carcinomas, have been reported in male rats receiving griseofulvin at levels of 2.0%, 1.0% and 0.2% of the diet, and in female rats receiving the two higher dose levels. Although studies in other animal species have not yielded evidence of tumorigenicity, these studies were not of adequate design to form a basis for conclusion in this regard. In subacute toxicity studies, orally administered griseofulvin produced hepatocellular necrosis in mice, but this has not been seen in other species. Disturbances in porphyrin metabolism have been reported in griseofulvin-treated laboratory animals. Griseofulvin has been reported to have a colchicine-like effect on mitosis and cocarcinogenicity with methylcholanthrene in cutaneous tumor induction in laboratory animals.

Usage in Pregnancy – see CONTRAINDICATIONS section.

Animal Reproduction Studies – It has been reported in the literature that griseofulvin was found to be embryotoxic and teratogenic on oral administration to pregnant rats. Pups with abnormalities have been reported in the litters of a few bitches treated with griseofulvin. Suppression of spermatogenesis has been reported to occur in rats, but investigation in man failed to confirm this.

PRECAUTIONS

Patients on prolonged therapy with any potent medication should be under close observation. Periodic monitoring of organ system function, including renal, hepatic and hematopoietic, should be done. Since griseofulvin is derived from species of *Penicillium,* the possibility of cross-sensitivity with penicillin exists; however, known penicillin-sensitive patients have been treated without difficulty. Since a photosensitivity reaction is occasionally associated with griseofulvin therapy, patients should be warned to avoid exposure to intense natural or artificial sunlight. Lupus erythematosus or lupus-like syndromes have been reported in patients receiving griseofulvin. Griseofulvin decreases the activity of warfarin-type anticoagulants so that patients receiving these drugs concomitantly may require dosage adjustment of the anticoagulant during and after griseofulvin therapy. Barbiturates usually depress griseofulvin activity and concomitant administration may require a dosage adjustment of the antifungal agent. There have been reports in the literature of possible interactions between griseofulvin and oral contraceptives. The effect of alcohol may be potentiated by griseofulvin, procuding such effects as tachycardia and flush.

ADVERSE REACTIONS

When adverse reactions occur, they are most commonly of the hypersensitivity type such as skin rashes, urticaria, erythema multiforme-like drug reactions, and rarely, angioneurotic edema, and may necessitate withdrawal of therapy and appropriate countermeasures. Paresthesias of the hands and feet have been reported rarely after extended therapy. Other side effects reported occasionally are oral thrush, nausea, vomiting, epigastric distress, diarrhea, headache, fatigue, dizziness, insomnia, mental confusion, and impairment of performance of routine activities. Proteinuria and leukopenia have been reported rarely. Administration of the drug should be discontinued if granulocytopenia occurs. When rare, serious reactions occur with griseofulvin, they are usually associated with high dosages, long periods of therapy, or both.

DOSAGE AND ADMINISTRATION

Accurate diagnosis of infecting organism is essential. Identification would be made either by direct microscopic examination of a mounting of infected tissue in a solution of potassium hydroxide or by culture on an appropriate medium. Medication must be continued until the infecting organism is completely eradicated as indicated by appropriate clinical or laboratory examination. Representative treatment periods are tinea capitis, 4 to 6 weeks; tinea corporis, 2 to 4 weeks; tinea pedis, 4 to 8 weeks; tinea unguium-depending on rate of growth-fingernails, at least 4 months; toenails, at least 6 months. General measures in regard to hygiene should be observed to control sources of infection or reinfection. Concomitant use of appropriate topical agents is usually required, particularly in treatment of tinea pedis. In some forms of athlete's foot, yeasts and bacteria may be involved as well as fungi. Griseofulvin will not eradicate the bacterial or monilial infection.

Adults: Daily administration of 375 mg (as a single dose or in divided doses) will give a satisfactory response in most patients with tinea corporis, tinea crurirs, and tinea capitis. For those fungal infections more difficult to eradicate, such as tinea pedis and tinea unguium, a divided dose of 750 mg is recommended.

Pediatric Use: Approximately 3.3 mg per pound of body weight per day of ultramicrosize griseofulvin is an effective dose for most pediatric patients. On this basis, the following dosage schedule is suggested:
Children weighing 35–60 pounds-125 mg to 187.5mg daily.
Children weighing over 60 pounds-187.5 mg to 375 mg daily.
Children and infants 2 years of age and younger-dosage has not been established. Clinical experience with griseofulvin in children with tinea capitis indicates that a single daily dose is effective. Clinical relapse will occur if the medication is not continued until the infecting organism is eradicated.

HOW SUPPLIED

Gris-PEG® (griseofulvin ultramicrosize) Tablets, 125 mg, white scored, elliptical-shaped, embossed "Gris-PEG" on one side and "125" on the other. Gris-PEG® (griseofulvin ultramicrosize) Tablets, 250 mg, white scored, capsule-shaped, embossed "Gris-PEG" on one side and "250" on the other. The 125 mg strength is available in bottles of 100 (NDC 0884-0763-04). The 250 mg strength is available in bottles of 100, and 500 (NDC 0884-0773-04, and NDC 0884-0773-50 respectively). Both strengths are film-coated.

Rx only

STORAGE

Store Gris-PEG® tablets at controlled room temperature 15°–30°C (59°–86°F) in tight, light-resistant containers.
Manufactured for:
PEDINOL PHARMACAL INC.
30 Banfi Plaza North, Farmingdale, NY 11735 U.S.A.
By:
NOVARTIS CONSUMER HEALTH INC.

LACTINOL-E® CRÈME ℞
LACTINOL® LOTION ℞
(lactic acid 10%)
For topical use only. Not for ophthalmic use.
℞ only.

DESCRIPTION

LACTINOL (lactic acid 10%) is indicated for moisturizing and softening dry, scaly skin (xerosis), ichthyosis vulgaris and itching associated with these conditions. Symptomatic relief of dry skin is provided by skin protectants containing hygroscopic substances (humectants) which increase skin moisture. Lactic acid, an alpha hydroxy acid, is reported to be one of the most effective naturally occurring humectants in the skin. The alpha-hydroxy acids (and their salts), in addition to having beneficial effects on dry skin, have also been shown to reduce excessive epidermal keratinization in patients with hyperkeratotic conditions (e.g., ichthyosis). Not for use in patients known to be sensitive to any of the ingredients in this product. Avoid contact with eyes, lips and mucous membranes. A mild, stinging, burning or peeling may occur on sensitive, inflamed or irritated skin areas. If irritation or sensitivity occurs, patient should discontinue use and notify their physician for appropriate therapy.

HOW SUPPLIED

Lactinol-E Crème is available in a 4 oz. (113.4g) plastic jar and 8 oz (226.8g) tube.
NDC 0884-4990-04 and NDC 0884-4990-08
Lactinol Lotion is available in a 12 oz. (354.84 mL) and 16 oz. (453.6 mL) bottle with pump.
NDC 0884-5292-12 and NDC 0884-5292-16
Store at controlled room temperature 15°–30° C (59°–86° F).

LAZERFORMALYDE® SOLUTION ℞

DESCRIPTION

Lazerformalyde Solution is a topical solution containing Formaldehyde 10% as a drying agent for pre and post surgical removal of warts or for cryosurgical treatment of warts where dryness is required. Safeguards against offensive odor and dries excessive moisture of feet.

HOW SUPPLIED

Available in 3 oz. (88.71 mL) plastic bottle with **roll-on** applicator. NDC 0884-3986-03
Store at controlled room temperature 15°–30°C (59°–86°F).

PEDI–BORO® SOAK PAKS OTC

DESCRIPTION

Pedi-Boro makes a soothing wet dressing of a modified Burow's Solution, Buffered. A mild astringent solution to aid in the relief of minor skin irritations due to allergies, poison ivy, insect bites, or athlete's foot, and as an aid in the relief of swelling associated with minor bruises. Dissolve one or two paks in a pint of water and prepare fresh daily.

HOW SUPPLIED

Box of 12 NDC 0884-1773-27
Box of 100 NDC 0884-1773-10

PEDI–DRI® TOPICAL POWDER ℞
(Nystatin Topical Powder USP)
For topical use only. Not for ophthalmic use.

DESCRIPTION

PEDI-DRI TOPICAL POWDER provides in each gram 100,000 USP nystatin units dispersed in talc.
Nystatin is an antibiotic which is both fungistatic and fungicidal *in vitro* against a wide variety of yeasts and yeast-like fungi, including *Candida albicans, C. parapsilosis, C. tropicalis, C. guilliermondi, C. pseudotropicalis, C. krusei, Torulopsis glabrata, Tricophyton rubrum, T. mentagrophytes.*
Nystatin acts by binding to sterols in the cell membrane of susceptible species resulting in a change in membrane permeability and the subsequent leakage of intracellular components. On repeated subculturing with increasing levels of nystatin., *Candida albicans* does not develop resistance to nystatin. Generally resistance to nystatin does not develop during therapy. However, other species of *Candida (C. tropicalis, C. guillermondi, C. krusei,* and *C. stellatoides)* become quite resistant on treatment with nystatin and simultaneously become cross resistant to amphotericin as well. This resistance is lost when the antibiotic is removed. Nystatin exhibits no appreciable activity against bacteria, protozoa, or viruses.
PEDI-DRI TOPICAL POWDER (Nystatin) is a topical preparation indicated in the treatment of cutaneous or mucocutaneous mycotic infections caused by Candida albicans and other susceptible Candida species.

HOW SUPPLIED

Available as 2 oz. of powder (56.7g) in a 6 oz. plastic squeeze bottle with shaker cap. NDC 0884-0396-02
Store at controlled room temperature 15°–30°C (59°–86°F).
Rx Only

UREACIN–10® LOTION OTC
UREACIN–20® CREME OTC

DESCRIPTION

Ureacin-10 Lotion and Ureacin-20 Creme are topical treatments for rough, dry, cracked, calloused skin.

HOW SUPPLIED

Ureacin-10®, 8 oz. (226.8g) plastic bottle w/pump. 0884-3249-08.
Ureacin-20®, 4 oz. (113.4g) plastic jar 0884-0449-04.
Store at controlled room temperature 15°–30°C (59°–86°F)

Person & Covey, Inc
616 ALLEN AVENUE
GLENDALE, CA 91221-5018

For Additional Information:
Telephone (800) 423-2341
Fax (818) 547-9821
E-Mail helpdesk@personandcovey.com

DRYSOL™ ℞
[drī-sōl]

A solution of Aluminum Chloride (Hexahydrate) 20% w/v in Anhydrous Ethyl Alcohol (S.D. Alcohol 40) 93%v/v

INDICATION

An aid in the management of hyperhidrosis (excess sweating).

WARNING

For external use only. Keep out of the reach of children. Do not apply Drysol to broken, irritated or recently shaved skin. Avoid contact with eyes. If contact occurs, wash eyes thoroughly with water. If irritation or sensitization occurs, discontinue use or contact a physician. Drysol may be harmful to cotton fibers or certain metals. Do not use near open flame. KEEP CAP TIGHTLY CLOSED WHEN NOT IN USE TO PREVENT EVAPORATION.

DIRECTIONS

To achieve optimum results this procedure should be followed: Drysol should only be applied to absolutely dry skin. Dry skin can be achieved by blow drying with a hair dryer on a warm setting for a few minutes. Medication should be kept on the skin for 6-8 hours, during which sweating does not occur. This means for best results, Drysol should be applied only before bedtime, since the sweat glands remain inactive during the tranquility of sleep.
HYPERHIDROSIS OF UNDERARMS (Axillae)
Apply Drysol evenly to dry skin of underarms. To minimize irritation let the alcohol evaporate. If needed, blow dry with a hair dryer on a cold air setting, leaving an evenly distributed film of the antiperspirant on the skin. Wear a T-Shirt while sleeping to prevent the medication from being rubbed off on bed linens. Do not apply Drysol to broken, irritated or recently shaved skin. Now check instructions under "next morning".
HYPERHIDROSIS OF THE PALMS (Hands)
Apply Drysol evenly to palm(s). Let the alcohol evaporate, leaving a thin film of antiperspirant on the skin. To keep the medication from being rubbed off during sleep, cover palm(s) with a sheet of saran wrap, held in place with cotton glove(s). Do not use adhesive tape. Now check instructions under "next morning".
HYPERHIDROSIS OF FEET (Bromhidrosis)
Apply Drysol evenly to sole(s). Let the alcohol evaporate, leaving a thin film of antiperspirant on the skin. To keep the medication from being rubbed off during sleep, cover sole(s) with a sheet of saran wrap, held in place with sock(s). Do not use adhesive tape. Now check instructions under "next morning".
HYPERHIDROSIS OF THE SCALP
Apply Drysol evenly to the scalp. Avoid contact with eyes. Let the alcohol evaporate, leaving a thin film of antiperspirant on the scalp. To keep the medication from being rubbed off during sleep, wear a plastic shower cap. Now check instructions under "next morning".
NEXT MORNING
Depending on the area being treated: Remove the T-shirt, glove(s), sock(s) or shower cap. Remove and discard saran wrap. Wash the treated area thoroughly with a mild soap or a mild shampoo to remove the residual antiperspirant and to prevent skin irritation as well as damage to dry clothing. Then towel dry the skin or scalp. Do not apply other deodorants or antiperspirants while using Drysol. Follow these procedures and repeat applications of Drysol for 2 or 3 nights, until the desired effect (lack of sweating) is achieved. Generally, after that, an application once or twice a week should maintain needed controlled protection from hyperhidrosis. Occasionally, there is some tingling or itching after application. Any irritation it might produce is temporary and will subside if application is avoided for a few days. Drysol is not absorbed but works locally on outer skin.

HOW SUPPLIED

37.5cc	Plastic bottle (NDC 0096-0707-37)
35cc	Plastic bottle with Dab-O-Matic applicator (NDC 0096-0707-35)
60cc	Plastic bottle with Dab-O-Matic applicator (NDC 0096-0707-60)

XERAC™ AC ℞
[zer-ac]

DESCRIPTION

A solution of Aluminum Chloride (Hexahydrate) 6.25%(w/v) in Anhydrous Ethyl Alcohol (S.D. Alcohol 40) 96%(v/v).

INDICATION

For topical application as an antiperspirant (anhidrotic).

Continued on next page

Xerac AC—Cont.

DIRECTIONS

Apply Xerac AC to the axillae at bedtime or as directed by physician. To help prevent irritation, the area should be completely dry prior to application. Do not apply Xerac AC to broken or irritated skin. Keep container tightly closed.

ADVERSE REACTIONS

Transient stinging or itching may occur. If intense, remove with soap and water.

WARNING

For external use only. Some users of this product will experience skin irritation. Keep out of the reach of children. Avoid contact with eyes. If irritation or sensitization occur, discontinue use or consult a physician. Xerac AC may be harmful to certain metals and fabrics. Keep away from open flame.

HOW SUPPLIED

35 cc plastic bottle Dab-O-Matic (NDC 0096-0709-35)
60cc plastic bottle Dab-O-Matic (NDC 0096-0708-60)

Pfizer Inc.

235 EAST 42ND STREET
NEW YORK, NY 10017-5755

For updates to the product information listed below, please check the Pfizer Web site: http://www.pfizer.com, or call (800) 438-1985. For complete product listing, please see the Manufacturers' Index.

For Medical Information, Contact:
(800) 438-1985
24 hours a day, seven days a week.

Distribution:
1855 Shelby Oaks Drive North
Memphis, TN 38134
(901) 387-5200
Customer Service:
(800) 533-4535
Pfizer companies include:
Agouron – see Agouron
Parke-Davis – see Parke-Davis
Pharmacia – see Pharmacia
G.D. Searle – see G.D. Searle

Product Identification Codes

To provide quick and positive identification of Pfizer Inc products, we have either a unique identifying number of the National Drug Code or the product name on all tablets or capsules.
In order that you may quickly identify a product by its code number, we have compiled below a numerical list of code numbers with their corresponding product names. We are also listing the code numbers by alphabetical order of products.

Numerical Listing

Product Ident.

Number	Product
152	**Norvasc® (amlodipine besylate) Tablets 2.5 mg**
153	**Norvasc® (amlodipine besylate) Tablets 5 mg**
154	**Norvasc® (amlodipine besylate) Tablets 10 mg**
155	**Glucotrol XL® (glipizide) Extended Release Tablets, 5 mg GITS**
156	**Glucotrol XL® (glipizide) Extended Release Tablets, 10 mg GITS**
162	**Glucotrol XL® (glipizide) Extended Release Tablets 2.5 mg GITS**
163	**Zyrtec-D 12 Hour® (cetirizine hydrochloride 5 mg and pseudoephedrine hydrochloride 120 mg) Extended Release Tablets**
E245	**Aricept® (donepezil HCl) Tablets, 5 mg**
E246	**Aricept® (donepezil HCl) Tablets, 10 mg**
305	**Zithromax® (azithromycin) Capsules 250 mg**
306	**Zithromax® (azithromycin) Z-Pak® (6 × 250-mg Tablets)**
306	**Zithromax® (azithromycin) Tablets, 250 mg**
307	**Zithromax® (azithromycin) Tri-Pak™ (3 × 500 mg Tablets)**
308	**Zithromax® (azithromycin) Tablets, 600 mg**
311	**Zithromax® (azithromycin for oral suspension) 300 mg (100 mg/5 mL)**
312	**Zithromax® (azithromycin for oral suspension) 600 mg (200 mg/5 mL)**
313	**Zithromax® (azithromycin for oral suspension) 900 mg (200 mg/5 mL)**
314	**Zithromax® (azithromycin for oral suspension) 1200 mg (200 mg/5 mL)**
315	**Zithromax® Injection (azithromycin) 500 mg Vial**
317	**Vfend® (voriconazole) Tablets, 50 mg**
318	**Vfend® (voriconazole) Tablets, 200 mg**
319	**Vfend® I.V. (voriconazole) 200 mg for Injection**
341	**Diflucan® (fluconazole) Tablets, 50 mg**
342	**Diflucan® (fluconazole) Tablets, 100 mg**
343	**Diflucan® (fluconazole) Tablets, 200 mg**
345	**Diflucan® (fluconazole for oral suspension) 40 mg/mL**
350	**Diflucan® (fluconazole) Tablets, 150 mg**
396	**Geodon® (ziprasidone HCl) Capsules 20 mg**
397	**Geodon® (ziprasidone HCl) Capsules 40 mg**
398	**Geodon® (ziprasidone HCl) Capsules 60 mg**
399	**Geodon® (ziprasidone HCl) Capsules 80 mg**
420	**Viagra® (sildenafil citrate) Tablets, 25 mg**
421	**Viagra® (sildenafil citrate) Tablets, 50 mg**
422	**Viagra® (sildenafil citrate) Tablets, 100 mg**
490	**Zoloft® (sertraline HCl) Tablets, 50 mg**
491	**Zoloft® (sertraline HCl) Tablets, 100 mg**
496	**Zoloft® (sertraline HCl) Tablets, 25 mg**
550	**Zyrtec® (cetirizine hydrochloride) Tablets, 5 mg**
551	**Zyrtec® (cetirizine hydrochloride) Tablets, 10 mg**
553	**Zyrtec® (cetirizine hydrochloride) Syrup, 5 mg/5 mL**

ARICEPT® ℞

[ă'rĭ-sĕpt]
(Donepezil Hydrochloride Tablets)

DESCRIPTION

ARICEPT® (donepezil hydrochloride) is a reversible inhibitor of the enzyme acetylcholinesterase, known chemically as (±)-2,3-dihydro-5,6-dimethoxy-2-[[1-(phenylmethyl)-4-piperidinyl]methyl]-1*H*-inden-1-one hydrochloride. Donepezil hydrochloride is commonly referred to in the pharmacological literature as E2020. It has an empirical formula of $C_{24}H_{29}NO_3HCl$ and a molecular weight of 415.96. Donepezil hydrochloride is a white crystalline powder and is freely soluble in chloroform, soluble in water and in glacial acetic acid, slightly soluble in ethanol and in acetonitrile and practically insoluble in ethyl acetate and in n-hexane.

ARICEPT® is available for oral administration in film-coated tablets containing 5 or 10 mg of donepezil hydrochloride. Inactive ingredients are lactose monohydrate, corn starch, microcrystalline cellulose, hydroxypropyl cellulose, and magnesium stearate. The film coating contains talc, polyethylene glycol, hypromellose and titanium dioxide. Additionally, the 10 mg tablet contains yellow iron oxide (synthetic) as a coloring agent.

CLINICAL PHARMACOLOGY

Current theories on the pathogenesis of the cognitive signs and symptoms of Alzheimer's Disease attribute some of them to a deficiency of cholinergic neurotransmission.
Donepezil hydrochloride is postulated to exert its therapeutic effect by enhancing cholinergic function. This is accomplished by increasing the concentration of acetylcholine through reversible inhibition of its hydrolysis by acetylcholinesterase. If this proposed mechanism of action is correct, donepezil's effect may lessen as the disease process advances and fewer cholinergic neurons remain functionally intact. There is no evidence that donepezil alters the course of the underlying dementing process.

Clinical Trial Data

The effectiveness of ARICEPT® as a treatment for Alzheimer's Disease is demonstrated by the results of two randomized, double-blind, placebo-controlled clinical investigations in patients with Alzheimer's Disease (diagnosed by NINCDS and DSM III-R criteria, Mini-Mental State Examination ≥ 10 and ≤ 26 and Clinical Dementia Rating of 1 or 2). The mean age of patients participating in ARICEPT® trials was 73 years with a range of 50 to 94. Approximately 62% of patients were women and 38% were men. The racial distribution was white 95%, black 3% and other races 2%.

Study Outcome Measures: In each study, the effectiveness of treatment with ARICEPT® was evaluated using a dual outcome assessment strategy.

The ability of ARICEPT® to improve cognitive performance was assessed with the cognitive subscale of the Alzheimer's Disease Assessment Scale (ADAS-cog), a multi-item instrument that has been extensively validated in longitudinal cohorts of Alzheimer's Disease patients. The ADAS-cog examines selected aspects of cognitive performance including elements of memory, orientation, attention, reasoning, language and praxis. The ADAS-cog scoring range is from 0 to 70, with higher scores indicating greater cognitive impairment. Elderly normal adults may score as low as 0 or 1, but it is not unusual for non-demented adults to score slightly higher.

The patients recruited as participants in each study had mean scores on the Alzheimer's Disease Assessment Scale (ADAS-cog) of approximately 26 units, with a range from 4 to 61. Experience gained in longitudinal studies of ambulatory patients with mild to moderate Alzheimer's Disease suggest that they gain 6 to 12 units a year on the ADAS-cog. However, lesser degrees of change are seen in patients with very mild or very advanced disease because the ADAS-cog is not uniformly sensitive to change over the course of the disease. The annualized rate of decline in the placebo patients participating in ARICEPT® trials was approximately 2 to 4 units per year.

The ability of ARICEPT® to produce an overall clinical effect was assessed using a Clinician's Interview Based Impression of Change that required the use of caregiver information, the CIBIC plus. The CIBIC plus is not a single instrument and is not a standardized instrument like the ADAS-cog. Clinical trials for investigational drugs have used a variety of CIBIC formats, each different in terms of depth and structure.

As such, results from a CIBIC plus reflect clinical experience from the trial or trials in which it was used and cannot be compared directly with the results of CIBIC plus evaluations from other clinical trials. The CIBIC plus used in ARICEPT® trials was a semi-structured instrument that was intended to examine four major areas of patient function: General, Cognitive, Behavioral and Activities of Daily Living. It represents the assessment of a skilled clinician based upon his/her observations at an interview with the patient, in combination with information supplied by a caregiver familiar with the behavior of the patient over the interval rated. The CIBIC plus is scored as a seven point categorical rating, ranging from a score of 1, indicating "markedly improved," to a score of 4, indicating "no change" to a score of 7, indicating "markedly worse." The CIBIC plus has not been systematically compared directly to assessments not using information from caregivers (CIBIC) or other global methods.

Thirty-Week Study

In a study of 30 weeks duration, 473 patients were randomized to receive single daily doses of placebo, 5 mg/day or 10 mg/day of ARICEPT®. The 30-week study was divided into a 24-week double-blind active treatment phase followed by a 6-week single-blind placebo washout period. The study was designed to compare 5 mg/day or 10 mg/day fixed doses of ARICEPT® to placebo. However, to reduce the likelihood of cholinergic effects, the 10 mg/day treatment was started following an initial 7-day treatment with 5 mg/day doses.

Effects on the ADAS-cog: Figure 1 illustrates the time course for the change from baseline in ADAS-cog scores for all three dose groups over the 30 weeks of the study. After 24 weeks of treatment, the mean differences in the ADAS-cog change scores for ARICEPT® treated patients compared to the patients on placebo were 2.8 and 3.1 units for the 5 mg/day and 10 mg/day treatments, respectively. These differences were statistically significant. While the treatment effect size may appear to be slightly greater for the 10 mg/day treatment, there was no statistically significant difference between the two active treatments.

Following 6 weeks of placebo washout, scores on the ADAS-cog for both the ARICEPT® treatment groups were indistinguishable from those patients who had received only placebo for 30 weeks. This suggests that the beneficial effects of ARICEPT® abate over 6 weeks following discontinuation of treatment and do not represent a change in the underlying disease. There was no evidence of a rebound effect 6 weeks after abrupt discontinuation of therapy.

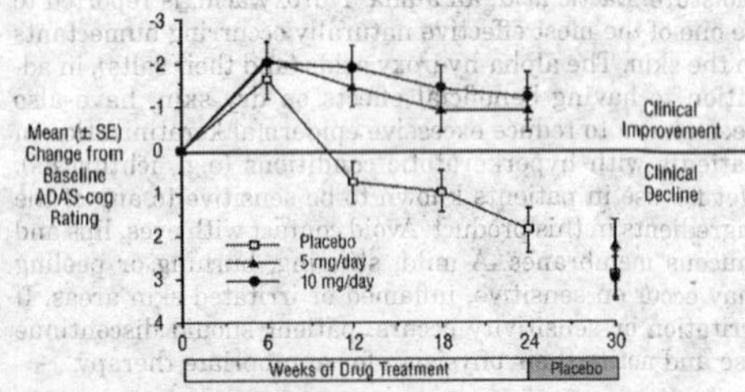

Figure 1. Time-course of the Change from Baseline in ADAS-cog Score for Patients Completing 24 Weeks of Treatment.

Figure 2 illustrates the cumulative percentages of patients from each of the three treatment groups who had attained the measure of improvement in ADAS-cog score shown on the X axis. Three change scores, (7-point and 4-point reductions from baseline or no change in score) have been identified for illustrative purposes and the percent of patients in each group achieving that result is shown in the inset table.
The curves demonstrate that both patients assigned to placebo and ARICEPT® have a wide range of responses, but that the active treatment groups are more likely to show the greater improvements. A curve for an effective treatment would be shifted to the left of the curve for placebo, while an ineffective or deleterious treatment would be superimposed

upon or shifted to the right of the curve for placebo, respectively.

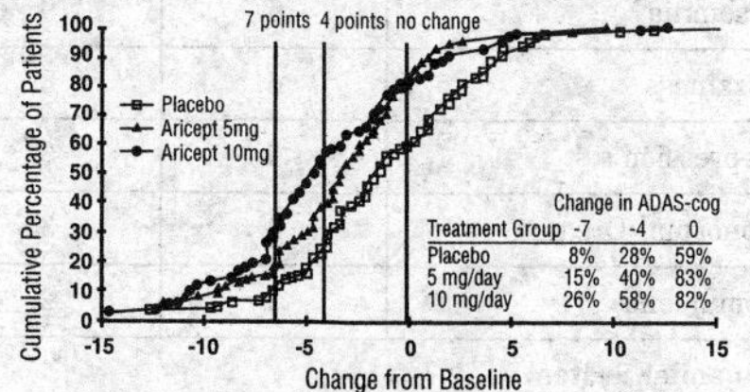

Figure 2. Cumulative Percentage of Patients Completing 24 Weeks of Double-blind Treatment with Specified Changes from Baseline ADAS-cog Scores. The Percentages of Randomized Patients who Completed the Study were: Placebo 80%, 5 mg/day 85% and 10 mg/day 68%.

Effects on the CIBIC plus: Figure 3 is a histogram of the frequency distribution of CIBIC plus scores attained by patients assigned to each of the three treatment groups who completed 24 weeks of treatment. The mean drug-placebo differences for these groups of patients were 0.35 units and 0.39 units for 5 mg/day and 10 mg/day of ARICEPT®, respectively. These differences were statistically significant. There was no statistically significant difference between the two active treatments.

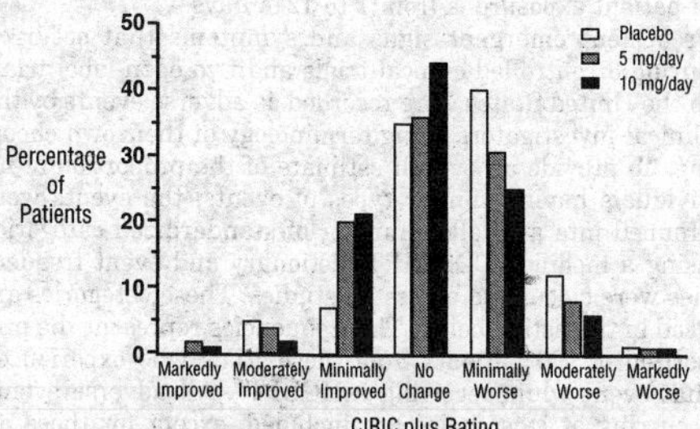

Figure 3. Frequency Distribution of CIBIC plus Scores at Week 24

Fifteen-Week Study

In a study of 15 weeks duration, patients were randomized to receive single daily doses of placebo or either 5 mg/day or 10 mg/day of ARICEPT® for 12 weeks, followed by a 3-week placebo washout period. As in the 30-week study, to avoid acute cholinergic effects, the 10 mg/day treatment followed an initial 7-day treatment with 5 mg/day doses.

Effects on the ADAS-Cog: Figure 4 illustrates the time course of the change from baseline in ADAS-cog scores for all three dose groups over the 15 weeks of the study. After 12 weeks of treatment, the differences in mean ADAS-cog change scores for the ARICEPT® treated patients compared to the patients on placebo were 2.7 and 3.0 units each, for the 5 and 10 mg/day ARICEPT® treatment groups respectively. These differences were statistically significant. The effect size for the 10 mg/day group may appear to be slightly larger than that for 5 mg/day. However, the differences between active treatments were not statistically significant.

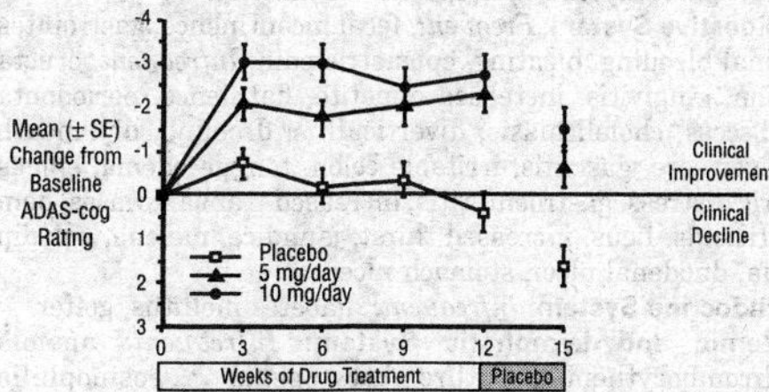

Figure 4. Time-course of the Change from Baseline in ADAS-cog Score for Patients Completing the 15-week Study.

Following 3 weeks of placebo washout, scores on the ADAS-cog for both the ARICEPT® treatment groups increased, indicating that discontinuation of ARICEPT® resulted in a loss of its treatment effect. The duration of this placebo washout period was not sufficient to characterize the rate of loss of the treatment effect, but, the 30-week study (see above) demonstrated that treatment effects associated with the use of ARICEPT® abate within 6 weeks of treatment discontinuation.

Figure 5 illustrates the cumulative percentages of patients from each of the three treatment groups who attained the measure of improvement in ADAS-cog score shown on the X axis. The same three change scores, (7-point and 4-point reductions from baseline or no change in score) as selected for the 30-week study have been used for this illustration. The percentages of patients achieving those results are shown in the inset table.

As observed in the 30-week study, the curves demonstrate that patients assigned to either placebo or to ARICEPT® have a wide range of responses, but that the ARICEPT® treated patients are more likely to show the greater improvements in cognitive performance.

[See figure 5 at top of next column]

Effects on the CIBIC plus: Figure 6 is a histogram of the frequency distribution of CIBIC plus scores attained by patients assigned to each of the three treatment groups who completed 12 weeks of treatment. The differences in mean scores for ARICEPT® treated patients compared to the pa-

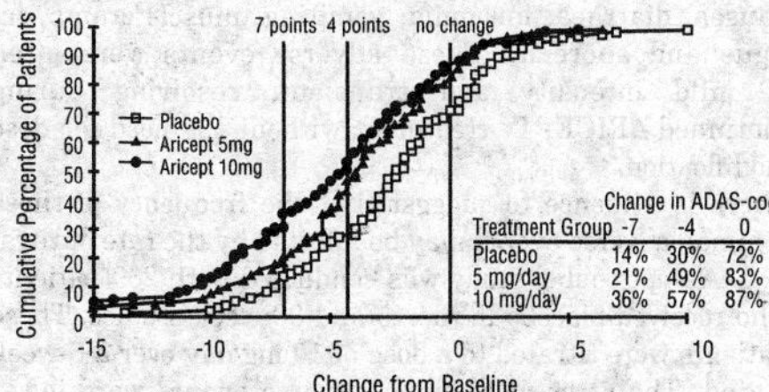

Figure 5. Cumulative Percentage of Patients with Specified Changes from Baseline ADAS-cog Scores. The Percentages of Randomized Patients Within Each Treatment Group Who Completed the Study Were: Placebo 93%, 5 mg/day 90% and 10 mg/day 82%.

tients on placebo at Week 12 were 0.36 and 0.38 units for the 5 mg/day and 10 mg/day treatment groups, respectively. These differences were statistically significant.

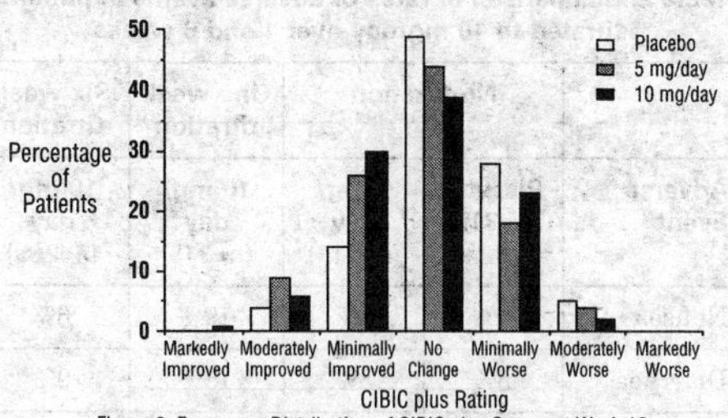

Figure 6. Frequency Distribution of CIBIC plus Scores at Week 12

In both studies, patient age, sex and race were not found to predict the clinical outcome of ARICEPT® treatment.

Clinical Pharmacokinetics

Donepezil is well absorbed with a relative oral bioavailability of 100% and reaches peak plasma concentrations in 3 to 4 hours. Pharmacokinetics are linear over a dose range of 1-10 mg given once daily. Neither food nor time of administration (morning vs. evening dose) influences the rate or extent of absorption. The elimination half life of donepezil is about 70 hours and the mean apparent plasma clearance (Cl/F) is 0.13 L/hr/kg. Following multiple dose administration, donepezil accumulates in plasma by 4-7 fold and steady state is reached within 15 days. The steady state volume of distribution is 12 L/kg. Donepezil is approximately 96% bound to human plasma proteins, mainly to albumins (about 75%) and $alpha_1$ - acid glycoprotein (about 21%) over the concentration range of 2-1000 ng/mL.

Donepezil is both excreted in the urine intact and extensively metabolized to four major metabolites, two of which are known to be active, and a number of minor metabolites, not all of which have been identified. Donepezil is metabolized by CYP 450 isoenzymes 2D6 and 3A4 and undergoes glucuronidation. Following administration of ^{14}C-labeled donepezil, plasma radioactivity, expressed as a percent of the administered dose, was present primarily as intact donepezil (53%) and as 6-O-desmethyl donepezil (11%), which has been reported to inhibit AChE to the same extent as donepezil *in vitro* and was found in plasma at concentrations equal to about 20% of donepezil. Approximately 57% and 15% of the total radioactivity was recovered in urine and feces, respectively, over a period of 10 days, while 28% remained unrecovered, with about 17% of the donepezil dose recovered in the urine as unchanged drug.

Special Populations:

Hepatic Disease: In a study of 10 patients with stable alcoholic cirrhosis, the clearance of ARICEPT® was decreased by 20% relative to 10 healthy age and sex matched subjects.

Renal Disease: In a study of 11 patients with moderate to severe renal impairment (Cl_{Cr} < 18 mL/min/1.73 m^2) the clearance of ARICEPT® did not differ from 11 age and sex matched healthy subjects.

Age: No formal pharmacokinetic study was conducted to examine age related differences in the pharmacokinetics of ARICEPT®. However, mean plasma ARICEPT® concentrations measured during therapeutic drug monitoring of elderly patients with Alzheimer's Disease are comparable to those observed in young healthy volunteers.

Gender and Race: No specific pharmacokinetic study was conducted to investigate the effects of gender and race on the disposition of ARICEPT®. However, retrospective pharmacokinetic analysis indicates that gender and race (Japanese and Caucasians) did not affect the clearance of ARICEPT®.

Drug-Drug Interactions

Drugs Highly Bound to Plasma Proteins: Drug displacement studies have been performed *in vitro* between this highly bound drug (96%) and other drugs such as furosemide, digoxin, and warfarin. ARICEPT® at concentrations of 0.3–10 µg/mL did not affect the binding of furosemide (5 µg/mL), digoxin (2 ng/mL), and warfarin (3 µg/mL) to human albumin. Similarly, the binding of ARICEPT® to human albumin was not affected by furosemide, digoxin and warfarin.

Effect of ARICEPT® on the Metabolism of Other Drugs: No *in vivo* clinical trials have investigated the effect of ARICEPT® on the clearance of drugs metabolized by CYP 3A4 (e.g. cisapride, terfenadine) or by CYP 2D6 (e.g. imipramine). However, *in vitro* studies show a low rate of binding to these enzymes (mean K_i about 50-130 µM), that, given the therapeutic plasma concentrations of donepezil (164 nM), indicates little likelihood of interference.

Whether ARICEPT® has any potential for enzyme induction is not known.

Formal pharmacokinetic studies evaluated the potential of ARICEPT® for interaction with theophylline, cimetidine, warfarin, digoxin and ketoconazole. No effects of ARICEPT® on the pharmacokinetics of these drugs were observed.

Effect of Other Drugs on the Metabolism of ARICEPT®: Ketoconazole and quinidine, inhibitors of CYP450, 3A4 and 2D6, respectively, inhibit donepezil metabolism *in vitro*. Whether there is a clinical effect of quinidine is not known. In a 7-day crossover study in 18 healthy volunteers, ketoconazole (200mg q.d.) increased mean donepezil (5mg q.d.) concentrations (AUC_{0-24} and C_{max}) by 36%. The clinical relevance of this increase in concentration is unknown.

Inducers of CYP 2D6 and CYP 3A4 (e.g., phenytoin, carbamazepine, dexamethasone, rifampin, and phenobarbital) could increase the rate of elimination of ARICEPT®.

Formal pharmacokinetic studies demonstrated that the metabolism of ARICEPT® is not significantly affected by concurrent administration of digoxin or cimetidine.

INDICATIONS AND USAGE

ARICEPT® is indicated for the treatment of mild to moderate dementia of the Alzheimer's type.

CONTRAINDICATIONS

ARICEPT® is contraindicated in patients with known hypersensitivity to donepezil hydrochloride or to piperidine derivatives.

WARNINGS

Anesthesia: ARICEPT®, as a cholinesterase inhibitor, is likely to exaggerate succinylcholine-type muscle relaxation during anesthesia.

Cardiovascular Conditions: Because of their pharmacological action, cholinesterase inhibitors may have vagotonic effects on the sinoatrial and atrioventricular nodes. This effect may manifest as bradycardia or heart block in patients both with and without known underlying cardiac conduction abnormalities. Syncopal episodes have been reported in association with the use of ARICEPT®.

Gastrointestinal Conditions: Through their primary action, cholinesterase inhibitors may be expected to increase gastric acid secretion due to increased cholinergic activity. Therefore, patients should be monitored closely for symptoms of active or occult gastrointestinal bleeding, especially those at increased risk for developing ulcers, e.g., those with a history of ulcer disease or those receiving concurrent nonsteroidal anti-inflammatory drugs (NSAIDS). Clinical studies of ARICEPT® have shown no increase, relative to placebo, in the incidence of either peptic ulcer disease or gastrointestinal bleeding.

ARICEPT®, as a predictable consequence of its pharmacological properties, has been shown to produce diarrhea, nausea and vomiting. These effects, when they occur, appear more frequently with the 10 mg/day dose than with the 5 mg/day dose. In most cases, these effects have been mild and transient, sometimes lasting one to three weeks, and have resolved during continued use of ARICEPT®.

Genitourinary: Although not observed in clinical trials of ARICEPT®, cholinomimetics may cause bladder outflow obstruction.

Neurological Conditions: Seizures: Cholinomimetics are believed to have some potential to cause generalized convulsions. However, seizure activity also may be a manifestation of Alzheimer's Disease.

Pulmonary Conditions: Because of their cholinomimetic actions, cholinesterase inhibitors should be prescribed with care to patients with a history of asthma or obstructive pulmonary disease.

PRECAUTIONS

Drug-Drug Interactions (see Clinical Pharmacology: Clinical Pharmacokinetics: Drug-drug Interactions)

Effect of ARICEPT® on the Metabolism of Other Drugs: No *in vivo* clinical trials have investigated the effect of ARICEPT® on the clearance of drugs metabolized by CYP 3A4 (e.g. cisapride, terfenadine) or by CYP 2D6 (e.g. imipramine). However, *in vitro* studies show a low rate of binding to these enzymes (mean K_i about 50-130 µM), that, given the therapeutic plasma concentrations of donepezil (164 nM), indicates little likelihood of interference.

Whether ARICEPT® has any potential for enzyme induction is not known.

Formal pharmacokinetic studies evaluated the potential of ARICEPT® for interaction with theophylline, cimetidine, warfarin, digoxin and ketoconazole. No effects of ARICEPT® on the pharmacokinetics of these drugs were observed.

Effect of Other Drugs on the Metabolism of ARICEPT®: Ketoconazole and quinidine, inhibitors of CYP450, 3A4 and 2D6, respectively, inhibit donepezil metabolism *in vitro*. Whether there is a clinical effect of quinidine is not known. In a 7-day crossover study in 18 healthy volunteers, ketoconazole (200mg q.d.) increased mean donepezil (5mg q.d.) concentrations (AUC_{0-24} and C_{max}) by 36%. The clinical relevance of this increase in concentration is unknown.

Inducers of CYP 2D6 and CYP 3A4 (e.g., phenytoin, carbamazepine, dexamethasone, rifampin, and phenobarbital) could increase the rate of elimination of ARICEPT®.

Formal pharmacokinetic studies demonstrated that the metabolism of ARICEPT® is not significantly affected by concurrent administration of digoxin or cimetidine.

Continued on next page

Aricept—Cont.

Use with Anticholinergics: Because of their mechanism of action, cholinesterase inhibitors have the potential to interfere with the activity of anticholinergic medications.

Use with Cholinomimetics and Other Cholinesterase Inhibitors: A synergistic effect may be expected when cholinesterase inhibitors are given concurrently with succinylcholine, similar neuromuscular blocking agents or cholinergic agonists such as bethanechol.

Carcinogenesis, Mutagenesis, Impairment of Fertility

No evidence of a carcinogenic potential was obtained in an 88-week carcinogenicity study of donepezil hydrochloride conducted in CD-1 mice at doses up to 180 mg/kg/day (approximately 90 times the maximum recommended human dose on a mg/m^2 basis), or in 104-week carcinogenicity study in Sprague-Dawley rats at doses up to 30 mg/kg/day (approximately 30 times the maximum recommended human dose on a mg/m^2 basis).

Donepezil was not mutagenic in the Ames reverse mutation assay in bacteria, or in a mouse lymphoma forward mutation assay *in vitro*. In the chromosome aberration test in cultures of Chinese hamster lung (CHL) cells, some clastogenic effects were observed. Donepezil was not clastogenic in the *in vivo* mouse micronucleus test and was not genotoxic in an *in vivo* unscheduled DNA synthesis assay in rats. Donepezil had no effect on fertility in rats at doses up to 10 mg/kg/day (approximately 8 times the maximum recommended human dose on a mg/m^2 basis).

Pregnancy

Pregnancy Category C: Teratology studies conducted in pregnant rats at doses up to 16 mg/kg/day (approximately 13 times the maximum recommended human dose on a mg/m^2 basis) and in pregnant rabbits at doses up to 10 mg/kg/day (approximately 16 times the maximum recommended human dose on a mg/m^2 basis) did not disclose any evidence for a teratogenic potential of donepezil. However, in a study in which pregnant rats were given up to 10 mg/kg/day (approximately 8 times the maximum recommended human dose on a mg/m^2 basis) from day 17 of gestation through day 20 postpartum, there was a slight increase in still births and a slight decrease in pup survival through day 4 postpartum at this dose; the next lower dose tested was 3 mg/kg/day. There are no adequate or well-controlled studies in pregnant women. ARICEPT® should be used during pregnancy only if the potential benefit justifies the potential risk to the fetus.

Nursing Mothers

It is not known whether donepezil is excreted in human breast milk. ARICEPT® has no indication for use in nursing mothers.

Pediatric Use

There are no adequate and well-controlled trials to document the safety and efficacy of ARICEPT® in any illness occurring in children.

Geriatric Use

Alzheimer's disease is a disorder occurring primarily in individuals over 55 years of age. The mean age of the patients enrolled in the clinical studies with ARICEPT® was 73 years; 80% of these patients were between 65 and 84 years old and 49% of the patients were at or above the age of 75. The efficacy and safety data presented in the clinical trials section were obtained from these patients. There were no clinically significant differences in most adverse events reported by patient groups ≥ 65 years old and < 65 years old.

ADVERSE REACTIONS

Adverse Events Leading to Discontinuation

The rates of discontinuation from controlled clinical trials of ARICEPT® due to adverse events for the ARICEPT® 5 mg/day treatment groups were comparable to those of placebo-treatment groups at approximately 5%. The rate of discontinuation of patients who received 7-day escalations from 5 mg/day to 10 mg/day, was higher at 13%.

The most common adverse events leading to discontinuation, defined as those occurring in at least 2% of patients and at twice the incidence seen in placebo patients, are shown in Table 1.

Table 1. Most Frequent Adverse Events Leading to Withdrawal from Controlled Clinical Trials by Dose Group

Dose Group	Placebo	5 mg/day ARICEPT®	10 mg/day ARICEPT®
Patients Randomized	355	350	315
Event/% Discontinuing			
Nausea	1%	1%	3%
Diarrhea	0%	<1%	3%
Vomiting	<1%	<1%	2%

Most Frequent Adverse Clinical Events Seen in Association with the Use of ARICEPT®

The most common adverse events, defined as those occurring at a frequency of at least 5% in patients receiving 10 mg/day and twice the placebo rate, are largely predicted by ARICEPT®'s cholinomimetic effects. These include nausea, diarrhea, insomnia, vomiting, muscle cramp, fatigue and anorexia. These adverse events were often of mild intensity and transient, resolving during continued ARICEPT® treatment without the need for dose modification.

There is evidence to suggest that the frequency of these common adverse events may be affected by the rate of titration. An open-label study was conducted with 269 patients who received placebo in the 15 and 30-week studies. These patients were titrated to a dose of 10 mg/day over a 6-week period. The rates of common adverse events were lower than those seen in patients titrated to 10 mg/day over one week in the controlled clinical trials and were comparable to those seen in patients on 5 mg/day.

See Table 2 for a comparison of the most common adverse events following one and six week titration regimens.

Table 2. Comparison of rates of adverse events in patients titrated to 10 mg/day over 1 and 6 weeks

	No titration		One week titration	Six week titration
Adverse Event	**Placebo (n=315)**	**5 mg/day (n=311)**	**10 mg/day (n=315)**	**10 mg/day (n=269)**
Nausea	6%	5%	19%	6%
Diarrhea	5%	8%	15%	9%
Insomnia	6%	6%	14%	6%
Fatigue	3%	4%	8%	3%
Vomiting	3%	3%	8%	5%
Muscle cramps	2%	6%	8%	3%
Anorexia	2%	3%	7%	3%

Adverse Events Reported in Controlled Trials

The events cited reflect experience gained under closely monitored conditions of clinical trials in a highly selected patient population. In actual clinical practice or in other clinical trials, these frequency estimates may not apply, as the conditions of use, reporting behavior, and the kinds of patients treated may differ. Table 3 lists treatment emergent signs and symptoms that were reported in at least 2% of patients in placebo-controlled trials who received ARICEPT® and for which the rate of occurrence was greater for ARICEPT® assigned than placebo assigned patients. In general, adverse events occurred more frequently in female patients and with advancing age.

Table 3. Adverse Events Reported in Controlled Clinical Trials in at Least 2% of Patients Receiving ARICEPT® and at a Higher Frequency than Placebo-treated Patients

Body System/ Adverse Event	Placebo (n=355)	ARICEPT® (n=747)
Percent of Patients with any Adverse Event	72	74
Body as a Whole		
Headache	9	10
Pain, various locations	8	9
Accident	6	7
Fatigue	3	5
Cardiovascular System		
Syncope	1	2
Digestive System		
Nausea	6	11
Diarrhea	5	10
Vomiting	3	5
Anorexia	2	4
Hemic and Lymphatic System		
Ecchymosis	3	4
Metabolic and Nutritional Systems		
Weight Decrease	1	3
Musculoskeletal System		
Muscle Cramps	2	6
Arthritis	1	2
Nervous System		
Insomnia	6	9
Dizziness	6	8
Depression	<1	3
Abnormal Dreams	0	3
Somnolence	<1	2
Urogenital System		
Frequent Urination	1	2

Other Adverse Events Observed During Clinical Trials

ARICEPT® has been administered to over 1700 individuals during clinical trials worldwide. Approximately 1200 of these patients have been treated for at least 3 months and more than 1000 patients have been treated for at least 6 months. Controlled and uncontrolled trials in the United States included approximately 900 patients. In regards to the highest dose of 10 mg/day, this population includes 650 patients treated for 3 months, 475 patients treated for 6 months and 116 patients treated for over 1 year. The range of patient exposure is from 1 to 1214 days.

Treatment emergent signs and symptoms that occurred during 3 controlled clinical trials and two open-label trials in the United States were recorded as adverse events by the clinical investigators using terminology of their own choosing. To provide an overall estimate of the proportion of individuals having similar types of events, the events were grouped into a smaller number of standardized categories using a modified COSTART dictionary and event frequencies were calculated across all studies. These categories are used in the listing below. The frequencies represent the proportion of 900 patients from these trials who experienced that event while receiving ARICEPT®. All adverse events occurring at least twice are included, except for those already listed in Tables 2 or 3, COSTART terms too general to be informative, or events less likely to be drug caused. Events are classified by body system and listed using the following definitions: *frequent adverse events* - those occurring in at least 1/100 patients; *infrequent adverse events* - those occurring in 1/100 to 1/1000 patients. These adverse events are not necessarily related to ARICEPT® treatment and in most cases were observed at a similar frequency in placebo-treated patients in the controlled studies. No important additional adverse events were seen in studies conducted outside the United States.

Body as a Whole: *Frequent:* influenza, chest pain, toothache; *Infrequent:* fever, edema face, periorbital edema, hernia hiatal, abscess, cellulitis, chills, generalized coldness, head fullness, listlessness.

Cardiovascular System: *Frequent:* hypertension, vasodilation, atrial fibrillation, hot flashes, hypotension; *Infrequent:* angina pectoris, postural hypotension, myocardial infarction, AV block (first degree), congestive heart failure, arteritis, bradycardia, peripheral vascular disease, supraventricular tachycardia, deep vein thrombosis.

Digestive System: *Frequent:* fecal incontinence, gastrointestinal bleeding, bloating, epigastric pain; *Infrequent:* eructation, gingivitis, increased appetite, flatulence, periodontal abscess, cholelithiasis, diverticulitis, drooling, dry mouth, fever sore, gastritis, irritable colon, tongue edema, epigastric distress, gastroenteritis, increased transaminases, hemorrhoids, ileus, increased thirst, jaundice, melena, polydipsia, duodenal ulcer, stomach ulcer.

Endocrine System: *Infrequent:* diabetes mellitus, goiter.

Hemic and Lymphatic System: *Infrequent:* anemia, thrombocythemia, thrombocytopenia, eosinophilia, erythrocytopenia.

Metabolic and Nutritional Disorders: *Frequent:* dehydration; *Infrequent:* gout, hypokalemia, increased creatine kinase, hyperglycemia, weight increase, increased lactate dehydrogenase.

Musculoskeletal System: *Frequent:* bone fracture; *Infrequent:* muscle weakness, muscle fasciculation.

Nervous System: *Frequent:* delusions, tremor, irritability, paresthesia, aggression, vertigo, ataxia, increased libido, restlessness, abnormal crying, nervousness, aphasia; *Infrequent:* cerebrovascular accident, intracranial hemorrhage, transient ischemic attack, emotional lability, neuralgia, coldness (localized), muscle spasm, dysphoria, gait abnormality, hypertonia, hypokinesia, neurodermatitis, numbness (localized), paranoia, dysarthria, dysphasia, hostility, decreased libido, melancholia, emotional withdrawal, nystagmus, pacing.

Respiratory System: *Frequent:* dyspnea, sore throat, bronchitis; *Infrequent:* epistaxis, post nasal drip, pneumonia, hyperventilation, pulmonary congestion, wheezing, hypoxia, pharyngitis, pleurisy, pulmonary collapse, sleep apnea, snoring.

Skin and Appendages: *Frequent:* pruritus, diaphoresis, urticaria; *Infrequent:* dermatitis, erythema, skin discoloration, hyperkeratosis, alopecia, fungal dermatitis, herpes zoster, hirsutism, skin striae, night sweats, skin ulcer.

Special Senses: *Frequent:* cataract, eye irritation, vision blurred; *Infrequent:* dry eyes, glaucoma, earache, tinnitus, blepharitis, decreased hearing, retinal hemorrhage, otitis externa, otitis media, bad taste, conjunctival hemorrhage, ear buzzing, motion sickness, spots before eyes.

Urogenital System: *Frequent:* urinary incontinence, nocturia; *Infrequent:* dysuria, hematuria, urinary urgency, metrorrhagia, cystitis, enuresis, prostate hypertrophy, pyelonephritis, inability to empty bladder, breast fibroadenosis, fibrocystic breast, mastitis, pyuria, renal failure, vaginitis.

Postintroduction Reports

Voluntary reports of adverse events temporally associated with ARICEPT® that have been received since market introduction that are not listed above, and that there is inadequate data to determine the causal relationship with the drug include the following: abdominal pain, agitation, cholecystitis, confusion, convulsions, hallucinations, heart block (all types), hemolytic anemia, hepatitis, hyponatremia, neuroleptic malignant syndrome, pancreatitis, and rash.

OVERDOSAGE

Because strategies for the management of overdose are continually evolving, it is advisable to contact a Poison Control Center to determine the latest recommendations for the management of an overdose of any drug.

As in any case of overdose, general supportive measures should be utilized. Overdosage with cholinesterase inhibitors can result in cholinergic crisis characterized by severe nausea, vomiting, salivation, sweating, bradycardia, hypotension, respiratory depression, collapse and convulsions. Increasing muscle weakness is a possibility and may result in death if respiratory muscles are involved. Tertiary anticholinergics such as atropine may be used as an antidote for ARICEPT® overdosage. Intravenous atropine sulfate titrated to effect is recommended: an initial dose of 1.0 to 2.0 mg IV with subsequent doses based upon clinical response. Atypical responses in blood pressure and heart rate have been reported with other cholinomimetics when coadministered with quaternary anticholinergics such as glycopyrrolate. It is not known whether ARICEPT® and/or its metabolites can be removed by dialysis (hemodialysis, peritoneal dialysis, or hemofiltration).

Dose-related signs of toxicity in animals included reduced spontaneous movement, prone position, staggering gait, lacrimation, clonic convulsions, depressed respiration, salivation, miosis, tremors, fasciculation and lower body surface temperature.

DOSAGE AND ADMINISTRATION

The dosages of ARICEPT® shown to be effective in controlled clinical trials are 5 mg and 10 mg administered once per day.

The higher dose of 10 mg did not provide a statistically significantly greater clinical benefit than 5 mg. There is a suggestion, however, based upon order of group mean scores and dose trend analyses of data from these clinical trials, that a daily dose of 10 mg of ARICEPT® might provide additional benefit for some patients. Accordingly, whether or not to employ a dose of 10 mg is a matter of prescriber and patient preference.

Evidence from the controlled trials indicates that the 10 mg dose, with a one week titration, is likely to be associated with a higher incidence of cholinergic adverse events than the 5 mg dose. In open label trials using a 6 week titration, the frequency of these same adverse events was similar between the 5 mg and 10 mg dose groups. Therefore, because steady state is not achieved for 15 days and because the incidence of untoward effects may be influenced by the rate of dose escalation, treatment with a dose of 10 mg should not be contemplated until patients have been on a daily dose of 5 mg for 4 to 6 weeks.

ARICEPT® should be taken in the evening, just prior to retiring. ARICEPT® can be taken with or without food.

HOW SUPPLIED

ARICEPT® is supplied as film-coated, round tablets containing either 5 mg or 10 mg of donepezil hydrochloride.

The 5 mg tablets are white. The strength, in mg (5), is debossed on one side and ARICEPT is debossed on the other side.

The 10 mg tablets are yellow. The strength, in mg (10), is debossed on one side and ARICEPT is debossed on the other side.

5 mg (White)	Bottles of 30 (NDC# 62856-245-30)
	Bottles of 90 (NDC# 62856-245-90)
	Unit Dose Blister Package 100 (10×10) (NDC# 62856-245-41)
10 mg (Yellow)	Bottles of 30 (NDC# 62856-246-30)
	Bottles of 90 (NDC# 62856-246-90)
	Unit Dose Blister Package 100 (10×10) (NDC# 62856-246-41)

Storage: Store at controlled room temperature, 15°C to 30°C (59°F to 86°F).

℞ only

ARICEPT® is a registered trademark of Eisai Co., Ltd.

Manufactured and Marketed by Eisai Inc., Teaneck, NJ 07666

Marketed by

Pfizer Inc, New York, NY 10017

200336

Revised April 2004

Shown in Product Identification Guide, page 329

CADUET® ℞

[*kă-dew-ĕt*]

(amlodipine besylate/atorvastatin calcium)

Tablets

DESCRIPTION

CADUET® (amlodipine besylate and atorvastatin calcium) tablets combine the long-acting calcium channel blocker amlodipine besylate with the synthetic lipid-lowering agent atorvastatin calcium.

The amlodipine besylate component of CADUET is chemically described as 3-Ethyl-5-methyl (±)-2-[(2-aminoethoxy)methyl]-4-(o-chlorophenyl)-1,4-dihydro-6-methyl-3,5-pyridinedicarboxylate, monobenzenesulphonate. Its empirical formula is $C_{20}H_{25}ClN_2O_5 \cdot C_6H_6O_3S$.

The atorvastatin calcium component of CADUET is chemically described as [R-(R*, R*)]-2-(4-fluorophenyl)-ß, δ-dihydroxy-5-(1-methylethyl)-3-phenyl-4-[(phenylamino)carbonyl]-1H-pyrrole-1-heptanoic acid, calcium salt (2:1) trihydrate. Its empirical formula is $(C_{33}H_{34}FN_2O_5)_2Ca \cdot 3H_2O$.

The structural formulae for amlodipine besylate and atorvastatin calcium are shown below.

Amlodipine besylate

Atorvastatin calcium

CADUET contains amlodipine besylate, a white to off-white crystalline powder, and atorvastatin calcium, also a white to off-white crystalline powder. Amlodipine besylate has a molecular weight of 567.1 and atorvastatin calcium has a molecular weight of 1209.42. Amlodipine besylate is slightly soluble in water and sparingly soluble in ethanol. Atorvastatin calcium is insoluble in aqueous solutions of pH 4 and below. Atorvastatin calcium is very slightly soluble in distilled water, pH 7.4 phosphate buffer, and acetonitrile; slightly soluble in ethanol, and freely soluble in methanol.

CADUET tablets are formulated for oral administration in the following strength combinations:

[See table 1 below]

Each tablet also contains calcium carbonate, croscarmellose sodium, microcrystalline cellulose, pregelatinized starch, polysorbate 80, hydroxypropyl cellulose, purified water, colloidal silicon dioxide (anhydrous), magnesium stearate, Opadry® II White 85F28751 (polyvinyl alcohol, titanium dioxide, PEG 3000 and talc) or Opadry® II Blue 85F10919 (polyvinyl alcohol, titanium dioxide, PEG 3000, talc and FD&C blue #2). Combinations of atorvastatin with 5 mg amlodipine are film coated white, and combinations of atorvastatin with 10 mg amlodipine are film coated blue.

CLINICAL PHARMACOLOGY

Mechanism of Action

CADUET

CADUET is a combination of two drugs, a dihydropyridine calcium antagonist (calcium ion antagonist or slow-channel blocker) amlodipine (antihypertensive/antianginal agent) and an HMG-CoA reductase inhibitor atorvastatin (cholesterol lowering agent). The amlodipine component of CADUET inhibits the transmembrane influx of calcium ions into vascular smooth muscle and cardiac muscle. The atorvastatin component of CADUET is a selective, competitive inhibitor of HMG-CoA reductase, the rate-limiting enzyme that converts 3-hydroxy-3-methylglutaryl-coenzyme A to mevalonate, a precursor of sterols, including cholesterol.

The Amlodipine Component of CADUET

Experimental data suggest that amlodipine binds to both dihydropyridine and nondihydropyridine binding sites. The contractile processes of cardiac muscle and vascular smooth muscle are dependent upon the movement of extracellular calcium ions into these cells through specific ion channels. Amlodipine inhibits calcium ion influx across cell membranes selectively, with a greater effect on vascular smooth muscle cells than on cardiac muscle cells. Negative inotropic effects can be detected *in vitro* but such effects have not been seen in intact animals at therapeutic doses. Serum calcium concentration is not affected by amlodipine. Within the physiologic pH range, amlodipine is an ionized compound (pKa=8.6), and its kinetic interaction with the calcium channel receptor is characterized by a gradual rate of association and dissociation with the receptor binding site, resulting in a gradual onset of effect.

Amlodipine is a peripheral arterial vasodilator that acts directly on vascular smooth muscle to cause a reduction in peripheral vascular resistance and reduction in blood pressure.

The precise mechanisms by which amlodipine relieves angina have not been fully delineated, but are thought to include the following:

Exertional Angina: In patients with exertional angina, amlodipine reduces the total peripheral resistance (afterload) against which the heart works and reduces the rate pressure product, and thus myocardial oxygen demand, at any given level of exercise.

Vasospastic Angina: Amlodipine has been demonstrated to block constriction and restore blood flow in coronary arteries and arterioles in response to calcium, potassium epinephrine, serotonin, and thromboxane A_2 analog in experimental animal models and in human coronary vessels *in vitro*. This inhibition of coronary spasm is responsible for the effectiveness of amlodipine in vasospastic (Prinzmetal's or variant) angina.

The Atorvastatin Component of CADUET

Cholesterol and triglycerides circulate in the bloodstream as part of lipoprotein complexes. With ultracentrifugation, these complexes separate into HDL (high-density lipoprotein), IDL (intermediate-density lipoprotein), LDL (low-density lipoprotein), and VLDL (very-low-density lipoprotein) fractions. Triglycerides (TG) and cholesterol in the liver are incorporated into VLDL and released into the plasma for delivery to peripheral tissues. LDL is formed from VLDL and is catabolized primarily through the high-affinity LDL receptor.

Clinical and pathologic studies show that elevated plasma levels of total cholesterol (total-C), LDL-cholesterol (LDL-C), and apolipoprotein B (apo B) promote human atherosclerosis and are risk factors for developing cardiovascular disease, while increased levels of HDL-C are associated with a decreased cardiovascular risk.

Epidemiologic investigations have established that cardiovascular morbidity and mortality vary directly with the level of total-C and LDL-C, and inversely with the level of HDL-C.

In animal models, atorvastatin lowers plasma cholesterol and lipoprotein levels by inhibiting HMG-CoA reductase and cholesterol synthesis in the liver and by increasing the number of hepatic LDL receptors on the cell-surface to enhance uptake and catabolism of LDL; atorvastatin also reduces LDL production and the number of LDL particles.

Atorvastatin reduces total-C, LDL-C, and apo B in patients with homozygous and heterozygous familial hypercholesterolemia (FH), nonfamilial forms of hypercholesterolemia, and mixed dyslipidemia. Atorvastatin also reduces VLDL-C and TG and produces variable increases in HDL-C and apolipoprotein A-1. Atorvastatin reduces total-C, LDL-C, VLDL-C, apo B, TG, and non-HDL-C, and increases HDL-C in patients with isolated hypertriglyceridemia. Atorvastatin reduces intermediate density lipoprotein cholesterol (IDL-C) in patients with dysbetalipoproteinemia.

The effect of atorvastatin on cardiovascular morbidity and mortality has not been determined.

Like LDL, cholesterol-enriched triglyceride-rich lipoproteins, including VLDL, intermediate density lipoprotein (IDL), and remnants, can also promote atherosclerosis. Elevated plasma triglycerides are frequently found in a triad with low HDL-C levels and small LDL particles, as well as in association with non-lipid metabolic risk factors for coronary heart disease. As such, total plasma TG has not consistently been shown to be an independent risk factor for CHD. Furthermore, the independent effect of raising HDL or lowering TG on the risk of coronary and cardiovascular morbidity and mortality has not been determined.

Pharmacokinetics and Metabolism

Absorption

Studies with amlodipine: After oral administration of therapeutic doses of amlodipine alone, absorption produces peak plasma concentrations between 6 and 12 hours. Abso-

Continued on next page

Table 1. CADUET Tablet Strengths

	5 mg/ 10 mg	5 mg/ 20 mg	5 mg/ 40 mg	5 mg/ 80 mg	10 mg/ 10 mg	10 mg/ 20 mg	10 mg/ 40 mg	10 mg/ 80 mg
amlodipine equivalent (mg)	5	5	5	5	10	10	10	10
atorvastatin equivalent (mg)	10	20	40	80	10	20	40	80

Caduet—Cont.

lute bioavailability has been estimated to be between 64 and 90%. The bioavailability of amlodipine when administered alone is not altered by the presence of food.

Studies with atorvastatin: After oral administration alone, atorvastatin is rapidly absorbed; maximum plasma concentrations occur within 1 to 2 hours. Extent of absorption increases in proportion to atorvastatin dose. The absolute bioavailability of atorvastatin (parent drug) is approximately 14% and the systemic availability of HMG-CoA reductase inhibitory activity is approximately 30%. The low systemic availability is attributed to presystemic clearance in gastrointestinal mucosa and/or hepatic first-pass metabolism. Although food decreases the rate and extent of drug absorption by approximately 25% and 9%, respectively, as assessed by Cmax and AUC, LDL-C reduction is similar whether atorvastatin is given with or without food. Plasma atorvastatin concentrations are lower (approximately 30% for Cmax and AUC) following evening drug administration compared with morning. However, LDL-C reduction is the same regardless of the time of day of drug administration (see **DOSAGE AND ADMINISTRATION**).

Studies with CADUET: Following oral administration of CADUET peak plasma concentrations of amlodipine and atorvastatin are seen at 6 to 12 hours and 1 to 2 hours post dosing, respectively. The rate and extent of absorption (bioavailability) of amlodipine and atorvastatin from CADUET are not significantly different from the bioavailability of amlodipine and atorvastatin administered separately (see above).

The bioavailability of amlodipine from CADUET was not affected by food. Although food decreases the rate and extent of absorption of atorvastatin from CADUET by approximately 32% and 11%, respectively, as it does with atorvastatin when given alone. LDL-C reduction is similar whether atorvastatin is given with or without food.

Distribution

Studies with amlodipine: *Ex vivo* studies have shown that approximately 93% of the circulating amlodipine drug is bound to plasma proteins in hypertensive patients. Steady-state plasma levels of amlodipine are reached after 7 to 8 days of consecutive daily dosing.

Studies with atorvastatin: Mean volume of distribution of atorvastatin is approximately 381 liters. Atorvastatin is ≥98% bound to plasma proteins. A blood/plasma ratio of approximately 0.25 indicates poor drug penetration into red blood cells. Based on observations in rats, atorvastatin calcium is likely to be secreted in human milk (see **CONTRAINDICATIONS, Pregnancy and Lactation,** and **PRECAUTIONS, Nursing Mothers**).

Metabolism

Studies with amlodipine: Amlodipine is extensively (about 90%) converted to inactive metabolites via hepatic metabolism.

Studies with atorvastatin: Atorvastatin is extensively metabolized to ortho- and parahydroxylated derivatives and various beta-oxidation products. *In vitro* inhibition of HMG-CoA reductase by ortho- and parahydroxylated metabolites is equivalent to that of atorvastatin. Approximately 70% of circulating inhibitory activity for HMG-CoA reductase is attributed to active metabolites. *In vitro* studies suggest the importance of atorvastatin metabolism by cytochrome P450 3A4, consistent with increased plasma concentrations of atorvastatin in humans following coadministration with erythromycin, a known inhibitor of this isozyme (see **PRECAUTIONS, Drug Interactions**). In animals, the ortho-hydroxy metabolite undergoes further glucuronidation.

Excretion

Studies with amlodipine: Elimination from the plasma is biphasic with a terminal elimination half-life of about 30-50 hours. Ten percent of the parent amlodipine compound and 60% of the metabolites of amlodipine are excreted in the urine.

Studies with atorvastatin: Atorvastatin and its metabolites are eliminated primarily in bile following hepatic and/or extra-hepatic metabolism; however, the drug does not appear to undergo enterohepatic recirculation. Mean plasma elimination half-life of atorvastatin in humans is approximately 14 hours, but the half-life of inhibitory activity for HMG-CoA reductase is 20 to 30 hours due to the contribution of active metabolites. Less than 2% of a dose of atorvastatin is recovered in urine following oral administration.

Special Populations

Geriatric

Studies with amlodipine: Elderly patients have decreased clearance of amlodipine with a resulting increase in AUC of approximately 40-60%, and a lower initial dose of amlodipine may be required.

Studies with atorvastatin: Plasma concentrations of atorvastatin are higher (approximately 40% for Cmax and 30% for AUC) in healthy elderly subjects (age ≥65 years) than in young adults. Clinical data suggest a greater degree of LDL-lowering at any dose of atorvastatin in the elderly population compared to younger adults (see **PRECAUTIONS** section, **Geriatric Use**).

Pediatric

Studies with amlodipine: Sixty-two hypertensive patients aged 6 to 17 years received doses of amlodipine between 1.25 mg and 20 mg. Weight-adjusted clearance and volume of distribution were similar to values in adults.

Studies with atorvastatin: Pharmacokinetic data in the pediatric population are not available.

Gender

Studies with atorvastatin: Plasma concentrations of atorvastatin in women differ from those in men (approximately 20% higher for Cmax and 10% lower for AUC); however, there is no clinically significant difference in LDL-C reduction with atorvastatin between men and women.

Renal Insufficiency

Studies with amlodipine: The pharmacokinetics of amlodipine are not significantly influenced by renal impairment. Patients with renal failure may therefore receive the usual initial amlodipine dose.

Studies with atorvastatin: Renal disease has no influence on the plasma concentrations or LDL-C reduction of atorvastatin; thus, dose adjustment of atorvastatin in patients with renal dysfunction is not necessary (see **DOSAGE AND ADMINISTRATION**).

Hemodialysis

While studies have not been conducted in patients with end-stage renal disease, hemodialysis is not expected to significantly enhance clearance of atorvastatin and/or amlodipine since both drugs are extensively bound to plasma proteins.

Hepatic Insufficiency

Studies with amlodipine: Elderly patients and patients with hepatic insufficiency have decreased clearance of amlodipine with a resulting increase in AUC of approximately 40-60%, and a lower initial dose may be required.

Studies with atorvastatin: In patients with chronic alcoholic liver disease, plasma concentrations of atorvastatin are markedly increased. Cmax and AUC are each 4-fold greater in patients with Childs-Pugh A disease. Cmax and AUC of atorvastatin are approximately 16-fold and 11-fold increased, respectively, in patients with Childs-Pugh B disease (see **CONTRAINDICATIONS**).

Heart Failure

Studies with amlodipine: In patients with moderate to severe heart failure, the increase in AUC for amlodipine was similar to that seen in the elderly and in patients with hepatic insufficiency.

Pharmacodynamics

Hemodynamic Effects of Amlodipine: Following administration of therapeutic doses to patients with hypertension, amlodipine produces vasodilation resulting in a reduction of supine and standing blood pressures. These decreases in blood pressure are not accompanied by a significant change in heart rate or plasma catecholamine levels with chronic dosing. Although the acute intravenous administration of amlodipine decreases arterial blood pressure and increases heart rate in hemodynamic studies of patients with chronic stable angina, chronic administration of oral amlodipine in clinical trials did not lead to clinically significant changes in heart rate or blood pressures in normotensive patients with angina.

With chronic once daily oral administration of amlodipine, antihypertensive effectiveness is maintained for at least 24 hours. Plasma concentrations correlate with effect in both young and elderly patients. The magnitude of reduction in blood pressure with amlodipine is also correlated with the height of pretreatment elevation; thus, individuals with moderate hypertension (diastolic pressure 105-114 mmHg) had about a 50% greater response than patients with mild hypertension (diastolic pressure 90-104 mmHg). Normotensive subjects experienced no clinically significant change in blood pressures (+1/–2 mmHg).

In hypertensive patients with normal renal function, therapeutic doses of amlodipine resulted in a decrease in renal vascular resistance and an increase in glomerular filtration rate and effective renal plasma flow without change in filtration fraction or proteinuria.

As with other calcium channel blockers, hemodynamic measurements of cardiac function at rest and during exercise (or pacing) in patients with normal ventricular function treated with amlodipine have generally demonstrated a small increase in cardiac index without significant influence on dP/dt or on left ventricular end diastolic pressure or volume. In hemodynamic studies, amlodipine has not been associated with a negative inotropic effect when administered in the therapeutic dose range to intact animals and man, even when co-administered with beta-blockers to man. Similar findings, however, have been observed in normals or well-compensated patients with heart failure with agents possessing significant negative inotropic effects.

Electrophysiologic Effects of Amlodipine: Amlodipine does not change sinoatrial nodal function or atrioventricular conduction in intact animals or man. In patients with chronic stable angina, intravenous administration of 10 mg did not significantly alter A-H and H-V conduction and sinus node recovery time after pacing. Similar results were obtained in patients receiving amlodipine and concomitant beta blockers. In clinical studies in which amlodipine was administered in combination with beta-blockers to patients with either hypertension or angina, no adverse effects on electrocardiographic parameters were observed. In clinical trials with angina patients alone, amlodipine therapy did not alter electrocardiographic intervals or produce higher degrees of AV blocks.

LDL-C Reduction with Atorvastatin: Atorvastatin as well as some of its metabolites are pharmacologically active in humans. The liver is the primary site of action and the principal site of cholesterol synthesis and LDL clearance. Drug dosage rather than systemic drug concentration correlates better with LDL-C reduction. Individualization of drug dosage should be based on therapeutic response (see **DOSAGE AND ADMINISTRATION**).

Clinical Studies

Clinical Studies with Amlodipine

Amlodipine Effects in Hypertension

Adult Patients: The antihypertensive efficacy of amlodipine has been demonstrated in a total of 15 double-blind, placebo-controlled, randomized studies involving 800 patients on amlodipine and 538 on placebo. Once daily administration produced statistically significant placebo-corrected reductions in supine and standing blood pressures at 24 hours postdose, averaging about 12/6 mmHg in the standing position and 13/7 mmHg in the supine position in patients with mild to moderate hypertension. Maintenance of the blood pressure effect over the 24-hour dosing interval was observed, with little difference in peak and trough effect. Tolerance was not demonstrated in patients studied for up to 1 year. The 3 parallel, fixed doses, dose response studies showed that the reduction in supine and standing blood pressures was dose-related within the recommended dosing range. Effects on diastolic pressure were similar in young and older patients. The effect on systolic pressure was greater in older patients, perhaps because of greater baseline systolic pressure. Effects were similar in black patients and in white patients.

Pediatric Patients: Two-hundred sixty-eight hypertensive patients aged 6 to 17 years were randomized first to amlodipine 2.5 or 5 mg once daily for 4 weeks and then randomized again to the same dose or to placebo for another 4 weeks. Patients receiving 5 mg amlodipine at the end of 8 weeks had lower blood pressure than those secondarily randomized to placebo. The magnitude of the treatment effect is difficult to interpret, but it is probably less than 5 mmHg systolic on the 5 mg dose. Adverse events were similar to those seen in adults.

Amlodipine Effects in Chronic Stable Angina: The effectiveness of 5–10 mg/day of amlodipine in exercise-induced angina has been evaluated in 8 placebo-controlled, double-blind clinical trials of up to 6 weeks duration involving 1038 patients (684 amlodipine, 354 placebo) with chronic stable angina. In 5 of the 8 studies, significant increases in exercise time (bicycle or treadmill) were seen with the 10 mg dose. Increases in symptom-limited exercise time averaged 12.8% (63 sec) for amlodipine 10 mg, and averaged 7.9% (38 sec) for amlodipine 5 mg. Amlodipine 10 mg also increased time to 1 mm ST segment deviation in several studies and decreased angina attack rate. The sustained efficacy of amlodipine in angina patients has been demonstrated over long-term dosing. In patients with angina, there were no clinically significant reductions in blood pressures (4/1 mmHg) or changes in heart rate (+0.3 bpm).

Amlodipine Effects in Vasospastic Angina: In a double-blind, placebo-controlled clinical trial of 4 weeks duration in 50 patients, amlodipine therapy decreased attacks by approximately 4/week compared with a placebo decrease of approximately 1/week ($p<0.01$). Two of 23 amlodipine and 7 of 27 placebo patients discontinued from the study due to lack of clinical improvement.

Amlodipine Effects in Patients with Congestive Heart Failure: Amlodipine has been compared to placebo in four 8–12 week studies of patients with NYHA class II/III heart failure, involving a total of 697 patients. In these studies, there was no evidence of worsened heart failure based on measures of exercise tolerance, NYHA classification, symptoms, or LVEF. In a long-term (follow-up at least 6 months, mean 13.8 months) placebo-controlled mortality/morbidity study of amlodipine 5–10 mg in 1153 patients with NYHA classes III (n=931) or IV (n=222) heart failure on stable doses of diuretics, digoxin, and ACE inhibitors, amlodipine had no effect on the primary endpoint of the study which was the combined endpoint of all-cause mortality and cardiac morbidity (as defined by life-threatening arrhythmia, acute myocardial infarction, or hospitalization for worsened heart failure), or on NYHA classification, or symptoms of heart failure. Total combined all-cause mortality and cardiac morbidity events were 222/571 (39%) for patients on amlodipine and 246/583 (42%) for patients on placebo; the cardiac morbid events represented about 25% of the endpoints in the study.

Another study (PRAISE-2) randomized patients with NYHA class III (80%) or IV (20%) heart failure without clinical symptoms or objective evidence of underlying ischemic disease, on stable doses of ACE inhibitor (99%), digitalis (99%) and diuretics (99%), to placebo (n=827) or amlodipine (n=827) and followed them for a mean of 33 months.

There was no statistically significant difference between amlodipine and placebo in the primary endpoint of all cause mortality (95% confidence limits from 8% reduction to 29% increase on amlodipine). With amlodipine there were more reports of pulmonary edema.

Clinical Studies with Atorvastatin

Atorvastatin Studies in Hypercholesterolemia (Heterozygous Familial and Nonfamilial) and Mixed Dyslipidemia (Fredrickson Types IIa and IIb*)*: Atorvastatin reduces total-C, LDL-C, VLDL-C, apo B, and TG, and increases HDL-C in patients with hypercholesterolemia and mixed dyslipidemia. Therapeutic response is seen within 2 weeks, and maximum response is usually achieved within 4 weeks and maintained during chronic therapy.

Atorvastatin is effective in a wide variety of patient populations with hypercholesterolemia, with and without hypertriglyceridemia, in men and women, and in the elderly.

In two multicenter, placebo-controlled, dose-response studies in patients with hypercholesterolemia, atorvastatin given as a single dose over 6 weeks significantly reduced total-C, LDL-C, apo B, and TG (pooled results are provided in Table 2).

[See table 2 at right]

In patients with *Fredrickson* Types IIa and IIb hyperlipoproteinemia pooled from 24 controlled trials, the median (25th and 75th percentile) percent changes from baseline in HDL-C for atorvastatin 10, 20, 40, and 80 mg were 6.4 (-1.4, 14), 8.7 (0, 17), 7.8 (0, 16), and 5.1 (-2.7, 15), respectively. Additionally, analysis of the pooled data demonstrated consistent and significant decreases in total-C, LDL-C, TG, total-C/HDL-C, and LDL-C/HDL-C.

In three multicenter, double-blind studies in patients with hypercholesterolemia, atorvastatin was compared to other HMG-CoA reductase inhibitors. After randomization, patients were treated for 16 weeks with either atorvastatin 10 mg per day or a fixed dose of the comparative agent (Table 3).

[See table 3 at right]

The impact on clinical outcomes of the differences in lipid-altering effects between treatments shown in Table 3 is not known. Table 3 does not contain data comparing the effects of atorvastatin 10 mg and higher doses of lovastatin, pravastatin, and simvastatin. The drugs compared in the studies summarized in the table are not necessarily interchangeable.

Atorvastatin Effects in Hypertriglyceridemia (Fredrickson Type IV): The response to atorvastatin in 64 patients with isolated hypertriglyceridemia treated across several clinical trials is shown in the table below. For the atorvastatin-treated patients, median (min, max) baseline TG level was 565 (267–1502).

[See table 4 at right]

Atorvastatin Effects in Dysbetalipoproteinemia (Fredrickson Type III): The results of an open-label crossover study of atorvastatin in 16 patients (genotypes: 14 apo E2/E2 and 2 apo E3/E2) with dysbetalipoproteinemia (*Fredrickson* Type III) are shown in the table below.

[See table 5 at right]

Atorvastatin Effects in Homozygous Familial Hypercholesterolemia: In a study without a concurrent control group, 29 patients ages 6 to 37 years with homozygous FH received maximum daily doses of 20 to 80 mg of atorvastatin. The mean LDL-C reduction in this study was 18%. Twenty-five patients with a reduction in LDL-C had a mean response of 20% (range of 7% to 53%, median of 24%); the remaining 4 patients had 7% to 24% increases in LDL-C. Five of the 29 patients had absent LDL-receptor function. Of these, 2 patients also had a portacaval shunt and had no significant reduction in LDL-C. The remaining 3 receptor-negative patients had a mean LDL-C reduction of 22%.

Atorvastatin Effects in Heterozygous Familial Hypercholesterolemic Pediatric Patients: In a double-blind, placebo-controlled study followed by an open-label phase, 187 boys and postmenarchal girls 10–17 years of age (mean age 14.1 years) with heterozygous FH or severe hypercholesterolemia were randomized to atorvastatin (n=140) or placebo (n=47) for 26 weeks and then all received atorvastatin for 26 weeks. Inclusion in the study required 1) a baseline LDL-C level ≥ 190 mg/dL or 2) a baseline LDL-C ≥ 160 mg/dL and positive family history of FH or documented premature cardiovascular disease in a first- or second-degree relative. The mean baseline LDL-C value was 218.6 mg/dL (range: 138.5-385.0 mg/dL) in the atorvastatin group compared to 230.0 mg/dL (range: 160.0-324.5 mg/dL) in placebo group. The dosage of atorvastatin (once daily) was 10 mg for the first 4 weeks and up-titrated to 20 mg if the LDL-C level was > 130 mg/dL. The number of atorvastatin-treated patients who required up-titration to 20 mg after Week 4 during the double-blind phase was 80 (57.1%).

Atorvastatin significantly decreased plasma levels of total-C, LDL-C, triglycerides, and apolipoprotein B during the 26 week double-blind phase (see Table 6).

[See table 6 at top of next page]

The mean achieved LDL-C value was 130.7 mg/dL (range: 70.0–242.0 mg/dL) in the atorvastatin group compared to 228.5 mg/dL (range: 152.0–385.0 mg/dL) in the placebo group during the 26 week double-blind phase.

The safety and efficacy of atorvastatin doses above 20 mg have not been studied in controlled trials in children. The long-term efficacy of atorvastatin therapy in childhood to reduce morbidity and mortality in adulthood has not been established.

Clinical Study of Combined Amlodipine and Atorvastatin in Patients with Hypertension and Dyslipidemia

In a double-blind, placebo-controlled study, a total of 1660 patients with co-morbid hypertension and dyslipidemia received once daily treatment with eight dose combinations of amlodipine and atorvastatin (5/10, 10/10, 5/20, 10/20, 5/40, 10/40, 5/80, or 10/80 mg), amlodipine alone (5 mg or 10 mg), atorvastatin alone (10 mg, 20 mg, 40 mg, or 80 mg) or placebo. In addition to concomitant hypertension and dyslipidemia, 15% of the patients had diabetes mellitus, 22% were smokers and 14% had a positive family history of cardiovascular disease. At eight weeks, all eight combination-treatment groups of amlodipine and atorvastatin demonstrated statistically significant dose-related reductions in systolic blood pressure (SBP), diastolic blood pressure (DBP) and LDL-C compared to placebo, with no overall modification of effect of either component on SBP, DBP and LDL-C (Table 7).

[See table 7 at top of next page]

Table 2. Dose-Response in Patients With Primary Hypercholesterolemia (Adjusted Mean % Change From Baseline)[a]

DOSE	N	TC	LDL-C	ApoB	TG	HDL-C	Non-HDL-C/ HDL-C
Placebo	21	4	4	3	10	-3	7
10	22	-29	-39	-32	-19	6	-34
20	20	-33	-43	-35	-26	9	-41
40	21	-37	-50	-42	-29	6	-45
80	23	-45	-60	-50	-37	5	-53

[a]Results are pooled from 2 dose-response studies.

Table 3. Mean Percent Change From Baseline at Endpoint (Double-Blind, Randomized, Active-Controlled Trials)

Treatment (Daily Dose)	N	Total-C	LDL-C	Apo B	TG	HDL-C	Non-HDL-C/ HDL-C
Study 1							
Atorvastatin 10 mg	707	-27[a]	-36[a]	-28[a]	-17[a]	+7	-37[a]
Lovastatin 20 mg	191	-19	-27	-20	- 6	+7	-28
95% CI for Diff[1]		-9.2, -6.5	-10.7, -7.1	-10.0, -6.5	-15.2, -7.1	-1.7, 2.0	-11.1, -7.1
Study 2							
Atorvastatin 10 mg	222	-25[b]	-35[b]	-27[b]	-17[b]	+6	-36[b]
Pravastatin 20 mg	77	-17	-23	-17	-9	+8	-28
95% CI for Diff[1]		-10.8, -6.1	-14.5, -8.2	-13.4, -7.4	-14.1, -0.7	-4.9, 1.6	-11.5, -4.1
Study 3							
Atorvastatin 10 mg	132	-29[c]	-37[c]	-34[c]	-23[c]	+7	-39[c]
Simvastatin 10 mg	45	-24	-30	-30	-15	+7	-33
95% CI for Diff[1]		-8.7, -2.7	-10.1, -2.6	-8.0, -1.1	-15.1, -0.7	-4.3, 3.9	-9.6, -1.9

[1] A negative value for the 95% CI for the difference between treatments favors atorvastatin for all except HDL-C, for which a positive value favors atorvastatin. If the range does not include 0, this indicates a statistically significant difference.
[a] Significantly different from lovastatin, ANCOVA, p ≤0.05
[b] Significantly different from pravastatin, ANCOVA, p ≤0.05
[c] Significantly different from simvastatin, ANCOVA, p ≤0.05

Table 4. Combined Patients With Isolated Elevated TG: Median (min, max) Percent Changes From Baseline

	Placebo (N=12)	Atorvastatin 10 mg (N=37)	Atorvastatin 20 mg (N=13)	Atorvastatin 80 mg (N=14)
Triglycerides	-12.4 (-36.6, 82.7)	-41.0 (-76.2, 49.4)	-38.7 (-62.7, 29.5)	-51.8 (-82.8, 41.3)
Total-C	-2.3 (-15.4, 24.4)	-28.2 (-44.9, -6.8)	-34.9 (-49.6, -15.2)	-44.4 (-63.5, -3.8)
LDL-C	3.6 (-31.3, 31.6)	-26.5 (-57.7, 9.8)	-30.4 (-53.9, 0.3)	-40.5 (-60.6, -13.8)
HDL-C	3.8 (-18.6, 13.4)	13.8 (-9.7, 61.5)	11.0 (-3.2, 25.2)	7.5 (-10.8, 37.2)
VLDL-C	-1.0 (-31.9, 53.2)	-48.8 (-85.8, 57.3)	-44.6 (-62.2, -10.8)	-62.0 (-88.2, 37.6)
non-HDL-C	-2.8 (-17.6, 30.0)	-33.0 (-52.1, -13.3)	-42.7 (-53.7, -17.4)	-51.5 (-72.9, -4.3)

Table 5. Open-Label Crossover Study of 16 Patients With Dysbetalipoproteinemia (*Fredrickson* Type III)

		Median % Change (min, max)	
	Median (min, max) at Baseline (mg/dL)	Atorvastatin 10 mg	Atorvastatin 80 mg
Total-C	442 (225, 1320)	-37 (-85, 17)	-58 (-90, -31)
Triglycerides	678 (273, 5990)	-39 (-92, -8)	-53 (-95, -30)
IDL-C + VLDL-C	215 (111, 613)	-32 (-76, 9)	-63 (-90, -8)
non-HDL-C	411 (218, 1272)	-43 (-87, -19)	-64 (-92, -36)

INDICATIONS AND USAGE

CADUET (amlodipine and atorvastatin) is indicated in patients for whom treatment with both amlodipine and atorvastatin is appropriate.

Amlodipine

1. Hypertension: Amlodipine is indicated for the treatment of hypertension. It may be used alone or in combination with other antihypertensive agents;

2. Chronic Stable Angina: Amlodipine is indicated for the treatment of chronic stable angina, for the treatment of confirmed or suspected vasospastic angina and for the treatment of hypertension. Amlodipine may be used alone or in combination with other antianginal or antihypertensive agents;

3. Vasospastic Angina (Prinzmetal's or Variant Angina): Amlodipine is indicated for the treatment of confirmed or suspected vasospastic angina. Amlodipine may be used as monotherapy or in combination with other antianginal drugs.

AND

Atorvastatin

1. Heterozygous Familial and Nonfamilial: Atorvastatin is indicated as an adjunct to diet to reduce elevated total-C, LDL-C, apo B, and TG levels and to increase HDL-C in patients with primary hypercholesterolemia (heterozygous familial and nonfamilial) and mixed dyslipidemia (*Fredrickson* Types IIa and IIb);

2. Elevated Serum TG Levels: Atorvastatin is indicated as an adjunct to diet for the treatment of patients with elevated serum TG levels (*Fredrickson* Type IV);

3. Primary Dysbetalipoproteinemia: Atorvastatin is indicated for the treatment of patients with primary dysbetalipoproteinemia (*Fredrickson* Type III) who do not respond adequately to diet;

4. Homozygous Familial Hypercholesterolemia: Atorvastatin is indicated to reduce total-C and LDL-C in patients with homozygous familial hypercholesterolemia as an adjunct to other lipid-lowering treatments (e.g., LDL apheresis) or if such treatments are unavailable;

5. Pediatric Patients: Atorvastatin is indicated as an adjunct to diet to reduce total-C, LDL-C, and apo B levels in boys and postmenarchal girls, 10 to 17 years of age, with heterozygous familial hypercholesterolemia if after an adequate trial of diet therapy the following findings are present:

a. LDL-C remains ≥ 190 mg/dL or

b. LDL-C remains ≥ 160 mg/dL and:

- there is a positive family history of premature cardiovascular disease or
- two or more other CVD risk factors are present in the pediatric patients.

Therapy with lipid-altering agents should be a component of multiple-risk-factor intervention in individuals at increased risk for atherosclerotic vascular disease due to hypercholesterolemia. Lipid-altering agents should be used, in addition to a diet restricted in saturated fat and cholesterol, only when the response to diet and other nonpharmacological measures has been inadequate (see *National Cholesterol*

Continued on next page

Caduet—Cont.

Education Program (NCEP) Guidelines, summarized in Table 8).

[See table 8 below]

After the LDL-C goal has been achieved, if the TG is still ≥ 200 mg/dL, non-HDL-C (total-C minus HDL-C) becomes a secondary target of therapy. Non-HDL-C goals are set 30 mg/dL higher than LDL-C goals for each risk category.

Prior to initiating therapy with atorvastatin, secondary causes for hypercholesterolemia (e.g., poorly controlled diabetes mellitus, hypothyroidism, nephrotic syndrome, dysproteinemias, obstructive liver disease, other drug therapy, and alcoholism) should be excluded, and a lipid profile performed to measure total-C, LDL-C, HDL-C, and TG. For patients with TG <400 mg/dL (<4.5 mmol/L), LDL-C can be estimated using the following equation: LDL-C = total-C - (0.20 x [TG] + HDL-C). For TG levels >400 mg/dL (>4.5 mmol/L), this equation is less accurate and LDL-C concentrations should be determined by ultracentrifugation.

The antidyslipidemic component of CADUET has not been studied in conditions where the major lipoprotein abnormality is elevation of chylomicrons (*Fredrickson* Types I and V).

The NCEP classification of cholesterol levels in pediatric patients with a familial history of hypercholesterolemia or premature cardiovascular disease is summarized below:

Table 9. NCEP Classification of Cholesterol Levels in Pediatric Patients

Category	Total-C (mg/dL)	LDL-C (mg/dL)
Acceptable	<170	<110
Borderline	170-199	110-129
High	≥200	≥130

CONTRAINDICATIONS

CADUET contains atorvastatin and is therefore contraindicated in patients with active liver disease or unexplained persistent elevations of serum transaminases.

CADUET is contraindicated in patients with known hypersensitivity to any component of this medication.

Pregnancy and Lactation

Atherosclerosis is a chronic process and discontinuation of lipid-lowering drugs during pregnancy should have little impact on the outcome of long-term therapy of primary hypercholesterolemia. Cholesterol and other products of cholesterol biosynthesis are essential components for fetal development (including synthesis of steroids and cell membranes). Since HMG-CoA reductase inhibitors decrease cholesterol synthesis and possibly the synthesis of other biologically active substances derived from cholesterol, they may cause fetal harm when administered to pregnant women. Therefore, HMG-CoA reductase inhibitors are contraindicated during pregnancy and in nursing mothers. CADUET, WHICH INCLUDES ATORVASTATIN, SHOULD BE ADMINISTERED TO WOMEN OF CHILDBEARING AGE ONLY WHEN SUCH PATIENTS ARE HIGHLY UNLIKELY TO CONCEIVE AND HAVE BEEN INFORMED OF THE POTENTIAL HAZARDS. If the patient becomes pregnant while taking this drug, therapy should be discontinued and the patient apprised of the potential hazard to the fetus.

WARNINGS

Increased Angina and/or Myocardial Infarction

Rarely, patients, particularly those with severe obstructive coronary artery disease, have developed documented increased frequency, duration and/or severity of angina or acute myocardial infarction on starting calcium channel blocker therapy or at the time of dosage increase. The mechanism of this effect has not been elucidated.

Liver Dysfunction

HMG-CoA reductase inhibitors, like some other lipid-lowering therapies, have been associated with biochemical abnormalities of liver function. **Persistent elevations (>3 times the upper limit of normal [ULN] occurring on 2 or more occasions) in serum transaminases occurred in 0.7% of patients who received atorvastatin in clinical trials. The incidence of these abnormalities was 0.2%, 0.2%, 0.6%, and 2.3% for 10, 20, 40, and 80 mg, respectively.**

In clinical trials in patients taking atorvastatin the following has been observed. One patient in clinical trials developed jaundice. Increases in liver function tests (LFT) in other patients were not associated with jaundice or other clinical signs or symptoms. Upon dose reduction, drug interruption, or discontinuation, transaminase levels returned to or near pretreatment levels without sequelae. Eighteen of 30 patients, with persistent LFT elevations continued treatment with a reduced dose of atorvastatin.

It is recommended that liver function tests be performed prior to and at 12 weeks following both the initiation of therapy and any elevation of dose, and periodically (e.g., semiannually) thereafter. Liver enzyme changes generally occur in the first 3 months of treatment with atorvastatin. Patients who develop increased transaminase levels should be monitored until the abnormalities resolve. Should an increase in ALT or AST of >3 times ULN persist, reduction of dose or withdrawal of CADUET is recommended.

CADUET should be used with caution in patients who consume substantial quantities of alcohol and/or have a history

Table 6. Lipid-altering Effects of Atorvastatin in Adolescent Boys and Girls with Heterozygous Familial Hypercholesterolemia or Severe Hypercholesterolemia (Mean Percent Change from Baseline at Endpoint in Intention-to-Treat Population)

DOSAGE	N	Total-C	LDL-C	HDL-C	TG	Apolipoprotein B
Placebo	47	-1.5	-0.4	-1.9	1.0	0.7
Atorvastatin	140	-31.4	-39.6	2.8	-12.0	-34.0

Table 7. Efficacy in Terms of Reduction in Blood Pressure and LDL-C: Efficacy of the Combined Treatments in Reducing Systolic BP

Parameter / Analysis		ATO 0 mg	ATO 10 mg	ATO 20 mg	ATO 40 mg	ATO 80 mg
AML 0 mg	Mean Change (mmHg)	-3.0	-4.5	-6.2	-6.2	-6.4
	Difference versus placebo (mmHg)	-	-1.5	-3.2	-3.2	-3.4
AML 5 mg	Mean change (mmHg)	-12.8	-13.7	-15.3	-12.7	-12.2
	Difference versus placebo (mmHg)	-9.8	-10.7	-12.3	-9.7	-9.2
AML 10 mg	Mean change (mmHg)	-16.2	-15.9	-16.1	-16.3	-17.6
	Difference versus placebo (mmHg)	-13.2	-12.9	-13.1	-13.3	-14.6

Efficacy of the Combined Treatments in Reducing Diastolic BP

Parameter / Analysis		ATO 0 mg	ATO 10 mg	ATO 20 mg	ATO 40 mg	ATO 80 mg
AML 0 mg	Mean change (mmHg)	-3.3	-4.1	-3.9	-5.1	-4.1
	Difference versus placebo (mmHg)	-	-0.8	-0.6	-1.8	-0.8
AML 5 mg	Mean change (mmHg)	-7.6	-8.2	-9.4	-7.3	-8.4
	Difference versus placebo (mmHg)	-4.3	-4.9	-6.1	-4.0	-5.1
AML 10 mg	Mean change (mmHg)	-10.4	-9.1	-10.6	-9.8	-11.1
	Difference versus placebo (mmHg)	-7.1	-5.8	-7.3	-6.5	-7.8

Efficacy of the Combined Treatments in Reducing LDL-C (% change)

Parameter / Analysis		ATO 0 mg	ATO 10 mg	ATO 20 mg	ATO 40 mg	ATO 80 mg
AML 0 mg	Mean % chg	-1.1	-33.4	-39.5	-43.1	-47.2
AML 5 mg	Mean % chg	-0.1	-38.7	-42.3	-44.9	-48.4
AML 10 mg	Mean % chg	-2.5	-36.6	-38.6	-43.2	-49.1

Table 8. NCEP Treatment Guidelines: LDL-C Goals and Cutpoints for Therapeutic Lifestyle Changes and Drug Therapy in Different Risk Categories

Risk Category	LDL Goal (mg/dL)	LDL Level at Which to Initiate Therapeutic Lifestyle Changes (mg/dL)	LDL Level at Which to Consider Drug Therapy (mg/dL)
CHD[a] or CHD risk equivalents (10-year risk >20%)	<100	≥100	≥130 (100-129: drug optional)[b]
2+ Risk Factors (10-year risk ≤20%)	<130	≥130	10-year risk 10%-20%: ≥130 10-year risk <10%: ≥ 160
0-1 Risk Factor[c]	<160	≥160	≥190 (160-189: LDL-lowering drug optional)

[a] CHD, coronary heart disease

[b] Some authorities recommend use of LDL-lowering drugs in this category if an LDL-C level of < 100 mg/dL cannot be achieved by therapeutic lifestyle changes. Others prefer use of drugs that primarily modify triglycerides and HDL-C, e.g., nicotinic acid or fibrate. Clinical judgement also may call for deferring drug therapy in this subcategory.

[c] Almost all people with 0-1 risk factor have 10-year risk <10%, thus, 10-year risk assessment in people with 0-1 risk factor is not necessary.

of liver disease. Active liver disease or unexplained persistent transaminase elevations are contraindications to the use of CADUET (see **CONTRAINDICATIONS**).

Skeletal Muscle

Rare cases of rhabdomyolysis with acute renal failure secondary to myoglobinuria have been reported with the atorvastatin component of CADUET and with other drugs in the HMG-CoA reductase inhibitor class.

Uncomplicated myalgia has been reported in atorvastatin-treated patients (see **ADVERSE REACTIONS**). Myopathy, defined as muscle aches or muscle weakness in conjunction with increases in creatine phosphokinase (CPK) values >10 times ULN, should be considered in any patient with diffuse myalgias, muscle tenderness or weakness, and/or marked elevation of CPK. Patients should be advised to report promptly unexplained muscle pain, tenderness or weakness, particularly if accompanied by malaise or fever. CADUET therapy should be discontinued if markedly elevated CPK levels occur or myopathy is diagnosed or suspected.

The risk of myopathy during treatment with drugs in the HMG-CoA reductase inhibitor class is increased with concurrent administration of cyclosporine, fibric acid derivatives, erythromycin, niacin, or azole antifungals. Physicians considering combined therapy with CADUET and fibric acid derivatives, erythromycin, immunosuppressive drugs, azole antifungals, or lipid-lowering doses of niacin should carefully weigh the potential benefits and risks and should carefully monitor patients for any signs or symptoms of muscle pain, tenderness, or weakness, particularly during the initial months of therapy and during any periods of upward dosage titration of either drug. Periodic creatine phosphokinase (CPK) determinations may be considered in such situations, but there is no assurance that such monitoring will prevent the occurrence of severe myopathy.

In patients taking CADUET, therapy should be temporarily withheld or discontinued in any patient with an acute, serious condition suggestive of a myopathy or having a risk factor predisposing to the development of renal failure secondary to rhabdomyolysis (e.g., severe acute infection, hypotension, major surgery, trauma, severe metabolic, endocrine and electrolyte disorders, and uncontrolled seizures).

PRECAUTIONS

General

Since the vasodilation induced by the amlodipine component of CADUET is gradual in onset, acute hypotension has rarely been reported after oral administration of amlodipine. Nonetheless, caution should be exercised when administering CADUET as with any other peripheral vasodilator particularly in patients with severe aortic stenosis.

Before instituting therapy with CADUET, an attempt should be made to control hypercholesterolemia with appropriate diet, exercise, and weight reduction in obese patients, and to treat other underlying medical problems (see **INDICATIONS AND USAGE**).

Use in Patients with Congestive Heart Failure

In general, calcium channel blockers should be used with caution in patients with heart failure. The amlodipine component of CADUET (5–10 mg per day) has been studied in a placebo-controlled trial of 1153 patients with NYHA Class III or IV heart failure (see **CLINICAL PHARMACOLOGY**) on stable doses of ACE inhibitor, digoxin, and diuretics. Follow-up was at least 6 months, with a mean of about 14 months. There was no overall adverse effect on survival or cardiac morbidity (as defined by life-threatening arrhythmia, acute myocardial infarction, or hospitalization for worsened heart failure). Amlodipine has been compared to placebo in four 8–12 week studies of patients with NYHA class II/III heart failure, involving a total of 697 patients. In these studies, there was no evidence of worsened heart failure based on measures of exercise tolerance, NYHA classification, symptoms, or LVEF.

Beta-Blocker Withdrawal

The amlodipine component of CADUET is not a beta-blocker and therefore gives no protection against the dangers of abrupt beta-blocker withdrawal; any such withdrawal should be by gradual reduction of the dose of beta-blocker.

Endocrine Function

HMG-CoA reductase inhibitors, such as the atorvastatin component of CADUET interfere with cholesterol synthesis and theoretically might blunt adrenal and/or gonadal steroid production. Clinical studies have shown that atorvastatin does not reduce basal plasma cortisol concentration or impair adrenal reserve. The effects of HMG-CoA reductase inhibitors on male fertility have not been studied in adequate numbers of patients. The effects, if any, on the pituitary-gonadal axis in premenopausal women are unknown. Caution should be exercised if an HMG-CoA reductase inhibitor is administered concomitantly with drugs that may decrease the levels or activity of endogenous steroid hormones, such as ketoconazole, spironolactone, and cimetidine.

CNS Toxicity

Studies with atorvastatin: Brain hemorrhage was seen in a female dog treated with atorvastatin calcium for 3 months at a dose equivalent to 120 mg atorvastatin/kg/day. Brain hemorrhage and optic nerve vacuolation were seen in another female dog that was sacrificed in moribund condition after 11 weeks of escalating doses of atorvastatin calcium equivalent to up to 280 mg atorvastatin/kg/day. The 120 mg/kg dose of atorvastatin resulted in a systemic exposure approximately 16 times the human plasma area-under-the-curve (AUC, 0–24 hours) based on the maximum human dose of 80 mg/day. A single tonic convulsion was seen in each of 2 male dogs (one treated with atorvastatin calcium at a dose equivalent to 10 mg atorvastatin/kg/day and one at a dose equivalent to 120 mg atorvastatin/kg/day) in a 2-year study. No CNS lesions have been observed in mice after chronic treatment for up to 2 years at doses of atorvastatin calcium equivalent to up to 400 mg atorvastatin/kg/day or in rats at doses equivalent to up to 100 mg atorvastatin/kg/day. These doses were 6 to 11 times (mouse) and 8 to 16 times (rat) the human AUC (0–24) based on the maximum recommended human dose of 80 mg atorvastatin/day.

CNS vascular lesions, characterized by perivascular hemorrhages, edema, and mononuclear cell infiltration of perivascular spaces, have been observed in dogs treated with other members of the HMG-CoA reductase class. A chemically similar drug in this class produced optic nerve degeneration (Wallerian degeneration of retinogeniculate fibers) in clinically normal dogs in a dose-dependent fashion at a dose that produced plasma drug levels about 30 times higher than the mean drug level in humans taking the highest recommended dose.

Information for Patients

Due to the risk of myopathy with drugs of the HMG-CoA reductase class, to which the atorvastatin component of CADUET belongs, patients should be advised to report promptly unexplained muscle pain, tenderness, or weakness, particularly if accompanied by malaise or fever.

Drug Interactions

Data from a drug-drug interaction study involving 10 mg of amlodipine and 80 mg of atorvastatin in healthy subjects indicate that the pharmacokinetics of amlodipine are not altered when the drugs are coadministered. The effect of amlodipine on the pharmacokinetics of atorvastatin showed no effect on the Cmax: 91% (90% confidence interval: 80 to 103%), but the AUC of atorvastatin increased by 18% (90% confidence interval: 109 to 127%) in the presence of amlodipine.

No drug interaction studies have been conducted with CADUET and other drugs, although studies have been conducted in the individual amlodipine and atorvastatin components, as described below:

Studies with Amlodipine:

In vitro data in human plasma indicate that amlodipine has no effect on the protein binding of drugs tested (digoxin, phenytoin, warfarin, and indomethacin).

Cimetidine: Co-administration of amlodipine with cimetidine did not alter the pharmacokinetics of amlodipine.

Maalox® (antacid): Co-administration of the antacid Maalox with a single dose of amlodipine had no significant effect on the pharmacokinetics of amlodipine.

Sildenafil: A single 100 mg dose of sildenafil (Viagra®) in subjects with essential hypertension had no effect on the pharmacokinetic parameters of amlodipine. When amlodipine and sildenafil were used in combination, each agent independently exerted its own blood pressure lowering effect.

Digoxin: Co-administration of amlodipine with digoxin did not change serum digoxin levels or digoxin renal clearance in normal volunteers.

Ethanol (alcohol): Single and multiple 10 mg doses of amlodipine had no significant effect on the pharmacokinetics of ethanol.

Warfarin: Co-administration of amlodipine with warfarin did not change the warfarin prothrombin response time.

In clinical trials, amlodipine has been safely administered with thiazide diuretics, beta-blockers, angiotensin-converting enzyme inhibitors, long-acting nitrates, sublingual nitroglycerin, digoxin, warfarin, non-steroidal anti-inflammatory drugs, antibiotics, and oral hypoglycemic drugs.

Studies with Atorvastatin:

The risk of myopathy during treatment with drugs of the HMG-CoA reductase class is increased with concurrent administration of cyclosporine, fibric acid derivatives, niacin (nicotinic acid), erythromycin, or azole antifungals (see **WARNINGS, Skeletal Muscle**).

Antacid: When atorvastatin and Maalox TC suspension were coadministered, plasma concentrations of atorvastatin decreased approximately 35%. However, LDL-C reduction was not altered.

Antipyrine: Because atorvastatin does not affect the pharmacokinetics of antipyrine, interactions with other drugs metabolized via the same cytochrome isozymes are not expected.

Colestipol: Plasma concentrations of atorvastatin decreased approximately 25% when colestipol and atorvastatin were coadministered. However, LDL-C reduction was greater when atorvastatin and colestipol were coadministered than when either drug was given alone.

Cimetidine: Atorvastatin plasma concentrations and LDL-C reduction were not altered by coadministration of cimetidine.

Digoxin: When multiple doses of atorvastatin and digoxin were coadministered, steady-state plasma digoxin concentrations increased by approximately 20%. Patients taking digoxin should be monitored appropriately.

Erythromycin: In healthy individuals, plasma concentrations of atorvastatin increased approximately 40% with co-administration of atorvastatin and erythromycin, a known inhibitor of cytochrome P450 3A4 (see **WARNINGS, Skeletal Muscle**).

Oral Contraceptives: Coadministration of atorvastatin and an oral contraceptive increased AUC values for norethindrone and ethinyl estradiol by approximately 30% and 20%. These increases should be considered when selecting an oral contraceptive for a woman taking CADUET.

Warfarin: Atorvastatin had no clinically significant effect on prothrombin time when administered to patients receiving chronic warfarin treatment.

Drug/Laboratory Test Interactions

None known.

Carcinogenesis, Mutagenesis, Impairment of Fertility

Studies with amlodipine: Rats and mice treated with amlodipine maleate in the diet for up to two years, at concentrations calculated to provide daily dosage levels of 0.5, 1.25, and 2.5 mg amlodipine/kg/day, showed no evidence of a carcinogenic effect of the drug. For the mouse, the highest dose was, on a mg/m² basis, similar to the maximum recommended human dose of 10 mg amlodipine/day*. For the rat, the highest dose level was, on a mg/m² basis, about twice the maximum recommended human dose*.

Mutagenicity studies conducted with amlodipine maleate revealed no drug related effects at either the gene or chromosome levels.

There was no effect on the fertility of rats treated orally with amlodipine maleate (males for 64 days and females for 14 days prior to mating) at doses up to 10 mg amlodipine/kg/day (8 times* the maximum recommended human dose of 10 mg/day on a mg/m² basis).

*Based on patient weight of 50 kg.

Studies with atorvastatin: In a 2-year carcinogenicity study with atorvastatin calcium in rats at dose levels equivalent to 10, 30, and 100 mg atorvastatin/kg/day, 2 rare tumors were found in muscle in high-dose females: in one, there was a rhabdomyosarcoma and, in another, there was a fibrosarcoma. This dose represents a plasma AUC (0-24) value of approximately 16 times the mean human plasma drug exposure after an 80 mg oral dose.

A 2-year carcinogenicity study in mice given atorvastatin calcium at dose levels equivalent to 100, 200, and 400 mg atorvastatin/kg/day resulted in a significant increase in liver adenomas in high-dose males and liver carcinomas in high-dose females. These findings occurred at plasma AUC (0-24) values of approximately 6 times the mean human plasma drug exposure after an 80 mg oral dose.

In vitro, atorvastatin was not mutagenic or clastogenic in the following tests with and without metabolic activation: the Ames test with *Salmonella typhimurium* and *Escherichia coli*, the HGPRT forward mutation assay in Chinese hamster lung cells, and the chromosomal aberration assay in Chinese hamster lung cells. Atorvastatin was negative in the *in vivo* mouse micronucleus test.

There were no effects on fertility when rats were given atorvastatin calcium at doses equivalent to up to 175 mg atorvastatin/kg/day (15 times the human exposure). There was aplasia and aspermia in the epididymides of 2 of 10 rats treated with atorvastatin calcium at a dose equivalent to 100 mg atorvastatin/kg/day for 3 months (16 times the human AUC at the 80 mg dose); testis weights were significantly lower at 30 and 100 mg/kg/day and epididymal weight was lower at 100 mg/kg/day. Male rats given the equivalent of 100 mg atorvastatin/kg/day for 11 weeks prior to mating had decreased sperm motility, spermatid head concentration, and increased abnormal sperm. Atorvastatin caused no adverse effects on semen parameters, or reproductive organ histopathology in dogs given doses of atorvastatin calcium equivalent to 10, 40, or 120 mg atorvastatin/kg/day for two years.

Pregnancy

Pregnancy Category X (see CONTRAINDICATIONS)

Safety in pregnant women has not been established with CADUET. CADUET should be administered to women of child-bearing potential only when such patients are highly unlikely to conceive and have been informed of the potential hazards. If the woman becomes pregnant while taking CADUET, it should be discontinued and the patient advised again as to the potential hazards to the fetus.

Studies with amlodipine: No evidence of teratogenicity or other embryo/fetal toxicity was found when pregnant rats and rabbits were treated orally with amlodipine maleate at doses up to 10 mg amlodipine/kg/day (respectively 8 times* and 23 times* the maximum recommended human dose of 10 mg/day on a mg/m² basis) during their respective periods of major organogenesis. However, litter size was significantly decreased (by about 50%) and the number of intrauterine deaths was significantly increased (about 5-fold) in rats receiving amlodipine maleate at 10 mg amlodipine/kg/day for 14 days before mating and throughout mating and gestation. Amlodipine maleate has been shown to prolong both the gestation period and the duration of labor in rats at this dose. There are no adequate and well-controlled studies in pregnant women.

*Based on patient weight of 50 kg.

Studies with atorvastatin: Atorvastatin crosses the rat placenta and reaches a level in fetal liver equivalent to that of maternal plasma. Atorvastatin was not teratogenic in rats at doses of atorvastatin calcium equivalent to up to 300 mg atorvastatin/kg/day or in rabbits at doses of atorvastatin calcium equivalent to up to 100 mg atorvastatin/kg/day. These doses resulted in multiples of about 30 times (rat) or 20 times (rabbit) the human exposure based on surface area (mg/m²).

In a study in rats given atorvastatin calcium at doses equivalent to 20, 100, or 225 mg atorvastatin/kg/day, from gestation day 7 through to lactation day 21 (weaning), there was decreased pup survival at birth, neonate, weaning, and maturity for pups of mothers dosed with 225 mg/kg/day. Body weight was decreased on days 4 and 21 for pups of mothers dosed at 100 mg/kg/day; pup body weight was decreased at birth and at days 4, 21, and 91 at 225 mg/kg/day. Pup development was delayed (rotorod performance at 100 mg/kg/day and acoustic startle at 225 mg/kg/day; pinnae detachment and eye opening at 225 mg/kg/day). These doses of atorvastatin correspond to 6 times (100 mg/kg) and 22 times (225 mg/kg) the human AUC at 80 mg/day.

Rare reports of congenital anomalies have been received following intrauterine exposure to HMG-CoA reductase inhibitors. There has been one report of severe congenital bony deformity, tracheo-esophageal fistula, and anal atresia (VATER association) in a baby born to a woman who took lovastatin with dextroamphetamine sulfate during the first trimester of pregnancy.

Continued on next page

Caduet—Cont.

Labor and Delivery

No studies have been conducted in pregnant women on the effect of CADUET, amlodipine or atorvastatin on the mother or the fetus during labor or delivery, or on the duration of labor or delivery. Amlodipine has been shown to prolong the duration of labor in rats.

Nursing Mothers

It is not known whether the amlodipine component of CADUET is excreted in human milk. Nursing rat pups taking atorvastatin had plasma and liver drug levels of 50% and 40%, respectively, of that in their mother's milk. Because of the potential for adverse reactions in nursing infants, women taking CADUET should not breast-feed (see **CONTRAINDICATIONS**).

Pediatric Use

There have been no studies conducted to determine the safety or effectiveness of CADUET in pediatric populations.

Studies with amlodipine: The effect of amlodipine on blood pressure in patients less than 6 years of age is not known.

Studies with atorvastatin: Safety and effectiveness in patients 10–17 years of age with heterozygous familial hypercholesterolemia have been evaluated in controlled clinical trials of 6 months duration in adolescent boys and postmenarchal girls. Patients treated with atorvastatin had an adverse experience profile generally similar to that of patients treated with placebo, the most common adverse experiences observed in both groups, regardless of causality assessment, were infections. **Doses greater than 20 mg have not been studied in this patient population.** In this limited controlled study, there was no detectable effect on growth or sexual maturation in boys or on menstrual cycle length in girls. See **CLINICAL PHARMACOLOGY, Clinical Studies** section; **ADVERSE REACTIONS,** *Pediatric Patients*; and **DOSAGE AND ADMINISTRATION,** *Pediatric Patients (10-17 years of age) with Heterozygous Familial Hypercholesterolemia*. Adolescent females should be counseled on appropriate contraceptive methods while on atorvastatin therapy (see **CONTRAINDICATIONS** and **PRECAUTIONS, Pregnancy**). **Atorvastatin has not been studied in controlled clinical trials involving pre-pubertal patients or patients younger than 10 years of age.**

Clinical efficacy with doses of atorvastatin up to 80 mg/day for 1 year have been evaluated in an uncontrolled study of patients with homozygous FH including 8 pediatric patients. See **CLINICAL PHARMACOLOGY, Clinical Studies,** *Atorvastatin Effects in Homozygous Familial Hypercholesterolemia*.

Geriatric Use

There have been no studies conducted to determine the safety or effectiveness of CADUET in geriatric populations.

In studies with amlodipine: Clinical studies of amlodipine did not include sufficient numbers of subjects aged 65 and over to determine whether they respond differently from younger subjects. Other reported clinical experience has not identified differences in responses between the elderly and younger patients. In general, dose selection of the amlodipine component of CADUET for an elderly patient should be cautious, usually starting at the low end of the dosing range, reflecting the greater frequency of decreased hepatic, renal, or cardiac function, and of concomitant disease or other drug therapy. Elderly patients have decreased clearance of amlodipine with a resulting increase of AUC of approximately 40-60%, and a lower initial dose may be required (see **DOSAGE AND ADMINISTRATION**).

In studies with atorvastatin: The safety and efficacy of atorvastatin (10-80 mg) in the geriatric population (≥65 years of age) was evaluated in the ACCESS study. In this 54-week open-label trial 1,958 patients initiated therapy with atorvastatin calcium 10 mg. Of these, 835 were elderly (≥65 years) and 1,123 were non-elderly. The mean change in LDL-C from baseline after 6 weeks of treatment with atorvastatin calcium 10 mg was −38.2% in the elderly patients versus −34.6% in the non-elderly group.

The rates of discontinuation in patients on atorvastatin due to adverse events were similar between the two age groups. There were no differences in clinically relevant laboratory abnormalities between the age groups.

ADVERSE REACTIONS

CADUET

CADUET (amlodipine besylate/atorvastatin calcium) has been evaluated for safety in 1092 patients in double-blind placebo controlled studies treated for co-morbid hypertension and dyslipidemia. In general, treatment with CADUET was well tolerated. For the most part, adverse experiences have been mild or moderate in severity. In clinical trials with CADUET, no adverse experiences peculiar to this combination have been observed. Adverse experiences are similar in terms of nature, severity, and frequency to those reported previously with amlodipine and atorvastatin.

The following information is based on the clinical experience with amlodipine and atorvastatin.

The Amlodipine Component of CADUET

Amlodipine has been evaluated for safety in more than 11,000 patients in U.S. and foreign clinical trials. In general, treatment with amlodipine was well tolerated at doses up to 10 mg daily. Most adverse reactions reported during therapy with amlodipine were of mild or moderate severity. In controlled clinical trials directly comparing amlodipine (N=1730) in doses up to 10 mg to placebo (N=1250), discontinuation of amlodipine due to adverse reactions was required in only about 1.5% of patients and was not significantly different from placebo (about 1%). The most common side effects are headache and edema. The incidence (%) of side effects which occurred in a dose related manner are as follows:

Adverse Event	amlodipine 2.5 mg N=275	amlodipine 5.0 mg N=296	amlodipine 10.0 mg N=268	Placebo N=520
Edema	1.8	3.0	10.8	0.6
Dizziness	1.1	3.4	3.4	1.5
Flushing	0.7	1.4	2.6	0.0
Palpitation	0.7	1.4	4.5	0.6

Other adverse experiences which were not clearly dose related but which were reported with an incidence greater than 1.0% in placebo-controlled clinical trials include the following:

Placebo-Controlled Studies

	amlodipine (%) (N=1730)	Placebo (%) (N=1250)
Headache	7.3	7.8
Fatigue	4.5	2.8
Nausea	2.9	1.9
Abdominal Pain	1.6	0.3
Somnolence	1.4	0.6

For several adverse experiences that appear to be drug and dose related, there was a greater incidence in women than men associated with amlodipine treatment as shown in the following table:

ADR	amlodipine M=% (N=1218)	amlodipine F=% (N=512)	Placebo M=% (N=914)	Placebo F=% (N=336)
Edema	5.6	14.6	1.4	5.1
Flushing	1.5	4.5	0.3	0.9
Palpitations	1.4	3.3	0.9	0.9
Somnolence	1.3	1.6	0.8	0.3

The following events occurred in ≤1% but >0.1% of patients treated with amlodipine in controlled clinical trials or under conditions of open trials or marketing experience where a causal relationship is uncertain; they are listed to alert the physician to a possible relationship:

Cardiovascular: arrhythmia (including ventricular tachycardia and atrial fibrillation), bradycardia, chest pain, hypotension, peripheral ischemia, syncope, tachycardia, postural dizziness, postural hypotension, vasculitis.

Central and Peripheral Nervous System: hypoesthesia, neuropathy peripheral, paresthesia, tremor, vertigo.

Gastrointestinal: anorexia, constipation, dyspepsia,** dysphagia, diarrhea, flatulence, pancreatitis, vomiting, gingival hyperplasia.

General: allergic reaction, asthenia,** back pain, hot flushes, malaise, pain, rigors, weight gain, weight decrease.

Musculoskeletal System: arthralgia, arthrosis, muscle cramps,** myalgia.

Psychiatric: sexual dysfunction (male** and female), insomnia, nervousness, depression, abnormal dreams, anxiety, depersonalization.

Respiratory System: dyspnea,** epistaxis.

Skin and Appendages: angioedema, erythema multiforme, pruritus,** rash,** rash erythematous, rash maculopapular.

**These events occurred in less than 1% in placebo-controlled trials, but the incidence of these side effects was between 1% and 2% in all multiple dose studies.

Special Senses: abnormal vision, conjunctivitis, diplopia, eye pain, tinnitus.

Urinary System: micturition frequency, micturition disorder, nocturia.

Autonomic Nervous System: dry mouth, sweating increased.

Metabolic and Nutritional: hyperglycemia, thirst.

Hemopoietic: leukopenia, purpura, thrombocytopenia.

The following events occurred in ≤0.1% of patients treated with amlodipine in controlled clinical trials or under conditions of open trials or marketing experience: cardiac failure, pulse irregularity, extrasystoles, skin discoloration, urticaria, skin dryness, alopecia, dermatitis, muscle weakness, twitching, ataxia, hypertonia, migraine, cold and clammy skin, apathy, agitation, amnesia, gastritis, increased appetite, loose stools, coughing, rhinitis, dysuria, polyuria, parosmia, taste perversion, abnormal visual accommodation, and xerophthalmia.

Other reactions occurred sporadically and cannot be distinguished from medications or concurrent disease states such as myocardial infarction and angina.

Amlodipine therapy has not been associated with clinically significant changes in routine laboratory tests. No clinically relevant changes were noted in serum potassium, serum glucose, total triglycerides, total cholesterol, HDL cholesterol, uric acid, blood urea nitrogen, or creatinine.

The following postmarketing event has been reported infrequently with amlodipine treatment where a causal relationship is uncertain: gynecomastia. In postmarketing experience, jaundice and hepatic enzyme elevations (mostly consistent with cholestasis or hepatitis) in some cases severe enough to require hospitalization have been reported in association with use of amlodipine.

Amlodipine has been used safely in patients with chronic obstructive pulmonary disease, well-compensated congestive heart failure, peripheral vascular disease, diabetes mellitus, and abnormal lipid profiles.

The Atorvastatin Component of CADUET

Atorvastatin is generally well-tolerated. Adverse reactions have usually been mild and transient. In controlled clinical studies of 2502 patients, <2% of patients were discontinued due to adverse experiences attributable to atorvastatin calcium. The most frequent adverse events thought to be related to atorvastatin calcium were constipation, flatulence, dyspepsia, and abdominal pain.

Clinical Adverse Experiences

Adverse experiences reported in ≥2% of patients in placebo-controlled clinical studies of atorvastatin, regardless of causality assessment, are shown in Table 10.

[See table 10 at left]

Table 10. Adverse Events in Placebo-Controlled Studies (% of Patients)

Body System/ Adverse Event	Placebo N=270	10 mg N=863	atorvastatin 20 mg N=36	40 mg N=79	80 mg N=94
BODY AS A WHOLE					
Infection	10.0	10.3	2.8	10.1	7.4
Headache	7.0	5.4	16.7	2.5	6.4
Accidental Injury	3.7	4.2	0.0	1.3	3.2
Flu Syndrome	1.9	2.2	0.0	2.5	3.2
Abdominal Pain	0.7	2.8	0.0	3.8	2.1
Back Pain	3.0	2.8	0.0	3.8	1.1
Allergic Reaction	2.6	0.9	2.8	1.3	0.0
Asthenia	1.9	2.2	0.0	3.8	0.0
DIGESTIVE SYSTEM					
Constipation	1.8	2.1	0.0	2.5	1.1
Diarrhea	1.5	2.7	0.0	3.8	5.3
Dyspepsia	4.1	2.3	2.8	1.3	2.1
Flatulence	3.3	2.1	2.8	1.3	1.1
RESPIRATORY SYSTEM					
Sinusitis	2.6	2.8	0.0	2.5	6.4
Pharyngitis	1.5	2.5	0.0	1.3	2.1
SKIN AND APPENDAGES					
Rash	0.7	3.9	2.8	3.8	1.1
MUSCULOSKELETAL SYSTEM					
Arthralgia	1.5	2.0	0.0	5.1	0.0
Myalgia	1.1	3.2	5.6	1.3	0.0

The following adverse events were reported, regardless of causality assessment, in patients treated with atorvastatin in clinical trials. The events in italics occurred in ≥2% of patients and the events in plain type occurred in <2% of patients.

Body as a Whole: *Chest pain*, face edema, fever, neck rigidity, malaise, photosensitivity reaction, generalized edema.

Digestive System: *Nausea*, gastroenteritis, liver function tests abnormal, colitis, vomiting, gastritis, dry mouth, rectal hemorrhage, esophagitis, eructation, glossitis, mouth ulceration, anorexia, increased appetite, stomatitis, biliary pain, cheilitis, duodenal ulcer, dysphagia, enteritis, melena, gum hemorrhage, stomach ulcer, tenesmus, ulcerative stomatitis, hepatitis, pancreatitis, cholestatic jaundice.

Respiratory System: *Bronchitis, rhinitis*, pneumonia, dyspnea, asthma, epistaxis.

Nervous System: *Insomnia, dizziness*, paresthesia, somnolence, amnesia, abnormal dreams, libido decreased, emotional lability, incoordination, peripheral neuropathy, torticollis, facial paralysis, hyperkinesia, depression, hypesthesia, hypertonia.

Musculoskeletal System: *Arthritis*, leg cramps, bursitis, tenosynovitis, myasthenia, tendinous contracture, myositis.

Skin and Appendages: Pruritus, contact dermatitis, alopecia, dry skin, sweating, acne, urticaria, eczema, seborrhea, skin ulcer.

Urogenital System: *Urinary tract infection*, urinary frequency, cystitis, hematuria, impotence, dysuria, kidney calculus, nocturia, epididymitis, fibrocystic breast, vaginal

hemorrhage, albuminuria, breast enlargement, metrorrhagia, nephritis, urinary incontinence, urinary retention, urinary urgency, abnormal ejaculation, uterine hemorrhage.
Special Senses: Amblyopia, tinnitus, dry eyes, refraction disorder, eye hemorrhage, deafness, glaucoma, parosmia, taste loss, taste perversion.
Cardiovascular System: Palpitation, vasodilatation, syncope, migraine, postural hypotension, phlebitis, arrhythmia, angina pectoris, hypertension.
Metabolic and Nutritional Disorders: *Peripheral edema*, hyperglycemia, creatine phosphokinase increased, gout, weight gain, hypoglycemia.
Hemic and Lymphatic System: Ecchymosis, anemia, lymphadenopathy, thrombocytopenia, petechia.
Postintroduction Reports with Atorvastatin
Adverse events associated with atorvastatin therapy reported since market introduction, that are not listed above, regardless of causality assessment, include the following: anaphylaxis, angioneurotic edema, bullous rashes (including erythema multiforme, Stevens-Johnson syndrome, and toxic epidermal necrolysis), and rhabdomyolysis.
Pediatric Patients (ages 10–17 years)
In a 26-week controlled study in boys and postmenarchal girls (n=140), the safety and tolerability profile of atorvastatin 10 to 20 mg daily was generally similar to that of placebo (see **CLINICAL PHARMACOLOGY, Clinical Studies** section and **PRECAUTIONS, Pediatric Use**).

OVERDOSAGE

There is no information on overdosage with CADUET in humans.
Information on Amlodipine
Single oral doses of amlodipine maleate equivalent to 40 mg amlodipine/kg and 100 mg amlodipine/kg in mice and rats, respectively, caused deaths. Single oral amlodipine maleate doses equivalent to 4 or more mg amlodipine/kg in dogs (11 or more times the maximum recommended clinical dose on a mg/m² basis) caused a marked peripheral vasodilation and hypotension.
Overdosage might be expected to cause excessive peripheral vasodilation with marked hypotension and possibly a reflex tachycardia. In humans, experience with intentional overdosage of amlodipine is limited. Reports of intentional overdosage include a patient who ingested 250 mg and was asymptomatic and was not hospitalized; another (120 mg) was hospitalized, underwent gastric lavage and remained normotensive; the third (105 mg) was hospitalized and had hypotension (90/50 mmHg) which normalized following plasma expansion. A patient who took 70 mg amlodipine and an unknown quantity of benzodiazepine in a suicide attempt developed shock which was refractory to treatment and died the following day with abnormally high benzodiazepine plasma concentration. A case of accidental drug overdose has been documented in a 19-month-old male who ingested 30 mg amlodipine (about 2 mg/kg). During the emergency room presentation, vital signs were stable with no evidence of hypotension, but a heart rate of 180 bpm. Ipecac was administered 3.5 hours after ingestion and on subsequent observation (overnight) no sequelae were noted.
If massive overdose should occur, active cardiac and respiratory monitoring should be instituted. Frequent blood pressure measurements are essential. Should hypotension occur, cardiovascular support including elevation of the extremities and the judicious administration of fluids should be initiated. If hypotension remains unresponsive to these conservative measures, administration of vasopressors (such as phenylephrine) should be considered with attention to circulating volume and urine output. Intravenous calcium gluconate may help to reverse the effects of calcium entry blockade. As amlodipine is highly protein bound, hemodialysis is not likely to be of benefit.
Information on Atorvastatin
There is no specific treatment for atorvastatin overdosage. In the event of an overdose, the patient should be treated symptomatically, and supportive measures instituted as required. Due to extensive drug binding to plasma proteins, hemodialysis is not expected to significantly enhance atorvastatin clearance.

DOSAGE AND ADMINISTRATION

Dosage of CADUET must be individualized on the basis of both effectiveness and tolerance for each individual component in the treatment of hypertension/angina and hyperlipidemia.
Amlodipine (Hypertension or angina)
Adults: The usual initial antihypertensive oral dose of amlodipine is 5 mg once daily with a maximum dose of 10 mg once daily. Small, fragile, or elderly individuals, or patients with hepatic insufficiency may be started on 2.5 mg once daily and this dose may be used when adding amlodipine to other antihypertensive therapy. Management of patients needing 2.5 mg amlodipine requires individual assessments of hypertension and therapy with the individual amlodipine component, since an amlodipine 2.5 mg CADUET tablet is not available.
Dosage should be adjusted according to each patient's need. In general, titration should proceed over 7 to 14 days so that the physician can fully assess the patient's response to each dose level. Titration may proceed more rapidly, however, if clinically warranted, provided the patient is assessed frequently.
The recommended dose of amlodipine for chronic stable or vasospastic angina is 5–10 mg, with the lower dose suggested in the elderly and in patients with hepatic insufficiency. Most patients will require 10 mg for adequate effect. See **ADVERSE REACTIONS** section for information related to dosage and side effects.
Children: The effective antihypertensive oral dose of amlodipine in pediatric patients ages 6-17 years is 2.5 mg to 5 mg once daily. Doses in excess of 5 mg daily have not been studied in pediatric patients. See **CLINICAL PHARMACOLOGY**.
Atorvastatin (Hyperlipidemia)
The patient should be placed on a standard cholesterol-lowering diet before receiving atorvastatin and should continue on this diet during treatment with atorvastatin.
Hypercholesterolemia (Heterozygous Familial and Nonfamilial) and Mixed Dyslipidemia (Fredrickson Types IIa and IIb)
The recommended starting dose of atorvastatin is 10 or 20 mg once daily. Patients who require a large reduction in LDL-C (more than 45%) may be started at 40 mg once daily. The dosage range of atorvastatin is 10 to 80 mg once daily. Atorvastatin can be administered as a single dose at any time of the day, with or without food. The starting dose and maintenance doses of atorvastatin should be individualized according to patient characteristics such as goal of therapy and response (see *NCEP Guidelines*, summarized in Table 8). After initiation and/or upon titration of atorvastatin, lipid levels should be analyzed within 2 to 4 weeks and dosage adjusted accordingly.
Since the goal of treatment is to lower LDL-C, the NCEP recommends that LDL-C levels be used to initiate and assess treatment response. Only if LDL-C levels are not available, should total-C be used to monitor therapy.
Heterozygous Familial Hypercholesterolemia in Pediatric Patients (10-17 years of age)
The recommended starting dose of atorvastatin is 10 mg/day; the maximum recommended dose is 20 mg/day (doses greater than 20 mg have not been studied in this patient population). Doses should be individualized according to the recommended goal of therapy (see NCEP Pediatric Panel Guidelines[1], **CLINICAL PHARMACOLOGY**, and **INDICATIONS AND USAGE**). Adjustments should be made at intervals of 4 weeks or more.
Homozygous Familial Hypercholesterolemia
The dosage of atorvastatin in patients with homozygous FH is 10 to 80 mg daily. Atorvastatin should be used as an adjunct to other lipid-lowering treatments (e.g., LDL apheresis) in these patients or if such treatments are unavailable.
Note: a 2.5/80 mg CADUET tablet is not available. Management of patients needing a 2.5/80 mg combination requires individual assessments of dyslipidemia and therapy with the individual components as a 2.5/80 mg CADUET tablet is not available.
Concomitant Therapy
Atorvastatin may be used in combination with a bile acid binding resin for additive effect. The combination of HMG-CoA reductase inhibitors and fibrates should generally be avoided (see **WARNINGS, Skeletal Muscle**, and **PRECAUTIONS, Drug Interactions** for other drug-drug interactions).
Dosage in Patients With Renal Insufficiency
Renal disease does not affect the plasma concentrations nor LDL-C reduction of atorvastatin; thus, dosage adjustment in patients with renal dysfunction is not necessary (see **CLINICAL PHARMACOLOGY, Pharmacokinetics**).
CADUET
CADUET may be substituted for its individually titrated components. Patients may be given the equivalent dose of CADUET or a dose of CADUET with increased amounts of amlodipine, atorvastatin or both for additional antianginal effects, blood pressure lowering, or lipid lowering effect.
CADUET may be used to provide additional therapy for patients already on one of its components. As initial therapy for one indication and continuation of treatment of the other, the recommended starting dose of CADUET should be selected based on the continuation of the component being used and the recommended starting dose for the added monotherapy.
CADUET may be used to initiate treatment in patients with hyperlipidemia and either hypertension or angina. The recommended starting dose of CADUET should be based on the appropriate combination of recommendations for the monotherapies. The maximum dose of the amlodipine component of CADUET is 10 mg once daily. The maximum dose of the atorvastatin component of CADUET is 80 mg once daily. See above for detailed information related to the dosing and administration of amlodipine and atorvastatin.

Table 11. CADUET Packaging Configurations

CADUET				
Package Configuration	Tablet Strength (amlodipine besylate/ atorvastatin calcium) mg	NDC #	Engraving	Tablet Color
Bottle of 30	5/10	0069-2150-30	CDT 051	White
Bottle of 30	5/20	0069-2170-30	CDT 052	White
Bottle of 30	5/40	0069-2190-30	CDT 054	White
Bottle of 30	5/80	0069-2260-30	CDT 058	White
Bottle of 30	10/10	0069-2160-30	CDT 101	Blue
Bottle of 30	10/20	0069-2180-30	CDT 102	Blue
Bottle of 30	10/40	0069-2250-30	CDT 104	Blue
Bottle of 30	10/80	0069-2270-30	CDT 108	Blue

[1] National Cholesterol Education Program (NCEP): Highlights of the Report of the Expert Panel on Blood Cholesterol Levels in Children Adolescents. *Pediatrics*. 89(3):495-501. 1992.

HOW SUPPLIED

CADUET® tablets contain amlodipine besylate and atorvastatin calcium equivalent to amlodipine and atorvastatin in the dose strengths described below.
CADUET tablets are differentiated by tablet color/size and are engraved with "Pfizer" on one side and a unique number on the other side. CADUET tablets are supplied for oral administration in the following strengths and package configurations:
[See table 11 above]
Store at 25°C (77°F); excursions permitted to 15-30°C (59-86°F) [see USP Controlled Room Temperature].
Rx only

Manufactured by:
Pfizer Ireland Pharmaceuticals
Dublin, Ireland
Distributed by
Pfizer Labs
Division of Pfizer Inc, NY, NY 10017
69-6113-00-0 **Issued January 2004**
Shown in Product Identification Guide, page 329

DIFLUCAN® ℞

[*dī-flew-kăn*]
(Fluconazole Tablets)
(Fluconazole Injection - for intravenous infusion only)
(Fluconazole for Oral Suspension)

DESCRIPTION

DIFLUCAN® (fluconazole), the first of a new subclass of synthetic triazole antifungal agents, is available as tablets for oral administration, as a powder for oral suspension and as a sterile solution for intravenous use in glass and in Viaflex® Plus plastic containers.
Fluconazole is designated chemically as 2,4-difluoro-α,α¹-bis(1H-1,2,4-triazol-l-ylmethyl) benzyl alcohol with an empirical formula of $C_{13}H_{12}F_2N_6O$ and molecular weight 306.3. The structural formula is:

[Structural formula: triazole–CH₂–C(OH)(2,4-difluorophenyl)–CH₂–triazole]

Fluconazole is a white crystalline solid which is slightly soluble in water and saline.
DIFLUCAN tablets contain 50, 100, 150, or 200 mg of fluconazole and the following inactive ingredients: microcrystalline cellulose, dibasic calcium phosphate anhydrous, povidone, croscarmellose sodium, FD&C Red No. 40 aluminum lake dye, and magnesium stearate.
DIFLUCAN for oral suspension contains 350 mg or 1400 mg of fluconazole and the following inactive ingredients: sucrose, sodium citrate dihydrate, citric acid anhydrous, sodium benzoate, titanium dioxide, colloidal silicon dioxide, xanthan gum and natural orange flavor. After reconstitution with 24 mL of distilled water or Purified Water (USP), each mL of reconstituted suspension contains 10 mg or 40 mg of fluconazole.
DIFLUCAN injection is an iso-osmotic, sterile, nonpyrogenic solution of fluconazole in a sodium chloride or dextrose diluent. Each mL contains 2 mg of fluconazole and

Continued on next page

Diflucan—Cont.

9 mg of sodium chloride or 56 mg of dextrose, hydrous. The pH ranges from 4.0 to 8.0 in the sodium chloride diluent and from 3.5 to 6.5 in the dextrose diluent. Injection volumes of 100 mL and 200 mL are packaged in glass and in Viaflex® Plus plastic containers.
The Viaflex® Plus plastic container is fabricated from a specially formulated polyvinyl chloride (PL 146® Plastic) (Viaflex and PL 146 are registered trademarks of Baxter International, Inc.). The amount of water that can permeate from inside the container into the overwrap is insufficient to affect the solution significantly. Solutions in contact with the plastic container can leach out certain of its chemical components in very small amounts within the expiration period, e.g., di-2-ethylhexylphthalate (DEHP), up to 5 parts per million. However, the suitability of the plastic has been confirmed in tests in animals according to USP biological tests for plastic containers as well as by tissue culture toxicity studies.

CLINICAL PHARMACOLOGY

Mode of Action
Fluconazole is a highly selective inhibitor of fungal cytochrome P-450 sterol C-14 alpha-demethylation. Mammalian cell demethylation is much less sensitive to fluconazole inhibition. The subsequent loss of normal sterols correlates with the accumulation of 14 alpha-methyl sterols in fungi and may be responsible for the fungistatic activity of fluconazole.

Pharmacokinetics and Metabolism
The pharmacokinetic properties of fluconazole are similar following administration by the intravenous or oral routes. In normal volunteers, the bioavailability of orally administered fluconazole is over 90% compared with intravenous administration. Bioequivalence was established between the 100 mg tablet and both suspension strengths when administered as a single 200 mg dose.
Peak plasma concentrations (Cmax) in fasted normal volunteers occur between 1 and 2 hours with a terminal plasma elimination half-life of approximately 30 hours (range: 20-50 hours) after oral administration.
In fasted normal volunteers, administration of a single oral 400 mg dose of DIFLUCAN (fluconazole) leads to a mean Cmax of 6.72 µg/mL (range: 4.12 to 8.08 µg/mL) and after single oral doses of 50-400 mg, fluconazole plasma concentrations and AUC (area under the plasma concentration-time curve) are dose proportional.
Administration of a single oral 150 mg tablet of DIFLUCAN (fluconazole) to ten lactating women resulted in a mean Cmax of 2.61 µg/mL (range: 1.57 to 3.65 µg/mL).
Steady-state concentrations are reached within 5-10 days following oral doses of 50-400 mg given once daily. Administration of a loading dose (on day 1) of twice the usual daily dose results in plasma concentrations close to steady-state by the second day. The apparent volume of distribution of fluconazole approximates that of total body water. Plasma protein binding is low (11-12%). Following either single- or multiple-oral doses for up to 14 days, fluconazole penetrates into all body fluids studied (see table below). In normal volunteers, saliva concentrations of fluconazole were equal to or slightly greater than plasma concentrations regardless of dose, route, or duration of dosing. In patients with bronchiectasis, sputum concentrations of fluconazole following a single 150 mg oral dose were equal to plasma concentrations at both 4 and 24 hours post dose. In patients with fungal meningitis, fluconazole concentrations in the CSF are approximately 80% of the corresponding plasma concentrations.
A single oral 150 mg dose of fluconazole administered to 27 patients penetrated into vaginal tissue, resulting in tissue: plasma ratios ranging from 0.94 to 1.14 over the first 48 hours following dosing.
A single oral 150 mg dose of fluconazole administered to 14 patients penetrated into vaginal fluid, resulting in fluid: plasma ratios ranging from 0.36 to 0.71 over the first 72 hours following dosing.

Tissue or Fluid	Ratio of Fluconazole Tissue (Fluid)/Plasma Concentration*
Cerebrospinal fluid†	0.5-0.9
Saliva	1
Sputum	1
Blister fluid	1
Urine	10
Normal skin	10
Nails	1
Blister skin	2
Vaginal tissue	1
Vaginal fluid	0.4-0.7

*Relative to concurrent concentrations in plasma in subjects with normal renal function.
†Independent of degree of meningeal inflammation.

In normal volunteers, fluconazole is cleared primarily by renal excretion, with approximately 80% of the administered dose appearing in the urine as unchanged drug. About 11% of the dose is excreted in the urine as metabolites.
The pharmacokinetics of fluconazole are markedly affected by reduction in renal function. There is an inverse relationship between the elimination half-life and creatinine clearance. The dose of DIFLUCAN may need to be reduced in patients with impaired renal function. (See **DOSAGE AND ADMINISTRATION.**) A 3-hour hemodialysis session decreases plasma concentrations by approximately 50%.
In normal volunteers, DIFLUCAN administration (doses ranging from 200 mg to 400 mg once daily for up to 14 days) was associated with small and inconsistent effects on testosterone concentrations, endogenous corticosteroid concentrations, and the ACTH-stimulated cortisol response.

Pharmacokinetics in Children
In children, the following pharmacokinetic data {Mean(%cv)} have been reported:
[See table above]

Age Studied	Dose (mg/kg)	Clearance (mL/min/kg)	Half-life (Hours)	Cmax (µg/mL)	Vdss (L/kg)
9 Months-13 years	Single-Oral 2 mg/kg	0.40 (38%) N=14	25.0	2.9 (22%) N=16	—
9 Months-13 years	Single-Oral 8 mg/kg	0.51 (60%) N=15	19.5	9.8 (20%) N=15	—
5-15 years	Multiple IV 2 mg/kg	0.49 (40%) N=4	17.4	5.5 (25%) N=5	0.722 (36%) N=4
5-15 years	Multiple IV 4 mg/kg	0.59 (64%) N=5	15.2	11.4 (44%) N=6	0.729 (33%) N=5
5-15 years	Multiple IV 8 mg/kg	0.66 (31%) N=7	17.6	14.1 (22%) N=8	1.069 (37%) N=7

Clearance corrected for body weight was not affected by age in these studies. Mean body clearance in adults is reported to be 0.23 (17%) mL/min/kg.
In premature newborns (gestational age 26 to 29 weeks), the mean (%cv) clearance within 36 hours of birth was 0.180 (35%, N=7) mL/min/kg, which increased with time to a mean of 0.218 (31%, N=9) mL/min/kg six days later and 0.333 (56%, N=4) mL/min/kg 12 days later. Similarly, the half-life was 73.6 hours, which decreased with time to a mean of 53.2 hours six days later and 46.6 hours 12 days later.

Drug Interaction Studies
Oral contraceptives: Oral contraceptives were administered as a single dose both before and after the oral administration of DIFLUCAN 50 mg once daily for 10 days in 10 healthy women. There was no significant difference in ethinyl estradiol or levonorgestrel AUC after the administration of 50 mg of DIFLUCAN. The mean increase in ethinyl estradiol AUC was 6% (range: –47 to 108%) and levonorgestrel AUC increased 17% (range: –33 to 141%).
In a second study, twenty-five normal females received daily doses of both 200 mg DIFLUCAN tablets or placebo for two, ten-day periods. The treatment cycles were one month apart with all subjects receiving DIFLUCAN during one cycle and placebo during the other. The order of study treatment was random. Single doses of an oral contraceptive tablet containing levonorgestrel and ethinyl estradiol were administered on the final treatment day (day 10) of both cycles. Following administration of 200 mg of DIFLUCAN, the mean percentage increase of AUC for levonorgestrel compared to placebo was 25% (range: -12 to 82%) and the mean percentage increase for ethinyl estradiol compared to placebo was 38% (range: -11 to 101%). Both of these increases were statistically significantly different from placebo.
Cimetidine: DIFLUCAN 100 mg was administered as a single oral dose alone and two hours after a single dose of cimetidine 400 mg to six healthy male volunteers. After the administration of cimetidine, there was a significant decrease in fluconazole AUC and Cmax. There was a mean ± SD decrease in fluconazole AUC of 13% ± 11% (range: –3.4 to –31%) and Cmax decreased 19% ± 14% (range: –5 to –40%). However, the administration of cimetidine 600 mg to 900 mg intravenously over a four-hour period (from one hour before to 3 hours after a single oral dose of DIFLUCAN 200 mg) did not affect the bioavailability or pharmacokinetics of fluconazole in 24 healthy male volunteers.
Antacid: Administration of Maalox® (20 mL) to 14 normal male volunteers immediately prior to a single dose of DIFLUCAN 100 mg had no effect on the absorption or elimination of fluconazole.
Hydrochlorothiazide: Concomitant oral administration of 100 mg DIFLUCAN and 50 mg hydrochlorothiazide for 10 days in 13 normal volunteers resulted in a significant increase in fluconazole AUC and Cmax compared to DIFLUCAN given alone. There was a mean ± SD increase in fluconazole AUC and Cmax of 45% ± 31% (range: 19 to 114%) and 43% ± 31% (range: 19 to 122%), respectively. These changes are attributed to a mean ± SD reduction in renal clearance of 30% ± 12% (range: –10 to –50%).
Rifampin: Administration of a single oral 200 mg dose of DIFLUCAN after 15 days of rifampin administered as 600 mg daily in eight healthy male volunteers resulted in a significant decrease in fluconazole AUC and a significant increase in apparent oral clearance of fluconazole. There was a mean ± SD reduction in fluconazole AUC of 23% ± 9% (range: –13 to –42%). Apparent oral clearance of fluconazole increased 32% ± 17% (range: 16 to 72%). Fluconazole half-life decreased from 33.4 ± 4.4 hours to 26.8 ± 3.9 hours. (See **PRECAUTIONS.**)
Warfarin: There was a significant increase in prothrombin time response (area under the prothrombin time-time curve) following a single dose of warfarin (15 mg) administered to 13 normal male volunteers following oral DIFLUCAN 200 mg administered daily for 14 days as compared to the administration of warfarin alone. There was a mean ± SD increase in the prothrombin time response (area under the prothrombin time-time curve) of 7% ± 4% (range: –2 to 13%). (See **PRECAUTIONS.**) Mean is based on data from 12 subjects as one of 13 subjects experienced a 2-fold increase in his prothrombin time response.
Phenytoin: Phenytoin AUC was determined after 4 days of phenytoin dosing (200 mg daily, orally for 3 days followed by 250 mg intravenously for one dose) both with and without the administration of fluconazole (oral DIFLUCAN 200 mg daily for 16 days) in 10 normal male volunteers. There was a significant increase in phenytoin AUC. The mean ± SD increase in phenytoin AUC was 88% ± 68% (range: 16 to 247%). The absolute magnitude of this interaction is unknown because of the intrinsically nonlinear disposition of phenytoin. (See **PRECAUTIONS.**)
Cyclosporine: Cyclosporine AUC and Cmax were determined before and after the administration of fluconazole 200 mg daily for 14 days in eight renal transplant patients who had been on cyclosporine therapy for at least 6 months and on a stable cyclosporine dose for at least 6 weeks. There was a significant increase in cyclosporine AUC, Cmax, Cmin (24-hour concentration), and a significant reduction in apparent oral clearance following the administration of fluconazole. The mean ± SD increase in AUC was 92% ± 43% (range: 18 to 147%). The Cmax increased 60% ± 48% (range: –5 to 133%). The Cmin increased 157% ± 96% (range: 33 to 360%). The apparent oral clearance decreased 45% ± 15% (range: –15 to –60%). (See **PRECAUTIONS.**)
Zidovudine: Plasma zidovudine concentrations were determined on two occasions (before and following fluconazole 200 mg daily for 15 days) in 13 volunteers with AIDS or ARC who were on a stable zidovudine dose for at least two weeks. There was a significant increase in zidovudine AUC following the administration of fluconazole. The mean ± SD increase in AUC was 20% ± 32% (range: –27 to 104%). The metabolite, GZDV, to parent drug ratio significantly decreased after the administration of fluconazole, from 7.6 ± 3.6 to 5.7 ± 2.2.
Theophylline: The pharmacokinetics of theophylline were determined from a single intravenous dose of aminophylline (6 mg/kg) before and after the oral administration of fluconazole 200 mg daily for 14 days in 16 normal male volunteers. There were significant increases in theophylline AUC, Cmax, and half-life with a corresponding decrease in clearance. The mean ± SD theophylline AUC increased 21% ± 16% (range: –5 to 48%). The Cmax increased 13% ± 17% (range: –13 to 40%). Theophylline clearance decreased 16% ± 11% (range: –32 to 5%). The half-life of theophylline increased from 6.6 ± 1.7 hours to 7.9 ± 1.5 hours. (See **PRECAUTIONS.**)
Terfenadine: Six healthy volunteers received terfenadine 60 mg BID for 15 days. Fluconazole 200 mg was administered daily from days 9 through 15. Fluconazole did not affect terfenadine plasma concentrations. Terfenadine acid metabolite AUC increased 36% ± 36% (range: 7 to 102%) from day 8 to day 15 with the concomitant administration of fluconazole. There was no change in cardiac repolarization as measured by Holter QTc intervals. Another study at a 400-mg and 800-mg daily dose of fluconazole demonstrated that DIFLUCAN taken in doses of 400 mg per day or greater significantly increases plasma levels of terfenadine when taken concomitantly. (See **CONTRAINDICATIONS** and **PRECAUTIONS.**)
Oral hypoglycemics: The effects of fluconazole on the pharmacokinetics of the sulfonylurea oral hypoglycemic agents tolbutamide, glipizide, and glyburide were evaluated in three placebo-controlled studies in normal volunteers. All subjects received the sulfonylurea alone as a single dose and again as a single dose following the administration of DIFLUCAN 100 mg daily for 7 days. In these three studies 22/46 (47.8%) of DIFLUCAN treated patients and 9/22 (40.1%) of placebo treated patients experienced symptoms consistent with hypoglycemia. (See **PRECAUTIONS.**)
Tolbutamide: In 13 normal male volunteers, there was significant increase in tolbutamide (500 mg single dose) AUC and Cmax following the administration of fluconazole. There was a mean ± SD increase in tolbutamide AUC of 26% ± 9% (range: 12 to 39%). Tolbutamide Cmax increased 11% ± 9% (range: –6 to 27%). (See **PRECAUTIONS.**)
Glipizide: The AUC and Cmax of glipizide (2.5 mg single dose) were significantly increased following the administration of fluconazole in 13 normal male volunteers.

There was a mean ± SD increase in AUC of 49% ± 13% (range: 27 to 73%) and an increase in Cmax of 19% ± 23% (range: –11 to 79%). (See **PRECAUTIONS**.)

Glyburide: The AUC and Cmax of glyburide (5 mg single dose) were significantly increased following the administration of fluconazole in 20 normal male volunteers. There was a mean ± SD increase in AUC of 44% ± 29% (range: –13 to 115%) and Cmax increased 19% ± 19% (range: –23 to 62%). Five subjects required oral glucose following the ingestion of glyburide after 7 days of fluconazole administration. (See **PRECAUTIONS**.)

Rifabutin: There have been published reports that an interaction exists when fluconazole is administered concomitantly with rifabutin, leading to increased serum levels of rifabutin. (See **PRECAUTIONS**.)

Tacrolimus: There have been published reports that an interaction exists when fluconazole is administered concomitantly with tacrolimus, leading to increased serum levels of tacrolimus. (See **PRECAUTIONS**.)

Cisapride: A preliminary report from a placebo-controlled, randomized multiple-dose study in subjects given fluconazole 200 mg daily and cisapride 20 mg four times daily starting after 7 days of fluconazole dosing found that fluconazole significantly increased the AUC and Cmax of cisapride both after single (AUC 102% and Cmax 92% increases) and multiple (AUC 192% and Cmax 153% increases) dosing of cisapride. Fluconazole significantly increased the QTc interval in subjects receiving cisapride 20 mg four times daily for 5 days. (See **CONTRAINDICATIONS** and **PRECAUTIONS**.)

Microbiology

Fluconazole exhibits *in vitro* activity against *Cryptococcus neoformans* and *Candida* spp. Fungistatic activity has also been demonstrated in normal and immunocompromised animal models for systemic and intracranial fungal infections due to *Cryptococcus neoformans* and for systemic infections due to *Candida albicans*.

In common with other azole antifungal agents, most fungi show a higher apparent sensitivity to fluconazole *in vivo* than *in vitro*. Fluconazole administered orally and/or intravenously was active in a variety of animal models of fungal infection using standard laboratory strains of fungi. Activity has been demonstrated against fungal infections caused by *Aspergillus flavus* and *Aspergillus fumigatus* in normal mice. Fluconazole has also been shown to be active in animal models of endemic mycoses, including one model of *Blastomyces dermatitidis* pulmonary infections in normal mice; one model of *Coccidioides immitis* intracranial infections in normal mice; and several models of *Histoplasma capsulatum* pulmonary infection in normal and immunosuppressed mice. The clinical significance of results obtained in these studies is unknown.

Oral fluconazole has been shown to be active in an animal model of vaginal candidiasis.

Concurrent administration of fluconazole and amphotericin B in infected normal and immunosuppressed mice showed the following results: a small additive antifungal effect in systemic infection with *C. albicans*, no interaction in intracranial infection with *Cr. neoformans*, and antagonism of the two drugs in systemic infection with *Asp. fumigatus*. The clinical significance of results obtained in these studies is unknown.

There have been reports of cases of superinfection with *Candida* species other than *C. albicans*, which are often inherently not susceptible to DIFLUCAN (e.g., *Candida krusei*). Such cases may require alternative antifungal therapy.

INDICATIONS AND USAGE

DIFLUCAN (fluconazole) is indicated for the treatment of:

1. Vaginal candidiasis (vaginal yeast infections due to *Candida*).
2. Oropharyngeal and esophageal candidiasis. In open noncomparative studies of relatively small numbers of patients, DIFLUCAN was also effective for the treatment of *Candida* urinary tract infections, peritonitis, and systemic *Candida* infections including candidemia, disseminated candidiasis, and pneumonia.
3. Cryptococcal meningitis. Before prescribing DIFLUCAN (fluconazole) for AIDS patients with cryptococcal meningitis, please see **CLINICAL STUDIES** section. Studies comparing DIFLUCAN to amphotericin B in non-HIV infected patients have not been conducted.

Prophylaxis. DIFLUCAN is also indicated to decrease the incidence of candidiasis in patients undergoing bone marrow transplantation who receive cytotoxic chemotherapy and/or radiation therapy.

Specimens for fungal culture and other relevant laboratory studies (serology, histopathology) should be obtained prior to therapy to isolate and identify causative organisms. Therapy may be instituted before the results of the cultures and other laboratory studies are known; however, once these results become available, anti-infective therapy should be adjusted accordingly.

CLINICAL STUDIES

Cryptococcal meningitis: In a multicenter study comparing DIFLUCAN (200 mg/day) to amphotericin B (0.3 mg/kg/day) for treatment of cryptococcal meningitis in patients with AIDS, a multivariate analysis revealed three pretreatment factors that predicted death during the course of therapy: abnormal mental status, cerebrospinal fluid cryptococcal antigen titer greater than 1:1024, and cerebrospinal fluid white blood cell count of less than 20 cells/mm^3. Mortality among high risk patients was 33% and 40% for amphotericin B and DIFLUCAN patients, respectively (p=0.58), with overall deaths 14% (9 of 63 subjects) and 18% (24 of 131 subjects) for the 2 arms of the study (p=0.48). Optimal doses and regimens for patients with acute cryptococcal meningitis and at high risk for treatment failure remain to be determined. (Saag, *et al.* N Engl J Med 1992; 326:83-9.)

Vaginal candidiasis: Two adequate and well-controlled studies were conducted in the U.S. using the 150 mg tablet. In both, the results of the fluconazole regimen were comparable to the control regimen (clotrimazole or miconazole intravaginally for 7 days) both clinically and statistically at the one month post-treatment evaluation.

The therapeutic cure rate, defined as a complete resolution of signs and symptoms of vaginal candidiasis (clinical cure), along with a negative KOH examination and negative culture for *Candida* (microbiologic eradication), was 55% in both the fluconazole group and the vaginal products group.

[See first table above]

	Fluconazole PO 150 mg tablet	Vaginal Product qhs × 7 days
Enrolled	448	422
Evaluable at Late Follow-up	347 (77%)	327 (77%)
Clinical cure	239/347 (69%)	235/327 (72%)
Mycologic erad.	213/347 (61%)	196/327 (60%)
Therapeutic cure	190/347 (55%)	179/327 (55%)

Approximately three-fourths of the enrolled patients had acute vaginitis (<4 episodes/12 months) and achieved 80% clinical cure, 67% mycologic eradication and 59% therapeutic cure when treated with a 150 mg DIFLUCAN tablet administered orally. These rates were comparable to control products. The remaining one-fourth of enrolled patients had recurrent vaginitis (≥4 episodes/12 months) and achieved 57% clinical cure, 47% mycologic eradication and 40% therapeutic cure. The numbers are too small to make meaningful clinical or statistical comparisons with vaginal products in the treatment of patients with recurrent vaginitis.

Substantially more gastrointestinal events were reported in the fluconazole group compared to the vaginal product group. Most of the events were mild to moderate. Because fluconazole was given as a single dose, no discontinuations occurred.

[See second table above]

Parameter	Fluconazole PO	Vaginal Products
Evaluable patients	448	422
With any adverse event	141 (31%)	112 (27%)
Nervous System	90 (20%)	69 (16%)
Gastrointestinal	73 (16%)	18 (4%)
With drug-related event	117 (26%)	67 (16%)
Nervous System	61 (14%)	29 (7%)
Headache	58 (13%)	28 (7%)
Gastrointestinal	68 (15%)	13 (3%)
Abdominal pain	25 (6%)	7 (2%)
Nausea	30 (7%)	3 (1%)
Diarrhea	12 (3%)	2 (<1%)
Application site event	0 (0%)	19 (5%)
Taste Perversion	6 (1%)	0 (0%)

Pediatric Studies

Oropharyngeal candidiasis: An open-label, comparative study of the efficacy and safety of DIFLUCAN (2-3 mg/kg/day) and oral nystatin (400,000 I.U. 4 times daily) in immunocompromised children with oropharyngeal candidiasis was conducted. Clinical and mycological response rates were higher in the children treated with fluconazole.

Clinical cure at the end of treatment was reported for 86% of fluconazole treated patients compared to 46% of nystatin treated patients. Mycologically, 76% of fluconazole treated patients had the infecting organism eradicated compared to 11% for nystatin treated patients.

	Fluconazole	Nystatin
Enrolled	96	90
Clinical Cure	76/88 (86%)	36/78 (46%)
Mycological eradication*	55/72 (76%)	6/54 (11%)

*Subjects without follow-up cultures for any reason were considered nonevaluable for mycological response.

The proportion of patients with clinical relapse 2 weeks after the end of treatment was 14% for subjects receiving DIFLUCAN and 16% for subjects receiving nystatin. At 4 weeks after the end of treatment the percentages of patients with clinical relapse were 22% for DIFLUCAN and 23% for nystatin.

CONTRAINDICATIONS

DIFLUCAN (fluconazole) is contraindicated in patients who have shown hypersensitivity to fluconazole or to any of its excipients. There is no information regarding cross-hypersensitivity between fluconazole and other azole antifungal agents. Caution should be used in prescribing DIFLUCAN to patients with hypersensitivity to other azoles. Coadministration of terfenadine is contraindicated in patients receiving DIFLUCAN (fluconazole) at multiple doses of 400 mg or higher based upon results of a multiple dose interaction study. Coadministration of cisapride is contraindicated in patients receiving DIFLUCAN (fluconazole). (See **CLINICAL PHARMACOLOGY: Drug Interaction Studies** and **PRECAUTIONS**.)

WARNINGS

(1) Hepatic injury: DIFLUCAN has been associated with rare cases of serious hepatic toxicity, including fatalities primarily in patients with serious underlying medical conditions. In cases of DIFLUCAN-associated hepatotoxicity, no obvious relationship to total daily dose, duration of therapy, sex or age of the patient has been observed.

DIFLUCAN hepatotoxicity has usually, but not always, been reversible on discontinuation of therapy. Patients who develop abnormal liver function tests during DIFLUCAN therapy should be monitored for the development of more severe hepatic injury. DIFLUCAN should be discontinued if clinical signs and symptoms consistent with liver disease develop that may be attributable to DIFLUCAN.

(2) Anaphylaxis: In rare cases, anaphylaxis has been reported.

(3) Dermatologic: Patients have rarely developed exfoliative skin disorders during treatment with DIFLUCAN. In patients with serious underlying diseases (predominantly AIDS and malignancy), these have rarely resulted in a fatal outcome. Patients who develop rashes during treatment with DIFLUCAN should be monitored closely and the drug discontinued if lesions progress.

PRECAUTIONS

General

Some azoles, including fluconazole, have been associated with prolongation of the QT interval on the electrocardiogram. During post-marketing surveillance, there have been very rare cases of QT prolongation and torsade de pointes in patients taking fluconazole. These reports included seriously ill patients with multiple confounding risk factors, such as structural heart disease, electrolyte abnormalities and concomitant medications that may have been contributory.

Fluconazole should be administered with caution to patients with these potentially proarrhythmic conditions.

Single Dose

The convenience and efficacy of the single dose oral tablet of fluconazole regimen for the treatment of vaginal yeast infections should be weighed against the acceptability of a higher incidence of drug related adverse events with DIFLUCAN (26%) versus intravaginal agents (16%) in U.S. comparative clinical studies. (See **ADVERSE REACTIONS** and **CLINICAL STUDIES**.)

Drug Interactions: (See **CLINICAL PHARMACOLOGY: Drug Interaction Studies** and **CONTRAINDICATIONS**.) Clinically or potentially significant drug interactions between DIFLUCAN and the following agents/classes have been observed. These are described in greater detail below:

Oral hypoglycemics
Coumarin-type anticoagulants
Phenytoin
Cyclosporine
Rifampin
Theophylline
Terfenadine
Cisapride
Astemizole
Rifabutin
Tacrolimus

Oral hypoglycemics: Clinically significant hypoglycemia may be precipitated by the use of DIFLUCAN with oral hypoglycemic agents; one fatality has been reported from hypoglycemia in association with combined DIFLUCAN and glyburide use. DIFLUCAN reduces the metabolism of tolbutamide, glyburide, and glipizide and increases the plasma concentration of these agents. When DIFLUCAN is used concomitantly with these or other sulfonylurea oral hypoglycemic agents, blood glucose concentrations should be carefully monitored and the dose of the sulfonylurea should be adjusted as necessary. (See **CLINICAL PHARMACOLOGY: Drug Interaction Studies.**)

Coumarin-type anticoagulants: Prothrombin time may be increased in patients receiving concomitant DIFLUCAN and coumarin-type anticoagulants. Careful monitoring of prothrombin time in patients receiving DIFLUCAN and

Continued on next page

Diflucan—Cont.

coumarin-type anticoagulants is recommended. (See **CLINICAL PHARMACOLOGY: Drug Interaction Studies.**)
Phenytoin: DIFLUCAN increases the plasma concentrations of phenytoin. Careful monitoring of phenytoin concentrations in patients receiving DIFLUCAN and phenytoin is recommended. (See **CLINICAL PHARMACOLOGY: Drug Interaction Studies.**)
Cyclosporine: DIFLUCAN may significantly increase cyclosporine levels in renal transplant patients with or without renal impairment. Careful monitoring of cyclosporine concentrations and serum creatinine is recommended in patients receiving DIFLUCAN and cyclosporine. (See **CLINICAL PHARMACOLOGY: Drug Interaction Studies.**)
Rifampin: Rifampin enhances the metabolism of concurrently administered DIFLUCAN. Depending on clinical circumstances, consideration should be given to increasing the dose of DIFLUCAN when it is administered with rifampin. (See **CLINICAL PHARMACOLOGY: Drug Interaction Studies.**)
Theophylline: DIFLUCAN increases the serum concentrations of theophylline. Careful monitoring of serum theophylline concentrations in patients receiving DIFLUCAN and theophylline is recommended. (See **CLINICAL PHARMACOLOGY: Drug Interaction Studies.**)
Terfenadine: Because of the occurrence of serious cardiac dysrhythmias secondary to prolongation of the QTc interval in patients receiving azole antifungals in conjunction with terfenadine, interaction studies have been performed. One study at a 200-mg daily dose of fluconazole failed to demonstrate a prolongation in QTc interval. Another study at a 400-mg and 800-mg daily dose of fluconazole demonstrated that DIFLUCAN taken in doses of 400 mg per day or greater significantly increases plasma levels of terfenadine when taken concomitantly. The combined use of fluconazole at doses of 400 mg or greater with terfenadine is contraindicated. (See **CONTRAINDICATIONS** and **CLINICAL PHARMACOLOGY: Drug Interaction Studies.**) The coadministration of fluconazole at doses lower than 400 mg/day with terfenadine should be carefully monitored.
Cisapride: There have been reports of cardiac events, including torsade de pointes in patients to whom fluconazole and cisapride were coadministered. The combined use of fluconazole with cisapride is contraindicated. (See **CONTRAINDICATIONS** and **CLINICAL PHARMACOLOGY: Drug Interaction Studies.**)
Astemizole: The use of fluconazole in patients concurrently taking astemizole or other drugs metabolized by the cytochrome P450 system may be associated with elevations in serum levels of these drugs. In the absence of definitive information, caution should be used when coadministering fluconazole. Patients should be carefully monitored.
Rifabutin: There have been reports of uveitis in patients to whom fluconazole and rifabutin were coadministered. Patients receiving rifabutin and fluconazole concomitantly should be carefully monitored. (See **CLINICAL PHARMACOLOGY: Drug Interaction Studies.**)
Tacrolimus: There have been reports of nephrotoxicity in patients to whom fluconazole and tacrolimus were coadministered. Patients receiving tacrolimus and fluconazole concomitantly should be carefully monitored. (See **CLINICAL PHARMACOLOGY: Drug Interaction Studies.**)
Fluconazole tablets coadministered with ethinyl estradiol- and levonorgestrel-containing oral contraceptives produced an overall mean increase in ethinyl estradiol and levonorgestrel levels; however, in some patients there were decreases up to 47% and 33% of ethinyl estradiol and levonorgestrel levels. (See **CLINICAL PHARMACOLOGY: Drug Interaction Studies.**) The data presently available indicate that the decreases in some individual ethinyl estradiol and levonorgestrel AUC values with fluconazole treatment are likely the result of random variation. While there is evidence that fluconazole can inhibit the metabolism of ethinyl estradiol and levonorgestrel, there is no evidence that fluconazole is a net inducer of ethinyl estradiol or levonorgestrel metabolism. The clinical significance of these effects is presently unknown.
Physicians should be aware that interaction studies with medications other than those listed in the **CLINICAL PHARMACOLOGY** section have not been conducted, but such interactions may occur.

Carcinogenesis, Mutagenesis and Impairment of Fertility
Fluconazole showed no evidence of carcinogenic potential in mice and rats treated orally for 24 months at doses of 2.5, 5 or 10 mg/kg/day (approximately 2-7× the recommended human dose). Male rats treated with 5 and 10 mg/kg/day had an increased incidence of hepatocellular adenomas.
Fluconazole, with or without metabolic activation, was negative in tests for mutagenicity in 4 strains of *S. typhimurium*, and in the mouse lymphoma L5178Y system. Cytogenetic studies *in vivo* (murine bone marrow cells, following oral administration of fluconazole) and *in vitro* (human lymphocytes exposed to fluconazole at 1000 µg/mL) showed no evidence of chromosomal mutations.
Fluconazole did not affect the fertility of male or female rats treated orally with daily doses of 5, 10 or 20 mg/kg or with parenteral doses of 5, 25 or 75 mg/kg, although the onset of parturition was slightly delayed at 20 mg/kg PO. In an intravenous perinatal study in rats at 5, 20 and 40 mg/kg, dystocia and prolongation of parturition were observed in a few dams at 20 mg/kg (approximately 5-15× the recommended human dose) and 40 mg/kg, but not at 5 mg/kg. The disturbances in parturition were reflected by a slight increase in the number of still-born pups and decrease of neonatal survival at these dose levels. The effects on parturition in rats are consistent with the species specific estrogen-lowering property produced by high doses of fluconazole. Such a hormone change has not been observed in women treated with fluconazole. (See **CLINICAL PHARMACOLOGY.**)

Pregnancy
Teratogenic Effects. Pregnancy Category C: Fluconazole was administered orally to pregnant rabbits during organogenesis in two studies, at 5, 10 and 20 mg/kg and at 5, 25, and 75 mg/kg, respectively. Maternal weight gain was impaired at all dose levels, and abortions occurred at 75 mg/kg (approximately 20-60× the recommended human dose); no adverse fetal effects were detected. In several studies in which pregnant rats were treated orally with fluconazole during organogenesis, maternal weight gain was impaired and placental weights were increased at 25 mg/kg. There were no fetal effects at 5 or 10 mg/kg; increases in fetal anatomical variants (supernumerary ribs, renal pelvis dilation) and delays in ossification were observed at 25 and 50 mg/kg and higher doses. At doses ranging from 80 mg/kg (approximately 20-60× the recommended human dose) to 320 mg/kg embryolethality in rats was increased and fetal abnormalities included wavy ribs, cleft palate and abnormal cranio-facial ossification. These effects are consistent with the inhibition of estrogen synthesis in rats and may be a result of known effects of lowered estrogen on pregnancy, organogenesis and parturition.
There are no adequate and well controlled studies in pregnant women. There have been reports of multiple congenital abnormalities in infants whose mothers were being treated for 3 or more months with high dose (400-800 mg/day) fluconazole therapy for coccidioidomycosis (an unindicated use). The relationship between fluconazole use and these events is unclear. DIFLUCAN should be used in pregnancy only if the potential benefit justifies the possible risk to the fetus.

Nursing Mothers
Fluconazole is secreted in human milk at concentrations similar to plasma. Therefore, the use of DIFLUCAN in nursing mothers is not recommended.

Pediatric Use
An open-label, randomized, controlled trial has shown DIFLUCAN to be effective in the treatment of oropharyngeal candidiasis in children 6 months to 13 years of age. (See **CLINICAL STUDIES.**)
The use of DIFLUCAN in children with cryptococcal meningitis, *Candida* esophagitis, or systemic *Candida* infections is supported by the efficacy shown for these indications in adults and by the results from several small noncomparative pediatric clinical studies. In addition, pharmacokinetic studies in children (see **CLINICAL PHARMACOLOGY**) have established a dose proportionality between children and adults. (See **DOSAGE AND ADMINISTRATION.**)
In a noncomparative study of children with serious systemic fungal infections, most of which were candidemia, the effectiveness of DIFLUCAN was similar to that reported for the treatment of candidemia in adults. Of 17 subjects with culture-confirmed candidemia, 11 of 14 (79%) with baseline symptoms (3 were asymptomatic) had a clinical cure; 13/15 (87%) of evaluable patients had a mycologic cure at the end of treatment but two of these patients relapsed at 10 and 18 days, respectively, following cessation of therapy.
The efficacy of DIFLUCAN for the suppression of cryptococcal meningitis was successful in 4 of 5 children treated in a compassionate-use study of fluconazole for the treatment of life-threatening or serious mycosis. There is no information regarding the efficacy of fluconazole for primary treatment of cryptococcal meningitis in children.
The safety profile of DIFLUCAN in children has been studied in 577 children ages 1 day to 17 years who received doses ranging from 1 to 15 mg/kg/day for 1 to 1,616 days. (See **ADVERSE REACTIONS.**)
Efficacy of DIFLUCAN has not been established in infants less than 6 months of age. (See **CLINICAL PHARMACOLOGY.**) A small number of patients (29) ranging in age from 1 day to 6 months have been treated safely with DIFLUCAN.

ADVERSE REACTIONS

In Patients Receiving a Single Dose for Vaginal Candidiasis:
During comparative clinical studies conducted in the United States, 448 patients with vaginal candidiasis were treated with DIFLUCAN, 150 mg single dose. The overall incidence of side effects possibly related to DIFLUCAN was 26%. In 422 patients receiving active comparative agents, the incidence was 16%. The most common treatment-related adverse events reported in the patients who received 150 mg single dose fluconazole for vaginitis were headache (13%), nausea (7%), and abdominal pain (6%). Other side effects reported with an incidence equal to or greater than 1% included diarrhea (3%), dyspepsia (1%), dizziness (1%), and taste perversion (1%). Most of the reported side effects were mild to moderate in severity. Rarely, angioedema and anaphylactic reaction have been reported in marketing experience.

In Patients Receiving Multiple Doses for Other Infections:
Sixteen percent of over 4000 patients treated with DIFLUCAN (fluconazole) in clinical trials of 7 days or more experienced adverse events. Treatment was discontinued in 1.5% of patients due to adverse clinical events and in 1.3% of patients due to laboratory test abnormalities.
Clinical adverse events were reported more frequently in HIV infected patients (21%) than in non-HIV infected patients (13%); however, the patterns in HIV infected and non-HIV infected patients were similar. The proportions of patients discontinuing therapy due to clinical adverse events were similar in the two groups (1.5%).
The following treatment-related clinical adverse events occurred at an incidence of 1% or greater in 4048 patients receiving DIFLUCAN for 7 or more days in clinical trials: nausea 3.7%, headache 1.9%, skin rash 1.8%, vomiting 1.7%, abdominal pain 1.7%, and diarrhea 1.5%.
The following adverse events have occurred under conditions where a causal association is probable:
Hepatobiliary: In combined clinical trials and marketing experience, there have been rare cases of serious hepatic reactions during treatment with DIFLUCAN. (See **WARNINGS.**) The spectrum of these hepatic reactions has ranged from mild transient elevations in transaminases to clinical hepatitis, cholestasis and fulminant hepatic failure, including fatalities. Instances of fatal hepatic reactions were noted to occur primarily in patients with serious underlying medical conditions (predominantly AIDS or malignancy) and often while taking multiple concomitant medications. Transient hepatic reactions, including hepatitis and jaundice, have occurred among patients with no other identifiable risk factors. In each of these cases, liver function returned to baseline on discontinuation of DIFLUCAN.
In two comparative trials evaluating the efficacy of DIFLUCAN for the suppression of relapse of cryptococcal meningitis, a statistically significant increase was observed in median AST (SGOT) levels from a baseline value of 30 IU/L to 41 IU/L in one trial and 34 IU/L to 66 IU/L in the other. The overall rate of serum transaminase elevations of more than 8 times the upper limit of normal was approximately 1% in fluconazole-treated patients in clinical trials. These elevations occurred in patients with severe underlying disease, predominantly AIDS or malignancies, most of whom were receiving multiple concomitant medications, including many known to be hepatotoxic. The incidence of abnormally elevated serum transaminases was greater in patients taking DIFLUCAN concomitantly with one or more of the following medications: rifampin, phenytoin, isoniazid, valproic acid, or oral sulfonylurea hypoglycemic agents.
Immunologic: In rare cases, anaphylaxis has been reported.
The following adverse events have occurred under conditions where a causal association is uncertain:
Cardiovascular: QT prolongation, torsade de pointes. (See **PRECAUTIONS.**)
Central Nervous System: Seizures.
Dermatologic: Exfoliative skin disorders including Stevens-Johnson syndrome and toxic epidermal necrolysis (see **WARNINGS**), alopecia.
Hematopoietic and *Lymphatic:* Leukopenia, including neutropenia and agranulocytosis, thrombocytopenia.
Metabolic: Hypercholesterolemia, hypertriglyceridemia, hypokalemia.

Adverse Reactions in Children:
In Phase II/III clinical trials conducted in the United States and in Europe, 577 pediatric patients, ages 1 day to 17 years were treated with DIFLUCAN at doses up to 15 mg/kg/day for up to 1,616 days. Thirteen percent of children experienced treatment related adverse events. The most commonly reported events were vomiting (5%), abdominal pain (3%), nausea (2%), and diarrhea (2%). Treatment was discontinued in 2.3% of patients due to adverse clinical events and in 1.4% of patients due to laboratory test abnormalities. The majority of treatment-related laboratory abnormalities were elevations of transaminases or alkaline phosphatase.

Percentage of Patients With Treatment-Related Side Effects

	Fluconazole (N=577)	Comparative Agents (N=451)
With any side effect	13.0	9.3
Vomiting	5.4	5.1
Abdominal pain	2.8	1.6
Nausea	2.3	1.6
Diarrhea	2.1	2.2

OVERDOSAGE

There has been one reported case of overdosage with DIFLUCAN (fluconazole). A 42-year-old patient infected with human immunodeficiency virus developed hallucinations and exhibited paranoid behavior after reportedly ingesting 8200 mg of DIFLUCAN. The patient was admitted to the hospital, and his condition resolved within 48 hours.
In the event of overdose, symptomatic treatment (with supportive measures and gastric lavage if clinically indicated) should be instituted.
Fluconazole is largely excreted in urine. A three-hour hemodialysis session decreases plasma levels by approximately 50%.
In mice and rats receiving very high doses of fluconazole, clinical effects in both species included decreased motility and respiration, ptosis, lacrimation, salivation, urinary incontinence, loss of righting reflex and cyanosis; death was sometimes preceded by clonic convulsions.

DOSAGE AND ADMINISTRATION

Dosage and Administration in Adults:
Single Dose
Vaginal candidiasis: The recommended dosage of DIFLUCAN for vaginal candidiasis is 150 mg as a single oral dose.

Multiple Dose

SINCE ORAL ABSORPTION IS RAPID AND ALMOST COMPLETE, THE DAILY DOSE OF DIFLUCAN (FLUCONAZOLE) IS THE SAME FOR ORAL (TABLETS AND SUSPENSION) AND INTRAVENOUS ADMINISTRATION. In general, a loading dose of twice the daily dose is recommended on the first day of therapy to result in plasma concentrations close to steady-state by the second day of therapy.

The daily dose of DIFLUCAN for the treatment of infections other than vaginal candidiasis should be based on the infecting organism and the patient's response to therapy. Treatment should be continued until clinical parameters or laboratory tests indicate that active fungal infection has subsided. An inadequate period of treatment may lead to recurrence of active infection. Patients with AIDS and cryptococcal meningitis or recurrent oropharyngeal candidiasis usually require maintenance therapy to prevent relapse.

Oropharyngeal candidiasis: The recommended dosage of DIFLUCAN for oropharyngeal candidiasis is 200 mg on the first day, followed by 100 mg once daily. Clinical evidence of oropharyngeal candidiasis generally resolves within several days, but treatment should be continued for at least 2 weeks to decrease the likelihood of relapse.

Esophageal candidiasis: The recommended dosage of DIFLUCAN for esophageal candidiasis is 200 mg on the first day, followed by 100 mg once daily. Doses up to 400 mg/day may be used, based on medical judgment of the patient's response to therapy. Patients with esophageal candidiasis should be treated for a minimum of three weeks and for at least two weeks following resolution of symptoms.

Systemic Candida infections: For systemic *Candida* infections including candidemia, disseminated candidiasis, and pneumonia, optimal therapeutic dosage and duration of therapy have not been established. In open, noncomparative studies of small numbers of patients, doses of up to 400 mg daily have been used.

Urinary tract infections and peritonitis: For the treatment of *Candida* urinary tract infections and peritonitis, daily doses of 50-200 mg have been used in open, noncomparative studies of small numbers of patients.

Cryptococcal meningitis: The recommended dosage for treatment of acute cryptococcal meningitis is 400 mg on the first day, followed by 200 mg once daily. A dosage of 400 mg once daily may be used, based on medical judgment of the patient's response to therapy. The recommended duration of treatment for initial therapy of cryptococcal meningitis is 10-12 weeks after the cerebrospinal fluid becomes culture negative. The recommended dosage of DIFLUCAN for suppression of relapse of cryptococcal meningitis in patients with AIDS is 200 mg once daily.

Prophylaxis in patients undergoing bone marrow transplantation: The recommended DIFLUCAN daily dosage for the prevention of candidiasis of patients undergoing bone marrow transplantation is 400 mg, once daily. Patients who are anticipated to have severe granulocytopenia (less than 500 neutrophils per cu mm) should start DIFLUCAN prophylaxis several days before the anticipated onset of neutropenia, and continue for 7 days after the neutrophil count rises above 1000 cells per cu mm.

Dosage and Administration in Children:

The following dose equivalency scheme should generally provide equivalent exposure in pediatric and adult patients:

Pediatric Patients	Adults
3 mg/kg	100 mg
6 mg/kg	200 mg
12* mg/kg	400 mg

*Some older children may have clearances similar to that of adults. Absolute doses exceeding 600 mg/day are not recommended.

Experience with DIFLUCAN in neonates is limited to pharmacokinetic studies in premature newborns. (See **CLINICAL PHARMACOLOGY**.) Based on the prolonged half-life seen in premature newborns (gestational age 26 to 29 weeks), these children, in the first two weeks of life, should receive the same dosage (mg/kg) as in older children, but administered every 72 hours. After the first two weeks, these children should be dosed once daily. No information regarding DIFLUCAN pharmacokinetics in full-term newborns is available.

Oropharyngeal candidiasis: The recommended dosage of DIFLUCAN for oropharyngeal candidiasis in children is 6 mg/kg on the first day, followed by 3 mg/kg once daily. Treatment should be administered for at least 2 weeks to decrease the likelihood of relapse.

Esophageal candidiasis: For the treatment of esophageal candidiasis, the recommended dosage of DIFLUCAN in children is 6 mg/kg on the first day, followed by 3 mg/kg once daily. Doses up to 12 mg/kg/day may be used based on medical judgment of the patient's response to therapy. Patients with esophageal candidiasis should be treated for a minimum of three weeks and for at least 2 weeks following the resolution of symptoms.

Systemic Candida infections: For the treatment of candidemia and disseminated *Candida* infections, daily doses of 6-12 mg/kg/day have been used in an open, noncomparative study of a small number of children.

Cryptococcal meningitis: For the treatment of acute cryptococcal meningitis, the recommended dosage is 12 mg/kg on the first day, followed by 6 mg/kg once daily. A dosage of 12 mg/kg once daily may be used, based on medical judgment of the patient's response to therapy. The recommended duration of treatment for initial therapy of cryptococcal meningitis is 10-12 weeks after the cerebrospinal fluid becomes culture negative. For suppression of relapse of cryptococcal meningitis in children with AIDS, the recommended dose of DIFLUCAN is 6 mg/kg once daily.

Dosage In Patients With Impaired Renal Function:

Fluconazole is cleared primarily by renal excretion as unchanged drug. There is no need to adjust single dose therapy for vaginal candidiasis because of impaired renal function. In patients with impaired renal function who will receive multiple doses of DIFLUCAN, an initial loading dose of 50 to 400 mg should be given. After the loading dose, the daily dose (according to indication) should be based on the following table:

Creatinine Clearance (mL/min)	Percent of Recommended Dose
>50	100%
≤50 (no dialysis)	50%
Regular dialysis	100% after each dialysis

These are suggested dose adjustments based on pharmacokinetics following administration of multiple doses. Further adjustment may be needed depending upon clinical condition.

When serum creatinine is the only measure of renal function available, the following formula (based on sex, weight, and age of the patient) should be used to estimate the creatinine clearance in adults:

$$\text{Males: } \frac{\text{Weight (kg)} \times (140\text{-age})}{72 \times \text{serum creatinine (mg/100 mL)}}$$

Females: 0.85 × above value

Although the pharmacokinetics of fluconazole has not been studied in children with renal insufficiency, dosage reduction in children with renal insufficiency should parallel that recommended for adults. The following formula may be used to estimate creatinine clearance in children:

$$K \times \frac{\text{linear length or height (cm)}}{\text{serum creatinine (mg/100 mL)}}$$

(Where K=0.55 for children older than 1 year and 0.45 for infants.)

Administration

DIFLUCAN may be administered either orally or by intravenous infusion. DIFLUCAN injection has been used safely for up to fourteen days of intravenous therapy. The intravenous infusion of DIFLUCAN should be administered at a maximum rate of approximately 200 mg/hour, given as a continuous infusion.

DIFLUCAN injections in glass and Viaflex® Plus plastic containers are intended only for intravenous administration using sterile equipment.

Parenteral drug products should be inspected visually for particulate matter and discoloration prior to administration whenever solution and container permit.

Do not use if the solution is cloudy or precipitated or if the seal is not intact.

Directions for Mixing the Oral Suspension

Prepare a suspension at time of dispensing as follows: tap bottle until all the powder flows freely. To reconstitute, add 24 mL of distilled water or Purified Water (USP) to fluconazole bottle and shake vigorously to suspend powder. Each bottle will deliver 35 mL of suspension. The concentrations of the reconstituted suspensions are as follows:

Fluconazole Content per Bottle	Concentration of Reconstituted Suspension
350 mg	10 mg/mL
1400 mg	40 mg/mL

Note: Shake oral suspension well before using. Store reconstituted suspension between 86°F (30°C) and 41°F (5°C) and discard unused portion after 2 weeks. Protect from freezing.

Directions for IV Use of DIFLUCAN in Viaflex® Plus Plastic Containers

Do not remove unit from overwrap until ready for use. The overwrap is a moisture barrier. The inner bag maintains the sterility of the product.

CAUTION: Do not use plastic containers in series connections. Such use could result in air embolism due to residual air being drawn from the primary container before administration of the fluid from the secondary container is completed.

To Open

Tear overwrap down side at slit and remove solution container. Some opacity of the plastic due to moisture absorption during the sterilization process may be observed. This is normal and does not affect the solution quality or safety. The opacity will diminish gradually. After removing overwrap, check for minute leaks by squeezing inner bag firmly. If leaks are found, discard solution as sterility may be impaired.

DO NOT ADD SUPPLEMENTARY MEDICATION.

Preparation for Administration:

1. Suspend container from eyelet support.
2. Remove plastic protector from outlet port at bottom of container.
3. Attach administration set. Refer to complete directions accompanying set.

HOW SUPPLIED

DIFLUCAN® Tablets: Pink trapezoidal tablets containing 50, 100 or 200 mg of fluconazole are packaged in bottles or unit dose blisters. The 150 mg fluconazole tablets are pink and oval shaped, packaged in a single dose unit blister.

DIFLUCAN® Tablets are supplied as follows:

DIFLUCAN® 50 mg Tablets: Engraved with "DIFLUCAN" and "50" on the front and "ROERIG" on the back.

NDC 0049-3410-30 Bottles of 30

DIFLUCAN® 100 mg Tablets: Engraved with "DIFLUCAN" and "100" on the front and "ROERIG" on the back.

NDC 0049-3420-30 Bottles of 30
NDC 0049-3420-41 Unit dose package of 100

DIFLUCAN® 150 mg Tablets: Engraved with "DIFLUCAN" and "150" on the front and "ROERIG" on the back.

NDC 0049-3500-79 Unit dose package of 1

DIFLUCAN® 200 mg Tablets: Engraved with "DIFLUCAN" and "200" on the front and "ROERIG" on the back.

NDC 0049-3430-30 Bottles of 30
NDC 0049-3430-41 Unit dose package of 100

Storage: Store tablets below 86°F (30°C).

DIFLUCAN® for Oral Suspension: DIFLUCAN® for oral suspension is supplied as an orange-flavored powder to provide 35 mL per bottle as follows:

NDC 0049-3440-19 Fluconazole 350 mg per bottle
NDC 0049-3450-19 Fluconazole 1400 mg per bottle

Storage: Store dry powder below 86°F (30°C). Store reconstituted suspension between 86°F (30°C) and 41°F (5°C) and discard unused portion after 2 weeks. Protect from freezing.

DIFLUCAN® Injections: DIFLUCAN® injections for intravenous infusion administration are formulated as sterile iso-osmotic solutions containing 2 mg/mL of fluconazole. They are supplied in glass bottles or in Viaflex® Plus plastic containers containing volumes of 100 mL or 200 mL affording doses of 200 mg and 400 mg of fluconazole, respectively. DIFLUCAN® injections in Viaflex® Plus plastic containers are available in both sodium chloride and dextrose diluents.

DIFLUCAN® Injections in Glass Bottles:

NDC 0049-3371-26 Fluconazole in Sodium Chloride Diluent 200 mg/100 mL × 6

NDC 0049-3372-26 Fluconazole in Sodium Chloride Diluent 400 mg/200 mL × 6

Storage: Store between 86°F (30°C) and 41°F (5°C). Protect from freezing.

DIFLUCAN® Injections in Viaflex® Plus Plastic Containers:

NDC 0049-3435-26 Fluconazole in Sodium Chloride Diluent 200 mg/100 mL × 6

NDC 0049-3436-26 Fluconazole in Sodium Chloride Diluent 400 mg/200 mL × 6

NDC 0049-3437-26 Fluconazole in Dextrose Diluent 200 mg/100 mL × 6

NDC 0049-3438-26 Fluconazole in Dextrose Diluent 400 mg/200 mL × 6

Storage: Store between 77°F (25°C) and 41°F (5°C). Brief exposure up to 104°F (40°C) does not adversely affect the product. Protect from freezing.

Rx only

Pfizer Roerig

Division of Pfizer Inc, NY, NY 10017

70-4526-00-8 Revised June 2003

Shown in Product Identification Guide, page 329

GEODON® ℞

[gē-ō-dōn]

(ziprasidone HCl)

GEODON® for Injection

(ziprasidone mesylate)

FOR IM USE ONLY

DESCRIPTION

GEODON® is available as GEODON Capsules (ziprasidone hydrochloride) for oral administration and as GEODON for Injection (ziprasidone mesylate) for intramuscular injection. Ziprasidone is an antipsychotic agent that is chemically unrelated to phenothiazine or butyrophenone antipsychotic agents. It has a molecular weight of 412.94 (free base), with the following chemical name: 5-[2-[4-(1,2-benzisothiazol-3-yl)-1-piperazinyl]ethyl]-6-chloro-1,3-dihydro-2*H*-indol-2-one. The empirical formula of $C_{21}H_{21}ClN_4OS$ (free base of ziprasidone) represents the following structural formula:

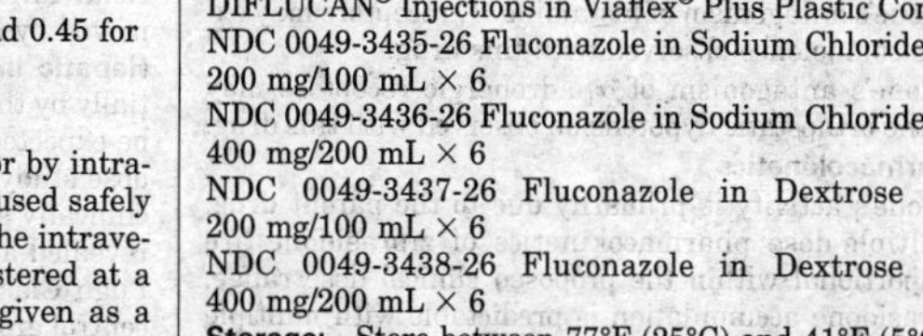

GEODON Capsules contain a monohydrochloride, monohydrate salt of ziprasidone. Chemically, ziprasidone hydrochloride monohydrate is 5-[2-[4-(1,2-benzisothiazol-3-yl)-1-piperazinyl]ethyl]-6-chloro-1,3-dihydro-2*H*-indol-2-one, monohydrochloride, monohydrate. The empirical formula is $C_{21}H_{21}ClN_4OS \cdot HCl \cdot H_2O$ and its molecular weight is 467.42. Ziprasidone hydrochloride monohydrate is a white to slightly pink powder.

Continued on next page

Geodon—Cont.

GEODON Capsules are supplied for oral administration in 20 mg (blue/white), 40 mg (blue/blue), 60 mg (white/white), and 80 mg (blue/white) capsules. GEODON Capsules contain ziprasidone hydrochloride monohydrate, lactose, pregelatinized starch, and magnesium stearate.

GEODON for Injection contains a lyophilized form of ziprasidone mesylate trihydrate. Chemically, ziprasidone mesylate trihydrate is 5-[2-[4-(1,2-benzisothiazol-3-yl)-1-piperazinyl]ethyl]-6-chloro-1,3-dihydro-2*H*-indol-2-one, methanesulfonate, trihydrate. The empirical formula is $C_{21}H_{21}ClN_4OS \bullet CH_3SO_3H \bullet 3H_2O$ and its molecular weight is 563.09.

GEODON for Injection is available in a single dose vial as ziprasidone mesylate (20 mg ziprasidone/mL when reconstituted according to label instructions - see **Preparation for Administration**) for intramuscular administration. Each mL of ziprasidone mesylate for injection (when reconstituted) contains 20 mg of ziprasidone and 4.7 mg of methanesulfonic acid solubilized by 294 mg of sulfobutylether β-cyclodextrin sodium (SBECD).

CLINICAL PHARMACOLOGY

Pharmacodynamics

Ziprasidone exhibited high *in vitro* binding affinity for the dopamine D_2 and D_3, the serotonin $5HT_{2A}$, $5HT_{2C}$, $5HT_{1A}$, $5HT_{1D}$, and α_1-adrenergic receptors (K_i s of 4.8, 7.2, 0.4, 1.3, 3.4, 2, and 10 nM, respectively), and moderate affinity for the histamine H_1 receptor (K_i=47 nM). Ziprasidone functioned as an antagonist at the D_2, $5HT_{2A}$, and $5HT_{1D}$ receptors, and as an agonist at the $5HT_{1A}$ receptor. Ziprasidone inhibited synaptic reuptake of serotonin and norepinephrine. No appreciable affinity was exhibited for other receptor/binding sites tested, including the cholinergic muscarinic receptor (IC_{50} >1 μM).

The mechanism of action of ziprasidone, as with other drugs having efficacy in schizophrenia, is unknown. However, it has been proposed that this drug's efficacy in schizophrenia is mediated through a combination of dopamine type 2 (D_2) and serotonin type 2 ($5HT_2$) antagonism. Antagonism at receptors other than dopamine and $5HT_2$ with similar receptor affinities may explain some of the other therapeutic and side effects of ziprasidone.

Ziprasidone's antagonism of histamine H_1 receptors may explain the somnolence observed with this drug.

Ziprasidone's antagonism of α_1-adrenergic receptors may explain the orthostatic hypotension observed with this drug.

Oral Pharmacokinetics

Ziprasidone's activity is primarily due to the parent drug. The multiple-dose pharmacokinetics of ziprasidone are dose-proportional within the proposed clinical dose range, and ziprasidone accumulation is predictable with multiple dosing. Elimination of ziprasidone is mainly via hepatic metabolism with a mean terminal half-life of about 7 hours within the proposed clinical dose range. Steady-state concentrations are achieved within one to three days of dosing. The mean apparent systemic clearance is 7.5 mL/min/kg. Ziprasidone is unlikely to interfere with the metabolism of drugs metabolized by cytochrome P450 enzymes.

Absorption: Ziprasidone is well absorbed after oral administration, reaching peak plasma concentrations in 6 to 8 hours. The absolute bioavailability of a 20 mg dose under fed conditions is approximately 60%. The absorption of ziprasidone is increased up to two-fold in the presence of food.

Distribution: Ziprasidone has a mean apparent volume of distribution of 1.5 L/kg. It is greater than 99% bound to plasma proteins, binding primarily to albumin and α_1-acid glycoprotein. The *in vitro* plasma protein binding of ziprasidone was not altered by warfarin or propranolol, two highly protein-bound drugs, nor did ziprasidone alter the binding of these drugs in human plasma. Thus, the potential for drug interactions with ziprasidone due to displacement is minimal.

Metabolism and Elimination: Ziprasidone is extensively metabolized after oral administration with only a small amount excreted in the urine (<1%) or feces (<4%) as unchanged drug. Ziprasidone is primarily cleared via three metabolic routes to yield four major circulating metabolites, benzisothiazole (BITP) sulphoxide, BITP-sulphone, ziprasidone sulphoxide, and S-methyl-dihydroziprasidone. Approximately 20% of the dose is excreted in the urine, with approximately 66% being eliminated in the feces. Unchanged ziprasidone represents about 44% of total drug-related material in serum. *In vitro* studies using human liver subcellular fractions indicate that S-methyl-dihydroziprasidone is generated in two steps. The data indicate that the reduction reaction is mediated by aldehyde oxidase and the subsequent methylation is mediated by thiol methyltransferase. *In vitro* studies using human liver microsomes and recombinant enzymes indicate that CYP3A4 is the major CYP contributing to the oxidative metabolism of ziprasidone. CYP1A2 may contribute to a much lesser extent. Based on *in vivo* abundance of excretory metabolites, less than one-third of ziprasidone metabolic clearance is mediated by cytochrome P450 catalyzed oxidation and approximately two-thirds via reduction by aldehyde oxidase. There are no known clinically relevant inhibitors or inducers of aldehyde oxidase.

Intramuscular Pharmacokinetics

Systemic Bioavailability: The bioavailability of ziprasidone administered intramuscularly is 100%. After intramuscular administration of single doses, peak serum concentrations typically occur at approximately 60 minutes post-dose or earlier and the mean half-life ($T_{½}$) ranges from two to five hours. Exposure increases in a dose-related manner and following three days of intramuscular dosing, little accumulation is observed.

Metabolism and Elimination: Although the metabolism and elimination of IM ziprasidone have not been systematically evaluated, the intramuscular route of administration would not be expected to alter the metabolic pathways.

Special Populations

Age and Gender Effects—In a multiple-dose (8 days of treatment) study involving 32 subjects, there was no difference in the pharmacokinetics of ziprasidone between men and women or between elderly (>65 years) and young (18 to 45 years) subjects. Additionally, population pharmacokinetic evaluation of patients in controlled trials has revealed no evidence of clinically significant age or gender-related differences in the pharmacokinetics of ziprasidone. Dosage modifications for age or gender are, therefore, not recommended.

Ziprasidone intramuscular has not been systematically evaluated in elderly patients (65 years and over).

Race—No specific pharmacokinetic study was conducted to investigate the effects of race. Population pharmacokinetic evaluation has revealed no evidence of clinically significant race-related differences in the pharmacokinetics of ziprasidone. Dosage modifications for race are, therefore, not recommended.

Smoking—Based on *in vitro* studies utilizing human liver enzymes, ziprasidone is not a substrate for CYP1A2; smoking should therefore not have an effect on the pharmacokinetics of ziprasidone. Consistent with these *in vitro* results, population pharmacokinetic evaluation has not revealed any significant pharmacokinetic differences between smokers and nonsmokers.

Renal Impairment—Because ziprasidone is highly metabolized, with less than 1% of the drug excreted unchanged, renal impairment alone is unlikely to have a major impact on the pharmacokinetics of ziprasidone. The pharmacokinetics of ziprasidone following 8 days of 20 mg BID dosing were similar among subjects with varying degrees of renal impairment (n=27), and subjects with normal renal function, indicating that dosage adjustment based upon the degree of renal impairment is not required. Ziprasidone is not removed by hemodialysis.

Hepatic Impairment—As ziprasidone is cleared substantially by the liver, the presence of hepatic impairment would be expected to increase the AUC of ziprasidone; a multiple-dose study at 20 mg BID for 5 days in subjects (n=13) with clinically significant (Childs-Pugh Class A and B) cirrhosis revealed an increase in AUC_{0-12} of 13% and 34% in Childs-Pugh Class A and B, respectively, compared to a matched control group (n=14). A half-life of 7.1 hours was observed in subjects with cirrhosis compared to 4.8 hours in the control group.

Intramuscular ziprasidone has not been systematically evaluated in elderly patients or in patients with hepatic or renal impairment. As the cyclodextrin excipient is cleared by renal filtration, ziprasidone intramuscular should be administered with caution to patients with impaired renal function.

Drug-Drug Interactions

An *in vitro* enzyme inhibition study utilizing human liver microsomes showed that ziprasidone had little inhibitory effect on CYP1A2, CYP2C9, CYP2C19, CYP2D6 and CYP3A4, and thus would not likely interfere with the metabolism of drugs primarily metabolized by these enzymes. *In vivo* studies have revealed no effect of ziprasidone on the pharmacokinetics of dextromethorphan, estrogen, progesterone, or lithium (see **Drug Interactions** under **PRECAUTIONS**).

In vivo studies have revealed an approximately 35% decrease in ziprasidone AUC by concomitantly administered carbamazepine, an approximately 35-40% increase in ziprasidone AUC by concomitantly administered ketoconazole, but no effect on ziprasidone's pharmacokinetics by cimetidine or antacid (see **Drug Interactions** under **PRECAUTIONS**).

Clinical Trials

The efficacy of oral ziprasidone in the treatment of schizophrenia was evaluated in 5 placebo-controlled studies, 4 short-term (4- and 6-week) trials and one long-term (52-week) trial. All trials were in inpatients, most of whom met DSM III-R criteria for schizophrenia. Each study included 2 to 3 fixed doses of ziprasidone as well as placebo. Four of the 5 trials were able to distinguish ziprasidone from placebo; one short-term study did not. Although a single fixed-dose haloperidol arm was included as a comparative treatment in one of the three short-term trials, this single study was inadequate to provide a reliable and valid comparison of ziprasidone and haloperidol.

Several instruments were used for assessing psychiatric signs and symptoms in these studies. The Brief Psychiatric Rating Scale (BPRS) and the Positive and Negative Syndrome Scale (PANSS) are both multi-item inventories of general psychopathology usually used to evaluate the effects of drug treatment in schizophrenia. The BPRS psychosis cluster (conceptual disorganization, hallucinatory behavior, suspiciousness, and unusual thought content) is considered a particularly useful subset for assessing actively psychotic schizophrenic patients. A second widely used assessment, the Clinical Global Impression (CGI), reflects the impression of a skilled observer, fully familiar with the manifestations of schizophrenia, about the overall clinical state of the patient. In addition, the Scale for Assessing Negative Symptoms (SANS) was employed for assessing negative symptoms in one trial.

The results of the oral ziprasidone trials follow:

(1) In a 4-week, placebo-controlled trial (n=139) comparing 2 fixed doses of ziprasidone (20 and 60 mg BID) with placebo, only the 60 mg BID dose was superior to placebo on the BPRS total score and the CGI severity score. This higher dose group was not superior to placebo on the BPRS psychosis cluster or on the SANS.

(2) In a 6-week, placebo-controlled trial (n=302) comparing 2 fixed doses of ziprasidone (40 and 80 mg BID) with placebo, both dose groups were superior to placebo on the BPRS total score, the BPRS psychosis cluster, the CGI severity score and the PANSS total and negative subscale scores. Although 80 mg BID had a numerically greater effect than 40 mg BID, the difference was not statistically significant.

(3) In a 6-week, placebo-controlled trial (n=419) comparing 3 fixed doses of ziprasidone (20, 60, and 100 mg BID) with placebo, all three dose groups were superior to placebo on the PANSS total score, the BPRS total score, the BPRS psychosis cluster, and the CGI severity score. Only the 100 mg BID dose group was superior to placebo on the PANSS negative subscale score. There was no clear evidence for a dose-response relationship within the 20 mg BID to 100 mg BID dose range.

(4) In a 4-week, placebo-controlled trial (n=200) comparing 3 fixed doses of ziprasidone (5, 20, and 40 mg BID), none of the dose groups was statistically superior to placebo on any outcome of interest.

(5) A study was conducted in chronic, symptomatically stable schizophrenic inpatients (n=294) randomized to 3 fixed doses of ziprasidone (20, 40, or 80 mg BID) or placebo and followed for 52 weeks. Patients were observed for "impending psychotic relapse," defined as CGI-improvement score of ≥6 (much worse or very much worse) and/or scores ≥6 (moderately severe) on the hostility or uncooperativeness items of the PANSS on two consecutive days. Ziprasidone was significantly superior to placebo in both time to relapse and rate of relapse, with no significant difference between the different dose groups.

There were insufficient data to examine population subsets based on age and race. Examination of population subsets based on gender did not reveal any differential responsiveness.

The efficacy of intramuscular ziprasidone in the management of agitated schizophrenic patients was established in two short-term, double-blind trials of schizophrenic subjects who were considered by the investigators to be "acutely agitated" and in need of IM antipsychotic medication. In addition, patients were required to have a score of 3 or more on at least 3 of the following items of the PANSS: anxiety, tension, hostility and excitement. Efficacy was evaluated by analysis of the area under the curve (AUC) of the Behavioural Activity Rating Scale (BARS) and Clinical Global Impression (CGI) severity rating. The BARS is a seven point scale with scores ranging from 1 (difficult or unable to rouse) to 7 (violent, requires restraint). Patients' scores on the BARS at baseline were mostly 5 (signs of overt activity [physical or verbal], calms down with instructions) and as determined by investigators, exhibited a degree of agitation that warranted intramuscular therapy. There were few patients with a rating higher than 5 on the BARS, as the most severely agitated patients were generally unable to provide informed consent for participation in pre-marketing clinical trials.

Both studies compared higher doses of ziprasidone intramuscular with a 2 mg control dose. In one study, the higher dose was 20 mg, which could be given up to 4 times in the 24 hours of the study, at interdose intervals of no less than 4 hours. In the other study, the higher dose was 10 mg, which could be given up to 4 times in the 24 hours of the study, at interdose intervals of no less than 2 hours.

The results of the intramuscular ziprasidone trials follow:

(1) In a one-day, double-blind, randomized trial (n=79) involving doses of ziprasidone intramuscular of 20 mg or 2 mg, up to QID, ziprasidone intramuscular 20 mg was statistically superior to ziprasidone intramuscular 2 mg, as assessed by AUC of the BARS at 0 to 4 hours, and by CGI severity at 4 hours and study endpoint.

(2) In another one-day, double-blind, randomized trial (n=117) involving doses of ziprasidone intramuscular of 10 mg or 2 mg, up to QID, ziprasidone intramuscular 10 mg was statistically superior to ziprasidone intramuscular 2 mg, as assessed by AUC of the BARS at 0 to 2 hours, but not by CGI severity.

INDICATIONS AND USAGE

Ziprasidone is indicated for the treatment of schizophrenia. When deciding among the alternative treatments available for this condition, the prescriber should consider the finding of ziprasidone's greater capacity to prolong the QT/QTc interval compared to several other antipsychotic drugs (see **WARNINGS**). Prolongation of the QTc interval is associated in some other drugs with the ability to cause torsade de pointes-type arrhythmia, a potentially fatal polymorphic ventricular tachycardia, and sudden death. In many cases this would lead to the conclusion that other drugs should be tried first. Whether ziprasidone will cause torsade de pointes or increase the rate of sudden death is not yet known (see **WARNINGS**).

The efficacy of oral ziprasidone was established in short-term (4- and 6-week) controlled trials of schizophrenic inpatients (see **CLINICAL PHARMACOLOGY**).

In a placebo-controlled trial involving the follow-up for up to 52 weeks of stable schizophrenic inpatients, GEODON was demonstrated to delay the time to and rate of relapse. The physician who elects to use GEODON for extended periods should periodically re-evaluate the long-term usefulness of the drug for the individual patient.

Ziprasidone intramuscular is indicated for the treatment of acute agitation in schizophrenic patients for whom treatment with ziprasidone is appropriate and who need intramuscular antipsychotic medication for rapid control of the agitation. "Psychomotor agitation" is defined in DSM-IV as "excessive motor activity associated with a feeling of inner tension." Schizophrenic patients experiencing agitation often manifest behaviors that interfere with their diagnosis and care, e.g., threatening behaviors, escalating or urgently distressing behavior, or self-exhausting behavior, leading clinicians to the use of intramuscular antipsychotic medications to achieve immediate control of the agitation. The efficacy of intramuscular ziprasidone for acute agitation in schizophrenia was established in single-day controlled trials of schizophrenic inpatients (see **CLINICAL PHARMACOLOGY**). Since there is no experience regarding the safety of administering ziprasidone intramuscular to schizophrenic patients already taking oral ziprasidone, the practice of co-administration is not recommended.

CONTRAINDICATIONS

QT Prolongation

Because of ziprasidone's dose-related prolongation of the QT interval and the known association of fatal arrhythmias with QT prolongation by some other drugs, ziprasidone is contraindicated in patients with a known history of QT prolongation (including congenital long QT syndrome), with recent acute myocardial infarction, or with uncompensated heart failure (see **WARNINGS**).

Pharmacokinetic/pharmacodynamic studies between ziprasidone and other drugs that prolong the QT interval have not been performed. An additive effect of ziprasidone and other drugs that prolong the QT interval cannot be excluded. Therefore, ziprasidone should not be given with dofetilide, sotalol, quinidine, other Class Ia and III anti-arrhythmics, mesoridazine, thioridazine, chlorpromazine, droperidol, pimozide, sparfloxacin, gatifloxacin, moxifloxacin, halofantrine, mefloquine, pentamidine, arsenic trioxide, levomethadyl acetate, dolasetron mesylate, probucol or tacrolimus. Ziprasidone is also contraindicated with drugs that have demonstrated QT prolongation as one of their pharmacodynamic effects and have this effect described in the full prescribing information as a contraindication or a boxed or bolded warning (see **WARNINGS**).

Hypersensitivity

Ziprasidone is contraindicated in individuals with a known hypersensitivity to the product.

WARNINGS

QT Prolongation and Risk of Sudden Death

Ziprasidone use should be avoided in combination with other drugs that are known to prolong the QTc interval (see CONTRAINDICATIONS, and see Drug Interactions under PRECAUTIONS). Additionally, clinicians should be alert to the identification of other drugs that have been consistently observed to prolong the QTc interval. Such drugs should not be prescribed with ziprasidone. Ziprasidone should also be avoided in patients with congenital long QT syndrome and in patients with a history of cardiac arrhythmias (see CONTRAINDICATIONS).

A study directly comparing the QT/QTc prolonging effect of oral ziprasidone with several other drugs effective in the treatment of schizophrenia was conducted in patient volunteers. In the first phase of the trial, ECGs were obtained at the time of maximum plasma concentration when the drug was administered alone. In the second phase of the trial, ECGs were obtained at the time of maximum plasma concentration while the drug was co-administered with an inhibitor of the CYP4503A4 metabolism of the drug.

In the first phase of the study, the mean change in QTc from baseline was calculated for each drug, using a sample-based correction that removes the effect of heart rate on the QT interval. The mean increase in QTc from baseline for ziprasidone ranged from approximately 9 to 14 msec greater than for four of the comparator drugs (risperidone, olanzapine, quetiapine, and haloperidol), but was approximately 14 msec less than the prolongation observed for thioridazine.

In the second phase of the study, the effect of ziprasidone on QTc length was not augmented by the presence of a metabolic inhibitor (ketoconazole 200 mg BID).

In placebo-controlled trials, oral ziprasidone increased the QTc interval compared to placebo by approximately 10 msec at the highest recommended daily dose of 160 mg. In clinical trials with oral ziprasidone, the electrocardiograms of 2/2988 (0.06%) patients who received GEODON and 1/440 (0.23%) patients who received placebo revealed QTc intervals exceeding the potentially clinically relevant threshold of 500 msec. In the ziprasidone-treated patients, neither case suggested a role of ziprasidone. One patient had a history of prolonged QTc and a screening measurement of 489 msec; QTc was 503 msec during ziprasidone treatment. The other patient had a QTc of 391 msec at the end of treatment with ziprasidone and upon switching to thioridazine experienced QTc measurements of 518 and 593 msec.

Some drugs that prolong the QT/QTc interval have been associated with the occurrence of torsade de pointes and with sudden unexplained death. The relationship of QT prolongation to torsade de pointes is clearest for larger increases (20 msec and greater) but it is possible that smaller QT/QTc prolongations may also increase risk, or increase it in susceptible individuals, such as those with hypokalemia, hypomagnesemia, or genetic predisposition. Although torsade de pointes has not been observed in association with the use of ziprasidone at recommended doses in premarketing studies, experience is too limited to rule out an increased risk.

A study evaluating the QT/QTc prolonging effect of intramuscular ziprasidone, with intramuscular haloperidol as a control, was conducted in patient volunteers. In the trial, ECGs were obtained at the time of maximum plasma concentration following two injections of ziprasidone (20 mg then 30 mg) or haloperidol (7.5 mg then 10 mg) given four hours apart. Note that a 30 mg dose of intramuscular ziprasidone is 50% higher than the recommended therapeutic dose. The mean change in QTc from baseline was calculated for each drug, using a sample-based correction that removes the effect of heart rate on the QT interval. The mean increase in QTc from baseline for ziprasidone was 4.6 msec following the first injection and 12.8 msec following the second injection. The mean increase in QTc from baseline for haloperidol was 6.0 msec following the first injection and 14.7 msec following the second injection. In this study, no patients had a QTc interval exceeding 500 msec.

As with other antipsychotic drugs and placebo, sudden unexplained deaths have been reported in patients taking ziprasidone at recommended doses. The premarketing experience for ziprasidone did not reveal an excess risk of mortality for ziprasidone compared to other antipsychotic drugs or placebo, but the extent of exposure was limited, especially for the drugs used as active controls and placebo. Nevertheless, ziprasidone's larger prolongation of QTc length compared to several other antipsychotic drugs raises the possibility that the risk of sudden death may be greater for ziprasidone than for other available drugs for treating schizophrenia. This possibility needs to be considered in deciding among alternative drug products (see INDICATIONS AND USAGE).

Certain circumstances may increase the risk of the occurrence of torsade de pointes and/or sudden death in association with the use of drugs that prolong the QTc interval, including (1) bradycardia; (2) hypokalemia or hypomagnesemia; (3) concomitant use of other drugs that prolong the QTc interval; and (4) presence of congenital prolongation of the QT interval.

It is recommended that patients being considered for ziprasidone treatment who are at risk for significant electrolyte disturbances, hypokalemia in particular, have baseline serum potassium and magnesium measurements. Hypokalemia (and/or hypomagnesemia) may increase the risk of QT prolongation and arrhythmia. Hypokalemia may result from diuretic therapy, diarrhea, and other causes. Patients with low serum potassium and/or magnesium should be repleted with those electrolytes before proceeding with treatment. It is essential to periodically monitor serum electrolytes in patients for whom diuretic therapy is introduced during ziprasidone treatment. Persistently prolonged QTc intervals may also increase the risk of further prolongation and arrhythmia, but it is not clear that routine screening ECG measures are effective in detecting such patients. Rather, ziprasidone should be avoided in patients with histories of significant cardiovascular illness, e.g., QT prolongation, recent acute myocardial infarction, uncompensated heart failure, or cardiac arrhythmia. Ziprasidone should be discontinued in patients who are found to have persistent QTc measurements >500 msec.

For patients taking ziprasidone who experience symptoms that could indicate the occurrence of torsade de pointes, e.g., dizziness, palpitations, or syncope, the prescriber should initiate further evaluation, e.g., Holter monitoring may be useful.

Neuroleptic Malignant Syndrome (NMS)

A potentially fatal symptom complex sometimes referred to as Neuroleptic Malignant Syndrome (NMS) has been reported in association with administration of antipsychotic drugs. Clinical manifestations of NMS are hyperpyrexia, muscle rigidity, altered mental status and evidence of autonomic instability (irregular pulse or blood pressure, tachycardia, diaphoresis, and cardiac dysrhythmia). Additional signs may include elevated creatinine phosphokinase, myoglobinuria (rhabdomyolysis), and acute renal failure.

The diagnostic evaluation of patients with this syndrome is complicated. In arriving at a diagnosis, it is important to exclude cases where the clinical presentation includes both serious medical illness (e.g., pneumonia, systemic infection, etc.) and untreated or inadequately treated extrapyramidal signs and symptoms (EPS). Other important considerations in the differential diagnosis include central anticholinergic toxicity, heat stroke, drug fever, and primary central nervous system (CNS) pathology.

The management of NMS should include: (1) immediate discontinuation of antipsychotic drugs and other drugs not essential to concurrent therapy; (2) intensive symptomatic treatment and medical monitoring; and (3) treatment of any concomitant serious medical problems for which specific treatments are available. There is no general agreement about specific pharmacological treatment regimens for NMS.

If a patient requires antipsychotic drug treatment after recovery from NMS, the potential reintroduction of drug therapy should be carefully considered. The patient should be carefully monitored, since recurrences of NMS have been reported.

Tardive Dyskinesia

A syndrome of potentially irreversible, involuntary, dyskinetic movements may develop in patients undergoing treatment with antipsychotic drugs. Although the prevalence of the syndrome appears to be highest among the elderly, especially elderly women, it is impossible to rely upon prevalence estimates to predict, at the inception of antipsychotic treatment, which patients are likely to develop the syndrome. Whether antipsychotic drug products differ in their potential to cause tardive dyskinesia is unknown.

The risk of developing tardive dyskinesia and the likelihood that it will become irreversible are believed to increase as the duration of treatment and the total cumulative dose of antipsychotic drugs administered to the patient increase. However, the syndrome can develop, although much less commonly, after relatively brief treatment periods at low doses.

There is no known treatment for established cases of tardive dyskinesia, although the syndrome may remit, partially or completely, if antipsychotic treatment is withdrawn. Antipsychotic treatment itself, however, may suppress (or partially suppress) the signs and symptoms of the syndrome and thereby may possibly mask the underlying process. The effect that symptomatic suppression has upon the long-term course of the syndrome is unknown.

Given these considerations, ziprasidone should be prescribed in a manner that is most likely to minimize the occurrence of tardive dyskinesia. Chronic antipsychotic treatment should generally be reserved for patients who suffer from a chronic illness that (1) is known to respond to antipsychotic drugs, and (2) for whom alternative, equally effective, but potentially less harmful treatments are not available or appropriate. In patients who do require chronic treatment, the smallest dose and the shortest duration of treatment producing a satisfactory clinical response should be sought. The need for continued treatment should be reassessed periodically.

If signs and symptoms of tardive dyskinesia appear in a patient on ziprasidone, drug discontinuation should be considered. However, some patients may require treatment with ziprasidone despite the presence of the syndrome.

Hyperglycemia and Diabetes Mellitus

Hyperglycemia, in some cases extreme and associated with ketoacidosis or hyperosmolar coma or death, has been reported in patients treated with atypical antipsychotics. There have been few reports of hyperglycemia or diabetes in patients treated with GEODON. Although fewer patients have been treated with GEODON, it is not known if this more limited experience is the sole reason for the paucity of such reports. Assessment of the relationship between atypical antipsychotic use and glucose abnormalities is complicated by the possibility of an increased background risk of diabetes mellitus in patients with schizophrenia and the increasing incidence of diabetes mellitus in the general population. Given these confounders, the relationship between atypical antipsychotic use and hyperglycemia-related adverse events is not completely understood. However, epidemiological studies, which did not include GEODON, suggest an increased risk of treatment-emergent hyperglycemia-related adverse events in patients treated with the atypical antipsychotics included in these studies. Because GEODON was not marketed at the time these studies were performed, it is not known if GEODON is associated with this increased risk. Precise risk estimates for hyperglycemia-related adverse events in patients treated with atypical antipsychotics are not available.

Patients with an established diagnosis of diabetes mellitus who are started on atypical antipsychotics should be monitored regularly for worsening of glucose control. Patients with risk factors for diabetes mellitus (e.g., obesity, family history of diabetes) who are starting treatment with atypical antipsychotics should undergo fasting blood glucose testing at the beginning of treatment and periodically during treatment. Any patient treated with atypical antipsychotics should be monitored for symptoms of hyperglycemia including polydipsia, polyuria, polyphagia, and weakness. Patients who develop symptoms of hyperglycemia during treatment with atypical antipsychotics should undergo fasting blood glucose testing. In some cases, hyperglycemia has resolved when the atypical antipsychotic was discontinued; however, some patients required continuation of antidiabetic treatment despite discontinuation of the suspect drug.

PRECAUTIONS

General

Rash—In premarketing trials with ziprasidone, about 5% of patients developed rash and/or urticaria, with discontinuation of treatment in about one-sixth of these cases. The occurrence of rash was related to dose of ziprasidone, although the finding might also be explained by the longer exposure time in the higher dose patients. Several patients with rash had signs and symptoms of associated systemic illness, e.g., elevated WBCs. Most patients improved promptly with adjunctive treatment with antihistamines or steroids and/or upon discontinuation of ziprasidone, and all patients experiencing these events were reported to recover completely. Upon appearance of rash for which an alternative etiology cannot be identified, ziprasidone should be discontinued.

Continued on next page

Geodon—Cont.

Orthostatic Hypotension—Ziprasidone may induce orthostatic hypotension associated with dizziness, tachycardia, and, in some patients, syncope, especially during the initial dose-titration period, probably reflecting its α_1-adrenergic antagonist properties. Syncope was reported in 0.6% of the patients treated with ziprasidone.

Ziprasidone should be used with particular caution in patients with known cardiovascular disease (history of myocardial infarction or ischemic heart disease, heart failure or conduction abnormalities), cerebrovascular disease or conditions which would predispose patients to hypotension (dehydration, hypovolemia, and treatment with antihypertensive medications).

Seizures—During clinical trials, seizures occurred in 0.4% of patients treated with ziprasidone. There were confounding factors that may have contributed to the occurrence of seizures in many of these cases. As with other antipsychotic drugs, ziprasidone should be used cautiously in patients with a history of seizures or with conditions that potentially lower the seizure threshold, e.g., Alzheimer's dementia. Conditions that lower the seizure threshold may be more prevalent in a population of 65 years or older.

Hyperprolactinemia—As with other drugs that antagonize dopamine D_2 receptors, ziprasidone elevates prolactin levels in humans. Increased prolactin levels were also observed in animal studies with this compound, and were associated with an increase in mammary gland neoplasia in mice; a similar effect was not observed in rats (see **Carcinogenesis**). Tissue culture experiments indicate that approximately one-third of human breast cancers are prolactin-dependent *in vitro*, a factor of potential importance if the prescription of these drugs is contemplated in a patient with previously detected breast cancer. Although disturbances such as galactorrhea, amenorrhea, gynecomastia, and impotence have been reported with prolactin-elevating compounds, the clinical significance of elevated serum prolactin levels is unknown for most patients. Neither clinical studies nor epidemiologic studies conducted to date have shown an association between chronic administration of this class of drugs and tumorigenesis in humans; the available evidence is considered too limited to be conclusive at this time.

Potential for Cognitive and Motor Impairment—Somnolence was a commonly reported adverse event in patients treated with ziprasidone. In the 4- and 6-week placebo-controlled trials, somnolence was reported in 14% of patients on ziprasidone compared to 7% of placebo patients. Somnolence led to discontinuation in 0.3% of patients in short-term clinical trials. Since ziprasidone has the potential to impair judgment, thinking, or motor skills, patients should be cautioned about performing activities requiring mental alertness, such as operating a motor vehicle (including automobiles) or operating hazardous machinery until they are reasonably certain that ziprasidone therapy does not affect them adversely.

Priapism—One case of priapism was reported in the premarketing database. While the relationship of the event to ziprasidone use has not been established, other drugs with alpha-adrenergic blocking effects have been reported to induce priapism, and it is possible that ziprasidone may share this capacity. Severe priapism may require surgical intervention.

Body Temperature Regulation—Although not reported with ziprasidone in premarketing trials, disruption of the body's ability to reduce core body temperature has been attributed to antipsychotic agents. Appropriate care is advised when prescribing ziprasidone for patients who will be experiencing conditions which may contribute to an elevation in core body temperature, e.g., exercising strenuously, exposure to extreme heat, receiving concomitant medication with anticholinergic activity, or being subject to dehydration.

Dysphagia—Esophageal dysmotility and aspiration have been associated with antipsychotic drug use. Aspiration pneumonia is a common cause of morbidity and mortality in elderly patients, in particular those with advanced Alzheimer's dementia. Ziprasidone and other antipsychotic drugs should be used cautiously in patients at risk for aspiration pneumonia.

Suicide—The possibility of a suicide attempt is inherent in psychotic illness and close supervision of high-risk patients should accompany drug therapy. Prescriptions for ziprasidone should be written for the smallest quantity of capsules consistent with good patient management in order to reduce the risk of overdose.

Use in Patients with Concomitant Illness—Clinical experience with ziprasidone in patients with certain concomitant systemic illnesses (see **Renal Impairment** and **Hepatic Impairment** under **CLINICAL PHARMACOLOGY, Special Populations**) is limited.

Ziprasidone has not been evaluated or used to any appreciable extent in patients with a recent history of myocardial infarction or unstable heart disease. Patients with these diagnoses were excluded from premarketing clinical studies. Because of the risk of QTc prolongation and orthostatic hypotension with ziprasidone, caution should be observed in cardiac patients (see **QTc Prolongation** under **WARNINGS** and **Orthostatic Hypotension** under **PRECAUTIONS**).

Information for Patients

Please refer to the patient package insert. To assure safe and effective use of GEODON, the information and instructions provided in the patient information should be discussed with patients.

Laboratory Tests

Patients being considered for ziprasidone treatment that are at risk of significant electrolyte disturbances should have baseline serum potassium and magnesium measurements. Low serum potassium and magnesium should be repleted before proceeding with treatment. Patients who are started on diuretics during ziprasidone therapy need periodic monitoring of serum potassium and magnesium. Ziprasidone should be discontinued in patients who are found to have persistent QTc measurements >500 msec (see **WARNINGS**).

Drug Interactions

Drug-drug interactions can be pharmacodynamic (combined pharmacologic effects) or pharmacokinetic (alteration of plasma levels). The risks of using ziprasidone in combination with other drugs have been evaluated as described below. All interactions studies have been conducted with oral ziprasidone. Based upon the pharmacodynamic and pharmacokinetic profile of ziprasidone, possible interactions could be anticipated:

Pharmacodynamic Interactions

(1) Ziprasidone should not be used with any drug that prolongs the QT interval (see **CONTRAINDICATIONS**).
(2) Given the primary CNS effects of ziprasidone, caution should be used when it is taken in combination with other centrally acting drugs.
(3) Because of its potential for inducing hypotension, ziprasidone may enhance the effects of certain antihypertensive agents.
(4) Ziprasidone may antagonize the effects of levodopa and dopamine agonists.

Pharmacokinetic Interactions

The Effect of Other Drugs on Ziprasidone

Carbamazepine—Carbamazepine is an inducer of CYP3A4; administration of 200 mg BID for 21 days resulted in a decrease of approximately 35% in the AUC of ziprasidone. This effect may be greater when higher doses of carbamazepine are administered.

Ketoconazole—Ketoconazole, a potent inhibitor of CYP3A4, at a dose of 400 mg QD for 5 days, increased the AUC and Cmax of ziprasidone by about 35-40%. Other inhibitors of CYP3A4 would be expected to have similar effects.

Cimetidine—Cimetidine at a dose of 800 mg QD for 2 days did not affect ziprasidone pharmacokinetics.

Antacid—The coadministration of 30 mL of Maalox® with ziprasidone did not affect the pharmacokinetics of ziprasidone.

In addition, population pharmacokinetic analysis of schizophrenic patients enrolled in controlled clinical trials has not revealed evidence of any clinically significant pharmacokinetic interactions with benztropine, propranolol, or lorazepam.

Effect of Ziprasidone on Other Drugs

In vitro studies revealed little potential for ziprasidone to interfere with the metabolism of drugs cleared primarily by CYP1A2, CYP2C9, CYP2C19, CYP2D6, and CYP3A4, and little potential for drug interactions with ziprasidone due to displacement (see **CLINICAL PHARMACOLOGY, Pharmacokinetics**).

Lithium—Ziprasidone at a dose of 40 mg BID administered concomitantly with lithium at a dose of 450 mg BID for 7 days did not affect the steady-state level or renal clearance of lithium.

Oral Contraceptives—Ziprasidone at a dose of 20 mg BID did not affect the pharmacokinetics of concomitantly administered oral contraceptives, ethinyl estradiol (0.03 mg) and levonorgestrel (0.15 mg).

Dextromethorphan—Consistent with *in vitro* results, a study in normal healthy volunteers showed that ziprasidone did not alter the metabolism of dextromethorphan, a CYP2D6 model substrate, to its major metabolite, dextrorphan. There was no statistically significant change in the urinary dextromethorphan/dextrorphan ratio.

Carcinogenesis, Mutagenesis, Impairment of Fertility

Carcinogenesis—Lifetime carcinogenicity studies were conducted with ziprasidone in Long Evans rats and CD-1 mice. Ziprasidone was administered for 24 months in the diet at doses of 2, 6, or 12 mg/kg/day to rats, and 50, 100, or 200 mg/kg/day to mice (0.1 to 0.6 and 1 to 5 times the maximum recommended human dose [MRHD] of 200 mg/day on a mg/m^2 basis, respectively). In the rat study, there was no evidence of an increased incidence of tumors compared to controls. In male mice, there was no increase in incidence of tumors relative to controls. In female mice, there were dose-related increases in the incidences of pituitary gland adenoma and carcinoma, and mammary gland adenocarcinoma at all doses tested (50 to 200 mg/kg/day or 1 to 5 times the MRHD on a mg/m^2 basis). Proliferative changes in the pituitary and mammary glands of rodents have been observed following chronic administration of other antipsychotic agents and are considered to be prolactin-mediated. Increases in serum prolactin were observed in a 1-month dietary study in female, but not male, mice at 100 and 200 mg/kg/day (or 2.5 and 5 times the MRHD on a mg/m^2 basis). Ziprasidone had no effect on serum prolactin in rats in a 5-week dietary study at the doses that were used in the carcinogenicity study. The relevance for human risk of the findings of prolactin-mediated endocrine tumors in rodents is unknown (see **Hyperprolactinemia** under **PRECAUTIONS, General**).

Mutagenesis—Ziprasidone was tested in the Ames bacterial mutation assay, the *in vitro* mammalian cell gene mutation mouse lymphoma assay, the *in vitro* chromosomal aberration assay in human lymphocytes, and the *in vivo* chromosomal aberration assay in mouse bone marrow. There was a reproducible mutagenic response in the Ames assay in one strain of *S. typhimurium* in the absence of metabolic activation. Positive results were obtained in both the *in vitro* mammalian cell gene mutation assay and the *in vitro* chromosomal aberration assay in human lymphocytes.

Impairment of Fertility—Ziprasidone was shown to increase time to copulation in Sprague-Dawley rats in two fertility and early embryonic development studies at doses of 10 to 160 mg/kg/day (0.5 to 8 times the MRHD of 200 mg/day on a mg/m^2 basis). Fertility rate was reduced at 160 mg/kg/day (8 times the MRHD on a mg/m^2 basis). There was no effect on fertility at 40 mg/kg/day (2 times the MRHD on a mg/m^2 basis). The effect on fertility appeared to be in the female since fertility was not impaired when males given 160 mg/kg/day (8 times the MRHD on a mg/m^2 basis) were mated with untreated females. In a 6-month study in male rats given 200 mg/kg/day (10 times the MRHD on a mg/m^2 basis) there were no treatment-related findings observed in the testes.

Pregnancy — Pregnancy Category C—In animal studies ziprasidone demonstrated developmental toxicity, including possible teratogenic effects at doses similar to human therapeutic doses. When ziprasidone was administered to pregnant rabbits during the period of organogenesis, an increased incidence of fetal structural abnormalities (ventricular septal defects and other cardiovascular malformations and kidney alterations) was observed at a dose of 30 mg/kg/day (3 times the MRHD of 200 mg/day on a mg/m^2 basis). There was no evidence to suggest that these developmental effects were secondary to maternal toxicity. The developmental no-effect dose was 10 mg/kg/day (equivalent to the MRHD on a mg/m^2 basis). In rats, embryofetal toxicity (decreased fetal weights, delayed skeletal ossification) was observed following administration of 10 to 160 mg/kg/day (0.5 to 8 times the MRHD on a mg/m^2 basis) during organogenesis or throughout gestation, but there was no evidence of teratogenicity. Doses of 40 and 160 mg/kg/day (2 and 8 times the MRHD on a mg/m^2 basis) were associated with maternal toxicity. The developmental no-effect dose was 5 mg/kg/day (0.2 times the MRHD on a mg/m^2 basis). There was an increase in the number of pups born dead and a decrease in postnatal survival through the first 4 days of lactation among the offspring of female rats treated during gestation and lactation with doses of 10 mg/kg/day (0.5 times the MRHD on a mg/m^2 basis) or greater. Offspring developmental delays and neurobehavioral functional impairment were observed at doses of 5 mg/kg/day (0.2 times the MRHD on a mg/m^2 basis) or greater. A no-effect level was not established for these effects.

There are no adequate and well-controlled studies in pregnant women. Ziprasidone should be used during pregnancy only if the potential benefit justifies the potential risk to the fetus.

Labor and Delivery—The effect of ziprasidone on labor and delivery in humans is unknown.

Nursing Mothers—It is not known whether, and if so in what amount, ziprasidone or its metabolites are excreted in human milk. It is recommended that women receiving ziprasidone should not breast feed.

Pediatric Use—The safety and effectiveness of ziprasidone in pediatric patients have not been established.

Geriatric Use—Of the approximately 4500 patients treated with ziprasidone in clinical studies, 2.4% (109) were 65 years of age or over. In general, there was no indication of any different tolerability of ziprasidone or for reduced clearance of ziprasidone in the elderly compared to younger adults. Nevertheless, the presence of multiple factors that might increase the pharmacodynamic response to ziprasidone, or cause poorer tolerance or orthostasis, should lead to consideration of a lower starting dose, slower titration, and careful monitoring during the initial dosing period for some elderly patients.

ADVERSE REACTIONS

The premarketing development program for oral ziprasidone included over 5400 patients and/or normal subjects exposed to one or more doses of ziprasidone. Of these 5400 subjects, over 4500 were patients who participated in multiple-dose effectiveness trials, and their experience corresponded to approximately 1733 patient years. The conditions and duration of treatment with ziprasidone included open-label and double-blind studies, inpatient and outpatient studies, and short-term and longer-term exposure. The premarketing development program for intramuscular ziprasidone included 570 patients and/or normal subjects who received one or more injections of ziprasidone. Over 325 of these subjects participated in trials involving the administration of multiple doses.

Adverse events during exposure were obtained by collecting voluntarily reported adverse experiences, as well as results of physical examinations, vital signs, weights, laboratory analyses, ECGs, and results of ophthalmologic examinations. Adverse experiences were recorded by clinical investigators using terminology of their own choosing. Consequently, it is not possible to provide a meaningful estimate of the proportion of individuals experiencing adverse events without first grouping similar types of events into a smaller number of standardized event categories. In the tables and tabulations that follow, standard COSTART dictionary terminology has been used to classify reported adverse events. The stated frequencies of adverse events represent the proportion of individuals who experienced, at least once, a treatment-emergent adverse event of the type listed. An event was considered treatment emergent if it occurred for the first time or worsened while receiving therapy following baseline evaluation.

Adverse Findings Observed in Short-Term, Placebo-Controlled Trials with Oral Ziprasidone

The following findings are based on a pool of two 6-week, and two 4-week placebo-controlled trials in which ziprasidone was administered in doses ranging from 10 to 200 mg/day.

Adverse Events Associated with Discontinuation of Treatment in Short-Term, Placebo-Controlled Trials of Oral Ziprasidone

Approximately 4.1% (29/702) of ziprasidone-treated patients in short-term, placebo-controlled studies discontinued treatment due to an adverse event, compared with about 2.2% (6/273) on placebo. The most common event associated with dropout was rash, including 7 dropouts for rash among ziprasidone patients (1%) compared to no placebo patients (see **PRECAUTIONS**).

Adverse Events Occurring at an Incidence of 1% or More Among Ziprasidone-Treated Patients in Short-Term, Oral, Placebo-Controlled Trials

Table 1 enumerates the incidence, rounded to the nearest percent, of treatment-emergent adverse events that occurred during acute therapy (up to 6 weeks) in predominantly schizophrenic patients, including only those events that occurred in 1% or more of patients treated with ziprasidone and for which the incidence in patients treated with ziprasidone was greater than the incidence in placebo-treated patients.

The prescriber should be aware that these figures cannot be used to predict the incidence of side effects in the course of usual medical practice where patient characteristics and other factors differ from those which prevailed in the clinical trials. Similarly, the cited frequencies cannot be compared with figures obtained from other clinical investigations involving different treatments, uses, and investigators. The cited figures, however, do provide the prescribing physician with some basis for estimating the relative contribution of drug and non-drug factors to the side effect incidence rate in the population studied.

In these studies, the most commonly observed adverse events associated with the use of ziprasidone (incidence of 5% or greater) and observed at a rate on ziprasidone at least twice that of placebo were somnolence (14%), extrapyramidal syndrome (5%), and respiratory disorder (8%).

Table 1. Treatment-Emergent Adverse Event Incidence In Short-Term Oral Placebo-Controlled Trials

	Percentage of Patients Reporting Event	
Body System/Adverse Event	Ziprasidone (N=702)	Placebo (N=273)
Body as a Whole		
Asthenia	5	3
Accidental Injury	4	2
Cardiovascular		
Tachycardia	2	1
Postural Hypotension	1	0
Digestive		
Nausea	10	7
Constipation	9	8
Dyspepsia	8	7
Diarrhea	5	4
Dry Mouth	4	2
Anorexia	2	1
Musculoskeletal		
Myalgia	1	0
Nervous		
Somnolence	14	7
Akathisia	8	7
Dizziness	8	6
Extrapyramidal Syndrome	5	1
Dystonia	4	2
Hypertonia	3	2
Respiratory		
Respiratory Disorder*	8	3
Rhinitis	4	2
Cough Increased	3	1
Skin and Appendages		
Rash	4	3
Fungal Dermatitis	2	1
Special Senses		
Abnormal Vision	3	2

*Cold symptoms and upper respiratory infection account for >90% of investigator terms pointing to "respiratory disorder".

Explorations for interactions on the basis of gender did not reveal any clinically meaningful differences in the adverse event occurrence on the basis of this demographic factor.

Dose Dependency of Adverse Events in Short-Term, Placebo-Controlled Trials

An analysis for dose response in this 4-study pool revealed an apparent relation of adverse event to dose for the following events: asthenia, postural hypotension, anorexia, dry mouth, increased salivation, arthralgia, anxiety, dizziness, dystonia, hypertonia, somnolence, tremor, rhinitis, rash, and abnormal vision.

Extrapyramidal Symptoms (EPS)—The incidence of reported EPS for ziprasidone-treated patients in the short-term, placebo-controlled trials was 5% vs. 1% for placebo. Objectively collected data from those trials on the Simpson Angus Rating Scale (for EPS) and the Barnes Akathisia Scale (for akathisia) did not generally show a difference between ziprasidone and placebo.

Vital Sign Changes—Ziprasidone is associated with orthostatic hypotension (see **PRECAUTIONS**).

Weight Gain—The proportions of patients meeting a weight gain criterion of ≥7% of body weight were compared in a pool of four 4- and 6-week placebo-controlled clinical trials, revealing a statistically significantly greater incidence of weight gain for ziprasidone (10%) compared to placebo (4%). A median weight gain of 0.5 kg was observed in ziprasidone patients compared to no median weight change in placebo patients. In this set of clinical trials, weight gain was reported as an adverse event in 0.4% and 0.4% of ziprasidone and placebo patients, respectively. During long-term therapy with ziprasidone, a categorization of patients at baseline on the basis of body mass index (BMI) revealed the greatest mean weight gain and highest incidence of clinically significant weight gain (>7% of body weight) in patients with low BMI (<23) compared to normal (23-27) or overweight patients (>27). There was a mean weight gain of 1.4 kg for those patients with a "low" baseline BMI, no mean change for patients with a "normal" BMI, and a 1.3 kg mean weight loss for patients who entered the program with a "high" BMI.

ECG Changes—Ziprasidone is associated with an increase in the QTc interval (see **WARNINGS**). Ziprasidone was associated with a mean increase in heart rate of 1.4 beats per minute compared to a 0.2 beats per minute decrease among placebo patients.

Other Adverse Events Observed During the Premarketing Evaluation of Oral Ziprasidone

Following is a list of COSTART terms that reflect treatment-emergent adverse events as defined in the introduction to the **ADVERSE REACTIONS** section reported by patients treated with ziprasidone at multiple doses >4 mg/day within the database of 3834 patients. All reported events are included except those already listed in Table 1 or elsewhere in labeling, those event terms that were so general as to be uninformative, events reported only once and that did not have a substantial probability of being acutely life-threatening, events that are part of the illness being treated or are otherwise common as background events, and events considered unlikely to be drug-related. It is important to emphasize that, although the events reported occurred during treatment with ziprasidone, they were not necessarily caused by it.

Events are further categorized by body system and listed in order of decreasing frequency according to the following definitions: frequent adverse events are those occurring in at least 1/100 patients (only those not already listed in the tabulated results from placebo-controlled trials appear in this listing); infrequent adverse events are those occurring in 1/100 to 1/1000 patients; rare events are those occurring in fewer than 1/1000 patients.

Body as a Whole: *Frequent:* abdominal pain, flu syndrome, fever, accidental fall, face edema, chills, photosensitivity reaction, flank pain, hypothermia, motor vehicle accident.

Cardiovascular System: *Frequent:* hypertension; *Infrequent:* bradycardia, angina pectoris, atrial fibrillation; *Rare:* first degree AV block, bundle branch block, phlebitis, pulmonary embolus, cardiomegaly, cerebral infarct, cerebrovascular accident, deep thrombophlebitis, myocarditis, thrombophlebitis.

Digestive System: *Frequent:* vomiting; *Infrequent:* rectal hemorrhage, dysphagia, tongue edema; *Rare:* gum hemorrhage, jaundice, fecal impaction, gamma glutamyl transpeptidase increased, hematemesis, cholestatic jaundice, hepatitis, hepatomegaly, leukoplakia of mouth, fatty liver deposit, melena.

Endocrine: *Rare:* hypothyroidism, hyperthyroidism, thyroiditis.

Hemic and Lymphatic System: *Infrequent:* anemia, ecchymosis, leukocytosis, leukopenia, eosinophilia, lymphadenopathy; *Rare:* thrombocytopenia, hypochromic anemia, lymphocytosis, monocytosis, basophilia, lymphedema, polycythemia, thrombocythemia.

Metabolic and Nutritional Disorders: *Infrequent:* thirst, transaminase increased, peripheral edema, hyperglycemia, creatine phosphokinase increased, alkaline phosphatase increased, hypercholesteremia, dehydration, lactic dehydrogenase increased, albuminuria, hypokalemia; *Rare:* BUN increased, creatinine increased, hyperlipemia, hypocholesteremia, hyperkalemia, hypochloremia, hypoglycemia, hyponatremia, hypoproteinemia, glucose tolerance decreased, gout, hyperchloremia, hyperuricemia, hypocalcemia, hypoglycemic reaction, hypomagnesemia, ketosis, respiratory alkalosis.

Musculoskeletal System: *Infrequent:* tenosynovitis; *Rare:* myopathy.

Nervous System: *Frequent:* agitation, tremor, dyskinesia, hostility, paresthesia, confusion, vertigo, hypokinesia, hyperkinesia, abnormal gait, oculogyric crisis, hypesthesia, ataxia, amnesia, cogwheel rigidity, delirium, hypotonia, akinesia, dysarthria, withdrawal syndrome, buccoglossal syndrome, choreoathetosis, diplopia, incoordination, neuropathy; *Rare:* myoclonus, nystagmus, torticollis, circumoral paresthesia, opisthotonos, reflexes increased, trismus.

Respiratory System: *Frequent:* dyspnea; *Infrequent:* pneumonia, epistaxis; *Rare:* hemoptysis, laryngismus.

Skin and Appendages: *Infrequent:* maculopapular rash, urticaria, alopecia, eczema, exfoliative dermatitis, contact dermatitis, vesiculobullous rash.

Special Senses: *Infrequent:* conjunctivitis, dry eyes, tinnitus, blepharitis, cataract, photophobia; *Rare:* eye hemorrhage, visual field defect, keratitis, keratoconjunctivitis.

Urogenital System: *Infrequent:* impotence, abnormal ejaculation, amenorrhea, hematuria, menorrhagia, female lactation, polyuria, urinary retention, metrorrhagia, male sexual dysfunction, anorgasmia, glycosuria; *Rare:* gynecomastia, vaginal hemorrhage, nocturia, oliguria, female sexual dysfunction, uterine hemorrhage.

Adverse Findings Observed in Trials of Intramuscular Ziprasidone

Adverse Events Occurring at an Incidence of 1% or More Among Ziprasidone-Treated Patients in Short-Term Trials of Intramuscular Ziprasidone

Table 2 enumerates the incidence, rounded to the nearest percent, of treatment-emergent adverse events that occurred during acute therapy with intramuscular ziprasidone in 1% or more of patients.

In these studies, the most commonly observed adverse events associated with the use of intramuscular ziprasidone (incidence of 5% or greater) and observed at a rate on intramuscular ziprasidone (in the higher dose groups) at least twice that of the lowest intramuscular ziprasidone group were headache (13%), nausea (12%), and somnolence (20%).

[See table 2 at bottom of next page]

DRUG ABUSE AND DEPENDENCE

Controlled Substance Class—Ziprasidone is not a controlled substance.

Physical and Psychological Dependence—Ziprasidone has not been systematically studied, in animals or humans, for its potential for abuse, tolerance, or physical dependence. While the clinical trials did not reveal any tendency for drug-seeking behavior, these observations were not systematic and it is not possible to predict on the basis of this limited experience the extent to which ziprasidone will be misused, diverted, and/or abused once marketed. Consequently, patients should be evaluated carefully for a history of drug abuse, and such patients should be observed closely for signs of ziprasidone misuse or abuse (e.g., development of tolerance, increases in dose, drug-seeking behavior).

OVERDOSAGE

Human Experience—In premarketing trials involving more than 5400 patients and/or normal subjects, accidental or intentional overdosage of oral ziprasidone was documented in 10 patients. All of these patients survived without sequelae. In the patient taking the largest confirmed amount, 3240 mg, the only symptoms reported were minimal sedation, slurring of speech, and transitory hypertension (200/95).

Management of Overdosage—In case of acute overdosage, establish and maintain an airway and ensure adequate oxygenation and ventilation. Intravenous access should be established and gastric lavage (after intubation, if patient is unconscious) and administration of activated charcoal together with a laxative should be considered. The possibility of obtundation, seizure, or dystonic reaction of the head and neck following overdose may create a risk of aspiration with induced emesis.

Cardiovascular monitoring should commence immediately and should include continuous electrocardiographic monitoring to detect possible arrhythmias. If antiarrhythmic therapy is administered, disopyramide, procainamide, and quinidine carry a theoretical hazard of additive QT-prolonging effects that might be additive to those of ziprasidone.

Hypotension and circulatory collapse should be treated with appropriate measures such as intravenous fluids. If

Continued on next page

Geodon—Cont.

sympathomimetic agents are used for vascular support, epinephrine and dopamine should not be used, since beta stimulation combined with α_1 antagonism associated with ziprasidone may worsen hypotension. Similarly, it is reasonable to expect that the alpha-adrenergic-blocking properties of bretylium might be additive to those of ziprasidone, resulting in problematic hypotension.

In cases of severe extrapyramidal symptoms, anticholinergic medication should be administered. There is no specific antidote to ziprasidone, and it is not dialyzable. The possibility of multiple drug involvement should be considered. Close medical supervision and monitoring should continue until the patient recovers.

DOSAGE AND ADMINISTRATION

When deciding among the alternative treatments available for schizophrenia, the prescriber should consider the finding of ziprasidone's greater capacity to prolong the QT/QTc interval compared to several other antipsychotic drugs (see **WARNINGS**).

Initial Treatment

GEODON® Capsules should be administered at an initial daily dose of 20 mg BID with food. In some patients, daily dosage may subsequently be adjusted on the basis of individual clinical status up to 80 mg BID. Dosage adjustments, if indicated, should generally occur at intervals of not less than 2 days, as steady-state is achieved within 1 to 3 days. In order to ensure use of the lowest effective dose, ordinarily patients should be observed for improvement for several weeks before upward dosage adjustment.

Efficacy in schizophrenia was demonstrated in a dose range of 20 to 100 mg BID in short-term, placebo-controlled clinical trials. There were trends toward dose response within the range of 20 to 80 mg BID, but results were not consistent. An increase to a dose greater than 80 mg BID is not generally recommended. The safety of doses above 100 mg BID has not been systematically evaluated in clinical trials.

Maintenance Treatment

While there is no body of evidence available to answer the question of how long a patient treated with ziprasidone should remain on it, systematic evaluation of ziprasidone has shown that its efficacy in schizophrenia is maintained for periods of up to 52 weeks at a dose of 20 to 80 mg BID (see **CLINICAL PHARMACOLOGY**). No additional benefit was demonstrated for doses above 20 mg BID. Patients should be periodically reassessed to determine the need for maintenance treatment.

Intramuscular Administration

The recommended dose is 10 to 20 mg administered as required up to a maximum dose of 40 mg per day. Doses of 10 mg may be administered every two hours; doses of 20 mg may be administered every four hours up to a maximum of 40 mg/day. Intramuscular administration of ziprasidone for more than three consecutive days has not been studied.

If long-term therapy is indicated, oral ziprasidone hydrochloride capsules should replace the intramuscular administration as soon as possible.

Since there is no experience regarding the safety of administering ziprasidone intramuscular to schizophrenic patients already taking oral ziprasidone, the practice of co-administration is not recommended.

Dosing in Special Populations

Oral: Dosage adjustments are generally not required on the basis of age, gender, race, or renal or hepatic impairment.

Intramuscular: Ziprasidone intramuscular has not been systematically evaluated in elderly patients or in patients with hepatic or renal impairment. As the cyclodextrin excipient is cleared by renal filtration, ziprasidone intramuscular should be administered with caution to patients with impaired renal function. Dosing adjustments are not required on the basis of gender or race.

Preparation for Administration

GEODON® for Injection (ziprasidone mesylate) should only be administered by intramuscular injection. Single-dose vials require reconstitution prior to administration; any unused portion should be discarded.

Add 1.2 mL of Sterile Water for Injection to the vial and shake vigorously until all the drug is dissolved. Each mL of reconstituted solution contains 20 mg ziprasidone. To administer a 10 mg dose, draw up 0.5 mL of the reconstituted solution. To administer a 20 mg dose, draw up 1.0 mL of the reconstituted solution. Since no preservative or bacteriostatic agent is present in this product, aseptic technique must be used in preparation of the final solution. This medicinal product must not be mixed with other medicinal products or solvents other than Sterile Water for Injection. Parenteral drug products should be inspected visually for particulate matter and discoloration prior to administration, whenever solution and container permit.

HOW SUPPLIED

GEODON® Capsules are differentiated by capsule color/size and are imprinted in black ink with "Pfizer" and a unique number. GEODON Capsules are supplied for oral administration in 20 mg (blue/white), 40 mg (blue/blue), 60 mg (white/white), and 80 mg (blue/white) capsules. They are supplied in the following strengths and package configurations:

GEODON® Capsules

Package Configuration	Capsule Strength (mg)	NDC Code	Imprint
Bottles of 60	20	NDC-0049-3960-60	396
Bottles of 60	40	NDC-0049-3970-60	397
Bottles of 60	60	NDC-0049-3980-60	398
Bottles of 60	80	NDC-0049-3990-60	399
Unit dose/80	20	NDC-0049-3960-41	396
Unit dose/80	40	NDC-0049-3970-41	397
Unit dose/80	60	NDC-0049-3980-41	398
Unit dose/80	80	NDC-0049-3990-41	399

Table 2. Treatment-Emergent Adverse Event Incidence In Short-Term Fixed-Dose Intramuscular Trials

Body System/Adverse Event	Percentage of Patients Reporting Event		
	Ziprasidone 2 mg (N=92)	Ziprasidone 10 mg (N=63)	Ziprasidone 20 mg (N=41)
Body as a Whole			
Headache	3	13	5
Injection Site Pain	9	8	7
Asthenia	2	0	0
Abdominal Pain	0	2	0
Flu Syndrome	1	0	0
Back Pain	1	0	0
Cardiovascular			
Postural Hypotension	0	0	5
Hypertension	2	0	0
Bradycardia	0	0	2
Vasodilation	1	0	0
Digestive			
Nausea	4	8	12
Rectal Hemorrhage	0	0	2
Diarrhea	3	3	0
Vomiting	0	3	0
Dyspepsia	1	3	2
Anorexia	0	2	0
Constipation	0	0	2
Tooth Disorder	1	0	0
Dry Mouth	1	0	0
Nervous			
Dizziness	3	3	10
Anxiety	2	0	0
Insomnia	3	0	0
Somnolence	8	8	20
Akathisia	0	2	0
Agitation	2	2	0
Extrapyramidal Syndrome	2	0	0
Hypertonia	1	0	0
Cogwheel Rigidity	1	0	0
Paresthesia	0	2	0
Personality Disorder	0	2	0
Psychosis	1	0	0
Speech Disorder	0	2	0
Respiratory			
Rhinitis	1	0	0
Skin and Appendages			
Furunculosis	0	2	0
Sweating	0	0	2
Urogenital			
Dysmenorrhea	0	2	0
Priapism	1	0	0

Storage and Handling—GEODON® Capsules should be stored at controlled room temperature, 15°-30°C (59°-86°F). GEODON® for Injection is available in a single dose vial as ziprasidone mesylate (20 mg ziprasidone/mL when reconstituted according to label instructions—see **Preparation for Administration**) for intramuscular administration. Each mL of ziprasidone mesylate for injection (when reconstituted) affords a colorless to pale pink solution that contains 20 mg of ziprasidone and 4.7 mg of methanesulfonic acid solubilized by 294 mg of sulfobutylether β-cyclodextrin sodium (SBECD).

GEODON® for Injection		
Package	Concentration	NDC Code
Single Use Vials	20 mg/mL	NDC-0049-3920-83

Storage and Handling—GEODON® for Injection should be stored at controlled room temperature, 15°-30°C (59°-86°F) in dry form. Protect from light. Following reconstitution, GEODON for Injection can be stored, when protected from light, for up to 24 hours at 15°-30°C (59°-86°F) or up to 7 days refrigerated, 2°-8°C (36°-46°F).

Rx only

Distributed by
Pfizer Roerig
Division of Pfizer Inc, NY, NY 10017
LAB-0273-3.0
Revised July 2004

Shown in Product Identification Guide, page 329

GLUCOTROL XL® ℞
(glipizide)
Extended Release Tablets
For Oral Use

DESCRIPTION

Glipizide is an oral blood-glucose-lowering drug of the sulfonylurea class.

The Chemical Abstracts name of glipizide is 1-cyclohexyl-3-[[p-[2-(5-methylpyrazinecarboxamido)ethyl] phenyl]sulfonyl]urea. The molecular formula is $C_{21}H_{27}N_5O_4S$; the molecular weight is 445.55; the structural formula is shown below:

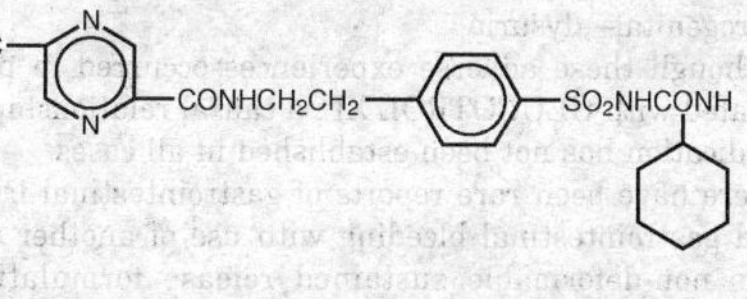

Glipizide is a whitish, odorless powder with a pKa of 5.9. It is insoluble in water and alcohols, but soluble in 0.1 *N* NaOH; it is freely soluble in dimethylformamide. GLUCOTROL XL® is a registered trademark for glipizide GITS. Glipizide GITS (Gastrointestinal Therapeutic System) is formulated as a once-a-day controlled release tablet for oral use and is designed to deliver 2.5, 5, or 10 mg of glipizide.

Inert ingredients in the 2.5 mg, 5 mg and 10 mg formulations are: polyethylene oxide, magnesium stearate, sodium chloride, red ferric oxide, cellulose acetate, polyethylene glycol, Opadry® blue (OY-LS-20921)(2.5 mg tablets), Opadry® white (YS-2-7063)(5 mg and 10 mg tablet) and black ink (S-1-8106).

System Components and Performance

GLUCOTROL XL Extended Release Tablet is similar in appearance to a conventional tablet. It consists, however, of an osmotically active drug core surrounded by a semipermeable membrane. The core itself is divided into two layers: an "active" layer containing the drug, and a "push" layer containing pharmacologically inert (but osmotically active) components. The membrane surrounding the tablet is permeable to water but not to drug or osmotic excipients. As water from the gastrointestinal tract enters the tablet, pressure increases in the osmotic layer and "pushes" against the drug layer, resulting in the release of drug through a small, laser-drilled orifice in the membrane on the drug side of the tablet.

The GLUCOTROL XL Extended Release Tablet is designed to provide a controlled rate of delivery of glipizide into the gastrointestinal lumen which is independent of pH or gastrointestinal motility. The function of the GLUCOTROL XL Extended Release Tablet depends upon the existence of an osmotic gradient between the contents of the bi-layer core and fluid in the GI tract. Drug delivery is essentially constant as long as the osmotic gradient remains constant, and then gradually falls to zero. The biologically inert components of the tablet remain intact during GI transit and are eliminated in the feces as an insoluble shell.

CLINICAL PHARMACOLOGY

Mechanism of Action: Glipizide appears to lower blood glucose acutely by stimulating the release of insulin from the pancreas, an effect dependent upon functioning beta cells in the pancreatic islets. Extrapancreatic effects also may play a part in the mechanism of action of oral sulfonylurea hypoglycemic drugs. Two extrapancreatic effects shown to be important in the action of glipizide are an increase in insulin sensitivity and a decrease in hepatic glucose production. However, the mechanism by which glipizide lowers blood glucose during long-term administration has not been clearly established. Stimulation of insulin secretion by glipizide in response to a meal is of major importance. The insulinotropic response to a meal is enhanced with GLUCOTROL XL administration in diabetic patients. The postprandial insulin and C-peptide responses continue to be enhanced after at least 6 months of treatment. In 2 randomized, double-blind, dose-response studies comprising a total of 347 patients, there was no significant increase in fasting insulin in all GLUCOTROL XL-treated patients combined compared to placebo, although minor elevations were observed at some doses. There was no increase in fasting insulin over the long term.

Some patients fail to respond initially, or gradually lose their responsiveness to sulfonylurea drugs, including glipizide. Alternatively, glipizide may be effective in some patients who have not responded or have ceased to respond to other sulfonylureas.

Effects on Blood Glucose

The effectiveness of GLUCOTROL XL Extended Release Tablets in type 2 diabetes at doses from 5-60 mg once daily has been evaluated in 4 therapeutic clinical trials each with long-term open extensions involving a total of 598 patients. Once daily administration of 5, 10 and 20 mg produced statistically significant reductions from placebo in hemoglobin A_{1C}, fasting plasma glucose and postprandial glucose in patients with mild to severe type 2 diabetes. In a pooled analysis of the patients treated with 5 mg and 20 mg, the relationship between dose and GLUCOTROL XL's effect of reducing hemoglobin A_{1C} was not established. However, in the case of fasting plasma glucose patients treated with 20 mg had a statistically significant reduction of fasting plasma glucose compared to the 5 mg-treated group.

The reductions in hemoglobin A_{1C} and fasting plasma glucose were similar in younger and older patients. Efficacy of GLUCOTROL XL was not affected by gender, race or weight (as assessed by body mass index). In long term extension trials, efficacy of GLUCOTROL XL was maintained in 81% of patients for up to 12 months.

In an open, two-way crossover study 132 patients were randomly assigned to either GLUCOTROL XL or Glucotrol® for 8 weeks and then crossed over to the other drug for an additional 8 weeks. GLUCOTROL XL administration resulted in significantly lower fasting plasma glucose levels and equivalent hemoglobin A_{1C} levels, as compared to Glucotrol.

Other Effects: It has been shown that GLUCOTROL XL therapy is effective in controlling blood glucose without deleterious changes in the plasma lipoprotein profiles of patients treated for type 2 diabetes.

In a placebo-controlled, crossover study in normal volunteers, glipizide had no antidiuretic activity, and, in fact, led to a slight increase in free water clearance.

Pharmacokinetics and Metabolism: Glipizide is rapidly and completely absorbed following oral administration in an immediate release dosage form. The absolute bioavailability of glipizide was 100% after single oral doses in patients with type 2 diabetes. Beginning 2 to 3 hours after administration of GLUCOTROL XL Extended Release Tablets, plasma drug concentrations gradually rise reaching maximum concentrations within 6 to 12 hours after dosing. With subsequent once daily dosing of GLUCOTROL XL Extended Release Tablets, effective plasma glipizide concentrations are maintained throughout the 24 hour dosing interval with less peak to trough fluctuation than that observed with twice daily dosing of immediate release glipizide. The mean relative bioavailability of glipizide in 21 males with type 2 diabetes after administration of 20 mg GLUCOTROL XL Extended Release Tablets, compared to immediate release Glucotrol (10 mg given twice daily), was 90% at steady-state. Steady-state plasma concentrations were achieved by at least the fifth day of dosing with GLUCOTROL XL Extended Release Tablets in 21 males with type 2 diabetes and patients younger than 65 years. Approximately 1 to 2 days longer were required to reach steady-state in 24 elderly (≥65 years) males and females with type 2 diabetes. No accumulation of drug was observed in patients with type 2 diabetes during chronic dosing with GLUCOTROL XL Extended Release Tablets. Administration of GLUCOTROL XL with food has no effect on the 2 to 3 hour lag time in drug absorption. In a single dose, food effect study in 21 healthy male subjects, the administration of GLUCOTROL XL immediately before a high fat breakfast resulted in a 40% increase in the glipizide mean Cmax value, which was significant, but the effect on the AUC was not significant. There was no change in glucose response between the fed and fasting state. Markedly reduced GI retention times of the GLUCOTROL XL tablets over prolonged periods (e.g., short bowel syndrome) may influence the pharmacokinetic profile of the drug and potentially result in lower plasma concentrations. In a multiple dose study in 26 males with type 2 diabetes, the pharmacokinetics of glipizide were linear over the dose range of 5 to 60 mg of GLUCOTROL XL in that the plasma drug concentrations increased proportionately with dose. In a single dose study in 24 healthy subjects, four 5 mg, two 10 mg, and one 20 mg GLUCOTROL XL Extended Release Tablets were bioequivalent. In a separate single dose study in 36 healthy subjects, four 2.5-mg GLUCOTROL XL Extended Release Tablets were bioequivalent to one 10-mg GLUCOTROL XL Extended Release Tablet.

Glipizide is eliminated primarily by hepatic biotransformation: less than 10% of a dose is excreted as unchanged drug in urine and feces; approximately 90% of a dose is excreted as biotransformation products in urine (80%) and feces (10%). The major metabolites of glipizide are products of aromatic hydroxylation and have no hypoglycemic activity. A minor metabolite which accounts for less than 2% of a dose, an acetylamino-ethyl benzene derivative, is reported to have 1/10 to 1/3 as much hypoglycemic activity as the parent compound. The mean total body clearance of glipizide was approximately 3 liters per hour after single intravenous doses in patients with type 2 diabetes. The mean apparent volume of distribution was approximately 10 liters. Glipizide is 98-99% bound to serum proteins, primarily to albumin. The mean terminal elimination half-life of glipizide ranged from 2 to 5 hours after single or multiple doses in patients with type 2 diabetes. There were no significant differences in the pharmacokinetics of glipizide after single dose administration to older diabetic subjects compared to younger healthy subjects. There is only limited information regarding the effects of renal impairment on the disposition of glipizide, and no information regarding the effects of hepatic disease. However, since glipizide is highly protein bound and hepatic biotransformation is the predominant route of elimination, the pharmacokinetics and/or pharmacodynamics of glipizide may be altered in patients with renal or hepatic impairment.

In mice no glipizide or metabolites were detectable autoradiographically in the brain or spinal cord of males or females, nor in the fetuses of pregnant females. In another study, however, very small amounts of radioactivity were detected in the fetuses of rats given labelled drug.

INDICATIONS AND USAGE

GLUCOTROL XL is indicated as an adjunct to diet for the control of hyperglycemia and its associated symptomatology in patients with type 2 diabetes formerly known as non-insulin-dependent diabetes mellitus (NIDDM) or maturity-onset diabetes, after an adequate trial of dietary therapy has proved unsatisfactory. GLUCOTROL XL is indicated when diet alone has been unsuccessful in correcting hyperglycemia, but even after the introduction of the drug in the patient's regimen, dietary measures should continue to be considered as important. In 12 week, well-controlled studies there was a maximal average net reduction in hemoglobin A_{1C} of 1.7% in absolute units between placebo-treated and GLUCOTROL XL-treated patients.

In initiating treatment for type 2 diabetes, diet should be emphasized as the primary form of treatment. Caloric restriction and weight loss are essential in the obese diabetic patient. Proper dietary management alone may be effective in controlling blood glucose and symptoms of hyperglycemia. The importance of regular physical activity should also be stressed, cardiovascular risk factors should be identified, and corrective measures taken where possible.

If this treatment program fails to reduce symptoms and/or blood glucose, the use of an oral sulfonylurea should be considered. If additional reduction of symptoms and/or blood glucose is required, the addition of insulin to the treatment regimen should be considered. Use of GLUCOTROL XL must be viewed by both the physician and patient as a treatment in addition to diet, and not as a substitute for diet or as a convenient mechanism for avoiding dietary restraint. Furthermore, loss of blood-glucose control on diet alone also may be transient, thus requiring only short-term administration of glipizide.

Some patients fail to respond initially or gradually lose their responsiveness to sulfonylurea drugs, including GLUCOTROL XL. In these cases, concomitant use of GLUCOTROL XL with other oral blood-glucose-lowering agents can be considered. Other approaches that can be considered include substitution of GLUCOTROL XL therapy with that of another oral blood-glucose-lowering agent or insulin. GLUCOTROL XL should be discontinued if it no longer contributes to glucose lowering. Judgment of response to therapy should be based on regular clinical and laboratory evaluations.

In considering the use of GLUCOTROL XL in asymptomatic patients, it should be recognized that controlling blood glucose in type 2 diabetes has not been definitely established to be effective in preventing the long-term cardiovascular or neural complications of diabetes. However, in insulin-dependent diabetes mellitus controlling blood glucose has been effective in slowing the progression of diabetic retinopathy, nephropathy, and neuropathy.

CONTRAINDICATIONS

Glipizide is contraindicated in patients with:

1. Known hypersensitivity to glipizide or any excipients in the GITS tablets.
2. Type 1 diabetes, diabetic ketoacidosis, with or without coma. This condition should be treated with insulin.

WARNINGS

SPECIAL WARNING ON INCREASED RISK OF CARDIOVASCULAR MORTALITY: The administration of oral hypoglycemic drugs has been reported to be associated with increased cardiovascular mortality as compared to treatment with diet alone or diet plus insulin. This warning is based on the study conducted by the University Group Diabetes Program (UGDP), a long-term prospective clinical trial de-

Continued on next page

Glucotrol XL—Cont.

signed to evaluate the effectiveness of glucose-lowering drugs in preventing or delaying vascular complications in patients with type 2 diabetes. The study involved 823 patients who were randomly assigned to one of four treatment groups (*Diabetes*, 19, SUPP. 2: 747–830, 1970).

UGDP reported that patients treated for 5 to 8 years with diet plus a fixed dose of tolbutamide (1.5 grams per day) had a rate of cardiovascular mortality approximately 2½ times that of patients treated with diet alone. A significant increase in total mortality was not observed, but the use of tolbutamide was discontinued based on the increase in cardiovascular mortality, thus limiting the opportunity for the study to show an increase in overall mortality. Despite controversy regarding the interpretation of these results, the findings of the UGDP study provide an adequate basis for this warning. The patient should be informed of the potential risks and advantages of glipizide and of alternative modes of therapy.

Although only one drug in the sulfonylurea class (tolbutamide) was included in this study, it is prudent from a safety standpoint to consider that this warning may also apply to other oral hypoglycemic drugs in this class, in view of their close similarities in mode of action and chemical structure.

As with any other non-deformable material, caution should be used when administering GLUCOTROL XL Extended Release Tablets in patients with preexisting severe gastrointestinal narrowing (pathologic or iatrogenic). There have been rare reports of obstructive symptoms in patients with known strictures in association with the ingestion of another drug in this non-deformable sustained release formulation.

PRECAUTIONS

General

Renal and Hepatic Disease: The pharmacokinetics and/or pharmacodynamics of glipizide may be affected in patients with impaired renal or hepatic function. If hypoglycemia should occur in such patients, it may be prolonged and appropriate management should be instituted.

GI Disease: Markedly reduced GI retention times of the GLUCOTROL XL Extended Release Tablets may influence the pharmacokinetic profile and hence the clinical efficacy of the drug.

Hypoglycemia: All sulfonylurea drugs are capable of producing severe hypoglycemia. Proper patient selection, dosage, and instructions are important to avoid hypoglycemic episodes. Renal or hepatic insufficiency may affect the disposition of glipizide and the latter may also diminish gluconeogenic capacity, both of which increase the risk of serious hypoglycemic reactions. Elderly, debilitated or malnourished patients, and those with adrenal or pituitary insufficiency are particularly susceptible to the hypoglycemic action of glucose-lowering drugs. Hypoglycemia may be difficult to recognize in the elderly, and in people who are taking beta-adrenergic blocking drugs. Hypoglycemia is more likely to occur when caloric intake is deficient, after severe or prolonged exercise, when alcohol is ingested, or when more than one glucose-lowering drug is used. Therapy with a combination of glucose-lowering agents may increase the potential for hypoglycemia.

Loss of Control of Blood Glucose: When a patient stabilized on any diabetic regimen is exposed to stress such as fever, trauma, infection, or surgery, a loss of control may occur. At such times, it may be necessary to discontinue glipizide and administer insulin.

The effectiveness of any oral hypoglycemic drug, including glipizide, in lowering blood glucose to a desired level decreases in many patients over a period of time, which may be due to progression of the severity of the diabetes or to diminished responsiveness to the drug. This phenomenon is known as secondary failure, to distinguish it from primary failure in which the drug is ineffective in an individual patient when first given. Adequate adjustment of dose and adherence to diet should be assessed before classifying a patient as a secondary failure.

Laboratory Tests: Blood and urine glucose should be monitored periodically. Measurement of hemoglobin A_{1C} may be useful.

Information for Patients: Patients should be informed that GLUCOTROL XL Extended Release Tablets should be swallowed whole. Patients should not chew, divide or crush tablets. Patients should not be concerned if they occasionally notice in their stool something that looks like a tablet. In the GLUCOTROL XL Extended Release Tablet, the medication is contained within a nonabsorbable shell that has been specially designed to slowly release the drug so the body can absorb it. When this process is completed, the empty tablet is eliminated from the body.

Patients should be informed of the potential risks and advantages of GLUCOTROL XL and of alternative modes of therapy. They should also be informed about the importance of adhering to dietary instructions, of a regular exercise program, and of regular testing of urine and/or blood glucose. The risks of hypoglycemia, its symptoms and treatment, and conditions that predispose to its development should be explained to patients and responsible family members. Primary and secondary failure also should be explained.

Drug Interactions: The hypoglycemic action of sulfonylureas may be potentiated by certain drugs including nonsteroidal anti-inflammatory agents and other drugs that are highly protein bound, salicylates, sulfonamides, chloramphenicol, probenecid, coumarins, monoamine oxidase inhibitors, and beta-adrenergic blocking agents. When such drugs are administered to a patient receiving glipizide, the patient should be observed closely for hypoglycemia. When such drugs are withdrawn from a patient receiving glipizide, the patient should be observed closely for loss of control. *In vitro* binding studies with human serum proteins indicate that glipizide binds differently than tolbutamide and does not interact with salicylate or dicumarol. However, caution must be exercised in extrapolating these findings to the clinical situation and in the use of glipizide with these drugs.

Certain drugs tend to produce hyperglycemia and may lead to loss of control. These drugs include the thiazides and other diuretics, corticosteroids, phenothiazines, thyroid products, estrogens, oral contraceptives, phenytoin, nicotinic acid, sympathomimetics, calcium channel blocking drugs, and isoniazid. When such drugs are administered to a patient receiving glipizide, the patient should be closely observed for loss of control. When such drugs are withdrawn from a patient receiving glipizide, the patient should be observed closely for hypoglycemia.

A potential interaction between oral miconazole and oral hypoglycemic agents leading to severe hypoglycemia has been reported. Whether this interaction also occurs with the intravenous, topical, or vaginal preparations of miconazole is not known. The effect of concomitant administration of Diflucan® (fluconazole) and Glucotrol has been demonstrated in a placebo-controlled crossover study in normal volunteers. All subjects received Glucotrol alone and following treatment with 100 mg of Diflucan® as a single daily oral dose for 7 days. The mean percentage increase in the Glucotrol AUC after fluconazole administration was 56.9% (range: 35 to 81%).

Carcinogenesis, Mutagenesis, Impairment of Fertility: A twenty month study in rats and an eighteen month study in mice at doses up to 75 times the maximum human dose revealed no evidence of drug-related carcinogenicity. Bacterial and *in vivo* mutagenicity tests were uniformly negative. Studies in rats of both sexes at doses up to 75 times the human dose showed no effects on fertility.

Pregnancy: Pregnancy Category C: Glipizide was found to be mildly fetotoxic in rat reproductive studies at all dose levels (5-50 mg/kg). This fetotoxicity has been similarly noted with other sulfonylureas, such as tolbutamide and tolazamide. The effect is perinatal and believed to be directly related to the pharmacologic (hypoglycemic) action of glipizide. In studies in rats and rabbits no teratogenic effects were found. There are no adequate and well controlled studies in pregnant women. Glipizide should be used during pregnancy only if the potential benefit justifies the potential risk to the fetus.

Because recent information suggests that abnormal blood-glucose levels during pregnancy are associated with a higher incidence of congenital abnormalities, many experts recommend that insulin be used during pregnancy to maintain blood-glucose levels as close to normal as possible.

Nonteratogenic Effects: Prolonged severe hypoglycemia (4 to 10 days) has been reported in neonates born to mothers who were receiving a sulfonylurea drug at the time of delivery. This has been reported more frequently with the use of agents with prolonged half-lives. If glipizide is used during pregnancy, it should be discontinued at least one month before the expected delivery date.

Nursing Mothers: Although it is not known whether glipizide is excreted in human milk, some sulfonylurea drugs are known to be excreted in human milk. Because the potential for hypoglycemia in nursing infants may exist, a decision should be made whether to discontinue nursing or to discontinue the drug, taking into account the importance of the drug to the mother. If the drug is discontinued and if diet alone is inadequate for controlling blood glucose, insulin therapy should be considered.

Pediatric Use: Safety and effectiveness in children have not been established.

Geriatric Use: Of the total number of patients in clinical studies of GLUCOTROL XL, 33 percent were 65 and over. Approximately 1-2 days longer were required to reach steady-state in the elderly. (See CLINICAL PHARMACOLOGY and DOSAGE AND ADMINISTRATION.) There were no overall differences in effectiveness or safety between younger and older patients, but greater sensitivity of some individuals cannot be ruled out. As such, it should be noted that elderly, debilitated or malnourished patients, and those with adrenal or pituitary insufficiency, are particularly susceptible to the hypoglycemic action of glucose-lowering drugs. Hypoglycemia may be difficult to recognize in the elderly. In addition, in elderly, debilitated or malnourished patients, and patients with impaired renal or hepatic function, the initial and maintenance dosing should be conservative to avoid hypoglycemic reactions.

ADVERSE REACTIONS

In U.S. controlled studies the frequency of serious adverse experiences reported was very low and causal relationship has not been established.

The 580 patients from 31 to 87 years of age who received GLUCOTROL XL Extended Release Tablets in doses from 5 mg to 60 mg in both controlled and open trials were included in the evaluation of adverse experiences. All adverse experiences reported were tabulated independently of their possible causal relation to medication.

Hypoglycemia: See PRECAUTIONS and OVERDOSAGE sections.

Only 3.4% of patients receiving GLUCOTROL XL Extended Release Tablets had hypoglycemia documented by a blood-glucose measurement <60 mg/dL and/or symptoms believed to be associated with hypoglycemia. In a comparative efficacy study of GLUCOTROL XL and Glucotrol, hypoglycemia occurred rarely with an incidence of less than 1% with both drugs.

In double-blind, placebo-controlled studies the adverse experiences reported with an incidence of 3% or more in GLUCOTROL XL-treated patients include:

Adverse Effect	GLUCOTROL XL (%) (N=278)	Placebo (%) (N=69)
Asthenia	10.1	13.0
Headache	8.6	8.7
Dizziness	6.8	5.8
Nervousness	3.6	2.9
Tremor	3.6	0.0
Diarrhea	5.4	0.0
Flatulence	3.2	1.4

The following adverse experiences occurred with an incidence of less than 3% in GLUCOTROL XL-treated patients:

Body as a whole—pain
Nervous system—insomnia, paresthesia, anxiety, depression and hypesthesia
Gastrointestinal—nausea, dyspepsia, constipation and vomiting
Metabolic—hypoglycemia
Musculoskeletal—arthralgia, leg cramps and myalgia
Cardiovascular—syncope
Skin—sweating and pruritus
Respiratory—rhinitis
Special senses—blurred vision
Urogenital—polyuria

Other adverse experiences occurred with an incidence of less than 1% in GLUCOTROL XL-treated patients:

Body as a whole—chills
Nervous system—hypertonia, confusion, vertigo, somnolence, gait abnormality and decreased libido
Gastrointestinal—anorexia and trace blood in stool
Metabolic—thirst and edema
Cardiovascular—arrhythmia, migraine, flushing and hypertension
Skin—rash and urticaria
Respiratory—pharyngitis and dyspnea
Special senses—pain in the eye, conjunctivitis and retinal hemorrhage
Urogenital—dysuria

Although these adverse experiences occurred in patients treated with GLUCOTROL XL, a causal relationship to the medication has not been established in all cases.

There have been rare reports of gastrointestinal irritation and gastrointestinal bleeding with use of another drug in this non-deformable sustained release formulation, although causal relationship to the drug is uncertain.

In post-marketing experience of GLUCOTROL XL, the additional adverse reaction of abdominal pain has been reported.

The following are adverse experiences reported with immediate release glipizide and other sulfonylureas, but have not been observed with GLUCOTROL XL:

Hematologic: Leukopenia, agranulocytosis, thrombocytopenia, hemolytic anemia, aplastic anemia, and pancytopenia have been reported with sulfonylureas.

Metabolic: Hepatic porphyria and disulfiram-like reactions have been reported with sulfonylureas. In the mouse, glipizide pretreatment did not cause an accumulation of acetaldehyde after ethanol administration. Clinical experience to date has shown that glipizide has an extremely low incidence of disulfiram-like alcohol reactions.

Endocrine Reactions: Cases of hyponatremia and the syndrome of inappropriate antidiuretic hormone (SIADH) secretion have been reported with glipizide and other sulfonylureas.

Laboratory Tests: The pattern of laboratory test abnormalities observed with glipizide was similar to that for other sulfonylureas. Occasional mild to moderate elevations of SGOT, LDH, alkaline phosphatase, BUN and creatinine were noted. One case of jaundice was reported. The relationship of these abnormalities to glipizide is uncertain, and they have rarely been associated with clinical symptoms.

OVERDOSAGE

There is no well-documented experience with GLUCOTROL XL overdosage in humans. There have been no known suicide attempts associated with purposeful overdosing with GLUCOTROL XL. In nonclinical studies the acute oral toxicity of glipizide was extremely low in all species tested (LD_{50} greater than 4 g/kg). Overdosage of sulfonylureas including glipizide can produce hypoglycemia. Mild hypoglycemic symptoms without loss of consciousness or neurologic findings should be treated aggressively with oral glucose and adjustments in drug dosage and/or meal patterns. Close monitoring should continue until the physician is assured that the patient is out of danger. Severe hypoglycemic reactions with coma, seizure, or other neurological impairment occur infrequently, but constitute medical emergencies requiring immediate hospitalization. If hypoglycemic coma is diagnosed or suspected, the patient should be given rapid intravenous injection of concentrated (50%) glucose solution. This should be followed by a continuous infusion of a more dilute (10%) glucose solution at a rate that will maintain the blood glucose at a level above 100 mg/dL. Patients should be closely monitored for a minimum of 24 to 48 hours since hypoglycemia may recur after apparent clinical recovery. Clearance of glipizide from plasma may be prolonged in persons with liver disease. Because of the extensive protein binding of glipizide, dialysis is unlikely to be of benefit.

DOSAGE AND ADMINISTRATION

There is no fixed dosage regimen for the management of diabetes mellitus with GLUCOTROL XL Extended Release Tablet or any other hypoglycemic agent. Glycemic control should be monitored with hemoglobin A_{1C} and/or blood-glucose levels to determine the minimum effective dose for the patient; to detect primary failure, i.e., inadequate lowering of blood glucose at the maximum recommended dose of medication; and to detect secondary failure, i.e., loss of an adequate blood-glucose-lowering response after an initial period of effectiveness. Home blood-glucose monitoring may also provide useful information to the patient and physician. Short-term administration of GLUCOTROL XL Extended Release Tablet may be sufficient during periods of transient loss of control in patients usually controlled on diet.

In general, GLUCOTROL XL should be given with breakfast.

Recommended Dosing: The usual starting dose of GLUCOTROL XL as initial therapy is 5 mg per day, given with breakfast. Those patients who may be more sensitive to hypoglycemic drugs may be started at a lower dose.

Dosage adjustment should be based on laboratory measures of glycemic control. While fasting blood-glucose levels generally reach steady-state following initiation or change in GLUCOTROL XL dosage, a single fasting glucose determination may not accurately reflect the response to therapy. In most cases, hemoglobin A_{1C} level measured at three month intervals is the preferred means of monitoring response to therapy.

Hemoglobin A_{1C} should be measured as GLUCOTROL XL therapy is initiated and repeated approximately three months later. If the result of this test suggests that glycemic control over the preceding three months was inadequate, the GLUCOTROL XL dose may be increased. Subsequent dosage adjustments should be made on the basis of hemoglobin A_{1C} levels measured at three month intervals. If no improvement is seen after three months of therapy with a higher dose, the previous dose should be resumed. Decisions which utilize fasting blood glucose to adjust GLUCOTROL XL therapy should be based on at least two or more similar, consecutive values obtained seven days or more after the previous dose adjustment.

Most patients will be controlled with 5 mg to 10 mg taken once daily. However, some patients may require up to the maximum recommended daily dose of 20 mg. While the glycemic control of selected patients may improve with doses which exceed 10 mg, clinical studies conducted to date have not demonstrated an additional group average reduction of hemoglobin A_{1C} beyond what was achieved with the 10 mg dose.

Based on the results of a randomized crossover study, patients receiving immediate release glipizide may be switched safely to GLUCOTROL XL Extended Release Tablets once-a-day at the nearest equivalent total daily dose. Patients receiving immediate release Glucotrol also may be titrated to the appropriate dose of GLUCOTROL XL starting with 5 mg once daily. The decision to switch to the nearest equivalent dose or to titrate should be based on clinical judgment.

In elderly patients, debilitated or malnourished patients, and patients with impaired renal or hepatic function, the initial and maintenance dosing should be conservative to avoid hypoglycemic reactions (see PRECAUTIONS section).

Combination Use:

When adding other blood-glucose-lowering agents to GLUCOTROL XL for combination therapy, the agent should be initiated at the lowest recommended dose, and patients should be observed carefully for hypoglycemia. Refer to the product information supplied with the oral agent for additional information.

When adding GLUCOTROL XL to other blood-glucose-lowering agents, GLUCOTROL XL can be initiated at 5 mg. Those patients who may be more sensitive to hypoglycemic drugs may be started at a lower dose. Titration should be based on clinical judgment.

Patients Receiving Insulin: As with other sulfonylurea-class hypoglycemics, many patients with stable type 2 diabetes receiving insulin may be transferred safely to treatment with GLUCOTROL XL Extended Release Tablets. When transferring patients from insulin to GLUCOTROL XL, the following general guidelines should be considered:

For patients whose daily insulin requirement is 20 units or less, insulin may be discontinued and GLUCOTROL XL therapy may begin at usual dosages. Several days should elapse between titration steps.

For patients whose daily insulin requirement is greater than 20 units, the insulin dose should be reduced by 50% and GLUCOTROL XL therapy may begin at usual dosages. Subsequent reductions in insulin dosage should depend on individual patient response. Several days should elapse between titration steps.

During the insulin withdrawal period, the patient should test urine samples for sugar and ketone bodies at least three times daily. Patients should be instructed to contact the prescriber immediately if these tests are abnormal. In some cases, especially when the patient has been receiving greater than 40 units of insulin daily, it may be advisable to consider hospitalization during the transition period.

Patients Receiving Other Oral Hypoglycemic Agents: As with other sulfonylurea-class hypoglycemics, no transition period is necessary when transferring patients to GLUCOTROL XL Extended Release Tablets. Patients should be observed carefully (1-2 weeks) for hypoglycemia when being transferred from longer half-life sulfonylureas (e.g., chlorpropamide) to GLUCOTROL XL due to potential overlapping of drug effect.

HOW SUPPLIED

GLUCOTROL XL® (glipizide) Extended Release Tablets are supplied as 2.5 mg, 5 mg, and 10 mg round, biconvex tablets and imprinted with black ink as follows:

2.5 mg tablets are blue and imprinted with "GLUCOTROL XL 2.5" on one side.

Bottles of 30: NDC 0049-1620-30

5 mg tablets are white and imprinted with "GLUCOTROL XL 5" on one side.

Bottles of 100: NDC 0049-1550-66
Bottles of 500: NDC 0049-1550-73

10 mg tablets are white and imprinted with "GLUCOTROL XL 10" on one side.

Bottles of 100: NDC 0049-1560-66
Bottles of 500: NDC 0049-1560-73

Recommended Storage: The tablets should be protected from moisture and humidity and stored at controlled room temperature, 59° to 86°F (15° to 30°C).

Rx only

Pfizer U.S. Pharmaceuticals
Pfizer Inc, NY, NY 10017
69-4951-00-9 Revised August 2003

Shown in Product Identification Guide, page 329

INSPRA™ ℞

[*ĭn-sprā̆*]
(eplerenone) tablets

DESCRIPTION

INSPRA™ contains eplerenone, a blocker of aldosterone binding at the mineralocorticoid receptor.

Eplerenone is chemically described as Pregn-4-ene-7,21-dicarboxylic acid, 9,11-epoxy-17-hydroxy-3-oxo-, γ-lactone, methyl ester, (7α,11α,17α)-. Its empirical formula is $C_{24}H_{30}O_6$ and it has a molecular weight of 414.50. The structural formula of eplerenone is represented below:

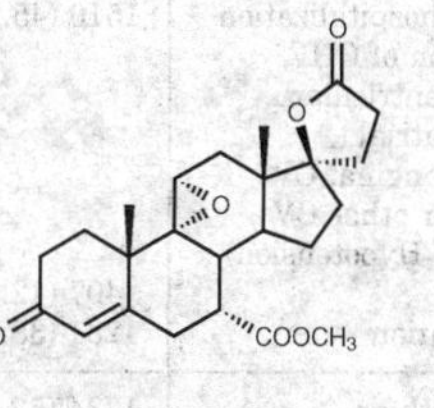

eplerenone

Eplerenone is an odorless, white to off-white crystalline powder. It is very slightly soluble in water, with its solubility essentially pH independent. The octanol/water partition coefficient of eplerenone is approximately 7.1 at pH 7.0.

INSPRA for oral administration contains 25 mg or 50 mg of eplerenone and the following inactive ingredients: lactose, microcrystalline cellulose, croscarmellose sodium, hypromellose, sodium lauryl sulfate, talc, magnesium stearate, titanium dioxide, polyethylene glycol, polysorbate 80, and iron oxide yellow and iron oxide red.

CLINICAL PHARMACOLOGY

Mechanism of Action

Eplerenone binds to the mineralocorticoid receptor and blocks the binding of aldosterone, a component of the renin-angiotensin-aldosterone-system (RAAS). Aldosterone synthesis, which occurs primarily in the adrenal gland, is modulated by multiple factors, including angiotensin II and non-RAAS mediators such as adrenocorticotropic hormone (ACTH) and potassium. Aldosterone binds to mineralocorticoid receptors in both epithelial (e.g., kidney) and nonepithelial (e.g., heart, blood vessels, and brain) tissues and increases blood pressure through induction of sodium reabsorption and possibly other mechanisms.

Eplerenone has been shown to produce sustained increases in plasma renin and serum aldosterone, consistent with inhibition of the negative regulatory feedback of aldosterone on renin secretion. The resulting increased plasma renin activity and aldosterone circulating levels do not overcome the effects of eplerenone.

Eplerenone selectively binds to recombinant human mineralocorticoid receptors relative to its binding to recombinant human glucocorticoid, progesterone and androgen receptors.

Pharmacokinetics

General: Eplerenone is cleared predominantly by cytochrome P450 (CYP) 3A4 metabolism, with an elimination half-life of 4 to 6 hours. Steady state is reached within 2 days. Absorption is not affected by food. Inhibitors of CYP3A4 (e.g., ketoconazole, saquinavir) increase blood levels of eplerenone.

Absorption and Distribution: Mean peak plasma concentrations of eplerenone are reached approximately 1.5 hours following oral administration. The absolute bioavailability of eplerenone is unknown. Both peak plasma levels (C_{max}) and area under the curve (AUC) are dose proportional for doses of 25 to 100 mg and less than proportional at doses above 100 mg.

The plasma protein binding of eplerenone is about 50% and it is primarily bound to alpha 1-acid glycoproteins. The apparent volume of distribution at steady state ranged from 43 to 90 L. Eplerenone does not preferentially bind to red blood cells.

Metabolism and Excretion: Eplerenone metabolism is primarily mediated via CYP3A4. No active metabolites of eplerenone have been identified in human plasma.

Less than 5% of an eplerenone dose is recovered as unchanged drug in the urine and feces. Following a single oral dose of radiolabeled drug, approximately 32% of the dose was excreted in the feces and approximately 67% was excreted in the urine. The elimination half-life of eplerenone is approximately 4 to 6 hours. The apparent plasma clearance is approximately 10 L/hr.

Special Populations

Age, Gender, and Race: The pharmacokinetics of eplerenone at a dose of 100 mg once daily have been investigated in the elderly (≥65 years), in males and females, and in blacks. The pharmacokinetics of eplerenone did not differ significantly between males and females. At steady state, elderly subjects had increases in C_{max} (22%) and AUC (45%) compared with younger subjects (18 to 45 years). At steady state, C_{max} was 19% lower and AUC was 26% lower in blacks. (See **PRECAUTIONS, Congestive Heart Failure Post-Myocardial Infarction and Hypertension, Geriatric Use** and **DOSAGE AND ADMINISTRATION, Hypertension.**)

Renal Insufficiency: The pharmacokinetics of eplerenone were evaluated in patients with varying degrees of renal insufficiency and in patients undergoing hemodialysis. Compared with control subjects, steady-state AUC and C_{max} were increased by 38% and 24%, respectively, in patients with severe renal impairment and were decreased by 26% and 3%, respectively, in patients undergoing hemodialysis. No correlation was observed between plasma clearance of eplerenone and creatinine clearance. Eplerenone is not removed by hemodialysis. (See **WARNINGS, Hyperkalemia in Patients Treated for Hypertension** and **PRECAUTIONS, Hyperkalemia in Patients Treated for Congestive Heart Failure Post-Myocardial Infarction and Congestive Heart Failure Post-Myocardial Infarction and Hypertension.**)

Hepatic Insufficiency: The pharmacokinetics of eplerenone 400 mg have been investigated in patients with moderate (Child-Pugh Class B) hepatic impairment and compared with normal subjects. Steady-state C_{max} and AUC of eplerenone were increased by 3.6% and 42%, respectively. (See **DOSAGE AND ADMINISTRATION, Hypertension.**)

Heart Failure: The pharmacokinetics of eplerenone 50 mg were evaluated in 8 patients with heart failure (NYHA classification II-IV) and 8 matched (gender, age, weight) healthy controls. Compared with the controls, steady state AUC and C_{max} in patients with stable heart failure were 38% and 30% higher, respectively.

Drug-Drug Interactions

(See **PRECAUTIONS, Congestive Heart Failure Post-Myocardial Infarction and Hypertension, Drug Interactions.**)

Drug-drug interaction studies were conducted with a 100 mg dose of eplerenone.

Eplerenone is metabolized primarily by CYP3A4. A potent inhibitor of CYP3A4 (ketoconazole) caused increased exposure of about 5-fold while less potent CYP3A4 inhibitors (erythromycin, saquinavir, verapamil, and fluconazole) gave approximately 2-fold increases. Grapefruit juice caused only a small increase (about 25%) in exposure. (See **PRECAUTIONS, Congestive Heart Failure Post-Myocardial Infarction and Hypertension, Drug Interactions** and **DOSAGE AND ADMINISTRATION, Hypertension.**)

Eplerenone is not an inhibitor of CYP1A2, CYP3A4, CYP2C19, CYP2C9, or CYP2D6. Eplerenone did not inhibit the metabolism of chlorzoxazone, diclofenac, methylphenidate, losartan, amiodarone, dexamethasone, mephobarbital, phenytoin, phenacetin, dextromethorphan, metoprolol, tolbutamide, amlodipine, astemizole, cisapride, 17α-ethinyl estradiol, fluoxetine, lovastatin, methylprednisolone, midazolam, nifedipine, simvastatin, triazolam, verapamil, and warfarin in vitro. Eplerenone is not a substrate or an inhibitor of P-Glycoprotein at clinically relevant doses.

No clinically significant drug-drug pharmacokinetic interactions were observed when eplerenone was administered with digoxin, warfarin, midazolam, cisapride, cyclosporine, simvastatin, glyburide, or oral contraceptives (norethindrone/ethinyl estradiol). St. Johns Wort (a CYP3A4 inducer) caused a small (about 30%) decrease in eplerenone AUC.

No significant changes in eplerenone pharmacokinetics were observed when eplerenone was administered with aluminum and magnesium-containing antacids.

CLINICAL STUDIES

Congestive Heart Failure Post-Myocardial Infarction

The eplerenone post-acute myocardial infarction heart failure efficacy and survival study (EPHESUS) was a multina-

Continued on next page

Inspra—Cont.

tional, multicenter, double-blind, randomized, placebo-controlled study in patients clinically stable 3-14 days after an acute myocardial infarction (MI) with left ventricular dysfunction (as measured by left ventricular ejection fraction [LVEF] ≤40%) and either diabetes or clinical evidence of congestive heart failure (CHF) (pulmonary congestion by exam or chest x-ray or S_3). Patients with CHF of valvular or congenital etiology, patients with unstable post-infarct angina, and patients with serum potassium >5.0 mEq/L or serum creatinine >2.5 mg/dL were to be excluded. Patients were allowed to receive standard post-MI drug therapy and to undergo revascularization by angioplasty or coronary artery bypass graft surgery.

Patients randomized to INSPRA were given an initial dose of 25 mg once daily and titrated to the target dose of 50 mg once daily after 4 weeks if serum potassium was < 5.0 mEq/L. Dosage was reduced or suspended anytime during the study if serum potassium levels were ≥ 5.5 mEq/L. (See **DOSAGE AND ADMINISTRATION, Congestive Heart Failure Post-Myocardial Infarction.**)

EPHESUS randomized 6,632 patients (9.3% U.S.) at 671 centers in 27 countries. The study population was primarily white (90%, with 1% black, 1% Asian, 6% Hispanic, 2% other) and male (71%). The mean age was 64 years (range, 22-94 years). The majority of patients had pulmonary congestion (75%) by exam or x-ray and were Killip Class II (64%). The mean ejection fraction was 33%. The average time to enrollment was 7 days post-MI. Medical histories prior to the index MI included hypertension (60%), coronary artery disease (62%), dyslipidemia (48%), angina (41%), type 2 diabetes (30%), previous MI (27%), and HF (15%).

The mean dose of INSPRA was 43 mg/day. Patients also received standard care including aspirin (92%), ACE inhibitors (90%), β-blockers (83%), nitrates (72%), loop diuretics (66%), or HMG-CoA reductase inhibitors (60%).

Patients were followed for an average of 16 months (range, 0-33 months). The ascertainment rate for vital status was 99.7%.

The co-primary endpoints for EPHESUS were (1) the time to death from any cause, and (2) the time to first occurrence of either cardiovascular (CV) mortality [defined as sudden cardiac death or death due to progression of congestive heart failure (CHF), stroke, or other CV causes] or CV hospitalization (defined as hospitalization for progression of CHF, ventricular arrhythmias, acute myocardial infarction, or stroke). For the co-primary endpoint for death from any cause, there were 478 deaths in the INSPRA group (14.4%) and 554 deaths in the placebo group (16.7%). The risk of death with INSPRA was reduced by 15% [hazard ratio equal to 0.85 (95% confidence interval 0.75 to 0.96; p = 0.008 by log rank test)]. Kaplan-Meier estimates of all-cause mortality are shown in Figure 1 and the components of mortality are provided in Table 1.

Figure 1. Kaplan-Meier Estimates of All-Cause Mortality

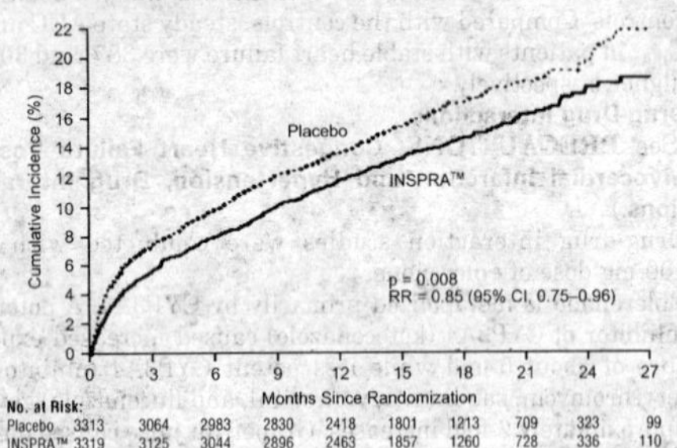

Table 1. Components of All-Cause Mortality in EPHESUS

	INSPRA™ (N=3319) n (%)	Placebo (N=3313) n (%)	Hazard Ratio	p-value
Death from any cause	478 (14.4)	554 (16.7)	0.85	0.008
CV Death	407 (12.3)	483 (14.6)	0.83	0.005
Non-CV Death	60 (1.8)	54 (1.6)		
Unknown or unwitnessed death	11 (0.3)	17 (0.5)		

Most CV deaths were attributed to sudden death, acute MI, and CHF.

The time to first event for the co-primary endpoint of CV death or hospitalization as defined above, was longer in the INSPRA group (hazard ratio 0.87, 95% confidence interval 0.79 to 0.95, p = 0.002). An analysis that included the time to first occurrence of CV mortality and all CV hospitalizations (atrial arrhythmia, angina, CV procedures, progression of CHF, MI, stroke, ventricular arrhythmia, or other CV causes) showed a smaller effect with a hazard ratio of 0.92 (95% confidence interval 0.86 to 0.99; p = 0.028). The combined endpoints, including combined all-cause hospitalization and mortality were driven primarily by CV mortality. The combined endpoints in EPHESUS, including all-cause hospitalization and all-cause mortality, are presented in Table 2.

Figure 2. Hazard Ratios of All-Cause Mortality by Subgroups

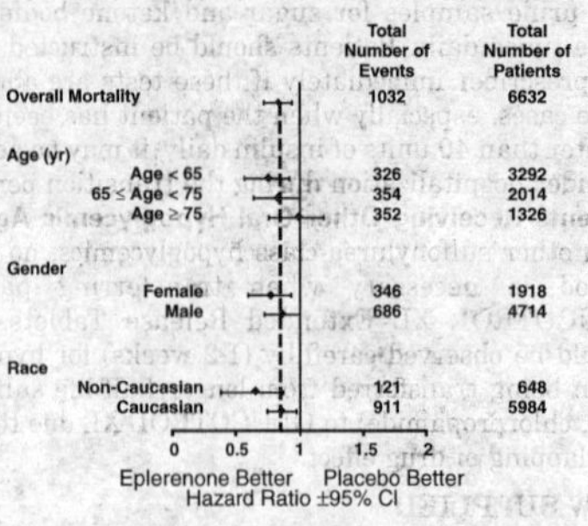

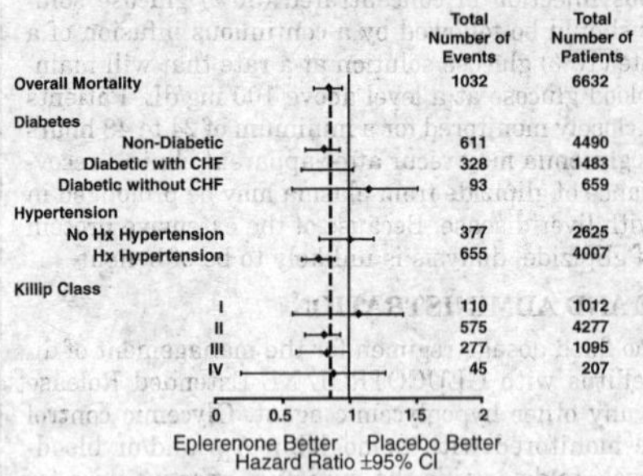

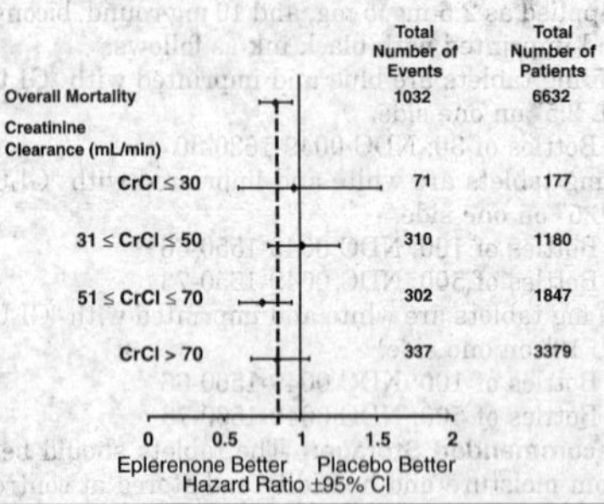

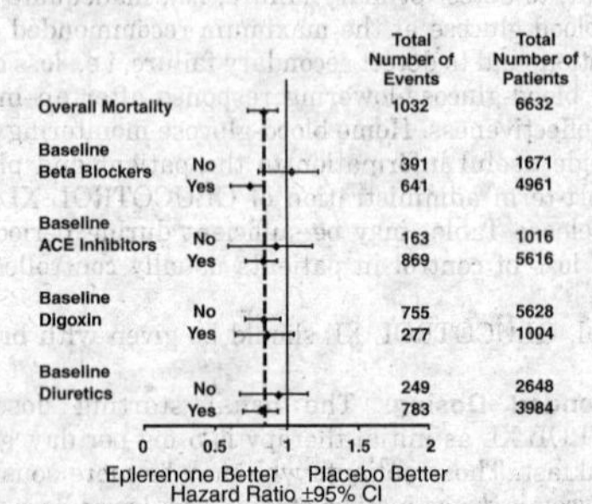

Table 2. Rates of Death or Hospitalization in EPHESUS

Event	INSPRA™ n (%)	Placebo n (%)
CV death or hospitalization for progression of CHF, stroke, MI or ventricular arrhythmia[1]	885 (26.7)	993 (30.0)
Death	407 (12.3)	483 (14.6)
Hospitalization	606 (18.3)	649 (19.6)
CV death or hospitalization for progression of CHF, stroke, MI, ventricular arrhythmia, atrial arrhythmia, angina, CV procedures, or other CV causes (PVD; Hypotension)	1516 (45.7)	1610 (48.6)
Death	407 (12.3)	483 (14.6)
Hospitalization	1281 (38.6)	1307 (39.5)
All-cause death or hospitalization	1734 (52.2)	1833 (55.3)
Death[1]	478 (14.4)	554 (16.7)
Hospitalization	1497 (45.1)	1530 (46.2)

[1]Co-Primary Endpoint.

Mortality hazard ratios varied for some subgroups as shown in Figure 2. Mortality hazard ratios appeared favorable for INSPRA for both genders and for all races or ethnic groups, although the numbers of non-caucasians were low (648, 10%). Patients with diabetes without clinical evidence of CHF and patients greater than 75 years did not appear to benefit from the use of INSPRA. Such subgroup analyses must be interpreted cautiously.

[See figure 2 above]

Analyses conducted for a variety of CV biomarkers did not confirm a mechanism of action by which mortality was reduced.

Hypertension

The safety and efficacy of INSPRA have been evaluated alone and in combination with other antihypertensive agents in clinical studies of 3091 hypertensive patients. The studies included 46% women, 14% blacks, and 22% elderly (age ≥65). The studies excluded patients with elevated baseline serum potassium (>5.0 mEq/L) and elevated baseline serum creatinine (generally >1.5 mg/dL in males and >1.3 mg/dL in females).

Two fixed-dose, placebo-controlled, 8- to 12-week monotherapy studies in patients with baseline diastolic blood pressures of 95 to 114 mm Hg were conducted to assess the antihypertensive effect of INSPRA. In these two studies, 611 patients were randomized to INSPRA and 140 patients to placebo. Patients received INSPRA in doses of 25 to 400 mg daily as either a single daily dose or divided into two daily doses. The mean placebo-subtracted reductions in trough cuff blood pressure achieved by INSPRA in these studies at doses up to 200 mg are shown in Figures 3 and 4.

Figure 3. INSPRA™ Dose Response – Trough Cuff SBP Placebo-Subtracted Adjusted Mean Change from Baseline in Hypertension Studies

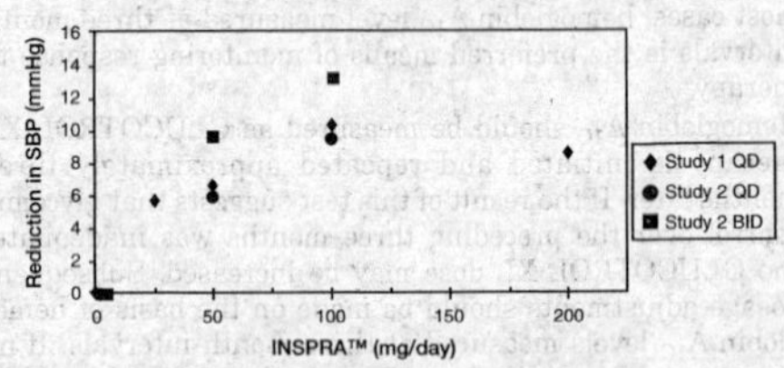

Figure 4. INSPRA™ Dose Response – Trough Cuff DBP Placebo-Subtracted Adjusted Mean Change from Baseline in Hypertension Studies

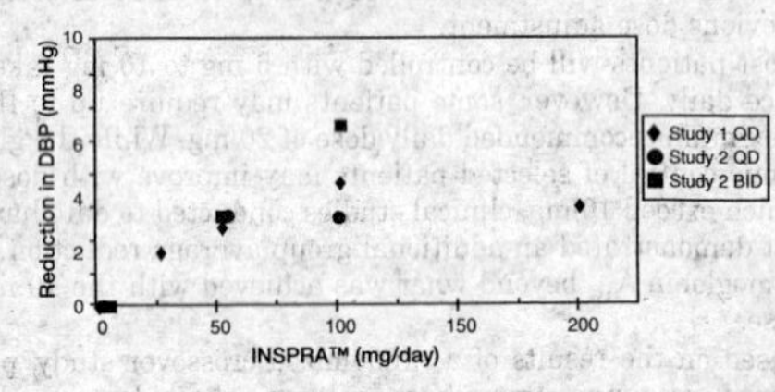

Patients treated with INSPRA 50 to 200 mg daily experienced significant decreases in sitting systolic and diastolic blood pressure at trough with differences from placebo of 6-13 mm Hg (systolic) and 3-7 mm Hg (diastolic). These effects were confirmed by assessments with 24-hour ambulatory blood pressure monitoring (ABPM). In these studies, assessments of 24-hour ABPM data demonstrated that INSPRA, administered once or twice daily, maintained antihypertensive efficacy over the entire dosing interval. However, at a total daily dose of 100 mg, INSPRA administered as 50 mg twice per day produced greater trough cuff (4/3 mm Hg) and ABPM (2/1 mm Hg) blood pressure reductions than 100 mg given once daily.

Blood pressure lowering was apparent within 2 weeks from the start of therapy with INSPRA, with maximal antihypertensive effects achieved within 4 weeks. Stopping INSPRA following treatment for 8 to 24 weeks in six studies did not lead to adverse event rates in the week following withdrawal of INSPRA greater than following placebo or active control withdrawal. Blood pressures in patients not taking other antihypertensives rose 1 week after withdrawal of INSPRA by about 6/3 mm Hg, suggesting that the antihypertensive effect of INSPRA was maintained through 8 to 24 weeks.

Blood pressure reductions with INSPRA in the two fixed-dose monotherapy studies and other studies using titrated doses, as well as concomitant treatments, were not significantly different when analyzed by age, gender, or race with one exception. In a study in patients with low renin hypertension, blood pressure reductions in blacks were smaller than those in whites during the initial titration period with INSPRA.

INSPRA has been studied concomitantly with treatment with ACE inhibitors, angiotensin II receptor antagonists, calcium channel blockers, beta blockers, and hydrochlorothiazide. When administered concomitantly with one of these drugs INSPRA usually produced its expected antihypertensive effects.

There was no significant change in average heart rate among patients treated with INSPRA in the combined clinical studies. No consistent effects of INSPRA on heart rate, QRS duration, or PR or QT interval were observed in 147 normal subjects evaluated for electrocardiographic changes during pharmacokinetic studies.

INDICATIONS AND USAGE

Congestive Heart Failure Post-Myocardial Infarction

INSPRA is indicated to improve survival of stable patients with left ventricular systolic dysfunction (ejection fraction ≤40%) and clinical evidence of congestive heart failure after an acute myocardial infarction. (See **CLINICAL STUDIES, Congestive Heart Failure Post-Myocardial Infarction.)**

Hypertension

INSPRA is indicated for the treatment of hypertension. INSPRA may be used alone or in combination with other antihypertensive agents. (See **CLINICAL STUDIES, Hypertension.**)

CONTRAINDICATIONS

INSPRA is contraindicated in all patients with the following:

- serum potassium >5.5 mEq/L at initiation
- creatinine clearance ≤30 mL/min
- concomitant use with the following potent CYP3A4 inhibitors: ketoconazole, itraconazole, nefazodone, troleandomycin, clarithromycin, ritonavir, and nelfinavir. Inspra should also not be used with other drugs noted in the **CONTRAINDICATIONS, WARNINGS** or **PRECAUTIONS** sections of their labeling to be potent CYP3A4 inhibitors. (See **CLINICAL PHARMACOLOGY, Drug-Drug Interactions; PRECAUTIONS, Congestive Heart Failure Post-Myocardial Infarction and Hypertension, Drug Interactions** and **DOSAGE AND ADMINISTRATION, Hypertension.**)

Hypertension

INSPRA is also contraindicated for the treatment of hypertension in patients with the following:

- type 2 diabetes with microalbuminuria
- serum creatinine >2.0 mg/dL in males or >1.8 mg/dL in females
- creatinine clearance <50 mL/min
- concomitant use of potassium supplements or potassium-sparing diuretics (amiloride, spironolactone, or triamterene)

(See **CLINICAL PHARMACOLOGY, Pharmacokinetics, Drug-Drug Interactions; WARNINGS, Hyperkalemia in Patients Treated for Hypertension; PRECAUTIONS, Congestive Heart Failure Post-Myocardial Infarction and Hypertension, Drug Interactions;** and **ADVERSE REACTIONS, Clinical Laboratory Test Findings, Hypertension, Potassium.**)

WARNINGS

Hyperkalemia in Patients Treated for Hypertension

The principal risk of INSPRA is hyperkalemia. Hyperkalemia can cause serious, sometimes fatal, arrhythmias. This risk can be minimized by patient selection, avoidance of certain concomitant treatments, and monitoring. For patient selection and avoidance of certain concomitant medications, see **CONTRAINDICATIONS; PRECAUTIONS, Congestive Heart Failure Post-Myocardial Infarction and Hypertension, Drug Interactions;** and **ADVERSE REACTIONS, Clinical Laboratory Test Findings, Congestive Heart Failure Post-Myocardial Infarction and Hypertension, Potassium.** Periodic monitoring is recommended in patients at risk for the development of hyperkalemia (including patients receiving concomitant ACE inhibitors or angiotensin II receptor antagonists) until the effect of INSPRA is established. Dose reduction of INSPRA has been shown to decrease potassium levels. (See **DOSAGE AND ADMINISTRATION, Congestive Heart Failure Post-Myocardial Infarction and Hypertension.**)

PRECAUTIONS

Hyperkalemia in Patients Treated for Congestive Heart Failure Post-Myocardial Infarction

The principal risk of INSPRA is hyperkalemia. Hyperkalemia can cause serious, sometimes fatal, arrhythmias. Patients who develop hyperkalemia (>5.5 mEq/L) may still benefit from INSPRA with proper dose adjustment. Hyperkalemia can be minimized by patient selection, avoidance of certain concomitant treatments, and periodic monitoring until the effect of INSPRA has been established. For patient selection and avoidance of certain concomitant medications, see **CONTRAINDICATIONS; PRECAUTIONS, Congestive Heart Failure Post-Myocardial Infarction and Hypertension, Drug Interactions;** and **ADVERSE REACTIONS, Clinical Laboratory Test Findings, Congestive Heart Failure Post-Myocardial Infarction, Potassium.** Dose reduction of INSPRA has been shown to decrease potassium levels. (See **DOSAGE AND ADMINISTRATION, Congestive Heart Failure Post-Myocardial Infarction.**)

Patients with CHF post MI who have serum creatinine levels >2.0 mg/dL (males) or >1.8 mg/dL (females) or creatinine clearance ≤50 mL/min should be treated with caution. The rates of hyperkalemia increased with declining renal function. (See **ADVERSE REACTIONS, Clinical Laboratory Test Findings, Congestive Heart Failure Post-Myocardial Infarction, Potassium.**)

Diabetic patients with CHF post-MI, including those with proteinuria, should also be treated with caution. The subset of patients in EPHESUS with both diabetes and proteinuria on the baseline urinalysis had increased rates of hyperkalemia. (See **ADVERSE REACTIONS Clinical Laboratory Test Findings, Congestive Heart Failure Post-Myocardial Infarction, Potassium.**)

Congestive Heart Failure Post-Myocardial Infarction and Hypertension

Impaired Hepatic Function: In 16 subjects with mild-to-moderate hepatic impairment who received 400 mg of eplerenone no elevations of serum potassium above 5.5 mEq/L were observed. The mean increase in serum potassium was 0.12 mEq/L in patients with hepatic impairment and 0.13 mEq/L in normal controls. The use of INSPRA in patients with severe hepatic impairment has not been evaluated. (See **DOSAGE AND ADMINISTRATION** and **CLINICAL PHARMACOLOGY, Special Populations.**)

Impaired Renal Function: (See **CONTRAINDICATIONS; WARNINGS;** and **PRECAUTIONS.**)

Information for Patients: Patients receiving INSPRA should be informed not to use potassium supplements, salt substitutes containing potassium, or contraindicated drugs without consulting the prescribing physician. (See **CONTRAINDICATIONS; WARNINGS;** and **PRECAUTIONS.**)

Drug Interactions:

Inhibitors of CYP3A4- Eplerenone metabolism is predominantly mediated via CYP3A4. A pharmacokinetic study evaluating the administration of a single dose of INSPRA 100 mg with ketoconazole 200 mg BID, a potent inhibitor of the CYP3A4 pathway, showed a 1.7-fold increase in C_{max} of eplerenone and a 5.4-fold increase in AUC of eplerenone. INSPRA should not be used with drugs described as strong inhibitors of CYP3A4 in their labeling. (See **CONTRAINDICATIONS.**)

Administration of eplerenone with other CYP3A4 inhibitors (e.g., erythromycin 500 mg BID, verapamil 240 mg QD, saquinavir 1200 mg TID, fluconazole 200 mg QD) resulted in increases in C_{max} of eplerenone ranging from 1.4- to 1.6-fold and AUC from 2.0- to 2.9-fold. (See **CLINICAL PHARMACOLOGY, Pharmacokinetics, Drug-Drug Interactions** and **DOSAGE AND ADMINISTRATION, Hypertension.**)

ACE Inhibitors and Angiotensin II Receptor Antagonists (Congestive Heart Failure Post-Myocardial Infarction)- In EPHESUS, 3020 (91%) patients receiving INSPRA 25 to 50 mg also received ACE inhibitors or angiotensin II receptor antagonists (ACEI/ARB). Rates of patients with maximum potassium levels >5.5 mEq/L were similar regardless of the use of ACEI/ARB.

ACE Inhibitors and Angiotensin II Receptor Antagonists (Hypertension)- In clinical studies of patients with hypertension, the addition of INSPRA 50 to 100 mg to ACE inhibitors and angiotensin II receptor antagonists increased mean serum potassium slightly (about 0.09-0.13 mEq/L). In a study in diabetics with microalbuminuria INSPRA 200 mg combined with the ACE inhibitor enalapril 10 mg increased the frequency of hyperkalemia (serum potassium >5.5 mEq/L) from 17% on enalapril alone to 38%. (See **CONTRAINDICATIONS.**)

Lithium- A drug interaction study of eplerenone with lithium has not been conducted. Lithium toxicity has been reported in patients receiving lithium concomitantly with diuretics and ACE inhibitors. Serum lithium levels should be monitored frequently if INSPRA is administered concomitantly with lithium.

Nonsteroidal Anti-Inflammatory Drugs (NSAIDs)- A drug interaction study of eplerenone with an NSAID has not been conducted. The administration of other potassium-sparing antihypertensives with NSAIDs has been shown to reduce the antihypertensive effect in some patients and result in severe hyperkalemia in patients with impaired renal function. Therefore, when INSPRA and NSAIDs are used concomitantly, patients should be observed to determine whether the desired effect on blood pressure is obtained.

Pregnancy:

Pregnancy Category B- There are no adequate and well-controlled studies in pregnant women. INSPRA should be used during pregnancy only if the potential benefit justifies the potential risk to the fetus.

Teratogenic Effects- Embryo-fetal development studies were conducted with doses up to 1000 mg/kg/day in rats and 300 mg/kg/day in rabbits (exposures up to 32 and 31 times the human AUC for the 100-mg/day therapeutic dose, respectively). No teratogenic effects were seen in rats or rabbits, although decreased body weight in maternal rabbits and increased rabbit fetal resorptions and post-implantation loss were observed at the highest administered dosage. Because animal reproduction studies are not always predictive of human response, INSPRA should be used during pregnancy only if clearly needed.

Nursing Mothers: The concentration of eplerenone in human breast milk after oral administration is unknown. However preclinical data show that eplerenone and/or metabolites are present in rat breast milk (0.85:1 [milkplasma] AUC ratio) obtained after a single oral dose. Peak concentrations in plasma and milk were obtained from 0.5 to 1 hour after dosing. Rat pups exposed by this route developed normally. Because many drugs are excreted in human milk and because of the unknown potential for adverse effects on the nursing infant, a decision should be made whether to discontinue nursing or discontinue the drug, taking into account the importance of the drug to the mother.

Pediatric Use: The safety and effectiveness of INSPRA has not been established in pediatric patients.

Geriatric Use:

Congestive Heart Failure Post-Myocardial Infarction- Of the total number of patients in EPHESUS, 3340 (50%) were 65 and over, while 1326 (20%) were 75 and over. Patients greater than 75 years did not appear to benefit from the use of INSPRA. (See **CLINICAL STUDIES, Congestive Heart Failure Post-Myocardial Infarction.)** No differences in overall incidence of adverse events were observed between elderly and younger patients. However, due to age-related decreases in creatinine clearance, the incidence of laboratory-documented hyperkalemia was increased in patients 65 and older. (See **PRECAUTIONS, Hyperkalemia in Patients Treated for Congestive Heart Failure.**)

Hypertension- Of the total number of subjects in clinical hypertension studies of INSPRA, 1123 (23%) were 65 and over, while 212 (4%) were 75 and over. No overall differences in safety or effectiveness were observed between elderly subjects and younger subjects.

Carcinogenesis, Mutagenesis, Impairment of Fertility: Eplerenone was non-genotoxic in a battery of assays including in vitro bacterial mutagenesis (Ames test in *Salmonella* spp. and *E. Coli*), in vitro mammalian cell mutagenesis (mouse lymphoma cells), in vitro chromosomal aberration (Chinese hamster ovary cells), in vivo rat bone marrow micronucleus formation, and in vivo/ex vivo unscheduled DNA synthesis in rat liver.

There was no drug-related tumor response in heterozygous P53 deficient mice when tested for 6 months at dosages up to 1000 mg/kg/day (systemic AUC exposures up to 9 times the exposure in humans receiving the 100-mg/day therapeutic dose). Statistically significant increases in benign thyroid tumors were observed after 2 years in both male and female rats when administered eplerenone 250 mg/kg/day (highest dose tested) and in male rats only at 75 mg/kg/day. These dosages provided systemic AUC exposures approximately 2 to 12 times higher than the average human therapeutic exposure at 100 mg/day. Repeat dose administration of eplerenone to rats increases the hepatic conjugation and clearance of thyroxin, which results in increased levels of TSH by a compensatory mechanism. Drugs that have produced thyroid tumors by this rodent-specific mechanism have not shown a similar effect in humans.

Male rats treated with eplerenone at 1000 mg/kg/day for 10 weeks (AUC 17 times that at the 100-mg/day human therapeutic dose) had decreased weights of seminal vesicles and epididymides and slightly decreased fertility. Dogs administered eplerenone at dosages of 15 mg/kg/day and higher (AUC 5 times that at the 100-mg/day human therapeutic dose) had dose-related prostate atrophy. The prostate atrophy was reversible after daily treatment for 1 year at 100 mg/kg/day. Dogs with prostate atrophy showed no decline in libido, sexual performance, or semen quality. Testicular weight and histology were not affected by eplerenone in any test animal species at any dosage.

ADVERSE REACTIONS

Congestive Heart Failure Post-Myocardial Infarction

In EPHESUS, safety was evaluated in 3307 patients treated with INSPRA and 3301 placebo-treated patients. The overall incidence of adverse events reported with INSPRA (78.9%) was similar to placebo (79.5%). Adverse events occurred at a similar rate regardless of age, gender, or race. Patients discontinued treatment due to an adverse event at similar rates in either treatment group (4.4% INSPRA vs. 4.3% placebo).

Adverse events that occurred more frequently in patients treated with INSPRA than placebo were hyperkalemia (3.4% vs 2.0%) and increased creatinine (2.4% vs 1.5%). Discontinuations due to hyperkalemia or abnormal renal function were less than 1.0% in both groups. Hypokalemia occurred less frequently in patients treated with INSPRA (0.6% vs. 1.6%).

The rates of sex hormone related adverse events are shown in Table 3.

Table 3. Rates of Sex Hormone Related Adverse Events in EPHESUS

	Rates in Males			Rates in Females
	Gyneco-mastia	Masto-dynia	Either	Abnormal Vaginal Bleeding
INSPRA™	0.4%	0.1%	0.5%	0.4%
Placebo	0.5%	0.1%	0.6%	0.4%

Hypertension

INSPRA has been evaluated for safety in 3091 patients treated for hypertension. A total of 690 patients were treated for over 6 months and 106 patients were treated for over 1 year.

Continued on next page

Inspra—Cont.

In placebo-controlled studies, the overall rates of adverse events were 47% with INSPRA and 45% with placebo. Adverse events occurred at a similar rate regardless of age, gender, or race. Therapy was discontinued due to an adverse event in 3% of patients treated with INSPRA and 3% of patients given placebo. The most common reasons for discontinuation of INSPRA were headache, dizziness, angina pectoris/myocardial infarction, and increased GGT. The adverse events that were reported at a rate of at least 1% of patients and at a higher rate in patients treated with INSPRA in daily doses of 25 to 400 mg versus placebo are shown in Table 4.

Table 4. Rates (%) of Adverse Events Occurring in Placebo-Controlled Hypertension Studies in ≥1% of Patients Treated with INSPRA™ (25 to 400 mg) and at a More Frequent Rate than in Placebo-Treated Patients

	INSPRA™ (n=945)	Placebo (n=372)
Metabolic		
Hypercholesterolemia	1	0
Hypertriglyceridemia	1	0
Digestive		
Diarrhea	2	1
Abdominal pain	1	0
Urinary		
Albuminuria	1	0
Respiratory		
Coughing	2	1
Central/Peripheral Nervous System		
Dizziness	3	2
Body as a Whole		
Fatigue	2	1
Influenza-like symptoms	2	1

Note: Adverse events that are too general to be informative or are very common in the treated population are excluded.

Gynecomastia and abnormal vaginal bleeding were reported with INSPRA but not with placebo. The rates of these sex hormone related adverse events are shown in Table 5. The rates increased slightly with increasing duration of therapy. In females, abnormal vaginal bleeding was also reported in 0.8% of patients on antihypertensive medications (other than spironolactone) in active control arms of the studies with INSPRA.

Table 5. Rates of Sex Hormone Related Adverse Events with INSPRA™ in Hypertension Clinical Studies

	Rates in Males			Rates in Females
	Gynecomastia	Mastodynia	Either	Abnormal Vaginal Bleeding
All controlled studies	0.5%	0.8%	1.0%	0.6%
Controlled studies lasting ≥ 6 months	0.7%	1.3%	1.6%	0.8%
Open label, long-term study	1.0%	0.3%	1.0%	2.1%

Clinical Laboratory Test Findings

Congestive Heart Failure Post-Myocardial Infarction:

Creatinine- Increases of more than 0.5 mg/dL were reported for 6.5% of patients administered INSPRA and for 4.9% of placebo-treated patients.

Potassium- In EPHESUS, the frequency of patients with changes in potassium (<3.5 mEq/L or >5.5 mEq/L or ≥6.0 mEq/L) receiving INSPRA compared with placebo are displayed in Table 6.

Table 6. Hypokalemia (<3.5 mEq/L) or Hyperkalemia (>5.5 or ≥6.0 mEq/L) in EPHESUS

Potassium (mEq/L)	INSPRA™ (N=3251) n (%)	Placebo (N=3237) n (%)
<3.5	273 (8.4)	424 (13.1)
>5.5	508 (15.6)	363 (11.2)
≥6.0	180 (5.5)	126 (3.9)

Table 7 shows the rates of hyperkalemia in EPHESUS as assessed by baseline renal function (creatinine clearance).

Table 7. Rates of Hyperkalemia (>5.5 mEq/L) in EPHESUS by Baseline Creatinine Clearance*

Baseline Creatinine Clearance	INSPRA™	Placebo
≤30 mL/min	31.5%	22.6%
31-50 mL/min	24.1%	12.7%
51-70 mL/min	16.9%	13.1%
>70 mL/min	10.8%	8.7%

* Estimated using the Cockroft-Gault formula.

Table 8 shows the rates of hyperkalemia in EPHESUS as assessed by two baseline characteristics: presence/absence of proteinuria from baseline urinalysis and presence/absence of diabetes. (See **PRECAUTIONS, Hyperkalemia in Patients Treated for Congestive Heart Failure.**)

Table 8. Rates of Hyperkalemia (>5.5 mEq/L) in EPHESUS by Proteinuria and History of Diabetes*

	INSPRA™	Placebo
Proteinuria, no Diabetes	16%	11%
Diabetes, no Proteinuria	18%	13%
Proteinuria and Diabetes	26%	16%

*Diabetes assessed as positive medical history at baseline; proteinuria assessed by positive dipstick urinalysis at baseline.

Hypertension:

Potassium- In placebo-controlled fixed-dose studies, the mean increases in serum potassium were dose related and are shown in Table 9 along with the frequencies of values >5.5 mEq/L.

Table 9. Changes in Serum Potassium in the Placebo-Controlled, Fixed-Dose Hypertension Studies of INSPRA™

Daily Dosage	n	Mean Change mEq/L	% >5.5 mEq/L
Placebo	194	0	1
25	97	0.08	0
50	245	0.14	0
100	193	0.09	1
200	139	0.19	1
400	104	0.36	8.7

Patients with both type 2 diabetes and microalbuminuria are at increased risk of developing persistent hyperkalemia. In a study in such patients taking INSPRA 200 mg, the frequencies of maximum serum potassium levels >5.5 mEq/L were 33% with INSPRA given alone and 38% when INSPRA was given with enalapril.

Rates of hyperkalemia increased with decreasing renal function. In all studies serum potassium elevations >5.5 mEq/L were observed in 10.4% of patients treated with INSPRA with baseline calculated creatinine clearance <70 mL/min, 5.6% of patients with baseline creatinine clearance of 70 to 100 mL/min, and 2.6% of patients with baseline creatinine clearance of >100 mL/min. (See **WARNINGS, Hyperkalemia in Patients Treated for Hypertension.**)

Sodium- Serum sodium decreased in a dose-related manner. Mean decreases ranged from 0.7 mEq/L at 50 mg daily to 1.7 mEq/L at 400 mg daily. Decreases in sodium (<135 mEq/L) were reported for 2.3% of patients administered INSPRA and 0.6% of placebo-treated patients.

Triglycerides- Serum triglycerides increased in a dose-related manner. Mean increases ranged from 7.1 mg/dL at 50 mg daily to 26.6 mg/dL at 400 mg daily. Increases in triglycerides (above 252 mg/dL) were reported for 15% of patients administered INSPRA and 12% of placebo-treated patients.

Cholesterol- Serum cholesterol increased in a dose-related manner. Mean changes ranged from a decrease of 0.4 mg/dL at 50 mg daily to an increase of 11.6 mg/dL at 400 mg daily. Increases in serum cholesterol values greater than 200 mg/dL were reported for 0.3% of patients administered INSPRA and 0% of placebo-treated patients.

Liver Function Tests- Serum alanine aminotransferase (ALT) and gamma glutamyl transpeptidase (GGT) increased in a dose-related manner. Mean increases ranged from 0.8 U/L at 50 mg daily to 4.8 U/L at 400 mg daily for ALT and 3.1 U/L at 50 mg daily to 11.3 U/L at 400 mg daily for GGT. Increases in ALT levels greater than 120 U/L (3 times upper limit of normal) were reported for 15/2259 patients administered INSPRA and 1/351 placebo-treated patients. Increases in ALT levels greater than 200 U/L (5 times upper limit of normal) were reported for 5/2259 of patients administered INSPRA and 1/351 placebo-treated patients. Increases of ALT greater than 120 U/L and bilirubin greater than 1.2 mg/dL were reported 1/2259 patients administered INSPRA and 0/351 placebo-treated patients. Hepatic failure was not reported in patients receiving INSPRA.

BUN/Creatinine- Serum creatinine increased in a dose-related manner. Mean increases ranged from 0.01 mg/dL at 50 mg daily to 0.03 mg/dL at 400 mg daily. Increases in blood urea nitrogen to greater than 30 mg/dL and serum creatinine to greater than 2 mg/dL were reported for 0.5% and 0.2%, respectively, of patients administered INSPRA and 0% of placebo-treated patients.

Uric Acid- Increases in uric acid to greater than 9 mg/dL were reported in 0.3% of patients administered INSPRA and 0% of placebo-treated patients.

OVERDOSAGE

No cases of human overdosage with eplerenone have been reported. Lethality was not observed in mice, rats, or dogs after single oral doses that provided C_{max} exposures at least 25 times higher than in humans receiving eplerenone 100 mg/day. Dogs showed emesis, salivation, and tremors at a C_{max} 41 times the human therapeutic C_{max}, progressing to sedation and convulsions at higher exposures.

The most likely manifestation of human overdosage would be anticipated to be hypotension or hyperkalemia. Eplerenone cannot be removed by hemodialysis. Eplerenone has been shown to bind extensively to charcoal. If symptomatic hypotension should occur, supportive treatment should be instituted. If hyperkalemia develops, standard treatment should be initiated.

DOSAGE AND ADMINISTRATION

Congestive Heart Failure Post-Myocardial Infarction

The recommended dose of INSPRA is 50 mg once daily. Treatment should be initiated at 25 mg once daily and titrated to the target dose of 50 mg once daily preferably within 4 weeks as tolerated by the patient. INSPRA may be administered with or without food.

Serum potassium should be measured before initiating INSPRA therapy, within the first week and at one month after the start of treatment or dose adjustment. Serum potassium should be assessed periodically thereafter. Factors such as patient characteristics and serum potassium levels may indicate that additional monitoring is appropriate. (See **PRECAUTIONS, Hyperkalemia in Patients Treated for Congestive Heart Failure** and **ADVERSE REACTIONS, Clinical Laboratory Test Findings, Congestive Heart Failure Post-Myocardial Infarction, Potassium.**) In EPHESUS, the majority of hyperkalemia was observed within the first three months after randomization. The dose should be adjusted based on the serum potassium level and the dose adjustment table shown in Table 10.

Table 10. Dose Adjustment in Congestive Heart Failure

Serum Potassium (mEq/L)	Action	Dose Adjustment
< 5.0	Increase	25mg QOD to 25mg QD 25mg QD to 50mg QD
5.0-5.4	Maintain	No adjustment
5.5-5.9	Decrease	50mg QD to 25mg QD 25mg QD to 25mg QOD 25mg QOD to withhold
≥ 6.0	Withhold	

Following withholding INSPRA due to serum potassium ≥6.0 mEq/L, INSPRA can be restarted at a dose of 25 mg QOD when serum potassium levels have fallen below 5.5 mEq/L.

Hypertension

INSPRA may be used alone or in combination with other antihypertensive agents. The recommended starting dose of INSPRA is 50 mg administered once daily. The full therapeutic effect of INSPRA is apparent within 4 weeks. For patients with an inadequate blood pressure response to 50 mg once daily the dosage of INSPRA should be increased to 50 mg twice daily. Higher dosages of INSPRA are not recommended either because they have no greater effect on blood pressure than 100 mg or because they are associated with an increased risk of hyperkalemia. (See **CLINICAL STUDIES, Hypertension.**)

No adjustment of the starting dose is recommended for the elderly or for patients with mild-to-moderate hepatic impairment. For patients receiving weak CYP3A4 inhibitors, such as erythromycin, saquinavir, verapamil, and fluconazole the starting dose should be reduced to 25 mg once daily. (See **CONTRAINDICATIONS** and **PRECAUTIONS, Congestive Heart Failure Post-Myocardial Infarction and Hypertension, Drug Interactions.**)

HOW SUPPLIED

INSPRA Tablets, 25 mg, are yellow diamond biconvex film-coated tablets. They are debossed with *Pfizer* on one side and *NSR* over *25* on the other. They are supplied as follows:

NDC Number	Size
0025-1710-01	Bottle of 30 tablets
0025-1710-02	Bottle of 90 tablets
0025-1710-03	Hospital Unit Dose

INSPRA Tablets, 50 mg, are yellow diamond biconvex film-coated tablets. They are debossed with *Pfizer* on one side and *NSR* over *50* on the other. They are supplied as follows:

NDC Number	Size
0025-1720-03	Bottle of 30 tablets
0025-1720-01	Bottle of 90 tablets

Store at 25°C (77°F); excursions permitted to 15-30°C (59-86°F) [See USP Controlled Room Temperature].
Rx only
U.S. Patent No. 4,559,332
INSPRA Tablets are manufactured for:
G.D. Searle LLC
October 2003
Distributed by
Pfizer
G.D. Searle LLC
Subsidiary of Pfizer Inc, NY, NY 10017
819 570 103A P04036-4

Shown in Product Identification Guide, page 329

NORVASC® ℞

[*nor'vask*]
(amlodipine besylate)
Tablets

DESCRIPTION

NORVASC® is the besylate salt of amlodipine, a long-acting calcium channel blocker.

NORVASC is chemically described as (R.S.) 3-ethyl-5-methyl-2-(2-aminoethoxymethyl)-4-(2-chlorophenyl)-1,4-dihydro-6-methyl-3,5-pyridinedicarboxylate benzenesulphonate. Its empirical formula is $C_{20}H_{25}ClN_2O_5 \bullet C_6H_6O_3S$, and its structural formula is:

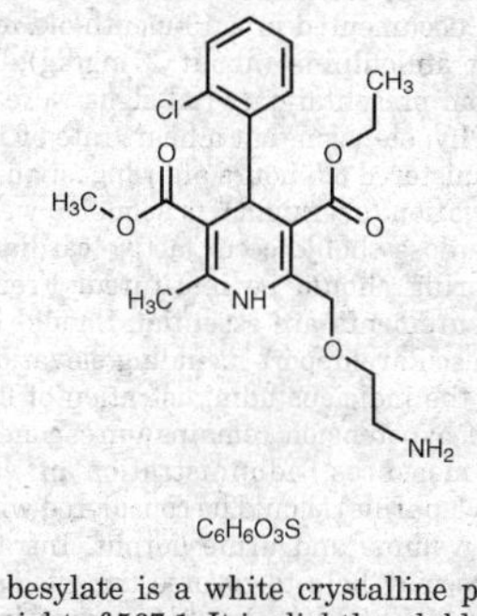

Amlodipine besylate is a white crystalline powder with a molecular weight of 567.1. It is slightly soluble in water and sparingly soluble in ethanol. NORVASC (amlodipine besylate) tablets are formulated as white tablets equivalent to 2.5, 5 and 10 mg of amlodipine for oral administration. In addition to the active ingredient, amlodipine besylate, each tablet contains the following inactive ingredients: microcrystalline cellulose, dibasic calcium phosphate anhydrous, sodium starch glycolate, and magnesium stearate.

CLINICAL PHARMACOLOGY

Mechanism of Action: NORVASC is a dihydropyridine calcium antagonist (calcium ion antagonist or slow-channel blocker) that inhibits the transmembrane influx of calcium ions into vascular smooth muscle and cardiac muscle. Experimental data suggest that NORVASC binds to both dihydropyridine and nondihydropyridine binding sites. The contractile processes of cardiac muscle and vascular smooth muscle are dependent upon the movement of extracellular calcium ions into these cells through specific ion channels. NORVASC inhibits calcium ion influx across cell membranes selectively, with a greater effect on vascular smooth muscle cells than on cardiac muscle cells. Negative inotropic effects can be detected *in vitro* but such effects have not been seen in intact animals at therapeutic doses. Serum calcium concentration is not affected by NORVASC. Within the physiologic pH range, NORVASC is an ionized compound (pKa=8.6), and its kinetic interaction with the calcium channel receptor is characterized by a gradual rate of association and dissociation with the receptor binding site, resulting in a gradual onset of effect.

NORVASC is a peripheral arterial vasodilator that acts directly on vascular smooth muscle to cause a reduction in peripheral vascular resistance and reduction in blood pressure.

The precise mechanisms by which NORVASC relieves angina have not been fully delineated, but are thought to include the following:

Exertional Angina: In patients with exertional angina, NORVASC reduces the total peripheral resistance (afterload) against which the heart works and reduces the rate pressure product, and thus myocardial oxygen demand, at any given level of exercise.

Vasospastic Angina: NORVASC has been demonstrated to block constriction and restore blood flow in coronary arteries and arterioles in response to calcium, potassium epinephrine, serotonin, and thromboxane A_2 analog in experimental animal models and in human coronary vessels *in vitro*. This inhibition of coronary spasm is responsible for the effectiveness of NORVASC in vasospastic (Prinzmetal's or variant) angina.

Pharmacokinetics and Metabolism: After oral administration of therapeutic doses of NORVASC, absorption produces peak plasma concentrations between 6 and 12 hours. Absolute bioavailability has been estimated to be between 64 and 90%. The bioavailability of NORVASC is not altered by the presence of food.

NORVASC is extensively (about 90%) converted to inactive metabolites via hepatic metabolism with 10% of the parent compound and 60% of the metabolites excreted in the urine. *Ex vivo* studies have shown that approximately 93% of the circulating drug is bound to plasma proteins in hypertensive patients. Elimination from the plasma is biphasic with a terminal elimination half-life of about 30-50 hours. Steady-state plasma levels of NORVASC are reached after 7 to 8 days of consecutive daily dosing.

The pharmacokinetics of NORVASC are not significantly influenced by renal impairment. Patients with renal failure may therefore receive the usual initial dose.

Elderly patients and patients with hepatic insufficiency have decreased clearance of amlodipine with a resulting increase in AUC of approximately 40-60%, and a lower initial dose may be required. A similar increase in AUC was observed in patients with moderate to severe heart failure.

Pediatric Patients: Sixty-two hypertensive patients aged greater than 6 years received doses of NORVASC between 1.25 mg and 20 mg. Weight-adjusted clearance and volume of distribution were similar to values in adults.

Pharmacodynamics: *Hemodynamics* Following administration of therapeutic doses to patients with hypertension, NORVASC produces vasodilation resulting in a reduction of supine and standing blood pressures. These decreases in blood pressure are not accompanied by a significant change in heart rate or plasma catecholamine levels with chronic dosing. Although the acute intravenous administration of amlodipine decreases arterial blood pressure and increases heart rate in hemodynamic studies of patients with chronic stable angina, chronic administration of oral amlodipine in clinical trials did not lead to clinically significant changes in heart rate or blood pressures in normotensive patients with angina.

With chronic once daily oral administration, antihypertensive effectiveness is maintained for at least 24 hours. Plasma concentrations correlate with effect in both young and elderly patients. The magnitude of reduction in blood pressure with NORVASC is also correlated with the height of pretreatment elevation; thus, individuals with moderate hypertension (diastolic pressure 105-114 mmHg) had about a 50% greater response than patients with mild hypertension (diastolic pressure 90-104 mmHg). Normotensive subjects experienced no clinically significant change in blood pressures (+1/−2 mmHg).

In hypertensive patients with normal renal function, therapeutic doses of NORVASC resulted in a decrease in renal vascular resistance and an increase in glomerular filtration rate and effective renal plasma flow without change in filtration fraction or proteinuria.

As with other calcium channel blockers, hemodynamic measurements of cardiac function at rest and during exercise (or pacing) in patients with normal ventricular function treated with NORVASC have generally demonstrated a small increase in cardiac index without significant influence on dP/dt or on left ventricular end diastolic pressure or volume. In hemodynamic studies, NORVASC has not been associated with a negative inotropic effect when administered in the therapeutic dose range to intact animals and man, even when co-administered with beta-blockers to man. Similar findings, however, have been observed in normals or well-compensated patients with heart failure with agents possessing significant negative inotropic effects.

Studies in Patients with Congestive Heart Failure: NORVASC has been compared to placebo in four 8-12 week studies of patients with NYHA class II/III heart failure, involving a total of 697 patients. In these studies, there was no evidence of worsened heart failure based on measures of exercise tolerance, NYHA classification, symptoms, or LVEF. In a long-term (follow-up at least 6 months, mean 13.8 months) placebo-controlled mortality/morbidity study of NORVASC 5-10 mg in 1153 patients with NYHA classes III (n=931) or IV (n=222) heart failure on stable doses of diuretics, digoxin, and ACE inhibitors, NORVASC had no effect on the primary endpoint of the study which was the combined endpoint of all-cause mortality and cardiac morbidity (as defined by life-threatening arrhythmia, acute myocardial infarction, or hospitalization for worsened heart failure), or on NYHA classification, or symptoms of heart failure. Total combined all-cause mortality and cardiac morbidity events were 222/571 (39%) for patients on NORVASC and 246/583 (42%) for patients on placebo; the cardiac morbid events represented about 25% of the endpoints in the study.

Another study (PRAISE-2) randomized patients with NYHA class III (80%) or IV (20%) heart failure without clinical symptoms or objective evidence of underlying ischemic disease, on stable doses of ACE inhibitor (99%), digitalis (99%) and diuretics (99%), to placebo (n=827) or NORVASC (n=827) and followed them for a mean of 33 months. There was no statistically significant difference between NORVASC and placebo in the primary endpoint of all cause mortality (95% confidence limits from 8% reduction to 29% increase on NORVASC). With NORVASC there were more reports of pulmonary edema.

Electrophysiologic Effects: NORVASC does not change sinoatrial nodal function or atrioventricular conduction in intact animals or man. In patients with chronic stable angina, intravenous administration of 10 mg did not significantly alter A-H and H-V conduction and sinus node recovery time after pacing. Similar results were obtained in patients receiving NORVASC and concomitant beta blockers. In clinical studies in which NORVASC was administered in combination with beta-blockers to patients with either hypertension or angina, no adverse effects on electrocardiographic parameters were observed. In clinical trials with angina patients alone, NORVASC therapy did not alter electrocardiographic intervals or produce higher degrees of AV blocks.

Effects in Hypertension

Adult Patients: The antihypertensive efficacy of NORVASC has been demonstrated in a total of 15 double-blind, placebo-controlled, randomized studies involving 800 patients on NORVASC and 538 on placebo. Once daily administration produced statistically significant placebo-corrected reductions in supine and standing blood pressures at 24 hours postdose, averaging about 12/6 mmHg in the standing position and 13/7 mmHg in the supine position in patients with mild to moderate hypertension. Maintenance of the blood pressure effect over the 24-hour dosing interval was observed, with little difference in peak and trough effect. Tolerance was not demonstrated in patients studied for up to 1 year. The 3 parallel, fixed dose, dose response studies showed that the reduction in supine and standing blood pressures was dose-related within the recommended dosing range. Effects on diastolic pressure were similar in young and older patients. The effect on systolic pressure was greater in older patients, perhaps because of greater baseline systolic pressure. Effects were similar in black patients and in white patients.

Pediatric Patients: Two hundred sixty-eight hypertensive patients aged 6 to 17 years were randomized first to NORVASC 2.5 or 5 mg once daily for 4 weeks and then randomized again to the same dose or to placebo for another 4 weeks. Patients receiving 5 mg at the end of 8 weeks had lower blood pressure than those secondarily randomized to placebo. The magnitude of the treatment effect is difficult to interpret, but it is probably less than 5 mmHg systolic on the 5 mg dose. Adverse events were similar to those seen in adults.

Effects in Chronic Stable Angina: The effectiveness of 5-10 mg/day of NORVASC in exercise-induced angina has been evaluated in 8 placebo-controlled, double-blind clinical trials of up to 6 weeks duration involving 1038 patients (684 NORVASC, 354 placebo) with chronic stable angina. In 5 of the 8 studies significant increases in exercise time (bicycle or treadmill) were seen with the 10 mg dose. Increases in symptom-limited exercise time averaged 12.8% (63 sec) for NORVASC 10 mg, and averaged 7.9% (38 sec) for NORVASC 5 mg. NORVASC 10 mg also increased time to 1 mm ST segment deviation in several studies and decreased angina attack rate. The sustained efficacy of NORVASC in angina patients has been demonstrated over long-term dosing. In patients with angina there were no clinically significant reductions in blood pressures (4/1 mmHg) or changes in heart rate (+0.3 bpm).

Effects in Vasospastic Angina: In a double-blind, placebo-controlled clinical trial of 4 weeks duration in 50 patients, NORVASC therapy decreased attacks by approximately 4/week compared with a placebo decrease of approximately 1/week ($p<0.01$). Two of 23 NORVASC and 7 of 27 placebo patients discontinued from the study due to lack of clinical improvement.

INDICATIONS AND USAGE

1. Hypertension

NORVASC is indicated for the treatment of hypertension. It may be used alone or in combination with other antihypertensive agents.

2. Chronic Stable Angina

NORVASC is indicated for the treatment of chronic stable angina. NORVASC may be used alone or in combination with other antianginal agents.

3. Vasospastic Angina (Prinzmetal's or Variant Angina)

NORVASC is indicated for the treatment of confirmed or suspected vasospastic angina. NORVASC may be used as monotherapy or in combination with other antianginal drugs.

CONTRAINDICATIONS

NORVASC is contraindicated in patients with known sensitivity to amlodipine.

WARNINGS

Increased Angina and/or Myocardial Infarction: Rarely, patients, particularly those with severe obstructive coronary artery disease, have developed documented increased frequency, duration and/or severity of angina or acute myocardial infarction on starting calcium channel blocker therapy or at the time of dosage increase. The mechanism of this effect has not been elucidated.

PRECAUTIONS

General: Since the vasodilation induced by NORVASC is gradual in onset, acute hypotension has rarely been reported after oral administration of NORVASC. Nonetheless, caution should be exercised when administering NORVASC as with any other peripheral vasodilator particularly in patients with severe aortic stenosis.

Continued on next page

Norvasc—Cont.

Use in Patients with Congestive Heart Failure: In general, calcium channel blockers should be used with caution in patients with heart failure. NORVASC (5-10 mg per day) has been studied in a placebo-controlled trial of 1153 patients with NYHA Class III or IV heart failure (see CLINICAL PHARMACOLOGY) on stable doses of ACE inhibitor, digoxin, and diuretics. Follow-up was at least 6 months, with a mean of about 14 months. There was no overall adverse effect on survival or cardiac morbidity (as defined by life-threatening arrhythmia, acute myocardial infarction, or hospitalization for worsened heart failure). NORVASC has been compared to placebo in four 8-12 week studies of patients with NYHA class II/III heart failure, involving a total of 697 patients. In these studies, there was no evidence of worsened heart failure based on measures of exercise tolerance, NYHA classification, symptoms, or LVEF.
Beta-Blocker Withdrawal: NORVASC is not a beta-blocker and therefore gives no protection against the dangers of abrupt beta-blocker withdrawal; any such withdrawal should be by gradual reduction of the dose of beta-blocker.
Patients with Hepatic Failure: Since NORVASC is extensively metabolized by the liver and the plasma elimination half-life (t 1/2) is 56 hours in patients with impaired hepatic function, caution should be exercised when administering NORVASC to patients with severe hepatic impairment.
Drug Interactions: *In vitro* data in human plasma indicate that NORVASC has no effect on the protein binding of drugs tested (digoxin, phenytoin, warfarin, and indomethacin).
Special Studies: Effect of other agents on NORVASC.
CIMETIDINE: Co-administration of NORVASC with cimetidine did not alter the pharmacokinetics of NORVASC.
GRAPEFRUIT JUICE: Co-administration of 240 mL of grapefruit juice with a single oral dose of amlodipine 10 mg in 20 healthy volunteers had no significant effect on the pharmacokinetics of amlodipine.
MAALOX (antacid): Co-administration of the antacid Maalox with a single dose of NORVASC had no significant effect on the pharmacokinetics of NORVASC.
SILDENAFIL: A single 100 mg dose of sildenafil (Viagra®) in subjects with essential hypertension had no effect on the pharmacokinetic parameters of NORVASC. When NORVASC and sildenafil were used in combination, each agent independently exerted its own blood pressure lowering effect.
Special Studies: Effect of NORVASC on other agents.
ATORVASTATIN: Co-administration of multiple 10 mg doses of NORVASC with 80 mg of atorvastatin resulted in no significant change in the steady state pharmacokinetic parameters of atorvastatin.
DIGOXIN: Co-administration of NORVASC with digoxin did not change serum digoxin levels or digoxin renal clearance in normal volunteers.
ETHANOL (alcohol): Single and multiple 10 mg doses of NORVASC had no significant effect on the pharmacokinetics of ethanol.
WARFARIN: Co-administration of NORVASC with warfarin did not change the warfarin prothrombin response time.
In clinical trials, NORVASC has been safely administered with thiazide diuretics, beta-blockers, angiotensin-converting enzyme inhibitors, long-acting nitrates, sublingual nitroglycerin, digoxin, warfarin, non-steroidal anti-inflammatory drugs, antibiotics, and oral hypoglycemic drugs.
Drug/Laboratory Test Interactions: None known.
Carcinogenesis, Mutagenesis, Impairment of Fertility: Rats and mice treated with amlodipine in the diet for two years, at concentrations calculated to provide daily dosage levels of 0.5, 1.25, and 2.5 mg/kg/day showed no evidence of carcinogenicity. The highest dose (for mice, similar to, and for rats twice* the maximum recommended clinical dose of 10 mg on a mg/m^2 basis) was close to the maximum tolerated dose for mice but not for rats.
Mutagenicity studies revealed no drug related effects at either the gene or chromosome levels.
There was no effect on the fertility of rats treated with amlodipine (males for 64 days and females 14 days prior to mating) at doses up to 10 mg/kg/day (8 times* the maximum recommended human dose of 10 mg on a mg/m^2 basis).
Pregnancy Category C: No evidence of teratogenicity or other embryo/fetal toxicity was found when pregnant rats or rabbits were treated orally with up to 10 mg/kg amlodipine (respectively 8 times* and 23 times* the maximum recommended human dose of 10 mg on a mg/m^2 basis) during their respective periods of major organogenesis. However, litter size was significantly decreased (by about 50%) and the number of intrauterine deaths was significantly increased (about 5-fold) in rats administered 10 mg/kg amlodipine for 14 days before mating and throughout mating and gestation. Amlodipine has been shown to prolong both the gestation period and the duration of labor in rats at this dose. There are no adequate and well-controlled studies in pregnant women. Amlodipine should be used during pregnancy only if the potential benefit justifies the potential risk to the fetus.

*Based on patient weight of 50 kg.

Nursing Mothers: It is not known whether amlodipine is excreted in human milk. In the absence of this information, it is recommended that nursing be discontinued while NORVASC is administered.
Pediatric Use: The effect of NORVASC on blood pressure in patients less than 6 years of age is not known.
Geriatric Use: Clinical studies of NORVASC did not include sufficient numbers of subjects aged 65 and over to determine whether they respond differently from younger subjects. Other reported clinical experience has not identified differences in responses between the elderly and younger patients. In general, dose selection for an elderly patient should be cautious, usually starting at the low end of the dosing range, reflecting the greater frequency of decreased hepatic, renal, or cardiac function, and of concomitant disease or other drug therapy. Elderly patients have decreased clearance of amlodipine with a resulting increase of AUC of approximately 40-60%, and a lower initial dose may be required (see **DOSAGE AND ADMINISTRATION**).

ADVERSE REACTIONS

NORVASC has been evaluated for safety in more than 11,000 patients in U.S. and foreign clinical trials. In general, treatment with NORVASC was well-tolerated at doses up to 10 mg daily. Most adverse reactions reported during therapy with NORVASC were of mild or moderate severity. In controlled clinical trials directly comparing NORVASC (N=1730) in doses up to 10 mg to placebo (N=1250), discontinuation of NORVASC due to adverse reactions was required in only about 1.5% of patients and was not significantly different from placebo (about 1%). The most common side effects are headache and edema. The incidence (%) of side effects which occurred in a dose related manner are as follows:

Adverse Event	2.5 mg N=275	5.0 mg N=296	10.0 mg N=268	Placebo N=520
Edema	1.8	3.0	10.8	0.6
Dizziness	1.1	3.4	3.4	1.5
Flushing	0.7	1.4	2.6	0.0
Palpitation	0.7	1.4	4.5	0.6

Other adverse experiences which were not clearly dose related but which were reported with an incidence greater than 1.0% in placebo-controlled clinical trials include the following:

Placebo-Controlled Studies

	NORVASC (%) (N=1730)	PLACEBO (%) (N=1250)
Headache	7.3	7.8
Fatigue	4.5	2.8
Nausea	2.9	1.9
Abdominal Pain	1.6	0.3
Somnolence	1.4	0.6

For several adverse experiences that appear to be drug and dose related, there was a greater incidence in women than men associated with amlodipine treatment as shown in the following table:

ADR	NORVASC M=% (N=1218)	NORVASC F=% (N=512)	PLACEBO M=% (N=914)	PLACEBO F=% (N=336)
Edema	5.6	14.6	1.4	5.1
Flushing	1.5	4.5	0.3	0.9
Palpitations	1.4	3.3	0.9	0.9
Somnolence	1.3	1.6	0.8	0.3

The following events occurred in ≤1% but >0.1% of patients in controlled clinical trials or under conditions of open trials or marketing experience where a causal relationship is uncertain; they are listed to alert the physician to a possible relationship:
Cardiovascular: arrhythmia (including ventricular tachycardia and atrial fibrillation), bradycardia, chest pain, hypotension, peripheral ischemia, syncope, tachycardia, postural dizziness, postural hypotension, vasculitis.
Central and Peripheral Nervous System: hypoesthesia, neuropathy peripheral, paresthesia, tremor, vertigo.
Gastrointestinal: anorexia, constipation, dyspepsia,** dysphagia, diarrhea, flatulence, pancreatitis, vomiting, gingival hyperplasia.
General: allergic reaction, asthenia,** back pain, hot flushes, malaise, pain, rigors, weight gain, weight decrease.
Musculoskeletal System: arthralgia, arthrosis, muscle cramps,** myalgia.
Psychiatric: sexual dysfunction (male** and female), insomnia, nervousness, depression, abnormal dreams, anxiety, depersonalization.
Respiratory System: dyspnea,** epistaxis.
Skin and Appendages: angioedema, erythema multiforme, pruritus,** rash,** rash erythematous, rash maculopapular.

**These events occurred in less than 1% in placebo-controlled trials, but the incidence of these side effects was between 1% and 2% in all multiple dose studies.

Special Senses: abnormal vision, conjunctivitis, diplopia, eye pain, tinnitus.
Urinary System: micturition frequency, micturition disorder, nocturia.
Autonomic Nervous System: dry mouth, sweating increased.
Metabolic and Nutritional: hyperglycemia, thirst.
Hemopoietic: leukopenia, purpura, thrombocytopenia.
The following events occurred in ≤0.1% of patients: cardiac failure, pulse irregularity, extrasystoles, skin discoloration, urticaria, skin dryness, alopecia, dermatitis, muscle weakness, twitching, ataxia, hypertonia, migraine, cold and clammy skin, apathy, agitation, amnesia, gastritis, increased appetite, loose stools, coughing, rhinitis, dysuria, polyuria, parosmia, taste perversion, abnormal visual accommodation, and xerophthalmia.
Other reactions occurred sporadically and cannot be distinguished from medications or concurrent disease states such as myocardial infarction and angina.
NORVASC therapy has not been associated with clinically significant changes in routine laboratory tests. No clinically relevant changes were noted in serum potassium, serum glucose, total triglycerides, total cholesterol, HDL cholesterol, uric acid, blood urea nitrogen, or creatinine.
The following postmarketing event has been reported infrequently where a causal relationship is uncertain: gynecomastia. In postmarketing experience, jaundice and hepatic enzyme elevations (mostly consistent with cholestasis or hepatitis) in some cases severe enough to require hospitalization have been reported in association with use of amlodipine.
NORVASC has been used safely in patients with chronic obstructive pulmonary disease, well-compensated congestive heart failure, peripheral vascular disease, diabetes mellitus, and abnormal lipid profiles.

OVERDOSAGE

Single oral doses of 40 mg/kg and 100 mg/kg in mice and rats, respectively, caused deaths. A single oral dose of 4 mg/kg or higher in dogs caused a marked peripheral vasodilation and hypotension.
Overdosage might be expected to cause excessive peripheral vasodilation with marked hypotension and possibly a reflex tachycardia. In humans, experience with intentional overdosage of NORVASC is limited. Reports of intentional overdosage include a patient who ingested 250 mg and was asymptomatic and was not hospitalized; another (120 mg) was hospitalized, underwent gastric lavage and remained normotensive; the third (105 mg) was hospitalized and had hypotension (90/50 mmHg) which normalized following plasma expansion. A patient who took 70 mg amlodipine and an unknown quantity of benzodiazepine in a suicide attempt developed shock which was refractory to treatment and died the following day with abnormally high benzodiazepine plasma concentration. A case of accidental drug overdose has been documented in a 19-month-old male who ingested 30 mg amlodipine (about 2 mg/kg). During the emergency room presentation, vital signs were stable with no evidence of hypotension, but a heart rate of 180 bpm. Ipecac was administered 3.5 hours after ingestion and on subsequent observation (overnight) no sequelae were noted.
If massive overdose should occur, active cardiac and respiratory monitoring should be instituted. Frequent blood pressure measurements are essential. Should hypotension occur, cardiovascular support including elevation of the extremities and the judicious administration of fluids should be initiated. If hypotension remains unresponsive to these conservative measures, administration of vasopressors (such as phenylephrine) should be considered with attention to circulating volume and urine output. Intravenous calcium gluconate may help to reverse the effects of calcium entry blockade. As NORVASC is highly protein bound, hemodialysis is not likely to be of benefit.

DOSAGE AND ADMINISTRATION

Adults: The usual initial antihypertensive oral dose of NORVASC is 5 mg once daily with a maximum dose of 10 mg once daily. Small, fragile, or elderly individuals, or patients with hepatic insufficiency may be started on 2.5 mg once daily and this dose may be used when adding NORVASC to other antihypertensive therapy.
Dosage should be adjusted according to each patient's need. In general, titration should proceed over 7 to 14 days so that the physician can fully assess the patient's response to each dose level. Titration may proceed more rapidly, however, if clinically warranted, provided the patient is assessed frequently.
The recommended dose for chronic stable or vasospastic angina is 5-10 mg, with the lower dose suggested in the elderly and in patients with hepatic insufficiency. Most patients will require 10 mg for adequate effect. See ADVERSE REACTIONS section for information related to dosage and side effects.
Children: The effective antihypertensive oral dose in pediatric patients ages 6-17 years is 2.5 mg to 5 mg once daily. Doses in excess of 5 mg daily have not been studied in pediatric patients. See **CLINICAL PHARMACOLOGY**.
Co-administration with Other Antihypertensive and/or Antianginal Drugs: NORVASC has been safely administered with thiazides, ACE inhibitors, beta-blockers, long-acting nitrates, and/or sublingual nitroglycerin.

HOW SUPPLIED

NORVASC®—2.5 mg Tablets (amlodipine besylate equivalent to 2.5 mg of amlodipine per tablet) are supplied as white, diamond, flat-faced, beveled edged engraved with "NORVASC" on one side and "2.5" on the other side and supplied as follows:

NDC 0069-1520-68	Bottle of 90

NORVASC®—5 mg Tablets (amlodipine besylate equivalent to 5 mg of amlodipine per tablet) are white, elongated octagon, flat-faced, beveled edged engraved with both "NORVASC" and "5" on one side and plain on the other side and supplied as follows:

NDC 0069-1530-68	Bottle of 90
NDC 0069-1530-41	Unit Dose package of 100
NDC 0069-1530-72	Bottle of 300

NORVASC®—10 mg Tablets (amlodipine besylate equivalent to 10 mg of amlodipine per tablet) are white, round, flat-faced, beveled edged engraved with both "NORVASC" and "10" on one side and plain on the other side and supplied as follows:

NDC 0069-1540-68 Bottle of 90
NDC 0069-1540-41 Unit Dose package of 100

Store bottles at controlled room temperature, 59° to 86°F (15° to 30°C) and dispense in tight, light-resistant containers (USP).

Rx only

Pfizer Labs
Division of Pfizer Inc, NY, NY 10017
70-4782-00-1
Revised June 2003

Shown in Product Identification Guide, page 329

REBIF® ℞

[rē-bîf]
(interferon beta-1a)

DESCRIPTION

Rebif® (interferon beta-1a) is a purified 166 amino acid glycoprotein with a molecular weight of approximately 22,500 daltons. It is produced by recombinant DNA technology using genetically engineered Chinese Hamster Ovary cells into which the human interferon beta gene has been introduced. The amino acid sequence of Rebif® is identical to that of natural fibroblast derived human interferon beta. Natural interferon beta and interferon beta-1a (Rebif®) are glycosylated with each containing a single N-linked complex carbohydrate moiety.

Using a reference standard calibrated against the World Health Organization natural interferon beta standard (Second International Standard for Interferon, Human Fibroblast GB 23 902 531), Rebif® has a specific activity of approximately 270 million international units (MIU) of antiviral activity per mg of interferon beta-1a determined specifically by an in vitro cytopathic effect bioassay using WISH cells and Vesicular Stomatitis virus. Rebif® 22 mcg and 44 mcg contains approximately 6 MIU or 12 MIU, respectively, of antiviral activity using this method.

Rebif® (interferon beta-1a) is formulated as a sterile solution in a prefilled syringe intended for subcutaneous (sc) injection. Each 0.5 mL (0.5 cc) of Rebif® contain either 22 mcg or 44 mcg of interferon beta-1a, 2 mg or 4 mg albumin (human) USP, 27.3 mg mannitol USP, 0.4 mg sodium acetate, Water for Injection USP.

CLINICAL PHARMACOLOGY

General

Interferons are a family of naturally occurring proteins that are produced by eukaryotic cells in response to viral infection and other biological inducers. Interferons possess immunomodulatory, antiviral and antiproliferative biological activities. They exert their biological effects by binding to specific receptors on the surface of cells. Three major groups of interferons have been distinguished: alpha, beta, and gamma. Interferons alpha and beta form the Type I interferons and interferon gamma is a Type II interferon. Type I interferons have considerably overlapping but also distinct biological activities. Interferon beta is produced naturally by various cell types including fibroblasts and macrophages. Binding of interferon beta to its receptors initiates a complex cascade of intracellular events that leads to the expression of numerous interferon-induced gene products and markers, including 2′, 5′-oligoadenylate synthetase, beta 2-microglobulin and neopterin, which may mediate some of the biological activities. The specific interferon-induced proteins and mechanisms by which interferon beta-1a exerts its effects in multiple sclerosis have not been fully defined.

Pharmacokinetics

The pharmacokinetics of Rebif® (interferon beta-1a) in people with multiple sclerosis have not been evaluated. In healthy volunteer subjects, a single subcutaneous (sc) injection of 60 mcg of Rebif® (liquid formulation), resulted in a peak serum concentration (C_{max}) of 5.1 ± 1.7 IU/mL (mean ± SD), with a median time of peak serum concentration (T_{max}) of 16 hours. The serum elimination half-life ($t_{1/2}$) was 69 ± 37 hours, and the area under the serum concentration versus time curve (AUC) from zero to 96 hours was 294 ± 81 IU·h/mL. Following every other day sc injections in healthy volunteer subjects, an increase in AUC of approximately 240% was observed, suggesting that accumulation of interferon beta-1a occurs after repeat administration. Total clearance is approximately 33-55 L/hour. There have been no observed gender-related effects on pharmacokinetic parameters. Pharmacokinetics of Rebif® in pediatric and geriatric patients or patients with renal or hepatic insufficiency have not been established.

Pharmacodynamics

Biological response markers (e.g., 2′, 5′-OAS activity, neopterin and beta 2-microglobulin) are induced by interferon beta-1a following parenteral doses administered to healthy volunteer subjects and to patients with multiple sclerosis. Following a single sc administration of 60 mcg of Rebif® intracellular 2′, 5′-OAS activity peaked between 12 to 24 hours and beta-2-microglobulin and neopterin serum concentrations showed a maximum at approximately 24 to 48 hours. All three markers remained elevated for up to four days. Administration of Rebif 22 mcg three times per week (tiw) inhibited mitogen-induced release of pro-inflammatory cytokines (IFN-γ, IL-1, IL-6, TNF-α and TNF-β) by peripheral blood mononuclear cells that, on average, was near double that observed with Rebif® administered once per week (qw) at either 22 or 66 mcg.

The relationships between serum interferon beta-1a levels and measurable pharmacodynamic activities to the mechanism(s) by which Rebif® exerts its effects in multiple sclerosis are unknown. No gender-related effects on pharmacodynamic parameters have been observed.

CLINICAL STUDIES

Two multicenter studies evaluated the safety and efficacy of Rebif® in patients with relapsing-remitting multiple sclerosis.

Study 1 was a randomized, double-blind, placebo controlled study in patients with multiple sclerosis for at least one year, Kurtzke Expanded Disability Status Scale (EDSS) scores ranging from 0 to 5, and at least 2 acute exacerbations in the previous 2 years.(1) Patients with secondary progressive multiple sclerosis were excluded from the study. Patients received sc injections of either placebo (n = 187), Rebif® 22 mcg (n = 189), or Rebif® 44 mcg (n = 184) administered tiw for two years. Doses of study agents were progressively increased to their target doses during the first 4 to 8 weeks for each patient in the study (see **DOSAGE AND ADMINISTRATION**).

The primary efficacy endpoint was the number of clinical exacerbations. Numerous secondary efficacy endpoints were also evaluated and included exacerbation-related parameters, effects of treatment on progression of disability and magnetic resonance imaging (MRI)-related parameters. Progression of disability was defined as an increase in the EDSS score of at least 1 point sustained for at least 3 months. Neurological examinations were completed every 3 months, during suspected exacerbations, and coincident with MRI scans. All patients underwent proton density T2-weighted (PD/T2) MRI scans at baseline and every 6 months. A subset of 198 patients underwent PD/T2 and T1-weighted gadolinium-enhanced (Gd)-MRI scans monthly for the first 9 months. Of the 560 patients enrolled, 533 (95%) provided 2 years of data and 502 (90%) received 2 years of study agent.

Study results are shown in Table 1 and Figure 1. Rebif® at doses of 22 mcg and 44 mcg administered sc tiw significantly reduced the number of exacerbations per patient as compared to placebo. Differences between the 22 mcg and 44 mcg groups were not significant (p >0.05).

The exact relationship between MRI findings and the clinical status of patients is unknown. Changes in lesion area often do not correlate with changes in disability progression. The prognostic significance of the MRI findings in these studies has not been evaluated.

[See table 1 above]

Table 1: Clinical and MRI Endpoints from Study 1

	Placebo	22 mcg tiw	44 mcg tiw
	n = 187	n = 189	n = 184
Exacerbation-related			
Mean number of exacerbations per patient over 2 years[1,2] (Percent reduction)	2.56	1.82** (29%)	1.73*** (32%)
Percent (%) of patients exacerbation-free at 2 years[3]	15%	25%*	32%***
Median time to first exacerbation (months)[1,4]	4.5	7.6**	9.6***
MRI	n = 172	n = 171	n = 171
Median percent (%) change of MRI PD-T2 lesion area at 2 years[5]	11.0	-1.2***	-3.8***
Median number of active lesions per patient per scan (PD/T2; 6 monthly)[5]	2.25	0.75***	0.5***

* p<0.05 compared to placebo
** p<0.001 compared to placebo
*** p<0.0001 compared to placebo
(1) Intent-to-treat analysis
(2) Poisson regression model adjusted for center and time on study
(3) Logistic regression adjusted for center. Patients lost to follow-up prior to an exacerbation were excluded from this analysis (n = 185, 183, and 184 for the placebo, 22 mcg tiw, and 44 mcg tiw groups, respectively)
(4) Cox proportional hazard model adjusted for center
(5) ANOVA on ranks adjusted for center. Patients with missing scans were excluded from this analysis

The time to onset of progression in disability sustained for three months was significantly longer in patients treated with Rebif® than in placebo-treated patients. The Kaplan-Meier estimates of the proportions of patients with sustained disability are depicted in Figure 1.

[See figure 1 at top of next column]

The safety and efficacy of treatment with Rebif® beyond 2 years have not been established.

Study 2 was a randomized, open-label, evaluator-blinded, active comparator study.(2) Patients with relapsing-remitting multiple sclerosis with EDSS scores ranging from 0 to 5.5, and at least 2 exacerbations in the previous 2 years were eligible for inclusion. Patients with secondary progressive multiple sclerosis were excluded from the study. Patients were randomized to treatment with Rebif® 44 mcg tiw by sc injection (n=339) or Avonex® 30 mcg qw by intramuscular (im) injection (n=338). Study duration was 48 weeks.

Figure 1: Proportions of Patients with Sustained Disability Progression

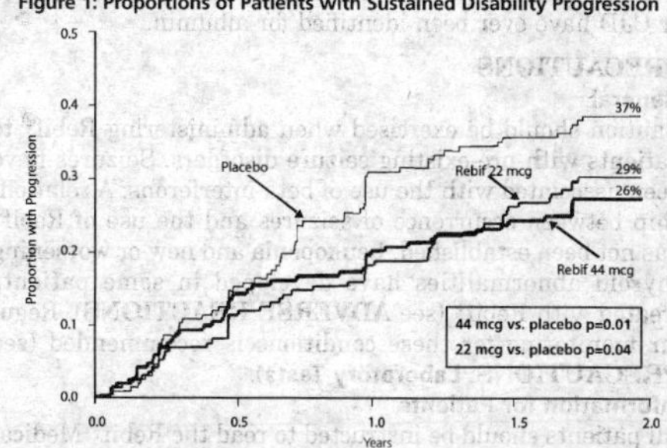

The primary efficacy endpoint was the proportion of patients who remained exacerbation-free at 24 weeks. The principal secondary endpoint was the mean number per patient per scan of combined unique active MRI lesions through 24 weeks, defined as any lesion that was T1 active or T2 active. Neurological examinations were performed every three months by a neurologist blinded to treatment assignment. Patient visits were conducted monthly, and mid-month telephone contacts were made to inquire about potential exacerbations. If an exacerbation was suspected, the patient was evaluated with a neurological examination. MRI scans were performed monthly and analyzed in a treatment–blinded manner.

Patients treated with Rebif® 44 mcg sc tiw were more likely to remain relapse-free at 24 and 48 weeks than were patients treated with Avonex® 30 mcg im qw (Table 2). This study does not support any conclusion regarding effects on the accumulation of physical disability.

[See table 2 at top of next page]

The adverse reactions over 48 weeks were generally similar between the two treatment groups. Exceptions included injection site disorders (83% of patients on Rebif® vs. 28% of patients on Avonex®), hepatic function disorders (18% on Rebif® vs. 10% on Avonex®), and leukopenia (6% on Rebif® vs. <1% on Avonex®), which were observed with greater frequency in the Rebif® group compared to the Avonex® group.

INDICATIONS AND USAGE

Rebif® (interferon-beta-1a) is indicated for the treatment of patients with relapsing forms of multiple sclerosis to decrease the frequency of clinical exacerbations and delay the accumulation of physical disability. Efficacy of Rebif® in chronic progressive multiple sclerosis has not been established.

CONTRAINDICATIONS

Rebif® (interferon beta-1a) is contraindicated in patients with a history of hypersensitivity to natural or recombinant interferon, human albumin, or any other component of the formulation.

WARNINGS

Depression

Rebif® (interferon beta-1a) should be used with caution in patients with depression, a condition that is common in people with multiple sclerosis. Depression, suicidal ideation, and suicide attempts have been reported to occur with increased frequency in patients receiving interferon compounds, including Rebif®. Patients should be advised to report immediately any symptoms of depression and/or suicidal ideation to the prescribing physician. If a patient develops depression, cessation of treatment with Rebif® should be considered.

Continued on next page

Rebif—Cont.

Hepatic Injury

A case of fulminant hepatic failure requiring liver transplantation in a patient who initiated Rebif® therapy while taking another potentially hepato-toxic medication has been reported from a non-U.S. postmarking source. Symptomatic hepatic dysfunction, primarily presenting as jaundice, has been reported as a rare complication of Rebif® use. Asymptomatic elevation of hepatic transaminases (particularly SGPT) is common with interferon therapy (see **ADVERSE REACTIONS**). Rebif® should be initiated with caution in patients with active liver disease, alcohol abuse, increased serum SGPT (> 2.5 times ULN), or a history of significant liver disease. Dose reduction should be considered if SGPT rises above times the upper limit of normal. The dose may be gradually re-escalated when enzyme levels have normalized. Treatment with Rebif® should be stopped if jaundice or other clinical symptoms of liver dysfunction appear.

Anaphylaxis

Anaphylaxis has been reported as a rare complication of Rebif® use. Other allergic reactions have included skin rash and urticaria, and have ranged from mild to severe without a clear relationship to dose or duration of exposure. Several allergic reactions, some severe, have occurred after prolonged use.

Albumin (Human)

This product contains albumin, a derivative of human blood. Based on effective donor screening and product manufacturing processes, it carries an extremely remote risk for transmission of viral diseases. A theoretical risk for transmission of Creutzfeldt-Jakob disease (CJD) also is considered extremely remote. No cases of transmission of viral diseases or CJD have ever been identified for albumin.

PRECAUTIONS

General

Caution should be exercised when administering Rebif® to patients with pre-existing seizure disorders. Seizures have been associated with the use of beta interferons. A relationship between occurrence of seizures and the use of Rebif® has not been established. Leukopenia and new or worsening thyroid abnormalities have developed in some patients treated with Rebif® (see **ADVERSE REACTIONS**). Regular monitoring for these conditions is recommended (see **PRECAUTIONS: Laboratory Tests**).

Information for Patients

All patients should be instructed to read the Rebif® Medication Guide supplied to them. Patients should be cautioned not to change the dosage or the schedule of administration without medical consultation.

Patients should be informed of the most common and the most severe adverse reactions associated with the use of Rebif® (see **WARNINGS** and **ADVERSE REACTIONS**). Patients should be advised of the symptoms associated with these conditions, and to report them to their physician.

Female patients should be cautioned about the abortifacient potential of Rebif® (see **PRECAUTIONS: Pregnancy**).

Patients should be instructed in the use of aseptic technique when administering Rebif®. Appropriate instruction for self-injection or injection by another person should be provided, including careful review of the Rebif® Medication Guide. If a patient is to self-administer Rebif®, the physical and cognitive ability of that patient to self-administer and properly dispose of syringes should be assessed. The initial injection should be performed under the supervision of an appropriately qualified health care professional. Patients should be advised of the importance of rotating sites of injection with each dose, to minimize the likelihood of severe injection site reactions or necrosis. A puncture-resistant container for disposal of used needles and syringes should be supplied to the patient along with instructions for safe disposal of full containers. Patients should be instructed in the technique and importance of proper syringe disposal and be cautioned against reuse of these items.

Laboratory Tests

In addition to those laboratory tests normally required for monitoring patients with multiple sclerosis, blood cell counts and liver function tests are recommended at regular intervals (1, 3, and 6 months) following introduction of Rebif® therapy and then periodically thereafter in the absence of clinical symptoms. Thyroid function tests are recommended every 6 months in patients with a history of thyroid dysfunction or as clinically indicated. Patients with myelosuppression may require more intensive monitoring of complete blood cell counts, with differential and platelet counts.

Drug Interactions

No formal drug interaction studies have been conducted with Rebif®. Due to its potential to cause neutropenia and lymphopenia, proper monitoring of patients is required if Rebif® is given in combination with myelosuppressive agents.

Carcinogenesis, Mutagenesis, Impairment of Fertility

Carcinogenesis: No carcinogenicity data for Rebif® are available in animals or humans.

Mutagenesis: Rebif® was not mutagenic when tested in the Ames bacterial test and in an *in vitro* cytogenetic assay in human lymphocytes in the presence and absence of metabolic activation.

Impairment of Fertility: No studies have been conducted to evaluate the effects of Rebif® on fertility in humans. In studies in normally cycling female cynomolgus monkeys given daily sc injections of Rebif® for six months at doses of up to 9 times the recommended weekly human dose (based on body surface area), no effects were observed on either menstrual cycling or serum estradiol levels. The validity of extrapolating doses used in animal studies to human doses is not established. In male monkeys, the same doses of Rebif® had no demonstrable adverse effects on sperm count, motility, morphology, or function.

Pregnancy Category C

Rebif® treatment has been associated with significant increases in embryolethal or abortifacient effects in cynomolgus monkeys administered doses approximately 2 times the cumulative weekly human dose (based on either body weight or surface area) either during the period of organogenesis (gestation day 21-89) or later in pregnancy. There were no fetal malformations or other evidence of teratogenesis noted in these studies. These effects are consistent with the abortifacient effects of other type I interferons. There are no adequate and well-controlled studies of Rebif® in pregnant women. However, in Studies 1 and 2, there were 2 spontaneous abortions observed and 5 fetuses carried to term among 7 women in the Rebif® groups. If a woman becomes pregnant or plans to become pregnant while taking Rebif®, she should be informed about the potential hazards to the fetus, and discontinuation of Rebif® should be considered.

A pregnancy registry has been established to monitor pregnancy outcomes of women exposed to Rebif® while pregnant. Health care providers are encouraged to register patients on line at rebifpregnancyregistry.com or by calling MS LifeLines at 1-877-44-REBIF (1-877-447-3243).

Nursing Mothers

It is not known whether Rebif® is excreted in human milk. Because many drugs are excreted in human milk, caution should be exercised when Rebif® is administered to a nursing woman.

Pediatric Use: The safety and effectiveness of Rebif® in pediatric patients have not been studied.

Geriatric Use: Clinical studies of Rebif® did not include sufficient numbers of subjects aged 65 and over to determine whether they respond differently than younger subjects. In general, dose selection for an elderly patient should be cautious, usually starting at the low end of the dosing range, reflecting the greater frequency of decreased hepatic, renal or cardiac function, and of concomitant disease or other drug therapy.

ADVERSE REACTIONS

The most frequently reported serious adverse reactions with Rebif® were psychiatric disorders including depression and suicidal ideation or attempt (see **WARNINGS**). The incidence of depression of any severity in the Rebif®-treated groups and placebo-treated group was approximately 25%. The most commonly reported adverse reactions were injection site disorders, influenza-like symptoms (headache, fatigue, fever, rigors, chest pain, back pain, myalgia), abdom-

Table 2: Clinical and MRI Results from Study 2

	Rebif®	Avonex®	Absolute Difference	Risk of relapse on Rebif® relative to Avonex®
Relapses	N=339	N=338		
Proportion of patients relapse-free at 24 weeks[1]	75%*	63%	12% (95% CI: 5%, 19%)	0.68 (95% CI: 0.54, 0.86)
Proportion of patients relapse-free at 48 weeks	62%**	52%	10% (95% CI: 2%, 17%)	0.81 (95% CI: 0.68, 0.96)
MRI (through 24 weeks)	N=325	N=325		
Median of the mean number of combined unique MRI lesions per patient per scan[2] (25th, 75th percentiles)	0.17* (0.00, 0.67)	0.33 (0.00, 1.25)		

* p <0.001, and ** p = 0.009, Rebif® compared to Avonex®

(1) Logistic regression model adjusted for treatment and center, intent to treat analysis

(2) Nonparametric ANCOVA model adjusted for treatment center, with baseline combined unique lesions as the single covariate.

Table 3. Adverse Reactions and Laboratory Abnormalities in Study 1

Body System Preferred Term	Placebo tiw (n=187)	Rebif® 22 mcg tiw (n=189)	Rebif® 44 mcg tiw (n=184)
BODY AS A WHOLE			
Influenza-like symptoms	51%	56%	59%
Headache	63%	65%	70%
Fatigue	36%	33%	41%
Fever	16%	25%	28%
Rigors	5%	6%	13%
Chest Pain	5%	6%	8%
Malaise	1%	4%	5%
INJECTION SITE DISORDERS			
Injection Site Reaction	39%	89%	92%
Injection Site Necrosis	0%	1%	3%
CENTRAL & PERIPH NERVOUS SYSTEM DISORDERS			
Hypertonia	5%	7%	6%
Coordination Abnormal	2%	5%	4%
Convulsions	2%	5%	4%
ENDOCRINE DISORDERS			
Thyroid Disorder	3%	4%	6%
GASTROINTESTINAL SYSTEM DISORDERS			
Abdominal Pain	17%	22%	20%
Dry Mouth	1%	1%	5%
LIVER AND BILIARY SYSTEM DISORDERS			
SGPT Increased	4%	20%	27%
SGOT Increased	4%	10%	17%
Hepatic Function Abnormal	2%	4%	9%
Bilirubinaemia	1%	3%	2%
MUSCULO-SKELETAL SYSTEM DISORDERS			
Myalgia	20%	25%	25%
Back Pain	20%	23%	25%
Skeletal Pain	10%	15%	10%
HEMATOLOGIC DISORDERS			
Leukopenia	14%	28%	36%
Lymphadenopathy	8%	11%	12%
Thrombocytopenia	2%	2%	8%
Anemia	3%	3%	5%
PSYCHIATRIC DISORDERS			
Somnolence	1%	4%	5%
SKIN DISORDERS			
Rash Erythematous	3%	7%	5%
Rash Maculo-Papular	2%	5%	4%
URINARY SYSTEM DISORDERS			
Micturition Frequency	4%	2%	7%
Urinary Incontinence	2%	4%	2%
VISION DISORDERS			
Vision Abnormal	7%	7%	13%
Xerophthalmia	0%	3%	1%

inal pain, depression, elevation of liver enzymes and hematologic abnormalities. The most frequently reported adverse reactions resulting in clinical intervention (e.g., discontinuation of Rebif®, adjustment in dosage, or the need for concomitant medication to treat an adverse reaction symptom) were injection site disorders, influenza-like symptoms, depression and elevation of liver enzymes (see **WARNINGS**).

In Study 1, 6 patients randomized to Rebif® 44 mcg tiw (3%), and 2 patients who received Rebif® 22 mcg tiw (1%) developed injection site necrosis during two years of therapy. Rebif® was continued in 7 patients and interrupted briefly in one patient. There was one report of injection site necrosis in Study 2 during 48 weeks of Rebif treatment. All events resolved with conservative management; none required skin debridement or grafting.

The rates of adverse reactions and association with Rebif® in patients with relapsing-remitting multiple sclerosis are drawn from the placebo-controlled study (n = 560) and the active comparator-controlled study (n = 339).

The population encompassed an age range from 18 to 55 years. Nearly three-fourths of the patients were female, and more than 90% were Caucasian, largely reflecting the general demographics of the population of patients with multiple sclerosis.

Because clinical trials are conducted under widely varying conditions, adverse reaction rates observed in the clinical trials of Rebif® cannot be directly compared to rates in the clinical trials of other drugs and may not reflect the rates observed in practice.

Table 3 enumerates adverse events and laboratory abnormalities that occurred at an incidence that was at least 2% more in either Rebif®-treated group than was observed in the placebo group.

[See table 3 on previous page]

The adverse reactions were generally similar in Studies 1 and 2, taking into account the disparity in study durations.

Immunogenicity

As with all therapeutic proteins, there is a potential for immunogenicity. In study 1, the presence of neutralizing antibodies (NAb) to Rebif® was determined by collecting and analyzing serum pre-study and at 6 month time intervals during the 2 years of the clinical trial. Serum NAb were detected in 59/189 (31%) and 45/184 (24%) of Rebif®-treated patients at the 22 mcg and 44 mcg tiw doses, respectively, at one or more times during the study. The clinical significance of the presence of NAb to Rebif® is unknown.

The data reflect the percentage of patients whose test results were considered positive for antibodies to Rebif® using an antiviral cytopathic effect assay, and are highly dependent on the sensitivity and specificity of the assay. Additionally, the observed incidence of NAb positivity in an assay may be influenced by several factors including sample handling, timing of sample collection, concomitant medications and underlying disease. For these reasons, comparison of the incidence of antibodies to Rebif® with the incidence of antibodies to other products may be misleading.

Anaphylaxis and other allergic reactions have been observed with the use of Rebif® (see **WARNINGS: Anaphylaxis**).

DRUG ABUSE AND DEPENDENCE

There is no evidence that abuse or dependence occurs with Rebif® therapy. However, the risk of dependence has not been systematically evaluated.

OVERDOSAGE

Safety of doses higher than 44 mcg sc tiw has not been adequately evaluated. The maximum amount of Rebif® that can be safely administered has not been determined.

DOSAGE AND ADMINISTRATION

Dosages of Rebif® shown to be safe and effective are 22 mcg and 44 mcg injected subcutaneously three times per week. Rebif® should be administered, if possible, at the same time (preferably in the late afternoon or evening) on the same three days (e.g., Monday, Wednesday, and Friday) at least 48 hours apart each week (see **CLINICAL STUDIES**). Generally, patients should be started at 20% of the prescribed dose tiw and increased over a 4-week period to the targeted dose, either 22 mcg or 44 mcg tiw (see **Table 4**). Following the administration of each dose, any residual product remaining in the syringe should be discarded in a safe and proper manner.

Table 4: Schedule for Patient Titration

	Recommended Titration (% of final dose)	Titration dose for Rebif® 22 mcg	Titration dose for Rebif® 44 mcg	Injection Volume
Weeks 1-2	20 %	4.4 mcg	8.8 mcg	0.1 mL
Weeks 3-4	50 %	11 mcg	22 mcg	0.25 mL
Weeks 5+	100 %	22 mcg	44 mcg	0.5 mL

Leukopenia or elevated liver function tests may necessitate dose reductions of 20-50% until toxicity is resolved (see **WARNINGS: Hepatic Injury, PRECAUTIONS: General**).

Rebif® is intended for use under the guidance and supervision of a physician. It is recommended that physicians or qualified medical personnel train patients in the proper technique for self-administering subcutaneous injections using the pre-filled syringe. Patients should be advised to rotate sites for sc injections (see **PRECAUTIONS: Information for Patients**). Concurrent use of analgesics and/or antipyretics may help ameliorate flu-like symptoms on treatment days. Rebif® should be inspected visually for particulate matter and discoloration prior to administration.

Stability and Storage

Rebif® should be stored refrigerated between 2-8°C (36-46°F). DO NOT FREEZE. If a refrigerator is not available, Rebif® may be stored at or below 25°C/77°F for up to 30 days and away from heat and light.

Do not use beyond the expiration date printed on packages. Rebif® contains no preservatives. Each syringe is intended for single use. Unused portions should be discarded.

HOW SUPPLIED

Rebif® is supplied as a sterile, preservative-free solution packaged in graduated, ready to use 0.5 mL pre-filled syringes with 27-gauge, 0.5 inch needle for subcutaneous injection. The following package presentations are available.

Rebif® (interferon beta -1a) 22 mcg Pre-filled syringe

— One Rebif® 22 mcg pre-filled syringe, NDC 44087-0022-1
— Twelve Rebif® 22 mcg pre-filled syringes, NDC 44087-0022-3

Rebif® (interferon beta -1a) 44 mcg Pre-filled syringe

— One Rebif® 44 mcg pre-filled syringe, NDC 44087-0044-1
— Twelve Rebif® 44 mcg pre-filled syringes, NDC 44087-0044-3

RX only.

REFERENCES

1. PRISMS Study Group. Randomized double-blind placebo-controlled study of interferon β-1a in relapsing/remitting multiple sclerosis. Lancet 1998; 352: 1498-1504.
2. Data on file.

Manufacturer: Serono, Inc. Rockland, MA 02370
U.S. License # 1574
Co-Marketed by:
Serono, Inc.
Rockland, MA 02370
Pfizer Inc.
New York, NY 10017
Revised: March 2004

*Avonex® is a registered trademark of Biogen, Inc.
N6700101B 04/04

RELPAX® ℞

[rĕl-păks]
(eletriptan hydrobromide)
Tablets

DESCRIPTION

RELPAX® (eletriptan) Tablets contain eletriptan hydrobromide, which is a selective 5-hydroxytryptamine 1B/1D (5-HT1B/1D) receptor agonist. Eletriptan is chemically designated as (R)-3-[(1-Methyl-2-pyrrolidinyl) methyl]-5-[2-(phenylsulfonyl)ethyl]-1H-indole, monohydrobromide, and it has the following chemical structure:

CH_3 . HBr

The empirical formula is $C_{22}H_{26}N_2O_2S$. HBr, representing a molecular weight of 463.40. Eletriptan hydrobromide is a white to light pale colored powder that is readily soluble in water.

Each RELPAX Tablet for oral administration contains 24.2 or 48.5 mg of eletriptan hydrobromide equivalent to 20 mg or 40 mg of eletriptan, respectively. Each tablet also contains the inactive ingredients microcrystalline cellulose NF, lactose NF, croscarmellose sodium NF, magnesium stearate NF, titanium dioxide USP, hypromellose, triacetin USP and FD&C Yellow No. 6 aluminum lake.

CLINICAL PHARMACOLOGY

Mechanism of Action: Eletriptan binds with high affinity to 5-HT_{1B}, 5-HT_{1D} and 5-HT_{1F} receptors, has modest affinity for 5-HT_{1A}, 5-HT_{1E}, 5-HT_{2B} and 5-HT_7 receptors, and little or no affinity for 5-HT_{2A}, 5-HT_{2C}, 5-HT_3, 5-HT_4, 5-HT_{5A} and 5-HT_6 receptors. Eletriptan has no significant affinity or pharmacological activity at adrenergic $alpha_1$, $alpha_2$, or beta; dopaminergic D_1 or D_2; muscarinic; or opioid receptors.

Two theories have been proposed to explain the efficacy of 5-HT receptor agonists in migraine. One theory suggests that activation of 5-HT_1 receptors located on intracranial blood vessels, including those on the arteriovenous anastomoses, leads to vasoconstriction, which is correlated with the relief of migraine headache. The other hypothesis suggests that activation of 5-HT_1 receptors on sensory nerve endings in the trigeminal system results in the inhibition of pro-inflammatory neuropeptide release.

In the anesthetized dog, eletriptan has been shown to reduce carotid arterial blood flow, with only a small increase in arterial blood pressure at high doses. While the effect on blood flow was selective for the carotid arterial bed, decreases in coronary artery diameter were observed. Eletriptan has also been shown to inhibit trigeminal nerve activity in the rat.

Pharmacokinetics:

Absorption: Eletriptan is well absorbed after oral administration with peak plasma levels occurring approximately 1.5 hours after dosing to healthy subjects. In patients with moderate to severe migraine the median T_{max} is 2.0 hours. The mean absolute bioavailability of eletriptan is approximately 50%. The oral pharmacokinetics are slightly more than dose proportional over the clinical dose range. The AUC and C_{max} of eletriptan are increased by approximately 20 to 30% following oral administration with a high fat meal.

Distribution: The volume of distribution of eletriptan following IV administration is 138L. Plasma protein binding is moderate and approximately 85%.

Metabolism: The N-demethylated metabolite of eletriptan is the only known active metabolite. This metabolite causes vasoconstriction similar to eletriptan in animal models. Though the half-life of the metabolite is estimated to be about 13 hours, the plasma concentration of the N-demethylated metabolite is 10-20% of parent drug and is unlikely to contribute significantly to the overall effect of the parent compound.

In vitro studies indicate that eletriptan is primarily metabolized by cytochrome P-450 enzyme CYP3A4 (see WARNINGS, DOSAGE AND ADMINISTRATION and CLINICAL PHARMACOLOGY: Drug Interactions).

Elimination: The terminal elimination half-life of eletriptan is approximately 4 hours. Mean renal clearance (CL_R) following oral administration is approximately 3.9 L/h. Non-renal clearance accounts for about 90% of the total clearance.

Special Populations:

Age: The pharmacokinetics of eletriptan are generally unaffected by age.

Eletriptan has been given to only 50 patients over the age of 65. Blood pressure was increased to a greater extent in elderly subjects than in young subjects. The pharmacokinetic disposition of eletriptan in the elderly is similar to that seen in younger adults (see PRECAUTIONS).

There is a statistically significant increased half-life (from about 4.4 hours to 5.7 hours) between elderly (65 to 93 years of age) and younger adult subjects (18 to 45 years of age) (see PRECAUTIONS).

Gender: The pharmacokinetics of eletriptan are unaffected by gender.

Race: A comparison of pharmacokinetic studies run in western countries with those run in Japan have indicated an approximate 35% reduction in the exposure of eletriptan in Japanese male volunteers compared to western males. Population pharmacokinetic analysis of two clinical studies indicates no evidence of pharmacokinetic differences between Caucasians and non Caucasian patients.

Menstrual Cycle: In a study of 16 healthy females, the pharmacokinetics of eletriptan remained consistent throughout the phases of the menstrual cycle.

Renal Impairment: There was no significant change in clearance observed in subjects with mild, moderate or severe renal impairment, though blood pressure elevations were observed in this population (see WARNINGS).

Hepatic Impairment: The effects of severe hepatic impairment on eletriptan metabolism have not been evaluated. Subjects with mild or moderate hepatic impairment demonstrated an increase in both AUC (34%) and half-life. The C_{max} was increased by 18% (see PRECAUTIONS and DOSAGE AND ADMINISTRATION).

Drug Interactions:

CYP3A4 inhibitors: *In vitro* studies have shown that eletriptan is metabolized by the CYP3A4 enzyme. A clinical study demonstrated about a 3-fold increase in C_{max} and about a 6-fold increase in the AUC of eletriptan when combined with ketoconazole. The half-life increased from 5 hours to 8 hours and the T_{max} increased from 2.8 hours to 5.4 hours. Another clinical study demonstrated about a 2-fold increase in C_{max} and about a 4-fold increase in AUC when erythromycin was co-administered with eletriptan. It has also been shown that co-administration of verapamil and eletriptan yields about a 2-fold increase in C_{max} and about a 3-fold increase in AUC of eletriptan, and that co-administration of fluconazole and eletriptan yields about a 1.4-fold increase in C_{max} and about a 2-fold increase in AUC of eletriptan.

Eletriptan should not be used within at least 72 hours of treatment with the following potent CYP3A4 inhibitors: ketoconazole, itraconazole, nefazodone, troleandomycin, clarithromycin, ritonavir and nelfinavir. Eletriptan should not be used within 72 hours with drugs that have demonstrated potent CYP3A4 inhibition and have this potent effect described in the CONTRAINDICATIONS, WARNINGS or PRECAUTIONS sections of their labeling (see WARNINGS and DOSAGE AND ADMINISTRATION).

Propranolol: The C_{max} and AUC of eletriptan were increased by 10 and 33% respectively in the presence of propranolol. No interactive increases in blood pressure were observed. No dosage adjustment appears to be needed for patients taking propranolol (see PRECAUTIONS).

The effect of eletriptan on other drugs: The effect of eletriptan on enzymes other than cytochrome P-450 has not been investigated. *In vitro* human liver microsome studies

Continued on next page

Relpax—Cont.

suggest that eletriptan has little potential to inhibit CYP1A2, 2C9, 2E1 and 3A4 at concentrations up to 100μM. While eletriptan has an effect on CYP2D6 at high concentration, this effect should not interfere with metabolism of other drugs when eletriptan is used at recommended doses. There is no *in vitro* or *in vivo* evidence that clinical doses of eletriptan will induce drug metabolizing enzymes. Therefore, eletriptan is unlikely to cause clinically important drug interactions mediated by these enzymes.

CLINICAL STUDIES

The efficacy of RELPAX in the acute treatment of migraines was evaluated in eight randomized, double-blind placebo-controlled studies. All eight studies used 40 mg. Seven studies evaluated an 80 mg dose and two studies included a 20 mg dose.

In all eight studies, randomized patients treated their headaches as outpatients. Seven studies enrolled adults and one study enrolled adolescents (age 11 to 17). Patients treated in the seven adult studies were predominantly female (85%) and Caucasian (94%) with a mean age of 40 years (range 18 to 78). In all studies, patients were instructed to treat a moderate to severe headache. Headache response, defined as a reduction in headache severity from moderate or severe pain to mild or no pain, was assessed up to 2 hours after dosing. Associated symptoms such as nausea, vomiting, photophobia and phonophobia were also assessed.

Maintenance of response was assessed for up to 24 hours post dose. In the adult studies, a second dose of RELPAX Tablets or other medication was allowed 2 to 24 hours after the initial treatment for both persistent and recurrent headaches. The incidence and time to use of these additional treatments were also recorded.

In the seven adult studies, the percentage of patients achieving headache response 2 hours after treatment was significantly greater among patients receiving RELPAX Tablets at all doses compared to those who received placebo. The two hour response rates from these controlled clinical studies are summarized in Table 1.

Table 1: Percentage of Patients with Headache Response (Mild or No Headache) 2 Hours Following Treatment

	Placebo	RELPAX 20 mg	RELPAX 40 mg	RELPAX 80 mg
Study 1	23.8% (n=126)	54.3%* (n=129)	65.0%* (n=117)	77.1%* (n=118)
Study 2	19.0% (n=232)	NA	61.6%* (n=430)	64.6%* (n=446)
Study 3	21.7% (n=276)	47.3%* (n=273)	61.9%* (n=281)	58.6%* (n=290)
Study 4	39.5% (n=86)	NA	62.3%* (n=175)	70.0%* (n=170)
Study 5	20.6% (n=102)	NA	53.9%* (n=206)	67.9%* (n=209)
Study 6	31.3% (n=80)	NA	63.9%* (n=169)	66.9%* (n=160)
Study 7	29.5% (n=122)	NA	57.5%* (n=492)	NA

* p value < 0.05 vs placebo
NA - Not Applicable

Comparisons of the performance of different drugs based upon results obtained in different clinical trials are never reliable. Because studies are generally conducted at different times, with different samples of patients, by different investigators, employing different criteria and/or different interpretations of the same criteria, under different conditions (dose, dosing regimen, etc.), quantitative estimates of treatment response and the timing of response may be expected to vary considerably from study to study.

The estimated probability of achieving an initial headache response within 2 hours following treatment is depicted in Figure 1.

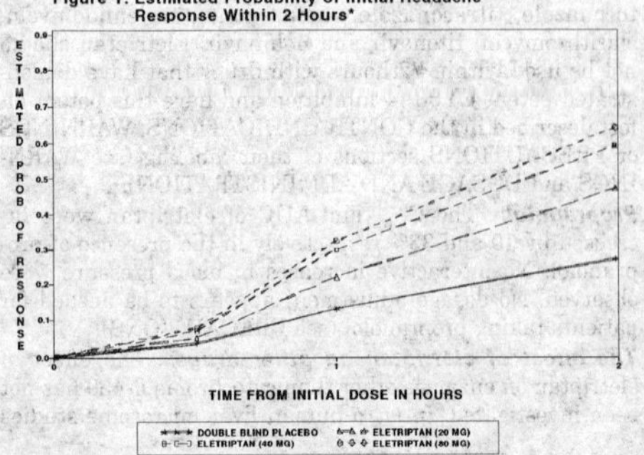

Figure 1: Estimated Probability of Initial Headache Response Within 2 Hours*

*Figure 1 shows the Kaplan-Meier plot of probability over time of obtaining headache response (no or mild pain) following treatment with eletriptan. The plot is based on 7 placebo-controlled, outpatient trials in adults providing evidence of efficacy (Studies 1 through 7). Patients not achieving headache response or taking additional treatment prior to 2 hours were censored at 2 hours.

For patients with migraine-associated photophobia, phonophobia, and nausea at baseline, there was a decreased incidence of these symptoms following administration of RELPAX as compared to placebo.

Two to 24 hours following the initial dose of study treatment, patients were allowed to use additional treatment for pain relief in the form of a second dose of study treatment or other medication. The estimated probability of taking a second dose or other medications for migraine over the 24 hours following the initial dose of study treatment is summarized in Figure 2.

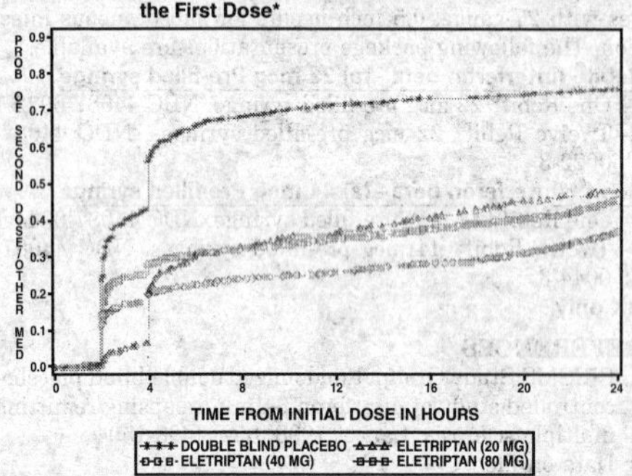

Figure 2: Estimated Probability of Taking a Second Dose/ Other Medication Over the 24 Hours Following the First Dose*

*This Kaplan-Meier plot is based on data obtained in 7 placebo-controlled trials in adults (Studies 1 through 7). Patients were instructed to take a second dose of study medication as follows: a) in the event of no response at 2 hours (studies 2 and 4-7) or at 4 hours (study 3); b) in the event of headache recurrence within 24 hours (studies 2-7). Patients not using additional treatments were censored at 24 hours. The plot includes both patients who had headache response at 2 hours and those who had no response to the initial dose. It should be noted that the protocols did not allow remedication within 2 hours post dose.

The efficacy of RELPAX was unaffected by the duration of attack; gender or age of the patient; relationship to menses; or concomitant use of estrogen replacement therapy/oral contraceptives or frequently used migraine prophylactic drugs.

In a single study in adolescents (n=274), there were no statistically significant differences between treatment groups. The headache response rate at 2 hours was 57% for both RELPAX 40 mg Tablets and placebo.

INDICATIONS AND USAGE

RELPAX is indicated for the acute treatment of migraine with or without aura in adults.

RELPAX is not intended for the prophylactic therapy of migraine or for use in the management of hemiplegic or basilar migraine (see CONTRAINDICATIONS). Safety and effectiveness of RELPAX Tablets have not been established for cluster headache, which is present in an older, predominantly male population.

CONTRAINDICATIONS

RELPAX Tablets should not be given to patients with ischemic heart disease (e.g., angina pectoris, history of myocardial infarction, or documented silent ischemia) or to patients who have symptoms, or findings consistent with ischemic heart disease, coronary artery vasospasm, including Prinzmetal's variant angina, or other significant underlying cardiovascular disease (see WARNINGS).

RELPAX Tablets should not be given to patients with cerebrovascular syndromes including (but not limited to) strokes of any type as well as transient ischemic attacks (see WARNINGS).

RELPAX Tablets should not be given to patients with peripheral vascular disease including (but not limited to) ischemic bowel disease (see WARNINGS).

Because RELPAX Tablets may increase blood pressure, it should not be given to patients with uncontrolled hypertension (see WARNINGS).

RELPAX Tablets should not be administered to patients with hemiplegic or basilar migraine.

RELPAX Tablets should not be used within 24 hours of treatment with another 5-HT$_1$ agonist, an ergotamine-containing or ergot-type medication such as dihydroergotamine (DHE) or methysergide.

RELPAX Tablets should not be used in patients with known hypersensitivity to eletriptan or any of its inactive ingredients.

RELPAX Tablets should not be given to patients with severe hepatic impairment.

WARNINGS

RELPAX Tablets should only be used where a clear diagnosis of migraine has been established.

CYP3A4 Inhibitors:

Eletriptan should not be used within at least 72 hours of treatment with the following potent CYP3A4 inhibitors: ketoconazole, itraconazole, nefazodone, troleandomycin, clarithromycin, ritonavir, and nelfinavir. Eletriptan should not be used within 72 hours with drugs that have demonstrated potent CYP3A4 inhibition and have this potent effect described in the CONTRAINDICATIONS, WARNINGS or PRECAUTIONS sections of their labeling (see CLINICAL PHARMACOLOGY: Drug Interactions and DOSAGE AND ADMINISTRATION).

In a coronary angiographic study of rapidly infused intravenous eletriptan to concentrations exceeding those achieved with 80 mg oral eletriptan in the presence of potent CYP3A4 inhibitors, a small dose-related decrease in coronary artery diameter similar to that seen with a 6 mg subcutaneous dose of sumatriptan was observed.

Risk of Myocardial Ischemia and/or Infarction and Other Cardiac Events: Because of the potential of 5-HT$_1$ agonists to cause coronary vasospasm, eletriptan should not be given to patients with documented ischemic or vasospastic coronary artery disease (CAD) (see CONTRAINDICATIONS). It is strongly recommended that eletriptan not be given to patients in whom unrecognized CAD is predicted by the presence of risk factors (e.g., hypertension, hypercholesterolemia, smoker, obesity, diabetes, strong family history of CAD, female with surgical or physiological menopause, or male over 40 years of age) unless a cardiovascular evaluation provides satisfactory clinical evidence that the patient is reasonably free of coronary artery and ischemic myocardial disease or other significant underlying cardiovascular disease. The sensitivity of cardiac diagnostic procedures to detect cardiovascular disease or predisposition to coronary artery vasospasm is modest, at best. If, during the cardiovascular evaluation, the patient's medical history, electrocardiographic, or other investigations reveal findings indicative of, or consistent with coronary artery vasospasm or myocardial ischemia, eletriptan should not be administered (see CONTRAINDICATIONS).

For patients with risk factors predictive of CAD, who are determined to have a satisfactory cardiovascular evaluation, it is strongly recommended that administration of the first dose of eletriptan take place in the setting of a physician's office or similar medically staffed and equipped facility unless the patient has previously received eletriptan. Because cardiac ischemia can occur in the absence of clinical symptoms, consideration should be given to obtaining on the first occasion of use an electrocardiogram (ECG) during the interval immediately following administration of RELPAX Tablets, in these patients with risk factors.

It is recommended that patients who are intermittent long-term users of 5-HT$_1$ agonists including RELPAX Tablets, and who have or acquire risk factors predictive of CAD, as described above, undergo periodic cardiovascular evaluation as they continue to use RELPAX Tablets.

The systematic approach described above is intended to reduce the likelihood that patients with unrecognized cardiovascular disease will be inadvertently exposed to eletriptan.

Cardiac Events and Fatalities Associated With 5-HT$_1$ Agonists: Serious adverse cardiac events, including acute myocardial infarction, life-threatening disturbances of cardiac rhythm, and death have been reported within a few hours following the administration of other 5-HT$_1$ agonists. Considering the extent of use of 5-HT$_1$ agonists in patients with migraine, the incidence of these events is extremely low.

Premarketing experience with eletriptan among the 7,143 unique individuals who received eletriptan during premarketing clinical trials: In a clinical pharmacology study, in subjects undergoing diagnostic coronary angiography, a subject with a history of angina, hypertension and hypercholesterolemia, receiving intravenous eletriptan (C_{max} of 127 ng/mL equivalent to 60 mg oral eletriptan), reported chest tightness and experienced angiographically documented coronary vasospasm with no ECG changes of ischemia. There was also one report of atrial fibrillation in a patient with a past history of atrial fibrillation.

Postmarketing experience with eletriptan: There was one report of myocardial infarction and death in a patient with cardiovascular risk factors (hypertension, hyperlipidemia, strong family history of CAD) in association with inappropriate concomitant use of eletriptan and sumatriptan. The uncontrolled nature of postmarketing surveillance, however, makes it impossible to determine definitively if the case was actually caused by eletriptan or to reliably assess causation in individual cases.

Cerebrovascular Events and Fatalities Associated With 5-HT$_1$ Agonists: Cerebral hemorrhage, subarachnoid hemorrhage, stroke, and other cerebrovascular events have been reported in patients treated with 5-HT$_1$ agonists, and some have resulted in fatalities. In a number of cases, it appears possible that the cerebrovascular events were primary, the agonist having been administered in the incorrect belief that the symptoms experienced were a consequence of migraine, when they were not. It should be noted that patients with migraine may be at increased risk of certain cerebrovascular events (e.g., stroke, hemorrhage, and transient ischemic attack).

Other Vasospasm-Related Events: 5-HT$_1$ agonists may cause vasospastic reactions other than coronary artery vasospasm. Both peripheral vascular ischemia and colonic ischemia with abdominal pain and bloody diarrhea have been reported with 5-HT$_1$ agonists.

Increase in Blood Pressure: Significant elevation in blood pressure, including hypertensive crisis, has been reported on rare occasion in patients receiving 5-HT$_1$ agonists with and without a history of hypertension. In clinical pharmacology studies, oral eletriptan (at doses of 60 mg or more) was shown to cause small, transient dose-related increases in blood pressure, predominantly diastolic, consistent with its mechanism of action and with other 5-$HT_{1B/1D}$ agonists. The effect was more pronounced in renally impaired and elderly subjects. A single patient with hepatic cirrhosis received eletriptan 80 mg and experienced a blood pressure of 220/96 mm Hg five hours after dosing. The treatment related event persisted for seven hours.

Eletriptan is contraindicated in patients with uncontrolled hypertension (see CONTRAINDICATIONS).

An 18% increase in mean pulmonary artery pressure was seen following dosing with another 5-HT_1 agonist in a study evaluating subjects undergoing cardiac catheterization.

PRECAUTIONS

General: As with other 5-HT_1 agonists, sensations of tightness, pain, pressure and heaviness have been reported after treatment with eletriptan in the precordium, throat, and jaw. Events that are localized to the chest, throat, neck and jaw have not been associated with arrhythmias or ischemic ECG changes in clinical trials; in a clinical pharmacology study of subjects undergoing diagnostic coronary angiography, one subject with a history of angina, hypertension and hypercholesterolemia, receiving intravenous eletriptan, reported chest tightness and experienced angiographically documented coronary vasospasm with no ECG changes of ischemia. Because 5-HT_1 agonists may cause coronary artery vasospasm, patients who experience signs or symptoms suggestive of angina following dosing should be evaluated for the presence of CAD or a predisposition to Prinzmetal's variant angina before receiving additional doses of medication, and should be monitored electrocardiographically if dosing is resumed and similar symptoms recur. Similarly, patients who experience other symptoms or signs suggestive of decreased arterial flow, such as ischemic bowel syndrome or Raynaud's syndrome following the use of any 5-HT_1 agonist are candidates for further evaluation (see CONTRAINDICATIONS and WARNINGS).

Hepatically Impaired Patients: The effects of severe hepatic impairment on eletriptan metabolism was not evaluated. Subjects with mild or moderate hepatic impairment demonstrated an increase in both AUC (34%) and half-life. The C_{max} was increased by 18%. Eletriptan should not be used in patients with severe hepatic impairment. No dose adjustment is necessary in mild to moderate impairment (see DOSAGE AND ADMINISTRATION).

Binding to Melanin-Containing Tissues: In rats treated with a single intravenous (3 mg/kg) dose of radiolabeled eletriptan, elimination of radioactivity from the retina was prolonged, suggesting that eletriptan and/or its metabolites may bind to the melanin of the eye. Because there could be accumulation in melanin-rich tissues over time, this raises the possibility that eletriptan could cause toxicity in these tissues after extended use. Although no systematic monitoring of ophthalmologic function was undertaken in clinical trials, and no specific recommendations for ophthalmologic monitoring are offered, prescribers should be aware of the possibility of long-term ophthalmologic effects.

Corneal Opacities: Transient corneal opacities were seen in dogs receiving oral eletriptan at 5 mg/kg and above. They were observed during the first week of treatment, but were not present thereafter despite continued treatment. Exposure at the no-effect dose level of 2.5 mg/kg was approximately equal to that achieved in humans at the maximum recommended daily dose.

Information for Patients: See PATIENT INFORMATION at the end of this labeling for the text of the separate leaflet provided for patients.

Laboratory Tests: No specific laboratory tests are recommended.

Drug Interactions:

Ergot-containing drugs: Ergot-containing drugs have been reported to cause prolonged vasospastic reactions. Because these effects may be additive, use of ergotamine-containing or ergot-type medications (like dihydroergotamine [DHE] or methysergide) and eletriptan within 24 hours of each other is not recommended (see CONTRAINDICATIONS).

CYP3A4 Inhibitors: Eletriptan is metabolized primarily by CYP3A4 (see WARNINGS regarding use with potent CYP3A4 inhibitors).

Monoamine Oxidase Inhibitors: Eletriptan is not a substrate for monoamine oxidase (MAO) enzymes, therefore there is no expectation of an interaction between eletriptan and MAO inhibitors.

Propranolol: The C_{max} and AUC of eletriptan were increased by 10 and 33% respectively in the presence of propranolol. No interactive increases in blood pressure were observed. No dosage adjustment appears to be needed for patients taking propranolol (see CLINICAL PHARMACOLOGY).

Selective serotonin reuptake inhibitors (SSRIs): SSRIs (e.g., fluoxetine, fluvoxamine, paroxetine, sertraline) have been reported, rarely, to cause weakness, hyperreflexia, and incoordination when coadministered with 5-HT_1 agonists. If concomitant treatment with eletriptan and an SSRI is clinically warranted, appropriate observation of the patient is advised.

Other 5-HT_1 agonists: Concomitant use of other 5-HT_1 agonists within 24 hours of RELPAX treatment is not recommended (see CONTRAINDICATIONS).

Drug/Laboratory Test Interactions: RELPAX Tablets are not known to interfere with commonly employed clinical laboratory tests.

Carcinogenesis: Lifetime carcinogenicity studies, 104 weeks in duration, were carried out in mice and rats by administering eletriptan in the diet. In rats, the incidence of testicular interstitial cell adenomas was increased at the high dose of 75 mg/kg/day. The estimated exposure (AUC) to parent drug at that dose was approximately 6 times that achieved in humans receiving the maximum recommended daily dose (MRDD) of 80 mg, and at the no-effect dose of 15 mg/kg/day it was approximately 2 times the human exposure at the MRDD. In mice, the incidence of hepatocellular adenomas was increased at the high dose of 400 mg/kg/day. The exposure to parent drug (AUC) at that dose was approximately 18 times that achieved in humans receiving the MRDD, and the AUC at the no-effect dose of 90 mg/kg/day was approximately 7 times the human exposure at the MRDD.

Mutagenesis: Eletriptan was not mutagenic in bacterial or mammalian cell assays *in vitro*, testing negative in the Ames reverse mutation test and the hypoxanthine-guanine phosphoribosyl transferase (HGPRT) mutation test in Chinese hamster ovary cells. It was not clastogenic in two *in vivo* mouse micronucleus assays. Results were equivocal in *in vitro* human lymphocyte clastogenicity tests, in which the incidence of polyploidy was increased in the absence of metabolic activation (-S9 conditions), but not in the presence of metabolic activation.

Impairment of Fertility: In a rat fertility and early embryonic development study, doses tested were 50, 100 and 200 mg/kg/day, resulting in systemic exposures to parent drug in rats, based on AUC, that were 4, 8 and 16 times MRDD, respectively, in males and 7, 14 and 28 times MRDD, respectively, in females. There was a prolongation of the estrous cycle at the 200 mg/kg/day dose due to an increase in duration of estrus, based on vaginal smears. There were also dose-related, statistically significant decreases in mean numbers of corpora lutea per dam at all 3 doses, resulting in decreases in mean numbers of implants and viable fetuses per dam. This suggests a partial inhibition of ovulation by eletriptan. There was no effect on fertility of males and no other effect on fertility of females.

Pregnancy: ***Pregnancy Category C:*** In reproductive toxicity studies in rats and rabbits, oral administration of eletriptan was associated with developmental toxicity (decreased fetal and pup weights and an increased incidence of fetal structural abnormalities). Effects on fetal and pup weights were observed at doses that were, on a mg/m^2 basis, 6 to 12 times greater than the clinical maximum recommended daily dose (MRDD) of 80 mg. The increase in structural alterations occurred in the rat and rabbit at doses that, on a mg/m^2 basis, were 12 times greater than (rat) and approximately equal to (rabbit) the MRDD.

When pregnant rats were administered eletriptan during the period of organogenesis at doses of 10, 30 or 100 mg/kg/day, fetal weights were decreased and the incidences of vertebral and sternebral variations were increased at 100 mg/kg/day (approximately 12 times the MRDD on a mg/m^2 basis). The 100 mg/kg dose was also maternally toxic, as evidenced by decreased maternal body weight gain during gestation. The no-effect dose for developmental toxicity in rats exposed during organogenesis was 30 mg/kg, which is approximately 4 times the MRDD on a mg/m^2 basis.

When doses of 5, 10 or 50 mg/kg/day were given to New Zealand White rabbits throughout organogenesis, fetal weights were decreased at 50 mg/kg, which is approximately 12 times the MRDD on a mg/m^2 basis. The incidences of fused sternebrae and vena cava deviations were increased in all treated groups. Maternal toxicity was not produced at any dose. A no-effect dose for developmental toxicity in rabbits exposed during organogenesis was not established, and the 5 mg/kg dose is approximately equal to the MRDD on a mg/m^2 basis.

There are no adequate and well-controlled studies in pregnant women; therefore, eletriptan should be used during pregnancy only if the potential benefit justifies the potential risk to the fetus.

Nursing Mothers: Eletriptan is excreted in human breast milk. In one study of 8 women given a single dose of 80 mg, the mean total amount of eletriptan in breast milk over 24 hours in this group was approximately 0.02% of the administered dose. The ratio of eletriptan mean concentration in breast milk to plasma was 1:4, but there was great variability. The resulting eletriptan concentration-time profile was similar to that seen in the plasma over 24 hours, with very low concentrations of drug (mean 1.7 ng/mL) still present in the milk 18-24 hours post dose. The N-desmethyl active metabolite was not measured in the breast milk. Caution should be exercised when RELPAX is administered to nursing women.

Pediatric Use: Safety and effectiveness of RELPAX Tablets in pediatric patients have not been established; therefore, RELPAX is not recommended for use in patients under 18 years of age.

The efficacy of RELPAX Tablets (40 mg) in patients 11-17 was not established in a randomized, placebo-controlled trial of 274 adolescent migraineurs (see CLINICAL STUDIES). Adverse events observed were similar in nature to those reported in clinical trials in adults. Postmarketing experience with other triptans includes a limited number of reports that describe pediatric patients who have experienced clinically serious adverse events that are similar in nature to those reported rarely in adults. Long-term safety of eletriptan was studied in 76 adolescent patients who received treatment for up to one year. A similar profile of adverse events to that of adults was observed. The long-term safety of eletriptan in pediatric patients has not been established.

Geriatric Use: Eletriptan has been given to only 50 patients over the age of 65. Blood pressure was increased to a greater extent in elderly subjects than in young subjects. The pharmacokinetic disposition of eletriptan in the elderly is similar to that seen in younger adults (see CLINICAL PHARMACOLOGY). In clinical trials, there were no apparent differences in efficacy or the incidence of adverse events between patients under 65 years of age and those 65 and above (n=50).

There is a statistically significantly increased half-life (from about 4.4 hours to 5.7 hours) between elderly (65 to 93 years of age) and younger adult subjects (18 to 45 years of age) (see CLINICAL PHARMACOLOGY).

ADVERSE REACTIONS

Serious cardiac events, including some that have been fatal, have occurred following the use of 5-HT_1 agonists. These events are extremely rare and most have been reported in patients with risk factors predictive of CAD. Events reported have included coronary artery vasospasm, transient myocardial ischemia, myocardial infarction, ventricular tachycardia, and ventricular fibrillation (see CONTRAINDICATIONS, WARNINGS and PRECAUTIONS).

Incidence in Controlled Clinical Trials:

Among 4,597 patients who treated the first migraine headache with RELPAX in short-term placebo-controlled trials, the most common adverse events reported with treatment with RELPAX were asthenia, nausea, dizziness, and somnolence. These events appear to be dose related.

In long-term open-label studies where patients were allowed to treat multiple migraine attacks for up to 1 year, 128 (8.3%) out of 1,544 patients discontinued treatment due to adverse events.

Table 2 lists adverse events that occurred in the subset of 5,125 migraineurs who received eletriptan doses of 20 mg, 40 mg and 80 mg or placebo in worldwide placebo-controlled clinical trials. The events cited reflect experience gained under closely monitored conditions of clinical trials in a highly selected patient population. In actual clinical practice or in other clinical trials, those frequency estimates may not apply, as the conditions of use, reporting behavior, and the kinds of patients treated may differ.

Only adverse events that were more frequent in a RELPAX treatment group compared to the placebo group with an incidence greater than or equal to 2% are included in Table 2.

Table 2: Adverse Experience Incidence in Placebo-Controlled Migraine Clinical Trials: Events Reported by ≥ 2% Patients Treated with RELPAX and More Than Placebo

Adverse Event Type	Placebo (n=988)	RELPAX 20 mg (n=431)	RELPAX 40 mg (n=1774)	RELPAX 80 mg (n=1932)
ATYPICAL SENSATIONS				
Paresthesia	2%	3%	3%	4%
Flushing/feeling of warmth	2%	2%	2%	2%
PAIN AND PRESSURE SENSATIONS				
Chest – tightness/pain/pressure	1%	1%	2%	4%
Abdominal – pain/discomfort/stomach pain/cramps/pressure	1%	1%	2%	2%
DIGESTIVE				
Dry mouth	2%	2%	3%	4%
Dyspepsia	1%	1%	2%	2%
Dysphagia – throat tightness/difficulty swallowing	0.2%	1%	2%	2%
Nausea	5%	4%	5%	8%
NEUROLOGICAL				
Dizziness	3%	3%	6%	7%
Somnolence	4%	3%	6%	7%
Headache	3%	4%	3%	4%
OTHER				
Asthenia	3%	4%	5%	10%

Continued on next page

Relpax—Cont.

RELPAX is generally well-tolerated. Across all doses, most adverse reactions were mild and transient. The frequency of adverse events in clinical trials did not increase when up to 2 doses of RELPAX were taken within 24 hours. The incidence of adverse events in controlled clinical trials was not affected by gender, age, or race of the patients. Adverse event frequencies were also unchanged by concomitant use of drugs commonly taken for migraine prophylaxis (e.g., SSRIs, beta blockers, calcium channel blockers, tricyclic antidepressants), estrogen replacement therapy and oral contraceptives.

Other Events Observed in Association With the Administration of RELPAX Tablets:

In the paragraphs that follow, the frequencies of less commonly reported adverse clinical events are presented. Because the reports include events observed in open studies, the role of RELPAX Tablets in their causation cannot be reliably determined. Furthermore, variability associated with adverse event reporting, the terminology used to describe adverse events, etc., limit the value of the quantitative frequency estimates provided. Event frequencies are calculated as the number of patients reporting an event divided by the total number of patients (N=4,719) exposed to RELPAX. All reported events are included except those already listed in Table 2, those too general to be informative, and those not reasonably associated with the use of the drug. Events are further classified within body system categories and enumerated in order of decreasing frequency using the following definitions: frequent adverse events are those occurring in at least 1/100 patients, infrequent adverse events are those occurring in 1/100 to 1/1000 patients and rare adverse events are those occurring in fewer than 1/1000 patients.

General: Frequent were back pain, chills and pain. Infrequent were face edema and malaise. Rare were abdomen enlarged, abscess, accidental injury, allergic reaction, fever, flu syndrome, halitosis, hernia, hypothermia, lab test abnormal, moniliasis, rheumatoid arthritis and shock.

Cardiovascular: Frequent was palpitation. Infrequent were hypertension, migraine, peripheral vascular disorder and tachycardia. Rare were angina pectoris, arrhythmia, atrial fibrillation, AV block, bradycardia, hypotension, syncope, thrombophlebitis, cerebrovascular disorder, vasospasm and ventricular arrhythmia.

Digestive: Infrequent were anorexia, constipation, diarrhea, eructation, esophagitis, flatulence, gastritis, gastrointestinal disorder, glossitis, increased salivation and liver function tests abnormal. Rare were gingivitis, hematemesis, increased appetite, rectal disorder, stomatitis, tongue disorder, tongue edema and tooth disorder.

Endocrine: Rare were goiter, thyroid adenoma and thyroiditis.

Hemic and Lymphatic: Rare were anemia, cyanosis, leukopenia, lymphadenopathy, monocytosis and purpura.

Metabolic: Infrequent were creatine phosphokinase increased, edema, peripheral edema and thirst. Rare were alkaline phosphatase increased, bilirubinemia, hyperglycemia, weight gain and weight loss.

Musculoskeletal: Infrequent were arthralgia, arthritis, arthrosis, bone pain, myalgia and myasthenia. Rare were bone neoplasm, joint disorder, myopathy and tenosynovitis.

Neurological: Frequent were hypertonia, hypesthesia and vertigo. Infrequent were abnormal dreams, agitation, anxiety, apathy, ataxia, confusion, depersonalization, depression, emotional lability, euphoria, hyperesthesia, hyperkinesia, incoordination, insomnia, nervousness, speech disorder, stupor, thinking abnormal and tremor. Rare were abnormal gait, amnesia, aphasia, catatonic reaction, dementia, diplopia, dystonia, hallucinations, hemiplegia, hyperalgesia, hypokinesia, hysteria, manic reaction, neuropathy, neurosis, oculogyric crisis, paralysis, psychotic depression, sleep disorder and twitching.

Respiratory: Frequent was pharyngitis. Infrequent were asthma, dyspnea, respiratory disorder, respiratory tract infection, rhinitis, voice alteration and yawn. Rare were bronchitis, choking sensation, cough increased, epistaxis, hiccup, hyperventilation, laryngitis, sinusitis and sputum increased.

Skin and Appendages: Frequent was sweating. Infrequent were pruritus, rash and skin disorder. Rare were alopecia, dry skin, eczema, exfoliative dermatitis, maculopapular rash, psoriasis, skin discoloration, skin hypertrophy and urticaria.

Special Senses: Infrequent was abnormal vision, conjunctivitis, ear pain, eye pain, lacrimation disorder, photophobia, taste perversion and tinnitus. Rare were abnormality of accommodation, dry eyes, ear disorder, eye hemorrhage, otitis media, parosmia and ptosis.

Urogenital: Infrequent were impotence, polyuria, urinary frequency and urinary tract disorder. Rare were breast pain, kidney pain, leukorrhea, menorrhagia, menstrual disorder and vaginitis.

DRUG ABUSE AND DEPENDENCE

Although the abuse potential of RELPAX has not been assessed, no abuse of, tolerance to, withdrawal from, or drug-seeking behavior was observed in patients who received RELPAX in clinical trials or their extensions. The 5-$HT_{1B/1D}$ agonists, as a class, have not been associated with drug abuse.

OVERDOSAGE

No significant overdoses in premarketing clinical trials have been reported. Volunteers (N=21) have received single doses of 120 mg without significant adverse effects. Daily doses of 160 mg were commonly employed in Phase III trials. Based on the pharmacology of the 5-$HT_{1B/1D}$ agonists, hypertension or other more serious cardiovascular symptoms could occur on overdose.

The elimination half-life of eletriptan is about 4 hours (see CLINICAL PHARMACOLOGY) and therefore monitoring of patients after overdose with eletriptan should continue for at least 20 hours, or longer should symptoms or signs persist.

There is no specific antidote to eletriptan. In cases of severe intoxication, intensive care procedures are recommended, including establishing and maintaining a patent airway, ensuring adequate oxygenation and ventilation, and monitoring and support of the cardiovascular system.

It is unknown what effect hemodialysis or peritoneal dialysis has on the serum concentration of eletriptan.

DOSAGE AND ADMINISTRATION

In controlled clinical trials, single doses of 20 mg and 40 mg were effective for the acute treatment of migraine in adults. A greater proportion of patients had a response following a 40 mg dose than following a 20 mg dose (see CLINICAL STUDIES). Individuals may vary in response to doses of RELPAX Tablets. The choice of dose should therefore be made on an individual basis. An 80 mg dose, although also effective, was associated with an increased incidence of adverse events. Therefore, the maximum recommended single dose is 40 mg.

If after the initial dose, headache improves but then returns, a repeat dose may be beneficial. If a second dose is required, it should be taken at least 2 hours after the initial dose. If the initial dose is ineffective, controlled clinical trials have not shown a benefit of a second dose to treat the same attack. The maximum daily dose should not exceed 80 mg.

The safety of treating an average of more than 3 headaches in a 30-day period has not been established.

CYP3A4 Inhibitors: Eletriptan is metabolized by the CYP3A4 enzyme. Eletriptan should not be used within at least 72 hours of treatment with the following potent CYP3A4 inhibitors: ketoconazole, itraconazole, nefazodone, troleandomycin, clarithromycin, ritonavir and nelfinavir. Eletriptan should not be used within 72 hours with drugs that have demonstrated potent CYP3A4 inhibition and have this potent effect described in the CONTRAINDICATIONS, WARNINGS or PRECAUTIONS sections of their labeling (see WARNINGS and CLINICAL PHARMACOLOGY: Drug Interactions).

Hepatic Impairment: The drug should not be given to patients with severe hepatic impairment since the effect of severe hepatic impairment on eletriptan metabolism was not evaluated. No dose adjustment is necessary in mild to moderate impairment (see CLINICAL PHARMACOLOGY, CONTRAINDICATIONS and PRECAUTIONS).

HOW SUPPLIED

RELPAX® Tablets of 20 mg and 40 mg eletriptan (base) as the hydrobromide. RELPAX Tablets are orange, round, convex shaped, film-coated tablets with appropriate debossing.

20 mg Tablets are identified with "REP20" on one side and "Pfizer" on the reverse. They are supplied in displays containing 2 folded blister cards with 6 tablets on each card (NDC 0049-2330-34).

40 mg Tablets are identified with "REP40" on one side and "Pfizer" on the reverse. They are supplied in displays containing 2 folded blister cards with 6 tablets on each card (NDC 0049-2340-34).

Store at 25°C (77°F); excursions permitted to 15-30°C (59-86°F) [see USP Controlled Room Temperature].

PATIENT SUMMARY OF INFORMATION

RELPAX®

(eletriptan hydrobromide)

Please read this information before you start taking RELPAX and each time you renew your prescription. Remember, this summary does not take the place of discussions with your doctor. You and your doctor should discuss RELPAX when you start taking your medication and at regular checkups.

What is RELPAX?

RELPAX is a prescription medicine used to treat migraine headaches in adults. RELPAX is not for other types of headaches.

What is a Migraine Headache?

Migraine is an intense, throbbing headache. You may have pain on one or both sides of your head. You may have nausea and vomiting, and be sensitive to light and noise. The pain and symptoms of a migraine headache can be worse than a common headache. Some women get migraines around the time of their menstrual period. Some people have visual symptoms before the headache, such as flashing lights or wavy lines, called an aura.

How Does RELPAX Work?

Treatment with RELPAX reduces swelling of blood vessels surrounding the brain. This swelling is associated with the headache pain of a migraine attack. RELPAX blocks the release of substances from nerve endings that cause more pain and other symptoms like nausea, and sensitivity to light and sound.

It is thought that these actions contribute to relief of your symptoms by RELPAX.

Who should not take RELPAX?

Do not take RELPAX if you:

- have uncontrolled high blood pressure.
- have heart disease or a history of heart disease.
- have hemiplegic or basilar migraine (if you are not sure about this, ask your doctor).
- have or had a stroke or problems with your blood circulation.
- have serious liver problems.
- have taken any of the following medicines in the last 24 hours: other "triptans" like almotriptan (Axert®), frovatriptan (Frova™), naratriptan (Amerge®), rizatriptan (Maxalt®), sumatriptan (Imitrex®), zolmitriptan (Zomig®); ergotamines like Bellegral-S®, Cafergot®, Ergoma®, Wigraine®; dihydroergotamine like D.H.E. 45® or Migranal®; or methysergide (Sansert®). These medicines have side effects similar to RELPAX.*
- have taken the following medicines within at least 72 hours: ketoconazole (Nizoral®), itraconazole (Sporonox®), nefazodone (Serzone®), troleandomycin (TAO®), clarithromycin (Biaxin®), ritonavir (Norvir®), and nelfinavir (Viracept®). These medicines may cause an increase in the amount of RELPAX in the blood.*
- are allergic to RELPAX or any of its ingredients. The active ingredient is eletriptan. The inactive ingredients are listed at the end of this leaflet.

Tell your doctor about all the medicines you take or plan to take, including prescription and non-prescription medicines, supplements, and herbal remedies. Your doctor will decide if you can take RELPAX with your other medicines.

Tell your doctor if you know that you have any of the following: risk factors for heart disease like high cholesterol, diabetes, smoking, obesity, menopause, or a family history of heart disease or stroke.

How should I take RELPAX?

RELPAX comes in 20 mg and 40 mg tablets. When you have a migraine headache, take your medicine as directed by your doctor.

- Take one RELPAX tablet as soon as you feel a migraine coming on.
- If your headache improves and then comes back after 2 hours, you can take a second tablet.
- If the first tablet did not help your headache at all, do not take a second tablet without talking with your doctor.
- Do not take more than two RELPAX tablets in any 24-hour period.

What are the possible side effects of RELPAX?

RELPAX is generally well tolerated. As with any medicine, people taking RELPAX may have side effects. The side effects are usually mild and do not last long.

The most common side effects of RELPAX are:

- dizziness
- nausea
- weakness
- tiredness
- pain or pressure sensation (e.g., in the chest or throat)

In very rare cases, patients taking triptans may experience serious side effects, including heart attacks. **Call your doctor right away** if you have:

- severe chest pains
- shortness of breath

This is not a complete list of side effects. Talk to your doctor if you develop any symptoms that concern you.

What to do in case of an overdose?

Call your doctor or poison control center or go to the ER.

General advice about RELPAX

Medicines are sometimes prescribed for conditions that are not mentioned in patient information leaflets. Do not use RELPAX for a condition for which it was not prescribed. Do not give RELPAX to other people, even if they have the same symptoms you have.

This leaflet summarizes the most important information about RELPAX. If you would like more information about RELPAX, talk with your doctor. You can ask your doctor or pharmacist for information on RELPAX that is written for health professionals. You can also call 1-866-4RELPAX (1-866-473-5729) or visit our web site at **www.RELPAX.com.**

What are the ingredients in RELPAX?

Active ingredient: eletriptan hydrobromide

Inactive ingredients: microcrystalline cellulose, lactose, croscarmellose sodium, magnesium stearate, titanium oxide, hypromellose, triacetin, and FD&C Yellow No. 6 aluminum lake.

Store RELPAX Tablets at room temperature 15-30°C (59-86°F).

*The brands listed are the trademarks of their respective owners and are not trademarks of Pfizer Inc.

Rx only

Distributed by
Pfizer Roerig
Division of Pfizer Inc, NY, NY 10017
70-5586-00-2 Revised September 2003

Shown in Product Identification Guide, page 329

RESCRIPTOR® ℞
[*rē-skrĭp'tōr*]
brand of delavirdine mesylate tablets

DESCRIPTION

RESCRIPTOR Tablets contain delavirdine mesylate, a synthetic non-nucleoside reverse transcriptase inhibitor of the human immunodeficiency virus type 1 (HIV-1). The chemical name of delavirdine mesylate is piperazine, 1-[3-[(1-methyl-ethyl)amino]-2-pyridinyl]-4-[[5-[(methylsulfonyl)-amino]-1H-indol-2-yl]carbonyl]-, monomethanesulfonate. Its molecular formula is $C_{22}H_{28}N_6O_3S \bullet CH_4O_3S$, and its molecular weight is 552.68. The structural formula is:

Delavirdine mesylate is an odorless white-to-tan crystalline powder. The aqueous solubility of delavirdine free base at 23° C is 2942 µg/mL at pH 1.0, 295 µg/mL at pH 2.0, and 0.81 µg/mL at pH 7.4.

Each RESCRIPTOR Tablet, for oral administration, contains 100 or 200 mg of delavirdine mesylate (henceforth referred to as delavirdine). Inactive ingredients consist of lactose, microcrystalline cellulose, croscarmellose sodium, magnesium stearate, colloidal silicon dioxide, and carnauba wax. In addition, the 100-mg tablet contains Opadry White YS-1-7000-E and the 200-mg tablet contains hypromellose, Opadry White YS-1-18202-A and Pharmaceutical Ink Black.

MICROBIOLOGY

Mechanism of Action: Delavirdine is a non-nucleoside reverse transcriptase inhibitor (NNRTI) of HIV-1. Delavirdine binds directly to reverse transcriptase (RT) and blocks RNA-dependent and DNA-dependent DNA polymerase activities. Delavirdine does not compete with template: primer or deoxynucleoside triphosphates. HIV-2 RT and human cellular DNA polymerases α, γ, or δ are not inhibited by delavirdine. In addition, HIV-1 group O, a group of highly divergent strains that are uncommon in North America, may not be inhibited by delavirdine.

***In Vitro* HIV-1 Susceptibility:** *In vitro* anti–HIV-1 activity of delavirdine was assessed by infecting cell lines of lymphoblastic and monocytic origin and peripheral blood lymphocytes with laboratory and clinical isolates of HIV-1. IC_{50} and IC_{90} values (50% and 90% inhibitory concentrations) for laboratory isolates (N=5) ranged from 0.005 to 0.030 µM and 0.04 to 0.10 µM, respectively. Mean IC_{50} of clinical isolates (N=74) was 0.038 µM (range 0.001 to 0.69 µM); 73 of 74 clinical isolates had an $IC_{50} \leq 0.18$ µM. The IC_{90} of 24 of these clinical isolates ranged from 0.05 to 0.10 µM. In drug combination studies of delavirdine with zidovudine, didanosine, zalcitabine, lamivudine, interferon-α, and protease inhibitors, additive to synergistic anti–HIV-1 activity was observed in cell culture. The relationship between the *in vitro* susceptibility of HIV-1 RT inhibitors and the inhibition of HIV replication in humans has not been established.

Drug Resistance: Phenotypic analyses of isolates from patients treated with RESCRIPTOR as monotherapy showed a 50-fold to 500-fold reduced susceptibility in 14 of 15 patients by week 8 of therapy. Genotypic analysis of HIV-1 isolates from patients receiving RESCRIPTOR plus zidovudine combination therapy (N=79) showed resistance conferring mutations in all isolates by week 24 of therapy. In RESCRIPTOR treated patients the mutations in RT occurred predominantly at amino acid positions 103 and less frequently at positions 181 and 236. In a separate study, an average of 86-fold increase in the zidovudine susceptibility of patient isolates (N=24) was observed after 24-weeks of RESCRIPTOR and zidovudine combination therapy. The clinical relevance of the phenotypic and the genotypic changes associated with RESCRIPTOR therapy has not been established.

Cross-resistance: RESCRIPTOR may confer cross-resistance to other non-nucleoside RT inhibitors when used alone or in combination. Mutations at positions 103 and/or 181 have been found in resistant virus during treatment with RESCRIPTOR and other non-nucleoside RT inhibitors. These mutations have been associated with cross-resistance among non-nucleoside RT inhibitors *in vitro*.

CLINICAL PHARMACOLOGY

Pharmacokinetics

Absorption and Bioavailability: Delavirdine is rapidly absorbed following oral administration, with peak plasma concentrations occurring at approximately one hour. Following administration of delavirdine 400 mg tid (n=67, HIV-1–infected patients), the mean ± SD steady-state peak plasma concentration (C_{max}) was 35 ± 20 µM (range 2 to 100 µM), systemic exposure (AUC) was 180 ± 100 µM • hr (range 5 to 515 µM • hr) and trough concentration (C_{min}) was 15 ± 10 µM (range 0.1 to 45 µM). The single-dose bioavailability of delavirdine tablets relative to an oral solution was 85 ± 25% (n=16, non-HIV–infected subjects). The single-dose bioavailability of delavirdine tablets (100 mg strength) was increased by approximately 20% when a slurry of drug was prepared by allowing delavirdine tablets to disintegrate in water before administration (n=16, non-HIV–infected subjects). The bioavailability of the 200 mg strength delavirdine tablets has not been evaluated when administered as a slurry, because they are not readily dispersed in water (see DOSAGE AND ADMINISTRATION).

Delavirdine may be administered with or without food. In a multiple-dose, crossover study, delavirdine was administered every eight hours with food or every eight hours, one hour before or two hours after a meal (n=13, HIV-1–infected patients). Patients remained on their typical diet throughout the study; meal content was not standardized. When multiple doses of delavirdine were administered with food, geometric mean C_{max} was reduced by approximately 25%, but AUC and C_{min} were not altered.

Distribution: Delavirdine is extensively bound (approximately 98%) to plasma proteins, primarily albumin. The percentage of delavirdine that is protein bound is constant over a delavirdine concentration range of 0.5 to 196 µM. In five HIV-1–infected patients whose total daily dose of delavirdine ranged from 600 to 1200 mg, cerebrospinal fluid concentrations of delavirdine averaged 0.4% ± 0.07% of the corresponding plasma delavirdine concentrations; this represents about 20% of the fraction not bound to plasma proteins. Steady-state delavirdine concentrations in saliva (n=5, HIV-1–infected patients who received delavirdine 400 mg tid) and semen (n=5 healthy volunteers who received delavirdine 300 mg tid) were about 6% and 2%, respectively, of the corresponding plasma delavirdine concentrations collected at the end of a dosing interval.

Metabolism and Elimination: Delavirdine is extensively converted to several inactive metabolites. Delavirdine is primarily metabolized by cytochrome P450 3A (CYP3A), but *in vitro* data suggest that delavirdine may also be metabolized by CYP2D6. The major metabolic pathways for delavirdine are N-desalkylation and pyridine hydroxylation. Delavirdine exhibits nonlinear steady-state elimination pharmacokinetics, with apparent oral clearance decreasing by about 22-fold as the total daily dose of delavirdine increases from 60 to 1200 mg/day. In a study of ^{14}C-delavirdine in six healthy volunteers who received multiple doses of delavirdine tablets 300 mg tid, approximately 44% of the radiolabeled dose was recovered in feces, and approximately 51% of the dose was excreted in urine. Less than 5% of the dose was recovered unchanged in urine. The parent plasma half-life of delavirdine increases with dose; mean half-life following 400 mg tid is 5.8 hours, with a range of 2 to 11 hours.

In vitro and *in vivo* studies have shown that delavirdine reduces CYP3A activity and inhibits its own metabolism. *In vitro* studies have also shown that delavirdine reduces CYP2C9, CYP2D6, and CYP2C19 activity. Inhibition of hepatic CYP3A activity by delavirdine is reversible within 1 week after discontinuation of drug.

Table 1. Pharmacokinetic Parameters for Coadministered Drugs in the Presence of Delavirdine.

Coadministered Drug	Dose of Coadministered Drug	Dose of RESCRIPTOR	n	% Change in Pharmacokinetic Parameters of Coadministered Drug (90% CI)		
				C_{max}	AUC	C_{min}
HIV-Protease Inhibitors						
Indinavir	400 mg tid × 7 days	400 mg tid × 7 days	28	↓36* (↓52- ↓14)	↔*	↑118* (↑16- ↑312)
	600 mg tid × 7 days	400 mg tid × 7 days	28	↔	↑53* (↑7- ↑120)	↑298* (↑104- ↑678)
Nelfinavir[†]	750 mg tid × 14 days	400 mg tid × 7 days	12	↑88 (↑66- ↑113)	↑107 (↑83- ↑135)	↑136 (↑103- ↑175)
Saquinavir	Soft gel capsule 1000 mg tid × 28 days	400 mg tid × 28 days	20	↑98[‡] (↑4- ↑277)	↑121[‡] (↑14- ↑340)	↑199[‡] (↑37- ↑553)
Nucleoside Reverse Transcriptase Inhibitors						
Didanosine (buffered tablets)	125 or 250 mg bid × 28 days	400 mg tid × 28 days	9	↓20[§] (↓44- ↑15)	↓21[§] (↓40- ↑5)	–
Zidovudine	200 mg tid for >38 days	100 mg qid to 400 mg tid for 8-10 days	34	↔	↔	–
Anti-infective Agents						
Clarithromycin	500 mg bid × 15 days	300 mg tid × 30 days	6	–	↑100	–
Rifabutin	300 mg qd for 15-99 days	400-1000 mg tid for 45-129 days	5	↑128 (↑71- ↑203)	↑230 (↑119- ↑396)	↑452 (↑246- ↑781)

↑ Indicates increase
↓ Indicates decrease
↔ Indicates no significant change
* Relative to indinavir 800 mg tid without RESCRIPTOR
† Plasma concentrations of the nelfinavir active metabolite (nelfinavir hydroxy-t-butylamide) were significantly reduced by delavirdine, which is more than compensated for by increased nelfinavir concentration
‡ Saquinavir soft gel capsule 1000 mg tid plus RESCRIPTOR 400 mg tid relative to saquinavir soft gel capsule 1200 mg tid without RESCRIPTOR
§ RESCRIPTOR taken with didanosine (buffered tablets) relative to doses of RESCRIPTOR and didanosine (buffered tablets) separated by at least 1 hr
– Indicates no data available

Special Populations

Hepatic or Renal Impairment: The pharmacokinetics of delavirdine in patients with hepatic or renal impairment have not been investigated (see PRECAUTIONS).

Age: The pharmacokinetics of delavirdine have not been adequately studied in patients <16 years or >65 years of age.

Gender: Data from population pharmacokinetics suggest that the plasma concentrations of delavirdine tend to be higher in females than in males. However, this difference is not considered to be clinically significant.

Race: No significant differences in the mean trough delavirdine concentrations were observed between different racial or ethnic groups.

Drug Interactions (see also PRECAUTIONS: Drug Interactions)

Specific drug interaction studies were performed with delavirdine and a number of drugs. Table 1 summarizes the effects of delavirdine on the geometric mean AUC, C_{max} and C_{min} of coadministered drugs. Table 2 shows the effects of coadministered drugs on the geometric mean AUC, C_{max} and C_{min} of delavirdine.

For information regarding clinical recommendations, see **CONTRAINDICATIONS, WARNINGS,** and **PRECAUTIONS: Drug Interactions.**

[See table 1 above]
[See table 2 at bottom of next page]

INDICATIONS AND USAGE

RESCRIPTOR Tablets are indicated for the treatment of HIV-1 infection in combination with at least 2 other active antiretroviral agents when therapy is warranted.

The following should be considered before initiating therapy with RESCRIPTOR in treatment-naive patients. There are insufficient data directly comparing RESCRIPTOR-containing antiretroviral regimens with currently preferred 3-drug regimens for initial treatment of HIV. In studies comparing regimens consisting of 2 NRTIs (currently considered suboptimal) to RESCRIPTOR plus 2 NRTIs, the proportion of patients receiving the RESCRIPTOR regimen who achieved and sustained an HIV-1 RNA level <400 copies/mL over one year of therapy was relatively low (see DESCRIPTION OF CLINICAL STUDIES).

Resistant virus emerges rapidly when RESCRIPTOR is administered as monotherapy. Therefore, RESCRIPTOR should always be administered in combination with other antiretroviral agents.

DESCRIPTION OF CLINICAL STUDIES

For clinical Studies 21 Part II and 13C described below, efficacy was evaluated by the percentage of patients with a

Continued on next page

Rescriptor—Cont.

plasma HIV RNA level <400 copies/mL through Week 52 as measured by the Roche Amplicor® HIV-1 Monitor (standard assay). An intent-to-treat analysis was performed where only subjects who achieved confirmed suppression and sustained it through Week 52 are regarded as responders. All other subjects (including never suppressed, discontinued, and those who rebounded after initial suppression of <400 copies/mL) are considered failures at Week 52. Results of an interim analysis of efficacy conducted for studies 21 Part II and 13C by independent Data and Safety Monitoring Boards (DSMBs) revealed that the triple therapy arms in both studies produced significantly greater antiviral benefit than the dual therapy arms, and early termination of the studies was recommended.

Study 21 Part II: Study 21 Part II was a double-blind, randomized, placebo-controlled trial comparing treatment with RESCRIPTOR (DLV; 400 mg tid), zidovudine (ZDV; 200 mg tid), and lamivudine (3TC; 150 mg bid) versus RESCRIPTOR (400 mg tid) and zidovudine (200 mg tid) versus zidovudine (200 mg tid) and lamivudine (150 mg bid) in 373 HIV-1–infected patients (mean age 35 years [range 17 to 67], 87% male and 60% Caucasian) who were antiretroviral treatment naive (84%) or had limited nucleoside experience (16%). Mean baseline CD_4 cell count was 359 cells/mm^3 and mean baseline plasma HIV RNA was 4.4 $\log_{10}$ copies/mL.

Results showed that the mean increase from baseline in CD_4 count at 52 weeks was 111 cells/mL for RESCRIPTOR + ZDV + 3TC, 27 cells/mL for RESCRIPTOR + ZDV, and 74 cells/mL for ZDV + 3TC.

The results of the intent-to-treat analysis of the percentage of patients with a plasma HIV RNA level <400 copies/mL are presented in Figure 1. HIV-1 RNA status and reasons for discontinuation of randomized treatment at 52 weeks are summarized in Table 3. Subjects who were never suppressed before discontinuation were placed in the discontinuation category.

Table 2. Pharmacokinetic Parameters for Delavirdine in the Presence of Coadministered Drugs

Coadministered Drug	Dose of Coadministered Drug	Dose of RESCRIPTOR	n	% Change in Delavirdine Pharmacokinetic Parameters (90% CI)		
				C_{max}	AUC	C_{min}
HIV-Protease Inhibitors						
Indinavir	400 or 600 mg tid × 7 days	400 mg tid × 7 days	81	No apparent changes based on a comparison to historical data		
Nelfinavir	750 mg tid × 7 days	400 mg tid × 14 days	7	↓27 (↓49-↑4)	↓31 (↓57-↑10)	↓33 (↓70-↑49)
Saquinavir	Soft gel capsule 1000 mg tid × 28 days	400 mg tid for 7-28 days	23	No apparent changes based on a comparison to historical data		
Nucleoside Reverse Transcriptase Inhibitors						
Didanosine (buffered tablets)	125 or 200 mg bid × 28 days	400 mg tid × 28 days	9	↓32* (↓48-↓11)	↓19* (↓37-↑6)	↔*
Zidovudine	200 mg tid for ≥ 7 days	400 mg tid for 7-14 days	42	No apparent changes based on a comparison to historical data		
Anti-infective Agents						
Clarithromycin	500 mg bid × 15 days	300 mg tid × 30 days	6	↔	↔	↔
Fluconazole	400 mg qd × 15 days	300 mg tid × 30 days	8	↔	↔	↔
Ketoconazole	Various	200-400 mg tid	26	–	–	↑50†
Rifabutin	300 mg qd × 14 days	400 mg tid × 28 days	7	↓72 (↓61-↓80)	↓82 (↓74-↓88)	↓94 (↓90-↓96)
Rifampin	600 mg qd × 15 days	400 mg tid × 30 days	7	↓90 (↓94-↓83)	↓97 (↓98-↓95)	↓100
Sulfamethoxazole or Trimethoprim & Sulfamethoxazole	Various	200-400 mg tid	311	–	–	↔†
Other						
Antacid (Maalox® TC)	20 mL	300 mg single dose	12	↓52 (↓68-↓29)	↓44 (↓58-↓27)	–
Fluoxetine	Various	200-400 mg tid	36	–	–	↑50†
Phenytoin, Phenobarbital, Carbamazepine	Various	300-400 mg tid	8	–	–	↓90†

↑ Indicates increase
↓ Indicates decrease
↔ Indicates no significant change
* RESCRIPTOR taken with didanosine (buffered tablets) relative to doses of RESCRIPTOR and didanosine (buffered tablets) separated by at least 1 hr
† Population pharmacokinetic data from efficacy studies
– Indicates no data available

Table 3: Outcomes of Randomized Treatment Through Week 52 for Protocol 21 Part 2

Outcome	ZDV + 3TC (N = 124) %	DLV + ZDV (N = 125) %	DLV + ZDV + 3TC (N = 124) %
HIV RNA <400 copies/mL*	14	2	45
HIV RNA ≥400 copies/mL†,‡	64	52	31
Discontinued due to adverse events‡	8	13	10
Discontinued due to other reasons‡,§	14	33	14

* Corresponds to rates at Week 52 in proportion curve
† Virologic failures at or before Week 52
‡ Considered to be treatment failure in the analysis
§ Includes discontinuations due to consent withdrawn, loss to follow-up, protocol violations, non-compliance, pregnancy, never treated, and other reasons

Figure 1
Percentage of Patients with HIV RNA Below 400 copies/mL
Standard PCR Assay
Protocol 21 Part 2
Intent-to-Treat Analysis

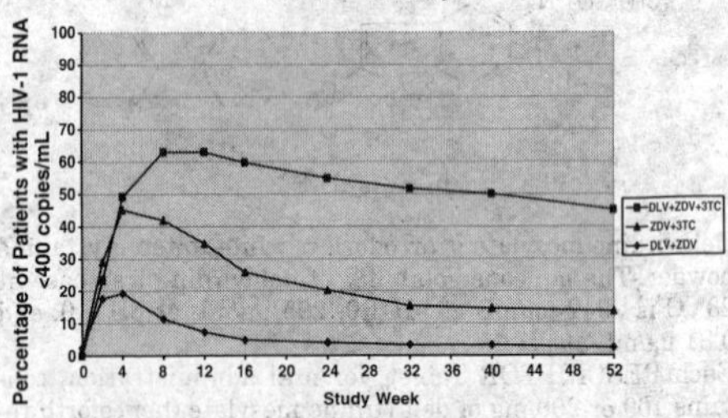

[See table 3 below]

Study 13C: Study 13C was a double-blind, randomized, placebo-controlled trial comparing treatment with RESCRIPTOR (400 mg tid), zidovudine (200 mg tid or 300 bid) and either didanosine (ddI; 200 mg bid), zalcitabine (ddC; 0.75 mg tid) or lamivudine (150 mg bid) versus zidovudine (200 mg tid or 300 mg bid) and either didanosine (200 mg bid), zalcitabine (0.75 mg tid) or lamivudine (150 mg bid) in 345 HIV-1–infected patients (mean age 35.8 years [range 18 to 72], 66% male and 63% Caucasian) who were antiretroviral treatment naive (63%) or had limited antiretroviral experience (37%). Mean baseline CD_4 cell count was 210 cells/mm^3 and mean baseline plasma HIV RNA was 4.9 $\log_{10}$ copies/mL.

Results showed that the mean increase from baseline in CD_4 count at 54 weeks was 102 cells/mL for RESCRIPTOR + ZDV + ddI or ddC or 3TC and 56 cells/mL for ZDV + ddI or ddC or 3TC.

Figure 2
Percentage of Patients with HIV RNA Below 400 copies/mL
Standard PCR Assay
Protocol 13C
Intent-to-Treat Analysis

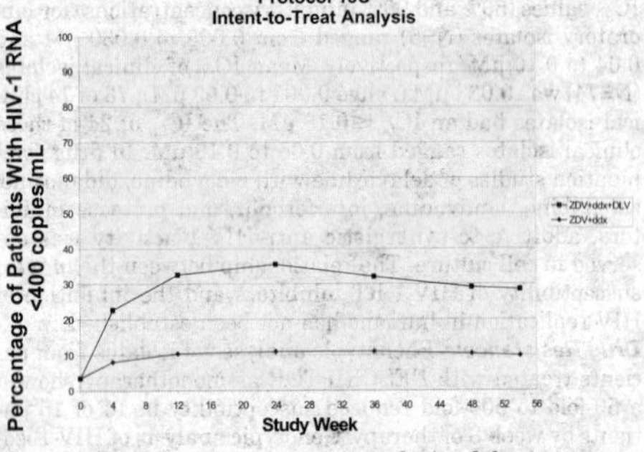

The results of the intent-to-treat analysis of the percentage of patients with a plasma HIV RNA level <400 copies/mL are presented in Figure 2. HIV-1 RNA status and reasons for discontinuation of randomized treatment at 54 weeks are summarized in Table 4. Subjects who were never suppressed before discontinuation were placed in the discontinuation category.

Table 4. Outcomes of Randomized Treatment Through Week 54 for Protocol 13C

Outcome	ZDV + ddx† (N = 173) %	ZDV + ddx + DLV (N = 172) %
HIV RNA <400 copies/mL*	10	29
HIV RNA ≥400 copies/mL§,‡	69	42
Discontinued due to adverse events§	7	12
Discontinued due to other reasons§‖	14	17

* Corresponds to rates at Week 54 in proportion curve
† ddx = ddI or ddC or 3TC
‡ Virologic failures at or before Week 54
§ Considered to be treatment failure in the analysis
‖ Includes discontinuations due to consent withdrawn, loss to follow-up, protocol violations, non-compliance, pregnancy, never treated, and other reasons

Results from several smaller supportive studies evaluating the use of RESCRIPTOR in treatment-naive patients suggest that it may have activity when used in combination with protease inhibitors and NRTIs in 3- or 4-drug combinations.

CONTRAINDICATIONS

RESCRIPTOR Tablets are contraindicated in patients with known hypersensitivity to any of its ingredients. Coadministration of RESCRIPTOR is contraindicated with drugs that are highly dependent on CYP3A for clearance and for which elevated plasma concentrations are associated with serious and/or life-threatening events. These drugs are listed in Table 5. **Also, see PRECAUTIONS, Table 6, Drugs That Should Not Be Coadministered With RESCRIPTOR.**

Table 5. Drugs That Are Contraindicated With RESCRIPTOR

Drug Class	Drugs Within Class That Are Contraindicated With RESCRIPTOR
Antihistamines	Astemizole, terfenadine
Ergot derivatives	Dihydroergotamine, ergonovine, ergotamine, methylergonovine
GI motility agent	Cisapride
Neuroleptic	Pimozide
Sedative/hypnotics	Alprazolam, midazolam, triazolam

WARNINGS

ALERT: Find out about medicines that should NOT be taken with RESCRIPTOR. This statement is included on the product's bottle label.

Drug Interactions

Because delavirdine may inhibit the metabolism of many different drugs (eg, antiarrhythmics, calcium channel blockers, sedative hypnotics, and others), **serious and/or life threatening drug interactions could result from inappropriate coadministration of some drugs with delavirdine.** In addition, some drugs may markedly reduce delavirdine plasma concentrations, resulting in suboptimal antiviral activity and subsequent emergence of drug resistance. All prescribers should become familiar with the following tables in this package insert: **Table 5, Drugs That Are Contraindicated With RESCRIPTOR; Table 6, Drugs That Should Not Be Coadministered With RESCRIPTOR; and Table 7, Established and Other Potentially Significant Drug Interactions: Alteration in Dose or Regimen May Be Recommended Based on Drug Interaction Studies or Predicted Interaction.** Additional details on drug interactions can be found in Tables 1 and 2 under the **CLINICAL PHARMACOLOGY** section.

Concomitant use of lovastatin or simvastatin with RESCRIPTOR is not recommended. Caution should be exercised if RESCRIPTOR is used concurrently with other HMG-CoA reductase inhibitors that are also metabolized by the CYP3A4 pathway (eg, atorvastatin or cerivastatin). The risk of myopathy including rhabdomyolysis may be increased when RESCRIPTOR is used in combination with these drugs.

Particular caution should be used when prescribing sildenafil in patients receiving RESCRIPTOR. Coadministration of sildenafil with RESCRIPTOR is expected to substantially increase sildenafil concentrations and may result in an increase in sildenafil-associated adverse events, including hypotension, visual changes, and priapism (see **PRECAUTIONS, Drug Interactions** and **Information for Patients**, and the complete prescribing information for sildenafil).

Concomitant use of St. John's wort (hypericum perforatum) or St. John's wort containing products and RESCRIPTOR is not recommended. Coadministration of St. John's wort with non-nucleoside reverse transcriptase inhibitors (NNRTIs), including RESCRIPTOR, is expected to substantially decrease NNRTI concentrations and may result in sub-optimal levels of RESCRIPTOR and lead to loss of virologic response and possible resistance to RESCRIPTOR or to the class of NNRTIs.

PRECAUTIONS

General: Delavirdine is metabolized primarily by the liver. Therefore, caution should be exercised when administering RESCRIPTOR Tablets to patients with impaired hepatic function.

Resistance/Cross-Resistance: Non-nucleoside reverse transcriptase inhibitors, when used alone or in combination, may confer cross-resistance to other non-nucleoside reverse transcriptase inhibitors.

Fat Redistribution: Redistribution/accumulation of body fat including central obesity, dorsocervical fat enlargement (buffalo hump), peripheral wasting, facial wasting, breast enlargement, and "cushingoid appearance" have been observed in patients receiving antiretroviral therapy. The mechanism and long-term consequences of these events are currently unknown. A causal relationship has not been established.

Skin Rash: Severe rash, including rare cases of erythema multiforme and Stevens-Johnson syndrome, has been reported in patients receiving RESCRIPTOR. Erythema multiforme and Stevens-Johnson syndrome were rarely seen in clinical trials and resolved after withdrawal of RESCRIPTOR. Any patient experiencing severe rash or rash accompanied by symptoms such as fever, blistering, oral lesions, conjunctivitis, swelling, and muscle or joint aches should discontinue RESCRIPTOR and consult a physician. Two cases of Stevens-Johnson syndrome have been reported through postmarketing surveillance out of a total of 339 surveillance reports.

In Studies 21 Part II and 13C (see **DESCRIPTION OF CLINICAL STUDIES**), rash (including maculopapular rash) was reported in more patients who were treated with RESCRIPTOR 400 mg tid (35% and 32%, respectively) than in those who were not treated with RESCRIPTOR (21% and 16%, respectively). The highest intensity of rash reported in these studies was severe (grade 3), which was observed in approximately 4% of patients treated with RESCRIPTOR in each study and in none of the patients who were not treated with RESCRIPTOR. Also in Studies 21 Part II and 13C, discontinuations due to rash were reported in more patients who received RESCRIPTOR 400 mg tid (3% and 4%, respectively) than in those who did not receive RESCRIPTOR (0% and 1%, respectively).

In most cases, the duration of the rash was less than two weeks and did not require dose reduction or discontinuation of RESCRIPTOR. Most patients were able to resume therapy after rechallenge with RESCRIPTOR following a treatment interruption due to rash. The distribution of the rash was mainly on the upper body and proximal arms, with decreasing intensity of the lesions on the neck and face, and progressively less on the rest of the trunk and limbs. Occurrence of a delavirdine-associated rash after one month is uncommon. Symptomatic relief has been obtained using diphenhydramine hydrochloride, hydroxyzine hydrochloride, and/or topical corticosteroids.

Information for Patients: A statement to patients and healthcare providers is included on the product's bottle label: **ALERT: Find out about medicines that should NOT be taken with RESCRIPTOR.** A patient package insert (PPI) for RESCRIPTOR is available for patient information.

Patients should be informed that RESCRIPTOR is not a cure for HIV-1 infection and that they may continue to acquire illnesses associated with HIV-1 infection, including opportunistic infections. Treatment with RESCRIPTOR has not been shown to reduce the incidence or frequency of such illnesses, and patients should be advised to remain under the care of a physician when using RESCRIPTOR.

Continued on next page

Table 6. Drugs That Should Not Be Coadministered With RESCRIPTOR

Drug Class: Drug Name	Clinical Comment
Anticonvulsant agents: phenytoin, phenobarbital, carbamazepine	May lead to loss of virologic response and possible resistance to RESCRIPTOR or to the class of non-nucleoside reverse transcriptase inhibitors.
Antihistamines: astemizole, terfenadine	CONTRAINDICATED due to potential for serious and/or life-threatening reactions such as cardiac arrhythmias.
Antimycobacterials: rifabutin,* rifampin*	May lead to loss of virologic response and possible resistance to RESCRIPTOR or to the class of non-nucleoside reverse transcriptase inhibitors or other coadministered antiviral agents.
Ergot Derivatives: dihydroergotamine, ergonovine, ergotamine, methylergonovine	CONTRAINDICATED due to potential for serious and/or life-threatening reactions such as acute ergot toxicity characterized by peripheral vasospasm and ischemia of the extremities and other tissues.
GI motility agent: cisapride	CONTRAINDICATED due to potential for serious and/or life-threatening reactions such as cardiac arrhythmias.
Herbal Products: St. John's wort (hypericum perforatum)	May lead to loss of virologic response and possible resistance to RESCRIPTOR or to the class of non-nucleoside reverse transcriptase inhibitors.
HMG-CoA reductase inhibitors: lovastatin, simvastatin	Potential for serious reactions such as risk of myopathy including rhabdomyolysis.
Neuroleptic: pimozide	CONTRAINDICATED due to potential for serious and/or life-threatening reactions such as cardiac arrhythmias.
Sedative/hypnotics: alprazolam, midazolam, triazolam	CONTRAINDICATED due to potential for serious and/or life-threatening reactions such as prolonged or increased sedation or respiratory depression.

*See **CLINICAL PHARMACOLOGY** for magnitude of interaction, Tables 1 and 2.

Table 7. Established and Other Potentially Significant Drug Interactions: Alteration in Dose or Regimen May Be Recommended Based on Drug Interaction Studies or Predicted Interaction

Concomitant Drug Class: Drug Name	Effect on Concentration of Delavirdine or Concomitant Drug	Clinical Comment
HIV-Antiviral Agents		
Amprenavir	↑ Amprenavir	Appropriate doses of this combination, with respect to safety, efficacy and pharmacokinetics, have not been established.
Didanosine*	↓ Delavirdine ↓ Didanosine	Administration of didanosine (buffered tablets) and RESCRIPTOR should be separated by at least one hour.
Indinavir*	↑ Indinavir	A dose reduction of indinavir to 600 mg tid should be considered when RESCRIPTOR and indinavir are coadministered.
Lopinavir/Ritonavir	↑ Lopinavir ↑ Ritonavir	Appropriate doses of this combination, with respect to safety, efficacy and pharmacokinetics, have not been established.
Nelfinavir*	↑ Nelfinavir ↓ Delavirdine	Appropriate doses of this combination, with respect to safety, efficacy and pharmacokinetics, have not been established. (See **CLINICAL PHARMACOLOGY:** Tables 1 and 2.)
Ritonavir	↑ Ritonavir	Appropriate doses of this combination, with respect to safety, efficacy and pharmacokinetics, have not been established.
Saquinavir*	↑ Saquinavir	A dose reduction of saquinavir (soft gelatin capsules) may be considered when RESCRIPTOR and saquinavir are coadministered. (See **CLINICAL PHARMACOLOGY:** Table 1.) Appropriate doses with respect to safety, efficacy and pharmacokinetics, have not been established.

(Table continued on next page)

Rescriptor—Cont.

Patients should be advised that the use of RESCRIPTOR has not been shown to reduce the risk of transmission of HIV-1.
Patients should be instructed that the major toxicity of RESCRIPTOR is rash and should be advised to promptly notify their physician should rash occur. The majority of rashes associated with RESCRIPTOR occur within 1 to 3 weeks after initiating treatment with RESCRIPTOR. The rash normally resolves in 3 to 14 days and may be treated symptomatically while therapy with RESCRIPTOR is continued. Any patient experiencing severe rash or rash accompanied by symptoms such as fever, blistering, oral lesions, conjunctivitis, swelling, and muscle or joint aches should discontinue medication and consult a physician.
Patients should be informed that redistribution or accumulation of body fat may occur in patients receiving antiretroviral therapy and that the cause and long-term health effects of these conditions are not known at this time.
Patients should be informed to take RESCRIPTOR every day as prescribed. Patients should not alter the dose of RESCRIPTOR without consulting their doctor. If a dose is missed, patients should take the next dose as soon as possible. However, if a dose is skipped, the patient should not double the next dose.
Patients with achlorhydria should take RESCRIPTOR with an acidic beverage (e.g., orange or cranberry juice). However, the effect of an acidic beverage on the absorption of delavirdine in patients with achlorhydria has not been investigated.
Patients taking both RESCRIPTOR and antacids should be advised to take them at least 1 hour apart.
Because RESCRIPTOR may interact with certain drugs, patients should be advised to report to their doctor the use of any prescription, nonprescription medication or herbal products, particularly St. John's wort.
Patients receiving sildenafil and RESCRIPTOR should be advised that they may be at an increased risk of sildenafil-associated adverse events, including hypotension, visual changes, and prolonged penile erection, and should promptly report any symptoms to their doctor.

Drug Interactions (see also CONTRAINDICATIONS, WARNINGS, and CLINICAL PHARMACOLOGY: Drug Interactions)
Delavirdine is an inhibitor of CYP3A isoform and other CYP isoforms to a lesser extent including CYP2C9, CYP2D6, and CYP2C19. Coadministration of RESCRIPTOR and drugs primarily metabolized by CYP3A (e.g., HMG-CoA reductase inhibitors, and sildenafil) may result in increased plasma concentrations of the coadministered drug that could increase or prolong both its therapeutic or adverse effects.
Delavirdine is metabolized primarily by CYP3A, but *in vitro* data suggest that delavirdine may also be metabolized by CYP2D6. Coadministration of RESCRIPTOR and drugs that induce CYP3A, such as rifampin, may decrease delavirdine plasma concentrations and reduce its therapeutic effect. Coadministration of RESCRIPTOR and drugs that inhibit CYP3A may increase delavirdine plasma concentrations. **(See Table 6, Drugs That Should Not Be Coadministered With RESCRIPTOR, and Table 7, Established and Other Potentially Significant Drug Interactions: Alteration in Dose or Regimen May Be Recommended Based on Drug Interaction Studies or Predicted Interaction.)**
[See table 6 at top of previous page]
[See table 7 on previous page and at left]

Table 7 *(cont.)*. Established and Other Potentially Significant Drug Interactions: Alteration in Dose or Regimen May Be Recommended Based on Drug Interaction Studies or Predicted Interaction

Concomitant Drug Class: Drug Name	Effect on Concentration of Delavirdine or Concomitant Drug	Clinical Comment
Other Agents		
Acid blockers: antacids*	↓ Delavirdine	Doses of an antacid and RESCRIPTOR should be separated by at least one hour, because the absorption of delavirdine is reduced when coadministered with antacids.
H_2Receptor antagonists: cimetidine, famotidine, nizatidine, ranitidine Proton pump inhibitors: omeprazole, lansoprazole		These agents increase gastric pH and may reduce the absorption of delavirdine. Although the effect of these drugs on delavirdine absorption has not been evaluated, chronic use of these drugs with RESCRIPTOR is not recommended.
Amphetamines	↑ Amphetamines	Use with caution.
Antiarrhythmics: bepridil	↑ Antiarrhythmics	Use with caution. Increased bepridil exposure may be associated with life-threatening reactions such as cardiac arrythmias.
Amiodarone, lidocaine (systemic), quinidine, flecainide, propafenone		Caution is warranted and therapeutic concentration monitoring is recommended, if available, for antiarrhythmics when coadministered with RESCRIPTOR.
Anticoagulant: warfarin	↑ Warfarin	It is recommended that INR (international normalized ratio) be monitored.
Anti-infective: clarithromycin*	↑ Clarithromycin	When coadministered with RESCRIPTOR, clarithromycin should be adjusted in patients with impaired renal function: • For patients with CL_{CR} 30 to 60 mL/min the dose of clarithromycin should be reduced by 50%. • For patients with CL_{CR} <30 mL/min the dose of clarithromycin should be reduced by 75%.
Dihydropyridine calcium channel blockers: amlodipine, diltiazem, felodipine, isradipine, nifedipine, nicardipine, nimodipine, nisoldipine, verapamil	↑ Dihydropyridine calcium channel blockers	Caution is warranted and clinical monitoring of patients is recommended.
Corticosteroid: dexamethasone	↓ Delavirdine	Use with caution. RESCRIPTOR may be less effective due to decreased delavirdine plasma concentrations in patients taking these agents concomitantly.
Erectile dysfunction agents: sildenafil	↑ Sildenafil	Sildenafil should not exceed a maximum single dose of 25 mg in a 48 hour period.
HMG-CoA reductase inhibitors: atorvastatin, cerivastatin, fluvastatin	↑ Atorvastatin ↑ Cerivastatin ↑ Fluvastatin	Use lowest possible dose of atorvastatin or cerivastatin, or fluvastatin with careful monitoring, or consider other HMG-CoA reductase inhibitors such as pravastatin in combination with RESCRIPTOR.
Immunosuppressants: cyclosporine, tacrolimus, rapamycin	↑ Immunosuppressants	Therapeutic concentration monitoring is recommended for immunosuppressant agents when coadministered with RESCRIPTOR.
Narcotic analgesic: methadone	↑ Methadone	Dosage of methadone may need to be decreased when coadministered with RESCRIPTOR.
Oral contraceptives: ethinyl estradiol	↑ Ethinyl estradiol	Concentrations of ethinyl estradiol may increase. However, the clinical significance is unknown.

↑ Indicates increase
↓ Indicates decrease
*See **CLINICAL PHARMACOLOGY** for magnitude of interaction, Tables 1 and 2.

Carcinogenesis, Mutagenesis and Impairment of Fertility: Delavirdine was negative in a battery of genetic toxicology tests which included an Ames assay, an *in vitro* rat hepatocyte unscheduled DNA synthesis assay, an *in vitro* chromosome aberration assay in human peripheral lymphocytes, an *in vitro* mutation assay in Chinese hamster ovary cells, and an *in vivo* micronucleus test in mice.
Lifetime carcinogenicity studies were conducted in rats at doses of 10, 32 and 100 mg/kg/day and in mice at doses of 62.5, 250 and 500 mg/kg/day for males and 62.5, 125 and 250 mg/kg/day for females. In rats, delavirdine was noncarcinogenic at maximally tolerated doses that produced exposures (AUC) up to 12 (male rats) and 9 (female rats) times human exposure at the recommended clinical dose. In mice, delavirdine produced significant increases in the incidence of hepatocellular adenoma/adenocarcinoma in both males and females, hepatocellular adenoma in females, and mesenchymal urinary bladder tumors in males. The systemic drug exposures (AUC) in female mice were 0.5- to 3-fold and in male mice 0.2- to 4-fold of those in humans at the recommended clinical dose. Given the lack of genotoxic activity of delavirdine, the relevance of urinary bladder and hepatocellular neoplasm in delavirdine-treated mice to humans is not known.
Delavirdine at doses of 20, 100, and 200 mg/kg/day did not cause impairment of fertility in rats when males were treated for 70 days and females were treated for 14 days prior to mating.

Pregnancy: Pregnancy Category C: Delavirdine has been shown to be teratogenic in rats. Delavirdine caused ventricular septal defects in rats at doses of 50, 100, and 200 mg/kg/day when administered during the period of organogenesis. The lowest dose of delavirdine that caused malformations produced systemic exposures in pregnant rats equal to or lower than the expected human exposure to RESCRIPTOR (C_{min} 15 µM) at the recommended dose. Exposure in rats approximately 5-fold higher than the expected human exposure resulted in marked maternal toxicity, embryotoxicity, fetal developmental delay, and reduced pup survival. Additionally, reduced pup survival on postpartum day 0 occurred at an exposure (mean C_{min}) approximately equal to the expected human exposure. Delavirdine was excreted in the milk of lactating rats at a concentration three to five times that of rat plasma.
Delavirdine at doses of 200 and 400 mg/kg/day administered during the period of organogenesis caused maternal toxicity, embryotoxicity and abortions in rabbits. The lowest dose of delavirdine that resulted in these toxic effects produced systemic exposures in pregnant rabbits approximately 6-fold higher than the expected human exposure to RESCRIPTOR (C_{min} 15 µM) at the recommended dose. The no-observed-adverse-effect dose in the pregnant rabbit was 100 mg/kg/day. Various malformations were observed at this dose, but the incidence of such malformations was not statistically significantly different from those observed in the control group. Systemic exposures in pregnant rabbits at a dose of 100 mg/kg/day were lower than those expected in humans at the recommended clinical dose. Malformations were not apparent at 200 and 400 mg/kg/day; however, only a limited number of fetuses were available for examination as a result of maternal and embryo death.
No adequate and well-controlled studies in pregnant women have been conducted. RESCRIPTOR should be used during pregnancy only if the potential benefit justifies the potential risk to the fetus. Of 9 pregnancies reported in premarketing clinical studies and postmarketing experience, a total of 10 infants were born (including 1 set of twins). Eight of the infants were born healthy. One infant was born HIV-positive but was otherwise healthy and with no congenital abnormalities detected, and 1 infant was born prematurely (34 to 35 weeks) with a small muscular ventricular septal defect that spontaneously resolved. The patient received approximately six weeks of treatment with delavirdine and zidovudine early in the course of the pregnancy.

Antiretroviral Pregnancy Registry: To monitor maternal-fetal outcomes of pregnant women exposed to RESCRIPTOR and other antiretroviral agents, an Antiretroviral Pregnancy Registry has been established. Physicians are encouraged to register patients by calling (800) 258-4263.

Nursing Mothers: The Centers for Disease Control and Prevention recommend that HIV-infected mothers not breast-feed their infants to avoid risking postnatal transmission of HIV. Because of both the potential for HIV transmission and any possible adverse reactions in nursing infants, **mothers should be instructed not to breast-feed if they are receiving RESCRIPTOR.**

Pediatric Use: Safety and effectiveness of delavirdine in combination with other antiretroviral agents have not been established in HIV-1–infected individuals younger than 16 years of age.

Geriatric Use: Clinical studies of RESCRIPTOR did not include sufficient numbers of subjects aged 65 and over to determine whether they respond differently from younger subjects. In general, caution should be taken when dosing RESCRIPTOR in elderly patients due to the greater frequency of decreased hepatic, renal or cardiac function and of concomitant disease or other drug therapy.

ADVERSE REACTIONS

The safety of RESCRIPTOR Tablets alone and in combination with other therapies has been studied in approximately 6,000 patients receiving RESCRIPTOR. The majority of adverse events were of mild or moderate (ie, ACTG grade 1 or 2) intensity. The most frequently reported drug-related adverse event (ie, events considered by the investigator to be related to the blinded study medication, or events with an unknown or missing causal relationship to the blinded medication) among patients receiving RESCRIPTOR was skin rash (see **Table 8** and **PRECAUTIONS: Skin Rash**).

[See table 8 at right]

Table 8. Percent of Patients With Treatment-Emergent Rash in Pivotal Trials (Studies 21 Part II and 13C)*

Percent of Patients with:	Description of Rash Grade†	RESCRIPTOR 400 mg TID (N = 412)	Control Group Patients (N = 295)
Grade 1 Rash	Erythema, pruritus	69 (16.7%)	35 (11.9%)
Grade 2 Rash	Diffuse maculopapular rash, dry desquamation	59 (14.3%)	17 (5.8%)
Grade 3 Rash	Vesiculation, moist desquamation, ulceration	18 (4.4%)	0 (0.0%)
Grade 4 Rash	Erythema multiforme, Stevens-Johnson syndrome, toxic epideral necrolysis, necrosis requiring surgery, exfoliative dermatitis	0 (0.0%)	0 (0.0%)
Rash of any Grade		146 (35.4%)	52 (17.6%)
Treatment discontinuation as a result of rash		13 (3.2%)	1 (0.3%)

*Includes events reported regardless of causality
† ACTG Toxicity Grading System; includes events reported as "rash", "maculopapular rash", and "urticaria".

Adverse events of moderate to severe intensity reported by at least 5% of evaluable patients in any treatment group in the pivotal trials, which includes patients receiving RESCRIPTOR in combination with zidovudine and/or lamivudine in Study 21 Part II for up to 98 weeks and in combination with zidovudine and either lamivudine, didanosine, or zalcitabine in Study 13C for up to 72 weeks are summarized in Table 9.

[See table 9 at right]

Table 9. Treatment-Emergent Events, Regardless of Causality, of Moderate-to-Severe or Life-Threatening Intensity Reported by at Least 5% of Evaluable* Patients in any Treatment Group

	Study 21 Part II			Study 13C	
Adverse Events	**ZDV + 3TC (N = 123)**	**400 mg tid RESCRIPTOR + ZDV (N = 123)**	**400 mg tid RESCRIPTOR + ZDV + 3TC (N = 119)**	**ZDV + ddI, ddC, or 3TC (N = 172)**	**400 mg tid RESCRIPTOR + ZDV + ddI, ddC, or 3TC (N = 170)**
	% of pts. (N)	% of pts. (N)	% of pts. (N)	% of pts. (N)	% of pts. (N)
Body as a Whole					
Abdominal pain, generalized	2.4 (3)	3.3 (4)	5.0 (6)	1.7 (3)	2.4 (4)
Asthenia/fatigue	16.3 (20)	15.4 (19)	16.0 (19)	8.1 (14)	5.3 (9)
Fever	2.4 (3)	1.6 (2)	3.4 (4)	6.4 (11)	7.1 (12)
Flu syndrome	4.9 (6)	7.3 (9)	5.0 (6)	5.2 (9)	2.4 (4)
Headache	14.6 (18)	12.2 (15)	16.8 (20)	12.8 (22)	11.2 (19)
Localized pain	4.9 (6)	5.7 (7)	5.0 (6)	2.9 (5)	1.8 (3)
Digestive					
Diarrhea	8.1 (10)	2.4 (3)	4.2 (5)	8.1 (14)	5.9 (10)
Nausea	17.1 (21)	20.3 (25)	16.8 (20)	9.3 (16)	14.7 (25)
Vomiting	8.9 (11)	4.9 (6)	2.5 (3)	4.1 (7)	6.5 (11)
Nervous					
Anxiety	1.6 (2)	2.4 (3)	6.7 (8)	4.1 (7)	3.5 (6)
Depressive symptoms	6.5 (8)	4.9 (6)	12.6 (15)	3.5 (6)	5.9 (10)
Insomnia	4.9 (6)	4.9 (6)	5.0 (6)	2.9 (5)	1.2 (2)
Respiratory					
Bronchitis	4.1 (5)	6.5 (8)	6.7 (8)	3.5 (6)	3.5 (6)
Cough	9.8 (12)	4.1 (5)	5.0 (6)	5.2 (9)	3.5 (6)
Pharyngitis	6.5 (8)	1.6 (2)	5.0 (6)	4.1 (7)	3.5 (6)
Sinusitis	8.9 (11)	7.3 (9)	5.0 (6)	2.3 (4)	1.2 (2)
Upper respiratory infection	11.4 (14)	6.5 (8)	7.6 (9)	8.7 (15)	4.7 (8)
Skin					
Rashes	3.3 (4)	19.5 (24)	13.4 (16)	7.6 (13)	18.8 (32)

*Evaluable patients in Study 21 Part II were those who received at least 1 dose of study medication and returned for at least 1 clinic study visit. Evaluable patients in Study 13C were those who received at least 1 dose of study medication.

Other adverse events that occurred in patients receiving RESCRIPTOR (in combination treatment) in all phase II and III studies, and considered possibly related to treatment, and of at least ACTG grade 2 in intensity are listed below by body system.

Body as a Whole: Abdominal cramps, abdominal distention, abdominal pain (localized), abscess, allergic reaction, chills, edema (generalized or localized), epidermal cyst, fever, infection, infection viral, lip edema, malaise, Mycobacterium tuberculosis infection, neck rigidity, sebaceous cyst, and redistribution/accumulation of body fat (see **PRECAUTIONS, Fat Redistribution**).

Cardiovascular System: Abnormal cardiac rate and rhythm, cardiac insufficiency, cardiomyopathy, hypertension, migraine, pallor, peripheral vascular disorder, and postural hypotension.

Digestive System: Anorexia, bloody stool, colitis, constipation, decreased appetite, diarrhea *(Clostridium difficile)*, diverticulitis, dry mouth, dyspepsia, dysphagia, enteritis at all levels, eructation, fecal incontinence, flatulence, gagging, gastroenteritis, gastroesophageal reflux, gastrointestinal bleeding, gastrointestinal disorder, gingivitis, gum hemorrhage, hepatomegaly, increased appetite, increased saliva, increased thirst, jaundice, mouth or tongue inflammation or ulcers, nonspecific hepatitis, oral/enteric moniliasis, pancreatitis, rectal disorder, sialadenitis, tooth abscess, and toothache.

Hemic and Lymphatic System: Adenopathy, bruising, eosinophilia, granulocytosis, leukopenia, pancytopenia, purpura, spleen disorder, thrombocytopenia, and prolonged prothrombin time.

Metabolic and Nutritional Disorders: Alcohol intolerance, amylase increased, bilirubinemia, hyperglycemia, hyperkalemia, hypertriglyceridemia, hyperuricemia, hypocalcemia, hyponatremia, hypophosphatemia, increased AST (SGOT), increased gamma glutamyl transpeptidase, increased lipase, increased serum alkaline phosphatase, increased serum creatinine, and weight increase or decrease.

Musculoskeletal System: Arthralgia or arthritis of single and multiple joints, bone disorder, bone pain, myalgia, tendon disorder, tenosynovitis, tetany, and vertigo.

Nervous System: Abnormal coordination, agitation, amnesia, change in dreams, cognitive impairment, confusion, decreased libido, disorientation, dizziness, emotional lability, euphoria, hallucination, hyperesthesia, hyperreflexia, hypertonia, hypesthesia, impaired concentration, manic symptoms, muscle cramp, nervousness, neuropathy, nystagmus, paralysis, paranoid symptoms, restlessness, sleep cycle disorder, somnolence, tingling, tremor, vertigo, and weakness.

Respiratory System: Chest congestion, dyspnea, epistaxis, hiccups, laryngismus, pneumonia, and rhinitis.

Skin and Appendages: Angioedema, dermal leukocytoclastic vasculitis, dermatitis, desquamation, diaphoresis, discolored skin, dry skin, erythema, erythema multiforme, folliculitis, fungal dermatitis, hair loss, herpes zoster or simplex, nail disorder, petechiae, non-application site pruritus, seborrhea, skin hypertrophy, skin disorder, skin nodule, Stevens-Johnson syndrome, urticaria, vesiculobullous rash, and wart.

Special Senses: Blepharitis, blurred vision, conjunctivitis, diplopia, dry eyes, ear pain, parosmia, otitis media, photophobia, taste perversion, and tinnitus.

Urogenital System: Amenorrhea, breast enlargement, calculi of the kidney, chromaturia, epididymitis, hematuria, hemospermia, impaired urination, impotence, kidney pain, metrorrhagia, nocturia, polyuria, proteinuria, testicular pain, urinary tract infection, and vaginal moniliasis.

Postmarketing Experience: Adverse event terms reported from postmarketing surveillance that were not reported in the phase II and III trials are presented below.

Digestive System: Hepatic failure.

Hemic and Lymphatic System: Hemolytic anemia.

Musculoskeletal System: Rhabdomyolysis.

Urogenital System: Acute kidney failure.

Laboratory Abnormalities: Marked laboratory abnormalities observed in at least 2% of patients during Studies 21 Part II and 13C are summarized in Table 10. Marked laboratory abnormalities are defined as any Grade 3 or 4 abnormality found in patients at any time during study.

[See table 10 at top of next page]

OVERDOSAGE

Human experience of acute overdose with RESCRIPTOR is limited.

Management of Overdosage: Treatment of overdosage with RESCRIPTOR should consist of general supportive measures, including monitoring of vital signs and observation of the patient's clinical status. There is no specific antidote for overdosage with RESCRIPTOR. If indicated, elimination of unabsorbed drug should be achieved by emesis or gastric lavage. Since delavirdine is extensively metabolized by the liver and is highly protein bound, dialysis is unlikely to result in significant removal of the drug.

DOSAGE AND ADMINISTRATION

The recommended dosage for RESCRIPTOR Tablets is 400 mg (four 100-mg or two 200-mg tablets) three times daily. RESCRIPTOR should be used in combination with

Continued on next page

Table 10. Marked Laboratory Abnormalities Reported by ≥2% of Patients

Adverse Events	Toxicity Limit	Study 21 Part II			Study 13C	
		ZDV + 3TC N = 123	400 mg tid RESCRIPTOR + ZDV N = 123	400 mg tid RESCRIPTOR + ZDV + 3TC N = 119	ZDV + ddI, ddC, or 3TC N = 172	400 mg tid RESCRIPTOR + ZDV + ddI, ddC, or 3TC N = 170
		% pts.	% pts.	% pts.	% pts.	% pts.
Hematology						
Hemoglobin	<7 mg/dL	4.1	2.5	0.9	1.7	2.9
Neutrophils	<750/mm^3	5.7	4.9	3.4	10.4	7.6
Prothrombin time (PT)	>1.5 × ULN	0	0	1.7	2.9	2.4
Activated partial thromboplastin (APTT)	>2.33 × ULN	0	0.8	0	5.8	2.4
Chemistry						
Alanine aminotransferase (ALT/SGPT)	>5 × ULN	2.5	4.1	5.1	3.5	4.1
Amylase	>2 × ULN	0.8	2.5	2.6	3.5	2.9
Aspartate aminotransferase (AST/SGOT)	>5 × ULN	1.6	2.5	3.4	3.5	2.3
Bilirubin	>2.5 × ULN	0.8	2.5	1.7	1.2	0
Gamma glutamyl transferase (GGT)	>5 × ULN	N/A	N/A	N/A	4.1	1.8
Glucose (hypo-/hyperglycemia)	<40 mg/dL >250 mg/dL	4.1	0.8	1.7	1.2	0.0

N/A = not applicable because no predose values were obtained for patients

Rescriptor—Cont.

other antiretroviral therapy. The complete prescribing information for other antiretroviral agents should be consulted for information on dosage and administration.
The 100-mg RESCRIPTOR Tablets may be dispersed in water prior to consumption. To prepare a dispersion, add four 100-mg RESCRIPTOR Tablets to at least 3 ounces of water, allow to stand for a few minutes, and then stir until a uniform dispersion occurs (see **CLINICAL PHARMACOLOGY: Pharmacokinetics: Absorption and Bioavailability**). The dispersion should be consumed promptly. The glass should be rinsed with water and the rinse swallowed to insure the entire dose is consumed. **The 200-mg tablets should be taken as intact tablets, because they are not readily dispersed in water.** Note: The 200-mg tablets are approximately one third smaller in size than the 100-mg tablets.
RESCRIPTOR Tablets may be administered with or without food (see **CLINICAL PHARMACOLOGY: Pharmacokinetics-Absorption and Bioavailability**). Patients with achlorhydria should take RESCRIPTOR with an acidic beverage (e.g., orange or cranberry juice). However, the effect of an acidic beverage on the absorption of delavirdine in patients with achlorhydria has not been investigated.
Patients taking both RESCRIPTOR and antacids should be advised to take them at least one hour apart.

HOW SUPPLIED

RESCRIPTOR Tablets are available as follows:
100 mg: white, capsule-shaped tablets marked with "U 3761".
Bottles of 360 tablets NDC 63010-020-36
200 mg: white, capsule-shaped tablets marked with "RESCRIPTOR 200 mg".
Bottles of 180 tablets NDC 63010-021-18
Store at controlled room temperature 20° to 25°C (68° to 77°F) [see USP]. Keep container tightly closed. Protect from high humidity.
Rx only

ANIMAL TOXICOLOGY

Toxicities among various organs and organ systems in rats, mice, rabbits, dogs, and monkeys were observed following the administration of delavirdine. Necrotizing vasculitis was the most significant toxicity that occurred in dogs when mean nadir serum concentrations of delavirdine were at least 7-fold higher than the expected human exposure to RESCRIPTOR (C_{min} 15 μM) at the recommended dose. Vasculitis in dogs was not reversible during a 2.5-month recovery period; however, partial resolution of the vascular lesion characterized by reduced inflammation, diminished necrosis, and intimal thickening occurred during this period. Other major target organs included the gastrointestinal tract, endocrine organs, liver, kidneys, bone marrow, lymphoid tissue, lung, and reproductive organs.
Agouron Pharmaceuticals, Inc.
La Jolla, CA 92037, USA

RESCRIPTOR is a registered trademark of Pharmacia & Upjohn Company.
L416-0001 Rev. 08/11/03
Shown in Product Identification Guide, page 329

SPIRIVA® HANDIHALER® ℞

[spĭ-rī-vă]
(tiotropium bromide inhalation powder)
FOR ORAL INHALATION ONLY

PRESCRIBING INFORMATION

DESCRIPTION

SPIRIVA® HandiHaler® (tiotropium bromide inhalation powder) consists of a capsule dosage form containing a dry powder formulation of SPIRIVA (tiotropium bromide) intended for oral inhalation only with the HandiHaler inhalation device.
Each light green, hard gelatin capsule contains 18 mcg tiotropium (equivalent to 22.5 mcg tiotropium bromide monohydrate) blended with lactose monohydrate as the carrier.
The dry powder formulation within the capsule is intended for oral inhalation only.
The active component of SPIRIVA is tiotropium. The drug substance, tiotropium bromide monohydrate, is an anticholinergic with specificity for muscarinic receptors. It is chemically described as (1α, 2β, 4β, 5α, 7β)-7-[(Hydroxydi-2-thienylacetyl)oxy]-9,9-dimethyl-3-oxa-9-azoniatricyclo [3.3.1.0^{2,4}]nonane bromide monohydrate. It is a synthetic, non-chiral, quaternary ammonium compound. Tiotropium bromide is a white or yellowish white powder. It is sparingly soluble in water and soluble in methanol.
The structural formula is:

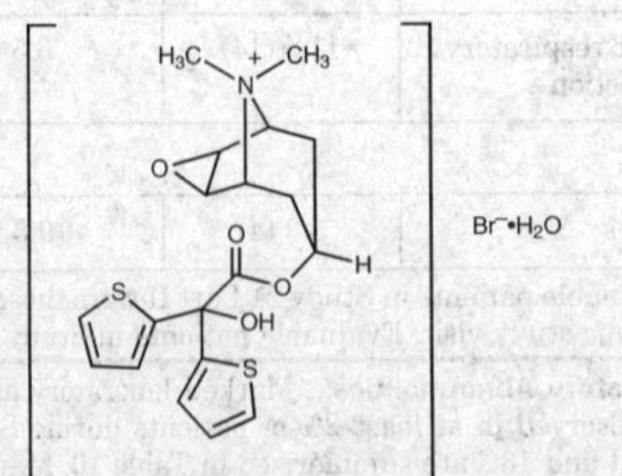

Tiotropium bromide (monohydrate) has a molecular mass of 490.4 and a molecular formula of $C_{19}H_{22}NO_4S_2Br \cdot H_2O$.
The HandiHaler is an inhalation device used to inhale the dry powder contained in the SPIRIVA capsule. The dry powder is delivered from the HandiHaler device at flow rates as low as 20 L/min. Under standardized *in vitro* testing, the HandiHaler device delivers a mean of 10.4 mcg tiotropium when tested at a flow rate of 39 L/min for 3.1 seconds (2L total). In a study of 26 adult patients with chronic obstructive pulmonary disease (COPD) and severely compromised lung function [mean FEV_1 1.02 L (range 0.45 to 2.24 L); 37.6% of predicted (range 16%–65%)], the median peak inspiratory flow (PIF) through the HandiHaler device was 30.0 L/min (range 20.4 to 45.6 L/min). The amount of drug delivered to the lungs will vary depending on patient factors such as inspiratory flow and peak inspiratory flow through the HandiHaler device, which may vary from patient to patient, and may vary with the exposure time of the capsule outside the blister pack.
For administration of SPIRIVA, a capsule is placed into the center chamber of the HandiHaler device. The capsule is pierced by pressing and releasing the button on the side of the inhalation device. The tiotropium formulation is dispersed into the air stream when the patient inhales through the mouthpiece. (see **Patient's Instructions For Use**)

CLINICAL PHARMACOLOGY

Mechanism of Action

Tiotropium is a long-acting, antimuscarinic agent, which is often referred to as an anticholinergic. It has similar affinity to the subtypes of muscarinic receptors, M_1 to M_5. In the airways, it exhibits pharmacological effects through inhibition of M_3-receptors at the smooth muscle leading to bronchodilation. The competitive and reversible nature of antagonism was shown with human and animal origin receptors and isolated organ preparations. In preclinical *in vitro* as well as *in vivo* studies prevention of methacholine-induced bronchoconstriction effects were dose-dependent and lasted longer than 24 hours. The bronchodilation following inhalation of tiotropium is predominantly a site-specific effect.

Pharmacokinetics

Tiotropium is administered by dry powder inhalation. In common with other inhaled drugs, the majority of the delivered dose is deposited in the gastrointestinal tract and, to a lesser extent, in the lung, the intended organ. Many of the pharmacokinetic data described below were obtained with higher doses than recommended for therapy.

Absorption:

Following dry powder inhalation by young healthy volunteers, the absolute bioavailability of 19.5% suggests that the fraction reaching the lung is highly bioavailable. It is expected from the chemical structure of the compound (quaternary ammonium compound) that tiotropium is poorly absorbed from the gastrointestinal tract. Food is not expected to influence the absorption of tiotropium for the same reason. Oral solutions of tiotropium have an absolute bioavailability of 2–3%. Maximum tiotropium plasma concentrations were observed five minutes after inhalation.

Distribution:

Tiotropium shows a volume of distribution of 32 L/kg indicating that the drug binds extensively to tissues. The drug is bound by 72% to plasma proteins. At steady state, peak tiotropium plasma levels in COPD patients were 17–19 pg/mL when measured 5 minutes after dry powder inhalation of an 18 mcg dose and decreased rapidly in a multi-compartmental manner. Steady state trough plasma concentrations were 3–4 pg/mL. Local concentrations in the lung are not known, but the mode of administration suggests substantially higher concentrations in the lung. Studies in rats have shown that tiotropium does not readily penetrate the blood-brain barrier.

Biotransformation:

The extent of biotransformation appears to be small. This is evident from a urinary excretion of 74% of unchanged substance after an intravenous dose to young healthy volunteers. Tiotropium, an ester, is nonenzymatically cleaved to the alcohol *N*-methylscopine and dithienylglycolic acid, neither of which bind to muscarinic receptors.
In vitro experiments with human liver microsomes and human hepatocytes suggest that a fraction of the administered dose (74% of an intravenous dose is excreted unchanged in the urine, leaving 25% for metabolism) is metabolized by cytochrome P450-dependent oxidation and subsequent glutathione conjugation to a variety of Phase II metabolites. This enzymatic pathway can be inhibited by CYP450 2D6 and 3A4 inhibitors, such as quinidine, ketoconazole, and gestodene. Thus, CYP450 2D6 and 3A4 are involved in the metabolic pathway that is responsible for the elimination of a small part of the administered dose. *In vitro* studies using human liver microsomes showed that tiotropium in supra-therapeutic concentrations does not inhibit CYP450 1A1, 1A2, 2B6, 2C9, 2C19, 2D6, 2E1, or 3A4.

Elimination:

The terminal elimination half-life of tiotropium is between 5 and 6 days following inhalation. Total clearance was 880 mL/min after an intravenous dose in young healthy volunteers with an inter-individual variability of 22%. Intravenously administered tiotropium is mainly excreted unchanged in urine (74%). After dry powder inhalation, urinary excretion is 14% of the dose, the remainder being mainly non-absorbed drug in the gut which is eliminated via the feces. The renal clearance of tiotropium exceeds the creatinine clearance, indicating active secretion into the urine. After chronic once-daily inhalation by COPD patients, pharmacokinetic steady state was reached after 2–3 weeks with no accumulation thereafter.

Drug Interactions:

An interaction study with tiotropium (14.4 mcg intravenous infusion over 15 minutes) and cimetidine 400 mg three times daily or ranitidine 300 mg once daily was conducted. Concomitant administration of cimetidine with tiotropium resulted in a 20% increase in the AUC_{0-4h}, a 28% decrease in the renal clearance of tiotropium and no significant change in the C_{max} and amount excreted in urine over 96 hours. Co-administration of tiotropium with ranitidine did not affect the pharmacokinetics of tiotropium. Therefore, no clinically significant interaction occurred between tiotropium and cimetidine or ranitidine.

Electrophysiology:
In a multicenter, randomized, double-blind trial that enrolled 198 patients with COPD, the number of subjects with changes from baseline-corrected QT interval of 30–60 msec was higher in the SPIRIVA group as compared with placebo. This difference was apparent using both the Bazett (QTcB) [20 (20%) patient vs. 12 (12%) patients] and Fredericia (QTcF) [16 (16%) patients vs. 1 (1%) patient] corrections of QT for heart rate. No patients in either group had either QTcB or QTcF of >500 msec. Other clinical studies with SPIRIVA did not detect an effect of the drug on QTc intervals.

Special Populations:
Elderly Patients:
As expected for drugs predominantly excreted renally, advanced age was associated with a decrease of tiotropium renal clearance (326 mL/min in COPD patients <58 years to 163 mL/min in COPD patients >70 years), which may be explained by decreased renal function. Tiotropium excretion in urine after inhalation decreased from 14% (young healthy volunteers) to about 7% (COPD patients). Plasma concentrations were numerically increased with advancing age within COPD patients (43% increase in AUC_{0-4} after dry powder inhalation), which was not significant when considered in relation to inter- and intra-individual variability. (See **DOSAGE AND ADMINISTRATION SECTION**)
Hepatically-impaired Patients:
The effects of hepatic impairment on the pharmacokinetics of tiotropium were not studied. However, hepatic insufficiency is not expected to have relevant influence on tiotropium pharmacokinetics. Tiotropium is predominantly cleared by renal elimination (74% in young healthy volunteers) and by simple non-enzymatic ester cleavage to products that do not bind to muscarinic receptors. (See **DOSAGE AND ADMINISTRATION SECTION**)
Renally-impaired Patients:
Since tiotropium is predominantly renally excreted, renal impairment was associated with increased plasma drug concentrations and reduced drug clearance after both intravenous infusion and dry powder inhalation. Mild renal impairment (CrCl 50–80 mL/min), which is often seen in elderly patients, increased tiotropium plasma concentrations (39% increase in AUC_{0-4} after intravenous infusion). In COPD patients with moderate to severe renal impairment (CrCl <50 mL/min), the intravenous administration of tiotropium resulted in doubling of the plasma concentrations (82% increase in AUC_{0-4}), which was confirmed by plasma concentrations after dry powder inhalation. (See **DOSAGE AND ADMINISTRATION** and **PRECAUTIONS** Sections)

CLINICAL STUDIES

The SPIRIVA HandiHaler clinical development program consisted of six phase 3 studies in 2,663 patients with COPD (1,308 receiving SPIRIVA): two 1-year, placebo-controlled studies, two 6-month, placebo-controlled studies and two 1-year, ipratropium-controlled studies. These studies enrolled patients who had a clinical diagnosis of COPD, were 40 years of age or older, had a history of smoking greater than 10 pack-years, had an FEV_1 less than or equal to 60 or 65% of predicted, and a ratio of FEV_1/FVC of less than or equal to 0.7.

In these studies, SPIRIVA, administered once-daily in the morning, provided improvement in lung function (forced expiratory volume in one second, FEV_1), with peak effect occurring within 3 hours following the first dose.

In the 1-year, placebo controlled trials, the mean improvement in FEV_1 at 30 minutes was 0.13 liters (13%) with a peak improvement of 0.24 liters (24%) relative to baseline after the first dose (day 1). Further improvements in FEV_1 and FVC were observed with pharmacodynamic steady state reached by day 8 with once-daily treatment. The mean peak improvement in FEV_1, relative to baseline, was 0.28 to 0.31 liters (28% to 31%), after 1 week (day 8) of once-daily treatment. Improvement of lung function was maintained for 24 hours after a single dose and consistently maintained over the 1-year treatment period with no evidence of tolerance.

In the two 6-month, placebo-controlled trials, serial spirometric evaluations were performed throughout daytime hours in Trial A (12 hours) and limited to 3 hours in Trial B. The serial FEV_1 values over 12 hours (Trial A) are displayed in Figure 1. These trials further support the improvement in pulmonary function (FEV_1) with SPIRIVA, which persisted over the spirometric observational period. Effectiveness was maintained for 24 hours after administration over the 6-month treatment period.

[See figure 1 above]

Results of each of the one-year ipratropium-controlled trials were similar to the results of the one-year placebo-controlled trials. The results of one of these trials are shown in Figure 2.

Figure 1: Mean FEV_1 Over Time (prior to and after administration of study drug) on Days 1 and 169 for Trial A (a Six-Month Placebo-Controlled Study)*

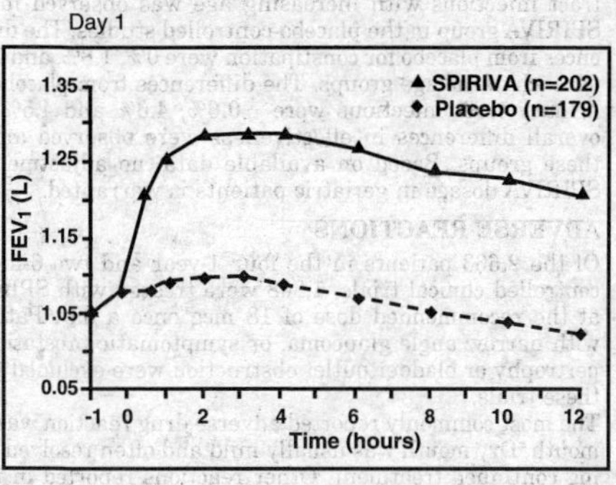

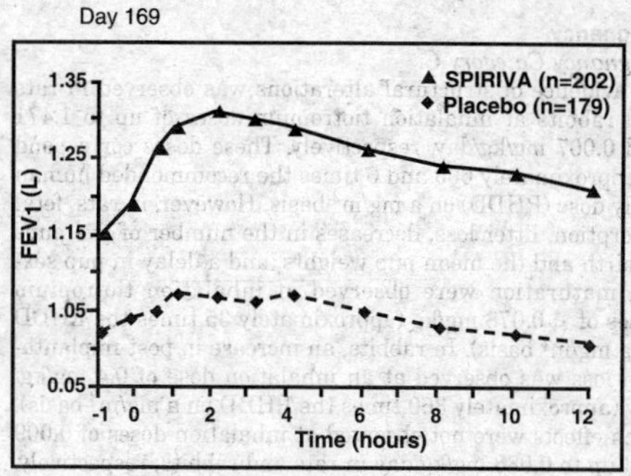

*Means adjusted for center, treatment, and baseline effect. On Day 169, a total of 183 and 149 patients in the SPIRIVA and placebo groups, respectively, completed the trial. The data for the remaining patients were imputed using last observation or least favorable observation carried forward.

Figure 2: Mean FEV_1 Over Time (0 to 6 hours postdose) on Days 1 and 92, respectively for one of the two Ipratropium-Controlled Studies*

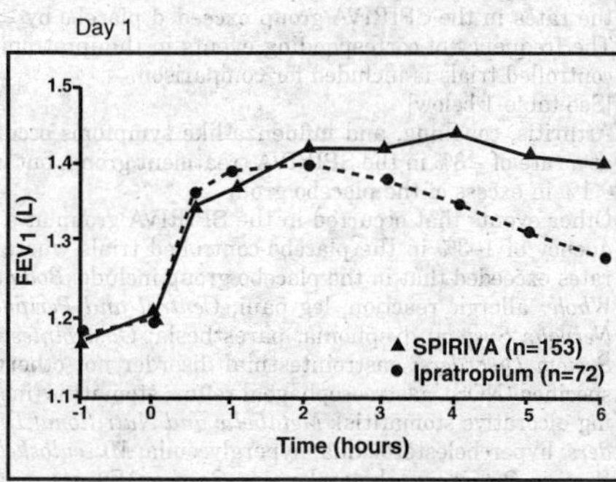

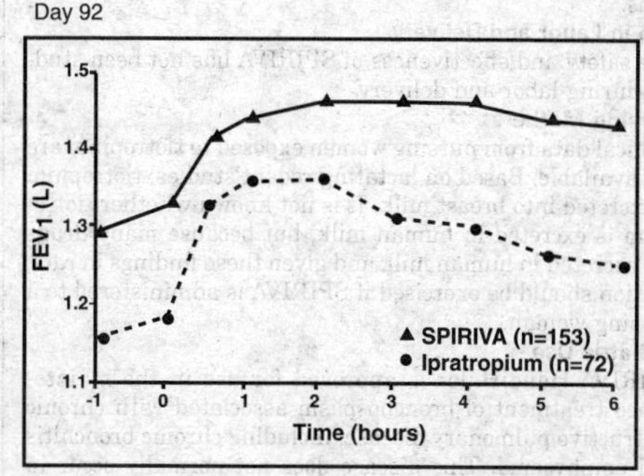

*Means adjusted for center, treatment, and baseline effect. On Day 92 (primary endpoint), a total of 151 and 69 patients in the SPIRIVA and ipratropium groups, respectively, completed through three months of observation.The data for the remaining patients were imputed using last observation or least favorable observation carried forward.

[See figure 2 above]

A randomized, placebo-controlled clinical study in 105 patients with COPD demonstrated that bronchodilation was maintained throughout the 24-hour dosing interval in comparison to placebo, regardless of whether SPIRIVA was administered in the morning or in the evening.

Throughout each week of the one-year treatment period in the two placebo-controlled trials, patients taking SPIRIVA had a reduced requirement for the use of rescue short-acting $beta_2$-agonists. Reduction in the use of rescue short-acting $beta_2$-agonists, as compared to placebo, was demonstrated in one of the two 6-month studies.

INDICATIONS AND USAGE

SPIRIVA HandiHaler is indicated for the long-term, once-daily, maintenance treatment of bronchospasm associated with chronic obstructive pulmonary disease (COPD), including chronic bronchitis and emphysema.

CONTRAINDICATIONS

SPIRIVA® HandiHaler® is contraindicated in patients with a history of hypersensitivity to atropine or its derivatives, including ipratropium, or to any component of this product.

WARNINGS

SPIRIVA HandiHaler is intended as a once-daily maintenance treatment for COPD and is not indicated for the initial treatment of acute episodes of bronchospasm, i.e., rescue therapy.

Immediate hypersensitivity reactions, including angioedema, may occur after administration of SPIRIVA. If such a reaction occurs, therapy with SPIRIVA should be stopped at once and alternative treatments should be considered.

Inhaled medicines, including SPIRIVA, may cause paradoxical bronchospasm. If this occurs, treatment with SPIRIVA should be stopped and other treatments considered.

PRECAUTIONS

General
As an anticholinergic drug, SPIRIVA may potentially worsen symptoms and signs associated with narrow-angle glaucoma, prostatic hyperplasia or bladder-neck obstruction and should be used with caution in patients with any of these conditions.

As a predominantly renally excreted drug, patients with moderate to severe renal impairment (creatinine clearance of ≤50 mL/min) treated with SPIRIVA should be monitored closely. (See **CLINICAL PHARMACOLOGY, Pharmacokinetics,** Special Populations: *Renally-impaired Patients*)

Information for Patients
It is important for patients to understand how to correctly administer SPIRIVA capsules using the HandiHaler inhalation device. (See **Patient's Instructions for Use**) SPIRIVA capsules should only be administered via the HandiHaler device and the HandiHaler device should not be used for administering other medications.

Capsules should always be stored in sealed blisters and only removed immediately before use. The blister strip should be carefully opened to expose only one capsule at a time. Open the blister foil as far as the *STOP* line to remove only one capsule at a time. The drug should be used immediately after the packaging over an individual capsule is opened, or else its effectiveness may be reduced. Capsules that are inadvertently exposed to air (i.e., not intended for immediate use) should be discarded.

Eye pain or discomfort, blurred vision, visual halos or colored images in association with red eyes from conjunctival congestion and corneal edema may be signs of acute narrow-angle glaucoma. Should any of these signs and symptoms develop, consult a physician immediately. Miotic eye drops alone are not considered to be effective treatment.

Care must be taken not to allow the powder to enter into the eyes as this may cause blurring of vision and pupil dilation.

SPIRIVA HandiHaler is a once-daily maintenance bronchodilator and should not be used for immediate relief of breathing problems, i.e., as a rescue medication.

Drug Interactions
SPIRIVA has been used concomitantly with other drugs commonly used in COPD without increases in adverse drug reactions. These include sympathomimetic bronchodilators, methylxanthines, and oral and inhaled steroids. However, the co-administration of SPIRIVA with other anticholinergic-containing drugs (e.g., ipratropium) has not been studied and is therefore not recommended.

Drug/Laboratory Test Interactions
None known.

Carcinogenesis, Mutagenesis, Impairment of Fertility
No evidence of tumorigenicity was observed in a 104-week inhalation study in rats at tiotropium doses up to 0.059 mg/kg/day, in an 83-week inhalation study in female mice at doses up to 0.145 mg/kg/day, and in a 101-week inhalation study in male mice at doses up to 0.002 mg/kg/day. These doses correspond to 25, 35, and 0.5 times the Recommended Human Daily Dose (RHDD) on a mg/m² basis, respectively. These dose multiples may be over-estimated due to difficulties in measuring deposited doses in animal inhalation studies.

Tiotropium bromide demonstrated no evidence of mutagenicity or clastogenicity in the following assays: the bacterial gene mutation assay, the V79 Chinese hamster cell mutagenesis assay, the chromosomal aberration assays in human lymphocytes *in vitro* and mouse micronucleus formation *in vivo*, and the unscheduled DNA synthesis in primary rat hepatocytes *in vitro* assay.

In rats, decreases in the number of corpora lutea and the percentage of implants were noted at inhalation tiotropium doses of 0.078 mg/kg/day or greater (approximately 35 times the RHDD on a mg/m² basis). No such effects were observed at 0.009 mg/kg/day (approximately 4 times than the RHDD on a mg/m² basis). The fertility index, however, was not affected at inhalation doses up to 1.689 mg/kg/day (approximately 760 times the RHDD on a mg/m² basis). These dose multiples may be over-estimated due to difficulties in measuring deposited doses in animal inhalation studies.

Continued on next page

Spiriva—Cont.

Pregnancy
Pregnancy Category C
No evidence of structural alterations was observed in rats and rabbits at inhalation tiotropium doses of up to 1.471 and 0.007 mg/kg/day, respectively. These doses correspond to approximately 660 and 6 times the recommended human daily dose (RHDD) on a mg/m² basis. However, in rats, fetal resorption, litter loss, decreases in the number of live pups at birth and the mean pup weights, and a delay in pup sexual maturation were observed at inhalation tiotropium doses of ≥ 0.078 mg/kg (approximately 35 times the RHDD on a mg/m² basis). In rabbits, an increase in post-implantation loss was observed at an inhalation dose of 0.4 mg/kg/day (approximately 360 times the RHDD on a mg/m² basis). Such effects were not observed at inhalation doses of 0.009 and up to 0.088 mg/kg/day in rats and rabbits, respectively. These doses correspond to approximately 4 and 80 times the RHDD on a mg/m² basis, respectively. These dose multiples may be over-estimated due to difficulties in measuring deposited doses in animal inhalation studies.
There are no adequate and well-controlled studies in pregnant women. SPIRIVA should be used during pregnancy only if the potential benefit justifies the potential risk to the fetus.

Use in Labor and Delivery
The safety and effectiveness of SPIRIVA has not been studied during labor and delivery.

Nursing Mothers
Clinical data from nursing women exposed to tiotropium are not available. Based on lactating rodent studies, tiotropium is excreted into breast milk. It is not known whether tiotropium is excreted in human milk, but because many drugs are excreted in human milk and given these findings in rats, caution should be exercised if SPIRIVA is administered to a nursing woman.

Pediatric Use
SPIRIVA HandiHaler is approved for use in the maintenance treatment of bronchospasm associated with chronic obstructive pulmonary disease, including chronic bronchitis and emphysema. This disease does not normally occur in children. The safety and effectiveness of SPIRIVA in pediatric patients have not been established.

Geriatric Use
Of the total number of patients who received SPIRIVA in the 1-year clinical trials, 426 were <65 years, 375 were 65–74 years and 105 were ≥75 years of age. Within each age subgroup, there were no differences between the proportion of patients with adverse events in the SPIRIVA and the comparator groups for most events. Dry mouth increased with age in the SPIRIVA group (differences from placebo were 9.0%, 17.1%, and 16.2% in the aforementioned age subgroups). A higher frequency of constipation and urinary tract infections with increasing age was observed in the SPIRIVA group in the placebo-controlled studies. The differences from placebo for constipation were 0%, 1.8%, and 7.8% for each of the age groups. The differences from placebo for urinary tract infections were −0.6%, 4.6% and 4.5%. No overall differences in effectiveness were observed among these groups. Based on available data, no adjustment of SPIRIVA dosage in geriatric patients is warranted.

ADVERSE REACTIONS

Of the 2,663 patients in the four 1-year and two 6-month controlled clinical trials, 1,308 were treated with SPIRIVA at the recommended dose of 18 mcg once a day. Patients with narrow angle glaucoma, or symptomatic prostatic hypertrophy or bladder outlet obstruction were excluded from these trials.
The most commonly reported adverse drug reaction was dry mouth. Dry mouth was usually mild and often resolved during continued treatment. Other reactions reported in individual patients and consistent with possible anticholinergic effects included constipation, increased heart rate, blurred vision, glaucoma, urinary difficulty, and urinary retention.
Four multicenter, 1-year, controlled studies evaluated SPIRIVA in patients with COPD. Table 1 shows all adverse events that occurred with a frequency of ≥3% in the SPIRIVA group in the 1-year placebo-controlled trials where the rates in the SPIRIVA group exceeded placebo by ≥1%. The frequency of corresponding events in the ipratropium-controlled trials is included for comparison.
[See table 1 below]
Arthritis, coughing, and influenza-like symptoms occurred at a rate of ≥3% in the SPIRIVA treatment group, but were <1% in excess of the placebo group.
Other events that occurred in the SPIRIVA group at a frequency of 1–3% in the placebo-controlled trials where the rates exceeded that in the placebo group include: *Body as a Whole:* allergic reaction, leg pain; *Central and Peripheral Nervous System:* dysphonia, paresthesia; *Gastrointestinal System Disorders:* gastrointestinal disorder not otherwise specified (NOS), gastroesophageal reflux, stomatitis (including ulcerative stomatitis); *Metabolic and Nutritional Disorders:* hypercholesterolemia, hyperglycemia; *Musculoskeletal System Disorders:* skeletal pain: *Cardiac Events:* angina pectoris (including aggravated angina pectoris); *Psychiatric Disorder:* depression; *Infections:* herpes zoster; *Respiratory System Disorder (Upper):* laryngitis; *Vision Disorder:* cataract. In addition, among the adverse events observed in the clinical trials with an incidence of <1% were atrial fibrillation, supraventricular tachycardia, angioedema, and urinary retention.
In the 1-year trials, the incidence of dry mouth, constipation, and urinary tract infection increased with age. (See **PRECAUTIONS, Geriatric Use**)

Table 1: Adverse Experience Incidence (% Patients) in One-Year-COPD Clinical Trials

Body System (Event)	Placebo-Controlled Trials		Ipratropium-Controlled Trials	
	SPIRIVA [n=550]	Placebo [n=371]	SPIRIVA [n=356]	Ipratropium [n=179]
Body as a Whole				
Accidents	13	11	5	8
Chest Pain (non-specific)	7	5	5	2
Edema, Dependent	5	4	3	5
Gastrointestinal System Disorders				
Abdominal Pain	5	3	6	6
Constipation	4	2	1	1
Dry Mouth	16	3	12	6
Dyspepsia	6	5	1	1
Vomiting	4	2	1	2
Musculoskeletal System				
Myalgia	4	3	4	3
Resistance Mechanism Disorders				
Infection	4	3	1	3
Moniliasis	4	2	3	2
Respiratory System (upper)				
Epistaxis	4	2	1	1
Pharyngitis	9	7	7	3
Rhinitis	6	5	3	2
Sinusitis	11	9	3	2
Upper Respiratory Tract Infection	41	37	43	35
Skin and Appendage Disorders				
Rash	4	2	2	2
Urinary System				
Urinary Tract Infection	7	5	4	2

Two multicenter, 6-month, controlled studies evaluated SPIRIVA in patients with COPD. The adverse events and the incidence rates were similar to those seen in the 1-year controlled trials.
In addition to adverse events identified during clinical trials, the following adverse reactions have been reported in the worldwide post-marketing experience: epistaxis, palpitations, pruritus, and urticaria.

OVERDOSAGE

High doses of tiotropium may lead to anticholinergic signs and symptoms. However, there were no systemic anticholinergic adverse effects following a single inhaled dose of up to 282 mcg tiotropium in 6 healthy volunteers. In a study of 12 healthy volunteers, bilateral conjunctivitis and dry mouth were seen following repeated once-daily inhalation of 141 mcg of tiotropium.
Acute intoxication by inadvertent oral ingestion of SPIRIVA capsules is unlikely since it is not well-absorbed systemically.
A case of overdose has been reported from post-marketing experience. A female patient was reported to have inhaled 30 capsules over a 2.5 day period, and developed altered mental status, tremors, abdominal pain, and severe constipation. The patient was hospitalized, SPIRIVA was discontinued, and the constipation was treated with an enema. The patient recovered and was discharged on the same day.
No mortality was observed at inhalation tiotropium doses up to 32.4 mg/kg in mice, 267.7 mg/kg in rats, and 0.6 mg/kg in dogs. These doses correspond to 7,3000, 120,000, and 850 times the recommended human daily dose on a mg/m² basis, respectively. These dose multiples may be over-estimated due to difficulties in measuring deposited doses in animal inhalation studies.

DOSAGE AND ADMINISTRATION

The recommended dosage of SPIRIVA HandiHaler is the inhalation of the contents of one SPIRIVA capsule, once-daily, with the HandiHaler inhalation device. (See **Patient's Instructions for Use**)
No dosage adjustment is required for geriatric, hepatically-impaired, or renally-impaired patients. However, patients with moderate to severe renal impairment given SPIRIVA should be monitored closely. (See **CLINICAL PHARMACOLOGY, Pharmacokinetics,** Special Populations and **PRECAUTIONS**)
SPIRIVA capsules are for inhalation only and must not be swallowed.

HOW SUPPLIED

SPIRIVA capsules, containing 18 mcg tiotropium, are light green, with TI01 printed on one side of the capsule and the Boehringer Ingelheim company logo on the other side.
The HandiHaler inhalation device is gray colored with a green button. It is imprinted with SPIRIVA HandiHaler (tiotropium bromide inhalation powder), the Boehringer Ingelheim company logo, and the Pfizer company logo. It is also imprinted to indicate that SPIRIVA capsules should not be stored in the HandiHaler device and that the HandiHaler device is only to be used with SPIRIVA capsules.
Six SPIRIVA capsules are packaged in an aluminum/PVC/aluminum blister card. One blister card consists of two blister strips, each containing 3 capsules and joined along a perforated-cut line. After using the first capsule, the 2 remaining capsules should be used over the next 2 consecutive days. Capsules should always be stored in the blister and only removed immediately before use. The foil lidding should only be peeled back as far as the *STOP* line printed on the blister foil to prevent exposure of more than one capsule. The drug should be used immediately after the packaging over an individual capsule is opened.
The following packages are available:
carton containing 6 SPIRIVA capsules (1 blister card) and 1 HandiHaler inhalation device (NDC 0597-0075-06)
carton containing 30 SPIRIVA capsules (5 blister cards) and 1 HandiHaler inhalation device (NDC 0597-0075-37)

Storage
Store at 25°C (77°F); excursions permitted to 15–30°C (59–86°F) [see USP Controlled Room Temperature].
The capsules should not be exposed to extreme temperature or moisture. Do not store capsules in the HandiHaler device.

℞ only

Manufactured by:
Boehringer Ingelheim Pharma GmbH & Co. KG
Ingelheim, Germany
Marketed by:
Boehringer Ingelheim Pharmaceuticals, Inc.
Ridgefield, CT 06877 USA
and
Pfizer Inc.
New York, NY 10017 USA
Address Medical Inquiries to:
www.Spiriva.com or (800) 542-6257
Licensed from Boehringer Ingelheim International GmbH.
SPIRIVA® and HandiHaler® are registered trademarks and are used under license from Boehringer Ingelheim International GmbH

Tiotropium bromide is covered by U.S. Patent No. 5,610,163 with other Patents Pending. The HandiHaler inhalation device is covered by U.S. Design Patient No. 355,029.
59873/US/1 January 2004

PATIENT'S INSTRUCTIONS FOR USE
Spiriva®
HandiHaler®
(tiotropium bromide
inhalation powder)
FOR ORAL INHALATION ONLY
Read all instructions before use.
This leaflet provides summary information about SPIRIVA capsules and the HandiHaler inhalation device. Before you start to take SPIRIVA or use the HandiHaler, read this leaflet carefully and keep it for future use. You should read the leaflet that comes with your prescription every time you refill it because there may be new information.
For more information, ask your health-care provider or pharmacist.
What should you know about SPIRIVA and HandiHaler?
Each SPIRIVA capsule contains a dry powder blend of active drug (18 mcg tiotropium) and lactose monohydrate as the carrier. The dry powder in the capsule is inhaled from the HandiHaler inhalation device. SPIRIVA capsules contain only a small amount of powder and as a result the capsule is only partially filled. When disposing of the capsule, you may notice that a tiny amount of this powder is left in the capsule. This is normal.
SPIRIVA is a once daily maintenance bronchodilator medicine that opens narrowed airways and helps keep them open for 24 hours. SPIRIVA HandiHaler should not be used for immediate relief of breathing problems, i.e., as a rescue medication.
SPIRIVA CAPSULES ARE INTENDED FOR ORAL INHALATION ONLY AND ARE TO BE USED ONLY WITH THE HANDIHALER INHALATION DEVICE.
SPIRIVA CAPSULES SHOULD NOT BE SWALLOWED.
The HandiHaler is an inhalation device that has been specially designed for use with SPIRIVA capsules. It must not be used to take any other medication.
Care must be taken not to allow the powder to enter into the eyes. If symptoms of eye pain, eye discomfort, blurred vision, visual halos, or colored images in association with red eyes occur, consult a physician immediately.
How do you take your dose of SPIRIVA using the HandiHaler?
Taking your dose of SPIRIVA, requires four main steps: Open the blister and the HandiHaler device, insert the SPIRIVA capsule, press the HandiHaler button, and inhale your medication. (See below for details.)

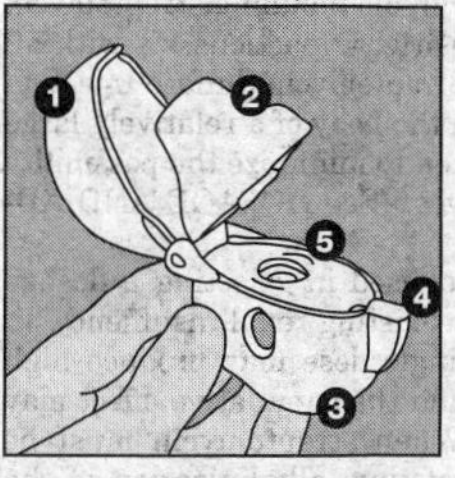

Become familiar with the components of the HandiHaler inhalation device:
1. dust cap
2. mouthpiece
3. base
4. piercing button
5. center chamber

Removing the SPIRIVA capsule from the blister.

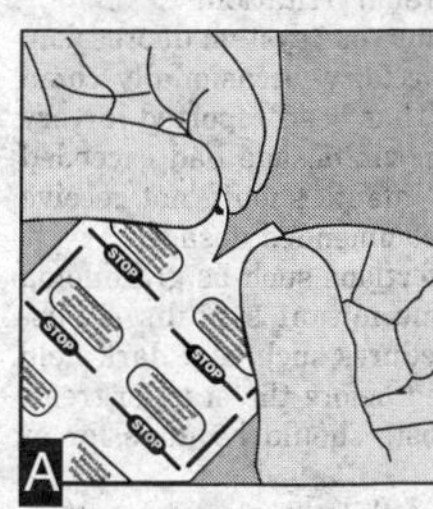

A) SPIRIVA capsules are packaged in a blister card. Each blister card consists of two blister strips, each containing 3 capsules and joined along a perforated-cut line. Prior to removing the first capsule from the blister card, separate the blister strips by tearing along the perforation. (Figure A)

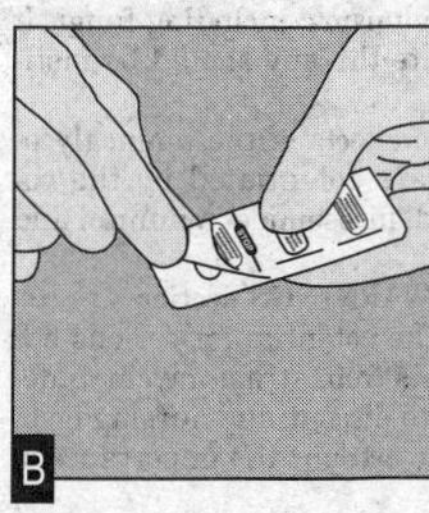

B) The blister should be carefully opened to expose only one capsule at a time. Immediately before you are ready to use your dose of SPIRIVA, peel back the aluminum foil using the tab until one capsule is fully visible. The foil lidding should only be peeled back as far as the ***STOP*** line printed on the blister foil to prevent exposure of more than one capsule. (Figure B)

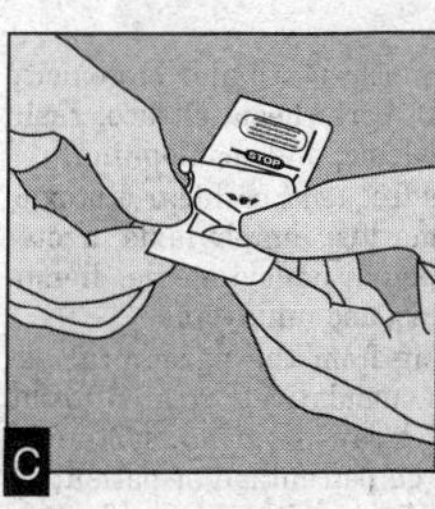

C) **Capsules should always be stored in the sealed blisters and only removed immediately before use. The drug should be used immediately after the packaging over an individual capsule is opened, or else its effectiveness may be reduced.** The blister strip should be carefully opened to expose one capsule at a time. After using the first capsule, the 2 remaining capsules should be used over the next 2 consecutive days. SPIRIVA capsules should always be stored in the blister. The blister should only be opened and the capsule removed immediately before use. If additional capsules are inadvertently exposed to air, they should not be used and should be discarded. (Figure C)
Do not store capsules in the HandiHaler device.
Opening the HandiHaler device and inserting the SPIRIVA capsule.

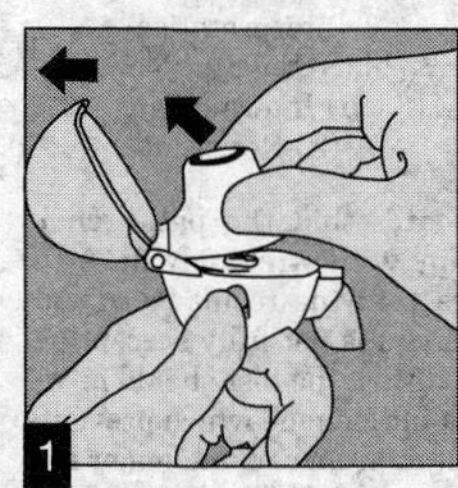

1) **OPEN:** Open the dust cap by pulling it upwards. Then open the mouthpiece. (Figure 1)

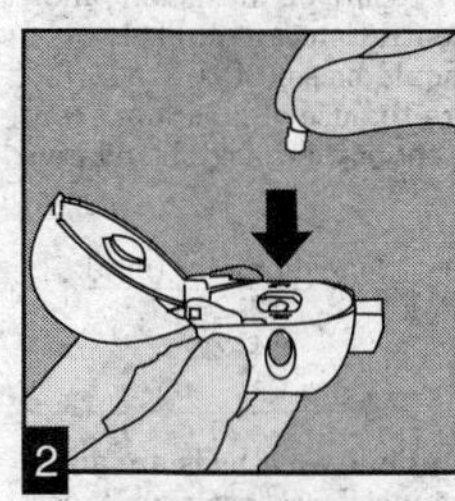

2) **INSERT:** Place the capsule in the center chamber. It does not matter which end of the capsule is placed in the chamber. (Figure 2)

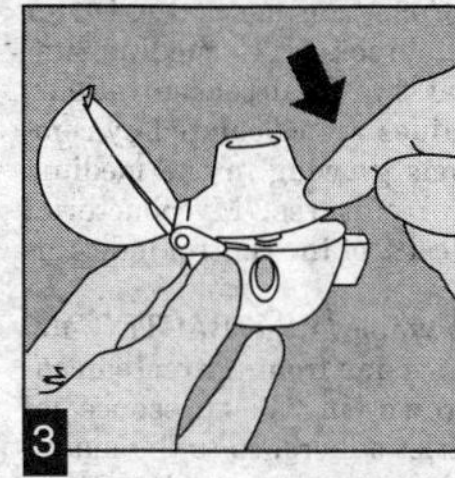

3) Close the mouthpiece **firmly until you hear a click,** leaving the dust cap open. (Figure 3)

Taking your dose of SPIRIVA.

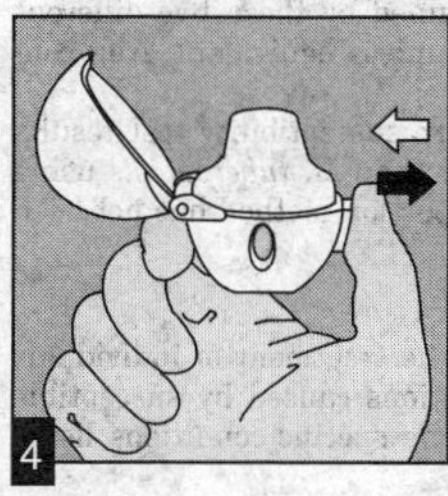

4) **PRESS: Hold the HandiHaler device with the mouthpiece upwards and press the piercing button completely in once, and release.** This makes holes in the capsule and allows the medication to be released when you breathe in. (Figure 4)

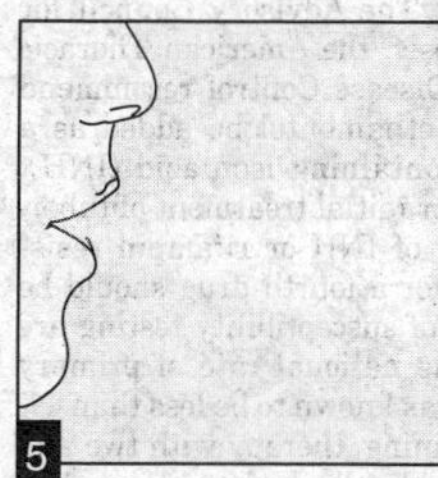

5) **Breathe out completely.** (Figure 5)
Important: Do not breathe into the mouthpiece at any time.

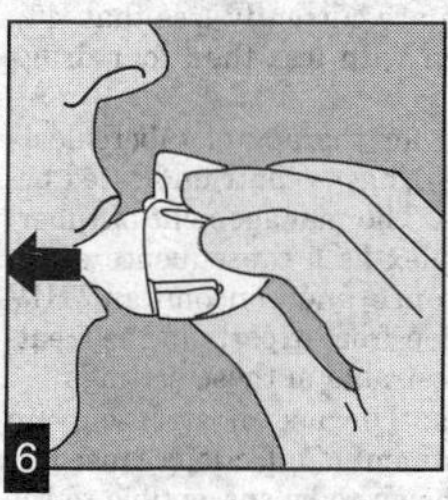

6) **INHALE:** Raise the HandiHaler device to your mouth and close your lips tightly around the mouthpiece. Keep your head in an upright position and breathe in slowly and deeply but at a rate **sufficient to hear the capsule vibrate.** Breathe in until your lungs are full; then hold your breath as long as is comfortable and at the same time take the HandiHaler device out of your mouth. Resume normal breathing. (Figure 6)

To ensure you get the full dose of SPIRIVA, you must repeat steps 5 and 6 once again.

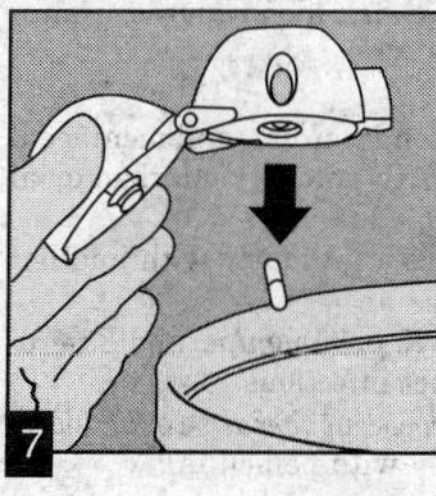

7) After you have finished taking your daily dose of SPIRIVA, open the mouthpiece again. Tip out the used capsule and dispose. (Figure 7)

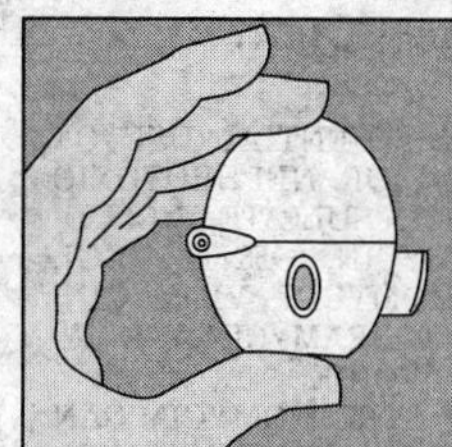

Close the mouthpiece and dust cap for storage of your HandiHaler device.

When and how should you clean your HandiHaler Device?

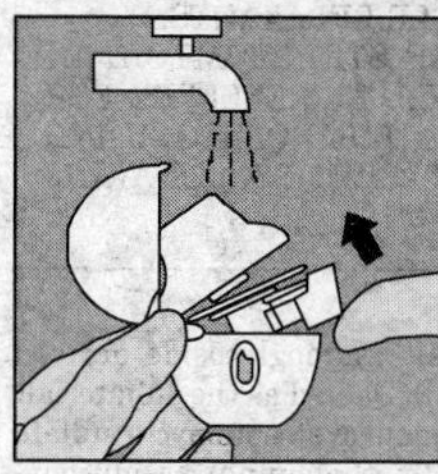

Normally, during a one-month period of use, the HandiHaler device does not need to be cleaned. However, if cleaning is needed the HandiHaler device can be cleaned as described below: Open the dust cap and mouthpiece. Open the base by lifting the piercing button. Rinse the complete inhaler with warm water to remove any powder. Do not use cleaning agents or detergents.
Dry the HandiHaler device thoroughly by tipping the excess water out on a paper towel and air-dry afterwards, leaving the dust cap, mouthpiece and base open. **It takes 24 hours to air dry, so clean it right after you use it and it will be ready for your next dose.** Do not use the HandiHaler device when it is wet.
If needed, the outside of the mouthpiece may be cleaned with a moist, but not wet tissue.
The HandiHaler device should not be placed in the dishwasher for cleaning.
Where should you store SPIRIVA capsules and the HandiHaler Device?
Store at 25°C (77°F); excursions permitted to 15–30°C (59–86°F) [see USP Controlled Room Temperature].
The capsules should not be exposed to extreme temperature or moisture. Do not store capsules in the HandiHaler.
As with all prescription medications, keep this out of the reach of children.
Tell your doctor before you use SPIRIVA HandiHaler:
if you may be pregnant or wish to become pregnant;
if you are a breastfeeding mother;
if you are taking any medications including eye drops, this includes those you can buy without a prescription;
if you have any other medical problems such as difficulty urinating or an enlarged prostate;
if you are allergic to any medications.
USE THIS PRODUCT AS DIRECTED, UNLESS INSTRUCTED TO DO OTHERWISE BY YOUR PHYSICIAN.
Manufactured by:
Boehringer Ingelheim Pharma GmbH & Co. KG
Ingelheim, Germany
Marketed by:
Boehringer Ingelheim Pharmaceuticals, Inc.
Ridgefield, CT 06877 USA
and
Pfizer Inc.
New York, NY 10017 USA
Licensed from Boehringer Ingelheim International GmbH.
SPIRIVA® and HandiHaler® are registered trademarks and are used under license from Boehringer Ingelheim International GmbH

Tiotropium bromide is covered by U.S. Patent No. 5,610,163 with other Patents Pending. The HandiHaler inhalation device is covered by U.S. Design Patient No. 355,029.
59873/US/1
January 2004
Shown in Product Identification Guide, page 329

STREPTOMYCIN SULFATE Injection, USP ℞
1 g/2.5 mL Ampoules
For Intramuscular Use Only

WARNING
THE RISK OF SEVERE NEUROTOXIC REACTIONS IS SHARPLY INCREASED IN PATIENTS WITH IMPAIRED RENAL FUNCTION OR PRE-RENAL AZOTEMIA. THESE INCLUDE DISTURBANCES OF VESTIBULAR AND COCHLEAR FUNCTION. OPTIC NERVE DYSFUNCTION, PERIPHERAL NEURITIS, ARACHNOIDITIS, AND ENCEPHALOPATHY MAY ALSO OCCUR. THE INCIDENCE OF CLINICALLY DETECTABLE, IRREVERSIBLE VESTIBULAR DAMAGE IS PARTICULARLY HIGH IN PATIENTS TREATED WITH STREPTOMYCIN.
RENAL FUNCTION SHOULD BE MONITORED CAREFULLY; PATIENTS WITH RENAL IMPAIRMENT AND/OR NITROGEN RETENTION SHOULD RECEIVE REDUCED DOSAGES. THE PEAK SERUM CONCENTRATION IN INDIVIDUALS WITH KIDNEY DAMAGE SHOULD NOT EXCEED 20 TO 25 MCG/ML.

Continued on next page

Streptomycin Sulfate—Cont.

THE CONCURRENT OR SEQUENTIAL USE OF OTHER NEUROTOXIC AND/OR NEPHROTOXIC DRUGS WITH STREPTOMYCIN SULFATE, INCLUDING NEOMYCIN, KANAMYCIN, GENTAMICIN, CEPHALORIDINE, PAROMOMYCIN, VIOMYCIN, POLYMYXIN B, COLISTIN, TOBRAMYCIN AND CYCLOSPORINE SHOULD BE AVOIDED.
THE NEUROTOXICITY OF STREPTOMYCIN CAN RESULT IN RESPIRATORY PARALYSIS FROM NEUROMUSCULAR BLOCKAGE, ESPECIALLY WHEN THE DRUG IS GIVEN SOON AFTER THE USE OF ANESTHESIA OR OF MUSCLE RELAXANTS.
THE ADMINISTRATION OF STREPTOMYCIN IN PARENTERAL FORM SHOULD BE RESERVED FOR PATIENTS WHERE ADEQUATE LABORATORY AND AUDIOMETRIC TESTING FACILITIES ARE AVAILABLE DURING THERAPY.

DESCRIPTION

Streptomycin is a water-soluble aminoglycoside derived from *Streptomyces griseus.* It is marketed as the sulfate salt of streptomycin. The chemical name of streptomycin sulfate is D-Streptamine, *O*-2-deoxy-2-(methylamino)-α-L-glucopyranosyl-(1→2)-*O*-5-deoxy-3-*C*-formyl-α-L-lyxofuranosyl-(1→4)-*N,N'*-bis(aminoiminomethyl)-, sulfate (2:3) (salt). The empirical formula for Streptomycin Sulfate is $(C_{21}H_{39}N_7O_{12})_2.3H_2SO_4$ and the molecular weight is 1457.38. It has the following structure:

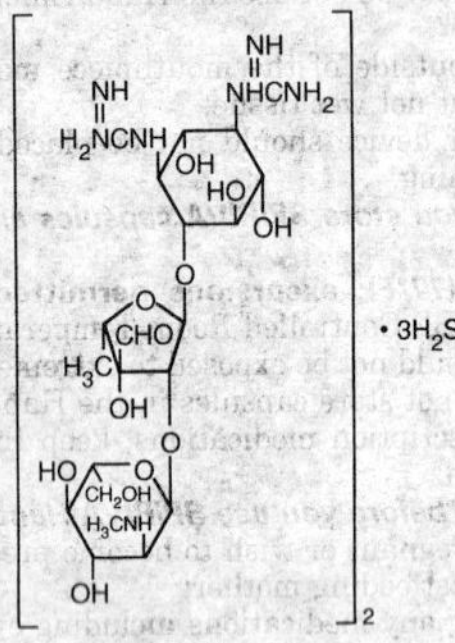

Streptomycin Sulfate Injection, 1 g/2.5 mL (400 mg/mL), is supplied as a sterile, nonpyrogenic solution for intramuscular use.
Each mL contains: Streptomycin sulfate equivalent to 400 mg of streptomycin, sodium citrate dihydrate 12 mg, phenol 0.25% w/v as preservative, sodium metabisulfite 2 mg in Water for Injection. pH range 5.0 to 8.0.

CLINICAL PHARMACOLOGY

Following intramuscular injection of 1 g of streptomycin, as the sulfate, a peak serum level of 25 to 50 mcg/mL is reached within 1 hour, diminishing slowly to about 50 percent after 5 to 6 hours.
Appreciable concentrations are found in all organ tissues except the brain. Significant amounts have been found in pleural fluid and tuberculous cavities. Streptomycin passes through the placenta with serum levels in the cord blood similar to maternal levels. Small amounts are excreted in milk, saliva, and sweat.
Streptomycin is excreted by glomerular filtration. In patients with normal kidney function, between 29% and 89% of a single 600 mg dose is excreted in the urine within 24 hours. Any reduction of glomerular function results in decreased excretion of the drug and concurrent rise in serum and tissue levels.

Microbiology
Streptomycin sulfate is a bactericidal antibiotic. It acts by interfering with normal protein synthesis.
Streptomycin has been shown to be active against most strains of the following organisms both *in vitro* and in clinical infection. (See INDICATIONS AND USAGE.):
Brucella (brucellosis),
Calymmatobacterium granulomatis (donovanosis, granuloma inguinale),
Escherichia coli, Proteus spp., Aerobacter aerogenes, Klebsiella pneumoniae, and *Enterococcus faecalis* in urinary tract infections,
Francisella tularensis,
Haemophilus ducreyi (chancroid),
Haemophilus influenzae (in respiratory, endocardial, and meningeal infections—concomitantly with another antibacterial agent),
Klebsiella pneumoniae pneumonia (concomitantly with another antibacterial agent),
Mycobacterium tuberculosis,
Pasteurella pestis
Streptococcus viridans, *Enterococcus faecalis* (in endocardial infections—concomitantly with penicillin).
SUSCEPTIBILITY TESTS: Diffusion Techniques
Quantitative methods that require measurement of zone diameters give the most precise estimate of the susceptibility of bacteria to antimicrobial agents. One such standard procedure[1] which has been recommended for use with disks to test susceptibility of organisms to streptomycin uses the 10 mcg streptomycin disk. Interpretation involves the correlation of the diameter obtained in the disk test with the minimum inhibitory concentration (MIC) for streptomycin. Reports from the laboratory giving results of the standard single disk susceptibility test with a 10 mcg streptomycin disk should be interpreted according to the following criteria:

Zone Diameter (mm)	Interpretation
≥15	(S) Susceptible
11–12	(I) Intermediate
≤10	(R) Resistant

A report of "Susceptible" indicates that the pathogen is likely to respond to monotherapy with streptomycin. A report of "Intermediate" indicates that the result be considered equivocal, and, if the organism is not fully susceptible to alternative clinically feasible drugs, the test should be repeated. This category provides a buffer zone which prevents small uncontrolled technical factors from causing major discrepancies in interpretations. A report of "Resistant" indicates that achievable drug concentrations are unlikely to be inhibitory and other therapy should be selected.
Standardized procedures require the use of laboratory control organisms. The 10 mcg streptomycin disk should give the following zone diameter:

Organism	Zone diameter (mm)
E. coli ATCC 25922	12–20
S. aureus ATCC 25923	14–22

Methods Section:
Two standardized *in vitro* susceptibility methods are available for testing streptomycin against *Mycobacterium tuberculosis* organisms. The agar proportion method (CDC or NCCLS M24–P) utilizes middlebrook 7H10 medium impregnated with streptomycin at two final concentrations, 2.0 and 10.0 mcg/mL. MIC_{90} values are calculated by comparing the quantity of organisms growing in the medium containing drug to the control cultures. Mycobacterial growth in the presence of drug ≥1% of the control indicates resistance.
The radiometric broth method employs the BACTEC 460 machine to compare the growth index from untreated control cultures to cultures grown in the presence of 6.0 mcg/mL of streptomycin. Strict adherence to the manufacturer's instructions for sample processing and data interpretation is required for this assay.
Susceptibility test results obtained by these two different methods cannot be compared unless equivalent drug concentrations are evaluated.
The clinical relevance of *in vitro* susceptibility test results for mycobacterial species other than *M. tuberculosis* using either the BACTEC or the proportion method has not been determined.

INDICATIONS AND USAGE

Streptomycin is indicated for the treatment of individuals with moderate to severe infections caused by susceptible strains of microorganisms in the specific conditions listed below:

1. Mycobacterium tuberculosis: The Advisory Council for the Elimination of Tuberculosis, the American Thoracic Society, and the Center for Disease Control recommend that either streptomycin or ethambutol be added as a fourth drug in a regimen containing isoniazid (INH), rifampin and pyrazinamide for initial treatment of tuberculosis unless the likelihood of INH or rifampin resistance is very low. The need for a fourth drug should be reassessed when the results of susceptibility testing are known. In the past when the national rate of primary drug resistance to isoniazid was known to be less than 4% and was either stable or declining, therapy with two and three drug regimens was considered adequate. If community rates of INH resistance are currently less than 4%, an initial treatment regimen with less than four drugs may be considered.

Streptomycin is also indicated for therapy of tuberculosis when one or more of the above drugs is contraindicated because of toxicity or intolerance. The management of tuberculosis has become more complex as a consequence of increasing rates of drug resistance and concomitant HIV infection. Additional consultation from experts in the treatment of tuberculosis may be desirable in those settings.

2. Non-tuberculosis infections: The use of streptomycin should be limited to the treatment of infections caused by bacteria which have been shown to be susceptible to the antibacterial effects of streptomycin and which are not amenable to therapy with less potentially toxic agents.

a. *Pasteurella pestis* (plague),
b. *Francisella tularensis* (tularemia),
c. *Brucella,*
d. *Calymmatobacterium granulomatis* (donovanosis, granuloma inguinale),
e. *H. ducreyi* (chancroid),
f. *H. influenzae* (in respiratory, endocardial, and meningeal infections—concomitantly with another antibacterial agent),
g. *K. pneumoniae* pneumonia (concomitantly with another antibacterial agent),
h. *E. coli, Proteus, A. aerogenes, K. pneumoniae,* and *Enterococcus faecalis* in urinary tract infections,
i. *Streptococcus* viridans, *Enterococcus faecalis* (in endocardial infections—concomitantly with penicillin),
j. Gram-negative bacillary bacteremia (concomitantly with another antibacterial agent).

CONTRAINDICATIONS

A history of clinically significant hypersensitivity to streptomycin is a contraindication to its use. Clinically significant hypersensitivity to other aminoglycosides may contraindicate the use of streptomycin because of the known cross-sensitivity of patients to drugs in this class.

WARNINGS

Ototoxicity: Both vestibular and auditory dysfunction can follow the administration of streptomycin. The degree of impairment is directly proportional to the dose and duration of streptomycin administration, to the age of the patient, to the level of renal function and to the amount of underlying existing auditory dysfunction. The ototoxic effects of the aminoglycosides, including streptomycin, are potentiated by the co-administration of ethacrynic acid, mannitol, furosemide and possibly other diuretics.
The vestibulotoxic potential of streptomycin exceeds that of its capacity for cochlear toxicity. Vestibular damage is heralded by headache, nausea, vomiting and disequilibrium. Early cochlear injury is demonstrated by the loss of high frequency hearing. Appropriate monitoring and early discontinuation of the drug may permit recovery prior to irreversible damage to the sensorineural cells.
Sulfites: Streptomycin contains sodium metabisulfite, a sulfite that may cause allergic type reactions including anaphylactic symptoms and life-threatening or less severe asthmatic episodes in certain susceptible people. The overall prevalence of sulfite sensitivity in the general population is unknown and probably low. Sulfite sensitivity is seen more frequently in asthmatic than in non-asthmatic people.
Pregnancy: Streptomycin can cause fetal harm when administered to a pregnant woman. Because streptomycin readily crosses the placental barrier, caution in use of the drug is important to prevent ototoxicity in the fetus. If this drug is used during pregnancy, or if the patient becomes pregnant while taking this drug, the patient should be apprised of the potential hazard to the fetus.

PRECAUTIONS

General: Baseline and periodic caloric stimulation tests and audiometric tests are advisable with extended streptomycin therapy. Tinnitus, roaring noises, or a sense of fullness in the ears indicates need for audiometric examination or termination of streptomycin therapy or both.
Care should be taken by individuals handling streptomycin for injection to avoid skin sensitivity reactions. As with all intramuscular preparations, Streptomycin Sulfate Injection should be injected well within the body of a relatively large muscle and care should be taken to minimize the possibility of damage to peripheral nerves. (See DOSAGE AND ADMINISTRATION.)
Extreme caution must be exercised in selecting a dosage regimen in the presence of preexisting renal insufficiency. In severely uremic patients a single dose may produce high blood levels for several days and the cumulative effect may produce ototoxic sequelae. When streptomycin must be given for prolonged periods of time alkalinization of the urine may minimize or prevent renal irritation.
A syndrome of apparent central nervous system depression, characterized by stupor and flaccidity, occasionally coma and deep respiratory depression, has been reported in very young infants in whom streptomycin dosage had exceeded the recommended limits. Thus, infants should not receive streptomycin in excess of the recommended dosage.
In the treatment of venereal infections such as granuloma inguinale, and chancroid, if concomitant syphilis is suspected, suitable laboratory procedures such as a dark field examination should be performed before the start of treatment, and monthly serologic tests should be done for at least four months.
As with other antibiotics, use of this drug may result in overgrowth of nonsusceptible organisms, including fungi. If superinfection occurs, appropriate therapy should be instituted.
Drug Interactions: The ototoxic effects of the aminoglycosides, including streptomycin, are potentiated by the co-administration of ethacrynic acid, furosemide, mannitol and possibly other diuretics.
Pregnancy: Category D: See WARNINGS section.
Nursing Mothers: Because of the potential for serious adverse reactions in nursing infants from streptomycin, a decision should be made whether to discontinue nursing or to discontinue the drug, taking into account the importance of the drug to the mother.
Pediatric Use: (See DOSAGE AND ADMINISTRATION.)

ADVERSE REACTIONS

The following reactions are common: vestibular ototoxicity (nausea, vomiting, and vertigo); paresthesia of face; rash; fever; urticaria; angioneurotic edema; and eosinophilia.
The following reactions are less frequent: cochlear ototoxicity (deafness); exfoliative dermatitis; anaphylaxis; azotemia; leucopenia; thrombocytopenia, pancytopenia; hemolytic anemia; muscular weakness; and amblyopia.
Vestibular dysfunction resulting from the parenteral administration of streptomycin is cumulatively related to the total daily dose. When 1.8 to 2 g/day are given, symptoms are likely to develop in the large percentage of patients—especially in the elderly or patients with impaired renal function—within four weeks. Therefore, it is recommended that caloric and audiometric tests be done prior to, during,

and following intensive therapy with streptomycin in order to facilitate detection of any vestibular dysfunction and/or impairment of hearing which may occur.

Vestibular symptoms generally appear early and usually are reversible with early detection and cessation of streptomycin administration. Two to three months after stopping the drug, gross vestibular symptoms usually disappear, except for the relative inability to walk in total darkness or on very rough terrain.

Although streptomycin is the least nephrotoxic of the aminoglycosides, nephrotoxicity does occur rarely.

Clinical judgment as to termination of therapy must be exercised when side effects occur.

DOSAGE AND ADMINISTRATION

Intramuscular Route Only

Adults: The preferred site is the upper outer quadrant of the buttock, (*i.e.,* gluteus maximus), or the mid-lateral thigh.

Children: It is recommended that intramuscular injections be given preferably in the mid-lateral muscles of the thigh. In infants and small children the periphery of the upper outer quadrant of the gluteal region should be used only when necessary, such as in burn patients, in order to minimize the possibility of damage to the sciatic nerve.

The deltoid area should be used only if well developed such as in certain adults and older children, and then only with caution to avoid radial nerve injury. Intramuscular injections should not be made into the lower and mid-third of the upper arm. As with all intramuscular injections, aspiration is necessary to help avoid inadvertent injection into a blood vessel.

Injection sites should be alternated. As higher doses or more prolonged therapy with streptomycin may be indicated for more severe or fulminating infections (endocarditis, meningitis, etc.), the physician should always take adequate measures to be immediately aware of any toxic signs or symptoms occurring in the patient as a result of streptomycin therapy.

1. TUBERCULOSIS: The standard regimen for the treatment of drug susceptible tuberculosis has been two months of INH, rifampin and pyrazinamide followed by four months of INH and rifampin (patients with concomitant infection with tuberculosis and HIV may require treatment for a longer period). When streptomycin is added to this regimen because of suspected or proven drug resistance (see **INDICATIONS AND USAGE** section), the recommended dosing for streptomycin is as follows:

	Daily	*Twice Weekly*	*Thrice Weekly*
Children	20–40 mg/kg Max 1 g	25–30 mg/kg Max 1.5 g	25–30 mg/kg Max 1.5 g
Adults	15 mg/kg Max 1 g	25–30 mg/kg Max 1.5 g	25–30 mg/kg Max 1.5 g

Streptomycin is usually administered daily as a single intramuscular injection. A total dose of not more than 120 g over the course of therapy should be given unless there are no other therapeutic options. In patients older than 60 years of age the drug should be used at a reduced dosage due to the risk of increased toxicity. (See **BOXED WARNING**).

Therapy with streptomycin may be terminated when toxic symptoms have appeared, when impending toxicity is feared, when organisms become resistant, or when full treatment effect has been obtained. The total period of drug treatment of tuberculosis is a minimum of 1 year; however, indications for terminating therapy with streptomycin may occur at any time as noted above.

2. TULAREMIA: One to 2 g daily in divided doses for 7 to 14 days until the patient is afebrile for 5 to 7 days.
3. PLAGUE: Two grams of streptomycin daily in two divided doses should be administered intramuscularly. A minimum of 10 days of therapy is recommended.
4. BACTERIAL ENDOCARDITIS:

   a. *Streptococcal endocarditis:* In penicillin-sensitive alpha and non-hemolytic streptococcal endocarditis (penicillin MIC≤0.1 mcg/mL), streptomycin may be used for 2-week treatment concomitantly with penicillin. The streptomycin regimen is 1 g b.i.d. for the first week, and 500 mg b.i.d. for the second week. If the patient is over 60 years of age, the dosage should be 500 mg b.i.d. for the entire 2-week period.

   b. *Enterococcal endocarditis:* Streptomycin in doses of 1 g b.i.d. for 2 weeks and 500 mg b.i.d. for an additional 4 weeks is given in combination with penicillin. Ototoxicity may require termination of the streptomycin prior to completion of the 6-week course of treatment.
5. CONCOMITANT USE WITH OTHER AGENTS: For concomitant use with other agents to which the infecting organism is also sensitive: Streptomycin is considered a second-line agent for the treatment of gram-negative bacillary bacteremia, meningitis, and pneumonia; brucellosis; granuloma inguinale; chancroid, and urinary tract infection.

For adults: 1 to 2 grams in divided doses every six to twelve hours for moderate to severe infections. Doses should generally not exceed 2 grams per day.

For children: 20 to 40 mg/kg/day (8 to 20 mg/lb/day) in divided doses every 6 to 12 hours. (Particular care should be taken to avoid excessive dosage in children.)

Parenteral drug products should be inspected visually for particulate matter and discoloration prior to administration, whenever solution and container permit.

HOW SUPPLIED

Streptomycin Sulfate Injection, USP is supplied in packages of 10 ampules (NDC 0049-0620-33). Each ampule contains streptomycin sulfate equivalent to 1 g of streptomycin in 2.5 mL.

Store under refrigeration at 36° to 46°F (2° to 8°C).

REFERENCES

[1] National Committee for Clinical Laboratory Standards. Performance Standards for Antimicrobial Disk Susceptibility Tests—Fourth Edition. Approved Standard NCCLS Document M2-A4. Vol. 10, No. 7. NCCLS, Villanova, PA 1990.

70-4895-44-0 Issued February 1998

Pfizer

Roerig

Division of Pfizer Inc, NY, NY 10017

TIKOSYN™ ℞

[*tĭk-ō-sĭn*]

(dofetilide)

Capsules

> To minimize the risk of induced arrhythmia, patients initiated or re-initiated on TIKOSYN should be placed for a minimum of 3 days in a facility that can provide calculations of creatinine clearance, continuous electrocardiographic monitoring, and cardiac resuscitation. For detailed instructions regarding dose selection, see **DOSAGE AND ADMINISTRATION**. TIKOSYN is available only to hospitals and prescribers who have received appropriate TIKOSYN dosing and treatment initiation education, see **DOSAGE AND ADMINISTRATION**.

DESCRIPTION

TIKOSYN (dofetilide) is an antiarrhythmic drug with Class III (cardiac action potential duration prolonging) properties. Its empirical formula is $C_{19}H_{27}N_3O_5S_2$ and it has a molecular weight of 441.6. The structural formula is

The chemical name for dofetilide is *N*-[4-[2-[methyl[2-[4-[(methylsulfonyl)amino]phenoxy]ethyl]amino]ethyl]phenyl]- methanesulfonamide.

Dofetilide is a white to off-white powder. It is very slightly soluble in water and propan-2-ol and is soluble in 0.1M aqueous sodium hydroxide, acetone and aqueous 0.1M hydrochloric acid.

TIKOSYN capsules contain the following inactive ingredients: microcrystalline cellulose, corn starch, colloidal silicon dioxide and magnesium stearate. TIKOSYN is supplied for oral administration in three dosage strengths: 125 mcg (0.125 mg) orange and white capsules, 250 mcg (0.25 mg) peach capsules, and 500 mcg (0.5 mg) peach and white capsules.

CLINICAL PHARMACOLOGY

Mechanism of Action

TIKOSYN (dofetilide) shows Vaughan Williams Class III antiarrhythmic activity. The mechanism of action is blockade of the cardiac ion channel carrying the rapid component of the delayed rectifier potassium current, I_{Kr}. At concentrations covering several orders of magnitude, dofetilide blocks only I_{Kr} with no relevant block of the other repolarizing potassium currents (e.g., I_{Ks}, I_{K1}). At clinically relevant concentrations, dofetilide has no effect on sodium channels (associated with Class I effect), adrenergic alpha-receptors, or adrenergic beta-receptors.

Electrophysiology

TIKOSYN (dofetilide) increases the monophasic action potential duration in a predictable, concentration-dependent manner, primarily due to delayed repolarization. This effect, and the related increase in effective refractory period, is observed in the atria and ventricles in both resting and paced electrophysiology studies. The increase in QT interval observed on the surface ECG is a result of prolongation of both effective and functional refractory periods in the His-Purkinje system and the ventricles.

Dofetilide did not influence cardiac conduction velocity and sinus node function in a variety of studies in patients with or without structural heart disease. This is consistent with a lack of effect of dofetilide on the PR interval and QRS width in patients with pre-existing heart block and/or sick sinus syndrome.

In patients, dofetilide terminates induced re-entrant tachyarrhythmias (e.g., atrial fibrillation/flutter and ventricular tachycardia) and prevents their re-induction. TIKOSYN does not increase the electrical energy required to convert electrically-induced ventricular fibrillation, and it significantly reduces the defibrillation threshold in patients with ventricular tachycardia and ventricular fibrillation undergoing implantation of a cardioverter-defibrillator device.

Hemodynamic Effects

In hemodynamic studies, TIKOSYN had no effect on cardiac output, cardiac index, stroke volume index, or systemic vascular resistance in patients with ventricular tachycardia, mild to moderate congestive heart failure or angina and either normal or low left ventricular ejection fraction. There was no evidence of a negative inotropic effect related to TIKOSYN therapy in patients with atrial fibrillation. There was no increase in heart failure in patients with significant left ventricular dysfunction (see **Safety in Patients with Structural Heart Disease: DIAMOND Studies**). In the overall clinical program, TIKOSYN did not affect blood pressure. Heart rate was decreased by 4–6 bpm in studies in patients.

Pharmacokinetics, General

Absorption and Distribution: The oral bioavailability of dofetilide is >90%, with maximal plasma concentrations occurring at about 2–3 hours in the fasted state. Oral bioavailability is unaffected by food or antacid. The terminal half life of TIKOSYN is approximately 10 hours; steady state plasma concentrations are attained within 2–3 days, with an accumulation index of 1.5 to 2.0. Plasma concentrations are dose proportional. Plasma protein binding of dofetilide is 60–70%, is independent of plasma concentration, and is unaffected by renal impairment. Volume of distribution is 3 L/kg.

Metabolism and Excretion: Approximately 80% of a single dose of dofetilide is excreted in urine, of which approximately 80% is excreted as unchanged dofetilide with the remaining 20% consisting of inactive or minimally active metabolites. Renal elimination involves both glomerular filtration and active tubular secretion (via the cation transport system, a process that can be inhibited by cimetidine, trimethoprim, prochlorperazine, megestrol and ketoconazole). *In vitro* studies with human liver microsomes show that dofetilide can be metabolized by CYP3A4, but it has a low affinity for this isoenzyme. Metabolites are formed by N-dealkylation and N-oxidation. There are no quantifiable metabolites circulating in plasma, but 5 metabolites have been identified in urine.

Pharmacokinetics in Special Populations

Renal Impairment: In volunteers with varying degrees of renal impairment and patients with arrhythmias, the clearance of dofetilide decreases with decreasing creatinine clearance. As a result, and as seen in clinical studies, the half-life of dofetilide is longer in patients with lower creatinine clearances. **Because increase in QT interval and the risk of ventricular arrhythmias are directly related to plasma concentrations of dofetilide, dosage adjustment based on calculated creatinine clearance is critically important** (see **DOSAGE AND ADMINISTRATION**). Patients with severe renal impairment (creatinine clearance <20 mL/min) were not included in clinical or pharmacokinetic studies (see **CONTRAINDICATIONS**).

Hepatic Impairment: There was no clinically significant alteration in the pharmacokinetics of dofetilide in volunteers with mild to moderate hepatic impairment (Child-Pugh class A and B) compared to age- and weight-matched healthy volunteers. Patients with severe hepatic impairment were not studied.

Patients with Heart Disease: Population pharmacokinetic analyses indicate that the plasma concentration of dofetilide in patients with supraventricular and ventricular arrhythmias, ischemic heart disease, or congestive heart failure are similar to those of healthy volunteers, after adjusting for renal function.

Elderly: After correction for renal function, clearance of dofetilide is not related to age.

Women: A population pharmacokinetic analysis showed that women have approximately 12–18% lower dofetilide oral clearances than men (14–22% greater plasma dofetilide levels), after correction for weight and creatinine clearance. In females, as in males, renal function was the single most important factor influencing dofetilide clearance. In normal female volunteers, hormone replacement therapy (a combination of conjugated estrogens and medroxyprogesterone) did not increase dofetilide exposure.

Drug-Drug Interactions (see PRECAUTIONS)

Dose-Response and Concentration Response for Increase in QT Interval

Increase in QT interval is directly related to dofetilide dose and plasma concentration. Figure 1 shows that the relationship in normal volunteers between dofetilide plasma concentrations and change in QTc is linear, with a positive slope of approximately 15–25 msec/(ng/mL) after the first dose and approximately 10–15 msec/(ng/mL) at Day 23 (reflecting a steady state of dosing). A linear relationship between mean QTc increase and dofetilide dose was also seen in patients with renal impairment, in patients with ischemic heart disease, and in patients with supraventricular and ventricular arrhythmias.

[See figure 1 at top of next column]

The relationship between dose, efficacy and the increase in QTc from baseline at steady state for the two randomized, placebo-controlled studies (described further below) is shown in Figure 2. The studies examined the effectiveness of TIKOSYN in conversion to sinus rhythm and maintenance of normal sinus rhythm after conversion in patients with atrial fibrillation/flutter of >1 week duration. As shown, both the probability of a patient's remaining in sinus rhythm at six months and the change in QTc from baseline at steady state of dosing increased in an approximately linear fashion with increasing dose of TIKOSYN.

Continued on next page

Tikosyn—Cont.

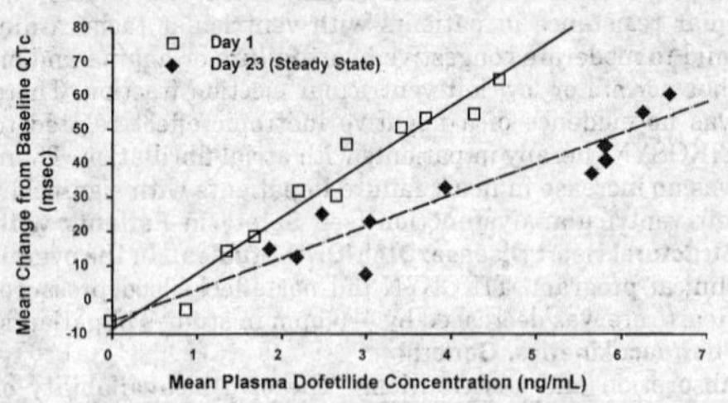

Figure 1: Mean QTc-Concentration Relationship in Young Volunteers Over 24 Days. Note: The range of dofetilide plasma concentrations achieved with the 500 mcg BID dose adjusted for creatinine clearance is 1-3.5 ng/mL.

Note that in these studies doses were modified by results of creatinine clearance measurement and in-hospital QTc prolongation.

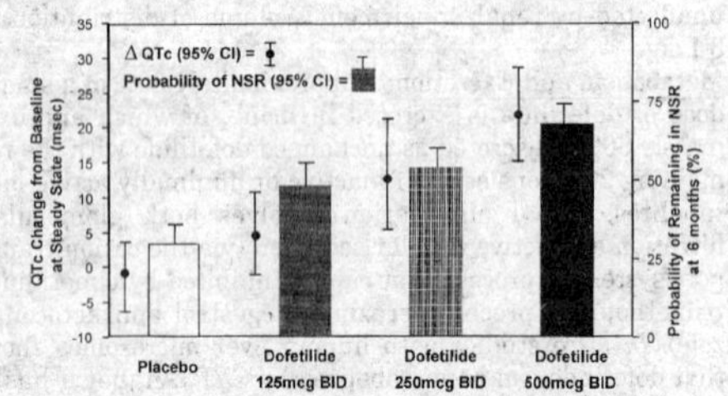

Figure 2: Relationship Between TIKOSYN Dose, QTc Increase and Maintenance of NSR.

CLINICAL STUDIES

Chronic Atrial Fibrillation and/or Atrial Flutter

Two randomized, parallel, double-blind, placebo controlled, dose-response trials evaluated the ability of TIKOSYN 1) to convert patients with atrial fibrillation or atrial flutter (AF/AFl) of more than 1 week duration to normal sinus rhythm (NSR) and 2) to maintain NSR (delay time to recurrence of AF/AFl) after drug-induced or electrical cardioversion. A total of 996 patients with a one week to two year history of atrial fibrillation/atrial flutter were enrolled. Both studies randomized patients to placebo or to doses of TIKOSYN 125 mcg, 250 mcg, 500 mcg or in one study a comparator drug, given twice a day (these doses were lowered based on calculated creatinine clearance and, in one of the studies, for QT interval or QTc). **All patients were started on therapy in a hospital where their ECG was monitored (see DOSAGE AND ADMINISTRATION).**

Patients were excluded from participation if they had had syncope within the past 6 months, AV block greater than first degree, MI or unstable angina within 1 month, cardiac surgery within 2 months, history of QT interval prolongation or polymorphic ventricular tachycardia associated with use of anti-arrhythmic drugs, QT interval or QTc >440 msec, serum creatinine >2.5 mg/mL, significant diseases of other organ systems; used cimetidine; or used drugs known to prolong the QT interval.

Both studies enrolled mostly Caucasians (over 90%), males (over 70%) and patients ≥65 years of age (over 50%). Most (>90%) were NYHA Functional Class I or II. Approximately one-half had structural heart disease (including ischemic heart disease, cardiomyopathies, and valvular disease) and about one-half were hypertensive. A substantial proportion of patients were on concomitant therapy, including digoxin (over 60%), diuretics (over 20%) and ACE inhibitors (over 30%). About 90% were on anticoagulants.

Acute conversion rates are shown in Table 1 for randomized doses (doses were adjusted for calculated creatinine clearance and, in Study 1, for QT interval or QTc). Of patients who converted pharmacologically, approximately 70% converted within 24–36 hours.

Table 1: Conversion of Atrial Fibrillation/Flutter to Normal Sinus Rhythm

	TIKOSYN Dose			
	125 mcg BID	250 mcg BID	500 mcg BID	Placebo
Study 1	5/82(6%)	8/82(10%)	23/77(30%)	1/84(1%)
Study 2	8/135(6%)	14/133(11%)	38/129(29%)	2/137(1%)

Patients who did not convert to NSR with randomized therapy within 48–72 hours had electrical cardioversion. Those patients remaining in NSR after conversion in hospital were continued on randomized therapy as outpatients (maintenance period) for up to one year unless they experienced a recurrence of atrial fibrillation/atrial flutter or withdrew for other reasons.

Table 2 shows, by randomized dose, the percentage of patients at 6 and 12 months in both studies, who remained on treatment in NSR and the percentage of patients who withdrew because of recurrence of AF/AFl or adverse events.

Table 2: Patient Status at 6 and 12 Months Post Randomization

	TIKOSYN Dose			
	125 mcg BID	250 mcg BID	500 mcg BID	Placebo
Study 1				
Randomized	82	82	77	84
Achieved NSR	60	61	61	68
6 months				
Still on treatment in NSR	38%	44%	52%	32%
D/C for recurrence	55%	49%	33%	63%
D/C for AEs	3%	3%	8%	4%
12 months				
Still on treatment in NSR	32%	26%	46%	22%
D/C for recurrence	58%	57%	36%	72%
D/C for AEs	7%	11%	8%	6%
Study 2				
Randomized	135	133	129	137
Achieved NSR	103	118	100	106
6 months				
Still on treatment in NSR	41%	49%	57%	22%
D/C for recurrence	48%	42%	27%	72%
D/C for AEs	9%	6%	10%	4%
12 months				
Still on treatment in NSR	25%	42%	49%	16%
D/C for recurrence	59%	47%	32%	76%
D/C for AEs	11%	6%	12%	5%

Please note that columns do not add up to 100% due to discontinuations for "other" reasons.

Table 3: P-Values and Median Time (days) to Recurrence of AF/AFl

	TIKOSYN Dose			
	125 mcg BID	250 mcg BID	500 mcg BID	Placebo
Study 1				
p-value vs placebo	P=0.21	P=0.10	P<0.001	
Median time to recurrence (days)	31	179	>365	27
Study 2				
p-value vs placebo	P=0.006	P<0.001	P<0.001	
Median time to recurrence (days)	182	>365	>365	34

Median time to recurrence of AF/AFl could not be estimated accurately for the 250 mcg BID treatment group in Study 2 and the 500 mcg BID treatment groups in Studies 1 and 2 because TIKOSYN maintained >50% of patients (51%, 58% and 66%, respectively) in NSR for the 12 months duration of the studies.

[See table 2 above]

Table 3 and Figures 3 and 4 show, by randomized dose, the effectiveness of TIKOSYN in maintaining NSR using Kaplan Meier analysis, which shows patients remaining on treatment.

[See table 3 above]

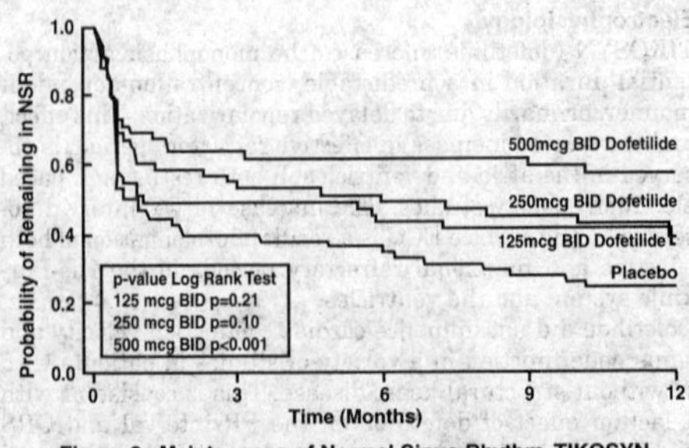

Figure 3: Maintenance of Normal Sinus Rhythm, TIKOSYN Regimen vs. Placebo (Study 1).

The point estimates of the probabilities of remaining in NSR at 6 and 12 months were 62% and 58% respectively for TIKOSYN 500 mcg BID, 50% and 37% for TIKOSYN 250 mcg BID, and 37% and 25% respectively on placebo.

[See figure 4 at top of next column]

The point estimates of the probabilities of remaining in NSR at 6 and 12 months were 71% and 66% respectively for

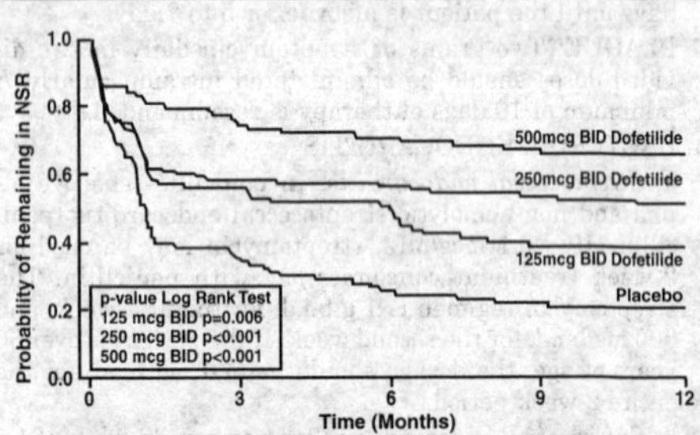

Figure 4: Maintenance of Normal Sinus Rhythm, TIKOSYN Regimen vs. Placebo (Study 2).

TIKOSYN 500 mcg BID, 56% and 51% for TIKOSYN 250 mcg BID, and 26% and 21% respectively on placebo.

In both studies, TIKOSYN resulted in a dose-related increase in the number of patients maintained in NSR at all time periods and delayed the time of recurrence of sustained AF. Data pooled from both studies show that there is a positive relationship between the probability of staying in NSR, TIKOSYN dose, and increase in QTc (see Figure 2 in **CLINICAL PHARMACOLOGY: Dose-Response and Concentration Response for QT Interval**).

Analysis of pooled data for patients randomized to a TIKOSYN dose of 500 mcg twice daily showed that maintenance of NSR was similar in both males and females, in both patients aged <65 years and patients ≥65 years of age, and in both patients with atrial flutter as a primary diagnosis and those with a primary diagnosis of atrial fibrillation.

During the period of in-hospital initiation of dosing, 23% of patients in Studies 1 and 2 had their dose adjusted downward on the basis of their calculated creatinine clearance, and 3% had their dose down-titrated due to increased QT interval or QTc. Increased QT interval or QTc led to discontinuation of therapy in 3% of patients.

Safety in Patients with Structural Heart Disease: DIAMOND Studies (The Danish Investigations of Arrhythmia and Mortality on Dofetilide)

The two DIAMOND studies were 3-year trials comparing the effects of TIKOSYN and placebo on mortality and morbidity in patients with impaired left ventricular function (ejection fraction ≤35%). Patients were treated for at least one year. One study was in patients with moderate to severe (60% NYHA Class III or IV) congestive heart failure (DIAMOND CHF) and the other was in patients with recent myocardial infarction (DIAMOND MI) (of whom 40% had NYHA Class III or IV heart failure). Both groups were at relatively high risk of sudden death. The DIAMOND trials were intended to determine whether TIKOSYN could reduce that risk. The trials did not demonstrate a reduction in mortality; however, they provide reassurance that, when initiated carefully, in a hospital or equivalent setting, TIKOSYN did not increase mortality in patients with structural heart disease, an important finding because other antiarrhythmics [notably the Class IC antiarrhythmics studied in the Cardiac Arrhythmia Suppression Trial (CAST) and a pure Class III antiarrhythmic, d-sotalol (SWORD)] have increased mortality in post-infarction populations. The DIAMOND trials therefore provide evidence of a method of safe use of TIKOSYN in a population susceptible to ventricular arrhythmias. In addition, the subset of patients with AF in the DIAMOND trials provide further evidence of safety in a population of patients with structural heart disease accompanying the AF. Note, however, that this AF population was given a lower (250 mcg BID) dose (see DIAMOND Patients with Atrial Fibrillation).

In both DIAMOND studies, patients were randomized to 500 mcg BID of TIKOSYN, but this was reduced to 250 mcg BID if calculated creatinine clearance was 40–60 mL/min, if patients had AF, or if QT interval prolongation (>550 msec or >20% increase from baseline) occurred after dosing. Dose reductions for reduced calculated creatinine clearance occurred in 47% and 45% of DIAMOND CHF and MI patients. Dose reductions for increased QT interval or QTc occurred in 5% and 7% of DIAMOND CHF and MI patients, respectively. Increased QT interval or QTc (>550 msec or >20% increase from baseline) resulted in discontinuation of 1.8% of patients in DIAMOND CHF and 2.5% of patients in DIAMOND MI.

In the DIAMOND studies all patients were hospitalized for at least 3 days after treatment was initiated and monitored by telemetry. Patients with QTc greater than 460 msec, second or third degree AV block (unless with pacemaker), resting heart rate <50 bpm, or prior history of polymorphic ventricular tachycardia were excluded.

DIAMOND CHF studied 1518 patients hospitalized with severe CHF who had confirmed impaired left ventricular function (ejection fraction ≤35%). Patients received a median duration of therapy of greater than one year. There were 311 deaths from all causes in patients randomized to TIKOSYN (n=762) and 317 deaths in patients randomized to placebo (n=756). The probability of survival at one year was 73% (95% CI: 70% – 76%) in the TIKOSYN group and 72% (95% CI: 69% – 75%) in the placebo group. Similar results were seen for cardiac deaths and arrhythmic deaths. Torsade de pointes occurred in 25/762 patients (3.3%) receiving TIKOSYN. The majority of cases (76%) occurred within the first 3 days of dosing. In all, 437/762 (57%) of patients on TIKOSYN and 459/756 (61%) on placebo required hospitalization. Of these, 229/762 (30%) of patients on TIKOSYN and 290/756 (38%) on placebo required hospitalization because of worsening heart failure.

DIAMOND MI studied 1510 patients hospitalized with recent myocardial infarction (2–7 days) who had confirmed impaired left ventricular function (ejection fraction ≤35%). Patients received a median duration of therapy of greater than one year. There were 230 deaths in patients randomized to TIKOSYN (n=749) and 243 deaths in patients randomized to placebo (n=761). The probability of survival at one year was 79% (95% CI: 76% – 82%) in the TIKOSYN group and 77% (95% CI: 74% – 80%) in the placebo group. Cardiac and arrhythmic mortality showed a similar result. Torsade de pointes occurred in 7/749 patients (0.9%) receiving TIKOSYN. Of these, 4 cases occurred within the first 3 days of dosing and 3 cases occurred between Day 4 and the conclusion of the study. In all, 371/749 (50%) of patients on TIKOSYN and 419/761 (55%) on placebo required hospitalization. Of these, 200/749 (27%) of patients on TIKOSYN and 205/761 (27%) on placebo required hospitalization because of worsening heart failure.

DIAMOND Patients with Atrial Fibrillation (the DIAMOND AF subpopulation). There were 506 patients in the two DIAMOND studies who had atrial fibrillation (AF) at entry to the studies (249 randomized to TIKOSYN and 257 randomized to placebo). DIAMOND AF patients randomized to TIKOSYN received 250 mcg BID; 65% of these patients had impaired renal function, so that 250 mcg BID represents the dose they would have received in the AF trials, which would give drug exposure similar to a person with normal renal function given 500 mcg BID. In the DIAMOND AF subpopulation there were 111 deaths (45%) in the 249 patients in the TIKOSYN group and 116 deaths (45%) in the 257 patients in the placebo group. Hospital readmission rates for any reason were 125/249 or 50% on TIKOSYN and 156/257 or 61% for placebo. Of these, readmission rates for worsening heart failure were 73/249 or 29% on TIKOSYN and 102/257 or 40% for placebo.

Of the 506 patients in the DIAMOND studies who had atrial fibrillation or flutter at baseline, 12% of patients in the TIKOSYN group and 2% of patients in the placebo group had converted to normal sinus rhythm after one month. In those patients converted to normal sinus rhythm, 79% of the TIKOSYN group and 42% of the placebo group remained in normal sinus rhythm for one year.

In the DIAMOND studies, although torsade de pointes occurred more frequently in the TIKOSYN-treated patients (see **ADVERSE REACTIONS**), TIKOSYN, given with an initial 3-day hospitalization and with dose modified for reduced creatinine clearance and increased QT interval, was not associated with an excess risk of mortality in these populations with structural heart disease in the individual studies or in an analysis of the combined studies. The presence of atrial fibrillation did not affect outcome.

INDICATIONS AND USAGE

Maintenance of Normal Sinus Rhythm (Delay in AF/AFl Recurrence)

TIKOSYN is indicated for the maintenance of normal sinus rhythm (delay in time to recurrence of atrial fibrillation/atrial flutter [AF/AFl]) in patients with atrial fibrillation/atrial flutter of greater than one week duration who have been converted to normal sinus rhythm. Because TIKOSYN can cause life threatening ventricular arrhythmias, it should be reserved for patients in whom atrial fibrillation/atrial flutter is highly symptomatic.

In general, antiarrhythmic therapy for atrial fibrillation/atrial flutter aims to prolong the time in normal sinus rhythm. Recurrence is expected in some patients. (See **CLINICAL TRIALS**.)

Conversion of Atrial Fibrillation/Flutter

TIKOSYN is indicated for the conversion of atrial fibrillation and atrial flutter to normal sinus rhythm.

TIKOSYN has not been shown to be effective in patients with paroxysmal atrial fibrillation.

CONTRAINDICATIONS

TIKOSYN is contraindicated in patients with congenital or acquired long QT syndromes. TIKOSYN should not be used in patients with a baseline QT interval or QTc >440 msec (500 msec in patients with ventricular conduction abnormalities). TIKOSYN is also contraindicated in patients with severe renal impairment (calculated creatinine clearance <20 mL/min).

The concomitant use of verapamil or the cation transport system inhibitors cimetidine, trimethoprim (alone or in combination with sulfamethoxazole) or ketoconazole with TIKOSYN is contraindicated (see **PRECAUTIONS, Drug-Drug Interactions**), as each of these drugs cause a substantial increase in dofetilide plasma concentrations. In addition, other known inhibitors of the renal cation transport system such as prochlorperazine and megestrol should not be used in patients on TIKOSYN.

TIKOSYN is also contraindicated in patients with a known hypersensitivity to the drug.

WARNINGS

Ventricular Arrhythmia: TIKOSYN (dofetilide) can cause serious ventricular arrhythmias, primarily torsade de pointes (TdP) type ventricular tachycardia, a polymorphic ventricular tachycardia associated with QT interval prolongation. QT interval prolongation is directly related to dofetilide plasma concentration. Factors such as reduced creatinine clearance or certain dofetilide drug interactions will increase dofetilide plasma concentration. The risk of TdP can be reduced by controlling the plasma concentration through adjustment of the initial dofetilide dose according to creatinine clearance and by monitoring the ECG for excessive increases in the QT interval.

Table 4: Summary of Torsade de Pointes in Patients Randomized to Dofetilide by Dose; Patients with Supraventricular Arrhythmias

	TIKOSYN Dose				
	<250 mcg BID	250 mcg BID	>250-500 mcg BID	>500 mcg BID	All Doses
Number of Patients	217	388	703	38	1346
Torsade de Pointes	0	1 (0.3%)	6 (0.9%)	4 (10.5%)	11 (0.8%)

Table 5: Incidence of Torsade de Pointes Before and After Introduction of Dosing According to Renal Function

	Total	Before	After
Population:	n/N %	n/N %	n/N %
Supraventricular Arrhythmias	11/1346 (0.8%)	6/193 (3.1%)	5/1153 (0.4%)
DIAMOND CHF	25/762 (3.3%)	7/148 (4.7%)	18/614 (2.9%)
DIAMOND MI	7/749 (0.9%)	3/101 (3.0%)	4/648 (0.6%)
DIAMOND AF	4/249 (1.6%)	0/43 (0%)	4/206 (1.9%)

Treatment with dofetilide must therefore be started only in patients placed for a minimum of three days in a facility that can provide electrocardiographic monitoring and in the presence of personnel trained in the management of serious ventricular arrhythmias. Calculation of the creatinine clearance for all patients must precede administration of the first dose of dofetilide. For detailed instructions regarding dose selection, see DOSAGE AND ADMINISTRATION.

The risk of dofetilide induced ventricular arrhythmia was assessed in three ways in clinical studies: 1) by description of the QT interval and its relation to the dose and plasma concentration of dofetilide; 2) by observing the frequency of TdP in TIKOSYN treated patients according to dose; 3) by observing the overall mortality rate in patients with atrial fibrillation and in patients with structural heart disease.

Relation of QT Interval to Dose: The QT interval increases linearly with increasing TIKOSYN dose (see Figures 1 and 2 in **CLINICAL PHARMACOLOGY: Dose-Response and Concentration Response for Increase in QT Interval**).

Frequency of Torsade de Pointes: In the supraventricular arrhythmia population (patients with AF and other supraventricular arrhythmias) the overall incidence of torsade de pointes was 0.8%. The frequency of TdP by dose is shown in Table 4. There were no cases of TdP on placebo.

[See table 4 above]

As shown in Table 5, the rate of TdP was reduced when patients were dosed according to their renal function (see **CLINICAL PHARMACOLOGY: Pharmacokinetics in Special Populations: Renal Impairment**, and **DOSAGE AND ADMINISTRATION**).

[See table 5 above]

The majority of the episodes of TdP occurred within the first three days of TIKOSYN therapy (10/11 events in the studies of patients with supraventricular arrhythmias; 19/25 and 4/7 events in DIAMOND CHF and DIAMOND MI, respectively; 2/4 events in the DIAMOND AF subpopulation).

Mortality: In a pooled survival analysis of patients in the supraventricular arrhythmia population (low prevalence of structural heart disease), deaths occurred in 0.9% (12/1346) of patients receiving TIKOSYN and 0.4% (3/677) in the placebo group. Adjusted for duration of therapy, primary diagnosis, age, gender, and prevalence of structural heart disease, the point estimate of the hazard ratio for the pooled studies (TIKOSYN/placebo) was 1.1 (95% CI: 0.3, 4.3). The DIAMOND CHF and MI trials examined mortality in patients with structural heart disease (ejection fraction ≤35%). In these large, double-blind studies, deaths occurred in 36% (541/1511) of TIKOSYN patients and 37% (560/1517) of placebo patients. In an analysis of 506 DIAMOND patients with atrial fibrillation/flutter at baseline, one year mortality on TIKOSYN was 31% vs. 32% on placebo (see **CLINICAL STUDIES**).

Because of the small number of events, an excess mortality due to TIKOSYN cannot be ruled out with confidence in the pooled survival analysis of placebo-controlled trials in patients with supraventricular arrhythmias. However, it is reassuring that in two large placebo-controlled mortality studies in patients with significant heart disease (DIAMOND CHF/MI), there were no more deaths in TIKOSYN-treated patients than in patients given placebo (see **CLINICAL STUDIES**).

Drug-Drug Interactions (see CONTRAINDICATIONS)

Because there is a linear relationship between dofetilide plasma concentration and QTc, concomitant drugs that interfere with the metabolism or renal elimination of dofetilide may increase the risk of arrhythmia (torsade de pointes). TIKOSYN is metabolized to a small degree by the CYP3A4 isoenzyme of the cytochrome P450 system and an inhibitor of this system could increase systemic dofetilide exposure. More important, dofetilide is eliminated by cationic renal secretion, and three inhibitors of this process have been shown to increase systemic dofetilide exposure. The magnitude of the effect on renal elimination by cimeti-

Continued on next page

Tikosyn—Cont.

dine, trimethoprim and ketoconazole (all contraindicated concomitant uses with dofetilide) suggests that all renal cation transport inhibitors should be contraindicated.

Use with Drugs that Prolong QT Interval and Antiarrhythmic Agents

The use of TIKOSYN in conjunction with other drugs that prolong the QT interval has not been studied and is not recommended. Such drugs include phenothiazines, cisapride, bepridil, tricyclic antidepressants, and certain oral macrolides. Class I or Class III antiarrhythmic agents should be withheld for at least three half-lives prior to dosing with TIKOSYN. In clinical trials, TIKOSYN was administered to patients previously treated with oral amiodarone only if serum amiodarone levels were below 0.3 mg/L or amiodarone had been withdrawn for at least three months.

PRECAUTIONS

Renal Impairment

The overall systemic clearance of dofetilide is decreased and plasma concentration increased with decreasing creatinine clearance. The dose of TIKOSYN must be adjusted based on creatinine clearance (see **DOSAGE AND ADMINISTRATION**). Patients undergoing dialysis were not included in clinical studies, and appropriate dosing recommendations for these patients are unknown. There is no information about the effectiveness of hemodialysis in removing dofetilide from plasma.

Hepatic Impairment

After adjustment for creatinine clearance, no additional dose adjustment is required for patients with mild or moderate hepatic impairment. Patients with severe hepatic impairment have not been studied. TIKOSYN should be used with particular caution in these patients.

Cardiac Conduction Disturbances

Animal and human studies have not shown any adverse effects of dofetilide on conduction velocity. No effect on AV nodal conduction following TIKOSYN treatment was noted in normal volunteers and in patients with 1st degree heart block. Patients with sick sinus syndrome or with 2nd or 3rd degree heart block were not included in the Phase 3 clinical trials unless a functioning pacemaker was present. TIKOSYN has been used safely in conjunction with pacemakers (53 patients in DIAMOND studies, 136 in trials in patients with ventricular and supraventricular arrhythmias).

Potassium-Depleting Diuretics

Hypokalemia or hypomagnesemia may occur with administration of potassium-depleting diuretics, increasing the potential for torsade de pointes. Potassium levels should be within the normal range prior to administration of TIKOSYN and maintained in the normal range during administration of TIKOSYN.

Information for Patients

Please refer patient to the patient package insert.

Prior to initiation of TIKOSYN therapy, the patient should be advised to read the patient package insert and reread it each time therapy is renewed in case the patient's status has changed. The patient should be fully instructed on the need for compliance with the recommended dosing of TIKOSYN and the potential for drug interactions, and the need for periodic monitoring of QTc and renal function to minimize the risk of serious abnormal rhythms.

Medications and Supplements: Assessment of patients' medication history should include all over-the-counter, prescription and herbal/natural preparations with emphasis on preparations that may affect the pharmacokinetics of TIKOSYN such as cimetidine (see **CONTRAINDICATIONS**), trimethoprim alone or in combination with sulfamethoxazole (see **CONTRAINDICATIONS**), prochlorperazine (see **CONTRAINDICATIONS**), megestrol (see **CONTRAINDICATIONS**), ketoconazole (see **CONTRAINDICATIONS**), other cardiovascular drugs (especially verapamil—see **CONTRAINDICATIONS**), phenothiazines, and tricyclic antidepressants (see **WARNINGS**). If a patient is taking TIKOSYN and requires anti-ulcer therapy, omeprazole, ranitidine or antacids (aluminum and magnesium hydroxides) should be used as alternatives to cimetidine, as these agents have no effect on the pharmacokinetics of TIKOSYN. Patients should be instructed to notify their health care providers of any change in over-the-counter, prescription or supplement use. If a patient is hospitalized or is prescribed a new medication for any condition, the patient must inform the health care provider of ongoing TIKOSYN therapy. Patients should also check with their health care provider and/or pharmacist prior to taking a new over-the-counter preparation.

Electrolyte Imbalance: If patients experience symptoms that may be associated with altered electrolyte balance, such as excessive or prolonged diarrhea, sweating, or vomiting or loss of appetite or thirst, these conditions should immediately be reported to their health care provider.

Dosing Schedule: Patients should be instructed NOT to double the next dose if a dose is missed. The next dose should be taken at the usual time.

Drug/Laboratory Test Interactions

None known.

Drug-Drug Interactions

Cimetidine: (see **CONTRAINDICATIONS**) Concomitant use of cimetidine is contraindicated. Cimetidine at 400 mg BID (the usual prescription dose) co-administered with TIKOSYN (500 mcg BID) for 7 days has been shown to increase dofetilide plasma levels by 58%. Cimetidine at doses of 100 mg BID (OTC dose) resulted in a 13% increase in dofetilide plasma levels (500 mcg single dose). No studies have been conducted at intermediate doses of cimetidine. If a patient requires TIKOSYN and anti-ulcer therapy, it is suggested that omeprazole, ranitidine, or antacids (aluminum and magnesium hydroxides) be used as alternatives to cimetidine, as these agents have no effect on the pharmacokinetic profile of TIKOSYN.

Verapamil: (see **CONTRAINDICATIONS**) Concomitant use of verapamil is contraindicated. Co-administration of TIKOSYN with verapamil resulted in increases in dofetilide peak plasma levels of 42%, although overall exposure to dofetilide was not significantly increased. In an analysis of the supraventricular arrhythmia and DIAMOND patient populations, the concomitant administration of verapamil with dofetilide was associated with a higher occurrence of torsade de pointes.

Ketoconazole: (see **CONTRAINDICATIONS**) Concomitant use of ketoconazole is contraindicated. Ketoconazole at 400 mg daily (the maximum approved prescription dose) co-administered with TIKOSYN (500 mcg BID) for 7 days has been shown to increase dofetilide Cmax by 53% in males and 97% in females, and AUC by 41% in males and 69% in females.

Trimethoprim Alone or in Combination with Sulfamethoxazole: (see **CONTRAINDICATIONS**) Concomitant use of trimethoprim alone or in combination with sulfamethoxazole is contraindicated. Trimethoprim 160 mg in combination with 800 mg sulfamethoxazole co-administered BID with TIKOSYN (500 mcg BID) for 4 days has been shown to increase dofetilide AUC by 103% and Cmax by 93%.

Potential Drug Interactions

Dofetilide is eliminated in the kidney by cationic secretion. Inhibitors of renal cationic secretion are contraindicated with TIKOSYN. In addition, drugs that are actively secreted via this route (e.g., triamterene, metformin and amiloride) should be co-administered with care as they might increase dofetilide levels.

Dofetilide is metabolized to a small extent by the CYP3A4 isoenzyme of the cytochrome P450 system. Inhibitors of the CYP3A4 isoenzyme could increase systemic dofetilide exposure. Inhibitors of this isoenzyme (e.g., macrolide antibiotics, azole antifungal agents, protease inhibitors, serotonin reuptake inhibitors, amiodarone, cannabinoids, diltiazem, grapefruit juice, nefazadone, norfloxacin, quinine, zafirlukast) should be cautiously coadministered with TIKOSYN as they can potentially increase dofetilide levels. Dofetilide is not an inhibitor of CYP3A4 nor of other cytochrome P450 isoenzymes (e.g., CYP2C9, CYP2D6) and is not expected to increase levels of drugs metabolized by CYP3A4.

Other Drug Interaction Information

Digoxin: Studies in healthy volunteers have shown that TIKOSYN does not affect the pharmacokinetics of digoxin. In patients, the concomitant administration of digoxin with dofetilide was associated with a higher occurrence of torsade de pointes. It is not clear whether this represents an interaction with TIKOSYN or the presence of more severe structural heart disease in patients on digoxin; structural heart disease is a known risk factor for arrhythmia. No increase in mortality was observed in patients taking digoxin as concomitant medication.

Other Drugs: In healthy volunteers, amlodipine, phenytoin, glyburide, ranitidine, omeprazole, hormone replacement therapy (a combination of conjugated estrogens and medroxyprogesterone), antacid (aluminum and magnesium hydroxides) and theophylline did not affect the pharmacokinetics of TIKOSYN. In addition, studies in healthy volunteers have shown that TIKOSYN does not affect the pharmacokinetics or pharmacodynamics of warfarin, or the pharmacokinetics of propranolol (40 mg twice daily), phenytoin, theophylline, or oral contraceptives.

Population pharmacokinetic analyses were conducted on plasma concentration data from 1445 patients in clinical trials to examine the effects of concomitant medications on clearance or volume of distribution of dofetilide. Concomitant medications were grouped as ACE inhibitors, oral anticoagulants, calcium channel blockers, beta blockers, cardiac glycosides, inducers of CYP3A4, substrates and inhibitors of CYP3A4, substrates and inhibitors of P-glycoprotein, nitrates, sulphonylureas, loop diuretics, potassium sparing diuretics, thiazide diuretics, substrates and inhibitors of tubular organic cation transport, and QTc-prolonging drugs. Differences in clearance between patients on these medications (at any occasion in the study) and those off medications varied between -16% and +3%. The mean clearances of dofetilide were 16% and 15% lower in patients on thiazide diuretics and inhibitors of tubular organic cation transport, respectively.

Carcinogenesis, Mutagenesis, Impairment of Fertility

Dofetilide had no genotoxic effects, with or without metabolic activation, based on the bacterial mutation assay and tests of cytogenetic aberrations *in vivo* in mouse bone marrow and *in vitro* in human lymphocytes. Rats and mice treated with dofetilide in the diet for two years showed no evidence of an increased incidence of tumors compared to controls. The highest dofetilide dose administered for 24 months was 10 mg/kg/day to rats and 20 mg/kg/day to mice. Mean dofetilide $AUCs_{(0-24hr)}$ at these doses were about 26 and 10 times, respectively, the maximum likely human AUC.

There was no effect on mating or fertility when dofetilide was administered to male and female rats at doses as high as 1.0 mg/kg/day, a dose that would be expected to provide a mean dofetilide AUC $_{(0-24hr)}$ about 3 times the maximum likely human AUC. Increased incidences of testicular atrophy and epididymal oligospermia and a reduction in testicular weight were, however, observed in other studies in rats. Reduced testicular weight and increased incidence of testicular atrophy were also consistent findings in dogs and mice. The no effect doses for these findings in chronic administration studies in these 3 species (3, 0.1 and 6 mg/kg/day) were associated with mean dofetilide AUCs that were about 4, 1.3 and 3 times the maximum likely human AUC, respectively.

Pregnancy Category C

Dofetilide has been shown to adversely affect *in utero* growth and survival of rats and mice when orally administered during organogenesis at doses of 2 or more mg/kg/day. Other than an increased incidence of non-ossified 5th metacarpal, and the occurrence of hydroureter and hydronephroses at doses as low as 1 mg/kg/day in the rat, structural anomalies associated with drug treatment were not observed in either species at doses below 2 mg/kg/day. The clearest drug-effect associations were for sternebral and vertebral anomalies in both species; cleft palate, adactyly, levocardia, dilation of cerebral ventricles, hydroureter, hydronephroses, and unossified metacarpal in the rat; and increased incidence of unossified calcaneum in the mouse. The "no observed adverse effect dose" in both species was 0.5 mg/kg/day. The mean dofetilide $AUCs_{(0-24hr)}$ at this dose in the rat and mouse are estimated to be about equal to the maximum likely human AUC and about half the likely human AUC, respectively. There are no adequate and well controlled studies in pregnant women. Therefore, dofetilide should only be administered to pregnant women where the benefit to the patient justifies the potential risk to the fetus.

Nursing Mothers

There is no information on the presence of dofetilide in breast milk. Patients should be advised not to breast feed an infant if they are taking TIKOSYN.

Geriatric Use

Of the total number of patients in clinical studies of TIKOSYN, 46% were 65 to 89 years old. No overall differences in safety, effect on QTc, or effectiveness were observed between elderly and younger patients. Because elderly patients are more likely to have decreased renal function with a reduced creatinine clearance, care must be taken in dose selection. (See **DOSAGE AND ADMINISTRATION**.)

Use in Women

Female patients constituted 32% of the patients in the placebo-controlled trials of TIKOSYN. As with other drugs that cause torsade de pointes, TIKOSYN was associated with a greater risk of torsade de pointes in female patients than in male patients. During the TIKOSYN clinical development program the risk of torsade de pointes in females was approximately 3 times the risk in males. Unlike torsade de pointes, the incidence of other ventricular arrhythmias was similar in female patients receiving TIKOSYN and patients receiving placebo. Although no study specifically investigated this risk, in post-hoc analyses, no increased mortality was observed in females on TIKOSYN compared to females on placebo.

Pediatric Use

The safety and effectiveness of TIKOSYN in children (<18 years old) has not been established.

ADVERSE REACTIONS

The TIKOSYN clinical program involved approximately 8,600 patients in 130 clinical studies of normal volunteers and patients with supraventricular and ventricular arrhythmias. TIKOSYN was administered to 5,194 patients, including two large, placebo-controlled mortality trials (DIAMOND CHF and DIAMOND MI) in which 1,511 patients received TIKOSYN for up to three years.

In the following section, adverse reaction data for cardiac arrhythmias and non-cardiac adverse reactions are presented separately for patients included in the supraventricular arrhythmia development program and for patients included in the DIAMOND CHF and MI mortality trials (see **CLINICAL STUDIES: Safety in Patients with Structural Heart Disease—DIAMOND Studies**, for a description of these trials).

In studies of patients with supraventricular arrhythmias a total of 1346 and 677 patients were exposed to TIKOSYN and placebo for 551 and 207 patient years, respectively. A total of 8.7% of patients in the dofetilide groups were discontinued from clinical trials due to adverse events compared to 8.0% in the placebo groups. The most frequent reason for discontinuation (>1%) was ventricular tachycardia (2.0% on dofetilide vs. 1.3% on placebo). The most frequent adverse events were headache, chest pain, and dizziness.

Serious Arrhythmias and Conduction Disturbances: Torsade de pointes is the only arrhythmia that showed a dose-response relationship to TIKOSYN treatment. It did not occur in placebo treated patients. The incidence of torsade de pointes in patients with supraventricular arrhythmias was 0.8% (11/1346) (see **WARNINGS**). The incidence of torsade de pointes in patients who were dosed according to the recommended dosing regimen (see **DOSAGE AND ADMINISTRATION**) was 0.8% (4/525). Table 6 shows the frequency by randomized dose of serious arrhythmias and conduction disturbances reported as adverse events in patients with supraventricular arrhythmias.

[See table 6 at top of next page]

In the DIAMOND trials a total of 1511 patients were exposed to TIKOSYN for 1757 patient years. The incidence of torsade de pointes was 3.3% in CHF patients and 0.9% in patients with a recent MI.

Table 7 shows the incidence of serious arrhythmias and conduction disturbances reported as adverse events in the DIAMOND subpopulation that had AF at entry to these trials. [See table 7 at right]

Other Adverse Reactions: Table 8 presents other adverse events reported with a frequency of >2% on TIKOSYN and reported numerically more frequently on TIKOSYN than on placebo in the studies of patients with supraventricular arrhythmias.

Table 8: Frequency of Adverse Events Occurring at >2% on TIKOSYN, and Numerically More Frequently on TIKOSYN than Placebo in Patients with Supraventricular Arrhythmias

	TIKOSYN	Placebo
Adverse Event	%	%
headache	11	9
chest pain	10	7
dizziness	8	6
respiratory tract infection	7	5
dyspnea	6	5
nausea	5	4
flu syndrome	4	2
insomnia	4	3
accidental injury	3	1
back pain	3	2
procedure (medical/ surgical/health service)	3	2
diarrhea	3	2
rash	3	2
abdominal pain	3	2

Adverse events reported at a rate >2% but no more frequently on TIKOSYN than on placebo were: angina pectoris, anxiety, arthralgia, asthenia, atrial fibrillation, complications (application, injection, incision, insertion, or device), hypertension, pain, palpitation, peripheral edema, supraventricular tachycardia, sweating, urinary tract infection, ventricular tachycardia.

The following adverse events have been reported with a frequency of ≤2% and numerically more frequently with TIKOSYN than placebo in patients with supraventricular arrhythmias: angioedema, bradycardia, cerebral ischemia, cerebrovascular accident, edema, facial paralysis, flaccid paralysis, heart arrest, increased cough, liver damage, migraine, myocardial infarct, paralysis, paresthesia, sudden death, and syncope.

The incidences of clinically significant laboratory test abnormalities in patients with supraventricular arrhythmias were similar for patients on TIKOSYN and those on placebo. No clinically relevant effects were noted in serum alkaline phosphatase, serum GGT, LDH, AST, ALT, total bilirubin, total protein, blood urea nitrogen, creatinine, serum electrolytes (calcium, chloride, glucose, magnesium, potassium, sodium) or creatine kinase. Similarly, no clinically relevant effects were observed in hematologic parameters.

In the DIAMOND population, adverse events other than those related to the post-infarction and heart failure patient population were generally similar to those seen in the supraventricular arrhythmia groups.

OVERDOSAGE

There is no known antidote to TIKOSYN; treatment of overdose should therefore be symptomatic and supportive. The most prominent manifestation of overdosage is likely to be excessive prolongation of the QT interval.

In cases of overdose cardiac monitoring should be initiated. Charcoal slurry may be given soon after overdosing but has been useful only when given within 15 minutes of TIKOSYN administration. Treatment of torsade de pointes or overdose may include administration of isoproterenol infusion, with or without cardiac pacing. Administration of intravenous magnesium sulfate may be effective in the management of torsade de pointes. Close medical monitoring and supervision should continue until the QT interval returns to normal levels.

Isoproterenol infusion into anesthetized dogs with cardiac pacing rapidly attenuates the dofetilide-induced prolongation of atrial and ventricular effective refractory periods in a dose-dependent manner. Magnesium sulfate, administered prophylactically either intravenously or orally in a dog model, was effective in the prevention of dofetilide-induced torsade de pointes ventricular tachycardia. Similarly, in man, intravenous magnesium sulfate may terminate torsade de pointes, irrespective of cause.

TIKOSYN overdose was rare in clinical studies; there were two reported cases of TIKOSYN overdose in the oral clinical program. One patient received very high multiples of the recommended dose (28 capsules), was treated with gastric aspiration 30 minutes later, and experienced no events. One patient inadvertently received two 500 mcg doses one hour apart and experienced ventricular fibrillation and cardiac arrest 2 hours after the second dose.

In the supraventricular arrhythmia population only 38 patients received doses greater than 500 mcg BID, all of whom received 750 mcg BID irrespective of creatinine clearance. In this very small patient population the incidence of torsade de pointes was 10.5% (4/38 patients), and the incidence of new ventricular fibrillation was 2.6% (1/38 patients).

Table 6: Incidence of Serious Arrhythmias and Conduction Disturbances in Patients with Supraventricular Arrhythmias

	TIKOSYN Dose				Placebo
Arrhythmia event:	<250 mcg BID N=217	250 mcg BID N=388	>250-500 mcg BID N=703	>500 mcg BID N=38	N=677
Ventricular arrhythmias* ^	3.7%	2.6%	3.4%	15.8%	2.7%
Ventricular fibrillation	0	0.3%	0.4%	2.6%	0.1%
Ventricular tachycardia^	3.7%	2.6%	3.3%	13.2%	2.5%
Torsade de pointes	0	0.3%	0.9%	10.5%	0
Various forms of block					
AV block	0.9%	1.5%	0.4%	0	0.3%
Bundle branch block	0	0.5%	0.1%	0	0.1%
Heart block	0	0.5%	0.1%	0	0.1%

* Patients with more than one arrhythmia are counted only once in this category.
^ Ventricular arrhythmias and ventricular tachycardia include all cases of torsade de pointes.

Table 7: Incidence of Serious Arrhythmias and Conduction Disturbances in Patients with AF at Entry to the DIAMOND Studies

	TIKOSYN	Placebo
	N=249	N=257
Ventricular arrhythmias*^	14.5%	13.6%
Ventricular fibrillation	4.8%	3.1%
Ventricular tachycardia^	12.4%	11.3%
Torsade de pointes	1.6%	0
Various forms of block		
AV block	0.8%	2.7%
(Left) bundle branch block	0	0.4%
Heart block	1.2%	0.8%

* Patients with more than one arrhythmia are counted only once in this category.
^ Ventricular arrhythmias and ventricular tachycardia include all cases of torsade de pointes.

$$\text{creatinine clearance (male)} = \frac{(140\text{-age}) \times \text{body weight in kg}}{72 \times \text{serum creatinine (mg/dL)}}$$

$$\text{creatinine clearance (female)} = \frac{(140\text{-age}) \times \text{body weight in kg} \times 0.85}{72 \times \text{serum creatinine (mg/dL)}}$$

DOSAGE AND ADMINISTRATION

- Therapy with TIKOSYN must be initiated (and, if necessary, re-initiated) in a setting that provides continuous electrocardiographic (ECG) monitoring and in the presence of personnel trained in the management of serious ventricular arrhythmias. Patients should continue to be monitored in this way for a minimum of three days. Additionally, patients should not be discharged within 12 hours of electrical or pharmacological conversion to normal sinus rhythm.
- **The dose of TIKOSYN must be individualized according to calculated creatinine clearance and QTc. (QT interval should be used if the heart rate is <60 beats per minute. There are no data on use of TIKOSYN when the heart rate is <50 beats per minute.)** The usual recommended dose of TIKOSYN is 500 mcg BID, as modified by the dosing algorithm described below. For consideration of a lower dose, see **Special Considerations** below.
- Patients with atrial fibrillation should be anticoagulated according to usual medical practice prior to electrical or pharmacological cardioversion. Anticoagulant therapy may be continued after cardioversion according to usual medical practice for the treatment of people with AF. Hypokalemia should be corrected before initiation of TIKOSYN therapy (see **WARNINGS, Ventricular Arrhythmia**).
- Patients to be discharged on TIKOSYN therapy from an in-patient setting as described above must have an adequate supply of TIKOSYN, at the patient's individualized dose, to allow uninterrupted dosing until the patient receives the first outpatient supply.
- TIKOSYN is distributed only to those hospitals and other appropriate institutions confirmed to have received applicable dosing and treatment initiation education programs. Inpatient and subsequent outpatient discharge and refill prescriptions are filled only upon confirmation that the prescribing physician has received applicable dosing and treatment initiation education programs. For this purpose, a list for use by pharmacists is maintained containing hospitals and physicians who have received one of the education programs.

Instructions for Individualized Dose Initiation

Initiation of TIKOSYN Therapy

Step 1. Electrocardiographic assessment: Prior to administration of the first dose, the QTc must be determined using an average of 5–10 beats. If the QTc is greater than 440 msec (500 msec in patients with ventricular conduction abnormalities), TIKOSYN is contraindicated. If heart rate is less than 60 beats per minute, QT interval should be used. Patients with heart rates <50 beats per minute have not been studied.

Step 2. Calculation of creatinine clearance: Prior to the administration of the first dose, the patient's creatinine clearance must be calculated using the following formula:
[See third table above]
When serum creatinine is given in µmol/L, divide the value by 88.4 (1 mg/dL = 88.4 µmol/L).

Step 3. Starting Dose: The starting dose of TIKOSYN is determined as follows:

Calculated Creatinine Clearance	TIKOSYN Dose
>60 mL/min	500 mcg twice daily
40–60 mL/min	250 mcg twice daily
20–<40 mL/min	125 mcg twice daily
<20 mL/min	Dofetilide is contraindicated in these patients

Step 4. Administer the adjusted TIKOSYN dose and begin continuous ECG monitoring.

Step 5. At 2–3 hours after administering the first dose of TIKOSYN, determine the QTc. If the QTc has increased by greater than 15% compared to the baseline established in Step 1 OR if the QTc is greater than 500 msec (550 msec in patients with ventricular conduction abnormalities), subsequent dosing should be adjusted as follows:

Continued on next page

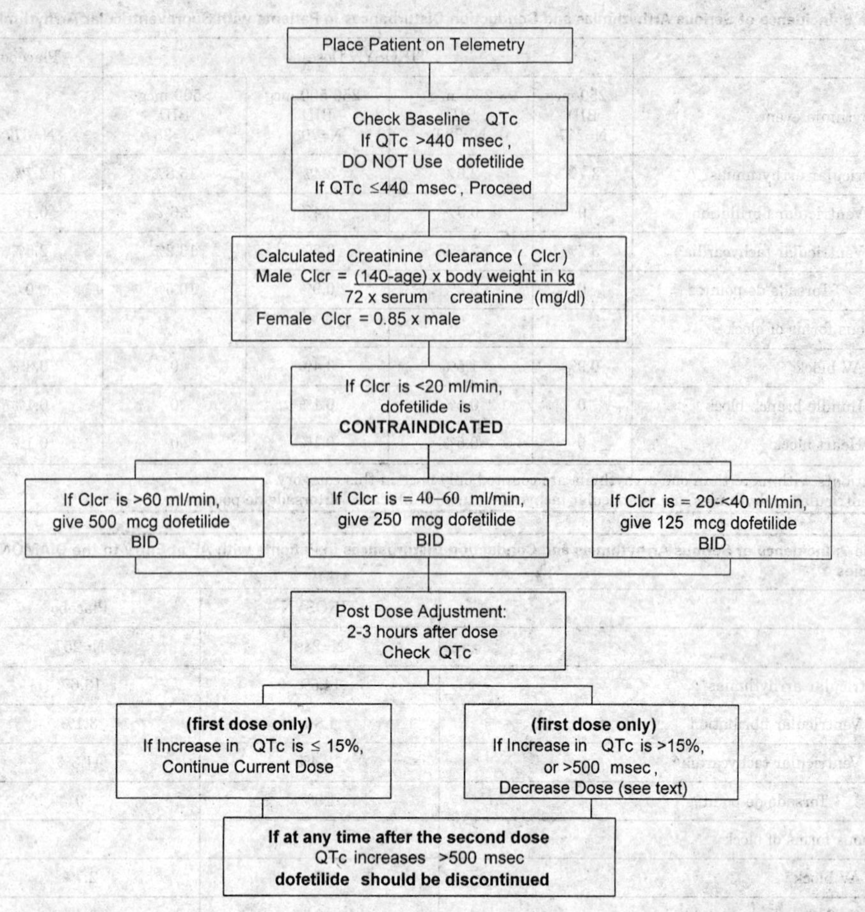

	125 mcg (0.125 mg)	250 mcg (0.25 mg)	500 mcg (0.5 mg)
Obverse:	TKN 125	TKN 250	TKN 500
Reverse	PFIZER	PFIZER	PFIZER
Bottle of 14	0069-5800-61	0069-5810-61	0069-5820-61
Bottle of 60	0069-5800-60	0069-5810-60	0069-5820-60
Unit dose / 40	0069-5800-43	0069-5810-43	0069-5820-43

Tikosyn—Cont.

If the Starting Dose Based on Creatinine Clearance is:	Then the Adjusted Dose (for QTc Prolongation) is:
500 mcg twice daily	250 mcg twice daily
250 mcg twice daily	125 mcg twice daily
125 mcg twice daily	125 mcg once a day

Step 6. At 2–3 hours after each subsequent dose of TIKOSYN, determine the QTc (for in-hospital doses 2–5). No further down titration of TIKOSYN based on QTc is recommended.

NOTE: If at any time after the second dose of TIKOSYN is given, the QTc is greater than 500 msec (550 msec in patients with ventricular conduction abnormalities) TIKOSYN should be discontinued.

Step 7. Patients are to be continuously monitored by ECG for a minimum of three days, or for a minimum of 12 hours after electrical or pharmacological conversion to normal sinus rhythm, whichever is greater.

The steps described above are summarized in the following diagram:

[See graphic above]

Maintenance of TIKOSYN Therapy

Renal function and QTc should be re-evaluated every three months or as medically warranted. If QTc exceeds 500 milliseconds (550 msec in patients with ventricular conduction abnormalities), TIKOSYN therapy should be discontinued and patients should be carefully monitored until QTc returns to baseline levels. If renal function deteriorates, adjust dose as described in **Initiation of TIKOSYN Therapy, Step 3.**

Special Considerations

Consideration of a Dose Lower than that Determined by the Algorithm: The dosing algorithm shown above should be used to determine the individualized dose of TIKOSYN. In clinical trials (see **CLINICAL STUDIES**), the highest dose of 500 mcg BID of TIKOSYN as modified by the dosing algorithm led to greater effectiveness than lower doses of 125 or 250 mcg BID as modified by the dosing algorithm. The risk of torsade de pointes, however, is related to dose as well as to patient characteristics (see **WARNINGS**). Physicians, in consultation with their patients, may therefore in some cases choose doses lower than determined by the algorithm. It is critically important that if at any time this lower dose is increased, the patient needs to be rehospitalized for three days. Previous toleration of higher doses does not eliminate the need for rehospitalization.

The maximum recommended dose in patients with a calculated creatinine clearance greater than 60 mL/min is 500 mcg BID; doses greater than 500 mcg BID have been associated with an increased incidence of torsade de pointes.

A patient who misses a dose should NOT double the next dose. The next dose should be taken at the usual time.

Cardioversion: If patients do not convert to normal sinus rhythm within 24 hours of initiation of TIKOSYN therapy, electrical conversion should be considered. Patients continuing on TIKOSYN after successful electrical cardioversion should continue to be monitored by electrocardiography for 12 hours post cardioversion, or a minimum of 3 days after initiation of TIKOSYN therapy, whichever is greater.

Switch to TIKOSYN from Class I or other Class III Antiarrhythmic Therapy

Before initiating TIKOSYN therapy, previous antiarrhythmic therapy should be withdrawn under careful monitoring for a minimum of three (3) plasma half-lives. Because of the unpredictable pharmacokinetics of amiodarone, TIKOSYN should not be initiated following amiodarone therapy until amiodarone plasma levels are below 0.3 mcg/mL or until amiodarone has been withdrawn for at least three months.

Stopping TIKOSYN Prior to Administration of Potentially Interacting Drugs

If TIKOSYN needs to be discontinued to allow dosing of other potentially interacting drug(s), a washout period of at least two days should be followed before starting the other drug(s).

HOW SUPPLIED

TIKOSYN™ 125 mcg (0.125 mg) capsules are supplied as No. 4 capsules with a light orange cap and white body, printed with TKN 125 PFIZER, and are available in:

TIKOSYN 250 mcg (0.25 mg) capsules are supplied as No. 4 capsules, peach cap and body, printed with TKN 250 PFIZER, and are available in:

TIKOSYN 500 mcg (0.5 mg) capsules are supplied as No. 2 capsules, peach cap and white body, printed with TKN 500 PFIZER, and are available in:

[See table above]

Store at controlled room temperature, 15° to 30°C (59° to 86°F).

PROTECT FROM MOISTURE AND HUMIDITY.

Dispense in tight containers (USP).

Rx only

Pfizer Labs
Division of Pfizer Inc, NY, NY 10017
69-5549-00-2 Issued December 1999

Shown in Product Identification Guide, page 329

UNASYN® ℞

[ew-nă-sĭn]

(ampicillin sodium/sulbactam sodium)

To reduce the development of drug-resistant bacteria and maintain the effectiveness of UNASYN® and other antibacterial drugs, UNASYN should be used only to treat or prevent infections that are proven or strongly suspected to be caused by bacteria.

DESCRIPTION

UNASYN is an injectable antibacterial combination consisting of the semisynthetic antibiotic ampicillin sodium and the beta-lactamase inhibitor sulbactam sodium for intravenous and intramuscular administration.

Ampicillin sodium is derived from the penicillin nucleus, 6-aminopenicillanic acid. Chemically, it is monosodium (2S, 5R, 6R)-6-[(R)-2-amino-2-phenylacetamido]-3,3-dimethyl-7-oxo-4-thia-1-azabicyclo[3.2.0]heptane-2-carboxylate and has a molecular weight of 371.39. Its chemical formula is $C_{16}H_{18}N_3NaO_4S$. The structural formula is:

Sulbactam sodium is a derivative of the basic penicillin nucleus. Chemically, sulbactam sodium is sodium penicillinate sulfone; sodium (2S, 5R)-3,3-dimethyl-7-oxo-4-thia- 1-azabicyclo [3.2.0] heptane-2-carboxylate 4,4-dioxide. Its chemical formula is $C_8H_{10}NNaO_5S$ with a molecular weight of 255.22. The structural formula is:

UNASYN, ampicillin sodium/sulbactam sodium parenteral combination, is available as a white to off-white dry powder for reconstitution. UNASYN dry powder is freely soluble in aqueous diluents to yield pale yellow to yellow solutions containing ampicillin sodium and sulbactam sodium equivalent to 250 mg ampicillin per mL and 125 mg sulbactam per mL. The pH of the solutions is between 8.0 and 10.0.

Dilute solutions (up to 30 mg ampicillin and 15 mg sulbactam per mL) are essentially colorless to pale yellow. The pH of dilute solutions remains the same.

1.5 g of UNASYN (1 g ampicillin as the sodium salt plus 0.5 g sulbactam as the sodium salt) parenteral contains approximately 115 mg (5 mEq) of sodium.

3 g of UNASYN (2 g ampicillin as the sodium salt plus 1 g sulbactam as the sodium salt) parenteral contains approximately 230 mg (10 mEq) of sodium.

CLINICAL PHARMACOLOGY

General: Immediately after completion of a 15-minute intravenous infusion of UNASYN, peak serum concentrations of ampicillin and sulbactam are attained. Ampicillin serum levels are similar to those produced by the administration of equivalent amounts of ampicillin alone. Peak ampicillin serum levels ranging from 109 to 150 mcg/mL are attained after administration of 2000 mg of ampicillin plus 1000 mg sulbactam and 40 to 71 mcg/mL after administration of 1000 mg ampicillin plus 500 mg sulbactam. The corresponding mean peak serum levels for sulbactam range from 48 to 88 mcg/mL and 21 to 40 mcg/mL, respectively. After an intramuscular injection of 1000 mg ampicillin plus 500 mg sulbactam, peak ampicillin serum levels ranging from 8 to 37 mcg/mL and peak sulbactam serum levels ranging from 6 to 24 mcg/mL are attained.

The mean serum half-life of both drugs is approximately 1 hour in healthy volunteers.

Approximately 75 to 85% of both ampicillin and sulbactam are excreted unchanged in the urine during the first 8 hours after administration of UNASYN to individuals with normal renal function. Somewhat higher and more prolonged serum levels of ampicillin and sulbactam can be achieved with the concurrent administration of probenecid.

In patients with impaired renal function the elimination kinetics of ampicillin and sulbactam are similarly affected, hence the ratio of one to the other will remain constant whatever the renal function. The dose of UNASYN in such patients should be administered less frequently in accordance with the usual practice for ampicillin (see DOSAGE and ADMINISTRATION).

Ampicillin has been found to be approximately 28% reversibly bound to human serum protein and sulbactam approximately 38% reversibly bound.
The following average levels of ampicillin and sulbactam were measured in the tissues and fluids listed:

TABLE A
Concentration of UNASYN in Various Body Tissues and Fluids

Fluid or Tissue	Dose (grams) Ampicillin/ Sulbactam	Concentration (mcg/mL or mcg/g) Ampicillin/ Sulbactam
Peritoneal Fluid	0.5/0.5 IV	7/14
Blister Fluid (Cantharides)	0.5/0.5 IV	8/20
Tissue Fluid	1/0.5 IV	8/4
Intestinal Mucosa	0.5/0.5 IV	11/18
Appendix	2/1 IV	3/40

Penetration of both ampicillin and sulbactam into cerebrospinal fluid in the presence of inflamed meninges has been demonstrated after IV administration of UNASYN.
The pharmacokinetics of ampicillin and sulbactam in pediatric patients receiving UNASYN are similar to those observed in adults. Immediately after a 15-minute infusion of 50 to 75 mg UNASYN/kg body weight, peak serum and plasma concentrations of 82 to 446 mcg ampicillin/mL and 44 to 203 mcg sulbactam/mL were obtained. Mean half-life values were approximately 1 hour.

MICROBIOLOGY

Ampicillin is similar to benzyl penicillin in its bactericidal action against susceptible organisms during the stage of active multiplication. It acts through the inhibition of cell wall mucopeptide biosynthesis. Ampicillin has a broad spectrum of bactericidal activity against many gram-positive and gram-negative aerobic and anaerobic bacteria. (Ampicillin is, however, degraded by beta-lactamases and therefore the spectrum of activity does not normally include organisms which produce these enzymes.)
A wide range of beta-lactamases found in microorganisms resistant to penicillins and cephalosporins have been shown in biochemical studies with cell free bacterial systems to be irreversibly inhibited by sulbactam. Although sulbactam alone possesses little useful antibacterial activity except against the *Neisseriaceae*, whole organism studies have shown that sulbactam restores ampicillin activity against beta-lactamase producing strains. In particular, sulbactam has good inhibitory activity against the clinically important plasmid mediated beta-lactamases most frequently responsible for transferred drug resistance. Sulbactam has no effect on the activity of ampicillin against ampicillin susceptible strains.
The presence of sulbactam in the UNASYN formulation effectively extends the antibiotic spectrum of ampicillin to include many bacteria normally resistant to it and to other beta-lactam antibiotics. Thus, UNASYN possesses the properties of a broad-spectrum antibiotic and a beta-lactamase inhibitor.
While *in vitro* studies have demonstrated the susceptibility of most strains of the following organisms, clinical efficacy for infections other than those included in the indications section has not been documented.
Gram-Positive Bacteria: *Staphylococcus aureus* (beta-lactamase and non-beta-lactamase producing), *Staphylococcus epidermidis* (beta-lactamase and non-beta-lactamase producing), *Staphylococcus saprophyticus* (beta-lactamase and non-beta-lactamase producing), *Streptococcus faecalis*† (Enterococcus), *Streptococcus pneumoniae*† (formerly *D. pneumoniae), Streptococcus pyogenes*†, *Streptococcus viridans*†.
Gram-Negative Bacteria: *Hemophilus influenzae* (beta-lactamase and non-beta-lactamase producing), *Moraxella (Branhamella) catarrhalis* (beta-lactamase and non-beta-lactamase producing), *Escherichia coli* (beta-lactamase and non-beta-lactamase producing), *Klebsiella* species (all known strains are beta-lactamase producing), *Proteus mirabilis* (beta-lactamase and non-beta-lactamase producing), *Proteus vulgaris, Providencia rettgeri, Providencia stuartii, Morganella morganii*, and *Neisseria gonorrhoeae* (beta-lactamase and non-beta-lactamase producing).
Anaerobes: *Clostridium* species†, *Peptococcus* species†, *Peptostreptococcus* species, *Bacteroides* species, including *B. fragilis*.
†These are not beta-lactamase producing strains and, therefore, are susceptible to ampicillin alone.
Susceptibility Testing
Diffusion Technique: For the Kirby-Bauer method of susceptibility testing, a 20 mcg (10 mcg ampicillin + 10 mcg sulbactam) diffusion disk should be used. The method is one outlined in the NCCLS publication M2-A4.[1] With this procedure, a report from the laboratory of "Susceptible" indicates that the infecting organism is likely to respond to UNASYN therapy and a report of "Resistant" indicates that the infecting organism is not likely to respond to therapy. An "Intermediate" susceptibility report suggests that the infecting organism would be susceptible to UNASYN if a higher dosage is used or if the infection is confined to tissues or fluids (e.g., urine) in which high antibiotic levels are attained.
Dilution Techniques: Broth or agar dilution methods may be used to determine the minimal inhibitory concentration (MIC) value for susceptibility of bacterial isolates to ampicillin/sulbactam. The method used is one outlined in the NCCLS publication M7-A2.[2] Tubes should be inoculated to contain 10^5 to 10^6 organisms/mL or plates "spotted" with 10^4 organisms.
The recommended dilution method employs a constant ampicillin/sulbactam ratio of 2:1 in all tubes with increasing concentrations of ampicillin. MIC's are reported in terms of ampicillin concentration in the presence of sulbactam at a constant 2 parts ampicillin to 1 part sulbactam.
[See table above]

Recommended ampicillin/sulbactam, Susceptibility Ranges[1,2,3]

	Resistant	Intermediate	Susceptible
Gram(-) and Staphylococcus			
Bauer/Kirby Zone Sizes	≤11 mm	12-13 mm	≥14 mm
MIC (mcg of ampicillin/mL)	≥32	16	≤ 8
Hemophilus influenzae			
Bauer/Kirby Zone Sizes	≤19	—	≥20
MIC (mcg of ampicillin/mL)	≥ 4	—	≤ 2

[1] The non-beta-lactamase producing organisms which are normally susceptible to ampicillin, such as *Streptococci*, will have similar zone sizes as for ampicillin disks.
[2] *Staphylococci* resistant to methicillin, oxacillin, or nafcillin must be considered resistant to UNASYN.
[3] The quality control cultures should have the following assigned daily ranges for ampicillin/sulbactam:

		Disks	Mode MIC (mcg/mL ampicillin/ mcg/mL sulbactam)
E. coli	(ATCC 25922)	20-24 mm	2/1
S. aureus	(ATCC 25923)	29-37 mm	0.12/0.06
E. coli	(ATCC 35218)	13-19 mm	8/4

INDICATIONS AND USAGE

UNASYN is indicated for the treatment of infections due to susceptible strains of the designated microorganisms in the conditions listed below.
Skin and Skin Structure Infections caused by beta-lactamase producing strains of *Staphylococcus aureus, Escherichia coli,* Klebsiella* spp.* (including *K. pneumoniae*), Proteus mirabilis,* Bacteroides fragilis,* Enterobacter* spp.,* and *Acinetobacter calcoaceticus.**
NOTE: For information on use in pediatric patients see PRECAUTIONS–Pediatric Use and CLINICAL STUDIES sections.
Intra-Abdominal Infections caused by beta-lactamase producing strains of *Escherichia coli, Klebsiella* spp. (including *K. pneumoniae*), Bacteroides* spp. (including *B. fragilis*), and *Enterobacter* spp.*
Gynecological Infections caused by beta-lactamase producing strains of *Escherichia coli,** and *Bacteroides* spp.* (including *B. fragilis**).
*Efficacy for this organism in this organ system was studied in fewer than 10 infections.
While UNASYN is indicated only for the conditions listed above, infections caused by ampicillin-susceptible organisms are also amenable to treatment with UNASYN due to its ampicillin content. Therefore, mixed infections caused by ampicillin-susceptible organisms and beta-lactamase producing organisms susceptible to UNASYN should not require the addition of another antibiotic.
Appropriate culture and susceptibility tests should be performed before treatment in order to isolate and identify the organisms causing infection and to determine their susceptibility to UNASYN.
Therapy may be instituted prior to obtaining the results from bacteriological and susceptibility studies, when there is reason to believe the infection may involve any of the beta-lactamase producing organisms listed above in the indicated organ systems. Once the results are known, therapy should be adjusted if appropriate.
To reduce the development of drug-resistant bacteria and maintain effectiveness of UNASYN and other antibacterial drugs, UNASYN should be used only to treat or prevent infections that are proven or strongly suspected to be caused by susceptible bacteria. When culture and susceptibility information are available, they should be considered in selecting or modifying antibacterial therapy. In the absence of such data, local epidemiology and susceptibility patterns may contribute to the empiric selection of therapy.

CONTRAINDICATIONS

The use of UNASYN is contraindicated in individuals with a history of hypersensitivity reactions to any of the penicillins.

WARNINGS

SERIOUS AND OCCASIONALLY FATAL HYPERSENSITIVITY (ANAPHYLACTIC) REACTIONS HAVE BEEN REPORTED IN PATIENTS ON PENICILLIN THERAPY. THESE REACTIONS ARE MORE APT TO OCCUR IN INDIVIDUALS WITH A HISTORY OF PENICILLIN HYPERSENSITIVITY AND/OR HYPERSENSITIVITY REACTIONS TO MULTIPLE ALLERGENS. THERE HAVE BEEN REPORTS OF INDIVIDUALS WITH A HISTORY OF PENICILLIN HYPERSENSITIVITY WHO HAVE EXPERIENCED SEVERE REACTIONS WHEN TREATED WITH CEPHALOSPORINS. BEFORE THERAPY WITH A PENICILLIN, CAREFUL INQUIRY SHOULD BE MADE CONCERNING PREVIOUS HYPERSENSITIVITY REACTIONS TO PENICILLINS, CEPHALOSPORINS, AND OTHER ALLERGENS. IF AN ALLERGIC REACTION OCCURS, UNASYN SHOULD BE DISCONTINUED AND THE APPROPRIATE THERAPY INSTITUTED.
SERIOUS ANAPHYLACTOID REACTIONS REQUIRE IMMEDIATE EMERGENCY TREATMENT WITH EPINEPHRINE. OXYGEN, INTRAVENOUS STEROIDS, AND AIRWAY MANAGEMENT, INCLUDING INTUBATION, SHOULD ALSO BE ADMINISTERED AS INDICATED.
Pseudomembranous colitis has been reported with nearly all antibacterial agents, including UNASYN, and has ranged in severity from mild to life-threatening. Therefore, it is important to consider this diagnosis in patients who present with diarrhea subsequent to the administration of antibacterial agents.
Treatment with antibacterial agents alters the normal flora of the colon and may permit overgrowth of clostridia. Studies indicate that toxin produced by *Clostridium difficile* is one primary cause of "antibiotic-associated colitis."
Mild cases of pseudomembranous colitis usually respond to drug discontinuation alone. In moderate to severe cases, consideration should be given to management with fluids and electrolytes, protein supplementation and treatment with an antibacterial drug clinically effective against *C. difficile* colitis.

PRECAUTIONS

General: A high percentage of patients with mononucleosis who receive ampicillin develop a skin rash. Thus, ampicillin class antibiotics should not be administered to patients with mononucleosis. In patients treated with UNASYN the possibility of superinfections with mycotic or bacterial pathogens should be kept in mind during therapy. If superinfections occur (usually involving *Pseudomonas* or *Candida*), the drug should be discontinued and/or appropriate therapy instituted.
Prescribing UNASYN in the absence of proven or strongly suspected bacterial infection or a prophylactic indication is unlikely to provide benefit to the patient and increases the risk of the development of drug-resistant bacteria.
Information for Patients: Patients should be counseled that antibacterial drugs including UNASYN should only be used to treat bacterial infections. They do not treat viral infections (e.g., the common cold). When UNASYN is prescribed to treat a bacterial infection, patients should be told that although it is common to feel better early in the course of therapy, the medication should be taken exactly as directed. Skipping doses or not completing the full course of therapy may (1) decrease the effectiveness of the immediate treatment and (2) increase the likelihood that bacteria will develop resistance and will not be treatable by UNASYN or other antibacterial drugs in the future.
Drug Interactions: Probenecid decreases the renal tubular secretion of ampicillin and sulbactam. Concurrent use of probenecid with UNASYN may result in increased and prolonged blood levels of ampicillin and sulbactam. The concurrent administration of allopurinol and ampicillin increases substantially the incidence of rashes in patients receiving both drugs as compared to patients receiving ampicillin alone. It is not known whether this potentiation of ampicillin rashes is due to allopurinol or the hyperuricemia present in these patients. There are no data with UNASYN and allopurinol administered concurrently. UNASYN and aminoglycosides should not be reconstituted together due to the *in vitro* inactivation of aminoglycosides by the ampicillin component of UNASYN.
Drug/Laboratory Test Interactions: Administration of UNASYN will result in high urine concentration of ampicillin. High urine concentrations of ampicillin may result in false positive reactions when testing for the presence of glucose in urine using Clinitest™, Benedict's Solution or Fehling's Solution. It is recommended that glucose tests based on enzymatic glucose oxidase reactions (such as Clinistix™ or Testape™) be used. Following administration of ampicillin to pregnant women, a transient decrease in plasma concentration of total conjugated estriol, estriol-glucuronide, conjugated estrone and estradiol has been noted. This effect may also occur with UNASYN.
Carcinogenesis, Mutagenesis, Impairment of Fertility: Long-term studies in animals have not been performed to evaluate carcinogenic or mutagenic potential.
Pregnancy
Pregnancy Category B: Reproduction studies have been performed in mice, rats, and rabbits at doses up to ten (10) times the human dose and have revealed no evidence of impaired fertility or harm to the fetus due to UNASYN. There

Continued on next page

Unasyn—Cont.

are, however, no adequate and well controlled studies in pregnant women. Because animal reproduction studies are not always predictive of human response, this drug should be used during pregnancy only if clearly needed. (See–Drug/Laboratory Test Interactions.)

Labor and Delivery: Studies in guinea pigs have shown that intravenous administration of ampicillin decreased the uterine tone, frequency of contractions, height of contractions, and duration of contractions. However, it is not known whether the use of UNASYN in humans during labor or delivery has immediate or delayed adverse effects on the fetus, prolongs the duration of labor, or increases the likelihood that forceps delivery or other obstetrical intervention or resuscitation of the newborn will be necessary.

Nursing Mothers: Low concentrations of ampicillin and sulbactam are excreted in the milk; therefore, caution should be exercised when UNASYN is administered to a nursing woman.

Pediatric Use: The safety and effectiveness of UNASYN have been established for pediatric patients one year of age and older for skin and skin structure infections as approved in adults. Use of UNASYN in pediatric patients is supported by evidence from adequate and well-controlled studies in adults with additional data from pediatric pharmacokinetic studies, a controlled clinical trial conducted in pediatric patients and post-marketing adverse events surveillance. (See **CLINICAL PHARMACOLOGY, INDICATIONS AND USAGE, ADVERSE REACTIONS, DOSAGE AND ADMINISTRATION,** and **CLINICAL STUDIES** sections.)

The safety and effectiveness of UNASYN have not been established for pediatric patients for intra-abdominal infections.

ADVERSE REACTIONS

Adult Patients: UNASYN is generally well tolerated. The following adverse reactions have been reported.

Local Adverse Reactions

Pain at IM injection site – 16%
Pain at IV injection site – 3%
Thrombophlebitis – 3%

Systemic Adverse Reactions

The most frequently reported adverse reactions were diarrhea in 3% of the patients and rash in less than 2% of the patients.

Additional systemic reactions reported in less than 1% of the patients were: itching, nausea, vomiting, candidiasis, fatigue, malaise, headache, chest pain, flatulence, abdominal distension, glossitis, urine retention, dysuria, edema, facial swelling, erythema, chills, tightness in throat, substernal pain, epistaxis and mucosal bleeding.

Pediatric Patients: Available safety data for pediatric patients treated with UNASYN demonstrate a similar adverse events profile to those observed in adult patients. Additionally, atypical lymphocytosis has been observed in one pediatric patient receiving UNASYN.

Adverse Laboratory Changes

Adverse laboratory changes without regard to drug relationship that were reported during clinical trials were:

Hepatic: Increased AST (SGOT), ALT (SGPT), alkaline phosphatase, and LDH.

Hematologic: Decreased hemoglobin, hematocrit, RBC, WBC, neutrophils, lymphocytes, platelets and increased lymphocytes, monocytes, basophils, eosinophils, and platelets.

Blood Chemistry: Decreased serum albumin and total proteins.

Renal: Increased BUN and creatinine.

Urinalysis: Presence of RBC's and hyaline casts in urine.

The following adverse reactions have been reported with ampicillin-class antibiotics and can also occur with UNASYN.

Gastrointestinal: Gastritis, stomatitis, black "hairy" tongue and enterocolitis. Onset of pseudomembranous colitis symptoms may occur during or after antibiotic treatment. (See WARNINGS.)

Hypersensitivity Reactions: Urticaria, erythema multiforme, and an occasional case of exfoliative dermatitis have been reported. These reactions may be controlled with antihistamines and, if necessary, systemic corticosteroids. Whenever such reactions occur, the drug should be discontinued, unless the opinion of the physician dictates otherwise. Serious and occasional fatal hypersensitivity (anaphylactic) reactions can occur with a penicillin. (See WARNINGS.)

Hematologic: In addition to the adverse laboratory changes listed above for UNASYN, agranulocytosis has been reported during therapy with penicillins. All of these reactions are usually reversible on discontinuation of therapy and are believed to be hypersensitivity phenomena. Some individuals have developed positive direct Coombs Tests during treatment with UNASYN, as with other beta-lactam antibiotics.

OVERDOSAGE

Neurological adverse reactions, including convulsions, may occur with the attainment of high CSF levels of beta-lactams. Ampicillin may be removed from circulation by hemodialysis. The molecular weight, degree of protein binding and pharmacokinetics profile of sulbactam suggest that this compound may also be removed by hemodialysis.

CLINICAL STUDIES

Skin and Skin Structure Infections in Pediatric Patients: Data from a controlled clinical trial conducted in pediatric patients provided evidence supporting the safety and efficacy of UNASYN for the treatment of skin and skin structure infections. Of 99 pediatric patients evaluable for clinical efficacy, 60 patients received a regimen containing intravenous UNASYN, and 39 patients received a regimen containing intravenous cefuroxime. This trial demonstrated similar outcomes (assessed at an appropriate interval after discontinuation of all antimicrobial therapy) for UNASYN- and cefuroxime-treated patients:

Therapeutic Regimen	Clinical Success	Clinical Failure
UNASYN	51/60 (85%)	9/60 (15%)
Cefuroxime	34/39 (87%)	5/39 (13%)

Most patients received a course of oral antimicrobials following initial treatment with intravenous administration of parenteral antimicrobials. The study protocol required that the following three criteria be met prior to transition from intravenous to oral antimicrobial therapy: 1) receipt of a minimum of 72 hours of intravenous therapy; 2) no documented fever for prior 24 hours; and 3) improvement or resolution of the signs and symptoms of infection.

The choice of oral antimicrobial agent used in this trial was determined by susceptibility testing of the original pathogen, if isolated, to oral agents available. The course of oral antimicrobial therapy should not routinely exceed 14 days.

DOSAGE AND ADMINISTRATION

UNASYN may be administered by either the IV or the IM routes.

For IV administration, the dose can be given by slow intravenous injection over at least 10-15 minutes or can also be delivered, in greater dilutions with 50-100 mL of a compatible diluent as an intravenous infusion over 15-30 minutes. UNASYN may be administered by deep intramuscular injection. (See Preparation for Intramuscular Injection.)

The recommended adult dosage of UNASYN is 1.5 g (1 g ampicillin as the sodium salt plus 0.5 g sulbactam as the sodium salt) to 3 g (2 g ampicillin as the sodium salt plus 1 g sulbactam as the sodium salt) every six hours. This 1.5 to 3 g range represents the total of ampicillin content plus the sulbactam content of UNASYN, and corresponds to a range of 1 g ampicillin/0.5 g sulbactam to 2 g ampicillin/1 g sulbactam. The total dose of sulbactam should not exceed 4 grams per day.

Pediatric Patients 1 Year of Age or Older: The recommended daily dose of UNASYN in pediatric patients is 300 mg per kg of body weight administered via intravenous infusion in equally divided doses every 6 hours. This 300 mg/kg/day dosage represents the total ampicillin content plus the sulbactam content of UNASYN, and corresponds to 200 mg ampicillin/100 mg sulbactam per kg per day. The safety and efficacy of UNASYN administered via intramuscular injection in pediatric patients have not been established. Pediatric patients weighing 40 kg or more should be dosed according to adult recommendations, and the total dose of sulbactam should not exceed 4 grams per day. The course of intravenous therapy should not routinely exceed 14 days. In clinical trials, most children received a course of oral antimicrobials following initial treatment with intravenous UNASYN. (See **CLINICAL STUDIES** section.)

Impaired Renal Function

In patients with impairment of renal function the elimination kinetics of ampicillin and sulbactam are similarly affected, hence the ratio of one to the other will remain constant whatever the renal function. The dose of UNASYN in such patients should be administered less frequently in accordance with the usual practice for ampicillin and according to the following recommendations:

UNASYN Dosage Guide For Patients With Renal Impairment

Creatinine Clearance (mL/min/1.73m²)	Ampicillin/Sulbactam Half-Life (Hours)	Recommended UNASYN Dosage
≥30	1	1.5-3.0 g q 6h-q 8h
15-29	5	1.5-3.0 g q 12h
5-14	9	1.5-3.0 g q 24h

When only serum creatinine is available, the following formula (based on sex, weight, and age of the patient) may be used to convert this value into creatinine clearance. The serum creatinine should represent a steady state of renal function.

$$\text{Males} \quad \frac{\text{weight (kg)} \times (140 - \text{age})}{72 \times \text{serum creatinine}}$$

$$\text{Females} \quad 0.85 \times \text{above value}$$

COMPATIBILITY, RECONSTITUTION AND STABILITY

UNASYN sterile powder is to be stored at or below 30°C (86°F) prior to reconstitution.

When concomitant therapy with aminoglycosides is indicated, UNASYN and aminoglycosides should be reconstituted and administered separately, due to the *in vitro* inactivation of aminoglycosides by any of the aminopenicillins.

DIRECTIONS FOR USE

General Dissolution Procedures: UNASYN sterile powder for intravenous and intramuscular use may be reconstituted with any of the compatible diluents described in this insert. Solutions should be allowed to stand after dissolution to allow any foaming to dissipate in order to permit visual inspection for complete solubilization.

Preparation for Intravenous Use

1.5 g and 3.0 g Bottles: UNASYN sterile powder in piggyback units may be reconstituted directly to the desired concentrations using any of the following parenteral diluents. Reconstitution of UNASYN, at the specified concentrations, with these diluents provide stable solutions for the time periods indicated in the following table: (After the indicated time periods, any unused portions of solutions should be discarded.)

[See table below]

Diluent	Maximum Concentration (mg/mL) UNASYN (Ampicillin/Sulbactam)	Use Periods
Sterile Water for Injection	45 (30/15)	8 hrs @ 25°C
	45 (30/15)	48 hrs @ 4°C
	30 (20/10)	72 hrs @ 4°C
0.9% Sodium Chloride Injection	45 (30/15)	8 hrs @ 25°C
	45 (30/15)	48 hrs @ 4°C
	30 (20/10)	72 hrs @ 4°C
5% Dextrose Injection	30 (20/10)	2 hrs @ 25°C
	30 (20/10)	4 hrs @ 4°C
	3 (2/1)	4 hrs @ 25°C
Lactated Ringer's Injection	45 (30/15)	8 hrs @ 25°C
	45 (30/15)	24 hrs @ 4°C
M/6 Sodium Lactate Injection	45 (30/15)	8 hrs @ 25°C
	45 (30/15)	8 hrs @ 4°C
5% Dextrose in 0.45% Saline	3 (2/1)	4 hrs @ 25°C
	15 (10/5)	4 hrs @ 4°C
10% Invert Sugar	3 (2/1)	4 hrs @ 25°C
	30 (20/10)	3 hrs @ 4°C

If piggyback bottles are unavailable, standard vials of UNASYN sterile powder may be used. Initially, the vials may be reconstituted with Sterile Water for Injection to yield solutions containing 375 mg UNASYN per mL (250 mg ampicillin/125 mg sulbactam per mL). An appropriate volume should then be immediately diluted with a suitable parenteral diluent to yield solutions containing 3 to 45 mg UNASYN per mL (2 to 30 mg ampicillin/1 to 15 mg sulbactam/per mL).

1.5 g ADD-Vantage® Vials: UNASYN in the ADD-Vantage® system is intended as a single dose for intravenous administration after dilution with the ADD-Vantage® Flexible Diluent Container containing 50 mL, 100 mL or 250 mL of 0.9% Sodium Chloride Injection, USP.

3 g ADD-Vantage® Vials: UNASYN in the ADD-Vantage® system is intended as a single dose for intravenous administration after dilution with the ADD-Vantage® Flexible Diluent Container containing 100 mL or 250 mL of 0.9% Sodium Chloride Injection, USP.

UNASYN in the ADD-Vantage® system is to be reconstituted with 0.9% Sodium Chloride Injection, USP only. See INSTRUCTIONS FOR USE OF THE ADD-Vantage® VIAL. Reconstitution of UNASYN, at the specified concentration, with 0.9% Sodium Chloride Injection, USP provides stable solutions for the time period indicated below:

Diluent	Maximum Concentration (mg/mL) UNASYN (Ampicillin/Sulbactam)	Use Period
0.9% Sodium Chloride Injection	30 (20/10)	8 hrs @ 25°C

In 0.9% Sodium Chloride Injection, USP

The final diluted solution of UNASYN should be completely administered *within 8 hours* in order to assure proper potency.

Preparation for Intramuscular Injection

1.5 g and 3.0 g Standard Vials: Vials for intramuscular use may be reconstituted with Sterile Water for Injection USP, 0.5% Lidocaine Hydrochloride Injection USP or 2% Lidocaine Hydrochloride Injection USP. Consult the following table for recommended volumes to be added to obtain solutions containing 375 mg UNASYN per mL (250 mg ampicillin/125 mg sulbactam per mL). Note: *Use only freshly prepared solutions and administer within one hour after preparation.*

UNASYN Vial Size	Volume of Diluent to be Added	Withdrawal Volume*
1.5 g	3.2 mL	4.0 mL
3.0 g	6.4 mL	8.0 mL

*There is sufficient excess present to allow withdrawal and administration of the stated volumes.

Animal Pharmacology: While reversible glycogenosis was observed in laboratory animals, this phenomenon was dose- and time-dependent and is not expected to develop at the therapeutic doses and corresponding plasma levels attained during the relatively short periods of combined ampicillin/sulbactam therapy in man.

HOW SUPPLIED

UNASYN® (ampicillin sodium/sulbactam sodium) is supplied as a sterile off-white dry powder in glass vials and piggyback bottles. The following packages are available:

Vials containing 1.5 g (NDC 0049-0013-83) equivalent of UNASYN (1 g ampicillin as the sodium salt plus 0.5 g sulbactam as the sodium salt)

Vials containing 3 g (NDC 0049-0014-83) equivalent of UNASYN (2 g ampicillin as the sodium salt plus 1 g sulbactam as the sodium salt)

Bottles containing 1.5 g (NDC 0049-0022-83) equivalent of UNASYN (1 g ampicillin as the sodium salt plus 0.5 g sulbactam as the sodium salt)

Bottles containing 3 g (NDC 0049-0023-83) equivalent of UNASYN (2 g ampicillin as the sodium salt plus 1 g sulbactam as the sodium salt)

Pharmacy Bulk Package containing 15 g (NDC 0049-0024-28) equivalent of UNASYN (10 g ampicillin as the sodium salt plus 5 g sulbactam as the sodium salt)

ADD-Vantage® vials containing 1.5 g (NDC 0049-0031-83) equivalent of UNASYN (1 g ampicillin as the sodium salt plus 0.5 g sulbactam as the sodium salt) are distributed by Pfizer Inc.

ADD-Vantage® vials containing 3 g (NDC 0049-0032-83) equivalent of UNASYN (2 g ampicillin as the sodium salt plus 1 g sulbactam as the sodium salt) are distributed by Pfizer Inc.

The 1.5 g UNASYN ADD-Vantage® vials are only to be used with Abbott Laboratories' ADD-Vantage® Flexible Diluent Container containing 0.9% Sodium Chloride Injection, USP, 50 mL, 100 mL, or 250 mL sizes.

The 3 g UNASYN ADD-Vantage® vials are only to be used with Abbott Laboratories' ADD-Vantage® Flexible Diluent Container containing 0.9% Sodium Chloride Injection, USP, 100 mL or 250 mL sizes.

INSTRUCTIONS FOR USE OF THE ADD-Vantage® VIAL

To Open Diluent Container: Peel overwrap from the corner and remove container. Some opacity of the plastic due to moisture absorption during the sterilization process may be observed. This is normal and does not affect the solution quality or safety. The opacity will diminish gradually.

To Assemble Vial and Flexible Diluent Container: (Use Aseptic Technique)

1. Remove the protective covers from the top of the vial and the vial port on the diluent container as follows:

a. To remove the breakaway vial cap, swing the pull ring over the top of the vial and pull down far enough to start the opening (see Figure 1), pull the ring approximately half way around the cap and then pull straight up to remove the cap (see Figure 2).

NOTE: Do not access vial with syringe.

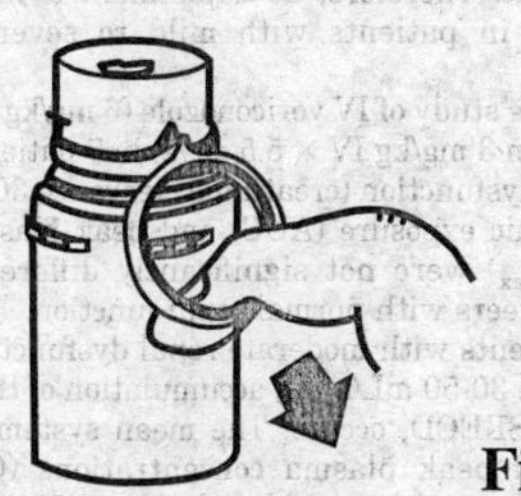

Fig. 1

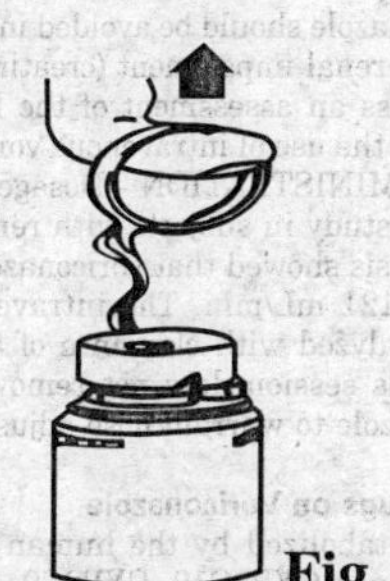

Fig. 2

b. To remove the vial port cover, grasp the tab on the pull ring, pull up to break the three tie strings, then pull back to remove the cover. (See Figure 3.)

2. Screw the vial into the vial port until it will go no further. THE VIAL MUST BE SCREWED IN TIGHTLY TO ASSURE A SEAL. This occurs approximately 1/2 turn (180°) after the first audible click. (See Figure 4.) The clicking sound does not assure a seal, the vial must be turned as far as it will go.

NOTE: Once vial is sealed, do not attempt to remove. (See Figure 4.)

3. Recheck the vial to assure that it is tight by trying to turn it further in the direction of assembly.

4. Label appropriately.

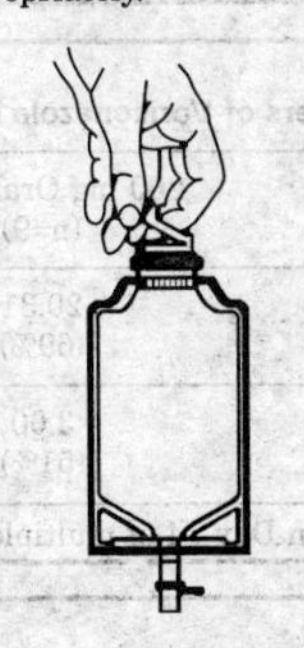

Fig. 3

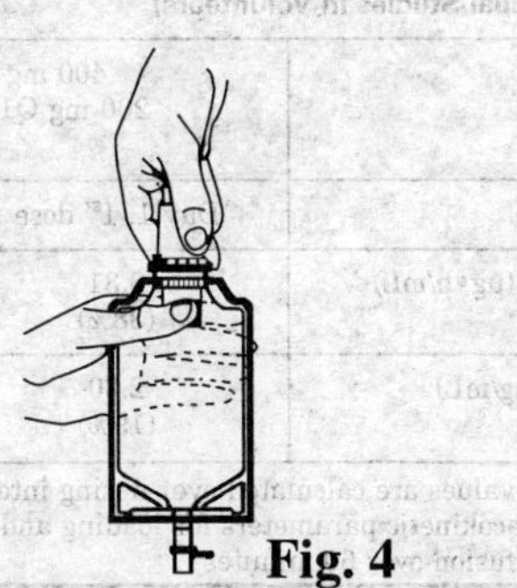

Fig. 4

To Prepare Admixture

1. Squeeze the bottom of the diluent container gently to inflate the portion of the container surrounding the end of the drug vial.
2. With the other hand, push the drug vial down into the container telescoping the walls of the container. Grasp the inner cap of the vial through the walls of the container. (See Figure 5.)
3. Pull the inner cap from the drug vial. (See Figure 6.) Verify that the rubber stopper has been pulled out, allowing the drug and diluent to mix.
4. Mix container contents thoroughly and use within the specified time.

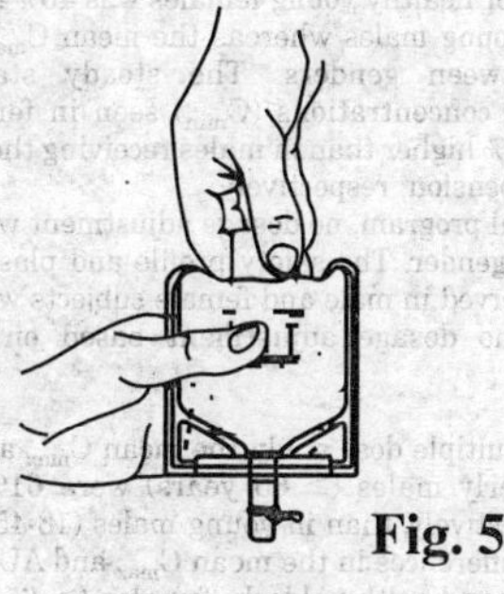

Fig. 5

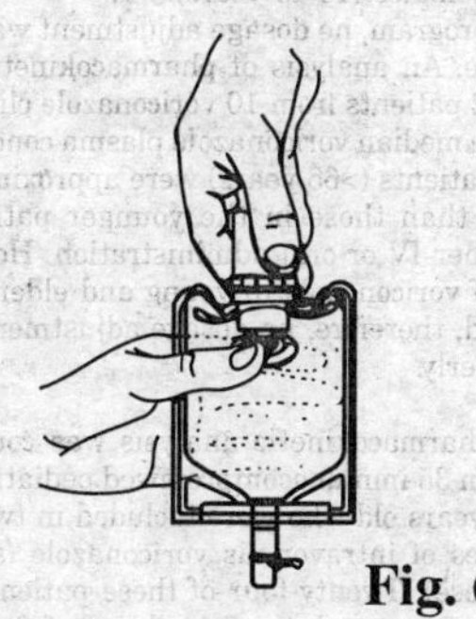

Fig. 6

REFERENCES

1. National Committee for Clinical Laboratory Standards, *Performance Standards for Antimicrobial Disk Susceptibility Tests*–Fourth Edition. Approved Standard NCCLS Document M2-A4, Vol. 10, No. 7 NCCLS, Villanova, PA, April 1990.
2. National Committee for Clinical Laboratory Standards, *Methods for Dilution Antimicrobial Susceptibility Tests for Bacteria that Grow Aerobically*, Second Edition. Approved Standard NCCLS Document M7-A2, Vol. 10, No. 8 NCCLS, Villanova, PA, April 1990.

Rx only

Pfizer Roerig
Division of Pfizer Inc, NY, NY 10017
70-4361-44-4 Revised September 2003

VFEND® I.V. ℞
[vee'fənd]
(voriconazole) for Injection
VFEND® Tablets ℞
(voriconazole)
VFEND® (voriconazole) for Oral Suspension ℞

DESCRIPTION

VFEND® (voriconazole), a triazole antifungal agent, is available as a lyophilized powder for solution for intravenous infusion, film-coated tablets for oral administration, and as a powder for oral suspension. The structural formula is:

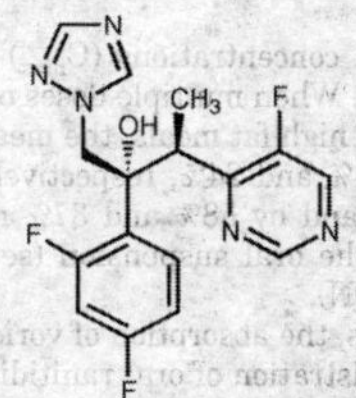

Voriconazole is designated chemically as (2R, 3S)-2-(2,4-difluorophenyl)-3-(5-fluoro-4-pyrimidinyl)-1-(1*H*-1,2,4-triazol-1-yl)-2-butanol with an empirical formula of $C_{16}H_{14}F_3N_5O$ and a molecular weight of 349.3.

Voriconazole drug substance is a white to light-colored powder.

VFEND I.V. is a white lyophilized powder containing nominally 200 mg voriconazole and 3200 mg sulfobutyl ether beta-cyclodextrin sodium in a 30 mL Type I clear glass vial.

VFEND I.V. is intended for administration by intravenous infusion. It is a single dose, unpreserved product. Vials containing 200 mg lyophilized voriconazole are intended for reconstitution with Water for Injection to produce a solution containing 10 mg/mL VFEND and 160 mg/mL of sulfobutyl ether beta-cyclodextrin sodium. The resultant solution is further diluted prior to administration as an intravenous infusion (see DOSAGE AND ADMINISTRATION).

VFEND Tablets contain 50 mg or 200 mg of voriconazole. The inactive ingredients include lactose monohydrate, pregelatinized starch, croscarmellose sodium, povidone, magnesium stearate and a coating containing hypromellose, titanium dioxide, lactose monohydrate and triacetin.

VFEND for Oral Suspension is a white to off-white powder providing a white to off-white orange-flavored suspension when reconstituted. Bottles containing 45 g powder for oral suspension are intended for reconstitution with water to produce a suspension containing 40 mg/mL voriconazole. The inactive ingredients include colloidal silicon dioxide, titanium dioxide, xanthan gum, sodium citrate dihydrate, sodium benzoate, anhydrous citric acid, natural orange flavor, and sucrose.

CLINICAL PHARMACOLOGY

Pharmacokinetics

General Pharmacokinetic Characteristics

The pharmacokinetics of voriconazole have been characterized in healthy subjects, special populations and patients. The pharmacokinetics of voriconazole are non-linear due to saturation of its metabolism. The interindividual variability of voriconazole pharmacokinetics is high. Greater than proportional increase in exposure is observed with increasing dose. It is estimated that, on average, increasing the oral dose in healthy subjects from 200 mg Q12h to 300 mg Q12h leads to a 2.5-fold increase in exposure (AUC_τ) while increasing the intravenous dose from 3 mg/kg Q12h to 4 mg/kg Q12h produces a 2.3-fold increase in exposure (Table 1).

[See table 1 at top of next page]

During oral administration of 200 mg or 300 mg twice daily for 14 days in patients at risk of aspergillosis (mainly patients with malignant neoplasms of lymphatic or hematopoietic tissue), the observed pharmacokinetic characteristics were similar to those observed in healthy subjects (Table 2).

[See table 2 at top of next page]

Sparse plasma sampling for pharmacokinetics was conducted in the therapeutic studies in patients aged 12-18 years. In 11 adolescent patients who received a mean voriconazole maintenance dose of 4 mg/kg IV, the median of the calculated mean plasma concentrations was 1.60 µg/mL (inter-quartile range 0.28 to 2.73 µg/mL). In 17 adolescent patients for whom mean plasma concentrations were calculated following a mean oral maintenance dose of 200 mg Q12h, the median of the calculated mean plasma concentrations was 1.16 µg/mL (inter-quartile range 0.85 to 2.14 µg/mL).

When the recommended intravenous or oral loading dose regimens are administered to healthy subjects, peak plasma concentrations close to steady state are achieved within the first 24 hours of dosing. Without the loading dose, accumulation occurs during twice-daily multiple dosing with steady-state peak plasma voriconazole concentrations being achieved by day 6 in the majority of subjects (Table 3).

Continued on next page

VFEND—Cont.

[See table 3 at right]

Steady state trough plasma concentrations with voriconazole are achieved after approximately 5 days of oral or intravenous dosing without a loading dose regimen. However, when an intravenous loading dose regimen is used, steady state trough plasma concentrations are achieved within one day.

Absorption

The pharmacokinetic properties of voriconazole are similar following administration by the intravenous and oral routes. Based on a population pharmacokinetic analysis of pooled data in healthy subjects (N=207), the oral bioavailability of voriconazole is estimated to be 96% (CV 13%). Bioequivalence was established between the 200 mg tablet and the 40 mg/mL oral suspension when administered as a 400 mg Q12h loading dose followed by a 200 mg Q12h maintenance dose.

Maximum plasma concentrations (C_{max}) are achieved 1-2 hours after dosing. When multiple doses of voriconazole are administered with high fat meals, the mean C_{max} and AUC_τ are reduced by 34% and 24%, respectively when administered as a tablet and by 58% and 37% respectively when administered as the oral suspension (see DOSAGE AND ADMINISTRATION).

In healthy subjects, the absorption of voriconazole is not affected by coadministration of oral ranitidine, cimetidine, or omeprazole, drugs that are known to increase gastric pH.

Distribution

The volume of distribution at steady state for voriconazole is estimated to be 4.6 L/kg, suggesting extensive distribution into tissues. Plasma protein binding is estimated to be 58% and was shown to be independent of plasma concentrations achieved following single and multiple oral doses of 200 mg or 300 mg (approximate range: 0.9-15 µg/mL). Varying degrees of hepatic and renal insufficiency do not affect the protein binding of voriconazole.

Metabolism

In vitro studies showed that voriconazole is metabolized by the human hepatic cytochrome P450 enzymes, CYP2C19, CYP2C9 and CYP3A4 (see CLINICAL PHARMACOLOGY - Drug Interactions).

In vivo studies indicated that CYP2C19 is significantly involved in the metabolism of voriconazole. This enzyme exhibits genetic polymorphism. For example, 15-20% of Asian populations may be expected to be poor metabolizers. For Caucasians and Blacks, the prevalence of poor metabolizers is 3-5%. Studies conducted in Caucasian and Japanese healthy subjects have shown that poor metabolizers have, on average, 4-fold higher voriconazole exposure (AUC_τ) than their homozygous extensive metabolizer counterparts. Subjects who are heterozygous extensive metabolizers have, on average, 2-fold higher voriconazole exposure than their homozygous extensive metabolizer counterparts.

The major metabolite of voriconazole is the N-oxide, which accounts for 72% of the circulating radiolabelled metabolites in plasma. Since this metabolite has minimal antifungal activity, it does not contribute to the overall efficacy of voriconazole.

Excretion

Voriconazole is eliminated via hepatic metabolism with less than 2% of the dose excreted unchanged in the urine. After administration of a single radiolabelled dose of either oral or IV voriconazole, preceded by multiple oral or IV dosing, approximately 80% to 83% of the radioactivity is recovered in the urine. The majority (>94%) of the total radioactivity is excreted in the first 96 hours after both oral and intravenous dosing.

As a result of non-linear pharmacokinetics, the terminal half-life of voriconazole is dose dependent and therefore not useful in predicting the accumulation or elimination of voriconazole.

Pharmacokinetic-Pharmacodynamic Relationships

Clinical Efficacy and Safety

In ten clinical trials, the median values for the average and maximum voriconazole plasma concentrations in individual patients across these studies (N=1121) was 2.51 µg/mL (inter-quartile range 1.21 to 4.44 µg/mL) and 3.79 µg/mL (inter-quartile range 2.06 to 6.31 µg/mL), respectively. A pharmacokinetic-pharmacodynamic analysis of patient data from 6 of these 10 clinical trials (N=280) could not detect a positive association between mean, maximum or minimum plasma voriconazole concentration and efficacy. However, PK/PD analyses of the data from all 10 clinical trials identified positive associations between plasma voriconazole concentrations and rate of both liver function test abnormalities and visual disturbances (see ADVERSE REACTIONS).

Electrocardiogram

A placebo-controlled, randomized, crossover study to evaluate the effect on the QT interval of healthy male and female volunteers was conducted with three single oral doses of voriconazole and ketoconazole. Serial ECGs and plasma samples were obtained at specified intervals over a 24-hour post dose observation period. The placebo-adjusted mean maximum increases in QTc from baseline after 800, 1200 and 1600 mg of voriconazole and after ketoconazole 800 mg were all <10 msec. Females exhibited a greater increase in QTc than males, although all mean changes were <10 msec. Age was not found to affect the magnitude of increase in QTc. No subject in any group had an increase in QTc of ≥60 msec from baseline. No subject experienced an interval

Table 1
Population Pharmacokinetic Parameters of Voriconazole in Volunteers

	200 mg Oral Q12h	300 mg Oral Q12h	3 mg/kg IV Q12h	4 mg/kg IV Q12h
AUC_τ* (µg•h/mL) (CV%)	19.86 (94%)	50.32 (74%)	21.81 (100%)	50.40 (83%)

*Mean AUC_τ are predicted values from population pharmacokinetic analysis of data from 236 volunteers

Table 2
Pharmacokinetic Parameters of Voriconazole in Patients at Risk for Aspergillosis

	200 mg Oral Q12h (n=9)	300 mg Oral Q12h (n=9)
AUC_τ* (µg•h/mL) (CV%)	20.31 (69%)	36.51 (45%)
C_{max}* (µg/mL) (CV%)	3.00 (51%)	4.66 (35%)

*Geometric mean values on Day 14 of multiple dosing in 2 cohorts of patients

Table 3
Pharmacokinetic Parameters of Voriconazole from Loading Dose and Maintenance Dose Regimens (Individual Studies in Volunteers)

	400 mg Q12h on Day 1, 200 mg Q12h on Days 2 to 10 (n=17)		6 mg/kg IV** Q12h on Day 1, 3 mg/kg IV Q12h on Days 2 to 10 (n=9)	
	Day 1, 1st dose	Day 10	Day 1, 1st dose	Day 10
AUC_τ* (µg•h/mL) (CV%)	9.31 (38%)	11.13 (103%)	13.22 (22%)	13.25 (58%)
C_{max} (µg/mL) (CV%)	2.30 (19%)	2.08 (62%)	4.70 (22%)	3.06 (31%)

*AUC_τ values are calculated over dosing interval of 12 hours
Pharmacokinetic parameters for loading and maintenance doses summarized for same cohort of volunteers
**IV infusion over 60 minutes

exceeding the potentially clinically relevant threshold of 500 msec. However, the QT effect of voriconazole combined with drugs known to prolong the QT interval is unknown. (See CONTRAINDICATIONS, PRECAUTIONS-Drug Interactions).

Pharmacokinetics in Special Populations

Gender

In a multiple oral dose study, the mean C_{max} and AUC_τ for healthy young females were 83% and 113% higher, respectively, than in healthy young males (18-45 years), after tablet dosing. In the same study, no significant differences in the mean C_{max} and AUC_τ were observed between healthy elderly males and healthy elderly females (≥65 years). In a similar study, after dosing with the oral suspension, the mean AUC for healthy young females was 45% higher than in healthy young males whereas the mean C_{max} was comparable between genders. The steady state trough voriconazole concentrations (C_{min}) seen in females were 100% and 91% higher than in males receiving the tablet and the oral suspension, respectively.

In the clinical program, no dosage adjustment was made on the basis of gender. The safety profile and plasma concentrations observed in male and female subjects were similar. Therefore, no dosage adjustment based on gender is necessary.

Geriatric

In an oral multiple dose study the mean C_{max} and AUC_τ in healthy elderly males (≥ 65 years) were 61% and 86% higher, respectively, than in young males (18-45 years). No significant differences in the mean C_{max} and AUC_τ were observed between healthy elderly females (≥ 65 years) and healthy young females (18-45 years).

In the clinical program, no dosage adjustment was made on the basis of age. An analysis of pharmacokinetic data obtained from 552 patients from 10 voriconazole clinical trials showed that the median voriconazole plasma concentrations in the elderly patients (>65 years) were approximately 80% to 90% higher than those in the younger patients (≤65 years) after either IV or oral administration. However, the safety profile of voriconazole in young and elderly subjects was similar and, therefore, no dosage adjustment is necessary for the elderly.

Pediatric

A population pharmacokinetic analysis was conducted on pooled data from 35 immunocompromised pediatric patients aged 2 to <12 years old who were included in two pharmacokinetic studies of intravenous voriconazole (single dose and multiple dose). Twenty-four of these patients received multiple intravenous maintenance doses of 3 mg/kg and 4 mg/kg. A comparison of the pediatric and adult population pharmacokinetic data revealed that the predicted average steady state plasma concentrations were similar at the maintenance dose of 4 mg/kg every 12 hours in children and 3 mg/kg every 12 hours in adults (medians of 1.19 µg/mL and 1.16 µg/mL in children and adults, respectively). (See PRECAUTIONS, Pediatric Use.)

Hepatic Insufficiency

After a single oral dose (200 mg) of voriconazole in 8 patients with mild (Child-Pugh Class A) and 4 patients with moderate (Child-Pugh Class B) hepatic insufficiency, the mean systemic exposure (AUC) was 3.2-fold higher than in age and weight matched controls with normal hepatic function. There was no difference in mean peak plasma concentrations (C_{max}) between the groups. When only the patients with mild (Child-Pugh Class A) hepatic insufficiency were compared to controls, there was still a 2.3-fold increase in the mean AUC in the group with hepatic insufficiency compared to controls.

In an oral multiple dose study, AUC_τ was similar in six subjects with moderate hepatic impairment (Child-Pugh Class B) given a lower maintenance dose of 100 mg twice daily compared to six subjects with normal hepatic function given the standard 200 mg twice daily maintenance dose. The mean peak plasma concentrations (C_{max}) were 20% lower in the hepatically impaired group.

It is recommended that the standard loading dose regimens be used but that the maintenance dose be halved in patients with mild to moderate hepatic cirrhosis (Child-Pugh Class A and B) receiving voriconazole. No pharmacokinetic data are available for patients with severe hepatic cirrhosis (Child-Pugh Class C) (see DOSAGE AND ADMINISTRATION).

Renal Insufficiency

In a single oral dose (200 mg) study in 24 subjects with normal renal function and mild to severe renal impairment, systemic exposure (AUC) and peak plasma concentration (C_{max}) of voriconazole were not significantly affected by renal impairment. Therefore, no adjustment is necessary for oral dosing in patients with mild to severe renal impairment.

In a multiple dose study of IV voriconazole (6 mg/kg IV loading dose × 2, then 3 mg/kg IV × 5.5 days) in 7 patients with moderate renal dysfunction (creatinine clearance 30-50 mL/min), the systemic exposure (AUC) and peak plasma concentrations (C_{max}) were not significantly different from those in 6 volunteers with normal renal function.

However, in patients with moderate renal dysfunction (creatinine clearance 30-50 mL/min), accumulation of the intravenous vehicle, SBECD, occurs. The mean systemic exposure (AUC) and peak plasma concentrations (C_{max}) of SBECD were increased by 4-fold and almost 50%, respectively, in the moderately impaired group compared to the normal control group.

Intravenous voriconazole should be avoided in patients with moderate or severe renal impairment (creatinine clearance <50 mL/min), unless an assessment of the benefit/risk to the patient justifies the use of intravenous voriconazole (see DOSAGE AND ADMINISTRATION - Dosage Adjustment).

A pharmacokinetic study in subjects with renal failure undergoing hemodialysis showed that voriconazole is dialyzed with clearance of 121 mL/min. The intravenous vehicle, SBECD, is hemodialyzed with clearance of 55 mL/min. A 4-hour hemodialysis session does not remove a sufficient amount of voriconazole to warrant dose adjustment.

Drug Interactions

Effects of Other Drugs on Voriconazole

Voriconazole is metabolized by the human hepatic cytochrome P450 enzymes CYP2C19, CYP2C9, and CYP3A4. Results of *in vitro* metabolism studies indicate that the affinity of voriconazole is highest for CYP2C19, followed by CYP2C9, and is appreciably lower for CYP3A4. Inhibitors or inducers of these three enzymes may increase or decrease voriconazole systemic exposure (plasma concentrations), respectively.

The systemic exposure to voriconazole is significantly reduced or is expected to be reduced by the concomitant administration of the following agents and their use is contraindicated:

***Rifampin* (potent CYP450 inducer):** Rifampin (600 mg once daily) decreased the steady state C_{max} and AUC_τ of voriconazole (200 mg Q12h × 7 days) by an average of 93% and 96%, respectively, in healthy subjects. Doubling the dose of voriconazole to 400 mg Q12h does not restore adequate exposure to voriconazole during coadministration with rifampin. **Coadministration of voriconazole and rifampin is contraindicated** (see CONTRAINDICATIONS, PRECAUTIONS - Drug Interactions).

***Ritonavir* (potent CYP450 inducer; CYP3A4 inhibitor and substrate):** Ritonavir (400 mg Q12h for 9 days) decreased the steady state C_{max} and AUC_τ of oral voriconazole (400 mg Q12h for 1 day, then 200 mg Q12h for 8 days) by an average of 66% and 82%, respectively, in healthy subjects. The effect of ritonavir (100 mg Q12h as used to inhibit CYP3A and increase concentrations of other antiretroviral drugs) on voriconazole concentrations has not been studied. Repeat oral administration of voriconazole (400 mg Q12h for 1 day, then 200 mg Q12h for 8 days) did not have a significant effect on steady state C_{max} and AUC_τ of ritonavir following repeat dose administration (400 mg Q12h for 9 days) in healthy subjects. **Coadministration of voriconazole and ritonavir (400 mg Q12h) is contraindicated** (see CONTRAINDICATIONS, PRECAUTIONS - Drug Interactions).

***Carbamazepine and long acting barbiturates* (potent CYP450 inducers):** Although not studied *in vitro* or *in vivo*, carbamazepine and long acting barbiturates (e.g. phenobarbital, mephobarbital) are likely to significantly decrease plasma voriconazole concentrations. **Coadministration of voriconazole with carbamazepine or long acting barbiturates is contraindicated** (see CONTRAINDICATIONS, PRECAUTIONS - Drug Interactions).

Minor or no significant pharmacokinetic interactions that do not require dosage adjustment:

***Cimetidine* (non-specific CYP450 inhibitor and increases gastric pH):** Cimetidine (400 mg Q12h × 8 days) increased voriconazole steady state C_{max} and AUC_τ by an average of 18% (90% CI: 6%, 32%) and 23% (90% CI: 13%, 33%), respectively, following oral doses of 200 mg Q12h × 7 days to healthy subjects.

***Ranitidine* (increases gastric pH):** Ranitidine (150 mg Q12h) had no significant effect on voriconazole C_{max} and AUC_τ following oral doses of 200 mg Q12h × 7 days to healthy subjects.

Macrolide antibiotics: Co-administration of **erythromycin** (CYP3A4 inhibitor;1g Q12h for 7 days) or **azithromycin** (500 mg qd for 3 days) with voriconazole 200 mg Q12h for 14 days had no significant effect on voriconazole steady state C_{max} and AUC_τ in healthy subjects. The effects of voriconazole on the pharmacokinetics of either erythromycin or azithromycin are not known.

Effects of Voriconazole on Other Drugs

In vitro studies with human hepatic microsomes show that voriconazole inhibits the metabolic activity of the cytochrome P450 enzymes CYP2C19, CYP2C9, and CYP3A4. In these studies, the inhibition potency of voriconazole for CYP3A4 metabolic activity was significantly less than that of two other azoles, ketoconazole and itraconazole. *In vitro* studies also show that the major metabolite of voriconazole, voriconazole N-oxide, inhibits the metabolic activity of CYP2C9 and CYP3A4 to a greater extent than that of CYP2C19. Therefore, there is potential for voriconazole and its major metabolite to increase the systemic exposure (plasma concentrations) of other drugs metabolized by these CYP450 enzymes.

The systemic exposure of the following drugs is significantly increased or is expected to be significantly increased by coadministration of voriconazole and their use is contraindicated:

***Sirolimus* (CYP3A4 substrate):** Repeat dose administration of oral voriconazole (400 mg Q12h for 1 day, then 200 mg Q12h for 8 days) increased the C_{max} and AUC of sirolimus (2 mg single dose) an average of 7-fold (90% CI: 5.7, 7.5) and 11-fold (90% CI: 9.9, 12.6), respectively, in healthy subjects. **Coadministration of voriconazole and sirolimus is contraindicated** (see CONTRAINDICATIONS, PRECAUTIONS - Drug Interactions).

***Terfenadine, astemizole, cisapride, pimozide and quinidine* (CYP3A4 substrates):** Although not studied *in vitro* or *in vivo*, concomitant administration of voriconazole with terfenadine, astemizole, cisapride, pimozide or quinidine may result in inhibition of the metabolism of these drugs. Increased plasma concentrations of these drugs can lead to QT prolongation and rare occurrences of *torsade de pointes*. **Coadministration of voriconazole and terfenadine, astemizole, cisapride, pimozide and quinidine is contraindicated** (see CONTRAINDICATIONS, PRECAUTIONS - Drug Interactions).

Ergot alkaloids: Although not studied *in vitro* or *in vivo*, voriconazole may increase the plasma concentration of ergot alkaloids (ergotamine and dihydroergotamine) and lead to ergotism. **Coadministration of voriconazole with ergot alkaloids is contraindicated** (see CONTRAINDICATIONS, PRECAUTIONS - Drug Interactions).

Coadministration of voriconazole with the following agents results in increased exposure or is expected to result in increased exposure to these drugs. Therefore, careful monitoring and/or dosage adjustment of these drugs is needed:

***Cyclosporine* (CYP3A4 substrate):** In stable renal transplant recipients receiving chronic cyclosporine therapy, concomitant administration of oral voriconazole (200 mg Q12h for 8 days) increased cyclosporine C_{max} and AUC_τ an average of 1.1 times (90% CI: 0.9, 1.41) and 1.7 times (90% CI: 1.5, 2.0), respectively, as compared to when cyclosporine was administered without voriconazole. When initiating therapy with voriconazole in patients already receiving cyclosporine, it is recommended that the cyclosporine dose be reduced to one-half of the original dose and followed with frequent monitoring of the cyclosporine blood levels. Increased cyclosporine levels have been associated with nephrotoxicity. When voriconazole is discontinued, cyclosporine levels should be frequently monitored and the dose increased as necessary (see PRECAUTIONS - Drug Interactions).

***Tacrolimus* (CYP3A4 substrate):** Repeat oral dose administration of voriconazole (400 mg Q12h × 1 day then 200 mg Q12h × 6 days) increased tacrolimus (0.1 mg/kg single dose) C_{max} and AUC_τ in healthy subjects by an average of 2-fold (90% CI: 1.9, 2.5) and 3-fold (90% CI: 2.7, 3.8), respectively. When initiating therapy with voriconazole in patients already receiving tacrolimus, it is recommended that the tacrolimus dose be reduced to one-third of the original dose and followed with frequent monitoring of the tacrolimus blood levels. Increased tacrolimus levels have been associated with nephrotoxicity. When voriconazole is discontinued, tacrolimus levels should be carefully monitored and the dose increased as necessary (see PRECAUTIONS - Drug Interactions).

***Warfarin* (CYP2C9 substrate):** Coadministration of voriconazole (300 mg Q12h × 12 days) with warfarin (30 mg single dose) significantly increased maximum prothrombin time by approximately 2-times that of placebo in healthy subjects. Close monitoring of prothrombin time or other suitable anti-coagulation tests is recommended if warfarin and voriconazole are coadministered and the warfarin dose adjusted accordingly (see PRECAUTIONS - Drug Interactions).

***Oral Coumarin Anticoagulants* (CYP2C9, CYP3A4 substrates):** Although not studied *in vitro* or *in vivo*, voriconazole may increase the plasma concentrations of coumarin anticoagulants and therefore may cause an increase in prothrombin time. If patients receiving coumarin preparations are treated simultaneously with voriconazole, the prothrombin time or other suitable anticoagulation tests should be monitored at close intervals and the dosage of anticoagulants adjusted accordingly (see PRECAUTIONS - Drug Interactions).

***Statins* (CYP3A4 substrates):** Although not studied clinically, voriconazole has been shown to inhibit lovastatin metabolism *in vitro* (human liver microsomes). Therefore, voriconazole is likely to increase the plasma concentrations of statins that are metabolized by CYP3A4. It is recommended that dose adjustment of the statin be considered during coadministration. Increased statin concentrations in plasma have been associated with rhabdomyolysis (see PRECAUTIONS - Drug Interactions).

***Benzodiazepines* (CYP3A4 substrates):** Although not studied clinically, voriconazole has been shown to inhibit midazolam metabolism *in vitro* (human liver microsomes). Therefore, voriconazole is likely to increase the plasma concentrations of benzodiazepines that are metabolized by CYP3A4 (e.g., midazolam, triazolam, and alprazolam) and lead to a prolonged sedative effect. It is recommended that dose adjustment of the benzodiazepine be considered during coadministration (see PRECAUTIONS - Drug Interactions).

***Calcium Channel Blockers* (CYP3A4 substrates):** Although not studied clinically, voriconazole has been shown to inhibit felodipine metabolism *in vitro* (human liver microsomes). Therefore, voriconazole may increase the plasma concentrations of calcium channel blockers that are metabolized by CYP3A4. Frequent monitoring for adverse events and toxicity related to calcium channel blockers is recommended during coadministration. Dose adjustment of the calcium channel blocker may be needed (see PRECAUTIONS - Drug Interactions).

***Sulfonylureas* (CYP2C9 substrates):** Although not studied *in vitro* or *in vivo*, voriconazole may increase plasma concentrations of sulfonylureas (e.g., tolbutamide, glipizide, and glyburide) and therefore cause hypoglycemia. Frequent monitoring of blood glucose and appropriate adjustment (i.e., reduction) of the sulfonylurea dosage is recommended during coadministration (see PRECAUTIONS - Drug Interactions).

***Vinca Alkaloids* (CYP3A4 substrates):** Although not studied *in vitro* or *in vivo*, voriconazole may increase the plasma concentrations of the vinca alkaloids (e.g., vincristine and vinblastine) and lead to neurotoxicity. Therefore, it is recommended that dose adjustment of the vinca alkaloid be considered.

No significant pharmacokinetic interactions were observed when voriconazole was coadministered with the following agents. Therefore, no dosage adjustment for these agents is recommended:

***Prednisolone* (CYP3A4 substrate):** Voriconazole (200 mg Q12h × 30 days) increased C_{max} and AUC of prednisolone (60 mg single dose) by an average of 11% and 34%, respectively, in healthy subjects.

***Digoxin* (P-glycoprotein mediated transport):** Voriconazole (200 mg Q12h × 12 days) had no significant effect on steady state C_{max} and AUC_τ of digoxin (0.25 mg once daily for 10 days) in healthy subjects.

***Mycophenolic acid* (UDP-glucuronyl transferase substrate):** Voriconazole (200 mg Q12h × 5 days) had no significant effect on the C_{max} and AUC_τ of mycophenolic acid and its major metabolite, mycophenolic acid glucuronide after administration of a 1 g single oral dose of mycophenolate mofetil.

Two-Way Interactions

Concomitant use of the following agents with voriconazole is contraindicated:

***Efavirenz*, a non-nucleoside reverse transcriptase inhibitor (CYP450 inducer; CYP3A4 inhibitor and substrate):** Steady state efavirenz (400 mg PO QD) decreased the steady state C_{max} and AUC_τ of voriconazole (400 mg PO Q12h for 1 day, then 200 mg PO Q12h for 8 days) by an average of 61% and 77%, respectively, in healthy subjects. Voriconazole at steady state (400 mg PO Q12h for 1 day, then 200 mg Q12h for 8 days) increased the steady state C_{max} and AUC_τ of efavirenz (400 mg PO QD for 9 days) by an average of 38% and 44%, respectively, in healthy subjects. **Coadministration of voriconazole and efavirenz is contraindicated** (see CONTRAINDICATIONS, PRECAUTIONS – Drug Interactions).

***Rifabutin* (potent CYP450 inducer):** Rifabutin (300 mg once daily) decreased the C_{max} and AUC_τ of voriconazole at 200 mg twice daily by an average of 67% (90% CI: 58%, 73%) and 79% (90% CI: 71%, 84%), respectively, in healthy subjects. During coadministration with rifabutin (300 mg once daily), the steady state C_{max} and AUC_τ of voriconazole following an increased dose of 400 mg twice daily were on average approximately 2-times higher, compared with voriconazole alone at 200 mg twice daily. Coadministration of voriconazole at 400 mg twice daily with rifabutin 300 mg twice daily increased the C_{max} and AUC_τ of rifabutin by an average of 3-times (90% CI: 2.2, 4.0) and 4-times (90% CI: 3.5, 5.4), respectively, compared to rifabutin given alone. **Coadministration of voriconazole and rifabutin is contraindicated.**

Significant drug interactions that may require dosage adjustment, frequent monitoring of drug levels and/or frequent monitoring of drug-related adverse events/toxicity:

***Phenytoin* (CYP2C9 substrate and potent CYP450 inducer):** Repeat dose administration of phenytoin (300 mg once daily) decreased the steady state C_{max} and AUC_τ of orally administered voriconazole (200 mg Q12h × 14 days) by an average of 50% and 70%, respectively, in healthy subjects. Administration of a higher voriconazole dose (400 mg Q12h × 7 days) with phenytoin (300 mg once daily) resulted in comparable steady state voriconazole C_{max} and AUC_τ estimates as compared to when voriconazole was given at 200 mg Q12h without phenytoin.

Phenytoin may be coadministered with voriconazole if the maintenance dose of voriconazole is increased from 4 mg/kg to 5 mg/kg intravenously every 12 hours or from 200 mg to 400 mg orally, every 12 hours (100 mg to 200 mg orally, every 12 hours in patients less than 40 kg) (see DOSAGE AND ADMINISTRATION).

Repeat dose administration of voriconazole (400 mg Q12h × 10 days) increased the steady state C_{max} and AUC_τ of phenytoin (300 mg once daily) by an average of 70% and 80%, respectively, in healthy subjects. The increase in phenytoin C_{max} and AUC when coadministered with voriconazole may be expected to be as high as 2-times the C_{max} and AUC estimates when phenytoin is given without voriconazole. Therefore, frequent monitoring of plasma phenytoin concentrations and phenytoin-related adverse effects is recommended when phenytoin is coadministered with voriconazole (see PRECAUTIONS - Drug Interactions).

***Omeprazole* (CYP2C19 inhibitor; CYP2C19 and CYP3A4 substrate):** Coadministration of omeprazole (40 mg once daily × 10 days) with oral voriconazole (400 mg Q12h × 1 day, then 200 mg Q12h × 9 days) increased the steady state C_{max} and AUC_τ of voriconazole by an average of 15% (90% CI: 5%, 25%) and 40% (90% CI: 29%, 55%), respectively, in healthy subjects. No dosage adjustment of voriconazole is recommended.

Coadministration of voriconazole (400 mg Q12h × 1 day, then 200 mg × 6 days) with omeprazole (40 mg once daily × 7 days) to healthy subjects significantly increased the steady state C_{max} and AUC_τ of omeprazole an average of 2-times (90% CI: 1.8, 2.6) and 4-times (90% CI: 3.3, 4.4), respectively, as compared to when omeprazole is given without voriconazole. When initiating voriconazole in patients already receiving omeprazole doses of 40 mg or greater, it is recommended that the omeprazole dose be reduced by one-half (see PRECAUTIONS - Drug Interactions).

The metabolism of other proton pump inhibitors that are CYP2C19 substrates may also be inhibited by voriconazole and may result in increased plasma concentrations of these drugs.

No significant pharmacokinetic interaction was seen and no dosage adjustment of these drugs is recommended:

***Indinavir* (CYP3A4 inhibitor and substrate):** Repeat dose administration of indinavir (800 mg TID for 10 days) had no significant effect on voriconazole C_{max} and AUC following repeat dose administration (200 mg Q12h for 17 days) in healthy subjects.

Repeat dose administration of voriconazole (200 mg Q12h for 7 days) did not have a significant effect on steady state C_{max} and AUC_τ of indinavir following repeat dose administration (800 mg TID for 7 days) in healthy subjects.

Two-Way Interactions Expected to be Significant Based on *In Vitro* and *In Vivo* Findings:

***Other HIV Protease Inhibitors* (CYP3A4 substrates and inhibitors):** *In vitro* studies (human liver microsomes) sug-

Continued on next page

VFEND—Cont.

gest that voriconazole may inhibit the metabolism of HIV protease inhibitors (e.g. saquinavir, amprenavir and nelfinavir). *In vitro* studies (human liver microsomes) also show that the metabolism of voriconazole may be inhibited by HIV protease inhibitors (e.g., saquinavir and amprenavir). Patients should be frequently monitored for drug toxicity during the coadministration of voriconazole and HIV protease inhibitors (see PRECAUTIONS - Drug Interactions).

***Other Non-Nucleoside Reverse Transcriptase Inhibitors (NNRTI)* (CYP3A4 substrates, inhibitors or CYP450 inducers):** *In vitro* studies (human liver microsomes) show that the metabolism of voriconazole may be inhibited by a NNRTI (e.g. delavirdine). The findings of a clinical voriconazole-efavirenz drug interaction study in healthy volunteers suggest that the metabolism of voriconazole may be induced by an NNRTI. This *in vivo* study also showed that voriconazole may inhibit the metabolism of a NNRTI. Efavirenz and voriconazole coadministration is contraindicated (see CLINICAL PHARMACOLOGY – Drug Interactions, CONTRAINDICATIONS, PRECAUTIONS – Drug Interactions). Patients should be frequently monitored for drug toxicity during the coadministration of voriconazole and other NNRTIs (e.g. nevirapine and delavirdine) (see PRECAUTIONS – Drug Interactions).

MICROBIOLOGY

Mechanism of Action

Voriconazole is a triazole antifungal agent. The primary mode of action of voriconazole is the inhibition of fungal cytochrome P-450-mediated 14 alpha-lanosterol demethylation, an essential step in fungal ergosterol biosynthesis. The accumulation of 14 alpha-methyl sterols correlates with the subsequent loss of ergosterol in the fungal cell wall and may be responsible for the antifungal activity of voriconazole. Voriconazole has been shown to be more selective for fungal cytochrome P-450 enzymes than for various mammalian cytochrome P-450 enzyme systems.

Activity *In Vitro* and *In Vivo*

Voriconazole has demonstrated *in vitro* activity against *Aspergillus* species (*A. fumigatus, A. flavus, A. niger* and *A. terreus*), *Candida* species (*C. albicans, C. glabrata* and *C. krusei*), *Scedosporium apiospermum* and *Fusarium* spp., including *Fusarium solani*. (see INDICATIONS AND USAGE, CLINICAL STUDIES).

In vitro susceptibility testing was performed according to the National Committee for Clinical Laboratory Standards (NCCLS) methods (M38-P for moulds and M27-A for yeasts). Voriconazole breakpoints have not been established for any fungi. The relationship between clinical outcome and *in vitro* susceptibility results remains to be elucidated. Voriconazole was active in normal and/or immunocompromised guinea pigs with systemic and/or pulmonary infections due to *A. fumigatus* (including an isolate with reduced susceptibility to itraconazole) or *Candida* species [*C.albicans* (including an isolate with reduced susceptibility to fluconazole), *C. krusei* and *C. glabrata*] in which the endpoints were prolonged survival of infected animals and/or reduction of mycological burden from target organs. In one experiment, voriconazole exhibited activity against *Scedosporium apiospermum* infections in immune competent guinea pigs.

Drug Resistance

Voriconazole drug resistance development has not been adequately studied *in vitro* against *Candida, Aspergillus, Scedosporium* and *Fusarium* species. The frequency of drug resistance development for the various fungi for which this drug is indicated is not known.

Fungal isolates exhibiting reduced susceptibility to fluconazole or itraconazole may also show reduced susceptibility to voriconazole, suggesting cross-resistance can occur among these azoles. The relevance of cross-resistance and clinical outcome has not been fully characterized. Clinical cases where azole cross-resistance is demonstrated may require alternative antifungal therapy.

INDICATIONS AND USAGE

VFEND is indicated for use in the treatment of the following fungal infections:

Invasive aspergillosis. In clinical trials, the majority of isolates recovered were *Aspergillus fumigatus*. There was a small number of cases of culture-proven disease due to species of *Aspergillus* other than *A. fumigatus* (see CLINICAL STUDIES, MICROBIOLOGY).

Esophageal candidiasis. (see CLINICAL STUDIES, MICROBIOLOGY).

Serious fungal infections caused by *Scedosporium apiospermum* (asexual form of *Pseudallescheria boydii*) and *Fusarium* spp. including *Fusarium solani*, in patients intolerant of, or refractory to, other therapy. (see CLINICAL STUDIES, MICROBIOLOGY).

Specimens for fungal culture and other relevant laboratory studies (including histopathology) should be obtained prior to therapy to isolate and identify causative organism(s). Therapy may be instituted before the results of the cultures and other laboratory studies are known. However, once these results become available, antifungal therapy should be adjusted accordingly.

CLINICAL STUDIES

Voriconazole, administered orally or parenterally, has been evaluated as primary or salvage therapy in 520 patients aged 12 years and older with infections caused by *Aspergillus* spp., *Fusarium* spp., and *Scedosporium* spp.

Invasive Aspergillosis

Voriconazole was studied in patients for primary therapy of invasive aspergillosis (randomized, controlled study 307/602), for primary and salvage therapy of aspergillosis (non-comparative study 304) and for treatment of patients with invasive aspergillosis who were refractory to, or intolerant of, other antifungal therapy (non-comparative study 309/604).

Study 307/602

The efficacy of voriconazole compared to amphotericin B in the primary treatment of acute invasive aspergillosis was demonstrated in 277 patients treated for 12 weeks in Study 307/602. The majority of study patients had underlying hematologic malignancies, including bone marrow transplantation. The study also included patients with solid organ transplantation, solid tumors, and AIDS. The patients were mainly treated for definite or probable invasive aspergillosis of the lungs. Other aspergillosis infections included disseminated disease, CNS infections and sinus infections. Diagnosis of definite or probable invasive aspergillosis was made according to criteria modified from those established by the National Institute of Allergy and Infectious Diseases Mycoses Study Group/European Organisation for Research and Treatment of Cancer (NIAID MSG/EORTC).

Voriconazole was administered intravenously with a loading dose of 6 mg/kg every 12 hours for the first 24 hours followed by a maintenance dose of 4 mg/kg every 12 hours for a minimum of seven days. Therapy could then be switched to the oral formulation at a dose of 200 mg Q12h. Median duration of IV voriconazole therapy was 10 days (range 2-90 days). After IV voriconazole therapy, the median duration of PO voriconazole therapy was 76 days (range 2-232 days).

Patients in the comparator group received conventional amphotericin B as a slow infusion at a daily dose of 1.0-1.5 mg/kg/day. Median duration of IV amphotericin therapy was 12 days (range 1-85 days). Treatment was then continued with other licensed antifungal therapy (OLAT), including itraconazole and lipid amphotericin B formulations. Although initial therapy with conventional amphotericin B was to be continued for at least two weeks, actual duration of therapy was at the discretion of the investigator. Patients who discontinued initial randomized therapy due to toxicity or lack of efficacy were eligible to continue in the study with OLAT treatment.

A satisfactory global response at 12 weeks (complete or partial resolution of all attributable symptoms, signs, radiographic/bronchoscopic abnormalities present at baseline) was seen in 53% of voriconazole treated patients compared to 32% of amphotericin B treated patients (Table 4). A benefit of voriconazole compared to amphotericin B on patient survival at Day 84 was seen with a 71% survival rate on voriconazole compared to 58% on amphotericin B (Table 4).

Table 4 also summarizes the response (success) based on mycological confirmation and species.

[See table 4 below]

Study Study 304

The results of this comparative trial (Study 307/602) confirmed the results of an earlier trial in the primary and salvage treatment of patients with acute invasive aspergillosis (Study 304). In this earlier study, an overall success rate of 52% (26/50) was seen in patients treated with voriconazole for primary therapy. Success was seen in 17/29 (59%) with *Aspergillus fumigatus* infections and 3/6 (50%) patients with infections due to non-*fumigatus* species [*A. flavus* (1/1); *A. nidulans* (0/2); *A. niger* (2/2); *A. terreus* (0/1)]. Success in patients who received voriconazole as salvage therapy is presented in Table 5.

Study 309/604

Additional data regarding response rates in patients who were refractory to, or intolerant of, other antifungal agents are also provided in Table 5. Overall mycological eradication for culture-documented infections due to *fumigatus* and non-*fumigatus* species of *Aspergillus* was 36/82 (44%) and 12/30 (40%), respectively, in voriconazole treated patients. Patients had various underlying diseases and species other than *A. fumigatus* contributed to mixed infections in some cases.

For patients who were infected with a single pathogen and were refractory to, or intolerant of, other antifungal agents, the satisfactory response rates for voriconazole in studies 304 and 309/604 are presented in Table 5.

Table 5 Combined Response Data in Salvage Patients with Single Aspergillus Species (Studies 304 and 309/604)

	Success n/N
A. fumigatus	43/97 (44%)
A. flavus	5/12
A. nidulans	1/3
A. niger	4/5
A. terreus	3/8
A. versicolor	0/1

Nineteen patients had more than one species of *Aspergillus* isolated. Success was seen in 4/17 (24%) of these patients.

Esophageal Candidiasis

The efficacy of oral voriconazole 200 mg bid compared to oral fluconazole 200 mg od in the primary treatment of esophageal candidiasis was demonstrated in Study 150-305, a double-blind, double-dummy, study in immunocompromised patients with endoscopically-proven esophageal candidiasis. Patients were treated for a median of 15 days (range 1 to 49 days). Outcome was assessed by repeat endoscopy at end of treatment (EOT). A successful response was defined as a normal endoscopy at EOT or at least a 1 grade improvement over baseline endoscopic score. For patients in the Intent To Treat (ITT) population with only a baseline endoscopy, a successful response was defined as symptomatic cure or improvement at EOT compared to

Table 4
Overall Efficacy and Success by Species in the Primary Treatment of Acute Invasive Aspergillosis Study 307/602

	Voriconazole	Ampho B[c]	Stratified Difference (95% CI)[d]
	n/N (%)	n/N (%)	
Efficacy as Primary Therapy			
Satisfactory Global Response[a]	76/144 (53)	42/133 (32)	21.8% (10.5%, 33.0%) $p<0.0001$
Survival at Day 84[b]	102/144 (71)	77/133 (58)	13.1% (2.1%, 24.2%)
Success by Species			
	Success n/N (%)		
Overall success	76/144 (53)	42/133 (32)	
Mycologically confirmed[e]	37/84 (44)	16/67 (24)	
Aspergillus spp.[f]			
A. fumigatus	28/63 (44)	12/47 (26)	
A. flavus	3/6	4/9	
A. terreus	2/3	0/3	
A. niger	1/4	0/9	
A. nidulans	1/1	0/0	

[a] Assessed by independent Data Review Committee (DRC)
[b] Proportion of subjects alive
[c] Amphotericin B followed by other licensed antifungal therapy
[d] Difference and corresponding 95% confidence interval are stratified by protocol
[e] Not all mycologically confirmed specimens were speciated
[f] Some patients had more than one species isolated at baseline

baseline. Voriconazole and fluconazole (200 mg od) showed comparable efficacy rates against esophageal candidiasis, as presented in Table 6.

[See table 6 at right]

Microbiologic success rates by *Candida* species are presented in Table 7.

[See table 7 at right]

Other Serious Fungal Pathogens

In pooled analyses of patients, voriconazole was shown to be effective against the following additional fungal pathogens: *Scedosporium apiospermum* - Successful response to voriconazole therapy was seen in 15 of 24 patients (63%). Three of these patients relapsed within 4 weeks, including 1 patient with pulmonary, skin and eye infections, 1 patient with cerebral disease, and 1 patient with skin infection. Ten patients had evidence of cerebral disease and 6 of these had a successful outcome (1 relapse). In addition, a successful response was seen in one of three patients with mixed organism infections.

Fusarium spp. - Nine of 21 (43%) patients were successfully treated with voriconazole. Of these nine patients, three had eye infections, one had an eye and blood infection, one had a skin infection, one had a blood infection alone, two had sinus infections, and one had disseminated infection (pulmonary, skin, hepatosplenic). Three of these patients (one with disseminated disease, one with an eye infection and one with a blood infection) had *Fusarium solani* and were complete successes. Two of these patients relapsed, one with a sinus infection and profound neutropenia and one post surgical patient with blood and eye infections.

CONTRAINDICATIONS

VFEND is contraindicated in patients with known hypersensitivity to voriconazole or its excipients. There is no information regarding cross-sensitivity between VFEND (voriconazole) and other azole antifungal agents. Caution should be used when prescribing VFEND to patients with hypersensitivity to other azoles.

Coadministration of the CYP3A4 substrates, terfenadine, astemizole, cisapride, pimozide or quinidine with VFEND are contraindicated since increased plasma concentrations of these drugs can lead to QT prolongation and rare occurrences of *torsade de pointes* (see CLINICAL PHARMACOLOGY - Drug Interactions, PRECAUTIONS - Drug Interactions).

Coadministration of VFEND with sirolimus is contraindicated because VFEND significantly increases sirolimus concentrations in healthy subjects (see CLINICAL PHARMACOLOGY - Drug Interactions, PRECAUTIONS - Drug Interactions).

Coadministration of VFEND with rifampin, carbamazepine and long-acting barbiturates is contraindicated since these drugs are likely to decrease plasma voriconazole concentrations significantly (see CLINICAL PHARMACOLOGY - Drug Interactions, PRECAUTIONS - Drug Interactions).

Coadministration of VFEND with ritonavir (400 mg Q12h) is contraindicated because ritonavir (400 mg Q12h) significantly decreases plasma voriconazole concentrations in healthy subjects. The effect of ritonavir (100 mg Q12h as used to inhibit CYP3A and increase concentrations of other antiretroviral drugs) on voriconazole concentrations has not been studied (see CLINICAL PHARMACOLOGY - Drug Interactions, PRECAUTIONS - Drug Interactions).

Coadministration of VFEND with efavirenz is contraindicated because efavirenz significantly decreases voriconazole plasma concentrations while VFEND also significantly increases efavirenz plasma concentrations (see CLINICAL PHARMACOLOGY - Drug Interactions, PRECAUTIONS - Drug Interactions).

Coadministration of VFEND with rifabutin is contraindicated since VFEND significantly increases rifabutin plasma concentrations and rifabutin also significantly decreases voriconazole plasma concentrations (see CLINICAL PHARMACOLOGY - Drug Interactions, PRECAUTIONS - Drug Interactions).

Coadministration of VFEND with ergot alkaloids (ergotamine and dihydroergotamine) is contraindicated because VFEND may increase the plasma concentration of ergot alkaloids, which may lead to ergotism.

WARNINGS

VISUAL DISTURBANCES: The effect of VFEND on visual function is not known if treatment continues beyond 28 days. If treatment continues beyond 28 days, visual function including visual acuity, visual field and color perception should be monitored **(see PRECAUTIONS – Information for Patients and ADVERSE EVENTS – Visual Disturbances).**

HEPATIC TOXICITY: In clinical trials, there have been uncommon cases of serious hepatic reactions during treatment with VFEND (including clinical hepatitis, cholestasis and fulminant hepatic failure, including fatalities). Instances of hepatic reactions were noted to occur primarily in patients with serious underlying medical conditions (predominantly hematological malignancy). Hepatic reactions, including hepatitis and jaundice, have occurred among patients with no other identifiable risk factors. Liver dysfunction has usually been reversible on discontinuation of therapy **(see PRECAUTIONS – Laboratory Tests and ADVERSE EVENTS – Clinical Laboratory Values).**

Monitoring of hepatic function: Liver function tests should be evaluated at the start of and during the course of VFEND therapy. Patients who develop abnormal liver function tests during VFEND therapy should be monitored for the development of more severe hepatic injury. Patient management should include laboratory evaluation of hepatic function (particularly liver function tests and bilirubin). Discontinuation of VFEND must be considered if clinical signs and symptoms consistent with liver disease develop that may be attributable to VFEND (see PRECAUTIONS - Laboratory Tests, DOSAGE AND ADMINISTRATION - Dosage Adjustment, ADVERSE EVENTS - Clinical Laboratory Tests).

Pregnancy Category D: Voriconazole can cause fetal harm when administered to a pregnant woman.

Voriconazole was teratogenic in rats (cleft palates, hydronephrosis/hydroureter) from 10 mg/kg (0.3 times the recommended maintenance dose (RMD) on a mg/m^2 basis) and embryotoxic in rabbits at 100 mg/kg (6 times the RMD). Other effects in rats included reduced ossification of sacral and caudal vertebrae, skull, pubic and hyoid bone, super numerary ribs, anomalies of the sternebrae and dilatation of the ureter/renal pelvis. Plasma estradiol in pregnant rats was reduced at all dose levels. Voriconazole treatment in rats produced increased gestational length and dystocia, which were associated with increased perinatal pup mortality at the 10 mg/kg dose. The effects seen in rabbits were an increased embryomortality, reduced fetal weight and increased incidences of skeletal variations, cervical ribs and extra sternebral ossification sites.

If this drug is used during pregnancy, or if the patient becomes pregnant while taking this drug, the patient should be apprised of the potential hazard to the fetus.

Table 6
Success Rates in Patients Treated for Esophageal Candidiasis

Population	Voriconazole	Fluconazole	Difference % (95% CI)[a]
PP[b]	113/115 (98.2%)	134/141 (95.0%)	3.2 (-1.1, 7.5)
ITT[c]	175/200 (87.5%)	171/191 (89.5%)	-2.0 (-8.3, 4.3)

[a] Confidence Interval for the difference (Voriconazole – Fluconazole) in success rates.
[b] PP (Per Protocol) patients had confirmation of *Candida* esophagitis by endoscopy, received at least 12 days of treatment, and had a repeat endoscopy at EOT (end of treatment).
[c] ITT (Intent to Treat) patients without endoscopy or clinical assessment at EOT were treated as failures.

Table 7
Clinical and mycological outcome by baseline pathogen in patients with esophageal candidiasis (Study 150-305).

Pathogen[a]	Voriconazole		Fluconazole	
	Favorable endoscopic response[b]	**Mycological eradication[b]**	**Favorable endoscopic response[b]**	**Mycological eradication[b]**
	Success/Total (%)	Eradication/Total (%)	Success/Total (%)	Eradication/Total (%)
C. albicans	134/140 (96%)	90/107 (84%)	147/156 (94%)	91/115 (79%)
C. glabrata	8/8 (100%)	4/7 (57%)	4/4 (100%)	1/4 (25%)
C. krusei	1/1	1/1	2/2 (100%)	0/0

[a]Some patients had more than one species isolated at baseline
[b]Patients with endoscopic and/or mycological assessment at end of therapy

Table 8 Effect of Other Drugs on Voriconazole Pharmacokinetics

Drug/Drug Class (Mechanism of Interaction by the Drug)	Voriconazole Plasma Exposure (C_{max} and AUC_τ after 200 mg Q12h)	Recommendations for Voriconazole Dosage Adjustment/Comments
Rifampin*, Efavirenz** and Rifabutin* (CYP450 Induction)	Significantly Reduced	**Contraindicated**
Ritonavir (400mg Q12h HIV Protease Inhibitor)** (CYP450 Induction)	Significantly Reduced	**Contraindicated** The effect of ritonavir (100 mg Q12h as used to inhibit CYP3A and increase concentrations of other antiretroviral drugs) on voriconazole concentrations has not been studied.
Carbamazepine (CYP450 Induction)	Not Studied *In Vivo* or *In Vitro*, but Likely to Result in Significant Reduction	**Contraindicated**
Long Acting Barbiturates (CYP450 Induction)	Not Studied *In Vivo* or *In Vitro*, but Likely to Result in Significant Reduction	**Contraindicated**
Phenytoin* (CYP450 Induction)	Significantly Reduced	Increase voriconazole maintenance dose from 4 mg/kg to 5 mg/kg IV every 12 hrs or from 200 mg to 400 mg orally every 12 hrs (100 mg to 200 mg orally every 12 hrs in patients weighing less than 40 kg)
Other HIV Protease Inhibitors (CYP3A4 Inhibition)	*In Vivo* Studies Showed No Significant Effects of Indinavir on Voriconazole Exposure *In Vitro* Studies Demonstrate Potential for Inhibition of Voriconazole Metabolism (Increased Plasma Exposure)	No dosage adjustment in the voriconazole dosage needed when coadministered with indinavir Frequent monitoring for adverse events and toxicity related to voriconazole when coadministered with other HIV protease inhibitors
Other NNRTIs*** (CYP3A4 Inhibition or CYP450 Induction)	*In Vitro* Studies Demonstrate Potential for Inhibition of Voriconazole Metabolism by Delaviridine and Other NNRTIs (Increased Plasma Exposure) A Voriconazole-Efavirenz Drug Interaction Study Demonstrates the Potential for the Metabolism of Voriconazole to be Induced by Efavirenz and Other NNRTIs (Decreased Plasma Exposure)	Frequent monitoring for adverse events and toxicity related to voriconazole Careful assessment of voriconazole effectiveness

*Results based on *in vivo* clinical studies generally following repeat oral dosing with 200 mg Q12h voriconazole to healthy subjects
**Results based on *in vivo* clinical study following repeat oral dosing with 400 mg Q12h for 1 day, then 200 mg Q12h for 8 days voriconazole to healthy subjects
***Non-Nucleoside Reverse Transcriptase Inhibitors

Continued on next page

VFEND—Cont.

Galactose intolerance: VFEND tablets contain lactose and should not be given to patients with rare hereditary problems of galactose intolerance, Lapp lactase deficiency or glucose-galactose malabsorption.

PRECAUTIONS

General

(See WARNINGS, DOSAGE AND ADMINISTRATION)

Some azoles, including voriconazole, have been associated with prolongation of the QT interval on the electrocardiogram. During clinical development and post-marketing surveillance, there have been rare cases of torsade de pointes in patients taking voriconazole. These reports involved seriously ill patients with multiple confounding risk factors, such as history of cardiotoxic chemotherapy, cardiomyopathy, hypokalemia and concomitant medications that may have been contributory.

Voriconazole should be administered with caution to patients with these potentially proarrhythmic conditions.

Rigorous attempts to correct potassium, magnesium and calcium should be made before starting voriconazole (see CLINICAL PHARMACOLOGY - Pharmacokinetic-pharmacodynamic Relationships - Electrocardiogram).

Infusion Related Reactions

During infusion of the intravenous formulation of voriconazole in healthy subjects, anaphylactoid-type reactions, including flushing, fever, sweating, tachycardia, chest tightness, dyspnea, faintness, nausea, pruritus and rash, have occurred uncommonly. Symptoms appeared immediately upon initiating the infusion. Consideration should be given to stopping the infusion should these reactions occur.

Information for Patients

Patients should be advised:

- that VFEND Tablets or Oral Suspension should be taken at least one hour before, or one hour following, a meal.
- **that they should not drive at night while taking VFEND. VFEND may cause changes to vision, including blurring and/or photophobia.**
- **that they should avoid potentially hazardous tasks, such as driving or operating machinery if they perceive any change in vision.**
- that strong, direct sunlight should be avoided during VFEND therapy.
- that VFEND for Oral Suspension contains sucrose and is not recommended for patients with rare hereditary problems of fructose intolerance, sucrase-isomaltase deficiency or glucose-galactose malabsorption.

Laboratory Tests

Electrolyte disturbances such as hypokalemia, hypomagnesemia and hypocalcemia should be corrected prior to initiation of VFEND therapy.

Patient management should include laboratory evaluation of renal (particularly serum creatinine) and hepatic function (particularly liver function tests and bilirubin).

Drug Interactions

Tables 8 and 9 provide a summary of significant drug interactions with voriconazole that either have been studied *in vivo* (clinically) or that may be expected to occur based on results of *in vitro* metabolism studies with human liver microsomes. For more details, see CLINICAL PHARMACOLOGY - Drug Interactions.

[See table 8 on previous page]

[See table 9 at right and on next page]

Patients with Hepatic Insufficiency

It is recommended that the standard loading dose regimens be used but that the maintenance dose be halved in patients with mild to moderate hepatic cirrhosis (Child-Pugh Class A and B) receiving VFEND (see CLINICAL PHARMACOLOGY - Hepatic Insufficiency, DOSAGE AND ADMINISTRATION - Hepatic Insufficiency).

VFEND has not been studied in patients with severe cirrhosis (Child-Pugh Class C). VFEND has been associated with elevations in liver function tests and clinical signs of liver damage, such as jaundice, and should only be used in patients with severe hepatic insufficiency if the benefit outweighs the potential risk. Patients with hepatic insufficiency must be carefully monitored for drug toxicity.

Patients with Renal Insufficiency

In patients with moderate to severe renal dysfunction (creatinine clearance <50 mL/min), accumulation of the intravenous vehicle, SBECD, occurs. Oral voriconazole should be administered to these patients, unless an assessment of the benefit/risk to the patient justifies the use of intravenous voriconazole. Serum creatinine levels should be closely monitored in these patients, and if increases occur, consideration should be given to changing to oral voriconazole therapy (see CLINICAL PHARMACOLOGY - Renal Insufficiency, DOSAGE AND ADMINISTRATION - Renal Insufficiency).

Renal Adverse Events

Acute renal failure has been observed in severely ill patients undergoing treatment with VFEND. Patients being treated with voriconazole are likely to be treated concomitantly with nephrotoxic medications and have concurrent conditions that may result in decreased renal function.

Monitoring of Renal Function

Patients should be monitored for the development of abnormal renal function. This should include laboratory evaluation, particularly serum creatinine.

Table 9 Effect of Voriconazole on Pharmacokinetics of Other Drugs

Drug/Drug Class (Mechanism of Interaction by Voriconazole)	Drug Plasma Exposure (C_{max} and AUC_τ)	Recommendations for Drug Dosage Adjustment/Comments
Sirolimus* (CYP3A4 Inhibition)	Significantly Increased	**Contraindicated**
Rifabutin* and Efavirenz** (CYP3A4 Inhibition)	Significantly Increased	**Contraindicated**
Ritonavir (400 mg Q12h HIV Protease Inhibitor)** (CYP3A4 Inhibition)	No significant effect of voriconazole on ritonavir C_{max} or AUC_τ	**Contraindicated** because of significant reduction of voriconazole C_{max} and AUC_τ
Terfenadine, Astemizole, Cisapride, Pimozide, Quinidine (CYP3A4 Inhibition)	Not Studied *In Vivo* or *In Vitro*, but Drug Plasma Exposure Likely to be Increased	**Contraindicated** because of potential for QT prolongation and rare occurrence of *torsade de pointes*
Ergot Alkaloids (CYP450 Inhibition)	Not Studied *In Vivo* or *In Vitro*, but Drug Plasma Exposure Likely to be Increased	**Contraindicated**
Cyclosporine* (CYP3A4 Inhibition)	AUC_τ Significantly Increased; No Significant Effect on C_{max}	When initiating therapy with VFEND in patients already receiving cyclosporine, reduce the cyclosporine dose to one-half of the starting dose and follow with frequent monitoring of cyclosporine blood levels. Increased cyclosporine levels have been associated with nephrotoxicity. When VFEND is discontinued, cyclosporine concentrations must be frequently monitored and the dose increased as necessary.
Tacrolimus* (CYP3A4 Inhibition)	Significantly Increased	When initiating therapy with VFEND in patients already receiving tacrolimus, reduce the tacrolimus dose to one-third of the starting dose and follow with frequent monitoring of tacrolimus blood levels. Increased tacrolimus levels have been associated with nephrotoxicity. When VFEND is discontinued, tacrolimus concentrations must be frequently monitored and the dose increased as necessary.
Phenytoin* (CYP2C9 Inhibition)	Significantly Increased	Frequent monitoring of phenytoin plasma concentrations and frequent monitoring of adverse effects related to phenytoin.
Warfarin* (CYP2C9 Inhibition)	Prothrombin Time Significantly Increased	Monitor PT or other suitable anticoagulation tests. Adjustment of warfarin dosage may be needed.
Omeprazole* (CYP2C19/3A4 Inhibition)	Significantly Increased	When initiating therapy with VFEND in patients already receiving omeprazole doses of 40 mg or greater, reduce the omeprazole dose by one-half. The metabolism of other proton pump inhibitors that are CYP2C19 substrates may also be inhibited by voriconazole and may result in increased plasma concentrations of other proton pump inhibitors.
Other HIV Protease Inhibitors (CYP3A4 Inhibition)	*In Vivo* Studies showed No Significant Effects on Indinavir Exposure *In Vitro* Studies Demonstrate Potential for Voriconazole to Inhibit Metabolism (Increased Plasma Exposure)	No dosage adjustment for indinavir when coadministered with VFEND Frequent monitoring for adverse events and toxicity related to other HIV protease inhibitors
Other NNRTIs*** (CYP3A4 Inhibition)	A Voriconazole-Efavirenz Drug Interaction Study Demonstrates the Potential for Voriconazole to Inhibit Metabolism of Other NNRTIs (Increased Plasma Exposure)	Frequent monitoring for adverse events and toxicity related to NNRTI
Benzodiazepines (CYP3A4 Inhibition)	*In Vitro* Studies Demonstrate Potential for Voriconazole to Inhibit Metabolism (Increased Plasma Exposure)	Frequent monitoring for adverse events and toxicity (i.e., prolonged sedation) related to benzodiazepines metabolized by CYP3A4 (e.g., midazolam, triazolam, alprazolam). Adjustment of benzodiazepine dosage may be needed.
HMG-CoA Reductase Inhibitors (Statins) (CYP3A4 Inhibition)	*In Vitro* Studies Demonstrate Potential for Voriconazole to Inhibit Metabolism (Increased Plasma Exposure)	Frequent monitoring for adverse events and toxicity related to statins. Increased statin concentrations in plasma have been associated with rhabdomyolysis. Adjustment of the statin dosage may be needed.

(Table continued on next page)

Dermatological Reactions

Patients have rarely developed serious cutaneous reactions, such as Stevens-Johnson syndrome, during treatment with VFEND. If patients develop a rash, they should be monitored closely and consideration given to discontinuation of VFEND. VFEND has been infrequently associated with photosensitivity skin reaction, especially during long-term therapy. It is recommended that patients avoid strong, direct sunlight during VFEND therapy.

Carcinogenesis, Mutagenesis, Impairment of Fertility

Two-year carcinogenicity studies were conducted in rats and mice. Rats were given oral doses of 6, 18 or 50 mg/kg

Table 9 *(cont.)* Effect of Voriconazole on Pharmacokinetics of Other Drugs

Drug/Drug Class (Mechanism of Interaction by Voriconazole)	Drug Plasma Exposure (C_{max} and AUC_τ)	Recommendations for Drug Dosage Adjustment/Comments
Dihydropyridine Calcium Channel Blockers (CYP3A4 Inhibition)	*In Vitro* Studies Demonstrate Potential for Voriconazole to Inhibit Metabolism (Increased Plasma Exposure)	Frequent monitoring for adverse events and toxicity related to calcium channel blockers. Adjustment of calcium channel blocker dosage may be needed.
Sulfonylurea Oral Hypoglycemics (CYP2C9 Inhibition)	Not Studied *In Vivo* or *In Vitro*, but Drug Plasma Exposure Likely to be Increased	Frequent monitoring of blood glucose and for signs and symptoms of hypoglycemia. Adjustment of oral hypoglycemic drug dosage may be needed.
Vinca Alkaloids (CYP3A4 Inhibition)	Not Studied *In Vivo* or *In Vitro*, but Drug Plasma Exposure Likely to be Increased	Frequent monitoring for adverse events and toxicity (i.e., neurotoxicity) related to vinca alkaloids. Adjustment of vinca alkaloid dosage may be needed.

*Results based on *in vivo* clinical studies generally following repeat oral dosing with 200 mg BID voriconazole to healthy subjects
**Results based on *in vivo* clinical study following repeat oral doing with 400 mg Q12h for 1 day, then 200 mg Q12h for 8 days voriconazole to healthy subjects
***Non-Nucleoside Reverse Transcriptase Inhibitors

Table 10
Treatment Emergent Adverse Events
Rate ≥ 1% or Adverse Events of Concern in All Therapeutic Studies
Possibly Related to Therapy or Causality Unknown

	All Therapeutic Studies	Protocol 305 (oral therapy)		Protocol 307/602 (IV/oral therapy)	
	Voriconazole N = 1493	Voriconazole N = 200	Fluconazole N = 191	Voriconazole N = 196	Ampho B** N = 185
	N (%)	N (%)	N (%)	N (%)	N (%)
Special Senses*					
Abnormal vision	307 (20.6)	31 (15.5)	8 (4.2)	55 (28.1)	1 (0.5)
Photophobia	36 (2.4)	5 (2.5)	2 (1.0)	7 (3.6)	0
Chromatopsia	20 (1.3)	2 (1.0)	0	2 (1.0)	0
Eye hemorrhage	3 (0.2)	0	0	0	0
Body as a Whole					
Fever	93 (6.2)	0	0	7 (3.6)	25 (13.5)
Chills	61 (4.1)	1 (0.5)	0	0	36 (19.5)
Headache	48 (3.2)	0	1 (0.5)	7 (3.6)	8 (4.3)
Abdominal pain	25 (1.7)	0	0	5 (2.6)	6 (3.2)
Chest pain	13 (0.9)	0	0	4 (2.0)	2 (1.1)
Cardiovascular System					
Tachycardia	37 (2.5)	0	0	5 (2.6)	5 (2.7)
Hypertension	29 (1.9)	0	0	1 (0.5)	2 (1.1)
Hypotension	26 (1.7)	1 (0.5)	0	1 (0.5)	3 (1.6)
Vasodilatation	23 (1.5)	0	0	2 (1.0)	2 (1.1)
Digestive System					
Nausea	88 (5.9)	2 (1.0)	3 (1.6)	14 (7.1)	29 (15.7)
Vomiting	71 (4.8)	2 (1.0)	1 (0.5)	11 (5.6)	18 (9.7)
Liver function tests abnormal	41 (2.7)	6 (3.0)	2 (1.0)	9 (4.6)	4 (2.2)
Diarrhea	16 (1.1)	0	0	3 (1.5)	6 (3.2)
Cholestatic jaundice	16 (1.1)	3 (1.5)	0	4 (2.0)	0
Dry mouth	15 (1.0)	0	1 (0.5)	3 (1.5)	0
Jaundice	3 (0.2)	1 (0.5)	0	0	0
Hemic and Lymphatic System					
Thrombocytopenia	7 (0.5)	0	1 (0.5)	2 (1.0)	2 (1.1)
Anemia	2 (0.1)	0	0	0	5 (2.7)
Leukopenia	4 (0.3)	0	0	1 (0.5)	0
Pancytopenia	1 (0.1)	0	0	0	0

(Table continued on next page)

voriconazole, or 0.2, 0.6, or 1.6 times the recommended maintenance dose (RMD) on a mg/m² basis. Hepatocellular adenomas were detected in females at 50 mg/kg and hepatocellular carcinomas were found in males at 6 and 50 mg/kg. Mice were given oral doses of 10, 30 or 100 mg/kg voriconazole, or 0.1, 0.4, or 1.4 times the RMD on a mg/m² basis. In mice, hepatocellular adenomas were detected in males and females and hepatocellular carcinomas were detected in males at 1.4 times the RMD of voriconazole.

Voriconazole demonstrated clastogenic activity (mostly chromosome breaks) in human lymphocyte cultures *in vitro*. Voriconazole was not genotoxic in the Ames assay, CHO assay, the mouse micronucleus assay or the DNA repair test (Unscheduled DNA Synthesis assay).

Voriconazole produced a reduction in the pregnancy rates of rats dosed at 50 mg/kg, or 1.6 times the RMD. This was statistically significant only in the preliminary study and not in a larger fertility study.

Teratogenic Effects

Pregnancy category D. See WARNINGS

Women of Childbearing Potential

Women of childbearing potential should use effective contraception during treatment.

Nursing Mothers

The excretion of voriconazole in breast milk has not been investigated. VFEND should not be used by nursing mothers unless the benefit clearly outweighs the risk.

Pediatric Use

Safety and effectiveness in pediatric patients below the age of 12 years have not been established.

A total of 22 patients aged 12-18 years with invasive aspergillosis were included in the therapeutic studies. Twelve out of 22 (55%) patients had successful response after treatment with a maintenance dose of voriconazole 4 mg/kg Q12h.

Sparse plasma sampling for pharmacokinetics in adolescents was conducted in the therapeutic studies (see CLINICAL PHARMACOLOGY - Pharmacokinetics, General Pharmacokinetic Characteristics).

Geriatric Use

In multiple dose therapeutic trials of voriconazole, 9.2% of patients were ≥ 65 years of age and 1.8% of patients were ≥ 75 years of age. In a study in healthy volunteers, the systemic exposure (AUC) and peak plasma concentrations (C_{max}) were increased in elderly males compared to young males. Pharmacokinetic data obtained from 552 patients from 10 voriconazole therapeutic trials showed that voriconazole plasma concentrations in the elderly patients were approximately 80% to 90% higher than those in younger patients after either IV or oral administration. However, the overall safety profile of the elderly patients was similar to that of the young so no dosage adjustment is recommended (see CLINICAL PHARMACOLOGY - Pharmacokinetics in Special Populations).

ADVERSE REACTIONS

Overview

The most frequently reported adverse events (all causalities) in the therapeutic trials were visual disturbances, fever, rash, vomiting, nausea, diarrhea, headache, sepsis, peripheral edema, abdominal pain, and respiratory disorder. The treatment-related adverse events which most often led to discontinuation of voriconazole therapy were elevated liver function tests, rash, and visual disturbances (see hepatic toxicity under WARNINGS and discussion of Clinical Laboratory Values and dermatological and visual adverse events below).

Discussion of Adverse Reactions

The data described in the table below reflect exposure to voriconazole in 1493 patients in the therapeutic studies. This represents a heterogeneous population, including immunocompromised patients, e.g., patients with hematological malignancy or HIV and non-neutropenic patients. This subgroup does not include healthy volunteers and patients treated in the compassionate use and non-therapeutic studies. This patient population was 62% male, had a mean age of 45.1 years (range 12-90, including 49 patients aged 12-18 years), and was 81% white and 9% black. Five hundred sixty-one patients had a duration of voriconazole therapy of greater than 12 weeks, with 136 patients receiving voriconazole for over six months. Table 10 includes all adverse events which were reported in therapeutic studies at an incidence of ≥1% as well as events of concern which occurred at an incidence of <1% during voriconazole therapy.

In study 307/602, 381 patients (196 on voriconazole, 185 on amphotericin B) were treated to compare voriconazole to amphotericin B followed by other licensed antifungal therapy in the primary treatment of patients with acute invasive aspergillosis. Study 305 evaluated the effects of oral voriconazole (200 patients) and oral fluconazole (191 patients) in the treatment of esophageal candidiasis. Laboratory test abnormalities for these studies are discussed under Clinical Laboratory Values below.

[See table 10 at left and on next page]

VISUAL DISTURBANCES: Voriconazole treatment-related visual disturbances are common. In clinical trials, approximately 30% of patients experienced altered/enhanced visual perception, blurred vision, color vision change and/or photophobia. The visual disturbances were generally mild and rarely resulted in discontinuation. Visual disturbances may be associated with higher plasma concentrations and/or doses.

The mechanism of action of the visual disturbance is unknown, although the site of action is most likely to be within the retina. In a study in healthy volunteers investigating the effect of 28-day treatment with voriconazole on retinal function, voriconazole caused a decrease in the electroreti-

Continued on next page

VFEND—Cont.

nogram (ERG) waveform amplitude, a decrease in the visual field, and an alteration in color perception. The ERG measures electrical currents in the retina. The effects were noted early in administration of voriconazole and continued through the course of study drug dosing. Fourteen days after end of dosing, ERG, visual fields and color perception returned to normal (see WARNINGS, PRECAUTIONS – Information For Patients).

Dermatological Reactions: Dermatological reactions were common in the patients treated with voriconazole. The mechanism underlying these dermatologic adverse events remains unknown. In clinical trials, rashes considered related to therapy were reported by 6% (86/1493) of voriconazole-treated patients. The majority of rashes were of mild to moderate severity. Cases of photosensitivity reactions appear to be more likely to occur with long-term treatment. Patients have rarely developed serious cutaneous reactions, including Stevens-Johnson syndrome, toxic epidermal necrolysis and erythema multiforme during treatment with VFEND. If patients develop a rash, they should be monitored closely and consideration given to discontinuation of VFEND. It is recommended that patients avoid strong, direct sunlight during VFEND therapy.

Less Common Adverse Events

The following adverse events occurred in <1% of all voriconazole-treated patients, including healthy volunteers and patients treated under compassionate use protocols (total N = 2090). This listing includes events where a causal relationship to voriconazole cannot be ruled out or those which may help the physician in managing the risks to the patients. The list does not include events included in Table 10 above and does not include every event reported in the voriconazole clinical program.

Body as a Whole: abdomen enlarged, allergic reaction, anaphylactoid reaction (see PRECAUTIONS), ascites, asthenia, back pain, cellulitis, edema, face edema, flank pain, flu syndrome, graft versus host reaction, granuloma, infection, bacterial infection, fungal infection, injection site pain, injection site infection/inflammation, mucous membrane disorder, multi-organ failure, pain, pelvic pain, peritonitis, sepsis, substernal chest pain

Cardiovascular: atrial arrhythmia, atrial fibrillation, AV block complete, bigeminy, bradycardia, bundle branch block, cardiomegaly, cardiomyopathy, cerebral hemorrhage, cerebral ischemia, cerebrovascular accident, congestive heart failure, deep thrombophlebitis, endocarditis, extrasystoles, heart arrest, myocardial infarction, nodal arrhythmia, palpitation, phlebitis, postural hypotension, pulmonary embolus, QT interval prolonged, supraventricular tachycardia, syncope, thrombophlebitis, vasodilatation, ventricular arrhythmia, ventricular fibrillation, ventricular tachycardia (including *torsade de pointes*)

Digestive: anorexia, cheilitis, cholecystitis, cholelithiasis, constipation, duodenal ulcer perforation, duodenitis, dyspepsia, dysphagia, esophageal ulcer, esophagitis, flatulence, gastroenteritis, gastrointestinal hemorrhage, GGT/LDH elevated, gingivitis, glossitis, gum hemorrhage, gum hyperplasia, hematemesis, hepatic coma, hepatic failure, hepatitis, intestinal perforation, intestinal ulcer, enlarged liver, melena, mouth ulceration, pancreatitis, parotid gland enlargement, periodontitis, proctitis, pseudomembranous colitis, rectal disorder, rectal hemorrhage, stomach ulcer, stomatitis, tongue edema

Endocrine: adrenal cortex insufficiency, diabetes insipidus, hyperthyroidism, hypothyroidism

Hemic and Lymphatic: agranulocytosis, anemia (macrocytic, megaloblastic, microcytic, normocytic), aplastic anemia, hemolytic anemia, bleeding time increased, cyanosis, DIC, ecchymosis, eosinophilia, hypervolemia, lymphadenopathy, lymphangitis, marrow depression, petechia, purpura, enlarged spleen, thrombotic thrombocytopenic purpura

Metabolic and Nutritional: albuminuria, BUN increased, creatine phosphokinase increased, edema, glucose tolerance decreased, hypercalcemia, hypercholesteremia, hyperglycemia, hyperkalemia, hypermagnesemia, hypernatremia, hyperuricemia, hypocalcemia, hypoglycemia, hyponatremia, hypophosphatemia, uremia

Musculoskeletal: arthralgia, arthritis, bone necrosis, bone pain, leg cramps, myalgia, myasthenia, myopathy, osteomalacia, osteoporosis

Nervous System: abnormal dreams, acute brain syndrome, agitation, akathisia, amnesia, anxiety, ataxia, brain edema, coma, confusion, convulsion, delirium, dementia, depersonalization, depression, diplopia, encephalitis, encephalopathy, euphoria, Extrapyramidal Syndrome, grand mal convulsion, Guillain-Barré syndrome, hypertonia, hypesthesia, insomnia, intracranial hypertension, libido decreased, neuralgia, neuropathy, nystagmus, oculogyric crisis, paresthesia, psychosis, somnolence, suicidal ideation, tremor, vertigo

Respiratory System: cough increased, dyspnea, epistaxis, hemoptysis, hypoxia, lung edema, pharyngitis, pleural effusion, pneumonia, respiratory disorder, respiratory distress syndrome, respiratory tract infection, rhinitis, sinusitis, voice alteration

Skin and Appendages: alopecia, angioedema, contact dermatitis, discoid lupus erythematosis, eczema, erythema multiforme, exfoliative dermatitis, fixed drug eruption, furunculosis, herpes simplex, melanosis, photosensitivity skin reaction, psoriasis, skin discoloration, skin disorder, skin dry, Stevens-Johnson syndrome, sweating, toxic epidermal necrolysis, urticaria

Table 10 *(cont.)*
Treatment Emergent Adverse Events
Rate ≥ 1% or Adverse Events of Concern in All Therapeutic Studies
Possibly Related to Therapy or Causality Unknown

	All Therapeutic Studies	**Protocol 305** (oral therapy)		**Protocol 307/602** (IV/oral therapy)	
	Voriconazole N = 1493	Voriconazole N = 200	Fluconazole N = 191	Voriconazole N = 196	Ampho B** N = 185
	N (%)	N (%)	N (%)	N (%)	N (%)
Metabolic and Nutritional Systems					
Alkaline phosphatase increased	54 (3.6)	10 (5.0)	3 (1.6)	6 (3.1)	4 (2.2)
Hepatic enzymes increased	28 (1.9)	3 (1.5)	0	7 (3.6)	5 (2.7)
SGOT increased	28 (1.9)	8 (4.0)	2 (1.0)	1 (0.5)	0
SGPT increased	27 (1.8)	6 (3.0)	2 (1.0)	3 (1.5)	1 (0.5)
Hypokalemia	24 (1.6)	0	0	1 (0.5)	36 (19.5)
Peripheral edema	16 (1.1)	1 (0.5)	0	7 (3.6)	9 (4.9)
Hypomagnesemia	16 (1.1)	0	0	2 (1.0)	10 (5.4)
Bilirubinemia	12 (0.8)	1 (0.5)	0	1 (0.5)	3 (1.6)
Creatinine increased	4 (0.3)	1 (0.5)	0	0	59 (31.9)
Nervous System					
Hallucinations	37 (2.5)	0	0	10 (5.1)	1 (0.5)
Dizziness	20 (1.3)	0	2 (1.0)	5 (2.6)	0
Skin and Appendages					
Rash	86 (5.8)	3 (1.5)	1 (0.5)	13 (6.6)	7 (3.8)
Pruritus	16 (1.1)	0	0	2 (1.0)	2 (1.1)
Maculopapular rash	17 (1.1)	3 (1.5)	0	1 (0.5)	0
Urogenital					
Kidney function abnormal	8 (0.5)	1 (0.5)	1 (0.5)	4 (2.0)	40 (21.6)
Acute kidney failure	7 (0.5)	0	0	0	11 (5.9)

* See WARNINGS – Visual Disturbances, PRECAUTIONS – Information For Patients
**Amphotericin B followed by other licensed antifungal therapy

Table 11
PROTOCOL 305
Clinically Significant Laboratory Test Abnormalities

	Criteria*	VORICONAZOLE	FLUCONAZOLE
		n/N (%)	n/N (%)
T. Bilirubin	>1.5× ULN	8/185 (4.3)	7/186 (3.8)
AST	>3.0× ULN	38/187 (20.3)	15/186 (8.1)
ALT	>3.0× ULN	20/187 (10.7)	12/186 (6.5)
Alk phos	>3.0× ULN	19/187 (10.2)	14/186 (7.5)

* Without regard to baseline value
n number of patients with a clinically significant abnormality while on study therapy
N total number of patients with at least one observation of the given lab test while on study therapy
ULN upper limit of normal

Special Senses: abnormality of accommodation, blepharitis, color blindness, conjunctivitis, corneal opacity, deafness, ear pain, eye pain, dry eyes, keratitis, keratoconjunctivitis, mydriasis, night blindness, optic atrophy, optic neuritis, otitis externa, papilledema, retinal hemorrhage, retinitis, scleritis, taste loss, taste perversion, tinnitus, uveitis, visual field defect

Urogenital: anuria, blighted ovum, creatinine clearance decreased, dysmenorrhea, dysuria, epididymitis, glycosuria, hemorrhagic cystitis, hematuria, hydronephrosis, impotence, kidney pain, kidney tubular necrosis, metrorrhagia, nephritis, nephrosis, oliguria, scrotal edema, urinary incontinence, urinary retention, urinary tract infection, uterine hemorrhage, vaginal hemorrhage

Clinical Laboratory Values

The overall incidence of clinically significant transaminase abnormalities in the voriconazole clinical program was 13.4% (200/1493) of patients treated with voriconazole. Increased incidence of liver function test abnormalities may be associated with higher plasma concentrations and/or doses. The majority of abnormal liver function tests either resolved during treatment without dose adjustment or following dose adjustment, including discontinuation of therapy.

Voriconazole has been infrequently associated with cases of serious hepatic toxicity including cases of jaundice and rare cases of hepatitis and hepatic failure leading to death. Most of these patients had other serious underlying conditions.

Liver function tests should be evaluated at the start of and during the course of VFEND therapy. Patients who develop abnormal liver function tests during VFEND therapy should be monitored for the development of more severe hepatic injury. Patient management should include laboratory evaluation of hepatic function (particularly liver function tests and bilirubin). Discontinuation of VFEND must be considered if clinical signs and symptoms consistent with liver disease develop that may be attributable to VFEND (see WARNINGS and PRECAUTIONS - Laboratory Tests).

Acute renal failure has been observed in severely ill patients undergoing treatment with VFEND. Patients being treated with voriconazole are likely to be treated concomitantly with nephrotoxic medications and have concurrent conditions that may result in decreased renal function. It is recommended that patients are monitored for the development of abnormal renal function. This should include laboratory evaluation, particularly serum creatinine.

Tables 11 and 12 show the number of patients with hypokalemia and clinically significant changes in renal and liver function tests in two randomized, comparative multicenter studies. In study 305, patients were randomized to either oral voriconazole or oral fluconazole to evaluate an indication other than invasive aspergillosis in immunocompromised patients. In study 307/602, patients with definite or probable invasive aspergillosis were randomized to either voriconazole or amphotericin B therapy.

[See table 11 above]

[See table 12 at right]

OVERDOSE

In clinical trials, there were three cases of accidental overdose. All occurred in pediatric patients who received up to five times the recommended intravenous dose of voriconazole. A single adverse event of photophobia of 10 minutes duration was reported.

There is no known antidote to voriconazole.

Voriconazole is hemodialyzed with clearance of 121 mL/min. The intravenous vehicle, SBECD, is hemodialyzed with clearance of 55 mL/min. In an overdose, hemodialysis may assist in the removal of voriconazole and SBECD from the body.

The minimum lethal oral dose in mice and rats was 300 mg/kg (equivalent to 4 and 7 times the recommended maintenance dose (RMD), based on body surface area). At this dose, clinical signs observed in both mice and rats included salivation, mydriasis, titubation (loss of balance while moving), depressed behavior, prostration, partially closed eyes, and dyspnea. Other signs in mice were convulsions, corneal opacification and swollen abdomen.

DOSAGE AND ADMINISTRATION

Administration

VFEND Tablets or Oral Suspension should be taken at least one hour before, or one hour following, a meal.

VFEND I.V. for Injection requires reconstitution to 10 mg/mL and subsequent dilution to 5 mg/mL or less prior to administration as an infusion, at a maximum rate of 3 mg/kg per hour over 1-2 hours (see Intravenous Administration).

NOT FOR IV BOLUS INJECTION

Electrolyte disturbances such as hypokalemia, hypomagnesemia and hypocalcemia should be corrected prior to initiation of VFEND therapy (see PRECAUTIONS).

Use In Adults

Invasive aspergillosis and serious fungal infections due to *Fusarium* spp. and *Scedosporium apiospermum*:

For the treatment of adults with invasive aspergillosis and infections due to *Fusarium* spp. and *Scedosporium apiospermum*, therapy must be initiated with the specified loading dose regimen of intravenous VFEND to achieve plasma concentrations on Day 1 that are close to steady state. On the basis of high oral bioavailability, switching between intravenous and oral administration is appropriate when clinically indicated (see CLINICAL PHARMACOLOGY). Once the patient can tolerate medication given by mouth, the oral tablet form or oral suspension form of VFEND may be utilized.

The recommended dosing regimen of VFEND is as follows:

Loading Dose Regimen	6 mg/kg IV every 12 hours (for the first 24 hours)	
Maintenance Dose	IV	Oral*
	4 mg/kg every 12 hours	200 mg every 12 hours

*Patients who weigh 40 kg or more should receive an oral maintenace dose of 200 mg VFEND every 12 hours. Adult patients who weigh less than 40 kg should receive an oral maintenance dose of 100 mg every 12 hours.

Dosage Adjustment

If patient response is inadequate, the oral maintenance dose may be increased from 200 mg every 12 hours to 300 mg every 12 hours. For adult patients weighing less than 40 kg, the oral maintenance dose may be increased from 100 mg every 12 hours to 150 mg every 12 hours.

If patients are unable to tolerate treatment, reduce the intravenous maintenance dose to 3 mg/kg every 12 hours and the oral maintenance dose by 50 mg steps to a minimum of 200 mg every 12 hours (or to 100 mg every 12 hours for adult patients weighing less than 40 kg).

Phenytoin may be coadministered with VFEND if the intravenous maintenance dose of VFEND is increased to 5 mg/kg every 12 hours, or the oral maintenance dose is increased from 200 mg to 400 mg every 12 hours (100 mg to 200 mg every 12 hours in adult patients weighing less than 40 kg) (see CLINICAL PHARMACOLOGY, PRECAUTIONS - Drug Interactions).

Duration of therapy should be based on the severity of the patient's underlying disease, recovery from immunosuppression, and clinical response.

Esophageal Candidiasis:

The recommended dosing regimen is an oral dose of 200 mg every 12 hours for patients who weigh 40 kg or more. Adult patients who weigh less than 40 kg should receive an oral dose of 100 mg every 12 hours. Patients should be treated for a minimum of 14 days and for at least 7 days following resolution of symptoms.

Use in Geriatric Patients

No dose adjustment is necessary for geriatric patients.

Use in Patients with Hepatic Insufficiency

In the clinical program, patients were included who had baseline liver function tests (ALT, AST) up to 5 times the upper limit of normal. No dose adjustment is necessary in patients with this degree of abnormal liver function, but continued monitoring of liver function tests for further elevations is recommended (see WARNINGS).

Table 12
PROTOCOL 307/602
Clinically Significant Laboratory Test Abnormalities

	Criteria*	VORICONAZOLE	AMPHOTERICIN B**
		n/N (%)	n/N (%)
T. Bilirubin	>1.5× ULN	35/180 (19.4)	46/173 (26.6)
AST	>3.0× ULN	21/180 (11.7)	18/174 (10.3)
ALT	>3.0× ULN	34/180 (18.9)	40/173 (23.1)
Alk phos	>3.0× ULN	29/181 (16.0)	38/173 (22.0)
Creatinine	>1.3× ULN	39/182 (21.4)	102/177 (57.6)
Potassium	<0.9× LLN	30/181 (16.6)	70/178 (39.3)

* Without regard to baseline value
** Amphotericin B followed by other licensed antifungal therapy
n number of patients with a clinically significant abnormality while on study therapy
N total number of patients with at least one observation of the given lab test while on study therapy
ULN upper limit of normal
LLN lower limit of normal

Table 13 Required Volumes of 10 mg/mL VFEND Concentrate

Body Weight (kg)	**Volume of VFEND Concentrate (10 mg/mL) required for:** 3 mg/kg dose (number of vials)	4 mg/kg dose (number of vials)	6 mg/kg dose (number of vials)
30	9.0 mL (1)	12 mL (1)	18 mL (1)
35	10.5 mL (1)	14 mL (1)	21 mL (2)
40	12.0 mL (1)	16 mL (1)	24 mL (2)
45	13.5 mL (1)	18 mL (1)	27 mL (2)
50	15.0 mL (1)	20 mL (1)	30 mL (2)
55	16.5 mL (1)	22 mL (2)	33 mL (2)
60	18.0 mL (1)	24 mL (2)	36 mL (2)
65	19.5 mL (1)	26 mL (2)	39 mL (2)
70	21.0 mL (2)	28 mL (2)	42 mL (3)
75	22.5 mL (2)	30 mL (2)	45 mL (3)
80	24.0 mL (2)	32 mL (2)	48 mL (3)
85	25.5 mL (2)	34 mL (2)	51 mL (3)
90	27.0 mL (2)	36 mL (2)	54 mL (3)
95	28.5 mL (2)	38 mL (2)	57 mL (3)
100	30.0 mL (2)	40 mL (2)	60 mL (3)

It is recommended that the standard loading dose regimens be used but that the maintenance dose be halved in patients with mild to moderate hepatic cirrhosis (Child-Pugh Class A and B).

VFEND has not been studied in patients with severe hepatic cirrhosis (Child-Pugh Class C) or in patients with chronic hepatitis B or chronic hepatitis C disease. VFEND has been associated with elevations in liver function tests and clinical signs of liver damage, such as jaundice, and should only be used in patients with severe hepatic insufficiency if the benefit outweighs the potential risk. Patients with hepatic insufficiency must be carefully monitored for drug toxicity.

Use in Patients with Renal Insufficiency

The pharmacokinetics of orally administered VFEND are not significantly affected by renal insufficiency. Therefore, no adjustment is necessary for oral dosing in patients with mild to severe renal impairment (see CLINICAL PHARMACOLOGY - Special Populations).

In patients with moderate or severe renal insufficiency (creatinine clearance <50 mL/min), accumulation of the intravenous vehicle, SBECD, occurs. Oral voriconazole should be administered to these patients, unless an assessment of the benefit/risk to the patient justifies the use of intravenous voriconazole. Serum creatinine levels should be closely monitored in these patients, and, if increases occur, consideration should be given to changing to oral voriconazole therapy (see DOSAGE and ADMINISTRATION).

Voriconazole is hemodialyzed with clearance of 121 mL/min. The intravenous vehicle, SBECD, is hemodialyzed with clearance of 55 mL/min. A 4-hour hemodialysis session does not remove a sufficient amount of voriconazole to warrant dose adjustment.

Intravenous Administration

VFEND I.V. For Injection:

Reconstitution

The powder is reconstituted with 19 mL of Water For Injection to obtain an extractable volume of 20 mL of clear concentrate containing 10 mg/mL of voriconazole. It is recommended that a standard 20 mL (non-automated) syringe be used to ensure that the exact amount (19.0 mL) of water for injection is dispensed. Discard the vial if a vacuum does not pull the diluent into the vial. Shake the vial until all the powder is dissolved.

Dilution

VFEND must be infused over 1-2 hours, at a concentration of 5 mg/mL or less. Therefore, the required volume of the 10 mg/mL VFEND concentrate should be further diluted as follows (appropriate diluents listed below):

1. Calculate the volume of 10 mg/mL VFEND concentrate required based on the patient's weight (see Table 13).
2. In order to allow the required volume of VFEND concentrate to be added, withdraw and discard at least an equal volume of diluent from the infusion bag or bottle to be used. The volume of diluent remaining in the bag or bottle should be such that when the 10 mg/mL VFEND concentrate is added, the final concentration is not less than 0.5 mg/mL nor greater than 5 mg/mL.
3. Using a suitable size syringe and aseptic technique, withdraw the required volume of VFEND concentrate from the appropriate number of vials and add to the infusion bag or bottle. DISCARD PARTIALLY USED VIALS.

The final VFEND solution must be infused over 1-2 hours at a maximum rate of 3 mg/kg per hour.

[See table 13 above]

VFEND I.V. for Injection is a single dose unpreserved sterile lyophile. Therefore, from a microbiological point of view, once reconstituted, the product should be used immediately. If not used immediately, in-use storage times and conditions prior to use are the responsibility of the user and should not be longer than 24 hours at 2° to 8°C (37° to 46°F). This medicinal product is for single use only and any unused solution should be discarded. Only clear solutions without particles should be used.

The reconstituted solution can be diluted with:
9 mg/mL (0.9%) Sodium Chloride USP
Lactated Ringers USP
5% Dextrose and Lactated Ringers USP
5% Dextrose and 0.45% Sodium Chloride, USP

Continued on next page

VFEND—Cont.

5% Dextrose USP
5% Dextrose and 20 mEq Potassium Chloride, USP
0.45% Sodium Chloride USP
5% Dextrose and 0.9% Sodium Chloride, USP

The compatibility of VFEND I.V. with diluents other than those described above is unknown (see Incompatibilities below).

Parenteral drug products should be inspected visually for particulate matter and discoloration prior to administration, whenever solution and container permit.

Incompatibilities:

VFEND I.V. must not be infused into the same line or cannula concomitantly with other drug infusions, including parenteral nutrition, e.g., Aminofusin 10% Plus. Aminofusin 10% Plus is physically incompatible, with an increase in subvisible particulate matter after 24 hours storage at 4°C.

Infusions of blood products must not occur simultaneously with VFEND I.V.

Infusions of total parenteral nutrition can occur simultaneously with VFEND I.V.

VFEND I.V. must not be diluted with 4.2% Sodium Bicarbonate Infusion. The mildly alkaline nature of this diluent caused slight degradation of VFEND after 24 hours storage at room temperature. Although refrigerated storage is recommended following reconstitution, use of this diluent is not recommended as a precautionary measure. Compatibility with other concentrations is unknown.

VFEND for Oral Suspension

Reconstitution

Tap the bottle to release the powder. Add 46 mL of water to the bottle. Shake the closed bottle vigorously for about 1 minute. Remove child-resistant cap and push bottle adaptor into the neck of the bottle. Replace the cap. Write the date of expiration of the reconstituted suspension on the bottle label (the shelf-life of the reconstituted suspension is 14 days at controlled room temperature 15-30°C (59-86°F)).

Instructions for use

Shake the closed bottle of reconstituted suspension for approximately 10 seconds before each use. The reconstituted oral suspension should only be administered using the oral dispenser supplied with each pack.

Incompatibilities

VFEND for Oral Suspension and the 40 mg/mL reconstituted oral suspension should not be mixed with any other medication or additional flavoring agent. It is not intended that the suspension be further diluted with water or other vehicles.

HOW SUPPLIED

Powder for Solution for Injection

VFEND I.V. for Injection is supplied in a single use vial as a sterile lyophilized powder equivalent to 200 mg VFEND and 3200 mg sulfobutyl ether beta-cyclodextrin sodium (SBECD).

Individually packaged vials of 200 mg VFEND I.V.
(NDC 0049-3190-28)

Tablets

VFEND 50 mg tablets - white, film-coated, round, debossed with "Pfizer" on one side and "VOR50" on the reverse.
Bottles of 30 (NDC 0049-3170-30)

VFEND 200 mg tablets – white, film-coated, capsule shaped, debossed with "Pfizer" on one side and "VOR200" on the reverse.
Bottles of 30 (NDC 0049-3180-30)

Powder for Oral Suspension

VFEND for Oral Suspension is supplied in 100 mL high density polyethylene (HDPE) bottles. Each bottle contains 45 g of powder for oral suspension. Following reconstitution, the volume of the suspension is 75 mL, providing a usable volume of 70 mL (40 mg voriconazole/mL). A 5 mL oral dispenser and a press-in bottle adaptor are also provided.
(NDC 0049-3160-44)

STORAGE

VFEND I.V. for injection unreconstituted-vials should be stored at 15°-30°C (59°-86°F) [see USP Controlled Room Temperature]. VFEND is a single dose unpreserved sterile lyophile. From a microbiological point of view, following reconstitution of the lyophile with Water for Injection, the reconstituted solution should be used immediately. If not used immediately, in-use storage times and conditions prior to use are the responsibility of the user and should not be longer than 24 hours at 2° to 8°C (36° to 46°F). Chemical and physical in-use stability has been demonstrated for 24 hours at 2° to 8°C (36° to 46°F). This medicinal product is for single use only and any unused solution should be discarded. Only clear solutions without particles should be used (see DOSAGE AND ADMINISTRATION - Intravenous Administration).

VFEND Tablets should be stored at 15°-30°C (59°-86°F) [see USP Controlled Room Temperature].

VFEND Powder for Oral Suspension should be stored at 2-8°C (36-46°F) (in a refrigerator) before reconstitution. The shelf-life of the powder for oral suspension is 18 months. The reconstituted suspension should be stored at 15-30°C (59-86°F) [see USP Controlled Room Temperature]. Do not refrigerate or freeze. Keep the container tightly closed. The shelf-life of the reconstituted suspension is 14 days. Any remaining suspension should be discarded 14 days after reconstitution.

REFERENCES

1. National Committee for Clinical Laboratory Standards. Reference method for broth dilution antifungal susceptibility testing of conidium-forming filamentous fungi. Approved Standard M38-P. National Committee for Clinical Laboratory Standards, Villanova, Pa.
2. National Committee for Clinical Laboratory Standards. Reference method for broth dilution antifungal susceptibility testing of yeasts. Approved Standard M27-A. National Committee for Clinical Laboratory Standards, Villanova, Pa.

Rx only **©2004 PFIZER INC**
Distributed by
Pfizer Roerig
Division of Pfizer Inc, NY, NY 10017
LAB-0271-8 Revised April 2004

Shown in Product Identification Guide, page 329

VIAGRA® ℞

[*vī-ă-grə*]
(sildenafil citrate)
Tablets

DESCRIPTION

VIAGRA®, an oral therapy for erectile dysfunction, is the citrate salt of sildenafil, a selective inhibitor of cyclic guanosine monophosphate (cGMP)-specific phosphodiesterase type 5 (PDE5).

Sildenafil citrate is designated chemically as 1-[[3-(6,7-dihydro-1-methyl-7-oxo-3-propyl-1*H*-pyrazolo[4,3-*d*]pyrimidin-5-yl)-4-ethoxyphenyl]sulfonyl]-4-methylpiperazine citrate and has the following structural formula:

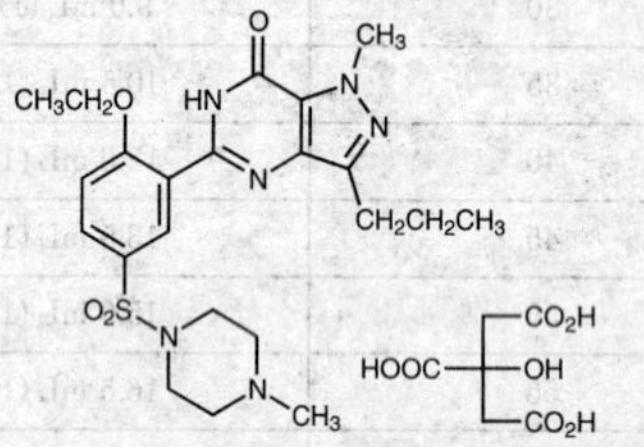

Sildenafil citrate is a white to off-white crystalline powder with a solubility of 3.5 mg/mL in water and a molecular weight of 666.7. VIAGRA (sildenafil citrate) is formulated as blue, film-coated rounded-diamond-shaped tablets equivalent to 25 mg, 50 mg and 100 mg of sildenafil for oral administration. In addition to the active ingredient, sildenafil citrate, each tablet contains the following inactive ingredients: microcrystalline cellulose, anhydrous dibasic calcium phosphate, croscarmellose sodium, magnesium stearate, hypromellose, titanium dioxide, lactose, triacetin, and FD & C Blue #2 aluminum lake.

CLINICAL PHARMACOLOGY

Mechanism of Action

The physiologic mechanism of erection of the penis involves release of nitric oxide (NO) in the corpus cavernosum during sexual stimulation. NO then activates the enzyme guanylate cyclase, which results in increased levels of cyclic guanosine monophosphate (cGMP), producing smooth muscle relaxation in the corpus cavernosum and allowing inflow of blood. Sildenafil has no direct relaxant effect on isolated human corpus cavernosum, but enhances the effect of nitric oxide (NO) by inhibiting phosphodiesterase type 5 (PDE5), which is responsible for degradation of cGMP in the corpus cavernosum. When sexual stimulation causes local release of NO, inhibition of PDE5 by sildenafil causes increased levels of cGMP in the corpus cavernosum, resulting in smooth muscle relaxation and inflow of blood to the corpus cavernosum. Sildenafil at recommended doses has no effect in the absence of sexual stimulation.

Studies *in vitro* have shown that sildenafil is selective for PDE5. Its effect is more potent on PDE5 than on other known phosphodiesterases (10-fold for PDE6, >80-fold for PDE1, >700-fold for PDE2, PDE3, PDE4, PDE7, PDE8, PDE9, PDE10, and PDE11). The approximately 4,000-fold selectivity for PDE5 versus PDE3 is important because PDE3 is involved in control of cardiac contractility. Sildenafil is only about 10-fold as potent for PDE5 compared to PDE6, an enzyme found in the retina which is involved in the phototransduction pathway of the retina. This lower selectivity is thought to be the basis for abnormalities related to color vision observed with higher doses or plasma levels (see **Pharmacodynamics**).

In addition to human corpus cavernosum smooth muscle, PDE5 is also found in lower concentrations in other tissues including platelets, vascular and visceral smooth muscle, and skeletal muscle. The inhibition of PDE5 in these tissues by sildenafil may be the basis for the enhanced platelet antiaggregatory activity of nitric oxide observed *in vitro*, an inhibition of platelet thrombus formation *in vivo* and peripheral arterial-venous dilatation *in vivo*.

Pharmacokinetics and Metabolism

VIAGRA is rapidly absorbed after oral administration, with absolute bioavailability of about 40%. Its pharmacokinetics are dose-proportional over the recommended dose range. It is eliminated predominantly by hepatic metabolism (mainly cytochrome P450 3A4) and is converted to an active metabolite with properties similar to the parent, sildenafil. The concomitant use of potent cytochrome P450 3A4 inhibitors (e.g., erythromycin, ketoconazole, itraconazole) as well as the nonspecific CYP inhibitor, cimetidine, is associated with increased plasma levels of sildenafil (see **DOSAGE AND ADMINISTRATION**). Both sildenafil and the metabolite have terminal half lives of about 4 hours.

Mean sildenafil plasma concentrations measured after the administration of a single oral dose of 100 mg to healthy male volunteers is depicted below:

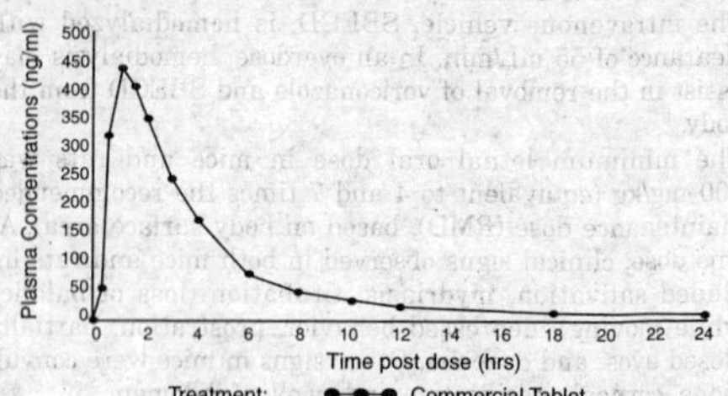

Figure 1: Mean Sildenafil Plasma Concentrations in Healthy Male Volunteers.

Absorption and Distribution: VIAGRA is rapidly absorbed. Maximum observed plasma concentrations are reached within 30 to 120 minutes (median 60 minutes) of oral dosing in the fasted state. When VIAGRA is taken with a high fat meal, the rate of absorption is reduced, with a mean delay in T_{max} of 60 minutes and a mean reduction in C_{max} of 29%. The mean steady state volume of distribution (Vss) for sildenafil is 105 L, indicating distribution into the tissues. Sildenafil and its major circulating N-desmethyl metabolite are both approximately 96% bound to plasma proteins. Protein binding is independent of total drug concentrations.

Based upon measurements of sildenafil in semen of healthy volunteers 90 minutes after dosing, less than 0.001% of the administered dose may appear in the semen of patients.

Metabolism and Excretion: Sildenafil is cleared predominantly by the CYP3A4 (major route) and CYP2C9 (minor route) hepatic microsomal isoenzymes. The major circulating metabolite results from N-desmethylation of sildenafil, and is itself further metabolized. This metabolite has a PDE selectivity profile similar to sildenafil and an *in vitro* potency for PDE5 approximately 50% of the parent drug. Plasma concentrations of this metabolite are approximately 40% of those seen for sildenafil, so that the metabolite accounts for about 20% of sildenafil's pharmacologic effects.

After either oral or intravenous administration, sildenafil is excreted as metabolites predominantly in the feces (approximately 80% of administered oral dose) and to a lesser extent in the urine (approximately 13% of the administered oral dose). Similar values for pharmacokinetic parameters were seen in normal volunteers and in the patient population, using a population pharmacokinetic approach.

Pharmacokinetics in Special Populations

Geriatrics: Healthy elderly volunteers (65 years or over) had a reduced clearance of sildenafil, with free plasma concentrations approximately 40% greater than those seen in healthy younger volunteers (18–45 years).

Renal Insufficiency: In volunteers with mild (CLcr=50-80 mL/min) and moderate (CLcr=30-49 mL/min) renal impairment, the pharmacokinetics of a single oral dose of VIAGRA (50 mg) were not altered. In volunteers with severe (CLcr=<30 mL/min) renal impairment, sildenafil clearance was reduced, resulting in approximately doubling of AUC and C_{max} compared to age-matched volunteers with no renal impairment.

Hepatic Insufficiency: In volunteers with hepatic cirrhosis (Child-Pugh A and B), sildenafil clearance was reduced, resulting in increases in AUC (84%) and C_{max} (47%) compared to age-matched volunteers with no hepatic impairment.

Therefore, age >65, hepatic impairment and severe renal impairment are associated with increased plasma levels of sildenafil. A starting oral dose of 25 mg should be considered in those patients (see **DOSAGE AND ADMINISTRATION**).

Pharmacodynamics

Effects of VIAGRA on Erectile Response: In eight double-blind, placebo-controlled crossover studies of patients with either organic or psychogenic erectile dysfunction, sexual stimulation resulted in improved erections, as assessed by an objective measurement of hardness and duration of erections (RigiScan®), after VIAGRA administration compared with placebo. Most studies assessed the efficacy of VIAGRA approximately 60 minutes post dose. The erectile response, as assessed by RigiScan®, generally increased with increasing sildenafil dose and plasma concentration. The time course of effect was examined in one study, showing an effect for up to 4 hours but the response was diminished compared to 2 hours.

Effects of VIAGRA on Blood Pressure: Single oral doses of sildenafil (100 mg) administered to healthy volunteers produced decreases in supine blood pressure (mean maximum decrease in systolic/diastolic blood pressure of 8.4/5.5 mmHg). The decrease in blood pressure was most notable approximately 1–2 hours after dosing, and was not different than placebo at 8 hours. Similar effects on blood pressure were noted with 25 mg, 50 mg and 100 mg of VIAGRA, therefore the effects are not related to dose or plasma levels within this dosage range. Larger effects were recorded among patients receiving concomitant nitrates (see

CONTRAINDICATIONS).

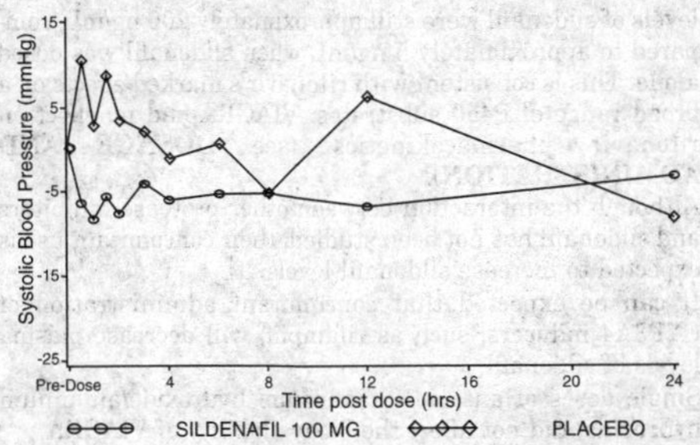

Figure 2: Mean Change from Baseline in Sitting Systolic Blood Pressure, Healthy Volunteers.

Effects of VIAGRA on Cardiac Parameters: Single oral doses of sildenafil up to 100 mg produced no clinically relevant changes in the ECGs of normal male volunteers.
Studies have produced relevant data on the effects of VIAGRA on cardiac output. In one small, open-label, uncontrolled, pilot study, eight patients with stable ischemic heart disease underwent Swan-Ganz catheterization. A total dose of 40 mg sildenafil was administered by four intravenous infusions.
The results from this pilot study are shown in Table 1; the mean resting systolic and diastolic blood pressures decreased by 7% and 10% compared to baseline in these patients. Mean resting values for right atrial pressure, pulmonary artery pressure, pulmonary artery occluded pressure and cardiac output decreased by 28%, 28%, 20% and 7% respectively. Even though this total dosage produced plasma sildenafil concentrations which were approximately 2 to 5 times higher than the mean maximum plasma concentrations following a single oral dose of 100 mg in healthy male volunteers, the hemodynamic response to exercise was preserved in these patients.
[See table 1 above]

TABLE 1. HEMODYNAMIC DATA IN PATIENTS WITH STABLE ISCHEMIC HEART DISEASE AFTER IV ADMINISTRATION OF 40 MG SILDENAFIL

Means ± SD	At rest				After 4 minutes of exercise			
	n	Baseline (B2)	n	Sildenafil (D1)	n	Baseline	n	Sildenafil
PAOP (mmHg)	8	8.1 ± 5.1	8	6.5 ± 4.3	8	36.0 ± 13.7	8	27.8 ± 15.3
Mean PAP (mmHg)	8	16.7 ± 4	8	12.1 ± 3.9	8	39.4 ± 12.9	8	31.7 ± 13.2
Mean RAP (mmHg)	7	5.7 ± 3.7	8	4.1 ± 3.7	–	–	–	–
Systolic SAP (mmHg)	8	150.4 ± 12.4	8	140.6 ± 16.5	8	199.5 ± 37.4	8	187.8 ± 30.0
Diastolic SAP (mmHg)	8	73.6 ± 7.8	8	65.9 ± 10	8	84.6 ± 9.7	8	79.5 ± 9.4
Cardiac output (L/min)	8	5.6 ± 0.9	8	5.2 ± 1.1	8	11.5 ± 2.4	8	10.2 ± 3.5
Heart rate (bpm)	8	67 ± 11.1	8	66.9 ± 12	8	101.9 ± 11.6	8	99.0 ± 20.4

In a double-blind study, 144 patients with erectile dysfunction and chronic stable angina limited by exercise, not receiving chronic oral nitrates, were randomized to a single dose of placebo or VIAGRA 100 mg 1 hour prior to exercise testing. The primary endpoint was time to limiting angina in the evaluable cohort. The mean times (adjusted for baseline) to onset of limiting angina were 423.6 and 403.7 seconds for sildenafil (N=70) and placebo, respectively. These results demonstrated that the effect of VIAGRA on the primary endpoint was statistically non-inferior to placebo.
Effects of VIAGRA on Vision: At single oral doses of 100 mg and 200 mg, transient dose-related impairment of color discrimination (blue/green) was detected using the Farnsworth-Munsell 100-hue test, with peak effects near the time of peak plasma levels. This finding is consistent with the inhibition of PDE6, which is involved in phototransduction in the retina. An evaluation of visual function at doses up to twice the maximum recommended dose revealed no effects of VIAGRA on visual acuity, intraocular pressure, or pupillometry.

Clinical Studies

In clinical studies, VIAGRA was assessed for its effect on the ability of men with erectile dysfunction (ED) to engage in sexual activity and in many cases specifically on the ability to achieve and maintain an erection sufficient for satisfactory sexual activity. VIAGRA was evaluated primarily at doses of 25 mg, 50 mg and 100 mg in 21 randomized, double-blind, placebo-controlled trials of up to 6 months in duration, using a variety of study designs (fixed dose, titration, parallel, crossover). VIAGRA was administered to more than 3,000 patients aged 19 to 87 years, with ED of various etiologies (organic, psychogenic, mixed) with a mean duration of 5 years. VIAGRA demonstrated statistically significant improvement compared to placebo in all 21 studies. The studies that established benefit demonstrated improvements in success rates for sexual intercourse compared with placebo.
The effectiveness of VIAGRA was evaluated in most studies using several assessment instruments. The primary measure in the principal studies was a sexual function questionnaire (the International Index of Erectile Function - IIEF) administered during a 4-week treatment-free run-in period, at baseline, at follow-up visits, and at the end of double-blind, placebo-controlled, at-home treatment. Two of the questions from the IIEF served as primary study endpoints; categorical responses were elicited to questions about (1) the ability to achieve erections sufficient for sexual intercourse and (2) the maintenance of erections after penetration. The patient addressed both questions at the final visit for the last 4 weeks of the study. The possible categorical responses to these questions were (0) no attempted intercourse, (1) never or almost never, (2) a few times, (3) sometimes, (4) most times, and (5) almost always or always. Also collected as part of the IIEF was information about other aspects of sexual function, including information on erectile function, orgasm, desire, satisfaction with intercourse, and overall sexual satisfaction. Sexual function data were also recorded by patients in a daily diary. In addition, patients were asked a global efficacy question and an optional partner questionnaire was administered.
The effect on one of the major end points, maintenance of erections after penetration, is shown in Figure 3, for the pooled results of 5 fixed-dose, dose-response studies of greater than one month duration, showing response according to baseline function. Results with all doses have been pooled, but scores showed greater improvement at the 50 and 100 mg doses than at 25 mg. The pattern of responses was similar for the other principal question, the ability to achieve an erection sufficient for intercourse. The titration studies, in which most patients received 100 mg, showed similar results. Figure 3 shows that regardless of the baseline levels of function, subsequent function in patients treated with VIAGRA was better than that seen in patients treated with placebo. At the same time, on-treatment function was better in treated patients who were less impaired at baseline.

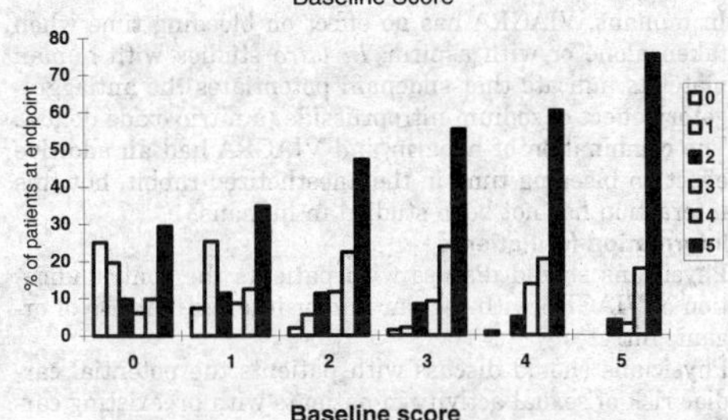

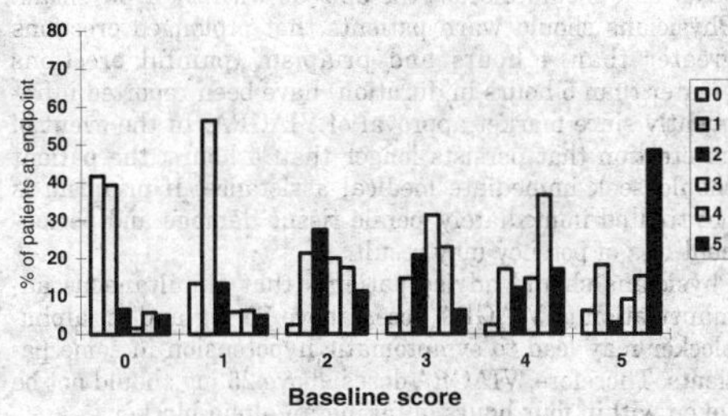

Figure 3. Effect of VIAGRA and Placebo on Maintenance of Erection by Baseline Score.

The frequency of patients reporting improvement of erections in response to a global question in four of the randomized, double-blind, parallel, placebo-controlled fixed dose studies (1797 patients) of 12 to 24 weeks duration is shown in Figure 4. These patients had erectile dysfunction at baseline that was characterized by median categorical scores of 2 (a few times) on principal IIEF questions. Erectile dysfunction was attributed to organic (58%; generally not characterized, but including diabetes and excluding spinal cord injury), psychogenic (17%), or mixed (24%) etiologies. Sixty-three percent, 74%, and 82% of the patients on 25 mg, 50 mg and 100 mg of VIAGRA, respectively, reported an improvement in their erections, compared to 24% on placebo. In the titration studies (n=644) (with most patients eventually receiving 100 mg), results were similar.
[See figure 4 at top of next column]

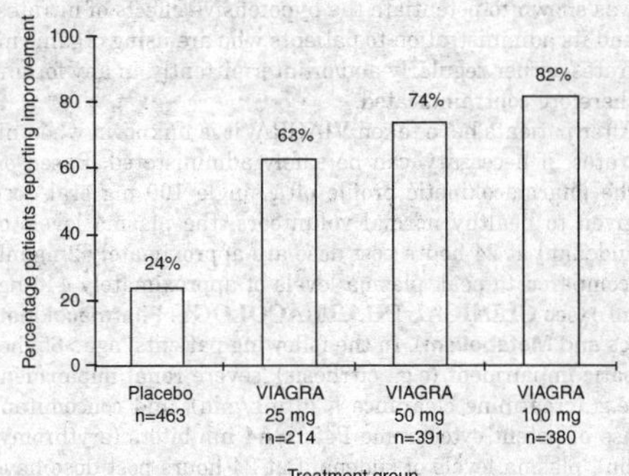

Figure 4. Percentage of Patients Reporting an Improvement in Erections.

The patients in studies had varying degrees of ED. One-third to one-half of the subjects in these studies reported successful intercourse at least once during a 4-week, treatment-free run-in period.
In many of the studies, of both fixed dose and titration designs, daily diaries were kept by patients. In these studies, involving about 1600 patients, analyses of patient diaries showed no effect of VIAGRA on rates of attempted intercourse (about 2 per week), but there was clear treatment-related improvement in sexual function: per patient weekly success rates averaged 1.3 on 50–100 mg of VIAGRA vs 0.4 on placebo; similarly, group mean success rates (total successes divided by total attempts) were about 66% on VIAGRA vs about 20% on placebo.
During 3 to 6 months of double-blind treatment or longer-term (1 year), open-label studies, few patients withdrew from active treatment for any reason, including lack of effectiveness. At the end of the long-term study, 88% of patients reported that VIAGRA improved their erections.
Men with untreated ED had relatively low baseline scores for all aspects of sexual function measured (again using a 5-point scale) in the IIEF. VIAGRA improved these aspects of sexual function: frequency, firmness and maintenance of erections; frequency of orgasm; frequency and level of desire; frequency, satisfaction and enjoyment of intercourse; and overall relationship satisfaction.
One randomized, double-blind, flexible-dose, placebo-controlled study included only patients with erectile dysfunction attributed to complications of diabetes mellitus (n=268). As in the other titration studies, patients were started on 50 mg and allowed to adjust the dose up to 100 mg or down to 25 mg of VIAGRA; all patients, however, were receiving 50 mg or 100 mg at the end of the study. There were highly statistically significant improvements on the two principal IIEF questions (frequency of successful penetration during sexual activity and maintenance of erections after penetration) on VIAGRA compared to placebo. On a global improvement question, 57% of VIAGRA patients reported improved erections versus 10% on placebo. Diary data indicated that on VIAGRA, 48% of intercourse attempts were successful versus 12% on placebo.
One randomized, double-blind, placebo-controlled, crossover, flexible-dose (up to 100 mg) study of patients with erectile dysfunction resulting from spinal cord injury (n=178) was conducted. The changes from baseline in scoring on the two end point questions (frequency of successful penetration during sexual activity and maintenance of erections after penetration) were highly statistically significantly in favor of VIAGRA. On a global improvement question, 83% of patients reported improved erections on VIAGRA versus 12% on placebo. Diary data indicated that on VIAGRA, 59% of attempts at sexual intercourse were successful compared to 13% on placebo.
Across all trials, VIAGRA improved the erections of 43% of radical prostatectomy patients compared to 15% on placebo.
Subgroup analyses of responses to a global improvement question in patients with psychogenic etiology in two fixed-dose studies (total n=179) and two titration studies (total n=149) showed 84% of VIAGRA patients reported improvement in erections compared with 26% of placebo. The changes from baseline in scoring on the two end point questions (frequency of successful penetration during sexual activity and maintenance of erections after penetration) were highly statistically significantly in favor of VIAGRA. Diary data in two of the studies (n=178) showed rates of successful intercourse per attempt of 70% for VIAGRA and 29% for placebo.
A review of population subgroups demonstrated efficacy regardless of baseline severity, etiology, race and age. VIAGRA was effective in a broad range of ED patients, including those with a history of coronary artery disease, hypertension, other cardiac disease, peripheral vascular dis-

Continued on next page

Viagra—Cont.

ease, diabetes mellitus, depression, coronary artery bypass graft (CABG), radical prostatectomy, transurethral resection of the prostate (TURP) and spinal cord injury, and in patients taking antidepressants/antipsychotics and antihypertensives/diuretics.
Analysis of the safety database showed no apparent difference in the side effect profile in patients taking VIAGRA with and without antihypertensive medication. This analysis was performed retrospectively, and was not powered to detect any pre-specified difference in adverse reactions.

INDICATION AND USAGE

VIAGRA is indicated for the treatment of erectile dysfunction.

CONTRAINDICATIONS

Consistent with its known effects on the nitric oxide/cGMP pathway (see **CLINICAL PHARMACOLOGY**), VIAGRA was shown to potentiate the hypotensive effects of nitrates, and its administration to patients who are using organic nitrates, either regularly and/or intermittently, in any form is therefore contraindicated.
After patients have taken VIAGRA, it is unknown when nitrates, if necessary, can be safely administered. Based on the pharmacokinetic profile of a single 100 mg oral dose given to healthy normal volunteers, the plasma levels of sildenafil at 24 hours post dose are approximately 2 ng/mL (compared to peak plasma levels of approximately 440 ng/mL) (see **CLINICAL PHARMACOLOGY: Pharmacokinetics and Metabolism**). In the following patients: age >65, hepatic impairment (e.g., cirrhosis), severe renal impairment (e.g., creatinine clearance <30 mL/min), and concomitant use of potent cytochrome P450 3A4 inhibitors (erythromycin), plasma levels of sildenafil at 24 hours post dose have been found to be 3 to 8 times higher than those seen in healthy volunteers. Although plasma levels of sildenafil at 24 hours post dose are much lower than at peak concentration, it is unknown whether nitrates can be safely coadministered at this time point.
VIAGRA is contraindicated in patients with a known hypersensitivity to any component of the tablet.

WARNINGS

There is a potential for cardiac risk of sexual activity in patients with preexisting cardiovascular disease. Therefore, treatments for erectile dysfunction, including VIAGRA, should not be generally used in men for whom sexual activity is inadvisable because of their underlying cardiovascular status.
VIAGRA has systemic vasodilatory properties that resulted in transient decreases in supine blood pressure in healthy volunteers (mean maximum decrease of 8.4/5.5 mmHg), (see **CLINICAL PHARMACOLOGY: Pharmacodynamics**). While this normally would be expected to be of little consequence in most patients, prior to prescribing VIAGRA, physicians should carefully consider whether their patients with underlying cardiovascular disease could be affected adversely by such vasodilatory effects, especially in combination with sexual activity.
Patients with the following underlying conditions can be particularly sensitive to the actions of vasodilators including VIAGRA – those with left ventricular outflow obstruction (e.g. aortic stenosis, idiopathic hypertrophic subaortic stenosis) and those with severely impaired autonomic control of blood pressure.
There is no controlled clinical data on the safety or efficacy of VIAGRA in the following groups; if prescribed, this should be done with caution.

- Patients who have suffered a myocardial infarction, stroke, or life-threatening arrhythmia within the last 6 months;
- Patients with resting hypotension (BP <90/50) or hypertension (BP >170/110);
- Patients with cardiac failure or coronary artery disease causing unstable angina;
- Patients with retinitis pigmentosa (a minority of these patients have genetic disorders of retinal phosphodiesterases).

Prolonged erection greater than 4 hours and priapism (painful erections greater than 6 hours in duration) have been reported infrequently since market approval of VIAGRA. In the event of an erection that persists longer than 4 hours, the patient should seek immediate medical assistance. If priapism is not treated immediately, penile tissue damage and permanent loss of potency could result.
The concomitant administration of the protease inhibitor ritonavir substantially increases serum concentrations of sildenafil (**11-fold increase in AUC**). If VIAGRA is prescribed to patients taking ritonavir, caution should be used. Data from subjects exposed to high systemic levels of sildenafil are limited. Visual disturbances occurred more commonly at higher levels of sildenafil exposure. Decreased blood pressure, syncope, and prolonged erection were reported in some healthy volunteers exposed to high doses of sildenafil (200–800 mg). To decrease the chance of adverse events in patients taking ritonavir, a decrease in sildenafil dosage is recommended (see **Drug Interactions, ADVERSE REACTIONS** and **DOSAGE AND ADMINISTRATION**).

PRECAUTIONS

General

The evaluation of erectile dysfunction should include a determination of potential underlying causes and the identification of appropriate treatment following a complete medical assessment.
Before prescribing VIAGRA, it is important to note the following:
Patients on multiple antihypertensive medications were included in the pivotal clinical trials for VIAGRA. In a separate drug interaction study, when amlodipine, 5 mg or 10 mg, and VIAGRA, 100 mg were orally administered concomitantly to hypertensive patients mean additional blood pressure reduction of 8 mmHg systolic and 7 mmHg diastolic were noted (see **Drug Interactions**).
When the alpha blocker doxazosin (4 mg) and VIAGRA (25 mg) were administered simultaneously to patients with benign prostatic hyperplasia (BPH), mean additional reductions of supine blood pressure of 7 mmHg systolic and 7 mmHg diastolic were observed. When higher doses of VIAGRA and doxazosin (4 mg) were administered simultaneously, there were infrequent reports of patients who experienced symptomatic postural hypotension within 1 to 4 hours of dosing. Simultaneous administration of VIAGRA to patients taking alpha-blocker therapy may lead to symptomatic hypotension in some patients. Therefore, VIAGRA doses above 25 mg should not be taken within 4 hours of taking an alpha-blocker.
The safety of VIAGRA is unknown in patients with bleeding disorders and patients with active peptic ulceration.
VIAGRA should be used with caution in patients with anatomical deformation of the penis (such as angulation, cavernosal fibrosis or Peyronie's disease), or in patients who have conditions which may predispose them to priapism (such as sickle cell anemia, multiple myeloma, or leukemia).
The safety and efficacy of combinations of VIAGRA with other treatments for erectile dysfunction have not been studied. Therefore, the use of such combinations is not recommended.
In humans, VIAGRA has no effect on bleeding time when taken alone or with aspirin. *In vitro* studies with human platelets indicate that sildenafil potentiates the antiaggregatory effect of sodium nitroprusside (a nitric oxide donor). The combination of heparin and VIAGRA had an additive effect on bleeding time in the anesthetized rabbit, but this interaction has not been studied in humans.

Information for Patients

Physicians should discuss with patients the contraindication of VIAGRA with regular and/or intermittent use of organic nitrates.
Physicians should discuss with patients the potential cardiac risk of sexual activity in patients with preexisting cardiovascular risk factors. Patients who experience symptoms (e.g., angina pectoris, dizziness, nausea) upon initiation of sexual activity should be advised to refrain from further activity and should discuss the episode with their physician.
Physicians should warn patients that prolonged erections greater than 4 hours and priapism (painful erections greater than 6 hours in duration) have been reported infrequently since market approval of VIAGRA. In the event of an erection that persists longer than 4 hours, the patient should seek immediate medical assistance. If priapism is not treated immediately, penile tissue damage and permanent loss of potency may result.
Physicians should advise patients that simultaneous administration of VIAGRA doses above 25 mg and an alpha-blocker may lead to symptomatic hypotension in some patients. Therefore, VIAGRA doses above 25 mg should not be taken within four hours of taking an alpha-blocker.
The use of VIAGRA offers no protection against sexually transmitted diseases. Counseling of patients about the protective measures necessary to guard against sexually transmitted diseases, including the Human Immunodeficiency Virus (HIV), may be considered.

Drug Interactions

Effects of Other Drugs on VIAGRA

***In vitro* studies:** Sildenafil metabolism is principally mediated by the cytochrome P450 (CYP) isoforms 3A4 (major route) and 2C9 (minor route). Therefore, inhibitors of these isoenzymes may reduce sildenafil clearance.
***In vivo* studies:** Cimetidine (800 mg), a nonspecific CYP inhibitor, caused a 56% increase in plasma sildenafil concentrations when coadministered with VIAGRA (50 mg) to healthy volunteers.
When a single 100 mg dose of VIAGRA was administered with erythromycin, a specific CYP3A4 inhibitor, at steady state (500 mg bid for 5 days), there was a 182% increase in sildenafil systemic exposure (AUC). In addition, in a study performed in healthy male volunteers, coadministration of the HIV protease inhibitor saquinavir, also a CYP3A4 inhibitor, at steady state (1200 mg tid) with VIAGRA (100 mg single dose) resulted in a 140% increase in sildenafil C_{max} and a 210% increase in sildenafil AUC. VIAGRA had no effect on saquinavir pharmacokinetics. Stronger CYP3A4 inhibitors such as ketoconazole or itraconazole would be expected to have still greater effects, and population data from patients in clinical trials did indicate a reduction in sildenafil clearance when it was coadministered with CYP3A4 inhibitors (such as ketoconazole, erythromycin, or cimetidine) (see **DOSAGE AND ADMINISTRATION**).
In another study in healthy male volunteers, coadministration with the HIV protease inhibitor ritonavir, which is a highly potent P450 inhibitor, at steady state (500 mg bid) with VIAGRA (100 mg single dose) resulted in a 300% (4-fold) increase in sildenafil C_{max} and a 1000% (11-fold) increase in sildenafil plasma AUC. At 24 hours the plasma levels of sildenafil were still approximately 200 ng/mL, compared to approximately 5 ng/mL when sildenafil was dosed alone. This is consistent with ritonavir's marked effects on a broad range of P450 substrates. VIAGRA had no effect on ritonavir pharmacokinetics (see **DOSAGE AND ADMINISTRATION**).
Although the interaction between other protease inhibitors and sildenafil has not been studied, their concomitant use is expected to increase sildenafil levels.
It can be expected that concomitant administration of CYP3A4 inducers, such as rifampin, will decrease plasma levels of sildenafil.
Single doses of antacid (magnesium hydroxide/aluminum hydroxide) did not affect the bioavailability of VIAGRA.
Pharmacokinetic data from patients in clinical trials showed no effect on sildenafil pharmacokinetics of CYP2C9 inhibitors (such as tolbutamide, warfarin), CYP2D6 inhibitors (such as selective serotonin reuptake inhibitors, tricyclic antidepressants), thiazide and related diuretics, ACE inhibitors, and calcium channel blockers. The AUC of the active metabolite, N-desmethyl sildenafil, was increased 62% by loop and potassium-sparing diuretics and 102% by nonspecific beta-blockers. These effects on the metabolite are not expected to be of clinical consequence.

Effects of VIAGRA on Other Drugs

***In vitro* studies:** Sildenafil is a weak inhibitor of the cytochrome P450 isoforms 1A2, 2C9, 2C19, 2D6, 2E1 and 3A4 (IC50 >150 µM). Given sildenafil peak plasma concentrations of approximately 1 µM after recommended doses, it is unlikely that VIAGRA will alter the clearance of substrates of these isoenzymes.
***In vivo* studies:** When VIAGRA 100 mg oral was coadministered with amlodipine, 5 mg or 10 mg oral, to hypertensive patients, the mean additional reduction on supine blood pressure was 8 mmHg systolic and 7 mmHg diastolic.
No significant interactions were shown with tolbutamide (250 mg) or warfarin (40 mg), both of which are metabolized by CYP2C9.
VIAGRA (50 mg) did not potentiate the increase in bleeding time caused by aspirin (150 mg).
VIAGRA (50 mg) did not potentiate the hypotensive effect of alcohol in healthy volunteers with mean maximum blood alcohol levels of 0.08%.
In a study of healthy male volunteers, sildenafil (100 mg) did not affect the steady state pharmacokinetics of the HIV protease inhibitors, saquinavir and ritonavir, both of which are CYP3A4 substrates.

Carcinogenesis, Mutagenesis, Impairment of Fertility

Sildenafil was not carcinogenic when administered to rats for 24 months at a dose resulting in total systemic drug exposure (AUCs) for unbound sildenafil and its major metabolite of 29- and 42-times, for male and female rats, respectively, the exposures observed in human males given the Maximum Recommended Human Dose (MRHD) of 100 mg. Sildenafil was not carcinogenic when administered to mice for 18–21 months at dosages up to the Maximum Tolerated Dose (MTD) of 10 mg/kg/day, approximately 0.6 times the MRHD on a mg/m^2 basis.
Sildenafil was negative in *in vitro* bacterial and Chinese hamster ovary cell assays to detect mutagenicity, and *in vitro* human lymphocytes and *in vivo* mouse micronucleus assays to detect clastogenicity.
There was no impairment of fertility in rats given sildenafil up to 60 mg/kg/day for 36 days to females and 102 days to males, a dose producing an AUC value of more than 25 times the human male AUC.
There was no effect on sperm motility or morphology after single 100 mg oral doses of VIAGRA in healthy volunteers.

Pregnancy, Nursing Mothers and Pediatric Use

VIAGRA is not indicated for use in newborns, children, or women.
Pregnancy Category B. No evidence of teratogenicity, embryotoxicity or fetotoxicity was observed in rats and rabbits which received up to 200 mg/kg/day during organogenesis. These doses represent, respectively, about 20 and 40 times the MRHD on a mg/m^2 basis in a 50 kg subject. In the rat pre- and postnatal development study, the no observed adverse effect dose was 30 mg/kg/day given for 36 days. In the nonpregnant rat the AUC at this dose was about 20 times human AUC. There are no adequate and well-controlled studies of sildenafil in pregnant women.
Geriatric Use: Healthy elderly volunteers (65 years or over) had a reduced clearance of sildenafil (see **CLINICAL PHARMACOLOGY: Pharmacokinetics in Special Populations**). Since higher plasma levels may increase both the efficacy and incidence of adverse events, a starting dose of 25 mg should be considered (see **DOSAGE AND ADMINISTRATION**).

ADVERSE REACTIONS

PRE-MARKETING EXPERIENCE:

VIAGRA was administered to over 3700 patients (aged 19–87 years) during clinical trials worldwide. Over 550 patients were treated for longer than one year.
In placebo-controlled clinical studies, the discontinuation rate due to adverse events for VIAGRA (2.5%) was not significantly different from placebo (2.3%). The adverse events were generally transient and mild to moderate in nature.
In trials of all designs, adverse events reported by patients receiving VIAGRA were generally similar. In fixed-dose studies, the incidence of some adverse events increased with

	25 mg	50 mg	100 mg
Obverse	VGR25	VGR50	VGR100
Reverse	PFIZER	PFIZER	PFIZER
Bottle of 30	NDC-0069-4200-30	NDC-0069-4210-30	NDC-0069-4220-30
Bottle of 100	N/A	NDC-0069-4210-66	NDC-0069-4220-66

dose. The nature of the adverse events in flexible-dose studies, which more closely reflect the recommended dosage regimen, was similar to that for fixed-dose studies.

When VIAGRA was taken as recommended (on an as-needed basis) in flexible-dose, placebo-controlled clinical trials, the following adverse events were reported:

TABLE 2. ADVERSE EVENTS REPORTED BY ≥2% OF PATIENTS TREATED WITH VIAGRA AND MORE FREQUENT ON DRUG THAN PLACEBO IN PRN FLEXIBLE-DOSE PHASE II/III STUDIES

Adverse Event	Percentage of Patients Reporting Event	
	VIAGRA N=734	PLACEBO N=725
Headache	16%	4%
Flushing	10%	1%
Dyspepsia	7%	2%
Nasal Congestion	4%	2%
Urinary Tract Infection	3%	2%
Abnormal Vision†	3%	0%
Diarrhea	3%	1%
Dizziness	2%	1%
Rash	2%	1%

† Abnormal Vision: Mild and transient, predominantly color tinge to vision, but also increased sensitivity to light or blurred vision. In these studies, only one patient discontinued due to abnormal vision.

Other adverse reactions occurred at a rate of >2%, but equally common on placebo: respiratory tract infection, back pain, flu syndrome, and arthralgia.

In fixed-dose studies, dyspepsia (17%) and abnormal vision (11%) were more common at 100 mg than at lower doses. At doses above the recommended dose range, adverse events were similar to those detailed above but generally were reported more frequently.

The following events occurred in <2% of patients in controlled clinical trials; a causal relationship to VIAGRA is uncertain. Reported events include those with a plausible relation to drug use; omitted are minor events and reports too imprecise to be meaningful:

Body as a whole: face edema, photosensitivity reaction, shock, asthenia, pain, chills, accidental fall, abdominal pain, allergic reaction, chest pain, accidental injury.

Cardiovascular: angina pectoris, AV block, migraine, syncope, tachycardia, palpitation, hypotension, postural hypotension, myocardial ischemia, cerebral thrombosis, cardiac arrest, heart failure, abnormal electrocardiogram, cardiomyopathy.

Digestive: vomiting, glossitis, colitis, dysphagia, gastritis, gastroenteritis, esophagitis, stomatitis, dry mouth, liver function tests abnormal, rectal hemorrhage, gingivitis.

Hemic and Lymphatic: anemia and leukopenia.

Metabolic and Nutritional: thirst, edema, gout, unstable diabetes, hyperglycemia, peripheral edema, hyperuricemia, hypoglycemic reaction, hypernatremia.

Musculoskeletal: arthritis, arthrosis, myalgia, tendon rupture, tenosynovitis, bone pain, myasthenia, synovitis.

Nervous: ataxia, hypertonia, neuralgia, neuropathy, paresthesia, tremor, vertigo, depression, insomnia, somnolence, abnormal dreams, reflexes decreased, hypesthesia.

Respiratory: asthma, dyspnea, laryngitis, pharyngitis, sinusitis, bronchitis, sputum increased, cough increased.

Skin and Appendages: urticaria, herpes simplex, pruritus, sweating, skin ulcer, contact dermatitis, exfoliative dermatitis.

Special Senses: mydriasis, conjunctivitis, photophobia, tinnitus, eye pain, deafness, ear pain, eye hemorrhage, cataract, dry eyes.

Urogenital: cystitis, nocturia, urinary frequency, breast enlargement, urinary incontinence, abnormal ejaculation, genital edema and anorgasmia.

POST-MARKETING EXPERIENCE:

Cardiovascular and cerebrovascular

Serious cardiovascular, cerebrovascular, and vascular events, including myocardial infarction, sudden cardiac death, ventricular arrhythmia, cerebrovascular hemorrhage, transient ischemic attack, hypertension, subarachnoid and intracerebral hemorrhages, and pulmonary hemorrhage have been reported post-marketing in temporal association with the use of VIAGRA. Most, but not all, of these patients had preexisting cardiovascular risk factors. Many of these events were reported to occur during or shortly after sexual activity, and a few were reported to occur shortly after the use of VIAGRA without sexual activity. Others were reported to have occurred hours to days after the use of VIAGRA and sexual activity. It is not possible to determine whether these events are related directly to VIAGRA, to sexual activity, to the patient's underlying cardiovascular disease, to a combination of these factors, or to other factors (see **WARNINGS** for further important cardiovascular information).

Other events

Other events reported post-marketing to have been observed in temporal association with VIAGRA and not listed in the pre-marketing adverse reactions section above include:

Nervous: seizure and anxiety.

Urogenital: prolonged erection, priapism (see **WARNINGS**) and hematuria.

Special Senses: diplopia, temporary vision loss/decreased vision, ocular redness or bloodshot appearance, ocular burning, ocular swelling/pressure, increased intraocular pressure, retinal vascular disease or bleeding, vitreous detachment/traction, paramacular edema and epistaxis.

OVERDOSAGE

In studies with healthy volunteers of single doses up to 800 mg, adverse events were similar to those seen at lower doses but incidence rates were increased.

In cases of overdose, standard supportive measures should be adopted as required. Renal dialysis is not expected to accelerate clearance as sildenafil is highly bound to plasma proteins and it is not eliminated in the urine.

DOSAGE AND ADMINISTRATION

For most patients, the recommended dose is 50 mg taken, as needed, approximately 1 hour before sexual activity. However, VIAGRA may be taken anywhere from 4 hours to 0.5 hour before sexual activity. Based on effectiveness and toleration, the dose may be increased to a maximum recommended dose of 100 mg or decreased to 25 mg. The maximum recommended dosing frequency is once per day.

The following factors are associated with increased plasma levels of sildenafil: age >65 (40% increase in AUC), hepatic impairment (e.g., cirrhosis, 80%), severe renal impairment (creatinine clearance <30 mL/min, 100%), and concomitant use of potent cytochrome P450 3A4 inhibitors [ketoconazole, itraconazole, erythromycin (182%), saquinavir (210%)]. Since higher plasma levels may increase both the efficacy and incidence of adverse events, a starting dose of 25 mg should be considered in these patients.

Ritonavir greatly increased the systemic level of sildenafil in a study of healthy, non-HIV infected volunteers (11-fold increase in AUC, see **Drug Interactions.**) Based on these pharmacokinetic data, it is recommended not to exceed a maximum single dose of 25 mg of VIAGRA in a 48 hour period.

VIAGRA was shown to potentiate the hypotensive effects of nitrates and its administration in patients who use nitric oxide donors or nitrates in any form is therefore contraindicated.

Simultaneous administration of VIAGRA doses above 25 mg and an alpha-blocker may lead to symptomatic hypotension in some patients. Doses of 50 mg or 100 mg of VIAGRA should not be taken within 4 hours of alpha-blocker administration. A 25 mg dose of VIAGRA may be taken at any time.

HOW SUPPLIED

VIAGRA® (sildenafil citrate) is supplied as blue, film-coated, rounded-diamond-shaped tablets containing sildenafil citrate equivalent to the nominally indicated amount of sildenafil as follows:

[See table above]

Recommended Storage: Store at 25°C (77°F); excursions permitted to 15-30°C (59-86°F) [see USP Controlled Room Temperature].

Rx only

Distributed by
Pfizer Labs
Division of Pfizer Inc, NY, NY 10017
69-5485-00-9 Revised August 2003

Shown in Product Identification Guide, page 329

VIRACEPT® ℞

[*vī-ră-cept*]
(nelfinavir mesylate)
TABLETS and ORAL POWDER

DESCRIPTION

VIRACEPT® (nelfinavir mesylate) is an inhibitor of the human immunodeficiency virus (HIV) protease. VIRACEPT Tablets are available for oral administration as a light blue, capsule-shaped tablet with a clear film coating in 250 mg strength (as nelfinavir free base) and as a white oval tablet with a clear film coating in 625 mg strength (as nelfinavir free base). Each tablet contains the following common inactive ingredients: calcium silicate, crospovidone, magnesium stearate, hypromellose, and triacetin. In addition, the 250 mg tablet contains FD&C blue #2 powder and the 625 mg tablet contains colloidal silicon dioxide. VIRACEPT Oral Powder is available for oral administration in a 50 mg/g strength (as nelfinavir free base) in bottles. The oral powder also contains the following inactive ingredients: microcrystalline cellulose, maltodextrin, dibasic potassium phosphate, crospovidone, hypromellose, aspartame, sucrose palmitate, and natural and artificial flavor. The chemical name for nelfinavir mesylate is [3*S*-[2(2*S**, 3*S**), 3α,4aβ,8aβ]]-*N*-(1,1-dimethylethyl)decahydro-2-[2-hydroxy-3-[(3-hydroxy-2-methylbenzoyl)amino]-4-(phenylthio)butyl]-3-isoquinoline carboxamide monomethanesulfonate (salt) and the molecular weight is 663.90 (567.79 as the free base). Nelfinavir mesylate has the following structural formula:

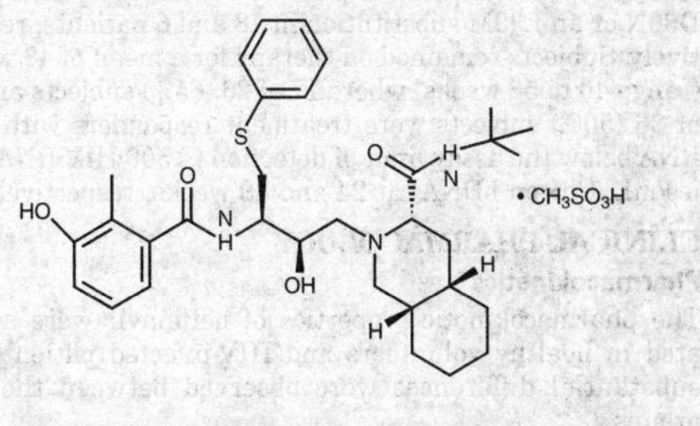

Nelfinavir mesylate is a white to off-white amorphous powder, slightly soluble in water at pH ≤4 and freely soluble in methanol, ethanol, 2-propanol propylene glycol.

MICROBIOLOGY

Mechanism of Action: Nelfinavir is an inhibitor of the HIV-1 protease. Inhibition of the viral protease prevents cleavage of the *gag* and *gag-pol* polyprotein resulting in the production of immature, non-infectious virus.

Antiviral Activity In Vitro: The antiviral activity of nelfinavir *in vitro* has been demonstrated in both acute and/or chronic HIV infections in lymphoblastoid cell lines, peripheral blood lymphocytes and monocytes/macrophages. Nelfinavir was found to be active against several laboratory strains and clinical isolates of HIV-1 and the HIV-2 strain ROD. The EC_{95} (95% effective concentration) of nelfinavir ranged from 7 to 196 nM. Drug combination studies with protease inhibitors showed nelfinavir had antagonistic interactions with indinavir, additive interactions with ritonavir or saquinavir and synergistic interactions with amprenavir and lopinavir. Minimal to no cellular cytotoxicity was observed with any of these protease inhibitors alone or in combination with nelfinavir. In combination with reverse transcriptase inhibitors, nelfinavir demonstrated additive (didanosine or stavudine) to synergistic (abacavir, delavirdine, efavirenz, lamivudine, nevirapine, tenofovir, zalcitabine or zidovudine) antiviral activity *in vitro* without enhanced cytotoxicity.

Drug Resistance: HIV-1 isolates with reduced susceptibility to nelfinavir have been selected *in vitro*. HIV isolates from selected patients treated with nelfinavir alone or in combination with reverse transcriptase inhibitors were monitored for phenotypic (n=19) and genotypic (n=195, 157 of which were evaluable) changes in clinical trials over a period of 2 to 82 weeks. One or more viral protease mutations at amino acid positions 30, 35, 36, 46, 71, 77 and 88 were detected in the HIV-1 of >10% of patients with evaluable isolates. The overall incidence of the D30N mutation in the viral protease of evaluable isolates (n=157) from patients receiving nelfinavir monotherapy or nelfinavir in combination with zidovudine and lamivudine or stavudine was 54.8%. The overall incidence of other mutations associated with primary protease inhibitor resistance was 9.6% for the L90M substitution whereas substitutions at 48, 82, or 84 were not observed. Of the 19 clinical isolates for which both phenotypic and genotypic analyses were performed, 9 showed reduced susceptibility (5- to 93-fold) to nelfinavir *in vitro*. All 9 patient isolates possessed one or more mutations in the viral protease gene. Amino acid position 30 appeared to be the most frequent mutation site.

Cross-resistance: Non-clinical Studies—Patient-derived recombinant HIV isolates containing the D30N mutation (n=4) and demonstrating high-level (>10-fold) NFV-resistance remained susceptible (<2.5-fold resistance) to amprenavir, indinavir, lopinavir, and saquinavir, *in vitro* Patient-derived recombinant HIV isolates containing the L90M mutation (n=8) demonstrated moderate to high-level resistance to NFV and had varying levels of susceptibility to amprenavir, indinavir, lopinavir, and saquinavir, *in vitro*. Most patient-derived recombinant isolates with phenotypic and genotypic evidence of reduced susceptibility (>2.5-fold) to amprenavir, indinavir, lopinavir, and/or saquinavir demonstrated high-level cross-resistance to nelfinavir, *in vitro*. Mutations associated with resistance to other PIs (e.g. G48V, V82A/F/T, I84V, L90M) appeared to confer high-level cross-resistance to NFV. Following ritonavir therapy 6 of 7 clinical isolates with decreased ritonavir susceptibility (8- to 113-fold) *in vitro* compared to baseline also exhibited decreased susceptibility to nelfinavir *in vitro* (5- to 40-fold). Cross-resistance between nelfinavir and reverse transcriptase inhibitors is unlikely because different enzyme targets are involved. Clinical isolates (n=5) with decreased sus-

Continued on next page

Viracept—Cont.

ceptibility to lamivudine, nevirapine or zidovudine remain fully susceptible to nelfinavir *in vitro*.

Clinical Studies—There have been no controlled or comparative studies evaluating the virologic response to subsequent protease inhibitor-containing regimens in patients who have demonstrated loss of virologic response to a nelfinavir-containing regimen. However, virologic response was evaluated in a single-arm prospective study of 26 patients with extensive prior antiretroviral experience with reverse transcriptase inhibitors (mean 2.9) who had received VIRACEPT for a mean duration of 59.7 weeks and were switched to a ritonavir (400 mg BID)/saquinavir hard-gel (400 mg BID) containing regimen after a prolonged period of VIRACEPT failure (median 48 weeks). Sequence analysis of HIV-1 isolates prior to switch demonstrated a D30N or an L90M substitution in 18 and 6 patients, respectively. Subjects remained on therapy for a mean of 48 weeks (range 40 to 56 weeks) where 17 of 26 (65%) subjects and 13 of 26 (50%) subjects were treatment responders with HIV RNA below the assay limit of detection (<500 HIV RNA copies/mL, Chiron bDNA) at 24 and 48 weeks, respectively.

CLINICAL PHARMACOLOGY

Pharmacokinetics

The pharmacokinetic properties of nelfinavir were evaluated in healthy volunteers and HIV-infected patients; no substantial differences were observed between the two groups.

Absorption: Pharmacokinetic parameters of nelfinavir (area under the plasma concentration-time curve during a 24-hour period at steady-state [AUC_{24}], peak plasma concentrations [C_{max}], morning and evening trough concentrations [C_{trough}]) from a pharmacokinetic study in HIV-positive patients after multiple dosing with 1250 mg (five 250 mg tablets) twice daily (BID) for 28 days (10 patients) and 750 mg (three 250 mg tablets) three times daily (TID) for 28 days (11 patients) are summarized in Table 1.

[See table 1 above]

The difference between morning and afternoon or evening trough concentrations for the TID and BID regimens was also observed in healthy volunteers who were dosed at precisely 8- or 12-hour intervals.

In healthy volunteers receiving a single 1250 mg dose, the 625 mg tablet was not bioequivalent to the 250 mg tablet formulation. Under fasted conditions (n=27), the AUC and C_{max} were 34% and 24% higher, respectively, for the 625 mg tablets. In a relative bioavailability assessment under fed conditions (n=28), the AUC was 24% higher for the 625 mg tablet; the C_{max} was comparable for both formulations. (See ADVERSE REACTIONS).

In healthy volunteers receiving a single 750 mg dose under fed conditions, nelfinavir concentrations were similar following administration of the 250 mg tablet and oral powder.

Effect of Food on Oral Absorption: Food increases nelfinavir exposure and decreases nelfinavir pharmacokinetic variability relative to the fasted state. In one study, healthy volunteers received a single dose of 1250 mg of VIRACEPT 250 mg tablets (5 tablets) under fasted or fed conditions (three different meals). In a second study, healthy volunteers received single doses of 1250 mg VIRACEPT (5 × 250 mg tablets) under fasted or fed conditions (two different fat content meals). The results from the two studies are summarized in Table 2 and Table 3 respectively.

[See table 2 above]
[See table 3 above]

Nelfinavir exposure can be increased by increasing the calorie or fat content in meals taken with VIRACEPT.

A food effect study has not been conducted with the 625 mg tablet. However, based on a cross-study comparison (n=26 fed vs. n=26 fasted) following single dose administration of nelfinavir 1250 mg, the magnitude of the food effect for the 625 mg nelfinavir tablet appears comparable to that of the 250 mg tablets. VIRACEPT should be taken with a meal.

Distribution: The apparent volume of distribution following oral administration of nelfinavir was 2-7 L/kg. Nelfinavir in serum is extensively protein-bound (>98%).

Metabolism: Unchanged nelfinavir comprised 82-86% of the total plasma radioactivity after a single oral 750 mg dose of ^{14}C-nelfinavir. *In vitro*, multiple cytochrome P-450 enzymes including CYP3A and CYP2C19 are responsible for metabolism of nelfinavir. One major and several minor oxidative metabolites were found in plasma. The major oxidative metabolite has *in vitro* antiviral activity comparable to the parent drug.

Elimination: The terminal half-life in plasma was typically 3.5 to 5 hours. The majority (87%) of an oral 750 mg dose containing ^{14}C-nelfinavir was recovered in the feces; fecal radioactivity consisted of numerous oxidative metabolites (78%) and unchanged nelfinavir (22%). Only 1-2% of the dose was recovered in urine, of which unchanged nelfinavir was the major component.

Special Populations

Hepatic Insufficiency: The multi-dose pharmacokinetics of nelfinavir have not been studied in HIV-positive patients with hepatic insufficiency.

Renal Insufficiency: The pharmacokinetics of nelfinavir have not been studied in patients with renal insufficiency; however, less than 2% of nelfinavir is excreted in the urine, so the impact of renal impairment on nelfinavir elimination should be minimal.

Gender and Race: No significant pharmacokinetic differences have been detected between males and females. Pharmacokinetic differences due to race have not been evaluated.

Pediatrics: The pharmacokinetics of nelfinavir have been investigated in 5 studies in pediatric patients from birth to 13 years of age either receiving VIRACEPT three times or twice daily. The dosing regimens and associated AUC_{24} values are summarized in Table 4.

[See table 4 above]

Table 1
Summary of a Pharmacokinetic Study in HIV-positive Patients with Multiple Dosing of 1250 mg BID for 28 days and 750 mg TID for 28 days

Regimen	AUC_{24} mg.h/L	C_{max} mg/L	C_{trough} Morning mg/L	C_{trough} Afternoon or Evening mg/L
1250 mg BID	52.8 ± 15.7	4.0 ± 0.8	2.2 ± 1.3	0.7 ± 0.4
750 mg TID	43.6 ± 17.8	3.0 ± 1.6	1.4 ± 0.6	1.0 ± 0.5

data are mean ± SD

Table 2
Increase in AUC, C_{max} and T_{max} for Nelfinavir in Fed State Relative to Fasted State Following 1250 mg VIRACEPT (5 × 250 mg tablets)

Number of Kcal	% Fat	Number of subjects	AUC fold increase	C_{max} fold increase	Increase in T_{max} (hr)
125	20	n=21	2.2	2.0	1.00
500	20	n=22	3.1	2.3	2.00
1000	50	n=23	5.2	3.3	2.00

Table 3
Increase in Nelfinavir AUC, C_{max} and T_{max} in Fed Low Fat (20%) versus High fat (50%) State Relative to Fasted State Following 1250 mg VIRACEPT (5 × 250 mg tablets)

Number of Kcal	% Fat	Number of Subjects	AUC fold increase	C_{max} fold increase	Increase in T_{max} (hr)
500	20	n=22	3.1	2.5	1.8
500	50	n=22	5.1	3.8	2.1

Table 4
Summary of Steady-state AUC_{24} of Nelfinavir in Pediatric Studies

Protocol No.	Dosing Regimen[1]	N[2]	Age	AUC_{24} (mg.hr/L) Arithmetic mean ± SD
AG1343-524	20 (19-28) mg/kg TID	14	2-13 years	56.1 ± 29.8
PACTG-725	55 (48-60) mg/kg BID	6	3-11 years	101.8 ± 56.1
PENTA 7	40 (34-43) mg/kg TID	4	2-9 months	33.8 ± 8.9
PENTA 7	75 (55-83) mg/kg BID	12	2-9 months	37.2 ± 19.2
PACTG-353	75 (14-56) mg/kg BID	10	6 weeks	44.1 ± 27.4
			1 week	45.8 ± 32.1

[1] Protocol specified dose (actual dose range)
[2] N: number of subjects with evaluable pharmacokinetic results
C_{trough} values are not presented in the table because they are not available for all studies

Table 5: Drug Interactions:
Changes in Pharmacokinetic Parameters for Coadministered Drug in the Presence of VIRACEPT

Coadministered Drug	Nelfinavir Dose	N	% Change of Coadministered Drug Pharmacokinetic Parameters[1] (90% CI): AUC	C_{max}	C_{min}
HIV-Protease Inhibitors					
Indinavir 800 mg Single Dose	750 mg q8h × 7 days	6	↑51% (↑29-↑77%)	↓10% (↓28-↑13%)	NA
Ritonavir 500 mg Single Dose	750 mg q8h × 5 doses	10	↔	↔	NA
Saquinavir 1200 mg Single Dose[2]	750 mg tid × 4 days	14	↑392% (↑291-↑521%)	↑179% (↑117-↑259%)	NA
Amprenavir 800 mg tid × 14 days	750 mg tid × 14 days	6	↔	↓14% (↓38-↑20%)	↑189% (↑52-↑448%)
Nucleoside Reverse Transcriptase Inhibitors					
Lamivudine 150 mg Single Dose	750 mg q8h × 7-10 days	11	↑10% (↑2-↑18%)	↑31% (↑9-↑56%)	
Stavudine 30-40 mg bid × 56 days	750 mg tid × 56 days	8		See footnote[3]	
Zidovudine 200 mg Single Dose	750 mg q8h × 7-10 days	11	↓35% (↓29-↓40%)	↓31% (↓13-↓46%)	NA

(Table continued on next page)

Table 5 *(cont.)*: Drug Interactions:
Changes in Pharmacokinetic Parameters for Coadministered Drug in the Presence of VIRACEPT

Coadministered Drug	Nelfinavir Dose	N	% Change of Coadministered Drug Pharmacokinetic Parameters[1] (90% CI)		
			AUC	C_{max}	C_{min}
Non-Nucleoside Reverse Transcriptase Inhibitors					
Efavirenz 600 mg qd × 7 days	750 mg q8h × 7 days	10	↓12% (↓31-↑12%)	↓12% (↓29-↑8%)	↓22% (↓54-↑32%)
Nevirapine 200 mg qd × 14 days[3] Followed by 200 mg bid × 14 days	750 mg tid × 36 days	23		See footnote[3]	
Delavirdine 400 mg q8h × 14 days	750 mg q8h × 7 days	7	↓31% (↓57-↑10%)	↓27% (↓49-↑4%)	↓33% (↓70-↑49%)
Anti-infective Agents					
Rifabutin 150 mg qd × 8 days[4]	750 mg q8h × 7-8 days[5]	12	↑83% (↑72-↑96%)	↑19% (↑11-↑28%)	↑177% (↑144-↑215%)
Rifabutin 300 mg qd × 8 days	750 mg q8h × 7-8 days	10	↑207% (↑161-↑263%)	↑146% (↑118-↑178%)	↑305% (↑245-↑375%)
Azithromycin 1200 mg Single Dose	750 mg tid × 11 days	12	↑112% (↑80-↑150%)	↑136% (↑77-↑215%)	NA
HMG-CoA Reductase Inhibitors					
Atorvastatin 10 mg qd × 28 days	1250 mg bid × 14 days	15	↑74% (↑41-↑116%)	↑122% (↑68-↑193%)	↑39% (↓21-↑145%)
Simvastatin 20 mg qd × 28 days	1250 mg bid × 14 days	16	↑505% (↑393-↑643%)	↑517% (↑367-↑715%)	ND
Other Agents					
Ethinyl estradiol 35 µg qd × 15 days	750 mg q8h × 7 days	12	↓47% (↓42-↓52%)	↓28% (↓16-↓37%)	↓62% (↓57-↓67%)
Norethindrone 0.4 mg qd × 15 days	750 mg q8h × 7 days	12	↓18% (↓13-↓23%)	↔	↓46% (↓38-↓53%)
Methadone 80 mg +/−21 mg qd[6] >1 month	1250 mg bid × 8 days	13	↓47% (↓42-↓51%)	↓46% (↓42-↓49%)	↓53% (↓49-↓57%)
Phenytoin 300 mg qd × 14 days[7]	1250 mg bid × 7 days	12	↓29% (↓17-↓39%)	↓21% (↓12-↓29%)	↓39% (↓27-↓49%)

NA: Not relevent for single-dose treatment; ND: Cannot be determined
[1]↑ indicates increase ↓ indicates decrease ↔ indicates no change (geometric mean exposure increased or decreased <10%)
[2]Using the soft-gelatin capsule formulation of saquinavir 1200 mg
[3]Based on non-definitive cross-study comparison, drug plasma concentrations appeared to be unaffected by coadministration
[4]Rifabutin 150 mg qd changes are relative to Rifabutin 300 mg qd × 8 days without coadministration with nelfinavir
[5]Comparable changes in rifabutin concentrations were observed with VIRACEPT 1250 mg q12h × 7 days
[6]Changes are reported for total plasma methadone; changes for the individual R-enantiomer and S-enantiomer were similar
[7]Phenytoin exposure measures are reported for total phenytoin exposure. The effect of nelfinavir on unbound phenytoin was similar

Table 6: Drug Interactions:
Change in Pharmacokinetic Parameters for Nelfinavir in the Presence of the Coadministered Drug

Coadministered Drug	Nelfinavir Dose	N	% Change of Nelfinavir Pharmacokinetic Parameters[1] (90% CI)		
			AUC	C_{max}	C_{min}
HIV-Protease Inhibitors					
Indinavir 800 mg q8h × 7 days	750 mg Single Dose	6	↑83% (↑42-↑137%)	↑31% (↑16-↑48%)	NA
Ritonavir 500 mg q12h × 3 doses	750 mg Single Dose	10	↑152% (↑96-↑224%)	↑44% (↑28-↑63%)	NA
Saquinavir 1200 mg tid × 4 days[2]	750 mg Single Dose	14	↑18% (↑7-↑30%)	↔	NA
Amprenavir 800 mg tid × 14 days	750 mg tid × 14 days	6		See footnote[3]	

(Table continued on next page)

Pharmacokinetic data are also available for 86 patients (age 2 to 12 years) who received VIRACEPT 25-35 mg/kg TID in Study AG1343-556. The pharmacokinetic data from Study AG1343-556 were more variable than data from other studies conducted in the pediatric population; the 95% confidence interval for AUC_{24} was 9 to 121 mg.hr/L.
Overall, use of VIRACEPT in the pediatric population is associated with highly variable drug exposure. The high variability may be due to inconsistent food intake in pediatric patients. (See PRECAUTIONS Pediatric Use; DOSAGE AND ADMINISTRATION.)

Geriatric Patients: The pharmacokinetics of nelfinavir have not been studied in patients over 65 years of age.
Drug Interactions (also see CONTRAINDICATIONS, WARNINGS, PRECAUTIONS: Drug Interactions)
CYP3A and CYP2C19 appear to be the predominant enzymes that metabolize nelfinavir in humans. The potential ability of nelfinavir to inhibit the major human cytochrome P450 enzymes (CYP3A, CYP2C19, CYP2D6, CYP2C9, CYP1A2 and CYP2E1) has been investigated *in vitro*. Only CYP3A was inhibited at concentrations in the therapeutic range. Specific drug interaction studies were performed with nelfinavir and a number of drugs. Table 5 summarizes the effects of nelfinavir on the geometric mean AUC, C_{max} and C_{min} of coadministered drugs. Table 6 shows the effects of coadministered drugs on the geometric mean AUC, C_{max} and C_{min} of nelfinavir.
[See table 5 on previous page and at left]
[See table 6 below and on next page]

For information regarding clinical recommendations see CONTRAINDICATIONS, WARNINGS, PRECAUTIONS: Drug Interactions.

INDICATIONS AND USAGE

VIRACEPT in combination with other antiretroviral agents is indicated for the treatment of HIV infection.

Description of Studies

In the clinical studies described below, efficacy was evaluated by the percent of patients with plasma HIV RNA < 400 copies/mL (Studies 511 and 542) or < 500 copies/mL (Study ACTG 364), using the Roche RT-PCR (Amplicor) HIV-1 Monitor or < 50 copies/mL, using the Roche HIV-1 Ultrasensitive assay (Study Avanti 3). In the analysis presented in each figure, patients who terminated the study early for any reason, switched therapy due to inadequate efficacy or who had a missing HIV-RNA measurement that was either preceded or followed by a measurement above the limit of assay quantification were considered to have HIV-RNA above 400 copies/mL, above 500 copies/mL, or above 50 copies/mL at subsequent time points, depending on the assay that was used.

a. Studies in Antiretroviral Treatment Naive Patients

Study 511: VIRACEPT + zidovudine + lamivudine versus zidovudine + lamivudine

Study 511 was a double-blind, randomized, placebo controlled trial comparing treatment with zidovudine (ZDV; 200 mg TID) and lamivudine (3TC; 150 mg BID) plus 2 doses of VIRACEPT (750 mg and 500 mg TID) to zidovudine (200 mg TID) and lamivudine (150 mg BID) alone in 297 antiretroviral naive HIV-1 infected patients (median age 35 years [range 21 to 63], 89% male and 78% Caucasian). Mean baseline CD4 cell count was 288 cells/mm³ and mean baseline plasma HIV RNA was 5.21 $\log_{10}$ copies/mL (160,394 copies/mL). The percent of patients with plasma HIV RNA <400 copies/mL and mean changes in CD4 cell count are summarized in Figures 1 and 2, respectively.

Figure 1
Study 511: Percentage of Patients With HIV RNA Below 400 Copies/mL

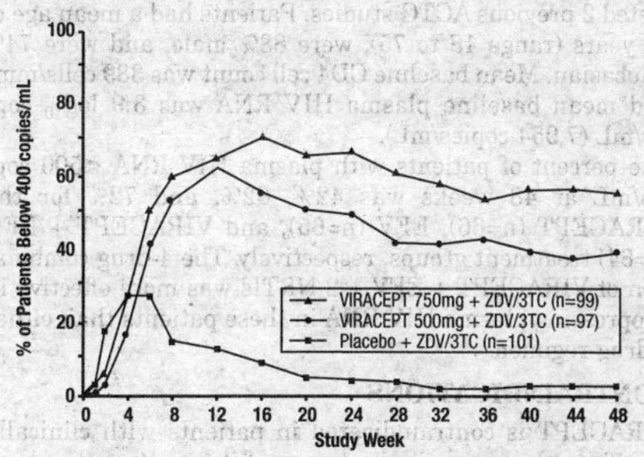

Figure 2
Study 511: Mean Change From Baseline in CD_4 Cell Counts

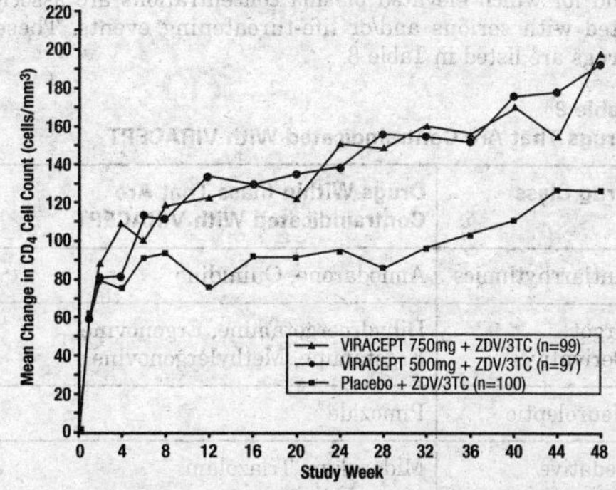

Study 542: VIRACEPT BID + stavudine + lamivudine compared to VIRACEPT TID + stavudine + lamivudine

Study 542 is an ongoing, randomized, open-label trial comparing the HIV RNA suppression achieved by VIRACEPT 1250 mg BID versus VIRACEPT 750 mg TID in patients also receiving stavudine (d4T; 30-40 mg BID) and lamivudine (3TC; 150 mg BID). Patients had a median age of 36 years (range 18 to 83), were 84% male, and were 91% Caucasian. Patients had received less than 6 months of therapy with nucleoside transcriptase inhibitors and were naïve to protease inhibitors. Mean baseline CD4 cell count was 296 cells/mm³ and mean baseline plasma HIV RNA was 5.0 $\log_{10}$ copies/mL (100,706 copies/mL).
Results showed that there was no significant difference in mean CD4 cell count among treatment groups; the mean increases from baseline for the BID and TID arms were 150 cells/mm³ at 24 weeks and approximately 200 cells/mm³ at 48 weeks.
The percent of patients with HIV RNA <400 copies/mL is summarized in Figure 3. The outcomes of patients through 48 weeks of treatment are summarized in Table 7.

Continued on next page

Viracept—Cont.

Figure 3
Study 542: Percentage of Patients With HIV RNA Below 400 Copies/mL

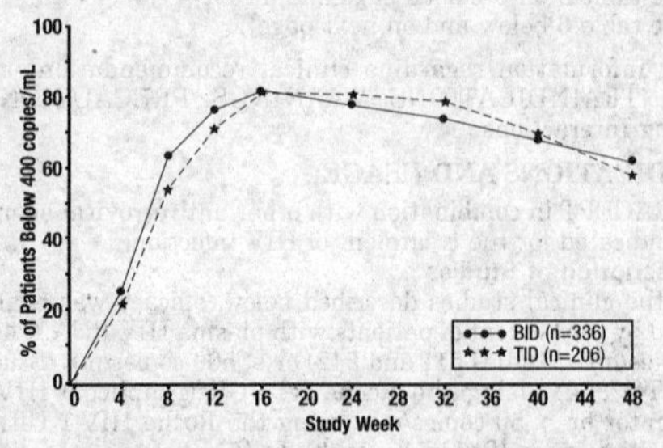

[See table 7 below]

Study Avanti 3: VIRACEPT TID + zidovudine + lamivudine compared to zidovudine + lamivudine

Study Avanti 3 was a placebo-controlled, randomized, double-blind study designed to evaluate the safety and efficacy of VIRACEPT (750 mg TID) in combination with zidovudine (ZDV; 300 mg BID) and lamivudine (3TC; 150 mg BID) (n=53) versus placebo in combination with ZDV and 3TC (n=52) administered to antiretroviral-naive patients with HIV infection and a CD4 cell count between 150 and 500 cells/µL. Patients had a mean age of 35 (range 22-59), were 89% male, and 88% Caucasian. Mean baseline CD4 cell count was 304 cells/mm^3 and mean baseline plasma HIV RNA was 4.8 log_{10} copies/mL (57,887 copies/mL). The percent of patients with plasma HIV RNA <50 copies/mL at 52 weeks was 54% for the VIRACEPT + ZDV + 3TC treatment group and 13% for the ZDV + 3TC treatment group.

b. Studies in Antiretroviral Treatment Experienced Patients

Study ACTG 364: VIRACEPT TID + 2NRTIs compared to efavirenz + 2NRTIs compared to VIRACEPT + efavirenz + 2NRTIs

Study ACTG 364 was a randomized, double-blind study that evaluated the combination of VIRACEPT 750 mg TID and/or efavirenz 600 mg QD with 2 NRTIs (either didanosine [ddI] + d4T, ddI + 3TC, or d4T + 3TC) in patients with prolonged prior nucleoside exposure who had completed 2 previous ACTG studies. Patients had a mean age of 41 years (range 18 to 75), were 88% male, and were 74% Caucasian. Mean baseline CD4 cell count was 389 cells/mm^3 and mean baseline plasma HIV RNA was 3.9 log_{10} copies/mL (7,954 copies/mL).

The percent of patients with plasma HIV RNA <500 copies/mL at 48 weeks was 42%, 62%, and 72% for the VIRACEPT (n=66), EFV (n=65), and VIRACEPT + EFV (n=64) treatment groups, respectively. The 4-drug combination of VIRACEPT + EFV + 2 NRTIs was more effective in suppressing plasma HIV RNA in these patients than either 3-drug regimen.

CONTRAINDICATIONS

VIRACEPT is contraindicated in patients with clinically significant hypersensitivity to any of its components.

Coadministration of VIRACEPT is contraindicated with drugs that are highly dependent on CYP3A for clearance and for which elevated plasma concentrations are associated with serious and/or life-threatening events. These drugs are listed in Table 8.

Table 8
Drugs That Are Contraindicated With VIRACEPT

Drug Class	Drugs Within Class That Are Contraindicated With VIRACEPT
Antiarrhythmics	Amiodarone, Quinidine
Ergot Derivatives	Dihydroergotamine, Ergonovine, Ergotamine, Methylergonovine
Neuroleptic	Pimozide
Sedative/ Hypnotics	Midazolam, Triazolam

WARNINGS

ALERT: Find out about medicines that should not be taken with VIRACEPT. This statement is included on the product's bottle label.

Drug Interactions (also see PRECAUTIONS)

Nelfinavir is an inhibitor of the CYP3A enzyme. Coadministration of VIRACEPT and drugs primarily metabolized by CYP3A may result in increased plasma concentrations of the other drug that could increase or prolong its therapeutic and adverse effects. Caution should be exercised when inhibitors of CYP3A, including VIRACEPT, are coadministered with drugs that are metabolized by CYP3A and that prolong the QT interval. (See ADVERSE REACTIONS; Post-Marketing Experience). Nelfinavir is metabolized by CYP3A and CYP2C19. Coadministration of VIRACEPT and drugs that induce CYP3A or CYP2C19 may decrease nelfinavir plasma concentrations and reduce its therapeutic effect. Coadministration of VIRACEPT and drugs that inhibit CYP3A or CYP2C19 may increase nelfinavir plasma concentrations. (Also see **PRECAUTIONS: Table 9: Drugs That Should Not Be Coadministered With VIRACEPT - Table 10: Established and Other Potentially Significant Drug Interactions With VIRACEPT.)**

Concomitant use of VIRACEPT with lovastatin or simvastatin is not recommended. Caution should be exercised if HIV protease inhibitors, including VIRACEPT, are used concurrently with other HMG-CoA reductase inhibitors that are also metabolized by the CYP3A pathway (e.g., atorvastatin). (Also see **Tables 5 and 6: Drug Interactions**). The risk of myopathy including rhabdomyolysis may be increased when protease inhibitors, including VIRACEPT, are used in combination with these drugs.

Particular caution should be used when prescribing sildenafil in patients receiving protease inhibitors, including

Table 6 *(cont.)*: Drug Interactions:
Change in Pharmacokinetic Parameters for Nelfinavir in the Presence of the Coadministered Drug

Coadministered Drug	Nelfinavir Dose	N	% Change of Nelfinavir Pharmacokinetic Parameters[1] (90% CI) AUC	C_{max}	C_{min}
Nucleoside Reverse Transcriptase Inhibitors					
Didanosine 200 mg Single Dose	750 mg Single Dose	9	↔	↔	NA
Zidovudine 200 mg + Lamivudine 150 mg Single Dose	750 mg q8h × 7-10 days	11	↔	↔	↔
Non-Nucleoside Reverse Transcriptase Inhibitors					
Efavirenz 600 mg qd × 7 days	750 mg q8h × 7 days	7	↑20% (↑8-↑34%)	↑21% (↑10-↑33%)	↔
Nevirapine 200 mg qd × 14 days Followed by 200 mg bid × 14 days	750 mg tid × 36 days	23	↔	↔	↓32% (↓50-↑5%)
Delavirdine 400 mg q8h × 7 days	750 mg q8h × 14 days	12	↑107% (↑83-↑135%)	↑88% (↑66-↑113%)	↑136% (↑103-↑175%)
Anti-infective Agents					
Ketoconazole 400 mg qd × 7 days	500 mg q8h × 5-6 days	12	↑35% (↑24–↑46%)	↑25% (↑11-↑40%)	↑14% (↓23-↑69%)
Rifabutin 150 mg qd × 8 days	750 mg q8h × 7-8 days	11	↓23% (↓14-↓31%)	↓18% (↓8-↓27%)	↓25% (↓8-↓39%)
	1250 mg q12h × 7-8 days	11	↔	↔	↓15% (↓43-↑27%)
Rifabutin 300 mg qd × 8 days	750 mg q8h × 7-8 days	10	↓32% (↓15-↓46%)	↓24% (↓10-↓36%)	↓53% (↓15-↓73%)
Rifampin 600 mg qd × 7 days	750 mg q8h × 5-6 days	12	↓83% (↓79-↓86%)	↓76% (↓69-↓82%)	↓92% (↓86-↓95%)
Azithromycin 1200 mg Single Dose	750 mg tid × 9 days	12	↓15% (↓7-↓22%)	↓10% (↓19-↑1%)	↓29% (↓19-↓38%)
HMG-CoA Reductase Inhibitors					
Atorvastatin 10 mg qd × 28 days	1250 mg bid × 14 days	15	See footnote[3]		
Simvastatin 20 mg qd × 28 days	1250 mg bid × 14 days	16	See footnote[3]		
Other Agents					
Methadone 80 mg +/-21 mg qd >1 month	1250 mg bid × 8 days	13	See footnote[3]		
Phenytoin 300 mg qd × 7 days	1250 mg bid × 14 days	15	↔	↔	↓18% (↓45-↑23%)

NA: Not relevent for single-dose treatment

[1] ↑ Indicates increase ↓ indicates decrease ↔ indicates no change (geometric mean exposure increased or decreased <10%)

[2] Using the soft-gelatin capsule formulation of saquinavir 1200 mg

[3] Based on non-definitive cross-study comparison, nelfinavir plasma concentrations appeared to be unaffected by co-administration

Table 7
Outcomes of Randomized Treatment Through 48 Weeks

Outcome	VIRACEPT 1250 mg BID Regimen	VIRACEPT 750 mg TID Regimen
Number of patients evaluable*	323	192
HIV RNA <400 copies/mL	198 (61%)	111 (58%)
HIV RNA ≥400 copies/mL	46 (14%)	22 (11%)
Discontinued due to VIRACEPT toxicity**	9 (3%)	2 (1%)
Discontinued due to other antiretroviral agents' Toxicity**	3 (1%)	3 (2%)
Others***	67 (21%)	54 (28%)

*Twelve patients in the BID arm and fourteen patients in the TID arm have not yet reached 48 weeks of therapy.

**These rates only reflect dose-limiting toxicities that were counted as the initial reason for treatment failure in the analysis (see ADVERSE REACTIONS for a description of the safety profile of these regimens).

***Consent withdrawn, lost to follow-up, intercurrent illness, noncompliance or missing data; all assumed as failures.

VIRACEPT. Coadministration of a protease inhibitor with sildenafil is expected to substantially increase sildenafil concentrations and may result in an increase in sildenafil-associated adverse events, including hypotension, visual changes, and priapism. (See PRECAUTIONS, Drug Interactions and Information for Patients, and the complete prescribing information for sildenafil.)
Concomitant use of St. John's wort (hypericum perforatum) or St. John's wort containing products and VIRACEPT is not recommended. Coadministration of St. John's wort with protease inhibitors, including VIRACEPT, is expected to substantially decrease protease inhibitor concentrations and may result in sub-optimal levels of VIRACEPT and lead to loss of virologic response and possible resistance to VIRACEPT or to the class of protease inhibitors.

Patients with Phenylketonuria
Patients with Phenylketonuria: VIRACEPT Oral Powder contains 11.2 mg phenylalanine per gram of powder.

Diabetes mellitus/Hyperglycemia
New onset diabetes mellitus, exacerbation of pre-existing diabetes mellitus and hyperglycemia have been reported during post-marketing surveillance in HIV-infected patients receiving protease inhibitor therapy. Some patients required either initiation or dose adjustments of insulin or oral hypoglycemic agents for treatment of these events. In some cases diabetic ketoacidosis has occurred. In those patients who discontinued protease inhibitor therapy, hyperglycemia persisted in some cases. Because these events have been reported voluntarily during clinical practice, estimates of frequency cannot be made and a causal relationship between protease inhibitor therapy and these events has not been established.

PRECAUTIONS

General
Nelfinavir is principally metabolized by the liver. Therefore, caution should be exercised when administering this drug to patients with hepatic impairment.

Resistance/Cross Resistance
HIV cross-resistance between protease inhibitors has been observed. (See MICROBIOLOGY.)

Hemophilia
There have been reports of increased bleeding, including spontaneous skin hematomas and hemarthrosis, in patients with hemophilia type A and B treated with protease inhibitors. In some patients, additional factor VIII was given. In more than half of the reported cases, treatment with protease inhibitors was continued or reintroduced. A causal relationship has not been established.

Fat Redistribution
Redistribution/accumulation of body fat including central obesity, dorsocervical fat enlargement (buffalo hump), peripheral wasting, facial wasting, breast enlargement, and "cushingoid appearance" have been observed in patients receiving antiretroviral therapy. The mechanism and long-term consequences of these events are currently unknown. A causal relationship has not been established.

Information For Patients
"A statement to patients and health care providers is included on the product's bottle label: **ALERT: Find out about medicines that should NOT be taken with VIRACEPT.** A Patient Package Insert (PPI) for VIRACEPT is available for patient information."
For optimal absorption, patients should be advised to take VIRACEPT with food (see CLINICAL PHARMACOLOGY: Pharmacokinetics and DOSAGE AND ADMINISTRATION).
Patients should be informed that VIRACEPT is not a cure for HIV infection and that they may continue to acquire illnesses associated with advanced HIV infection, including opportunistic infections.
Patients should be told that there is currently no data demonstrating that VIRACEPT therapy can reduce the risk of transmitting HIV to others through sexual contact or blood contamination.
Patients should be told that sustained decreases in plasma HIV RNA have been associated with a reduced risk of progression to AIDS and death. Patients should be advised to take VIRACEPT and other concomitant antiretroviral therapy every day as prescribed. Patients should not alter the dose or discontinue therapy without consulting with their doctor. If a dose of VIRACEPT is missed, patients should take the dose as soon as possible and then return to their normal schedule. However, if a dose is skipped, the patient should not double the next dose.
Patients should be informed that VIRACEPT Tablets are film-coated and that this film-coating is intended to make the tablets easier to swallow.
The most frequent adverse event associated with VIRACEPT is diarrhea, which can usually be controlled with non-prescription drugs, such as loperamide, which slow gastrointestinal motility.
Patients should be informed that redistribution or accumulation of body fat may occur in patients receiving antiretroviral therapy and that the cause and long term health effects of these conditions are not known at this time.
VIRACEPT may interact with some drugs, therefore, patients should be advised to report to their doctor the use of any other prescription, non-prescription medication or herbal products, particularly St. John's wort.
Patients receiving oral contraceptives should be instructed that alternate or additional contraceptive measures should be used during therapy with VIRACEPT.
Patients receiving sildenafil and nelfinavir should be advised that they may be at an increased risk of sildenafil-associated adverse events including hypotension, visual changes, and prolonged penile erection, and should promptly report any symptoms to their doctor.

Drug Interactions (Also see CONTRAINDICATIONS, WARNINGS, CLINICAL PHARMACOLOGY: Drug Interactions).
Nelfinavir is an inhibitor of CYP3A. Coadministration of VIRACEPT and drugs primarily metabolized by CYP3A (e.g., dihydropyridine calcium channel blockers, HMG-CoA reductase inhibitors, immunosuppressants and sildenafil) may result in increased plasma concentrations of the other drug that could increase or prolong both its therapeutic and adverse effects. (See Tables 9 and 10). Nelfinavir is metabolized by CYP3A and CYP2C19. Coadministration of VIRACEPT and drugs that induce CYP3A or CYP2C19, such as rifampin, may decrease nelfinavir plasma concentrations and reduce its therapeutic effect. Coadministration of VIRACEPT and drugs that inhibit CYP3A or CYP2C19 may increase nelfinavir plasma concentrations.
Drug interaction studies reveal no clinically significant drug interactions between nelfinavir and didanosine, lamivudine, stavudine, zidovudine, efavirenz, nevirapine, or ketoconazole and no dose adjustments are needed. In the case of didanosine, it is recommended that didanosine be administered on an empty stomach; therefore, nelfinavir should be administered with food one hour after or more than 2 hours before didanosine.
Based on known metabolic profiles, clinically significant drug interactions are not expected between VIRACEPT and dapsone, trimethoprim/sulfamethoxazole, or itraconazole.

Table 9
Drugs That Should Not Be Coadministered With VIRACEPT

Drug Class: Drug Name	Clinical Comment
Antiarrhythmics: amiodarone, quinidine	CONTRAINDICATED due to potential for serious and/or life threatening reactions such as cardiac arrhythmias.
Antimycobacterial: rifampin	May lead to loss of virologic response and possible resistance to VIRACEPT or other coadministered antiretroviral agents.
Ergot Derivatives: dihydroergotamine, ergonovine, ergotamine, methylergonovine	CONTRAINDICATED due to potential for serious and/or life threatening reactions such as acute ergot toxicity characterized by peripheral vasospasm and ischemia of the extremities and other tissues.
Herbal Products: St. John's wort (hypericum perforatum)	May lead to loss of virologic response and possible resistance to VIRACEPT or other coadministered antiretroviral agents.
HMG-CoA Reductase Inhibitors: lovastatin, simvastatin	Potential for serious reactions such as risk of myopathy including rhabdomyolysis.
Neuroleptic: pimozide	CONTRAINDICATED due to potential for serious and/or life threatening reactions such as cardiac arrhythmias.
Sedative/Hypnotics: midazolam, triazolam	CONTRAINDICTED due to potential for serious and/or life threatening reactions such as prolonged or increased sedation or respiratory depression.

[See table 10 at top of next page]

Carcinogenesis, Mutagenesis, Impairment of Fertility
Carcinogenicity studies in mice and rats were conducted with nelfinavir at oral doses up to 1000 mg/kg/day. No evidence of a tumorigenic effect was noted in mice at systemic exposures (C_{max}) up to 9-fold those measured in humans at the recommended therapeutic dose (750 mg TID or 1250 mg BID). In rats, thyroid follicular cell adenomas and carcinomas were increased in males at 300 mg/kg/day and higher and in females at 1000 mg/kg/day. Systemic exposures (C_{max}) at 300 and 1000 mg/kg/day were 1- to 3-fold, respectively, those measured in humans at the recommended therapeutic dose. Repeated administration of nelfinavir to rats produced effects consistent with hepatic microsomal enzyme induction and increased thyroid hormone disposition; these effects predispose rats, but not humans, to thyroid follicular cell neoplasms. Nelfinavir showed no evidence of mutagenic or clastogenic activity in a battery of *in vitro* and *in vivo* genetic toxicology assays. These studies included bacterial mutation assays in *S. typhimurium* and *E. coli*, a mouse lymphoma tyrosine kinase assay, a chromosomal aberration assay in human lymphocytes, and an *in vivo* mouse bone marrow micronucleus assay.
Nelfinavir produced no effects on either male or female mating and fertility or embryo survival in rats at systemic exposures comparable to the human therapeutic exposure.

Pregnancy—Pregnancy Category B
There were no effects on fetal development or maternal toxicity when nelfinavir was administered to pregnant rats at systemic exposures (AUC) comparable to human exposure. Administration of nelfinavir to pregnant rabbits resulted in no fetal development effects up to a dose at which a slight decrease in maternal body weight was observed; however, even at the highest dose evaluated, systemic exposure in rabbits was significantly lower than human exposure. Additional studies in rats indicated that exposure to nelfinavir in females from mid-pregnancy through lactation had no effect on the survival, growth, and development of the offspring to weaning. Subsequent reproductive performance of these offspring was also not affected by maternal exposure to nelfinavir. However, there are no adequate and well-controlled studies in pregnant women taking VIRACEPT. Because animal reproduction studies are not always predictive of human response, VIRACEPT should be used during pregnancy only if clearly needed.
Antiretroviral Pregnancy Registry: (APR): To monitor maternal-fetal outcomes of pregnant women exposed to VIRACEPT and other antiretroviral agents, an Antiretroviral Pregnancy Registry has been established. Physicians are encouraged to register patients by calling (800) 258-4263.

Nursing Mothers
The Centers for Disease Control and Prevention recommends that HIV-infected mothers not breast-feed their infants to avoid risking postnatal transmission of HIV. Studies in lactating rats have demonstrated that nelfinavir is excreted in milk. Because of both the potential for HIV transmission and the potential for serious adverse reactions in nursing infants, **mothers should be instructed not to breast-feed if they are receiving VIRACEPT.**

Pediatric Use
The safety and effectiveness of VIRACEPT have been established in patients from 2 to 13 years of age. The use of VIRACEPT in these age groups is supported by evidence from adequate and well-controlled studies of VIRACEPT in adults and pharmacokinetic studies and studies supporting activity in pediatric patients. In patients less than 2 years of age, VIRACEPT was found to be safe at the doses studied, but a reliably effective dose could not be established (see CLINICAL PHARMACOLOGY: Special Populations, ADVERSE REACTIONS: Pediatric Population, and DOSAGE AND ADMINISTRATION: Pediatric Patients).
The following issues should be considered when initiating VIRACEPT in pediatric patients:

- In pediatric patients $\geq$ 2 years of age receiving VIRACEPT as part of triple combination antiretroviral therapy in randomized studies, the proportion of patients achieving a HIV RNA level <400 copies/mL through 48 weeks ranged from 26% to 42%.
- Response rates in children <2 years of age appeared to be poorer than those in patients $\geq$ 2 years of age in some studies.
- Highly variable drug exposure remains a significant problem in the use of VIRACEPT in pediatric patients. Unpredictable drug exposure may be exacerbated in pediatric patients because of increased clearance compared to adults and difficulties with compliance and adequate food intake with dosing. Pharmacokinetic results from the pediatric studies are reported in Table 4 (see Clinical Pharmacology, Special Populations).

Study 556 was a randomized, double-blind, placebo-controlled trial with VIRACEPT or placebo coadministered with ZDV and ddI in 141 HIV-positive children who had received minimal antiretroviral therapy. The mean age of the children was 3.9 years. 94 (67%) children were between 2-12 years, and 47 (33%) were < 2 years of age. The mean baseline HIV RNA value was 5.0 log for all patients and the mean CD4 cell count 886 cells/mm^3 for all patients. The efficacy of VIRACEPT measured by HIV RNA <400 at 48 weeks in children $\geq$ 2 years of age was 26% compared to 2% of placebo patients (p=0.0008). In the children < 2 years of age, only 1 of 27 and 2 of 20 maintained an undetectable HIV RNA level at 48 weeks for placebo and VIRACEPT patients respectively.
PACTG 377 was an open-label study that randomized 181 HIV treatment-experienced pediatric patients to receive: d4T+NVP+RTV, d4T+3TC+NFV, or d4T+3TC+NVP+NFV with NFV given on a TID schedule. The median age was 5.9 years and 46% were male. At baseline the median HIV RNA was 4.4 log and median CD4 cell count was 690 cells/mm^3. Substudy PACTG 725 evaluated d4T+3TC+NFV with NFV given on a BID schedule. The proportion of patients with detectable viral load at baseline achieving HIV RNA <400 copies/mL at 48 weeks was: 41% for d4T+NVP+RTV, 42% for d4T+3TC+NFV, 30% for d4T+NVP+NFV, and 52% for d4T+3TC+NVP+NFV. No significant clinical differences were identified between patients receiving VIRACEPT in BID or TID schedules.
VIRACEPT has been evaluated in 2 studies of young infants. The PENTA 7 study was an open-label study to evaluate the toxicity, tolerability, pharmacokinetics, and activity of NFV+d4T+ddI in 20 HIV-infected infants less than 12 weeks of age. PACTG 353 evaluated the pharmacokinetics and safety of VIRACEPT in infants born to HIV-infected women receiving NFV as part of combination therapy during pregnancy.

Geriatric Use
Clinical studies of VIRACEPT did not include sufficient numbers of subjects aged 65 and over to determine whether they respond differently from younger subjects.

Continued on next page

Viracept—Cont.

ADVERSE REACTIONS

The safety of VIRACEPT was studied in over 5000 patients who received drug either alone or in combination with nucleoside analogues. The majority of adverse events were of mild intensity. The most frequently reported adverse event among patients receiving VIRACEPT was diarrhea, which was generally of mild to moderate intensity. The frequency of nelfinavir-associated diarrhea may be increased in patients receiving the 625 mg tablet because of the increased bioavailability of this formulation.

Drug-related clinical adverse experiences of moderate or severe intensity in ≥2% of patients treated with VIRACEPT coadministered with d4T and 3TC (Study 542) for up to 48 weeks or with ZDV plus 3TC (Study 511) for up to 24 weeks are presented in Table 11.

[See table 11 below]

Adverse events occurring in less than 2% of patients receiving VIRACEPT in all phase II/III clinical trials and considered at least possibly related or of unknown relationship to treatment and of at least moderate severity are listed below.

Body as a Whole: abdominal pain, accidental injury, allergic reaction, asthenia, back pain, fever, headache, malaise, pain, and redistribution/accumulation of body fat (see PRECAUTIONS, Fat Redistribution).

Digestive System: anorexia, dyspepsia, epigastric pain, gastrointestinal bleeding, hepatitis, mouth ulceration, pancreatitis and vomiting.

Hemic/Lymphatic System: anemia, leukopenia and thrombocytopenia.

Metabolic/Nutritional System: increases in alkaline phosphatase, amylase, creatine phosphokinase, lactic dehydrogenase, SGOT, SGPT and gamma glutamyl transpeptidase; hyperlipemia, hyperuricemia, hyperglycemia, hypoglycemia, dehydration, and liver function tests abnormal.

Musculoskeletal System: arthralgia, arthritis, cramps, myalgia, myasthenia and myopathy.

Nervous System: anxiety, depression, dizziness, emotional lability, hyperkinesia, insomnia, migraine, paresthesia, seizures, sleep disorder, somnolence and suicide ideation.

Respiratory System: dyspnea, pharyngitis, rhinitis, and sinusitis.

Skin/Appendages: dermatitis, folliculitis, fungal dermatitis, maculopapular rash, pruritus, sweating, and urticaria.

Special Senses: acute iritis and eye disorder.

Urogenital System: kidney calculus, sexual dysfunction and urine abnormality.

Post-Marketing Experience

The following additional adverse experiences have been reported from postmarketing surveillance as at least possibly related or of unknown relationship to VIRACEPT:

Body as a Whole: hypersensitivity reactions (including bronchospasm, moderate to severe rash, fever and edema)

Cardiovascular System: QTc prolongation, torsades de pointes

Digestive System: jaundice

Metabolic/Nutritional System: bilirubinemia, metabolic acidosis

Laboratory Abnormalities

The percentage of patients with marked laboratory abnormalities in Studies 542 and 511 are presented in Table 12. Marked laboratory abnormalities are defined as a Grade 3 or 4 abnormality in a patient with a normal baseline value or a Grade 4 abnormality in a patient with a Grade 1 abnormality at baseline.

[See table 12 at top of next page]

Pediatric Population

VIRACEPT has been studied in approximately 400 pediatric patients in clinical trials from birth to 13 years of age. The adverse event profile seen during pediatric clinical trials was similar to that for adults.

The most commonly reported drug-related, treatment-emergent adverse events reported in the pediatric studies included: diarrhea, leukopenia/neutropenia, rash, anorexia and abdominal pain. Diarrhea, regardless of assigned relationship to study drug, was reported in 39% to 47% of pediatric patients receiving VIRACEPT in 2 of the larger treatment trials. Leukopenia/neutropenia was the laboratory abnormality most commonly reported as a significant event across the pediatric studies.

OVERDOSAGE

Human experience of acute overdose with VIRACEPT is limited. There is no specific antidote for overdose with VIRACEPT. If indicated, elimination of unabsorbed drug should be achieved by emesis or gastric lavage. Administration of activated charcoal may also be used to aid removal of unabsorbed drug. Since nelfinavir is highly protein bound, dialysis is unlikely to significantly remove drug from blood.

DOSAGE AND ADMINISTRATION

Adults: The recommended dose is 1250 mg (five 250 mg tablets or two 625 mg tablets) twice daily or 750 mg (three 250 mg tablets) three times daily. VIRACEPT should be taken with a meal. Patients unable to swallow the 250 or 625 mg tablets may dissolve the tablets in a small amount of water. Once dissolved, patients should mix the cloudy liquid well, and consume it immediately. The glass should be rinsed with water and the rinse swallowed to ensure the entire dose is consumed.

Pediatric Patients (2-13 years): In children 2 years of age and older, the recommended oral dose of VIRACEPT oral

Table 10
Established and Other Potentially Significant Drug Interactions: Alteration in Dose or Regimen May Be Recommended Based on Drug Interaction Studies (see CLINICAL PHARMACOLOGY, for Magnitude of Interaction, Tables 4 and 5)

Concomitant Drug Class: Drug Name	Effect on Concentration	Clinical Comment
	HIV-Antiviral Agents	
Protease Inhibitors: indinavir ritonavir saquinavir	↑ nelfinavir ↑ indinavir ↑ nelfinavir ↑ saquinavir	Appropriate doses for these combinations, with respect to safety and efficacy, have not been established.
Non-nucleoside Reverse Transcriptase inhibitors: delavirdine nevirapine	↑ nelfinavir ↓ delavirdine ↓ nelfinavir (C_{min})	Appropriate doses for these combinations, with respect to safety and efficacy, have not been established.
Nucleoside Reverse Transcriptase Inhibitor: didanosine		It is recommended that didanosine be administered on an empty stomach; therefore, didanosine should be given one hour before or two hours after VIRACEPT (given with food).
	Other Agents	
Anti-Convulsants: carbamazepine phenobarbital	↓ nelfinavir	May decrease nelfinavir plasma concentrations. VIRACEPT may not be effective due to decreased nelfinavir plasma concentrations in patients taking these agents concomitantly.
Anti-Convulsant: phenytoin	↓ phenytoin	Phenytoin plasma/serum concentrations should be monitored; phenytoin dose may require adjustment to compensate for altered phenytoin concentration.
Anti-Mycobacterial: rifabutin	↑ rifabutin ↓ nelfinavir (750 mg TID) ↔nelfinavir (1250 mg BID)	It is recommended that the dose of rifabutin be reduced to one-half the usual dose when administered with VIRACEPT; 1250 mg BID is the preferred dose of VIRACEPT when coadministered with rifabutin.
Erectile Dysfunction Agent: sildenafil	↑ sildenafil	Sildenafil should not exceed a maximum single dose of 25 mg in a 48 hour period.
HMG-CoA Reductase Inhibitor: atorvastatin	↑ atorvastatin	Use lowest possible dose of atorvastatin with careful monitoring, or consider other HMG-CoA reductase inhibitors such as pravastatin or fluvastatin in combination with VIRACEPT.
Immunosuppressants: cyclosporine tacrolimus sirolimus	↑ immuno-suppressants	Plasma concentrations may be increased by VIRACEPT.
Narcotic Analgesic: methadone	↓ methadone	Dosage of methadone may need to be increased when coadministered with VIRACEPT.
Oral Contraceptive: ethinyl estradiol	↓ ethinyl estradiol	Alternative or additional contraceptive measures should be used when oral contraceptives and VIRACEPT are coadministered.
Macrolide Antibiotic: azithromycin	↑ azithromycin	Dose adjustment of azithromycin is not recommended, but close monitoring for known side effects such as liver enzyme abnormalities and hearing impairment is warranted.

Table 11
Percentage of Patients with Treatment-Emergent[1] Adverse Events of Moderate or Severe Intensity Reported in ≥ 2% of Patients

	Study 511 24 weeks			Study 542 48 weeks	
Adverse Events	Placebo + ZDV/3TC (n=101)	500 mg TID VIRACEPT + ZDV/3TC (n=97)	750 mg TID VIRACEPT + ZDV/3TC (n=100)	1250 mg BID VIRACEPT + d4T/3TC (n=344)	750 mg TID VIRACEPT + d4T/3TC (n=210)
Digestive System					
Diarrhea	3%	14%	20%	20%	15%
Nausea	4%	3%	7%	3%	3%
Flatulence	0	5%	2%	1%	1%
Skin/Appendages					
Rash	1%	1%	3%	2%	1%

[1] Includes those adverse events at least possibly related to study drug or of unknown relationship and excludes concurrent HIV conditions

Table 12
Percentage of Patients by Treatment Group With Marked Laboratory Abnormalities[1] in > 2% of Patients

	Study 511			Study 542	
	Placebo + ZDV/3TC (n=101)	500 mg TID VIRACEPT + ZDV/3TC (n=97)	750 mg TID VIRACEPT + ZDV/3TC (n=100)	1250 mg BID VIRACEPT + d4T/3TC (n=344)	750 mg TID VIRACEPT + d4T/3TC (n=210)
Hematology					
Hemoglobin	6%	3%	2%	0	0
Neutrophils	4%	3%	5%	2%	1%
Lymphocytes	1%	6%	1%	1%	0
Chemistry					
ALT (SGPT)	6%	1%	1%	2%	1%
AST (SGOT)	4%	1%	0	2%	1%
Creatine Kinase	7%	2%	2%	NA	NA

[1] Marked laboratory abnormalities are defined as a shift from Grade 0 at baseline to at least Grade 3 or from Grade 1 to Grade 4

Table 14
Dosing Table for Children ≥2 years of age (powder)

Body Weight		Twice Daily (BID) 45-55 mg/kg		Three Times Daily (TID) 25-35 mg/kg	
Kg.	Lbs.	Scoops of powder (50 mg/1 g)	Teaspoons[1] of Powder	Scoops of powder (50 mg/1 g)	Teaspoons[1] of Powder
9.0 to <10.5	20 to <23	10	2½	6	1½
10.5 to <12	23 to <26.5	11	2¾	7	1¾
12 to <14	26.5 to <31	13	3¼	8	2
14 to <16	31 to <35	15	3¾	9	2¼
16 to <18	35 to <39.5	Not recommended[2]	Not recommended[2]	10	2½
18 to <23	39.5 to <50.5	Not recommended[2]	Not recommended[2]	12	3
≥23	≥50.5	Not recommended[2]	Not recommended[2]	15	3¾

[1] If a teaspoon is used to measure VIRACEPT oral powder, 1 level teaspoon contains 200 mg of VIRACEPT (4 level scoops equals 1 level teaspoon)
[2] Use VIRACEPT 250 mg tablet

powder or 250 mg tablets is 45 to 55 mg/kg twice daily or 25 to 35 mg/kg three times daily. All doses should be taken **with a meal**. Doses higher than the adult maximum dose of 2500 mg per day have not been studied in children. For children unable to take tablets, VIRACEPT Oral Powder may be administered. The oral powder may be mixed with a small amount of water, milk, formula, soy formula, soy milk or dietary supplements; once mixed, the entire contents must be consumed in order to obtain the full dose. If the mixture is not consumed immediately, it must be stored under refrigeration, but storage must not exceed 6 hours. Acidic food or juice (e.g., orange juice, apple juice or apple sauce) are not recommended to be used in combination with VIRACEPT, because the combination may result in a bitter taste. VIRACEPT Oral Powder should not be reconstituted with water in its original container.

The healthcare provider should assess appropriate formulation and dosage for each patient. Crushed 250 mg tablets can be used in lieu of powder. Tables 13 and 14 provide dosing guidelines for VIRACEPT tablets and powder based on age and body weight.

Table 13
Dosing Table for Children ≥ 2 years of age (tablets)

Body Weight		Twice Daily (BID) 45-55 mg/kg ≥ 2 years	Three Times Daily (TID) 25-35 mg/kg ≥ 2 years
Kg.	Lbs.	# of tablets (250 mg)	# of tablets (250 mg)
10–12	22–26.4	2	1
13–18	28.6–39.6	3	2
19–20	41.8–44	4	2
≥21	≥46.2	4-5[1]	3[2]

[1] For BID dosing, the maximum dose per day is 5 tablets BID
[2] For TID dosing, the maximum dose per day is 3 tablets TID

[See table 14 above]

HOW SUPPLIED

VIRACEPT (nelfinavir mesylate) 250 mg: Light blue, capsule-shaped tablets with a clear film coating engraved with "VIRACEPT" on one side and "250 mg" on the other.

Bottles of 300, 250 mg tablets .... NDC 63010-010-30

VIRACEPT (nelfinavir mesylate) 625 mg: White oval tablet with a clear film coating engraved with "V" on one side and "625" on the other.

Bottles of 120, 625 mg tablets .... NDC 63010-027-70

VIRACEPT (nelfinavir mesylate) Oral Powder is available as a 50 mg/g off-white powder containing 50 mg (as nelfinavir free base) in each level scoopful (1 gram).

Multiple use bottles of 144 grams of powder with scoop .... NDC 63010-011-90

VIRACEPT TABLETS AND ORAL POWDER SHOULD BE STORED AT 15° TO 30°C (59° TO 86°F).

Keep container tightly closed. Dispense in original container.

℞ only

VIRACEPT and Agouron are registered trademarks of Agouron Pharmaceuticals, Inc.

LAB-0174-10 Revised May 2004

Shown in Product Identification Guide, page 330

ZITHROMAX® ℞

[*zĭth-rō-măks*]
(azithromycin tablets)
and
(azithromycin for oral suspension)

To reduce the development of drug-resistant bacteria and maintain the effectiveness of ZITHROMAX® (azithromycin) and other bacterial drugs, ZITHROMAX (azithromycin) should be used only to treat or prevent infections that are proven or strongly suspected to be caused by bacteria.

DESCRIPTION

ZITHROMAX (azithromycin tablets and azithromycin for oral suspension) contain the active ingredient azithromycin, an azalide, a subclass of macrolide antibiotics, for oral administration. Azithromycin has the chemical name (*2R,3S,4R,5R,8R, 10R,11R,12S,13S,14R*)- 13-[(2,6-dideoxy-3-*C*-methyl-3-*O*-methyl-α-*L*-*ribo*-hexopyranosyl)oxy]-2-ethyl-3,4,10-trihydroxy-3,5,6,8,10,12,14-heptamethyl-11-[[3,4,6-trideoxy-3-(dimethylamino)-β-*D*-*xylo*-hexopyranosyl]oxy]-1-oxa-6-azacyclopentadecan-15-one. Azithromycin is derived from erythromycin; however, it differs chemically from erythromycin in that a methyl-substituted nitrogen atom is incorporated into the lactone ring. Its molecular formula is $C_{38}H_{72}N_2O_{12}$, and its molecular weight is 749.00. Azithromycin has the following structural formula:

Azithromycin, as the dihydrate, is a white crystalline powder with a molecular formula of $C_{38}H_{72}N_2O_{12}•2H_2O$ and a molecular weight of 785.0.

ZITHROMAX is supplied for oral administration as film-coated, modified capsular shaped tablets containing azithromycin dihydrate equivalent to either 250 mg or 500 mg azithromycin and the following inactive ingredients: dibasic calcium phosphate anhydrous, pregelatinized starch, sodium croscarmellose, magnesium stearate, sodium lauryl sulfate, hypromellose, lactose, titanium dioxide, triacetin and D&C Red #30 aluminum lake.

ZITHROMAX for oral suspension is supplied in bottles containing azithromycin dihydrate powder equivalent to 300 mg, 600 mg, 900 mg, or 1200 mg azithromycin per bottle and the following inactive ingredients: sucrose; sodium phosphate, tribasic, anhydrous; hydroxypropyl cellulose; xanthan gum; FD&C Red #40; and spray dried artificial cherry, creme de vanilla and banana flavors. After constitution, each 5 mL of suspension contains 100 mg or 200 mg of azithromycin.

CLINICAL PHARMACOLOGY

Pharmacokinetics

Following oral administration of a single 500 mg dose (two 250 mg tablets) to 36 fasted healthy male volunteers, the mean (SD) pharmacokinetic parameters were AUC_{0-72} = 4.3 (1.2) µg•h/mL; C_{max} = 0.5 (0.2) µg/mL; T_{max} = 2.2 (0.9) hours.

With a regimen of 500 mg (two 250 mg capsules*) on day 1, followed by 250 mg daily (one 250 mg capsule) on days 2 through 5, the pharmacokinetic parameters of azithromycin in plasma in healthy young adults (18-40 years of age) are portrayed in the chart below. C_{min} and C_{max} remained essentially unchanged from day 2 through day 5 of therapy.

Pharmacokinetic Parameters (Mean)	Total n=12 Day 1	Day 5
C_{max} (µg/mL)	0.41	0.24
T_{max} (h)	2.5	3.2
AUC_{0-24} (µg•h/mL)	2.6	2.1
C_{min} (µg/mL)	0.05	0.05
Urinary Excret. (% dose)	4.5	6.5

*Azithromycin 250 mg tablets are bioequivalent to 250 mg capsules in the fasted state. Azithromycin 250 mg capsules are no longer commercially available.

In a two-way crossover study, 12 adult healthy volunteers (6 males, 6 females) received 1,500 mg of azithromycin administered in single daily doses over either 5 days (two 250 mg tablets on day 1, followed by one 250 mg tablet on days 2-5) or 3 days (500 mg per day for days 1-3). Due to limited serum samples on day 2 (3-day regimen) and days 2-4 (5-day regimen), the serum concentration-time profile of each subject was fit to a 3-compartment model and the $AUC_{0-\infty}$ for the fitted concentration profile was comparable between the 5-day and 3-day regimens.

[See first table at top of next page]

Median azithromycin exposure (AUC_{0-288}) in mononuclear (MN) and polymorphonuclear (PMN) leukocytes following either the 5-day or 3-day regimen was more than a 1000-fold and 800-fold greater than in serum, respectively. Administration of the same total dose with either the 5-day or 3-day regimen may be expected to provide comparable concentrations of azithromycin within MN and PMN leukocytes.

Two azithromycin 250 mg tablets are bioequivalent to a single 500 mg tablet.

Absorption

The absolute bioavailability of azithromycin 250 mg capsules is 38%.

In a two-way crossover study in which 12 healthy subjects received a single 500 mg dose of azithromycin (two 250 mg tablets) with or without a high fat meal, food was shown to increase C_{max} by 23% but had no effect on AUC.

When azithromycin suspension was administered with food to 28 adult healthy male subjects, C_{max} increased by 56% and AUC was unchanged.

The AUC of azithromycin was unaffected by co-administration of an antacid containing aluminum and magnesium hydroxide with azithromycin capsules; however, the C_{max} was reduced by 24%. Administration of cimetidine (800 mg) two hours prior to azithromycin had no effect on azithromycin absorption.

Continued on next page

Zithromax Tabs/O.S.—Cont.

Distribution

The serum protein binding of azithromycin is variable in the concentration range approximating human exposure, decreasing from 51% at 0.02 μg/mL to 7% at 2 μg/mL.

Following oral administration, azithromycin is widely distributed throughout the body with an apparent steady-state volume of distribution of 31.1 L/kg. Greater azithromycin concentrations in tissues than in plasma or serum were observed. High tissue concentrations should not be interpreted to be quantitatively related to clinical efficacy. The antimicrobial activity of azithromycin is pH related and appears to be reduced with decreasing pH. However, the extensive distribution of drug to tissues may be relevant to clinical activity.

Selected tissue (or fluid) concentration and tissue (or fluid) to plasma/serum concentration ratios are shown in the following table:

[See second table at right]

The extensive tissue distribution was confirmed by examination of additional tissues and fluids (bone, ejaculum, prostate, ovary, uterus, salpinx, stomach, liver, and gallbladder). As there are no data from adequate and well-controlled studies of azithromycin treatment of infections in these additional body sites, the clinical importance of these tissue concentration data is unknown.

Following a regimen of 500 mg on the first day and 250 mg daily for 4 days, only very low concentrations were noted in cerebrospinal fluid (less than 0.01 μg/mL) in the presence of non-inflamed meninges.

Metabolism

In vitro and *in vivo* studies to assess the metabolism of azithromycin have not been performed.

Elimination

Plasma concentrations of azithromycin following single 500 mg oral and i.v. doses declined in a polyphasic pattern with a mean apparent plasma clearance of 630 mL/min and terminal elimination half-life of 68 hours. The prolonged terminal half-life is thought to be due to extensive uptake and subsequent release of drug from tissues.

Biliary excretion of azithromycin, predominantly as unchanged drug, is a major route of elimination. Over the course of a week, approximately 6% of the administered dose appears as unchanged drug in urine.

Special Populations

Renal Insufficiency

Azithromycin pharmacokinetics were investigated in 42 adults (21 to 85 years of age) with varying degrees of renal impairment. Following the oral administration of a single 1,000 mg dose of azithromycin, mean C_{max} and AUC_{0-120} increased by 5.1% and 4.2%, respectively in subjects with mild to moderate renal impairment (GFR 10 to 80 mL/min) compared to subjects with normal renal function (GFR >80 mL/min). The mean C_{max} and AUC_{0-120} increased 61% and 35%, respectively in subjects with severe renal impairment (GFR <10 mL/min) compared to subjects with normal renal function (GFR >80 mL/min). (See **DOSAGE AND ADMINISTRATION**.)

Hepatic Insufficiency

The pharmacokinetics of azithromycin in subjects with hepatic impairment have not been established.

Gender

There are no significant differences in the disposition of azithromycin between male and female subjects. No dosage adjustment is recommended based on gender.

Geriatric Patients

When studied in healthy elderly subjects aged 65 to 85 years, the pharmacokinetic parameters of azithromycin in elderly men were similar to those in young adults; however, in elderly women, although higher peak concentrations (increased by 30 to 50%) were observed, no significant accumulation occurred.

Pediatric Patients

In two clinical studies, azithromycin for oral suspension was dosed at 10 mg/kg on day 1, followed by 5 mg/kg on days 2 through 5 to two groups of pediatric patients (aged 1-5 years and 5-15 years, respectively). The mean pharmacokinetic parameters on day 5 were C_{max}=0.216 μg/mL, T_{max}=1.9 hours, and AUC_{0-24}=1.822 μg•hr/mL for the 1- to 5-year-old group and were C_{max}=0.383 μg/mL, T_{max}=2.4 hours, and AUC_{0-24}=3.109 μg•hr/mL for the 5- to 15-year-old group.

Two clinical studies were conducted in 68 pediatric patients aged 3-16 years to determine the pharmacokinetics and safety of azithromycin for oral suspension. Azithromycin was administered following a low-fat breakfast.

The first study consisted of 35 pediatric patients treated with 20 mg/kg/day (maximum daily dose 500 mg) for 3 days of whom 34 patients were evaluated for pharmacokinetics.

In the second study, 33 pediatric patients received doses of 12 mg/kg/day (maximum daily dose 500 mg) for 5 days of whom 31 patients were evaluated for pharmacokinetics.

In both studies, azithromycin concentrations were determined over a 24 hour period following the last daily dose. Patients weighing above 25.0 kg in the 3-day study or 41.7 kg in the 5-day study received the maximum adult daily dose of 500 mg. Eleven patients (weighing 25.0 kg or less) in the first study and 17 patients (weighing 41.7 kg or less) in the second study received a total dose of 60 mg/kg. The following table shows pharmacokinetic data in the subset of pediatric patients who received a total dose of 60 mg/kg.

Pharmackoinetic Parameter [mean (SD)]	3-Day Regimen		5-Day Regimen	
	Day 1	Day 3	Day 1	Day 5
C_{max} (serum, μg/mL)	0.44 (0.22)	0.54 (0.25)	0.43 (0.20)	0.24 (0.06)
Serum $AUC_{0-\infty}$ (μg•hr/mL)	17.4 (6.2)*		14.9 (3.1)*	
Serum $T_{½}$	71.8 hr		68.9 hr	

*Total AUC for the entire 3-day and 5-day regimens

AZITHROMYCIN CONCENTRATIONS FOLLOWING A 500 mg DOSE (TWO 250 mg CAPSULES) IN ADULTS[1]

TISSUE OR FLUID	TIME AFTER DOSE (h)	TISSUE OR FLUID CONCENTRATION (μg/g or μg/mL)	CORRESPONSING PLASMA OR SERUM LEVEL (μg/mL)	TISSUE (FLUID) PLASMA (SERUM) RATIO
SKIN	72-96	0.4	0.012	35
LUNG	72-96	4.0	0.012	>100
SPUTUM*	2-4	1.0	0.64	2
SPUTUM**	10-12	2.9	0.1	30
TONSIL***	9-18	4.5	0.03	>100
TONSIL***	180	0.9	0.006	>100
CERVIX****	19	2.8	0.04	70

[1] Azithromycin tissue concentrations were originally determined using 250 mg capsules.
* Sample was obtained 2–4 hours after the first dose.
** Sample was obtained 10–12 hours after the first dose.
*** Dosing regimen of two doses of 250 mg each, separated by 12 hours.
**** Sample was obtained 19 hours after a single 500 mg dose.

Pharmacokinetic Parameter [mean (SD)]	3-Day Regimen (20 mg/kg × 3 days)	5-Day Regimen (12 mg/kg × 5 days)
n	11	17
C_{max} (μg/mL)	1.1 (0.4)	0.5 (0.4)
T_{max} (hr)	2.7 (1.9)	2.2 (0.8)
AUC_{0-24} (μg•hr/mL)	7.9 (2.9)	3.9 (1.9)

The similarity of the overall exposure ($AUC_{0-\infty}$) between the 3-day and 5-day regimens in pediatric patients is unknown. Single dose pharmacokinetics in pediatric patients given doses of 30 mg/kg have not been studied. (See **DOSAGE AND ADMINISTRATION**.)

Drug-Drug Interactions

Drug interaction studies were performed with azithromycin and other drugs likely to be co-administered. The effects of co-administration of azithromycin on the pharmacokinetics of other drugs are shown in Table 1 and the effect of other drugs on the pharmacokinetics of azithromycin are shown in Table 2.

Co-administration of azithromycin at therapeutic doses had a modest effect on the pharmacokinetics of the drugs listed in Table 1. No dosage adjustment of drugs listed in Table 1 is recommended when co-administered with azithromycin.

Co-administration of azithromycin with efavirenz or fluconazole had a modest effect on the pharmacokinetics of azithromycin. Nelfinavir significantly increased the C_{max} and AUC of azithromycin. No dosage adjustment of azithromycin is recommended when administered with drugs listed in Table 2. (See **PRECAUTIONS - Drug Interactions.**)

[See table 1 at bottom of next page]

Mean rifabutin concentrations one-half day after the last dose of rifabutin were 60 ng/mL when co-administered with azithromycin and 71 ng/mL when co-administered with placebo.

[See table 2 at top of page 2668]

Microbiology: Azithromycin acts by binding to the 50S ribosomal subunit of susceptible microorganisms and, thus, interfering with microbial protein synthesis. Nucleic acid synthesis is not affected.

Azithromycin concentrates in phagocytes and fibroblasts as demonstrated by *in vitro* incubation techniques. Using such methodology, the ratio of intracellular to extracellular concentration was >30 after one hour incubation. *In vivo* studies suggest that concentration in phagocytes may contribute to drug distribution to inflamed tissues.

Azithromycin has been shown to be active against most isolates of the following microorganisms, both *in vitro* and in clinical infections as described in the **INDICATIONS AND USAGE** section.

Aerobic and facultative gram-positive microorganisms

Staphylococcus aureus
Streptococcus agalactiae
Streptococcus pneumoniae
Streptococcus pyogenes

NOTE: Azithromycin demonstrates cross-resistance with erythromycin-resistant gram-positive strains. Most strains of *Enterococcus faecalis* and methicillin-resistant staphylococci are resistant to azithromycin.

Aerobic and facultative gram-negative microorganisms

Haemophilus ducreyi
Haemophilus influenzae
Moraxella catarrhalis
Neisseria gonorrhoeae

"Other" microorganisms

Chlamydia pneumoniae
Chlamydia trachomatis
Mycoplasma pneumoniae

Beta-lactamase production should have no effect on azithromycin activity.

The following *in vitro* data are available, **but their clinical significance is unknown.**

At least 90% of the following microorganisms exhibit an *in vitro* minimum inhibitory concentration (MIC) less than or equal to the susceptible breakpoints for azithromycin. However, the safety and effectiveness of azithromycin in treating clinical infections due to these microorganisms have not been established in adequate and well-controlled trials.

Aerobic and facultative gram-positive microorganisms

Streptococci (Groups C, F, G)
Viridans group streptococci

Aerobic and facultative gram-negative microorganisms

Bordetella pertussis
Legionella pneumophila

Anaerobic microorganisms

Peptostreptococcus species
Prevotella bivia

"Other" microorganisms

Ureaplasma urealyticum

Susceptibility Testing Methods:

When available, the results of *in vitro* susceptibility test results for antimicrobial drugs used in resident hospitals should be provided to the physician as periodic reports which describe the susceptibility profile of nosocomial and community-acquired pathogens. These reports may differ from susceptibility data obtained from outpatient use, but could aid the physician in selecting the most effective antimicrobial.

Dilution techniques:

Quantitative methods are used to determine antimicrobial minimum inhibitory concentrations (MICs). These MICs provide estimates of the susceptibility of bacteria to antimicrobial compounds. The MICs should be determined using a standardized procedure. Standardized procedures are based on a dilution method[1,3] (broth or agar) or equivalent with standardized inoculum concentrations and standardized concentrations of azithromycin powder. The MIC values should be interpreted according to criteria provided in Table 1.

Diffusion techniques:

Quantitative methods that require measurement of zone diameters also provide reproducible estimates of the susceptibility of bacteria to antimicrobial compounds. One such standardized procedure[2,3] requires the use of standardized inoculum concentrations. This procedure uses paper disks impregnated with 15-μg azithromycin to test the susceptibility of microorganisms to azithromycin. The disk diffusion interpretive criteria are provided in Table 1.

[See table 1 on page 2668]

No interpretive criteria have been established for testing *Neisseria gonorrhoeae*. This species is not usually tested.

A report of "susceptible" indicates that the pathogen is likely to be inhibited if the antimicrobial compound reaches the concentrations usually achievable. A report of "intermediate" indicates that the result should be considered equivocal, and, if the microorganism is not fully susceptible to alternative, clinically feasible drugs, the test should be repeated. This category implies possible clinical applicability in body sites where the drug is physiologically concentrated or in situations where high dosage of drug can be used. This category also provides a buffer zone which prevents small uncontrolled technical factors from causing major discrepancies in interpretation. A report of "resistant" indicates that the pathogen is not likely to be inhibited if the antimicrobial compound reaches the concentrations usually achievable; other therapy should be selected.

QUALITY CONTROL:

Standardized susceptibility test procedures require the use of quality control microorganisms to control the technical aspects of the test procedures. Standard azithromycin powder should provide the following range of values noted in Table 2. Quality control microorganisms are specific strains of organisms with intrinsic biological properties. QC strains are very stable strains which will give a standard and repeatable susceptibility pattern. The specific strains used for microbiological quality control are not clinically significant.

[See table 2 at top of next page]

INDICATIONS AND USAGE

ZITHROMAX (azithromycin) is indicated for the treatment of patients with mild to moderate infections (pneumonia: see **WARNINGS**) caused by susceptible strains of the designated microorganisms in the specific conditions listed below. As recommended dosages, durations of therapy and applicable patient populations vary among these infections, please see **DOSAGE AND ADMINISTRATION** for specific dosing recommendations.

Adults:

Acute bacterial exacerbations of chronic obstructive pulmonary disease due to *Haemophilus influenzae, Moraxella catarrhalis* or *Streptococcus pneumoniae.*

Acute bacterial sinusitis due to *Haemophilus influenzae, Moraxella catarrhalis* or *Streptococcus pneumoniae.*

Community-**acquired pneumonia** due to *Chlamydia pneumoniae, Haemophilus influenzae, Mycoplasma pneumoniae* or *Streptococcus pneumoniae* in patients appropriate for oral therapy.

NOTE: Azithromycin should not be used in patients with pneumonia who are judged to be inappropriate for oral therapy because of moderate to severe illness or risk factors such as any of the following:

patients with cystic fibrosis,

patients with nosocomially acquired infections,

patients with known or suspected bacteremia,

patients requiring hospitalization,

elderly or debilitated patients, or

patients with significant underlying health problems that may compromise their ability to respond to their illness (including immunodeficiency or functional asplenia).

Pharyngitis/tonsillitis caused by *Streptococcus pyogenes* as an alternative to first-line therapy in individuals who cannot use first-line therapy.

NOTE: Penicillin by the intramuscular route is the usual drug of choice in the treatment of *Streptococcus*

Table 1. Drug Interactions: Pharmacokinetic Parameters for Co-administered Drugs in the Presence of Azithromycin

Co-administered Drug	Dose of Co-administered Drug	Dose of Azithromycin	n	Ratio (with/without azithromycin) of Co-administered Drug Pharmacokinetic Parameters (90% CI); No Effect = 1.00	
				Mean C_{max}	Mean AUC
Atrovastatin	10 mg/day × 8 days	500 mg/day PO on days 6-8	12	0.83 (0.63 to 1.08)	1.01 (0.81 to 1.25)
Carbamazepine	200 mg/day × 2 days, then 200 mg BID × 18 days	500 mg/day PO for days 16-18	7	0.97 (0.88 to 1.06)	0.96 (0.88 to 1.06)
Cetirizine	20 mg/day × 11 days	500 mg PO on day 7, then 250 mg day on days 8-11	14	1.03 (0.93 to 1.14)	1.02 (0.92 to 1.13)
Didanosine	200 mg PO BID × 21 days	1,200 mg/day PO on days 8-21	6	1.44 (0.85 to 2.43)	1.14 (0.83 to 1.57)
Efavirenz	400 mg/day × 7 days	600 mg PO on day 7	14	1.04*	0.95*
Fluconazole	200 mg PO single dose	1,200 mg PO single dose	18	1.04 (0.98 to 1.11)	1.01 (0.97 to 1.05)
Indinavir	800 mg TID × 5 days	1,200 mg PO on day 5	18	0.96 (0.86 to 1.08)	0.90 (0.81 to 1.00)
Midazolam	15 mg PO on day 3	500 mg/day PO × 3 days	12	1.27 (0.89 to 1.81)	1.26 (1.01 to 1.56)
Nelfinavir	750 mg TID × 11 days	1,200 mg PO on day 9	14	0.90 (0.81 to 1.01)	0.85 (0.78 to 0.93)
Rifabutin	300 mg/day × 10 days	500 mg PO on day 1, then 250 mg/day on days 2-10	6	See footnote below	NA
Sildenafil	100 mg on days 1 and 4	500 mg/day PO × 3 days	12	1.16 (0.86 to 1.57)	0.92 (0.75 to 1.12)
Theophylline	4 mg/kg IV on days 1, 11, 25	500 mg PO on day 7, 250 mg/ day on days 8-11	10	1.19 (1.02 to 1.40)	1.02 (0.86 to 1.22)
Theophylline	300 mg PO BID × 15 days	500 mg PO on day 6, then 250 mg/day on days 7-10	8	1.09 (0.92 to 1.29)	1.08 (0.89 to 1.31)
Triazolam	0.125 mg on day 2	500 mg PO on day 1, then 250 mg/day on day 2	12	1.06*	1.02*
Trimethoprim/Sulfamethoxazole	160 mg/800 mg/day PO × 7 days	1,200 mg PO on day 7	12	0.85 (0.75 to 0.97)/ 0.90 (0.78 to 1.03)	0.87 (0.80 to 0.95)/ 0.96 (0.88 to 1.03)
Zidovudine	500 mg/day PO × 21 days	600 mg/day PO × 14 days	5	1.12 (0.42 to 3.02)	0.94 (0.52 to 1.70)
Zidovudine	500 mg/day PO × 21 days	1,200 mg/day PO × 14 days	4	1.31 (0.43 to 3.97)	1.30 (0.69 to 2.43)

NA - Not Available
* - 90% Confidence interval not reported

pyogenes infection and the prophylaxis of rheumatic fever. ZITHROMAX is often effective in the eradication of susceptible strains of *Streptococcus pyogenes* from the nasopharynx. Because some strains are resistant to ZITHROMAX, susceptibility tests should be performed when patients are treated with ZITHROMAX. Data establishing efficacy of azithromycin in subsequent prevention of rheumatic fever are not available.

Uncomplicated skin and skin structure infections due to *Staphylococcus aureus, Streptococcus pyogenes,* or *Streptococcus agalactiae.* Abscesses usually require surgical drainage.

Urethritis and cervicitis due to *Chlamydia trachomatis* or *Neisseria gonorrhoeae.*

Genital ulcer disease in men due to *Haemophilus ducreyi* (chancroid). Due to the small number of women included in clinical trials, the efficacy of azithromycin in the treatment of chancroid in women has not been established.

ZITHROMAX, at the recommended dose, should not be relied upon to treat syphilis. Antimicrobial agents used in high doses for short periods of time to treat non-gonococcal urethritis may mask or delay the symptoms of incubating syphilis. All patients with sexually-transmitted urethritis or cervicitis should have a serologic test for syphilis and appropriate cultures for gonorrhea performed at the time of diagnosis. Appropriate antimicrobial therapy and follow-up tests for these diseases should be initiated if infection is confirmed.

Appropriate culture and susceptibility tests should be performed before treatment to determine the causative organism and its susceptibility to azithromycin. Therapy with ZITHROMAX may be initiated before results of these tests are known; once the results become available, antimicrobial therapy should be adjusted accordingly.

To reduce the development of drug-resistant bacteria and maintain the effectiveness of ZITHROMAX (azithromycin) and other antibacterial drugs, ZITHROMAX (azithromycin) should be used only to treat or prevent infections that are proven or strongly suspected to be caused by susceptible bacteria. When culture and susceptibility information are available, they should be considered in selecting or modifying antibacterial therapy. In the absence of such data, local epidemiology and susceptibility patterns may contribute to the empiric selection of therapy.

Pediatric Patients: (See **PRECAUTIONS—Pediatric Use** and **CLINICAL STUDIES IN PEDIATRIC PATIENTS.**)

Acute otitis media caused by *Haemophilus influenzae, Moraxella catarrhalis* or *Streptococcus pneumoniae.* (For specific dosage recommendation, see **DOSAGE AND ADMINISTRATION.**)

Community-acquired pneumonia due to *Chlamydia pneumoniae, Haemophilus influenzae, Mycoplasma pneumoniae* or *Streptococcus pneumoniae* in patients appropriate for oral therapy. (For specific dosage recommendation, see **DOSAGE AND ADMINISTRATION.**)

NOTE: Azithromycin should not be used in pediatric patients with pneumonia who are judged to be inappropriate for oral therapy because of moderate to severe illness or risk factors such as any of the following:

patients with cystic fibrosis,

patients with nosocomially acquired infections,

patients with known or suspected bacteremia,

patients requiring hospitalization, or

patients with significant underlying health problems that may compromise their ability to respond to their illness (including immunodeficiency or functional asplenia).

Pharyngitis/tonsillitis caused by *Streptococcus pyogenes* as an alternative to first-line therapy in individuals who cannot use first-line therapy. (For specific dosage recommendation, see **DOSAGE AND ADMINISTRATION.**)

NOTE: Penicillin by the intramuscular route is the usual drug of choice in the treatment of *Streptococcus pyogenes* infection and the prophylaxis of rheumatic fever. ZITHROMAX is often effective in the eradication of susceptible strains of *Streptococcus pyogenes* from the nasopharynx. Because some strains are resistant to ZITHROMAX, susceptibility tests should be performed when patients are treated with ZITHROMAX. Data establishing efficacy of azithromycin in subsequent prevention of rheumatic fever are not available.

Appropriate culture and susceptibility tests should be performed before treatment to determine the causative organism and its susceptibility to azithromycin. Therapy with ZITHROMAX may be initiated before results of these tests are known; once the results become available, antimicrobial therapy should be adjusted accordingly.

CONTRAINDICATIONS

ZITHROMAX is contraindicated in patients with known hypersensitivity to azithromycin, erythromycin or any macrolide antibiotic.

WARNINGS

Serious allergic reactions, including angioedema, anaphylaxis, and dermatologic reactions including Stevens Johnson Syndrome and toxic epidermal necrolysis have been reported rarely in patients on azithromycin therapy. Although rare, fatalities have been reported. (See **CONTRAINDICATIONS.**) Despite initially successful symptomatic treatment of the allergic symptoms, when symptomatic therapy was discontinued, the allergic symptoms **recurred soon thereafter in some patients without further azithromycin**

Continued on next page

Zithromax Tabs/O.S.—Cont.

exposure. These patients required prolonged periods of observation and symptomatic treatment. The relationship of these episodes to the long tissue half-life of azithromycin and subsequent prolonged exposure to antigen is unknown at present.

If an allergic reaction occurs, the drug should be discontinued and appropriate therapy should be instituted. Physicians should be aware that reappearance of the allergic symptoms may occur when symptomatic therapy is discontinued.

In the treatment of pneumonia, azithromycin has only been shown to be safe and effective in the treatment of community-acquired pneumonia due to *Chlamydia pneumoniae*, *Haemophilus influenzae*, *Mycoplasma pneumoniae* or *Streptococcus pneumoniae* in patients appropriate for oral therapy. Azithromycin should not be used in patients with pneumonia who are judged to be inappropriate for oral therapy because of moderate to severe illness or risk factors such as any of the following: patients with cystic fibrosis, patients with nosocomially acquired infections, patients with known or suspected bacteremia, patients requiring hospitalization, elderly or debilitated patients, or patients with significant underlying health problems that may compromise their ability to respond to their illness (including immunodeficiency or functional asplenia).

Pseudomembranous colitis has been reported with nearly all antibacterial agents and may range in severity from mild to life-threatening. Therefore, it is important to consider this diagnosis in patients who present with diarrhea subsequent to the administration of antibacterial agents.

Treatment with antibacterial agents alters the normal flora of the colon and may permit overgrowth of clostridia. Studies indicate that a toxin produced by *Clostridium difficile* is a primary cause of "antibiotic-associated colitis."

After the diagnosis of pseudomembranous colitis has been established, therapeutic measures should be initiated. Mild cases of pseudomembranous colitis usually respond to discontinuation of the drug alone. In moderate to severe cases, consideration should be given to management with fluids and electrolytes, protein supplementation, and treatment with an antibacterial drug clinically effective against *Clostridium difficile* colitis.

PRECAUTIONS

General: Because azithromycin is principally eliminated via the liver, caution should be exercised when azithromycin is administered to patients with impaired hepatic function. Due to the limited data in subjects with GFR <10 mL/min, caution should be exercised when prescribing azithromycin in these patients. (See **CLINICAL PHARMACOLOGY – Special Populations – Renal Insufficiency.**)

Prolonged cardiac repolarization and QT interval, imparting a risk of developing cardiac arrhythmia and *torsades de pointes*, have been seen in treatment with other macrolides. A similar effect with azithromycin cannot be completely ruled out in patients at increased risk for prolonged cardiac repolarization.

Prescribing ZITHROMAX (azithromycin) in the absence of a proven or strongly suspected bacterial infection or a prophylactic indication is unlikely to provide benefit to the patient and increases the risk of the development of drug-resistant bacteria.

Information for Patients:

ZITHROMAX tablets and oral suspension can be taken with or without food.

Patients should also be cautioned not to take aluminum- and magnesium-containing antacids and azithromycin simultaneously.

The patient should be directed to discontinue azithromycin immediately and contact a physician if any signs of an allergic reaction occur.

Patients should be counseled that antibacterial drugs including ZITHROMAX (azithromycin) should only be used to treat bacterial infections. They do not treat viral infections (e.g., the common cold). When ZITHROMAX (azithromycin) is prescribed to treat a bacterial infection, patients should be told that although it is common to feel better early in the course of the therapy, the medication should be taken exactly as directed. Skipping doses or not completing the full course of therapy may (1) decrease the effectiveness of the immediate treatment and (2) increase the likelihood that bacteria will develop resistance and will not be treatable by ZITHROMAX (azithromycin) or other antibacterial drugs in the future.

Drug Interactions:

Co-administration of nelfinavir at steady-state with a single oral dose of azithromycin resulted in increased azithromycin serum concentrations. Although a dose adjustment of azithromycin is not recommended when administered in combination with nelfinavir, close monitoring for known side effects of azithromycin, such as liver enzyme abnormalities and hearing impairment, is warranted. (See **ADVERSE REACTIONS.**)

Azithromycin did not affect the prothrombin time response to a single dose of warfarin. However, prudent medical practice dictates careful monitoring of prothrombin time in all patients treated with azithromycin and warfarin concomitantly. Concurrent use of macrolides and warfarin in clinical practice has been associated with increased anticoagulant effects.

Table 2. Drug Interactions: Pharmacokinetic Parameters for Azithromycin in the Presence of Co-administered Drugs (See **PRECAUTIONS—Drug Interactions.**)

Co-administered Drug	Dose of Co-administered Drug	Dose of Azithromycin	n	Ratio (with/without co-administered drug) of Azithromycin Pharmacokinetic Parameters (90% CI); No Effect = 1.00	
				Mean C_{max}	Mean AUC
Efavirenz	400 mg/day × 7 days	600 mg PO on day 7	14	1.22 (1.04 to 1.42)	0.92*
Fluconazole	200 mg PO single dose	1,200 mg PO single dose	18	0.82 (0.66 to 1.02)	1.07 (0.94 to 1.22)
Nelfinavir	750 mg TID × 11 days	1,200 mg PO on day 9	14	2.36 (1.77 to 3.15)	2.12 (1.80 to 2.50)
Rifabutin	300 mg/day × 10 days	500 mg PO on day 1, then 250 mg/day on days 2-10	6	See footnote below	NA

NA – Not available

* - 90% Confidence interval not reported

Mean azithromycin concentrations one day after the last dose were 53 ng/mL when coadministered with 300 mg daily rifabutin and 49 ng/mL when coadministered with placebo.

Table 1. Susceptibility Interpretive Criteria for Azithromycin
Susceptibility Test Result Interpretive Criteria

Pathogen	Minimum Inhibitory Concentrations (μg/mL)			Disk Diffusion (zone diameters in mm)		
	S	I	R[a]	S	I	R[a]
Haemophilus spp.	≤ 4	—	—	≥ 12	—	—
Staphylococcus aureus	≤ 2	4	≥ 8	≥ 18	14-17	≤ 13
Streptococci including *S. pneumoniae*[b]	≤ 0.5	1	≥ 2	≥ 18	14-17	≤ 13

[a]The current absence of data on resistant strains precludes defining any category other than "susceptible." If strains yield MIC results other than susceptible, they should be submitted to a reference laboratory for further testing.

[b]Susceptibility of streptococci including *S. pneumoniae* to azithromycin and other macrolides can be predicted by testing erythromycin.

Table 2. Acceptable Quality Control Ranges for Azithromycin

QC Strain	Minimum Inhibitory Concentrations (μg/mL)	Disk Diffusion (zone diameters in mm)
Haemophilus influenzae ATCC 49247	1.0-4.0	13-21
Staphylococcus aureus ATCC 29213	0.5-2.0	
Staphylococcus aureus ATCC 25923		21-26
Streptococcus pneumoniae ATCC 49619	0.06-0.25	19-25

Drug interaction studies were performed with azithromycin and other drugs likely to be co-administered. (See **CLINICAL PHARMACOLOGY—Drug-Drug Interactions.**) When used in therapeutic doses, azithromycin had a modest effect on the pharmacokinetics of atorvastatin, carbamazepine, cetirizine, didanosine, efavirenz, fluconazole, indinavir, midazolam, rifabutin, sildenafil, theophylline (intravenous and oral), triazolam, trimethoprim/sulfamethoxazole or zidovudine. Co-administration with efavirenz, or fluconazole had a modest effect on the pharmacokinetics of azithromycin. No dosage adjustment of either drug is recommended when azithromycin is coadministered with any of the above agents.

Interactions with the drugs listed below have not been reported in clinical trials with azithromycin; however, no specific drug interaction studies have been performed to evaluate potential drug-drug interaction. Nonetheless, they have been observed with macrolide products. Until further data are developed regarding drug interactions when azithromycin and these drugs are used concomitantly, careful monitoring of patients is advised:

Digoxin–elevated digoxin concentrations.

Ergotamine or dihydroergotamine–acute ergot toxicity characterized by severe peripheral vasospasm and dysesthesia.

Terfenadine, cyclosporine, hexobarbital and phenytoin concentrations.

Laboratory Test Interactions: There are no reported laboratory test interactions.

Carcinogenesis, Mutagenesis, Impairment of Fertility: Long-term studies in animals have not been performed to evaluate carcinogenic potential. Azithromycin has shown no mutagenic potential in standard laboratory tests: mouse lymphoma assay, human lymphocyte clastogenic assay, and mouse bone marrow clastogenic assay. No evidence of impaired fertility due to azithromycin was found.

Pregnancy: Teratogenic Effects. Pregnancy Category B: Reproduction studies have been performed in rats and mice at doses up to moderately maternally toxic dose concentrations (i.e., 200 mg/kg/day). These doses, based on a mg/m^2 basis, are estimated to be 4 and 2 times, respectively, the human daily dose of 500 mg. In the animal studies, no evidence of harm to the fetus due to azithromycin was found. There are, however, no adequate and well-controlled studies in pregnant women. Because animal reproduction studies are not always predictive of human response, azithromycin should be used during pregnancy only if clearly needed.

Nursing Mothers: It is not known whether azithromycin is excreted in human milk. Because many drugs are excreted in human milk, caution should be exercised when azithromycin is administered to a nursing woman.

Pediatric Use: (See **CLINICAL PHARMACOLOGY, INDICATIONS AND USAGE,** and **DOSAGE AND ADMINISTRATION.**)

Acute Otitis Media (total dosage regimen: 30 mg/kg, see **DOSAGE AND ADMINISTRATION**): Safety and effectiveness in the treatment of pediatric patients with otitis media under 6 months of age have not been established.

Acute Bacterial Sinusitis (dosage regimen: 10 mg/kg on Days 1-3): Safety and effectiveness in the treatment of pediatric patients with acute bacterial sinusitis under 6 months of age have not been established. Use of Zithromax® for the treatment of acute bacterial sinusitis pediatric patients (6 months of age or greater) is supported by adequate and well-controlled studies in adults, similar pathophysiology of acute sinusitis in adults and pediatric patients, and studies of acute otitis media in pediatric patients.

Community-Acquired Pneumonia (dosage regimen: 10 mg/kg on Day 1 followed by 5 mg/kg on Days 2-5): Safety and effectiveness in the treatment of pediatric patients with community-acquired pneumonia under 6 months of age have not been established. Safety and effectiveness for pneumonia due to *Chlamydia pneumoniae* and *Mycoplasma pneumoniae* were documented in pediatric clinical trials. Safety and effectiveness for pneumonia due to *Haemophilus influenzae* and *Streptococcus pneumoniae* were not documented bacteriologically in the pediatric clinical trial due to difficulty in obtaining specimens. Use of azithromycin for these two microorganisms is supported, however, by evidence from adequate and well-controlled studies in adults.

Pharyngitis/Tonsillitis (dosage regimen: 12 mg/kg on Days 1-5): Safety and effectiveness in the treatment of pediatric patients with pharyngitis/tonsillitis under 2 years of age have not been established.

Studies evaluating the use of repeated courses of therapy have not been conducted. (See **CLINICAL PHARMACOLOGY and ANIMAL TOXICOLOGY.**)

Geriatric Use: Pharmacokinetic parameters in older volunteers (65–85 years old) were similar to those in younger volunteers (18–40 years old) for the 5-day therapeutic regimen. Dosage adjustment does not appear to be necessary for older patients with normal renal and hepatic function receiving treatment with this dosage regimen. (See **CLINICAL PHARMACOLOGY**.)

In multiple-dose clinical trials of oral azithromycin, 9% of patients were at least 65 years of age (458/4949) and 3% of patients (144/4949) were at least 75 years of age. No overall differences in safety or effectiveness were observed between these subjects and younger subjects, and other reported clinical experience has not identified differences in response between the elderly and younger patients, but greater sensitivity of some older individuals cannot be ruled out.

ZITHROMAX 250 mg tablets contain 0.9 mg of sodium per tablet.

ZITHROMAX 500 mg tablets contain 1.8 mg of sodium per tablet.

ZITHROMAX for oral suspension 100 mg/5 mL contains 3.7 mg of sodium per 5 mL of constituted solution.

ZITHROMAX for oral suspension 200 mg/5 mL contains 7.4 mg of sodium per 5 mL of constituted solution.

ADVERSE REACTIONS

In clinical trials, most of the reported side effects were mild to moderate in severity and were reversible upon discontinuation of the drug. Potentially serious side effects of angioedema and cholestatic jaundice were reported rarely. Approximately 0.7% of the patients (adults and pediatric patients) from the 5-day multiple-dose clinical trials discontinued ZITHROMAX (azithromycin) therapy because of treatment-related side effects. In adults given 500 mg/day for 3 days, the discontinuation rate due to treatment-related side effects was 0.6%. In clinical trials in pediatric patients given 30 mg/kg, either as a single dose or over 3 days, discontinuation from the trials due to treatment-related side effects was approximately 1%. (See **DOSAGE AND ADMINISTRATION**.) Most of the side effects leading to discontinuation were related to the gastrointestinal tract, e.g., nausea, vomiting, diarrhea, or abdominal pain. (See **CLINICAL STUDIES IN PEDIATRIC PATIENTS**.)

Clinical:

Adults:

Multiple-dose regimens: Overall, the most common treatment-related side effects in adult patients receiving multiple-dose regimens of ZITHROMAX were related to the gastrointestinal system with diarrhea/loose stools (4-5%), nausea (3%) and abdominal pain (2-3%) being the most frequently reported.

No other treatment-related side effects occurred in patients on the multiple-dose regimens of ZITHROMAX with a frequency greater than 1%. Side effects that occurred with a frequency of 1% or less included the following:

Cardiovascular: Palpitations, chest pain.

Gastrointestinal: Dyspepsia, flatulence, vomiting, melena and cholestatic jaundice.

Genitourinary: Monilia, vaginitis and nephritis.

Nervous System: Dizziness, headache, vertigo and somnolence.

General: Fatigue.

Allergic: Rash, pruritus, photosensitivity and angioedema.

Single 1-gram dose regimen: Overall, the most common side effects in patients receiving a single-dose regimen of 1 gram of ZITHROMAX were related to the gastrointestinal system and were more frequently reported than in patients receiving the multiple-dose regimen.

Side effects that occurred in patients on the single one-gram dosing regimen of ZITHROMAX with a frequency of 1% or greater included diarrhea/loose stools (7%), nausea (5%), abdominal pain (5%), vomiting (2%), dyspepsia (1%) and vaginitis (1%).

Single 2-gram dose regimen: Overall, the most common side effects in patients receiving a single 2-gram dose of ZITHROMAX were related to the gastrointestinal system. Side effects that occurred in patients in this study with a frequency of 1% or greater included nausea (18%), diarrhea/loose stools (14%), vomiting (7%), abdominal pain (7%), vaginitis (2%), dyspepsia (1%) and dizziness (1%). The majority of these complaints were mild in nature.

Pediatric Patients:

Single and Multiple-dose regimens: The types of side effects in pediatric patients were comparable to those seen in adults, with different incidence rates for the dosage regimens recommended in pediatric patients.

Acute Otitis Media: For the recommended total dosage regimen of 30 mg/kg, the most frequent side effects (≥1%) attributed to treatment were diarrhea, abdominal pain, vomiting, nausea and rash. (See **DOSAGE AND ADMINISTRATION** and **CLINICAL STUDIES IN PEDIATRIC PATIENTS**.)

The incidence, based on dosing regimen, is described in the table below:

[See first table above]

Community-Acquired Pneumonia: For the recommended dosage regimen of 10 mg/kg on Day 1 followed by 5 mg/kg on Days 2-5, the most frequent side effects attributed to treatment were diarrhea/loose stools, abdominal pain, vomiting, nausea and rash.

The incidence is described in the table below:

[See second table above]

Pharyngitis/tonsillitis: For the recommended dosage regimen of 12 mg/kg on Days 1–5, the most frequent side effects attributed to treatment were diarrhea, vomiting, abdominal pain, nausea and headache.

The incidence is described in the table below:

Dosage Regimen	Diarrhea, %	Abdominal Pain, %	Vomiting, %	Nausea, %	Rash, %
1-day	4.3%	1.4%	4.9%	1.0%	1.0%
3-day	2.6%	1.7%	2.3%	0.4%	0.6%
5-day	1.8%	1.2%	1.1%	0.5%	0.4%

Dosage Regimen	Diarrhea/Loose stools, %	Abdominal Pain, %	Vomiting, %	Nausea, %	Rash, %
5-day	5.8%	1.9%	1.9%	1.9%	1.6%

Dosage Regimen	Diarrhea, %	Abdominal Pain, %	Vomiting, %	Nausea, %	Rash, %	Headache, %
5-day	5.4%	3.4%	5.6%	1.8%	0.7%	1.1%

Infection*	Recommended Dose/Duration of Therapy
Community-acquired pneumonia (mild severity) Pharyngitis/tonsillitis (second line therapy) Skin/skin structure (uncomplicated)	500 mg as a single dose on Day 1, followed by 250 mg once daily on Days 2 through 5.
Acute bacterial exacerbations of chronic obstructive pulmonary disease (mild to moderate)	500 mg QD × 3 days OR 500 mg as a single dose on Day 1, followed by 250 mg once daily on Days 2 through 5.
Acute bacterial sinusitis	500 mg QD × 3 days
Genital ulcer disease (chancroid)	One single 1 gram dose
Non-gonococcal urethritis and cervicitis	One single 1 gram dose
Gonococcal urethritis and cervicitis	One single 2 gram dose

*DUE TO THE INDICATED ORGANISMS (See **INDICATIONS AND USAGE.**)

[See third table above]

With any of the treatment regimens, no other treatment-related side effects occurred in pediatric patients treated with ZITHROMAX with a frequency greater than 1%. Side effects that occurred with a frequency of 1% or less included the following:

Cardiovascular: Chest pain.

Gastrointestinal: Dyspepsia, constipation, anorexia, enteritis, flatulence, gastritis, jaundice, loose stools and oral moniliasis.

Hematologic and Lymphatic: Anemia and leukopenia.

Nervous System: Headache (otitis media dosage), hyperkinesia, dizziness, agitation, nervousness and insomnia.

General: Fever, face edema, fatigue, fungal infection, malaise and pain.

Allergic: Rash and allergic reaction.

Respiratory: Cough increased, pharyngitis, pleural effusion and rhinitis.

Skin and Appendages: Eczema, fungal dermatitis, pruritus, sweating, urticaria and vesiculobullous rash.

Special Senses: Conjunctivitis.

Post-Marketing Experience:

Adverse events reported with azithromycin during the post-marketing period in adult and/or pediatric patients for which a causal relationship may not be established include:

Allergic: Arthralgia, edema, urticaria and angioedema.

Cardiovascular: Arrhythmias including ventricular tachycardia and hypotension. There have been rare reports of QT prolongation and *torsades de pointes*.

Gastrointestinal: Anorexia, constipation, dyspepsia, flatulence, vomiting/diarrhea rarely resulting in dehydration, pseudomembranous colitis, pancreatitis, oral candidiasis and rare reports of tongue discoloration.

General: Asthenia, paresthesia, fatigue, malaise and anaphylaxis (rarely fatal).

Genitourinary: Interstitial nephritis and acute renal failure and vaginitis.

Hematopoietic: Thrombocytopenia.

Liver/Biliary: Abnormal liver function including hepatitis and cholestatic jaundice, as well as rare cases of hepatic necrosis and hepatic failure, some of which have resulted in death.

Nervous System: Convulsions, dizziness/vertigo, headache, somnolence, hyperactivity, nervousness, agitation and syncope.

Psychiatric: Aggressive reaction and anxiety.

Skin/Appendages: Pruritus, rarely serious skin reactions including erythema multiforme, Stevens Johnson Syndrome and toxic epidermal necrolysis.

Special Senses: Hearing disturbances including hearing loss, deafness and/or tinnitus and rare reports of taste perversion.

Laboratory Abnormalities:

Adults:

Clinically significant abnormalities (irrespective of drug relationship) occurring during the clinical trials were reported as follows: with an incidence of greater than 1%: decreased hemoglobin, hematocrit, lymphocytes, neutrophils and blood glucose; elevated serum creatine phosphokinase, potassium, ALT, GGT, AST, BUN, creatinine, blood glucose, platelet count, lymphocytes, neutrophils and eosinophils; with an incidence of less than 1%: leukopenia, neutropenia, decreased sodium, potassium, platelet count, elevated monocytes, basophils, bicarbonate, serum alkaline phosphatase, bilirubin, LDH and phosphate. The majority of subjects with elevated serum creatinine also had abnormal values at baseline.

When follow-up was provided, changes in laboratory tests appeared to be reversible.

In multiple-dose clinical trials involving more than 5000 patients, four patients discontinued therapy because of treatment-related liver enzyme abnormalities and one because of a renal function abnormality.

Pediatric Patients:

One, Three and Five Day Regimens

Laboratory data collected from comparative clinical trials employing two 3-day regimens (30 mg/kg or 60 mg/kg in divided doses over 3 days), or two 5-day regimens (30 mg/kg or 60 mg/kg in divided doses over 5 days) were similar for regimens of azithromycin and all comparators combined, with most clinically significant laboratory abnormalities occurring at incidences of 1-5%. Laboratory data for patients receiving 30 mg/kg as a single dose were collected in one single center trial. In that trial, an absolute neutrophil count between 500-1500 cells/mm^3 was observed in 10/64 patients receiving 30 mg/kg as a single dose, 9/62 patients receiving 30 mg/kg given over 3 days, and 8/63 comparator patients. No patient had an absolute neutrophil count <500 cells/mm^3. (See **DOSAGE AND ADMINISTRATION**.)

In multiple-dose clinical trials involving approximately 4700 pediatric patients, no patients discontinued therapy because of treatment-related laboratory abnormalities.

DOSAGE AND ADMINISTRATION

(See **INDICATIONS AND USAGE** and **CLINICAL PHARMACOLOGY.**)

Adults:

[See fourth table above]

ZITHROMAX® tablets can be taken with or without food.

Renal Insufficiency:

No dosage adjustment is recommended for subjects with renal impairment (GFR ≤80 mL/min). The mean AUC_{0-120} was similar in subjects with GFR 10-80 mL/min compared to subjects with normal renal function, whereas it increased 35% in subjects with GFR <10 mL/min compared to subjects with normal renal function. Caution should be exercised when azithromycin is administered to subjects with severe renal impairment. (See **CLINICAL PHARMACOLOGY, Special Populations, Renal Insufficiency**.)

Hepatic Insufficiency:

The pharmacokinetics of azithromycin in subjects with hepatic impairment have not been established. No dose adjustment recommendations can be made in patients with impaired hepatic function (See **CLINICAL PHARMACOLOGY, Special Populations, Hepatic Insufficiency**.)

No dosage adjustment is recommended based on age or gender. (See **CLINICAL PHARMACOLOGY, Special Populations**.)

Pediatric Patients:

ZITHROMAX for oral suspension can be taken with or without food.

Acute Otitis Media: The recommended dose of ZITHROMAX for oral suspension for the treatment of pediatric patients with acute otitis media is 30 mg/kg given as a single dose or 10 mg/kg once daily for 3 days or 10 mg/kg as a single dose on the first day followed by 5 mg/kg/day on Days 2 through 5. (See chart below.)

Acute Bacterial Sinusitis: The recommended dose of ZITHROMAX® for oral suspension for the treatment of pediatric patients with acute bacterial sinusitis is 10 mg/kg once daily for 3 days. (See chart below.)

Continued on next page

Zithromax Tabs/O.S.—Cont.

Community-Acquired Pneumonia: The recommended dose of ZITHROMAX for oral suspension for the treatment of pediatric patients with community-acquired pneumonia is 10 mg/kg as a single dose on the first day followed by 5 mg/kg on Days 2 through 5. (See chart below.)

[See first table at right]

[See second table at right]

[See third table at right]

The safety of re-dosing azithromycin in pediatric patients who vomit after receiving 30 mg/kg as a single dose has not been established. In clinical studies involving 487 patients with acute otitis media given a single 30 mg/kg dose of azithromycin, eight patients who vomited within 30 minutes of dosing were re-dosed at the same total dose.

Pharyngitis/Tonsillitis: The recommended dose of ZITHROMAX for children with pharyngitis/tonsillitis is 12 mg/kg once daily for 5 days. (See chart below.)

[See first table at top of next page]

Constituting instructions for ZITHROMAX Oral Suspension, 300, 600, 900, 1200 mg bottles. The table below indicates the volume of water to be used for constitution:

[See second table at top of next page]

Shake well before each use. Oversized bottle provides shake space. Keep tightly closed.

After mixing, store suspension at 5° to 30°C (41° to 86°F) and use within 10 days. Discard after full dosing is completed.

HOW SUPPLIED

ZITHROMAX 250 mg tablets are supplied as pink modified capsular shaped, engraved, film-coated tablets containing azithromycin dihydrate equivalent to 250 mg of azithromycin. ZITHROMAX 250 mg tablets are engraved with "PFIZER" on one side and "306" on the other. These are packaged in bottles and blister cards of 6 tablets (Z-PAKS®) as follows:

Bottles of 30	NDC 0069-3060-30
Boxes of 3 (Z-PAKS® of 6)	NDC 0069-3060-75
Unit Dose package of 50	NDC 0069-3060-86

ZITHROMAX 500 mg tablets are supplied as pink modified capsular shaped, engraved, film-coated tablets containing azithromycin dihydrate equivalent to 500 mg of azithromycin. ZITHROMAX 500 mg tablets are engraved with "Pfizer" on one side and "ZTM500" on the other. These are packaged in bottles and blister cards of 3 tablets (TRI-PAKS™) as follows:

Bottles of 30	NDC 0069-3070-30
Boxes of 3 (TRI-PAKS™ of 3 tablets)	NDC 0069-3070-75
Unit Dose package of 50	NDC 0069-3070-86

ZITHROMAX tablets should be stored between 15° to 30°C (59° to 86°F).

ZITHROMAX for oral suspension after constitution contains a flavored suspension. ZITHROMAX® for oral suspension is supplied to provide 100 mg/5 mL or 200 mg/5 mL suspension in bottles as follows:

Azithromycin contents per bottle	NDC
300 mg	0069-3110-19
600 mg	0069-3120-19
900 mg	0069-3130-19
1200 mg	0069-3140-19

See **DOSAGE AND ADMINISTRATION** for constitution instructions with each bottle type.

Storage: Store dry powder below 30°C (86°F). Store constituted suspension between 5° to 30°C (41° to 86°F) and discard when full dosing is completed.

CLINICAL STUDIES (See INDICATIONS AND USAGE and Pediatric Use.)

Pediatric Patients

From the perspective of evaluating pediatric clinical trials, Days 11-14 were considered on-therapy evaluations because of the extended half-life of azithromycin. Day 11-14 data are provided for clinical guidance. Day 24-32 evaluations were considered the primary test of cure endpoint.

Acute Otitis Media

Safety and efficacy using azithromycin 30 mg/kg given over 5 days

Protocol 1

In a double-blind, controlled clinical study of acute otitis media performed in the United States, azithromycin (10 mg/kg on Day 1 followed by 5 mg/kg on Days 2-5) was compared to amoxicillin/clavulanate potassium (4:1). For the 553 patients who were evaluated for clinical efficacy, the clinical success rate (i.e., cure plus improvement) at the Day 11 visit was 88% for azithromycin and 88% for the control agent. For the 521 patients who were evaluated at the Day 30 visit, the clinical success rate was 73% for azithromycin and 71% for the control agent.

In the safety analysis of the above study, the incidence of treatment-related adverse events, primarily gastrointestinal, in all patients treated was 9% with azithromycin and 31% with the control agent. The most common side effects were diarrhea/loose stools (4% azithromycin vs. 20% control), vomiting (2% azithromycin vs. 7% control), and abdominal pain (2% azithromycin vs. 5% control).

PEDIATRIC DOSAGE GUIDELINES FOR OTITIS MEDIA, ACUTE BACTERIAL SINUSITIS AND COMMUNITY-ACQUIRED PNEUMONIA
(Age 6 months and above, see PRECAUTIONS—Pediatric Use.)
Based on Body Weight

OTITIS MEDIA AND COMMUNITY-ACQUIRED PNEUMONIA: (5-Day Regimen)*

Dosing Calculated on 10 mg/kg/day Day 1 and 5 mg/kg/day Days 2 to 5.

Weight		100 mg/5 mL		200 mg/5 mL		Total mL per Treatment Course	Total mg per Treatment Course
Kg	Lbs.	Day 1	Days 2–5	Day 1	Days 2–5		
5	11	2.5 mL (½ tsp)	1.25 mL (¼ tsp)			7.5 mL	150 mg
10	22	5 mL (1 tsp)	2.5 mL (½ tsp)			15 mL	300 mg
20	44			5 mL (1 tsp)	2.5 mL (½ tsp)	15 mL	600 mg
30	66			7.5 mL (1½ tsp)	3.75 mL (¾ tsp)	22.5 mL	900 mg
40	88			10 mL (2 tsp)	5 mL (1 tsp)	30 mL	1200 mg
50 and above	110 and above			12.5 mL (2½ tsp)	6.25 mL (1¼ tsp)	37.5 mL	1500 mg

*Effectiveness of the 3-day or 1-day regimen in pediatric patients with community-acquired pneumonia has not been established.

OTITIS MEDIA AND ACUTE BACTERIAL SINUSITIS: (3-Day Regimen)*

Dosing Calculated on 10 mg/kg/day

Weight		100 mg/5 mL	200 mg/5 mL	Total mL per Treatment Course	Total mg per Treatment Course
Kg	Lbs.	Day 1–3	Day 1–3		
5	11	2.5 mL (½ tsp)		7.5 mL	150 mg
10	22	5 mL (1 tsp)		15 mL	300 mg
20	44		5 mL (1 tsp)	15 mL	600 mg
30	66		7.5 mL (1½ tsp)	22.5 mL	900 mg
40	88		10 mL (2 tsp)	30 mL	1200 mg
50 and above	110 and above		12.5 mL (2½ tsp)	37.5 mL	1500 mg

*Effectiveness of the 5-day or 1-day regimen in pediatric patients with acute bacterial sinusitis has not been established.

OTITIS MEDIA: (1-Day Regimen)

Dosing Calculated on 30 mg/kg as a single dose

Weight		200 mg/5 mL	Total mL per Treatment Course	Total mg per Treatment Course
Kg	Lbs.	Day 1		
5	11	3.75 mL (¾ tsp)	3.75 mL	150 mg
10	22	7.5 mL (1½ tsp)	7.5 mL	300 mg
20	44	15 mL (3 tsp)	15 mL	600 mg
30	66	22.5 mL (4½ tsp)	22.5 mL	900 mg
40	88	30 mL (6 tsp)	30 mL	1200 mg
50 and above	110 and above	37.5 mL (7½ tsp)	37.5 mL	1500 mg

Protocol 2

In a non-comparative clinical and microbiologic trial performed in the United States, where significant rates of beta-lactamase producing organisms (35%) were found, 131 patients were evaluable for clinical efficacy. The combined clinical success rate (i.e., cure and improvement) at the Day 11 visit was 84% for azithromycin. For the 122 patients who were evaluated at the Day 30 visit, the clinical success rate was 70% for azithromycin.

Microbiologic determinations were made at the pre-treatment visit. Microbiology was not reassessed at later visits. The following presumptive bacterial/clinical cure outcomes (i.e., clinical success) were obtained from the evaluable group:

Presumed Bacteriologic Eradication

	Day 11 Azithromycin	Day 30 Azithromycin
S. pneumoniae	61/74 (82%)	40/56 (71%)
H. influenzae	43/54 (80%)	30/47 (64%)
M. catarrhalis	28/35 (80%)	19/26 (73%)
S. pyogenes	11/11 (100%)	7/7
Overall	177/217 (82%)	97/137 (73%)

In the safety analysis of this study, the incidence of treatment-related adverse events, primarily gastrointestinal, in all patients treated was 9%. The most common side effect was diarrhea (4%).

Protocol 3
In another controlled comparative clinical and microbiologic study of otitis media performed in the United States, azithromycin was compared to amoxicillin/clavulanate potassium (4:1). This study utilized two of the same investigators as Protocol 2 (above), and these two investigators enrolled 90% of the patients in Protocol 3. For this reason, Protocol 3 was not considered to be an independent study. Significant rates of beta-lactamase producing organisms (20%) were found. Ninety-two (92) patients were evaluable for clinical and microbiologic efficacy. The combined clinical success rate (i.e., cure and improvement) of those patients with a baseline pathogen at the Day 11 visit was 88% for azithromycin vs. 100% for control; at the Day 30 visit, the clinical success rate was 82% for azithromycin vs. 80% for control.
Microbiologic determinations were made at the pre-treatment visit. Microbiology was not reassessed at later visits. At the Day 11 and Day 30 visits, the following presumptive bacterial/clinical cure outcomes (i.e., clinical success) were obtained from the evaluable group:
[See third table at right]
In the safety analysis of the above study, the incidence of treatment-related adverse events, primarily gastrointestinal, in all patients treated was 4% with azithromycin and 31% with the control agent. The most common side effect was diarrhea/loose stools (2% azithromycin vs. 29% control).

Safety and efficacy using azithromycin 30 mg/kg given over 3 days
Protocol 4
In a double-blind, controlled, randomized clinical study of acute otitis media in pediatric patients from 6 months to 12 years of age, azithromycin (10 mg/kg per day for 3 days) was compared to amoxicillin/clavulanate potassium (7:1) in divided doses q12h for 10 days. Each patient received active drug and placebo matched for the comparator.
For the 366 patients who were evaluated for clinical efficacy at the Day 12 visit, the clinical success rate (i.e., cure plus improvement) was 83% for azithromycin and 88% for the control agent. For the 362 patients who were evaluated at the Day 24–28 visit, the clinical success rate was 74% for azithromycin and 69% for the control agent.
In the safety analysis of the above study, the incidence of treatment-related adverse events, primarily gastrointestinal, in all patients treated was 10.6% with azithromycin and 20.0% with the control agent. The most common side effects were diarrhea/loose stools (5.9% azithromycin vs. 14.6% control), vomiting (2.1% azithromycin vs. 1.1% control), and rash (0.0% azithromycin vs. 4.3% control).

Safety and efficacy using azithromycin 30 mg/kg given as a single dose
Protocol 5
A double blind, controlled, randomized trial was performed at nine clinical centers. Pediatric patients from 6 months to 12 years of age were randomized 1:1 to treatment with either azithromycin (given at 30 mg/kg as a single dose on Day 1) or amoxicillin/clavulanate potassium (7:1), divided q12h for 10 days. Each child received active drug, and placebo matched for the comparator.
Clinical response (Cure, Improvement, Failure) was evaluated at End of Therapy (Day 12–16) and Test of Cure (Day 28–32). Safety was evaluated throughout the trial for all treated subjects. For the 321 subjects who were evaluated at End of Treatment, the clinical success rate (cure plus improvement) was 87% for azithromycin, and 88% for the comparator. For the 305 subjects who were evaluated at Test of Cure, the clinical success rate was 75% for both azithromycin and the comparator.
In the safety analysis, the incidence of treatment-related adverse events, primarily gastrointestinal, was 16.8% with azithromycin, and 22.5% with the comparator. The most common side effects were diarrhea (6.4% with azithromycin vs. 12.7% with the comparator), vomiting (4% with each agent), rash (1.7% with azithromycin vs. 5.2% with the comparator) and nausea (1.7% with azithromycin vs. 1.2% with the comparator).
Protocol 6
In a non-comparative clinical and microbiological trial, 248 patients from 6 months to 12 years of age with documented acute otitis media were dosed with a single oral dose of azithromycin (30 mg/kg on Day 1).
For the 240 patients who were evaluable for clinical modified Intent-to-Treat (MITT) analysis, the clinical success rate (i.e., cure plus improvement) at Day 10 was 89% and for the 242 patients evaluable at Day 24–28, the clinical success rate (cure) was 85%.

Presumed Bacteriologic Eradication

	Day 10	Day 24-28
S. pneumoniae	70/76 (92%)	67/76 (88%)
H. influenzae	30/42 (71%)	28/44 (64%)
M. catarrhalis	10/10 (100%)	10/10 (100%)
Overall	110/128 (86%)	105/130 (81%)

In the safety analysis of this study, the incidence of treatment-related adverse events, primarily gastrointestinal, in all the subjects treated was 12.1%. The most common side effects were vomiting (5.6%), diarrhea (3.2%), and abdominal pain (1.6%).

Pharyngitis/Tonsillitis
In three double-blind controlled studies, conducted in the United States, azithromycin (12 mg/kg once a day for 5 days) was compared to penicillin V (250 mg three times a day for 10 days) in the treatment of pharyngitis due to documented Group A β-hemolytic streptococci (GABHS or *S. pyogenes*). Azithromycin was clinically and microbiologically statistically superior to penicillin at Day 14 and Day 30 with the following clinical success (i.e., cure and improvement) and bacteriologic efficacy rates (for the combined evaluable patient with documented GABHS):
[See fourth table above]
Approximately 1% of azithromycin-susceptible *S. pyogenes* isolates were resistant to azithromycin following therapy.
The incidence of treatment-related adverse events, primarily gastrointestinal, in all patients treated was 18% on azithromycin and 13% on penicillin. The most common side effects were diarrhea/loose stools (6% azithromycin vs. 2% penicillin), vomiting (6% azithromycin vs. 4% penicillin), and abdominal pain (3% azithromycin vs. 1% penicillin).

PEDIATRIC DOSAGE GUIDELINES FOR PHARYNGITIS/TONSILLITIS
(Age 2 years and above, see PRECAUTIONS—Pediatric Use.)
Based on Body Weight

PHARYNGITIS/TONSILLITIS: (5-Day Regimen)

Dosing Calculated on 12 mg/kg/day for 5 days.

Weight		200 mg/5 mL	Total mL per Treatment Course	Total mg per Treatment Course
Kg	Lbs.	Day 1–5		
8	18	2.5 mL (½ tsp)	12.5 mL	500 mg
17	37	5 mL (1 tsp)	25 mL	1000 mg
25	55	7.5 mL (1½ tsp)	37.5 mL	1500 mg
33	73	10 mL (2 tsp)	50 mL	2000 mg
40	88	12.5 mL (2½ tsp)	62.5 mL	2500 mg

Amount of water to be added	Total volume after constitution (azithromycin content)	Azithromycin concentration after constitution
9 mL (300 mg)	15 mL (300 mg)	100 mg/5 mL
9 mL (600 mg)	15 mL (600 mg)	200 mg/5 mL
12 mL (900 mg)	22.5 mL (900 mg)	200 mg/5 mL
15 mL (1200 mg)	30 mL (1200 mg)	200 mg/5 mL

Presumed Bacteriologic Eradication

	Day 11		Day 30	
	Azithromycin	Control	Azithromycin	Control
S. pneumoniae	25/29 (86%)	26/26 (100%)	22/28 (79%)	18/22 (82%)
H. influenzae	9/11 (82%)	9/9	8/10 (80%)	6/8
M. catarrhalis	7/7	5/5	5/5	2/3
S. pyogenes	2/2	5/5	2/2	4/4
Overall	43/49 (88%)	45/45 (100%)	37/45 (82%)	30/37 (81%)

Three U.S. Streptococcal Pharyngitis Studies
Azithromycin vs. Penicillin V
EFFICACY RESULTS

	Day 14	Day 30
Bacteriologic Eradication:		
Azithromycin	323/340 (95%)	255/330 (77%)
Penicillin V	242/332 (73%)	206/325 (63%)
Clinical Success (Cure plus improvement):		
Azithromycin	336/343 (98%)	310/330 (94%)
Penicillin V	284/338 (84%)	241/325 (74%)

Adult Patients
Acute Bacterial Exacerbations of Chronic Obstructive Pulmonary Disease
In a randomized, double-blind controlled clinical trial of acute exacerbation of chronic bronchitis (AECB), azithromycin (500 mg once daily for 3 days) was compared with clarithromycin (500 mg twice daily for 10 days). The primary endpoint of this trial was the clinical cure rate at Day 21–24. For the 304 patients analyzed in the modified intent to treat analysis at the Day 21–24 visit, the clinical cure rate for 3 days of azithromycin was 85% (125/147) compared to 82% (129/157) for 10 days of clarithromycin.
The following outcomes were the clinical cure rates at the Day 21–24 visit for the bacteriologically evaluable patients by pathogen:

Pathogen	Azithromycin (3 Days)	Clarithromycin (10 Days)
S. pneumoniae	29/32 (91%)	21/27 (78%)
H. influenzae	12/14 (86%)	14/16 (88%)
M. catarrhalis	11/12 (92%)	12/15 (80%)

In the safety analysis of this study, the incidence of treatment-related adverse events, primarily gastrointestinal, were comparable between treatment arms (25% with azithromycin and 29% with clarithromycin). The most common side effects were diarrhea, nausea and abdominal pain with comparable incidence rates for each symptom of 5-9% between the two treatment arms. (See **ADVERSE REACTIONS**.)

Acute Bacterial Sinusitis
In a randomized, double blind, double-dummy controlled clinical trial of acute bacterial sinusitis, azithromycin (500 mg once daily for 3 days) was compared with amoxicillin/clavulanate (500/125 mg tid for 10 days). Clinical response assessments were made at Day 10 and Day 28. The primary endpoint of this trial was prospectively defined as the clinical cure rate at Day 28. For the 594 patients analyzed in the modified intent to treat analysis at the Day 10 visit, the clinical cure rate for 3 days azithromycin was 88% (268/303) compared to 85% (248/291) for 10 days of amoxicillin/clavulanate. For the 586 patients analyzed in the modified intent to treat analysis at the Day 28 visit, the clinical cure rate for 3 days of azithromycin was 71.5% (213/298) compared to 71.5% (206/288), with a 97.5% confidence interval of –8.4 to 8.3, for 10 days of amoxicillin/clavulanate.
In the safety analysis of this study, the overall incidence of treatment-related adverse events, primarily gastrointestinal, was lower in the azithromycin treatment arm (31%) than in the amoxicillin/clavulanate arm (51%). The most common side effects were diarrhea (17% in the azithromycin arm vs. 32% in the amoxicillin/clavulanate arm), and nausea (7% in the azithromycin arm vs. 12% in the amoxicillin/clavulanate arm). (See **ADVERSE REACTIONS**).
In an open label, noncomparative study requiring baseline transantral sinus punctures the following outcomes were the clinical success rates at the Day 7 and Day 28 visits for the modified intent to treat patients administered 500 mg of azithromycin once daily for 3 days with the following pathogens:

Pathogen	Azithromycin (500 mg per day for 3 Days)	
	Day 7	*Day 28*
S. pneumoniae	23/26 (88%)	21/25 (84%)
H. influenzae	28/32 (87%)	24/32 (75%)
M. catarrhalis	14/15 (93%)	13/15 (87%)

The overall incidence of treatment-related adverse events in the noncomparative study was 21% in modified intent to treat patients treated with azithromycin at 500 mg once daily for 3 days with the most common side effects being diarrhea (9%), abdominal pain (4%) and nausea (3%). (See **ADVERSE REACTIONS**).

ANIMAL TOXICOLOGY
Phospholipidosis (intracellular phospholipid accumulation) has been observed in some tissues of mice, rats, and dogs given multiple doses of azithromycin. It has been demonstrated in numerous organ systems (e.g., eye, dorsal root ganglia, liver, gallbladder, kidney, spleen, and pancreas) in dogs treated with azithromycin at doses which, expressed on the basis of mg/m^2, are approximately equal to the recommended adult human dose, and in rats treated at doses

Continued on next page

Zithromax Tabs/O.S.—Cont.

approximately one-sixth of the recommended adult human dose. This effect has been shown to be reversible after cessation of azithromycin treatment. Phospholipidosis has been observed to a similar extent in the tissues of neonatal rats and dogs given daily doses of azithromycin ranging from 10 days to 30 days. Based on the pharmacokinetic data, phospholipidosis has been seen in the rat (30 mg/kg dose) at observed C_{max} value of 1.3 µg/mL (six times greater than the observed C_{max} of 0.216 µg/mL at the pediatric dose of 10 mg/kg). Similarly, it has been shown in the dog (10 mg/kg dose) at observed C_{max} value of 1.5 µg/mL (seven times greater than the observed same C_{max} and drug dose in the studied pediatric population). On a mg/m^2 basis, 30 mg/kg dose in the neonatal rat (135 mg/m^2) and 10 mg/kg dose in the neonatal dog (79 mg/m^2) are approximately 0.5 and 0.3 times, respectively, the recommended dose in the pediatric patients with an average body weight of 25 kg. Phospholipidosis, similar to that seen in the adult animals, is reversible after cessation of azithromycin treatment. The significance of these findings for animals and for humans is unknown.

REFERENCES:

1. National Committee for Clinical Laboratory Standards, *Methods for Dilution Antimicrobial Susceptibility Tests for Bacteria That Grow Aerobically* – Fifth Edition. Approved Standard NCCLS Document M7-A5, Vol. 20, No. 2 (ISBN 1-56238-394-9). NCCLS, 940 West Valley Road, Suite 1400, Wayne, PA 19087-1898, January 2000.
2. National Committee for Clinical Laboratory Standards, *Performance Standards for Antimicrobial Disk Susceptibility Tests* – Seventh Edition. Approved Standard NCCLS Document M2-A7, Vol. 20, No. 1 (ISBN 1-56238-393-0). NCCLS, 940 West Valley Road, Suite 1400, Wayne, PA 19087-1898, January 2000.
3. National Committee for Clinical Laboratory Standards. *Performance Standards for Antimicrobial Susceptibility Testing* – Eleventh Informational Supplement. NCCLS Document M100-S11, Vol. 21, No. 1 (ISBN 1-56238-426-0). NCCLS, 940 West Valley Road, Suite 1400, Wayne, PA 19087-1898, January 2001.

Rx only

Licensed from Pliva

Distributed by:
Pfizer Labs
Division of Pfizer Inc, NY, NY 10017
70-5179-00-4 Revised January 2004

Shown in Product Identification Guide, page 330

ZITHROMAX® ℞
[*zĭth'rō-măks*]
(azithromycin capsules)
(azithromycin tablets)
and (azithromycin for oral suspension)

To reduce the development of drug-resistant bacteria and maintain the effectiveness of Zithromax® (azithromycin) and other antibacterial drugs, Zithromax (azithromycin) should be used only to treat or prevent infections that are proven or strongly suspected to be caused by bacteria.

DESCRIPTION

ZITHROMAX® (azithromycin capsules, azithromycin tablets and azithromycin for oral suspension) contain the active ingredient azithromycin, an azalide, a subclass of macrolide antibiotics, for oral administration. Azithromycin has the chemical name *(2R,3S,4R,5R,8R,10R,11R,12S,13S,14R)*-13-[(2,6-dideoxy-3-*C*-methyl-3-*O*-methyl-α-*L*-*ribo*-hexopyranosyl)oxy]-2-ethyl-3,4,10-trihydroxy-3,5,6,8,10,12,14-heptamethyl-11-[[3,4,6-trideoxy-3-(dimethylamino)-β-*D*-*xylo*-hexopyranosyl]oxy]-1-oxa-6-azacyclopentadecan-15-one. Azithromycin is derived from erythromycin; however, it differs chemically from erythromycin in that a methyl-substituted nitrogen atom is incorporated into the lactone ring. Its molecular formula is $C_{38}H_{72}N_2O_{12}$, and its molecular weight is 749.0. Azithromycin has the following structural formula:

Azithromycin, as the dihydrate, is a white crystalline powder with a molecular formula of $C_{38}H_{72}N_2O_{12} \cdot 2H_2O$ and a molecular weight of 785.0.

ZITHROMAX® capsules contain azithromycin dihydrate equivalent to 250 mg of azithromycin. The capsules are supplied in red opaque hard-gelatin capsules (containing FD&C Red #40). They also contain the following inactive ingredients: anhydrous lactose, corn starch, magnesium stearate, and sodium lauryl sulfate.

MEAN (CV%) PK PARAMETER

DOSE/DOSAGE FORM (serum, except as indicated)	Subjects	Day No.	C_{max} (µg/mL)	T_{max} (hr)	C_{24} (µg/mL)	ACU (µg•hr/mL)	$T_{½}$ (hr)	Urinary Excretion (% of dose)
500 mg/250 mg capsule	12	Day 1	0.41	2.5	0.05	2.6[a]	—	4.5
and 250 mg on Days 2-5	12	Day 5	0.24	3.2	0.05	2.1[a]	—	6.5
1200 mg/600 mg tablets	12	Day 1	0.66	2.5	0.074	6.8[b]	40	—
%CV			(62%)	(79%)	(49%)	(64%)	(33%)	
600 mg tablet/day	7	1	0.33	2.0	0.039	2.4[a]		
%CV			25%	(50%)	(36%)	(19%)		
	7	22	0.55	2.1	0.14	5.8[a]	84.5	—
%CV			(18%)	(52%)	(26%)	(25%)		—
600 mg tablet/day (leukocytes)	7	22	252	10.9	146	4763[a]	82.8	—
%CV			(49%)	(28%)	(33%)	(42%)	—	—

[a]AUC_{0-24}; [b]0-last.

AZITHROMYCIN CONCENTRATIONS FOLLOWING TWO 250 mg (500 mg) CAPSULES IN ADULTS

TISSUE OR FLUID	TIME AFTER DOSE (h)	TISSUE OR FLUID CONCENTRATION (µg/g or µg/mL)[1]	CORRESPONDING PLASMA OR SERUM LEVEL (µg/mL)	TISSUE (FLUID) PLASMA (SERUM) RATIO[1]
SKIN	72-96	0.4	0.012	35
LUNG	72-96	4.0	0.012	>100
SPUTUM*	2-4	1.0	0.64	2
SPUTUM**	10-12	2.9	0.1	30
TONSIL***	9-18	4.5	0.03	>100
TONSIL***	180	0.9	0.006	>100
CERVIX****	19	2.8	0.04	70

[1] High tissue concentrations should not be interpreted to be quantitatively related to clinical efficacy. The antimicrobial activity of azithromycin is pH related. Azithromycin is concentrated in cell lysosomes which have a low intraorganelle pH, at which the drug's activity is reduced. However, the extensive distribution of drug to tissues may be relevant to clinical activity.
* Sample was obtained 2-4 hours after the first dose
** Sample was obtained 10-12 hours after the first dose.
*** Dosing regimen of 2 doses of 250 mg each, separated by 12 hours.
**** Sample was obtained 19 hours after a single 500 mg dose.

ZITHROMAX® tablets contain azithromycin dihydrate equivalent to 600 mg azithromycin. The tablets are supplied as white, modified oval-shaped, film-coated tablets. They also contain the following inactive ingredients: dibasic calcium phosphate anhydrous, pregelatinized starch, sodium croscarmellose, magnesium stearate, sodium lauryl sulfate and an aqueous film coat consisting of hypromellose, titanium dioxide, lactose and triacetin.

ZITHROMAX® for oral suspension is supplied in a single dose packet containing azithromycin dihydrate equivalent to 1 g azithromycin. It also contains the following inactive ingredients: colloidal silicon dioxide, sodium phosphate tribasic, anhydrous; spray dried artificial banana flavor, spray dried artificial cherry flavor, and sucrose.

CLINICAL PHARMACOLOGY

Pharmacokinetics: Following oral administration, azithromycin is rapidly absorbed and widely distributed throughout the body. Rapid distribution of azithromycin into tissues and high concentration within cells result in significantly higher azithromycin concentrations in tissues than in plasma or serum. The 1 g single dose packet is bioequivalent to four 250 mg capsules.

The pharmacokinetic parameters of azithromycin in plasma after dosing as per labeled recommendations in healthy young adults and asymptomatic HIV-seropositive adults (age 18-40 years old) are portrayed in the following chart:

[See first table above]

In these studies (500 mg Day 1, 250 mg Days 2–5), there was no significant difference in the disposition of azithromycin between male and female subjects. Plasma concentrations of azithromycin following single 500 mg oral and i.v. doses declined in a polyphasic pattern resulting in an average terminal half-life of 68 hours. With a regimen of 500 mg on Day 1 and 250 mg/day on Days 2–5, C_{min} and C_{max} remained essentially unchanged from Day 2 through Day 5 of therapy. However, without a loading dose, azithromycin C_{min} levels required 5 to 7 days to reach steady-state.

In asymptomatic HIV-seropositive adult subjects receiving 600-mg ZITHROMAX® tablets once daily for 22 days, steady state azithromycin serum levels were achieved by Day 15 of dosing.

When azithromycin capsules were administered with food, the rate of absorption (C_{max}) of azithromycin was reduced by 52% and the extent of absorption (AUC) by 43%.

When the oral suspension of azithromycin was administered with food, the C_{max} increased by 46% and the AUC by 14%.

The absolute bioavailability of two 600 mg tablets was 34% (CV=56%). Administration of two 600 mg tablets with food increased C_{max} by 31% (CV=43%) while the extent of absorption (AUC) was unchanged (mean ratio of AUCs=1.00; CV=55%).

The AUC of azithromycin in 250 mg capsules was unaffected by coadministration of an antacid containing aluminum and magnesium hydroxide with ZITHROMAX® (azithromycin); however, the C_{max} was reduced by 24%. Administration of cimetidine (800 mg) two hours prior to azithromycin had no effect on azithromycin absorption.

When studied in healthy elderly subjects from age 65 to 85 years, the pharmacokinetic parameters of azithromycin (500 mg Day 1, 250 mg Days 2-5) in elderly men were similar to those in young adults; however, in elderly women, although higher peak concentrations (increased by 30 to 50%) were observed, no significant accumulation occurred.

The high values in adults for apparent steady-state volume of distribution (31.1 L/kg) and plasma clearance (630 mL/min) suggest that the prolonged half-life is due to extensive uptake and subsequent release of drug from tissues. Selected tissue (or fluid) concentration and tissue (or fluid) to plasma/serum concentration ratios are shown in the following table:

[See second table above]

The extensive tissue distribution was confirmed by examination of additional tissues and fluids (bone, ejaculum, prostate, ovary, uterus, salpinx, stomach, liver, and gallbladder). As there are no data from adequate and well-controlled studies of azithromycin treatment of infections in these additional body sites, the clinical significance of these tissue concentration data is unknown.

Following a regimen of 500 mg on the first day and 250 mg daily for 4 days, only very low concentrations were noted in cerebrospinal fluid (less than 0.01 µg/mL) in the presence of non-inflamed meninges.

Following oral administration of a single 1200 mg dose (two 600 mg tablets), the mean maximum concentration in pe-

ripheral leukocytes was 140 μg/mL. Concentrations remained above 32 μg/mL for approximately 60 hr. The mean half-lives for 6 males and 6 females were 34 hr and 57 hr, respectively. Leukocyte to plasma C_{max} ratios for males and females were 258 (±77%) and 175 (±60%), respectively, and the AUC ratios were 804 (±31%) and 541 (±28%), respectively. The clinical relevance of these findings is unknown.
Following oral administration of multiple daily doses of 600 mg (1 tablet/day) to asymptomatic HIV-seropositive adults, mean maximum concentration in peripheral leukocytes was 252 μg/mL (±49%). Trough concentrations in peripheral leukocytes at steady-state averaged 146 μg/mL (±33%). The mean leukocyte to serum C_{max} ratio was 456 (±38%) and the mean leukocyte to serum AUC ratio was 816 (±31%). The clinical relevance of these findings is unknown.
The serum protein binding of azithromycin is variable in the concentration range approximating human exposure, decreasing from 51% at 0.02 μg/mL to 7% at 2 μg/mL. Biliary excretion of azithromycin, predominantly as unchanged drug, is a major route of elimination. Over the course of a week, approximately 6% of the administered dose appears as unchanged drug in urine.
There are no pharmacokinetic data available from studies in hepatically- or renally-impaired individuals.
The effect of azithromycin on the plasma levels or pharmacokinetics of theophylline administered in multiple doses adequate to reach therapeutic steady-state plasma levels is not known. (See PRECAUTIONS.)
Mechanism of Action: Azithromycin acts by binding to the 50S ribosomal subunit of susceptible microorganisms and, thus, interfering with microbial protein synthesis. Nucleic acid synthesis is not affected.
Azithromycin concentrates in phagocytes and fibroblasts as demonstrated by *in vitro* incubation techniques. Using such methodology, the ratio of intracellular to extracellular concentration was >30 after one hour incubation. *In vivo* studies suggest that concentration in phagocytes may contribute to drug distribution to inflamed tissues.
Microbiology:
Azithromycin has been shown to be active against most strains of the following microorganisms, both *in vitro* and in clinical infections as described in the INDICATIONS AND USAGE section.
Aerobic Gram-Positive Microorganisms
Staphylococcus aureus
Streptococcus agalactiae
Streptococcus pneumoniae
Streptococcus pyogenes
NOTE: Azithromycin demonstrates cross-resistance with erythromycin-resistant gram-positive strains. Most strains of *Enterococcus faecalis* and methicillin-resistant staphylococci are resistant to azithromycin.
Aerobic Gram-Negative Microorganisms
Haemophilus influenzae
Moraxella catarrhalis
"Other" Microorganisms
Chlamydia trachomatis
Beta-lactamase production should have no effect on azithromycin activity.
Azithromycin has been shown to be active *in vitro* and in the prevention and treatment of disease caused by the following microorganisms:
Mycobacteria
Mycobacterium avium complex (MAC) consisting of:
Mycobacterium avium
Mycobacterium intracellulare.
The following *in vitro* data are available, *but their clinical significance is unknown.*
Azithromycin exhibits *in vitro* minimal inhibitory concentrations (MICs) of 2.0 μg/mL or less against most (≥90%) strains of the following microorganisms; however, the safety and effectiveness of azithromycin in treating clinical infections due to these microorganisms have not been established in adequate and well-controlled trials.
Aerobic Gram-Positive Microorganisms
Streptococci (Groups C, F, G)
Viridans group streptococci
Aerobic Gram-Negative Microorganisms
Bordetella pertussis
Campylobacter jejuni
Haemophilus ducreyi
Legionella pneumophila
Anaerobic Microorganisms
Bacteroides bivius
Clostridium perfringens
Peptostreptococcus species
"Other" Microorganisms
Borrelia burgdorferi
Mycoplasma pneumoniae
Treponema pallidum
Ureaplasma urealyticum
Susceptibility Testing of Bacteria Excluding Mycobacteria
The *in vitro* potency of azithromycin is markedly affected by the pH of the microbiological growth medium during incubation. Incubation in a 10% CO_2 atmosphere will result in lowering of media pH (7.2 to 6.6) within 18 hours and in an apparent reduction of the *in vitro* potency of azithromycin. Thus, the initial pH of the growth medium should be 7.2-7.4, and the CO_2 content of the incubation atmosphere should be as low as practical.
Azithromycin can be solubilized for *in vitro* susceptibility testing by dissolving in a minimum amount of 95% ethanol and diluting to working concentration with water.

Dilution Techniques:
Quantitative methods are used to determine minimal inhibitory concentrations that provide reproducible estimates of the susceptibility of bacteria to antimicrobial compounds. One such standardized procedure uses a standardized dilution method[1] (broth, agar or microdilution) or equivalent with azithromycin powder. The MIC values should be interpreted according to the following criteria:

MIC (μg/mL)	Interpretation
≤ 2	Susceptible (S)
4	Intermediate (I)
≥ 8	Resistant (R)

A report of "Susceptible" indicates that the pathogen is likely to respond to monotherapy with azithromycin. A report of "Intermediate" indicates that the result should be considered equivocal, and, if the microorganism is not fully susceptible to alternative, clinically feasible drugs, the test should be repeated. This category also provides a buffer zone which prevents small uncontrolled technical factors from causing major discrepancies in interpretation. A report of "Resistant" indicates that usually achievable drug concentrations are unlikely to be inhibitory and that other therapy should be selected.
Measurement of MIC or MBC and achieved antimicrobial compound concentrations may be appropriate to guide therapy in some infections. (See CLINICAL PHARMACOLOGY section for further information on drug concentrations achieved in infected body sites and other pharmacokinetic properties of this antimicrobial drug product.)
Standardized susceptibility test procedures require the use of laboratory control microorganisms. Standard azithromycin powder should provide the following MIC values:

Microorganism	MIC (μg/mL)
Escherichia coli ATCC 25922	2.0-8.0
Enterococcus faecalis ATCC 29212	1.0-4.0
Staphylococcus aureus ATCC 29213	0.25-1.0

Diffusion Techniques:
Quantitative methods that require measurement of zone diameters also provide reproducible estimates of the susceptibility of bacteria to antimicrobial compounds. One such standardized procedure[2] that has been recommended for use with disks to test the susceptibility of microorganisms to azithromycin uses the 15-μg azithromycin disk. Interpretation involves the correlation of the diameter obtained in the disk test with the minimal inhibitory concentration (MIC) for azithromycin.
Reports from the laboratory providing results of the standard single-disk susceptibility test with a 15 μg azithromycin disk should be interpreted according to the following criteria:

Zone Diameter (mm)	Interpretation
≥ 18	(S) Susceptible
14-17	(I) Intermediate
≤ 13	(R) Resistant

Interpretation should be as stated above for results using dilution techniques.
As with standardized dilution techniques, diffusion methods require the use of laboratory control microorganisms. The 15-μg azithromycin disk should provide the following zone diameters in these laboratory test quality control strains:

Microorganism	Zone Diameter (mm)
Staphylococcus aureus ATCC 25923	21-26

***In Vitro* Activity of Azithromycin Against Mycobacteria.**
Azithromycin has demonstrated *in vitro* activity against *Mycobacterium avium* complex (MAC) organisms. While gene probe techniques may be used to distinguish between *M. avium* and *M. intracellulare*, many studies only reported results on *M. avium* complex (MAC) isolates. Azithromycin has also been shown to be active against phagocytized *M. avium* complex (MAC) organisms in mouse and human macrophage cell cultures as well as in the beige mouse infection model.
Various *in vitro* methodologies employing broth or solid media at different pHs, with and without oleic acid-albumin dextrose-catalase (OADC), have been used to determine azithromycin MIC values for *Mycobacterium avium* complex strains. In general, azithromycin MIC values decreased 4 to 8 fold as the pH of Middlebrook 7H11 agar media increased from 6.6 to 7.4. At pH 7.4, azithromycin MIC values determined with Mueller-Hinton agar were 4 fold higher than that observed with Middlebrook 7H12 media at the same pH. Utilization of oleic acid-albumin-dextrose-catalase (OADC) in these assays has been shown to further alter MIC values. The relationship between azithromycin and clarithromycin MIC values has not been established. In general, azithromycin MIC values were observed to be 2 to 32 fold higher than clarithromycin independent of the susceptibility method employed.
The ability to correlate MIC values and plasma drug levels is difficult as azithromycin concentrates in macrophages and tissues. (See CLINICAL PHARMACOLOGY)
Drug Resistance:
Complete cross-resistance between azithromycin and clarithromycin has been observed with *Mycobacterium avium* complex (MAC) isolates. In most isolates, a single point mutation at a position that is homologous to the *Escherichia coli* positions 2058 or 2059 on the 23S rRNA gene is the mechanism producing this cross-resistance pattern.[3,4] *Mycobacterium avium* complex (MAC) isolates exhibiting cross-resistance show an increase in azithromycin MICs to ≥128 μg/mL with clarithromycin MICs increasing to ≥32 μg/mL. These MIC values were determined employing the radiometric broth dilution susceptibility testing method with Middlebrook 7H12 medium. The clinical significance of azithromycin and clarithromycin cross-resistance is not fully understood at this time but preclinical data suggest that reduced activity to both agents will occur after *M. avium* complex strains produce the 23S rRNA mutation.
Susceptibility testing for *Mycobacterium avium* complex (MAC):
The disk diffusion techniques and dilution methods for susceptibility testing against Gram-positive and Gram-negative bacteria should not be used for determining azithromycin MIC values against mycobacteria. *In vitro* susceptibility testing methods and diagnostic products currently available for determining minimal inhibitory concentration (MIC) values against *Mycobacterium avium* complex (MAC) organisms have not been standardized or validated. Azithromycin MIC values will vary depending on the susceptibility testing method employed, composition and pH of media and the utilization of nutritional supplements. Breakpoints to determine whether clinical isolates of *M. avium* or *M. intracellulare* are susceptible or resistant to azithromycin have not been established.
The clinical relevance of azithromycin *in vitro* susceptibility test results for other mycobacterial species, including *Mycobacterium tuberculosis*, using any susceptibility testing method has not been determined.

INDICATIONS AND USAGE
ZITHROMAX® (azithromycin) is indicated for the treatment of patients with mild to moderate infections (pneumonia: see WARNINGS) caused by susceptible strains of the designated microorganisms in the specific conditions listed below.
Lower Respiratory Tract:
Acute bacterial exacerbations of chronic obstructive pulmonary disease due to *Haemophilus influenzae, Moraxella catarrhalis,* or *Streptococcus pneumoniae.*
Community-acquired pneumonia of mild severity due to *Streptococcus pneumoniae* or *Haemophilus influenzae* in patients appropriate for outpatient oral therapy.
NOTE: Azithromycin should not be used in patients with pneumonia who are judged to be inappropriate for outpatient oral therapy because of moderate to severe illness or risk factors such as any of the following:
patients with nosocomially acquired infections,
patients with known or suspected bacteremia,
patients requiring hospitalization,
elderly or debilitated patients, or
patients with significant underlying health problems that may compromise their ability to respond to their illness (including immunodeficiency or functional asplenia).
Upper Respiratory Tract:
Streptococcal pharyngitis/tonsillitis–As an alternative to first line therapy of acute pharyngitis/tonsillitis due to *Streptococcus pyogenes* occurring in individuals who cannot use first line therapy.
NOTE: Penicillin is the usual drug of choice in the treatment of *Streptococcus pyogenes* infection and the prophylaxis of rheumatic fever. ZITHROMAX® is often effective in the eradication of susceptible strains of *Streptococcus pyogenes* from the nasopharynx. Data establishing efficacy of azithromycin in subsequent prevention of rheumatic fever are not available.
Skin and Skin Structure
Uncomplicated skin and skin structure infections due to *Staphylococcus aureus, Streptococcus pyogenes,* or *Streptococcus agalactiae.* Abscesses usually require surgical drainage.
Sexually Transmitted Diseases
Non-gonococcal urethritis and cervicitis due to *Chlamydia trachomatis.*
ZITHROMAX®, at the recommended dose, should not be relied upon to treat gonorrhea or syphilis. Antimicrobial agents used in high doses for short periods of time to treat non-gonococcal urethritis may mask or delay the symptoms of incubating gonorrhea or syphilis. All patients with sexually-transmitted urethritis or cervicitis should have a serologic test for syphilis and appropriate cultures for gonorrhea performed at the time of diagnosis. Appropriate antimicrobial therapy and follow-up tests for these diseases should be initiated if infection is confirmed.
Appropriate culture and susceptibility tests should be performed before treatment to determine the causative organism and its susceptibility to azithromycin. Therapy with ZITHROMAX® may be initiated before results of these tests are known; once the results become available, antimicrobial therapy should be adjusted accordingly.
To reduce the development of drug-resistant bacteria and maintain the effectiveness of Zithromax (azithromycin) and other antibacterial drugs, Zithromax (azithromycin) should be used only to treat or prevent infections that are proven or strongly suspected to be caused by susceptible bacteria. When culture and susceptibility information are available, they should be considered in selecting or modifying antibac-

Continued on next page

Zithromax Caps/Tabs/O.S.—Cont.

terial therapy. In the absence of such data, local epidemiology and susceptibility patterns may contribute to the empiric selection of therapy.

Mycobacterial Infections

Prophylaxis of Disseminated *Mycobacterium avium* complex (MAC) Disease

ZITHROMAX®, taken alone or in combination with rifabutin at its approved dose, is indicated for the prevention of disseminated *Mycobacterium avium* complex (MAC) disease in persons with advanced HIV infection. (See DOSAGE AND ADMINISTRATION, CLINICAL STUDIES)

Treatment of Disseminated *Mycobacterium avium* complex (MAC) Disease

ZITHROMAX®, taken in combination with ethambutol, is indicated for the treatment of disseminated MAC infections in persons with advanced HIV infection. (See DOSAGE AND ADMINISTRATION, CLINICAL STUDIES)

CONTRAINDICATIONS

ZITHROMAX® is contraindicated in patients with known hypersensitivity to azithromycin, erythromycin, or any macrolide antibiotic.

WARNINGS

Rare serious allergic reactions, including angioedema and anaphylaxis, have been reported rarely in patients on azithromycin therapy. (See **CONTRAINDICATIONS**.) Despite initially successful symptomatic treatment of the allergic symptoms, when symptomatic therapy was discontinued, the allergic symptoms **recurred soon thereafter in some patients without further azithromycin exposure**. These patients required prolonged periods of observation and symptomatic treatment. The relationship of these episodes to the long tissue half-life of azithromycin and subsequent prolonged exposure to antigen is unknown at present. If an allergic reaction occurs, the drug should be discontinued and appropriate therapy should be instituted. Physicians should be aware that reappearance of the allergic symptoms may occur when symptomatic therapy is discontinued.

In the treatment of pneumonia, azithromycin has only been shown to be safe and effective in the treatment of community-acquired pneumonia of mild severity due to *Streptococcus pneumoniae* or *Haemophilus influenzae* in patients appropriate for outpatient oral therapy. Azithromycin should not be used in patients with pneumonia who are judged to be inappropriate for outpatient oral therapy because of moderate to severe illness or risk factors such as any of the following: patients with nosocomially acquired infections, patients with known or suspected bacteremia, patients requiring hospitalization, elderly or debilitated patients, or patients with significant underlying health problems that may compromise their ability to respond to their illness (including immunodeficiency or functional asplenia).

Pseudomembranous colitis has been reported with nearly all antibacterial agents and may range in severity from mild to life-threatening. Therefore, it is important to consider this diagnosis in patients who present with diarrhea subsequent to the administration of antibacterial agents.

Treatment with antibacterial agents alters the normal flora of the colon and may permit overgrowth of clostridia. Studies indicate that a toxin produced by *Clostridium difficile* is a primary cause of "antibiotic-associated colitis."

After the diagnosis of pseudomembranous colitis has been established, therapeutic measures should be initiated. Mild cases of pseudomembranous colitis usually respond to discontinuation of the drug alone. In moderate to severe cases, consideration should be given to management with fluids and electrolytes, protein supplementation, and treatment with an antibacterial drug clinically effective against *Clostridium difficile* colitis.

PRECAUTIONS

General: Because azithromycin is principally eliminated via the liver, caution should be exercised when azithromycin is administered to patients with impaired hepatic function. There are no data regarding azithromycin usage in patients with renal impairment; thus, caution should be exercised when prescribing azithromycin in these patients.

Prolonged cardiac repolarization and QT interval, imparting a risk of developing cardiac arrhythmia and *torsades de pointes*, have been seen in treatment with other macrolides. A similar effect with azithromycin cannot be completely ruled out in patients at increased risk for prolonged cardiac repolarization.

Prescribing Zithromax (azithromycin) in the absence of a proven or strongly suspected bacterial infection or a prophylactic indication is unlikely to provide benefit to the patient and increases the risk of the development of drug-resistant bacteria.

Information for Patients:

Patients should be cautioned to take ZITHROMAX® capsules at least one hour prior to a meal or at least two hours after a meal. Azithromycin capsules should not be taken with food.

ZITHROMAX® tablets may be taken with or without food. However, increased tolerability has been observed when tablets are taken with food.

ZITHROMAX® for oral suspension in single 1 g packets can be taken with or without food after constitution.

Patients should also be cautioned not to take aluminum- and magnesium-containing antacids and azithromycin simultaneously.

The patient should be directed to discontinue azithromycin immediately and contact a physician if any signs of an allergic reaction occur.

Patients should be counseled that antibacterial drugs including Zithromax (azithromycin) should only be used to treat bacterial infections. They do not treat viral infections (e.g., the common cold). When Zithromax (azithromycin) is prescribed to treat bacterial infection, patients should be told that although it is common to feel better early in the course of therapy, the medication should be taken exactly as directed. Skipping doses or not completing the full course of therapy may (1) decrease the effectiveness of the immediate treatment and (2) increase the likelihood that bacteria will develop resistance and will not be treatable by Zithromax (azithromycin) or other antibacterial drugs in the future.

Drug Interactions: Aluminum- and magnesium-containing antacids reduce the peak serum levels (rate) but not the AUC (extent) of azithromycin (500 mg) absorption.

Administration of cimetidine (800 mg) two hours prior to azithromycin had no effect on azithromycin (500 mg) absorption.

A single oral dose of 1200 mg azithromycin (2 x 600 mg ZITHROMAX® tablets) did not alter the pharmacokinetics of a single 800 mg oral dose of fluconazole in healthy adult subjects.

Total exposure (AUC) and half-life of azithromycin following the single oral tablet dose of 1200 mg were unchanged and the reduction in Cmax was not significant (mean decrease of 18%) by coadministration with 800 mg fluconazole.

A single oral dose of 1200 mg azithromycin (2 x 600 mg ZITHROMAX® tablets) had no significant effect on the pharmacokinetics of indinavir (800 mg indinavir tid for 5 days) in healthy adult subjects.

Coadministration of a single oral dose of 1200 mg azithromycin (2 x 600 mg ZITHROMAX® tablets) with steady-state nelfinavir (750 mg tid) to healthy adult subjects produced a decrease of approximately 15% in mean $AUC_{0\text{-}8}$ of nelfinavir and its M8 metabolite. Mean Cmax of nelfinavir and its M8 metabolite were not significantly affected. No dosage adjustment of nelfinavir is required when nelfinavir is coadministered with azithromycin.

Coadministration of nelfinavir (750 mg tid) at steady state with a single oral dose of 1200 mg azithromycin increased the mean $AUC_{0\text{-}\infty}$ of azithromycin by approximately a factor of 2-times (range of up to 4 times) of that when azithromycin was given alone. The mean Cmax of azithromycin was also increased by approximately a factor of 2-times (range of up to 5 times) of that when azithromycin was given alone. Dose adjustment of azithromycin is not recommended. However, when administered in conjunction with nelfinavir, close monitoring for known side effects of azithromycin, such as liver enzyme abnormalities and hearing impairment, is warranted. (See ADVERSE REACTIONS.)

Following administration of trimethoprim/sulfamethoxazole DS (160 mg/800 mg) for 7 days to healthy adult subjects, coadministration of 1200 mg azithromycin (2 x 600 mg ZITHROMAX® tablets) on the 7th day had no significant effects on peak concentrations (C_{max}), total exposure (AUC), and the urinary excretion of either trimethoprim or sulfamethoxazole.

Coadministration of trimethoprim/sulfamethoxazole DS for 7 days had no significant effect on the peak concentration (C_{max}) and total exposure (AUC) of azithromycin following administration of the single 1200 mg tablet dose to healthy adult subjects.

Administration of a 600 mg single oral dose of azithromycin had no effect on the pharmacokinetics of efavirenz given at 400 mg doses for 7 days to healthy adult subjects.

Efavirenz, when administered at a dose of 400 mg for seven days produced a 22% increase in the C_{max} of azithromycin administered as a 600 mg single oral dose, while the AUC of azithromycin was not affected.

Azithromycin (500 mg Day 1, 250 mg Days 2-5) did not affect the plasma levels or pharmacokinetics of theophylline administered as a single intravenous dose. The effect of azithromycin on the plasma levels or pharmacokinetics of theophylline administered in multiple doses resulting in therapeutic steady-state levels of theophylline is not known. However, concurrent use of macrolides and theophylline has been associated with increases in the serum concentrations of theophylline. Therefore, until further data are available, prudent medical practice dictates careful monitoring of plasma theophylline levels in patients receiving azithromycin and theophylline concomitantly.

Azithromycin (500 mg Day 1, 250 mg Days 2-5) did not affect the prothrombin time response to a single dose of warfarin. However, prudent medical practice dictates careful monitoring of prothrombin time in all patients treated with azithromycin and warfarin concomitantly. Concurrent use of macrolides and warfarin in clinical practice has been associated with increased anticoagulant effects.

Dose adjustments are not indicated when azithromycin and zidovudine are coadministered. When zidovudine (100 mg q3h x5) was coadministered with daily azithromycin (600 mg, n=5 or 1200 mg, n=7), mean C_{max}, AUC and Clr increased by 26% (CV 54%), 10% (CV 26%) and 38% (CV 114%), respectively. The mean AUC of phosphorylated zidovudine increased by 75% (CV 95%), while zidovudine glucuronide C_{max} and AUC increased by less than 10%. In another study, addition of 1 gram azithromycin per week to a regimen of 10 mg/kg daily zidovudine resulted in 25% (CV 70%) and 13% (CV 37%) increases in zidovudine C_{max} and AUC, respectively. Zidovudine glucuronide mean C_{max} and AUC increased by 16% (CV 61%) and 8.0% (CV 32%), respectively.

Doses of 1200 mg/day azithromycin for 14 days in 6 subjects increased C_{max} of concurrently administered didanosine (200 mg *q*.12h) by 44% (54% CV) and AUC by 14% (23% CV). However, none of these changes were significantly different from those produced in a parallel placebo control group of subjects.

Preliminary data suggest that coadministration of azithromycin and rifabutin did not markedly affect the mean serum concentrations of either drug. Administration of 250 mg azithromycin daily for 10 days (500 mg on the first day) produced mean concentrations of azithromycin 1 day after the last dose of 53 ng/mL when coadministered with 300 mg daily rifabutin and 49 mg/mL when coadministered with placebo. Mean concentrations 5 days after the last dose were 23 ng/mL and 21 ng/mL in the two groups of subjects. Administration of 300 mg rifabutin for 10 days produced mean concentrations of rifabutin one half day after the last dose of 60 mg/ml when coadministered with daily 250 mg azithromycin and 71 ng/mL when coadministered with placebo. Mean concentrations 5 days after the last dose were 8.1 ng/mL and 9.2 ng/mL in the two groups of subjects.

The following drug interactions have not been reported in clinical trials with azithromycin; however, no specific drug interaction studies have been performed to evaluate potential drug-drug interaction. Nonetheless, they have been observed with macrolide products. Until further data are developed regarding drug interactions when azithromycin and these drugs are used concomitantly, careful monitoring of patients is advised:

Digoxin–elevated digoxin levels.

Ergotamine or dihydroergotamine–acute ergot toxicity characterized by severe peripheral vasospasm and dysesthesia.

Triazolam–decrease the clearance of triazolam and thus may increase the pharmacologic effect of triazolam.

Drugs metabolized by the cytochrome P^{450} system–elevations of serum carbamazepine, cyclosporine, hexobarbital, and phenytoin levels.

Laboratory Test Interactions: There are no reported laboratory test interactions.

Carcinogenesis, Mutagenesis, Impairment of Fertility: Long-term studies in animals have not been performed to evaluate carcinogenic potential. Azithromycin has shown no mutagenic potential in standard laboratory tests: mouse lymphoma assay, human lymphocyte clastogenic assay, and mouse bone marrow clastogenic assay.

Pregnancy: Teratogenic Effects. Pregnancy Category B: Reproduction studies have been performed in rats and mice at doses up to moderately maternally toxic dose levels (i.e., 200 mg/kg/day). These doses, based on a mg/m^2 basis, are estimated to be 4 and 2 times, respectively, the human daily dose of 500 mg.

With regard to the MAC treatment dose of 600 mg daily, on a mg/m^2/day basis, the doses in rats and mice are approximately 3.3 and 1.7 times the human dose, respectively.

With regard to the MAC prophylaxis dose of 1200 mg weekly, on a mg/m^2/day basis, the doses in rats and mice are approximately 2 and 1 times the human dose, respectively.

No evidence of impaired fertility or harm to the fetus due to azithromycin was found. There are, however, no adequate and well-controlled studies in pregnant women. Because animal reproduction studies are not always predictive of human response, azithromycin should be used during pregnancy only if clearly needed.

Nursing Mothers: It is not known whether azithromycin is excreted in human milk. Because many drugs are excreted in human milk, caution should be exercised when azithromycin is administered to a nursing woman.

Pediatric Use:

In controlled clinical studies, azithromycin has been administered to pediatric patients ranging in age from 6 months to 12 years. For information regarding the use of ZITHROMAX (azithromycin for oral suspension) in the treatment of pediatric patients, please refer to the INDICATIONS AND USAGE and DOSAGE AND ADMINISTRATION sections of the prescribing information for ZITHROMAX (azithromycin for oral suspension) 100 mg/5 mL and 200 mg/5 mL bottles.

Safety in HIV-Infected Pediatric Patients: Safety and efficacy of azithromycin for the prevention or treatment of MAC in HIV-infected children have not been established. Safety data are available for 72 children 5 months to 18 years of age (mean 7 years) who received azithromycin for treatment of opportunistic infections. The mean duration of therapy was 242 days (range 3-2004 days) at doses of <1 to 52 mg/kg/day (mean 12 mg/kg/day). Adverse events were similar to those observed in the adult population, most of which involved the gastrointestinal tract. Treatment related reversible hearing impairment in children was observed in 4 subjects (5.6%). Two (2.8%) children prematurely discontinued treatment due to side effects: one due to back pain and one due to abdominal pain, hot and cold flushes, dizziness, headache, and numbness. A third child discontinued due to a laboratory abnormality (eosinophilia). The protocols upon which these data are based specified a daily dose of 10-20 mg/kg/day (oral and/or i.v.) of azithromycin.

Geriatric Use: Pharmacokinetic parameters in older volunteers (65-85 years old) were similar to those in younger volunteers (18-40 years old) for the 5-day therapeutic regimen. Dosage adjustment does not appear to be necessary for older patients with normal renal and hepatic function receiving treatment with this dosage regimen. (See CLINICAL PHARMACOLOGY.)

In multiple-dose clinical trials of oral azithromycin, 9% of patients were at least 65 years of age (458/4949) and 3% of patients (144/4949) were at least 75 years of age. No overall differences in safety or effectiveness were observed between these subjects and younger subjects, and other reported clinical experience has not identified differences in responses between the elderly and younger patients, but greater sensitivity of some older individuals cannot be ruled out.

ZITHROMAX® 600 mg tablets contain 2.1 mg of sodium per tablet. ZITHROMAX® for oral suspension 1 gram single-dose packets contain 37.0 mg of sodium per packet.

Geriatric Patients with Opportunistic Infections, Including *Mycobacterium avium* complex (MAC) Disease: Safety data are available for 30 patients (65-94 years old) treated with azithromycin at doses >300 mg/day for a mean of 207 days. These patients were treated for a variety of opportunistic infections, including MAC. The side effect profile was generally similar to that seen in younger patients, except for a higher incidence of side effects relating to the gastrointestinal system and to reversible impairment of hearing. (See DOSAGE AND ADMINISTRATION.)

ADVERSE REACTIONS

In clinical trials, most of the reported side effects were mild to moderate in severity and were reversible upon discontinuation of the drug. Approximately 0.7% of the patients from the multiple-dose clinical trials discontinued ZITHROMAX® (azithromycin) therapy because of treatment-related side effects. Most of the side effects leading to discontinuation were related to the gastrointestinal tract, e.g., nausea, vomiting, diarrhea, or abdominal pain. Rarely but potentially serious side effects were angioedema and cholestatic jaundice.

Clinical:

Multiple-dose regimen:

Overall, the most common side effects in adult patients receiving a multiple-dose regimen of ZITHROMAX® were related to the gastrointestinal system with diarrhea/loose stools (5%), nausea (3%), and abdominal pain (3%) being the most frequently reported.

No other side effects occurred in patients on the multiple-dose regimen of ZITHROMAX® with a frequency greater than 1%. Side effects that occurred with a frequency of 1% or less included the following:

Cardiovascular: Palpitations, chest pain.

Gastrointestinal: Dyspepsia, flatulence, vomiting, melena, and cholestatic jaundice.

Genitourinary: Monilia, vaginitis, and nephritis.

Nervous System: Dizziness, headache, vertigo, and somnolence.

General: Fatigue.

Allergic: Rash, photosensitivity, and angioedema.

Chronic therapy with 1200 mg weekly regimen: The nature of side effects seen with the 1200 mg weekly dosing regimen for the prevention of *Mycobacterium avium* infection in severely immunocompromised HIV-infected patients were similar to those seen with short term dosing regimens. (See CLINICAL STUDIES.)

Chronic therapy with 600 mg daily regimen combined with ethambutol: The nature of side effects seen with the 600 mg daily dosing regimen for the treatment of *Mycobacterium avium* complex infection in severely immunocompromised HIV-infected patients were similar to those seen with short term dosing regimens. Five percent of patients experienced reversible hearing impairment in the pivotal clinical trial for the treatment of disseminated MAC in patients with AIDS. Hearing impairment has been reported with macrolide antibiotics, especially at higher doses. Other treatment related side effects occurring in >5% of subjects and seen at any time during a median of 87.5 days of therapy include: abdominal pain (14%), nausea (14%), vomiting (13%), diarrhea (12%), flatulence (5%), headache (5%) and abnormal vision (5%). Discontinuations from treatment due to laboratory abnormalities or side effects considered related to study drug occurred in 8/88 (9.1%) of subjects.

Single 1-gram dose regimen: Overall, the most common side effects in patients receiving a single-dose regimen of 1 gram of ZITHROMAX® were related to the gastrointestinal system and were more frequently reported than in patients receiving the multiple-dose regimen.

Side effects that occurred in patients on the single one-gram dosing regimen of ZITHROMAX® with a frequency of 1% or greater included diarrhea/loose stools (7%), nausea (5%), abdominal pain (5%), vomiting (2%), dyspepsia (1%), and vaginitis (1%).

Post-Marketing Experience:

Adverse events reported with azithromycin during the post-marketing period in adult and/or pediatric patients for which a causal relationship may not be established include:

Allergic: Arthralgia, edema, urticaria, angioedema.

Cardiovascular: Arrhythmias including ventricular tachycardia, hypotension. There have been rare reports of QT prolongation and *torsades de pointes*.

Gastrointestinal: Anorexia, constipation, dyspepsia, flatulence, vomiting/diarrhea rarely resulting in dehydration, pseudomembranous colitis, pancreatitis, oral candidiasis and rare reports of tongue discoloration.

Cumulative Incidence Rate, %: Placebo (n=89)

Month	MAC Free and Alive	MAC	Adverse Experience	Lost to Follow-up
6	69.7	13.5	6.7	10.1
12	47.2	19.1	15.7	18.0
18	37.1	22.5	18.0	22.5

Cumulative Incidence Rate, %: Azithromycin (n=85)

Month	MAC Free and Alive	MAC	Adverse Experience	Lost to Follow-up
6	84.7	3.5	9.4	2.4
12	63.5	8.2	16.5	11.8
18	44.7	11.8	25.9	17.6

Cumulative Incidence Rate, %: Rifabutin (n=223)

Month	MAC Free and Alive	MAC	Adverse Experience	Lost to Follow-up
6	83.4	7.2	8.1	1.3
12	60.1	15.2	16.1	8.5
18	40.8	21.5	24.2	13.5

Cumulative Incidence Rate, %: Azithromycin (n=223)

Month	MAC Free and Alive	MAC	Adverse Experience	Lost to Follow-up
6	85.2	3.6	5.8	5.4
12	65.5	7.6	16.1	10.8
18	45.3	12.1	23.8	18.8

Cumulative Incidence Rate, %: Azithromycin/Rifabutin Combination (n=218)

Month	MAC Free and Alive	MAC	Adverse Experience	Lost to Follow-up
6	89.4	1.8	5.5	3.2
12	71.6	2.8	15.1	10.6
18	49.1	6.4	29.4	15.1

General: Asthenia, paresthesia, fatigue, malaise and anaphylaxis (rarely fatal).

Genitourinary: Interstitial nephritis and acute renal failure, vaginitis.

Hematopoietic: Thrombocytopenia.

Liver/Biliary: Abnormal liver function including hepatitis and cholestatic jaundice, as well as rare cases of hepatic necrosis and hepatic failure, some of which have resulted in death.

Nervous System: Convulsions, dizziness/vertigo, headache, somnolence, hyperactivity, nervousness, agitation and syncope.

Psychiatric: Aggressive reaction and anxiety.

Skin/Appendages: Pruritus, rarely serious skin reactions including erythema multiforme, Stevens Johnson Syndrome, and toxic epidermal necrolysis.

Special Senses: Hearing disturbances including hearing loss, deafness, and/or tinnitus, rare reports of taste perversion.

Laboratory Abnormalities:

Significant abnormalities (irrespective of drug relationship) occurring during the clinical trials were reported as follows: With an incidence of 1-2%, elevated serum creatine phosphokinase, potassium, ALT (SGPT), GGT, and AST (SGOT). With an incidence of less than 1%, leukopenia, neutropenia, decreased platelet count, elevated serum alkaline phosphatase, bilirubin, BUN, creatinine, blood glucose, LDH, and phosphate.

When follow-up was provided, changes in laboratory tests appeared to be reversible.

In multiple-dose clinical trials involving more than 3000 patients, 3 patients discontinued therapy because of treatment-related liver enzyme abnormalities and 1 because of a renal function abnormality.

In a phase I drug interaction study performed in normal volunteers, 1 of 6 subjects given the combination of azithromycin and rifabutin, 1 of 7 given rifabutin alone and 0 of 6 given azithromycin alone developed a clinically significant neutropenia (<500 cells/mm^3).

Laboratory abnormalities seen in clinical trials for the prevention of disseminated *Mycobacterium avium* disease in severely immunocompromised HIV-infected patients are presented in the CLINICAL STUDIES section.

Chronic therapy (median duration: 87.5 days, range: 1-229 days) that resulted in laboratory abnormalities in >5% subjects with normal baseline values in the pivotal trial for treatment of disseminated MAC in severely immunocompromised HIV infected patients treated with azithromycin 600 mg daily in combination with ethambutol include: a reduction in absolute neutrophils to <50% of the lower limit of normal (10/52, 19%) and an increase to five times the upper limit of normal in alkaline phosphatase (3/35, 9%). These findings in subjects with normal baseline values are similar when compared to all subjects for analyses of neutrophil reductions (22/75 [29%]) and elevated alkaline phosphatase (16/80 [20%]). Causality of these laboratory abnormalities due to the use of study drug has not been established.

DOSAGE AND ADMINISTRATION

(See INDICATIONS AND USAGE.)

ZITHROMAX® capsules should be given at least 1 hour before or 2 hours after a meal. ZITHROMAX® capsules should not be mixed with or taken with food.

ZITHROMAX® for oral suspension (single dose 1 g packet) can be taken with or without food after constitution. Not for pediatric use. For pediatric suspension, please refer to the INDICATIONS AND USAGE and DOSAGE AND ADMINISTRATION sections of the prescribing information for ZITHROMAX (azithromycin for oral suspension) 100 mg/5 mL and 200 mg/5 mL bottles.

ZITHROMAX® tablets may be taken without regard to food. However, increased tolerability has been observed when tablets are taken with food.

The recommended dose of ZITHROMAX® for the treatment of individuals 16 years of age and older with mild to moderate acute bacterial exacerbations of chronic obstructive pulmonary disease, pneumonia, pharyngitis/tonsillitis (as second line therapy), and uncomplicated skin and skin structure infections due to the indicated organisms is: 500 mg as a single dose on the first day followed by 250 mg once daily on Days 2 through 5 for a total dose of 1.5 grams of ZITHROMAX®.

The recommended dose of ZITHROMAX® for the treatment of non-gonococcal urethritis and cervicitis due to *C. trachomatis* is: a single 1 gram (1000 mg) dose of ZITHROMAX®. This dose can be administered as four 250 mg capsules or as one single dose packet (1 g).

Prevention of Disseminated MAC Infections

The recommended dose of ZITHROMAX® for the prevention of disseminated *Mycobacterium avium* complex (MAC) disease is: 1200 mg taken once weekly. This dose of ZITHROMAX® may be combined with the approved dosage regimen of rifabutin.

Treatment of Disseminated MAC Infections

ZITHROMAX® should be taken at a daily dose of 600 mg, in combination with ethambutol at the recommended daily dose of 15 mg/kg. Other antimycobacterial drugs that have shown *in vitro* activity against MAC may be added to the regimen of azithromycin plus ethambutol at the discretion of the physician or health care provider.

DIRECTIONS FOR ADMINISTRATION OF ZITHROMAX® for oral suspension in the single dose packet (1 g): The entire contents of the packet should be mixed thoroughly with two ounces (approximately 60 mL) of water. Drink the entire contents immediately; add an additional two ounces of water, mix, and drink to assure complete consumption of dosage. **The single dose packet should not be used to admin-**

Continued on next page

INCIDENCE OF ONE OR MORE TREATMENT RELATED* ADVERSE EVENTS IN HIV INFECTED PATIENTS RECEIVING PROPHYLAXIS FOR DISSEMINATED MAC OVER APPROXIMATELY 1 YEAR**

	Study 155		Study 174		
	Placebo (N=91)	Azithromycin 1200 mg weekly (N=89)	Azithromycin 1200 mg weekly (N=233)	Rifabutin 300 mg daily (N=236)	Azithromycin + Rifabutin (N=224)
Mean Duration of Therapy (days)	303.8	402.9	315	296.1	344.4
Discontinuation of Therapy	2.3	8.2	13.5	15.9	22.7
Autonomic Nervous System					
Mouth Dry	0	0	0	3.0	2.7
Central Nervous System					
Dizziness	0	1.1	3.9	1.7	0.4
Headache	0	0	3.0	5.5	4.5
Gastrointestinal					
Diarrhea	15.4	52.8	50.2	19.1	50.9
Loose Stools	6.6	19.1	12.9	3.0	9.4
Abdominal Pain	6.6	27	32.2	12.3	31.7
Dyspepsia	1.1	9	4.7	1.7	1.8
Flatulence	4.4	9	10.7	5.1	5.8
Nausea	11	32.6	27.0	16.5	28.1
Vomiting	1.1	6.7	9.0	3.8	5.8
General					
Fever	1.1	0	2.1	4.2	4.9
Fatigue	0	2.2	3.9	2.1	3.1
Malaise	0	1.1	0.4	0	2.2
Musculoskeletal					
Arthralgia	0	0	3.0	4.2	7.1
Psychiatric					
Anorexia	1.1	0	2.1	2.1	3.1
Skin & Appendages					
Pruritus	3.3	0	3.9	3.4	7.6
Rash	3.2	3.4	8.1	9.4	11.1
Skin discoloration	0	0	0	2.1	2.2
Special Senses					
Tinnitus	4.4	3.4	0.9	1.3	0.9
Hearing Decreased	2.2	1.1	0.9	0.4	0
Uveitis	0	0	0.4	1.3	1.8
Taste Perversion	0	0	1.3	2.5	1.3

* Includes those events considered possibly or probably related to study drug
** >2% adverse event rates for any group (except uveitis).

Prophylaxis Against Disseminated MAC Abnormal Laboratory Values*

		Placebo		Azithromycin 1200 mg weekly		Rifabutin 300 mg daily		Azithromycin & Rifabutin	
Hemoglobin	<8 g/dl	1/51	2%	4/170	2%	4/114	4%	8/107	8%
Platelet Count	≤50 × 10³/mm³	1/71	1%	4/260	2%	2/182	1%	6/181	3%
WBC Count	<1 × 10³/mm³	0/8	0%	2/70	3%	2/47	4%	0/43	0%
Neutrophils	<500/mm³	0/26	0%	4/106	4%	3/82	4%	2/78	3%
SGOT	>5 × ULN[a]	1/41	2%	8/158	5%	3/121	3%	6/114	5%
SGPT	>5 × ULN	0/49	0%	8/166	5%	3/130	2%	5/117	4%
Alk Phos	>5 × ULN	1/80	1%	4/247	2%	2/172	1%	3/164	2%

[a]=Upper Limit of Normal
*excludes subjects outside of the relevant normal range at baseline

Zithromax Caps/Tabs/O.S.—Cont.

ister doses other than 1000 mg of azithromycin. This packet not for pediatric use.

HOW SUPPLIED

ZITHROMAX® capsules (imprinted with "Pfizer 305") are supplied in red opaque hard-gelatin capsules containing azithromycin dihydrate equivalent to 250 mg of azithromycin. These are packaged in bottles and blister cards of 6 capsules (Z-PAKS®) as follows:

Bottles of 50 NDC 0069-3050-50
Boxes of 3 (Z-PAKS® of 6) NDC 0069-3050-34
Unit Dose package of 50 NDC 0069-3050-86

Store capsules below 30°C (86°F).

ZITHROMAX® 600 mg tablets (engraved on front with "PFIZER" and on back with "308") are supplied as white, modified oval-shaped, film-coated tablets containing azithromycin dihydrate equivalent to 600 mg azithromycin. These are packaged in bottles of 30 tablets. ZITHROMAX® tablets are supplied as follows:

Bottles of 30 NDC 0069-3080-30

Tablets should be stored at or below 30°C (86°F).

ZITHROMAX® for oral suspension is supplied in single dose packets containing azithromycin dihydrate equivalent to 1 gram of azithromycin as follows:

Boxes of 10 Single Dose Packets (1 g) NDC 0069-3051-07
Boxes of 3 Single Dose Packets (1 g) NDC 0069-3051-75

Store single dose packets between 5° and 30°C (41° and 86°F).

CLINICAL STUDIES IN PATIENTS WITH ADVANCED HIV INFECTION FOR THE PREVENTION AND TREATMENT OF DISEASE DUE TO DISSEMINATED *MYCOBACTERIUM AVIUM* COMPLEX (MAC)

(See INDICATIONS AND USAGE):

Prevention of Disseminated MAC Disease

Two randomized, double blind clinical trials were performed in patients with CD4 counts <100 cells/μL. The first study (155) compared azithromycin (1200 mg once weekly) to placebo and enrolled 182 patients with a mean CD4 count of 35 cells/μL. The second study (174) randomized 723 patients to either azithromycin (1200 mg once weekly), rifabutin (300 mg daily) or the combination of both. The mean CD4 count was 51 cells/μL. The primary endpoint in these studies was disseminated MAC disease. Other endpoints included the incidence of clinically significant MAC disease and discontinuations from therapy for drug-related side effects.

MAC bacteremia

In trial 155, 85 patients randomized to receive azithromycin and 89 patients randomized to receive placebo met study entrance criteria. Cumulative incidences at 6, 12 and 18 months of the possible outcomes are in the following table:

[See first table at top of previous page]

The difference in the one year cumulative incidence rates of disseminated MAC disease (placebo–azithromycin) is 10.9%. This difference is statistically significant (p=0.037) with a 95% confidence interval for this difference of (0.8%, 20.9%). The comparable number of patients experiencing adverse events and the fewer number of patients lost to follow-up on azithromycin should be taken into account when interpreting the significance of this difference.

In trial 174, 223 patients randomized to receive rifabutin, 223 patients randomized to receive azithromycin, and 218 patients randomized to receive both rifabutin and azithromycin met study entrance criteria. Cumulative incidences at 6, 12 and 18 months of the possible outcomes are recorded in the following table:

[See second table at top of previous page]

Comparing the cumulative one year incidence rates, azithromycin monotherapy is at least as effective as rifabutin monotherapy. The difference (rifabutin–azithromycin) in the one year rates (7.6%) is statistically significant (p=0.022) with an adjusted 95% confidence interval (0.9%, 14.3%). Additionally, azithromycin/rifabutin combination therapy is more effective than rifabutin alone. The difference (rifabutin–azithromycin/rifabutin) in the cumulative one year incidence rates (12.5%) is statistically significant (p<0.001) with an adjusted 95% confidence interval of (6.6%, 18.4%). The comparable number of patients experiencing adverse events and the fewer number of patients lost to follow-up on rifabutin should be taken into account when interpreting the significance of this difference.

In Study 174, sensitivity testing[5] was performed on all available MAC isolates from subjects randomized to either azithromycin, rifabutin or the combination. The distribution of MIC values for azithromycin from susceptibility testing of the breakthrough isolates was similar between study arms. As the efficacy of azithromycin in the treatment of disseminated MAC has not been established, the clinical relevance of these *in vitro* MICs as an indicator of susceptibility or resistance is not known.

Clinically Significant Disseminated MAC Disease

In association with the decreased incidence of bacteremia, patients in the groups randomized to either azithromycin alone or azithromycin in combination with rifabutin showed reductions in the signs and symptoms of disseminated MAC disease, including fever or night sweats, weight loss and anemia.

Discontinuations From Therapy For Drug-Related Side Effects

In Study 155, discontinuations for drug-related toxicity occurred in 8.2% of subjects treated with azithromycin and 2.3% of those given placebo (p=0.121). In Study 174, more subjects discontinued from the combination of azithromycin and rifabutin (22.7%) than from azithromycin alone (13.5%; p=0.026) or rifabutin alone (15.9%; p=0.209).

Safety

As these patients with advanced HIV disease were taking multiple concomitant medications and experienced a variety of intercurrent illnesses, it was often difficult to attribute adverse events to study medication. Overall, the nature of side effects seen on the weekly dosage regimen of azithromycin over a period of approximately one year in patients with advanced HIV disease was similar to that previously reported for shorter course therapies.

[See first table at left]

Side effects related to the gastrointestinal tract were seen more frequently in patients receiving azithromycin than in those receiving placebo or rifabutin. In Study 174, 86% of diarrheal episodes were mild to moderate in nature with discontinuation of therapy for this reason occurring in only 9/233 (3.8%) of patients.

Changes in Laboratory Values

In these immunocompromised patients with advanced HIV infection, it was necessary to assess laboratory abnormalities developing on study with additional criteria if baseline values were outside the relevant normal range.

[See second table at left]

Treatment of Disseminated MAC Disease

One randomized, double blind clinical trial (Study 189) was performed in patients with disseminated MAC. In this trial, 246 HIV infected patients with disseminated MAC received either azithromycin 250 mg qd (N=65), azithromycin 600 mg qd (N=91) or clarithromycin 500 mg bid (N=90), each administered with ethambutol 15 mg/kg qd, for 24 weeks. Patients were cultured and clinically assessed every 3 weeks through week 12 and monthly thereafter through week 24. After week 24, patients were switched to any open label therapy at the discretion of the investigator and followed every 3 months through the last follow up visit of the trial. Patients were followed from the baseline visit for a period of up to 3.7 years (median: 9 months). MAC isolates recovered during study treatment or post-treatment were obtained whenever possible.

The primary endpoint was sterilization by week 24. Sterilization was based on data from the central laboratory, and was defined as two consecutive observed negative blood cultures for MAC, independent of missing culture data between the two negative observations. Analyses were performed on all randomized patients who had a positive baseline culture for MAC.

The azithromycin 250 mg arm was discontinued after an interim analysis at 12 weeks showed a significantly lower clearance of bacteremia compared to clarithromycin 500 mg bid.

Efficacy results for the azithromycin 600 mg qd and clarithromycin 500 mg bid treatment regimens are described in the following table:

Response to therapy of patients taking ethambutol and either azithromycin 600 mg qd or clarithromycin 500 mg bid

	Azithromycin 600 mg qd	Clarithromycin 500 mg bid	**95.1% CI on difference
Patients with positive culture at baseline	68	57	
Week 24			
Two consecutive negative blood cultures*	31/68 (46%)	32/57 (56%)	[-28, 7]
Mortality	16/68 (24%)	15/57 (26%)	[-18, 13]

*Primary endpoint

**[95% confidence interval] on difference in rates (azithromycin-clarithromycin)

The primary endpoint, rate of sterilization of blood cultures (two consecutive negative cultures) at 24 weeks, was lower in the azithromycin 600 mg qd group than in the clarithromycin 500 mg bid group.

Sterilization by Baseline Colony Count

Within both treatment groups, the sterilization rates at week 24 decreased as the range of MAC cfu/mL increased.

	Azithromycin 600 mg (N=68)	Clarithromycin 500 mg bid (N=57)
Groups Stratified by MAC Colony Counts at Baseline	No. (%) Subjects in Stratified Group Sterile at Week 24	No. (%) Subjects in Stratified Group Sterile at Week 24
≤ 10 cfu/mL	10/15 (66.7%)	12/17 (70.6%)
11-100 cfu/mL	13/28 (46.4%)	13/19 (68.4%)
101-1,000 cfu/mL	7/19 (36.8%)	5/13 (38.5%)
1,001-10,000 cfu/mL	1/5 (20.0%)	1/5 (20%)
>10,000 cfu/mL	0/1 (0.0%)	1/3 (33.3%)

Susceptibility Pattern of MAC Isolates:

Susceptibility testing was performed on MAC isolates recovered at baseline, at the time of breakthrough on therapy or during post-therapy follow-up. The T100 radiometric broth method was employed to determine azithromycin and clarithromycin MIC values. Azithromycin MIC values ranged from <4 to >256 µg/mL and clarithromycin MICs ranged from <1 to >32 µg/mL. The individual MAC susceptibility results demonstrated that azithromycin MIC values could be 4 to 32 fold higher than clarithromycin MIC values. During study treatment and post-treatment follow up for up to 3.7 years (median: 9 months) in study 189, a total of 6/68 (9%) and 6/57 (11%) of the patients randomized to azithromycin 600 mg daily and clarithromycin 500 mg bid, respectively, developed MAC blood culture isolates that had a sharp increase in MIC values. All twelve MAC isolates had azithromycin MIC's ≥256 µg/mL and clarithromycin MIC's >32 µg/mL. These high MIC values suggest development of drug resistance. However, at this time, specific breakpoints for separating susceptible and resistant MAC isolates have not been established for either macrolide.

ANIMAL TOXICOLOGY

Phospholipidosis (intracellular phospholipid binding) has been observed in some tissues of mice, rats, and dogs given multiple doses of azithromycin. It has been demonstrated in numerous organ systems (e.g., eye, dorsal root ganglia, liver, gallbladder, kidney, spleen, and pancreas) in dogs administered doses which, based on pharmacokinetics, are as low as 2 times greater than the recommended adult human dose and in rats at doses comparable to the recommended adult human dose. This effect has been reversible after cessation of azithromycin treatment. The significance of these findings for humans is unknown.

REFERENCES

1. National Committee for Clinical Laboratory Standards. Methods for Dilution Antimicrobial Susceptibility Tests for Bacteria that Grow Aerobically–Third Edition. Approved Standard NCCLS Document M7-A3, Vol. 13, No. 25, NCCLS, Villanova, PA, December 1993.
2. National Committee for Clinical Laboratory Standards. Performance Standards for Antimicrobial Disk Susceptibility Tests–Fifth Edition. Approved Standard NCCLS Document M2-A5, Vol. 13, No. 24, NCCLS, Villanova, PA, December 1993.
3. Dunne MW, Foulds G, Retsema JA. Rationale for the use of azithromycin as *Mycobacterium avium* chemoprophylaxis. *American J Medicine* 1997; 102(5C):37-49.
4. Meier A, Kirshner P, Springer B, et al. Identification of mutations in 23S rRNA gene of clarithromycin-resistant *Mycobacterium intracellulare. Antimicrob Agents Chemother.* 1994;38:381-384.
5. Methodology per Inderlied CB, et al. Determination of *In Vitro* Susceptibility of *Mycobacterium avium* Complex Isolates to Antimicrobial Agents by Various Methods. *Antimicrob Agents Chemother* 1987; 31:1697-1702.

Rx only

Licensed from Pliva

Distributed by:
Pfizer Labs
Division of Pfizer Inc, NY, NY 10017
69-4763-00-9 Revised October 2003

Shown in Product Identification Guide, page 330

ZITHROMAX® ℞

[zĭth-ro-măks]

(azithromycin for injection)

For IV infusion only

To reduce the development of drug-resistant bacteria and maintain the effectiveness of ZITHROMAX® (azithromycin) and other bacterial drugs, ZITHROMAX (azithromycin) should be used only to treat or prevent infections that are proven or strongly suspected to be caused by bacteria.

Plasma concentrations (µg/mL ± S.D.) after the last daily intravenous infusion of 500 mg azithromycin

Infusion Concentration, Duration	Time after starting the infusion (hr)								
	0.5	1	2	3	4	6	8	12	24
2 mg/mL, 1 hr[a]	2.98 ±1.12	3.63 ±1.73	0.60 ±0.31	0.40 ±0.23	0.33 ±0.16	0.26 ±0.14	0.27 ±0.15	0.20 ±0.12	0.20 ±0.15
1 mg/mL, 3 hr[b]	0.91 ±0.13	1.02 ±0.11	1.14 ±0.13	1.13 ±0.16	0.32 ±0.05	0.28 ±0.04	0.27 ±0.03	0.22 ±0.02	0.18 ±0.02

a = 500 mg (2 mg/mL) for 2-5 days in Community-acquired pneumonia patients.
b = 500 mg (1 mg/mL) for 5 days in healthy subjects.

DESCRIPTION

ZITHROMAX (azithromycin for injection) contains the active ingredient azithromycin, an azalide, a subclass of macrolide antibiotics, for intravenous injection. Azithromycin has the chemical name (*2R,3S,4R,5R,8R,10R,11R,12S,13S,14R*)-13-[(2,6-dideoxy-3-*C*-methyl-3-*O*-methyl-α-*L*-*ribo*-hexopyranosyl)oxy]-2-ethyl-3,4,10-trihydroxy-3,5,6,8,10,12,14-heptamethyl-11-[[3,4,6-trideoxy-3-(dimethylamino)-β-*D*-*xylo*-hexopyranosyl]oxy]-1-oxa-6-azacyclopentadecan-15-one. Azithromycin is derived from erythromycin; however, it differs chemically from erythromycin in that a methyl-substituted nitrogen atom is incorporated into the lactone ring. Its molecular formula is $C_{38}H_{72}N_2O_{12}$, and its molecular weight is 749.00. Azithromycin has the following structural formula:

Azithromycin, as the dihydrate, is a white crystalline powder with a molecular formula of $C_{38}H_{72}N_2O_{12} \cdot 2H_2O$ and a molecular weight of 785.0.

ZITHROMAX (azithromycin for injection) consists of azithromycin dihydrate and the following inactive ingredients: citric acid and sodium hydroxide. ZITHROMAX (azithromycin for injection) is supplied in lyophilized form in a 10-mL vial equivalent to 500 mg of azithromycin for intravenous administration. Reconstitution, according to label directions, results in approximately 5 mL of ZITHROMAX for intravenous injection with each mL containing azithromycin dihydrate equivalent to 100 mg of azithromycin.

CLINICAL PHARMACOLOGY

Pharmacokinetics

In patients hospitalized with community-acquired pneumonia receiving single daily one-hour intravenous infusions for 2 to 5 days of 500 mg azithromycin at a concentration of 2 mg/mL, the mean C_{max} ± S.D. achieved was 3.63 ± 1.60 µg/mL, while the 24-hour trough level was 0.20 ± 0.15 µg/mL, and the AUC_{24} was 9.60 ± 4.80 µg•h/mL.

The mean C_{max}, 24-hour trough and AUC_{24} values were 1.14 ± 0.14 µg/mL, 0.18 ± 0.02 µg/mL, and 8.03 ±0.86 µg•h/mL, respectively, in normal volunteers receiving a 3-hour intravenous infusion of 500 mg azithromycin at a concentration of 1 mg/mL. Similar pharmacokinetic values were obtained in patients hospitalized with community-acquired pneumonia that received the same 3-hour dosage regimen for 2-5 days.

[See table above]

The average CL_t and V_d values were 10.18 mL/min/kg and 33.3 L/kg, respectively, in 18 normal volunteers receiving 1000 to 4000-mg doses given as 1 mg/mL over 2 hours.

Comparison of the plasma pharmacokinetic parameters following the 1st and 5th daily doses of 500 mg intravenous azithromycin showed only an 8% increase in C_{max} but a 61% increase in AUC_{24} reflecting a threefold rise in C_{24} trough levels.

Following single oral doses of 500 mg azithromycin (two 250 mg capsules) to 12 healthy volunteers, C_{max}, trough level, and AUC_{24} were reported to be 0.41 µg/mL, 0.05 µg/mL, and 2.6 µg•h/mL, respectively. These oral values are approximately 38%, 83%, and 52% of the values observed following a single 500-mg I.V. 3-hour infusion (C_{max}: 1.08 µg/mL, trough: 0.06 µg/mL, and AUC^{24}: 5.0 µg•h/mL). Thus, plasma concentrations are higher following the intravenous regimen throughout the 24-hour interval. The pharmacokinetic parameters on day 5 of azithromycin 250-mg capsules following a 500-mg oral loading dose to healthy young adults (age 18-40 years old) were as follows: C_{max}: 0.24 µg/mL, AUC_{24}: 2.1 µg•h/mL. Azithromycin 250 mg capsules are no longer commercially available. Azithromycin 250 mg tablets are bioequivalent to 250 mg capsules in the fasting state.

Median azithromycin exposure (AUC_{0-288}) in mononuclear (MN) and polymorphonuclear (PMN) leukocytes following 1,500 mg of oral azithromycin, administered in single daily doses over either 5 days (two 250 mg tablets on day 1, followed by one 250 mg tablet on days 2-5) or 3 days (500 mg per day for days 1-3) to 12 healthy volunteers, was more than a 1000-fold and 800-fold greater than in serum, respectively.

Distribution:

The serum protein binding of azithromycin is variable in the concentration range approximating human exposure, decreasing from 51% at 0.02 µg/mL to 7% at 2 µg/mL.

Tissue concentrations have not been obtained following intravenous infusions of azithromycin. Selected tissue (or fluid) concentration and tissue (or fluid) to plasma/serum concentration ratios following oral administration of azithromycin are shown in the following table:

[See first table at top of next page]

Tissue levels were determined following a single oral dose of 500 mg azithromycin in 7 gynecological patients. Approximately 17 hours after dosing, azithromycin concentrations were 2.7 µg/g in ovarian tissue, 3.5 µg/g in uterine tissue, and 3.3 µg/g in salpinx. Following a regimen of 500 mg on the first day followed by 250 mg daily for 4 days, concentrations in the cerebrospinal fluid were less than 0.01 µg/mL in the presence of non-inflamed meninges.

Metabolism

In vitro and *in vivo* studies to assess the metabolism of azithromycin have not been performed.

Elimination

Plasma concentrations of azithromycin following single 500 mg oral and i.v. doses declined in a polyphasic pattern with a mean apparent plasma clearance of 630 mL/min and terminal elimination half-life of 68 hours. The prolonged terminal half-life is thought to be due to extensive uptake and subsequent release of drug from tissues.

In a multiple-dose study in 12 normal volunteers utilizing a 500-mg (1 mg/mL) one-hour intravenous-dosage regimen for five days, the amount of administered azithromycin dose excreted in urine in 24 hours was about 11% after the 1st dose and 14% after the 5th dose. These values are greater than the reported 6% excreted unchanged urine after oral administration of azithromycin. Biliary excretion is a major route of elimination for unchanged drug, following oral administration.

Special Populations

Renal Insufficiency

Azithromycin pharmacokinetics were investigated in 42 adults (21 to 85 years of age) with varying degrees of renal impairment. Following the oral administration of a single 1,000 mg dose of azithromycin, mean C_{max} and AUC_{0-120} increased by 5.1% and 4.2%, respectively in subjects with mild to moderate renal impairment (GFR 10 to 80 mL/min) compared to subjects with normal renal function (GFR >80 mL/min). The mean C_{max} and AUC_{0-120} increased 61% and 35%, respectively in subjects with severe renal impairment (GFR <10 mL/min) compared to subjects with normal renal function (GFR >80 mL/min). (See **DOSAGE AND ADMINISTRATION**.)

Hepatic Insufficiency

The pharmacokinetics of azithromycin in subjects with hepatic impairment have not been established.

Gender

There are no significant differences in the disposition of azithromycin between male and female subjects. No dosage adjustment is recommended based on gender.

Geriatric Patients

Pharmacokinetic studies with intravenous azithromycin have not been performed in older volunteers. Pharmacokinetics of azithromycin following oral administration in older volunteers (65-85 years old) were similar to those in younger volunteers (18-40 years old) for the 5-day therapeutic regimen.

Pediatric Patients

Pharmacokinetic studies with intravenous azithromycin have not been performed in children.

Drug-Drug Interactions

Drug interaction studies were performed with oral azithromycin and other drugs likely to be co-administered. The effects of co-administration of azithromycin on the pharmacokinetics of other drugs are shown in Table 1 and the effect of other drugs on the pharmacokinetics of azithromycin are shown in Table 2.

Co-administration of azithromycin at therapeutic doses had a modest effect on the pharmacokinetics of the drugs listed in Table 1. No dosage adjustment of drugs listed in Table 1 is recommended when co-administered with azithromycin.

Co-administration of azithromycin with efavirenz or fluconazole had a modest effect on the pharmacokinetics of azithromycin. Nelfinavir significantly increased the C_{max} and AUC of azithromycin. No dosage adjustment of azithromycin is recommended when administered with drugs listed in Table 2. (See **PRECAUTIONS - Drug Interactions.)**

Continued on next page

Zithromax IV—Cont.

[See second table at right]

Mean rifabutin concentrations one-half day after the last dose rifabutin were 60 ng/mL when co-administered with azithromycin and 71 ng/mL when co-administered with placebo.

[See table 2 at bottom of next page]

Microbiology: Azithromycin acts by binding to the 50S ribosomal subunit of susceptible microorganisms and, thus, interfering with microbial protein synthesis. Nucleic acid synthesis is not affected.

Azithromycin concentrates in phagocytes and fibroblasts as demonstrated by *in vitro* incubation techniques. Using such methodology, the ratio of intracellular to extracellular concentration was >30 after one hour incubation. *In vivo* studies suggest that concentration in phagocytes may contribute to drug distribution to inflamed tissues.

Azithromycin has been shown to be active against most isolates of the following microorganisms, both *in vitro* and in clinical infections as described in the **INDICATIONS AND USAGE** section of the package insert for ZITHROMAX (azithromycin for injection).

Aerobic and facultative gram-positive microorganisms
Staphylococcus aureus
Streptococcus pneumoniae

NOTE: Azithromycin demonstrates cross-resistance with erythromycin-resistant gram-positive strains. Most strains of *Enterococcus faecalis* and methicillin-resistant staphylococci are resistant to azithromycin.

Aerobic and facultative gram-negative microorganisms
Haemophilus influenzae
Moraxella catarrhalis
Neisseria gonorrhoeae

"Other" microorganisms
Chlamydia pneumoniae
Chlamydia trachomatis
Legionella pneumophila
Mycoplasma hominis
Mycoplasma pneumoniae

Beta-lactamase production should have no effect on azithromycin activity.

Azithromycin has been shown to be active against most strains of the following microorganisms, both *in vitro* and in clinical infections as described in the **INDICATIONS AND USAGE** section of the package insert for ZITHROMAX (azithromycin tablets) and ZITHROMAX (azithromycin for oral suspension).

Aerobic and facultative gram-positive microorganisms
Staphylococcus aureus
Streptococcus agalactiae
Streptococcus pneumoniae
Streptococcus pyogenes

Aerobic and facultative gram-negative microorganisms
Haemophilus ducreyi
Haemophilus influenzae
Moraxella catarrhalis
Neisseria gonorrhoeae

"Other" microorganisms
Chlamydia pneumoniae
Chlamydia trachomatis
Mycoplasma pneumoniae

Beta-lactamase production should have no effect on azithromycin activity.

The following *in vitro* data are available, **but their clinical significance is unknown.**

At least 90% of the following microorganisms exhibit an *in vitro* minimum inhibitory concentration (MIC) less than or equal to the susceptible breakpoints for azithromycin. However, the safety and effectiveness of azithromycin in treating clinical infections due to these microorganisms have not been established in adequate and well-controlled clinical trials.

Aerobic and facultative gram-positive microorganisms
Streptococci (Groups C, F, G)
Viridans group streptococci

Aerobic and facultative gram-negative microorganisms
Bordetella pertussis

Anaerobic microorganisms
Peptostreptococcus species
Prevotella bivia

"Other" microorganisms
Ureaplasma urealyticum

Beta-lactamase production should have no effect on azithromycin activity.

Susceptibility Testing Methods:

When available, the results of *in vitro* susceptibility test results for antimicrobial drugs used in resident hospitals should be provided to the physician as periodic reports which describe the susceptibility profile of nosocomial and community-acquired pathogens. These reports may differ from susceptibility data obtained from outpatient use, but could aid the physician in selecting the most effective antimicrobial.

Dilution techniques:

Quantitative methods are used to determine antimicrobial minimum inhibitory concentrations (MICs). These MICs provide estimates of the susceptibility of bacteria to antimicrobial compounds. The MICs should be determined using a standardized procedure. Standardized procedures are based on a dilution method[1,3] (broth or agar) or equivalent with standardized inoculum concentrations and standardized concentrations of azithromycin powder. The MIC values should be interpreted according to criteria provided in Table 1.

Diffusion techniques:

Quantitative methods that require measurement of zone diameters also provide reproducible estimates of the susceptibility of bacteria to antimicrobial compounds. One such standardized procedure[2,3] requires the use of standardized inoculum concentrations. This procedure uses paper disks impregnated with 15-μg azithromycin to test the susceptibility of microorganisms to azithromycin. The disk diffusion interpretive criteria are provided in Table 1.

AZITHROMYCIN CONCENTRATIONS FOLLOWING A 500 mg DOSE (TWO 250 mg CAPSULES) IN ADULTS

TISSUE OR FLUID	TIME AFTER DOSE (h)	TISSUE OR FLUID CONCENTRATION (μg/g or μg/mL)[1]	CORRESPONDING PLASMA OR SERUM LEVEL (μg/mL)	TISSUE (FLUID) PLASMA (SERUM) RATIO[1]
SKIN	72-96	0.4	0.012	35
LUNG	72-96	4.0	0.012	>100
SPUTUM*	2-4	1.0	0.64	2
SPUTUM**	10-12	2.9	0.1	30
TONSIL***	9-18	4.5	0.03	>100
TONSIL***	180	0.9	0.006	>100
CERVIX****	19	2.8	0.04	70

[1]High tissue concentrations should not be interpreted to be quantitatively related to clinical efficacy. The antimicrobial activity of azithromycin is pH related and appears to be reduced with decreasing pH. However, the extensive distribution of drug to tissues may be relevant to clinical activity.

* Sample was obtained 2-4 hours after the first dose.
** Sample was obtained 10-12 hours after the first dose.
*** Dosing regimen of 2 doses of 250 mg each, separated by 12 hours.
**** Sample was obtained 19 hours after a single 500 mg dose.

Table 1. Drug Interactions: Pharmacokinetic Parameters for Co-administered Drugs in the Presence of Azithromycin

Co-administered Drug	Dose of Co-administered Drug	Dose of Azithromycin	n	Ratio (with/without azithromycin) of Co-administered Drug Pharmacokinetic Parameters (90% CI); No Effect = 1.00 Mean C_{max}	Mean AUC
Atorvastatin	10 mg/day × 8 days	500 mg/day PO on days 6-8	12	0.83 (0.63 to 1.08)	1.01 (0.81 to 1.25)
Carbamazepine	200 mg/day × 2 days, then 200 mg BID × 18 days	500 mg/day PO for days 16-18	7	0.97 (0.88 to 1.06)	0.96 (0.88 to 1.06)
Cetirizine	20 mg/day × 11 days	500 mg PO on day 7, then 250 mg/day on days 8-11	14	1.03 (0.93 to 1.14)	1.02 (0.92 to 1.13)
Didanosine	200 mg PO BID × 21 days	1,200 mg/day PO on days 8-21	6	1.44 (0.85 to 2.43)	1.14 (0.83 to 1.57)
Efavirenz	400 mg/day × 7 days	600 mg PO on day 7	14	1.04*	0.95*
Fluconazole	200 mg PO single dose	1,200 mg PO single dose	18	1.04 (0.98 to 1.11)	1.01 (0.97 to 1.05)
Indinavir	800 mg TID × 5 days	1,200 mg PO on day 5	18	0.96 (0.86 to 1.08)	0.90 (0.81 to 1.00)
Midazolam	15 mg PO on day 3	500 mg/day PO × 3 days	12	1.27 (0.89 to 1.81)	1.26 (1.01 to 1.56)
Nelfinavir	750 mg TID × 11 days	1,200 mg PO on day 9	14	0.90 (0.81 to 1.01)	0.85 (0.78 to 0.93)
Rifabutin	300 mg/day × 10 days	500 mg PO on day 1, then 250 mg/day on days 2-10	6	See footnote below	NA
Sildenafil	100 mg on days 1 and 4	500 mg/day PO × 3 days	12	1.16 (0.86 to 1.57)	0.92 (0.75 to 1.12)
Theophylline	4 mg/kg IV on days 1, 11, 25	500 mg PO on day 7, 250 mg/day on days 8-11	10	1.19 (1.02 to 1.40)	1.02 (0.86 to 1.22)
Theophylline	300 mg PO BID × 15 days	500 mg PO on day 6, then 250 mg/day on days 7-10	8	1.09 (0.92 to 1.29)	1.08 (0.89 to 1.31)
Triazolam	0.125 mg on day 2	500 mg PO on day 1, then 250 mg/day on day 2	12	1.06*	1.02*
Trimethoprim/ Sulfamethoxazole	160 mg/800 mg/day PO × 7 days	1,200 mg PO on day 7	12	0.85 (0.75 to 0.97)/ 0.90 (0.78 to 1.03)	0.87 (0.80 to 0.95)/ 0.96 (0.88 to 1.03)
Zidovudine	500 mg/day PO × 21 days	600 mg/day PO × 14 days	5	1.12 (0.42 to 3.02)	0.94 (0.52 to 1.70)
Zidovudine	500 mg/day PO × 21 days	1,200 mg/day PO × 14 days	4	1.31 (0.43 to 3.97)	1.30 (0.69 to 2.43)

NA - Not Available
* - 90% Confidence interval not reported

[See table 1 below]
No interpretive criteria have been established for testing *Neisseria gonorrhoeae*. This species is not usually tested.
A report of "susceptible" indicates that the pathogen is likely to be inhibited if the antimicrobial compound reaches the concentrations usually achievable. A report of "intermediate" indicates that the result should be considered equivocal, and, if the microorganism is not fully susceptible to alternative, clinically feasible drugs, the test should be repeated. This category implies possible clinical applicability in body sites where the drug is physiologically concentrated or in situations where high dosage of drug can be used. This category also provides a buffer zone which prevents small uncontrolled technical factors from causing major discrepancies in interpretation. A report of "resistant" indicates that the pathogen is not likely to be inhibited if the antimicrobial compound reaches the concentrations usually achievable; other therapy should be selected.
QUALITY CONTROL:
Standardized susceptibility test procedures require the use of quality control microorganisms to control the technical aspects of the test procedures. Standard azithromycin powder should provide the following range of values noted in Table 2. Quality control microorganisms are specific strains of organisms with intrinsic biological properties. QC strains are very stable strains which will give a standard and repeatable susceptibility pattern. The specific strains used for microbiological quality control are not clinically significant.

Table 2. Acceptable Quality Control Ranges for Azithromycin

QC Strain	Minimum Inhibitory Concentrations (µg/mL)	Disk Diffusion (zone diameters in mm)
Haemophilus influenzae ATCC 49247	1.0-4.0	13-21
Staphylococcus aureus ATCC 29213	0.5-2.0	
Staphylococcus aureus ATCC 25923		21-26
Streptococcus pneumoniae ATCC 49619	0.06-0.25	19-25

INDICATIONS AND USAGE
ZITHROMAX (azithromycin for injection) is indicated for the treatment of patients with infections caused by susceptible strains of the designated microorganisms in the conditions listed below. As recommended dosages, durations of therapy, and applicable patient populations vary among these infections, please see **DOSAGE AND ADMINISTRATION** for dosing recommendations.
Community-acquired pneumonia due to *Chlamydia pneumoniae, Haemophilus influenzae, Legionella pneumophila, Moraxella catarrhalis, Mycoplasma pneumoniae, Staphylococcus aureus,* or *Streptococcus pneumoniae* in patients who require initial intravenous therapy.
Pelvic inflammatory disease due to *Chlamydia trachomatis, Neisseria gonorrhoeae,* or *Mycoplasma hominis* in patients who require initial intravenous therapy. If anaerobic microorganisms are suspected of contributing to the infection, an antimicrobial agent with anaerobic activity should be administered in combination with ZITHROMAX.
ZITHROMAX® (azithromycin for injection) should be followed by ZITHROMAX by the oral route as required. (See **DOSAGE AND ADMINISTRATION.**)
Appropriate culture and susceptibility tests should be performed before treatment to determine the causative microorganism and its susceptibility to azithromycin. Therapy with ZITHROMAX may be initiated before results of these tests are known; once the results become available, antimicrobial therapy should be adjusted accordingly.
To reduce the development of drug-resistant bacteria and maintain the effectiveness of ZITHROMAX (azithromycin) and other antibacterial drugs, ZITHROMAX (azithromycin) should be used only to treat or prevent infections that are proven or strongly suspected to be caused by susceptible bacteria. When culture and susceptibility information are available, they should be considered in selecting or modifying antibacterial therapy. In the absence of such data, local epidemiology and susceptibility patterns may contribute to the empiric selection of therapy.

CONTRAINDICATIONS
ZITHROMAX is contraindicated in patients with known hypersensitivity to azithromycin, erythromycin, or any macrolide antibiotic.

WARNINGS
Serious allergic reactions, including angioedema, anaphylaxis, and dermatologic reactions including Stevens Johnson Syndrome and toxic epidermal necrolysis have been reported rarely in patients on azithromycin therapy. Although rare, fatalities have been reported. (See **CONTRAINDICATIONS.**) Despite initially successful symptomatic treatment of the allergic symptoms, when symptomatic therapy was discontinued, the allergic symptoms **recurred soon thereafter in some patients without further azithromycin exposure.** These patients required prolonged periods of observation and symptomatic treatment. The relationship of these episodes to the long tissue half-life of azithromycin and subsequent prolonged exposure to antigen is unknown at present.
If an allergic reaction occurs, the drug should be discontinued and appropriate therapy should be instituted. Physicians should be aware that reappearance of the allergic symptoms may occur when symptomatic therapy is discontinued.
Pseudomembranous colitis has been reported with nearly all antibacterial agents and may range in severity from mild to life-threatening. Therefore, it is important to consider this diagnosis in patients who present with diarrhea subsequent to the administration of antibacterial agents.
Treatment with antibacterial agents alters the normal flora of the colon and may permit overgrowth of clostridia. Studies indicate that a toxin produced by *Clostridium difficile* is a primary cause of "antibiotic-associated colitis."
After the diagnosis of pseudomembranous colitis has been established, therapeutic measures should be initiated. Mild cases of pseudomembranous colitis usually respond to discontinuation of the drug alone. In moderate to severe cases, consideration should be given to management with fluids and electrolytes, protein supplementation, and treatment with an antibacterial drug clinically effective against *Clostridium difficile* colitis.

PRECAUTIONS
General: Because azithromycin is principally eliminated via the liver, caution should be exercised when azithromycin is administered to patients with impaired hepatic function. Due to the limited data in subjects with GFR <10 mL/min, caution should be exercised when prescribing azithromycin in these patients. (See **CLINICAL PHARMACOLOGY - Special Populations - Renal Insufficiency.**)
ZITHROMAX (azithromycin for injection) should be reconstituted and diluted as directed and administered as an intravenous infusion over not less than 60 minutes. (See **DOSAGE AND ADMINISTRATION.**)
Local I.V. site reactions have been reported with the intravenous administration of azithromycin. The incidence and severity of these reactions were the same when 500 mg azithromycin were given over 1 hour (2 mg/mL as 250 mL infusion) or over 3 hours (1 mg/mL as 500 mL infusion). (See **ADVERSE REACTIONS.**) All volunteers who received infusate concentrations above 2.0 mg/mL experienced local I.V. site reactions and, therefore, higher concentrations should be avoided.
Prolonged cardiac repolarization and QT interval, imparting a risk of developing cardiac arrhythmia and *torsades de pointes*, have been seen in treatment with other macrolides. A similar effect with azithromycin cannot be completely ruled out in patients at increased risk for prolonged cardiac repolarization.
Prescribing ZITHROMAX (azithromycin) in the absence of a proven or strongly suspected bacterial infection or a prophylactic indication is unlikely to provide benefit to the patient and increases the risk of the development of drug-resistant bacteria.
Information for Patients:
Patients should be directed to discontinue azithromycin and contact a physician if any signs of an allergic reaction occur.
Patients should be counseled that antibacterial drugs including ZITHROMAX (azithromycin) should only be used to treat bacterial infections. They do not treat viral infections (e.g., the common cold). When ZITHROMAX (azithromycin) is prescribed to treat a bacterial infection, patients should be told that although it is common to feel better early in the course of the therapy, the medication should be taken exactly as directed. Skipping doses or not completing the full course of therapy may (1) decrease the effectiveness of the immediate treatment and (2) increase the likelihood that bacteria will develop resistance and will not be treatable by ZITHROMAX (azithromycin) or other antibacterial drugs in the future.
Drug Interactions: Co-administration of nelfinavir at steady-state with a single oral dose of azithromycin resulted in increased azithromycin serum concentrations. Although a dose adjustment of azithromycin is not recommended when administered in combination with nelfinavir, close monitoring for known side effects of azithromycin, such as liver enzyme abnormalities and hearing impairment, is warranted. (See **ADVERSE REACTIONS.**)
Azithromycin given by the oral route did not affect the prothrombin time response to a single dose of warfarin. However, prudent medical practice dictates careful monitoring of prothrombin time in all patients treated with azithromycin and warfarin concomitantly. Concurrent use of macrolides and warfarin in clinical practice has been associated with increased anticoagulant effects.
Drug interaction studies were performed with azithromycin and other drugs likely to be co-administered. (See CLINICAL PHARMACOLOGY-Drug-Drug Interactions.) When used in therapeutic doses, azithromycin had a modest effect on the pharmacokinetics of atorvastatin, carbamazepine, cetirizine, didanosine, efavirenz, fluconazole, indinavir, midazolam, rifabutin, sildenafil, theophylline (intravenous and oral), triazolam, trimethoprim/sulfamethoxazole or zidovudine. Co-administration with efavirenz or fluconazole had a modest effect on the pharmacokinetics of azithromycin. No dosage adjustment of either drug is recommended when azithromycin is coadministered with any of these agents.
Interactions with the drugs listed below have not been reported in clinical trials with azithromycin; however, no specific drug interaction studies have been performed to evaluate potential drug-drug interaction. Nonetheless, they have been observed with macrolide products. Until further data are developed regarding drug interactions when azithromycin and these drugs are used concomitantly, careful monitoring of patients is advised:

- Digoxin - elevated digoxin concentrations.
- Ergotamine or dihydroergotamine - acute ergot toxicity characterized by severe peripheral vasospasm and dysesthesia.
- Terfenadine, cyclosporine, hexobarbital and phenytoin - elevated concentrations.

Laboratory Test Interactions: There are no reported laboratory test interactions.
Carcinogenesis, Mutagenesis, Impairment of Fertility: Long-term studies in animals have not been performed to evaluate carcinogenic potential. Azithromycin has shown no mutagenic potential in standard laboratory tests: mouse

Table 2. Drug Interactions: Pharmacokinetic Parameters for Azithromycin in the Presence of Co-administered Drugs (See **PRECAUTIONS - Drug Interactions.**)

Co-administered Drug	Dose of Co-administered Drug	Dose of Azithromycin	n	Ratio (with/without co-administered drug) of Azithromycin Pharmacokinetic Parameters (90% CI); No Effect = 1.00	
				Mean C_{max}	Mean AUC
Efavirenz	400 mg/day × 7 days	600 mg PO on day 7	14	1.22 (1.04 to 1.42)	0.92*
Fluconazole	200 mg PO single dose	1,200 mg PO single dose	18	0.82 (0.66 to 1.02)	1.07 (0.94 to 1.22)
Nelfinavir	750 mg TID × 11 days	1,200 mg PO on day 9	14	2.36 (1.77 to 3.15)	2.12 (1.80 to 2.50)
Rifabutin	300 mg/day × 10 days	500 mg PO on day 1, then 250 mg/day on days 2-10	6	See footnote below	NA

NA – Not available
* - 90% Confidence interval not reported
Mean azithromycin concentrations one day after the last dose were 53 ng/mL when coadministered with 300 mg daily rifabutin and 49 ng/mL when coadministered with placebo.

Table 1. Susceptibility Interpretive Criteria for Azithromycin Susceptibility Test Result Interpretive Criteria

Pathogen	Minimum Inhibitory Concentrations (µg/mL)			Disk Diffusion (zone diameters in mm)		
	S	I	R[a]	S	I	R[a]
Haemophilus spp.	≤ 4	--	--	≥ 12	--	--
Staphylococcus aureus	≤ 2	4	≥ 8	≥ 18	14-17	≤ 13
Streptococci including S. pneumoniae[b]	≤ 0.5	1	≥ 2	≥ 18	14-17	≤ 13

[a] The current absence of data on resistant strains precludes defining any category other than "susceptible". If strains yield MIC results other than susceptible, they should be submitted to a reference laboratory for further testing.
[b] Susceptibility of streptococci including *S. pneumoniae* to azithromycin and other macrolides can be predicted by testing erythromycin.

Continued on next page

Zithromax IV—Cont.

lymphoma assay, human lymphocyte clastogenic assay, and mouse bone marrow clastogenic assay. No evidence of impaired fertility due to azithromycin was found.

Pregnancy: Teratogenic Effects. Pregnancy Category B: Reproduction studies have been performed in rats and mice at doses up to moderately maternally toxic dose concentrations (i.e., 200 mg/kg/day by the oral route). These doses, based on a mg/m^2 basis, are estimated to be 4 and 2 times, respectively, the human daily dose of 500 mg by the oral route. In the animal studies, no evidence of harm to the fetus due to azithromycin was found. There are, however, no adequate and well-controlled studies in pregnant women. Because animal reproduction studies are not always predictive of human response, azithromycin should be used during pregnancy only if clearly needed.

Nursing Mothers: It is not known whether azithromycin is excreted in human milk. Because many drugs are excreted in human milk, caution should be exercised when azithromycin is administered to a nursing woman.

Pediatric Use: Safety and effectiveness of azithromycin for injection in children or adolescents under 16 years have not been established. In controlled clinical studies, azithromycin has been administered to pediatric patients (age 6 months to 16 years) by the oral route. For information regarding the use of ZITHROMAX (azithromycin for oral suspension) in the treatment of pediatric patients, refer to the **INDICATIONS AND USAGE** and **DOSAGE AND ADMINISTRATION** sections of the prescribing information for ZITHROMAX (azithromycin for oral suspension) 100 mg/5 mL and 200 mg/5 mL bottles.

Geriatric Use: Pharmacokinetic studies with intravenous azithromycin have not been performed in older volunteers. Pharmacokinetics of azithromycin following oral administration in older volunteers (65-85 years old) were similar to those in younger volunteers (18-40 years old) for the 5-day therapeutic regimen.

In multiple-dose clinical trials of intravenous azithromycin in the treatment of community-acquired pneumonia, 45% of patients (188/414) were at least 65 years of age and 22% of patients (91/414) were at least 75 years of age. No overall differences in safety were observed between these subjects and younger subjects in terms of adverse events, laboratory abnormalities, and discontinuations. Similar decreases in clinical response were noted in azithromycin- and comparator-treated patients with increasing age.

ZITHROMAX (azithromycin for injection) contains 114 mg (4.96 mEq) of sodium per vial. At the usual recommended doses, patients would receive 114 mg (4.96 mEq) of sodium. The geriatric population may respond with a blunted natriuresis to salt loading. The total sodium content from dietary and non-dietary sources may be clinically important with regard to such diseases as congestive heart failure.

ADVERSE REACTIONS

In clinical trials of intravenous azithromycin for community-acquired pneumonia, in which 2-5 I.V. doses were given, most of the reported side effects were mild to moderate in severity and were reversible upon discontinuation of the drug. The majority of patients in these trials had one or more comorbid diseases and were receiving concomitant medications. Approximately 1.2% of the patients discontinued intravenous ZITHROMAX therapy, and a total of 2.4% discontinued azithromycin therapy by either the intravenous or oral route because of clinical or laboratory side effects.

In clinical trials conducted in patients with pelvic inflammatory disease, in which 1-2 I.V. doses were given, 2% of women who received monotherapy with azithromycin and 4% who received azithromycin plus metronidazole discontinued therapy due to clinical side effects.

Clinical side effects leading to discontinuations from these studies were most commonly gastrointestinal (abdominal pain, nausea, vomiting, diarrhea), and rashes; laboratory side effects leading to discontinuation were increases in transaminase levels and/or alkaline phosphatase levels.

Clinical:

Overall, the most common side effects associated with treatment in adult patients who received I.V./P.O. ZITHROMAX in studies of community-acquired pneumonia were related to the gastrointestinal system with diarrhea/loose stools (4.3%), nausea (3.9%), abdominal pain (2.7%), and vomiting (1.4%) being the most frequently reported. Approximately 12% of patients experienced a side effect related to the intravenous infusion; most common were pain at the injection site (6.5%) and local inflammation (3.1%).

The most common side effects associated with treatment in adult women who received I.V./P.O. ZITHROMAX® in studies of pelvic inflammatory disease were related to the gastrointestinal system. Diarrhea (8.5%) and nausea (6.6%) were most commonly reported, followed by vaginitis (2.8%), abdominal pain (1.9%), anorexia (1.9%), rash and pruritus (1.9%). When azithromycin was co-administered with metronidazole in these studies, a higher proportion of women experienced side effects of nausea (10.3%), abdominal pain (3.7%), vomiting (2.8%), application site reaction, stomatitis, dizziness, or dyspnea (all at 1.9%).

No other side effects occurred in patients on the multiple dose I.V./P.O. regimen of ZITHROMAX® in these studies with a frequency greater than 1%.

Side effects that occurred with a frequency of 1% or less included the following:

Gastrointestinal: dyspepsia, flatulence, mucositis, oral moniliasis, and gastritis
Nervous System: headache, somnolence
Allergic: bronchospasm
Special Senses: taste perversion

Post-Marketing Experience:

Adverse events reported with azithromycin during the post-marketing period in adult and/or pediatric patients for which a causal relationship may not be established include:

Allergic: Arthralgia, edema, urticaria and angioedema.
Cardiovascular: Arrhythmias including ventricular tachycardia and hypotension. There have been rare reports of QT prolongation and *torsades de pointes*.
Gastrointestinal: Anorexia, constipation, dyspepsia, flatulence, vomiting/diarrhea rarely resulting in dehydration, pseudomembranous colitis, pancreatitis, oral candidiasis and rare reports of tongue discoloration.
General: Asthenia, paresthesia, fatigue, malaise and anaphylaxis (rarely fatal).
Genitourinary: Interstitial nephritis and acute renal failure and vaginitis.
Hematopoietic: Thrombocytopenia.
Liver/Biliary: Abnormal liver function including hepatitis and cholestatic jaundice, as well as rare cases of hepatic necrosis and hepatic failure, some of which have resulted in death.
Nervous System: Convulsions, dizziness/vertigo, headache, somnolence, hyperactivity, nervousness, agitation and syncope.
Psychiatric: Aggressive reaction and anxiety.
Skin/Appendages: Pruritus, rarely serious skin reactions including erythema multiforme, Stevens-Johnson Syndrome and toxic epidermal necrolysis.
Special Senses: Hearing disturbances including hearing loss, deafness and/or tinnitus and rare reports of taste perversion.

Laboratory Abnormalities:

Significant abnormalities (irrespective of drug relationship) occurring during the clinical trials were reported as follows:
with an incidence of 4-6%, elevated ALT (SGPT), AST (SGOT), creatinine
with an incidence of 1-3%, elevated LDH, bilirubin
with an incidence of less than 1%, leukopenia, neutropenia, decreased platelet count, and elevated serum alkaline phosphatase

When follow-up was provided, changes in laboratory tests appeared to be reversible.

In multiple-dose clinical trials involving more than 750 patients treated with ZITHROMAX (I.V./P.O.), less than 2% of patients discontinued azithromycin therapy because of treatment-related liver enzyme abnormalities.

DOSAGE AND ADMINISTRATION

(See INDICATIONS AND USAGE and CLINICAL PHARMACOLOGY.)

The recommended dose of ZITHROMAX (azithromycin for injection) for the treatment of adult patients with community-acquired pneumonia due to the indicated organisms is: 500 mg as a single daily dose by the intravenous route for at least two days. Intravenous therapy should be followed by azithromycin by the oral route at a single, daily dose of 500 mg, administered as two 250-mg tablets to complete a 7- to 10-day course of therapy. The timing of the switch to oral therapy should be done at the discretion of the physician and in accordance with clinical response.

The recommended dose of ZITHROMAX (azithromycin) for the treatment of adult patients with pelvic inflammatory disease due to the indicated organisms is: 500 mg as a single daily dose by the intravenous route for one or two days. Intravenous therapy should be followed by azithromycin by the oral route at a single, daily dose of 250 mg to complete a 7-day course of therapy. The timing of the switch to oral therapy should be done at the discretion of the physician and in accordance with clinical response. If anaerobic microorganisms are suspected of contributing to the infection, an antimicrobial agent with anaerobic activity should be administered in combination with ZITHROMAX.

Renal Insufficiency:

No dosage adjustment is recommended for subjects with renal impairment (GFR $\leq$ 80 mL/min). The mean AUC_{0-120} was similar in subjects with GFR 10-80 mL/min compared to subjects with normal renal function, whereas it increased 35% in subjects with GFR <10 mL/min compared to subjects with normal renal function. Caution should be exercised when azithromycin is administered to subjects with severe renal impairment. (See **CLINICAL PHARMACOLOGY, Special Populations, Renal Insufficiency.**)

Hepatic Insufficiency:

The pharmacokinetics of azithromycin in subjects with hepatic impairment have not been established. No dose adjustment recommendations can be made in patients with impaired hepatic function (See **CLINICAL PHARMACOLOGY, Special Populations, Hepatic Insufficiency.**)

No dosage adjustment is recommended based on age or gender. (See **CLINICAL PHARMACOLOGY, Special Populations.**)

The infusate concentration and rate of infusion for ZITHROMAX (azithromycin for injection) should be either 1 mg/mL over 3 hours or 2 mg/mL over 1 hour.

Preparation of the solution for intravenous administration is as follows:

Reconstitution

Prepare the initial solution of ZITHROMAX (azithromycin for injection) by adding 4.8 mL of Sterile Water For Injection to the 500 mg vial and shaking the vial until all of the drug is dissolved. Since ZITHROMAX (azithromycin for injection) is supplied under vacuum, it is recommended that a standard 5 mL (non-automated) syringe be used to ensure that the exact amount of 4.8 mL of Sterile Water is dispensed. Each mL of reconstituted solution contains 100 mg azithromycin. Reconstituted solution is stable for 24 hours when stored below 30°C or 86°F.

Parenteral drug products should be inspected visually for particulate matter prior to administration. If particulate matter is evident in reconstituted fluids, the drug solution should be discarded.

Dilute this solution further prior to administration as instructed below.

Dilution

To provide azithromycin over a concentration range of 1.0-2.0 mg/mL, transfer 5 mL of the 100 mg/mL azithromycin solution into the appropriate amount of any of the diluents listed below:

Normal Saline (0.9% sodium chloride)
1/2 Normal Saline (0.45% sodium chloride)
5% Dextrose in Water
Lactated Ringer's Solution
5% Dextrose in 1/2 Normal Saline (0.45% sodium chloride) with 20 mEq KCl
5% Dextrose in Lactated Ringer's Solution
5% Dextrose in 1/3 Normal Saline (0.3% sodium chloride)
5% Dextrose in 1/2 Normal Saline (0.45% sodium chloride)
Normosol®-M in 5% Dextrose
Normosol®-R in 5% Dextrose

When used with the Vial-Mate™ drug reconstitution device, please reference the Vial-Mate™ instructions for assembly and reconstitution.

Final Infusion Solution Concentration (mg/mL)	Amount of Diluent (mL)
1.0 mg/mL	500 mL
2.0 mg/mL	250 mL

It is recommended that a 500-mg dose of ZITHROMAX (azithromycin for injection), diluted as above, be infused over a period of not less than 60 minutes.

ZITHROMAX (azithromycin for injection) should not be given as a bolus or as an intramuscular injection.

Other intravenous substances, additives, or medications should not be added to ZITHROMAX (azithromycin for injection), or infused simultaneously through the same intravenous line.

Storage

When diluted according to the instructions (1.0 mg/mL to 2.0 mg/mL), ZITHROMAX (azithromycin for injection) is stable for 24 hours at or below room temperature (30°C or 86°F), or for 7 days if stored under refrigeration (5°C or 41°F).

HOW SUPPLIED

ZITHROMAX® (azithromycin for injection) is supplied in lyophilized form under a vacuum in a 10-mL vial equivalent to 500 mg of azithromycin for intravenous administration. Each vial also contains sodium hydroxide and 413.6 mg citric acid.

These are packaged as follows:

10 vials of 500 mg	NDC 0069-3150-83
10 vials of 500 mg with 1 Vial-Mate™ Adaptor each	NDC 0069-3150-14

CLINICAL STUDIES

Community-Acquired Pneumonia

In a controlled study of community-acquired pneumonia performed in the U.S., azithromycin (500 mg as a single daily dose by the intravenous route for 2-5 days, followed by 500 mg/day by the oral route to complete 7-10 days therapy) was compared to cefuroxime (2250 mg/day in three divided doses by the intravenous route for 2-5 days followed by 1000 mg/day in two divided doses by the oral route to complete 7-10 days therapy), with or without erythromycin. For the 291 patients who were evaluable for clinical efficacy, the clinical outcome rates, i.e., cure, improved, and success (cure + improved) among the 277 patients seen at 10-14 days post-therapy were as follows:

Clinical Outcome	Azithromycin	Comparator
Cure	46%	44%
Improved	32%	30%
Success (Cure + Improved)	78%	74%

In a separate, uncontrolled clinical and microbiological trial performed in the U.S., 94 patients with community-acquired pneumonia who received azithromycin in the same regimen were evaluable for clinical efficacy. The clinical outcome rates, i.e., cure, improved, and success (cure + improved) among the 84 patients seen at 10-14 days post-therapy were as follows:

Clinical Outcome	Azithromycin
Cure	60%
Improved	29%
Success (Cure + Improved)	89%

Microbiological determinations in both trials were made at the pre-treatment visit and, where applicable, were reassessed at later visits. Serological testing was done on baseline and final visit specimens. The following combined presumptive bacteriological eradication rates were obtained from the evaluable groups:

Combined Bacteriological Eradication Rates for Azithromycin:

(at last completed visit)	Azithromycin
S. pneumoniae	64/67 (96%)[a]
H. influenzae	41/43 (95%)
M. catarrhalis	9/10
S. aureus	9/10

[a] Nineteen of twenty-four patients (79%) with positive blood cultures for *S. pneumoniae* were cured (intent to treat analysis) with eradication of the pathogen.

The presumed bacteriological outcomes at 10-14 days post-therapy for patients treated with azithromycin with evidence (serology and/or culture) of atypical pathogens for both trials were as follows:

Evidence of Infection	Total	Cure	Improved	Cure + Improved
Mycoplasma pneumoniae	18	11 (61%)	5 (28%)	16 (89%)
Chlamydia pneumoniae	34	15 (44%)	13 (38%)	28 (82%)
Legionella pneumophila	16	5 (31%)	8 (50%)	13 (81%)

ANIMAL TOXICOLOGY

Phospholipidosis (intracellular phospholipid accumulation) has been observed in some tissues of mice, rats, and dogs given multiple doses of azithromycin. It has been demonstrated in numerous organ systems (e.g., eye, dorsal root ganglia, liver, gallbladder, kidney, spleen, and pancreas) in dogs treated with azithromycin at doses which, expressed on the basis of mg/m^2, are approximately equal to the recommended adult human dose, and in rats treated at doses approximately one-sixth of the recommended adult human dose. This effect has been shown to be reversible after cessation of azithromycin treatment. Phospholipidosis has been observed to a similar extent in the tissues of neonatal rats and dogs given daily doses of azithromycin ranging from 10 days to 30 days. Based on the pharmacokinetic data, phospholipidosis has been seen in the rat (30 mg/kg dose) at observed C_{max} value of 1.3 µg/mL (six times greater than the observed C_{max} of 0.216 µg/mL at the pediatric dose of 10 mg/kg). Similarly, it has been shown in the dog (10 mg/kg dose) at observed C_{max} value of 1.5 µg/mL (seven times greater than the observed same C_{max} and drug dose in the studied pediatric population). On a mg/m^2 basis, 30 mg/kg dose in the neonatal rat (135 mg/m^2) and 10 mg/kg dose in the neonatal dog (79 mg/m^2) are approximately 0.45 and 0.3 times, respectively, the recommended dose in the pediatric patients with an average body weight of 25 kg. Phospholipidosis, similar to that seen in the adult animals, is reversible after cessation of azithromycin treatment. The significance of these findings for animals and for humans is unknown.

REFERENCES

1. National Committee for Clinical Laboratory Standards, *Methods for Dilution Antimicrobial Susceptibility Tests for Bacteria That Grow Aerobically* – Fifth Edition. Approved Standard NCCLS Document M7-A5, Vol. 20, No. 2 (ISBN 1-56238-394-9). NCCLS, 940 West Valley Road, Suite 1400, Wayne, PA 19087-1898, January, 2000.
2. National Committee for Clinical Laboratory Standards, *Performance Standards for Antimicrobial Disk Susceptibility Tests* - Seventh Edition. Approved Standard NCCLS Document M2-A7, Vol. 20, No. 1 (ISBN 1-56238-393-0). NCCLS, 940 West Valley Road, Suite 1400, Wayne, PA 19087-1898, January, 2000.
3. National Committee for Clinical Laboratory Standards. *Performance Standards for Antimicrobial Susceptibility Testing* – Eleventh Informational Supplement. NCCLS Document M100-S11, Vol. 21, No. 1 (ISBN 1-56238-426-0). NCCLS, 940 West Valley Road, Suite 1400, Wayne, PA 19087-1898, January, 2001.

Rx only

Licensed from Pliva

Distributed by:
Pfizer Labs
Division of Pfizer Inc
NY, NY 10017
70-5191-00-8 Revised October 2003

ZOLOFT® ℞

[zō-lŏft]

(sertraline hydrochloride)
Tablets and Oral Concentrate

DESCRIPTION

ZOLOFT® (sertraline hydrochloride) is a selective serotonin reuptake inhibitor (SSRI) for oral administration. It has a molecular weight of 342.7. Sertraline hydrochloride has the following chemical name: (1S-cis)-4-(3,4-dichlorophenyl)-1,2,3,4-tetrahydro-N-methyl-1-naphthalenamine hydrochloride. The empirical formula $C_{17}H_{17}NCl_2 \bullet HCl$ is represented by the following structural formula:

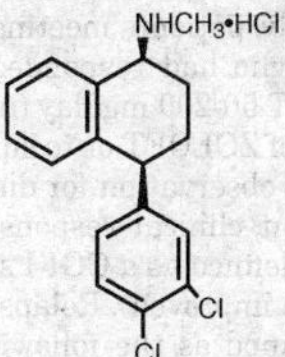

Sertraline hydrochloride is a white crystalline powder that is slightly soluble in water and isopropyl alcohol, and sparingly soluble in ethanol.

ZOLOFT is supplied for oral administration as scored tablets containing sertraline hydrochloride equivalent to 25, 50 and 100 mg of sertraline and the following inactive ingredients: dibasic calcium phosphate dihydrate, D & C Yellow #10 aluminum lake (in 25 mg tablet), FD & C Blue #1 aluminum lake (in 25 mg tablet), FD & C Red #40 aluminum lake (in 25 mg tablet), FD & C Blue #2 aluminum lake (in 50 mg tablet), hydroxypropyl cellulose, hypromellose, magnesium stearate, microcrystalline cellulose, polyethylene glycol, polysorbate 80, sodium starch glycolate, synthetic yellow iron oxide (in 100 mg tablet), and titanium dioxide.

ZOLOFT oral concentrate is available in a multidose 60 mL bottle. Each mL of solution contains sertraline hydrochloride equivalent to 20 mg of sertraline. The solution contains the following inactive ingredients: glycerin, alcohol (12%), menthol, butylated hydroxytoluene (BHT). The oral concentrate must be diluted prior to administration (see PRECAUTIONS, Information for Patients and DOSAGE AND ADMINISTRATION).

CLINICAL PHARMACOLOGY

Pharmacodynamics

The mechanism of action of sertraline is presumed to be linked to its inhibition of CNS neuronal uptake of serotonin (5HT). Studies at clinically relevant doses in man have demonstrated that sertraline blocks the uptake of serotonin into human platelets. *In vitro* studies in animals also suggest that sertraline is a potent and selective inhibitor of neuronal serotonin reuptake and has only very weak effects on norepinephrine and dopamine neuronal reuptake. *In vitro* studies have shown that sertraline has no significant affinity for adrenergic ($alpha_1$, $alpha_2$, beta), cholinergic, GABA, dopaminergic, histaminergic, serotonergic ($5HT_{1A}$, $5HT_{1B}$, $5HT_2$), or benzodiazepine receptors; antagonism of such receptors has been hypothesized to be associated with various anticholinergic, sedative, and cardiovascular effects for other psychotropic drugs. The chronic administration of sertraline was found in animals to downregulate brain norepinephrine receptors, as has been observed with other drugs effective in the treatment of major depressive disorder. Sertraline does not inhibit monoamine oxidase.

Pharmacokinetics

Systemic Bioavailability–In man, following oral once-daily dosing over the range of 50 to 200 mg for 14 days, mean peak plasma concentrations (Cmax) of sertraline occurred between 4.5 to 8.4 hours post-dosing. The average terminal elimination half-life of plasma sertraline is about 26 hours. Based on this pharmacokinetic parameter, steady-state sertraline plasma levels should be achieved after approximately one week of once-daily dosing. Linear dose-proportional pharmacokinetics were demonstrated in a single dose study in which the Cmax and area under the plasma concentration time curve (AUC) of sertraline were proportional to dose over a range of 50 to 200 mg. Consistent with the terminal elimination half-life, there is an approximately two-fold accumulation, compared to a single dose, of sertraline with repeated dosing over a 50 to 200 mg dose range. The single dose bioavailability of sertraline tablets is approximately equal to an equivalent dose of solution.

In a relative bioavailability study comparing the pharmacokinetics of 100 mg sertraline as the oral solution to a 100 mg sertraline tablet in 16 healthy adults, the solution to tablet ratio of geometric mean AUC and Cmax values were 114.8% and 120.6%, respectively. 90% confidence intervals (CI) were within the range of 80-125% with the exception of the upper 90% CI limit for Cmax which was 126.5%.

The effects of food on the bioavailability of the sertraline tablet and oral concentrate were studied in subjects administered a single dose with and without food. For the tablet, AUC was slightly increased when drug was administered with food but the Cmax was 25% greater, while the time to reach peak plasma concentration (Tmax) decreased from 8 hours post-dosing to 5.5 hours. For the oral concentrate, Tmax was slightly prolonged from 5.9 hours to 7.0 hours with food.

Metabolism–Sertraline undergoes extensive first pass metabolism. The principal initial pathway of metabolism for sertraline is N-demethylation. N-desmethylsertraline has a plasma terminal elimination half-life of 62 to 104 hours. Both *in vitro* biochemical and *in vivo* pharmacological testing have shown N-desmethylsertraline to be substantially less active than sertraline. Both sertraline and N-desmethylsertraline undergo oxidative deamination and subsequent reduction, hydroxylation, and glucuronide conjugation. In a study of radiolabeled sertraline involving two healthy male subjects, sertraline accounted for less than 5% of the plasma radioactivity. About 40-45% of the administered radioactivity was recovered in urine in 9 days. Unchanged sertraline was not detectable in the urine. For the same period, about 40-45% of the administered radioactivity was accounted for in feces, including 12-14% unchanged sertraline.

Desmethylsertraline exhibits time-related, dose dependent increases in AUC (0-24 hour), Cmax and Cmin, with about a 5-9 fold increase in these pharmacokinetic parameters between day 1 and day 14.

Protein Binding–*In vitro* protein binding studies performed with radiolabeled ^3H-sertraline showed that sertraline is highly bound to serum proteins (98%) in the range of 20 to 500 ng/mL. However, at up to 300 and 200 ng/mL concentrations, respectively, sertraline and N-desmethylsertraline did not alter the plasma protein binding of two other highly protein bound drugs, viz., warfarin and propranolol (see PRECAUTIONS).

Pediatric Pharmacokinetics–Sertraline pharmacokinetics were evaluated in a group of 61 pediatric patients (29 aged 6-12 years, 32 aged 13-17 years) with a DSM-III-R diagnosis of major depressive disorder or obsessive-compulsive disorder. Patients included both males (N=28) and females (N=33). During 42 days of chronic sertraline dosing, sertraline was titrated up to 200 mg/day and maintained at that dose for a minimum of 11 days. On the final day of sertraline 200 mg/day, the 6-12 year old group exhibited a mean sertraline AUC (0-24 hr) of 3107 ng-hr/mL, mean Cmax of 165 ng/mL, and mean half-life of 26.2 hr. The 13-17 year old group exhibited a mean sertraline AUC (0-24 hr) of 2296 ng-hr/mL, mean Cmax of 123 ng/mL, and mean half-life of 27.8 hr. Higher plasma levels in the 6-12 year old group were largely attributable to patients with lower body weights. No gender associated differences were observed. By comparison, a group of 22 separately studied adults between 18 and 45 years of age (11 male, 11 female) received 30 days of 200 mg/day sertraline and exhibited a mean sertraline AUC (0-24 hr) of 2570 ng-hr/mL, mean Cmax of 142 ng/mL, and mean half-life of 27.2 hr. Relative to the adults, both the 6-12 year olds and the 13-17 year olds showed about 22% lower AUC (0-24 hr) and Cmax values when plasma concentration was adjusted for weight. These data suggest that pediatric patients metabolize sertraline with slightly greater efficiency than adults. Nevertheless, lower doses may be advisable for pediatric patients given their lower body weights, especially in very young patients, in order to avoid excessive plasma levels (see DOSAGE AND ADMINISTRATION).

Age–Sertraline plasma clearance in a group of 16 (8 male, 8 female) elderly patients treated for 14 days at a dose of 100 mg/day was approximately 40% lower than in a similarly studied group of younger (25 to 32 y.o.) individuals. Steady-state, therefore, should be achieved after 2 to 3 weeks in older patients. The same study showed a decreased clearance of desmethylsertraline in older males, but not in older females.

Liver Disease–As might be predicted from its primary site of metabolism, liver impairment can affect the elimination of sertraline. In patients with chronic mild liver impairment (N=10, 8 patients with Child-Pugh scores of 5-6 and 2 patients with Child-Pugh scores of 7-8) who received 50 mg sertraline per day maintained for 21 days, sertraline clearance was reduced, resulting in approximately 3-fold greater exposure compared to age-matched volunteers with no hepatic impairment (N=10). The exposure to desmethylsertraline was approximately 2-fold greater compared to age-matched volunteers with no hepatic impairment. There were no significant differences in plasma protein binding observed between the two groups. The effects of sertraline in patients with moderate and severe hepatic impairment have not been studied. The results suggest that the use of sertraline in patients with liver disease must be approached with caution. If sertraline is administered to patients with liver impairment, a lower or less frequent dose should be used (see PRECAUTIONS and DOSAGE AND ADMINISTRATION).

Renal Disease–Sertraline is extensively metabolized and excretion of unchanged drug in urine is a minor route of elimination. In volunteers with mild to moderate (CLcr=30-60 mL/min), moderate to severe (CLcr=10-29 mL/min) or severe (receiving hemodialysis) renal impairment (N=10 each group), the pharmacokinetics and protein binding of 200 mg sertraline per day maintained for 21 days were not altered compared to age-matched volunteers (N=12) with no renal impairment. Thus sertraline multiple dose pharmacokinetics appear to be unaffected by renal impairment (see PRECAUTIONS).

Clinical Trials

Major Depressive Disorder–The efficacy of ZOLOFT as a treatment for major depressive disorder was established in two placebo-controlled studies in adult outpatients meeting DSM-III criteria for major depressive disorder. Study 1 was an 8-week study with flexible dosing of ZOLOFT in a range of 50 to 200 mg/day; the mean dose for completers was 145 mg/day. Study 2 was a 6-week fixed-dose study, including ZOLOFT doses of 50, 100, and 200 mg/day. Overall, these studies demonstrated ZOLOFT to be superior to placebo on the Hamilton Depression Rating Scale and the Clinical Global Impression Severity and Improvement scales. Study 2 was not readily interpretable regarding a dose response relationship for effectiveness.

Study 3 involved depressed outpatients who had responded by the end of an initial 8-week open treatment phase on ZOLOFT 50-200 mg/day. These patients (N=295) were randomized to continuation for 44 weeks on double-blind ZOLOFT 50-200 mg/day or placebo. A statistically significantly lower relapse rate was observed for patients taking ZOLOFT compared to those on placebo. The mean dose for completers was 70 mg/day.

Continued on next page

Zoloft—Cont.

Analyses for gender effects on outcome did not suggest any differential responsiveness on the basis of sex.

Obsessive-Compulsive Disorder (OCD)–The effectiveness of ZOLOFT in the treatment of OCD was demonstrated in three multicenter placebo-controlled studies of adult outpatients (Studies 1-3). Patients in all studies had moderate to severe OCD (DSM-III or DSM-III-R) with mean baseline ratings on the Yale–Brown Obsessive-Compulsive Scale (YBOCS) total score ranging from 23 to 25.

Study 1 was an 8-week study with flexible dosing of ZOLOFT in a range of 50 to 200 mg/day; the mean dose for completers was 186 mg/day. Patients receiving ZOLOFT experienced a mean reduction of approximately 4 points on the YBOCS total score which was significantly greater than the mean reduction of 2 points in placebo-treated patients.

Study 2 was a 12-week fixed-dose study, including ZOLOFT doses of 50, 100, and 200 mg/day. Patients receiving ZOLOFT doses of 50 and 200 mg/day experienced mean reductions of approximately 6 points on the YBOCS total score which were significantly greater than the approximately 3 point reduction in placebo-treated patients.

Study 3 was a 12-week study with flexible dosing of ZOLOFT in a range of 50 to 200 mg/day; the mean dose for completers was 185 mg/day. Patients receiving ZOLOFT experienced a mean reduction of approximately 7 points on the YBOCS total score which was significantly greater than the mean reduction of approximately 4 points in placebo-treated patients.

Analyses for age and gender effects on outcome did not suggest any differential responsiveness on the basis of age or sex.

The effectiveness of ZOLOFT for the treatment of OCD was also demonstrated in a 12-week, multicenter, placebo-controlled, parallel group study in a pediatric outpatient population (children and adolescents, ages 6-17). Patients receiving ZOLOFT in this study were initiated at doses of either 25 mg/day (children, ages 6-12) or 50 mg/day (adolescents, ages 13-17), and then titrated over the next four weeks to a maximum dose of 200 mg/day, as tolerated. The mean dose for completers was 178 mg/day. Dosing was once a day in the morning or evening. Patients in this study had moderate to severe OCD (DSM-III-R) with mean baseline ratings on the Children's Yale-Brown Obsessive-Compulsive Scale (CYBOCS) total score of 22. Patients receiving sertraline experienced a mean reduction of approximately 7 units on the CYBOCS total score which was significantly greater than the 3 unit reduction for placebo patients. Analyses for age and gender effects on outcome did not suggest any differential responsiveness on the basis of age or sex.

In a longer-term study, patients meeting DSM-III-R criteria for OCD who had responded during a 52-week single-blind trial on ZOLOFT 50-200 mg/day (n=224) were randomized to continuation of ZOLOFT or to substitution of placebo for up to 28 weeks of observation for discontinuation due to relapse or insufficient clinical response. Response during the single-blind phase was defined as a decrease in the YBOCS score of ≥ 25% compared to baseline and a CGI-I of 1 (very much improved), 2 (much improved) or 3 (minimally improved). Relapse during the double-blind phase was defined as the following conditions being met (on three consecutive visits for 1 and 2, and for visit 3 for condition 3): (1) YBOCS score increased by ≥ 5 points, to a minimum of 20, relative to baseline; (2) CGI-I increased by ≥ one point; and (3) worsening of the patient's condition in the investigator's judgment, to justify alternative treatment. Insufficient clinical response indicated a worsening of the patient's condition that resulted in study discontinuation, as assessed by the investigator. Patients receiving continued ZOLOFT treatment experienced a significantly lower rate of discontinuation due to relapse or insufficient clinical response over the subsequent 28 weeks compared to those receiving placebo. This pattern was demonstrated in male and female subjects.

Panic Disorder–The effectiveness of ZOLOFT in the treatment of panic disorder was demonstrated in three double-blind, placebo-controlled studies (Studies 1-3) of adult outpatients who had a primary diagnosis of panic disorder (DSM-III-R), with or without agoraphobia.

Studies 1 and 2 were 10-week flexible dose studies. ZOLOFT was initiated at 25 mg/day for the first week, and then patients were dosed in a range of 50-200 mg/day on the basis of clinical response and toleration. The mean ZOLOFT doses for completers to 10 weeks were 131 mg/day and 144 mg/day, respectively, for Studies 1 and 2. In these studies, ZOLOFT was shown to be significantly more effective than placebo on change from baseline in panic attack frequency and on the Clinical Global Impression Severity of Illness and Global Improvement scores. The difference between ZOLOFT and placebo in reduction from baseline in the number of full panic attacks was approximately 2 panic attacks per week in both studies.

Study 3 was a 12-week fixed-dose study, including ZOLOFT doses of 50, 100, and 200 mg/day. Patients receiving ZOLOFT experienced a significantly greater reduction in panic attack frequency than patients receiving placebo. Study 3 was not readily interpretable regarding a dose response relationship for effectiveness.

Subgroup analyses did not indicate that there were any differences in treatment outcomes as a function of age, race, or gender.

In a longer-term study, patients meeting DSM-III-R criteria for Panic Disorder who had responded during a 52-week open trial on ZOLOFT 50-200 mg/day (n=183) were randomized to continuation of ZOLOFT or to substitution of placebo for up to 28 weeks of observation for discontinuation due to relapse or insufficient clinical response. Response during the open phase was defined as a CGI-I score of 1 (very much improved) or 2 (much improved). Relapse during the double-blind phase was defined as the following conditions being met on three consecutive visits: (1) CGI-I ≥ 3; (2) meets DSM-III-R criteria for Panic Disorder; (3) number of panic attacks greater than at baseline. Insufficient clinical response indicated a worsening of the patient's condition that resulted in study discontinuation, as assessed by the investigator. Patients receiving continued ZOLOFT treatment experienced a significantly lower rate of discontinuation due to relapse or insufficient clinical response over the subsequent 28 weeks compared to those receiving placebo. This pattern was demonstrated in male and female subjects.

Posttraumatic Stress Disorder (PTSD)–The effectiveness of ZOLOFT in the treatment of PTSD was established in two multicenter placebo-controlled studies (Studies 1-2) of adult outpatients who met DSM-III-R criteria for PTSD. The mean duration of PTSD for these patients was 12 years (Studies 1 and 2 combined) and 44% of patients (169 of the 385 patients treated) had secondary depressive disorder.

Studies 1 and 2 were 12-week flexible dose studies. ZOLOFT was initiated at 25 mg/day for the first week, and patients were then dosed in the range of 50-200 mg/day on the basis of clinical response and toleration. The mean ZOLOFT dose for completers was 146 mg/day and 151 mg/day, respectively for Studies 1 and 2. Study outcome was assessed by the Clinician-Administered PTSD Scale Part 2 (CAPS) which is a multi-item instrument that measures the three PTSD diagnostic symptom clusters of reexperiencing/intrusion, avoidance/numbing, and hyperarousal as well as the patient-rated Impact of Event Scale (IES) which measures intrusion and avoidance symptoms. ZOLOFT was shown to be significantly more effective than placebo on change from baseline to endpoint on the CAPS, IES and on the Clinical Global Impressions (CGI) Severity of Illness and Global Improvement scores. In two additional placebo-controlled PTSD trials, the difference in response to treatment between patients receiving ZOLOFT and patients receiving placebo was not statistically significant. One of these additional studies was conducted in patients similar to those recruited for Studies 1 and 2, while the second additional study was conducted in predominantly male veterans.

As PTSD is a more common disorder in women than men, the majority (76%) of patients in these trials were women (152 and 139 women on sertraline and placebo versus 39 and 55 men on sertraline and placebo; Studies 1 and 2 combined). Post hoc exploratory analyses revealed a significant difference between ZOLOFT and placebo on the CAPS, IES and CGI in women, regardless of baseline diagnosis of comorbid major depressive disorder, but essentially no effect in the relatively smaller number of men in these studies. The clinical significance of this apparent gender interaction is unknown at this time. There was insufficient information to determine the effect of race or age on outcome.

In a longer-term study, patients meeting DSM-III-R criteria for PTSD who had responded during a 24-week open trial on ZOLOFT 50-200 mg/day (n=96) were randomized to continuation of ZOLOFT or to substitution of placebo for up to 28 weeks of observation for relapse. Response during the open phase was defined as a CGI-I of 1 (very much improved) or 2 (much improved), and a decrease in the CAPS-2 score of > 30% compared to baseline. Relapse during the double-blind phase was defined as the following conditions being met on two consecutive visits: (1) CGI-I ≥ 3; (2) CAPS-2 score increased by ≥ 30% and by ≥ 15 points relative to baseline; and (3) worsening of the patient's condition in the investigator's judgment. Patients receiving continued ZOLOFT treatment experienced significantly lower relapse rates over the subsequent 28 weeks compared to those receiving placebo. This pattern was demonstrated in male and female subjects.

Premenstrual Dysphoric Disorder (PMDD) – The effectiveness of ZOLOFT for the treatment of PMDD was established in two double-blind, parallel group, placebo-controlled flexible dose trials (Studies 1 and 2) conducted over 3 menstrual cycles. Patients in Study 1 met DSM-III-R criteria for Late Luteal Phase Dysphoric Disorder (LLPDD), the clinical entity now referred to as Premenstrual Dysphoric Disorder (PMDD) in DSM-IV. Patients in Study 2 met DSM-IV criteria for PMDD. Study 1 utilized daily dosing throughout the study, while Study 2 utilized luteal phase dosing for the 2 weeks prior to the onset of menses. The mean duration of PMDD symptoms for these patients was approximately 10.5 years in both studies. Patients on oral contraceptives were excluded from these trials; therefore, the efficacy of sertraline in combination with oral contraceptives for the treatment of PMDD is unknown.

Efficacy was assessed with the Daily Record of Severity of Problems (DRSP), a patient-rated instrument that mirrors the diagnostic criteria for PMDD as identified in the DSM-IV, and includes assessments for mood, physical symptoms, and other symptoms. Other efficacy assessments included the Hamilton Depression Rating Scale (HAMD-17), and the Clinical Global Impression Severity of Illness (CGI-S) and Improvement (CGI-I) scores.

In Study 1, involving n=251 randomized patients, ZOLOFT treatment was initiated at 50 mg/day and administered daily throughout the menstrual cycle. In subsequent cycles, patients were dosed in the range of 50-150 mg/day on the basis of clinical response and toleration. The mean dose for completers was 102 mg/day. ZOLOFT administered daily throughout the menstrual cycle was significantly more effective than placebo on change from baseline to endpoint on the DRSP total score, the HAMD-17 total score, and the CGI-S score, as well as the CGI-I score at endpoint.

In Study 2, involving n=281 randomized patients, ZOLOFT treatment was initiated at 50 mg/day in the late luteal phase (last 2 weeks) of each menstrual cycle and then discontinued at the onset of menses. In subsequent cycles, patients were dosed in the range of 50-100 mg/day in the luteal phase of each cycle, on the basis of clinical response and toleration. Patients who were titrated to 100 mg/day received 50 mg/day for the first 3 days of the cycle, then 100 mg/day for the remainder of the cycle. The mean ZOLOFT dose for completers was 74 mg/day. ZOLOFT administered in the late luteal phase of the menstrual cycle was significantly more effective than placebo on change from baseline to endpoint on the DRSP total score and the CGI-S score, as well as the CGI-I score at endpoint.

There was insufficient information to determine the effect of race or age on outcome in these studies.

Social Anxiety Disorder – The effectiveness of ZOLOFT in the treatment of social anxiety disorder (also known as social phobia) was established in two multicenter placebo-controlled studies (Study 1 and 2) of adult outpatients who met DSM-IV criteria for social anxiety disorder.

Study 1 was a 12-week, multicenter, flexible dose study comparing ZOLOFT (50-200 mg/day) to placebo, in which ZOLOFT was initiated at 25 mg/day for the first week. Study outcome was assessed by (a) the Liebowitz Social Anxiety Scale (LSAS), a 24-item clinician administered instrument that measures fear, anxiety and avoidance of social and performance situations, and by (b) the proportion of responders as defined by the Clinical Global Impression of Improvement (CGI-I) criterion of CGI-I ≤ 2 (very much or much improved). ZOLOFT was statistically significantly more effective than placebo as measured by the LSAS and the percentage of responders.

Study 2 was a 20-week, multicenter, flexible dose study that compared ZOLOFT (50-200 mg/day) to placebo. Study outcome was assessed by the (a) Duke Brief Social Phobia Scale (BSPS), a multi-item clinician-rated instrument that measures fear, avoidance and physiologic response to social or performance situations, (b) the Marks Fear Questionnaire Social Phobia Subscale (FQ-SPS), a 5-item patient-rated instrument that measures change in the severity of phobic avoidance and distress, and (c) the CGI-I responder criterion of ≤ 2. ZOLOFT was shown to be statistically significantly more effective than placebo as measured by the BSPS total score and fear, avoidance and physiologic factor scores, as well as the FQ-SPS total score, and to have significantly more responders than placebo as defined by the CGI-I.

Subgroup analyses did not suggest differences in treatment outcome on the basis of gender. There was insufficient information to determine the effect of race or age on outcome.

In a longer-term study, patients meeting DSM-IV criteria for social anxiety disorder who had responded while assigned to ZOLOFT (CGI-I of 1 or 2) during a 20-week placebo-controlled trial on ZOLOFT 50-200 mg/day were randomized to continuation of ZOLOFT or to substitution of placebo for up to 24 weeks of observation for relapse. Relapse was defined as ≥ 2 point increase in the Clinical Global Impression – Severity of Illness (CGI-S) score compared to baseline or study discontinuation due to lack of efficacy. Patients receiving ZOLOFT continuation treatment experienced a statistically significantly lower relapse rate over this 24-week study than patients randomized to placebo substitution.

INDICATIONS AND USAGE

Major Depressive Disorder–ZOLOFT® (sertraline hydrochloride) is indicated for the treatment of major depressive disorder.

The efficacy of ZOLOFT in the treatment of a major depressive episode was established in six to eight week controlled trials of outpatients whose diagnoses corresponded most closely to the DSM-III category of major depressive disorder (see Clinical Trials under CLINICAL PHARMACOLOGY).

A major depressive episode implies a prominent and relatively persistent depressed or dysphoric mood that usually interferes with daily functioning (nearly every day for at least 2 weeks); it should include at least 4 of the following 8 symptoms: change in appetite, change in sleep, psychomotor agitation or retardation, loss of interest in usual activities or decrease in sexual drive, increased fatigue, feelings of guilt or worthlessness, slowed thinking or impaired concentration, and a suicide attempt or suicidal ideation.

The antidepressant action of ZOLOFT in hospitalized depressed patients has not been adequately studied.

The efficacy of ZOLOFT in maintaining an antidepressant response for up to 44 weeks following 8 weeks of open-label acute treatment (52 weeks total) was demonstrated in a placebo-controlled trial. The usefulness of the drug in patients receiving ZOLOFT for extended periods should be re-evaluated periodically (see Clinical Trials under CLINICAL PHARMACOLOGY).

Obsessive-Compulsive Disorder–ZOLOFT is indicated for the treatment of obsessions and compulsions in patients with obsessive-compulsive disorder (OCD), as defined in the DSM-III-R; i.e., the obsessions or compulsions cause marked distress, are time-consuming, or significantly interfere with social or occupational functioning.

The efficacy of ZOLOFT was established in 12-week trials with obsessive-compulsive outpatients having diagnoses of obsessive-compulsive disorder as defined according to DSM-III or DSM-III-R criteria (see Clinical Trials under CLINICAL PHARMACOLOGY).

Obsessive-compulsive disorder is characterized by recurrent and persistent ideas, thoughts, impulses, or images (obsessions) that are ego-dystonic and/or repetitive, purposeful, and intentional behaviors (compulsions) that are recognized by the person as excessive or unreasonable.

The efficacy of ZOLOFT in maintaining a response, in patients with OCD who responded during a 52-week treatment phase while taking ZOLOFT and were then observed for relapse during a period of up to 28 weeks, was demonstrated in a placebo-controlled trial (see Clinical Trials under CLINICAL PHARMACOLOGY). Nevertheless, the physician who elects to use ZOLOFT for extended periods should periodically re-evaluate the long-term usefulness of the drug for the individual patient (see DOSAGE AND ADMINISTRATION).

Panic Disorder–ZOLOFT is indicated for the treatment of panic disorder, with or without agoraphobia, as defined in DSM-IV. Panic disorder is characterized by the occurrence of unexpected panic attacks and associated concern about having additional attacks, worry about the implications or consequences of the attacks, and/or a significant change in behavior related to the attacks.

The efficacy of ZOLOFT was established in three 10-12 week trials in panic disorder patients whose diagnoses corresponded to the DSM-III-R category of panic disorder (see Clinical Trials under CLINICAL PHARMACOLOGY).

Panic disorder (DSM-IV) is characterized by recurrent unexpected panic attacks, i.e., a discrete period of intense fear or discomfort in which four (or more) of the following symptoms develop abruptly and reach a peak within 10 minutes: (1) palpitations, pounding heart, or accelerated heart rate; (2) sweating; (3) trembling or shaking; (4) sensations of shortness of breath or smothering; (5) feeling of choking; (6) chest pain or discomfort; (7) nausea or abdominal distress; (8) feeling dizzy, unsteady, lightheaded, or faint; (9) derealization (feelings of unreality) or depersonalization (being detached from oneself); (10) fear of losing control; (11) fear of dying; (12) paresthesias (numbness or tingling sensations); (13) chills or hot flushes.

The efficacy of ZOLOFT in maintaining a response, in patients with panic disorder who responded during a 52-week treatment phase while taking ZOLOFT and were then observed for relapse during a period of up to 28 weeks, was demonstrated in a placebo-controlled trial (see Clinical Trials under CLINICAL PHARMACOLOGY). Nevertheless, the physician who elects to use ZOLOFT for extended periods should periodically re-evaluate the long-term usefulness of the drug for the individual patient (see DOSAGE AND ADMINISTRATION).

Posttraumatic Stress Disorder (PTSD)–ZOLOFT (sertraline hydrochloride) is indicated for the treatment of posttraumatic stress disorder.

The efficacy of ZOLOFT in the treatment of PTSD was established in two 12-week placebo-controlled trials of outpatients whose diagnosis met criteria for the DSM-III-R category of PTSD (see Clinical Trials under CLINICAL PHARMACOLOGY).

PTSD, as defined by DSM-III-R/IV, requires exposure to a traumatic event that involved actual or threatened death or serious injury, or threat to the physical integrity of self or others, and a response which involves intense fear, helplessness, or horror. Symptoms that occur as a result of exposure to the traumatic event include reexperiencing of the event in the form of intrusive thoughts, flashbacks or dreams, and intense psychological distress and physiological reactivity on exposure to cues to the event; avoidance of situations reminiscent of the traumatic event, inability to recall details of the event, and/or numbing of general responsiveness manifested as diminished interest in significant activities, estrangement from others, restricted range of affect, or sense of foreshortened future; and symptoms of autonomic arousal including hypervigilance, exaggerated startle response, sleep disturbance, impaired concentration, and irritability or outbursts of anger. A PTSD diagnosis requires that the symptoms are present for at least a month and that they cause clinically significant distress or impairment in social, occupational, or other important areas of functioning.

The efficacy of ZOLOFT in maintaining a response in patients with PTSD for up to 28 weeks following 24 weeks of open-label treatment was demonstrated in a placebo-controlled trial. Nevertheless, the physician who elects to use ZOLOFT for extended periods should periodically re-evaluate the long-term usefulness of the drug for the individual patient (see DOSAGE AND ADMINISTRATION).

Premenstrual Dysphoric Disorder (PMDD) – ZOLOFT is indicated for the treatment of premenstrual dysphoric disorder (PMDD).

The efficacy of ZOLOFT in the treatment of PMDD was established in 2 placebo-controlled trials of female outpatients treated for 3 menstrual cycles who met criteria for the DSM-III-R/IV category of PMDD (see Clinical Trials under CLINICAL PHARMACOLOGY).

The essential features of PMDD include markedly depressed mood, anxiety or tension, affective lability, and persistent anger or irritability. Other features include decreased interest in activities, difficulty concentrating, lack of energy, change in appetite or sleep, and feeling out of control. Physical symptoms associated with PMDD include breast tenderness, headache, joint and muscle pain, bloating and weight gain. These symptoms occur regularly during the luteal phase and remit within a few days following onset of menses; the disturbance markedly interferes with work or school or with usual social activities and relationships with others. In making the diagnosis, care should be taken to rule out other cyclical mood disorders that may be exacerbated by treatment with an antidepressant.

The effectiveness of ZOLOFT in long-term use, that is, for more than 3 menstrual cycles, has not been systematically evaluated in controlled trials. Therefore, the physician who elects to use ZOLOFT for extended periods should periodically re-evaluate the long-term usefulness of the drug for the individual patient (see DOSAGE AND ADMINISTRATION).

Social Anxiety Disorder – ZOLOFT (sertraline hydrochloride) is indicated for the treatment of social anxiety disorder, also known as social phobia.

The efficacy of ZOLOFT in the treatment of social anxiety disorder was established in two placebo-controlled trials of outpatients with a diagnosis of social anxiety disorder as defined by DSM-IV criteria (see Clinical Trials under CLINICAL PHARMACOLOGY).

Social anxiety disorder, as defined by DSM-IV, is characterized by marked and persistent fear of social or performance situations involving exposure to unfamiliar people or possible scrutiny by others and by fears of acting in a humiliating or embarrassing way. Exposure to the feared social situation almost always provokes anxiety and feared social or performance situations are avoided or else are endured with intense anxiety or distress. In addition, patients recognize that the fear is excessive or unreasonable and the avoidance and anticipatory anxiety of the feared situation is associated with functional impairment or marked distress.

The efficacy of ZOLOFT in maintaining a response in patients with social anxiety disorder for up to 24 weeks following 20 weeks of ZOLOFT treatment was demonstrated in a placebo-controlled trial. Physicians who prescribe ZOLOFT for extended periods should periodically re-evaluate the long-term usefulness of the drug for the individual patient (see Clinical Trials under CLINICAL PHARMACOLOGY).

CONTRAINDICATIONS

All Dosage Forms of ZOLOFT:

Concomitant use in patients taking monoamine oxidase inhibitors (MAOIs) is contraindicated (see WARNINGS). Concomitant use in patients taking pimozide is contraindicated (see PRECAUTIONS).

ZOLOFT is contraindicated in patients with a hypersensitivity to sertraline or any of the inactive ingredients in ZOLOFT.

Oral Concentrate:

ZOLOFT oral concentrate is contraindicated with ANTABUSE (disulfiram) due to the alcohol content of the concentrate.

WARNINGS

Cases of serious sometimes fatal reactions have been reported in patients receiving ZOLOFT® (sertraline hydrochloride), a selective serotonin reuptake inhibitor (SSRI), in combination with a monoamine oxidase inhibitor (MAOI). Symptoms of a drug interaction between an SSRI and an MAOI include: hyperthermia, rigidity, myoclonus, autonomic instability with possible rapid fluctuations of vital signs, mental status changes that include confusion, irritability, and extreme agitation progressing to delirium and coma. These reactions have also been reported in patients who have recently discontinued an SSRI and have been started on an MAOI. Some cases presented with features resembling neuroleptic malignant syndrome. Therefore, ZOLOFT should not be used in combination with an MAOI, or within 14 days of discontinuing treatment with an MAOI. Similarly, at least 14 days should be allowed after stopping ZOLOFT before starting an MAOI.

PRECAUTIONS

General

Activation of Mania/Hypomania–During premarketing testing, hypomania or mania occurred in approximately 0.4% of ZOLOFT® (sertraline hydrochloride) treated patients.

Weight Loss–Significant weight loss may be an undesirable result of treatment with sertraline for some patients, but on average, patients in controlled trials had minimal, 1 to 2 pound weight loss, versus smaller changes on placebo. Only rarely have sertraline patients been discontinued for weight loss.

Seizure–ZOLOFT has not been evaluated in patients with a seizure disorder. These patients were excluded from clinical studies during the product's premarket testing. No seizures were observed among approximately 3000 patients treated with ZOLOFT in the development program for major depressive disorder. However, 4 patients out of approximately 1800 (220<18 years of age) exposed during the development program for obsessive-compulsive disorder experienced seizures, representing a crude incidence of 0.2%. Three of these patients were adolescents, two with a seizure disorder and one with a family history of seizure disorder, none of whom were receiving anticonvulsant medication. Accordingly, ZOLOFT should be introduced with care in patients with a seizure disorder.

Suicide–The possibility of a suicide attempt is inherent in major depressive disorder and may persist until significant remission occurs. Close supervision of high risk patients should accompany initial drug therapy. Prescriptions for ZOLOFT should be written for the smallest quantity of tablets consistent with good patient management, in order to reduce the risk of overdose.

Because of the well-established comorbidity between OCD, panic disorder, PTSD, PMDD or social anxiety disorder and major depressive disorder, the same precautions observed when treating patients with major depressive disorder should be observed when treating patients with OCD, panic disorder, PTSD, PMDD or social anxiety disorder.

Weak Uricosuric Effect–ZOLOFT® (sertraline hydrochloride) is associated with a mean decrease in serum uric acid of approximately 7%. The clinical significance of this weak uricosuric effect is unknown.

Use in Patients with Concomitant Illness–Clinical experience with ZOLOFT in patients with certain concomitant systemic illness is limited. Caution is advisable in using ZOLOFT in patients with diseases or conditions that could affect metabolism or hemodynamic responses.

ZOLOFT has not been evaluated or used to any appreciable extent in patients with a recent history of myocardial infarction or unstable heart disease. Patients with these diagnoses were excluded from clinical studies during the product's premarket testing. However, the electrocardiograms of 774 patients who received ZOLOFT in double-blind trials were evaluated and the data indicate that ZOLOFT is not associated with the development of significant ECG abnormalities.

ZOLOFT is extensively metabolized by the liver. In patients with chronic mild liver impairment, sertraline clearance was reduced, resulting in increased AUC, Cmax and elimination half-life. The effects of sertraline in patients with moderate and severe hepatic impairment have not been studied. The use of sertraline in patients with liver disease must be approached with caution. If sertraline is administered to patients with liver impairment, a lower or less frequent dose should be used (see CLINICAL PHARMACOLOGY and DOSAGE AND ADMINISTRATION).

Since ZOLOFT is extensively metabolized, excretion of unchanged drug in urine is a minor route of elimination. A clinical study comparing sertraline pharmacokinetics in healthy volunteers to that in patients with renal impairment ranging from mild to severe (requiring dialysis) indicated that the pharmacokinetics and protein binding are unaffected by renal disease. Based on the pharmacokinetic results, there is no need for dosage adjustment in patients with renal impairment (see CLINICAL PHARMACOLOGY).

Interference with Cognitive and Motor Performance–In controlled studies, ZOLOFT did not cause sedation and did not interfere with psychomotor performance. (See **Information for Patients.**)

Hyponatremia–Several cases of hyponatremia have been reported and appeared to be reversible when ZOLOFT was discontinued. Some cases were possibly due to the syndrome of inappropriate antidiuretic hormone secretion. The majority of these occurrences have been in elderly individuals, some in patients taking diuretics or who were otherwise volume depleted.

Platelet Function–There have been rare reports of altered platelet function and/or abnormal results from laboratory studies in patients taking ZOLOFT. While there have been reports of abnormal bleeding or purpura in several patients taking ZOLOFT, it is unclear whether ZOLOFT had a causative role.

Information for Patients

Physicians are advised to discuss the following issues with patients for whom they prescribe ZOLOFT:

Patients should be told that although ZOLOFT has not been shown to impair the ability of normal subjects to perform tasks requiring complex motor and mental skills in laboratory experiments, drugs that act upon the central nervous system may affect some individuals adversely. Therefore, patients should be told that until they learn how they respond to ZOLOFT they should be careful doing activities when they need to be alert, such as driving a car or operating machinery.

Patients should be told that although ZOLOFT has not been shown in experiments with normal subjects to increase the mental and motor skill impairments caused by alcohol, the concomitant use of ZOLOFT and alcohol is not advised.

Patients should be told that while no adverse interaction of ZOLOFT with over-the-counter (OTC) drug products is known to occur, the potential for interaction exists. Thus, the use of any OTC product should be initiated cautiously according to the directions of use given for the OTC product.

Patients should be advised to notify their physician if they become pregnant or intend to become pregnant during therapy.

Patients should be advised to notify their physician if they are breast feeding an infant.

ZOLOFT oral concentrate is contraindicated with ANTABUSE (disulfiram) due to the alcohol content of the concentrate.

ZOLOFT Oral Concentrate contains 20 mg/mL of sertraline (as the hydrochloride) as the active ingredient and 12% alcohol. ZOLOFT Oral Concentrate must be diluted before use. Just before taking, use the dropper provided to remove the required amount of ZOLOFT Oral Concentrate and mix with 4 oz (1/2 cup) of water, ginger ale, lemon/lime soda, lemonade or orange juice ONLY. Do not mix ZOLOFT Oral Concentrate with anything other

Continued on next page

Zoloft—Cont.

than the liquids listed. The dose should be taken immediately after mixing. Do not mix in advance. At times, a slight haze may appear after mixing; this is normal. Note that caution should be exercised for persons with latex sensitivity, as the dropper dispenser contains dry natural rubber.

Laboratory Tests

None.

Drug Interactions

Potential Effects of Coadministration of Drugs Highly Bound to Plasma Proteins–Because sertraline is tightly bound to plasma protein, the administration of ZOLOFT® (sertraline hydrochloride) to a patient taking another drug which is tightly bound to protein (e.g., warfarin, digitoxin) may cause a shift in plasma concentrations potentially resulting in an adverse effect. Conversely, adverse effects may result from displacement of protein bound ZOLOFT by other tightly bound drugs.

In a study comparing prothrombin time AUC (0-120 hr) following dosing with warfarin (0.75 mg/kg) before and after 21 days of dosing with either ZOLOFT (50-200 mg/day) or placebo, there was a mean increase in prothrombin time of 8% relative to baseline for ZOLOFT compared to a 1% decrease for placebo ($p<0.02$). The normalization of prothrombin time for the ZOLOFT group was delayed compared to the placebo group. The clinical significance of this change is unknown. Accordingly, prothrombin time should be carefully monitored when ZOLOFT therapy is initiated or stopped.

Cimetidine–In a study assessing disposition of ZOLOFT (100 mg) on the second of 8 days of cimetidine administration (800 mg daily), there were significant increases in ZOLOFT mean AUC (50%), Cmax (24%) and half-life (26%) compared to the placebo group. The clinical significance of these changes is unknown.

CNS Active Drugs–In a study comparing the disposition of intravenously administered diazepam before and after 21 days of dosing with either ZOLOFT (50 to 200 mg/day escalating dose) or placebo, there was a 32% decrease relative to baseline in diazepam clearance for the ZOLOFT group compared to a 19% decrease relative to baseline for the placebo group ($p<0.03$). There was a 23% increase in Tmax for desmethyldiazepam in the ZOLOFT group compared to a 20% decrease in the placebo group ($p<0.03$). The clinical significance of these changes is unknown.

In a placebo-controlled trial in normal volunteers, the administration of two doses of ZOLOFT did not significantly alter steady-state lithium levels or the renal clearance of lithium.

Nonetheless, at this time, it is recommended that plasma lithium levels be monitored following initiation of ZOLOFT therapy with appropriate adjustments to the lithium dose.

In a controlled study of a single dose (2 mg) of pimozide, 200 mg sertraline (q.d.) co-administration to steady state was associated with a mean increase in pimozide AUC and Cmax of about 40%, but was not associated with any changes in EKG. Since the highest recommended pimozide dose (10 mg) has not been evaluated in combination with sertraline, the effect on QT interval and PK parameters at doses higher than 2 mg at this time are not known. While the mechanism of this interaction is unknown, due to the narrow therapeutic index of pimozide and due to the interaction noted at a low dose of pimozide, concomitant administration of ZOLOFT and pimozide should be contraindicated (see CONTRAINDICATIONS).

The risk of using ZOLOFT in combination with other CNS active drugs has not been systematically evaluated. Consequently, caution is advised if the concomitant administration of ZOLOFT and such drugs is required.

There is limited controlled experience regarding the optimal timing of switching from other drugs effective in the treatment of major depressive disorder, obsessive-compulsive disorder, panic disorder, posttraumatic stress disorder, premenstrual dysphoric disorder and social anxiety disorder to ZOLOFT. Care and prudent medical judgment should be exercised when switching, particularly from long-acting agents. The duration of an appropriate washout period which should intervene before switching from one selective serotonin reuptake inhibitor (SSRI) to another has not been established.

Monoamine Oxidase Inhibitors–See CONTRAINDICATIONS and WARNINGS.

Drugs Metabolized by P450 3A4–In three separate *in vivo* interaction studies, sertraline was co-administered with cytochrome P450 3A4 substrates, terfenadine, carbamazepine, or cisapride under steady-state conditions. The results of these studies indicated that sertraline did not increase plasma concentrations of terfenadine, carbamazepine, or cisapride. These data indicate that sertraline's extent of inhibition of P450 3A4 activity is not likely to be of clinical significance. Results of the interaction study with cisapride indicate that sertraline 200 mg (q.d.) induces the metabolism of cisapride (cisapride AUC and Cmax were reduced by about 35%).

Drugs Metabolized by P450 2D6–Many drugs effective in the treatment of major depressive disorder, e.g., the SSRIs, including sertraline, and most tricyclic antidepressant drugs effective in the treatment of major depressive disorder inhibit the biochemical activity of the drug metabolizing isozyme cytochrome P450 2D6 (debrisoquin hydroxylase), and, thus, may increase the plasma concentrations of co-administered drugs that are metabolized by P450 2D6. The drugs for which this potential interaction is of greatest concern are those metabolized primarily by 2D6 and which have a narrow therapeutic index, e.g., the tricyclic antidepressant drugs effective in the treatment of major depressive disorder and the Type 1C antiarrhythmics propafenone and flecainide. The extent to which this interaction is an important clinical problem depends on the extent of the inhibition of P450 2D6 by the antidepressant and the therapeutic index of the co-administered drug. There is variability among the drugs effective in the treatment of major depressive disorder in the extent of clinically important 2D6 inhibition, and in fact sertraline at lower doses has a less prominent inhibitory effect on 2D6 than some others in the class. Nevertheless, even sertraline has the potential for clinically important 2D6 inhibition. Consequently, concomitant use of a drug metabolized by P450 2D6 with ZOLOFT may require lower doses than usually prescribed for the other drug. Furthermore, whenever ZOLOFT is withdrawn from co-therapy, an increased dose of the co-administered drug may be required (see Tricyclic Antidepressant Drugs Effective in the Treatment of Major Depressive Disorder under PRECAUTIONS).

Sumatriptan–There have been rare postmarketing reports describing patients with weakness, hyperreflexia, and incoordination following the use of a selective serotonin reuptake inhibitor (SSRI) and sumatriptan. If concomitant treatment with sumatriptan and an SSRI (e.g., citalopram, fluoxetine, fluvoxamine, paroxetine, sertraline) is clinically warranted, appropriate observation of the patient is advised.

Tricyclic Antidepressant Drugs Effective in the Treatment of Major Depressive Disorder (TCAs)–The extent to which SSRI–TCA interactions may pose clinical problems will depend on the degree of inhibition and the pharmacokinetics of the SSRI involved. Nevertheless, caution is indicated in the co-administration of TCAs with ZOLOFT, because sertraline may inhibit TCA metabolism. Plasma TCA concentrations may need to be monitored, and the dose of TCA may need to be reduced, if a TCA is co-administered with ZOLOFT (see Drugs Metabolized by P450 2D6 under PRECAUTIONS).

Hypoglycemic Drugs–In a placebo-controlled trial in normal volunteers, administration of ZOLOFT for 22 days (including 200 mg/day for the final 13 days) caused a statistically significant 16% decrease from baseline in the clearance of tolbutamide following an intravenous 1000 mg dose. ZOLOFT administration did not noticeably change either the plasma protein binding or the apparent volume of distribution of tolbutamide, suggesting that the decreased clearance was due to a change in the metabolism of the drug. The clinical significance of this decrease in tolbutamide clearance is unknown.

Atenolol–ZOLOFT (100 mg) when administered to 10 healthy male subjects had no effect on the beta-adrenergic blocking ability of atenolol.

Digoxin–In a placebo-controlled trial in normal volunteers, administration of ZOLOFT for 17 days (including 200 mg/day for the last 10 days) did not change serum digoxin levels or digoxin renal clearance.

Microsomal Enzyme Induction–Preclinical studies have shown ZOLOFT to induce hepatic microsomal enzymes. In clinical studies, ZOLOFT was shown to induce hepatic enzymes minimally as determined by a small (5%) but statistically significant decrease in antipyrine half-life following administration of 200 mg/day for 21 days. This small change in antipyrine half-life reflects a clinically insignificant change in hepatic metabolism.

Electroconvulsive Therapy–There are no clinical studies establishing the risks or benefits of the combined use of electroconvulsive therapy (ECT) and ZOLOFT.

Alcohol–Although ZOLOFT did not potentiate the cognitive and psychomotor effects of alcohol in experiments with normal subjects, the concomitant use of ZOLOFT and alcohol is not recommended.

Carcinogenesis–Lifetime carcinogenicity studies were carried out in CD-1 mice and Long-Evans rats at doses up to 40 mg/kg/day. These doses correspond to 1 times (mice) and 2 times (rats) the maximum recommended human dose (MRHD) on a mg/m^2 basis. There was a dose-related increase of liver adenomas in male mice receiving sertraline at 10-40 mg/kg (0.25-1.0 times the MRHD on a mg/m^2 basis). No increase was seen in female mice or in rats of either sex receiving the same treatments, nor was there an increase in hepatocellular carcinomas. Liver adenomas have a variable rate of spontaneous occurrence in the CD-1 mouse and are of unknown significance to humans. There was an increase in follicular adenomas of the thyroid in female rats receiving sertraline at 40 mg/kg (2 times the MRHD on a mg/m^2 basis); this was not accompanied by thyroid hyperplasia. While there was an increase in [illegible] nomas in rats receiving sertraline at 10-40 mg/kg (0.5-2.0 times the MRHD on a mg/m^2 basis) compared to placebo controls, this effect was not clearly drug related.

Mutagenesis–Sertraline had no genotoxic effects, with or without metabolic activation, based on the following assays: bacterial mutation assay; mouse lymphoma mutation assay; and tests for cytogenetic aberrations *in vivo* in mouse bone marrow and *in vitro* in human lymphocytes.

Impairment of Fertility–A decrease in fertility was seen in one of two rat studies at a dose of 80 mg/kg (4 times the maximum recommended human dose on a mg/m^2 basis).

Pregnancy–Pregnancy Category C–Reproduction studies have been performed in rats and rabbits at doses up to 80 mg/kg/day and 40 mg/kg/day, respectively. These doses correspond to approximately 4 times the maximum recommended human dose (MRHD) on a mg/m^2 basis. There was no evidence of teratogenicity at any dose level. When pregnant rats and rabbits were given sertraline during the period of organogenesis, delayed ossification was observed in fetuses at doses of 10 mg/kg (0.5 times the MRHD on a mg/m^2 basis) in rats and 40 mg/kg (4 times the MRHD on a mg/m^2 basis) in rabbits. When female rats received sertraline during the last third of gestation and throughout lactation, there was an increase in the number of stillborn pups and in the number of pups dying during the first 4 days after birth. Pup body weights were also decreased during the first four days after birth. These effects occurred at a dose of 20 mg/kg (1 times the MRHD on a mg/m^2 basis). The no effect dose for rat pup mortality was 10 mg/kg (0.5 times the MRHD on a mg/m^2 basis). The decrease in pup survival was shown to be due to *in utero* exposure to sertraline. The clinical significance of these effects is unknown. There are no adequate and well-controlled studies in pregnant women. ZOLOFT® (sertraline hydrochloride) should be used during pregnancy only if the potential benefit justifies the potential risk to the fetus.

Labor and Delivery–The effect of ZOLOFT on labor and delivery in humans is unknown.

Nursing Mothers–It is not known whether, and if so in what amount, sertraline or its metabolites are excreted in human milk. Because many drugs are excreted in human milk, caution should be exercised when ZOLOFT is administered to a nursing woman.

Pediatric Use–The efficacy of ZOLOFT for the treatment of obsessive-compulsive disorder was demonstrated in a 12-week, multicenter, placebo-controlled study with 187 outpatients ages 6-17 (see Clinical Trials under CLINICAL PHARMACOLOGY). The efficacy of ZOLOFT in pediatric patients with major depressive disorder, panic disorder, PTSD, PMDD or social anxiety disorder has not been established.

The safety of ZOLOFT use in children and adolescents with OCD, ages 6-18, was evaluated in a 12-week, multicenter, placebo-controlled study with 187 outpatients, ages 6-17, and in a flexible dose, 52 week open extension study of 137 patients, ages 6-18, who had completed the initial 12-week, double-blind, placebo-controlled study. ZOLOFT was administered at doses of either 25 mg/day (children, ages 6-12) or 50 mg/day (adolescents, ages 13-18) and then titrated in weekly 25 mg/day or 50 mg/day increments, respectively, to a maximum dose of 200 mg/day based upon clinical response. The mean dose for completers was 157 mg/day. In the acute 12 week pediatric study and in the 52 week study, ZOLOFT had an adverse event profile generally similar to that observed in adults.

Sertraline pharmacokinetics were evaluated in 61 pediatric patients between 6 and 17 years of age with major depressive disorder or OCD and revealed similar drug exposures to those of adults when plasma concentration was adjusted for weight (see Pharmacokinetics under CLINICAL PHARMACOLOGY).

Approximately 600 patients with major depressive disorder or OCD between 6 and 17 years of age have received ZOLOFT in clinical trials, both controlled and uncontrolled. The adverse event profile observed in these patients was generally similar to that observed in adult studies with ZOLOFT (see ADVERSE REACTIONS). As with other SSRIs, decreased appetite and weight loss have been observed in association with the use of ZOLOFT. In a pooled analysis of two 10-week, double-blind, placebo-controlled, flexible dose (50-200 mg) outpatient trials for major depressive disorder (n=373), there was a difference in weight change between sertraline and placebo of roughly 1 kilogram, for both children (ages 6-11) and adolescents (ages 12-17), in both cases representing a slight weight loss for sertraline compared to a slight gain for placebo. At baseline the mean weight for children was 39.0 kg for sertraline and 38.5 kg for placebo. At baseline the mean weight for adolescents was 61.4 kg for sertraline and 62.5 kg for placebo. There was a bigger difference between sertraline and placebo in the proportion of outliers for clinically important weight loss in children than in adolescents. For children, about 7% had a weight loss > 7% of body weight compared to none of the placebo patients; for adolescents, about 2% had a weight loss > 7% of body weight compared to about 1% of the placebo patients. A subset of these patients who completed the randomized controlled trials (sertraline n=99, placebo n=122) were continued into a 24-week, flexible-dose, open-label, extension study. A mean weight loss of approximately 0.5 kg was seen during the first eight weeks of treatment for subjects with first exposure to sertraline during the open-label extension study, similar to mean weight loss observed among sertralinetreated subjects during the first eight weeks of the randomized controlled trials. The subjects continuing in the open label study began gaining weight compared to baseline by week 12 of sertraline treatment. Those subjects who completed 34 weeks of sertraline treatment (10 weeks in a placebo controlled trial + 24 weeks open label, n=68) had weight gain that was similar to that expected using data from age-adjusted peers. Regular monitoring of weight and growth is recommended if treatment of a pediatric patient with an SSRI is to be continued long term. Safety and effectiveness in pediatric patients below the age of 6 have not been established.

The risks, if any, that may be associated with ZOLOFT's use beyond 1 year in children and adolescents with OCD or major depressive disorder have not been systematically as-

TABLE 1
MOST COMMON TREATMENT-EMERGENT ADVERSE EVENTS: INCIDENCE IN PLACEBO-CONTROLLED CLINICAL TRIALS

	Percentage of Patients Reporting Event													
	Major Depressive Disorder/Other*		OCD		Panic Disorder		PTSD		PMDD Daily Dosing		PMDD Luteal Phase Dosing(2)		Social Anxiety Disorder	
Body System/ Adverse Event	**ZOLOFT (N=861)**	**Placebo (N=853)**	**ZOLOFT (N=533)**	**Placebo (N=373)**	**ZOLOFT (N=430)**	**Placebo (N=275)**	**ZOLOFT (N=374)**	**Placebo (N=376)**	**ZOLOFT (N=121)**	**Placebo (N=122)**	**ZOLOFT (N=136)**	**Placebo (N=127)**	**ZOLOFT (N=344)**	**Placebo (N=268)**
Autonomic Nervous System Disorders														
Ejaculation Failure(1)	7	<1	17	2	19	1	11	1	N/A	N/A	N/A	N/A	14	–
Mouth Dry	16	9	14	9	15	10	11	6	6	3	10	3	12	4
Sweating Increased	8	3	6	1	5	1	4	2	6	<1	3	0	11	2
Centr. & Periph. Nerv. System Disorders														
Somnolence	13	6	15	8	15	9	13	9	7	<1	2	0	9	6
Tremor	11	3	8	1	5	1	5	1	2	0	<1	<1	9	3
Dizziness	12	7	17	9	10	10	8	5	6	3	7	5	14	6
General														
Fatigue	11	8	14	10	11	6	10	5	16	7	10	<1	12	6
Pain	1	2	3	1	3	3	4	6	6	<1	3	2	1	3
Malaise	<1	1	1	1	7	14	10	10	9	5	7	5	8	3
Gastrointestinal Disorders														
Abdominal Pain	2	2	5	5	6	7	6	5	7	<1	3	3	5	5
Anorexia	3	2	11	2	7	2	8	2	3	2	5	0	6	3
Constipation	8	6	6	4	7	3	3	3	2	3	1	2	5	3
Diarrhea/Loose Stools	18	9	24	10	20	9	24	15	13	3	13	7	21	8
Dyspepsia	6	3	10	4	10	8	6	6	7	2	7	3	13	5
Nausea	26	12	30	11	29	18	21	11	23	9	13	3	22	8
Psychiatric Disorders														
Agitation	6	4	6	3	6	2	5	5	2	<1	1	0	4	2
Insomnia	16	9	28	12	25	18	20	11	17	11	12	10	25	10
Libido Decreased	1	<1	11	2	7	1	7	2	11	2	4	2	9	3

(1)Primarily ejaculatory delay. Denominator used was for male patients only (N=271 ZOLOFT major depressive disorder/other*; N=271 placebo major depressive disorder/other*; N=296 ZOLOFT OCD; N=219 placebo OCD; N=216 ZOLOFT panic disorder; N=134 placebo panic disorder; N=130 ZOLOFT PTSD; N=149 placebo PTSD; No male patients in PMDD studies; N=205 ZOLOFT social anxiety disorder; N=153 placebo social anxiety disorder).
*Major depressive disorder and other premarketing controlled trials.
(2)The luteal phase and daily dosing PMDD trials were not designed for making direct comparisons between the two dosing regimens. Therefore, a comparison between the two dosing regimens of the PMDD trials of incidence rates shown in Table 1 should be avoided.

sessed. The prescriber should be mindful that the evidence relied upon to conclude that sertraline is safe for use in children and adolescents derives from clinical studies that were 10 to 52 weeks in duration and from the extrapolation of experience gained with adult patients. In particular, there are no studies that directly evaluate the effects of long-term sertraline use on the growth, development, and maturation of children and adolescents. Although there is no affirmative finding to suggest that sertraline possesses a capacity to adversely affect growth, development or maturation, the absence of such findings is not compelling evidence of the absence of the potential of sertraline to have adverse effects in chronic use.

Geriatric Use–U.S. geriatric clinical studies of ZOLOFT in major depressive disorder included 663 ZOLOFT-treated subjects ≥ 65 years of age, of those, 180 were ≥ 75 years of age. No overall differences in the pattern of adverse reactions were observed in the geriatric clinical trial subjects relative to those reported in younger subjects (see ADVERSE REACTIONS), and other reported experience has not identified differences in safety patterns between the elderly and younger subjects. As with all medications, greater sensitivity of some older individuals cannot be ruled out. There were 947 subjects in placebo-controlled geriatric clinical studies of ZOLOFT in major depressive disorder. No overall differences in the pattern of efficacy were observed in the geriatric clinical trial subjects relative to those reported in younger subjects.

Other Adverse Events in Geriatric Patients. In 354 geriatric subjects treated with ZOLOFT in placebo-controlled trials, the overall profile of adverse events was generally similar to that shown in Tables 1 and 2. Urinary tract infection was the only adverse event not appearing in Tables 1 and 2 and reported at an incidence of at least 2% and at a rate greater than placebo in placebo-controlled trials.

As with other SSRIs, ZOLOFT has been associated with cases of clinically significant hyponatremia in elderly patients (see Hyponatremia under PRECAUTIONS).

ADVERSE REACTIONS

During its premarketing assessment, multiple doses of ZOLOFT were administered to over 4000 adult subjects as of February 18, 2000. The conditions and duration of exposure to ZOLOFT varied greatly, and included (in overlapping categories) clinical pharmacology studies, open and double-blind studies, uncontrolled and controlled studies, inpatient and outpatient studies, fixed-dose and titration studies, and studies for multiple indications, including major depressive disorder, OCD, panic disorder, PTSD, PMDD and social anxiety disorder.

Untoward events associated with this exposure were recorded by clinical investigators using terminology of their own choosing. Consequently, it is not possible to provide a meaningful estimate of the proportion of individuals experiencing adverse events without first grouping similar types of untoward events into a smaller number of standardized event categories.

In the tabulations that follow, a World Health Organization dictionary of terminology has been used to classify reported adverse events. The frequencies presented, therefore, represent the proportion of the over 4000 adult individuals exposed to multiple doses of ZOLOFT who experienced a treatment-emergent adverse event of the type cited on at least one occasion while receiving ZOLOFT. An event was considered treatment-emergent if it occurred for the first time or worsened while receiving therapy following baseline evaluation. It is important to emphasize that events reported during therapy were not necessarily caused by it.

The prescriber should be aware that the figures in the tables and tabulations cannot be used to predict the incidence of side effects in the course of usual medical practice where patient characteristics and other factors differ from those that prevailed in the clinical trials. Similarly, the cited frequencies cannot be compared with figures obtained from other clinical investigations involving different treatments, uses, and investigators. The cited figures, however, do provide the prescribing physician with some basis for estimating the relative contribution of drug and nondrug factors to the side effect incidence rate in the population studied.

Incidence in Placebo-Controlled Trials–Table 1 enumerates the most common treatment-emergent adverse events associated with the use of ZOLOFT (incidence of at least 5% for ZOLOFT and at least twice that for placebo within at least one of the indications) for the treatment of adult patients with major depressive disorder/other*, OCD, panic disorder, PTSD, PMDD and social anxiety disorder in placebo-controlled clinical trials. Most patients in major depressive disorder/other*, OCD, panic disorder, PTSD and social anxiety disorder studies received doses of 50 to 200 mg/day. Patients in the PMDD study with daily dosing throughout the menstrual cycle received doses of 50 to 150 mg/day, and in the PMDD study with dosing during the luteal phase of the menstrual cycle received doses of 50 to 100 mg/day. Table 2 enumerates treatment-emergent adverse events that occurred in 2% or more of adult patients treated with ZOLOFT and with incidence greater than placebo who participated in controlled clinical trials comparing ZOLOFT with placebo in the treatment of major depressive disorder/other*, OCD, panic disorder, PTSD, PMDD and social anxiety disorder. Table 2 provides combined data for the pool of studies that are provided separately by indication in Table 1.

[See table 1 above]

Continued on next page

Zoloft—Cont.

TABLE 2
TREATMENT-EMERGENT ADVERSE EVENTS: INCIDENCE IN PLACEBO-CONTROLLED CLINICAL TRIALS
Percentage of Patients Reporting Event
Major Depressive Disorder/Other*, OCD, Panic Disorder, PTSD, PMDD and Social Anxiety Disorder combined

Body System/Adverse Event**	ZOLOFT (N=2799)	Placebo (N=2394)
Autonomic Nervous System Disorders		
Ejaculation Failure(1)	14	1
Mouth Dry	14	8
Sweating Increased	7	2
Centr. & Periph. Nerv. System Disorders		
Somnolence	13	7
Dizziness	12	7
Headache	25	23
Paresthesia	2	1
Tremor	8	2
Disorders of Skin and Appendages		
Rash	3	2
Gastrointestinal Disorders		
Anorexia	6	2
Constipation	6	4
Diarrhea/Loose Stools	20	10
Dyspepsia	8	4
Nausea	25	11
Vomiting	4	2
General		
Fatigue	12	7
Psychiatric Disorders		
Agitation	5	3
Anxiety	4	3
Insomnia	21	11
Libido Decreased	6	2
Nervousness	5	4
Special Senses		
Vision Abnormal	3	2

(1)Primarily ejaculatory delay. Denominator used was for male patients only (N=1118 ZOLOFT; N=926 placebo).
*Major depressive disorder and other premarketing controlled trials.
**Included are events reported by at least 2% of patients taking ZOLOFT except the following events, which had an incidence on placebo greater than or equal to ZOLOFT: abdominal pain, back pain, flatulence, malaise, pain, pharyngitis, respiratory disorder, upper respiratory tract infection.

Associated with Discontinuation in Placebo-Controlled Clinical Trials
Table 3 lists the adverse events associated with discontinuation of ZOLOFT® (sertraline hydrochloride) treatment (incidence at least twice that for placebo and at least 1% for ZOLOFT in clinical trials) in major depressive disorder/other*, OCD, panic disorder, PTSD, PMDD and social anxiety disorder.
[See table 3 below]

Male and Female Sexual Dysfunction with SSRIs
Although changes in sexual desire, sexual performance and sexual satisfaction often occur as manifestations of a psychiatric disorder, they may also be a consequence of pharmacologic treatment. In particular, some evidence suggests that selective serotonin reuptake inhibitors (SSRIs) can cause such untoward sexual experiences. Reliable estimates of the incidence and severity of untoward experiences involving sexual desire, performance and satisfaction are difficult to obtain, however, in part because patients and physicians may be reluctant to discuss them. Accordingly, estimates of the incidence of untoward sexual experience and performance cited in product labeling, are likely to underestimate their actual incidence.
Table 4 below displays the incidence of sexual side effects reported by at least 2% of patients taking ZOLOFT in placebo-controlled trials.

TABLE 4

Adverse Event	ZOLOFT	Placebo
Ejaculation failure* (primarily delayed ejaculation)	14%	1%
Decreased libido**	6%	1%

* Denominator used was for male patients only (N=1118 ZOLOFT; N=926 placebo)
** Denominator used was for male and female patients (N=2799 ZOLOFT; N=2394 placebo)

There are no adequate and well-controlled studies examining sexual dysfunction with sertraline treatment.
Priapism has been reported with all SSRIs.
While it is difficult to know the precise risk of sexual dysfunction associated with the use of SSRIs, physicians should routinely inquire about such possible side effects.

Other Adverse Events in Pediatric Patients–In over 600 pediatric patients treated with ZOLOFT, the overall profile of adverse events was generally similar to that seen in adult studies. However, the following adverse events, from controlled trials, not appearing in Tables 1 and 2, were reported at an incidence of at least 2% and occurred at a rate of at least twice the placebo rate (N=281 patients treated with ZOLOFT): fever, hyperkinesia, urinary incontinence, aggressive reaction, sinusitis, epistaxis and purpura.

Other Events Observed During the Premarketing Evaluation of ZOLOFT® (sertraline hydrochloride)–Following is a list of treatment-emergent adverse events reported during premarketing assessment of ZOLOFT in clinical trials (over 4000 adult subjects) except those already listed in the previous tables or elsewhere in labeling.
In the tabulations that follow, a World Health Organization dictionary of terminology has been used to classify reported adverse events. The frequencies presented, therefore, represent the proportion of the over 4000 adult individuals exposed to multiple doses of ZOLOFT who experienced an event of the type cited on at least one occasion while receiving ZOLOFT. All events are included except those already listed in the previous tables or elsewhere in labeling and those reported in terms so general as to be uninformative and those for which a causal relationship to ZOLOFT treatment seemed remote. It is important to emphasize that although the events reported occurred during treatment with ZOLOFT, they were not necessarily caused by it. Events are further categorized by body system and listed in order of decreasing frequency according to the following definitions: frequent adverse events are those occurring on one or more occasions in at least 1/100 patients; infrequent adverse events are those occurring in 1/100 to 1/1000 patients; rare events are those occurring in fewer than 1/1000 patients. Events of major clinical importance are also described in the PRECAUTIONS section.

Autonomic Nervous System Disorders–*Frequent:* impotence; *Infrequent:* flushing, increased saliva, cold clammy skin, mydriasis; *Rare:* pallor, glaucoma, priapism, vasodilation.
Body as a Whole–General Disorders–*Rare:* allergic reaction, allergy.
Cardiovascular–*Frequent:* palpitations, chest pain; *Infrequent:* hypertension, tachycardia, postural dizziness, postural hypotension, periorbital edema, peripheral edema, hypotension, peripheral ischemia, syncope, edema, dependent edema; *Rare:* precordial chest pain, substernal chest pain, aggravated hypertension, myocardial infarction, cerebrovascular disorder.
Central and Peripheral Nervous System Disorders–*Frequent:* hypertonia, hypoesthesia; *Infrequent:* twitching, confusion, hyperkinesia, vertigo, ataxia, migraine, abnormal coordination, hyperesthesia, leg cramps, abnormal gait, nystagmus, hypokinesia; *Rare:* dysphonia, coma, dyskinesia, hypotonia, ptosis, choreoathetosis, hyporeflexia.
Disorders of Skin and Appendages–*Infrequent:* pruritus, acne, urticaria, alopecia, dry skin, erythematous rash, photosensitivity reaction, maculopapular rash; *Rare:* follicular rash, eczema, dermatitis, contact dermatitis, bullous eruption, hypertrichosis, skin discoloration, pustular rash.
Endocrine Disorders–*Rare:* exophthalmos, gynecomastia.
Gastrointestinal Disorders–*Frequent:* appetite increased; *Infrequent:* dysphagia, tooth caries aggravated, eructation, esophagitis, gastroenteritis; *Rare:* melena, glossitis, gum hyperplasia, hiccup, stomatitis, tenesmus, colitis, diverticulitis, fecal incontinence, gastritis, rectum hemorrhage, hemorrhagic peptic ulcer, proctitis, ulcerative stomatitis, tongue edema, tongue ulceration.
General–*Frequent:* back pain, asthenia, malaise, weight increase; *Infrequent:* fever, rigors, generalized edema; *Rare:* face edema, aphthous stomatitis.
Hearing and Vestibular Disorders–*Rare:* hyperacusis, labyrinthine disorder.
Hematopoietic and Lymphatic–*Rare:* anemia, anterior chamber eye hemorrhage.

TABLE 3
MOST COMMON ADVERSE EVENTS ASSOCIATED WITH DISCONTINUATION IN PLACEBO-CONTROLLED CLINICAL TRIALS

Adverse Event	Major Depressive Disorder/ Other*, OCD, Panic Disorder, PTSD, PMDD and Social Anxiety Disorder combined (N=2799)	Major Depressive Disorder/ Other* (N=861)	OCD (N=533)	Panic Disorder (N=430)	PTSD (N=374)	PMDD Daily Dosing (N=121)	PMDD Luteal Phase Dosing (N=136)	Social Anxiety Disorder (N=344)
Abdominal Pain	–	–	–	–	–	–	–	1%
Agitation	–	1%	–	2%	–	–	–	–
Anxiety	–	–	–	–	–	–	–	2%
Diarrhea/Loose Stools	2%	2%	2%	1%	–	2%	–	–
Dizziness	–	–	1%	–	–	–	–	–
Dry Mouth	–	1%	–	–	–	–	–	–
Dyspepsia	–	–	–	1%	–	–	–	–
Ejaculation Failure(1)	1%	1%	1%	2%	–	N/A	N/A	2%
Fatigue	–	–	–	–	–	–	–	2%
Headache	1%	2%	–	–	1%	–	–	2%
Hot Flushes	–	–	–	–	–	–	1%	–
Insomnia	2%	1%	3%	2%	–	–	1%	3%
Nausea	3%	4%	3%	3%	2%	2%	1%	2%
Nervousness	–	–	–	–	–	2%	–	–
Palpitation	–	–	–	–	–	–	1%	–
Somnolence	1%	1%	2%	2%	–	–	–	–
Tremor	–	2%	–	–	–	–	–	–

(1)Primarily ejaculatory delay. Denominator used was for male patients only (N=271 major depressive disorder/other*; N=296 OCD; N=216 panic disorder; N=130 PTSD; No male patients in PMDD studies; N=205 social anxiety disorder).
*Major depressive disorder and other premarketing controlled trials.

Liver and Biliary System Disorders–*Rare:* abnormal hepatic function.

Metabolic and Nutritional Disorders–*Infrequent:* thirst; *Rare:* hypoglycemia, hypoglycemia reaction.

Musculoskeletal System Disorders–*Frequent:* myalgia; *Infrequent:* arthralgia, dystonia, arthrosis, muscle cramps, muscle weakness.

Psychiatric Disorders–*Frequent:* yawning, other male sexual dysfunction, other female sexual dysfunction; *Infrequent:* depression, amnesia, paroniria, teeth-grinding, emotional lability, apathy, abnormal dreams, euphoria, paranoid reaction, hallucination, aggressive reaction, aggravated depression, delusions; *Rare:* withdrawal syndrome, suicide ideation, libido increased, somnambulism, illusion.

Reproductive–*Infrequent:* menstrual disorder, dysmenorrhea, intermenstrual bleeding, vaginal hemorrhage, amenorrhea, leukorrhea; *Rare:* female breast pain, menorrhagia, balanoposthitis, breast enlargement, atrophic vaginitis, acute female mastitis.

Respiratory System Disorders–*Frequent:* rhinitis; *Infrequent:* coughing, dyspnea, upper respiratory tract infection, epistaxis, bronchospasm, sinusitis; *Rare:* hyperventilation, bradypnea, stridor, apnea, bronchitis, hemoptysis, hypoventilation, laryngismus, laryngitis.

Special Senses–*Frequent:* tinnitus; *Infrequent:* conjunctivitis, earache, eye pain, abnormal accommodation; *Rare:* xerophthalmia, photophobia, diplopia, abnormal lacrimation, scotoma, visual field defect.

Urinary System Disorders–*Infrequent:* micturition frequency, polyuria, urinary retention, dysuria, nocturia, urinary incontinence; *Rare:* cystitis, oliguria, pyelonephritis, hematuria, renal pain, strangury.

Laboratory Tests–In man, asymptomatic elevations in serum transaminases (SGOT [or AST] and SGPT [or ALT]) have been reported infrequently (approximately 0.8%) in association with ZOLOFT® (sertraline hydrochloride) administration. These hepatic enzyme elevations usually occurred within the first 1 to 9 weeks of drug treatment and promptly diminished upon drug discontinuation.

ZOLOFT therapy was associated with small mean increases in total cholesterol (approximately 3%) and triglycerides (approximately 5%), and a small mean decrease in serum uric acid (approximately 7%) of no apparent clinical importance.

The safety profile observed with ZOLOFT treatment in patients with major depressive disorder, OCD, panic disorder, PTSD, PMDD and social anxiety disorder is similar.

Other Events Observed During the Postmarketing Evaluation of ZOLOFT–Reports of adverse events temporally associated with ZOLOFT that have been received since market introduction, that are not listed above and that may have no causal relationship with the drug, include the following: acute renal failure, anaphylactoid reaction, angioedema, blindness, optic neuritis, cataract, increased coagulation times, bradycardia, AV block, atrial arrhythmias, QT-interval prolongation, ventricular tachycardia (including torsade de pointes-type arrhythmias), hypothyroidism, agranulocytosis, aplastic anemia and pancytopenia, leukopenia, thrombocytopenia, lupus-like syndrome, serum sickness, hyperglycemia, galactorrhea, hyperprolactinemia, neuroleptic malignant syndrome-like events, extrapyramidal symptoms, oculogyric crisis, serotonin syndrome, psychosis, pulmonary hypertension, severe skin reactions, which potentially can be fatal, such as Stevens-Johnson syndrome, vasculitis, photosensitivity and other severe cutaneous disorders, rare reports of pancreatitis, and liver events—clinical features (which in the majority of cases appeared to be reversible with discontinuation of ZOLOFT) occurring in one or more patients include: elevated enzymes, increased bilirubin, hepatomegaly, hepatitis, jaundice, abdominal pain, vomiting, liver failure and death.

DRUG ABUSE AND DEPENDENCE

Controlled Substance Class–ZOLOFT® (sertraline hydrochloride) is not a controlled substance.

Physical and Psychological Dependence–In a placebo-controlled, double-blind, randomized study of the comparative abuse liability of ZOLOFT, alprazolam, and d-amphetamine in humans, ZOLOFT did not produce the positive subjective effects indicative of abuse potential, such as euphoria or drug liking, that were observed with the other two drugs. Premarketing clinical experience with ZOLOFT did not reveal any tendency for a withdrawal syndrome or any drug-seeking behavior. In animal studies ZOLOFT does not demonstrate stimulant or barbiturate-like (depressant) abuse potential. As with any CNS active drug, however, physicians should carefully evaluate patients for history of drug abuse and follow such patients closely, observing them for signs of ZOLOFT misuse or abuse (e.g., development of tolerance, incrementation of dose, drug-seeking behavior).

OVERDOSAGE

Human Experience–Of 1,027 cases of overdose involving sertraline hydrochloride worldwide, alone or with other drugs, there were 72 deaths (circa 1999).

Among 634 overdoses in which sertraline hydrochloride was the only drug ingested, 8 resulted in fatal outcome, 75 completely recovered, and 27 patients experienced sequelae after overdosage to include alopecia, decreased libido, diarrhea, ejaculation disorder, fatigue, insomnia, somnolence and serotonin syndrome. The remaining 524 cases had an unknown outcome. The most common signs and symptoms associated with non-fatal sertraline hydrochloride overdosage were somnolence, vomiting, tachycardia, nausea, dizziness, agitation and tremor.

The largest known ingestion was 13.5 grams in a patient who took sertraline hydrochloride alone and subsequently recovered. However, another patient who took 2.5 grams of sertraline hydrochloride alone experienced a fatal outcome.

Other important adverse events reported with sertraline hydrochloride overdose (single or multiple drugs) include bradycardia, bundle branch block, coma, convulsions, delirium, hallucinations, hypertension, hypotension, manic reaction, pancreatitis, QT-interval prolongation, serotonin syndrome, stupor and syncope.

Overdose Management–Treatment should consist of those general measures employed in the management of overdosage with any antidepressant.

Ensure an adequate airway, oxygenation and ventilation. Monitor cardiac rhythm and vital signs. General supportive and symptomatic measures are also recommended. Induction of emesis is not recommended. Gastric lavage with a large-bore orogastric tube with appropriate airway protection, if needed, may be indicated if performed soon after ingestion, or in symptomatic patients.

Activated charcoal should be administered. Due to large volume of distribution of this drug, forced diuresis, dialysis, hemoperfusion and exchange transfusion are unlikely to be of benefit. No specific antidotes for sertraline are known.

In managing overdosage, consider the possibility of multiple drug involvement. The physician should consider contacting a poison control center on the treatment of any overdose. Telephone numbers for certified poison control centers are listed in the *Physicians' Desk Reference*® (PDR®).

DOSAGE AND ADMINISTRATION

Initial Treatment

Dosage for Adults

Major Depressive Disorder and Obsessive-Compulsive Disorder–ZOLOFT treatment should be administered at a dose of 50 mg once daily.

Panic Disorder, Posttraumatic Stress Disorder and Social Anxiety Disorder–ZOLOFT treatment should be initiated with a dose of 25 mg once daily. After one week, the dose should be increased to 50 mg once daily.

While a relationship between dose and effect has not been established for major depressive disorder, OCD, panic disorder, PTSD or social anxiety disorder, patients were dosed in a range of 50-200 mg/day in the clinical trials demonstrating the effectiveness of ZOLOFT for the treatment of these indications. Consequently, a dose of 50 mg, administered once daily, is recommended as the initial therapeutic dose. Patients not responding to a 50 mg dose may benefit from dose increases up to a maximum of 200 mg/day. Given the 24 hour elimination half-life of ZOLOFT, dose changes should not occur at intervals of less than 1 week.

Premenstrual Dysphoric Disorder–ZOLOFT treatment should be initiated with a dose of 50 mg/day, either daily throughout the menstrual cycle or limited to the luteal phase of the menstrual cycle, depending on physician assessment.

While a relationship between dose and effect has not been established for PMDD, patients were dosed in the range of 50-150 mg/day with dose increases at the onset of each new menstrual cycle (see Clinical Trials under CLINICAL PHARMACOLOGY). Patients not responding to a 50 mg/day dose may benefit from dose increases (at 50 mg increments/menstrual cycle) up to 150 mg/day when dosing daily throughout the menstrual cycle, or 100 mg/day when dosing during the luteal phase of the menstrual cycle. If a 100 mg/day dose has been established with luteal phase dosing, a 50 mg/day titration step for three days should be utilized at the beginning of each luteal phase dosing period.

ZOLOFT should be administered once daily, either in the morning or evening.

Dosage for Pediatric Population (Children and Adolescents)

Obsessive-Compulsive Disorder–ZOLOFT treatment should be initiated with a dose of 25 mg once daily in children (ages 6-12) and at a dose of 50 mg once daily in adolescents (ages 13-17).

While a relationship between dose and effect has not been established for OCD, patients were dosed in a range of 25-200 mg/day in the clinical trials demonstrating the effectiveness of ZOLOFT for pediatric patients (6-17 years) with OCD. Patients not responding to an initial dose of 25 or 50 mg/day may benefit from dose increases up to a maximum of 200 mg/day. For children with OCD, their generally lower body weights compared to adults should be taken into consideration in advancing the dose, in order to avoid excess dosing. Given the 24 hour elimination half-life of ZOLOFT, dose changes should not occur at intervals of less than 1 week.

ZOLOFT should be administered once daily, either in the morning or evening.

Dosage for Hepatically Impaired Patients

The use of sertraline in patients with liver disease should be approached with caution. The effects of sertraline in patients with moderate and severe hepatic impairment have not been studied. If sertraline is administered to patients with liver impairment, a lower or less frequent dose should be used (see CLINICAL PHARMACOLOGY and PRECAUTIONS).

Maintenance/Continuation/Extended Treatment

Major Depressive Disorder–It is generally agreed that acute episodes of major depressive disorder require several months or longer of sustained pharmacologic therapy beyond response to the acute episode. Systematic evaluation of ZOLOFT has demonstrated that its antidepressant efficacy is maintained for periods of up to 44 weeks following 8 weeks of initial treatment at a dose of 50-200 mg/day (mean dose of 70 mg/day) (see Clinical Trials under CLINICAL PHARMACOLOGY). It is not known whether the dose of ZOLOFT needed for maintenance treatment is identical to the dose needed to achieve an initial response. Patients should be periodically reassessed to determine the need for maintenance treatment.

Posttraumatic Stress Disorder–It is generally agreed that PTSD requires several months or longer of sustained pharmacological therapy beyond response to initial treatment. Systematic evaluation of ZOLOFT has demonstrated that its efficacy in PTSD is maintained for periods of up to 28 weeks following 24 weeks of treatment at a dose of 50-200 mg/day (see Clinical Trials under CLINICAL PHARMACOLOGY). It is not known whether the dose of ZOLOFT needed for maintenance treatment is identical to the dose needed to achieve an initial response. Patients should be periodically reassessed to determine the need for maintenance treatment.

Social Anxiety Disorder–Social anxiety disorder is a chronic condition that may require several months or longer of sustained pharmacological therapy beyond response to initial treatment. Systematic evaluation of ZOLOFT has demonstrated that its efficacy in social anxiety disorder is maintained for periods of up to 24 weeks following 20 weeks of treatment at a dose of 50-200 mg/day (see Clinical Trials under CLINICAL PHARMACOLOGY). Dosage adjustments should be made to maintain patients on the lowest effective dose and patients should be periodically reassessed to determine the need for long-term treatment.

Obsessive-Compulsive Disorder and Panic Disorder–It is generally agreed that OCD and Panic Disorder require several months or longer of sustained pharmacological therapy beyond response to initial treatment. Systematic evaluation of continuing ZOLOFT for periods of up to 28 weeks in patients with OCD and Panic Disorder who have responded while taking ZOLOFT during initial treatment phases of 24 to 52 weeks of treatment at a dose range of 50-200 mg/day has demonstrated a benefit of such maintenance treatment (see Clinical Trials under CLINICAL PHARMACOLOGY). It is not known whether the dose of ZOLOFT needed for maintenance treatment is identical to the dose needed to achieve an initial response. Nevertheless, patients should be periodically reassessed to determine the need for maintenance treatment.

Premenstrual Dysphoric Disorder–The effectiveness of ZOLOFT in long-term use, that is, for more than 3 menstrual cycles, has not been systematically evaluated in controlled trials. However, as women commonly report that symptoms worsen with age until relieved by the onset of menopause, it is reasonable to consider continuation of a responding patient. Dosage adjustments, which may include changes between dosage regimens (e.g., daily throughout the menstrual cycle versus during the luteal phase of the menstrual cycle), may be needed to maintain the patient on the lowest effective dosage and patients should be periodically reassessed to determine the need for continued treatment.

Switching Patients to or from a Monoamine Oxidase Inhibitor–At least 14 days should elapse between discontinuation of an MAOI and initiation of therapy with ZOLOFT. In addition, at least 14 days should be allowed after stopping ZOLOFT before starting an MAOI (see CONTRAINDICATIONS and WARNINGS).

ZOLOFT Oral Concentrate

ZOLOFT Oral Concentrate contains 20 mg/mL of sertraline (as the hydrochloride) as the active ingredient and 12% alcohol. ZOLOFT Oral Concentrate must be diluted before use. Just before taking, use the dropper provided to remove the required amount of ZOLOFT Oral Concentrate and mix with 4 oz (1/2 cup) of water, ginger ale, lemon/lime soda, lemonade or orange juice ONLY. Do not mix ZOLOFT Oral Concentrate with anything other than the liquids listed. The dose should be taken immediately after mixing. Do not mix in advance. At times, a slight haze may appear after mixing; this is normal. Note that caution should be exercised for patients with latex sensitivity, as the dropper dispenser contains dry natural rubber.

ZOLOFT Oral Concentrate is contraindicated with ANTABUSE (disulfiram) due to the alcohol content of the concentrate.

HOW SUPPLIED

ZOLOFT® (sertraline hydrochloride) capsular-shaped scored tablets, containing sertraline hydrochloride equivalent to 25, 50 and 100 mg of sertraline, are packaged in bottles.

ZOLOFT® 25 mg Tablets: light green film coated tablets engraved on one side with ZOLOFT and on the other side scored and engraved with 25 mg.

NDC 0049-4960-50	Bottles of 50

ZOLOFT® 50 mg Tablets: light blue film coated tablets engraved on one side with ZOLOFT and on the other side scored and engraved with 50 mg.

NDC 0049-4900-66	Bottles of 100
NDC 0049-4900-73	Bottles of 500
NDC 0049-4900-94	Bottles of 5000
NDC 0049-4900-41	Unit Dose Packages of 100

ZOLOFT® 100 mg Tablets: light yellow film coated tablets engraved on one side with ZOLOFT and on the other side scored and engraved with 100 mg.

Continued on next page

Zoloft—Cont.

NDC 0049-4910-66 Bottles of 100
NDC 0049-4910-73 Bottles of 500
NDC 0049-4910-94 Bottles of 5000
NDC 0049-4910-41 Unit Dose Packages of 100

Store at 25°C (77°F); excursions permitted to 15°-30°C (59°-86°F) [see USP Controlled Room Temperature].

ZOLOFT® Oral Concentrate: ZOLOFT Oral Concentrate is a clear, colorless solution with a menthol scent containing sertraline hydrochloride equivalent to 20 mg of sertraline per mL and 12% alcohol. It is supplied as a 60 mL bottle with an accompanying calibrated dropper.

NDC 0049-4940-23 Bottles of 60 mL

Store at 25°C (77°F); excursions permitted to 15° - 30°C (59° - 86°F) [see USP Controlled Room Temperature].

Rx only

Distributed by
Pfizer Roerig
Division of Pfizer Inc, NY, NY 10017
69-4721-00-7 Revised September 2003

Shown in Product Identification Guide, page 330

ZYRTEC® ℞

[*zər'tĕk*]
(cetirizine hydrochloride)
Tablets, Chewable Tablets and Syrup
For Oral Use

DESCRIPTION

Cetirizine hydrochloride, the active component of ZYRTEC® tablets and syrup, is an orally active and selective H_1-receptor antagonist. The chemical name is (±) - [2- [4- [(4- chlorophenyl)phenylmethyl] -1- piperazinyl] ethoxy]acetic acid, dihydrochloride. Cetirizine hydrochloride is a racemic compound with an empirical formula of $C_{21}H_{25}ClN_2O_3 \bullet 2HCl$. The molecular weight is 461.82 and the chemical structure is shown below:

Cetirizine hydrochloride is a white, crystalline powder and is water soluble. ZYRTEC tablets are formulated as white, film-coated, rounded-off rectangular shaped tablets for oral administration and are available in 5 and 10 mg strengths. Inactive ingredients are: lactose; magnesium stearate; povidone; titanium dioxide; hypromellose; polyethylene glycol; and corn starch.

ZYRTEC chewable tablets are formulated as purple round tablets for oral administration and are available in 5 and 10 mg strengths. Inactive ingredients of the chewable tablets are: acesulfame potassium; artificial grape flavor; betadex, NF; blue dye; colloidal silicon dioxide; lactose monohydrate; magnesium stearate; mannitol; microcrystalline cellulose; natural flavor; red dye (carmine).

ZYRTEC syrup is a colorless to slightly yellow syrup containing cetirizine hydrochloride at a concentration of 1 mg/mL (5 mg/5 mL) for oral administration. The pH is between 4 and 5. The inactive ingredients of the syrup are: banana flavor; glacial acetic acid; glycerin; grape flavor; methylparaben; propylene glycol; propylparaben; sodium acetate; sugar syrup; and water.

CLINICAL PHARMACOLOGY

Mechanism of Actions: Cetirizine, a human metabolite of hydroxyzine, is an antihistamine; its principal effects are mediated via selective inhibition of peripheral H_1 receptors. The antihistaminic activity of cetirizine has been clearly documented in a variety of animal and human models. *In vivo* and *ex vivo* animal models have shown negligible anticholinergic and antiserotonergic activity. In clinical studies, however, dry mouth was more common with cetirizine than with placebo. *In vitro* receptor binding studies have shown no measurable affinity for other than H_1 receptors. Autoradiographic studies with radiolabeled cetirizine in the rat have shown negligible penetration into the brain. *Ex vivo* experiments in the mouse have shown that systemically administered cetirizine does not significantly occupy cerebral H_1 receptors.

Pharmacokinetics:

Absorption: Cetirizine was rapidly absorbed with a time to maximum concentration (Tmax) of approximately 1 hour following oral administration of tablets, chewable tablets or syrup in adults. Comparable bioavailability was found between the tablet and syrup dosage forms. Comparable bioavailability was also found between the ZYRTEC tablet and the ZYRTEC chewable tablet taken with or without water. When healthy volunteers were administered multiple doses of cetirizine (10 mg tablets once daily for 10 days), a mean peak plasma concentration (Cmax) of 311 ng/mL was observed. No accumulation was observed. Cetirizine pharmacokinetics were linear for oral doses ranging from 5 to 60 mg. Food had no effect on the extent of exposure (AUC) of the cetirizine tablet or chewable tablet, but Tmax was delayed by 1.7 hours and 2.8 hours respectively, and Cmax was decreased by 23% and 37%, respectively in the presence of food.

Distribution: The mean plasma protein binding of cetirizine is 93%, independent of concentration in the range of 25-1000 ng/mL, which includes the therapeutic plasma levels observed.

Metabolism: A mass balance study in 6 healthy male volunteers indicated that 70% of the administered radioactivity was recovered in the urine and 10% in the feces. Approximately 50% of the radioactivity was identified in the urine as unchanged drug. Most of the rapid increase in peak plasma radioactivity was associated with parent drug, suggesting a low degree of first-pass metabolism. Cetirizine is metabolized to a limited extent by oxidative O-dealkylation to a metabolite with negligible antihistaminic activity. The enzyme or enzymes responsible for this metabolism have not been identified.

Elimination: The mean elimination half-life in 146 healthy volunteers across multiple pharmacokinetic studies was 8.3 hours and the apparent total body clearance for cetirizine was approximately 53 mL/min.

Interaction Studies

Pharmacokinetic interaction studies with cetirizine in adults were conducted with pseudoephedrine, antipyrine, ketoconazole, erythromycin and azithromycin. No interactions were observed. In a multiple dose study of theophylline (400 mg once daily for 3 days) and cetirizine (20 mg once daily for 3 days), a 16% decrease in the clearance of cetirizine was observed. The disposition of theophylline was not altered by concomitant cetirizine administration.

Special Populations

Pediatric Patients: When pediatric patients aged 7 to 12 years received a single, 5-mg oral cetirizine capsule, the mean Cmax was 275 ng/mL. Based on cross-study comparisons, the weight-normalized, apparent total body clearance was 33% greater and the elimination half-life was 33% shorter in this pediatric population than in adults. In pediatric patients aged 2 to 5 years who received 5 mg of cetirizine, the mean Cmax was 660 ng/mL. Based on cross-study comparisons, the weight-normalized apparent total body clearance was 81 to 111% greater and the elimination half-life was 33 to 41% shorter in this pediatric population than in adults. In pediatric patients aged 6 to 23 months who received a single dose of 0.25 mg/kg cetirizine oral solution (mean dose 2.3 mg), the mean Cmax was 390 ng/mL. Based on cross-study comparisons, the weight-normalized, apparent total body clearance was 304% greater and the elimination half-life was 63% shorter in this pediatric population compared to adults. The average AUC(0-t) in children 6 months to <2 years of age receiving the maximum dose of cetirizine solution (2.5 mg twice a day) is expected to be two-fold higher than that observed in adults receiving a dose of 10 mg cetirizine tablets once a day.

Geriatric Patients: Following a single, 10-mg oral dose, the elimination half-life was prolonged by 50% and the apparent total body clearance was 40% lower in 16 geriatric subjects with a mean age of 77 years compared to 14 adult subjects with a mean age of 53 years. The decrease in cetirizine clearance in these elderly volunteers may be related to decreased renal function.

A dosing adjustment may be necessary in patients 77 years of age and older (see **DOSAGE AND ADMINISTRATION**).

Effect of Gender: The effect of gender on cetirizine pharmacokinetics has not been adequately studied.

Effect of Race: No race-related differences in the kinetics of cetirizine have been observed.

Renal Impairment: The kinetics of cetirizine were studied following multiple, oral, 10-mg daily doses of cetirizine for 7 days in 7 normal volunteers (creatinine clearance 89-128 mL/min), 8 patients with mild renal function impairment (creatinine clearance 42-77 mL/min) and 7 patients with moderate renal function impairment (creatinine clearance 11-31 mL/min). The pharmacokinetics of cetirizine were similar in patients with mild impairment and normal volunteers. Moderately impaired patients had a 3-fold increase in half-life and a 70% decrease in clearance compared to normal volunteers.

Patients on hemodialysis (n=5) given a single, 10-mg dose of cetirizine had a 3-fold increase in half-life and a 70% decrease in clearance compared to normal volunteers. Less than 10% of the administered dose was removed during the single dialysis session.

Dosing adjustment is necessary in patients with moderate or severe renal impairment and in patients on dialysis (see **DOSAGE AND ADMINISTRATION**).

Hepatic Impairment: Sixteen patients with chronic liver diseases (hepatocellular, cholestatic, and biliary cirrhosis), given 10 or 20 mg of cetirizine as a single, oral dose had a 50% increase in half-life along with a corresponding 40% decrease in clearance compared to 16 healthy subjects.

Dosing adjustment may be necessary in patients with hepatic impairment (see **DOSAGE AND ADMINISTRATION**).

Pharmacodynamics: Studies in 69 adult normal volunteers (aged 20 to 61 years) showed that ZYRTEC at doses of 5 and 10 mg strongly inhibited the skin wheal and flare caused by the intradermal injection of histamine. The onset of this activity after a single 10-mg dose occurred within 20 minutes in 50% of subjects and within one hour in 95% of subjects; this activity persisted for at least 24 hours. ZYRTEC at doses of 5 and 10 mg also strongly inhibited the wheal and flare caused by intradermal injection of histamine in 19 pediatric volunteers (aged 5 to 12 years) and the activity persisted for at least 24 hours. In a 35-day study in children aged 5 to 12, no tolerance to the antihistaminic (suppression of wheal and flare response) effects of ZYRTEC was found. In 10 infants 7 to 25 months of age who received 4 to 9 days of cetirizine in an oral solution (0.25 mg/kg bid), there was a 90% inhibition of histamine-induced (10 mg/mL) cutaneous wheal and 87% inhibition of the flare 12 hours after administration of the last dose. The clinical relevance of this suppression of histamine-induced wheal and flare response on skin testing is unknown.

The effects of intradermal injection of various other mediators or histamine releasers were also inhibited by cetirizine, as was response to a cold challenge in patients with cold-induced urticaria. In mildly asthmatic subjects, ZYRTEC at 5 to 20 mg blocked bronchoconstriction due to nebulized histamine, with virtually total blockade after a 20-mg dose. In studies conducted for up to 12 hours following cutaneous antigen challenge, the late phase recruitment of eosinophils, neutrophils and basophils, components of the allergic inflammatory response, was inhibited by ZYRTEC at a dose of 20 mg.

In four clinical studies in healthy adult males, no clinically significant mean increases in QTc were observed in ZYRTEC treated subjects. In the first study, a placebo-controlled crossover trial, ZYRTEC was given at doses up to 60 mg per day, 6 times the maximum clinical dose, for 1 week, and no significant mean QTc prolongation occurred. In the second study, a crossover trial, ZYRTEC 20 mg and erythromycin (500 mg every 8 hours) were given alone and in combination. There was no significant effect on QTc with the combination or with ZYRTEC alone. In the third trial, also a crossover study, ZYRTEC 20 mg and ketoconazole (400 mg per day) were given alone and in combination. ZYRTEC caused a mean increase in QTc of 9.1 msec from baseline after 10 days of therapy. Ketoconazole also increased QTc by 8.3 msec. The combination caused an increase of 17.4 msec, equal to the sum of the individual effects. Thus, there was no significant drug interaction on QTc with the combination of ZYRTEC and ketoconazole. In the fourth study, a placebo-controlled parallel trial, ZYRTEC 20 mg was given alone or in combination with azithromycin (500 mg as a single dose on the first day followed by 250 mg once daily). There was no significant increase in QTc with ZYRTEC 20 mg alone or in combination with azithromycin.

In a four-week clinical trial in pediatric patients aged 6 to 11 years, results of randomly obtained ECG measurements before treatment and after 2 weeks of treatment showed that ZYRTEC 5 or 10 mg did not increase QTc versus placebo. In a one week clinical trial (N=86) of ZYRTEC syrup (0.25 mg/kg bid) compared with placebo in pediatric patients 6 to 11 months of age, ECG measurements taken within 3 hours of the last dose did not show any ECG abnormalities or increases in QTc interval in either group compared to baseline assessments. Data from other studies where ZYRTEC was administered to patients 6-23 months of age were consistent with the findings in this study.

The effects of ZYRTEC on the QTc interval at doses higher than 10 mg have not been studied in children less than 12 years of age.

In a six-week, placebo-controlled study of 186 patients (aged 12 to 64 years) with allergic rhinitis and mild to moderate asthma, ZYRTEC 10 mg once daily improved rhinitis symptoms and did not alter pulmonary function. In a two-week, placebo-controlled clinical trial, a subset analysis of 65 pediatric (aged 6 to 11 years) allergic rhinitis patients with asthma showed ZYRTEC did not alter pulmonary function. These studies support the safety of administering ZYRTEC to pediatric and adult allergic rhinitis patients with mild to moderate asthma.

Clinical Studies: Nine multicenter, randomized, double-blind, clinical trials comparing cetirizine 5 to 20 mg to placebo in patients 12 years and older with seasonal or perennial allergic rhinitis were conducted in the United States. Five of these showed significant reductions in symptoms of allergic rhinitis, 3 in seasonal allergic rhinitis (1 to 4 weeks in duration) and 2 in perennial allergic rhinitis for up to 8 weeks in duration. Two 4-week multicenter, randomized, double-blind, clinical trials comparing cetirizine 5 to 20 mg to placebo in patients with chronic idiopathic urticaria were also conducted and showed significant improvement in symptoms of chronic idiopathic urticaria. In general, the 10-mg dose was more effective than the 5-mg dose and the 20-mg dose gave no added effect. Some of these trials included pediatric patients aged 12 to 16 years. In addition, four multicenter, randomized, placebo-controlled, double-blind 2-4 week trials in 534 pediatric patients aged 6 to 11 years with seasonal allergic rhinitis were conducted in the United States at doses up to 10 mg.

INDICATIONS AND USAGE

Seasonal Allergic Rhinitis: ZYRTEC is indicated for the relief of symptoms associated with seasonal allergic rhinitis due to allergens such as ragweed, grass and tree pollens in adults and children 2 years of age and older. Symptoms treated effectively include sneezing, rhinorrhea, nasal pruritus, ocular pruritus, tearing, and redness of the eyes.

Perennial Allergic Rhinitis: ZYRTEC is indicated for the relief of symptoms associated with perennial allergic rhinitis due to allergens such as dust mites, animal dander and molds in adults and children 6 months of age and older. Symptoms treated effectively include sneezing, rhinorrhea, postnasal discharge, nasal pruritus, ocular pruritus, and tearing.

Chronic Urticaria: ZYRTEC is indicated for the treatment of the uncomplicated skin manifestations of chronic idiopathic urticaria in adults and children 6 months of age and older. It significantly reduces the occurrence, severity, and duration of hives and significantly reduces pruritus.

CONTRAINDICATIONS

ZYRTEC is contraindicated in those patients with a known hypersensitivity to it or any of its ingredients or hydroxyzine.

PRECAUTIONS

Activities Requiring Mental Alertness: In clinical trials, the occurrence of somnolence has been reported in some patients taking ZYRTEC; due caution should therefore be exercised when driving a car or operating potentially dangerous machinery. Concurrent use of ZYRTEC with alcohol or other CNS depressants should be avoided because additional reductions in alertness and additional impairment of CNS performance may occur.

Drug-Drug Interactions: No clinically significant drug interactions have been found with theophylline at a low dose, azithromycin, pseudoephedrine, ketoconazole, or erythromycin. There was a small decrease in the clearance of cetirizine caused by a 400-mg dose of theophylline; it is possible that larger theophylline doses could have a greater effect.

Carcinogenesis, Mutagenesis and Impairment of Fertility: In a 2-year carcinogenicity study in rats, cetirizine was not carcinogenic at dietary doses up to 20 mg/kg (approximately 15 times the maximum recommended daily oral dose in adults on a mg/m^2 basis, or approximately 7 times the maximum recommended daily oral dose in infants on a mg/m^2 basis). In a 2-year carcinogenicity study in mice, cetirizine caused an increased incidence of benign liver tumors in males at a dietary dose of 16 mg/kg (approximately 6 times the maximum recommended daily oral dose in adults on a mg/m^2 basis, or approximately 3 times the maximum recommended daily oral dose in infants on a mg/m^2 basis). No increase in the incidence of liver tumors was observed in mice at a dietary dose of 4 mg/kg (approximately 2 times the maximum recommended daily oral dose in adults on a mg/m^2 basis, or approximately equivalent to the maximum recommended daily oral dose in infants on a mg/m^2 basis). The clinical significance of these findings during long-term use of ZYRTEC is not known.

Cetirizine was not mutagenic in the Ames test, and not clastogenic in the human lymphocyte assay, the mouse lymphoma assay, and *in vivo* micronucleus test in rats.

In a fertility and general reproductive performance study in mice, cetirizine did not impair fertility at an oral dose of 64 mg/kg (approximately 25 times the maximum recommended daily oral dose in adults on a mg/m^2 basis).

Pregnancy Category B: In mice, rats, and rabbits, cetirizine was not teratogenic at oral doses up to 96, 225, and 135 mg/kg, respectively (approximately 40, 180 and 220 times the maximum recommended daily oral dose in adults on a mg/m^2 basis). There are, however, no adequate and well-controlled studies in pregnant women. Because animal reproduction studies are not always predictive of human response, ZYRTEC should be used during pregnancy only if clearly needed.

Nursing Mothers: In mice, cetirizine caused retarded pup weight gain during lactation at an oral dose in dams of 96 mg/kg (approximately 40 times the maximum recommended daily oral dose in adults on a mg/m^2 basis). Studies in beagle dogs indicated that approximately 3% of the dose was excreted in milk. Cetirizine has been reported to be excreted in human breast milk. Because many drugs are excreted in human milk, use of ZYRTEC in nursing mothers is not recommended.

Geriatric Use: Of the total number of patients in clinical studies of ZYRTEC, 186 patients were 65 years and older, and 39 patients were 75 years and older. No overall differences in safety were observed between these patients and younger patients, but greater sensitivity of some older individuals cannot be ruled out. With regard to efficacy, clinical studies of ZYRTEC for each approved indication did not include sufficient numbers of patients aged 65 years and older to determine whether they respond differently than younger patients.

ZYRTEC is known to be substantially excreted by the kidney, and the risk of toxic reactions to this drug may be greater in patients with impaired renal function. Because elderly patients are more likely to have decreased renal function, care should be taken in dose selection, and it may be useful to monitor renal function. (See **Geriatric Patients** and **Renal Impairment** subsections in **CLINICAL PHARMACOLOGY**).

Pediatric Use: The safety of ZYRTEC has been demonstrated in pediatric patients aged 6 months to 11 years. The safety of ZYRTEC, at daily doses of 5 or 10 mg, has been demonstrated in 376 pediatric patients aged 6 to 11 years in placebo-controlled trials lasting up to four weeks and in 254 patients in a non-placebo-controlled 12-week trial. The safety of cetirizine has been demonstrated in 168 patients aged 2 to 5 years in placebo-controlled trials of up to 4 weeks duration. On a mg/kg basis, most of the 168 patients received between 0.2 and 0.4 mg/kg of cetirizine HCl. The safety of cetirizine in 399 patients aged 12 to 24 months has been demonstrated in a placebo-controlled 18-month trial, in which the average dose was 0.25 mg/kg bid, corresponding to a range of 4 to 11 mg/day. The safety of ZYRTEC syrup has been demonstrated in 42 patients aged 6 to 11 months in a placebo-controlled 7-day trial. The prescribed dose was 0.25 mg/kg bid, which corresponded to a mean of 4.5 mg/day, with a range of 3.4 to 6.2 mg/day.

The effectiveness of ZYRTEC for the treatment of allergic rhinitis and chronic idiopathic urticaria in pediatric patients aged 6 months to 11 years is based on an extrapolation of the demonstrated efficacy of ZYRTEC in adults with these conditions and the likelihood that the disease course, pathophysiology and the drug's effect are substantially similar between these two populations. Efficacy is extrapolated down to 6 months of age for perennial allergic rhinitis and down to 2 years of age for seasonal allergic rhinitis because these diseases are thought to occur down to these ages in children. The recommended doses for the pediatric population are based on cross-study comparisons of the pharmacokinetics and pharmacodynamics of cetirizine in adult and pediatric subjects and on the safety profile of cetirizine in both adult and pediatric patients at doses equal to or higher than the recommended doses. The cetirizine AUC and Cmax in pediatric subjects aged 6 to 23 months who received a mean of 2.3 mg in a single dose, and in subjects aged 2 to 5 years who received a single dose of 5 mg of cetirizine syrup and in pediatric subjects aged 6 to 11 years who received a single dose of 10 mg of cetirizine syrup were estimated to be intermediate between that observed in adults who received a single dose of 10 mg of cetirizine tablets and those who received a single dose of 20 mg of cetirizine tablets.

The safety and effectiveness of cetirizine in pediatric patients under the age of 6 months have not been established.

ADVERSE REACTIONS

Controlled and uncontrolled clinical trials conducted in the United States and Canada included more than 6000 patients aged 12 years and older, with more than 3900 receiving ZYRTEC at doses of 5 to 20 mg per day. The duration of treatment ranged from 1 week to 6 months, with a mean exposure of 30 days.

Most adverse reactions reported during therapy with ZYRTEC were mild or moderate. In placebo-controlled trials, the incidence of discontinuations due to adverse reactions in patients receiving ZYRTEC 5 or 10 mg was not significantly different from placebo (2.9% vs. 2.4%, respectively).

The most common adverse reaction in patients aged 12 years and older that occurred more frequently on ZYRTEC than placebo was somnolence. The incidence of somnolence associated with ZYRTEC was dose related, 6% in placebo, 11% at 5 mg and 14% at 10 mg. Discontinuations due to somnolence for ZYRTEC were uncommon (1.0% on ZYRTEC vs. 0.6% on placebo). Fatigue and dry mouth also appeared to be treatment-related adverse reactions. There were no differences by age, race, gender or by body weight with regard to the incidence of adverse reactions.

Table 1 lists adverse experiences in patients aged 12 years and older which were reported for ZYRTEC 5 and 10 mg in controlled clinical trials in the United States and that were more common with ZYRTEC than placebo.

Table 1.
Adverse Experiences Reported in Patients Aged 12 Years and Older in Placebo-Controlled United States ZYRTEC Trials (Maximum Dose of 10 mg) at Rates of 2% or Greater (Percent Incidence)

Adverse Experience	ZYRTEC (N=2034)	Placebo (N=1612)
Somnolence	13.7	6.3
Fatigue	5.9	2.6
Dry Mouth	5.0	2.3
Pharyngitis	2.0	1.9
Dizziness	2.0	1.2

In addition, headache and nausea occurred in more than 2% of the patients, but were more common in placebo patients. Pediatric studies were also conducted with ZYRTEC. More than 1300 pediatric patients aged 6 to 11 years with more than 900 treated with ZYRTEC at doses of 1.25 to 10 mg per day were included in controlled and uncontrolled clinical trials conducted in the United States. The duration of treatment ranged from 2 to 12 weeks. Placebo-controlled trials up to 4 weeks duration included 168 pediatric patients aged 2 to 5 years who received cetirizine, the majority of whom received single daily doses of 5 mg. A placebo-controlled trial 18 months in duration included 399 patients aged 12 to 24 months treated with cetirizine (0.25 mg/kg bid), and another placebo-controlled trial of 7 days duration included 42 patients aged 6 to 11 months who were treated with cetirizine (0.25 mg/kg bid).

The majority of adverse reactions reported in pediatric patients aged 2 to 11 years with ZYRTEC were mild or moderate. In placebo-controlled trials, the incidence of discontinuations due to adverse reactions in pediatric patients receiving up to 10 mg of ZYRTEC was uncommon (0.4% on ZYRTEC vs. 1.0% on placebo).

Table 2 lists adverse experiences which were reported for ZYRTEC 5 and 10 mg in pediatric patients aged 6 to 11 years in placebo-controlled clinical trials in the United States and were more common with ZYRTEC than placebo. Of these, abdominal pain was considered treatment-related and somnolence appeared to be dose-related, 1.3% in placebo, 1.9% at 5 mg and 4.2% at 10 mg. The adverse experiences reported in pediatric patients aged 2 to 5 years in placebo-controlled trials were qualitatively similar in nature and generally similar in frequency to those reported in trials with children aged 6 to 11 years.

In the placebo-controlled trials of pediatric patients 6 to 24 months of age, the incidences of adverse experiences were similar in the cetirizine and placebo treatment groups in each study. Somnolence occurred with essentially the same frequency in patients who received cetirizine and patients who received placebo. In a study of 1 week duration in children 6-11 months of age, patients who received cetirizine exhibited greater irritability/fussiness than patients on placebo. In a study of 18 months duration in patients 12 months and older, insomnia occurred more frequently in patients who received cetirizine compared to patients who received placebo (9.0% v. 5.3%). In those patients who received 5 mg or more per day of cetirizine as compared to patients who received placebo, fatigue (3.6% v. 1.3%) and malaise (3.6% v. 1.8%) occurred more frequently.

Table 2.
Adverse Experiences Reported in Pediatric Patients Aged 6 to 11 Years in Placebo-Controlled United States ZYRTEC Trials (5 or 10 mg Dose) Which Occurred at a Frequency of ≥2% in Either the 5-mg or the 10-mg ZYRTEC Group, and More Frequently Than in the Placebo Group

Adverse Experiences	Placebo (N=309)	ZYRTEC 5 mg (N=161)	ZYRTEC 10 mg (N=215)
Headache	12.3%	11.0%	14.0%
Pharyngitis	2.9%	6.2%	2.8%
Abdominal pain	1.9%	4.4%	5.6%
Coughing	3.9%	4.4%	2.8%
Somnolence	1.3%	1.9%	4.2%
Diarrhea	1.3%	3.1%	1.9%
Epistaxis	2.9%	3.7%	1.9%
Bronchospasm	1.9%	3.1%	1.9%
Nausea	1.9%	1.9%	2.8%
Vomiting	1.0%	2.5%	2.3%

The following events were observed infrequently (less than 2%), in either 3982 adults and children 12 years and older or in 659 pediatric patients aged 6 to 11 years who received ZYRTEC in U.S. trials, including an open adult study of six months duration. A causal relationship of these infrequent events with ZYRTEC administration has not been established.

Autonomic Nervous System: anorexia, flushing, increased salivation, urinary retention.

Cardiovascular: cardiac failure, hypertension, palpitation, tachycardia.

Central and Peripheral Nervous Systems: abnormal coordination, ataxia, confusion, dysphonia, hyperesthesia, hyperkinesia, hypertonia, hypoesthesia, leg cramps, migraine, myelitis, paralysis, paresthesia, ptosis, syncope, tremor, twitching, vertigo, visual field defect.

Gastrointestinal: abnormal hepatic function, aggravated tooth caries, constipation, dyspepsia, eructation, flatulence, gastritis, hemorrhoids, increased appetite, melena, rectal hemorrhage, stomatitis including ulcerative stomatitis, tongue discoloration, tongue edema.

Genitourinary: cystitis, dysuria, hematuria, micturition frequency, polyuria, urinary incontinence, urinary tract infection.

Hearing and Vestibular: deafness, earache, ototoxicity, tinnitus.

Metabolic/Nutritional: dehydration, diabetes mellitus, thirst.

Musculoskeletal: arthralgia, arthritis, arthrosis, muscle weakness, myalgia.

Psychiatric: abnormal thinking, agitation, amnesia, anxiety, decreased libido, depersonalization, depression, emotional lability, euphoria, impaired concentration, insomnia, nervousness, paroniria, sleep disorder.

Respiratory System: bronchitis, dyspnea, hyperventilation, increased sputum, pneumonia, respiratory disorder, rhinitis, sinusitis, upper respiratory tract infection.

Reproductive: dysmenorrhea, female breast pain, intermenstrual bleeding, leukorrhea, menorrhagia, vaginitis.

Reticuloendothelial: lymphadenopathy.

Skin: acne, alopecia, angioedema, bullous eruption, dermatitis, dry skin, eczema, erythematous rash, furunculosis, hyperkeratosis, hypertrichosis, increased sweating, maculopapular rash, photosensitivity reaction, photosensitivity toxic reaction, pruritus, purpura, rash, seborrhea, skin disorder, skin nodule, urticaria.

Special Senses: parosmia, taste loss, taste perversion.

Vision: blindness, conjunctivitis, eye pain, glaucoma, loss of accommodation, ocular hemorrhage, xerophthalmia.

Continued on next page

Zyrtec—Cont.

Body as a Whole: accidental injury, asthenia, back pain, chest pain, enlarged abdomen, face edema, fever, generalized edema, hot flashes, increased weight, leg edema, malaise, nasal polyp, pain, pallor, periorbital edema, peripheral edema, rigors.

Occasional instances of transient, reversible hepatic transaminase elevations have occurred during cetirizine therapy. Hepatitis with significant transaminase elevation and elevated bilirubin in association with the use of ZYRTEC has been reported.

Post-Marketing Experience

In the post-marketing period, the following additional rare, but potentially severe adverse events have been reported: aggressive reaction, anaphylaxis, cholestasis, convulsions, glomerulonephritis, hallucinations, hemolytic anemia, hepatitis, orofacial dyskinesia, severe hypotension, stillbirth, suicidal ideation, suicide and thrombocytopenia.

DRUG ABUSE AND DEPENDENCE

There is no information to indicate that abuse or dependency occurs with ZYRTEC.

OVERDOSAGE

Overdosage has been reported with ZYRTEC. In one adult patient who took 150 mg of ZYRTEC, the patient was somnolent but did not display any other clinical signs or abnormal blood chemistry or hematology results. In an 18 month old pediatric patient who took an overdose of ZYRTEC (approximately 180 mg), restlessness and irritability were observed initially; this was followed by drowsiness. Should overdose occur, treatment should be symptomatic or supportive, taking into account any concomitantly ingested medications. There is no known specific antidote to ZYRTEC. ZYRTEC is not effectively removed by dialysis, and dialysis will be ineffective unless a dialyzable agent has been concomitantly ingested. The acute minimal lethal oral doses were 237 mg/kg in mice (approximately 95 times the maximum recommended daily oral dose in adults on a mg/m^2 basis, or approximately 40 times the maximum recommended daily oral dose in infants on a mg/m^2 basis) and 562 mg/kg in rats (approximately 460 times the maximum recommended daily oral dose in adults on a mg/m^2 basis, or approximately 190 times the maximum recommended daily oral dose in infants on a mg/m^2 basis). In rodents, the target of acute toxicity was the central nervous system, and the target of multiple-dose toxicity was the liver.

DOSAGE AND ADMINISTRATION

ZYRTEC can be taken without regard to food consumption. ZYRTEC is available as 5 mg and 10 mg tablets, 1 mg/mL syrup, and 5 mg and 10 mg chewable tablets which can be taken with or without water.

Adults and Children 12 Years and Older: The recommended initial dose of ZYRTEC is 5 mg or 10 mg per day in adults and children 12 years and older, depending on symptom severity. Most patients in clinical trials started at 10 mg. ZYRTEC is given as a single daily dose. The time of administration may be varied to suit individual patient needs.

Children 6 to 11 Years: The recommended initial dose of ZYRTEC in children aged 6 to 11 years is 5 mg or 10 mg once daily depending on symptom severity. The time of administration may be varied to suit individual patient needs.

Children 2 to 5 Years: The recommended initial dose of ZYRTEC in children aged 2 to 5 years is 2.5 mg (½ teaspoon) syrup once daily. The dosage in this age group can be increased to a maximum dose of 5 mg per day given as 1 teaspoon syrup once a day or one ½ teaspoon syrup given every 12 hours, or one 5 mg chewable tablet once a day.

Children 6 months to <2 years: The recommended dose of ZYRTEC syrup in children 6 months to 23 months of age is 2.5 mg (½ teaspoon) once daily. The dose in children 12 to 23 months of age can be increased to a maximum dose of 5 mg per day, given as ½ teaspoon (2.5 mg) every 12 hours. Syrup is recommended for children under the age of 2 years.

Dose Adjustment for Renal and Hepatic Impairment: In patients 12 years of age and older with decreased renal function (creatinine clearance 11-31 mL/min), patients on hemodialysis (creatinine clearance less than 7 mL/min), and in hepatically impaired patients, a dose of 5 mg once daily is recommended. Similarly, pediatric patients aged 6 to 11 years with impaired renal or hepatic function should use the lower recommended dose. Because of the difficulty in reliably administering doses of less than 2.5 mg (½ teaspoon) of ZYRTEC syrup and in the absence of pharmacokinetic and safety information for cetirizine in children below the age of 6 years with impaired renal or hepatic function, its use in this impaired patient population is not recommended.

Dose Adjustment for Geriatric Patients: In patients 77 years of age and older, a dose of 5 mg once daily is recommended.

HOW SUPPLIED

ZYRTEC® tablets are white, film-coated, rounded-off rectangular shaped containing 5 mg or 10 mg cetirizine hydrochloride.

5 mg tablets are engraved with "ZYRTEC" on one side and "5" on the other.
Bottles of 100: NDC 0069-5500-66
10 mg tablets are engraved with "ZYRTEC" on one side and "10" on the other.
Bottles of 100: NDC 0069-5510-66

STORAGE: Store at 20-25°C (68-77°F); excursions permitted to 15-30°C (59-86°F) [see USP Controlled Room Temperature].

ZYRTEC chewable tablets are purple round tablets containing 5 mg or 10 mg cetirizine hydrochloride. The tablets are packaged in blister cards as follows:

5 mg tablets are engraved with "ZYRTEC C5" on one side.
Boxes of 3 (Blister Cards of 10) NDC 0069-1440-03
10 mg tablets are engraved with "ZYRTEC C10" on one side.
Boxes of 3 (Blister Cards of 10) NDC 0069-1450-03

STORAGE: Store at 20-25°C (68-77°F); excursions permitted to 15-30°C (59-86°F) [see USP Controlled Room Temperature].

ZYRTEC syrup is colorless to slightly yellow with a banana-grape flavor. Each teaspoon (5 mL) contains 5 mg cetirizine hydrochloride. ZYRTEC syrup is supplied as follows:

120 mL amber glass bottles NDC 0069-5530-47
1 pint amber glass bottles NDC 0069-5530-93

STORAGE: Store at 20-25°C (68-77°F) excursions permitted to 15-30°C (59-86°F) [see USP Controlled Room Temperature]; **or Store refrigerated, 2-8°C (36-46°F).**

Cetirizine is licensed from UCB Pharma, Inc.

Rx only **©2004 PFIZER INC**

Manufactured/Marketed by
Pfizer Labs
Division of Pfizer Inc, NY, NY 10017
Marketed by
UCB Pharma, Inc.
Smyrna, GA 30080
70-4573-00-8 Revised March 2004

Shown in Product Identification Guide, page 330

ZYRTEC-D 12 HOUR® ℞

(cetirizine hydrochloride 5 mg and pseudoephedrine hydrochloride 120 mg)
Extended Release Tablets
For Oral Use

DESCRIPTION

ZYRTEC-D 12 HOUR™ (cetirizine hydrochloride 5 mg and pseudoephedrine hydrochloride 120 mg) Extended Release Tablets for oral administration contain 5 mg of cetirizine hydrochloride for immediate release and 120 mg of pseudoephedrine hydrochloride for extended release in a bilayer tablet. Tablets also contain as inactive ingredients: colloidal silicon dioxide, croscarmellose sodium, hypromellose, lactose monohydrate, magnesium stearate, microcrystalline cellulose.

Cetirizine hydrochloride, one of the two active components of ZYRTEC-D 12 HOUR Extended Release Tablets, is an orally active and selective H_1-receptor antagonist. The chemical name is (+/–)- [2-[4-[(4-chlorophenyl)phenylmethyl]-1-piperazinyl] ethoxy] acetic acid, dihydrochloride. Cetirizine hydrochloride is a racemic compound with an empirical formula of $C_{21}H_{25}ClN_2O_3 \cdot 2HCl$. The molecular weight is 461.82. Cetirizine hydrochloride is a white, crystalline powder and is water-soluble. The chemical structure is shown below:

Cl HC—N N—O—OH O • 2 HCl

Pseudoephedrine hydrochloride, the other active ingredient of ZYRTEC-D 12 HOUR Extended Release Tablets, is an adrenergic (vasoconstrictor) agent with the chemical name (1S.2S)-2-methylamino-1-phenyl-1-propanol hydrochloride. The molecular weight is 201.70. The molecular formula is $C_{10}H_{15}NO \cdot HCl$. Pseudoephedrine hydrochloride occurs as fine, white to off-white crystals or powder, having a faint characteristic odor. It is very soluble in water, freely soluble in alcohol, and sparingly soluble in chloroform. The chemical structure is shown below:

H OH H N CH₃ • HCl H₃C H

CLINICAL PHARMACOLOGY

Mechanisms of Action: Cetirizine, a metabolite of hydroxyzine, is an antihistamine; its principal effects are mediated via selective inhibition of H_1 receptors. The antihistaminic activity of cetirizine has been clearly documented in a variety of animal and human models. *In vivo* and *Ex vivo* animal models have shown negligible anticholinergic and antiserotonergic activity. In clinical trials, however, dry mouth was more common with cetirizine than with placebo. *In vitro* receptor binding studies have shown no measurable affinity for other than H_1 receptors. Autoradiographic studies with radiolabeled cetirizine in the rat have shown negligible penetration into the brain. *Ex vivo* experiments in the mouse have shown that systemically administered cetirizine does not significantly occupy cerebral H_1 receptors.

Pseudoephedrine hydrochloride is an orally active sympathomimetic amine and exerts a decongestant action on the nasal mucosa. Pseudoephedrine hydrochloride is recognized as an effective agent for the relief of nasal congestion due to allergic rhinitis. Pseudoephedrine produces peripheral effects similar to those of ephedrine and central effects similar to, but less intense than, amphetamines. It has the potential for excitatory side effects.

Pharmacokinetics:

Absorption: The bioavailability of cetirizine hydrochloride and pseudoephedrine hydrochloride from ZYRTEC-D 12 HOUR Extended Release Tablets is not significantly different from that achieved with separate administration of a cetirizine 5 mg tablet and a pseudoephedrine 120 mg extended release caplet. Co-administration of cetirizine and pseudoephedrine does not significantly affect the bioavailability of either component.

Following a single dose of the ZYRTEC-D 12 HOUR Extended Release Tablet, a mean peak plasma concentration (Cmax) of 114 ng/mL at a time (Tmax) of 2.2 hours postdose was observed for cetirizine and a mean Cmax of 309 ng/mL at a Tmax of 4.4 hours postdose was observed for pseudoephedrine.

When healthy volunteers were administered multiple doses of the ZYRTEC-D 12 HOUR Extended Release Tablet to reach steady-state concentrations (cetirizine hydrochloride 5 mg and pseudoephedrine hydrochloride 120 mg twice daily for seven days), a mean Cmax of 178 ng/mL was observed for cetirizine and 526 ng/mL for pseudoephedrine.

Food had no significant effect on the extent of cetirizine absorption (AUC), but Tmax was delayed by 1.8 hours and Cmax was decreased by 30%. Food had no significant effect on the pharmacokinetics of pseudoephedrine. ZYRTEC-D 12 HOUR Extended Release Tablets may be given with or without food (see **DOSAGE AND ADMINISTRATION**).

Distribution: The mean plasma protein binding of cetirizine is 93%, independent of concentration in the range of 25-1000 ng/mL, which includes the therapeutic plasma levels observed. The apparent volume of distribution (V/F) of pseudoephedrine has been reported to be 2.6-3.3 L/kg. No plasma protein binding data in humans are available.

Metabolism: A human mass balance study of cetirizine in 6 healthy male volunteers indicated that 70% of the administered radioactivity was recovered in the urine and 10% in the feces. Approximately 50% of the radioactivity was identified in the urine as unchanged drug. Most of the rapid increase in peak plasma radioactivity was associated with parent drug, suggesting low first pass metabolism. Cetirizine is metabolized to a limited extent by oxidative O-dealkylation to a metabolite with negligible antihistaminic activity. The enzyme or enzymes responsible for this metabolism have not been identified.

One to seven percent of the pseudoephedrine dose appeared to be metabolized to norpseudoephedrine by N-demethylation after a single dose.

Elimination: After administration of the ZYRTEC-D 12 HOUR Extended Release Tablet, the mean elimination half-life of cetirizine was 7.9 hours and the mean elimination half-life of pseudoephedrine was 6.0 hours.

It was reported that 0.4-0.7% of the pseudoephedrine dose was estimated to be excreted in the breast milk over 24 hours after a single dose. The pattern of the relative milk/plasma drug concentration profile showed that pseudoephedrine concentrations in milk were 2- to 3-fold higher than those in plasma.

Drug Interactions

Pharmacokinetic interaction trials with cetirizine in adults were conducted with pseudoephedrine, antipyrine, ketoconazole, erythromycin and azithromycin. No interactions were observed. In a multiple dose study of theophylline (400 mg once daily for 3 days) and cetirizine (20 mg once daily for 3 days), a 16% decrease in the clearance of cetirizine was observed. The disposition of theophylline was not altered by concomitant cetirizine administration.

Special Populations

Pediatrics: Although cetirizine pharmacokinetics have been studied in children, ZYRTEC-D 12 HOUR Extended Release Tablets contain 120 mg of pseudoephedrine hydrochloride, which exceeds the recommended dose for patients less than 12 years of age. Therefore, ZYRTEC-D 12 HOUR Extended Release Tablets are not recommended for patients under 12 years of age.

Geriatrics: Following a single, 10-mg oral dose of cetirizine, the elimination half-life was prolonged by 50% and the apparent total body clearance was 40% lower in 16 geriatric subjects with a mean age of 77 years compared to 14 adult subjects with a mean age of 53 years. The decrease in cetirizine clearance in these elderly volunteers may be related to decreased renal function.

The pharmacokinetics of pseudoephedrine has not been adequately studied in geriatric subjects.

Gender: The effect of gender on cetirizine or pseudoephedrine pharmacokinetics has not been adequately studied.

Race: The effect of race on cetirizine or pseudoephedrine pharmacokinetics has not been adequately studied.

Renal Impairment: The kinetics of cetirizine were studied following multiple, oral, 10-mg daily doses of cetirizine for 7 days in 7 normal volunteers (creatinine clearance 89-128 mL/min), 8 patients with mild renal function impairment (creatinine clearance 42-77 mL/min) and 7 patients with moderate renal function impairment (creatinine clearance 11-31 mL/min). The pharmacokinetics of cetirizine were similar in patients with mild impairment and normal volunteers. Moderately impaired patients had a 3-fold increase in half-life and a 70% decrease in clearance compared to normal volunteers.

Patients on hemodialysis (n=5) given a single, 10-mg dose of cetirizine had a 3-fold increase in half-life and a 70% decrease in clearance compared to normal volunteers. Less than 10% of the administered dose was removed during the single dialysis session.

About 55-75% of an administered dose of pseudoephedrine hydrochloride is excreted unchanged in the urine; the remainder is apparently metabolized in the liver. Therefore, pseudoephedrine may accumulate in patients with renal insufficiency.

Dosing adjustment is necessary in patients with moderate or severe renal impairment and in patients on dialysis (see **DOSAGE AND ADMINISTRATION**).

Hepatic Impairment: Sixteen patients with chronic liver diseases (hepatocellular, cholestatic, and biliary cirrhosis), given 10 or 20 mg of cetirizine as a single, oral dose had a 50% increase in half-life along with a corresponding 40% decrease in clearance compared to 16 healthy subjects.

The effect of hepatic impairment on pseudoephedrine pharmacokinetics is unknown.

Dosing adjustment may be necessary in patients with hepatic impairment (see **DOSAGE AND ADMINISTRATION**).

Pharmacodynamics: Trials in 69 adult normal volunteers (aged 20-61 years) showed that cetirizine at doses of 5 and 10 mg inhibited the skin wheal and flare caused by the intradermal injection of histamine. The onset of this activity after a single 10-mg dose occurred within 20 minutes in 50% of subjects and within one hour in 95% of subjects; this activity persisted for at least 24 hours. The effects of intradermal injection of various other mediators or histamine releasers were also inhibited by cetirizine. In mildly asthmatic subjects, cetirizine at 5 to 20 mg blocked bronchoconstriction due to nebulized histamine, with virtually total blockade after a 20 mg dose. In trials conducted for up to 12 hours following cutaneous antigen challenge, the late phase recruitment of eosinophils, neutrophils and basophils, components of the allergic inflammatory response, was inhibited by cetirizine at a dose of 20 mg. The clinical significance of these findings is not known.

In four clinical trials in healthy adult males, no clinically significant mean increases in QTc were observed in cetirizine treated subjects. In the first study, a placebo-controlled crossover trial, cetirizine was given at doses up to 60 mg per day, 6 times the maximum clinical dose, for 1 week, and no significant mean QTc prolongation occurred. In the second study, a crossover trial, cetirizine 20 mg and erythromycin (500 mg every 8 hours) were given alone and in combination. There was no significant effect on QTc with the combination or with cetirizine alone. In the third trial, also a crossover study, cetirizine 20 mg and ketoconazole (400 mg per day) were given alone and in combination. Cetirizine caused a mean increase in QTc of 9.1 msec from baseline after 10 days of therapy. Ketoconazole also increased QTc by 8.3 msec. The combination caused an increase of 17.4 msec, equal to the sum of the individual effects. Thus, there was no significant drug interaction on QTc with the combination of cetirizine and ketoconazole. In the fourth study, a placebo-controlled parallel trial, cetirizine 20 mg was given alone or in combination with azithromycin (500 mg as a single dose on the first day followed by 250 mg once daily). There was no significant increase in QTc with cetirizine 20 mg alone or in combination with azithromycin.

In a six-week, placebo-controlled study of 186 patients (aged 12-64 years) with allergic rhinitis and mild to moderate asthma, cetirizine 10 mg once daily improved rhinitis symptoms and did not alter pulmonary function. This study supports the safety of administering cetirizine to allergic rhinitis patients with mild to moderate asthma.

Clinical Trials:

ZYRTEC-D 12 HOUR Extended Release Tablets: Two multicenter, randomized, double-blind, placebo-controlled clinical trials (n = 1094 and n = 1000) comparing ZYRTEC-D 12 HOUR Extended Release Tablets (cetirizine hydrochloride 5 mg and pseudoephedrine hydrochloride 120 mg) to active control and placebo for two weeks in patients 12 years and older with seasonal allergic rhinitis were conducted in the United States. In the two trials, 390 patients were aged 12 to 17 years. The primary efficacy measure in both trials was the mean change from baseline in the subject-rated Total Symptom Severity Complex (TSSC) score, which included the following symptoms: sneezing, runny nose, itchy nose, itchy eyes, watery eyes, postnasal drip, and nasal congestion. In both trials patients who received ZYRTEC-D showed a significant reduction in the TSSC score compared to those who received placebo.

Zyrtec Tablets: Nine multicenter, randomized, double-blind, clinical trials comparing cetirizine 5 to 20 mg to placebo in patients 12 years and older with seasonal or perennial allergic rhinitis were conducted in the United States. Five of these showed significant reductions in symptoms of allergic rhinitis, 3 in seasonal allergic rhinitis (1 to 4 weeks in duration) and 2 in perennial allergic rhinitis for up to 8 weeks in duration. In general, the 10 mg dose was more effective than the 5 mg dose and the 20 mg dose gave no added effect. Some of these trials included pediatric patients aged 12 to 16 years.

INDICATIONS AND USAGE

ZYRTEC-D 12 HOUR Extended Release Tablets should be administered when both the antihistaminic properties of cetirizine hydrochloride and the nasal decongestant properties of pseudoephedrine hydrochloride are desired.

ZYRTEC-D 12 HOUR Extended Release Tablets are indicated for the relief of nasal and non-nasal symptoms associated with seasonal or perennial allergic rhinitis in adults and children 12 years of age and older.

CONTRAINDICATIONS

ZYRTEC-D 12 HOUR Extended Release Tablets are contraindicated in patients with a known hypersensitivity to any of its ingredients or to hydroxyzine.

Due to its pseudoephedrine component, ZYRTEC-D 12 HOUR Extended Release Tablets are contraindicated in patients with narrow-angle glaucoma or urinary retention, and in patients receiving monoamine oxidase (MAO) inhibitor therapy or within fourteen (14) days of stopping such treatment (see **PRECAUTIONS, Drug Interactions** section). It is also contraindicated in patients with severe hypertension, or severe coronary artery disease, and in those who have shown hypersensitivity or idiosyncrasy to its components, to adrenergic agents, or to other drugs of similar chemical structures. Manifestations of patient idiosyncrasy to adrenergic agents include insomnia, dizziness, weakness, tremor, or arrhythmias.

WARNINGS

Sympathomimetic amines should be used judiciously and sparingly in patients with hypertension, diabetes mellitus, ischemic heart disease, increased intraocular pressure, hyperthyroidism, renal impairment, or prostatic hypertrophy (see **CONTRAINDICATIONS**). Sympathomimetic amines may produce central nervous system stimulation with convulsions or cardiovascular collapse with accompanying hypotension. The elderly are more likely to have adverse reactions to sympathomimetic amines.

PRECAUTIONS

Due to its pseudoephedrine component, ZYRTEC-D 12 HOUR Extended Release Tablets should be used with caution in patients with hypertension, diabetes mellitus, ischemic heart disease, increased intraocular pressure, hyperthyroidism, renal impairment, or prostatic hypertrophy (see **WARNINGS** and **CONTRAINDICATIONS**). Patients with decreased renal function should be given a lower initial dose (one tablet per day) because they have reduced elimination of cetirizine and pseudoephedrine (see **CLINICAL PHARMACOLOGY** and **DOSAGE AND ADMINISTRATION**).

Activities Requiring Mental Alertness: In clinical trials, the occurrence of somnolence has been reported in some patients taking cetirizine or ZYRTEC-D 12 HOUR Extended Release Tablets; due caution should therefore be exercised when driving a car or operating potentially dangerous machinery after taking ZYRTEC-D 12 HOUR Extended Release Tablets. Concurrent use of ZYRTEC-D 12 HOUR Extended Release Tablets with alcohol or other CNS depressants should be avoided because additional reductions in alertness and additional impairment of CNS performance may occur.

Drug Interactions: Cetirizine hydrochloride and pseudoephedrine hydrochloride do not influence the pharmacokinetics of each other when administered concomitantly.

No clinically significant drug interactions have been found with cetirizine and theophylline at a low dose, azithromycin, ketoconazole, or erythromycin. There was a small decrease in the clearance of cetirizine caused by a 400 mg dose of theophylline; it is possible that larger theophylline doses could have a greater effect.

Due to the pseudoephedrine component, ZYRTEC-D 12 HOUR Extended Release Tablets are contraindicated in patients taking monoamine oxidase (MAO) inhibitors and for 14 days after stopping use of an MAO inhibitor. Concomitant use with antihypertensive drugs that interfere with sympathetic activity (e.g., methyldopa, mecamylamine, and reserpine) may reduce their antihypertensive effects. Increased ectopic pacemaker activity can occur when pseudoephedrine is used concomitantly with digitalis. Care should be taken in the administration of ZYRTEC-D 12 HOUR Extended Release Tablets concomitantly with other sympathomimetic amines because combined effects on the cardiovascular system may be harmful to the patient (see **WARNINGS**).

Carcinogenesis, Mutagenesis and Impairment of Fertility: There are no carcinogenicity trials of pseudoephedrine and cetirizine in combination.

Cetirizine: In a 2-year study in rats, cetirizine was not carcinogenic at dietary doses up to 20 mg/kg (approximately 15 times the maximum recommended daily dose in adults on a mg/m^2 basis). In a 2-year study in mice, cetirizine caused an increased incidence of benign liver tumors in males at a dietary dose of 16 mg/kg (approximately 6 times the maximum recommended daily dose in adults on a mg/m^2 basis). No increase in the incidence of liver tumors was observed in mice at a dietary dose of 4 mg/kg (approximately 2 times the maximum recommended daily dose in adults on a mg/m^2 basis). The clinical significance of these findings during long-term use of ZYRTEC-D 12 HOUR Extended Release Tablets is not known.

Pseudoephedrine: Two-year studies in rats and mice conducted under the auspices of the National Toxicology Program (NTP) demonstrated no evidence of carcinogenic potential with ephedrine sulfate, a structurally related drug with pharmacological properties similar to pseudoephedrine, at dietary doses up to 10 and 27 mg/kg, respectively (approximately 1/3 and 1/2, respectively, the maximum recommended daily dose of pseudoephedrine in adults on a mg/m^2 basis).

Cetirizine was not mutagenic in the Ames test or mouse lymphoma test and not clastogenic in the human lymphocyte assay or the *in vivo* rodent micronucleus test. Likewise, the combination of cetirizine and pseudoephedrine in a 1:24 ratio was not mutagenic or clastogenic in these tests. However, the Ames and mouse lymphoma assays did not strictly adhere to test standards.

In a reproductive toxicity study in rats, combination oral doses of cetirizine and pseudoephedrine up to 6/154 mg/kg (approximately 5 times the maximum recommended daily dose in adults on a mg/m^2 basis) had no effect on fertility.

Pregnancy Category C: In rats, the combination of cetirizine and pseudoephedrine caused developmental toxicity when administered orally at 6/154 mg/kg (approximately 5 times the maximum recommended daily dose in adults on a mg/m^2 basis). When rats were dosed throughout pregnancy with oral doses of cetirizine/pseudoephedrine, 6/154 mg/kg increased the number of fetal skeletal malformations (rib distortions) and variants (unossified sternebrae). When dosing was continued through lactation, 6/154 mg/kg also decreased the viability and weight gain of offspring. These effects were not observed at 1.6/38 mg/kg (approximately equivalent to the maximum recommended daily dose in adults on a mg/m^2 basis). No embryofetal toxicity was observed when rabbits were dosed throughout organogenesis with oral doses of cetirizine/pseudoephedrine of up to 6/154 mg/kg (approximately 10 times the maximum recommended daily dose in adults on a mg/m^2 basis). Because there are no adequate and well-controlled trials in pregnant women, ZYRTEC-D 12 HOUR Extended Release Tablets should be used during pregnancy only if the potential benefit justifies the potential risk to the fetus.

Nursing Mothers: In rats the combination of cetirizine/pseudoephedrine decreased the viability and weight gain of offspring when administered orally to dams throughout pregnancy and lactation at 6/154 mg/kg (approximately 5 times the maximum recommended daily dose in adults on a mg/m^2 basis). This effect was not observed at 1.6/38 mg/kg (approximately equivalent to the maximum recommended daily dose in adults on a mg/m^2 basis). For cetirizine administered alone, studies in dogs indicate that approximately 3% of the dose is excreted in milk, and cetirizine has been reported to be excreted in human breast milk. For pseudoephedrine administered alone, 0.4-0.7% of the dose has been reported to be excreted in human breast milk.

Because cetirizine and pseudoephedrine are excreted in milk, use of ZYRTEC-D 12 HOUR Extended Release Tablets in nursing mothers is not recommended.

Geriatric Use: Clinical trials of ZYRTEC-D 12 HOUR Extended Release Tablets did not include sufficient numbers of patients aged 65 and over to determine whether they respond differently from younger subjects. Other reported clinical experience has not identified differences in responses between the elderly and younger patients, although the elderly are more likely to have adverse reactions to sympathomimetic amines. In general, dosing in an elderly patient should be cautious, reflecting the greater frequency of decreased hepatic, renal, or cardiac function, and of concomitant disease or other drug therapy.

The cetirizine and pseudoephedrine components of ZYRTEC-D 12 HOUR Extended Release Tablets are known to be substantially excreted by the kidney, and the risk of toxic reactions to this drug may be greater in patients with impaired renal function. Because elderly patients are more likely to have decreased renal function, care should be taken in dose selection, and it may be useful to monitor renal function (see **CLINICAL PHARMACOLOGY**).

Cetirizine: Of the total number of subjects in clinical trials of cetirizine alone, 186 were 65 years and over, while 39 were 75 years and over. No overall differences in safety were observed between these subjects and younger subjects, and other reported experience has not identified differences in responses between the elderly and younger patients, but greater sensitivity of some older individuals cannot be ruled out. With regard to efficacy, clinical trials of cetirizine for each approved indication did not include sufficient numbers of subjects aged 65 years and over to determine whether they respond differently than younger patients.

Pediatric Use: ZYRTEC-D 12 HOUR Extended Release Tablets contain 120 mg of pseudoephedrine hydrochloride in an extended release formulation. This dose of pseudoephedrine exceeds the recommended dose for pediatric patients under 12 years of age. Therefore, clinical trials of ZYRTEC-D 12 HOUR Extended Release Tablets have not been conducted in patients under 12 years of age.

ADVERSE REACTIONS

ZYRTEC-D 12 HOUR Extended Release Tablets

In two double-blind, placebo-controlled trials (n = 2094) in which 701 patients with seasonal allergic rhinitis were treated with ZYRTEC-D 12 HOUR Extended Release Tablets (cetirizine hydrochloride 5 mg and pseudoephedrine hydrochloride 120 mg) twice daily for two weeks, the percent of patients who withdrew prematurely due to adverse events was 2.0% in the ZYRTEC-D group, compared with 1.1% in the placebo group. All adverse events that were reported by greater than 1% of patients in the ZYRTEC-D group are listed in Table 1.

Continued on next page

Zyrtec-D—Cont.

TABLE 1. ADVERSE EXPERIENCES REPORTED IN PATIENTS AGED 12 YEARS AND OLDER IN SEASONAL ALLERGIC RHINITIS TRIALS OF ZYRTEC-D 12 HOUR EXTENDED RELEASE TABLETS AT RATES OF 1% OR GREATER (PERCENT INCIDENCE)

ADVERSE EXPERIENCE	ZYRTEC-D (n = 701)	PLACEBO (n = 696)
Insomnia	4.0	0.6
Dry Mouth	3.6	0.4
Fatigue	2.4	0.9
Somnolence	1.9	0.1
Pharyngitis	1.7	1.1
Epistaxis	1.1	0.9
Accidental Injury	1.1	0.4
Dizziness	1.1	0.1
Sinusitis	1.0	0.6

ZYRTEC Tablets

Controlled and uncontrolled clinical trials of cetirizine conducted in the United States and Canada included more than 6000 patients aged 12 years and older, with more than 3900 receiving cetirizine at doses of 5 to 20 mg per day. The duration of treatment ranged from 1 week to 6 months, with a mean exposure of 30 days.

Most adverse reactions reported during therapy with cetirizine were mild or moderate. In placebo-controlled trials, the incidence of discontinuations due to adverse reactions in patients receiving cetirizine 5 mg or 10 mg was not significantly different from placebo (2.9% vs. 2.4%, respectively). The most common adverse reaction in patients aged 12 years and older that occurred more frequently on cetirizine than placebo was somnolence. The incidence of somnolence associated with cetirizine was dose related, 6% in placebo, 11% at 5 mg and 14% at 10 mg. Discontinuations due to somnolence for cetirizine were uncommon (1.0% on cetirizine vs. 0.6% on placebo). Fatigue and dry mouth also appeared to be treatment-related adverse reactions. There were no differences by age, race, gender or by body weight with regard to the incidence of adverse reactions.

Table 2 lists adverse experiences in patients aged 12 years and older that were reported for cetirizine 5 and 10 mg in controlled clinical trials in the United States and were more common with cetirizine than placebo.

TABLE 2.
ADVERSE EXPERIENCES REPORTED IN PATIENTS AGED 12 YEARS AND OLDER IN PLACEBO-CONTROLLED UNITED STATES CETIRIZINE TRIALS (MAXIMUM DOSE OF 10 MG) AT RATES OF 2% OR GREATER (PERCENT INCIDENCE)

ADVERSE EXPERIENCE	CETIRIZINE (N=2034)	PLACEBO (N=1612)
Somnolence	13.7	6.3
Fatigue	5.9	2.6
Dry Mouth	5.0	2.3
Pharyngitis	2.0	1.9
Dizziness	2.0	1.2

In addition, headache and nausea occurred in more than 2% of the patients, but were more common in placebo patients. The following events were observed infrequently (less than 2%), in 3982 adults and children 12 years and older or in 659 pediatric (6 to 11 years) patients who received cetirizine in U.S. trials, including an open study of six months duration. A causal relationship of these infrequent events with cetirizine administration has not been established.

Autonomic Nervous System: anorexia, flushing, increased salivation, urinary retention.

Cardiovascular: cardiac failure, hypertension, palpitation, tachycardia.

Central and Peripheral Nervous Systems: abnormal coordination, ataxia, confusion, dysphonia, hyperesthesia, hyperkinesia, hypertonia, hypoesthesia, leg cramps, migraine, myelitis, paralysis, paresthesia, ptosis, syncope, tremor, twitching, vertigo, visual field defect.

Gastrointestinal: abnormal hepatic function, aggravated tooth caries, constipation, dyspepsia, eructation, flatulence, gastritis, hemorrhoids, increased appetite, melena, rectal hemorrhage, stomatitis including ulcerative stomatitis, tongue discoloration, tongue edema.

Genitourinary: cystitis, dysuria, hematuria, micturition frequency, polyuria, urinary incontinence, urinary tract infection.

Hearing and Vestibular: deafness, earache, ototoxicity, tinnitus.

Metabolic/Nutritional: dehydration, diabetes mellitus, thirst.

Musculoskeletal: arthralgia, arthritis, arthrosis, muscle weakness, myalgia.

Psychiatric: abnormal thinking, agitation, amnesia, anxiety, decreased libido, depersonalization, depression, emotional lability, euphoria, impaired concentration, insomnia, nervousness, paroniria, sleep disorder.

Respiratory System: bronchitis, dyspnea, hyperventilation, increased sputum, pneumonia, respiratory disorder, rhinitis, sinusitis, upper respiratory tract infection.

Reproductive: dysmenorrhea, female breast pain, intermenstrual bleeding, leukorrhea, menorrhagia, vaginitis.

Reticuloendothelial: lymphadenopathy.

Skin: acne, alopecia, angioedema, bullous eruption, dermatitis, dry skin, eczema, erythematous rash, furunculosis, hyperkeratosis, hypertrichosis, increased sweating, maculopapular rash, photosensitivity reaction, photosensitivity toxic reaction, pruritus, purpura, rash, seborrhea, skin disorder, skin nodule, urticaria.

Special Senses: parosmia, taste loss, taste perversion.

Vision: blindness, conjunctivitis, eye pain, glaucoma, loss of accommodation, ocular hemorrhage, xerophthalmia.

Body as a Whole: accidental injury, asthenia, back pain, chest pain, enlarged abdomen, face edema, fever, generalized edema, hot flashes, increased weight, leg edema, malaise, nasal polyp, pain, pallor, periorbital edema, peripheral edema, rigors.

Occasional instances of transient, reversible hepatic transaminase elevations have occurred during cetirizine therapy. Hepatitis with significant transaminase elevation and elevated bilirubin in association with the use of cetirizine has been reported.

In foreign marketing experience or experience in the post market period, the following additional rare, but potentially severe adverse events have been reported: anaphylaxis, cholestasis, glomerulonephritis, hemolytic anemia, hepatitis, orofacial dyskinesia, severe hypotension, stillbirth, thrombocytopenia, aggressive reaction and convulsions.

Pseudoephedrine Hydrochloride

Pseudoephedrine hydrochloride may cause mild CNS stimulation in hypersensitive patients. Nervousness, excitability, restlessness, dizziness, weakness, or insomnia may occur. Headache, nausea, drowsiness, tachycardia, palpitation, pressor activity, and cardiac arrhythmias have been reported. Sympathomimetic drugs have also been associated with other untoward effects such as fear, anxiety, tenseness, tremor, hallucinations, seizures, pallor, respiratory difficulty, dysuria, and cardiovascular collapse.

OVERDOSAGE

Information regarding acute overdosage is limited to experience with cetirizine alone and the marketing history of pseudoephedrine hydrochloride.

Overdosage has been reported with cetirizine. In one adult patient who took 150 mg of cetirizine, the patient was somnolent but did not display any other clinical signs or abnormal blood chemistry or hematology results. In an 18-month-old pediatric patient who took an overdose of cetirizine (approximately 180 mg), restlessness and irritability were observed initially; this was followed by drowsiness. Should overdose occur, treatment should be symptomatic or supportive, taking into account any concomitantly ingested medications. There is no known specific antidote to cetirizine. Cetirizine is not effectively removed by dialysis, and dialysis will be ineffective unless a dialyzable agent has been concomitantly ingested. The acute minimal lethal oral doses in mice and rats were 237 and 562 mg/kg, respectively (approximately 95 and 460 times the maximum recommended daily dose in adults on a mg/m^2 basis). In rodents, the target of acute toxicity was the central nervous system, and the target of multiple-dose toxicity was the liver.

In large doses, sympathomimetics may give rise to giddiness, headache, nausea, vomiting, sweating, thirst, tachycardia, precordial pain, palpitations, difficulty in micturition, muscular weakness and tenseness, anxiety, restlessness, and insomnia. Many patients can present a toxic psychosis with delusions and hallucinations. Some may develop cardiac arrhythmias, circulatory collapse, convulsions, coma and respiratory failure.

DOSAGE AND ADMINISTRATION

Adults and Children 12 Years of Age and Older: The recommended dose of ZYRTEC-D 12 HOUR Extended Release Tablets is one tablet twice daily for adults and children 12 years of age and older. ZYRTEC-D 12 HOUR Extended Release Tablets may be given with or without food.

Dose Adjustment for Renal and Hepatic Impairment: In patients with decreased renal function (creatinine clearance 11-31 mL/min), patients on hemodialysis (creatinine clearance less than 7 mL/min), and in hepatically impaired patients, a dose of one tablet once daily is recommended (see **CLINICAL PHARMACOLOGY** and **PRECAUTIONS**).

ZYRTEC-D 12 HOUR Extended Release Tablets should be swallowed whole, and should not be broken or chewed.

HOW SUPPLIED

ZYRTEC-D 12 HOUR™ Extended Release Tablets are white, round, biconvex, bilayer tablets containing 5 mg cetirizine hydrochloride in an immediate release layer and 120 mg pseudoephedrine hydrochloride in an extended release layer. ZYRTEC-D 12 HOUR Extended Release Tablets are supplied in high-density polyethylene bottles of 100 tablets fitted with polypropylene child-resistant closures (NDC 0069-1630-66).

ZYRTEC-D 12 HOUR Extended Release Tablets are engraved with ZYRTEC-D on one side.

STORAGE: ***Store at 20-25°C (68-77°F); excursions permitted to 15-30°C (59-86°F) [see USP Controlled Room Temperature]***

Cetirizine is licensed from UCB Pharma, Inc.

Manufactured/Distributed by
Pfizer Labs
Division of Pfizer Inc., NY, NY 10017
Marketed by
UCB Pharma, Inc.
Smyrna, GA 30080
69-5723-00-3 Revised August 2003

Shown in Product Identification Guide, page 330

Pharmaceutical Associates, Inc.

A Subsidiary of Beach Products, Inc.
201 DELAWARE STREET
GREENVILLE, SC 29605

Direct Inquiries to:
Clete Harmon, Vice President, Q.A.
PH: (800) 845-8210
(864) 277-7282
FAX: (864) 236-0116

HOSPITAL UNIT DOSE / TRADE PACKAGE

NDC Prefix: 00121-

PRODUCT LISTING

ACETAMINOPHEN ORAL SOLUTION USP OTC
(160 mg per 5 mL)
Unit Dose 5 mL, 10.15 mL, and 20.3 mL

ACETAMINOPHEN and CODEINE PHOSPHATE ORAL SOLUTION USP CV ℞
(120 mg/12 mg per 5 mL)
Unit Dose 5 mL, 10 mL, 12.5 mL, and 15 mL
Bottles of 4 fl oz and 16 fl oz

ALUMINUM HYDROXIDE GEL USP OTC
(320 mg per 5 mL)
Unit Dose 30 mL
Bottles of 12 fl oz and 16 fl oz

ALUMINUM HYDROXIDE GEL CONCENTRATE OTC
(600 mg per 5 mL)
Bottles of 12 fl oz

AMANTADINE HYDROCHLORIDE SYRUP USP ℞
(50 mg per 5 mL)
Unit Dose 10 mL
Bottles of 16 fl oz

CHLORAL HYDRATE SYRUP USP CIV ℞
(500 mg per 5 mL)
Unit Dose 5 mL
Bottles of 16 fl oz

CIMETIDINE HYDROCHLORIDE ORAL SOLUTION ℞
(300 mg per 5 mL)
Bottles of 8 fl oz

DIPHENHYDRAMINE HYDROCHLORIDE ELIXIR USP ℞
(12.5 mg per 5 mL)
Unit Dose 5 mL, 10 mL, and 20 mL

DOCUSATE SODIUM LIQUID OTC
(50 mg per 5 mL)
Unit Dose 10 mL and 25 mL
Bottles of 16 fl oz

DOCUSATE SODIUM SYRUP USP OTC
(20 mg per 5 mL)
Unit Dose 25 mL
Bottles of 16 fl oz

ETHOSUXIMIDE SYRUP ℞
(250 mg per 5 mL)
Bottles of 16 fl oz

FERROUS SULFATE LIQUID OTC
(300 mg per 5 mL)
Unit Dose 5 mL

FLUOXETINE ORAL SOLUTION USP ℞
(20 mg per 5 mL)
Unit Dose 5 mL
Bottles of 4 fl oz

FLUPHENAZINE HYDROCHLORIDE ELIXIR USP ℞
(2.5 mg per 5 mL)
Bottles of 60 mL and 16 fl oz

FLUPHENAZINE HYDROCHLORIDE ORAL SOLUTION USP Concentrate ℞
(5 mg per 1 mL)
Bottles of 4 fl oz

GUAIFENESIN SYRUP USP OTC
(100 mg per 5 mL)
Unit Dose 5 mL, 10 mL, and 15 mL
Bottles of 4 fl oz

GUAIFENESIN SYRUP with CODEINE CV OTC
(100 mg/10 mg per 5 mL)
Unit Dose 5 mL and 10 mL
Bottles of 4 fl oz and 16 fl oz

GUAIFENESIN SYRUP and DEXTROMETHORPHAN OTC
(100 mg/10 mg per 5 mL)
Unit Dose 5 mL and 10 mL
Bottles of 4 fl oz

HALOPERIDOL ORAL SOLUTION USP Concentrate ℞
(2 mg per 1 mL)
Unit Dose 5 mL
Bottles of 4 fl oz

HYDROCODONE BITARTRATE and ACETAMINOPHEN ORAL SOLUTION CIII ℞
(7.5 mg/500 mg per 15 mL)
Unit Dose 5 mL, 10 mL and 15 mL
Bottles of 4 fl oz and 16 fl oz

HYDROCODONE BITARTRATE and GUAIFENESIN EXPECTORANT CIII ℞
(5 mg/100 mg per 5 mL)
Bottles of 16 fl oz

LACTULOSE SOLUTION USP ℞
(10 g per 15 mL)
Unit Dose 15 mL and 30 mL
Bottles of 8 fl oz, 16 fl oz, and 32 fl oz

MAG-AL LIQUID OTC
(1200 mg/1200 mg per 30 mL)
Unit Dose 30 mL

MAG-AL Plus with Simethicone OTC
(1200 mg/1200 mg/120 mg per 30 mL)
Unit Dose 30 mL

MAG-AL Plus XS with Simethicone OTC
(2400 mg/2400 mg/240 mg per 30 mL)
Unit Dose 30 mL

METOCLOPRAMIDE ORAL SOLUTION USP ℞
(5 mg per 5 mL)
Unit Dose 10 mL
Bottles of 16 fl oz

MILK OF MAGNESIA USP OTC
(400 mg per 5 mL)
Unit Dose 30 mL

MILK OF MAGNESIA CONCENTRATE OTC
(2400 mg per 10 mL)
Unit Dose 10 mL

MINERAL OIL OTC
Unit Dose 30 mL

NORTRIPTYLINE HYDROCHLORIDE ORAL SOLUTION USP ℞
(10 mg per 5 mL)
Bottles of 16 fl oz

OXYBUTYNIN CHLORIDE SYRUP USP ℞
(5 mg per 5 mL)
Unit Dose 5 mL
Bottles of 16 fl oz

PERPHENAZINE ORAL SOLUTION USP Concentrate ℞
(16 mg per 5 mL)
Bottles of 4 fl oz

PHENOBARBITAL ELIXIR CIV ℞
(20 mg per 5 mL)
Unit Dose 5 mL, 7.5 mL, and 15 mL

POTASSIUM CHLORIDE ORAL SOLUTION USP 10% ℞
(20 mEq per 15 mL)
Unit Dose 15 mL and 30 mL

POTASSIUM CHLORIDE ORAL SOLUTION USP 20% ℞
(40 mEq per 15 mL)
Unit Dose 15 mL

POTASSIUM CITRATE and CITRIC ACID ORAL SOLUTION USP ℞
(1100 mg/334 mg per 5 mL)
Bottles of 16 fl oz

PREDNISOLONE SODIUM PHOSPHATE ORAL SOLUTION ℞
(6.7 mg per 5 mL) 5 mg base
Unit Dose 5 mL
Bottles of 4 fl oz

PREDNISOLONE SYRUP USP ℞
(15 mg per 5 mL)
Unit Dose 5 mL
Bottles of 8 fl oz and 16 fl oz

PROMETHAZINE HYDROCHLORIDE and CODEINE PHOSPHATE SYRUP CV ℞
(6.25 mg/10 mg per 5 mL)
Unit Dose 5 mL
Bottles of 16 fl oz

PSEUDOEPHEDRINE HYDROCHLORIDE SYRUP USP OTC
(30 mg per 5 mL)
Bottles of 4 fl oz

RANITIDINE HYDROCHLORIDE SYRUP USP ℞
(150 mg per 10 mL)
Unit Dose 10 mL

SODIUM CITRATE and CITRIC ACID ORAL SOLUTION USP ℞
(500 mg/334 mg per 5 mL)
Unit Dose 15 mL and 30 mL
Bottles of 16 fl oz

SORBITOL SOLUTION USP OTC
(70% w/w)
Unit Dose 30 mL
Bottles of 16 fl oz

SORE THROAT SPRAY OTC
(Phenol 1.4%) Cherry
Bottles of 6 fl oz

SUCRALFATE SUSPENSION ℞
(1 g per 10 mL)
Unit Dose 10 mL

TRICITRATES ORAL SOLUTION ℞
(550 mg/500 mg/334 mg per 5 mL)
Bottles of 16 fl oz

TRIHEXYPHENIDYL HYDROCHLORIDE ELIXIR USP ℞
(2 mg per 5 mL)
Unit Dose 5 mL
Bottles of 16 fl oz

VALPROIC ACID SYRUP USP ℞
(250 mg per 5 mL)
Unit Dose 5 mL
Bottles of 16 fl oz

Pharmacia & Upjohn

A DIVISION OF PFIZER
235 EAST 42ND STREET
NEW YORK, NY 10017-5755

For updates to the product information listed below, please check the Pfizer Web site: http://www.pfizer.com, or call (800) 438-1985. For complete product listing, please see the Manufacturers' Index.

For Medical Information, Contact:
(800) 438-1985
24 hours a day, seven days a week

Distribution:
1855 Shelby Oaks Drive North
Memphis, TN 38134
(901) 387-5200
Customer Service:
(800) 533-4535

PRODUCT IDENTIFICATION

Prescription capsules and tablets manufactured by Pharmacia & Upjohn Company are imprinted with one or a combination of the following: (1) Product trademark, (2) Dosage strength, (3) "Adria," "Pharmacia," "Upjohn," "U," or the code "KP." That portion of the National Drug Code (NDC) number that indicates product and strength.

A list of oral solid dosage forms with NDC product identification numbers is provided below.

Code #	Product	Strength
01	**DOSTINEX®** Tablets (cabergoline tablets)	0.5 mg
02	**MIRAPEX®** Tablets (pramipexole dihydrochloride tablets)	0.125 mg
04	**MIRAPEX®** Tablets (pramipexole dihydrochloride tablets)	0.25 mg
06	**MIRAPEX®** Tablets (pramipexole dihydrochloride tablets)	1 mg
08	**MIRAPEX®** Tablets (pramipexole dihydrochloride tablets)	0.5 mg
29	**XANAX®** Tablets (alprazolam tablets, USP) *See Product Identification Guide*	0.25 mg
37	**MIRAPEX®** Tablets (pramipexole dihydrochloride tablets) *See Product Identification Guide*	1.5 mg
55	**XANAX®** Tablets (alprazolam tablets, USP) *See Product Identification Guide*	0.5 mg
90	**XANAX®** Tablets (alprazolam tablets, USP) *See Product Identification Guide*	1 mg
94	**XANAX®** Tablets (alprazolam tablets, USP) *See Product Identification Guide*	2 mg
225	**CLEOCIN HCl®** Capsules (clindamycin hydrochloride capsules, USP) *See Product Identification Guide*	150 mg
331	**CLEOCIN HCl®** Capsules (clindamycin hydrochloride capsules, USP) *See Product Identification Guide*	75 mg
395	**CLEOCIN HCl®** Capsules (clindamycin hydrochloride capsules, USP) *See Product Identification Guide*	300 mg
617	**VANTIN®** Tablets (cefpodoxime proxetil tablets)	100 mg
618	**VANTIN®** Tablets (cefpodoxime proxetil tablets)	200 mg
4541	**DETROL®** Tablets (tolterodine tartrate tablets) *See Product Identification Guide*	1 mg
4544	**DETROL®** Tablets (tolterodine tartrate tablets) *See Product Identification Guide*	2 mg
5190	**DETROL® LA** Capsules (tolterodine tartrate extended release capsules) *See Product Identification Guide*	2 mg
5191	**DETROL® LA** Capsules (tolterodine tartrate extended release capsules) *See Product Identification Guide*	4 mg

AROMASIN® ℞
[*ărō-mă-sĭn*]
(exemestane tablets)

DESCRIPTION

AROMASIN® Tablets for oral administration contain 25 mg of exemestane, an irreversible, steroidal aromatase inactivator. Exemestane is chemically described as 6-methylenandrosta-1,4-diene-3,17-dione. Its molecular formula is $C_{20}H_{24}O_2$ and its structural formula is as follows:

The active ingredient is a white to slightly yellow crystalline powder with a molecular weight of 296.41. Exemestane is freely soluble in N, N-dimethylformamide, soluble in methanol, and practically insoluble in water.

Each AROMASIN Tablet contains the following inactive ingredients: mannitol, crospovidone, polysorbate 80, hypromellose, colloidal silicon dioxide, microcrystalline cellulose, sodium starch glycolate, magnesium stearate, simethicone, polyethylene glycol 6000, sucrose, magnesium carbonate, titanium dioxide, methylparaben, and polyvinyl alcohol.

CLINICAL PHARMACOLOGY

Mechanism of Action

Breast cancer cell growth may be estrogen-dependent. Aromatase is the principal enzyme that converts androgens to estrogens both in pre- and postmenopausal women. While the main source of estrogen (primarily estradiol) is the ovary in premenopausal women, the principal source of circulating estrogens in postmenopausal women is from conversion of adrenal and ovarian androgens (androstenedione and testosterone) to estrogens (estrone and estradiol) by the aromatase enzyme in peripheral tissues. Estrogen deprivation through aromatase inhibition is an effective and selective treatment for some postmenopausal patients with hormone-dependent breast cancer.

Exemestane is an irreversible, steroidal aromatase inactivator, structurally related to the natural substrate androstenedione. It acts as a false substrate for the aromatase enzyme, and is processed to an intermediate that binds irreversibly to the active site of the enzyme causing its inactivation, an effect also known as "suicide inhibition." Exemestane significantly lowers circulating estrogen concentrations in postmenopausal women, but has no detectable effect on adrenal biosynthesis of corticosteroids or aldosterone. Exemestane has no effect on other enzymes involved in the steroidogenic pathway up to a concentration at least 600 times higher than that inhibiting the aromatase enzyme.

Pharmacokinetics

Following oral administration to healthy postmenopausal women, exemestane is rapidly absorbed. After maximum plasma concentration is reached, levels decline polyexponentially with a mean terminal half-life of about 24 hours. Exemestane is extensively distributed and is cleared from the systemic circulation primarily by metabolism. The pharmacokinetics of exemestane are dose proportional after single (10 to 200 mg) or repeated oral doses (0.5 to 50 mg). Following repeated daily doses of exemestane 25 mg, plasma concentrations of unchanged drug are similar to levels measured after a single dose.

Pharmacokinetic parameters in postmenopausal women with advanced breast cancer following single or repeated doses have been compared with those in healthy, postmenopausal women. Exemestane appeared to be more rapidly absorbed in the women with breast cancer than in the healthy women, with a mean t_{max} of 1.2 hours in the women with breast cancer and 2.9 hours in the healthy women. After repeated dosing, the average oral clearance in women with advanced breast cancer was 45% lower than the oral clearance in healthy postmenopausal women, with corresponding higher systemic exposure. Mean AUC values following repeated doses in women with breast cancer (75.4 ng•h/mL) were about twice those in healthy women (41.4 ng•h/mL).

Absorption: Following oral administration of radiolabeled exemestane, at least 42% of radioactivity was absorbed from the gastrointestinal tract. Exemestane plasma levels increased by approximately 40% after a high-fat breakfast.

Distribution: Exemestane is distributed extensively into tissues. Exemestane is 90% bound to plasma proteins and the fraction bound is independent of the total concentration. Albumin and α_1-acid glycoprotein both contribute to the binding. The distribution of exemestane and its metabolites into blood cells is negligible.

Metabolism and Excretion: Following administration of radiolabeled exemestane to healthy postmenopausal women, the cumulative amounts of radioactivity excreted in urine and feces were similar (42 ± 3% in urine and 42 ± 6% in feces over a 1-week collection period). The amount of drug excreted unchanged in urine was less than 1% of the dose. Exemestane is extensively metabolized, with levels of the unchanged drug in plasma accounting for less than 10% of the total radioactivity. The initial steps in the metabolism of

Continued on next page

Aromasin—Cont.

exemestane are oxidation of the methylene group in position 6 and reduction of the 17-keto group with subsequent formation of many secondary metabolites. Each metabolite accounts only for a limited amount of drug-related material. The metabolites are inactive or inhibit aromatase with decreased potency compared with the parent drug. One metabolite may have androgenic activity (see Pharmacodynamics, Other Endocrine Effects). Studies using human liver preparations indicate that cytochrome P-450 3A4 (CYP 3A4) is the principal isoenzyme involved in the oxidation of exemestane.

Special Populations

Geriatric: Healthy postmenopausal women aged 43 to 68 years were studied in the pharmacokinetic trials. Age-related alterations in exemestane pharmacokinetics were not seen over this age range.

Gender: The pharmacokinetics of exemestane following administration of a single, 25-mg tablet to fasted healthy males (mean age 32 years) were similar to the pharmacokinetics of exemestane in fasted healthy postmenopausal women (mean age 55 years).

Race: The influence of race on exemestane pharmacokinetics has not been evaluated.

Hepatic Insufficiency: The pharmacokinetics of exemestane have been investigated in subjects with moderate or severe hepatic insufficiency (Childs-Pugh B or C). Following a single 25-mg oral dose, the AUC of exemestane was approximately 3 times higher than that observed in healthy volunteers (see PRECAUTIONS).

Renal Insufficiency: The AUC of exemestane after a single 25-mg dose was approximately 3 times higher in subjects with moderate or severe renal insufficiency (creatinine clearance <35 mL/min/1.73 m^2) compared with the AUC in healthy volunteers (see PRECAUTIONS).

Pediatric: The pharmacokinetics of exemestane have not been studied in pediatric patients.

Drug-Drug Interactions

Exemestane is metabolized by cytochrome P-450 3A4 (CYP 3A4) and aldoketoreductases. It does not inhibit any of the major CYP isoenzymes, including CYP 1A2, 2C9, 2D6, 2E1, and 3A4. In a clinical pharmacokinetic study, ketoconazole showed no significant influence on the pharmacokinetics of exemestane. Although no other formal drug-drug interaction studies have been conducted, significant effects on exemestane clearance by CYP isoenzymes inhibitors appear unlikely. In a pharmacokinetic interaction study of 10 healthy postmenopausal volunteers pretreated with potent CYP 3A4 inducer rifampicin 600 mg daily for 14 days followed by a single dose of exemestane 25 mg, the mean plasma Cmax and $AUC_{0-\infty}$ of exemestane were decreased by 41% and 54%, respectively (see PRECAUTIONS AND DOSAGE AND ADMINISTRATION).

Pharmacodynamics

Effect on Estrogens: Multiple doses of exemestane ranging from 0.5 to 600 mg/day were administered to postmenopausal women with advanced breast cancer. Plasma estrogen (estradiol, estrone, and estrone sulfate) suppression was seen starting at a 5-mg daily dose of exemestane, with a maximum suppression of at least 85% to 95% achieved at a 25-mg dose. Exemestane 25 mg daily reduced whole body aromatization (as measured by injecting radiolabeled androstenedione) by 98% in postmenopausal women with breast cancer. After a single dose of exemestane 25 mg, the maximal suppression of circulating estrogens occurred 2 to 3 days after dosing and persisted for 4 to 5 days.

Effect on Corticosteroids: In multiple-dose trials of doses up to 200 mg daily, exemestane selectivity was assessed by examining its effect on adrenal steroids. Exemestane did not affect cortisol or aldosterone secretion at baseline or in response to ACTH at any dose. Thus, no glucocorticoid or mineralocorticoid replacement therapy is necessary with exemestane treatment.

Other Endocrine Effects: Exemestane does not bind significantly to steroidal receptors, except for a slight affinity for the androgen receptor (0.28% relative to dihydrotestosterone). The binding affinity of its 17-dihydrometabolite for the androgen receptor, however, is 100-times that of the parent compound. Daily doses of exemestane up to 25 mg had no significant effect on circulating levels of testosterone, androstenedione, dehydroepiandrosterone sulfate, or 17-hydroxyprogesterone. Increases in testosterone and androstenedione levels have been observed at daily doses of 200 mg or more. A dose-dependent decrease in sex hormone binding globulin (SHBG) has been observed with daily exemestane doses of 2.5 mg or higher. Slight, nondose-dependent increases in serum luteinizing hormone (LH) and follicle-stimulating hormone (FSH) levels have been observed even at low doses as a consequence of feedback at the pituitary level.

CLINICAL STUDIES

Exemestane 25 mg administered once daily was evaluated in a randomized double-blind, multicenter, multinational comparative study and in two multicenter single-arm studies of postmenopausal women with advanced breast cancer who had disease progression after treatment with tamoxifen for metastatic disease or as adjuvant therapy. Some patients also have received prior cytotoxic therapy, either as adjuvant treatment or for metastatic disease.

The primary purpose of the three studies was evaluation of objective response rate (complete response [CR] and partial response [PR]). Time to tumor progression and overall survival were also assessed in the comparative trial. Response rates were assessed based on World Health Organization (WHO) criteria, and in the comparative study, were submitted to an external review committee that was blinded to patient treatment. In the comparative study, 769 patients were randomized to receive AROMASIN (exemestane tablets) 25 mg once daily (N = 366) or megestrol acetate 40 mg four times daily (N = 403). Demographics and baseline characteristics are presented in Table 1.

[See table 1 above]

Table 1. Demographics and Baseline Characteristics from the Comparative Study of Postmenopausal Women with Advanced Breast Cancer Whose Disease Had Progressed after Tamoxifen Therapy

Parameter	AROMASIN (N = 366)	Megestrol Acetate (N = 403)
Median Age (range)	65 (35-89)	65 (30-91)
ECOG Performance Status		
0	167 (46%)	187 (46%)
1	162 (44%)	172 (43%)
2	34 (9%)	42 (10%)
Receptor Status		
ER and/or PgR +	246 (67%)	274 (68%)
ER and PgR unknown	116 (32%)	128 (32%)
Responders to prior tamoxifen	68 (19%)	85 (21%)
NE for response to prior tamoxifen	46 (13%)	41 (10%)
Site of Metastasis		
Visceral ± other sites	207 (57%)	239 (59%)
Bone only	61 (17%)	73 (18%)
Soft tissue only	54 (15%)	51 (13%)
Bone & soft tissue	43 (12%)	38 (9%)
Measurable Disease	287 (78%)	314 (78%)
Prior Tamoxifen Therapy		
Adjuvant or Neoadjuvant	145 (40%)	152 (38%)
Advanced Disease, Outcome		
CR, PR or SD≥ 6 months	179 (49%)	210 (52%)
SD< 6 months, PD or NE	42 (12%)	41 (10%)
Prior Chemotherapy		
For advanced disease ± adjuvant	58 (16%)	67 (17%)
Adjuvant only	104 (28%)	108 (27%)
No chemotherapy	203 (56%)	226 (56%)

The efficacy results from the comparative study are shown in Table 2. The objective response rates observed in the two treatment arms showed that AROMASIN was not different from megestrol acetate. Response rates for exemestane from the two single-arm trials were 23.4% and 28.1%.

[See table 2 above]

Table 2. Efficacy Results from the Comparative Study of Postmenopausal Women with Advanced Breast Cancer Whose Disease Had Progressed after Tamoxifen Therapy

Response Characteristics	AROMASIN (N=366)		Megestrol Acetate (N=403)
Objective Response Rate = CR+ PR (%)	15.0		12.4
Difference in Response Rate (AR-MA)		2.6	
95% C. I.		7.5, -2.3	
CR (%)	2.2		1.2
PR (%)	12.8		11.2
SD ≥ 24 Weeks (%)	21.3		21.1
Median Duration of Response (weeks)	76.1		71.0
Median TTP (weeks)	20.3		16.6
Hazard Ratio (AR-MA)		0.84	

Abbreviations: CR = complete response, PR = partial response, SD = stable disease (no change), TTP = time to tumor progression, C. I. = confidence interval, MA = megestrol acetate, AR = AROMASIN

There were too few deaths occurring across treatment groups to draw conclusions on overall survival differences. The Kaplan-Meier curve for time to tumor progression in the comparative study is shown in Figure 1.

Figure 1. Time to Tumor Progression in the Comparative Study of Postmenopausal Women With Advanced Breast Cancer Whose Disease Had Progressed After Tamoxifen Therapy

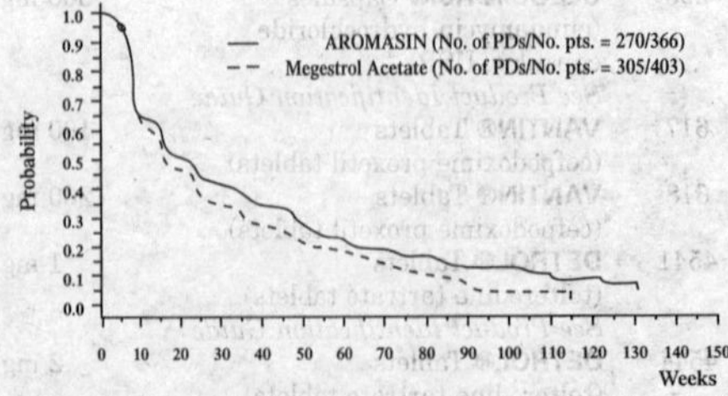

INDICATIONS AND USAGE

AROMASIN Tablets are indicated for the treatment of advanced breast cancer in postmenopausal women whose disease has progressed following tamoxifen therapy.

CONTRAINDICATIONS

AROMASIN Tablets are contraindicated in patients with a known hypersensitivity to the drug or to any of the excipients.

WARNINGS

AROMASIN Tablets may cause fetal harm when administered to a pregnant woman. Radioactivity related to ^{14}C-exemestane crossed the placenta of rats following oral administration of 1 mg/kg exemestane. The concentration of exemestane and its metabolites was approximately equivalent in maternal and fetal blood. When rats were administered exemestane from 14 days prior to mating until either days 15 or 20 of gestation, and resuming for the 21 days of lactation, an increase in placental weight was seen at 4 mg/kg/day (approximately 1.5 times the recommended human daily dose on a mg/m^2 basis). Prolonged gestation and abnormal or difficult labor was observed at doses equal to or greater than 20 mg/kg/day. Increased resorption, reduced number of live fetuses, decreased fetal weight, and retarded ossification were also observed at these doses. No malformations were noted when exemestane was administered to pregnant rats during the organogenesis period at doses up to 810 mg/kg/day (approximately 320 times the recommended human dose on a mg/m^2 basis). Daily doses of exemestane, given to rabbits during organogenesis caused a decrease in placental weight at 90 mg/kg/day (approximately 70 times the recommended human daily dose on a mg/m^2 basis). Abortions, an increase in resorptions, and a reduction in fetal body weight were seen at 270 mg/kg/day. There was no increase in the incidence of malformations in rabbits at doses up to 270 mg/kg/day (approximately 210 times the recommended human dose on a mg/m^2 basis).

There are no studies in pregnant women using AROMASIN. AROMASIN is indicated for postmenopausal women. If there is exposure to AROMASIN during pregnancy, the patient should be apprised of the potential hazard to the fetus and potential risk for loss of the pregnancy.

PRECAUTIONS

General. AROMASIN Tablets should not be administered to premenopausal women. AROMASIN should not be coadministered with estrogen-containing agents as these could interfere with its pharmacologic action.

Hepatic Insufficiency. The pharmacokinetics of exemestane have been investigated in subjects with moderate or severe hepatic insufficiency (Childs-Pugh B or C). Following a single 25-mg oral dose, the AUC of exemestane was approximately 3 times higher than that observed in healthy volunteers. The safety of chronic dosing in patients with moderate or severe hepatic impairment has not been studied. Based on experience with exemestane at repeated doses up to 200 mg daily that demonstrated a moderate increase in non-life threatening adverse events, dosage adjustment does not appear to be necessary.

Renal Insufficiency. The AUC of exemestane after a single 25-mg dose was approximately 3 times higher in subjects with moderate or severe renal insufficiency (creatinine clearance <35 mL/min/1.73 m^2) compared with the AUC in healthy volunteers. The safety of chronic dosing in patients with moderate or severe renal impairment has not been studied. Based on experience with exemestane at repeated doses up to 200 mg daily that demonstrated a moderate increase in non-life threatening adverse events, dosage adjustment does not appear to be necessary.

Laboratory Tests. Approximately 20% of patients receiving exemestane in clinical studies, experienced Common Toxicity Criteria (CTC) grade 3 or 4 lymphocytopenia. Of these patients, 89% had a pre-exisiting lower grade lymphopenia. Forty percent of patients either recovered or improved to a lesser severity while on treatment. Patients did not have a significant increase in viral infections, and no opportunistic infections were observed. Elevations of serum levels of AST, ALT, alkaline phosphatase and gamma glutamyl transferase > 5 times the upper value of the normal range (i.e., ≥ CTC grade 3) have been rarely reported but appear mostly attributable to the underlying presence of liver and/or bone metastases. In the comparative study, CTC grade 3 or 4 elevation of gamma glutamyl transferase without documented evidence of liver metastasis was reported in 2.7% of patients treated with AROMASIN and in 1.8% of patients treated with megestrol acetate.

Drug Interactions. Exemestane is extensively metabolized by CYP 3A4, but coadministration of ketoconazole, a potent inhibitor of CYP 3A4, has no significant effect on exemestane pharmacokinetics. Significant pharmacokinetic interactions mediated by inhibition of CYP isoenzymes therefore appear unlikely. Co-medications that induce CYP 3A4 (e.g. rifampicin, phenytoin, carbamazepine, Phenobarbital, or St. John's wort) may significantly decrease exposure to exemestane. Dose modification is recommended for patients who are also receiving a potent CYP 3A4 inducer (see DOSAGE AND ADMINISTRATION and CLINICAL PHARMACOLOGY).

Drug/Laboratory Tests Interactions. No clinically relevant changes in the results of clinical laboratory tests have been observed.

Carcinogenesis, Mutagenesis, Impairment of Fertility. Carcinogenicity studies have not been conducted with exemestane. Exemestane was not mutagenic in bacteria (Ames test) or mammalian cells (V79 Chinese hamster lung cells). Exemestane was clastogenic in human lymphocytes in vitro without metabolic activation but was not clastogenic in vivo (micronucleus assay in mouse bone marrow). Exemestane did not increase unscheduled DNA synthesis in rat hepatocytes.

Untreated female rats showed reduced fertility when mated to males treated with 500 mg/kg/day exemestane (approximately 200 times the recommended human dose on a mg/m^2 basis) for 63 days prior to and during cohabitation. Exemestane given to female rats 14 days prior to mating and through day 15 or 20 of gestation increased the placental weights at 4 mg/kg/day (approximately 1.5 times the human dose on a mg/m^2 basis). Exemestane showed no effects on female fertility parameters (e.g., ovarian function, mating behavior, conception rate) in rats given doses up to 20 mg/kg/day (approximately 8 times the human dose on a mg/m^2 basis), but mean litter size was decreased at this dose. In general toxicology studies, changes in the ovary, including hyperplasia, an increase in ovarian cysts and a decrease in corpora lutea were observed with variable frequency in mice, rats and dogs at doses that ranged from 3-20 times the human dose on a mg/m^2 basis.

Pregnancy. Pregnancy Category D. See WARNINGS.

Nursing Mothers. AROMASIN is only indicated in postmenopausal women. However, radioactivity related to exemestane appeared in rat milk within 15 minutes of oral administration of radiolabeled exemestane. Concentrations of exemestane and its metabolites were approximately equivalent in the milk and plasma of rats for 24 hours after a single oral dose of 1 mg/kg ^{14}C-exemestane. It is not known whether exemestane is excreted in human milk. Because many drugs are excreted in human milk, caution should be exercised if a nursing woman is inadvertently exposed to AROMASIN (see WARNINGS).

Pediatric Use. The safety and effectiveness of AROMASIN in pediatric patients have not been established.

Geriatric Use. The use of AROMASIN in geriatric patients does not require special precautions.

ADVERSE REACTIONS

A total of 1058 patients were treated with exemestane 25 mg once daily in the clinical trials program. Exemestane was generally well tolerated, and adverse events were usually mild to moderate. Only one death was considered possibly related to treatment with exemestane; an 80-year-old woman with known coronary artery disease had a myocardial infarction with multiple organ failure after 9 weeks on study treatment. In the clinical trials program, only 3% of the patients discontinued treatment with exemestane because of adverse events, mainly within the first 10 weeks of treatment; late discontinuations because of adverse events were uncommon (0.3%).

In the comparative study, adverse reactions were assessed for 358 patients treated with AROMASIN and 400 patients treated with megestrol acetate. Fewer patients receiving AROMASIN discontinued treatment because of adverse events than those treated with megestrol acetate (2% vs. 5%). Adverse events that were considered drug related or of indeterminate cause included hot flashes (13% vs. 5%), nausea (9% vs. 5%), fatigue (8% vs. 10%), increased sweating (4% vs. 8%), and increased appetite (3% vs. 6%). The proportion of patients experiencing an excessive weight gain (>10% of their baseline weight) was significantly higher with megestrol acetate than with AROMASIN (17% vs. 8%). Table 3 shows the adverse events of all CTC grades, regardless of causality, reported in 5% or greater of patients in the study treated either with AROMASIN or megestrol acetate.

Table 3. Incidence (%) of Adverse Events of all Grades* and Causes Occurring in ≥5% of Patients in Each Treatment Arm in the Comparative Study

Event	AROMASIN 25 mg once daily (N=358)	Megestrol Acetate 40 mg QID (N=400)
Autonomic Nervous		
Increased sweating	6	9
Body as a Whole		
Fatigue	22	29
Hot flashes	13	6
Pain	13	13
Influenza-like symptoms	6	5
Edema (includes edema, peripheral edema, leg edema)	7	6
Cardiovascular		
Hypertension	5	6
Nervous		
Depression	13	9
Insomnia	11	9
Anxiety	10	11
Dizziness	8	6
Headache	8	7
Gastrointestinal		
Nausea	18	12
Vomiting	7	4
Abdominal pain	6	11
Anorexia	6	5
Constipation	5	8
Diarrhea	4	5
Increased appetite	3	6
Respiratory		
Dyspnea	10	15
Coughing	6	7

* Graded according to Common Toxicity Criteria

Less frequent adverse events of any cause (from 2% to 5%) reported in the comparative study for patients receiving AROMASIN 25 mg once daily were fever, generalized weakness, paresthesia, pathological fracture, bronchitis, sinusitis, rash, itching, urinary tract infection, and lymphedema.

Additional adverse events of any cause observed in the overall clinical trials program (N = 1058) in 5% or greater of patients treated with exemestane 25 mg once daily but not in the comparative study included pain at tumor sites (8%), asthenia (6%) and fever (5%). Adverse events of any cause reported in 2% to 5% of all patients treated with exemestane 25 mg in the overall clinical trials program but not in the comparative study included chest pain, hypoesthesia, confusion, dyspepsia, arthralgia, back pain, skeletal pain, infection, upper respiratory tract infection, pharyngitis, rhinitis, and alopecia.

OVERDOSAGE

Clinical trials have been conducted with exemestane given as a single dose to healthy female volunteers at doses as high as 800 mg and daily for 12 weeks to postmenopausal women with advanced breast cancer at doses as high as 600 mg. These dosages were well tolerated. There is no specific antidote to overdosage and treatment must be symptomatic. General supportive care, including frequent monitoring of vital signs and close observation of the patient, is indicated.

A male child (age unknown) accidentally ingested a 25-mg tablet of exemestane. The initial physical examination was normal, but blood tests performed 1 hour after ingestion indicated leucocytosis (WBC 25000/mm^3 with 90% neutrophils). Blood tests were repeated 4 days after the incident and were normal. No treatment was given.

In mice, mortality was observed after a single oral dose of exemestane of 3200 mg/kg, the lowest dose tested (about 640 times the recommended human dose on a mg/m^2 basis). In rats and dogs, mortality was observed after single oral doses of exemestane of 5000 mg/kg (about 2000 times the recommended human dose on a mg/m^2 basis) and of 3000 mg/kg (about 4000 times the recommended human dose on a mg/m^2 basis), respectively.

Convulsions were observed after single doses of exemestane of 400 mg/kg and 3000 mg/kg in mice and dogs (approximately 80 and 4000 times the recommended human dose on a mg/m^2 basis), respectively.

DOSAGE AND ADMINISTRATION

The recommended dose of AROMASIN Tablets is 25 mg once daily after a meal. Treatment with AROMASIN should continue until tumor progression is evident.

For patients receiving AROMASIN with a potent CYP 3A4 inducer such as rifampicin or phenytoin, the recommended dose of AROMASIN is 50 mg once daily after a meal.

The safety of chronic dosing in patients with moderate or severe hepatic or renal impairment has not been studied. Based on experience with exemestane at repeated doses up to 200 mg daily that demonstrated a moderate increase in non-life threatening adverse events, dosage adjustment does not appear to be necessary (see CLINICAL PHARMACOLOGY, Special Populations and PRECAUTIONS).

HOW SUPPLIED

AROMASIN Tablets are round, biconvex, and off-white to slightly gray. Each tablet contains 25 mg of exemestane. The tablets are printed on one side with the number "7663" in black. AROMASIN is packaged in HDPE bottles with a child-resistant screw cap, supplied in packs of 30 tablets.

30-tablet HDPE bottle NDC 0009-7663-04

Store at 25°C (77°F); excursions permitted to 15°-30°C (59°-86°F) [see USP Controlled Room Temperature].

℞ only MADE IN ITALY

Manufactured for: Pharmacia & Upjohn Company
A subsidiary of Pharmacia Corporation
Kalamazoo, Michigan 49001, USA

By: Pharmacia Italia S.p.A.
Ascoli Piceno, Italy

Revised March 2004 420079800 817 885 003

Shown in Product Identification Guide, page 330

BEXTRA® ℞

[bĕks'tră]

valdecoxib tablets

DESCRIPTION

Valdecoxib is chemically designated as 4-(5-methyl-3-phenyl-4-isoxazolyl) benzenesulfonamide and is a diaryl substituted isoxazole. It has the following chemical structure:

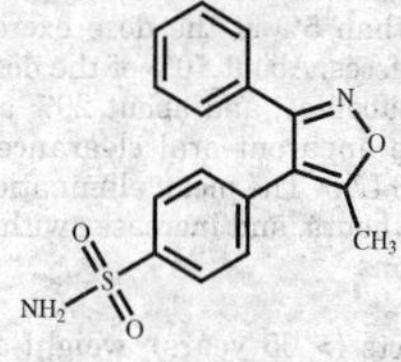

Valdecoxib

The empirical formula for valdecoxib is $C_{16}H_{14}N_2O_3S$, and the molecular weight is 314.36. Valdecoxib is a white crystalline powder that is relatively insoluble in water (10 µg/mL) at 25°C and pH 7.0, soluble in methanol and ethanol, and freely soluble in organic solvents and alkaline (pH=12) aqueous solutions.

BEXTRA Tablets for oral administration contain either 10 mg or 20 mg of valdecoxib. Inactive ingredients include lactose monohydrate, microcrystalline cellulose, pregelatinized starch, croscarmellose sodium, magnesium stearate, hypromellose, polyethylene glycol, polysorbate 80, and titanium dioxide.

CLINICAL PHARMACOLOGY

Mechanism of Action

Valdecoxib is a nonsteroidal anti-inflammatory drug (NSAID) that exhibits anti-inflammatory, analgesic and antipyretic properties in animal models. The mechanism of action is believed to be due to inhibition of prostaglandin synthesis primarily through inhibition of cyclooxygenase-2 (COX-2). At therapeutic plasma concentrations in humans valdecoxib does not inhibit cyclooxygenase-1 (COX-1).

Pharmacokinetics

Absorption

Valdecoxib achieves maximal plasma concentrations in approximately 3 hours. The absolute bioavailability of valdecoxib is 83% following oral administration of BEXTRA compared to intravenous infusion of valdecoxib.

Dose proportionality was demonstrated after single doses (1-400 mg) of valdecoxib. With multiple doses (up to 100 mg/day for 14 days), valdecoxib exposure as measured by the AUC, increases in a more than proportional manner at doses above 10 mg BID. Steady state plasma concentrations of valdecoxib are achieved by day 4.

The steady state pharmacokinetic parameters of valdecoxib in healthy male subjects are shown in Table 1.

Table 1
Mean (SD) Steady State Pharmacokinetic Parameters

Steady State Pharmacokinetic Parameters after Valdecoxib 10 mg Once Daily for 14 Days	Healthy Male Subjects (n=8, 20 to 42 yr.)
$AUC_{(0-24hr)}$ (hr•ng/mL)	1479.0 (291.9)
C_{max} (ng/mL)	161.1 (48.1)
T_{max} (hr)	2.25 (0.71)
C_{min} (ng/mL)	21.9 (7.68)
Elimination Half-life (hr)	8.11 (1.32)

Continued on next page

Bextra—Cont.

No clinically significant age or gender differences were seen in pharmacokinetic parameters that would require dosage adjustments.

Effect of Food and Antacid

BEXTRA can be taken with or without food. Food had no significant effect on either the peak plasma concentration (C_{max}) or extent of absorption (AUC) of valdecoxib when BEXTRA was taken with a high fat meal. The time to peak plasma concentration (T_{max}), however, was delayed by 1-2 hours. Administration of BEXTRA with antacid (aluminum/magnesium hydroxide) had no significant effect on either the rate or extent of absorption of valdecoxib.

Distribution

Plasma protein binding for valdecoxib is about 98% over the concentration range (21–2384 ng/mL). Steady state apparent volume of distribution (Vss/F) of valdecoxib is approximately 86 L after oral administration. Valdecoxib and its active metabolite preferentially partition into erythrocytes with a blood to plasma concentration ratio of about 2.5:1. This ratio remains approximately constant with time and therapeutic blood concentrations.

Metabolism

In humans, valdecoxib undergoes extensive hepatic metabolism involving both P450 isoenzymes (3A4 and 2C9) and non-P450 dependent pathways (i.e., glucuronidation). Concomitant administration of BEXTRA with known CYP 3A4 and 2C9 inhibitors (e.g., fluconazole and ketoconazole) can result in increased plasma exposure of valdecoxib (see PRECAUTIONS — Drug Interactions).

One active metabolite of valdecoxib has been identified in human plasma at approximately 10% the concentration of valdecoxib. This metabolite, which is a less potent COX-2 specific inhibitor than the parent, also undergoes extensive metabolism and constitutes less than 2% of the valdecoxib dose excreted in the urine and feces. Due to its low concentration in the systemic circulation, it is not likely to contribute significantly to the efficacy profile of BEXTRA.

Excretion

Valdecoxib is eliminated predominantly via hepatic metabolism with less than 5% of the dose excreted unchanged in the urine and feces. About 70% of the dose is excreted in the urine as metabolites, and about 20% as valdecoxib N-glucuronide. The apparent oral clearance (CL/F) of valdecoxib is about 6 L/hr. The mean elimination half-life ($T_{1/2}$) ranges from 8-11 hours, and increases with age.

Special Populations

Geriatric

In elderly subjects (> 65 years), weight-adjusted steady state plasma concentrations ($AUC_{(0-12hr)}$) are about 30% higher than in young subjects. No dose adjustment is needed based on age.

Pediatric

BEXTRA has not been investigated in pediatric patients below 18 years of age.

Race

Pharmacokinetic differences due to race have not been identified in clinical and pharmacokinetic studies conducted to date.

Hepatic Insufficiency

Valdecoxib plasma concentrations are significantly increased (130%) in patients with moderate (Child-Pugh Class B) hepatic impairment. In clinical trials, doses of BEXTRA above those recommended have been associated with fluid retention. Hence, treatment with BEXTRA should be initiated with caution in patients with mild to moderate hepatic impairment and fluid retention. The use of BEXTRA in patients with severe hepatic impairment (Child-Pugh Class C) is not recommended.

Renal Insufficiency

The pharmacokinetics of valdecoxib have been studied in patients with varying degrees of renal impairment. Because renal elimination of valdecoxib is not important to its disposition, no clinically significant changes in valdecoxib clearance were found even in patients with severe renal impairment or in patients undergoing renal dialysis. In patients undergoing hemodialysis the plasma clearance (CL/F) of valdecoxib was similar to the CL/F found in healthy elderly subjects (CL/F about 6 to 7 L/hr) with normal renal function (based on creatinine clearance).

NSAIDs have been associated with worsening renal function and use in advanced renal disease is not recommended (see PRECAUTIONS – Renal Effects).

Drug Interactions

For quantitative information on the following drug interaction studies, see **PRECAUTIONS — Drug Interactions**.

General

Valdecoxib undergoes both P450 (CYP) dependent and non-P450 dependent (glucuronidation) metabolism. In vitro studies indicate that valdecoxib is not a significant inhibitor of CYP 1A2, 3A4, or 2D6 and is a weak inhibitor of CYP 2C9 and a weak to moderate inhibitor of CYP 2C19 at therapeutic concentrations. The P450-mediated metabolic pathway of valdecoxib predominantly involves the 3A4 and 2C9 isozymes. Using prototype inhibitors and substrates of these isozymes, the following results were obtained. Coadministration of a known inhibitor of CYP 2C9/3A4 (fluconazole) and a CYP 3A4 inhibitor (ketoconazole) enhanced the total plasma exposure (AUC) of valdecoxib. Coadministration of valdecoxib with a CYP 3A4 inducer (phenytoin) decreased total plasma exposure (AUC) of valdecoxib. (See PRECAUTIONS – Drug Interactions.)

Coadministration of valdecoxib with warfarin (a CYP 2C9 substrate) caused a small, but statistically significant increase in plasma exposures of R-warfarin and S-warfarin, and also in the pharmacodynamic effects (International Normalized Ratio - INR) of warfarin. (See PRECAUTIONS – Drug Interactions.)

Coadministration of valdecoxib with diazepam (a CYP 2C19/3A4 substrate) resulted in increased exposure of diazepam, but not its major metabolite, desmethyldiazepam. (See PRECAUTIONS – Drug Interactions.)

Coadministration of valdecoxib with glyburide (a CYP 2C9 substrate) (40 mg valdecoxib QD with 10 mg glyburide BID) resulted in increased exposure of glyburide. (See PRECAUTIONS – Drug Interactions.)

Coadministration of valdecoxib with an oral contraceptive, 1 mg norethindrone/0.035 mg ethinyl estradiol (CYP 3A4 substrates), resulted in increased exposure of both norethindrone and ethinyl estradiol. (See PRECAUTIONS – Drug Interactions.)

Coadministration of valdecoxib with omeprazole (a CYP 3A4/2C19 substrate) caused an increase in omeprazole exposure. (See PRECAUTIONS – Drug Interactions.)

Coadministration of valdecoxib with dextromethorphan (a CYP 2D6/3A4 substrate) resulted in an increase in dextromethorphan plasma levels above those seen in subjects with normal levels of CYP 2D6. Even so these levels were almost 5-fold lower than those seen in CYP 2D6 poor metabolizers. (See PRECAUTIONS – Drug Interactions.)

Coadministration of valdecoxib with phenytoin (a CYP 2C9/2C19 substrate) did not affect the pharmacokinetics of phenytoin.

Coadministration of valdecoxib, or its injectable prodrug, with substrates of CYP 2C9 (propofol) and CYP 3A4 (midazolam, alfentanil, fentanyl) did not inhibit the metabolism of these substrates.

CLINICAL STUDIES

The efficacy and clinical utility of BEXTRA Tablets have been demonstrated in osteoarthritis (OA), rheumatoid arthritis (RA) and in the treatment of primary dysmenorrhea.

Osteoarthritis

BEXTRA was evaluated for treatment of the signs and symptoms of osteoarthritis of the knee or hip, in five double-blind, randomized, controlled trials in which 3918 patients were treated for 3 to 6 months. BEXTRA was shown to be superior to placebo in improvement in three domains of OA symptoms: (1) the WOMAC (Western Ontario and McMaster Universities) osteoarthritis index, a composite of pain, stiffness and functional measures in OA, (2) the overall patient assessment of pain, and (3) the overall patient global assessment. The two 3-month pivotal trials in OA generally showed changes statistically significantly different from placebo, and comparable to the naproxen control, in measures of these domains for the 10 mg/day dose. No additional benefit was seen with a valdecoxib 20-mg daily dose.

Rheumatoid Arthritis

BEXTRA demonstrated significant reduction compared to placebo in the signs and symptoms of RA, as measured by the ACR (American College of Rheumatology) 20 improvement, a composite defined as both improvement of 20% in the number of tender and number of swollen joints, and a 20% improvement in three of the following five: patient global, physician global, patient pain, patient function assessment, and C-reactive protein (CRP). BEXTRA was evaluated for treatment of the signs and symptoms of rheumatoid arthritis in four double-blind, randomized, controlled studies in which 3444 patients were treated for 3 to 6 months. The two 3-month pivotal trials compared valdecoxib to naproxen and placebo. The results for the ACR20 responses in these trials are shown below (Table 2). Trials of BEXTRA in rheumatoid arthritis allowed concomitant use of corticosteroids and/or disease-modifying anti-rheumatic drugs (DMARDs), such as methotrexate, gold salts, and hydroxychloroquine. No additional benefit was seen with a valdecoxib 20-mg daily dose.

Table 2
ACR20 Response Rate (%) in Rheumatoid Arthritis

	Study 1	Study 2
BEXTRA 10 mg/day	49%** (103/209)	46%** (103/226)
BEXTRA 20 mg/day	48%** (102/212)	47%* (103/219)
Naproxen 500 mg BID	44%* (100/225)	53%** (115/219)
Placebo	32% (70/222)	32% (71/220)

* p<0.01; ** p<0.001 compared to placebo

Primary Dysmenorrhea

BEXTRA was compared to naproxen sodium 550 mg in two placebo-controlled studies of women with moderate to severe primary dysmenorrhea. The onset of analgesia was within 60 minutes for BEXTRA 20 mg. The onset, magnitude, and duration of analgesic effect with BEXTRA 20 mg were comparable to naproxen sodium 550 mg.

Safety Studies

Gastrointestinal (GI) Endoscopy Studies with Therapeutic Doses: Scheduled upper GI endoscopic evaluations were performed with BEXTRA at doses of 10 and 20 mg daily in over 800 OA patients who were enrolled into two randomized 3-month studies using active comparators and placebo controls (Study 3 and Study 4). These studies enrolled patients free of endoscopic ulcers at baseline and compared rates of endoscopic ulcers, defined as any gastroduodenal ulcer seen endoscopically provided it was of "unequivocal depth" and at least 3 mm in diameter.

In both studies, BEXTRA 10 mg daily was associated with a statistically significant lower incidence of endoscopic gastroduodenal ulcers over the study period compared to the active comparators. Figure 1 summarizes the incidence of gastroduodenal ulcers in Studies 3 and 4 for the placebo, valdecoxib, and active control arms.

Figure 1
Incidence of Endoscopically Observed Gastroduodenal Ulcers in OA Patients

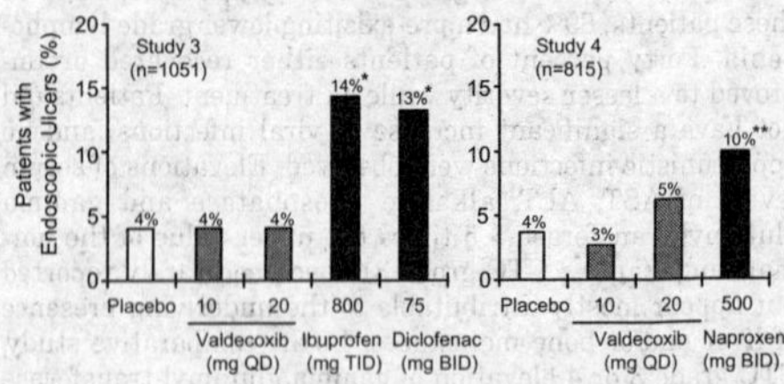

* Significantly different vs placebo and both valdecoxib treatment groups; p<0.05
** Significantly different vs placebo and valdecoxib 10 mg; p<0.05

Safety Study with Supratherapeutic Doses: Scheduled upper GI endoscopic evaluations were performed in a randomized 6-month study of 1217 patients with OA and RA comparing valdecoxib 20 mg BID (40 mg daily) and 40 mg BID (80 mg daily) (4 to 8 times the recommended therapeutic dose) to naproxen 500 mg BID (Study 5). This study also formally assessed renal events as a primary outcome with supratherapeutic doses of BEXTRA. The renal endpoint was defined as any of the following: new/increase in edema, new/increase in congestive heart failure, increase in blood pressure (BP; >20 mm Hg systolic, >10 mm Hg diastolic), new/increase in BP treatment, new/increase in diuretic therapy, creatinine increase over 30% (or >1.2 mg/dL if baseline <0.9 mg/dL), BUN increase over 200% or >50 mg/dL, 24-hr urinary protein increase to >500 mg (if baseline 0-150 mg or >750 if baseline 151-300 or >1000 if baseline 301-500), serum potassium increase to >6 mEq/L, or serum sodium decrease to <130 mEq/L.

Figure 2 summarizes the incidence rates of gastroduodenal ulcers and renal events that were seen in Study 5. BEXTRA 40 mg daily and 80 mg daily were associated with a statistically significant lower incidence of endoscopic gastroduodenal ulcers over the study period compared to naproxen. The incidence of renal events was significantly different between the BEXTRA 80 mg daily group and naproxen. The clinical relevance of renal events observed with supratherapeutic doses (4 to 8 times the recommended therapeutic dose) of BEXTRA is not known (see PRECAUTIONS – Renal Effects).

Figure 2
Incidence of Endoscopic Gastroduodenal Ulcers and Renal Events in the High-dose Safety Study

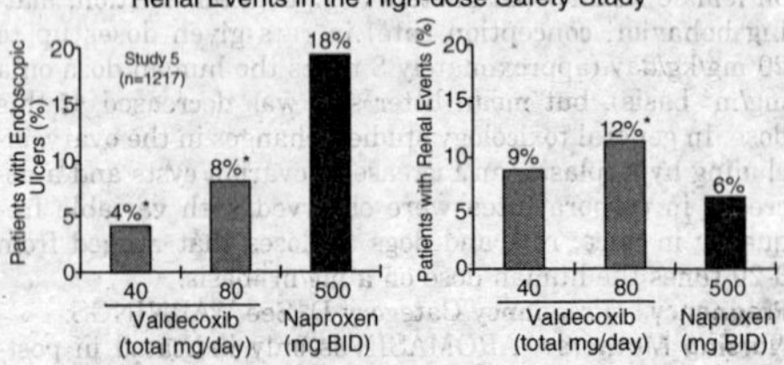

* Significantly different vs naproxen, p<0.05

Renal Safety at the Therapeutic Chronic Dose: The renal effects of valdecoxib compared with placebo and conventional NSAIDs were also assessed by prospectively designed pooled analyses of renal events data (see definition above — Supratherapeutic Doses) from five placebo- and active-controlled 12-week arthritis trials that included 995 OA or RA patients given valdecoxib 10 mg daily. The incidence of renal events observed in this analysis with valdecoxib 10 mg daily (3%), ibuprofen 800 mg TID (7%), naproxen 500 mg BID (2%) and diclofenac 75 mg BID (4%) were significantly higher than placebo-treated patients (1%). In all treatment groups, the majority of renal events were either due to the occurrence of edema or worsening BP.

Gastrointestinal Ulcers in High-Risk Patients: Subset analyses were performed of patients with risk factors (age, concomitant low-dose aspirin use, history of prior ulcer disease) enrolled in four upper GI endoscopic studies. Table 3 summarizes the trends seen.

[See table 3 at bottom of next page]

The correlation between findings of endoscopic studies, and the incidence of clinically significant serious upper GI events has not been established.

Platelets: In four clinical studies with young and elderly (≥65 years) subjects, single and multiple doses up to 7 days of BEXTRA 10 to 40 mg BID had no effect on platelet aggregation.

INDICATIONS AND USAGE

BEXTRA Tablets are indicated:

- For relief of the signs and symptoms of osteoarthritis and adult rheumatoid arthritis.
- For the treatment of primary dysmenorrhea.

CONTRAINDICATIONS

BEXTRA should not be given to patients who have demonstrated allergic-type reactions to sulfonamides. BEXTRA Tablets are contraindicated in patients with known hypersensitivity to valdecoxib. BEXTRA should not be given to patients who have experienced asthma, urticaria, or allergic-type reactions after taking aspirin or NSAIDs. Severe, rarely fatal, anaphylactic-like reactions to NSAIDs are possible in such patients (see WARNINGS — Anaphylactoid Reactions, and PRECAUTIONS — Preexisting Asthma).

WARNINGS

Gastrointestinal (GI) Effects — Risk of GI Ulceration, Bleeding, and Perforation

Serious gastrointestinal toxicity such as bleeding, ulceration and perforation of the stomach, small intestine or large intestine can occur at any time with or without warning symptoms in patients treated with nonsteroidal anti-inflammatory drugs (NSAIDs). Minor gastrointestinal problems such as dyspepsia are common and may also occur at any time during NSAID therapy. Therefore, physicians and patients should remain alert for ulceration and bleeding even in the absence of previous GI tract symptoms. Patients should be informed about the signs and symptoms of serious GI toxicity and the steps to take if they occur. The utility of periodic laboratory monitoring has not been demonstrated, nor has it been adequately assessed. Only one in five patients who develop a serious upper GI adverse event on NSAID therapy is symptomatic. It has been demonstrated that upper GI ulcers, gross bleeding or perforation caused by NSAIDs appear to occur in approximately 1% of patients treated for 3 to 6 months and 2-4% of patients treated for one year. These trends continue, thus increasing the likelihood of developing a serious GI event at some time during the course of therapy. However, even short-term therapy is not without risk.

NSAIDs should be prescribed with extreme caution in patients with a prior history of ulcer disease or gastrointestinal bleeding. Most spontaneous reports of fatal GI events are in elderly or debilitated patients and therefore special care should be taken in treating this population. For high risk patients, alternate therapies that do not involve NSAIDs should be considered.

Studies have shown that patients with a *prior history of peptic ulcer disease and/or gastrointestinal bleeding* and who use NSAIDs, have a greater than 10-fold higher risk for developing a GI bleed than patients with neither of these risk factors. In addition to a past history of ulcer disease, pharmacoepidemiological studies have identified several other co-therapies or co-morbid conditions that may increase the risk for GI bleeding such as: treatment with oral corticosteroids, treatment with anticoagulants, longer duration of NSAID therapy, smoking, alcoholism, older age, and poor general health status. (See CLINICAL STUDIES — Safety Studies.)

Serious Skin Reactions

Serious skin reactions, including exfoliative dermatitis, Stevens-Johnson syndrome, and toxic epidermal necrolysis, have been reported through postmarketing surveillance in patients receiving BEXTRA (see ADVERSE REACTIONS—Postmarketing Experience). Fatalities due to Stevens-Johnson syndrome and toxic epidermal necrolysis have been reported. BEXTRA should be discontinued at the first appearance of skin rash or any other sign of hypersensitivity.

Anaphylactoid Reactions

In postmarketing experience, cases of hypersensitivity reactions (anaphylactic reactions and angioedema) have been reported in patients receiving BEXTRA (see ADVERSE REACTIONS—Postmarketing Experience). These cases have occurred in patients with and without a history of allergic-type reactions to sulfonamides (see CONTRAINDICATIONS). BEXTRA should not be given to patients with the aspirin triad. This symptom complex typically occurs in asthmatic patients who experience rhinitis with or without nasal polyps, or who exhibit severe, potentially fatal bronchospasm after taking aspirin or other NSAIDs (see CONTRAINDICATIONS and PRECAUTIONS — Pre-existing Asthma). Emergency help should be sought in cases where an anaphylactoid reaction occurs.

Advanced Renal Disease

No information is available regarding the safe use of BEXTRA Tablets in patients with advanced kidney disease. Therefore, treatment with BEXTRA is not recommended in these patients. If therapy with BEXTRA must be initiated, close monitoring of the patient's kidney function is advisable (see PRECAUTIONS — Renal Effects).

Pregnancy

In late pregnancy, BEXTRA should be avoided because it may cause premature closure of the ductus arteriosus.

PRECAUTIONS

General

BEXTRA Tablets cannot be expected to substitute for corticosteroids or to treat corticosteroid insufficiency. Abrupt discontinuation of corticosteroids may lead to exacerbation of corticosteroid-responsive illness. Patients on prolonged corticosteroid therapy should have their therapy tapered slowly if a decision is made to discontinue corticosteroids.

The pharmacological activity of valdecoxib in reducing fever and inflammation may diminish the utility of these diagnostic signs in detecting complications of presumed noninfectious, painful conditions.

Hepatic Effects

Borderline elevations of one or more liver tests may occur in up to 15% of patients taking NSAIDs. Notable elevations of ALT or AST (approximately three or more times the upper limit of normal) have been reported in approximately 1% of patients in clinical trials with NSAIDs. These laboratory abnormalities may progress, may remain unchanged, or may remain transient with continuing therapy. Rare cases of severe hepatic reactions, including jaundice and fatal fulminant hepatitis, liver necrosis and hepatic failure (some with fatal outcome) have been reported with NSAIDs. In controlled clinical trials of valdecoxib, the incidence of borderline (defined as 1.2- to 3.0-fold) elevations of liver tests was 8.0% for valdecoxib and 8.4% for placebo, while approximately 0.3% of patients taking valdecoxib, and 0.2% of patients taking placebo, had notable (defined as greater than 3-fold) elevations of ALT or AST.

A patient with symptoms and/or signs suggesting liver dysfunction, or in whom an abnormal liver test has occurred, should be monitored carefully for evidence of the development of a more severe hepatic reaction while on therapy with BEXTRA. If clinical signs and symptoms consistent with liver disease develop, or if systemic manifestations occur (e.g., eosinophilia, rash), BEXTRA should be discontinued.

Renal Effects

Long-term administration of NSAIDs has resulted in renal papillary necrosis and other renal injury. Renal toxicity has also been seen in patients in whom renal prostaglandins have a compensatory role in the maintenance of renal perfusion. In these patients, administration of a nonsteroidal anti-inflammatory drug may cause a dose-dependent reduction in prostaglandin formation and, secondarily, in renal blood flow, which may precipitate overt renal decompensation. Patients at greatest risk of this reaction are those with impaired renal function, heart failure, liver dysfunction, those taking diuretics and Angiotensin Converting Enzyme (ACE) inhibitors, and the elderly. Discontinuation of NSAID therapy is usually followed by recovery to the pretreatment state.

Caution should be used when initiating treatment with BEXTRA in patients with considerable dehydration. It is advisable to rehydrate patients first and then start therapy with BEXTRA. Caution is also recommended in patients with preexisting kidney disease. (See WARNINGS — Advanced Renal Disease.)

Hematological Effects

Anemia is sometimes seen in patients receiving BEXTRA. Patients on long-term treatment with BEXTRA should have their hemoglobin or hematocrit checked if they exhibit any signs or symptoms of anemia.

BEXTRA does not generally affect platelet counts, prothrombin time (PT), or activated partial thromboplastin time (APTT), and does not appear to inhibit platelet aggregation at indicated dosages (See CLINICAL STUDIES — Safety Studies — Platelets).

Table 3

Incidence of Endoscopic Gastroduodenal Ulcers in Patients With and Without Selected Risk Factors

	Placebo-controlled Studies		Active-controlled Studies			
Risk Factor	Placebo	Valdecoxib (10-20 mg daily)	Valdecoxib (10-80 mg daily)	Ibuprofen 800 mg TID	Naproxen 500 mg BID	Diclofenac 75 mg BID
Age						
<65 yrs	3.7% (8/219)	3.5% (17/484)	3.7% (48/1306)	8.2% (9/110)	12.8% (51/397)	13.2% (34/258)
≥65 yrs	5.8% (8/137)	4.6% (12/262)	7.6% (43/568)	21.6% (16/74)	22.0% (33/150)	18.2% (25/137)
Concomitant Low Dose Aspirin Use						
no	4.4% (13/298)	3.2% (21/650)	3.8% (64/1671)	9.8% (15/153)	16.0% (75/468)	12.8% (45/351)
yes	5.2% (3/58)	8.3% (8/96)	13.3% (27/203)	32.3% (10/31)	11.4% (9/79)	31.8% (14/44)
History of Ulcer Disease						
no	4.4% (14/317)	3.4% (22/647)	4.1% (68/1666)	13.8% (22/160)	13.3% (63/475)	14.7% (52/354)
yes	5.1% (2/39)	7.1% (7/99)	11.1% (23/208)	12.5% (3/24)	29.2% (21/72)	17.1% (7/41)

No statistical conclusions can be drawn from these comparisons.

Fluid Retention and Edema

Fluid retention and edema have been observed in some patients taking BEXTRA (see ADVERSE REACTIONS). Therefore, BEXTRA should be used with caution in patients with fluid retention, hypertension, or heart failure.

Preexisting Asthma

Patients with asthma may have aspirin-sensitive asthma. The use of aspirin in patients with aspirin-sensitive asthma has been associated with severe bronchospasm, which can be fatal. Since cross reactivity, including bronchospasm, between aspirin and other nonsteroidal anti-inflammatory drugs has been reported in such aspirin-sensitive patients, BEXTRA should not be administered to patients with this form of aspirin sensitivity and should be used with caution in patients with preexisting asthma.

Information for Patients

BEXTRA can cause GI discomfort and, rarely, more serious GI side effects, which may result in hospitalization and even fatal outcomes. Although serious GI tract ulcerations and bleeding can occur without warning symptoms, patients should be alert for the signs and symptoms of ulcerations and bleeding, and should ask for medical advice when observing any indicative sign or symptoms. Patients should be apprised of the importance of this follow-up (see WARNINGS — Gastrointestinal (GI) Effects — Risk of GI Ulceration, Bleeding, and Perforation).

Patients should report to their physicians, signs or symptoms of gastrointestinal ulceration or bleeding, skin rash, weight gain, or edema.

Patients should be informed of the warning signs and symptoms of hepatotoxicity (e.g., nausea, fatigue, lethargy, pruritus, jaundice, right upper quadrant tenderness, and flu-like symptoms). If these occur, patients should be instructed to stop therapy and seek immediate medical attention.

Patients should also be instructed to seek immediate emergency help in the case of an anaphylactoid reaction (see WARNINGS — Anaphylactoid Reactions).

In late pregnancy, BEXTRA should be avoided because it may cause premature closure of the ductus arteriosus.

Laboratory Tests

Because serious GI tract ulcerations and bleeding can occur without warning symptoms, physicians should monitor for signs and symptoms of GI bleeding.

Drug Interactions

The drug interaction studies with valdecoxib were performed both with valdecoxib and a rapidly hydrolyzed intravenous prodrug form. The results from trials using the intravenous prodrug are reported in this section as they relate to the role of valdecoxib in drug interactions.

General: In humans, valdecoxib metabolism is predominantly mediated via CYP 3A4 and 2C9 with glucuronidation being a further (20%) route of metabolism. In vitro studies indicate that valdecoxib is a moderate inhibitor of CYP 2C19 (IC50 = 6 µg/mL or 19 µM) and 2C9 (IC50 = 13 µg/mL or 41 µM), and a weak inhibitor of CYP 2D6 (IC50 = 31 µg/mL or 100 µM) and 3A4 (IC50 = 44 µg/mL or 141 µM).

Aspirin: Concomitant administration of aspirin with valdecoxib may result in an increased risk of GI ulceration and complications compared to valdecoxib alone. Because of its lack of anti-platelet effect valdecoxib is not a substitute for aspirin for cardiovascular prophylaxis.

In a parallel group drug interaction study comparing the intravenous prodrug form of valdecoxib at 40 mg BID (n=10) vs placebo (n=9), valdecoxib had no effect on in vitro aspirin-mediated inhibition of arachidonate- or collagen-stimulated platelet aggregation.

Methotrexate: Valdecoxib 10 mg BID did not show a significant effect on the plasma exposure or renal clearance of methotrexate.

ACE-inhibitors: Reports suggest that NSAIDs may diminish the antihypertensive effect of ACE-inhibitors. This interaction should be given consideration in patients taking BEXTRA concomitantly with ACE-inhibitors.

Furosemide: Clinical studies, as well as post-marketing observations, have shown that NSAIDs can reduce the natriuretic effect of furosemide and thiazides in some patients. This response has been attributed to inhibition of renal prostaglandin synthesis.

Anticonvulsants (Phenytoin): Steady state plasma exposure (AUC) of valdecoxib (40 mg BID for 12 days) was decreased by 27% when coadministered with multiple doses (300 mg QD for 12 days) of phenytoin (a CYP 3A4 inducer). Patients already stabilized on valdecoxib should be closely monitored for loss of symptom control with phenytoin coadministration. Valdecoxib did not have a statistically significant effect on the pharmacokinetics of phenytoin (a CYP 2C9 and CYP 2C19 substrate).

Drug interaction studies with other anticonvulsants have not been conducted. Routine monitoring should be performed when therapy with BEXTRA is either initiated or discontinued in patients on anticonvulsant therapy.

Dextromethorphan: Dextromethorphan is primarily metabolized by CYP 2D6 and to a lesser extent by 3A4. Coadministration with valdecoxib (40 mg BID for 7 days) resulted in a significant increase in dextromethorphan plasma levels suggesting that, at these doses, valdecoxib is a weak inhibitor of 2D6. Even so, dextromethorphan plasma concentrations in the presence of high doses of valdecoxib were almost 5-fold lower than those seen in CYP 2D6 poor metabolizers suggesting that dose adjustment is not necessary.

Continued on next page

Bextra—Cont.

Lithium: Valdecoxib 40 mg BID for 7 days produced significant decreases in lithium serum clearance (25%) and renal clearance (30%) with a 34% higher serum exposure compared to lithium alone. Lithium serum concentrations should be monitored closely when initiating or changing therapy with BEXTRA in patients receiving lithium. Lithium carbonate (450 mg BID for 7 days) had no effect on valdecoxib pharmacokinetics.

Warfarin: The effect of valdecoxib on the anticoagulant effect of warfarin (1-8 mg/day) was studied in healthy subjects by coadministration of BEXTRA 40 mg BID for 7 days. Valdecoxib caused a statistically significant increase in plasma exposures of R-warfarin and S-warfarin (12% and 15%, respectively), and in the pharmacodynamic effects (prothrombin time, measured as INR) of warfarin. While mean INR values were only slightly increased with coadministration of valdecoxib, the day-to-day variability in individual INR values was increased. Anticoagulant therapy should be monitored, particularly during the first few weeks, after initiating therapy with BEXTRA in patients receiving warfarin or similar agents.

Fluconazole and Ketoconazole: Ketoconazole and fluconazole are predominantly CYP 3A4 and 2C9 inhibitors, respectively. Concomitant single dose administration of valdecoxib 20 mg with multiple doses of ketoconazole and fluconazole produced a significant increase in exposure of valdecoxib. Plasma exposure (AUC) to valdecoxib was increased 62% when coadministered with fluconazole and 38% when coadministered with ketoconazole.

Glyburide: Glyburide is a CYP 2C9 substrate. Coadministration of valdecoxib (10 mg BID for 7 days) with glyburide (5 mg QD or 10 mg BID) did not affect the pharmacokinetics (exposure) of glyburide. Coadministration of valdecoxib 40 mg BID (day 1) and 40 mg QD (days 2-7) with glyburide (5 mg QD) did not affect either the pharmacokinetics (exposure) or the pharmacodynamics (blood glucose and insulin levels) of glyburide. Coadministration of valdecoxib 40 mg BID (day 1) and 40 mg QD (days 2-7) with glyburide (10 mg glyburide BID) resulted in 21% increase in glyburide $AUC_{(0-12hr)}$ and a 16% increase in glyburide C_{max} leading to a 16% decrease in glucose $AUC_{(0-24hr)}$. Insulin parameters were not affected. Because changes in glucose concentrations with valdecoxib coadministration were within the normal variability and individual glucose concentrations were above or near 70 mg/dL, dose adjustment for glyburide (5 mg QD and 10 mg BID) with valdecoxib coadministration (up to 40 mg QD) is not indicated. Coadministration of glyburide with doses higher than 40 mg valdecoxib (e.g., 40 mg BID) has not been studied.

Omeprazole: Omeprazole is a CYP 3A4 substrate and CYP 2C19 substrate and inhibitor. Valdecoxib steady state plasma concentrations (40 mg BID) were not affected significantly with multiple doses of omeprazole (40 mg QD). Coadministration with valdecoxib increased exposure of omeprazole (AUC) by 46%. Drugs whose absorption is sensitive to pH may be negatively impacted by concomitant administration of omeprazole and valdecoxib. However, because higher doses (up to 360 mg QD) of omeprazole are tolerated in Zollinger-Ellison (ZE) patients, no dose adjustment for omeprazole is recommended at current doses. Coadministration of valdecoxib with doses higher than 40 mg QD omeprazole has not been studied.

Oral Contraceptives: Valdecoxib (40 mg BID) did not induce the metabolism of the combination oral contraceptive norethindrone/ethinyl estradiol (1 mg/0.035 mg combination, Ortho-Novum 1/35®). Coadministration of valdecoxib and Ortho-Novum 1/35® increased the exposure of norethindrone and ethinyl estradiol by 20% and 34%, respectively. Although there is little risk for loss of contraceptive efficacy, the clinical significance of these increased exposures in terms of safety is not known. These increased exposures of norethindrone and ethinyl estradiol should be taken into consideration when selecting an oral contraceptive for women taking valdecoxib.

Diazepam: Diazepam (Valium®) is a CYP 3A4 and CYP 2C19 substrate. Plasma exposure of diazepam (10 mg BID) was increased by 28% following administration of valdecoxib (40 mg BID) for 12 days, while plasma exposure of valdecoxib (40 mg BID) was not substantially increased following administration of diazepam (10 mg BID) for 12 days. Although the magnitude of changes in diazepam plasma exposure when coadministered with valdecoxib were not sufficient to warrant dosage adjustments, patients may experience enhanced sedative side effects caused by increased exposure of diazepam under this circumstance. Patients should be cautioned against engaging in hazardous activities requiring complete mental alertness such as operating machinery or driving a motor vehicle.

Carcinogenesis, Mutagenesis, Impairment of Fertility

Valdecoxib was not carcinogenic in rats given oral doses up to 7.5 mg/kg/day for males and 1.5 mg/kg/day for females (equivalent to approximately 2- to 6-fold human exposure at 20 mg QD as measured by the $AUC_{(0-24hr)}$) or in mice given oral doses up to 25 mg/kg/day for males and 50 mg/kg/day for females (equivalent to approximately 0.6- to 2.4-fold human exposure at 20 mg QD as measured by the $AUC_{(0-24hr)}$) for two years.

Valdecoxib was not mutagenic in an Ames test or a mutation assay in Chinese hamster ovary (CHO) cells, nor was it clastogenic in a chromosome aberration assay in CHO cells or in an *in vivo* micronucleus test in rat bone marrow.

Table 4

Adverse Events with Incidence ≥ 2.0% in Valdecoxib Treatment Groups: Controlled Arthritis Trials of Three Months or Longer

		(Total Daily Dose)				
		Valdecoxib		Diclofenac	Ibuprofen	Naproxen
Adverse Event	**Placebo**	**10 mg**	**20 mg**	**150 mg**	**2400 mg**	**1000 mg**
Number Treated	973	1214	1358	711	207	766
Autonomic Nervous System Disorders						
Hypertension	0.6	1.6	2.1	2.5	2.4	1.7
Body as a Whole						
Back pain	1.6	1.6	2.7	2.8	1.4	1.0
Edema peripheral	0.7	2.4	3.0	3.2	2.9	2.1
Influenza-like symptoms	2.2	2.0	2.2	3.1	2.9	2.0
Injury accidental	2.8	4.0	3.7	3.9	3.9	3.0
Central and Peripheral Nervous System Disorders						
Dizziness	2.1	2.6	2.7	4.2	3.4	2.7
Headache	7.1	4.8	8.5	6.6	4.3	5.5
Gastrointestinal System Disorders						
Abdominal fullness	2.0	2.1	1.9	3.0	2.9	2.5
Abdominal pain	6.3	7.0	8.2	17.0	8.2	10.1
Diarrhea	4.2	5.4	6.0	10.8	3.9	4.7
Dyspepsia	6.3	7.9	8.7	13.4	15.0	12.9
Flatulence	4.1	2.9	3.5	3.1	7.7	5.4
Nausea	5.9	7.0	6.3	8.4	7.7	8.7
Musculoskeletal System Disorders						
Myalgia	1.6	2.0	1.9	2.4	2.4	1.4
Respiratory System Disorders						
Sinusitis	2.2	2.6	1.8	1.1	3.4	3.4
Upper respiratory tract infection	6.0	6.7	5.7	6.3	4.3	6.4
Skin and Appendages Disorders						
Rash	1.0	1.4	2.1	1.5	0.5	1.4

Valdecoxib did not impair male rat fertility at oral doses up to 9.0 mg/kg/day (equivalent to approximately 3- to 6-fold human exposure at 20 mg QD as measured by the $AUC_{(0-24hr)}$). In female rats, a decrease in ovulation with increased pre- and post-implantation loss resulted in decreased live embryos/fetuses at doses ≥2 mg/kg/day (equivalent to approximately 2-fold human exposure at 20 mg QD as measured by the $AUC_{(0-24hr)}$ for valdecoxib). The effects on female fertility were reversible. This effect is expected with inhibition of prostaglandin synthesis and is not the result of irreversible alteration of female reproductive function.

Pregnancy

Teratogenic Effects: Pregnancy Category C.

The incidence of fetuses with skeletal anomalies such as semi-bipartite thoracic vertebra centra and fused sternebrae was slightly higher in rabbits at an oral dose of 40 mg/kg/day (equivalent to approximately 72-fold human exposures at 20 mg QD as measured by the $AUC_{(0-24hr)}$) throughout organogenesis. Valdecoxib was not teratogenic in rabbits up to an oral dose of 10 mg/kg/day (equivalent to approximately 8-fold human exposures at 20 mg QD as measured by the $AUC_{(0-24hr)}$).

Valdecoxib was not teratogenic in rats up to an oral dose of 10 mg/kg/day (equivalent to approximately 19-fold human exposure at 20 mg QD as measured by the $AUC_{(0-24hr)}$). There are no studies in pregnant women. However, valdecoxib crosses the placenta in rats and rabbits. BEXTRA should be used during pregnancy only if the potential benefit justifies the potential risk to the fetus.

Non-Teratogenic Effects: Valdecoxib caused increased pre- and post-implantation loss with reduced live fetuses at oral doses ≥10 mg/kg/day (equivalent to approximately 19-fold human exposure at 20 mg QD as measured by the $AUC_{(0-24hr)}$) in rats and an oral dose of 40 mg/kg/day (equivalent to approximately 72-fold human exposure at 20 mg QD as measured by the $AUC_{(0-24hr)}$) in rabbits throughout organogenesis. In addition, reduced neonatal survival and decreased neonatal body weight when rats were treated with valdecoxib at oral doses ≥6 mg/kg/day (equivalent to approximately 7-fold human exposure at 20 mg QD as measured by the $AUC_{(0-24hr)}$) throughout organogenesis and lactation period. No studies have been conducted to evaluate the effect of valdecoxib on the closure of the ductus arteriosus in humans. Therefore, as with other drugs known to inhibit prostaglandin synthesis, use of BEXTRA during the third trimester of pregnancy should be avoided.

Labor and Delivery

Valdecoxib produced no evidence of delayed labor or parturition at oral doses up to 10 mg/kg/day in rats (equivalent to approximately 19-fold human exposure at 20 mg QD as measured by the $AUC_{(0-24hr)}$). The effects of BEXTRA on labor and delivery in pregnant women are unknown.

Nursing Mothers

Valdecoxib and its active metabolite are excreted in the milk of lactating rats. It is not known whether this drug is excreted in human milk. Because many drugs are excreted in human milk, and because of the potential for adverse reactions in nursing infants from BEXTRA, a decision should be made whether to discontinue nursing or to discontinue the drug, taking into account the importance of the drug to the mother and the importance of nursing to the infant.

Pediatric Use

Safety and effectiveness of BEXTRA in pediatric patients below the age of 18 years have not been evaluated.

Geriatric Use

Of the patients who received BEXTRA in arthritis clinical trials of three months duration, or greater, approximately 2100 were 65 years of age or older, including 570 patients who were 75 years or older. No overall differences in effectiveness were observed between these patients and younger patients.

ADVERSE REACTIONS

Of the patients treated with BEXTRA Tablets in controlled arthritis trials, 2665 were patients with OA, and 2684 were patients with RA. More than 4000 patients have received a chronic total daily dose of BEXTRA 10 mg or more. More than 2800 patients have received BEXTRA 10 mg/day, or more, for at least 6 months and 988 of these have received BEXTRA for at least 1 year.

Osteoarthritis and Rheumatoid Arthritis

Table 4 lists all adverse events, regardless of causality, that occurred in ≥2.0% of patients receiving BEXTRA 10 and 20 mg/day in studies of three months or longer from 7 controlled studies conducted in patients with OA or RA that included a placebo and/or a positive control group.

[See table 4 above]

In these placebo- and active-controlled clinical trials, the discontinuation rate due to adverse events was 7.5% for arthritis patients receiving valdecoxib 10 mg daily, 7.9% for arthritis patients receiving valdecoxib 20 mg daily and 6.0% for patients receiving placebo.

In the seven controlled OA and RA studies, the following adverse events occurred in 0.1 - 1.9% of patients treated with BEXTRA 10 - 20 mg daily, regardless of causality.

Application site disorders: Cellulitis, dermatitis contact

Cardiovascular: Aggravated hypertension, aneurysm, angina pectoris, arrhythmia, cardiomyopathy, congestive heart failure, coronary artery disorder, heart murmur, hypotension

Central, peripheral nervous system: Cerebrovascular disorder, hypertonia, hypoesthesia, migraine, neuralgia, neuropathy, paresthesia, tremor, twitching, vertigo

Endocrine: Goiter

Female reproductive: Amenorrhea, dysmenorrhea, leukorrhea, mastitis, menstrual disorder, menorrhagia, menstrual bloating, vaginal hemorrhage

Gastrointestinal: Abnormal stools, constipation, diverticulosis, dry mouth, duodenal ulcer, duodenitis, eructation, esophagitis, fecal incontinence, gastric ulcer, gastritis, gastroenteritis, gastroesophageal reflux, hematemesis, hematochezia, hemorrhoids, hemorrhoids bleeding, hiatal hernia, melena, stomatitis, stool frequency increased, tenesmus, tooth disorder, vomiting

General: Allergy aggravated, allergic reaction, asthenia, chest pain, chills, cyst NOS, edema generalized, face edema, fatigue, fever, hot flushes, halitosis, malaise, pain, periorbital swelling, peripheral pain

Hearing and vestibular: Ear abnormality, earache, tinnitus

Heart rate and rhythm: Bradycardia, palpitation, tachycardia

Hemic: Anemia

Liver and biliary system: Hepatic function abnormal, hepatitis, ALT increased, AST increased

Male reproductive: Impotence, prostatic disorder

Metabolic and nutritional: Alkaline phosphatase increased, BUN increased, CPK increased, creatinine increased, diabetes mellitus, glycosuria, gout, hypercholesterolemia, hyperglycemia, hyperkalemia, hyperlipemia, hyperuricemia, hypocalcemia, hypokalemia, LDH increased, thirst increased, weight decrease, weight increase, xerophthalmia

Musculoskeletal: Arthralgia, fracture accidental, neck stiffness, osteoporosis, synovitis, tendonitis

Neoplasm: Breast neoplasm, lipoma, malignant ovarian cyst

Platelets (bleeding or clotting): Ecchymosis, epistaxis, hematoma NOS, thrombocytopenia

Psychiatric: Anorexia, anxiety, appetite increased, confusion, depression, depression aggravated, insomnia, nervousness, morbid dreaming, somnolence
Resistance mechanism disorders: Herpes simplex, herpes zoster, infection fungal, infection soft tissue, infection viral, moniliasis, moniliasis genital, otitis media
Respiratory: Abnormal breath sounds, bronchitis, bronchospasm, coughing, dyspnea, emphysema, laryngitis, pneumonia, pharyngitis, pleurisy, rhinitis
Skin and appendages: Acne, alopecia, dermatitis, dermatitis fungal, eczema, photosensitivity allergic reaction, pruritus, rash erythematous, rash maculopapular, rash psoriaform, skin dry, skin hypertrophy, skin ulceration, sweating increased, urticaria
Special senses: Taste perversion
Urinary system: Albuminuria, cystitis, dysuria, hematuria, micturition frequency increased, pyuria, urinary incontinence, urinary tract infection
Vascular: Claudication intermittent, hemangioma acquired, varicose vein
Vision: Blurred vision, cataract, conjunctival hemorrhage, conjunctivitis, eye pain, keratitis, vision abnormal
White cell and RES disorders: Eosinophilia, leukopenia, leukocytosis, lymphadenopathy, lymphangitis, lymphopenia
Other serious adverse events that were reported rarely (estimated <0.1%) in clinical trials, regardless of causality, in patients taking BEXTRA:
Autonomic nervous system disorders: Hypertensive encephalopathy, vasospasm
Cardiovascular: Abnormal ECG, aortic stenosis, atrial fibrillation, carotid stenosis, coronary thrombosis, heart block, heart valve disorders, mitral insufficiency, myocardial infarction, myocardial ischemia, pericarditis, syncope, thrombophlebitis, unstable angina, ventricular fibrillation
Central, peripheral nervous system: Convulsions
Endocrine: Hyperparathyroidism
Female reproductive: Cervical dysplasia
Gastrointestinal: Appendicitis, colitis with bleeding, dysphagia, esophageal perforation, gastrointestinal bleeding, ileus, intestinal obstruction, peritonitis
Hemic: Lymphoma-like disorder, pancytopenia
Liver and biliary system: Cholelithiasis
Metabolic: Dehydration
Musculoskeletal: Pathological fracture, osteomyelitis
Neoplasm: Benign brain neoplasm, bladder carcinoma, carcinoma, gastric carcinoma, prostate carcinoma, pulmonary carcinoma
Platelets (bleeding or clotting): Embolism, pulmonary embolism, thrombosis
Psychiatric: Manic reaction, psychosis
Renal: Acute renal failure
Resistance mechanism disorders: Sepsis
Respiratory: Apnea, pleural effusion, pulmonary edema, pulmonary fibrosis, pulmonary infarction, pulmonary hemorrhage, respiratory insufficiency
Skin: Basal cell carcinoma, malignant melanoma
Urinary system: Pyelonephritis, renal calculus
Vision: Retinal detachment

Postmarketing Experience

The following reactions have been identified during postmarketing use of BEXTRA. These reactions have been chosen for inclusion either due to their seriousness, reporting frequency, possible causal relationship to BEXTRA, or a combination of these factors. Because these reactions were reported voluntarily from a population of uncertain size, it is not possible to reliably estimate their frequency or establish a causal relationship to drug exposure.
General: Hypersensitivity reactions (including anaphylactic reactions and angioedema)
Skin and appendages: Erythema multiforme, exfoliative dermatitis, Stevens-Johnson syndrome, toxic epidermal necrolysis

OVERDOSAGE

Symptoms following acute NSAID overdoses are usually limited to lethargy, drowsiness, nausea, vomiting, and epigastric pain, which are generally reversible with supportive care. Gastrointestinal bleeding can occur. Hypertension, acute renal failure, respiratory depression and coma may occur, but are rare.
Anaphylactoid reactions have been reported with therapeutic ingestion of NSAIDs, and may occur following an overdose.
Patients should be managed by symptomatic and supportive care following an NSAID overdose. There are no specific antidotes. Hemodialysis removed only about 2% of administered valdecoxib from the systemic circulation of 8 patients with end-stage renal disease and, based on its degree of plasma protein binding (>98%), dialysis is unlikely to be useful in overdose. Forced diuresis, alkalinization of urine, or hemoperfusion also may not be useful due to high protein binding.

DOSAGE AND ADMINISTRATION

Osteoarthritis and Adult Rheumatoid Arthritis

The recommended dose of BEXTRA Tablets for the relief of the signs and symptoms of arthritis is 10 mg once daily.

Primary Dysmenorrhea

The recommended dose of BEXTRA Tablets for treatment of primary dysmenorrhea is 20 mg twice daily, as needed.

HOW SUPPLIED

BEXTRA Tablets 10 mg are white, film-coated, and capsule-shaped, debossed "10" on one side with a four pointed star shape on the other, supplied as:

NDC Number	Size
0025-1975-31	Bottle of 100
0025-1975-51	Bottle of 500
0025-1975-34	Carton of 100 unit dose

BEXTRA Tablets 20 mg are white, film-coated, and capsule-shaped, debossed "20" on one side with a four pointed star shape on the other, supplied as:

NDC Number	Size
0025-1980-31	Bottle of 100
0025-1980-51	Bottle of 500
0025-1980-34	Carton of 100 unit dose

Store at 25°C (77°F); excursions permitted to 15-30°C (59-86°F) [See USP Controlled Room Temperature]
Rx only
Revised: May 2004
Manufactured for:
G.D. Searle LLC
A subsidiary of Pharmacia Corporation
Chicago, IL 60680, USA
Pfizer Inc
New York, NY 10017, USA
by: Searle Ltd.
Caguas, PR 00725
LAB-0266-4.0

Shown in Product Identification Guide, page 330

CAMPTOSAR® ℞

irinotecan hydrochloride injection
For Intravenous Use Only

WARNINGS

CAMPTOSAR Injection should be administered only under the supervision of a physician who is experienced in the use of cancer chemotherapeutic agents. Appropriate management of complications is possible only when adequate diagnostic and treatment facilities are readily available.
CAMPTOSAR can induce both early and late forms of diarrhea that appear to be mediated by different mechanisms. Both forms of diarrhea may be severe. Early diarrhea (occurring during or shortly after infusion of CAMPTOSAR) may be accompanied by cholinergic symptoms of rhinitis, increased salivation, miosis, lacrimation, diaphoresis, flushing, and intestinal hyperperistalsis that can cause abdominal cramping. Early diarrhea and other cholinergic symptoms may be prevented or ameliorated by atropine (see PRECAUTIONS, General). Late diarrhea (generally occurring more than 24 hours after administration of CAMPTOSAR) can be life threatening since it may be prolonged and may lead to dehydration, electrolyte imbalance, or sepsis. Late diarrhea should be treated promptly with loperamide. Patients with diarrhea should be carefully monitored and given fluid and electrolyte replacement if they become dehydrated or antibiotic therapy if they develop ileus, fever, or severe neutropenia (see WARNINGS). Administration of CAMPTOSAR should be interrupted and subsequent doses reduced if severe diarrhea occurs (see DOSAGE AND ADMINISTRATION).
Severe myelosuppression may occur (see WARNINGS).

DESCRIPTION

CAMPTOSAR Injection (irinotecan hydrochloride injection) is an antineoplastic agent of the topoisomerase I inhibitor class. Irinotecan hydrochloride was clinically investigated as CPT-11.
CAMPTOSAR is supplied as a sterile, pale yellow, clear, aqueous solution. It is available in two single-dose sizes: 2 mL-fill vials contain 40 mg irinotecan hydrochloride and 5 mL-fill vials contain 100 mg irinotecan hydrochloride. Each milliliter of solution contains 20 mg of irinotecan hydrochloride (on the basis of the trihydrate salt), 45 mg of sorbitol NF powder, and 0.9 mg of lactic acid, USP. The pH of the solution has been adjusted to 3.5 (range, 3.0 to 3.8) with sodium hydroxide or hydrochloric acid. CAMPTOSAR is intended for dilution with 5% Dextrose Injection, USP (D5W), or 0.9% Sodium Chloride Injection, USP, prior to intravenous infusion. The preferred diluent is 5% Dextrose Injection, USP.
Irinotecan hydrochloride is a semisynthetic derivative of camptothecin, an alkaloid extract from plants such as *Camptotheca acuminata*. The chemical name is ***(S)***-4,11-diethyl-3,4,12,14-tetrahydro-4-hydroxy-3,14-dioxo-1***H***-pyrano[3′,4′:6,7]-indolizino[1,2-b]quinolin-9-yl-[1,4′-bipiperidine]-1′-carboxylate, monohydrochloride, trihydrate. Its structural formula is as follows:

Irinotecan Hydrochloride

Irinotecan hydrochloride is a pale yellow to yellow crystalline powder, with the empirical formula $C_{33}H_{38}N_4O_6 \cdot HCl \cdot 3H_2O$ and a molecular weight of 677.19. It is slightly soluble in water and organic solvents.

CLINICAL PHARMACOLOGY

Irinotecan is a derivative of camptothecin. Camptothecins interact specifically with the enzyme topoisomerase I which relieves torsional strain in DNA by inducing reversible single-strand breaks. Irinotecan and its active metabolite SN-38 bind to the topoisomerase I-DNA complex and prevent religation of these single-strand breaks. Current research suggests that the cytotoxicity of irinotecan is due to double-strand DNA damage produced during DNA synthesis when replication enzymes interact with the ternary complex formed by topoisomerase I, DNA, and either irinotecan or SN-38. Mammalian cells cannot efficiently repair these double-strand breaks.
Irinotecan serves as a water-soluble precursor of the lipophilic metabolite SN-38. SN-38 is formed from irinotecan by carboxylesterase-mediated cleavage of the carbamate bond between the camptothecin moiety and the dipiperidino side chain. SN-38 is approximately 1000 times as potent as irinotecan as an inhibitor of topoisomerase I purified from human and rodent tumor cell lines. In vitro cytotoxicity assays show that the potency of SN-38 relative to irinotecan varies from 2- to 2000-fold. However, the plasma area under the concentration versus time curve (AUC) values for SN-38 are 2% to 8% of irinotecan and SN-38 is 95% bound to plasma proteins compared to approximately 50% bound to plasma proteins for irinotecan (see Pharmacokinetics). The precise contribution of SN-38 to the activity of CAMPTOSAR is thus unknown. Both irinotecan and SN-38 exist in an active lactone form and an inactive hydroxy acid anion form. A pH-dependent equilibrium exists between the two forms such that an acid pH promotes the formation of the lactone, while a more basic pH favors the hydroxy acid anion form.
Administration of irinotecan has resulted in antitumor activity in mice bearing cancers of rodent origin and in human carcinoma xenografts of various histological types.

Pharmacokinetics

After intravenous infusion of irinotecan in humans, irinotecan plasma concentrations decline in a multiexponential manner, with a mean terminal elimination half-life of about 6 to 12 hours. The mean terminal elimination half-life of the active metabolite SN-38 is about 10 to 20 hours. The half-lives of the lactone (active) forms of irinotecan and SN-38 are similar to those of total irinotecan and SN-38, as the lactone and hydroxy acid forms are in equilibrium.
Over the recommended dose range of 50 to 350 mg/m^2, the AUC of irinotecan increases linearly with dose; the AUC of SN-38 increases less than proportionally with dose. Maximum concentrations of the active metabolite SN-38 are generally seen within 1 hour following the end of a 90-minute infusion of irinotecan. Pharmacokinetic parameters for irinotecan and SN-38 following a 90-minute infusion of irinotecan at dose levels of 125 and 340 mg/m^2 determined in two clinical studies in patients with solid tumors are summarized in Table 1:
[See table 1 at top of next page]
Irinotecan exhibits moderate plasma protein binding (30% to 68% bound). SN-38 is highly bound to human plasma proteins (approximately 95% bound). The plasma protein to which irinotecan and SN-38 predominantly binds is albumin.
Metabolism and Excretion: The metabolic conversion of irinotecan to the active metabolite SN-38 is mediated by carboxylesterase enzymes and primarily occurs in the liver. SN-38 subsequently undergoes conjugation to form a glucuronide metabolite. SN-38 glucuronide had 1/50 to 1/100 the activity of SN-38 in cytotoxicity assays using two cell lines in vitro. The disposition of irinotecan has not been fully elucidated in humans. The urinary excretion of irinotecan is 11% to 20%; SN-38, <1%; and SN-38 glucuronide, 3%. The cumulative biliary and urinary excretion of irinotecan and its metabolites (SN-38 and SN-38 glucuronide) over a period of 48 hours following administration of irinotecan in two patients ranged from approximately 25% (100 mg/m^2) to 50% (300 mg/m^2).

Pharmacokinetics in Special Populations

Geriatric: In studies using the weekly schedule, the terminal half-life of irinotecan was 6.0 hours in patients who were 65 years or older and 5.5 hours in patients younger than 65 years. Dose-normalized $AUC_{0\text{-}24}$ for SN-38 in patients who were at least 65 years of age was 11% higher than in patients younger than 65 years. No change in the starting dose is recommended for geriatric patients receiving the weekly dosage schedule of irinotecan. The pharmacokinetics of irinotecan given once every 3 weeks has not been studied in the geriatric population; a lower starting dose is recommended in patients 70 years or older based on clinical toxicity experience with this schedule (see DOSAGE AND ADMINISTRATION).
Pediatric: Information regarding the pharmacokinetics of irinotecan is not available.
Gender: The pharmacokinetics of irinotecan do not appear to be influenced by gender.
Race: The influence of race on the pharmacokinetics of irinotecan has not been evaluated.
Hepatic Insufficiency: The influence of hepatic insufficiency on the pharmacokinetic characteristics of irinotecan and its metabolites has not been formally studied. Among patients with known hepatic tumor involvement (a majority

Continued on next page

Table 1. Summary of Mean (± Standard Deviation) Irinotecan and SN-38 Pharmacokinetic Parameters in Patients with Solid Tumors

Dose (mg/m^2)	Irinotecan					SN-38		
	C_{max} (ng/mL)	AUC_{0-24} (ng·h/mL)	$t_{1/2}$ (h)	V_z (L/m^2)	CL ($L/h/m^2$)	C_{max} (ng/mL)	AUC_{0-24} (ng·h/mL)	$t_{1/2}$ (h)
125 (N=64)	1,660 ±797	10,200 ±3,270	5.8[a] ±0.7	110 ±48.5	13.3 ±6.01	26.3 ±11.9	229 ±108	10.4[a] ±3.1
340 (N=6)	3,392 ±874	20,604 ±6,027	11.7[b] ±1.0	234 ±69.6	13.9 ±4.0	56.0 ±28.2	474 ±245	21.0[b] ±4.3

C_{max} - Maximum plasma concentration
AUC_{0-24} - Area under the plasma concentration-time curve from time 0 to 24 hours after the end of the 90-minute infusion
$t_{1/2}$ - Terminal elimination half-life
V_z - Volume of distribution of terminal elimination phase
CL - Total systemic clearance
[a] Plasma specimens collected for 24 hours following the end of the 90-minute infusion.
[b] Plasma specimens collected for 48 hours following the end of the 90-minute infusion. Because of the longer collection period, these values provide a more accurate reflection of the terminal elimination half-lives of irinotecan and SN-38.

Table 2. Combination Dosage Schedule: Study Results

	Study 1			Study 2	
	Irinotecan + Bolus 5-FU/LV weekly×4 q 6 weeks	**Bolus 5-FU/LV daily×5 q 4 weeks**	**Irinotecan weekly×4 q 6 weeks**	**Irinotecan + Infusional 5-FU/LV**	**Infusional 5-FU/LV**
Number of Patients	231	226	226	198	187
Demographics and Treatment Administration					
Female/Male (%)	34/65	45/54	35/64	33/67	47/53
Median Age in years (range)	62 (25-85)	61 (19-85)	61 (30-87)	62 (27-75)	59 (24-75)
Performance Status (%)					
0	39	41	46	51	51
1	46	45	46	42	41
2	15	13	8	7	8
Primary Tumor (%)					
Colon	81	85	84	55	65
Rectum	17	14	15	45	35
Median Time from Diagnosis to Randomization (months, range)	1.9 (0-161)	1.7 (0-203)	1.8 (0.1-185)	4.5 (0-88)	2.7 (0-104)
Prior Adjuvant 5-FU Therapy (%)					
No	89	92	90	74	76
Yes	11	8	10	26	24
Median Duration of Study Treatment[a] (months)	5.5	4.1	3.9	5.6	4.5
Median Relative Dose Intensity (%)[a]					
Irinotecan	72	—	75	87	—
5-FU	71	86	—	86	93
Efficacy Results					
Confirmed Objective Tumor Response Rate[b] (%)	39	21 (p<0.0001)[c]	18	35	22 (p<0.005)[c]
Median Time to Tumor Progression[d] (months)	7.0	4.3 (p=0.004)[d]	4.2	6.7	4.4 (p<0.001)[d]
Median Survival (months)	14.8	12.6 (p<0.05)[d]	12.0	17.4	14.1 (p<0.05)[d]

[a] Study 1: N=225 (irinotecan/5-FU/LV), N=219 (5-FU/LV), N=223 (irinotecan)
Study 2: N=199 (irinotecan/5-FU/LV), N=186 (5-FU/LV)
[b] Confirmed ≥4 to 6 weeks after first evidence of objective response
[c] Chi-square test
[d] Log-rank test

Camptosar—Cont.

of patients), irinotecan and SN-38 AUC values were somewhat higher than values for patients without liver metastases (see PRECAUTIONS).

Renal Insufficiency: The influence of renal insufficiency on the pharmacokinetics of irinotecan has not been evaluated.

Drug-Drug Interactions

In a phase 1 clinical study involving irinotecan, 5-fluorouracil (5-FU), and leucovorin (LV) in 26 patients with solid tumors, the disposition of irinotecan was not substantially altered when the drugs were co-administered. Although the C_{max} and AUC_{0-24} of SN-38, the active metabolite, were reduced (by 14% and 8%, respectively) when irinotecan was followed by 5-FU and LV administration compared with when irinotecan was given alone, this sequence of administration was used in the combination trials and is recommended (see DOSAGE AND ADMINISTRATION). Formal in vivo or in vitro drug interaction studies to evaluate the influence of irinotecan on the disposition of 5-FU and LV have not been conducted.

Possible pharmacokinetic interactions of CAMPTOSAR with other concomitantly administered medications have not been formally investigated.

CLINICAL STUDIES

Irinotecan has been studied in clinical trials in combination with 5-fluorouracil (5-FU) and leucovorin (LV) and as a single agent (see DOSAGE AND ADMINISTRATION). When given as a component of combination-agent treatment, irinotecan was either given with a weekly schedule of bolus 5-FU/LV or with an every-2-week schedule of infusional 5-FU/LV. Weekly and a once-every-3-week dosage schedules were used for the single-agent irinotecan studies. Clinical studies of combination and single-agent use are described below.

First-Line Therapy in Combination with 5-FU/LV for the Treatment of Metastatic Colorectal Cancer

Two phase 3, randomized, controlled, multinational clinical trials support the use of CAMPTOSAR Injection as first-line treatment of patients with metastatic carcinoma of the colon or rectum. In each study, combinations of irinotecan with 5-FU and LV were compared with 5-FU and LV alone. Study 1 compared combination irinotecan/bolus 5-FU/LV therapy given weekly with a standard bolus regimen of 5-FU/LV alone given daily for 5 days every 4 weeks; an irinotecan-alone treatment arm given on a weekly schedule was also included. Study 2 evaluated two different methods of administering infusional 5-FU/LV, with or without irinotecan. In both studies, concomitant medications such as antiemetics, atropine, and loperamide were given to patients for prophylaxis and/or management of symptoms from treatment. In Study 2, a 7-day course of fluoroquinolone antibiotic prophylaxis was given in patients whose diarrhea persisted for greater than 24 hours despite loperamide or if they developed a fever in addition to diarrhea. Treatment with oral fluoroquinolone was also initiated in patients who developed an absolute neutrophil count (ANC) $<500/mm^3$, even in the absence of fever or diarrhea. Patients in both studies also received treatment with intravenous antibiotics if they had persistent diarrhea or fever or if ileus developed.

In both studies, the combination of irinotecan/5-FU/LV therapy resulted in significant improvements in objective tumor response rates, time to tumor progression, and survival when compared with 5-FU/LV alone. These differences in survival were observed in spite of second-line therapy in a majority of patients on both arms, including crossover to irinotecan-containing regimens in the control arm. Patient characteristics and major efficacy results are shown in Table 2.

[See table 2 at left]

Improvement was noted with irinotecan-based combination therapy relative to 5-FU/LV when response rates and time to tumor progression were examined across the following demographic and disease-related subgroups (age, gender, ethnic origin, performance status, extent of organ involvement with cancer, time from diagnosis of cancer, prior adjuvant therapy, and baseline laboratory abnormalities). Figures 1 and 2 illustrate the Kaplan-Meier survival curves for the comparison of irinotecan/5-FU/LV versus 5-FU/LV in Studies 1 and 2, respectively.

Figure 1. Survival First-Line Irinotecan/5-FU/LV vs 5-FU/LV Study 1

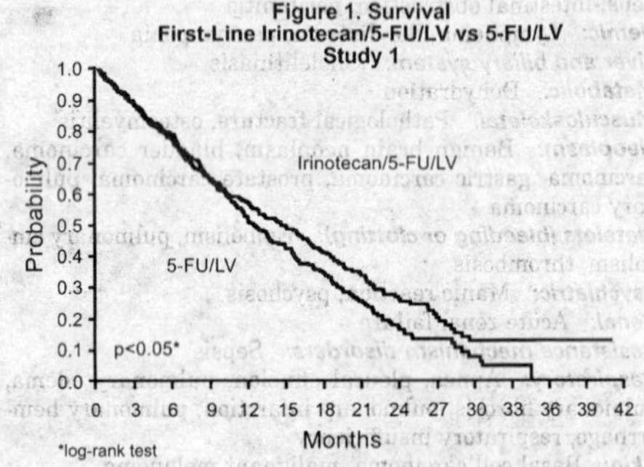

Figure 2. Survival First-Line Irinotecan/5-FU/LV vs 5-FU/LV Study 2

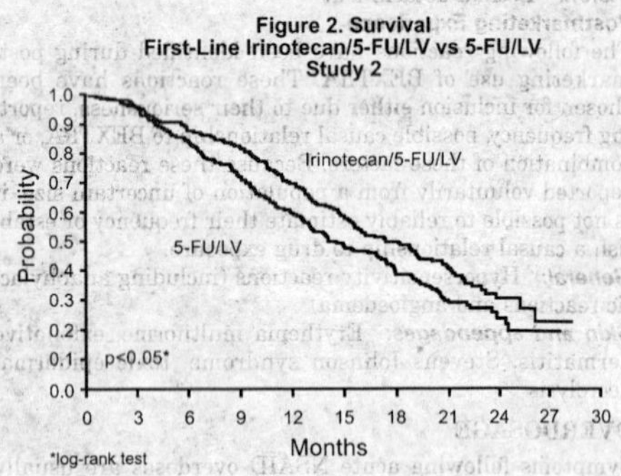

Second-Line Treatment for Recurrent or Progressive Metastatic Colorectal Cancer After 5-FU-Based Treatment

Weekly Dosage Schedule

Data from three open-label, single-agent, clinical studies, involving a total of 304 patients in 59 centers, support the use of CAMPTOSAR in the treatment of patients with metastatic cancer of the colon or rectum that has recurred or progressed following treatment with 5-FU-based therapy. These studies were designed to evaluate tumor response rate and do not provide information on actual clinical benefit, such as effects on survival and disease-related symptoms. In each study, CAMPTOSAR was administered in repeated 6-week cycles consisting of a 90-minute intravenous infusion once weekly for 4 weeks, followed by a 2-week rest period. Starting doses of CAMPTOSAR in these trials were 100, 125, or 150 mg/m^2, but the 150-mg/m^2 dose was poorly tolerated (due to unacceptably high rates of grade 4 late diarrhea and febrile neutropenia). Study 1 enrolled 48 patients and was conducted by a single investigator at several regional hospitals. Study 2 was a multicenter study conducted by the North Central Cancer Treatment Group. All 90 patients enrolled in Study 2 received a starting dose of 125 mg/m^2. Study 3 was a multicenter study that enrolled 166 patients from 30 institutions. The initial dose in Study 3 was 125 mg/m^2 but was reduced to 100 mg/m^2 because the toxicity seen at the 125-mg/m^2 dose was perceived to be greater than that seen in previous studies. All patients in these studies had metastatic colorectal cancer, and the majority had disease that recurred or progressed following a

5-FU-based regimen administered for metastatic disease. The results of the individual studies are shown in Table 3. [See table 3 at right]

In the intent-to-treat analysis of the pooled data across all three studies, 193 of the 304 patients began therapy at the recommended starting dose of 125 mg/m^2. Among these 193 patients, 2 complete and 27 partial responses were observed, for an overall response rate of 15.0% (95% Confidence Interval [CI], 10.0% to 20.1%) at this starting dose. A considerably lower response rate was seen with a starting dose of 100 mg/m^2. The majority of responses were observed within the first two cycles of therapy, but responses did occur in later cycles of treatment (one response was observed after the eighth cycle). The median response duration for patients beginning therapy at 125 mg/m^2 was 5.8 months (range, 2.6 to 15.1 months). Of the 304 patients treated in the three studies, response rates to CAMPTOSAR were similar in males and females and among patients older and younger than 65 years. Rates were also similar in patients with cancer of the colon or cancer of the rectum and in patients with single and multiple metastatic sites. The response rate was 18.5% in patients with a performance status of 0 and 8.2% in patients with a performance status of 1 or 2. Patients with a performance status of 3 or 4 have not been studied. Over half of the patients responding to CAMPTOSAR had not responded to prior 5-FU. Patients who had received previous irradiation to the pelvis responded to CAMPTOSAR at approximately the same rate as those who had not previously received irradiation.

Once-Every-3-Week Dosage Schedule

Single-Arm Studies: Data from an open-label, single-agent, single-arm, multicenter, clinical study involving a total of 132 patients support a once every-3-week dosage schedule of irinotecan in the treatment of patients with metastatic cancer of the colon or rectum that recurred or progressed following treatment with 5-FU. Patients received a starting dose of 350 mg/m^2 given by 30-minute intravenous infusion once every 3 weeks. Among the 132 previously treated patients in this trial, the intent-to-treat response rate was 12.1% (95% CI, 7.0% to 18.1%).

Randomized Trials: Two multicenter, randomized, clinical studies further support the use of irinotecan given by the once-every-3-week dosage schedule in patients with metastatic colorectal cancer whose disease has recurred or progressed following prior 5-FU therapy. In the first study, second-line irinotecan therapy plus best supportive care was compared with best supportive care alone. In the second study, second-line irinotecan therapy was compared with infusional 5-FU-based therapy. In both studies, irinotecan was administered intravenously at a starting dose of 350 mg/m^2 over 90 minutes once every 3 weeks. The starting dose was 300 mg/m^2 for patients who were 70 years and older or who had a performance status of 2. The highest total dose permitted was 700 mg. Dose reductions and/or administration delays were permitted in the event of severe hematologic and/or nonhematologic toxicities while on treatment. Best supportive care was provided to patients in both arms of Study 1 and included antibiotics, analgesics, corticosteroids, transfusions, psychotherapy, or any other symptomatic therapy as clinically indicated. In both studies, concomitant medications such as antiemetics, atropine, and loperamide were given to patients for prophylaxis and/or management of symptoms from treatment. If late diarrhea persisted for greater than 24 hours despite loperamide, a 7-day course of fluoroquinolone antibiotic prophylaxis was given. Patients in the control arm of the second study received one of the following 5-FU regimens: (1) LV, 200 mg/m^2 IV over 2 hours; followed by 5-FU, 400 mg/m^2 IV bolus; followed by 5-FU, 600 mg/m^2 continuous IV infusion over 22 hours on days 1 and 2 every 2 weeks; (2) 5-FU, 250 to 300 mg/m^2/day protracted continuous IV infusion until toxicity; (3) 5-FU, 2.6 to 3 g/m^2 IV over 24 hours every week for 6 weeks with or without LV, 20 to 500 mg/m^2/day every week IV for 6 weeks with 2-week rest between cycles. Patients were to be followed every 3 to 6 weeks for 1 year.

A total of 535 patients were randomized in the two studies at 94 centers. The primary endpoint in both studies was survival. The studies demonstrated a significant overall survival advantage for irinotecan compared with best supportive care (p=0.0001) and infusional 5-FU-based therapy (p=0.035) as shown in Figures 3 and 4. In Study 1, median survival for patients treated with irinotecan was 9.2 months compared with 6.5 months for patients receiving best supportive care. In Study 2, median survival for patients treated with irinotecan was 10.8 months compared with 8.5 months for patients receiving infusional 5-FU-based therapy. Multiple regression analyses determined that patients' baseline characteristics also had a significant effect on survival. When adjusted for performance status and other baseline prognostic factors, survival among patients treated with irinotecan remained significantly longer than in the control populations (p=0.001 for Study 1 and p=0.017 for Study 2). Measurements of pain, performance status, and weight loss were collected prospectively in the two studies; however, the plan for the analysis of these data was defined retrospectively. When comparing irinotecan with best supportive care in Study 1, this analysis showed a statistically significant advantage for irinotecan, with longer time to development of pain (6.9 months versus 2.0 months), time to performance status deterioration (5.7 months versus 3.3

Table 3. Weekly Dosage Schedule: Study Results

	Study			
	1	2	3	
Number of Patients	48	90	64	102
Starting Dose (mg/m^2/wk × 4)	125[a]	125	125	100
Demographics and Treatment Administration				
Female/Male (%)	46/54	36/64	50/50	51/49
Median Age in years (range)	63 (29–78)	63 (32–81)	61 (42–84)	64 (25–84)
Ethnic Origin (%)				
White	79	96	81	91
African American	12	4	11	5
Hispanic	8	0	8	2
Oriental/Asian	0	0	0	2
Performance Status (%)				
0	60	38	59	44
1	38	48	33	51
2	2	14	8	5
Primary Tumor (%)				
Colon	100	71	89	87
Rectum	0	29	11	8
Unknown	0	0	0	5
Prior 5-FU Therapy (%)				
For Metastatic Disease	81	66	73	68
≤ 6 months after Adjuvant	15	7	27	28
> 6 months after Adjuvant	2	16	0	2
Classification Unknown	2	12	0	3
Prior Pelvic/Abdominal Irradiation (%)				
Yes	3	29	0	0
Other	0	9	2	4
None	97	62	98	96
Duration of Treatment with CAMPTOSAR (median, months)	5	4	4	3
Relative Dose Intensity[b] (median %)	74	67	73	81
Efficacy				
Confirmed Objective Response Rate (%)[c] (95% CI)	21 (9.3–32.3)	13 (6.3–20.4)	14 (5.5–22.6)	9 (3.3–14.3)
Time to Response (median, months)	2.6	1.5	2.8	2.8
Response Duration (median, months)	6.4	5.9	5.6	6.4
Survival (median, months)	10.4	8.1	10.7	9.3
1-Year Survival (%)	46	31	45	43

[a] Nine patients received 150 mg/m^2 as a starting dose; two (22.2%) responded to CAMPTOSAR.
[b] Relative dose intensity for CAMPTOSAR based on planned dose intensity of 100, 83.3, and 66.7 mg/m^2/wk corresponding with 150, 125, and 100 mg/m^2 starting doses, respectively.
[c] Confirmed ≥ 4 to 6 weeks after first evidence of objective response.

months), and time to > 5% weight loss (6.4 months versus 4.2 months). Additionally, 33.3% (33/99) of patients with a baseline performance status of 1 or 2 showed an improvement in performance status when treated with irinotecan versus 11.3% (7/62) of patients receiving best supportive care (p=0.002). Because of the inclusion of patients with non-measurable disease, intent-to-treat response rates could not be assessed.

Figure 3. Survival
Second-Line Irinotecan vs Best Supportive Care (BSC)
Study 1

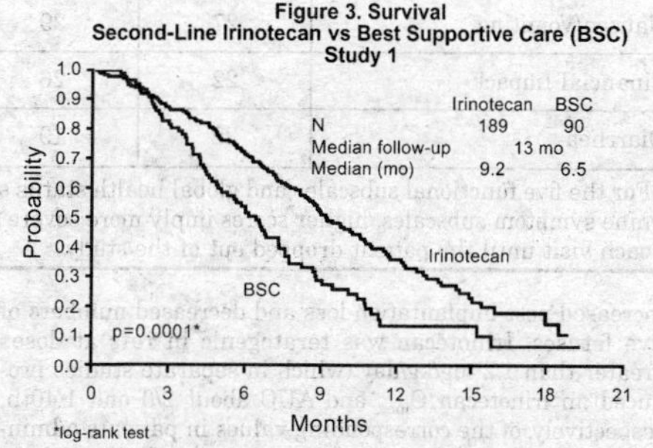

[See figure 4 at top of next column]

In the two randomized studies, the EORTC QLQ-C30 instrument was utilized. At the start of each cycle of therapy, patients completed a questionnaire consisting of 30 questions, such as "Did pain interfere with daily activities?" (1 = Not at All, to 4 = Very Much) and "Do you have any trouble taking a long walk?" (Yes or No). The answers from the 30 questions were converted into 15 subscales, that were scored from 0 to 100, and the global health status subscale that was derived from two questions about the patient's sense of general well being in the past week. In addition to

Figure 4. Survival
Second-Line Irinotecan vs Infusional 5-FU
Study 2

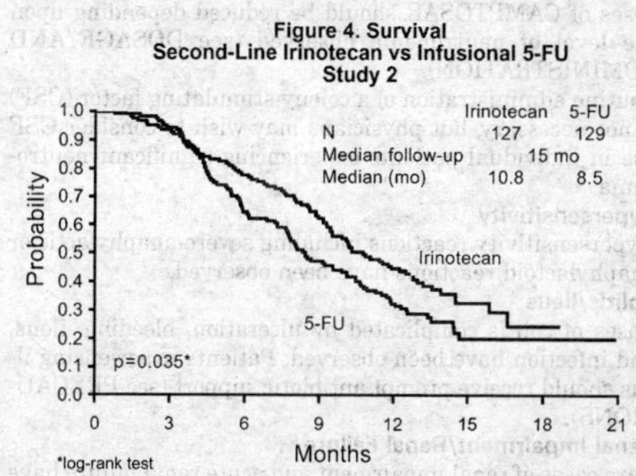

the global health status subscale, there were five functional (i.e., cognitive, emotional, social, physical, role) and nine symptom (i.e., fatigue, appetite loss, pain assessment, insomnia, constipation, dyspnea, nausea/vomiting, financial impact, diarrhea) subscales. The results as summarized in Table 5 are based on patients' worst post-baseline scores. In Study 1, a multivariate analysis and univariate analyses of the individual subscales were performed and corrected for multivariate testing. Patients receiving irinotecan reported significantly better results for the global health status, on two of five functional subscales, and on four of nine symptom subscales. As expected, patients receiving irinotecan noted significantly more diarrhea than those receiving best supportive care. In Study 2, the multivariate analysis on all 15 subscales did not indicate a statistically significant difference between irinotecan and infusional 5-FU.

[See table 4 at top of next page]
[See table 5 on next page]

Continued on next page

Camptosar—Cont.

INDICATIONS AND USAGE

CAMPTOSAR Injection is indicated as a component of first-line therapy in combination with 5-fluorouracil and leucovorin for patients with metastatic carcinoma of the colon or rectum. CAMPTOSAR is also indicated for patients with metastatic carcinoma of the colon or rectum whose disease has recurred or progressed following initial fluorouracil-based therapy.

CONTRAINDICATIONS

CAMPTOSAR Injection is contraindicated in patients with a known hypersensitivity to the drug.

WARNINGS

General

Outside of a well-designed clinical study, CAMPTOSAR Injection should not be used in combination with the "Mayo Clinic" regimen of 5-FU/LV (administration for 4–5 consecutive days every 4 weeks) because of reports of increased toxicity, including toxic deaths. CAMPTOSAR should be used as recommended (see DOSAGE AND ADMINISTRATION, Table 10).

In patients receiving either irinotecan/5-FU/LV or 5-FU/LV in the clinical trials, higher rates of hospitalization, neutropenic fever, thromboembolism, first-cycle treatment discontinuation, and early deaths were observed in patients with a baseline performance status of 2 than in patients with a baseline performance status of 0 or 1.

Diarrhea

CAMPTOSAR can induce both early and late forms of diarrhea that appear to be mediated by different mechanisms. Early diarrhea (occurring during or shortly after infusion of CAMPTOSAR) is cholinergic in nature. It is usually transient and only infrequently is severe. It may be accompanied by symptoms of rhinitis, increased salivation, miosis, lacrimation, diaphoresis, flushing, and intestinal hyperperistalsis that can cause abdominal cramping. Early diarrhea and other cholinergic symptoms may be prevented or ameliorated by administration of atropine (see PRECAUTIONS, General, for dosing recommendations for atropine). Late diarrhea (generally occurring more than 24 hours after administration of CAMPTOSAR) can be life threatening since it may be prolonged and may lead to dehydration, electrolyte imbalance, or sepsis. Late diarrhea should be treated promptly with loperamide (see PRECAUTIONS, Information for Patients, for dosing recommendations for loperamide). Patients with diarrhea should be carefully monitored, should be given fluid and electrolyte replacement if they become dehydrated, and should be given antibiotic support if they develop ileus, fever, or severe neutropenia. After the first treatment, subsequent weekly chemotherapy treatments should be delayed in patients until return of pretreatment bowel function for at least 24 hours without need for antidiarrhea medication. If grade 2, 3, or 4 late diarrhea occurs subsequent doses of CAMPTOSAR should be decreased within the current cycle (see DOSAGE AND ADMINISTRATION).

Neutropenia

Deaths due to sepsis following severe neutropenia have been reported in patients treated with CAMPTOSAR. Neutropenic complications should be managed promptly with antibiotic support (see PRECAUTIONS). Therapy with CAMPTOSAR should be temporarily omitted during a cycle of therapy if neutropenic fever occurs or if the absolute neutrophil count drops $<1000/mm^3$. After the patient recovers to an absolute neutrophil count $\geq 1000/mm^3$, subsequent doses of CAMPTOSAR should be reduced depending upon the level of neutropenia observed (see DOSAGE AND ADMINISTRATION).

Routine administration of a colony-stimulating factor (CSF) is not necessary, but physicians may wish to consider CSF use in individual patients experiencing significant neutropenia.

Hypersensitivity

Hypersensitivity reactions including severe anaphylactic or anaphylactoid reactions have been observed.

Colitis/Ileus

Cases of colitis complicated by ulceration, bleeding, ileus, and infection have been observed. Patients experiencing ileus should receive prompt antibiotic support (see PRECAUTIONS).

Renal Impairment/Renal Failure

Rare cases of renal impairment and acute renal failure have been identified, usually in patients who became volume depleted from severe vomiting and/or diarrhea.

Thromboembolism

Thromboembolic events have been observed in patients receiving irinotecan-containing regimens; the specific cause of these events has not been determined.

Pregnancy

CAMPTOSAR may cause fetal harm when administered to a pregnant woman. Radioactivity related to ^{14}C-irinotecan crosses the placenta of rats following intravenous administration of 10 mg/kg (which in separate studies produced an irinotecan C_{max} and AUC about 3 and 0.5 times, respectively, the corresponding values in patients administered 125 mg/m^2). Administration of 6 mg/kg/day intravenous irinotecan to rats (which in separate studies produced an irinotecan C_{max} and AUC about 2 and 0.2 times, respectively, the corresponding values in patients administered 125 mg/m^2) and rabbits (about one-half the recommended human weekly starting dose on a mg/m^2 basis) during the period of organogenesis, is embryotoxic as characterized by increased post-implantation loss and decreased numbers of live fetuses. Irinotecan was teratogenic in rats at doses greater than 1.2 mg/kg/day (which in separate studies produced an irinotecan C_{max} and AUC about 2/3 and 1/40th, respectively, of the corresponding values in patients administered 125 mg/m^2) and in rabbits at 6.0 mg/kg/day (about one-half the recommended human weekly starting dose on a mg/m^2 basis). Teratogenic effects included a variety of external, visceral, and skeletal abnormalities. Irinotecan administered to rat dams for the period following organogenesis through weaning at doses of 6 mg/kg/day caused decreased learning ability and decreased female body weights in the offspring. There are no adequate and well-controlled studies of irinotecan in pregnant women. If the drug is used during pregnancy, or if the patient becomes pregnant while receiving this drug, the patient should be apprised of the potential hazard to the fetus. Women of childbearing potential should be advised to avoid becoming pregnant while receiving treatment with CAMPTOSAR.

Table 4. Once-Every-3-Week Dosage Schedule: Study Results

	Study 1		Study 2	
	Irinotecan	BSC[a]	Irinotecan	5-FU
Number of Patients	189	90	127	129
Demographics and Treatment Administration				
Female/Male (%)	32/68	42/58	43/57	35/65
Median Age in years (range)	59 (22–75)	62 (34–75)	58 (30–75)	58 (25–75)
Performance Status (%)				
0	47	31	58	54
1	39	46	35	43
2	14	23	8	3
Primary Tumor (%)				
Colon	55	52	57	62
Rectum	45	48	43	38
Prior 5-FU Therapy (%)				
For Metastatic Disease	70	63	58	68
As Adjuvant Treatment	30	37	42	32
Prior Irradiation (%)	26	27	18	20
Duration of Study Treatment (median, months) (Log-rank test)	4.1	—	4.2 (p=0.02)	2.8
Relative Dose Intensity (median %)[b]	94	—	95	81–99
Survival				
Survival (median, months) (Log-rank test)	9.2 (p=0.0001)	6.5	10.8 (p=0.035)	8.5

[a] BSC = best supportive care

[b] Relative dose intensity for irinotecan based on planned dose intensity of 116.7 and 100 mg/m^2/wk corresponding with 350 and 300 mg/m^2 starting doses, respectively.

Table 5. EORTC QLQ-C30: Mean Worst Post-Baseline Score[a]

QLQ-C30 Subscale	Study 1			Study 2		
	Irinotecan	BSC	p-value	Irinotecan	5-FU	p-value
Global Health Status	47	37	0.03	53	52	0.9
Functional Scales						
Cognitive	77	68	0.07	79	83	0.9
Emotional	68	64	0.4	64	68	0.9
Social	58	47	0.06	65	67	0.9
Physical	60	40	0.0003	66	66	0.9
Role	53	35	0.02	54	57	0.9
Symptom Scales						
Fatigue	51	63	0.03	47	46	0.9
Appetite Loss	37	57	0.0007	35	38	0.9
Pain Assessment	41	56	0.009	38	34	0.9
Insomnia	39	47	0.3	39	33	0.9
Constipation	28	41	0.03	25	19	0.9
Dyspnea	31	40	0.2	25	24	0.9
Nausea/Vomiting	27	29	0.5	25	16	0.09
Financial Impact	22	26	0.5	24	15	0.3
Diarrhea	32	19	0.01	32	22	0.2

[a] For the five functional subscales and global health status subscale, higher scores imply better functioning, whereas, on the nine symptom subscales, higher scores imply more severe symptoms. The subscale scores of each patient were collected at each visit until the patient dropped out of the study.

PRECAUTIONS

General

Care of Intravenous Site: CAMPTOSAR Injection is administered by intravenous infusion. Care should be taken to avoid extravasation, and the infusion site should be monitored for signs of inflammation. Should extravasation occur, flushing the site with sterile water and applications of ice are recommended.

Premedication with Antiemetics: Irinotecan is emetigenic. It is recommended that patients receive premedication with antiemetic agents. In clinical studies of the weekly dosage schedule, the majority of patients received 10 mg of dexamethasone given in conjunction with another type of antiemetic agent, such as a 5-HT^3 blocker (e.g., ondansetron or granisetron). Antiemetic agents should be given on the day of treatment, starting at least 30 minutes before administration of CAMPTOSAR. Physicians should also consider providing patients with an antiemetic regimen (e.g., prochlorperazine) for subsequent use as needed.

Treatment of Cholinergic Symptoms: Prophylactic or therapeutic administration of 0.25 to 1 mg of intravenous or subcutaneous atropine should be considered (unless clinically contraindicated) in patients experiencing rhinitis, increased salivation, miosis, lacrimation, diaphoresis, flushing, abdominal cramping, or diarrhea (occurring during or shortly after infusion of CAMPTOSAR). These symptoms are expected to occur more frequently with higher irinotecan doses.

Patients at Particular Risk: In patients receiving either irinotecan/5-FU/LV or 5-FU/LV in the clinical trials, higher rates of hospitalization, neutropenic fever, thromboembolism, first-cycle treatment discontinuation, and early deaths were observed in patients with a baseline performance status of 2 than in patients with a baseline performance status of 0 or 1. Patients who had previously received pelvic/abdominal radiation and elderly patients with comorbid conditions should be closely monitored.

The use of CAMPTOSAR in patients with significant hepatic dysfunction has not been established. In clinical trials of either dosing schedule, irinotecan was not administered to patients with serum bilirubin >2.0 mg/dL, or transaminase >3 times the upper limit of normal if no liver metastasis, or transaminase >5 times the upper limit of normal with liver metastasis. However in clinical trials of the weekly dosage schedule, it has been noted that patients with modestly elevated baseline serum total bilirubin levels (1.0 to 2.0 mg/dL) have had a significantly greater likelihood of experiencing first-cycle grade 3 or 4 neutropenia than those with bilirubin levels that were less than 1.0 mg/dL (50.0% [19/38] versus 17.7% [47/226]; $p<0.001$). Patients with abnormal glucuronidation of bilirubin, such as those with Gilbert's syndrome, may also be at greater risk of myelosuppression when receiving therapy with CAMPTOSAR. An association between baseline bilirubin elevations and an increased risk of late diarrhea has not been observed in studies of the weekly dosage schedule.

Table 6. Study 1: Percent (%) of Patients Experiencing Clinically Relevant Adverse Events in Combination Therapies[a]

Adverse Event	Study 1 Irinotecan + Bolus 5-FU/LV weekly × 4 q 6 weeks N=225		Bolus 5-FU/LV daily × 5 q 4 weeks N=219		Irinotecan weekly × 4 q 6 weeks N=223	
	Grade 1–4	Grade 3&4	Grade 1–4	Grade 3&4	Grade 1–4	Grade 3&4
TOTAL Adverse Events	100	53.3	100	45.7	99.6	45.7
GASTROINTESTINAL						
Diarrhea						
late	84.9	22.7	69.4	13.2	83.0	31.0
grade 3	—	15.1	—	5.9	—	18.4
grade 4	—	7.6	—	7.3	—	12.6
early	45.8	4.9	31.5	1.4	43.0	6.7
Nausea	79.1	15.6	67.6	8.2	81.6	16.1
Abdominal pain	63.1	14.6	50.2	11.5	67.7	13.0
Vomiting	60.4	9.7	46.1	4.1	62.8	12.1
Anorexia	34.2	5.8	42.0	3.7	43.9	7.2
Constipation	41.3	3.1	31.5	1.8	32.3	0.4
Mucositis	32.4	2.2	76.3	16.9	29.6	2.2
HEMATOLOGIC						
Neutropenia	96.9	53.8	98.6	66.7	96.4	31.4
grade 3	—	29.8	—	23.7	—	19.3
grade 4	—	24.0	—	42.5	—	12.1
Leukopenia	96.9	37.8	98.6	23.3	96.4	21.5
Anemia	96.9	8.4	98.6	5.5	96.9	4.5
Neutropenic fever	—	7.1	—	14.6	—	5.8
Thrombocytopenia	96.0	2.6	98.6	2.7	96.0	1.7
Neutropenic infection	—	1.8	—	0	—	2.2
BODY AS A WHOLE						
Asthenia	70.2	19.5	64.4	11.9	69.1	13.9
Pain	30.7	3.1	26.9	3.6	22.9	2.2
Fever	42.2	1.7	32.4	3.6	43.5	0.4
Infection	22.2	0	16.0	1.4	13.9	0.4
METABOLIC & NUTRITIONAL						
↑ Bilirubin	87.6	7.1	92.2	8.2	83.9	7.2
DERMATOLOGIC						
Exfoliative dermatitis	0.9	0	3.2	0.5	0	0
Rash	19.1	0	26.5	0.9	14.3	0.4
Alopecia[b]	43.1	—	26.5	—	46.1	—
RESPIRATORY						
Dyspnea	27.6	6.3	16.0	0.5	22.0	2.2
Cough	26.7	1.3	18.3	0	20.2	0.4
Pneumonia	6.2	2.7	1.4	1.0	3.6	1.3
NEUROLOGIC						
Dizziness	23.1	1.3	16.4	0	21.1	1.8
Somnolence	12.4	1.8	4.6	1.8	9.4	1.3
Confusion	7.1	1.8	4.1	0	2.7	0
CARDIOVASCULAR						
Vasodilation	9.3	0.9	5.0	0	9.0	0
Hypotension	5.8	1.3	2.3	0.5	5.8	1.7
Thromboembolic events[c]	9.3	—	11.4	—	5.4	—

[a] Severity of adverse events based on NCI CTC (version 1.0)
[b] Complete hair loss = Grade 2
[c] Includes angina pectoris, arterial thrombosis, cerebral infarct, cerebrovascular accident, deep thrombophlebitis, embolus lower extremity, heart arrest, myocardial infarct, myocardial ischemia, peripheral vascular disorder, pulmonary embolus, sudden death, thrombophlebitis, thrombosis, vascular disorder.

Information for Patients

Patients and patients' caregivers should be informed of the expected toxic effects of CAMPTOSAR, particularly of its gastrointestinal complications, such as nausea, vomiting, abdominal cramping, diarrhea, and infection. Each patient should be instructed to have loperamide readily available and to begin treatment for late diarrhea (generally occurring more than 24 hours after administration of CAMPTOSAR) at the first episode of poorly formed or loose stools or the earliest onset of bowel movements more frequent than normally expected for the patient. One dosage regimen for loperamide used in clinical trials consisted of the following (Note: This dosage regimen exceeds the usual dosage recommendations for loperamide.): 4 mg at the first onset of late diarrhea and then 2 mg every 2 hours until the patient is diarrhea-free for at least 12 hours. During the night, the patient may take 4 mg of loperamide every 4 hours. Premedication with loperamide is not recommended. The use of drugs with laxative properties should be avoided because of the potential for exacerbation of diarrhea. Patients should be advised to contact their physician to discuss any laxative use.

Patients should be instructed to contact their physician or nurse if any of the following occur: diarrhea for the first time during treatment; black or bloody stools; symptoms of dehydration such as lightheadedness, dizziness, or faintness; inability to take fluids by mouth due to nausea or vomiting; inability to get diarrhea under control within 24 hours; or fever or evidence of infection.

Patients should be alerted to the possibility of alopecia.

Laboratory Tests

Careful monitoring of the white blood cell count with differential, hemoglobin, and platelet count is recommended before each dose of CAMPTOSAR.

Drug Interactions

The adverse effects of CAMPTOSAR, such as myelosuppression and diarrhea, would be expected to be exacerbated by other antineoplastic agents having similar adverse effects.

Patients who have previously received pelvic/abdominal irradiation are at increased risk of severe myelosuppression following the administration of CAMPTOSAR. The concurrent administration of CAMPTOSAR with irradiation has not been adequately studied and is not recommended.

Lymphocytopenia has been reported in patients receiving CAMPTOSAR, and it is possible that the administration of dexamethasone as antiemetic prophylaxis may have enhanced the likelihood of this effect. However, serious opportunistic infections have not been observed, and no complications have specifically been attributed to lymphocytopenia.

Hyperglycemia has also been reported in patients receiving CAMPTOSAR. Usually, this has been observed in patients with a history of diabetes mellitus or evidence of glucose intolerance prior to administration of CAMPTOSAR. It is probable that dexamethasone, given as antiemetic prophylaxis, contributed to hyperglycemia in some patients.

The incidence of akathisia in clinical trials of the weekly dosage schedule was greater (8.5%, 4/47 patients) when prochlorperazine was administered on the same day as CAMPTOSAR than when these drugs were given on separate days (1.3%, 1/80 patients). The 8.5% incidence of akathisia, however, is within the range reported for use of prochlorperazine when given as a premedication for other chemotherapies.

It would be expected that laxative use during therapy with CAMPTOSAR would worsen the incidence or severity of diarrhea, but this has not been studied.

In view of the potential risk of dehydration secondary to vomiting and/or diarrhea induced by CAMPTOSAR, the physician may wish to withhold diuretics during dosing with CAMPTOSAR and, certainly, during periods of active vomiting or diarrhea.

Drug-Laboratory Test Interactions

There are no known interactions between CAMPTOSAR and laboratory tests.

Carcinogenesis, Mutagenesis & Impairment of Fertility

Long-term carcinogenicity studies with irinotecan were not conducted. Rats were, however, administered intravenous doses of 2 mg/kg or 25 mg/kg irinotecan once per week for 13 weeks (in separate studies, the 25 mg/kg dose produced an irinotecan C_{max} and AUC that were about 7.0 times and 1.3 times the respective values in patients administered 125 mg/m^2 weekly) and were then allowed to recover for 91 weeks. Under these conditions, there was a significant linear trend with dose for the incidence of combined uterine horn endometrial stromal polyps and endometrial stromal sarcomas. Neither irinotecan nor SN-38 was mutagenic in the in vitro Ames assay. Irinotecan was clastogenic both in vitro (chromosome aberrations in Chinese hamster ovary cells) and in vivo (micronucleus test in mice). No significant adverse effects on fertility and general reproductive performance were observed after intravenous administration of irinotecan in doses of up to 6 mg/kg/day to rats and rabbits. However, atrophy of male reproductive organs was observed after multiple daily irinotecan doses both in rodents at 20 mg/kg (which in separate studies produced an irinotecan C_{max} and AUC about 5 and 1 times, respectively, the corresponding values in patients administered 125 mg/m^2 weekly) and dogs at 0.4 mg/kg (which in separate studies produced an irinotecan C_{max} and AUC about one-half and 1/15th, respectively, the corresponding values in patients administered 125 mg/m^2 weekly).

Pregnancy

Pregnancy Category D—see WARNINGS.

Nursing Mothers

Radioactivity appeared in rat milk within 5 minutes of intravenous administration of radiolabeled irinotecan and was concentrated up to 65-fold at 4 hours after administration relative to plasma concentrations. Because many drugs are excreted in human milk and because of the potential for serious adverse reactions in nursing infants, it is recommended that nursing be discontinued when receiving therapy with CAMPTOSAR.

Pediatric Use

The safety and effectiveness of CAMPTOSAR in pediatric patients have not been established.

Geriatric Use

Patients greater than 65 years of age should be closely monitored because of a greater risk of late diarrhea in this population (see CLINICAL PHARMACOLOGY, Pharmacokinetics in Special Populations and ADVERSE REACTIONS, Overview of Adverse Events). The starting dose of CAMPTOSAR in patients 70 years and older for the once-every-3-week-dosage schedule should be 300 mg/m^2 (see DOSAGE AND ADMINISTRATION).

Continued on next page

Camptosar—Cont.

ADVERSE REACTIONS

First-Line Combination Therapy

A total of 955 patients with metastatic colorectal cancer received the recommended regimens of irinotecan in combination with 5-FU/LV, 5-FU/LV alone, or irinotecan alone. In the two phase 3 studies, 370 patients received irinotecan in combination with 5-FU/LV, 362 patients received 5-FU/LV alone, and 223 patients received irinotecan alone. (See Table 10 in DOSAGE AND ADMINISTRATION for recommended combination-agent regimens.)

In Study 1, 49 (7.3%) patients died within 30 days of last study treatment: 21 (9.3%) received irinotecan in combination with 5-FU/LV, 15 (6.8%) received 5-FU/LV alone, and 13 (5.8%) received irinotecan alone. Deaths potentially related to treatment occurred in 2 (0.9%) patients who received irinotecan in combination with 5-FU/LV (2 neutropenic fever/sepsis), 3 (1.4%) patients who received 5-FU/LV alone (1 neutropenic fever/sepsis, 1 CNS bleeding during thrombocytopenia, 1 unknown) and 2 (0.9%) patients who received irinotecan alone (2 neutropenic fever). Deaths from any cause within 60 days of first study treatment were reported for 15 (6.7%) patients who received irinotecan in combination with 5-FU/LV, 16 (7.3%) patients who received 5-FU/LV alone, and 15 (6.7%) patients who received irinotecan alone. Discontinuations due to adverse events were reported for 17 (7.6%) patients who received irinotecan in combination with 5-FU/LV, 14 (6.4%) patients who received 5-FU/LV alone, and 26 (11.7%) patients who received irinotecan alone.

In Study 2, 10 (3.5%) patients died within 30 days of last study treatment: 6 (4.1%) received irinotecan in combination with 5-FU/LV and 4 (2.8%) received 5-FU/LV alone. There was one potentially treatment-related death, which occurred in a patient who received irinotecan in combination with 5-FU/LV (0.7%, neutropenic sepsis). Deaths from any cause within 60 days of first study treatment were reported for 3 (2.1%) patients who received irinotecan in combination with 5-FU/LV and 2 (1.4%) patients who received 5-FU/LV alone. Discontinuations due to adverse events were reported for 9 (6.2%) patients who received irinotecan in combination with 5-FU/LV and 1 (0.7%) patient who received 5-FU/LV alone.

The most clinically significant adverse events for patients receiving irinotecan-based therapy were diarrhea, nausea, vomiting, neutropenia, and alopecia. The most clinically significant adverse events for patients receiving 5-FU/LV therapy were diarrhea, neutropenia, neutropenic fever, and mucositis. In Study 1, grade 4 neutropenia, neutropenic fever (defined as grade 2 fever and grade 4 neutropenia), and mucositis were observed less often with weekly irinotecan/5-FU/LV than with monthly administration of 5-FU/LV.

Tables 6 and 7 list the clinically relevant adverse events reported in Studies 1 and 2, respectively.

[See table 6 at top of previous page]

[See table 7 below]

Second-Line Single-Agent Therapy

Weekly Dosage Schedule

In three clinical studies evaluating the weekly dosage schedule, 304 patients with metastatic carcinoma of the colon or rectum that had recurred or progressed following 5-FU-based therapy were treated with CAMPTOSAR. Seventeen of the patients died within 30 days of the administration of CAMPTOSAR; in five cases (1.6%, 5/304), the deaths were potentially drug-related. These five patients experienced a constellation of medical events that included known effects of CAMPTOSAR. One of these patients died of neutropenic sepsis without fever. Neutropenic fever occurred in nine (3.0%) other patients; these patients recovered with supportive care.

One hundred nineteen (39.1%) of the 304 patients were hospitalized a total of 156 times because of adverse events; 81 (26.6%) patients were hospitalized for events judged to be related to administration of CAMPTOSAR. The primary reasons for drug-related hospitalization were diarrhea, with or without nausea and/or vomiting (18.4%); neutropenia/leukopenia, with or without diarrhea and/or fever (8.2%); and nausea and/or vomiting (4.9%).

Table 8. Adverse Events Occurring in >10% of 304 Previously Treated Patients with Metastatic Carcinoma of the Colon or Rectum[a]

Body System & Event	% of Patients Reporting: NCI Grades 1–4	% of Patients Reporting: NCI Grades 3 & 4
GASTROINTESTINAL		
Diarrhea (late)[b]	88	31
7–9 stools/day (grade 3)	—	(16)
≥10 stools/day (grade 4)	—	(14)
Nausea	86	17
Vomiting	67	12
Anorexia	55	6
Diarrhea (early)[c]	51	8
Constipation	30	2
Flatulence	12	0
Stomatitis	12	1
Dyspepsia	10	0
HEMATOLOGIC		
Leukopenia	63	28
Anemia	60	7
Neutropenia	54	26
500 to <1000/mm^3 (grade 3)	—	(15)
<500/mm^3 (grade 4)	—	(12)
BODY AS A WHOLE		
Asthenia	76	12
Abdominal cramping/pain	57	16
Fever	45	1
Pain	24	2
Headache	17	1
Back pain	14	2
Chills	14	0
Minor infection[d]	14	0
Edema	10	1
Abdominal Enlargement	10	0
METABOLIC & NUTRITIONAL		
↓ Body weight	30	1
Dehydration	15	4
↑ Alkaline phosphatase	13	4
↑ SGOT	10	1
DERMATOLOGIC		
Alopecia	60	NA[e]
Sweating	16	0
Rash	13	1
RESPIRATORY		
Dyspnea	22	4
↑ Coughing	17	0
Rhinitis	16	0
NEUROLOGIC		
Insomnia	19	0
Dizziness	15	0
CARDIOVASCULAR		
Vasodilation (flushing)	11	0

[a] Severity of adverse events based on NCI CTC (version 1.0)

[b] Occurring >24 hours after administration of CAMPTOSAR

[c] Occurring ≤24 hours after administration of CAMPTOSAR

[d] Primarily upper respiratory infections

[e] Not applicable; complete hair loss = NCI grade 2

Table 7. Study 2: Percent (%) of Patients Experiencing Clinically Relevant Adverse Events in Combination Therapies[a]

Adverse Event	Study 2: Irinotecan + 5-FU/LV Infusional d 1&2 q 2 weeks N=145		5-FU/LV Infusional d 1&2 q 2 weeks N=143	
	Grade 1–4	Grade 3&4	Grade 1–4	Grade 3&4
TOTAL Adverse Events	100	72.4	100	39.2
GASTROINTESTINAL				
Diarrhea				
late	72.4	14.4	44.8	6.3
grade 3	—	10.3	—	4.2
grade 4	—	4.1	—	2.1
Cholinergic syndrome[b]	28.3	1.4	0.7	0
Nausea	66.9	2.1	55.2	3.5
Abdominal pain	17.2	2.1	16.8	0.7
Vomiting	44.8	3.5	32.2	2.8
Anorexia	35.2	2.1	18.9	0.7
Constipation	30.3	0.7	25.2	1.4
Mucositis	40.0	4.1	28.7	2.8
HEMATOLOGIC				
Neutropenia	82.5	46.2	47.9	13.4
grade 3	—	36.4	—	12.7
grade 4	—	9.8	—	0.7
Leukopenia	81.3	17.4	42.0	3.5
Anemia	97.2	2.1	90.9	2.1
Neutropenic fever	—	3.4	—	0.7
Thrombocytopenia	32.6	0	32.2	0
Neutropenic infection	—	2.1	—	0
BODY AS A WHOLE				
Asthenia	57.9	9.0	48.3	4.2
Pain	64.1	9.7	61.5	8.4
Fever	22.1	0.7	25.9	0.7
Infection	35.9	7.6	33.6	3.5
METABOLIC & NUTRITIONAL				
↑ Bilirubin	19.1	3.5	35.9	10.6
DERMATOLOGIC				
Hand & foot syndrome	10.3	0.7	12.6	0.7
Cutaneous signs	17.2	0.7	20.3	0
Alopecia[c]	56.6	—	16.8	—
RESPIRATORY				
Dyspnea	9.7	1.4	4.9	0
CARDIOVASCULAR				
Hypotension	3.4	1.4	0.7	0
Thromboembolic events[d]	11.7	—	5.6	—

[a] Severity of adverse events based on NCI CTC (version 1.0)

[b] Includes rhinitis, increased salivation, miosis, lacrimation, diaphoresis, flushing, abdominal cramping or diarrhea (occurring during or shortly after infusion of irinotecan).

[c] Complete hair loss = Grade 2

[d] Includes angina pectoris, arterial thrombosis, cerebral infarct, cerebrovascular accident, deep thrombophlebitis, embolus lower extremity, heart arrest, myocardial infarct, myocardial ischemia, peripheral vascular disorder, pulmonary embolus, sudden death, thrombophlebitis, thrombosis, vascular disorder.

Table 9. Percent of Patients Experiencing Grade 3 & 4 Adverse Events in Comparative Studies of Once-Every-3-Week Irinotecan Therapy[a]

Adverse Event	Study 1: Irinotecan N=189	Study 1: BSC[b] N=90	Study 2: Irinotecan N=127	Study 2: 5-FU N=129
TOTAL Grade 3/4 Adverse Events	79	67	69	54
GASTROINTESTINAL				
Diarrhea	22	6	22	11
Vomiting	14	8	14	5
Nausea	14	3	11	4
Abdominal pain	14	16	9	8
Constipation	10	8	8	6
Anorexia	5	7	6	4
Mucositis	2	1	2	5
HEMATOLOGIC				
Leukopenia/ Neutropenia	22	0	14	2
Anemia	7	6	6	3

Hemorrhage	5	3	1	3
Thrombocytopenia	1	0	4	2
Infection				
without grade 3/4 neutropenia	8	3	1	4
with grade 3/4 neutropenia	1	0	2	0
Fever				
without grade 3/4 neutropenia	2	1	2	0
with grade 3/4 neutropenia	2	0	4	2
BODY AS A WHOLE				
Pain	19	22	17	13
Asthenia	15	19	13	12
METABOLIC & NUTRITIONAL				
Hepatic[c]	9	7	9	6
DERMATOLOGIC				
Hand & foot syndrome	0	0	0	5
Cutaneous signs[d]	2	0	1	3
RESPIRATORY[e]	10	8	5	7
NEUROLOGIC[f]	12	13	9	4
CARDIOVASCULAR[g]	9	3	4	2
OTHER[h]	32	28	12	14

[a] Severity of adverse events based on NCI CTC (version 1.0)
[b] BSC = best supportive care
[c] Hepatic includes events such as ascites and jaundice
[d] Cutaneous signs include events such as rash
[e] Respiratory includes events such as dyspnea and cough
[f] Neurologic includes events such as somnolence
[g] Cardiovascular includes events such as dysrhythmias, ischemia, and mechanical cardiac dysfunction
[h] Other includes events such as accidental injury, hepatomegaly, syncope, vertigo, and weight loss

Adjustments in the dose of CAMPTOSAR were made during the cycle of treatment and for subsequent cycles based on individual patient tolerance. The first dose of at least one cycle of CAMPTOSAR was reduced for 67% of patients who began the studies at the 125-mg/m^2 starting dose. Within-cycle dose reductions were required for 32% of the cycles initiated at the 125-mg/m^2 dose level. The most common reasons for dose reduction were late diarrhea, neutropenia, and leukopenia. Thirteen (4.3%) patients discontinued treatment with CAMPTOSAR because of adverse events. The adverse events in Table 8 are based on the experience of the 304 patients enrolled in the three studies described in the CLINICAL STUDIES, Studies Evaluating the Weekly Dosage Schedule, section.

Once-Every-3-Week Dosage Schedule

A total of 535 patients with metastatic colorectal cancer whose disease had recurred or progressed following prior 5-FU therapy participated in the two phase 3 studies: 316 received irinotecan, 129 received 5-FU, and 90 received best supportive care. Eleven (3.5%) patients treated with irinotecan died within 30 days of treatment. In three cases (1%, 3/316), the deaths were potentially related to irinotecan treatment and were attributed to neutropenic infection, grade 4 diarrhea, and asthenia, respectively. One (0.8%, 1/129) patient treated with 5-FU died within 30 days of treatment; this death was attributed to grade 4 diarrhea. Hospitalizations due to serious adverse events (whether or not related to study treatment) occurred at least once in 60% (188/316) of patients who received irinotecan, 63% (57/90) who received best supportive care, and 39% (50/129) who received 5-FU-based therapy. Eight percent of patients treated with irinotecan and 7% treated with 5-FU-based therapy discontinued treatment due to adverse events.

Of the 316 patients treated with irinotecan, the most clinically significant adverse events (all grades, 1–4) were diarrhea (84%), alopecia (72%), nausea (70%), vomiting (62%), cholinergic symptoms (47%), and neutropenia (30%). Table 9 lists the grade 3 and 4 adverse events reported in the patients enrolled to all treatment arms of the two studies described in the CLINICAL STUDIES, Studies Evaluating the Once-Every-3-Week Dosage Schedule, section.

Overview of Adverse Events

Gastrointestinal: Nausea, vomiting, and diarrhea are common adverse events following treatment with CAMPTOSAR and can be severe. When observed, nausea and vomiting usually occur during or shortly after infusion of CAMPTOSAR. In the clinical studies testing the every 3-week-dosage schedule, the median time to the onset of late diarrhea was 5 days after irinotecan infusion. In the clinical studies evaluating the weekly dosage schedule, the median time to onset of late diarrhea was 11 days following administration of CAMPTOSAR. For patients starting treatment at the 125-mg/m^2 weekly dose, the median duration of any grade of late diarrhea was 3 days. Among those patients treated at the 125-mg/m^2 weekly dose who experienced grade 3 or 4 late diarrhea, the median duration of the entire episode of diarrhea was 7 days. The frequency of grade 3 or 4 late diarrhea was somewhat greater in patients starting treatment at 125 mg/m^2 than in patients given a 100-mg/m^2 weekly starting dose (34% [65/193] versus 23% [24/102]; p=0.08). The frequency of grade 3 and 4 late diarrhea by age was significantly greater in patients ≥65 years than in patients <65 years (40% [53/133] versus 23% [40/171]; p=0.002). In one study of the weekly dosage treatment, the frequency of grade 3 and 4 late diarrhea was significantly greater in male than in female patients (43% [25/58] versus 16% [5/32]; p=0.01), but there were no gender differences in the frequency of grade 3 and 4 late diarrhea in the other two studies of the weekly dosage treatment schedule. Colonic ulceration, sometimes with gastrointestinal bleeding, has been observed in association with administration of CAMPTOSAR.

Hematology: CAMPTOSAR commonly causes neutropenia, leukopenia (including lymphocytopenia), and anemia. Serious thrombocytopenia is uncommon. When evaluated in the trials of weekly administration, the frequency of grade 3 and 4 neutropenia was significantly higher in patients who received previous pelvic/abdominal irradiation than in those who had not received such irradiation (48% [13/27] versus 24% [67/277]; p=0.04). In these same studies, patients with baseline serum total bilirubin levels of 1.0 mg/dL or more also had a significantly greater likelihood of experiencing first-cycle grade 3 or 4 neutropenia than those with bilirubin levels that were less than 1.0 mg/dL (50% [19/38] versus 18% [47/266]; p<0.001). There were no significant differences in the frequency of grade 3 and 4 neutropenia by age or gender. In the clinical studies evaluating the weekly dosage schedule, neutropenic fever (concurrent NCI grade 4 neutropenia and fever of grade 2 or greater) occurred in 3% of the patients; 6% of patients received G-CSF for the treatment of neutropenia. NCI grade 3 or 4 anemia was noted in 7% of the patients receiving weekly treatment; blood transfusions were given to 10% of the patients in these trials.

Table 10. Combination-Agent Dosage Regimens & Dose Modifications[a]

Regimen 1 6-wk cycle with bolus 5-FU/LV (next cycle begins on day 43)	CAMPTOSAR LV 5-FU	125 mg/m^2 IV over 90 min, d 1,8,15,22 20 mg/m^2 IV bolus, d 1,8,15,22 500 mg/m^2 IV bolus, d 1,8,15,22		
		Starting Dose & Modified Dose Levels (mg/m^2)		
		Starting Dose	Dose Level −1	Dose Level −2
	CAMPTOSAR	125	100	75
	LV	20	20	20
	5-FU	500	400	300
Regimen 2 6-wk cycle with infusional 5-FU/LV (next cycle begins on day 43)	CAMPTOSAR LV 5-FU Bolus 5-FU Infusion[b]	180 mg/m^2 IV over 90 min, d 1,15,29 200 mg/m^2 IV over 2 h, d 1,2,15,16,29,30 400 mg/m^2 IV bolus, d 1,2,15,16,29,30 600 mg/m^{2}IV over 22 h, d 1,2,15,16,29,30		
		Starting Dose & Modified Dose Levels (mg/m^2)		
		Starting Dose	Dose Level −1	Dose Level −2
	CAMPTOSAR	180	150	120
	LV	200	200	200
	5-FU Bolus	400	320	240
	5-FU Infusion[b]	600	480	360

[a] Dose reductions beyond dose level −2 by decrements of ≈20% may be warranted for patients continuing to experience toxicity. Provided intolerable toxicity does not develop, treatment with additional cycles may be continued indefinitely as long as patients continue to experience clinical benefit.
[b] Infusion follows bolus administration.

Table 11. Recommended Dose Modifications for CAMPTOSAR/5-Fluorouracil (5-FU)/Leucovorin (LV) Combination Schedules

Patients should return to pre-treatment bowel function without requiring antidiarrhea medications for at least 24 hours before the next chemotherapy administration. A new cycle of therapy should not begin until the granulocyte count has recovered to ≥ 1500/mm^3, and the platelet count has recovered to ≥ 100,000/mm^3, and treatment-related diarrhea is fully resolved. Treatment should be delayed 1 to 2 weeks to allow for recovery from treatment-related toxicities. If the patient has not recovered after a 2-week delay, consideration should be given to discontinuing therapy.

Toxicity NCI CTC Grade[a] (Value)	During a Cycle of Therapy	At the Start of Subsequent Cycles of Therapy[b]
No toxicity	Maintain dose level	Maintain dose level
Neutropenia		
1 (1500 to 1999/mm^3)	Maintain dose level	Maintain dose level
2 (1000 to 1499/mm^3)	↓ 1 dose level	Maintain dose level
3 (500 to 999/mm^3)	Omit dose until resolved to ≤ grade 2, then ↓ 1 dose level	↓ 1 dose level
4 (<500/mm^3)	Omit dose until resolved to ≤ grade 2, then ↓ 2 dose levels	↓ 2 dose levels
Neutropenic fever	Omit dose until resolved, then ↓ 2 dose levels	
Other hematologic toxicities	Dose modifications for leukopenia or thrombocytopenia during a cycle of therapy and at the start of subsequent cycles of therapy are also based on NCI toxicity criteria and are the same as recommended for neutropenia above.	
Diarrhea		
1 (2–3 stools/day > pretx[c])	Delay dose until resolved to baseline, then give same dose	Maintain dose level
2 (4–6 stools/day > pretx)	Omit dose until resolved to baseline, then ↓ 1 dose level	Maintain dose level
3 (7–9 stools/day > pretx)	Omit dose until resolved to baseline, then ↓ 1 dose level	↓ 1 dose level
4 (≥10 stools/day > pretx)	Omit dose until resolved to baseline, then ↓ 2 dose levels	↓ 2 dose levels
Other nonhematologic toxicities[d]		
1	Maintain dose level	Maintain dose level
2	Omit dose until resolved to ≤ grade 1, then ↓ 1 dose level	Maintain dose level
3	Omit dose until resolved to ≤ grade 2, then ↓ 1 dose level	↓ 1 dose level
4	Omit dose until resolved to ≤ grade 2, then ↓ 2 dose levels *For mucositis/stomatitis decrease only 5-FU, not CAMPTOSAR*	↓ 2 dose levels *For mucositis/stomatitis decrease only 5-FU, not CAMPTOSAR*

[a] National Cancer Institute Common Toxicity Criteria (version 1.0)
[b] Relative to the starting dose used in the previous cycle
[c] Pretreatment
[d] Excludes alopecia, anorexia, asthenia

Continued on next page

Camptosar—Cont.

Body as a Whole: Asthenia, fever, and abdominal pain are generally the most common events of this type.
Cholinergic Symptoms: Patients may have cholinergic symptoms of rhinitis, increased salivation, miosis, lacrimation, diaphoresis, flushing, and intestinal hyperperistalsis that can cause abdominal cramping and early diarrhea. If these symptoms occur, they manifest during or shortly after drug infusion. They are thought to be related to the anticholinesterase activity of the irinotecan parent compound and are expected to occur more frequently with higher irinotecan doses.
Hepatic: In the clinical studies evaluating the weekly dosage schedule, NCI grade 3 or 4 liver enzyme abnormalities were observed in fewer than 10% of patients. These events typically occur in patients with known hepatic metastases.
Dermatologic: Alopecia has been reported during treatment with CAMPTOSAR. Rashes have also been reported but did not result in discontinuation of treatment.
Respiratory: Severe pulmonary events are infrequent. In the clinical studies evaluating the weekly dosage schedule, NCI grade 3 or 4 dyspnea was reported in 4% of patients. Over half the patients with dyspnea had lung metastases; the extent to which malignant pulmonary involvement or other preexisting lung disease may have contributed to dyspnea in these patients is unknown.
Neurologic: Insomnia and dizziness can occur, but are not usually considered to be directly related to the administration of CAMPTOSAR. Dizziness may sometimes represent symptomatic evidence of orthostatic hypotension in patients with dehydration.
Cardiovascular: Vasodilation (flushing) may occur during administration of CAMPTOSAR. Bradycardia may also occur, but has not required intervention. These effects have been attributed to the cholinergic syndrome sometimes observed during or shortly after infusion of CAMPTOSAR. Thromboembolic events have been observed in patients receiving CAMPTOSAR; the specific cause of these events has not been determined.

Other Non-U.S. Clinical Trials
Irinotecan has been studied in over 1100 patients in Japan. Patients in these studies had a variety of tumor types, including cancer of the colon or rectum, and were treated with several different doses and schedules. In general, the types of toxicities observed were similar to those seen in U.S. trials with CAMPTOSAR. There is some information from Japanese trials that patients with considerable ascites or pleural effusions were at increased risk for neutropenia or diarrhea. A potentially life-threatening pulmonary syndrome, consisting of dyspnea, fever, and a reticulonodular pattern on chest x-ray, was observed in a small percentage of patients in early Japanese studies. The contribution of irinotecan to these preliminary events was difficult to assess because these patients also had lung tumors and some had preexisting nonmalignant pulmonary disease. As a result of these observations, however, clinical studies in the United States have enrolled few patients with compromised pulmonary function, significant ascites, or pleural effusions.

Post-Marketing Experience
The following events have been identified during post-marketing use of CAMPTOSAR in clinical practice. Cases of colitis complicated by ulceration, bleeding, ileus, or infection have been observed. There have been rare cases of renal impairment and acute renal failure, generally in patients who became infected and/or volume depleted from severe gastrointestinal toxicities (see WARNINGS).
Hypersensitivity reactions including severe anaphylactic or anaphylactoid reactions have also been observed (see WARNINGS).

OVERDOSAGE

In U.S. phase 1 trials, single doses of up to 345 mg/m^2 of irinotecan were administered to patients with various cancers. Single doses of up to 750 mg/m^2 of irinotecan have been given in non-U.S. trials. The adverse events in these patients were similar to those reported with the recommended dosage and regimen. There is no known antidote for overdosage of CAMPTOSAR. Maximum supportive care should be instituted to prevent dehydration due to diarrhea and to treat any infectious complications.

DOSAGE AND ADMINISTRATION

Combination-Agent Dosage

Dosage Regimens

CAMPTOSAR Injection in Combination with 5-Fluorouracil (5-FU) and Leucovorin (LV)
CAMPTOSAR should be administered as an intravenous infusion over 90 minutes (see Preparation of Infusion Solution). For all regimens, the dose of LV should be administered immediately after CAMPTOSAR, with the administration of 5-FU to occur immediately after receipt of LV. CAMPTOSAR should be used as recommended; the currently recommended regimens are shown in Table 10.
Dosing for patients with bilirubin >2 mg/dL cannot be recommended since such patients were not included in clinical studies. It is recommended that patients receive premedication with antiemetic agents. Prophylactic or therapeutic administration of atropine should be considered in patients experiencing cholinergic symptoms. See PRECAUTIONS, General.

Dose Modifications
Patients should be carefully monitored for toxicity and assessed prior to each treatment. Doses of CAMPTOSAR and

Table 13. Recommended Dose Modifications for Single-Agent Schedules[a]

A new cycle of therapy should not begin until the granulocyte count has recovered to ≥1500/mm³, and the platelet count has recovered to ≥100,000/mm³, and treatment-related diarrhea is fully resolved. Treatment should be delayed 1 to 2 weeks to allow for recovery from treatment-related toxicities. If the patient has not recovered after a 2-week delay, consideration should be given to discontinuing CAMPTOSAR.

Worst Toxicity NCI Grade[b] (Value)	During a Cycle of Therapy	At the Start of the Next Cycles of Therapy (After Adequate Recovery), Compared with the Starting Dose in the Previous Cycle[a]	
	Weekly	Weekly	Once Every 3 Weeks
No toxicity	Maintain dose level	↑ 25 mg/m^2 up to a maximum dose of 150 mg/m^2	Maintain dose level
Neutropenia			
1 (1500 to 1999/mm^3)	Maintain dose level	Maintain dose level	Maintain dose level
2 (1000 to 1499/mm^3)	↓ 25 mg/m^2	Maintain dose level	Maintain dose level
3 (500 to 999/mm^3)	Omit dose until resolved to ≤ grade 2, then ↓ 25 mg/m^2	↓ 25 mg/m^2	↓ 50 mg/m^2
4 (<500/mm^3)	Omit dose until resolved to ≤ grade 2, then ↓ 50 mg/m^2	↓ 50 mg/m^2	↓ 50 mg/m^2
Neutropenic fever	Omit dose until resolved, then ↓ 50 mg/m^2 when resolved	↓ 50 mg/m^2	↓ 50 mg/m^2
Other hematologic toxicities	Dose modifications for leukopenia, thrombocytopenia, and anemia during a cycle of therapy and at the start of subsequent cycles of therapy are also based on NCI toxicity criteria and are the same as recommended for neutropenia above.		
Diarrhea			
1 (2–3 stools/day > pretx[c])	Maintain dose level	Maintain dose level	Maintain dose level
2 (4–6 stools/day > pretx)	↓ 25 mg/m^2	Maintain dose level	Maintain dose level
3 (7–9 stools/day > pretx)	Omit dose until resolved to ≤ grade 2, then ↓ 25 mg/m^2	↓ 25 mg/m^2	↓ 50 mg/m^2
4 (≥ 10 stools/day > pretx)	Omit dose until resolved to ≤ grade 2, then ↓ 50 mg/m^2	↓ 50 mg/m^2	↓ 50 mg/m^2
Other nonhematologic toxicities[d]			
1	Maintain dose level	Maintain dose level	Maintain dose level
2	↓ 25 mg/m^2	↓ 25 mg/m^2	↓ 50 mg/m^2
3	Omit dose until resolved to ≤ grade 2, then ↓ 25 mg/m^2	↓ 25 mg/m^2	↓ 50 mg/m^2
4	Omit dose until resolved to ≤ grade 2, then ↓ 50 mg/m^2	↓ 50 mg/m^2	↓ 50 mg/m^2

[a] All dose modifications should be based on the worst preceding toxicity
[b] National Cancer Institute Common Toxicity Criteria (version 1.0)
[c] Pretreatment
[d] Excludes alopecia, anorexia, asthenia

5-FU should be modified as necessary to accommodate individual patient tolerance to treatment. Based on the recommended dose-levels described in Table 10, Combination-Agent Dosage Regimens & Dose Modifications, subsequent doses should be adjusted as suggested in Table 11, Recommended Dose Modifications for Combination Schedules. All dose modifications should be based on the worst preceding toxicity. After the first treatment, patients with active diarrhea should return to pre-treatment bowel function without requiring antidiarrhea medications for at least 24 hours before the next chemotherapy administration.
A new cycle of therapy should not begin until the toxicity has recovered to NCI grade 1 or less. Treatment may be delayed 1 to 2 weeks to allow for recovery from treatment-related toxicity. If the patient has not recovered, consideration should be given to discontinuing therapy. Provided intolerable toxicity does not develop, treatment with additional cycles of CAMPTOSAR/5-FU/LV may be continued indefinitely as long as patients continue to experience clinical benefit.
[See table 10 at top of previous page]
[See table 11 on previous page]

Single-Agent Dosage Schedules

Dosage Regimens
CAMPTOSAR should be administered as an intravenous infusion over 90 minutes for both the weekly and once-every-3-week dosage schedules (see Preparation of Infusion Solution). Single-agent dosage regimens are shown in Table 12. A reduction in the starting dose by one dose level of CAMPTOSAR may be considered for patients with any of the following conditions: age ≥65 years, prior pelvic/abdominal radiotherapy, performance status of 2, or increased bilirubin levels. Dosing for patients with bilirubin >2 mg/dL cannot be recommended since such patients were not included in clinical studies.
It is recommended that patients receive premedication with antiemetic agents. Prophylactic or therapeutic administration of atropine should be considered in patients experiencing cholinergic symptoms. See PRECAUTIONS, General.

Dose Modifications
Patients should be carefully monitored for toxicity and doses of CAMPTOSAR should be modified as necessary to accommodate individual patient tolerance to treatment. Based on recommended dose-levels described in Table 12, Single-Agent Regimens of CAMPTOSAR and Dose Modifications, subsequent doses should be adjusted as suggested in Table 13, Recommended Dose Modifications for Single-Agent Schedules. All dose modifications should be based on the worst preceding toxicity.

A new cycle of therapy should not begin until the toxicity has recovered to NCI grade 1 or less. Treatment may be delayed 1 to 2 weeks to allow for recovery from treatment-related toxicity. If the patient has not recovered, consideration should be given to discontinuing this combination therapy. Provided intolerable toxicity does not develop, treatment with additional cycles of CAMPTOSAR may be continued indefinitely as long as patients continue to experience clinical benefit.

Table 12. Single-Agent Regimens of CAMPTOSAR and Dose Modifications

Weekly Regimen[a]	125 mg/m^2 IV over 90 min, d 1,8,15,22 then 2-wk rest		
	Starting Dose & Modified Dose Levels[c] (mg/m^2)		
	Starting Dose	Dose Level −1	Dose Level −2
	125	100	75
Once-Every-3-Week Regimen[b]	350 mg/m^2 IV over 90 min, once every 3 wks[c]		
	Starting Dose & Modified Dose Levels (mg/m^2)		
	Starting Dose	Dose Level −1	Dose Level −2
	350	300	250

[a] Subsequent doses may be adjusted as high as 150 mg/m^2 or to as low as 50 mg/m^2 in 25 to 50 mg/m^2 decrements depending upon individual patient tolerance.
[b] Subsequent doses may be adjusted as low as 200 mg/m^2 in 50 mg/m^2 decrements depending upon individual patient tolerance.
[c] Provided intolerable toxicity does not develop, treatment with additional cycles may be continued indefinitely as long as patients continue to experience clinical benefit.

[See table 13 above]

Preparation & Administration Precautions
As with other potentially toxic anticancer agents, care should be exercised in the handling and preparation of infusion solutions prepared from CAMPTOSAR Injection. The use of gloves is recommended. If a solution of CAMPTOSAR

contacts the skin, wash the skin immediately and thoroughly with soap and water. If CAMPTOSAR contacts the mucous membranes, flush thoroughly with water. Several published guidelines for handling and disposal of anticancer agents are available.[1–7]

Preparation of Infusion Solution

Inspect vial contents for particulate matter and repeat inspection when drug product is withdrawn from vial into syringe.

CAMPTOSAR Injection must be diluted prior to infusion. CAMPTOSAR should be diluted in 5% Dextrose Injection, USP, (preferred) or 0.9% Sodium Chloride Injection, USP, to a final concentration range of 0.12 to 2.8 mg/mL. In most clinical trials, CAMPTOSAR was administered in 250 mL to 500 mL of 5% Dextrose Injection, USP.

The solution is physically and chemically stable for up to 24 hours at room temperature (approximately 25°C) and in ambient fluorescent lighting. Solutions diluted in 5% Dextrose Injection, USP, and stored at refrigerated temperatures (approximately 2° to 8°C), and protected from light are physically and chemically stable for 48 hours. Refrigeration of admixtures using 0.9% Sodium Chloride Injection, USP, is not recommended due to a low and sporadic incidence of visible particulates. Freezing CAMPTOSAR and admixtures of CAMPTOSAR may result in precipitation of the drug and should be avoided. Because of possible microbial contamination during dilution, it is advisable to use the admixture prepared with 5% Dextrose Injection, USP, within 24 hours if refrigerated (2° to 8°C, 36° to 46°F). In the case of admixtures prepared with 5% Dextrose Injection, USP, or Sodium Chloride Injection, USP, the solutions should be used within 6 hours if kept at room temperature (15° to 30°C, 59° to 86°F).

Other drugs should not be added to the infusion solution. Parenteral drug products should be inspected visually for particulate matter and discoloration prior to administration whenever solution and container permit.

HOW SUPPLIED

Each mL of CAMPTOSAR Injection contains 20 mg irinotecan (on the basis of the trihydrate salt); 45 mg sorbitol; and 0.9 mg lactic acid. When necessary, pH has been adjusted to 3.5 (range, 3.0 to 3.8) with sodium hydroxide or hydrochloric acid.

CAMPTOSAR Injection is available in single-dose amber glass vials in the following package sizes:

2 mL	NDC 0009-7529-02
5 mL	NDC 0009-7529-01

This is packaged in a backing/plastic blister to protect against inadvertent breakage and leakage. The vial should be inspected for damage and visible signs of leaks before removing the backing/plastic blister. If damaged, incinerate the unopened package.

Store at controlled room temperature 15° to 30°C (59° to 86°F). Protect from light. It is recommended that the vial (and backing/plastic blister) should remain in the carton until the time of use.

Rx only

REFERENCES

1. Recommendations for the Safe Handling of Parenteral Antineoplastic Drugs. NIH Publication No. 83-2621. For sale by the Superintendent of Documents, U.S. Government Printing Office, Washington, DC 20402.
2. AMA Council Report. Guidelines for handling parenteral antineoplastics. JAMA 1985;253(11):1590–2.
3. National Study Commission on Cytotoxic Exposure. Recommendations for handling cytotoxic agents. Available from Louis P. Jeffrey, ScD, Chairman, National Study Commission on Cytotoxic Exposure, Massachusetts College of Pharmacy and Allied Health Sciences, 179 Longwood Avenue, Boston, MA 02115.
4. Clinical Oncological Society of Australia. Guidelines and recommendations for safe handling of antineoplastic agents. Med J Australia 1983;1:426–8.
5. Jones RB, et. al. Safe handling of chemotherapeutic agents: a report from the Mount Sinai Medical Center. CA-A Cancer J for Clinicians 1983;Sept./Oct.:258–63.
6. American Society of Hospital Pharmacists Technical Assistance Bulletin on handling cytotoxic and hazardous drugs. Am J Hosp Pharm 1990;47:1033–49.
7. Controlling Occupational Exposure to Hazardous Drugs (OSHA Work-Practice Guidelines). Am J Health-Syst Pharm 1996;53:1669–85.

Manufactured by Pharmacia & Upjohn Company
A subsidiary of Pharmacia Corporation
Kalamazoo, Michigan 49001, USA
Licensed from Yakult Honsha Co., LTD, Japan, and Daiichi Pharmaceutical Co., LTD, Japan
Revised May 2002 816 907 113
692839

CAVERJECT IMPULSE® ℞

[kă-vər-jĕkt]

Dual Chamber System
alprostadil for injection
For Intracavernosal Use

DESCRIPTION

CAVERJECT contains alprostadil as the naturally occurring form of prostaglandin E_1 (PGE_1) and is designated chemically as (11α,13E,15S)-11,15-dihydroxy-9-oxoprost-13-en-1-oic acid. The molecular weight is 354.49.

Alprostadil is a white to off-white crystalline powder with a melting point between 115° and 116°C. Its solubility at 35°C is 8000 micrograms (mcg) per 100 milliliter double distilled water.

The structural formula of alprostadil is represented below:

[Structural formula: O, C–OH, HO, OH]

CAVERJECT IMPULSE is available as a disposable, single-dose, dual chamber syringe system. The system includes a glass cartridge which contains sterile, freeze-dried alprostadil in the front chamber and sterile bacteriostatic water for injection in the rear chamber. The alprostadil is reconstituted with the sterile bacteriostatic water just before injection. CAVERJECT IMPULSE is available in two strengths for intracavernosal administration:

10 microgram—The reconstituted solution has a volume of 0.64 mL. The delivered volume, 0.5 mL, contains 10 micrograms (mcg) of alprostadil, 324.7 mcg of alpha cyclodextrin, 45.4 mg of lactose, 23.5 mcg of sodium citrate, and 4.45 mg of benzyl alcohol.

20 microgram—The reconstituted solution has a volume of 0.64 mL. The delivered volume, 0.5 mL, contains 20 micrograms (mcg) of alprostadil, 649.3 mcg of alpha cyclodextrin, 45.4 mg of lactose, 23.5 mcg of sodium citrate, and 4.45 mg of benzyl alcohol.

When necessary, the pH of the alprostadil for injection was adjusted with hydrochloric acid and/or sodium hydroxide before lyophilization.

CLINICAL PHARMACOLOGY

Alprostadil has a wide variety of pharmacological actions; vasodilation and inhibition of platelet aggregation are among the most notable of these effects. In most animal species tested, alprostadil relaxed retractor penis and corpus cavernosum urethrae *in vitro*. Alprostadil also relaxed isolated preparations of human corpus cavernosum and spongiosum, as well as cavernous arterial segments contracted by either noradrenaline or $PGF_{2\alpha}$ *in vitro*. In pigtail monkeys (*Macaca nemestrina*), alprostadil increased cavernous arterial blood flow *in vivo*. The degree and duration of cavernous smooth muscle relaxation in this animal model was dose-dependent.

Alprostadil induces erection by relaxation of trabecular smooth muscle and by dilation of cavernosal arteries. This leads to expansion of lacunar spaces and entrapment of blood by compressing the venules against the tunica albuginea, a process referred to as the corporal veno-occlusive mechanism.

Pharmacokinetics

Absorption: For the treatment of erectile dysfunction, alprostadil is administered by injection into the corpora cavernosa. The absolute bioavailability of alprostadil has not been determined.

Distribution: Following intracavernosal injection of 20 mcg alprostadil, mean peripheral plasma concentrations of alprostadil at 30 and 60 minutes after injection (89 and 102 picograms/mL, respectively) were not significantly greater than baseline levels of endogenous alprostadil (96 picograms/mL). Plasma levels of alprostadil were measured using a radioimmunoassay method. Alprostadil is bound in plasma primarily to albumin (81% bound) and to a lesser extent I-globulin IV-4 fraction (55% bound). No significant binding to erythrocytes or white blood cells was observed.

Metabolism: Alprostadil is rapidly converted to compounds, which are further metabolized prior to excretion. Following intravenous administration, approximately 80% of circulating alprostadil is metabolized in one pass through the lungs, primarily by beta- and omega-oxidation. Hence, any alprostadil entering the systemic circulation following intracavernosal injection is very rapidly metabolized. Following intracavernosal injection of 20 mcg alprostadil, peripheral levels of the major circulating metabolite, 13,14-dihydro-15-oxo-PGE_1, increased to reach a peak 30 minutes after injection and returned to pre-dose levels by 60 minutes after injection.

Excretion: The metabolites of alprostadil are excreted primarily by the kidney, with almost 90% of an administered intravenous dose excreted in urine within 24 hours post-dose. The remainder of the dose is excreted in the feces. There is no evidence of tissue retention of alprostadil or its metabolites following intravenous administration.

Pharmacokinetics in Special Populations

Geriatric: The potential effect of age on the pharmacokinetics of alprostadil has not been formally evaluated. In patients with acute respiratory distress syndrome (ARDS), the mean (± SD) pulmonary extraction of alprostadil was 72% ± 15% in 11 elderly patients aged 65 years or older (mean, 71 ± 6 years) and 65% ± 20% in 6 young patients aged 35 years or younger (mean, 28 ± 5 years).

Pediatric: Alprostadil plasma concentrations were measured in 10 neonates (gestational age of 34 weeks in 2 infants and 38 to 40 weeks in 8 infants) receiving steady-state intravenous infusions of alprostadil to treat underlying cardiac malformations. Infusion rates of alprostadil ranged from 5 to 50 (median, 45) nanograms/kilogram/minute, resulting in alprostadil plasma concentrations ranging between 22 and 530 (median, 56) picograms/mL. The wide range of alprostadil plasma concentrations in neonates reflects high variability in individual clearances of alprostadil in this patient population.

Gender: The potential influence of gender on the pharmacokinetics of alprostadil has not been formally studied in healthy subjects. Two studies determined the pulmonary extraction of alprostadil following intravascular administration in 23 patients with ARDS. The mean (± SD) pulmonary extraction was 66% ± 20% in 17 male patients and 69% ± 18% in 6 female patients, suggesting that the pharmacokinetics of alprostadil are not influenced by gender.

Race: The potential influence of race in the pharmacokinetics of alprostadil has not been formally evaluated.

Renal and Hepatic Insufficiency: The pharmacokinetics of alprostadil have not been formally studied in patients with renal or hepatic insufficiency.

Pulmonary Disease: The pulmonary extraction of alprostadil following intravascular administration was reduced by 15% (66 ± 3.2% vs. 78 ± 2.4%) in patients with ARDS compared with a control group of patients with normal respiratory function who were undergoing cardiopulmonary bypass surgery. Pulmonary clearance was found to vary as a function of cardiac output and pulmonary intrinsic clearance in a group of 14 patients with ARDS or at risk of developing ARDS following trauma or sepsis. In this study, the extraction efficiency of alprostadil ranged from subnormal (11%) to normal (90%), with an overall mean of 67%.

Drug-Drug Interactions: The potential for pharmacokinetic drug-drug interactions between alprostadil and other agents has not been formally studied.

CLINICAL STUDIES

The safety and efficacy of CAVERJECT Sterile Powder was investigated in men with a diagnosis of erectile dysfunction due to psychogenic, vasculogenic, neurogenic, and/or mixed etiology in two well-controlled studies (Study 1 and Study 2) and in one 6-month open-label study (Study 3).

Study 1: One hundred fifty-three men with a mean age of 53 years (range 23-69 years) were enrolled. The study had three phases: a 2.5 week double-blind, in-office randomized crossover phase in which each man received placebo or 2.5 mcg, 5 mcg, 7.5 mcg, or 10 mcg of CAVERJECT Sterile Powder; a 2 week open-label, in-office dose-titration phase to identify the optimum home-use dose (the latter dose was defined as a dose inducing an erection sufficient for penetration and lasting ≤ 60 minutes); and a 4-week open-label, self-injection phase. In the double-blind phase, each dose of CAVERJECT was significantly more effective than placebo by clinical evaluation ("full penile rigidity") and by RigiScan criteria (≥ 70% rigidity for at least 10 minutes); there was no response to placebo. The percentage of responders increased with increasing doses of CAVERJECT. The overall response in the dose-ranging phases was 76% (117/153) by clinical evaluation and 51% (78/152) by RigiScan criteria. The optimum dose for self-injection ranged from 1.25 to 65 mcg (median 20 mcg). Seventy-three percent of the injections in 102 men who self-injected CAVERJECT resulted in satisfactory intercourse. Seventy-five percent of the patients remained on the dose identified during the dose-ranging phase; 17% and 8% of the patients slightly decreased or increased the dose, respectively. The mean duration of erection per injection was 70.8 minutes.

Study 2: Two hundred ninety-six men with a mean age of 53.8 years (range 21-74 years) were enrolled in this parallel-design, double-blind study. The men were randomly assigned to one of five groups and received either a single dose of placebo, 2.5 mcg, 5 mcg, 10 mcg, or 20 mcg of CAVERJECT Sterile Powder. No patient responded to placebo. The differences in the response rates in both the clinical and the RigiScan evaluations between each of the doses of CAVERJECT and placebo were statistically significant. There was also a statistically significant dose-response relationship with higher clinical response rates and higher RigiScan response rates with increasing doses of CAVERJECT (with exception of the 10-mcg dose). The mean duration of erection after injection ranged from 12 minutes after the 2.5-mcg dose to 44 minutes after the 20-mcg dose and the relationship was linear ($p = .025$, linear regression analysis).

Study 3: The safety and efficacy of CAVERJECT Sterile Powder was evaluated in a 6-month, open-label study in 683 men with a mean age of 58 years (range 20-79 years). The optimum dose of CAVERJECT was established by titration in 89% of men (606/683). Four hundred seventy-one men (69%) completed the 6-month study. At the start of the study, the mean dose was 17.7 mcg of CAVERJECT and at the end of the study it was 20.7 mcg. Eighty-seven percent of the 13,762 injections of CAVERJECT, administered by self-injection by the men in the study, resulted in satisfactory sexual activity. The mean duration of erection was 67.5 minutes.

The formulation of alprostadil contained in CAVERJECT IMPULSE includes the inactive excipient alpha cyclodextrin. This formulation was compared with CAVERJECT Sterile Powder in 87 men in a single-blind, crossover study designed to evaluate efficacy and safety. The doses used by the patients in the study ranged from 2.5 mcg to 20 mcg and were the same for both formulations. The efficacy of the two formulations was shown to be comparable, as assessed by the 30-point erectile function (EF) domain score from the International Index of Erectile Function (IIEF) and by a physician-assessment score for erectile response. The mean EF domain scores for CAVERJECT Sterile Powder and the

Continued on next page

Caverject Impulse—Cont.

formulation contained in CAVERJECT IMPULSE were 26.6 (SD=5.3) and 27.6 (SD=3.8), respectively. The mean physician's assessment scores for CAVERJECT Sterile Powder and the formulation contained in CAVERJECT IMPULSE were 2.6 (SD=0.6) and 2.7 (SD=0.5), respectively, based on a scale of 0 (no tumescence) to 3 (full rigidity).

INDICATION AND USAGE

CAVERJECT (CAVERJECT IMPULSE, CAVERJECT Sterile Powder, and CAVERJECT Injection) is indicated for the treatment of erectile dysfunction due to neurogenic, vasculogenic, psychogenic, or mixed etiology.

Intracavernosal CAVERJECT is also indicated as an adjunct to other diagnostic tests in the diagnosis of erectile dysfunction.

CONTRAINDICATIONS

CAVERJECT should not be used in patients who have a known hypersensitivity to the drug, in patients who have conditions that might predispose them to priapism, such as sickle cell anemia or trait, multiple myeloma, or leukemia, or in patients with anatomical deformation of the penis, such as angulation, cavernosal fibrosis, or Peyronie's disease. Patients with penile implants should not be treated with CAVERJECT.

CAVERJECT is intended for use in adult men only.

CAVERJECT is not indicated for use in children or newborns.

CAVERJECT should not be used in men for whom sexual activity is inadvisable or contraindicated.

WARNINGS

Prolonged erection defined as erection lasting > 4 to ≤ 6 hours in duration occurred in 4% of 1,861 patients treated up to 18 months in studies of CAVERJECT Sterile Powder. The incidence of priapism (erections lasting > 6 hours in duration) was 0.4% with the same length of use. Pharmacologic intervention and/or aspiration of blood from the corpora cavernosum was performed in 2 of the 7 patients with priapism. To minimize the chances of prolonged erection or priapism, CAVERJECT should be titrated slowly to the lowest effective dose (see DOSAGE AND ADMINISTRATION). The patient must be instructed to immediately report to his prescribing physician, or, if unavailable, to seek immediate medical assistance for any erection that persists longer than 4 hours. If priapism is not treated immediately, penile tissue damage and permanent loss of potency may result.

PRECAUTIONS

General Precautions

1. CAVERJECT IMPULSE is designed for one use only. Following a single use, the injection device and any remaining solution should be properly discarded.
2. The overall incidence of penile fibrosis, including Peyronie's disease, reported in clinical studies with CAVERJECT Sterile Powder was 3%. In one self-injection clinical study where duration of use was up to 18 months, the incidence of fibrosis was 7.8%.
   Regular follow-up of patients, with careful examination of the penis, is strongly recommended to detect signs of penile fibrosis. Treatment with CAVERJECT should be discontinued in patients who develop penile angulation, cavernosal fibrosis, or Peyronie's disease.
3. Intracavernous injections of CAVERJECT can lead to increased peripheral blood levels of PGE_1 and its metabolites, especially in those patients with significant corpora cavernosa venous leakage. Increased peripheral blood levels of PGE_1 and its metabolites may lead to hypotension and/or dizziness.
4. Patients on anticoagulants, such as warfarin or heparin, may have increased propensity for bleeding after intracavernosal injection.
5. Underlying treatable medical causes of erectile dysfunction should be diagnosed and treated prior to initiation of therapy with CAVERJECT.
6. The safety and efficacy of combinations of CAVERJECT and other vasoactive agents have not been systematically studied. Therefore, the use of such combinations is not recommended.
7. CAVERJECT IMPULSE uses a superfine (29 gauge) needle. As with all superfine needles, the possibility of needle breakage exists. Careful instruction in proper patient handling and injection techniques may minimize the potential for needle breakage.
8. The patient should be instructed not to re-use or to share needles or syringes. As with all prescription medicines, the patient should not allow anyone else to use his medicine.

Information for the Patient:

To ensure safe and effective use of CAVERJECT, the patient should be thoroughly instructed and trained in the self-injection technique before he begins intracavernosal treatment with CAVERJECT at home. The desirable dose should be established in the physician's office.

Any reconstituted solution with precipitates or discoloration should be discarded. The CAVERJECT IMPULSE syringe system is designed for one use only and should be discarded after use. The device and the needle must be properly discarded after use. Needles must not be re-used or shared with other persons. Patient instructions for administration are included in each package of CAVERJECT IMPULSE.

The dose of CAVERJECT that is established in the physician's office should not be changed by the patient without consulting the physician. The patient may expect an erection to occur within 5 to 20 minutes. A standard treatment goal is to produce an erection lasting no longer than 1 hour. Generally, CAVERJECT should be used no more than 3 times per week, with at least 24 hours between each use.

Patients should be aware of possible side effects of therapy with CAVERJECT; the most frequently occurring is penile pain after injection, usually mild to moderate in severity. A potentially serious adverse reaction with intracavernosal therapy is priapism. Accordingly, the patient should be instructed to contact the physician's office immediately or, if unavailable, to seek immediate medical assistance if an erection persists for longer than 4 hours.

The patient should report any penile pain that was not present before or that increased in intensity, as well as the occurrence of nodules or hard tissue in the penis to his physician as soon as possible. As with any injection, an infection is a possibility. Patients should be instructed to report to the physician any penile redness, swelling, tenderness or curvature of the erect penis. The patient must visit the physician's office for regular checkups for assessment of the therapeutic benefit and safety of treatment with CAVERJECT.

Note: Use of intracavernosal CAVERJECT offers no protection from the transmission of sexually transmitted diseases. Individuals who use CAVERJECT should be counseled about the protective measures that are necessary to guard against the spread of sexually transmitted diseases, including the human immunodeficiency virus (HIV).

The injection of CAVERJECT can induce a small amount of bleeding at the site of injection (see ADVERSE REACTIONS section hematoma, ecchymosis, hemorrhage at the site of injection). In patients infected with blood-borne diseases, this could increase the risk of transmission of blood-borne diseases between partners.

In clinical trials, concomitant use of agents such as antihypertensive drugs, diuretics, antidiabetic agents (including insulin), or non-steroidal anti-inflammatory drugs had no effect on the efficacy or safety of CAVERJECT.

Carcinogenesis, Mutagenesis, and Impairment of Fertility:

Long-term carcinogenicity studies have not been conducted. Rat reproductive studies indicate that alprostadil at doses of up to 0.2 mg/kg/day does not adversely affect or alter rat spermatogenesis, providing a 200-fold margin of safety compared with the usual human doses. The following battery of mutagenicity assays revealed no potential for mutagenesis: bacterial mutation (Ames), alkaline elution, rat micronucleus, sister chromatid exchange, CHO/HGPRT mammalian cell forward gene mutation, and unscheduled DNA synthesis (UDS).

A 1-year irritancy study was conducted in three groups of 5 male Cynomolgus monkeys injected intracavernosally twice weekly with either vehicle or 3 or 8.25 mcg of alprostadil/injection. An additional two groups of 6 monkeys each were injected with vehicle or with 8.25 mcg/injection twice weekly as described previously plus they received multiple doses during weeks 44, 48, and 52. Three monkeys from each group were retained for a 4-week recovery period. There was no evidence of drug-related penile irritancy or nonpenile tissue lesions, which could be directly related to alprostadil. The irritancy, which was noted for control and treated monkeys, was considered to be a result of the injection procedure itself, and any lesions noted were shown to be reversible. At the end of the 4-week recovery period, the histological changes in the penis had regressed.

Pregnancy, Nursing Mothers, and Pediatric Use:

CAVERJECT is not indicated for use in pediatric patients or women.

Geriatric Use:

A total of 341 subjects included in clinical studies were 65 and older. No overall differences in safety and effectiveness were observed between these subjects and younger subjects, and the other reported clinical experience has not identified differences in responses between elderly and younger patients, but decreased sensitivity of some older individuals cannot be ruled out.

ADVERSE REACTIONS

Local Adverse Reactions: The following local adverse reaction information was derived from controlled and uncontrolled studies of CAVERJECT Sterile Powder, including an uncontrolled 18-month safety study.

Local Adverse Reactions Reported by ≥ 1% of Patients Treated with CAVERJECT Sterile Powder for up to 18 Months*

Event	CAVERJECT N = 1861
Penile pain	37%
Prolonged erection	4%
Penile fibrosis**	3%
Injection site hematoma	3%
Penis disorder***	3%
Injection site ecchymosis	2%
Penile rash	1%
Penile edema	1%

* Except for penile pain (2%), no significant local adverse reactions were reported by 294 patients who received 1 to 3 injections of placebo.

** See General Precautions.

*** Includes numbness, yeast infection, irritation, sensitivity, phimosis, pruritus, erythema, venous leak, penile skin tear, strange feeling of penis, discoloration of penile head, itch at tip of penis.

Penile Pain: Penile pain after intracavernosal administration of CAVERJECT was reported at least once by 37% of patients in clinical studies of up to 18 months in duration. In the majority of the cases, penile pain was rated mild or moderate in intensity. Three percent of patients discontinued treatment because of penile pain. The frequency of penile pain was 2% in 294 patients who received 1 to 3 injections of placebo.

Prolonged Erection/Priapism: In clinical trials, prolonged erection was defined as an erection that lasted for 4 to 6 hours; priapism was defined as erection that lasted 6 hours or longer. The frequency of prolonged erection after intracavernosal administration of CAVERJECT was 4%, while the frequency of priapism was 0.4% (see WARNINGS).

Hematoma/Ecchymosis: The frequency of hematoma and ecchymosis was 3% and 2%, respectively. In most cases, hematoma/ecchymosis was judged to be a complication of a faulty injection technique. Accordingly, proper instruction of the patient in self-injection is of importance to minimize the potential of hematoma/ecchymosis (see DOSAGE AND ADMINISTRATION).

The following local adverse reactions were reported by fewer than 1% of patients after injection of CAVERJECT: balanitis, injection site hemorrhage, injection site inflammation, injection site itching, injection site swelling, injection site edema, urethral bleeding, penile warmth, numbness, yeast infection, irritation, sensitivity, phimosis, pruritus, erythema, venous leak, painful erection, and abnormal ejaculation.

Systemic Adverse Events: The following systemic adverse event information was derived from controlled and uncontrolled studies of CAVERJECT Sterile Powder, including an uncontrolled 18-month safety study.

Systemic Adverse Events Reported by ≥ 1% of Patients Treated with CAVERJECT Sterile Powder for up to 18 Months*

Body System/Reaction	CAVERJECT N = 1861
Cardiovascular System	
Hypertension	2%
Central Nervous System	
Headache	2%
Dizziness	1%
Musculoskeletal System	
Back pain	1%
Respiratory System	
Upper respiratory infection	4%
Flu syndrome	2%
Sinusitis	2%
Nasal congestion	1%
Cough	1%
Urogenital System	
Prostatic Disorder**	2%
Miscellaneous	
Localized pain***	2%
Trauma****	2%

* No significant adverse events were reported by 294 patients who received 1 to 3 injections of placebo.

** Prostatitis, pain, hypertrophy, enlargement

*** Pain in various anatomical structures other than injection site

**** Injuries, fractures, abrasions, lacerations, dislocations

The following systemic events, which were reported for < 1% of patients in clinical studies, were judged by investigators to be possibly related to use of CAVERJECT: testicular pain, scrotal disorder, scrotal edema, hematuria, testicular disorder, impaired urination, urinary frequency, urinary urgency, pelvic pain, hypotension, vasodilation, peripheral vascular disorder, supraventricular extrasystoles, vasovagal reactions, hypesthesia, non-generalized weakness, diaphoresis, rash, non-application site pruritus, skin neoplasm, nausea, dry mouth, increased serum creatinine, leg cramps, and mydriasis.

Hemodynamic changes, manifested as decreases in blood pressure and increases in pulse rate, were observed during clinical studies, principally at doses above 20 mcg and above 30 mcg of alprostadil, respectively, and appeared to be dose-dependent. However, these changes were usually clinically unimportant; only three patients discontinued the treatment because of symptomatic hypotension.

CAVERJECT had no clinically important effect on serum or urine laboratory tests.

The safety of CAVERJECT IMPULSE was evaluated in a study that compared the formulation of alprostadil for injection contained in CAVERJECT IMPULSE with the formulation contained in CAVERJECT Sterile Powder. The doses used by the 87 patients in this crossover study were the same for both formulations. The number and type of events reported for CAVERJECT IMPULSE were consistent between formulations in this study and in other controlled and uncontrolled studies with CAVERJECT Sterile Powder.

OVERDOSAGE

Overdosage was not observed in clinical trials with CAVERJECT. If intracavernous overdose of CAVERJECT occurs, the patient should be under medical supervision until any systemic effects have resolved and/or until penile detumescence has occurred. Symptomatic treatment of any systemic symptoms would be appropriate.

DOSAGE AND ADMINISTRATION

The dose of CAVERJECT should be individualized for each patient by careful titration under supervision by the physician. In clinical studies, patients were treated with CAVERJECT Sterile Powder in doses ranging from 0.2 to 140 mcg; however, since 99% of patients received doses of 60 mcg or less, doses of greater than 60 mcg are not recommended. In general, the lowest possible effective dose should always be employed. In clinical studies, over 80% of patients experienced an erection sufficient for sexual intercourse after intracavernosal injection of CAVERJECT.

Initial Titration in Physician's Office:

Erectile Dysfunction of Vasculogenic, Psychogenic, or Mixed Etiology. Dosage titration should be initiated at 2.5 mcg of alprostadil. The 10 mcg strength of CAVERJECT IMPULSE is designed to allow delivery of a 2.5 mcg dose of alprostadil (see General Procedure for Solution Preparation). If there is a partial response at 2.5 mcg, the dose may be increased by 2.5 mcg to a dose of 5 mcg within 1 hour. No more than 2 doses during initial titration should be given within a 24-hour period. If additional titration is required, doses in increments of 5 to 10 mcg may be given at least 24 hours apart until the dose that produces an erection suitable for intercourse and not exceeding a duration of 1 hour is reached. If there is no response to the initial 2.5-mcg dose, the second dose may be increased to 7.5 mcg within 1 hour. No more than 2 doses during initial titration should be given within a 24-hour period. If additional titration is required, doses in increments of 5 to 10 mcg may be given at least 24 hours apart. The patient must stay in the physician's office until complete detumescence occurs.

Erectile Dysfunction of Pure Neurogenic Etiology (Spinal Cord Injury). Dosage titration should be initiated at 1.25 mcg of alprostadil. Because CAVERJECT IMPULSE is designed to deliver doses of 2.5 mcg or greater (see General Procedure for Solution Preparation), CAVERJECT Sterile Powder or CAVERJECT Injection may be used for an initial dose of 1.25 mcg. The initial dose may be increased by 1.25 mcg to a dose of 2.5 mcg within 1 hour. No more than 2 doses during initial titration should be given within a 24-hour period. If additional titration is required, a dose of 5 mcg may be given during the next 24 hours. Thereafter, doses in increments of 5 mcg may be given at least 24 hours apart until the dose that produces an erection suitable for intercourse and not exceeding a duration of 1 hour is reached. The patient must stay in the physician's office until complete detumescence occurs.

The majority of patients (56%) in one clinical study involving 579 patients with erectile dysfunction of various etiologies were titrated to doses of greater than 5 mcg but less than or equal to 20 mcg. The mean dose at the end of the titration phase was 17.8 mcg of alprostadil.

Maintenance Therapy:

The first injections of CAVERJECT must be done at the physician's office by medically trained personnel. Self-injection therapy by the patient should be started only after the patient is properly instructed and well trained in the self-injection technique. The physician should make a careful assessment of the patient's skills and competence with this procedure. The intracavernosal injection must be done under sterile conditions. The site of injection is usually along the dorso-lateral aspect of the proximal third of the penis. Visible veins should be avoided. The side of the penis that is injected and the site of injection must be alternated; the injection site must be cleansed with an alcohol swab.

The dose of CAVERJECT that is selected for self-injection treatment should provide the patient with an erection that is satisfactory for sexual intercourse and that is maintained for no longer than 1 hour. If the duration of erection is longer than 1 hour, the dose of CAVERJECT should be reduced. Self-injection therapy for use at home should be initiated at the dose that was determined in the physician's office; however, dose adjustment, if required (up to 57% of patients in one clinical study), should be made only after consultation with the physician. The dose should be adjusted in accordance with the titration guidelines described above. The effectiveness of CAVERJECT for long-term use of up to 6 months has been documented in an uncontrolled, self-injection study. The mean dose of CAVERJECT Sterile Powder at the end of 6 months was 20.7 mcg in this study. CAVERJECT IMPULSE in the 10 mcg strength is designed to deliver a minimum dose of 2.5 mcg and a maximum dose of 10 mcg. CAVERJECT IMPULSE in the 20 mcg strength is designed to deliver a minimum dose of 5 mcg and a maximum dose of 20 mcg. The physician should determine the most suitable formulation of CAVERJECT for the individual patient (CAVERJECT IMPULSE, CAVERJECT Sterile Powder, or CAVERJECT Injection).

Careful and continuous follow-up of the patient while in the self-injection program must be exercised. This is especially true for the initial self-injections, since adjustments in the dose of CAVERJECT may be needed. The recommended frequency of injection is no more than 3 times weekly, with at least 24 hours between each dose. All formulations of CAVERJECT are intended for single use only and should be discarded after use. The user should be instructed in the proper disposal of the injection materials (e.g., device, needles).

While on self-injection treatment, it is recommended that the patient visit the prescribing physician's office every 3 months. At that time, the efficacy and safety of the therapy should be assessed, and the dose of CAVERJECT should be adjusted, if needed.

CAVERJECT as an Adjunct to the Diagnosis of Erectile Dysfunction:

In the simplest diagnostic test for erectile dysfunction (pharmacologic testing), patients are monitored for the occurrence of an erection after an intracavernosal injection of CAVERJECT. Extensions of this testing are the use of CAVERJECT as an adjunct to laboratory investigations, such as duplex or Doppler imaging, ^{133}Xenon washout tests, radioisotope penogram, and penile arteriography, to allow visualization and assessment of penile vasculature. For any of these tests, a single dose of CAVERJECT that induces an erection with firm rigidity should be used.

General Procedure for Solution Preparation:

CAVERJECT IMPULSE consists of a disposable, single-dose, dual-chamber syringe system. The system includes a glass cartridge, which contains sterile, freeze-dried alprostadil in the front chamber and sterile bacteriostatic water for injection in the rear chamber. Following proper reconstitution instructions, the 10 mcg strength syringe can deliver up to 0.5 mL of solution. Each 0.5 mL of solution contains 10 mcg of alprostadil, 324.7 mcg of alpha cyclodextrin, 45.4 mg of lactose, 23.5 mcg of sodium citrate, and 4.45 mg of benzyl alcohol. The delivery device can be set to deliver a solution volume of 0.125, 0.25, 0.375, or 0.50 mL to enable administration of 2.5, 5, 7.5, or 10 mcg of alprostadil. Following proper reconstitution instructions, the 20 mcg strength syringe can deliver up to 0.5 mL of solution. Each 0.5 mL of solution contains 20 mcg of alprostadil, 649.3 mcg of alpha cyclodextrin, 45.4 mg of lactose, 23.5 mcg of sodium citrate, and 4.45 mg of benzyl alcohol. The delivery device can be set to deliver a solution volume of 0.125, 0.25, 0.375, or 0.50 mL to enable administration of 5, 10, 15, or 20 mcg of alprostadil. After reconstitution, the solution of CAVERJECT should be used within 24 hours when stored at or below 25°C (77°F). Parenteral drug products should be inspected visually for particulate matter and discoloration prior to administration whenever the solution and container permit. The product should not be used if particulate matter or discoloration are present. Following a single use, the injection device and any remaining solution should be properly discarded.

Caution: CAVERJECT IMPULSE is for single use only. Do not use any remaining CAVERJECT solution.

HOW SUPPLIED

CAVERJECT IMPULSE is supplied as a disposable, single-dose, dual chamber syringe system. The system includes a glass cartridge, which contains sterile, freeze-dried alprostadil in the front chamber and sterile bacteriostatic water for reconstitution in the rear chamber. The syringes contain either 12.8 or 25.6 mcg of alprostadil to allow delivery of a maximum of 10 or 20 mcg/0.5mL. Store the unreconstituted product at 25°C (77°F); excursions permitted to 15° to 30°C (59° to 86°F) [see USP Controlled Room Temperature].

When reconstituted and used as directed, the deliverable amount for the 10 mcg strength is 10 mcg/0.5 mL or an increment of 10 mcg/0.5 mL, 2.5 mcg/0.125 mL, 5 mcg/0.25 mL, or 7.5 mcg/0.375 mL of alprostadil and the deliverable amount for the 20 microgram strength is 20 mcg/0.5 mL or an increment of 20 mcg/0.5 mL, 5 mcg/ 0.125 mL, 10 mcg/0.250 mL, or 15 mcg/0.375 mL of alprostadil. The reconstituted solution should be used within 24 hours when stored at or below 25°C (77°F).

CAVERJECT IMPULSE is supplied in a carton containing 2 blister trays. Each blister tray contains one dual chamber syringe system, one needle and 2 alcohol swabs. It is available in the following strengths:

10 mcg	NDC 0009-5181-01
20 mcg	NDC 0009-5182-01

CAVERJECT is also available as follows:

CAVERJECT Sterile Powder (alprostadil for injection) packaged in vials, 6 vials per carton

10 mcg	NDC 0009-3778-05
20 mcg	NDC 0009-3701-05
40 mcg	NDC 0009-7686-04

CAVERJECT Sterile Powder (alprostadil for injection) vials with diluent syringe, 6 syringe systems per carton

5 mcg	NDC 0009-7212-03
10 mcg	NDC 0009-3778-08
20 mcg	NDC 0009-3701-01

CAVERJECT Injection ([alprostadil injection] aqueous), 5 ampoules per carton

10 mcg (10 mcg/mL)	NDC 0009-7655-02
20 mcg (20 mcg/mL)	NDC 0009-7654-02
40 mcg (40 mcg/2mL)	NDC 0009-7650-02

℞ only

MADE IN SWEDEN

Manufactured for:
Pharmacia & Upjohn Company
A subsidiary of Pharmacia Corporation
Kalamazoo, MI 49001, USA
By:
Pharmacia AB
Stockholm, Sweden
September 2003
819 369 001
1-001-481

Patient Instructions For:
Caverject *impulse*®

Dual Chamber System
alprostadil for injection

Read this information carefully before using CAVERJECT [KAV-er-jeckt]. Read the information you get each time you renew your prescription, in case anything has changed. This is a summary and does not replace talking with your doctor when you start this medication and at check-ups. If you have any questions or concerns, talk to your doctor about them.

What is CAVERJECT?

CAVERJECT is a medicine to treat male impotence (erectile dysfunction). CAVERJECT is injected into a specific area of the penis and should produce an erection in 5 to 20 minutes. The erection should last for no longer than 1 hour.

CAVERJECT IMPULSE is for one use only and should be thrown away properly after a single use.

CAVERJECT does not protect you from sexually transmitted diseases (STDs), such as HIV (the virus that causes AIDS). In addition, small amounts of bleeding at the injection site can increase the risk of passing diseases carried by the blood, such as HIV.

What are the causes of and treatments for impotence?

There are several causes of impotence. These include medications that you may be taking for other conditions, poor blood circulation in the penis, nerve damage, emotional problems, too much smoking or alcohol use, use of street drugs, and hormonal problems. Often, impotence is due to more than one cause.

Treatments for impotence include switching medications if you are taking a medication that causes impotence, prescription medications, medical devices that produce an erection, surgical procedures to correct blood flow in the penis, penile implants, and psychological counseling.

You should not stop taking any prescription medications, unless told to do so by your doctor.

The use of other medical treatments for impotence in combination with CAVERJECT is not recommended. Discuss any concerns you may have about combination treatment with your doctor.

Who should not use CAVERJECT?

Do not use CAVERJECT if you have certain conditions that might cause long-lasting erections (lasting more than 4 hours). Long-lasting erections may cause penis damage. These conditions include:

- sickle cell anemia or trait
- leukemia
- tumor of the bone marrow (multiple myeloma)

Do not use CAVERJECT if you

- have a penile implant
- have an abnormally formed penis
- have other penis problems
- were told by your doctor not to have sex

Women and children should not use CAVERJECT.

How should I use CAVERJECT?

You will be treated with CAVERJECT in your doctor's office to find out what dose is best for you. After that, you can inject it yourself at home. Do not use it more than 3 times a week. There should be at least 24 hours between doses. See your doctor for regular check-ups to be sure CAVERJECT is not causing damage and that it is working as well as possible.

See the section "Instructions for Use" at the end of this leaflet for details about how to use CAVERJECT.

What are the possible side effects of CAVERJECT?

About 4 in 100 men who use CAVERJECT may get erections that last more than 4 hours. These can cause serious and permanent damage. **Call your doctor or seek professional help immediately if you still have an erection 4 hours after injection.**

The most common side effect of CAVERJECT is mild to moderate pain after injection. About one-third of patients report this effect.

You may get a small amount of bleeding at the injection site. This is more likely if you have a medical condition or are taking a medicine that interferes with blood clotting.

Call your doctor if you notice any redness, lumps, swelling, tenderness, or curving of the erect penis. Also, tell your doctor about any penis pain you did not have before or other penis problems you have.

There is a possibility of needle breakage with use of CAVERJECT IMPULSE. To best avoid breaking the needle, you should pay careful attention to your doctor's instructions and try to handle the device properly. If the needle breaks during injection and you are able to see and grasp the broken end, you should remove it and contact your doctor. If you cannot see or cannot grasp the broken end, you should promptly contact your doctor.

How should I store CAVERJECT IMPULSE?

1. Unmixed packages of CAVERJECT IMPULSE should be stored at room temperature. Temperatures between 59° to 86°F (15° to 30°C) are allowed. Avoid storing CAVERJECT IMPULSE at very high and very low temperatures.
2. During travel, do not let the medicine freeze or be stored at a temperature above 77°F (25°C). For example, do not store it in checked luggage during air travel or leave it in a closed automobile.
3. After mixing, CAVERJECT IMPULSE should be used within 24 hours. It should be kept at a temperature of 77°F or below during this storage time.

Continued on next page

Caverject Impulse—Cont.

General advice about prescription medicines
Medicines are sometimes prescribed for purposes other than those listed in a Patient Information Leaflet. If you have any concerns about CAVERJECT, ask your doctor. Your doctor or pharmacist can give you information about CAVERJECT that was written for health care professionals. Do not use CAVERJECT for a condition for which it was not prescribed. Do not share CAVERJECT with other people. You can get more information about impotence (erectile dysfunction) and its treatment from the National Institutes of Health (Washington, DC), the American Foundation for Urological Diseases (Baltimore, MD), or the Impotence Institute of America (Washington, DC).

INSTRUCTIONS FOR USE
Before you use CAVERJECT, your doctor must train you in how to prepare and give the injection properly.
Before using CAVERJECT, talk to your doctor about what to expect when using it, possible side effects, and what to do if side effects occur. Your dose has been selected for your individual needs. Do not change your dose without consulting your doctor. If you are not sure of the volume or dose to be used, talk to your doctor or pharmacist.
Follow these instructions exactly to prepare and inject a sterile (germ-free) dose of CAVERJECT.
Supplies Needed
CAVERJECT IMPULSE is packaged with a needle for injection (Figure A) and alcohol swab.

Figure A

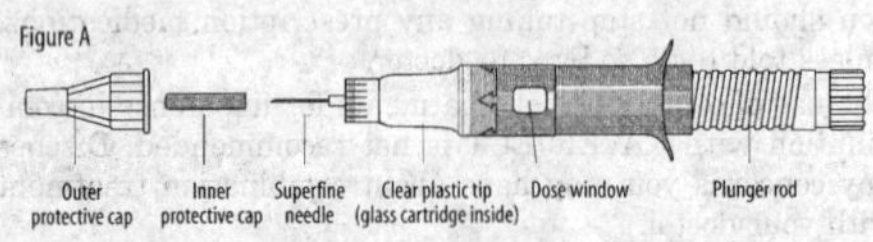

CAVERJECT IMPULSE is available in 10 and 20 mcg strengths.
MAKE SURE YOU HAVE THE RIGHT STRENGTH OF CAVERJECT IMPULSE.
Prepare the Dose
1. Wash your hands thoroughly and dry them with a clean towel.
2. Remove the device, needle, and alcohol swabs from the blistered tray.
3. Using one of the alcohol swabs, clean the rubber membrane at the tip of the syringe (Figure B).

Figure B

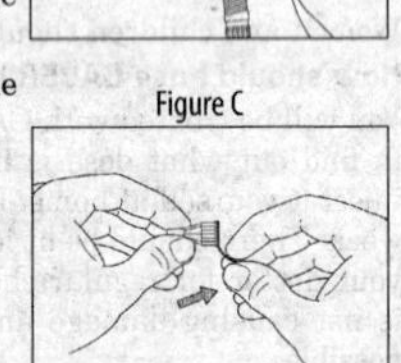

4. Peel the paper lid from the needle (Figure C).

Figure C

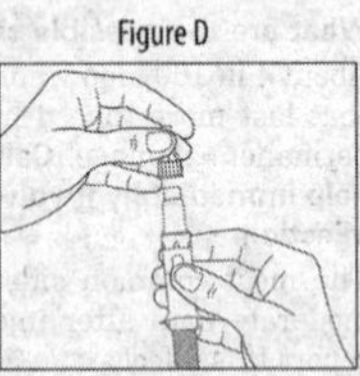

5. Attach the needle to the device by pressing the needle on to the tip of the device and turning clockwise until the needle is firmly in place. Remove the outer protective cap from the needle (Figure D).

Figure D

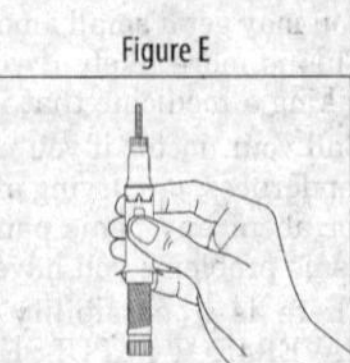

6. Hold the device with the needle pointing upward. The white plunger rod is in the extended position (Figure E).

Figure E

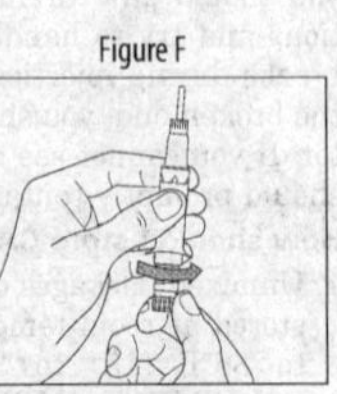

7. Turn the plunger rod slowly clockwise until it stops. This automatically mixes the alprostadil powder and the diluent. Turn the device upside down several times to make sure the solution is evenly mixed. The solution should be clear. Do not use it if it is cloudy or contains particles (Figure F).

Figure F

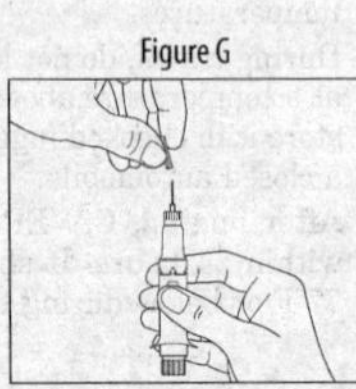

8. Hold the device with the needle upward and carefully remove the inner protective cap from the needle (Figure G).

Figure G

9. Keeping the device upright, press the plunger rod as far as it will go. A few drops will appear at the needlepoint and the solution will be free of bubbles although typically there may be some very small bubbles at the side of the glass cartridge (Figure H).

Figure H

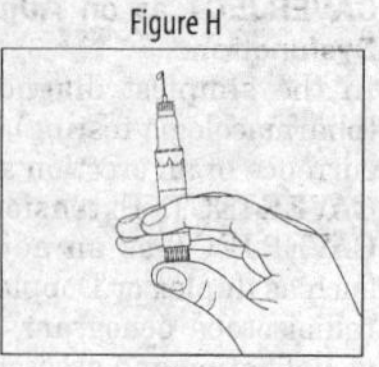

10. Turn the end of the plunger rod clockwise slowly to choose the dose your physician has determined is appropriate for you. The number that appears in the window shows the dose in micrograms. If the number is higher than your prescribed dose, continue to turn the plunger rod clockwise slowly until you reach the correct dose (Figure I).

Figure I

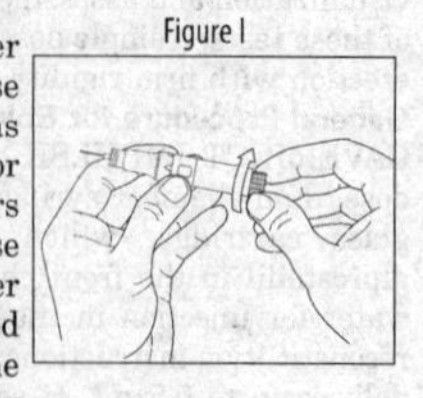

11. Set the device down on a level surface making sure the needle is not in contact with the surface.

Select Injection Site
1. CAVERJECT IMPULSE will be injected into a corpus cavernosum (spongy tissue) of the penis. One corpus cavernosum runs the length of the right side of the penis. Another corpus cavernosum runs the length of the left side of the penis (see Figures J and K).

Figure J

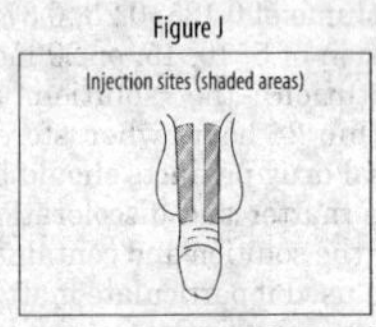

Figure K

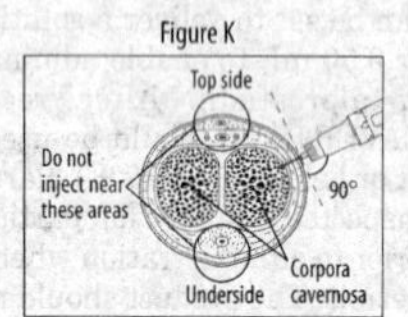

2. Choose an injection site on one side of the shaft of the penis as shown in Figure J. **Avoid visible veins.**
3. **With each use of CAVERJECT, alternate the side of the penis and vary the site of injection.**

Inject Your Dose of CAVERJECT
1. You should be sitting upright or slightly reclined when injecting CAVERJECT.
2. Holding the head of your penis with your thumb and forefinger, stretch your penis lengthwise along your thigh so that the skin is tight and you can clearly see the selected injection site.
3. Clean the injection site with a new alcohol swab. Do not discard this swab, you will need to use it again (see step 6).
4. Reposition the penis firmly against your thigh as in step 2 to keep it from moving during the injection.
5. Holding the device between your thumb and index finger, push the needle into the selected site through the skin and into the tissue as far as it will go. Push the plunger rod as far as it will go so the entire dose is injected (Figure L). If the injection solution does not flow easily, move the needle slightly and push as before. When using a dose less than the full capacity, a small amount of liquid will remain in the device.

Figure L

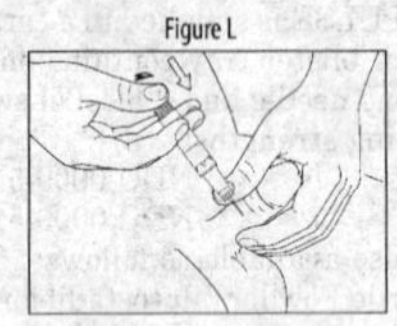

6. Grasp the device and pull the needle out of your penis. **Push on the injection site with the alcohol swab for about 5 minutes or until any bleeding stops.**
7. Carefully replace the outer protective cap on the needle.

Disposal of Injection Materials
After use, dispose of all injection materials safely. Your pharmacist may be able to supply a disposal box especially for disposable injection devices. **As with all prescription medicines, do not allow anyone else to use your medicine.**
℞ only
MADE IN SWEDEN
Manufactured for:
Pharmacia & Upjohn Company
A subsidiary of Pharmacia Corporation
Kalamazoo, MI 49001, USA
By:
Pharmacia AB
Stockholm, Sweden
September 2003
819 369 001
1-001-481
Shown in Product Identification Guide, page 330

CLEOCIN HCL® ℞
[klē-ō-sĭn]
(clindamycin hydrochloride)
capsules, USP

To reduce the development of drug-resistant bacteria and maintain the effectiveness of CLEOCIN HCl and other antibacterial drugs, CLEOCIN HCl should be used only to treat or prevent infections that are proven or strongly suspected to be caused by bacteria.

WARNING
Pseudomembranous colitis has been reported with nearly all antibacterial agents, including clindamycin, and may range in severity from mild to life-threatening. Therefore, it is important to consider this diagnosis in patients who present with diarrhea subsequent to the administration of antibacterial agents.
Because clindamycin therapy has been associated with severe colitis which may end fatally, it should be reserved for serious infections where less toxic antimicrobial agents are inappropriate, as described in the **INDICATIONS AND USAGE** section. It should not be used in patients with nonbacterial infections such as most upper respiratory tract infections. Treatment with antibacterial agents alters the normal flora of the colon and may permit over-growth of clostridia. Studies indicate that a toxin produced by *Clostridium difficile* is one primary cause of "antibiotic-associated colitis".
After the diagnosis of pseudomembranous colitis has been established, therapeutic measures should be initiated. Mild cases of pseudomembranous colitis usually respond to drug discontinuation alone. In moderate to severe cases, consideration should be given to management with fluids and electrolytes, protein supplementation, and treatment with an antibacterial drug clinically effective against *C. difficile* colitis.
Diarrhea, colitis, and pseudomembranous colitis have been observed to begin up to several weeks following cessation of therapy with clindamycin.

DESCRIPTION
Clindamycin hydrochloride is the hydrated hydrochloride salt of clindamycin. Clindamycin is a semisynthetic antibiotic produced by a 7(S)-chloro-substitution of the 7(R)-hydroxyl group of the parent compound lincomycin.
CLEOCIN HCl Capsules contain clindamycin hydrochloride equivalent to 75 mg, 150 mg or 300 mg of clindamycin.
Inactive ingredients: **75 mg**—corn starch, FD&C blue no. 1, FD&C yellow no. 5, gelatin, lactose, magnesium stearate and talc; **150 mg**—corn starch, FD&C blue no. 1, FD&C yellow no. 5, gelatin, lactose, magnesium stearate, talc and titanium dioxide; **300 mg**—corn starch, FD&C blue no. 1, gelatin, lactose, magnesium stearate, talc and titanium dioxide.
The structural formula is represented below:

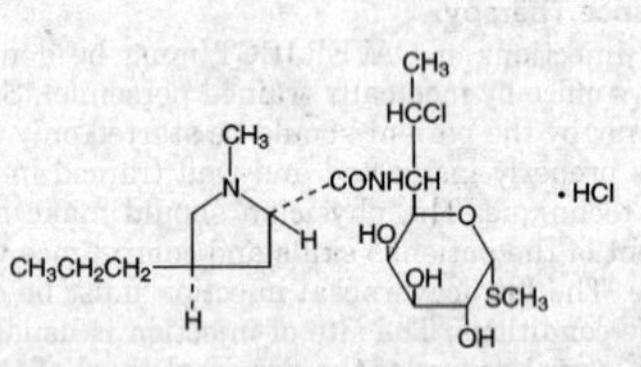

The chemical name for clindamycin hydrochloride is Methyl 7-chloro-6,7,8-trideoxy-6-(1-methyl-*trans*-4-propyl-L-2-pyrrolidinecarboxamido)-1-thio-L-*threo*-α-D-*galacto*-octopyranoside monohydrochloride.

CLINICAL PHARMACOLOGY
Microbiology: Clindamycin has been shown to have *in vitro* activity against isolates of the following organisms:
Aerobic gram-positive cocci, including:
Staphylococcus aureus
Staphylococcus epidermidis
(penicillinase and nonpenicillinase producing strains). When tested by *in vitro* methods some staphylococcal strains originally resistant to erythromycin rapidly develop resistance to clindamycin.
Streptococci (except *Streptococcus faecalis*)
Pneumococci
Anaerobic gram-negative bacilli, including:
Bacteroides species (including *Bacteroides fragilis* group and *Bacteroides melaninogenicus* group)
Fusobacterium species
Anaerobic gram-positive nonsporeforming bacilli, including:
Propionibacterium
Eubacterium
Actinomyces species
Anaerobic and microaerophilic gram-positive cocci, including:
Peptococcus species
Peptostreptococcus species
Microaerophilic streptococci
Clostridia: Clostridia are more resistant than most anaerobes to clindamycin. Most *Clostridium perfringens* are susceptible, but other species, eg, *Clostridium sporogenes* and *Clostridium tertium* are frequently resistant to clindamycin. Susceptibility testing should be done.
Cross resistance has been demonstrated between clindamycin and lincomycin.
Antagonism has been demonstrated between clindamycin and erythromycin.

Human Pharmacology: Serum level studies with a 150 mg oral dose of clindamycin hydrochloride in 24 normal adult volunteers showed that clindamycin was rapidly absorbed after oral administration. An average peak serum level of 2.50 mcg/mL was reached in 45 minutes; serum levels averaged 1.51 mcg/mL at 3 hours and 0.70 mcg/mL at 6 hours. Absorption of an oral dose is virtually complete (90%), and the concomitant administration of food does not appreciably modify the serum concentrations; serum levels have been uniform and predictable from person to person and dose to dose. Serum level studies following multiple doses of CLEOCIN HCl for up to 14 days show no evidence of accumulation or altered metabolism of drug.

Serum half-life of clindamycin is increased slightly in patients with markedly reduced renal function. Hemodialysis and peritoneal dialysis are not effective in removing clindamycin from the serum.

Concentrations of clindamycin in the serum increased linearly with increased dose. Serum levels exceed the MIC (minimum inhibitory concentration) for most indicated organisms for at least six hours following administration of the usually recommended doses. Clindamycin is widely distributed in body fluids and tissues (including bones). The average biological half-life is 2.4 hours. Approximately 10% of the bioactivity is excreted in the urine and 3.6% in the feces; the remainder is excreted as bioinactive metabolites. Doses of up to 2 grams of clindamycin per day for 14 days have been well tolerated by healthy volunteers, except that the incidence of gastrointestinal side effects is greater with the higher doses.

No significant levels of clindamycin are attained in the cerebrospinal fluid, even in the presence of inflamed meninges. Pharmacokinetic studies in elderly volunteers (61–79 years) and younger adults (18–39 years) indicate that age alone does not alter clindamycin pharmacokinetics (clearance, elimination half-life, volume of distribution, and area under the serum concentration-time curve) after IV administration of clindamycin phosphate. After oral administration of clindamycin hydrochloride, elimination half-life is increased to approximately 4.0 hours (range 3.4–5.1 h) in the elderly compared to 3.2 hours (range 2.1–4.2 h) in younger adults. The extent of absorption, however, is not different between age groups and no dosage alteration is necessary for the elderly with normal hepatic function and normal (age-adjusted) renal function[1].

INDICATIONS AND USAGE

Clindamycin is indicated in the treatment of serious infections caused by susceptible anaerobic bacteria.

Clindamycin is also indicated in the treatment of serious infections due to susceptible strains of streptococci, pneumococci, and staphylococci. Its use should be reserved for penicillin-allergic patients or other patients for whom, in the judgment of the physician, a penicillin is inappropriate. Because of the risk of colitis, as described in the WARNING box, before selecting clindamycin the physician should consider the nature of the infection and the suitability of less toxic alternatives (eg, erythromycin).

Anaerobes: Serious respiratory tract infections such as empyema, anaerobic pneumonitis and lung abscess; serious skin and soft tissue infections; septicemia; intra-abdominal infections such as peritonitis and intra-abdominal abscess (typically resulting from anaerobic organisms resident in the normal gastrointestinal tract); infections of the female pelvis and genital tract such as endometritis, nongonococcal tuboovarian abscess, pelvic cellulitis and postsurgical vaginal cuff infection.

Streptococci: Serious respiratory tract infections; serious skin and soft tissue infections.

Staphylococci: Serious respiratory tract infections; serious skin and soft tissue infections.

Pneumococci: Serious respiratory tract infections.

Bacteriologic studies should be performed to determine the causative organisms and their susceptibility to clindamycin.

***In Vitro* Susceptibility Testing:** A standardized disk testing procedure* is recommended for determining susceptibility of aerobic bacteria to clindamycin. A description is contained in the CLEOCIN® Susceptibility Disk insert. Using this method, the laboratory can designate isolates as resistant, intermediate, or susceptible. Tube or agar dilution methods may be used for both anaerobic and aerobic bacteria. When the directions in the CLEOCIN® Susceptibility Powder insert are followed, an MIC of 1.6 mcg/mL may be considered susceptible; MICs of 1.6 to 4.8 mcg/mL may be considered intermediate and MICs greater than 4.8 mcg/mL may be considered resistant.

---

*Bauer AW, Kirby WMM, Sherris JC, et al: Antibiotic susceptibility testing by a standardized single disc method. *Am J Clin Pathol* **45**:493-496, 1966. Standardized disc susceptibility test. *Federal Register* **37**:20527-29, 1972.

CLEOCIN Susceptibility Disks 2 mcg. See package insert for use.

CLEOCIN Susceptibility Powder 20 mg. See package insert for use.

For anaerobic bacteria the minimal inhibitory concentration (MIC) of clindamycin can be determined by agar dilution and broth dilution (including microdilution) techniques. If MICs are not determined routinely, the disk broth method is recommended for routine use. THE KIRBY-BAUER DISK DIFFUSION METHOD AND ITS INTERPRETIVE STANDARDS ARE NOT RECOMMENDED FOR ANAEROBES.

To reduce the development of drug-resistant bacteria and maintain the effectiveness of CLEOCIN HCl and other antibacterial drugs, CLEOCIN HCl should be used only to treat or prevent infections that are proven or strongly suspected to be caused by susceptible bacteria. When culture and susceptibility information are available, they should be considered in selecting or modifying antibacterial therapy. In the absence of such data, local epidemiology and susceptibility patterns may contribute to the empiric selection of therapy.

CONTRAINDICATIONS

CLEOCIN HCl is contraindicated in individuals with a history of hypersensitivity to preparations containing clindamycin or lincomycin.

WARNINGS

See WARNING box.

Pseudomembranous colitis has been reported with nearly all antibacterial agents, including clindamycin, and may range in severity from mild to life-threatening. Therefore, it is important to consider this diagnosis in patients who present with diarrhea subsequent to the administration of antibacterial agents.

Treatment with antibacterial agents alters the normal flora of the colon and may permit overgrowth of clostridia. Studies indicate that a toxin produced by *Clostridium difficile* is one primary cause of "antibiotic-associated colitis".

After the diagnosis of pseudomembranous colitis has been established, therapeutic measures should be initiated. Mild cases of pseudomembranous colitis usually respond to drug discontinuation alone. In moderate to severe cases, consideration should be given to management with fluids and electrolytes, protein supplementation, and treatment with an antibacterial drug clinically effective against *C. difficile* colitis.

A careful inquiry should be made concerning previous sensitivities to drugs and other allergens.

Usage in Meningitis—Since clindamycin does not diffuse adequately into the cerebrospinal fluid, the drug should not be used in the treatment of meningitis.

PRECAUTIONS

General

Review of experience to date suggests that a subgroup of older patients with associated severe illness may tolerate diarrhea less well. When clindamycin is indicated in these patients, they should be carefully monitored for change in bowel frequency.

CLEOCIN HCl should be prescribed with caution in individuals with a history of gastrointestinal disease, particularly colitis.

CLEOCIN HCl should be prescribed with caution in atopic individuals.

Indicated surgical procedures should be performed in conjunction with antibiotic therapy.

The use of CLEOCIN HCl occasionally results in overgrowth of nonsusceptible organisms—particularly yeasts. Should superinfections occur, appropriate measures should be taken as indicated by the clinical situation.

Clindamycin dosage modification may not be necessary in patients with renal disease. In patients with moderate to severe liver disease, prolongation of clindamycin half-life has been found. However, it was postulated from studies that when given every eight hours, accumulation should rarely occur. Therefore, dosage modification in patients with liver disease may not be necessary. However, periodic liver enzyme determinations should be made when treating patients with severe liver disease.

The 75 mg and 150 mg capsules contain FD&C yellow no. 5 (tartrazine) which may cause allergic-type reactions (including bronchial asthma) in certain susceptible individuals. Although the overall incidence of FD&C yellow no. 5 (tartrazine) sensitivity in the general population is low, it is frequently seen in patients who also have aspirin hypersensitivity.

Prescribing CLEOCIN HCl in the absence of a proven or strongly suspected bacterial infection or a prophylactic indication is unlikely to provide benefit to the patient and increases the risk of the development of drug-resistant bacteria.

Information for Patients

Patients should be counseled that antibacterial drugs including CLEOCIN HCl should only be to treat bacterial infections. They do not treat viral infections (e.g., the common cold). When CLEOCIN HCl is prescribed to treat a bacterial infection, patients should be told that although it is common to feel better early in the course of therapy, the medication should be taken exactly as directed. Skipping doses or not completing the full course of therapy may (1) decrease the effectiveness of the immediate treatment and (2) increase the likelihood that bacteria will develop resistance and will not be treatable by CLEOCIN HCl or other antibacterial drugs in the future.

Laboratory Tests

During prolonged therapy, periodic liver and kidney function tests and blood counts should be performed.

Drug Interactions

Clindamycin has been shown to have neuromuscular blocking properties that may enhance the action of other neuromuscular blocking agents. Therefore, it should be used with caution in patients receiving such agents.

Antagonism has been demonstrated between clindamycin and erythromycin *in vitro*. Because of possible clinical significance, these two drugs should not be administered concurrently.

Carcinogenesis, Mutagenesis, Impairment of Fertility

Long term studies in animals have not been performed with clindamycin to evaluate carcinogenic potential. Genotoxicity tests performed included a rat micronucleus test and an Ames Salmonella reversion test. Both tests were negative. Fertility studies in rats treated orally with up to 300 mg/kg/day (approximately 1.6 times the highest recommended adult human dose based on mg/m^2) revealed no effects on fertility or mating ability.

Pregnancy: Teratogenic effects

Pregnancy category B

Reproduction studies performed in rats and mice using oral doses of clindamycin up to 600 mg/kg/day (3.2 and 1.6 times the highest recommended adult human dose based on mg/m^2, respectively) or subcutaneous doses of clindamycin up to 250 mg/kg/day (1.3 and 0.7 times the highest recommended adult human dose based on mg/m^2, respectively) revealed no evidence of teratogenicity.

There are, however, no adequate and well-controlled studies in pregnant women. Because animal reproduction studies are not always predictive of the human response, this drug should be used during pregnancy only if clearly needed.

Nursing Mothers

Clindamycin has been reported to appear in breast milk in the range of 0.7 to 3.8 mcg/mL.

Pediatric Use

When CLEOCIN HCl is administered to the pediatric population (birth to 16 years), appropriate monitoring of organ system functions is desirable.

Geriatric Use

Clinical studies of clindamycin did not include sufficient numbers of patients age 65 and over to determine whether they respond differently from younger patients. However, other reported clinical experience indicates that antibiotic-associated colitis and diarrhea (due to *Clostridium difficile*) seen in association with most antibiotics occur more frequently in the elderly >60 years) and may be more severe. These patients should be carefully monitored for the development of diarrhea.

Pharmacokinetic studies with clindamycin have shown no clinically important differences between young and elderly subjects with normal hepatic function and normal (age-adjusted) renal function after oral or intravenous administration.

ADVERSE REACTIONS

The following reactions have been reported with the use of clindamycin.

Gastrointestinal: Abdominal pain, pseudomembranous colitis, esophagitis, nausea, vomiting and diarrhea (see **WARNING** box). The onset of pseudomembranous colitis symptoms may occur during or after antibacterial treatment (see **WARNINGS**).

Hypersensitivity Reactions: Generalized mild to moderate morbilliform-like (maculopapular) skin rashes are the most frequently reported adverse reactions. Vesiculobullous rashes, as well as urticaria, have been observed during drug therapy. Rare instances of erythema multiforme, some resembling Stevens-Johnson syndrome, and a few cases of anaphylactoid reactions have also been reported.

Skin and Mucous Membranes: Pruritus, vaginitis, and rare instances of exfoliative dermatitis have been reported. (See *Hypersensitivity Reactions.*)

Liver: Jaundice and abnormalities in liver function tests have been observed during clindamycin therapy.

Renal: Although no direct relationship of clindamycin to renal damage has been established, renal dysfunction as evidenced by azotemia, oliguria, and/or proteinuria has been observed in rare instances.

Hematopoietic: Transient neutropenia (leukopenia) and eosinophilia have been reported. Reports of agranulocytosis and thrombocytopenia have been made. No direct etiologic relationship to concurrent clindamycin therapy could be made in any of the foregoing.

Musculoskeletal: Rare instances of polyarthritis have been reported.

OVERDOSAGE

Significant mortality was observed in mice at an intravenous dose of 855 mg/kg and in rats at an oral or subcutaneous dose of approximately 2618 mg/kg. In the mice, convulsions and depression were observed.

Hemodialysis and peritoneal dialysis are not effective in removing clindamycin from the serum.

DOSAGE AND ADMINISTRATION

If significant diarrhea occurs during therapy, this antibiotic should be discontinued (see **WARNING** box).

Adults: *Serious infections*—150 to 300 mg every 6 hours. *More severe infections*—300 to 450 mg every 6 hours. **Pediatric Patients:** *Serious infections*—8 to 16 mg/kg/day (4 to 8 mg/lb/day) divided into three or four equal doses. *More severe infections*—16 to 20 mg/kg/day (8 to 10 mg/lb/day) divided into three or four equal doses.

To avoid the possibility of esophageal irritation, CLEOCIN HCl Capsules should be taken with a full glass of water.

Serious infections due to anaerobic bacteria are usually treated with CLEOCIN PHOSPHATE® Sterile Solution. However, in clinically appropriate circumstances, the physician may elect to initiate treatment or continue treatment with CLEOCIN HCI Capsules.

Continued on next page

Cleocin HCl—Cont.

In cases of β-hemolytic streptococcal infections, treatment should continue for at least 10 days.

HOW SUPPLIED

CLEOCIN HCl Capsules are available in the following strengths, colors and sizes:

75 mg Green	
Bottles of 100	NDC 0009-0331-02
150 mg Light Blue and Green	
Bottles of 16	NDC 0009-0225-01
Bottles of 100	NDC 0009-0225-02
Unit dose package of 100	NDC 0009-0225-03
300 mg Light Blue	
Bottles of 16	NDC 0009-0395-13
Bottles of 100	NDC 0009-0395-14
Unit dose package of 100	NDC 0009-0395-02

Store at controlled room temperature 20° to 25° C (68° to 77° F) [see USP].

ANIMAL TOXICOLOGY

One year oral toxicity studies in Spartan Sprague-Dawley rats and beagle dogs at dose levels up to 300 mg/kg/day (approximately 1.6 and 5.4 times the highest recommended adult human dose based on mg/m², respectively) have shown clindamycin to be well tolerated. No appreciable difference in pathological findings has been observed between groups of animals treated with clindamycin and comparable control groups. Rats receiving clindamycin hydrochloride at 600 mg/kg/day (approximately 3.2 times the highest recommended adult human dose based on mg/m²) for 6 months tolerated the drug well; however, dogs dosed at this level (approximately 10.8 times the highest recommended adult human dose based on mg/m²) vomited, would not eat, and lost weight.

℞ only

REFERENCE

1. Smith RB, Phillips JP: Evaluation of CLEOCIN HCl and CLEOCIN Phosphate in an Aged Population. Upjohn TR 8147-82-9122-021, December 1982.

Made in Canada for
Pharmacia & Upjohn Company
A subsidiary of Pharmacia Corporation
Kalamazoo, MI 49001, USA
By Patheon YM, Inc.
Toronto, Ontario
M3B 1Y5
Canada
Revised September 2003 810 570 927
692851

Shown in Product Identification Guide, page 330

DEPO-MEDROL® ℞

(methylprednisolone acetate)
injectable suspension, USP

Not For Intravenous Use

DESCRIPTION

DEPO-MEDROL Sterile Aqueous Suspension contains methylprednisolone acetate which is the 6-methyl derivative of prednisolone. Methylprednisolone acetate is a white or practically white, odorless, crystalline powder which melts at about 215° with some decomposition. It is soluble in dioxane, sparingly soluble in acetone, in alcohol, in chloroform, and in methanol, and slightly soluble in ether. It is practically insoluble in water. The chemical name for methylprednisolone acetate is pregna-1,4-diene-3,20-dione, 21-(acetyloxy)-11,17-dihydroxy-6-methyl-, (6α, 11β)-and the molecular weight is 416.51. The structural formula is:

DEPO-MEDROL is an anti-inflammatory glucocorticoid for intramuscular, intrasynovial, soft tissue or intralesional injection. It is available in three strengths: 20 mg/mL; 40 mg/mL; 80 mg/mL.

Each mL of these preparations contains:

Methylprednisolone acetate	20 mg	40 mg	80 mg
Polyethylene glycol 3350	29.5 mg	29.1 mg	28.2 mg
Polysorbate 80	1.97 mg	1.94 mg	1.88 mg
Monobasic sodium phosphate	6.9 mg	6.8 mg	6.59 mg
Dibasic sodium phosphate USP	1.44 mg	1.42 mg	1.37 mg
Benzyl alcohol added as a preservative	9.3 mg	9.16 mg	8.88 mg

Sodium Chloride was added to adjust tonicity.

When necessary, pH was adjusted with sodium hydroxide and/or hydrochloric acid.

The pH of the finished product remains within the USP specified range; ie, 3.5 to 7.0.

ACTIONS

Naturally occurring glucocorticoids (hydrocortisone), which also have salt retaining properties, are used in replacement therapy in adrenocortical deficiency states. Their synthetic analogs are used primarily for their potent anti-inflammatory effects in disorders of many organ systems.

Glucocorticoids cause profound and varied metabolic effects. In addition, they modify the body's immune response to diverse stimuli.

As of November, 1990, the formulation for DEPO-MEDROL Sterile Aqueous Suspension was revised. In a bioavailability study with thirty subjects, the new formulation was found to be more bioavailable than the previous formulation. An increase in the extent of methylprednisolone absorption was observed for the new formulation as indicated by significantly increased values for area under the serum methylprednisolone concentration curve and maximum serum methylprednisolone concentration (see table below). No difference in elimination half-life ($t_{1/2}$, calculated from the mean terminal elimination rate) was observed between the two formulations. No medically meaningful differences between the two formulations were seen in relation to vital signs, safety laboratory analyses, formulation effects, local tolerance, or side effects. This increase in absorption is not considered clinically significant.

	Previous Formulation	*Current Formulation*
AUC 0–240 hrs	1053 (47.3)*	1286 (39.2)
(ng × hr/mL)	[133–2297]**	[208–2225]
C_{MAX} (ng/mL)	8.98 (65.9)	11.8 (44.1)
	[0–28.5]	[3.37–23.4]
$t_{1/2}$ (hr)	139	139
	[46–990]	[58–866]

* Coefficient of variation (%)
** Range of values

INDICATIONS

A. FOR INTRAMUSCULAR ADMINISTRATION

When oral therapy is not feasible and the strength, dosage form, and route of administration of the drug reasonably lend the preparation to the treatment of the condition, the intramuscular use of DEPO-MEDROL Sterile Aqueous Suspension is indicated as follows:

1. Endocrine Disorders
- Primary or secondary adrenocortical insufficiency (hydrocortisone or cortisone is the drug of choice; synthetic analogs may be used in conjunction with mineralocorticoids where applicable; in infancy, mineralocorticoid supplementation is of particular importance)
- Acute adrenocortical insufficiency (hydrocortisone or cortisone is the drug of choice; mineralocorticoid supplementation may be necessary, particularly when synthetic analogs are used)
- Preoperatively and in the event of serious trauma or illness, in patients with known adrenal insufficiency or when adrenocortical reserve is doubtful:
- Congenital adrenal hyperplasia
- Hypercalcemia associated with cancer
- Nonsuppurative thyroiditis

2. Rheumatic Disorders

As adjunctive therapy for short-term administration (to tide the patient over an acute episode or exacerbation) in:
- Post-traumatic osteoarthritis
- Synovitis of osteoarthritis
- Rheumatoid arthritis, including juvenile rheumatoid arthritis (selected cases may require low-dose maintenance therapy)
- Acute and subacute bursitis
- Epicondylitis
- Acute nonspecific tenosynovitis
- Acute gouty arthritis
- Psoriatic arthritis
- Ankylosing spondylitis

3. Collagen Diseases

During an exacerbation or as maintenance therapy in selected cases of:
- Systemic lupus erythematosus
- Systemic dermatomyositis (polymyositis)
- Acute rheumatic carditis

4. Dermatologic Diseases
- Pemphigus
- Severe erythema multiforme (Stevens-Johnson syndrome)
- Exfoliative dermatitis
- Bullous dermatitis herpetiformis
- Severe seborrheic dermatitis
- Severe psoriasis
- Mycosis fungoides

5. Allergic States

Control of severe or incapacitating allergic conditions intractable to adequate trials of conventional treatment in:
- Bronchial asthma
- Contact dermatitis
- Atopic dermatitis
- Serum sickness
- Seasonal or perennial allergic rhinitis
- Drug hypersensitivity reactions
- Urticarial transfusion reactions
- Acute noninfectious laryngeal edema (epinephrine is the drug of first choice)

6. Ophthalmic Diseases

Severe acute and chronic allergic and inflammatory processes involving the eye, such as:
- Herpes zoster ophthalmicus
- Iritis, iridocyclitis
- Chorioretinitis
- Diffuse posterior uveitis and choroiditis
- Optic neuritis
- Sympathetic ophthalmia
- Anterior segment inflammation
- Allergic conjunctivitis
- Allergic corneal marginal ulcers
- Keratitis

7. Gastrointestinal Diseases

To tide the patient over a critical period of the disease in:
- Ulcerative colitis (systemic therapy)
- Regional enteritis (systemic therapy)

8. Respiratory Diseases
- Symptomatic sarcoidosis
- Berylliosis
- Fulminating or disseminated pulmonary tuberculosis when used concurrently with appropriate antituberculous chemotherapy
- Loeffler's syndrome not manageable by other means
- Aspiration pneumonitis

9. Hematologic Disorders
- Acquired (autoimmune) hemolytic anemia
- Secondary thrombocytopenia in adults
- Erythroblastopenia (RBC anemia)
- Congenital (erythroid) hypoplastic anemia

10. Neoplastic Diseases

For palliative management of:
- Leukemias and lymphomas in adults
- Acute leukemia of childhood

11. Edematous States

To induce diuresis or remission of proteinuria in the nephrotic syndrome, without uremia, of the idiopathic type or that due to lupus erythematosus

12. Nervous System

Acute exacerbations of multiple sclerosis

13. Miscellaneous
- Tuberculous meningitis with subarachnoid block or impending block when used concurrently with appropriate antituberculous chemotherapy
- Trichinosis with neurologic or myocardial involvement

B. FOR INTRASYNOVIAL OR SOFT TISSUE ADMINISTRATION (See WARNINGS).

DEPO-MEDROL is indicated as adjunctive therapy for short-term administration (to tide the patient over an acute episode or exacerbation) in:
- Synovitis of osteoarthritis
- Rheumatoid arthritis
- Acute and subacute bursitis
- Acute gouty arthritis
- Epicondylitis
- Acute nonspecific tenosynovitis
- Post-traumatic osteoarthritis

C. FOR INTRALESIONAL ADMINISTRATION

DEPO-MEDROL is indicated for intralesional use in the following conditions:
- Keloids
- Localized hypertrophic, infiltrated, inflammatory lesions of:
  - lichen planus, psoriatic plaques, granuloma annulare, and lichen simplex chronicus (neurodermatitis)
  - Discoid lupus erythematosus
  - Necrobiosis lipoidica diabeticorum
  - Alopecia areata

DEPO-MEDROL also may be useful in cystic tumors of an aponeurosis or tendon (ganglia).

CONTRAINDICATIONS

DEPO-MEDROL Sterile Aqueous Suspension is contraindicated for intrathecal administration. Reports of severe medical events have been associated with this route of administration. DEPO-MEDROL is contraindicated for use in premature infants because the formulation contains benzyl alcohol. Benzyl alcohol has been reported to be associated with a fatal "gasping syndrome" in premature infants. DEPO-MEDROL is also contraindicated in systemic fungal infections and patients with known hypersensitivity to the product and its constituents.

WARNINGS

This product contains benzyl alcohol which is potentially toxic when administered locally to neural tissue.

Multidose use of DEPO-MEDROL Sterile Aqueous Suspension from a single vial requires special care to avoid contamination. Although initially sterile, any multidose use of vials may lead to contamination unless strict aseptic technique is observed. Particular care, such as use of disposable sterile syringes and needles is necessary.

While crystals of adrenal steroids in the dermis suppress inflammatory reactions, their presence may cause disintegration of the cellular elements and physiochemical changes in the ground substance of the connective tissue. The resultant infrequently occurring dermal and/or subdermal changes may form depressions in the skin at the injec-

tion site. The degree to which this reaction occurs will vary with the amount of adrenal steroid injected. Regeneration is usually complete within a few months or after all crystals of the adrenal steroid have been absorbed.

In order to minimize the incidence of dermal and subdermal atrophy, care must be exercised not to exceed recommended doses in injections. Multiple small injections into the area of the lesion should be made whenever possible. The technique of intrasynovial and intramuscular injection should include precautions against injection or leakage into the dermis. Injection into the deltoid muscle should be avoided because of a high incidence of subcutaneous atrophy.

It is critical that, during administration of DEPO-MEDROL, appropriate technique be used and care taken to assure proper placement of drug.

In patients on corticosteroid therapy subjected to any unusual stress, increased dosage of rapidly acting corticosteroids before, during, and after the stressful situation is indicated.

Corticosteroids may mask some signs of infection, and new infections may appear during their use. There may be decreased resistance and inability to localize infection when corticosteroids are used. Infections with any pathogen including viral, bacterial, fungal, protozoan or helminthic infections, in any location of the body, may be associated with the use of corticosteroids alone or in combination with other immunosuppressive agents that affect cellular immunity, humoral immunity, or neutrophil function.[1]

These infections may be mild, but can be severe and at times fatal. With increasing doses of corticosteroids, the rate of occurrence of infectious complications increases.[2] Do not use intra-articularly, intrabursally or for intratendinous administration for *local* effect in the presence of acute infection.

Prolonged use of corticosteroids may produce posterior subcapsular cataracts, glaucoma with possible damage to the optic nerves, and may enhance the establishment of secondary ocular infections due to fungi or viruses.

Usage in pregnancy. Since adequate human reproduction studies have not been done with corticosteroids, the use of these drugs in pregnancy, nursing mothers, or women of childbearing potential requires that the possible benefits of the drug be weighed against the potential hazards to the mother and embryo or fetus. Infants born of mothers who have received substantial doses of corticosteroids during pregnancy should be carefully observed for signs of hypoadrenalism.

Average and large doses of cortisone or hydrocortisone can cause elevation of blood pressure, salt and water retention, and increased excretion of potassium. These effects are less likely to occur with the synthetic derivatives except when used in large doses. Dietary salt restriction and potassium supplementation may be necessary. All corticosteroids increase calcium excretion.

Administration of live or live, attenuated vaccines is contraindicated in patients receiving immunosuppressive doses of corticosteroids. Killed or inactivated vaccines may be administered to patients receiving immunosuppressive doses of corticosteroids; however, the response to such vaccines may be diminished. Indicated immunization procedures may be undertaken in patients receiving nonimmunosuppressive doses of corticosteroids.

The use of DEPO-MEDROL in active tuberculosis should be restricted to those cases of fulminating or disseminated tuberculosis in which the corticosteroid is used for the management of the disease in conjunction with appropriate antituberculous regimen.

If corticosteroids are indicated in patients with latent tuberculosis or tuberculin reactivity, close observation is necessary as reactivation of the disease may occur. During prolonged corticosteroid therapy, these patients should receive chemoprophylaxis.

Because rare instances of anaphylactoid reactions have occurred in patients receiving parenteral corticosteroid therapy, appropriate precautionary measures should be taken prior to administration, especially when the patient has a history of allergy to any drug.

Persons who are on drugs which suppress the immune system are more susceptible to infections than healthy individuals. Chicken pox and measles, for example, can have a more serious or even fatal course in non-immune children or adults on corticosteroids. In such children or adults who have not had these diseases, particular care should be taken to avoid exposure. How the dose, route and duration of corticosteroid administration affects the risk of developing a disseminated infection is not known. The contribution of the underlying disease and/or prior corticosteroid treatment to the risk is also not known. If exposed to chicken pox, prophylaxis with varicella zoster immune globulin (VZIG) may be indicated. If exposed to measles, prophylaxis with pooled intramuscular immunoglobulin (IG) may be indicated. (See the respective package inserts for complete VZIG and IG prescribing information.) If chicken pox develops, treatment with antiviral agents may be considered. Similarly, corticosteroids should be used with great care in patients with known or suspected Strongyloides (threadworm) infestation. In such patients, corticosteroid-induced immunosuppression may lead to Strongyloides hyperinfection and dissemination with widespread larval migration, often accompanied by severe enterocolitis and potentially fatal gram-negative septicemia.

PRECAUTIONS

General precautions

Drug-induced secondary adrenocortical insufficiency may be minimized by gradual reduction of dosage. This type of relative insufficiency may persist for months after discontinuation of therapy; therefore, in any situation of stress occurring during that period, hormone therapy should be reinstituted. Since mineralocorticoid secretion may be impaired, salt and/or a mineralocorticoid should be administered concurrently.

When multidose vials are used, special care to prevent contamination of the contents is essential. There is some evidence that benzalkonium chloride is not an adequate antiseptic for sterilizing DEPO-MEDROL Sterile Aqueous Suspension multidose vials. A povidone-iodine solution or similar product is recommended to cleanse the vial top prior to aspiration of contents. (See WARNINGS.)

There is an enhanced effect of corticosteroids in patients with hypothyroidism and in those with cirrhosis.

Corticosteroids should be used cautiously in patients with ocular herpes simplex for fear of corneal perforation.

The lowest possible dose of corticosteroid should be used to control the condition under treatment, and when reduction in dosage is possible, the reduction must be gradual.

Psychic derangements may appear when corticosteroids are used, ranging from euphoria, insomnia, mood swings, personality changes, and severe depression to frank psychotic manifestations. Also, existing emotional instability or psychotic tendencies may be aggravated by corticosteroids.

Steroids should be used with caution in nonspecific ulcerative colitis, if there is a probability of impending perforation, abscess or other pyogenic infection. Caution must also be used in diverticulitis, fresh intestinal anastomoses, active or latent peptic ulcer, renal insufficiency, hypertension, osteoporosis, and myasthenia gravis, when steroids are used as direct or adjunctive therapy.

Growth and development of infants and children on prolonged corticosteroid therapy should be carefully followed.

Kaposi's sarcoma has been reported to occur in patients receiving corticosteroid therapy. Discontinuation of corticosteroids may result in clinical remission.

The following additional precautions apply for parenteral corticosteroids. Intrasynovial injection of a corticosteroid may produce systemic as well as local effects.

Appropriate examination of any joint fluid present is necessary to exclude a septic process.

A marked increase in pain accompanied by local swelling, further restriction of joint motion, fever, and malaise are suggestive of septic arthritis. If this complication occurs and the diagnosis of sepsis is confirmed, appropriate antimicrobial therapy should be instituted.

Local injection of a steroid into a previously infected joint is to be avoided.

Corticosteroids should not be injected into unstable joints.

The slower rate of absorption by intramuscular administration should be recognized.

Although controlled clinical trials have shown corticosteroids to be effective in speeding the resolution of acute exacerbations of multiple sclerosis, they do not show that corticosteroids affect the ultimate outcome or natural history of the disease. The studies do show that relatively high doses of corticosteroids are necessary to demonstrate a significant effect. (See DOSAGE AND ADMINISTRATION.)

Since complications of treatment with glucocorticoids are dependent on the size of the dose and the duration of treatment, a risk/benefit decision must be made in each individual case as to dose and duration of treatment and as to whether daily or intermittent therapy should be used.

DRUG INTERACTIONS:

The pharmacokinetic interactions listed below are potentially clinically important. Mutual inhibition of metabolism occurs with concurrent use of cyclosporin and methylprednisolone; therefore, it is possible that adverse events associated with the individual use of either drug may be more apt to occur. Convulsions have been reported with concurrent use of methylprednisolone and cyclosporin. Drugs that induce hepatic enzymes such as phenobarbital, phenytoin and rifampin may increase the clearance of methylprednisolone and may require increases in methylprednisolone dose to achieve the desired response. Drugs such as troleandomycin and ketoconazole may inhibit the metabolism of methylprednisolone and thus decrease its clearance. Therefore, the dose of methylprednisolone should be titrated to avoid steroid toxicity.

Methylprednisolone may increase the clearance of chronic high dose aspirin. This could lead to decreased salicylate serum levels or increase the risk of salicylate toxicity when methylprednisolone is withdrawn. Aspirin should be used cautiously in conjunction with corticosteroids in patients suffering from hypoprothrombinemia.

The effect of methylprednisolone on oral anticoagulants is variable. There are reports of enhanced as well as diminished effects of anticoagulant when given concurrently with corticosteroids. Therefore, coagulation indices should be monitored to maintain the desired anticoagulant effect.

Information for the Patient

Persons who are on immunosuppressant doses of corticosteroids should be warned to avoid exposure to chicken pox or measles. Patients should also be advised that if they are exposed, medical advice should be sought without delay.

ADVERSE REACTIONS

Fluid and electrolyte disturbances

Sodium retention
Fluid retention
Congestive heart failure in susceptible patients
Potassium loss
Hypokalemic alkalosis
Hypertension

Musculoskeletal

Muscle weakness
Steroid myopathy
Loss of muscle mass
Osteoporosis
Tendon rupture, particularly of the Achilles tendon
Vertebral compression fractures
Aseptic necrosis of femoral and humeral heads
Pathologic fracture of long bones

Gastrointestinal

Peptic ulcer with possible subsequent perforation and hemorrhage
Pancreatitis
Abdominal distention
Ulcerative esophagitis
Increases in alanine transaminase (ALT, SGPT), aspartate transaminase (AST, SGOT), and alkaline phosphatase have been observed following corticosteroid treatment. These changes are usually small, not associated with any clinical syndrome and are reversible upon discontinuation.

Dermatologic

Impaired wound healing
Thin fragile skin
Petechiae and ecchymoses
Facial erythema
Increased sweating
May suppress reactions to skin tests

Neurological

Convulsions
Increased intracranial pressure with papilledema (pseudotumor cerebri) usually after treatment
Vertigo
Headache

Endocrine

Menstrual irregularities
Development of Cushingoid state
Suppression of growth in children
Secondary adrenocortical and pituitary unresponsiveness, particularly in times of stress, as in trauma, surgery or illness
Decreased carbohydrate tolerance
Manifestations of latent diabetes mellitus
Increased requirements for insulin or oral hypoglycemic agents in diabetes

Ophthalmic

Posterior subcapsular cataracts
Increased intraocular pressure
Glaucoma
Exophthalmos

Metabolic

Negative nitrogen balance due to protein catabolism

The following *additional* adverse reactions are related to parenteral corticosteroid therapy:

Anaphylactic reaction
Allergic or hypersensitivity reactions
Urticaria
Hyperpigmentation or hypopigmentation
Subcutaneous and cutaneous atrophy
Sterile abscess
Injection site infections following non-sterile administration (see WARNINGS)
Postinjection flare, following intrasynovial use
Charcot-like arthropathy

Adverse Reactions Reported with the Following Routes of Administration

Intrathecal/Epidural

Arachnoiditis
Meningitis
Paraparesis/paraplegia
Sensory disturbances
Bowel/bladder dysfunction
Headache
Seizures

Intranasal

Temporary/permanent visual impairment including blindness
Allergic reactions
Rhinitis

Ophthalmic

Temporary/permanent visual impairment including blindness
Increased intraocular pressure
Ocular and periocular inflammation including allergic reactions
Infection
Residue or slough at injection site

Miscellaneous injection sites (scalp, tonsillar fauces, sphenopalatine ganglion)-blindness

DOSAGE AND ADMINISTRATION

Because of possible physical incompatibilities, DEPO-MEDROL Sterile Aqueous Suspension should not be diluted or mixed with other solutions.

A. Administration for Local Effect

Therapy with DEPO-MEDROL does not obviate the need for the conventional measures usually employed. Although

Continued on next page

Depo-Medrol—Cont.

this method of treatment will ameliorate symptoms, it is in no sense a cure and the hormone has no effect on the cause of the inflammation.

1. Rheumatoid and Osteoarthritis. The dose for intra-articular administration depends upon the size of the joint and varies with the severity of the condition in the individual patient. In chronic cases, injections may be repeated at intervals ranging from one to five or more weeks depending upon the degree of relief obtained from the initial injection. The doses in the following table are given as a general guide:

Size of Joint	*Examples*	*Range of Dosage*
Large	Knees Ankles Shoulders	20 to 80 mg
Medium	Elbows Wrists	10 to 40 mg
Small	Metacarpophalangeal Interphalangeal Sternoclavicular Acromioclavicular	4 to 10 mg

Procedure: It is recommended that the anatomy of the joint involved be reviewed before attempting intra-articular injection. In order to obtain the full anti-inflammatory effect it is important that the injection be made into the synovial space. Employing the same sterile technique as for a lumbar puncture, a sterile 20 to 24 gauge needle (on a dry syringe) is quickly inserted into the synovial cavity. Procaine infiltration is elective. The aspiration of only a few drops of joint fluid proves the joint space has been entered by the needle. *The injection site for each joint is determined by that location where the synovial cavity is most superficial and most free of large vessels and nerves.* With the needle in place, the aspirating syringe is removed and replaced by a second syringe containing the desired amount of DEPO-MEDROL. The plunger is then pulled outward slightly to aspirate synovial fluid and to make sure the needle is still in the synovial space. After injection, the joint is moved gently a few times to aid mixing of the synovial fluid and the suspension. The site is covered with a small sterile dressing.

Suitable sites for intra-articular injection are the knee, ankle, wrist, elbow, shoulder, phalangeal, and hip joints. Since difficulty is not infrequently encountered in entering the hip joint, precautions should be taken to avoid any large blood vessels in the area. Joints not suitable for injection are those that are anatomically inaccessible such as the spinal joints and those like the sacroiliac joints that are devoid of synovial space. Treatment failures are most frequently the result of failure to enter the joint space. Little or no benefit follows injection into surrounding tissue. If failures occur when injections into the synovial spaces are certain, as determined by aspiration of fluid, repeated injections are usually futile. Local therapy does not alter the underlying disease process, and whenever possible comprehensive therapy including physiotherapy and orthopedic correction should be employed.

Following intra-articular steroid therapy, care should be taken to avoid overuse of joints in which symptomatic benefit has been obtained. Negligence in this matter may permit an increase in joint deterioration that will more than offset the beneficial effects of the steroid.

Unstable joints should not be injected. Repeated intra-articular injection may in some cases result in instability of the joint. X-ray follow-up is suggested in selected cases to detect deterioration.

If a local anesthetic is used prior to injection of DEPO-MEDROL, the anesthetic package insert should be read carefully and all the precautions observed.

2. Bursitis. The area around the injection site is prepared in a sterile way and a wheal at the site made with 1 percent procaine hydrochloride solution. A 20 to 24 gauge needle attached to a dry syringe is inserted into the bursa and the fluid aspirated. The needle is left in place and the aspirating syringe changed for a small syringe containing the desired dose. After injection, the needle is withdrawn and a small dressing applied.

3. Miscellaneous: Ganglion, Tendinitis, Epicondylitis. In the treatment of conditions such as tendinitis or tenosynovitis, care should be taken, following application of a suitable antiseptic to the overlying skin, to inject the suspension into the tendon sheath rather than into the substance of the tendon. The tendon may be readily palpated when placed on a stretch. When treating conditions such as epicondylitis, the area of greatest tenderness should be outlined carefully and the suspension infiltrated into the area. For ganglia of the tendon sheaths, the suspension is injected directly into the cyst. In many cases, a single injection causes a marked decrease in the size of the cystic tumor and may effect disappearance. The usual sterile precautions should be observed, of course, with each injection.

The dose in the treatment of the various conditions of the tendinous or bursal structures listed above varies with the condition being treated and ranges from 4 to 30 mg. In recurrent or chronic conditions, repeated injections may be necessary.

4. Injections for Local Effect in Dermatologic Conditions. Following cleansing with an appropriate antiseptic such as 70% alcohol, 20 to 60 mg of the suspension is injected into the lesion. It may be necessary to distribute doses ranging from 20 to 40 mg by repeated local injections in the case of large lesions. Care should be taken to avoid injection of sufficient material to cause blanching since this may be followed by a small slough. One to four injections are usually employed, the intervals between injections varying with the type of lesion being treated and the duration of improvement produced by the initial injection.

When multidose vials are used, special care to prevent contamination of the contents is essential. (See WARNINGS.)

B. Administration for Systemic Effect.

The intramuscular dosage will vary with the condition being treated. When employed as a temporary substitute for oral therapy, a single injection during each 24-hour period of a dose of the suspension equal to the total daily oral dose of MEDROL® Tablets (methylprednisolone) is usually sufficient. When a prolonged effect is desired, the weekly dose may be calculated by multiplying the daily oral dose by 7 and given as a single intramuscular injection.

Dosage must be individualized according to the severity of the disease and response of the patient. For infants and children, the recommended dosage will have to be reduced, but dosage should be governed by the severity of the condition rather than by strict adherence to the ratio indicated by age or body weight.

Hormone therapy is an adjunct to, and not a replacement for, conventional therapy. Dosage must be decreased or discontinued gradually when the drug has been administered for more than a few days. The severity, prognosis and expected duration of the disease and the reaction of the patient to medication are primary factors in determining dosage. If a period of spontaneous remission occurs in a chronic condition, treatment should be discontinued. Routine laboratory studies, such as urinalysis, two-hour postprandial blood sugar, determination of blood pressure and body weight, and a chest X-ray should be made at regular intervals during prolonged therapy. Upper GI X-rays are desirable in patients with an ulcer history or significant dyspepsia.

In patients with the **adrenogenital syndrome,** a single intramuscular injection of 40 mg every two weeks may be adequate. For maintenance of patients with **rheumatoid arthritis,** the weekly intramuscular dose will vary from 40 to 120 mg. The usual dosage for patients with **dermatologic lesions** benefited by systemic corticoid therapy is 40 to 120 mg of methylprednisolone acetate administered intramuscularly at weekly intervals for one to four weeks. In acute severe dermatitis due to poison ivy, relief may result within 8 to 12 hours following intramuscular administration of a single dose of 80 to 120 mg. In chronic contact dermatitis repeated injections at 5 to 10 day intervals may be necessary. In seborrheic dermatitis, a weekly dose of 80 mg may be adequate to control the condition.

Following intramuscular administration of 80 to 120 mg to asthmatic patients, relief may result within 6 to 48 hours and persist for several days to two weeks. Similarly in patients with allergic rhinitis (hay fever) an intramuscular dose of 80 to 120 mg may be followed by relief of coryzal symptoms within six hours persisting for several days to three weeks.

If signs of stress are associated with the condition being treated, the dosage of the suspension should be increased. If a rapid hormonal effect of maximum intensity is required, the intravenous administration of highly soluble methylprednisolone sodium succinate is indicated.

Multiple Sclerosis

In treatment of acute exacerbations of multiple sclerosis daily doses of 200 mg of prednisolone for a week followed by 80 mg every other day for 1 month have been shown to be effective (4 mg of methylprednisolone is equivalent to 5 mg of prednisolone).

HOW SUPPLIED

DEPO-MEDROL Sterile Aqueous Suspension is available in the following strengths and package sizes:

20 mg per mL	
5 mL multidose vials	NDC 0009-0274-01
40 mg per mL	
5 mL multidose vials	NDC 0009-0280-02
25 × 5 mL multidose vials	NDC 0009-0280-51
10 mL multidose vials	NDC 0009-0280-03
25 × 10 mL multidose vials	NDC 0009-0280-52
80 mg per mL	
5 mL multidose vials	NDC 0009-0306-02
25 × 5 mL multidose vials	NDC 0009-0306-12

Store at controlled room temperature 20° to 25°C (68° to 77°F) [see USP].

REFERENCES

1. Fekety R. Infections associated with corticosteroids and immunosuppressive therapy. In: Gorbach SL, Bartlett JG, Blacklow NR, eds. *Infectious Diseases.* Philadelphia: WBSaunders Company 1992:1050–1.
2. Stuck AE, Minder CE, Frey FJ. Risk of infectious complications in patients taking glucocorticoids. *Rev Infect Dis* 1989:11(6):954–63.

℞ only

Pharmacia & Upjohn Company, A subsidiary of Pharmacia Corporation 810 341 328
Kalamazoo, Michigan 49001, USA 691211
Revised June 2002

DEPO-MEDROL® ℞

methylprednisolone acetate
injectable suspension, USP
Single-Dose Vial
Not For Intravenous Use

DESCRIPTION

DEPO-MEDROL Sterile Aqueous Suspension contains methylprednisolone acetate which is the 6-methyl derivative of prednisolone. Methylprednisolone acetate is a white or practically white, odorless, crystalline powder which melts at about 215° with some decomposition. It is soluble in dioxane, sparingly soluble in acetone, in alcohol, in chloroform, and in methanol, and slightly soluble in ether. It is practically insoluble in water. The chemical name for methylprednisolone acetate is pregna-1,4-diene-3,20-dione, 21-(acetyloxy)-11,17-dihydroxy-6-methyl-,(6α,11β)-and the molecular weight is 416.51. The structural formula is:

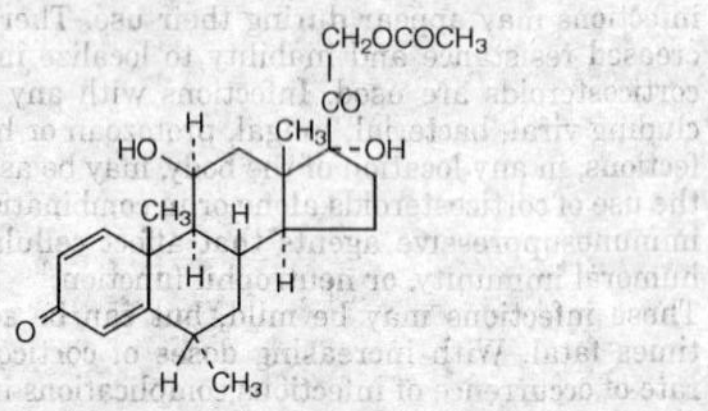

DEPO-MEDROL is an anti-inflammatory glucocorticoid for intramuscular, intrasynovial, soft tissue or intralesional injection. It is available as single-dose vials in two strengths: 40 mg/mL; 80 mg/mL.

Methylprednisolone acetate	**40 mg**	**80 mg**
Polyethylene glycol 3350	29 mg	28 mg
Myristyl-gamma-picolinium chloride	0.195 mg	0.189 mg

Sodium Chloride was added to adjust tonicity.

When necessary, pH was adjusted with sodium hydroxide and/or hydrochloric acid.

The pH of the finished product remains within the USP specified range; ie, 3.5 to 7.0.

ACTIONS

Naturally occurring glucocorticoids (hydrocortisone), which also have salt retaining properties, are used in replacement therapy in adrenocortical deficiency states. Their synthetic analogs are used primarily for their potent anti-inflammatory effects in disorders of many organ systems.

Glucocorticoids cause profound and varied metabolic effects. In addition, they modify the body's immune response to diverse stimuli.

INDICATIONS

A. FOR INTRAMUSCULAR ADMINISTRATION

When oral therapy is not feasible and the strength, dosage form, and route of administration of the drug reasonably lend the preparation to the treatment of the condition, the intramuscular use of DEPO-MEDROL Sterile Aqueous Suspension is indicated as follows:

1. Endocrine Disorders

Primary or secondary adrenocortical insufficiency (hydrocortisone or cortisone is the drug of choice; synthetic analogs may be used in conjunction with mineralocorticoids where applicable; in infancy, mineralocorticoid supplementation is of particular importance)

Acute adrenocortical insufficiency (hydrocortisone or cortisone is the drug of choice; mineralocorticoid supplementation may be necessary, particularly when synthetic analogs are used)

Preoperatively and in the event of serious trauma or illness, in patients with known adrenal insufficiency or when adrenocortical reserve is doubtful:

Congenital adrenal hyperplasia

Hypercalcemia associated with cancer

Nonsuppurative thyroiditis

2. Rheumatic Disorders

As adjunctive therapy for short-term administration (to tide the patient over an acute episode or exacerbation) in:

Post-traumatic osteoarthritis

Synovitis of osteoarthritis

Rheumatoid arthritis, including juvenile rheumatoid arthritis (selected cases may require low-dose maintenance therapy)

Acute and subacute bursitis

Epicondylitis

Acute nonspecific tenosynovitis

Acute gouty arthritis

Psoriatic arthritis

Ankylosing spondylitis

3. Collagen Diseases

During an exacerbation or as maintenance therapy in selected cases of:

Systemic lupus erythematosus

Systemic dermatomyositis (polymyositis)

Acute rheumatic carditis

4. Dermatologic Diseases

Pemphigus

Severe erythema multiforme (Stevens-Johnson syndrome)

Exfoliative dermatitis

Bullous dermatitis herpetiformis
Severe seborrheic dermatitis
Severe psoriasis
Mycosis fungoides

5. Allergic States
Control of severe or incapacitating allergic conditions intractable to adequate trials of conventional treatment in:
Bronchial asthma
Contact dermatitis
Atopic dermatitis
Serum sickness
Seasonal or perennial allergic rhinitis
Drug hypersensitivity reactions
Urticarial transfusion reactions
Acute noninfectious laryngeal edema (epinephrine is the drug of first choice)

6. Ophthalmic Diseases
Severe acute and chronic allergic and inflammatory processes involving the eye, such as:
Herpes zoster ophthalmicus
Iritis, iridocyclitis
Chorioretinitis
Diffuse posterior uveitis and choroiditis
Optic neuritis
Sympathetic ophthalmia
Anterior segment inflammation
Allergic conjunctivitis
Allergic corneal marginal ulcers
Keratitis

7. Gastrointestinal Diseases
To tide the patient over a critical period of the disease in:
Ulcerative colitis (systemic therapy)
Regional enteritis (systemic therapy)

8. Respiratory Diseases
Symptomatic sarcoidosis
Berylliosis
Fulminating or disseminated pulmonary tuberculosis when used concurrently with appropriate antituberculous chemotherapy
Loeffler's syndrome not manageable by other means
Aspiration pneumonitis

9. Hematologic Disorders
Acquired (autoimmune) hemolytic anemia
Secondary thrombocytopenia in adults
Erythroblastopenia (RBC anemia)
Congenital (erythroid) hypoplastic anemia

10. Neoplastic Diseases
For palliative management of:
Leukemias and lymphomas in adults
Acute leukemia of childhood

11. Edematous States
To induce diuresis or remission of proteinuria in the nephrotic syndrome, without uremia, of the idiopathic type or that due to lupus erythematosus

12. Nervous System
Acute exacerbations of multiple sclerosis

13. Miscellaneous
Tuberculous meningitis with subarachnoid block or impending block when used concurrently with appropriate antituberculous chemotherapy
Trichinosis with neurologic or myocardial involvement

B. FOR INTRASYNOVIAL OR SOFT TISSUE ADMINISTRATION (See WARNINGS).
DEPO-MEDROL is indicated as adjunctive therapy for short-term administration (to tide the patient over an acute episode or exacerbation) in:
Synovitis of osteoarthritis
Rheumatoid arthritis
Acute and subacute bursitis
Acute gouty arthritis
Epicondylitis
Acute nonspecific tenosynovitis
Post-traumatic osteoarthritis

C. FOR INTRALESIONAL ADMINISTRATION
DEPO-MEDROL is indicated for intralesional use in the following conditions:
Keloids
Localized hypertrophic, infiltrated, inflammatory lesions of: lichen planus, psoriatic plaques, granuloma annulare, and lichen simplex chronicus (neurodermatitis)
Discoid lupus erythematosus
Necrobiosis lipoidica diabeticorum
Alopecia areata
DEPO-MEDROL also may be useful in cystic tumors of an aponeurosis or tendon (ganglia).

CONTRAINDICATIONS

DEPO-MEDROL Sterile Aqueous Suspension is contraindicated for intrathecal administration. This formulation of methylprednisolone acetate has been associated with reports of severe medical events when administered by this route. DEPO-MEDROL is also contraindicated in systemic fungal infections and patients with known hypersensitivity to the product and its constituents.

WARNINGS

This product is not suitable for multi-dose use. Following administration of the desired dose, any remaining suspension should be discarded.

While crystals of adrenal steroids in the dermis suppress inflammatory reactions, their presence may cause disintegration of the cellular elements and physiochemical changes in the ground substance of the connective tissue. The resultant infrequently occurring dermal and/or subdermal changes may form depressions in the skin at the injection site. The degree to which this reaction occurs will vary with the amount of adrenal steroid injected. Regeneration is usually complete within a few months or after all crystals of the adrenal steroid have been absorbed.

In order to minimize the incidence of dermal and subdermal atrophy, care must be exercised not to exceed recommended doses in injections. Multiple small injections into the area of the lesion should be made whenever possible. The technique of intrasynovial and intramuscular injection should include precautions against injection or leakage into the dermis. Injection into the deltoid muscle should be avoided because of a high incidence of subcutaneous atrophy.

It is critical that, during administration of DEPO-MEDROL, appropriate technique be used and care taken to assure proper placement of drug.

In patients on corticosteroid therapy subjected to any unusual stress, increased dosage of rapidly acting corticosteroids before, during, and after the stressful situation is indicated.

Corticosteroids may mask some signs of infection, and new infections may appear during their use. There may be decreased resistance and inability to localize infection when corticosteroids are used. Infections with any pathogen including viral, bacterial, fungal, protozoan or helminthic infections, in any location of the body, may be associated with the use of corticosteroids alone or in combination with other immunosuppressive agents that affect cellular immunity, humoral immunity, or neutrophil function.[1]

These infections may be mild, but can be severe and at times fatal. With increasing doses of corticosteroids, the rate of occurrence of infectious complications increases.[2] Do not use intra-articularly, intrabursally or for intratendinous administration for *local* effect in the presence of acute infection.

Prolonged use of corticosteroids may produce posterior subcapsular cataracts, glaucoma with possible damage to the optic nerves, and may enhance the establishment of secondary ocular infections due to fungi or viruses.

Usage in pregnancy. Since adequate human reproduction studies have not been done with corticosteroids, the use of these drugs in pregnancy, nursing mothers, or women of childbearing potential requires that the possible benefits of the drug be weighed against the potential hazards to the mother and embryo or fetus. Infants born of mothers who have received substantial doses of corticosteroids during pregnancy should be carefully observed for signs of hypoadrenalism.

Average and large doses of cortisone or hydrocortisone can cause elevation of blood pressure, salt and water retention, and increased excretion of potassium. These effects are less likely to occur with the synthetic derivatives except when used in large doses. Dietary salt restriction and potassium supplementation may be necessary. All corticosteroids increase calcium excretion.

Administration of live or live, attenuated vaccines is contraindicated in patients receiving immunosuppressive doses of corticosteroids. Killed or inactivated vaccines may be administered to patients receiving immunosuppressive doses of corticosteroids; however, the response to such vaccines may be diminished. Indicated immunization procedures may be undertaken in patients receiving nonimmunosuppressive doses of corticosteroids.

The use of DEPO-MEDROL in active tuberculosis should be restricted to those cases of fulminating or disseminated tuberculosis in which the corticosteroid is used for the management of the disease in conjunction with appropriate antituberculous regimen.

If corticosteroids are indicated in patients with latent tuberculosis or tuberculin reactivity, close observation is necessary as reactivation of the disease may occur. During prolonged corticosteroid therapy, these patients should receive chemoprophylaxis.

Because rare instances of anaphylactoid reactions have occurred in patients receiving parenteral corticosteroid therapy, appropriate precautionary measures should be taken prior to administration, especially when the patient has a history of allergy to any drug.

Persons who are on drugs which suppress the immune system are more susceptible to infections than healthy individuals. Chicken pox and measles, for example, can have a more serious or even fatal course in non-immune children or adults on corticosteroids. In such children or adults who have not had these diseases, particular care should be taken to avoid exposure. How the dose, route and duration of corticosteroid administration affects the risk of developing a disseminated infection is not known. The contribution of the underlying disease and/or prior corticosteroid treatment to the risk is also not known. If exposed to chicken pox, prophylaxis with varicella zoster immune globulin (VZIG) may be indicated. If exposed to measles, prophylaxis with pooled intramuscular immunoglobulin (IG) may be indicated. (See the respective package inserts for complete VZIG and IG prescribing information.) If chicken pox develops, treatment with antiviral agents may be considered. Similarly, corticosteroids should be used with great care in patients with known or suspected Strongyloides (threadworm) infestation. In such patients, corticosteroid-induced immunosuppression may lead to Strongyloides hyperinfection and dissemination with widespread larval migration, often accompanied by severe enterocolitis and potentially fatal gram-negative septicemia.

PRECAUTIONS

General precautions

Drug-induced secondary adrenocortical insufficiency may be minimized by gradual reduction of dosage. This type of relative insufficiency may persist for months after discontinuation of therapy; therefore, in any situation of stress occurring during that period, hormone therapy should be reinstituted. Since mineralocorticoid secretion may be impaired, salt and/or a mineralocorticoid should be administered concurrently.

There is an enhanced effect of corticosteroids in patients with hypothyroidism and in those with cirrhosis.

Corticosteroids should be used cautiously in patients with ocular herpes simplex for fear of corneal perforation.

The lowest possible dose of corticosteroid should be used to control the condition under treatment, and when reduction in dosage is possible, the reduction must be gradual.

Psychic derangements may appear when corticosteroids are used, ranging from euphoria, insomnia, mood swings, personality changes, and severe depression to frank psychotic manifestations. Also, existing emotional instability or psychotic tendencies may be aggravated by corticosteroids.

Steroids should be used with caution in nonspecific ulcerative colitis, if there is a probability of impending perforation, abscess or other pyogenic infection. Caution must also be used in diverticulitis, fresh intestinal anastomoses, active or latent peptic ulcer, renal insufficiency, hypertension, osteoporosis, and myasthenia gravis, when steroids are used as direct or adjunctive therapy.

Growth and development of infants and children on prolonged corticosteroid therapy should be carefully followed.

Kaposi's sarcoma has been reported to occur in patients receiving corticosteroid therapy. Discontinuation of corticosteroids may result in clinical remission.

The following additional precautions apply for parenteral corticosteroids. Intrasynovial injection of a corticosteroid may produce systemic as well as local effects.

Appropriate examination of any joint fluid present is necessary to exclude a septic process.

A marked increase in pain accompanied by local swelling, further restriction of joint motion, fever, and malaise are suggestive of septic arthritis. If this complication occurs and the diagnosis of sepsis is confirmed, appropriate antimicrobial therapy should be instituted.

Local injection of a steroid into a previously infected joint is to be avoided.

Corticosteroids should not be injected into unstable joints.

The slower rate of absorption by intramuscular administration should be recognized.

Although controlled clinical trials have shown corticosteroids to be effective in speeding the resolution of acute exacerbations of multiple sclerosis, they do not show that corticosteroids affect the ultimate outcome or natural history of the disease. The studies do show that relatively high doses of corticosteroids are necessary to demonstrate a significant effect. (See DOSAGE AND ADMINISTRATION.)

Since complications of treatment with glucocorticoids are dependent on the size of the dose and the duration of treatment, a risk/benefit decision must be made in each individual case as to dose and duration of treatment and as to whether daily or intermittent therapy should be used.

DRUG INTERACTIONS

The pharmacokinetic interactions listed below are potentially clinically important. Mutual inhibition of metabolism occurs with concurrent use of cyclosporin and methylprednisolone; therefore, it is possible that adverse events associated with the individual use of either drug may be more apt to occur. Convulsions have been reported with concurrent use of methylprednisolone and cyclosporin. Drugs that induce hepatic enzymes such as phenobarbital, phenytoin and rifampin may increase the clearance of methylprednisolone and may require increases in methylprednisolone dose to achieve the desired response. Drugs such as troleandomycin and ketoconazole may inhibit the metabolism of methylprednisolone and thus decrease its clearance. Therefore, the dose of methylprednisolone should be titrated to avoid steroid toxicity. Methylprednisolone may increase the clearance of chronic high dose aspirin. This could lead to decreased salicylate serum levels or increase the risk of salicylate toxicity when methylprednisolone is withdrawn. Aspirin should be used cautiously in conjunction with corticosteroids in patients suffering from hypoprothrombinemia. The effect of methylprednisolone on oral anticoagulants is variable. There are reports of enhanced as well as diminished effects of anticoagulant when given concurrently with corticosteroids. Therefore, coagulation indices should be monitored to maintain the desired anticoagulant effect.

Information for the Patient

Persons who are on immunosuppressant doses of corticosteroids should be warned to avoid exposure to chicken pox or measles. Patients should also be advised that if they are exposed, medical advice should be sought without delay.

ADVERSE REACTIONS

Fluid and electrolyte disturbances
Sodium retention
Fluid retention
Congestive heart failure in susceptible patients
Potassium loss
Hypokalemic alkalosis
Hypertension

Continued on next page

Depo-Medrol Single-Dose—Cont.

Musculoskeletal
Muscle weakness
Steroid myopathy
Loss of muscle mass
Osteoporosis
Tendon rupture, particularly of the Achilles tendon
Vertebral compression fractures
Aseptic necrosis of femoral and humeral heads
Pathologic fracture of long bones
Gastrointestinal
Peptic ulcer with possible subsequent perforation and hemorrhage
Pancreatitis
Abdominal distention
Ulcerative esophagitis
Increases in alanine transaminase (ALT, SGPT), aspartate transaminase (AST, SGOT), and alkaline phosphatase have been observed following corticosteroid treatment. These changes are usually small, not associated with any clinical syndrome and are reversible upon discontinuation.
Dermatologic
Impaired wound healing
Thin fragile skin
Petechiae and ecchymoses
Facial erythema
Increased sweating
May suppress reactions to skin tests
Neurological
Convulsions
Increased intracranial pressure with papilledema (pseudotumor cerebri) usually after treatment
Vertigo
Headache
Endocrine
Menstrual irregularities
Development of Cushingoid state
Suppression of growth in children
Secondary adrenocortical and pituitary unresponsiveness, particularly in times of stress, as in trauma, surgery or illness
Decreased carbohydrate tolerance
Manifestations of latent diabetes mellitus
Increased requirements for insulin or oral hypoglycemic agents in diabetes
Ophthalmic
Posterior subcapsular cataracts
Increased intraocular pressure
Glaucoma
Exophthalmos
Metabolic
Negative nitrogen balance due to protein catabolism
The following *additional* adverse reactions are related to parenteral corticosteroid therapy:
Anaphylactic reaction
Allergic or hypersensitivity reactions
Urticaria
Injection site infections following non-sterile administration (see WARNINGS)
Postinjection flare, following intrasynovial use
Charcot-like arthropathy
Hyperpigmentation or hypopigmentation
Subcutaneous and cutaneous atrophy
Sterile abscess
Adverse Reactions Reported with the Following Routes of Administration
Intrathecal/Epidural
Arachnoiditis
Meningitis
Paraparesis/paraplegia
Sensory disturbances
Bowel/bladder dysfunction
Headache
Seizures
Intranasal
Temporary/permanent visual impairment including blindness
Allergic reactions
Rhinitis
Ophthalmic
Temporary/permanent visual impairment including blindness
Increased intraocular pressure
Ocular and periocular inflammation including allergic reactions
Infection
Residue or slough at injection site
Miscellaneous injection sites (scalp, tonsillar fauces, sphenopalatine ganglion) blindness

DOSAGE AND ADMINISTRATION

Because of possible physical incompatibilities, DEPO-MEDROL Sterile Aqueous Suspension should not be diluted or mixed with other solutions.

A. Administration for Local Effect
Therapy with DEPO-MEDROL does not obviate the need for the conventional measures usually employed. Although this method of treatment will ameliorate symptoms, it is in no sense a cure and the hormone has no effect on the cause of the inflammation.
1. Rheumatoid and Osteoarthritis. The dose for intra-articular administration depends upon the size of the joint and varies with the severity of the condition in the individual patient. In chronic cases, injections may be repeated at intervals ranging from one to five or more weeks depending upon the degree of relief obtained from the initial injection. The doses in the following table are given as a general guide:

Size of Joint	*Examples*	*Range of Dosage*
Large	Knees Ankles Shoulders	20 to 80 mg
Medium	Elbows Wrists	10 to 40 mg
Small	Metacarpophalangeal Interphalangeal Sternoclavicular Acromioclavicular	4 to 10 mg

Procedure: It is recommended that the anatomy of the joint involved be reviewed before attempting intra-articular injection. In order to obtain the full anti-inflammatory effect it is important that the injection be made into the synovial space. Employing the same sterile technique as for a lumbar puncture, a sterile 20 to 24 gauge needle (on a dry syringe) is quickly inserted into the synovial cavity. Procaine infiltration is elective. The aspiration of only a few drops of joint fluid proves the joint space has been entered by the needle. *The injection site for each joint is determined by that location where the synovial cavity is most superficial and most free of large vessels and nerves.* With the needle in place, the aspirating syringe is removed and replaced by a second syringe containing the desired amount of DEPO-MEDROL. The plunger is then pulled outward slightly to aspirate synovial fluid and to make sure the needle is still in the synovial space. After injection, the joint is moved gently a few times to aid mixing of the synovial fluid and the suspension. The site is covered with a small sterile dressing.
Suitable sites for intra-articular injection are the knee, ankle, wrist, elbow, shoulder, phalangeal, and hip joints. Since difficulty is not infrequently encountered in entering the hip joint, precautions should be taken to avoid any large blood vessels in the area. Joints not suitable for injection are those that are anatomically inaccessible such as the spinal joints and those like the sacroiliac joints that are devoid of synovial space. Treatment failures are most frequently the result of failure to enter the joint space. Little or no benefit follows injection into surrounding tissue. If failures occur when injections into the synovial spaces are certain, as determined by aspiration of fluid, repeated injections are usually futile. Local therapy does not alter the underlying disease process, and whenever possible comprehensive therapy including physiotherapy and orthopedic correction should be employed.
Following intra-articular steroid therapy, care should be taken to avoid overuse of joints in which symptomatic benefit has been obtained. Negligence in this matter may permit an increase in joint deterioration that will more than offset the beneficial effects of the steroid.
Unstable joints should not be injected. Repeated intra-articular injection may in some cases result in instability of the joint. X-ray follow-up is suggested in selected cases to detect deterioration.
If a local anesthetic is used prior to injection of DEPO-MEDROL, the anesthetic package insert should be read carefully and all the precautions observed.
2. Bursitis. The area around the injection site is prepared in a sterile way and a wheal at the site made with 1 percent procaine hydrochloride solution. A 20 to 24 gauge needle attached to a dry syringe is inserted into the bursa and the fluid aspirated. The needle is left in place and the aspirating syringe changed for a small syringe containing the desired dose. After injection, the needle is withdrawn and a small dressing applied.
3. Miscellaneous: Ganglion, Tendinitis, Epicondylitis. In the treatment of conditions such as tendinitis or tenosynovitis, care should be taken, following application of a suitable antiseptic to the overlying skin, to inject the suspension into the tendon sheath rather than into the substance of the tendon. The tendon may be readily palpated when placed on a stretch. When treating conditions such as epicondylitis, the area of greatest tenderness should be outlined carefully and the suspension infiltrated into the area. For ganglia of the tendon sheaths, the suspension is injected directly into the cyst. In many cases, a single injection causes a marked decrease in the size of the cystic tumor and may effect disappearance. The usual sterile precautions should be observed of course, with each injection.
The dose in the treatment of the various conditions of the tendinous or bursal structures listed above varies with the condition being treated and ranges from 4 to 30 mg. In recurrent or chronic conditions, repeated injections may be necessary.
4. Injections for Local Effect in Dermatologic Conditions. Following cleansing with an appropriate antiseptic such as 70% alcohol, 20 to 60 mg of the suspension is injected into the lesion. It may be necessary to distribute doses ranging from 20 to 40 mg by repeated local injections in the case of large lesions. Care should be taken to avoid injection of sufficient material to cause blanching since this may be followed by a small slough. One to four injections are usually employed, the intervals between injections varying with the type of lesion being treated and the duration of improvement produced by the initial injection.

B. Administration for Systemic Effect.
The intramuscular dosage will vary with the condition being treated. When employed as a temporary substitute for oral therapy, a single injection during each 24-hour period of a dose of the suspension equal to the total daily oral dose of MEDROL® Tablets (methylprednisolone) is usually sufficient. When a prolonged effect is desired, the weekly dose may be calculated by multiplying the daily oral dose by 7 and given as a single intramuscular injection.
Dosage must be individualized according to the severity of the disease and response of the patient. For infants and children, the recommended dosage will have to be reduced, but dosage should be governed by the severity of the condition rather than by strict adherence to the ratio indicated by age or body weight.
Hormone therapy is an adjunct to, and not a replacement for, conventional therapy. Dosage must be decreased or discontinued gradually when the drug has been administered for more than a few days. The severity, prognosis and expected duration of the disease and the reaction of the patient to medication are primary factors in determining dosage. If a period of spontaneous remission occurs in a chronic condition, treatment should be discontinued. Routine laboratory studies, such as urinalysis, two-hour postprandial blood sugar, determination of blood pressure and body weight, and a chest X-ray should be made at regular intervals during prolonged therapy. Upper GI X-rays are desirable in patients with an ulcer history or significant dyspepsia.
In patients with the **adrenogenital syndrome**, a single intramuscular injection of 40 mg every two weeks may be adequate. For maintenance of patients with **rheumatoid arthritis**, the weekly intramuscular dose will vary from 40 to 120 mg. The usual dosage for patients with **dermatologic lesions** benefited by systemic corticoid therapy is 40 to 120 mg of methylprednisolone acetate administered intramuscularly at weekly intervals for one to four weeks. In acute severe dermatitis due to poison ivy, relief may result within 8 to 12 hours following intramuscular administration of a single dose of 80 to 120 mg. In chronic contact dermatitis repeated injections at 5 to 10 day intervals may be necessary. In seborrheic dermatitis, a weekly dose of 80 mg may be adequate to control the condition.
Following intramuscular administration of 80 to 120 mg to asthmatic patients, relief may result within 6 to 48 hours and persist for several days to two weeks. Similarly in patients with allergic rhinitis (hay fever) an intramuscular dose of 80 to 120 mg may be followed by relief of coryzal symptoms within six hours persisting for several days to three weeks.
If signs of stress are associated with the condition being treated, the dosage of the suspension should be increased. If a rapid hormonal effect of maximum intensity is required, the intravenous administration of highly soluble methylprednisolone sodium succinate is indicated.
Multiple Sclerosis
In treatment of acute exacerbations of multiple sclerosis daily doses of 200 mg of prednisolone for a week followed by 80 mg every other day for 1 month have been shown to be effective (4 mg of methylprednisolone is equivalent to 5 mg of prednisolone).

HOW SUPPLIED

DEPO-MEDROL Sterile Aqueous Suspension is available as single-dose vials in the following strengths and package sizes:

40 mg per mL	
1 mL vials	NDC 0009-3073-01
25 × 1 mL vials	NDC 0009-3073-03
80 mg per mL	
1 mL vials	NDC 0009-3475-01
25 × 1 mL vials	NDC 0009-3475-03

Store at controlled room temperature 20° to 25°C (68° to 77°F) [see USP].

REFERENCES

[1] Fekety R. Infections associated with corticosteroids and immunosuppressive therapy. In: Gorbach SL, Bartlett JG, Blacklow NR, eds. *Infectious Diseases.* Philadelphia: WB Saunders Company 1992:1050-1.
[2] Stuck AE, Minder CE, Frey FJ. Risk of infectious complications in patients taking glucocorticoids. *Rev Infect Dis* 1989:11(6):954-63.

℞ only

Pharmacia & Upjohn Company, a subsidiary of Pharmacia Corporation
Kalamazoo, Michigan 49001, USA 815 027 311
Revised March 2003 691211

DEPO-PROVERA® CONTRACEPTIVE INJECTION ℞

[*dĕ-pō prō-vĕ-ră*]
medroxyprogesterone acetate injectable suspension, USP

Patients should be counseled that this product does not protect against HIV infection (AIDS) and other sexually transmitted diseases.

DESCRIPTION

DEPO-PROVERA Contraceptive Injection contains medroxyprogesterone acetate, a derivative of progesterone, as its active ingredient. Medroxyprogesterone acetate is active by the parenteral and oral routes of administration. It is a white to off-white, odorless crystalline powder that is stable in air and that melts between 200°C and 210°C. It is freely soluble in chloroform, soluble in acetone and dioxane, sparingly soluble in alcohol and methanol, slightly soluble in ether, and insoluble in water.

The chemical name for medroxyprogesterone acetate is pregn-4-ene-3,20-dione, 17-(acetyloxy)-6-methyl-, (6ϵ)-. The structural formula is as follows:

medroxyprogesterone acetate

DEPO-PROVERA Contraceptive Injection for intramuscular (IM) injection is available in vials and prefilled syringes, each containing 1 mL of medroxyprogesterone acetate sterile aqueous suspension 150 mg/mL.

Each mL contains:

Medroxyprogesterone acetate	150 mg
Polyethylene glycol 3350	28.9 mg
Polysorbate 80	2.41 mg
Sodium chloride	8.68 mg
Methylparaben	1.37 mg
Propylparaben	0.150 mg
Water for injection	qs

When necessary, pH is adjusted with sodium hydroxide or hydrochloric acid, or both.

CLINICAL PHARMACOLOGY

DEPO-PROVERA Contraceptive Injection (medroxyprogesterone acetate), when administered at the recommended dose to women every 3 months, inhibits the secretion of gonadotropins which, in turn, prevents follicular maturation and ovulation and results in endometrial thinning. These actions produce its contraceptive effect.

Following a single 150 mg IM dose of DEPO-PROVERA Contraceptive Injection, medroxyprogesterone acetate concentrations, measured by an extracted radioimmunoassay procedure, increase for approximately 3 weeks to reach peak plasma concentrations of 1 to 7 ng/mL. The levels then decrease exponentially until they become undetectable (<100 pg/mL) between 120 to 200 days following injection. Using an unextracted radioimmunoassay procedure for the assay of medroxyprogesterone acetate in serum, the apparent half-life for medroxyprogesterone acetate following IM administration of DEPO-PROVERA Contraceptive Injection is approximately 50 days.

Women with lower body weights conceive sooner than women with higher body weights after discontinuing DEPO-PROVERA Contraceptive Injection.

The effect of hepatic and/or renal disease on the pharmacokinetics of DEPO-PROVERA Contraceptive Injection is unknown.

INDICATIONS AND USAGE

DEPO-PROVERA Contraceptive Injection is indicated only for the prevention of pregnancy. To ensure that DEPO-PROVERA Contraceptive Injection is not administered inadvertently to a pregnant woman, the first injection must be given **ONLY** during the first 5 days of a normal menstrual period; **ONLY** within the first 5-days postpartum if not breast-feeding, and if exclusively breast-feeding, **ONLY** at the sixth postpartum week. The efficacy of DEPO-PROVERA Contraceptive Injection depends on adherence to the recommended dosage schedule (see DOSAGE AND ADMINISTRATION). It is a long-term injectable contraceptive in women when administered at 3-month (13-week) intervals. Dosage does not need to be adjusted for body weight.

In five clinical studies using DEPO-PROVERA Contraceptive Injection, the 12-month failure rate for the group of women treated with DEPO-PROVERA Contraceptive Injection was zero (no pregnancies reported) to 0.7 by Life-Table method. Pregnancy rates with contraceptive measures are typically reported for only the first year of use as shown in Table 1. Except for intrauterine devices (IUD), implants, sterilization, and DEPO-PROVERA Contraceptive Injection, the efficacy of these contraceptive measures depends in part on the reliability of use. The effectiveness of DEPO-PROVERA Contraceptive Injection is dependent on the patient returning every 3 months (13 weeks) for reinjection.

Table 1
Lowest Expected and Typical Failure Rates*
Expressed as Percent of Women Experiencing an Accidental Pregnancy in the First Year of Continuous Use

Method	Lowest Expected	Typical
Injectable progestogen		
DEPO-PROVERA	0.3	0.3
Implants		
Norplant (6 capsules)	0.2†	0.2†
Female sterilization	0.2	0.4
Male sterilization	0.1	0.15
Pill		3
Combined	0.1	
Progestogen only	0.5	
IUD		3
Progestasert	2	
Copper T 380A	0.8	
Condom	2	12
Diaphragm	6	18
Cap	6	18
Spermicides	3	21
Sponge		
Parous women	9	28
Nulliparous women	6	18
Periodic abstinence	1-9	20
Withdrawal	4	18
No method	85	85

Source: Trussell et al[1]

*Lowest expected - when used exactly as directed.
Typical - includes those not following directions exactly.

†from Norplant® package insert

CONTRAINDICATIONS

1. Known or suspected pregnancy or as a diagnostic test for pregnancy.
2. Undiagnosed vaginal bleeding.
3. Known or suspected malignancy of breast.
4. Active thrombophlebitis, or current or past history of thromboembolic disorders, or cerebral vascular disease.
5. Liver dysfunction or disease.
6. Known hypersensitivity to DEPO-PROVERA Contraceptive Injection (medroxyprogesterone acetate or any of its other ingredients).

WARNINGS

1. *Bleeding Irregularities*

Most women using DEPO-PROVERA Contraceptive Injection experience disruption of menstrual bleeding patterns. Altered menstrual bleeding patterns include irregular or unpredictable bleeding or spotting, or rarely, heavy or continuous bleeding. If abnormal bleeding persists or is severe, appropriate investigation should be instituted to rule out the possibility of organic pathology, and appropriate treatment should be instituted when necessary.

As women continue using DEPO-PROVERA Contraceptive Injection, fewer experience irregular bleeding and more experience amenorrhea. By month 12 amenorrhea was reported by 55% of women, and by month 24 amenorrhea was reported by 68% of women using DEPO-PROVERA Contraceptive Injection.[2]

2. *Bone Mineral Density Changes*

Use of DEPO-PROVERA Contraceptive Injection may be considered among the risk factors for development of osteoporosis. The rate of bone loss is greatest in the early years of use and then subsequently approaches the normal rate of age related fall.

3. *Cancer Risks*

Long-term case-controlled surveillance of users of DEPO-PROVERA Contraceptive Injection found slight or no increased overall risk of breast cancer[3] and no overall increased risk of ovarian,[4] liver,[5] or cervical[6] cancer and a prolonged, protective effect of reducing the risk of endometrial[7] cancer in the population of users.

A pooled analysis[14] from two case-control studies, the World Health Organization Study[3] and the New Zealand Study[13], reported the relative risk (RR) of breast cancer for women who had ever used DEPO-PROVERA Contraceptive Injection as 1.1 (95% confidence interval (CI) 0.97 to 1.4). Overall, there was no increase in risk with increasing duration of use of DEPO-PROVERA Contraceptive Injection. The RR of breast cancer for women of all ages who had initiated use of DEPO-PROVERA Contraceptive Injection within the previous 5 years was estimated to be 2.0 (95% CI 1.5 to 2.8).

The World Health Organization Study[3], a component of the pooled analysis[14] described above, showed an increased RR of 2.19 (95% CI 1.23 to 3.89) of breast cancer associated with use of DEPO-PROVERA Contraceptive Injection in women whose first exposure to drug was within the previous 4 years and who were under 35 years of age. However, the overall RR for ever-users of DEPO-PROVERA Contraceptive Injection was only 1.2 (95% CI 0.96 to 1.52).

[**NOTE**: A RR of 1.0 indicates neither an increased nor a decreased risk of cancer associated with the use of the drug, relative to no use of the drug. In the case of the subpopulation with a RR of 2.19, the 95% CI is fairly wide and does not include the value of 1.0, thus inferring an increased risk of breast cancer in the defined subgroup relative to nonusers. The value of 2.19 means that women whose first exposure to drug was within the previous 4 years and who are under 35 years of age have a 2.19-fold (95% CI 1.23 to 3.89-fold) increased risk of breast cancer relative to nonusers. The National Cancer Institute[8] reports an average annual incidence rate for breast cancer for US women, all races, age 30 to 34 years of 26.7 per 100,000. A RR of 2.19, thus, increases the possible risk from 26.7 to 58.5 cases per 100,000 women. The attributable risk, thus, is 31.8 per 100,000 women per year.]

A statistically insignificant increase in RR estimates of invasive squamous-cell cervical cancer has been associated with the use of DEPO-PROVERA Contraceptive Injection in women who were first exposed before the age of 35 years (RR 1.22 to 1.28 and 95% CI 0.93 to 1.70). The overall, nonsignificant relative rate of invasive squamous-cell cervical cancer in women who ever used DEPO-PROVERA Contraceptive Injection was estimated to be 1.11 (95% CI 0.96 to 1.29). No trends in risk with duration of use or times since initial or most recent exposure were observed.

4. *Thromboembolic Disorders*

The physician should be alert to the earliest manifestations of thrombotic disorders (thrombophlebitis, pulmonary embolism, cerebrovascular disorders, and retinal thrombosis). Should any of these occur or be suspected, the drug should not be readministered.

5. *Ocular Disorders*

Medication should not be readministered pending examination if there is a sudden partial or complete loss of vision or if there is a sudden onset of proptosis, diplopia, or migraine. If examination reveals papilledema or retinal vascular lesions, medication should not be readministered.

6. *Unexpected Pregnancies*

To ensure that DEPO-PROVERA Contraceptive Injection is not administered inadvertently to a pregnant woman, the first injection must be given **ONLY** during the first 5 days of a normal menstrual period; **ONLY** within the first 5-days postpartum if not breast-feeding, and if exclusively breast-feeding, **ONLY** at the sixth postpartum week (see DOSAGE AND ADMINISTRATION).

Neonates from unexpected pregnancies that occur 1 to 2 months after injection of DEPO-PROVERA Contraceptive Injection may be at an increased risk of low birth weight, which, in turn, is associated with an increased risk of neonatal death. The attributable risk is low because such pregnancies are uncommon.[9,10]

A significant increase in incidence of polysyndactyly and chromosomal anomalies was observed among infants of users of DEPO-PROVERA Contraceptive Injection, the former being most pronounced in women under 30 years of age. The unrelated nature of these defects, the lack of confirmation from other studies, the distant preconceptual exposure to DEPO-PROVERA Contraceptive Injection, and the chance effects due to multiple statistical comparisons, make a causal association unlikely.[11]

Neonates exposed to medroxyprogesterone acetate *in utero* and followed to adolescence, showed no evidence of any adverse effects on their health including their physical, intellectual, sexual, or social development.

Several reports suggest an association between intrauterine exposure to progestational drugs in the first trimester of pregnancy and genital abnormalities in male and female fetuses. The risk of hypospadias (five to eight per 1,000 male births in the general population) may be approximately doubled with exposure to these drugs. There are insufficient data to quantify the risk to exposed female fetuses, but because some of these drugs induce mild virilization of the external genitalia of the female fetus and because of the increased association of hypospadias in the male fetus, it is prudent to avoid the use of these drugs during the first trimester of pregnancy.

To ensure that DEPO-PROVERA Contraceptive Injection is not administered inadvertently to a pregnant woman, it is important that the first injection be given only during the first 5 days after the onset of a normal menstrual period within 5 days postpartum if not breast-feeding and if breast-feeding, at the sixth week postpartum (see DOSAGE AND ADMINISTRATION).

7. *Ectopic Pregnancy*

Health-care providers should be alert to the possibility of an ectopic pregnancy among women using DEPO-PROVERA Contraceptive Injection who become pregnant or complain of severe abdominal pain.

8. *Lactation*

Detectable amounts of drug have been identified in the milk of mothers receiving DEPO-PROVERA Contraceptive Injection. In nursing mothers treated with DEPO-PROVERA Contraceptive Injection, milk composition, quality, and amount are not adversely affected. Neonates and infants exposed to medroxyprogesterone from breast milk have been studied for developmental and behavioral effects through puberty. No adverse effects have been noted.

Continued on next page

Depo-Provera Contraceptive—Cont.

9. Anaphylaxis and Anaphylactoid Reaction
Anaphylaxis and anaphylactoid reaction have been reported with the use of DEPO-PROVERA Contraceptive Injection. If an anaphylactic reaction occurs appropriate therapy should be instituted. Serious anaphylactic reactions require emergency medical treatment.

PRECAUTIONS

GENERAL

1. Physical Examination
It is good medical practice for all women to have annual history and physical examinations, including women using DEPO-PROVERA Contraceptive Injection. The physical examination, however, may be deferred until after initiation of DEPO-PROVERA if requested by the woman and judged appropriate by the clinician. The physical examination should include special reference to blood pressure, breasts, abdomen and pelvic organs, including cervical cytology and relevant laboratory tests. In case of undiagnosed, persistent or recurrent abnormal vaginal bleeding, appropriate measures should be conducted to rule out malignancy. Women with a strong family history of breast cancer or who have breast nodules should be monitored with particular care.

2. Fluid Retention
Because progestational drugs may cause some degree of fluid retention, conditions that might be influenced by this condition, such as epilepsy, migraine, asthma, and cardiac or renal dysfunction, require careful observation.

3. Weight Changes
There is a tendency for women to gain weight while on therapy with DEPO-PROVERA Contraceptive Injection. From an initial average body weight of 136 lb, women who completed 1 year of therapy with DEPO-PROVERA Contraceptive Injection gained an average of 5.4 lb. Women who completed 2 years of therapy gained an average of 8.1 lb. Women who completed 4 years gained an average of 13.8 lb. Women who completed 6 years gained an average of 16.5 lb. Two percent of women withdrew from a large-scale clinical trial because of excessive weight gain.

4. Return of Fertility
DEPO-PROVERA Contraceptive Injection has a prolonged contraceptive effect. In a large US study of women who discontinued use of DEPO-PROVERA Contraceptive Injection to become pregnant, data are available for 61% of them. Based on Life-Table analysis of these data, it is expected that 68% of women who do become pregnant may conceive within 12 months, 83% may conceive within 15 months, and 93% may conceive within 18 months from the last injection. The median time to conception for those who do conceive is 10 months following the last injection with a range of 4 to 31 months, and is unrelated to the duration of use. No data are available for 39% of the patients who discontinued DEPO-PROVERA Contraceptive Injection to become pregnant and who were lost to follow-up or changed their mind.

5. CNS Disorders and Convulsions
Patients who have a history of psychic depression should be carefully observed and the drug not be readministered if the depression recurs.
There have been a few reported cases of convulsions in patients who were treated with DEPO-PROVERA Contraceptive Injection. Association with drug use or pre-existing conditions is not clear.

6. Carbohydrate Metabolism
A decrease in glucose tolerance has been observed in some patients on DEPO-PROVERA Contraceptive Injection treatment. The mechanism of this decrease is obscure. For this reason, diabetic patients should be carefully observed while receiving such therapy.

7. Liver Function
If jaundice develops, consideration should be given to not readministering the drug.

8. Protection Against Sexually Transmitted Diseases
Patients should be counseled that this product does not protect against HIV infection (AIDS) and other sexually transmitted diseases.

DRUG INTERACTIONS
Aminoglutethimide administered concomitantly with the DEPO-PROVERA Contraceptive Injection may significantly depress the serum concentrations of medroxyprogesterone acetate.[12] Users of DEPO-PROVERA Contraceptive Injection should be warned of the possibility of decreased efficacy with the use of this or any related drugs.

LABORATORY TEST INTERACTIONS
The pathologist should be advised of progestin therapy when relevant specimens are submitted.
The following laboratory tests may be affected by progestins including DEPO-PROVERA Contraceptive Injection:

(a) Plasma and urinary steroid levels are decreased (eg, progesterone, estradiol, pregnanediol, testosterone, cortisol).
(b) Gonadotropin levels are decreased.
(c) Sex-hormone-binding-globulin concentrations are decreased.
(d) Protein-bound iodine and butanol extractable protein-bound iodine may increase.
T_3-uptake values may decrease.
(e) Coagulation test values for prothrombin (Factor II), and Factors VII, VIII, IX, and X may increase.
(f) Sulfobromophthalein and other liver function test values may be increased.
(g) The effects of medroxyprogesterone acetate on lipid metabolism are inconsistent. Both increases and decreases in total cholesterol, triglycerides, low-density lipoprotein (LDL) cholesterol, and high-density lipoprotein (HDL) cholesterol have been observed in studies.

CARCINOGENESIS
See "WARNINGS" section 3.

PREGNANCY
Pregnancy Category X. See "WARNINGS" section 6.

NURSING MOTHERS
See "WARNINGS" section 8.

PEDIATRIC USE
Safety and effectiveness in pediatric patients have not been established. See "WARNINGS" section 6.

INFORMATION FOR THE PATIENT
See Patient Labeling.
Patient labeling is included with each single-dose vial and pre-filled syringe of DEPO-PROVERA Contraceptive Injection to help describe its characteristics to the patient. It is recommended that prospective users be given this labeling and be informed about the risks and benefits associated with the use of DEPO-PROVERA Contraceptive Injection, as compared with other forms of contraception or with no contraception at all. It is recommended that physicians or other health-care providers responsible for those patients advise them at the beginning of treatment that their menstrual cycle may be disrupted and that irregular and unpredictable bleeding or spotting results, and that this usually decreases to the point of amenorrhea as treatment with DEPO-PROVERA Contraceptive Injection continues, without other therapy being required.

ADVERSE REACTIONS

In the largest clinical trial with DEPO-PROVERA Contraceptive Injection, over 3,900 women, who were treated for up to 7 years, reported the following adverse reactions, which may or may not be related to the use of DEPO-PROVERA Contraceptive Injection.
The following adverse reactions were reported by more than 5% of subjects:

Menstrual irregularities (bleeding or amenorrhea, or both)
Abdominal pain or discomfort
Weight changes
Dizziness
Headache
Asthenia (weakness or fatigue)
Nervousness

Adverse reactions reported by 1% to 5% of subjects using DEPO-PROVERA Contraceptive Injection were:

Decreased libido or anorgasmia
Pelvic pain
Backache
Breast pain
Leg cramps
No hair growth or alopecia
Depression
Bloating
Nausea
Rash
Insomnia
Edema
Leukorrhea
Hot flashes
Acne
Arthralgia
Vaginitis

Events reported by fewer than 1% of subjects included: galactorrhea, melasma, chloasma, convulsions, changes in appetite, gastrointestinal disturbances, jaundice, genitourinary infections, vaginal cysts, dyspareunia, paresthesia, chest pain, pulmonary embolus, allergic reactions, anemia, drowsiness, syncope, dyspnea and asthma, tachycardia, fever, excessive sweating and body odor, dry skin, chills, increased libido, excessive thirst, hoarseness, pain at injection site, blood dyscrasia, rectal bleeding, changes in breast size, breast lumps or nipple bleeding, axillary swelling, breast cancer, prevention of lactation, sensation of pregnancy, lack of return to fertility, paralysis, facial palsy, scleroderma, osteoporosis, uterine hyperplasia, cervical cancer, varicose veins, dysmenorrhea, hirsutism, unexpected pregnancy, thrombophlebitis, deep vein thrombosis.
In addition, voluntary reports have been received of anaphylaxis and anaphylactoid reaction with use of DEPO-PROVERA Contraceptive Injection.

DOSAGE AND ADMINISTRATION

Both the 1 mL vial and the 1 mL prefilled syringe of DEPO-PROVERA Contraceptive Injection should be vigorously shaken just before use to ensure that the dose being administered represents a uniform suspension.
The recommended dose is 150 mg of DEPO-PROVERA Contraceptive Injection every 3 months (13 weeks) administered by deep, IM injection in the gluteal or deltoid muscle. To ensure the patient is not pregnant at the time of the first injection, the first injection **MUST** be given **ONLY** during the first 5 days of a normal menstrual period; **ONLY** within the first 5-days postpartum if not breast-feeding; and if exclusively breast-feeding, **ONLY** at the sixth postpartum week. If the time interval between injections is greater than 13 weeks, the physician should determine that the patient is not pregnant before administering the drug. The efficacy of DEPO-PROVERA Contraceptive Injection depends on adherence to the dosage schedule of administration.

HOW SUPPLIED

DEPO-PROVERA Contraceptive Injection (medroxyprogesterone acetate sterile aqueous suspension 150 mg/mL) is available as:

NDC 0009-0746-30	1 mL vial
NDC 0009-0746-35	25 × 1 mL vials
NDC 0009-7376-01	1 mL prefilled syringe
NDC 0009-7376-02	6 × 1 mL prefilled syringes
NDC 0009-7376-03	24 × 1 mL prefilled syringes

DEPO-PROVERA Contraceptive Injection prefilled syringes are available packaged with 22-gauge × 1 1/2 inch BD SafetyGlide™ Needles in the following presentations:

NDC 0009-7376-04	1 mL prefilled syringe
NDC 0009-7376-05	6 × 1 mL prefilled syringes
NDC 0009-7376-06	24 × 1 mL prefilled syringes

Store at controlled room temperature 20° to 25°C (68° to 77°F) [see USP].

REFERENCES

1. Trussell J, Hatcher RA, Cates W Jr, Stewart FH, Kost K. A guide to interpreting contraceptive efficacy studies. Obstet Gynecol. 1990; *76*:558-567.
2. Schwallie PC, Assenzo JR. Contraceptive use-efficacy study utilizing medroxyprogesterone acetate administered as an intramuscular injection once every 90 days. Fertil Steril. 1973; *24*:331-339.
3. WHO Collaborative Study of Neoplasia and Steroid Contraceptives. Breast cancer and depot-medroxyprogesterone acetate: a multi-national study. Lancet. 1991; *338*:833-838.
4. WHO Collaborative Study of Neoplasia and Steroid Contraceptives. Depot-medroxyprogesterone acetate (DMPA) and risk of epithelial ovarian cancer. Int J Cancer. 1991; *49*:191-195.
5. WHO Collaborative Study of Neoplasia and Steroid Contraceptives. Depot-medroxyprogesterone acetate (DMPA) and risk of liver cancer. Int J Cancer. 1991; *49*: 182-185.
6. WHO Collaborative Study of Neoplasia and Steroid Contraceptives. Depot-medroxyprogesterone acetate (DMPA) and risk of invasive squamous-cell cervical cancer. Contraception. 1992; *45*:299-312.
7. WHO Collaborative Study of Neoplasia and Steroid Contraceptives. Depot-medroxyprogesterone acetate (DMPA) and risk of endometrial cancer. Int J Cancer. 1991; *49*:186-190.
8. Surveillance, Epidemiology, and End Results: Incidence and Mortality Data, 1973–1977. National Cancer Institute Monograph, 57: June 1981. (NIH publication No. 81-2330).
9. Gray RH, Pardthaisong T. *In Utero* exposure to steroid contraceptives and survival during infancy. Am J Epidemiol. 1991; *134*:804-811.
10. Pardthaisong T, Gray RH. *In Utero* exposure to steroid contraceptives and outcome of pregnancy. Am J Epidemiol. 1991; *134*:795-803.
11. Pardthaisong T, Gray RH, McDaniel EB, Chandacham A. Steroid contraceptive use and pregnancy outcome. Teratology. 1988; *38*:51-58.
12. Van Deijk WA, Biljham GH, Mellink WAM, Meulenberg PMM. Influence of aminoglutethimide on plasma levels of medroxyprogesterone acetate: its correlation with serum cortisol. Cancer Treatment Reports. 1985; *69*:1, 85-90.
13. Paul C, Skegg DCG, Spears GFS. Depot medroxyprogesterone (Depo-Provera) and risk of breast cancer. Br Med J. 1989; *299*:759-762.
14. Skegg DCG, Noonan EA, Paul C, Spears GFS, Meirik O, Thomas DB. Depot Medroxyprogesterone Acetate and Breast Cancer: A Pooled Analysis from the World Health Organization and New Zealand Studies. JAMA. 1995; *273(10)*:799-804.

℞ only

DEPO-PROVERA Contraceptive Injection 1 mL vials are manufactured by:
Pharmacia & Upjohn Company
Kalamazoo, MI 49001, USA
DEPO-PROVERA Contraceptive Injection 1 mL prefilled syringes are manufactured by:
Pharmacia & Upjohn, N.V./S.A.
Puurs, Belgium
for:
Pharmacia & Upjohn Company
A subsidiary of Pharmacia Corporation
Kalamazoo, MI 49001, USA
Revised July 2003 815 461 714
692843

DEPO-PROVERA® ℞

[*dĕ-pō prō-vĕ-ră*]

medroxyprogesterone acetate injectable suspension, USP

DESCRIPTION

DEPO-PROVERA Sterile Aqueous Suspension contains medroxyprogesterone acetate, which is a derivative of progesterone and is active by the parenteral and oral routes of administration. It is a white to off-white, odorless crystalline powder, stable in air, melting between 200° and 210° C.

It is freely soluble in chloroform, soluble in acetone and in dioxane, sparingly soluble in alcohol and methanol, slightly soluble in ether and insoluble in water.

The chemical name for medroxyprogesterone acetate is Pregn-4-ene-3,20-dione, 17-(acetyloxy)-6-methyl-, (6α)-. The structural formula is:

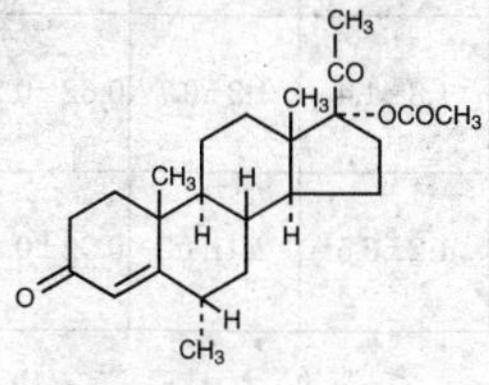

medroxyprogesterone acetate

DEPO-PROVERA for intramuscular injection is available as 400 mg/mL medroxyprogesterone acetate. Each mL of the 400 mg/mL suspension contains:

Medroxyprogesterone acetate	400 mg
Polyethylene glycol 3350	20.3 mg
Sodium sulfate anhydrous	11 mg
with	
Myristyl-gamma-picolinium chloride	1.69 mg
added as preservative	

When necessary, pH was adjusted with sodium hydroxide and/or hydrochloric acid.

ACTIONS

Medroxyprogesterone acetate, administered parenterally in the recommended doses to women with adequate endogenous estrogen, transforms proliferative endometrium into secretory endometrium.

Medroxyprogesterone acetate inhibits (in the usual dose range) the secretion of pituitary gonadotropin which, in turn, prevents follicular maturation and ovulation.

Because of its prolonged action and the resulting difficulty in predicting the time of withdrawal bleeding following injection, medroxyprogesterone acetate is not recommended in secondary amenorrhea or dysfunctional uterine bleeding. In these conditions oral therapy is recommended.

INDICATIONS AND USES

Adjunctive therapy and palliative treatment of inoperable, recurrent, and metastatic endometrial or renal carcinoma.

CONTRAINDICATIONS

1. Known or suspected pregnancy or as a diagnostic test for pregnancy
2. Undiagnosed vaginal bleeding
3. Known or suspected malignancy of breast
4. Active thrombophlebitis, or current or past history of thromboembolic disorders, or cerebral vascular disease
5. Liver dysfunction or disease
6. Known sensitivity to DEPO-PROVERA (medroxyprogesterone acetate or any of its other ingredients).

WARNINGS

1. *Pregnancy* The use of progestational drugs during the first four months of pregnancy is not recommended. Progestational agents have been used beginning with the first trimester of pregnancy in attempts to prevent abortion but there is no evidence that such use is effective. Furthermore, the use of progestational agents, with their uterine-relaxant properties, in patients with fertilized defective ova may cause a delay in spontaneous abortion.

2. *Intrauterine Exposure* Several reports suggest an association between intrauterine exposure to progestational drugs in the first trimester of pregnancy and genital abnormalities in male and female fetuses. The risk of hypospadias (5 to 8 per 1,000 male births in the general population) may be approximately doubled with exposure to these drugs. There are insufficient data to quantify the risk to exposed female fetuses, but insofar as some of these drugs induce mild virilization of the external genitalia of the female fetus, and because of the increased association of hypospadias in the male fetus, it is prudent to avoid the use of these drugs during the first trimester of pregnancy.

If the patient is exposed to DEPO-PROVERA Sterile Aqueous Suspension during the first four months of pregnancy or if she becomes pregnant while taking this drug, she should be apprised of the potential risks to the fetus.

3. *Thromboembolic Disorders* The physician should be alert to the earliest manifestations of thrombotic disorder (thrombophlebitis, cerebrovascular disorder, pulmonary embolism, and retinal thrombosis). Should any of these occur or be suspected, the drug should be discontinued immediately.

4. *Ocular Disorders* Medication should be discontinued pending examination if there is a sudden partial or complete loss of vision, or if there is a sudden onset of proptosis, diplopia or migraine. If examination reveals papilledema or retinal vascular lesions, medication should be withdrawn.

5. *Lactation* Detectable amounts of drug have been identified in the milk of mothers receiving progestational drugs. The effect of this on the nursing infant has not been determined.

6. *Multi-dose Use* Multi-dose use of DEPO-PROVERA Sterile Aqueous Suspension from a single vial requires special care to avoid contamination. Although initially sterile, any multi-dose use of vials may lead to contamination unless strict aseptic technique is observed.

PRECAUTIONS

1. *Physical Examination* It is good medical practice for all women to have annual history and physical examinations, including women using DEPO-PROVERA Sterile Aqueous Suspension. The physical examination, however, may be deferred until after initiation of DEPO-PROVERA if requested by the woman and judged appropriate by the clinician. The physical examination should include special reference to blood pressure, breasts, abdomen and pelvic organs, including cervical cytology and relevant laboratory tests. In case of undiagnosed, persistent or recurrent abnormal vaginal bleeding, appropriate measures should be conducted to rule out malignancy. Women with a strong family history of breast cancer or who have breast nodules should be monitored with particular care.

2. *Fluid Retention* Because progestational drugs may cause some degree of fluid retention, conditions which might be influenced by this condition, such as epilepsy, migraine, asthma, cardiac or renal dysfunction, require careful observation.

3. *Vaginal Bleeding* In cases of breakthrough bleeding, as in all cases of irregular bleeding per vaginum, nonfunctional causes should be borne in mind and adequate diagnostic measures undertaken.

4. *Depression* Patients who have a history of psychic depression should be carefully observed and the drug discontinued if the depression recurs to a serious degree.

5. *Masking of Climacteric* The age of the patient constitutes no absolute limiting factor although treatment with progestin may mask the onset of the climacteric.

6. *Use with Estrogen* Studies of the addition of a progestin product to an estrogen replacement regimen for seven or more days of a cycle of estrogen administration have reported a lowered incidence of endometrial hyperplasia. Morphological and biochemical studies of endometria suggest that 10-13 days of a progestin are needed to provide maximal maturation of the endometrium and to eliminate any hyperplastic changes. Whether this will provide protection from endometrial carcinoma has not been clearly established.

There are possible risks which may be associated with the inclusion of progestin in estrogen replacement regimen, including adverse effects on carbohydrate and lipid metabolism. The dosage used may be important in minimizing these adverse effects.

A decrease in glucose tolerance has been observed in a small percentage of patients on estrogen-progestin combination treatment. The mechanism of this decrease is obscure. For this reason, diabetic patients should be carefully observed while receiving such therapy.

7. *Prolonged Use* The effect of prolonged use of DEPO-PROVERA Sterile Aqueous Suspension at the recommended doses on pituitary, ovarian, adrenal, hepatic, and uterine function is not known.

8. *Multi-dose Use* When multi-dose vials are used, special care to prevent contamination of the contents is essential. There is some evidence that benzalkonium chloride is not an adequate antiseptic for sterilizing DEPO-PROVERA Sterile Aqueous Suspension multi-dose vials. A povidone-iodine solution or similar product is recommended to cleanse the vial top prior to aspiration of contents. (See WARNINGS)

DRUG INTERACTIONS

Aminoglutethimide administered concomitantly with DEPO-PROVERA Sterile Aqueous Suspension may significantly depress the serum concentrations of medroxyprogesterone acetate. DEPO-PROVERA users should be warned of the possibility of decreased efficacy with the use of this or any related drugs.

LABORATORY TEST INTERACTIONS

The pathologist should be advised of progestin therapy when relevant specimens are submitted. The following laboratory tests may be affected by progestins including DEPO-PROVERA Sterile Aqueous Suspension:

a) Plasma and urinary steroid levels are decreased (e.g. progesterone, estradiol, pregnanediol, testosterone, cortisol).
b) Gonadotropin levels are decreased.
c) Sex-hormone binding globulin concentrations are decreased.
d) Protein bound iodine and butanol extractable protein bound iodine may increase. T_3 uptake values may decrease.
e) Coagulation test values for prothrombin (Factor II), and Factors VII, VIII, IX, and X may increase.
f) Sulfobromophthalein and other liver function test values may be increased.
g) The effects of medroxyprogesterone acetate on lipid metabolism are inconsistent. Both increases and decreases in total cholesterol, triglycerides, low-density lipoprotein (LDL) cholesterol, and high-density lipoprotein (HDL) cholesterol have been observed in studies.

CARCINOGENESIS, MUTAGENESIS, IMPAIRMENT OF FERTILITY

Long-term intramuscular administration of Medroxyprogesterone acetate (MPA) has been shown to produce mammary tumors in beagle dogs. There is no evidence of a carcinogenic effect associated with the oral administration of MPA to rats and mice. Medroxyprogesterone acetate was not mutagenic in a battery of *in vitro* or *in vivo* genetic toxicity assays.

Medroxyprogesterone acetate at high doses is an antifertility drug and high doses would be expected to impair fertility until the cessation of treatment.

INFORMATION FOR THE PATIENT

See Patient Information at end of insert.

ADVERSE REACTIONS

— (See WARNINGS for possible adverse effects on the fetus)
— breakthrough bleeding
— spotting
— change in menstrual flow
— amenorrhea
— headache
— nervousness
— dizziness
— edema
— change in weight (increase or decrease)
— changes in cervical erosion and cervical secretions
— cholestatic jaundice, including neonatal jaundice
— breast tenderness and galactorrhea
— skin sensitivity reactions consisting of urticaria, pruritus, edema and generalized rash
— acne, alopecia and hirsutism
— rash (allergic) with and without pruritis
— anaphylactoid reactions and anaphylaxis
— mental depression
— pyrexia
— fatigue
— insomnia
— nausea
— somnolence

In a few instances there have been undesirable sequelae at the site of injection, such as residual lump, change in color of skin, or sterile abscess.

A statistically significant association has been demonstrated between use of estrogen-progestin combination drugs and pulmonary embolism and cerebral thrombosis and embolism. For this reason patients on progestin therapy should be carefully observed. There is also evidence suggestive of an association with neuro-ocular lesions, e.g. retinal thrombosis and optic neuritis.

The following adverse reactions have been observed in patients receiving estrogen-progestin combination drugs:
— rise in blood pressure in susceptible individuals
— premenstrual syndrome
— changes in libido
— changes in appetite
— cystitis-like syndrome
— headache
— nervousness
— fatigue
— backache
— hirsutism
— loss of scalp hair
— erythema multiforma
— erythema nodosum
— hemorrhagic eruption
— itching
— dizziness

The following laboratory results may be altered by the use of estrogen-progestin combination drugs:
— increased sulfobromophthalein retention and other hepatic function tests
— coagulation tests: increase in prothrombin factors VII, VIII, IX, and X
— metyrapone test
— pregnanediol determinations
— thyroid function: increase in PBI, and butanol extractable protein bound iodine and decrease in T_3 uptake values

DOSAGE AND ADMINISTRATION

The suspension is intended for intramuscular administration only.

Endometrial or renal carcinoma—doses of 400 mg to 1000 mg of DEPO-PROVERA Sterile Aqueous Suspension per week are recommended initially. If improvement is noted within a few weeks or months and the disease appears stabilized, it may be possible to maintain improvement with as little as 400 mg per month. Medroxyprogesterone acetate is not recommended as primary therapy, but as adjunctive and palliative treatment in advanced inoperable cases including those with recurrent or metastatic disease.

When multi-dose vials are used, special care to prevent contamination of the contents is essential (See WARNINGS).

HOW SUPPLIED

DEPO-PROVERA Sterile Aqueous Suspension is available as 400 mg/mL in 2.5 mL vials.

The text of the patient insert for progestational drugs is set forth below.

PATIENT INFORMATION

DEPO-PROVERA Sterile Aqueous Suspension is a progestational drug. The information below is required by the U.S. Food and Drug Administration to be provided to all patients taking such products. This information relates only to the risk to the unborn child associated with use of progestational drugs during pregnancy. For further information on the use, side effects, and other risks associated with this product, ask your doctor.

WARNING FOR WOMEN

Progesterone or progesterone-like drugs have been used to prevent miscarriage in the first few months of pregnancy.

Continued on next page

Depo-Provera—Cont.

No adequate evidence is available to show that they are effective for this purpose. Furthermore, most cases of early miscarriage are due to causes which could not be helped by these drugs.

There is an increased risk of minor birth defects in children whose mothers take this drug during the first 4 months of pregnancy. Several reports suggest an association between mothers who take these drugs in the first trimester of pregnancy and genital abnormalities in male and female babies. The risk to the male baby is the possibility of being born with a condition in which the opening of the penis is on the underside rather than the tip of the penis (hypospadias). Hypospadias occurs in about 5 to 8 per 1000 male births and is about doubled with exposure to these drugs. There is not enough information to quantify the risk to exposed female fetuses, but enlargement of the clitoris and fusion of the labia may occur, although rarely.

Therefore, since drugs of this type may induce mild masculinization of the external genitalia of the female fetus, as well as hypospadias in the male fetus, it is wise to avoid using the drug during the first trimester of pregnancy.

These drugs have been used as a test for pregnancy but such use is no longer considered safe because of possible damage to a developing baby. Also, more rapid methods for testing for pregnancy are now available.

If you take DEPO-PROVERA Sterile Aqueous Suspension and later find you were pregnant when you took it, be sure to discuss this with your doctor as soon as possible.

℞ only

Pharmacia & Upjohn Company
A subsidiary of Pharmacia Corporation
Kalamazoo, Michigan 49001, U.S.A.

Revised March 2003 810 597 314
692166

DETROL® ℞
tolterodine tartrate tablets

DESCRIPTION

DETROL Tablets contain tolterodine tartrate. The active moiety, tolterodine, is a muscarinic receptor antagonist. The chemical name of tolterodine tartrate is (R)-2-[3-[bis(1-methylethyl)-amino]-1-phenylpropyl]-4-methylphenol [R-(R*,R*)]-2,3-dihydroxybutanedioate (1:1) (salt). The empirical formula of tolterodine tartrate is $C_{26}H_{37}NO_7$, and its molecular weight is 475.6. The structural formula of tolterodine tartrate is represented below:

Tolterodine tartrate is a white, crystalline powder. The pKa value is 9.87 and the solubility in water is 12 mg/mL. It is soluble in methanol, slightly soluble in ethanol, and practically insoluble in toluene. The partition coefficient (Log D) between n-octanol and water is 1.83 at pH 7.3.

DETROL Tablets for oral administration contain 1 or 2 mg of tolterodine tartrate. The inactive ingredients are colloidal anhydrous silica, calcium hydrogen phosphate dihydrate, cellulose microcrystalline, hypromellose, magnesium stearate, sodium starch glycolate (pH 3.0 to 5.0), stearic acid, and titanium dioxide.

CLINICAL PHARMACOLOGY

Tolterodine is a competitive muscarinic receptor antagonist. Both urinary bladder contraction and salivation are mediated via cholinergic muscarinic receptors.

After oral administration, tolterodine is metabolized in the liver, resulting in the formation of the 5-hydroxymethyl derivative, a major pharmacologically active metabolite. The 5-hydroxymethyl metabolite, which exhibits an antimuscarinic activity similar to that of tolterodine, contributes significantly to the therapeutic effect. Both tolterodine and the 5-hydroxymethyl metabolite exhibit a high specificity for muscarinic receptors, since both show negligible activity or affinity for other neurotransmitter receptors and other potential cellular targets, such as calcium channels.

Tolterodine has a pronounced effect on bladder function. Effects on urodynamic parameters before and 1 and 5 hours after a single 6.4-mg dose of tolterodine immediate release were determined in healthy volunteers. The main effects of tolterodine at 1 and 5 hours were an increase in residual urine, reflecting an incomplete emptying of the bladder, and a decrease in detrusor pressure. These findings are consistent with an antimuscarinic action on the lower urinary tract.

Pharmacokinetics

Absorption: In a study with ^{14}C-tolterodine solution in healthy volunteers who received a 5-mg oral dose, at least 77% of the radiolabeled dose was absorbed. Tolterodine immediate release is rapidly absorbed, and maximum serum concentrations (C_{max}) typically occur within 1 to 2 hours after dose administration. C_{max} and area under the concentration-time curve (AUC) determined after dosage of tolterodine immediate release are dose-proportional over the range of 1 to 4 mg.

Table 1. Summary of Mean (±SD) Pharmacokinetic Parameters of Tolterodine and its Active Metabolite (5-hydroxymethyl metabolite) in Healthy Volunteers

	Tolterodine					5-Hydroxymethyl Metabolite			
Phenotype (CYP2D6)	t_{max} (h)	C_{max}* (µg/L)	C_{avg}* (µg/L)	$t_{1/2}$ (h)	CL/F (L/h)	t_{max} (h)	C_{max}* (µg/L)	C_{avg}* (µg/L)	$t_{1/2}$ (h)
Single-dose									
EM	1.6±1.5	1.6±1.2	0.50±0.35	2.0±0.7	534±697	1.8±1.4	1.8±0.7	0.62±0.26	3.1±0.7
PM	1.4±0.5	10±4.9	8.3±4.3	6.5±1.6	17±7.3	-†	-	-	-
Multiple-dose									
EM	1.2±0.5	2.6±2.8	0.58±0.54	2.2±0.4	415±377	1.2±0.5	2.4±1.3	0.92±0.46	2.9±0.4
PM	1.9±1.0	19±7.5	12±5.1	9.6±1.5	11±4.2	-	-	-	-

* Parameter was dose-normalized from 4 mg to 2 mg.
C_{max} = Maximum plasma concentration; t_{max} = Time of occurrence of C_{max};
C_{avg} = Average plasma concentration; $t_{1/2}$ = Terminal elimination half-life; CL/F = Apparent oral clearance.
EM = Extensive metabolizers; PM = Poor metabolizers.
†- = not applicable.

Table 2. 95% Confidence Intervals (CI) for the Difference between DETROL (2 mg bid) and Placebo for the Mean Change at Week 12 from Baseline in Study 007

	DETROL (SD) N=514	Placebo (SD) N=508	Difference (95% CI)
Number of Incontinence Episodes per Week			
Mean baseline	23.2	23.3	
Mean change from baseline	-10.6 (17)	-6.9 (15)	-3.7 (-5.7, -1.6)
Number of Micturitions per 24 Hours			
Mean baseline	11.1	11.3	
Mean change from baseline	-1.7 (3.3)	-1.2 (2.9)	-0.5* (-0.9, -0.1)
Volume Voided per Micturition (mL)			
Mean baseline	137	136	
Mean change from baseline	29 (47)	14 (41)	15* (9, 21)

SD = Standard Deviation.
*The difference between DETROL and placebo was statistically significant.

Effect of Food: Food intake increases the bioavailability of tolterodine (average increase 53%), but does not affect the levels of the 5-hydroxymethyl metabolite in extensive metabolizers. This change is not expected to be a safety concern and adjustment of dose is not needed.

Distribution: Tolterodine is highly bound to plasma proteins, primarily α_1-acid glycoprotein. Unbound concentrations of tolterodine average 3.7% ± 0.13% over the concentration range achieved in clinical studies. The 5-hydroxymethyl metabolite is not extensively protein bound, with unbound fraction concentrations averaging 36% ± 4.0%. The blood to serum ratio of tolterodine and the 5-hydroxymethyl metabolite averages 0.6 and 0.8, respectively, indicating that these compounds do not distribute extensively into erythrocytes. The volume of distribution of tolterodine following administration of a 1.28-mg intravenous dose is 113 ± 26.7 L.

Metabolism: Tolterodine is extensively metabolized by the liver following oral dosing. The primary metabolic route involves the oxidation of the 5-methyl group and is mediated by the cytochrome P450 2D6 (CYP2D6) and leads to the formation of a pharmacologically active 5-hydroxymethyl metabolite. Further metabolism leads to formation of the 5-carboxylic acid and *N*-dealkylated 5-carboxylic acid metabolites, which account for 51% ± 14% and 29% ± 6.3% of the metabolites recovered in the urine, respectively.

Variability in Metabolism: A subset (about 7%) of the population is devoid of CYP2D6, the enzyme responsible for the formation of the 5-hydroxymethyl metabolite of tolterodine. The identified pathway of metabolism for these individuals ("poor metabolizers") is dealkylation via cytochrome P450 3A4 (CYP3A4) to *N*-dealkylated tolterodine. The remainder of the population is referred to as "extensive metabolizers." Pharmacokinetic studies revealed that tolterodine is metabolized at a slower rate in poor metabolizers than in extensive metabolizers; this results in significantly higher serum concentrations of tolterodine and in negligible concentrations of the 5-hydroxymethyl metabolite.

Excretion: Following administration of a 5-mg oral dose of ^{14}C-tolterodine solution to healthy volunteers, 77% of radioactivity was recovered in urine and 17% was recovered in feces in 7 days. Less than 1% (<2.5% in poor metabolizers) of the dose was recovered as intact tolterodine, and 5% to 14% (<1% in poor metabolizers) was recovered as the active 5-hydroxymethyl metabolite.

A summary of mean (± standard deviation) pharmacokinetic parameters of tolterodine immediate release and the 5-hydroxymethyl metabolite in extensive (EM) and poor (PM) metabolizers is provided in Table 1. These data were obtained following single- and multiple-doses of tolterodine 4 mg administered twice daily to 16 healthy male volunteers (8 EM, 8 PM).

[See table 1 above]

Pharmacokinetics in Special Populations

Age: In Phase 1, multiple-dose studies in which tolterodine immediate release 4 mg (2 mg bid) was administered, serum concentrations of tolterodine and of the 5-hydroxymethyl metabolite were similar in healthy elderly volunteers (aged 64 through 80 years) and healthy young volunteers (aged less than 40 years). In another Phase 1 study, elderly volunteers (aged 71 through 81 years) were given tolterodine immediate release 2 or 4 mg (1 or 2 mg bid). Mean serum concentrations of tolterodine and the 5-hydroxymethyl metabolite in these elderly volunteers were approximately 20% and 50% higher, respectively, than reported in young healthy volunteers. However, no overall differences were observed in safety between older and younger patients on tolterodine in Phase 3, 12-week, controlled clinical studies; therefore, no tolterodine dosage adjustment for elderly patients is recommended (see **PRECAUTIONS, Geriatric Use**).

Pediatric: The pharmacokinetics of tolterodine have not been established in pediatric patients.

Gender: The pharmacokinetics of tolterodine immediate release and the 5-hydroxymethyl metabolite are not influenced by gender. Mean C_{max} of tolterodine (1.6 mg/L in males versus 2.2 mg/L in females) and the active 5-hydroxymethyl metabolite (2.2 mg/L in males versus 2.5 mg/L in females) are similar in males and females who were administered tolterodine immediate release 2 mg. Mean AUC values of tolterodine (6.7 µg•h/L in males versus 7.8 µg•h/L in females) and the 5-hydroxymethyl metabolite (10 µg•h/L in males versus 11 µg•h/L in females) are also similar. The elimination half-life of tolterodine for both males and females is 2.4 hours, and the half-life of the 5-hydroxymethyl metabolite is 3.0 hours in females and 3.3 hours in males.

Race: Pharmacokinetic differences due to race have not been established.

Renal Insufficiency: Renal impairment can significantly alter the disposition of tolterodine immediate release and its metabolites. In a study conducted in patients with creatinine clearance between 10 and 30 mL/min, tolterodine immediate release and the 5-hydroxymethyl metabolite levels were approximately 2-3 fold higher in patients with renal impairment than in healthy volunteers. Exposure levels of other metabolites of tolterodine (eg, tolterodine acid, *N*-dealkylated tolterodine acid, *N*-dealkylated tolterodine, and *N*-dealkylated hydroxylated tolterodine) were significantly higher (10-30 fold) in renally impaired patients as compared to the healthy volunteers. The recommended dosage for patients with significantly reduced renal function is DETROL 1 mg twice daily (see **PRECAUTIONS, General**).

Hepatic Insufficiency: Liver impairment can significantly alter the disposition of tolterodine immediate release. In a study conducted in cirrhotic patients, the elimination half-life of tolterodine immediate release was longer in cirrhotic patients (mean, 7.8 hours) than in healthy, young, and elderly volunteers (mean, 2 to 4 hours). The clearance of orally administered tolterodine was substantially lower in cirrhotic patients (1.0 ± 1.7 L/h/kg) than in the healthy volunteers (5.7 ± 3.8 L/h/kg). The recommended dose for patients with significantly reduced hepatic function is DETROL 1 mg twice daily (see **PRECAUTIONS, General**).

Drug-Drug Interactions

Fluoxetine: Fluoxetine is a selective serotonin reuptake inhibitor and a potent inhibitor of CYP2D6 activity. In a study to assess the effect of fluoxetine on the pharmacokinetics of tolterodine immediate release and its metabolites, it was observed that fluoxetine significantly inhibited the metabolism of tolterodine immediate release in extensive metabolizers, resulting in a 4.8-fold increase in tolterodine AUC. There was a 52% decrease in C_{max} and a 20% decrease in AUC of the 5-hydroxymethyl metabolite. Fluoxetine thus alters the pharmacokinetics in patients who would otherwise be extensive metabolizers of tolterodine immediate release to resemble the pharmacokinetic profile in poor metabolizers. The sums of unbound serum concentrations of tolterodine immediate release and the 5-hydroxymethyl metabolite are only 25% higher during the interaction. No dose adjustment is required when DETROL and fluoxetine are coadministered.

Other Drugs Metabolized by Cytochrome P450 Isoenzymes: Tolterodine immediate release does not cause clinically significant interactions with other drugs metabolized by the major drug metabolizing CYP enzymes. In vivo drug-interaction data show that tolterodine immediate release does not result in clinically relevant inhibition of CYP1A2, 2D6, 2C9, 2C19, or 3A4 as evidenced by lack of influence on the marker drugs caffeine, debrisoquine, S-warfarin, and omeprazole. In vitro data show that tolterodine immediate release is a competitive inhibitor of CYP2D6 at high concentrations (Ki 1.05 μM), while tolterodine immediate release as well as the 5-hydroxymethyl metabolite are devoid of any significant inhibitory potential regarding the other isoenzymes.

CYP3A4 Inhibitors: The effect of 200 mg daily dose of ketoconazole on the pharmacokinetics of tolterodine immediate release was studied in 8 healthy volunteers, all of whom were poor metabolizers (see **Pharmacokinetics**, Variability in Metabolism for discussion of poor metabolizers). In the presence of ketoconazole, the mean C_{max} and AUC of tolterodine increased by 2 and 2.5 fold, respectively. Based on these findings, other potent CYP3A inhibitors such as other azole antifungals (eg, itraconazole, miconazole) or macrolide antibiotics (eg, erythromycin, clarithromycin) or cyclosporine or vinblastine may also lead to increases of tolterodine plasma concentrations (see **PRECAUTIONS** and **DOSAGE AND ADMINISTRATION**).

Warfarin: In healthy volunteers, coadministration of tolterodine immediate release 4 mg (2 mg bid) for 7 days and a single dose of warfarin 25 mg on day 4 had no effect on prothrombin time, Factor VII suppression, or on the pharmacokinetics of warfarin.

Oral Contraceptives: Tolterodine immediate release 4 mg (2 mg bid) had no effect on the pharmacokinetics of an oral contraceptive (ethinyl estradiol 30 mg/levonorgestrel 150 mg) as evidenced by the monitoring of ethinyl estradiol and levonorgestrel over a 2-month cycle in healthy female volunteers.

Diuretics: Coadministration of tolterodine immediate release up to 8 mg (4 mg bid) for up to 12 weeks with diuretic agents, such as indapamide, hydrochlorothiazide, triamterene, bendroflumethiazide, chlorothiazide, methylchlorothiazide, or furosemide, did not cause any adverse electrocardiographic (ECG) effects.

CLINICAL STUDIES

DETROL Tablets were evaluated for the treatment of overactive bladder with symptoms of urge urinary incontinence, urgency, and frequency in four randomized, double-blind, placebo-controlled, 12-week studies. A total of 853 patients received DETROL 2 mg twice daily and 685 patients received placebo. The majority of patients were Caucasian (95%) and female (78%), with a mean age of 60 years (range, 19 to 93 years). At study entry, nearly all patients perceived they had urgency and most patients had increased frequency of micturitions and urge incontinence. These characteristics were well balanced across treatment groups for the studies.

The efficacy endpoints for study 007 (see Table 2) included the change from baseline for:

- Number of incontinence episodes per week
- Number of micturitions per 24 hours (averaged over 7 days)
- Volume of urine voided per micturition (averaged over 2 days)

The efficacy endpoints for studies 008, 009, and 010 (see Table 3) were identical to the above endpoints with the exception that the number of incontinence episodes was per 24 hours (averaged over 7 days).

[See table 2 at top of previous page]
[See table 3 above]

Table 3. 95% Confidence Intervals (CI) for the Difference between DETROL (2 mg bid) and Placebo for the Mean Change at Week 12 from Baseline in Studies 008, 009, 010

Study		DETROL (SD)	Placebo (SD)	Difference (95% CI)
Number of Incontinence Episodes per 24 Hours				
008	Number of patients	93	40	
	Mean baseline	2.9	3.3	
	Mean change from baseline	-1.3 (3.2)	-0.9 (1.5)	0.5 (-1.3,0.3)
009	Number of patients	116	55	
	Mean baseline	3.6	3.5	
	Mean change from baseline	-1.7 (2.5)	-1.3 (2.5)	-0.4 (-1.0,0.2)
010	Number of patients	90	50	
	Mean baseline	3.7	3.5	
	Mean change from baseline	-1.6 (2.4)	-1.1 (2.1)	-0.5 (-1.1,0.1)
Number of Micturitions per 24 Hours				
008	Number of patients	118	56	
	Mean baseline	11.5	11.7	
	Mean change from baseline	-2.7 (3.8)	-1.6 (3.6)	-1.2*(-2.0,-0.4)
009	Number of patients	128	64	
	Mean baseline	11.2	11.3	
	Mean change from baseline	-2.3 (2.1)	-1.4 (2.8)	-0.9* (-1.5,-0.3)
010	Number of patients	108	56	
	Mean baseline	11.6	11.6	
	Mean change from baseline	-1.7 (2.3)	-1.4 (2.8)	-0.38 (-1.1,0.3)
Volume Voided per Micturition (mL)				
008	Number of patients	118	56	
	Mean baseline	166	157	
	Mean change from baseline	38 (54)	6 (42)	32* (18,46)
009	Number of patients	129	64	
	Mean baseline	155	158	
	Mean change from baseline	36 (50)	10 (47)	26* (14,38)
010	Number of patients	108	56	
	Mean baseline	155	160	
	Mean change from baseline	31 (45)	13 (52)	18* (4,32)

SD = Standard Deviation.
*The difference between DETROL and placebo was statistically significant.

INDICATIONS AND USAGE

DETROL Tablets are indicated for the treatment of overactive bladder with symptoms of urge urinary incontinence, urgency, and frequency.

CONTRAINDICATIONS

DETROL Tablets are contraindicated in patients with urinary retention, gastric retention, or uncontrolled narrow-angle glaucoma. DETROL is also contraindicated in patients who have demonstrated hypersensitivity to the drug or its ingredients.

PRECAUTIONS

General

Risk of Urinary Retention and Gastric Retention: DETROL Tablets should be administered with caution to patients with clinically significant bladder outflow obstruction because of the risk of urinary retention and to patients with gastrointestinal obstructive disorders, such as pyloric stenosis, because of the risk of gastric retention (see **CONTRAINDICATIONS**).

Controlled Narrow-Angle Glaucoma: DETROL should be used with caution in patients being treated for narrow-angle glaucoma.

Reduced Hepatic and Renal Function: For patients with significantly reduced hepatic function or renal function, the recommended dose of DETROL is 1 mg twice daily (see **CLINICAL PHARMACOLOGY**, **Pharmacokinetics in Special Populations**).

Information for Patients

Patients should be informed that antimuscarinic agents such as DETROL may produce the following effects: blurred vision, dizziness, or drowsiness.

Drug Interactions

CYP3A4 Inhibitors: Ketoconazole, an inhibitor of the drug metabolizing enzyme CYP3A4, significantly increased plasma concentrations of tolterodine when coadministered to subjects who were poor metabolizers (see **CLINICAL PHARMACOLOGY**, Variability in Metabolism and **Drug-Drug Interactions**). For patients receiving ketoconazole or other potent CYP3A4 inhibitors such as other azole anitfungals (eg, itraconazole, miconazole) or macrolide antibiotics (eg, erythromycin, clarithromycin) or cyclosporine or vinblastine, the recommended dose of DETROL is 1 mg twice daily.

Drug-Laboratory-Test Interactions

Interactions between tolterodine and laboratory tests have not been studied.

Carcinogenesis, Mutagenesis, Impairment of Fertility

Carcinogenicity studies with tolterodine were conducted in mice and rats. At the maximum tolerated dose in mice (30 mg/kg/day), female rats (20 mg/kg/day), and male rats (30 mg/kg/day), AUC values obtained for tolterodine were 355, 291, and 462 mg•h/L, respectively. In comparison, the human AUC value for a 2-mg dose administered twice daily is estimated at 34 mg•h/L. Thus, tolterodine exposure in the carcinogenicity studies was 9- to 14-fold higher than expected in humans. No increase in tumors was found in either mice or rats.

No mutagenic effects of tolterodine were detected in a battery of in vitro tests, including bacterial mutation assays (Ames test) in 4 strains of *Salmonella typhimurium* and in 2 strains of *Escherichia coli*, a gene mutation assay in L5178Y mouse lymphoma cells, and chromosomal aberration tests in human lymphocytes. Tolterodine was also negative in vivo in the bone marrow micronucleus test in the mouse.

In female mice treated for 2 weeks before mating and during gestation with 20 mg/kg/day (corresponding to AUC value of about 500 mg•h/L), neither effects on reproductive performance or fertility were seen. Based on AUC values, the systemic exposure was about 15-fold higher in animals than in humans. In male mice, a dose of 30 mg/kg/day did not induce any adverse effects on fertility.

Pregnancy

Pregnancy Category C. At oral doses of 20 mg/kg/day (approximately 14 times the human exposure), no anomalies or malformations were observed in mice. When given at doses of 30 to 40 mg/kg/day, tolterodine has been shown to be embryolethal, reduce fetal weight, and increase the incidence of fetal abnormalities (cleft palate, digital abnormalities, intra-abdominal hemorrhage, and various skeletal abnormalities, primarily reduced ossification) in mice. At these doses, the AUC values were about 20- to 25-fold higher than in humans. Rabbits treated subcutaneously at a dose of 0.8 mg/kg/day achieved an AUC of 100 mg•h/L, which is about 3-fold higher than that resulting from the human dose. This dose did not result in any embryotoxicity or teratogenicity. There are no studies of tolterodine in pregnant women. Therefore, DETROL should be used during pregnancy only if the potential benefit for the mother justifies the potential risk to the fetus.

Nursing Mothers

Tolterodine is excreted into the milk in mice. Offspring of female mice treated with tolterodine 20 mg/kg/day during the lactation period had slightly reduced body-weight gain. The offspring regained the weight during the maturation phase. It is not known whether tolterodine is excreted in human milk; therefore, DETROL should not be administered during nursing. A decision should be made whether to discontinue nursing or to discontinue DETROL in nursing mothers.

Pediatric Use

The safety and effectiveness of DETROL in pediatric patients have not been established.

Geriatric Use

Of the 1120 patients who were treated in the four Phase 3, 12-week clinical studies of DETROL, 474 (42%) were 65 to 91 years of age. No overall differences in safety were observed between the older and younger patients (see **CLINICAL PHARMACOLOGY**, **Pharmacokinetics in Special Populations**).

ADVERSE REACTIONS

The Phase 2 and 3 clinical trial program for DETROL Tablets included 3071 patients who were treated with DETROL (N=2133) or placebo (N=938). The patients were treated with 1, 2, 4, or 8 mg/day for up to 12 months. No differences in the safety profile of tolterodine were identified based on age, gender, race, or metabolism.

The data described below reflect exposure to DETROL 2 mg bid in 986 patients and to placebo in 683 patients exposed for 12 weeks in five Phase 3, controlled clinical studies. Because clinical trials are conducted under widely varying conditions, adverse reaction rates observed in the clinical trials of a drug cannot be directly compared to rates in the clinical trials of another drug and may not reflect the rates observed in practice. The adverse reaction information from clinical trials does, however, provide a basis for identifying the adverse events that appear to be related to drug use and approximating rates.

Sixty-six percent of patients receiving DETROL 2 mg bid reported adverse events versus 56% of placebo patients. The most common adverse events reported by patients receiving DETROL were dry mouth, headache, constipation, vertigo/dizziness, and abdominal pain. Dry mouth, constipation, abnormal vision (accommodation abnormalities), urinary retention, and xerophthalmia are expected side effects of antimuscarinic agents.

Dry mouth was the most frequently reported adverse event for patients treated with DETROL 2 mg bid in the Phase 3

Continued on next page

Table 4. Incidence* (%) of Adverse Events Exceeding Placebo Rate and Reported in >1% of Patients Treated with DETROL Tablets (2 mg bid) in 12-week, Phase 3 Clinical Studies

Body System	Adverse Event	% DETROL N=986	% Placebo N=683
Autonomic Nervous	accommodation abnormal	2	1
	dry mouth	35	10
General	chest pain	2	1
	fatigue	4	3
	headache	7	5
	influenza-like symptoms	3	2
Central/Peripheral Nervous	vertigo/dizziness	5	3
Gastrointestinal	abdominal pain	5	3
	constipation	7	4
	diarrhea	4	3
	dyspepsia	4	1
Urinary	dysuria	2	1
Skin/Appendages	dry skin	1	0
Musculoskeletal	arthralgia	2	1
Vision	xerophthalmia	3	2
Psychiatric	somnolence	3	2
Metabolic/Nutritional	weight gain	1	0
Resistance Mechanism	infection	1	0

*in nearest integer.

Detrol—Cont.

clinical studies, occurring in 34.8% of patients treated with DETROL and 9.8% of placebo-treated patients. One percent of patients treated with DETROL discontinued treatment due to dry mouth.

The frequency of discontinuation due to adverse events was highest during the first 4 weeks of treatment. Seven percent of patients treated with DETROL 2 mg bid discontinued treatment due to adverse events versus 6% of placebo patients. The most common adverse events leading to discontinuation of DETROL were dizziness and headache.

Three percent of patients treated with DETROL 2 mg bid reported a serious adverse event versus 4% of placebo patients. Significant ECG changes in QT and QTc have not been demonstrated in clinical-study patients treated with DETROL 2 mg bid. Table 4 lists the adverse events reported in 1% or more of the patients treated with DETROL 2 mg bid in the 12-week studies. The adverse events are reported regardless of causality.

[See table 4 above]

Postmarketing Surveillance

The following events have been reported in association with tolterodine use in clinical practice: anaphylactoid reactions, including angioedema; tachycardia; palpations; peripheral edema; and hallucinations. Because these spontaneously reported events are from the worldwide postmarketing experience, the frequency of events and the role of tolterodine in their causation cannot be reliably determined.

OVERDOSAGE

A 27-month-old child who ingested 5 to 7 DETROL Tablets 2 mg was treated with a suspension of activated charcoal and was hospitalized overnight with symptoms of dry mouth. The child fully recovered.

Management of Overdosage

Overdosage with DETROL can potentially result in severe central anticholinergic effects and should be treated accordingly.

ECG monitoring is recommended in the event of overdosage. In dogs, changes in the QT interval (slight prolongation of 10% to 20%) were observed at a suprapharmacologic dose of 4.5 mg/kg, which is about 68 times higher than the recommended human dose. In clinical trials of normal volunteers and patients, QT interval prolongation was not observed with tolterodine immediate release at doses up to 4 mg twice daily (higher doses were not evaluated).

DOSAGE AND ADMINISTRATION

The initial recommended dose of DETROL Tablets is 2 mg twice daily. The dose may be lowered to 1 mg twice daily based on individual response and tolerability. For patients with significantly reduced hepatic or renal function or who are currently taking drugs that are potent inhibitors of CYP3A4, the recommended dose of DETROL is 1 mg twice daily (see **PRECAUTIONS, General** and **PRECAUTIONS, Drug Interactions**).

HOW SUPPLIED

DETROL Tablets 1 mg (white, round, biconvex, film-coated tablets engraved with arcs above and below the letters "TO") and **DETROL Tablets 2 mg** (white, round, biconvex, film-coated tablets engraved with arcs above and below the letters "DT") are supplied as follows:

Bottles of 60
1 mg NDC 0009-4541-02
2 mg NDC 0009-4544-02

Bottles of 500
1 mg NDC 0009-4541-03
2 mg NDC 0009-4544-03

Unit Dose Pack of 140
1 mg NDC 0009-4541-01
2 mg NDC 0009-4544-01

Store at 25°C (77°F); excursions permitted to 15-30°C (59-86°F) [see USP Controlled Room Temperature] (DTL).

℞ only

US Patent No. 5,382,600

Pharmacia & Upjohn Company
A subsidiary of Pharmacia Corporation
Kalamazoo, MI 49001, USA
Revised July 2003

817 413 008
692167

Shown in Product Identification Guide, page 330

DETROL® LA ℞

[*dĕ-trōl*]
(tolterodine tartrate extended release capsules)

DESCRIPTION

DETROL LA Capsules contain tolterodine tartrate. The active moiety, tolterodine, is a muscarinic receptor antagonist. The chemical name of tolterodine tartrate is (R)-N,N-diisopropyl-3-(2-hydroxy-5-methylphenyl)-3-phenylpropanamine L-hydrogen tartrate. The empirical formula of tolterodine tartrate is $C_{26}H_{37}NO_7$, and its molecular weight is 475.6. The structural formula of tolterodine tartrate is represented below.

Tolterodine tartrate is a white, crystalline powder. The pKa value is 9.87 and the solubility in water is 12 mg/mL. It is soluble in methanol, slightly soluble in ethanol, and practically insoluble in toluene. The partition coefficient (Log D) between n-octanol and water is 1.83 at pH 7.3.

DETROL LA for oral administration contains 2 mg or 4 mg of tolterodine tartrate. Inactive ingredients are sucrose, starch, hypromellose, ethylcellulose, medium chain triglycerides, oleic acid, gelatin, and FD&C Blue #2. The 2-mg capsules also contain yellow iron oxide. Both capsule strengths are imprinted with a pharmaceutical grade printing ink that contains shellac glaze, titanium dioxide, propylene glycol, and simethicone.

CLINICAL PHARMACOLOGY

Tolterodine is a competitive muscarinic receptor antagonist. Both urinary bladder contraction and salivation are mediated via cholinergic muscarinic receptors.

After oral administration, tolterodine is metabolized in the liver, resulting in the formation of the 5-hydroxymethyl derivative, a major pharmacologically active metabolite. The 5-hydroxymethyl metabolite, which exhibits an antimuscarinic activity similar to that of tolterodine, contributes significantly to the therapeutic effect. Both tolterodine and the 5-hydroxymethyl metabolite exhibit a high specificity for muscarinic receptors, since both show negligible activity or affinity for other neurotransmitter receptors and other potential cellular targets, such as calcium channels.

Tolterodine has a pronounced effect on bladder function. Effects on urodynamic parameters before and 1 and 5 hours after a single 6.4-mg dose of tolterodine immediate release were determined in healthy volunteers. The main effects of tolterodine at 1 and 5 hours were an increase in residual urine, reflecting an incomplete emptying of the bladder, and a decrease in detrusor pressure. These findings are consistent with an antimuscarinic action on the lower urinary tract.

Pharmacokinetics

Absorption: In a study with ^{14}C-tolterodine solution in healthy volunteers who received a 5-mg oral dose, at least 77% of the radiolabeled dose was absorbed. C_{max} and area under the concentration-time curve (AUC) determined after dosage of tolterodine immediate release are dose-proportional over the range of 1 to 4 mg. Based on the sum of unbound serum concentrations of tolterodine and the 5-hydroxymethyl metabolite ("active moiety"), the AUC of tolterodine extended release 4 mg daily is equivalent to tolterodine immediate release 4 mg (2 mg bid). C_{max} and C_{min} levels of tolterodine extended release are about 75% and 150% of tolterodine immediate release, respectively. Maximum serum concentrations of tolterodine extended release are observed 2 to 6 hours after dose administration.

Effect of Food: There is no effect of food on the pharmacokinetics of tolterodine extended release.

Distribution: Tolterodine is highly bound to plasma proteins, primarily α_1-acid glycoprotein. Unbound concentrations of tolterodine average 3.7% ± 0.13% over the concentration range achieved in clinical studies. The 5-hydroxymethyl metabolite is not extensively protein bound, with unbound fraction concentrations averaging 36% ± 4.0%. The blood to serum ratio of tolterodine and the 5-hydroxymethyl metabolite averages 0.6 and 0.8, respectively, indicating that these compounds do not distribute extensively into erythrocytes. The volume of distribution of tolterodine following administration of a 1.28-mg intravenous dose is 113 ± 26.7 L.

Metabolism: Tolterodine is extensively metabolized by the liver following oral dosing. The primary metabolic route involves the oxidation of the 5-methyl group and is mediated by the cytochrome P450 2D6 (CYP2D6) and leads to the formation of a pharmacologically active 5-hydroxymethyl metabolite. Further metabolism leads to formation of the 5-carboxylic acid and *N*-dealkylated 5-carboxylic acid metabolites, which account for 51% ± 14% and 29% ± 6.3% of the metabolites recovered in the urine, respectively.

Variability in Metabolism: A subset (about 7%) of the Caucasian population is devoid of CYP2D6, the enzyme responsible for the formation of the 5-hydroxymethyl metabolite of tolterodine. The identified pathway of metabolism for these individuals ("poor metabolizers") is dealkylation via cytochrome P450 3A4 (CYP3A4) to *N*-dealkylated tolterodine. The remainder of the population is referred to as "extensive metabolizers." Pharmacokinetic studies revealed that tolterodine is metabolized at a slower rate in poor metabolizers than in extensive metabolizers; this results in significantly higher serum concentrations of tolterodine and in negligible concentrations of the 5-hydroxymethyl metabolite.

Excretion: Following administration of a 5-mg oral dose of ^{14}C-tolterodine solution to healthy volunteers, 77% of radioactivity was recovered in urine and 17% was recovered in feces in 7 days. Less than 1% (<2.5% in poor metabolizers) of the dose was recovered as intact tolterodine, and 5% to 14% (<1% in poor metabolizers) was recovered as the active 5-hydroxymethyl metabolite.

A summary of mean (± standard deviation) pharmacokinetic parameters of tolterodine extended release and the 5-hydroxymethyl metabolite in extensive (EM) and poor (PM) metabolizers is provided in Table 1. These data were obtained following single and multiple doses of tolterodine extended release administered daily to 17 healthy male volunteers (13 EM, 4 PM).

[See table 1 at top of next page]

Pharmacokinetics in Special Populations

Age: In Phase 1, multiple-dose studies in which tolterodine immediate release 4 mg (2 mg bid) was administered, serum concentrations of tolterodine and of the 5-hydroxy metabolite were similar in healthy elderly volunteers (aged 64 through 80 years) and healthy young volunteers (aged less than 40 years). In another Phase 1 study, elderly volunteers (aged 71 through 81 years) were given tolterodine immediate release 2 or 4 mg (1 or 2 mg bid). Mean serum concentrations of tolterodine and the 5-hydroxymethyl metabolite in these elderly volunteers were approximately 20% and 50% higher, respectively, than reported in young healthy volunteers. However, no overall differences were observed in safety between older and younger patients on tolterodine in the Phase 3, 12-week, controlled clinical studies; therefore, no tolterodine dosage adjustment for elderly patients is recommended (see **PRECAUTIONS, Geriatric Use**).

Pediatric: Efficacy in the pediatric population has not been demonstrated.

The pharmacokinetics of tolterodine extended release capsules have been evaluated in pediatric patients ranging in age from 11-15 years. The dose-plasma concentration relationship was linear over the range of doses assessed. Parent/metabolite ratios differed according to CYP2D6 metabolizer status: EMs had low serum concentrations of tolterodine and high concentrations of the active 5-hydroxymethyl metabolite, while PMs had high concentrations of tolterodine and negligible active metabolite concentrations.

Gender: The pharmacokinetics of tolterodine immediate release and the 5-hydroxymethyl metabolite are not influenced by gender. Mean C_{max} of tolterodine immediate release (1.6 µg/L in males versus 2.2 µg/L in females) and the active 5-hydroxymethyl metabolite (2.2 µg/L in males versus 2.5 µg/L in females) are similar in males and females who were administered tolterodine immediate release 2 mg. Mean AUC values of tolterodine (6.7 µg•h/L in males versus 7.8 µg•h/L in females) and the 5-hydroxymethyl metabolite (10 µg•h/L in males versus 11 µg•h/L in females) are also similar. The elimination half-life of tolterodine immediate release for both males and females is 2.4 hours, and the half-life of the 5-hydroxymethyl metabolite is 3.0 hours in females and 3.3 hours in males.

Race: Pharmacokinetic differences due to race have not been established.

Renal Insufficiency: Renal impairment can significantly alter the disposition of tolterodine immediate release and its metabolites. In a study conducted in patients with creatinine clearance between 10 and 30 mL/min, tolterodine immediate release and the 5-hydroxymethyl metabolite levels were approximately 2-3 fold higher in patients with renal impairment than in healthy volunteers. Exposure levels of other metabolites of tolterodine (eg, tolterodine acid, *N*-dealkylated tolterodine acid, *N*-dealkylated tolterodine and *N*-dealkylated hydroxy tolterodine) were significantly higher (10-30 fold) in renally impaired patients as compared to the healthy volunteers. The recommended dose for patients with significantly reduced renal function is tolterodine 2 mg daily (see **PRECAUTIONS, General**).

Hepatic Insufficiency: Liver impairment can significantly alter the disposition of tolterodine immediate release. In a study of tolterodine immediate release conducted in cirrhotic patients, the elimination half-life of tolterodine immediate release was longer in cirrhotic patients (mean, 7.8 hours) than in healthy, young, and elderly volunteers (mean, 2 to 4 hours). The clearance of orally administered tolterodine immediate release was substantially lower in cirrhotic patients (1.0 ± 1.7 L/h/kg) than in the healthy volunteers (5.7 ± 3.8 L/h/kg). The recommended dose for patients with significantly reduced hepatic function is tolterodine 2 mg daily (see **PRECAUTIONS, General**).

Drug-Drug Interactions

Fluoxetine: Fluoxetine is a selective serotonin reuptake inhibitor and a potent inhibitor of CYP2D6 activity. In a study to assess the effect of fluoxetine on the pharmacokinetics of tolterodine immediate release and its metabolites, it was observed that fluoxetine significantly inhibited the metabolism of tolterodine immediate release in extensive metabolizers, resulting in a 4.8-fold increase in tolterodine AUC. There was a 52% decrease in C_{max} and a 20% decrease in AUC of the 5-hydroxymethyl metabolite. Fluoxetine thus alters the pharmacokinetics in patients who would otherwise be extensive metabolizers of tolterodine immediate release to resemble the pharmacokinetic profile in poor metabolizers. The sums of unbound serum concentrations of tolterodine immediate release and the 5-hydroxymethyl metabolite are only 25% higher during the interaction. No dose adjustment is required when tolterodine and fluoxetine are coadministered.

Other Drugs Metabolized by Cytochrome P450 Isoenzymes: Tolterodine immediate release does not cause clinically significant interactions with other drugs metabolized by the major drug metabolizing CYP enzymes. In vivo drug-interaction data show that tolterodine immediate release does not result in clinically relevant inhibition of CYP1A2, 2D6, 2C9, 2C19, or 3A4 as evidenced by lack of influence on the marker drugs caffeine, debrisoquine, S-warfarin, and omeprazole. In vitro data show that tolterodine immediate release is a competitive inhibitor of CYP2D6 at high concentrations (Ki 1.05 µM), while tolterodine immediate release as well as the 5-hydroxymethyl metabolite are devoid of any significant inhibitory potential regarding the other isoenzymes.

CYP3A4 Inhibitors: The effect of a 200-mg daily dose of ketoconazole on the pharmacokinetics of tolterodine immediate release was studied in 8 healthy volunteers, all of whom were poor metabolizers (see **Pharmacokinetics**, Variability in Metabolism for discussion of poor metabolizers). In the presence of ketoconazole, the mean C_{max} and AUC of tolterodine increased by 2 and 2.5 fold, respectively. Based on these findings, other potent CYP3A4 inhibitors such as other azole antifungals (eg, itraconazole, miconazole) or macrolide antibiotics (eg, erythromycin, clarithromycin) or cyclosporine or vinblastine may also lead to increases of tolterodine plasma concentrations (see **PRECAUTIONS** and **DOSAGE AND ADMINISTRATION**).

Warfarin: In healthy volunteers, coadministration of tolterodine immediate release 4 mg (2 mg bid) for 7 days and a single dose of warfarin 25 mg on day 4 had no effect on prothrombin time, Factor VII suppression, or on the pharmacokinetics of warfarin.

Oral Contraceptives: Tolterodine immediate release 4 mg (2 mg bid) had no effect on the pharmacokinetics of an oral contraceptive (ethinyl estradiol 30 µg/levonorgestrel 150 µg) as evidenced by the monitoring of ethinyl estradiol and levonorgestrel over a 2-month period in healthy female volunteers.

Diuretics: Coadministration of tolterodine immediate release up to 8 mg (4 mg bid) for up to 12 weeks with diuretic agents, such as indapamide, hydrochlorothiazide, triamterene, bendroflumethiazide, chlorothiazide, methylchlorothiazide, or furosemide, did not cause any adverse electrocardiographic (ECG) effects.

Table 1. Summary of Mean (±SD) Pharmacokinetic Parameters of Tolterodine Extended Release and its Active Metabolite (5-hydroxymethyl metabolite) in Healthy Volunteers

	Tolterodine				5-hydroxymethyl metabolite			
	t_{max}† (h)	C_{max} (µg/L)	C_{avg} (µg/L)	t1/2 (h)	t_{max}† (h)	C_{max} (µg/L)	C_{avg} (µg/L)	t1/2 (h)
Single dose 4 mg* EM	4 (2-6)	1.3 (0.8)	0.8 (0.57)	8.4 (3.2)	4 (3-6)	1.6 (0.5)	1.0 (0.32)	8.8 (5.9)
Multiple dose 4 mg EM	4 (2-6)	3.4 (4.9)	1.7 (2.8)	6.9 (3.5)	4 (2-6)	2.7 (0.90)	1.4 (0.6)	9.9 (4.0)
PM	4 (3-6)	19 (16)	13 (11)	18 (16)	— ‡	—	—	—

*Parameter dose-normalized from 8 to 4 mg for the single-dose data.
C_{max} = Maximum serum concentration; t_{max} = Time of occurrence of C_{max};
C_{avg} = Average serum concentration; t1/2 = Terminal elimination half-life.
†Data presented as median (range).
‡ = not applicable.

Table 2. 95% Confidence Intervals (CI) for the Difference between DETROL LA (4 mg daily) and Placebo for Mean Change at Week 12 from Baseline*

	DETROL LA (n=507)	Placebo (n=508) †	Treatment Difference, vs Placebo (95% CI)
Number of incontinence episodes/week			
Mean Baseline	22.1	23.3	
Mean Change from Baseline	−11.8 (SD 17.8)	−6.9 (SD 15.4)	−4.8 ‡ (−6.9, −2.8)
Number of micturitions/day			
Mean Baseline	10.9	11.3	
Mean Change from Baseline	−1.8 (SD 3.4)	−1.2 (SD 2.9)	−0.6 ‡ (−1.0, −0.2)
Volume Voided per micturition (mL)			
Mean Baseline	141	136	
Mean Change from Baseline	34 (SD 51)	14 (SD 41)	20 ‡ (14, 26)

SD = Standard Deviation.
* Intent-to-treat analysis.
† 1 to 2 patients missing in placebo group for each efficacy parameter.
‡ The difference between DETROL LA and placebo was statistically significant.

CLINICAL STUDIES

DETROL LA Capsules 2 mg were evaluated in 29 patients in a Phase 2 dose-effect study. DETROL LA 4 mg was evaluated for the treatment of overactive bladder with symptoms of urge urinary incontinence and frequency in a randomized, placebo-controlled, multicenter, double-blind, Phase 3, 12-week study. A total of 507 patients received DETROL LA 4 mg once daily in the morning and 508 received placebo. The majority of patients were Caucasian (95%) and female (81%), with a mean age of 61 years (range, 20 to 93 years). In the study, 642 patients (42%) were 65 to 93 years of age. The study included patients known to be responsive to tolterodine immediate release and other anticholinergic medications, however, 47% of patients never received prior pharmacotherapy for overactive bladder. At study entry, 97% of patients had at least 5 urge incontinence episodes per week and 91% of patients had 8 or more micturitions per day. The primary efficacy endpoint was change in mean number of incontinence episodes per week at week 12 from baseline. Secondary efficacy endpoints included change in mean number of micturitions per day and mean volume voided per micturition at week 12 from baseline.

[See table 2 above]

INDICATIONS AND USAGE

DETROL LA Capsules are once daily extended release capsules indicated for the treatment of overactive bladder with symptoms of urge urinary incontinence, urgency, and frequency.

CONTRAINDICATIONS

DETROL LA Capsules are contraindicated in patients with urinary retention, gastric retention, or uncontrolled narrow-angle glaucoma. DETROL LA is also contraindicated in patients who have demonstrated hypersensitivity to the drug or its ingredients.

PRECAUTIONS

General

Risk of Urinary Retention and Gastric Retention: DETROL LA Capsules should be administered with caution to patients with clinically significant bladder outflow obstruction because of the risk of urinary retention and to patients with gastrointestinal obstructive disorders, such as pyloric stenosis, because of the risk of gastric retention (see **CONTRAINDICATIONS**).

Controlled Narrow-Angle Glaucoma: DETROL LA should be used with caution in patients being treated for narrow-angle glaucoma.

Reduced Hepatic and Renal Function: For patients with significantly reduced hepatic function or renal function, the recommended dose for DETROL LA is 2 mg daily (see **CLINICAL PHARMACOLOGY, Pharmacokinetics in Special Populations**).

Information for Patients

Patients should be informed that antimuscarinic agents such as DETROL LA may produce the following effects: blurred vision, dizziness, or drowsiness.

Drug Interactions

CYP3A4 Inhibitors: Ketoconazole, an inhibitor of the drug metabolizing enzyme CYP3A4, significantly increased plasma concentrations of tolterodine when coadministered to subjects who were poor metabolizers (see **CLINICAL PHARMACOLOGY,** Variability in Metabolism and **Drug-Drug Interactions**). For patients receiving ketoconazole or other potent CYP3A4 inhibitors such as other azole antifungals (eg, itraconazole, miconazole) or macrolide antibiotics (eg, erythromycin, clarithromycin) or cyclosporine or vinblastine, the recommended dose of DETROL LA is 2 mg daily.

Drug-Laboratory-Test Interactions

Interactions between tolterodine and laboratory tests have not been studied.

Carcinogenesis, Mutagenesis, Impairment of Fertility

Carcinogenicity studies with tolterodine immediate release were conducted in mice and rats. At the maximum tolerated dose in mice (30 mg/kg/day), female rats (20 mg/kg/day), and male rats (30 mg/kg/day), AUC values obtained for tolterodine were 355, 291, and 462 µg•h/L, respectively. In comparison, the human AUC value for a 2-mg dose administered twice daily is estimated at 34 µg•h/L. Thus, tolterodine exposure in the carcinogenicity studies was 9- to 14-fold higher than expected in humans. No increase in tumors was found in either mice or rats.

No mutagenic effects of tolterodine were detected in a battery of in vitro tests, including bacterial mutation assays (Ames test) in 4 strains of *Salmonella typhimurium* and in 2 strains of *Escherichia coli*, a gene mutation assay in L5178Y mouse lymphoma cells, and chromosomal aberration tests in human lymphocytes. Tolterodine was also negative in vivo in the bone marrow micronucleus test in the mouse.

In female mice treated for 2 weeks before mating and during gestation with 20 mg/kg/day (corresponding to AUC value of about 500 µg•h/L), neither effects on reproductive performance or fertility were seen. Based on AUC values, the systemic exposure was about 15-fold higher in animals than in humans. In male mice, a dose of 30 mg/kg/day did not induce any adverse effects on fertility.

Pregnancy

Pregnancy Category C. At oral doses of 20 mg/kg/day (approximately 14 times the human exposure), no anomalies or malformations were observed in mice. When given at doses of 30 to 40 mg/kg/day, tolterodine has been shown to be embryolethal and reduce fetal weight, and increase the incidence of fetal abnormalities (cleft palate, digital abnormalities, intra abdominal hemorrhage, and various skeletal abnormalities, primarily reduced ossification) in mice. At

Continued on next page

Table 3. Incidence* (%) of Adverse Events Exceeding Placebo Rate and Reported in ≥1% of Patients Treated with DETROL LA (4 mg daily) in a 12-week, Phase 3 Clinical Trial

Body System	Adverse Event	% DETROL LA n=505	% Placebo n=507
Autonomic Nervous	dry mouth	23	8
General	headache	6	4
	fatigue	2	1
Central/Peripheral Nervous	dizziness	2	1
Gastrointestinal	constipation	6	4
	abdominal pain	4	2
	dyspepsia	3	1
Vision	xerophthalmia	3	2
	vision abnormal	1	0
Psychiatric	somnolence	3	2
	anxiety	1	0
Respiratory	sinusitis	2	1
Urinary	dysuria	1	0

* in nearest integer.

Bottle of 30		Bottles of 500	
2 mg Capsules	NDC 0009-5190-01	2 mg Capsules	NDC 0009-5190-03
4 mg Capsules	NDC 0009-5191-01	4 mg Capsules	NDC 0009-5191-03
Bottles of 90		Unit Dose Blisters	
2 mg Capsules	NDC 0009-5190-02	2 mg Capsules	NDC 0009-5190-04
4 mg Capsules	NDC 0009-5191-02	4 mg Capsules	NDC 0009-5191-04

Detrol LA—Cont.

these doses, the AUC values were about 20- to 25-fold higher than in humans. Rabbits treated subcutaneously at a dose of 0.8 mg/kg/day achieved an AUC of 100 μg•h/L, which is about 3-fold higher than that resulting from the human dose. This dose did not result in any embryotoxicity or teratogenicity. There are no studies of tolterodine in pregnant women. Therefore, DETROL LA should be used during pregnancy only if the potential benefit for the mother justifies the potential risk to the fetus.

Nursing Mothers

Tolterodine immediate release is excreted into the milk in mice. Offspring of female mice treated with tolterodine 20 mg/kg/day during the lactation period had slightly reduced bodyweight gain. The offspring regained the weight during the maturation phase. It is not known whether tolterodine is excreted in human milk; therefore, DETROL LA should not be administered during nursing. A decision should be made whether to discontinue nursing or to discontinue DETROL LA in nursing mothers.

Pediatric Use

Efficacy in the pediatric population has not been demonstrated.

A total of 710 pediatric patients (486 on DETROL LA, 224 on placebo) aged 5-10 with urinary frequency and urge incontinence were studied in two phase 3 randomized, placebo-controlled, double-blind, 12-week studies. The percentage of patients with urinary tract infections was higher in patients treated with DETROL LA (6.6%) compared to patients who received placebo (4.5%). Aggressive, abnormal and hyperactive behavior and attention disorders occurred in 2.9% of children treated with DETROL LA compared to 0.9% of children treated with placebo.

Geriatric Use

No overall differences in safety were observed between the older and younger patients treated with tolterodine (see **CLINICAL PHARMACOLOGY, Pharmacokinetics in Special Populations**).

ADVERSE REACTIONS

The Phase 2 and 3 clinical trial program for DETROL LA Capsules included 1073 patients who were treated with DETROL LA (n=537) or placebo (n=536). The patients were treated with 2, 4, 6, or 8 mg/day for up to 15 months. Because clinical trials are conducted under widely varying conditions, adverse reaction rates observed in the clinical trials of a drug cannot be directly compared to rates in the clinical trials of another drug and may not reflect the rates observed in practice. The adverse reaction information from clinical trials does, however, provide a basis for identifying the adverse events that appear to be related to drug use and for approximating rates. The data described below reflect exposure to DETROL LA 4 mg once daily every morning in 505 patients and to placebo in 507 patients exposed for 12 weeks in the Phase 3, controlled clinical study.

Adverse events were reported in 52% (n=263) of patients receiving DETROL LA and in 49% (n=247) of patients receiving placebo. The most common adverse events reported by patients receiving DETROL LA were dry mouth, headache, constipation, and abdominal pain. Dry mouth was the most frequently reported adverse event for patients treated with DETROL LA occurring in 23.4% of patients treated with DETROL LA and 7.7% of placebo-treated patients. Dry mouth, constipation, abnormal vision (accommodation abnormalities), urinary retention, and dry eyes are expected side effects of antimuscarinic agents. A serious adverse event was reported by 1.4% (n=7) of patients receiving DETROL LA and by 3.6% (n=18) of patients receiving placebo.

The frequency of discontinuation due to adverse events was highest during the first 4 weeks of treatment. Similar percentages of patients treated with DETROL LA or placebo discontinued treatment due to adverse events. Treatment was discontinued due to adverse events and dry mouth was reported as an adverse event in 2.4% (n=12) of patients treated with DETROL LA and in 1.2% (n=6) of patients treated with placebo.

Table 3 lists the adverse events reported in 1% or more of patients treated with DETROL LA 4 mg once daily in the 12-week study. The adverse events were reported regardless of causality.

[See table 3 above]

Postmarketing Surveillance

The following events have been reported in association with tolterodine use in clinical practice: anaphylactoid reactions, including angioedema; tachycardia; palpitations; peripheral edema; and hallucinations. Because these spontaneously reported events are from the worldwide postmarketing experience, the frequency of events and the role of tolterodine in their causation cannot be reliably determined.

OVERDOSAGE

A 27-month-old child who ingested 5 to 7 tolterodine immediate release tablets 2 mg was treated with a suspension of activated charcoal and was hospitalized overnight with symptoms of dry mouth. The child fully recovered.

Management of Overdosage

Overdosage with DETROL LA Capsules can potentially result in severe central anticholinergic effects and should be treated accordingly.

ECG monitoring is recommended in the event of overdosage. In dogs, changes in the QT interval (slight prolongation of 10% to 20%) were observed at a suprapharmacologic dose of 4.5 mg/kg, which is about 68 times higher than the recommended human dose. In clinical trials of normal volunteers and patients, QT interval prolongation was not observed with tolterodine immediate release at doses up to 8 mg (4 mg bid) and higher doses were not evaluated.

DOSAGE AND ADMINISTRATION

The recommended dose of DETROL LA Capsules are 4 mg daily. DETROL LA should be taken once daily with liquids and swallowed whole. The dose may be lowered to 2 mg daily based on individual response and tolerability, however, limited efficacy data is available for DETROL LA 2 mg (see **CLINICAL STUDIES**).

For patients with significantly reduced hepatic or renal function or who are currently taking drugs that are potent inhibitors of CYP3A4, the recommended dose of DETROL LA is 2 mg daily (see **CLINICAL PHARMACOLOGY** and **PRECAUTIONS, Drug Interactions**).

HOW SUPPLIED

DETROL LA Capsules 2 mg are blue-green with symbol and 2 printed in white ink. DETROL LA Capsules 4 mg are blue with symbol and 4 printed in white ink. DETROL LA Capsules are supplied as follows:

[See second table above]

Store at 25°C (77°F); excursions permitted to 15-30°C (59-86°F) [see USP Controlled Room Temperature].

Protect from light.

℞ **only**

U.S. Patent No. 5,382,600

Manufactured for
Pharmacia & Upjohn Company
A subsidiary of Pharmacia Corporation
Kalamazoo, MI 49001, USA
By
International Processing Corporation
Winchester, Kentucky 40391, USA
Revised April 2004
818 229 007
692167
4688-76

Shown in Product Identification Guide, page 330

DOSTINEX® ℞

(cabergoline tablets)

DESCRIPTION

DOSTINEX Tablets contain cabergoline, a dopamine receptor agonist. The chemical name for cabergoline is 1-[(6-allylergolin-8β-yl)-carbonyl]-1-[3-(dimethylamino)propyl]-3-ethylurea. Its empirical formula is $C_{26}H_{37}N_5O_2$, and its molecular weight is 451.62. The structural formula is as follows:

Cabergoline is a white powder soluble in ethyl alcohol, chloroform, and N, N-dimethylformamide (DMF); slightly soluble in 0.1N hydrochloric acid; very slightly soluble in n-hexane; and insoluble in water.

DOSTINEX Tablets, for oral administration, contain 0.5 mg of cabergoline. Inactive ingredients consist of leucine, USP, and lactose, NF.

CLINICAL PHARMACOLOGY

Mechanism of Action: The secretion of prolactin by the anterior pituitary is mainly under hypothalmic inhibitory control, likely exerted through release of dopamine by tuberoinfundibular neurons. Cabergoline is a long-acting dopamine receptor agonist with a high affinity for D_2 receptors. Results of in vitro studies demonstrate that cabergoline exerts a direct inhibitory effect on the secretion of prolactin by rat pituitary lactotrophs. Cabergoline decreased serum prolactin levels in reserpinized rats. Receptor-binding studies indicate that cabergoline has low affinity for dopamine D_1, α_1- and α_2-adrenergic, and 5-HT_1- and 5-HT_2-serotonin receptors.

Clinical Studies: The prolactin-lowering efficacy of DOSTINEX was demonstrated in hyperprolactinemic women in two randomized, double-blind, comparative studies, one with placebo and the other with bromocriptine. In the placebo-controlled study (placebo n=20; cabergoline n=168), DOSTINEX produced a dose-related decrease in serum prolactin levels with prolactin normalized after 4 weeks of treatment in 29%, 76%, 74% and 95% of the patients receiving 0.125, 0.5, 0.75, and 1.0 mg twice weekly respectively.

In the 8-week, double-blind period of the comparative trial with bromocriptine (cabergoline n=223; bromocriptine n=236 in the intent-to-treat analysis), prolactin was normalized in 77% of the patients treated with DOSTINEX at 0.5 mg twice weekly compared with 59% of those treated with bromocriptine at 2.5 mg twice daily. Restoration of menses occurred in 77% of the women treated with DOSTINEX, compared with 70% of those treated with bromocriptine. Among patients with galactorrhea, this symptom disappeared in 73% of those treated with DOSTINEX compared with 56% of those treated with bromocriptine.

Pharmacokinetics

Absorption: Following single oral doses of 0.5 mg to 1.5 mg given to 12 healthy adult volunteers, mean peak plasma levels of 30 to 70 picograms (pg)/mL of cabergoline were observed within 2 to 3 hours. Over the 0.5-to-7 mg dose range, cabergoline plasma levels appeared to be dose-proportional in 12 healthy adult volunteers and nine adult parkinsonian patients. A repeat-dose study in 12 healthy volunteers suggests that steady-state levels following a once-weekly dosing schedule are expected to be twofold to threefold higher than after a single dose. The absolute bioavailability of cabergoline is unknown. A significant fraction of the administered dose undergoes a first-pass effect. The elimination half-life of cabergoline estimated from urinary data of 12 healthy subjects ranged between 63 to 69 hours. The prolonged prolactin-lowering effect of cabergoline may be related to its slow elimination and long half-life.

Distribution: In animals, based on total radioactivity, cabergoline (and/or its metabolites) has shown extensive tissue distribution. Radioactivity in the pituitary exceeded that in plasma by >100-fold and was eliminated with a half-life of approximately 60 hours. This finding is consistent with the long-lasting prolactin-lowering effect of the drug. Whole body autoradiography studies in pregnant rats showed no fetal uptake but high levels in the uterine wall. Significant radioactivity (parent plus metabolites) detected in the milk of lactating rats suggests a potential for exposure to nursing infants. The drug is extensively distributed throughout the body. Cabergoline is moderately bound (40% to 42%) to human plasma proteins in a concentration-independent manner. Concomitant dosing of highly protein-bound drugs is unlikely to affect its disposition.

Metabolism: In both animals and humans, cabergoline is extensively metabolized, predominately via hydrolysis of the acylurea bond or the urea moiety. Cytochrome P-450 mediated metabolism appears to be minimal. Cabergoline does not cause enzyme induction and/or inhibition in the rat. Hydrolysis of the acylurea or urea moiety abolishes the prolactin-lowering effect of cabergoline, and major metabolites identified thus far do not contribute to the therapeutic effect.

Excretion: After oral dosing of radioactive cabergoline to five healthy volunteers, approximately 22% and 60% of the dose was excreted within 20 days in the urine and feces, respectively. Less than 4% of the dose was excreted unchanged in the urine. Nonrenal and renal clearances for cabergoline are about 3.2 L/min and 0.08 L/min, respectively. Urinary excretion in hyperprolactinemic patients was similar.

Special Populations

Renal Insufficiency: The pharmacokinetics of cabergoline were not altered in 12 patients with moderate-to-severe renal insufficiency as assessed by creatinine clearance.

Hepatic Insufficiency: In 12 patients with mild-to-moderate hepatic dysfunction (Child-Pugh score ≤10), no effect on mean cabergoline C_{max} or area under the plasma concentration curve (AUC) was observed. However, patients with severe insufficiency (Child-Pugh score >10) show a substantial increase in the mean cabergoline C_{max} and AUC, and thus necessitate caution.

Elderly: Effect of age on the pharmacokinetics of cabergoline has not been studied.

Food-Drug Interaction

In 12 healthy adult volunteers, food did not alter cabergoline kinetics.

Pharmacodynamics

Dose response with inhibition of plasma prolactin, onset of maximal effect, and duration of effect has been documented following single cabergoline doses to healthy volunteers (0.05 to 1.5 mg) and hyperprolactinemic patients (0.3 to 1 mg). In volunteers, prolactin inhibition was evident at doses >0.2 mg, while doses ≥0.5 mg caused maximal suppression in most subjects. Higher doses produce prolactin suppression in a greater proportion of subjects and with an earlier onset and longer duration of action. In 12 healthy volunteers, 0.5, 1, and 1.5 mg doses resulted in complete prolactin inhibition, with a maximum effect within 3 hours in 92% to 100% of subjects after the 1 and 1.5 mg doses compared with 50% of subjects after the 0.5 mg dose.

In hyperprolactinemic patients (N=51), the maximal prolactin decrease after a 0.6 mg single dose of cabergoline was comparable to 2.5 mg bromocriptine; however, the duration of effect was markedly longer (14 days vs 24 hours). The time to maximal effect was shorter for bromocriptine than cabergoline (6 hours vs 48 hours).

In 72 healthy volunteers, single or multiple doses (up to 2 mg) of cabergoline resulted in selective inhibition of prolactin with no apparent effect on other anterior pituitary hormones (GH, FSH, LH, ACTH, and TSH) or cortisol.

INDICATIONS AND USAGE

DOSTINEX Tablets are indicated for the treatment of hyperprolactinemic disorders, either idiopathic or due to pituitary adenomas.

CONTRAINDICATIONS

DOSTINEX Tablets are contraindicated in patients with uncontrolled hypertension or known hypersensitivity to ergot derivatives.

WARNINGS

Dopamine agonists in general should not be used in patients with pregnancy-induced hypertension, for example, preeclampsia and eclampsia, unless the potential benefit is judged to outweigh the possible risk.

PRECAUTIONS

General: Initial doses higher than 1.0 mg may produce orthostatic hypotension. Care should be exercised when administering DOSTINEX with other medications known to lower blood pressure.

Postpartum Lactation Inhibition or Suppression: DOSTINEX is not indicated for the inhibition or suppression of physiologic lactation. Use of bromocriptine, another dopamine agonist for this purpose, has been associated with cases of hypertension, stroke, and seizures.

Hepatic Impairment: Since cabergoline is extensively metabolized by the liver, caution should be used, and careful monitoring exercised, when administering DOSTINEX to patients with hepatic impairment.

Information for Patients: A patient should be instructed to notify her physician if she suspects she is pregnant, becomes pregnant, or intends to become pregnant during therapy. A pregnancy test should be done if there is any suspicion of pregnancy and continuation of treatment should be discussed with her physician.

Drug Interactions: DOSTINEX should not be administered concurrently with D_2-antagonists, such as phenothiazines, butyrophenones, thioxanthines, or metoclopramide.

Carcinogenesis, Mutagenesis, Impairment of Fertility: Carcinogenicity studies were conducted in mice and rats with cabergoline given by gavage at doses up to 0.98 mg/kg/day and 0.32 mg/kg/day, respectively. These doses are 7 times and 4 times the maximum recommended human dose calculated on a body surface area basis using total mg/m^2/week in rodents and mg/m^2/week for a 50 kg human.

There was a slight increase in the incidence of cervical and uterine leiomyomas and uterine leiomyosarcomas in mice. In rats, there was a slight increase in malignant tumors of the cervix and uterus and interstitial cell adenomas. The occurrence of tumors in female rodents may be related to the prolonged suppression of prolactin secretion because prolactin is needed in rodents for the maintenance of the corpus luteum. In the absence of prolactin, the estrogen/progesterone ratio is increased, thereby increasing the risk for uterine tumors. In male rodents, the decrease in serum prolactin levels was associated with an increase in serum luteinizing hormone, which is thought to be a compensatory effect to maintain testicular steroid synthesis. Since these hormonal mechanisms are thought to be species-specific, the relevance of these tumors to humans is not known.

The mutagenic potential of cabergoline was evaluated and found to be negative in a battery of in vitro tests. These tests included the bacterial mutation (Ames) test with *Salmonella typhimurium*, the gene mutation assay with *Schizosaccharomyces pombe* P_1 and V79 Chinese hamster cells, DNA damage and repair in *Saccharomyces cerevisiae* D_4, and chromosomal aberrations in human lymphocytes. Cabergoline was also negative in the bone marrow micronucleus test in the mouse.

In female rats, a daily dose of 0.003 mg/kg for 2 weeks prior to mating and throughout the mating period inhibited conception. This dose represents approximately 1/28 the maximum recommended human dose calculated on a body surface area basis using total mg/m^2/week in rats and mg/m^2/week for a 50 kg human.

Pregnancy: Teratogenic Effects: Category B. Reproduction studies have been performed with cabergoline in mice, rats, and rabbits administered by gavage.

(Multiples of the maximum recommended human dose in this section are calculated on a body surface area basis using total mg/m^2/week for animals and mg/m^2/week for a 50 kg human.)

There were maternotoxic effects but no teratogenic effects in mice given cabergoline at doses up to 8 mg/kg/day (approximately 55 times the maximum recommended human dose) during the period of organogenesis.

A dose of 0.012 mg/kg/day (approximately 1/7 the maximum recommended human dose) during the period of organogenesis in rats caused an increase in post-implantation embryofetal losses. These losses could be due to the prolactin inhibitory properties of cabergoline in rats. At daily doses of 0.5 mg/kg/day (approximately 19 times the maximum recommended human dose) during the period of organogenesis in the rabbit, cabergoline caused maternotoxicity characterized by a loss of body weight and decreased food consumption. Doses of 4 mg/kg/day (approximately 150 times the maximum recommended human dose) during the period of organogenesis in the rabbit caused an increased occurrence of various malformations. However, in another study in rabbits, no treatment-related malformations or embryofetotoxicity were observed at doses up to 8 mg/kg/day (approximately 300 times the maximum recommended human dose).

In rats, doses higher than 0.003 mg/kg/day (approximately 1/28 the maximum recommended human dose) from 6 days before parturition and throughout the lactation period inhibited growth and caused death of offspring due to decreased milk secretion.

There are, however, no adequate and well-controlled studies in pregnant women. Because animal reproduction studies are not always predictive of human response, this drug should be used during pregnancy only if clearly needed.

Nursing Mothers: It is not known whether this drug is excreted in human milk. Because many drugs are excreted in human milk and because of the potential for serious adverse reactions in nursing infants from cabergoline, a decision should be made whether to discontinue nursing or to discontinue the drug, taking into account the importance of the drug to the mother. Use of DOSTINEX for the inhibition or suppression of physiologic lactation is not recommended (see PRECAUTIONS section).

The prolactin-lowering action of cabergoline suggests that it will interfere with lactation. Due to this interference with lactation, DOSTINEX should not be given to women postpartum who are breastfeeding or who are planning to breastfeed.

Pediatric Use: Safety and effectiveness of DOSTINEX in pediatric patients have not been established.

Geriatric Use: Clinical studies of DOSTINEX did not include sufficient numbers of subjects aged 65 and over to determine whether they respond differently from younger patients. Other reported clinical experience has not identified differences in responses between the elderly and younger patients. In general, dose selection for an elderly patient should be cautious, usually starting at the low end of the dosing range, reflecting the greater frequency of decreased hepatic, renal, or cardiac function, and of concomitant disease or other drug therapy.

ADVERSE REACTIONS

The safety of DOSTINEX Tablets has been evaluated in more than 900 patients with hyperprolactinemic disorders. Most adverse events were mild or moderate in severity.

In a 4-week, double-blind, placebo-controlled study, treatment consisted of placebo or cabergoline at fixed doses of 0.125, 0.5, 0.75, or 1.0 mg twice weekly. Doses were halved during the first week. Since a possible dose-related effect was observed for nausea only, the four cabergoline treatment groups have been combined. The incidence of the most common adverse events during the placebo-controlled study is presented in the following table.

Incidence of Reported Adverse Events During the 4-Week, Double-Blind, Placebo-Controlled Trial

Adverse Event*	Cabergoline (n=168) 0.125 to 1 mg two times a week	Placebo (n=20)
	Number (percent)	
Gastrointestinal		
Nausea	45 (27)	4 (20)
Constipation	16 (10)	0
Abdominal pain	9 (5)	1 (5)
Dyspepsia	4 (2)	0
Vomiting	4 (2)	0
Central and Peripheral Nervous System		
Headache	43 (26)	5 (25)
Dizziness	25 (15)	1 (5)
Paresthesia	2 (1)	0
Vertigo	2 (1)	0
Body As a Whole		
Asthenia	15 (9)	2 (10)
Fatigue	12 (7)	0
Hot flashes	2 (1)	1 (5)
Psychiatric		
Somnolence	9 (5)	1 (5)
Depression	5 (3)	1 (5)
Nervousness	4 (2)	0
Autonomic Nervous System		
Postural hypotension	6 (4)	0
Reproductive—Female		
Breast pain	2 (1)	0
Dysmenorrhea	2 (1)	0
Vision		
Abnormal vision	2 (1)	0

*Reported at ≥1% for cabergoline

In the 8-week, double-blind period of the comparative trial with bromocriptine, DOSTINEX (at a dose of 0.5 mg twice weekly) was discontinued because of an adverse event in 4 of 221 patients (2%) while bromocriptine (at a dose of 2.5 mg two times a day) was discontinued in 14 of 231 patients (6%). The most common reasons for discontinuation from DOSTINEX were headache, nausea and vomiting (3, 2 and 2 patients respectively); the most common reasons for discontinuation from bromocriptine were nausea, vomiting, headache, and dizziness or vertigo (10, 3, 3, and 3 patients respectively). The incidence of the most common adverse events during the double-blind portion of the comparative trial with bromocriptine is presented in the following table.

Incidence of Reported Adverse Events During the 8-week, Double-Blind Period of the Comparative Trial With Bromocriptine

Adverse Event*	Cabergoline (n=221)	Bromocriptine (n=231)
	Number (percent)	
Gastrointestinal		
Nausea	63 (29)	100 (43)
Constipation	15 (7)	21 (9)
Abdominal pain	12 (5)	19 (8)
Dyspepsia	11 (5)	16 (7)
Vomiting	9 (4)	16 (7)

Continued on next page

Dostinex—Cont.

Dry mouth	5 (2)	2 (1)
Diarrhea	4 (2)	7 (3)
Flatulence	4 (2)	3 (1)
Throat irritation	2 (1)	0
Toothache	2 (1)	0
Central and Peripheral Nervous System		
Headache	58 (26)	62 (27)
Dizziness	38 (17)	42 (18)
Vertigo	9 (4)	10 (4)
Paresthesia	5 (2)	6 (3)
Body As a Whole		
Asthenia	13 (6)	15 (6)
Fatigue	10 (5)	18 (8)
Syncope	3 (1)	3 (1)
Influenza-like symptoms	2 (1)	0
Malaise	2 (1)	0
Periorbital edema	2 (1)	2 (1)
Peripheral edema	2 (1)	1
Psychiatric		
Depression	7 (3)	5 (2)
Somnolence	5 (2)	5 (2)
Anorexia	3 (1)	3 (1)
Anxiety	3 (1)	3 (1)
Insomnia	3 (1)	2 (1)
Impaired concentration	2 (1)	1
Nervousness	2 (1)	5 (2)
Cardiovascular		
Hot flashes	6 (3)	3 (1)
Hypotension	3 (1)	4 (2)
Dependent edema	2 (1)	1
Palpitation	2 (1)	5 (2)
Reproductive—Female		
Breast pain	5 (2)	8 (3)
Dysmenorrhea	2 (1)	1
Skin and Appendages		
Acne	3 (1)	0
Pruritus	2 (1)	1
Musculoskeletal		
Pain	4 (2)	6 (3)
Arthralgia	2 (1)	0
Respiratory		
Rhinitis	2 (1)	9 (4)
Vision		
Abnormal vision	2 (1)	2 (1)

*Reported at ≥1% for cabergoline

Other adverse events that were reported at an incidence of <1.0% in the overall clinical studies follow.

Body As a Whole: facial edema, influenza-like symptoms, malaise

Cardiovascular System: hypotension, syncope, palpitations

Digestive System: dry mouth, flatulence, diarrhea, anorexia

Metabolic and Nutritional System: weight loss, weight gain

Nervous System: somnolence, nervousness, paresthesia, insomnia, anxiety

Respiratory System: nasal stuffiness, epistaxis

Skin and Appendages: acne, pruritus

Special Senses: abnormal vision

Urogenital System: dysmenorrhea, increased libido

The safety of cabergoline has been evaluated in approximately 1,200 patients with Parkinson's disease in controlled and uncontrolled studies at dosages of up to 11.5 mg/day which greatly exceeds the maximum recommended dosage of cabergoline for hyperprolactinemic disorders. In addition to the adverse events that occurred in the patients with hyperprolactinemic disorders, the most common adverse events in patients with Parkinson's disease were dyskinesia, hallucinations, confusion, and peripheral edema. Heart failure, pleural effusion, pulmonary fibrosis, and gastric or duodenal ulcer occurred rarely. One case of constrictive pericarditis has been reported.

OVERDOSAGE

Overdosage might be expected to produce nasal congestion, syncope, or hallucinations. Measures to support blood pressure should be taken if necessary.

DOSAGE AND ADMINISTRATION

The recommended dosage of DOSTINEX Tablets for initiation of therapy is 0.25 mg twice a week. Dosage may be increased by 0.25 mg twice weekly up to a dosage of 1 mg twice a week according to the patient's serum prolactin level.

Dosage increases should not occur more rapidly than every 4 weeks, so that the physician can assess the patient's response to each dosage level. If the patient does not respond adequately, and no additional benefit is observed with higher doses, the lowest dose that achieved maximal response should be used and other therapeutic approaches considered.

After a normal serum prolactin level has been maintained for 6 months, DOSTINEX may be discontinued, with periodic monitoring of the serum prolactin level to determine whether or when treatment with DOSTINEX should be reinstituted. The durability of efficacy beyond 24 months of therapy with DOSTINEX has not been established.

HOW SUPPLIED

DOSTINEX Tablets are white, scored, capsule-shaped tablets containing 0.5 mg cabergoline. Each tablet is scored on one side and has the letter P and the letter U on either side of the breakline. The other side of the tablet is engraved with the number 700.

DOSTINEX is available as follows:

Bottles of 8 tablets NDC 0013-7001-12

STORAGE

Store at controlled room temperature 20° to 25° C (68° to 77° F) [see USP].

℞ only

U.S. Patent No. 4,526,892.

Manufactured for: Pharmacia & Upjohn Company
A subsidiary of Pharmacia Corporation
Kalamazoo, MI 49001, USA

by: Pharmacia Italia S.p.A.
Milan, Italy

816 989 103 **N. 320006104.00.8** Revised March 2003

Shown in Product Identification Guide, page 330

ELLENCE® ℞

[ĕl-ĕns]

(epirubicin hydrochloride injection)

> **WARNING**
>
> 1. Severe local tissue necrosis will occur if there is extravasation during administration (See PRECAUTIONS). Epirubicin must not be given by the intramuscular or subcutaneous route.
> 2. Myocardial toxicity, manifested in its most severe form by potentially fatal congestive heart failure (CHF), may occur either during therapy with epirubicin or months to years after termination of therapy. The probability of developing clinically evident CHF is estimated as approximately 0.9% at a cumulative dose of 550 mg/m^2, 1.6% at 700 mg/m^2, and 3.3% at 900 mg/m^2. In the adjuvant treatment of breast cancer, the maximum cumulative dose used in clinical trials was 720 mg/m^2. The risk of developing CHF increases rapidly with increasing total cumulative doses of epirubicin in excess of 900 mg/m^2; this cumulative dose should only be exceeded with extreme caution. Active or dormant cardiovascular disease, prior or concomitant radiotherapy to the mediastinal/pericardial area, previous therapy with other anthracyclines or anthracenediones, or concomitant use of other cardiotoxic drugs may increase the risk of cardiac toxicity. Cardiac toxicity with ELLENCE may occur at lower cumulative doses whether or not cardiac risk factors are present.
> 3. Secondary acute myelogenous leukemia (AML) has been reported in patients with breast cancer treated with anthracyclines, including epirubicin. The occurrence of refractory secondary leukemia is more common when such drugs are given in combination with DNA-damaging antineoplastic agents, when patients have been heavily pretreated with cytotoxic drugs, or when doses of anthracyclines have been escalated. The cumulative risk of developing treatment-related AML, in 3844 patients with breast cancer who received adjuvant treatment with epirubicin-containing regimens, was estimated as 0.2% at 3 years and 0.8% at 5 years.
> 4. Dosage should be reduced in patients with impaired hepatic function (see DOSAGE AND ADMINISTRATION).
> 5. Severe myelosuppression may occur.
> 6. Epirubicin should be administered only under the supervision of a physician who is experienced in the use of cancer chemotherapeutic agents.

DESCRIPTION

ELLENCE Injection (epirubicin hydrochloride injection) is an anthracycline cytotoxic agent, intended for intravenous administration. ELLENCE is supplied as a sterile, clear, red solution and is available in polypropylene vials containing 50 and 200 mg of epirubicin hydrochloride as a preservative-free, ready-to-use solution. Each milliliter of solution contains 2 mg of epirubicin hydrochloride. Inactive ingredients include sodium chloride, USP, and water for injection, USP. The pH of the solution has been adjusted to 3.0 with hydrochloric acid, NF.

Epirubicin hydrochloride is the 4-epimer of doxorubicin and is a semi-synthetic derivative of daunorubicin. The chemical name is (8S- ***cis***)-10-[(3-amino-2,3,6-trideoxy-α-L- ***arabino***-hexopyranosyl)oxy]-7,8,9,10- tetrahydro-6,8,11-trihydroxy-8-(hydroxyacetyl)-1-methoxy-5,12-naphthacenedione hydrochloride. The active ingredient is a red-orange hygroscopic powder, with the empirical formula $C_{27}H_{29}NO_{11}$ HCl and a molecular weight of 579.95. The structural formula is as follows:

CLINICAL PHARMACOLOGY

Epirubicin is an anthracycline cytotoxic agent. Although it is known that anthracyclines can interfere with a number of biochemical and biological functions within eukaryotic cells, the precise mechanisms of epirubicin's cytotoxic and/or antiproliferative properties have not been completely elucidated.

Epirubicin forms a complex with DNA by intercalation of its planar rings between nucleotide base pairs, with consequent inhibition of nucleic acid (DNA and RNA) and protein synthesis. Such intercalation triggers DNA cleavage by topoisomerase II, resulting in cytocidal activity. Epirubicin also inhibits DNA helicase activity, preventing the enzymatic separation of double-stranded DNA and interfering with replication and transcription. Epirubicin is also involved in oxidation/reduction reactions by generating cytotoxic free radicals. The antiproliferative and cytotoxic activity of epirubicin is thought to result from these or other possible mechanisms.

Epirubicin is cytotoxic in vitro to a variety of established murine and human cell lines and primary cultures of human tumors. It is also active in vivo against a variety of murine tumors and human xenografts in athymic mice, including breast tumors.

Pharmacokinetics

Epirubicin pharmacokinetics are linear over the dose range of 60 to 150 mg/m^2 and plasma clearance is not affected by the duration of infusion or administration schedule. Pharmacokinetic parameters for epirubicin following 6- to 10-minute, single-dose intravenous infusions of epirubicin at doses of 60 to 150 mg/m^2 in patients with solid tumors are shown in Table 1. The plasma concentration declined in a triphasic manner with mean half-lives for the alpha, beta, and gamma phases of about 3 minutes, 2.5 hours, and 33 hours, respectively.

[See table 1 below]

Distribution. Following intravenous administration, epirubicin is rapidly and widely distributed into the tissues. Binding of epirubicin to plasma proteins, predominantly albumin, is about 77% and is not affected by drug concentration. Epirubicin also appears to concentrate in red blood cells; whole blood concentrations are approximately twice those of plasma.

Metabolism. Epirubicin is extensively and rapidly metabolized by the liver and is also metabolized by other organs and cells, including red blood cells. Four main metabolic routes have been identified:

Table 1. Summary of Mean (±SD) Pharmacokinetic Parameters in Patients[1] with Solid Tumors Receiving Intravenous Epirubicin 60 to 150 mg/m^2

Dose[2] (mg/m^2)	C_{max}[3] (μg/mL)	AUC[4] (μg · h/mL)	t ½[5] (hours)	CL[6] (L/hour)	Vss[7] (L/kg)
60	5.7 ± 1.6	1.6 ± 0.2	35.3 ± 9	65 ± 8	21 ± 2
75	5.3 ± 1.5	1.7 ± 0.3	32.1 ± 5	83 ± 14	27 ± 11
120	9.0 ± 3.5	3.4 ± 0.7	33.7 ± 4	65 ± 13	23 ± 7
150	9.3 ± 2.9	4.2 ± 0.8	31.1 ± 6	69 ± 13	21 ± 7

[1] Advanced solid tumor cancers, primarily of the lung
[2] N=6 patients per dose level
[3] Plasma concentration at the end of 6 to 10 minute infusion
[4] Area under the plasma concentration curve
[5] Half-life of terminal phase
[6] Plasma clearance
[7] Steady state volume of distribution

(1) reduction of the C-13 keto-group with the formation of the 13(S)-dihydro derivative, epirubicinol;
(2) conjugation of both the unchanged drug and epirubicinol with glucuronic acid; (3) loss of the amino sugar moiety through a hydrolytic process with the formation of the doxorubicin and doxorubicinol aglycones; and (4) loss of the amino sugar moiety through a redox process with the formation of the 7-deoxy-doxorubicin aglycone and 7-deoxydoxorubicinol aglycone. Epirubicinol has in vitro cytotoxic activity one-tenth that of epirubicin. As plasma levels of epirubicinol are lower than those of the unchanged drug, they are unlikely to reach in vivo concentrations sufficient for cytotoxicity. No significant activity or toxicity has been reported for the other metabolites.

Excretion. Epirubicin and its major metabolites are eliminated through biliary excretion and, to a lesser extent, by urinary excretion. Mass-balance data from 1 patient found about 60% of the total radioactive dose in feces (34%) and urine (27%). These data are consistent with those from 3 patients with extrahepatic obstruction and percutaneous drainage, in whom approximately 35% and 20% of the administered dose were recovered as epirubicin or its major metabolites in bile and urine, respectively, in the 4 days after treatment.

Pharmacokinetics in Special Populations

Age. A population analysis of plasma data from 36 cancer patients (13 males and 23 females, 20 to 73 years) showed that age affects plasma clearance of epirubicin in female patients. The predicted plasma clearance for a female patient of 70 years of age was about 35% lower than that for a female patient of 25 years of age. An insufficient number of males > 50 years of age were included in the study to draw conclusions about age-related alterations in clearance in males. Although a lower epirubicin starting dose does not appear necessary in elderly female patients, and was not used in clinical trials, particular care should be taken in monitoring toxicity when epirubicin is administered to female patients > 70 years of age. (See PRECAUTIONS).

Gender. In patients ≤ 50 years of age, mean clearance values in adult male and female patients were similar. The clearance of epirubicin is decreased in elderly women (see Pharmacokinetics in Special Populations - Age).

Pediatric. The pharmacokinetics of epirubicin in pediatric patients have not been evaluated.

Race. The influence of race on the pharmacokinetics of epirubicin has not been evaluated.

Hepatic Impairment. Epirubicin is eliminated by both hepatic metabolism and biliary excretion and clearance is reduced in patients with hepatic dysfunction. In a study of the effect of hepatic dysfunction, patients with solid tumors were classified into 3 groups. Patients in Group 1 (n=22) had serum AST (SGOT) levels above the upper limit of normal (median: 93 IU/L) and normal serum bilirubin levels (median: 0.5 mg/dL) and were given epirubicin doses of 12.5 to 90 mg/m^2. Patients in Group 2 had alterations in both serum AST (median: 175 IU/L) and bilirubin levels (median: 2.7 mg/dL) and were treated with an epirubicin dose of 25 mg/m^2 (n=8). Their pharmacokinetics were compared to those of patients with normal serum AST and bilirubin values, who received epirubicin doses of 12.5 to 120 mg/m^2. The median plasma clearance of epirubicin was decreased compared to patients with normal hepatic function by about 30% in patients in Group 1 and by 50% in patients in Group 2. Patients with more severe hepatic impairment have not been evaluated. (See WARNINGS and DOSAGE AND ADMINISTRATION.)

Renal Impairment. No significant alterations in the pharmacokinetics of epirubicin or its major metabolite, epirubicinol, have been observed in patients with serum creatinine < 5 mg/dL. A 50% reduction in plasma clearance was reported in four patients with serum creatinine ≥ 5 mg/dL (see WARNINGS and DOSAGE AND ADMINISTRATION). Patients on dialysis have not been studied.

Drug-Drug Interactions

Taxanes. Coadministration of paclitaxel or docetaxel did not affect the pharmacokinetics of epirubicin when given immediately following the taxane.

Cimetidine. Coadministration of cimetidine (400 mg twice daily for 7 days starting 5 days before chemotherapy) increased the mean AUC of epirubicin (100 mg/m^2) by 50% and decreased its plasma clearance by 30% (see PRECAUTIONS).

Drugs metabolized by cytochrome P-450 enzymes. No systematic in vitro or in vivo evaluation has been performed to examine the potential for inhibition or induction by epirubicin of oxidative cytochrome P-450 isoenzymes.

CLINICAL STUDIES

Two randomized, open-label, multicenter studies evaluated the use of ELLENCE Injection 100 to 120 mg/m^2 in combination with cyclophosphamide and fluorouracil for the adjuvant treatment of patients with axiliary-node-positive breast cancer and no evidence of distant metastatic disease (Stage II or III). Study MA-5 evaluated 120 mg/m^2 of epirubicin per course in combination with cyclophosphamide and fluorouracil (CEF-120 regimen). This study randomized premenopausal and perimenopausal women with one or more positive lymph nodes to an epirubicin-containing CEF-120 regimen or to a CMF regimen. Study GFEA-05 evaluated the use of 100 mg/m^2 of epirubicin per course in combination with fluorouracil and cyclophosphamide (FEC-100). This study randomized pre- and postmenopausal women to the FEC-100 regimen or to a lower-dose FEC-50 regimen. In the GFEA-05 study, eligible patients were either required to have ≥ 4 nodes involved with tumor or, if only 1 to 3 nodes were positive, to have negative estrogen- and progesterone-receptors and a histologic tumor grade of 2 or 3. A total of 1281 women participated in these studies. Patients with T4 tumors were not eligible for either study. Table 2 shows the treatment regimens that the patients received.

[See table 2 above]

Table 2. Treatment Regimens Used in Phase 3 Studies of Patients with Early Breast Cancer

	Treatment Groups	Agent	Regimen
MA-5[1] N=716	**CEF-120** (total, 6 cycles)[2] N=356	Cyclophosphamide	75 mg/m^2 PO, d 1-14, q 28 days
		ELLENCE	60 mg/m^2 IV, d 1 & 8, q 28 days
		Fluorouracil	500 mg/m^2 IV, d 1 & 8, q 28 days
	CMF (total, 6 cycles) N=360	Cyclophosphamide	100 mg/m^{2}PO, d 1-14, q 28 days
		Methotrexate	40 mg/m^2 IV, d 1 & 8, q 28 days
		Fluorouracil	600 mg/m^2 IV, d 1 & 8, q 28 days
GFEA-05[3] N=565	**FEC-100** (total, 6 cycles) N=276	Fluorouracil	500 mg/m^{2}IV, d 1, q 21 days
		ELLENCE	100 mg/m^2 IV, d 1, q 21 days
		Cyclophosphamide	500 mg/m^2 IV, d 1, q 21 days
	FEC-50 (total, 6 cycles) N=289	Fluorouracil	500 mg/m^{2}IV, d 1, q 21 days
		ELLENCE	50 mg/m^2 IV, d 1, q 21 days
		Cyclophosphamide	500 mg/m^2 IV, d 1, 21 days
	Tamoxifen 30 mg daily × 3 years, postmenopausal women, any receptor status		

[1] In women who underwent lumpectomy, breast irradiation was to be administered after completion of study chemotherapy.
[2] Patients also received prophylactic antibiotic therapy with trimethoprim-sulfamethoxazole or fluroquinolone for the duration of their chemotherapy.
[3] All women were to receive breast irradiation after the completion of chemotherapy.

In the MA-5 trial, the median age of the study population was 45 years. Approximately 60% of patients had 1 to 3 involved nodes and approximately 40% had ≥ 4 nodes involved with tumor. In the GFEA-05 study, the median age was 51 years and approximately half of the patients were postmenopausal. About 17% of the study population had 1 to 3 positive nodes and 80% of patients had ≥ 4 involved lymph nodes. Demographic and tumor characteristics were well-balanced between treatment arms in each study.

The efficacy endpoints of relapse-free survival (RFS) and overall survival (OS) were analyzed using Kaplan-Meier methods in the intent-to-treat (ITT) patient populations in each study. Results for endpoints are described in terms of the outcomes at 5 years. In Study MA-5, epirubicin-containing combination therapy (CEF-120) showed significantly longer 5-year RFS than CMF (62% versus 53%; stratified log rank p=0.013). The overall reduction in risk of relapse was 24%. The 5-year OS was also greater for the epirubicin-containing CEF-120 regimen than for the CMF regimen (77% versus 70%; stratified log rank p=0.043; nonstratified log rank p=0.13). The overall relative reduction in the risk of death was 29%.

In Study GFEA-05, patients treated with the higher-dose epirubicin regimen (FEC-100) had a significantly longer 5-year RFS (65% versus 52%, log rank p=0.007) and OS (76% versus 65%, log rank p=0.007) than patients given the lower dose regimen (FEC-50). The overall reduction in risk of relapse was 32%. The relative reduction in the risk of death was 31%.

Although the trials were not powered for subset analyses, improvement in RFS and OS were observed both in patients with 1-3 nodes positive and in those with ≥ 4 nodes positive for tumor involvement when comparing the CEF-120 or FEC-100 groups with the control groups. In addition, in the GFEA-05 study, similar improvements in RFS and OS were observed in both pre- and postmenopausal women treated with FEC-100 compared to FEC-50. Efficacy results for the two studies are shown in Table 3.

[See table 3 above]

Table 3. Efficacy Results from Phase 3 Studies of Patients with Early Breast Cancer*

	MA-5 Study		GFEA-05 Study	
	CEF-120 N=356	CMF N=360	FEC-100 N=276	FEC-50 N=289
RFS at 5 yrs (%)	62	53	65	52
Log-rank Test	(stratified p=0.013)		(p=0.007)	
OS at 5 yrs	77	70	76	65
Log-rank Test	(stratified p=0.043) (unstratified p=0.13)		(p=0.007)	

*Based on Kaplan-Meier estimates

The Kaplan-Meier curves for RFS and OS from Study MA-5 are shown in Figures 1 and 2 and those for Study GFEA-05 are shown in Figures 3 and 4.

[See figures 1 through 4 at top of next page]

INDICATIONS AND USAGE

ELLENCE Injection is indicated as a component of adjuvant therapy in patients with evidence of axillary node tumor involvement following resection of primary breast cancer.

CONTRAINDICATIONS

Patients should not be treated with ELLENCE Injection if they have any of the following conditions: baseline neutrophil count < 1500 cells/mm^3; severe myocardial insufficiency, recent myocardial infarction, severe arrhythmias; previous treatment with anthracyclines up to the maximum cumulative dose; hypersensitivity to epirubicin, other anthracyclines, or anthracenediones; or severe hepatic dysfunction (see WARNINGS and DOSAGE AND ADMINISTRATION).

WARNINGS

ELLENCE Injection should be administered only under the supervision of qualified physicians experienced in the use of cytotoxic therapy. Before beginning treatment with epirubicin, patients should recover from acute toxicities (such as stomatitis, neutropenia, thrombocytopenia, and generalized infections) of prior cytotoxic treatment. Also, initial treatment with ELLENCE should be preceded by a careful baseline assessment of blood counts; serum levels of total bilirubin, AST, and creatinine; and cardiac function as measured by left ventricular ejection function (LVEF). Patients should be carefully monitored during treatment for possible clinical complications due to myelosuppression. Supportive care may be necessary for the treatment of severe neutropenia and severe infectious complications. Monitoring for potential cardiotoxicity is also important, especially with greater cumulative exposure to epirubicin.

Hematologic Toxicity. A dose-dependent, reversible leukopenia and/or neutropenia is the predominant manifestation of hematologic toxicity associated with epirubicin and represents the most common acute dose-limiting toxicity of this drug. In most cases, the white blood cell (WBC) nadir is reached 10 to 14 days from drug administration. Leukopenia/neutropenia is usually transient, with WBC and neutrophil counts generally returning to normal values by Day 21 after drug administration. As with other cytotoxic agents, ELLENCE at the recommended dose in combination with cyclophosphamide and fluorouracil can produce severe leukopenia and neutropenia. Severe thrombocytopenia and anemia may also occur. Clinical consequences of severe myelosuppression include fever, infection, septicemia, septic shock, hemorrhage, tissue hypoxia, symptomatic anemia, or death. If myelosuppressive complications occur, appropriate supportive measures (e.g., intravenous antibiotics, colony-stimulating factors, transfusions) may be required. Myelosuppression requires careful monitoring. Total and differential WBC, red blood cell (RBC), and platelet counts should be assessed before and during each cycle of therapy with ELLENCE.

Cardiac Function. Cardiotoxicity is a known risk of anthracycline treatment. Anthracycline-induced cardiac toxicity may be manifested by early (or acute) or late (delayed) events. Early cardiac toxicity of epirubicin consists mainly of sinus tachycardia and/or ECG abnormalities such as nonspecific ST-T wave changes, but tachyarrhythmias, including premature ventricular contractions and ventricular tachycardia, bradycardia, as well as atrioventricular and bundle-branch block have also been reported. These effects do not usually predict subsequent development of delayed

Continued on next page

Ellence—Cont.

cardiotoxicity, are rarely of clinical importance, and are generally not considered an indication for the suspension of epirubicin treatment. Delayed cardiac toxicity results from a characteristic cardiomyopathy that is manifested by reduced LVEF and/or signs and symptoms of congestive heart failure (CHF) such as tachycardia, dyspnea, pulmonary edema, dependent edema, hepatomegaly, ascites, pleural effusion, gallop rhythm. Life-threatening CHF is the most severe form of anthracycline-induced cardiomyopathy. This toxicity appears to be dependent on the cumulative dose of ELLENCE and represents the cumulative dose-limiting toxicity of the drug. If it occurs, delayed cardiotoxicity usually develops late in the course of therapy with ELLENCE or within 2 to 3 months after completion of therapy, but later events (several months to years after treatment termination) have been reported.

In a retrospective survey, including 9144 patients, mostly with solid tumors in advanced stages, the probability of developing CHF increased with increasing cumulative doses of ELLENCE (Figure 5). The estimated risk of epirubicin-treated patients developing clinically evident CHF was 0.9% at a cumulative dose of 550 mg/m^2, 1.6% at 700 mg/m^2, and 3.3% at 900 mg/m^2. The risk of developing CHF in the absence of other cardiac risk factors increased steeply after an epirubicin cumulative dose of 900 mg/m^2.

Figure 5. Risk of CHF in 9144 Patients Treated with Epirubicin

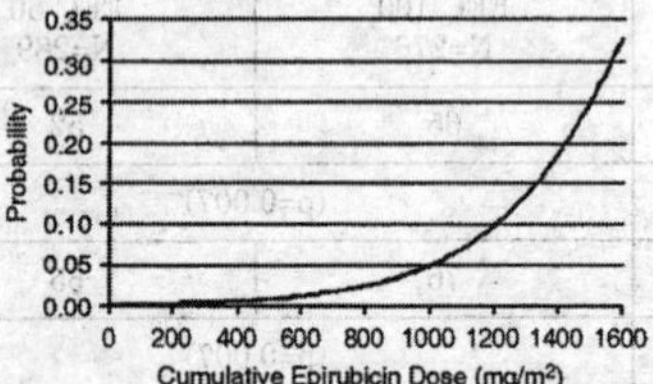

In another retrospective survey of 469 epirubicin-treated patients with metastatic or early breast cancer, the reported risk of CHF was comparable to that observed in the larger study of over 9000 patients.

Given the risk of cardiomyopathy, a cumulative dose of 900 mg/m^2 ELLENCE should be exceeded only with extreme caution. Risk factors (active or dormant cardiovascular disease, prior or concomitant radiotherapy to the mediastinal/pericardial area, previous therapy with other anthracyclines or anthracenediones, concomitant use of other drugs with the ability to suppress cardiac contractility) may increase the risk of cardiac toxicity. Although not formally tested, it is probable that the toxicity of epirubicin and other anthracyclines or anthracenediones is additive. Cardiac toxicity with ELLENCE may occur at lower cumulative doses whether or not cardiac risk factors are present. Although endomyocardial biopsy is recognized as the most sensitive diagnostic tool to detect anthracycline-induced cardiomyopathy, this invasive examination is not practically performed on a routine basis. Electrocardiogram (ECG) changes such as dysrhythmias, a reduction of the QRS voltage, or a prolongation beyond normal limits of the systolic time interval may be indicative of anthracycline-induced cardiomyopathy, but ECG is not a sensitive or specific method for following anthracycline-related cardiotoxicity. The risk of serious cardiac impairment may be decreased through regular monitoring of LVEF during the course of treatment with prompt discontinuation of ELLENCE at the first sign of impaired function. The preferred method for repeated assessment of cardiac function is evaluation of LVEF measured by multi-gated radionuclide angiography (MUGA) or echocardiography (ECHO). A baseline cardiac evaluation with an ECG and a MUGA scan or an ECHO is recommended, especially in patients with risk factors for increased cardiac toxicity. Repeated MUGA or ECHO determinations of LVEF should be performed, particularly with higher, cumulative anthracycline doses. The technique used for assessment should be consistent through follow-up. In patients with risk factors, particularly prior anthracycline or anthracenedione use, the monitoring of cardiac function must be particularly strict and the risk-benefit of continuing treatment with ELLENCE in patients with impaired cardiac function must be carefully evaluated.

Secondary Leukemia. The occurrence of secondary acute myelogenous leukemia, with or without a preleukemic phase, has been reported in patients treated with anthracyclines. Secondary leukemia is more common when such drugs are given in combination with DNA-damaging antineoplastic agents, when patients have been heavily pretreated with cytotoxic drugs, or when doses of the anthracyclines have been escalated. These leukemias can have a short 1- to 3- year latency period. An analysis of 3844 patients who received adjuvant treatment with epirubicin in controlled clinical trials, showed a cumulative risk of secondary acute myelogenous leukemia of about 0.2% (approximate 95% CI, 0.05-0.4) at 3 years and approximately 0.8% (approximate 95% CI, 0.3-1.2) at 5 years. ELLENCE is mutagenic, clastogenic, and carcinogenic in animals (see next section, Carcinogenesis, Mutagenesis and Impairment of Fertility).

Carcinogenesis, Mutagenesis & Impairment of Fertility. Treatment-related acute myelogenous leukemia has been reported in women treated with epirubicin-based adjuvant chemotherapy regimens (see above section, WARNINGS, Secondary Leukemia). Conventional long-term animal studies to evaluate the carcinogenic potential of epirubicin have not been conducted, but intravenous administration of a single 3.6 mg/kg epirubicin dose to female rats (about 0.2 times the maximum recommended human dose on a body surface area basis) approximately doubled the incidence of mammary tumors (primarily fibroadenomas) observed at 1 year. Administration of 0.5 mg/kg epirubicin intravenously to rats (about 0.025 times the maximum recommended human dose on a body surface area basis) every 3 weeks for ten doses increased the incidence of subcutaneous fibromas in males over an 18-month observation period. In addition, subcutaneous administration of 0.75 or 1.0 mg/kg/day (about 0.015 times the maximum recommended human dose on a body surface area basis) to newborn rats for 4 days on both the first and tenth day after birth for a total of eight doses increased the incidence of animals with tumors compared to controls during a 24-month observation period.

Epirubicin was mutagenic in vitro to bacteria (Ames test) either in the presence or absence of metabolic activation and to mammalian cells (HGPRT assay in V79 Chinese hamster lung fibroblasts) in the absence but not in the presence of metabolic activation. Epirubicin was clastogenic in vitro (chromosome aberrations in human lymphocytes) both in the presence and absence of metabolic activation and was also clastogenic in vivo (chromosome aberration in mouse bone marrow).

In fertility studies in rats, males were given epirubicin daily for 9 weeks and mated with females that were given epirubicin daily for 2 weeks prior to mating and through Day 7 of gestation. When 0.3 mg/kg/day (about 0.015 times the maximum recommended human single dose on a body surface area basis) was administered to both sexes, no pregnancies resulted. No effects on mating behavior or fertility were observed at 0.1 mg/kg/day, but male rats had atrophy of the testes and epididymis, and reduced spermatogenesis. The 0.1 mg/kg/day dose also caused embryolethality. An increased incidence of fetal growth retardation was observed in these studies at 0.03 mg/kg/day (about 0.0015 times the maximum recommended human single dose on a body surface area basis). Multiple daily doses of epirubicin to rabbits and dogs also caused atrophy of male reproductive organs. Single 20.5 and 12 mg/kg doses of intravenous epirubicin caused testicular atrophy in mice and rats, respectively (both approximately 0.5 times the maximum recommended human dose on a body surface area basis). A single dose of 16.7 mg/kg epirubicin caused uterine atrophy in rats.

Although experimental data are not available, ELLENCE could induce chromosomal damage in human spermatozoa due to its genotoxic potential. Men undergoing treatment with ELLENCE should use effective contraceptive methods. ELLENCE may cause irreversible amenorrhea (premature menopause) in premenopausal women.

Liver Function. The major route of elimination of epirubicin is the hepatobiliary system (see CLINICAL PHARMACOLOGY, Pharmacokinetics in Special Populations). Serum total bilirubin and AST levels should be evaluated before and during treatment with ELLENCE. Patients with elevated bilirubin or AST may experience slower clearance of drug with an increase in overall toxicity. Lower doses are recommended in these patients (see DOSAGE AND ADMINISTRATION). Patients with severe hepatic impairment have not been evaluated; therefore, epirubicin should not be used in this patient population.

Renal Function. Serum creatinine should be assessed before and during therapy. Dosage adjustment is necessary in patients with serum creatinine >5 mg/dL (see DOSAGE AND ADMINISTRATION). Patients undergoing dialysis have not been studied.

Tumor-Lysis Syndrome. As with other cytotoxic agents, ELLENCE may induce hyperuricemia as a consequence of the extensive purine catabolism that accompanies drug-induced rapid lysis of highly chemosensitive neoplastic cells (tumor lysis syndrome). Other metabolic abnormalities may also occur. While not generally a problem in patients with breast cancer, physicians should consider the potential for tumor-lysis syndrome in potentially susceptible patients and should consider monitoring serum uric acid, potassium, calcium, phosphate, and creatinine immediately after initial chemotherapy administration. Hydration, urine alkalinization, and prophylaxis with allopurinol to prevent hyperuricemia may minimize potential complications of tumor-lysis syndrome.

Pregnancy - Category D. ELLENCE may cause fetal harm when administered to a pregnant woman. Administration of 0.8 mg/kg/day intravenously of epirubicin to rats (about 0.04 times the maximum recommended single human dose on a body surface area basis) during Days 5 to 15 of gestation was embryotoxic (increased resorptions and post-implantation loss) and caused fetal growth retardation (decreased body weight), but was not teratogenic up to this dose. Administration of 2 mg/kg/day intravenously of epirubicin to rats (about 0.1 times the maximum recommended single human dose on a body surface area basis) on Days 9 and 10 of gestation was embryotoxic (increased late resorptions, post-implantation losses, and dead fetuses; and decreased live fetuses), retarded fetal growth (decreased body weight), and caused decreased placental weight. This dose was also teratogenic, causing numerous external (anal atresia, misshapen tail, abnormal genital tubercle), visceral (primarily gastrointestinal, urinary, and cardiovascular systems), and skeletal (deformed long bones and girdles, rib abnormalities, irregular spinal ossification) malformations. Administration of intravenous epirubicin to rabbits at doses up to 0.2 mg/kg/day (about 0.02 times the maximum recommended single human dose on a body surface area basis) during Days 6 to 18 of gestation was not embryotoxic or teratogenic, but a maternally toxic dose of 0.32 mg/kg/day increased abortions and delayed ossification. Administration of a maternally toxic intravenous dose of 1 mg/kg/day epirubicin to rabbits (about 0.1 times the maximum recommended single human dose on a body surface area basis) on Days 10 to 12 of gestation induced abortion, but no other signs of embryofetal toxicity or teratogenicity were observed. When doses up to 0.5 mg/kg/day epirubicin were administered to rat dams from Day 17 of gestation to Day 21 after delivery (about 0.025 times the maximum recommended single human dose on a body surface area basis), no permanent changes were observed in the development, functional activity, behavior, or reproductive performance of the offspring.

There are no adequate and well-controlled studies in pregnant women. Two pregnancies have been reported in women taking epirubicin. A 34-year-old woman, 28 weeks pregnant at her diagnosis of breast cancer, was treated with cyclophosphamide and epirubicin every 3 weeks for 3 cycles. She received the last dose at 34 weeks of pregnancy and delivered a healthy baby at 35 weeks. A second 34-year-old woman with breast cancer metastatic to the liver was randomized to FEC-50 but was removed from study because of pregnancy. She experienced a spontaneous abortion. If epirubicin is used during pregnancy, or if the patient becomes pregnant while taking this drug, the patient should be apprised of the potential hazard to the fetus. Women of childbearing potential should be advised to avoid becoming pregnant.

Figure 1. Relapse-Free Survival in Study MA-5

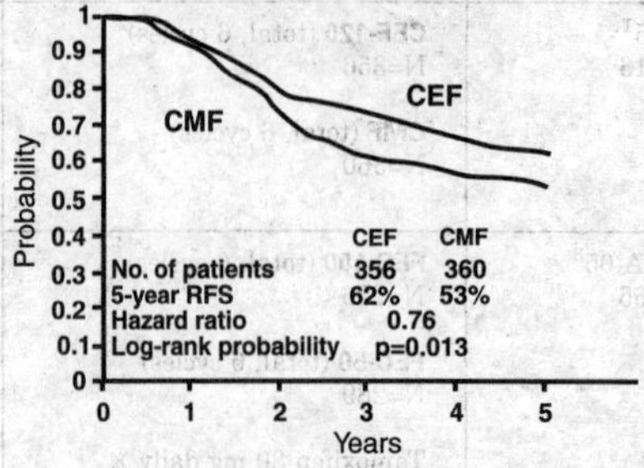

Figure 2. Overall Survival in Study MA-5

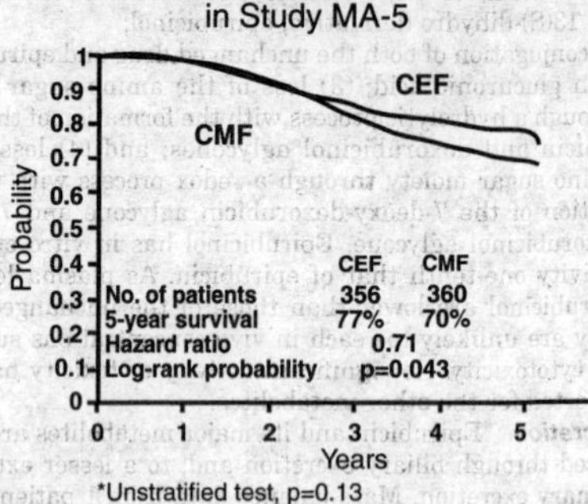

*Unstratified test, p=0.13

Figure 3. Relapse-Free Survival in Study GFEA-05

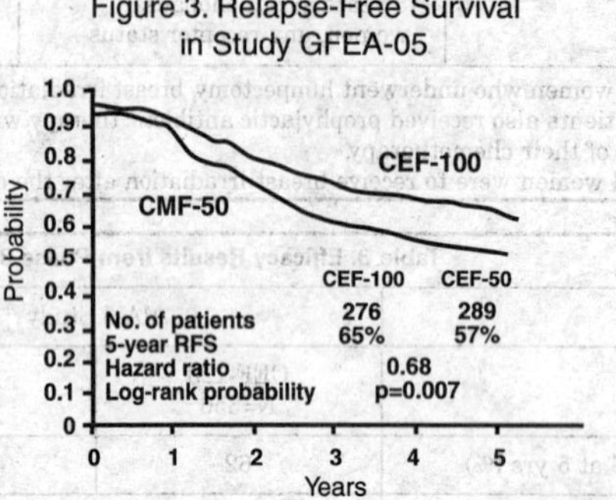

Figure 4. Overall Survival in Study GFEA-0

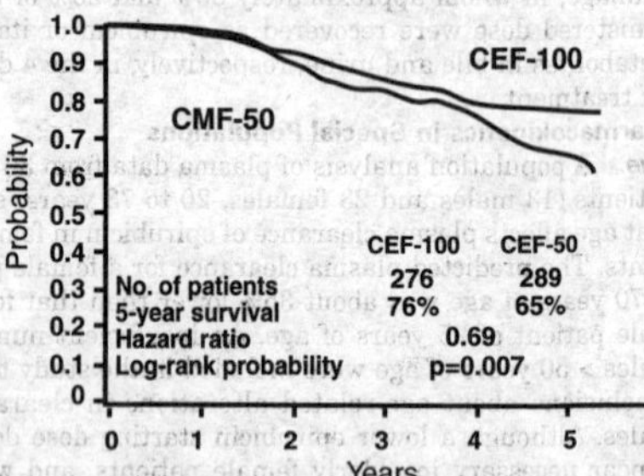

PRECAUTIONS

General

ELLENCE Injection is administered by intravenous infusion. Venous sclerosis may result from an injection into a small vessel or from repeated injections into the same vein. Extravasation of epirubicin during the infusion may cause local pain, severe tissue lesions (vesication, severe cellulitis) and necrosis. It is recommended that ELLENCE be slowly administered into the tubing of a freely running intravenous infusion, usually between 3 and 20 minutes depending upon dosage and volume of the infusion solution (see DOSAGE AND ADMINISTRATION, Preparation of Infusion Solution). If possible, veins over joints or in extremities with compromised venous or lymphatic drainage should be avoided. A burning or stinging sensation may be indicative of perivenous infiltration, and the infusion should be immediately terminated and restarted in another vein. Perivenous infiltration may occur without causing pain.

Facial flushing, as well as local erythematous streaking along the vein, may be indicative of excessively rapid administration. It may precede local phlebitis or thrombophlebitis.

Patients administered the 120-mg/m² regimen of ELLENCE as a component of combination chemotherapy should also receive prophylactic antibiotic therapy with trimethoprim-sulfamethoxazole (e.g., Septra®, Bactrim®) or a fluoroquinolone (see CLINICAL STUDIES, Early Breast Cancer, and DOSAGE AND ADMINISTRATION).

Epirubicin is emetigenic. Antiemetics may reduce nausea and vomiting; prophylactic use of antiemetics should be considered before administration of ELLENCE, particularly when given in conjunction with other emetigenic drugs.

As with other anthracyclines, administration of ELLENCE after previous radiation therapy may induce an inflammatory recall reaction at the site of the irradiation.

As with other cytotoxic agents, thrombophlebitis and thromboembolic phenomena, including pulmonary embolism (in some cases fatal) have been coincidentally reported with the use of epirubicin.

Information for Patients

Patients should be informed of the expected adverse effects of epirubicin, including gastrointestinal symptoms (nausea, vomiting, diarrhea, and stomatitis) and potential neutropenic complications. Patients should consult their physician if vomiting, dehydration, fever, evidence of infection, symptoms of CHF, or injection-site pain occurs following therapy with ELLENCE. Patients should be informed that they will almost certainly develop alopecia. Patients should be advised that their urine may appear red for 1 to 2 days after administration of ELLENCE and that they should not be alarmed. Patients should understand that there is a risk of irreversible myocardial damage associated with treatment with ELLENCE, as well as a risk of treatment-related leukemia. Because epirubicin may induce chromosomal damage in sperm, men undergoing treatment with ELLENCE should use effective contraceptive methods. Women treated with ELLENCE may develop irreversible amenorrhea, or premature menopause.

Laboratory Testing

See WARNINGS. Blood counts, including absolute neutrophil counts, and liver function should be assessed before and during each cycle of therapy with epirubicin. Repeated evaluations of LVEF should be performed during therapy.

Drug Interactions

ELLENCE when used in combination with other cytotoxic drugs may show on-treatment additive toxicity, especially hematologic and gastrointestinal effects.

Concomitant use of ELLENCE with other cardioactive compounds that could cause heart failure (e.g., calcium channel blockers), requires close monitoring of cardiac function throughout treatment.

There are few data regarding the coadministration of radiation therapy and epirubicin. In adjuvant trials of epirubicin-containing CEF-120 or FEC-100 chemotherapies, breast irradiation was delayed until after chemotherapy was completed. This practice resulted in no apparent increase in local breast cancer recurrence relative to published accounts in the literature. A small number of patients received epirubicin-based chemotherapy concomitantly with radiation therapy but had chemotherapy interrupted in order to avoid potential overlapping toxicities. It is likely that use of epirubicin with radiotherapy may sensitize tissues to the cytotoxic actions of irradiation. Administration of ELLENCE after previous radiation therapy may induce an inflammatory recall reaction at the site of the irradiation.

Epirubicin is extensively metabolized by the liver. Changes in hepatic function induced by concomitant therapies may affect epirubicin metabolism, pharmacokinetics, therapeutic efficacy, and/or toxicity.

Cimetidine increased the AUC of epirubicin by 50%. Cimetidine treatment should be stopped during treatment with ELLENCE (see CLINICAL PHARMACOLOGY).

Drug-Laboratory Test Interactions

There are no known interactions between ELLENCE and laboratory tests.

Carcinogenesis, Mutagenesis & Impairment of Fertility

See WARNINGS.

Pregnancy

Pregnancy Category D - see WARNINGS.

Nursing Mothers

Epirubicin was excreted into the milk of rats treated with 0.50 mg/kg/day of epirubicin during peri- and postnatal periods. It is not known whether epirubicin is excreted in human milk. Because many drugs, including other anthracyclines, are excreted in human milk and because of the potential for serious adverse reactions in nursing infants from epirubicin, mothers should discontinue nursing prior to taking this drug.

Table 4. Clinically Relevant Acute Adverse Events in Patients with Early Breast Cancer

Event	FEC-100/CEF-120 (N = 620) Grades 1-4	FEC-100/CEF-120 (N = 620) Grades 3/4	FEC-50 (N = 280) Grades 1-4	FEC-50 (N = 280) Grades 3/4	CMF (N = 360) Grades 1-4	CMF (N = 360) Grades 3/4
Hematologic						
Leukopenia	80.3	58.6	49.6	1.5	98.1	60.3
Neutropenia	80.3	67.2	53.9	10.5	95.8	78.1
Anemia	72.2	5.8	12.9	0	70.9	0.9
Thrombocytopenia	48.8	5.4	4.6	0	51.4	3.6
Endocrine						
Amenorrhea	71.8	0	69.3	0	67.7	0
Hot flashes	38.9	4.0	5.4	0	69.1	6.4
Body as a Whole						
Lethargy	45.8	1.9	1.1	0	72.7	0.3
Fever	5.2	0	1.4	0	4.5	0
Gastrointestinal						
Nausea/vomiting	92.4	25.0	83.2	22.1	85.0	6.4
Mucositis	58.5	8.9	9.3	0	52.9	1.9
Diarrhea	24.8	0.8	7.1	0	50.7	2.8
Anorexia	2.9	0	1.8	0	5.8	0.3
Infection						
Infection	21.5	1.6	15.0	0	25.9	0.6
Febrile neutropenia	NA	6.1	0	0	NA	1.1
Ocular						
Conjunctivitis/keratitis	14.8	0	1.1	0	38.4	0
Skin						
Alopecia	95.5	56.6	69.6	19.3	84.4	6.7
Local toxicity	19.5	0.3	2.5	0.4	8.1	0
Rash/itch	8.9	0.3	1.4	0	14.2	0
Skin changes	4.7	0	0.7	0	7.2	0

FEC & CEF = cyclophosphamide + epirubicin + fluorouracil; CMF = cyclophosphamide + methotrexate + flurouracil

NA = not available

Table 5. Long-Term Adverse Events in Patients with Early Breast Cancer

Event	FEC-100/CEF-120 (N=620)	FEC-50 (N=280)	CMF (N=360)
	% of Patients		
Cardiac toxicity			
Asymptomatic drops in LVEF	1.8	1.4	0.8
CHF	1.5	0.4	0.3
Leukemia			
AML	0.8	0	0.3

Geriatric Use

Although a lower starting dose of ELLENCE was not used in trials in elderly female patients, particular care should be taken in monitoring toxicity when ELLENCE is administered to female patients ≥ 70 years of age. (See CLINICAL PHARMACOLOGY, Pharmacokinetics in Special Populations).

Pediatric Use

The safety and effectiveness of epirubicin in pediatric patients have not been established in adequate and well-controlled clinical trials. Pediatric patients may be at greater risk for anthracycline-induced acute manifestations of cardiotoxicity and for chronic CHF.

ADVERSE REACTIONS

On-Study Events

Integrated safety data are available from two studies (Studies MA-5 and GFEA-05, see CLINICAL STUDIES) evaluating epirubicin-containing combination regimens in patients with early breast cancer. Of the 1260 patients treated in these studies, 620 patients received the higher-dose epirubicin regimen (FEC-100/CEF-120), 280 patients received the lower-dose epirubicin regimen (FEC-50), and 360 patients received CMF. Serotonin-specific antiemetic therapy and colony-stimulating factors were not used in these trials. Clinically relevant acute adverse events are summarized in Table 4.

[See table 4 above]

Grade 1 or 2 changes in transaminase levels were observed but were more frequently seen with CMF than with CEF.

Delayed Events

Table 5 describes the incidence of delayed adverse events in patients participating in the MA-5 and GFEA-05 trials.

[See table 5 above]

Two cases of acute lymphoid leukemia (ALL) were also observed in patients receiving epirubicin. However, an association between anthracyclines such as epirubicin and ALL has not been clearly established.

Overview of Acute and Delayed Toxicities

Hematologic—See WARNINGS.

Gastrointestinal. A dose-dependent mucositis (mainly oral stomatitis, less often esophagitis) may occur in patients treated with epirubicin. Clinical manifestations of mucositis may include a pain or burning sensation, erythema, erosions, ulcerations, bleeding, or infections. Mucositis generally appears early after drug administration and, if severe, may progress over a few days to mucosal ulcerations; most patients recover from this adverse event by the third week of therapy. Hyperpigmentation of the oral mucosa may also occur.

Nausea, vomiting, and occasionally diarrhea and abdominal pain can also occur. Severe vomiting and diarrhea may produce dehydration. Antiemetics may reduce nausea and vomiting; prophylactic use of antiemetics should be considered before therapy (see PRECAUTIONS).

Cutaneous and Hypersensitivity Reactions. Alopecia occurs frequently, but is usually reversible, with hair regrowth occurring within 2 to 3 months from the termination of therapy. Flushes, skin and nail hyperpigmentation, photosensitivity, and hypersensitivity to irradiated skin (radiation-recall reaction) have been observed. Urticaria and anaphylaxis have been reported in patients treated with epirubicin; signs and symptoms of these reactions may vary from skin rash and pruritus to fever, chills, and shock.

Cardiovascular—See WARNINGS.

Secondary Leukemia—See WARNINGS

Injection-Site Reactions—See PRECAUTIONS.

OVERDOSAGE

A 36-year-old man with non-Hodgkin's lymphoma received a daily 95 mg/m² dose of ELLENCE Injection for 5 consecutive days. Five days later, he developed bone marrow aplasia, grade 4 mucositis, and gastrointestinal bleeding. No signs of acute cardiac toxicity were observed. He was treated with antibiotics, colony-stimulating factors, and antifungal agents, and recovered completely. A 63-year-old woman with breast cancer and liver metastasis received a single 320 mg/m² dose of ELLENCE. She was hospitalized

Continued on next page

Ellence—Cont.

with hyperthermia and developed multiple organ failure (respiratory and renal), with lactic acidosis, increased lactate dehydrogenase, and anuria. Death occurred within 24 hours after administration of ELLENCE. Additional instances of administration of doses higher than recommended have been reported at doses ranging from 150 to 250 mg/m^2. The observed adverse events in these patients were qualitatively similar to known toxicities of epirubicin. Most of the patients recovered with appropriate supportive care.

If an overdose occurs, supportive treatment (including antibiotic therapy, blood and platelet transfusions, colony-stimulating factors, and intensive care as needed) should be provided until the recovery of toxicities. Delayed CHF has been observed months after anthracycline administration. Patients must be observed carefully over time for signs of CHF and provided with appropriate supportive therapy.

DOSAGE AND ADMINISTRATION

ELLENCE Injection is administered to patients by intravenous infusion. ELLENCE is given in repeated 3- to 4-week cycles. The total dose of ELLENCE may be given on Day 1 of each cycle or divided equally and given on Days 1 and 8 of each cycle. The recommended dosages of ELLENCE are as follows:

Starting Doses

The recommended starting dose of ELLENCE is 100 to 120 mg/m^2. The following regimens were used in the trials supporting use of ELLENCE as a component of adjuvant therapy in patients with axillary-node positive breast cancer:

[See table below]

Patients administered the 120-mg/m^2 regimen of ELLENCE also received prophylactic antibiotic therapy with trimethoprim-sulfamethoxazole (e.g., Septra®, Bactrim®) or a fluoroquinolone.

Bone Marrow Dysfunction. Consideration should be given to administration of lower starting doses (75-90 mg/m^2) for heavily pretreated patients, patients with pre-existing bone marrow depression, or in the presence of neoplastic bone marrow infiltration (see WARNINGS and PRECAUTIONS).

Hepatic Dysfunction. Definitive recommendations regarding use of ELLENCE in patients with hepatic dysfunction are not available because patients with hepatic abnormalities were excluded from participation in adjuvant trials of FEC-100/CEF-120 therapy. In patients with elevated serum AST or serum total bilirubin concentrations, the following dose reductions were recommended in clinical trials, although few patients experienced hepatic impairment:

- Bilirubin 1.2 to 3 mg/dL or AST 2 to 4 times upper limit of normal
  1/2 of recommended starting dose
- Bilirubin > 3 mg/dL or AST > 4 times upper limit of normal
  1/4 of recommended starting dose

Information regarding experience in patients with hepatic dysfunction is provided in CLINICAL PHARMACOLOGY, Pharmacokinetics In Special Populations.

Renal Dysfunction. While no specific dose recommendation can be made based on the limited available data in patients with renal impairment, lower doses should be considered in patients with severe renal impairment (serum creatinine > 5 mg/dL).

Dose Modifications

Dosage adjustments after the first treatment cycle should be made based on hematologic and nonhematologic toxicities. Patients experiencing during treatment cycle nadir platelet counts <50,000/mm^3, absolute neutrophil counts (ANC) <250/mm^3, neutropenic fever, or Grades 3/4 nonhematologic toxicity should have the Day 1 dose in subsequent cycles reduced to 75% of the Day 1 dose given in the current cycle. Day 1 chemotherapy in subsequent courses of treatment should be delayed until platelet counts are ≥100,000/mm^3, ANC ≥1500/mm^3, and nonhematologic toxicities have recovered to ≤ Grade 1.

For patients receiving a divided dose of ELLENCE (Day 1 and Day 8), the Day 8 dose should be 75% of Day 1 if platelet counts are 75,000-100,000/mm^3 and ANC is 1000 to 1499/mm^3. If Day 8 platelet counts are <75,000/mm^3, ANC <1000/mm^3, or Grade 3/4 nonhematologic toxicity has occurred, the Day 8 dose should be omitted.

Preparation & Administration Precautions

Parenteral drug products should be inspected visually for particulate matter and discoloration prior to administration, whenever solution and container permit. Procedures normally used for proper handling and disposal of anticancer drugs should be considered for use with ELLENCE. Several guidelines on this subject have been published.[1-8]

Protective measures. The following protective measures should be taken when handling ELLENCE:

- Personnel should be trained in appropriate techniques for reconstitution and handling.
- Pregnant staff should be excluded from working with this drug.
- Personnel handling ELLENCE should wear protective clothing: goggles, gowns and disposable gloves and masks.
- A designated area should be defined for syringe preparation (preferably under a laminar flow system), with the work surface protected by disposable, plastic-backed, absorbent paper.
- All items used for reconstitution, administration or cleaning (including gloves) should be placed in high-risk, waste-disposal bags for high temperature incineration.

Spillage or leakage should be treated with dilute sodium hypochlorite (1% available chlorine) solution, preferably by soaking, and then water. All contaminated and cleaning materials should be placed in high-risk, waste-disposal bags for incineration. Accidental contact with the skin or eyes should be treated immediately by copious lavage with water, or soap and water, or sodium bicarbonate solution. However, do not abrade the skin by using a scrub brush. Medical attention should be sought. Always wash hands after removing gloves.

Incompatibilities. Prolonged contact with any solution of an alkaline pH should be avoided as it will result in hydrolysis of the drug. ELLENCE should not be mixed with heparin or fluorouracil due to chemical incompatibility that may lead to precipitation.

ELLENCE can be used in combination with other antitumor agents, but it is not recommended that it be mixed with other drugs in the same syringe.

Preparation of Infusion Solution

ELLENCE is provided as a preservative-free, ready-to-use solution.

ELLENCE should be administered into the tubing of a freely flowing intravenous infusion (0.9% sodium chloride or 5% glucose solution). The usual infusion time ranges between 3 and 20 minutes depending upon dosage and volume of the infusion solution. This technique is intended to minimize the risk of thrombosis or perivenous extravasation, which could lead to severe cellulitis, vesication, or tissue necrosis. A direct push injection is not recommended due to the risk of extravasation, which may occur even in the presence of adequate blood return upon needle aspiration. Venous sclerosis may result from injection into small vessels or repeated injections into the same vein (see PRECAUTIONS). ELLENCE should be used within 24 hours of first penetration of the rubber stopper. Discard any unused solution.

HOW SUPPLIED

ELLENCE Injection is available in polypropylene single-use vials containing 2 mg epirubicin hydrochloride per mL as a sterile, preservative-free, ready-to-use solution in the following strengths:

50 mg/25 mL single-use vial	NDC 0009-5091-01
200 mg/100 mL single-use vial	NDC 0009-5093-01

Store refrigerated between 2°C and 8°C (36°F and 46°F). Do not freeze. Protect from light. Discard unused portion.

℞ only

US Patent No. 5,977,082

Manufactured for: Pharmacia & Upjohn Company, A subsidiary of Pharmacia Corporation, Kalamazoo, MI 49001 USA

By: Pharmacia (Perth) Pty Limited, Bentley WA 6102 Australia

April 2003 817 911 105
692532

REFERENCES

1. ONS Clinical Practice Committee. Cancer Chemotherapy Guidelines and Recommendations for Practice. Pittsburgh, PA: Oncology Nursing Society; 1999: 32-41.
2. Recommendations for the Safe Handling of Parenteral Antineoplastic Drugs. Washington, DC: Division of Safety, Clinical Center Pharmacy Department and Cancer Nursing Services, National Institutes of Health; 1992 US Dept of Health and Human Services. Public Health Service Publication NIH 92-2621.
3. AMA Council on Scientific Affairs. Guidelines for Handling Parenteral Antineoplastics. JAMA 1985; 253(11): 1590-1592.
4. National Study Commission on Cytotoxic Exposure - Recommendations for Handling of Cytotoxic Agents. 1987. Available from Louis P. Jeffrey, ScD., Chairman, National Study Commission on Cytotoxic Exposure, Massachusetts College of Pharmacy and Allied Health Sciences, 179 Longwood Avenue, Boston, MA 02115.
5. Clinical Oncology Society of Australia, Guidelines and Recommendations for Safe Handling of Antineoplastic Agents. Med J Australia 1983; 1:426-428.
6. Jones RB, Frank R, Mass T. Safe Handling of Chemotherapeutic Agents: A Report from the Mount Sinai Medical Center. CA-A Cancer J for Clin [illegible]
7. American Society of Hospital Pharmacists. ASHP Technical Assistance Bulletin on Handling Cytotoxic and Hazardous Drugs. Am J Hosp Pharm 1990; 47:1033-1049.
8. Controlling Occupational Exposure to Hazardous Drugs (OSHA Work-Practice Guidelines). Am J Health-Syst Pharm 1996; 53:1669-1685.

Jun 2003 PAM274AC

CEF-120:	Cyclophosphamide	75 mg/m^2 PO D 1-14
	ELLENCE	60 mg/m^2 IV D 1, 8
	5-Fluorouracil	500 mg/m^2 IV D 1, 8
	Repeated every 28 days for 6 cycles	
FEC-100:	5-Fluorouracil	500 mg/m^2
	ELLENCE	100 mg/m^2
	Cyclophosphamide	500 mg/m^2
	All drugs administered intravenously on Day 1 and repeated every 21 days for 6 cycles	

ESTRING® ℞

[ĕ-strĭng]

(estradiol vaginal ring)

2 mg

PHYSICIAN'S LEAFLET

1. ESTROGENS HAVE BEEN REPORTED TO INCREASE THE RISK OF ENDOMETRIAL CARCINOMA IN POSTMENOPAUSAL WOMEN.
   Close clinical surveillance of all women taking estrogens is important. Adequate diagnostic measures, including endometrial sampling when indicated, should be undertaken to rule out malignancy in all cases of undiagnosed persistent or recurring abnormal vaginal bleeding. There is no evidence that "natural" estrogens are more or less hazardous than "synthetic" estrogens at equi-estrogenic doses.
2. ESTROGENS SHOULD NOT BE USED DURING PREGNANCY.
   There is no indication for estrogen therapy during pregnancy or during immediate postpartum period. Estrogens are ineffective for the prevention or treatment of threatened or habitual abortion. Estrogens are not indicated for the prevention of postpartum breast engorgement.
   Estrogen therapy during pregnancy is associated with an increased risk of congenital defects in the reproductive organs of the fetus, and possibly other birth defects. Studies of women who received diethylstilbestrol (DES) during pregnancy have shown that female offspring have an increased risk of vaginal adenosis, squamous cell dysplasia of the uterine cervix, and clear cell vaginal cancer later in life; male offspring have an increased risk of urogenital abnormalities and possibly testicular cancer later in life. The 1985 DES Task Force concluded that the use of DES during pregnancy is associated with a subsequent increased risk of breast cancer in the mothers, although a causal relationship remains unproven and the observed level of excess risk is similar to that for a number of other breast cancer risk factors.

DESCRIPTION

ESTRING (estradiol vaginal ring) is a slightly opaque ring with a whitish core containing a drug reservoir of 2 mg estradiol. Estradiol, silicone polymers and barium sulfate are combined to form the ring. When placed in the vagina, ESTRING releases estradiol, approximately 7.5 µg/24 hours, in a consistent stable manner over 90 days. ESTRING has the following dimensions: outer diameter 55 mm; cross-sectional diameter 9 mm; core diameter 2 mm. One ESTRING should be inserted into the upper third of the vaginal vault, to be worn continuously for three months. Estradiol is chemically described as estra-1,3,5(10)-triene-3,17β-diol. The molecular formula of estradiol is $C_{18}H_{24}O_2$ and the structural formula is:

CH$_3$ OH HO

The molecular weight of estradiol is 272.39.

CLINICAL PHARMACOLOGY

Pharmacokinetics

ABSORPTION

Estrogens used in therapeutics are well absorbed through the skin, mucous membranes, and the gastrointestinal (GI) tract. The vaginal delivery of estrogens circumvents first-pass metabolism possibly reducing the induction of several other hepatic proteins.

In a Phase I study of 14 postmenopausal women, the insertion of ESTRING (estradiol vaginal ring) rapidly increased serum estradiol (E_2) levels attesting to the rapid absorption of estradiol via the vaginal mucosa. The time to attain peak serum estradiol levels (T_{max}) was 0.5 to 1 hour. Peak serum estradiol concentrations post-initial burst declined rapidly over the next 24 hours and were virtually indistinguishable from the baseline mean (range: 5 to 22 pg/mL). Serum levels of estradiol and estrone (E_1) over the following 12 weeks during which the ring was maintained in the vaginal vault remained relatively unchanged (see Table 1).

The initial estradiol peak post-application of the second ring in the same women resulted in ~38% lower C_{max}, apparently due to reduced systemic absorption via the revitalized vaginal epithelium. The relative systemic exposure from the initial peak of ESTRING accounted for approximately 4% of the total estradiol exposure over the 12 week period.

The constant and stable release of estradiol from ESTRING was demonstrated in a Phase II study of 166 - 222 postmenopausal women who inserted up to four rings consecutively at three month intervals. Low dose systemic delivery of estradiol from ESTRING resulted in mean steady state serum estradiol estimates of 7.8, 7.0, 7.0, 8.1 pg/mL at weeks 12, 24, 36, and 48, respectively. Similar reproducibility is also seen in levels of estrone. Lower systemic exposure to estradiol and estrone is further supported by serum levels measured during a pivotal Phase III study.

In post-menopausal women, mean dose of estradiol systemically absorbed unchanged from ESTRING is ~8% [95% CI: 2.8–12.8%] of the daily amount released locally. Low systemic exposure to estradiol and estrone resulting from ESTRING should elicit lower estrogen-dependent effects.

DISTRIBUTION

Circulating, unbound estrogens are known to modulate pharmacological response. Estrogens circulate in blood bound to sex-hormone binding globulin (SHBG) and albumin. A dynamic equilibrium exists between the conjugated and the unconjugated forms of estradiol and estrone, which undergo rapid interconversion.

METABOLISM

Exogenously delivered or endogenously derived estrogens are primarily metabolized in the liver to estrone and estriol, which are also found in the systemic circulation. Estrogen metabolites are primarily excreted in the urine as glucuronides and sulphates. Of the several estrogen metabolites, urinary estrone and estrone sulphate (E_1S), post-ESTRING use, are in the normal post-menopausal range.

EXCRETION

Mean percent dose excreted in the 24-hour urine as estradiol, 4 and 12 weeks post-application of ESTRING in a Phase I study was 5 and 8%, respectively, of the daily released amount.

Drug-Drug Interactions

No formal *drug-drug* interactions studies have been done with ESTRING. It is anticipated that lower exposure to systemic estrogens may reduce the potential for drug interactions thus maintaining the benefit to risk ratio of concomitant drugs.

[See table 1 above]

Pharmacodynamics

In-vivo, estrogens diffuse through cell membranes, distribute throughout the cell, bind to and activate the estrogen receptors, thereby eliciting their biological effects. Estrogen receptors have been identified in tissues of the reproductive tract, breast, pituitary, hypothalamus, liver and bone of women. ESTRING delivers estradiol constantly at a mean rate of ~ 7.5 µg/24 hours for a period of up to 90 days. Its use in post-menopausal patients in Phase I and II studies showed no apparent effects on systemic levels of hepatic protein SHBG, or FSH. Lowering of the pretreatment vaginal pH from a mean of 6.0 to a mean of 4.6 (as found in fertile women) over the 12 to 48 week treatment period, and improvements evident in the vaginal mucosal epithelium seen in all studies attest to the local dynamic effects of estrogens.

INDICATIONS AND USAGE

ESTRING (estradiol vaginal ring) is indicated for the treatment of urogenital symptoms associated with post-menopausal atrophy of the vagina (such as dryness, burning, pruritus and dyspareunia) and/or the lower urinary tract (urinary urgency and dysuria).

CLINICAL STUDIES

Two pivotal controlled studies have demonstrated the efficacy of ESTRING (estradiol vaginal ring) in the treatment of post-menopausal urogenital symptoms due to estrogen deficiency.

In a U.S. study where ESTRING was compared with conjugated estrogens vaginal cream, no difference in efficacy between the treatment groups was found with respect to improvement in the physician's global assessment of vaginal symptoms (83% and 82% of patients receiving ESTRING and cream, respectively) and in the patient's global assessment of vaginal symptoms (83% and 82% of patients receiving ESTRING and cream, respectively) after 12 weeks of treatment. In an Australian study, ESTRING was also compared with conjugated estrogens vaginal cream and no difference in the physician's assessment of improvement of vaginal mucosal atrophy (79% and 75% for ESTRING and cream, respectively) or in the patient's assessment of improvement in vaginal dryness (82% and 76% for ESTRING and cream, respectively) after 12 weeks of treatment.

In the U.S. study, symptoms of dysuria and urinary urgency improved in 74% and 65%, respectively, of patients receiving ESTRING as assessed by the patient. In the Australian study, symptoms of dysuria and urinary urgency improved in 90% and 71%, respectively, of patients receiving ESTRING as assessed by the patient.

In both studies, ESTRING and conjugated estrogens vaginal cream had a similar ability to reduce vaginal pH levels and to mature the vaginal mucosa (as measured cytologically using the maturation index and/or the maturation value) after 12 weeks of treatment. In supportive studies, ESTRING was also shown to have a similar significant treatment effect on the maturation of the urethral mucosa.

Endometrial overstimulation, as evaluated in non-hysterectomized patients participating in the U.S. study by the progestogen challenge test and pelvic sonogram, was reported for none of the 58 (0%) patients receiving ESTRING and 4 of the 35 patients (11%) receiving conjugated estrogens vaginal cream.

Of the U.S. women who completed 12 weeks of treatment, 95% rated product comfort for ESTRING as excellent or very good compared with 65% of patients receiving conjugated estrogens vaginal cream, 95% of ESTRING patients judged the product to be very easy or easy to use compared with 88% of cream patients, and 82% gave ESTRING an overall rating of excellent or very good compared with 58% for the cream.

TABLE 1: PHARMACOKINETIC MEAN ESTIMATES FOLLOWING ESTRING APPLICATION

Estrogen	C_{max} (pg/mL)	$C_{ss\text{-}48\ hr}$ (pg/mL)	$C_{ss\text{-}4w}$ (pg/mL)	$C_{ss\text{-}12w}$ (pg/mL)
Estradiol (E_2)	63.2[a]	11.2	9.5	8.0
Baseline-adjusted E_2[b]	55.6	3.6	2.0	0.4
Estrone (E_1)	66.3	52.5	43.8	47.0
Baseline-adjusted E_1	20.0	6.2	-2.4	0.8

[a] n=14
[b] Based on means

CONTRAINDICATIONS

1. Estrogens should not be used in women with any of the following conditions:
   a. Known or suspected pregnancy (see **BOXED WARNING**).
   b. Undiagnosed abnormal genital bleeding.
   c. Known or suspected cancer of the breast.
   d. Known or suspected estrogen-dependent neoplasia.
2. ESTRING (estradiol vaginal ring) should not be used in patients hypersensitive to any of its ingredients.

WARNINGS

1. **Breast cancer.**
   While the majority of studies have not shown an increased risk of breast cancer in women who have ever used estrogen replacement therapy, some have reported a moderately increased risk (relative risks of 1.3 to 2.0) in those taking higher doses or those taking lower doses for prolonged periods of time, especially in excess of ten years. Other studies have not shown this relationship.
2. **Other.**
   Congenital lesions with malignant potential, gallbladder disease, cardiovascular disease, elevated blood pressure and hypercalcemia have been associated with systemic estrogen treatment.

PRECAUTIONS

A. General

1. **Use of Progestins.**
   It is common practice with systemic administration of estrogen to add progestin for ten or more days during a cycle to lower the incidence of endometrial proliferation or hyperplasia. From the available clinical data, it seems unlikely that ESTRING would have adverse effects on the endometrium. Furthermore, addition of progestins to a patient being treated with ESTRING is not expected to result in vaginal bleeding.
2. **Physical Examination.**
   A complete medical and family history should be taken prior to the initiation of any estrogen therapy. The pretreatment and periodic physical examinations should include special reference to blood pressure, breasts, abdomen, and pelvic organs and should include a Papanicolaou smear. As a general rule, estrogen should not be prescribed for longer than one year without reexamining the patient.
3. **Uterine Bleeding and Mastodynia.**
   Although uncommon with ESTRING, certain patients may develop undesirable manifestations of estrogenic stimulation, such as abnormal uterine bleeding and mastodynia.
4. **Liver Disease.**
   ESTRING should be used with caution in patients with impaired liver function.
5. **Location of ESTRING.**
   Some women have experienced moving or gliding of ESTRING within the vagina. Instances of ESTRING being expelled from the vagina in connection with moving the bowels, strain, or constipation have been reported. If this occurs, ESTRING can be rinsed in lukewarm water and reinserted into the vagina by the patient.
6. **Vaginal Irritation.**
   ESTRING may not be suitable for women with narrow, short, or stenosed vaginas. Narrow vagina, vaginal stenosis, prolapse, and vaginal infections are conditions that make the vagina more susceptible to ESTRING-caused irritation or ulceration. Women with signs or symptoms of vaginal irritation should alert their physician.
7. **Vaginal Infection.**
   Vaginal infection is generally more common in postmenopausal women due to the lack of the normal flora of fertile women, especially lactobacillus, and the subsequent higher pH. Vaginal infections should be treated with appropriate antimicrobial therapy before initiation of ESTRING. If a vaginal infection develops during use of ESTRING, then ESTRING should be removed and reinserted only after the infection has been appropriately treated.
8. **Other.**
   Hypercoagulability and hyperlipidemia have been reported in women on other types of estrogen replacement therapy but, these have not been seen with ESTRING patients.
   Fluid retention is another known risk factor with estrogen therapy and may be harmful to patients with asthma, epilepsy, migraine and cardiac or renal dysfunction. ESTRING treatment has not been associated with any indication of increase in body weight up to 48 weeks of treatment.

B. Information for the Patient.

See text of **Information for Patients** which appears at the end of this insert.

C. Drug-Drug and Drug-Laboratory Interactions.

It is recommended that ESTRING be removed during treatment with other vaginally administered preparations.

Drug-drug and drug-laboratory interactions have been reported with estrogen administration overall, but were not observed in clinical trials with ESTRING. However, the possibility of the following interactions should be considered when treating patients with ESTRING.

1. Accelerated prothrombin time, partial thromboplastin time, and platelet aggregation time; increased platelet count; increased factors II, VII antigen, VIII antigen, VIII coagulant activity, IX, X, XII, VII-X complex, II-VII-X complex, and beta-thromboglobulin; decreased levels of anti-factor Xa and antithrombin III, decreased antithrombin III activity; increased levels of fibrinogen and fibrinogen activity; increased plasminogen antigen and activity.
2. Increased plasma HDL and HDL-2 subfraction concentrations, reduced LDL cholesterol concentration, increased triglycerides levels.

D. Carcinogenesis, Mutagenesis, and Impairment of Fertility.

Long term continuous administration of natural and synthetic estrogens in certain animal species increases the frequency of carcinomas of the breast, uterus, cervix, vagina, and liver (see **CONTRAINDICATIONS** and **BOXED WARNING**).

E. Pregnancy Category X.

Estrogens should not be used during pregnancy (see **CONTRAINDICATIONS** and **BOXED WARNING**).

F. Nursing Mothers.

This product is not intended for nursing mothers. As a general principle, the administration of any drug to nursing mothers should be done only when clearly necessary since many drugs are excreted in human milk. In addition, estrogen administration to nursing mothers has been shown to decrease the quantity and quality of the milk.

G. Geriatric Use.

Of the total number of subjects in clinical studies of ESTRING (including subjects treated with ESTRING, placebo, and comparator drug; n=951), 25% were 65 and over, while 4% were 75 and over. No overall differences in safety or effectiveness were observed between these subjects and younger subjects, and other reported clinical experience has not identified differences in responses between the elderly and younger patients, but greater sensitivity of some older individuals cannot be ruled out.

ADVERSE REACTIONS

The biological safety of the silicone elastomer has been studied in various *in vitro* and *in vivo* test models. The results show that the silicone elastomer is non-toxic, non-pyrogenic, non-irritating, and non-sensitizing. Long-term implantation induced encapsulation equal to or less than the negative control (polyethylene) used in the USP test. No toxic reaction or tumor formation was observed with the silicone elastomer.

In general, ESTRING (estradiol vaginal ring) was well tolerated. In the two pivotal controlled studies, discontinuation of treatment due to an adverse event was required by 5.4% of patients receiving ESTRING and 3.9% of patients receiving conjugated estrogens vaginal cream. The most common reasons for withdrawal from ESTRING treatment due to an adverse event were vaginal discomfort and gastrointestinal symptoms.

The adverse events reported with a frequency of 3% or greater in the two pivotal controlled studies by patients receiving ESTRING or conjugated estrogens vaginal cream are listed in Table 2.

[See table 2 at top of next page]

Other adverse events (listed alphabetically) occurring at a frequency of 1 to 3% in the two pivotal controlled studies by patients receiving ESTRING include: anxiety, bronchitis, chest pain, cystitis, dermatitis, diarrhea, dyspepsia, dysuria, flatulence, gastritis, genital eruption, genital pruritus, hemorrhoids, leg edema, migraine, otitis media, skin hypertrophy, syncope, toothache, tooth disorder, urinary incontinence.

The following additional adverse events were reported at least once by patients receiving ESTRING in the worldwide clinical program, which includes controlled and uncontrolled studies. A causal relationship with ESTRING has not been established.

Body as a Whole: allergic reaction

CNS/Peripheral Nervous System: dizziness

Gastrointestinal: enlarged abdomen, vomiting

Continued on next page

Estring—Cont.

Metabolic/Nutritional Disorders: weight decrease or increase
Psychiatric: depression, decreased libido, nervousness
Reproductive: breast engorgement, breast enlargement, intermenstrual bleeding, genital edema, vulval disorder
Skin/Appendages: pruritus, pruritus ani
Urinary: micturition frequency, urethral disorder
Vascular: thrombophlebitis
Vision: abnormal vision

OVERDOSAGE

Given the nature and design of ESTRING (estradiol vaginal ring), it is unlikely that overdosage will occur. However, should overdosage occur, it may manifest itself as nausea, vomiting, and/or vaginal bleeding. Serious ill effects have not been reported following acute ingestion of large doses of estrogen-containing oral contraceptives by young children.

DOSAGE AND ADMINISTRATION

One ESTRING (estradiol vaginal ring) is to be inserted as deeply as possible into the upper one-third of the vaginal vault. The ring is to remain in place continuously for three months, after which it is to be removed and, if appropriate, replaced by a new ring. The need to continue treatment should be assessed at 3 or 6 month intervals.
Should the ring be removed or fall out at any time during the 90-day treatment period, the ring should be rinsed in lukewarm water and re-inserted by the patient, or, if necessary, by a physician or nurse.
Retention of the ring for greater than 90 days does not represent overdosage but will result in progressively greater underdosage with the attendant risk of loss of efficacy and increasing risk of vaginal infections and/or erosions.

Instructions for Use

ESTRING (estradiol vaginal ring) insertion
The ring should be pressed into an oval and inserted into the upper third of the vaginal vault. The exact position is not critical. When ESTRING is in place, the patient should not feel anything. If the patient feels discomfort, ESTRING is probably not far enough inside. Gently push ESTRING further into the vagina.

ESTRING use
ESTRING should be left in place continuously for 90 days and then, if continuation of therapy is deemed appropriate, replaced by a new ESTRING.
The patient should not feel ESTRING when it is in place and it should not interfere with sexual intercourse. Straining at defecation may make ESTRING move down in the lower part of the vagina. If so, it may be pushed up again with a finger.
If ESTRING is expelled totally from the vagina, it should be rinsed in lukewarm water and reinserted by the patient (or doctor/nurse if necessary).

ESTRING removal
ESTRING may be removed by hooking a finger through the ring and pulling it out.
For patient instructions, see **Information for Patients**.

HOW SUPPLIED

Each ESTRING (estradiol vaginal ring) is individually packaged in a heat-sealed rectangular pouch consisting of three layers, from outside to inside: polyester, aluminum foil, and low density polyethylene, respectively. The pouch is provided with a tear-off notch on one side.
NDC 0013-2150-36 ESTRING (estradiol vaginal ring) 2 mg - available in single packs.
STORAGE—Store at controlled room temperature 15° to 30° C (59° to 86° F).
℞ only

INFORMATION FOR PATIENTS

INTRODUCTION

This leaflet describes when and how to use ESTRING (estradiol vaginal ring), and the risks and benefits of estrogen treatment. Please read this information carefully before starting treatment.
Estrogens have important benefits but also some risks. You must decide, with your doctor, whether the risks to you of estrogen use are acceptable because of their benefits. If you use estrogens, check with your doctor to be sure you are using the dose that is appropriate for you, and that you don't use them longer than necessary. How long you need to use estrogens should be decided by you and your doctor.

1. ESTROGENS INCREASE THE RISK OF CANCER OF THE UTERUS IN WOMEN WHO HAVE HAD THEIR MENOPAUSE ("CHANGE OF LIFE")
If you use any estrogen-containing drug, it is important to visit your doctor regularly and report any unusual vaginal bleeding right away. Vaginal bleeding after menopause may be a warning sign of uterine cancer. Your doctor should evaluate any unusual vaginal bleeding to find out the cause.

2. ESTROGENS SHOULD NOT BE USED DURING PREGNANCY
Estrogens do not prevent miscarriage (spontaneous abortion) and are not needed in the days following childbirth. If you take estrogens during pregnancy, your unborn child has a greater than usual chance of having birth defects. The risk of developing these defects is small, but clearly larger than the risk in children whose mothers did not take estrogens during pregnancy. These birth defects may affect the baby's urinary system and sex organs. Daughters born to mothers who took DES (an estrogen drug) have a higher than usual chance of developing cancer of the vagina or cervix when they become teenagers or young adults. Sons may have a higher than usual chance of developing cancer of the testicles when they become teenagers or young adults.

Table 2: Adverse Events Reported by 3% or More of Patients Receiving Either ESTRING or Conjugated Estrogens Vaginal Cream in Two Pivotal Controlled Studies

ADVERSE EVENT	Estring (n=257) %	Conjugated Estrogens Vaginal Cream (n=129) %
Musculoskeletal		
Back Pain	6	8
Arthritis	4	2
Arthralgia	3	5
Skeletal Pain	2	4
CNS/Peripheral Nervous System		
Headache	13	16
Psychiatric		
Insomnia	4	0
Gastrointestinal		
Abdominal Pain	4	2
Nausea	3	2
Respiratory		
Upper Respiratory Tract Infection	5	6
Sinusitis	4	3
Pharyngitis	1	3
Urinary		
Urinary Tract Infection	2	7
Female Reproductive		
Leukorrhea	7	3
Vaginitis	5	2
Vaginal Discomfort/Pain	5	5
Vaginal Hemorrhage	4	5
Asymptomatic Genital Bacterial Growth	4	6
Breast Pain	1	7
Resistance Mechanisms		
Genital Moniliasis	6	7
Body as a Whole		
Flu-Like Symptoms	3	2
Hot Flushes	2	3
Allergy	1	4
Miscellaneous		
Family Stress	2	3

USES OF ESTROGEN

Estrogens are hormones made by the ovaries of women during their reproductive years. Between ages 45 and 55, the ovaries normally stop making estrogens. This leads to a drop in body estrogen levels which causes the "change of life" or menopause (the end of monthly menstrual periods).
If both ovaries are removed during an operation before natural menopause takes place, the sudden drop in estrogen levels results in what is known as "surgically induced menopause."
When the estrogen levels begin dropping, some women develop very uncomfortable symptoms, such as feelings of warmth in the face, neck, and chest, or sudden intense episodes of heat and sweating ("hot flashes" or "hot flushes"). Using estrogen drugs can help the body adjust to lower estrogen levels and reduce these symptoms. ESTRING DOES NOT PROVIDE ENOUGH ESTROGEN TO REDUCE THESE SYMPTOMS.
The declining estrogen levels associated with advancing age after menopause may also result in thinning and drying of the tissue in the urinary tract and vagina (urogenital atrophy). Vaginal symptoms of this condition include dryness in the vagina (atrophic vaginitis), genital itching and burning, and pain with intercourse. Urinary symptoms may include urinary urgency and pain on urination. Small amounts of estrogen delivered directly to the local tissue can be used to help reduce these symptoms.

USE OF ESTRING (estradiol vaginal ring)

ESTRING is a local estrogen therapy designed to relieve vaginal and urinary symptoms of postmenopausal estrogen deficiency for a full 90 days. ESTRING exerts its effect locally in the lower urogenital tract and has not been shown to have significant effects in other estrogen-sensitive organs or tissues of the body. Consequently, ESTRING PROVIDES RELIEF OF LOCAL SYMPTOMS OF MENOPAUSE ONLY.

DESCRIPTION

ESTRING (estradiol vaginal ring) contains a drug reservoir of 2 mg of the estrogen, estradiol, in its core.
ESTRING releases estradiol into the vagina in a consistent, stable manner for 90 days. The soft, flexible ring is placed in the upper third of the vagina (by the physician or the patient) and worn continuously for 90 days, then removed and replaced if continuation of therapy is indicated.

WHO SHOULD NOT USE ESTRING
(estradiol vaginal ring)

ESTRING should not be used:

During pregnancy (see **Boxed Warning**).
Women who are definitely postmenopausal cannot become pregnant. Women who believe they are postmenopausal because their menstrual cycles have recently stopped should confirm that they are not pregnant before using any form of estrogen-containing drug. Using estrogens while pregnant may cause the unborn child to have birth defects. Estrogens do not prevent miscarriage.

In the presence of unusual vaginal bleeding which has not been evaluated by a doctor (see Boxed Warning).
Unusual vaginal bleeding after menopause can be a warning sign of cancer of the uterus. Estrogens may increase the risk of cancer of the uterus in women who have had their menopause ("change of life"). If you use any estrogen-containing drug, it is important to visit your doctor regularly and report any unusual vaginal bleeding right away. Your doctor should evaluate any unusual vaginal bleeding to find out the cause.

If there is a history of certain types of cancer.
Estrogens may increase the risk of certain types of cancer. In general, ESTRING should not be used in women who have ever had cancer of the breast or uterus.

During treatment for vaginal infection with vaginal antimicrobial therapy.
It is recommended that ESTRING be discontinued while other vaginal medications are being used to treat a vaginal infection. Use of ESTRING can be resumed after termination of the other vaginal medication, and after first consulting with a physician.

After childbirth or when breast-feeding a baby.
ESTRING should not be used to try to stop the breasts from filling with milk after a baby is born. Women who are breast-feeding should avoid using any drugs because many drugs pass through to the baby in the milk. While nursing a baby, drugs should only be taken on the advice of your healthcare giver.

POSSIBLE RISKS FROM TREATMENT WITH ESTROGENS

The following risk factors apply to estrogens in general:

Cancer of the uterus.
Estrogens increase the risk of developing a condition (endometrial hyperplasia) that may lead to cancer of the lining of the uterus (endometrial cancer). The risk of endometrial cancer is greater in estrogen users than nonusers. Studies have shown that this increased risk depends on estrogen dose, duration of treatment, and treatment regimen.
If the uterus has been removed (total hysterectomy), there is no danger of developing cancer of the uterus.

Cancer of the breast.
Most studies have not shown a higher risk of breast cancer in women who have ever used estrogens. However, some studies have reported that breast cancer developed more often (up to twice the usual rate) in women who used estrogens for long periods of time (especially more than 10 years), or who used higher doses for shorter time periods.
Regular breast examinations by a health professional and monthly self-examination are recommended for all women.

Gallbladder disease and abnormal blood clotting.
Gallbladder disease and abnormal blood clotting are risk factors associated with medium to high doses of estrogen. Most studies of low dose estrogen usage by women do not show an increased risk of these complications, and to date have not been seen with ESTRING (estradiol vaginal ring) treatment.

SIDE EFFECTS

Like all medications, ESTRING (estradiol vaginal ring) may cause side effects. The most frequently reported side effect is increased vaginal secretions. Many of these vaginal secretions are like those that occur normally prior to menopause and indicate that ESTRING is working. Vaginal secretions that are associated with a bad odor, vaginal itching, or other signs of vaginal infection are NOT normal and may indicate a risk or a cause for concern.
Other side effects may include vaginal discomfort, abdominal pain, or genital itching.

Estrogens in General.
In addition to the risks listed above, the following side effects have been reported with estrogen use:
— Nausea and vomiting.
— Breast tenderness or enlargement.
— Enlargement of benign tumors ("fibroids") of the uterus.
— Retention of excess fluid. This may worsen some conditions, such as asthma, epilepsy, migraine, heart disease, or kidney disease.
— Spotty darkening of the skin, particularly on the face.

REDUCING RISK OF ESTROGEN USE
If you use estrogens, you may reduce your risks by doing these things:

See your doctor regularly.
While you are using estrogens, it is important to visit your doctor at least once a year for a check-up. If you develop vaginal bleeding while taking estrogens, call your doctor — you may need further evaluation. If members of your family have had breast cancer or if you have ever had breast lumps or an abnormal mammogram (breast X-ray), you may need to have more frequent breast examinations.

Reassess your need for estrogens.
You and your doctor should reevaluate whether or not you still need estrogens at least every 6 months.

Be alert for warning signs.
If any of these warning signals (or any other unusual symptoms) happen while you are using estrogens, call your doctor immediately:
- Abnormal bleeding from the vagina (possible uterine cancer).
- Pains in the calves or chest, sudden shortness of breath, or coughing blood (possible clot in the legs, heart, or lungs).
- Severe headache or vomiting, dizziness, faintness, changes in vision or speech, weakness or numbness of an arm or leg (possible clot in the brain or eye).
- Breast lumps (possible breast cancer; ask your doctor or health professional to show you how to examine your breasts monthly).
- Yellowing of skin or eyes (possible liver problem).
- Pain, swelling, or tenderness in the abdomen (possible gallbladder problem).

OTHER INFORMATION
1. Estrogens increase the risk of developing a condition (endometrial hyperplasia) that may lead to cancer of the lining of the uterus. Progestin, another hormone drug, is usually prescribed with higher-dose estrogen preparations to lower the risk of developing endometrial hyperplasia. Progestins are not usually needed for women using ESTRING (estradiol vaginal ring) alone.
2. Some women have experienced moving or sliding of ESTRING within the vagina. If this happens, ESTRING can be gently pushed back into position with a clean finger. Instances of ESTRING slipping out of the vagina have been infrequent and were usually associated with moving the bowels, straining, or constipation within the first few weeks of treatment. If this occurs, ESTRING can be washed with lukewarm (NOT hot) water and reinserted. If this happens repeatedly, you should consult with your doctor or healthcare giver and determine whether continued treatment is appropriate for you.
3. ESTRING may not be suitable for women with narrow, short, or stenosed (constricted) vaginas. A narrow vagina, vaginal stenosis (constriction), significant prolapse, and vaginal infections are conditions that make the vagina more susceptible to irritation or ulceration caused by ESTRING. Women with signs or symptoms of vaginal irritation should alert their doctor or healthcare giver.
4. Vaginal infection is generally more common in postmenopausal women. Vaginal infections should be treated with appropriate antimicrobial therapy before initiation of ESTRING. If a vaginal infection develops during use of ESTRING, then ESTRING should be removed and re-inserted only after the infection has been appropriately treated. See your doctor or healthcare giver if you have vaginal discomfort or suspect you have a vaginal infection.
5. Your doctor has prescribed this drug for you and you alone. Do not give the drug to anyone else.
6. Keep this and all drugs out of the reach of children.
7. This leaflet provides a summary of important information about ESTRING. If you want more information, ask your doctor or pharmacist to show you the professional labeling. The professional labeling is also published in a book called the "Physicians' Desk Reference®", which is available in book stores and public libraries. Generic drugs carry virtually the same labeling information as their brand name versions.

HOW SUPPLIED
Each ESTRING (estradiol vaginal ring) is individually packaged in a heat-sealed rectangular pouch. The pouch is provided with a tear-off notch on one side.
NDC 0013-2150-36 ESTRING (estradiol vaginal ring) 2 mg available in single units.
Storage: Store at controlled room temperature 15° to 30° C (59° to 86° F).
℞ only

A Patient Guide to ESTRING (estradiol vaginal ring) 2 mg Insertion and Removal

FEMALE ANATOMY

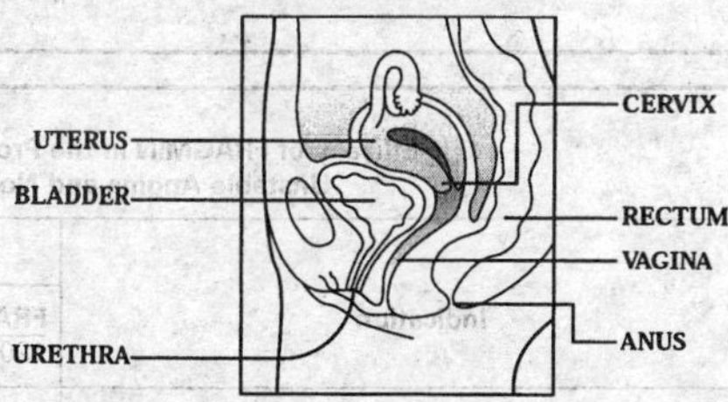

ESTRING INSERTION
ESTRING can be inserted and removed by you or your doctor. To insert ESTRING yourself, choose the position that is most comfortable for you: standing with one leg up, squatting, or lying down.

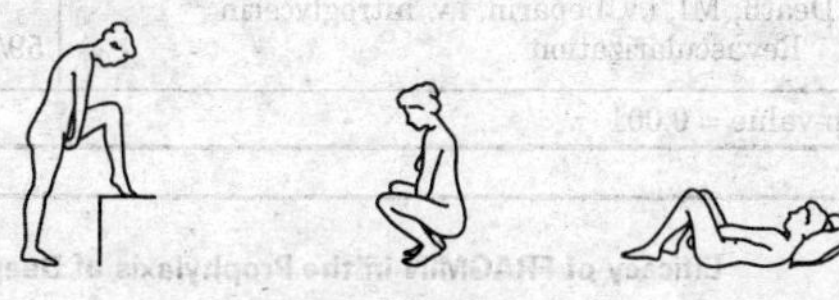

1. After washing and drying your hands, remove ESTRING from its pouch using the tear-off notch on the side. (Since the ring becomes slippery when wet, be sure your hands are dry before handling it.)
2. Hold ESTRING between your thumb and index finger and press the opposite sides of the ring together as shown.

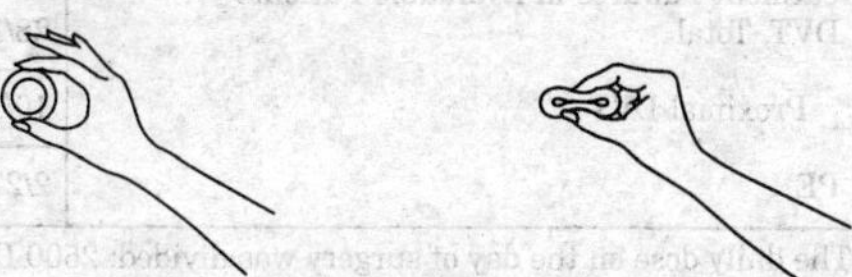

3. Gently push the compressed ring into your vagina as far as you can.

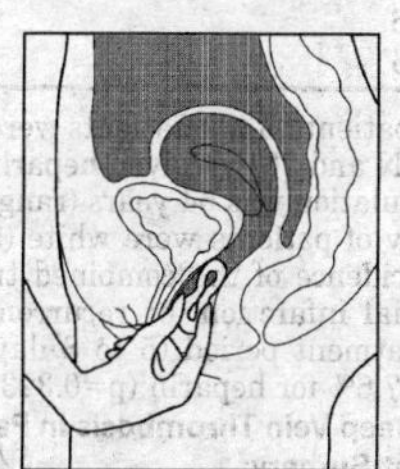

ESTRING PLACEMENT
The exact position of ESTRING is not critical, as long as it is placed in the upper third of the vagina.

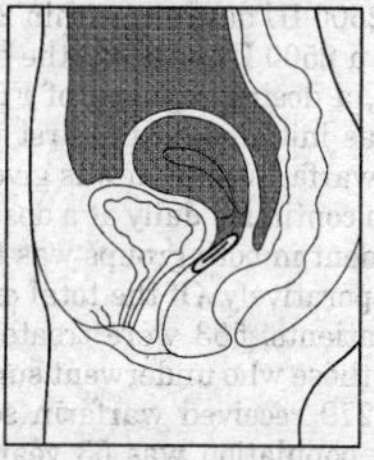

When ESTRING is in place, you should not feel anything. If you feel uncomfortable, ESTRING is probably not far enough inside. Use your finger to gently push ESTRING further into your vagina.
There is no danger of ESTRING being pushed too far up in the vagina or getting lost. ESTRING can only be inserted as far as the end of the vagina, where the cervix (the narrow, lower end of the uterus) will block ESTRING from going any further (see diagram of Female Anatomy).

ESTRING USE
Once inserted, ESTRING should remain in place in the vagina for 90 days.
Most women and their partners experience no discomfort with ESTRING in place during intercourse, so it is NOT necessary that the ring be removed. If ESTRING should cause you or your partner any discomfort, you may remove it prior to intercourse (see ESTRING Removal, below). Be sure to reinsert ESTRING as soon as possible afterwards.
ESTRING may slide down into the lower part of the vagina as a result of the abdominal pressure or straining that sometimes accompanies constipation. If this should happen, gently guide ESTRING back into place with your finger.
There have been rare reports of ESTRING falling out in some women following intense straining or coughing. If this should occur, simply wash ESTRING with lukewarm (NOT hot) water and reinsert it.

ESTRING DRUG DELIVERY
Once in the vagina, ESTRING begins to release estradiol immediately. ESTRING will continue to release a low, continuous dose of estradiol for the full 90 days it remains in place.

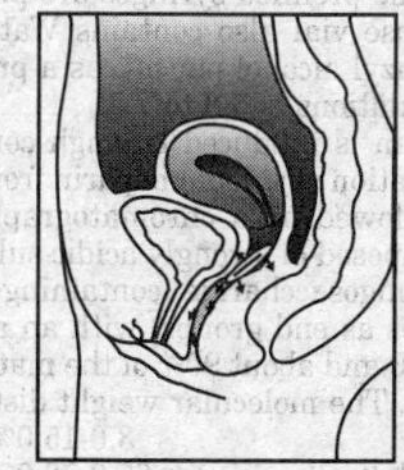

It will take about 2 to 3 weeks to restore the tissue of the vagina and urinary tract to a healthier condition and to feel the full effect of ESTRING in relieving vaginal and urinary symptoms. If your symptoms persist for more than a few weeks after beginning ESTRING therapy, contact your doctor.
One of the most frequently reported effects associated with the use of ESTRING is an increase in vaginal secretions. These secretions are like those that occur normally prior to menopause and indicate that ESTRING is working. However, if the secretions are associated with a bad odor or vaginal itching or discomfort, be sure to contact your doctor.

ESTRING REMOVAL
After 90 days there will no longer be enough estradiol in the ring to maintain its full effect in relieving your vaginal or urinary symptoms. ESTRING should be removed at that time and replaced with a new ESTRING, if your doctor determines that you need to continue your therapy.
To remove ESTRING:
1. Wash and dry your hands thoroughly.
2. Assume a comfortable position, either standing with one leg up, squatting, or lying down.
3. Loop your finger through the ring and gently pull it out.
4. Discard the used ring in a waste receptacle. (Do not flush ESTRING).

If you have any additional questions about removing ESTRING, contact your doctor or healthcare giver.
Manufactured for: Pharmacia & Upjohn Company
By: QPharma AB
Mulmör, Sweden
A subsidiary of Pharmacia Corporation
Kalamazoo, MI 49001, USA
818 049 001
Revised July 2002

FRAGMIN® ℞
[frăg-mĭn]
dalteparin sodium injection
For *Subcutaneous* Use Only

SPINAL/EPIDURAL HEMATOMAS
When neuraxial anesthesia (epidural/spinal anesthesia) or spinal puncture is employed, patients anticoagulated or scheduled to be anticoagulated with low molecular weight heparins or heparinoids for prevention of thromboembolic complications are at risk of developing an epidural or spinal hematoma which can result in long-term or permanent paralysis.
The risk of these events is increased by the use of indwelling epidural catheters for administration of analgesia or by the concomitant use of drugs affecting hemostasis such as non steroidal anti-inflammatory drugs (NSAIDs), platelet inhibitors, or other anticoagulants. The risk also appears to be increased by traumatic or repeated epidural or spinal puncture.
Patients should be frequently monitored for signs and symptoms of neurological impairment. If neurological compromise is noted, urgent treatment is necessary.
The physician should consider the potential benefit versus risk before neuraxial intervention in patients anticoagulated or to be anticoagulated for thromboprophylaxis (also see **WARNINGS, Hemorrhage** and **PRECAUTIONS, Drug Interactions**).

DESCRIPTION
FRAGMIN Injection (dalteparin sodium injection) is a sterile, low molecular weight heparin. It is available in single-dose, prefilled syringes preassembled with a needle guard device, and multiple-dose vials. With reference to the W.H.O. First International Low Molecular Weight Heparin Reference Standard, each syringe contains either 2500, 5000, 7500, or 10,000 anti-Factor Xa international units (IU), equivalent to 16, 32, 48, or 64 mg dalteparin sodium, respectively. Each vial contains either 10,000 or 25,000 anti-Factor Xa IU per 1 mL (equivalent to 64 or 160 mg dalteparin sodium, respectively), for a total of 95,000 anti-Factor Xa IU per vial.

Continued on next page

Fragmin—Cont.

Each prefilled syringe also contains Water for Injection and sodium chloride, when required, to maintain physiologic ionic strength. The prefilled syringes are preservative free. Each multiple-dose vial also contains Water for Injection and 14 mg of benzyl alcohol per mL as a preservative. The pH of both formulations is 5.0 to 7.5.

Dalteparin sodium is produced through controlled nitrous acid depolymerization of sodium heparin from porcine intestinal mucosa followed by a chromatographic purification process. It is composed of strongly acidic sulphated polysaccharide chains (oligosaccharide, containing 2,5-anhydro-D-mannitol residues as end groups) with an average molecular weight of 5000 and about 90% of the material within the range 2000-9000. The molecular weight distribution is:

< 3000 daltons	3.0-15.0%
3000 to 8000 daltons	65.0-78.0%
> 8000 daltons	14.0-26.0%

Structural Formula

[See chemical structure above]

R_2, R_3, CH_2OR, OH OR, OR NHR_1, n, CH_2OR, CH_2OH, HO

R = H or SO_3Na
R_1 = $COCH_3$ or SO_3Na
R_2 = H R_3 = COONa
or
R_2 = COONa R_3 = H

n = 3–20

CLINICAL PHARMACOLOGY

Dalteparin is a low molecular weight heparin with antithrombotic properties. It acts by enhancing the inhibition of Factor Xa and thrombin by antithrombin. In man, dalteparin potentiates preferentially the inhibition of coagulation Factor Xa, while only slightly affecting clotting time, e.g., activated partial thromboplastin time (APTT).

Pharmacodynamics:

Doses of FRAGMIN Injection of up to 10,000 anti-Factor Xa IU administered subcutaneously as a single dose or two 5000 IU doses 12 hours apart to healthy subjects do not produce a significant change in platelet aggregation, fibrinolysis, or global clotting tests such as prothrombin time (PT), thrombin time (TT) or APTT. Subcutaneous (s.c.) administration of doses of 5000 IU bid of FRAGMIN for seven consecutive days to patients undergoing abdominal surgery did not markedly affect APTT, Platelet Factor 4 (PF4), or lipoprotein lipase.

Pharmacokinetics:

Mean peak levels of plasma anti-Factor Xa activity following single s.c. doses of 2500, 5000 and 10,000 IU were 0.19 ± 0.04, 0.41 ± 0.07 and 0.82 ± 0.10 IU/mL, respectively, and were attained in about 4 hours in most subjects. Absolute bioavailability in healthy volunteers, measured as the anti-Factor Xa activity, was 87 ± 6%. Increasing the dose from 2500 to 10,000 IU resulted in an overall increase in anti-Factor Xa AUC that was greater than proportional by about one-third.

Peak anti-Factor Xa activity increased more or less linearly with dose over the same dose range. There appeared to be no appreciable accumulation of anti-Factor Xa activity with twice-daily dosing of 100 IU/kg s.c. for up to 7 days.

The volume of distribution for dalteparin anti-Factor Xa activity was 40 to 60 mL/kg. The mean plasma clearances of dalteparin anti-Factor Xa activity in normal volunteers following single intravenous bolus doses of 30 and 120 anti-Factor Xa IU/kg were 24.6 ± 5.4 and 15.6 ± 2.4 mL/hr/kg, respectively. The corresponding mean disposition half-lives are 1.47 ± 0.3 and 2.5 ± 0.3 hours.

Following intravenous doses of 40 and 60 IU/kg, mean terminal half-lives were 2.1 ± 0.3 and 2.3 ± 0.4 hours, respectively. Longer apparent terminal half-lives (3 to 5 hours) are observed following s.c. dosing, possibly due to delayed absorption. In patients with chronic renal insufficiency requiring hemodialysis, the mean terminal half-life of anti-Factor Xa activity following a single intravenous dose of 5000 IU FRAGMIN was 5.7 ± 2.0 hours, i.e. considerably longer than values observed in healthy volunteers, therefore, greater accumulation can be expected in these patients.

CLINICAL TRIALS

Prophylaxis of Ischemic Complications in Unstable Angina and Non-Q-Wave Myocardial Infarction:

In a double-blind, randomized, placebo-controlled clinical trial, patients who recently experienced unstable angina with EKG changes or non-Q-wave myocardial infarction (MI) were randomized to FRAGMIN Injection 120 IU/kg every 12 hours subcutaneously (s.c.) or placebo every 12 hours s.c. In this trial, unstable angina was defined to include only angina with EKG changes. All patients, except when contraindicated, were treated concurrently with aspirin (75 mg once daily) and beta blockers. Treatment was initiated within 72 hours of the event (the majority of patients received treatment within 24 hours) and continued for 5 to 8 days. A total of 1506 patients were enrolled and treated; 746 received FRAGMIN and 760 received placebo. The mean age of the study population was 68 years (range 40 to 90 years) and the majority of patients were white (99.7%) and male (63.9%). The combined incidence of the double endpoint of death or myocardial infarction was lower for FRAGMIN compared with placebo at 6 days after initiation of therapy. These results were observed in an analysis of all-randomized and all-treated patients. The combined incidence of death, MI, need for intravenous (i.v.) heparin or i.v. nitroglycerin, and revascularization was also lower for FRAGMIN than for placebo (see Table 1).

[See table above]

Table 1
Efficacy of FRAGMIN in the Prophylaxis of Ischemic Complications in Unstable Angina and Non-Q-Wave Myocardial Infarction

Indication	Dosing Regimen	
	FRAGMIN 120 IU/kg/12 hr s.c.	Placebo q 12 hr s.c.
All Treated Unstable Angina and Non-Q-Wave MI Patients	746	760
Primary Endpoints – 6 day timepoint Death, MI	13/741 (1.8%)[1]	36/757 (4.8%)
Secondary Endpoints – 6 day timepoint Death, MI, i.v. heparin, i.v. nitroglycerin, Revascularization	59/739 (8.0%)[1]	106/756 (14.0%)

[1] p-value = 0.001

In a second randomized, controlled trial designed to evaluate long-term treatment with FRAGMIN (days 6 to 45), data were also collected comparing 1-week (5 to 8 days) treatment of FRAGMIN 120 IU/kg every 12 hours s.c. with heparin at an APTT-adjusted dosage. All patients, except when contraindicated, were treated concurrently with aspirin (100 to 165 mg per day). Of the total enrolled study population of 1499 patients, 1482 patients were treated; 751 received FRAGMIN and 731 received heparin. The mean age of the study population was 64 years (range 25 to 92 years) and the majority of patients were white (96.0%) and male (64.2%). The incidence of the combined triple endpoint of death, myocardial infarction, or recurrent angina during this 1-week treatment period (5 to 8 days) was 9.3% for FRAGMIN and 7.6% for heparin (p=0.323).

Prophylaxis of Deep Vein Thrombosis in Patients Following Hip Replacement Surgery:

In an open-label randomized study, FRAGMIN 5000 IU administered once daily s.c. was compared with warfarin sodium, administered orally, in patients undergoing hip replacement surgery. Treatment with FRAGMIN was initiated with a 2500 IU dose s.c. within 2 hours before surgery, followed by a 2500 IU dose s.c. the evening of the day of surgery. Then, a dosing regimen of FRAGMIN 5000 IU s.c. once daily was initiated on the first postoperative day. The first dose of warfarin sodium was given the evening before surgery, then continued daily at a dose adjusted for INR 2.0 to 3.0. Treatment in both groups was then continued for 5 to 9 days postoperatively. Of the total enrolled study population of 580 patients, 553 were treated and 550 underwent surgery. Of those who underwent surgery, 271 received FRAGMIN and 279 received warfarin sodium. The mean age of the study population was 63 years (range 20 to 92 years) and the majority of patients were white (91.1%) and female (52.9%). The incidence of deep vein thrombosis (DVT), any vein, as determined by evaluable venography, was significantly lower for the group treated with FRAGMIN compared with patients treated with warfarin sodium (28/192 vs 49/190; p=0.006) [see Table 2].

[See table 2 above]

Table 2
Efficacy of FRAGMIN in the Prophylaxis of Deep Vein Thrombosis Following Hip Replacement Surgery

Indication	Dosing Regimen	
	FRAGMIN 5000 IU qd[1] s.c.	Warfarin Sodium qd[2] oral
All Treated Hip Replacement Surgery Patients	271	279
Treatment Failures in Evaluable Patients DVT, Total	28/192 (14.6%)[3]	49/190 (25.8%)
Proximal DVT	10/192 (5.2%)[4]	16/190 (8.4%)
PE	2/271 (0.7%)	2/279 (0.7%)

[1] The daily dose on the day of surgery was divided: 2500 IU was given two hours before surgery and again in the evening of the day of surgery.
[2] Warfarin sodium dosage was adjusted to maintain a prothrombin time index of 1.4 to 1.5, corresponding to an International Normalized Ratio (INR) of approximately 2.5.
[3] p-value = 0.006
[4] p-value = 0.185

In a second single-center, double-blind study of patients undergoing hip replacement surgery, FRAGMIN 5000 IU once daily s.c. starting the evening before surgery, was compared with heparin 5000 U s.c. tid, starting the morning of surgery. Treatment in both groups was continued for up to 9 days postoperatively. Of the total enrolled study population of 140 patients, 139 were treated and 136 underwent surgery. Of those who underwent surgery, 67 received FRAGMIN and 69 received heparin. The mean age of the study population was 69 years (range 42 to 87 years) and the majority of patients were female (58.8%). In the intent-to-treat analysis, the incidence of proximal DVT was significantly lower for patients treated with FRAGMIN compared with patients treated with heparin (6/67 vs 18/69; p=0.012). Further, the incidence of pulmonary embolism detected by lung scan was also significantly lower in the group treated with FRAGMIN (9/67 vs 19/69; p=0.032).

A third multi-center, double-blind, randomized study evaluated a postoperative dosing regimen of FRAGMIN for thromboprophylaxis following total hip replacement surgery. Patients received either FRAGMIN or warfarin sodium, randomized into one of three treatment groups. One group of patients received the first dose of FRAGMIN 2500 IU s.c. within 2 hours before surgery, followed by another dose of FRAGMIN 2500 IU s.c. at least 4 hours (6.6 ± 2.3 hr) after surgery. Another group received the first dose of FRAGMIN 2500 IU s.c. at least 4 hours (6.6 ± 2.4 hr) after surgery. Then, **both** of these groups began a dosing regimen of FRAGMIN 5000 IU once daily s.c. on postoperative day 1. The third group of patients received warfarin sodium the evening of the day of surgery, then continued daily at a dose adjusted for INR 2.0 to 3.0. Treatment for all groups was continued for 4 to 8 days postoperatively, after which time all patients underwent bilateral venography.

In the total enrolled study population of 1501 patients, 1472 patients were treated; 496 received FRAGMIN (first dose before surgery), 487 received FRAGMIN (first dose after surgery) and 489 received warfarin sodium. The mean age of the study population was 63 years (range 18 to 91 years) and the majority of patients were white (94.4%) and female (51.8%).

Administration of the first dose of FRAGMIN after surgery was as effective in reducing the incidence of thromboembolic events as administration of the first dose of FRAGMIN before surgery (44/336 vs 37/338; p=0.448). Both dosing regimens of FRAGMIN were more effective than warfarin sodium in reducing the incidence of thromboembolic events following hip replacement surgery.

Prophylaxis of Deep Vein Thrombosis Following Abdominal Surgery in Patients at Risk for Thromboembolic Complications:

Abdominal surgery patients at risk include those who are over 40 years of age, obese, undergoing surgery under general anesthesia lasting longer than 30 minutes, or who have additional risk factors such as malignancy or a history of deep vein thrombosis or pulmonary embolism.

FRAGMIN administered once daily s.c. beginning prior to surgery and continuing for 5 to 10 days after surgery, was shown to reduce the risk of DVT in patients at risk for thromboembolic complications in two double-blind, randomized, controlled clinical trials performed in patients undergoing major abdominal surgery. In the first study, a total of 204 patients were enrolled and treated; 102 received FRAGMIN and 102 received placebo. The mean age of the study population was 64 years (range 40 to 98 years) and the majority of patients were female (54.9%). In the second study, a total of 391 patients were enrolled and treated; 195 received FRAGMIN and 196 received heparin. The mean

age of the study population was 59 years (range 30 to 88 years) and the majority of patients were female (51.9%). As summarized in the following tables, FRAGMIN 2500 IU was superior to placebo and similar to heparin in reducing the risk of DVT (see Tables 3 and 4).
[See table 3 at right]
[See table 4 at right]
In a third double-blind, randomized study performed in patients undergoing major abdominal surgery with malignancy, FRAGMIN 5000 IU once daily was compared with FRAGMIN 2500 IU once daily. Treatment was continued for 6 to 8 days. A total of 1375 patients were enrolled and treated; 679 received FRAGMIN 5000 IU and 696 received 2500 IU. The mean age of the combined groups was 71 years (range 40 to 95 years). The majority of patients were female (51.0%). The study showed that FRAGMIN 5000 IU once daily was more effective than FRAGMIN 2500 IU once daily in reducing the risk of DVT in patients undergoing abdominal surgery with malignancy (see Table 5).
[See table 5 at right]

Prophylaxis of Deep Vein Thrombosis in Medical Patients at Risk for Thromboembolic Complications Due to Severely Restricted Mobility During Acute Illness:
In a double-blind, multi-center, randomized, placebo-controlled clinical trial, general medical patients with severely restricted mobility who were at risk of venous thromboembolism were randomized to receive either FRAGMIN 5000 IU or placebo s.c. once daily during Days 1 to 14 of the study. The primary endpoint was evaluated at Day 21, and the follow-up period was up to Day 90. These patients had an acute medical condition requiring a projected hospital stay of at least 4 days, and were confined to bed during waking hours. The study included patients with congestive heart failure (NYHA Class III or IV), acute respiratory failure not requiring ventilatory support, and the following acute conditions with at least one risk factor occurring in > 1% of treated patients: acute infection (excluding septic shock), acute rheumatic disorder, acute lumbar or sciatic pain, vertebral compression, or acute arthritis of the lower extremities. Risk factors include > 75 years of age, cancer, previous DVT/PE, obesity and chronic venous insufficiency. A total of 3681 patients were enrolled and treated: 1848 received FRAGMIN and 1833 received placebo. The mean age of the study population was 69 years (range 26 to 99 years), 92.1% were white and 51.9% were female. The primary efficacy endpoint was defined as at least one of the following within Days 1 to 21 of the study: asymptomatic DVT (diagnosed by compression ultrasound), a confirmed symptomatic DVT, a confirmed pulmonary embolism or sudden death.
When given at a dose of 5000 IU once a day s.c., FRAGMIN significantly reduced the incidence of thromboembolic events including verified DVT by Day 21 (see Table 6). The prophylactic effect was sustained through Day 90.
[See table 6 at top of next page]

INDICATIONS AND USAGE
FRAGMIN Injection is indicated for the prophylaxis of ischemic complications in unstable angina and non-Q-wave myocardial infarction, when concurrently administered with aspirin therapy (as described in CLINICAL TRIALS, Prophylaxis of Ischemic Complications in Unstable Angina and Non-Q-Wave Myocardial Infarction).
FRAGMIN is also indicated for the prophylaxis of deep vein thrombosis (DVT), which may lead to pulmonary embolism (PE):
- In patients undergoing hip replacement surgery;
- In patients undergoing abdominal surgery who are at risk for thromboembolic complications;
- In medical patients who are at risk for thromboembolic complications due to severely restricted mobility during acute illness.

CONTRAINDICATIONS
FRAGMIN Injection is contraindicated in patients with known hypersensitivity to the drug, active major bleeding, or thrombocytopenia associated with positive ***in vitro*** tests for anti-platelet antibody in the presence of FRAGMIN.
Patients undergoing regional anesthesia should not receive FRAGMIN for unstable angina or non-Q-wave myocardial infarction due to an increased risk of bleeding associated with the dosage of FRAGMIN recommended for unstable angina and non-Q-wave myocardial infarction.
Patients with known hypersensitivity to heparin or pork products should not be treated with FRAGMIN.

WARNINGS
FRAGMIN Injection is not intended for intramuscular administration.
FRAGMIN cannot be used interchangeably (unit for unit) with unfractionated heparin or other low molecular weight heparins.
FRAGMIN should be used with extreme caution in patients with history of heparin-induced thrombocytopenia.
Hemorrhage:
FRAGMIN, like other anticoagulants, should be used with extreme caution in patients who have an increased risk of hemorrhage, such as those with severe uncontrolled hypertension, bacterial endocarditis, congenital or acquired bleeding disorders, active ulceration and angiodysplastic gastrointestinal disease, hemorrhagic stroke, or shortly after brain, spinal or ophthalmological surgery.
Spinal or epidural hematomas can occur with the associated use of low molecular weight heparins or heparinoids and neuraxial (spinal/epidural) anesthesia or spinal puncture, which can result in long-term or permanent paralysis. The risk of these events is higher with the use of indwelling epidural catheters or concomitant use of additional drugs affecting hemostasis such as NSAIDs (see boxed WARNING and ADVERSE REACTIONS, Ongoing Safety Surveillance).
As with other anticoagulants, bleeding can occur at any site during therapy with FRAGMIN. An unexpected drop in hematocrit or blood pressure should lead to a search for a bleeding site.
Thrombocytopenia:
In clinical trials, thrombocytopenia with platelet counts of < 100,000/mm^3 and < 50,000/mm^3 occurred in < 1% and < 1%, respectively. In clinical practice, rare cases of thrombocytopenia with thrombosis have also been observed.
Thrombocytopenia of any degree should be monitored closely. Heparin-induced thrombocytopenia can occur with the administration of FRAGMIN. The incidence of this complication is unknown at present.
Miscellaneous:
The multiple-dose vial of FRAGMIN contains benzyl alcohol as a preservative. Benzyl alcohol has been reported to be associated with a fatal "Gasping Syndrome" in premature infants. Because benzyl alcohol may cross the placenta, FRAGMIN preserved with benzyl alcohol should not be used in pregnant women (see **PRECAUTIONS, Pregnancy Category B, Nonteratogenic Effects**).

PRECAUTIONS
General:
FRAGMIN Injection should not be mixed with other injections or infusions unless specific compatibility data are available that support such mixing.
FRAGMIN should be used with caution in patients with bleeding diathesis, thrombocytopenia or platelet defects; severe liver or kidney insufficiency, hypertensive or diabetic retinopathy, and recent gastrointestinal bleeding.
If a thromboembolic event should occur despite dalteparin prophylaxis, FRAGMIN should be discontinued and appropriate therapy initiated.
Drug Interactions:
FRAGMIN should be used with care in patients receiving oral anticoagulants, platelet inhibitors, and thrombolytic agents because of increased risk of bleeding (see **PRECAUTIONS, Laboratory Tests**). Aspirin, unless contraindicated, is recommended in patients treated for unstable angina or non-Q-wave myocardial infarction (see **DOSAGE AND ADMINISTRATION**).
Laboratory Tests:
Periodic routine complete blood counts, including platelet count, and stool occult blood tests are recommended during the course of treatment with FRAGMIN. No special monitoring of blood clotting times (e.g., APTT) is needed.
When administered at recommended prophylaxis doses, routine coagulation tests such as Prothrombin Time (PT) and Activated Partial Thromboplastin Time (APTT) are relatively insensitive measures of FRAGMIN activity and, therefore, unsuitable for monitoring.
Drug/Laboratory Test Interactions:
Elevations of Serum Transaminases:
Asymptomatic increases in transaminase levels (SGOT/AST and SGPT/ALT) greater than three times the upper limit of normal of the laboratory reference range have been reported in 1.7 and 4.3%, respectively, of patients during treatment with FRAGMIN. Similar significant increases in transaminase levels have also been observed in patients treated with heparin and other low molecular weight heparins. Such elevations are fully reversible and are rarely associated with increases in bilirubin. Since transaminase determinations

Table 3
Efficacy of FRAGMIN in the Prophylaxis of Deep Vein Thrombosis Following Abdominal Surgery

Indication	Dosing Regimen	
	FRAGMIN 2500 IU qd s.c.	**Placebo** qd s.c.
All Treated Abdominal Surgery Patients	102	102
Treatment Failures in Evaluable Patients Total Thromboembolic Events	4/91 (4.4%)[1]	16/91 (17.6%)
Proximal DVT	0	5/91 (5.5%)
Distal DVT	4/91 (4.4%)	11/91 (12.1%)
PE	0	2/91 (2.2%)[2]

[1] p-value = 0.008
[2] Both patients also had DVT, 1 proximal and 1 distal

Table 4
Efficacy of FRAGMIN in the Prophylaxis of Deep Vein Thrombosis Following Abdominal Surgery

Indication	Dosing Regimen	
	FRAGMIN 2500 IU qd s.c.	**Heparin** 5000 U bid s.c.
All Treated Abdominal Surgery Patients	195	196
Treatment Failures in Evaluable Patients Total Thromboembolic Events	7/178 (3.9%)[1]	7/174 (4.0%)
Proximal DVT	3/178 (1.7%)	4/174 (2.3%)
Distal DVT	3/178 (1.7%)	3/174 (1.7%)
PE	1/178 (0.6%)	0

[1] p-value = 0.74

Table 5
Efficacy of FRAGMIN in the Prophylaxis of Deep Vein Thrombosis Following Abdominal Surgery

Indication	Dosing Regimen	
	FRAGMIN 2500 IU qd s.c.	**FRAGMIN** 5000 IU qd s.c.
All Treated Abdominal Surgery Patients[1]	696	679
Treatment Failures in Evaluable Patients Total Thromboembolic Events	99/656 (15.1%)[2]	60/645 (9.3%)
Proximal DVT	18/657 (2.7%)	14/646 (2.2%)
Distal DVT	80/657 (12.2%)	41/646 (6.3%)
PE Fatal	1/674 (0.1%)	1/669 (0.1%)
Non-fatal	2	4

[1] Major abdominal surgery with malignancy
[2] p-value = 0.001

Continued on next page

Fragmin—Cont.

are important in the differential diagnosis of myocardial infarction, liver disease and pulmonary emboli, elevations that might be caused by drugs like FRAGMIN should be interpreted with caution.

Carcinogenicity, Mutagenesis, Impairment of Fertility:
Dalteparin sodium has not been tested for its carcinogenic potential in long-term animal studies. It was not mutagenic in the ***in vitro*** Ames Test, mouse lymphoma cell forward mutation test and human lymphocyte chromosomal aberration test and in the ***in vivo*** mouse micronucleus test. Dalteparin sodium at subcutaneous doses up to 1200 IU/kg (7080 IU/m²) did not affect the fertility or reproductive performance of male and female rats.

Pregnancy: Pregnancy Category B.

Teratogenic Effects:
Reproduction studies with dalteparin sodium at intravenous doses up to 2400 IU/kg (14,160 IU/m²) in pregnant rats and 4800 IU/kg (40,800 IU/m²) in pregnant rabbits did not produce any evidence of impaired fertility or harm to the fetuses. There are, however, no adequate and well-controlled studies in pregnant women. Because animal reproduction studies are not always predictive of human response, this drug should be used during pregnancy only if clearly needed.

Nonteratogenic Effects:
Cases of "Gasping Syndrome" have occurred when large amounts of benzyl alcohol have been administered (99-404 mg/kg/day). The 9.5 mL multiple-dose vial of FRAGMIN contains 14 mg/mL of benzyl alcohol.

Nursing Mothers:
It is not known whether dalteparin sodium is excreted in human milk. Because many drugs are excreted in human milk, caution should be exercised when FRAGMIN is administered to a nursing mother.

Pediatric Use:
Safety and effectiveness in pediatric patients have not been established.

Geriatric Use:
Of the total number of patients in clinical studies of FRAGMIN, 5204 patients were 65 years of age or older and 2123 were 75 or older. No overall differences in effectiveness were observed between these subjects and younger subjects. Some studies suggest that the risk of bleeding increases with age. Postmarketing surveillance and literature reports have not revealed additional differences in the safety of FRAGMIN between elderly and younger patients. Careful attention to dosing intervals and concomitant medications (especially antiplatelet medications) is advised, particularly in geriatric patients with low body weight (< 45 kg) and those predisposed to decreased renal function (see also **CLINICAL PHARMACOLOGY** and **General** and **Drug Interactions** subsections of **PRECAUTIONS**).

ADVERSE REACTIONS

Hemorrhage:
The incidence of hemorrhagic complications during treatment with FRAGMIN Injection has been low. The most commonly reported side effect is hematoma at the injection site. The incidence of bleeding may increase with higher doses; however, in abdominal surgery patients with malignancy, no significant increase in bleeding was observed when comparing FRAGMIN 5000 IU to either FRAGMIN 2500 IU or low dose heparin.

In a trial comparing FRAGMIN 5000 IU once daily to FRAGMIN 2500 IU once daily in patients undergoing surgery for malignancy, the incidence of bleeding events was 4.6% and 3.6%, respectively (n.s.). In a trial comparing FRAGMIN 5000 IU once daily to heparin 5000 U twice daily, the incidence of bleeding events was 3.2% and 2.7%, respectively (n.s.) in the malignancy subgroup.

Unstable Angina and Non-Q-Wave Myocardial Infarction:
Table 7 summarizes major bleeding events that occurred with FRAGMIN, heparin, and placebo in clinical trials of unstable angina and non-Q-wave myocardial infarction.
[See table 7 above]

Hip Replacement Surgery:
Table 8 summarizes: 1) all major bleeding events and, 2) other bleeding events possibly or probably related to treatment with FRAGMIN (preoperative dosing regimen), warfarin sodium, or heparin in two hip replacement surgery clinical trials.
[See table 8 at right]

Six of the patients treated with FRAGMIN experienced seven major bleeding events. Two of the events were wound hematoma (one requiring reoperation), three were bleeding from the operative site, one was intraoperative bleeding due to vessel damage, and one was gastrointestinal bleeding. None of the patients experienced retroperitoneal or intracranial hemorrhage nor died of bleeding complications.

In the third hip replacement surgery clinical trial, the incidence of major bleeding events was similar in all three treatment groups: 3.6% (18/496) for patients who started FRAGMIN before surgery; 2.5% (12/487) for patients who started FRAGMIN after surgery; and 3.1% (15/489) for patients treated with warfarin sodium.

Abdominal Surgery:
Table 9 summarizes bleeding events that occurred in clinical trials which studied FRAGMIN 2500 and 5000 IU administered once daily to abdominal surgery patients.
[See table 9 at right]

Medical Patients with Severely Restricted Mobility During Acute Illness:
Table 10 summarizes major bleeding events that occurred in a clinical trial of medical patients with severely restricted mobility during acute illness.

Table 6
Efficacy of FRAGMIN in the Prophylaxis of Deep Vein Thrombosis in Medical Patients with Severely Restricted Mobility During Acute Illness

Indication	Dosing Regimen	
	FRAGMIN 5000 IU qd s.c.	Placebo qd s.c.
All Treated Medical Patients During Acute Illness	1848	1833
Treatment failure in evaluable patients (Day 21)[1] DVT, PE, or sudden death	42/1518 (2.77%)[2]	73/1473 (4.96%)
Total thromboembolic events (Day 21)	37/1513 (2.45%)	70/1470 (4.76%)
Total DVT	32/1508 (2.12%)	64/1464 (4.37%)
Proximal DVT	29/1518 (1.91%)	60/1474 (4.07%)
Symptomatic VTE	10/1759 (0.57%)	17/1740 (0.98%)
PE	5/1759 (0.28%)	6/1740 (0.34%)
Sudden Death	5/1829 (0.27%)	3/1807 (0.17%)

[1] Defined as DVT (diagnosed by compression ultrasound at Day 21 + 3), confirmed symptomatic DVT, confirmed PE or sudden death.
[2] p-value = 0.0015

Table 7
Major Bleeding Events in Unstable Angina and Non-Q-Wave Myocardial Infarction

Indication	Dosing Regimen		
Unstable Angina and Non-Q-Wave MI	FRAGMIN 120 IU/kg/12 hr s.c.[1]	Heparin i.v. and s.c.[2]	Placebo q 12 hr s.c.
Major Bleeding Events[3,4]	15/1497 (1.0%)	7/731 (1.0%)	4/760 (0.5%)

[1] Treatment was administered for 5 to 8 days.
[2] Heparin i.v. infusion for at least 48 hours, APPT 1.5 to 2 times control, then 12,500 U s.c. every 12 hours for 5 to 8 days.
[3] Aspirin (75 to 165 mg per day) and beta blocker therapies were administered concurrently.
[4] Bleeding events were considered major if: 1) accompanied by a decrease in hemoglobin of ≥2 g/dL in connection with clinical symptoms; 2) a transfusion was required; 3) bleeding led to interruption of treatment or death; or 4) intracranial bleeding.

Table 8
Bleeding Events Following Hip Replacement Surgery

Indication	FRAGMIN vs Warfarin Sodium		FRAGMIN vs Heparin	
	Dosing Regimen		Dosing Regimen	
Hip Replacement Surgery	FRAGMIN 5000 IU qd s.c. (n=274[2])	Warfarin Sodium[1] oral (n=279)	FRAGMIN 5000 IU qd s.c. (n=69[4])	Heparin 5000 U tid s.c. (n=69)
Major Bleeding Events[3]	7/274 (2.6%)	1/279 (0.4%)	0	3/69 (4.3%)
Other Bleeding Events[5]				
Hematuria	8/274 (2.9%)	5/279 (1.8%)	0	0
Wound Hematoma	6/274 (2.2%)	0	0	0
Injection Site Hematoma	3/274 (1.1%)	NA	2/69 (2.9%)	7/69 (10.1%)

[1] Warfarin sodium dosage was adjusted to maintain a prothrombin time index of 1.4 to 1.5, corresponding to an International Normalized Ratio (INR) of approximately 2.5.
[2] Includes three treated patients who did not undergo a surgical procedure.
[3] A bleeding event was considered major if: 1) hemorrhage caused a significant clinical event, 2) it was associated with a hemoglobin decrease of ≥2 g/dL or transfusion of 2 or more units of blood products, 3) it resulted in reoperation due to bleeding, or 4) it involved retroperitoneal or intracranial hemorrhage.
[4] Includes two treated patients who did not undergo a surgical procedure.
[5] Occurred at a rate of at least 2% in the group treated with FRAGMIN 5000 IU once daily.

Table 9
Bleeding Events Following Abdominal Surgery

Indication	FRAGMIN vs Heparin				FRAGMIN vs Placebo		FRAGMIN vs FRAGMIN	
	Dosing Regimen				Dosing Regimen		Dosing Regimen	
Abdominal Surgery	FRAGMIN 2500 IU qd s.c.	Heparin 5000 U bid s.c.	FRAGMIN 5000 IU qd s.c.	Heparin 5000 U bid s.c.	FRAGMIN 2500 IU qd s.c.	Placebo qd s.c.	FRAGMIN 2500 IU qd s.c.	FRAGMIN 5000 IU qd s.c.
Postoperative Transfusions	26/459 (5.7%)	36/454 (7.9%)	81/508 (15.9%)	63/498 (12.7%)	14/182 (7.7%)	13/182 (7.1%)	89/1025 (8.7%)	125/1033 (12.1%)
Wound Hematoma	16/467 (3.4%)	18/467 (3.9%)	12/508 (2.4%)	6/498 (1.2%)	2/79 (2.5%)	2/77 (2.6%)	1/1030 (0.1%)	4/1039 (0.4%)
Reoperation Due to Bleeding	2/392 (0.5%)	3/392 (0.8%)	4/508 (0.8%)	2/498 (0.4%)	1/79 (1.3%)	1/78 (1.3%)	2/1030 (0.2%)	13/1038 (1.3%)
Injection Site Hematoma	1/466 (0.2%)	5/464 (1.1%)	36/506 (7.1%)	47/493 (9.5%)	8/172 (4.7%)	2/174 (1.1%)	36/1026 (3.5%)	57/1035 (5.5%)

[See table 10 at top of next page]

Three of the major bleeding events that occurred by Day 21 were fatal, all due to gastrointestinal hemorrhage (two patients in the group treated with FRAGMIN and one in the group receiving placebo). Two deaths occurred after Day 21: one patient in the placebo group died from a subarachnoid hemorrhage that started on Day 55, and one patient died on day 71 (two months after receiving the last dose of FRAGMIN) from a subdural hematoma.

Thrombocytopenia: See WARNINGS: Thrombocytopenia.

Table 10
Bleeding Events in Medical Patients with Severely Restricted Mobility During Acute Illness

Indication	Dosing Regimen	
Medical Patients with Severely Restricted Mobility	**FRAGMIN** 5000 IU qd s.c.	**Placebo** qd s.c.
Major Bleeding Events[1] at Day 14	8/1848 (0.43%)	0/1833 (0%)
Major Bleeding Events[1] at Day 21	9/1848 (0.49%)	3/1833 (0.16%)

[1] A bleeding event was considered major if: 1) it was accompanied by a decrease in hemoglobin of ≥ 2 g/dL in connection with clinical symptoms; 2) intraocular, spinal/epidural, intracranial, or retroperitoneal bleeding; 3) required transfusion of ≥ 2 units of blood products; 4) required significant medical or surgical intervention; or 5) led to death.

Table 11
Volume of FRAGMIN to be Administered by Patient Weight, Based on 9.5 mL Vial (10,000 IU/mL)

Patient weight (lb)	< 110	110 to 131	132 to 153	154 to 175	176 to 197	≥ 198
Patient weight (kg)	< 50	50 to 59	60 to 69	70 to 79	80 to 89	≥ 90
Volume of FRAGMIN (mL)	0.55	0.65	0.75	0.90	1.00	1.00

Table 12
Dosing Options for Patients Undergoing Hip Replacement Surgery

	Dose of FRAGMIN to be Given Subcutaneously			
Timing of First Dose of FRAGMIN	**10 to 14 Hours Before Surgery**	**Within 2 Hours Before Surgery**	**4 to 8 Hours After Surgery[1]**	**Postoperative Period[2]**
Postoperative Start	—	—	2500 IU[3]	5000 IU qd
Preoperative Start - Day of Surgery	—	2500 IU	2500 IU[3]	5000 IU qd
Preoperative Start - Evening Before Surgery[4]	5000 IU	—	5000 IU	5000 IU qd

[1] Or later, if hemostasis has not been achieved.
[2] Up to 14 days of treatment was well tolerated in controlled clinical trials, where the usual duration of treatment was 5 to 10 days postoperatively.
[3] Allow a minimum of 6 hours between this dose and the dose to be given on Postoperative Day 1. Adjust the timing of the dose on Postoperative Day 1 accordingly.
[4] Allow approximately 24 hours between doses.

Other:
Allergic Reactions:
Allergic reactions (i.e., pruritus, rash, fever, injection site reaction, bulleous eruption) and skin necrosis have occurred rarely. A few cases of anaphylactoid reactions have been reported.
Local Reactions:
Pain at the injection site, the only non-bleeding event determined to be possibly or probably related to treatment with FRAGMIN and reported at a rate of at least 2% in the group treated with FRAGMIN, was reported in 4.5% of patients treated with FRAGMIN 5000 IU qd vs 11.8% of patients treated with heparin 5000 U bid in the abdominal surgery trials. In the hip replacement trials, pain at injection site was reported in 12% of patients treated with FRAGMIN 5000 IU qd vs 13% of patients treated with heparin 5000 U tid.
Ongoing Safety Surveillance:
Since first international market introduction in 1985, there have been nine reports of epidural or spinal hematoma formation with concurrent use of dalteparin sodium and spinal/epidural anesthesia or spinal puncture. Five of the nine patients had post-operative indwelling epidural catheters placed for analgesia or received additional drugs affecting hemostasis. The hematomas caused long-term or permanent paralysis (partial or complete) in seven of these cases. One patient experienced temporary paraplegia but made a full recovery, and one patient had no neurological deficit. Because these events were reported voluntarily from a population of unknown size, estimates of frequency cannot be made.

OVERDOSAGE

Symptoms/Treatment:
An excessive dosage of FRAGMIN Injection may lead to hemorrhagic complications. These may generally be stopped by the slow intravenous injection of protamine sulfate (1% solution), at a dose of 1 mg protamine for every 100 anti-Xa IU of FRAGMIN given. A second infusion of 0.5 mg protamine sulfate per 100 anti-Xa IU of FRAGMIN may be administered if the APTT measured 2 to 4 hours after the first infusion remains prolonged. Even with these additional doses of protamine, the APTT may remain more prolonged than would usually be found following administration of conventional heparin. In all cases, the anti-Factor Xa activity is never completely neutralized (maximum about 60 to 75%).

Particular care should be taken to avoid overdosage with protamine sulfate. Administration of protamine sulfate can cause severe hypotensive and anaphylactoid reactions. Because fatal reactions, often resembling anaphylaxis, have been reported with protamine sulfate, it should be given only when resuscitation techniques and treatment of anaphylactic shock are readily available. For additional information, consult the labeling of Protamine Sulfate Injection, USP, products. A single subcutaneous dose of 100,000 IU/kg of FRAGMIN to mice caused a mortality of 8% (1/12) whereas 50,000 IU/kg was a non-lethal dose. The observed sign was hematoma at the site of injection.

DOSAGE AND ADMINISTRATION

Unstable Angina and Non-Q-Wave Myocardial Infarction:
In patients with unstable angina or non-Q-wave myocardial infarction, the recommended dose of FRAGMIN Injection is 120 IU/kg of body weight, but not more than 10,000 IU, subcutaneously (s.c.) every 12 hours with concurrent oral aspirin (75 to 165 mg once daily) therapy. Treatment should be continued until the patient is clinically stabilized. The usual duration of administration is 5 to 8 days. Concurrent aspirin therapy is recommended except when contraindicated. Table 11 lists the volume of FRAGMIN, based on the 9.5 mL multiple-dose vial (10,000 IU/mL), to be administered for a range of patient weights.
[See table 11 above]
Hip Replacement Surgery:
Table 12 presents the dosing options for patients undergoing hip replacement surgery. The usual duration of administration is 5 to 10 days after surgery; up to 14 days of treatment with FRAGMIN have been well tolerated in clinical trials.
[See table 12 above]
Abdominal Surgery:
In patients undergoing abdominal surgery with a risk of thromboembolic complications, the recommended dose of FRAGMIN is 2500 IU administered by s.c. injection once daily, starting 1 to 2 hours prior to surgery and repeated once daily postoperatively. The usual duration of administration is 5 to 10 days.

In patients undergoing abdominal surgery associated with a high risk of thromboembolic complications, such as malignant disorder, the recommended dose of FRAGMIN is 5000 IU s.c. the evening before surgery, then once daily postoperatively. The usual duration of administration is 5 to 10 days. Alternatively, in patients with malignancy, 2500 IU of FRAGMIN can be administered s.c. 1 to 2 hours before surgery followed by 2500 IU s.c. 12 hours later, and then 5000 IU once daily postoperatively. The usual duration of administration is 5 to 10 days.

Dosage adjustment and routine monitoring of coagulation parameters are not required if the dosage and administration recommendations specified above are followed.

Medical Patients with Severely Restricted Mobility During Acute Illness:
In medical patients with severely restricted mobility during acute illness, the recommended dose of FRAGMIN is 5000 IU administered by s.c. injection once daily. In clinical trials, the usual duration of administration was 12 to 14 days.
Administration:
FRAGMIN is administered by subcutaneous injection. It must not be administered by intramuscular injection.
Subcutaneous injection technique: Patients should be sitting or lying down and FRAGMIN administered by deep s.c. injection. FRAGMIN may be injected in a U-shape area around the navel, the upper outer side of the thigh or the upper outer quadrangle of the buttock. The injection site should be varied daily. When the area around the navel or the thigh is used, using the thumb and forefinger, you **must** lift up a fold of skin while giving the injection. The entire length of the needle should be inserted at a 45 to 90 degree angle.
Parenteral drug products should be inspected visually for particulate matter and discoloration prior to administration, whenever solution and container permit.
After first penetration of the rubber stopper, store the multiple-dose vials at room temperature for up to 2 weeks. Discard any unused solution after 2 weeks.
Instructions for using the prefilled single-dose syringes preassembled with needle guard devices:

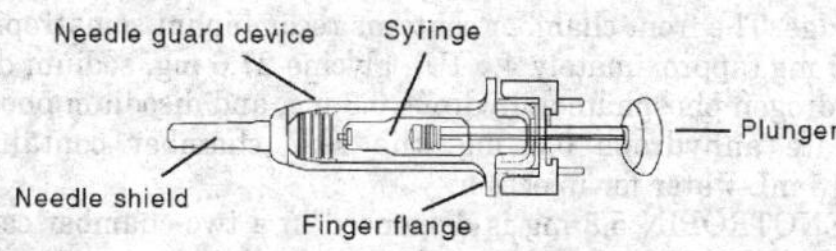

Fixed dose syringes: To ensure delivery of the full dose, do not expel the air bubble from the prefilled syringe before injection. Hold the syringe assembly by the open sides of the device. Remove the needle shield. Insert the needle into the injection area as instructed above. Depress the plunger of the syringe while holding the finger flange **until the entire dose has been given.** The needle guard will **not** be activated unless the **entire** dose has been given. Remove needle from the patient. Let go of the plunger and allow syringe to move up inside the device until the entire needle is guarded. Discard the syringe assembly in approved containers.
Graduated syringes: Hold the syringe assembly by the open sides of the device. Remove the needle shield. With the needle pointing up, prepare the syringe by expelling the air bubble and then continuing to push the plunger to the desired dose or volume, discarding the extra solution in an appropriate manner. Insert the needle into the injection area as instructed above. Depress the plunger of the syringe while holding the finger flange **until the entire dose remaining in the syringe has been given.** The needle guard will **not** be activated unless the **entire** dose has been given. Remove needle from the patient. Let go of the plunger and allow syringe to move up inside the device until the entire needle is guarded. Discard the syringe assembly in approved containers.

HOW SUPPLIED

FRAGMIN Injection is available in the following strengths and package sizes:
0.2 mL single-dose prefilled syringe, affixed with a 27-gauge × 1/2 inch needle and preassembled with UltraSafe Passive™ Needle Guard* devices.
Package of 10:
2500 anti-Factor Xa IU NDC 0013-2406-91
5000 anti-Factor Xa IU NDC 0013-2426-91
0.3 mL single-dose prefilled syringe, affixed with a 27-gauge × 1/2 inch needle and preassembled with UltraSafe Passive™ Needle Guard* devices.
Package of 10:
7500 anti-Factor Xa IU NDC 0013-2426-01
1.0 mL single-dose graduated syringe, affixed with a 27-gauge × 1/2 inch needle and preassembled with UltraSafe Passive™ Needle Guard* devices.
Package of 10:
10,000 anti-Factor Xa IU NDC 0013-5190-01
3.8 mL multiple-dose vial:
25,000 anti-Factor Xa IU/mL NDC 0013-5191-01 (95,000 anti-Factor Xa IU/vial)
9.5 mL multiple-dose vial:
10,000 anti-Factor Xa IU/mL NDC 0013-2436-06 (95,000 anti-Factor Xa IU/vial)
Store at controlled room temperature 20° to 25°C (68° to 77°F) [see USP].
℞ only
U.S. Patent 4,303,651

*UltraSafe Passive™ Needle Guard is a trademark of Safety Syringes, Inc.
Manufactured for: Pharmacia & Upjohn Company
A subsidiary of Pharmacia Corporation
Kalamazoo, MI 49001, USA

Continued on next page

Fragmin—Cont.

By: Vetter Pharma-Fertigung
Ravensburg, Germany
(prefilled syringes)
Pharmacia N.V./S.A.
Puurs, Belgium
(multiple-dose vial)

818 312 112 Revised March 2004
5R7216

GENOTROPIN® ℞

[*gen-ō" trō-pĭn*]
somatropin [rDNA origin] for injection
In a Two-Chamber Cartridge

DESCRIPTION

GENOTROPIN Lyophilized Powder contains somatropin [rDNA origin], which is a polypeptide hormone of recombinant DNA origin. It has 191 amino acid residues and a molecular weight of 22,124 daltons. The amino acid sequence of the product is identical to that of human growth hormone of pituitary origin (somatropin). GENOTROPIN is synthesized in a strain of *Escherichia coli* that has been modified by the addition of the gene for human growth hormone. GENOTROPIN is a sterile white lyophilized powder intended for subcutaneous injection.

GENOTROPIN 1.5 mg is dispensed in a two-chamber cartridge. The front chamber contains recombinant somatropin 1.5 mg (approximately 4.5 IU), glycine 27.6 mg, sodium dihydrogen phosphate anhydrous 0.3 mg, and disodium phosphate anhydrous 0.3 mg; the rear chamber contains 1.13 mL water for injection.

GENOTROPIN 5.8 mg is dispensed in a two-chamber cartridge. The front chamber contains recombinant somatropin 5.8 mg (approximately 17.4 IU), glycine 2.2 mg, mannitol 1.8 mg, sodium dihydrogen phosphate anhydrous 0.32 mg, and disodium phosphate anhydrous 0.31 mg; the rear chamber contains 0.3% m-Cresol (as a preservative) and mannitol 45 mg in 1.14 mL water for injection.

GENOTROPIN 13.8 mg is dispensed in a two-chamber cartridge. The front chamber contains recombinant somatropin 13.8 mg (approximately 41.4 IU), glycine 2.3 mg, mannitol 14.0 mg, sodium dihydrogen phosphate anhydrous 0.47 mg, and disodium phosphate anhydrous 0.46 mg; the rear chamber contains 0.3% m-Cresol (as a preservative) and mannitol 32 mg in 1.13 mL water for injection.

GENOTROPIN MINIQUICK® is dispensed as a single-use syringe device containing a two-chamber cartridge. GENOTROPIN MINIQUICK is available as individual doses of 0.2 mg to 2.0 mg in 0.2-mg increments. The front chamber contains recombinant somatropin 0.22 to 2.2 mg (approximately 0.66 to 6.6 IU), glycine 0.23 mg, mannitol 1.14 mg, sodium dihydrogen phosphate 0.05 mg, and disodium phosphate anhydrous 0.027 mg; the rear chamber contains mannitol 12.6 mg in water for injection 0.275 mL.

GENOTROPIN is a highly purified preparation. The reconstituted recombinant somatropin solution has an osmolality of approximately 300 mOsm/kg, and a pH of approximately 6.7. The concentration of the reconstituted solution varies by strength and presentation (see HOW SUPPLIED).

CLINICAL PHARMACOLOGY

In vitro, preclinical, and clinical tests have demonstrated that GENOTROPIN Lyophilized Powder is therapeutically equivalent to human growth hormone of pituitary origin and achieves similar pharmacokinetic profiles in normal adults. In pediatric patients who have growth hormone deficiency (GHD) or Prader-Willi syndrome (PWS), or who were born small for gestational age (SGA), treatment with GENOTROPIN stimulates linear growth. In patients with GHD or PWS, treatment with GENOTROPIN also normalizes concentrations of IGF-I (Insulin-like Growth Factor-I/Somatomedin C). In adults with GHD, treatment with GENOTROPIN results in reduced fat mass, increased lean body mass, metabolic alterations that include beneficial changes in lipid metabolism, and normalization of IGF-I concentrations.

In addition, the following actions have been demonstrated for GENOTROPIN and/or somatropin.

1. Tissue Growth

A. *Skeletal Growth:* GENOTROPIN stimulates skeletal growth in pediatric patients with GHD, PWS, or SGA. The measurable increase in body length after administration of GENOTROPIN results from an effect on the epiphyseal plates of long bones. Concentrations of IGF-I, which may play a role in skeletal growth, are generally low in the serum of pediatric patients with GHD, PWS, or SGA, but tend to increase during treatment with GENOTROPIN. Elevations in mean serum alkaline phosphatase concentration are also seen.

B. *Cell Growth:* It has been shown that there are fewer skeletal muscle cells in short-statured pediatric patients who lack endogenous growth hormone as compared with the normal pediatric population. Treatment with somatropin results in an increase in both the number and size of muscle cells.

2. Protein Metabolism

Linear growth is facilitated in part by increased cellular protein synthesis. Nitrogen retention, as demonstrated by decreased urinary nitrogen excretion and serum urea nitrogen, follows the initiation of therapy with GENOTROPIN.

3. Carbohydrate Metabolism

Pediatric patients with hypopituitarism sometimes experience fasting hypoglycemia that is improved by treatment with GENOTROPIN. Large doses of growth hormone may impair glucose tolerance.

4. Lipid Metabolism

In GHD patients, administration of somatropin has resulted in lipid mobilization, reduction in body fat stores, and increased plasma fatty acids.

5. Mineral Metabolism

Somatropin induces retention of sodium, potassium, and phosphorus. Serum concentrations of inorganic phosphate are increased in patients with GHD after therapy with GENOTROPIN. Serum calcium is not significantly altered by GENOTROPIN. Growth hormone could increase calciuria.

6. Body Composition

Adult GHD patients treated with GENOTROPIN at the recommended adult dose (see DOSAGE AND ADMINISTRATION) demonstrate a decrease in fat mass and an increase in lean body mass. When these alterations are coupled with the increase in total body water, the overall effect of GENOTROPIN is to modify body composition, an effect that is maintained with continued treatment.

PHARMACOKINETICS

Absorption

Following a 0.03 mg/kg subcutaneous (SC) injection in the thigh of 1.3 mg/mL GENOTROPIN to adult GHD patients, approximately 80% of the dose was systemically available as compared with that available following intravenous dosing. Results were comparable in both male and female patients. Similar bioavailability has been observed in healthy adult male subjects.

In healthy adult males, following an SC injection in the thigh of 0.03 mg/kg, the extent of absorption (AUC) of a concentration of 5.3 mg/mL GENOTROPIN was 35% greater than that for 1.3 mg/mL GENOTROPIN. The mean (± standard deviation) peak (C_{max}) serum levels were 23.0 (± 9.4) ng/mL and 17.4 (± 9.2) ng/mL, respectively.

In a similar study involving pediatric GHD patients, 5.3 mg/mL GENOTROPIN yielded a mean AUC that was 17% greater than that for 1.3 mg/mL GENOTROPIN. The mean C_{max} levels were 21.0 ng/mL and 16.3 ng/mL, respectively.

Adult GHD patients received two single SC doses of 0.03 mg/kg of GENOTROPIN at a concentration of 1.3 mg/mL, with a one- to four-week washout period between injections. Mean C_{max} levels were 12.4 ng/mL (first injection) and 12.2 ng/mL (second injection), achieved at approximately six hours after dosing.

There are no data on the bioequivalence between the 12-mg/mL formulation and either the 1.3-mg/mL or the 5.3-mg/mL formulations.

Distribution

The mean volume of distribution of GENOTROPIN following administration to GHD adults was estimated to be 1.3 (± 0.8) L/kg.

Metabolism

The metabolic fate of GENOTROPIN involves classical protein catabolism in both the liver and kidneys. In renal cells, at least a portion of the breakdown products are returned to the systemic circulation. The mean terminal half-life of intravenous GENOTROPIN in normal adults is 0.4 hours, whereas subcutaneously administered GENOTROPIN has a half-life of 3.0 hours in GHD adults. The observed difference is due to slow absorption from the subcutaneous injection site.

Excretion

The mean clearance of subcutaneously administered GENOTROPIN in 16 GHD adult patients was 0.3 (± 0.11) L/hrs/kg.

Special Populations

Pediatric: The pharmacokinetics of GENOTROPIN are similar in GHD pediatric and adult patients.

Gender: No gender studies have been performed in pediatric patients; however, in GHD adults, the absolute bioavailability of GENOTROPIN was similar in males and females.

Race: No studies have been conducted with GENOTROPIN to assess pharmacokinetic differences among races.

Renal or hepatic insufficiency: No studies have been conducted with GENOTROPIN in these patient populations.

[See table 1 below]

Table 1
Mean SC Pharmacokinetic Parameters in Adult GHD Patients

	Bioavailability (%) (N=15)	T_{max} (hours) (N=16)	CL/F (L/hr/kg) (N=16)	Vss/F (L/kg) (N=16)	$T_{1/2}$ (hours) (N=16)
Mean (± SD)	80.5 *	5.9 (± 1.65)	0.3 (± 0.11)	1.3 (± 0.80)	3.0 (± 1.44)
95% CI	70.5 – 92.1	5.0 – 6.7	0.2 – 0.4	0.9 – 1.8	2.2 – 3.7

T_{max} = time of maximum plasma concentration
CL/F = plasma clearance
Vss/F = volume of distribution
$T_{½}$ = terminal half-life
SD = standard deviation
CI = confidence interval

*The absolute bioavailability was estimated under the assumption that the log-transformed data follow a normal distribution. The mean and standard deviation of the log-transformed data were mean = 0.22 (± 0.241).

CLINICAL STUDIES

Adult Patients with Growth Hormone Deficiency (GHD)

GENOTROPIN Lyophilized Powder was compared with placebo in six randomized clinical trials involving a total of 172 adult GHD patients. These trials included a 6-month double-blind treatment period, during which 85 patients received GENOTROPIN and 87 patients received placebo, followed by an open-label treatment period in which participating patients received GENOTROPIN for up to a total of 24 months. GENOTROPIN was administered as a daily SC injection at a dose of 0.04 mg/kg/week for the first month of treatment and 0.08 mg/kg/week for subsequent months.

Beneficial changes in body composition were observed at the end of the 6-month treatment period for the patients receiving GENOTROPIN as compared with the placebo patients. Lean body mass, total body water, and lean/fat ratio increased while total body fat mass and waist circumference decreased. These effects on body composition were maintained when treatment was continued beyond 6 months. Bone mineral density declined after 6 months of treatment but returned to baseline values after 12 months of treatment.

Pediatric Patients with Prader-Willi Syndrome (PWS)

The safety and efficacy of GENOTROPIN in the treatment of pediatric patients with Prader-Willi syndrome (PWS) were evaluated in two randomized, open-label, controlled clinical trials. Patients received either GENOTROPIN or no treatment for the first year of the studies, while all patients received GENOTROPIN during the second year. GENOTROPIN was administered as a daily SC injection, and the dose was calculated for each patient every 3 months. In Study 1, the treatment group received GENOTROPIN at a dose of 0.24 mg/kg/week during the entire study. During the second year, the control group received GENOTROPIN at a dose of 0.48 mg/kg/week. In Study 2, the treatment group received GENOTROPIN at a dose of 0.36 mg/kg/week during the entire study. During the second year, the control group received GENOTROPIN at a dose of 0.36 mg/kg/week.

Patients who received GENOTROPIN showed significant increases in linear growth during the first year of study, compared with patients who received no treatment (see Table 2). Linear growth continued to increase in the second year, when both groups received treatment with GENOTROPIN.

[See table 2 at bottom of next page]

Changes in body composition were also observed in the patients receiving GENOTROPIN (see Table 3). These changes included a decrease in the amount of fat mass, and increases in the amount of lean body mass and the ratio of lean-to-fat tissue, while changes in body weight were similar to those seen in patients who received no treatment. Treatment with GENOTROPIN did not accelerate bone age, compared with patients who received no treatment.

[See table 3 at bottom of next page]

Pediatric Patients Born Small for Gestational Age (SGA) Who Fail to Manifest Catch-up Growth by Age 2

The safety and efficacy of GENOTROPIN in the treatment of children born small for gestational age (SGA) were evaluated in 4 randomized, open-label, controlled clinical trials. Patients (age range of 2 to 8 years) were observed for 12 months before being randomized to receive either GENOTROPIN (two doses per study, most often 0.24 and 0.48 mg/kg/week) as a daily SC injection or no treatment for the first 24 months of the studies. After 24 months in the studies, all patients received GENOTROPIN.

Patients who received any dose of GENOTROPIN showed significant increases in growth during the first 24 months of study, compared with patients who received no treatment (see Table 4). Children receiving 0.48 mg/kg/week demonstrated a significant improvement in height standard deviation score (SDS) compared with children treated with 0.24 mg/kg/week. Both of these doses resulted in a slower but constant increase in growth between months 24 to 72 (data not shown).

[See table 4 at bottom of next page]

INDICATIONS AND USAGE

GENOTROPIN Lyophilized Powder is indicated for:

- Long-term treatment of pediatric patients who have growth failure due to an inadequate secretion of endogenous growth hormone.

- Long-term treatment of pediatric patients who have growth failure due to Prader-Willi syndrome (PWS). The diagnosis of PWS should be confirmed by appropriate genetic testing (see CONTRAINDICATIONS).
- Long-term treatment of growth failure in children born small for gestational age (SGA) who fail to manifest catch-up growth by age 2.

Other causes of short stature in pediatric patients should be excluded.

- Long-term replacement therapy in adults with growth hormone deficiency (GHD) of either childhood- or adult-onset etiology. GHD should be confirmed by an appropriate growth hormone stimulation test.

CONTRAINDICATIONS

GENOTROPIN Lyophilized Powder should not be used when there is any evidence of neoplastic activity. Intracranial lesions must be inactive and antitumor therapy complete prior to the institution of therapy. GENOTROPIN should be discontinued if there is evidence of tumor growth. Growth hormone should not be used for growth promotion in pediatric patients with fused epiphyses.

Growth hormone should not be initiated to treat patients with acute critical illness due to complications following open heart or abdominal surgery, multiple accidental trauma, or to patients having acute respiratory failure. Two placebo-controlled clinical trials in non-growth hormone deficient adult patients (n=522) with these conditions revealed a significant increase in mortality (41.9% vs 19.3%) among somatropin treated patients (doses 5.3 to 8 mg/day) compared to those receiving placebo (see WARNINGS).

Growth hormone is contraindicated in patients with Prader-Willi syndrome who are severely obese or have severe respiratory impairment (see WARNINGS).

WARNINGS

The 5.8-mg and 13.8-mg presentations of GENOTROPIN Lyophilized Powder contain m-Cresol as a preservative. These products should not be used by patients with a known sensitivity to this preservative. The GENOTROPIN 1.5-mg and GENOTROPIN MINIQUICK presentations are preservative-free (see HOW SUPPLIED).

See CONTRAINDICATIONS for information on increased mortality in patients with acute critical illnesses in intensive care units due to complications following open heart or abdominal surgery, multiple accidental trauma, or with acute respiratory failure. The safety of continuing growth hormone treatment in patients receiving replacement doses for approved indications who concurrently develop these illnesses has not been established. Therefore, the potential benefit of treatment continuation with growth hormone in patients having acute critical illnesses should be weighed against the potential risk.

There have been reports of fatalities after initiating therapy with growth hormone in pediatric patients with Prader-Willi syndrome who had one or more of the following risk factors: severe obesity, history of upper airway obstruction or sleep apnea, or unidentified respiratory infection. Male patients with one or more of these factors may be at greater risk than females. Patients with Prader-Willi syndrome should be evaluated for signs of upper airway obstruction and sleep apnea before initiation of treatment with growth hormone. If during treatment with growth hormone patients show signs of upper airway obstruction (including onset of or increased snoring) and/or new onset sleep apnea, treatment should be interrupted. All patients with Prader-Willi syndrome treated with growth hormone should also have effective weight control and be monitored for signs of respiratory infections, which should be diagnosed as early as possible and treated aggressively (see CONTRAINDICATIONS).

Table 2
Efficacy of GENOTROPIN in Pediatric Patients with Prader-Willi Syndrome (Mean ± SD)

	Study 1		Study 2	
	GENOTROPIN (0.24 mg/kg/week) n=15	Untreated Control n=12	GENOTROPIN (0.36 mg/kg/week) n=7	Untreated Control n=9
Linear growth (cm)				
Baseline height	112.7 ± 14.9	109.5 ± 12.0	120.3 ± 17.5	120.5 ± 11.2
Growth from months 0 to 12	11.6* ± 2.3	5.0 ± 1.2	10.7* ± 2.3	4.3 ± 1.5
Height Standard Deviation Score (SDS) for age				
Baseline SDS	-1.6 ± 1.3	-1.8 ± 1.5	-2.6 ± 1.7	-2.1 ± 1.4
SDS at 12 months	-0.5† ± 1.3	-1.9 ± 1.4	-1.4† ± 1.5	-2.2 ± 1.4

* p ≤ 0.001
† p ≤ 0.002 (when comparing SDS change at 12 months)

Table 3
Effect of GENOTROPIN on Body Composition in Pediatric Patients with Prader-Willi Syndrome (Mean ± SD)

	GENOTROPIN n=14	Untreated Control n=10
Fat mass (kg)		
Baseline	12.3 ± 6.8	9.4 ± 4.9
Change from months 0 to 12	-0.9* ± 2.2	2.3 ± 2.4
Lean body mass (kg)		
Baseline	15.6 ± 5.7	14.3 ± 4.0
Change from months 0 to 12	4.7* ± 1.9	0.7 ± 2.4
Lean body mass/Fat mass		
Baseline	1.4 ± 0.4	1.8 ± 0.8
Change from months 0 to 12	1.0* ± 1.4	-0.1 ± 0.6
Body weight (kg)†		
Baseline	27.2 ± 12.0	23.2 ± 7.0
Change from months 0 to 12	3.7‡ ± 2.0	3.5 ± 1.9

* p < 0.005
† n=15 for the group receiving GENOTROPIN; n=12 for the Control group
‡ n.s.

Table 4
Efficacy of GENOTROPIN in Children Born Small for Gestational Age (Mean ± SD)

	GENOTROPIN (0.24 mg/kg/week) n=76	GENOTROPIN (0.48 mg/kg/week) n=93	Untreated Control n=40
Height Standard Deviation Score (SDS)			
Baseline SDS	-3.2 ± 0.8	-3.4 ± 1.0	-3.1 ± 0.9
SDS at 24 months	-0.2 ± 0.8	-1.7 ± 1.0	-2.9 ± 0.9
Change in SDS from baseline to month 24	1.2* ± 0.5	1.7*† ± 0.6	0.1 ± 0.3

* p = 0.0001 vs Untreated Control group
† p = 0.0001 vs group treated with GENOTROPIN 0.24 mg/kg/week

PRECAUTIONS

General

Treatment with GENOTROPIN Lyophilized Powder, as with other growth hormone preparations, should be directed by physicians who are experienced in the diagnosis and management of patients with GHD or Prader-Willi syndrome (PWS), or those who were born small for gestational age (SGA).

Patients and caregivers who will administer GENOTROPIN in medically unsupervised situations should receive appropriate training and instruction on the proper use of GENOTROPIN from the physician or other suitably qualified health professional.

Patients with GHD secondary to an intracranial lesion should be examined frequently for progression or recurrence of the underlying disease process. Review of literature reports of pediatric use of somatropin replacement therapy reveals no relationship between this therapy and recurrence of central nervous system (CNS) tumors. In adults, it is unknown whether there is any relationship between somatropin treatment and CNS tumor recurrence.

Patients should be monitored carefully for any malignant transformation of skin lesions.

Caution should be used if growth hormone is administered to patients with diabetes mellitus, and insulin dosage may need to be adjusted. Patients with diabetes or glucose intolerance should be monitored closely during treatment with GENOTROPIN. Patients with risk factors for glucose intolerance, such as obesity (including obese patients with PWS) or a family history of Type II diabetes, should be monitored closely as well. Because growth hormone may induce a state of insulin resistance, patients should be observed for evidence of glucose intolerance.

In patients with hypopituitarism (multiple hormonal deficiencies) standard hormonal replacement therapy should be monitored closely when treatment with GENOTROPIN is instituted. Hypothyroidism may develop during treatment with GENOTROPIN, and inadequate treatment of hypothyroidism may prevent optimal response to GENOTROPIN. Therefore, patients should have periodic thyroid function tests and be treated with thyroid hormone when indicated.

Pediatric patients with endocrine disorders, including GHD, have a higher incidence of slipped capital femoral epiphyses. Any pediatric patient with the onset of a limp or complaints of hip or knee pain during growth hormone therapy should be evaluated.

Progression of scoliosis can occur in patients who experience rapid growth. Because growth hormone increases growth rate, patients with a history of scoliosis who are treated with growth hormone should be monitored for progression of scoliosis. However, growth hormone has not been shown to increase the incidence of scoliosis. Scoliosis is commonly seen in untreated patients with PWS. Physicians should be alert to this abnormality, which may manifest during growth hormone therapy.

Intracranial hypertension (IH) with papilledema, visual changes, headache, nausea and/or vomiting has been reported in a small number of patients treated with growth hormone products. Symptoms usually occurred within the first 8 weeks of the initiation of growth hormone therapy. In all reported cases, IH-associated signs and symptoms resolved after termination of therapy or a reduction of the growth hormone dose. Funduscopic examination of patients is recommended at the initiation, and periodically during the course of, growth hormone therapy. Patients with PWS may be at increased risk for development of IH.

Before continuing treatment as an adult, a post-pubertal GHD patient who received growth hormone replacement therapy in childhood should be reevaluated with proper testing as described in INDICATIONS AND USAGE. If continued treatment is appropriate, GENOTROPIN should be administered at the reduced dose level recommended for adult GHD patients.

Drug Interactions

Concomitant glucocorticoid treatment may inhibit the growth-promoting effect of growth hormone. Pediatric GHD patients with coexisting ACTH deficiency should have their glucocorticoid replacement dose carefully adjusted to avoid an inhibitory effect on growth (see also PRECAUTIONS - General). Limited published data indicate that growth hormone treatment increases cytochrome P450 (CP450) mediated antipyrine clearance in man. These data suggest that growth hormone administration may alter the clearance of compounds known to be metabolized by CP450 liver enzymes (e.g. corticosteroids, sex steroids, anticonvulsants, cyclosporine). Careful monitoring is advisable when growth hormone is administered in combination with other drugs known to be metabolized by CP450 liver enzymes.

Carcinogenesis, Mutagenesis, Impairment of Fertility

Carcinogenicity studies have not been conducted with rhGH. No potential mutagenicity of rhGH was revealed in a battery of tests including induction of gene mutations in bacteria (the Ames test), gene mutations in mammalian cells grown in vitro (mouse L5178Y cells), and chromosomal damage in intact animals (bone marrow cells in rats). See PREGNANCY section for effect on fertility.

Continued on next page

Genotropin—Cont.

Pregnancy: Pregnancy Category B

Reproduction studies carried out with GENOTROPIN at doses of 0.3, 1, and 3.3 mg/kg/day administered SC in the rat and 0.08, 0.3, and 1.3 mg/kg/day administered intramuscularly in the rabbit (highest doses approximately 24 times and 19 times the recommended human therapeutic levels, respectively, based on body surface area) resulted in decreased maternal body weight gains but were not teratogenic. In rats receiving SC doses during gametogenesis and up to 7 days of pregnancy, 3.3 mg/kg/day (approximately 24 times human dose) produced anestrus or extended estrus cycles in females and fewer and less motile sperm in males. When given to pregnant female rats (days 1 to 7 of gestation) at 3.3 mg/kg/day a very slight increase in fetal deaths was observed. At 1 mg/kg/day (approximately seven times human dose) rats showed slightly extended estrus cycles, whereas at 0.3 mg/kg/day no effects were noted.

In perinatal and postnatal studies in rats, GENOTROPIN doses of 0.3, 1, and 3.3 mg/kg/day produced growth-promoting effects in the dams but not in the fetuses. Young rats at the highest dose showed increased weight gain during suckling but the effect was not apparent by 10 weeks of age. No adverse effects were observed on gestation, morphogenesis, parturition, lactation, postnatal development, or reproductive capacity of the offsprings due to GENOTROPIN. There are, however, no adequate and well-controlled studies in pregnant women. Because animal reproduction studies are not always predictive of human response, this drug should be used during pregnancy only if clearly needed.

Nursing Mothers

There have been no studies conducted with GENOTROPIN in nursing mothers. It is not known whether this drug is excreted in human milk. Because many drugs are excreted in human milk, caution should be exercised when GENOTROPIN is administered to a nursing woman.

Geriatric Use

The safety and effectiveness of GENOTROPIN in patients aged 65 and over has not been evaluated in clinical studies. Elderly patients may be more sensitive to the action of GENOTROPIN and may be more prone to develop adverse reactions.

ADVERSE REACTIONS

As with all protein drugs, a small number of patients may develop antibodies to the protein. Growth hormone antibody with binding lower than 2 mg/L has not been associated with growth attenuation. In some cases when binding capacity is > 2 mg/L, interference with growth response has been observed.

In 419 pediatric patients evaluated in clinical studies with GENOTROPIN Lyophilized Powder, 244 had been treated previously with GENOTROPIN or other growth hormone preparations and 175 had received no previous growth hormone therapy. Antibodies to growth hormone (anti-hGH antibodies) were present in six previously treated patients at baseline. Three of the six became negative for anti-hGH antibodies during 6 to 12 months of treatment with GENOTROPIN. Of the remaining 413 patients, eight (1.9%) developed detectable anti-hGH antibodies during treatment with GENOTROPIN; none had an antibody binding capacity > 2 mg/L. There was no evidence that the growth response to GENOTROPIN was affected in these antibody-positive patients.

Preparations of GENOTROPIN contain a small amount of periplasmic *Escherichia coli* peptides (PECP). Anti-PECP antibodies are found in a small number of patients treated with GENOTROPIN, but these appear to be of no clinical significance.

In clinical studies with GENOTROPIN in pediatric GHD patients, the following events were reported infrequently: injection site reactions, including pain or burning associated with the injection, fibrosis, nodules, rash, inflammation, pigmentation, or bleeding; lipoatrophy; headache; hematuria; hypothyroidism; and mild hyperglycemia.

Leukemia has been reported in a small number of pediatric patients who have been treated with growth hormone, including growth hormone of pituitary origin and recombinant somatropin. The relationship, if any, between leukemia and growth hormone therapy is uncertain.

In two clinical studies with GENOTROPIN in pediatric patients with Prader-Willi syndrome, the following drug-related events were reported: edema, aggressiveness, arthralgia, benign intracranial hypertension, hair loss, headache, and myalgia.

In clinical studies of 273 pediatric patients born small for gestational age treated with GENOTROPIN, the following clinically significant events were reported: mild transient hyperglycemia, one patient with benign intracranial hypertension, two patients with central precocious puberty, two patients with jaw prominence, and several patients with aggravation of pre-existing scoliosis, injection site reactions, and self-limited progression of pigmented nevi. Anti-hGH antibodies were not detected in any of the patients treated with GENOTROPIN.

In clinical trials with GENOTROPIN in 1,145 GHD adults, the majority of the adverse events consisted of mild to moderate symptoms of fluid retention, including peripheral swelling, arthralgia, pain and stiffness of the extremities, peripheral edema, myalgia, paresthesia, and hypoesthesia. These events were reported early during therapy, and tended to be transient and/or responsive to dosage reduction.

Table 5 displays the adverse events reported by 5% or more of adult GHD patients in clinical trials after various durations of treatment with GENOTROPIN. Also presented are the corresponding incidence rates of these adverse events in placebo patients during the 6-month double-blind portion of the clinical trials.

[See table 5 below]

In expanded post-trial extension studies, diabetes mellitus developed in 12 of 3,031 patients (0.4%) during treatment with GENOTROPIN. All 12 patients had predisposing factors, e.g., elevated glycated hemoglobin levels and/or marked obesity, prior to receiving GENOTROPIN. Of the 3,031 patients receiving GENOTROPIN, 61 (2%) developed symptoms of carpal tunnel syndrome, which lessened after dosage reduction or treatment interruption (52) or surgery (9). Other adverse events that have been reported include generalized edema and hypoesthesia.

OVERDOSAGE

There is little information on acute or chronic overdosage with GENOTROPIN Lyophilized Powder. Intravenously administered growth hormone has been shown to result in an acute decrease in plasma glucose. Subsequently, hyperglycemia was seen. It is thought that the same effect might occur on rare occasions with a high dosage of GENOTROPIN administered SC. Long-term overdosage may result in signs and symptoms of acromegaly consistent with overproduction of growth hormone.

DOSAGE AND ADMINISTRATION

The dosage of GENOTROPIN Lyophilized Powder must be adjusted for the individual patient. The weekly dose should be divided into 6 or 7 **subcutaneous** injections. GENOTROPIN may be given in the thigh, buttocks, or abdomen; the site of SC injections should be rotated daily to help prevent lipoatrophy.

Pediatric GHD Patients: Generally, a dose of 0.16 to 0.24 mg/kg body weight/week is recommended.

Pediatric PWS Patients: Generally, a dose of 0.24 mg/kg body weight/week is recommended.

Pediatric SGA Patients: Generally, a dose of 0.48 mg/kg body weight/week is recommended.

Adult GHD Patients: The recommended dosage at the start of therapy is not more than 0.04 mg/kg/week. The dose may be increased at 4- to 8-week intervals according to individual patient requirements to a maximum of 0.08 mg/kg/week, depending upon patient tolerance of treatment. Clinical response, side effects, and determination of age-adjusted serum IGF-I may be used as guidance in dose titration. This approach will tend to result in weight-adjusted doses that are larger for women compared with men and smaller for older and obese patients.

GENOTROPIN must not be injected intravenously.

GENOTROPIN is supplied in a two-chamber cartridge, with the lyophilized powder in the front chamber and a diluent in the rear chamber. A reconstitution device is used to mix the diluent and powder.

Follow the directions for reconstitution provided with each device. **Do not shake;** shaking may cause denaturation of the active ingredient.

All parenteral drug products should be inspected visually for particulate matter and discoloration prior to administration, whenever solution and container permit. If the solution is cloudy, the contents **MUST NOT** be injected.

Patients and caregivers who will administer GENOTROPIN in medically unsupervised situations should receive appropriate training and instruction on the proper use of GENOTROPIN from the physician or other suitably qualified health professional.

STABILITY AND STORAGE

Except as noted below, store GENOTROPIN Lyophilized Powder under refrigeration at 2° to 8°C (36° to 46°F). Do not freeze. Protect from light.

The 1.5-mg cartridge of GENOTROPIN contains a diluent with no preservative. After reconstitution, the cartridge may be stored under refrigeration for up to 24 hours. Use only once and discard any remaining solution.

The 5.8-mg and 13.8-mg cartridges of GENOTROPIN contain a diluent with a preservative. Thus, after reconstitution, they may be stored under refrigeration for up to 21 days.

The GENOTROPIN MINIQUICK Growth Hormone Delivery Device should be refrigerated prior to dispensing, but may be stored at or below 25°C (77°F) for up to three months after dispensing. The diluent has no preservative. After reconstitution, the GENOTROPIN MINIQUICK may be stored under refrigeration for up to 24 hours before use. The GENOTROPIN MINIQUICK should be used only once and then discarded.

HOW SUPPLIED

GENOTROPIN Lyophilized Powder is available in the following packages:

1.5-mg two-chamber cartridge (without preservative)
concentration of 1.3 mg/mL (approximately 4 IU/mL)
Pre-assembled in a GENOTROPIN INTRA-MIX® Growth Hormone Reconstitution Device and packaged with a pressure release needle
Package of 5 NDC 0013-2606-94

5.8-mg two-chamber cartridge (with preservative)
concentration of 5 mg/mL (approximately 15 IU/mL)
For use with the GENOTROPIN PEN® 5 Growth Hormone Delivery Device and/or the GENOTROPIN MIXER™ Growth Hormone Reconstitution Device
Package of 5 NDC 0013-2626-94
Package of 1 NDC 0013-2626-81
Pre-assembled in a GENOTROPIN INTRA-MIX Growth Hormone Reconstitution Device and packaged with a pressure release needle
Package of 5 NDC 0013-2616-94
Package of 1 NDC 0013-2616-81

13.8-mg two-chamber cartridge (with preservative)
concentration of 12 mg/mL (approximately 36 IU/mL)
For use with the GENOTROPIN PEN 12 Growth Hormone Delivery Device and/or the GENOTROPIN MIXER Growth Hormone Reconstitution Device
Package of 5 NDC 0013-2646-94
Package of 1 NDC 0013-2646-81

Manufactured by: Pharmacia AB
Stockholm, Sweden
or
Vetter Pharma-Fertigung GmbH & Co. KG
Langenargen, Germany

GENOTROPIN MINIQUICK Growth Hormone Delivery Device containing a two-chamber cartridge of GENOTROPIN (without preservative)

After reconstitution, each GENOTROPIN MINIQUICK delivers a fixed volume of 0.25 mL, regardless of strength. Available in the following strengths, each in a package of 7:

0.2 mg	NDC 0013-2649-02
0.4 mg	NDC 0013-2650-02
0.6 mg	NDC 0013-2651-02
0.8 mg	NDC 0013-2652-02
1.0 mg	NDC 0013-2653-02
1.2 mg	NDC 0013-2654-02
1.4 mg	NDC 0013-2655-02
1.6 mg	NDC 0013-2656-02
1.8 mg	NDC 0013-2657-02
2.0 mg	NDC 0013-2658-02

Please see accompanying directions for use of the reconstitution and/or delivery device.

Manufactured by: Pharmacia AB
Stockholm, Sweden

Rx only

Manufactured for: Pharmacia & Upjohn Company
A subsidiary of Pharmacia Corporation
Kalamazoo, MI 49001, USA

Revised February 2004
818 279 005

Table 5
Adverse Events Reported by ≥ 5% of 1,145 Adult GHD Patients During Clinical Trials of GENOTROPIN and Placebo, Grouped by Duration of Treatment

	Double Blind Phase		Open Label Phase GENOTROPIN		
Adverse Event	**Placebo 0-6 mo. n = 572 % Patients**	**GENOTROPIN 0-6 mo. n = 573 % Patients**	**6-12 mo. n = 504 % Patients**	**12-18 mo. n = 63 % Patients**	**18-24 mo. n = 60 % Patients**
Swelling, peripheral	5.1	17.5*	5.6	0	1.7
Arthralgia	4.2	17.3*	6.9	6.3	3.3
Upper respiratory infection	14.5	15.5	13.1	15.9	13.3
Pain, extremities	5.9	14.7*	6.7	1.6	3.3
Edema, peripheral	2.6	10.8*	3.0	0	0
Paresthesia	1.9	9.6*	2.2	3.2	0
Headache	7.7	9.9	6.2	0	0
Stiffness of extremities	1.6	7.9*	2.4	1.6	0
Fatigue	3.8	5.8	4.6	6.3	1.7
Myalgia	1.6	4.9*	2.0	4.8	6.7
Back pain	4.4	2.8	3.4	4.8	5.0

* Increased significantly when compared to placebo, $P \leq .025$: Fisher's Exact Test (one-sided)
n = number of patients receiving treatment during the indicated period.
% = percentage of patients who reported the event during the indicated period.

IDAMYCIN PFS® ℞

[īd-ă-mī-sĭn]

(idarubicin hydrochloride injection)

℞ only

FOR INTRAVENOUS USE ONLY

WARNINGS

1. IDAMYCIN PFS Injection should be given slowly into a freely flowing intravenous infusion. It must never be given intramuscularly or subcutaneously. Severe local tissue necrosis can occur if there is extravasation during administration.
2. As is the case with other anthracyclines the use of IDAMYCIN PFS can cause myocardial toxicity leading to congestive heart failure. Cardiac toxicity is more common in patients who have received prior anthracyclines or who have pre-existing cardiac disease.
3. As is usual with antileukemic agents, severe myelosuppression occurs when IDAMYCIN PFS is used at effective therapeutic doses.
4. It is recommended that IDAMYCIN PFS be administered only under the supervision of a physician who is experienced in leukemia chemotherapy and in facilities with laboratory and supportive resources adequate to monitor drug tolerance and protect and maintain a patient compromised by drug toxicity. The physician and institution must be capable of responding rapidly and completely to severe hemorrhagic conditions and/or overwhelming infection.
5. Dosage should be reduced in patients with impaired hepatic or renal function. (See DOSAGE AND ADMINISTRATION.)

DESCRIPTION

IDAMYCIN PFS Injection contains idarubicin hydrochloride and is a sterile, semi-synthetic, preservative-free solution (PFS) antineoplastic anthracycline for intravenous use. Chemically, idarubicin hydrochloride is 5, 12-Naphthacenedione, 9-acetyl-7-[(3-amino-2,3,6-trideoxy-α-L-*lyxo*-hexopyranosyl)oxy]-7,8,9,10-tetrahydro-6,9,11-trihydroxyhydrochloride, (7S-*cis*). The structural formula is as follows:

$C_{26}H_{27}NO_9 \cdot HCl$ M.W. 533.96

IDAMYCIN PFS is a sterile, red-orange, isotonic parenteral preservative-free solution, available in 5 mL (5 mg), 10 mL (10 mg) and 20 mL (20 mg) single-use-only vials.

Each mL contains Idarubicin HCl, USP 1 mg and the following inactive ingredients: Glycerin, USP 25 mg and Water for Injection, USP q.s. Hydrochloric Acid, NF is used to adjust the pH to a target of 3.5.

CLINICAL PHARMACOLOGY

Mechanism of Action

Idarubicin hydrochloride is a DNA-intercalating analog of daunorubicin which has an inhibitory effect on nucleic acid synthesis and interacts with the enzyme topoisomerase II. The absence of a methoxy group at position 4 of the anthracycline structure gives the compound a high lipophilicity which results in an increased rate of cellular uptake compared with other anthracyclines.

Pharmacokinetics

General Pharmacokinetics: Pharmacokinetic studies have been performed in adult leukemia patients with normal renal and hepatic function following intravenous administration of 10 to 12 mg/m² of idarubicin daily for 3 to 4 days as a single agent or combined with cytarabine. The plasma concentrations of idarubicin are best described by a two or three compartment open model. The elimination rate of idarubicin from plasma is slow with an estimated mean terminal half-life of 22 hours (range, 4 to 48 hours) when used as a single agent and 20 hours (range, 7 to 38 hours) when used in combination with cytarabine. The elimination of the primary active metabolite, idarubicinol, is considerably slower than that of the parent drug with an estimated mean terminal half-life that exceeds 45 hours; hence, its plasma levels are sustained for a period greater than 8 days.

Distribution: The disposition profile shows a rapid distributive phase with a very high volume of distribution presumably reflecting extensive tissue binding. Studies of cellular (nucleated blood and bone marrow cells) drug concentrations in leukemia patients have shown that peak cellular idarubicin concentrations are reached a few minutes after injection. Concentrations of idarubicin and idarubicinol in nucleated blood and bone marrow cells are more than a hundred times the plasma concentrations. Idarubicin disappearance rates in plasma and cells were comparable with a terminal half-life of about 15 hours. The terminal half-life of idarubicinol in cells was about 72 hours. The extent of drug and metabolite accumulation predicted in leukemia patients for Days 2 and 3 of dosing, based on the mean plasma levels and half-life obtained after the first dose, is 1.7- and 2.3-fold, respectively, and suggests no change in kinetics following a daily × 3 regimen. The percentages of idarubicin and idarubicinol bound to human plasma proteins averaged 97% and 94%, respectively, at concentrations similar to maximum plasma levels obtained in the pharmacokinetic studies. The binding is concentration independent. The plasma clearance is twice the expected hepatic plasma flow indicating extensive extrahepatic metabolism.

Metabolism: The primary active metabolite formed is idarubicinol. As idarubicinol has cytotoxic activity, it presumably contributes to the effects of idarubicin.

Elimination: The drug is eliminated predominately by biliary and to a lesser extent by renal excretion, mostly in the form of idarubicinol.

Pharmacokinetics in Special Populations

Pediatric Patients: Idarubicin studies in pediatric leukemia patients, at doses of 4.2 to 13.3 mg/m²/day × 3, suggest dose independent kinetics. There is no difference between the half-lives of the drug following daily × 3 or weekly × 3 administration. Cerebrospinal fluid (CSF) levels of idarubicin and idarubicinol were measured in pediatric leukemia patients treated intravenously. Idarubicin was detected in 2 of 21 CSF samples (0.14 and 1.57 ng/mL), while idarubicinol was detected in 20 of these 21 CSF samples obtained 18 to 30 hours after dosing (mean = 0.51 ng/mL; range, 0.22 to 1.05 ng/mL). The clinical relevance of these findings is unknown.

Hepatic and Renal Impairment: The pharmacokinetics of idarubicin have not been evaluated in leukemia patients with hepatic impairment. It is expected that in patients with moderate or severe hepatic dysfunction, the metabolism of idarubicin may be impaired and lead to higher systemic drug levels. The disposition of idarubicin may be also affected by renal impairment. Therefore, a dose reduction should be considered in patients with hepatic and/or renal impairment (see DOSAGE AND ADMINISTRATION).

Drug-Drug Interactions

No formal drug interaction studies have been performed.

CLINICAL STUDIES

Four prospective randomized studies, three U.S. and one Italian, have been conducted to compare the efficacy and safety of idarubicin (IDR) to that of daunorubicin (DNR), each in combination with cytarabine as induction therapy in previously untreated adult patients with acute myeloid leukemia (AML). These data are summarized in the following table and demonstrate significantly greater complete remission rates for the IDR regimen in two of the three U.S. studies and significantly longer overall survival for the IDR regimen in two of the three U.S. studies.

[See table above]

	Induction[a] Regimen Dose in mg/m²- Daily × 3 Days		Complete Remission Rate, All Pts Randomized		Median Survival (Days) All Pts Randomized	
	IDR	DNR	IDR	DNR	IDR	DNR
U.S. (IND Studies)						
1. MSKCC* (Age ≤ 60 years)	12[b]	50[b]	51/65⁺ (78%)	38/65 (58%)	508⁺	435
2. SEG** (Age ≥ 15 years)	12[c]	45[c]	76/111⁺ (69%)	65/119 (55%)	328	277
3. U.S. Multicenter (Age ≥ 18 years)	13[c]	45[c]	68/101 (67%)	66/113 (58%)	393⁺	281
Foreign (non-IND study)						
GIMEMA*** (Age ≥ 55 years)	12[c]	45[c]	49/124 (40%)	49/125 (39%)	87	169

*Memorial Sloan Kettering Cancer Center

**Southeastern Cancer Study Group

***Gruppo Italiano Malattie Ematologiche Maligne dell' Adulto

⁺ Overall $p < 0.05$, unadjusted for prognostic factors or multiple endpoints

[a] Patients who had persistent leukemia after the first induction course received a second course

[b] Cytarabine 25 mg/m² bolus IV followed by 200 mg/m² daily × 5 days by continuous infusion

[c] Cytarabine 100 mg/m² daily × 7 days by continuous infusion

There is no consensus regarding optional regimens to be used for consolidation; however, the following consolidation regimens were used in U.S. controlled trials. Patients received the same anthracycline for consolidation as was used for induction.

Studies 1 and 3 utilized 2 courses of consolidation therapy consisting of idarubicin 12 or 13 mg/m² daily for 2 days, respectively (or DNR 50 or 45 mg/m² daily for 2 days), and cytarabine, either 25 mg/m² by IV bolus followed by 200 mg/m² daily by continuous infusion for 4 days (Study 1), or 100 mg/m² daily for 5 days by continuous infusion (Study 3). A rest period of 4 to 6 weeks is recommended prior to initiation of consolidation and between the courses. Hematologic recovery is mandatory prior to initiation of each consolidation course.

Study 2 utilized 3 consolidation courses, administered at intervals of 21 days or upon hematologic recovery. Each course consisted of idarubicin 15 mg/m² IV for 1 dose (or DNR 50 mg/m² IV for 1 dose), cytarabine 100 mg/m² every 12 hours for 10 doses and 6-thioguanine 100 mg/m² orally for 10 doses. If severe myelosuppression occurred, subsequent courses were given with 25% reduction in the doses of all drugs. In addition, this study included 4 courses of maintenance therapy (2 days of the same anthracycline as was used in induction and 5 days of cytarabine).

Toxicities and duration of aplasia were similar during induction on the 2 arms in the U.S. studies except for an increase in mucositis on the IDR arm in one study. During consolidation, duration of aplasia on the IDR arm was longer in all three studies and mucositis was more frequent in two studies. During consolidation, transfusion requirements were higher on the IDR arm in the two studies in which they were tabulated, and patients on the IDR arm in Study 3 spent more days on IV antibiotics (Study 3 used a higher dose of idarubicin).

The benefit of consolidation and maintenance therapy in prolonging the duration of remission and survival is not proven.

Intensive maintenance with idarubicin is not recommended in view of the considerable toxicity (including deaths in remission) experienced by patients during the maintenance phase of Study 2.

A higher induction death rate was noted in patients on the IDR arm in the Italian trial. Since this was not noted in patients of similar age in the U.S. trials, one may speculate that it was due to a difference in the level of supportive care.

INDICATIONS AND USAGE

IDAMYCIN PFS Injection in combination with other approved antileukemic drugs is indicated for the treatment of acute myeloid leukemia (AML) in adults. This includes French-American-British (FAB) classifications M1 through M7.

WARNINGS

Idarubicin is intended for administration under the supervision of a physician who is experienced in leukemia chemotherapy.

Idarubicin is a potent bone marrow suppressant. Idarubicin should not be given to patients with pre-existing bone marrow suppression induced by previous drug therapy or radiotherapy unless the benefit warrants the risk.

Severe myelosuppression will occur in all patients given a therapeutic dose of this agent for induction, consolidation or maintenance. Careful hematologic monitoring is required. Deaths due to infection and/or bleeding have been reported during the period of severe myelosuppression. Facilities with laboratory and supportive resources adequate to monitor drug tolerability and protect and maintain a patient compromised by drug toxicity should be available. It must be possible to treat rapidly and completely a severe hemorrhagic condition and/or a severe infection.

Pre-existing heart disease and previous therapy with anthracyclines at high cumulative doses or other potentially cardiotoxic agents are co-factors for increased risk of idarubicin-induced cardiac toxicity and the benefit to risk ratio of idarubicin therapy in such patients should be weighed before starting treatment with idarubicin.

Myocardial toxicity as manifested by potentially fatal congestive heart failure, acute life-threatening arrhythmias or other cardiomyopathies may occur following therapy with idarubicin. Appropriate therapeutic measures for the management of congestive heart failure and/or arrhythmias are indicated.

Cardiac function should be carefully monitored during treatment in order to minimize the risk of cardiac toxicity of the type described for other anthracycline compounds. The risk of such myocardial toxicity may be higher following concomitant or previous radiation to the mediastinal-pericardial area or in patients with anemia, bone marrow depression, infections, leukemic pericarditis and/or myocarditis. While there are no reliable means for predicting congestive heart failure, cardiomyopathy induced by anthracyclines is usually associated with a decrease of the left ventricular ejection fraction (LVEF) from pretreatment baseline values.

Since hepatic and/or renal function impairment can affect the disposition of idarubicin, liver and kidney function should be evaluated with conventional clinical laboratory tests (using serum bilirubin and serum creatinine as indicators) prior to and during treatment. In a number of Phase III clinical trials, treatment was not given if bilirubin and/or creatinine serum levels exceeded 2 mg%. However, in one Phase III trial, patients with bilirubin levels between 2.6 and 5 mg% received the anthracycline with a 50% reduction in dose. Dose reduction of idarubicin should be considered if the bilirubin and/or creatinine levels are above the normal range. (See DOSAGE AND ADMINISTRATION.)

Continued on next page

Idamycin PFS—Cont.

Pregnancy Category D—Idarubicin was embryotoxic and teratogenic in the rat at a dose of 1.2 mg/m^2/day or one tenth the human dose, which was nontoxic to dams. Idarubicin was embryotoxic but not teratogenic in the rabbit even at a dose of 2.4 mg/m^2/day or two tenths the human dose, which was toxic to dams. There is no conclusive information about idarubicin adversely affecting human fertility or causing teratogenesis. There has been one report of a fetal fatality after maternal exposure to idarubicin during the second trimester.

There are no adequate and well-controlled studies in pregnant women. If idarubicin is to be used during pregnancy, or if the patient becomes pregnant during therapy, the patient should be apprised of the potential hazard to the fetus. Women of childbearing potential should be advised to avoid pregnancy.

PRECAUTIONS

General

Therapy with idarubicin requires close observation of the patient and careful laboratory monitoring. Hyperuricemia secondary to rapid lysis of leukemic cells may be induced. Appropriate measures must be taken to prevent hyperuricemia and to control any systemic infection before beginning therapy.

Extravasation of idarubicin can cause severe local tissue necrosis. Extravasation may occur with or without an accompanying stinging or burning sensation even if blood returns well on aspiration of the infusion needle. If signs or symptoms of extravasation occur the injection or infusion should be terminated immediately and restarted in another vein. (See DOSAGE AND ADMINISTRATION.)

Laboratory Tests

Frequent complete blood counts and monitoring of hepatic and renal function tests are recommended.

Carcinogenesis, Mutagenesis, Impairment of Fertility

Formal long-term carcinogenicity studies have not been conducted with idarubicin. Idarubicin and related compounds have been shown to have mutagenic and carcinogenic properties when tested in experimental models (including bacterial systems, mammalian cells in culture and female Sprague-Dawley rats).

In male dogs given 1.8 mg/m^2/day 3 times/week (about one seventh the weekly human dose on a mg/m^2 basis) for 13 weeks, or 3 times the human dose, testicular atrophy was observed with inhibition of spermatogenesis and sperm maturation with few or no mature sperm. These effects were not readily reversed after a recovery of 8 weeks.

Pregnancy Category D

(See WARNINGS.)

Nursing Mothers

It is not known whether this drug is excreted in human milk. Because many drugs are excreted in human milk and because of the potential for serious adverse reactions in nursing infants from idarubicin, mothers should discontinue nursing prior to taking this drug.

Pediatric Use

Safety and effectiveness in children have not been established.

Geriatric Use

Patients over 60 years of age who were undergoing induction therapy experienced congestive heart failure, serious arrhythmias, chest pain, myocardial infarction, and asymptomatic declines in LVEF More frequently than younger patients (see ADVERSE REACTIONS).

ADVERSE REACTIONS

Approximately 550 patients with AML have received idarubicin in combination with cytarabine in controlled clinical trials worldwide. In addition, over 550 patients with acute leukemia have been treated in uncontrolled trials utilizing idarubicin as a single agent or in combination. The table below lists the adverse experiences reported in U.S. Study 2 (see CLINICAL STUDIES) and is representative of the experiences in other studies. These adverse experiences constitute all reported or observed experiences, including those not considered to be drug related. Patients undergoing induction therapy for AML are seriously ill due to their disease, are receiving multiple transfusions, and concomitant medications including potentially toxic antibiotics and antifungal agents. The contribution of the study drug to the adverse experience profile is difficult to establish.

Induction Phase	Percentage of Patients	
	IDR	DNR
Adverse Experiences	(N=110)	(N=118)
Infection	95%	97%
Nausea & Vomiting	82%	80%
Hair Loss	77%	72%
Abdominal Cramps/Diarrhea	73%	68%
Hemorrhage	63%	65%
Mucositis	50%	55%
Dermatologic	46%	40%
Mental Status	41%	34%
Pulmonary-Clinical	39%	39%
Fever (not elsewhere classified)	26%	28%
Headache	20%	24%
Cardiac-Clinical	16%	24%
Neurologic-Peripheral Nerves	7%	9%
Pulmonary Allergy	2%	4%
Seizure	4%	5%
Cerebellar	4%	4%

The duration of aplasia and incidence of mucositis were greater on the IDR arm than the DNR arm, especially during consolidation in some U.S. controlled trials (see CLINICAL STUDIES).

The following information reflects experience based on U.S. controlled clinical trials.

Myelosuppression

Severe myelosuppression is the major toxicity associated with idarubicin therapy, but this effect of the drug is required in order to eradicate the leukemic clone. During the period of myelosuppression, patients are at risk of developing infection and bleeding which may be life-threatening or fatal.

Gastrointestinal

Nausea and/or vomiting, mucositis, abdominal pain and diarrhea were reported frequently, but were severe (equivalent to WHO Grade 4) in less than 5% of patients. Severe enterocolitis with perforation has been reported rarely. The risk of perforation may be increased by instrumental intervention. The possibility of perforation should be considered in patients who develop severe abdominal pain and appropriate steps for diagnosis and management should be taken.

Dermatologic

Alopecia was reported frequently and dermatologic reactions including generalized rash, urticaria and a bullous erythrodermatous rash of the palms and soles have occurred. The dermatologic reactions were usually attributed to concomitant antibiotic therapy. Local reactions including hives at the injection site have been reported. Recall of skin reaction due to prior radiotherapy has occurred with idarubicin administration.

Hepatic and Renal

Changes in hepatic and renal function tests have been observed. These changes were usually transient and occurred in the setting of sepsis and while patients were receiving potentially hepatotoxic and nephrotoxic antibiotics and antifungal agents. Severe changes in renal function (equivalent to WHO Grade 4) occurred in no more than 1% of patients, while severe changes in hepatic function (equivalent to WHO Grade 4) occurred in less than 5% of patients.

Cardiac

Congestive heart failure (frequently attributed to fluid overload), serious arrhythmias including atrial fibrillation, chest pain, myocardial infarction and asymptomatic declines in LVEF have been reported in patients undergoing induction therapy for AML. Myocardial insufficiency and arrhythmias were usually reversible and occurred in the setting of sepsis, anemia and aggressive intravenous fluid administration. The events were reported more frequently in patients over age 60 years and in those with pre-existing cardiac disease.

OVERDOSAGE

There is no known antidote to idarubicin. Two cases of fatal overdosage in patients receiving therapy for AML have been reported. The doses were 135 mg/m^2 over 3 days and 45 mg/m^2 of idarubicin and 90 mg/m^2 of daunorubicin over a three day period.

It is anticipated that overdosage with idarubicin will result in severe and prolonged myelosuppression and possibly in increased severity of gastrointestinal toxicity. Adequate supportive care including platelet transfusions, antibiotics and symptomatic treatment of mucositis is required. The effect of acute overdose on cardiac function is not fully known, but severe arrhythmia occurred in 1 of the 2 patients exposed. It is anticipated that very high doses of idarubicin may cause acute cardiac toxicity and may be associated with a higher incidence of delayed cardiac failure.

Disposition studies with idarubicin in patients undergoing dialysis have not been carried out. The profound multicompartment behavior, extensive extravascular distribution and tissue binding, coupled with the low unbound fraction available in the plasma pool make it unlikely that therapeutic efficacy or toxicity would be altered by conventional peritoneal or hemodialysis.

DOSAGE AND ADMINISTRATION (See WARNINGS)

For induction therapy in adult patients with AML the following dose schedule is recommended:

IDAMYCIN PFS Injection 12 mg/m^2 daily for 3 days by slow (10 to 15 min) intravenous injection in combination with cytarabine. The cytarabine may be given as 100 mg/m^2 daily by continuous infusion for 7 days or as cytarabine 25 mg/m^2 intravenous bolus followed by cytarabine 200 mg/m^2 daily for 5 days continuous infusion. In patients with unequivocal evidence of leukemia after the first induction course, a second course may be administered. Administration of the second course should be delayed in patients who experience severe mucositis, until recovery from this toxicity has occurred, and a dose reduction of 25% is recommended. In patients with hepatic and/or renal impairment, a dose reduction of IDAMYCIN PFS should be considered. IDAMYCIN PFS should not be administered if the bilirubin level exceeds 5 mg%. (See WARNINGS.)

The benefit of consolidation in prolonging the duration of remissions and survival is not proven. There is no consensus regarding optional regimens to be used for consolidation. (See CLINICAL STUDIES for doses used in U.S. Clinical studies.)

Preparation and Administration Precautions

Caution in handling the solution must be exercised as skin reactions associated with IDAMYCIN PFS may occur. Skin accidentally exposed to IDAMYCIN PFS should be washed thoroughly with soap and water and if the eyes are involved, standard irrigation techniques should be used immediately. The use of goggles, gloves, and protective gowns is recommended during preparation and administration of the drug.

Care in the administration of IDAMYCIN PFS will reduce the chance of perivenous infiltration. It may also decrease the chance of local reactions such as urticaria and erythematous streaking. During intravenous administration of IDAMYCIN PFS extravasation may occur with or without an accompanying stinging or burning sensation even if blood returns well on aspiration of the infusion needle. If any signs or symptoms of extravasation have occurred, the injection or infusion should be immediately terminated and restarted in another vein. If it is known or suspected that subcutaneous extravasation has occurred, it is recommended that intermittent ice packs (1/2 hour immediately, then 1/2 hour 4 times per day for 3 days) be placed over the area of extravasation and that the affected extremity be elevated. Because of the progressive nature of extravasation reactions, the area of injection should be frequently examined and plastic surgery consultation obtained early if there is any sign of a local reaction such as pain, erythema, edema or vesication. If ulceration begins or there is severe persistent pain at the site of extravasation, early wide excision of the involved area should be considered.

IDAMYCIN PFS should be administered slowly (over 10 to 15 minutes) into the tubing of a freely running intravenous infusion of Sodium Chloride Injection, USP (0.9%) or 5% Dextrose Injection, USP. The tubing should be attached to a Butterfly needle or other suitable device and inserted preferably into a large vein.

Incompatibility

Unless specific compatibility data are available, IDAMYCIN PFS should not be mixed with other drugs. Precipitation occurs with heparin. Prolonged contact with any solution of an alkaline pH will result in degradation of the drug.

Parenteral drug products should be inspected visually for particulate matter and discoloration prior to administration whenever solution and containers permit.

Handling and Disposal—Procedures for handling and disposal of anticancer drugs should be considered. Several guidelines on this subject have been published.[1–8] There is no general agreement that all of the procedures recommended in the guidelines are necessary or appropriate.

HOW SUPPLIED

IDAMYCIN PFS Injection (idarubicin hydrochloride injection)

Single Dose Glass Vials: Sterile single use only, contains no preservative.

NDC 0013-2200-01 5 mg/5 mL vial (1 mg/mL), single vials.
NDC 0013-2201-01 10 mg/10 mL vial (1 mg/mL), single vials.
NDC 0013-2202-01 20 mg/20 mL vial (1 mg/mL), single vials.

Single Dose Cytosafe™ Vials: Sterile single use only, contains no preservative.

NDC 0013-2576-91 5 mg/5 mL vial (1 mg/mL), single vials.
NDC 0013-2586-91 10 mg/10 mL vial (1 mg/mL), single vials.
NDC 0013-2596-91 20 mg/20 mL vial (1 mg/mL), single vials.

Store under refrigeration 2° to 8°C (36° to 46°F), and protect from light. Retain in carton until time of use.

Manufactured for: Pharmacia & Upjohn Company
A subsidiary of Pharmacia Corporation
Kalamazoo, MI 49001, USA
by: Pharmacia Italia S.p.A.
Milan, Italy
(glass vials)
Pharmacia (Perth) Pty Limited
Bentley, WA 6102, Australia
(polypropylene vials)

REFERENCES

1. ONS Clinical Practice Committee. Cancer Chemotherapy Guidelines and Recommendations for Practice. Pittsburgh, PA: Oncology Nursing Society. 1999: 32-41.
2. Recommendations for the Safe Handling of Parenteral Antineoplastic Drugs. Washington, DC; Division of Safety, Clinical Center Pharmacy Department and Cancer Nursing Services, National Institutes of Health; 1992. US Department of Health and Human Services, Public Health Service Publication NIH 92-2621.
3. AMA Council on Scientific Affairs. Guidelines for Handling Parenteral Antineoplastics. JAMA. 1985; 253: 1590-1591.
4. National Study Commission on Cytotoxic Exposure - Recommendations for Handling Cytotoxic Agents. 1987. Available from Louis P. Jeffrey, Sc.D., Chairman, National Study Commission on Cytotoxic Exposure, Massachusetts College of Pharmacy and Allied Health Sciences, 179 Longwood Avenue, Boston, MA 02115.
5. Clinical Oncological Society of Australia: Guidelines and Recommendations for Safe Handling of Antineoplastic Agents. Med J Australia. 1983; 1:426-428.
6. Jones RB, Frank R, Mass T. Safe Handling of Chemotherapeutic Agents: A Report from the Mount Sinai Medical Center. CA Cancer J Clin. 1983; 33: 258-263.
7. American Society of Hospital Pharmacists. ASHP Technical Assistance Bulletin on Handling Cytotoxic and Hazardous Drugs. Am J Hosp Pharm. 1990; 47:1033-1049.

8. Controlling Occupational Exposure to Hazardous Drugs (OSHA Work-Practice Guidelines). Am J Health-Syst Pharm. 1996; 53: 1669-1685.

N. 320006368.00.4 817 166 108 Revised May 2003

LUNELLE™ Monthly Contraceptive Injection ℞

medroxyprogesterone acetate and estradiol cypionate injectable suspension

Patients should be counseled that this product does not protect against HIV infection (AIDS) and other sexually transmitted diseases.

DESCRIPTION

LUNELLE™ Monthly Contraceptive Injection contains medroxyprogesterone acetate and estradiol cypionate as its active ingredients. The chemical name for medroxyprogesterone acetate is pregn-4-ene-3,20-dione,17-(acetyloxy)-6-methyl-(6α)-. The empirical formula is $C_{24}H_{34}O_4$ and its molecular weight is 386.53. Medroxyprogesterone acetate is a white to off-white, odorless crystalline powder that is stable in air and melts between 200°C and 210°C. It is freely soluble in chloroform, soluble in acetone and dioxane, sparingly soluble in alcohol and methanol, slightly soluble in ether, and practically insoluble in water. The chemical name for estradiol cypionate is estra-1,3,5,(10)-triene-3,17-diol,(17β)-,17-cyclopentanepropanoate. Estradiol cypionate is a white to off-white crystalline powder that melts between 149°C and 153°C. It is soluble in alcohol, acetone, chloroform, and dioxane; sparingly soluble in vegetable oils; and practically insoluble in water. The empirical formula is $C_{26}H_{36}O_3$ and its molecular weight is 396.57. The structural formulas for these ingredients are represented below:

Medroxyprogesterone Acetate

Estradiol Cypionate

LUNELLE™ Monthly Contraceptive Injection is available as a 0.5 mL aqueous suspension and contains 25 mg medroxyprogesterone acetate and 5 mg estradiol cypionate. Inactive ingredients are 0.9 mg methylparaben, 14.28 mg polyethylene glycol, 0.95 mg polysorbate 80, 0.1 mg propylparaben, 4.28 mg sodium chloride, and sterile water for injection.

CLINICAL PHARMACOLOGY

LUNELLE™ Monthly Contraceptive Injection (medroxyprogesterone acetate and estradiol cypionate injectable suspension) when administered at the recommended dose to women every month inhibits the secretion of gonadotropins, which, in turn, prevents follicular maturation and ovulation. Although the primary mechanism of this action is inhibition of ovulation, other possible mechanisms of action include thickening and a reduction in volume of cervical mucus (which decrease sperm penetration) and thinning of the endometrium (which may reduce the likelihood of implantation).

Pharmacokinetics

Steady-state pharmacokinetic parameters of medroxyprogesterone acetate (MPA) and 17β-estradiol (E_2), the parent active moiety of estradiol cypionate (E_2C), following the third monthly injection of LUNELLE™ Monthly Contraceptive Injection are shown in Table 1.

[See table 1 above]

Absorption: Absorption of MPA and E_2 from the injection site is prolonged after an intramuscular injection of LUNELLE™ Monthly Contraceptive Injection. The time to maximum plasma concentration (T_{max}) typically occurs within 1 to 10 days postinjection for MPA and 1 to 7 days postinjection for E_2. The peak concentrations (C_{max}) generally range from 0.94 to 2.17 ng/mL for MPA and from 140 to 480 pg/mL for E_2. The PK profile of E_2 following administration of LUNELLE™ Monthly Contraceptive Injection is shown in Figure 1a.

[See figure 1a at top of next column]

[See figure 1b at top of next column]

Berne RM, Levy MN, 1988.

Effect of Injection Site: AUC_{0-28} for MPA values were statistically significantly higher following injection of LUNELLE™ Monthly Contraceptive Injection into the arm as compared to the anterior thigh (average increase was approximately 25%). The mean MPA C_{max} was higher but not

Table 1. Pharmacokinetic Parameters of Medroxyprogesterone Acetate (MPA) and Estradiol (17β-E_2) after the 3rd Monthly Injection of LUNELLE™ Monthly Contraceptive Injection in 14 Surgically Sterile Women

		C_{max} (ng/mL)	T_{max} (day)	AUC_{0-28} (ng•day/mL)	$AUC_{0-\infty}$ (ng•day/mL)	$t_{1/2}$ (day)
MPA	Mean	1.25	3.5	21.51	33.65	14.7
	Min	0.94	1.0	14.44	22.02	6.2
	Max	2.17	10.0	27.00	49.09	36.0
17β-E_2	Mean	0.25	2.1	2.74	2.99	8.4
	Min	0.14	1.0	1.65	1.65	2.6
	Max	0.48	7.0	3.56	3.89	20.4

C_{max} = peak serum concentration; T_{max} = time when C_{max} is observed; AUC_{0-28}= area under the concentration-time curve over 28 days; $t_{1/2}$= terminal half-life; 1 nanogram = 10^3 picogram.

Figure 1a. Mean (SD) Serum Concentration-Time Profile of 17β-Estradiol (E_2) after the 3rd Monthly IM Injection of LUNELLE™ Monthly Contraceptive Injection in 14 Surgically Sterile Females

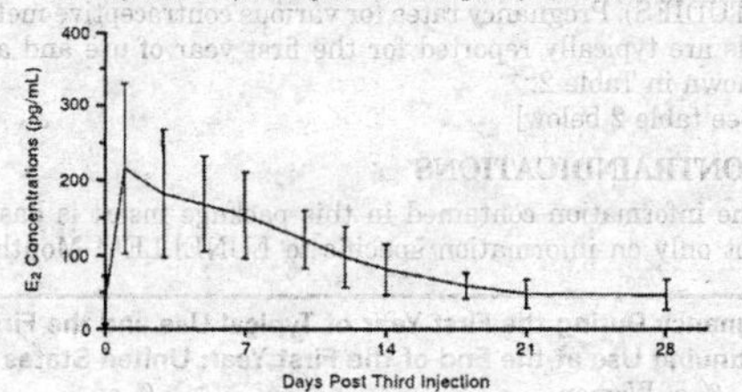

Figure 1b. Plasma E_2 Hormone Profile of the Normal Menstrual Cycle

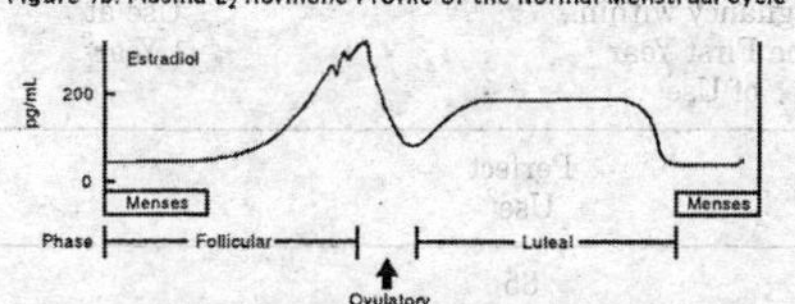

statistically significant (average increase 6 to 12%) when LUNELLE™ Monthly Contraceptive Injection was injected into the arm compared with the C_{max} observed after injection into the hip or the anterior thigh. However, the average MPA trough (C_{min}) concentrations and the half-lives were comparable for the three injection sites. E_2 concentrations were not measured.

Distribution: Plasma protein binding of MPA averages 86%. MPA binding occurs primarily to serum albumin; no binding of MPA occurs with sex-hormone-binding globulin (SHBG). Estrogens circulate in blood bound to albumin, SHBG, α1-glycoproteins, and transcortin. Estradiol is primarily bound to SHBG and albumin and approximately 3% remains unbound. Unbound estrogens are known to modulate pharmacologic response.

Metabolism: MPA is extensively metabolized. Its metabolism primarily involves ring A and/or side-chain reduction, loss of the acetyl group, hydroxylation in the 2-, 6-, and 21-positions or a combination of these positions, resulting in numerous derivatives. E_2C undergoes ester hydrolysis after intramuscular injection of LUNELLE™ Monthly Contraceptive Injection, releasing the parent, active compound E_2. Exogenously delivered or endogenously derived E_2 is primarily metabolized to estrone and estriol, both of which are metabolized to their sulfate and glucuronide forms.

Elimination: Residual MPA concentrations at the end of a monthly injection of LUNELLE™ Monthly Contraceptive Injection are generally below 0.5 ng/mL, consistent with its apparent elimination half-life of 15 days. Most MPA metabolites are excreted in the urine as glucuronide conjugates with only small amounts excreted as sulfates. Following the peak concentration, serum E_2 levels typically decline to 100 pg/mL by day 14 and are consistent with the apparent elimination half-life of 7 to 8 days. Estrogen metabolites are primarily excreted in the urine as glucuronides and sulfates.

Return of Ovulation: Return of ovulation correlated to some extent with MPA AUC_{0-84} days. Additionally, body weight and site of injection affected the AUC of MPA. AUC_{0-28} values are significantly higher when LUNELLE™ Monthly Contraceptive Injection is injected into the arm compared to the anterior thigh muscle and into women with BMI ≤28 kg/m^2 compared to those with BMI >28 kg/m^2. Consequently, return of ovulation may be delayed in women with BMI ≤28 kg/m^2 who receive an injection in the arm.

Pharmacokinetics in Subpopulations

Race: The pharmacokinetics of MPA and E_2 has been evaluated in different populations in separate studies. With the exception of one study in Thai women that demonstrated relatively higher C_{max} and shorter T_{max} values indicating more rapid absorption of both MPA and E_2, the pharmacokinetics of MPA and E_2 after the administration of LUNELLE™ Monthly Contraceptive Injection were similar in women from various ethnic backgrounds. Although pharmacokinetic differences were observed, the contraceptive efficacy was similar among all women of all ethnic backgrounds studied. Following discontinuation, ovulation returned earlier in Thai women.

Pediatric: Safety and efficacy of LUNELLE™ Monthly Contraceptive Injection have been established in women of reproductive age. Safety and efficacy are expected to be the same for postpubertal adolescents under 16 years of age and users 16 years of age and older. Use of this product before menarche is not indicated.

Geriatric: LUNELLE™ Monthly Contraceptive Injection is intended for use in healthy women desiring contraception; studies in geriatric women have not been conducted.

Effect of Body Weight: No dosage adjustment is necessary based on body weight. The effect of body weight on the pharmacokinetics of MPA was assessed in a subset of women (n = 77, body mass index ranged from 18 to 45.5 kg/m^2) enrolled in a Phase 3 trial. AUC_{0-28} values for MPA were significantly higher in thinner women with body mass index ≤28 kg/m^2 (average increase was approximately 20%) when compared to that in heavier women with body mass index > 28 kg/m^2. The mean MPA C_{max} was higher (average increase 42%) in thin/normal women with body mass index ≤28 kg/m^2 compared with heavier women with body mass index > 28 kg/m^2. The range of MPA trough (C_{min}) concentrations and the half-lives were comparable for both groups.

Hepatic Insufficiency: No formal studies have evaluated the effect of hepatic disease on the disposition of LUNELLE™ Monthly Contraceptive Injection. However, steroid hormones may be poorly metabolized in patients with impaired liver function. (See CONTRAINDICATIONS.)

Renal Insufficiency: No formal studies have evaluated the effect of renal disease on the pharmacokinetics of LUNELLE™ Monthly Contraceptive Injection. However, since both steroidal components of LUNELLE™ Monthly Contraceptive Injection are almost exclusively eliminated by hepatic metabolism, no dosage adjustment is necessary in women with renal dysfunction.

Drug-Drug Interactions

No formal drug-drug interaction studies were conducted with LUNELLE™ Monthly Contraceptive Injection. Aminoglutethimide administered concomitantly with LUNELLE™ Monthly Contraceptive Injection may significantly depress the serum concentrations of MPA. Users of LUNELLE™ Monthly Contraceptive Injection should be warned of the possibility of decreased efficacy with the use of this or any related drugs. (See PRECAUTIONS, DRUG INTERACTIONS.)

CLINICAL STUDIES

LUNELLE™ Monthly Contraceptive Injection has been studied for safety and efficacy in various comparative and introductory clinical trials around the world. One US study was performed with the goal of describing bleeding patterns in women using LUNELLE™ Monthly Contraceptive Injection compared to women using a standard oral contraceptive product. The group of LUNELLE™ Monthly Contraceptive Injection users in this study was 67.9% White, 15.5% Hispanic, 13.6% Black, 2.4% Asian, and 0.6% other.

In the clinical trials, reported 12-month pregnancy rates have been low (≤0.2%). Due to certain limitations of the available data (loss to follow-up, lack of pregnancy testing, use of barrier contraceptive products, and concomitant medications, etc.), a precise estimate of the failure rate is not possible, but is likely in the range of 0.1 to 1%.

The bleeding pattern over one year of use for LUNELLE™ Monthly Contraceptive Injection was examined in the US trial. Bleeding patterns during the last three months (months 9-12) of LUNELLE™ Monthly Contraceptive Injection use were compared with a concurrent group of standard oral contraceptive users. During this last three-month reference period, 58.6% of women using LUNELLE™ Monthly Contraceptive Injection experienced altered bleeding patterns (compared to 23.7% in the comparison group). See also WARNINGS, BLEEDING IRREGULARITIES. The one-year Life Table bleeding-related discontinuation rate for LUNELLE™ Monthly Contraceptive Injection was 6.1% for 782 participants in a US trial of up to 15 months duration. Bleeding patterns did not predict discontinuation from this large clinical trial.

Continued on next page

Lunelle—Cont.

Bleeding data from the US trial was re-analyzed based on injection intervals of 23 to 33 days. During the first injection interval, withdrawal bleeding lasted for more than 7 days in 42% of women, including 16% whose bleeding exceeded 10 days. The remaining 58% experienced bleeding for 7 days or less. Withdrawal bleeding began between days 20 and 25 (median 21) after initial injection in 48% of women using LUNELLE™ Monthly Contraceptive Injection.

At the end of one year of treatment, withdrawal bleeding lasted for more than 7 days in 29% of women, including 7% whose bleeding exceeded 10 days. The remaining 71% experienced bleeding 7 days or less in duration. Fifty percent of patients experienced withdrawal bleeding that began within 21–25 days (median 22) after their previous injection.

In any given injection interval, approximately 75% of women experienced a single withdrawal bleeding episode, without additional breakthrough bleeding or spotting, during that interval. In any given injection interval, approximately 15% of women experienced no bleeding and 10% experienced bleeding or spotting at various times in that injection interval.

In the US trial, weight gain was the most common adverse event leading to discontinuation of LUNELLE™ Monthly Contraceptive Injection (5.7% LUNELLE™ Monthly Contraceptive Injection group vs. 0.9% in the oral contraceptive comparator group). Weight change over 12 months in the LUNELLE™ Monthly Contraceptive Injection group ranged from 48 pounds lost to 49 pounds gained. Mean body weight change in the LUNELLE™ Monthly Contraceptive Injection group was a gain of 4 pounds after 13 injections and a gain of 5 pounds after 15 injections. Wide variability in individual weight gain or loss was observed; however, an increasing percentage of LUNELLE™ Monthly Contraceptive Injection users exhibited weight change in excess of 10 and 20 pounds with continued treatment. See also PRECAUTIONS, Weight Change.

INDICATIONS AND USAGE

LUNELLE™ Monthly Contraceptive Injection is indicated for the prevention of pregnancy.

The efficacy of LUNELLE™ Monthly Contraceptive Injection is dependent on adherence to the recommended dosage schedule (e.g., intramuscular injections every 28 to 30 days, not to exceed 33 days). To ensure that LUNELLE™ Monthly Contraceptive Injection is not administered inadvertently to a pregnant woman, the first injection should be given during the first 5 days of a normal menstrual period. LUNELLE™ Monthly Contraceptive Injection should be administered no earlier than 4 weeks after delivery if not breastfeeding or 6 weeks after delivery if breastfeeding (see NURSING MOTHERS).

Several clinical trials of LUNELLE™ Monthly Contraceptive Injection have reported 12-month failure rates of < 1% by Life Table analysis (see also CLINICAL STUDIES). Pregnancy rates for various contraceptive methods are typically reported for the first year of use and are shown in Table 2.

[See table 2 below]

CONTRAINDICATIONS

The information contained in this package insert is based not only on information specific to LUNELLE™ Monthly Contraceptive Injection, but also on studies carried out in women who used injectable progestin-only contraceptives (medroxyprogesterone acetate) or oral contraceptives with higher doses of both estrogens and progestogens than those in common use today. The effect of long-term use of hormonal contraceptives with formulations having lower doses of both estrogens and progestogens remains to be determined.

LUNELLE™ Monthly Contraceptive Injection should not be used in women with any of the following conditions or circumstances.

- Known or suspected pregnancy.
- Thrombophlebitis or thromboembolic disorders.
- A past history of deep-vein thrombophlebitis or thromboembolic disorders.
- Cerebral vascular or coronary artery disease.
- Undiagnosed abnormal genital bleeding.
- Liver dysfunction or disease, such as history of hepatic adenoma or carcinoma; history of cholestatic jaundice of pregnancy or jaundice with prior hormonal contraceptive use including severe pruritus of pregnancy.
- Carcinoma of the endometrium, breast, or other known or suspected estrogen-dependent neoplasia.
- Known hypersensitivity to any of the ingredients contained in LUNELLE™ Monthly Contraceptive Injection.
- Heavy smoking (≥15 cigarettes per day) and over age 35.
- Severe hypertension.
- Diabetes with vascular involvement.
- Headaches with focal neurological symptoms.
- Valvular heart disease with complications.

WARNINGS

Cigarette smoking increases the risk of serious cardiovascular side effects from contraceptives containing estrogen. This risk increases with age and with heavy smoking (15 or more cigarettes per day) and is quite marked in women over 35 years of age. Women who use LUNELLE™ Monthly Contraceptive Injection should be strongly advised not to smoke.

The use of oral contraceptives is associated with increased risks of several serious conditions including myocardial infarction, thromboembolism, stroke, hepatic neoplasia, and gallbladder disease, although the risk of serious morbidity or mortality is very small in healthy women without underlying risk factors. The risk of morbidity and mortality increases significantly in the presence of other underlying risk factors such as hypertension, hyperlipidemias, obesity, and diabetes.

Practitioners prescribing LUNELLE™ Monthly Contraceptive Injection should be familiar with the following information relating to these risks.

Throughout this labeling, epidemiological studies reported are of two types: retrospective or case control studies and prospective or cohort studies. Case control studies provide a measure of the relative risk of a disease, namely, a ratio of the incidence of a disease among oral contraceptive users to that among non-users. The relative risk does not provide information on the actual clinical occurrence of a disease. Cohort studies provide a measure of attributable risk, which is the difference in the incidence of disease between oral contraceptive users and non-users. The attributable risk does provide information about the actual occurrence of a disease in the population. For further information, the reader is referred to a text on epidemiological methods.

1. THROMBOEMBOLIC DISORDERS AND OTHER VASCULAR PROBLEMS

a. Myocardial Infarction

An increased risk of myocardial infarction has been attributed to oral contraceptive use. This risk is primarily in smokers or women with other underlying risk factors for coronary artery disease such as hypertension, hypercholesterolemia, morbid obesity, and diabetes. The relative risk of heart attack for current oral contraceptive users has been estimated to be two to six. The risk is very low in women under the age of 30.

Smoking in combination with oral contraceptive use has been shown to contribute substantially to the incidence of myocardial infarctions in women in their mid-thirties or older with smoking accounting for the majority of excess cases. Mortality rates associated with circulatory disease have been shown to increase substantially in smokers over 35 years of age and older and non-smokers over 40 years of age who use oral contraceptives (see Table 3).

[See table 3 at top of next page]

Oral contraceptives may compound the effects of well-known risk factors, such as hypertension, diabetes, hyperlipidemias, age, and obesity. In particular, some progestogens are known to decrease high density lipoproteins (HDL) cholesterol and cause glucose intolerance, while estrogens may create a state of hyperinsulinism. Oral contraceptives have been shown to increase blood pressure among users (see WARNINGS, No. 9). Similar effects on risk factors have been associated with an increased risk of heart disease. LUNELLE™ Monthly Contraceptive Injection must be used with caution in women with cardiovascular disease risk factors.

b. Thromboembolism

An increased risk of thromboembolic and thrombotic diseases associated with the use of oral contraceptives is well established. Case control studies have found the relative risk of users compared with non-users to be 3 for the first

Table 2. Percentage of Women Experiencing an Unintended Pregnancy During the First Year of Typical Use and the First Year of Perfect Use of Contraception and the Percentage Continuing Use at the End of the First Year: United States

Method	% of Women Experiencing an Unintended Pregnancy within the First Year of Use: Typical Use[1]	Perfect Use[2]	% of Women Continuing Use at 1 Year[3]
Chance[4]	85	85	
Spermicides[5]	26	6	40
Periodic Abstinence	25		63
Calendar		9	
Ovulation Method		3	
Symptothermal[6]		2	
Post-ovulation		1	
Cap[7]			
Parous Women	40	26	42
Nulliparous Women	20	9	56
Sponge			
Parous Women	40	20	42
Nulliparous Women	20	9	56
Diaphragm[7]	20	6	56
Withdrawal	19	4	
Condom[8]			
Female (Reality)	21	5	56
Male	14	3	61
Pill	5		71
Progestin only		0.5	
Combined		0.1	
IUD			
Progesterone T	2.0	1.5	81
Copper T 380A	0.8	0.6	78
LNg 20	0.1	0.1	81
Depo-Provera	0.3	0.3	70
Norplant and Norplant-2	0.05	0.05	88
Female Sterilization	0.5	0.5	100
Male Sterilization	0.15	0.10	100

Emergency Contraceptive Pills: Treatment initiated within 72 hours after unprotected intercourse reduces the risk of pregnancy by at least 75%.[9]

Lactational Amenorrhea Method: LAM is a highly effective, temporary method of contraception.[10]

Adapted from Hatcher et al., 1998.

[1] Among typical couples who initiate use of a method (not necessarily for the first time), the percentage who experience an accidental pregnancy during the first year if they do not stop use for any other reason.

[2] Among couples who initiate use of a method (not necessarily for the first time) and who use it perfectly (both consistently and correctly), the percentage who experience an accidental pregnancy during the first year if they do not stop use for any other reason.

[3] Among couples attempting to avoid pregnancy, the percentage who continue to use a method for 1 year.

[4] The percentages becoming pregnant in columns (2) and (3) are based on data from populations where contraception is not used and from women who cease using contraception in order to become pregnant. Among such populations, about 89% become pregnant within 1 year. This estimate was lowered slightly (to 85%) to represent the percentages who would become pregnant within 1 year among women now relying on reversible methods of contraception if they abandoned contraception altogether.

[5] Foams, creams, gels, vaginal suppositories, and vaginal film.

[6] Cervical mucus (ovulation) method supplemented by calendar in the pre-ovulatory and basal body temperature in the post-ovulatory phases.

[7] With spermicidal cream or jelly.

[8] Without spermicides.

[9] The treatment schedule is one dose within 72 hours after unprotected intercourse, and a second dose 12 hours after the first dose. The Food and Drug Administration has declared the following brands of oral contraceptives to be safe and effective for emergency contraception: Ovral (1 dose is 2 white pills), Alesse (1 dose is 5 pink pills), Nordette or Levlen (1 dose is 4 light-orange pills), Lo/Ovral (1 dose is 4 white pills), Triphasil or Tri-Levlen (1 dose is 4 yellow pills).

[10] However, to maintain effective protection against pregnancy, another method of contraception must be used as soon as menstruation resumes, the frequency or duration of breastfeeds is reduced, bottle feeds are introduced, or the baby reaches 6 months of age.

episode of superficial venous thrombosis, 4 to 11 for deep vein thrombosis or pulmonary embolism, and 1.5 to 6 for women with predisposing conditions for venous thromboembolic disease. Cohort studies have shown the relative risk to be somewhat lower, about 3 for new cases and about 4.5 for new cases requiring hospitalization. The risk of thromboembolic disease due to oral contraceptives is not related to length of use and disappears after pill use is stopped.

A two- to four-fold increase in relative risk of post-operative thromboembolic complications has been reported with the use of oral contraceptives. The relative risk of venous thrombosis in women who have predisposing conditions is twice that of women without such medical conditions. If feasible, oral contraceptives should be discontinued at least 4 weeks prior to and for 2 weeks after elective surgery of a type associated with an increase in risk of thromboembolism and during and following prolonged immobilization. Since the immediate postpartum period is also associated with an increased risk of thromboembolism, oral contraceptives and other combined hormonal contraceptives such as LUNELLE™ Monthly Contraceptive Injection, should be started no earlier than 4 weeks after delivery.

The clinician should be alert to the earliest manifestations of thrombotic disorders (thrombophlebitis, pulmonary embolism, cerebrovascular disorders, and retinal thrombosis). Should any of these occur or be suspected, LUNELLE™ Monthly Contraceptive Injection should not be readministered.

c. Cerebrovascular Disease

Oral contraceptives have been shown to increase both the relative and attributable risks of cerebrovascular events (thrombotic and hemorrhagic strokes), although, in general, the risk is greatest among older (> 35 years), hypertensive women who also smoke. Hypertension was found to be a risk factor for both users and non-users, for both types of strokes, while smoking interacted to increase the risk for hemorrhagic stroke.

The relative risk of thrombotic strokes has been shown to range from 3 for normotensive users to 14 for users with severe hypertension. The relative risk of hemorrhagic stroke is reported to be 1.2 for non-smokers who used oral contraceptives, 2.6 for smokers who did not use oral contraceptives, 7.6 for smokers who used oral contraceptives, 1.8 for normotensive users, and 25.7 for users with severe hypertension. The attributable risk is also greater in older women.

d. Dose-related Risk of Vascular Disease

A positive association has been observed between the amount of estrogen and progestogen in oral contraceptives and the risk of vascular disease. A decline in serum HDL has been reported with many progestational agents. A decline in serum HDL has been associated with an increased incidence of ischemic heart disease. Because estrogens increase HDL cholesterol, the net effect of an oral contraceptive depends on a balance achieved between doses of estrogen and progestogen and the type of progestogens used in the contraceptives. The activity and amount of both hormones should be considered in the choice of a hormonal contraceptive.

e. Persistence of Risk of Vascular Disease

There are two studies which have shown persistence of risk of vascular disease for ever-users of oral contraceptives. In a study in the United States, the risk of developing myocardial infarction after discontinuing oral contraceptives persists for at least 9 years for women 40-49 years who had used oral contraceptives for five or more years, but this increased risk was not demonstrated in other age groups. In another study in Great Britain, the risk of developing cerebrovascular disease persisted for at least 6 years after discontinuation of oral contraceptives, although excess risk was very small. However, both studies were performed with oral contraceptive formulations containing 50 micrograms or more of estrogen.

2. ESTIMATES OF MORTALITY FROM CONTRACEPTIVE USE

One study gathered data from a variety of sources that have estimated the mortality rate associated with different methods of contraception at different ages (see Table 4). These estimates include the combined risk of death associated with contraceptive methods plus the risk attributable to pregnancy in the event of method failure. Each method of contraception has its specific benefits and risks. The study concluded that with the exception of oral contraceptive users 35 years and older who smoke, and oral contraceptive users 40 years and older who do not smoke, mortality associated with all methods of birth control is low and below that associated with childbirth.

The observation of a possible increase in risk of mortality with age for oral contraceptive users is based on data gathered in the 1970s, but not reported until 1983. However, current clinical practice involves the use of lower estrogen-dose formulations combined with careful restriction of oral contraceptive use to women who do not have the various risk factors listed in this labeling.

Because of these changes in practice and because of some limited new data that suggest the risk of cardiovascular disease with the use of oral contraceptives may now be less than previously observed, the Fertility and Maternal Health Drugs Advisory Committee was asked to review the topic in 1989. The Committee concluded that although cardiovascular disease risk may be increased with oral contraceptive use after age 40 in healthy non-smoking women (even with the newer low-dose formulations), there are also greater potential health risks associated with pregnancy in

Table 3. Circulatory Disease Mortality Rates per 100,000 Women Years by Age, Smoking Status and Oral Contraceptive Use

Age (y)	Ever-Users Non-smokers	Ever-Users Smokers	Controls Non-smokers	Controls Smokers
15-24	0.0	10.5	0.0	0.0
25-34	4.4	14.2	2.7	4.2
35-44	21.5	63.4	6.4	15.2
45+	52.4	206.7	11.4	27.9

Adapted from Layde PM, Beral V., 1981.

Table 4. Annual Number of Birth-Related or Method-Related Deaths Associated with Control of Fertility per 100,000 Non-sterile Women, by Fertility Control Method According to Age

Method of Control & Outcome	Range of Ages (years)					
	15-19	20-24	25-29	30-34	35-39	40-44
No fertility control*	7.0	7.4	9.1	14.8	25.7	28.2
Oral hormonal contraceptives** (non-smoker)	0.3	0.5	0.9	1.9	13.8	31.6
Oral hormonal contraceptives** (smoker)	2.2	3.4	6.6	13.5	51.1	117.2
IUD**	0.8	0.8	1.0	1.0	1.4	1.4
Condom*	1.1	1.6	0.7	0.2	0.3	0.4
Diaphragm/spermicide*	1.9	1.2	1.2	1.3	2.2	2.8
Periodic abstinence	2.5	1.6	1.6	1.7	2.9	3.6

Adapted from Ory HW. 1983.
* Deaths are birth-related
** Deaths are method-related

older women and with the alternative surgical and medical procedures that may be necessary if such women do not have access to effective and acceptable means of contraception. Therefore, the Committee recommended that the benefits of oral contraceptive use by healthy non-smoking women over age 40 may outweigh the possible risks. Women of all ages who take oral contraceptives should take a product which contains the lowest amount of estrogen and progestogen that is effective.

[See table 4 above]

3. CARCINOMA OF THE REPRODUCTIVE ORGANS AND BREASTS

Numerous epidemiological studies have been performed on the incidence of breast, endometrial, ovarian, and cervical cancer in women using oral contraceptives. Although the risk of breast cancer may be slightly increased among current and recent users of combined oral contraceptives, this excess risk decreases over time after product discontinuation, and by 10 years after cessation the increased risk disappears. In addition, breast cancers diagnosed in current or ever-oral contraceptive users tend to be less invasive than in non-users.

The risk of breast cancer does not increase with duration of use, and no relationships have been found with dose or type of steroid. The patterns of risk are also similar regardless of a woman's reproductive history or her family breast cancer history. The sub-group for whom risk has been found to be significantly elevated is women who first used combined oral contraceptives before age 20, but because breast cancer is so rare at these young ages, the number of cases attributable to this early combined oral contraceptive use is extremely small.

Women who currently have or have had breast cancer should not use combined hormonal contraceptives because breast cancer is a hormonally sensitive tumor.

Long-term case-controlled surveillance of users of depot medroxyprogesterone acetate (DMPA) found slight or no increased overall risk of breast cancer. A pooled analysis from two case-control studies, the World Health Organization (WHO) Study and the New Zealand Study, reported the relative risk of breast cancer for women who had ever used DMPA as 1.1. Overall, there was no increase in risk with increasing duration of use of DMPA. The relative risk of breast cancer for women of all ages who had initiated use of DMPA within the previous 5 years was estimated to be 2.0. The WHO Study, a component of the pooled analysis described above, showed an increased relative risk of 2.19 of breast cancer associated with use of DMPA in women whose first exposure to drug was within the previous 4 years and who were under 35 years of age. However, the overall relative risk for ever-users of DMPA was only 1.2.

Some studies suggest that oral contraceptive use has been associated with an increase in the risk of cervical intraepithelial neoplasia in some populations of women. However, there continues to be controversy about the extent to which such findings may be due to differences in sexual behavior and other factors.

A statistically insignificant increase in relative risk estimates of invasive squamous-cell cervical cancer has been associated with the use of DMPA in women who were first exposed before the age of 35 years. The overall, non-significant relative rate of invasive squamous-cell cervical cancer in women who ever used DMPA was estimated to be 1.11. No trends in risk with duration of use or times since initial or most recent exposure were observed.

In spite of many studies of the relationship between oral contraceptive use and breast and cervical cancers, a cause and effect relationship has not been established. No long-term studies have been conducted with LUNELLE™ Monthly Contraceptive Injection to evaluate risk for carcinoma of the reproductive organs.

4. HEPATIC NEOPLASIA

Benign hepatic adenomas are associated with oral contraceptive use, although the incidence of benign tumors is rare in the United States. Indirect calculations have estimated the attributable risk to be in the range of 3.3 cases per 100,000 cases for users, a risk that increases after 4 or more years of use. Rupture of benign, hepatic adenomas may cause death through intra-abdominal hemorrhage.

Studies from Britain have shown an increased risk of developing hepatocellular carcinoma in long-term (> 8 years) oral contraceptive users. However, these cancers are extremely rare in the United States and the attributable risk (the excess incidence) of liver cancers in oral contraceptive users approaches less than one per million users.

5. OCULAR LESIONS

There have been clinical case reports of retinal thrombosis associated with the use of oral contraceptives. LUNELLE™ Monthly Contraceptive Injection should be discontinued if there is unexplained partial or complete loss of vision, onset of proptosis or diplopia, papilledema, or retinal vascular lesions. Appropriate diagnostic and therapeutic measures should be undertaken immediately.

6. HORMONAL CONTRACEPTIVE USE BEFORE OR DURING PREGNANCY

The use of hormonal contraceptives during pregnancy is not indicated.

Extensive epidemiological studies have revealed no increased risk of birth defects in women who have used oral contraceptives prior to pregnancy. Studies also do not suggest a teratogenic effect, particularly in so far as cardiac anomalies and limb reduction defects are concerned, when oral contraceptives are taken inadvertently during early pregnancy.

Pregnancies occurring in women receiving injectable progestin-only contraceptives are uncommon. Neonates from unexpected pregnancies that occurred 1 to 2 months after injection of DMPA may be at an increased risk of low birth weight, which, in turn, is associated with an increased risk of neonatal death. A significant increase in incidence of polysyndactyly and chromosomal anomalies was observed among infants of users of DMPA, the former being most pronounced in women under 30 years of age. The unrelated nature of these defects, the lack of confirmation from other studies, the distant preconceptual exposure to DMPA, and the chance effects due to multiple statistical comparisons, make a causal association unlikely.

Continued on next page

Lunelle—Cont.

Neonates exposed to MPA in utero and followed to adolescence, showed no evidence of any adverse effects on their health including their physical, intellectual, sexual or social development.
Several reports suggest an association between intrauterine exposure to progestational drugs in the first trimester of pregnancy and genital abnormalities in male and female fetuses. The risk of hypospadias (five to eight per 1,000 male births in the general population) may be approximately doubled with exposure to these drugs. There are insufficient data to quantify the risk to exposed female fetuses, but because some of these drugs induce mild virilization of the external genitalia of the female fetus and because of the increased association of hypospadias in the male fetus, these drugs should be avoided during pregnancy.
Unexpected pregnancies occurring in women receiving LUNELLE™ Monthly Contraceptive Injection are uncommon and have not shown congenital malformations or other adverse events.
The administration of combined hormonal contraceptives, such as LUNELLE™ Monthly Contraceptive Injection, to induce withdrawal bleeding should not be used as a test for pregnancy. LUNELLE™ Monthly Contraceptive Injection should not be used during pregnancy to treat threatened or habitual abortion. It is recommended that for any patient who has missed two consecutive periods, pregnancy should be considered before initiating or continuing LUNELLE™ Monthly Contraceptive Injection. If the patient has exceeded the prescribed injection interval (> 33 days) for LUNELLE™ Monthly Contraceptive Injection, the possibility of pregnancy should be ruled out before another injection is administered.

7. GALLBLADDER DISEASE
Combined hormonal contraceptives may worsen existing gallbladder disease and may accelerate the development of this disease in previously asymptomatic women. Women with a history of combined hormonal contraceptive-related cholestasis are more likely to have the condition recur with subsequent combined hormonal contraceptive use.
In a study of 782 women taking LUNELLE™ Monthly Contraceptive Injection for up to 15 cycles, cholecystitis and cholelithiasis were the only serious adverse events judged to be possibly related to the study drug. They were reported as an adverse event in five subjects, and three subjects required cholecystectomy.

8. CARBOHYDRATE AND LIPID METABOLIC EFFECTS
Combined hormonal or progestin-only contraceptives have been shown to cause glucose intolerance in some users. However, in the non-diabetic woman, combined hormonal contraceptives appear to have no effect on fasting blood glucose. Pre-diabetic and diabetic patients should be carefully observed while receiving therapy with LUNELLE™ Monthly Contraceptive Injection.
A small proportion of women may have persistent hypertriglyceridemia while using oral contraceptives. Changes in serum triglycerides and lipoprotein levels have been reported in oral contraceptive users.

9. ELEVATED BLOOD PRESSURE
An increase in blood pressure has been reported in women taking oral contraceptives and this increase is more likely in older oral contraceptive users and with continued use. Data from the Royal College of General Practitioners and subsequent randomized trials have shown that the incidence of hypertension increases with increasing concentrations of progestogens. In a US clinical study, no increase in mean blood pressure was observed over 15 months use of LUNELLE™ Monthly Contraceptive Injection.
Women with a history of hypertension or hypertension-related diseases, or renal disease should be encouraged to use another method of contraception. If women elect to use combined hormonal contraceptives such as LUNELLE™ Monthly Contraceptive Injection, they should be monitored closely and if significant elevation of blood pressure occurs, LUNELLE™ Monthly Contraceptive Injection should be discontinued. For most women, elevated blood pressure will return to normal after stopping oral contraceptives, and there is no difference in the occurrence of hypertension among former and never-users.

10. HEADACHE
The onset or exacerbation of migraine or development of headache with a new pattern which is recurrent, persistent, or severe requires evaluation of the cause before further injections of LUNELLE™ Monthly Contraceptive Injection are given.

11. BLEEDING IRREGULARITIES
Most women using LUNELLE™ Monthly Contraceptive Injection (58.6%) experienced alteration of menstrual bleeding patterns, including 4.1% amenorrhea, after one year of use. Altered bleeding patterns include frequent bleeding, irregular bleeding, prolonged bleeding, infrequent bleeding, and amenorrhea. As women continued using LUNELLE™ Monthly Contraceptive Injection, the percent experiencing frequent or prolonged bleeding decreased, while the percent experiencing amenorrhea increased. The percent of women experiencing irregular bleeding remained fairly constant at approximately 30% throughout the first year of use.
Regardless of the bleeding pattern, subsequent injections should be given 1 month (28 to 30 days, not to exceed 33 days) after the previous injection, unless discontinuation is medically indicated.
If abnormal bleeding associated with LUNELLE™ Monthly Contraceptive Injection persists or is severe, appropriate investigation should be instituted to rule out the possibility of organic pathology, and appropriate treatment should be instituted when necessary. In the event of amenorrhea, pregnancy should be ruled out.

12. BONE MINERAL DENSITY CHANGES
Use of injectable progestogen-only methods may be considered among the risk factors for development of osteoporosis. The rate of bone loss is greatest in the early years of use and then subsequently approaches the normal rate of age-related fall. Formal studies on the effect of bone mineral density changes in women receiving LUNELLE™ Monthly Contraceptive Injection have not been conducted.

13. ANAPHYLAXIS AND ANAPHYLACTOID REACTION
Anaphylaxis and anaphylactoid reactions have been reported with the components of LUNELLE™ Monthly Contraceptive Injection. Allergic reactions occurring in women using LUNELLE™ Monthly Contraceptive Injection have been mainly dermatologic, not respiratory, in nature. If an anaphylactic reaction occurs, appropriate therapy should be instituted. Serious anaphylactic reactions require emergency medical treatment.

PRECAUTIONS

1. **General. Patients should be counseled that this product does not protect against HIV infection (AIDS) and other sexually transmitted diseases.**
2. **Physical Examination.** It is good medical practice for all women to have an annual history and physical examination, including women using combined hormonal contraceptives. The physical examination should include special reference to blood pressure, breasts, abdomen and pelvic organs, including cervical cytology, and relevant laboratory tests. In case of undiagnosed, persistent, or recurrent abnormal vaginal bleeding, appropriate measures should be conducted to rule out malignancy. Women with a strong family history of breast cancer or who have breast nodules should be monitored with particular care.
3. **Weight Change.** In a study of 782 women using LUNELLE™ Monthly Contraceptive Injection for up to 15 cycles, 5.7% of participants discontinued due to weight gain. Weight gain was the most common adverse event leading to discontinuation of the drug. Women gained an average of 4 pounds during the first year, and an additional 2 pounds during the second year, of LUNELLE™ Monthly Contraceptive Injection use. The range of weight change during the first year of LUNELLE™ Monthly Contraceptive Injection use was 48 pounds lost to 49 pounds gained. The following table shows the range of weight changes seen for women continuing use up to 24 cycles.

Weight Change	12 Cycles (n=469)	15 Cycles (n=433)	24 Cycles (n=111)
Lost >20 pounds	1%	2%	5%
Lost >10 to 20 pounds	6%	6%	7%
Gained >10 to 20 pounds	19%	24%	14%
Gained >20 pounds	5%	7%	23%

4. **Lipid Disorders.** Women who are being treated for hyperlipidemias should be followed closely if they use combined hormonal contraceptives. Some progestogens may elevate LDL levels and may render the control of hyperlipidemias more difficult.
5. **Liver Function.** If jaundice develops in any woman receiving combined hormonal contraceptives, the medication should be discontinued. Steroid hormones may be poorly metabolized in patients with impaired liver function.
6. **Fluid Retention.** Progestogens and/or estrogens may cause some degree of fluid retention; therefore, caution should be used in treating any patient with a pre-existing medical condition that might be adversely affected by fluid retention.
7. **Contact Lenses.** Contact lens wearers who develop visual changes or changes in lens tolerance should be assessed by an ophthalmologist.
8. **Emotional Disorders.** Patients becoming significantly depressed while taking combined hormonal contraceptives should stop the medication and use an alternative method of contraception in an attempt to determine whether the symptom is drug-related. Women with a history of depression should be carefully observed and consideration should be given to the discontinuation of LUNELLE™ Monthly Contraceptive Injection if depression recurs to a serious degree.

DRUG INTERACTIONS

1. Effects of Other Drugs on MPA
Aminoglutethamide may decrease the serum concentration of MPA. Users of LUNELLE™ Monthly Contraceptive Injection should be informed of the possibility of decreased effectiveness with the use of this or any related drug. (See CLINICAL PHARMACOLOGY, Drug-Drug Interactions.)

2. Effects of Other Drugs on Combined Hormonal Contraceptives
Rifampin. Metabolism of some synthetic estrogens (e.g., ethinyl estradiol) and progestins (e.g., norethindrone) is increased by rifampin. A reduction in contraceptive effectiveness and an increase in menstrual irregularities have been associated with concomitant use of rifampin.
Anticonvulsants. Anticonvulsants such as phenobarbital, phenytoin, and carbamazepine have been shown to increase the metabolism of some synthetic estrogens and progestins, which could result in a reduction of contraceptive effectiveness.
Antibiotics. Pregnancy while taking oral contraceptives has been reported when the oral contraceptives were administered with antimicrobials such as ampicillin, tetracycline, and griseofulvin. However, clinical pharmacokinetic studies have not demonstrated any consistent effects of antibiotics (other than rifampin) on plasma concentrations of synthetic steroids.
Herbal products. Herbal products containing St. John's Wort (hypericum perforatum) may induce hepatic enzymes (cytochrome P450) and p-glycoprotein transporter and may reduce the effectiveness of contraceptive steroids. This may also result in breakthrough bleeding.
Other. Ascorbic acid and acetominophen may increase plasma concentrations of some synthetic estrogens, possibly by inhibition of conjugation. A reduction in contraceptive effectiveness and an increased incidence of menstrual irregularities has been suggested with phenylbutazone.

3. Effects of Combined Hormonal Contraceptives on Other Drugs
Combined hormonal contraceptives containing some synthetic estrogens (e.g., ethinyl estradiol) may inhibit the metabolism of other compounds. Increased plasma concentrations of cyclosporine, prednisolone and theophylline have been reported with concomitant administration of oral contraceptives. In addition, oral contraceptives may induce the conjugation of other compounds. Decreased plasma concentrations of acetominophen and increased clearance of temazepam, salicylic acid, morphine and clofibric acid have been noted when these drugs were administered with oral contraceptives.

4. Drug Interactions with Laboratory Tests
Certain endocrine and liver function tests and blood components may be affected by combined hormonal contraceptives:

a. Increased prothrombin and factors VII, VIII, IX, and X; decreased antithrombin 3; increased norepinephrine-induced platelet aggregability.
b. Increased thyroid binding globulin (TBG) leading to increased circulating total thyroid hormone, as measured by protein-bound iodine (PBI). T4 by column or by radioimmunoassay. Free T3 resin uptake is decreased, reflecting the elevated TBG, free T4 concentration is unaltered.
c. Other binding proteins may be elevated in serum.
d. Sex-hormone-binding-globulins are increased and result in elevated levels of total circulating sex steroids and corticoids: however, free or biologically active levels remain unchanged.
e. Triglycerides may be increased.
f. Glucose tolerance may be decreased.
g. Serum folate levels may be depressed by combined hormonal contraceptive therapy. This may be of clinical significance if a woman becomes pregnant shortly after discontinuing combined hormonal contraceptives.

The pathologist should be advised of progestogen and estrogen therapy when relevant tissue specimens are submitted. The following laboratory tests may be affected by progestins including LUNELLE™ Monthly Contraceptive Injection:

a. Plasma and urinary steroid levels are decreased (e.g., progesterone, estradiol, pregnanediol, testosterone, cortisol).
b. Gonadotropin levels are decreased.
c. Sex-hormone-binding-globulin concentrations are decreased.
d. Sulfobromophthalein and other liver function test values may be increased.

CARCINOGENESIS, MUTAGENESIS, IMPAIRMENT OF FERTILITY
See WARNINGS section.

PREGNANCY
Pregnancy Category X. See CONTRAINDICATIONS and WARNINGS.

Return of Ovulation and Fertility
Ovulation (signaled by a rise in serum progesterone concentrations ≥4.7 ng/mL) was observed 63 to 112 days after the third monthly injection of LUNELLE™ Monthly Contraceptive Injection in 11 of 14 women participating in a pharmacodynamic study. The remaining three women had not ovulated by day 85 and were lost to follow-up.
In a study of 21 women who received LUNELLE™ Monthly Contraceptive Injection for 3 months, 52% ovulated during the first post-treatment month, and 71% during the second post-treatment month. In another study of 10 women receiving long term administration (2 years of treatment) of LUNELLE™ Monthly Contraceptive Injection, 60% ovulated by the third post-treatment month.
A study of 70 women who discontinued LUNELLE™ Monthly Contraceptive Injection to become pregnant demonstrated that more than 50% achieved fertility within 6 months after discontinuation, and 83% did so by 1 year.

NURSING MOTHERS
The effects of LUNELLE™ Monthly Contraceptive Injection in nursing mothers have not been evaluated and are unknown. However, estrogen administration to nursing mothers has been shown to decrease the quantity and quality of breast milk. Small amounts of combined hormonal contraceptive steroids have been identified in the milk of nursing

mothers and a few adverse effects on the child have been reported, including jaundice and breast enlargement. Long-term follow-up of children whose mothers used combined hormonal contraceptives while breastfeeding has shown no deleterious effects. However, women who are breastfeeding should not start taking combined hormonal contraceptives until six weeks postpartum.

PEDIATRIC USE

Safety and efficacy of LUNELLE™ Monthly Contraceptive Injection have been established in women of reproductive age. Safety and efficacy are expected to be the same for post-pubertal adolescents under 16 years of age and users 16 years of age and older. Use of this product before menarche is not indicated.

INFORMATION FOR PATIENTS

Patients should be given a copy of the patient labeling prior to administration of LUNELLE™ Monthly Contraceptive Injection.

Patients should be advised that the contraceptive efficacy of LUNELLE™ Monthly Contraceptive Injection depends on receiving injections monthly (28 to 30 days, not to exceed 33 days). The injection schedule must be measured by the number of days, not by bleeding episodes. It is recommended that for any patient who has missed two consecutive menstrual periods, pregnancy should be considered before initiating or continuing LUNELLE™ Monthly Contraceptive Injection. Thereafter, a woman who has continued amenorrhea while using LUNELLE™ Monthly Contraceptive Injection and who has received her injections according to the recommended dosing schedule may continue to receive subsequent injections each month after the previous injection (not to exceed 33 days), unless discontinuation is medically indicated. All patients presenting for a follow-up injection of LUNELLE™ Monthly Contraceptive Injection after day 33 should use a barrier method of contraception and should not receive another injection of LUNELLE™ Monthly Contraceptive Injection until pregnancy has been ruled out.

Patients should be advised that menstrual bleeding patterns are likely to be disrupted with use of LUNELLE™ Monthly Contraceptive Injection. A few patients may experience amenorrhea. Irregular bleeding that occurs after a regular bleeding pattern has emerged should be investigated. In the presence of excessive or prolonged bleeding, other causes should be investigated and consideration should be given to alternative methods of contraception.

Patients should be counseled that this product does not protect against HIV infection (AIDS) and other sexually transmitted diseases.

ADVERSE REACTIONS

An increased risk of the following serious adverse reactions has been associated with the use of combined hormonal contraceptives (see CONTRAINDICATIONS and WARNINGS).

- Arterial thromboembolism
- Cerebral hemorrhage
- Cerebral thrombosis
- Gallbladder disease
- Hepatic adenomas or benign liver tumors
- Hypertension
- Myocardial infarction
- Pulmonary embolism
- Thrombophlebitis

The following adverse reactions have been reported in patients receiving LUNELLE™ Monthly Contraceptive Injection and are believed to be drug-related:

- Abdominal pain
- Acne
- Alopecia
- Amenorrhea
- Asthenia
- Breast tenderness/pain
- Decreased libido
- Depression
- Dizziness
- Dysmenorrhea
- Emotional lability
- Enlarged abdomen
- Headache
- Menorrhagia
- Metrorrhagia
- Nausea
- Nervousness
- Vaginal moniliasis
- Vulvovaginal disorder
- Weight gain

There is evidence of an association between the following conditions and the use of combined hormonal contraceptives, although additional confirmatory studies are needed:

- Mesenteric thrombosis
- Retinal thrombosis

The following additional adverse reactions have been reported in users of combined hormonal contraceptives, and are believed to be drug-related:

- Anaphylactic reactions
- Breast changes: enlargement, secretion
- Cervical changes
- Cholestatic jaundice
- Corneal curvature changes (i.e., steepening)
- Diminution in lactation when given immediately postpartum
- Edema
- Intolerance to contact lenses
- Melasma that may persist
- Migraine
- Rash (allergic)
- Reduced carbohydrate tolerance

Percentage of Women Experiencing an Unintended Pregnancy During the First Year of Typical Use and the First Year of Perfect Use of Contraception and the Percentage Continuing Use at the End of the First Year: United States

Method	% of Women Experiencing an Unintended Pregnancy within the First Year of Use: Typical Use[1]	Perfect Use[2]	% of Women Continuing Use at 1 Year[3]
Chance[4]	85	85	
Spermicides[5]	26	6	40
Periodic Abstinence	25		63
Calendar		9	
Ovulation Method		3	
Symptothermal[6]		2	
Post-ovulation		1	
Cap[7]			
Parous Women	40	26	42
Nulliparous Women	20	9	56
Sponge			
Parous Women	40	20	42
Nulliparous Women	20	9	56
Diaphragm[7]	20	6	56
Withdrawal	19	4	
Condom[8]			
Female (Reality)	21	5	56
Male	14	3	61
Pill	5		71
Progestin only		0.5	
Combined		0.1	
IUD			
Progesterone T	2.0	1.5	81
Copper T 380A	0.8	0.6	78
LNg 20	0.1	0.1	81
Depo-Provera	0.3	0.3	70
Norplant and Norplant-2	0.05	0.05	88
Female Sterilization	0.5	0.5	100
Male Sterilization	0.15	0.10	100

Emergency Contraceptive Pills: Treatment initiated within 72 hours after unprotected intercourse reduces the risk of pregnancy by at least 75%.[9]

Lactational Amenorrhea Method: LAM is a highly effective, temporary method of contraception.[10]

Adapted from Hatcher et al., 1998.

[1] Among *typical* couples who initiate use of a method (not necessarily for the first time), the percentage who experience an accidental pregnancy during the first year if they do not stop use for any other reason.

[2] Among couples who initiate use of a method (not necessarily for the first time) and who use it *perfectly* (both consistently and correctly), the percentage who experience an accidental pregnancy during the first year if they do not stop use for any other reason.

[3] Among couples attempting to avoid pregnancy, the percentage who continue to use a method for 1 year.

[4] The percentages becoming pregnant in columns (2) and (3) are based on data from populations where contraception is not used and from women who cease using contraception in order to become pregnant. Among such populations, about 89% become pregnant within 1 year. This estimate was lowered slightly (to 85%) to represent the percentages who would become pregnant within 1 year among women now relying on reversible methods of contraception if they abandoned contraception altogether.

[5] Foams, creams, gels, vaginal suppositories, and vaginal film.

[6] Cervical mucus (ovulation) method supplemented by calendar in the pre-ovulatory and basal body temperature in the post-ovulatory phases.

[7] With spermicidal cream or jelly.

[8] Without spermicides.

[9] The treatment schedule is one dose within 72 hours after unprotected intercourse, and a second dose 12 hours after the first dose. The Food and Drug Administration has declared the following brands of oral contraceptives to be safe and effective for emergency contraception: Ovral (1 dose is 2 white pills), Alesse (1 dose is 5 pink pills), Nordette or Levlen (1 dose is 4 light-orange pills), Lo/Ovral (1 dose is 4 white pills), Triphasil or Tri-Levlen (1 dose is 4 yellow pills).

[10] However, to maintain effective protection against pregnancy, another method of contraception must be used as soon as menstruation resumes, the frequency or duration of breastfeeds is reduced, bottle feeds are introduced, or the baby reaches 6 months of age.

- Temporary infertility after treatment discontinuation
- Weight decrease

The following additional adverse reactions have been reported in users of combined hormonal contraceptives, and the association has been neither confirmed nor refuted:

- Budd-Chiari syndrome
- Cataracts
- Changes in appetite
- Changes in libido
- Colitis
- Cystitis-like syndrome
- Erythema multiforme
- Erythema nodosum
- Hemolytic uremic syndrome
- Hemorrhagic eruption
- Hirsutism
- Impaired renal function
- Premenstrual syndrome
- Porphyria
- Vaginitis

The most frequent adverse events (reported by 1% or more patients) leading to discontinuation in various trials of women using LUNELLE™ Monthly Contraceptive Injection were weight gain, menorrhagia, amenorrhea, metrorrhagia, vaginal spotting, emotional lability, acne, breast tenderness/pain, headache, dysmenorrhea, nausea, and depression.

OVERDOSAGE

Overdosage of a Progestin/estrogen drug combination may cause nausea and vomiting, and vaginal bleeding or other menstrual irregularities in females.

DOSAGE AND ADMINISTRATION

LUNELLE™ Monthly Contraceptive Injection is effective for contraception during the first cycle of use when administered as recommended.

The recommended dose of LUNELLE™ Monthly Contraceptive Injection is 0.5 mL administered by intramuscular injection, into the deltoid, gluteus maximus, or anterior thigh. The aqueous suspension must be vigorously shaken just before use to ensure a uniform suspension of 25 mg medroxyprogesterone acetate and 5 mg estradiol cypionate.

First Injection

- Within first 5 days of the onset of a normal menstrual period, **or**
- Within 5 days of a complete first trimester abortion, **or**
- No earlier than 4 weeks postpartum if not breastfeeding.
- No earlier than 6 weeks postpartum if breastfeeding.

Second and Subsequent Injections

- Monthly (28 to 30 days) after previous injection, not to exceed 33 days.
- If the patient has not adhered to the prescribed schedule (greater than 33 days since last injection), pregnancy should be considered and she should not receive another injection until pregnancy is ruled out.
- Shortening the injection interval could lead to a change in menstrual pattern.

Continued on next page

Lunelle—Cont.

• Do not use bleeding episodes to guide the injection schedule.

Switching from other Methods of Contraception

When switching from other contraceptive methods, LUNELLE™ Monthly Contraceptive Injection should be given in a manner that ensures continuous contraceptive coverage based upon the mechanism of action of both methods, e.g., patients switching from oral contraceptives should have their first injection of LUNELLE™ Monthly Contraceptive Injection within 7 days after taking their last active pill.

HOW SUPPLIED

LUNELLE™ Monthly Contraceptive Injection (25 mg medroxyprogesterone acetate and 5 mg estradiol cypionate per 0.5 mL sterile aqueous injectable suspension) is available in vials and prefilled syringes. Each vial or prefilled syringe contains enough product to deliver 0.5 mL for single-dose administration. It is available in the following packages:

NDC 0009-3484-04	1 × 0.5 mL vial
NDC 0009-3484-10	3 × 0.5 mL vials
NDC 0009-3484-05	25 × 0.5 mL vials
NDC 0009-3484-06	1 × 0.5 mL prefilled syringe
NDC 0009-3484-07	3 × 0.5 mL prefilled syringe
NDC 0009-3484-08	6 × 0.5 mL prefilled syringe
NDC 0009-3484-09	24 × 0.5 mL prefilled syringe

Store at 20°-25°C (68°-77°F); excursions permitted to 15-30°C (59-86°F) [see USP Controlled Room Temperature].

℞ only

References available upon request.

Manufactured for: Pharmacia & Upjohn Company
A subsidiary of Pharmacia Corporation
Kalamazoo, MI 49001, USA
by: Pharmacia NV/SA
Puurs, Belgium
(prefilled syringes)
Pharmacia & Upjohn Company
Kalamazoo, MI 49001, USA
(vials)

Revised July 2001 817 821 001
692804
3484-04

Patient Information About
LUNELLE™ Monthly Contraceptive Injection

medroxyprogesterone acetate and estradiol cypionate injectable suspension

PHARMACIA

LUNELLE™ Monthly Contraceptive Injection (like all hormonal contraceptives) is intended to prevent pregnancy. It does not protect against HIV infection (AIDS) and other sexually transmitted diseases.

Every woman who considers using hormonal contraceptives must understand the benefits and risks of this type of birth control. This sheet contains important information about hormonal contraceptives that you need in order to decide if LUNELLE™ Monthly Contraceptive Injection is a good type of birth control for you. Please read this sheet carefully and ask your health care provider to help you compare LUNELLE™ Monthly Contraceptive Injection with other methods of birth control. This sheet is not meant to take the place of careful discussions with your health care provider. You should discuss the information provided in this sheet with him or her, both when you first start taking LUNELLE™ Monthly Contraceptive Injection and during your revisits. You should also follow your health care provider's advice with regard to regular check-ups while you are on LUNELLE™ Monthly Contraceptive Injection.

WHAT IS LUNELLE™ MONTHLY CONTRACEPTIVE INJECTION?

LUNELLE™ Monthly Contraceptive Injection is a type of hormonal birth control that is given as an injection (a shot) in your arm, thigh, or buttock once a month to prevent pregnancy. It contains hormones which have effects similar to the natural hormones, estrogen and progesterone, produced in your body. Similar combinations of hormones are found in some oral contraceptives also known as "birth control pills" or "the pill." When you receive your injections once a month as prescribed, LUNELLE™ Monthly Contraceptive Injection is as effective as birth control pills. When given according to the prescribed schedule, LUNELLE™ Monthly Contraceptive Injection is effective in preventing pregnancy during the cycle in which it is given. Clinical studies have shown that when women receive LUNELLE™ Monthly Contraceptive Injection according to the recommended schedule, the failure rate of this method of birth control is less than 1% per year.

The following table shows the typical failure rates for other methods of birth control during the first year of use:

[See table at top of previous page]

WHO SHOULD NOT TAKE LUNELLE™ MONTHLY CONTRACEPTIVE INJECTION

Cigarette smoking increases the risk of serious cardiovascular side effects from hormonal contraceptive use. This risk increases with age and with heavy smoking (15 or more cigarettes per day) and is quite marked in women over 35 years of age. Women who use hormonal contraceptives are strongly advised not to smoke.

Some women should not use hormonal contraceptives. For example, you should not take LUNELLE™ Monthly Contraceptive Injection if you are pregnant or think you may be pregnant. You should also not use LUNELLE™ Monthly Contraceptive Injection if you have any of the following conditions:

- A history of heart attack or stroke
- Blood clots in the legs (thrombophlebitis), lungs (pulmonary embolism), or eyes
- A history of blood clots in the deep veins of your legs
- Chest pain (angina pectoris)
- Known or suspected breast cancer or cancer of the lining of the uterus, cervix or vagina
- Unexplained vaginal bleeding (until a diagnosis is reached by your doctor)
- Yellowing of the whites of the eyes or of the skin (jaundice) during pregnancy or during previous use of the pill or other hormonal contraceptives
- Liver tumor (benign or cancerous)
- Known or suspected pregnancy
- Allergy to any of the ingredients contained in LUNELLE™ Monthly Contraceptive Injection
- Over age 35 and smoke 15 or more cigarettes per day

Tell your health care provider if you have ever had any of these conditions. Your health care provider can recommend a safer method of birth control.

OTHER CONSIDERATIONS BEFORE TAKING LUNELLE™ MONTHLY CONTRACEPTIVE INJECTION

For the majority of women, hormonal contraceptives can be taken safely. But there are some women who are at high risk of developing certain serious diseases that can be life-threatening or may cause temporary or permanent disability. Tell your health care provider if you have:

- Breast nodules, fibrocystic disease of the breast, an abnormal breast x-ray or mammogram, strong family history of breast cancer
- Diabetes
- Elevated cholesterol or triglycerides
- High blood pressure
- Migraine or other headaches or epilepsy
- Mental depression
- Gallbladder, heart or kidney disease
- History of scanty or irregular menstrual periods
- Smoke, especially if 35 years or older

Women with any of these conditions should be checked often by their health care provider if they choose to use LUNELLE™ Monthly Contraceptive Injection.

Also, be sure to inform your doctor or health care provider if you smoke or are on any medications.

RISKS OF TAKING HORMONAL CONTRACEPTIVES

1. Risk of developing blood clots, heart attacks, and strokes

Blood clots and blockage of blood vessels are the most serious side effects of taking hormonal contraceptives. In particular, blood clots can occur in the legs and can travel to the lungs and can cause sudden blocking of the vessel carrying blood to the lungs. Rarely, clots occur in the blood vessels of the eye and may cause blindness, double vision, or impaired vision.

If you take hormonal contraceptives such as LUNELLE™ Monthly Contraceptive Injection and need elective surgery, need to stay in bed for a prolonged illness, or have recently had a baby, you may be at risk of developing blood clots. You should consult your doctor about stopping hormonal contraceptives three to four weeks before surgery and not taking hormonal contraceptives for two weeks after surgery or during bed rest. You should also not take hormonal contraceptives soon after delivery of a baby. It is advisable to wait for at least four weeks after delivery before using hormonal contraceptives such as LUNELLE™ Monthly Contraceptive Injection. (See also the section on Breast Feeding in GENERAL PRECAUTIONS.)

Hormonal contraceptives may also increase the tendency to develop strokes (stoppage or rupture of blood vessels in the brain) and angina pectoris and heart attacks (blockage of blood vessels in the heart). Any of these conditions can cause death or disability.

Smoking greatly increases the possibility of developing blood clots or suffering heart attacks and strokes. Furthermore, smoking and the use of hormonal contraceptives greatly increase the chances of developing and dying of heart disease, particularly if you are over 35 years of age.

2. Gallbladder disease

Hormonal contraceptive users probably have a greater risk than non-users of having gallbladder disease.

3. Liver tumors

In rare cases, hormonal contraceptives can cause benign but dangerous liver tumors. These benign liver tumors can rupture and cause fatal internal bleeding. In addition, a possible but not definite association has been found with hormonal contraceptives and liver cancers in two studies, in which a few women who developed these very rare cancers were found to have used hormonal contraceptives for long periods. However, liver cancers are extremely rare. The chance of developing liver cancer from using hormonal contraceptives is thus even rarer.

4. Cancer of the reproductive organs and breasts

There is, at present, no confirmed evidence that oral hormonal contraceptives increase the risk of cancer of the reproductive organs in human studies. Studies to date of women taking the pill have reported conflicting findings on whether pill use increases the risk of developing cancer of the breast. Most of the studies on breast cancer and pill use have found no overall increase in the risk of developing breast cancer, although some studies have reported an increased risk of developing breast cancer in certain groups of women.

Some studies have found an increase in the incidence of cancer of the cervix in women who use oral hormonal contraceptives. However, this finding may be related to factors other than the use of oral hormonal contraceptives.

Studies have found that women who used injectable hormonal contraceptives (Depo-Provera Contraceptive Injection) had no increased overall risk of developing cancer of the breast, ovary, uterus, or cervix. However, women under 35 years of age whose first exposure to Depo-Provera Contraceptive Injection was within the previous 4 to 5 years may have a slightly increased risk of developing breast cancer similar to that seen with oral contraceptives.

Women who use hormonal contraceptives and have a strong family history of breast cancer or who have breast nodules or abnormal mammogram should be closely followed by their doctors.

5. Changes in bone mineral density

Use of injectable hormonal contraceptives containing the progesterone-type hormone found in LUNELLE™ Monthly Contraceptive Injection may be associated with a decrease in the amount of mineral stored in your bones. This could increase your risk of developing bone fractures. The rate of bone mineral loss is greatest in the early years of use of this type of contraceptive, but after that, it begins to resemble the normal rate of age-related bone mineral loss.

Formal studies on the effect of bone mineral density changes in women receiving LUNELLE™ Monthly Contraceptive Injection have not been conducted.

6. Allergic reactions

Severe allergic reactions have been reported in some women using injectable hormonal contraceptives containing the progesterone-type hormone found in LUNELLE™ Monthly Contraceptive Injection. Allergic reactions occurring in women using LUNELLE™ Monthly Contraceptive Injection have been mainly skin reactions, and not respiratory in nature. Serious allergic reactions require emergency medical treatment.

ESTIMATED RISK OF DEATH FROM A BIRTH CONTROL METHOD OR PREGNANCY

All methods of birth control and pregnancy are associated with a risk of developing certain diseases that may lead to disability or death. An estimate of the number of deaths associated with different methods of birth control and pregnancy has been calculated and is shown in the following table.

[See table above]

Annual Number of Birth-Related or Method-Related Deaths Associated with Control of Fertility per 100,000 Non-sterile Women, by Fertility Control Method According to Age

Method of Control & Outcome	Range of Ages (years)					
	15-19	20-24	25-29	30-34	35-39	40-44
No fertility control*	7.0	7.4	9.1	14.8	25.7	28.2
Oral hormonal contraceptives** (non-smoker)	0.3	0.5	0.9	1.9	13.8	31.6
Oral hormonal contraceptives** (smoker)	2.2	3.4	6.6	13.5	51.1	117.2
IUD**	0.8	0.8	1.0	1.0	1.4	1.4
Condom*	1.1	1.6	0.7	0.2	0.3	0.4
Diaphragm/spermicide*	1.9	1.2	1.2	1.3	2.2	2.8
Periodic abstinence	2.5	1.6	1.6	1.7	2.9	3.6

* Deaths are birth-related
**Deaths are method-related

In the above table, the risk of death from any birth control method is less than the risk of childbirth, except for oral hormonal contraceptive users over the age of 35 who smoke and oral hormonal contraceptive users over the age of 40 even if they do not smoke. It can be seen in the table that for women aged 15 to 39, the risk of death was highest with pregnancy (7–26 deaths per 100,000 women, depending on age). Among oral hormonal contraceptive users who do not smoke, the risk of death is always lower than that associated with pregnancy for any age group, although over the age of 40, the risk increases to 32 deaths per 100,000 women, compared to 28 associated with pregnancy at that age. However, for oral hormonal contraceptive users who smoke and are over the age of 35, the estimated number of deaths exceeds those for other methods of birth control. If a woman is over the age of 40 and smokes, her estimated risk of death is four times higher (117/100,000 women) than the estimated risk associated with pregnancy (28/100,000 women) in that age group.

An Advisory Committee of the FDA discussed this issue in 1989 and recommended that the benefits of oral contraceptive use by healthy, non-smoking women over 40 years of age may outweigh the possible risks. However, women of all ages are cautioned to use the lowest dose oral contraceptive that is effective, and are strongly advised not to smoke.

WARNING SIGNALS

If any of these adverse effects occur while you are taking LUNELLE™ Monthly Contraceptive Injection, call your doctor immediately:

- Sharp chest pain, coughing of blood, or sudden shortness of breath (indicating a possible clot in the lung)
- Pain in the calf (indicating a possible clot in the leg)
- Crushing chest pain or heaviness in the chest (indicating a possible heart attack)
- Sudden severe headache or vomiting, dizziness or fainting, disturbances of vision or speech, weakness, or numbness in an arm or leg (indicating a possible stroke)
- Sudden partial or complete loss of vision (indicating a possible clot in the eye)
- Breast lumps (indicating possible breast cancer or fibrocystic disease of the breast; ask your doctor or health care provider to show you how to examine your breasts)
- Severe pain or tenderness in the abdominal area (indicating a possibly ruptured liver tumor, ovarian cyst, or pregnancy outside the uterus)
- Difficulty in sleeping, weakness, lack of energy, fatigue, or change in mood (possibly indicating severe depression)
- Jaundice or a yellowing of the skin or eyeballs, accompanied frequently by fever, fatigue, loss of appetite, dark-colored urine, or light-colored bowel movements (indicating possible liver problems)
- Persistent pain, pus, or bleeding at the injection site
- Unusually heavy vaginal bleeding

SIDE EFFECTS OF LUNELLE™ MONTHLY CONTRACEPTIVE INJECTION

1. Vaginal bleeding

Most women using LUNELLE™ Monthly Contraceptive Injection experience alteration of menstrual bleeding. Bleeding patterns may vary from a single monthly bleed to no bleeding at all or slight staining between menstrual periods to frequent, prolonged, and/or unpredictable bleeding. In any given injection interval, approximately 50% of women using LUNELLE™ Monthly Contraceptive Injection experience withdrawal bleeding that begins 20–25 days after the injection. Withdrawal bleeding lasts more than 7 days in 42% of women during the first month of use and in 29% of women at the end of one year of use. In any given injection interval, approximately 15% of women may have no bleeding at all and 10% may experience bleeding or spotting at various times in the cycle. Irregular bleeding often occurs during the first few months of LUNELLE™ Monthly Contraceptive Injection use and may persist with continued use in up to one third of women. Your menstrual blood flow may be heavier or lighter, and there may be no bleeding, fewer days of bleeding, or more days of bleeding than what you have previously experienced. Such bleeding usually does not indicate any serious problems. If an altered bleeding pattern persists or the bleeding is severe, discuss it with your health care provider. There is also a small risk that (painful) cramps may be associated with bleeding.

2. Weight change

Weight gain is a common side effect in women using LUNELLE™ Monthly Contraceptive Injection. The average expected weight gain is 4 pounds in the first year of use. Some women gain more than 10 to 20 pounds in the first year. Women have gained as much as 49 pounds or lost as much as 48 pounds in one year of use. Clinical trials showed wide variability in individual weight change with an increasing percentage of LUNELLE™ Monthly Contraceptive Injection users experiencing weight change in excess of 10 and 20 pounds with continued treatment.

3. Contact lenses

If you wear contact lenses and notice a change in vision or an inability to wear your lenses, contact your doctor or health care provider.

4. Fluid retention

Hormonal contraceptives may cause edema (fluid retention) with swelling of the fingers or ankles and may raise your blood pressure. If you experience fluid retention, contact your doctor or health care provider.

5. Other side effects

Other side effects may include breast pain or tenderness, acne, change in appetite, nausea, headache, nervousness, depression, mood changes, changes in sexual desire, dizziness, loss of scalp hair, rash, and vaginal infections.

If any of these side effects bother you, call your health care provider.

GENERAL PRECAUTIONS

1. Missed periods and use of hormonal contraceptives before or during early pregnancy.

You may not menstruate regularly after you receive an injection of LUNELLE™ Monthly Contraceptive Injection. If you have received your injections regularly and miss one menstrual period, be sure to inform your health care provider. The risk of unexpected pregnancy for women receiving injectable contraceptives as scheduled is very low. If you have not received your injections as scheduled and missed a menstrual period, or if you missed two consecutive menstrual periods, you may be pregnant. Check with your health care provider immediately to determine whether you are pregnant. Do not continue the injections until you are sure you are not pregnant, but use another method of contraception.

There is no conclusive evidence that oral hormonal contraceptive use is associated with an increase in birth defects, when taken inadvertently during early pregnancy. Nevertheless, hormonal contraceptives should not be used during pregnancy.

With Depo-Provera Contraceptive Injection, there have been reports of an increased risk of low birth weight and neonatal infant death or other health problems in infants conceived close to the time of injection. However, these pregnancies are uncommon. Children exposed in the womb to one of the hormones found in LUNELLE™ Monthly Contraceptive Injection (MPA), and followed to adolescence, showed no evidence of any adverse effects on their health including their physical, mental, sexual or social development.

If you think you may have become pregnant while using LUNELLE™ Monthly Contraceptive Injection, see your health care provider as soon as possible. You should check with your health care provider about risks to your unborn child from any medication taken during pregnancy.

2. While breast feeding

If you are breast feeding, consult your health care provider before starting hormonal contraceptives, including LUNELLE™ Monthly Contraceptive Injection. Some of the drugs in hormonal contraceptives are passed on to the child in breast milk. A few adverse effects on the child have been reported, including yellowing of the skin (jaundice) and breast enlargement. In addition, hormonal contraceptives may decrease the amount and quality of your milk. To insure the best quantity and quality of your breast milk, you should wait until 6 weeks after childbirth before you start using LUNELLE™ Monthly Contraceptive Injection. If possible, do not use hormonal contraceptives while breast feeding.

Breast feeding provides only partial protection from becoming pregnant and this partial protection decreases significantly as you breast feed for longer periods of time. You should use another method of contraception while breast feeding and consider starting hormonal contraceptives only after you have weaned your child completely.

3. Laboratory tests

If you are scheduled for any laboratory tests, tell your doctor you are taking a hormonal contraceptive. Certain blood tests may be affected by hormonal contraceptives.

4. Drug interactions

Certain drugs may interact with hormonal contraceptives to make them less effective in preventing pregnancy or cause a change in bleeding patterns. Such drugs include aminoglutethimide, rifampin, drugs used for epilepsy such as barbiturates (for example, phenobarbital), carbamazepine, and phenytoin (Dilantin is one brand of this drug), phenylbutazone (Butazolidin is one brand), herbal products containing St. John's Wort (hypericum perforatum), and possibly certain antibiotics. You may need to use an additional contraception method when you take drugs which can make hormonal contraceptives less effective. Drug interaction studies have not been conducted with LUNELLE™ Monthly Contraceptive Injection.

5. Sexually transmitted diseases

This product (like all hormonal contraceptives) is intended to prevent pregnancy. It does not protect against transmission of HIV (AIDS) and other sexually transmitted diseases such as chlamydia, genital herpes, genital warts, gonorrhea, hepatitis B, and syphilis.

6. Weight change

LUNELLE™ Monthly Contraceptive Injection may cause weight gain of more than 10 pounds.

WHEN DO I GET MY LUNELLE™ MONTHLY CONTRACEPTIVE INJECTION?

LUNELLE™ Monthly Contraceptive Injection can only be effective if you receive your injections at the proper times.

First Injection

- Within the first 5 days of the start of your normal menstrual period.
- If you are presently using another type of birth control, your health care provider will decide the best time for you to start LUNELLE™ Monthly Contraceptive Injection. This will help make sure you have continued contraceptive coverage.
- If you have recently been pregnant or had a baby, discuss with your health care provider the best time for you to start LUNELLE™ Monthly Contraceptive Injection.

Next Injections

- LUNELLE™ Monthly Contraceptive Injection must be given monthly, every 28 to 30 days and no later than 33 days after your last injection.
  The time for your next injection is determined by the number of days since your previous injection, and not by the timing or amount of your menstrual bleeding.
  Even if you do not have any menstrual bleeding, you should still return once a month for your injection of LUNELLE™ Monthly Contraceptive Injection.
- It is important that you receive each of your next injections at the right time. If you cannot receive your injection on time, contact your health care provider to receive an earlier injection.

What Happens if I Miss an Injection or Wait Longer than 33 Days Between Injections?

- You could become pregnant if you miss your injection or wait longer than 33 days between injections. The more days you wait, the greater the risk that you could become pregnant.
- Ask your health care provider to recommend another type of birth control (such as condoms or a spermicide) for you to use.
- Talk with your health care provider to find out when you should receive your next injection of LUNELLE™ Monthly Contraceptive Injection.
- Your health care provider may do a test to make sure you are not pregnant before giving you your next injection of LUNELLE™ Monthly Contraceptive Injection.

Pregnancy Due to Failure with LUNELLE™ Monthly Contraceptive Injection

The incidence of failure with LUNELLE™ Monthly Contraceptive Injection resulting in pregnancy is less than 1 percent (i.e., one pregnancy per 100 women per year) if given every month as directed. If you think that you may be pregnant, be sure to call your health care provider.

What If I Want to Become Pregnant?

You will need to stop your monthly injections of LUNELLE™ Monthly Contraceptive Injection. Most women begin to produce eggs again (and could become pregnant) about two to three months after their last injection.

There may be some delay in becoming pregnant after you stop using hormonal contraceptives, including LUNELLE™ Monthly Contraceptive Injection, especially if you had irregular menstrual cycles before you started using hormonal contraceptives. There does not appear to be any increase in birth defects in newborn babies when pregnancy occurs soon after stopping hormonal contraceptives.

OVERDOSAGE

Serious ill effects have not been reported following ingestion of large doses of oral hormonal contraceptives by young children. Overdosage may cause nausea and withdrawal bleeding in females. In case of overdosage, contact your health care provider or pharmacist.

OTHER INFORMATION

Your health care provider will take a medical and family history before prescribing hormonal contraceptives. You should receive yearly physical examinations by your health care provider. Be sure to inform your health care provider if there is a family history of any of the conditions listed previously in this leaflet. Be sure to keep all appointments with your health care provider, because this is a time to determine if there are early signs of side effects of hormonal contraceptive use. If you want more information about hormonal contraceptives, ask your health care provider or pharmacist for a more technical leaflet called the Prescribing Information that you may wish to read.

Each 0.5 mL dose of LUNELLE™ Monthly Contraceptive Injection contains:

Active Ingredients: medroxyprogesterone acetate (25 mg), estradiol cypionate (5 mg)

Inactive Ingredients: methylparaben (0.9 mg), polyethylene glycol (14.28 mg), polysorbate 80 (0.95 mg), propylparaben (0.1 mg), sodium chloride (4.28 mg), sterile water for injection

Manufactured for: Pharmacia & Upjohn Company
A subsidiary of Pharmacia Corporation
Kalamazoo, MI 49001, USA
by: Pharmacia NV/SA
Puurs, Belgium
(prefilled syringes)
Pharmacia & Upjohn Company
Kalamazoo, MI 49001, USA
(vials)

Revised July 2001 817 821 001
692804
3484-04

MIRAPEX® ℞

[mĭ-ră-pĕks]

pramipexole dihydrochloride tablets

DESCRIPTION

MIRAPEX Tablets contain pramipexole, a dopamine agonist indicated for the treatment of the signs and symptoms of idiopathic Parkinson's disease. The chemical name of pramipexole dihydrochloride is (*S*)-2-amino-4,5,6,7-tetrahydro-6-(propylamino)benzothiazole dihydrochloride mono-

Continued on next page

Mirapex—Cont.

hydrate. Its empirical formula is $C_{10}H_{17}N_3S \cdot 2\ HCl \cdot H_2O$, and its molecular weight is 302.27.
The structural formula is:

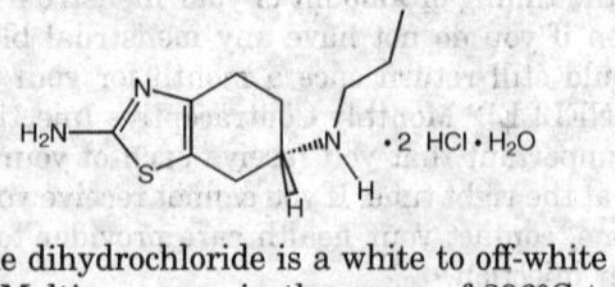

Pramipexole dihydrochloride is a white to off-white powder substance. Melting occurs in the range of 296°C to 301°C, with decomposition. Pramipexole dihydrochloride is more than 20% soluble in water, about 8% in methanol, about 0.5% in ethanol, and practically insoluble in dichloromethane.
MIRAPEX Tablets, for oral administration, contain 0.125 mg, 0.25 mg, 0.5 mg, 1.0 mg, or 1.5 mg of pramipexole dihydrochloride monohydrate. Inactive ingredients consist of mannitol, corn starch, colloidal silicon dioxide, povidone, and magnesium stearate.

CLINICAL PHARMACOLOGY

Pramipexole is a nonergot dopamine agonist with high relative in vitro specificity and full intrinsic activity at the D_2 subfamily of dopamine receptors, binding with higher affinity to D_3 than to D_2 or D_4 receptor subtypes. The relevance of D_3 receptor binding in Parkinson's disease is unknown.
The precise mechanism of action of pramipexole as a treatment for Parkinson's disease is unknown, although it is believed to be related to its ability to stimulate dopamine receptors in the striatum. This conclusion is supported by electrophysiologic studies in animals that have demonstrated that pramipexole influences striatal neuronal firing rates via activation of dopamine receptors in the striatum and the substantia nigra, the site of neurons that send projections to the striatum.

Pharmacokinetics

Pramipexole is rapidly absorbed, reaching peak concentrations in approximately 2 hours. The absolute bioavailability of pramipexole is greater than 90%, indicating that it is well absorbed and undergoes little presystemic metabolism. Food does not affect the extent of pramipexole absorption, although the time of maximum plasma concentration (T_{max}) is increased by about 1 hour when the drug is taken with a meal.
Pramipexole is extensively distributed, having a volume of distribution of about 500 L (coefficient of variation [CV]=20%). It is about 15% bound to plasma proteins. Pramipexole distributes into red blood cells as indicated by an erythrocyte-to-plasma ratio of approximately 2.
Pramipexole displays linear pharmacokinetics over the clinical dosage range. Its terminal half-life is about 8 hours in young healthy volunteers and about 12 hours in elderly volunteers (see CLINICAL PHARMACOLOGY, Pharmacokinetics in Special Population). Steady-state concentrations are achieved within 2 days of dosing.
Metabolism and elimination: Urinary excretion is the major route of pramipexole elimination, with 90% of a pramipexole dose recovered in urine, almost all as unchanged drug. Nonrenal routes may contribute to a small extent to pramipexole elimination, although no metabolites have been identified in plasma or urine. The renal clearance of pramipexole is approximately 400 mL/min (CV=25%), approximately three times higher than the glomerular filtration rate. Thus, pramipexole is secreted by the renal tubules, probably by the organic cation transport system.

Pharmacokinetics in Special Populations

Because therapy with pramipexole is initiated at a subtherapeutic dosage and gradually titrated upward according to clinical tolerability to obtain the optimum therapeutic effect, adjustment of the initial dose based on gender, weight, or age is not necessary. However, renal insufficiency, which can cause a large decrease in the ability to eliminate pramipexole, may necessitate dosage adjustment (see CLINICAL PHARMACOLOGY, Renal Insufficiency).
Gender: Pramipexole clearance is about 30% lower in women than in men, but most of this difference can be accounted for by differences in body weight. There is no difference in half-life between males and females.
Age: Pramipexole clearance decreases with age as the half-life and clearance are about 40% longer and 30% lower, respectively, in elderly (aged 65 years or older) compared with young healthy volunteers (aged less than 40 years). This difference is most likely due to the well-known reduction in renal function with age, since pramipexole clearance is correlated with renal function, as measured by creatinine clearance (see CLINICAL PHARMACOLOGY, Renal Insufficiency).
Parkinson's disease patients: A cross-study comparison of data suggests that the clearance of pramipexole may be reduced by about 30% in Parkinson's disease patients compared with healthy elderly volunteers. The reason for this difference appears to be reduced renal function in Parkinson's disease patients, which may be related to their poorer general health. The pharmacokinetics of pramipexole were comparable between early and advanced Parkinson's disease patients.
Pediatric: The pharmacokinetics of pramipexole in the pediatric population have not been evaluated.
Hepatic insufficiency: The influence of hepatic insufficiency on pramipexole pharmacokinetics has not been evaluated. Because approximately 90% of the recovered dose is excreted in the urine as unchanged drug, hepatic impairment would not be expected to have a significant effect on pramipexole elimination.
Renal insufficiency: The clearance of pramipexole was about 75% lower in patients with severe renal impairment (creatinine clearance approximately 20 mL/min) and about 60% lower in patients with moderate impairment (creatinine clearance approximately 40 mL/min) compared with healthy volunteers. A lower starting and maintenance dose is recommended in these patients (see PRECAUTIONS and DOSAGE AND ADMINISTRATION). In patients with varying degrees of renal impairment, pramipexole clearance correlates well with creatinine clearance. Therefore, creatinine clearance can be used as a predictor of the extent of decrease in pramipexole clearance. Pramipexole clearance is extremely low in dialysis patients, as a negligible amount of pramipexole is removed by dialysis. Caution should be exercised when administering pramipexole to patients with renal disease.

CLINICAL STUDIES

The effectiveness of MIRAPEX Tablets in the treatment of Parkinson's disease was evaluated in a multinational drug development program consisting of seven randomized, controlled trials. Three were conducted in patients with early Parkinson's disease who were not receiving concomitant levodopa, and four were conducted in patients with advanced Parkinson's disease who were receiving concomitant levodopa. Among these seven studies, three studies provide the most persuasive evidence of pramipexole's effectiveness in the management of patients with Parkinson's disease who were and were not receiving concomitant levodopa. Two of these three trials enrolled patients with early Parkinson's disease (not receiving levodopa), and one enrolled patients with advanced Parkinson's disease who were receiving maximally tolerated doses of levodopa.
In all studies, the Unified Parkinson's Disease Rating Scale (UPDRS), or one or more of its subparts, served as the primary outcome assessment measure. The UPDRS is a four-part multi-item rating scale intended to evaluate mentation (part I), activities of daily living (part II), motor performance (part III), and complications of therapy (part IV).
Part II of the UPDRS contains 13 questions relating to activities of daily living (ADL), which are scored from 0 (normal) to 4 (maximal severity) for a maximum (worst) score of 52. Part III of the UPDRS contains 27 questions (for 14 items) and is scored as described for part II. It is designed to assess the severity of the cardinal motor findings in patients with Parkinson's disease (eg, tremor, rigidity, bradykinesia, postural instability, etc), scored for different body regions, and has a maximum (worst) score of 108.

Studies in Patients With Early Parkinson's Disease

Patients (N=599) in the two studies of early Parkinson's disease had a mean disease duration of 2 years, limited or no prior exposure to levodopa (generally none in the preceding 6 months), and were not experiencing the "on-off" phenomenon and dyskinesia characteristic of later stages of the disease.
One of the two early Parkinson's disease studies (N=335) was a double-blind, placebo-controlled, parallel trial consisting of a 7-week dose-escalation period and a 6-month maintenance period. Patients could be on selegiline, anticholinergics, or both, but could not be on levodopa products or amantadine. Patients were randomized to MIRAPEX or placebo. Patients treated with MIRAPEX had a starting daily dose of 0.375 mg and were titrated to a maximally tolerated dose, but no higher than 4.5 mg/day in three divided doses. At the end of the 6-month maintenance period, the mean improvement from baseline on the UPDRS part II (ADL) total score was 1.9 in the group receiving MIRAPEX and -0.4 in the placebo group, a difference that was statistically significant. The mean improvement from baseline on the UPDRS part III total score was 5.0 in the group receiving MIRAPEX and -0.8 in the placebo group, a difference that was also statistically significant. A statistically significant difference between groups in favor of MIRAPEX was seen beginning at week 2 of the UPDRS part II (maximum dose 0.75 mg/day) and at week 3 of the UPDRS part III (maximum dose 1.5 mg/day).
The second early Parkinson's disease study (N=264) was a double-blind, placebo-controlled, parallel trial consisting of a 6-week dose-escalation period and a 4-week maintenance period. Patients could be on selegiline, anticholinergics, amantadine, or any combination of these, but could not be on levodopa products. Patients were randomized to 1 of 4 fixed doses of MIRAPEX (1.5 mg, 3.0 mg, 4.5 mg, or 6.0 mg per day) or placebo. At the end of the 4-week maintenance period, the mean improvement from baseline on the UPDRS part II total score was 1.8 in the patients treated with MIRAPEX, regardless of assigned dose group, and 0.3 in placebo-treated patients. The mean improvement from baseline on the UPDRS part III total score was 4.2 in patients treated with MIRAPEX and 0.6 in placebo-treated patients. No dose-response relationship was demonstrated. The between-treatment differences on both parts of the UPDRS were statistically significant in favor of MIRAPEX for all doses.
No differences in effectiveness based on age or gender were detected. There were too few non-Caucasian patients to evaluate the effect of race. Patients receiving selegiline or anticholinergics had responses similar to patients not receiving these drugs.

Studies in Patients With Advanced Parkinson's Disease

In the advanced Parkinson's disease study, the primary assessments were the UPDRS and daily diaries that quantified amounts of "on" and "off" time.
Patients in the advanced Parkinson's disease study (N=360) had a mean disease duration of 9 years, had been exposed to levodopa for long periods of time (mean 8 years), used concomitant levodopa during the trial, and had "on-off" periods.
The advanced Parkinson's disease study was a double-blind, placebo-controlled, parallel trial consisting of a 7-week dose-escalation period and a 6-month maintenance period. Patients were all treated with concomitant levodopa products and could additionally be on concomitant selegiline, anticholinergics, amantadine, or any combination. Patients treated with MIRAPEX had a starting dose of 0.375 mg/day and were titrated to a maximally tolerated dose, but no higher than 4.5 mg/day in three divided doses. At selected times during the 6-month maintenance period, patients were asked to record the amount of "off," "on," or "on with dyskinesia" time per day for several sequential days. At the end of the 6-month maintenance period, the mean improvement from baseline on the UPDRS part II total score was 2.7 in the group treated with MIRAPEX and 0.5 in the placebo group, a difference that was statistically significant. The mean improvement from baseline on the UPDRS part III total score was 5.6 in the group treated with MIRAPEX and 2.8 in the placebo group, a difference that was statistically significant. A statistically significant difference between groups in favor of MIRAPEX was seen at week 3 of the UPDRS part II (maximum dose 1.5 mg/day) and at week 2 of the UPDRS part III (maximum dose 0.75 mg/day). Dosage reduction of levodopa was allowed during this study if dyskinesia (or hallucinations) developed; levodopa dosage reduction occurred in 76% of patients treated with MIRAPEX versus 54% of placebo patients. On average, the levodopa dose was reduced 27%.
The mean number of "off" hours per day during baseline was 6 hours for both treatment groups. Throughout the trial, patients treated with MIRAPEX had a mean of 4 "off" hours per day, while placebo-treated patients continued to experience 6 "off" hours per day.
No differences in effectiveness based on age or gender were detected. There were too few non-Caucasian patients to evaluate the effect of race.

INDICATIONS AND USAGE

MIRAPEX Tablets are indicated for the treatment of the signs and symptoms of idiopathic Parkinson's disease.
The effectiveness of MIRAPEX was demonstrated in randomized, controlled trials in patients with early Parkinson's disease who were not receiving concomitant levodopa therapy as well as in patients with advanced disease on concomitant levodopa (see CLINICAL STUDIES).

CONTRAINDICATIONS

MIRAPEX Tablets are contraindicated in patients who have demonstrated hypersensitivity to the drug or its ingredients.

WARNINGS

Falling Asleep During Activities of Daily Living:

Patients treated with MIRAPEX have reported falling asleep while engaged in activities of daily living, including the operation of motor vehicles which sometimes resulted in accidents. Although many of these patients reported somnolence while on MIRAPEX, some perceived that they had no warning signs such as excessive drowsiness, and believed that they were alert immediately prior to the event. Some of these events have been reported as late as one year after the initiation of treatment.
Somnolence is a common occurrence in patients receiving MIRAPEX at doses above 1.5 mg/day. Many clinical experts believe that falling asleep while engaged in activities of daily living always occurs in a setting of pre-existing somnolence, although patients may not give such a history. For this reason, prescribers should continually reassess patients for drowsiness or sleepiness, especially since some of the events occur well after the start of treatment. Prescribers should also be aware that patients may not acknowledge drowsiness or sleepiness until directly questioned about drowsiness or sleepiness during specific activities.
Before initiating treatment with MIRAPEX, patients should be advised of the potential to develop drowsiness and specifically asked about factors that may increase the risk with MIRAPEX such as concomitant sedating medications, the presence of sleep disorders, and concomitant medications that increase pramipexole plasma levels (e.g., cimetidine—see PRECAUTIONS, Drug Interactions). If a patient develops significant daytime sleepiness or episodes of falling asleep during activities that require active participation (e.g., conversations, eating, etc.), MIRAPEX should ordinarily be discontinued. If a decision is made to continue MIRAPEX, patients should be advised to not drive and to avoid other potentially dangerous activities. While dose reduction clearly reduces the degree of somnolence, there is insufficient information to establish that dose reduction will eliminate episodes of falling asleep while engaged in activities of daily living.
Symptomatic Hypotension: Dopamine agonists, in clinical studies and clinical experience, appear to impair the systemic regulation of blood pressure, with resulting orthostatic hypotension, especially during dose escalation. Parkinson's disease patients, in addition, appear to have an impaired capacity to respond to an orthostatic challenge. For these reasons, Parkinson's disease patients being treated with dopaminergic agonists ordinarily require careful monitoring for signs and symptoms of orthostatic hypo-

tension, especially during dose escalation, and should be informed of this risk (see PRECAUTIONS, Information for Patients).

In clinical trials of pramipexole, however, and despite clear orthostatic effects in normal volunteers, the reported incidence of clinically significant orthostatic hypotension was not greater among those assigned to MIRAPEX Tablets than among those assigned to placebo. This result is clearly unexpected in light of the previous experience with the risks of dopamine agonist therapy.

While this finding could reflect a unique property of pramipexole, it might also be explained by the conditions of the study and the nature of the population enrolled in the clinical trials. Patients were very carefully titrated, and patients with active cardiovascular disease or significant orthostatic hypotension at baseline were excluded.

Hallucinations: In the three double-blind, placebo-controlled trials in early Parkinson's disease, hallucinations were observed in 9% (35 of 388) of patients receiving MIRAPEX, compared with 2.6% (6 of 235) of patients receiving placebo. In the four double-blind, placebo-controlled trials in advanced Parkinson's disease, where patients received MIRAPEX and concomitant levodopa, hallucinations were observed in 16.5% (43 of 260) of patients receiving MIRAPEX compared with 3.8% (10 of 264) of patients receiving placebo. Hallucinations were of sufficient severity to cause discontinuation of treatment in 3.1% of the early Parkinson's disease patients and 2.7% of the advanced Parkinson's disease patients compared with about 0.4% of placebo patients in both populations.

Age appears to increase the risk of hallucinations attributable to pramipexole. In the early Parkinson's disease patients, the risk of hallucinations was 1.9 times greater than placebo in patients younger than 65 years and 6.8 times greater than placebo in patients older than 65 years. In the advanced Parkinson's disease patients, the risk of hallucinations was 3.5 times greater than placebo in patients younger than 65 years and 5.2 times greater than placebo in patients older than 65 years.

PRECAUTIONS

Rhabdomyolysis: A single case of rhabdomyolysis occurred in a 49-year-old male with advanced Parkinson's disease treated with MIRAPEX Tablets. The patient was hospitalized with an elevated CPK (10,631 IU/L). The symptoms resolved with discontinuation of the medication.

Renal: Since pramipexole is eliminated through the kidneys, caution should be exercised when prescribing MIRAPEX to patients with renal insufficiency (see DOSAGE AND ADMINISTRATION).

Dyskinesia: MIRAPEX may potentiate the dopaminergic side effects of levodopa and may cause or exacerbate preexisting dyskinesia. Decreasing the dose of levodopa may ameliorate this side effect.

Retinal pathology in albino rats: Pathologic changes (degeneration and loss of photoreceptor cells) were observed in the retina of albino rats in the 2-year carcinogenicity study. While retinal degeneration was not diagnosed in pigmented rats treated for 2 years, a thinning in the outer nuclear layer of the retina was slightly greater in rats given drug compared with controls. Evaluation of the retinas of albino mice, monkeys, and minipigs did not reveal similar changes. The potential significance of this effect in humans has not been established, but cannot be disregarded because disruption of a mechanism that is universally present in vertebrates (ie, disk shedding) may be involved (see ANIMAL TOXICOLOGY).

Events Reported With Dopaminergic Therapy

Although the events enumerated below have not been reported in association with the use of pramipexole in its development program, they are associated with the use of other dopaminergic drugs. The expected incidence of these events, however, is so low that even if pramipexole caused these events at rates similar to those attributable to other dopaminergic therapies, it would be unlikely that even a single case would have occurred in a cohort of the size exposed to pramipexole in studies to date.

Withdrawal-emergent hyperpyrexia and confusion: Although not reported with pramipexole in the clinical development program, a symptom complex resembling the neuroleptic malignant syndrome (characterized by elevated temperature, muscular rigidity, altered consciousness, and autonomic instability), with no other obvious etiology, has been reported in association with rapid dose reduction, withdrawal of, or changes in antiparkinsonian therapy.

Fibrotic complications: Although not reported with pramipexole in the clinical development program, cases of retroperitoneal fibrosis, pulmonary infiltrates, pleural effusion, and pleural thickening have been reported in some patients treated with ergot-derived dopaminergic agents. While these complications may resolve when the drug is discontinued, complete resolution does not always occur.

Although these adverse events are believed to be related to the ergoline structure of these compounds, whether other, nonergot derived dopamine agonists can cause them is unknown.

Information for Patients: Patients should be instructed to take MIRAPEX only as prescribed.

Patients should be alerted to the potential sedating effects associated with MIRAPEX, including somnolence and the possibility of falling asleep while engaged in activities of daily living. Since somnolence is a frequent adverse event with potentially serious consequences, patients should neither drive a car nor engage in other potentially dangerous activities until they have gained sufficient experience with MIRAPEX to gauge whether or not it affects their mental and/or motor performance adversely. Patients should be advised that if increased somnolence or new episodes of falling asleep during activities of daily living (e.g., watching television, passenger in a car, etc.) are experienced at any time during treatment, they should not drive or participate in potentially dangerous activities until they have contacted their physician. Because of possible additive effects, caution should be advised when patients are taking other sedating medications or alcohol in combination with MIRAPEX and when taking concomitant medications that increase plasma levels of pramipexole (e.g., cimetidine).

Patients should be informed that hallucinations can occur and that the elderly are at a higher risk than younger patients with Parkinson's disease.

Patients may develop postural (orthostatic) hypotension, with or without symptoms such as dizziness, nausea, fainting or blackouts, and sometimes, sweating. Hypotension may occur more frequently during initial therapy. Accordingly, patients should be cautioned against rising rapidly after sitting or lying down, especially if they have been doing so for prolonged periods and especially at the initiation of treatment with MIRAPEX.

Because the teratogenic potential of pramipexole has not been completely established in laboratory animals, and because experience in humans is limited, patients should be advised to notify their physicians if they become pregnant or intend to become pregnant during therapy (see PRECAUTIONS, Pregnancy).

Because of the possibility that pramipexole may be excreted in breast milk, patients should be advised to notify their physicians if they intend to breast-feed or are breast-feeding an infant.

If patients develop nausea, they should be advised that taking MIRAPEX with food may reduce the occurrence of nausea.

Laboratory Tests: During the development of MIRAPEX, no systematic abnormalities on routine laboratory testing were noted. Therefore, no specific guidance is offered regarding routine monitoring; the practitioner retains responsibility for determining how best to monitor the patient in his or her care.

Drug Interactions

Carbidopa/levodopa: Carbidopa/levodopa did not influence the pharmacokinetics of pramipexole in healthy volunteers (N=10). Pramipexole did not alter the extent of absorption (AUC) or the elimination of carbidopa/levodopa, although it caused an increase in levodopa C_{max} by about 40% and a decrease in T_{max} from 2.5 to 0.5 hours.

Selegiline: In healthy volunteers (N=11), selegiline did not influence the pharmacokinetics of pramipexole.

Amantadine: Population pharmacokinetic analysis suggests that amantadine is unlikely to alter the oral clearance of pramipexole (N=54).

Cimetidine: Cimetidine, a known inhibitor of renal tubular secretion of organic bases via the cationic transport system, caused a 50% increase in pramipexole AUC and a 40% increase in half-life (N=12).

Probenecid: Probenecid, a known inhibitor of renal tubular secretion of organic acids via the anionic transporter, did not noticeably influence pramipexole pharmacokinetics (N=12).

Other drugs eliminated via renal secretion: Population pharmacokinetic analysis suggests that coadministration of drugs that are secreted by the cationic transport system (eg, cimetidine, ranitidine, diltiazem, triamterene, verapamil, quinidine, and quinine) decreases the oral clearance of pramipexole by about 20%, while those secreted by the anionic transport system (eg, cephalosporins, penicillins, indomethacin, hydrochlorothiazide, and chlorpropamide) are likely to have little effect on the oral clearance of pramipexole.

CYP interactions: Inhibitors of cytochrome P450 enzymes would not be expected to affect pramipexole elimination because pramipexole is not appreciably metabolized by these enzymes in vivo or in vitro. Pramipexole does not inhibit CYP enzymes CYP1A2, CYP2C9, CYP2C19, CYP2E1, and CYP3A4. Inhibition of CYP2D6 was observed with an apparent Ki of 30 µM, indicating that pramipexole will not inhibit CYP enzymes at plasma concentrations observed following the highest recommended clinical dose (1.5 mg tid).

Dopamine antagonists: Since pramipexole is a dopamine agonist, it is possible that dopamine antagonists, such as the neuroleptics (phenothiazines, butyrophenones, thioxanthenes) or metoclopramide, may diminish the effectiveness of MIRAPEX.

Drug/Laboratory Test Interactions: There are no known interactions between MIRAPEX and laboratory tests.

Carcinogenesis, Mutagenesis, Impairment of Fertility: Two-year carcinogenicity studies with pramipexole have been conducted in mice and rats. Pramipexole was administered in the diet to Chbb:NMRI mice at doses of 0.3, 2, and 10 mg/kg/day (0.3, 2.2, and 11 times the highest recommended clinical dose [1.5 mg tid] on a mg/m^2 basis). Pramipexole was administered in the diet to Wistar rats at 0.3, 2, and 8 mg/kg/day (plasma AUCs equal to 0.3, 2.5, and 12.5 times the AUC in humans receiving 1.5 mg tid). No significant increases in tumors occurred in either species.

Pramipexole was not mutagenic or clastogenic in a battery of assays, including the in vitro Ames assay, V79 gene mutation assay for HGPRT mutants, chromosomal aberration assay in Chinese hamster ovary cells, and in vivo mouse micronucleus assay.

In rat fertility studies, pramipexole at a dose of 2.5 mg/kg/day (5.4 times the highest clinical dose on a mg/m^2 basis), prolonged estrus cycles and inhibited implantation. These effects were associated with reductions in serum levels of prolactin, a hormone necessary for implantation and maintenance of early pregnancy in rats.

Pregnancy: Pregnancy Category C. When pramipexole was given to female rats throughout pregnancy, implantation was inhibited at a dose of 2.5 mg/kg/day (5.4 times the highest clinical dose on a mg/m^2 basis). Administration of 1.5 mg/kg/day of pramipexole to pregnant rats during the period of organogenesis (gestation days 7 through 16) resulted in a high incidence of total resorption of embryos. The plasma AUC in rats dosed at this level was 4.3 times the AUC in humans receiving 1.5 mg tid. These findings are thought to be due to the prolactin-lowering effect of pramipexole, since prolactin is necessary for implantation and maintenance of early pregnancy in rats (but not rabbits or humans). Because of pregnancy disruption and early embryonic loss in these studies, the teratogenic potential of pramipexole could not be adequately evaluated. There was no evidence of adverse effects on embryo-fetal development following administration of up to 10 mg/kg/day to pregnant rabbits during organogenesis (plasma AUC was 71 times that in humans receiving 1.5 mg tid). Postnatal growth was inhibited in the offspring of rats treated with 0.5 mg/kg/day (approximately equivalent to the highest clinical dose on a mg/m^2 basis) or greater during the latter part of pregnancy and throughout lactation.

There are no studies of pramipexole in human pregnancy. Because animal reproduction studies are not always predictive of human response, pramipexole should be used during pregnancy only if the potential benefit outweighs the potential risk to the fetus.

Nursing Mothers: A single-dose, radio-labeled study showed that drug-related materials were excreted into the breast milk of lactating rats. Concentrations of radioactivity in milk were three to six times higher than concentrations in plasma at equivalent time points.

Other studies have shown that pramipexole treatment resulted in an inhibition of prolactin secretion in humans and rats.

It is not known whether this drug is excreted in human milk. Because many drugs are excreted in human milk and because of the potential for serious adverse reactions in nursing infants from pramipexole, a decision should be made as to whether to discontinue nursing or to discontinue the drug, taking into account the importance of the drug to the mother.

Pediatric Use: The safety and efficacy of MIRAPEX in pediatric patients has not been established.

Geriatric Use: Pramipexole total oral clearance was approximately 30% lower in subjects older than 65 years compared with younger subjects, because of a decline in pramipexole renal clearance due to an age-related reduction in renal function. This resulted in an increase in elimination half-life from approximately 8.5 hours to 12 hours. In clinical studies, 38.7% of patients were older than 65 years. There were no apparent differences in efficacy or safety between older and younger patients, except that the relative risk of hallucination associated with the use of MIRAPEX was increased in the elderly.

ADVERSE EVENTS

During the premarketing development of pramipexole, patients with either early or advanced Parkinson's disease were enrolled in clinical trials. Apart from the severity and duration of their disease, the two populations differed in their use of concomitant levodopa therapy. Patients with early disease did not receive concomitant levodopa therapy during treatment with pramipexole; those with advanced Parkinson's disease all received concomitant levodopa treatment. Because these two populations may have differential risks for various adverse events, this section will, in general, present adverse-event data for these two populations separately.

Because the controlled trials performed during premarketing development all used a titration design, with a resultant confounding of time and dose, it was impossible to adequately evaluate the effects of dose on the incidence of adverse events.

Early Parkinson's Disease

In the three double-blind, placebo-controlled trials of patients with early Parkinson's disease, the most commonly observed adverse events (>5%) that were numerically more frequent in the group treated with MIRAPEX Tablets were nausea, dizziness, somnolence, insomnia, constipation, asthenia, and hallucinations.

Approximately 12% of 388 patients with early Parkinson's disease and treated with MIRAPEX who participated in the double-blind, placebo-controlled trials discontinued treatment due to adverse events compared with 11% of 235 patients who received placebo. The adverse events most commonly causing discontinuation of treatment were related to the nervous system (hallucinations [3.1% on MIRAPEX vs 0.4% on placebo]; dizziness [2.1% on MIRAPEX vs 1% on placebo]; somnolence [1.6% on MIRAPEX vs 0% on placebo]; extrapyramidal syndrome [1.6% on MIRAPEX vs 6.4% on placebo]; headache and confusion [1.3% and 1.0%, respectively, on MIRAPEX vs 0% on placebo]); and gastrointestinal system (nausea [2.1% on MIRAPEX vs 0.4% on placebo]).

Continued on next page

Mirapex—Cont.

Adverse-event incidence in controlled clinical studies in early Parkinson's disease: Table 1 lists treatment-emergent adverse events that occurred in the double-blind, placebo-controlled studies in early Parkinson's disease that were reported by ≥1% of patients treated with MIRAPEX and were numerically more frequent than in the placebo group. In these studies, patients did not receive concomitant levodopa. Adverse events were usually mild or moderate in intensity.

The prescriber should be aware that these figures cannot be used to predict the incidence of adverse events in the course of usual medical practice where patient characteristics and other factors differ from those that prevailed in the clinical studies. Similarly, the cited frequencies cannot be compared with figures obtained from other clinical investigations involving different treatments, uses, and investigators. However, the cited figures do provide the prescribing physician with some basis for estimating the relative contribution of drug and nondrug factors to the adverse-event incidence rate in the population studied.

Table 1
Treatment-Emergent Adverse-Event* Incidence in Double-Blind, Placebo-Controlled Trials in Early Parkinson's Disease (Events ≥1% of Patients Treated With MIRAPEX and Numerically More Frequent Than in the Placebo Group)

Body System/ Adverse Event	MIRAPEX N=388	Placebo N=235
Body as a Whole		
Asthenia	14	12
General edema	5	3
Malaise	2	1
Reaction unevaluable	2	1
Fever	1	0
Digestive System		
Nausea	28	18
Constipation	14	6
Anorexia	4	2
Dysphagia	2	0
Metabolic & Nutritional System		
Peripheral edema	5	4
Decreased weight	2	0
Nervous System		
Dizziness	25	24
Somnolence	22	9
Insomnia	17	12
Hallucinations	9	3
Confusion	4	1
Amnesia	4	2
Hypesthesia	3	1
Dystonia	2	1
Akathisia	2	0
Thinking abnormalities	2	0
Decreased libido	1	0
Myoclonus	1	0
Special Senses		
Vision abnormalities	3	0
Urogenital System		
Impotence	2	1

*Patients may have reported multiple adverse experiences during the study or at discontinuation; thus, patients may be included in more than one category.

Other events reported by 1% or more of patients with early Parkinson's disease and treated with MIRAPEX but reported equally or more frequently in the placebo group were infection, accidental injury, headache, pain, tremor, back pain, syncope, postural hypotension, hypertonia, depression, abdominal pain, anxiety, dyspepsia, flatulence, diarrhea, rash, ataxia, dry mouth, extrapyramidal syndrome, leg cramps, twitching, pharyngitis, sinusitis, sweating, rhinitis, urinary tract infection, vasodilation, flu syndrome, increased saliva, tooth disease, dyspnea, increased cough, gait abnormalities, urinary frequency, vomiting, allergic reaction, hypertension, pruritis, hypokinesia, increased creatine PK, nervousness, dream abnormalities, chest pain, neck pain, paresthesia, tachycardia, vertigo, voice alteration, conjunctivitis, paralysis, accommodation abnormalities, tinnitus, diplopia, and taste perversions.

In a fixed-dose study in early Parkinson's disease, occurrence of the following events increased in frequency as the dose increased over the range from 1.5 mg/day to 6 mg/day: postural hypotension, nausea, constipation, somnolence, and amnesia. The frequency of these events was generally 2-fold greater than placebo for pramipexole doses greater than 3 mg/day. The incidence of somnolence with pramipexole at a dose of 1.5 mg/day was comparable to that reported for placebo.

Advanced Parkinson's Disease

In the four double-blind, placebo-controlled trials of patients with advanced Parkinson's disease, the most commonly observed adverse events (>5%) that were numerically more frequent in the group treated with MIRAPEX and concomitant levodopa were postural (orthostatic) hypotension, dyskinesia, extrapyramidal syndrome, insomnia, dizziness, hallucinations, accidental injury, dream abnormalities, confusion, constipation, asthenia, somnolence, dystonia, gait abnormality, hypertonia, dry mouth, amnesia, and urinary frequency.

Approximately 12% of 260 patients with advanced Parkinson's disease who received MIRAPEX and concomitant levodopa in the double-blind, placebo-controlled trials discontinued treatment due to adverse events compared with 16% of 264 patients who received placebo and concomitant levodopa. The events most commonly causing discontinuation of treatment were related to the nervous system (hallucinations [2.7% on MIRAPEX vs 0.4% on placebo]; dyskinesia [1.9% on MIRAPEX vs 0.8% on placebo]; extrapyramidal syndrome [1.5% on MIRAPEX vs 4.9% on placebo]; dizziness [1.2% on MIRAPEX vs 1.5% on placebo]; confusion [1.2% on MIRAPEX vs 2.3% on placebo]); and cardiovascular system (postural [orthostatic] hypotension [2.3% on MIRAPEX vs 1.1% on placebo]).

Adverse-event incidence in controlled clinical studies in advanced Parkinson's disease: Table 2 lists treatment-emergent adverse events that occurred in the double-blind, placebo-controlled studies in advanced Parkinson's disease that were reported by ≥1% of patients treated with MIRAPEX and were numerically more frequent than in the placebo group. In these studies, MIRAPEX or placebo was administered to patients who were also receiving concomitant levodopa. Adverse events were usually mild or moderate in intensity.

The prescriber should be aware that these figures cannot be used to predict the incidence of adverse events in the course of usual medical practice where patient characteristics and other factors differ from those that prevailed in the clinical studies. Similarly, the cited frequencies cannot be compared with figures obtained from other clinical investigations involving different treatments, uses, and investigators. However, the cited figures do provide the prescribing physician with some basis for estimating the relative contribution of drug and nondrug factors to the adverse-events incidence rate in the population studied.

Table 2
Treatment-Emergent Adverse-Event* Incidence in Double-Blind, Placebo-Controlled Trials in Advanced Parkinson's Disease (Events ≥ 1% of Patients Treated With MIRAPEX and Numerically More Frequent Than in the Placebo Group)

Body System/ Adverse Event	MIRAPEX† N=260	Placebo† N=264
Body as a Whole		
Accidental injury	17	15
Asthenia	10	8
General edema	4	3
Chest pain	3	2
Malaise	3	2
Cardiovascular System		
Postural hypotension	53	48
Digestive System		
Constipation	10	9
Dry mouth	7	3
Metabolic & Nutritional System		
Peripheral edema	2	1
Increased creatine PK	1	0
Musculoskeletal System		
Arthritis	3	1
Twitching	2	0
Bursitis	2	0
Myasthenia	1	0
Nervous System		
Dyskinesia	47	31
Extrapyramidal syndrome	28	26
Insomnia	27	22
Dizziness	26	25
Hallucinations	17	4
Dream abnormalities	11	10
Confusion	10	7
Somnolence	9	6
Dystonia	8	7
Gait abnormalities	7	5
Hypertonia	7	6
Amnesia	6	4
Akathisia	3	2
Thinking abnormalities	3	2
Paranoid reaction	2	0
Delusions	1	0
Sleep disorders	1	0
Respiratory System		
Dyspnea	4	3
Rhinitis	3	1
Pneumonia	2	0
Skin & Appendages		
Skin disorders	2	1
Special Senses		
Accommodation abnormalities	4	2
Vision abnormalities	3	1
Diplopia	1	0
Urogenital System		
Urinary frequency	6	3
Urinary tract infection	4	3
Urinary incontinence	2	1

*Patients may have reported multiple adverse experiences during the study or at discontinuation; thus, patients may be included in more than one category.
† Patients received concomitant levodopa.

Other events reported by 1% or more of patients with advanced Parkinson's disease and treated with MIRAPEX but reported equally or more frequently in the placebo group were nausea, pain, infection, headache, depression, tremor, hypokinesia, anorexia, back pain, dyspepsia, flatulence, ataxia, flu syndrome, sinusitis, diarrhea, myalgia, abdominal pain, anxiety, rash, paresthesia, hypertension, increased saliva, tooth disorder, apathy, hypotension, sweating, vasodilation, vomiting, increased cough, nervousness, pruritus, hypesthesia, neck pain, syncope, arthralgia, dysphagia, palpitations, pharyngitis, vertigo, leg cramps, conjunctivitis, and lacrimation disorders.

Adverse Events; Relationship to Age, Gender, and Race: Among the treatment-emergent adverse events in patients treated with MIRAPEX, hallucination appeared to exhibit a positive relationship to age. No gender-related differences were observed. Only a small percentage (4%) of patients enrolled were non-Caucasian, therefore, an evaluation of adverse events related to race is not possible.

Other Adverse Events Observed During All Phase 2 and 3 Clinical Trials: MIRAPEX has been administered to 1,408 individuals during all clinical trials (Parkinson's disease and other patient populations), 648 of whom were in seven double-blind, placebo-controlled Parkinson's disease trials. During these trials, all adverse events were recorded by the clinical investigators using terminology of their own choosing. To provide a meaningful estimate of the proportion of individuals having adverse events, similar types of events were grouped into a smaller number of standardized categories using modified COSTART dictionary terminology. These categories are used in the listing below. The events listed below occurred in less than 1% of the 1,408 individuals exposed to MIRAPEX and occurred on at least two occasions (on one occasion if the event was serious). All reported events, except those already listed above, are included, without regard to determination of a causal relationship to MIRAPEX.

Events are listed within body-system categories in order of decreasing frequency.

Body as a whole: enlarged abdomen, death, fever, suicide attempt.

Cardiovascular system: peripheral vascular disease, myocardial infarction, angina pectoris, atrial fibrillation, heart failure, arrhythmia, atrial arrhythmia, pulmonary embolism.

Digestive system: thirst.

Musculoskeletal system: joint disorder, myasthenia.

Nervous system: agitation, CNS stimulation, hyperkinesia, psychosis, convulsions.

Respiratory system: pneumonia.

Special senses: cataract, eye disorder, glaucoma.

Urogenital system: dysuria, abnormal ejaculation, prostate cancer, hematuria, prostate disorder.

Falling Asleep During Activities of Daily Living: Patients treated with MIRAPEX have reported falling asleep while engaged in activities of daily living, including operation of a motor vehicle which sometimes resulted in accidents (see bolded WARNING).

DRUG ABUSE AND DEPENDENCE

Pramipexole is not a controlled substance.

Pramipexole has not been systematically studied in animals or humans for its potential for abuse, tolerance, or physical dependence. However, in a rat model on cocaine self-administration, pramipexole had little or no effect.

OVERDOSAGE

There is no clinical experience with massive overdosage. One patient, with a 10-year history of schizophrenia, took 11 mg/day of pramipexole for 2 days; this is two to three times the protocol recommended daily dose. No adverse events were reported related to the increased dose. Blood pressure remained stable although pulse rate increased to between 100 and 120 beats/minute. The patient withdrew from the study at the end of week 2 due to lack of efficacy. There is no known antidote for overdosage of a dopamine agonist. If signs of central nervous system stimulation are present, a phenothiazine or other butyrophenone neuroleptic agent may be indicated; the efficacy of such drugs in reversing the effects of overdosage has not been assessed. Management of overdose may require general supportive measures along with gastric lavage, intravenous fluids, and electrocardiogram monitoring.

DOSAGE AND ADMINISTRATION

In all clinical studies, dosage was initiated at a subtherapeutic level to avoid intolerable adverse effects and orthostatic hypotension. MIRAPEX should be titrated gradually in all patients. The dosage should be increased to achieve a maximum therapeutic effect, balanced against the principal side effects of dyskinesia, hallucinations, somnolence, and dry mouth.

Dosing in Patients With Normal Renal Function

Initial Treatment: Dosages should be increased gradually from a starting dose of 0.375 mg/day given in three divided doses and should not be increased more frequently than every 5 to 7 days. A suggested ascending dosage schedule that was used in clinical studies is shown in the following table:

Ascending Dosage Schedule of MIRAPEX

Week	Dosage (mg)	Total Daily Dose (mg)
1	0.125 tid	0.375
2	0.25 tid	0.75
3	0.5 tid	1.50
4	0.75 tid	2.25
5	1.0 tid	3.0
6	1.25 tid	3.75
7	1.5 tid	4.50

Maintenance Treatment: MIRAPEX Tablets were effective and well tolerated over a dosage range of 1.5 to 4.5 mg/day administered in equally divided doses three times per day with or without concomitant levodopa (approximately 800 mg/day).

In a fixed-dose study in early Parkinson's disease patients, doses of 3 mg, 4.5 mg, and 6 mg per day of MIRAPEX were not shown to provide any significant benefit beyond that achieved at a daily dose of 1.5 mg/day. However, in the same fixed-dose study, the following adverse events were dose related: postural hypotension, nausea, constipation, somnolence, and amnesia. The frequency of these events was generally 2-fold greater than placebo for pramipexole doses greater than 3 mg/day. The incidence of somnolence reported with pramipexole at a dose of 1.5 mg/day was comparable to placebo.

When MIRAPEX is used in combination with levodopa, a reduction of the levodopa dosage should be considered. In a controlled study in advanced Parkinson's disease, the dosage of levodopa was reduced by an average of 27% from baseline.

Patients with Renal Impairment

Pramipexole Dosage in the Renally Impaired

Renal Status	Starting Dose (mg)	Maximum Dose (mg)
Normal to mild impairment (creatinine Cl > 60 mL/min)	0.125 tid	1.5 tid
Moderate impairment (creatinine Cl = 35 to 59 mL/min)	0.125 bid	1.5 bid
Severe impairment (creatinine Cl = 15 to 34 mL/min)	0.125 qd	1.5 qd
Very severe impairment (creatinine Cl < 15 mL/min and hemodialysis patients)	The use of MIRAPEX has not been adequately studied in this group of patients.	

Discontinuation of Treatment: It is recommended that MIRAPEX be discontinued over a period of 1 week; in some studies, however, abrupt discontinuation was uneventful.

HOW SUPPLIED

MIRAPEX Tablets are available as follows:

0.125 mg: white, round tablet with "U" on one side and "2" on the reverse side.
Bottles of 63 NDC 0009-0002-02

0.25 mg: white, oval, scored tablet with "U" twice on one side and "4" twice on the reverse side.
Bottles of 90 NDC 0009-0004-02
Unit dose packages of 100 NDC 0009-0004-06

0.5 mg: white, oval, scored tablet with "U" twice on one side and "8" twice on the reverse side.
Bottles of 90 NDC 0009-0008-02
Unit dose packages of 100 NDC 0009-0008-03

1 mg: white, round, scored tablet with "U" twice on one side and "6" twice on the reverse side.
Bottles of 90 NDC 0009-0006-02
Unit dose packages of 100 NDC 0009-0006-06

1.5 mg: white, round, scored tablet with "U" twice on one side and "37" twice on the reverse side.
Bottles of 90 NDC 0009-0037-02
Unit dose packages of 100 NDC 0009-0037-06

Store at 25°C (77°F); excursions permitted to 15°–30°C (59°–86°F) [see USP Controlled Room Temperature]. Protect from light.

℞ only

ANIMAL TOXICOLOGY

Retinal Pathology in Albino Rats

Pathologic changes (degeneration and loss of photoreceptor cells) were observed in the retina of albino rats in the 2-year carcinogenicity study with pramipexole. These findings were first observed during week 76 and were dose dependent in animals receiving 2 or 8 mg/kg/day (plasma AUCs equal to 2.5 and 12.5 times the AUC in humans that received 1.5 mg tid). In a similar study of pigmented rats with 2 years exposure to pramipexole at 2 or 8 mg/kg/day, retinal degeneration was not diagnosed. Animals given drug had thinning in the outer nuclear layer of the retina that was only slightly greater than that seen in control rats utilizing morphometry.

Investigative studies demonstrated that pramipexole reduced the rate of disk shedding from the photoreceptor rod cells of the retina in albino rats, which was associated with enhanced sensitivity to the damaging effects of light. In a comparative study, degeneration and loss of photoreceptor cells occurred in albino rats after 13 weeks of treatment with 25 mg/kg/day of pramipexole (54 times the highest clinical dose on a mg/m^2 basis) and constant light (100 lux) but not in pigmented rats exposed to the same dose and higher light intensities (500 lux). Thus, the retina of albino rats is considered to be uniquely sensitive to the damaging effects of pramipexole and light. Similar changes in the retina did not occur in a 2-year carcinogenicity study in albino mice treated with 0.3, 2, or 10 mg/kg/day (0.3, 2.2 and 11 times the highest clinical dose on a mg/m^2 basis). Evaluation of the retinas of monkeys given 0.1, 0.5, or 2.0 mg/kg/day of pramipexole (0.4, 2.2, and 8.6 times the highest clinical dose on a mg/m^2 basis) for 12 months and minipigs given 0.3, 1, or 5 mg/kg/day of pramipexole for 13 weeks also detected no changes.

The potential significance of this effect in humans has not been established, but cannot be disregarded because disruption of a mechanism that is universally present in vertebrates (ie, disk shedding) may be involved.

Fibro-osseous Proliferative Lesions in Mice

An increased incidence of fibro-osseous proliferative lesions occurred in the femurs of female mice treated for 2 years with 0.3, 2.0, or 10 mg/kg/day (0.3, 2.2, and 11 times the highest clinical dose on a mg/m^2 basis). Lesions occurred at a lower rate in control animals. Similar lesions were not observed in male mice or rats and monkeys of either sex that were treated chronically with pramipexole. The significance of this lesion to humans is not known.

Pharmacia & Upjohn Company
A subsidiary of Pharmacia Corporation
Kalamazoo, Michigan 49001, USA
Revised June 2003 817 017 208
692167

Shown in Product Identification Guide, page 330

R-GENE® 10 ℞

[r-jĕn]

10% Arginine Hydrochloride Injection, USP
For Intravenous Use

DESCRIPTION

Each 100 mL of R-Gene® 10 (10% Arginine Hydrochloride Injection, USP) for intravenous use contains 10 g of L-Arginine Hydrochloride, USP in Water for Injection, USP. L-arginine is a naturally occurring amino acid.

R-Gene® 10 is hypertonic (950 mOsmol/liter) and contains 47.5 mEq of chloride ion per 100 mL of solution. The pH is adjusted to 5.6 (5.0-6.5) with arginine base or hydrochloric acid.

CLINICAL PHARMACOLOGY

Intravenous infusion of R-Gene® 10 often induces a pronounced rise in the plasma level of human growth hormone (HGH) in subjects with intact pituitary function. This rise is usually diminished or absent in patients with impairment of this function.

Expected Plasma Levels of HGH in ng/mL

Patient	Control Range	Range of Peak Response to Arginine
Normal	0-6	10-30
Pituitary deficient	0-4	0-10

These ranges are based on the mean values of plasma HGH levels calculated from the data of several clinical investigators and reflect their experiences with various methods of radioimmunoassay. Upon gaining experience with this diagnostic test, each clinician will establish his/her own ranges for control and peak levels of HGH.

L-arginine is a normal metabolite in animals and man and has a low order of toxicity.

INDICATIONS AND USAGE

R-Gene® 10 is indicated as an intravenous stimulant to the pituitary for the release of human growth hormone in patients where the measurement of pituitary reserve for HGH can be of diagnostic usefulness. It can be used as a diagnostic aid in such conditions as panhypopituitarism, pituitary dwarfism, chromophobe adenoma, postsurgical craniopharyngioma, hypophysectomy, pituitary trauma, acromegaly, gigantism and problems of growth and stature.

If the insulin hypoglycemia test has indicated a deficiency of pituitary reserve for HGH, a test with R-Gene® 10 is advisable to confirm the negative response. This can be done after a waiting period of one day. As patients may not respond to R-Gene® 10 (10% Arginine Hydrochloride Injection, USP) during the first test, the unresponsive patient should be tested again to confirm the negative result. A second test can be performed after a waiting period of one day. Some patients who respond to R-Gene® 10 do not respond to insulin and vice versa. The rate of false positive responses for R-Gene® 10 is approximately 32%, and the rate of false negatives is approximately 27%.

CONTRAINDICATIONS

The administration of R-Gene® 10 is contraindicated in persons having highly allergic tendencies.

WARNINGS

There have been two reports of possible overdosage of R-Gene® 10 in children. EXTREME CAUTION MUST BE EXERCISED WHEN INFUSING R-GENE® 10 INTO PEDIATRIC PATIENTS. OVERDOSAGE OF R-GENE® 10 IN PEDIATRIC PATIENTS CAN RESULT IN HYPERCHLOREMIC METABOLIC ACIDOSIS, CEREBRAL EDEMA, OR POSSIBLY DEATH.

R-Gene® 10 should always be administered by intravenous injection because of its hypertonicity.

A suitable antihistaminic drug should be available in the event that an allergic reaction occurs.

R-Gene® 10 is a diagnostic aid and is not intended for therapeutic use.

PRECAUTIONS

General

R-Gene® 10 is a hypertonic (950 mOsmol/liter) and acidic (average pH of 5.6) solution that can irritate tissues. Care should be used to insure administration of R-Gene® 10 through a patent catheter within a patent vein. Excessive rates of infusion may result in local irritation and in flushing, nausea, or vomiting. Inadequate dosing or prolongation of the infusion period may diminish the stimulus to the pituitary and nullify the test.

The arginine in R-Gene® 10 can be metabolized resulting in nitrogen-containing products for excretion. The effect of an acute amino acid or nitrogen burden upon patients with impairment of renal function should be considered when R-Gene® 10 is to be administered.

The chloride content of R-Gene® 10 is 47.5 mEq per 100 mL of solution, and the effect of infusing this amount of chloride into patients with electrolyte imbalance should be evaluated before the test is undertaken.

It should be noted that the basal and post stimulation levels of growth hormone are elevated in patients who are pregnant or are taking oral contraceptives.

Carcinogenesis, mutagenesis, and impairment of fertility

Long term animal studies have not been performed to evaluate the carcinogenic potential, the mutagenic potential or the effect on fertility of intravenously administered R-Gene® 10.

Pregnancy Category B

Reproduction studies have been performed in rabbits and mice at doses 12 times the human dose and have revealed no evidence of impaired fertility or harm to the fetus due to R-Gene® 10 (10% Arginine Hydrochloride Injection, USP). There have been no adequate or well controlled studies for the use of R-Gene® 10 in pregnant women. Because animal reproduction studies are not always predictive of human response, this drug should not be used during pregnancy.

Continued on next page

R-Gene 10—Cont.

Nursing Mothers

It is not known whether intravenous administration of R-Gene® 10 could result in significant quantities of arginine in breast milk. Systemically administered amino acids are secreted into breast milk in quantities not likely to have a deleterious effect on the infant. Nevertheless, caution should be exercised when R-Gene® 10 is to be administered to nursing women.

Geriatric Use

Clinical studies of arginine did not include a sufficient number of subjects aged 65 and over to determine whether they respond differently from younger subjects. Other reported clinical experience has not identified differences in responses between the elderly and younger patients.

ADVERSE REACTIONS

Adverse reactions associated with 1670 infusions in premarketing studies were as follows:

Non-specific side effects consisting of nausea, vomiting, headache, flushing, numbness and local venous irritation were reported in approximately 3% of the patients.

One patient had an allergic reaction which was manifested as a confluent macular rash with reddening and swelling of the hands and face. The rash subsided rapidly after the infusion was terminated and 50 mg of diphenhydramine were administered. One patient had an apparent decrease in platelet count from 150,000 to 60,000. One patient with a history of acrocyanosis had an exacerbation of this condition following infusion of R-Gene® 10.

OVERDOSAGE

An overdosage may cause a transient metabolic acidosis with hyperventilation. The acidosis will be compensated and the base deficit will return to normal following completion of the infusion. If the condition persists, the deficit should be determined and corrected by a calculated dose of an alkalizing agent. See "WARNINGS" for information about overdosage in pediatric patients.

DOSAGE AND ADMINISTRATION

The intravenous dose for adults is 300 mL (30 g arginine hydrochloride) of R-Gene® 10. The intravenous dose for children is 5 mL (0.5 g arginine hydrochloride) per kilogram of body weight of R-Gene® 10.

The intravenous infusion of R-Gene® 10 is a part of the test for measurement of pituitary reserve of human growth hormone and, for successful administration of the test, clinical conditions and procedures should be as follows:

1. The test should be scheduled in the morning following a normal night's sleep, and an overnight fast should continue through the test period.
2. Patients must be placed at bed rest for at least 30 minutes before the infusion begins. Care should be taken to minimize apprehension and distress. This is particularly important in children.
3. R-Gene® 10 (10% Arginine Hydrochloride Injection, USP) should be infused through an indwelling needle or soft catheter placed in an antecubital vein or other suitable vein. Blood samples should be taken by venipuncture from the contra-lateral arm.
4. A desirable schedule for drawing blood samples is at –30, 0, 30, 60, 90, 120 and 150 minutes.
5. R-Gene® 10 should be infused beginning at zero time at a uniform rate which will permit the recommended dose to be administered in 30 minutes.
6. Blood samples should be promptly centrifuged and the plasma stored at –20°C until assayed by one of the published radioimmunoassay procedures.
7. Diagnostic test results showing a deficiency of pituitary reserve for HGH should be confirmed by a second test with R-Gene® 10, or one may elect to confirm with the insulin hypoglycemia test. A waiting period of one day is advised between tests.

Parenteral drug products should be inspected visually for particulate matter and discoloration prior to administration whenever solution and container permit.

HOW SUPPLIED

R-Gene® 10 is supplied as a 300 mL fill in 500 mL containers.

NDC 0009-0436-24

Exposure of pharmaceutical products to heat should be minimized. Avoid excessive heat. It is recommended that the product be stored at room temperature (25°C); however, brief exposure up to 40°C does not adversely affect the product. Solution that has been frozen must not be used.

Manufactured for
Pharmacia & Upjohn Company
A subsidiary of Pharmacia Corporation
Kalamazoo, Michigan 49001, USA
By
Fresenius Kabi Clayton, L.P.
Clayton, NC 27520 USA
R-Gene® is a registered trademark of Pharmacia AB.

Directions for Use of I.V. Container

The important feature of this container is that **it is a closed system.** That is, **no** unfiltered air comes in contact with the solution. The spike is thrust through a solid stopper, the air enters through a bacterial air filter, and only filtered air enters the bottle then or during the infusion. The rubber stopper surface beneath the metal seal is sterile.

A special air-inletting, air-filtering set with a bacterial air filter is required. **No airway needle is needed.**

1. **Use only if solution is clear and seal is intact.** Carefully examine bottle for evidence of damage, e.g., dents or other evidence of damage to metal cap, small cracks, dents in seal, or areas of dried powder on exterior. **Do not administer contents if such damage is found.**
2. Remove tamperproof metal seal and metal disc from bottle to expose rubber stopper, taking care that you do not contaminate the target site of the stopper with fingers, hair, clothing, etc. **Immediately** perform step #3.
3. With shut-off clamp closed, remove sterility protector from spike of administration set and immediately insert set with a quick thrust into center of stopper with bottle upright on table. (Push straight in — don't twist — twisting may cause stopper coring.)
4. Promptly invert bottle to automatically establish fluid level in drip chamber and to check for vacuum by observing rising filtered air bubbles. **Discard bottle if there is no vacuum or if the solution is not clear.**
5. Clear tubing of air. Proceed with infusion.

CAUTION: While the top of the rubber stopper is sterile, as soon as the seal and disc are removed the stopper is exposed. The longer the time between removal of the seal and disc and the piercing of the stopper, the greater the chance of contamination of the stopper.

NOTE: When medication is to be added to the bottle:

A. See #1 and #2 above.

B. Add medications before attaching administration set. Vacuum should be observed at this point, by sucking in of additive container content, since vacuum may be lost during this procedure and not observable during administration set insertion.

C. If medications have been placed in bottle through stopper, it is recommended that the face of the stopper be swabbed immediately before piercing with administration set.

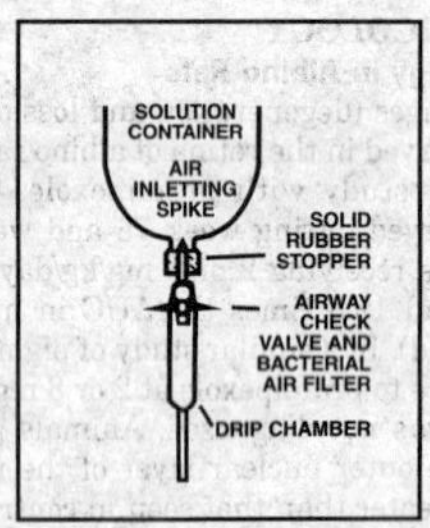

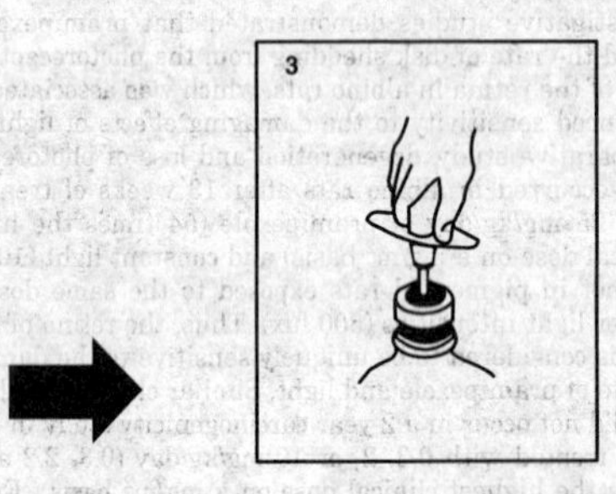

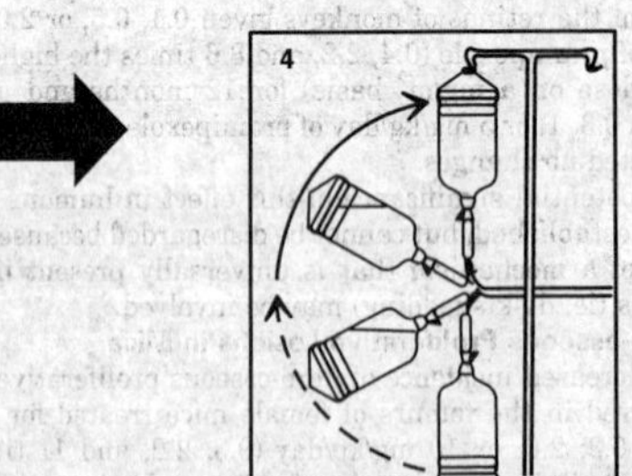

CONTINUED USE OF SOLUTIONS AND SETS

Procedure differs with every hospital for the length of time solutions and administration sets may be used continuously. Some recommend change of both every 8 hours, others recommend change of both every 24 hours, and others recommend change of solutions every 8 hours and change of sets every 24 hours. The shorter the period of use the less the possibility of multiplication of organisms inadvertently introduced.

74-3624-16
(Revised August 2003)

SOMAVERT® ℞

[SOM-ah-vert]
pegvisomant for injection
℞ only

DESCRIPTION

SOMAVERT contains pegvisomant for injection, an analog of human growth hormone (GH) that has been structurally altered to act as a GH receptor antagonist.

Pegvisomant is a protein of recombinant DNA origin containing 191 amino acid residues to which several polyethylene glycol (PEG) polymers are covalently bound (predominantly 4 to 6 PEG/protein molecule). The molecular weight of the protein of pegvisomant is 21,998 Daltons. The molecular weight of the PEG portion of pegvisomant is approximately 5000 Daltons. The predominant molecular weights of pegvisomant are thus approximately 42,000, 47,000, and 52,000 Daltons. The schematic shows the amino acid sequence of the pegvisomant protein (PEG polymers are shown attached to the 5 most probable attachment sites). Pegvisomant is synthesized by a specific strain of *Escherichia coli* bacteria that has been genetically modified by the addition of a plasmid that carries a gene for GH receptor antagonist. Biological potency is determined using a cell proliferation bioassay.

[See graphic at top of next page]

SOMAVERT is supplied as a sterile, white lyophilized powder intended for subcutaneous injection after reconstitution with 1 mL of Sterile Water for Injection, USP. SOMAVERT is available in single-dose sterile vials containing 10, 15, or 20 mg of pegvisomant protein (approximately 10, 15, and 20 U activity, respectively). Vials containing 10, 15, and 20 mg of pegvisomant protein correspond to approximately 21, 32, and 43 mg pegvisomant, respectively. Each vial also contains 1.36 mg of glycine, 36.0 mg of mannitol, 1.04 mg of sodium phosphate dibasic anhydrous, and 0.36 mg of sodium phosphate monobasic monohydrate.

SOMAVERT is supplied in packages that include a plastic vial containing diluent. Sterile Water for Injection, USP, is a sterile, nonpyrogenic preparation of water for injection that contains no bacteriostat, antimicrobial agent, or added buffer, and is supplied in single-dose containers to be used as a diluent.

CLINICAL PHARMACOLOGY

Mechanism of Action

Pegvisomant selectively binds to growth hormone (GH) receptors on cell surfaces, where it blocks the binding of endogenous GH, and thus interferes with GH signal transduction. Inhibition of GH action results in decreased serum concentrations of insulin-like growth factor-I (IGF-I), as well as other GH-responsive serum proteins, including IGF binding protein-3 (IGFBP-3), and the acid-labile subunit (ALS).

Pharmacokinetics

Absorption: Following subcutaneous administration, peak serum pegvisomant concentrations are not generally attained until 33 to 77 hours after administration. The mean extent of absorption of a 20-mg subcutaneous dose was 57%, relative to a 10-mg intravenous dose.

Distribution: The mean apparent volume of distribution of pegvisomant is 7 L (12% coefficient of variation), suggesting that pegvisomant does not distribute extensively into tissues. After a single subcutaneous administration, exposure (C_{max}, AUC) to pegvisomant increases disproportionately with increasing dose. Mean ± SEM serum pegvisomant concentrations after 12 weeks of therapy with daily doses of 10, 15, and 20 mg were 6600 ± 1330; 16,000 ± 2200; and 27,000 ± 3100 ng/mL, respectively.

Metabolism and Elimination: The pegvisomant molecule contains covalently bound polyethylene glycol polymers in order to reduce the clearance rate. Clearance of pegvisomant following multiple doses is lower than seen following a single dose. The mean total body systemic clearance of pegvisomant following multiple doses is estimated to range between 36 to 28 mL/h for subcutaneous doses ranging from 10 to 20 mg/day, respectively. Clearance of pegvisomant was found to increase with body weight. Pegvisomant is eliminated from serum with a mean half-life of approximately 6 days following either single or multiple doses. Less than 1% of administered drug is recovered in the urine over 96 hours. The elimination route of pegvisomant has not been studied in humans.

Drug-Drug Interactions

In clinical studies, patients on opioids often needed higher serum pegvisomant concentrations to achieve appropriate IGF-I suppression compared with patients not receiving opioids. The mechanism of this interaction is not known (see **PRECAUTIONS, Drug Interactions**).

Special Populations

Renal: No pharmacokinetic studies have been conducted in patients with renal insufficiency.

Hepatic: No pharmacokinetic studies have been conducted in patients with hepatic insufficiency.

Geriatric: No pharmacokinetic studies have been conducted in elderly subjects.

Pediatric: No pharmacokinetic studies have been conducted in pediatric subjects.

Gender: No gender effect on the pharmacokinetics of pegvisomant was found in a population pharmacokinetic analysis.

Race: The effect of race on the pharmacokinetics of pegvisomant has not been studied.

CLINICAL STUDIES

One hundred twelve patients with acromegaly previously treated with surgery, radiation therapy, and/or medical therapies participated in a 12-week, randomized, double-blind, multi-center study comparing placebo and SOMAVERT. Following withdrawal from previous medical therapy, the 80 patients randomized to treatment with SOMAVERT received a subcutaneous (SC) loading dose, followed by 10, 15, or 20 mg/day SC. The three groups that received SOMAVERT showed dose-dependent reductions in serum levels of IGF-I, free IGF-I, IGFBP-3, and ALS compared with placebo at all post-baseline visits (Figure 1 and Table 1).

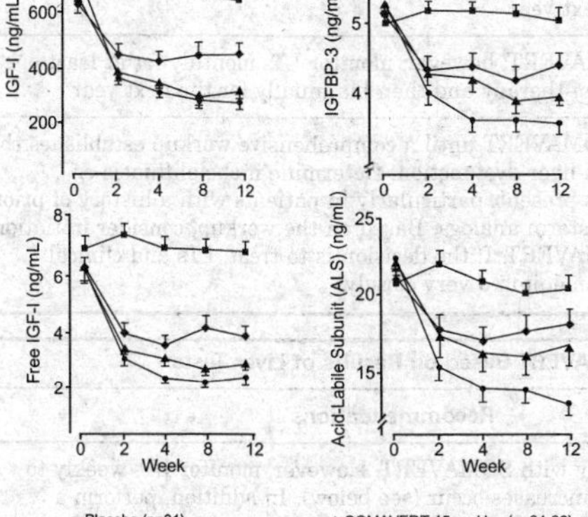

Figure 1. Effects of SOMAVERT on Serum Markers (Mean ± Standard Error)

After 12 weeks of treatment, serum IGF-I levels were normalized in 10%, 39%, 75%, and 82% of subjects treated with placebo, 10, 15, or 20 mg/day of SOMAVERT, respectively (Figure 2).

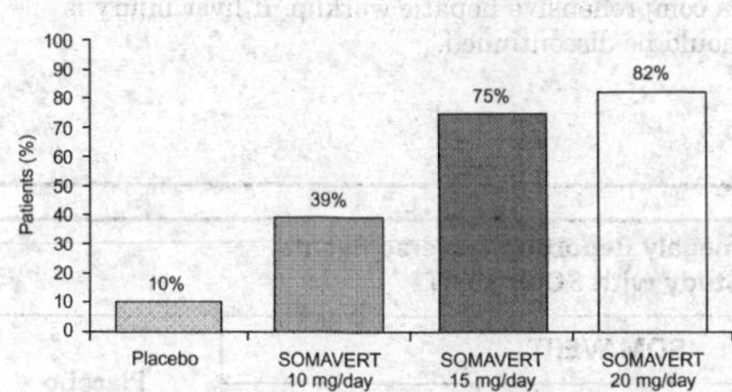

Figure 2. Percent of Patients Whose IGF-I Levels Normalized at Week 12

Table 2 shows the effect of treatment with SOMAVERT on ring size (standard jeweler's sizes converted to a numeric score ranging from 1 to 63), and on both the total and individual scores for signs and symptoms of acromegaly. Each individual score (for soft-tissue swelling, arthralgia, headache, perspiration and fatigue) was based on a nine-point ordinal rating scale (0 = absent and 8 = severe and incapacitating), and the total score was derived from the sum of the individual scores. Mean baseline scores were as follows: ring size = 47.1; total signs and symptoms = 15.2; soft tissue swelling = 2.5; arthralgia = 3.2; headache = 2.4; perspiration = 3.3; and fatigue = 3.7.

[See table 1 at right]
[See table 2 at right]

Ring size at week 12 was smaller (improved) in the groups treated with 15 or 20 mg of SOMAVERT, compared with placebo. The mean total score for signs and symptoms at week 12 was lower (improved) in each of the groups treated with SOMAVERT, compared with the group treated with placebo.

Serum growth hormone (GH) concentrations, as measured by research assays using antibodies that do not cross-react with pegvisomant (see **PRECAUTIONS Drug/Laboratory Test Interactions**), rise within two weeks of beginning treatment with SOMAVERT. The largest GH response was seen in patients treated with doses of SOMAVERT greater than 20 mg/day. This effect is presumably the result of diminished inhibition of GH secretion as IGF-I levels fall. As shown in Figure 3, when patients with acromegaly were given a loading dose of SOMAVERT followed by a fixed daily dose, this rise in GH was inversely proportional to the fall in IGF-I and generally stabilized by week 2. Serum GH concentrations also remained stable in patients treated with SOMAVERT for up to 18 months.

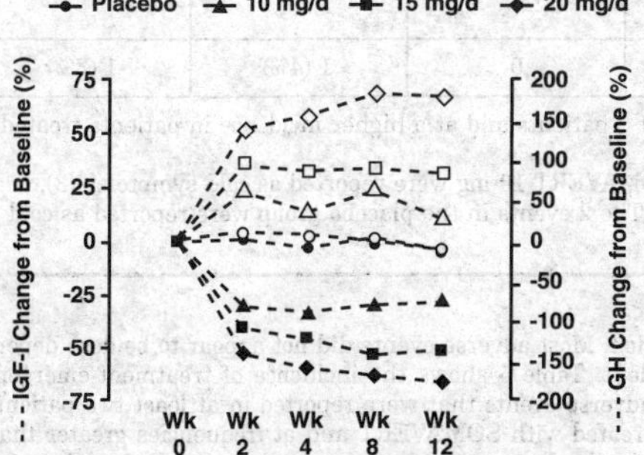

Figure 3. Percent Change in Serum GH and IGF-I Concentrations

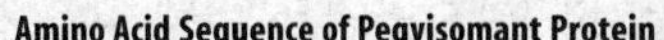

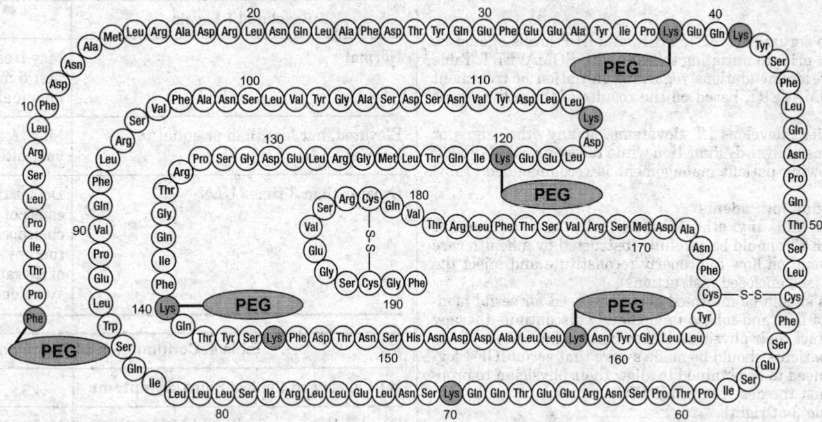

Stippled residues indicate PEG attachment sites (Phe_1, Lys_{38}, Lys_{41}, Lys_{70}, Lys_{115}, Lys_{120}, Lys_{140}, Lys_{145}, Lys_{158})

Table 1. Mean Percent Change from Baseline in IGF-I at Week 12 for Intent-to-Treat Population

	SOMAVERT			
	10 mg/day n=26	**15 mg/day n=26**	**20 mg/day n=28**	**Placebo n=31**
Mean percent change from baseline in IGF-1 (SD)	−27 (28)	−48 (26)	−63 (21)	−4.0 (17)
SOMAVERT minus Placebo (95% CI for treatment difference)	−23* (−35, −11)	−44* (−56, −33)	−59* (−68, −49)	

* P<0.01

Table 2. Mean Change from Baseline (SD) at Week 12 for Ring Size and Signs and Symptoms of Acromegaly

	SOMAVERT			
	10 mg/day n=26	**15 mg/day n=24-25**	**20 mg/day n=26-27**	**Placebo n=30**
Ring size	−0.8 (1.6)	−1.9 (2.0)	−2.5 (3.3)	−0.1 (2.3)
Total score for signs and symptoms of acromegaly	−2.5 (4.3)	−4.4 (5.9)	−4.7 (4.7)	1.3 (6.0)
Soft-tissue swelling	−0.7 (1.6)	−1.2 (2.3)	−1.3 (1.3)	0.3 (2.3)
Arthralgia	−0.3 (1.8)	−0.5 (2.5)	−0.4 (2.1)	0.1 (1.8)
Headache	−0.4 (1.6)	−0.3 (1.4)	−0.3 (2.0)	0.1 (1.7)
Perspiration	−0.6 (1.6)	−1.1 (1.3)	−1.7 (1.6)	0.1 (1.7)
Fatigue	−0.5 (1.4)	−1.3 (1.7)	−1.0 (1.6)	0.7 (0.5)

Another cohort of 38 patients with acromegaly was treated with SOMAVERT in a long-term, open-label, dose-titration study and received at least 12 consecutive months of daily dosing with SOMAVERT (mean = 55 weeks). The mean (± standard deviation) IGF-I concentration at baseline in this cohort was 917 (± 356) ng/mL after withdrawal from previous medical therapy, falling to 268 (± 134) ng/mL at the end of treatment with SOMAVERT. Thirty-five of the 38 patients (92%) achieved a normal (age-adjusted) IGF-I concentration. After the first visit at which a normal IGF-I concentration was observed, IGF-I levels remained within the normal range at 92% of all subsequent visits over a mean duration of one year.

INDICATIONS AND USAGE

SOMAVERT is indicated for the treatment of acromegaly in patients who have had an inadequate response to surgery and/or radiation therapy and/or other medical therapies, or for whom these therapies are not appropriate. The goal of treatment is to normalize serum IGF-I levels.

CONTRAINDICATIONS

SOMAVERT is contraindicated in patients with a history of hypersensitivity to any of its components. The stopper on the vial of SOMAVERT contains latex.

PRECAUTIONS

General

Tumor Growth: Tumors that secrete growth hormone (GH) may expand and cause serious complications. Therefore, all patients with these tumors, including those who are receiving SOMAVERT, should be carefully monitored with periodic imaging scans of the sella turcica. During clinical studies of SOMAVERT, two patients manifested progressive tumor growth. Both patients had, at baseline, large globular tumors impinging on the optic chiasm, which had been relatively resistant to previous anti-acromegalic therapies. Overall, mean tumor size was unchanged during the course of treatment with SOMAVERT in the clinical studies.

Glucose Metabolism: GH opposes the effects of insulin on carbohydrate metabolism by decreasing insulin sensitivity; thus, glucose tolerance may increase in some patients treated with SOMAVERT. Although none of the acromegalic patients with diabetes mellitus who were treated with SOMAVERT during the clinical studies had clinically relevant hypoglycemia, these patients should be carefully monitored and doses of anti-diabetic drugs reduced as necessary.

GH Deficiency: A state of functional GH deficiency may result from administration of SOMAVERT, despite the presence of elevated serum GH levels. Therefore, during treatment with SOMAVERT, patients should be carefully observed for the clinical signs and symptoms of a GH-deficient state, and serum IGF-I concentrations should be monitored and maintained within the age-adjusted normal range (by adjustment of the dose of SOMAVERT).

Liver Tests (LTs)

Elevations of serum concentrations of alanine aminotransferase (ALT) and aspartate aminotransferase (AST) greater than 10 times the upper limit of normal (ULN) were reported in two patients (0.8%) exposed to SOMAVERT during pre-marketing clinical studies. One patient was rechallenged with SOMAVERT, and the recurrence of elevated transaminase levels suggested a probable causal relationship between administration of the drug and the elevation in liver enzymes. A liver biopsy performed on the second patient was consistent with chronic hepatitis of unknown etiology. In both patients, the transaminase elevations normalized after discontinuation of the drug.

During the pre-marketing clinical studies, the incidence of elevations in ALT greater than 3 times but less than or equal to 10 times the ULN in patients treated with SOMAVERT and placebo were 1.2% and 2.1%, respectively. Elevations in ALT and AST levels were not associated with increased levels of serum total bilirubin (TBIL) and alkaline phosphatase (ALP), with the exception of two patients with minimal associated increases in ALP levels (i.e., less than 3 times ULN). The transaminase elevations did not appear to be related to the dose of SOMAVERT administered, generally occurred within 4 to 12 weeks of initiation of therapy, and were not associated with any identifiable biochemical, phenotypic, or genetic predictors.

Continued on next page

Somavert—Cont.

Baseline serum ALT, AST, TBIL, and ALP levels should be obtained prior to initiating therapy with SOMAVERT. Table 3 lists recommendations regarding initiation of treatment with SOMAVERT, based on the results of these liver tests (LTs).

If a patient develops LT elevations, or any other signs or symptoms of liver dysfunction while receiving SOMAVERT, the following patient management is recommended (Table 4).

Information for Patients

Patients and any other persons who may administer SOMAVERT should be carefully instructed by a health care professional on how to properly reconstitute and inject the product (see enclosed instructions).

Patients should be informed about the need for serial monitoring of LTs, and told to immediately discontinue therapy and contact their physician if they become jaundiced. In addition, patients should be made aware that serial IGF-I levels will need to be obtained to allow their physician to properly adjust the dose of SOMAVERT.

[See table 3 at right]

[See table 4 at right]

Table 3. Initiation of Treatment with SOMAVERT Based on Results of Liver Tests

Baseline LT Levels	Recommendations
Normal	May treat with SOMAVERT. Monitor LTs at monthly intervals during the first 6 months of treatment, quarterly for the next 6 months, and then biannually for the next year.
Elevated, but less than or equal to 3 times ULN	May treat with SOMAVERT; however, monitor LTs monthly for at least one year after initiation of therapy and then biannually for the next year.
Greater than 3 times ULN	Do not treat with SOMAVERT until a comprehensive workup establishes the cause of the patient's liver dysfunction. Determine if cholelithiasis or choledocholithiasis is present, particularly in patients with a history of prior therapy with somatostatin analogs. Based on the workup, consider initiation of therapy with SOMAVERT. If the decision is to treat, LTs and clinical symptoms should be monitored very closely.

Table 4. Continuation of Treatment with SOMAVERT Based on Results of Liver Tests

LT Levels and Clinical Signs/Symptoms	Recommendations
Greater than or equal to 3 but less than 5 times ULN (without signs/symptoms of hepatitis or other liver injury, or increase in serum TBIL)	May continue therapy with SOMAVERT. However, monitor LTs weekly to determine if further increases occur (see below). In addition, perform a comprehensive hepatic workup to discern if an alternative cause of liver dysfunction is present.
At least 5 times ULN, or transaminase elevations at least 3 times ULN associated with any increase in serum TBIL (with or without signs/symptoms of hepatitis or other liver injury)	Discontinue SOMAVERT immediately. Perform a comprehensive hepatic workup, including serial LTs, to determine if and when serum levels return to normal. If LTs normalize (regardless of whether an alternative cause of the liver dysfunction is discovered), consider cautious reinitiation of therapy with SOMAVERT, with frequent LT monitoring.
Signs or symptoms suggestive of hepatitis or other liver injury (e.g., jaundice, bilirubinuria, fatigue, nausea, vomiting, right upper quadrant pain, ascites, unexplained edema, easy bruisability)	Immediately perform a comprehensive hepatic workup. If liver injury is confirmed, the drug should be discontinued.

Laboratory Tests

Liver Tests: Recommendations for monitoring LTs are stated above (see **PRECAUTIONS, Liver Tests [LTs]**).

IGF-I Levels: Treatment with SOMAVERT should be evaluated by monitoring serum IGF-I concentrations four to six weeks after therapy is initiated or any dose adjustments are made and at least every six months after IGF-I levels have normalized. The goals of treatment should be to maintain a patient's serum IGF-I concentration within the age-adjusted normal range and to control the signs and symptoms of acromegaly.

GH Levels: Pegvisomant interferes with the measurement of serum GH concentrations by commercially available GH assays (see **Drug/Laboratory Test Interactions**). Furthermore, even when accurately determined, GH levels usually increase during therapy with SOMAVERT. Therefore, treatment with SOMAVERT should not be adjusted based on serum GH concentrations.

Drug Interactions

Acromegalic patients with diabetes mellitus being treated with insulin and/or oral hypoglycemic agents may require dose reductions of these therapeutic agents after the initiation of therapy with SOMAVERT.

In clinical studies, patients on opioids often needed higher serum pegvisomant concentrations to achieve appropriate IGF-I suppression compared with patients not receiving opioids. The mechanism of this interaction is not known.

Drug/Laboratory Test Interactions

Pegvisomant has significant structural similarity to GH, which causes it to cross-react in commercially available GH assays. Because serum concentrations of pegvisomant at therapeutically effective doses are generally 100 to 1000 times higher than endogenous serum GH levels seen in patients with acromegaly, commercially available GH assays will overestimate true GH levels. Treatment with SOMAVERT should therefore not be monitored or adjusted based on serum GH concentrations reported from these assays. Instead, monitoring and dose adjustments should only be based on serum IGF-I levels.

Carcinogenesis, Mutagenesis, Impairment of Fertility

Standard two-year rodent bioassays have not been performed with pegvisomant. Pegvisomant was not mutagenic in the Ames assay or clastogenic in the *in vitro* chromosomal aberration test in human lymphocytes. Pegvisomant was found to have no effect on fertility and reproductive performance of female rabbits at subcutaneous doses up to 10 mg/kg/day (10 times the maximum human therapeutic exposure based on body surface area, mg/m^2).

Pregnancy: Pregnancy Category B

Early embryonic development and teratology studies were conducted in pregnant rabbits with pegvisomant at subcutaneous doses of 1, 3, and 10 mg/kg/day.There was no evidence of teratogenic effects associated with pegvisomant treatment during organogenesis. At the 10-mg/kg/day dose (10 times the maximum human therapeutic dose based on body surface area), a reproducible, slight increase in post-implantation loss was observed in both studies. There are no adequate and well-controlled studies in pregnant women. Because animal reproduction studies are not always predictive of human responses, SOMAVERT should be used during pregnancy only if clearly needed.

Nursing Mothers

It is not known whether pegvisomant is excreted in human milk. Because many drugs are excreted in milk, caution should be exercised when SOMAVERT is administered to a nursing woman.

Pediatric Use

The safety and effectiveness of SOMAVERT in pediatric patients have not been established.

Geriatric Use

Clinical studies of SOMAVERT did not include sufficient numbers of subjects aged 65 and over to determine whether they respond differently from younger subjects. In general, dose selection for an elderly patient should be cautious, usually starting at the low end of the dosing range, reflecting the greater frequency of decreased hepatic, renal, or cardiac function, and of concomitant disease or other drug therapy.

ADVERSE REACTIONS

Laboratory Changes

Elevations of serum concentrations of ALT and AST greater than ten times the ULN were reported in two subjects (0.8%) exposed to SOMAVERT in pre-approval clinical studies (see **PRECAUTIONS, Liver Tests [LTs]**).

Table 5. Number of Patients (%) with Acromegaly Reporting Adverse Events in a 12-week Placebo-controlled Study with SOMAVERT*

Event	SOMAVERT 10 mg/day n=26	SOMAVERT 15 mg/day n=26	SOMAVERT 20 mg/day n=28	Placebo n=32
Body as a whole				
Infection†	6 (23%)	0	0	2 (6%)
Pain	2 (8%)	1 (4%)	4 (14%)	2 (6%)
Injection site reaction	2 (8%)	1 (4%)	3 (11%)	0
Accidental injury	2 (8%)	1 (4%)	0	1 (3%)
Back pain	2 (8%)	0	1 (4%)	1 (3%)
Flu syndrome	1 (4%)	3 (12%)	2 (7%)	0
Chest pain	1 (4%)	2 (8%)	0	0
Digestive				
Abnormal liver function tests	3 (12%)	1 (4%)	1 (4%)	1 (3%)
Diarrhea	1 (4%)	0	4 (14%)	1 (3%)
Nausea	0	2 (8%)	4 (14%)	1 (3%)
Nervous				
Dizziness	2 (8%)	1 (4%)	1 (4%)	2 (6%)
Paresthesia	0	0	2 (7%)	2 (6%)
Metabolic and nutritional disorders				
Peripheral edema	2 (8%)	0	1 (4%)	0
Cardiovascular				
Hypertension	0	2 (8%)	0	0
Respiratory				
Sinusitis	2 (8%)	0	1 (4%)	1 (3%)

* Table includes only those events that were reported in at least 2 patients and at a higher incidence in patients treated with SOMAVERT than in patients treated with placebo.

† The 6 events coded as "infection" in the group treated with SOMAVERT 10 mg were reported as cold symptoms (3), upper respiratory infection (1), blister (1), and ear infection (1). The 2 events in the placebo group were reported as cold symptoms (1) and chest infection (1).

General

Nine acromegalic patients (9.6%) withdrew from premarketing clinical studies because of adverse events, including two patients with marked transaminase elevations (see **PRECAUTIONS, Liver Tests [LTs]**), one patient with lipohypertrophy at the injection sites, and one patient with substantial weight gain. The majority of reported adverse events were of mild to moderate intensity and limited duration. Most adverse events did not appear to be dose dependent. Table 5 shows the incidence of treatment-emergent adverse events that were reported in at least two patients treated with SOMAVERT and at frequencies greater than placebo during the 12-week, placebo-controlled study.

Immunogenicity

In pre-marketing clinical studies, approximately 17% of the patients developed low titer, non-neutralizing anti-GH antibodies. Although the presence of these antibodies did not appear to impact the efficacy of SOMAVERT, the long-term clinical significance of these antibodies is not known. No assay for anti-pegvisomant antibodies is commercially available for patients receiving SOMAVERT.

[See table 5 at top of previous page]

OVERDOSAGE

In one reported incident of acute overdose with SOMAVERT during pre-marketing clinical studies, a patient self-administered 80 mg/day for seven days. The patient experienced a slight increase in fatigue, had no other complaints, and demonstrated no significant clinical laboratory abnormalities.

In cases of overdose, administration of SOMAVERT should be discontinued and not resumed until IGF-I levels return to within or above the normal range.

Drug Abuse and Dependence

Available data do not demonstrate drug-abuse potential or psychological dependence with SOMAVERT. Radiolabeled pegvisomant does not cross the blood-brain barrier in rats.

DOSAGE AND ADMINISTRATION

A loading dose of 40 mg of SOMAVERT should be administered subcutaneously under physician supervision. The patient should then be instructed to begin daily subcutaneous injections of 10 mg of SOMAVERT. Serum IGF-I concentrations should be measured every four to six weeks, at which time the dosage of SOMAVERT should be adjusted in 5-mg increments if IGF-I levels are still elevated (or 5-mg decrements if IGF-I levels have decreased below the normal range). While the goals of therapy are to achieve (and then maintain) serum IGF-I concentrations within the age-adjusted normal range and to alleviate the signs and symptoms of acromegaly, titration of dosing should be based on IGF-I levels. It is unknown whether patients who remain symptomatic while achieving normalized IGF-I levels would benefit from increased dosing with SOMAVERT.

The maximum daily maintenance dose should not exceed 30 mg.

SOMAVERT is supplied as a lyophilized powder. Each vial of SOMAVERT should be reconstituted with 1 mL of the diluent provided in the package (Sterile Water for Injection, USP). Instructions regarding reconstitution and administration are included in the package of SOMAVERT and should be closely followed.To prepare the solution, withdraw 1 mL of Sterile Water for Injection, USP and inject it into the vial of SOMAVERT, aiming the stream of liquid against the glass wall. Hold the vial between the palms of both hands and gently roll it to dissolve the powder. **DO NOT SHAKE THE VIAL**, as this may cause denaturation of pegvisomant. Discard the diluent vial containing the remaining water for injection. After reconstitution, each vial of SOMAVERT contains 10, 15, or 20 mg of pegvisomant protein in one mL of solution. Parenteral drug products should be inspected visually for particulate matter and discoloration prior to administration.The solution should be clear after reconstitution. If the solution is cloudy, do not inject it. Only one dose should be administered from each vial. SOMAVERT should be administered within six hours after reconstitution.

HOW SUPPLIED

SOMAVERT is available in single-dose, sterile glass vials in the following strengths:

10 mg (as protein) vial NDC 0009-5176-01
15 mg (as protein) vial NDC 0009-5178-01
20 mg (as protein) vial NDC 0009-5180-01

Each package of SOMAVERT also includes a single-dose LifeShield® plastic fliptop vial containing 10 mL of Sterile Water for Injection, USP.

The stopper on the vial of SOMAVERT contains latex.

Storage

Prior to reconstitution, SOMAVERT should be stored in a refrigerator at 2 to 8°C (36 to 46°F). Protect from freezing. After reconstitution, SOMAVERT should be administered within six hours. Only one dose should be administered from each vial.

Manufactured for:
Pharmacia & Upjohn Company
A subsidiary of Pharmacia Corporation
Kalamazoo, MI 49001, USA
by:
Abbott Laboratories
North Chicago, IL 60064, USA
U.S. Patent Nos. 5,350,836; 5,681,809; 5,849,535; 5,958,879; 6,057,292; 6,583,115.
Revised June 2003

818 727 001
692842

TRELSTAR™ DEPOT 3.75 mg ℞

[*trel-star*]

triptorelin pamoate for injectable suspension

DESCRIPTION

TRELSTAR™ DEPOT contains a pamoate salt of triptorelin, and triptorelin is a synthetic decapeptide agonist analog of luteinizing hormone releasing hormone (LHRH or GnRH) with greater potency than the naturally occurring LHRH. The chemical name of triptorelin pamoate is 5-oxo-L-prolyl-L-histidyl-L-tryptophyl-L-seryl-L-tyrosyl-D-tryptophyl-L-leucyl-L-arginyl-L-prolylglycine amide (pamoate salt); the empirical formula is $C_{64}H_{82}N_{18}O_{13} \bullet C_{23}H_{16}O_6$ and the molecular weight is 1699.9. The structural formula is shown below.

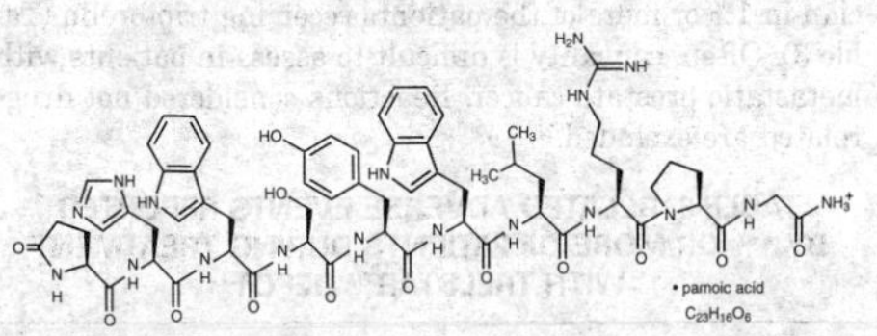

• pamoic acid
$C_{23}H_{16}O_6$

TRELSTAR™ DEPOT is a sterile, lyophilized biodegradable micro-granule formulation supplied as a single-dose vial containing triptorelin pamoate (3.75 mg as the peptide base), 170 mg poly-*d,l*-lactide-co-glycolide, 85 mg mannitol USP, 30 mg carboxymethylcellulose sodium USP, 2 mg polysorbate 80 NF. When 2 mL sterile water for injection is added to the vial containing **TRELSTAR™ DEPOT** and mixed, a suspension is formed which is intended as a monthly intramuscular injection.

CLINICAL PHARMACOLOGY

Mechanism of Action

Triptorelin is a potent inhibitor of gonadotropin secretion when given continuously and in therapeutic doses. Following the first administration, there is a transient surge in circulating levels of luteinizing hormone (LH), follicle-stimulating hormone (FSH), testosterone, and estradiol (see ADVERSE REACTIONS). After chronic and continuous administration, usually 2 to 4 weeks after initiation of therapy, a sustained decrease in LH and FSH secretion and marked reduction of testicular and ovarian steroidogenesis is observed. In men, a reduction of serum testosterone concentration to a level typically seen in surgically castrated men is obtained. Consequently, the result is that tissues and functions that depend on these hormones for maintenance become quiescent. These effects are usually reversible after cessation of therapy.

Following a single intramuscular (IM) injection of **TRELSTAR™ DEPOT** to healthy male volunteers, serum testosterone levels first increased, peaking on day 4, and declined thereafter to low levels by week 4. Similar testosterone profiles were observed in patients with advanced prostate cancer, when injected with **TRELSTAR™ DEPOT**. In healthy volunteers, testosterone serum levels returned to near baseline by week 8.

Pharmacokinetics

Results of pharmacokinetic investigations conducted in healthy men indicate that after intravenous (IV) bolus administration, triptorelin is distributed and eliminated according to a 3-compartment model and corresponding half-lives are approximately 6 minutes, 45 minutes, and 3 hours.

Absorption: Triptorelin pamoate is not active when given orally. Intramuscular injection of the depot formulation provides plasma concentrations of triptorelin over a period of 1 month. The pharmacokinetic parameters following a single IM injection of 3.75 mg of **TRELSTAR™ DEPOT** to 20 healthy male volunteers are listed in Table 1. The plasma concentrations declined to 0.084 ng/mL at 4 weeks.

TABLE 1. PHARMACOKINETIC PARAMETERS FOLLOWING INTRAMUSCULAR ADMINISTRATION OF TRELSTAR™ DEPOT TO HEALTHY MALE VOLUNTEERS

Dose (No. of subjects)	C_{max} (ng/mL)	T_{max} (h)	$AUC_{0\text{-}28d}$ (h•ng/mL)	F (%)[3] (No. of days)
3.75 mg (n=20)	28.43 ± 7.31[1]	1.0 (1.0-3.0)[2]	223.15 ± 46.96[1]	83 (28 d)

[1] Mean ± SD
[2] Median (range)
[3] Computed as the mean AUC of the study divided by the mean AUC of healthy volunteers corrected for dose where AUC=36.1 h·ng/mL and 500 µg IV bolus dose of triptorelin was administered.

Distribution: The volume of distribution following an IV bolus dose of 0.5 mg of triptorelin peptide was 30-33 L in healthy male volunteers. There is no evidence that triptorelin, at clinically relevant concentrations, binds to plasma proteins.

TABLE 2. PHARMACOKINETIC PARAMETERS (MEAN ± SD) IN HEALTHY VOLUNTEERS AND SPECIAL POPULATIONS

Group	C_{max} (ng/mL)	AUC_{inf} (h•ng/mL)	Cl_p (mL/min)	Cl_{renal} (mL/min)	$t_{1/2}$ (h)	Cl_{creat} (mL/min)
6 healthy male volunteers	48.2±11.8	36.1±5.8	211.9±31.6	90.6±35.3	2.81±1.21	149.9±7.3
6 males with moderate renal impairment	45.6±20.5	69.9±24.6	120.0±45.0	23.3±17.6	6.56±1.25	39.7±22.5
6 males with severe renal impairment	46.5±14.0	88.0±18.4	88.6±19.7	4.3±2.9	7.65±1.25	8.9±6.0
6 males with liver disease	54.1±5.3	131.9±18.1	57.8±8.0	35.9±5.0	7.58±1.17	89.9±15.1

Metabolism: The metabolism of triptorelin in humans is unknown, but is unlikely to involve hepatic microsomal enzymes (cytochrome P-450). However, the effect of triptorelin on the activity of other drug metabolizing enzymes is unknown. Thus far, no metabolites of triptorelin have been identified. Pharmacokinetic data suggest that C-terminal fragments produced by tissue degradation are either completely degraded in the tissues, or rapidly degraded in plasma, or cleared by the kidneys.

Excretion: Triptorelin is eliminated by both the liver and the kidneys. Following IV administration of 0.5 mg triptorelin peptide to 6 healthy male volunteers with a creatinine clearance of 149.9 mL/min, 41.7% of the dose was excreted in urine as intact peptide with a total triptorelin clearance of 211.9 mL/min. This percentage increased to 62.3% in patients with liver disease who have a lower creatinine clearance (89.9 mL/min). It has also been observed that the nonrenal clearance of triptorelin (patient anuric, Cl_{creat} =0) was 76.2 mL/min, thus indicating that the nonrenal elimination of triptorelin is mainly dependent on the liver (see Special Populations).

[See table 2 above]

Special Populations:

Renal and Hepatic Impairment: After an IV injection of 0.5 mg triptorelin peptide, the two distribution half-lives were unaffected by renal and hepatic impairment, but renal insufficiency led to a decrease in total triptorelin clearance proportional to the decrease in creatinine clearance as well as an increase in volume of distribution and consequently an increase in elimination half-life (Table 2). The decrease in triptorelin clearance was more pronounced in subjects with liver insufficiency, but the half-life was prolonged similarly in subjects with renal insufficiency, since the volume of distribution was only minimally increased.

Age and Race: The effects of age and race on triptorelin pharmacokinetics have not been systematically studied. However, pharmacokinetic data obtained in young healthy male volunteers aged 20 to 22 years with an elevated creatinine clearance (approximately 150 mL/min) indicates that triptorelin was eliminated twice as fast in this young population (see Special Populations, Renal and Hepatic Impairment) as compared to patients with moderate renal insufficiency. This is related to the fact that triptorelin clearance is partly corelated to total creatinine clearance, which is well known to decrease with age.

Pharmacokinetic Drug-Drug Interactions: No pharmacokinetic drug-drug interaction studies have been conducted with triptorelin (see PRECAUTIONS, Drug Interactions).

Clinical Trials

TRELSTAR™ DEPOT was studied in a randomized, active control trial of 277 men with advanced prostate cancer. The clinical trial population consisted of 59.9% Caucasian, 39.3% Black, and 0.8% Other. There was no difference observed with triptorelin response between racial groups. Men were between 47 and 89 years of age (71 mean). Patients received either **TRELSTAR™ DEPOT** or an approved GnRH agonist monthly for 9 months. The primary efficacy endpoints were both achievement of castration by Day 29 and maintenance of castration from Day 57 through Day 253.

Castration levels of serum testosterone (≤1.735 nmol/L) were achieved in 91.2% of **TRELSTAR™ DEPOT** patients at Day 29 and in 97.7% of patients at Day 57.

Maintenance of castration levels of serum testosterone from Day 57 through Day 253 was found in 96.4% of **TRELSTAR™ DEPOT** patients.

The presence of an acute-on-chronic flare phenomenon was also studied as a secondary efficacy endpoint. Serum LH levels were measured at 2 hours after repeat **TRELSTAR™ DEPOT** administration on Days 85 and 169. One hundred twenty-four of 126 evaluable patients (98.4%) on Day 85 had a serum LH level of ≤1.0 IU/L at 2 hours after dosing, indicating desensitization of the pituitary gonadotroph receptors.

INDICATIONS AND USAGE

TRELSTAR™ DEPOT is indicated in the palliative treatment of advanced prostate cancer. It offers an alternative treatment for prostate cancer when orchiectomy or estrogen administration are either not indicated or unacceptable to the patient.

CONTRAINDICATIONS

TRELSTAR™ DEPOT is contraindicated in individuals with a known hypersensitivity to triptorelin or any other compo-

Continued on next page

Trelstar—Cont.

nent of the product, other LHRH agonists or LHRH. Three postmarketing reports of anaphylactic shock and seven postmarketing reports of angioedema related to triptorelin administration have been reported since 1986 (see WARNINGS).

TRELSTAR™ DEPOT may cause fetal harm when administered to a pregnant woman.

WARNINGS

Initially, triptorelin, like other LHRH agonists, causes a transient increase in serum testosterone levels. As a result, isolated cases of worsening of signs and symptoms of prostate cancer during the first weeks of treatment have been reported with LHRH agonists. Patients may experience worsening of symptoms or onset of new symptoms, including bone pain, neuropathy, hematuria, or urethral or bladder outlet obstruction. Cases of spinal cord compression, which may contribute to paralysis with or without fatal complications, have been reported with LHRH agonists.

If spinal cord compression or renal impairment develops, standard treatment of these complications should be instituted, and in extreme cases an immediate orchiectomy considered.

TRELSTAR™ DEPOT should not be administered to individuals who are hypersensitive to triptorelin, other LHRH agonists, or LHRH. In the event of a hypersensitivity reaction, therapy with **TRELSTAR™ DEPOT** should be discontinued immediately and the appropriate supportive and symptomatic care should be administered.

PRECAUTIONS

General: Patients with metastatic vertebral lesions and/or with upper or lower urinary tract obstruction should be closely observed during the first few weeks of therapy (see WARNINGS). Hypersensitivity and anaphylactic reactions have been reported with triptorelin as with other LHRH agonists (see CONTRAINDICATIONS and WARNINGS).

Laboratory Tests: Response to **TRELSTAR™ DEPOT** should be monitored by measuring serum levels of testosterone and prostate-specific antigen.

Drug Interactions: No drug-drug interaction studies involving triptorelin have been conducted. In the absence of relevant data and as a precaution, hyperprolactinemic drugs should not be prescribed concomitantly with **TRELSTAR™ DEPOT** since hyperprolactinemia reduces the number of pituitary GnRH receptors.

Drug/Laboratory Test Interactions: Chronic or continuous administration of triptorelin in therapeutic doses results in suppression of the pituitary-gonadal axis. Diagnostic tests of the pituitary-gonadal function conducted during treatment and after cessation of therapy may therefore be misleading.

Pregnancy, Teratogenic Effects: **Pregnancy Category X (see CONTRAINDICATIONS). TRELSTAR™ DEPOT** is contraindicated in women who are or may become pregnant while receiving the drug. Studies in pregnant rats administered triptorelin at doses of 2, 10, and 100 µg/kg/day (approximately equivalent to 0.2, 0.8, and 8 times the recommended human therapeutic dose based on body surface area) during the period of organogenesis displayed maternal toxicity and embryotoxicity, but no fetotoxicity or teratogenicity. Similarly, no teratogenic effects were observed when mice were administered doses of 2, 20, and 200 µg/kg/day (approximately equivalent to 0.1, 0.7, and 7 times the recommended human therapeutic dose based on body surface area). If this drug is used during pregnancy or if the patient becomes pregnant while taking this drug, she should be apprised of the potential hazard to the fetus.

Carcinogenesis, Mutagenesis, Impairment of Fertility: In rats, doses of 120, 600, and 3000 µg/kg given every 28 days (approximately 0.3, 2.0, and 8 times the recommended human therapeutic dose based on body surface area) resulted in increased mortality with a drug treatment period of 13-19 months. The incidence of benign and malignant pituitary tumors and histiosarcomas were increased in a dose related manner. No oncogenic effect was observed in mice administered triptorelin for 18 months at doses up to 6000 µg/kg every 28 days (approximately 8 times the human therapeutic dose based on body surface area).

Mutagenicity studies performed with triptorelin using bacterial and mammalian systems (in vitro Ames test and chromosomal aberration test in CHO cells and an in vivo mouse micronucleus test) provided no evidence of mutagenic potential.

After 60 days of treatment followed by a minimum of four estrus cycles prior to mating, triptorelin, at doses of 2, 20, and 200 µg/kg/day in saline (approximately 0.2, 2.0, and 16 times the recommended human therapeutic dose based on body surface area) or 20 µg/kg/day in slow release microspheres, had no effect on the fertility or general reproductive performance of female rats. Treatment did not elicit embryotoxicity, teratogenicity, or any effects on the development of the offspring (F_1 generation) or their reproductive performance.

No studies were conducted to assess the effect of triptorelin on male fertility.

Geriatric Use: Prostate cancer occurs primarily in an older patient population. Clinical studies with **TRELSTAR™ DEPOT** have been conducted primarily in patients ≥65 years.

Nursing Mothers: It is not known whether **TRELSTAR™ DEPOT** is excreted in human milk. Because many drugs are excreted in human milk, and because the effects of **TRELSTAR™ DEPOT** on lactation and/or the breastfed child have not been determined, **TRELSTAR™ DEPOT** should not be used by nursing mothers.

Pediatric Use: **TRELSTAR™ DEPOT** has not been studied in pediatric patients.

ADVERSE REACTIONS

In the majority of patients, testosterone levels increased above baseline during the first week following the initial injection, declining thereafter to baseline levels or below by the end of the second week of treatment. The transient increase in testosterone levels may be associated with temporary worsening of disease signs and symptoms, including bone pain, hematuria, and bladder outlet obstruction. Isolated cases of spinal cord compression with weakness or paralysis of the lower extremities have occurred (see WARNINGS).

In a controlled, comparative clinical trial, the following adverse reactions were reported to have a possible or probable relationship to therapy as ascribed by the treating physician in 1% or more of the patients receiving triptorelin (Table 3). Often, causality is difficult to assess in patients with metastatic prostate cancer. Reactions considered not drug-related are excluded.

TABLE 3. RELATED ADVERSE EVENTS REPORTED BY 1% OR MORE OF PATIENTS DURING TREATMENT WITH TRELSTAR™ DEPOT

Adverse Event	TRELSTAR™ DEPOT N=140 N	%
Application Site Disorders		
Injection site pain	5	3.6
Body As A Whole		
Hot flushes*	82	58.6
Pain	3	2.1
Leg pain	3	2.1
Fatigue	3	2.1
Cardiovascular		
Hypertension	5	3.6
Central and Peripheral Nervous System Disorders		
Headache	7	5.0
Dizziness	2	1.4
Gastrointestinal Disorders		
Diarrhea	2	1.4
Vomiting	3	2.1
Musculoskeletal System Disorders		
Skeletal pain	17	12.1
Psychiatric		
Insomnia	3	2.1
Impotence*	10	7.1
Emotional lability	2	1.4
Red Blood Cell Disorders		
Anemia	2	1.4
Skin and Appendages Disorders		
Pruritus	2	1.4
Urinary System		
Urinary retention	2	1.4
Urinary tract infection	2	1.4

* Expected pharmacologic consequences of testosterone suppression.

Changes in Laboratory Values During Treatment: There were no clinically meaningful changes in laboratory values during or following therapy with **TRELSTAR™ DEPOT**.

OVERDOSAGE

The pharmacological properties of triptorelin and its mode of administration make accidental or intentional overdosage unlikely. There were no reported overdoses in clinical trials. In single dose toxicity studies in mice and rats, the subcutaneous LD_{50} of triptorelin was 400 mg/kg in mice and 250 mg/kg in rats, approximately 7000 and 4000 times, respectively, the usual human dose. If overdosage occurs however, therapy should be discontinued immediately and the appropriate supportive and symptomatic treatment administered.

DOSAGE AND ADMINISTRATION

TRELSTAR™ DEPOT *Must Be Administered Under the Supervision of a Physician.*

The recommended dose of **TRELSTAR™ DEPOT** is 3.75 mg incorporated in a depot formulation and is administered monthly as a single intramuscular injection. The lyophilized microgranules are to be reconstituted **in sterile water. No other diluent should be used.** Reconstitute in accord with the following:

For **TRELSTAR™ DEPOT**:

1) Using a syringe fitted with a sterile 20-gauge needle, withdraw 2 mL **sterile water** for injection, USP, and after removing the flip-off seal from the vial, inject into the vial.
2) Shake well to thoroughly disperse particles to obtain a uniform suspension. The suspension will appear milky.
3) Withdraw the entire content of the reconstituted suspension into the syringe and inject it immediately.
   The suspension should be discarded if not used immediately after reconstitution.

As with other drugs administered by intramuscular injection, the injection site should be altered periodically.

For the **TRELSTAR™ DEPOT** Debioclip™ single-dose delivery system:

1. Remove the Tyvek® cover from the blister pack.
2. Remove the vial from its case. Remove the flip-off vial cover and place the vial in the vertical position.
3. Hold the lower part of the **TRELSTAR™ DEPOT** Debioclip™ and press it firmly onto the top of the vial (See Figure).
4. Hold firmly the syringe barrel. Push the finger grip in the direction of the vial as far as it will go (until you hear a click).
5. Take the plunger rod and screw it into the upper joint of the syringe.
6. Press the plunger rod to release the contents of the syringe into the vial.
7. Mix and withdraw the contents of the vial into the syringe.
8. Remove the syringe from the **TRELSTAR™ DEPOT** Debioclip™.
9. Inject the patient in either buttock with the contents of the syringe.

The suspension should be discarded if not used immediately after reconstitution.

As with other drugs administered by intramuscular injection, the injection site should be altered periodically.

Dosage Adjustments: Patients with renal or hepatic impairment showed 2- to 4-fold higher exposure than young healthy males. The clinical consequences of this increase, as well as the potential need for dose adjustment, is unknown.

HOW SUPPLIED

TRELSTAR™ DEPOT (NDC 0009-7664-01) is supplied in a single-dose vial with a flip-off seal containing sterile lyophilized triptorelin pamoate microgranules equivalent to 3.75 mg triptorelin peptide base, incorporated in a biodegradable copolymer of lactic and glycolic acids. A single dose vial of **TRELSTAR™ DEPOT** contains triptorelin pamoate (3.75 mg as peptide base units), poly-*d,l*-lactide-co-glycolide (170 mg), mannitol, USP (85 mg), carboxymethylcellulose sodium, USP (30 mg), and polysorbate 80, NF (2 mg).

TRELSTAR™ DEPOT (NDC 0009-5219-01) is also supplied in the **TRELSTAR™ DEPOT** Debioclip™ single-dose delivery system consisting of a vial with a flip-off seal containing sterile lyophilized triptorelin pamoate microgranules equivalent to 3.75 mg of triptorelin peptide base, incorporated in a biodegradable copolymer of lactic and glycolic acids, and a pre-filled syringe containing 2 mL sterile water for injection, USP.

When mixed with sterile water for injection, **TRELSTAR™ DEPOT** is administered every 28 days as a single intramuscular injection.

Store at 20-25°C (68-77°F); excursions permitted to 15-30°C (59-86°F) [see USP Controlled Room Temperature].

℞ only

U.S. Patent No.: 5,134,122; 5,225,205; 5,192,741.

™ - Trademark

Manufactured for:
Pharmacia & Upjohn Company
Kalamazoo, MI 49001, USA
by:
Debio RP
CH-1920 Martigny, Switzerland

818 916 002
Revised: November 2001 692166

VANTIN® ℞

[văn-tĭn]

Tablets and Oral Suspension
cefpodoxime proxetil tablets and
cefpodoxime proxetil for oral suspension, USP
For Oral Use Only

DESCRIPTION

Cefpodoxime proxetil is an orally administered, extended spectrum, semi-synthetic antibiotic of the cephalosporin class. The chemical name is (RS)-1(isopropoxycarbonyloxy) ethyl (+)-(6R,7R)-7-[2- (2-amino-4-thiazolyl)-2-{(Z)methoxyimino}acetamido]-3-methoxymethyl-8-oxo-5-thia-1-azabicyclo [4.2.0] oct-2-ene-2-carboxylate.

Its empirical formula is $C_{21}H_{27}N_5O_9S_2$ and its structural formula is represented below:

The molecular weight of cefpodoxime proxetil is 557,6.

Cefpodoxime proxetil is a prodrug; its active metabolite is cefpodoxime. All doses of cefpodoxime proxetil in this insert are expressed in terms of the active cefpodoxime moiety. The drug is supplied both as film-coated tablets and as flavored granules for oral suspension.

VANTIN Tablets contain cefpodoxime proxetil equivalent to 100 mg or 200 mg of cefpodoxime activity and the following inactive ingredients: carboxymethylcellulose calcium, carnauba wax, FD&C Yellow No. 6, hydroxypropylcellulose, hypromellose, lactose hydrous, magnesium stearate, propylene glycol, sodium lauryl sulfate and titanium dioxide. In addition, the 100 mg film-coated tablets contain D&C Yellow No. 10 and the 200 mg film-coated tablets contain FD&C Red No. 40.

Each 5 mL of VANTIN Oral Suspension contains cefpodoxime proxetil equivalent to 50 mg or 100 mg of cefpodoxime activity after constitution and the following inactive ingredients: artificial flavorings, butylated hydroxy anisole (BHA), carboxymethylcellulose sodium, microcrystalline cellulose, carrageenan, citric acid, colloidal silicon dioxide, croscarmellose sodium, hydroxypropylcellulose, lactose, maltodextrin, natural flavorings, propylene glycol alginate, sodium citrate, sodium benzoate, starch, sucrose, and vegetable oil.

CLINICAL PHARMACOLOGY

Absorption and Excretion:

Cefpodoxime proxetil is a prodrug that is absorbed from the gastrointestinal tract and de-esterified to its active metabolite, cefpodoxime. Following oral administration of 100 mg of cefpodoxime proxetil to fasting subjects, approximately 50% of the administered cefpodoxime dose was absorbed systemically. Over the recommended dosing range (100 to 400 mg), approximately 29 to 33% of the administered cefpodoxime dose was excreted unchanged in the urine in 12 hours. There is minimal metabolism of cefpodoxime *in vivo*.

Effects of Food:

The extent of absorption (mean AUC) and the mean peak plasma concentration increased when film-coated tablets were administered with food. Following a 200 mg tablet dose taken with food, the AUC was 21 to 33% higher than under fasting conditions, and the peak plasma concentration averaged 3.1 mcg/mL in fed subjects versus 2.6 mcg/mL in fasted subjects. Time to peak concentration was not significantly different between fed and fasted subjects.

When a 200 mg dose of the suspension was taken with food, the extent of absorption (mean AUC) and mean peak plasma concentration in fed subjects were not significantly different from fasted subjects, but the rate of absorption was slower with food (48% increase in T_{max}).

Pharmacokinetics of Cefpodoxime Proxetil Film-coated Tablets:

Over the recommended dosing range, (100 to 400 mg), the rate and extent of cefpodoxime absorption exhibited dose-dependency; dose-normalized C_{max} and AUC decreased by up to 32% with increasing dose. Over the recommended dosing range, the T_{max} was approximately 2 to 3 hours and the $T_{1/2}$ ranged from 2.09 to 2.84 hours. Mean C_{max} was 1.4 mcg/mL for the 100 mg dose, 2.3 mcg/mL for the 200 mg dose, and 3.9 mcg/mL for the 400 mg dose. In patients with normal renal function, neither accumulation nor significant changes in other pharmacokinetic parameters were noted following multiple oral doses of up to 400 mg Q 12 hours. [See first table above]

Pharmacokinetics of Cefpodoxime Proxetil Suspension:

In adult subjects, a 100 mg dose of oral suspension produced an average peak cefpodoxime concentration of approximately 1.5 mcg/mL (range: 1.1 to 2.1 mcg/mL), which is equivalent to that reported following administration of the 100 mg tablet. Time to peak plasma concentration and area under the plasma concentration-time curve (AUC) for the oral suspension were also equivalent to those produced with film-coated tablets in adults following a 100 mg oral dose.

The pharmacokinetics of cefpodoxime were investigated in 29 patients aged 1 to 17 years. Each patient received a single, oral, 5 mg/kg dose of cefpodoxime oral suspension. Plasma and urine samples were collected for 12 hours after dosing. The plasma levels reported from this study are as follows:

[See second table above]

Distribution:

Protein binding of cefpodoxime ranges from 22 to 33% in serum and from 21 to 29% in plasma.

Skin Blister:

Following multiple-dose administration every 12 hours for 5 days of 200 mg or 400 mg cefpodoxime proxetil, the mean maximum cefpodoxime concentration in skin blister fluid averaged 1.6 and 2.8 mcg/mL, respectively. Skin blister fluid

CEFPODOXIME PLASMA LEVELS (mcg/mL) IN FASTED ADULTS AFTER FILM-COATED TABLET ADMINISTRATION (Single Dose)

Dose (cefpodoxime equivalents)	Time after oral ingestion 1hr	2hr	3hr	4hr	6hr	8hr	12hr
100 mg	0.98	1.4	1.3	1.0	0.59	0.29	0.08
200 mg	1.5	2.2	2.2	1.8	1.2	0.62	0.18
400 mg	2.2	3.7	3.8	3.3	2.3	1.3	0.38

CEFPODOXIME PLASMA LEVELS (mcg/mL) IN FASTED PATIENTS (1 to 17 YEARS OF AGE) AFTER SUSPENSION ADMINISTRATION

Dose (cefpodoxime equivalents)	Time after oral ingestion 1hr	2hr	3hr	4hr	6hr	8hr	12hr
5 mg/kg[1]	1.4	2.1	2.1	1.7	0.90	0.40	0.090

[1] Dose did not exceed 200 mg.

cefpodoxime levels at 12 hours after dosing averaged 0.2 and 0.4 mcg/mL for the 200 mg and 400 mg multiple-dose regimens, respectively.

Tonsil Tissue:

Following a single, oral 100 mg cefpodoxime proxetil film-coated tablet, the mean maximum cefpodoxime concentration in tonsil tissue averaged 0.24 mcg/g at 4 hours post-dosing and 0.09 mcg/g at 7 hours post-dosing. Equilibrium was achieved between plasma and tonsil tissue within 4 hours of dosing. No detection of cefpodoxime in tonsillar tissue was reported 12 hours after dosing. These results demonstrated that concentrations of cefpodoxime exceeded the MIC_{90} of *S. pyogenes* for at least 7 hours after dosing of 100 mg of cefpodoxime proxetil.

Lung Tissue:

Following a single, oral 200 mg cefpodoxime proxetil film-coated tablet, the mean maximum cefpodoxime concentration in lung tissue averaged 0.63 mcg/g at 3 hours post-dosing, 0.52 mcg/g at 6 hours post-dosing, and 0.19 mcg/g at 12 hours post-dosing. The results of this study indicated that cefpodoxime penetrated into lung tissue and produced sustained drug concentrations for at least 12 hours after dosing at levels that exceeded the MIC_{90} for *S. pneumoniae* and *H. influenzae*.

CSF:

Adequate data on CSF levels of cefpodoxime are not available.

Effects of Decreased Renal Function:

Elimination of cefpodoxime is reduced in patients with moderate to severe renal impairment (< 50mL/min creatinine clearance). (See **PRECAUTIONS** and **DOSAGE AND ADMINISTRATION**.) In subjects with mild impairment of renal function (50 to 80 mL/min creatinine clearance), the average plasma half-life of cefpodoxime was 3.5 hours. In subjects with moderate (30 to 49 mL/min creatinine clearance) or severe renal impairment (5 to 29 mL/min creatinine clearance), the half-life increased to 5.9 and 9.8 hours, respectively. Approximately 23% of the administered dose was cleared from the body during a standard 3-hour hemodialysis procedure.

Effect of Hepatic Impairment (cirrhosis):

Absorption was somewhat diminished and elimination unchanged in patients with cirrhosis. The mean cefpodoxime $T_{½}$ and renal clearance in cirrhotic patients were similar to those derived in studies of healthy subjects. Ascites did not appear to affect values in cirrhotic subjects. No dosage adjustment is recommended in this patient population.

Pharmacokinetics in Elderly Subjects:

Elderly subjects do not require dosage adjustments unless they have diminished renal function. (See **PRECAUTIONS**.) In healthy geriatric subjects, cefpodoxime half-life in plasma averaged 4.2 hours (vs 3.3 in younger subjects) and urinary recovery averaged 21% after a 400 mg dose was administered every 12 hours. Other pharmacokinetic parameters (C_{max}, AUC, and T_{max}) were unchanged relative to those observed in healthy young subjects.

Microbiology:

Cefpodoxime is active against a wide-spectrum of Gram-positive and Gram-negative bacteria.

Cefpodoxime is stable in the presence of beta-lactamase enzymes. As a result, many organisms resistant to penicillins and cephalosporins, due to their production of beta lactamase, may be susceptible to cefpodoxime. Cefpodoxime is inactivated by certain extended spectrum beta-lactamases. The bactericidal activity of cefpodoxime results from its inhibition of cell wall synthesis.

Cefpodoxime has been shown to be active against most strains of the following microorganisms, both *in vitro* and in clinical infections, as described in the **INDICATIONS AND USAGE** section.

Aerobic Gram-positive microorganisms:

Staphylococcus aureus (including penicillinase-producing strains)

NOTE: Cefpodoxime is inactive against methicillin-resistant staphylococci.

Staphylococcus saprophyticus

Streptococcus pneumoniae (excluding penicillin-resistant strains)

Streptococcus pyogenes

Aerobic Gram-negative microorganisms:

Escherichia coli

Klebsiella pneumoniae

Proteus mirabilis

Haemophilus influenzae (including beta-lactamase producing strains)

Moraxella (Branhamella) catarrhalis

Neisseria gonorrhoeae (including penicillinase-producing strains)

The following *in vitro* data are available, but their clinical significance is unknown. Cefpodoxime exhibits *in vitro* minimum inhibitory concentrations (MICs) of ≤ 2.0 mcg/mL against most (≥90%) of isolates of the following microorganisms. However, the safety and efficacy of cefpodoxime in treating clinical infections due to these microorganisms have not been established in adequate and well controlled clinical trials.

Aerobic Gram-positive microorganisms:

Streptococcus agalactiae

Streptococcus spp. (Groups C, F, G)

NOTE: Cefpodoxime is inactive against enterococci.

Aerobic Gram-negative microorganisms:

Citrobacter diversus

Klebsiella oxytoca

Proteus vulgaris

Providencia rettgeri

Haemophilus parainfluenzae

NOTE: Cefpodoxime is inactive against most strains of Pseudomonas and Enterobacter.

Anaerobic Gram-positive microorganisms:

Peptostreptococcus magnus

SUSCEPTIBILITY TESTING

Dilution Techniques: Quantitative methods are used to determine antimicrobial inhibitory concentrations (MICs). These MICs provide estimates of the susceptibility of microorganisms to antimicrobial compounds. The MICs should be determined using a standardized procedure. Standardized procedures are based on dilution methods[1,2] (broth or agar) or equivalent using standardized inoculum concentrations, and standardized concentrations of cefpodoxime from a powder of known potency. The MIC values should be interpreted according to the following criteria:

For Susceptibility Testing of *Enterobacteriaceae* and *Staphylococcus* spp.

MIC (mcg/mL)	Interpretation
≤ 2.0	Susceptible (S)
4.0	Intermediate (I)
≥ 8.0	Resistant (R)

For Susceptibility Testing of *Haemophilus* spp.[a]

MIC (mcg/mL)	Interpretation[b]
≤ 2.0	Susceptible (S)

[a] The interpretive criteria for *Haemophilus* spp. is applicable only to broth microdilution susceptibility testing done with Haemophilus Test Medium (HTM) broth.[2]

[b] "Intermediate" and "Resistant" categories have not been determined.

For Susceptibility Testing of *Neisseria gonorrhoeae*.[c]

MIC (mcg/mL)	Interpretation[d]
≤ 0.5	Susceptible (S)

[c] The interpretive value for *N. gonorroheae* is applicable only to agar dilution susceptibility testing done with *Neisseria gonorrhoeae* susceptibility test medium.[2]

[d] "Intermediate" and "Resistant" categories have not been determined.

For Susceptibility Testing of *Streptococcus pneumoniae*.

MIC (mcg/mL)	Interpretation[e]
≤ 0.5	Susceptible (S)
1.0	Intermediate (I)
≥ 2.0	Resistant (R)

[e] The interpretive value for *S. pneumoniae* is applicable only to broth microdilution susceptibility testing done with cation-adjusted Mueller-Hinton broth with lysed horse blood (LHB) (2-5% v/v).[2]

For Susceptibility Testing of *Streptococcus* spp. other than *Streptococcus pneumoniae*.[f]

A streptococcal isolate that is susceptible to penicillin (MIC ≤ 0.12 mcg/mL) can be considered susceptible to cefpodoxime for approved indications, and need not be tested against cefpodoxime.

Continued on next page

Vantin—Cont.

[f] The interpretive value for *Streptococcus* spp. is applicable only to broth microdilution susceptibility testing done with cation-adjusted Mueller-Hinton broth with lysed horse blood (LHB) (2-5% v/v).[2]

A report of "Susceptible" indicates that the pathogen is likely to be inhibited if the concentration of the antimicrobial compound in the blood reaches usually achievable levels. A report of "Intermediate" indicates that the results should be considered equivocal, and, if the microorganism is not fully susceptible to alternative, clinically feasible drugs, the test should be repeated. This category implies possible clinical applicability in body sites where the drug is physiologically concentrated or in situations where high dosage of drug can be used. This category also provides a buffer zone which prevents small technical factors from causing major discrepancies in interpretation. A report of "Resistant" indicates that the pathogen is not likely to be inhibited if the antimicrobial compound in the blood reaches the concentrations usually achievable; other therapy should be selected.

Quality Control

A standardized susceptibility test procedure requires the use of laboratory control organisms to control the technical aspects of the laboratory procedures. Standard cefpodoxime powder should provide the following MIC values with the indicated quality control strains:

Microorganism (ATCC®#)	MIC Range (mcg/mL)
Escherichia coli (25922)	0.25 - 1.0
Staphylococcus aureus (29213)	1.0 - 8.0
Haemophilus influenzae (49247)	0.25 - 1.0[g]
Neisseria gonorrhoeae (49226)	0.03 - 0.12[h]
Streptococcus pneumoniae(49619)[j]	0.03 - 0.12[i]

[g] These quality control ranges are applicable to tests performed by a broth microdilution procedure using Haemophilus Test Medium (HTM).

[h] These quality control ranges are applicable to tests performed by agar dilution only using GC agar base with 1% defined growth supplement.

[i] These quality control ranges are applicable to tests performed by the broth microdilution method only using cation-adjusted Mueller-Hinton broth with 2 to 5% lysed horse blood.

[j] When susceptibility testing *Streptococcus pneumoniae* or *Streptococcus* spp. this quality control strain should be tested.

Diffusion Techniques: Quantitative methods that require measurement of zone diameters also provide reproducible estimates of the susceptibility of bacteria to antimicrobial compounds. One such standardized procedure[3] requires the use of standardized inoculum concentrations. This procedure uses paper disks impregnated with 10 mcg cefpodoxime to test the susceptibility of microorganisms to cefpodoxime. Reports from the laboratory providing results of the standard single-disk susceptibility test with a 10 mcg cefpodoxime disk should be interpreted according to the following criteria:

For Susceptibility Testing of *Enterobacteriaceae* and *Staphylococcus* spp.

Zone Diameter (mm)	Interpretation
≥ 21	Susceptible (S)
18-20	Intermediate (I)
≤ 17	Resistant (R)

For Susceptibility Testing of *Haemophilus* spp.[k]

Zone Diameter (mm)	Interpretation[l]
≥ 21	Susceptible (S)

[k] The zone diameter for *Haemophilus spp.* is applicable only to tests performed on Haemophilus Test Medium (HTM) agar incubated under 5% CO_2.[2]

[l] "Intermediate" and "Resistant" criteria have not been determined.

For Susceptibility Testing of *Neisseria gonorrhoeae*.[m]

Zone Diameter (mm)	Interpretation[n]
≥ 29	Susceptible (S)

[m] The zone diameter for *N. gonorrhoeae* is applicable only to tests performed on GC agar base and 1% defined growth supplement incubated under 5% CO_2.[2]

[n] "Intermediate" and "Resistant" categories have not been determined.

For Susceptibility Testing of *Streptococcus pneumoniae*.[o]

Isolates of pneumococci with oxacillin zone sizes of ≥20 mm are susceptible (MIC ≤ 0.06 mcg/mL) to penicillin and can be considered susceptible to cefpodoxime for approved indications, and cefpodoxime need not be tested.

[o] The zone diameter for *S. pneumoniae* is applicable only to tests performed on Mueller-Hinton agar with 5% sheep blood incubated in 5% CO_2.[2]

For Susceptibility Testing of *Streptococcus* spp. other than *Streptococcus pneumoniae*.[p]

A streptococcal isolate that is susceptible to penicillin (zone diameter ≥ 28 mm) can be considered susceptible to cefpodoxime for approved indications, and cefpodoxime need not be tested.

[p] The zone diameter for *Streptococcus* spp. is applicable only to tests performed on Mueller-Hinton agar with 5% sheep blood incubated in 5% CO_2.[2]

Quality Control

As with standardized dilution techniques, diffusion methods require the use of laboratory control microorganisms that are used to control the technical aspects of the laboratory procedures. For the diffusion technique, the 10 mcg cefpodoxime disk should provide the following zone diameters with the quality control strains listed below:

Microorganism (ATCC®#)	Zone Diameter Range (mm)
Escherichia coli (25922)	23-28
Staphylococcus aureus (25923)	19-25
Haemophilus influenzae (49247)	25-31[q]
Neisseria gonorrhoeae (49226)	35-43[r]
Streptococcus pneumoniae(49619)[t]	28-34[s]

[q] This zone diameter range is only applicable to tests performed on Haemophilus Test Medium (HTM) agar incubated in 5% CO_2.

[r] This zone diameter range is only applicable to tests performed on GC agar base and 1% defined growth supplement incubated in 5% CO_2.

[s] This zone diameter range is only applicable to tests performed on Mueller-Hinton agar supplemented with 5% defibrinated sheep blood, incubated in 5% CO_2.

[t] This organism is to be used for quality control testing for both *S. pneumoniae* and *Streptococcus* spp.

ATCC® is a registered trademark of the American Type Culture Collection.

INDICATIONS AND USAGE

Cefpodoxime proxetil is indicated for the treatment of patients with mild to moderate infections caused by susceptible strains of the designated microorganisms in the conditions listed below. **Recommended dosages, durations of therapy, and applicable patient populations vary among these infections. Please see DOSAGE AND ADMINISTRATION for specific recommendations.**

Acute otitis media caused by *Streptococcus pneumoniae*, (excluding penicillin-resistant strains), *Streptococcus pyogenes, Haemophilus influenzae* (including beta-lactamase-producing strains), or *Moraxella (Branhamella) catarrhalis* (including beta-lactamase producing strains).

Pharyngitis and/or tonsillitis caused by *Streptococcus pyogenes*.

NOTE: Only penicillin by the intramuscular route of administration has been shown to be effective in the prophylaxis of rheumatic fever. Cefpodoxime proxetil is generally effective in the eradication of streptococci from the oropharynx. However, data establishing the efficacy of cefpodoxime proxetil for the prophylaxis of subsequent rheumatic fever are not available.

Community-acquired pneumonia caused by *S. pneumoniae* or *H. influenzae* (including beta-lactamase-producing strains).

Acute bacterial exacerbation of chronic bronchitis caused by *S. pneumoniae, H. influenzae* (non-beta-lactamase-producing strains only), or *M. catarrhalis*. Data are insufficient at this time to establish efficacy in patients with acute bacterial exacerbations of chronic bronchitis caused by beta-lactamase-producing strains of *H. influenzae*.

Acute, uncomplicated urethral and cervical gonorrhea caused by *Neisseria gonorrhoeae* (including penicillinase-producing strains).

Acute, uncomplicated ano-rectal infections in women due to *Neisseria gonorrhoeae* (including penicillinase-producing strains).

NOTE: The efficacy of cefpodoxime in treating male patients with rectal infections caused by *N. gonorrhoeae* has not been established. Data do not support the use of cefpodoxime proxetil in the treatment of pharyngeal infections due to *N. gonorrhoeae* in men or women.

Uncomplicated skin and skin structure infections caused by *Staphylococcus aureus* (including penicillinase-producing strains) or *Streptococcus pyogenes*. Abscesses should be surgically drained as clinically indicated.

NOTE: In clinical trials, successful treatment of uncomplicated skin and skin structure infections was dose-related. The effective therapeutic dose for skin infections was higher than those used in other recommended indications. (See **DOSAGE AND ADMINISTRATION**.)

Acute maxillary sinusitis caused by *Haemophilus influenzae* (including beta-lactamase producing strains), *Streptococcus pneumoniae*, and *Moraxella catarrhalis*.

Uncomplicated urinary tract infections (cystitis) caused by *Escherichia coli, Klebsiella pneumoniae, Proteus mirabilis*, or *Staphylococcus saprophyticus*.

NOTE: In considering the use of cefpodoxime proxetil in the treatment of cystitis, cefpodoxime proxetil's lower bacterial eradication rates should be weighed against the increased eradication rates and different safety profiles of some other classes of approved agents. (See **CLINICAL STUDIES** section.)

Appropriate specimens for bacteriological examination should be obtained in order to isolate and identify causative organisms and to determine their susceptibility to cefpodoxime. Therapy may be instituted while awaiting the results of these studies. Once these results become available, antimicrobial therapy should be adjusted accordingly.

CONTRAINDICATIONS

Cefpodoxime proxetil is contraindicated in patients with a known allergy to cefpodoxime or to the cephalosporin group of antibiotics.

WARNINGS

BEFORE THERAPY WITH CEFPODOXIME PROXETIL IS INSTITUTED, CAREFUL INQUIRY SHOULD BE MADE TO DETERMINE WHETHER THE PATIENT HAS HAD PREVIOUS HYPERSENSITIVITY REACTIONS TO CEFPODOXIME, OTHER CEPHALOSPORINS, PENICILLINS, OR OTHER DRUGS. IF CEFPODOXIME IS TO BE ADMINISTERED TO PENICILLIN SENSITIVE PATIENTS, CAUTION SHOULD BE EXERCISED BECAUSE CROSS HYPERSENSITIVITY AMONG BETA-LACTAM ANTIBIOTICS HAS BEEN CLEARLY DOCUMENTED AND MAY OCCUR IN UP TO 10% OF PATIENTS WITH A HISTORY OF PENICILLIN ALLERGY. IF AN ALLERGIC REACTION TO CEFPODOXIME PROXETIL OCCURS, DISCONTINUE THE DRUG. SERIOUS ACUTE HYPERSENSITIVITY REACTIONS MAY REQUIRE TREATMENT WITH EPINEPHRINE AND OTHER EMERGENCY MEASURES, INCLUDING OXYGEN, INTRAVENOUS FLUIDS, INTRAVENOUS ANTIHISTAMINE, AND AIRWAY MANAGEMENT, AS CLINICALLY INDICATED. PSEUDOMEMBRANOUS COLITIS HAS BEEN REPORTED WITH NEARLY ALL ANTIBACTERIAL AGENTS, INCLUDING CEFPODOXIME, AND MAY RANGE IN SEVERITY FROM MILD TO LIFE-THREATENING. THEREFORE, IT IS IMPORTANT TO CONSIDER THIS DIAGNOSIS IN PATIENTS WHO PRESENT WITH DIARRHEA SUBSEQUENT TO THE ADMINISTRATION OF ANTIBACTERIAL AGENTS.

Extreme caution should be observed when using this product in patients at increased risk for antibiotic-induced, pseudomembranous colitis because of exposure to institutional settings, such as nursing homes or hospitals with endemic *C. difficile*.

Treatment with broad-spectrum antibiotics, including cefpodoxime proxetil, alters the normal flora of the colon and may permit overgrowth of clostridia. Studies indicate a toxin produced by *Clostridium difficile* is the primary cause of "antibiotic-associated colitis".

After the diagnosis of pseudomembranous colitis has been established, therapeutic measures should be initiated. Mild cases of pseudomembranous colitis usually respond to drug discontinuation alone. In moderate to severe cases, consideration should be given to management with fluids and electrolytes, protein supplementation, and treatment with an oral antibacterial drug effective against *C. difficile*.

A concerted effort to monitor for *C. difficile* in cefpodoxime-treated patients with diarrhea was undertaken because of an increased incidence of diarrhea associated with *C. difficile* in early trials in normal subjects. *C. difficile* organisms or toxin was reported in 10% of the cefpodoxime-treated adult patients with diarrhea; however, no specific diagnosis of pseudomembranous colitis was made in these patients.

In post-marketing experience outside the United States, reports of pseudomembranous colitis associated with the use of cefpodoxime proxetil have been received.

PRECAUTIONS

General:

In patients with transient or persistent reduction in urinary output due to renal insufficiency, the total daily dose of cefpodoxime proxetil should be reduced because high and prolonged serum antibiotic concentrations can occur in such individuals following usual doses. Cefpodoxime, like other cephalosporins, should be administered with caution to patients receiving concurrent treatment with potent diuretics. (See **DOSAGE AND ADMINISTRATION**.)

As with other antibiotics, prolonged use of cefpodoxime proxetil may result in overgrowth of non-susceptible organisms. Repeated evaluation of the patient's condition is essential. If superinfection occurs during therapy, appropriate measures should be taken.

Drug Interactions:

Antacids: Concomitant administration of high doses of antacids (sodium bicarbonate and aluminum hydroxide) or H_2 blockers reduces peak plasma levels by 24% to 42% and the extent of absorption by 27% to 32%, respectively. The rate of absorption is not altered by these concomitant medications. Oral anti-cholinergics (e.g., propantheline) delay peak plasma levels (47% increase in T_{max}), but do not affect the extent of absorption (AUC).

Probenecid: As with other beta-lactam antibiotics, renal excretion of cefpodoxime was inhibited by probenecid and resulted in an approximately 31% increase in AUC and 20% increase in peak cefpodoxime plasma levels.

Nephrotoxic drugs: Although nephrotoxicity has not been noted when cefpodoxime proxetil was given alone, close monitoring of renal function is advised when cefpodoxime proxetil is administered concomitantly with compounds of known nephrotoxic potential.

Drug/Laboratory Test Interactions:

Cephalosporins, including cefpodoxime proxetil, are known to occasionally induce a positive direct Coombs' test.

Carcinogenesis, Mutagenesis, Impairment of Fertility:

Long-term animal carcinogenesis studies of cefpodoxime proxetil have not been performed. Mutagenesis studies of cefpodoxime, including the Ames test both with and without metabolic activation, the chromosome aberration test, the unscheduled DNA synthesis assay, mitotic recombination and gene conversion, the forward gene mutation assay and the *in vivo* micronucleus test, were all negative. No untoward effects on fertility or reproduction were noted when 100 mg/kg/day or less (2 times the human dose based on mg/m^2) was administered orally to rats.

Pregnancy - Teratogenic Effects:

Pregnancy Category B

Cefpodoxime proxetil was neither teratogenic nor embryocidal when administered to rats during organogenesis at doses up to 100 mg/kg/day (2 times the human dose based on mg/m^2) or to rabbits at doses up to 30 mg/kg/day (1-2 times the human dose based on mg/m^2).

There are, however, no adequate and well-controlled studies of cefpodoxime proxetil use in pregnant women. Because animal reproduction studies are not always predictive of human response, this drug should be used during pregnancy only if clearly needed.

Labor and Delivery:

Cefpodoxime proxetil has not been studied for use during labor and delivery. Treatment should only be given if clearly needed.

Nursing Mothers:

Cefpodoxime is excreted in human milk. In a study of 3 lactating women, levels of cefpodoxime in human milk were 0%, 2% and 6% of concomitant serum levels at 4 hours following a 200 mg oral dose of cefpodoxime proxetil. At 6 hours post-dosing, levels were 0%, 9% and 16% of concomitant serum levels. Because of the potential for serious reactions in nursing infants, a decision should be made whether to discontinue nursing or to discontinue the drug, taking into account the importance of the drug to the mother.

Pediatric Use:

Safety and efficacy in infants less than 2 months of age have not been established.

Geriatric Use:

Of the 3338 patients in multiple-dose clinical studies of cefpodoxime proxetil film-coated tablets, 521 (16%) were 65 and over, while 214 (6%) were 75 and over. No overall differences in effectiveness or safety were observed between the elderly and younger patients. In healthy geriatric subjects with normal renal function, cefpodoxime half-life in plasma averaged 4.2 hours and urinary recovery averaged 21% after a 400 mg dose was given every 12 hours for 15 days. Other pharmacokinetic parameters were unchanged relative to those observed in healthy younger subjects.

Dose adjustment in elderly patients with normal renal function is not necessary.

ADVERSE REACTIONS

Clinical Trials:

Film-coated Tablets (Multiple dose):

In clinical trials using **multiple doses** of cefpodoxime proxetil film-coated tablets, 4696 patients were treated with the recommended dosages of cefpodoxime (100 to 400 mg Q 12 hours). There were no deaths or permanent disabilities thought related to drug toxicity. One-hundred twenty-nine (2.7%) patients discontinued medication due to adverse events thought possibly- or probably-related to drug toxicity. Ninety-three (52%) of the 178 patients who discontinued therapy (whether thought related to drug therapy or not) did so because of gastrointestinal disturbances, nausea, vomiting, or diarrhea. The percentage of cefpodoxime proxetil-treated patients who discontinued study drug because of adverse events was significantly greater at a dose of 800 mg daily than at a dose of 400 mg daily or at a dose of 200 mg daily. Adverse events thought possibly- or probably-related to cefpodoxime in multiple dose clinical trials (N=4696 cefpodoxime-treated patients) were:

Incidence Greater Than 1%:

Diarrhea 7.0%

Diarrhea or loose stools were dose related: decreasing from 10.4% of patients receiving 800 mg per day to 5.7% for those receiving 200 mg per day. Of patients with diarrhea, 10% had *C. difficile* organism or toxin in the stool. (See **WARNINGS.**)

Nausea	3.3%
Vaginal Fungal Infections	1.0%
Vulvovaginal Infections	1.3%
Abdominal Pain	1.2%
Headache	1.0%

Incidence Less Than 1%: By body system in decreasing order:

Clinical Studies

Adverse events thought possibly- or probably-related to cefpodoxime proxetil that occurred in **less than 1%** of patients (N=4696)

Body - fungal infections, abdominal distention, malaise, fatigue, asthenia, fever, chest pain, back pain, chills, generalized pain, abnormal microbiological tests, moniliasis, abscess, allergic reaction, facial edema, bacterial infections, parasitic infections, localized edema, localized pain.

Cardiovascular - congestive heart failure, migraine, palpitations, vasodilation, hematoma, hypertension, hypotension.

Digestive - vomiting, dyspepsia, dry mouth, flatulence, decreased appetite, constipation, oral moniliasis, anorexia, eructation, gastritis, mouth ulcers, gastrointestinal disorders, rectal disorders, tongue disorders, tooth disorders, increased thirst, oral lesions, tenesmus, dry throat, toothache.

Hemic and Lymphatic - anemia.

Metabolic and Nutritional - dehydration, gout, peripheral edema, weight increase.

Musculo-skeletal - myalgia.

Nervous - dizziness, insomnia, somnolence, anxiety, shakiness, nervousness, cerebral infarction, change in dreams, impaired concentration, confusion, nightmares, paresthesia, vertigo.

Adults and Adolescents (age 12 years and older):

Type of Infection	Total Daily Dose	Dose Frequency	Duration
Pharyngitis and/or tonsillitis	200 mg	100 mg Q 12 hours	5 to 10 days
Acute community-acquired pneumonia	400 mg	200 mg Q 12 hours	14 days
Acute bacterial exacerbations of chronic bronchitis	400 mg	200 mg Q 12 hours	10 days
Uncomplicated gonorrhea (men and women) and rectal gonococcal infections (women)	200 mg	single dose	
Skin and skin structure	800 mg	400 mg Q 12 hours	7 to 14 days
Acute maxillary sinusitis	400 mg	200 mg Q 12 hours	10 days
Uncomplicated urinary tract infection	200 mg	100 mg Q 12 hours	7 days

Respiratory - asthma, cough, epistaxis, rhinitis, wheezing, bronchitis, dyspnea, pleural effusion, pneumonia, sinusitis.

Skin - urticaria, rash, pruritus non-application site, diaphoresis, maculopapular rash, fungal dermatitis, desquamation, dry skin non-application site, hair loss, vesiculobullous rash, sunburn.

Special Senses - taste alterations, eye irritation, taste loss, tinnitus.

Urogenital - hematuria, urinary tract infections, metrorrhagia, dysuria, urinary frequency, nocturia, penile infection, proteinuria, vaginal pain.

Granules for Oral Suspension (Multiple dose):

In clinical trials using multiple doses of cefpodoxime proxetil granules for oral suspension, 2128 pediatric patients (93% of whom were less than 12 years of age) were treated with the recommended dosages of cefpodoxime (10 mg/kg/day Q 24 hours or divided Q 12 hours to a maximum equivalent adult dose). There were no deaths or permanent disabilities in any of the patients in these studies. Twenty-four patients (1.1%) discontinued medication due to adverse events thought possibly- or probably-related to study drug. Primarily, these discontinuations were for gastrointestinal disturbances, usually diarrhea, vomiting, or rashes.

Adverse events thought possibly- or probably-related, or of unknown relationship to cefpodoxime proxetil for oral suspension in multiple dose clinical trials (N=2128 patients treated with cefpodoxime) were:

Incidence Greater Than 1%:

Diarrhea 6.0%

The incidence of diarrhea in infants and toddlers (age 1 month to 2 years) was 12.8%

Diaper rash/Fungal skin rash 2.0% (includes moniliasis)

The incidence of diaper rash in infants and toddlers was 8.5%.

Other skin rashes	1.8%
Vomiting	2.3%

Incidence Less Than 1%:

Body: Localized abdominal pain, abdominal cramp, headache, monilia, generalized abdominal pain, asthenia, fever, fungal infection.

Digestive: Nausea, monilia, anorexia, dry mouth, stomatitis, pseudomembranous colitis.

Hemic & Lymphatic: Thrombocythemia, positive direct Coombs' test, eosinophilia, leukocytosis, leukopenia, prolonged partial thromboplastin time, thrombocytopenic purpura.

Metabolic & Nutritional: Increased SGPT.

Musculo-Skeletal: Myalgia.

Nervous: Hallucination, hyperkinesia, nervousness, somnolence.

Respiratory: Epistaxis, rhinitis.

Skin: Skin moniliasis, urticaria, fungal dermatitis, acne, exfoliative dermatitis, maculopapular rash.

Special Senses: Taste perversion.

Film-coated Tablets (Single dose):

In clinical trials using **a single dose** of cefpodoxime proxetil film-coated tablets, 509 patients were treated with the recommended dosage of cefpodoxime (200 mg). There were no deaths or permanent disabilities thought related to drug toxicity in these studies.

Adverse events thought possibly- or probably-related to cefpodoxime in single dose clinical trials conducted in the United States were:

Incidence Greater Than 1%:

Nausea	1.4%
Diarrhea	1.2%

Incidence Less Than 1%:

Central Nervous System: Dizziness, headache, syncope.

Dermatologic: Rash.

Genital: Vaginitis.

Gastrointestinal: Abdominal pain.

Psychiatric: Anxiety.

Laboratory Changes

Significant laboratory changes that have been reported in adult and pediatric patients in clinical trials of cefpodoxime proxetil, without regard to drug relationship, were:

Hepatic: Transient increases in AST (SGOT), ALT (SGPT), GGT, alkaline phosphatase, bilirubin, and LDH.

Hematologic: Eosinophilia, leukocytosis, lymphocytosis, granulocytosis, basophilia, monocytosis, thrombocytosis, decreased hemoglobin, decreased hematocrit, leukopenia, neutropenia, lymphocytopenia, thrombocytopenia, thrombocythemia, positive Coombs' test, and prolonged PT, and PTT.

Serum Chemistry: Hyperglycemia, hypoglycemia, hypoalbuminemia, hypoproteinemia, hyperkalemia, and hyponatremia.

Renal: Increases in BUN and creatinine.

Most of these abnormalities were transient and not clinically significant.

Post-marketing Experience:

The following serious adverse experiences have been reported: allergic reactions including Stevens-Johnson syndrome, toxic epidermal necrolysis, erythema multiforme and serum sickness-like reactions, pseudomembranous colitis, bloody diarrhea with abdominal pain, ulcerative colitis, rectorrhagia with hypotension, anaphylactic shock, acute liver injury, *in utero* exposure with miscarriage, purpuric nephritis, pulmonary infiltrate with eosinophilia, and eyelid dermatitis.

One death was attributed to pseudomembranous colitis and disseminated intravascular coagulation.

Cephalosporin Class Labeling:

In addition to the adverse reactions listed above which have been observed in patients treated with cefpodoxime proxetil, the following adverse reactions and altered laboratory tests have been reported for cephalosporin class antibiotics:

Adverse Reactions and Abnormal Laboratory Tests: Renal dysfunction, toxic nephropathy, hepatic dysfunction including cholestasis, aplastic anemia, hemolytic anemia, serum sickness-like reaction, hemorrhage, agranulocytosis, and pancytopenia.

Several cephalosporins have been implicated in triggering seizures, particularly in patients with renal impairment when the dosage was not reduced. (See **DOSAGE AND ADMINISTRATION** and **OVERDOSAGE.**) If seizures associated with drug therapy occur, the drug should be discontinued. Anticonvulsant therapy can be given if clinically indicated.

OVERDOSAGE

In acute rodent toxicity studies, a single 5 g/kg oral dose produced no adverse effects.

In the event of serious toxic reaction from overdosage, hemodialysis or peritoneal dialysis may aid in the removal of cefpodoxime from the body, particularly if renal function is compromised.

The toxic symptoms following an overdose of beta-lactam antibiotics may include nausea, vomiting, epigastric distress, and diarrhea.

DOSAGE AND ADMINISTRATION

(See INDICATIONS AND USAGE for indicated pathogens.)

FILM-COATED TABLETS:

VANTIN Tablets should be administered orally with food to enhance absorption. (See **CLINICAL PHARMACOLOGY.**)

The recommended dosages, durations of treatment, and applicable patient population are as described in the following chart:

[See table above]

GRANULES FOR ORAL SUSPENSION:

VANTIN Oral Suspension may be given without regard to food. The recommended dosages, durations of treatment, and applicable patient populations are as described in the following chart:

[See first table at top of next page]

Patients with Renal Dysfunction:

For patients with severe renal impairment (< 30 mL/min creatinine clearance), the dosing intervals should be increased to Q 24 hours. In patients maintained on hemodialysis, the dose frequency should be 3 times/week after hemodialysis.

When only the serum creatinine level is available, the following formula (based on sex, weight, and age of the patient) may be used to estimate creatinine clearance (mL/min). For this estimate to be valid, the serum creatinine level should represent a steady state of renal function.

$$\text{Males: (mL/min)} \quad \frac{\text{Weight (kg)} \times (140 - \text{age})}{72 \times \text{serum creatinine (mg/100 mL)}}$$

Females: (mL/min) 0.85 × above value

Patients with Cirrhosis:

Cefpodoxime pharmacokinetics in cirrhotic patients (with or without ascites) are similar to those in healthy subjects. Dose adjustment is not necessary in this population.

Continued on next page

Adults and Adolescents (age 12 years and older):

Type of Infection	Total Daily Dose	Dose Frequency	Duration
Pharyngitis and/or tonsillitis	200 mg	100 mg Q 12 hours	5 to 10 days
Acute community-acquired pneumonia	400 mg	200 mg Q 12 hours	14 days
Uncomplicated gonorrhea (men and women) and rectal gonococcal infections (women)	200 mg	single dose	
Skin and skin structure	800 mg	400 mg Q 12 hours	7 to 14 days
Acute maxillary sinusitis	400 mg	200 mg Q 12 hours	10 days
Uncomplicated urinary tract infection	200 mg	100 mg Q 12 hours	7 days

Infants and Pediatric Patients (age 2 months through 12 years):

Type of Infection	Total Daily Dose	Dose Frequency	Duration
Acute otitis media	10 mg/kg/day (Max 400 mg/day)	5 mg/kg Q 12 h (Max 200 mg/dose)	5 days
Pharyngitis and/or tonsillitis	10 mg/kg/day (Max 200 mg/day)	5 mg/kg/dose Q 12 h (Max 100 mg/dose)	5 to 10 days
Acute maxillary sinusitis	10 mg/kg/day (Max 400 mg/kg/day)	5 mg/kg Q 12 hours (Max 200 mg/dose)	10 days

Constitution Directions For Oral Suspension

Constituted Volume	Final Concentration	Directions
50 mL	50 mg per 5 mL	Suspend in a total of 29 mL of distilled water. Method: First, shake the bottle to loosen granules. Then add the water in two approximately equal portions, shaking vigorously after each aliquot of water.
75 mL	50 mg per 5 mL	Suspend in a total of 44 mL of distilled water. Method: First, shake the bottle to loosen granules. Then add the water in two approximately equal portions, shaking vigorously after each aliquot of water.
100 mL	50 mg per 5 mL	Suspend in a total of 58 mL of distilled water. Method: First, shake the bottle to loosen granules. Then add the water in two approximately equal portions, shaking vigorously after each aliquot of water.
50 mL	100 mg per 5 mL	Suspend in a total of 29 mL of distilled water. Method: First, shake the bottle to loosen granules. Then add the water in two approximately equal portions, shaking vigorously after each aliquot of water.
75 mL	100 mg per 5 mL	Suspend in a total of 43 mL of distilled water. Method: First, shake the bottle to loosen granules. Then add the water in two approximately equal portions, shaking vigorously after each aliquot of water.
100 mL	100 mg per 5 mL	Suspend in a total of 57 mL of distilled water. Method: First, shake the bottle to loosen granules. Then add the water in two approximately equal portions, shaking vigorously after each aliquot of water.

Vantin—Cont.

Preparation of Suspension:
[See second table above]
After mixing, the suspension should be stored in a refrigerator, 2° to 8°C (36° to 46°F). Shake well before using. Keep container tightly closed. The mixture may be used for 14 days. Discard unused portion after 14 days.

HOW SUPPLIED

VANTIN Tablets are available in the following strengths (cefpodoxime equivalent), colors, and sizes:

100 mg, (light orange, elliptical, debossed with U3617)

Bottles of 20	NDC 0009-3617-01
Bottles of 100	NDC 0009-3617-02
Unit dose packs of 100	NDC 0009-3617-03

200 mg, (coral red, elliptical, debossed with U3618)

Bottles of 20	NDC 0009-3618-01
Bottles of 100	NDC 0009-3618-02
Unit dose packs of 100	NDC 0009-3618-03

Store tablets at controlled room temperature 20° to 25°C (68° to 77°F) [see USP]. Replace cap securely after each opening. Protect unit dose packs from excessive moisture.
VANTIN Oral Suspension provides the equivalent of 50 mg or 100 mg cefpodoxime per 5 mL suspension (when constituted as directed) and is available in lemon creme flavor in the following sizes:

50 mg/5 mL

100-mL suspension	NDC 0009-3531-01
75-mL suspension	NDC 0009-3531-02
50-mL suspension	NDC 0009-3531-03

100 mg/5 mL

100-mL suspension	NDC 0009-3615-01
75-mL suspension	NDC 0009-3615-02
50-mL suspension	NDC 0009-3615-03

Store unsuspended granules at controlled room temperature 20° to 25°C (68° to 77°F) [see USP].
Directions for mixing are included on the label. After mixing, suspension should be stored in a refrigerator, 2° to 8°C (36° to 46°F). Shake well before using. Keep container tightly closed. The mixture may be used for 14 days. Discard unused portion after 14 days.

REFERENCES

1. NCCLS. Methods for dilution antimicrobial susceptibility tests for bacteria that grow aerobically - fourth edition; Approved standard. NCCLS document M7-A4 (ISBN 1-56238-309-4). NCCLS, 940 West Valley Rd., Suite 1400, Wayne, PA 19087-1898, 1997.
2. NCCLS. Performance standards for antimicrobial susceptibility testing; Eighth informational supplement. NCCLS document M100-S8 (ISBN 1-56238-337-x). NCCLS, 940 West Valley Rd., Suite 1400, Wayne, PA 19087-1898, 1998.
3. NCCLS. Performance standards for antimicrobial disk susceptibility tests - sixth edition; Approved standard. NCCLS document M2-A6 (ISBN 1-56238-306-6). NCCLS, 940 West Valley Rd., Suite 1400, Wayne, PA 19087-1898, 1997.

CLINICAL TRIALS

Cystitis

In two double-blind, 2:1 randomized, comparative trials performed in adults in the United States, cefpodoxime proxetil was compared to other beta-lactam antibiotics. In these studies, the following bacterial eradication rates were obtained at 5 to 9 days after therapy:

Pathogen	Cefpodoxime	Comparator
E. coli	200/243 (82%)	99/123 (80%)
Other pathogens	34/42 (81%)	23/28 (82%)
K. pneumoniae		
P. mirabilis		
S. saprophyticus		
TOTAL	234/285 (82%)	122/151 (81%)

In these studies, clinical cure rates and bacterial eradication rates for cefpodoxime proxetil were comparable to the comparator agents; however, the clinical cure rates and bacteriologic eradication rates were lower than those observed with some other classes of approved agents for cystitis.

Acute Otitis Media Studies

In controlled studies of acute otitis media performed in the United States, where significant rates of beta-lactamase-producing organisms were found, cefpodoxime proxetil was compared to cefixime. In these studies, using very strict evaluability criteria and microbiologic and clinical response criteria at the 4 to 21 day post-therapy follow-up, the following presumptive bacterial eradication/clinical success outcomes (cured and improved) were obtained.

Pathogen	Cefpodoxime Proxetil 5 mg/kg Q 12h × 5 d	Cefixime
S. pneumoniae	88/122 (72%)	72/124 (58%)
H. influenzae	50/76 (66%)	61/81 (75%)
M. catarrhalis	22/39 (56%)	23/41 (56%)
S. pyogenes	20/25 (80%)	13/23 (57%)
Clinical succes rate	171/254 (67%)	165/258 (64%)

℞ only
U.S. Patent No. 4,668,783.
Licensed from Sankyo Company, Ltd., Japan

Made by: Pharmacia N.V./S.A., Puurs - Belgium
For: Pharmacia & Upjohn Company, A subsidiary of Pharmacia Corporation, Kalamazoo, Michigan 49001, USA
Revised August 2003 815 267 317
5R6847
Shown in Product Identification Guide, page 330

XALATAN® ℞

[*ză-lă-tăn*]
(latanoprost ophthalmic solution)
0.005% (50 µg/mL)

DESCRIPTION

Latanoprost is a prostaglandin $F_{2\alpha}$ analogue. Its chemical name is isopropyl - (Z)- 7 [(1R,2R,3R,5S) 3,5-dihydroxy-2-[(3R)-3-hydroxy-5-phenylpentyl] cyclopentyl] -5-heptenoate. Its molecular formula is $C_{26}H_{40}O_5$ and its chemical structure is:

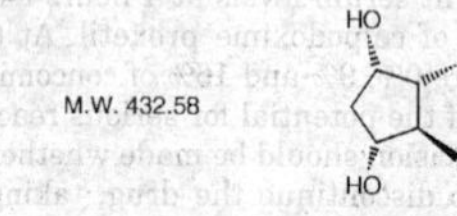

M.W. 432.58

Latanoprost is a colorless to slightly yellow oil that is very soluble in acetonitrile and freely soluble in acetone, ethanol, ethyl acetate, isopropanol, methanol and octanol. It is practically insoluble in water.
XALATAN Sterile Ophthalmic Solution (latanoprost ophthalmic solution) is supplied as a sterile, isotonic, buffered aqueous solution of latanoprost with a pH of approximately 6.7 and an osmolality of approximately 267 mOsmol/kg. Each mL of XALATAN contains 50 micrograms of latanoprost. Benzalkonium chloride, 0.02% is added as a preservative. The inactive ingredients are: sodium chloride, sodium dihydrogen phosphate monohydrate, disodium hydrogen phosphate anhydrous and water for injection. One drop contains approximately 1.5 µg of latanoprost.

CLINICAL PHARMACOLOGY

Mechanism of Action

Latanoprost is a prostanoid selective FP receptor agonist that is believed to reduce the intraocular pressure (IOP) by increasing the outflow of aqueous humor. Studies in animals and man suggest that the main mechanism of action is increased uveoscleral outflow. Elevated IOP represents a major risk factor for glaucomatous field loss. The higher the level of IOP, the greater the likelihood of optic nerve damage and visual field loss.

Pharmacokinetics/Pharmacodynamics

Absorption: Latanoprost is absorbed through the cornea where the isopropyl ester prodrug is hydrolyzed to the acid form to become biologically active. Studies in man indicate that the peak concentration in the aqueous humor is reached about two hours after topical administration.
Distribution: The distribution volume in humans is 0.16 ± 0.02 L/kg. The acid of latanoprost can be measured in aqueous humor during the first 4 hours, and in plasma only during the first hour after local administration.
Metabolism: Latanoprost, an isopropyl ester prodrug, is hydrolyzed by esterases in the cornea to the biologically active acid. The active acid of latanoprost reaching the systemic circulation is primarily metabolized by the liver to the 1,2-dinor and 1,2,3,4-tetranor metabolites via fatty acid β-oxidation.
Excretion: The elimination of the acid of latanoprost from human plasma is rapid ($t_{1/2}$ =17 min) after both intravenous and topical administration. Systemic clearance is approximately 7 mL/min/kg. Following hepatic β-oxidation, the metabolites are mainly eliminated via the kidneys. Approximately 88% and 98% of the administered dose is recovered in the urine after topical and intravenous dosing, respectively.

Animal Studies

In monkeys, latanoprost has been shown to induce increased pigmentation of the iris. The mechanism of increased pigmentation seems to be stimulation of melanin production in melanocytes of the iris, with no proliferative changes observed. The change in iris color may be permanent.
Ocular administration of latanoprost at a dose of 6 µg/eye/day (4 times the daily human dose) to cynomolgus monkeys has also been shown to induce increased palpebral fissure. This effect was reversible upon discontinuation of the drug.

INDICATIONS AND USAGE

XALATAN Sterile Ophthalmic Solution is indicated for the reduction of elevated intraocular pressure in patients with open-angle glaucoma or ocular hypertension.

CLINICAL STUDIES

Patients with mean baseline intraocular pressure of 24 – 25 mmHg who were treated for 6 months in multi-center, randomized, controlled trials demonstrated 6 – 8 mmHg reductions in intraocular pressure. This IOP reduction with XALATAN Sterile Ophthalmic Solution 0.005% dosed once daily was equivalent to the effect of timolol 0.5% dosed twice daily.
A 3-year open-label, prospective safety study with a 2-year extension phase was conducted to evaluate the progression

of increased iris pigmentation with continuous use of XALATAN once-daily as adjunctive therapy in 519 patients with open-angle glaucoma. The analysis was based on observed-cases population of the 380 patients who continued in the extension phase.
Results showed that the onset of noticeable increased iris pigmentation occurred within the first year of treatment for the majority of the patients who developed noticeable increased iris pigmentation. Patients continued to show signs of increasing iris pigmentation throughout the five years of the study. Observation of increased iris pigmentation did not affect the incidence, nature or severity of adverse events (other than increased iris pigmentation) recorded in the study. IOP reduction was similar regardless of the development of increased iris pigmentation during the study.

CONTRAINDICATIONS

Known hypersensitivity to latanoprost, benzalkonium chloride or any other ingredients in this product.

WARNINGS

XALATAN Sterile Ophthalmic Solution has been reported to cause changes to pigmented tissues. The most frequently reported changes have been increased pigmentation of the iris, periorbital tissue (eyelid) and eyelashes, and growth of eyelashes. Pigmentation is expected to increase as long as XALATAN is administered. After discontinuation of XALATAN, pigmentation of the iris is likely to be permanent while pigmentation of the periorbital tissue and eyelash changes have been reported to be reversible in some patients. Patients who receive treatment should be informed of the possibility of increased pigmentation. The effects of increased pigmentation beyond 5 years are not known.

PRECAUTIONS

General: XALATAN Sterile Ophthalmic Solution may gradually increase the pigmentation of the iris. The eye color change is due to increased melanin content in the stromal melanocytes of the iris rather than to an increase in the number of melanocytes. This change may not be noticeable for several months to years (see **WARNINGS**). Typically, the brown pigmentation around the pupil spreads concentrically towards the periphery of the iris and the entire iris or parts of the iris become more brownish. Neither nevi nor freckles of the iris appear to be affected by treatment. While treatment with XALATAN can be continued in patients who develop noticeably increased iris pigmentation, these patients should be examined regularly.
During clinical trials, the increase in brown iris pigment has not been shown to progress further upon discontinuation of treatment, but the resultant color change may be permanent.
Eyelid skin darkening, which may be reversible, has been reported in association with the use of XALATAN (see **WARNINGS**).
XALATAN may gradually change eyelashes and vellus hair in the treated eye; these changes include increased length, thickness, pigmentation, the number of lashes or hairs, and misdirected growth of eyelashes. Eyelash changes are usually reversible upon discontinuation of treatment.
XALATAN should be used with caution in patients with a history of intraocular inflammation (iritis/uveitis) and should generally not be used in patients with active intraocular inflammation.
Macular edema, including cystoid macular edema, has been reported during treatment with XALATAN. These reports have mainly occurred in aphakic patients, in pseudophakic patients with a torn posterior lens capsule, or in patients with known risk factors for macular edema. XALATAN should be used with caution in patients who do not have an intact posterior capsule or who have known risk factors for macular edema.
There is limited experience with XALATAN in the treatment of angle closure, inflammatory or neovascular glaucoma.
There have been reports of bacterial keratitis associated with the use of multiple-dose containers of topical ophthalmic products. These containers had been inadvertently contaminated by patients who, in most cases, had a concurrent corneal disease or a disruption of the ocular epithelial surface (see **PRECAUTIONS**, *Information for Patients*).
Contact lenses should be removed prior to the administration of XALATAN, and may be reinserted 15 minutes after administration (see **PRECAUTIONS**, *Information for Patients*).
Information for Patients (see **WARNINGS** and **PRECAUTIONS**): Patients should be advised about the potential for increased brown pigmentation of the iris, which may be permanent. Patients should also be informed about the possibility of eyelid skin darkening, which may be reversible after discontinuation of XALATAN.
Patients should also be informed of the possibility of eyelash and vellus hair changes in the treated eye during treatment with XALATAN. These changes may result in a disparity between eyes in length, thickness, pigmentation, number of eyelashes or vellus hairs, and/or direction of eyelash growth. Eyelash changes are usually reversible upon discontinuation of treatment.
Patients should be instructed to avoid allowing the tip of the dispensing container to contact the eye or surrounding structures because this could cause the tip to become contaminated by common bacteria known to cause ocular infections. Serious damage to the eye and subsequent loss of vision may result from using contaminated solutions.
Patients also should be advised that if they develop an intercurrent ocular condition (e.g., trauma, or infection) or have ocular surgery, they should immediately seek their physician's advice concerning the continued use of the multiple-dose container.
Patients should be advised that if they develop any ocular reactions, particularly conjunctivitis and lid reactions, they should immediately seek their physician's advice.
Patients should also be advised that XALATAN contains benzalkonium chloride, which may be absorbed by contact lenses. Contact lenses should be removed prior to administration of the solution. Lenses may be reinserted 15 minutes following administration of XALATAN.
If more than one topical ophthalmic drug is being used, the drugs should be administered at least five (5) minutes apart.
Drug Interactions: In vitro studies have shown that precipitation occurs when eye drops containing thimerosal are mixed with XALATAN. If such drugs are used they should be administered at least five (5) minutes apart.
Carcinogenesis, Mutagenesis, Impairment of Fertility: Latanoprost was not mutagenic in bacteria, in mouse lymphoma or in mouse micronucleus tests.
Chromosome aberrations were observed *in vitro* with human lymphocytes.
Latanoprost was not carcinogenic in either mice or rats when administered by oral gavage at doses of up to 170 µg/kg/day (approximately 2,800 times the recommended maximum human dose) for up to 20 and 24 months, respectively.
Additional *in vitro* and *in vivo* studies on unscheduled DNA synthesis in rats were negative. Latanoprost has not been found to have any effect on male or female fertility in animal studies.
Pregnancy: Teratogenic Effects: Pregnancy Category C. Reproduction studies have been performed in rats and rabbits. In rabbits an incidence of 4 of 16 dams had no viable fetuses at a dose that was approximately 80 times the maximum human dose, and the highest nonembryocidal dose in rabbits was approximately 15 times the maximum human dose. There are no adequate and well-controlled studies in pregnant women. XALATAN should be used during pregnancy only if the potential benefit justifies the potential risk to the fetus.
Nursing Mothers: It is not known whether this drug or its metabolites are excreted in human milk. Because many drugs are excreted in human milk, caution should be exercised when XALATAN is administered to a nursing woman.
Pediatric Use: Safety and effectiveness in pediatric patients have not been established.
Geriatric Use: No overall differences in safety or effectiveness have been observed between elderly and younger patients.

ADVERSE REACTIONS

Adverse events referred to in other sections of this insert:
Eyelash changes (increased length, thickness, pigmentation, and number of lashes); eyelid skin darkening; intraocular inflammation (iritis/uveitis); iris pigmentation changes; and macular edema, including cystoid macular edema (see **WARNINGS** and **PRECAUTIONS**).

Controlled Clinical Trials:
The ocular adverse events and ocular signs and symptoms reported in 5 to 15% of the patients on XALATAN Sterile Ophthalmic Solution in the three 6-month, multi-center, double-masked, active-controlled trials were blurred vision, burning and stinging, conjunctival hyperemia, foreign body sensation, itching, increased pigmentation of the iris, and punctate epithelial keratopathy.
Local conjunctival hyperemia was observed; however, less than 1% of the patients treated with XALATAN required discontinuation of therapy because of intolerance to conjunctival hyperemia.
In addition to the above listed ocular events/signs and symptoms, the following were reported in 1 to 4% of the patients: dry eye, excessive tearing, eye pain, lid crusting, lid discomfort/pain, lid edema, lid erythema, and photophobia.
The following events were reported in less than 1% of the patients: conjunctivitis, diplopia and discharge from the eye.
During clinical studies, there were extremely rare reports of the following: retinal artery embolus, retinal detachment, and vitreous hemorrhage from diabetic retinopathy.
The most common systemic adverse events seen with XALATAN were upper respiratory tract infection/cold/flu, which occurred at a rate of approximately 4%. Chest pain/angina pectoris, muscle/joint/back pain, and rash/allergic skin reaction each occurred at a rate of 1 to 2%.

Clinical Practice:
The following events have been identified during post-marketing use of XALATAN in clinical practice. Because they are reported voluntarily from a population of unknown size, estimates of frequency cannot be made. The events, which have been chosen for inclusion due to either their seriousness, frequency of reporting, possible causal connection to XALATAN, or a combination of these factors, include: asthma and exacerbation of asthma; corneal edema and erosions; dyspnea; eyelash and vellus hair changes (increased length, thickness, pigmentation, and number); eyelid skin darkening; herpes keratitis; intraocular inflammation (iritis/uveitis); keratitis; macular edema, including cystoid macular edema; misdirected eyelashes sometimes resulting in eye irritation; and toxic epidermal necrolysis.

OVERDOSAGE

Apart from ocular irritation and conjunctival or episcleral hyperemia, the ocular effects of latanoprost administered at high doses are not known. Intravenous administration of large doses of latanoprost in monkeys has been associated with transient bronchoconstriction; however, in 11 patients with bronchial asthma treated with latanoprost, bronchoconstriction was not induced. Intravenous infusion of up to 3 µg/kg in healthy volunteers produced mean plasma concentrations 200 times higher than during clinical treatment and no adverse reactions were observed. Intravenous dosages of 5.5 to 10 µg/kg caused abdominal pain, dizziness, fatigue, hot flushes, nausea and sweating.
If overdosage with XALATAN Sterile Ophthalmic Solution occurs, treatment should be symptomatic.

DOSAGE AND ADMINISTRATION

The recommended dosage is one drop (1.5 µg) in the affected eye(s) once daily in the evening.
The dosage of XALATAN Sterile Ophthalmic Solution should not exceed once daily since it has been shown that more frequent administration may decrease the intraocular pressure lowering effect.
Reduction of the intraocular pressure starts approximately 3 to 4 hours after administration and the maximum effect is reached after 8 to 12 hours.
XALATAN may be used concomitantly with other topical ophthalmic drug products to lower intraocular pressure. If more than one topical ophthalmic drug is being used, the drugs should be administered at least five (5) minutes apart.

HOW SUPPLIED

XALATAN Sterile Ophthalmic Solution is a clear, isotonic, buffered, preserved colorless solution of latanoprost 0.005% (50 µg/mL). It is supplied as a 2.5 mL solution in a 5 mL clear low density polyethylene bottle with a clear low density polyethylene dropper tip, a turquoise high density polyethylene screw cap, and a tamper-evident clear low density polyethylene overcap.

2.5 mL fill, 0.005% (50 µg/mL)
Package of 1 bottle NDC 0013-8303-04

Storage: Protect from light. Store unopened bottle(s) under refrigeration at 2° to 8°C (36° to 46°F). During shipment to the patient, the bottle may be maintained at temperatures up to 40°C (104°F) for a period not exceeding 8 days. Once a bottle is opened for use, it may be stored at room temperature up to 25°C (77°F) for 6 weeks.
℞ only
U.S. Patent Nos. 4,599,353; 5,296,504 and 5,422,368.
Manufactured for:
Pharmacia & Upjohn Company
A subsidiary of Pharmacia Corporation
Kalamazoo, MI 49001, USA
By:
Cardinal Health
Woodstock, IL 60098, USA
Revised September 2003 818 057 207
691211

XANAX® Ⓒ ℞
alprazolam tablets, USP

DESCRIPTION

XANAX Tablets contain alprazolam which is a triazolo analog of the 1,4 benzodiazepine class of central nervous system-active compounds.
The chemical name of alprazolam is 8-Chloro-1-methyl-6-phenyl-4H-s-triazolo [4,3-α] [1,4] benzodiazepine.
The structural formula is represented below:

Alprazolam is a white crystalline powder, which is soluble in methanol or ethanol but which has no appreciable solubility in water at physiological pH.
Each XANAX Tablet, for oral administration, contains 0.25, 0.5, 1 or 2 mg of alprazolam.
XANAX Tablets, 2 mg, are multi-scored and may be divided as shown below:
[See figure at top of next column]
Inactive ingredients: Cellulose, corn starch, docusate sodium, lactose, magnesium stearate, silicon dioxide and sodium benzoate. In addition, the 0.5 mg tablet contains FD&C Yellow No. 6 and the 1 mg tablet contains FD&C Blue No. 2.

CLINICAL PHARMACOLOGY

CNS agents of the 1,4 benzodiazepine class presumably exert their effects by binding at stereo specific receptors at several sites within the central nervous system. Their exact

Continued on next page

Xanax—Cont.

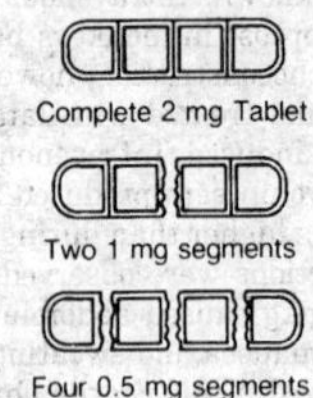

Complete 2 mg Tablet

Two 1 mg segments

Four 0.5 mg segments

mechanism of action is unknown. Clinically, all benzodiazepines cause a dose-related central nervous system depressant activity varying from mild impairment of task performance to hypnosis.

Following oral administration, alprazolam is readily absorbed. Peak concentrations in the plasma occur in one to two hours following administration. Plasma levels are proportionate to the dose given; over the dose range of 0.5 to 3.0 mg, peak levels of 8.0 to 37 ng/mL were observed. Using a specific assay methodology, the mean plasma elimination half-life of alprazolam has been found to be about 11.2 hours (range: 6.3–26.9 hours) in healthy adults.

The predominant metabolites are α-hydroxy-alprazolam and a benzophenone derived from alprazolam. The biological activity of α-hydroxy-alprazolam is approximately one-half that of alprazolam. The benzophenone metabolite is essentially inactive. Plasma levels of these metabolites are extremely low, thus precluding precise pharmacokinetic description. However, their half-lives appear to be of the same order of magnitude as that of alprazolam. Alprazolam and its metabolites are excreted primarily in the urine.

The ability of alprazolam to induce human hepatic enzyme systems has not yet been determined. However, this is not a property of benzodiazepines in general. Further, alprazolam did not affect the prothrombin or plasma warfarin levels in male volunteers administered sodium warfarin orally.

In vitro, alprazolam is bound (80 percent) to human serum protein.

Changes in the absorption, distribution, metabolism and excretion of benzodiazepines have been reported in a variety of disease states including alcoholism, impaired hepatic function and impaired renal function. Changes have also been demonstrated in geriatric patients. A mean half-life of alprazolam of 16.3 hours has been observed in healthy elderly subjects (range: 9.0–26.9 hours, n=16) compared to 11.0 hours (range: 6.3–15.8 hours, n=16) in healthy adult subjects. In patients with alcoholic liver disease the half-life of alprazolam ranged between 5.8 and 65.3 hours (mean: 19.7 hours, n=17) as compared to between 6.3 and 26.9 hours (mean=11.4 hours, n=17) in healthy subjects. In an obese group of subjects the half-life of alprazolam ranged between 9.9 and 40.4 hours (mean=21.8 hours, n=12) as compared to between 6.3 and 15.8 hours (mean=10.6 hours, n=12) in healthy subjects.

Because of its similarity to other benzodiazepines, it is assumed that alprazolam undergoes transplacental passage and that it is excreted in human milk.

INDICATIONS AND USAGE

XANAX Tablets (alprazolam) are indicated for the management of anxiety disorder (a condition corresponding most closely to the APA Diagnostic and Statistical Manual [DSM-III-R] diagnosis of generalized anxiety disorder) or the short-term relief of symptoms of anxiety. Anxiety or tension associated with the stress of everyday life usually does not require treatment with an anxiolytic.

Generalized anxiety disorder is characterized by unrealistic or excessive anxiety and worry (apprehensive expectation) about two or more life circumstances, for a period of six months or longer, during which the person has been bothered more days than not by these concerns. At least 6 of the following 18 symptoms are often present in these patients: *Motor Tension* (trembling, twitching, or feeling shaky; muscle tension, aches, or soreness; restlessness; easy fatigability); *Autonomic Hyperactivity* (shortness of breath or smothering sensations; palpitations or accelerated heart rate; sweating, or cold clammy hands; dry mouth; dizziness or light-headedness; nausea, diarrhea, or other abdominal distress; flushes or chills; frequent urination; trouble swallowing or 'lump in throat'); *Vigilance and Scanning* (feeling keyed up or on edge; exaggerated startle response; difficulty concentrating or 'mind going blank' because of anxiety; trouble falling or staying asleep; irritability). These symptoms must not be secondary to another psychiatric disorder or caused by some organic factor.

Anxiety associated with depression is responsive to XANAX.

XANAX is also indicated for the treatment of panic disorder, with or without agoraphobia.

Studies supporting this claim were conducted in patients whose diagnoses corresponded closely to the DSM-III-R criteria for panic disorder (see CLINICAL STUDIES).

Panic disorder is an illness characterized by recurrent panic attacks. The panic attacks, at least initially, are unexpected. Later in the course of this disturbance certain situations, eg, driving a car or being in a crowded place, may become associated with having a panic attack. These panic attacks are not triggered by situations in which the person is the focus of others' attention (as in social phobia). The diagnosis requires four such attacks within a four week period, or one or more attacks followed by at least a month of persistent fear of having another attack. The panic attacks must be characterized by at least four of the following symptoms: dyspnea or smothering sensations; dizziness, unsteady feelings, or faintness; palpitations or tachycardia; trembling or shaking; sweating; choking; nausea or abdominal distress; depersonalization or derealization; paresthesias; hot flashes or chills; chest pain or discomfort; fear of dying; fear of going crazy or of doing something uncontrolled. At least some of the panic attack symptoms must develop suddenly, and the panic attack symptoms must not be attributable to some known organic factors. Panic disorder is frequently associated with some symptoms of agoraphobia.

Demonstrations of the effectiveness of XANAX by systematic clinical study are limited to four months duration for anxiety disorder and four to ten weeks duration for panic disorder; however, patients with panic disorder have been treated on an open basis for up to eight months without apparent loss of benefit. The physician should periodically reassess the usefulness of the drug for the individual patient.

CONTRAINDICATIONS

XANAX Tablets are contraindicated in patients with known sensitivity to this drug or other benzodiazepines. XANAX may be used in patients with open angle glaucoma who are receiving appropriate therapy, but is contraindicated in patients with acute narrow angle glaucoma.

XANAX is contraindicated with ketoconazole and itraconazole, since these medications significantly impair the oxidative metabolism mediated by cytochrome P450 3A (CYP 3A) (see WARNINGS and PRECAUTIONS – Drug Interactions).

WARNINGS

Dependence and withdrawal reactions, including seizures:
Certain adverse clinical events, some life-threatening, are a direct consequence of physical dependence to XANAX. These include a spectrum of withdrawal symptoms; the most important is seizure (see DRUG ABUSE AND DEPENDENCE). Even after relatively short-term use at the doses recommended for the treatment of transient anxiety and anxiety disorder (ie, 0.75 to 4.0 mg per day), there is some risk of dependence. Spontaneous reporting system data suggest that the risk of dependence and its severity appear to be greater in patients treated with doses greater than 4 mg/day and for long periods (more than 12 weeks). However, in a controlled postmarketing discontinuation study of panic disorder patients, the duration of treatment (three months compared to six months) had no effect on the ability of patients to taper to zero dose. In contrast, patients treated with doses of XANAX greater than 4 mg/day had more difficulty tapering to zero dose than those treated with less than 4 mg/day.

The importance of dose and the risks of XANAX as a treatment for panic disorder:
Because the management of panic disorder often requires the use of average daily doses of XANAX above 4 mg, the risk of dependence among panic disorder patients may be higher than that among those treated for less severe anxiety. Experience in randomized placebo-controlled discontinuation studies of patients with panic disorder showed a high rate of rebound and withdrawal symptoms in patients treated with XANAX compared to placebo treated patients.

Relapse or return of illness was defined as a return of symptoms characteristic of panic disorder (primarily panic attacks) to levels approximately equal to those seen at baseline before active treatment was initiated. Rebound refers to a return of symptoms of panic disorder to a level substantially greater in frequency, or more severe in intensity than seen at baseline. Withdrawal symptoms were identified as those which were generally not characteristic of panic disorder and which occurred for the first time more frequently during discontinuation than at baseline.

In a controlled clinical trial in which 63 patients were randomized to XANAX and where withdrawal symptoms were specifically sought, the following were identified as symptoms of withdrawal: heightened sensory perception, impaired concentration, dysosmia, clouded sensorium, paresthesias, muscle cramps, muscle twitch, diarrhea, blurred vision, appetite decrease and weight loss. Other symptoms, such as anxiety and insomnia, were frequently seen during discontinuation, but it could not be determined if they were due to return of illness, rebound or withdrawal.

In a larger database comprised of both controlled and uncontrolled studies in which 641 patients received XANAX, discontinuation-emergent symptoms which occurred at a rate of over 5% in patients treated with XANAX and at a greater rate than the placebo treated group were as follows:

DISCONTINUATION EMERGENT SYMPTOM INCIDENCE
Percentage of 641 XANAX-Treated Panic Disorder Patients Reporting Events

Body System/Event			
Neurologic		**Gastrointestinal**	
Insomnia	29.5	Nausea/Vomiting	16.5
Light-headedness	19.3	Diarrhea	13.6
Abnormal involuntary movement	17.3	Decreased salivation	10.6
Headache	17.0	**Metabolic-Nutritional**	
Muscular twitching	6.9	Weight loss	13.3
Impaired coordination	6.6	Decreased appetite	12.8
Muscle tone disorders	5.9		
Weakness	5.8	**Dermatological**	
Psychiatric		Sweating	14.4
Anxiety	19.2		
Fatigue and Tiredness	18.4	**Cardiovascular**	
Irritability	10.5	Tachycardia	12.2
Cognitive disorder	10.3		
Memory impairment	5.5	**Special Senses**	
Depression	5.1	Blurred vision	10.0
Confusional state	5.0		

From the studies cited, it has not been determined whether these symptoms are clearly related to the dose and duration of therapy with XANAX in patients with panic disorder.

In two controlled trials of six to eight weeks duration where the ability of patients to discontinue medication was measured, 71%–93% of XANAX treated patients tapered completely off therapy compared to 89%–96% of placebo treated patients. In a controlled postmarketing discontinuation study of panic disorder patients, the duration of treatment (three months compared to six months) had no effect on the ability of patients to taper to zero dose.

Seizures attributable to XANAX were seen after drug discontinuance or dose reduction in 8 of 1980 patients with panic disorder or in patients participating in clinical trials where doses of XANAX greater than 4 mg/day for over 3 months were permitted. Five of these cases clearly occurred during abrupt dose reduction, or discontinuation from daily doses of 2 to 10 mg. Three cases occurred in situations where there was not a clear relationship to abrupt dose reduction or discontinuation. In one instance, seizure occurred after discontinuation from a single dose of 1 mg after tapering at a rate of 1 mg every three days from 6 mg daily. In two other instances, the relationship to taper is indeterminate; in both of these cases the patients had been receiving doses of 3 mg daily prior to seizure. The duration of use in the above 8 cases ranged from 4 to 22 weeks. There have been occasional voluntary reports of patients developing seizures while apparently tapering gradually from XANAX. The risk of seizure seems to be greatest 24–72 hours after discontinuation (see DOSAGE AND ADMINISTRATION for recommended tapering and discontinuation schedule).

Status epilepticus and its treatment:
The medical event voluntary reporting system shows that withdrawal seizures have been reported in association with the discontinuation of XANAX. In most cases, only a single seizure was reported; however, multiple seizures and status epilepticus were reported as well. Ordinarily, the treatment of status epilepticus of any etiology involves use of intravenous benzodiazepines plus phenytoin or barbiturates, maintenance of a patent airway and adequate hydration. For additional details regarding therapy, consultation with an appropriate specialist may be considered.

Interdose Symptoms:
Early morning anxiety and emergence of anxiety symptoms between doses of XANAX have been reported in patients with panic disorder taking prescribed maintenance doses of XANAX. These symptoms may reflect the development of tolerance or a time interval between doses which is longer than the duration of clinical action of the administered dose. In either case, it is presumed that the prescribed dose is not sufficient to maintain plasma levels above those needed to prevent relapse, rebound or withdrawal symptoms over the entire course of the interdosing interval. In these situations, it is recommended that the same total daily dose be given divided as more frequent administrations (see DOSAGE AND ADMINISTRATION).

Risk of dose reduction:
Withdrawal reactions may occur when dosage reduction occurs for any reason. This includes purposeful tapering, but also inadvertent reduction of dose (eg, the patient forgets, the patient is admitted to a hospital, etc.). Therefore, the dosage of XANAX should be reduced or discontinued gradually (see DOSAGE AND ADMINISTRATION).

XANAX Tablets are not of value in the treatment of psychotic patients and should not be employed in lieu of appropriate treatment for psychosis. Because of its CNS depressant effects, patients receiving XANAX should be cautioned against engaging in hazardous occupations or activities requiring complete mental alertness such as operating machinery or driving a motor vehicle. For the same reason, patients should be cautioned about the simultaneous ingestion of alcohol and other CNS depressant drugs during treatment with XANAX.

Benzodiazepines can potentially cause fetal harm when administered to pregnant women. If XANAX is used during pregnancy, or if the patient becomes pregnant while taking this drug, the patient should be apprised of the potential hazard to the fetus. Because of experience with other members of the benzodiazepine class, XANAX is assumed to be capable of causing an increased risk of congenital abnormalities when administered to a pregnant woman during the first trimester. Because use of these drugs is rarely a matter of urgency, their use during the first trimester should almost always be avoided. The possibility that a woman of childbearing potential may be pregnant at the time of institution of therapy should be considered. Patients should be advised that if they become pregnant during therapy or intend to become pregnant they should communicate with their physicians about the desirability of discontinuing the drug.

Alprazolam interaction with drugs that inhibit metabolism via cytochrome P450 3A: The initial step in alprazolam metabolism is hydroxylation catalyzed by cytochrome P450 3A (CYP 3A). Drugs that inhibit this metabolic pathway may have a profound effect on the clearance of alprazolam.

Consequently, alprazolam should be avoided in patients receiving very potent inhibitors of CYP 3A. With drugs inhibiting CYP 3A to a lesser but still significant degree, alprazolam should be used only with caution and consideration of appropriate dosage reduction. For some drugs, an interaction with alprazolam has been quantified with clinical data; for other drugs, interactions are predicted from *in vitro* data and/or experience with similar drugs in the same pharmacologic class.

The following are examples of drugs known to inhibit the metabolism of alprazolam and/or related benzodiazepines, presumably through inhibition of CYP 3A.

Potent CYP 3A inhibitors:

Azole antifungal agents—Although *in vivo* interaction data with alprazolam are not available, ketoconazole and itraconazole are potent CYP 3A inhibitors and the coadministration of alprazolam with them is not recommended. Other azole-type antifungal agents should also be considered potent CYP 3A inhibitors and the coadministration of alprazolam with them is not recommended (see CONTRAINDICATIONS).

Drugs demonstrated to be CYP 3A inhibitors on the basis of clinical studies involving alprazolam (caution and consideration of appropriate alprazolam dose reduction are recommended during coadministration with the following drugs):

Nefazodone—Coadministration of nefazodone increased alprazolam concentration two-fold.

Fluvoxamine—Coadministration of fluvoxamine approximately doubled the maximum plasma concentration of alprazolam, decreased clearance by 49%, increased half-life by 71%, and decreased measured psychomotor performance.

Cimetidine—Coadministration of cimetidine increased the maximum plasma concentration of alprazolam by 86%, decreased clearance by 42%, and increased half-life by 16%.

Other drugs possibly affecting alprazolam metabolism:

Other drugs possibly affecting alprazolam metabolism by inhibition of CYP 3A are discussed in the PRECAUTIONS section (see PRECAUTIONS—Drug Interactions).

ANXIETY DISORDERS

	Treatment-Emergent Symptom Incidence†		Incidence of Intervention Because of Symptom
	XANAX	PLACEBO	XANAX
Number of Patients	565	505	565
% of Patients Reporting:			
Central Nervous System			
Drowsiness	41.0	21.6	15.1
Light-headedness	20.8	19.3	1.2
Depression	13.9	18.1	2.4
Headache	12.9	19.6	1.1
Confusion	9.9	10.0	0.9
Insomnia	8.9	18.4	1.3
Nervousness	4.1	10.3	1.1
Syncope	3.1	4.0	*
Dizziness	1.8	0.8	2.5
Akathisia	1.6	1.2	*
Tiredness/Sleepiness	*	*	1.8
Gastrointestinal			
Dry Mouth	14.7	13.3	0.7
Constipation	10.4	11.4	0.9
Diarrhea	10.1	10.3	1.2
Nausea/Vomiting	9.6	12.8	1.7
Increased Salivation	4.2	2.4	*
Cardiovascular			
Tachycardia/Palpitations	7.7	15.6	0.4
Hypotension	4.7	2.2	*
Sensory			
Blurred Vision	6.2	6.2	0.4
Musculoskeletal			
Rigidity	4.2	5.3	*
Tremor	4.0	8.8	0.4
Cutaneous			
Dermatitis/Allergy	3.8	3.1	0.6
Other			
Nasal Congestion	7.3	9.3	*
Weight Gain	2.7	2.7	*
Weight Loss	2.3	3.0	*

**None reported*

†Events reported by 1% or more of XANAX patients are included.

PRECAUTIONS

General: If XANAX Tablets are to be combined with other psychotropic agents or anticonvulsant drugs, careful consideration should be given to the pharmacology of the agents to be employed, particularly with compounds which might potentiate the action of benzodiazepines (see DRUG INTERACTIONS).

As with other psychotropic medications, the usual precautions with respect to administration of the drug and size of the prescription are indicated for severely depressed patients or those in whom there is reason to expect concealed suicidal ideation or plans.

It is recommended that the dosage be limited to the smallest effective dose to preclude the development of ataxia or oversedation which may be a particular problem in elderly or debilitated patients. (See DOSAGE AND ADMINISTRATION.) The usual precautions in treating patients with impaired renal, hepatic or pulmonary function should be observed. There have been rare reports of death in patients with severe pulmonary disease shortly after the initiation of treatment with XANAX. A decreased systemic alprazolam elimination rate (eg, increased plasma half-life) has been observed in both alcoholic liver disease patients and obese patients receiving XANAX (see CLINICAL PHARMACOLOGY).

Episodes of hypomania and mania have been reported in association with the use of XANAX in patients with depression.

Alprazolam has a weak uricosuric effect. Although other medications with weak uricosuric effect have been reported to cause acute renal failure, there have been no reported instances of acute renal failure attributable to therapy with XANAX.

Information for Patients:

For all users of XANAX:

To assure safe and effective use of benzodiazepines, all patients prescribed XANAX should be provided with the following guidance. In addition, panic disorder patients, for whom doses greater than 4 mg/day are typically prescribed, should be advised about the risks associated with the use of higher doses.

1. Inform your physician about any alcohol consumption and medicine you are taking now, including medication you may buy without a prescription. Alcohol should generally not be used during treatment with benzodiazepines.
2. Not recommended for use in pregnancy. Therefore, inform your physician if you are pregnant, if you are planning to have a child, or if you become pregnant while you are taking this medication.
3. Inform your physician if you are nursing.
4. Until you experience how this medication affects you, do not drive a car or operate potentially dangerous machinery, etc.
5. Do not increase the dose even if you think the medication "does not work anymore" without consulting your physician. Benzodiazepines, even when used as recommended, may produce emotional and/or physical dependence.
6. Do not stop taking this medication abruptly or decrease the dose without consulting your physician, since withdrawal symptoms can occur.

Additional advice for panic disorder patients:

The use of XANAX at doses greater than 4 mg/day, often necessary to treat panic disorder, is accompanied by risks that you need to carefully consider. When used at doses greater than 4 mg/day, which may or may not be required for your treatment, XANAX has the potential to cause severe emotional and physical dependence in some patients and these patients may find it exceedingly difficult to terminate treatment. In two controlled trials of six to eight weeks duration where the ability of patients to discontinue medication was measured, 7 to 29% of patients treated with XANAX did not completely taper off therapy. In a controlled postmarketing discontinuation study of panic disorder patients, the patients treated with doses of XANAX greater than 4 mg/day had more difficulty tapering to zero dose than patients treated with less than 4 mg/day. In all cases, it is important that your physician help you discontinue this medication in a careful and safe manner to avoid overly extended use of XANAX.

In addition, the extended use at doses greater than 4 mg/day appears to increase the incidence and severity of withdrawal reactions when XANAX is discontinued. These are generally minor but seizure can occur, especially if you reduce the dose too rapidly or discontinue the medication abruptly. Seizure can be life-threatening.

Laboratory Tests: Laboratory tests are not ordinarily required in otherwise healthy patients.

Drug Interactions: The benzodiazepines, including alprazolam, produce additive CNS depressant effects when co-administered with other psychotropic medications, anticonvulsants, antihistaminics, ethanol and other drugs which themselves produce CNS depression.

The steady state plasma concentrations of imipramine and desipramine have been reported to be increased an average of 31% and 20%, respectively, by the concomitant administration of XANAX Tablets in doses up to 4 mg/day. The clinical significance of these changes is unknown.

Drugs that inhibit alprazolam metabolism via cytochrome P450 3A: The initial step in alprazolam metabolism is hydroxylation catalyzed by cytochrome P450 3A (CYP 3A). Drugs which inhibit this metabolic pathway may have a profound effect on the clearance of alprazolam (see CONTRAINDICATIONS and WARNINGS for additional drugs of this type).

Drugs demonstrated to be CYP 3A inhibitors of possible clinical significance on the basis of clinical studies involving alprazolam (caution is recommended during coadministration with alprazolam):

Fluoxetine—Coadministration of fluoxetine with alprazolam increased the maximum plasma concentration of alprazolam by 46%, decreased clearance by 21%, increased half-life by 17%, and decreased measured psychomotor performance.

Propoxyphene—Coadministration of propoxyphene decreased the maximum plasma concentration of alprazolam by 6%, decreased clearance by 38%, and increased half-life by 58%.

Oral Contraceptives—Coadministration of oral contraceptives increased the maximum plasma concentration of alprazolam by 18%, decreased clearance by 22%, and increased half-life by 29%.

Drugs and other substances demonstrated to be CYP 3A inhibitors on the basis of clinical studies involving benzodiazepines metabolized similarly to alprazolam or on the basis of in vitro studies with alprazolam or other benzodiazepines (caution is recommended during coadministration with alprazolam): Available data from clinical studies of benzodiazepines other than alprazolam suggest a possible drug interaction with alprazolam for the following: diltiazem, isoniazid, macrolide antibiotics such as erythromycin and clarithromycin, and grapefruit juice. Data from *in vitro* studies of alprazolam suggest a possible drug interaction with alprazolam for the following: sertraline and paroxetine. Data from *in vitro* studies of benzodiazepines other than alprazolam suggest a possible drug interaction for the following: ergotamine, cyclosporine, amiodarone, nicardipine, and nifedipine. Caution is recommended during the coadministration of any of these with alprazolam (see WARNINGS).

Drug/Laboratory Test Interactions: Although interactions between benzodiazepines and commonly employed clinical laboratory tests have occasionally been reported, there is no consistent pattern for a specific drug or specific test.

Carcinogenesis, Mutagenesis, Impairment of Fertility: No evidence of carcinogenic potential was observed during 2-year bioassay studies of alprazolam in rats at doses up to 30 mg/kg/day (150 times the maximum recommended daily human dose of 10 mg/day) and in mice at doses up to 10 mg/kg/day (50 times the maximum recommended daily human dose).

Alprazolam was not mutagenic in the rat micronucleus test at doses up to 100 mg/kg, which is 500 times the maximum recommended daily human dose of 10 mg/day. Alprazolam also was not mutagenic *in vitro* in the DNA Damage/Alkaline Elution Assay or the Ames Assay.

Alprazolam produced no impairment of fertility in rats at doses up to 5 mg/kg/day, which is 25 times the maximum recommended daily human dose of 10 mg/day.

Pregnancy: Teratogenic Effects: Pregnancy Category D: (See WARNINGS Section).

Nonteratogenic Effects: It should be considered that the child born of a mother who is receiving benzodiazepines may be at some risk for withdrawal symptoms from the drug during the postnatal period. Also, neonatal flaccidity and respiratory problems have been reported in children born of mothers who have been receiving benzodiazepines.

Labor and Delivery: XANAX has no established use in labor or delivery.

Nursing Mothers: Benzodiazepines are known to be excreted in human milk. It should be assumed that alprazolam is as well. Chronic administration of diazepam to nursing mothers has been reported to cause their infants to become lethargic and to lose weight. As a general rule, nursing should not be undertaken by mothers who must use XANAX.

Continued on next page

Xanax—Cont.

Pediatric Use: Safety and effectiveness of XANAX in individuals below 18 years of age have not been established.

Geriatric Use: The elderly may be more sensitive to the effects of benzodiazepines. They exhibit higher plasma alprazolam concentrations due to reduced clearance of the drug as compared with a younger population receiving the same doses. The smallest effective dose of XANAX should be used in the elderly to preclude the development of ataxia and oversedation (see CLINICAL PHARMACOLOGY and DOSAGE AND ADMINISTRATION).

ADVERSE REACTIONS

Side effects to XANAX Tablets, if they occur, are generally observed at the beginning of therapy and usually disappear upon continued medication. In the usual patient, the most frequent side effects are likely to be an extension of the pharmacological activity of alprazolam, eg, drowsiness or light-headedness.

The data cited in the two tables below are estimates of untoward clinical event incidence among patients who participated under the following clinical conditions: relatively short duration (ie, four weeks) placebo-controlled clinical studies with dosages up to 4 mg/day of XANAX (for the management of anxiety disorders or for the short-term relief of the symptoms of anxiety) and short-term (up to ten weeks) placebo-controlled clinical studies with dosages up to 10 mg/day of XANAX in patients with panic disorder, with or without agoraphobia.

These data cannot be used to predict precisely the incidence of untoward events in the course of usual medical practice where patient characteristics, and other factors often differ from those in clinical trials. These figures cannot be compared with those obtained from other clinical studies involving related drug products and placebo as each group of drug trials are conducted under a different set of conditions.

Comparison of the cited figures, however, can provide the prescriber with some basis for estimating the relative contributions of drug and non-drug factors to the untoward event incidence in the population studied. Even this use must be approached cautiously, as a drug may relieve a symptom in one patient but induce it in others. (For example, an anxiolytic drug may relieve dry mouth [a symptom of anxiety] in some subjects but induce it [an untoward event] in others.)

Additionally, for anxiety disorders the cited figures can provide the prescriber with an indication as to the frequency with which physician intervention (eg, increased surveillance, decreased dosage or discontinuation of drug therapy) may be necessary because of the untoward clinical event.

[See table at top of previous page]

In addition to the relatively common (ie, greater than 1%) untoward events enumerated in the table above, the following adverse events have been reported in association with the use of benzodiazepines: dystonia, irritability, concentration difficulties, anorexia, transient amnesia or memory impairment, loss of coordination, fatigue, seizures, sedation, slurred speech, jaundice, musculoskeletal weakness, pruritus, diplopia, dysarthria, changes in libido, menstrual irregularities, incontinence and urinary retention.

PANIC DISORDER

	Treatment-Emergent Symptom Incidence*	
	XANAX	PLACEBO
Number of Patients	1388	1231
% of Patients Reporting:		
Central Nervous System		
Drowsiness	76.8	42.7
Fatigue and Tiredness	48.6	42.3
Impaired Coordination	40.1	17.9
Irritability	33.1	30.1
Memory Impairment	33.1	22.1
Light-headedness/Dizziness	29.8	36.9
Insomnia	29.4	41.8
Headache	29.2	35.6
Cognitive Disorder	28.8	20.5
Dysarthria	23.3	6.3
Anxiety	16.6	24.9
Abnormal Involuntary Movement	14.8	21.0
Decreased Libido	14.4	8.0
Depression	13.8	14.0
Confusional State	10.4	8.2
Muscular Twitching	7.9	11.8
Increased Libido	7.7	4.1
Change in Libido (Not Specified)	7.1	5.6
Weakness	7.1	8.4
Muscle Tone Disorders	6.3	7.5
Syncope	3.8	4.8
Akathisia	3.0	4.3
Agitation	2.9	2.6
Disinhibition	2.7	1.5
Paresthesia	2.4	3.2
Talkativeness	2.2	1.0
Vasomotor Disturbances	2.0	2.6
Derealization	1.9	1.2
Dream Abnormalities	1.8	1.5
Fear	1.4	1.0
Feeling Warm	1.3	0.5
Gastrointestinal		
Decreased Salivation	32.8	34.2
Constipation	26.2	15.4
Nausea/Vomiting	22.0	31.8
Diarrhea	20.6	22.8
Abdominal Distress	18.3	21.5
Increased Salivation	5.6	4.4
Cardio-Respiratory		
Nasal Congestion	17.4	16.5
Tachycardia	15.4	26.8
Chest Pain	10.6	18.1
Hyperventilation	9.7	14.5
Upper Respiratory Infection	4.3	3.7
Sensory		
Blurred Vision	21.0	21.4
Tinnitus	6.6	10.4
Musculoskeletal		
Muscular Cramps	2.4	2.4
Muscle Stiffness	2.2	3.3
Cutaneous		
Sweating	15.1	23.5
Rash	10.8	8.1
Other		
Increased Appetite	32.7	22.8
Decreased Appetite	27.8	24.1
Weight Gain	27.2	17.9
Weight Loss	22.6	16.5
Micturition Difficulties	12.2	8.6
Menstrual Disorders	10.4	8.7
Sexual Dysfunction	7.4	3.7
Edema	4.9	5.6
Incontinence	1.5	0.6
Infection	1.3	1.7

**Events reported by 1% or more of XANAX patients are included.*

In addition to the relatively common (ie, greater than 1%) untoward events enumerated in the table above, the following adverse events have been reported in association with the use of XANAX: seizures, hallucinations, depersonalization, taste alterations, diplopia, elevated bilirubin, elevated hepatic enzymes, and jaundice.

There have also been reports of withdrawal seizures upon rapid decrease or abrupt discontinuation of XANAX Tablets (see WARNINGS).

To discontinue treatment in patients taking XANAX, the dosage should be reduced slowly in keeping with good medical practice. It is suggested that the daily dosage of XANAX be decreased by no more than 0.5 mg every three days (see DOSAGE AND ADMINISTRATION). Some patients may benefit from an even slower dosage reduction. In a controlled postmarketing discontinuation study of panic disorder patients which compared this recommended taper schedule with a slower taper schedule, no difference was observed between the groups in the proportion of patients who tapered to zero dose; however, the slower schedule was associated with a reduction in symptoms associated with a withdrawal syndrome.

Panic disorder has been associated with primary and secondary major depressive disorders and increased reports of suicide among untreated patients. Therefore, the same precaution must be exercised when using doses of XANAX greater than 4 mg/day in treating patients with panic disorders as is exercised with the use of any psychotropic drug in treating depressed patients or those in whom there is reason to expect concealed suicidal ideation or plans.

As with all benzodiazepines, paradoxical reactions such as stimulation, increased muscle spasticity, sleep disturbances, hallucinations and other adverse behavioral effects such as agitation, rage, irritability, and aggressive or hostile behavior have been reported rarely. In many of the spontaneous case reports of adverse behavioral effects, patients were receiving other CNS drugs concomitantly and/or were described as having underlying psychiatric conditions. Should any of the above events occur, alprazolam should be discontinued. Isolated published reports involving small numbers of patients have suggested that patients who have borderline personality disorder, a prior history of violent or aggressive behavior, or alcohol or substance abuse may be at risk for such events. Instances of irritability, hostility, and intrusive thoughts have been reported during discontinuation of alprazolam in patients with post-traumatic stress disorder.

Laboratory analyses were performed on patients participating in the clinical program for XANAX. The following incidences of abnormalities shown below were observed in patients receiving XANAX and in patients in the corresponding placebo group. Few of these abnormalities were considered to be of physiological signficance.

	XANAX		PLACEBO	
	Low	High	Low	High
Hematology				
Hematocrit	*	*	*	*
Hemoglobin	*	*	*	*
Total WBC Count	1.4	2.3	1.0	2.0
Neutrophil Count	2.3	3.0	4.2	1.7
Lymphocyte Count	5.5	7.4	5.4	9.5
Monocyte Count	5.3	2.8	6.4	*
Eosinophil Count	3.2	9.5	3.3	7.2
Basophil Count	*	*	*	*
Urinalysis				
Albumin	–	*	–	*
Sugar	–	*	–	*
RBC/HPF	–	3.4	–	5.0
WBC/HPF	–	25.7	–	25.9
Blood Chemistry				
Creatinine	2.2	1.9	3.5	1.0
Bilirubin	*	1.6	*	*
SGOT	*	3.2	1.0	1.8
Alkaline Phosphatase	*	1.7	*	1.8

**Less than 1%*

When treatment with XANAX is protracted, periodic blood counts, urinalysis and blood chemistry analyses are advisable.

Minor changes in EEG patterns, usually low-voltage fast activity have been observed in patients during therapy with XANAX and are of no known signficance.

Post Introduction Reports: Various adverse drug reactions have been reported in association with the use of XANAX since market introduction. The majority of these reactions were reported through the medical event voluntary reporting system. Because of the spontaneous nature of the reporting of medical events and the lack of controls, a causal relationship to the use of XANAX cannot be readily determined. Reported events include: liver enzyme elevations, hepatitis, hepatic failure, Stevens-Johnson syndrome, hyperprolactinemia, gynecomastia and galactorrhea.

DRUG ABUSE AND DEPENDENCE

Physical and Psychological Dependence: Withdrawal symptoms similar in character to those noted with sedative/hypnotics and alcohol have occurred following discontinuance of benzodiazepines, including XANAX. The symptoms can range from mild dysphoria and insomnia to a major syndrome that may include abdominal and muscle cramps, vomiting, sweating, tremors and convulsions. Distinguishing between withdrawal emergent signs and symptoms and the recurrence of illness is often difficult in patients undergoing dose reduction. The long term strategy for treatment of these phenomena will vary with their cause and the therapeutic goal. When necessary, immediate management of withdrawal symptoms requires re-institution of treatment at doses of XANAX sufficient to suppress symptoms. There have been reports of failure of other benzodiazepines to fully suppress these withdrawal symptoms. These failures have been attributed to incomplete cross-tolerance but may also reflect the use of inadequate dosing regimen of the substituted benzodiazepine or the effects of concomitant medications.

While it is difficult to distinguish withdrawal and recurrence for certain patients, the time course and the nature of the symptoms may be helpful. A withdrawal syndrome typically includes the occurrence of new symptoms, tends to appear toward the end of taper or shortly after discontinuation, and will decrease with time. In recurring panic disorder, symptoms similar to those observed before treatment may recur either early or late, and they will persist.

While the severity and incidence of withdrawal phenomena appear to be related to dose and duration of treatment, withdrawal symptoms, including seizures, have been reported after only brief therapy with XANAX at doses within the recommended range for the treatment of anxiety (eg, 0.75 to 4 mg/day). Signs and symptoms of withdrawal are often more prominent after rapid decrease of dosage or abrupt discontinuance. The risk of withdrawal seizures may be increased at doses above 4 mg/day (see WARNINGS).

Patients, especially individuals with a history of seizures or epilepsy, should not be abruptly discontinued from any CNS depressant agent, including XANAX. It is recommended that all patients on XANAX who require a dosage reduction be gradually tapered under close supervision (see WARNINGS and DOSAGE AND ADMINISTRATION).

Psychological dependence is a risk with all benzodiazepines, including XANAX. The risk of psychological dependence may also be increased at doses greater than 4 mg/day and with longer term use, and this risk is further increased in patients with a history of alcohol or drug abuse. Some patients have experienced considerable difficulty in tapering and discontinuing from XANAX, especially those receiving higher doses for extended periods. Addiction-prone individuals should be under careful surveillance when receiving XANAX. As with all anxiolytics, repeat prescriptions should be limited to those who are under medical supervision.

Controlled Substance Class: Alprazolam is a controlled substance under the Controlled Substance Act by the Drug Enforcement Administration and XANAX Tablets have been assigned to Schedule IV.

OVERDOSAGE

Manifestations of alprazolam overdosage include somnolence, confusion, impaired coordination, diminished reflexes and coma. Death has been reported in association with overdoses of alprazolam by itself, as it has with other benzodiazepines. In addition, fatalities have been reported in patients who have overdosed with a combination of a single benzodiazepine, including alprazolam, and alcohol; alcohol levels seen in some of these patients have been lower than those usually associated with alcohol-induced fatality.

The acute oral LD_{50} in rats is 331–2171 mg/kg. Other experiments in animals have indicated that cardiopulmonary collapse can occur following massive intravenous doses of alprazolam (over 195 mg/kg; 975 times the maximum recommended daily human dose of 10 mg/day). Animals could be resuscitated with positive mechanical ventilation and the intravenous infusion of norepinephrine bitartrate.

Animal experiments have suggested that forced diuresis or hemodialysis are probably of little value in treating overdosage.

General Treatment of Overdose: Overdosage reports with XANAX Tablets are limited. As in all cases of drug overdosage, respiration, pulse rate, and blood pressure should be monitored. General supportive measures should be employed, along with immediate gastric lavage. Intravenous fluids should be administered and an adequate airway maintained. If hypotension occurs, it may be combated by the use of vasopressors. Dialysis is of limited value. As with the management of intentional overdosing with any drug, it should be borne in mind that multiple agents may have been ingested.

Flumazenil, a specific benzodiazepine receptor antagonist, is indicated for the complete or partial reversal of the sedative effects of benzodiazepines and may be used in situations when an overdose with a benzodiazepine is known or suspected. Prior to the administration of flumazenil, necessary measures should be instituted to secure airway, ventilation and intravenous access. Flumazenil is intended as an adjunct to, not as a substitute for, proper management of benzodiazepine overdosage. Patients treated with flumazenil should be monitored for re-sedation, respiratory depression, and other residual benzodiazepine effects for an appropriate period after treatment. **The prescriber should be aware of a risk of seizure in association with flumazenil treatment, particularly in long-term benzodiazepine users and in cyclic antidepressant overdose.** The complete flumazenil package insert including CONTRAINDICATIONS, WARNINGS and PRECAUTIONS should be consulted prior to use.

DOSAGE AND ADMINISTRATION

Dosage should be individualized for maximum beneficial effect. While the usual daily dosages given below will meet the needs of most patients, there will be some who require doses greater than 4 mg/day. In such cases, dosage should be increased cautiously to avoid adverse effects.

Anxiety disorders and transient symptoms of anxiety:

Treatment for patients with anxiety should be initiated with a dose of 0.25 to 0.5 mg given three times daily. The dose may be increased to achieve a maximum therapeutic effect, at intervals of 3 to 4 days, to a maximum daily dose of 4 mg, given in divided doses. The lowest possible effective dose should be employed and the need for continued treatment reassessed frequently. The risk of dependence may increase with dose and duration of treatment.

In elderly patients, in patients with advanced liver disease or in patients with debilitating disease, the usual starting dose is 0.25 mg, given two or three times daily. This may be gradually increased if needed and tolerated. The elderly may be especially sensitive to the effects of benzodiazepines. If side effects occur at the recommended starting dose, the dose may be lowered.

In all patients, dosage should be reduced gradually when discontinuing therapy or when decreasing the daily dosage. Although there are no systematically collected data to support a specific discontinuation schedule, it is suggested that the daily dosage be decreased by no more than 0.5 mg every three days. Some patients may require an even slower dosage reduction.

Panic disorder:

The successful treatment of many panic disorder patients has required the use of XANAX at doses greater than 4 mg daily. In controlled trials conducted to establish the efficacy of XANAX in panic disorder, doses in the range of 1 to 10 mg daily were used. The mean dosage employed was approximately 5 to 6 mg daily. Among the approximately 1700 patients participating in the panic disorder development program, about 300 received XANAX in dosages of greater than 7 mg/day, including approximately 100 patients who received maximum dosages of greater than 9 mg/day. Occasional patients required as much as 10 mg a day to achieve a successful response.

Generally, therapy should be initiated at a low dose to minimize the risk of adverse responses in patients especially sensitive to the drug. Thereafter, the dose can be increased at intervals equal to at least 5 times the elimination half-life (about 11 hours in young patients, about 16 hours in elderly patients). Longer titration intervals should probably be used because the maximum therapeutic response may not occur until after the plasma levels achieve steady state. Dose should be advanced until an acceptable therapeutic response (ie, a substantial reduction in or total elimination of panic attacks) is achieved, intolerance occurs, or the maximum recommended dose is attained. For patients receiving doses greater than 4 mg/day, periodic reassessment and consideration of dosage reduction is advised. In a controlled postmarketing dose-response study, patients treated with doses of XANAX greater than 4 mg/day for three months were able to taper to 50% of their total maintenance dose without apparent loss of clinical benefit. Because of the danger of withdrawal, abrupt discontinuation of treatment should be avoided. (See WARNINGS, PRECAUTIONS, DRUG ABUSE AND DEPENDENCE).

The following regimen is one that follows the principles outlined above:

Treatment may be initiated with a dose of 0.5 mg three times daily. Depending on the response, the dose may be increased at intervals of 3 to 4 days in increments of no more than 1 mg per day. Slower titration to the dose levels greater than 4 mg/day may be advisable to allow full expression of the pharmacodynamic effect of XANAX. To lessen the possibility of interdose symptoms, the times of administration should be distributed as evenly as possible throughout the waking hours, that is, on a three or four times per day schedule.

The necessary duration of treatment for panic disorder patients responding to XANAX is unknown. After a period of extended freedom from attacks, a carefully supervised tapered discontinuation may be attempted, but there is evidence that this may often be difficult to accomplish without recurrence of symptoms and/or the manifestation of withdrawal phenomena.

In any case, reduction of dose must be undertaken under close supervision and must be gradual. If significant withdrawal symptoms develop, the previous dosing schedule should be reinstituted and, only after stabilization, should a less rapid schedule of discontinuation be attempted. In a controlled postmarketing discontinuation study of panic disorder patients which compared this recommended taper schedule with a slower taper schedule, no difference was observed between the groups in the proportion of patients who tapered to zero dose; however, the slower schedule was associated with a reduction in symptoms associated with a withdrawal syndrome. It is suggested that the dose be reduced by no more than 0.5 mg every three days, with the understanding that some patients may benefit from an even more gradual discontinuation. Some patients may prove resistant to all discontinuation regimens.

HOW SUPPLIED

XANAX Tablets are available as follows:

0.25 mg (white, oval, scored, imprinted "XANAX 0.25")

Bottles of 100	NDC 0009-0029-01
Reverse Numbered	
Unit Dose (100)	NDC 0009-0029-46
Bottles of 500	NDC 0009-0029-02
Bottles of 1000	NDC 0009-0029-14

0.5 mg (peach, oval, scored, imprinted "XANAX 0.5")

Bottles of 100	NDC 0009-0055-01
Reverse Numbered	
Unit Dose (100)	NDC 0009-0055-46
Bottles of 500	NDC 0009-0055-03
Bottles of 1000	NDC 0009-0055-15

1 mg (blue, oval, scored, imprinted "XANAX 1.0")

Bottles of 100	NDC 0009-0090-01
Bottles of 500	NDC 0009-0090-04
Bottles of 1000	NDC 0009-0090-13

2 mg (white, oblong, multi-scored, imprinted "XANAX" on one side and "2" on the reverse side)

Bottles of 100	NDC 0009-0094-01
Bottles of 500	NDC 0009-0094-03

Store at controlled room temperature 20° to 25°C (68° to 77°F) [see USP].

℞ only

ANIMAL STUDIES

When rats were treated with alprazolam at 3, 10, and 30 mg/kg/day (15 to 150 times the maximum recommended human dose) orally for 2 years, a tendency for a dose related increase in the number of cataracts was observed in females and a tendency for a dose related increase in corneal vascularization was observed in males. These lesions did not appear until after 11 months of treatment.

CLINICAL STUDIES

Anxiety Disorders:

XANAX Tablets were compared to placebo in double blind clinical studies (doses up to 4 mg/day) in patients with a diagnosis of anxiety or anxiety with associated depressive symptomatology. XANAX was significantly better than placebo at each of the evaluation periods of these four week studies as judged by the following psychometric instruments: Physician's Global Impressions, Hamilton Anxiety Rating Scale, Target Symptoms, Patient's Global Impressions and Self-Rating Symptom Scale.

Panic Disorder:

Support for the effectiveness of XANAX in the treatment of panic disorder came from three short-term, placebo-controlled studies (up to 10 weeks) in patients with diagnoses closely corresponding to DSM-III-R criteria for panic disorder.

The average dose of XANAX was 5–6 mg/day in two of the studies, and the doses of XANAX were fixed at 2 and 6 mg/day in the third study. In all three studies, XANAX was superior to placebo on a variable defined as "the number of patients with zero panic attacks" (range, 37–83% met this criterion), as well as on a global improvement score. In two of the three studies, XANAX was superior to placebo on a variable defined as "change from baseline on the number of panic attacks per week" (range, 3.3–5.2), and also on a phobia rating scale. A subgroup of patients who were improved on XANAX during short-term treatment in one of these trials was continued on an open basis up to eight months, without apparent loss of benefit.

Pharmacia & Upjohn Company
A subsidiary of Pharmacia Corporation
Kalamazoo, Michigan 49001, USA 811 557 929
Revised December 2001 692167

Shown in Product Identification Guide, page 330

XANAX XR® Ⓒ ℞

[*ză-nĕks*]

alprazolam extended-release tablets

DESCRIPTION

XANAX XR Tablets contain alprazolam which is a triazolo analog of the 1,4 benzodiazepine class of central nervous system-active compounds.

The chemical name of alprazolam is 8-chloro-1-methyl-6-phenyl-4*H*-*s*-triazolo [4,3-α] [1,4] benzodiazepine. The molecular formula is $C_{17}H_{13}ClN_4$ which corresponds to a molecular weight of 308.76.

The structural formula is represented to the right:

Alprazolam is a white crystalline powder, which is soluble in methanol or ethanol but which has no appreciable solubility in water at physiological pH.

Each XANAX XR extended-release tablet, for oral administration, contains 0.5 mg, 1 mg, 2 mg, or 3 mg of alprazolam. The inactive ingredients are lactose, magnesium stearate, colloidal silicon dioxide, and hypromellose. In addition, the 1 mg and 3 mg tablets contain D & C yellow No. 10 and the 2 mg and 3 mg tablets contain FD&C blue No. 2.

CLINICAL PHARMACOLOGY

Pharmacodynamics

CNS agents of the 1,4 benzodiazepine class presumably exert their effects by binding at stereospecific receptors at several sites within the central nervous system. Their exact mechanism of action is unknown. Clinically, all benzodiazepines cause a dose-related central nervous system depressant activity varying from mild impairment of task performance to hypnosis.

Pharmacokinetics

Absorption

Following oral administration of XANAX (immediate-release) Tablets, alprazolam is readily absorbed. Peak concentrations in the plasma occur in one to two hours following administration. Plasma levels are proportional to the dose given; over the dose range of 0.5 to 3.0 mg, peak levels of 8.0 to 37 ng/mL were observed. Using a specific assay methodology, the mean plasma elimination half-life of alprazolam has been found to be about 11.2 hours (range: 6.3-26.9 hours) in healthy adults.

The mean absolute bioavailability of alprazolam from XANAX XR Tablets is approximately 90%, and the relative bioavailability compared to XANAX Tablets is 100%. The bioavailability and pharmacokinetics of alprazolam following administration of XANAX XR Tablets are similar to that for XANAX Tablets, with the exception of a slower rate of absorption. The slower absorption rate results in a relatively constant concentration that is maintained between 5 and 11 hours after the dosing. The pharmacokinetics of alprazolam and two of its major active metabolites (4-hydroxyalprazolam and α-hydroxyalprazolam) are linear, and concentrations are proportional up to the recommended maximum daily dose of 10 mg given once daily. Multiple dose studies indicate that the metabolism and elimination of alprazolam are similar for the immediate-release and the extended-release products.

Food has a significant influence on the bioavailability of XANAX XR Tablets. A high-fat meal given up to 2 hours before dosing with XANAX XR Tablets increased the mean C_{max} by about 25%. The effect of this meal on T_{max} depended on the timing of the meal, with a reduction in T_{max} by about 1/3 for subjects eating immediately before dosing and an increase in T_{max} by about 1/3 for subjects eating 1 hour or more after dosing. The extent of exposure (AUC) and elimination half-life ($t_{1/2}$) were not affected by eating.

There were significant differences in absorption rate for the XANAX XR Tablet, depending on the time of day administered, with the C_{max} increased by 30% and the T_{max} decreased by an hour following dosing at night, compared to morning dosing.

Distribution

The apparent volume of distribution of alprazolam is similar for XANAX XR and XANAX Tablets. In vitro, alprazolam is bound (80%) to human serum protein. Serum albumin accounts for the majority of the binding.

Metabolism

Alprazolam is extensively metabolized in humans, primarily by cytochrome P450 3A4 (CYP3A4), to two major metabolites in the plasma: 4-hydroxyalprazolam and α-hydroxyalprazolam. A benzophenone derived from alprazolam is also found in humans. Their half-lives appear to be similar to that of alprazolam. The pharmacokinetic parameters at steady-state for the two hydroxylated metabolites of alprazolam (4-hydroxyalprazolam and α-hydroxyalprazolam) were similar for XANAX and XANAX XR Tablets, indicating that the metabolism of alprazolam is not affected by absorption rate. The plasma concentrations of 4-hydroxyalprazolam and α-hydroxyalprazolam relative to unchanged alprazolam concentration after both XANAX XR and XANAX Tablets were always less than 10% and 4%, respectively. The reported relative potencies in benzodiazepine receptor binding experiments and in animal models of induced seizure inhibition are 0.20 and 0.66, respectively, for 4-hydroxyalprazolam and α-hydroxyalprazolam. Such low concentrations and the lesser potencies of 4-hydroxyalprazolam and α-hydroxyalprazolam suggest that they are unlikely to contribute much to the pharmacological effects of alprazolam. The benzophenone metabolite is essentially inactive.

Continued on next page

Xanax XR—Cont.

Elimination

Alprazolam and its metabolites are excreted primarily in the urine. The mean plasma elimination half-life of alprazolam following administration of XANAX XR Tablet ranges from 10.7-15.8 hours in healthy adults.

Special Populations

While pharmacokinetic studies have not been performed in special populations with XANAX XR Tablets, the factors (such as age, gender, hepatic or renal impairment) that would affect the pharmacokinetics of alprazolam after the administration of XANAX Tablets would not be expected to be different with the administration of XANAX XR Tablets. Changes in the absorption, distribution, metabolism, and excretion of benzodiazepines have been reported in a variety of disease states including alcoholism, impaired hepatic function, and impaired renal function. Changes have also been demonstrated in geriatric patients. A mean half-life of alprazolam of 16.3 hours has been observed in healthy elderly subjects (range: 9.0-26.9 hours, n=16) compared to 11.0 hours (range: 6.3-15.8 hours, n=16) in healthy adult subjects. In patients with alcoholic liver disease the half-life of alprazolam ranged between 5.8 and 65.3 hours (mean: 19.7 hours, n=17) as compared to between 6.3 and 26.9 hours (mean=11.4 hours, n=17) in healthy subjects. In an obese group of subjects the half-life of alprazolam ranged between 9.9 and 40.4 hours (mean=21.8 hours, n=12) as compared to between 6.3 and 15.8 hours (mean=10.6 hours, n=12) in healthy subjects.

Because of its similarity to other benzodiazepines, it is assumed that alprazolam undergoes transplacental passage and that it is excreted in human milk.

Race—Maximal concentrations and half-life of alprazolam are approximately 15% and 25% higher in Asians compared to Caucasians.

Pediatrics—The pharmacokinetics of alprazolam after administration of the XANAX XR Tablet in pediatric patients have not been studied.

Gender—Gender has no effect on the pharmacokinetics of alprazolam.

Cigarette Smoking—Alprazolam concentrations may be reduced by up to 50% in smokers compared to non-smokers.

Drug-Drug Interactions

Alprazolam is primarily eliminated by metabolism via cytochrome P450 3A (CYP3A). Most of the interactions that have been documented with alprazolam are with drugs that inhibit or induce CYP3A4.

Compounds that are potent inhibitors of CYP3A would be expected to increase plasma alprazolam concentrations. Drug products that have been studied in vivo, along with their effect on increasing alprazolam AUC, are as follows: ketoconazole, 3.98 fold; itraconazole, 2.70 fold; nefazodone, 1.98 fold; fluvoxamine, 1.96 fold; and erythromycin, 1.61 fold (see CONTRAINDICATIONS, WARNINGS, and PRECAUTIONS–Drug Interactions).

CYP3A inducers would be expected to decrease alprazolam concentrations and this has been observed in vivo. The oral clearance of alprazolam (given in a 0.8 mg single dose) was increased from 0.90±0.21 mL/min/kg to 2.13±0.54 mL/min/kg and the elimination $t_{1/2}$ was shortened (from 17.1±4.9 to 7.7±1.7 h) following administration of 300 mg/day carbamazepine for 10 days (see PRECAUTIONS–Drug Interactions). However, the carbamazepine dose used in this study was fairly low compared to the recommended doses (1000–1200 mg/day); the effect at usual carbamazepine doses is unknown.

The ability of alprazolam to induce or inhibit human hepatic enzyme systems has not been determined. However, this is not a property of benzodiazepines in general. Further, alprazolam did not affect the prothrombin or plasma warfarin levels in male volunteers administered sodium warfarin orally.

CLINICAL EFFICACY TRIALS

The efficacy of XANAX XR Tablets in the treatment of panic disorder was established in two 6-week, placebo-controlled studies of XANAX XR in patients with panic disorder.

In two 6-week, flexible-dose, placebo-controlled studies in patients meeting DSM-III criteria for panic disorder, patients were treated with XANAX XR in a dose range of 1 to 10 mg/day, on a once-a-day basis. The effectiveness of XANAX XR was assessed on the basis of changes in various measures of panic attack frequency, on various measures of the Clinical Global Impression, and on the Overall Phobia Scale. In all, there were seven primary efficacy measures in these studies, and XANAX XR was superior to placebo on all seven outcomes in both studies. The mean dose of XANAX XR at the last treatment visit was 4.2 mg/day in the first study and 4.6 mg/day in the second.

In addition, there were two 8-week, fixed-dose, placebo-controlled studies of XANAX XR in patients with panic disorder, involving fixed XANAX XR doses of 4 and 6 mg/day, on a once-a-day basis, that did not show a benefit for either dose of XANAX XR.

The longer-term efficacy of XANAX XR in panic disorder has not been systematically evaluated.

Analyses of the relationship between treatment outcome and gender did not suggest any differential responsiveness on the basis of gender.

INDICATIONS AND USAGE

XANAX XR Tablets are indicated for the treatment of panic disorder, with or without agoraphobia.

This claim is supported on the basis of two positive studies with XANAX XR conducted in patients whose diagnoses corresponded closely to the DSM-III-R/IV criteria for panic disorder (see CLINICAL STUDIES).

Panic disorder (DSM-IV) is characterized by recurrent unexpected panic attacks, ie, a discrete period of intense fear or discomfort in which four (or more) of the following symptoms develop abruptly and reach a peak within 10 minutes: (1) palpitations, pounding heart, or accelerated heart rate; (2) sweating; (3) trembling or shaking; (4) sensations of shortness of breath or smothering; (5) feeling of choking; (6) chest pain or discomfort; (7) nausea or abdominal distress; (8) feeling dizzy, unsteady, lightheaded, or faint; (9) derealization (feelings of unreality) or depersonalization (being detached from oneself); (10) fear of losing control; (11) fear of dying; (12) paresthesias (numbness or tingling sensations); (13) chills or hot flushes.

The longer-term efficacy of XANAX XR has not been systematically evaluated. Thus, the physician who elects to use this drug for periods longer than 8 weeks should periodically reassess the usefulness of the drug for the individual patient.

CONTRAINDICATIONS

XANAX XR Tablets are contraindicated in patients with known sensitivity to this drug or other benzodiazepines. XANAX XR may be used in patients with open angle glaucoma who are receiving appropriate therapy, but is contraindicated in patients with acute narrow angle glaucoma.

XANAX XR is contraindicated with ketoconazole and itraconazole, since these medications significantly impair the oxidative metabolism mediated by cytochrome P450 3A (CYP3A) (see CLINICAL PHARMACOLOGY, WARNINGS and PRECAUTIONS–Drug Interactions).

WARNINGS

Dependence and Withdrawal Reactions, Including Seizures

Certain adverse clinical events, some life-threatening, are a direct consequence of physical dependence to alprazolam. These include a spectrum of withdrawal symptoms; the most important is seizure (see DRUG ABUSE AND DEPENDENCE). Even after relatively short-term use at doses of $\leq$ 4 mg/day, there is some risk of dependence. Spontaneous reporting system data suggest that the risk of dependence and its severity appear to be greater in patients treated with doses greater than 4 mg/day and for long periods (more than 12 weeks). However, in a controlled postmarketing discontinuation study of panic disorder patients who received XANAX Tablets, the duration of treatment (3 months compared to 6 months) had no effect on the ability of patients to taper to zero dose. In contrast, patients treated with doses of XANAX Tablets greater than 4 mg/day had more difficulty tapering to zero dose than those treated with less than 4 mg/day.

Relapse or return of illness was defined as a return of symptoms characteristic of panic disorder (primarily panic attacks) to levels approximately equal to those seen at baseline before active treatment was initiated. Rebound refers to a return of symptoms of panic disorder to a level substantially greater in frequency, or more severe in intensity than seen at baseline. Withdrawal symptoms were identified as those which were generally not characteristic of panic disorder and which occurred for the first time more frequently during discontinuation than at baseline.

The rate of relapse, rebound, and withdrawal in patients with panic disorder who received XANAX XR Tablets has not been systematically studied. Experience in randomized placebo-controlled discontinuation studies of patients with panic disorder who received XANAX Tablets showed a high rate of rebound and withdrawal symptoms compared to placebo treated patients.

In a controlled clinical trial in which 63 patients were randomized to XANAX Tablets and where withdrawal symptoms were specifically sought, the following were identified as symptoms of withdrawal: heightened sensory perception, impaired concentration, dysosmia, clouded sensorium, paresthesias, muscle cramps, muscle twitch, diarrhea, blurred vision, appetite decrease, and weight loss. Other symptoms, such as anxiety and insomnia, were frequently seen during discontinuation, but it could not be determined if they were due to return of illness, rebound, or withdrawal.

In two controlled trials of 6 to 8 weeks duration where the ability of patients to discontinue medication was measured, 71%-93% of patients treated with XANAX Tablets tapered completely off therapy compared to 89%-96% of placebo treated patients. In a controlled postmarketing discontinuation study of panic disorder patients treated with XANAX Tablets, the duration of treatment (3 months compared to 6 months) had no effect on the ability of patients to taper to zero dose.

Seizures were reported for three patients in panic disorder clinical trials with XANAX XR. In two cases, the patients had completed 6 weeks of treatment with XANAX XR 6 mg/day before experiencing a single seizure. In one case, the patient abruptly discontinued XANAX XR, and in both cases, alcohol intake was implicated. The third case involved multiple seizures after the patient completed treatment with XANAX XR 4 mg/day and missed taking the medication on the first day of taper. All three patients recovered without sequelae.

Seizures have also been observed in association with dose reduction or discontinuation of XANAX Tablets, the immediate release form of alprazolam. Seizures attributable to XANAX were seen after drug discontinuance or dose reduction in 8 of 1980 patients with panic disorder or in patients participating in clinical trials where doses of XANAX greater than 4 mg/day for over 3 months were permitted. Five of these cases clearly occurred during abrupt dose reduction, or discontinuation from daily doses of 2 to 10 mg. Three cases occurred in situations where there was not a clear relationship to abrupt dose reduction or discontinuation. In one instance, seizure occurred after discontinuation from a single dose of 1 mg after tapering at a rate of 1 mg every three days from 6 mg daily. In two other instances, the relationship to taper is indeterminate; in both of these cases the patients had been receiving doses of 3 mg daily prior to seizure. The duration of use in the above 8 cases ranged from 4 to 22 weeks. There have been occasional voluntary reports of patients developing seizures while apparently tapering gradually from XANAX. The risk of seizure seems to be greatest 24-72 hours after discontinuation (see DOSAGE AND ADMINISTRATION for recommended tapering and discontinuation schedule).

Status Epilepticus

The medical event voluntary reporting system shows that withdrawal seizures have been reported in association with the discontinuation of XANAX Tablets. In most cases, only a single seizure was reported; however, multiple seizures and status epilepticus were reported as well.

Interdose Symptoms

Early morning anxiety and emergence of anxiety symptoms between doses of XANAX Tablets have been reported in patients with panic disorder taking prescribed maintenance doses. These symptoms may reflect the development of tolerance or a time interval between doses which is longer than the duration of clinical action of the administered dose. In either case, it is presumed that the prescribed dose is not sufficient to maintain plasma levels above those needed to prevent relapse, rebound, or withdrawal symptoms over the entire course of the interdosing interval.

Risk of Dose Reduction

Withdrawal reactions may occur when dosage reduction occurs for any reason. This includes purposeful tapering, but also inadvertent reduction of dose (eg, the patient forgets, the patient is admitted to a hospital). Therefore, the dosage of XANAX XR should be reduced or discontinued gradually (see DOSAGE AND ADMINISTRATION).

CNS Depression and Impaired Performance

Because of its CNS depressant effects, patients receiving XANAX XR should be cautioned against engaging in hazardous occupations or activities requiring complete mental alertness such as operating machinery or driving a motor vehicle. For the same reason, patients should be cautioned about the simultaneous ingestion of alcohol and other CNS depressant drugs during treatment with XANAX XR.

Risk of Fetal Harm

Benzodiazepines can potentially cause fetal harm when administered to pregnant women. If alprazolam is used during pregnancy, or if the patient becomes pregnant while taking this drug, the patient should be apprised of the potential hazard to the fetus. Because of experience with other members of the benzodiazepine class, alprazolam is assumed to be capable of causing an increased risk of congenital abnormalities when administered to a pregnant woman during the first trimester. Because use of these drugs is rarely a matter of urgency, their use during the first trimester should almost always be avoided. The possibility that a woman of childbearing potential may be pregnant at the time of institution of therapy should be considered. Patients should be advised that if they become pregnant during therapy or intend to become pregnant they should communicate with their physicians about the desirability of discontinuing the drug.

Alprazolam Interaction With Drugs That Inhibit Metabolism Via Cytochrome P450 3A

The initial step in alprazolam metabolism is hydroxylation catalyzed by cytochrome P450 3A (CYP3A). Drugs that inhibit this metabolic pathway may have a profound effect on the clearance of alprazolam. Consequently, alprazolam should be avoided in patients receiving very potent inhibitors of CYP3A. With drugs inhibiting CYP3A to a lesser but still significant degree, alprazolam should be used only with caution and consideration of appropriate dosage reduction. For some drugs, an interaction with alprazolam has been quantified with clinical data; for other drugs, interactions are predicted from in vitro data and/or experience with similar drugs in the same pharmacologic class.

The following are examples of drugs known to inhibit the metabolism of alprazolam and/or related benzodiazepines, presumably through inhibition of CYP3A.

Potent CYP3A Inhibitors

Azole antifungal agents—Ketoconazole and itraconazole are potent CYP3A inhibitors and have been shown in vivo to increase plasma alprazolam concentrations 3.98 fold and 2.70 fold, respectively. The coadministration of alprazolam with these agents is not recommended. Other azole-type antifungal agents should also be considered potent CYP3A inhibitors and the coadministration of alprazolam with them is not recommended (see CONTRAINDICATIONS).

Drugs demonstrated to be CYP3A inhibitors on the basis of clinical studies involving alprazolam (caution and consideration of appropriate alprazolam dose reduction are recommended during coadministration with the following drugs)

Nefazodone—Coadministration of nefazodone increased alprazolam concentration two-fold.

Fluvoxamine—Coadministration of fluvoxamine approximately doubled the maximum plasma concentration of alprazolam, decreased clearance by 49%, increased half-life by 71%, and decreased measured psychomotor performance.
Cimetidine—Coadministration of cimetidine increased the maximum plasma concentration of alprazolam by 86%, decreased clearance by 42%, and increased half-life by 16%.
Other Drugs Possibly Affecting Alprazolam Metabolism
Other drugs possibly affecting alprazolam metabolism by inhibition of CYP3A are discussed in the PRECAUTIONS section (see PRECAUTIONS–Drug Interactions).

PRECAUTIONS

General

Suicide
As with other psychotropic medications, the usual precautions with respect to administration of the drug and size of the prescription are indicated for severely depressed patients or those in whom there is reason to expect concealed suicidal ideation or plans. Panic disorder has been associated with primary and secondary major depressive disorders and increased reports of suicide among untreated patients.
Mania
Episodes of hypomania and mania have been reported in association with the use of XANAX Tablets in patients with depression.
Uricosuric Effect
Alprazolam has a weak uricosuric effect. Although other medications with weak uricosuric effect have been reported to cause acute renal failure, there have been no reported instances of acute renal failure attributable to therapy with alprazolam.
Use in Patients with Concomitant Illness
It is recommended that the dosage be limited to the smallest effective dose to preclude the development of ataxia or oversedation which may be a particular problem in elderly or debilitated patients (see DOSAGE AND ADMINISTRATION). The usual precautions in treating patients with impaired renal, hepatic, or pulmonary function should be observed. There have been rare reports of death in patients with severe pulmonary disease shortly after the initiation of treatment with XANAX Tablets. A decreased systemic alprazolam elimination rate (eg, increased plasma half-life) has been observed in both alcoholic liver disease patients and obese patients receiving XANAX Tablets (see CLINICAL PHARMACOLOGY).

Information for Patients

To assure safe and effective use of XANAX XR, the physician should provide the patient with the following guidance.
1. Inform your physician about any alcohol consumption and medicine you are taking now, including medication you may buy without a prescription. Alcohol should generally not be used during treatment with benzodiazepines.
2. Not recommended for use in pregnancy. Therefore, inform your physician if you are pregnant, if you are planning to have a child, or if you become pregnant while you are taking this medication.
3. Inform your physician if you are nursing.
4. Until you experience how this medication affects you, do not drive a car or operate potentially dangerous machinery, etc.
5. Do not increase the dose even if you think the medication "does not work anymore" without consulting your physician. Benzodiazepines, even when used as recommended, may produce emotional and/or physical dependence.
6. Do not stop taking this medication abruptly or decrease the dose without consulting your physician, since withdrawal symptoms can occur.
7. Some patients may find it very difficult to discontinue treatment with XANAX XR due to severe emotional and physical dependence. Discontinuation symptoms, including possible seizures, may occur following discontinuation from any dose, but the risk may be increased with extended use at doses greater than 4 mg/day, especially if discontinuation is too abrupt. It is important that you seek advice from your physician to discontinue treatment in a careful and safe manner. Proper discontinuation will help to decrease the possibility of withdrawal reactions that can range from mild reactions to severe reactions such as seizure.

Laboratory Tests

Laboratory tests are not ordinarily required in otherwise healthy patients. However, when treatment is protracted, periodic blood counts, urinalysis, and blood chemistry analyses are advisable in keeping with good medical practice.

Drug Interactions

Use with Other CNS Depressants
If XANAX XR Tablets are to be combined with other psychotropic agents or anticonvulsant drugs, careful consideration should be given to the pharmacology of the agents to be employed, particularly with compounds which might potentiate the action of benzodiazepines. The benzodiazepines, including alprazolam, produce additive CNS depressant effects when coadministered with other psychotropic medications, anticonvulsants, antihistaminics, ethanol and other drugs which themselves produce CNS depression.
Use with Imipramine and Desipramine
The steady state plasma concentrations of imipramine and desipramine have been reported to be increased an average of 31% and 20%, respectively, by the concomitant administration of XANAX Tablets in doses up to 4 mg/day. The clinical significance of these changes is unknown.
Drugs that inhibit alprazolam metabolism via cytochrome P450 3A
The initial step in alprazolam metabolism is hydroxylation catalyzed by cytochrome P450 3A (CYP3A). Drugs which inhibit this metabolic pathway may have a profound effect on the clearance of alprazolam (see CONTRAINDICATIONS and WARNINGS for additional drugs of this type).
Drugs demonstrated to be CYP3A inhibitors of possible clinical significance on the basis of clinical studies involving alprazolam (caution is recommended during coadministration with alprazolam)
Fluoxetine—Coadministration of fluoxetine with alprazolam increased the maximum plasma concentration of alprazolam by 46%, decreased clearance by 21%, increased half-life by 17%, and decreased measured psychomotor performance.
Propoxyphene—Coadministration of propoxyphene decreased the maximum plasma concentration of alprazolam by 6%, decreased clearance by 38%, and increased half-life by 58%.
Oral Contraceptives—Coadministration of oral contraceptives increased the maximum plasma concentration of alprazolam by 18%, decreased clearance by 22%, and increased half-life by 29%.
Drugs and other substances demonstrated to be CYP3A inhibitors on the basis of clinical studies involving benzodiazepines metabolized similarly to alprazolam or on the basis of in vitro studies with alprazolam or other benzodiazepines (caution is recommended during coadministration with alprazolam)
Available data from clinical studies of benzodiazepines other than alprazolam suggest a possible drug interaction with alprazolam for the following: diltiazem, isoniazid, macrolide antibiotics such as erythromycin and clarithromycin, and grapefruit juice. Data from in vitro studies of alprazolam suggest a possible drug interaction with alprazolam for the following: sertraline and paroxetine. However, data from an in vivo drug interaction study involving a single dose of alprazolam 1 mg and steady state doses of sertraline (50 to 150 mg/day) did not reveal any clinically significant changes in the pharmacokinetics of alprazolam. Data from in vitro studies of benzodiazepines other than alprazolam suggest a possible drug interaction for the following: ergotamine, cyclosporine, amiodarone, nicardipine, and nifedipine. Caution is recommended during the coadministration of any of these with alprazolam (see WARNINGS).
Drugs demonstrated to be inducers of CYP3A
Carbamazepine can increase alprazolam metabolism and therefore can decrease plasma levels of alprazolam.

Drug/Laboratory Test Interactions

Although interactions between benzodiazepines and commonly employed clinical laboratory tests have occasionally been reported, there is no consistent pattern for a specific drug or specific test.

Carcinogenesis, Mutagenesis, Impairment of Fertility

No evidence of carcinogenic potential was observed during 2-year bioassay studies of alprazolam in rats at doses up to 30 mg/kg/day (150 times the maximum recommended daily human dose of 10 mg/day) and in mice at doses up to 10 mg/kg/day (50 times the maximum recommended daily human dose).
Alprazolam was not mutagenic in the rat micronucleus test at doses up to 100 mg/kg, which is 500 times the maximum recommended daily human dose of 10 mg/day. Alprazolam also was not mutagenic in vitro in the DNA Damage/Alkaline Elution Assay or the Ames Assay.
Alprazolam produced no impairment of fertility in rats at doses up to 5 mg/kg/day, which is 25 times the maximum recommended daily human dose of 10 mg/day.

Pregnancy

Teratogenic Effects: Pregnancy Category D: (see WARNINGS section).
Nonteratogenic Effects: It should be considered that the child born of a mother who is receiving benzodiazepines may be at some risk for withdrawal symptoms from the drug during the postnatal period. Also, neonatal flaccidity and respiratory problems have been reported in children born of mothers who have been receiving benzodiazepines.

Labor and Delivery

Alprazolam has no established use in labor or delivery.

Nursing Mothers

Benzodiazepines are known to be excreted in human milk. It should be assumed that alprazolam is as well. Chronic administration of diazepam to nursing mothers has been reported to cause their infants to become lethargic and to lose weight. As a general rule, nursing should not be undertaken by mothers who must use alprazolam.

Pediatric Use

Safety and effectiveness of alprazolam in individuals below 18 years of age have not been established.

Geriatric Use

The elderly may be more sensitive to the effects of benzodiazepines. They exhibit higher plasma alprazolam concentrations due to reduced clearance of the drug as compared with a younger population receiving the same doses. The smallest effective dose of alprazolam should be used in the elderly to preclude the development of ataxia and oversedation (see CLINICAL PHARMACOLOGY and DOSAGE AND ADMINISTRATION).

ADVERSE REACTIONS

The information included in the subsection on Adverse Events Observed in Short-Term, Placebo-Controlled Trials with XANAX XR Tablets is based on pooled data of five 6- and 8-week placebo-controlled clinical studies in panic disorder.
Adverse event reports were elicited either by general inquiry or by checklist, and were recorded by clinical investigators using terminology of their own choosing. The stated frequencies of adverse events represent the proportion of individuals who experienced, at least once, a treatment-emergent adverse event of the type listed. An event was considered treatment emergent if it occurred for the first time or worsened during therapy following baseline evaluation. In the tables and tabulations that follow, standard MedDRA terminology (version 4.0) was used to classify reported adverse events.

Adverse Events Observed in Short-Term, Placebo-Controlled Trials of XANAX XR

Adverse Events Reported as Reasons for Discontinuation of Treatment in Placebo-Controlled Trials
Approximately 17% of the 531 patients who received XANAX XR in placebo-controlled clinical trials for panic disorder had at least one adverse event that led to discontinuation compared to 8% of 349 placebo-treated patients. The most common events leading to discontinuation and considered to be drug-related (ie, leading to discontinuation in at least 1% of the patients treated with XANAX XR at a rate at least twice that of placebo) are shown in the following table.

Common Adverse Events Leading to Discontinuation of Treatment in Placebo-Controlled Trials

System Organ Class/Adverse Event	Percentage of Patients Discontinuing Due to Adverse Events	
	XANAX XR (n=531)	Placebo (n=349)
Nervous system disorders		
Sedation	7.5	0.6
Somnolence	3.2	0.3
Dysarthria	2.1	0
Coordination abnormal	1.9	0.3
Memory impairment	1.5	0.3
General disorders/administration site conditions		
Fatigue	1.7	0.6
Psychiatric disorders		
Depression	2.5	1.2

Adverse Events Occurring at an Incidence of 1% or More Among Patients Treated with XANAX XR
The prescriber should be aware that adverse event incidence cannot be used to predict the incidence of adverse events in the course of usual medical practice where patient characteristics and other factors differ from those which prevailed in the clinical trials. Similarly, the cited frequencies cannot be compared with event incidence obtained from other clinical investigations involving different treatments, uses, and investigators. The cited values, however, do provide the prescribing physician with some basis for estimating the relative contribution of drug and non-drug factors to the adverse event incidence rate in the population studied. The following table shows the incidence of treatment-emergent adverse events that occurred during 6- to 8-week placebo-controlled trials in 1% or more of patients treated with XANAX XR where the incidence in patients treated with XANAX XR was greater than the incidence in placebo-treated patients. The most commonly observed adverse events in panic disorder patients treated with XANAX XR (incidence of 5% or greater and at least twice the incidence in placebo patients) were: sedation, somnolence, memory impairment, dysarthria, coordination abnormal, ataxia, libido decreased (see table).

Treatment-Emergent Adverse Events: Incidence in Short-Term, Placebo-Controlled Clinical Trials with XANAX XR

System Organ Class/Adverse Event	Percentage of Patients Reporting Adverse Event	
	XANAX XR (n=531)	Placebo (n=349)
Nervous system disorders		
Sedation	45.2	22.6
Somnolence	23.0	6.0
Memory impairment	15.4	6.9
Dysarthria	10.9	2.6
Coordination abnormal	9.4	0.9
Mental impairment	7.2	5.7
Ataxia	7.2	3.2
Disturbance in attention	3.2	0.6
Balance impaired	3.2	0.6
Paresthesia	2.4	1.7

Continued on next page

Xanax XR—Cont.

Dyskinesia	1.7	1.4
Hypoesthesia	1.3	0.3
Hypersomnia	1.3	0
General disorders/ administration site conditions		
Fatigue	13.9	9.2
Lethargy	1.7	0.6
Infections and infestations		
Influenza	2.4	2.3
Upper respiratory tract infections	1.9	1.7
Psychiatric disorders		
Depression	12.1	9.2
Libido decreased	6.0	2.3
Disorientation	1.5	0
Confusion	1.5	0.9
Depressed mood	1.3	0.3
Anxiety	1.1	0.6
Metabolism and nutrition disorders		
Appetite decreased	7.3	7.2
Appetite increased	7.0	6.0
Anorexia	1.5	0
Gastrointestinal disorders		
Dry mouth	10.2	9.7
Constipation	8.1	4.3
Nausea	6.0	3.2
Pharyngolaryngeal pain	3.2	2.6
Investigations		
Weight increased	5.1	4.3
Weight decreased	4.3	3.7
Injury, poisoning, and procedural complications		
Road traffic accident	1.5	0
Reproductive system and breast disorders		
Dysmenorrhea	3.6	2.9
Sexual dysfunction	2.4	1.1
Premenstrual syndrome	1.7	0.6
Musculoskeletal and connective tissue disorders		
Arthralgia	2.4	0.6
Myalgia	1.5	1.1
Pain in limb	1.1	0.3
Vascular disorders		
Hot flushes	1.5	1.4
Respiratory, thoracic, and mediastinal disorders		
Dyspnea	1.5	0.3
Rhinitis allergic	1.1	0.6
Skin and subcutaneous tissue disorders		
Pruritis	1.1	0.9

Other Adverse Events Observed During the Premarketing Evaluation of XANAX XR Tablets

Following is a list of MedDRA terms that reflect treatment-emergent adverse events reported by 531 patients with panic disorder treated with XANAX XR. All potentially important reported events are included except those already listed in the above table or elsewhere in labeling, those events for which a drug cause was remote, those event terms that were so general as to be uninformative, and those events that occurred at rates similar to background rates in the general population. It is important to emphasize that, although the events reported occurred during treatment with XANAX XR, they were not necessarily caused by the drug. Events are further categorized by body system and listed in order of decreasing frequency according to the following definitions: frequent adverse events are those occurring on 1 or more occasions in at least 1/100 patients; infrequent adverse events are those occurring in less than 1/100 patients but at least 1/1000 patients; rare events are those occurring in fewer than 1/1000 patients.

Cardiac disorders: *Frequent:* palpitation; *Infrequent:* sinus tachycardia

Ear and Labyrinth disorders: *Frequent:* Vertigo; *Infrequent:* tinnitus, ear pain

Eye disorders: *Frequent:* blurred vision; *Infrequent:* mydriasis, photophobia

Gastrointestinal disorders: *Frequent:* diarrhea, vomiting, dyspepsia, abdominal pain; *Infrequent:* dysphagia, salivary hypersecretion

General disorders and administration site conditions: *Frequent:* malaise, weakness, chest pains; *Infrequent:* fall, pyrexia, thirst, feeling hot and cold, edema, feeling jittery, sluggishness, asthenia, feeling drunk, chest tightness, increased energy, feeling of relaxation, hangover, loss of control of legs, rigors

Musculoskeletal and connective tissue disorders: *Frequent:* back pain, muscle cramps, muscle twitching

Nervous system disorders: *Frequent:* headache, dizziness, tremor; *Infrequent:* amnesia, clumsiness, syncope, hypotonia, seizures, depressed level of consciousness, sleep apnea syndrome, sleep talking, stupor

Psychiatric system disorders: *Frequent:* irritability, insomnia, nervousness, derealization, libido increased, restlessness, agitation, depersonalization, nightmare; *Infrequent:* abnormal dreams, apathy, aggression, anger, bradyphrenia, euphoric mood, logorrhea, mood swings, dysphonia, hallucination, homicidal ideation, mania, hypomania, impulse control, psychomotor retardation, suicidal ideation

Renal and urinary disorders: *Frequent:* difficulty in micturition; *Infrequent:* urinary frequency, urinary incontinence

Respiratory, thoracic, and mediastinal disorders: *Frequent:* nasal congestion, hyperventilation; *Infrequent:* choking sensation, epistaxis, rhinorrhea

Skin and subcutaneous tissue disorders: *Frequent:* sweating increased; *Infrequent:* clamminess, rash, urticaria

Vascular disorders: *Infrequent:* hypotension

The categories of adverse events reported in the clinical development program for XANAX Tablets in the treatment of panic disorder differ somewhat from those reported for XANAX XR Tablets because the clinical trials with XANAX Tablets and XANAX XR Tablets used different standard medical nomenclature for reporting the adverse events. Nevertheless, the types of adverse events reported in the clinical trials with XANAX Tablets were generally the same as those reported in the clinical trials with XANAX XR Tablets.

Discontinuation-Emergent Adverse Events Occurring at an Incidence of 5% or More Among Patients Treated with XANAX XR

The following table shows the incidence of discontinuation-emergent adverse events that occurred during short-term, placebo-controlled trials in 5% or more of patients treated with XANAX XR where the incidence in patients treated with XANAX XR was two times greater than the incidence in placebo-treated patients.

Discontinuation-Emergent Symptoms: Incidence in Short-Term, Placebo-Controlled Trials with XANAX XR

System Organ Class/Adverse Event	Percentage of Patients Reporting Adverse Event	
	XANAX XR (n=422)	Placebo (n=261)
Nervous system disorders		
Tremor	28.2	10.7
Headache	26.5	12.6
Hypoesthesia	7.8	2.3
Paresthesia	7.1	2.7
Psychiatric disorders		
Insomnia	24.2	9.6
Nervousness	21.8	8.8
Depression	10.9	5.0
Derealization	8.0	3.8
Anxiety	7.8	2.7
Depersonalization	5.7	1.9
Gastrointestinal disorders		
Diarrhea	12.1	3.1
Respiratory, thoracic and mediastinal disorders		
Hyperventilation	8.5	2.7
Metabolism and nutrition disorders		
Appetite decreased	9.5	3.8
Musculoskeletal and connective tissue disorders		
Muscle twitching	7.4	2.7
Vascular disorders		
Hot flushes	5.9	2.7

There have also been reports of withdrawal seizures upon rapid decrease or abrupt discontinuation of alprazolam (see WARNINGS).

To discontinue treatment in patients taking XANAX XR Tablets, the dosage should be reduced slowly in keeping with good medical practice. It is suggested that the daily dosage of XANAX XR Tablets be decreased by no more than 0.5 mg every three days (see DOSAGE AND ADMINISTRATION). Some patients may benefit from an even slower dosage reduction. In a controlled postmarketing discontinuation study of panic disorder patients which compared this recommended taper schedule with a slower taper schedule, no difference was observed between the groups in the proportion of patients who tapered to zero dose; however, the slower schedule was associated with a reduction in symptoms associated with a withdrawal syndrome.

As with all benzodiazepines, paradoxical reactions such as stimulation, increased muscle spasticity, sleep disturbances, hallucinations, and other adverse behavioral effects such as agitation, rage, irritability, and aggressive or hostile behavior have been reported rarely. In many of the spontaneous case reports of adverse behavioral effects, patients were receiving other CNS drugs concomitantly and/or were described as having underlying psychiatric conditions. Should any of the above events occur, alprazolam should be discontinued. Isolated published reports involving small numbers of patients have suggested that patients who have borderline personality disorder, a prior history of violent or aggressive behavior, or alcohol or substance abuse may be at risk for such events. Instances of irritability, hostility, and intrusive thoughts have been reported during discontinuation of alprazolam in patients with posttraumatic stress disorder.

Post Introduction Reports

Various adverse drug reactions have been reported in association with the use of XANAX Tablets since market introduction. The majority of these reactions were reported through the medical event voluntary reporting system. Because of the spontaneous nature of the reporting of medical events and the lack of controls, a causal relationship to the use of XANAX Tablets cannot be readily determined. Reported events include: liver enzyme elevations, hepatitis, hepatic failure, Stevens-Johnson syndrome, hyperprolactinemia, gynecomastia, and galactorrhea.

DRUG ABUSE AND DEPENDENCE

Physical and Psychological Dependence

Withdrawal symptoms similar in character to those noted with sedative/hypnotics and alcohol have occurred following discontinuance of benzodiazepines, including alprazolam. The symptoms can range from mild dysphoria and insomnia to a major syndrome that may include abdominal and muscle cramps, vomiting, sweating, tremors, and convulsions. Distinguishing between withdrawal emergent signs and symptoms and the recurrence of illness is often difficult in patients undergoing dose reduction. The long-term strategy for treatment of these phenomena will vary with their cause and the therapeutic goal. When necessary, immediate management of withdrawal symptoms requires re-institution of treatment at doses of alprazolam sufficient to suppress symptoms. There have been reports of failure of other benzodiazepines to fully suppress these withdrawal symptoms. These failures have been attributed to incomplete cross-tolerance but may also reflect the use of an inadequate dosing regimen of the substituted benzodiazepine or the effects of concomitant medications.

While it is difficult to distinguish withdrawal and recurrence for certain patients, the time course and the nature of the symptoms may be helpful. A withdrawal syndrome typically includes the occurrence of new symptoms, tends to appear toward the end of taper or shortly after discontinuation, and will decrease with time. In recurring panic disorder, symptoms similar to those observed before treatment may recur either early or late, and they will persist.

While the severity and incidence of withdrawal phenomena appear to be related to dose and duration of treatment, withdrawal symptoms, including seizures, have been reported after only brief therapy with alprazolam at doses within the recommended range for the treatment of anxiety (eg, 0.75 to 4 mg/day). Signs and symptoms of withdrawal are often more prominent after rapid decrease of dosage or abrupt discontinuance. The risk of withdrawal seizures may be increased at doses above 4 mg/day (see WARNINGS).

Patients, especially individuals with a history of seizures or epilepsy, should not be abruptly discontinued from any CNS depressant agent, including alprazolam. It is recommended that all patients on alprazolam who require a dosage reduction be gradually tapered under close supervision (see WARNINGS and DOSAGE AND ADMINISTRATION).

Psychological dependence is a risk with all benzodiazepines, including alprazolam. The risk of psychological dependence may also be increased at doses greater than 4 mg/day and with longer term use, and this risk is further increased in patients with a history of alcohol or drug abuse. Some patients have experienced considerable difficulty in tapering and discontinuing from alprazolam, especially those receiving higher doses for extended periods. Addiction-prone individuals should be under careful surveillance when receiving alprazolam. As with all anxiolytics, repeat prescriptions should be limited to those who are under medical supervision.

Controlled Substance Class

Alprazolam is a controlled substance under the Controlled Substance Act by the Drug Enforcement Administration and XANAX XR Tablets have been assigned to Schedule IV.

OVERDOSAGE

Clinical Experience

Overdosage reports with XANAX Tablets are limited. Manifestations of alprazolam overdosage include somnolence, confusion, impaired coordination, diminished reflexes, and coma. Death has been reported in association with overdoses of alprazolam by itself, as it has with other benzodiazepines. In addition, fatalities have been reported in patients who have overdosed with a combination of a single benzodiazepine, including alprazolam, and alcohol; alcohol levels seen in some of these patients have been lower than those usually associated with alcohol-induced fatality.

Animal experiments have suggested that forced diuresis or hemodialysis are probably of little value in treating overdosage.

General Treatment of Overdose
As in all cases of drug overdosage, respiration, pulse rate, and blood pressure should be monitored. General supportive measures should be employed, along with immediate gastric lavage. Intravenous fluids should be administered and an adequate airway maintained. If hypotension occurs, it may be combated by the use of vasopressors. Dialysis is of limited value. As with the management of intentional overdosing with any drug, it should be borne in mind that multiple agents may have been ingested.
Flumazenil, a specific benzodiazepine receptor antagonist, is indicated for the complete or partial reversal of the sedative effects of benzodiazepines and may be used in situations when an overdose with a benzodiazepine is known or suspected. Prior to the administration of flumazenil, necessary measures should be instituted to secure airway, ventilation, and intravenous access. Flumazenil is intended as an adjunct to, not as a substitute for, proper management of benzodiazepine overdose. Patients treated with flumazenil should be monitored for re-sedation, respiratory depression, and other residual benzodiazepine effects for an appropriate period after treatment. **The prescriber should be aware of a risk of seizure in association with flumazenil treatment, particularly in long-term benzodiazepine users and in cyclic antidepressant overdose.** The complete flumazenil package insert including CONTRAINDICATIONS, WARNINGS, and PRECAUTIONS should be consulted prior to use.

DOSAGE AND ADMINISTRATION

XANAX XR Tablets may be administered once daily, preferably in the morning. The tablets should be taken intact; they should not be chewed, crushed, or broken.
The suggested total daily dose ranges between 3 to 6 mg/day. Dosage should be individualized for maximum beneficial effect. While the suggested total daily dosages given will meet the needs of most patients, there will be some patients who require doses greater than 6 mg/day. In such cases, dosage should be increased cautiously to avoid adverse effects.
Dosing in Special Populations
In elderly patients, in patients with advanced liver disease, or in patients with debilitating disease, the usual starting dose of XANAX XR is 0.5 mg once daily. This may be gradually increased if needed and tolerated (see Dose Titration). The elderly may be especially sensitive to the effects of benzodiazepines.
Dose Titration
Treatment with XANAX XR may be initiated with a dose of 0.5 mg to 1 mg once daily. Depending on the response, the dose may be increased at intervals of 3 to 4 days in increments of no more than 1 mg/day. Slower titration to the dose levels may be advisable to allow full expression of the pharmacodynamic effect of XANAX XR.
Generally, therapy should be initiated at a low dose to minimize the risk of adverse responses in patients especially sensitive to the drug. Dose should be advanced until an acceptable therapeutic response (ie, a substantial reduction in or total elimination of panic attacks) is achieved, intolerance occurs, or the maximum recommended dose is attained.
Dose Maintenance
In controlled trials conducted to establish the efficacy of XANAX XR Tablets in panic disorder, doses in the range of 1 to 10 mg/day were used. Most patients showed efficacy in the dose range of 3 to 6 mg/day. Occasional patients required as much as 10 mg/day to achieve a successful response.
The necessary duration of treatment for panic disorder patients responding to XANAX XR is unknown. However, periodic reassessment is advised. After a period of extended freedom from attacks, a carefully supervised tapered discontinuation may be attempted, but there is evidence that this may often be difficult to accomplish without recurrence of symptoms and/or the manifestation of withdrawal phenomena.
Dose Reduction
Because of the danger of withdrawal, abrupt discontinuation of treatment should be avoided (see WARNINGS, PRECAUTIONS, DRUG ABUSE AND DEPENDENCE).
In all patients, dosage should be reduced gradually when discontinuing therapy or when decreasing the daily dosage. Although there are no systematically collected data to support a specific discontinuation schedule, it is suggested that the daily dosage be decreased by no more than 0.5 mg every three days. Some patients may require an even slower dosage reduction.
In any case, reduction of dose must be undertaken under close supervision and must be gradual. If significant withdrawal symptoms develop, the previous dosing schedule should be reinstituted and, only after stabilization, should a less rapid schedule of discontinuation be attempted. In a controlled postmarketing discontinuation study of panic disorder patients which compared this recommended taper schedule with a slower taper schedule, no difference was observed between the groups in the proportion of patients who tapered to zero dose; however, the slower schedule was associated with a reduction in symptoms associated with a withdrawal syndrome. It is suggested that the dose be reduced by no more than 0.5 mg every three days, with the understanding that some patients may benefit from an even more gradual discontinuation. Some patients may prove resistant to all discontinuation regimens.
Switch from XANAX (immediate-release) Tablets to XANAX XR (extended-release) Tablets
Patients who are currently being treated with divided doses of XANAX (immediate-release) Tablets, for example 3 to 4 times a day, may be switched to XANAX XR Tablets at the same total daily dose taken once daily. If the therapeutic response after switching is inadequate, the dosage may be titrated as outlined above.

HOW SUPPLIED

XANAX XR (extended-release) Tablets are available as follows:
0.5 mg (white, pentagonal-shaped tablets debossed with an "X" on one side and "0.5" on the other side)
Bottles of 60 NDC 0009-0057-07
1 mg (yellow, square-shaped tablets debossed with an "X" on one side and "1" on the other side)
Bottles of 60 NDC 0009-0059-07
2 mg (blue, round-shaped tablets debossed with an "X" on one side and "2" on the other side)
Bottles of 60 NDC 0009-0066-07
3 mg (green, triangular-shaped tablets debossed with an "X" on one side and "3" on the other side)
Bottles of 60 NDC 0009-0068-07
Store at 25°C (77°F); excursions permitted to 15-30°C (59-86°F) [see USP Controlled Room Temperature].
Rx only

ANIMAL STUDIES

When rats were treated with alprazolam at 3, 10, and 30 mg/kg/day (15 to 150 times the maximum recommended human dose) orally for 2 years, a tendency for a dose related increase in the number of cataracts was observed in females and a tendency for a dose related increase in corneal vascularization was observed in males. These lesions did not appear until after 11 months of treatment.
Pharmacia & Upjohn Company
A subsidiary of Pharmacia Corporation
Kalamazoo, Michigan 49001, USA
April 2004 819 612 001
692842

Shown in Product Identification Guide, page 330

ZINECARD® ℞
[zĭ-nĕ-kard]
dexrazoxane for injection

DESCRIPTION

ZINECARD® (dexrazoxane for injection) is a sterile, pyrogen-free lyophilizate intended for intravenous administration. It is a cardioprotective agent for use in conjunction with doxorubicin.
Chemically, dexrazoxane is (S)-4,4′-(1-methyl-1,2-ethanediyl)bis-2,6piperazinedione. The structural formula is as follows:

$C_{11}H_{16}N_4O_4$ M.W. 268.28

Dexrazoxane, a potent intracellular chelating agent is a derivative of EDTA. Dexrazoxane is a whitish crystalline powder which melts at 191° to 197°C. It is sparingly soluble in water and 0.1 N HCl, slightly soluble in ethanol and methanol and practically insoluble in nonpolar organic solvents. The pK_a is 2.1. Dexrazoxane has an octanol/water partition coefficient of 0.025 and degrades rapidly above a pH of 7.0.
ZINECARD is available in 250 mg and 500 mg single use only vials.
Each **250 mg vial** contains dexrazoxane hydrochloride equivalent to 250 mg dexrazoxane. Hydrochloric Acid, NF is added for pH adjustment. When reconstituted as directed with the 25 mL vial of 0.167 Molar (M/6) Sodium Lactate Injection, USP diluent provided, each mL contains: 10 mg dexrazoxane. The pH of the resultant solution is 3.5 to 5.5.
Each **500 mg vial** contains dexrazoxane hydrochloride equivalent to 500 mg dexrazoxane. Hydrochloric Acid, NF is added for pH adjustment. When reconstituted as directed with the 50 mL vial of 0.167 Molar (M/6) Sodium Lactate Injection, USP diluent provided, each mL contains: 10 mg dexrazoxane. The pH of the resultant solution is 3.5 to 5.5.

CLINICAL PHARMACOLOGY

Mechanism of Action: The mechanism by which ZINECARD exerts its cardioprotective activity is not fully understood. Dexrazoxane is a cyclic derivative of EDTA that readily penetrates cell membranes. Results of laboratory studies suggest that dexrazoxane is converted intracellularly to a ring-opened chelating agent that interferes with iron-mediated free radical generation thought to be responsible, in part, for anthracycline induced cardiomyopathy.
Pharmacokinetics: The pharmacokinetics of dexrazoxane have been studied in advanced cancer patients with normal renal and hepatic function. Generally, the pharmacokinetics of dexrazoxane can be adequately described by a two-compartment open model with first-order elimination. Dexrazoxane has been administered as a 15 minute infusion over a dose-range of 60 to 900 mg/m² with 60 mg/m² of doxorubicin, and at a fixed dose of 500 mg/m² with 50 mg/m² doxorubicin. The disposition kinetics of dexrazoxane are dose-independent, as shown by linear relationship between the area under plasma concentration-time curves and administered doses ranging from 60 to 900 mg/m². The mean peak plasma concentration of dexrazoxane was 36.5 µg/mL at the end of the 15 minute infusion of a 500 mg/m² dose of ZINECARD administered 15 to 30 minutes prior to the 50 mg/m² doxorubicin dose. The important pharmacokinetic parameters of dexrazoxane are summarized in the following table.
[See table below]
Following a rapid distributive phase (~0.2 to 0.3 hours), dexrazoxane reaches post-distributive equilibrium within two to four hours. The estimated steady-state volume of distribution of dexrazoxane suggests its distribution primarily in the total body water (25 L/m²). The mean systemic clearance and steady-state volume of distribution of dexrazoxane in two Asian female patients at 500 mg/m² dexrazoxane along with 50 mg/m² doxorubicin were 15.15 L/h/m² and 36.27 L/m², respectively, but their elimination half-life and renal clearance of dexrazoxane were similar to those of the ten Caucasian patients from the same study. Qualitative metabolism studies with ZINECARD have confirmed the presence of unchanged drug, a diacid-diamide cleavage product, and two monoacid-monoamide ring products in the urine of animals and man. The metabolite levels were not measured in the pharmacokinetic studies.
Urinary excretion plays an important role in the elimination of dexrazoxane. Forty-two percent of the 500 mg/m² dose of ZINECARD was excreted in the urine.
Protein Binding: *In vitro* studies have shown that ZINECARD is not bound to plasma proteins.
Special Populations:
Pediatric: The pharmacokinetics of ZINECARD have not been evaluated in pediatric patients.
Gender: Analysis of pooled data from two pharmacokinetic studies indicate that male patients have a lower mean clearance value than female patients (110 mL/min/m² versus 133 mL/min/m²). This gender effect is not clinically relevant.
Renal insufficiency: The pharmacokinetics of ZINECARD have not been evaluated in patients with renal impairment.
Hepatic insufficiency: The pharmacokinetics of ZINECARD have not been evaluated in patients with hepatic impairment. The ZINECARD dose is dependent upon the dose of doxorubicin (see **DOSAGE AND ADMINISTRATION**). Since a doxorubicin dose reduction is recommended in the presence of hyperbilirubinemia, the ZINECARD dosage is proportionately reduced in patients with hepatic impairment.
Drug Interactions: There was no significant change in the pharmacokinetics of doxorubicin (50 mg/m²) and its predominant metabolite, doxorubicinol, in the presence of dexrazoxane (500 mg/m²) in a crossover study in cancer patients.
Clinical Studies: The ability of ZINECARD to prevent/reduce the incidence and severity of doxorubicin-induced cardiomyopathy was demonstrated in three prospectively randomized placebo-controlled studies. In these studies, patients were treated with a doxorubicin-containing regimen and either ZINECARD or placebo starting with the first course of chemotherapy. There was no restriction on the cumulative dose of doxorubicin. Cardiac function was assessed by measurement of the left ventricular ejection fraction (LVEF), utilizing resting multigated nuclear medicine (MUGA) scans, and by clinical evaluations. Patients receiving ZINECARD had significantly smaller mean decreases from baseline in LVEF and lower incidences of congestive heart failure than the control group. The difference in decline from baseline in LVEF was evident beginning with a cumulative doxorubicin dose of 150 mg/m² and reached statistical significance in patients who received ≥400 mg/m² of doxorubicin. In addition to evaluating the effect of ZINECARD on cardiac function, the studies also assessed the effect of the addition of ZINECARD on the antitumor efficacy of the chemotherapy regimens. In one study (the largest of three breast cancer studies) patients with advanced breast cancer receiving fluorouracil, doxorubicin and

Continued on next page

SUMMARY OF MEAN (%CV[a]) DEXRAZOXANE PHARMACOKINETIC PARAMETERS AT A DOSAGE RATIO OF 10:1 OF ZINECARD: DOXORUBICIN

Dose Doxorubicin (mg/m²)	Dose Zinecard (mg/m²)	Number of Subjects	Elimination Half-Life (h)	Plasma Clearance (L/h/m²)	Renal Clearance (L/h/m²)	[b]Volume of Distribution (L/m²)
50	500	10	2.5 (16)	7.88 (18)	3.35 (36)	22.4 (22)
60	600	5	2.1 (29)	6.25 (31)	—	22.0 (55)

[a] Coefficient of variation
[b] Steady-state volume of distribution

Zinecard—Cont.

cyclophosphamide (FAC) with ZINECARD had a lower response rate (48% vs 63%; p=0.007) and a shorter time to progression than patients who received FAC + placebo, although the survival of patients who did or did not receive ZINECARD with FAC was similar.

Two of the randomized breast cancer studies evaluating the efficacy and safety of FAC with either ZINECARD or placebo were amended to allow patients on the placebo arm who had attained a cumulative dose of doxorubicin of 300 mg/m^2 (six courses of FAC) to receive FAC with open-label ZINECARD for each subsequent course. This change in design allowed examination of whether there was a cardioprotective effect of ZINECARD even when it was started after substantial exposure to doxorubicin.

Retrospective historical analyses were then performed to compare the likelihood of heart failure in patients to whom ZINECARD was added to the FAC regimen after they had received six (6) courses of FAC (and who then continued treatment with FAC therapy) with the heart failure rate in patients who had received six (6) courses of FAC and continued to receive this regimen without added ZINECARD. These analyses showed that the risk of experiencing a cardiac event (see Table 1 for definition) at a given cumulative dose of doxorubicin above 300 mg/m^2 was substantially greater in the 99 patients who did *not* receive ZINECARD beginning with their seventh course of FAC than in the 102 patients who did receive ZINECARD (See Figure 1).

Table 1

The development of cardiac events is shown by:

1. Development of congestive heart failure, defined as having two or more of the following:
   a. Cardiomegaly by X-ray
   b. Basilar Rales
   c. S3 Gallop
   d. Paroxysmal nocturnal dyspnea and/or orthopnea and/or significant dyspnea on exertion.
2. Decline from baseline in LVEF by ≥10% and to below the lower limit of normal for the institution.
3. Decline in LVEF by ≥20% from baseline value.
4. Decline in LVEF to ≥5% below lower limit of normal for the institution.

Figure 1 displays the risk of developing congestive heart failure by cumulative dose of doxorubicin in patients who received ZINECARD starting with their seventh course of FAC compared to patients who did not. Patients unprotected by ZINECARD had a 13 times greater risk of developing congestive heart failure. Overall, 3% of patients treated with ZINECARD developed CHF compared with 22% of patients not receiving ZINECARD.

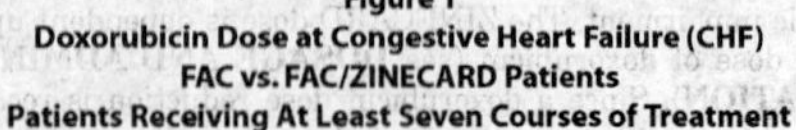

Figure 1
Doxorubicin Dose at Congestive Heart Failure (CHF)
FAC vs. FAC/ZINECARD Patients
Patients Receiving At Least Seven Courses of Treatment

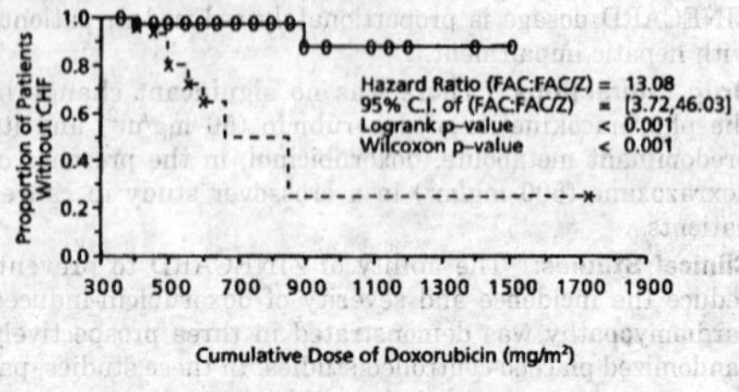

Because of its cardioprotective effect, ZINECARD permitted a greater percentage of patients to be treated with extended doxorubicin therapy. Figure 2 shows the number of patients still on treatment at increasing cumulative doses.

Figure 2
Cumulative Number of Patients On Treatment
FAC vs. FAC/ZINECARD Patients
Patients Receiving at Least Seven Courses of Treatment

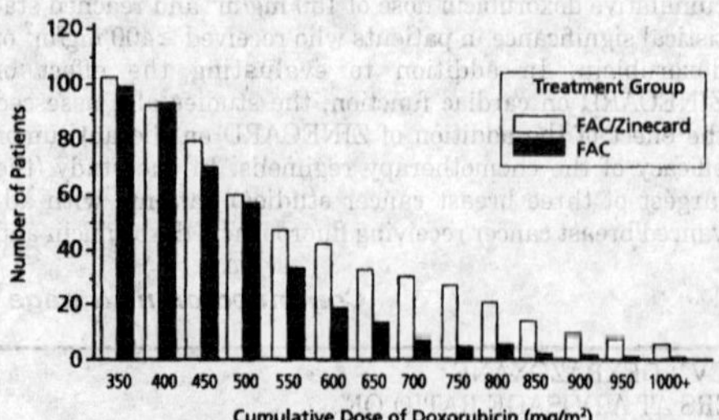

In addition to evaluating the cardioprotective efficacy of ZINECARD in this setting, the time to tumor progression and survival of these two groups of patients were also compared. There was a similar time to progression in the two groups and survival was at least as long for the group of patients that received ZINECARD starting with their seventh course, i.e., starting after a cumulative dose of doxorubicin of 300 mg/m^2. These time to progression and survival data should be interpreted with caution, however,

TABLE 2

ADVERSE EXPERIENCE	PERCENTAGE (%) OF BREAST CANCER PATIENTS WITH ADVERSE EXPERIENCE			
	FAC + ZINECARD		FAC + PLACEBO	
	Courses 1-6 N = 413	Courses ≥ 7 N = 102	Courses 1-6 N = 458	Course ≥ 7 N = 99
Alopecia	94	100	97	98
Nausea	77	51	84	60
Vomiting	59	42	72	49
Fatigue/Malaise	61	48	58	55
Anorexia	42	27	47	38
Stomatitis	34	26	41	28
Fever	34	22	29	18
Infection	23	19	18	21
Diarrhea	21	14	24	7
Pain on Injection	12	13	3	0
Sepsis	17	12	14	9
Neurotoxicity	17	10	13	5
Streaking/Erythema	5	4	4	2
Phlebitis	6	3	3	5
Esophagitis	6	3	7	4
Dysphagia	8	0	10	5
Hemorrhage	2	3	2	1
Extravasation	1	3	1	2
Urticaria	2	2	2	0
Recall Skin Reaction	1	1	2	0

because they are based on comparisons of groups entered sequentially in the studies and are not comparisons of prospectively randomized patients.

INDICATIONS AND USAGE

ZINECARD is indicated for reducing the incidence and severity of cardiomyopathy associated with doxorubicin administration in women with metastatic breast cancer who have received a cumulative doxorubicin dose of 300 mg/m^2 and who will continue to receive doxorubicin therapy to maintain tumor control. It is not recommended for use with the initiation of doxorubicin therapy (see **WARNINGS**).

CONTRAINDICATIONS

ZINECARD should not be used with chemotherapy regimens that do not contain an anthracycline.

WARNINGS

ZINECARD may add to the myelosuppression caused by chemotherapeutic agents. There is some evidence that the use of dexrazoxane concurrently with the initiation of fluorouracil, doxorubicin and cyclophosphamide (FAC) therapy interferes with the antitumor efficacy of the regimen, and this use is not recommended. In the largest of three breast cancer trials, patients who received dexrazoxane starting with their first cycle of FAC therapy had a lower response rate (48% vs 63%; p=0.007) and shorter time to progression than patients who did not receive dexrazoxane (see **Clinical Studies** section of **CLINICAL PHARMACOLOGY**). Therefore, ZINECARD should only be used in those patients who have received a cumulative doxorubicin dose of 300 mg/m^2 and are continuing with doxorubicin therapy.

Although clinical studies have shown that patients receiving FAC with ZINECARD may receive a higher cumulative dose of doxorubicin before experiencing cardiac toxicity than patients receiving FAC without ZINECARD, the use of ZINECARD in patients who have already received a cumulative dose of doxorubicin of 300 mg/m^2 without ZINECARD, does not eliminate the potential for anthracycline induced cardiac toxicity. Therefore, cardiac function should be carefully monitored.

Secondary malignancies (primarily acute myeloid leukemia) have been reported in patients treated chronically with oral razoxane. Razoxane is the racemic mixture, of which dexrazoxane is the S(+)-enantiomer. In these patients, the total cumulative dose of razoxane ranged from 26 to 480 grams and the duration of treatment was from 42 to 319 weeks. One case of T-cell lymphoma, a case of B-cell lymphoma and six to eight cases of cutaneous basal cell or squamous cell carcinoma have also been reported in patients treated with razoxane.

PRECAUTIONS

General

Doxorubicin should not be given prior to the intravenous injection of ZINECARD. ZINECARD should be given by slow I.V. push or rapid drip intravenous infusion from a bag. Doxorubicin should be given within 30 minutes after beginning the infusion with ZINECARD. (See **DOSAGE AND ADMINISTRATION**).

As ZINECARD will always be used with cytotoxic drugs, patients should be monitored closely. While the myelosuppressive effects of ZINECARD at the recommended dose are mild, additive effects upon the myelosuppressive activity of chemotherapeutic agents may occur.

Laboratory tests

As ZINECARD may add to the myelosuppressive effects of cytotoxic drugs, frequent complete blood counts are recommended. (See **ADVERSE REACTIONS**).

Drug Interactions

ZINECARD does not influence the pharmacokinetics of doxorubicin. **Carcinogenesis, Mutagenesis, Impairment of Fertility** (see **WARNINGS** section for information on human carcinogenicity) - No long-term carcinogenicity studies have been carried out with dexrazoxane in animals. Dexrazoxane was not mutagenic in the Ames test but was found to be clastogenic to human lymphocytes *in vitro* and to mouse bone marrow erythrocytes *in vivo* (micronucleus test).

The possible adverse effects of ZINECARD on the fertility of humans and experimental animals, male or female, have not been adequately studied. Testicular atrophy was seen with dexrazoxane administration at doses as low as 30 mg/kg weekly for 6 weeks in rats (1/3 the human dose on a mg/m^2 basis) and as low as 20 mg/kg weekly for 13 weeks in dogs (approximately equal to the human dose on a mg/m^2 basis).

Pregnancy - *Pregnancy Category C* - Dexrazoxane was maternotoxic at doses of 2 mg/kg (1/40 the human dose on a mg/m^2 basis) and embryotoxic and teratogenic at 8 mg/kg (approximately 1/10 the human dose on a mg/m^2 basis) when given daily to pregnant rats during the period of organogenesis. Teratogenic effects in the rat included imperforate anus, microphthalmia, and anophthalmia. In offspring allowed to develop to maturity, fertility was impaired in the male and female rats treated in utero during organogenesis at 8 mg/kg. In rabbits, doses of 5 mg/kg (approximately 1/10 the human dose on a mg/m^2 basis) daily during the period of organogenesis were maternotoxic and dosages of 20 mg/kg (1/2 the human dose on a mg/m^2 basis) were embryotoxic and teratogenic. Teratogenic effects in the rabbit included several skeletal malformations such as short tail, rib and thoracic malformations, and soft tissue variations including subcutaneous, eye and cardiac hemorrhagic areas, as well as agenesis of the gallbladder and of the intermediate lobe of the lung. There are no adequate and well-controlled studies in pregnant women. ZINECARD should be used during pregnancy only if the potential benefit justifies the potential risk to the fetus.

Nursing Mothers - It is not known whether dexrazoxane is excreted in human milk. Because many drugs are excreted in human milk and because of the potential for serious adverse reactions in nursing infants exposed to dexrazoxane, mothers should be advised to discontinue nursing during dexrazoxane therapy.

Pediatric Use - Safety and effectiveness of dexrazoxane in pediatric patients have not been established.

Geriatric Use - Clinical studies of ZINECARD did not include sufficient numbers of subjects aged 65 and over to determine whether they respond differently from younger subjects. Other reported clinical experience has not identified differences in responses between the elderly and younger patients. In general, elderly patients should be treated with caution due to the greater frequency of decreased hepatic, renal, or cardiac function, and concomitant disease or other drug therapy.

ADVERSE REACTIONS

ZINECARD at a dose of 500 mg/m^2 has been administered in combination with FAC in randomized, placebo-controlled, double-blind studies to patients with metastatic breast cancer. The dose of doxorubicin was 50 mg/m^2 in each of the trials. Courses were repeated every three weeks, provided recovery from toxicity had occurred. Table 2 below lists the incidence of adverse experiences for patients receiving FAC with either ZINECARD or placebo in the breast cancer studies. Adverse experiences occurring during courses 1 through 6 are displayed for patients receiving ZINECARD or placebo with FAC beginning with their first course of therapy (column 1 & 3, respectively). Adverse experiences occurring at course 7 and beyond for patients who received placebo with FAC during the first six courses and who then received either ZINECARD or placebo with FAC are also displayed (column 2 & 4, respectively).

[See table at top of previous page]

The adverse experiences listed above are likely attributable to the FAC regimen with the exception of pain on injection that was observed mainly on the ZINECARD arm.

Myelosuppression

Patients receiving FAC with ZINECARD experienced more severe leucopenia, granulocytopenia and thrombocytopenia at nadir than patients receiving FAC without ZINECARD, but recovery counts were similar for the two groups of patients.

Hepatic and Renal

Some patients receiving FAC + ZINECARD or FAC + placebo experienced marked abnormalities in hepatic or renal function tests, but the frequency and severity of abnormalities in bilirubin, alkaline phosphatase, BUN, and creatinine were similar for patients receiving FAC with or without ZINECARD.

OVERDOSAGE

There have been no instances of drug overdose in the clinical studies sponsored by either Pharmacia & Upjohn Company or the National Cancer Institute. The maximum dose administered during the cardioprotective trials was 1000 mg/m^2 every three weeks.

Disposition studies with ZINECARD have not been conducted in cancer patients undergoing dialysis, but retention of a significant dose fraction (>0.4) of the unchanged drug in the plasma pool, minimal tissue partitioning or binding, and availability of greater than 90% of the systemic drug levels in the unbound form suggest that it could be removed using conventional peritoneal or hemodialysis.

There is no known antidote for dexrazoxane. Instances of suspected overdose should be managed with good supportive care until resolution of myelosuppression and related conditions is complete. Management of overdose should include treatment of infections, fluid regulation, and maintenance of nutritional requirements.

DOSAGE AND ADMINISTRATION

The recommended dosage ratio of ZINECARD:doxorubicin is 10:1 (eg, 500 mg/m^2 ZINECARD:50 mg/m^2 doxorubicin). Since a doxorubicin dose reduction is recommended in the presence of hyperbilirubinemia, the ZINECARD dosage should be proportionately reduced (maintaining the 10:1 ratio) in patients with hepatic impairment. ZINECARD must be reconstituted with 0.167 Molar (M/6) Sodium Lactate Injection, USP, to give a concentration of 10 mg ZINECARD for each mL of sodium lactate. The reconstituted solution should be given by slow I.V. push or rapid drip intravenous infusion from a bag. After completing the infusion of ZINECARD, and prior to a total elapsed time of 30 minutes (from the beginning of the ZINECARD infusion), the intravenous injection of doxorubicin should be given.

Reconstituted ZINECARD, when transferred to an empty infusion bag, is stable for 6 hours from the time of reconstitution when stored at controlled room temperature, 15° to 30°C (59° to 86°F) or under refrigeration, 2° to 8°C (36° to 46°F). DISCARD UNUSED SOLUTIONS.

The reconstituted ZINECARD solution may be diluted with either 0.9% Sodium Chloride Injection, USP or 5.0% Dextrose Injection, USP to a concentration range of 1.3 to 5.0 mg/mL in intravenous infusion bags. The resultant solutions are stable for 6 hours when stored at controlled room temperature, 15° to 30°C (59° to 86°F) or under refrigeration, 2° to 8°C (36° to 46°F). DISCARD UNUSED SOLUTIONS.

Incompatibility

ZINECARD should not be mixed with other drugs.

Parenteral drug products should be inspected visually for particulate matter and discoloration prior to administration, whenever solution and container permit.

Handling and Disposal: Caution in the handling and preparation of the reconstituted solution must be exercised and the use of gloves is recommended. If ZINECARD powder or solutions contact the skin or mucosae, immediately wash thoroughly with soap and water.

Procedures normally used for proper handling and disposal of anticancer drugs should be considered for use with ZINECARD. Several guidelines on this subject have been published.[1-8] There is no general agreement that all of the procedures recommended in the guidelines are necessary or appropriate.

HOW SUPPLIED

ZINECARD® (dexrazoxane for injection) is available in the following strengths as sterile, pyrogen-free lyophilizates.

NDC 0013-8715-62

250 mg single dose vial with a red flip-top seal, packaged in single vial packs. (This package also contains a 25 mL vial of 0.167 Molar (M/6) Sodium Lactate Injection, USP.)

NDC 0013-8725-89

500 mg single dose vial with a blue flip-top seal, packaged in single vial packs. (This package also contains a 50 mL vial of 0.167 Molar (M/6) Sodium Lactate Injection, USP.)

Store at 25°C (77°F); excursions permitted to 15° to 30°C (59° to 86°F) [see USP Controlled Room Temperature]. Reconstituted solutions of ZINECARD are stable for 6 hours at controlled room temperature or under refrigeration, 2° to 8°C (36° to 46°F). DISCARD UNUSED SOLUTIONS.

℞ only

REFERENCES:

1. ONS Clinical Practice Committee. Cancer Chemotherapy Guidelines and Recommendations for Practice. Pittsburgh, PA: Oncology Nursing Society. 1999; 32-41.
2. Recommendations for the Safe Handling of Parenteral Antineoplastic Drugs. Washington, DC: Division of Safety, Clinical Center Pharmacy Department and Cancer Nursing Services, National Institutes of Health; 1992. US Dept of Health and Human Services, Public Health Service Publication NIH 92-2621.
3. AMA Council on Scientific Affairs. Guidelines for Handling Parenteral Antineoplastics. *JAMA.* 1985; 253: 1590-1591.
4. National Study Commission on Cytotoxic Exposure-Recommendations for Handling Cytotoxic Agents. 1987. Available from Louis P. Jeffrey, Sc.D., Chairman, National Study Commission on Cytotoxic Exposure, Massachusetts College of Pharmacy and Allied Health Sciences, 179 Longwood Avenue, Boston, MA 02115.
5. Clinical Oncological Society of Australia. Guidelines and Recommendations for Safe Handling of Antineoplastic Agents. *Med J Australia.* 1983; 1:426-428.
6. Jones RB, Frank R, Mass T. Safe Handling of Chemotherapeutic Agents: A Report from the Mount Sinai Medical Center. CA - *A Cancer J for Clin.* 1983; 33: 258-263.
7. American Society of Hospital Pharmacists. ASHP Technical Assistance Bulletin on Handling Cytotoxic and Hazardous Drugs. *Am J Hosp Pharm.* 1990; 47:1033-1049.
8. Controlling Occupational Exposure to Hazardous Drugs. (OSHA Work Practice Guidelines.) *Am J Health-Syst Pharm.* 1996; 53: 1669-1685.

Manufactured for: Pharmacia & Upjohn Company
A subsidiary of Pharmacia Corporation
Kalamazoo, MI 49001, USA
By: Cardinal Health
Albuquerque, NM 87109, USA
Revised: September 2003 817 546 003

ZYVOX™ ℞

[zī-vŏks]

linezolid injection
linezolid tablets
linezolid for oral suspension

To reduce the development of drug-resistant bacteria and maintain the effectiveness of ZYVOX formulations and other antibacterial drugs, ZYVOX should be used only to treat or prevent infections that are proven or strongly suspected to be caused by bacteria.

DESCRIPTION

ZYVOX I.V. Injection, ZYVOX Tablets, and ZYVOX for Oral Suspension contain linezolid, which is a synthetic antibacterial agent of the oxazolidinone class. The chemical name for linezolid is (S)-N-[[3-[3-Fluoro-4-(4-morpholinyl)phenyl]-2-oxo-5-oxazolidinyl] methyl]-acetamide.

The empirical formula is $C_{16}H_{20}FN_3O_4$. Its molecular weight is 337.35, and its chemical structure is represented below:

[chemical structure of linezolid]

ZYVOX I.V. Injection is supplied as a ready-to-use sterile isotonic solution for intravenous infusion. Each mL contains 2 mg of linezolid. Inactive ingredients are sodium citrate, citric acid, and dextrose in an aqueous vehicle for intravenous administration. The sodium (Na^+) content is 0.38 mg/mL (5 mEq per 300-mL bag; 3.3 mEq per 200-mL bag; and 1.7 mEq per 100-mL bag).

ZYVOX Tablets for oral administration contain 400 mg or 600 mg linezolid as film-coated compressed tablets. Inactive ingredients are corn starch, microcrystalline cellulose, hydroxypropylcellulose, sodium starch glycolate, magnesium stearate, hydroxypropyl methylcellulose, polyethylene glycol, titanium dioxide, and carnauba wax. The sodium (Na^+) content is 1.95 mg per 400-mg tablet and 2.92 mg per 600-mg tablet (0.1 mEq per tablet, regardless of strength).

ZYVOX for Oral Suspension is supplied as an orange-flavored granule/powder for constitution into a suspension for oral administration. Following constitution, each 5 mL contains 100 mg of linezolid. Inactive ingredients are sucrose, citric acid, sodium citrate, microcrystalline cellulose and carboxymethylcellulose sodium, aspartame, xanthan gum, mannitol, sodium benzoate, colloidal silicon dioxide, sodium chloride, and flavors (see **PRECAUTIONS, Information for Patients**). The sodium (Na^+) content is 8.52 mg per 5 mL (0.4 mEq per 5 mL).

CLINICAL PHARMACOLOGY

Pharmacokinetics

The mean pharmacokinetic parameters of linezolid in adults after single and multiple oral and intravenous (IV) doses are summarized in Table 1. Plasma concentrations of linezolid at steady-state after oral doses of 600 mg given every 12 hours (q12h) are shown in Figure 1.

[See table 1 at top of next page]

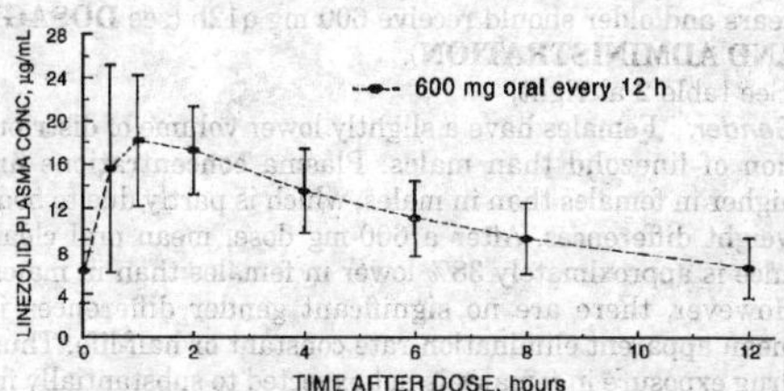

Figure 1. Plasma Concentrations of Linezolid in Adults at Steady-State Following Oral Dosing Every 12 Hours (Mean±Standard Deviation, n=16)

Absorption: Linezolid is rapidly and extensively absorbed after oral dosing. Maximum plasma concentrations are reached approximately 1 to 2 hours after dosing, and the absolute bioavailability is approximately 100%. Therefore, linezolid may be given orally or intravenously without dose adjustment.

Linezolid may be administered without regard to the timing of meals. The time to reach the maximum concentration is delayed from 1.5 hours to 2.2 hours and C_{max} is decreased by about 17% when high fat food is given with linezolid. However, the total exposure measured as $AUC_{0-\infty}$ values is similar under both conditions.

Distribution: Animal and human pharmacokinetic studies have demonstrated that linezolid readily distributes to well-perfused tissues. The plasma protein binding of linezolid is approximately 31% and is concentration-independent. The volume of distribution of linezolid at steady-state averaged 40 to 50 liters in healthy adult volunteers.

Linezolid concentrations have been determined in various fluids from a limited number of subjects in Phase 1 volunteer studies following multiple dosing of linezolid. The ratio of linezolid in saliva relative to plasma was 1.2 to 1 and for sweat relative to plasma was 0.55 to 1.

Metabolism: Linezolid is primarily metabolized by oxidation of the morpholine ring, which results in two inactive ring-opened carboxylic acid metabolites: the aminoethoxyacetic acid metabolite (A), and the hydroxyethyl glycine metabolite (B). Formation of metabolite B is mediated by a non-enzymatic chemical oxidation mechanism in vitro. Linezolid is not an inducer of cytochrome P450 (CYP) in rats, and it has been demonstrated from in vitro studies that linezolid is not detectably metabolized by human cytochrome P450 and it does not inhibit the activities of clinically significant human CYP isoforms (1A2, 2C9, 2C19, 2D6, 2E1, 3A4).

Excretion: Nonrenal clearance accounts for approximately 65% of the total clearance of linezolid. Under steady-state conditions, approximately 30% of the dose appears in the urine as linezolid, 40% as metabolite B, and 10% as metabolite A. The renal clearance of linezolid is low (average 40 mL/min) and suggests net tubular reabsorption. Virtually no linezolid appears in the feces, while approximately 6% of the dose appears in the feces as metabolite B, and 3% as metabolite A.

A small degree of nonlinearity in clearance was observed with increasing doses of linezolid, which appears to be due to lower renal and nonrenal clearance of linezolid at higher concentrations. However, the difference in clearance was small and was not reflected in the apparent elimination half-life.

Special Populations

Geriatric: The pharmacokinetics of linezolid are not significantly altered in elderly patients (65 years or older). Therefore, dose adjustment for geriatric patients is not necessary.

Pediatric: The pharmacokinetics of linezolid following a single IV dose were investigated in pediatric patients ranging in age from birth through 17 years (including premature and full-term neonates), in healthy adolescent subjects

Continued on next page

Zyvox—Cont.

ranging in age from 12 through 17 years, and in pediatric patients ranging in age from 1 week through 12 years. The pharmacokinetic parameters of linezolid are summarized in Table 2 for the pediatric populations studied and healthy adult subjects after administration of single IV doses.

The C_{max} and the volume of distribution (V_{ss}) of linezolid are similar regardless of age in pediatric patients. However, clearance of linezolid varies as a function of age. With the exclusion of pre-term neonates less than one week of age, clearance is most rapid in the youngest age groups ranging from >1 week old to 11 years, resulting in lower single-dose systemic exposure (AUC) and shorter half-life as compared with adults. As age of pediatric patients increases, the clearance of linezolid gradually decreases, and by adolescence mean clearance values approach those observed for the adult population. There is wider inter-subject variability in linezolid clearance and systemic drug exposure (AUC) across all pediatric age groups as compared with adults.

Similar mean daily AUC values were observed in pediatric patients from birth to 11 years of age dosed every 8 hours (q8h) relative to adolescents or adults dosed every 12 hours (q12h). Therefore, the dosage for pediatric patients up to 11 years of age should be 10 mg/kg q8h. Pediatric patients 12 years and older should receive 600 mg q12h (see **DOSAGE AND ADMINISTRATION**).

[See table 2 at right]

Gender: Females have a slightly lower volume of distribution of linezolid than males. Plasma concentrations are higher in females than in males, which is partly due to body weight differences. After a 600-mg dose, mean oral clearance is approximately 38% lower in females than in males. However, there are no significant gender differences in mean apparent elimination-rate constant or half-life. Thus, drug exposure in females is not expected to substantially increase beyond levels known to be well tolerated. Therefore, dose adjustment by gender does not appear to be necessary.

Renal Insufficiency: The pharmacokinetics of the parent drug, linezolid, are not altered in patients with any degree of renal insufficiency; however, the two primary metabolites of linezolid may accumulate in patients with renal insufficiency, with the amount of accumulation increasing with the severity of renal dysfunction (see Table 3). The clinical significance of accumulation of these two metabolites has not been determined in patients with severe renal insufficiency. Because similar plasma concentrations of linezolid are achieved regardless of renal function, no dose adjustment is recommended for patients with renal insufficiency. However, given the absence of information on the clinical significance of accumulation of the primary metabolites, use of linezolid in patients with renal insufficiency should be weighed against the potential risks of accumulation of these metabolites. Both linezolid and the two metabolites are eliminated by dialysis. No information is available on the effect of peritoneal dialysis on the pharmacokinetics of linezolid. Approximately 30% of a dose was eliminated in a 3-hour dialysis session beginning 3 hours after the dose of linezolid was administered; therefore, linezolid should be given after hemodialysis.

[See table 3 at top of next page]

Hepatic Insufficiency: The pharmacokinetics of linezolid are not altered in patients (n=7) with mild-to-moderate hepatic insufficiency (Child-Pugh class A or B). On the basis of the available information, no dose adjustment is recommended for patients with mild-to-moderate hepatic insufficiency. The pharmacokinetics of linezolid in patients with severe hepatic insufficiency have not been evaluated.

Drug-Drug Interactions

Drugs Metabolized by Cytochrome P450: Linezolid is not an inducer of cytochrome P450 (CYP) in rats. It is not detectably metabolized by human cytochrome P450 and it does not inhibit the activities of clinically significant human CYP isoforms (1A2, 2C9, 2C19, 2D6, 2E1, 3A4). Therefore, no CYP450-induced drug interactions are expected with linezolid. Concurrent administration of linezolid does not substantially alter the pharmacokinetic characteristics of (S)-warfarin, which is extensively metabolized by CYP2C9. Drugs such as warfarin and phenytoin, which are CYP2C9 substrates, may be given with linezolid without changes in dosage regimen.

Antibiotics:

Aztreonam: The pharmacokinetics of linezolid or aztreonam are not altered when administered together.

Gentamicin: The pharmacokinetics of linezolid or gentamicin are not altered when administered together.

Monoamine Oxidase Inhibition: Linezolid is a reversible, nonselective inhibitor of monoamine oxidase. Therefore, linezolid has the potential for interaction with adrenergic and serotonergic agents.

Adrenergic Agents: A significant pressor response has been observed in normal adult subjects receiving linezolid and tyramine doses of more than 100 mg. Therefore, patients receiving linezolid need to avoid consuming large amounts of foods or beverages with high tyramine content (see **PRECAUTIONS, Information for Patients**).

A reversible enhancement of the pressor response of either pseudoephedrine HCl (PSE) or phenylpropanolamine HCl (PPA) is observed when linezolid is administered to healthy normotensive subjects (see **PRECAUTIONS, Drug Interactions**). A similar study has not been conducted in hypertensive patients. The interaction studies conducted in normotensive subjects evaluated the blood pressure and heart rate

Table 1. Mean (Standard Deviation) Pharmacokinetic Parameters of Linezolid in Adults

Dose of Linezolid	C_{max} µg/mL	C_{min} µg/mL	T_{max} hrs	AUC* µg • h/mL	$t_{1/2}$ hrs	CL mL/min
400 mg tablet						
single dose†	8.10 (1.83)	—	1.52 (1.01)	55.10 (25.00)	5.20 (1.50)	146 (67)
every 12 hours	11.00 (4.37)	3.08 (2.25)	1.12 (0.47)	73.40 (33.50)	4.69 (1.70)	110 (49)
600 mg tablet						
single dose	12.70 (3.96)	—	1.28 (0.66)	91.40 (39.30)	4.26 (1.65)	127 (48)
every 12 hours	21.20 (5.78)	6.15 (2.94)	1.03 (0.62)	138.00 (42.10)	5.40 (2.06)	80 (29)
600 mg IV injection‡						
single dose	12.90 (1.60)	—	0.50 (0.10)	80.20 (33.30)	4.40 (2.40)	138 (39)
every 12 hours	15.10 (2.52)	3.68 (2.36)	0.51 (0.03)	89.70 (31.00)	4.80 (1.70)	123 (40)
600 mg oral suspension						
single dose	11.00 (2.76)	—	0.97 (0.88)	80.80 (35.10)	4.60 (1.71)	141 (45)

*AUC for single dose = $AUC_{0-\infty}$; for multiple-dose = $AUC_{0-\tau}$

† Data dose-normalized from 375 mg

‡ Data dose-normalized from 625 mg, IV dose was given as 0.5-hour infusion.

C_{max} = Maximum plasma concentration; C_{min} = Minimum plasma concentration; T_{max} = Time to C_{max}; AUC = Area under concentration-time curve; $t_{1/2}$ = Elimination half-life; CL = Systemic clearance

Table 2. Pharmacokinetic Parameters of Linezolid in Pediatrics and Adults Following a Single Intravenous Infusion of 10 mg/kg or 600 mg Linezolid (Mean: (%CV); [Min, Max Values])

Age Group	C_{max} µg/mL	V_{ss} L/kg	AUC* µg·h/mL	$t_{1/2}$ hrs	CL mL/min/kg
Neonatal Patients					
Pre-term** <1 week (N=9)†	12.7 (30%) [9.6, 22.2]	0.81 (24%) [0.43, 1.05]	108 (47%) [41, 191]	5.6 (46%) [2.4, 9.8]	2.0 (52%) [0.9, 4.0]
Full-term*** <1 week (N=10)†	11.5 (24%) [8.0, 18.3]	0.78 (20%) [0.45, 0.96]	55 (47%) [19, 103]	3.0 (55%) [1.3, 6.1]	3.8 (55%) [1.5, 8.8]
Full-term*** ≥1 week to ≤28 days (N=10)†	12.9 (28%) [7.7, 21.6]	0.66 (29%) [0.35, 1.06]	34 (21%) [23, 50]	1.5 (17%) [1.2, 1.9]	5.1 (22%) [3.3, 7.2]
Infant Patients					
> 28 days to < 3 Months (N=12)†	11.0 (27%) [7.2, 18.0]	0.79 (26%) [0.42, 1.08]	33 (26%) [17, 48]	1.8 (28%) [1.2, 2.8]	5.4 (32%) [3.5, 9.9]
Pediatric Patients					
3 months through 11 years† (N=59)	15.1 (30%) [6.8, 36.7]	0.69 (28%) [0.31, 1.50]	58 (54%) [19, 153]	2.9 (53%) [0.9, 8.0]	3.8 (53%) [1.0, 8.5]
Adolescent Subjects and Patients					
12 through 17 years‡ (N=36)	16.7 (24%) [9.9, 28.9]	0.61 (15%) [0.44, 0.79]	95 (44%) [32, 178]	4.1 (46%) [1.3, 8.1]	2.1 (53%) [0.9, 5.2]
Adult Subjects§ (N=29)	12.5 (21%) [8.2, 19.3]	0.65 (16%) [0.45, 0.84]	91 (33%) [53, 155]	4.9 (35%) [1.8, 8.3]	1.7 (34%) [0.9, 3.3]

* AUC = Single dose $AUC_{0-\infty}$

** In this data set, "pre-term" is defined as <34 weeks gestational age (Note: Only 1 patient enrolled was pre-term with a postnatal age between 1 week and 28 days)

*** In this data set, "full-term" is defined as ≥34 weeks gestational age

† Dose of 10 mg/kg

‡ Dose of 600 mg or 10 mg/kg up to a maximum of 600 mg

§ Dose normalized to 600 mg

C_{max}= Maximum plasma concentration; V_{ss}=Volume of distribution; AUC = Area under concentration-time curve;
$t_{1/2}$ = Apparent elimination half-life; CL = Systemic clearance normalized for body weight

effects of placebo, PPA or PSE alone, linezolid alone, and the combination of steady-state linezolid (600 mg q12h for 3 days) with two doses of PPA (25 mg) or PSE (60 mg) given 4 hours apart. Heart rate was not affected by any of the treatments. Blood pressure was increased with both combination treatments. Maximum blood pressure levels were seen 2 to 3 hours after the second dose of PPA or PSE, and returned to baseline 2 to 3 hours after peak. The results of the PPA study follow, showing the mean (and range) maximum systolic blood pressure in mm Hg: placebo = 121 (103 to 158); linezolid alone = 120 (107 to 135); PPA alone = 125 (106 to 139); PPA with linezolid = 147 (129 to 176). The results from the PSE study were similar to those in the PPA study. The mean maximum increase in systolic blood pressure over baseline was 32 mm Hg (range: 20-52 mm Hg) and 38 mm Hg (range: 18-79 mm Hg) during co-administration of linezolid with pseudoephedrine or phenylpropanolamine, respectively.

Serotonergic Agents: The potential drug-drug interaction with dextromethorphan was studied in healthy volunteers. Subjects were administered dextromethorphan (two 20-mg doses given 4 hours apart) with or without linezolid. No serotonin syndrome effects (confusion, delirium, restlessness, tremors, blushing, diaphoresis, hyperpyrexia) have been observed in normal subjects receiving linezolid and dextromethorphan. The effects of other serotonin re-uptake inhibitors have not been studied.

MICROBIOLOGY

Linezolid is a synthetic antibacterial agent of a new class of antibiotics, the oxazolidinones, which has clinical utility in the treatment of infections caused by aerobic Gram-positive bacteria. The in vitro spectrum of activity of linezolid also includes certain Gram-negative bacteria and anaerobic bacteria. Linezolid inhibits bacterial protein synthesis through a mechanism of action different from that of other antibacterial agents; therefore, cross-resistance between linezolid and other classes of antibiotics is unlikely. Linezolid binds to a site on the bacterial 23S ribosomal RNA of the 50S subunit and prevents the formation of a functional 70S initiation complex, which is an essential component of the bacterial translation process. The results of time-kill studies have shown linezolid to be bacteriostatic against enterococci and staphylococci. For streptococci, linezolid was found to be bactericidal for the majority of strains.

In clinical trials, resistance to linezolid developed in 6 patients infected with *Enterococcus faecium* (4 patients received 200 mg q12h, lower than the recommended dose, and 2 patients received 600 mg q12h). In a compassionate use program, resistance to linezolid developed in 8 patients with *E. faecium* and in 1 patient with *Enterococcus faecalis*. All patients had either unremoved prosthetic devices or undrained abscesses. Resistance to linezolid occurs in vitro at a frequency of 1×10^{-9} to 1×10^{-11}. In vitro studies have shown that point mutations in the 23S rRNA are associated with linezolid resistance. Reports of vancomycin-resistant *E. faecium* becoming resistant to linezolid during its clinical use have been published.[1] In one report nosocomial spread of vancomycin- and linezolid-resistant *E. faecium* occurred[2]. There has been a report of *Staphylococcus aureus* (methicillin-resistant) developing resistance to linezolid during its clinical use.[3] The linezolid resistance in these organisms was associated with a point mutation in the 23S rRNA (substitution of thymine for guanine at position 2576) of the organism. When antibiotic-resistant organisms are encountered in the hospital, it is important to emphasize infection control policies.[4,5] Resistance to linezolid has not been reported in *Streptococcus* spp., including *Streptococcus pneumoniae.*

In vitro studies have demonstrated additivity or indifference between linezolid and vancomycin, gentamicin, rifampin, imipenem-cilastatin, aztreonam, ampicillin, or streptomycin.

Linezolid has been shown to be active against most isolates of the following microorganisms, both in vitro and in clinical infections, as described in the **INDICATIONS AND USAGE** section.

Aerobic and facultative Gram-positive microorganisms
Enterococcus faecium (vancomycin-resistant strains only)
Staphylococcus aureus (including methicillin-resistant strains)
Streptococcus agalactiae
Streptococcus pneumoniae (including multi-drug resistant isolates [MDRSP]*)
Streptococcus pyogenes

The following in vitro data are available, but their clinical significance is unknown. At least 90% of the following microorganisms exhibit an in vitro minimum inhibitory concentration (MIC) less than or equal to the susceptible breakpoint for linezolid. However, the safety and effectiveness of linezolid in treating clinical infections due to these microorganisms have not been established in adequate and well-controlled clinical trials.

*MDRSP refers to isolates resistant to two or more of the following antibiotics: penicillin, second-generation cephalosporins, macrolides, tetracycline, and trimethoprim/sulfamethoxazole.

Aerobic and facultative Gram-positive microorganisms
Enterococcus faecalis (including vancomycin-resistant strains)
Enterococcus faecium (vancomycin-susceptible strains)
Staphylococcus epidermidis (including methicillin-resistant strains)
Staphylococcus haemolyticus
Viridans group streptococci

Aerobic and facultative Gram-negative microorganisms
Pasteurella multocida

Susceptibility Testing Methods

NOTE: Susceptibility testing by dilution methods requires the use of linezolid susceptibility powder.

When available, the results of in vitro susceptibility tests should be provided to the physician as periodic reports which describe the susceptibility profile of nosocomial and community-acquired pathogens. These reports should aid the physician in selecting the most effective antimicrobial.

Dilution Techniques: Quantitative methods are used to determine antimicrobial minimum inhibitory concentrations (MICs). These MICs provide estimates of the susceptibility of bacteria to antimicrobial compounds. The MICs should be determined using a standardized procedure. Standardized procedures are based on a dilution method[6,7] (broth or agar) or equivalent with standardized inoculum concentrations and standardized concentrations of linezolid powder. The MIC values should be interpreted according to criteria provided in Table 4.

Diffusion Techniques: Quantitative methods that require measurement of zone diameters also provide reproducible estimates of the susceptibility of bacteria to antimicrobial compounds. One such standardized procedure[7,8] requires the use of standardized inoculum concentrations. This procedure uses paper disks impregnated with 30 μg of linezolid to test the susceptibility of microorganisms to linezolid. The disk diffusion interpretive criteria are provided in Table 4.
[See table 4 above]

A report of "Susceptible" indicates that the pathogen is likely to be inhibited if the antimicrobial compound in the blood reaches the concentrations usually achievable. A report of "Intermediate" indicates that the result should be considered equivocal, and, if the microorganism is not fully susceptible to alternative, clinically feasible drugs, the test should be repeated. This category implies possible clinical applicability in body sites where the drug is physiologically concentrated or in situations where high dosage of drug can be used. This category also provides a buffer zone which prevents small uncontrolled technical factors from causing major discrepancies in interpretation. A report of "Resistant" indicates that the pathogen is not likely to be inhibited if the antimicrobial compound in the blood reaches the concentrations usually achievable; other therapy should be selected.

Quality Control

Standardized susceptibility test procedures require the use of quality control microorganisms to control the technical aspects of the test procedures. Standard linezolid powder should provide the following range of values noted in Table 5. **NOTE:** Quality control microorganisms are specific strains of organisms with intrinsic biological properties relating to resistance mechanisms and their genetic expression within bacteria; the specific strains used for microbiological quality control are not clinically significant.
[See table 5 at right]

INDICATIONS AND USAGE

ZYVOX formulations are indicated in the treatment of the following infections caused by susceptible strains of the designated microorganisms (see **PRECAUTIONS, Pediatric Use** and **DOSAGE AND ADMINISTRATION**).

Table 3. Mean (Standard Deviation) AUCs and Elimination Half-lives of Linezolid and Metabolites A and B in Patients with Varying Degrees of Renal Insufficiency After a Single 600-mg Oral Dose of Linezolid

Parameter	Healthy Subjects CL_{CR} > 80 mL/min	Moderate Renal Impairment 30 < CL_{CR} < 80 mL/min	Severe Renal Impairment 10 < CL_{CR} < 30 mL/min	Hemodialysis-Dependent Off Dialysis*	Hemodialysis-Dependent On Dialysis
Linezolid					
$AUC_{0-\infty}$, μg h/mL	110 (22)	128 (53)	127 (66)	141 (45)	83 (23)
$t_{1/2}$, hours	6.4 (2.2)	6.1 (1.7)	7.1 (3.7)	8.4 (2.7)	7.0 (1.8)
Metabolite A					
AUC_{0-48}, μg h/mL	7.6 (1.9)	11.7 (4.3)	56.5 (30.6)	185 (124)	68.8 (23.9)
$t_{1/2}$, hours	6.3 (2.1)	6.6 (2.3)	9.0 (4.6)	NA	NA
Metabolite B					
AUC_{0-48}, μg h/mL	30.5 (6.2)	51.1 (38.5)	203 (92)	467 (102)	239 (44)
$t_{1/2}$, hours	6.6 (2.7)	9.9 (7.4)	11.0 (3.9)	NA	NA

* between hemodialysis sessions
NA = Not applicable

Table 4. Susceptibility Interpretive Criteria for Linezolid

Pathogen	MIC (μg/mL) S	MIC I	MIC R	Disk Diffusion (mm) S	Disk I	Disk R
Enterococcus spp	≤ 2	4	≥8	≥ 23	21-22	≤20
Staphylococcus spp[a]	≤4	—	—	≥ 21	—	—
Streptococcus pneumoniae[a]	≤2[b]	—	—	≥ 21[c]	—	—
Streptococcus spp other than *S pneumoniae*[a]	≤2[b]	—	—	≥ 21[c]	—	—

Susceptibility Interpretive Criteria: Minimal Inhibitory Concentrations (MIC in μg/mL); Disk Diffusion (Zone Diameters in mm)

[a] The current absence of data on resistant strains precludes defining any categories other than "Susceptible." Strains yielding test results suggestive of a "nonsusceptible" category should be retested, and if the result is confirmed, the isolate should be submitted to a reference laboratory for further testing.
[b] These interpretive standards for *S. pneumoniae* and *Streptococcus* spp. other than *S. pneumoniae* are applicable only to tests performed by broth microdilution using cation-adjusted Mueller-Hinton broth with 2 to 5% lysed horse blood inoculated with a direct colony suspension and incubated in ambient air at 35°C for 20 to 24 hours.
[c] These zone diameter interpretive standards are applicable only to tests performed using Mueller-Hinton agar supplemented with 5% defibrinated sheep blood inoculated with a direct colony suspension and incubated in 5% CO_2 at 35°C for 20 to 24 hours.

Table 5. Acceptable Quality Control Ranges for Linezolid to be Used in Validation of Susceptibility Test Results

QC Strain	Minimum Inhibitory Concentration (MIC in μg/mL)	Disk Diffusion (Zone Diameters in mm)
Enterococcus faecalis ATCC 29212	1 - 4	Not applicable
Staphylococcus aureus ATCC 29213	1 - 4	Not applicable
Staphylococcus aureus ATCC 25923	Not applicable	25 - 32
Streptococcus pneumoniae ATCC 49619[d]	0.50 - 2[e]	25 - 34[f]

(Acceptable Quality Control Ranges)

[d] This organism may be used for validation of susceptibility test results when testing *Streptococcus* spp. other than *S. pneumoniae.*
[e] This quality control range for *S. pneumoniae* is applicable only to tests performed by broth microdilution using cation-adjusted Mueller-Hinton broth with 2 to 5% lysed horse blood inoculated with a direct colony suspension and incubated in ambient air at 35°C for 20 to 24 hours.
[f] This quality control zone diameter range is applicable only to tests performed using Mueller-Hinton agar supplemented with 5% defibrinated sheep blood inoculated with a direct colony suspension and incubated in 5% CO_2 at 35°C for 20 to 24 hours.

Vancomycin-Resistant *Enterococcus faecium* infections, including cases with concurrent bacteremia (see **CLINICAL STUDIES**).

Nosocomial pneumonia caused by *Staphylococcus aureus* (methicillin-susceptible and -resistant strains), or *Streptococcus pneumoniae* (including multi-drug resistant strains [MDRSP]). Combination therapy may be clinically indicated if the documented or presumptive pathogens include Gram-negative organisms (see **CLINICAL STUDIES**).

Complicated skin and skin structure infections, including diabetic foot infections, without concomitant osteomyelitis, caused by *Staphylococcus aureus* (methicillin-susceptible and -resistant strains), *Streptococcus pyogenes*, or *Streptococcus agalactiae.* ZYVOX has not been studied in the treatment of decubitus ulcers. Combination therapy may be clinically indicated if the documented or presumptive pathogens include Gram-negative organisms (see **CLINICAL STUDIES**).

Uncomplicated skin and skin structure infections caused by *Staphylococcus aureus* (methicillin-susceptible only) or *Streptococcus pyogenes.*

Community-acquired pneumonia caused by *Streptococcus pneumoniae* (including multi-drug resistant strains [MDRSP]*), including cases with concurrent bacteremia, or *Staphylococcus aureus* (methicillin-susceptible strains only).

To reduce the development of drug-resistant bacteria and maintain the effectiveness of ZYVOX and other antibacterial drugs, ZYVOX should be used only to treat or prevent infections that are proven or strongly suspected to be caused by susceptible bacteria. When culture and suscepti-

Continued on next page

Zyvox—Cont.

bility information are available, they should be considered in selecting or modifying antibacterial therapy. In the absence of such data, local epidemiology and susceptibility patterns may contribute to the empiric selection of therapy.

*MDRSP refers to isolates resistant to two or more of the following antibiotics: penicillin, second-generation cephalosporins, macrolides, tetracycline, and trimethoprim/sulfamethoxazole.

CONTRAINDICATIONS

ZYVOX formulations are contraindicated for use in patients who have known hypersensitivity to linezolid or any of the other product components.

WARNINGS

Myelosuppression (including anemia, leukopenia, pancytopenia, and thrombocytopenia) has been reported in patients receiving linezolid. In cases where the outcome is known, when linezolid was discontinued, the affected hematologic parameters have risen toward pretreatment levels. Complete blood counts should be monitored weekly in patients who receive linezolid, particularly in those who receive linezolid for longer than two weeks, those with preexisting myelosuppression, those receiving concomitant drugs that produce bone marrow suppression, or those with a chronic infection who have received previous or concomitant antibiotic therapy. Discontinuation of therapy with linezolid should be considered in patients who develop or have worsening myelosuppression.

In adult and juvenile dogs and rats, myelosuppression, reduced extramedullary hematopoiesis in spleen and liver, and lymphoid depletion of thymus, lymph nodes, and spleen were observed (see **ANIMAL PHARMACOLOGY**).

Pseudomembranous colitis has been reported with nearly all antibacterial agents, including ZYVOX, and may range in severity from mild to life-threatening. Therefore, it is important to consider this diagnosis in patients who present with diarrhea subsequent to the administration of any antibacterial agent.

Treatment with antibacterial agents alters the normal flora of the colon and may permit overgrowth of clostridia. Studies indicated that a toxin produced by *Clostridium difficile* is a primary cause of "antibiotic-associated colitis."

After the diagnosis of pseudomembranous colitis has been established, appropriate therapeutic measures should be initiated. Mild cases of pseudomembranous colitis usually respond to drug discontinuation alone. In moderate to severe cases, consideration should be given to management with fluids and electrolytes, protein supplementation, and treatment with an antibacterial agent clinically effective against *Clostridium difficile*.

PRECAUTIONS

General

Lactic acidosis has been reported with the use of ZYVOX. In reported cases, patients experienced repeated episodes of nausea and vomiting. Patients who develop recurrent nausea or vomiting, unexplained acidosis, or a low bicarbonate level while receiving ZYVOX should receive immediate medical evaluation.

The use of antibiotics may promote the overgrowth of nonsusceptible organisms. Should superinfection occur during therapy, appropriate measures should be taken.

ZYVOX has not been studied in patients with uncontrolled hypertension, pheochromocytoma, carcinoid syndrome, or untreated hyperthyroidism.

The safety and efficacy of ZYVOX formulations given for longer than 28 days have not been evaluated in controlled clinical trials.

Prescribing ZYVOX in the absence of a proven or strongly suspected bacterial infection or a prophylactic indication is unlikely to provide benefit to the patient and increases the risk of the development of drug-resistant bacteria.

Information for Patients

Patients should be advised that:

- ZYVOX may be taken with or without food.
- They should inform their physician if they have a history of hypertension.
- Large quantities of foods or beverages with high tyramine content should be avoided while taking ZYVOX. Quantities of tyramine consumed should be less than 100 mg per meal. Foods high in tyramine content include those that may have undergone protein changes by aging, fermentation, pickling, or smoking to improve flavor, such as aged cheeses (0 to 15 mg tyramine per ounce); fermented or air-dried meats (0.1 to 8 mg tyramine per ounce); sauerkraut (8 mg tyramine per 8 ounces); soy sauce (5 mg tyramine per 1 teaspoon); tap beers (4 mg tyramine per 12 ounces); red wines (0 to 6 mg tyramine per 8 ounces). The tyramine content of any protein-rich food may be increased if stored for long periods or improperly refrigerated.[9,10]
- They should inform their physician if taking medications containing pseudoephedrine HCl or phenylpropanolamine HCl, such as cold remedies and decongestants.
- They should inform their physician if taking serotonin re-uptake inhibitors or other antidepressants.
- *Phenylketonurics:* Each 5 mL of the 100 mg/5 mL ZYVOX for Oral Suspension contains 20 mg phenylalanine. The other ZYVOX formulations do not contain phenylalanine. Contact your physician or pharmacist.

Table 7. Incidence (%) of Drug-Related Adverse Events Occurring in >1% of Adult Patients Treated with ZYVOX in Comparator-Controlled Clinical Trials

	Uncomplicated Skin and Skin Structure Infections		All Other Indications	
Adverse Event	ZYVOX 400 mg PO q12h (n=548)	Clarithromycin 250 mg PO q12h (n=537)	ZYVOX 600 mg q12h (n=1498)	All Other Comparators* (n=1464)
% of patients with 1 drug-related adverse event	25.4	19.6	20.4	14.3
% of patients discontinuing due to drug-related adverse events†	3.5	2.4	2.1	1.7
Diarrhea	5.3	4.8	4.0	2.7
Nausea	3.5	3.5	3.3	1.8
Headache	2.7	2.2	1.9	1.0
Taste alteration	1.8	2.0	0.9	0.2
Vaginal moniliasis	1.6	1.3	1.0	0.4
Fungal infection	1.5	0.2	0.1	<0.1
Abnormal liver function tests	0.4	0	1.3	0.5
Vomiting	0.9	0.4	1.2	0.4
Tongue discoloration	1.1	0	0.2	0
Dizziness	1.1	1.5	0.4	0.3
Oral moniliasis	0.4	0	1.1	0.4

*Comparators included cefpodoxime proxetil 200 mg PO q12h; ceftriaxone 1 g IV q12h; dicloxacillin 500 mg PO q6h; oxacillin 2 g IV q6h; vancomycin 1 g IV q12h.

† The most commonly reported drug-related adverse events leading to discontinuation in patients treated with ZYVOX were nausea, headache, diarrhea, and vomiting.

Patients should be counseled that antibacterial drugs including ZYVOX should only be used to treat bacterial infections. They do not treat viral infections (e.g., the common cold).

When ZYVOX is prescribed to treat a bacterial infection, patients should be told that although it is common to feel better early in the course of therapy, the medication should be taken exactly as directed. Skipping doses or not completing the full course of therapy may (1) decrease the effectiveness of the immediate treatment and (2) increase the likelihood that bacteria will develop resistance and will not be treatable by ZYVOX or other antibacterial drugs in the future.

Drug Interactions (see also CLINICAL PHARMACOLOGY, Drug-Drug Interactions)

Monoamine Oxidase Inhibition: Linezolid is a reversible, nonselective inhibitor of monoamine oxidase. Therefore, linezolid has the potential for interaction with adrenergic and serotonergic agents.

Adrenergic Agents: Some individuals receiving ZYVOX may experience a reversible enhancement of the pressor response to indirect-acting sympathomimetic agents, vasopressor or dopaminergic agents. Commonly used drugs such as phenylpropanolamine and pseudoephedrine have been specifically studied. Initial doses of adrenergic agents, such as dopamine or epinephrine, should be reduced and titrated to achieve the desired response.

Serotonergic Agents: Co-administration of linezolid and serotonergic agents was not associated with serotonin syndrome in phase 1, 2 or 3 studies. Spontaneous reports of serotonin syndrome occurring with co-administration of ZYVOX and serotonergic agents have occurred. Physicians should be alert to the possibility of signs and symptoms of serotonin syndrome (cognitive dysfunction, hyperpyrexia, hyperreflexia, incoordination) in patients receiving concomitant serotonergic agents.

Drug-Laboratory Test Interactions

There are no reported drug-laboratory test interactions.

Carcinogenesis, Mutagenesis, Impairment of Fertility

Lifetime studies in animals have not been conducted to evaluate the carcinogenic potential of linezolid. Neither mutagenic nor clastogenic potential was found in a battery of tests including: assays for mutagenicity (Ames bacterial reversion and CHO cell mutation), an in vitro unscheduled DNA synthesis (UDS) assay, an in vitro chromosome aberration assay in human lymphocytes, and an in vivo mouse micronucleus assay.

Linezolid did not affect the fertility or reproductive performance of adult female rats. It reversibly decreased fertility and reproductive performance in adult male rats when given at doses ≥50 mg/kg/day, with exposures approximately equal to or greater than the expected human exposure level (exposure comparisons are based on AUCs). The reversible fertility effects were mediated through altered spermatogenesis. Affected spermatids contained abnormally formed and oriented mitochondria and were non-viable. Epithelial cell hypertrophy and hyperplasia in the epididymis was observed in conjunction with decreased fertility. Similar epididymal changes were not seen in dogs.

In sexually mature male rats exposed to drug as juveniles, mildly decreased fertility was observed following treatment with linezolid through most of their period of sexual development (50 mg/kg/day from days 7 to 36 of age, and 100 mg/kg/day from days 37 to 55 of age), with exposures up to 1.7-fold greater than mean AUCs observed in pediatric patients aged 3 months to 11 years. Decreased fertility was not observed with shorter treatment periods, corresponding to exposure in utero through the early neonatal period (gestation day 6 through postnatal day 5), neonatal exposure (postnatal days 5 to 21), or to juvenile exposure (postnatal days 22 to 35). Reversible reductions in sperm motility and altered sperm morphology were observed in rats treated from postnatal day 22 to 35.

Pregnancy

Teratogenic Effects. Pregnancy Category C: Linezolid was not teratogenic in mice or rats at exposure levels 6.5-fold (in mice) or equivalent to (in rats) the expected human exposure level, based on AUCs. However, embryo and fetal toxicities were seen (see **Non-teratogenic Effects**). There are no adequate and well-controlled studies in pregnant women. ZYVOX should be used during pregnancy only if the potential benefit justifies the potential risk to the fetus.

Non-teratogenic Effects

In mice, embryo and fetal toxicities were seen only at doses that caused maternal toxicity (clinical signs and reduced body weight gain). A dose of 450 mg/kg/day (6.5-fold the estimated human exposure level based on AUCs) correlated with increased postimplantational embryo death, including total litter loss, decreased fetal body weights, and an increased incidence of costal cartilage fusion.

In rats, mild fetal toxicity was observed at 15 and 50 mg/kg/day (exposure levels 0.22-fold to approximately equivalent to the estimated human exposure, respectively based on AUCs). The effects consisted of decreased fetal body weights and reduced ossification of sternebrae, a finding often seen in association with decreased fetal body weights. Slight maternal toxicity, in the form of reduced body weight gain, was seen at 50 mg/kg/day.

When female rats were treated with 50 mg/kg/day (approximately equivalent to the estimated human exposure based on AUCs) of linezolid during pregnancy and lactation, survival of pups was decreased on postnatal days 1 to 4. Male and female pups permitted to mature to reproductive age, when mated, showed an increase in preimplantation loss.

Nursing Mothers

Linezolid and its metabolites are excreted in the milk of lactating rats. Concentrations in milk were similar to those in maternal plasma. It is not known whether linezolid is excreted in human milk. Because many drugs are excreted in human milk, caution should be exercised when ZYVOX is administered to a nursing woman.

Pediatric Use

The safety and effectiveness of ZYVOX for the treatment of pediatric patients with the following infections are supported by evidence from adequate and well-controlled studies in adults, pharmacokinetic data in pediatric patients, and additional data from a comparator-controlled study of Gram-positive infections in pediatric patients ranging in age from birth through 11 years (see **INDICATIONS AND USAGE** and **CLINICAL STUDIES**):

- nosocomial pneumonia
- complicated skin and skin structure infections
- community-acquired pneumonia (also supported by evidence from an uncontrolled study in patients ranging in age from 8 months through 12 years)
- vancomycin-resistant *Enterococcus faecium* infections

The safety and effectiveness of ZYVOX for the treatment of pediatric patients with the following infection have been established in a comparator-controlled study in pediatric patients ranging in age from 5 through 17 years (see **CLINICAL STUDIES**):

- uncomplicated skin and skin structure infections caused by *Staphylococcus aureus* (methicillin-susceptible strains only) or *Streptococcus pyogenes*

The C_{max} and the volume of distribution (V_{ss}) of linezolid are similar regardless of age in pediatric patients. However, linezolid clearance is a function of age. Excluding neonates less than a week of age, clearance is most rapid in the youngest age groups ranging from >1 week old to 11 years, resulting in lower single-dose systemic exposure (AUC) and shorter half-life as compared with adults. As age of pediatric patients increases, the clearance of linezolid gradually decreases, and by adolescence, mean clearance values approach those observed for the adult population. There is wider inter-subject variability in linezolid clearance and in systemic drug exposure (AUC) across all pediatric age groups as compared with adults.

Similar mean daily AUC values were observed in pediatric patients from birth to 11 years of age dosed q8h relative to adolescents or adults dosed q12h. Therefore, the dosage for pediatric patients up to 11 years of age should be 10 mg/kg q8h. Pediatric patients 12 years and older should receive 600 mg q12h.

Recommendations for the dosage regimen for pre-term neonates less than 7 days of age (gestational age less than 34 weeks) are based on pharmacokinetic data from 9 pre-term neonates. Most of these pre-term neonates have lower systemic linezolid clearance values and larger AUC values than many full-term neonates and older infants. Therefore, these pre-term neonates should be initiated with a dosing regimen of 10 mg/kg q12h. Consideration may be given to the use of a 10 mg/kg q8h regimen in neonates with a sub-optimal clinical response. All neonatal patients should receive 10 mg/kg q8h by 7 days of life (see **CLINICAL PHARMACOLOGY, Special Populations, Pediatric** and **DOSAGE AND ADMINISTRATION**).

In limited clinical experience, 5 out of 6 (83%) pediatric patients with infections due to Gram-positive pathogens with MICs of 4 µg/mL treated with ZYVOX had clinical cures. However, pediatric patients exhibit wider variability in linezolid clearance and systemic exposure (AUC) compared with adults. In pediatric patients with a sub-optimal clinical response, particularly those with pathogens with MIC of 4 µg/mL, lower systemic exposure, site and severity of infection, and the underlying medical condition should be considered when assessing clinical response (see **CLINICAL PHARMACOLOGY, Special Populations, Pediatric** and **DOSAGE AND ADMINISTRATION**).

Geriatric Use

Of the 2046 patients treated with ZYVOX in phase 3 comparator-controlled clinical trials, 589 (29%) were 65 years or older and 253 (12%) were 75 years or older. No overall differences in safety or effectiveness were observed between these patients and younger patients.

ANIMAL PHARMACOLOGY

Target organs of linezolid toxicity were similar in juvenile and adult rats and dogs. Dose- and time-dependent myelosuppression, as evidenced by bone marrow hypocellularity/decreased hematopoiesis, decreased extramedullary hematopoiesis in spleen and liver, and decreased levels of circulating erythrocytes, leukocytes, and platelets have been seen in animal studies. Lymphoid depletion occurred in thymus, lymph nodes, and spleen. Generally, the lymphoid findings were associated with anorexia, weight loss, and suppression of body weight gain, which may have contributed to the observed effects. These effects were observed at exposure levels that are comparable to those observed in some human subjects. The hematopoietic and lymphoid effects were reversible, although in some studies, reversal was incomplete within the duration of the recovery period.

ADVERSE REACTIONS

Adult Patients

The safety of ZYVOX formulations was evaluated in 2046 adult patients enrolled in seven phase 3 comparator-controlled clinical trials, who were treated for up to 28 days. In these studies, 85% of the adverse events reported with ZYVOX were described as mild to moderate in intensity. Table 6 shows the incidence of adverse events reported in at least 2% of patients in these trials. The most common adverse events in patients treated with ZYVOX were diarrhea (incidence across studies: 2.8% to 11.0%), headache (incidence across studies: 0.5% to 11.3%), and nausea (incidence across studies: 3.4% to 9.6%).

Table 6. Incidence (%) of Adverse Events Reported in ≥2% of Adult Patients in Comparator-Controlled Clinical Trials with ZYVOX

Event	ZYVOX (n=2046)	All Comparators* (n=2001)
Diarrhea	8.3	6.3
Headache	6.5	5.5
Nausea	6.2	4.6
Vomiting	3.7	2.0
Insomnia	2.5	1.7
Constipation	2.2	2.1
Rash	2.0	2.2
Dizziness	2.0	1.9
Fever	1.6	2.1

*Comparators included cefpodoxime proxetil 200 mg PO q12h; ceftriaxone 1 g IV q12h; clarithromycin 250 mg PO q12h; dicloxacillin 500 mg PO q6h; oxacillin 2 g IV q6h; vancomycin 1 g IV q12h.

Other adverse events reported in phase 2 and phase 3 studies included oral moniliasis, vaginal moniliasis, hypertension, dyspepsia, localized abdominal pain, pruritus, and tongue discoloration.

Table 7 shows the incidence of drug-related adverse events reported in at least 1% of adult patients in these trials by dose of ZYVOX.

[See table 7 at top of previous page]

Pediatric Patients

The safety of ZYVOX formulations was evaluated in 215 pediatric patients ranging in age from birth through 11 years, and in 248 pediatric patients aged 5 through 17 years (146 of these 248 were age 5 through 11 and 102 were age 12 to 17). These patients were enrolled in two phase 3 comparator-controlled clinical trials and were treated for up to 28 days. In these studies, 83% and 99%, respectively, of

Continued on next page

Table 8. Incidence (%) of Adverse Events Reported in ≥2% of Pediatric Patients Treated with ZYVOX in Comparator-Controlled Clinical Trials

	Uncomplicated Skin and Skin Structure Infections*		All Other Indications†	
Event	ZYVOX (n=248)	Cefadroxil (n = 251)	ZYVOX (n = 215)	Vancomycin (n=101)
Fever	2.9	3.6	14.1	14.1
Diarrhea	7.8	8.0	10.8	12.1
Vomiting	2.9	6.4	9.4	9.1
Sepsis	0	0	8.0	7.1
Rash	1.6	1.2	7.0	15.2
Headache	6.5	4.0	0.9	0
Anemia	0	0	5.6	7.1
Thrombocytopenia	0	0	4.7	2.0
Upper respiratory infection	3.7	5.2	4.2	1.0
Nausea	3.7	3.2	1.9	0
Dyspnea	0	0	3.3	1.0
Reaction at site of injection or of vascular catheter	0	0	3.3	5.1
Trauma	3.3	4.8	2.8	2.0
Pharyngitis	2.9	1.6	0.5	1.0
Convulsion	0	0	2.8	2.0
Hypokalemia	0	0	2.8	3.0
Pneumonia	0	0	2.8	2.0
Thrombocythemia	0	0	2.8	2.0
Cough	2.4	4.0	0.9	0
Generalized abdominal pain	2.4	2.8	0.9	2.0
Localized abdominal pain	2.4	2.8	0.5	1.0
Apnea	0	0	2.3	2.0
Gastrointestinal bleeding	0	0	2.3	1.0
Generalized edema	0	0	2.3	1.0
Loose stools	1.6	0.8	2.3	3.0
Localized pain	2.0	1.6	0.9	0
Skin disorder	2.0	0	0.9	1.0

*Patients 5 through 11 years of age received ZYVOX 10 mg/kg PO q12h or cefadroxil 15 mg/kg PO q12h. Patients 12 years or older received ZYVOX 600 mg PO q12h or cefadroxil 500 mg PO q12h.

† Patients from birth through 11 years of age received ZYVOX 10 mg/kg IV/PO q8h or vancomycin 10 to 15 mg/kg IV q6-24h, depending on age and renal clearance.

Table 9. Incidence (%) of Drug-related Adverse Events Occurring in >1% of Pediatric Patients (and >1 Patient) in Either Treatment Group in Comparator-Controlled Clinical Trials

	Uncomplicated Skin and Skin Structure Infections*		All Other Indications†	
Event	ZYVOX (n=248)	Cefadroxil (n=251)	ZYVOX (n=215)	Vancomycin (n=101)
% of patients with ≥1 drug-related adverse event	19.2	14.1	18.8	34.3
% of patients discontinuing due to a drug-related adverse event	1.6	2.4	0.9	6.1
Diarrhea	5.7	5.2	3.8	6.1

(Table continued on next page)

Zyvox—Cont.

Table 9 *(cont.)*. Incidence (%) of Drug-related Adverse Events Occurring in >1% of Pediatric Patients (and >1 Patient) in Either Treatment Group in Comparator-Controlled Clinical Trials

Event	Uncomplicated Skin and Skin Structure Infections*		All Other Indications†	
	ZYVOX (n=248)	Cefadroxil (n=251)	ZYVOX (n=215)	Vancomycin (n=101)
Nausea	3.3	2.0	1.4	0
Headache	2.4	0.8	0	0
Loose stools	1.2	0.8	1.9	0
Thrombocytopenia	0	0	1.9	0
Vomiting	1.2	2.4	1.9	1.0
Generalized abdominal pain	1.6	1.2	0	0
Localized abdominal pain	1.6	1.2	0	0
Anemia	0	0	1.4	1.0
Eosinophilia	0.4	0.4	1.4	0
Rash	0.4	1.2	1.4	7.1
Vertigo	1.2	0.4	0	0
Oral moniliasis	0	0	0.9	4.0
Fever	0	0	0.5	3.0
Pruritus at non-application site	0.4	0	0	2.0
Anaphylaxis	0	0	0	10.1‡

* Patients 5 through 11 years of age received ZYVOX 10 mg/kg PO q12h or cefadroxil 15 mg/kg PO q12h. Patients 12 years or older received ZYVOX 600 mg PO q12h or cefadroxil 500 mg PO q12h.
† Patients from birth through 11 years of age received ZYVOX 10 mg/kg IV/PO q8h or vancomycin 10 to 15 mg/kg IV q6-24h, depending on age and renal clearance.
‡ These reports were of 'red-man syndrome', which were coded as anaphylaxis.

the adverse events reported with ZYVOX were described as mild to moderate in intensity. In the study of hospitalized pediatric patients (birth through 11 years) with Gram-positive infections, who were randomized 2 to 1 (linezolid: vancomycin), mortality was 6.0% (13/215) in the linezolid arm and 3.0% (3/101) in the vancomycin arm. However, given the severe underlying illness in the patient population, no causality could be established. Table 8 shows the incidence of adverse events reported in at least 2% of pediatric patients treated with ZYVOX in these trials.
[See table 8 at top of previous page]
Table 9 shows the incidence of drug-related adverse events reported in more than 1% of pediatric patients (and more than 1 patient) in either treatment group in the comparator-controlled phase 3 trials.
[See table 9 on previous page and at right]

Laboratory Changes

ZYVOX has been associated with thrombocytopenia when used in doses up to and including 600 mg every 12 hours for up to 28 days. In phase 3 comparator-controlled trials, the percentage of adult patients who developed a substantially low platelet count (defined as less than 75% of lower limit of normal and/or baseline) was 2.4% (range among studies: 0.3 to 10.0%) with ZYVOX and 1.5% (range among studies: 0.4 to 7.0%) with a comparator. In a study of hospitalized pediatric patients ranging in age from birth through 11 years, the percentage of patients who developed a substantially low platelet count (defined as less than 75% of lower limit of normal and/or baseline) was 12.9% with ZYVOX and 13.4% with vancomycin. In an outpatient study of pediatric patients aged from 5 through 17 years, the percentage of patients who developed a substantially low platelet count was 0% with ZYVOX and 0.4% with cefadroxil. Thrombocytopenia associated with the use of ZYVOX appears to be dependent on duration of therapy, (generally greater than 2 weeks of treatment). The platelet counts for most patients returned to the normal range/baseline during the follow-up period. No related clinical adverse events were identified in phase 3 clinical trials in patients developing thrombocytopenia. Bleeding events were identified in thrombocytopenic patients in a compassionate use program for ZYVOX; the role of linezolid in these events cannot be determined (see **WARNINGS**).

Changes seen in other laboratory parameters, without regard to drug relationship, revealed no substantial differences between ZYVOX and the comparators. These changes were generally not clinically significant, did not lead to discontinuation of therapy, and were reversible. The incidence of adult and pediatric patients with at least one substantially abnormal hematologic or serum chemistry value is presented in Tables 10, 11, 12, and 13.
[See table 10 at right]
[See table 11 at right]
[See table 12 on next page]
[See table 13 on next page]

Table 10. Percent of Adult Patients who Experienced at Least One Substantially Abnormal* Hematology Laboratory Value in Comparator-Controlled Clinical Trials with ZYVOX

Laboratory Assay	Uncomplicated Skin and Skin Structure Infections		All Other Indications	
	ZYVOX 400 mg q12h	Clarithromycin 250 mg q12h	ZYVOX 600 mg q12h	All Other Comparators†
Hemoglobin (g/dL)	0.9	0.0	7.1	6.6
Platelet count ($\times 10^3/mm^3$)	0.7	0.8	3.0	1.8
WBC ($\times 10^3/mm^3$)	0.2	0.6	2.2	1.3
Neutrophils ($\times 10^3/mm^3$)	0.0	0.2	1.1	1.2

* <75% (<50% for neutrophils) of Lower Limit of Normal (LLN) for values normal at baseline;
<75% (<50% for neutrophils) of LLN and of baseline for values abnormal at baseline.
† Comparators included cefpodoxime proxetil 200 mg PO q12h; ceftriaxone 1 g IV q12h; dicloxacillin 500 mg PO q6h; oxacillin 2 g IV q6h; vancomycin 1 g IV q12h.

Table 11. Percent of Adult Patients who Experienced at Least One Substantially Abnormal* Serum Chemistry Laboratory Value in Comparator-Controlled Clinical Trials with ZYVOX

Laboratory Assay	Uncomplicated Skin and Skin Structure Infections		All Other Indications	
	ZYVOX 400 mg q12h	Clarithromycin 250 mg q12h	ZYVOX 600 mg q12h	All Other Comparators†
AST (U/L)	1.7	1.3	5.0	6.8
ALT (U/L)	1.7	1.7	9.6	9.3
LDH (U/L)	0.2	0.2	1.8	1.5
Alkaline phosphatase (U/L)	0.2	0.2	3.5	3.1
Lipase (U/L)	2.8	2.6	4.3	4.2
Amylase (U/L)	0.2	0.2	2.4	2.0
Total bilirubin (mg/dL)	0.2	0.0	0.9	1.1
BUN (mg/dL)	0.2	0.0	2.1	1.5
Creatinine (mg/dL)	0.2	0.0	0.2	0.6

* >2 × Upper Limit of Normal (ULN) for values normal at baseline;
>2 × ULN and >2× baseline for values abnormal at baseline.
† Comparators included cefpodoxime proxetil 200 mg PO q12h; ceftriaxone 1 g IV q12h; dicloxacillin 500 mg PO q6h; oxacillin 2 g IV q6h; vancomycin 1 g IV q12h.

Postmarketing Experience

Myelosuppression (including anemia, leukopenia, pancytopenia, and thrombocytopenia) has been reported during postmarketing use of ZYVOX (see **WARNINGS**). Neuropathy (peripheral, optic) has been reported in patients treated with ZYVOX. Lactic acidosis has been reported with the use of ZYVOX (see **PRECAUTIONS**). Although these reports have primarily been in patients treated for longer than the maximum recommended duration of 28 days, these events have also been reported in patients receiving shorter courses of therapy. Serotonin syndrome has been reported in patients receiving concomitant serotonergic agents and ZYVOX (see **PRECAUTIONS**). These events have been chosen for inclusion due to either their seriousness, frequency of reporting, possible causal connection to ZYVOX, or a combination of these factors. Because they are reported voluntarily from a population of unknown size, estimates of frequency cannot be made and causal relationship cannot be precisely established.

OVERDOSAGE

In the event of overdosage, supportive care is advised, with maintenance of glomerular filtration. Hemodialysis may facilitate more rapid elimination of linezolid. In a phase 1 clinical trial, approximately 30% of a dose of linezolid was removed during a 3-hour hemodialysis session beginning 3 hours after the dose of linezolid was administered. Data are not available for removal of linezolid with peritoneal dialysis or hemoperfusion. Clinical signs of acute toxicity in animals were decreased activity and ataxia in rats and vomiting and tremors in dogs treated with 3000 mg/kg/day and 2000 mg/kg/day, respectively.

DOSAGE AND ADMINISTRATION

The recommended dosage for ZYVOX formulations for the treatment of infections is described in Table 14.
[See table 14 at bottom of next page]
Adult patients with infection due to MRSA should be treated with ZYVOX 600 mg q12h.

In limited clinical experience, 5 out of 6 (83%) pediatric patients with infections due to Gram-positive pathogens with MICs of 4 µg/mL treated with ZYVOX had clinical cures. However, pediatric patients exhibit wider variability in linezolid clearance and systemic exposure (AUC) compared with adults. In pediatric patients with a sub-optimal clinical response, particularly those with pathogens with MIC of 4 µg/mL, lower systemic exposure, site and severity of infection, and the underlying medical condition should be considered when assessing clinical response (see **CLINICAL PHARMACOLOGY, Special Populations, Pediatric** and **PRECAUTIONS, Pediatric Use**).

In controlled clinical trials, the protocol-defined duration of treatment for all infections ranged from 7 to 28 days. Total treatment duration was determined by the treating physician based on site and severity of the infection, and on the patient's clinical response.

No dose adjustment is necessary when switching from intravenous to oral administration. Patients whose therapy is started with ZYVOX I.V. Injection may be switched to either ZYVOX Tablets or Oral Suspension at the discretion of the physician, when clinically indicated.

Intravenous Administration

ZYVOX I.V. Injection is supplied in single-use, ready-to-use infusion bags (see **HOW SUPPLIED** for container sizes). Parenteral drug products should be inspected visually for particulate matter prior to administration. Check for minute leaks by firmly squeezing the bag. If leaks are detected, discard the solution, as sterility may be impaired.

ZYVOX I.V. Injection should be administered by intravenous infusion over a period of 30 to 120 minutes. **Do not use this intravenous infusion bag in series connections.** Additives should not be introduced into this solution. If ZYVOX I.V. Injection is to be given concomitantly with another drug, each drug should be given separately in accordance with the recommended dosage and route of administration for each product. In particular, physical incompatibilities resulted when ZYVOX I.V. Injection was combined with the following drugs during simulated Y-site administration: amphotericin B, chlorpromazine HCl, diazepam, pentamidine isothionate, erythromycin lactobionate, phenytoin sodium, and trimethoprim-sulfamethoxazole. Additionally, chemical incompatibility resulted when ZYVOX I.V. Injection was combined with ceftriaxone sodium.

If the same intravenous line is used for sequential infusion of several drugs, the line should be flushed before and after infusion of ZYVOX I.V. Injection with an infusion solution compatible with ZYVOX I.V. Injection and with any other drug(s) administered via this common line (see **Compatible Intravenous Solutions**).

Compatible Intravenous Solutions

5% Dextrose Injection, USP
0.9% Sodium Chloride Injection, USP
Lactated Ringer's Injection, USP

Keep the infusion bags in the overwrap until ready to use. Store at room temperature. Protect from freezing. ZYVOX I.V. Injection may exhibit a yellow color that can intensify over time without adversely affecting potency.

Constitution of Oral Suspension

ZYVOX for Oral Suspension is supplied as a powder/granule for constitution. Gently tap bottle to loosen powder. Add a total of 123 mL distilled water in two portions. After adding the first half, shake vigorously to wet all of the powder. Then add the second half of the water and shake vigorously to obtain a uniform suspension. After constitution, each 5 mL of the suspension contains 100 mg of linezolid. Before using, gently mix by inverting the bottle 3 to 5 times. **DO NOT SHAKE.** Store constituted suspension at room temperature. Use within 21 days after constitution.

Table 12. Percent of Pediatric Patients who Experienced at Least One Substantially Abnormal* Hematology Laboratory Value in Comparator-Controlled Clinical Trials with ZYVOX

Laboratory Assay	Uncomplicated Skin and Skin Structure Infections†		All Other Indications‡	
	ZYVOX	Cefadroxil	ZYVOX	Vancomycin
Hemoglobin (g/dL)	0.0	0.0	15.7	12.4
Platelet count (× 10³/mm³)	0.0	0.4	12.9	13.4
WBC (× 10³/mm³)	0.8	0.8	12.4	10.3
Neutrophils (× 10³/mm³)	1.2	0.8	5.9	4.3

* <75% (<50% for neutrophils) of Lower Limit of Normal (LLN) for values normal at baseline; <75% (<50% for neutrophils) of LLN and <75% (<50% for neutrophils, <90% for hemoglobin if baseline <LLN) of baseline for values abnormal at baseline.
† Patients 5 through 11 years of age received ZYVOX 10 mg/kg PO q12h or cefadroxil 15 mg/kg PO q12h. Patients 12 years or older received ZYVOX 600 mg PO q12h or cefadroxil 500 mg PO q12h.
‡ Patients from birth through 11 years of age received ZYVOX 10 mg/kg IV/PO q8h or vancomycin 10 to 15 mg/kg IV q6-24h, depending on age and renal clearance.

Table 13. Percent of Pediatric Patients who Experienced at Least One Substantially Abnormal* Serum Chemistry Laboratory Value in Comparator-Controlled Clinical Trials with ZYVOX

Laboratory Assay	Uncomplicated Skin and Skin Structure Infections†		All Other Indications‡	
	ZYVOX	Cefadroxil	ZYVOX	Vancomycin
ALT (U/L)	0.0	0.0	10.1	12.5
Lipase (U/L)	0.4	1.2	—	—
Amylase (U/L)	—	—	0.6	1.3
Total bilirubin (mg/dL)	—	—	6.3	5.2
Creatinine (mg/dL)	0.4	0.0	2.4	1.0

* >2 × Upper Limit of Normal (ULN) for values normal at baseline; >2 × ULN and >2 (>1.5 for total bilirubin) × baseline for values abnormal at baseline.
† Patients 5 through 11 years of age received ZYVOX 10 mg/kg PO q12h or cefadroxil 15 mg/kg PO q12h. Patients 12 years or older received ZYVOX 600 mg PO q12h or cefadroxil 500 mg PO q12h.
‡ Patients from birth through 11 years of age received ZYVOX 10 mg/kg IV/PO q8h or vancomycin 10 to 15 mg/kg IV q6-24h, depending on age and renal clearance.

Table 14. Dosage Guidelines for ZYVOX

Infection*	Dosage and Route of Administration: Pediatric Patients† (Birth through 11 Years of Age)	Dosage and Route of Administration: Adults and Adolescents (12 Years and Older)	Recommended Duration of Treatment (consecutive days)
Complicated skin and skin structure infections	10 mg/kg IV or oral‡ q8h	600 mg IV or oral‡ q12h	10 to 14
Community-acquired pneumonia, including concurrent bacteremia			
Nosocomial pneumonia			
Vancomycin-resistant *Enterococcus faecium* infections, including concurrent bacteremia	10 mg/kg IV or oral‡ q8h	600 mg IV or oral‡ q12h	14 to 28
Uncomplicated skin and skin structure infections	<5 yrs: 10 mg/kg oral‡ q8h 5-11 yrs: 10 mg/kg oral‡ q12h	Adults: 400 mg oral‡ q12h Adolescents: 600 mg oral‡ q12h	10 to 14

*Due to the designated pathogens (see **INDICATIONS AND USAGE**)
† **Neonates <7 days:** Most pre-term neonates <7 days of age (gestational age <34 weeks) have lower systemic linezolid clearance values and larger AUC values than many full-term neonates and older infants. These neonates should be initiated with a dosing regimen of 10 mg/kg q12h. Consideration may be given to the use of 10 mg/kg q8h regimen in neonates with a sub-optimal clinical response. All neonatal patients should receive 10 mg/kg q8h by 7 days of life (see **CLINICAL PHARMACOLOGY, Special Populations, Pediatric**).
‡ Oral dosing using either ZYVOX Tablets or ZYVOX for Oral Suspension.

HOW SUPPLIED

Injection

ZYVOX I.V. Injection is available in single-use, ready-to-use flexible plastic infusion bags in a foil laminate overwrap. The infusion bags and ports are latex-free. The infusion bags are available in the following package sizes:

100 mL bag (200 mg linezolid) NDC 0009-5137-01
200 mL bag (400 mg linezolid) NDC 0009-5139-01
300 mL bag (600 mg linezolid) NDC 0009-5140-01

Tablets

ZYVOX Tablets are available as follows:

400 mg (white, oblong, film-coated tablets printed with "ZYVOX 400mg")
100 tablets in HDPE bottle NDC 0009-5134-01
20 tablets in HDPE bottle NDC 0009-5134-02
Unit dose packages of 30 tablets NDC 0009-5134-03

600 mg (white, capsule-shaped, film-coated tablets printed with "ZYVOX 600 mg")
100 tablets in HDPE bottle NDC 0009-5135-01
20 tablets in HDPE bottle NDC 0009-5135-02
Unit dose packages of 30 tablets NDC 0009-5135-03

Oral Suspension

ZYVOX for Oral Suspension is available as a dry, white to off-white, orange-flavored granule/powder. When constituted as directed, each bottle will contain 150 mL of a suspension providing the equivalent of 100 mg of linezolid per each 5 mL. ZYVOX for Oral Suspension is supplied as follows:

100 mg/5 mL in 240-mL glass bottles NDC 0009-5136-01

Storage of ZYVOX Formulations

Store at 25°C (77°F); excursions permitted to 15-30°C (59-86°F) [see USP Controlled Room Temperature]. Protect from light. Keep bottles tightly closed to protect from moisture. It is recommended that the infusion bags be kept in the overwrap until ready to use. Protect infusion bags from freezing.

CLINICAL STUDIES

Adults

Vancomycin-Resistant Enterococcal Infections

Adult patients with documented or suspected vancomycin-resistant enterococcal infection were enrolled in a randomized, multi-center, double-blind trial comparing a high dose of ZYVOX (600 mg) with a low dose of ZYVOX (200 mg) given every 12 hours (q12h) either intravenously (IV) or orally for 7 to 28 days. Patients could receive concomitant aztreonam or aminoglycosides. There were 79 patients randomized to high-dose linezolid and 66 to low-dose linezolid. The intent-to-treat (ITT) population with documented vancomycin-resistant enterococcal infection at baseline consisted of 65 patients in the high-dose arm and 52 in the low-dose arm.

The cure rates for the ITT population with documented vancomycin-resistant enterococcal infection at baseline are presented in Table 15 by source of infection. These cure rates do not include patients with missing or indeterminate outcomes. The cure rate was higher in the high-dose arm than in the low-dose arm, although the difference was not statistically significant at the 0.05 level.

Table 15. Cure Rates at the Test-of-Cure Visit for ITT Adult Patients with Documented Vancomycin-Resistant Enterococcal Infections at Baseline

Source of Infection	Cured: ZYVOX 600 mg q12h n/N (%)	Cured: ZYVOX 200 mg q12h n/N (%)
Any site	39/58 (67)	24/46 (52)
Any site with associated bacteremia	10/17 (59)	4/14 (29)
Bacteremia of unknown origin	5/10 (50)	2/7 (29)
Skin and skin structure	9/13 (69)	5/5 (100)
Urinary tract	12/19 (63)	12/20 (60)
Pneumonia	2/3 (67)	0/1 (0)
Other*	11/13 (85)	5/13 (39)

*Includes sources of infection such as hepatic abscess, biliary sepsis, necrotic gall bladder, pericolonic abscess, pancreatitis, and catheter-related infection.

Nosocomial Pneumonia

Adult patients with clinically and radiologically documented nosocomial pneumonia were enrolled in a randomized, multi-center, double-blind trial. Patients were treated for 7 to 21 days. One group received ZYVOX I.V. Injection

Continued on next page

Zyvox—Cont.

600 mg q12h, and the other group received vancomycin 1 g q12h IV. Both groups received concomitant aztreonam (1 to 2 g every 8 hours IV), which could be continued if clinically indicated. There were 203 linezolid-treated and 193 vancomycin-treated patients enrolled in the study. One hundred twenty-two (60%) linezolid-treated patients and 103 (53%) vancomycin-treated patients were clinically evaluable. The cure rates in clinically evaluable patients were 57% for linezolid-treated patients and 60% for vancomycin-treated patients. The cure rates in clinically evaluable patients with ventilator-associated pneumonia were 47% for linezolid-treated patients and 40% for vancomycin-treated patients. A modified intent-to-treat (MITT) analysis of 94 linezolid-treated patients and 83 vancomycin-treated patients included subjects who had a pathogen isolated before treatment. The cure rates in the MITT analysis were 57% in linezolid-treated patients and 46% in vancomycin-treated patients. The cure rates by pathogen for microbiologically evaluable patients are presented in Table 16.

Table 16. Cure Rates at the Test-of-Cure Visit for Microbiologically Evaluable Adult Patients with Nosocomial Pneumonia

Pathogen	Cured	
	ZYVOX n/N (%)	Vancomycin n/N (%)
Staphylococcus aureus	23/38 (61)	14/23 (61)
Methicillin-resistant *S. aureus*	13/22 (59)	7/10 (70)
Streptococcus pneumoniae	9/9 (100)	9/10 (90)

Pneumonia caused by multi-drug resistant *S.pneumoniae* (MDRSP*)

ZYVOX was studied for the treatment of community-acquired (CAP) and hospital-acquired (HAP) pneumonia due to MDRSP by pooling clinical data from seven comparative and non-comparative Phase 2 and Phase 3 studies involving adult and pediatric patients. The pooled MITT population consisted of all patients with *S.pneumoniae* isolated at baseline; the pooled ME population consisted of patients satisfying criteria for microbiologic evaluability. The pooled MITT population with CAP included 15 patients (41%) with severe illness (risk classes IV and V) as assessed by a prediction rule[11]. The pooled clinical cure rates for patients with CAP due to MDRSP were 35/48 (73%) in the MITT and 33/36 (92%) in the ME populations respectively. The pooled clinical cure rates for patients with HAP due to MDRSP were 12/18 (67%) in the MITT and 10/12 (83%) in the ME populations respectively.

Table 17. Clinical cure rates for 36 microbiologically-evaluable patients with CAP due to MDRSP* who were treated with ZYVOX (stratified by antibiotic susceptibility)

Susceptibility Screening	Clinical Cure	
	n/N[a]	(%)
Penicillin-resistant	14/16	88
2nd generation cephalosporin-resistant[b]	19/22	86
Macrolide-resistant[c]	29/30	97
Tetracycline-resistant	22/24	92
Trimethoprim/ sulfamethoxazole-resistant	18/21	86

a) n= pooled number of patients treated successfully; N= pooled number of patients having MDRSP isolates that exhibited resistance to the listed antibiotic
b) 2nd-generation cephalosporin tested was cefuroxime
c) macrolide tested was erythromycin

*MDRSP refers to isolates resistant to two or more of the following antibiotics: penicillin, second-generation cephalosporins, macrolides, tetracycline, and trimethoprim/sulfamethoxazole.

Complicated Skin and Skin Structure Infections

Adult patients with clinically documented complicated skin and skin structure infections were enrolled in a randomized, multi-center, double-blind, double-dummy trial comparing study medications administered IV followed by medications given orally for a total of 10 to 21 days of treatment. One group of patients received ZYVOX I.V. Injection 600 mg q12h followed by ZYVOX Tablets 600 mg q12h; the other group received oxacillin 2 g every 6 hours (q6h) IV followed by dicloxacillin 500 mg q6h orally. Patients could receive concomitant aztreonam if clinically indicated. There were 400 linezolid-treated and 419 oxacillin-treated patients enrolled in the study. Two hundred forty-five (61%) linezolid-treated patients and 242 (58%) oxacillin-treated patients were clinically evaluable. The cure rates in clinically evaluable patients were 90% in linezolid-treated patients and 85% in oxacillin-treated patients. A modified intent-to-treat (MITT) analysis of 316 linezolid-treated patients and 313 oxacillin-treated patients included subjects who met all criteria for study entry. The cure rates in the MITT analysis were 86% in linezolid-treated patients and 82% in oxacillin-treated patients. The cure rates by pathogen for microbiologically evaluable patients are presented in Table 18.

Table 18. Cure Rates at the Test-of-Cure Visit for Microbiologically Evaluable Adult Patients with Complicated Skin and Skin Structure Infections

Pathogen	Cured	
	ZYVOX n/N (%)	Oxacillin/ Dicloxacillin n/N (%)
Staphylococcus aureus	73/83 (88)	72/84 (86)
Methicillin-resistant *S. aureus*	2/3 (67)	0/0 (-)
Streptococcus agalactiae	6/6 (100)	3/6 (50)
Streptococcus pyogenes	18/26 (69)	21/28 (75)

A separate study provided additional experience with the use of ZYVOX in the treatment of methicillin-resistant *Staphylococcus aureus* (MRSA) infections. This was a randomized, open-label trial in hospitalized adult patients with documented or suspected MRSA infection.

One group of patients received ZYVOX I.V. Injection 600 mg q12h followed by ZYVOX Tablets 600 mg q12h. The other group of patients received vancomycin 1 g q12h IV. Both groups were treated for 7 to 28 days, and could receive concomitant aztreonam or gentamicin if clinically indicated. The cure rates in microbiologically evaluable patients with MRSA skin and skin structure infection were 26/33 (79%) for linezolid-treated patients and 24/33 (73%) for vancomycin-treated patients.

Diabetic Foot Infections

Adult diabetic patients with clinically documented complicated skin and skin structure infections ("diabetic foot infections") were enrolled in a randomized (2:1 ratio), multi-center, open-label trial comparing study medications administered IV or orally for a total of 14 to 28 days of treatment. One group of patients received ZYVOX 600 mg q12h IV or orally; the other group received ampicillin/sulbactam 1.5 to 3 g IV or amoxicillin/clavulanate 500 to 875 mg every 8 to 12 hours (q8-12h) orally. In countries where ampicillin/sulbactam is not marketed, amoxicillin/clavulanate 500 mg to 2 g every 6 hours (q6h) was used for the intravenous regimen. Patients in the comparator group could also be treated with vancomycin 1 g q12h IV if MRSA was isolated from the foot infection. Patients in either treatment group who had Gram-negative bacilli isolated from the infection site could also receive aztreonam 1 to 2 g q8-12h IV. All patients were eligible to receive appropriate adjunctive treatment methods, such as debridement and off-loading, as typically required in the treatment of diabetic foot infections, and most patients received these treatments. There were 241 linezolid-treated and 120 comparator-treated patients in the intent-to-treat (ITT) study population. Two hundred twelve (86%) linezolid-treated patients and 105 (85%) comparator-treated patients were clinically evaluable. In the ITT population, the cure rates were 68.5% (165/241) in linezolid-treated patients and 64% (77/120) in comparator-treated patients, where those with indeterminate and missing outcomes were considered failures. The cure rates in the clinically evaluable patients (excluding those with indeterminate and missing outcomes) were 83% (159/192) and 73% (74/101) in the linezolid- and comparator-treated patients, respectively. A critical post-hoc analysis focused on 121 linezolid-treated and 60 comparator-treated patients who had a Gram-positive pathogen isolated from the site of infection or from blood, who had less evidence of underlying osteomyelitis than the overall study population, and who did not receive prohibited antimicrobials. Based upon that analysis, the cure rates were 71% (86/121) in the linezolid-treated patients and 63% (38/60) in the comparator-treated patients. None of the above analyses were adjusted for the use of adjunctive therapies. The cure rates by pathogen for microbiologically evaluable patients are presented in Table 19.

Table 19. Cure Rates at the Test-of-Cure Visit for Microbiologically Evaluable Adult Patients with Diabetic Foot Infections

Pathogen	Cured	
	ZYVOX n/N (%)	Comparator n/N (%)
Staphylococcus aureus	49/63 (78)	20/29 (69)
Methicillin-resistant *S. aureus*	12/17 (71)	2/3 (67%)
Streptococcus agalactiae	25/29 (86)	9/16 (56)

Pediatric Patients

Infections Due to Gram-positive Organisms

A safety and efficacy study provided experience on the use of ZYVOX in pediatric patients for the treatment of nosocomial pneumonia, complicated skin and skin structure infections, catheter-related bacteremia, bacteremia of unidentified source, and other infections due to Gram-positive bacterial pathogens, including methicillin-resistant and -susceptible *Staphylococcus aureus* and vancomycin-resistant *Enterococcus faecium*. Pediatric patients ranging in age from birth through 11 years with infections caused by the documented or suspected Gram-positive organisms were enrolled in a randomized, open-label, comparator-controlled trial. One group of patients received ZYVOX I.V. Injection 10 mg/kg every 8 hours (q8h) followed by ZYVOX for Oral Suspension 10 mg/kg q8h. A second group received vancomycin 10 to 15 mg/kg IV every 6 to 24 hours, depending on age and renal clearance. Patients who had confirmed VRE infections were placed in a third arm of the study and received ZYVOX 10 mg/kg q8h IV and/or orally. All patients were treated for a total of 10 to 28 days and could receive concomitant Gram-negative antibiotics if clinically indicated. In the intent-to-treat (ITT) population, there were 206 patients randomized to linezolid and 102 patients randomized to vancomycin. One hundred seventeen (57%) linezolid-treated patients and 55 (54%) vancomycin-treated patients were clinically evaluable. The cure rates in ITT patients were 81% in patients randomized to linezolid and 83% in patients randomized to vancomycin (95% Confidence Interval of the treatment difference; –13%, 8%). The cure rates in clinically evaluable patients were 91% in linezolid-treated patients and 91% in vancomycin-treated patients (95% CI; -11%, 11%). Modified intent-to-treat (MITT) patients included ITT patients who, at baseline, had a Gram-positive pathogen isolated from the site of infection or from blood. The cure rates in MITT patients were 80% in patients randomized to linezolid and 90% in patients randomized to vancomycin (95% CI; -23%, 3%). The cure rates for ITT, MITT, and clinically evaluable patients are presented in Table 20, and cure rates by pathogen for microbiologically evaluable patients are provided in Table 21.

[See table 20 above]

Table 20. Cure Rates at the Test-of-Cure Visit for Intent to Treat, Modified Intent to Treat, and Clinically Evaluable Pediatric Patients by Baseline Diagnosis

Population	ITT		MITT*		Clinically Evaluable	
	ZYVOX n/N (%)	Vancomycin n/N (%)	ZYVOX n/N (%)	Vancomycin n/N (%)	ZYVOX n/N (%)	Vancomycin n/N (%)
Any diagnosis	150/186 (81)	69/83 (83)	86/108 (80)	44/49 (90)	106/117 (91)	49/54 (91)
Bacteremia of unidentified source	22/29 (76)	11/16 (69)	8/12 (67)	7/8 (88)	14/17 (82)	7/9 (78)
Catheter-related bacteremia	30/41 (73)	8/12 (67)	25/35 (71)	7/10 (70)	21/25 (84)	7/9 (78)
Complicated skin and skin structure infections	61/72 (85)	31/34 (91)	37/43 (86)	22/23 (96)	46/49 (94)	26/27 (96)
Nosocomial pneumonia	13/18 (72)	11/12 (92)	5/6 (83)	4/4 (100)	7/7 (100)	5/5 (100)
Other infections	24/26 (92)	8/9 (89)	11/12 (92)	4/4 (100)	18/19 (95)	4/4 (100)

* MITT = ITT patients with an isolated Gram-positive pathogen at baseline

Table 21. Cure Rates at the Test-of-Cure Visit for Microbiologically Evaluable Pediatric Patients with Infections due to Gram-positive Pathogens

Pathogen	Microbiologically Evaluable	
	ZYVOX n/N (%)	Vancomycin n/N (%)
Vancomycin-resistant *Enterococcus faecium*	1/1 (100)	0/0 (-)
Staphylococcus aureus	36/38 (95)	23/24 (96)
Methicillin-resistant *S. aureus*	16/17 (94)	9/9 (100)
Streptococcus pyogenes	2/2 (100)	1/2 (50)

REFERENCES

1. Gonzales RD, PC Schreckenberger, MB Graham, et al. Infections due to vancomycin-resistant *Enterococcus faecium* resistant to linezolid. The Lancet 2001;357:1179.
2. Herrero IA, NC Issa, R Patel. Nosocomial spread of linezolid-resistant, vancomycin-resistant *Enterococcus faecium.* The New England Journal of Medicine 2002;346:867-869.
3. Tsiodras S, HS Gold, G Sakoulas, et al. Linezolid resistance in a clinical isolate of *Staphylococcus aureus.* The Lancet 2001;358:207-208.
4. Goldman DA, RA Weinstein, RP Wenzel, et al. Strategies to prevent and control the emergence and spread of antimicrobial-resistant microorganisms in hospitals. A challenge to hospital leadership. The Journal of the American Medical Association 1996;275:234-240.
5. Centers for Disease Control and Prevention. Guideline for hand hygiene in health-care settings: Recommendations of the Healthcare Infection Control Practices Advisory Committee and the HIPAC/SHEA/APIC/IDSA Hand Hygiene Task Force. Morbidity and Mortality Weekly Report 2002;51 (RR-16).
6. National Committee for Clinical Laboratory Standards. Methods for Dilution Antimicrobial Susceptibility Tests for Bacteria that Grow Aerobically. Fifth Edition. Approved Standard NCCLS Document M7-A5, Vol. 20, No. 2, NCCLS, Wayne, PA, January 2000.
7. National Committee for Clinical Laboratory Standards. Twelfth Informational Supplement. Approved NCCLS Document M100-S12, Vol. 21, No. 1, NCCLS, Wayne, PA, January 2002.
8. National Committee for Clinical Laboratory Standards. Performance Standards for Antimicrobial Disk Susceptibility Tests. Seventh Edition. Approved Standard NCCLS Document M2-A7, Vol. 20, No. 1, NCCLS, Wayne, PA, January 2000.
9. Walker SE et al. Tyramine content of previously restricted foods in monoamine oxidase inhibitor diets. Journal of Clinical Psychopharmacology 1996;16(5): 383-388.
10. DaPrada M et al. On tyramine, food, beverages and the reversible MAO inhibitor moclobemide. Journal of Neural Transmission 1988; [Supplement] 26:31-56.
11. Fine MJ, Auble TE, Yealy DM, et al. A Prediction Rule to Identify Low-Risk Patients with Community-acquired Pneumonia. The New England Journal of Medicine. 1997;336 (4):243-250.

Rx only
US Patent No. 5,688,792

Injection
Manufactured for: Pharmacia & Upjohn Company
A subsidiary of Pharmacia Corporation
Kalamazoo, Michigan 49001
By: Fresenius Kabi Norge AS
Halden, Norway

Tablets and Oral Suspension
Manufactured by: Pharmacia & Upjohn Company
A subsidiary of Pharmacia Corporation
Kalamazoo, Michigan 49001

Revised July 2004 LAB-0139-7.0

Shown in Product Identification Guide, page 330

IDENTIFICATION PROBLEM?
Turn to the **Product Identification Guide,** where you'll find more than 1600 products pictured in actual size and full color.

Pharmanex, LLC

75 WEST CENTER STREET
PROVO, UT 84601

For Technical Information and Product Support:
1-888-742-7626
www.pharmanex.com

Founded in 1994, Pharmanex is a science-based developer and marketer of natural, preventive healthcare products. Pharmanex® products are researched and developed by an internal staff of more than 75 scientists and Ph.D.s, as well as through an advisory network of professionals from institutions across the United States and around the world. All Pharmanex® products are subjected to a stringent, scientific analysis known as the Pharmanex® 6S Quality Manufacturing Process. Pharmanex® products are distributed through independent sales representatives. For more information about Pharmanex® product availability, visit the company Web site at www.pharmanex.com.

CORDYMAX® Cs-4® OTC

***Cordyceps sinensis* mushroom mycelia**
525 mg capsules
Dietary Supplement

DESCRIPTION

CordyMax® Cs-4® (Patent Pending) is a dietary supplement used to reduce symptoms of fatigue, and to promote vitality and overall well-being.* It is an exclusive fermentation product derived from the mycelia of the principal fungal strain (*Paecilomyces hepiali* Chen Cs-4) isolated from the renowned *Cordyceps sinensis* mushroom. In humans and animals, CordyMax substantially increases the serum levels of the enzyme superoxide dismutase (SOD).* This enhancement of the enzyme's proven ability to scavenge the free radicals associated with age-related oxidative cellular damage may explain the traditional use of the mushroom as a dietary supplement to improve vitality, energy, and quality of life.*

INGREDIENTS

Each capsule of CordyMax contains 525 mg of the fermentation product of mycelia (*Paecilomyces hepiali* Chen, Cs-4) isolated from the mushroom *Cordyceps sinensis* (Berk.) Sacc., and is scientifically standardized to contain a minimum of 0.14% adenosine and 5% mannitol (an indicatory of polysaccharide content).

RECOMMENDED USE

As a dietary supplement, take two 525 mg capsules bid or tid with water or food. Optimal results typically take 3 to 6 weeks.

SAFETY

With the exception of one case of allergic skin reaction, no other adverse reactions have been reported. During clinical trails in China, some subjects noted a mild sensation of thirst, and one subject noted slight nausea. All subjects considered these effects quite tolerable. No cases of CNS effects have been reported. No contraindications were identified based on Chinese human studies. CordyMax is non-mutagenic and non-teratogenic.

WARNINGS

CordyMax has not been evaluated in children and should only be used by adults. Pregnant and breastfeeding mothers should consult a physician prior to use. Consult a physician prior to use if using anticoagulants, MAO inhibitors, or any other prescription medication.

HOW SUPPLIED

CordyMax capsules of 525 mg each are supplied in 120 count bottles, and can be purchased from independent distributors and select pharmacies.

CORTITROL™ OTC

Stress Control Formula
348 mg capsules
Dietary Supplement

DESCRIPTION

Cortitrol™ Stress Control Formula is a dietary supplement developed to help the body modulate healthy levels of cortisol.* Cortitrol is a patent-pending cortisol-balancing dietary supplement that combines natural ingredients that have been scientifically shown to have direct cortisol-managing effects. Ingredients included in Cortitrol that may have cortisol-managing effects include magnolia bark (*Magnolia officinalis*), epimedium (*Epimedium koreanum*), theanine, beta sitosterol and phosphatidylserine.*

INGREDIENTS

Each capsule of Cortitrol contains 133 mg of Magnolia bark (*Magnolia officinalis*), standardized to 2% Honokiol – a constituent with known anxiolytic properties, 100 mg Epimedium (*Epimedium koreanum*) Water Extract 6:1, 66.7 mg L-Theanine (from *Camellia sinensis*) Extract 70:1 (TheaPure™), 40 mg Beta Sitosterol, and 8.3 mg Phosphatidylserine.

RECOMMENDED USE

As a dietary supplement, take two to three 348 mg capsules qd. Take two 348 mg capsules with evening meal. For optimal results take an additional 348 mg capsule with your morning meal.

SAFETY

Cortitrol is safe and well tolerated at the recommended dosage. L-theanine has been approved in Japan for unlimited use in all foods, except infant foods, after favorable toxicology studies. There are no limitations to duration of administration or known adverse drug interactions.

WARNINGS

Cortitrol has not been evaluated in children and should only be used by adults. Pregnant and breastfeeding mothers should consult a physician prior to use. Consult a physician prior to use if using any prescription medication. Because Cortitrol is indicated for stress relief, consult a physician if you are taking prescription "anti-stress" medications such as anxiolytics, sedatives, or hypnotics. Consult a physician if you are taking other CNS depressants, tricyclic antidepressants, anti-epileptics, muscle relaxants, anticoagulants, corticosteroids and quinalone antibiotics. Use of L-theanine concomitantly with chemotherapeutic agents must be done under medical supervision. L-theanine may enhance the effects of doxorubicin, idarubicin, adriamycin, and picarubicin and may ameliorate some of their side effects. This supplement should be discontinued two weeks prior to surgery.

HOW SUPPLIED

Cortitrol capsules of 348 mg each are supplied in 60 count bottles, and can be purchased from independent distributors and select pharmacies.

LIFEPAK® OTC

Multivitamin/mineral/phytonutrient supplement
Multinutrient capsules in packets
Dietary Supplement

DESCRIPTION

LifePak® is the most comprehensive micronutrient supplement, delivering the optimum types and amounts of vitamins, minerals, trace elements, antioxidants, and phytonutrients for general health and well-being.* LifePak addresses all common nutrient deficiencies, such as vitamins A, E, B6, the bone nutrients calcium and magnesium, and the minerals iron and zinc; provides the key anti-aging nutrients such as alpha-lipoic acid, vitamins C, E, and B12, folic acid, flavonoids, and mixed carotenoids that promote cellular protection and regeneration; and supports cardiovascular health, bone metabolism, and normal immune function.* The amounts of vitamins and minerals included in LifePak were chosen not only to prevent vitamin and mineral deficiencies, but also to correct any pre-existing deficiencies with regular use.* LifePak is intended for the general adult population. Pharmanex also offers LifePak Women® for premenopausal women, LifePak PreNatal® for pregnant and lactating women, and LifePak Prime® for men over age 40 and postmenopausal women.

INGREDIENTS

LifePak provides 39 vitamins, minerals, trace elements, antioxidants, and phytonutrients, which are provided in two daily packets. For a detailed ingredient list call Pharmanex at 1-800-487-1000 or visit www.pharmanex.com.

RECOMMENDED USE

As a dietary supplement, take the contents of one LifePak packet bid with water or food.

SAFETY

All individual nutrient levels in LifePak are documented to be safe and clinical studies showed no adverse effects due to LifePak supplementation. The daily amounts of all vitamins and minerals are well below the No-Observed Adverse Effect Levels (NOAEL) established by the Council for Responsible Nutrition (CRN) in 1997 and the Upper Limits (UL) established by the Food and Nutrition Board of the National Research Council. The other nutrients in LifePak, including the phytonutrients, are added in amounts that can be obtained from diets high in fruits and vegetables (5-10 servings/day) or other commonly consumed foods and beverages.

WARNINGS

Keep this product out of reach of children. Accidental overdose of iron-containing products is a leading cause of fatal poisoning in children under six years of age. In case of accidental overdose, call a doctor or poison control center immediately. Consult a physician prior to use of taking a prescription medication. Discontinue use of this product 2 weeks prior to and after surgery.

HOW SUPPLIED

Each box provides 60 individual packets, or the equivalent of a one-month supply, and can be purchased from independent distributors and select pharmacies.

Continued on next page

OPTIMUM OMEGA OTC
EPA & DHA Fish Oils
1000 mg capsules
Dietary Supplement

DESCRIPTION
Optimum Omega is a dietary supplement containing a combination of the pure omega 3 fatty acids (including EPA and DHA) to promote normal heart function, immune health, and joint health.* Omega 3 fatty acids are considered essential fatty acids and are necessary for normal growth, healthy skin, arteries, nerves, and metabolism. Fish oils are excellent sources of omega 3 fatty acids. Omega 3 (n-3) fatty acids in fish oil are highly unsaturated and may easily undergo oxidation. The vitamin E present in Optimum Omega has antioxidant properties that help prevent the pro-oxidant effects of fish oil, and also provides nutritional benefit.*

INGREDIENTS
Two softgel capsules of Optimum Omega contain 1000 mg of Marine Lipid Concentrate (300 mg of EPA, 200 mg of DHA, and 100 mg of other Omega 3 Fatty Acids), 10 IU of Vitamin E (as D-Alpha Tocopherol), and 2 mg of Deodorized Garlic Oil, the amount found in 200 mg of fresh garlic bulb.

RECOMMENDED USE
As a dietary supplement, take 1 softgel capsule bid with water and food.

SAFETY
Fish oil is a food. Adverse effects with diabetics, such as increased plasma glucose, LDL cholesterol, and glycosylated hemoglobin have been observed with large, perhaps excessive doses of omega-3 fatty acids, in the range of 4–10g/day.

WARNINGS
Keep this product out of reach of children. If you are pregnant or lactating, consult a physician prior to use. Consult a physician if taking anticoagulants, or any other prescription medication. Discontinue use of this product 2 weeks prior to and after surgery.

HOW SUPPLIED
Optimum Omega softgel capsules of 1000 mg each are supplied in 60 count bottles, and can be purchased from independent distributors and select pharmacies.

REISHIMAX GLP® OTC
Standardized Reishi Mushroom Extract
500 mg capsules
Dietary Supplement

DESCRIPTION
ReishiMax GLp® is a proprietary, standardized extract of Reishi (*Ganoderma lucidum*) mushroom. ReishiMax supports healthy immune system function by stimulating cell-mediated immunity with a proprietary standardized Reishi formula.* ReishiMax is intended for adults who wish to maintain a healthy immune system; who smoke or who are frequently exposed to environmental pollutants; who do not get enough sleep; or who are under constant stress.*

INGREDIENTS
ReishiMax is composed of Reishi fruiting bodies and cracked spores. The key active constituents found in Reishi include polysaccharides (beta-1,3-glucans) and triterpenes (ganoderic acids and others). Other ingredients naturally found in Reishi include nucleosides, fatty acids (oleic acid), and amino acids. The active ingredients in ReishiMax are standardized to 6% triterpenes and 13.5% polysaccharides. ReishiMax also contains a 1% extract of 100% cracked spores.

RECOMMENDED USE
Take one to two capsules of ReishiMax bid with food and liquid. For optimal health benefits, take one (1) capsule twice daily for health maintenance, and two (2) capsules twice daily for immune modulation.

SAFETY
ReishiMax is safe and well tolerated at the recommended dosage. In animal studies, Reishi has been shown to be non-carcinogenic, has not produced hepatic toxicity, and has not impaired growth or development. In high doses (1.5 to 1.9 grams/day), some people have experienced temporary symptoms of sleepiness, thirst, rashes, bloating, frequent urination, abnormal sweating, and loose stools.

WARNINGS
Keep out of reach of children. If you are pregnant or nursing, or taking a prescription medication, consult a physician before using this product. Consult a physician if you are concurrently using anticoagulants, receiving immunosuppressive therapies or have an immune disorder. Individuals with known fungal allergies should be cautious when taking Reishi. Discontinue use of this product 2 weeks prior to and after surgery.

HOW SUPPLIED
ReishiMax is supplied in a 15-30 day supply of 60 capsules, and can be purchased from independent distributors and select pharmacies. Each capsule contains 495 mg of standardized Reishi mushroom extract and 5 mg of Reishi cracked spores.

TĒGREEN 97® OTC
Standardized Green Tea Polyphenol Extract
250 mg capsules
Dietary Supplement

DESCRIPTION
Tēgreen 97® is a standardized, caffeine-free polyphenol extract of the fresh leaves of the tea plant *Camellia sinensis.* The major components of Tēgreen are polyphenols, which have proven free radical scavenging and antioxidant properties. The polyphenols with the most active antioxidant activity are the catechins, specifically epigallocatechin gallate (EGCg) and epigallocatechin (EGC).*

INGREDIENTS
Each 250 mg capsule of proprietary Tēgreen contains a 20:1 extract of green tea leaves (*Camellia sinensis*) standardized to a minimum 97% pure polyphenols including 162 mg catechins, of which 95 mg is EGCg, 37 mg is ECG, and 15 mg is EGC. Tēgreen 97 is decaffeinated (<0.5 mg).

RECOMMENDED USE
As a dietary supplement, take one to four 250 mg capsules qd; preferably one to two each morning and evening with food. Each capsule provides the green tea polyphenols typically found in approximately 7 cups of high-quality brewed green tea.

SAFETY
Not known to be associated with any significant side effects or toxicity. Since Tēgreen contains only trace amounts of caffeine (approximately 1-1.3 mg/capsule), it should not produce the stimulant caused by the consumption of caffeine-containing beverages.

WARNINGS
Tēgreen has not been evaluated in children and should only be used by adults. Pregnant or breastfeeding mothers should consult a physician prior to use. Consult a physician prior to use if taking anticoagulants, or other prescription medications. Discontinue use of this product 2 weeks prior to and after surgery.

HOW SUPPLIED
Tēgreen capsules of 250 mg each are supplied in 30 and 120 count bottles, and can be purchased from independent distributors and select pharmacies.

***These statements have not been evaluated by the Food and Drug Administration. This product is not intended to diagnose, treat, cure or prevent any disease.**

PolyMedica Pharmaceuticals (U.S.A.), Inc.
11 STATE STREET
WOBURN, MA 01801

For Medical Emergencies Contact:
Peter Etzel or Patricia Collins
(781) 933-2020
FAX: (781) 933-7992

ANESTACON® ℞
(lidocaine hydrochloride jelly, USP) 2%

DESCRIPTION
Each mL contains: Active: Lidocaine Hydrochloride 20 mg/ml (2%). Vehicle: Hydroxypropyl Methylcellulose 10 mg (1%). Preservative: Benzalkonium Chloride 0.1 mg (0.01%). Inactive: Sodium Chloride, Hydrochloric Acid and/or Sodium Hydroxide (to adjust pH to 6.0–7.0), Purified Water. The resulting mixture maximizes contact with mucosa and provides lubrication for instrumentation.

HOW SUPPLIED
In 15 ml. unit-dose for **SINGLE PATIENT USE.**

B & O SUPPRETTES® CII ℞
(Belladonna and Opium) Rectal Suppositories

DESCRIPTION
Each B&O SUPPRETTE® contains (in the water-soluble NEOCERA® Suppository Base for rectal administration):
B&O No. 15A: Powdered opium* 30 mg (0.46 gr) and Powdered Belladonna Extract 16.2 mg (equivalent to 0.21 mg or 0.0032 gr belladonna alkaloids).
B&O No. 16A: Powdered opium* 60 mg (0.92 gr) and Powdered Belladonna Extract 16.2 mg (equivalent to 0.21 mg or 0.0032 gr belladonna alkaloids).

Store at room temperature. DO NOT REFRIGERATE.

HOW SUPPLIED
In strip packaged units of 12.

CYSTOSPAZ® ℞
(hyoscyamine) Tablets

DESCRIPTION
CYSTOSPAZ® is a pale blue uncoated tablet for oral administration. Each tablet contains: hyoscyamine 0.15 mg.

HOW SUPPLIED
Bottles of 100 light blue tablets imprinted "**W 2225**".

URISED® ℞

DESCRIPTION
URISED® is a dark blue, round, tablet for oral administration. Each tablet contains: Methenamine 40.8 mg, Phenyl Salicylate 18.1 mg, Methylene Blue 5.4 mg, Benzoic Acid 4.5 mg, Atropine Sulfate 0.03 mg and Hyoscyamine (as the sulfate) 0.03 mg.

HOW SUPPLIED
Bottles of 100 blue tablets imprinted "**W 2183**".

PRAECIS PHARMACEUTICALS INCORPORATED
830 WINTER STREET
WALTHAM, MA 02451-1420

Direct Inquiries to:
Telephone: 781-795-4100
For Medical Information, Consumer Inquiries, Adverse Drug Experiences & Medical Emergencies
Telephone: 866-753-6294
E-mail: medinfo@praecis.com
Internet: http://www.praecis.com
For Sales and Ordering
Telephone: 866-753-6294
Internet: http://www.plenaxis.com

PLENAXIS® ℞
[*plen-AK-sis*]
(abarelix for injectable suspension)

WARNING
Immediate-onset systemic allergic reactions, some resulting in hypotension and syncope, have occurred after administration of Plenaxis®. These immediate-onset reactions have been reported to occur following any administration of Plenaxis®, including after the initial dose. The cumulative risk of such a reaction increases with the duration of treatment (see WARNINGS). Following each injection of Plenaxis®, patients should be observed for at least 30 minutes in the office and in the event of an allergic reaction, managed appropriately.

- **Only physicians who have enrolled in the Plenaxis® PLUS Program (Plenaxis® User Safety Program), based on their attestation of qualifications and acceptance of prescribing responsibilities, may prescribe Plenaxis® (See DOSAGE AND ADMINISTRATION and HOW SUPPLIED).**
- **Plenaxis® is indicated for the palliative treatment of men with advanced symptomatic prostate cancer, in whom LHRH agonist therapy is not appropriate and who refuse surgical castration, and have one or more of the following: (1) risk of neurological compromise due to metastases, (2) ureteral or bladder outlet obstruction due to local encroachment or metastatic disease, or (3) severe bone pain from skeletal metastases persisting on narcotic analgesia.**
- **The effectiveness of Plenaxis® in suppressing serum testosterone to castrate levels decreases with continued dosing in some patients (see CLINICAL PHARMACOLOGY, Pharmacodynamics). Effectiveness beyond 12 months has not been established. Treatment failure can be detected by measuring serum total testosterone concentrations just prior to administration on Day 29 and every 8 weeks thereafter (see WARNINGS).**

DESCRIPTION
Abarelix for injectable suspension (Plenaxis®) is a synthetic decapeptide with potent antagonistic activity against natu-

rally occurring gonadotropin releasing-hormone (GnRH). Plenaxis® inhibits gonadotropin and related androgen production by directly and competitively blocking GnRH receptors in the pituitary.

Abarelix is chemically described as acetyl-D-β-naphthylalanyl-D-4-chlorophenylalanyl-D-3-pyridylalanyl-L-seryl-L-N-methyl-tyrosyl-D-asparagyl-L-leucyl-L-N(ε)-isopropyl-lysyl-L-prolyl-D-alanyl-amide. It is initially manufactured as an acetate water complex and converted to a carboxymethylcellulose (CMC) water complex in manufacturing the drug product. The molecular weight for abarelix anhydrous free base is 1416.06.

The structural formula for abarelix peptide is:

[See chemical structure above]

Abarelix for injectable suspension is supplied as a white to off-white sterile dry powder which, when mixed with the diluent, 0.9% Sodium Chloride Injection, USP, becomes a depot suspension intended for intramuscular (IM) injection.

The single-dose vial contains 113 mg of anhydrous free base abarelix peptide (net) supplied in an abarelix CMC complex. This complex also contains 19.1 to 31 mg of CMC. After the vial is reconstituted with 2.2 mL of 0.9% sodium chloride injection, 2 mL is administered to deliver a dose of 100 mg of abarelix (net) as the abarelix CMC complex at a pH of 5±1.

CLINICAL PHARMACOLOGY

Mechanism of Action

Abarelix exerts its pharmacological action by directly suppressing luteinizing hormone (LH) and follicle stimulating hormone (FSH) secretion and thereby reducing the secretion of testosterone by the testes. Due to the direct inhibition of the secretion of LH by abarelix, there is no initial increase in serum testosterone concentrations.

Saturation binding studies revealed that [^{125}I]-abarelix has a very high affinity (K_D = 0.1 nM) for the rat pituitary LHRH receptor.

PHARMACOKINETICS

A single dose (100 mg IM) of Plenaxis® was given to 14 healthy male volunteers 52 to 75 years of age, with body weight of 61.6 to 110.5 kg, and the pharmacokinetic information is provided in Table 1:

Table 1. Mean ± SD Pharmacokinetic Parameter Values of 100 mg of Plenaxis® Following a Single IM Injection (n = 14)

C_{max} (ng/mL)	T_{max} (days)	$AUC_{0-\infty}$ (ng • day/mL)	CL/F (L/day)	$t_{1/2}$ (days)
43.4 ± 32.3	3.0 ± 2.9	500 ± 96	208 ± 48	13.2 ± 3.2

Absorption

Following IM administration of 100 mg of Plenaxis®, abarelix is absorbed slowly with a mean peak concentration of 43.4 ng/mL observed approximately 3 days after the injection.

Distribution

The apparent volume of distribution during the terminal phase determined after IM administration of Plenaxis® was 4040 ± 1607 liters, implying that abarelix probably distributes extensively within the body.

Metabolism

In vitro hepatocyte (rat, monkey, human) studies and *in vivo* studies in rats and monkeys showed that the major metabolites of abarelix were formed via hydrolysis of peptide bonds. No significant oxidative or conjugated metabolites of abarelix were found either *in vitro* or *in vivo*. There is no evidence of cytochrome P-450 involvement in the metabolism of abarelix.

Excretion

In humans, approximately 13% of unchanged abarelix was recovered in urine after a 15 μg/kg IM injection; there were no detectable metabolites in urine. Renal clearance of abarelix was 14.4 L/day (or 10 mL/min) after administration of 100 mg Plenaxis®.

Pharmacodynamics:

Effects of Plenaxis® on Serum Testosterone: The effectiveness of Plenaxis® in suppressing serum testosterone was studied in two randomized, open-label, active-comparator trials. Patients were not those with advanced symptomatic prostate cancer. They were randomized in a 2:1 ratio to Plenaxis® 100 mg IM versus LHRH agonist (Study 1) or to Plenaxis® versus LHRH agonist + nonsteroidal antiandrogen (Study 2). Plenaxis® was administered IM on Days 1, 15, 29 (Week 4), then every 4 weeks thereafter for at least 6 months (24 weeks). LHRH agonist and nonsteroidal antiandrogen were administered in standard fashion. After completing 6 months of treatment, patients could continue randomized treatment for an additional 6 months.

Avoidance of testosterone surge: In both studies combined, 100% (348/348) of Plenaxis® patients and 16% (28/172) of comparator patients avoided a testosterone surge.

Attainment of medical castration: The percentage of patients who attained serum testosterone concentration ≤50 ng/dL on Study Days 2, 4, 8, 15 and 29 are summarized in the table below:

Table 2. Percentage of patients who attained medical castration (serum testosterone concentration ≤50 ng/dL) in Studies 1 and 2.

Plenaxis®		
Day	Total N	% Castrate
2	339	24%
4	333	56%
8	348	70%
15	347	73%
29	347	94%

Attainment and maintenance of medical castration: Successful response was defined as attainment of medical castration on Day 29 and maintenance through Day 85 (where no **two** consecutive serum testosterone concentrations between Days 29 and 85 were greater than 50 ng/dL). In Study 1, 92% of Plenaxis® patients responded and 96% of LHRH agonist patients responded. In Study 2, 93% of Plenaxis® patients and 95% of LHRH agonist + nonsteroidal antiandrogen patients responded.

However, when failure was defined as any observed serum testosterone > 50 ng/dL (including transient elevations) just prior to dosing on Day 29 and every 28 days thereafter, effectiveness of testosterone suppression decreased over time. Results of this analysis are summarized in Table 3.

Table 3. Percentage of patients who attained and maintained medical castration; [no serum testosterone >50 ng/dL just prior to dosing on Day 29 and every 28 days thereafter]

	Study 1	N	Study 2	N
Day	Plenaxis®		Plenaxis®	
85	84%	176	92%	164
169	75%	166	87%	155
365	62%	93	71%	86

Effects of Plenaxis® on Cardiac Electrophysiology: In a single, active-controlled, clinical study comparing Plenaxis® to LHRH agonist + nonsteroidal antiandrogen, periodic electrocardiograms were performed. Both therapies prolonged the mean Fridericia-corrected QT interval by >10 msec from baseline. In approximately 20% of patients in both groups, there were either changes from baseline QTc of >30 msec, or end-of-treatment QTc values exceeding 450 msec. Similar results were observed in 2 other Phase 3 studies with Plenaxis® and the active-control treatments. It is unclear whether these changes were directly related to study drugs, to androgen deprivation therapy, or to other variables.

Special Populations

Race

Data from Hispanics, Blacks and Caucasians demonstrated that race appeared to have no influence on the pharmacokinetics of Plenaxis®.

Renal and Hepatic Insufficiency

The pharmacokinetics of Plenaxis® in hepatically and/or renally impaired patients have not been determined.

Pediatric Use

There have been no studies of Plenaxis® in pediatric patients.

CLINICAL STUDIES

One study of Plenaxis® was conducted in 81 men with advanced symptomatic prostate cancer who were at risk for clinical exacerbation ("clinical flare") if treated with an LHRH agonist. The objective of this open-label, multicenter, uncontrolled, single-arm study was to demonstrate that such patients could avoid orchiectomy through at least 12 weeks of treatment. In this trial, treatment was to be given for at least 6 months with the option to continue treatment in an extension trial.

Of the 81 patients who enrolled, 9 patients from one site were excluded from the efficacy analysis due to inadequate documentation by the study investigator. The specific reasons given for enrollment of the 72 patients were: bone pain from prostate cancer skeletal metastases (n = 31); an enlarged prostate gland or pelvic mass causing bladder neck outlet obstruction (n = 25); bilateral retroperitoneal adenopathy with ureteral obstruction (n = 9); impending neurological compromise from spinal, spinal cord, or epidural metastases (n = 6); or other (n = 1). The median age was 73 years, range 40 to 94 years. There were 62 Caucasians, 6 African Americans and 4 Hispanics.

Plenaxis® 100 mg was administered via IM injection on Days 1, 15 and 29, then every 4 weeks thereafter. Twelve patients discontinued prior to Day 169 for the following reasons: adverse event (n=2), voluntary withdrawal (n=3), death (n=4), and "other" (n=3). Sixty patients were treated for at least 24 weeks; in the extension phase, 33 patients for at least 48 weeks and 15 patients for at least 96 weeks. None (0%) of the 72 patients required orchiectomy while being treated with Plenaxis®, including the extension phase (median combined duration of therapy was 40 weeks). However, 2 patients were withdrawn before week 12 for treatment-related adverse events (immediate-onset systemic allergic reactions consisting of urticaria, and urticaria and pruritis, respectively) and received alternate therapy. In this trial, medical castration (defined as serum total testosterone concentration ≤50 ng/dL) was achieved in 57 of the 72 patients (79%) by Day 8, and by 68 of 71 patients (96%) by Week 4.

Although the study was not designed to assess specific clinical outcomes, the following were observed:

- None (0) of 8 patients with vertebral or epidural metastases and without neurological symptoms developed neurological symptoms.
- Ten of 13 patients with bladder outlet obstruction and a bladder drainage catheter had the catheter removed by 12 weeks.
- Eleven of 15 patients with pain due to skeletal metastases were able to reduce the potency, dose and/or frequency of narcotic analgesia at 12 weeks.

INDICATIONS AND USAGE

Plenaxis® is indicated for the palliative treatment of men with advanced symptomatic prostate cancer, in whom LHRH agonist therapy is not appropriate and who refuse surgical castration, and have one or more of the following: (1) risk of neurological compromise due to metastases, (2) ureteral or bladder outlet obstruction due to local encroachment or metastatic disease, or (3) severe bone pain from skeletal metastases persisting on narcotic analgesia.

CONTRAINDICATIONS

Plenaxis® is contraindicated in those patients with a known hypersensitivity to any of the components in abarelix for injectable suspension.

Plenaxis® is not indicated in women or pediatric patients. In addition, Plenaxis® may cause fetal harm if administered to a pregnant woman.

WARNINGS

Immediate-Onset Systemic Allergic Reactions (See Boxed Warnings)

In the clinical trial of patients with advanced, symptomatic prostate cancer, 3 of 81 (3.7%) patients experienced an immediate-onset systemic allergic reaction within minutes of receiving Plenaxis®. The allergic reactions were urticaria (Day 15), urticaria and pruritis (Day 29), and hypotension and syncope (Day 141). Patients should be monitored for at least 30 minutes after each injection of Plenaxis®. In the event of an allergic reaction associated with hypotension and/or syncope, appropriate supportive measures such as leg elevation, oxygen, IV fluids, antihistamines, corticosteroids, and epinephrine (alone or in combination) should be employed.

From all the prostate cancer clinical trials with Plenaxis® (mostly in men without advanced, symptomatic disease), immediate-onset systemic allergic reactions (occurring within 30 minutes of dosing), were observed in 1.1% (15/1397) of patients dosed with Plenaxis®. In 14/15 patients who experienced an allergic reaction, each developed symptoms within 8 minutes of injection. The cumulative risk of such a reaction increased with duration of treatment. The cumulative rates (and 95% confidence intervals) on Days 56, 141, 365 and 676 were 0.51%, (0.13%, 0.88%) 0.80% (0.30%, 1.29%), 1.24% (0.43%, 2.04%) and 2.91% (0.87%, 4.95%), respectively. Seven patients experienced hypotension or syncope as part of their allergic reaction, representing 0.5% of all patients. The cumulative rates (and 95% confidence intervals) for these types of reactions on Days 56, 141, 365, and 617 after the initial dose were 0.22% (0.0%, 0.46%), 0.32% (0.0%, 0.64%), 0.61% (0.0%, 1.24%) and 1.67% (0.07, 3.28%), respectively.

Decrease in Effectiveness With Continued Dosing

A decrease in overall effectiveness with increased duration of treatment, as measured by failure to maintain suppression of serum testosterone below 50 ng/dL, was noted **(see Clinical Pharmacology, Pharmacodynamics)**. Treatment

Continued on next page

Plenaxis—Cont.

failure can be detected by measuring serum total testosterone concentrations just prior to administration on Day 29 after the initial dose and every 8 weeks thereafter.

Prolongation of the QT Interval

Because Plenaxis® may prolong the QT interval **(see Clinical Pharmacology, Pharmacodynamics)**, physicians should carefully consider whether the risks of Plenaxis® outweigh the benefits in patients with baseline QTc values >450 msec (e.g. congenital QT prolongation) and in patients taking Class IA (e.g. quinidine, procainamide) or Class III (e.g. amiodarone, sotalol) antiarrhythmic medications.

PRECAUTIONS

General

Decreased effectiveness in patients >225 pounds: The decrease in overall effectiveness of Plenaxis® with increased duration of treatment is greater in patients who weigh more than 225 pounds. Strict monitoring of serum testosterone in these patients is warranted.

Monitoring of liver function: Clinically meaningful transaminase elevations were observed in some patients who received Plenaxis® or comparator drugs. Serum transaminase levels should be obtained before starting treatment with Plenaxis® and periodically during treatment **(see Adverse Reactions)**.

Decrease in bone mineral density: Extended treatment with GnRH antagonists and LHRH agonists may result in a decrease in bone mineral density.

Drug Interactions

No formal drug/drug interaction studies with Plenaxis® were performed. Cytochrome P-450 is not known to be involved in the metabolism of Plenaxis®. Plenaxis® is highly bound to plasma proteins (96 to 99%).

Laboratory Tests

Response to Plenaxis® should be monitored by measuring serum total testosterone concentrations just prior to administration on Day 29 and every 8 weeks thereafter **(see WARNINGS)**. Serum transaminase levels should be obtained before starting treatment with Plenaxis® and periodically during treatment. Periodic measurement of serum PSA levels may also be considered.

Geriatric Use

Prostate cancer occurs primarily in an older patient population. Clinical studies with Plenaxis® have been conducted primarily in patients ≥ 65 years of age. No difference in the safety profile, when examined as a function of age, was apparent.

Pediatric Use

The safety and effectiveness of Plenaxis® in pediatric patients have not been studied. Plenaxis® is not indicated for use in pediatric patients.

Carcinogenesis, Mutagenesis, Impairment of Fertility

Plenaxis® was not carcinogenic to mice or rats when administered as a subcutaneous depot every 28 days for 2 years at doses up to 300 mg/kg in mice and 100 mg/kg in rats. Systemic drug exposures, as measured by mean C_{max}, were approximately 210–278-fold for mice and 21–32-fold for rats the human exposure following subcutaneous depot administration of 100 mg.

Plenaxis® was not mutagenic in the *in vitro* bacterial Ames assay or forward mutation assay in mouse lymphoma, or clastogenic in the *in vivo* mouse micronucleus assay.

No effects on mating or fertility in male and female rats given 1 mg/kg subcutaneous Plenaxis®, a dose 0.114-fold the human therapeutic dose of 100 mg based on body surface area. Mating and fertility were significantly decreased at doses of 3 and 10 mg/kg (0.34-fold and 1.135-fold, respectively, the human therapeutic dose of 100 mg based on body surface area), but the effects were reversible.

Pregnancy Category X (see **CONTRAINDICATIONS**)

Embryolethality occurred in pregnant rats administered a single subcutaneous dose of Plenaxis® up to 3 mg/kg (0.228-fold the human therapeutic dose of 100 mg based on body surface area). In rabbits a dose-related increase in fetal resorptions and reduced viability was observed at doses up to 30 mg/kg (6.81-fold the human therapeutic dose of 100 mg based on body surface area). No teratogenic effects were observed in rats or rabbits up to doses of 3 mg/kg or 30 mg/kg, respectively. A no-observable-adverse-effect-level (NOAEL) dose was 0.3 mg/kg (approximately 0.034-fold the human therapeutic dose of 100 mg based on body surface area) in rats and <0.01 mg/kg (<0.0023-fold the human therapeutic dose of 100 mg based on body surface area) in rabbits.

Nursing Mothers

It is not known whether Plenaxis® is excreted in human milk. Because many drugs are excreted in human milk, and because the effects of Plenaxis® on lactation and/or the breastfed child have not been determined, Plenaxis® should not be used by nursing mothers.

ADVERSE REACTIONS

Immediate-Onset Systemic Allergic Reactions: See **BOXED WARNINGS** and **WARNINGS**

In the single study of Plenaxis® conducted in men with advanced symptomatic prostate cancer, adverse events reported by ≥10% of patients are listed in Table 4. Adverse events are listed without regard to causality. Causality is often difficult to assess in elderly patients with multiple comorbidities and prostate cancer.

Table 4. Adverse Events in ≥10% of Patients in the Advanced Symptomatic Prostate Cancer Study (without regard for causality).

Preferred Term	Plenaxis® N=81 n (%)
Hot flushes*	64 (79)
Sleep disturbance*	36 (44)
Pain	25 (31)
Breast enlargement*	24 (30)
Breast pain/nipple tenderness*	16 (20)
Back pain	14 (17)
Constipation	12 (15)
Peripheral edema	12 (15)
Dizziness	10 (12)
Headache	10 (12)
Upper respiratory tract infection	10 (12)
Diarrhea	9 (11)
Dysuria	8 (10)
Fatigue	8 (10)
Micturition frequency	8 (10)
Nausea	8 (10)
Urinary retention	8 (10)
Urinary tract infection	8 (10)

*Pharmacological consequence of androgen deprivation

Changes in Laboratory Values

Clinically meaningful increases in serum transaminases were seen in a small percentage of patients in both treatment groups in each active-controlled Plenaxis® study. In Study 1 and Study 2 combined, the percentage of Plenaxis® patients reporting serum ALT >2.5 times upper limit of normal or >200 U/L was 8.2% and 1.8%, respectively. The percentage reporting serum AST >2.5 times upper limit of normal or >200 U/L was 3.1% and 0.8%, respectively. Similar results were reported for active comparators.

Slight decrease in hemoglobin, a pharmacological consequence of castration, were observed in patients receiving Plenaxis® and active comparator. Mean increases in serum triglycerides of approximately 10% were seen in Plenaxis®-treated patients.

OVERDOSAGE

The maximum tolerated dose of Plenaxis® has not been determined. The maximum dose used in clinical studies was 150 mg. There have been no reports of accidental overdose with Plenaxis®.

DOSAGE AND ADMINISTRATION

For safety reasons, Plenaxis® is approved with marketing restrictions. Only physicians who attest to the following qualifications and accept the following responsibilities, and on that basis enroll in PRAECIS PHARMACEUTICALS INCORPORATED's Plenaxis® **PLUS** Program should prescribe Plenaxis®. PRAECIS PHARMACEUTICALS INCORPORATED and its agents will provide Plenaxis® to physicians enrolled in the Plenaxis® **PLUS** Program.

To enroll, physicians must attest that they are able and willing to:

- diagnose and manage advanced symptomatic prostate cancer.
- diagnose and treat allergic reactions, including anaphylaxis.
- have access to medication and equipment necessary to treat allergic reactions, including anaphylaxis.
- have patients observed for development of allergic reactions for 30 minutes following each administration of Plenaxis®.
- understand the risks and benefits of palliative treatment with Plenaxis®, including information from the Package Insert, Patient Information, and the Physician Attestation.
- educate the patients on the risks and benefits of treatment with Plenaxis® and obtain the patient's signature on the Patient Information signature page, sign it, and place the original signed form in the patient's medical record, and give a copy of the Patient Information leaflet with the signed page to the patient.
- report serious adverse events, such as any immediate-onset systemic allergic event (including anaphylaxis, hypotension, and syncope) as soon as possible to PRAECIS PHARMACEUTICALS INCORPORATED at 1-866-PLENAXIS (1-866-753-6294) or to the Food and Drug Administration's MedWatch Program at 1-800-FDA-1088.
- understand that they may withdraw their enrollment in the Plenaxis® Prescribing Program by a written statement submitted to PRAECIS PHARMACEUTICALS INCORPORATED (contact information below) or that PRAECIS PHARMACEUTICALS INCORPORATED may withdraw physicians from the Plenaxis® PLUS Program if they do not meet the agreed upon responsibilities.

To enroll in the Plenaxis® Prescribing Program call 1-866-PLENAXIS (1-866-753-6294) or visit **www.plenaxisplus.com**.

Dose: The recommended dose of Plenaxis® is 100 mg administered intramuscularly to the buttock on Day 1, 15, 29 (week 4) and every 4 weeks thereafter. Treatment failure can be detected by measuring serum testosterone concentrations just prior to Plenaxis® administration, beginning on Day 29 and every 8 weeks thereafter.

Directions for Reconstituting and Administering Plenaxis®

Read the instructions completely before performing reconstitution.

The sterile powder for suspension is to be reconstituted in accordance with the following directions:

Reconstitution Instructions for 1 Vial of Plenaxis® to Provide a 100 mg (50 mg/mL) Dose as a Single IM Injection

Use aseptic technique throughout.

1 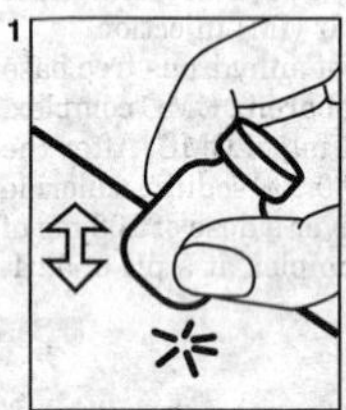

Prior to reconstitution, gently shake the vial of Plenaxis® (abarelix for injectable suspension). Hold the vial at an angle (45 degrees) and tap lightly on table to break up any caking.

Withdraw 2.2 mL of 0.9% Sodium Chloride Inj., USP using the enclosed 18 G × 1½″ needle and a 3 cc syringe. Discard the remaining diluent.

(Picture 1)

2 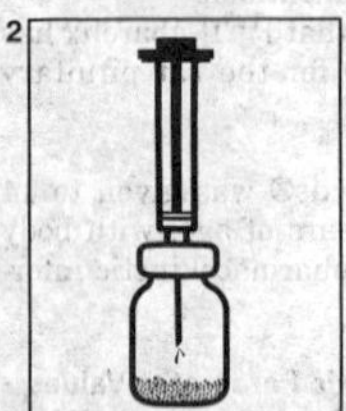

Keeping the vial **upright**, insert the needle all the way into the vial and inject the diluent **quickly**.

Before withdrawing the needle, remove **2.2** mL of air. Shake immediately.

(Picture 2)

3 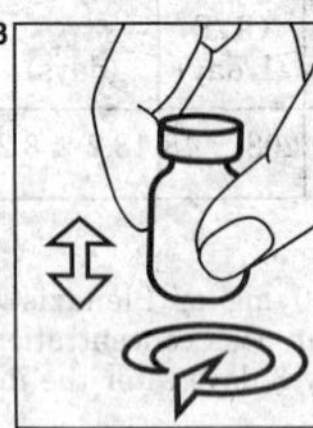

Shake for approximately 15 seconds. Allow the vial to stand for approximately 2 minutes. Tap the vial to **reduce foaming** and swirl the vial occasionally.

Again, **shake** for approximately 15 seconds. Allow the vial to stand for approximately 2 minutes. Tap the vial to **reduce foaming** and swirl the vial occasionally.

(Picture 3)

4 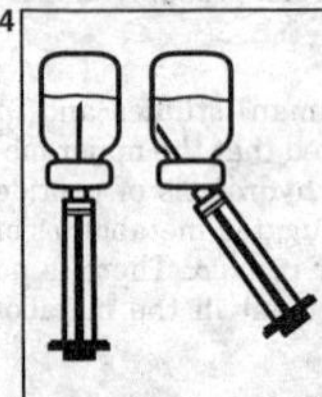

Do not reinject the air into the vial. Locate a **second injection spot** on the stopper, and then insert the 18 G needle. Invert the vial and draw up some of the suspension into the syringe and **without removing the needle from the vial reinject it at any remaining solids in the vial. Repeat the process until all solids are dispersed.**

Swirl the vial before withdrawal and withdraw **the entire contents (at least 2 mL)** by positioning the needle at a 45 degree angle as shown in the picture.

(Picture 4)

5 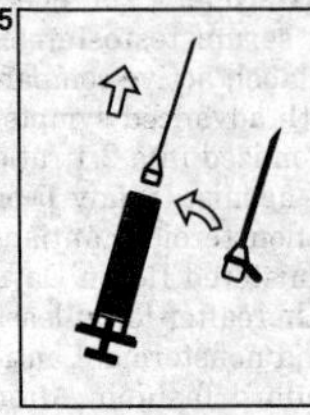

Pull the plunger back to recover the residual suspension in the 18 G × 1½″ needle.

Exchange the 18 G × 1½″ needle with the enclosed 22 G × 1½″ Safety Glide™ injection needle.

(Picture 5)

6 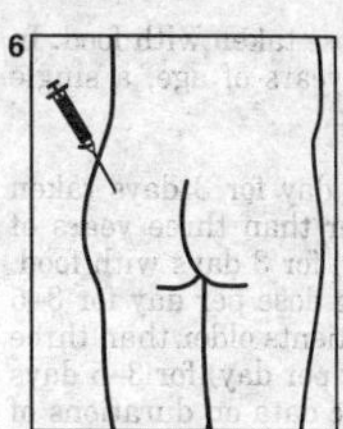

Insert the needle at the desired injection site, pull the plunger back to check for back-flow of blood. If blood flows into the syringe, do not inject at this site. Select another injection site.
Deliver the entire reconstituted suspension intramuscularly **immediately.**
(Picture 6)

Observe the patient for after injection for 30 minutes for any sign of an allergic-type response.

Plenaxis® does not contain a preservative and should be administered within 1 hour following reconstitution.

STORAGE
Store at 25°C (77°F), excursions permitted to 15–30°C (59–86°F), USP Controlled Room Temperature.

HOW SUPPLIED
The physician must attest to meeting the qualifications and accepting the responsibilities in the **DOSAGE AND ADMINISTRATION** section of this package insert by submitting the Physician's Attestation form to PRAECIS PHARMACEUTICALS INCORPORATED to be enrolled in the Plenaxis® **PLUS** Program. PRAECIS PHARMACEUTICALS INCORPORATED and its agents will only provide Plenaxis® to physicians enrolled in the Plenaxis® Prescribing Program. Plenaxis® vials are not to be resold or redistributed.
Plenaxis® (abarelix for injectable suspension) is supplied as a single-dose, preservative-free vial containing 113 mg of abarelix (anhydrous free base peptide) as an abarelix CMC complex, a sterile powder (NDC 68158-149-01) which, when reconstituted with 2.2 mL of 0.9% sodium chloride solution, yields a 2 mL delivered dose of 100 mg (50 mg/mL). Each single use dispensing pack also contains: a single-use 10 mL diluent vial of 0.9% Sodium Chloride Injection, USP, one 3 cc syringe with an 18 gauge 11/2 inch needle and one 22 gauge 1½ inch Safety Glide™ injection needle.

PRAECIS
PRAECIS PHARMACEUTICALS INCORPORATED
830 Winter Street
Waltham, MA 02451
1-877-PRAECIS (1-877-772-3247)

Issue Date: August 2004 02-01

Presutti Laboratories, Inc.

1685 WINNETKA CIRCLE
ROLLING MEADOWS, IL 60008-1372

Direct Inquiries to:
Toll Free: (888) 405-7800
Telephone: (847) 483-6050
Fax: (847) 788-9192

TINDAMAX™ ℞
[tĭn-dă-măx]
(tinidazole tablets)

Carcinogenicity has been seen in mice and rats treated chronically with another agent in the nitroimidazole class (metronidazole). (See PRECAUTIONS). Although such data have not been reported for tinidazole, unnecessary use of tinidazole should be avoided. Its use should be reserved for the conditions described in INDICATIONS AND USAGE.

DESCRIPTION
Tinidazole is a synthetic antiprotozoal agent. It is 1-[2-(ethylsulfonyl)ethyl]-2-methyl-5-nitroimidazole, a second-generation 2-methyl-5-nitroimidazole, which has the following chemical structure:

O_2N–[imidazole ring, N]–CH_3 ; N–CH_2–CH_2–SO_2–CH_2–CH_3

Tindamax pink film-coated oral tablets contain 500 mg or 250 mg of tinidazole. Inactive ingredients include croscarmellose sodium, FD&C Red 40 lake, FD&C Yellow 6 lake, hypromellose, magnesium stearate, microcrystalline cellulose, polydextrose, polyethylene glycol, pregelatinized corn starch, titanium dioxide and triacetin.

CLINICAL PHARMACOLOGY
Absorption
After oral administration, tinidazole is rapidly and completely absorbed. A bioavailability study of Tindamax tablets was conducted in adult healthy volunteers. All subjects received a single oral dose of 2 g (four 500 mg tablets) of tinidazole following an overnight fast. Oral administration of four 500 mg tablets of Tindamax under fasted conditions produced a mean peak plasma concentration (C_{max}) of 47.7 (±7.5) µg/mL with a mean time to peak concentration (T_{max}) of 1.6 (±0.7) hours and a mean area under the plasma concentration-time curve (AUC, 0-∞) of 901.6 (± 126.5) µg•hr/mL at 72 hours. The elimination half-life (T½) was 13.2 (±1.4) hours. Mean plasma levels decreased to 14.3 µg/mL at 24 hours, 3.8 µg/mL at 48 hours and 0.8 µg/mL at 72 hours following administration. Steady-state conditions are reached in 2½ - 3 days of multi-day dosing. Administration of Tindamax tablets with food resulted in a delay in T_{max} of approximately 2 hours and a decline in C_{max} of approximately 10%, compared to fasted conditions. However, administration of Tindamax with food did not affect AUC or T½ in this study.
In healthy volunteers, administration of crushed Tindamax tablets in artificial cherry syrup, prepared as described below, after an overnight fast has no effect on any pharmacokinetic parameter as compared to tablets swallowed whole under fasted conditions.
Procedure for extemporaneous pharmacy compounding of the oral suspension: Four 500 mg oral tablets were ground to a fine powder with a mortar and pestle. Approximately 10 mL of cherry syrup were added to the powder and mixed until smooth. The suspension was transferred to a graduated amber container. Several small rinses of cherry syrup were used to transfer any remaining drug in the mortar to the final suspension for a final volume of 30 mL. The suspension of crushed tablets in artificial cherry syrup (Humco®) is stable for 7 days at room temperature. When this suspension is used, it should be shaken well before each administration.
Distribution
Tinidazole is distributed into virtually all tissues and body fluids and also crosses the blood-brain barrier. The apparent volume of distribution is about 50 liters. Plasma protein binding of tinidazole is 12%. Tinidazole crosses the placental barrier and is secreted in breast milk (see **PRECAUTIONS/Pregnancy** and **PRECAUTIONS/Nursing mothers**).
Metabolism
Tinidazole, like metronidazole, is significantly metabolized in humans prior to excretion. Tinidazole is partly metabolized by oxidation, hydroxylation and conjugation. Tinidazole is the major drug-related constituent in plasma after human treatment, along with a small amount of the 2-hydroxymethyl metabolite.
Tinidazole is biotransformed mainly by CYP3A4. In an *in vitro* metabolic drug interaction study, tinidazole concentrations of up to 75 µg/mL did not inhibit the enzyme activities of CYP1A2, CYP2B6, CYP2C9, CYP2D6, CYP2E1 and CYP3A4.
The potential of tinidazole to induce the metabolism of other drugs has not been evaluated.
Elimination
The plasma half-life of tinidazole is approximately 12–14 hours. Tinidazole is excreted by the liver and the kidneys. Tinidazole is excreted in the urine mainly as unchanged drug (approximately 20–25% of the administered dose). Approximately 12% of the drug is excreted in the feces.
Pharmacokinetics in Special Populations
Patients with impaired renal function: The pharmacokinetics of tinidazole in patients with severe renal impairment (CrCL < 22 mL/min) are not significantly different from the pharmacokinetics seen in healthy subjects. However, during hemodialysis, clearance of tinidazole is significantly increased; the half-life is reduced from 12.0 hours to 4.9 hours. Approximately 43% of the amount present in the body is eliminated during a 6-hour hemodialysis session. The pharmacokinetics of tinidazole in patients undergoing routine continuous peritoneal dialysis have not been investigated. (See **DOSAGE AND ADMINISTRATION**).
Patients with impaired hepatic function: There are no data on tinidazole pharmacokinetics in patients with impaired hepatic function. Reduction of metabolic elimination of metronidazole, a chemically-related nitroimidazole, in patients with hepatic dysfunction has been reported in several studies. (See **DOSAGE AND ADMINISTRATION**).

MICROBIOLOGY
Mechanism of Action: Tinidazole is an antiprotozoal agent. The nitro group of tinidazole is reduced by cell extracts of *Trichomonas*. The free nitro radical generated as a result of this reduction may be responsible for the antiprotozoal activity. The mechanism by which tinidazole exhibits activity against *Giardia* and *Entamoeba* species is not known.
Activity *in vitro* and *in vivo*: Tinidazole demonstrates activity both *in vitro* and in clinical infections against the following protozoa:
Trichomonas vaginalis
Giardia duodenalis (also termed G. lamblia)
Entamoeba histolytica
Tinidazole does not appear to have activity against most strains of vaginal lactobacilli.
Susceptibility Tests
For protozoal parasites, standardized tests do not exist for use in clinical microbiology laboratories.
Drug Resistance
The development of resistance to tinidazole by *T. vaginalis*, *G. duodenalis* or *E. histolytica* has not been examined.
Cross-resistance
Approximately 38% of *T. vaginalis* isolates exhibiting reduced susceptibility to metronidazole also show reduced susceptibility to tinidazole *in vitro*. The clinical significance of such an effect is not known.

INDICATIONS AND USAGE
Trichomoniasis: Tindamax oral tablets are indicated for the treatment of trichomoniasis caused by T. vaginalis in both female and male patients. The organism should be identified by appropriate diagnostic procedures. Because trichomoniasis is a sexually transmitted disease with potentially serious sequelae, partners of infected patients should be treated simultaneously in order to prevent re-infection.
Giardiasis: Tindamax oral tablets are indicated for the treatment of giardiasis caused by *G. duodenalis* (also termed *G. lamblia*) in both adults and pediatric patients older than three years of age.
Amebiasis: Tindamax oral tablets are indicated for the treatment of intestinal amebiasis and amebic liver abscess caused by *E. histolytica* in both adults and pediatric patients older than three years of age. It is not indicated in the treatment of asymptomatic cyst passage.

CONTRAINDICATIONS
Tindamax (tinidazole) is contraindicated in patients with hypersensitivity to tinidazole, any component of the tablet, or other nitroimidazole derivatives. Tindamax is contraindicated during the first trimester of pregnancy. See **PRECAUTIONS/Nursing mothers**.

WARNINGS
Convulsive seizures and peripheral neuropathy, the latter characterized mainly by numbness or paresthesia of an extremity, have been reported in patients treated with nitroimidazole drugs including tinidazole and metronidazole. The appearance of abnormal neurologic signs demands the prompt discontinuation of Tindamax therapy. Tinidazole should be administered with caution to patients with central nervous system diseases.

PRECAUTIONS
General:
Tinidazole is a nitroimidazole and should be used with caution in patients with evidence of or history of blood dyscrasia.
The disposition of tinidazole in patients with hepatic impairment has not been evaluated. Patients with severe hepatic disease metabolize nitroimidazoles slowly, with resultant accumulation of parent drug in the plasma. Accordingly, for patients with hepatic dysfunction, usual recommended doses of tinidazole should be administered cautiously.
Known or previously unrecognized candidiasis may present more prominent symptoms during therapy with tinidazole and requires treatment with an antifungal agent.
Information for patients:
Tindamax tablets should be taken with food (see **DOSAGE AND ADMINISTRATION**).
Alcoholic beverages should be avoided while taking Tindamax and for three days afterward (see **PRECAUTIONS/Drug interactions**).
Laboratory tests:
Tinidazole, like metronidazole, may produce transient leukopenia and neutropenia; however, no persistent hematological abnormalities attributable to tinidazole have been observed in clinical studies. Total and differential leukocyte counts are recommended if retreatment is necessary.
Drug interactions:
Although not studied specifically for tinidazole, the following drug interactions were reported for metronidazole, a chemically-related nitroimidazole. Therefore, these drug interactions may occur with tinidazole.
Potential effect of tinidazole on other drugs
Warfarin and other oral coumarin anticoagulants. As with other nitroimidazole derivatives, tinidazole may enhance the effect of warfarin and other coumarin anticoagulants, resulting in a prolongation of prothrombin time. This potential interaction should be considered when tinidazole is prescribed for patients on this type of anticoagulant therapy. The dosage of oral anticoagulants may need to be adjusted during tinidazole co-administration and up to 8 days after discontinuation.
Alcohols, Disulfiram. Alcoholic beverages and preparations containing ethanol or propylene glycol should be avoided during tinidazole therapy and for three days afterward because abdominal cramps, nausea, vomiting, headaches and flushing may occur. Psychotic reactions have been reported in alcoholic patients using metronidazole and disulfiram concurrently. Though no similar reactions have been reported with tinidazole, tinidazole should not be given to patients who have taken disulfiram within the last two weeks.
Lithium. Metronidazole has been reported to elevate serum lithium levels. It is not known if tinidazole shares this property with metronidazole, but consideration should be given to measuring serum lithium and creatinine levels after several days of simultaneous lithium and tinidazole treatment to detect potential lithium intoxication.
Phenytoin, Fosphenytoin. Fosphenytoin is a pro-drug of phenytoin. Concomitant administration of oral metronidazole and intravenous phenytoin was reported to result in prolongation of the half-life and reduction in the clearance of phenytoin. Metronidazole did not significantly affect the pharmacokinetics of orally-administered phenytoin.

Continued on next page

Tindamax—Cont.

Cyclosporine, Tacrolimus. There are several case reports suggesting that metronidazole has the potential to increase the levels of cyclosporine and tacrolimus. During tinidazole co-administration with either of these drugs, the patient should be monitored for signs of calcineurin-inhibitor associated toxicities.
Fluorouracil. Metronidazole was shown to decrease the clearance of fluorouracil, resulting in an increase in side-effects without an increase in therapeutic benefits. If the concomitant use of tinidazole and fluorouracil cannot be avoided, the patient should be monitored for fluorouracil-associated toxicities.
Potential effect of other drugs on tinidazole
Simultaneous administration of tinidazole with drugs that induce liver microsomal enzymes (cytochrome P-450) such as *phenobarbital, rifampin, phenytoin* and *fosphenytoin* (a pro-drug of phenytoin) may accelerate the elimination of tinidazole, decreasing the plasma level of tinidazole. Simultaneous administration of drugs that inhibit the activity of liver microsomal enzymes, such as *cimetidine* and *ketoconazole,* may prolong the half-life and decrease the plasma clearance of tinidazole, increasing the plasma level of tinidazole.
Cholestyramine. Cholestyramine was shown to decrease the oral bioavailability of metronidazole by 21%. Thus, it is advisable to separate dosing of cholestyramine and tinidazole to minimize any potential effect on the oral bioavailability of tinidazole.
Oxytetracycline. Oxytetracycline was reported to antagonize the therapeutic effect of metronidazole.
Drug/Laboratory test interactions: Tinidazole, like metronidazole, may interfere with certain types of determinations of serum chemistry values, such as aspartate aminotransferase (AST, SGOT), alanine aminotransferase (ALT, SGPT), lactate dehydrogenase (LDH), triglycerides, and hexokinase glucose. Values of zero may be observed. All of the assays in which interference has been reported involve enzymatic coupling of the assay to oxidation-reduction of nicotinamide adenine dinucleotide ($NAD^+ \leftrightarrow NADH$). Potential interference is due to the similarity of absorbance peaks of NADH and tinidazole.
Carcinogenesis, Mutagenesis, Impairment of fertility: Metronidazole, a chemically-related nitroimidazole, has been reported to be carcinogenic in mice and rats but not hamsters. In several studies metronidazole showed evidence of pulmonary, hepatic and lymphatic tumorigenesis in mice and mammary and hepatic tumors in female rats. Tinidazole carcinogenicity studies in rats, mice or hamsters have not been reported.
Tinidazole was mutagenic in the TA 100, *S. typhimurium* tester strain both with and without the metabolic activation system and was negative for mutagenicity in the TA 98 strain. Mutagenicity results were mixed (positive and negative) in the TA 1535, 1537 and 1538 strains. Tinidazole was also mutagenic in a tester strain of *Klebsiella pneumonia.* Tinidazole was negative for mutagenicity in a mammalian cell culture system utilizing Chinese hamster lung V79 cells (HGPRT test system) and negative for genotoxicity in the Chinese hamster ovary (CHO) sister chromatid exchange assay. Tinidazole was positive for *in vivo* genotoxicity in the mouse micronucleus assay.
In a 60-day fertility study, tinidazole reduced fertility and produced testicular histopathology in male rats at a 600 mg/kg/day dose level (approximately 3-fold the highest human therapeutic dose based upon body surface area conversions). Spermatogenic effects resulted from 300 and 600 mg/kg/day dose levels. The no observed adverse effect level for testicular and spermatogenic effects was 100 mg/kg/day (approximately 0.5-fold the highest human therapeutic dose based upon body surface area conversions). This effect is characteristic of agents in the 5-nitroimidazole class.
Pregnancy:
Teratogenic effects: Pregnancy Category C
The use of tinidazole in pregnant patients has not been studied. Since tinidazole crosses the placental barrier and enters fetal circulation it should not be administered to pregnant patients in the first trimester. Embryo-fetal developmental toxicity studies in pregnant mice indicated no embryo-fetal toxicity or malformations at the highest dose level of 2,500 mg/kg (approximately 6.3-fold the highest human therapeutic dose based upon body surface area conversions). In a study with pregnant rats a slightly higher incidence of fetal mortality was observed at a maternal dose of 500 mg/kg (2.5-fold the highest human therapeutic dose based upon body surface area conversions). No biologically relevant neonatal developmental effects were observed in rat neonates following maternal doses as high as 600 mg/kg (3-fold the highest human therapeutic dose based upon body surface area conversions). Because animal reproduction studies are not always predictive of human response and because there is some evidence of mutagenic potential, the use of tinidazole during pregnancy requires that the potential benefits of the drug be weighed against the possible risks to both the mother and the fetus. (See **CONTRAINDICATIONS**).
Nursing mothers: Tinidazole is excreted in breast milk in concentrations similar to those seen in serum. Tinidazole can be detected in breast milk for up to 72 hours following administration. Interruption of breast-feeding is recommended during tinidazole therapy and for three days following the last dose.
Pediatric use: Other than for use in the treatment of giardiasis and amebiasis in pediatric patients older than three years of age, safety and effectiveness of tinidazole in pediatric patients have not been established.
Geriatric use: Clinical studies of tinidazole did not include sufficient numbers of subjects aged 65 and over to determine whether they respond differently from younger subjects. In general, dose selection for an elderly patient should be cautious, reflecting the greater frequency of decreased hepatic, renal, or cardiac function, and of concomitant disease or other drug therapy.

ADVERSE REACTIONS

Among 3,669 patients treated with a single 2 g dose of tinidazole, in both controlled and uncontrolled trichomoniasis and giardiasis clinical studies, adverse effects were reported by 11.0% of patients. For multi-day dosing in controlled and uncontrolled amebiasis studies, adverse effects were reported by 13.8% of 1,765 patients. Reported adverse effects from clinical trials have generally been mild and self-limiting. Common (≥ 1% incidence) adverse effects reported by body system are as follows. (Note: Data described below are pooled from studies with variable designs and safety evaluations.)

	2 g	Multi-day dose
GI		
Metallic/bitter taste	3.7%	6.3%
Nausea	3.2%	4.5%
Anorexia	1.5%	2.5%
Dyspepsia/cramps/epigastric discomfort	1.8%	1.4%
Vomiting	1.5%	0.9%
Constipation	0.4%	1.4%
CNS		
Weakness/fatigue/malaise	2.1%	1.1%
Dizziness	1.1%	0.5%
Other		
Headache	1.3%	0.7%
Total patients with adverse effects	11.0% (403/3669)	13.8% (244/1765)

Other adverse effects reported with tinidazole include:
Central Nervous System: Two serious adverse reactions reported include convulsions and transient peripheral neuropathy including numbness and paresthesia. Other CNS reports include vertigo, ataxia, giddiness, insomnia, drowsiness.
Gastrointestinal: tongue discoloration, stomatitis, diarrhea
Hypersensitivity: urticaria, pruritis, rash, flushing, sweating, dryness of mouth, fever, burning sensation, thirst, salivation, angioedema
Renal: darkened urine
Cardiovascular: palpitations
Hematopoietic: transient neutropenia, transient leukopenia
Other: candida overgrowth, increased vaginal discharge, oral candidiasis, hepatic abnormalities including raised transaminase level, arthralgias, myalgias, arthritis
Rare reported adverse effects include bronchospasm, dypsnea, coma, confusion, depression, furry tongue, pharyngitis and reversible thrombocytopenia.
Adverse Reactions in Pediatric Patients: Among 6 pooled pediatric studies, 287 patients between the ages of 4 months and 11 years were evaluated. Adverse events reported in pediatric patients taking tinidazole were similar in nature and frequency to adult findings including nausea, vomiting, diarrhea, taste change, anorexia and abdominal pain.

OVERDOSAGE

There are no reported overdoses with tinidazole in humans. In acute studies with mice and rats, the LD_{50} for mice was generally > 3,600 mg/kg for oral administration and was > 2,300 mg/kg for intraperitoneal administration. In rats, the LD_{50} was > 2,000 mg/kg for both oral and intraperitoneal administration.
Treatment of overdosage
There is no specific antidote for the treatment of overdosage with tinidazole; therefore, treatment should be symptomatic and supportive. Gastric lavage may be helpful. Hemodialysis can be considered because approximately 43% of the amount present in the body is eliminated during a 6-hour hemodialysis session.

DOSAGE AND ADMINISTRATION

As with metronidazole, it is advisable to take tinidazole with food to minimize the incidence of epigastric discomfort and other gastrointestional side-effects. Food does not affect the oral bioavailability of tinidazole.
Trichomoniasis: In both females and males, a single 2 g oral dose taken with food. Since trichomoniasis is a sexually transmitted disease, sexual partners should be treated with the same dose and at the same time.
Giardiasis: In adults, a single 2 g dose taken with food. In pediatric patients older than three years of age, a single dose of 50 mg/kg (up to 2 g) with food.
Amebiasis:
Intestinal: In adults, a 2 g dose per day for 3 days taken with food. In pediatric patients older than three years of age, 50 mg/kg/day (up to 2 g per day) for 3 days with food.
Amebic liver abscess: In adults, a 2 g dose per day for 3–5 days taken with food. In pediatric patients older than three years of age, 50 mg/kg/day (up to 2 g per day) for 3–5 days with food. There are limited pediatric data on durations of therapy exceeding 3 days, although a small number of children were treated for 5 days without reported adverse events. Children should be closely monitored when treatment durations exceed 3 days.
Pediatric Administration: For those unable to swallow tablets, Tindamax (tinidazole) tablets may be crushed in artificial cherry syrup, to be taken with food. See **CLINICAL PHARMACOLOGY** for procedure for extemporaneous pharmacy compounding of the oral suspension, as used in clinical pharmacology studies.
Patients with impaired renal function: Tinidazole pharmacokinetics in patients with significantly impaired renal function are not significantly different than those seen in healthy subjects. Therefore, no dose adjustments are necessary in these patients.
Patients undergoing hemodialysis: During hemodialysis, clearance of tinidazole is significantly increased; the half-life is reduced from 12.0 hours to 4.9 hours. Approximately 43% of the amount present in the body is eliminated during a 6-hour hemodialysis session. Thus, if tinidazole is administered on a day when dialysis is performed, it is recommended that an additional dose of tinidazole equivalent to one-half of the recommended dose be administered after the end of the hemodialysis.
The pharmacokinetics of tinidazole in patients undergoing routine continuous peritoneal dialysis have not been investigated. (See **CLINICAL PHARMACOLOGY/Special Populations**).
Patients with impaired hepatic function: There are no data on tinidazole pharmacokinetics in patients with impaired hepatic function. Reduction of metabolic elimination of metronidazole, a chemically-related nitroimidazole, in patients with hepatic dysfunction has been reported in several studies. In the absence of data on tinidazole, usually recommended doses of tinidazole should be administered cautiously in such patients.

HOW SUPPLIED

Tindamax 500 mg tablets are pink, caplet-shaped, film-coated, scored tablets, with P L debossed on one side and 500 on the other, supplied in bottles with child-resistant caps as:
NDC 66378-500-20 Bottle of 20
NDC 66378-500-60 Bottle of 60
Tindamax 250 mg tablets are pink, round, film-coated, scored tablets, with P L debossed on one side and 250 on the other, supplied in bottles with child-resistant caps as:
NDC 66378-250-40 Bottle of 40
NDC 66378-250-44 Bottle of 100
Storage and stability
Store at controlled room temperature 20–25° C (68–77° F); excursions permitted to 15–30° C (59–86° F) [see USP]. Protect contents from light.

CLINICAL STUDIES

Trichomoniasis
Tinidazole (2 g single oral dose) use in trichomoniasis has been well documented in 34 published reports from the world literature involving over 2,800 patients treated with tinidazole. In four published, blinded, randomized, comparative studies of the 2 g tinidazole single oral dose where efficacy was assessed by culture at time points post-treatment ranging from one week to one month, reported cure rates ranged from 92% (37/40) to 100% (65/65) (n=172 total subjects). In four published, blinded, randomized, comparative studies where efficacy was assessed by wet mount between 7–14 days post-treatment, reported cure rates ranged from 80% (8/10) to 100% (16/16) (n=116 total subjects). In these studies, tinidazole was superior to placebo and comparable to other anti-trichomonal drugs. The single oral 2 g tinidazole dose was also assessed in four open-label trials in men (one comparative to metronidazole and 3 single-arm studies). Parasitological evaluation of the urine was performed both pre- and post-treatment and reported cure rates ranged from 83% (25/30) to 100% (80/80) (n=142 total subjects).
Giardiasis
Tinidazole (2 g single dose) use in giardiasis has been documented in 19 published reports from the world literature involving over 1,600 patients (adults and pediatric patients). In eight controlled studies involving a total of 619 subjects of whom 299 were given the 2 g × 1 day (50 mg/kg × 1 day in pediatric patients) oral dose of tinidazole, reported cure rates ranged from 80% (40/50) to 100% (15/15). In three of these trials where the comparator was 2 to 3 days of various doses of metronidazole, reported cure rates for metronidazole were 76% (19/25) to 93% (14/15). Data comparing a single 2 g dose of tinidazole to usually recommended 5–7 days of metronidazole are limited.
Intestinal Amebiasis
Tinidazole use in intestinal amebiasis has been documented in 26 published reports from the world literature involving over 1,400 patients. Most reports utilized tinidazole 2 g/day × 3 days. In four published, randomized, controlled studies (1 investigator single-blind, 3 open-label) of the 2 g/day × 3 days oral dose of tinidazole, reported cure rates after three

days of therapy among a total of 220 subjects ranged from 86% (25/29) to 93% (25/27).

Amebic Liver Abscess

Tinidazole use in amebic liver abscess has been documented in 18 published reports from the world literature involving over 470 patients. Most reports utilized tinidazole 2 g/day × 2–5 days. In seven published, randomized, controlled studies (1 double-blind, 1 single-blind, 5 open-label) of the 2 g/day × 2-5 days oral dose of tinidazole accompanied by aspiration of the liver abscess when clinically necessary, reported cure rates among 133 subjects ranged from 81% (17/21) to 100% (16/16). Four of these studies utilized at least 3 days of tinidazole.

Manufactured for Presutti Laboratories, Inc., Arlington Heights, IL 60004 by Mikart, Inc., Atlanta, GA.

Revised: May 14, 2004

Rx Only

Procaps Laboratories, Inc.

Formerly YOURVITAMINS, INC.
430 PARKSON ROAD
HENDERSON, NV 89015

For Sales Inquiries:
800-800-1200 weekdays

For Product Information:
Research Department
702-564-9000 weekdays

www.Cholox.com
PDR@Cholox.com

CHOLOX is a family of six Cholesterol-lowering formulas, three of which are prescription (below) and three of which are non-prescription (see the PDR for NonPrescription Drugs). All CHOLOX formulas are clinically proven and designed to reduce Total and LDL Cholesterol levels, while each of the CHOLOX RX also includes Homocysteine-lowering factors.

CHOLOX RX ℞

[*ko-les-ta-kar*]

A blend of Cholesterol- and Homocysteine-lowering factors.

DESCRIPTION

CHOLOX RX is clinically proven to support heart health by helping to reduce Total Cholesterol and LDL Cholesterol levels. Medical experts recognize that Total Cholesterol and LDL Cholesterol levels are controllable risk factors for heart disease. The FDA recognizes that the active ingredient in CHOLOX RX provides a safe, natural means of lowering Total and LDL Cholesterol, thereby reducing heart disease risk. This natural Cholesterol-lowering ingredient possesses absolutely no side effects. Clinical studies have consistently proven that including adequate amounts of CHOLOX RX's active ingredient in the diet helps to significantly lower Total Cholesterol and LDL Cholesterol. *According to the FDA, consuming at least 400 mgs of plant sterols twice daily with meals for a total daily intake of at least 800 mgs, as part of a diet low in saturated fat and cholesterol, may reduce the risk of heart disease.* Clinical studies have demonstrated a 10–20% reduction in LDL Cholesterol with consumption of 800 milligrams of phytosterols daily and consumption of 1,000 to 3,000 mgs daily yielding more substantial reductions. CHOLOX RX also contains therapeutic levels of Folic Acid, Vitamins B12 and B6 to help maintain healthy levels of Homocysteine, since research has shown that high levels of Homocysteine may play a role in the development of heart disease, blood clots and vascular spasm.

COMPOSITION

CHOLOX RX contains the following per 1 capsule and 8 capsule dosage respectively:

Proprietary Phytosterols	400 mg	3,200 mg
Vitamin B6	5 mg	40 mg
Vitamin B12	50 mcg	400 mcg
Folic Acid	125 mcg	1,000 mcg

Other Ingredients: Gelatin Capsule, Vegetable Magnesium Stearate, Vegetable Stearine and Silicon Dioxide.

MECHANISM OF ACTION

Cholesterol Reduction. Plant sterols are structurally similar to both cholesterol and bile salts, yet unlike cholesterol and bile salts, phytosterols are poorly absorbed from the GI tract. This causes phytosterols to interfere with both endogenous and exogenous cholesterol and bile salt absorption by limiting solubility and competing for transport at the intestinal absorption sites. The result of these mechanisms is to divert significant amounts of cholesterol and bile salts out of the body thereby safely and naturally reducing Total Cholesterol and LDL Cholesterol levels.

Homocysteine Reduction. Normal protein metabolism results in the intermediate byproduct, homocysteine. Clinical studies have shown that elevated homocysteine levels are associated with atherosclerosis and heart disease risk. Vitamins B12, B6, and Folic Acid have been shown to effectively reduce elevated levels of homocysteine. Vitamin B12 and Folic Acid are involved in the re-methylation pathway of homocysteine back into methionine, while Vitamin B6 is required for the trans-sulfuration of homocysteine into the amino acids cysteine and taurine.

INDICATIONS AND USAGE

For individuals who seek to naturally lower Total Cholesterol and LDL Cholesterol without side effects or health risks. CHOLOX RX can be used effectively in conjunction with or independent from cholesterol-lowering prescription medications. As with any cholesterol reduction regime, CHOLOX RX is most effective when part of a high-fiber diet containing reduced levels of cholesterol and saturated fat.

PRECAUTIONS

Those with a potential B12 deficiency or Pernicious Anemia should not consume large amounts of folic acid without the supervision of a physician. High folic acid supplementation may mask the symptoms of B12 deficiency, potentially resulting in neurological damage.

DOSAGE AND ADMINISTRATION

Consume 1 to 3 capsules with each meal or snack depending on the amount of food consumed. With small meals or snacks consume 1 capsule and with larger meals 2 or 3 capsules. Consume at least 2 capsules per day; however, there is no additional benefit from consuming more than 8 capsules daily. The largest reduction in Total and LDL Cholesterol is experienced as the dosage increases from 2 to 8 capsules daily with optimum reductions achieved with 4 to 6 capsules daily. CHOLOX RX is most effective when taken with food – 30 minutes before or no more than 60 minutes after eating.

HOW SUPPLIED

Available in blister-packs of 90, 180 and 360 gelatin capsules containing beige powder.

REFERENCES

Available at www.Cholox.com.

CHOLOX COMPLETE RX

A blend of Cholesterol- and Homocysteine-lowering factors plus Fiber, Gamma Vitamin E, Essential Omega-3 Oils and Phosphatidyl Choline.

DESCRIPTION

CHOLOX COMPLETE RX is clinically proven to support heart health by helping to reduce Total Cholesterol and LDL Cholesterol levels. Medical experts recognize that higher Total Cholesterol and LDL Cholesterol levels are controllable risk factors for heart disease. The FDA recognizes that the active ingredient in CHOLOX COMPLETE RX provides a safe, natural means of lowering Total and LDL Cholesterol, thereby reducing heart disease risk. This natural Cholesterol- lowering ingredient possesses absolutely no side effects. Clinical studies have consistently proven that including adequate amounts of CHOLOX COMPLETE RX's active ingredient in the diet helps to significantly lower Total Cholesterol and LDL Cholesterol. *According to the FDA, consuming at least 400 mgs of plant sterols twice daily with meals for a total daily intake of at least 800 mgs, as part of a diet low in saturated fat and cholesterol, may reduce the risk of heart disease.* Clinical studies have demonstrated a 10–20% reduction in LDL Cholesterol with consumption of 800 milligrams of phytosterols daily and consumption of 1,000 to 3,000 mgs daily yielding more substantial reductions. CHOLOX COMPLETE RX also contains therapeutic levels of Folic Acid, Vitamins B12 and B6 to help maintain healthy levels of Homocysteine, since research has shown that high levels of Homocysteine may play a role in the development of heart disease, blood clots and vascular spasm. CHOLOX COMPLETE RX also includes Omega-3 Fatty Acids, including a balanced blend of EPA and DHA from fish oils, as well as high levels of Alpha Linolenic Acid from Flax Seed Oil. CHOLOX COMPLETE RX also provides high levels of Vitamin E from a balanced blend of natural Tocopherols with particular emphasis on the superior antioxidant protection of Gamma and Alpha Tocopherol. Lastly, CHOLOX COMPLETE RX also includes high levels of Phosphatidyl Choline.

COMPOSITION

CHOLOX COMPLETE RX contains the following per 1 packet and 4 packet dosage respectively:

Proprietary Phytosterols	1 gram	4 grams
Psyllium	1.5 grams	6 grams
Vitamin B6	10 mg	40 mg
Vitamin B12	100 mcg	400 mcg
Folic Acid	250 mcg	1,000 mcg
Vitamin E	67 IU	267 IU
Total Tocopherols	231 mg	925 mg
Gamma Tocopherol	133 mg	533 mg
Alpha Tocopherol	45 mg	179 mg
Beta/Delta Tocopherol	53 mg	212 mg
Soy Lecithin Oil	233 mg	932 mg
Phosphatidyl Choline	82 mg	326 mg
Fish Oil	120 mg	480 mg
DHA	34 mg	134 mg
EPA	34 mg	134 mg
Flax Seed Oil	120 mg	480 mg
Alpha-Linolenic Acid	84 mg	336 mg

Other Ingredients: Vegetable Magnesium Stearate, Vegetable Stearine, Silicon Dioxide, Peppermint Oil and Spearmint Oil.

MECHANISM OF ACTION

Cholesterol Reduction. Plant sterols are structurally similar to both cholesterol and bile salts, yet unlike cholesterol and bile salts, phytosterols are poorly absorbed from the GI tract. This causes phytosterols to interfere with both endogenous and exogenous cholesterol and bile salt absorption by limiting solubility and competing for transport at the intestinal absorption sites. The result of these mechanisms is to divert significant amounts of cholesterol and bile salts out of the body thereby safely and naturally reducing Total Cholesterol and LDL Cholesterol levels.

Homocysteine Reduction. Normal protein metabolism results in the intermediate byproduct, homocysteine. Clinical studies have shown that elevated homocysteine levels are associated with atherosclerosis and heart disease risk. Vitamins B12, B6, and Folic Acid have been shown to effectively reduce elevated levels of homocysteine. Vitamin B12 and Folic Acid are involved in the re-methylation pathway of homocysteine back into methionine, while Vitamin B6 is required for the trans-sulfuration of homocysteine into the amino acids cysteine and taurine.

INDICATIONS AND USAGE

For individuals who seek to naturally lower Total Cholesterol and LDL Cholesterol without side effects or health risks. CHOLOX COMPLETE RX can be used effectively in conjunction with or independent from cholesterol-lowering prescription medications. As with any cholesterol reduction regime, CHOLOX COMPLETE RX is most effective when part of a high-fiber diet containing reduced levels of cholesterol and saturated fat.

PRECAUTIONS

Those with a potential B12 deficiency or Pernicious Anemia should not consume large amounts of folic acid without the supervision of a physician. High folic acid supplementation may mask the symptoms of B12 deficiency, potentially resulting in neurological damage.

DOSAGE AND ADMINISTRATION

Consume 1 packet with each of your day's largest meals. Consume at least 2 packets per day; however, there is no additional benefit from consuming more than 4 packets per day. The largest reduction in Total and LDL Cholesterol is experienced as the dosage increases from 2 to 4 packets daily with optimum reductions achieved with 2 or 3 packets daily. CHOLOX COMPLETE RX is most effective when taken with food – 30 minutes before or no more than 60 minutes after eating.

HOW SUPPLIED

Available in bottles of 60 and 180 packets. Each packet contains 6 gelatin capsules containing beige powder and 1 gelatin capsule containing amber liquid.

REFERENCES

Available at www.Cholox.com.

CHOLOX COMPLETE RX MULTIVITAMIN

A Cholesterol- and Homocysteine-lowering multivitamin plus Gamma Vitamin E, Essential Omega-3 oils and Phosphatidyl Choline.

DESCRIPTION

See CHOLOX COMPLETE RX above. CHOLOX COMPLETE RX MULTIVITAMIN includes the additional support of a comprehensive medium potency multi-vitamin-mineral formula.

COMPOSITION

CHOLOX COMPLETE RX MULTIVITAMIN contains the following per 1 packet and 4 packet dosage respectively:

Vitamin A	1,250 IU	5,000 IU
Vitamin C	125 mg	500 mg
Vitamin D	150 IU	600 IU
Vitamin E	67 IU	267 IU
Total Tocopherols	231 mg	925 mg
Gamma Tocopherol	133 mg	533 mg
Alpha Tocopherol	45 mg	179 mg
Beta/Delta Tocopherol	53 mg	212 mg
Vitamin B1	5 mg	20 mg
Vitamin B2	5 mg	20 mg
Niacin	5.5 mg	22 mg
Vitamin B6	10 mg	40 mg
Folic Acid	250 mcg	1,000 mcg
Vitamin B12	100 mcg	400 mcg
Biotin	75 mcg	300 mcg
Pantothenic Acid	5 mg	20 mg
Calcium	200 mg	800 mg
Magnesium	100 mg	400 mg
Zinc	7.5 mg	30 mg
Selenium	60 mcg	240 mcg
Copper	750 mcg	3 mg
Manganese	250 mcg	1,000 mcg
Chromium	60 mcg	240 mcg
Molybdenum	12.5 mcg	50 mcg
Boron	125 mcg	500 mcg
Vanadium	12.5 mcg	50 mcg
Lutein	250 mcg	1,000 mcg
Lycopene	250 mcg	1,000 mcg
Astaxanthin	62.5 mcg	250 mcg
Proprietary Phytosterols	1 gram	4 grams

Continued on next page

Cholox RX—Cont.

Psyllium	1.75 grams	7 grams
Soy Lecithin Oil	233 mg	932 mg
Phosphatidyl Choline	82 mg	326 mg
Fish Oil	120 mg	480 mg
DHA	34 mg	134 mg
EPA	34 mg	134 mg
Flax Seed Oil	120 mg	480 mg
Alpha-Linolenic Acid	84 mg	336 mg

Other Ingredients: Vegetable Magnesium Stearate, Vegetable Stearine, Silicon Dioxide, Peppermint Oil and Spearmint Oil.

MECHANISM OF ACTION
See CHOLOX COMPLETE RX above.

INDICATIONS AND USAGE
See CHOLOX COMPLETE RX above.

PRECAUTIONS
See CHOLOX COMPLETE RX above.

DOSAGE AND ADMINISTRATION
See CHOLOX COMPLETE RX above.

HOW SUPPLIED
See CHOLOX COMPLETE RX above.

REFERENCES
Available at www.CHOLOX.com.

Procter & Gamble

P.O. BOX 599
CINCINNATI, OH 45201

Direct Inquiries to:
Consumer Relations
800-832-3064
For Medical Emergencies:
Call Collect: (513) 636-5107

CHILDREN'S VICKS® NYQUIL® OTC
COLD/COUGH RELIEF
Antihistamine/Nasal Decongestant/ Cough Suppressant

Children's NyQuil was specially formulated with three effective ingredients to relieve nighttime cough, nasal congestion, and runny nose so children can rest. Children's NyQuil® is alcohol free and analgesic free and has a pleasant cherry flavor.

Drug Facts:

ACTIVE INGREDIENTS **Purpose:**
(per tablespoon, 15 ml)
Chlorpheniramine maleate
2 mg .... Antihistamine
Dextromethorphan HBr
15 mg .... Cough suppressant
Pseudoephedrine HCl
30 mg .... Nasal decongestant

USES
Temporarily relieves cold symptoms:
- cough due to minor throat and bronchial irritation
- sneezing
- runny nose
- nasal congestion

WARNINGS
Failure to follow these warnings could result in serious consequences.
Do not use
- if you are now taking a prescription monoamine oxidase inhibitor (MAOI) (certain drugs for depression, psychiatric or emotional conditions, or Parkinson's disease), or for 2 weeks after stopping the MAOI durg. If you do not know if your prescription drug contains an MAOI, ask a doctor or pharmacist before taking this product.

Ask a doctor before use if you have:
- heart disease
- a breathing problem or chronic cough that lasts or as occurs with smoking, asthma, chronic bronchitis or emphysema
- thyroid disease
- diabetes
- glaucoma
- high blood pressure
- cough that occurs with too much phlegm (mucus)
- a sodium-restricted diet
- trouble urinating due to enlarged prostate gland

Ask a doctor or pharmacist before use if you are taking sedatives or tranquilizers.
When using this product:
- **do not use more than directed**
- excitability may occur, especially in children
- drowsiness may occur
- avoid alcoholic drinks
- be careful when driving a motor vehicle or operating machinery
- alcohol, sedatives, and tranquilizers may increase drowsiness

Stop use and ask a doctor if:
- you get nervous, dizzy or sleepless
- symptoms do not get better within 7 days or accompanied by a fever
- cough lasts more than 7 days, comes back, or occurs with fever, rash, or headache that lasts.

These could be signs of a serious condition.

If pregnant or breast-feeding, ask a health professional before use.
Keep out of reach of children. In case of overdose, get medical help or contact a Poison Control Center right away. Quick medical attention is critical for adults as well as for children even if you do not notice any signs or symptoms.

DIRECTIONS
- use tablespoon (TBSP) or dose cup
- do not exceed 4 doses per 24 hours

under 6 yrs. .... ask a doctor
6–11 yrs. .... 1 TBSP or 15 ml every 6 hours
12 yrs. & older .... 2 TBSP or 30 ml every 6 hours

OTHER INFORMATION
- **each tablespoon contains** sodium 71 mg
- store at room temperature

INACTIVE INGREDIENTS
Citric acid, flavor, potassium sorbate, propylene glycol, purified water, FD&C red 40, sodium citrate, sucrose.

HOW SUPPLIED
Available in 4 FL OZ (118 ml) and 6 FL OZ (177 ml) plastic bottles with child-resistant, tamper-evident cap and a calibrated medicine cup.
Questions? 1-800-362-1683 www.vicks.com
Exp. Date: See Bottom. 42434744
Dist. by Procter & Gamble, Cincinnati OH 45202.

HEAD & SHOULDERS CLASSIC CLEAN DANDRUFF SHAMPOO OTC

Head & Shoulders Classic Clean Dandruff Shampoo for normal/oily hair offers effective control of persistent dandruff and beautiful hair from a pleasant-to-use formula. Double-blind, expert-graded testing have proven that it reduces dandruff very effectively. It is also gentle enough to use every day for clean, manageable hair.
The formula ingredients below are for Classic Clean version. Head & Shoulders is also available in a Classic Clean 2-in-1 version for increased manageability and hair damage prevention. The key formula difference is increased dimethicone conditioner and substitution of Polyquaternium-10 polymer instead of Guar Hydroxypropyltrimonium Chloride.

Drug Facts
ACTIVE INGREDIENT **Purpose**
Pyrithione zinc 1% Anti-dandruff

USES
helps prevent recurrence of flaking and itching associated with dandruff

WARNINGS
For external use only
When using this product
- avoid contact with eyes. If contact occurs, rinse eyes thoroughly with water.

Stop use and ask a doctor if
- condition worsens or does not improve after regular use of this product as directed.

Keep this and all drugs out of reach of children. If swallowed, get medical help or contact a Poison Control Center right away.

DIRECTIONS
- for maximum dandruff control, use every time you shampoo.
- wet hair.
- massage onto scalp
- rinse.
- repeat if desired.
- for best results use <u>at least</u> twice a week or as directed by a doctor.

Inactive Ingredients
Water, sodium laureth sulfate, sodium lauryl sulfate, cocamide MEA, glycol distearate, zinc carbonate, dimethicone, fragrance, cetyl alcohol, guar hydroxypropyltrimonium chloride, magnesium sulfate, sodium benzoate, magnesium carbonate hydroxide, ammonium laureth sulfate, benzyl alcohol, sodium chloride, methylchloroisothiazolinone, blue no. 1, methylisothiazolinone, sodium xylenesulfonate

HOW SUPPLIED
Head & Shoulders Classic Clean Dandruff Shampoo is available in 2.0 FL, 6.8 FL OZ, 13.5 FL OZ, 25.4 FL OZ, 33.9 FL OZ unbreakable plastic bottles.
***Questions [or comments]?* 1-800-723-9569**

HEAD & SHOULDERS DRY SCALP CARE DANDRUFF SHAMPOO OTC

Head & Shoulders Dry Scalp Care Dandruff Shampoo offers effective control of persistent dandruff and beautiful hair from a pleasant-to-use formula. Double-blind, expert-graded testing have proven that it reduces dandruff very effectively. It is also gentle enough to use every day for clean, manageable hair.
The formula ingredients below are for Dry Scalp version. Head & Shoulders is also available in a conditioning Smooth & Silky 2-in-1 version whose primary formula difference is the addition of Guar Hydroxypropyltrimonium Chloride.

Drug Facts
ACTIVE INGREDIENT **Purpose**
Pyrithione zinc 1% Anti-dandruff

USES
Helps prevent recurrence of flaking and itching associated with dandruff

WARNINGS
For external use only
When using this product
- avoid contact with eyes. If contact occurs, rinse eyes thoroughly with water.

Stop use and ask a doctor if
- condition worsens or does not improve after regular use of this product as directed.

Keep this and all drugs out of reach of children. If swallowed, get medical help or contact a Poison Control Center right away.

DIRECTIONS
- for maximum dandruff control, use every time you shampoo.
- wet hair.
- massage onto scalp.
- rinse.
- repeat if desired.
- for best results use <u>at least</u> twice a week or as directed by a doctor.

Inactive Ingredients
Water, sodium laureth sulfate, sodium lauryl sulfate, cocamide MEA, zinc carbonate, glycol distearate, dimethicone, fragrance, cetyl alcohol, polyquaternium-10, magnesium sulfate, sodium benzoate, magnesium carbonate hydroxide, ammonium laureth sulfate, benzyl alcohol, sodium chloride, methylchloroisothiazolinone, methylisothiazolinone, sodium xylenesulfonate, aloe barbadensis leaf extract, anthemis nobilis flower oil, tocopheryl acetate

HOW SUPPLIED
Head & Shoulders Dry Scalp Care Dandruff Shampoo is available in 6.8 FL OZ, 13.5 FL OZ, 25.4 FL OZ, 33.9 FL OZ unbreakable plastic bottles.
***Questions [or comments]?* 1-800-723-9569**

HEAD & SHOULDERS® INTENSIVE TREATMENT DANDRUFF AND SEBORRHEIC DERMATITIS SHAMPOO OTC

Head & Shoulders Intensive Treatment Dandruff and Seborrheic Dermatitis Shampoo offers effective control of persistent dandruff and beautiful hair from a pleasant-to-use formula. Double-blind, expert-graded testing have proven that it reduces dandruff very effectively. It is also gentle enough to use every day for clean, manageable hair.

Drug Facts
ACTIVE INGREDIENT **Purpose**
Selenium Sulfide 1% Anti-dandruff
Anti-seborrheic dermatitis

USES
Helps stop itching, flaking, scaling, irritation and redness associated with dandruff and seborrheic dermatitis.

WARNINGS
For external use only
Ask a doctor before use if you have a condition that covers a large portion of the body.
When using this product
- avoid contact with eyes. If contact occurs, rinse eyes thoroughly with water.

Stop use and ask a doctor if
- condition worsens or does not improve after regular use of this product as directed.

Keep this and all drugs out of reach of children. If swallowed, get medical help or contact a Poison Control Center right away.

DIRECTIONS
- wet hair.
- massage onto scalp
- rinse thoroughly
- for best results use <u>at least</u> twice a week or as directed by a doctor.
- caution: if used on bleached, tinted, grey, or permed hair, rinse for 5 minutes
- for maximum dandruff control, use every time you shampoo

INACTIVE INGREDIENTS
Water, Ammonium laureth sulfate, Ammonium lauryl sulfate, Glycol distearate, Cocamide MEA, Fragrance, Dimethicone, Tricetylmonium chloride, Ammonium xylenesulfonate, Cetyl alcohol, DMDM hydantoin, Sodium chloride, Stearyl alcohol, Hydroxypropyl methylcellulose, FD&C red no. 4

HOW SUPPLIED

Head & Shoulders Intensive Treatment Dandruff and Seborrheic Dermatitis Shampoo is available in 13.5 FL OZ unbreakable plastic bottles.

***Questions [or comments]?* 1-800-723-9569**

METAMUCIL® FIBER LAXATIVE OTC

[*met uh-mü sil*]

(psyllium husk)

***Also see Metamucil Dietary Fiber Supplement** in PDR for Nonprescription Drugs*

DESCRIPTION

Metamucil contains psyllium husk (from the plant *Plantago ovata*), a bulk forming, natural therapeutic fiber for restoring and maintaining regularity when recommended by a physician. Metamucil contains no chemical stimulants and does not disrupt normal bowel function. Each dose of Metamucil powder and Metamucil Fiber Wafers contains approximately 3.4 grams of psyllium husk (or 2.4 grams of soluble fiber). Each dose of Metamucil capsules fiber laxative (5 capsules) contains approximately 2.6 grams of psyllium husk (or 2.0 grams of soluble fiber). Inactive ingredients, sodium, calcium, potassium, calories, carbohydrate, dietary fiber, and phenylalanine content are shown in the following table for all versions and flavors. Metamucil Smooth Texture Sugar-Free Regular Flavor and Metamucil capsules contains no sugar and no artificial sweeteners; Metamucil Smooth Texture Sugar-Free Orange Flavor contains aspartame (phenylalanine content per dose is 25 mg). Metamucil powdered products and Metamucil capsules are gluten-free. Metamucil Fiber Wafers contain gluten: Apple Crisp contains 0.7g/dose, Cinnamon Spice contains 0.5g/dose. Each two-wafer dose contains 5 grams of fat.

ACTIONS

The active ingredient in Metamucil is psyllium husk, a natural fiber which promotes elimination due to its bulking effect in the colon. This bulking effect is due to both the water-holding capacity of undigested fiber and the increased bacterial mass following partial fiber digestion. These actions result in enlargement of the lumen of the colon, and softer stool, thereby decreasing intraluminal pressure and straining, and speeding colonic transit in constipated patients.

INDICATIONS

Metamucil is indicated for the treatment of occasional constipation, and when recommended by a physician, for chronic constipation and constipation associated with irritable bowel syndrome, diverticulosis, hemorrhoids, convalescence, senility and pregnancy. Pregnancy: Category B. If considering use of Metamucil as part of a cholesterol-lowering program, see **Metamucil Dietary Fiber Supplement** in Dietary Supplement Section.

Drug Facts

Active Ingredient:

(in each DOSE) Purpose:

Psyllium husk
approximately 3.4 g .... Fiber therapy for regularity

For Metamucil capsules each dose of 5 capsules contains approximately 2.6 gm of psyllium husk.

USES

- effective in treating occasional constipation and restoring regularity

WARNINGS

Choking: Taking this product without adequate fluid may cause it to swell and block your throat or esophagus and may cause choking. Do not take this product if you have difficulty in swallowing. If you experience chest pain, vomiting, or difficulty in swallowing or breathing after taking this product, seek immediate medical attention.

Allergy alert: This product may cause allergic reaction in people sensitive to inhaled or ingested psyllium.

Ask a doctor before use if you have:

- a sudden change in bowel habits persisting for 2 weeks
- abdominal pain, nausea or vomiting

Stop use and ask a doctor if:

- constipation lasts more than 7 days
- rectal bleeding occurs

These may be signs of a serious condition.

Keep out of reach of children. In case of overdose, get medical help or contact a Poison Control Center right away.

DIRECTIONS

For Powders: Put one dose into an empty glass. Fill glass with at least 8 oz of water or your favorite beverage. Stir briskly and drink promptly. If mixture thickens, add more liquid and stir. Mix this product (child or adult dose) with at least 8 ounces (a full glass) of water or other fluid. For capsules: Take product with 8 oz of liquid (swallow 1 capsule at a time) up to 3 times daily. Take this product with at least 8 oz (a full glass) of liquid. For Wafers: Take this product (child or adult dose) with at least 8 ounces (a full glass) of liquid. Taking these products without enough liquid may cause choking. See choking warning.

Adults 12 yrs. & older	Powders: 1 dose in 8 oz of liquid. Capsules: 5 capsules with 8 oz of liquid (swallow one capsule at a time). Wafers: 1 dose with 8 oz of liquid. Take at the first sign of irregularity; can be taken up to 3 times daily. Generally produces effect in 12 – 72 hours.
6 – 11 yrs.	Powders: ½ adult dose in 8 oz of liquid. Wafers: 1 wafer with 8 oz of liquid. Can be taken up to 3 times daily. Capsules: consider use of powder or wafer products
Under 6 yrs.	consult a doctor

Laxatives, including bulk fibers, may affect how well other medicines work. If you are taking a prescription medicine by mouth, take this product at least 2 hours before or 2 hours after the prescribed medicine. As your body adjusts to increased fiber intake, you may experience changes in bowel habits or minor bloating. **New Users:** Start with 1 dose per day; gradually increase to 3 doses per day as necessary.

Other Information:

- **Each product contains:** sodium (See table for amount/dose)
- **PHENYLKETONURICS: Smooth Texture Sugar Free Orange product contains phenylalanine** 25 mg per dose
- Each product contains a 100% natural, therapeutic fiber

Inactive Ingredients: See tableNotice to Health Care Professionals:

To minimize the potential for allergic reaction, health care professionals who frequently dispense powdered psyllium products should avoid inhaling airborne dust while dispensing these products.

Handling and Dispensing: To minimize generating airborne dust, spoon product from the canister into a glass according to label directions.

HOW SUPPLIED

Powder: canisters and cartons of single-dose packets. Capsules: 100, 160 and 300 count bottles. Wafers: cartons of single dose packets. (See table)

[See table below]

***Questions?* 1-800-983-4237**

Continued on next page

Metamucil Fiber Laxative/Dietary Fiber Supplement

Versions/Flavors	Ingredients (alphabetical order)	Sodium mg/ dose	Calcium mg/ dose	Potassium mg/ dose	Calories kcal/ dose	Total Carbohydrate g/dose	Dietary Fiber/ (Soluble) g/dose	Dosage (Weight in gms)	How Supplied
Smooth Texture Orange Flavor Metamucil Powder	Citric Acid, FD&C Yellow #6, Natural and Artificial Flavor, Psyllium Husk, Sucrose	5	7	30	45	12	3 (2.4)	1 rounded tablespoon ~12g	Canisters: Doses: 48, 72, 114; Cartons: 30 single-dose packets.
Smooth Texture Sugar-Free Orange Flavor Metamucil Powder	Aspartame, Citric Acid, FD&C Yellow #6, Maltodextrin, Natural and Artificial Flavor, Psyllium Husk	5	7	30	20	5	3 (2.4)	1 rounded teaspoon ~5.8g	Canisters: Doses: 30, 48, 72, 114, 180; Cartons: 30 single-dose packets.
Smooth Texture Sugar-Free Unflavored Metamucil Powder	Citric Acid, Maltodextrin, Psyllium Husk	4	7	30	20	5	3 (2.4)	1 rounded teaspoon ~5.4g	Canisters: Doses: 48, 72 114.
Coarse Milled Unflavored Metamucil Powder	Psyllium Husk, Sucrose	3	6	30	25	7	3 (2.4)	1 rounded teaspoon ~7g	Canisters: Doses: 48, 72 114.
Coarse Milled Orange Flavor Metamucil Powder	Citric Acid, FD&C Yellow #6, Natural and Artificial Flavor, Psyllium Husk, Sucrose	5	6	30	40	11	3 (2.4)	1 rounded tablespoon ~11g	Canisters: Doses: 48,72 114.
Metamucil Capsules	Caramel color, FD&C Blue No. 1 Aluminum Lake, FD&C Red No. 40 Aluminum Lake, FD&C Yellow No. 6 Aluminum Lake, gelatin, polysorbate 80, psyllium husk	0	5	0	10	3	3 (2.4)	6 capsules 3.2g	Bottles: 100 ct, 160 ct, 300 ct
Fiber Laxative Wafers									
Apple Metamucil Wafers	(1)	20	14	60	120	17	6	2 wafers 24 g	Cartons: 12 doses
Cinnamon Metamucil Wafers	(2)	20	14	60	120	17	6	2 wafers 24 g	Cartons: 12 doses

(1) ascorbic acid, brown sugar, cinnamon, corn oil, corn starch, fructose, lecithin, molasses, natural and artificial flavors, oat hull fiber, psyllium husk, sodium bicarbonate, sucrose, water, wheat flour

(2) ascorbic acid, cinnamon, corn oil, corn starch, fructose, lecithin, molasses, natural and artificial flavors, nutmeg, oat hull fiber, oats, psyllium husk, sodium bicarbonate, sucrose, water, wheat flour

PEDIATRIC VICKS® 44e® OTC

Cough & Chest Congestion Relief
Cough suppressant/Expectorant

- Non-drowsy
- Alcohol-free
- Aspirin-free

Drug Facts:

ACTIVE INGREDIENTS

(per 15 ml tablespoon) Purpose:
Dextromethorphan
HBr 10 mg .... Cough suppressant
Guaifenesin 100mg .... Expectorant

USES

- temporarily relieves cough due to the common cold
- helps loosen phlegm and thin bronchial secretions to rid bronchial passageways of bothersome mucus

WARNINGS

Do not use

- if you are now taking a prescription monoamine oxidase inhibitor (MAOI) (certain drugs for depression, psychiatric or emotional conditions, or Parkinson's disease), or for 2 weeks after stopping the MAOI drug. If you do not know if your prescription drug contains an MAOI, ask a doctor or pharmacist before taking this product.

Ask a doctor before use if you have:

- a sodium restricted diet
- cough that occurs with too much phlegm (mucus)
- persistent or chronic cough such as occurs with smoking, asthma, chronic bronchitis or emphysema

Stop use and ask a doctor if:

- cough lasts more than 7 days, comes back, or occurs with fever, rash, or headache that lasts. These could be signs of a serious condition.

If pregnant or breast-feeding, ask a health professional before use.

Keep out of reach of children. In case of overdose, get medical help or contact a Poison Control Center right away.

DIRECTIONS

- use tablespoon (TBSP) or dose cup
- do not exceed 6 doses per 24 hours

Under 2 yrs.	ask a doctor
2–5 yrs.	½ TBSP (7½ ml) every 4 hours
6–11 yrs.	1 TBSP (15 ml) every 4 hours
12 yrs.& older	2 TBSP (30 ml) every 4 hours

OTHER INFORMATION

- **each tablespoon contains** sodium 30 mg
- store at room temperature

INACTIVE INGREDIENTS

Carboxymethylcellulose sodium, citric acid, FD&C red no. 40, flavor, high fructose corn syrup, polyethylene oxide, polyoxyl 40 stearate, propylene glycol, purified water, saccharin sodium, sodium benzoate, sodium citrate.

HOW SUPPLIED

4 FL OZ (118 ml) plastic bottles. A calibrated dose cup accompanies each bottle.

TAMPER EVIDENT: Do not use if imprinted shrinkband is missing or broken.

***Questions?* 1-800-342-6844 www.vicks.com**

Dist. by Procter & Gamble, Cincinnati OH 45202.
US Pat 5,458,879 42434802

PEDIATRIC VICKS® 44m® OTC

Cough & Cold Relief
Cough Suppressant/Nasal Decongestant/Antihistamine

- Alcohol-free
- Aspirin-free

Drug Facts:

ACTIVE INGREDIENTS

(per 15 ml tablespoon) Purpose:
Chlorpheniramine maleate
2 mg .... Antihistamine
Dextromethorphan HBr
15 mg .... Cough suppressant
Pseudoephedrine HCl
30 mg .... Nasal decongestant

USES

Temporarily relieves cough/cold symptoms

- cough
- sneezing
- runny nose
- nasal congestion

WARNINGS

Failure to follow these warnings could result in serious consequences.

Do not use:

- if you are now taking a prescription monoamine oxidase inhibitor (MAOI) (certain drugs for depression, psychiatric or emotional conditions, or Parkinson's disease), or for 2 weeks after stopping the MAOI drug. If you do not know if your prescription drug contains an MAOI, ask a doctor or pharmacist before taking this product.

Ask a doctor before use if you have:

- heart disease
- a sodium restricted diet
- a breathing problem or chronic cough that lasts or occurs with smoking, asthma, chronic bronchitis or emphysema
- thyroid disease
- diabetes
- glaucoma
- high blood pressure
- cough that occurs with too much phlegm (mucus)
- trouble urinating due to enlarged prostate gland

Ask a doctor or pharmicist before use if you are taking sedatives or tranquilizers.

When using this product:

- **do not use more than directed**
- excitability may occur, especially in children
- drowsiness may occur
- avoid alcoholic drinks
- be careful when driving a motor vehicle or operating machinery
- alcohol, sedatives, and tranquilizers may increase drowsiness

Stop use and ask a doctor if:

- you get nervous, dizzy or sleepless
- symptoms do not get better within 7 days or are accompanied by a fever.
- cough last more than 7 days, comes back, or occurs with fever, rash, or headache that lasts
These could be signs of a serious condition.

If pregnant or breast-feeding, ask a health professional before use.

Keep out of reach of children. In case of overdose, get medical help or contact a Poison Control Center right away.

DIRECTIONS

- use tablespoon (TBSP) or dose cup
- do not exceed 4 doses per 24 hours

Under 6 yrs.	ask a doctor
6–11 yrs.	1 TBSP or 15 ml every 6 hours
12 yrs. & older	2 TBSP or 30 ml every 6 hours

OTHER INFORMATION

- **each tablespoon contains** sodium 30 mg
- store at room temperature

INACTIVE INGREDIENTS

Carboxymethylcellulose sodium, citric acid, FD&C red 40, flavor, high fructose corn syrup, polyethylene oxide, polyoxyl 40 stearate, propylene glycol, purified water, saccharin sodium, sodium benzoate, sodium citrate.

HOW SUPPLIED

4 FL OZ (118 ml) plastic bottles. A calibrated dose cup accompanies each bottle.

TAMPER EVIDENT: Do not use if imprinted shrinkband is missing or broken.

***Questions?* 1-800-342-6844 www.vicks.com**

Dist. by Procter & Gamble, Cincinnati OH 45202.
US Pat 5,458,879 42434743

PEPTO-BISMOL® OTC

ORIGINAL LIQUID,
MAXIMUM STRENGTH LIQUID,
ORIGINAL AND CHERRY FLAVOR CHEWABLE TABLETS
AND EASY-TO-SWALLOW CAPLETS
For upset stomach, indigestion, heartburn, nausea and diarrhea.

Multi-symptom Pepto-Bismol® contains bismuth subsalicylate and is the only leading OTC stomach remedy clinically proven effective for both upper and lower GI symptoms. It has been clinically proven in double-blind placebo-controlled trials for relief of upset stomach symptoms and diarrhea.

ACTIVE INGREDIENT

(per tablespoon/per tablet/per caplet)
Original Liquid/Tablets/Caplets
Bismuth subsalicylate 262 mg
Maximum Strength Liquid
Bismuth subsalicylate 525 mg

INACTIVE INGREDIENTS

[Original Liquid] benzoic acid, flavor, magnesium aluminum silicate, methylcellulose, red 22, red 28, saccharin sodium, salicylic acid, sodium salicylate, sorbic acid, water

[Maximum Strength Liquid] benzoic acid, flavor, magnesium aluminum silicate, methylcellulose, red 22, red 28, saccharin sodium, salicylic acid, sodium salicylate, sorbic acid, water

[Original Tablets] calcium carbonate, flavor, magnesium stearate, mannitol, povidone, red 27 aluminum lake, saccharin sodium, talc

[Cherry Tablets] adipic acid, calcium carbonate, flavor, magnesium stearate, mannitol, povidone, red 27 aluminum lake, red 40 aluminum lake, saccharin sodium, talc

[Caplets] calcium carbonate, magnesium stearate, mannitol, microcrystalline cellulose, polysorbate 80, povidone, red 27 aluminum lake, silicon dioxide, sodium starch glycolate.

Other Information:

Sodium Content
Original Liquid—each Tbsp contains: sodium 6 mg • low sodium
Maximum Strength Liquid—each Tbsp contains: sodium 6 mg • low sodium
Chewable Tablets—each Original or Cherry Flavor Tablet contains: sodium less than 1 mg • very low sodium
Caplets—each Caplet contains: sodium 2 mg • low sodium

Salicylate Content
Original Liquid—each Tbsp contains: salicylate 130 mg
Maximum Strength Liquid—each Tbsp contains: salicylate 236 mg
Chewable Tablets—each tablet contains:
[original] salicylate 102 mg
[cherry] salicylate 99 mg
Caplets—each caplet contains: salicylate 99 mg
All Forms are sugar free.

INDICATIONS

- relieves upset stomach symptoms (i.e., indigestion, heartburn, nausea and fullness caused by over-indulgence in food and drink) without constipating; and,
- controls diarrhea.

ACTIONS

For upset stomach symptoms, the active ingredient is believed to work via a topical effect on the stomach mucosa. For diarrhea, it is believed to work by several mechanisms in the gastrointestinal tract, including: 1) normalizing fluid movement via an antisecretory merchanism, 2) binding bacterial toxins and 3) antimicrobial activity.

WARNINGS

Reye's syndrome: Children and teenagers who have or are recovering from chicken pox or flu-like symptoms should not use this product. When using this product, if changes in behavior with nausea and vomiting occur, consult a doctor because these symptoms could be an early sign of Reye's syndrome, a rare but serious illness.

Allergy alert: Contains salicylate. Do not take if you are

- allergic to salicylates (including aspirin)
- taking other salicylate products

Do not use if you have

- an ulcer
- a bleeding problem
- bloody or black stool

Ask a doctor before use if you have

- fever
- mucus in the stool

Ask a doctor or pharmacist before use if you are taking any drug for

- anticoagulation (thinning the blood)
- diabetes
- gout
- arthritis

When using this product a temporary, but harmless, darkening of the stool and/or tongue may occur

Stop use and ask a doctor if

- symptoms get worse
- ringing in the ears or loss of hearing occurs
- diarrhea lasts more than 2 days

If pregnant or breast feeding, ask a health professional before use.

Keep out of reach of children. In case of overdose, get medical help or contact a Poison Control Center right away.

Notes: May cause a temporary and harmless darkening of the tongue or stool. Stool darkening should not be confused with melena.

While no lead is intentionally added to Pepto-Bismol, this product contains certain ingredients that are mined from the ground and thus contain small amounts of naturally occurring lead. For example, bismuth, contained in the active ingredient of Pepto-Bismol, is mined and therefore contains some naturally occurring lead. The small amounts of naturally occurring lead in Pepto-Bismol are low in comparison to average daily lead exposure; this is for the information of healthcare professionals. Pepto-Bismol is indicated for treatment of acute upset stomach symptoms and diarrhea. It is not intended for chronic use.

OVERDOSAGE

In case of overdose, patients are advised to contact a physician or Poison Control Center. Emesis induced by ipecac syrup is indicated in large ingestions provided ipecac can be administered within one hour of ingestion. Activated charcoal should be administered after gastric emptying. Patients should be evaluated for signs and symptoms of salicylate toxicity.

DIRECTIONS

Pepto-Bismol® Original Liquid, Original & Cherry Flavor Chewable Tablets, and Caplets

[Original Liquid]

- shake well before using
- for accurate dosing, use dose cup

[Original Tablet, Cherry Tablets]

- chew or dissolve in mouth

[Caplets]

- swallow with water, do not chew

- adults and children 12 years and over: 1 dose (2 Tbsp or 30 ml; 2 tablets or 2 caplets) every 1/2 to 1 hour as needed
- do not exceed 8 doses (16 Tbsp or 240 ml) in 24 hours
- use until diarrhea stops but not more than 2 days
- children under 12 years: ask a doctor
- drink plenty of clear fluids to help prevent dehydration caused by diarrhea

Pepto-Bismol® Maximum Strength Liquid
- shake well before use
- for accurate dosing, use dose cup
- adults and children 12 years and over: 1 dose (2 Tbsp 30 ml) every 1 hour as needed
- do not exceed 4 doses (8 Tbsp or 120 ml) in 24 hours
- use until diarrhea stops but not more than 2 days
- children under 12 years: ask a doctor
- drink plenty of clear fluids to help prevent dehydration caused by diarrhea

HOW SUPPLIED

Pepto-Bismol® Original and Maximum Strength Liquids are pink. Pepto-Bismol® Original Liquid is available in: 4, 8, 12 and 16 fl oz bottles. Pepto-Bismol® Maximum Strength Liquid is available in: 4, 8 and 12 fl oz bottles. Pepto-Bismol® Original and Cherry Flavor Tablets are pink, round, chewable tablets imprinted with a debossed triangle and "Pepto-Bismol" on one side. Tablets are available in: boxes of 30 and 48. Pepto-Bismol® Caplets are pink and imprinted with "Pepto-Bismol" on one side. Caplets are available in bottles of 24 and 40.
- avoid excessive heat (over 104°F or 40°C)
- protect liquids from freezing

Questions: 1-800-717-3786
www.pepto-bismol.com

PRILOSEC OTC™ OTC

[prī-lō-sĕk]
Acid Reducer
(Procter & Gamble)

Drug Facts:

ACTIVE INGREDIENTS

Omeprazole magnesium delayed-release tablet 20.6 mg (equivalent to 20 mg omeprazole)

USES
- treats frequent heartburn (occurs 2 or more days a week)
- not intended for immediate relief of heartburn; this drug may take 1 to 4 days for full effect

WARNINGS

Allergy Alert: Do not use if you are allergic to omeprazole

Do not use if you have
- trouble or pain swallowing food
- vomiting with blood
- bloody or black stools

These may be signs of a serious condition. See your doctor.

Ask a doctor before use if you have
- had heartburn over 3 months. This may be a sign of a more serious condition.
- heartburn **with lightheadedness, sweating or dizziness**
- chest pain or shoulder pain with shortness of breath; sweating; pain spreading to arms, neck or shoulders; or lightheadedness
- frequent **chest pain**
- frequent wheezing, particularly with heartburn
- unexplained weight loss
- nausea or vomiting
- stomach pain

Ask a doctor or pharmacist before use if you are taking
- warfarin (blood-thinning medicine)
- prescription antifungal or anti-yeast medicines
- diazepam (anxiety medicine)
- digoxin (heart medicine)

Stop use and ask a doctor if
- your heartburn continues or worsens
- you need to take this product for more than 14 days
- you need to take more than 1 course of treatment every 4 months

If pregnant or breast feeding, ask a health professional before use.

Keep out of reach of children. In case of overdose, get medical help or contact a Poison Control Center right away.

DIRECTIONS
- adults 18 years of age and older
- this product is to be used once a day (every 24 hours), every day for 14 days
- it may take 1 to 4 days for full effect, although some people get complete relief of symptoms within 24 hours

14-Day Course of Treatment
- swallow 1 tablet with a glass of water before eating in the morning
- take every day for 14 days
- do not take more than 1 tablet a day
- do not chew or crush the tablets
- do not crush tablets in food
- do not use for more than 14 days unless directed by your doctor

Repeated 14-Day Courses (if needed)
- you may repeat a 14-day course every 4 months
- **do not take for more than 14 days or more often than every 4 months unless directed by a doctor**
- children under 18 years of age: ask a doctor

OTHER INFORMATION
- read the directions, warnings and package insert before use
- keep the carton and package insert. They contain important information.
- store at 20-25°C (68-77°F)
- keep product out of high heat and humidity
- protect product from moisture

INACTIVE INGREDIENTS

Glyceryl monostearate, hydroxypropyl cellulose, hypromellose, iron oxide, magnesium stearate, methacrylic acid copolymer, microcrystalline cellulose, paraffin, polyethylene glycol 6000, polysorbate 80, polyvinylpyrrolidone, sodium stearate fumarate, starch, sucrose, talc, titanium dioxide, triethyl citrate

HOW SUPPLIED

Available in: 2-count child-resistant sample pouches and 14-count, 28-count and 42-count boxes containing child-resistant blister-packs (1, 2, and 3 14 day courses of treatment, respectively). Tablets are pink with a *P* debossing.

Questions: 1-800-289-9181
Manufactured by AstraZeneca
Dist. by Procter & Gamble, Cincinnatil OH 45202

THERMACARE® OTC

[thərm' ă-kār]
Therapeutic Heat Wraps
with Air-Activated Heat Discs

USES

Back/Hip Wrap: Provides temporary relief of minor muscular back aches and pains associated with overexertion, joint strains, sprains, and arthritis.
Neck to Arm Wrap: Provides temporary relief of minor muscular and joint aches and pains associated with overexertion, strains, sprains and arthritis.
Menstrual Patch: Provides temporary relief of minor menstrual cramp pain and associated back ache.

WARNINGS

Do not microwave or attempt to reheat this product to avoid risk of fire. This product has the potential to cause skin irritation or burns. Heat discs contain iron (~2 grams) which can be harmful if ingested. If ingested, rinse mouth with water and call a Poison Control Center right away. If the heat disc contents contact your skin or eyes, rinse right away with water.

Do not use: On broken or damaged skin
- with medicated lotions, creams, or ointments
- on areas of bruising or swelling that have occurred within 48 hours
- on people unable to remove the product, including children and infants
- on areas of the body where heat cannot be felt
- with other forms of heat.

Ask a doctor before use if you have diabetes, poor circulation, rheumatoid arthritis or are pregnant.

When using this product: It is normal to experience temporary skin redness after removing the wrap. If your skin is still red after a few hours, stop using ThermaCare until the redness goes away completely. To reduce the risk of prolonged redness in the future, we recommend you: (a) wear for a shorter period of time, (b) wear looser clothing over wrap, (c) wear over a thin layer of clothing
- Periodically check your skin: (a) if your skin is sensitive to heat, (b) if your tolerance to heat has decreased over the years, (c) when wearing a tight fitting belt or waistband
- Consider wearing during the day before deciding to use during sleep.

Stop use and ask a doctor if:
- after 7 days of product use (4 days for menstrual product) the pain you are treating gets worse or remains unchanged. This could be a sign of a more serious condition
- you experience any discomfort, swelling, rash or other changes in your skin that persist where the wrap is worn

Keep out of reach of children and pets.

For maximum effectiveness, we recommend you wear ThermaCare for 8 hours. Do not use for more than 8 hours in any 24 hour period.

DIRECTIONS

Tear open the pouch when ready to use. It may take up to 30 minutes for ThermaCare to reach its therapeutic temperature. For maximum effectiveness, we recommend you wear ThermaCare for the full 8 hours. Do not use for more than 8 hours in any 24 hour period OR for more than 7 days in a row (4 days in a row for menstrual product).

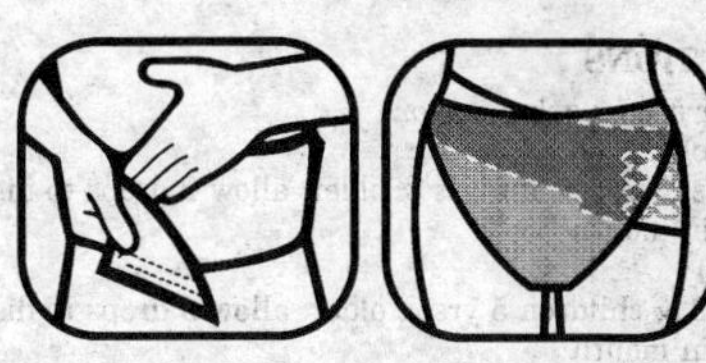

Place on pain area on lower back or hip with darker discs toward skin. Attach firmly.

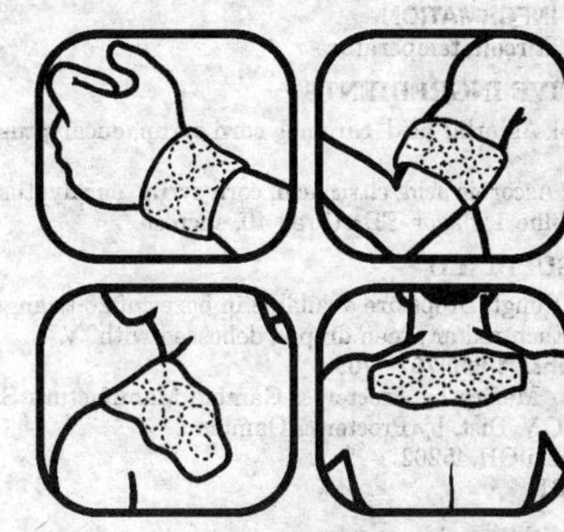

Peel away paper to reveal adhesive side. Place on pain area with adhesive side toward skin. Attach firmly.

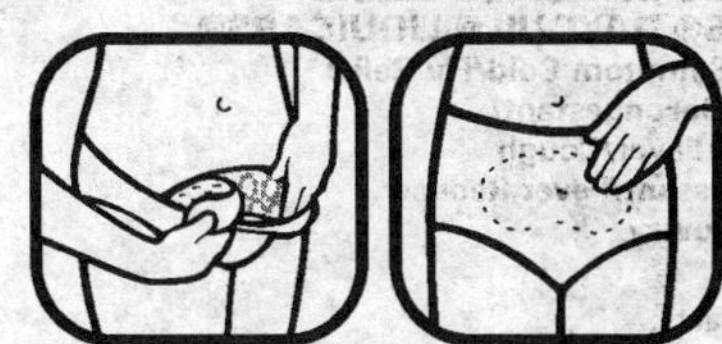

Peel away paper to reveal adhesive side. Place on pain area with adhesive side toward panties. Attach firmly.

HOW SUPPLIED

Back/Hip Wrap: Available in trial size of 1 L/XL or in boxes of 2 S/M or L/XL wraps.
Neck to Arm: Available in boxes of 3 wraps.
Menstrual: Available in boxes of 3 patches.

INGREDIENTS

Heat cells contain activated charcoal, iron powder, sodium chloride, sodium thiosulfate and water.

VICKS® Cough Drops OTC

Menthol Cough Suppressant/Oral Anesthetic
Menthol and Cherry Flavors

CONSUMER INFORMATION: Vicks Cough Drops provide fast and effective relief. Each drop contains effective medicine to suppress your impulse to cough as it dissolves into a soothing syrup to relieve your sore throat.

Drug Facts:

ACTIVE INGREDIENT

Menthol:

ACTIVE INGREDIENT (per drop)	**Purpose:**
Menthol flavor	
Menthol 3.3 mg	Cough suppressant/ oral anesthetic

Cherry flavor:

ACTIVE INGREDIENT (per drop)	**Purpose:**
Menthol 1.7 mg	Cough suppressant/ oral anesthetic

USES

Temporarily relieves:
- sore throat
- coughs due to colds or inhaled irritants

WARNINGS

Ask a doctor before use if you have:
- cough associated with excessive phlegm (mucus)
- persistent or chronic cough such as those caused by asthma, emphysema, or smoking
- a severe sore throat accompanied by difficulty in breathing or that lasts more than 2 days
- a sore throat accompanied or followed by fever, headache, rash, swelling, nausea or vomiting

Stop use and ask a doctor if:
- you need to use more than 7 days
- cough lasts more than 7 days, comes back, or occurs with fever, rash, or headache that lasts. These could be the signs of a serious condition.

If pregnant or breast-feeding, ask a health professional before use.

Keep out of reach of children.

Continued on next page

Vicks Cough Drops—Cont.

DIRECTIONS

- under 5 yrs.: ask a doctor

(menthol)

- adults & children 5 yrs & older: allow 2 drops to dissolve slowly in mouth

(cherry)

- adults & children 5 yrs & older: allow 3 drops to dissolve slowly in mouth

Cough: may be repeated every hour.
Sore Throat: may be repeated every 2 hours.

OTHER INFORMATION

- store at room temperature

INACTIVE INGREDIENTS

Menthol: Ascorbic acid, caramel, corn syrup, eucalyptus oil, sucrose.
Cherry: Ascorbic acid, citric acid, corn syrup, eucalyptus oil, FD&C blue 1, flavor, FD&C red 40, sucrose.

HOW SUPPLIED

Vicks® Cough Drops are available in boxes of 20 triangular drops. Each red or green drop is debossed with "V."
Questions? 1-800-707-1709
Made in Mexico by Procter & Gamble Manufactura S. de R.I. de C.V. Dist. by Procter & Gamble
Cincinnati OH 45202
50144381

VICKS® DAYQUIL® LIQUID OTC
VICKS® DAYQUIL® LIQUICAPS® OTC

Multi-Symptom Cold/Flu Relief
Nasal Decongestant/
Pain Reliever/Cough
Suppressant/Fever Reducer
Non-drowsy

Drug Facts:

ACTIVE INGREDIENTS

LIQUID:

ACTIVE INGREDIENTS **Purpose:**

(per 15 ml tablespoon)
Acetaminophen
325 mg .... Pain reliever/fever reducer
Dextromethorphan HBr
15 mg .... Cough suppressant
Pseudoephedrine HCl
30 mg .... Nasal decongestant

LIQUICAP®:

ACTIVE INGREDIENTS **Purpose:**

(per softgel)
Acetaminophen
325 mg .... Pain reliever/fever reducer
Dextromethorphan HBr
15 mg .... Cough suppressant
Pseudoephedrine HCl
30 mg .... Nasal decongestant

USES

Temporarily relieves common cold/flu symptoms:

- nasal congestion
- cough due to minor throat and bronchial irritation
- sore throat
- headache
- minor aches and pains
- fever

WARNINGS

Failure to follow these warnings could result in serious consequences.
Alcohol warning: If you consume 3 or more alcoholic drinks every day, ask your doctor whether you should take acetaminophen or other pain relievers/fever reducers. Acetaminophen may cause liver damage.
Sore throat warning: If sore throat is severe, persists more than 2 days, is accompanied by fever, nausea, rash or vomiting, consult a doctor promptly.
Do not use • with other medicines containing acetaminophen • if you are now taking a prescription monoamine oxidase inhibitor (MAOI) (certain drugs for depression, psychiatric or emotional conditions, or Parkinson's disease), or for 2 weeks after stopping the MAOI drug. If you do not know if your prescription drug contains an MAOI, ask a doctor or pharmacist before taking this product.
Ask a doctor before use if you have:

- heart disease
- thyroid disease
- diabetes
- persistent or chronic cough such as occurs with smoking, asthma, or emphysema
- high blood pressure
- cough that occurs with too much phlegm (mucus)
- trouble urinating due to enlarged prostate gland
- sodium-restricted diet (Specific to DayQuil Liquid only)

When using this product:

- **do not use more than directed**

Stop use and ask a doctor if:

- you get nervous, dizzy or sleepless
- fever gets worse or lasts more than 3 days
- new symptoms occur
- redness or swelling is present
- symptoms do not get better within 7 days or are accompanied by a fever
- cough lasts more than 7 days, comes back, or occurs with fever, rash, or headache that lasts. These could be the signs of a serious condition.

If pregnant or breast-feeding, ask a health professional before use.
Keep out of reach of children. Overdose warning: Taking more than the recommended dose can cause serious health problems. In case of overdose, get medical help or contact a Poison Control Center right away. Quick medical attention is critical for adults as well as for children even if you do not notice any signs or symptoms.

DIRECTIONS

- take only as recommended – see Overdose warning

LIQUID:

- use tablespoon (TBSP) or dose cup
- do not exceed 4 doses per 24 hours

Children under 12 years .... ask a doctor
12 yrs. & older .... 2 TBSP or 30 ml
every 6 hours

- If taking NyQuil® and DayQuil, limit total to 4 doses per 24 hours.

LIQUICAP:

- take only as recommended – see **Overdose Warning**
- do not exceed 4 doses per 24 hours

Children under 12 years .... ask a doctor
12 yrs. & older .... 2 softgels with water
every 6 hours

- If taking NyQuil® and DayQuil, limit total to 4 doses per 24 hours.

OTHER INFORMATION

LIQUID:

- **each tablespoon contains** sodium 71 mg
- store at room temperature

LIQUICAP:

- store at room temperature

INACTIVE INGREDIENTS

LIQUID: Citric acid, FD&C yellow 6, flavor, glycerin, polyethylene glycol, propylene glycol, purified water, saccharin sodium, sodium citrate, sucrose.
LIQUICAP: FD&C red 40, FD&C yellow 6, gelatin, glycerin, polyethylene glycol, povidone, propylene glycol, purified water, sorbitol special.

HOW SUPPLIED

Available in: **LIQUID** 6 FL OZ (177 ml) and 10 FL OZ (295 ml) plastic bottles with child-resistant, tamper-evident cap and a calibrated medicine cup.
LIQUICAP: in 2-count, 12-count 40-count and 60-count child-resistant packages and 20-nonchild-resistant packages. Each softgel is imprinted: "DayQ"
LIQUID:
TAMPER EVIDENT: Do not use if imprinted shrinkband is missing or broken.
LIQUICAP, 12-count, 40-count and 60-count
TAMPER EVIDENT: This package is safety sealed and child resistant. Use only if blisters are intact. If difficult to open, use scissors.
LIQUICAP, 20-count:
This Package for households without young children.
TAMPER EVIDENT: Use only if blisters are intact. If difficult to open, use scissors.
***Questions?* 1-800-251-3374** www.vicks.com
Made in Canada
Dist. by Procter & Gamble
Cincinnati OH 45202
42435018

VICKS® 44® COUGH RELIEF OTC

Dextromethorphan HBr/
Cough Suppressant
Alcohol 5%

- Maximum Strength
- Non-Drowsy
- For Adults & Children

Drug Facts:

ACTIVE INGREDIENT

(per 15 ml tablespoon) **Purpose**
Dextromethorphan HBr
30 mg .... Cough suppressant

USES

Temporarily relieves cough due to minor throat and bronchial irritation associated with a cold

WARNING

Do not use if you are now taking a prescription monoamine oxidase inhibitor (MAOI) (certain drugs for depression, psychiatric or emotional conditions, or Parkinson's disease), or for 2 weeks after stopping the MAOI drug. If you do not know if your prescription drug contains an MAOI, ask a doctor or pharmacist before taking this product.
Ask a doctor before use if you have:

- cough that occurs with too much phlegm (mucus)
- persistent or chronic cough such as occurs with smoking, asthma, or emphysema

Stop use and ask a doctor if:

- cough lasts more than 7 days, comes back, or occurs with fever, rash, or headache that lasts. These could be signs of a serious condition.

If pregnant or breast feeding, ask a health professional before use.
Keep out of reach of children. In case of overdose, get medical help or contact a Poison Control Center right away.

DIRECTIONS

- use teaspoon (tsp), tablespoon (TBSP) or dose cup
- do not exceed 4 doses per 24 hours

Under 6 yrs. .... ask a doctor
6–11 yrs. .... 1½ tsp (7½ ml)
every 6-8 hours
12 yrs. & older .... 1 TBSP (15 ml)
every 6-8 hours

OTHER INFORMATION

- **each tablespoon contains** sodium 31 mg
- store at room temperature

INACTIVE INGREDIENTS

Alcohol, FD&C blue no.1, FD&C red 40, carboxymethylcellulose sodium, citric acid, flavor, high fructose corn syrup, polyethylene oxide, polyoxyl 40 stearate, propylene glycol, purified water, saccharin sodium, sodium benzoate, sodium citrate.

HOW SUPPLIED

Available in 4 FL OZ (118 ml) 6 FL OZ (177 ml) plastic bottle. A calibrated dose cup accompanies each bottle.
TAMPER EVIDENT: Do not use if imprinted shrinkband is missing or broken.
Questions? 1-800-342-6844 www.vicks.com
Dist. by Procter & Gamble, Cincinnati, OH 45202.
US Pat 5,458,879 42434792

VICKS® 44D® OTC

COUGH & HEAD CONGESTION RELIEF
Cough Suppressant/
Nasal Decongestant
Alcohol 5%

- Maximum Strength
- Non-Drowsy
- For Adults & Children

Drug Facts:

ACTIVE INGREDIENTS

(per 15 ml tablespoon) **Purpose:**
Dextromethorphan HBr
30 mg .... Cough suppressant
Pseudoephedrine HCl
60 mg .... Nasal decongestant

USES

Temporarily relieves these cold symptoms

- cough
- nasal congestion

WARNINGS

Failure to follow these warnings could result in serious consequences.
Do not use if you are now taking a prescription monoamine oxidase inhibitor (MAOI) (certain drugs for depression, psychiatric or emotional conditions, or Parkinson's disease), or for 2 weeks after stopping the MAOI drug. If you do not know if your prescription drug contains an MAOI, ask a doctor or pharmacist before taking this product.
Ask a doctor before use if you have:

- heart disease
- cough that lasts or is chronic such as occurs with smoking, asthma, or emphysema
- thyroid disease
- diabetes
- high blood pressure
- cough that occurs with too much phlegm (mucus)
- trouble urinating due to enlarged prostate gland

When using this product do not take more than directed.
Stop use and ask a doctor if:

- symptoms do not get better within 7 days or are accompanied by fever.
- you get nervous, dizzy or sleepless
- cough lasts more than 7 days, comes back, or occurs with fever, rash, or headache that lasts.
These could be signs of a serious condition.

If pregnant or breast-feeding, ask a health professional before use.
Keep out of reach of children. In case of overdose, get medical help or contact a Poison Control Center right away.

DIRECTIONS

- use teaspoon (tsp), tablespoon (TBSP) or dose cup
- do not exceed 4 doses in a 24 hour period

Under 6 yrs. .... ask a doctor
6–11 yrs. .... $1^1/_2$ tsp ($7^1/_2$ ml)
every 6 hours
12 yrs. & older .... 1 TBSP (15 ml)
every 6 hours

OTHER INFORMATION

- **each tablespoonful contains** sodium 31 mg
- store at room temperature

Inactive Ingredients: Alcohol, FD&C blue no. 1, carboxymethylcellulose sodium, citric acid, flavor, high fructose corn syrup, polyethylene oxide, polyoxyl 40 stearate, propylene glycol, purified water, FD&C red no. 40, saccharin sodium, sodium benzoate, sodium citrate.

HOW SUPPLIED

Available in 1 FL OZ (30 ml) 4 FL OZ (118 ml) 6 FL OZ (177 ml) and 8 FL OZ (236 ml) plastic bottles. A calibrated dose cup accompanies each bottle.

TAMPER EVIDENT: Do not use if imprinted shrinkband is missing or broken.

Question? 1-800-342-6844 www.vicks.com

Dist. by Procter & Gamble, Cincinnati OH 45202.

US Pat 5,458,879 42434796

Shown in Product Identification Guide, page 522

VICKS® 44E® OTC

Cough & Chest Congestion Relief
Cough Suppressant/Expectorant
Alcohol 5%

- Non-Drowsy
- For Adults & Children

Drug Facts:

ACTIVE INGREDIENTS

(per 15 ml tablespoon) **Purpose:**

Dextromethorphan HBr
20 mg .... Cough suppressant

Guaifenesin
200 mg .... Expectorant

USES

- temporarily relieves cough due to the common cold
- helps loosen phlegm and thin bronchial secretions to rid the bronchial passageways of bothersome mucus

WARNINGS

Do not use

- if you are now taking a prescription monoamine oxidase inhibitor (MAOI) (certain drugs for depression, psychiatric or emotional conditions, or Parkinson's disease), or for 2 weeks after stopping the MAOI drug. If you do not know if your prescription drug contains an MAOI, ask a doctor or pharmacist before taking this product.

Ask a doctor before use if you have:

- a sodium restricted diet
- persistent or chronic cough such as occurs with smoking, asthma, chronic bronchitis or emphysema
- cough that occurs with too much phlegm (mucus)

Stop use and ask a doctor if:

- cough lasts more than 7 days, comes back, or occurs with fever, rash, or headache that lasts. These could be signs of a serious condition.

If pregnant or breast-feeding, ask a health professional before use.

Keep out of reach of children. In case of overdose, get medical help or contact a Poison Control Center right away.

DIRECTIONS

- use teaspoon (tsp), tablespoon (TBSP) or dose cup
- do not exceed 6 doses per 24 hours

Under 6 yrs.	ask a doctor
6–11 yrs.	1½ tsp (7½ ml) every 4 hours
12 yrs. & older.	1 TBSP (15 ml) every 4 hours

OTHER INFORMATION

- **each tablespoon contains** sodium 31 mg
- store at room temperature

INACTIVE INGREDIENTS

Alcohol, FD&C blue 1, carboxymethylcellulose sodium, citric acid, flavor, high fructose corn syrup, polyethylene oxide, polyoxyl 40 stearate, propylene glycol, purified water, FD&C red no. 40, saccharin sodium, sodium benzoate, sodium citrate.

HOW SUPPLIED

Available in 4 FL OZ (118 ml) 6 FL OZ (177 ml) and 8 FL OZ (236 ml) plastic bottles. A calibrated dose cup accompanies each bottle.

TAMPER EVIDENT: Do not use if imprinted shrinkband is missing or broken.

Questions? 1-800-342-6844 www.vicks.com

Dist. by Procter & Gamble, Cincinnati OH 45202.

US Pat 5,458,879 42434800

Shown in Product Identification Guide, page 522

VICKS® 44M® OTC

COUGH, COLD & FLU RELIEF
Cough Suppressant/Nasal Decongestant/Antihistamine/Pain Reliever–Fever Reducer
Alcohol 10%

Maximum strength cough formula

Drug Facts:

ACTIVE INGREDIENTS

(per 5 ml teaspoon) **Purpose:**

Acetaminophen
162.5 mg .... Pain reliever/fever reducer

Chlorpheniramine maleate
1 mg .... Antihistamine

Dextromethorphan HBr
7.5 mg .... Cough suppressant

Pseudoephedrine HCl
15 mg .... Nasal decongestant

USES

Temporarily relieves cough/cold/flu symptoms

- cough due to minor throat and bronchial irritation
- sneezing
- headache
- sore throat
- fever
- runny nose
- nasal congestion

WARNINGS

Failure to follow these warnings could result in serious consequences.

Alcohol warning If you consume 3 or more alcoholic drinks every day, ask your doctor whether you should take acetaminophen or other pain relievers/fever reducers. Acetaminophen may cause liver damage.

Sore throat warning If sore throat is severe, persists more than two days, is accompanied or followed by a fever, headache, rash, nausea or vomiting, consult a doctor promptly.

Do not use • with other medicines containing acetaminophen if you are now taking a prescription monoamine oxidase inhibitor (MAOI) (certain drugs for depression, psychiatric or emotional conditions, or Parkinson's disease), or for 2 weeks after stopping the MAOI drug. If you do not know if your prescription drug contains an MAOI, ask a doctor or pharmacist before taking this product.

Ask a doctor before use if you have:

- heart disease
- breathing problems or chronic cough such as occurs with smoking, asthma, chronic bronchitis or emphysema
- thyroid disease
- diabetes
- glaucoma
- high blood pressure
- cough that occurs with too much phlegm (mucus)
- trouble urinating due to enlarged prostate gland

Ask a doctor or pharmacist before use if you are taking sedatives or tranquilizers.

When using this product:

- **do not use more than directed**
- excitability may occur, especially in children
- drowsiness may occur
- avoid alcoholic drinks
- be careful when driving a motor vehicle or operating machinery
- alcohol, sedatives, and tranquilizers may increase drowsiness

Stop use and ask a doctor if:

- you get nervous, dizzy or sleepless
- fever gets worse or lasts more than 3 days
- new symptoms occur
- redness or swelling is present
- symptoms do not get better within 7 days or are accompanied by fever
- cough lasts more than 7 days, comes back, or occurs with fever, rash, or headache that lasts.
These could be signs of a serious condition.

If pregnant or breast-feeding, ask a health professional before use.

Keep out of reach of children.

Overdose Warning: Taking more than recommended dose can cause serious health problems. In case of overdose, get medical help or contact a Poison Control Center right away. Quick medical attention is critical for adults as well as for children even if you do not notice any signs or symptoms.

DIRECTIONS

- take only as recommended—see **Overdose Warning**
- use teaspoon or dose cup
- do not exceed 4 doses per 24 hours
- children 12 and under: ask a doctor.
- 12 yrs. & older: take 4 teaspoons (20 ml) every 6 hours.

OTHER INFORMATION

- **each teaspoon contains** sodium 8 mg
- store at room temperature

INACTIVE INGREDIENTS

Alcohol, FD&C blue 1, carboxymethylcellulose sodium, citric acid, flavor, high fructose corn syrup, polyethylene glycol, polyethylene oxide, propylene glycol, purified water, FD&C red 40, saccharin sodium, sodium citrate.

HOW SUPPLIED

Available in 4 FL OZ (118 ml) 6 FL OZ (177 ml) and 8 FL OZ (236 ml) plastic bottles. A calibrated dose cup accompanies each bottle.

TAMPER EVIDENT: Do not use if imprinted shrinkband is missing or broken.

Not recommended for children.

Questions? 1-800-342-6844 www.vicks.com

Dist. by Procter & Gamble, Cincinnati OH 45202.

US Pat 5,458,879 42434741

Shown in Product Identification Guide, page 522

VICKS® NYQUIL® COUGH OTC

Antihistamine
Cough Suppressant
All Night Cough Relief
Cherry Flavor

alcohol 10%

Drug Facts:

ACTIVE INGREDIENTS **Purpose:**

(per 15 ml tablespoon)

Dextromethorphan HBr
15 mg .... Cough suppressant

Doxylamine succinate
6.25 mg .... Antihistamine

USES

Temporarily relieves cold symptoms

- cough
- runny nose and sneezing

WARNINGS

Do not use if you are now taking a prescription monoamine oxidase inhibitor (MAOI) (certain drugs for depression, psychiatric or emotional conditions, or Parkinson's disease), or for 2 weeks after stopping the MAOI drug. If you do not know if your prescription drug contains an MAOI, ask a doctor or pharmacist before taking this product.

Ask a doctor before use if you have:

- asthma
- emphysema
- breathing problems
- excessive phlegm (mucus)
- glaucoma
- chronic bronchitis
- persistent or chronic cough
- cough associated with smoking
- trouble urinating due to enlarged prostate gland

Ask a doctor or pharmacist before use if you are: taking sedatives or tranquilizers.

When using this product:

- **do not use more than directed**
- marked drowsiness may occur
- avoid alcoholic drinks
- excitability may occur, especially in children
- be careful when driving a motor vehicle or operating machinery
- alcohol, sedatives, and tranquilizers may increase drowsiness

Stop use and ask a doctor if:

- cough lasts more than 7 days, comes back, or occurs with fever, rash, or headache that lasts.

These could be signs of a serious condition.

If pregnant or breast-feeding, ask a health professional before use.

Keep out of reach of children. In case of overdose, get medical help or contact a Poison Control Center right away.

DIRECTIONS

[1 oz bottle] use tablespoon (TBSP)
Use tablespoon (TBSP) or dose cup

- do not exceed 4 doses per 24 hours

Under 12 yrs.	ask a doctor
12 yrs. and older	2 TBSP or 30 ml every 6 hours

[6 & 10 oz bottle, twin, quad pack]

- if taking NyQuil and DayQuil®, limit total to 4 doses per day.

Other Information:

- **each tablespoon contains** sodium 17 mg
- store at room temperature

INACTIVE INGREDIENTS

Alcohol, F&C blue no. 1, citric acid, flavor, high fructose corn syrup, polyethylene glycol, propylene glycol, purified water, FD&C red no. 40, saccharin sodium, sodium citrate

HOW SUPPLIED

Available in 1 FL OZ (30 ml) 6 FL OZ (177 ml), 10 FL OZ (295 ml) plastic bottles with child-resistant, tamper-evident cap and calibrated Medicine cup.

TAMPER EVIDENT: Do not use if imprinted shrinkband is missing or broken.

***Questions?* 1-800-362-1683 www.vicks.com**

Dist. by Procter & Gamble,
Cincinnati OH 45202. 42437885

VICKS® NYQUIL® LIQUICAPS®
VICKS® NYQUIL® LIQUID OTC

(Original and Cherry)
Multi-Symptom Cold/Flu Relief
Antihistamine/Cough Suppressant/Pain Reliever/Nasal Decongestant/Fever Reducer

Liquid (Original and Cherry)—alcohol 10%

Drug Facts:

ACTIVE INGREDIENTS

LiquiCaps®:

ACTIVE INGREDIENTS **Purpose:**

(per softgel)

Acetaminophen
325 mg .... Pain reliever/fever reducer

Continued on next page

Vicks Nyquil LiquiCaps—Cont.

Dextromethorphan HBr
15 mg .... Cough suppressant
Doxylamine succinate
6.25 mg .... Antihistamine
Pseudoephedrine HCl
30 mg .... Nasal decongestant

Liquid (Original and Cherry):
Active Ingredients: **Purpose:**
(per 15 ml tablespoon)
Acetaminophen
500 mg .... Pain reliever/fever reducer
Dextromethorphan HBr
15 mg .... Cough suppressant
Doxylamine succinate
6.25 mg .... Antihistamine
Pseudoephedrine HCl
30 mg .... Nasal decongestant

USES

LiquiCaps®:
Temporarily relieves these common cold/flu symptoms:
- nasal congestion
- cough due to minor throat & bronchial irritation
- sore throat
- headache
- minor aches and pains
- fever
- runny nose and sneezing

Liquid (Original and Cherry):
Temporarily relieves these common cold/flu symptoms:
- minor aches and pains
- headache
- sore throat
- fever
- runny nose and sneezing
- nasal congestion
- cough due to minor throat and bronchial irritation

WARNINGS

Failure to follow these warnings could result in serious consequences.

Alcohol warning If you consume 3 or more alcoholic drinks every day, ask your doctor whether you should take acetaminophen or other pain relievers/fever reducers. Acetaminophen may cause liver damage.

Sore throat warning If sore throat is severe, persists more than 2 days, is accompanied or followed by fever, rash, nausea, or vomiting, consult a doctor promptly.

Do not use • with other medications containing acetaminophen • if you are now taking a prescription monoamine oxidase inhibitor (MAOI) (certain drugs for depression, psychiatric or emotional conditions, or Parkinson's disease), or for 2 weeks after stopping the MAOI drug. If you do not know if your prescription drug contains an MAOI, ask a doctor or pharmacist before taking this product.

Ask a doctor before use if you have:
- heart disease
- a breathing problem or chronic cough such as occurs with smoking, asthma, chronic bronchitis, or emphysema
- thyroid disease
- diabetes
- glaucoma
- high blood pressure
- cough that occurs with too much phlegm (mucus)
- chronic bronchitis

Ask a doctor or pharmacist before use if you are taking sedatives or tranquilizers.

When using this product
- **do not use more than directed**
- excitability may occur, especially in children
- marked drowsiness may occur
- avoid alcoholic drinks
- be careful when driving a motor vehicle or operating machinery
- alcohol, sedatives, and tranquilizers may increase drowsiness

Stop use and ask a doctor if:
- symptoms do not get better within 7 days or are accompanied by fever.
- you get nervous, dizzy or sleepless
- fever gets worse or lasts more than 3 days
- new symptoms occur
- swelling or redness is present.
- cough lasts more than 7 days, comes back, or occurs with fever, rash, or headache that lasts. These could be signs of a serious condition.

If pregnant or breast-feeding, ask a health professional before use.

Keep out of reach of children.

OVERDOSE WARNING Taking more than the recommended dose can cause serious health problems. In case of overdose, get medical help or contact a Poison Control Center right away. Quick medical attention is critical for adults as well as for children even if you do not notice any signs or symptoms.

DIRECTIONS

LiquiCaps®:
- take only as recommended – see **Overdose warning**
- children under 12 yrs.: ask a doctor.
- do not exceed 4 doses per 24 hours
- 12 yrs and older . . . . 2 softgels with water every 4 to 6 hours
- If taking NyQuil and DayQuil®, limit total to 4 doses per 24 hours.

Liquid (Original and cherry):

AGE	DOSAGE
take only as recommended – see **Overdose warning**	
use tablespoon (TBSP) or dose cup	
do not exceed 4 doses per 24 hours	
children under 12	ask a doctor
adults and children 12 years and over	2 TBSP (30 ml) every 6 hours
If taking NyQuil and DayQuil®, limit total to 4 doses per 24 hours.	

OTHER INFORMATION

LiquiCaps®:
- store at room temperature

Liquid (Original and Cherry):
- **each tablespoon contains** sodium 17 mg
- store at room temperature

INACTIVE INGREDIENTS

LiquiCaps®: FD&C Blue no. 1, gelatin, glycerin, polyethylene glycol, povidone, propylene glycol, purified water, sorbitol special, D&C Yellow no. 10.

Liquid (Original): Alcohol, citric acid, flavor, FD&C Green no. 3, high fructose corn syrup, polyethylene glycol, propylene glycol, purified water, saccharin sodium, sodium citrate, yellow 6, D&C Yellow 10.

Liquid (Cherry): Alcohol, FD&C Blue 1, citric acid, flavor, high fructose corn syrup, polyethylene glycol, propylene glycol, purified water, FD&C Red 40, saccharin sodium, sodium citrate.

HOW SUPPLIED

LiquiCaps®: Available in 2-count 12-count, 40-count and 60-count child resistant blister packages. Each softgel is imprinted: "NyQ".

Liquid: Available in 1 FL OZ (30 ml) 6 and 10 FL OZ (177 ml and 295 ml, respectively) plastic bottles with child-resistant, tamper-evident cap and calibrated medicine cup.

LiquiCaps®: 12- and 36-ct
TAMPER EVIDENT: This package is safety sealed and child resistant. Use only if blisters are intact. If difficult to open, use scissors.
LiquiCaps, 20-count:
This package for households without young children.
TAMPER EVIDENT: Use only if blisters are intact. If difficult to open, use scissors.
Liquid (Original and cherry):
TAMPER EVIDENT: Do not use if imprinted shrinkband is missing or broken.
***Questions?* 1-800-362-1683** www.vicks.com
Liqui Caps®:
Made in Canada
Dist. by Procter & Gamble,
Cincinnati OH 45202.
©2001 42435017
Liquid (Original): Dist. by Procter & Gamble
Cincinnati OH 45202 42434786
Liquid (Cherry): Dist. by Procter & Gamble
Cincinnati OH 45202 42434789

Shown in Product Identification Guide, page 523

VICKS® SINEX® [NASAL SPRAY] OTC

[Ultra Fine Mist] for Sinus Relief
[sī 'nĕx]
Phenylephrine HCl Nasal Decongestant

Drug Facts:

ACTIVE INGREDIENTS **Purpose:**
Phenylephrine
HCl 0.5% .... Nasal decongestant

USES

Temporarily relieves sinus/nasal congestion due to
- colds
- hay fever
- upper respiratory allergies
- sinusitis

WARNINGS

Ask a doctor before use if you have:
- heart disease
- thyroid disease
- diabetes
- high blood pressure
- trouble urinating due to enlarged prostate gland

When using this product:
- **do not exceed recommended dosage**
- use of this container by more than one person may cause infection
- temporary burning, stinging, sneezing, or increased nasal discharge may occur
- frequent or prolonged use may cause nasal congestion to recur or worsen

Stop use and ask a doctor if:
- symptoms persist for more than 3 days

If pregnant or breast-feeding, ask a health professional before use.

Keep out of reach of children. In case of accidental ingestion, get medical help or contact a poison control center right away.

DIRECTIONS

Nasal Spray:
- under 12 yrs. ask a doctor
- adults & children 12 yrs. & older: 2 or 3 sprays in each nostril without tilting your head, not more often than every 4 hours.

Ultra Fine Mist: Remove protective cap. Before using for the first time, prime the pump by firmly depressing its rim several times. Hold container with thumb at base and nozzle between first and second fingers. Without tilting your head, insert nozzle into nostril. Fully depress rim with a firm, even stroke and inhale deeply.
- under 12 yrs.: ask a doctor
- adults & children 12 yrs. & older: 2 or 3 sprays in each nostril, not more often than every 4 hours.

OTHER INFORMATION
- store at room temperature

INACTIVE INGREDIENTS

Benzalkonium chloride, camphor, chlorhexidine gluconate, citric acid, disodium EDTA, eucalyptol, menthol, purified water, tyloxapol

HOW SUPPLIED

Available in $^1/_2$ FL OZ (14.7 ml) plastic squeeze bottle and $^1/_2$ FL OZ (14.7 ml) measured dose Ultra Fine mist pump. Note: This container is properly filled when approximately half full. Air space equal to one half of volume is necessary to propel the fine spray.
TAMPER EVIDENT:
Do not use if imprinted shrinkband is missing or broken.
Questions? 1-800-873-8276
Nasal Spray 42436771
Ultra Fine Mist 42436765
Dist. by Procter & Gamble
Cincinnati OH 45202

VICKS® SINEX® OTC

[sī 'nĕx]
12-HOUR [Nasal Spray]
[Ultra Fine Mist] for Sinus Relief
Oxymetazoline HCl
Nasal Decongestant

Drug Facts:

ACTIVE INGREDIENTS **Purpose:**
Oxymetazoline HCl
0.05% .... Nasal decongestant

Uses: Temporarily relieves sinus/nasal congestion due to
- colds
- hay fever
- upper respiratory allergies
- sinusitis

WARNINGS

Ask a doctor before use if you have:
- heart disease
- thyroid disease
- diabetes
- high blood pressure
- trouble urinating due to enlarged prostate gland

When using this product:
- **do not exceed recommended dosage**
- temporary burning, stinging, sneezing, or increased nasal discharge may occur
- frequent or prolonged use may cause nasal congestion to recur or worsen
- use of this container by more than one person may cause infection

Stop use and ask a doctor if:
- symptoms persist for more than 3 days

If pregnant or breast-feeding, ask a health professional before use.

Keep out of reach of children. In case of accidental ingestion, get medical help or contact a poison control center right away.

DIRECTIONS

Nasal Spray:
- under 6 yrs: ask a doctor
- adults & children 6 yrs. & older (with adult supervision): 2 or 3 sprays in each nostril without tilting your head, not more often than every 10 to 12 hours. Do not exceed 2 doses in 24 hours.

Ultra Fine Mist: Remove protective cap. Before using for the first time, prime the pump by firmly depressing its rim several times. Hold container with thumb at base and nozzle between first and second fingers. Without tilting your head, insert nozzle into nostril. Fully depress rim with a firm, even stroke and inhale deeply.

• under 6 yrs.: ask a doctor
• adults & children 6 yrs. & older (with adult supervision): 2 or 3 sprays in each nostril, not more often than every 10 to 12 hours. Do not exceed 2 doses in 24 hours.

OTHER INFORMATION
• store at room temperature

INACTIVE INGREDIENTS
Benzalkonium chloride, camphor, chlorhexidine gluconate, disodium EDTA, eucalyptol, menthol, potassium phosphate, purified water, sodium chloride, sodium phosphate, tyloxapol.

HOW SUPPLIED
Available in ½ FL OZ (14.7 ml) plastic squeeze bottle and ½ FL OZ (14.7 ml) measured-dose Ultra Fine mist pump.
TAMPER EVIDENT: Do not use if imprinted shrinkband is missing or broken.
Nasal Spray 42436768
Ultra Fine Mist 42436763
***Questions?* 1-800-873-8276**
Dist. by
Procter & Gamble,
Cincinnati OH 45202

VICKS® VAPOR INHALER — OTC
Levmetamfetamine/Nasal Decongestant

Drug Facts:

ACTIVE INGREDIENTS — **Purpose:**
(per inhaler)
Levmetamfetamine
50 mg .... Nasal decongestant

USES
Temporarily relieves nasal congestion due to:
• a cold
• hay fever or other upper respiratory allergies
• sinusitis

WARNINGS
When using this product:
• **do not exceed recommended dosage**
• temporary burning, stinging, sneezing, or increased nasal discharge may occur
• frequent or prolonged use may cause nasal congestion to recur or worsen
• do not use for more than 7 days
• do not use container by more than one person as it may spread infection
• use only as directed
Stop use and ask a doctor if:
• symptoms persist
If pregnant or breast-feeding, ask a health professional before use.
Keep out of reach of children. If swallowed, get medical help or contact a poison control center right away.

DIRECTIONS
The product delivers in each 800 ml air 0.04 to 0.15 mg of levmetamfetamine.
• do not use more often than every 2 hours
• under 6 yrs.: ask a doctor
• 6–11 yrs.: with adult supervision, 1 inhalation in each nostril.
• 12 yrs. & older: 2 inhalation in each nostril.

OTHER INFORMATION
• store at room temperature
• keep inhaler tightly closed.
• This inhaler is effective for a minimum of 3 months after first use.

INACTIVE INGREDIENTS
Bornyl acetate, camphor, lavender oil, menthol.

HOW SUPPLIED
Available as a cylindrical plastic nasal inhaler.
Net weight: 0.007 OZ (198 mg).
TAMPER EVIDENT: Use only if imprinted wrap is intact.
***Questions?* 1-800-873-8276 www.vicks.com**
Dist. by Procter & Gamble, Cincinnati OH 45202. ©2001 42438038

VICKS® VAPORUB® — OTC
VICKS® VAPORUB® CREAM
(greaseless)
[*vā ′pō-rub*]
Cough Suppressant/Nasal Decongestant/Topical Analgesic

Drug Facts:

ACTIVE INGREDIENTS
Vicks® VapoRub®:
Active Ingredients: — **Purpose:**
Camphor 4.8% .... Cough suppressant, & topical analgesic
Eucalyptus oil 1.2% .... Cough suppressant
Menthol 2.6% .... Cough suppressant & topical analgesic

Vicks® VapoRub® Cream:
ACTIVE INGREDIENTS — **Purpose:**
Camphor 4.8% .... Cough suppressant & topical analgesic
Eucalyptus oil 1.2% .... Cough suppressant
Menthol 2.8% .... Cough suppressant & topical analgesic

USES
• On chest & throat temporarily relieves cough due to the common cold
• on muscles and joints, temporarily relieves minor aches & pains

WARNINGS
Failure to follow these warnings could result in serious consequences.
For external use only; avoid contact with eyes.
Do not use:
• by mouth
• with tight bandages
• in nostrils
• on wounds or damaged skin
Ask a doctor before use if you have:
• cough that occurs with too much phlegm (mucus)
• persistent or chronic cough such as occurs with smoking, asthma or emphysema
When using this product do not:
• **heat**
• **microwave**
• **add to hot water or any container where heating water. May cause splattering and result in burns.**
Stop use and ask a doctor if:
• muscle aches and pains persist more than 7 days or come back
• cough lasts more than 7 days, comes back, or occurs with fever, rash, or headache that lasts.
These could be signs of a serious condition.
If pregnant or breast-feeding, ask a health professional before use.
Keep out of reach of children. In case of accidental ingestion, get medical help or contact a Poison Control Center right away.

DIRECTIONS
• **See important warnings under "When using this product"**
• children under 2 years: ask a doctor
• adults and children 2 years and over: Rub a thick layer on chest & throat or rub on sore aching muscles. If desired, cover with a soft cloth but keep clothing loose. Repeat up to three times per 24 hours or as directed by a doctor.

Other Information:
• store at room temperature

INACTIVE INGREDIENTS
Vicks® VapoRub®: Cedarleaf oil, nutmeg oil, special petrolatum, thymol, turpentine oil
Vicks® VapoRub® Cream: Carbomer 954, cedarleaf oil, cetyl alcohol, cetyl palmitate, cyclomethicone copolyol, dimethicone copolyol, dimethicone, EDTA, glycerin, imidazolidinyl urea, isopropyl palmitate, methylparaben, nutmeg oil, peg-100 stearate, propylparaben, purified water, sodium hydroxide, stearic acid, stearyl alcohol, thymol, titanium dioxide, turpentine oil

HOW SUPPLIED
Vicks VapoRub®: Available in 1.76 oz (50 g) 3.53 oz (100 g) and 6 oz (170 g) plastic jars
Vicks® VapoRub® Cream: Available in 2.99 oz (85 g) tube 1/6 oz pouch.
Questions? 1-800-873-8276
www.vicks.com
Vicks® VapoRub® 50142932
Vicks® VapoRub® Cream 50117758
US Pat. 5,322,689
Made in Mexico by Procter & Gamble
Manufactura, S. de R.L. de C.V.
Dist. by Procter & Gamble,
Cincinnati OH 45202

VICKS® VAPOSTEAM® — OTC
[*vā ′pō ″stēm*]
Liquid Medication for Hot Steam Vaporizers. Camphor/Cough Suppressant

Drug Facts:

ACTIVE INGREDIENT — **Purpose:**
Camphor 6.2% .... Cough suppressant

USES
Temporarily relieves cough associated with a cold.

WARNINGS
Failure to follow these warnings could result in serious consequences.
For external use only
Flammable Keep away from fire or flame. For steam inhalation only.
Ask a doctor before use if you have:
• a persistent or chronic cough such as occurs with smoking, emphysema or asthma
• cough that occurs with too much phlegm (mucus)
When using this product, do not
• **heat**
• **microwave**
• **use near an open flame**
• **take by mouth**
• **direct steam from the vaporizer too close to the face**
• **add to hot water or any container where heating water except when adding to cold water only in a hot steam vaporizer. May cause splattering and result in burns.**
Stop use and ask a doctor if:
• cough lasts more than 7 days, comes back, or occurs with fever, rash, or headache that lasts.
These could be signs of a serious condition.
Keep out of reach of children. In case of eye exposure (flush eyes with water); or in case of accidental ingestion, seek medical help or contact a Poison Control Center right away.

DIRECTIONS
see important warnings under "When using this product"
• under 2 yrs.: ask a doctor
• adults & children 2 yrs. & older: use 1 tablespoon of solution for each quart of water or 1½ teaspoonsful of solution for each pint of water
• add solution directly to cold water only in a hot steam vaporizer
• follow manufacturer's directions for using vaporizer.
• Breathe in medicated vapors.
• May be repeated up to 3 times a day.
Other Information:
• Close container tightly and store at room temperature away from heat

INACTIVE INGREDIENTS
Alcohol 78%, cedarleaf oil, eucalyptus oil, laureth-7, menthol, nutmeg oil, poloxamer 124, silicone.

HOW SUPPLIED
Available in 4 FL OZ (118 ml) and 8 FL OZ (235 ml) bottles.
Questions? 1-800-873-8276
Made in Mexico by Procter & Gamble
Manufactura S. de R.L. de C.V.
Dist. by Procter & Gamble
Cincinnati OH 45202
50144018

Procter & Gamble Pharmaceuticals, Inc.
**HEALTH CARE RESEARCH CENTER
8700 MASON MONTGOMERY RD
MASON, OH 45040-9462**

Direct Inquiries to:
Customer Service
(800) 448-4878

For Medical Information Contact:
Medical Communication Services
(800) 836-0658
Fax: (800) 438-0138
or write
Procter & Gamble Pharmaceuticals, Inc.
Medical Communication Services
Health Care Research Center
P.O. Box 8006
Mason, OH 45040-8006

In Emergencies:
Medical Communications
(800) 836-0658

For Product Information:
www.pgpharma.com

ACTONEL® — ℞
[*ăkt′ō-nĕl*]
(risedronate sodium tablets)

DESCRIPTION
ACTONEL (risedronate sodium tablets) is a pyridinyl bisphosphonate that inhibits osteoclast-mediated bone resorption and modulates bone metabolism. Each ACTONEL tablet for oral administration contains the equivalent of 5, 30, or 35 mg of anhydrous risedronate sodium in the form of the hemi-pentahydrate with small amounts of monohydrate. The empirical formula for risedronate sodium hemi-pentahydrate is $C_7H_{10}NO_7P_2Na \bullet 2.5\ H_2O$. The chemical name of risedronate sodium is [1-hydroxy-2-(3-pyridinyl) ethylidene]bis[phosphonic acid] monosodium salt. The chemical

Continued on next page

Actonel—Cont.

structure of risedronate sodium hemi-pentahydrate is the following:

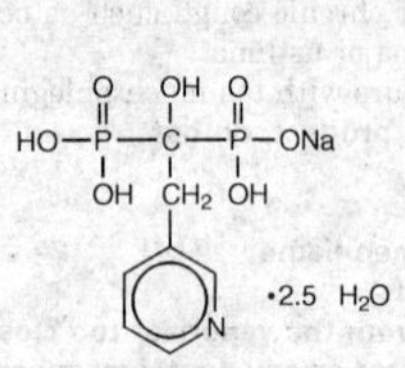

Molecular Weight:
Anhydrous: 305.10
Hemi-pentahydrate: 350.13

Risedronate sodium is a fine, white to off-white, odorless, crystalline powder. It is soluble in water and in aqueous solutions, and essentially insoluble in common organic solvents.

Inactive Ingredients:

Crospovidone, ferric oxide red (35-mg tablets only), ferric oxide yellow (5 and 35-mg tablets only), hydroxypropyl cellulose, hydroxypropyl methylcellulose, lactose monohydrate, magnesium stearate, microcrystalline cellulose, polyethylene glycol, silicon dioxide, titanium dioxide.

CLINICAL PHARMACOLOGY

Mechanism of Action:

ACTONEL has an affinity for hydroxyapatite crystals in bone and acts as an antiresorptive agent. At the cellular level, ACTONEL inhibits osteoclasts. The osteoclasts adhere normally to the bone surface, but show evidence of reduced active resorption (e.g., lack of ruffled border). Histomorphometry in rats, dogs, and minipigs showed that ACTONEL treatment reduces bone turnover (activation frequency, i.e., the rate at which bone remodeling sites are activated) and bone resorption at remodeling sites.

Pharmacokinetics:

Absorption:

Absorption after an oral dose is relatively rapid (t_{max} ~1 hour) and occurs throughout the upper gastrointestinal tract. The fraction of the dose absorbed is independent of dose over the range studied (single dose, 2.5 to 30 mg; multiple dose, 2.5 to 5 mg). Steady-state conditions in the serum are observed within 57 days of daily dosing. Mean absolute oral bioavailability of the 30-mg tablet is 0.63% (90% CI: 0.54% to 0.75%) and is comparable to a solution. The extent of absorption of a 30-mg dose (three 10-mg tablets) when administered 0.5 hours before breakfast is reduced by 55% compared to dosing in the fasting state (no food or drink for 10 hours prior to or 4 hours after dosing). Dosing 1 hour prior to breakfast reduces the extent of absorption by 30% compared to dosing in the fasting state. Dosing either 0.5 hours prior to breakfast or 2 hours after dinner (evening meal) results in a similar extent of absorption. ACTONEL is effective when administered at least 30 minutes before breakfast.

Distribution:

The mean steady-state volume of distribution is 6.3 L/kg in humans. Human plasma protein binding of drug is about 24%. Preclinical studies in rats and dogs dosed intravenously with single doses of [^{14}C] risedronate indicate that approximately 60% of the dose is distributed to bone. The remainder of the dose is excreted in the urine. After multiple oral dosing in rats, the uptake of risedronate in soft tissues was in the range of 0.001% to 0.01%.

Metabolism:

There is no evidence of systemic metabolism of risedronate.

Elimination:

Approximately half of the absorbed dose is excreted in urine within 24 hours, and 85% of an intravenous dose is recovered in the urine over 28 days. Mean renal clearance is 105 mL/min (CV = 34%) and mean total clearance is 122 mL/min (CV = 19%), with the difference primarily reflecting nonrenal clearance or clearance due to adsorption to bone. The renal clearance is not concentration dependent, and there is a linear relationship between renal clearance and creatinine clearance. Unabsorbed drug is eliminated unchanged in feces. Once risedronate is absorbed, the serum concentration-time profile is multi-phasic, with an initial half-life of about 1.5 hours and a terminal exponential half-life of 480 hours. This terminal half-life is hypothesized to represent the dissociation of risedronate from the surface of bone.

Special Populations:

Pediatric:

Risedronate pharmacokinetics have not been studied in patients <18 years of age.

Gender:

Bioavailability and pharmacokinetics following oral administration are similar in men and women.

Geriatric:

Bioavailability and disposition are similar in elderly (>60 years of age) and younger subjects. No dosage adjustment is necessary.

Race:

Pharmacokinetic differences due to race have not been studied.

Renal Insufficiency:

Risedronate is excreted unchanged primarily via the kidney. As compared to persons with normal renal function, the renal clearance of risedronate was decreased by about 70% in patients with creatinine clearance of approximately 30 mL/min. ACTONEL is not recommended for use in patients with severe renal impairment (creatinine clearance <30 mL/min) because of lack of clinical experience. No dosage adjustment is necessary in patients with a creatinine clearance ≥30 mL/min.

Hepatic Insufficiency:

No studies have been performed to assess risedronate's safety or efficacy in patients with hepatic impairment. Risedronate is not metabolized in rat, dog, and human liver preparations. Insignificant amounts (<0.1% of intravenous dose) of drug are excreted in the bile in rats. Therefore, dosage adjustment is unlikely to be needed in patients with hepatic impairment.

Pharmacodynamics:

Treatment and Prevention of Osteoporosis in Postmenopausal Women:

Osteoporosis is characterized by decreased bone mass and increased fracture risk, most commonly at the spine, hip, and wrist.

The diagnosis can be confirmed by the finding of low bone mass, evidence of fracture on x-ray, a history of osteoporotic fracture, or height loss or kyphosis indicative of vertebral fracture. Osteoporosis occurs in both men and women but is more common among women following menopause. In healthy humans, bone formation and resorption are closely linked; old bone is resorbed and replaced by newly-formed bone. In postmenopausal osteoporosis, bone resorption exceeds bone formation, leading to bone loss and increased risk of bone fracture. After menopause, the risk of fractures of the spine and hip increases; approximately 40% of 50 year-old women will experience an osteoporosis-related fracture during their remaining lifetimes. After experiencing 1 osteoporosis-related fracture, the risk of future fracture increases 5-fold compared to the risk among a non-fractured population.

ACTONEL treatment decreases the elevated rate of bone turnover that is typically seen in postmenopausal osteoporosis. In clinical trials, administration of ACTONEL to postmenopausal women resulted in decreases in biochemical markers of bone turnover, including urinary deoxypyridinoline/creatinine and urinary collagen cross-linked N-telopeptide (markers of bone resorption) and serum bone specific alkaline phosphatase (a marker of bone formation). At the 5-mg dose, decreases in deoxypyridinoline/creatinine were evident within 14 days of treatment. Changes in bone formation markers were observed later than changes in resorption markers, as expected, due to the coupled nature of bone resorption and bone formation; decreases in bone specific alkaline phosphatase of about 20% were evident within 3 months of treatment. Bone turnover markers reached a nadir of about 40% below baseline values by the sixth month of treatment and remained stable with continued treatment for up to 3 years. Bone turnover is decreased as early as 14 days and maximally within about 6 months of treatment, with achievement of a new steady-state that more nearly approximates the rate of bone turnover seen in premenopausal women. In a 1-year study comparing daily versus weekly oral dosing regimens of ACTONEL for the treatment of osteoporosis in postmenopausal women, ACTONEL 5-mg daily and ACTONEL 35-mg once a week decreased urinary collagen cross-linked N-telopeptide by 60% and 61%, respectively. In addition, serum bone-specific alkaline phosphatase was also reduced by 42% and 41% in the ACTONEL 5-mg daily and ACTONEL 35-mg once a week groups, respectively. ACTONEL is not an estrogen and does not have the benefits and risks of estrogen therapy.

As a result of the inhibition of bone resorption, asymptomatic and usually transient decreases from baseline in serum calcium (<1%) and serum phosphate (<3%) and compensatory increases in serum PTH levels (<30%) were observed within 6 months in patients in osteoporosis clinical trials. There were no significant differences in serum calcium, phosphate, or PTH levels between the ACTONEL and placebo groups at 3 years. In a 1-year study comparing daily versus weekly oral dosing regimens of ACTONEL in postmenopausal women, the mean changes from baseline at 12 months were similar between the ACTONEL 5-mg daily and ACTONEL 35-mg once a week groups, respectively, for serum calcium (0.4% and 0.7%), phosphate (-3.8% and -2.6%) and PTH (6.4% and 4.2%).

Glucocorticoid-Induced Osteoporosis:

Sustained use of glucocorticoids is commonly associated with development of osteoporosis and resulting fractures (especially vertebral, hip, and rib). It occurs in both males and females of all ages. The relative risk of a hip fracture in patients on >7.5 mg/day prednisone is more than doubled (RR = 2.27); the relative risk of vertebral fracture is increased 5-fold (RR = 5.18). Bone loss occurs most rapidly during the first 6 months of therapy with persistent but slowing bone loss for as long as glucocorticoid therapy continues. Osteoporosis occurs as a result of inhibited bone formation and increased bone resorption resulting in net bone loss. ACTONEL decreases bone resorption without directly inhibiting bone formation.

In two 1-year clinical trials in the treatment and prevention of glucocorticoid-induced osteoporosis, ACTONEL 5 mg decreased urinary collagen cross-linked N-telopeptide (a marker of bone resorption), and serum bone specific alkaline phosphatase (a marker of bone formation) by 50% to 55% and 25% to 30%, respectively, within 3 to 6 months after initiation of therapy.

Paget's Disease:

Paget's disease of bone is a chronic, focal skeletal disorder characterized by greatly increased and disordered bone remodeling. Excessive osteoclastic bone resorption is followed by osteoblastic new bone formation, leading to the replacement of the normal bone architecture by disorganized, enlarged, and weakened bone structure.

Clinical manifestations of Paget's disease range from no symptoms to severe bone pain, bone deformity, pathological fractures, and neurological disorders. Serum alkaline phosphatase, the most frequently used biochemical marker of disease activity, provides an objective measure of disease severity and response to therapy.

In pagetic patients treated with ACTONEL 30 mg/day for 2 months, bone turnover returned to normal in a majority of patients as evidenced by significant reductions in serum alkaline phosphatase (a marker of bone formation), and in urinary hydroxyproline/creatinine and deoxypyridinoline/creatinine (markers of bone resorption). Radiographic structural changes of bone lesions, especially improvement of a majority of lesions with an osteolytic front in weight-bearing bones, were also observed after ACTONEL treatment. In addition, histomorphometric data provide further support that ACTONEL can lead to a more normal bone structure in these patients.

Radiographs taken at baseline and after 6 months from patients treated with ACTONEL 30 mg daily demonstrate that ACTONEL decreases the extent of osteolysis in both the appendicular and axial skeleton. Osteolytic lesions in the lower extremities improved or were unchanged in 15/16 (94%) of assessed patients; 9/16 (56%) patients showed clear improvement in osteolytic lesions. No evidence of new fractures was observed.

CLINICAL STUDIES

Treatment of Osteoporosis in Postmenopausal Women:

The fracture efficacy of ACTONEL 5 mg daily in the treatment of postmenopausal osteoporosis was demonstrated in 2 large, randomized, placebo-controlled, double-blind studies that enrolled a total of almost 4000 postmenopausal women under similar protocols. The Multinational study (VERT MN) (ACTONEL 5 mg, n = 408) was conducted primarily in Europe and Australia; a second study was conducted in North America (VERT NA) (ACTONEL 5 mg, n = 821). Patients were selected on the basis of radiographic evidence of previous vertebral fracture, and therefore, had established disease. The average number of prevalent vertebral fractures per patient at study entry was 4 in VERT MN, and 2.5 in VERT NA, with a broad range of baseline bone mineral density (BMD) levels. All patients in these studies received supplemental calcium 1000 mg/day. Patients with low vitamin D levels (approximately 40 nmol/L or less) also received supplemental vitamin D 500 IU/day.

Positive effects of ACTONEL treatment on BMD were also demonstrated in each of 2 large, randomized, placebo-controlled trials (BMD MN and BMD NA) in which almost 1200 postmenopausal women (ACTONEL 5 mg, n = 394) were recruited on the basis of low lumbar spine bone mass (more than 2 SD below the premenopausal mean) rather than a history of vertebral fracture.

ACTONEL 35-mg once a week (n = 485) was shown to be therapeutically equivalent to ACTONEL 5-mg daily (n = 480) in a 1-year, double-blind, multicenter study of postmenopausal women with osteoporosis. In the primary efficacy analysis of completers, the mean increases from baseline in lumbar spine BMD at 1 year were 4.0% (3.7, 4.3; 95% confidence interval [CI]) in the 5-mg daily group (n = 391) and 3.9% (3.6, 4.3; 95% CI) in the 35-mg once a week group (n = 387) and the mean difference between 5 mg daily and 35 mg weekly was 0.1%(-0.42, 0.55; 95% CI). The results of the intent-to-treat analysis with the last observation carried forward were consistent with the primary efficacy analysis of completers. The 2 treatment groups were also similar with regard to BMD increases at other skeletal sites.

The safety and efficacy of once weekly ACTONEL 35 mg in women without osteoporosis are currently being studied, but data are not yet available.

Effect on Vertebral Fractures:

Fractures of previously undeformed vertebrae (new fractures) and worsening of pre-existing vertebral fractures were diagnosed radiographically; some of these fractures were also associated with symptoms (i.e., clinical fractures). Spinal radiographs were scheduled annually and prospectively planned analyses were based on the time to a patient's first diagnosed fracture. The primary endpoint for these studies was the incidence of new and worsening vertebral fractures across the period of 0 to 3 years. ACTONEL 5 mg daily significantly reduced the incidence of new and worsening vertebral fractures and of new vertebral fractures in both VERT NA and VERT MN at all time points (Table 1). The reduction in risk seen in the subgroup of patients who had 2 or more vertebral fractures at study entry was similar to that seen in the overall study population.

[See table 1 at top of next page]

Effect on Osteoporosis-Related Nonvertebral Fractures:

In VERT MN and VERT NA, a prospectively planned efficacy endpoint was defined consisting of all radiographically confirmed fractures of skeletal sites accepted as associated with osteoporosis. Fractures at these sites were collectively referred to as osteoporosis-related nonvertebral fractures. ACTONEL 5 mg daily significantly reduced the incidence of nonvertebral osteoporosis-related fractures over 3 years in VERT NA (8% vs. 5%; relative risk reduction 39%) and reduced the fracture incidence in VERT MN from 16% to 11%. There was a significant reduction from 11% to 7% when the studies were combined, with a corresponding 36% reduction in relative risk. Figure 1 shows the overall results as well as the results at the individual skeletal sites for the combined studies.

Figure 1
Nonvertebral Osteoporosis-Related Fractures Cumulative Incidence Over 3 Years Combined VERT MN and VERT NA

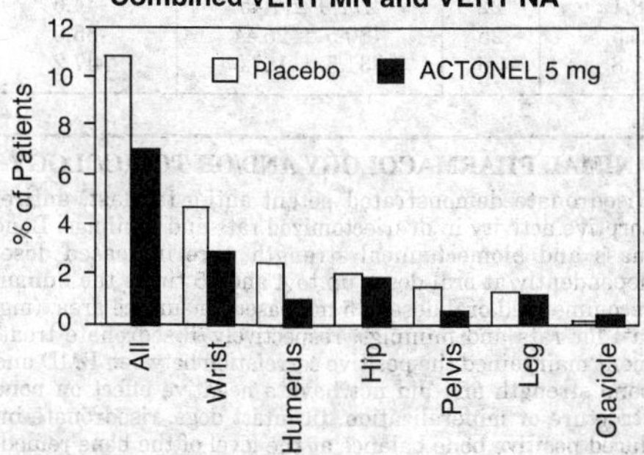

Effect on Height:
In the two 3-year osteoporosis treatment studies, standing height was measured yearly by stadiometer. Both ACTONEL and placebo-treated groups lost height during the studies. Patients who received ACTONEL had a statistically significantly smaller loss of height than those who received placebo. In VERT MN, the median annual height change was -1.3 mm/yr in the ACTONEL 5-mg daily group compared to -2.4 mm/yr in the placebo group. In VERT NA, the median annual height change was -0.7 mm/yr in the ACTONEL 5-mg daily group compared to -1.1 mm/yr in the placebo group.
Effect on Bone Mineral Density:
The results of 4 randomized, placebo-controlled trials in women with postmenopausal osteoporosis (VERT MN, VERT NA, BMD MN, BMD NA) demonstrate that ACTONEL 5 mg daily increases BMD at the spine, hip, and wrist compared to the effects seen with placebo. Table 2 displays the significant increases in BMD seen at the lumbar spine, femoral neck, femoral trochanter, and midshaft radius in these trials compared to placebo. Thus, overall ACTONEL reverses the loss of BMD, a central factor in the progression of osteoporosis. In both VERT studies (VERT MN and VERT NA), ACTONEL 5 mg daily produced increases in lumbar spine BMD that were progressive over the 3 years of treatment, and were statistically significant relative to baseline and to placebo at 6 months and at all later time points.
[See table 2 at right]
Histology/Histomorphometry:
Bone biopsies from 110 postmenopausal women were obtained at endpoint. Patients had received daily ACTONEL (2.5 mg or 5 mg) or placebo for 2 to 3 years. Histologic evaluation (n = 103) showed no osteomalacia, impaired bone mineralization, or other adverse effects on bone in ACTONEL-treated women. These findings demonstrate that bone formed during ACTONEL administration is of normal quality. The histomorphometric parameter mineralizing surface, an index of bone turnover, was assessed based upon baseline and post-treatment biopsy samples from 23 patients treated with ACTONEL 5 mg and 21 treated with placebo. Mineralizing surface decreased moderately in ACTONEL-treated patients (median percent change: ACTONEL 5 mg, -74%; placebo, -21%), consistent with the known effects of treatment on bone turnover.

Prevention of Osteoporosis in Postmenopausal Women:
ACTONEL 5 mg daily prevented bone loss in a majority of postmenopausal women (age range 42 to 63 years) within 3 years of menopause in a 2-year, double-blind, placebo-controlled study in 383 patients (ACTONEL 5 mg, n = 129). All patients in this study received supplemental calcium 1000 mg/day. Increases in BMD were observed as early as 3 months following initiation of ACTONEL treatment. ACTONEL 5 mg produced significant mean increases in BMD at the lumbar spine, femoral neck, and trochanter compared to placebo at the end of the study (Figure 2). ACTONEL 5 mg daily was also effective in patients with lower baseline lumbar spine BMD (more than 1 SD below the premenopausal mean) and in those with normal baseline lumbar spine BMD. Bone mineral density at the distal radius decreased in both ACTONEL and placebo-treated women following 1 year of treatment.
[See figure 2 at top of next column]
Combined Administration with Hormone Replacement Therapy:
The effects of combining ACTONEL 5 mg daily with conjugated estrogen 0.625 mg daily (n = 263) were compared to the effects of conjugated estrogen alone (n = 261) in a 1-year, randomized, double-blind study of women ages 37 to 82 years, who were on average 14 years postmenopausal. The BMD results for this study are presented in Table 3.

Table 1
The Effect of ACTONEL on the Risk of Vertebral Fractures

	Proportion of Patients with Fracture (%)[a]			
VERT NA	Placebo n = 678	ACTONEL 5 mg n = 696	Absolute Risk Reduction (%)	Relative Risk Reduction (%)
New and Worsening				
0-1 Year	7.2	3.9	3.3	49
0-2 Years	12.8	8.0	4.8	42
0-3 Years	18.5	13.9	4.6	33
New				
0-1 Year	6.4	2.4	4.0	65
0-2 Years	11.7	5.8	5.9	55
0-3 Years	16.3	11.3	5.0	41
VERT MN	Placebo n = 346	ACTONEL 5 mg n = 344	Absolute Risk Reduction (%)	Relative Risk Reduction (%)
New and Worsening				
0-1 Year	15.3	8.2	7.1	50
0-2 Years	28.3	13.9	14.4	56
0-3 Years	34.0	21.8	12.2	46
New				
0-1 Year	13.3	5.6	7.7	61
0-2 Years	24.7	11.6	13.1	59
0-3 Years	29.0	18.1	10.9	49

[a]Calculated by Kaplan-Meier methodology.

Table 2
Mean Percent Increase in BMD from Baseline in Patients Taking ACTONEL 5 mg or Placebo at Endpoint[a]

	VERT MN[b]		VERT NA[b]		BMD MN[c]		BMD NA[c]	
	Placebo n = 323	5 mg n = 323	Placebo n = 599	5 mg n = 606	Placebo n = 161	5 mg n = 148	Placebo n = 191	5 mg n = 193
Lumbar Spine	1.0	6.6	0.8	5.0	0.0	4.0	0.2	4.8
Femoral Neck	-1.4	1.6	-1.0	1.4	-1.1	1.3	0.1	2.4
Femoral Trochanter	-1.9	3.9	-0.5	3.0	-0.6	2.5	1.3	4.0
Midshaft Radius	-1.5*	0.2*	-1.2*	0.1*	ND		ND	

[a] The endpoint value is the value at the study's last time point for all patients who had BMD measured at that time; otherwise the last postbaseline BMD value prior to the study's last time point is used.
[b] The duration of the studies was 3 years.
[c] The duration of the studies was 1.5 to 2 years.
*BMD of the midshaft radius was measured in a subset of centers in VERT MN (placebo, n = 222; 5 mg, n = 214) and VERT NA (placebo, n = 310; 5 mg, n = 306)
ND = analysis not done

Figure 2
Change in BMD from Baseline 2-Year Prevention Study

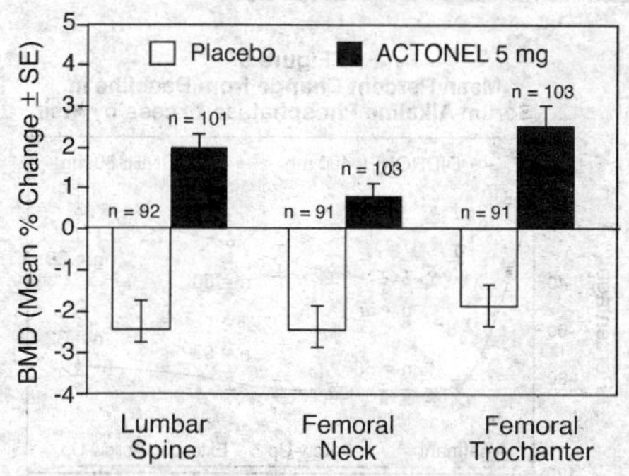

Table 3
Percent Change from Baseline in BMD After 1 Year of Treatment

	Estrogen 0.625 mg n = 261	ACTONEL 5 mg + Estrogen 0.625 mg n = 263
Lumbar Spine	4.6 ± 0.20	5.2 ± 0.23
Femoral Neck	1.8 ± 0.25	2.7 ± 0.25
Femoral Trochanter	3.2 ± 0.28	3.7 ± 0.25
Midshaft Radius	0.4 ± 0.14	0.7 ± 0.17
Distal Radius	1.7 ± 0.24	1.6 ± 0.28

Values shown are mean (± SEM) percent change from baseline.

Histology/Histomorphometry:
Bone biopsies from 53 postmenopausal women were obtained at endpoint. Patients had received ACTONEL 5 mg plus estrogen or estrogen alone once daily for 1 year. Histologic evaluation (n = 47) demonstrated that the bone of patients treated with ACTONEL plus estrogen was of normal lamellar structure and normal mineralization. The histomorphometric parameter mineralizing surface, a measure of bone turnover, was assessed based upon baseline and post-treatment biopsy samples from 12 patients treated with ACTONEL plus estrogen and 12 treated with estrogen alone. Mineralizing surface decreased in both treatment groups (median percent change: ACTONEL plus estrogen, -79%; estrogen alone, -50%), consistent with the known effects of these agents on bone turnover.

Glucocorticoid-Induced Osteoporosis:
Bone Mineral Density:
Two 1-year, double-blind, placebo-controlled trials in patients who were taking ≥7.5 mg/day of prednisone or equivalent demonstrated that ACTONEL 5 mg once daily was effective in the prevention and treatment of glucocorticoid-induced osteoporosis in men and women who were either initiating or continuing glucocorticoid therapy.
The prevention study enrolled 228 patients (ACTONEL 5 mg, n = 76) (18 to 85 years of age), each of whom had initiated glucocorticoid therapy (mean daily dose of prednisone 21 mg) within the previous 3 months (mean duration of use prior to study 1.8 months) for rheumatic, skin, and pulmonary diseases. The mean lumbar spine BMD was normal at baseline (average T score 0.684). All patients in this study received supplemental calcium 500 mg/day. By the third month of treatment, and continuing through the year-long treatment, the placebo group experienced losses in BMD at the lumbar spine, femoral neck, and trochanter, while BMD was maintained or increased in the ACTONEL 5-mg group. At each skeletal site there were statistically significant differences between the ACTONEL 5-mg group and the placebo group at all timepoints (Months 3, 6, 9, and 12). The treatment differences increased with continued treatment. Although BMD increased at the distal radius in the ACTONEL 5-mg group compared to the placebo group, the difference was not statistically significant. The differences between placebo and ACTONEL 5 mg after 1 year were 3.8% at the lumbar spine, 4.1% at the femoral neck, and 4.6% at the trochanter, as shown in Figure 3. The results at these skeletal sites were similar to the overall results when the subgroups of men and postmenopausal women, but not premenopausal women, were analyzed separately. ACTONEL was effective at the lumbar spine, femoral neck, and trochanter regardless of age (<65 vs. ≥65), gender, prior and concomitant glucocorticoid dose, or baseline BMD. Positive treatment effects were also observed in patients taking glucocorticoids for a broad range of rheumatologic disorders, the most common of which were rheumatoid arthritis, temporal arteritis, and polymyalgia rheumatica.

Continued on next page

Actonel—Cont.

The treatment study of similar design enrolled 290 patients (ACTONEL 5 mg, n = 100) (19 to 85 years of age) with continuing, long-term (≥6 months) use of glucocorticoids (mean duration of use prior to study 60 months; mean daily dose of prednisone 15 mg) for rheumatic, skin, and pulmonary diseases. The baseline mean lumbar spine BMD was low (1.63 SD below the young healthy population mean), with 28% of the patients more than 2.5 SD below the mean. All patients in this study received supplemental calcium 1000 mg/day and vitamin D 400 IU/day.

After 1 year of treatment, the BMD of the placebo group was within ±1% of baseline levels at the lumbar spine, femoral neck, and trochanter. ACTONEL 5 mg increased BMD at the lumbar spine (2.9%), femoral neck (1.8%), and trochanter (2.4%). The differences between ACTONEL and placebo were 2.7% at the lumbar spine, 1.9% at the femoral neck, and 1.6% at the trochanter as shown in Figure 4. The differences were statistically significant for the lumbar spine and femoral neck, but not at the femoral trochanter. ACTONEL was similarly effective on lumbar spine BMD regardless of age (<65 vs. ≥65), gender, or pre-study glucocorticoid dose. Positive treatment effects were also observed in patients taking glucocorticoids for a broad range of rheumatologic disorders, the most common of which were rheumatoid arthritis, temporal arteritis, and polymyalgia rheumatica.

Figure 3
Change in BMD from Baseline Patients Recently Initiating Glucocorticoid Therapy

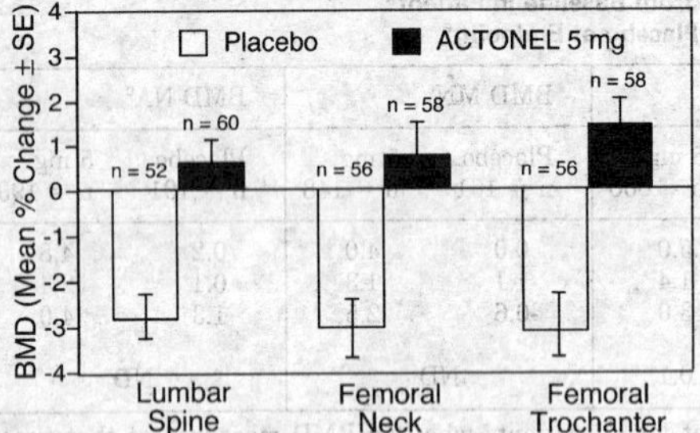

Figure 4
Change in BMD from Baseline Patients on Long-Term Glucocorticoid Therapy

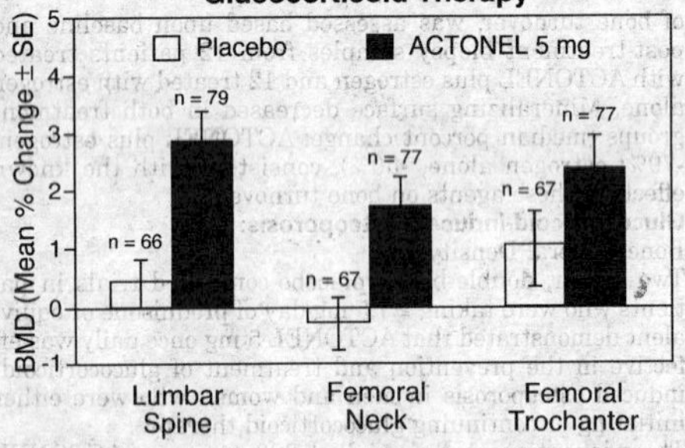

Vertebral Fractures:

In the prevention study of patients initiating glucocorticoids, the incidence of vertebral fractures at 1 year was reduced from 17% in the placebo group to 6% in the ACTONEL group. In the treatment study of patients continuing glucocorticoids, the incidence of vertebral fractures was reduced from 15% in the placebo group to 5% in the ACTONEL group (Figure 5). The statistically significant reduction in vertebral fracture incidence in the analysis of the combined studies corresponded to an absolute risk reduction of 11% and a relative risk reduction of 70%. All vertebral fractures were diagnosed radiographically; some of these fractures also were associated with symptoms (i.e., clinical fractures).

[See figure 5 at top of next column]

Histology/Histomorphometry:

Bone biopsies from 40 patients on glucocorticoid therapy were obtained at endpoint. Patients had received daily ACTONEL (2.5 mg or 5 mg) or placebo for 1 year. Histologic evaluation (n = 33) showed that bone formed during treatment with ACTONEL was of normal lamellar structure and normal mineralization, with no bone or marrow abnormalities observed. The histomorphometric parameter mineralizing surface, a measure of bone turnover, was assessed based upon baseline and post-treatment biopsy samples from 10 patients treated with ACTONEL 5 mg. Mineralizing surface decreased 24% (median percent change) in these patients. Only a small number of placebo-treated patients had both baseline and post-treatment biopsy samples, precluding a meaningful quantitative assessment.

Treatment of Paget's Disease:

The efficacy of ACTONEL was demonstrated in 2 clinical studies involving 120 men and 65 women. In a double-blind, active-controlled study of patients with moderate-to-severe Paget's disease (serum alkaline phosphatase levels of at least 2 times the upper limit of normal), patients were treated with ACTONEL 30 mg daily for 2 months or Didronel® (etidronate disodium) 400 mg/day for 6 months. At Day 180, 77% (43/56) of ACTONEL-treated patients achieved normalization of serum alkaline phosphatase levels, compared to 10.5% (6/57) of patients treated with Didronel (p<0.001). At Day 540, 16 months after discontinuation of therapy, 53% (17/32) of ACTONEL-treated patients and 14% (4/29) of Didronel-treated patients with available data remained in biochemical remission.

During the first 180 days of the active-controlled study, 85% (51/60) of ACTONEL-treated patients demonstrated a ≥75% reduction from baseline in serum alkaline phosphatase excess (difference between measured level and midpoint of the normal range) with 2 months of treatment compared to 20% (12/60) in the Didronel-treated group with 6 months of treatment (p<0.001). Changes in serum alkaline phosphatase excess over time (shown in Figure 6) were significant following only 30 days of treatment, with a 36% reduction in serum alkaline phosphatase excess at that time compared to only a 6% reduction seen with Didronel treatment at the same time point (p<0.01).

Table 4
Mean Percent Reduction from Baseline at Day 180 in Total Serum Alkaline Phosphatase Excess by Disease Severity

Subgroup: Baseline Disease Severity (AP)	ACTONEL 30 mg n	ACTONEL 30 mg Baseline Serum AP (U/L)*	ACTONEL 30 mg Mean % Reduction	DIDRONEL 400 mg n	DIDRONEL 400 mg Baseline Serum AP (U/L)*	DIDRONEL 400 mg Mean % Reduction
>2, <3× ULN	32	271.6 ± 5.3	-88.1	22	277.9 ± 7.45	-44.6
≥3, <7× ULN	14	475.3 ± 28.8	-87.5	25	480.5 ± 26.44	-35.0
≥7× ULN	8	1336.5 ± 134.19	-81.8	6	1331.5 ± 167.58	-47.2

*Values shown are mean ± SEM; ULN = upper limit of normal.

Figure 5
Incidence of Vertebral Fractures in Patients Initiating or Continuing Glucocorticoid Therapy

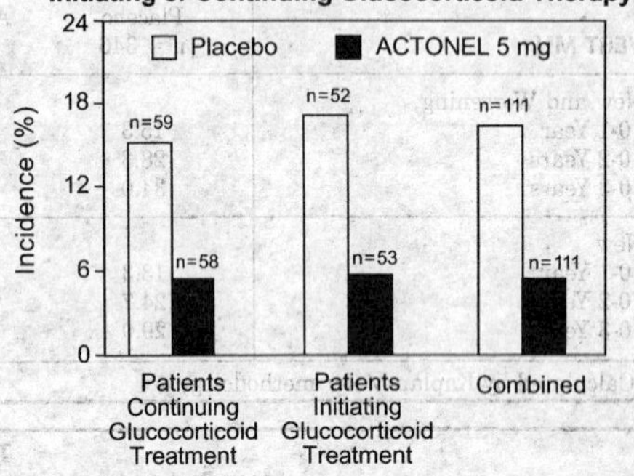

Figure 6
Mean Percent Change from Baseline in Serum Alkaline Phosphatase Excess by Visit

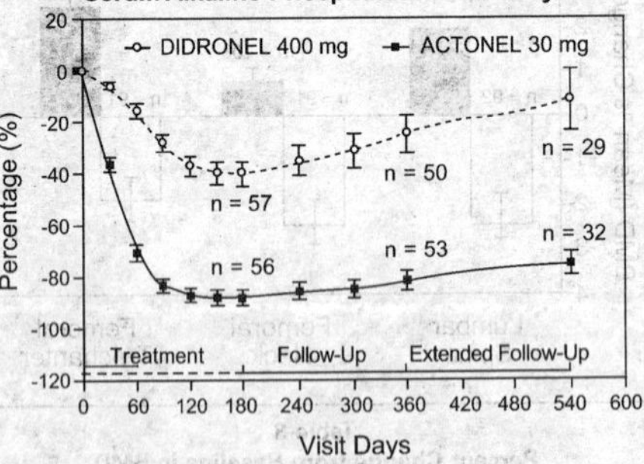

Response to ACTONEL therapy was similar in patients with mild to very severe Paget's disease. Table 4 shows the mean percent reduction from baseline at Day 180 in excess serum alkaline phosphatase in patients with mild, moderate, or severe disease.

[See table 4 above]

Response to ACTONEL therapy was similar between patients who had previously received anti-pagetic therapy and those who had not. In the active-controlled study, 4 patients previously non-responsive to 1 or more courses of anti-pagetic therapy (calcitonin, Didronel) responded to treatment with ACTONEL 30 mg daily (defined by at least a 30% change from baseline). Each of these patients achieved at least 90% reduction from baseline in serum alkaline phosphatase excess, with 3 patients achieving normalization of serum alkaline phosphatase levels.

Histomorphometry of the bone was studied in 14 patients with bone biopsies: 9 patients had biopsies from pagetic bone lesions and 5 patients from non-pagetic bone. The bone biopsy results in non-pagetic bone did not reveal osteomalacia, impairment of bone remodeling, or induction of a significant decline in bone turnover in patients treated with ACTONEL.

ANIMAL PHARMACOLOGY AND/OR TOXICOLOGY

Risedronate demonstrated potent anti-osteoclast, antiresorptive activity in ovariectomized rats and minipigs. Bone mass and biomechanical strength were increased dose-dependently at oral doses up to 4 and 25 times the human recommended oral dose of 5 mg based on surface area, (mg/m²) for rats and minipigs, respectively. Risedronate treatment maintained the positive correlation between BMD and bone strength and did not have a negative effect on bone structure or mineralization. In intact dogs, risedronate induced positive bone balance at the level of the bone remodeling unit at oral doses ranging from 0.35 to 1.4 times the human 5-mg dose based on surface area (mg/m²).

In dogs treated with an oral dose of 1 mg/kg/day (approximately 5 times the human 5-mg dose based on surface area, mg/m²), risedronate caused a delay in fracture healing of the radius. The observed delay in fracture healing is similar to other bisphosphonates. This effect did not occur at a dose of 0.1 mg/kg/day (approximately 0.5 times the human 5-mg dose based on surface area, mg/m²).

The Schenk rat assay, based on histologic examination of the epiphyses of growing rats after drug treatment, demonstrated that risedronate did not interfere with bone mineralization even at the highest dose tested (5 mg/kg/day, subcutaneously), which was approximately 3500 times the lowest antiresorptive dose (1.5 mcg/kg/day in this model) and approximately 8 times the human 5-mg dose based on surface area (mg/m²). This indicates that ACTONEL administered at the therapeutic dose is unlikely to induce osteomalacia.

INDICATIONS AND USAGE

Postmenopausal Osteoporosis:

ACTONEL is indicated for the treatment and prevention of osteoporosis in postmenopausal women.

Treatment of Osteoporosis:

In postmenopausal women with osteoporosis, ACTONEL increases BMD and reduces the incidence of vertebral fractures and a composite endpoint of nonvertebral osteoporosis-related fractures (see **CLINICAL STUDIES**). Osteoporosis may be confirmed by the presence or history of osteoporotic fracture, or by the finding of low bone mass (for example, at least 2 SD below the premenopausal mean).

Prevention of Osteoporosis:

ACTONEL may be considered in postmenopausal women who are at risk of developing osteoporosis and for whom the desired clinical outcome is to maintain bone mass and to reduce the risk of fracture.

Factors such as family history of osteoporosis, previous fracture, smoking, BMD (at least 1 SD below the premenopausal mean), high bone turnover, thin body frame, Caucasian or Asian race, and early menopause are associated with an increased risk of developing osteoporosis and fractures. The presence of these risk factors may be important when considering the use of ACTONEL for prevention of osteoporosis.

Glucocorticoid-Induced Osteoporosis:

ACTONEL is indicated for the prevention and treatment of glucocorticoid-induced osteoporosis in men and women who are either initiating or continuing systemic glucocorticoid treatment (daily dosage equivalent to 7.5 mg or greater of prednisone) for chronic diseases. Patients treated with glucocorticoids should receive adequate amounts of calcium and vitamin D.

Paget's Disease:

ACTONEL is indicated for treatment of Paget's disease of bone (osteitis deformans). Treatment is indicated in patients with Paget's disease of bone (1) who have a level of serum alkaline phosphatase at least 2 times the upper limit of normal, or (2) who are symptomatic, or (3) who are at risk for future complications from their disease, to induce remission (normalization of serum alkaline phosphatase).

CONTRAINDICATIONS

- Hypocalcemia (see **PRECAUTIONS, General**)
- Known hypersensitivity to any component of this product
- Inability to stand or sit upright for at least 30 minutes

WARNINGS

Bisphosphonates may cause upper gastrointestinal disorders such as dysphagia, esophagitis, and esophageal or gastric ulcer (see **PRECAUTIONS**).

PRECAUTIONS

General:

Hypocalcemia and other disturbances of bone and mineral metabolism should be effectively treated before starting ACTONEL therapy. Adequate intake of calcium and vitamin D is important in all patients, especially in patients with Paget's disease in whom bone turnover is significantly elevated. ACTONEL is not recommended for use in patients with severe renal impairment (creatinine clearance <30 mL/min).

Bisphosphonates have been associated with gastrointestinal disorders such as dysphagia, esophagitis, and esophageal or gastric ulcers. This association has been reported for bisphosphonates in postmarketing experience, but has not been found in most pre-approval clinical trials, including those conducted with ACTONEL. Patients should be advised that taking the medication according to the instructions is important to minimize the risk of these events. They should take ACTONEL with sufficient plain water (6 to 8 oz) to facilitate delivery to the stomach, and should not lie down for 30 minutes after taking the drug.

Glucocorticoid-Induced Osteoporosis:
The risk versus benefit of ACTONEL for the prevention and treatment of glucocorticoid-induced osteoporosis at daily doses of glucocorticoids <7.5 mg of prednisone or equivalent has not been established. Before initiating treatment, the hormonal status of both men and women should be ascertained and appropriate replacement considered.
The efficacy of ACTONEL for this indication has been established in studies of 1-year duration. The efficacy of ACTONEL beyond 1 year has not been studied.

Information for Patients:
The patient should be informed to pay particular attention to the dosing instructions as clinical benefits may be compromised by failure to take the drug according to instructions. Specifically, ACTONEL should be taken at least 30 minutes before the first food or drink of the day other than water.
To facilitate delivery to the stomach, and thus reduce the potential for esophageal irritation, patients should take ACTONEL while in an upright position (sitting or standing) with a full glass of plain water (6 to 8 oz). Patients should not lie down for 30 minutes after taking the medication (see **PRECAUTIONS, General**). Patients should not chew or suck on the tablet because of a potential for oropharyngeal irritation.
Patients should be instructed that if they develop symptoms of esophageal disease (such as difficulty or pain upon swallowing, retrosternal pain or severe persistent or worsening heartburn) they should consult their physician before continuing ACTONEL.
Patients should be instructed that if they miss a dose of ACTONEL 35-mg once a week, they should take 1 tablet on the morning after they remember and return to taking 1 tablet once a week, as originally scheduled on their chosen day. Patients should not take 2 tablets on the same day.
Patients should receive supplemental calcium and vitamin D if dietary intake is inadequate (see **PRECAUTIONS, General**). Calcium supplements or calcium-, aluminum-, and magnesium-containing medications may interfere with the absorption of ACTONEL and should be taken at a different time of the day, as with food.
Weight-bearing exercise should be considered along with the modification of certain behavioral factors, such as excessive cigarette smoking, and/or alcohol consumption, if these factors exist.
Physicians should instruct their patients to read the Patient Information before starting therapy with ACTONEL 5 mg or 35 mg and to re-read it each time the prescription is renewed.

Drug Interactions:
No specific drug-drug interaction studies were performed. Risedronate is not metabolized and does not induce or inhibit hepatic microsomal drug-metabolizing enzymes (Cytochrome P450).
Calcium Supplements/Antacids:
Co-administration of ACTONEL and calcium, antacids, or oral medications containing divalent cations will interfere with the absorption of ACTONEL.
Hormone Replacement Therapy:
One study of about 500 early postmenopausal women has been conducted to date in which treatment with ACTONEL (5 mg/day) plus estrogen replacement therapy was compared to estrogen replacement therapy alone. Exposure to study drugs was approximately 12 to 18 months and the primary endpoint was change in BMD. If considered appropriate, ACTONEL may be used concomitantly with hormone replacement therapy.
Aspirin/Nonsteroidal Anti-Inflammatory Drugs (NSAIDs):
Of over 5700 patients enrolled in the ACTONEL Phase 3 osteoporosis studies, aspirin use was reported by 31% of patients, 24% of whom were regular users (3 or more days per week). Forty-eight percent of patients reported NSAID use, 21% of whom were regular users. Among regular aspirin or NSAID users, the incidence of upper gastrointestinal adverse experiences in ACTONEL-treated patients (24.5%) was similar to that in placebo-treated patients (24.8%).
H_2 Blockers and Proton Pump Inhibitors (PPIs):
Of over 5700 patients enrolled in the ACTONEL Phase 3 osteoporosis studies, 21% used H_2 blockers and/or PPIs. Among these patients, the incidence of upper gastrointestinal adverse experiences in the ACTONEL-treated patients was similar to that in placebo-treated patients.

Drug/Laboratory Test Interactions:
Bisphosphonates are known to interfere with the use bone-imaging agents. Specific studies with ACTONEL have not been performed.

Carcinogenesis, Mutagenesis, Impairment of Fertility:
Carcinogenesis:
In a 104-week carcinogenicity study, rats were administered daily oral doses up to 24 mg/kg/day (approximately 7.7 times the maximum recommended human daily dose of 30 mg based on surface area, mg/m^2). There were no significant drug-induced tumor findings in male or female rats. The high dose male group of 24 mg/kg/day was terminated early in the study (Week 93) due to excessive toxicity, and data from this group were not included in the statistical evaluation of the study results. In an 80-week carcinogenicity study, mice were administered daily oral doses up to 32 mg/kg/day (approximately 6.4 times the 30-mg/day human dose based on surface area, mg/m^2). There were no significant drug-induced tumor findings in male or female mice.
Mutagenesis:
Risedronate did not exhibit genetic toxicity in the following assays: *In vitro* bacterial mutagenesis in *Salmonella* and *E. coli* (Ames assay), mammalian cell mutagenesis in CHO/HGPRT assay, unscheduled DNA synthesis in rat hepatocytes and an assessment of chromosomal aberrations *in vivo* in rat bone marrow. Risedronate was positive in a chromosomal aberration assay in CHO cells at highly cytotoxic concentrations (>675 mcg/mL, survival of 6% to 7%). When the assay was repeated at doses exhibiting appropriate cell survival (29%), there was no evidence of chromosomal damage.
Impairment of Fertility:
In female rats, ovulation was inhibited at an oral dose of 16 mg/kg/day (approximately 5.2 times the 30-mg/day human dose based on surface area, mg/m^2). Decreased implantation was noted in female rats treated with doses ≥7 mg/kg/day (approximately 2.3 times the 30-mg/day human dose based on surface area, mg/m^2). In male rats, testicular and epididymal atrophy and inflammation were noted at 40 mg/kg/day (approximately 13 times the 30-mg/day human dose based on surface area, mg/m^2). Testicular atrophy was also noted in male rats after 13 weeks of treatment at oral doses of 16 mg/kg/day (approximately 5.2 times the 30-mg/day human dose based on surface area, mg/m^2). There was moderate-to-severe spermatid maturation block after 13 weeks in male dogs at an oral dose of 8 mg/kg/day (approximately 8 times the 30-mg/day human dose based on surface area, mg/m^2). These findings tended to increase in severity with increased dose and exposure time.

Pregnancy:
Pregnancy Category C: Survival of neonates was decreased in rats treated during gestation with oral doses ≥16 mg/kg/day (approximately 5.2 times the 30-mg/day human dose based on surface area, mg/m^2). Body weight was decreased in neonates from dams treated with 80 mg/kg (approximately 26 times the 30-mg/day human dose based on surface area, mg/m^2). In rats treated during gestation, the number of fetuses exhibiting incomplete ossification of sternebrae or skull was statistically significantly increased at 7.1 mg/kg/day (approximately 2.3 times the 30-mg/day human dose based on surface area, mg/m^2). Both incomplete ossification and unossified sternebrae were increased in rats treated with oral doses ≥16 mg/kg/day (approximately 5.2 times the 30-mg/day human dose based on surface area, mg/m^2). A low incidence of cleft palate was observed in fetuses from female rats treated with oral doses ≥3.2 mg/kg/day (approximately 1 time the 30-mg/day human dose based on surface area, mg/m^2). The relevance of this finding to human use of ACTONEL is unclear. No significant fetal ossification effects were seen in rabbits treated with oral doses up to 10 mg/kg/day during gestation (approximately 6.7 times the 30-mg/day human dose based on surface area, mg/m^2). However, in rabbits treated with 10 mg/kg/day, 1 of 14 litters were aborted and 1 of 14 litters were delivered prematurely.
Similar to other bisphosphonates, treatment during mating and gestation with doses as low as 3.2 mg/kg/day (approximately 1 time the 30-mg/day human dose based on surface area, mg/m^2) has resulted in periparturient hypocalcemia and mortality in pregnant rats allowed to deliver.
Bisphosphonates are incorporated into the bone matrix, from which they are gradually released over periods of weeks to years. The amount of bisphosphonate incorporation into adult bone, and hence, the amount available for release back into the systemic circulation, is directly related to the dose and duration of bisphosphonate use. There are no data on fetal risk in humans. However, there is a theoretical risk of fetal harm, predominantly skeletal, if a woman becomes pregnant after completing a course of bisphosphonate therapy. The impact of variables such as time between cessation of bisphosphonate therapy to conception, the particular bisphosphonate used, and the route of administration (intravenous versus oral) on this risk has not been studied.
There are no adequate and well-controlled studies of ACTONEL in pregnant women. ACTONEL should be used during pregnancy only if the potential benefit justifies the potential risk to the mother and fetus.

Nursing Women:
Risedronate was detected in feeding pups exposed to lactating rats for a 24-hour period post-dosing, indicating a small degree of lacteal transfer. It is not known whether risedronate is excreted in human milk. Because many drugs are excreted in human milk and because of the potential for serious adverse reactions in nursing infants from bisphosphonates, a decision should be made whether to discontinue nursing or to discontinue the drug, taking into account the importance of the drug to the mother.

Pediatric Use:
Safety and effectiveness in pediatric patients have not been established.

Geriatric Use:
Of the patients receiving ACTONEL in postmenopausal osteoporosis studies (see **CLINICAL STUDIES**), 47% were between 65 and 75 years of age, and 17% were over 75. The corresponding proportions were 26% and 11% in glucocorticoid-induced osteoporosis trials, and 40% and 26% in Paget's disease trials. No overall differences in efficacy or safety were observed between these patients and younger patients but greater sensitivity of some older individuals cannot be ruled out.

Use in Men:
Safety and effectiveness have been demonstrated in clinical studies in men receiving ACTONEL both for Paget's disease and for treatment and prevention of glucocorticoid-induced osteoporosis. However, the safety and effectiveness in men for osteoporosis due to other causes have not been established.

ADVERSE REACTIONS

Osteoporosis:
ACTONEL has been studied in over 5700 patients enrolled in the Phase 3 glucocorticoid-induced osteoporosis clinical trials and in postmenopausal osteoporosis trials of up to 3-years duration. The overall adverse event profile of ACTONEL 5 mg in these studies was similar to that of placebo. Most adverse events were either mild or moderate and did not lead to discontinuation from the study. The incidence of serious adverse events in the placebo group was 24.9% and in the ACTONEL 5-mg group was 26.3%. The percentage of patients who withdrew from the study due to adverse events was 14.4% and 13.5% for the placebo and ACTONEL 5-mg groups, respectively. Table 5 lists adverse events from the Phase 3 osteoporosis trials reported in ≥2% of patients and in more ACTONEL-treated patients than placebo-treated patients. Adverse events are shown without attribution of causality.

Table 5
Adverse Events Occurring at a Frequency ≥2% and in More ACTONEL-Treated Patients than Placebo-Treated Patients Combined Phase 3 Osteoporosis Trials

Body System	Placebo % (N = 1914)	ACTONEL 5 mg % (N = 1916)
Body as a Whole		
Infection	29.7	29.9
Back Pain	23.6	26.1
Pain	13.1	13.6
Abdominal Pain	9.4	11.6
Neck Pain	4.5	5.3
Asthenia	4.3	5.1
Chest Pain	4.9	5.0
Neoplasm	3.0	3.3
Hernia	2.5	2.9
Cardiovascular		
Hypertension	9.0	10.0
Cardiovascular Disorder	1.7	2.5
Angina Pectoris	2.4	2.5
Digestive		
Nausea	10.7	10.9
Diarrhea	9.6	10.6
Flatulence	4.2	4.6
Gastritis	2.3	2.5
Gastrointestinal Disorder	2.1	2.3
Rectal Disorder	1.9	2.2
Tooth Disorder	2.0	2.1
Hemic and Lymphatic		
Ecchymosis	4.0	4.3
Anemia	1.9	2.4
Musculoskeletal		
Arthralgia	21.1	23.7
Joint Disorder	5.4	6.8
Myalgia	6.3	6.6
Bone Pain	4.3	4.6
Bone Disorder	3.2	4.0
Leg Cramps	2.6	3.5
Bursitis	2.9	3.0
Tendon Disorder	2.5	3.0
Nervous		
Depression	6.2	6.8
Dizziness	5.4	6.4
Insomnia	4.5	4.7
Anxiety	3.0	4.3
Neuralgia	3.5	3.8
Vertigo	3.2	3.3
Hypertonia	2.1	2.2
Paresthesia	1.8	2.1
Respiratory		
Pharyngitis	5.0	5.8
Rhinitis	5.0	5.7
Dyspnea	3.2	3.8
Pneumonia	2.6	3.1
Skin and Appendages		
Rash	7.2	7.7
Pruritus	2.2	3.0
Skin Carcinoma	1.8	2.0
Special Senses		
Cataract	5.4	5.9
Conjunctivitis	2.8	3.1
Otitis Media	2.4	2.5

Continued on next page

Actonel—Cont.

Urogenital		
Urinary Tract Infection	9.7	10.9
Cystitis	3.5	4.1

Duodenitis and glossitis have been reported uncommonly (0.1% to 1%). There have been rare reports (<0.1%) of abnormal liver function tests.

Laboratory Test Findings:

Asymptomatic and small decreases were observed in serum calcium and phosphorus levels. Overall, mean decreases of 0.8% in serum calcium and of 2.7% in phosphorus were observed at 6 months in patients receiving ACTONEL. Throughout the Phase 3 studies, serum calcium levels below 8 mg/dL were observed in 18 patients, 9 (0.5%) in each treatment arm (ACTONEL and placebo). Serum phosphorus levels below 2 mg/dL were observed in 14 patients, 11 (0.6%) treated with ACTONEL and 3 (0.2%) treated with placebo.

Endoscopic Findings:

ACTONEL clinical studies enrolled over 5700 patients, many with pre-existing gastrointestinal disease and concomitant use of NSAIDs or aspirin. Investigators were encouraged to perform endoscopies in any patients with moderate-to-severe gastrointestinal complaints, while maintaining the blind. These endoscopies were ultimately performed on equal numbers of patients between the treated and placebo groups [75 (14.5%) placebo; 75 (11.9%) ACTONEL]. Across treatment groups, the percentage of patients with normal esophageal, gastric, and duodenal mucosa on endoscopy was similar (20% placebo, 21% ACTONEL). The number of patients who withdrew from the studies due to the event prompting endoscopy was similar across treatment groups. Positive findings on endoscopy were also generally comparable across treatment groups. There was a higher number of reports of mild duodenitis in the ACTONEL group, however there were more duodenal ulcers in the placebo group. Clinically important findings (perforations, ulcers, or bleeding) among this symptomatic population were similar between groups (51% placebo; 39% ACTONEL).

Once-a-week Dosing:

In a 1-year, double-blind, multicenter study comparing ACTONEL 5-mg daily and ACTONEL 35-mg once a week in postmenopausal women, the overall safety and tolerability profiles of the 2 oral dosing regimens were similar. Table 6 lists the adverse events in ≥2% of patients from this trial. Events are shown without attribution of causality.

Table 6
Adverse Events Occurring in ≥ 2% of Patients of Either Treatment Group in the Daily vs. Weekly Osteoporosis Treatment Study in Postmenopausal Women

Body System	5 mg Daily ACTONEL % (N = 480)	35 mg Weekly ACTONEL % (N = 485)
Body as a Whole		
Infection	19.0	20.6
Accidental Injury	10.6	10.7
Pain	7.7	9.9
Back Pain	9.2	8.7
Flu Syndrome	7.1	8.5
Abdominal Pain	7.3	7.6
Headache	7.3	7.2
Overdose	6.9	6.8
Asthenia	3.5	5.4
Chest Pain	2.3	2.7
Allergic Reaction	1.9	2.5
Neoplasm	0.8	2.1
Neck Pain	2.7	1.2
Cardiovascular System		
Hypertension	5.8	4.9
Syncope	0.6	2.1
Vasodilatation	2.3	1.4
Digestive System		
Constipation	12.5	12.2
Dyspepsia	6.9	7.6
Nausea	8.5	6.2
Diarrhea	6.3	4.9
Gastroenteritis	3.8	3.5
Flatulence	3.3	3.1
Colitis	0.8	2.5
Gastrointestinal Disorder	1.9	2.5
Vomiting	1.9	2.5
Dry Mouth	2.5	1.4
Metabolic and Nutritional Disorders		
Peripheral Edema	4.2	1.6
Musculoskeletal System		
Arthralgia	11.5	14.2
Traumatic Bone Fracture	5.0	6.4
Myalgia	4.6	6.2
Arthritis	4.8	4.1
Bursitis	1.3	2.5
Bone Pain	2.9	1.4
Nervous System		
Dizziness	5.8	4.9
Anxiety	0.6	2.7
Depression	2.3	2.3
Vertigo	2.1	1.6
Respiratory System		
Bronchitis	2.3	4.9
Sinusitis	4.6	4.5
Pharyngitis	4.6	2.9
Cough Increased	3.1	2.5
Pneumonia	0.8	2.5
Rhinitis	2.3	2.1
Skin and Appendages		
Rash	3.1	4.1
Pruritus	1.9	2.3
Special Senses		
Cataract	2.9	1.9
Urogenital System		
Urinary Tract Infection	2.9	5.2

Paget's Disease:

ACTONEL has been studied in 392 patients with Paget's disease of bone. As in trials of ACTONEL for other indications, the adverse experiences reported in the Paget's disease trials have generally been mild or moderate, have not required discontinuation of treatment, and have not appeared to be related to patient age, gender, or race.

In a double-blind, active-controlled study, the adverse event profile was similar for ACTONEL and Didronel: 6.6% (4/61) of patients treated with ACTONEL 30 mg/day for 2 months discontinued treatment due to adverse events, compared to 8.2% (5/61) of patients treated with Didronel 400 mg/day for 6 months.

Table 7
Adverse Events Reported in ≥2% of ACTONEL-Treated Patients* in Phase 3 Paget's Disease Trials

Body System	30 mg/day × 2 months ACTONEL % (n = 61)	400 mg/day × 6 months DIDRONEL % (n = 61)
Body as a Whole		
Flu Syndrome	9.8	1.6
Chest Pain	6.6	3.3
Asthenia	4.9	0.0
Neoplasm	3.3	1.6
Gastrointestinal		
Diarrhea	19.7	14.8
Abdominal Pain	11.5	8.2
Nausea	9.8	9.8
Constipation	6.6	8.2
Belching	3.3	1.6
Colitis	3.3	3.3
Metabolic and Nutritional Disorders		
Peripheral Edema	8.2	6.6
Musculoskeletal		
Arthralgia	32.8	29.5
Bone Pain	4.9	4.9
Leg Cramps	3.3	3.3
Myasthenia	3.3	0.0
Nervous		
Headache	18.0	16.4
Dizziness	6.6	4.9
Respiratory		
Bronchitis	3.3	4.9
Sinusitis	4.9	1.6
Skin and Appendages		
Rash	11.5	8.2
Special Senses		
Amblyopia	3.3	3.3
Tinnitus	3.3	3.3
Dry Eye	3.3	0.0

*Considered to be possibly or probably causally related in at least one patient.

Three patients who received ACTONEL 30 mg/day experienced acute iritis in 1 supportive study. All 3 patients recovered from their events; however, in 1 of these patients, the event recurred during ACTONEL treatment and again during treatment with pamidronate. All patients were effectively treated with topical steroids.

Post-marketing Experience:

Very rare hypersensitivity and skin reactions, including angioedema, generalized rash and bullous skin reactions, some severe.

OVERDOSAGE

Decreases in serum calcium and phosphorus following substantial overdose may be expected in some patients. Signs and symptoms of hypocalcemia may also occur in some of these patients. Milk or antacids containing calcium should be given to bind ACTONEL and reduce absorption of the drug.

In cases of substantial overdose, gastric lavage may be considered to remove unabsorbed drug. Standard procedures that are effective for treating hypocalcemia, including the administration of calcium intravenously, would be expected to restore physiologic amounts of ionized calcium and to relieve signs and symptoms of hypocalcemia.

Lethality after single oral doses was seen in female rats at 903 mg/kg and male rats at 1703 mg/kg. The minimum lethal dose in mice and rabbits was 4000 mg/kg and 1000 mg/kg. These values represent 320 to 620 times the 30-mg human dose based on surface area (mg/m^2).

DOSAGE AND ADMINISTRATION

ACTONEL should be taken at least 30 minutes before the first food or drink of the day other than water.

To facilitate delivery to the stomach, ACTONEL should be swallowed while the patient is in an upright position and with a full glass of plain water (6 to 8 oz). Patients should not lie down for 30 minutes after taking the medication (see **PRECAUTIONS, General**).

Patients should receive supplemental calcium and vitamin D if dietary intake is inadequate (see **PRECAUTIONS, General**). Calcium supplements and calcium-, aluminum-, and magnesium-containing medications may interfere with the absorption of ACTONEL and should be taken at a different time of the day. ACTONEL is not recommended for use in patients with severe renal impairment (creatinine clearance <30 mL/min). No dosage adjustment is necessary in patients with a creatinine clearance ≥30 mL/min or in the elderly.

Treatment of Postmenopausal Osteoporosis (see INDICATIONS AND USAGE):

The recommended regimen is:

- one 5-mg tablet orally, taken daily

or

- one 35-mg tablet orally, taken once a week

Prevention of Postmenopausal Osteoporosis (see INDICATIONS AND USAGE):

- The recommended regimen is one 5-mg tablet orally, taken daily
- Alternatively, one 35-mg tablet orally, taken once a week may be considered

Treatment and Prevention of Glucocorticoid-Induced Osteoporosis (see INDICATIONS AND USAGE):

The recommended regimen is:

- one 5-mg tablet orally, taken daily

Paget's Disease (see INDICATIONS AND USAGE):

The recommended treatment regimen is 30 mg orally once daily for 2 months. Retreatment may be considered (following post-treatment observation of at least 2 months) if relapse occurs, or if treatment fails to normalize serum alkaline phosphatase. For retreatment, the dose and duration of therapy are the same as for initial treatment. No data are available on more than 1 course of retreatment.

HOW SUPPLIED

ACTONEL is available as follows:

5-mg film-coated, oval, yellow tablets with RSN on 1 face and 5 mg on the other.

NDC 0149-0471-01 bottle of 30

5-mg film-coated, oval, yellow tablets with RSN on 1 face and 5 mg on the other.

NDC 0149-0471-03 bottle of 2000

30-mg film-coated, oval, white tablets with RSN on 1 face and 30 mg on the other.

NDC 0149-0470-01 bottle of 30

35-mg film-coated, oval, orange tablets with RSN on 1 face and 35 mg on the other.

NDC 0149-0472-01 dose pack of 4

Store at controlled room temperature 20°-25°C (68°-77°F) [See USP].

Sold under U.S. patent No. 5,583,122; 6,096,342 and 6,165,513

Mfg. by: Procter & Gamble Pharmaceuticals
Cincinnati, OH 45202, or
OSG Norwich Pharmaceuticals, Inc.
North Norwich, NY 13814
Dist. by: Procter & Gamble Pharmaceuticals, TM Owner
Cincinnati, OH 45202
Marketed with:
Aventis Pharmaceuticals Inc.
Kansas City, MO 64137
JULY 2004

Shown in Product Identification Guide, page 330

ASACOL® ℞

[āce 'ah-kol]
(mesalamine)
Delayed-Release Tablets

DESCRIPTION

Each **Asacol** delayed-release tablet for oral administration contains 400 mg of mesalamine, an anti-inflammatory drug. The **Asacol** delayed-release tablets are coated with acrylic based resin, Eudragit S (methacrylic acid copolymer B, NF), which dissolves at pH 7 or greater, releasing mesalamine in the terminal ileum and beyond for topical anti-inflammatory action in the colon. Mesalamine has the chemical name 5-amino-2-hydroxybenzoic acid; its structural formula is:

COOH
OH
H_2N

Molecular Weight: 153.1
Molecular Formula: $C_7H_7NO_3$

Inactive Ingredients: Each tablet contains colloidal silicon dioxide, dibutyl phthalate, edible black ink, iron oxide red, iron oxide yellow, lactose, magnesium stearate, methacrylic acid copolymer B (Eudragit S), polyethylene glycol, povidone, sodium starch glycolate, and talc.

CLINICAL PHARMACOLOGY

Mesalamine is thought to be the major therapeutically active part of the sulfasalazine molecule in the treatment of ulcerative colitis. Sulfasalazine is converted to equimolar amounts of sulfapyridine and mesalamine by bacterial action in the colon. The usual oral dose of sulfasalazine for active ulcerative colitis is 3 to 4 grams daily in divided doses, which provides 1.2 to 1.6 grams of mesalamine to the colon.

The mechanism of action of mesalamine (and sulfasalazine) is unknown, but appears to be topical rather than systemic. Mucosal production of arachidonic acid (AA) metabolites, both through the cyclooxygenase pathways, i.e., prostanoids, and through the lipoxygenase pathways, i.e., leukotrienes (LTs) and hydroxyeicosatetraenoic acids (HETEs), is increased in patients with chronic inflammatory bowel disease, and it is possible that mesalamine diminishes inflammation by blocking cyclooxygenase and inhibiting prostaglandin (PG) production in the colon.

Pharmacokinetics: **Asacol** tablets are coated with an acrylic-based resin that delays release of mesalamine until it reaches the terminal ileum and beyond. This has been demonstrated in human studies conducted with radiological and serum markers. Approximately 28% of the mesalamine in **Asacol** tablets is absorbed after oral ingestion, leaving the remainder available for topical action and excretion in the feces. Absorption of mesalamine is similar in fasted and fed subjects. The absorbed mesalamine is rapidly acetylated in the gut mucosal wall and by the liver. It is excreted mainly by the kidney as N-acetyl-5-aminosalicylic acid.

Mesalamine from orally administered **Asacol** tablets appears to be more extensively absorbed than the mesalamine released from sulfasalazine. Maximum plasma levels of mesalamine and N-acetyl-5-aminosalicylic acid following multiple **Asacol** doses are about 1.5 to 2 times higher than those following an equivalent dose of mesalamine in the form of sulfasalazine. Combined mesalamine and N-acetyl-5-aminosalicylic acid AUC's and urine drug dose recoveries following multiple doses of **Asacol** tablets are about 1.3 to 1.5 times higher than those following an equivalent dose of mesalamine in the form of sulfasalazine.

The t_{max} for mesalamine and its metabolite, N-acetyl-5-aminosalicylic acid, is usually delayed, reflecting the delayed release, and ranges from 4 to 12 hours. The half-lives of elimination ($t1/2_{elm}$) for mesalamine and N-acetyl-5-aminosalicylic acid are usually about 12 hours, but are variable, ranging from 2 to 15 hours. There is a large intersubject variability in the plasma concentrations of mesalamine and N-acetyl-5-aminosalicylic acid and in their elimination half-lives following administration of **Asacol** tablets.

Clinical Studies:

Mildly to moderately active ulcerative colitis: Two placebo-controlled studies have demonstrated the efficacy of **Asacol** tablets in patients with mildly to moderately active ulcerative colitis. In one randomized, double-blind, multi-center trial of 158 patients, **Asacol** doses of 1.6 g/day and 2.4 g/day were compared to placebo. At the dose of 2.4 g/day, **Asacol** tablets reduced the disease activity, with 21 of 43 (49%) **Asacol** patients showing improvement in sigmoidoscopic appearance of the bowel compared to 12 of 44 (27%) placebo patients ($p = 0.048$). In addition, significantly more patients in the **Asacol** 2.4 g/day group showed improvement in rectal bleeding and stool frequency. The 1.6 g/day dose did not produce consistent evidence of effectiveness.

In a second randomized, double-blind, placebo-controlled clinical trial of 6 weeks duration in 87 ulcerative colitis patients, **Asacol** tablets, at a dose of 4.8 g/day, gave sigmoidoscopic improvement in 28 of 38 (74%) patients compared to 10 of 38 (26%) placebo patients ($p < 0.001$). Also, more patients in the **Asacol** 4.8 g/day group showed improvement in overall symptoms.

Maintenance of remission of ulcerative colitis: A 6-month, randomized, double-blind, placebo-controlled, multi-center study involved 264 patients treated with **Asacol** 0.8 g/day (n = 90), 1.6 g/day (n = 87), or placebo (n = 87). The proportion of patients treated with 0.8 g/day who maintained endoscopic remission was not statistically significant compared to placebo. In the intention to treat (ITT) analysis of all 174 patients treated with **Asacol** 1.6 g/day or placebo, **Asacol** maintained endoscopic remission of ulcerative colitis in 61 of 87 (70.1%) of patients, compared to 42 of 87 (48.3%) of placebo recipients ($p = 0.005$).

A pooled efficacy analysis of 4 maintenance trials compared **Asacol**, at doses of 0.8 g/day to 2.8 g/day, with sulfasalazine, at doses of 2 g/day to 4 g/day (n = 200). Treatment success was 59 of 98 (59%) for **Asacol** and 70 of 102 (69%) for sulfasalazine, a non-significant difference.

Study to assess the effect on male fertility: The effect of **Asacol** (mesalamine) on sulfasalazine-induced impairment of male fertility was examined in an open-label study. Nine patients (age < 40 years) with chronic ulcerative colitis in clinical remission on sulfasalazine 2 g/day to 3 g/day were crossed over to an equivalent **Asacol** dose (0.8 g/day to 1.2 g/day) for 3 months. Improvement in sperm count ($p < 0.02$) and morphology ($p < 0.02$) occurred in all cases. Improvement in sperm motility ($p < 0.001$) occurred in 8 of the 9 patients.

INDICATIONS AND USAGE

Asacol tablets are indicated for the treatment of mildly to moderately active ulcerative colitis and for the maintenance of remission of ulcerative colitis.

CONTRAINDICATIONS

Asacol tablets are contraindicated in patients with hypersensitivity to salicylates or to any of the components of the **Asacol** tablet.

PRECAUTIONS

General: Patients with pyloric stenosis may have prolonged gastric retention of **Asacol** tablets which could delay release of mesalamine in the colon.

Exacerbation of the symptoms of colitis has been reported in 3% of **Asacol**-treated patients in controlled clinical trials. This acute reaction, characterized by cramping, abdominal pain, bloody diarrhea, and occasionally by fever, headache, malaise, pruritus, rash, and conjunctivitis, has been reported after the initiation of **Asacol** tablets as well as other mesalamine products. Symptoms usually abate when **Asacol** tablets are discontinued.

Some patients who have experienced a hypersensitivity reaction to sulfasalazine may have a similar reaction to **Asacol** tablets or to other compounds which contain or are converted to mesalamine.

Renal: Renal impairment, including minimal change nephropathy, and acute and chronic interstitial nephritis, has been reported in patients taking **Asacol** tablets as well as other compounds which contain or are converted to mesalamine. In animal studies (rats, dogs), the kidney is the principal target organ for toxicity. At doses of approximately 750 mg/kg to 1000 mg/kg [15 to 20 times the administered recommended human dose (based on a 50 kg person) on a mg/kg basis and 3 to 4 times on a mg/m^2 basis], mesalamine causes renal papillary necrosis. **Therefore, caution should be exercised when using Asacol (or other compounds which contain or are converted to mesalamine or its metabolites) in patients with known renal dysfunction or history of renal disease. It is recommended that all patients have an evaluation of renal function prior to initiation of Asacol tablets and periodically while on Asacol therapy.**

Information for Patients: Patients should be instructed to swallow the **Asacol** tablets whole, taking care not to break the outer coating. The outer coating is designed to remain intact to protect the active ingredient and thus ensure mesalamine availability for action in the colon. In 2% to 3% of patients in clinical studies, intact or partially intact tablets have been reported in the stool. If this occurs repeatedly, patients should contact their physician.

Patients with ulcerative colitis should be made aware that ulcerative colitis rarely remits completely, and that the risk of relapse can be substantially reduced by continued administration of **Asacol** at a maintenance dosage.

Drug Interactions: There are no known drug interactions.

Carcinogenesis, Mutagenesis, Impairment of Fertility: Dietary mesalamine was not carcinogenic in rats at doses as high as 480 mg/kg/day, or in mice at 2000 mg/kg/day. These doses are 2.4 and 5.1 times the maximum recommended human maintenance dose of **Asacol** of 1.6 g/day (32 mg/kg/day if 50 kg body weight assumed or 1184 mg/m^2), respectively, based on body surface area. Mesalamine was negative in the Ames assay for mutagenesis, negative for induction of sister chromatid exchanges (SCE) and chromosomal aberrations in Chinese hamster ovary cells *in vitro*, and negative for induction of micronuclei (MN) in mouse bone marrow polychromatic erythrocytes. Mesalamine, at oral doses up to 480 mg/kg/day, had no adverse effect on fertility or reproductive performance of male and female rats.

Pregnancy: Teratogenic Effects: Pregnancy Category B: Reproduction studies in rats and rabbits at oral doses up to 480 mg/kg/day have revealed no evidence of teratogenic effects or fetal toxicity due to mesalamine. There are, however, no adequate and well-controlled studies in pregnant women. Because animal reproduction studies are not always predictive of human response, this drug should be used during pregnancy only if clearly needed.

Nursing Mothers: Low concentrations of mesalamine and higher concentrations of its N-acetyl metabolite have been detected in human breast milk. While the clinical significance of this has not been determined, caution should be exercised when mesalamine is administered to a nursing woman.

Pediatric Use: Safety and effectiveness of **Asacol** tablets in pediatric patients have not been established.

Geriatric Use: Clinical studies of **Asacol** did not include sufficient numbers of subjects aged 65 and over to determine whether they respond differently from younger subjects. Other reported clinical experience has not identified differences in responses between the elderly and younger patients. In general, the greater frequency of decreased hepatic, renal, or cardiac function, and of concomitant disease or other drug therapy in elderly patients should be considered when prescribing **Asacol**. Reports from uncontrolled clinical studies and post-marketing reporting systems suggest a higher incidence of blood dyscrasias, i.e., agranulocytosis, neutropenia, pancytopenia, in subjects receiving **Asacol** who are 65 years or older. Caution should be taken to closely monitor blood cell counts during drug therapy.

This drug is known to be substantially excreted by the kidney, and the risk of toxic reactions to this drug may be greater in patients with impaired renal function. Because elderly patients are more likely to have decreased renal function, care should be taken when prescribing this drug therapy. As stated in the PRECAUTIONS section, it is recommended that all patients have an evaluation of renal function prior to initiation of **Asacol** tablets and periodically while on **Asacol** therapy.

ADVERSE REACTIONS

Asacol tablets have been evaluated in 3685 inflammatory bowel disease patients (most patients with ulcerative colitis) in controlled and open-label studies. Adverse events seen in clinical trials with **Asacol** tablets have generally been mild and reversible. Adverse events presented in the following sections may occur regardless of length of therapy and similar events have been reported in short- and long-term studies and in the post-marketing setting.

In two short-term (6 weeks) placebo-controlled clinical studies involving 245 patients, 155 of whom were randomized to **Asacol** tablets, five (3.2%) of the **Asacol** patients discontinued **Asacol** therapy because of adverse events as compared to two (2.2%) of the placebo patients. Adverse reactions leading to withdrawal from **Asacol** tablets included (each in one patient): diarrhea and colitis flare; dizziness, nausea, joint pain, and headache; rash, lethargy and constipation; dry mouth, malaise, lower back discomfort, mild disorientation, mild indigestion and cramping; headache, nausea, aching, vomiting, muscle cramps, a stuffy head, plugged ears, and fever.

Adverse events occurring in **Asacol**-treated patients at a frequency of 2% or greater in the two short-term, double-blind, placebo-controlled trials mentioned above are listed in Table 1 below. Overall, the incidence of adverse events seen with **Asacol** tablets was similar to placebo.

Table 1
Frequency (%) of Common Adverse Events Reported in Ulcerative Colitis Patients Treated with **Asacol** Tablets or Placebo in Short-Term (6-Week) Double-Blind Controlled Studies

	Percent of Patients with Adverse Events	
Event	Placebo (n = 87)	**Asacol** tablets (n = 152)
Headache	36	35
Abdominal pain	14	18
Eructation	15	16
Pain	8	14
Nausea	15	13
Pharyngitis	9	11
Dizziness	8	8
Asthenia	15	7
Diarrhea	9	7
Back pain	5	7
Fever	8	6
Rash	3	6
Dyspepsia	1	6
Rhinitis	5	5
Arthralgia	3	5
Hypertonia	3	5
Vomiting	2	5
Constipation	1	5
Flatulence	7	3
Dysmenorrhea	3	3
Chest pain	2	3
Chills	2	3
Flu syndrome	2	3
Peripheral edema	2	3
Myalgia	1	3
Sweating	1	3
Colitis exacerbation	0	3
Pruritus	0	3
Acne	1	2
Increased cough	1	2
Malaise	1	2
Arthritis	0	2
Conjunctivitis	0	2
Insomnia	0	2

Of these adverse events, only rash showed a consistently higher frequency with increasing **Asacol** dose in these studies.

In a 6-month placebo-controlled maintenance trial involving 264 patients, 177 of whom were randomized to **Asacol** tablets, six (3.4%) of the **Asacol** patients discontinued **Asacol** therapy because of adverse events, as compared to four (4.6%) of the placebo patients. Adverse reactions leading to withdrawal from **Asacol** tablets included (each in one patient): anxiety; headache; pruritus; decreased libido; rheumatoid arthritis; and stomatitis and asthenia.

In the 6-month placebo-controlled maintenance trial, the incidence of adverse events seen with **Asacol** tablets was similar to that seen with placebo. In addition to events listed in Table 1, the following adverse events occurred in **Asacol**-treated patients at a frequency of 2% or greater in this study: abdominal enlargement, anxiety, bronchitis, ear disorder, ear pain, gastroenteritis, gastrointestinal hemorrhage, infection, joint disorder, migraine, nervousness, paresthesia, rectal disorder, rectal hemorrhage, sinusitis, stool abnormalities, tenesmus, urinary frequency, vasodilation, and vision abnormalities.

In 3342 patients in uncontrolled clinical studies, the following adverse events occurred at a frequency of 5% or greater and appeared to increase in frequency with increasing dose: asthenia, fever, flu syndrome, pain, abdominal pain, back

Continued on next page

Asacol—Cont.

pain, flatulence, gastrointestinal bleeding, arthralgia, and rhinitis.

In addition to the adverse events listed above, the following events have been reported in clinical studies, literature reports, and postmarketing use of products which contain (or have been metabolized to) mesalamine. Because many of these events were reported voluntarily from a population of unknown size, estimates of frequency cannot be made. These events have been chosen for inclusion due to their seriousness or potential causal connection to mesalamine:

Body as a Whole: Neck pain, facial edema, edema, lupus-like syndrome.

Cardiovascular: Pericarditis (rare), myocarditis (rare).

Gastrointestinal: Anorexia, pancreatitis, gastritis, increased appetite, cholecystitis, dry mouth, oral ulcers, perforated peptic ulcer (rare), bloody diarrhea. There have been rare reports of hepatotoxicity including, jaundice, cholestatic jaundice, hepatitis, and possible hepatocellular damage including liver necrosis and liver failure. Some of these cases were fatal. Asymptomatic elevations of liver enzymes which usually resolve during continued use or with discontinuation of the drug have also been reported. One case of Kawasaki-like syndrome which included changes in liver enzymes was also reported.

Hematologic: Agranulocytosis (rare), aplastic anemia (rare), thrombocytopenia, eosinophilia, leukopenia, anemia, lymphadenopathy.

Musculoskeletal: Gout.

Nervous: Depression, somnolence, emotional lability, hyperesthesia, vertigo, confusion, tremor, peripheral neuropathy (rare), transverse myelitis (rare), Guillain-Barré syndrome (rare).

Respiratory/Pulmonary: Eosinophilic pneumonia, interstitial pneumonitis, asthma exacerbation, pleuritis.

Skin: Alopecia, psoriasis (rare), pyoderma gangrenosum (rare), dry skin, erythema nodosum, urticaria.

Special Senses: Eye pain, taste perversion, blurred vision, tinnitus.

Urogenital: Interstitial nephritis (See also Renal subsection in PRECAUTIONS), minimal change nephropathy (See also Renal subsection in PRECAUTIONS), dysuria, urinary urgency, hematuria, epididymitis, menorrhagia.

Laboratory Abnormalities: Elevated AST (SGOT) or ALT (SGPT), elevated alkaline phosphatase, elevated GGT, elevated LDH, elevated bilirubin, elevated serum creatinine and BUN.

DRUG ABUSE AND DEPENDENCY

Abuse: None reported.

Dependency: Drug dependence has not been reported with chronic administration of mesalamine.

OVERDOSAGE

Two cases of pediatric overdosage have been reported. A 3-year-old male who ingested 2 grams of **Asacol** tablets was treated with ipecac and activated charcoal; no adverse events occurred. Another 3-year-old male, approximately 16 kg, ingested an unknown amount of a maximum of 24 grams of **Asacol** crushed in solution (i.e., uncoated mesalamine); he was treated with orange juice and activated charcoal, and experienced no adverse events. In dogs, single doses of 6 grams of delayed-release **Asacol** tablets resulted in renal papillary necrosis but were not fatal. This was approximately 12.5 times the recommended human dose (based on a dose of 2.4 g/day in a 50 kg person). Single oral doses of uncoated mesalamine in mice and rats of 5000 mg/kg and 4595 mg/kg, respectively, or of 3000 mg/kg in cynomolgus monkeys, caused significant lethality.

DOSAGE AND ADMINISTRATION

For the treatment of mildly to moderately active ulcerative colitis: The usual dosage in adults is two 400-mg tablets to be taken three times a day for a total daily dose of 2.4 grams for a duration of 6 weeks.

For the maintenance of remission of ulcerative colitis: The recommended dosage in adults is 1.6 grams daily, in divided doses. Treatment duration in the prospective, well-controlled trial was 6 months.

HOW SUPPLIED

Asacol tablets are available as red-brown, capsule-shaped tablets containing 400 mg mesalamine and imprinted "Asacol NE" in black.

NDC 0149-0752-15 Bottle of 180

Store at controlled room temperature 20°-25°C (68°-77°F) [See USP].

Procter & Gamble Pharmaceuticals
Cincinnati, OH 45202
under license from Medeva Pharma Schweiz AG
registered trademark owner.
Made in Germany, D-64331 Weiterstadt
U.S. Patent Nos. 5,541,170 and 5,541,171
REVISED March 2004

Shown in Product Identification Guide, page 330

DANTRIUM® ℞

[*dăn-trē-um*]
(dantrolene sodium)
Capsules

Dantrium (dantrolene sodium) has a potential for hepatotoxicity, and should not be used in conditions other than those recommended. Symptomatic hepatitis (fatal and non-fatal) has been reported at various dose levels of the drug. The incidence reported in patients taking up to 400 mg/day is much lower than in those taking doses of 800 mg or more per day. Even sporadic short courses of these higher dose levels within a treatment regimen markedly increased the risk of serious hepatic injury. Liver dysfunction as evidenced by blood chemical abnormalities alone (liver enzyme elevations) has been observed in patients exposed to **Dantrium** for varying periods of time. Overt hepatitis has occurred at varying intervals after initiation of therapy, but has been most frequently observed between the third and twelfth month of therapy. The risk of hepatic injury appears to be greater in females, in patients over 35 years of age, and in patients taking other medication(s) in addition to **Dantrium** (dantrolene sodium). **Dantrium** should be used only in conjunction with appropriate monitoring of hepatic function including frequent determination of SGOT or SGPT. If no observable benefit is derived from the administration of **Dantrium** after a total of 45 days, therapy should be discontinued. The lowest possible effective dose for the individual patient should be prescribed.

DESCRIPTION

The chemical formula of **Dantrium** (dantrolene sodium) is hydrated 1-[[[5-(4-nitrophenyl)-2-furanyl]methylene] amino]-2, 4-imidazolidinedione sodium salt. It is an orange powder, slightly soluble in water, but due to its slightly acidic nature the solubility increases somewhat in alkaline solution. The anhydrous salt has a molecular weight of 336. The hydrated salt contains approximately 15% water (3-1/2 moles) and has a molecular weight of 399. The structural formula for the hydrated salt is:

O_2N—(phenyl)—(furan)—CH=N—N(imidazolidinedione) NNa • xH_2O

Dantrium is supplied in capsules of 25 mg, 50 mg, and 100 mg.

Inactive Ingredients: Each capsule contains edible black ink, FD&C Yellow No. 6, gelatin, lactose, magnesium stearate, starch, synthetic iron oxide red, synthetic iron oxide yellow, talc, and titanium dioxide.

CLINICAL PHARMACOLOGY

In isolated nerve-muscle preparation, **Dantrium** has been shown to produce relaxation by affecting the contractile response of the skeletal muscle at a site beyond the myoneural junction, directly on the muscle itself. In skeletal muscle, **Dantrium** dissociates the excitation-contraction coupling, probably by interfering with the release of Ca^{++} from the sarcoplasmic reticulum. This effect appears to be more pronounced in fast muscle fibers as compared to slow ones, but generally affects both. A central nervous system effect occurs, with drowsiness, dizziness, and generalized weakness occasionally present. Although **Dantrium** does not appear to directly affect the CNS, the extent of its indirect effect is unknown. The absorption of **Dantrium** after oral administration in humans is incomplete and slow but consistent, and dose-related blood levels are obtained. The duration and intensity of skeletal muscle relaxation is related to the dosage and blood levels. The mean biologic half-life of **Dantrium** in adults is 8.7 hours after a 100-mg dose. Specific metabolic pathways in the degradation and elimination of **Dantrium** in human subjects have been established. Metabolic patterns are similar in adults and pediatric patients. In addition to the parent compound, dantrolene, which is found in measurable amounts in blood and urine, the major metabolites noted in body fluids are the 5-hydroxy analog and the acetamido analog. Since **Dantrium** is probably metabolized by hepatic microsomal enzymes, enhancement of its metabolism by other drugs is possible. However, neither phenobarbital nor diazepam appears to affect **Dantrium** metabolism.

Clinical experience in the management of fulminant human malignant hyperthermia, as well as experiments conducted in malignant hyperthermia susceptible swine, have revealed that the administration of intravenous dantrolene, combined with indicated supportive measures, is effective in reversing the hypermetabolic process of malignant hyperthermia. Known differences between human and swine malignant hyperthermia are minor. The prophylactic administration of oral or intravenous dantrolene to malignant hyperthermia susceptible swine will attenuate or prevent the development of signs of malignant hyperthermia in a manner dependent upon the dosage of dantrolene administered and the intensity of the malignant hyperthermia triggering stimulus. Limited clinical experience with the administration of oral dantrolene to patients judged malignant hyperthermia susceptible, when combined with clinical experience in the use of intravenous dantrolene for the treatment of malignant hyperthermia and data derived from the above cited animal model experiments, suggests that oral dantrolene will also attenuate or prevent the development of signs of human malignant hyperthermia, provided that currently accepted practices in the management of such patients are adhered to (see **INDICATIONS AND USAGE**); intravenous dantrolene should also be available for use should the signs of malignant hyperthermia appear.

INDICATIONS AND USAGE

In Chronic Spasticity: **Dantrium** is indicated in controlling the manifestations of clinical spasticity resulting from upper motor neuron disorders (e.g., spinal cord injury, stroke, cerebral palsy, or multiple sclerosis). It is of particular benefit to the patient whose functional rehabilitation has been retarded by the sequelae of spasticity. Such patients must have presumably reversible spasticity where relief of spasticity will aid in restoring residual function. **Dantrium** is not indicated in the treatment of skeletal muscle spasm resulting from rheumatic disorders.

If improvement occurs, it will ordinarily occur within the dosage titration (see **DOSAGE AND ADMINISTRATION**), and will be manifested by a decrease in the severity of spasticity and the ability to resume a daily function not quite attainable without **Dantrium.**

Occasionally, subtle but meaningful improvement in spasticity may occur with **Dantrium** therapy. In such instances, information regarding improvement should be solicited from the patient and those who are in constant daily contact and attendance with him. Brief withdrawal of **Dantrium** for a period of 2 to 4 days will frequently demonstrate exacerbation of the manifestations of spasticity and may serve to confirm a clinical impression.

A decision to continue the administration of **Dantrium** on a long-term basis is justified if introduction of the drug into the patient's regimen:

- produces a significant reduction in painful and/or disabling spasticity such as clonus, or
- permits a significant reduction in the intensity and/or degree of nursing care required, or
- rids the patient of any annoying manifestation of spasticity considered important by the patient himself.

In Malignant Hyperthermia: Oral **Dantrium** is also indicated preoperatively to prevent or attenuate the development of signs of malignant hyperthermia in known, or strongly suspect, malignant hyperthermia susceptible patients who require anesthesia and/or surgery. Currently accepted clinical practices in the management of such patients must still be adhered to (careful monitoring for early signs of malignant hyperthermia, minimizing exposure to triggering mechanisms and prompt use of intravenous dantrolene sodium and indicated supportive measures should signs of malignant hyperthermia appear); see also the package insert for **Dantrium®** (dantrolene sodium) **Intravenous.**

Oral **Dantrium** should be administered following a malignant hyperthermic crisis to prevent recurrence of the signs of malignant hyperthermia.

CONTRAINDICATIONS

Active hepatic disease, such as hepatitis and cirrhosis, is a contraindication for use of **Dantrium. Dantrium** is contraindicated where spasticity is utilized to sustain upright posture and balance in locomotion or whenever spasticity is utilized to obtain or maintain increased function.

WARNINGS

It is important to recognize that fatal and non-fatal liver disorders of an idiosyncratic or hypersensitivity type may occur with **Dantrium** therapy.

At the start of **Dantrium** therapy, it is desirable to do liver function studies (SGOT, SGPT, alkaline phosphatase, total bilirubin) for a baseline or to establish whether there is preexisting liver disease. If baseline liver abnormalities exist and are confirmed, there is a clear possibility that the potential for **Dantrium** hepatotoxicity could be enhanced, although such a possibility has not yet been established.

Liver function studies (e.g., SGOT or SGPT) should be performed at appropriate intervals during **Dantrium** therapy. If such studies reveal abnormal values, therapy should generally be discontinued. Only where benefits of the drug have been of major importance to the patient, should reinitiation or continuation of therapy be considered. Some patients have revealed a return to normal laboratory values in the face of continued therapy while others have not.

If symptoms compatible with hepatitis, accompanied by abnormalities in liver function tests or jaundice appear, **Dantrium** should be discontinued. If caused by **Dantrium** and detected early, the abnormalities in liver function characteristically have reverted to normal when the drug was discontinued. **Dantrium** therapy has been reinstituted in a few patients who have developed clinical and/or laboratory evidence of hepatocellular injury. If such reinstitution of therapy is done, it should be attempted only in patients who clearly need **Dantrium** and only after previous symptoms and laboratory abnormalities have cleared. The patient should be hospitalized and the drug should be restarted in very small and gradually increasing doses. Laboratory monitoring should be frequent and the drug should be withdrawn immediately if there is any indication of recurrent liver involvement. Some patients have reacted with unmistakable signs of liver abnormality upon administration of a challenge dose, while others have not.

Dantrium should be used with particular caution in females and in patients over 35 years of age in view of apparent greater likelihood of drug-induced, potentially fatal, hepatocellular disease in these groups.

Carcinogenesis, Mutagenesis, Impairment of Fertility: Long-term safety of **Dantrium** in humans has not been established. Chronic studies in rats, dogs, and monkeys at dosages greater than 30 mg/kg/day showed growth or weight depression and signs of hepatopathy and possible occlusion nephropathy, all of which were reversible upon cessation of treatment. Sprague-Dawley female rats fed dantrolene sodium for 18 months at dosage levels of 15, 30, and 60 mg/kg/day showed an increased incidence of benign and malignant mammary tumors compared with concurrent controls. At the highest dose level, there was an increase in the incidence of benign hepatic lymphatic neoplasms. In a 30-month study at the same dose levels also in Sprague-Dawley rats, dantrolene sodium produced a decrease in the time of onset of mammary neoplasms. Female rats at the highest dose level showed an increased incidence of hepatic lymphangiomas and hepatic angiosarcomas.

The only drug-related effect seen in a 30-month study in Fischer-344 rats was a dose-related reduction in the time of onset of mammary and testicular tumors. A 24-month study in HaM/ICR mice revealed no evidence of carcinogenic activity. Carcinogenicity in humans cannot be fully excluded, so that this possible risk of chronic administration must be weighed against the benefits of the drug (i.e., after a brief trial) for the individual patient.

Dantrolene sodium has produced positive results in the Ames S. Typhimurium bacterial mutagenesis assay in the presence and absence of a liver activating system.

Pregnancy: Pregnancy Category C: **Dantrium** has been shown to be embryocidal in the rabbit and has been shown to decrease pup survival in the rat when given at doses seven times the human oral dose. There are no adequate and well-controlled studies in pregnant women (see Labor and Delivery subheading for information regarding placental transfer of the drug). **Dantrium** capsules should be used during pregnancy only if the potential benefit justifies the potential risk to the fetus.

Labor and Delivery: In one non-randomized open-label study, 21 term pregnant patients received prophylactic oral **Dantrium** 100 mg per day for 2 to 10 days prior to delivery. Dantrolene readily crossed the placenta with maternal and fetal whole blood levels approximately equal at delivery; neonatal levels then fell approximately 50% per day for 2 days before declining sharply. No neonatal respiratory and neuromuscular side effects were detected at low dose. More data, at higher doses, are needed before more definitive conclusions can be made.

Nursing Mothers: **Dantrium** should not be used in nursing mothers.

Usage in Pediatric Patients: The long-term safety of **Dantrium** in pediatric patients under the age of 5 years has not been established. Because of the possibility that adverse effects of the drug could become apparent only after many years, a benefit-risk consideration of the long-term use of **Dantrium** is particularly important in pediatric patients.

Drug Interactions: Drowsiness may occur with **Dantrium** therapy, and the concomitant administration of CNS depressants such as sedatives and tranquilizing agents may result in further drowsiness.

While a definite drug interaction with estrogen therapy has not yet been established, caution should be observed if the two drugs are to be given concomitantly. Hepatotoxicity has occurred more often in women over 35 years of age receiving concomitant estrogen therapy.

Cardiovascular collapse in patients treated simultaneously with verapamil and dantrolene sodium is rare. The combination of therapeutic doses of intravenous dantrolene sodium and verapamil in halothane/α-chloralose anesthetized swine has resulted in ventricular fibrillation and cardiovascular collapse in association with marked hyperkalemia. Until the relevance of these findings to humans is established, the combination of dantrolene sodium and calcium channel blockers is not recommended during the management of malignant hyperthermia.

Administration of **Dantrium** may potentiate vecuronium-induced neuromuscular block.

PRECAUTIONS

Dantrium should be used with caution in patients with impaired pulmonary function, particularly those with obstructive pulmonary disease, and in patients with severely impaired cardiac function due to myocardial disease. It should be used with caution in patients with a history of previous liver disease or dysfunction (see **WARNINGS**).

Information for Patients: Patients should be cautioned against driving a motor vehicle or participating in hazardous occupations while taking **Dantrium**. Caution should be exercised in the concomitant administration of tranquilizing agents.

Dantrium might possibly evoke a photosensitivity reaction; patients should be cautioned about exposure to sunlight while taking it.

ADVERSE REACTIONS

The most frequently occurring side effects of **Dantrium** have been drowsiness, dizziness, weakness, general malaise, fatigue, and diarrhea. These are generally transient, occurring early in treatment, and can often be obviated by beginning with a low dose and increasing dosage gradually until an optimal regimen is established. Diarrhea may be severe and may necessitate temporary withdrawal of **Dantrium** therapy. If diarrhea recurs upon readministration of **Dantrium**, therapy should probably be withdrawn permanently.

Other less frequent side effects, listed according to system, are:

Gastrointestinal: Constipation, rarely progressing to signs of intestinal obstruction, GI bleeding, anorexia, swallowing difficulty, gastric irritation, abdominal cramps, nausea and/or vomiting.

Hepatobiliary: Hepatitis (see **WARNINGS**).

Neurologic: Speech disturbance, seizure, headache, lightheadedness, visual disturbance, diplopia, alteration of taste, insomnia, drooling.

Cardiovascular: Tachycardia, erratic blood pressure, phlebitis, heart failure.

Hematologic: Aplastic anemia, leukopenia, lymphocytic lymphoma, thrombocytopenia.

Psychiatric: Mental depression, mental confusion, increased nervousness.

Urogenital: Increased urinary frequency, crystalluria, hematuria, difficult erection, urinary incontinence and/or nocturia, difficult urination and/or urinary retention.

Integumentary: Abnormal hair growth, acne-like rash, pruritus, urticaria, eczematoid eruption, sweating.

Musculoskeletal: Myalgia, backache.

Respiratory: Feeling of suffocation, respiratory depression.

Special Senses: Excessive tearing.

Hypersensitivity: Pleural effusion with pericarditis, anaphylaxis.

Other: Chills and fever.

The published literature has included some reports of **Dantrium** use in patients with Neuroleptic Malignant Syndrome (NMS). **Dantrium** capsules are not indicated for the treatment of NMS and patients may expire despite treatment with **Dantrium** capsules.

DRUG ABUSE AND DEPENDENCE

Drug abuse and dependency potential has not been evaluated in human or animal studies.

OVERDOSE

Symptoms which may occur in case of overdose include, but are not limited to, muscular weakness and alterations in the state of consciousness (e.g. lethargy, coma), vomiting, diarrhea, and crystalluria. For acute overdose, general supportive measures should be employed along with immediate gastric lavage.

Intravenous fluids should be administered in fairly large quantities to avert the possibility of crystalluria. An adequate airway should be maintained and artificial resuscitation equipment should be at hand. Electrocardiographic monitoring should be instituted, and the patient carefully observed. To date, no experience has been reported with dialysis and its value in Dantrium overdose is not known.

DOSAGE AND ADMINISTRATION

For Use in Chronic Spasticity: Prior to the administration of **Dantrium**, consideration should be given to the potential response to treatment. A decrease in spasticity sufficient to allow a daily function not otherwise attainable should be the therapeutic goal of treatment with **Dantrium**. Refer to **INDICATIONS AND USAGE** section for description of response to be anticipated.

It is important to establish a therapeutic goal (regain and maintain a specific function such as therapeutic exercise program, utilization of braces, transfer maneuvers, etc.) before beginning **Dantrium** therapy. Dosage should be increased until the maximum performance compatible with the dysfunction due to underlying disease is achieved. No further increase in dosage is then indicated.

Usual Dosage: It is important that the dosage be titrated and individualized for maximum effect. The lowest dose compatible with optimal response is recommended.

In view of the potential for liver damage in long-term **Dantrium** *use, therapy should be stopped if benefits are not evident within 45 days.*

Adults: The following gradual titration schedule is suggested. Some patients will not respond until higher daily dosage is achieved. Each dosage level should be maintained for seven days to determine the patient's response. If no further benefit is observed at the next higher dose, dosage should be decreased to the previous lower dose.

25 mg once daily for seven days, then
25 mg t.i.d. for seven days
50 mg t.i.d. for seven days
100 mg t.i.d.

Therapy with a dose four times daily may be necessary for some individuals. Doses higher than 100 mg four times daily should not be used. (See Box Warning.)

Pediatric Patients: The following gradual titration schedule is suggested. Some patients will not respond until higher daily dosage is achieved. Each dosage level should be maintained for seven days to determine the patient's response. If no further benefit is observed at the next higher dose, dosage should be decreased to the previous lower dose.

0.5 mg/kg once daily for seven days, then
0.5 mg/kg t.i.d. for seven days
1 mg/kg t.i.d. for seven days
2 mg/kg t.i.d.

Therapy with a dose four times daily may be necessary for some individuals. Doses higher than 100 mg four times daily should not be used. (See Box Warning.)

For Malignant Hyperthermia:

Preoperatively: Administer 4 to 8 mg/kg/day of oral **Dantrium** in 3 or 4 divided doses for one or two days prior to surgery, with the last dose being given approximately 3 to 4 hours before scheduled surgery with a minimum of water. This dosage will usually be associated with skeletal muscle weakness and sedation (sleepiness or drowsiness); adjustment can usually be made within the recommended dosage range to avoid incapacitation or excessive gastrointestinal irritation (including nausea and/or vomiting).

Post Crisis Follow-up: Oral **Dantrium** should also be administered following a malignant hyperthermia crisis, in doses of 4 to 8 mg/kg per day in four divided doses, for a one to three day period to prevent recurrence of the manifestations of malignant hyperthermia.

HOW SUPPLIED

Dantrium (dantrolene sodium) is available in:

25-mg opaque, orange and tan capsules:
NDC 0149-0030-05 bottle of 100
NDC 0149-0030-66 bottle of 500
50-mg opaque, orange and tan capsules:
NDC 0149-0031-05 bottle of 100
100-mg opaque, orange and tan capsules:
NDC 0149-0033-05 bottle of 100

Avoid excessive heat (over 104°F or 40°C).

Address medical inquiries to Procter & Gamble Pharmaceuticals, Medical Communications Department, PO Box 8006, Mason, Ohio 45040-8006.

REVISED SEPTEMBER 2002

DANTRIUM® INTRAVENOUS ℞

[*dăn trē ŭm*]

(dantrolene sodium for injection)

DESCRIPTION

Dantrium Intravenous is a sterile, non-pyrogenic, lyophilized formulation of dantrolene sodium for injection. **Dantrium Intravenous** is supplied in 70 mL vials containing 20 mg dantrolene sodium, 3000 mg mannitol, and sufficient sodium hydroxide to yield a pH of approximately 9.5 when reconstituted with 60 mL sterile water for injection USP (without a bacteriostatic agent).

Dantrium is classified as a direct-acting skeletal muscle relaxant. Chemically, **Dantrium** is hydrated 1-[[[5-(4-nitrophenyl)-2-furanyl]methylene]amino]-2,4-imidazolidinedione sodium salt. The structural formula for the hydrated salt is:

O_2N–(phenyl)–(furan)–CH = N – N(imidazolidinedione, NNa) $\cdot xH_2O$

The hydrated salt contains approximately 15% water (3-1/2 moles) and has a molecular weight of 399. The anhydrous salt (dantrolene) has a molecular weight of 336.

CLINICAL PHARMACOLOGY

In isolated nerve-muscle preparation, **Dantrium** has been shown to produce relaxation by affecting the contractile response of the muscle at a site beyond the myoneural junction. In skeletal muscle, **Dantrium** dissociates the excitation-contraction coupling, probably by interfering with the release of Ca^{++} from the sarcoplasmic reticulum. The administration of intravenous **Dantrium** to human volunteers is associated with loss of grip strength and weakness in the legs, as well as subjective CNS complaints (see also PRECAUTIONS, Information for Patients). Information concerning the passage of **Dantrium** across the blood-brain barrier is not available.

In the anesthetic-induced malignant hyperthermia syndrome, evidence points to an intrinsic abnormality of skeletal muscle tissue. In affected humans, it has been postulated that "triggering agents" (e.g., general anesthetics and depolarizing neuromuscular blocking agents) produce a change within the cell which results in an elevated myoplasmic calcium. This elevated myoplasmic calcium activates acute cellular catabolic processes that cascade to the malignant hyperthermia crisis.

It is hypothesized that addition of **Dantrium** to the "triggered" malignant hyperthermic muscle cell reestablishes a normal level of ionized calcium in the myoplasm. Inhibition of calcium release from the sarcoplasmic reticulum by **Dantrium** reestablishes the myoplasmic calcium equilibrium, increasing the percentage of bound calcium. In this way, physiologic, metabolic, and biochemical changes associated with the malignant hyperthermia crisis may be reversed or attenuated. Experimental results in malignant hyperthermia susceptible swine show that prophylactic administration of intravenous or oral dantrolene prevents or attenuates the development of vital sign and blood gas changes characteristic of malignant hyperthermia in a dose related manner. The efficacy of intravenous dantrolene in the treatment of human and porcine malignant hyperthermia crisis, when considered along with prophylactic experiments in malignant hyperthermia susceptible swine, lends support to prophylactic use of oral or intravenous dantrolene in malignant hyperthermia susceptible humans. When prophylactic intravenous dantrolene is administered as directed, whole blood concentrations remain at a near steady state level for 3 or more hours after the infusion is completed. Clinical experience has shown that early vital sign and/or blood gas changes characteristic of malignant hyperthermia may appear during or after anesthesia and surgery despite the prophylactic use of dantrolene and adherence to currently accepted patient management practices. These signs are compatible with attenuated malignant hyperthermia and respond to the administration of

Continued on next page

Dantrium Intravenous—Cont.

additional i.v. dantrolene (see DOSAGE AND ADMINISTRATION). The administration of the recommended prophylactic dose of intravenous dantrolene to healthy volunteers was not associated with clinically significant cardiorespiratory changes.
Specific metabolic pathways for the degradation and elimination of **Dantrium** in humans have been established. Dantrolene is found in measurable amounts in blood and urine. Its major metabolites in body fluids are 5-hydroxy dantrolene and an acetylamino metabolite of dantrolene. Another metabolite with an unknown structure appears related to the latter. **Dantrium** may also undergo hydrolysis and subsequent oxidation forming nitrophenylfuroic acid.
The mean biologic half-life of **Dantrium** after intravenous administration is variable, between 4 to 8 hours under most experimental conditions. Based on assays of whole blood and plasma, slightly greater amounts of dantrolene are associated with red blood cells than with the plasma fraction of blood. Significant amounts of dantrolene are bound to plasma proteins, mostly albumin, and this binding is readily reversible.
Cardiopulmonary depression has not been observed in malignant hyperthermia susceptible swine following the administration of up to 7.5 mg/kg i.v. dantrolene. This is twice the amount needed to maximally diminish twitch response to single supramaximal peripheral nerve stimulation (95% inhibition). A transient, inconsistent, depressant effect on gastrointestinal smooth muscles has been observed at high doses.

INDICATIONS AND USAGE

Dantrium Intravenous is indicated, along with appropriate supportive measures, for the management of the fulminant hypermetabolism of skeletal muscle characteristic of malignant hyperthermia crises in patients of all ages. **Dantrium Intravenous** should be administered by continuous rapid intravenous push as soon as the malignant hyperthermia reaction is recognized (i.e., tachycardia, tachypnea, central venous desaturation, hypercarbia, metabolic acidosis, skeletal muscle rigidity, increased utilization of anesthesia circuit carbon dioxide absorber, cyanosis and mottling of the skin, and, in many cases, fever).
Dantrium Intravenous is also indicated preoperatively, and sometimes postoperatively, to prevent or attenuate the development of clinical and laboratory signs of malignant hyperthermia in individuals judged to be malignant hyperthermia susceptible.

CONTRAINDICATIONS

None.

WARNINGS

The use of **Dantrium Intravenous** *in the management of malignant hyperthermia crisis is not a substitute for previously known supportive measures. These measures must be individualized, but it will usually be necessary to discontinue the suspect triggering agents, attend to increased oxygen requirements, manage the metabolic acidosis, institute cooling when necessary, monitor urinary output, and monitor for electrolyte imbalance.*
Since the effect of disease state and other drugs on **Dantrium** related skeletal muscle weakness, including possible respiratory depression, cannot be predicted, patients who receive i.v. **Dantrium** preoperatively should have vital signs monitored.
If patients judged malignant hyperthermia susceptible are administered intravenous or oral **Dantrium** preoperatively, anesthetic preparation must still follow a standard malignant hyperthermia susceptible regimen, including the avoidance of known triggering agents. Monitoring for early clinical and metabolic signs of malignant hyperthermia is indicated because attenuation of malignant hyperthermia, rather than prevention, is possible. These signs usually call for the administration of additional i.v. dantrolene.

PRECAUTIONS

General: Care must be taken to prevent extravasation of **Dantrium** solution into the surrounding tissues due to the high pH of the intravenous formulation.
When mannitol is used for prevention or treatment of late renal complications of malignant hyperthermia, the 3 g of mannitol needed to dissolve each 20 mg vial of i.v. **Dantrium** should be taken into consideration.
Information for Patients: Based upon data in human volunteers, it will sometimes be appropriate to tell patients who receive **Dantrium Intravenous** that decrease in grip strength and weakness of leg muscles, especially walking down stairs, can be expected postoperatively. In addition, symptoms such as "lightheadedness" may be noted. Since some of these symptoms may persist for up to 48 hours, patients must not operate an automobile or engage in other hazardous activity during this time. Caution is also indicated at meals on the day of administration because difficulty swallowing and choking has been reported. Caution should be exercised in the concomitant administration of tranquilizing agents.
Hepatotoxicity seen with **Dantrium Capsules: Dantrium** (dantrolene sodium) has a potential for hepatotoxicity, and should not be used in conditions other than those recommended. Symptomatic hepatitis (fatal and non-fatal) has been reported at various dose levels of the drug. The incidence reported in patients taking up to 400 mg/day is much lower than in those taking doses of 800 mg or more per day. Even sporadic short courses of these higher dose levels within a treatment regimen markedly increased the risk of serious hepatic injury. Liver dysfunction as evidenced by blood chemical abnormalities alone (liver enzyme elevations) has been observed in patients exposed to **Dantrium** for varying periods of time. Overt hepatitis has occurred at varying intervals after initiation of therapy, but has been most frequently observed between the third and twelfth month of therapy. The risk of hepatic injury appears to be greater in females, in patients over 35 years of age, and in patients taking other medication(s) in addition to **Dantrium** (dantrolene sodium). **Dantrium** should be used only in conjunction with appropriate monitoring of hepatic function including frequent determination of SGOT or SGPT.
Fatal and non-fatal liver disorders of an idiosyncratic or hypersensitivity type may occur with **Dantrium** therapy.
Drug Interactions: Dantrium is metabolized by the liver, and it is theoretically possible that its metabolism may be enhanced by drugs known to induce hepatic microsomal enzymes. However, neither phenobarbital nor diazepam appears to affect **Dantrium** metabolism. Binding to plasma protein is not significantly altered by diazepam, diphenylhydantoin, or phenylbutazone. Binding to plasma proteins is reduced by warfarin and clofibrate and increased by tolbutamide.
Cardiovascular collapse in patients treated simultaneously with verapamil and dantrolene sodium is rare. The combination of therapeutic doses of intravenous dantrolene sodium and verapamil in halothane/alpha-chloralose anesthetized swine has resulted in ventricular fibrillation and cardiovascular collapse in association with marked hyperkalemia. It is recommended that the combination of intravenous dantrolene sodium and calcium channel blockers, such as verapamil, not be used together during the management of malignant hyperthermia crisis until the relevance of these findings to humans is established.
Administration of dantrolene may potentiate vecuronium-induced neuromuscular block.
Carcinogenesis, Mutagenesis, and Impairment of Fertility: Sprague-Dawley female rats fed **Dantrium** for 18 months at dosage levels of 15, 30, and 60 mg/kg/day showed an increased incidence of benign and malignant mammary tumors compared with concurrent controls. At the highest dose level (approximately the same as the maximum recommended daily dose on a mg/m^2 basis), there was an increase in the incidence of benign hepatic lymphatic neoplasms. In a 30-month study in Sprague-Dawley rats fed dantrolene sodium, the highest dose level (approximately the same as the maximum recommended daily dose on a mg/m^2 basis) produced a decrease in the time of onset of mammary neoplasms. Female rats at the highest dose level showed an increased incidence of hepatic lymphangiomas and hepatic angiosarcomas.
The only drug-related effect seen in a 30-month study in Fischer-344 rats was a dose-related reduction in the time of onset of mammary and testicular tumors. A 24-month study in HaM/ICR mice revealed no evidence of carcinogenic activity.
The significance of carcinogenicity data relative to use of **Dantrium** in humans is unknown.
Dantrolene sodium has produced positive results in the Ames *S. Typhimurium* bacterial mutagenesis assay in the presence and absence of a liver activating system.
Dantrolene sodium administered to male and female rats at dose levels up to 45 mg/kg/day (approximately 1.4 times the maximum recommended daily dose on a mg/m^2 basis) showed no adverse effects on fertility or general reproductive performance.
Pregnancy: Pregnancy Category C: **Dantrium** has been shown to be embryocidal in the rabbit and has been shown to decrease pup survival in the rat when given at doses seven times the human oral dose. There are no adequate and well-controlled studies in pregnant women. **Dantrium Intravenous** should be used during pregnancy only if the potential benefit justifies the potential risk to the fetus.
Labor and Delivery: In one uncontrolled study, 100 mg per day of prophylactic oral **Dantrium** was administered to term pregnant patients awaiting labor and delivery. Dantrolene readily crossed the placenta, with maternal and fetal whole blood levels approximately equal at delivery; neonatal levels then fell approximately 50% per day for 2 days before declining sharply. No neonatal respiratory and neuromuscular side effects were detected at low dose. More data, at higher doses, are needed before more definitive conclusions can be made.

ADVERSE REACTIONS

There have been occasional reports of death following malignant hyperthermia crisis even when treated with intravenous dantrolene; incidence figures are not available (the pre-dantrolene mortality of malignant hyperthermia crisis was approximately 50%). Most of these deaths can be accounted for by late recognition, delayed treatment, inadequate dosage, lack of supportive therapy, intercurrent disease and/or the development of delayed complications such as renal failure or disseminated intravascular coagulopathy. In some cases there are insufficient data to completely rule out therapeutic failure of dantrolene.
There are rare reports of fatality in malignant hyperthermia crisis, despite initial satisfactory response to i.v. dantrolene, which involve patients who could not be weaned from dantrolene after initial treatment.
The administration of intravenous **Dantrium** to human volunteers is associated with loss of grip strength and weakness in the legs, as well as drowsiness and dizziness.
The following adverse reactions are in approximate order of severity:
There are rare reports of pulmonary edema developing during the treatment of malignant hyperthermia crisis in which the diluent volume and mannitol needed to deliver i.v. dantrolene possibly contributed.
There have been reports of thrombophlebitis following administration of intravenous dantrolene; actual incidence figures are not available.
There have been rare reports of urticaria and erythema possibly associated with the administration of i.v. **Dantrium**. There has been one case of anaphylaxis.
None of the serious reactions occasionally reported with long-term oral **Dantrium**, such as hepatitis, seizures, and pleural effusion with pericarditis, have been reasonably associated with short-term **Dantrium Intravenous** therapy.
The following events have been reported in patients receiving oral dantrolene: aplastic anemia, leukopenia, lymphocytic lymphoma, and heart failure. (See package insert for **Dantrium** (dantrolene sodium) **Capsules** for a complete listing of adverse reactions.)
The published literature has included some reports of **Dantrium** use in patients with Neuroleptic Malignant Syndrome (NMS). **Dantrium Intravenous** is not indicated for the treatment of NMS and patients may expire despite treatment with **Dantrium Intravenous**.

OVERDOSAGE

Because **Dantrium Intravenous** must be administered at a low concentration in a large volume of fluid, acute toxicity of **Dantrium** could not be assessed in animals. In 14-day (subacute) studies, the intravenous formulation of **Dantrium** was relatively non-toxic to rats at doses of 10 mg/kg/day and 20 mg/kg/day. While 10 mg/kg/day in dogs for 14 days evoked little toxicity, 20 mg/kg/day for 14 days caused hepatic changes of questionable biologic significance.
Symptoms which may occur in case of overdose include, but are not limited to, muscular weakness and alterations in the state of consciousness (e.g., lethargy, coma), vomiting, diarrhea, and crystalluria.
For acute overdosage, general supportive measures should be employed.
Intravenous fluids should be administered in fairly large quantities to avert the possibility of crystalluria. An adequate airway should be maintained and artificial resuscitation equipment should be at hand. Electrocardiographic monitoring should be instituted, and the patient carefully observed. The value of dialysis in **Dantrium** overdose is not known.

DOSAGE AND ADMINISTRATION

As soon as the malignant hyperthermia reaction is recognized, all anesthetic agents should be discontinued; the administration of 100% oxygen is recommended. **Dantrium Intravenous** should be administered by continuous rapid intravenous push beginning at a minimum dose of 1 mg/kg, and continuing until symptoms subside or the maximum cumulative dose of 10 mg/kg has been reached.
If the physiologic and metabolic abnormalities reappear, the regimen may be repeated. It is important to note that administration of **Dantrium Intravenous** should be continuous until symptoms subside. The effective dose to reverse the crisis is directly dependent upon the individuals degree of susceptibility to malignant hyperthermia, the amount and time of exposure to the triggering agent, and the time elapsed between onset of the crisis and initiation of treatment.
Pediatric Dose: Experience to date indicates that the dose of **Dantrium Intravenous** for pediatric patients is the same as for adults.
Preoperatively: Dantrium Intravenous and/or **Dantrium Capsules** may be administered preoperatively to patients judged malignant hyperthermia susceptible as part of the overall patient management to prevent or attenuate the development of clinical and laboratory signs of malignant hyperthermia.

Dantrium Intravenous: The recommended prophylactic dose of **Dantrium Intravenous** is 2.5 mg/kg, starting approximately 1–1/4 hours before anticipated anesthesia and infused over approximately 1 hour. This dose should prevent or attenuate the development of clinical and laboratory signs of malignant hyperthermia provided that the usual precautions, such as avoidance of established malignant hyperthermia triggering agents, are followed. Additional **Dantrium Intravenous** may be indicated during anesthesia and surgery because of the appearance of early clinical and/or blood gas signs of malignant hyperthermia or because of prolonged surgery (see also CLINICAL PHARMACOLOGY, WARNINGS, and PRECAUTIONS). Additional doses must be individualized.

Oral Administration of Dantrium Capsules: Administer 4 to 8 mg/kg/day of oral **Dantrium** in three or four divided doses for 1 or 2 days prior to surgery, with the last dose being given with a minimum of water approximately 3 to 4 hours before scheduled surgery. Adjustment can usually be made within the recommended dosage range to avoid incapacitation (weakness, drowsiness, etc.) or excessive gastrointestinal irritation (nausea and/or vomiting). See also the package insert for **Dantrium Capsules**.

Post Crisis Follow-Up: Dantrium Capsules, 4 to 8 mg/kg/day, in four divided doses should be administered for 1 to 3 days following a malignant hyperthermia crisis to prevent recurrence of the manifestations of malignant hyperthermia.

Intravenous **Dantrium** may be used postoperatively to prevent or attenuate the recurrence of signs of malignant hyperthermia when oral **Dantrium** administration is not practical. The i.v. dose of **Dantrium** in the postoperative period must be individualized, starting with 1 mg/kg or more as the clinical situation dictates.

PREPARATION

Each vial of **Dantrium Intravenous** should be reconstituted by adding 60 mL of *sterile water for injection USP (without a bacteriostatic agent), and the vial shaken until the solution is clear.* 5% Dextrose Injection USP, 0.9% Sodium Chloride Injection USP, and other acidic solutions are not compatible with **Dantrium Intravenous** and should not be used. The contents of the vial must be *protected from direct light and used within 6 hours* after reconstitution. Store reconstituted solutions at controlled room temperature (59°F to 86°F or 15°C to 30°C).

Reconstituted **Dantrium Intravenous** should *not* be transferred to large glass bottles for prophylactic infusion due to precipitate formation observed with the use of some glass bottles as reservoirs.

For prophylactic infusion, the required number of individual vials of **Dantrium Intravenous** should be reconstituted as outlined above. The contents of individual vials are then transferred to a larger volume sterile intravenous plastic bag. Stability data on file at Procter & Gamble Pharmaceuticals indicate commercially available sterile plastic bags are acceptable drug delivery devices. However, it is recommended that the prepared infusion be inspected carefully for cloudiness and/or precipitation prior to dispensing and administration. Such solutions should not be used. While stable for 6 hours, it is recommended that the infusion be prepared immediately prior to the anticipated dosage administration time.

Parenteral drug products should be inspected visually for particulate matter and discoloration prior to administration.

HOW SUPPLIED

Dantrium Intravenous (**NDC** 0149-0734-02) is available in vials containing a sterile lyophilized mixture of 20 mg dantrolene sodium, 3000 mg mannitol, and sufficient sodium hydroxide to yield a pH of approximately 9.5 when reconstituted with 60 mL sterile water for injection USP (without a bacteriostatic agent).

Store unreconstituted product at controlled room temperature (59°F to 86°F or 15°C to 30°C) and avoid prolonged exposure to light.

Address medical inquiries to Procter & Gamble Pharmaceuticals, Medical Communications Department, PO Box 8006, Mason, Ohio 45040-8006.

To place an order, call Procter & Gamble Pharmaceuticals Customer Service 800-448-4878.

Mfg. by: Ben Venue Laboratories
Bedford, OH 44146
Dist. By: **Procter & Gamble Pharmaceuticals,** TM Owner,
Cincinnati, Ohio 45202
REVISED MAY 2001

DIDRONEL® ℞

[dī'drō-nĕl]
(etidronate disodium)

DESCRIPTION

Didronel tablets contain either 200 mg or 400 mg of etidronate disodium, the disodium salt of (1-hydroxyethylidene) diphosphonic acid, for oral administration. This compound, also known as EHDP, regulates bone metabolism. It is a white powder, highly soluble in water, with a molecular weight of 250 and the following structural formula:

ONa OH ONa
HO—P—C—P—OH
O CH₃ O

Inactive Ingredients: Each tablet contains magnesium stearate, microcrystalline cellulose, and starch.

CLINICAL PHARMACOLOGY

Didronel acts primarily on bone. It can inhibit the formation, growth, and dissolution of hydroxyapatite crystals and their amorphous precursors by chemisorption to calcium phosphate surfaces. Inhibition of crystal resorption occurs at lower doses than are required to inhibit crystal growth. Both effects increase as the dose increases.

Didronel is not metabolized. The amount of drug absorbed after an oral dose is approximately 3%. In normal subjects, plasma half-life ($t_{1/2}$ of etidronate, based on non-compartmental pharmacokinetics is 1 to 6 hours. Within 24 hours, approximately half the absorbed dose is excreted in urine; the remainder is distributed to bone compartments from which it is slowly eliminated. Animal studies have yielded bone clearance estimates up to 165 days. In humans, the residence time on bone may vary due to such factors as specific metabolic condition and bone type. Unabsorbed drug is excreted intact in the feces. Preclinical studies indicate etidronate disodium does not cross the blood-brain barrier. **Didronel** therapy does not adversely affect serum levels of parathyroid hormone or calcium.

Paget's Disease: Paget's disease of bone (osteitis deformans) is an idiopathic, progressive disease characterized by abnormal and accelerated bone metabolism in one or more bones. Signs and symptoms may include bone pain and/or deformity, neurologic disorders, elevated cardiac output and other vascular disorders, and increased serum alkaline phosphatase and/or urinary hydroxyproline levels. Bone fractures are common in patients with Paget's disease.

Didronel slows accelerated bone turnover (resorption and accretion) in pagetic lesions and, to a lesser extent, in normal bone. This has been demonstrated histologically, scintigraphically, biochemically, and through calcium kinetic and balance studies. Reduced bone turnover is often accompanied by symptomatic improvement, including reduced bone pain. Also, the incidence of pagetic fractures may be reduced, and elevated cardiac output and other vascular disorders may be improved by **Didronel** therapy.

Heterotopic Ossification: Heterotopic ossification, also referred to as myositis ossificans (circumscripta, progressiva or traumatica), ectopic calcification, periarticular ossification, or paraosteoarthropathy, is characterized by metaplastic osteogenesis. It usually presents with signs of localized inflammation or pain, elevated skin temperature, and redness. When tissues near joints are involved, functional loss may also be present.

Heterotopic ossification may occur for no known reason as in myositis ossificans progressiva or may follow a wide variety of surgical, occupational, and sports trauma (e.g., hip arthroplasty, spinal cord injury, head injury, burns, and severe thigh bruises). Heterotopic ossification has also been observed in non-traumatic conditions (e.g., infections of the central nervous system, peripheral neuropathy, tetanus, biliary cirrhosis, Peyronie's disease, as well as in association with a variety of benign and malignant neoplasms).

Clinical trials have demonstrated the efficacy of **Didronel** in heterotopic ossification following total hip replacement, or due to spinal cord injury.

— *Heterotopic ossification complicating total hip replacement* typically develops radiographically 3 to 8 weeks postoperatively in the pericapsular area of the affected hip joint. The overall incidence is about 50%; about one-third of these cases are clinically significant.
— *Heterotopic ossification due to spinal cord injury* typically develops radiographically 1 to 4 months after injury. It occurs below the level of injury, usually at major joints. The overall incidence is about 40%; about one-half of these cases are clinically significant.

Didronel chemisorbs to calcium hydroxyapatite crystals and their amorphous precursors, blocking the aggregation, growth, and mineralization of these crystals. This is thought to be the mechanism by which **Didronel** prevents or retards heterotopic ossification. There is no evidence **Didronel** affects mature heterotopic bone.

INDICATIONS AND USAGE

Didronel is indicated for the treatment of symptomatic Paget's disease of bone and in the prevention and treatment of heterotopic ossification following total hip replacement or due to spinal cord injury. **Didronel** is not approved for the treatment of osteoporosis.

Paget's Disease: **Didronel** is indicated for the treatment of symptomatic Paget's disease of bone. **Didronel** therapy usually arrests or significantly impedes the disease process as evidenced by:

— Symptomatic relief, including decreased pain and/or increased mobility (experienced by 3 out of 5 patients).
— Reductions in serum alkaline phosphatase and urinary hydroxyproline levels (30% or more in 4 out of 5 patients).
— Histomorphometry showing reduced numbers of osteoclasts and osteoblasts, and more lamellar bone formation.
— Bone scans showing reduced radionuclide uptake at pagetic lesions.

In addition, reductions in pagetically elevated cardiac output and skin temperature have been observed in some patients.

In many patients, the disease process will be suppressed for a period of at least 1 year following cessation of therapy. The upper limit of this period has not been determined.

The effects of the **Didronel** treatment in patients with asymptomatic Paget's disease have not been studied. However, **Didronel** treatment of such patients may be warranted if extensive involvement threatens irreversible neurologic damage, major joints, or major weight-bearing bones.

Heterotopic Ossification: **Didronel** is indicated in the prevention and treatment of heterotopic ossification following total hip replacement or due to spinal cord injury.

Didronel reduces the incidence of clinically important heterotopic bone by about two-thirds. Among those patients who form heterotopic bone, **Didronel** retards the progression of immature lesions and reduces the severity by at least half. Follow-up data (at least 9 months posttherapy) suggest these benefits persist.

In total hip replacement patients, **Didronel** does not promote loosening of the prosthesis or impede trochanteric reattachment.

In spinal cord injury patients, **Didronel** does not inhibit fracture healing or stabilization of the spine.

CONTRAINDICATIONS

Didronel tablets are contraindicated in patients with known hypersensitivity to etidronate disodium or in patients with clinically overt osteomalacia.

WARNINGS

Paget's Disease: In Paget's patients the response to therapy may be of slow onset and continue for months after **Didronel** therapy is discontinued. Dosage should not be increased prematurely. A 90-day drug-free interval should be provided between courses of therapy.

Heterotopic Ossification: No specific warnings.

PRECAUTIONS

General: Patients should maintain an adequate nutritional status, particularly an adequate intake of calcium and vitamin D.

Therapy has been withheld from some patients with enterocolitis since diarrhea may be experienced, particularly at higher doses.

Didronel is not metabolized and is excreted intact via the kidney. Hyperphosphatemia may occur at doses of 10 to 20 mg/kg/day, apparently as a result of drug-related increases in tubular reabsorption of phosphate. Serum phosphate levels generally return to normal 2 to 4 weeks posttherapy. There is no experience to specifically guide treatment in patients with impaired renal function. **Didronel** dosage should be reduced when reductions in glomerular filtration rates are present. Patients with renal impairment should be closely monitored. In approximately 10% of patients in clinical trials of **Didronel® I. V. Infusion** (etidronate disodium) for hypercalcemia of malignancy, occasional, mild-to-moderate abnormalities in renal function (increases of > 0.5 mg/dl serum creatinine) were observed during or immediately after treatment.

Didronel suppresses bone turnover, and may retard mineralization of osteoid laid down during the bone accretion process. These effects are dose and time dependent. Osteoid, which may accumulate noticeably at doses of 10 to 20 mg/kg/day, mineralizes normally posttherapy. In patients with fractures, especially of long bones, it may be advisable to delay or interrupt treatment until callus is evident.

Paget's Disease: In Paget's patients, treatment regimens exceeding the recommended (see DOSAGE AND ADMINISTRATION daily maximum dose of 20 mg/kg or continuous administration of medication for periods greater than 6 months may be associated with osteomalacia and an increased risk of fracture.

Long bones predominantly affected by lytic lesions, particularly in those patients unresponsive to **Didronel** therapy, may be especially prone to fracture.

Patients with predominantly lytic lesions should be monitored radiographically and biochemically to permit termination of **Didronel** in those patients unresponsive to treatment.

Drug Interactions: There have been isolated reports of patients experiencing increases in their prothrombin times when etidronate was added to warfarin therapy. The majority of these reports concerned variable elevations in prothrombin times without clinically significant sequelae. Although the relevance of these reports and any mechanism of coagulation alterations is unclear, patients on warfarin should have their prothrombin time monitored.

Carcinogenesis: Long-term studies in rats have indicated that **Didronel** is not carcinogenic.

Pregnancy: Teratogenic Effects: Pregnancy Category C. In teratology and developmental toxicity studies conducted in rats and rabbits treated with dosages of up to 100 mg/kg (5 to 20 times the clinical dose), no adverse or teratogenic effects have been observed in the offspring. Etidronate disodium has been shown to cause skeletal abnormalities in rats when given at oral dose levels of 300 mg/kg (15 to 60 times the human dose). Other effects on the offspring (including decreased live births) are at dosages that cause significant toxicity in the parent generation and are 25 to 200 times the human dose. The skeletal effects are thought to be the result of the pharmacological effects of the drug on bone. Bisphosphonates are incorporated into the bone matrix, from where they are gradually released over periods of weeks to years. The extent of bisphosphonate incorporation into adult bone, and hence, the amount available for release back into the systemic circulation, is directly related to the total dose and duration of bisphosphonate use. Although there are no data on fetal risk in humans, bisphosphonates do cause fetal harm in animals, and animal data suggest that uptake of bisphosphonates into fetal bone is greater than into maternal bone. Therefore, there is a theoretical risk of fetal harm (e.g., skeletal and other abnormalities) if a woman becomes pregnant after completing a course of bisphosphonate therapy. The impact of variables such as time between cessation of bisphosphonate therapy to conception, the particular bisphosphonate used, and the route of administration (intravenous versus oral) on this risk has not been established.

There are no adequate and well-controlled studies in pregnant women. **Didronel** (etidronate disodium) should be used during pregnancy only if the potential benefit justifies the potential risk to the fetus.

Nursing Mothers: It is not known whether this drug is excreted in human milk. Because many drugs are excreted in human milk, caution should be exercised when **Didronel** is administered to a nursing woman.

Pediatric Use: Safety and effectiveness in pediatric patients have not been established. Pediatric patients have been treated with **Didronel**, at doses recommended for adults, to prevent heterotopic ossifications or soft tissue calcifications. A rachitic syndrome has been reported infrequently at doses of 10 mg/kg/day and more for prolonged periods approaching or exceeding a year. The epiphyseal

Continued on next page

Didronel—Cont.

radiologic changes associated with retarded mineralization of new osteoid and cartilage, and occasional symptoms reported, have been reversible when medication is discontinued.

Geriatric Use: Clinical studies of **Didronel** did not include sufficient numbers of subjects aged 65 and over to determine whether they respond differently from younger subjects. Other reported clinical experience has not identified differences in responses between elderly and younger patients. In general, dose selection for an elderly patient should be cautious, reflecting the greater frequency of decreased hepatic, renal, or cardiac function, and of concomitant disease or other drug therapy. This drug is known to be substantially excreted by the kidney, and the risk of toxic reactions to this drug may be greater in patients with impaired renal function. Because elderly patients are more likely to have decreased renal function, care should be taken when prescribing this drug therapy. As stated in **PRECAUTIONS**, **Didronel** dosage should be reduced when reductions in glomerular filtration rates are present. In addition, patients with renal impairment should be closely monitored.

ADVERSE REACTIONS

The incidence of gastrointestinal complaints (diarrhea, nausea) is the same for **Didronel** at 5 mg/kg/day as for placebo, about 1 patient in 15. At 10 to 20 mg/kg/day the incidence may increase to 2 or 3 in 10. These complaints are often alleviated by dividing the total daily dose.

Paget's Disease: In Paget's patients, increased or recurrent bone pain at pagetic sites, and/or the onset of pain at previously asymptomatic sites has been reported. At 5 mg/kg/day about 1 patient in 10 (versus 1 in 15 in the placebo group) report these phenomena. At higher doses the incidence rises to about 2 in 10. When therapy continues, pain resolves in some patients but persists in others.

Heterotopic Ossification: No specific adverse reactions.

Worldwide Postmarketing Experience: The worldwide postmarketing experience for etidronate disodium reflects its use in the following approved indications: Paget's disease, heterotopic ossification, and hypercalcemia of malignancy. It also reflects the use of etidronate disodium for osteoporosis where approved in countries outside the US. Other adverse events that have been reported and were thought to be possibly related to etidronate disodium include the following: alopecia; arthropathies, including arthralgia and arthritis; bone fracture; esophagitis; glossitis; hypersensitivity reactions, including angioedema, follicular eruption, macular rash, maculopapular rash, pruritus, a single case of Stevens-Johnson syndrome, and urticaria; osteomalacia; neuropsychiatric events, including amnesia, confusion, depression, and hallucination; and paresthesias.

In patients receiving etidronate disodium, there have been rare reports of agranulocytosis, pancytopenia, and a report of leukopenia with recurrence on rechallenge. In addition, there have been rare reports of exacerbation of asthma. Exacerbation of existing peptic ulcer disease has been reported in a few patients. In one patient, perforation also occurred.

In osteoporosis clinical trials, headache, gastritis, leg cramps, and arthralgia occurred at a significantly greater incidence in patients who received etidronate as compared with those who received placebo.

OVERDOSAGE

Clinical experience with acute **Didronel** overdosage is extremely limited. Decreases in serum calcium following substantial overdosage may be expected in some patients. Signs and symptoms of hypocalcemia also may occur in some of these patients. Some patients may develop vomiting. In one event, an 18-year-old female who ingested an estimated single dose of 4000 to 6000 mg (67 to 100 mg/kg) of **Didronel** was reported to be mildly hypocalcemic (7.52 mg/dl) and experienced paresthesia of the fingers. Hypocalcemia resolved 6 hours after lavage and treatment with intravenous calcium gluconate. A 92-year-old female who accidentally received 1600 mg of etidronate disodium per day for 3.5 days experienced marked diarrhea and required treatment for electrolyte imbalance. Orally administered etidronate disodium may cause hematologic abnormalities in some patients (see **ADVERSE REACTIONS**).

Etidronate disodium suppresses bone turnover and may retard mineralization of osteoid laid down during the bone accretion process. These effects are dose and time dependent. Osteoid which may accumulate noticeably at doses of 10 to 20 mg/kg/day of chronic, continuous dosing mineralizes normally posttherapy.

Prolonged continuous treatment (chronic overdosage) has been reported to cause nephrotic syndrome and fracture.

Gastric lavage may remove unabsorbed drug. Standard procedures for treating hypocalcemia, including the administration of Ca^{++} intravenously, would be expected to restore physiologic amounts of ionized calcium and relieve signs and symptoms of hypocalcemia. Such treatment has been effective.

DOSAGE AND ADMINISTRATION

Didronel should be taken as a single, oral dose. However, should gastrointestinal discomfort occur, the dose may be divided. To maximize absorption, patients should avoid taking the following items within two hours of dosing:

- Food, especially food high in calcium, such as milk or milk products.
- Vitamins with mineral supplements or antacids which are high in metals such as calcium, iron, magnesium, or aluminum.

***Paget's Disease:* Initial Treatment Regimens:** 5 to 10 mg/kg/day, not to exceed 6 months, or 11 to 20 mg/kg/day, not to exceed 3 months.

The recommended initial dose is 5 mg/kg/day for a period not to exceed 6 months. Doses above 10 mg/kg/day should be reserved for when 1) lower doses are ineffective or 2) there is an overriding need to suppress rapid bone turnover (especially when irreversible neurologic damage is possible) or reduce elevated cardiac output. Doses in excess of 20 mg/kg/day are not recommended.

Retreatment Guidelines: Retreatment should be initiated only after 1) a **Didronel**-free period of at least 90 days and 2) there is biochemical, symptomatic or other evidence of active disease process. It is advisable to monitor patients every 3 to 6 months although some patients may go drug free for extended periods. Retreatment regimens are the same as for initial treatment. For most patients the original dose will be adequate for retreatment. If not, consideration should be given to increasing the dose within the recommended guidelines.

Heterotopic Ossification: The following treatment regimens have been shown to be effective:

- Total Hip Replacement Patients: 20 mg/kg/day for 1 month before and 3 months after surgery (4 months total).
- Spinal Cord Injured Patients: 20 mg/kg/day for 2 weeks followed by 10 mg/kg/day for 10 weeks (12 weeks total). **Didronel** therapy should begin as soon as medically feasible following the injury, preferably prior to evidence of heterotopic ossification.

Retreatment has not been studied.

HOW SUPPLIED

Didronel is available as 200-mg, white, rectangular tablets with "P & G" on one face and "402" on the other.

NDC 0149-0405-60 bottle of 60

400-mg, white, scored, capsule-shaped tablets with "N E" on one face and "406" on the other.

NDC 0149-0406-60 bottle of 60

Avoid excessive heat (over 104°F or 40°C).

Mfg. by: OSG Norwich
Pharmaceuticals, Inc.
North Norwich, NY 13814
Dist. by:
Procter & Gamble Pharmaceuticals,
TM Owner, Cincinnati, OH 45202
REVISED MAY 2003

Shown in Product Identification Guide, page 330

The Purdue Frederick Company

ONE STAMFORD FORUM
STAMFORD, CT 06901-3431

For Medical Information Contact:
888-726-7535
Adverse Drug Experiences:
888-726-7535
Customer Service:
800-877-5666
FAX 800-877-3210

OxyContin® 10 mg Tablets
OxyContin® 20 mg Tablets
OxyContin® 40 mg Tablets
OxyContin® 80 mg Tablets
OxyContin® 160 mg Tablets
see listing under Purdue Pharma L.P., page 2537

OxyIR® Capsules—see listing under Purdue Pharma L.P., page 2541

BETADINE® SKIN CLEANSER OTC

[*bā 'tăh-dīn "*]
(povidone-iodine, 7.5%)

BETADINE Skin Cleanser, a sudsing, antiseptic bactericidal, liquid cleanser, forms a rich, golden lather.

INDICATIONS

Disinfectant hand wash and skin cleanser; significantly reduces bacteria on the skin; used routinely for general hygiene; virtually nonirritating, nonstaining to skin.

DIRECTIONS

Wet skin and apply a sufficient amount for lather to cover all surfaces; wash vigorously for at least 15 seconds; rinse and dry thoroughly.

WARNINGS

For external use only.

Do not use this product if you are sensitive to iodine or other product ingredients, in the eyes, over large areas of the body, or for longer than 1 week unless directed by a doctor. Ask a doctor before use if you have deep or puncture wounds, serious burns, or animal bites.

Stop using this product and ask a doctor if redness, irritation, swelling, or pain continues or increases, or infection occurs. **Keep out of reach of children.** If swallowed, get medical help or contact a Poison Control Center right away.

HOW SUPPLIED

4 fl. oz. plastic bottles.

NOTE

Blue stains on starched linen will wash off with soap and water.

BETADINE® SOLUTION OTC

[*bā 'tăh-dīn "*]
(povidone-iodine,10%)
Topical Antiseptic Bactericide

INDICATIONS

For preparation of the skin prior to surgery. Helps reduce bacteria that potentially can cause skin infection.

ADMINISTRATION

Clean the area. Apply product to the operative site prior to surgery. May be covered with a bandage.

WARNINGS

For external use only.

Do not use in the eyes or if you are allergic to povidone iodine or any other ingredient in this preparation.

Stop use and ask a doctor if irritation, sensitization, or allergic reaction occurs. In preoperative prepping, avoid "pooling" beneath the patient. Prolonged exposure to wet solution may cause irritation or, rarely, severe skin reactions. **Keep out of reach of children.** If swallowed, get medical help or contact a Poison Control Center right away.

HOW SUPPLIED

$^1/_2$ oz., 4 oz., 8 oz., 16 oz. (1 pt.), 32 oz. (1 qt.) and 1 gal. plastic bottles.

BETADINE® SURGICAL SCRUB OTC

[*bā 'tăh-dīn "*]
(povidone-iodine, 7.5%)
Topical Antiseptic Bactericide/Virucide

INDICATIONS

A broad-spectrum antiseptic, bactericidal, sudsing skin cleanser for pre- and postoperative scrubbing or washing by hospital operating room personnel; for preparation of the skin prior to surgery; for hand washing to reduce bacteria on the skin; for preoperative use on patients; and general use as an antiseptic microbicide in physician's office. Forms rich, golden lather.

DIRECTIONS

A. **Surgical hand scrub:**
Wet hands with water.
Pour about 5 cc (1 teaspoonful) of Scrub on the palm of the hand and spread over both hands.
Without adding more water, scrub thoroughly for about 5 minutes.
Use a brush if desired. Clean thoroughly under fingernails.
Add a little water and develop copious suds. Rinse thoroughly under running water.
Repeat the entire procedure using another 5 cc of Scrub.

B. **Patient pre-operative skin preparation:**
After the skin is shaved, wet with water.
Apply Scrub (1 cc is sufficient to cover an area of 20–30 square inches), develop lather and scrub thoroughly for about five minutes.
Rinse off using sterile gauze saturated with water.
The area may be painted with BETADINE® Solution and allowed to dry.

WARNINGS

For external use only. Do not use this product in the eyes.

Stop use and ask a doctor if irritation and redness develop, in rare instances of local irritation or sensitivity. Do not heat prior to application. Prolonged exposure to wet solution may cause irritation or, rarely, severe skin reactions. In pre-operative prepping, avoid "pooling" beneath the patient. **Keep out of reach of children.** If swallowed, get medical help or contact a Poison Control Center right away.

SUPPLIED

4 oz. plastic bottle, 16 oz. (1 pint) plastic bottle with and without pump, 32 oz. (1 quart) and 1 gal. plastic bottles.

BETASEPT® Surgical Scrub OTC
[*bă 'tăh-sĕp-t"*]
(chlorhexidine gluconate) 4%

ACTION AND USES

BETASEPT Surgical Scrub (chlorhexidine gluconate) is an antiseptic/antimicrobial skin cleanser for hand scrubbing or washing by operating room personnel, for hand-washing by medical personnel, for pre-operative skin preparation, and for skin wound and general skin cleansing.

BETASEPT Surgical Scrub provides rapid bactericidal action and has a persistent antimicrobial effect against a wide range of microorganisms.

ADVANTAGES

BETASEPT Surgical Scrub is formulated in a highly viscous base which can help reduce waste and per-use cost during prepping and hand-washing. No pink tint has been added.

DIRECTIONS FOR USE

Surgical Hand Scrub:

Wet hands and forearms with water. Scrub for 3 minutes with about 5 mL of BETASEPT Surgical Scrub and a wet brush, paying particular attention to the nails, cuticles and interdigital spaces. A separate nail cleaner may be used. Rinse thoroughly. Wash for an additional 3 minutes with 5 mL of BETASEPT Surgical Scrub and rinse under running water. Dry thoroughly.

Personnel Hand Wash:

Wet hands with water. Dispense about 5 mL of BETASEPT Surgical Scrub into cupped hands and wash in a vigorous manner for 15 seconds. Rinse and dry thoroughly.

Pre-Operative Skin Preparation:

Apply BETASEPT Surgical Scrub liberally to surgical site and swab for at least 2 minutes. Dry with a sterile towel. Repeat procedure for an additional 2 minutes and again dry with a sterile towel.

Skin Wound and General Skin Cleansing:

Wounds which involve more than the superficial layers of the skin should not be routinely treated with BETASEPT Surgical Scrub. BETASEPT Surgical Scrub should not be used for repeated general skin cleansing of large body areas except in those patients whose underlying condition makes it necessary to reduce the bacterial population of the skin. To use, thoroughly rinse the area to be cleansed with water. Apply the minimum amount of BETASEPT Surgical Scrub necessary to cover the skin or wound area and wash gently. Rinse again thoroughly.

WARNINGS

FOR EXTERNAL USE ONLY. KEEP OUT OF EYES, EARS AND MOUTH, BETASEPT SURGICAL SCRUB SHOULD NOT BE USED AS A PRE-OPERATIVE SKIN PREPARATION OF THE FACE OR HEAD, MISUSE OF PRODUCTS CONTAINING CHLORHEXIDINE GLUCONATE HAS BEEN REPORTED TO CAUSE SERIOUS AND PERMANENT EYE INJURY WHEN IT HAS BEEN PERMITTED TO ENTER AND REMAIN IN THE EYE DURING SURGICAL PROCEDURES. IF BETASEPT SURGICAL SCRUB SHOULD CONTACT THESE AREAS, RINSE OUT PROMPTLY AND THOROUGHLY WITH WATER.

Avoid contact with meninges. Betasept Surgical Scrub should not be used by persons who have sensitivity to it or its components. Chlorhexidine gluconate has been reported to cause deafness when instilled in the middle ear through perforated ear drums. Irritation, sensitization and generalized allergic reactions have been reported with chlorhexidine-containing products, especially in the genital areas. If adverse reactions occur, discontinue use immediately and if severe, contact a physician. Keep this and all drugs out of the reach of children. In case of accidental ingestion, seek professional assistance or contact a Poison Control Center immediately.

Avoid excessive heat (above 104°F).

HOW SUPPLIED

BETASEPT® Surgical Scrub 4% is packaged in 1 gallon, 32 oz., 32 oz. with pump, 16 oz., 8 oz., and 4 oz. plastic bottles.

MS CONTIN® Ⓒ℞
[*ms-kŏn'-tĭn*]
(Morphine Sulfate Controlled-Release) Tablets
15 mg 30 mg 60 mg 100 mg 200 mg*

***200 mg for use in opioid-tolerant patients only**

OT00001C
300519-0B-001

DESCRIPTION

Chemically, morphine sulfate is 7,8-didehydro-4,5α-epoxy-17-methylmorphinan-3,6α-diol sulfate (2:1) (salt) pentahydrate and has the following structural formula:

[See chemical structure at top of next column]

Each MS CONTIN 15 mg Controlled-Release Tablet contains: 15 mg Morphine sulfate USP. Inactive ingredients: cetostearyl alcohol, FD&C blue No. 2, hydroxyethyl cellulose, hydroxypropyl methylcellulose, lactose, magnesium stearate, talc, titanium dioxide, and other ingredients.

Each MS CONTIN 30 mg Controlled-Release Tablet contains: 30 mg Morphine sulfate USP. Inactive ingredients: cetostearyl alcohol, D&C red No. 7, FD&C blue No. 1, hydroxyethyl cellulose, hydroxypropyl methylcellulose, lactose, magnesium stearate, talc, titanium dioxide, and other ingredients.

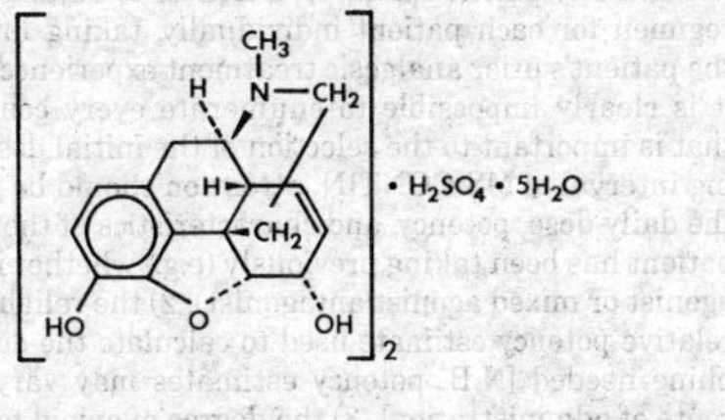

$[\ldots]_2 \cdot H_2SO_4 \cdot 5H_2O$

Each MS CONTIN 60 mg Controlled-Release Tablet contains: 60 mg Morphine sulfate USP. Inactive ingredients: cetostearyl alcohol, D&C red No. 30, D&C yellow No. 10, hydroxyethyl cellulose, hydroxypropyl methylcellulose, lactose, magnesium stearate, talc, titanium dioxide, and other ingredients.

Each MS CONTIN 100 mg Controlled-Release Tablet contains: 100 mg Morphine sulfate USP. Inactive ingredients: cetostearyl alcohol, hydroxyethyl cellulose, hydroxypropyl methylcellulose, magnesium stearate, synthetic black iron oxide, talc, titanium dioxide, and other ingredients.

MS CONTIN 200 mg Tablets*
(For use in opioid-tolerant patients only)
Each MS CONTIN 200 mg Controlled-Release Tablet* contains: 200 mg Morphine sulfate USP. Inactive ingredients: cetostearyl alcohol, D&C yellow No. 10, FD&C blue No. 1, hydroxyethyl cellulose, hydroxypropyl cellulose, hydroxypropyl methylcellulose, magnesium stearate, polyethylene glycol, talc, and titanium dioxide.

***FOR USE IN OPIOID-TOLERANT PATIENTS ONLY**

CLINICAL PHARMACOLOGY

Pharmacokinetics and Metabolism

MS CONTIN is a controlled-release tablet containing morphine sulfate. Following oral administration of a given dose of morphine, the amount ultimately absorbed is essentially the same whether the source is MS CONTIN or a conventional formulation. Morphine is released from MS CONTIN somewhat more slowly than from conventional oral preparations. Because of pre-systemic elimination (i.e., metabolism in the gut wall and liver) only about 40% of the administered dose reaches the central compartment.

Once absorbed, morphine is distributed to skeletal muscle, kidneys, liver, intestinal tract, lungs, spleen, and brain. Morphine also crosses the placental membranes and has been found in breast milk.

Although a small fraction (less than 5%) of morphine is demethylated, for all practical purposes, virtually all morphine is converted to glucuronide metabolites; among these, morphine-3-glucuronide is present in the highest plasma concentration following oral administration.

The glucuronide system has a very high capacity and is not easily saturated even in disease. Therefore, rate of delivery of morphine to the gut and liver should not influence the total and, probably, the relative quantities of the various metabolites formed. Moreover, even if rate affected the relative amounts of each metabolite formed, it should be unimportant clinically because morphine's metabolites are ordinarily inactive.

The following pharmacokinetic parameters show considerable inter-subject variation but are representative of average values reported in the literature. The volume of distribution (Vd) for morphine is 4 liters per kilogram, and its terminal elimination half-life is normally 2 to 4 hours.

Following the administration of conventional oral morphine products, approximately fifty percent of the morphine that will reach the central compartment intact reaches it within 30 minutes. Following the administration of an equal amount of MS CONTIN to normal volunteers, however, this extent of absorption occurs, on average, after 1.5 hours.

The possible effect of food upon the systemic bioavailability of MS CONTIN has not been systematically evaluated for all strengths. Data from at least one study suggests that concurrent administration of MS CONTIN with a fatty meal may cause a slight decrease in peak plasma concentration.

Variation in the physical/mechanical properties of a formulation of an oral morphine drug product can affect both its absolute bioavailability and its absorption rate constant (k_a). The formulation employed in MS CONTIN has not been shown to affect morphine's oral bioavailability, but does decrease its apparent k_a. Other basic pharmacokinetic parameters (e.g., volume of distribution [Vd], elimination rate constant [k_e], clearance [Cl]), are unchanged as they are fundamental properties of morphine in the organism. However, in chronic use, the possibility that shifts in metabolite to parent drug ratios may occur cannot be excluded.

When immediate-release oral morphine or MS CONTIN is given on a fixed dosing regimen, steady-state is achieved in about a day.

For a given dose and dosing interval, the AUC and average blood concentration of morphine at steady-state (Css) will be independent of the specific type of oral formulation administered so long as the formulations have the same absolute bioavailability. The absorption rate of a formulation will, however, affect the maximum (C_{max}) and minimum (C_{min}) blood levels and the times of their occurrence.

Pharmacodynamics

The effects described below are common to all morphine-containing products.

Central Nervous System

The principal actions of therapeutic value of morphine are analgesia and sedation (i.e., sleepiness and anxiolysis).

The precise mechanism of the analgesic action is unknown. However, specific CNS opiate receptors and endogenous compounds with morphine-like activity have been identified throughout the brain and spinal cord and are likely to play a role in the expression of analgesic effects.

Morphine produces respiratory depression by direct action on brain stem respiratory centers. The mechanism of respiratory depression involves a reduction in the responsiveness of the brain stem respiratory centers to increases in carbon dioxide tension, and to electrical stimulation.

Morphine depresses the cough reflex by direct effect on the cough center in the medulla. Antitussive effects may occur with doses lower than those usually required for analgesia.

Morphine causes miosis, even in total darkness. Pinpoint pupils are a sign of narcotic overdose but are not pathognomonic (e.g., pontine lesions of hemorrhagic or ischemic origins may produce similar findings). Marked mydriasis rather than miosis may be seen with worsening hypoxia.

Gastrointestinal Tract and Other Smooth Muscle

Gastric, biliary, and pancreatic secretions are decreased by morphine. Morphine causes a reduction in motility associated with an increase in tone in the antrum of the stomach and duodenum. Digestion of food in the small intestine is delayed and propulsive contractions are decreased. Propulsive peristaltic waves in the colon are decreased, while tone is increased to the point of spasm. The end result is constipation. Morphine can cause a marked increase in biliary tract pressure as a result of spasm of sphincter of Oddi.

Cardiovascular System

Morphine produces peripheral vasodilation which may result in orthostatic hypotension. Release of histamine can occur and may contribute to narcotic-induced hypotension. Manifestations of histamine release and/or peripheral vasodilation may include pruritus, flushing, red eyes, and sweating.

Plasma Level-Analgesia Relationships

In any particular patient, both analgesic effects and plasma morphine concentrations are related to the morphine dose.

In non-tolerant individuals, plasma morphine concentration-efficacy relationships have been demonstrated and suggest that opiate receptors occupy effector compartments, leading to a lag-time, or hysteresis, between rapid changes in plasma morphine concentrations and the effects of such changes. The most direct and predictable concentration-effect relationships can, therefore, be expected at distribution equilibrium and/or steady-state conditions. In general, the minimum effective analgesic concentration in the plasma of non-tolerant patients ranges from approximately 5 to 20 ng/mL.

While plasma morphine-efficacy relationships can be demonstrated in non-tolerant individuals, they are influenced by a wide variety of factors and are not generally useful as a guide to the clinical use of morphine. The effective dose in opioid-tolerant patients may be 10-50 times as great (or greater) than the appropriate dose for opioid-naive individuals. Dosages of morphine should be chosen and must be titrated on the basis of clinical evaluation of the patient and the balance between therapeutic and adverse effects.

For any fixed dose and dosing interval, MS CONTIN will have at steady-state, a lower C_{max} and a higher C_{min} than conventional morphine. This is a potential advantage; a reduced fluctuation in morphine concentration during the dosing interval should keep morphine blood levels more centered within the theoretical "therapeutic window." (Fluctuation for a dosing interval is defined as [C_{max}-C_{min}]/[Css-average].) On the other hand, the degree of fluctuation in serum morphine concentration might conceivably affect other phenomena. For example, reduced fluctuations in blood morphine concentrations might influence the rate of tolerance induction.

The elimination of morphine occurs primarily as renal excretion of 3-morphine glucuronide. A small amount of the glucuronide conjugate is excreted in the bile, and there is some minor enterohepatic recycling. Because morphine is primarily metabolized to inactive metabolites, the effects of renal disease on morphine's elimination are not likely to be pronounced. However, as with any drug, caution should be taken to guard against unanticipated accumulation if renal and/or hepatic function is seriously impaired.

INDICATIONS AND USAGE

MS CONTIN is a controlled-release oral morphine formulation indicated for the relief of moderate to severe pain. It is intended for use in patients who require repeated dosing with potent opioid analgesics over periods of more than a few days.

The MS CONTIN 200 mg tablet strength is a high dose, controlled-release, oral morphine formulation indicated for the relief of pain in opioid-tolerant patients only.

CONTRAINDICATIONS

MS CONTIN is contraindicated in patients with known hypersensitivity to the drug, in patients with respiratory depression in the absence of resuscitative equipment, and in patients with acute or severe bronchial asthma.

MS CONTIN is contraindicated in any patient who has or is suspected of having a paralytic ileus.

Continued on next page

MS Contin—Cont.

WARNINGS

(See also: **CLINICAL PHARMACOLOGY**)

Impaired Respiration

Respiratory depression is the chief hazard of all morphine preparations. Respiratory depression occurs most frequently in the elderly and debilitated patients as well as in those suffering from conditions accompanied by hypoxia or hypercapnia when even moderate therapeutic doses may dangerously decrease pulmonary ventilation.

Morphine should be used with extreme caution in patients with chronic obstructive pulmonary disease or cor pulmonale, and in patients having a substantially decreased respiratory reserve, hypoxia, hypercapnia, or pre-existing respiratory depression. In such patients, even usual therapeutic doses of morphine may decrease respiratory drive while simultaneously increasing airway resistance to the point of apnea.

Head Injury and Increased Intracranial Pressure

The respiratory depressant effects of morphine with carbon dioxide retention and secondary elevation of cerebrospinal fluid pressure may be markedly exaggerated in the presence of head injury, other intracranial lesions, or pre-existing increase in intracranial pressure. Morphine produces effects which may obscure neurologic signs of further increases in pressure in patients with head injuries.

Hypotensive Effect

MS CONTIN, like all opioid analgesics, may cause severe hypotension in an individual whose ability to maintain his blood pressure has already been compromised by a depleted blood volume, or a concurrent administration of drugs such as phenothiazines or general anesthetics. (See also: **PRECAUTIONS; Drug Interactions.**) MS CONTIN may produce orthostatic hypotension in ambulatory patients.

MS CONTIN, like all opioid analgesics, should be administered with caution to patients in circulatory shock, since vasodilation produced by the drug may further reduce cardiac output and blood pressure.

Interactions with other CNS Depressants

MS CONTIN, like all opioid analgesics, should be used with great caution and in reduced dosage in patients who are concurrently receiving other central nervous system depressants including sedatives or hypnotics, general anesthetics, phenothiazines, other tranquilizers, and alcohol because respiratory depression, hypotension, and profound sedation or coma may result.

Interactions with Mixed Agonist/Antagonist Opioid Analgesics

From a theoretical perspective, agonist/antagonist analgesics (i.e., pentazocine, nalbuphine, butorphanol, and buprenorphine) should NOT be administered to a patient who has received or is receiving a course of therapy with a pure opioid agonist analgesic. In these patients, mixed agonist/antagonist analgesics may reduce the analgesic effect or may precipitate withdrawal symptoms.

Drug Dependence

Morphine can produce drug dependence and has a potential for being abused. Tolerance as well as psychological and physical dependence may develop upon repeated administration. Physical dependence, however, is not of paramount importance in the management of terminally ill patients or any patients in severe pain. Abrupt cessation or a sudden reduction in dose after prolonged use may result in withdrawal symptoms. After prolonged exposure to opioid analgesics, if withdrawal is necessary, it must be undertaken gradually. (See **DRUG ABUSE AND DEPENDENCE.**)

Infants born to mothers physically dependent on opioid analgesics may also be physically dependent and exhibit respiratory depression and withdrawal symptoms. (See **DRUG ABUSE AND DEPENDENCE.**)

Other

Although extremely rare, cases of anaphylaxis have been reported.

PRECAUTIONS (See also: CLINICAL PHARMACOLOGY)

Special precautions regarding MS CONTIN 200 mg Tablets

MS CONTIN 200 mg Tablets are for use only in opioid-tolerant patients requiring daily morphine equivalent dosages of 400 mg or more. Care should be taken in its prescription and patients should be instructed against use by individuals other than the patient for whom it was prescribed, as this may have severe medical consequences for that individual.

General

MS CONTIN® is intended for use in patients who require more than several days continuous treatment with a potent opioid analgesic. The controlled-release nature of the formulation allows it to be administered on a more convenient schedule than conventional immediate-release oral morphine products. (See **CLINICAL PHARMACOLOGY: Pharmacokinetics and Metabolism.**) However, MS CONTIN does not release morphine continuously over the course of a dosing interval. The administration of single doses of MS CONTIN on a q12h dosing schedule will result in higher peak and lower trough plasma levels than those that occur when an identical daily dose of morphine is administered using conventional oral formulations on a q4h regimen. The clinical significance of greater fluctuations in morphine plasma level has not been systematically evaluated. (See **DOSAGE AND ADMINISTRATION.**)

As with any potent opioid, it is critical to adjust the dosing regimen for each patient individually, taking into account the patient's prior analgesic treatment experience. Although it is clearly impossible to enumerate every consideration that is important to the selection of the initial dose and dosing interval of MS CONTIN, attention should be given to 1) the daily dose, potency, and characteristics of the opioid the patient has been taking previously (e.g., whether it is a pure agonist or mixed agonist/antagonist), 2) the reliability of the relative potency estimate used to calculate the dose of morphine needed [N.B. potency estimates may vary with the route of administration], 3) the degree of opioid tolerance, if any, and 4) the general condition and medical status of the patient.

Selection of patients for treatment with MS CONTIN should be governed by the same principles that apply to the use of morphine or other potent opioid analgesics. Specifically, the increased risks associated with its use in the following populations should be considered: the elderly or debilitated and those with severe impairment of hepatic, pulmonary, or renal function; myxedema or hypothyroidism; adrenocortical insufficiency (e.g., Addison's Disease); CNS depression or coma; toxic psychosis; prostatic hypertrophy, or urethral stricture; acute alcoholism; delirium tremens; kyphoscoliosis, or inability to swallow.

The administration of morphine, like all opioid analgesics, may obscure the diagnosis or clinical course in patients with acute abdominal conditions.

Morphine may aggravate pre-existing convulsions in patients with convulsive disorders. Morphine should be used with caution in patients about to undergo surgery of the biliary tract since it may cause spasm of the sphincter of Oddi. Similarly, morphine should be used with caution in patients with acute pancreatitis secondary to biliary tract disease.

Information for Patients

If clinically advisable, patients receiving MS CONTIN should be given the following instructions by the physician:

1. Appropriate pain management requires changes in the dose to maintain best pain control. Patients should be advised of the need to contact their physician if pain control is inadequate, but not to change the dose of MS CONTIN without consulting their physician.
2. Morphine may impair mental and/or physical ability required for the performance of potentially hazardous tasks (e.g., driving, operating machinery). Patients started on MS CONTIN or whose dose has been changed should refrain from dangerous activity until it is established that they are not adversely affected.
3. Morphine should not be taken with alcohol or other CNS depressants (sleep aids, tranquilizers) because additive effects including CNS depression may occur. A physician should be consulted if other prescription medications are currently being used or are prescribed for future use.
4. For women of childbearing potential who become or are planning to become pregnant, a physician should be consulted regarding analgesics and other drug use.
5. Upon completion of therapy, it may be appropriate to taper the morphine dose, rather than abruptly discontinue it.
6. While psychological dependence ("addiction") to morphine used in the treatment of pain is very rare, morphine is one of a class of drugs known to be abused and should be handled accordingly.
7. The MS CONTIN 200 mg Tablet is for use only in opioid-tolerant patients requiring daily morphine equivalent dosages of 400 mg or more. Special care must be taken to avoid accidental ingestion or the use by individuals (including children) other than the patient for whom it was originally prescribed, as such unsupervised use may have severe, even fatal, consequences.

Drug Interactions (See also: **WARNINGS**)

The concomitant use of other central nervous system depressants including sedatives or hypnotics, general anesthetics, phenothiazines, tranquilizers, and alcohol may produce additive depressant effects. Respiratory depression, hypotension, and profound sedation or coma may occur. When such combined therapy is contemplated, the dose of one or both agents should be reduced. Opioid analgesics, including MS CONTIN, may enhance the neuromuscular blocking action of skeletal muscle relaxants and produce an increased degree of respiratory depression.

Carcinogenicity/Mutagenicity/Impairment of Fertility

Studies of morphine sulfate in animals to evaluate the drug's carcinogenic and mutagenic potential or the effect on fertility have not been conducted.

Pregnancy

Teratogenic Effects - CATEGORY C

Adequate animal studies on reproduction have not been performed to determine whether morphine affects fertility in males or females. There are no well-controlled studies in women, but marketing experience does not include any evidence of adverse effects on the fetus following routine (short-term) clinical use of morphine sulfate products. Although there is no clearly defined risk, such experience cannot exclude the possibility of infrequent or subtle damage to the human fetus.

MS CONTIN® should be used in pregnant women only when clearly needed. (See also: **PRECAUTIONS: Labor and Delivery, and DRUG ABUSE AND DEPENDENCE.**)

Nonteratogenic Effects

Infants born from mothers who have been taking morphine chronically may exhibit withdrawal symptoms.

Labor and Delivery

MS CONTIN is not recommended for use in women during and immediately prior to labor. Occasionally, opioid analgesics may prolong labor through actions which temporarily reduce the strength, duration, and frequency of uterine contractions. However, this effect is not consistent and may be offset by an increased rate of cervical dilatation which tends to shorten labor.

Neonates whose mothers received opioid analgesics during labor should be observed closely for signs of respiratory depression. A specific narcotic antagonist, naloxone, should be available for reversal of narcotic-induced respiratory depression in the neonate.

Nursing Mothers

Low levels of *morphine* have been detected in the breast milk. Withdrawal symptoms can occur in breast-feeding infants when maternal administration of morphine sulfate is stopped. Ordinarily, nursing should not be undertaken while a patient is receiving MS CONTIN since morphine may be excreted in the milk.

Pediatric Use

Use of MS CONTIN has not been evaluated systematically in children.

Geriatric Use

Clinical studies of MS CONTIN did not include sufficient numbers of subjects aged 65 and over to determine whether they respond differently from younger subjects. Other reported clinical experience has not identified differences in responses between the elderly and younger patients. In general, dose selection for an elderly patient should be cautious, usually starting at the low end of the dosing range, reflecting the greater frequency of decreased hepatic, renal, or cardiac function, and of concomitant disease or other drug therapy.

ADVERSE REACTIONS

The adverse reactions caused by morphine are essentially those observed with other opioid analgesics. They include the following major hazards: respiratory depression, apnea, and to a lesser degree, circulatory depression, respiratory arrest, shock, and cardiac arrest.

Most Frequently Observed

Constipation, lightheadedness, dizziness, sedation, nausea, vomiting, sweating, dysphoria, and euphoria.

Some of these effects seem to be more prominent in ambulatory patients and in those not experiencing severe pain. Some adverse reactions in ambulatory patients may be alleviated if the patient lies down.

Less Frequently Observed Reactions

Central Nervous System: Weakness, headache, agitation, tremor, uncoordinated muscle movements, seizure, alterations of mood (nervousness, apprehension, depression, floating feelings), dreams, muscle rigidity, transient hallucinations and disorientation, visual disturbances, insomnia, increased intracranial pressure

Gastrointestinal: Dry mouth, biliary tract spasm, laryngospasm, anorexia, diarrhea, cramps, taste alteration, constipation, ileus, intenstinal obstruction, increases in hepatic enzymes.

Cardiovascular: Flushing of the face, chills, tachycardia, bradycardia, palpitation, faintness, syncope, hypotension, hypertension

Genitourinary: Urine retention or hesitance, reduced libido and/or potency

Dermatologic: Pruritus, urticaria, other skin rashes, edema, diaphoresis

Other: Antidiuretic effect, paresthesia, muscle tremor, blurred vision, nystagmus, diplopia, miosis, anaphylaxis

DRUG ABUSE AND DEPENDENCE

Opioid analgesics may cause psychological and physical dependence (see **WARNINGS**). Physical dependence results in withdrawal symptoms in patients who abruptly discontinue the drug or may be precipitated through the administration of drugs with narcotic antagonist activity, e.g., naloxone or mixed agonist/antagonist analgesics (pentazocine, etc.; see also **OVERDOSAGE**). Physical dependence usually does not occur to a clinically significant degree until after several weeks of continued narcotic usage. Tolerance, in which increasingly large doses are required in order to produce the same degree of analgesia, is initially manifested by a shortened duration of analgesic effect, and, subsequently, by decreases in the intensity of analgesia.

In chronic-pain patients, and in narcotic-tolerant cancer patients, the administration of MS CONTIN should be guided by the degree of tolerance manifested. Physical dependence, per se, is not ordinarily a concern when one is dealing with opioid-tolerant patients whose pain and suffering is associated with an irreversible illness.

If MS CONTIN is abruptly discontinued, a moderate to severe abstinence syndrome may occur. The opioid agonist abstinence syndrome is characterized by some or all of the following: restlessness, lacrimation, rhinorrhea, yawning, perspiration, gooseflesh, restless sleep or "yen", and mydriasis during the first 24 hours. These symptoms often increase in severity and over the next 72 hours may be accompanied by increasing irritability, anxiety, weakness, twitching and spasms of muscles; kicking movements; severe backache, abdominal and leg pains; abdominal and muscle cramps; hot and cold flashes, insomnia; nausea, anorexia, vomiting, intestinal spasm, diarrhea; coryza and repetitive sneezing; increase in body temperature, blood pressure, respiratory rate and heart rate. Because of excessive loss of fluids through sweating, vomiting, and diarrhea, there is usually marked weight loss, dehydration, ketosis, and disturbances in acid-base balance. Cardiovascular collapse can occur. Without treatment most observable symptoms disappear in 5-14 days; however, there appears to be a phase of secondary or chronic abstinence which may last for 2-6 months characterized by insomnia, irritability, and muscular aches.

If treatment of physical dependence of patients on MS CONTIN is necessary, the patient may be detoxified by gradual reduction of the dosage. Gastrointestinal disturbances or dehydration should be treated accordingly.

OVERDOSAGE

Acute overdosage with morphine is manifested by respiratory depression, somnolence progressing to stupor or coma, skeletal muscle flaccidity, cold and clammy skin, constricted pupils, and, sometimes, bradycardia, hypotension and death.

In the treatment of overdosage, primary attention should be given to the re-establishment of a patent airway and institution of assisted or controlled ventilation. The pure opioid antagonist, naloxone, is a specific antidote against respiratory depression which results from opioid overdose. Naloxone (usually 0.4 to 2.0 mg) should be administered intravenously; however, because its duration of action is relatively short, the patient must be carefully monitored until spontaneous respiration is reliably re-established. If the response to naloxone is suboptimal or not sustained, additional naloxone may be administered, as needed, or given by continuous infusion to maintain alertness and respiratory function; however, there is no information available about the cumulative dose of naloxone that may be safely administered.

Naloxone should not be administered in the absence of clinically significant respiratory or circulatory depression secondary to morphine overdose. Naloxone should be administered cautiously to persons who are known or suspected to be physically dependent on MS CONTIN. In such cases, an abrupt or complete reversal of narcotic effects may precipitate an acute abstinence syndrome.

Note: In an individual physically dependent on opioids, administration of the usual dose of the antagonist will precipitate an acute withdrawal syndrome. The severity of the withdrawal syndrome produced will depend on the degree of physical dependence and the dose of the antagonist administered. Use of a narcotic antagonist in such a person should be avoided. If necessary to treat serious respiratory depression in the physically dependent patient, the antagonist should be administered with care and by titration with smaller than usual doses of the antagonist.

Supportive measures (including oxygen, vasopressors) should be employed in the management of circulatory shock and pulmonary edema accompanying overdose as indicated. Cardiac arrest or arrhythmias may require cardiac massage or defibrillation.

DOSAGE AND ADMINISTRATION

(See also: **CLINICAL PHARMACOLOGY, WARNINGS,** and **PRECAUTIONS** sections)

MS CONTIN TABLETS ARE TO BE TAKEN WHOLE, AND ARE NOT TO BE BROKEN, CHEWED, OR CRUSHED.

TAKING BROKEN, CHEWED, OR CRUSHED MS CONTIN TABLETS COULD LEAD TO THE RAPID RELEASE AND ABSORPTION OF A POTENTIALLY TOXIC DOSE OF MORPHINE.

MS CONTIN is intended for use in patients who require more than several days continuous treatment with a potent opioid analgesic. The controlled-release nature of the formulation allows it to be administered on a more convenient schedule than conventional immediate-release oral morphine products. (See **CLINICAL PHARMACOLOGY: Pharmacokinetics and Metabolism.**) However, MS CONTIN does not release morphine continuously over the course of a dosing interval. The administration of single doses of MS CONTIN on a q12h dosing schedule will result in higher peak and lower trough plasma levels than those that occur when an identical daily dose of morphine is administered using conventional oral formulations on a q4h regimen. The clinical significance of greater fluctuations in morphine plasma level has not been systematically evaluated.

As with any potent opioid drug product, it is critical to adjust the dosing regimen for each patient individually, taking into account the patient's prior analgesic treatment experience. Although it is clearly impossible to enumerate every consideration that is important to the selection of initial dose and dosing interval of MS CONTIN, attention should be given to 1) the daily dose, potency, and precise characteristics of the opioid the patient has been taking previously (e.g., whether it is a pure agonist or mixed agonist/antagonist), 2) the reliability of the relative potency estimate used to calculate the dose of morphine needed [N.B. potency estimates may vary with the route of administration], 3) the degree of opioid tolerance, if any, and 4) the general condition and medical status of the patient.

The following dosing recommendations, therefore, can only be considered suggested approaches to what is actually a series of clinical decisions in the management of the pain of an individual patient.

Conversion from Conventional Oral Morphine to MS CONTIN

A patient's daily morphine requirement is established using immediate-release oral morphine (dosing every 4 to 6 hours). The patient is then converted to MS CONTIN in either of two ways: 1) by administering one-half of the patient's 24-hour requirement as MS CONTIN on an every 12-hour schedule; or, 2) by administering one-third of the patient's daily requirement as MS CONTIN on an every eight hour schedule. With either method, dose and dosing interval is then adjusted as needed (see discussion below). The 15 mg tablet should be used for initial conversion for patients whose total daily requirement is expected to be less than 60 mg. The 30 mg tablet strength is recommended for patients with a daily morphine requirement of 60 to 120 mg. When the total daily dose is expected to be greater than 120 mg, the appropriate combination of tablet strengths should be employed.

Conversion from Parenteral Morphine or Other Opioids (Parenteral or Oral) to MS CONTIN

MS CONTIN can be administered as the initial oral morphine drug product; in this case, however, particular care must be exercised in the conversion process. Because of uncertainty about, and intersubject variation in, relative estimates of opioid potency and cross tolerance, initial dosing regimens should be conservative; that is, an underestimation of the 24-hour oral morphine requirement is preferred to an overestimate. To this end, initial individual doses of MS CONTIN should be estimated conservatively. In patients whose daily morphine requirements are expected to be less than or equal to 120 mg per day, the 30 mg tablet strength is recommended for the initial titration period. Once a stable dose regimen is reached, the patient can be converted to the 60 mg or 100 mg tablet strength, or an appropriate combination of tablet strengths, if desired.

Estimates of the relative potency of opioids are only approximate and are influenced by route of administration, individual patient differences, and possibly, by an individual's medical condition. Consequently, it is difficult to recommend any fixed rule for converting a patient to MS CONTIN directly. The following general points should be considered, however.

1. *Parenteral to oral morphine ratio:* Estimates of the oral to parenteral potency of morphine vary. Some authorities suggest that a dose of oral morphine only three times the daily parenteral morphine requirement may be sufficient in chronic use settings.

2. *Other parenteral or oral opioids to oral morphine:* Because there is lack of systematic evidence bearing on these types of analgesic substitutions, specific recommendations are not possible.

Physicians are advised to refer to published relative potency data, keeping in mind that such ratios are only approximate. In general, it is safer to underestimate the daily dose of MS CONTIN required and rely upon ad hoc supplementation to deal with inadequate analgesia. (See discussion which follows.)

Use of MS CONTIN as the First Opioid Analgesic

There has been no systematic evaluation of MS CONTIN as an initial opioid analgesic in the management of pain. Because it may be more difficult to titrate a patient using a controlled-release morphine, it is ordinarily advisable to begin treatment using an immediate-release formulation.

Considerations in the Adjustment of Dosing Regimens

Whatever the approach, if signs of excessive opioid effects are observed early in a dosing interval, the next dose should be reduced. If this adjustment leads to inadequate analgesia, that is, "breakthrough" pain occurs late in the dosing interval, the dosing interval may be shortened. Alternatively, a supplemental dose of a short-acting analgesic may be given. As experience is gained, adjustments can be made to obtain an appropriate balance between pain relief, opioid side effects, and the convenience of the dosing schedule.

In adjusting dosing requirements, it is recommended that the dosing interval never be extended beyond 12 hours because the administration of very large single doses may lead to acute overdose. (N.B. MS CONTIN is a controlled-release formulation; it does not release morphine continuously over the dosing interval.)

For patients with low daily morphine requirements, the 15 mg tablet should be used.

Special Instructions for MS CONTIN® 200 mg Tablets (For use in opioid-tolerant patients only.)

The MS CONTIN 200 mg tablet is for use only in opioid-tolerant patients requiring daily morphine equivalent dosages of 400 mg or more. It is recommended that this strength be reserved for patients that have already been titrated to a stable analgesic regimen using lower strengths of MS CONTIN or other opioids.

Conversion from MS CONTIN to Parenteral Opioids

When converting a patient from MS CONTIN to parenteral opioids, it is best to assume that the parenteral to oral potency is high. NOTE THAT THIS IS THE CONVERSE OF THE STRATEGY USED WHEN THE DIRECTION OF CONVERSION IS FROM THE PARENTERAL TO ORAL FORMULATIONS. IN BOTH CASES, HOWEVER, THE AIM IS TO ESTIMATE THE NEW DOSE CONSERVATIVELY. For example, to estimate the required 24-hour dose of morphine for IM use, one could employ a conversion of 1 mg of morphine IM for every 6 mg of morphine as MS CONTIN. Of course, the IM 24-hour dose would have to be divided by six and administered on a q4h regimen. This approach is recommended because it is least likely to cause overdose.

SAFETY AND HANDLING

MS CONTIN TABLETS ARE TO BE TAKEN WHOLE, AND ARE NOT TO BE BROKEN, CHEWED, OR CRUSHED. TAKING BROKEN, CHEWED, OR CRUSHED MS CONTIN TABLETS COULD LEAD TO THE RAPID RELEASE AND ABSORPTION OF A POTENTIALLY TOXIC DOSE OF MORPHINE.

The MS CONTIN 200 mg tablet strength is for use only in opioid-tolerant patients requiring daily morphine equivalent dosages of 400 mg or more. This strength is potentially toxic if accidentally ingested and patients and their families should be instructed to take special care to avoid accidental or intentional ingestion by individuals other than those for whom the medication was originally prescribed.

HOW SUPPLIED

NDC 0034-0514-10: MS CONTIN (morphine sulfate controlled-release tablets) 15 mg are supplied in opaque plastic bottles containing 100 tablets.

NDC 0034-0514-12: MS CONTIN (morphine sulfate controlled-release tablets) 15 mg are supplied in opaque plastic bottles containing 120 tablets.

NDC 0034-0514-90: MS CONTIN (morphine sulfate controlled-release tablets) 15 mg are supplied in opaque plastic bottles containing 500 tablets.

NDC 0034-0515-50: MS CONTIN (morphine sulfate controlled-release tablets) 30 mg are supplied in opaque plastic bottles containing 50 tablets.

NDC 0034-0515-10: MS CONTIN (morphine sulfate controlled-release tablets) 30 mg are supplied in opaque plastic bottles containing 100 tablets.

NDC 0034-0515-12: MS CONTIN (morphine sulfate controlled-release tablets) 30 mg are supplied in opaque plastic bottles containing 120 tablets.

NDC 0034-0515-45: MS CONTIN (morphine sulfate controlled-release tablets) 30 mg are supplied in opaque plastic bottles containing 250 tablets.

NDC 0034-0515-90: MS CONTIN (morphine sulfate controlled-release tablets) 30 mg are supplied in opaque plastic bottles containing 500 tablets.

NDC 0034-0516-10: MS CONTIN (morphine sulfate controlled-release tablets) 60 mg are supplied in opaque plastic bottles containing 100 tablets.

NDC 0034-0516-12: MS CONTIN (morphine sulfate controlled-release tablets) 60 mg are supplied in opaque plastic bottles containing 120 tablets.

NDC 0034-0516-90: MS CONTIN (morphine sulfate controlled-release tablets) 60 mg are supplied in opaque plastic bottles containing 500 tablets.

NDC 0034-0517-10: MS CONTIN (morphine sulfate controlled-release tablets) 100 mg are supplied in opaque plastic bottles containing 100 tablets.

NDC 0034-0517-12: MS CONTIN (morphine sulfate controlled-release tablets) 100 mg are supplied in opaque plastic bottles containing 120 tablets.

NDC 0034-0517-90: MS CONTIN (morphine sulfate controlled-release tablets) 100 mg are supplied in opaque plastic bottles containing 500 tablets.

NDC 0034-0513-10: MS CONTIN (morphine sulfate controlled-release tablets) 200 mg are supplied in opaque plastic bottles containing 100 tablets.

NDC 0034-0513-12:: MS CONTIN (morphine sulfate controlled-release tablets) 200 mg are supplied in opaque plastic bottles containing 120 tablets.

15 mg: Each round, blue-colored, film-coated tablet bears the symbol PF on one side and M 15 on the other side.

30 mg: Each round, lavender-colored, film-coated tablet bears the symbol PF on one side and M 30 on the other side.

60 mg: Each round, orange-colored, film-coated tablet bears the symbol PF on one side and M 60 on the other side.

100 mg: Each round, gray-colored, film-coated tablet bears the symbol PF on one side and 100 on the other side.

200 mg: Each capsule-shaped, green-colored, film-coated tablet bears the symbol PF on one side and M 200 on the other side.

Store at controlled room temperature 15°-30°C (59°-86°F). Dispense in a tight, light-resistant container.

CAUTION

DEA Order Form Required.

The Purdue Frederick Company
Stamford, CT 06901-3431

January 14, 2003 OT00001C
300519-0B-001

Shown in Product Identification Guide, page 330

MSIR® Ⓒ℞
Oral Solution Concentrate*
(morphine sulfate)

WARNING: DRUG CONCENTRATE—CHECK DOSAGE AND MEASURE ACCURATELY.

MSIR® Ⓒ℞
Immediate-Release Oral Tablets
(morphine sulfate)

***This product contains dry natural rubber**

DESCRIPTION

Chemically, morphine sulfate is 7,8 didehydro-4,5 α-epoxy-17-methylmorphinan-3,6 α-diol sulfate (2:1) (salt) pentahydrate and has the following structural formula:

[See chemical structure at top of next column]

MSIR Oral Solution Concentrate

Each 1 mL of MSIR Oral Solution Concentrate contains:

Morphine Sulfate .... 20 mg

Continued on next page

MSIR—Cont.

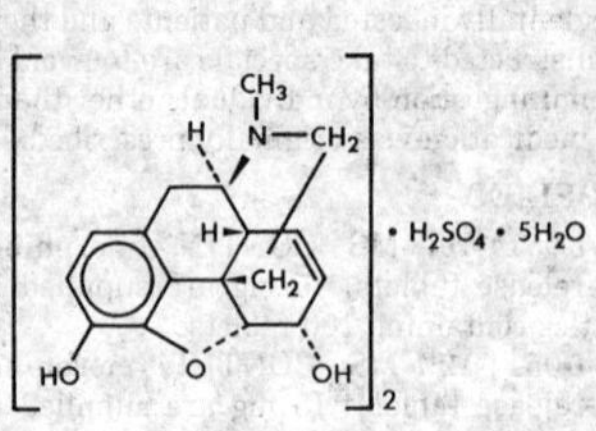

Inactive Ingredients: edetate disodium, purified water and sodium benzoate.

MSIR Tablets

Each MSIR Tablet for oral administration contains:

Morphine Sulfate .... 15 or 30 mg

Inactive Ingredients: croscarmellose sodium, lactose, magnesium stearate, microcrystalline cellulose and talc.

CLINICAL PHARMACOLOGY

Metabolism and Pharmacokinetics

MSIR Oral Solution Concentrate and MSIR Tablets containing morphine sulfate are for oral administration and are conventional immediate-release products. Only about 40% of the administered dose reaches the central compartment because of pre-systemic elimination (i.e., metabolism in the gut wall and liver).

Once absorbed, morphine is distributed to skeletal muscle, kidneys, liver, intestinal tract, lungs, spleen, and brain. Morphine also crosses the placental membranes and has been found in breast milk.

Although a small fraction (less than 5%) of morphine is demethylated, for all practical purposes virtually all morphine is converted to glucuronide metabolites; among these, morphine-3-glucuronide is present in the highest plasma concentration following oral administration.

The glucuronide system has a very high capacity and is not easily saturated even in disease. Therefore, rate of delivery of morphine to the gut and liver should not influence the total and, probably, the relative quantities of the various metabolites formed. Moreover, even if rate affected the relative amounts of each metabolite formed, it should be unimportant clinically because morphine's metabolites are ordinarily inactive.

The following pharmacokinetic parameters show considerable intersubject variation but are representative of average values reported in the literature. The volume of distribution (Vd) for morphine is 4 liters per kilogram, and its terminal elimination half-life is approximately 2 to 4 hours. Following the administration of conventional oral morphine products, approximately 50% of the morphine that will reach the central compartment intact reaches it within 30 minutes.

Variation in the physical/mechanical properties of a formulation of an oral morphine drug product can affect both its absolute bioavailability and its absorption rate constant (k_a). The basic pharmacokinetic parameters (e.g., volume of distribution [Vd], elimination rate constant [k_e], clearance [Cl]) are fundamental properties of morphine in the organism. However, in chronic use, the possibility that shifts in metabolite to parent drug ratios may occur cannot be excluded.

When immediate-release oral morphine is given on a fixed dosing regimen, steady-state is achieved in about a day.

For a given dose and dosing interval, the AUC and average blood concentration of morphine at steady-state (Css) will be independent of the specific type of oral formulation administered so long as the formulations have the same absolute bioavailability. The absorption rate of a formulation will, however, affect the maximum (C_{max}) and minimum (C_{min}) blood levels and the times of their occurrence.

While there is no predictable relationship between morphine blood levels and analgesic response, effective analgesia will not occur below some minimum blood level in a given patient. The minimum effective blood level for analgesia will vary among patients, especially among patients who have been previously treated with potent mu (μ) agonist opioids. Similarly, there is no predictable relationship between blood morphine concentration and untoward clinical responses; again, however, higher concentrations are more likely to be toxic than lower ones.

The elimination of morphine occurs primarily as renal excretion of 3-morphine glucuronide. A small amount of the glucuronide conjugate is excreted in the bile, and there is some minor enterohepatic recycling.

The elimination half-life of morphine is reported to vary between 2 and 4 hours. Thus, steady-state is probably achieved on most regimens within a day. Because morphine is primarily metabolized to inactive metabolites, the effects of renal disease on morphine's elimination are not likely to be pronounced. However, as with any drug, caution should be taken to guard against unanticipated accumulation if renal and/or hepatic function is seriously impaired.

Individual differences in the metabolism of morphine suggest that MSIR Oral Solution, Concentrate and MSIR Tablets be dosed conservatively according to the dosing initiation and titration recommendations in the **DOSAGE AND ADMINISTRATION** section.

PHARMACODYNAMICS

The effects described below are common to all morphine-containing products.

Central Nervous System

The principal actions of therapeutic value of morphine are analgesia and sedation (i.e., sleepiness and anxiolysis).

The precise mechanism of analgesic action is unknown. However, specific CNS opiate receptors and endogenous compounds with morphine-like activity have been identified throughout the brain and spinal cord and are likely to play a role in the expression of analgesic effects.

Morphine produces respiratory depression by direct action on brain stem respiratory centers. The mechanism of respiratory depression involves a reduction in the responsiveness of the brain stem respiratory centers to increases in carbon dioxide tension, and to electrical stimulation.

Morphine depresses the cough reflex by direct effect on the cough center in the medulla. Antitussive effects may occur with doses lower than those usually required for analgesia.

Morphine causes miosis, even in total darkness. Pinpoint pupils are a sign of narcotic overdose but are not pathognomonic (e.g., pontine lesions of hemorrhagic or ischemic origins may produce similar findings). Marked mydriasis rather than miosis may be seen with worsening hypoxia.

Gastrointestinal Tract and Other Smooth Muscle

Gastric, biliary and pancreatic secretions are decreased by morphine. Morphine causes a reduction in motility associated with an increase in tone in the antrum of the stomach and duodenum. Digestion of food in the small intestine is delayed and propulsive contractions are decreased. In addition, propulsive peristaltic waves in the colon are decreased, while tone is increased to the point of spasm. The end result is constipation. Morphine can cause a marked increase in biliary tract pressure as a result of spasm of the sphincter of Oddi.

Cardiovascular System

Morphine produces peripheral vasodilation which may result in orthostatic hypotension. Release of histamine can occur and may contribute to narcotic-induced hypotension. Manifestations of histamine release and/or peripheral vasodilation may include pruritus, flushing, red eyes, and sweating.

INDICATIONS AND USAGE

MSIR Oral Solution Concentrate and MSIR Tablets are indicated for the relief of moderate to severe pain.

CONTRAINDICATIONS

MSIR Oral Solution Concentrate and MSIR Tablets are contraindicated in patients with known hypersensitivity to the drug, in patients with respiratory depression in the absence of resuscitative equipment, and in patients with acute or severe bronchial asthma.

MSIR Oral Solution Concentrate and MSIR Tablets are contraindicated in any patient who has or is suspected of having a paralytic ileus.

WARNINGS

(See also: **CLINICAL PHARMACOLOGY**)

Impaired Respiration

Respiratory depression is the chief hazard of all morphine preparations. Respiratory depression occurs most frequently in elderly and debilitated patients, and those suffering from conditions accompanied by hypoxia or hypercapnia when even moderate therapeutic doses may dangerously decrease pulmonary ventilation.

Morphine should be used with extreme caution in patients with chronic obstructive pulmonary disease or cor pulmonale, and in patients having a substantially decreased respiratory reserve, hypoxia, hypercapnia, or pre-existing respiratory depression. In such patients, even usual therapeutic doses of morphine may decrease respiratory drive while simultaneously increasing airway resistance to the point of apnea.

Head Injury and Increased Intracranial Pressure

The respiratory depressant effects of morphine with carbon dioxide retention and secondary elevation of cerebrospinal fluid pressure may be markedly exaggerated in the presence of head injury, other intracranial lesions, or pre-existing increase in intracranial pressure. Morphine produces effects which may obscure neurologic signs of further increase in pressure in patients with head injuries.

Hypotensive Effects

MSIR Oral Solution Concentrate and MSIR Tablets, like all opioid analgesics, may cause severe hypotension in an individual whose ability to maintain his blood pressure has already been compromised by a depleted blood volume, or a concurrent administration of drugs such as phenothiazines, or general anesthetics. (See also: **PRECAUTIONS: Drug Interactions.**) MSIR Oral Solution Concentrate and MSIR Tablets may produce orthostatic hypotension in ambulatory patients.

MSIR Oral Solution Concentrate and MSIR Tablets, like all opioid analgesics, should be administered with caution to patients in circulatory shock, since vasodilation produced by the drug may further reduce cardiac output and blood pressure.

Interactions with Other CNS Depressants

MSIR Oral Solution Concentrate and MSIR Tablets, like all opioid analgesics, should be used with great caution and in reduced dosage in patients who are concurrently receiving other central nervous system depressants including sedatives or hypnotics, general anesthetics, phenothiazines, other tranquilizers and alcohol, because respiratory depression, hypotension and profound sedation or coma may result.

Interactions with Mixed Agonist/Antagonist Opioid Analgesics

From a theoretical perspective, agonist/antagonist analgesics (i.e., pentazocine, nalbuphine, butorphanol, and buprenorphine) should NOT be administered to a patient who has received or is receiving a course of therapy with a pure agonist opioid analgesic. In these patients, mixed agonist-antagonist analgesics may reduce the analgesic effect or may precipitate withdrawal symptoms.

Drug Dependence

Morphine can produce drug dependence and has a potential for being abused. Tolerance and psychological and physical dependence may develop upon repeated administration. Physical dependence, however, is not of paramount importance in the management of terminally ill patients or any patient in severe pain. Abrupt cessation or a sudden reduction in dose after prolonged use may result in withdrawal symptoms. After prolonged exposure to opioid analgesics, if withdrawal is necessary, it must be undertaken gradually. (See **DRUG ABUSE AND DEPENDENCE**).

Infants born to mothers physically dependent on opioid analgesics may also be physically dependent and exhibit respiratory depression and withdrawal symptoms. (See **DRUG ABUSE AND DEPENDENCE**).

PRECAUTIONS

(See also: **CLINICAL PHARMACOLOGY**)

General

MSIR Oral Solution Concentrate and MSIR Tablets are intended for use in patients who require a potent opioid analgesic for relief of moderate to severe pain.

Selection of patients for treatment with MSIR Oral Solution Concentrate and MSIR Tablets should be governed by the same principles that apply to the use of morphine and other potent opioid analgesics. Specifically, the increased risks associated with its use in the following populations should be considered: the elderly or debilitated and those with severe impairment of hepatic, pulmonary, or renal function; myxedema or hypothyroidism; adrenocortical insufficiency (e.g., Addison's Disease); CNS depression or coma; toxic psychoses; prostatic hypertrophy or urethral stricture; acute alcoholism; delirium tremens; kyphoscoliosis, or inability to swallow.

The administration of morphine, like all opioid analgesics, may obscure the diagnosis or clinical course in patients with acute abdominal conditions.

Morphine may aggravate pre-existing convulsions in patients with convulsive disorders.

Morphine should be used with caution in patients about to undergo surgery of the biliary tract, since it may cause spasm of the sphincter of Oddi. Similarly, morphine should be used with caution in patients with acute pancreatitis secondary to biliary tract disease.

Information for Patients

If clinically advisable, patients receiving MSIR Oral Solution Concentrate and MSIR Tablets should be given the following instructions by the physician.

1. Morphine may produce physical and/or psychological dependence. For this reason, the dose of the drug should not be adjusted without consulting a physician.
2. Morphine may impair mental and/or physical ability required for the performance of potentially hazardous tasks (e.g., driving, operating machinery).
3. Morphine should not be taken with alcohol or other CNS depressants (sleep aids, tranquilizers) because additive effects including CNS depression may occur. A physician should be consulted if other prescription medications are currently being used or are prescribed for future use.
4. For women of childbearing potential who become or are planning to become pregnant, a physician should be consulted regarding analgesics and other drug use.

Drug Interactions (See also **WARNINGS**)

The concomitant use of other central nervous system depressants including sedatives or hypnotics, general anesthetics, phenothiazines, tranquilizers and alcohol may produce additive depressant effects. Respiratory depression, hypotension and profound sedation or coma may occur. When such combined therapy is contemplated, the dose of one or both agents should be reduced. Opioid analgesics, including MSIR Oral Solution Concentrate and MSIR Tablets may enhance the neuromuscular blocking action of skeletal muscle relaxants and produce an increased degree of respiratory depression.

Carcinogenicity/Mutagenicity/Impairment of Fertility

Studies of morphine sulfate in animals to evaluate the drug's carcinogenic and mutagenic potential or the effect on fertility have not been conducted.

Pregnancy

Teratogenic effects—*Category C:* Adequate animal studies on reproduction have not been performed to determine whether morphine affects fertility in males or females. There are no well-controlled studies in women, but marketing experience does not include any evidence of adverse effects on the fetus following routine (short-term) clinical use of morphine sulfate products. Although there is no clearly defined risk, such experience cannot exclude the possibility of infrequent or subtle damage to the human fetus. MSIR Oral Solution Concentrate and MSIR Tablets should be used in pregnant women only when clearly needed. (See also: **PRECAUTIONS: Labor and Delivery**, and **DRUG ABUSE AND DEPENDENCE.**)

Nonteratogenic effects: Infants born from mothers who have been taking morphine chronically may exhibit withdrawal symptoms.

Labor and Delivery

MSIR Oral Solution Concentrate and MSIR Tablets are not recommended for use in women during and immediately prior to labor. Occasionally, opioid analgesics may prolong labor through actions which temporarily reduce the strength, duration, and frequency of uterine contractions. However, this effect is not consistent and may be offset by an increased rate of cervical dilatation which tends to shorten labor.

Neonates whose mothers received opioid analgesics during labor should be observed closely for signs of respiratory depression. A specific narcotic antagonist, naloxone, should be available for reversal of narcotic-induced respiratory depression in the neonate.

Nursing Mothers

Low levels of morphine have been detected in human milk. Withdrawal symptoms can occur in breast-feeding infants when maternal administration of morphine sulfate is stopped. Nursing should not be undertaken while a patient is receiving MSIR Oral Solution Concentrate and MSIR Tablets since morphine may be excreted in the milk.

Pediatric Use

MSIR Oral Solution Concentrate and MSIR Tablets have not been evaluated systematically in children.

ADVERSE REACTIONS

The adverse reactions caused by morphine are essentially the same as those observed with other opioid analgesics. They include the following major hazards: respiratory depression, apnea, and to a lesser degree, circulatory depression; respiratory arrest, shock, and cardiac arrest.

Most Frequently Observed

Constipation, lightheadedness, dizziness, sedation, nausea, vomiting, sweating, dysphoria, and euphoria.

Some of these effects seem to be more prominent in ambulatory patients and in those not experiencing severe pain. Some adverse reactions in ambulatory patients may be alleviated if the patient lies down.

Less Frequently Observed Reactions

Central Nervous System: Weakness, headache, agitation, tremor, uncoordinated muscle movements, seizure, alterations of mood (nervousness, apprehension, depression, floating feelings), dreams, muscle rigidity, transient hallucinations and disorientation, visual disturbances, insomnia, and increased intracranial pressure.

Gastrointestinal: Dry mouth, biliary tract spasm, laryngospasm, anorexia, diarrhea, cramps, taste alterations, ileus, and intestinal obstruction.

Cardiovascular: Flushing of the face, chills, tachycardia, bradycardia, palpitation, faintness, syncope, hypotension and hypertension.

Genitourinary: Urinary retention or hesitance, reduced libido and/or potency.

Dermatologic: Pruritus, urticaria, other skin rashes, edema and diaphoresis.

Other: Antidiuretic effect, paresthesia, muscle tremor, blurred vision, nystagmus, diplopia miosis, and anaphylaxis.

DRUG ABUSE AND DEPENDENCE

Opioid analgesics may cause psychological and physical dependence. (See **WARNINGS**). Physical dependence results in withdrawal symptoms in patients who abruptly discontinue the drug or may be precipitated through the administration of drugs with narcotic antagonist activity, e.g., naloxone or mixed agonist/antagonist analgesics (pentazocine, etc.: see also **OVERDOSAGE**). Physical dependence usually does not occur to a clinically significant degree until after several weeks of continued narcotic usage. Tolerance, in which increasingly large doses are required in order to produce the same degree of analgesia, is initially manifested by a shortened duration of analgesic effect, and, subsequently, by decreases in the intensity of analgesia.

In chronic-pain patients and in narcotic-tolerant cancer patients, the administration of MSIR Oral Solution Concentrate and MSIR Tablets should be guided by the degree of tolerance manifested. Physical dependence, per se, is not ordinarily a concern when one is dealing with opioid-tolerant patients whose pain and suffering is associated with an irreversible illness.

If MSIR Oral Solution Concentrate and MSIR Tablets are abruptly discontinued, a moderate to severe abstinence syndrome may occur. The opioid agonist abstinence syndrome is characterized by some or all of the following: restlessness, lacrimation, rhinorrhea, yawning, perspiration, cutis anserina, restless sleep known as the "yen" and mydriasis during the first 24 hours. These symptoms often increase in severity and over the next 72 hours may be accompanied by increasing irritability, anxiety, weakness, twitching and spasms of muscles; kicking movements; severe backache, abdominal and leg pains; abdominal and muscle cramps; hot and cold flashes; insomnia; nausea, anorexia, vomiting, intestinal spasm, diarrhea; coryza and repetitive sneezing; and increase in body temperature, blood pressure, respiratory rate, and heart rate. Because of excessive loss of fluids through sweating, vomiting and diarrhea, there is usually marked weight loss, dehydration, ketosis, and disturbances in acid-base balance. Cardiovascular collapse can occur. Without treatment, most observable symptoms disappear in 5–14 days; however, there appears to be a phase of secondary or chronic abstinence which may last for 2–6 months, characterized by insomnia, irritability, and muscular aches.

If treatment of physical dependence on MSIR Oral Solution Concentrate and MSIR Tablets is necessary, the patient may be detoxified by gradual reduction of the dosage. Gastrointestinal disturbances or dehydration should be treated accordingly.

OVERDOSAGE

Acute overdosage with morphine is manifested by respiratory depression, somnolence progressing to stupor or coma, skeletal muscle flaccidity, cold and clammy skin, constricted pupils, and, sometimes, bradycardia, hypotension and death.

In the treatment of overdosage, primary attention should be given to the re-establishment of a patent airway and institution of assisted or controlled ventilation. The pure opioid antagonist, naloxone, is a specific antidote against respiratory depression which results from opioid overdose. Naloxone (usually 0.4 to 2.0 mg) should be administered intravenously; however, because its duration of action is relatively short, the patient must be carefully monitored until spontaneous respiration is reliably re-established. If the response to naloxone is suboptimal or not sustained, additional naloxone may be re-administered, as needed, or given by continuous infusion to maintain alertness and respiratory function; however, there is no information available about the cumulative dose of naloxone that may be safely administered.

Naloxone should not be administered in the absence of clinically significant respiratory or circulatory depression secondary to morphine overdose. Naloxone should be administered cautiously to persons who are known or suspected to be physically dependent on morphine. In such cases, an abrupt or complete reversal of narcotic effects may precipitate an acute abstinence syndrome.

Note: In an individual physically dependent on opioids, administration of the usual dose of the antagonist will precipitate an acute withdrawal syndrome. The severity of the withdrawal syndrome produced will depend on the degree of physical dependence and the dose of the antagonist administered. Use of a narcotic antagonist in such a person should be avoided. If necessary to treat serious respiratory depression in the physically dependent patient the antagonist should be administered with extreme care and by titration with smaller than usual doses of the antagonist.

Supportive measures (including oxygen, vasopressors) should be employed in the management of circulatory shock and pulmonary edema accompanying overdose as indicated. Cardiac arrest or arrhythmias may require cardiac massage or defibrillation.

DOSAGE AND ADMINISTRATION

(See also: **CLINICAL PHARMACOLOGY, WARNINGS** and **PRECAUTIONS** sections)

WARNING: DRUG CONCENTRATE—CHECK DOSAGE AND MEASURE ACCURATELY.

Dosage of morphine is a patient-dependent variable, which must be individualized according to patient metabolism, age and disease state, and also response to morphine. Each patient should be maintained at the lowest dosage level that will produce acceptable analgesia. As the patient's well-being improves after successful relief of moderate to severe pain, periodic reduction of dosage and/or extension of dosing interval should be attempted to minimize exposure to morphine.

Usual Adult Oral Dose: 5 to 30 mg every four (4) hours or as directed by physician, administered either as MSIR Oral Solution Concentrate or MSIR Tablets. For control of pain in terminal illness, it is recommended that the appropriate dose of MSIR Oral Solution Concentrate or MSIR Tablets be given on a regularly scheduled basis every four hours at the minimum dose to achieve acceptable analgesia. If converting a patient from another narcotic to morphine sulfate on the basis of standard equivalence tables, a 1 to 3 ratio of parenteral to oral morphine equivalence is suggested. This ratio is conservative and may underestimate the amount of morphine required. If this is the case, the dose of MSIR Oral Solution Concentrate and MSIR Tablets should be gradually increased to achieve acceptable analgesia and tolerable side effects.

HOW SUPPLIED

MSIR (morphine sulfate) Oral Solution Concentrate:

20 mg per 1 mL unflavored, clear, colorless liquid

NDC 0034-0523-01: plastic bottle with child-resistant dropper in 30 mL size.

NDC 0034-0523-02: plastic bottle with child-resistant dropper in 120 mL size.

Discard opened bottle of Oral Solution after 90 days. **Protect from light.**

MSIR (morphine sulfate) Tablets:

15 mg round, white scored tablets

NDC 0034-0518-10: opaque plastic bottle containing 100 tablets. Each tablet bears the symbol PF on the scored side and MI 15 on the other side.

30 mg capsule-shaped, white scored tablets

NDC 0034-0519-10: opaque plastic bottle containing 100 tablets. Each tablet bears the symbol PF on the scored side and MI 30 on the other side.

Store MSIR Oral Solution Concentrate and MSIR Tablets at 25°C (77°F); excursions permitted between 15°–30°C (59°–86°F).

CAUTION

DEA Order Form Required.

The Purdue Frederick Company
Stamford, CT 06901-3431
March 17, 2004
IT00318B 091930-0D-001

Shown in Product Identification Guide, page 330

SENOKOT® TABLETS — OTC

[*sĕn' ō-kŏt*]

(standardized senna concentrate)

Natural Vegetable Laxative Ingredient

SENOKOT-S® Tablets — OTC

(standardized senna concentrate and docusate sodium)

Natural Vegetable Laxative Ingredient/Stool Softener Combination

INDICATIONS

Relieves occasional constipation (irregularity).

Senokot Laxatives provide a virtually colon-specific action which is gentle, effective and predictable, generally producing bowel movement in 6 to 12 hours.

SENOKOT Tablets contain a natural vegetable laxative ingredient standardized for uniform action.

SENOKOT has been found to be effective even in many previously intractable cases of functional constipation. SENOKOT preparations may aid in rehabilitation of the constipated patient by facilitating regular elimination. SENOKOT preparations enjoy patient acceptance. Numerous and extensive clinical studies show their high degree of effectiveness in several types of functional constipation: geriatric and postpartum, drug-induced, pediatric, as well as in functional constipation concurrent with heart disease or anorectal surgery.

SENOKOT-S Tablets are designed to relieve both aspects of functional constipation—bowel inertia and hard, dry stools. They provide a stimulant combined with a classic stool softener, standardized senna concentrate gently stimulates the colon while docusate sodium softens the stool for smoother and easier evacuation. This coordinated dual action of the two ingredients results in colon-specific, predictable laxative effect, generally producing bowel movement in 6 to 12 hours. Flexibility of dosage permits adjustment to individual requirements. SENOKOT-S Tablets are suitable for relief of postsurgical and postpartum constipation, and effectively relieve drug-induced constipation.

DESCRIPTION

SENOKOT Tablets: Each tablet contains 8.6 mg sennosides.

Active Ingredient: Standardized Senna Concentrate.

Inactive Ingredients: Croscarmellose sodium, Dicalcium phosphate, Hypromellose, Magnesium stearate, Microcrystalline cellulose, Mineral oil.

SENOKOT-S Tablets: Each tablet contains 8.6 mg sennosides and 50 mg of docusate sodium. Active Ingredients: Docusate Sodium and Standardized Senna Concentrate.

Inactive Ingredients: Carnauba wax, Colloidal silicon dioxide, Croscarmellose sodium, Dicalcium phosphate, D&C Yellow #10, FD&C Yellow #6, Hypromellose, Magnesium stearate, Microcrystalline cellulose, PEG 8000, Sodium benzoate, Stearic acid, Titanium dioxide.

RECOMMENDED DOSAGE

(or as directed by a doctor): Take preferably at bedtime. Dosing for Senokot Tablets is available for children as young as 2 years. For children under 2 years of age, consult a physician.

SENOKOT® Tablets and SENOKOT-S® Tablets:

Recommended Dosage (or as directed by a doctor):

Take preferably at bedtime.

AGE	STARTING	MAXIMUM
Adults and children 12 years of age and over	2 tablets once a day	4 tablets twice a day
6 to under 12 years of age	1 tablet once a day	2 tablets twice a day
2 to under 6 years of age	$^1/_2$ tablet once a day	1 tablet twice a day
Under 2 years	Ask a doctor	

WARNINGS

Do not use laxative products for longer than 1 week unless directed by a doctor.

Ask a doctor before use if you have stomach pain, nausea, vomiting, or noticed a sudden change in bowel habits that continues over a period of 2 weeks.

Stop use and ask a doctor if you have rectal bleeding or fail to have a bowel movement after use of a laxative. These may indicate a serious condition.

If pregnant or breast-feeding, ask a health professional before use. Keep out of reach of children. In case of overdose, get medical help or contact a Poison Control Center right away.

HOW SUPPLIED

Senokot Tablets: Blister packs of 20. Bottles of 50 and 100. Unit Strip Packs in boxes of 100 tablets: each tablet individually sealed.

Continued on next page

Senokot—Cont.

Senokot-S Tablets: Blister packs of 10. Bottles of 30 and 60, and Unit Strip Boxes of 100 tablets.

UNIPHYL® Tablets ℞

[*ūnĭ-fĭl*]

(theophylline, anhydrous)

400 mg and 600 mg

UNICONTIN®

Controlled-Release System

OT00987

300945-0A

DESCRIPTION

Uniphyl® (theophylline, anhydrous) Tablets in a controlled-release system allows a 24-hour dosing interval for appropriate patients.

Theophylline is structurally classified as a methylxanthine. It occurs as a white, odorless, crystalline powder with a bitter taste. Anhydrous theophylline has the chemical name 1H-Purine-2,6-dione, 3,7-dihydro-1,3-dimethyl-, and is represented by the following structural formula:

The molecular formula of anhydrous theophylline is $C_7H_8N_4O_2$ with a molecular weight of 180.17.

Each controlled-release tablet for oral administration, contains 400 or 600 mg of anhydrous theophylline.

Inactive Ingredients: cetostearyl alcohol, hydroxyethyl cellulose, magnesium stearate, povidone and talc.

CLINICAL PHARMACOLOGY

Mechanism of Action: Theophylline has two distinct actions in the airways of patients with reversible obstruction; smooth muscle relaxation (i.e., bronchodilation) and suppression of the response of the airways to stimuli (i.e., non-bronchodilator prophylactic effects). While the mechanisms of action of theophylline are not known with certainty, studies in animals suggest that bronchodilatation is mediated by the inhibition of two isozymes of phosphodiesterase (PDE III and, to a lesser extent, PDE IV) while non-bronchodilator prophylactic actions are probably mediated through one or more different molecular mechanisms, that do not involve inhibition of PDE III or antagonism of adenosine receptors. Some of the adverse effects associated with theophylline appear to be mediated by inhibition of PDE III (e.g., hypotension, tachycardia, headache, and emesis) and adenosine receptor antagonism (e.g., alterations in cerebral blood flow).

Theophylline increases the force of contraction of diaphragmatic muscles. This action appears to be due to enhancement of calcium uptake through an adenosine-mediated channel.

Serum Concentration-Effect Relationship: Bronchodilation occurs over the serum theophylline concentration range of 5–20 mcg/mL. Clinically important improvement in symptom control has been found in most studies to require peak serum theophylline concentrations >10 mcg/mL, but patients with mild disease may benefit from lower concentrations. At serum theophylline concentrations >20 mcg/mL, both the frequency and severity of adverse reactions increase. In general, maintaining peak serum theophylline concentrations between 10 and 15 mcg/mL will achieve most of the drug's potential therapeutic benefit while minimizing the risk of serious adverse events.

Pharmacokinetics

Overview: Theophylline is rapidly and completely absorbed after oral administration in solution or immediate-release solid oral dosage form. Theophylline does not undergo any appreciable pre-systemic elimination, distributes freely into fat-free tissues and is extensively metabolized in the liver.

The pharmacokinetics of theophylline vary widely among similar patients and cannot be predicted by age, sex, body weight or other demographic characteristics. In addition, certain concurrent illnesses and alterations in normal physiology (see Table I) and co-administration of other drugs (see Table II) can significantly alter the pharmacokinetic characteristics of theophylline. Within-subject variability in metabolism has also been reported in some studies, especially in acutely ill patients. It is, therefore, recommended that serum theophylline concentrations be measured frequently in acutely ill patients (e.g., at 24-hr intervals) and periodically in patients receiving long-term therapy, e.g., at 6–12 month intervals. More frequent measurements should be made in the presence of any condition that may significantly alter theophylline clearance (see **PRECAUTIONS, Laboratory Tests**).

[See table I below]

Absorption: Uniphyl® administered in the fed state is completely absorbed after oral administration.

In a single-dose crossover study, two 400 mg Uniphyl Tablets were administered to 19 normal volunteers in the morning or evening immediately following the same standardized meal (769 calories consisting of 97 grams carbohydrates, 33 grams protein and 27 grams fat). There was no evidence of dose dumping nor were there any significant differences in pharmacokinetic parameters attributable to time of drug administration. On the morning arm, the pharmacokinetic parameters were AUC=241.9±83.0 mcg hr/mL, C_{max}=9.3±2.0 mcg/mL, T_{max}=12.8±4.2 hours. On the evening arm, the pharmacokinetic parameters were AUC=219.7±83.0 mcg hr/mL, C_{max}=9.2±2.0 mcg/mL, T_{max}=12.5±4.2 hours.

A study in which Uniphyl 400 mg Tablets were administered to 17 fed adult asthmatics produced similar theophylline level-time curves when administered in the morning or evening. Serum levels were generally higher in the evening regimen but there were no statistically significant differences between the two regimens.

	MORNING	**EVENING**
AUC (0–24 hrs) (mcg hr/mL)	236.0±76.7	256.0±80.4
C_{max} (mcg/mL)	14.5±4.1	16.3±4.5
C_{min} (mcg/mL)	5.5±2.9	5.0±2.5
T_{max} (hours)	8.1±3.7	10.1±4.1

A single-dose study in 15 normal fasting male volunteers whose theophylline inherent mean elimination half-life was verified by a liquid theophylline product to be 6.9±2.5 (SD) hours were administered two or three 400 mg Uniphyl® Tablets. The relative bioavailability of Uniphyl given in the fasting state in comparison to an immediate-release product was 59%. Peak serum theophylline levels occurred at 6.9±5.2 (SD) hours, with a normalized (to 800 mg) peak level being 6.2±2.1 (SD). The apparent elimination half-life for the 400 mg Uniphyl Tablets was 17.2±5.8 (SD) hours.

Steady-state pharmacokinetics were determined in a study in 12 fasted patients with chronic reversible obstructive pulmonary disease. All were dosed with two 400 mg Uniphyl Tablets given once daily in the morning and a reference controlled-release BID product administered as two 200 mg tablets given 12 hours apart. The pharmacokinetic parameters obtained for Uniphyl Tablets given at doses of 800 mg once daily in the morning were virtually identical to the corresponding parameters for the reference drug when given as 400 mg BID. In particular, the AUC, C_{max} and C_{min} values obtained in this study were as follows:

	Uniphyl Tablets 800 mg Q24h±SD	**Reference Drug 400 mg Q12h±SD**
AUC, (0–24 hours), mcg hr/mL	288.9±21.5	283.5±38.4
C_{max}, mcg/mL	15.7±2.8	15.2±2.1
C_{min}, mcg/mL	7.9±1.6	7.8±1.7
C_{max}-C_{min} diff.	7.7±1.5	7.4±1.5

Single-dose studies in which subjects were fasted for twelve (12) hours prior to and an additional four (4) hours following dosing, demonstrated reduced bioavailability as compared to dosing with food. One single-dose study in 20 normal volunteers dosed with two (2) 400 mg tablets in the morning, compared dosing under these fasting conditions with dosing immediately prior to a standardized breakfast (769 calories, consisting of 97 grams carbohydrates, 33 grams protein and 27 grams fat). Under fed conditions, the pharmacokinetic parameters were: AUC=231.7±92.4 mcg hr/mL, C_{max}=8.4±2.6 mcg/mL, T_{max}=17.3±6.7 hours. Under fasting conditions, these parameters were AUC=141.2±6.53 mcg hr/mL, C_{max}=5.5±1.5 mcg/mL, T_{max}=6.5±2.1 hours.

Another single-dose study in 21 normal male volunteers, dosed in the evening, compared fasting to a standardized high calorie, high fat meal (870–1,020 calories, consisting of 33 grams protein, 55–75 grams fat, 58 grams carbohydrates). In the fasting arm subjects received one Uniphyl® 400 mg Tablet at 8 p.m. after an eight hour fast followed by a further four hour fast. In the fed arm, subjects were again dosed with one 400 mg Uniphyl Tablet, but at 8 p.m. immediately after the high fat content standardized meal cited above. The pharmacokinetic parameters (normalized to 800 mg) fed were AUC=221.8±40.9 mcg hr/mL, C_{max}=10.9±1.7 mcg/mL, T_{max}=11.8±2.2 hours. In the fasting arm, the pharmacokinetic parameters (normalized to 800 mg) were AUC=146.4±40.9 mcg hr/mL, C_{max}=6.7±1.7 mcg/mL, T_{max}=7.3±2.2 hours.

Thus, administration of single Uniphyl doses to healthy normal volunteers, under prolonged fasted conditions (at least 10 hour overnight fast before dosing followed by an additional four (4) hour fast after dosing) results in decreased bioavailability. However, there was no failure of this

TABLE I. Mean and range of total body clearance and half-life of theophylline related to age and altered physiological states.¶

Population Characteristics	**Total body clearance* mean (range)†† (mL/kg/min)**	**Half-life mean (range)†† (hr)**
Age		
Premature neonates		
postnatal age 3–15 days	0.29 (0.09–0.49)	30 (17–43)
postnatal age 25–57 days	0.64 (0.04–1.2)	20 (9.4–30.6)
Term infants		
postnatal age 1–2 days	NR†	25.7 (25–26.5)
postnatal age 3–30 weeks	NR†	11 (6–29)
Children		
1–4 years	1.7 (0.5–2.9)	3.4 (1.2–5.6)
4–12 years	1.6 (0.8–2.4)	NR†
13–15 years	0.9 (0.48–1.3)	NR†
6–17 years	1.4 (0.2–2.6)	3.7 (1.5–5.9)
Adults (16–60 years)		
otherwise healthy non-smoking asthmatics	0.65 (0.27–1.03)	8.7 (6.1–12.8)
Elderly (>60 years)		
non-smokers with normal cardiac, liver, and renal function	0.41 (0.21–0.61)	9.8 (1.6–18)
Concurrent illness or altered physiological state		
Acute pulmonary edema	0.33** (0.07–2.45)	19** (3.1–82)
COPD->60 years, stable non-smoker >1 year	0.54 (0.44–0.64)	11 (9.4–12.6)
COPD with cor pulmonale	0.48 (0.08–0.88)	NR†
Cystic fibrosis (14–28 years)	1.25 (0.31–2.2)	6.0 (1.8–10.2)
Fever associated with acute viral respiratory illness (children 9–15 years)	NR†	7.0 (1.0–13)
Liver disease		
cirrhosis	0.31** (0.1–0.7)	32** (10–56)
acute hepatitis	0.35 (0.25–0.45)	19.2 (16.6–21.8)
cholestasis	0.65 (0.25–1.45)	14.4 (5.7–31.8)
Pregnancy		
1st trimester	NR†	8.5 (3.1–13.9)
2nd trimester	NR†	8.8 (3.8–13.8)
3rd trimester	NR†	13.0 (8.4–17.6)
Sepsis with multi-organ failure	0.47 (0.19–1.9)	18.8 (6.3–24.1)
Thyroid disease		
hypothyroid	0.38 (0.13–0.57)	11.8 (8.2–25)
hyperthyroid	0.8 (0.68–0.97)	4.5 (3.7–5.6)

¶ For various North American patient populations from literature reports. Different rates of elimination and consequent dosage requirements have been observed among other peoples.

* Clearance represents the volume of blood completely cleared of theophylline by the liver in one minute. Values listed were generally determined at serum theophylline concentrations <20 mcg/mL; clearance may decrease and half-life may increase at higher serum concentrations due to non-linear pharmacokinetics.

†† Reported range or estimated range (mean ±2 SD) where actual range not reported.

† NR = not reported or not reported in a comparable format.

** Median

Note: In addition to the factors listed above, theophylline clearance is increased and half-life decreased by low carbohydrate/high protein diets, parenteral nutrition, and daily consumption of charcoal-broiled beef. A high carbohydrate/low protein diet can decrease the clearance and prolong the half-life of theophylline.

delivery system leading to a sudden and unexpected release of a large quantity of theophylline with Uniphyl Tablets even when they are administered with a high fat, high calorie meal.

Similar studies were conducted with the 600 mg Uniphyl Tablet. A single-dose study in 24 subjects with an established theophylline clearance of ≤ 4 L/hr, compared the pharmacokinetic evaluation of one 600 mg Uniphyl Tablet and one and one-half 400 mg Uniphyl Tablets under fed (using a standard high fat diet) and fasted conditions. The results of this 4-way randomized crossover study demonstrate the bioequivalence of the 400 mg and 600 mg Uniphyl Tablets. Under fed conditions, the pharmacokinetic results for the one and one-half 400 mg tablets were AUC=214.64±55.88 mcg hr/mL, C_{max}=10.58±2.21 mcg/mL and T_{max}=9.00±2.64 hours, and for the 600 mg tablet were AUC=207.85±48.9 mcg hr/mL, C_{max}=10.39±1.91 mcg/mL and T_{max}=9.58±1.86 hours. Under fasted conditions the pharmacokinetic results for the one and one-half 400 mg tablets were AUC=191.85±51.1 mcg hr/mL, C_{max}= 7.37±1.83 mcg/mL and T_{max}=8.08±4.39 hours; and for the 600 mg tablet were AUC=199.39±70.27 mcg hr/mL, C_{max}=7.66±2.09 mcg/mL and T_{max}=9.67±4.89 hours.

In this study the mean fed/fasted ratios for the one and one-half 400 mg tablets and the 600 mg tablet were about 112% and 104%, respectively.

In another study, the bioavailability of the 600 mg Uniphyl Tablet was examined with morning and evening administration. This single-dose, crossover study in 22 healthy males was conducted under fed (standard high fat diet) conditions. The results demonstrated no clinically significant difference in the bioavailability of the 600 mg Uniphyl Tablet administered in the morning or in the evening. The results were: AUC=233.6±45.1 mcg hr/mL, C_{max}=10.6±1.3 mcg/mL and T_{max}=12.5±3.2 hours with morning dosing; AUC=209.8±46.2 mcg hr/mL, C_{max}=9.7±1.4 mcg/mL and T_{max}=13.7±3.3 hours with evening dosing. The PM/AM ratio was 89.3%.

The absorption characteristics of Uniphyl® Tablets (theophylline, anhydrous) have been extensively studied. A steady-state crossover bioavailability study in 22 normal males compared two Uniphyl 400 mg Tablets administered q24h at 8 a.m. immediately after breakfast with a reference controlled-release theophylline product administered BID in fed subjects at 8 a.m. immediately after breakfast and 8 p.m. immediately after dinner (769 calories, consisting of 97 grams carbohydrates, 33 grams protein and 27 grams fat). The pharmacokinetic parameters for Uniphyl 400 mg Tablets under these steady-state conditions were AUC=203.3±87.1 mcg hr/mL, C_{max}=12.1±3.8 mcg/mL, C_{min}=4.50±3.6, T_{max}=8.8±4.6 hours. For the reference BID product, the pharmacokinetic parameters were AUC=219.2±88.4 mcg hr/mL, C_{max} =11.0±4.1 mcg/mL, C_{min}=7.28±3.5, T_{max}=6.9±3.4 hours. The mean percent fluctuation [$(C_{max}-C_{min}/C_{min})\times 100$]=169% for the once-daily regimen and 51% for the reference product BID regimen.

The bioavailability of the 600 mg Uniphyl Tablet was further evaluated in a multiple dose, steady-state study in 26 healthy males comparing the 600 mg Tablet to one and one-half 400 mg Uniphyl Tablets. All subjects had previously established theophylline clearances of ≤ 4 L/hr and were dosed once-daily for 6 days under fed conditions. The results showed no clinically significant difference between the 600 mg and one and one-half 400 mg Uniphyl Tablet regimens. Steady-state results were:

	600 MG TABLET FED	600 MG (ONE + ONE-HALF 400 MG TABLETS) FED
AUC 0–24hrs (mcg hr/mL)	209.77±51.04	212.32±56.29
C_{max} (mcg/mL)	12.91±2.46	13.17±3.11
C_{min} (mcg/mL)	5.52±1.79	5.39±1.95
T_{max} (hours)	8.62±3.21	7.23±2.35
Percent Fluctuation	183.73±54.02	179.72±28.86

The bioavailability ratio for the 600/400 mg tablets was 98.8%. Thus, under all study conditions the 600 mg tablet is bioequivalent to one and one-half 400 mg tablets.

Studies demonstrate that as long as subjects were either consistently fed or consistently fasted, there is similar bioavailability with once-daily administration of Uniphyl Tablets whether dosed in the morning or evening.

Distribution: Once theophylline enters the systemic circulation, about 40% is bound to plasma protein, primarily albumin. Unbound theophylline distributes throughout body water, but distributes poorly into body fat. The apparent volume of distribution of theophylline is approximately 0.45 L/kg (range 0.3–0.7 L/kg) based on ideal body weight. Theophylline passes freely across the placenta, into breast milk and into the cerebrospinal fluid (CSF). Saliva theophylline concentrations approximate unbound serum concentrations, but are not reliable for routine or therapeutic monitoring unless special techniques are used. An increase in the volume of distribution of theophylline, primarily due to reduction in plasma protein binding, occurs in premature neonates, patients with hepatic cirrhosis, uncorrected acidemia, the elderly and in women during the third trimester of pregnancy. In such cases, the patient may show signs of toxicity at total (bound+unbound) serum concentrations of theophylline in the therapeutic range (10–20 mcg/mL) due to elevated concentrations of the pharmacologically active unbound drug. Similarly, a patient with decreased theophylline binding may have a sub-therapeutic total drug concentration while the pharmacologically active unbound concentration is in the therapeutic range. If only total serum theophylline concentration is measured, this may lead to an unnecessary and potentially dangerous dose increase. In patients with reduced protein binding, measurement of unbound serum theophylline concentration provides a more reliable means of dosage adjustment than measurement of total serum theophylline concentration. Generally, concentrations of unbound theophylline should be maintained in the range of 6–12 mcg/mL.

Metabolism: Following oral dosing, theophylline does not undergo any measurable first-pass elimination. In adults and children beyond one year of age, approximately 90% of the dose is metabolized in the liver. Biotransformation takes place through demethylation to 1-methylxanthine and 3-methylxanthine and hydroxylation to 1,3-dimethyluric acid. 1-methylxanthine is further hydroxylated, by xanthine oxidase, to 1-methyluric acid. About 6% of a theophylline dose is N-methylated to caffeine. Theophylline demethylation to 3-methylxanthine is catalyzed by cytochrome P-450 1A2, while cytochromes P-450 2E1 and P-450 3A3 catalyze the hydroxylation to 1,3-dimethyluric acid. Demethylation to 1-methylxanthine appears to be catalyzed either by cytochrome P-450 1A2 or a closely related cytochrome. In neonates, the N-demethylation pathway is absent while the function of the hydroxylation pathway is markedly deficient. The activity of these pathways slowly increases to maximal levels by one year of age.

Caffeine and 3-methylxanthine are the only theophylline metabolites with pharmacologic activity. 3-methylxanthine has approximately one tenth the pharmacologic activity of theophylline and serum concentrations in adults with normal renal function are <1 mcg/mL. In patients with end-stage renal disease, 3-methylxanthine may accumulate to concentrations that approximate the unmetabolized theophylline concentration. Caffeine concentrations are usually undetectable in adults regardless of renal function. In neonates, caffeine may accumulate to concentrations that approximate the unmetabolized theophylline concentration and thus, exert a pharmacologic effect.

Both the N-demethylation and hydroxylation pathways of theophylline biotransformation are capacity-limited. Due to the wide intersubject variability of the rate of theophylline metabolism, non-linearity of elimination may begin in some patients at serum theophylline concentrations <10 mcg/mL. Since this non-linearity results in more than proportional changes in serum theophylline concentrations with changes in dose, it is advisable to make increases or decreases in dose in small increments in order to achieve desired changes in serum theophylline concentrations (see **DOSAGE AND ADMINISTRATION**, Table VI). Accurate prediction of dose-dependency of theophylline metabolism in patients *a priori* is not possible, but patients with very high initial clearance rates (i.e., low steady-state serum theophylline concentrations at above average doses) have the greatest likelihood of experiencing large changes in serum theophylline concentration in response to dosage changes.

Excretion: In neonates, approximately 50% of the theophylline dose is excreted unchanged in the urine. Beyond the first three months of life, approximately 10% of the theophylline dose is excreted unchanged in the urine. The remainder is excreted in the urine mainly as 1,3-dimethyluric acid (35–40%), 1-methyluric acid (20–25%) and 3-methylxanthine (15–20%). Since little theophylline is excreted unchanged in the urine and since active metabolites of theophylline (i.e., caffeine, 3-methylxanthine) do not accumulate to clinically significant levels even in the face of end-stage renal disease, no dosage adjustment for renal insufficiency is necessary in adults and children >3 months of age. In contrast, the large fraction of the theophylline dose excreted in the urine as unchanged theophylline and caffeine in neonates requires careful attention to dose reduction and frequent monitoring of serum theophylline concentrations in neonates with reduced renal function (See **WARNINGS**).

Serum Concentrations at Steady-State: After multiple doses of theophylline, steady-state is reached in 30–65 hours (average 40 hours) in adults. At steady-state, on a dosage regimen with 24-hour intervals, the expected mean trough concentration is approximately 50% of the mean peak concentration, assuming a mean theophylline half-life of 8 hours. The difference between peak and trough concentrations is larger in patients with more rapid theophylline clearance. In these patients administration of Uniphyl® may be required more frequently (every 12 hours).

Special Populations (See Table I for mean clearance and half-life values)

Geriatric: The clearance of theophylline is decreased by an average of 30% in healthy elderly adults (>60 yrs) compared to healthy young adults. Careful attention to dose reduction and frequent monitoring of serum theophylline concentrations are required in elderly patients (see **WARNINGS**).

Pediatrics: The clearance of theophylline is very low in neonates (see **WARNINGS**). Theophylline clearance reaches maximal values by one year of age, remains relatively constant until about 9 years of age and then slowly decreases by approximately 50% to adult values at about age 16. Renal excretion of unchanged theophylline in neonates amounts to about 50% of the dose, compared to about 10% in children older than three months and in adults. Careful attention to dosage selection and monitoring of serum theophylline concentrations are required in pediatric patients (see **WARNINGS** and **DOSAGE AND ADMINISTRATION**).

Gender: Gender differences in theophylline clearance are relatively small and unlikely to be of clinical significance. Significant reduction in theophylline clearance, however, has been reported in women on the 20th day of the menstrual cycle and during the third trimester of pregnancy.

Race: Pharmacokinetic differences in theophylline clearance due to race have not been studied.

Renal Insufficiency: Only a small fraction, e.g., about 10%, of the administered theophylline dose is excreted unchanged in the urine of children greater than three months of age and adults. Since little theophylline is excreted unchanged in the urine and since active metabolites of theophylline (i.e., caffeine, 3-methylxanthine) do not accumulate to clinically significant levels even in the face of end-stage renal disease, no dosage adjustment for renal insufficiency is necessary in adults and children >3 months of age. In contrast, approximately 50% of the administered theophylline dose is excreted unchanged in the urine in neonates. Careful attention to dose reduction and frequent monitoring of serum theophylline concentrations are required in neonates with decreased renal function (see **WARNINGS**).

Hepatic Insufficiency: Theophylline clearance is decreased by 50% or more in patients with hepatic insufficiency (e.g., cirrhosis, acute hepatitis, cholestasis). Careful attention to dose reduction and frequent monitoring of serum theophylline concentrations are required in patients with reduced hepatic function (see **WARNINGS**).

Congestive Heart Failure (CHF): Theophylline clearance is decreased by 50% or more in patients with CHF. The extent of reduction in theophylline clearance in patients with CHF appears to be directly correlated to the severity of the cardiac disease. Since theophylline clearance is independent of liver blood flow, the reduction in clearance appears to be due to impaired hepatocyte function rather than reduced perfusion. Careful attention to dose reduction and frequent monitoring of serum theophylline concentrations are required in patients with CHF (see **WARNINGS**).

Smokers: Tobacco and marijuana smoking appears to increase the clearance of theophylline by induction of metabolic pathways. Theophylline clearance has been shown to increase by approximately 50% in young adult tobacco smokers and by approximately 80% in elderly tobacco smokers compared to non-smoking subjects. Passive smoke exposure has also been shown to increase theophylline clearance by up to 50%. Abstinence from tobacco smoking for one week causes a reduction of approximately 40% in theophylline clearance. Careful attention to dose reduction and frequent monitoring of serum theophylline concentrations are required in patients who stop smoking (see **WARNINGS**). Use of nicotine gum has been shown to have no effect on theophylline clearance.

Fever: Fever, regardless of its underlying cause, can decrease the clearance of theophylline. The magnitude and duration of the fever appear to be directly correlated to the degree of decrease of theophylline clearance. Precise data are lacking, but a temperature of 39°C (102°F) for at least 24 hours is probably required to produce a clinically significant increase in serum theophylline concentrations. Children with rapid rates of theophylline clearance (i.e., those who require a dose that is substantially larger than average [e.g., >22 mg/kg/day]) to achieve a therapeutic peak serum theophylline concentration when afebrile) may be at greater risk of toxic effects from decreased clearance during sustained fever. Careful attention to dose reduction and frequent monitoring of serum theophylline concentrations are required in patients with sustained fever (see **WARNINGS**).

Miscellaneous: Other factors associated with decreased theophylline clearance include the third trimester of pregnancy, sepsis with multiple organ failure, and hypothyroidism. Careful attention to dose reduction and frequent monitoring of serum theophylline concentrations are required in patients with any of these conditions (see **WARNINGS**). Other factors associated with increased theophylline clearance include hyperthyroidism and cystic fibrosis.

Clinical Studies: In patients with chronic asthma, including patients with severe asthma requiring inhaled corticosteroids or alternate-day oral corticosteroids, many clinical studies have shown that theophylline decreases the frequency and severity of symptoms, including nocturnal exacerbations, and decreases the "as needed" use of inhaled $beta_2$ agonists. Theophylline has also been shown to reduce the need for short courses of daily oral prednisone to relieve exacerbations of airway obstruction that are unresponsive to bronchodilators in asthmatics.

In patients with chronic obstructive pulmonary disease (COPD), clinical studies have shown that theophylline decreases dyspnea, air trapping, the work of breathing, and improves contractility of diaphragmatic muscles with little or no improvement in pulmonary function measurements.

INDICATIONS AND USAGE

Theophylline is indicated for the treatment of the symptoms and reversible airflow obstruction associated with chronic asthma and other chronic lung diseases, e.g., emphysema and chronic bronchitis.

Continued on next page

Uniphyl—Cont.

CONTRAINDICATIONS

Uniphyl® is contraindicated in patients with a history of hypersensitivity to theophylline or other components in the product.

WARNINGS

Concurrent Illness: Theophylline should be used with extreme caution in patients with the following clinical conditions due to the increased risk of exacerbation of the concurrent condition:

Active peptic ulcer disease
Seizure disorders
Cardiac arrhythmias (not including bradyarrhythmias)

Conditions That Reduce Theophylline Clearance: There are several readily identifiable causes of reduced theophylline clearance. ***If the total daily dose is not appropriately reduced in the presence of these risk factors, severe and potentially fatal theophylline toxicity can occur.*** Careful consideration must be given to the benefits and risks of theophylline use and the need for more intensive monitoring of serum theophylline concentrations in patients with the following risk factors:

Age

Neonates (term and premature)
Children <1 year
Elderly (>60 years)

Concurrent Diseases

Acute pulmonary edema
Congestive heart failure
Cor-pulmonale
Fever; ≥102° for 24 hours or more; or lesser temperature elevations for longer periods
Hypothyroidism
Liver disease; cirrhosis, acute hepatitis
Reduced renal function in infants <3 months of age
Sepsis with multi-organ failure
Shock

Cessation of Smoking

Drug Interactions: Adding a drug that inhibits theophylline metabolism (e.g., cimetidine, erythromycin, tacrine) or stopping a concurrently administered drug that enhances theophylline metabolism (e.g., carbamazepine, rifampin). (See **PRECAUTIONS, Drug Interactions**, Table II).

When Signs or Symptoms of Theophylline Toxicity Are Present:

Whenever a patient receiving theophylline develops nausea or vomiting, particularly repetitive vomiting, or other signs or symptoms consistent with theophylline toxicity (even if another cause may be suspected), additional doses of theophylline should be withheld and a serum theophylline concentration measured immediately. Patients should be instructed not to continue any dosage that causes adverse effects and to withhold subsequent doses until the symptoms have resolved, at which time the healthcare professional may instruct the patient to resume the drug at a lower dosage (see **DOSAGE AND ADMINISTRATION**, Dosing Guidelines, Table VI).

Dosage Increases: Increases in the dose of theophylline should not be made in response to an acute exacerbation of symptoms of chronic lung disease since theophylline provides little added benefit to inhaled $beta_2$-selective agonists and systemically administered corticosteroids in this circumstance and increases the risk of adverse effects. A peak steady-state serum theophylline concentration should be measured before increasing the dose in response to persistent chronic symptoms to ascertain whether an increase in dose is safe. Before increasing the theophylline dose on the basis of a low serum concentration, the healthcare professional should consider whether the blood sample was obtained at an appropriate time in relationship to the dose and whether the patient has adhered to the prescribed regimen (see **PRECAUTIONS, Laboratory Tests**).

As the rate of theophylline clearance may be dose-dependent (i.e., steady-state serum concentrations may increase disproportionately to the increase in dose), an increase in dose based upon a sub-therapeutic serum concentration measurement should be conservative. In general, limiting dose increases to about 25% of the previous total daily dose will reduce the risk of unintended excessive increases in serum theophylline concentration (see **DOSAGE AND ADMINISTRATION**, Table VI).

PRECAUTIONS

General: Careful consideration of the various interacting drugs and physiologic conditions that can alter theophylline clearance and require dosage adjustment should occur prior to initiation of theophylline therapy, prior to increases in theophylline dose, and during follow up (see **WARNINGS**). The dose of theophylline selected for initiation of therapy should be low and, ***if tolerated,*** increased slowly over a period of a week or longer with the final dose guided by monitoring serum theophylline concentrations and the patient's clinical response (see **DOSAGE AND ADMINISTRATION**, Table V).

Monitoring Serum Theophylline Concentrations: Serum theophylline concentration measurements are readily available and should be used to determine whether the dosage is appropriate. Specifically, the serum theophylline concentration should be measured as follows:

1. When initiating therapy to guide final dosage adjustment after titration.
2. Before making a dose increase to determine whether the serum concentration is sub-therapeutic in a patient who continues to be symptomatic.
3. Whenever signs or symptoms of theophylline toxicity are present.
4. Whenever there is a new illness, worsening of a chronic illness or a change in the patient's treatment regimen that may alter theophylline clearance (e.g., fever >102°F sustained for ≥24 hours, hepatitis, or drugs listed in Table II are added or discontinued).

To guide a dose increase, the blood sample should be obtained at the time of the expected peak serum theophylline concentration; 12 hours after an evening dose or 9 hours after a morning dose at steady-state. For most patients, steady-state will be reached after 3 days of dosing when no doses have been missed, no extra doses have been added, and none of the doses have been taken at unequal intervals. A trough concentration (i.e., at the end of the dosing interval) provides no additional useful information and may lead to an inappropriate dose increase since the peak serum theophylline concentration can be two or more times greater than the trough concentration with an immediate-release formulation. If the serum sample is drawn more than 12 hours after the evening dose, or more than 9 hours after a morning dose, the results must be interpreted with caution since the concentration may not be reflective of the peak concentration. In contrast, when signs or symptoms of theophylline toxicity are present, a serum sample should be obtained as soon as possible, analyzed immediately, and the result reported to the healthcare professional without delay. In patients in whom decreased serum protein binding is suspected (e.g., cirrhosis, women during the third trimester of pregnancy), the concentration of unbound theophylline should be measured and the dosage adjusted to achieve an unbound concentration of 6–12 mcg/mL.

Saliva concentrations of theophylline cannot be used reliably to adjust dosage without special techniques.

Effects on Laboratory Tests: As a result of its pharmacological effects, theophylline at serum concentrations within the 10–20 mcg/mL range modestly increases plasma glucose (from a mean of 88 mg% to 98 mg%), uric acid (from a mean of 4 mg/dL to 6 mg/dL), free fatty acids (from a mean of 451 µEq/L to 800 µEq/L, total cholesterol (from a mean of 140 vs 160 mg/dL), HDL (from a mean of 36 to 50 mg/dL), HDL/LDL ratio (from a mean of 0.5 to 0.7), and urinary free cortisol excretion (from a mean of 44 to 63 mcg/24 hr). Theophylline at serum concentrations within the 10–20 mcg/mL range may also transiently decrease serum concentrations of triiodothyronine (144 before, 131 after one week and 142 ng/dL after 4 weeks of theophylline). The clinical importance of these changes should be weighed against the potential therapeutic benefit of theophylline in individual patients.

Information for Patients: The patient (or parent/caregiver) should be instructed to seek medical advice whenever nausea, vomiting, persistent headache, insomnia or rapid heartbeat occurs during treatment with theophylline, even if another cause is suspected. The patient should be instructed to contact their healthcare professional if they develop a new illness, especially if accompanied by a persistent fever, if they experience worsening of a chronic illness, if they start or stop smoking cigarettes or marijuana, or if another healthcare professional adds a new medication or discontinues a previously prescribed medication. Patients should be informed that theophylline interacts with a wide variety of drugs (see Table II). The dietary supplement St. John's Wort (Hypericum perforatum) should not be taken at the same time as theophylline, since it may result in decreased theophylline levels. If patients are already taking St. John's Wort and theophylline together, they should consult their healthcare professional before stopping the St. John's Wort, since their theophylline concentrations may rise when this is done, resulting in toxicity. Patients should be instructed to inform all healthcare professionals involved in their care that they are taking theophylline, especially when a medication is being added or deleted from their treatment. Patients should be instructed to not alter the dose, timing of the dose, or frequency of administration without first consulting their healthcare professional. If a dose is missed, the patient should be instructed to take the next dose at the usually scheduled time and to not attempt to make up for the missed dose.

Uniphyl® Tablets can be taken once a day in the morning or evening. It is recommended that Uniphyl be taken with meals. Patients should be advised that if they choose to take Uniphyl with food it should be taken consistently with food and if they take it in a fasted condition it should routinely be taken fasted. It is important that the product whenever dosed be dosed consistently with or without food.

Uniphyl Tablets are not to be chewed or crushed because it may lead to a rapid release of theophylline with the potential for toxicity. The scored tablet may be split. Patients receiving Uniphyl Tablets may pass an intact matrix tablet in the stool or via colostomy. These matrix tablets usually contain little or no residual theophylline.

Drug Interactions: Theophylline interacts with a wide variety of drugs. The interaction may be pharmacodynamic, i.e., alterations in the therapeutic response to theophylline or another drug or occurrence of adverse effects without a change in serum theophylline concentration. More frequently, however, the interaction is pharmacokinetic, i.e., the rate of theophylline clearance is altered by another drug resulting in increased or decreased serum theophylline concentrations. Theophylline only rarely alters the pharmacokinetics of other drugs.

The drugs listed in Table II have the potential to produce clinically significant pharmacodynamic or pharmacokinetic interactions with theophylline. The information in the "Effect" column of Table II assumes that the interacting drug is being added to a steady-state theophylline regimen. If theophylline is being initiated in a patient who is already taking a drug that inhibits theophylline clearance (e.g., cimetidine, erythromycin), the dose of theophylline required to achieve a therapeutic serum theophylline concentration will be smaller. Conversely, if theophylline is being initiated in a patient who is already taking a drug that enhances theophylline clearance (e.g., rifampin), the dose of theophylline required to achieve a therapeutic serum theophylline concentration will be larger. Discontinuation of a concomitant drug that increases theophylline clearance will result in accumulation of theophylline to potentially toxic levels, unless the theophylline dose is appropriately reduced. Discontinuation of a concomitant drug that inhibits theophylline clearance will result in decreased serum theophylline concentrations, unless the theophylline dose is appropriately increased.

The drugs listed in Table III have either been documented not to interact with theophylline or do not produce a clinically significant interaction (i.e., <15% change in theophylline clearance).

The listing of drugs in Tables II and III are current as of February 9, 1995. New interactions are continuously being reported for theophylline, especially with new chemical entities. **The healthcare professional should not assume that a drug does not interact with theophylline if it is not listed in Table II.** Before addition of a newly available drug in a patient receiving theophylline, the package insert of the new drug and/or the medical literature should be consulted to determine if an interaction between the new drug and theophylline has been reported.

[See table at top of next page]

Table III. Drugs that have been documented not to interact with theophylline or drugs that produce no clinically significant interaction with theophylline.*

albuterol, systemic and inhaled	mebendazole
amoxicillin	medroxyprogesterone
ampicillin, with or without sulbactam	methylprednisolone
atenolol	metronidazole
azithromycin	metoprolol
caffeine, dietary ingestion	nadolol
cefaclor	nifedipine
co-trimoxazole (trimethoprim and sulfamethoxazole)	nizatidine
diltiazem	norfloxacin
dirithromycin	ofloxacin
enflurane	omeprazole
famotidine	prednisone, prednisolone
felodipine	ranitidine
finasteride	rifabutin
hydrocortisone	roxithromycin
isoflurane	sorbitol (purgative doses do not inhibit theophylline absorption)
isoniazid	sucralfate
isradipine	terbutaline, systemic
influenza vaccine	terfenadine
ketoconazole	tetracycline
lomefloxacin	tocainide

*Refer to **PRECAUTIONS, Drug Interactions** for information regarding table.

Drug-Food Interactions: The bioavailability of Uniphyl® Tablets (theophylline, anhydrous) has been studied with co-administration of food. In three single-dose studies, subjects given Uniphyl 400 mg or 600 mg Tablets with a standardized high-fat meal were compared to fasted conditions. Under fed conditions, the peak plasma concentration and bioavailability were increased; however, a precipitous increase in the rate and extent of absorption was not evident (see **Pharmacokinetics**, Absorption). The increased peak and extent of absorption under fed conditions suggests that dosing should be ideally administered consistently either with or without food.

The Effect of Other Drugs on Theophylline Serum Concentration Measurements: Most serum theophylline assays in clinical use are immunoassays which are specific for theophylline. Other xanthines such as caffeine, dyphylline, and pentoxifylline are not detected by these assays. Some drugs (e.g., cefazolin, cephalothin), however, may interfere with certain HPLC techniques. Caffeine and xanthine metabolites in neonates or patients with renal dysfunction may cause the reading from some dry reagent office methods to be higher than the actual serum theophylline concentration.

Carcinogenesis, Mutagenesis, and Impairment of Fertility: Long term carcinogenicity studies have been carried out in mice (oral doses 30–150 mg/kg) and rats (oral doses 5–75 mg/kg). Results are pending.

Theophylline has been studied in Ames salmonella, *in vivo* and *in vitro* cytogenetics, micronucleus and Chinese hamster ovary test systems and has not been shown to be genotoxic.

In a 14 week continuous breeding study, theophylline, administered to mating pairs of $B6C3F_1$ mice at oral doses of 120, 270 and 500 mg/kg (approximately 1.0–3.0 times the human dose on a mg/m^2 basis) impaired fertility, as evidenced by decreases in the number of live pups per litter,

TABLE II. Clinically significant drug interactions with theophylline.*

Drug	Type of Interaction	Effect**
Adenosine	Theophylline blocks adenosine receptors.	Higher doses of adenosine may be required to achieve desired effect.
Alcohol	A single large dose of alcohol (3 mL/kg of whiskey) decreases theophylline clearance for up to 24 hours.	30% increase
Allopurinol	Decreases theophylline clearance at allopurinol doses ≥ 600 mg/day.	25% increase
Aminoglutethimide	Increases theophylline clearance by induction of microsomal enzyme activity.	25% decrease
Carbamazepine	Similar to aminoglutethimide.	30% decrease
Cimetidine	Decreases theophylline clearance by inhibiting cytochrome P450 1A2.	70% increase
Ciprofloxacin	Similar to cimetidine.	40% increase
Clarithromycin	Similar to erythromycin.	25% increase
Diazepam	Benzodiazepines increase CNS concentrations of adenosine, a potent CNS depressant, while theophylline blocks adenosine receptors.	Larger diazepam doses may be required to produce desired level of sedation. Discontinuation of theophylline without reduction of diazepam dose may result in respiratory depression.
Disulfiram	Decreases theophylline clearance by inhibiting hydroxylation and demethylation.	50% increase
Enoxacin	Similar to cimetidine.	300% increase
Ephedrine	Synergistic CNS effects.	Increased frequency of nausea, nervousness, and insomnia.
Erythromycin	Erythromycin metabolite decreases theophylline clearance by inhibiting cytochrome P450 3A3.	35% increase. Erythromycin steady-state serum concentrations decrease by a similar amount.
Estrogen	Estrogen containing oral contraceptives decrease theophylline clearance in a dose-dependent fashion. The effect of progesterone on theophylline clearance is unknown.	30% increase
Flurazepam	Similar to diazepam.	Similar to diazepam.
Fluvoxamine	Similar to cimetidine.	Similar to cimetidine.
Halothane	Halothane sensitizes the myocardium to catecholamines, theophylline increases release of endogenous catecholamines.	Increased risk of ventricular arrhythmias.
Interferon, human recombinant alpha-A	Decreases theophylline clearance.	100% increase
Isoproterenol (IV)	Increases theophylline clearance.	20% decrease
Ketamine	Pharmacologic	May lower theophylline seizure threshold.
Lithium	Theophylline increases renal lithium clearance.	Lithium dose required to achieve a therapeutic serum concentration increased an average of 60%.
Lorazepam	Similar to diazepam.	Similar to diazepam.
Methotrexate (MTX)	Decreases theophylline clearance.	20% increase after low dose MTX, higher dose MTX may have a greater effect.
Mexiletine	Similar to disulfiram.	80% increase
Midazolam	Similar to diazepam.	Similar to diazepam.
Moricizine	Increases theophylline clearance.	25% decrease
Pancuronium	Theophylline may antagonize non-depolarizing neuromuscular blocking effects; possibly due to phosphodiesterase inhibition.	Larger dose of pancuronium may be required to achieve neuromuscular blockade.
Pentoxifylline	Decreases theophylline clearance.	30% increase
Phenobarbital (PB)	Similar to aminoglutethimide.	25% decrease after two weeks of concurrent PB.
Phenytoin	Phenytoin increases theophylline clearance by increasing microsomal enzyme activity. Theophylline decreases phenytoin absorption.	Serum theophylline and phenytoin concentrations decrease about 40%.
Propafenone	Decreases theophylline clearance and pharmacologic interaction.	40% increase. Beta-2 blocking effect may decrease efficacy of theophylline.
Propranolol	Similar to cimetidine and pharmacologic interaction.	100% increase. Beta-2 blocking effect may decrease efficacy of theophylline.
Rifampin	Increases theophylline clearance by increasing cytochrome P450 1A2 and 3A3 activity.	20–40% decrease
St. John's Wort (Hypericum Perforatum)	Decrease in theophylline plasma concentrations.	Higher doses of theophylline may be required to achieve desired effect. Stopping St. John's Wort may result in theophylline toxicity.
Sulfinpyrazone	Increases theophylline clearance by increasing demethylation and hydroxylation. Decreases renal clearance of theophylline.	20% decrease
Tacrine	Similar to cimetidine, also increases renal clearance of theophylline.	90% increase
Thiabendazole	Decreases theophylline clearance.	190% increase
Ticlopidine	Decreases theophylline clearance.	60% increase
Troleandomycin	Similar to erythromycin.	33–100% increase depending on troleandomycin dose.
Verapamil	Similar to disulfiram.	20% increase

***Refer to PRECAUTIONS, Drug Interactions for further information regarding table.**
****Average effect on steady-state theophylline concentration or other clinical effect for pharmacologic interactions. Individual patients may experience larger changes in serum theophylline concentration than the value listed.**

decreases in the mean number of litters per fertile pair, and increases in the gestation period at the high dose as well as decreases in the proportion of pups born alive at the mid and high dose. In 13 week toxicity studies, theophylline was administered to F344 rats and B6C3F$_1$ mice at oral doses of 40–300 mg/kg (approximately 2.0 times the human dose on a mg/m^2 basis). At the high dose, systemic toxicity was observed in both species including decreases in testicular weight.

Pregnancy: Teratogenic Effects: Category C: In studies in which pregnant mice, rats and rabbits were dosed during the period of organogenesis, theophylline produced teratogenic effects.

In studies with mice, a single intraperitoneal dose at and above 100 mg/kg (approximately equal to the maximum recommended oral dose for adults on a mg/m^2 basis) during organogenesis produced cleft palate and digital abnormalities. Micromelia, micrognathia, clubfoot, subcutaneous hematoma, open eyelids, and embryolethality were observed at doses that are approximately 2 times the maximum recommended oral dose for adults on a mg/m^2 basis.

In a study with rats dosed from conception through organogenesis, an oral dose of 150 mg/kg/day (approximately 2 times the maximum recommended oral dose for adults on a mg/m^2 basis) produced digital abnormalities. Embryolethality was observed with a subcutaneous dose of 200 mg/kg/day (approximately 4 times the maximum recommended oral dose for adults on a mg/m^2 basis).

In a study in which pregnant rabbits were dosed throughout organogenesis, an intravenous dose of 60 mg/kg/day (approximately 2 times the maximum recommended oral dose for adults on a mg/m^2 basis), which caused the death of one doe and clinical signs in others, produced cleft palate and was embryolethal. Doses at and above 15 mg/kg/day (less than the maximum recommended oral dose for adults on a mg/m^2 basis) increased the incidence of skeletal variations. There are no adequate and well-controlled studies in pregnant women. Theophylline should be used during pregnancy only if the potential benefit justifies the potential risk to the fetus.

Nursing Mothers: Theophylline is excreted into breast milk and may cause irritability or other signs of mild toxicity in nursing human infants. The concentration of theophylline in breast milk is about equivalent to the maternal serum concentration. An infant ingesting a liter of breast milk containing 10–20 mcg/mL of theophylline per day is likely to receive 10–20 mg of theophylline per day. Serious adverse effects in the infant are unlikely unless the mother has toxic serum theophylline concentrations.

Pediatric Use: Theophylline is safe and effective for the approved indications in pediatric patients. The maintenance dose of theophylline must be selected with caution in pediatric patients since the rate of theophylline clearance is highly variable across the pediatric age range (see **CLINICAL PHARMACOLOGY,** Table I, **WARNINGS,** and **DOSAGE AND ADMINISTRATION,** Table V).

Geriatric Use: Elderly patients are at a significantly greater risk of experiencing serious toxicity from theophylline than younger patients due to pharmacokinetic and pharmacodynamic changes associated with aging. The clearance of theophylline is decreased by an average of 30% in healthy elderly adults (>60 yrs) compared to healthy young adults. Theophylline clearance may be further reduced by concomitant diseases prevalent in the elderly, which further impair clearance of this drug and have the potential to increase serum levels and potential toxicity. These conditions include impaired renal function, chronic obstructive pulmonary disease, congestive heart failure, hepatic disease and an increased prevalence of use of certain medications (see **PRECAUTIONS: Drug Interactions**) with the potential for pharmacokinetic and pharmacodynamic interaction. Protein binding may be decreased in the elderly resulting in an increased proportion of the total serum theophylline concentration in the pharmacologically active unbound form. Elderly patients also appear to be more sensitive to the toxic effects of theophylline after chronic overdosage than younger patients. Careful attention to dose reduction and frequent monitoring of serum theophylline concentrations are required in elderly patients (see **PRECAUTIONS, Monitoring Serum Theophylline Concentrations,** and **DOSAGE AND ADMINISTRATION**). The maximum daily dose of theophylline in patients greater than 60 years of age ordinarily should not exceed 400 mg/day unless the patient continues to be symptomatic and the peak steady-state serum theophylline concentration is <10 mcg/mL (see **DOSAGE AND ADMINISTRATION**). Theophylline doses greater than 400 mg/d should be prescribed with caution in elderly patients.

ADVERSE REACTIONS

Adverse reactions associated with theophylline are generally mild when peak serum theophylline concentrations are <20 mcg/mL and mainly consist of transient caffeine-like adverse effects such as nausea, vomiting, headache, and insomnia. When peak serum theophylline concentrations exceed 20 mcg/mL, however, theophylline produces a wide range of adverse reactions including persistent vomiting, cardiac arrhythmias, and intractable seizures which can be lethal (see **OVERDOSAGE**). The transient caffeine-like adverse reactions occur in about 50% of patients when theophylline therapy is initiated at doses higher than recommended initial doses (e.g., >300 mg/day in adults and >12 mg/kg/day in children beyond >1 year of age). During the initiation of theophylline therapy, caffeine-like adverse effects may transiently alter patient behavior, especially in school age children, but this response rarely persists. Initiation of theophylline therapy at a low dose with subsequent slow titration to a predetermined age-related maximum dose will significantly reduce the frequency of these tran-

Continued on next page

Uniphyl—Cont.

sient adverse effects (see **DOSAGE AND ADMINISTRATION**, Table V). In a small percentage of patients (<3% of children and <10% of adults) the caffeine-like adverse effects persist during maintenance therapy, even at peak serum theophylline concentrations within the therapeutic range (i.e., 10–20 mcg/mL). Dosage reduction may alleviate the caffeine-like adverse effects in these patients, however, persistent adverse effects should result in a reevaluation of the need for continued theophylline therapy and the potential therapeutic benefit of alternative treatment.

Other adverse reactions that have been reported at serum theophylline concentrations <20 mcg/mL include diarrhea, irritability, restlessness, fine skeletal muscle tremors, and transient diuresis. In patients with hypoxia secondary to COPD, multifocal atrial tachycardia and flutter have been reported at serum theophylline concentrations ≥ 15 mcg/mL. There have been a few isolated reports of seizures at serum theophylline concentrations <20 mcg/mL in patients with an underlying neurological disease or in elderly patients. The occurrence of seizures in elderly patients with serum theophylline concentrations <20 mcg/mL may be secondary to decreased protein binding resulting in a larger proportion of the total serum theophylline concentration in the pharmacologically active unbound form. The clinical characteristics of the seizures reported in patients with serum theophylline concentrations <20 mcg/mL have generally been milder than seizures associated with excessive serum theophylline concentrations resulting from an overdose (i.e., they have generally been transient, often stopped without anticonvulsant therapy, and did not result in neurological residua).

Table IV. Manifestations of theophylline toxicity.*

	Percentage of patients reported with sign or symptom			
	Acute Overdose (Large Single Ingestion)		Chronic Overdosage (Multiple Excessive Doses)	
Sign/Symptom	Study 1 (n=157)	Study 2 (n=14)	Study 1 (n=92)	Study 2 (n=102)
Asymptomatic	NR**	0	NR**	6
Gastrointestinal				
Vomiting	73	93	30	61
Abdominal Pain	NR**	21	NR**	12
Diarrhea	NR**	0	NR**	14
Hematemesis	NR**	0	NR**	2
Metabolic/Other				
Hypokalemia	85	79	44	43
Hyperglycemia	98	NR**	18	NR**
Acid/base disturbance	34	21	9	5
Rhabdomyolysis	NR**	7	NR**	0
Cardiovascular				
Sinus tachycardia	100	86	100	62
Other supraventricular tachycardias	2	21	12	14
Ventricular premature beats	3	21	10	19
Atrial fibrillation or flutter	1	NR**	12	NR**
Multifocal atrial tachycardia	0	NR**	2	NR**
Ventricular arrhythmias with hemodynamic instability	7	14	40	0
Hypotension/shock	NR**	21	NR**	8
Neurologic				
Nervousness	NR**	64	NR**	21
Tremors	38	29	16	14
Disorientation	NR**	7	NR**	11
Seizures	5	14	14	5
Death	3	21	10	4

*These data are derived from two studies in patients with serum theophylline concentrations >30 mcg/mL. In the first study (Study #1—Shanon, *Ann Intern Med* 1993; 119:1161–67), data were prospectively collected from 249 consecutive cases of theophylline toxicity referred to a regional poison center for consultation. In the second study (Study #2—Sessler, *Am J Med* 1990;88:567–76), data were retrospectively collected from 116 cases with serum theophylline concentrations >30 mcg/mL among 6000 blood samples obtained for measurement of serum theophylline concentrations in three emergency departments. Differences in the incidence of manifestations of theophylline toxicity between the two studies may reflect sample selection as a result of study design (e.g., in Study #1, 48% of the patients had acute intoxications versus only 10% in Study #2) and different methods of reporting results.

**NR=Not reported in a comparable manner.

OVERDOSAGE

General: The chronicity and pattern of theophylline overdosage significantly influences clinical manifestations of toxicity, management and outcome. There are two common presentations: (1) *acute overdose*, i.e., ingestion of a single large excessive dose (>10 mg/kg), as occurs in the context of an attempted suicide or isolated medication error, and (2) *chronic overdosage*, i.e., ingestion of repeated doses that are excessive for the patient's rate of theophylline clearance. The most common causes of chronic theophylline overdosage include patient or caregiver error in dosing, healthcare professional prescribing of an excessive dose or a normal dose in the presence of factors known to decrease the rate of theophylline clearance, and increasing the dose in response to an exacerbation of symptoms without first measuring the serum theophylline concentration to determine whether a dose increase is safe.

Severe toxicity from theophylline overdose is a relatively rare event. In one health maintenance organization, the frequency of hospital admissions for chronic overdosage of theophylline was about 1 per 1000 person-years exposure. In another study, among 6000 blood samples obtained for measurement of serum theophylline concentration, for any reason, from patients treated in an emergency department, 7% were in the 20–30 mcg/mL range and 3% were >30 mcg/mL. Approximately two-thirds of the patients with serum theophylline concentrations in the 20–30 mcg/mL range had one or more manifestations of toxicity while >90% of patients with serum theophylline concentrations >30 mcg/mL were clinically intoxicated. Similarly, in other reports, serious toxicity from theophylline is seen principally at serum concentrations >30 mcg/mL.

Several studies have described the clinical manifestations of theophylline overdose and attempted to determine the factors that predict life-threatening toxicity. In general, patients who experience an acute overdose are less likely to experience seizures than patients who have experienced a chronic overdosage, unless the peak serum theophylline concentration is >100 mcg/mL. After a chronic overdosage, generalized seizures, life-threatening cardiac arrhythmias, and death may occur at serum theophylline concentrations >30 mcg/mL. The severity of toxicity after chronic overdosage is more strongly correlated with the patient's age than the peak serum theophylline concentration; patients >60 years are at the greatest risk for severe toxicity and mortality after a chronic overdosage. Pre-existing or concurrent disease may also significantly increase the susceptibility of a patient to a particular toxic manifestation, e.g., patients with neurologic disorders have an increased risk of seizures and patients with cardiac disease have an increased risk of cardiac arrhythmias for a given serum theophylline concentration compared to patients without the underlying disease.

The frequency of various reported manifestations of theophylline overdose according to the mode of overdose are listed in Table IV.

Other manifestations of theophylline toxicity include increases in serum calcium, creatine kinase, myoglobin and leukocyte count, decreases in serum phosphate and magnesium, acute myocardial infarction, and urinary retention in men with obstructive uropathy.

Seizures associated with serum theophylline concentrations >30 mcg/mL are often resistant to anticonvulsant therapy and may result in irreversible brain injury if not rapidly controlled. Death from theophylline toxicity is most often secondary to cardiorespiratory arrest and/or hypoxic encephalopathy following prolonged generalized seizures or intractable cardiac arrhythmias causing hemodynamic compromise.

Overdose Management: General Recommendations for Patients with Symptoms of Theophylline Overdose or Serum Theophylline Concentrations >30 mcg/mL (Note: Serum theophylline concentrations may continue to increase after presentation of the patient for medical care.)

1. While simultaneously instituting treatment, contact a regional poison center to obtain updated information and advice on individualizing the recommendations that follow.
2. Institute supportive care, including establishment of intravenous access, maintenance of the airway, and electrocardiographic monitoring.
3. Treatment of seizures Because of the high morbidity and mortality associated with theophylline-induced seizures, treatment should be rapid and aggressive. Anticonvulsant therapy should be initiated with an intravenous benzodiazepine, e.g., diazepam, in increments of 0.1–0.2 mg/kg every 1–3 minutes until seizures are terminated. Repetitive seizures should be treated with a loading dose of phenobarbital (20 mg/kg infused over 30–60 minutes). Case reports of theophylline overdose in humans and animal studies suggest that phenytoin is ineffective in terminating theophylline-induced seizures. The doses of benzodiazepines and phenobarbital required to terminate theophylline-induced seizures are close to the doses that may cause severe respiratory depression or respiratory arrest; the healthcare professional should therefore be prepared to provide assisted ventilation. Elderly patients and patients with COPD may be more susceptible to the respiratory depressant effects of anticonvulsants. Barbiturate-induced coma or administration of general anesthesia may be required to terminate repetitive seizures or status epilepticus. General anesthesia should be used with caution in patients with theophylline overdose because fluorinated volatile anesthetics may sensitize the myocardium to endogenous catecholamines released by theophylline. Enflurane appears less likely to be associated with this effect than halothane and may, therefore, be safer. Neuromuscular blocking agents alone should not be used to terminate seizures since they abolish the musculoskeletal manifestations without terminating seizure activity in the brain.
4. Anticipate Need for Anticonvulsants In patients with theophylline overdose who are at high risk for theophylline-induced seizures, e.g., patients with acute overdoses and serum theophylline concentrations >100 mcg/mL or chronic overdosage in patients >60 years of age with serum theophylline concentrations >30 mcg/mL, the need for anticonvulsant therapy should be anticipated. A benzodiazepine such as diazepam should be drawn into a syringe and kept at the patient's bedside and medical personnel qualified to treat seizures should be immediately available. In selected patients at high risk for theophylline-induced seizures, consideration should be given to the administration of prophylactic anticonvulsant therapy. Situations where prophylactic anticonvulsant therapy should be considered in high risk patients include anticipated delays in instituting methods for extracorporeal removal of theophylline (e.g., transfer of a high risk patient from one healthcare facility to another for extracorporeal removal) and clinical circumstances that significantly interfere with efforts to enhance theophylline clearance (e.g., a neonate where dialysis may not be technically feasible or a patient with vomiting unresponsive to antiemetics who is unable to tolerate multiple-dose oral activated charcoal). In animal studies, prophylactic administration of phenobarbital, but not phenytoin, has been shown to delay the onset of theophylline-induced generalized seizures and to increase the dose of theophylline required to induce seizures (i.e., markedly increases the LD_{50}). Although there are no controlled studies in humans, a loading dose of intravenous phenobarbital (20 mg/kg infused over 60 minutes) may delay or prevent life-threatening seizures in high risk patients while efforts to enhance theophylline clearance are continued. Phenobarbital may cause respiratory depression, particularly in elderly patients and patients with COPD.
5. Treatment of cardiac arrhythmias Sinus tachycardia and simple ventricular premature beats are not harbingers of life-threatening arrhythmias, they do not require treatment in the absence of hemodynamic compromise, and they resolve with declining serum theophylline concentrations. Other arrhythmias, especially those associated with hemodynamic compromise, should be treated with antiarrhythmic therapy appropriate for the type of arrhythmia.
6. Gastrointestinal decontamination Oral activated charcoal (0.5 g/kg up to 20 g and repeat at least once 1–2 hours after the first dose) is extremely effective in blocking the absorption of theophylline throughout the gastrointestinal tract, even when administered several hours after ingestion. If the patient is vomiting, the charcoal should be administered through a nasogastric tube or after administration of an antiemetic. Phenothiazine antiemetics such as prochlorperazine or perphenazine should be avoided since they can lower the seizure threshold and frequently cause dystonic reactions. A single dose of sorbitol may be used to promote stooling to facilitate removal of theophylline bound to charcoal from the gastrointestinal tract. Sorbitol, however, should be dosed with caution since it is a potent purgative which can cause profound fluid and electrolyte abnormalities, particularly after multiple doses. Commercially available fixed combinations of liquid charcoal and sorbitol should be avoided in young children and after the first dose in adolescents and adults since they do not allow for individualization of charcoal and sorbitol dosing. Ipecac syrup should be avoided in theophylline overdoses. Although ipecac induces emesis, it does not reduce the absorption of theophylline unless administered within 5 minutes of ingestion and even then is less effective than oral activated charcoal. Moreover, ipecac induced emesis may persist for several hours after a single dose and significantly decrease the retention and the effectiveness of oral activated charcoal.
7. Serum Theophylline Concentration Monitoring The serum theophylline concentration should be measured immediately upon presentation, 2–4 hours later, and then at sufficient intervals, e.g., every 4 hours, to guide treatment decisions and to assess the effectiveness of therapy. Serum theophylline concentrations may continue to increase after presentation of the patient for medical care as a result of continued absorption of theophylline from the gastrointestinal tract. Serial monitoring of serum theophylline serum concentrations should be continued until it is clear that the concentration is no longer rising and has returned to non-toxic levels.
8. General Monitoring Procedures Electrocardiographic monitoring should be initiated on presentation and continued until the serum theophylline level has returned to a non-toxic level. Serum electrolytes and glucose should be measured on presentation and at appropriate intervals indicated by clinical circumstances. Fluid and electrolyte abnormalities should be promptly corrected. **Monitoring and treatment should be continued until the serum concentration decreases below 20 mcg/mL.**
9. Enhance clearance of theophylline Multiple-dose oral activated charcoal (e.g., 0.5 mg/kg up to 20 g, every two hours) increases the clearance of theophylline at least twofold by adsorption of theophylline secreted into gastrointestinal fluids. Charcoal must be retained in, and pass through, the gastrointestinal tract to be effective; emesis should therefore be controlled by administration of appropriate antiemetics. Alternatively, the charcoal

can be administered continuously through a nasogastric tube in conjunction with appropriate antiemetics. A single dose of sorbitol may be administered with the activated charcoal to promote stooling to facilitate clearance of the adsorbed theophylline from the gastrointestinal tract. Sorbitol alone does not enhance clearance of theophylline and should be dosed with caution to prevent excessive stooling which can result in severe fluid and electrolyte imbalances. Commercially available fixed combinations of liquid charcoal and sorbitol should be avoided in young children and after the first dose in adolescents and adults since they do not allow for individualization of charcoal and sorbitol dosing. In patients with intractable vomiting, extracorporeal methods of theophylline removal should be instituted (see **OVERDOSAGE, Extracorporeal Removal**).

Specific Recommendations

Acute Overdose

A. Serum Concentration >20<30 mcg/mL
  1. Administer a single dose of oral activated charcoal.
  2. Monitor the patient and obtain a serum theophylline concentration in 2–4 hours to insure that the concentration is not increasing.

B. Serum Concentration >30<100 mcg/mL
  1. Administer multiple dose oral activated charcoal and measures to control emesis.
  2. Monitor the patient and obtain serial theophylline concentrations every 2–4 hours to gauge the effectiveness of therapy and to guide further treatment decisions.
  3. Institute extracorporeal removal if emesis, seizures, or cardiac arrhythmias cannot be adequately controlled (see **OVERDOSAGE, Extracorporeal Removal**).

C. Serum Concentration >100 mcg/mL
  1. Consider prophylactic anticonvulsant therapy.
  2. Administer multiple-dose oral activated charcoal and measures to control emesis.
  3. Consider extracorporeal removal, even if the patient has not experienced a seizure (see **OVERDOSAGE, Extracorporeal Removal**).
  4. Monitor the patient and obtain serial theophylline concentrations every 2–4 hours to gauge the effectiveness of therapy and to guide further treatment decisions.

Chronic Overdosage

A. Serum Concentration >20<30 mcg/mL (with manifestations of theophylline toxicity)
  1. Administer a single dose of oral activated charcoal.
  2. Monitor the patient and obtain a serum theophylline concentration in 2–4 hours to insure that the concentration is not increasing.

B. Serum Concentration >30 mcg/mL in patients <60 years of age
  1. Administer multiple-dose oral activated charcoal and measures to control emesis.
  2. Monitor the patient and obtain serial theophylline concentrations every 2–4 hours to gauge the effectiveness of therapy and to guide further treatment decisions.
  3. Institute extracorporeal removal if emesis, seizures, or cardiac arrhythmias cannot be adequately controlled (see **OVERDOSAGE, Extracorporeal Removal**).

C. Serum Concentration >30 mcg/mL in patients ≥ 60 years of age
  1. Consider prophylactic anticonvulsant therapy.
  2. Administer multiple-dose oral activated charcoal and measures to control emesis.
  3. Consider extracorporeal removal even if the patient has not experienced a seizure (see **OVERDOSAGE, Extracorporeal Removal**).
  4. Monitor the patient and obtain serial theophylline concentrations every 2–4 hours to gauge the effectiveness of therapy and to guide further treatment decisions.

Extracorporeal Removal: Increasing the rate of theophylline clearance by extracorporeal methods may rapidly decrease serum concentrations, but the risks of the procedure must be weighed against the potential benefit. Charcoal hemoperfusion is the most effective method of extracorporeal removal, increasing theophylline clearance up to six-fold, but serious complications, including hypotension, hypocalcemia, platelet consumption and bleeding diatheses may occur. Hemodialysis is about as efficient as multiple-dose oral activated charcoal and has a lower risk of serious complications than charcoal hemoperfusion. Hemodialysis should be considered as an alternative when charcoal hemoperfusion is not feasible and multiple-dose oral charcoal is ineffective because of intractable emesis. Serum theophylline concentrations may rebound 5–10 mcg/mL after discontinuation of charcoal hemoperfusion or hemodialysis due to redistribution of theophylline from the tissue compartment. Peritoneal dialysis is ineffective for theophylline removal; exchange transfusions in neonates have been minimally effective.

DOSAGE AND ADMINISTRATION

Uniphyl® 400 or 600 mg Tablets can be taken once a day in the morning or evening. It is recommended that Uniphyl be taken with meals. Patients should be advised that if they choose to take Uniphyl with food it should be taken consistently with food and if they take it in a fasted condition it should routinely be taken fasted. It is important that the product whenever dosed be dosed consistently with or without food.

Uniphyl® Tablets are not to be chewed or crushed because it may lead to a rapid release of theophylline with the potential for toxicity. The scored tablet may be split. Infrequently, patients receiving Uniphyl 400 or 600 mg Tablets may pass an intact matrix tablet in the stool or via colostomy. These matrix tablets usually contain little or no residual theophylline.

Stabilized patients, 12 years of age or older, who are taking an immediate-release or controlled-release theophylline product may be transferred to once-daily administration of 400 mg or 600 mg Uniphyl Tablets on a mg-for-mg basis.

It must be recognized that the peak and trough serum theophylline levels produced by the once-daily dosing may vary from those produced by the previous product and/or regimen.

General Considerations: The steady-state peak serum theophylline concentration is a function of the dose, the dosing interval, and the rate of theophylline absorption and clearance in the individual patient. Because of marked individual differences in the rate of theophylline clearance, the dose required to achieve a peak serum theophylline concentration in the 10–20 mcg/mL range varies fourfold among otherwise similar patients in the absence of factors known to alter theophylline clearance (e.g., 400–1600 mg/day in adults <60 years old and 10–36 mg/kg/day in children 1–9 years old). For a given population there is no single theophylline dose that will provide both safe and effective serum concentrations for all patients. Administration of the median theophylline dose required to achieve a therapeutic serum theophylline concentration in a given population may result in either sub-therapeutic or potentially toxic serum theophylline concentrations in individual patients. For example, at a dose of 900 mg/d in adults <60 years or 22 mg/kg/d in children 1–9 years, the steady-state peak serum theophylline concentration will be <10 mcg/mL in about 30% of patients, 10–20 mcg/mL in about 50% and 20–30 mcg/mL in about 20% of patients. **The dose of theophylline must be individualized on the basis of peak serum theophylline concentration measurements in order to achieve a dose that will provide maximum potential benefit with minimal risk of adverse effects.**

Transient caffeine-like adverse effects and excessive serum concentrations in slow metabolizers can be avoided in most patients by starting with a sufficiently low dose and slowly increasing the dose, if judged to be clinically indicated, in small increments (See Table V). Dose increases should only be made if the previous dosage is well tolerated and at intervals of no less than 3 days to allow serum theophylline concentrations to reach the new steady-state. Dosage adjustment should be guided by serum theophylline concentration measurement (see **PRECAUTIONS, Laboratory Tests** and **DOSAGE AND ADMINISTRATION**, Table VI). Healthcare providers should instruct patients and caregivers to discontinue any dosage that causes adverse effects, to withhold the medication until these symptoms are gone and to then resume therapy at a lower, previously tolerated dosage (see **WARNINGS**).

If the patient's symptoms are well controlled, there are no apparent adverse effects, and no intervening factors that might alter dosage requirements (see **WARNINGS** and **PRECAUTIONS**), serum theophylline concentrations should be monitored at 6 month intervals for rapidly growing children and at yearly intervals for all others. In acutely ill patients, serum theophylline concentrations should be monitored at frequent intervals, e.g., every 24 hours.

Theophylline distributes poorly into body fat, therefore, mg/kg dose should be calculated on the basis of ideal body weight.

Table V contains theophylline dosing titration schema recommended for patients in various age groups and clinical circumstances. Table VI contains recommendations for theophylline dosage adjustment based upon serum theophylline concentrations. **Application of these general dosing recommendations to individual patients must take into account the unique clinical characteristics of each patient. In general, these recommendations should serve as the upper limit for dosage adjustments in order to decrease the risk of potentially serious adverse events associated with unexpected large increases in serum theophylline concentration.**

Table V. Dosing initiation and titration (as anhydrous theophylline).*

A. Children (12–15 years) and adults (16–60 years) without risk factors for impaired clearance.

Titration Step	Children <45 kg	Children >45 kg and adults
1. Starting Dosage	12–14 mg/kg/day up to a maximum of 300 mg/day admin. QD*	300–400 mg/day[1] admin. QD*
2. After 3 days, if tolerated, increase dose to:	16 mg/kg/day up to a maximum of 400 mg/day admin. QD*	400–600 mg/day[1] admin. QD*
3. After 3 more days, if tolerated and if needed increase dose to:	20 mg/kg/day up to a maximum of 600 mg/day admin. QD*	As with all theophylline products, doses greater than 600 mg should be titrated according to blood level (See Table VI)

[1]If caffeine-like adverse effects occur, then consideration should be given to a lower dose and titrating the dose more slowly (see **ADVERSE REACTIONS**).

B. Patients With Risk Factors For Impaired Clearance, The Elderly (>60 Years), And Those In Whom It Is Not Feasible To Monitor Serum Theophylline Concentrations:

In children 12–15 years of age, the theophylline dose should not exceed 16 mg/kg/day up to a maximum of 400 mg/day in the presence of risk factors for reduced theophylline clearance (see **WARNINGS**) or if it is not feasible to monitor serum theophylline concentrations.

In adolescents ≥ 16 years and adults, including the elderly, the theophylline dose should not exceed 400 mg/day in the presence of risk factors for reduced theophylline clearance (see **WARNINGS**) or if it is not feasible to monitor serum theophylline concentrations.

*Patients with more rapid metabolism clinically identified by higher than average dose requirements, should receive a smaller dose more frequently (every 12 hours) to prevent breakthrough symptoms resulting from low trough concentrations before the next dose.

Table VI. Dosage adjustment guided by serum theophylline concentration.

Peak Serum Concentration	Dosage Adjustment
<9.9 mcg/mL	If symptoms are not controlled and current dosage is tolerated, increase dose about 25%. Recheck serum concentration after three days for further dosage adjustment
10–14.9 mcg/mL	If symptoms are controlled and current dosage is tolerated, maintain dose and recheck serum concentration at 6–12 month intervals.¶ If symptoms are not controlled and current dosage is tolerated consider adding additional medication(s) to treatment regimen.
15–19.9 mcg/mL	Consider 10% decrease in dose to provide greater margin of safety even if current dosage is tolerated.¶
20–24.9 mcg/mL	Decrease dose by 25% even if no adverse effects are present. Recheck serum concentration after 3 days to guide further dosage adjustment.
25–30 mcg/mL	Skip next dose and decrease subsequent doses at least 25% even if no adverse effects are present. Recheck serum concentration after 3 days to guide further dosage adjustment. If symptomatic, consider whether overdose treatment is indicated (see recommendations for chronic overdosage).
>30 mcg/mL	Treat overdose as indicated (see recommendations for chronic overdosage). If theophylline is subsequently resumed, decrease dose by at least 50% and recheck serum concentration after 3 days to guide further dosage adjustment.

¶ Dose reduction and/or serum theophylline concentration measurement is indicated whenever adverse effects are present, physiologic abnormalities that can reduce theophylline clearance occur (e.g., sustained fever), or a drug that interacts with theophylline is added or discontinued (see **WARNINGS**).

HOW SUPPLIED

Uniphyl® (theophylline, anhydrous) Controlled-Release Tablets 400 mg are supplied in white, opaque plastic, child-resistant bottles containing 100 tablets (NDC 67781-251-01) or 500 tablets (NDC 67781-251-05). Each round, white 400 mg tablet bears the symbol PF on the scored side and U400 on the other side.

Uniphyl® (theophylline, anhydrous) Controlled-Release Tablets 600 mg are supplied in white, opaque plastic, child-resistant bottles containing 100 tablets (NDC 67781-252-01). Each rectangular, concave, white 600 mg tablet bears the symbol PF on the scored side and U 600 on the other side.

Store at 25°C (77°F); excursions permitted between 15°–30°C (59°–86°F).

Dispense in a tight, light-resistant container.

Dist. by: Purdue Pharmaceutical Products L.P.
Stamford, CT 06901-3431
March 17, 2004
OT00987
300945-0A

Shown in Product Identification Guide, page 331

Continued on next page

EDUCATIONAL MATERIAL

www.senokot.com provides dosing information for the Senokot® products family of laxatives, as well as patient education about constipation and its causes. A special section on toilet training, written by a pediatrician, describes the popular child-centered approach.

Website containing pain management information for healthcare professionals and patients. Available at **www.partnersagainstpain.com**

Website containing general information on all Purdue products can be obtained at **www.purduepharma.com.**

Website containing information about constipation and the Colace® and Peri-Colace® brand stool softeners is available at **www.colacecapsules.com**

EDUCATIONAL MATERIAL

Laxative Protocol Sheets English version (00PS77) and Spanish version (0PS125) 1 page (pad of 25)
Available to physicians, nurses and pharmacists

Purdue Pharma L.P.

ONE STAMFORD FORUM
STAMFORD, CT 06901-3431

For Medical Inquiries:
888-726-7535
Adverse Drug Experiences:
888-726-7535
Customer Service:
800-877-5666
FAX 800-877-3210

MS Contin® Tablets—see listing under The Purdue Frederick Company, page 2524

MSIR® Immediate-Release Oral Tablets—see listing under The Purdue Frederick Company, page 2527

MSIR® Oral Solution Concentrate—see listing under The Purdue Frederick Company, page 2527

OXYCONTIN® Ⓒ℞

[*ŏks' ē-kŏn-tĭn*]
(Oxycodone HCl Controlled-Release) Tablets
10 mg 20 mg 40 mg 80 mg* 160 mg*

***80 mg and 160 mg for use in opioid-tolerant patients only**

OT00367D
300514-0C-001

WARNING:

OxyContin is an opioid agonist and a Schedule II controlled substance with an abuse liability similar to morphine.

Oxycodone can be abused in a manner similar to other opioid agonists, legal or illicit. This should be considered when prescribing or dispensing OxyContin in situations where the physician or pharmacist is concerned about an increased risk of misuse, abuse, or diversion.

OxyContin Tablets are a controlled-release oral formulation of oxycodone hydrochloride indicated for the management of moderate to severe pain when a continuous, around-the-clock analgesic is needed for an extended period of time.

OxyContin Tablets are NOT intended for use as a prn analgesic.

OxyContin 80 mg and 160 mg Tablets ARE FOR USE IN OPIOID-TOLERANT PATIENTS ONLY. These tablet strengths may cause fatal respiratory depression when administered to patients not previously exposed to opioids.

OxyContin TABLETS ARE TO BE SWALLOWED WHOLE AND ARE NOT TO BE BROKEN, CHEWED, OR CRUSHED. TAKING BROKEN, CHEWED, OR CRUSHED OxyContin TABLETS LEADS TO RAPID RELEASE AND ABSORPTION OF A POTENTIALLY FATAL DOSE OF OXYCODONE.

DESCRIPTION

OxyContin® (oxycodone hydrochloride controlled-release) Tablets are an opioid analgesic supplied in 10 mg, 20 mg, 40 mg, 80 mg, and 160 mg tablet strengths for oral administration. The tablet strengths describe the amount of oxycodone per tablet as the hydrochloride salt. The structural formula for oxycodone hydrochloride is as follows:

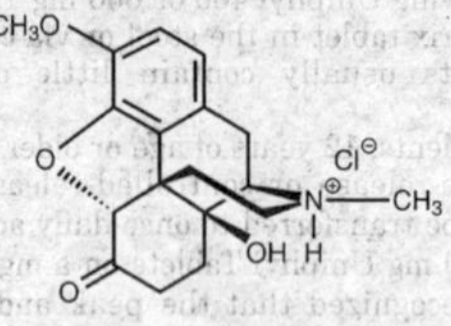

The chemical formula is 4, 5α-epoxy-14-hydroxy-3-methoxy-17-methylmorphinan-6-one hydrochloride.

Oxycodone is a white, odorless crystalline powder derived from the opium alkaloid, thebaine. Oxycodone hydrochloride dissolves in water (1 g in 6 to 7 mL). It is slightly soluble in alcohol (octanol water partition coefficient 0.7). The tablets contain the following inactive ingredients: ammonio methacrylate copolymer, hypromellose, lactose, magnesium stearate, polyethylene glycol 400, povidone, sodium hydroxide, sorbic acid, stearyl alcohol, talc, titanium dioxide, and triacetin.

The 10 mg tablets also contain: hydroxypropyl cellulose.

The 20 mg tablets also contain: polysorbate 80 and red iron oxide.

The 40 mg tablets also contain: polysorbate 80 and yellow iron oxide.

The 80 mg tablets also contain: FD&C blue No. 2, hydroxypropyl cellulose, and yellow iron oxide.

The 160 mg tablets also contain: FD&C blue No. 2 and polysorbate 80.

CLINICAL PHARMACOLOGY

Oxycodone is a pure agonist opioid whose principal therapeutic action is analgesia. Other members of the class known as opioid agonists include substances such as morphine, hydromorphone, fentanyl, codeine, and hydrocodone. Pharmacological effects of opioid agonists include anxiolysis, euphoria, feelings of relaxation, respiratory depression, constipation, miosis, and cough suppression, as well as analgesia. Like all pure opioid agonist analgesics, with increasing doses there is increasing analgesia, unlike with mixed agonist/antagonists or non-opioid analgesics, where there is a limit to the analgesic effect with increasing doses. With pure opioid agonist analgesics, there is no defined maximum dose; the ceiling to analgesic effectiveness is imposed only by side effects, the more serious of which may include somnolence and respiratory depression.

Central Nervous System

The precise mechanism of the analgesic action is unknown. However, specific CNS opioid receptors for endogenous compounds with opioid-like activity have been identified throughout the brain and spinal cord and play a role in the analgesic effects of this drug.

Oxycodone produces respiratory depression by direct action on brain stem respiratory centers. The respiratory depression involves both a reduction in the responsiveness of the brain stem respiratory centers to increases in carbon dioxide tension and to electrical stimulation.

Oxycodone depresses the cough reflex by direct effect on the cough center in the medulla. Antitussive effects may occur with doses lower than those usually required for analgesia.

Oxycodone causes miosis, even in total darkness. Pinpoint pupils are a sign of opioid overdose but are not pathognomonic (e.g., pontine lesions of hemorrhagic or ischemic origin may produce similar findings). Marked mydriasis rather than miosis may be seen with hypoxia in the setting of OxyContin® overdose (See **OVERDOSAGE**).

Gastrointestinal Tract And Other Smooth Muscle

Oxycodone causes a reduction in motility associated with an increase in smooth muscle tone in the antrum of the stomach and duodenum. Digestion of food in the small intestine is delayed and propulsive contractions are decreased. Propulsive peristaltic waves in the colon are decreased, while tone may be increased to the point of spasm resulting in constipation. Other opioid-induced effects may include a reduction in gastric, biliary and pancreatic secretions, spasm of sphincter of Oddi, and transient elevations in serum amylase.

Cardiovascular System

Oxycodone may produce release of histamine with or without associated peripheral vasodilation. Manifestations of histamine release and/or peripheral vasodilation may include pruritus, flushing, red eyes, sweating, and/or orthostatic hypotension.

Concentration – Efficacy Relationships

Studies in normal volunteers and patients reveal predictable relationships between oxycodone dosage and plasma oxycodone concentrations, as well as between concentration and certain expected opioid effects, such as pupillary constriction, sedation, overall "drug effect", analgesia and feelings of "relaxation".

As with all opioids, the minimum effective plasma concentration for analgesia will vary widely among patients, especially among patients who have been previously treated with potent agonist opioids. As a result, patients must be treated with individualized titration of dosage to the desired effect. The minimum effective analgesic concentration of oxycodone for any individual patient may increase over time due to an increase in pain, the development of a new pain syndrome and/or the development of analgesic tolerance.

Concentration – Adverse Experience Relationships

OxyContin® Tablets are associated with typical opioid-related adverse experiences. There is a general relationship between increasing oxycodone plasma concentration and increasing frequency of dose-related opioid adverse experiences such as nausea, vomiting, CNS effects, and respiratory depression. In opioid-tolerant patients, the situation is altered by the development of tolerance to opioid-related side effects, and the relationship is not clinically relevant.

As with all opioids, the dose must be individualized (see **DOSAGE AND ADMINISTRATION**), because the effective analgesic dose for some patients will be too high to be tolerated by other patients.

PHARMACOKINETICS AND METABOLISM

The activity of OxyContin Tablets is primarily due to the parent drug oxycodone. OxyContin Tablets are designed to provide controlled delivery of oxycodone over 12 hours.

Breaking, chewing or crushing OxyContin Tablets eliminates the controlled delivery mechanism and results in the rapid release and absorption of a potentially fatal dose of oxycodone.

Oxycodone release from OxyContin Tablets is pH independent. Oxycodone is well absorbed from OxyContin Tablets with an oral bioavailability of 60% to 87%. The relative oral bioavailability of OxyContin to immediate-release oral dosage forms is 100%. Upon repeated dosing in normal volunteers in pharmacokinetic studies, steady-state levels were achieved within 24-36 hours. Dose proportionality and/or bioavailability has been established for the 10 mg, 20 mg, 40 mg, 80 mg, and 160 mg tablet strengths for both peak plasma levels (C_{max}) and extent of absorption (AUC). Oxycodone is extensively metabolized and eliminated primarily in the urine as both conjugated and unconjugated metabolites. The apparent elimination half-life of oxycodone following the administration of OxyContin® was 4.5 hours compared to 3.2 hours for immediate-release oxycodone.

Absorption

About 60% to 87% of an oral dose of oxycodone reaches the central compartment in comparison to a parenteral dose. This high oral bioavailability is due to low pre-systemic and/or first-pass metabolism. In normal volunteers, the t½ of absorption is 0.4 hours for immediate-release oral oxycodone. In contrast, OxyContin Tablets exhibit a biphasic absorption pattern with two apparent absorption half-lives of 0.6 and 6.9 hours, which describes the initial release of oxycodone from the tablet followed by a prolonged release.

Plasma Oxycodone by Time

Dose proportionality has been established for the 10 mg, 20 mg, 40 mg, and 80 mg tablet strengths for both peak plasma concentrations (C_{max}) and extent of absorption (AUC) (see Table 1 below). Another study established that the 160 mg tablet is bioequivalent to 2 × 80 mg tablets as well as to 4 × 40 mg for both peak plasma concentrations (C_{max}) and extent of absorption (AUC) (see Table 2 below). Given the short half-life of elimination of oxycodone from OxyContin®, steady-state plasma concentrations of oxycodone are achieved within 24-36 hours of initiation of dosing with OxyContin Tablets. In a study comparing 10 mg of OxyContin every 12 hours to 5 mg of immediate-release oxycodone every 6 hours, the two treatments were found to be equivalent for AUC and C_{max}, and similar for C_{min} (trough) concentrations. There was less fluctuation in plasma concentrations for the OxyContin Tablets than for the immediate-release formulation.

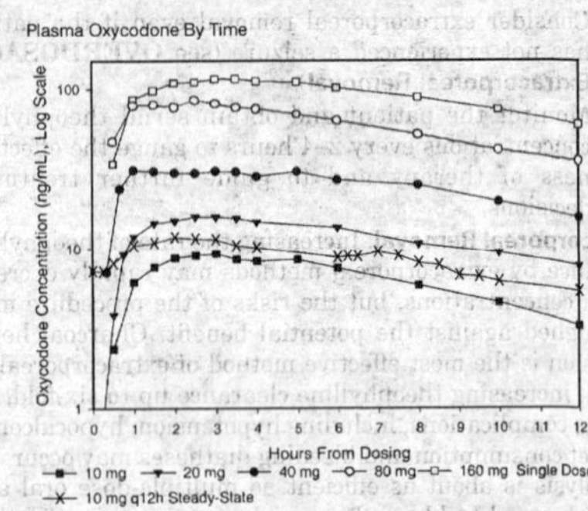

[See table 1 at bottom of next page]
[See table 2 at bottom of next page]

OxyContin® is NOT INDICATED FOR RECTAL ADMINISTRATION. Data from a study involving 21 normal volunteers show that OxyContin Tablets administered per rectum resulted in an AUC 39% greater and a C_{max} 9% higher than tablets administered by mouth. Therefore, there is an increased risk of adverse events with rectal administration.

Food Effects

Food has no significant effect on the extent of absorption of oxycodone from OxyContin. However, the peak plasma concentration of oxycodone increased by 25% when a OxyContin 160 mg Tablet was administered with a high-fat meal.

Distribution

Following intravenous administration, the volume of distribution (Vss) for oxycodone was 2.6 L/kg. Oxycodone binding to plasma protein at 37°C and a pH of 7.4 was about 45%.

Once absorbed, oxycodone is distributed to skeletal muscle, liver, intestinal tract, lungs, spleen, and brain. Oxycodone has been found in breast milk (see **PRECAUTIONS**).

Metabolism

Oxycodone hydrochloride is extensively metabolized to noroxycodone, oxymorphone, and their glucuronides. The major circulating metabolite is noroxycodone with an AUC ratio of 0.6 relative to that of oxycodone. Noroxycodone is reported to be a considerably weaker analgesic than oxycodone. Oxymorphone, although possessing analgesic activity, is present in the plasma only in low concentrations. The correlation between oxymorphone concentrations and opioid effects was much less than that seen with oxycodone plasma concentrations. The analgesic activity profile of other metabolites is not known.

The formation of oxymorphone, but not noroxycodone, is mediated by cytochrome P450 2D6 and, as such, its formation can, in theory, be affected by other drugs (see **Drug-Drug Interactions**).

Excretion

Oxycodone and its metabolites are excreted primarily via the kidney. The amounts measured in the urine have been reported as follows: free oxycodone up to 19%; conjugated oxycodone up to 50%; free oxymorphone 0%; conjugated oxymorphone $\leq$ 14%; both free and conjugated noroxycodone have been found in the urine but not quantified. The total plasma clearance was 0.8 L/min for adults.

Special Populations

Elderly

The plasma concentrations of oxycodone are only nominally affected by age, being 15% greater in elderly as compared to young subjects.

Gender

Female subjects have, on average, plasma oxycodone concentrations up to 25% higher than males on a body weight adjusted basis. The reason for this difference is unknown.

Renal Impairment

Data from a pharmacokinetic study involving 13 patients with mild to severe renal dysfunction (creatinine clearance <60 mL/min) show peak plasma oxycodone and noroxycodone concentrations 50% and 20% higher, respectively, and AUC values for oxycodone, noroxycodone, and oxymorphone 60%, 50%, and 40% higher than normal subjects, respectively. This is accompanied by an increase in sedation but not by differences in respiratory rate, pupillary constriction, or several other measures of drug effect. There was an increase in t½ of elimination for oxycodone of only 1 hour (see **PRECAUTIONS**).

Hepatic Impairment

Data from a study involving 24 patients with mild to moderate hepatic dysfunction show peak plasma oxycodone and noroxycodone concentrations 50% and 20% higher, respectively, than normal subjects. AUC values are 95% and 65% higher, respectively. Oxymorphone peak plasma concentrations and AUC values are lower by 30% and 40%. These differences are accompanied by increases in some, but not other, drug effects. The t½ elimination for oxycodone increased by 2.3 hours (see **PRECAUTIONS**).

Drug-Drug Interactions (see PRECAUTIONS)

Oxycodone is metabolized in part by cytochrome P450 2D6 to oxymorphone which represents less than 15% of the total administered dose. This route of elimination may be blocked by a variety of drugs (e.g., certain cardiovascular drugs including amiodarone and quinidine as well as polycyclic antidepressants). However, in a study involving 10 subjects using quinidine, a known inhibitor of cytochrome P450 2D6, the pharmacodynamic effects of oxycodone were unchanged.

Pharmacodynamics

A single-dose, double-blind, placebo- and dose-controlled study was conducted using OxyContin® (10, 20, and 30 mg) in an analgesic pain model involving 182 patients with moderate to severe pain. Twenty and 30 mg of OxyContin were superior in reducing pain compared with placebo, and this difference was statistically significant. The onset of analgesic action with OxyContin occurred within 1 hour in most patients following oral administration.

CLINICAL TRIALS

A double-blind placebo-controlled, fixed-dose, parallel group, two-week study was conducted in 133 patients with chronic, moderate to severe pain, who were judged as having inadequate pain control with their current therapy. In this study, 20 mg OxyContin q12h but not 10 mg OxyContin q12h decreased pain compared with placebo, and this difference was statistically significant.

INDICATIONS AND USAGE

OxyContin Tablets are a controlled-release oral formulation of oxycodone hydrochloride indicated for the management of moderate to severe pain when a continuous, around-the-clock analgesic is needed for an extended period of time.

OxyContin is **NOT** intended for use as a prn analgesic.

Physicians should individualize treatment in every case, initiating therapy at the appropriate point along a progression from non-opioid analgesics, such as non-steroidal anti-inflammatory drugs and acetaminophen to opioids in a plan of pain management such as outlined by the World Health Organization, the Agency for Healthcare Research and Quality (formerly known as the Agency for Health Care Policy and Research), the Federation of State Medical Boards Model Guidelines, or the American Pain Society.

OxyContin is not indicated for pain in the immediate post-operative period (the first 12–24 hours following surgery), or if the pain is mild, or not expected to persist for an extended period of time. OxyContin is only indicated for postoperative use if the patient is already receiving the drug prior to surgery or if the postoperative pain is expected to be moderate to severe and persist for an extended period of time. Physicians should individualize treatment, moving from parenteral to oral analgesics as appropriate. (See American Pain Society guidelines.)

CONTRAINDICATIONS

OxyContin® is contraindicated in patients with known hypersensitivity to oxycodone, or in any situation where opioids are contraindicated. This includes patients with significant respiratory depression (in unmonitored settings or the absence of resuscitative equipment), and patients with acute or severe bronchial asthma or hypercarbia. OxyContin is contraindicated in any patient who has or is suspected of having paralytic ileus.

WARNINGS

OXYCONTIN TABLETS ARE TO BE SWALLOWED WHOLE AND ARE NOT TO BE BROKEN, CHEWED, OR CRUSHED. TAKING BROKEN, CHEWED, OR CRUSHED OXYCONTIN TABLETS LEADS TO RAPID RELEASE AND ABSORPTION OF A POTENTIALLY FATAL DOSE OF OXYCODONE.

TABLE 1
Mean [% coefficient variation]

Regimen/ Dosage Form	AUC (ng•hr/mL)†	C_{max} (ng/mL)	T_{max} (hrs)	Trough Conc. (ng/mL)
Single Dose 10 mg OxyContin	100.7 [26.6]	10.6 [20.1]	2.7 [44.1]	n.a.
20 mg OxyContin	207.5 [35.9]	21.4 [36.6]	3.2 [57.9]	n.a.
40 mg OxyContin	423.1 [33.3]	39.3 [34.0]	3.1 [77.4]	n.a.
80 mg OxyContin*	1085.5 [32.3]	98.5 [32.1]	2.1 [52.3]	n.a.
Multiple Dose 10 mg OxyContin Tablets q12h	103.6 [38.6]	15.1 [31.0]	3.2 [69.5]	7.2 [48.1]
5 mg immediate-release q6h	99.0 [36.2]	15.5 [28.8]	1.6 [49.7]	7.4 [50.9]

TABLE 2
Mean [% coefficient variation]

Regimen/ Dosage Form	AUC_∞ (ng•hr/mL)†	C_{max} (ng/mL)	T_{max} (hrs)	Trough Conc. (ng/mL)
Single Dose 4×40 mg OxyContin*	1935.3 [34.7]	152.0 [28.9]	2.56 [42.3]	n.a.
2×80 mg OxyContin*	1859.3 [30.1]	153.4 [25.1]	2.78 [69.3]	n.a.
1×160 mg OxyContin*	1856.4 [30.5]	156.4 [24.8]	2.54 [36.4]	n.a.

†for single-dose AUC=$AUC_{0\text{-inf}}$; for multiple-dose AUC=$AUC_{0\text{-T}}$
*data obtained while volunteers received naltrexone which can enhance absorption.

OxyContin 80 mg and 160 mg Tablets ARE FOR USE IN OPIOID-TOLERANT PATIENTS ONLY. These tablet strengths may cause fatal respiratory depression when administered to patients not previously exposed to opioids.

OxyContin 80 mg and 160 mg Tablets are for use only in opioid-tolerant patients requiring daily oxycodone equivalent dosages of 160 mg or more for the 80 mg tablet and 320 mg or more for the 160 mg tablet. Care should be taken in the prescribing of these tablet strengths. Patients should be instructed against use by individuals other than the patient for whom it was prescribed, as such inappropriate use may have severe medical consequences, including death.

Misuse, Abuse and Diversion of Opioids

Oxycodone is an opioid agonist of the morphine-type. Such drugs are sought by drug abusers and people with addiction disorders and are subject to criminal diversion.

Oxycodone can be abused in a manner similar to other opioid agonists, legal or illicit. This should be considered when prescribing or dispensing OxyContin in situations where the physician or pharmacist is concerned about an increased risk of misuse, abuse, or diversion.

OxyContin has been reported as being abused by crushing, chewing, snorting, or injecting the dissolved product. These practices will result in the uncontrolled delivery of the opioid and pose a significant risk to the abuser that could result in overdose and death (see **WARNINGS** and **DRUG ABUSE AND ADDICTION**).

Concerns about abuse, addiction, and diversion should not prevent the proper management of pain. The development of addiction to opioid analgesics in properly managed patients with pain has been reported to be rare. However, data are not available to establish the true incidence of addiction in chronic pain patients.

Healthcare professionals should contact their State Professional Licensing Board, or State Controlled Substances Authority for information on how to prevent and detect abuse or diversion of this product.

Interactions with Alcohol and Drugs of Abuse

Oxycodone may be expected to have additive effects when used in conjunction with alcohol, other opioids, or illicit drugs that cause central nervous system depression.

DRUG ABUSE AND ADDICTION

OxyContin® is a mu-agonist opioid with an abuse liability similar to morphine and is a Schedule II controlled substance. Oxycodone, like morphine and other opioids used in analgesia, can be abused and is subject to criminal diversion.

Drug addiction is characterized by compulsive use, use for non-medical purposes, and continued use despite harm or risk of harm. Drug addiction is a treatable disease, utilizing a multi-disciplinary approach, but relapse is common.

"Drug-seeking" behavior is very common in addicts and drug abusers. Drug-seeking tactics include emergency calls or visits near the end of office hours, refusal to undergo appropriate examination, testing or referral, repeated "loss" of prescriptions, tampering with prescriptions and reluctance to provide prior medical records or contact information for other treating physician(s). "Doctor shopping" to obtain additional prescriptions is common among drug abusers and people suffering from untreated addiction.

Abuse and addiction are separate and distinct from physical dependence and tolerance. Physicians should be aware that addiction may not be accompanied by concurrent tolerance and symptoms of physical dependence in all addicts. In addition, abuse of opioids can occur in the absence of true addiction and is characterized by misuse for non-medical purposes, often in combination with other psychoactive substances. OxyContin, like other opioids, has been diverted for non-medical use. Careful record-keeping of prescribing information, including quantity, frequency, and renewal requests is strongly advised.

Proper assessment of the patient, proper prescribing practices, periodic re-evaluation of therapy, and proper dispensing and storage are appropriate measures that help to limit abuse of opioid drugs.

OxyContin consists of a dual-polymer matrix, intended for oral use only. Abuse of the crushed tablet poses a hazard of overdose and death. This risk is increased with concurrent abuse of alcohol and other substances. With parenteral abuse, the tablet excipients, especially talc, can be expected to result in local tissue necrosis, infection, pulmonary granulomas, and increased risk of endocarditis and valvular heart injury. Parenteral drug abuse is commonly associated with transmission of infectious diseases such as hepatitis and HIV.

Respiratory Depression

Respiratory depression is the chief hazard from oxycodone, the active ingredient in OxyContin®, as with all opioid agonists. Respiratory depression is a particular problem in elderly or debilitated patients, usually following large initial doses in non-tolerant patients, or when opioids are given in conjunction with other agents that depress respiration.

Oxycodone should be used with extreme caution in patients with significant chronic obstructive pulmonary disease or cor pulmonale, and in patients having a substantially decreased respiratory reserve, hypoxia, hypercapnia, or pre-existing respiratory depression. In such patients, even usual therapeutic doses of oxycodone may decrease respiratory drive to the point of apnea. In these patients alterna-

Continued on next page

OxyContin—Cont.

tive non-opioid analgesics should be considered, and opioids should be employed only under careful medical supervision at the lowest effective dose.

Head Injury

The respiratory depressant effects of opioids include carbon dioxide retention and secondary elevation of cerebrospinal fluid pressure, and may be markedly exaggerated in the presence of head injury, intracranial lesions, or other sources of pre-existing increased intracranial pressure. Oxycodone produces effects on pupillary response and consciousness which may obscure neurologic signs of further increases in intracranial pressure in patients with head injuries.

Hypotensive Effect

OxyContin may cause severe hypotension. There is an added risk to individuals whose ability to maintain blood pressure has been compromised by a depleted blood volume, or after concurrent administration with drugs such as phenothiazines or other agents which compromise vasomotor tone. Oxycodone may produce orthostatic hypotension in ambulatory patients. Oxycodone, like all opioid analgesics of the morphine-type, should be administered with caution to patients in circulatory shock, since vasodilation produced by the drug may further reduce cardiac output and blood pressure.

PRECAUTIONS

General

Opioid analgesics have a narrow therapeutic index in certain patient populations, especially when combined with CNS depressant drugs, and should be reserved for cases where the benefits of opioid analgesia outweigh the known risks of respiratory depression, altered mental state, and postural hypotension.

Use of OxyContin® is associated with increased potential risks and should be used only with caution in the following conditions: acute alcoholism; adrenocortical insufficiency (e.g., Addison's disease); CNS depression or coma; delirium tremens; debilitated patients; kyphoscoliosis associated with respiratory depression; myxedema or hypothyroidism; prostatic hypertrophy or urethral stricture; severe impairment of hepatic, pulmonary or renal function; and toxic psychosis.

The administration of oxycodone may obscure the diagnosis or clinical course in patients with acute abdominal conditions. Oxycodone may aggravate convulsions in patients with convulsive disorders, and all opioids may induce or aggravate seizures in some clinical settings.

Interactions with other CNS Depressants

OxyContin should be used with caution and started in a reduced dosage (1/3 to 1/2 of the usual dosage) in patients who are concurrently receiving other central nervous system depressants including sedatives or hypnotics, general anesthetics, phenothiazines, other tranquilizers, and alcohol. Interactive effects resulting in respiratory depression, hypotension, profound sedation, or coma may result if these drugs are taken in combination with the usual doses of OxyContin.

Interactions with Mixed Agonist/Antagonist Opioid Analgesics

Agonist/antagonist analgesics (i.e., pentazocine, nalbuphine, and butorphanol) should be administered with caution to a patient who has received or is receiving a course of therapy with a pure opioid agonist analgesic such as oxycodone. In this situation, mixed agonist/antagonist analgesics may reduce the analgesic effect of oxycodone and/or may precipitate withdrawal symptoms in these patients.

Ambulatory Surgery and Postoperative Use

OxyContin is not indicated for pre-emptive analgesia (administration pre-operatively for the management of postoperative pain).

OxyContin is not indicated for pain in the immediate postoperative period (the first 12 to 24 hours following surgery) for patients not previously taking the drug, because its safety in this setting has not been established.

OxyContin is not indicated for pain in the postoperative period if the pain is mild or not expected to persist for an extended period of time.

OxyContin is only indicated for postoperative use if the patient is already receiving the drug prior to surgery or if the postoperative pain is expected to be moderate to severe and persist for an extended period of time. Physicians should individualize treatment, moving from parenteral to oral analgesics as appropriate (See American Pain Society guidelines).

Patients who are already receiving OxyContin® Tablets as part of ongoing analgesic therapy may be safely continued on the drug if appropriate dosage adjustments are made considering the procedure, other drugs given, and the temporary changes in physiology caused by the surgical intervention (see **DOSAGE AND ADMINISTRATION**).

OxyContin and other morphine-like opioids have been shown to decrease bowel motility. Ileus is a common postoperative complication, especially after intra-abdominal surgery with opioid analgesia. Caution should be taken to monitor for decreased bowel motility in postoperative patients receiving opioids. Standard supportive therapy should be implemented.

Use in Pancreatic/Biliary Tract Disease

Oxycodone may cause spasm of the sphincter of Oddi and should be used with caution in patients with biliary tract disease, including acute pancreatitis. Opioids like oxycodone may cause increases in the serum amylase level.

Tolerance and Physical Dependence

Tolerance is the need for increasing doses of opioids to maintain a defined effect such as analgesia (in the absence of disease progression or other external factors). Physical dependence is manifested by withdrawal symptoms after abrupt discontinuation of a drug or upon administration of an antagonist. Physical dependence and tolerance are not unusual during chronic opioid therapy.

The opioid abstinence or withdrawal syndrome is characterized by some or all of the following: restlessness, lacrimation, rhinorrhea, yawning, perspiration, chills, myalgia, and mydriasis. Other symptoms also may develop, including: irritability, anxiety, backache, joint pain, weakness, abdominal cramps, insomnia, nausea, anorexia, vomiting, diarrhea, or increased blood pressure, respiratory rate, or heart rate.

In general, opioids should not be abruptly discontinued (see **DOSAGE AND ADMINISTRATION: Cessation of Therapy**).

Information for Patients/Caregivers

If clinically advisable, patients receiving OxyContin Tablets or their caregivers should be given the following information by the physician, nurse, pharmacist, or caregiver:

1. Patients should be aware that OxyContin Tablets contain oxycodone, which is a morphine-like substance.
2. Patients should be advised that OxyContin Tablets were designed to work properly only if swallowed whole. OxyContin Tablets will release all their contents at once if broken, chewed, or crushed, resulting in a risk of fatal overdose.
3. Patients should be advised to report episodes of breakthrough pain and adverse experiences occurring during therapy. Individualization of dosage is essential to make optimal use of this medication.
4. Patients should be advised not to adjust the dose of OxyContin® without consulting the prescribing professional.
5. Patients should be advised that OxyContin may impair mental and/or physical ability required for the performance of potentially hazardous tasks (e.g., driving, operating heavy machinery).
6. Patients should not combine OxyContin with alcohol or other central nervous system depressants (sleep aids, tranquilizers) except by the orders of the prescribing physician, because dangerous additive effects may occur, resulting in serious injury or death.
7. Women of childbearing potential who become, or are planning to become, pregnant should be advised to consult their physician regarding the effects of analgesics and other drug use during pregnancy on themselves and their unborn child.
8. Patients should be advised that OxyContin is a potential drug of abuse. They should protect it from theft, and it should never be given to anyone other than the individual for whom it was prescribed.
9. Patients should be advised that they may pass empty matrix "ghosts" (tablets) via colostomy or in the stool, and that this is of no concern since the active medication has already been absorbed.
10. Patients should be advised that if they have been receiving treatment with OxyContin for more than a few weeks and cessation of therapy is indicated, it may be appropriate to taper the OxyContin dose, rather than abruptly discontinue it, due to the risk of precipitating withdrawal symptoms. Their physician can provide a dose schedule to accomplish a gradual discontinuation of the medication.
11. Patients should be instructed to keep OxyContin in a secure place out of the reach of children. When OxyContin is no longer needed, the unused tablets should be destroyed by flushing down the toilet.

Use in Drug and Alcohol Addiction

OxyContin is an opioid with no approved use in the management of addictive disorders. Its proper usage in individuals with drug or alcohol dependence, either active or in remission, is for the management of pain requiring opioid analgesia.

Drug-Drug Interactions

Opioid analgesics, including OxyContin®, may enhance the neuromuscular blocking action of skeletal muscle relaxants and produce an increased degree of respiratory depression.

Oxycodone is metabolized in part to oxymorphone via cytochrome P450 2D6. While this pathway may be blocked by a variety of drugs (e.g., certain cardiovascular drugs including amiodarone and quinidine as well as polycyclic antidepressants), such blockade has not yet been shown to be of clinical significance with this agent. Clinicians should be aware of this possible interaction, however.

Use with CNS Depressants

OxyContin, like all opioid analgesics, should be started at 1/3 to 1/2 of the usual dosage in patients who are concurrently receiving other central nervous system depressants including sedatives or hypnotics, general anesthetics, phenothiazines, centrally acting anti-emetics, tranquilizers, and alcohol because respiratory depression, hypotension, and profound sedation or coma may result. No specific interaction between oxycodone and monoamine oxidase inhibitors has been observed, but caution in the use of any opioid in patients taking this class of drugs is appropriate.

Carcinogenesis, Mutagenesis, Impairment of Fertility

Studies of oxycodone to evaluate its carcinogenic potential have not been conducted.

Oxycodone was not mutagenic in the following assays: Ames Salmonella and E. coli test with and without metabolic activation at doses of up to 5000 μg, chromosomal aberration test in human lymphocytes in the absence of metabolic activation at doses of up to 1500 μg/mL and with activation 48 hours after exposure at doses of up to 5000 μg/mL, and in the in vivo bone marrow micronucleus test in mice (at plasma levels of up to 48 μg/mL). Oxycodone was clastogenic in the human lymphocyte chromosomal assay in the presence of metabolic activation in the human chromosomal aberration test (at greater than or equal to 1250 μg/mL) at 24 but not 48 hours of exposure and in the mouse lymphoma assay at doses of 50 μg/mL or greater with metabolic activation and at 400 μg/mL or greater without metabolic activation.

Pregnancy

Teratogenic Effects — Category B: Reproduction studies have been performed in rats and rabbits by oral administration at doses up to 8 mg/kg and 125 mg/kg, respectively. These doses are 3 and 46 times a human dose of 160 mg/day, based on mg/kg basis. The results did not reveal evidence of harm to the fetus due to oxycodone. There are, however, no adequate and well-controlled studies in pregnant women. Because animal reproduction studies are not always predictive of human response, this drug should be used during pregnancy only if clearly needed.

Labor and Delivery

OxyContin® is not recommended for use in women during and immediately prior to labor and delivery because oral opioids may cause respiratory depression in the newborn. Neonates whose mothers have been taking oxycodone chronically may exhibit respiratory depression and/or withdrawal symptoms, either at birth and/or in the nursery.

Nursing Mothers

Low concentrations of oxycodone have been detected in breast milk. Withdrawal symptoms can occur in breast-feeding infants when maternal administration of an opioid analgesic is stopped. Ordinarily, nursing should not be undertaken while a patient is receiving OxyContin because of the possibility of sedation and/or respiratory depression in the infant.

Pediatric Use

Safety and effectiveness of OxyContin have not been established in pediatric patients below the age of 18. **It must be remembered that OxyContin Tablets cannot be crushed or divided for administration.**

Geriatric Use

In controlled pharmacokinetic studies in elderly subjects (greater than 65 years) the clearance of oxycodone appeared to be slightly reduced. Compared to young adults, the plasma concentrations of oxycodone were increased approximately 15% (see **PHARMACOKINETICS AND METABOLISM**). Of the total number of subjects (445) in clinical studies of OxyContin, 148 (33.3%) were age 65 and older (including those age 75 and older) while 40 (9.0%) were age 75 and older. In clinical trials with appropriate initiation of therapy and dose titration, no untoward or unexpected side effects were seen in the elderly patients who received OxyContin. Thus, the usual doses and dosing intervals are appropriate for these patients. As with all opioids, the starting dose should be reduced to 1/3 to 1/2 of the usual dosage in debilitated, non-tolerant patients. Respiratory depression is the chief hazard in elderly or debilitated patients, usually following large initial doses in non-tolerant patients, or when opioids are given in conjunction with other agents that depress respiration.

Laboratory Monitoring

Due to the broad range of plasma concentrations seen in clinical populations, the varying degrees of pain, and the development of tolerance, plasma oxycodone measurements are usually not helpful in clinical management. Plasma concentrations of the active drug substance may be of value in selected, unusual or complex cases.

Hepatic Impairment

A study of OxyContin in patients with hepatic impairment indicates greater plasma concentrations than those with normal function. The initiation of therapy at 1/3 to 1/2 the usual doses and careful dose titration is warranted.

Renal Impairment

In patients with renal impairment, as evidenced by decreased creatinine clearance (<60 mL/min), the concentrations of oxycodone in the plasma are approximately 50% higher than in subjects with normal renal function. Dose initiation should follow a conservative approach. Dosages should be adjusted according to the clinical situation.

Gender Differences

In pharmacokinetic studies, opioid-naive females demonstrate up to 25% higher average plasma concentrations and greater frequency of typical opioid adverse events than males, even after adjustment for body weight. The clinical relevance of a difference of this magnitude is low for a drug intended for chronic usage at individualized dosages, and there was no male/female difference detected for efficacy or adverse events in clinical trials.

ADVERSE REACTIONS

The safety of OxyContin® was evaluated in double-blind clinical trials involving 713 patients with moderate to severe pain of various etiologies. In open-label studies of cancer pain, 187 patients received OxyContin in total daily doses ranging from 20 mg to 640 mg per day. The average total daily dose was approximately 105 mg per day.

Serious adverse reactions which may be associated with OxyContin Tablet therapy in clinical use are those observed with other opioid analgesics, including respiratory depression, apnea, respiratory arrest, and (to an even lesser degree) circulatory depression, hypotension, or shock (see **OVERDOSAGE**).

The non-serious adverse events seen on initiation of therapy with OxyContin are typical opioid side effects. These events are dose-dependent, and their frequency depends upon the dose, the clinical setting, the patient's level of opioid tolerance, and host factors specific to the individual. They should be expected and managed as a part of opioid analgesia. The most frequent (>5%) include: constipation, nausea, somnolence, dizziness, vomiting, pruritus, headache, dry mouth, sweating, and asthenia.

In many cases the frequency of these events during initiation of therapy may be minimized by careful individualization of starting dosage, slow titration, and the avoidance of large swings in the plasma concentrations of the opioid. Many of these adverse events will cease or decrease in intensity as OxyContin therapy is continued and some degree of tolerance is developed.

Clinical trials comparing OxyContin with immediate-release oxycodone and placebo revealed a similar adverse event profile between OxyContin and immediate-release oxycodone. The most common adverse events (>5%) reported by patients at least once during therapy were:

TABLE 3

	OxyContin (n=227) (%)	Immediate-Release (n=225) (%)	Placebo (n=45) (%)
Constipation	(23)	(26)	(7)
Nausea	(23)	(27)	(11)
Somnolence	(23)	(24)	(4)
Dizziness	(13)	(16)	(9)
Pruritus	(13)	(12)	(2)
Vomiting	(12)	(14)	(7)
Headache	(7)	(8)	(7)
Dry Mouth	(6)	(7)	(2)
Asthenia	(6)	(7)	–
Sweating	(5)	(6)	(2)

The following adverse experiences were reported in OxyContin®-treated patients with an incidence between 1% and 5%. In descending order of frequency they were anorexia, nervousness, insomnia, fever, confusion, diarrhea, abdominal pain, dyspepsia, rash, anxiety, euphoria, dyspnea, postural hypotension, chills, twitching, gastritis, abnormal dreams, thought abnormalities, and hiccups.

The following adverse reactions occurred in less than 1% of patients involved in clinical trials or were reported in postmarketing experience.

General: accidental injury, chest pain, facial edema, malaise, neck pain, pain, and symptoms associated with either an anaphylactic or anaphylactoid reaction

Cardiovascular: migraine, syncope, vasodilation, ST depression

Digestive: dysphagia, eructation, flatulence, gastrointestinal disorder, increased appetite, nausea and vomiting, stomatitis, ileus

Hemic and Lymphatic: lymphadenopathy

Metabolic and Nutritional: dehydration, edema, hyponatremia, peripheral edema, syndrome of inappropriate antidiuretic hormone secretion, thirst

Nervous: abnormal gait, agitation, amnesia, depersonalization, depression, emotional lability, hallucination, hyperkinesia, hypesthesia, hypotonia, malaise, paresthesia, seizures, speech disorder, stupor, tinnitus, tremor, vertigo, withdrawal syndrome with or without seizures

Respiratory: cough increased, pharyngitis, voice alteration

Skin: dry skin, exfoliative dermatitis, urticaria

Special Senses: abnormal vision, taste perversion

Urogenital: amenorrhea, decreased libido, dysuria, hematuria, impotence, polyuria, urinary retention, urination impaired

OVERDOSAGE

Acute overdosage with oxycodone can be manifested by respiratory depression, somnolence progressing to stupor or coma, skeletal muscle flaccidity, cold and clammy skin, constricted pupils, bradycardia, hypotension, and death.

Deaths due to overdose have been reported with abuse and misuse of OxyContin®, by ingesting, inhaling, or injecting the crushed tablets. Review of case reports has indicated that the risk of fatal overdose is further increased when OxyContin is abused concurrently with alcohol or other CNS depressants, including other opioids.

In the treatment of oxycodone overdosage, primary attention should be given to the re-establishment of a patent airway and institution of assisted or controlled ventilation. Supportive measures (including oxygen and vasopressors) should be employed in the management of circulatory shock and pulmonary edema accompanying overdose as indicated. Cardiac arrest or arrhythmias may require cardiac massage or defibrillation.

The pure opioid antagonists such as naloxone or nalmefene are specific antidotes against respiratory depression from opioid overdose. Opioid antagonists should not be administered in the absence of clinically significant respiratory or circulatory depression secondary to oxycodone overdose. In patients who are physically dependent on any opioid agonist including OxyContin, an abrupt or complete reversal of opioid effects may precipitate an acute abstinence syndrome. The severity of the withdrawal syndrome produced will depend on the degree of physical dependence and the dose of the antagonist administered. Please see the prescribing information for the specific opioid antagonist for details of their proper use.

DOSAGE AND ADMINISTRATION

General Principles

OXYCONTIN IS AN OPIOID AGONIST AND A SCHEDULE II CONTROLLED SUBSTANCE WITH AN ABUSE LIABILITY SIMILAR TO MORPHINE. OXYCODONE, LIKE MORPHINE AND OTHER OPIOIDS USED IN ANALGESIA, CAN BE ABUSED AND IS SUBJECT TO CRIMINAL DIVERSION.

OXYCONTIN TABLETS ARE TO BE SWALLOWED WHOLE AND ARE NOT TO BE BROKEN, CHEWED, OR CRUSHED. TAKING BROKEN, CHEWED, OR CRUSHED OXYCONTIN® TABLETS LEADS TO RAPID RELEASE AND ABSORPTION OF A POTENTIALLY FATAL DOSE OF OXYCODONE.

One OxyContin 160 mg tablet is comparable to two 80 mg tablets when taken on an empty stomach. With a high-fat meal, however, there is a 25% greater peak plasma concentration following one 160 mg tablet. Dietary caution should be taken when patients are initially titrated to 160 mg tablets (see DOSAGE AND ADMINISTRATION).

In treating pain it is vital to assess the patient regularly and systematically. Therapy should also be regularly reviewed and adjusted based upon the patient's own reports of pain and side effects and the health professional's clinical judgment.

OxyContin Tablets are a controlled-release oral formulation of oxycodone hydrochloride indicated for the management of moderate to severe pain when a continuous, around-the-clock analgesic is needed for an extended period of time. The controlled-release nature of the formulation allows OxyContin to be effectively administered every 12 hours (see **CLINICAL PHARMACOLOGY; PHARMACOKINETICS AND METABOLISM**). While symmetric (same dose AM and PM), around-the-clock, q12h dosing is appropriate for the majority of patients, some patients may benefit from asymmetric (different dose given in AM than in PM) dosing, tailored to their pain pattern. It is usually appropriate to treat a patient with only one opioid for around-the-clock therapy.

Physicians should individualize treatment using a progressive plan of pain management such as outlined by the World Health Organization, the American Pain Society and the Federation of State Medical Boards Model Guidelines. Healthcare professionals should follow appropriate pain management principles of careful assessment and ongoing monitoring (see **BOXED WARNING**).

Initiation of Therapy

It is critical to initiate the dosing regimen for each patient individually, taking into account the patient's prior opioid and non-opioid analgesic treatment. Attention should be given to:

(1) the general condition and medical status of the patient;
(2) the daily dose, potency, and kind of the analgesic(s) the patient has been taking;
(3) the reliability of the conversion estimate used to calculate the dose of oxycodone;
(4) the patient's opioid exposure and opioid tolerance (if any);
(5) special safety issues associated with conversion to OxyContin® doses at or exceeding 160 mg q12h (see **Special instructions for OxyContin 80 mg and 160 mg Tablets**); and
(6) the balance between pain control and adverse experiences.

Care should be taken to use low initial doses of OxyContin in patients who are not already opioid-tolerant, especially those who are receiving concurrent treatment with muscle relaxants, sedatives, or other CNS active medications (see **PRECAUTIONS: Drug-Drug Interactions**).

For initiation of OxyContin therapy for patients previously taking opioids, the conversion ratios from Foley, KM. [NEJM, 1985; 313:84-95], found below, are a reasonable starting point, although not verified in well-controlled, multiple-dose trials.

Experience indicates a reasonable starting dose of OxyContin for patients who are taking non-opioid analgesics and require continuous around-the-clock therapy for an extended period of time is 10 mg q12h. If a non-opioid analgesic is being provided, it may be continued. OxyContin should be individually titrated to a dose that provides adequate analgesia and minimizes side effects.

1. Using standard conversion ratio estimates (see Table 4 below), multiply the mg/day of the previous opioids by the appropriate multiplication factors to obtain the equivalent total daily dose of oral oxycodone.
2. When converting from oxycodone, divide the 24-hour oxycodone dose in half to obtain the twice a day (q12h) dose of OxyContin.
3. Round down to a dose which is appropriate for the tablet strengths available (10 mg, 20 mg, 40 mg, 80 mg, and 160 mg tablets).
4. Discontinue all other around-the-clock opioid drugs when OxyContin therapy is initiated.
5. No fixed conversion ratio is likely to be satisfactory in all patients, especially patients receiving large opioid doses. The recommended doses shown in Table 4 are only a starting point, and close observation and frequent titration are indicated until patients are stable on the new therapy.

TABLE 4
Multiplication Factors for Converting the Daily Dose of Prior Opioids to the Daily Dose of Oral Oxycodone*
(Mg/Day Prior Opioid × Factor = Mg/Day Oral Oxycodone)

	Oral Prior Opioid	Parenteral Prior Opioid
Oxycodone	1	—
Codeine	0.15	—
Hydrocodone	0.9	—
Hydromorphone	4	20
Levorphanol	7.5	15
Meperidine	0.1	0.4
Methadone	1.5	3
Morphine	0.5	3

***To be used only for conversion to oral oxycodone.** For patients receiving high-dose parenteral opioids, a more conservative conversion is warranted. For example, for high-dose parenteral morphine, use 1.5 instead of 3 as a multiplication factor.

In all cases, supplemental analgesia should be made available in the form of a suitable short-acting analgesic.

OxyContin® can be safely used concomitantly with usual doses of non-opioid analgesics and analgesic adjuvants, provided care is taken to select a proper initial dose (see **PRECAUTIONS**).

Conversion from Transdermal Fentanyl to OxyContin

Eighteen hours following the removal of the transdermal fentanyl patch, OxyContin treatment can be initiated. Although there has been no systematic assessment of such conversion, a conservative oxycodone dose, approximately 10 mg q12h of OxyContin, should be initially substituted for each 25 µg/hr fentanyl transdermal patch. The patient should be followed closely for early titration, as there is very limited clinical experience with this conversion.

Managing Expected Opioid Adverse Experiences

Most patients receiving opioids, especially those who are opioid-naive, will experience side effects. Frequently the side effects from OxyContin are transient, but may require evaluation and management. Adverse events such as constipation should be anticipated and treated aggressively and prophylactically with a stimulant laxative and/or stool softener. Patients do not usually become tolerant to the constipating effects of opioids.

Other opioid-related side effects such as sedation and nausea are usually self-limited and often do not persist beyond the first few days. If nausea persists and is unacceptable to the patient, treatment with antiemetics or other modalities may relieve these symptoms and should be considered.

Patients receiving OxyContin® may pass an intact matrix "ghost" in the stool or via colostomy. These ghosts contain little or no residual oxycodone and are of no clinical consequence.

Individualization of Dosage

Once therapy is initiated, pain relief and other opioid effects should be frequently assessed. Patients should be titrated to adequate effect (generally mild or no pain with the regular use of no more than two doses of supplemental analgesia per 24 hours). Patients who experience breakthrough pain may require dosage adjustment or rescue medication. Because steady-state plasma concentrations are approximated within 24 to 36 hours, dosage adjustment may be carried out every 1 to 2 days. It is most appropriate to increase the q12h dose, not the dosing frequency. There is no clinical information on dosing intervals shorter than q12h. As a guideline, except for the increase from 10 mg to 20 mg q12h, the total daily oxycodone dose usually can be increased by 25% to 50% of the current dose at each increase.

If signs of excessive opioid-related adverse experiences are observed, the next dose may be reduced. If this adjustment leads to inadequate analgesia, a supplemental dose of immediate-release oxycodone may be given. Alternatively, non-opioid analgesic adjuvants may be employed. Dose adjustments should be made to obtain an appropriate balance between pain relief and opioid-related adverse experiences.

If significant adverse events occur before the therapeutic goal of mild or no pain is achieved, the events should be treated aggressively. Once adverse events are under control, upward titration should continue to an acceptable level of pain control.

During periods of changing analgesic requirements, including initial titration, frequent contact is recommended between physician, other members of the healthcare team, the patient and the caregiver/family.

Special Instructions for OxyContin 80 mg and 160 mg Tablets (For use in opioid-tolerant patients only.)

OxyContin 80 mg and 160 mg Tablets are for use only in opioid-tolerant patients requiring daily oxycodone equivalent dosages of 160 mg or more for the 80 mg tablet and 320 mg or more for the 160 mg tablet. Care should be taken in the prescribing of these tablet strengths. Patients should be instructed against use by individuals other than the patient for whom it was prescribed, as such inappropriate use may have severe medical consequences, including death.

One OxyContin® 160 mg tablet is comparable to two 80 mg tablets when taken on an empty stomach. With a high-fat meal, however, there is a 25% greater peak plasma concen-

Continued on next page

OxyContin—Cont.

tration following one 160 mg tablet. Dietary caution should be taken when patients are initially titrated to 160 mg tablets.

Supplemental Analgesia

Most patients given around-the-clock therapy with controlled-release opioids may need to have immediate-release medication available for exacerbations of pain or to prevent pain that occurs predictably during certain patient activities (incident pain).

Maintenance of Therapy

The intent of the titration period is to establish a patient-specific q12h dose that will maintain adequate analgesia with acceptable side effects for as long as pain relief is necessary. Should pain recur then the dose can be incrementally increased to re-establish pain control. The method of therapy adjustment outlined above should be employed to re-establish pain control.

During chronic therapy, especially for non-cancer pain syndromes, the continued need for around-the-clock opioid therapy should be reassessed periodically (e.g., every 6 to 12 months) as appropriate.

Cessation of Therapy

When the patient no longer requires therapy with OxyContin Tablets, doses should be tapered gradually to prevent signs and symptoms of withdrawal in the physically dependent patient.

Conversion from OxyContin to Parenteral Opioids

To avoid overdose, conservative dose conversion ratios should be followed.

SAFETY AND HANDLING

OxyContin Tablets are solid dosage forms that contain oxycodone which is a controlled substance. Like morphine, oxycodone is controlled under Schedule II of the Controlled Substances Act.

OxyContin has been targeted for theft and diversion by criminals. Healthcare professionals should contact their State Professional Licensing Board or State Controlled Substances Authority for information on how to prevent and detect abuse or diversion of this product.

HOW SUPPLIED

OxyContin® (oxycodone hydrochloride controlled-release) Tablets 10 mg are round, unscored, white-colored, convex tablets imprinted with OC on one side and 10 on the other. They are supplied as follows:

NDC 59011-100-10: child-resistant closure, opaque plastic bottles of 100

NDC 59011-100-25: unit dose packaging with 25 individually numbered tablets per card; one card per glue end carton

OxyContin® (oxycodone hydrochloride controlled-release) Tablets 20 mg are round, unscored, pink-colored, convex tablets imprinted with OC on one side and 20 on the other. They are supplied as follows:

NDC 59011-103-10: child-resistant closure, opaque plastic bottles of 100

NDC 59011-103-25: unit dose packaging with 25 individually numbered tablets per card; one card per glue end carton

OxyContin® (oxycodone hydrochloride controlled-release) Tablets 40 mg are round, unscored, yellow-colored, convex tablets imprinted with OC on one side and 40 on the other. They are supplied as follows:

NDC 59011-105-10: child-resistant closure, opaque plastic bottles of 100

NDC 59011-105-25: unit dose packaging with 25 individually numbered tablets per card; one card per glue end carton

OxyContin® (oxycodone hydrochloride controlled-release) Tablets 80 mg are round, unscored, green-colored, convex tablets imprinted with OC on one side and 80 on the other. They are supplied as follows:

NDC 59011-107-10: child-resistant closure, opaque plastic bottles of 100

NDC 59011-107-25: unit dose packaging with 25 individually numbered tablets per card; one card per glue end carton

OxyContin® (oxycodone hydrochloride controlled-release) Tablets 160 mg are caplet-shaped, unscored, blue-colored, convex tablets imprinted with OC on one side and 160 on the other. They are supplied as follows:

NDC 59011-109-10: child-resistant closure, opaque plastic bottles of 100

NDC 59011-109-25: unit dose packaging with 25 individually numbered tablets per card; one card per glue end carton

Store at 25°C (77°F); excursions permitted between 15°-30°C (59°-86°F).

Dispense in tight, light-resistant container.

Healthcare professionals can telephone Purdue Pharma's Medical Services Department (1-888-726-7535) for information on this product.

CAUTION

DEA Order Form Required.

Purdue Pharma L.P., Stamford, CT 06901-3431

U.S. Patent Numbers 4,861,598; 4,970,075; 5,266,331; 5,508,042; 5,549,912; and 5,656,295

July 30, 2003

OT00367D 300514-0C-001

PATIENT INFORMATION

OXYCONTIN® CII

(OXYCODONE HCl CONTROLLED-RELEASE) TABLETS

OxyContin® Tablets, 10 mg
OxyContin® Tablets, 20 mg
OxyContin® Tablets, 40 mg
OxyContin® Tablets, 80 mg
OxyContin® Tablets, 160 mg

Read this information carefully before you take OxyContin® (ox-e-CON-tin) tablets. Also read the information you get with your refills. There may be something new. This information does not take the place of talking with your doctor about your medical condition or your treatment. Only you and your doctor can decide if OxyContin is right for you. Share the important information in this leaflet with members of your household.

What Is The Most Important Information I Should Know About OxyContin®?

- **Use OxyContin the way your doctor tells you to.**
- **Use OxyContin only for the condition for which it was prescribed.**
- **OxyContin is not for occasional ("as needed") use.**
- **Swallow the tablets whole.** Do not break, crush, dissolve, or chew them before swallowing. OxyContin® works properly over 12 hours only when swallowed whole. **If a tablet is broken, crushed, dissolved, or chewed, the entire 12 hour dose will be absorbed into your body all at once. This can be dangerous, causing an overdose, and possibly death.**
- **Keep OxyContin® out of the reach of children.** Accidental overdose by a child is dangerous and may result in death.
- **Prevent theft and misuse.** OxyContin contains a narcotic painkiller that can be a target for people who abuse prescription medicines. Therefore, keep your tablets in a secure place, to protect them from theft. Never give them to anyone else. Selling or giving away this medicine is dangerous and against the law.

What is OxyContin®?

OxyContin® is a tablet that comes in several strengths and contains the medicine oxycodone (ox-e-KOE-done). This medicine is a painkiller like morphine. OxyContin treats moderate to severe pain that is expected to last for an extended period of time. Use OxyContin regularly during treatment. It contains enough medicine to last for up to twelve hours.

Who Should Not Take OxyContin®?

Do not take OxyContin® if

- your doctor did not prescribe OxyContin® for you.
- your pain is mild or will go away in a few days.
- your pain can be controlled by occasional use of other painkillers.
- you have severe asthma or severe lung problems.
- you have had a severe allergic reaction to codeine, hydrocodone, dihydrocodeine, or oxycodone (such as Tylox, Tylenol with Codeine, or Vicodin). A severe allergic reaction includes a severe rash, hives, breathing problems, or dizziness.
- you had surgery less than 12–24 hours ago and you were not taking OxyContin just before surgery.

Your doctor should know about all your medical conditions before deciding if OxyContin is right for you and what dose is best. Tell your doctor about all of your medical problems, especially the ones listed below:

- trouble breathing or lung problems
- head injury
- liver or kidney problems
- adrenal gland problems, such as Addison's disease
- convulsions or seizures
- alcoholism
- hallucinations or other severe mental problems
- past or present substance abuse or drug addiction

If any of these conditions apply to you, and you haven't told your doctor, then you should tell your doctor before taking OxyContin.

If you are pregnant or plan to become pregnant, talk with your doctor. OxyContin may not be right for you. **Tell your doctor if you are breast feeding.** OxyContin will pass through the milk and may harm the baby.

Tell your doctor about all the medicines you take, including prescription and non-prescription medicines, vitamins, and herbal supplements. They may cause serious medical problems when taken with OxyContin, especially if they cause drowsiness.

How Should I Take OxyContin®?

- **Follow your doctor's directions exactly.** Your doctor may change your dose based on your reactions to the medicine. Do not change your dose unless your doctor tells you to change it. Do not take OxyContin more often than prescribed.
- **Swallow the tablets whole. Do not break, crush, dissolve, or chew before swallowing. If the tablets are not whole, your body will absorb too much medicine at one time. This can lead to serious problems, including overdose and death.**
- **If you miss a dose,** take it as soon as possible. If it is almost time for your next dose, skip the missed dose and go back to your regular dosing schedule. Do not take 2 doses at once unless your doctor tells you to.
- **In case of overdose,** call your local emergency number or Poison Control Center right away.
- **Review your pain regularly with your doctor** to determine if you still need OxyContin.
- **You may see tablets in your stools (bowel movements).** Do not be concerned. Your body has already absorbed the medicine.

If you continue to have pain or bothersome side effects, call your doctor.

Stopping OxyContin. Consult your doctor for instructions on how to stop this medicine slowly to avoid uncomfortable symptoms. You should not stop taking OxyContin all at once if you have been taking it for more than a few days.

After you stop taking OxyContin, flush the unused tablets down the toilet.

What Should I Avoid While Taking OxyContin®?

- **Do not drive, operate heavy machinery, or participate in any other possibly dangerous activities** until you know how you react to this medicine. OxyContin can make you sleepy.
- **Do not drink alcohol while using OxyContin. It may increase the chance of getting dangerous side effects.**
- **Do not take other medicines without your doctor's approval.** Other medicines include prescription and non-prescription medicines, vitamins, and supplements. Be especially careful about products that make you sleepy.

What are the Possible Side Effects of OxyContin®?

Call your doctor or get medical help right away if

- your breathing slows down
- you feel faint, dizzy, confused, or have any other unusual symptoms

Some of the common side effects of OxyContin® are nausea, vomiting, dizziness, drowsiness, constipation, itching, dry mouth, sweating, weakness, and headache. Some of these side effects may decrease with continued use.

There is a risk of abuse or addiction with narcotic painkillers. If you have abused drugs in the past, you may have a higher chance of developing abuse or addiction again while using OxyContin. We do not know how often patients with continuing (chronic) pain become addicted to narcotics, but the risk has been reported to be small.

These are not all the possible side effects of OxyContin. For a complete list, ask your doctor or pharmacist.

General Advice About OxyContin

- Do not use OxyContin for conditions for which it was not prescribed.
- Do not give OxyContin to other people, even if they have the same symptoms you have. Sharing is illegal and may cause severe medical problems, including death.

This leaflet summarizes the most important information about OxyContin. If you would like more information, talk with your doctor. Also, you can ask your pharmacist or doctor for information about OxyContin that is written for health professionals.

℞ Only

Purdue Pharma L.P., Stamford, CT 06901-3431

July 30, 2003

OT00367D 300514-0C-001

Shown in Product Identification Guide, page 330

OXYIR® CII ℞

[*ŏx'-ē-i'-r'*]

(oxycodone hydrochloride)

Immediate-Release Oral Capsules

5 mg

OXYFAST® CII ℞

[*ŏx-ē-făst'*]

(oxycodone hydrochloride)

Oral CONCENTRATE Solution*

20 mg/1mL

***This product contains dry natural rubber**

OT00623A 061430-0C-001

DESCRIPTION

Oxycodone is 14-hydroxydihydrocodeinone, a white odorless crystalline powder which is derived from the opium alkaloid, thebaine, and may be represented by the following structural formula:

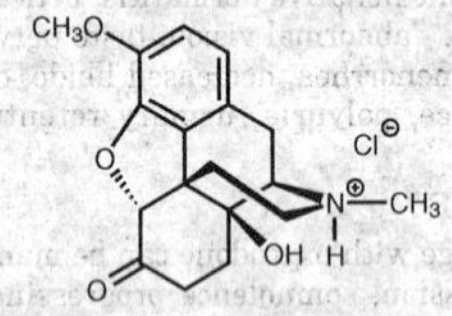

OxyIR® Oral Capsules

Each 5 mg of OxyIR Capsules contains:

Oxycodone hydrochloride .... 5 mg

Inactive ingredients: FD&C blue No. 2, FD&C yellow No. 6, gelatin, hypromellose, maize starch, polyethylene glycol, polysorbate 80, red iron oxide, silicon dioxide, sodium laurel sulfate, sucrose, titanium dioxide, and yellow iron oxide.

OxyFast® Oral CONCENTRATE Solution

Each 1 mL of OxyFast **Concentrate** Solution contains:

Oxycodone hydrochloride .... 20 mg

Inactive ingredients: Citric acid, D&C yellow #10, sodium benzoate, sodium citrate, sodium saccharine and water.

ACTIONS

The analgesic ingredient, oxycodone, is a semisynthetic narcotic with multiple actions qualitatively similar to those of morphine; the most prominent of these involve the central nervous system and organs composed of smooth muscle. The principal actions of therapeutic value of oxycodone are analgesia and sedation.

CLINICAL PHARMACOLOGY

Central Nervous System

Oxycodone is a pure agonist opioid whose principal therapeutic action is analgesia. Other therapeutic effects of oxycodone include anxiolysis, euphoria, and feelings of relaxation. Like all pure opioid agonists, there is no ceiling effect to analgesia, such as is seen with partial agonists or non-opioid analgesics.

The precise mechanism of the analgesic action is unknown. However, specific CNS opioid receptors for endogenous compounds with opioid-like activity have been identified throughout the brain and spinal cord and play a role in the analgesic effects of this drug.

Oxycodone produces respiratory depression by direct action on brain stem respiratory centers. The respiratory depression involves both a reduction in the responsiveness of the brain stem respiratory centers to increases in carbon dioxide tension and to electrical stimulation.

Oxycodone depresses the cough reflex by direct effect on the cough center in the medulla. Antitussive effects may occur with doses lower than those usually required for analgesia. Oxycodone causes miosis, even in total darkness. Pinpoint pupils are a sign of opioid overdose but are not pathognomonic. Marked mydriasis rather than miosis may be seen due to hypoxia in overdose situations.

Gastrointestinal Tract and Other Smooth Muscle

Oxycodone causes a reduction in motility associated with an increase in smooth muscle tone in the antrum of the stomach and duodenum. Digestion of food in the small intestine is delayed and propulsive contractions are decreased. Propulsive peristaltic waves in the colon are decreased, while tone may be increased to the point of spasm resulting in constipation. Other opioid-induced effects may include a reduction in gastric, biliary, and pancreatic secretions, spasm of sphincter of Oddi, and transient elevations in serum amylase.

Cardiovascular System

Oxycodone may produce release of histamine with or without associated peripheral vasodilation. Manifestations of histamine release and/or peripheral vasodilation may include pruritus, flushing, red eyes, sweating, and/or orthostatic hypotension.

Concentration—Effect Relationships (PHARMACODYNAMICS)

Studies in normal volunteers and patients reveal predictable relationships between oxycodone dosage and plasma oxycodone concentrations, as well as between concentration and certain expected opioid effects. In normal volunteers these include pupillary constriction, sedation and overall "drug effect" and in patients, analgesia and feelings of "relaxation." In non-tolerant patients, analgesia is not usually seen at a plasma oxycodone concentration of less than 5–10 ng/mL.

As with all opioids, the minimum effective plasma concentration for analgesia will vary widely among patients, especially among patients who have been previously treated with potent agonist opioids. As a result, patients need to be treated with individualized titration of dosage to the desired effect. The minimum effective analgesic concentration of oxycodone for any individual patient may increase with repeated dosing due to an increase in pain and/or the development of tolerance.

Concentration—Adverse Experience Relationships

OxyIR Capsules and OxyFast **CONCENTRATE** Solution are associated with typical opioid-related adverse experiences similar to those seen with all opioids. There is a general relationship between increasing oxycodone plasma concentration and increasing frequency of dose-related opioid adverse experiences such as nausea, vomiting, CNS effects, and respiratory depression. In opioid-tolerant patients, the situation is altered by the development of tolerance to opioid-related side effects, and the relationship is poorly understood.

As with all opioids, the dose must be individualized (see **DOSAGE AND ADMINISTRATION**), because the effective analgesic dose for some patients will be too high to be tolerated by other patients.

INDICATIONS AND USAGE

For the relief of moderate to moderately severe pain.

CONTRAINDICATIONS

OxyIR and OxyFast are contraindicated in patients with known hypersensitivity to oxycodone, or in any situation where opioids are contraindicated. This includes patients with significant respiratory depression (in unmonitored settings or the absence of resuscitative equipment), and patients with acute or severe bronchial asthma or hypercarbia. OxyIR and OxyFast are contraindicated in any patient who has or is suspected of having paralytic ileus.

WARNINGS

Respiratory Depression

Respiratory depression is the chief hazard from all opioid agonist preparations. Respiratory depression occurs most frequently in elderly or debilitated patients, usually following large initial doses in non-tolerant patients, or when opioids are given in conjunction with other agents that depress respiration.

Oxycodone should be used with extreme caution in patients with significant chronic obstructive pulmonary disease or cor pulmonale, and in patients having a substantially decreased respiratory reserve, hypoxia, hypercapnia, or preexisting respiratory depression. In such patients, even usual therapeutic doses of oxycodone may decrease respiratory drive to the point of apnea. In these patients alternative non-opioid analgesics should be considered, and opioids should be employed only under careful medical supervision at the lowest effective dose.

Hypotensive Effect

OxyIR® Capsules and OxyFast® **CONCENTRATE** Solution, like all opioid analgesics, may cause severe hypotension in an individual whose ability to maintain blood pressure has been compromised by a depleted blood volume, or after concurrent administration with drugs such as phenothiazines or other agents which compromise vasomotor tone. OxyIR and OxyFast may produce orthostatic hypotension in ambulatory patients. OxyIR and OxyFast, like all opioid analgesics, should be administered with caution to patients in circulatory shock, since vasodilation produced by the drug may further reduce cardiac output and blood pressure.

Drug Dependence: Oxycodone can produce drug dependence of the morphine type, and therefore, has the potential for being abused. Psychic dependence, physical dependence and tolerance may develop upon repeated administration of this drug, and it should be prescribed and administered with the same degree of caution appropriate to the use of other oral narcotic-containing medications. Like other narcotic-containing medications, this drug is subject to the Federal Controlled Substances Act.

Usage in Ambulatory Patients

Oxycodone may impair the mental and/or physical abilities required for the performance of potential hazardous tasks such as driving a car or operating machinery. The patient using this drug should be cautioned accordingly.

Interaction with Other Central Nervous System Depressants

Patients receiving other narcotic analgesics, general anesthetics, phenothiazines, other tranquilizers, sedative-hypnotics or other CNS depressants (including alcohol) concomitantly with oxycodone hydrochloride may exhibit an additive CNS depression. When such combined therapy is contemplated, the dose of one or both agents should be reduced.

Usage in Pregnancy

Safe use in pregnancy has not been established relative to possible adverse effects on fetal development. Therefore, this drug should not be used in pregnant women unless, in the judgment of the physician, the potential benefits outweigh the possible hazards.

Usage in Children

This drug should not be administered to children.

PRECAUTIONS

Special Precautions Regarding OxyFast Oral CONCENTRATE 20 mg/1 mL Solution

OxyFast 20 mg/1 mL solution is a highly concentrated solution. Care should be taken in the prescription and dispensing of this solution strength. Patients should be instructed against use by individuals other than the patient, as inappropriate use may cause acute overdosage.

General

Opioid analgesics given on a fixed-dosage schedule have a narrow therapeutic index in certain patient populations, especially when combined with other drugs, and should be reserved for cases where the benefits of opioid analgesia outweigh the known risks of respiratory depression, altered mental state, and postural hypotension.

Use of OxyIR® and OxyFast® is associated with increased potential risks and should be used only with caution in the following conditions: acute alcoholism; adrenocortical insufficiency (e.g., Addison's disease); CNS depression or coma; delirium tremens; debilitated patients; kyphoscoliosis associated with respiratory depression; myxedema or hypothyroidism; prostatic hypertrophy or urethral stricture; severe impairment of hepatic, pulmonary or renal function; and toxic psychosis.

The administration of oxycodone, like all opioid analgesics, may obscure the diagnosis or clinical course in patients with acute abdominal conditions. Oxycodone may aggravate convulsions in patients with convulsive disorders, and all opioids may induce or aggravate seizures in some clinical settings.

Interactions with Mixed Agonist/Antagonist Opioid Analgesics

Agonist/antagonist and partial agonist analgesics (i.e., pentazocine, nalbuphine, butorphanol and buprenorphine) should be administered with caution to a patient who has received or is receiving a course of therapy with a pure opioid agonist analgesic such as oxycodone. In this situation, mixed agonist/antagonist and partial agonist analgesics may reduce the analgesic effect of oxycodone and/or may precipitate withdrawal symptoms in these patients.

Use in Pancreatic/Biliary Tract Disease

Oxycodone may cause spasm of the sphincter of Oddi and should be used with caution in patients with biliary tract disease, including acute pancreatitis. Opioids like oxycodone may cause increases in the serum amylase level.

Head Injury and Increased Intracranial Pressure

The respiratory depressant effects of opioids and their capacity to elevate cerebrospinal fluid pressure may be markedly exaggerated in the presence of head injury, other intracranial lesions, or a pre-existing increase in intracranial pressure. Furthermore, opioids produce adverse reactions which may obscure the clinical course of patients with head injuries.

Acute Abdominal Conditions

The administration of this drug or other opioids may obscure the diagnosis or clinical course in patients with acute abdominal conditions.

Information for Patients/Caregivers

If clinically advisable, patients receiving OxyIR (immediate-release) Capsules or OxyFast **CONCENTRATE** Solution or their caregivers should be given the following information by the physician, nurse, pharmacist or caregiver:

1. Patients should be advised not to adjust the dose of this drug without consulting the prescribing professional.
2. Patients should be advised that this drug may impair mental and/or physical ability required for the performance of potentially hazardous tasks (e.g., driving, operating heavy machinery).
3. Patients should not combine this drug with alcohol or other central nervous system depressants (sleep aids, tranquilizers) except by the orders of the prescribing physician, because additive effects may occur.
4. Women of childbearing potential who become, or are planning to become, pregnant should be advised to consult their physician regarding the effects of analgesics and other drug use during pregnancy on themselves and their unborn child.
5. Patients should be advised that this drug is a potential drug of abuse. They should protect it from theft, and it should never be given to anyone other than the individual for whom it was prescribed.
6. Patients should be advised that if they have been receiving treatment with this drug for more than a few weeks and cessation of therapy is indicated, it may be appropriate to taper this drug dose, rather than abruptly discontinue it, due to the risk of precipitating withdrawal symptoms. Their physician can provide a dose schedule to accomplish a gradual discontinuation of the medication.

Laboratory Monitoring

Due to the broad range of plasma concentrations seen in clinical populations, the varying degrees of pain, and the development of tolerance, plasma oxycodone measurements are usually not helpful in clinical management. Plasma concentrations of the active drug substance may be of value in selected, unusual, or complex cases.

Use in Drug and Alcohol Addiction

OxyIR and OxyFast are opioids with no approved use in the management of addictive disorders. Its proper usage in individuals with drug or alcohol dependence, either active or in remission, is for the management of pain requiring opioid analgesia.

Drug-Drug Interactions

The CNS depressant effects of oxycodone hydrochloride may be additive with that of other CNS depressants. See **WARNINGS.**

Opioid analgesics, including OxyIR and OxyFast may enhance the neuromuscular blocking action of skeletal muscle relaxants and produce an increased degree of respiratory depression.

Oxycodone is metabolized in part to oxymorphone via CYP2D6. While this pathway may be blocked by a variety of drugs (e.g., certain cardiovascular drugs and antidepressants), such blockade has not yet been shown to be of clinical significance with this agent. Clinicians should be aware of this possible interaction, however.

Mutagenicity/Carcinogenicity

Oxycodone was not mutagenic in the following assays: Ames Salmonella and E. Coli test with and without metabolic activation at doses of up to 5000 µg, chromosomal aberration test in human lymphocytes in the absence of metabolic activation at doses of up to 1500 µg/mL and with activation 48 hours after exposure at doses of up to 5000 µg/mL, and in the in vivo bone marrow micronucleus test in mice (at plasma levels of up to 48 µg/mL). Mutagenic results occurred in the presence of metabolic activation in the human chromosomal aberration test (at greater than or equal to 1250 µg/mL) at 24 but not 48 hours of exposure and in the mouse lymphoma assay at doses of 50 µg/mL or greater with metabolic activation and at 400 µg/mL or greater without metabolic activation. The data from these tests indicate that the genotoxic risk to humans may be considered low.

Studies of oxycodone in animals to evaluate its carcinogenic potential have not been conducted owing to the length of clinical experience with the drug substance.

Pregnancy

Teratogenic Effects—Category B: Reproduction studies have been performed in rats and rabbits by oral administration at doses up to 8 mg/kg (48 mg/m^2) and 125 mg/kg (1375 mg/m^2), respectively. These doses are 3 and 47 times a human dose of 160 mg/day (90 mg/m^2), based on mg/kg of a 60 kg adult (0.5 and 15 times this human dose based upon mg/m^2). The results did not reveal evidence of harm to the fetus due to oxycodone. There are, however, no adequate and well-controlled studies in pregnant women. Because animal reproduction studies are not always predictive of human response, this drug should be used during pregnancy only if clearly needed.

Nonteratogenic Effects—Neonates whose mothers have been taking oxycodone chronically may exhibit respiratory depression and/or withdrawal symptoms, either at birth and/or in the nursery.

Labor and Delivery

OxyIR® and OxyFast® are not recommended for use in women during and immediately prior to labor and delivery because oral opioids may cause respiratory depression in the newborn.

Nursing Mothers

Low concentrations of oxycodone have been detected in breast milk. Withdrawal symptoms can occur in breast-feeding infants when maternal administration of an opioid

Continued on next page

OxyIR/OxyFast—Cont.

analgesic is stopped. Ordinarily, nursing should not be undertaken while a patient is receiving OxyIR or OxyFast since oxycodone may be excreted in the milk.

Pediatric Use

Safety and effectiveness in pediatric patients have not been established.

Special Risk Patients

This drug should be given with caution to certain patients such as the elderly or debilitated, and those with severe impairment of hepatic or renal function, hypothyroidism, Addison's disease and prostatic hypertrophy, or urethral stricture.

ADVERSE REACTIONS

The most frequently observed reactions include light-headedness, dizziness, sedation, nausea, and vomiting. These effects seem to be more prominent in ambulatory than in nonambulatory patients, and some of these adverse reactions may be alleviated if the patient lies down. Many of these adverse events will cease or decrease in intensity as oxycodone therapy is continued and some degree of tolerance is developed.

Other adverse reactions include euphoria, dysphoria, constipation, skin rash and pruritus.

DRUG ABUSE AND DEPENDENCE (Addiction)

Oxycodone products are common targets for both drug abusers and drug addicts.

Drug addiction (drug dependence, psychological dependence) is characterized by a preoccupation with the procurement, hoarding, and abuse of drugs for non-medicinal purposes. Drug dependence is treatable, utilizing a multidisciplinary approach, but relapse is common. Iatrogenic "addiction" to opioids legitimately used in the management of pain is very rare. "Drug seeking" behavior is very common to addicts. Tolerance and physical dependence in pain patients are not signs of psychological dependence. Preoccupation with achieving adequate pain relief can be appropriate behavior in a patient with poor pain control. Most chronic pain patients limit their intake of opioids to achieve a balance between the benefits of the drug and dose-limiting side effects. Physicians should be aware that psychological dependence may not be accompanied by concurrent tolerance and symptoms of physical dependence in all addicts. In addition, abuse of opioids can occur in the absence of true psychological dependence and is characterized by misuse for non-medical purposes, often in combination with other psychoactive substances.

MANAGEMENT OF OVERDOSAGE

Signs and Symptoms

Serious overdose of oxycodone hydrochloride is characterized by respiratory depression (a decrease in respiratory rate and/or tidal volume, Cheyne-Stokes respiration, cyanosis), extreme somnolence progressing to stupor or coma, skeletal muscle flaccidity, cold and clammy skin, and sometimes bradycardia and hypotension. In severe overdosage, apnea, circulatory collapse, cardiac arrest, and death may occur.

Treatment

Primary attention should be given to the re-establishment of adequate respiratory exchange through provision of a patent airway and the institution of assisted or controlled ventilation. The narcotic antagonist naloxone is a specific antidote against respiratory depression which may result from overdosage or unusual sensitivity to narcotics, including oxycodone. Therefore, an appropriate dose of naloxone (usual initial adult dose: 0.4 mg) should be administered, preferably by the intravenous route, simultaneously with efforts at respiratory resuscitation. Since the duration of action of oxycodone may exceed that of the antagonist, the patient should be kept under continued surveillance and repeated doses of the antagonist should be administered as needed to maintain adequate respiration. An antagonist should not be administered in the absence of clinically significant respiratory or cardiovascular depression.

Oxygen, intravenous fluids, vasopressors, and other supportive measures should be employed as indicated.

Gastric emptying may be useful in removing unabsorbed drug.

DOSAGE AND ADMINISTRATION

Special Precautions Regarding OxyFast Oral CONCENTRATE 20 mg/1 mL Solution

OxyFast 20 mg/1 mL solution is a highly concentrated solution. Care should be taken in the prescription and dispensing of this solution strength. Patients should be instructed against use by individuals other than the patient, as inappropriate use may cause acute overdosage.

Dosage should be adjusted to the severity of the pain and the response of the patient. It may occasionally be necessary to exceed the usual dosage recommended below in cases of more severe pain or in those patients who have become tolerant to the analgesic effects of opioids. This drug is given orally. The usual adult dosage is 5 mg every 6 hours as needed for pain.

Nurse/Patient Instructions

Fill dropper to the level of the prescribed dose (1.0 mL=20 mg; 0.75 mL=15 mg; 0.5 mL=10 mg and 0.25 mL=5 mg). For ease of administration, add dose to approximately 30 mL (1 Fl Oz) or more of juice or other liquid. May also be added to applesauce, pudding or other semi-solid foods. The drug-food mixture should be used immediately and not stored for future use.

HOW SUPPLIED

OxyIR® (oxycodone hydrochloride) Immediate-Release Oral Capsules:

5 mg capsules, Cap: Beige Imprinted with O-IR; Body: Orange Imprinted with PF 5mg

NDC 59011-201-10: Opaque plastic bottle containing 100 capsules

OxyFast (oxycodone hydrochloride) Oral CONCENTRATE Solution

20 mg per 1 mL clear yellow liquid

NDC 59011-225-20: Plastic bottle with child-resistant dropper in 30 mL size.

Discard opened bottle of oral solution after 90 days.

Store OxyFast Oral **CONCENTRATE** solutions and OxyIR (oxycodone hydrochloride) capsules at 25°C (77°F); excursions permitted between 15°-30°C (59°-86°F).

CAUTION

DEA Order Form Required.

Printed in USA

Purdue Pharma L.P., Stamford, CT 06901-3431

August 4, 2003

OT00623A 061430-0C-001

Shown in Product Identification Guide, page 331

EDUCATIONAL MATERIAL

Website containing pain management information for healthcare professionals and patients. Available at www.partnersagainstpain.com

Please contact your local Purdue sales representative to order the following: Opioid Documentation Kit CD-ROM (PAP 047), Pain Management Kit CD-ROM (PAP 005), "How to Stop Drug Diversion and Protect Your Practice" brochure (PPXX01), and "How to Stop Drug Diversion and Protect Your Pharmacy" brochure (PPXX02).

Purdue Pharmaceutical Products L.P.

ONE STAMFORD FORUM
STAMFORD CT 06901-3431

For Medical Inquiries:
888-726-7535
Adverse Drug Experiences:
888-726-7535
Customer Service:
800-877-5666
FAX 800-877-3210

SPECTRACEF® ℞

[spĕk'trə-sĕf]
cefditoren pivoxil
200 mg Tablets
OT00617B 300780-0B-001

To reduce the development of drug-resistant bacteria and maintain the effectiveness of SPECTRACEF and other antibacterial drugs, SPECTRACEF should be used only to treat infections that are proven or strongly suspected to be caused by bacteria.

DESCRIPTION

SPECTRACEF tablets contain cefditoren pivoxil, a semisynthetic cephalosporin antibiotic for oral administration. It is a prodrug which is hydrolyzed by esterases during absorption, and the drug is distributed in the circulating blood as active cefditoren.

Chemically, cefditoren pivoxil is (-)-(6R,7R)-2,2-dimethylpropionyloxymethyl 7-[(Z)-2-(2-aminothiazol-4-yl)-2-methoxyiminoacetamido]-3-[(Z)-2-(4-methylthiazol-5-yl)ethenyl]-8-oxo-5-thia-1-azabicyclo[4.2.0]oct-2-ene-2-carboxylate. The empirical formula is $C_{25}H_{28}N_6O_7S_3$ and the molecular weight is 620.73. The structural formula of cefditoren pivoxil is shown below:

cefditoren pivoxil

The amorphous form of cefditoren pivoxil developed for clinical use is a light yellow powder. It is freely soluble in dilute hydrochloric acid and soluble at levels equal to 6.06 mg/mL in ethanol and <0.1 mg/mL in water.

SPECTRACEF® (cefditoren pivoxil) tablets contain 200 mg of cefditoren as cefditoren pivoxil and the following inactive ingredients: croscarmellose sodium, D-mannitol, hydroxypropyl cellulose, hypromellose, magnesium stearate, sodium caseinate (a milk protein), and sodium tripolyphosphate. The tablet coating contains carnauba wax, hypromellose, polyethylene glycol, and titanium dioxide. Tablets are printed with ink containing D&C Red No. 27, FD&C Blue No. 1, propylene glycol, and shellac.

CLINICAL PHARMACOLOGY

Pharmacokinetics

Absorption

Oral Bioavailability

Following oral administration, cefditoren pivoxil is absorbed from the gastrointestinal tract and hydrolyzed to cefditoren by esterases. Maximal plasma concentrations (C_{max}) of cefditoren under fasting conditions average 1.8 ± 0.6 µg/mL following a single 200 mg dose and occur 1.5 to 3 hours following dosing. Less than dose-proportional increases in C_{max} and area under the concentration-time curve (AUC) were observed at doses of 400 mg and above. Cefditoren does not accumulate in plasma following twice daily administration to subjects with normal renal function. Under fasting conditions, the estimated absolute bioavailability of cefditoren pivoxil is approximately 14%. The absolute bioavailability of cefditoren pivoxil administered with a low fat meal (693 cal, 14 g fat, 122 g carb, 23 g protein) is 16.1 ± 3.0%.

Food Effect

Administration of cefditoren pivoxil following a high fat meal (858 cal, 64 g fat, 43 g carb, 31 g protein) resulted in a 70% increase in mean AUC and a 50% increase in mean C_{max} compared to administration of cefditoren pivoxil in the fasted state. After a high fat meal, the C_{max} averaged 3.1 ± 1.0 µg/mL following a single 200 mg dose of cefditoren pivoxil and 4.4 ± 0.9 µg/mL following a 400 mg dose. Cefditoren AUC and C_{max} values from studies conducted with a moderate fat meal (648 cal, 27 g fat, 73 g carb, 29 g protein) are similar to those obtained following a high fat meal.

Distribution

The mean volume of distribution at steady state (V_{ss}) of cefditoren is 9.3 ± 1.6 L. Binding of cefditoren to plasma proteins averages 88% from *in vitro* determinations, and is concentration-independent at cefditoren concentrations ranging from 0.05 to 10 µg/mL. Cefditoren is primarily bound to human serum albumin and its binding is decreased when serum albumin concentrations are reduced. Binding to α-1-acid glycoprotein ranges from 3.3 to 8.1%. Penetration into red blood cells is negligible.

Skin blister fluid

Maximal concentrations of cefditoren in suction-induced blister fluid were observed 4 to 6 hours following administration of a 400 mg dose of cefditoren pivoxil with a mean of 1.1 ± 0.42 µg/mL. Mean blister fluid AUC values were 56 ± 15% of corresponding plasma concentrations.

Tonsil tissue

In fasted patients undergoing elective tonsillectomy, the mean concentration of cefditoren in tonsil tissue 2 to 4 hours following administration of a 200 mg dose of cefditoren pivoxil was 0.18 ± 0.07 µg/g. Mean tonsil tissue concentrations of cefditoren were 12 ± 3% of the corresponding serum concentrations.

Cerebrospinal Fluid (CSF)

Data on the penetration of cefditoren into human cerebrospinal fluid are not available.

Metabolism and Excretion

Cefditoren is eliminated from the plasma, with a mean terminal elimination half-life ($t_{1/2}$) of 1.6 ± 0.4 hours in young healthy adults. Cefditoren is not appreciably metabolized. After absorption, cefditoren is mainly eliminated by excretion into the urine, with a renal clearance of approximately 4-5 L/h. Studies with the renal tubular transport blocking agent probenecid indicate that tubular secretion, along with glomerular filtration is involved in the renal elimination of cefditoren. Cefditoren renal clearance is reduced in patients with renal insufficiency. (See Special Populations, *Renal Insufficiency* and *Hemodialysis*.)

Hydrolysis of cefditoren pivoxil to its active component, cefditoren, results in the formation of pivalate. Following multiple doses of cefditoren pivoxil, greater than 70% of the pivalate is absorbed. Pivalate is mainly eliminated (>99%) through renal excretion, nearly exclusively as pivaloylcarnitine. Following a 200 mg BID regimen for 10 days, the mean decrease in plasma concentrations of total carnitine was 18.1 ± 7.2 nmole/mL, representing a 39% decrease in plasma carnitine concentrations. Following a 400 mg BID regimen for 14 days, the mean decrease in plasma concentrations of carnitine was 33.3 ± 9.7 nmole/mL, representing a 63% decrease in plasma carnitine concentrations. Plasma concentrations of carnitine returned to the normal control range within 7 to 10 days after discontinuation of cefditoren pivoxil. (See **PRECAUTIONS**, **General** and **CONTRAINDICATIONS**.)

Special Populations

Geriatric

The effect of age on the pharmacokinetics of cefditoren was evaluated in 48 male and female subjects aged 25 to 75 years given 400 mg cefditoren pivoxil BID for 7 days. Physiological changes related to increasing age increased the extent of cefditoren exposure in plasma, as evidenced by a 26% higher C_{max} and a 33% higher AUC for subjects aged ≥ 65 years compared with younger subjects. The rate of elimination of cefditoren from plasma was lower in subjects aged ≥ 65 years, with $t_{1/2}$ values 16-26% longer than for younger subjects. Renal clearance of cefditoren in subjects aged ≥ 65 years was 20-24% lower than in younger subjects. These changes could be attributed to age-related changes in creatinine clearance. No dose adjustments are necessary for elderly patients with normal (for their age) renal function.

Gender

The effect of gender on the pharmacokinetics of cefditoren was evaluated in 24 male and 24 female subjects given 400 mg cefditoren pivoxil BID for 7 days. The extent of exposure in plasma was greater in females than in males, as evidenced by a 14% higher C_{max} and a 16% higher AUC for females compared to males. Renal clearance of cefditoren in females was 13% lower than in males. These differences could be attributed to gender-related differences in lean body mass. No dose adjustments are necessary for gender.

Renal Insufficiency

Cefditoren pharmacokinetics were investigated in 24 adult subjects with varying degrees of renal function following administration of cefditoren pivoxil 400 mg BID for 7 days. Decreased creatinine clearance (CL_{cr}) was associated with an increase in the fraction of unbound cefditoren in plasma and a decrease in the cefditoren elimination rate, resulting in greater systemic exposure in subjects with renal impairment. The unbound C_{max} and AUC were similar in subjects with mild renal impairment (CL_{cr}: 50-80 mL/min/1.73 m^2) compared to subjects with normal renal function (CL_{cr}: >80 mL/min/1.73 m^2). Moderate (CL_{cr}: 30-49 mL/min/1.73 m^2) or severe (CL_{cr}: <30 mL/min/1.73 m^2) renal impairment increased the extent of exposure in plasma, as evidenced by mean unbound C_{max} values 90% and 114% higher and AUC values 232% and 324% higher than that for subjects with normal renal function. The rate of elimination from plasma was lower in subjects with moderate or severe renal impairment, with respective mean $t_{1/2}$ values of 2.7 and 4.7 hours. No dose adjustment is necessary for patients with mild renal impairment (CL_{cr}: 50–80 mL/min/1.73 m^2). It is recommended that not more than 200 mg BID be administered to patients with moderate renal impairment (CL_{cr}: 30–49 mL/min/1.73 m^2) and 200 mg QD be administered to patients with severe renal impairment (CL_{cr}: <30 mL/min/1.73 m^2). (See **DOSAGE AND ADMINISTRATION.**)

Hemodialysis

Cefditoren pharmacokinetics investigated in six adult subjects with end-stage renal disease (ESRD) undergoing hemodialysis given a single 400 mg dose of cefditoren pivoxil were highly variable. The mean $t_{1/2}$ was 4.7 hours and ranged from 1.5 to 15 hours. Hemodialysis (4 hours duration) removed approximately 30% of cefditoren from systemic circulation but did not change the apparent terminal elimination half-life. The appropriate dose for ESRD patients has not been determined. (See **DOSAGE AND ADMINISTRATION.**)

Hepatic Disease

Cefditoren pharmacokinetics were evaluated in six adult subjects with mild hepatic impairment (Child-Pugh Class A) and six with moderate hepatic impairment (Child-Pugh Class B). Following administration of cefditoren pivoxil 400 mg BID for 7 days in these subjects, mean C_{max} and AUC values were slightly (<15%) greater than those observed in normal subjects. No dose adjustments are necessary for patients with mild or moderate hepatic impairment (Child-Pugh Class A or B). The pharmacokinetics of cefditoren in subjects with severe hepatic impairment (Child-Pugh Class C) have not been studied.

Microbiology

Cefditoren is a cephalosporin with antibacterial activity against gram-positive and gram-negative pathogens. The bactericidal activity of cefditoren results from the inhibition of cell wall synthesis via affinity for penicillin-binding proteins (PBPs). Cefditoren is stable in the presence of a variety of β-lactamases, including penicillinases and some cephalosporinases.

Cefditoren has been shown to be active against most strains of the following bacteria, both *in vitro* and in clinical infections, as described in the **INDICATIONS AND USAGE** section.

Aerobic Gram-Positive Microorganisms

Staphylococcus aureus (methicillin-susceptible strains, including β-lactamase-producing strains)

Note: Cefditoren is inactive against methicillin-resistant *Staphylococcus aureus*

Streptococcus pneumoniae (penicillin-susceptible strains only)

Streptococcus pyogenes

Aerobic Gram-Negative Microorganisms

Haemophilus influenzae (including β-lactamase-producing strains)

Haemophilus parainfluenzae (including β-lactamase-producing strains)

Moraxella catarrhalis (including β-lactamase-producing strains)

The following *in vitro* data are available, **but their clinical significance is unknown.** Cefditoren exhibits *in vitro* minimum inhibitory concentrations (MICs) of ≤0.125 μg/mL against most (≥ 90%) strains of the following bacteria; however, the safety and effectiveness of cefditoren in treating clinical infections due to these bacteria have not been established in adequate and well-controlled clinical trials.

Aerobic Gram-Positive Microorganisms

Streptococcus agalactiae

Streptococcus Groups C and G

Streptococcus, viridans group (penicillin-susceptible and -intermediate strains)

Susceptibility Tests

Dilution Techniques

Quantitative methods that are used to determine MICs provide reproducible estimates of the susceptibility of bacteria to antimicrobial compounds. The MICs should be determined using a standardized procedure. Standardized procedures are based on dilution methods[1] (broth) or equivalent with standardized inoculum concentrations and standardized concentrations of cefditoren powder. The MIC values obtained should be interpreted according to the following criteria:

For testing *Haemophilus* spp.[a] and *Streptococcus* spp. including *S. pneumoniae*[b]:

Clinical Isolates	MIC (μg/mL)	Interpretation
S. pneumoniae	≤ 0.125	Susceptible (S)
	0.250	Intermediate (I)
	≥ 0.50	Resistant (R)
Haemophilus spp.	≤ 0.125	Susceptible (S)
	0.250	Intermediate (I)
	≥ 0.50	Resistant (R)
S. pyogenes	≤ 0.125	Susceptible (S)

[a] This interpretive standard is applicable only to broth microdilution susceptibility tests with *Haemophilus* spp. using *Haemophilus* Test Medium (HTM).[1]

[b] These interpretive standards are applicable only to broth microdilution susceptibility tests with *Streptococcus* spp. using cation-adjusted Mueller-Hinton broth with 2-5% lysed horse blood.[1]

Susceptibility test criteria cannot be established for *S. aureus.*

A report of "Susceptible" indicates that the pathogen is likely to be inhibited if the antimicrobial compound in the blood reaches the concentration usually achievable. A report of "Intermediate" indicates that the result should be considered equivocal, and, if the microorganism is not fully susceptible to alternative, clinically feasible drugs, the test should be repeated. This category implies possible clinical applicability in body sites where the drug is physiologically concentrated or in situations where high dosage of drug can be used. This category also provides a buffer zone that prevents small, uncontrolled technical factors from causing major discrepancies in interpretation. A report of "Resistant" indicates that the pathogen is not likely to be inhibited if the antimicrobial compound in the blood reaches the concentration usually achievable and that other therapy should be selected.

Standardized susceptibility test procedures require the use of laboratory control bacterial strains to control the technical aspects of the laboratory procedures. Standard cefditoren powder should provide the following MICs with these quality control strains:

Microorganisms	MIC Ranges (μg/mL)
Streptococcus pneumoniae[a] ATCC 49619	0.016-0.12
Haemophilus influenzae[b] ATCC 49766	0.004-0.016
Haemophilus influenzae[b] ATCC 49247	0.06-0.25

[a] This quality control range is applicable to only *S. pneumoniae* ATCC 49619 tested by a microdilution procedure using cation-adjusted Mueller-Hinton broth with 2-5% lysed horse blood.[1]

[b] This quality control range is applicable to only *H. influenzae* ATCC 49247 and ATCC 49766 tested by a microdilution procedure using HTM.[1]

INDICATIONS AND USAGE

SPECTRACEF® (cefditoren pivoxil) is indicated for the treatment of mild to moderate infections in adults and adolescents (12 years of age or older) which are caused by susceptible strains of the designated microorganisms in the conditions listed below.

Acute Bacterial Exacerbation of Chronic Bronchitis caused by *Haemophilus influenzae* (including β-lactamase-producing strains), *Haemophilus parainfluenzae* (including β-lactamase-producing strains), *Streptococcus pneumoniae* (penicillin-susceptible strains only), or *Moraxella catarrhalis* (including β-lactamase-producing strains).

Community-Acquired Pneumonia caused by *Haemophilus influenzae* (including β-lactamase-producing strains), *Haemophilus parainfluenzae* (including β-lactamase-producing strains), *Streptococcus pneumoniae* (penicillin-susceptible strains only), or *Moraxella catarrhalis* (including β-lactamase-producing strains).

Pharyngitis/Tonsillitis caused by *Streptococcus pyogenes.* NOTE: SPECTRACEF is effective in the eradication of *Streptococcus pyogenes* from the oropharynx. SPECTRACEF has not been studied for the prevention of rheumatic fever following *Streptococcus pyogenes* pharyngitis/tonsillitis. Only intramuscular penicillin has been demonstrated to be effective for the prevention of rheumatic fever.

Uncomplicated Skin and Skin-Structure Infections caused by *Staphylococcus aureus* (including β-lactamase-producing strains) or *Streptococcus pyogenes.*

To reduce the development of drug-resistant bacteria and maintain the effectiveness of SPECTRACEF and other antibacterial drugs, SPECTRACEF should be used only to treat infections that are proven or strongly suspected to be caused by susceptible bacteria. When culture and susceptibility information are available, they should be considered in selecting or modifying antibacterial therapy. In the absence of such data, local epidemiology and susceptibility patterns may contribute to the empiric selection of therapy.

CONTRAINDICATIONS

SPECTRACEF is contraindicated in patients with known allergy to the cephalosporin class of antibiotics or any of its components.

SPECTRACEF is contraindicated in patients with carnitine deficiency or inborn errors of metabolism that may result in clinically significant carnitine deficiency, because use of SPECTRACEF causes renal excretion of carnitine. (See **PRECAUTIONS, General.**)

SPECTRACEF® tablets contain sodium caseinate, a milk protein. Patients with milk protein hypersensitivity (not lactose intolerance) should not be administered SPECTRACEF.

WARNINGS

BEFORE THERAPY WITH SPECTRACEF (CEFDITOREN PIVOXIL) IS INSTITUTED, CAREFUL INQUIRY SHOULD BE MADE TO DETERMINE WHETHER THE PATIENT HAS HAD PREVIOUS HYPERSENSITIVITY REACTIONS TO CEFDITOREN PIVOXIL, OTHER CEPHALOSPORINS, PENICILLINS, OR OTHER DRUGS. IF CEFDITOREN PIVOXIL IS TO BE GIVEN TO PENICILLIN-SENSITIVE PATIENTS, CAUTION SHOULD BE EXERCISED BECAUSE CROSS-HYPERSENSITIVITY AMONG β-LACTAM ANTIBIOTICS HAS BEEN CLEARLY DOCUMENTED AND MAY OCCUR IN UP TO 10% OF PATIENTS WITH A HISTORY OF PENICILLIN ALLERGY. IF AN ALLERGIC REACTION TO CEFDITOREN PIVOXIL OCCURS, THE DRUG SHOULD BE DISCONTINUED. SERIOUS ACUTE HYPERSENSITIVITY REACTIONS MAY REQUIRE TREATMENT WITH EPINEPHRINE AND OTHER EMERGENCY MEASURES, INCLUDING OXYGEN, INTRAVENOUS FLUIDS, INTRAVENOUS ANTIHISTAMINES, CORTICOSTEROIDS, PRESSOR AMINES, AND AIRWAY MANAGEMENT, AS CLINICALLY INDICATED.

Pseudomembranous colitis has been reported with nearly all antibacterial agents, including cefditoren pivoxil, and may range in severity from mild to life-threatening. Therefore, it is important to consider this diagnosis in patients who present with diarrhea subsequent to the administration of antibacterial agents.

Treatment with antibacterial agents alters normal flora of the colon and may permit overgrowth of clostridia. Studies indicate that a toxin produced by *Clostridium difficile* (*C. difficile*) is a primary cause of antibiotic-associated colitis.

After the diagnosis of pseudomembranous colitis has been established, appropriate therapeutic measures should be initiated. Mild cases of pseudomembranous colitis usually respond to drug discontinuation alone. In moderate to severe cases, consideration should be given to management with fluids and electrolytes, protein supplementation, and treatment with an antibacterial drug clinically effective against *C. difficile* colitis.

PRECAUTIONS

General

Prescribing SPECTRACEF® in the absence of a proven or strongly suspected bacterial infection or a prophylactic indication is unlikely to provide benefit to the patient and increases the risk of the development of drug-resistant bacteria.

SPECTRACEF is not recommended when prolonged antibiotic treatment is necessary, since other pivalate-containing compounds have caused clinical manifestations of carnitine deficiency when used over a period of months. No clinical effects of carnitine decrease have been associated with short-term treatment. The effects on carnitine concentrations of repeat short-term courses of SPECTRACEF are not known.

In community-acquired pneumonia patients (N=192, mean age 50.3 ± 17.2 years) given a 200 mg BID regimen for 14 days, the mean decrease in serum concentrations of total carnitine while on therapy was 13.8 ± 10.8 nmole/mL, representing a 30% decrease in serum carnitine concentrations. In community-acquired pneumonia patients (N=192, mean age 51.3 ± 17.8 years) given a 400 mg BID regimen for 14 days, the mean decrease in serum concentrations of total carnitine while on therapy was 21.5 ± 13.1 nmole/mL, representing a 46% decrease in serum carnitine concentrations. Plasma concentrations of carnitine returned to the normal control range within 7 days after discontinuation of cefditoren pivoxil. Comparable decreases in carnitine were observed in healthy volunteers (mean age 33.6 ± 7.4 years) following a 200 mg or 400 mg BID regimen. (See **CLINICAL PHARMACOLOGY.**) Community-acquired pneumonia clinical trials demonstrated no adverse events attributable to decreases in serum carnitine concentrations.

However, some sub-populations (e.g., patients with renal impairment, patients with decreased muscle mass) may be

Continued on next page

Spectracef—Cont.

at increased risk for reductions in serum carnitine concentrations during cefditoren pivoxil therapy. Furthermore, the appropriate dose in patients with end-stage renal disease has not been determined. (See **DOSAGE AND ADMINISTRATION, Patients with Renal Insufficiency).**

As with other antibiotics, prolonged treatment may result in the possible emergence and overgrowth of resistant organisms. Careful observation of the patient is essential. If superinfection occurs during therapy, appropriate alternative therapy should be administered.

Cephalosporins may be associated with a fall in prothrombin activity. Those at risk include patients with renal or hepatic impairment, or poor nutritional state, as well as patients receiving a protracted course of antimicrobial therapy, and patients previously stabilized on anticoagulant therapy. Prothrombin time should be monitored in patients at risk and exogenous vitamin K administered as indicated. In clinical trials, there was no difference between cefditoren and comparator cephalosporins in the incidence of increased prothrombin time.

Information for Patients

Patients should be counseled that antibacterial drugs including SPECTRACEF should only be used to treat bacterial infections. They do not treat viral infections (e.g., the common cold). When SPECTRACEF is prescribed to treat a bacterial infection, patients should be told that although it is common to feel better early in the course of therapy, the medication should be taken exactly as directed. Skipping doses or not completing the full course of therapy may (1) decrease the effectiveness of the immediate treatment and (2) increase the likelihood that bacteria will develop resistance and will not be treatable by SPECTRACEF or other antibacterial drugs in the future.

SPECTRACEF® (cefditoren pivoxil) should be taken with meals to enhance absorption.

SPECTRACEF may be taken concomitantly with oral contraceptives.

It is not recommended that SPECTRACEF be taken concomitantly with antacids or other drugs taken to reduce stomach acids. (See **PRECAUTIONS, Drug Interactions.**)

SPECTRACEF tablets contain sodium caseinate, a milk protein. Patients with milk protein hypersensitivity (not lactose intolerance) should not be administered SPECTRACEF.

Drug Interactions

Oral Contraceptives

Multiple doses of cefditoren pivoxil had no effect on the pharmacokinetics of ethinyl estradiol, the estrogenic component in most oral contraceptives.

Antacids

Co-administration of a single dose of an antacid which contained both magnesium (800 mg) and aluminum (900 mg) hydroxides reduced the oral absorption of a single 400 mg dose of cefditoren pivoxil administered following a meal, as evidenced by a 14% decrease in mean C_{max} and an 11% decrease in mean AUC. Although the clinical significance is not known, it is not recommended that cefditoren pivoxil be taken concomitantly with antacids.

H_2-Receptor Antagonists

Co-administration of a single dose of intravenously administered famotidine (20 mg) reduced the oral absorption of a single 400 mg dose of cefditoren pivoxil administered following a meal, as evidenced by a 27% decrease in mean C_{max} and a 22% decrease in mean AUC. Although the clinical significance is not known, it is not recommended that cefditoren pivoxil be taken concomitantly with H_2 receptor antagonists.

Probenecid

As with other β-lactam antibiotics, co-administration of probenecid with cefditoren pivoxil resulted in an increase in the plasma exposure of cefditoren, with a 49% increase in mean C_{max}, a 122% increase in mean AUC, and a 53% increase in $t_{1/2}$.

Drug/Laboratory Test Interactions

Cephalosporins are known to occasionally induce a positive direct Coombs' test. A false-positive reaction for glucose in the urine may occur with copper reduction tests (Benedict's or Fehling's solution or with CLINITEST® tablets), but not with enzyme-based tests for glycosuria (e.g., CLINISTIX®, TES-TAPE®). As a false-negative result may occur in the ferricyanide test, it is recommended that either the glucose oxidase or hexokinase method be used to determine blood/plasma glucose levels in patients receiving cefditoren pivoxil.

Carcinogenesis, Mutagenesis, Impairment of Fertility

No long-term animal carcinogenicity studies have been conducted with cefditoren pivoxil. Cefditoren pivoxil was not mutagenic in the Ames bacterial reverse mutation assay, or in the mouse lymphoma mutation assay at the hypoxanthine-guanine phosphoribosyltransferase locus. In Chinese hamster lung cells, chromosomal aberrations were produced by cefditoren pivoxil, but not by cefditoren. Subsequent studies showed that the chromosome aberrations were due to the release of formaldehyde from the pivoxil ester moiety in the *in vitro* assay system. Neither cefditoren nor cefditoren pivoxil produced chromosomal aberrations when tested in an *in vitro* human peripheral blood lymphocyte assay, or in the *in vivo* mouse micronucleus assay. Cefditoren pivoxil did not induce unscheduled DNA syntheses when tested.

Treatment-Related Adverse Events in Trials in Adults and Adolescent Patients ≥ 12 Years

		SPECTRACEF 200 mg BID (N=2675)	SPECTRACEF 400 mg BID (N=2159)	COMPARATORS[a] (N=2648)
Incidence ≥ 1%	Diarrhea	11%	15%	8%
	Nausea	4%	6%	5%
	Headache	3%	2%	2%
	Abdominal Pain	2%	2%	1%
	Vaginal Moniliasis	3%[b]	6%[c]	6%[d]
	Dyspepsia	1%	2%	2%
	Vomiting	1%	1%	2%

[a]includes amoxicillin/clavulanate, cefadroxil monohydrate, cefuroxime axetil, cefpodoxime proxetil, clarithromycin, and penicillin

[b]1428 females

[c]1135 females

[d]1461 females

In rats, fertility and reproduction were not affected by cefditoren pivoxil at oral doses up to 1000 mg/kg/day, approximately 24 times a human dose of 200 mg BID based on mg/m^2/day.

Pregnancy-Teratogenic Effects

Pregnancy Category B

Cefditoren pivoxil was not teratogenic up to the highest doses tested in rats and rabbits. In rats, this dose was 1000 mg/kg/day, which is approximately 24 times a human dose of 200 mg BID based on mg/m^2/day. In rabbits, the highest dose tested was 90 mg/kg/day, which is approximately four times a human dose of 200 mg BID based on mg/m^2/day. This dose produced severe maternal toxicity and resulted in fetal toxicity and abortions.

In a postnatal development study in rats, cefditoren pivoxil produced no adverse effects on postnatal survival, physical and behavioral development, learning abilities, and reproductive capability at sexual maturity when tested at doses of up to 750 mg/kg/day, the highest dose tested. This is approximately 18 times a human dose of 200 mg BID based on mg/m^2/day.

There are, however, no adequate and well-controlled studies in pregnant women. Because animal reproductive studies are not always predictive of human response, this drug should be used during pregnancy only if clearly needed.

Labor and Delivery

Cefditoren pivoxil has not been studied for use during labor and delivery.

Nursing Mothers

Cefditoren was detected in the breast milk of lactating rats. Because many drugs are excreted in human breast milk, caution should be exercised when cefditoren pivoxil is administered to nursing women.

Pediatric Use

Use of cefditoren pivoxil is not recommended for pediatric patients less than 12 years of age. The safety and efficacy of cefditoren pivoxil tablets in this population, including any effects of altered carnitine concentration, have not been established (See **PRECAUTIONS, General**).

Geriatric Use

Of the 2675 patients in clinical studies who received cefditoren pivoxil 200 mg BID, 308 (12%) were >65 years of age. Of the 2159 patients in clinical studies who received cefditoren pivoxil 400 mg BID, 307 (14%) were >65 years of age. No clinically significant differences in effectiveness or safety were observed between older and younger patients. No dose adjustments are necessary in geriatric patients with normal (for their age) renal function. This drug is known to be substantially excreted by the kidney, and the risk of toxic reactions to this drug may be greater in patients with impaired renal function. Because elderly patients are more likely to have decreased renal function, care should be taken in dose selection, and it may be useful to monitor renal function. (See **DOSAGE AND ADMINISTRATION.**)

ADVERSE EVENTS

Clinical Trials – SPECTRACEF® (cefditoren pivoxil) Tablets (Adults and Adolescent Patients ≥ 12 Years of Age)

In clinical trials, 4834 adult and adolescent patients have been treated with the recommended doses of cefditoren pivoxil tablets (200 mg or 400 mg BID). Most adverse events were mild and self-limiting. No deaths or permanent disabilities have been attributed to cefditoren.

The following adverse events were thought by the investigators to be possibly, probably, or definitely related to cefditoren tablets in multiple-dose clinical trials:

[See table above]

The overall incidence of adverse events, and in particular diarrhea, increased with the higher recommended dose of SPECTRACEF.

Treatment related adverse events experienced by <1% but >0.1% of patients who received 200 mg or 400 mg BID of cefditoren pivoxil were abnormal dreams, allergic reaction, anorexia, asthenia, asthma, coagulation time increased, constipation, dizziness, dry mouth, eructation, face edema, fever, flatulence, fungal infection, gastrointestinal disorder, hyperglycemia, increased appetite, insomnia, leukopenia, leukorrhea, liver function test abnormal, myalgia, nervousness, oral moniliasis, pain, peripheral edema, pharyngitis, pseudomembranous colitis, pruritus, rash, rhinitis, sinusitis, somnolence, stomatitis, sweating, taste perversion, thirst, thrombocythemia, urticaria, and vaginitis. Pseudomembranous colitis symptoms may begin during or after antibiotic treatment. (See **WARNINGS.**)

Sixty-one of 2675 (2%) patients who received 200 mg BID and 69 of 2159 (3%) patients who received 400 mg BID of cefditoren pivoxil discontinued medication due to adverse events thought by the investigators to be possibly, probably, or definitely associated with cefditoren therapy. The discontinuations were primarily for gastrointestinal disturbances, usually diarrhea or nausea. Diarrhea was the reason for discontinuation in 19 of 2675 (0.7%) patients who received 200 mg BID and in 31 of 2159 (1.4%) patients who received 400 mg BID of cefditoren pivoxil.

Changes in laboratory parameters of possible clinical significance, without regard to drug relationship and which occurred in ≥ 1% of patients who received cefditoren pivoxil 200 mg or 400 mg BID, were hematuria (3.0% and 3.1%), increased urine white blood cells (2.3% and 2.3%), decreased hematocrit (2.1% and 2.2%), and increased glucose (1.8% and 1.1%). Those events which occurred in <1% but >0.1% of patients included the following: increased/decreased white blood cells, increased eosinophils, decreased neutrophils, increased lymphocytes, increased platelet count, decreased hemoglobin, decreased sodium, increased potassium, decreased chloride, decreased inorganic phosphorus, decreased calcium, increased SGPT/ALT, increased SGOT/AST, increased cholesterol, decreased albumin, proteinuria, and increased BUN. It is not known if these abnormalities were caused by the drug or the underlying condition being treated.

Cephalosporin Class Adverse Reactions

In addition to the adverse reactions listed above which have been observed in patients treated with cefditoren pivoxil, the following adverse reactions and altered laboratory test results have been reported for cephalosporin class antibiotics:

Adverse Reactions: Allergic reactions, anaphylaxis, drug fever, Stevens-Johnson syndrome, serum sickness-like reaction, erythema multiforme, toxic epidermal necrolysis, colitis, renal dysfunction, toxic nephropathy, reversible hyperactivity, hypertonia, hepatic dysfunction including cholestasis, aplastic anemia, hemolytic anemia, hemorrhage, and superinfection.

Altered Laboratory Tests: Prolonged prothrombin time, positive direct Coombs' test, false-positive test for urinary glucose, elevated alkaline phosphatase, elevated bilirubin, elevated LDH, increased creatinine, pancytopenia, neutropenia, and agranulocytosis.

Several cephalosporins have been implicated in triggering seizures, particularly in patients with renal impairment when the dosage was not reduced. (See **DOSAGE AND ADMINISTRATION.**) If seizures associated with drug therapy occur, the drug should be discontinued. Anticonvulsant therapy can be given if clinically indicated.

Postmarketing Experience

The following adverse experiences, regardless of their relationship to cefditoren pivoxil, have been reported during extensive postmarketing experience, beginning with approval in Japan in 1994: pneumonia interstitial, eosinophilic pneumonia acute, acute renal failure, arthralgia, thrombocytopenia.

OVERDOSAGE

Information on cefditoren pivoxil overdosage in humans is not available. However, with other β-lactam antibiotics, adverse effects following overdosage have included nausea, vomiting, epigastric distress, diarrhea, and convulsions. Hemodialysis may aid in the removal of cefditoren from the body, particularly if renal function is compromised (30% reduction of plasma concentrations following 4 hours of hemodialysis). Treat overdosage symptomatically and institute supportive measures as required.

In acute animal toxicity studies, cefditoren pivoxil when tested at the limit oral doses of 5100 mg/kg in rats and up to 2000 mg/kg in dogs did not exhibit any health effects of concern. Certain effects, such as diarrhea and soft stool lasting for a few days were observed in some animals as expected with most oral antibiotics due to inhibition of intestinal microflora.

DOSAGE AND ADMINISTRATION

(See **INDICATIONS AND USAGE** for Indicated Pathogens.)

SPECTRACEF® (cefditoren pivoxil) Dosage and Administration* Adults and Adolescents (≥ 12 Years)

Type of Infection	Dosage	Duration (days)
Community-Acquired Pneumonia	400 mg BID	14
Acute Bacterial Exacerbation of Chronic Bronchitis	400 mg BID	
Pharyngitis/Tonsillitis		10
Uncomplicated Skin and Skin Structure Infections	200 mg BID	

*Should be taken with meals

Patients with Renal Insufficiency

No dose adjustment is necessary for patients with mild renal impairment (CL_{cr}: 50-80 mL/min/1.73 m^2). It is recommended that not more than 200 mg BID be administered to patients with moderate renal impairment (CL_{cr}: 30-49 mL/min/1.73 m^2) and 200 mg QD be administered to patients with severe renal impairment (CL_{cr}: <30 mL/min/1.73 m^2). The appropriate dose in patients with end-stage renal disease has not been determined.

Patients with Hepatic Disease

No dose adjustments are necessary for patients with mild or moderate hepatic impairment (Child-Pugh Class A or B). The pharmacokinetics of cefditoren have not been studied in patients with severe hepatic impairment (Child-Pugh Class C).

HOW SUPPLIED

SPECTRACEF® (cefditoren pivoxil) tablets containing cefditoren pivoxil equivalent to 200 mg of cefditoren are available as white, elliptical, film-coated tablets imprinted with Purdue 200 mg in blue. These tablets are available in a multi-dose tamper-evident container as follows:

NDC 67781-181-60 Bottles of 60

Store at 25°C (77°F); excursions permitted to 15°-30°C (59°-86°F). [See USP Controlled Room Temperature.] Protect from light and moisture.

Dispense in a tight, light-resistant container.

Healthcare professionals can telephone Purdue's Medical Services Department (1-888-726-7535) for information on this product.

REFERENCES

1. National Committee for Clinical Laboratory Standards. *Methods for Dilution Antimicrobial Susceptibility Tests for Bacteria That Grow Aerobically – Fifth Edition*; Approved Standard, NCCLS Document M7-A5, Vol. 20, No. 2, NCCLS, Wayne, PA, January, 2000.

Rx Only

Manufactured by:
Ceph International, Inc.
Carolina, Puerto Rico 00985
Distributed by:
Purdue Pharmaceutical Products L.P.
Stamford, CT 06901-3431
U.S. Patent Nos. 4,839,350; 4,918,068; and 5,958,915
August 4, 2003
OT00617B
300780-0B-001

Shown in Product Identification Guide, page 331

Purdue Products L.P.

ONE STAMFORD FORUM
STAMFORD CT 06901-3431

FOR MEDICAL INFORMATION CONTACT:
(888) 726-7535
Adverse Drug Experiences:
(888) 726-7535
Customer Service:
(800) 877-5666
FAX: (800) 877-3210

COLACE® CAPSULES 50 MG OTC

[kōlās]
docusate sodium

DESCRIPTION

Colace® (docusate sodium) is a stool softener laxative

Active Ingredient: Colace® Capsules 50 mg. contains 50 mg of docusate sodium

Inactive Ingredients: D&C Red No. 33, FD&C Red No. 40, gelatin, glycerin, polyethylene glycol 400, propylene glycol, sorbitol

USES

Relieves occasional constipation (irregularity). Generally produces a bowel movement in 12 to 72 hours.

WARNINGS

Do not use if you are presently taking mineral oil, unless told to do so by a doctor. Ask a doctor before use if you have stomach pain, nausea, vomiting, or noticed a sudden change in bowel habits that lasts over 2 weeks. Stop use and ask a doctor if you have rectal bleeding or fail to have a bowel movement after use of a laxative. These could be signs of a serious condition. Stop use and ask a doctor if you need to use a laxative for more than 1 week. If pregnant or breast-feeding, ask a health professional before use.

Keep out of reach of children. In case of overdose, get medical help or contact a Poison Control Center right away.

DOSAGE

doses may be taken as a single daily dose or in divided doses

adults and children 12 years and over	take 1–6 capsules daily
children 2 to under 12 years of age	take 1–3 capsules daily
children under 2 years	ask a doctor

Other information

Each capsule contains sodium 3 mg.
VERY LOW SODIUM
store at 25°C (77°F); excursions permitted between 15°-30°C (59°-86°F).

HOW SUPPLIED

Capsules: Boxes of 10. Bottles of 30 and 60.

 www.colacecapsules.com

COLACE® CAPSULES 100 mg OTC

[kō lās]
docusate sodium

DESCRIPTION

Colace® (docusate sodium) is a stool softener laxative

Active Ingredient: Colace® Capsules 100 mg. contains 100 mg of docusate sodium

Inactive Ingredients: D&C Red No. 33, FD&C Red No. 40, FD&C Yellow No. 6, gelatin, glycerin, methylparaben, polyethylene glycol 400, propylene glycol, propylparaben, sorbitol, titanium dioxide

USES

Relieves occasional constipation (irregularity). Generally produces a bowel movement in 12 to 72 hours.

WARNINGS

Do not use if you are presently taking mineral oil, unless told to do so by a doctor. Ask a doctor before use if you have stomach pain, nausea, vomiting, or noticed a sudden change in bowel habits that lasts over 2 weeks. Stop use and ask a doctor if you have rectal bleeding or fail to have a bowel movement after use of a laxative. These could be signs of a serious condition. Stop use and ask a doctor if you need to use a laxative for more than 1 week. If pregnant or breast-feeding, ask a health professional before use.

Keep out of reach of children. In case of overdose, get medical help or contact a Poison Control Center right away.

DOSAGE

doses may be taken as a single daily dose or in divided doses

adults and children 12 years and over	take 1–3 capsules daily
children 2 to under 12 years of age	take 1 capsule daily
children under 2 years	ask a doctor

Other information

Each capsule contains sodium 5 mg.
VERY LOW SODIUM
store at 25°C (77°F); excursions permitted between 15°–30°C (59°–86°F).
Keep tightly closed.

HOW SUPPLIED

Capsules: Boxes of 10. Bottles of 30, 60 and 250.

 www.colacecapsules.com

COLACE® Glycerin, USP 1.2 grams per dose OTC

[kō lās]
Laxative for infants and children
glycerin

DESCRIPTION

Colace® (glycerin) Suppositories – laxative for infants and children

Active Ingredient (per suppository): Colace® Suppositories contains glycerin, USP 1.2 grams

Inactive Ingredients: purified water, sodium hydroxide, stearic acid

USES

Relieves occasional constipation (irregularity). Generally produces a bowel movement in 1/4 to 1 hour.

WARNINGS

For rectal use only. Do not give laxative products for longer than 1 week unless told to do so by a doctor. Ask a doctor before use if your child has stomach pain, nausea, vomiting, a sudden change in bowel habits that lasts over 2 weeks. When using this product your child may have rectal discomfort or a burning sensation. Stop use and ask a doctor if your child has rectal bleeding or fails to have a bowel movement after use of a laxative. These could be signs of a serious condition. **Keep out of reach of children.** If swallowed, get medical help or contact a Poison Control Center right away.

DOSAGE

children 2 to under 6 years of age	insert 1 suppository well into the rectum and retain for 15 minutes. it need not melt to produce laxative action. Do not exceed 1 suppository daily or as directed by a doctor.
children under 2	ask a doctor

Other Information

• avoid excessive heat. Keep tightly closed.

HOW SUPPLIED

Infants and Children Suppositories: Jars of 12 and 24.

COLACE® Glycerin, USP 2.1 grams per dose OTC

[kō lās]
Laxative for adults and children
glycerin

DESCRIPTION

Colace® (glycerin) Suppositories—laxative for adults and children

Active Ingredient (per suppository): Colace® Suppositories contains glycerin, USP 2.1 grams

Inactive Ingredients: purified water, sodium hydroxide, stearic acid

USES

Relieves occasional constipation (irregularity). Generally produces a bowel movement in 1/4 to 1 hour.

WARNINGS

For rectal use only. Do not use laxative products for longer than 1 week unless told to do so by a doctor. Ask a doctor before use if you have stomach pain, nausea, vomiting, noticed a sudden change in bowel habits that lasts over 2 weeks. When using this product you may have rectal discomfort or a burning sensation. Stop use and ask a doctor if you have rectal bleeding or fail to have a bowel movement after use of a laxative. These could be signs of a serious condition. If pregnant or breast-feeding, ask a health professional before use. **Keep out of reach of children.** If swallowed, get medical help or contact a Poison Control Center right away.

DOSAGE

adults and children 6 years of age and over	Insert 1 suppository well into the rectum and retain for 15 minutes; it need not melt to produce laxative action. Do not exceed 1 suppository daily or as directed by a doctor.
children under 6 years	use Colace® Suppositories for infants and children

Other information

avoid excessive heat. Keep tightly closed.

Continued on next page

Colace Glycerin 2.1 g—Cont.

HOW SUPPLIED

Adults and Children Suppositories: Jars of 12, 24, 48, 100.

COLACE® LIQUID 1% SOLUTION OTC

[kō lās]
docusate sodium

DESCRIPTION

Colace® (docusate sodium) is a stool softener laxative

Active Ingredient: Colace® Liquid 1% Solution. Each mL contains 10 mg of docusate sodium

Inactive Ingredients: citric acid, D&C Red No. 33, methylparaben, poloxamer, polyethylene glycol 400, propylene glycol, propylparaben, purified water, sodium citrate, vanillin

USES

Relieves occasional constipation (irregularity). Generally produces a bowel movement in 12 to 72 hours.

WARNINGS

Do not use if you are presently taking mineral oil, unless told to do so by a doctor. Ask a doctor before use if you have stomach pain, nausea, vomiting, or noticed a sudden change in bowel habits that lasts over 2 weeks. Stop use and ask a doctor if you have rectal bleeding or fail to have a bowel movement after use of a laxative. These could be signs of a serious condition. Stop use and ask a doctor if you need to use a laxative for more than 1 week. If pregnant or breast-feeding, ask a health professional before use. **Keep out of reach of children.** In case of overdose, get medical help or contact a Poison Control Center right away.

DOSAGE

Doses must be given in a 6–8 oz glass of milk or fruit juice, or in infant's formula to prevent throat irritation

adults and children 12 years of age and over	take 5–15 mL once or twice a day
children 2 to under 12 years of age	take 5–15 mL once a day
children under 2 years	ask a doctor

Other information

sodium content 1 mg/mL VERY LOW SODIUM
store at 25°C (77°F); excursions permitted between 15°–30°C (59°–86°F).
Keep tightly closed.
calibration mark on dropper measures a 1 mL dose

HOW SUPPLIED

Liquid: Bottle (30 mL)

MINERAL OIL OTC

DESCRIPTION

Intestinal lubricant laxative. Odorless, tasteless, crystal clear.
Active ingredient: mineral oil
Inactive ingredient: di-alpha-tocopherol

ACTIONS AND USES

Relieves occasional constipation (irregularity). Generally produces a bowel movement in 6 to 8 hours.

WARNINGS

Take only at bedtime and do not take with meals. **Do not use:** for longer than 1 week, if you are presently taking a stool softener laxative, if you are pregnant, in children under 12 years of age, in bedridden patients, in persons with difficulty swallowing. **Ask a doctor before use if you have:** stomach pain, nausea, vomiting, noticed a sudden change in bowel habits that lasts over 2 weeks. **Stop use and ask a doctor** if you have rectal bleeding or fail to have a bowel movement after use of a laxative. These could be signs of a serious condition. **If you are breast-feeding,** ask a health professional before use. **Keep out of reach of children.** In case of overdose, get medical help or contact a Poison Control Center right away.

ADMINISTRATION AND DOSAGE

Adults and children 12 years of age or over take 1–3 tablespoonfuls at bedtime or as directed by a doctor.

HOW SUPPLIED

Liquid: Bottles of 6 oz. and 16 oz.
Note: Store between 20°–25°C (68°–77°F); excursions permitted between 15°–30°C (59°–86°F). Keep tightly closed. Protect from sunlight.

PERI-COLACE® TABLETS OTC

[pě-rē-kō-lās]
docusate sodium and standardized senna concentrate

DESCRIPTION

Peri-Colace® (docusate sodium and standardized senna concentrate) is a combination stimulant laxative and stool softener
Peri-Colace® Tablets contains the following:
Active Ingredient: contains 50 mg of docusate sodium and 8.6 mg of sennosides
Inactive Ingredients: carnauba wax, colloidal silicon dioxide, croscarmellose sodium, dicalcium phosphate, FD&C Blue No. 2, FD&C Red No. 40, hypromellose, magnesium stearate, microcrystalline cellulose, PEG 400, sodium benzoate, stearic acid, titanium dioxide

USES

Relieves occasional constipation (irregularity). Generally produces bowel movement in 6 to 12 hours.

WARNINGS

Do not use laxative products for longer than 1 week unless told to do so by a doctor; if you are presently taking mineral oil, unless told to do so by a doctor. Ask a doctor before use if you have stomach pain, nausea, vomiting, noticed a sudden change in bowel habits that lasts over 2 weeks. Stop use and ask a doctor if you have rectal bleeding or fail to have a bowel movement after use of a laxative. These could be signs of a serious condition. If pregnant or breast-feeding, ask a health professional before use. **Keep out of reach of children.** In case of overdose, get medical help or contact a Poison Control Center right away.

DOSAGE

doses may be taken as a single daily dose or in divided doses preferably in the evening

adults and children 12 years and over	take 2–4 tablets daily
children 6 to under 12 years of age	take 1–2 tablets daily
children 2 to under 6 years of age	take up to 1 tablet daily
children under 2	ask a doctor

Other information

each tablet contains: sodium 4 mg VERY LOW SODIUM
store at 25°C (77°F); excursions permitted between 15°–30°C (59°–86°F).
Keep tightly closed.

HOW SUPPLIED

Tablets: Box of 10. Bottles of 30 and 60.

Questcor Pharmaceuticals, Inc.

3260 WHIPPLE ROAD
UNION CITY, CA 94587

Direct Inquiries to:
(510) 400-0700
FAX: (510) 400-0799
www.questcor.com

ETHAMOLIN® ℞

[ĕ-tham-ō-lin]
(ethanolamine oleate)
Injection, 5%
For Local Intravenous Use Only

GLOFIL®-125 ℞

[glōw-fill]
Sodium Iothalamate I-125
Injection, USP

H.P. ACTHAR® Gel ℞

(REPOSITORY CORTICOTROPIN INJECTION)

NASCOBAL® ℞

(Cyanocobalamin, USP)
Gel for Intranasal Administration
500 mcg/0.1 mL
Rx Only

Reckitt Benckiser Pharmaceuticals Inc.

10710 MIDLOTHIAN TURNPIKE
RICHMOND, VA 23235

Direct Inquiries to:
Reckitt Benckiser Pharmaceuticals, Inc.
Tel: (800) 444-7599
Fax: (804) 379-1215

For Medical Information/Emergencies Generally:
Tel: (877) 782-6966 or
www.Suboxone.com
Emergencies:
Tel: (804) 423-7089
Fax: (804) 379-1215

Order Fulfillment
(866) 282-2107

BUPRENEX® Ⓒ ℞

[būp 'rĕn-ex]
(buprenorphine hydrochloride)
Injectable

DESCRIPTION

Buprenex (buprenorphine hydrochloride) is a narcotic under the Controlled Substances Act due to its chemical derivation from thebaine. Chemically, it is 17-(cyclopropylmethyl)-α-(1, 1-dimethylethyl)-4, 5-epoxy-18, 19-dihydro-3-hydroxy-6-methoxy-α-methyl-6, 14-ethenomorphinan-7-methanol, hydrochloride [5α, 7α(S)]. Buprenorphine hydrochloride is a white powder, weakly acidic and with limited solubility in water. Buprenex is a clear, sterile, injectable agonist-antagonist analgesic intended for intravenous or intramuscular administration. Each ml of Buprenex contains 0.324 mg buprenorphine hydrochloride (equivalent to 0.3 mg buprenorphine), 50 mg anhydrous dextrose, water for injection and HCl to adjust pH. Buprenorphine hydrochloride has the molecular formula, $C_{29}H_{41}NO_4HCl$, and the following structure:

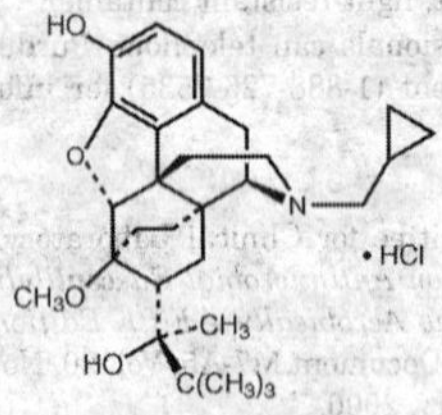

Molecular weight: 504.09

CLINICAL PHARMACOLOGY

Buprenex is a parenteral opioid analgesic with 0.3mg Buprenex being approximately equivalent to 10 mg morphine sulfate in analgesic and respiratory depressant effects in adults. Pharmacological effects occur as soon as 15 minutes after intramuscular injection and persist for 6 hours or longer. Peak pharmacologic effects usually are observed at 1 hour. When used intravenously, the times to onset and peak effect are shortened.
The limits of sensitivity of available analytical methodology precluded demonstration of bioequivalence between intramuscular and intravenous routes of administration. In post-operative adults, pharmacokinetic studies have shown elimination half-lives ranging from 1.2–7.2 hours (mean 2.2 hours) after intravenous administration of 0.3mg of buprenorphine. A single, ten-patient, pharmacokinetic study of doses of 3μg/kg in children (age 5–7 years) showed a high inter-patient variability, but suggests that the clearance of the drug may be higher in children than in adults. This is supported by at least one repeat-dose study in post-operative pain that showed an optimal inter-dose interval of 4–5 hours in pediatric patients as opposed to the recommended 6–8 hours in adults.
Buprenorphine, in common with morphine and other phenolic opioid analgesics, is metabolized by the liver and its clearance is related to hepatic blood flow. Studies in patients anesthetized with 0.5% halothane have shown that this anesthetic decreases hepatic blood flow by about 30%.
Mechanism of Analgesic Action: Buprenex exerts its analgesic effect via high affinity binding to μ subclass opiate receptors in the central nervous system. Although Buprenex may be classified as a partial agonist, under the conditions of recommended use it behaves very much like classical μ agonists such as morphine. One unusual property of Buprenex observed in *in vitro* studies is its very slow rate of dissociation from its receptor. This could account for its longer duration of action than morphine, the unpredictability of its reversal by opioid antagonists, and its low level of manifest physical dependence.
Narcotic Antagonist Activity: Buprenorphine demonstrates narcotic antagonist activity and has been shown to be equipotent with naloxone as an antagonist of morphine in the mouse tail flick test.

Cardiovascular Effects: Buprenex may cause a decrease or, rarely, an increase in pulse rate and blood pressure in some patients.
Effects on Respiration: Under usual conditions of use in adults, both Buprenex and morphine show similar dose-related respiratory depressant effects. At adult therapeutic doses, Buprenex (0.3mg buprenorphine) can decrease respiratory rate in an equivalent manner to an equianalgesic dose of morphine (10mg). (See WARNINGS.)

INDICATIONS AND USAGE

Buprenex is indicated for the relief of moderate to severe pain.

CONTRAINDICATIONS

Buprenex should not be administered to patients who have been shown to be hypersensitive to the drug.

WARNINGS

Impaired Respiration: As with other potent opioids, clinically significant respiratory depression may occur within the recommended dose range in patients receiving therapeutic doses of buprenorphine. Buprenex should be used with caution in patients with compromised respiratory function (e.g., chronic obstructive pulmonary disease, cor pulmonale, decreased respiratory reserve, hypoxia, hypercapnia, or preexisting respiratory depression). Particular caution is advised if Buprenex is administered to patients taking or recently receiving drugs with CNS/respiratory depressant effects. In patients with the physical and/or pharmacological risk factors above, the dose should be reduced by approximately one-half.

NALOXONE MAY NOT BE EFFECTIVE IN REVERSING THE RESPIRATORY DEPRESSION PRODUCED BY BUPRENEX. THEREFORE, AS WITH OTHER POTENT OPIOIDS, THE PRIMARY MANAGEMENT OF OVERDOSE SHOULD BE THE REESTABLISHMENT OF ADEQUATE VENTILATION WITH MECHANICAL ASSISTANCE OF RESPIRATION, IF REQUIRED.

Interaction with Other Central Nervous System Depressants: Patients receiving Buprenex in the presence of other narcotic analgesics, general anesthetics, antihistamines, benzodiazepines, phenothiazines, other tranquilizers, sedative/hypnotics or other CNS depressants (including alcohol) may exhibit increased CNS depression. When such combined therapy is contemplated, it is particularly important that the dose of one or both agents be reduced.
Head Injury and Increased Intracranial Pressure: Buprenex, like other potent analgesics, may itself elevate cerebrospinal fluid pressure and should be used with caution in head injury, intracranial lesions and other circumstances where cerebrospinal pressure may be increased. Buprenex can produce miosis and changes in the level of consciousness which may interfere with patient evaluation.
Use in Ambulatory Patients: Buprenex may impair the mental or physical abilities required for the performance of potentially dangerous tasks such as driving a car or operating machinery. Therefore, Buprenex should be administered with caution to ambulatory patients who should be warned to avoid such hazards.
Use in Narcotic-Dependent Patients: Because of the narcotic antagonist activity of Buprenex, use in the physically dependent individual may result in withdrawal effects.

PRECAUTIONS

General: Buprenex should be administered with caution in the elderly, debilitated patients, in children and those with severe impairment of hepatic, pulmonary, or renal function; myxedema or hypothyroidism; adrenal cortical insufficiency (e.g., Addison's disease); CNS depression or coma; toxic psychoses; prostatic hypertrophy or urethral stricture; acute alcoholism; delirium tremens; or kyphoscoliosis.
Because Buprenex is metabolized by the liver, the activity of Buprenex may be increased and/or extended in those individuals with impaired hepatic function or those receiving other agents known to decrease hepatic clearance.
Buprenex has been shown to increase intracholedochal pressure to a similar degree as other opioid analgesics, and thus should be administered with caution to patients with dysfunction of the biliary tract.
Information for Patients: The effects of Buprenex, particularly drowsiness, may be potentiated by other centrally acting agents such as alcohol or benzodiazepines. It is particularly important that in these circumstances patients must not drive or operate machinery. Buprenex has some pharmacologic effects similar to morphine which in susceptible patients may lead to self-administration of the drug when pain no longer exists. Patients must not exceed the dosage of Buprenex prescribed by their physician. Patients should be urged to consult their physician if other prescription medications are currently being used or are prescribed for future use.
Drug Interactions: Drug interactions common to other potent opioid analgesics also may occur with Buprenex. Particular care should be taken when Buprenex is used in combination with central nervous system depressant drugs (see WARNINGS). Although specific information is not presently available, caution should be exercised when Buprenex is used in combination with MAO inhibitors. There have been reports of respiratory and cardiovascular collapse in patients who received therapeutic doses of diazepam and Buprenex. A suspected interaction between Buprenex and phenprocoumon resulting in purpura has been reported.
CYP3A4 Inhibitors: Since the metabolism of buprenorphine is mediated by the CYP3A4 isozyme, coadministration of drugs that inhibit CYP3A4 activity may cause decreased clearance of buprenorphine. Thus patients coadministered with inhibitors of CYP3A4 such as macrolide antibiotics (e.g., erythromycin), azole antifungal agents (e.g., ketoconazole), and protease inhibitors (e.g., ritanovir) while receiving Buprenex should be carefully monitored and dosage adjustment made if warranted.
CYP3A4 Inducers: Cytochrome P450 inducers, such as rifampin, carbamazepine, and phenytoin, induce metabolism and as such may cause increased clearance of buprenorphine. Caution is advised when administering Buprenex to patients receiving these medications and if necessary dose adjustments should be considered
Carcinogenesis, Mutagenesis and Impairment of Fertility:
Carcinogenesis: Carcinogenicity studies were conducted in Sprague-Dawley rats and CD-1 mice. Buprenorphine was administered in the diet at doses of 0.6, 5.5, and 56 mg/kg/day for 27 months in rats. These doses were approximately equivalent to 5.7, 52 and 534 times the recommended human dose (1.2 mg) on a mg/m^2 body surface area basis. Statistically significant dose-related increases in testicular interstitial (Leydig's) cell tumors occurred, according to the trend test adjusted for survival. Pair-wise comparison of the high dose against control failed to show statistical significance. In the mouse study, buprenorphine was administered in the diet at doses of 8, 50, and 100 mg/kg/day for 86 weeks. The high dose was approximately equivalent to 477 times the recommended human dose (1.2 mg) on a mg/m^2 basis. Buprenorphine was not carcinogenic in mice.
Mutagenesis: Buprenorphine was studied in a series of tests. Results were negative in Chinese hamster bone marrow and spermatogonia cells, and negative in mouse lymphoma L5178Y assay. Results were equivocal in the Ames test: negative in studies in two laboratories, but positive in frame shift mutation at high dose (5 mg/plate) in a third study.
Impairment of Fertility: Reproduction studies of buprenorphine in rats demonstrated no evidence of impaired fertility at daily oral doses up to 80 mg/kg (approximately 763 times the recommended human daily dose of 1.2 mg on a mg/m^2 basis) or up to 5mg/kg I.M. or S.C. (approximately 48 times the recommended human daily dose of 1.2 mg on a mg/m^2 basis)
Pregnancy: Pregnancy Category C.
Teratogenic effects: Buprenorphine was not teratogenic in rats or rabbits after I.M. or S.C. doses up to 5 mg/kg/day (approximately 48 and 95 times the recommended human daily dose of 1.2 mg on a mg/m^2 basis), I.V. doses up to 0.8 mg/kg/day (approximately 8 times and 15 times the recommended human daily dose of 1.2 mg on a mg/m^2 basis), or oral doses up to 160 mg/kg/day in rats (approximately 1525 times the recommended human daily dose of 1.2 mg on a mg/m^2 basis) and 25 mg/kg/day in rabbits (approximately 475 times the recommended human daily dose of 1.2 mg on a mg/m^2 basis). Significant increases in skeletal abnormalities (e.g. extra thoracic vertebra or thoraco-lumbar ribs) were noted in rats after S.C. administration of 1 mg/kg/day and up (approximately 9.5 times the recommended human daily dose of 1.2 mg on a mg/m^2 basis) and in rabbits after I.M. administration of 5 mg/kg/day (approximately 95 times the recommended human daily dose of 1.2 mg on a mg/m^2 basis), but these increases were not statistically significant. Increases in skeletal abnormalities after oral administration were not observed in rats, and increases in rabbits (1–25 mg/kg/day) were not statistically significant.
There are no adequate and well-controlled studies in pregnant women. Buprenex should be used during pregnancy only if the potential benefit justifies the potential risk to the fetus.
Labor and Delivery: The safety of Buprenex given during labor and delivery has not been established.
Nursing Mothers: An apparent lack of milk production during general reproduction studies with buprenorphine in rats caused decreased viability and lactation indices. Use of high doses of sublingual buprenorphine in pregnant women showed that buprenorprhine passes into the mother's milk. Breast-feeding is therefore not advised in nursing mothers treated with Buprenex.
Pediatric Use: The safety and effectiveness of Buprenex have been established for children between 2 and 12 years of age. Use of Buprenex in children is supported by evidence from adequate and well controlled trials of Buprenex in adults, with additional data from studies of 960 children ranging in age from 9 months to 18 years of age. Data is available from a pharmacokinetic study, several controlled clinical trials, and several large post-marketing studies and case series. The available information provides reasonable evidence that Buprenex may be used safely in children ranging from 2–12 years of age, and that it is of similar effectiveness in children as in adults.

ADVERSE REACTIONS

The most frequent side effect in clinical studies involving 1,133 patients was sedation which occurred in approximately two-thirds of the patients. Although sedated, these patients could easily be aroused to an alert state.
Other less frequent adverse reactions occurring in 5–10% of the patients were:
Nausea
Dizziness/Vertigo
Occurring in 1–5% of the patients:
Sweating
Hypotension
Vomiting
Miosis
Headache
Nausea/Vomiting
Hypoventilation
The following adverse reactions were reported to have occurred in less than 1% of the patients:
CNS Effect: confusion, blurred vision, euphoria, weakness/fatigue, dry mouth, nervousness, depression, slurred speech, paresthesia.
Cardiovascular: hypertension, tachycardia, bradycardia.
Gastrointestinal: constipation.
Respiratory: dyspnea, cyanosis.
Dermatological: pruritus.
Ophthalmological: diplopia, visual abnormalities.
Miscellaneous: injection site reaction, urinary retention, dreaming, flushing/warmth, chills/cold, tinnitus, conjunctivitis, Wenckebach block, and psychosis.
Other effects observed infrequently include malaise, hallucinations, depersonalization, coma, dyspepsia, flatulence, apnea, rash, amblyopia, tremor, and pallor.

The following reactions have been reported to occur rarely: loss of appetite, dysphoria/agitation, diarrhea, urticaria, and convulsions/lack of muscle coordination.

Allergic Reactions: Cases of acute and chronic hypersensitivity to buprenorphine have been reported both in clinical trials and in the postmarketing experience of Buprenex and other buprenorphine- containing products. The most common signs and symptoms include rashes, hives, and pruritus. Cases of bronchospasm, angioneurotic edema, and anaphylactic shock have been reported. A history of hypersensitivity to buprenorphine is a contraindication to Buprenex.
In the United Kingdom, buprenorphine hydrochloride was made available under monitored release regulation during the first year of sale, and yielded data from 1,736 physicians on 9,123 patients (17,120 administrations). Data on 240 children under the age of 18 years were included in this monitored release program. No important new adverse effects attributable to buprenorphine hydrochloride were observed.

DRUG ABUSE AND DEPENDENCE

Buprenorphine hydrochloride is a partial agonist of the morphine type; i.e., it has certain opioid properties which may lead to psychic dependence of the morphine type due to an opiate-like euphoric component of the drug. Direct dependence studies have shown little physical dependence upon withdrawal of the drug. However, caution should be used in prescribing to individuals who are known to be drug abusers or ex-narcotic addicts. The drug may not substitute in acutely dependent narcotic addicts due to its antagonist component and may induce withdrawal symptoms.

OVERDOSAGE

Manifestations: Clinical experience with Buprenex overdosage has been insufficient to define the signs of this condition at this time. Although the antagonist activity of buprenorphine may become manifest at doses somewhat above the recommended therapeutic range, doses in the recommended therapeutic range may produce clinically significant respiratory depression in certain circumstances. (See WARNINGS.)
Treatment: The respiratory and cardiac status of the patients should be monitored carefully. Primary attention should be given to the reestablishment of adequate respiratory exchange through provision of a patent airway and institution of assisted or controlled ventilation. Oxygen, intravenous fluids, vasopressors, and other supportive measures should be employed as indicated. Doxapram, a respiratory stimulant, may be used. **NALOXONE MAY NOT BE EFFECTIVE IN REVERSING THE RESPIRATORY DEPRESSION PRODUCED BY BUPRENEX. THEREFORE, AS WITH OTHER POTENT OPIOIDS, THE PRIMARY MANAGEMENT OF OVERDOSE SHOULD BE THE REESTABLISHMENT OF ADEQUATE VENTILATION WITH MECHANICAL ASSISTANCE OF RESPIRATION, IF REQUIRED.**

DOSAGE AND ADMINISTRATION

Adults: The usual dosage for persons 13 years of age and over is 1 ml Buprenex (0.3 mg buprenorphine) given by deep intramuscular or slow (over at least 2 minutes) intravenous injection at up to 6-hour intervals, as needed. Repeat once (up to 0.3 mg) if required, 30 to 60 minutes after initial dosage, giving consideration to previous dose pharmacokinetics, and thereafter only as needed. In high-risk patients (e.g., elderly, debilitated, presence of respiratory disease, etc.) and/or in patients where other CNS depressants are present, such as in the immediate postoperative period, the dose should be reduced by approximately one-half. Extra caution should be exercised with the intravenous route of administration, particularly with the initial dose.
Occasionally, it may be necessary to administer single doses of up to 0.6 mg to adults depending on the severity of the pain and the response of the patient. This dose should only be given I.M. and only to adult patients who are not in a high risk category (see WARNINGS and PRECAUTIONS). At this time, there are insufficient data to recommend single doses greater than 0.6 mg for long-term use.
Children: Buprenex has been used in children 2–12 years of age at doses between 2–6 micrograms/kg of body weight given every 4–6 hours. There is insufficient experience to recommend a dose in infants below the age of two years, single doses greater than 6 micrograms/kg of body weight,

Continued on next page

Buprenex—Cont.

or the use of a repeat or second dose at 30–60 minutes (such as is used in adults). Since there is some evidence that not all children clear buprenorphine faster than adults, fixed interval or "round-the-clock" dosing should not be undertaken until the proper inter-dose interval has been established by clinical observation of the child. Physicians should recognize that, as with adults, some pediatric patients may not need to be remedicated for 6–8 hours.

Safety and Handling: Buprenex is supplied in sealed ampules and poses no known environmental risk to health care providers. Accidental dermal exposure should be treated by removal of any contaminated clothing and rinsing the affected area with water.

Buprenex is a potent narcotic, and like all drugs of this class has been associated with abuse and dependence among health care providers. To control the risk of diversion, it is recommended that measures appropriate to the health care setting be taken to provide rigid accounting, control of wastage, and restriction of access.

Parenteral drug products should be inspected visually for particulate matter and discoloration prior to administration, whenever solution and container permit.

HOW SUPPLIED

Buprenex (buprenorphine hydrochloride) is supplied in clear glass snap-ampuls of 1 ml (0.3 mg buprenorphine).

NDC 12496-0757-1

Avoid excessive heat (over 104°F or 40°C). Protect from prolonged exposure to light.

Manufactured by:
Reckitt Benckiser Healthcare (UK) Ltd
Hull, England HU8 7DS
UK

Distributed by:
Reckitt Benckiser Pharmaceuticals Inc.
Richmond, VA 23235

Buprenex ® is a trademark of Reckitt & Colman (Overseas) Limited.

REVISED November 2002

Shown in Product Identification Guide, page 331

SUBOXONE ℂⅢ ℞

*[sə*box'ōne]

(buprenorphine HCl and naloxone HCl dihydrate sublingual tablets)

SUBUTEX ℂⅢ ℞

[səb'ūtex]

(buprenorphine HCl sublingual tablets)

℞ only

Under the Drug Addiction Treatment Act of 2000 (DATA) codified at 21 U.S.C. 823(g), prescription use of this product in the treatment of opioid dependence is limited to physicians who meet certain qualifying requirements, and have notified the Secretary of Health and Human Services (HHS) of their intent to prescribe this product for the treatment of opioid dependence.

DESCRIPTION

SUBOXONE sublingual tablets contain buprenorphine HCl and naloxone HCl dihydrate at a ratio of 4:1 buprenorphine: naloxone (ratio of free bases).

SUBUTEX sublingual tablets contain buprenorphine HCl.

Buprenorphine is a partial agonist at the mu-opioid receptor and an antagonist at the kappa-opioid receptor. Naloxone is an antagonist at the mu-opioid receptor.

Buprenorphine is a Schedule III narcotic under the Controlled Substances Act.

Buprenorphine hydrochloride is a white powder, weakly acidic with limited solubility in water (17mg/mL). Chemically, buprenorphine is 17-(cyclopropylmethyl)-α-(1,1-dimethylethyl)-4, 5-epoxy-18, 19-dihydro-3-hydroxy-6-methoxy-α-methyl-6, 14-ethenomorphinan-7-methanol, hydrochloride [5α, 7α(S)]-. Buprenorphine hydrochloride has the molecular formula $C_{29}H_{41}NO_4HCl$ and the molecular weight is 504.10.

HO O N •HCl CH_3O HO CH_3 $C(CH_3)_3$

Naloxone hydrochloride is a white to slightly off-white powder and is soluble in water, in dilute acids and in strong alkali. Chemically, naloxone is 17-Allyl-4,5 α-epoxy-3, 14-dihydroxymorphinan-6-one hydrochloride. Naloxone hydrochloride has the molecular formula $C_{19}H_{21}NO_4HCl\ .2H_2O$ and the molecular weight is 399.87.

[See chemical structure at top of next column]

SUBOXONE is an uncoated **hexagonal orange tablet** intended for sublingual administration. It is available in two dosage strengths, 2mg buprenorphine with 0.5mg naloxone, and 8mg buprenorphine with 2mg naloxone free bases.

HO O N OH O • HCl • 2 H_2O

Each tablet also contains lactose, mannitol, cornstarch, povidone K30, citric acid, sodium citrate, FD&C Yellow No.6 color, magnesium stearate, and the tablets also contain Acesulfame K sweetener and a lemon/lime flavor.

SUBUTEX is an uncoated **oval white tablet** intended for sublingual administration. It is available in two dosage strengths, 2mg buprenorphine and 8mg buprenorphine free base. Each tablet also contains lactose, mannitol, cornstarch, povidone K30, citric acid, sodium citrate and magnesium stearate.

CLINICAL PHARMACOLOGY

Subjective Effects:

Comparisons of buprenorphine with full agonists such as methadone and hydromorphone suggest that sublingual buprenorphine produces typical opioid agonist effects which are limited by a ceiling effect.

In non-dependent subjects, acute sublingual doses of SUBOXONE tablets produced opioid agonist effects, which reached a maximum between doses of 8 mg and 16mg of SUBUTEX. The effects of 16mg SUBOXONE were similar to those produced by 16mg SUBUTEX (buprenorphine alone).

Opioid agonist ceiling effects were also observed in a double-blind, parallel group, dose ranging comparison of single doses of buprenorphine sublingual solution (1, 2, 4, 8, 16, or 32 mg), placebo, and a full agonist control at various doses. The treatments were given in ascending dose order at intervals of at least one week to 16 opioid-experienced, non-dependent subjects. Both drugs produced typical opioid agonist effects. For all the measures for which the drugs produced an effect, buprenorphine produced a dose-related response but, in each case, there was a dose that produced no further effect. In contrast, the highest dose of the full agonist control always produced the greatest effects. Agonist objective rating scores remained elevated for the higher doses of buprenorphine (8-32 mg) longer than for the lower doses and did not return to baseline until 48 hours after drug administrations. The onset of effects appeared more rapidly with buprenorphine than with the full agonist control, with most doses nearing peak effect after 100 minutes for buprenorphine compared to 150 minutes for the full agonist control.

Physiologic Effects:

Buprenorphine in intravenous (2mg, 4mg, 8mg, 12mg and 16 mg) and sublingual (12mg) doses has been administered to non-dependent subjects to examine cardiovascular, respiratory and subjective effects at doses comparable to those used for treatment of opioid dependence. Compared with placebo, there were no statistically significant differences among any of the treatment conditions for blood pressure, heart rate, respiratory rate, O_2 saturation or skin temperature across time. Systolic BP was higher in the 8 mg group than placebo (3 hour AUC values). Minimum and maximum effects were similar across all treatments. Subjects remained responsive to low voice and responded to computer prompts. Some subjects showed irritability, but no other changes were observed.

The respiratory effects of sublingual buprenorphine were compared with the effects of methadone in a double-blind, parallel group, dose ranging comparison of single doses of buprenorphine sublingual solution (1, 2, 4, 8, 16, or 32 mg) and oral methadone (15, 30, 45, or 60 mg) in non-dependent, opioid-experienced volunteers. In this study, hypoventilation not requiring medical intervention was reported more frequently after buprenorphine doses of 4 mg and higher than after methadone. Both drugs decreased O_2 saturation to the same degree.

Effect of Naloxone:

Physiologic and subjective effects following acute sublingual administration of SUBOXONE and SUBUTEX tablets were similar at equivalent dose levels of buprenorphine. Naloxone, in the SUBOXONE formulation, had no clinically significant effect when administered by the sublingual route, although blood levels of the drug were measurable. SUBOXONE, when administered sublingually even to an opioid-dependent population, was recognized as an opioid agonist, whereas when administered intramuscularly, combinations of buprenorphine with naloxone produced opioid antagonist actions similar to naloxone. In methadone-maintained patients and heroin-dependent subjects, intravenous administration of buprenorphine/naloxone combinations precipitated opioid withdrawal and was perceived as unpleasant and dysphoric. In morphine-stabilized subjects, intravenously administered combinations of buprenorphine with naloxone produced opioid antagonist and withdrawal effects that were ratio-dependent; the most intense withdrawal effects were produced by 2:1 and 4:1 ratios, less intense by an 8:1 ratio. SUBOXONE tablets contain buprenorphine with naloxone at a ratio of 4:1.

Pharmacokinetics:

Absorption:

Plasma levels of buprenorphine increased with the sublingual dose of SUBUTEX and SUBOXONE, and plasma levels of naloxone increased with the sublingual dose of SUBOXONE (Table 1). There was a wide inter-patient variability in the sublingual absorption of buprenorphine and naloxone, but within subjects the variability was low. Both C_{max} and AUC of buprenorphine increased in a linear fashion with the increase in dose (in the range of 4 to 16 mg), although the increase was not directly dose-proportional.

Naloxone did not affect the pharmacokinetics of buprenorphine and both SUBUTEX and SUBOXONE deliver similar plasma concentrations of buprenorphine. The levels of naloxone were too low to assess dose-proportionality. At the three naloxone doses of 1 mg, 2 mg, and 4 mg, levels above the limit of quantitation (0.05 ng/mL) were not detected beyond 2 hours in seven of eight subjects. In one individual, at the 4mg dose, the last measurable concentration was at 8 hours. Within each subject (for most of the subjects), across the doses there was a trend toward an increase in naloxone concentrations with increase in dose. Mean peak naloxone levels ranged from 0.11 to 0.28ng/ml in the dose range of 1-4 mg.

Table 1. Pharmacokinetic parameters of buprenorphine after the administration of 4 mg, 8mg, and 16 mg Suboxone® doses and 16mg Subutex® dose (mean (%CV)).

Pharmacokinetic Parameter	Suboxone® 4 mg	Suboxone® 8 mg	Suboxone® 16 mg	Subutex® 16 mg
C_{max}, ng/mL	1.84 (39)	3.0 (51)	5.95 (38)	5.47 (23)
AUC_{0-48}, hour*ng/mL	12.52 (35)	20.22 (43)	34.89 (33)	32.63 (25)

Distribution:

Buprenorphine is approximately 96% protein bound, primarily to alpha and beta globulin.

Naloxone is approximately 45% protein bound, primarily to albumin.

Metabolism:

Buprenorphine undergoes both N-dealkylation to norbuprenorphine and glucuronidation. The N-dealkylation pathway is mediated by cytochrome P-450 3A4 isozyme. Norbuprenorphine, an active metabolite, can further undergo glucuronidation.

Naloxone undergoes direct glucuronidation to naloxone 3-glucuronide as well as N-dealkylation, and reduction of the 6-oxo group.

Elimination:

A mass balance study of buprenorphine showed complete recovery of radiolabel in urine (30%) and feces (69%) collected up to 11 days after dosing. Almost all of the dose was accounted for in terms of buprenorphine, norbuprenorphine, and two unidentified buprenorphine metabolites. In urine, most of buprenorphine and norbuprenorphine was conjugated (buprenorphine, 1% free and 9.4% conjugated; norbuprenorphine, 2.7% free and 11% conjugated). In feces, almost all of the buprenorphine and norbuprenorphine were free (buprenorphine, 33% free and 5% conjugated; norbuprenorphine, 21% free and 2% conjugated).

Buprenorphine has a mean elimination half-life from plasma of 37 h.

Naloxone has a mean elimination half-life from plasma of 1.1 h.

Special Populations:

Hepatic Disease:

The effect of hepatic impairment on the pharmacokinetics of buprenorphine and naloxone is unknown. Since both drugs are extensively metabolized, the plasma levels will be expected to be higher in patients with moderate and severe hepatic impairment. However, it is not known whether both drugs are affected to the same degree. Therefore, in patients with hepatic impairment dosage should be adjusted and patients should be observed for symptoms of precipitated opioid withdrawal.

Renal Disease:

No differences in buprenorphine pharmacokinetics were observed between 9 dialysis-dependent and 6 normal patients following intravenous administration of 0.3mg buprenorphine.

The effects of renal failure on naloxone pharmacokinetics are unknown.

Drug-drug interactions:

CYP 3A4 Inhibitors and Inducers: A pharmacokinetic interaction study of ketoconazole (400 mg/day), a potent inhibitor of CYP 3A4, in 12 patients stabilized on SUBOXONE [8mg (n=1) or 12mg (n=5) or 16mg (n=6)] resulted in increases in buprenorphine mean Cmax values (from 4.3 to 9.8, 6.3 to 14.4 and 9.0 to 17.1) and mean AUC values (from 30.9 to 46.9, 41.9 to 83.2 and 52.3 to 120) respectively. Subjects receiving SUBUTEX or SUBOXONE should be closely monitored and may require dose-reduction if inhibitors of CYP 3A4 such as azole antifungal agents (e.g. ketoconazole), macrolide antibiotics (e.g., erythromycin) and HIV protease inhibitors (e.g. ritonavir, indinavir and saquinavir) are co-administered. The interaction of buprenorphine with CYP 3A4 inducers has not been investigated; therefore it is recommended that patients receiving SUBUTEX or SUBOXONE should be closely monitored if inducers of CYP 3A4 (e.g. phenobarbital, carbamazepine, phenytoin, rifampicin) are co-administered (SEE WARNINGS).

CLINICAL STUDIES

Clinical data on the safety and efficacy of SUBOXONE and SUBUTEX are derived from studies of buprenorphine sublingual tablet formulations, with and without naloxone, and from studies of sublingual administration of a more bioavailable ethanolic solution of buprenorphine.

SUBOXONE tablets have been studied in 575 patients, SUBUTEX tablets in 1834 patients and buprenorphine sublingual solutions in 2470 patients. A total of 1270 females have received buprenorphine in clinical trials. Dosing recommendations are based on data from one trial of both tablet formulations and two trials of the ethanolic solution. All trials used buprenorphine in conjunction with psychosocial counseling as part of a comprehensive addiction treatment program. There have been no clinical studies conducted to assess the efficacy of buprenorphine as the only component of treatment.

In a double blind placebo- and active controlled study, 326 heroin-addicted subjects were randomly assigned to either SUBOXONE 16 mg per day, 16 mg SUBUTEX per day or placebo tablets. For subjects randomized to either active treatment, dosing began with one 8 mg tablet of SUBUTEX on Day 1, followed by 16 mg (two 8 mg tablets) of SUBUTEX on Day 2. On Day 3, those randomized to receive SUBOXONE were switched to the combination tablet. Subjects randomized to placebo received one placebo tablet on Day 1 and two placebo tablets per day thereafter for four weeks. Subjects were seen daily in the clinic (Monday through Friday) for dosing and efficacy assessments. Take-home doses were provided for weekends. Subjects were instructed to hold the medication under the tongue for approximately 5 to 10 minutes until completely dissolved. Subjects received one hour of individual counseling per week and a single session of HIV education. The primary study comparison was to assess the efficacy of SUBUTEX and SUBOXONE individually against placebo. The percentage of thrice-weekly urine samples that were negative for non-study opioids was statistically higher for both SUBUTEX and SUBOXONE, than for placebo.

In a double-blind, double-dummy, parallel-group study comparing buprenorphine ethanolic solution to a full agonist active control, 162 subjects were randomized to receive the ethanolic sublingual solution of buprenorphine at 8 mg/day (a dose which is roughly comparable to a dose of 12 mg/day of SUBUTEX or SUBOXONE), or two relatively low doses of active control, one of which was low enough to serve as an alternative to placebo, during a 3-10 day induction phase, a 16-week maintenance phase and a 7-week detoxification phase. Buprenorphine was titrated to maintenance dose by Day 3; active control doses were titrated more gradually.

Maintenance dosing continued through Week 17, and then medications were tapered by approximately 20-30% per week over Weeks 18-24, with placebo dosing for the last two weeks. Subjects received individual and/or group counseling weekly.

Based on retention in treatment and the percentage of thrice-weekly urine samples negative for non-study opioids, buprenorphine was more effective than the low dose of the control, in keeping heroin addicts in treatment and in reducing their use of opioids while in treatment. The effectiveness of buprenorphine, 8 mg per day was similar to that of the moderate active control dose, but equivalence was not demonstrated.

In a dose-controlled, double-blind, parallel-group, 16-week study, 731 subjects were randomized to receive one of four doses of buprenorphine ethanolic solution. Buprenorphine was titrated to maintenance doses over 1-4 days (Table 2) and continued for 16 weeks. Subjects received at least one session of AIDS education and additional counseling ranging from one hour per month to one hour per week, depending on site.

Table 2. Doses of Sublingual Buprenorphine Solution used for Induction in a Double-Blind Dose Ranging Study

Target Dose of Buprenorphine*	Induction Dose			Maintenance dose
	Day 1	Day 2	Day 3	
1 mg	1 mg	1 mg	1 mg	1 mg
4 mg	2 mg	4 mg	4 mg	4 mg
8 mg	2 mg	4 mg	8 mg	8 mg
16 mg	2 mg	4 mg	8 mg	16 mg

*Sublingual solution. Doses in this table cannot necessarily be delivered in tablet form, but for comparison purposes:
2 mg solution would be roughly equivalent to 3 mg tablet
4 mg solution would be roughly equivalent to 6 mg tablet
8 mg solution would be roughly equivalent to 12 mg tablet
16 mg solution would be roughly equivalent to 24 mg tablet

Based on retention in treatment and the percentage of thrice-weekly urine samples negative for non-study opioids, the three highest tested doses were superior to the 1mg dose. Therefore, this study showed that a range of buprenorphine doses may be effective. The 1mg dose of buprenorphine sublingual solution can be considered to be somewhat lower than a 2 mg tablet dose. The other doses used in the study encompass a range of tablet doses from approximately 6 mg to approximately 24 mg.

INDICATIONS AND USAGE

SUBOXONE and SUBUTEX are indicated for the treatment of opioid dependence.

CONTRAINDICATIONS

SUBOXONE and SUBUTEX should not be administered to patients who have been shown to be hypersensitive to buprenorphine, and SUBOXONE should not be administered to patients who have been shown to be hypersensitive to naloxone.

WARNINGS

Respiratory Depression:

Significant respiratory depression has been associated with buprenorphine, particularly by the intravenous route. A number of deaths have occurred when addicts have intravenously misused buprenorphine, usually with benzodiazepines concomitantly. Deaths have also been reported in association with concomitant administration of buprenorphine with other depressants such as alcohol or other opioids. Patients should be warned of the potential danger of the self-administration of benzodiazepines or other depressants while under treatment with SUBUTEX or SUBOXONE.

IN THE CASE OF OVERDOSE, THE PRIMARY MANAGEMENT SHOULD BE THE RE-ESTABLISHMENT OF ADEQUATE VENTILATION WITH MECHANICAL ASSISTANCE OF RESPIRATION, IF REQUIRED. NALOXONE MAY NOT BE EFFECTIVE IN REVERSING ANY RESPIRATORY DEPRESSION PRODUCED BY BUPRENORPHINE.

SUBOXONE and SUBUTEX should be used with caution in patients with compromised respiratory function (e.g., chronic obstructive pulmonary disease, cor pulmonale, decreased respiratory reserve, hypoxia, hypercapnia, or preexisting respiratory depression).

CNS Depression:

Patients receiving buprenorphine in the presence of other narcotic analgesics, general anesthetics, benzodiazepines, phenothiazines, other tranquilizers, sedative/hypnotics or other CNS depressants (including alcohol) may exhibit increased CNS depression. When such combined therapy is contemplated, reduction of the dose of one or both agents should be considered.

Dependence:

Buprenorphine is a partial agonist at the mu-opiate receptor and chronic administration produces dependence of the opioid type, characterized by withdrawal upon abrupt discontinuation or rapid taper. The withdrawal syndrome is milder than seen with full agonists, and may be delayed in onset

Hepatitis, hepatic events:

Cases of cytolytic hepatitis and hepatitis with jaundice have been observed in the addict population receiving buprenorphine both in clinical trials and in post-marketing adverse event reports. The spectrum of abnormalities ranges from transient asymptomatic elevations in hepatic transaminases to case reports of hepatic failure, hepatic necrosis, hepatorenal syndrome, and hepatic encephalopathy. In many cases, the presence of pre-existing liver enzyme abnormalities, infection with hepatitis B or hepatitis C virus, concomitant usage of other potentially hepatotoxic drugs, and ongoing injecting drug use may have played a causative or contributory role. In other cases, insufficient data were available to determine the etiology of the abnormality. The possibility exists that buprenorphine had a causative or contributory role in the development of the hepatic abnormality in some cases. Measurements of liver function tests prior to initiation of treatment is recommended to establish a baseline. Periodic monitoring of liver function tests during treatment is also recommended. A biological and etiological evaluation is recommended when a hepatic event is suspected. Depending on the case, the drug should be carefully discontinued to prevent withdrawal symptoms and a return to illicit drug use, and strict monitoring of the patient should be initiated.

Allergic Reactions:

Cases of acute and chronic hypersensitivity to buprenorphine have been reported both in clinical trials and in the post-marketing experience. The most common signs and symptoms include rashes, hives, and pruritus. Cases of bronchospasm, angioneurotic edema, and anaphylactic shock have been reported. A history of hypersensitivity to buprenorphine is a contraindication to Subutex or Suboxone use. A history of hypersensitivity to naloxone is a contraindication to Suboxone use.

Use in Ambulatory Patients:

SUBOXONE and SUBUTEX may impair the mental or physical abilities required for the performance of potentially dangerous tasks such as driving a car or operating machinery, especially during drug induction and dose adjustment. Patients should be cautioned about operating hazardous machinery, including automobiles, until they are reasonably certain that buprenorphine therapy does not adversely affect their ability to engage in such activities. Like other opioids, SUBOXONE and SUBUTEX may produce orthostatic hypotension in ambulatory patients.

Head Injury and Increased Intracranial Pressure:

SUBOXONE and SUBUTEX, like other potent opioids, may elevate cerebrospinal fluid pressure and should be used with caution in patients with head injury, intracranial lesions and other circumstances where cerebrospinal pressure may be increased. SUBOXONE and SUBUTEX can produce miosis and changes in the level of consciousness that may interfere with patient evaluation.

Opioid withdrawal effects:

Because it contains naloxone, SUBOXONE is highly likely to produce marked and intense withdrawal symptoms if misused parenterally by individuals dependent on opioid agonists such as heroin, morphine, or methadone. Sublingually, SUBOXONE may cause opioid withdrawal symptoms in such persons if administered before the agonist effects of the opioid have subsided.

PRECAUTIONS

General:

SUBOXONE and SUBUTEX should be administered with caution in elderly or debilitated patients and those with severe impairment of hepatic, pulmonary, or renal function; myxedema or hypothyroidism, adrenal cortical insufficiency (e.g., Addison's disease); CNS depression or coma; toxic psychoses; prostatic hypertrophy or urethral stricture; acute alcoholism; delirium tremens; or kyphoscoliosis.

The effect of hepatic impairment on the pharmacokinetics of buprenorphine and naloxone is unknown. Since both drugs are extensively metabolized, the plasma levels will be expected to be higher in patients with moderate and severe hepatic impairment. However, it is not known whether both drugs are affected to the same degree. Therefore, dosage should be adjusted and patients should be watched for symptoms of precipitated opioid withdrawal.

Buprenorphine has been shown to increase intracholedochal pressure, as do other opioids, and thus should be administered with caution to patients with dysfunction of the biliary tract.

As with other mu-opioid receptor agonists, the administration of SUBOXONE or SUBUTEX may obscure the diagnosis or clinical course of patients with acute abdominal conditions.

Drug Interactions:

Buprenorphine is metabolized to norbuprenorphine by cytochrome CYP 3A4. Because CYP 3A4 inhibitors may increase plasma concentrations of buprenorphine, patients already on CYP 3A4 inhibitors such as azole antifungals (e.g. ketoconazole), macrolide antibiotics (e.g. erythromycin), and HIV protease inhibitors (e.g. ritonavir, indinavir and saquinavir) should have their dose of SUBUTEX or SUBOXONE adjusted.

Based on anecdotal reports, there may be an interaction between buprenorphine and benzodiazepines. There have been a number of reports in the post-marketing experience of coma and death associated with the concomitant intravenous misuse of buprenorphine and benzodiazepines by addicts. In many of these cases, buprenorphine was misused by self-injection of crushed SUBUTEX tablets. SUBUTEX and SUBOXONE should be prescribed with caution to patients on benzodiazepines or other drugs that act on the central nervous system, regardless of whether these drugs are taken on the advice of a physician or are taken as drugs of abuse. Patients should be warned of the potential danger of the intravenous self-administration of benzodiazepines while under treatment with SUBOXONE or SUBUTEX.

Information for Patients:

Patients should inform their family members that, in the event of emergency, the treating physician or emergency room staff should be informed that the patient is physically dependent on narcotics and that the patient is being treated with SUBOXONE or SUBUTEX.

Patients should be cautioned that a serious overdose and death may occur if benzodiazepines, sedatives, tranquilizers, antidepressants, or alcohol are taken at the same time as SUBOXONE or SUBUTEX.

SUBOXONE and SUBUTEX may impair the mental or physical abilities required for the performance of potentially dangerous tasks such as driving a car or operating machinery, especially during drug induction and dose adjustment. Patients should be cautioned about operating hazardous machinery, including automobiles, until they are reasonably certain that buprenorphine therapy does not adversely affect their ability to engage in such activities. Like other opioids, SUBOXONE and SUBUTEX may produce orthostatic hypotension in ambulatory patients.

Patients should consult their physician if other prescription medications are currently being used or are prescribed for future use.

Carcinogenesis, Mutagenesis and Impairment of Fertility:

Carcinogenicity: Carcinogenicity data on SUBOXONE are not available. Carcinogenicity studies of buprenorphine were conducted in Sprague-Dawley rats and CD-1 mice. Buprenorphine was administered in the diet to rats at doses of 0.6, 5.5, and 56 mg/kg/day (estimated exposure was approximately 0.4, 3 and 35 times the recommended human daily sublingual dose of 16 mg on a mg/m^2 basis) for 27 months. Statistically significant dose-related increases in testicular interstitial (Leydig's) cell tumors occurred, according to the trend test adjusted for survival. Pair-wise comparison of the high dose against control failed to show statistical significance. In an 86-week study in CD-1 mice, buprenorphine was not carcinogenic at dietary doses up to 100 mg/kg/day (estimated exposure was approximately 30

Continued on next page

Suboxone/Subutex—Cont.

times the recommended human daily sublingual dose of 16 mg on a mg/m^2 basis).

Mutagenicity:

SUBOXONE: The 4:1 combination of buprenorphine and naloxone was not mutagenic in a bacterial mutation assay (Ames test) using four strains of *S. typhimurium* and two strains of *E. coli*. The combination was not clastogenic in an *in vitro* cytogenetic assay in human lymphocytes, or in an intravenous micronucleus test in the rat.

SUBUTEX: Buprenorphine was studied in a series of tests utilizing gene, chromosome, and DNA interactions in both prokaryotic and eukaryotic systems. Results were negative in yeast (*Saccharomyces cerevisiae*) for recombinant, gene convertant, or forward mutations; negative in *Bacillus subtilis* "rec" assay, negative for clastogenicity in CHO cells, Chinese hamster bone marrow and spermatogonia cells, and negative in the mouse lymphoma L5178Y assay. Results were equivocal in the Ames test: negative in studies in two laboratories, but positive for frame shift mutation at a high dose (5mg/plate) in a third study. Results were positive in the Green-Tweets (*E. coli*) survival test, positive in a DNA synthesis inhibition (DSI) test with testicular tissue from mice, for both in vivo and in vitro incorporation of [^{3}H]thymidine, and positive in unscheduled DNA synthesis (UDS) test using testicular cells from mice.

Impairment of Fertility:

SUBOXONE: Dietary administration of SUBOXONE in the rat at dose levels of 500 ppm or greater (equivalent to approximately 47 mg/kg/day or greater; estimated exposure was approximately 28 times the recommended human daily sublingual dose of 16 mg on a mg/m^2 basis) produced a reduction in fertility demonstrated by reduced female conception rates. A dietary dose of 100 ppm (equivalent to approximately 10 mg/kg/day; estimated exposure was approximately 6 times the recommended human daily sublingual dose of 16 mg on a mg/m^2 basis) had no adverse effect on fertility.

SUBUTEX: Reproduction studies of buprenorphine in rats demonstrated no evidence of impaired fertility at daily oral doses up to 80mg/kg/day (estimated exposure was approximately 50 times the recommended human daily sublingual dose of 16 mg on a mg/m^2 basis) or up to 5mg/kg/day *im* or *sc* (estimated exposure was approximately 3 times the recommended human daily sublingual dose of 16 mg on a mg/m^2 basis).

Pregnancy:

Pregnancy Category C:

Teratogenic effects:

SUBOXONE: Effects on embryo-fetal development were studied in Sprague-Dawley rats and Russian white rabbits following oral (1:1) and intramuscular (3:2) administration of mixtures of buprenorphine and naloxone. Following oral administration to rats and rabbits, no teratogenic effects were observed at doses up to 250 mg/kg/day and 40 mg/kg/day, respectively (estimated exposure was approximately 150 times and 50 times, respectively, the recommended human daily sublingual dose of 16 mg on a mg/m^2 basis). No definitive drug-related teratogenic effects were observed in rats and rabbits at intramuscular doses up to 30 mg/kg/day (estimated exposure was approximately 20 times and 35 times, respectively, the recommended human daily dose of 16 mg on a mg/m^2 basis). Acephalus was observed in one rabbit fetus from the low-dose group and omphacele was observed in two rabbit fetuses from the same litter in the mid-dose group; no findings were observed in fetuses from the high-dose group. Following oral administration to the rat, dose-related post-implantation losses, evidenced by increases in the numbers of early resorptions with consequent reductions in the numbers of fetuses, were observed at doses of 10 mg/kg/day or greater (estimated exposure was approximately 6 times the recommended human daily sublingual dose of 16 mg on a mg/m^2 basis). In the rabbit, increased post-implantation losses occurred at an oral dose of 40 mg/kg/day. Following intramuscular administration in the rat and the rabbit, post-implantation losses, as evidenced by decreases in live fetuses and increases in resorptions, occurred at 30 mg/kg/day.

SUBUTEX: Buprenorphine was not teratogenic in rats or rabbits after *im* or *sc* doses up to 5 mg/kg/day (estimated exposure was approximately 3 and 6 times, respectively, the recommended human daily sublingual dose of 16 mg on a mg/m^2 basis), after *iv* doses up to 0.8 mg/kg/day (estimated exposure was approximately 0.5 times and equal to, respectively, the recommended human daily sublingual dose of 16 mg on a mg/m^2 basis), or after oral doses up to 160 mg/kg/day in rats (estimated exposure was approximately 95 times the recommended human daily sublingual dose of 16 mg on a mg/m^2 basis) and 25 mg/kg/day in rabbits (estimated exposure was approximately 30 times the recommended human daily sublingual dose of 16 mg on a mg/m^2 basis). Significant increases in skeletal abnormalities (e.g., extra thoracic vertebra or thoraco-lumbar ribs) were noted in rats after *sc* administration of 1 mg/kg/day and up (estimated exposure was approximately 0.6 times the recommended human daily sublingual dose of 16 mg on a mg/m^2 basis), but were not observed at oral doses up to 160 mg/kg/day. Increases in skeletal abnormalities in rabbits after *im* administration of 5 mg/kg/day (estimated exposure was approximately 6 times the recommended human daily sublingual dose of 16 mg on a mg/m^2 basis) or oral administration of 1 mg/kg/day or greater (estimated exposure was approximately equal to the recommended human daily sublingual dose of 16 mg on a mg/m^2 basis) were not statistically significant.

In rabbits, buprenorphine produced statistically significant pre-implantation losses at oral doses of 1 mg/kg/day or greater and post-implantation losses that were statistically significant at *iv* doses of 0.2 mg/kg/day or greater (estimated exposure was approximately 0.3 times the recommended human daily sublingual dose of 16 mg on a mg/m^2 basis).

There are no adequate and well-controlled studies of SUBOXONE or SUBUTEX in pregnant women. SUBOXONE or SUBUTEX should only be used during pregnancy if the potential benefit justifies the potential risk to the fetus.

Non-teratogenic effects:

Dystocia was noted in pregnant rats treated *im* with buprenorphine 5 mg/kg/day (approximately 3 times the recommended human daily sublingual dose of 16 mg on a mg/m^2 basis). Both fertility and peri- and postnatal development studies with buprenorphine in rats indicated increases in neonatal mortality after oral doses of 0.8 mg/kg/day and up (approximately 0.5 times the recommended human daily sublingual dose of 16 mg on a mg/m^2 basis), after *im* doses of 0.5 mg/kg/day and up (approximately 0.3 times the recommended human daily sublingual dose of 16 mg on a mg/m^2 basis), and after *sc* doses of 0.1 mg/kg/day and up (approximately 0.06 times the recommended human daily sublingual dose of 16 mg on a mg/m^2 basis). Delays in the occurrence of righting reflex and startle response were noted in rat pups at an oral dose of 80 mg/kg/day (approximately 50 times the recommended human daily sublingual dose of 16 mg on a mg/m^2 basis).

Neonatal Withdrawal:

Neonatal withdrawal has been reported in the infants of women treated with SUBUTEX during pregnancy. From post-marketing reports, the time to onset of neonatal withdrawal symptoms ranged from Day 1 to Day 8 of life with most occurring on Day 1. Adverse events associated with neonatal withdrawal syndrome included hypertonia, neonatal tremor, neonatal agitation, and myoclonus. There have been rare reports of convulsions and in one case, apnea and bradycardia were also reported.

Nursing Mothers:

An apparent lack of milk production during general reproduction studies with buprenorphine in rats caused decreased viability and lactation indices. Use of high doses of sublingual buprenorphine in pregnant women showed that buprenorphine passes into the mother's milk. Breast-feeding is therefore not advised in mothers treated with SUBUTEX or SUBOXONE.

Pediatric Use:

SUBOXONE and SUBUTEX are not recommended for use in pediatric patients. The safety and effectiveness of SUBOXONE and SUBUTEX in patients below the age of 16 have not been established.

ADVERSE REACTIONS

The safety of SUBOXONE has been evaluated in 497 opioid-dependent subjects. The prospective evaluation of SUBOXONE was supported by clinical trials using SUBUTEX (buprenorphine tablets without naloxone) and other trials using buprenorphine sublingual solutions. In total, safety data are available from 3214 opioid-dependent subjects exposed to buprenorphine at doses in the range used in treatment of opioid addiction.

Few differences in adverse event profile were noted between SUBOXONE and SUBUTEX or buprenorphine administered as a sublingual solution.

In a comparative study, adverse event profiles were similar for subjects treated with 16 mg SUBOXONE or 16mg SUBUTEX. The following adverse events were reported to occur by at least 5% of patients in a 4-week study (Table 3). [See table 3 at left]

The adverse event profile of buprenorphine was also characterized in the dose-controlled study of buprenorphine solution, over a range of doses in four months of treatment. Table 4 shows adverse events reported by at least 5% of subjects in any dose group in the dose-controlled study.

[See table 4 on next page]

Table 3. Adverse Events (≥5%) by Body System and Treatment Group in a 4-week Study

Body System/Adverse Event (COSTART Terminology)	N (%) SUBOXONE 16 mg/day N = 107	N (%) SUBUTEX 16 mg/day N = 103	N (%) Placebo N = 107
Body As A Whole			
Asthenia	7 (6.5%)	5 (4.9%)	7 (6.5%)
Chills	8 (7.5%)	8 (7.8%)	8 (7.5%)
Headache	39 (36.4%)	30 (29.1%)	24 (22.4%)
Infection	6 (5.6%)	12 (11.7%)	7 (6.5%)
Pain	24 (22.4%)	19 (18.4%)	20 (18.7%)
Pain Abdomen	12 (11.2%)	12 (11.7%)	7 (6.5%)
Pain Back	4 (3.7%)	8 (7.8%)	12 (11.2%)
Withdrawal Syndrome	27 (25.2%)	19 (18.4%)	40 (37.4%)
Cardiovascular System			
Vasodilation	10 (9.3%)	4 (3.9%)	7 (6.5%)
Digestive System			
Constipation	13 (12.1%)	8 (7.8%)	3 (2.8%)
Diarrhea	4 (3.7%)	5 (4.9%)	16 (15.0%)
Nausea	16 (15.0%)	14 (13.6%)	12 (11.2%)
Vomiting	8 (7.5%)	8 (7.8%)	5 (4.7%)
Nervous System			
Insomnia	15 (14.0%)	22 (21.4%)	17 (15.9%)
Respiratory System			
Rhinitis	5 (4.7%)	10 (9.7%)	14 (13.1%)
Skin And Appendages			
Sweating	15 (14.0%)	13 (12.6%)	11 (10.3%)

DRUG ABUSE AND DEPENDENCE

SUBOXONE and SUBUTEX are controlled as Schedule III narcotics under the Controlled Substances Act.

Buprenorphine is a partial agonist at the mu-opioid receptor and chronic administration produces dependence of the opioid type, characterized by moderate withdrawal upon abrupt discontinuation or rapid taper. The withdrawal syndrome is milder than seen with full agonists, and may be delayed in onset (SEE WARNINGS).

Neonatal withdrawal has been reported in the infants of women treated with SUBUTEX during pregnancy (See PRECAUTIONS)

SUBOXONE contains naloxone and if misused parenterally, is highly likely to produce marked and intense withdrawal symptoms in subjects dependent on other opioid agonists.

OVERDOSAGE

Manifestations:

Manifestations of acute overdose include pinpoint pupils, sedation, hypotension, respiratory depression and death.

Treatment:

The respiratory and cardiac status of the patient should be monitored carefully. In the event of depression of respiratory or cardiac function, primary attention should be given to the re-establishment of adequate respiratory exchange through provision of a patent airway and institution of assisted or controlled ventilation. Oxygen, intravenous fluids, vasopressors, and other supportive measures should be employed as indicated.

IN THE CASE OF OVERDOSE, THE PRIMARY MANAGEMENT SHOULD BE THE RE-ESTABLISHMENT OF ADEQUATE VENTILATION WITH MECHANICAL ASSISTANCE OF RESPIRATION, IF REQUIRED. NALOXONE MAY NOT BE EFFECTIVE IN REVERSING ANY RESPIRATORY DEPRESSION PRODUCED BY BUPRENORPHINE.

High doses of naloxone hydrochloride, 10-35 mg/70 kg may be of limited value in the management of buprenorphine overdose. Doxapram (a respiratory stimulant) also has been used.

DOSAGE AND ADMINISTRATION

SUBUTEX or SUBOXONE is administered sublingually as a single daily dose in the range of 12 to 16 mg/day. When taken sublingually, SUBOXONE and SUBUTEX have similar clinical effects and are interchangeable. There are no adequate and well-controlled studies using SUBOXONE as initial medication. SUBUTEX contains no naloxone and is preferred for use during induction. Following induction, SUBOXONE, due to the presence of naloxone, is preferred when clinical use includes unsupervised administration. The use of SUBUTEX for unsupervised administration should be limited to those patients who cannot tolerate SUBOXONE, for example those patients who have been shown to be hypersensitive to naloxone.

Method of administration:

SUBOXONE and SUBUTEX tablets should be placed under the tongue until they are dissolved. For doses requiring the use of more than two tablets, patients are advised to either place all the tablets at once or alternatively (if they cannot fit in more than two tablets comfortably) place two tablets at a time under the tongue. Either way, the patients should continue to hold the tablets under the tongue until they dissolve; swallowing the tablets reduces the bioavailability of the drug. To ensure consistency in bioavailability, patients should follow the same manner of dosing with continued use of the product.

Induction:

Prior to induction, consideration should be given to the type of opioid dependence (i.e. long- or short-acting opioid), the time since last opioid use, and the degree or level of opioid dependence. To avoid precipitating withdrawal, induction with SUBUTEX should be undertaken when objective and clear signs of withdrawal are evident.

In a one-month study of SUBOXONE tablets induction was conducted with SUBUTEX tablets. Patients received 8mg of SUBUTEX on day 1 and 16mg SUBUTEX on day 2. From day 3 onward, patients received SUBOXONE tablets at the same buprenorphine dose as day 2. Induction in the studies of buprenorphine solution was accomplished over 3-4 days, depending on the target dose. In some studies, gradual induction over several days led to a high rate of drop-out of buprenorphine patients during the induction period. Therefore it is recommended that an adequate maintenance dose, titrated to clinical effectiveness, should be achieved as rapidly as possible to prevent undue opioid withdrawal symptoms.

Patients taking heroin or other short-acting opioids:

At treatment initiation, the dose of SUBUTEX should be administered at least 4 hours after the patient last used opioids or preferably when early signs of opioid withdrawal appear.

Patients on methadone or other long-acting opioids:

There is little controlled experience with the transfer of methadone-maintained patients to buprenorphine. Available evidence suggests that withdrawal symptoms are possible during induction to buprenorphine treatment. Withdrawal appears more likely in patients maintained on higher doses of methadone (>30mg) and when the first buprenorphine dose is administered shortly after the last methadone dose.

Maintenance:

SUBOXONE is the preferred medication for maintenance treatment due to the presence of naloxone in the formulation.

Adjusting the dose until the maintenance dose is achieved:

The recommended target dose of SUBOXONE is 16 mg/day. Clinical studies have shown that 16mg of SUBUTEX or SUBOXONE is a clinically effective dose compared with placebo and indicate that doses as low as 12 mg may be effective in some patients. The dosage of SUBOXONE should be progressively adjusted in increments/decrements of 2mg or 4mg to a level that holds the patient in treatment and suppresses opioid withdrawal effects. This is likely to be in the range of 4mg to 24mg per day depending on the individual.

Reducing dosage and stopping treatment:

The decision to discontinue therapy with SUBOXONE or SUBUTEX after a period of maintenance or brief stabilization should be made as part of a comprehensive treatment plan. Both gradual and abrupt discontinuation have been used, but no controlled trials have been undertaken to determine the best method of dose taper at the end of treatment.

Table 4. Adverse Events (≥5%) by Body System and Treatment Group in a 16-week Study

Body System/Adverse Event (COSTART Terminology)	Buprenorphine Dose*				
	Very Low* (N=184)	Low* (N=180)	Moderate* (N=186)	High* (N=181)	Total* (N=731)
	N (%)	N (%)	N (%)	N (%)	N (%)
Body as a Whole					
Abscess	9 (5%)	2 (1%)	3 (2%)	2 (1%)	16 (2%)
Asthenia	26 (14%)	28 (16%)	26 (14%)	24 (13%)	104 (14%)
Chills	11 (6%)	12 (7%)	9 (5%)	10 (6%)	42 (6%)
Fever	7 (4%)	2 (1%)	2 (1%)	10 (6%)	21 (3%)
Flu Syndrome	4 (2%)	13 (7%)	19 (10%)	8 (4%)	44 (6%)
Headache	51 (28%)	62 (34%)	54 (29%)	53 (29%)	220 (30%)
Infection	32 (17%)	39 (22%)	38 (20%)	40 (22%)	149 (20%)
Injury Accidental	5 (3%)	10 (6%)	5 (3%)	5 (3%)	25 (3%)
Pain	47 (26%)	37 (21%)	49 (26%)	44 (24%)	177 (24%)
Pain Back	18 (10%)	29 (16%)	28 (15%)	27 (15%)	102 (14%)
Withdrawal Syndrome	45 (24%)	40 (22%)	41 (22%)	36 (20%)	162 (22%)
Digestive System					
Constipation	10 (5%)	23 (13%)	23 (12%)	26 (14%)	82 (11%)
Diarrhea	19 (10%)	8 (4%)	9 (5%)	4 (2%)	40 (5%)
Dyspepsia	6 (3%)	10 (6%)	4 (2%)	4 (2%)	24 (3%)
Nausea	12 (7%)	22 (12%)	23 (12%)	18 (10%)	75 (10%)
Vomiting	8 (4%)	6 (3%)	10 (5%)	14 (8%)	38 (5%)
Nervous System					
Anxiety	22 (12%)	24 (13%)	20 (11%)	25 (14%)	91 (12%)
Depression	24 (13%)	16 (9%)	25 (13%)	18 (10%)	83 (11%)
Dizziness	4 (2%)	9 (5%)	7 (4%)	11 (6%)	31 (4%)
Insomnia	42 (23%)	50 (28%)	43 (23%)	51 (28%)	186 (25%)
Nervousness	12 (7%)	11 (6%)	10 (5%)	13 (7%)	46 (6%)
Somnolence	5 (3%)	13 (7%)	9 (5%)	11 (6%)	38 (5%)
Respiratory System					
Cough Increase	5 (3%)	11 (6%)	6 (3%)	4 (2%)	26 (4%)
Pharyngitis	6 (3%)	7 (4%)	6 (3%)	9 (5%)	28 (4%)
Rhinitis	27 (15%)	16 (9%)	15 (8%)	21 (12%)	79 (11%)
Skin and Appendages					
Sweat	23 (13%)	21 (12%)	20 (11%)	23 (13%)	87 (12%)
Special Senses					
Runny Eyes	13 (7%)	9 (5%)	6 (3%)	6 (3%)	34 (5%)

*Sublingual solution. Doses in this table cannot necessarily be delivered in tablet form, but for comparison purposes:
"Very low" dose (1 mg solution) would be less than a tablet dose of 2 mg
"Low" dose (4mg solution) approximates a 6 mg tablet dose
"Moderate" dose (8mg solution) approximates a 12 mg tablet dose
"High" dose (16mg solution) approximates a 24 mg tablet dose

HOW SUPPLIED

SUBOXONE is supplied as sublingual tablets in white HDPE bottles:

Hexagonal orange tablets containing 2mg buprenorphine with 0.5mg naloxone
NDC 12496-1283-2 30 tablets per bottle
Hexagonal orange tablets containing 8mg buprenorphine with 2mg naloxone
NDC 12496-1306-2 30 tablets per bottle
Store at 25°C (77°F), excursions permitted to 15-30°C (59–86°F) [see USP Controlled Room Temperature]

SUBUTEX is supplied as sublingual tablets in white HDPE bottles:

Oval white tablets containing 2mg buprenorphine
NDC 12496-1278-2 30 tablets per bottle
Oval white tablets containing 8mg buprenorphine
NDC 12496-1310-2 30 tablets per bottle
Store at 25°C (77°F), excursions permitted to 15-30°C (59-86°F) [see USP Controlled Room Temperature]

Manufactured by:
Reckitt Benckiser Healthcare (UK) Ltd
Hull, UK, HU8 7DS
Distributed by:
Reckitt Benckiser Pharmaceuticals, Inc.
Richmond, VA 23235

Shown in Product Identification Guide, page 331

Reliant Pharmaceuticals

110 ALLEN ROAD
LIBERTY CORNER, NJ 07938

Direct Inquiries to:
(908) 580-1200

AXID® ℞

[*ăk-sĭd*]
(nizatidine) Oral Solution

DESCRIPTION

Nizatidine (USP) is a histamine H_2-receptor antagonist. Chemically, it is N-[2-[[[2-[(dimethylamino)methyl]-4-thiazolyl]methyl]thio]ethyl]-N′-methyl-2-nitro-1,1-ethenediamine.

The structural formula is as follows:
[See chemical structure at top of next column]

Nizatidine has the empirical formula $C_{12}H_{21}N_5O_2S_2$ representing a molecular weight of 331.47. It is an off-white to buff crystalline solid that is soluble in water. Nizatidine has a bitter taste and mild sulfur-like odor.

Continued on next page

Axid—Cont.

Nizatidine

Axid Oral Solution is formulated as a clear, yellow, oral solution with bubble gum flavor and each 1 mL contains 15 mg of nizatidine. Axid Oral Solution also contains the inactive ingredients methylparaben, propylparaben, glycerin, sodium alginate, purified water, sodium chloride, saccharin sodium, sodium citrate dihydrate, citric acid anhydrous, sucrose, bubble gum flavor, artificial sweetness enhancer, and sodium hydroxide.

CLINICAL PHARMACOLOGY IN ADULTS

Nizatidine is a competitive, reversible inhibitor of histamine at the histamine H_2-receptors, particularly those in the gastric parietal cells.

Antisecretory Activity—1. Effects on Acid Secretion: Nizatidine significantly inhibited nocturnal gastric acid secretion for up to 12 hours. Nizatidine also significantly inhibited gastric acid secretion stimulated by food, caffeine, betazole, and pentagastrin (Table 1).

[See table 1 at right]

2. Effects on Other Gastrointestinal Secretions—Pepsin: Oral administration of 75 to 300 mg of nizatidine did not affect pepsin activity in gastric secretions. Total pepsin output was reduced in proportion to the reduced volume of gastric secretions.

Intrinsic Factor: Oral administration of 75 to 300 mg of nizatidine increased betazole-stimulated secretion of intrinsic factor.

Serum Gastrin Concentration: Nizatidine had no effect on basal serum gastrin concentration. No rebound of gastrin secretion was observed when food was ingested 12 hours after administration of nizatidine.

3. Other Pharmacologic Actions—

a. Hormones: Nizatidine was not shown to affect the serum concentrations of gonadotropins, prolactin, growth hormone, antidiuretic hormone, cortisol, triiodo-thyronine, thyroxin, testosterone, 5 α-dihydro-testosterone, androstenedione, or estradiol.

b. Nizatidine had no demonstrable antiandrogenic action.

4. Pharmacokinetics—The absolute oral bioavailability of nizatidine exceeds 70%. Peak plasma concentrations (700 to 1,800 µg/L for a 150-mg dose and 1,400 to 3,600 µg/L for a 300-mg dose) occur from 0.5 to 3 hours following the dose. Plasma concentrations 12 hours after administration are less than 10 µg/L. The elimination half-life is 1 to 2 hours, plasma clearance is 40 to 60 L/h, and the volume of distribution is 0.8 to 1.5 L/kg. Because of the short half-life and rapid clearance of nizatidine, accumulation of the drug would not be expected in individuals with normal renal function who take either 300 mg once daily at bedtime or 150 mg twice daily. Nizatidine exhibits dose proportionality over the recommended dose range.

The oral bioavailability of nizatidine is unaffected by concomitant ingestion of the anticholinergic propantheline. Antacids consisting of aluminum and magnesium hydroxides with simethicone decrease the absorption of nizatidine by about 10%. With food, the AUC and C_{max} increase by approximately 10%. In humans, less than 7% of an oral dose is metabolized as N2-monodesmethylnizatidine, an H_2-receptor antagonist, which is the principal metabolite excreted in the urine. Other likely metabolites are the N2-oxide (less than 5% of the dose) and the S-oxide (less than 6% of the dose).

More than 90% of an orally administered dose of nizatidine is excreted in the urine within 12 hours. About 60% of an oral dose is excreted as unchanged drug. Renal clearance is about 500 mL/min, which indicates excretion by active tubular secretion. Less than 6% of an administered dose is eliminated in the feces.

Moderate to severe renal impairment significantly prolongs the half-life and decreases the clearance of nizatidine. In individuals who are functionally anephric, the half-life is 3.5 to 11 hours, and the plasma clearance is 7 to 14 L/h. To avoid accumulation of the drug in individuals with clinically significant renal impairment, the amount and/or frequency of doses of nizatidine should be reduced in proportion to the severity of dysfunction (see Dosage and Administration).

Approximately 35% of nizatidine is bound to plasma protein, mainly to α_1-acid glycoprotein. Warfarin, diazepam, acetaminophen, propantheline, phenobarbital, and propranolol did not affect plasma protein binding of nizatidine in vitro.

At a dose of 150 mg, the Axid Oral Solution (15 mg/mL) is bioequivalent to nizatidine capsules.

CLINICAL PHARMACOLOGY IN PEDIATRIC PATIENTS

Pharmacokinetics

Table 2 presents pharmacokinetic data of nizatidine administered orally to adolescents with gastroesophageal reflux (GER) and healthy adults. Pharmacokinetic parameters for adolescent patients ages 12 to 18 years are comparable to those obtained for adults.

[See table 2 above]

Pharmacodynamics

Pharmacodynamics of nizatidine were evaluated in 48 pediatric patients. These data suggest that gastric acid suppression is similar to that observed in adult studies (Table 3).

Table 1. Effect of Oral Nizatidine on Gastric Acid Secretion

	Time After Dose (h)	% Inhibition of Gastric Acid Output by Dose (mg)				
		20-50	75	100	150	300
Nocturnal	Up to 10	57	–	73	–	90
Betazole	Up to 3	–	93	–	100	99
Pentagastrin	Up to 6	–	25	–	64	67
Meal	Up to 4	41	64	–	98	97
Caffeine	Up to 3	–	73	–	65	96

Table 2. Pharmacokinetics of Oral Nizatidine

Age Range	Formulation	Dose	C_{max} (ng/mL)	T_{max} (h)	$AUC_{0-\infty}$ (ng•h/mL)	CL_F (L/h)	Vd_F (L)	$T_{1/2}$ (h)
12-18 yr	Capsule	150 mg SD	1422.9	1.3	3764.2	41.0	71.4	1.2
Adolescents with GER		150 mg SS	1480.2	1.4	3776.1	41.1	74.2	1.3
Healthy	Capsule	150 mg SD	1367.6	1.0	3703.1	41.9	83.4	1.4
Adults	Oral Solution	150 mg SD	1340.6	0.8	3610.9	43.0	86.4	1.4
	Apple Juice	150 mg SD	762.8	1.3	2694.1	57.5	142.3	1.7

SD=single dose SS=steady state

Administration of nizatidine capsules in apple juice results in 27% reduction of nizatidine bioavailability.

Table 4. Healing Response of Ulcers to Nizatidine

	Nizalidine 300 mg h.s. Number Entered	Healed/ Evaluable	Nizalidine 150 mg b.i.d. Number Entered	Healed/ Evaluable	Placebo Number Entered	Healed/ Evaluable
STUDY 1						
Week 2			276	93/265 (35%)*	279	55/260 (21%)
Week 4				198/259 (76%)*		95/243 (39%)
STUDY 2						
Week 2	108	24/103 (23%)*	106	27/101 (27%)*	101	9/93 (10%)
Week 4		65/97 (67%)*		66/97 (68%)*		24/84 (29%)
STUDY 3						
Week 2	92	22/90 (24%)†			98	13/92 (14%)
Week 4		62/85 (61%)*				29/88 (33%)
Week 8		68/83 (82%)*				39/79 (49%)

*$P<0.01$ as compared with placebo.
†$P<0.05$ as compared with placebo.

Table 3. Pharmacodynamics of Oral Nizatidine

Age	% Time pH>3	% Time pH>4	$AUEC_{0\text{-}12h}$ (pH•h)
12-18 years	57	42	41.4
Adults	31	19	34.8

Clinical Trials (Adults)—1. Active Duodenal Ulcer: In multicenter, double-blind, placebo-controlled studies in the United States, endoscopically diagnosed duodenal ulcers healed more rapidly following administration of nizatidine, 300 mg h.s. or 150 mg b.i.d., than with placebo (Table 4). Lower doses, such as 100 mg h.s., had slightly lower effectiveness.

[See table 4 above]

2. Maintenance of Healed Duodenal Ulcer: Treatment with a reduced dose of nizatidine has been shown to be effective as maintenance therapy following healing of active duodenal ulcers. In multicenter, double-blind, placebo-controlled studies conducted in the United States, 150 mg of nizatidine taken at bedtime resulted in a significantly lower incidence of duodenal ulcer recurrence in patients treated for up to 1 year (Table 5).

Table 5. Percentage of Ulcers Recurring by 3, 6, and 12 Months in Double-Blind Studies Conducted in the United States

Month	Nizatidine, 150 mg h.s.	Placebo
3	13% (28/208)*	40% (82/204)
6	24% (45/188)*	57% (106/187)
12	34% (57/166)*	64% (112/175)

*$P<0.001$ as compared with placebo.

3. Gastroesophageal Reflux Disease (GERD): In 2 multicenter, double-blind, placebo-controlled clinical trials performed in the United States and Canada, nizatidine was more effective than placebo in improving endoscopically diagnosed esophagitis and in healing erosive and ulcerative esophagitis.

In patients with erosive or ulcerative esophagitis, 150 mg b.i.d. of nizatidine given to 88 patients compared with placebo in 98 patients in Study 1 yielded a higher healing rate at 3 weeks (16% vs 7%) and at 6 weeks (32% vs 16%, $P<0.05$). Of 99 patients on nizatidine and 94 patients on placebo, Study 2 at the same dosage yielded similar results at 6 weeks (21% vs 11%, $P<0.05$) and at 12 weeks (29% vs 13%, $P<0.01$).

In addition, relief of associated heartburn was greater in patients treated with nizatidine. Patients treated with nizatidine consumed fewer antacids than did patients treated with placebo.

4. Active Benign Gastric Ulcer: In a multicenter, double-blind, placebo-controlled study conducted in the United States and Canada, endoscopically diagnosed benign gastric ulcers healed significantly more rapidly following administration of nizatidine than of placebo (Table 6).

Table 6.

Week	Treatment	Healing Rate	vs. Placebo P-value*
4	Nizatidine 300 mg h.s.	52/153 (34%)	0.342
	Nizatidine 150 mg b.i.d.	65/151 (43%)	0.022
	Placebo	48/151 (32%)	
8	Nizatidine 300 mg h.s.	99/153 (65%)	0.011
	Nizatidine 150 mg b.i.d.	105/151 (70%)	<0.001
	Placebo	78/151 (52%)	

*P-values are one-sided, obtained by Chi-square test, and not adjusted for multiple comparisons.

In a multicenter, double-blind, comparator-controlled study in Europe, healing rates for patients receiving nizatidine (300 mg h.s. or 150 mg b.i.d.) were equivalent to rates for patients receiving a comparator drug, and statistically superior to historical placebo control rates.

INDICATIONS AND USAGE

Axid Oral Solution is indicated for up to 8 weeks for the treatment of active duodenal ulcer. In most patients, the ulcer will heal within 4 weeks.

Axid Oral Solution is indicated for maintenance therapy for duodenal ulcer patients at a reduced dosage of 150 mg h.s. after healing of an active duodenal ulcer. The consequences of continuous therapy with nizatidine for longer than 1 year are not known.

Axid Oral Solution is indicated for up to 12 weeks for the treatment of endoscopically diagnosed esophagitis, including erosive and ulcerative esophagitis, and associated heartburn due to GERD.

Axid Oral Solution is indicated for up to 8 weeks for the treatment of active benign gastric ulcer. Before initiating therapy, care should be taken to exclude the possibility of malignant gastric ulceration.

In pediatric patients, Axid Oral Solution is indicated for ages 12 years and older. Axid Oral Solution is indicated for up to 12 weeks for the treatment of endoscopically diagnosed esophagitis, including erosive and ulcerative esophagitis, and associated heartburn due to GERD.

CONTRAINDICATION

Axid Oral Solution is contraindicated in patients with known hypersensitivity to the drug. Because cross-sensitivity in this class of compounds has been observed, H_2-receptor antagonists, including nizatidine, should not be administered to patients with a history of hypersensitivity to other H_2-receptor antagonists.

PRECAUTIONS

General—1. Symptomatic response to nizatidine therapy does not preclude the presence of gastric malignancy.

2. Because nizatidine is excreted primarily by the kidney, dosage should be reduced in patients with moderate to severe renal insufficiency (see Dosage and Administration).

3. Pharmacokinetic studies in patients with hepatorenal syndrome have not been done. Part of the dose of nizatidine is metabolized in the liver. In patients with normal renal function and uncomplicated hepatic dysfunction, the disposition of nizatidine is similar to that in normal subjects.

Laboratory Tests—False-positive tests for urobilinogen with Multistix® may occur during therapy with nizatidine.

Drug Interactions—No interactions have been observed between nizatidine and theophylline, chlordiazepoxide, lorazepam, lidocaine, phenytoin, and warfarin. Nizatidine does not inhibit the cytochrome P-450-linked drug-metabolizing enzyme system; therefore, drug interactions mediated by inhibition of hepatic metabolism are not expected to occur. In patients given very high doses (3,900 mg) of aspirin daily, increases in serum salicylate levels were seen when nizatidine, 150 mg b.i.d., was administered concurrently.

Carcinogenesis, Mutagenesis, Impairment of Fertility—A 2-year oral carcinogenicity study in rats with doses as high as 500 mg/kg/day (about 13 times the recommended human dose based on body surface area) showed no evidence of a carcinogenic effect. There was a dose-related increase in the density of enterochromaffin-like (ECL) cells in the gastric oxyntic mucosa. In a 2-year study in mice, there was no evidence of a carcinogenic effect in male mice; although hyperplastic nodules of the liver were increased in the high-dose males as compared with placebo. Female mice given the high dose of nizatidine (2,000 mg/kg/day, about 27 times the recommended human dose based on body surface area) showed marginally statistically significant increases in hepatic carcinoma and hepatic nodular hyperplasia with no numerical increase seen in any of the other dose groups. The rate of hepatic carcinoma in the high-dose animals was within the historical control limits seen for the strain of mice used. The female mice were given a dose larger than the maximum tolerated dose, as indicated by excessive (30%) weight decrement as compared with concurrent controls and evidence of mild liver injury (transaminase elevations). The occurrence of a marginal finding at high dose only in animals given an excessive and somewhat hepatotoxic dose, with no evidence of a carcinogenic effect in rats, male mice, and female mice (given up to 360 mg/kg/day, about 5 times the recommended human dose based on body surface area), and a negative mutagenicity battery are not considered evidence of a carcinogenic potential for nizatidine.

Nizatidine was not mutagenic in a battery of tests performed to evaluate its potential genetic toxicity, including bacterial mutation tests, unscheduled DNA synthesis, sister chromatid exchange, mouse lymphoma assay, chromosome aberration tests, and a micronucleus test.

In a 2-generation, perinatal and postnatal fertility study in rats, doses of nizatidine up to 650 mg/kg/day (about 17.5 times the recommended human dose based on body surface area) produced no adverse effects on the reproductive performance of parental animals or their progeny.

Pregnancy—Teratogenic Effects—Pregnancy Category B—Oral reproduction studies in pregnant rats at doses up to 1500 mg/kg/day (about 40.5 times the recommended human dose based on body surface area) and in pregnant rabbits at doses up to 275 mg/kg/day (about 14.6 times the recommended human dose based on body surface area) have revealed no evidence of impaired fertility or harm to the fetus due to nizatidine. There are, however, no adequate and well-controlled studies in pregnant women. Because animal reproduction studies are not always predictive of human response, this drug should be used during pregnancy only if clearly needed.

Nursing Mothers—Studies conducted in lactating women have shown that 0.1% of the administered oral dose of nizatidine is secreted in human milk in proportion to plasma concentrations. Because of the growth depression in pups reared by lactating rats treated with nizatidine, a decision should be made whether to discontinue nursing or discontinue the drug, taking into account the importance of the drug to the mother.

Pediatric Use—Effectiveness in pediatric patients <12 years of age has not been established. Use of nizatidine in pediatric patients from 12 to 18 years of age is supported by evidence from published pediatric literature, adequate and well-controlled published studies in adults, and by the following adequate and well-controlled studies in pediatric patients: (see DOSAGE AND ADMINISTRATION)

Clinical Trials (Pediatric). In randomized studies, nizatidine was administered to pediatric patients for up to eight weeks, using age appropriate formulations. A total of 230 pediatric patients from 2 to 18 years of age were administered nizatidine at a dose of either 2.5 mg/kg b.i.d, or 5.0 mg/kg b.i.d, (patients 12 years and under) or 150 mg b.i.d (12 to 18 years). Patients were required to have either symptomatic, clinically suspected or endoscopically diagnosed GERD with age-relevant symptoms. In patients 2 to 18 years of age, nizatidine was found generally safe and well-tolerated. In these studies in patients 12 years and older, nizatidine was found to reduce the severity and frequency of GERD symptoms, improve physical well-being, and reduce the frequency of supplemental antacid consumption. No efficacy in pediatric patients <12 years of age has been established. Clinical studies in patients 2 to 12 years of age with GERD, demonstrated no difference in either symptom improvements or healing rates between nizatidine and placebo or between different doses of nizatidine.

Geriatric Use—Of the 955 patients in clinical studies who were treated with nizatidine, 337 (35.3%) were 65 and older. No overall differences in safety or effectiveness were observed between these and younger subjects. Other reported clinical experience has not identified differences in responses between the elderly and younger patients, but greater sensitivity of some older individuals cannot be ruled out.

This drug is known to be substantially excreted by the kidney, and the risk of toxic reactions to this drug may be greater in patients with impaired renal function. Because elderly patients are more likely to have decreased renal function, care should be taken in dose selection, and it may be useful to monitor renal function (see Dosage and Administration).

ADVERSE REACTIONS IN ADULTS

Worldwide, controlled clinical trials of nizatidine included over 6,000 patients given nizatidine in studies of varying durations. Placebo-controlled trials in the United States and Canada included over 2,600 patients given nizatidine and over 1,700 given placebo. Among the adverse events in these placebo-controlled trials, anemia (0.2% vs 0%) and urticaria (0.5% vs 0.1%) were significantly more common in the nizatidine group.

Incidence in Placebo-Controlled Clinical Trials in the United States and Canada—Table 7 lists adverse events that occurred at a frequency of 1% or more among nizatidine-treated patients who participated in placebo-controlled trials. The cited figures provide some basis for estimating the relative contribution of drug and non-drug factors to the side-effect incidence rate in the population studied.

Table 7.
Incidence of Treatment-Emergent Adverse Events in Placebo-Controlled Clinical Trials in the United States and Canada

Body System/ Adverse Event*	Percentage of Patients Reporting Event: Nizatidine (N=2,694)	Placebo (N=1,729)
Body as a Whole		
Headache	16.6	15.6
Pain	4.2	3.8
Asthenia	3.1	2.9
Chest pain	2.3	2.1
Infection	1.7	1.1
Injury, accident	1.2	0.9
Digestive		
Diarrhea	7.2	6.9
Dry mouth	1.4	1.3
Tooth disorder	1.0	0.8
Musculoskeletal		
Myalgia	1.7	1.5
Nervous		
Dizziness	4.6	3.8
Insomnia	2.7	3.4
Abnormal dreams	1.9	1.9
Somnolence	1.9	1.6
Anxiety	1.8	1.4
Nervousness	1.1	0.8
Respiratory		
Rhinitis	9.8	9.6
Pharyngitis	3.3	3.1
Sinusitis	2.4	2.1
Cough, increased	2.0	2.0
Skin and Appendages		
Rash	1.9	2.1
Pruritis	1.7	1.3
Special Senses		
Amblyopia	1.0	0.9

*Events reported by at least 1% of nizatidine-treated patients are included.

A variety of less common events were also reported; it was not possible to determine whether these were caused by nizatidine.

Hepatic—Hepatocellular injury, evidenced by elevated liver enzyme tests (SGOT [AST], SGPT [ALT], or alkaline phosphatase), occurred in some patients and was possibly or probably related to nizatidine. In some cases, there was marked elevation of SGOT, SGPT enzymes (greater than 500 IU/L) and, in a single instance, SGPT was greater than 2,000 IU/L.The overall rate of occurrences of elevated liver enzymes and elevations to 3 times the upper limit of normal, however, did not significantly differ from the rate of liver enzyme abnormalities in placebo-treated patients. All abnormalities were reversible after discontinuation of nizatidine. Since market introduction, hepatitis and jaundice have been reported. Rare cases of cholestatic or mixed hepatocellular and cholestatic injury with jaundice have been reported with reversal of the abnormalities after discontinuation of nizatidine.

Cardiovascular—In clinical pharmacology studies, short episodes of asymptomatic ventricular tachycardia occurred in 2 individuals administered nizatidine and in 3 untreated subjects.

CNS—Rare cases of reversible mental confusion have been reported.

Endocrine—Clinical pharmacology studies and controlled clinical trials showed no evidence of antiandrogenic activity due to nizatidine. Impotence and decreased libido were reported with similar frequency by patients who received nizatidine and by those given placebo. Rare reports of gynecomastia occurred.

Hematologic—Anemia was reported significantly more frequently in nizatidine-than in placebo-treated patients. Fatal thrombocytopenia was reported in a patient who was treated with nizatidine and another H_2-receptor antagonist. On previous occasions, this patient had experienced thrombocytopenia while taking other drugs. Rare cases of thrombocytopenic purpura have been reported.

Integumental—Sweating and urticaria were reported significantly more frequently in nizatidine than in placebo-treated patients. Rash and exfoliative dermatitis were also reported. Vasculitis has been reported rarely.

Hypersensitivity—As with other H_2-receptor antagonists, rare cases of anaphylaxis following administration of nizatidine have been reported. Rare episodes of hypersensitivity reactions (eg, bronchospasm, laryngeal edema, rash, and eosinophilia) have been reported.

Body as a Whole—Serum sickness-like reactions have occurred rarely in conjunction with nizatidine use.

Genitourinary—Reports of impotence have occurred.

Other—Hyperuricemia unassociated with gout or nephrolithiasis was reported. Eosinophilia, fever, and nausea related to nizatidine administration have been reported.

ADVERSE REACTIONS (PEDIATRIC)

In controlled clinical trials in pediatric patients (age 2 to 18 years), nizatidine was found to be generally safe and well tolerated. The principal adverse experiences (> 5%) were pyrexia, nasopharyngitis, diarrhea, vomiting, irritability, nasal congestion and cough. Most adverse events were mild or moderate in severity. Mild elevations in serum transaminase (1-2 × ULN) were noted in some patients. One subject experienced a seizure by EEG diagnosis after taking Axid Oral Solution 2.5 mg/kg b.i.d. for 23 days. The adverse reactions reported for nizatidine may also occur with Axid Oral Solution.

OVERDOSAGE

Overdoses of nizatidine have been reported rarely. The following is provided to serve as a guide should such an overdose be encountered.

Signs and Symptoms—There is little clinical experience with overdosage of nizatidine in humans. Test animals that received large doses of nizatidine have exhibited cholinergic-type effects, including lacrimation, salivation, emesis, miosis, and diarrhea. Single oral doses of 800 mg/kg in dogs and of 1,200 mg/kg in monkeys were not lethal. Intravenous median lethal doses in the rat and mouse were 301 mg/kg and 232 mg/kg respectively.

In the two 8-week pediatric exposure trials of nizatidine in 256 pediatric patients, there were no cases of deliberate overdosage. In one study of nizatidine 10 mg/kg/day, drug compliance rates up to 7.5% above 100% compliance were not associated with clinically significant adverse events.

Treatment—To obtain up-to-date information about the treatment of overdose, a good resource is your certified Regional Poison Control Center. Telephone numbers of certified Poison Control Centers are listed in the *Physicians' Desk Reference (PDR)*. In managing overdosage, consider the possibility of multiple drug overdoses, interaction among drugs, and unusual drug kinetics in your patient.

If overdosage occurs, use of activated charcoal, emesis, or lavage should be considered along with clinical monitoring and supportive therapy. The ability of hemodialysis to remove nizatidine from the body has not been conclusively demonstrated; however, due to its large volume of distribution, nizatidine is not expected to be efficiently removed from the body by this method.

DOSAGE AND ADMINISTRATION

Active Duodenal Ulcer—The recommended oral dosage for adults is 300 mg once daily at bedtime. An alternative dosage regimen is 150 mg twice daily.

Maintenance of Healed Duodenal Ulcer—The recommended oral dosage for adults is 150 mg once daily at bedtime.

Gastroesophageal Reflux Disease—The recommended oral dosage in adults for the treatment of erosions, ulcerations, and associated heartburn is 150 mg twice daily.

Active Benign Gastric Ulcer—The recommended oral dosage is 300 mg given either as 150 mg twice daily or 300 mg once daily at bedtime. Prior to treatment, care should be taken to exclude the possibility of malignant gastric ulceration.

Each mL of Axid Oral Solution contains 15 mg of nizatidine. In adults, Axid Oral Solution may be substituted for any of the above indications using equivalent doses of the oral solution.

Continued on next page

Axid—Cont.

Pediatric Dosing—Each mL of oral solution contains 15 mg of nizatidine. Axid Oral Solution is indicated for pediatric patients 12 years of age or older. For pediatric patients 12 years of age and older, the dosage of nizatidine is 150 mg b.i.d. (2 tsp, b.i.d.)

The following dosage recommendations are provided:

Erosive Esophagitis—For pediatric patients 12 years or older, the dosage is 150 mg b.i.d. (300 mg/d). The maximum daily dose for nizatidine PO is 300 mg/d. The dosing duration may be up to eight weeks.

Gastroesophageal Reflux Disease—For pediatric patients 12 years or older, the dosage is 150 mg b.i.d. (300 mg/d). The maximum daily dose for nizatidine PO is 300 mg/d. The dosing duration may be up to eight weeks.

Dosage Adjustment for Patients With Moderate to Severe Renal Insufficiency—The dose for patients with renal dysfunction should be reduced as follows:

Active Duodenal Ulcer, GERD, and Benign Gastric Ulcer

Creatine Clearance	Dose
20-50 mL/min	150 mg daily
<20 mL/min	150 mg every other day

Maintenance Therapy

Creatine Clearance	Dose
20-50 mL/min	150 mg every other day
<20 mL/min	150 mg every 3 days

Some elderly patients may have creatinine clearances of less than 50 mL/min, and, based on pharmacokinetic data in patients with renal impairment, the dose for such patients should be reduced accordingly. The clinical effects of this dosage reduction in patients with renal failure have not been evaluated.

Based on the pharmacokinetic data in elderly patients with renal impairment, pediatric patients with creatinine clearances less than 50 mL/min should have their dose of nizatidine reduced accordingly. The clinical effects of this dose reduction in pediatric patients with renal failure have not been evaluated.

HOW SUPPLIED

Axid (nizatidine) Oral Solution 15 mg/mL is formulated as a clear, yellow, oral solution with bubble gum flavor, available as:

Bottles of 480 mL (16 fl. oz.) – NDC# 65726-147-62

Store at 25°C (77°F); excursions permitted to 15° - 30°C (59° - 86°F) [see USP Controlled Room Temperature] and dispense in tight, light-resistant container.

Rx only

June 2004

Reliant PHARMACEUTICALS, INC.

Manufactured for:
Reliant Pharmaceuticals, Inc.
Liberty Corner, NJ 07938, USA
By:
Lyne Laboratories, Inc.
Brockton, MA 02301, USA

Address Medical Inquiries to:
Reliant Pharmaceuticals, Inc.
Medical Affairs
110 Allen Road
Liberty Corner, NJ 07938, USA
PRINTED IN USA

114F700

Shown in Product Identification Guide, page 331

DYNACIRC CR® ℞

[dī' nă-sŭrk CR]
(isradipine)
Controlled Release Tablets
Rx only

DESCRIPTION

DynaCirc CR® contains isradipine, a calcium antagonist. It is available for once-daily oral administration as a controlled release 5 mg and 10 mg tablet for DynaCirc CR® (isradipine). DynaCirc CR® is a registered trademark for isradipine GITS (Gastrointestinal Therapeutic System) tablets.

The structural formula of isradipine is:

$C_{19}H_{21}N_3O_5$ Mol. wt. 371.39

Chemically, isradipine is 3,5-Pyridinedicarboxylic acid, 4-(4-benzofurazanyl)-1,4-dihydro-2,6-dimethyl-, methyl 1-methylethyl ester. Isradipine is a yellow, fine crystalline powder which is odorless or has a faint characteristic odor. Isradipine is practically insoluble in water (<10 mg/L at 37°C), but is soluble in ethanol and freely soluble in acetone, chloroform and methylene chloride.

Active Ingredient: isradipine

Inactive Ingredients: butylated hydroxytoluene; cellulose acetate; hydroxypropyl methylcellulose; magnesium stearate; polyethylene glycol; polyethylene oxide; polysorbate 80; propylene glycol; red ferric oxide; silicon dioxide; sodium chloride; titanium dioxide; yellow ferric oxide.

System Components and Performance

Isradipine is delivered from the DynaCirc CR® (isradipine) Controlled Release Tablet as follows: a semipermeable membrane surrounds an osmotically active drug core. The core is composed of two layers: an "active" layer containing the drug, and a pharmacologically inert but osmotically active "push" layer. After ingestion, the tablet overcoating is quickly dissipated in the gastrointestinal tract, allowing water to enter the tablet through the semipermeable membrane. The polyethylene oxide polymer swells in the osmotic ("push") layer and exerts pressure against the "active" drug layer, releasing isradipine as a fine suspension through the laser-drilled tablet orifice which has been positioned on the "active" drug layer side. Drug delivery is essentially constant as long as the osmotic gradient remains constant and, after either 5 mg or 10 mg of isradipine is released, gradually falls to a negligible amount. The controlled rate of drug delivery into the gastrointestinal lumen is independent of pH or gastrointestinal motility. The delivery of isradipine in DynaCirc CR® (isradipine) Controlled Release Tablets depends on the existence of an osmotic gradient between the contents of the bilayer core and the fluid in the GI tract. The biologically inert core of the tablet remains intact and, unless it becomes trapped, is eliminated in the feces.

CLINICAL PHARMACOLOGY

Mechanism of Action

Isradipine is a dihydropyridine calcium channel blocker. It binds to calcium channels with high affinity and specificity and inhibits calcium flux into cardiac and smooth muscle. The effects observed in mechanistic experiments *in vitro* and studied in intact animals and man are compatible with this mechanism of action and are typical of the class.

Except for diuretic activity, the mechanism of which is not clearly understood, the pharmacodynamic effects of isradipine observed in whole animals can also be explained by calcium channel blocking activity, especially dilating effects in arterioles which reduce systemic resistance and lower blood pressure, with a small increase in resting heart rate. Although like other dihydropyridine calcium channel blockers, isradipine has negative inotropic effects *in vitro*, studies conducted in intact anesthetized animals have shown that the vasodilating effect occurs at doses lower than those which affect contractility. In patients with normal ventricular function, isradipine's afterload reducing properties lead to some increase in cardiac output.

Effects in patients with impaired ventricular function have not been fully studied.

Clinical Effects

In randomized, placebo-controlled, double-blind, clinical trials, DynaCirc CR® (isradipine) Controlled Release Tablets have been shown to have antihypertensive effects proportional to doses between 5 and 20 mg, administered once daily. DynaCirc CR® (isradipine) produced statistically significant reductions in supine and standing blood pressure, compared with placebo, 24 hours postdose. The endpoint results of one parallel group dose-ranging trial showed mean responses 24 hours after ingestion of DynaCirc CR® (isradipine) (systolic/diastolic) −5.2/−2.8, −13.4/−9.7, −15.6/−10.2 and −15.5/−11.8 mmHg, for 5, 10, 15 and 20 mg doses, respectively, change from baseline greater than concurrent placebo. The antihypertensive effect of any one dose begins in about 2 hours and reaches a peak at about 8–10 hours postdose. At the recommended starting dose (5 mg) the trough response (24 hours after dosing) was about 76% that of the peak. At doses of 10, 15 and 20 mg, the trough blood pressure response was about equal to that at peak effect. In association with the fall in blood pressure, resting heart rate is slightly increased, on average from 1–3 beats/minute. The antihypertensive response to DynaCirc CR® (isradipine) has not been detected to be influenced by gender or age.

Hemodynamics

In man, peripheral vasodilation produced by immediate-release DynaCirc® (isradipine) is reflected by decreased systemic vascular resistance and increased cardiac output. Hemodynamic studies conducted in patients with normal left ventricular function produced, following intravenous isradipine administration, increases in cardiac index, stroke volume index, coronary sinus blood flow, heart rate and peak positive left ventricular dP/dt. Systemic, coronary, and pulmonary vascular resistance was decreased. These studies were conducted with doses of isradipine which produced clinically significant decreases in blood pressure. The clinical consequences of these hemodynamic effects, if any, have not been evaluated.

Effects on heart rate are variable, dependent upon rate of administration and presence of underlying cardiac condition. While increases in both peak positive dP/dt and LV ejection fraction are seen when intravenous isradipine is given, it is impossible to conclude that these represent a positive inotropic effect due to simultaneous changes in preload and afterload. In patients with coronary artery disease undergoing atrial pacing during cardiac catheterization, intravenous isradipine diminished abnormalities of systolic performance. In patients with moderate left ventricular dysfunction, oral and intravenous isradipine in doses which reduce blood pressure by 12%–30%, resulted in improvement in cardiac index without increase in heart rate, and with no change or reduction in pulmonary capillary wedge pressure. Combination of isradipine and propranolol did not significantly affect left ventricular dP/dt max. The clinical consequences of these effects have not been evaluated.

Electrophysiologic Effects

In general, no detrimental effects on the cardiac conduction system were seen with the use of immediate-release DynaCirc® (isradipine). Electrophysiologic studies were conducted on patients with normal sinus and atrioventricular node function. Intravenous isradipine in doses which reduce systolic blood pressure did not affect PR, QRS, AH* or HV* intervals.

No changes were seen in Wenckebach cycle length, atrial, and ventricular refractory periods. Slight prolongation of QT_c interval of 3% was seen in one study. Effects on sinus node recovery time (CSNRT) were mild or not seen.

In patients with sick sinus syndrome, at doses which significantly reduced blood pressure, intravenous isradipine resulted in no depressant effect on sinus and atrioventricular node function.

*AH = conduction time from low right atrium to His bundle deflection, or AV nodal conduction time; HV = conduction time through His bundle and the bundle branch-Purkinje system.

Pharmacokinetics and Metabolism

With the immediate-release formulation DynaCirc® (isradipine) Capsules, 90%–95% of the orally administered dose is absorbed. Because of the biotransformation of isradipine during its first-pass through the portal circulation, the bioavailability of DynaCirc CR® (isradipine) ranges from 15%–24%. Isradipine is 95% bound to plasma proteins.

Peak concentrations of approximately 1 ng/mL/mg dosed occur about 1.5 hours after DynaCirc® (isradipine) Capsules administration. The elimination of isradipine is biphasic with an early half-life of 1½–2 hours, and a terminal half-life of about 8 hours, resulting in trough concentrations of about 0.1 ng/mL/mg dosed of immediate-release DynaCirc® (isradipine) Capsules.

In single dose studies of DynaCirc CR® (isradipine) Controlled Release Tablets, after a 2–3 hour lag time, concentrations of isradipine plateau between 7 and 18 hours post-dosing (reaching a C_{max} of 3–4 ng/mL with an AUC of 62–73 ng•h/mL for a 10 mg dose) and then a concentration >50% of the peak exists for 17–20 hours.

There is no evidence of dose dumping either in the presence or absence of food. Food has been shown to decrease the extent of bioavailability of DynaCirc CR® (isradipine) by up to 25%.

The pharmacokinetics of DynaCirc CR® (isradipine) Controlled Release Tablets are linear over the dose range of 5–20 mg, in that the plasma drug concentrations are proportional to the dose administered.

Isradipine is completely metabolized prior to excretion, and no unchanged drug is detected in the urine. The major routes of isradipine metabolism are ring oxidation of the dihydropyridine moiety to give the corresponding pyridine, and ester cleavage, with or without concomitant oxidation of the dihydropyridine moiety, giving the corresponding carboxylic acids. The cytochrome P-450 IIIA4 system is implicated in the formation of these metabolites, which are hemodynamically inactive. Approximately 60%–65% of an administered dose is excreted in the urine and 25%–30% in the feces. With immediate-release DynaCirc® (isradipine), mild renal impairment (creatinine clearance 30–80 mL/min) increases the AUC of isradipine by 45%. Progressive deterioration reverses this trend, and patients with severe renal failure (creatinine clearance <10 mL/min) who have been on hemodialysis show a 20%–50% lower AUC than healthy volunteers. In elderly patients administered DynaCirc® (isradipine) Capsules, C_{max} and AUC are increased by 13% and 40%, respectively; in patients with hepatic impairment, C_{max} and AUC are increased by 32% and 52%, respectively (*see DOSAGE AND ADMINISTRATION*).

INDICATIONS AND USAGE

Hypertension

DynaCirc CR® (isradipine) is indicated in the management of hypertension. It may be used alone or concurrently with thiazide-type diuretics.

CONTRAINDICATIONS

DynaCirc CR® (isradipine) is contraindicated in individuals who have shown hypersensitivity to any of the ingredients in the formulation.

WARNINGS

None

PRECAUTIONS

General

Blood Pressure: Because DynaCirc CR® (isradipine) decreases peripheral resistance, like other calcium blockers DynaCirc CR® (isradipine) may occasionally produce symptomatic hypotension. However, symptoms like syncope and severe dizziness have rarely been reported in hypertensive patients administered DynaCirc CR® (isradipine), particularly at the initial recommended doses (*see DOSAGE AND ADMINISTRATION*).

Use in Patients with Congestive Heart Failure: Although acute hemodynamic studies in patients with congestive heart failure have shown that immediate-release DynaCirc® (isradipine) reduced afterload without impairing myocardial contractility, it has a negative inotropic effect at high doses *in vitro* and possibly in some patients.

Caution should be exercised when using DynaCirc CR® (isradipine) in congestive heart failure patients, particularly in combination with a beta-blocker.

Peripheral Edema: Peripheral edema, when it occurs, is usually mild to moderate in severity. It is a localized phenomenon thought to be associated with vasodilation of arterioles and other small blood vessels, and not due to left ventricular dysfunction or generalized fluid retention. Peripheral edema is dose-related with an incidence ranging from approximately 9% at 5 mg; 13% at 10 mg; 16% at 15 mg; and 36% at the highest dose studied (20 mg once-daily). With patients whose hypertension is complicated by congestive heart failure, care should be taken to differentiate this edema from the effects of decreasing left ventricular function. Although the frequency of edema is correlated with dose, no DynaCirc CR® (isradipine) treated patients discontinued the short-term (6 weeks or less), placebo-controlled hypertension studies as a result of edema. Less than 5% of DynaCirc CR® (isradipine) treated patients in long-term studies discontinued due to edema.

Other: As with any other non-deformable material, caution should be used when administering DynaCirc CR® (isradipine) in patients with pre-existing severe gastrointestinal narrowing (pathologic or iatrogenic). There have been reports of obstructive symptoms in patients with known strictures associated with ingestion of other GITS products.

Information for Patients: DynaCirc CR® (isradipine) Controlled Release Tablets should be swallowed whole. Do not chew, divide or crush tablets. Do not be concerned if you occasionally notice in your stool something resembling a tablet. In DynaCirc CR® (isradipine), the medication is contained within a nonabsorbable shell that has been specially designed to slowly release the drug for your body to absorb. When this process is completed, the empty tablet shell is eliminated in the stool.

Drug Interactions

Nitroglycerin: Immediate-release DynaCirc® (isradipine) has been safely coadministered with nitroglycerin.

Hydrochlorothiazide: A study in normal healthy volunteers has shown that concomitant administration of immediate-release DynaCirc® (isradipine) and hydrochlorothiazide does not result in altered pharmacokinetics of either drug. In a study in hypertensive patients, addition of isradipine to existing hydrochlorothiazide therapy did not result in any unexpected adverse effects, and isradipine had an additional antihypertensive effect.

Propranolol: In a single dose study in normal volunteers using immediate-release DynaCirc® (isradipine), co-administration of propranolol had a small effect on the rate but no effect on the extent of isradipine bioavailability. Significant increases in AUC (27%) and C_{max} (58%) and decreases in t_{max} (23%) of propranolol were noted in this study.

Digoxin: The concomitant administration of immediate-release DynaCirc® (isradipine) and digoxin in a single-dose pharmacokinetic study did not affect renal, non-renal and total body clearance of digoxin.

Fentanyl Anesthesia: Severe hypotension has been reported during fentanyl anesthesia with concomitant use of a beta blocker and a calcium channel blocker. An increased volume of circulating fluids might be required if such an interaction were to occur.

Carcinogenesis, Mutagenesis, Impairment of Fertility

Treatment of male rats for 2 years with 2.5, 12.5, or 62.5 mg/kg/day isradipine admixed with the diet (approximately 6, 31, and 156 times the maximum recommended daily dose based on a 50 kg man) resulted in dose dependent increases in the incidence of benign Leydig cell tumors and testicular hyperplasia relative to untreated control animals. These findings, which were replicated in a subsequent experiment, may have been indirectly related to an effect of isradipine on circulating gonadotropin levels in the rats; a comparable endocrine effect was not evident in male patients receiving therapeutic doses of the drug on a chronic basis. Treatment of mice for two years with 2.5, 15, or 80 mg/kg/day isradipine in the diet (approximately 6, 38, and 200 times the maximum recommended dose based on a 50 kg man) showed no evidence of oncogenicity. There was no evidence of mutagenic potential based on the results of a battery of mutagenic tests. No effect on fertility was observed in male and female rats treated with up to 60 mg/kg/day isradipine.

Pregnancy

Pregnancy Category C: Isradipine was administered orally to rats and rabbits during organogenesis. Treatment of pregnant rats with doses of 6, 20, or 60 mg/kg/day produced a significant reduction in maternal weight gain during treatment with the highest dose (150 times the maximum recommended human daily dose) but with no lasting effects on the mother or the offspring. Treatment of pregnant rabbits with doses of 1, 3, or 10 mg/kg/day (2.5, 7.5, and 25 times the maximum recommended human daily dose) produced decrements in maternal body weight gain and increased fetal resorption at the two higher doses. There was no evidence of embryotoxicity at doses which were not maternotoxic and no evidence of teratogenicity at any dose tested. In a peri/postnatal administration study in rats, reduced maternal body weight gain during late pregnancy at oral doses of 20 and 60 mg/kg/day isradipine was associated with reduced birth weights and decreased peri and postnatal pup survival.

There are no adequate and well controlled studies in pregnant women. The use of DynaCirc® CR (isradipine) during pregnancy should only be considered if the potential benefit outweighs potential risks.

Most Frequently Reported Newly-Occurring Adverse Reactions in Dose-Response Study

Adverse Reactions (Excluding Non-Drug Related)	DynaCirc CR® (isradipine) 5 mg (N=79)	10 mg (N=79)	15 mg (N=82)	20 mg (N=78)	Placebo Group (N=83)
Headache	13.9%	12.7%	18.3%	10.3%	15.7%
Edema	8.9%	12.7%	15.9%	35.9%	3.6%
Dizziness	5.1%	6.3%	3.7%	6.4%	2.4%
Constipation	3.8%	1.3%	1.2%	2.6%	0.0%
Fatigue	2.5%	7.6%	3.7%	3.8%	2.4%
Flushing	2.5%	3.8%	1.2%	1.3%	1.2%
Abdominal Discomfort	1.3%	5.1%	3.7%	5.1%	1.2%
Rash	1.3%	1.3%	0.0%	2.6%	0.0%

Adverse Experience	DynaCirc® (isradipine) All Doses	2.5 mg b.i.d.	5 mg b.i.d.†	10 mg b.i.d.††	Placebo (N=297) %	Active Controls* (N=414) %
Headache	13.7	12.6	10.7	22.0	14.1	9.4
Dizziness	7.3	8.0	5.3	3.4	4.4	8.2
Edema	7.2	3.5	8.7	8.5	3.0	2.9
Palpitations	4.0	1.0	4.7	5.1	1.4	1.5
Fatigue	3.9	2.5	2.0	8.5	0.3	6.3
Flushing	2.6	3.0	2.0	5.1	0.0	1.2
Chest Pain	2.4	2.5	2.7	1.7	2.4	2.9
Nausea	1.8	1.0	2.7	5.1	1.7	3.1
Dyspnea	1.8	0.5	2.7	3.4	1.0	2.2
Abdominal Discomfort	1.7	0.0	3.3	1.7	1.7	3.9
Tachycardia	1.5	1.0	1.3	3.4	0.3	0.5
Rash	1.5	1.5	2.0	1.7	0.3	0.7
Pollakiuria	1.5	2.0	1.3	3.4	0.0	<1.0
Weakness	1.2	0.0	0.7	0.0	0.0	1.2
Vomiting	1.1	1.0	1.3	0.0	0.3	0.2
Diarrhea	1.1	0.0	2.7	3.4	2.0	1.9

†Initial dose of 2.5 mg b.i.d. followed by maintenance dose of 5.0 mg b.i.d.

††Initial dose of 2.5 mg b.i.d. followed by sequential titration to 5.0 mg b.i.d., 7.5 mg b.i.d., and maintenance dose of 10.0 mg b.i.d.

*Propranolol, prazosin, hydrochlorothiazide, enalapril, captopril.

Nursing Mothers

It is not known whether DynaCirc® (isradipine) is excreted in human milk. Because many drugs are excreted in human milk, and because of the potential for adverse effects of DynaCirc® (isradipine) on nursing infants, a decision should be made as to whether to discontinue nursing or discontinue the drug, taking into account the importance of the drug to the mother.

Pediatric Use

Safety and effectiveness have not been established in children.

ADVERSE REACTIONS

In a controlled clinical trial with DynaCirc CR® (isradipine), dose-related edema occurred at an incidence of approximately 9% at 5 mg; 13% at 10mg; 16% at 15 mg; and 36% at the highest dose studied (20 mg), was mild to moderate in severity, and was not related to age or gender.

The incidences of elicited or volunteered adverse reactions (excluding non-drug related) in the following tables are based on 6-week multicenter, placebo-controlled, double-blind hypertension studies. Less than 1% of DynaCirc CR® (isradipine) or placebo-treated patients discontinued from these studies due to adverse reactions.

The most common adverse experiences (≥1.0%) reported with DynaCirc CR® (isradipine) in a dose-response study are shown in the following table. There were no discontinuations of patients treated with DynaCirc CR® (isradipine) in this study due to these common side effects.

[See first table above]

The table below shows elicited or volunteered adverse experiences for DynaCirc CR® (isradipine) treated patients in two 6-week, placebo-controlled, multicenter studies, at doses from 5–20 mg, and considered by the investigator to be at least possibly drug related. The results for DynaCirc CR® (isradipine) treated patients are presented for all doses pooled together (reported by at least 1.0% of active drug treated patients). The incidence of adverse reactions are listed below:

Adverse Reactions (Excluding Non-Drug Related)	Treatment Group: DynaCirc CR® (isradipine) (N=422)	Placebo (N=186)
Edema	15.2%	2.2%
Headache	13.0%	12.4%
Dizziness	4.7%	2.7%
Fatigue	4.3%	2.2%
Abdominal Discomfort	2.8%	0.5%
Flushing	1.9%	0.5%
Constipation	1.7%	0.0%
Palpitations	1.2%	0.0%
Nausea	1.2%	1.6%
Abdominal Distention	1.2%	0.0%

The following adverse experiences were reported in 0.5%–1.0% or less of DynaCirc CR® (isradipine) or immediate-release DynaCirc® (isradipine) treated patients in hypertensive studies, or were noted in postmarketing experience with immediate-release DynaCirc® (isradipine) Capsules. More serious events are shown in italics. The relationship of these adverse experiences to isradipine administration is uncertain.

Skin: pruritus, *urticaria*

Musculoskeletal: backache/pain, joint pain, neck pain/sore/stiff, legs ache/pain, cramps of legs/feet

Respiratory: dyspnea, nasal congestion, cough

Cardiovascular: epistaxis, tachycardia, chest pain, shortness of breath, hypotension, *syncope, atrial or ventricular fibrillation, myocardial infarction, heart failure*

Gastrointestinal: diarrhea, vomiting, appetite increased or decreased

Urogenital: pollakiuria, impotence, dysuria, nocturia

Central Nervous: drowsiness, insomnia, lethargy, nervousness, libido decrease/frigidity, impotence, depression, *paresthesia* (which includes numbness and tingling), *transient ischemic attack, stroke*

Autonomic: dry mouth, hyperhidrosis, visual disturbance

Miscellaneous: weight gain, throat discomfort, *drug fever, leukopenia, elevated liver function tests*

No gastrointestinal bleeding has been reported in clinical trials with DynaCirc® CR (isradipine) Controlled Release Tablets.

In a long-term (one-year) DynaCirc CR® (isradipine) open-label, hypertension trial, the adverse events reported were generally the same as those seen in the short-term placebo-controlled studies. About 6% of DynaCirc CR® (isradipine) treated patients discontinued the long-term trial due to adverse reactions.

With immediate-release DynaCirc® (isradipine) Capsules, most of the adverse experiences were transient, mild, and related to vasodilatory effects. The following table shows the most common adverse events reported in U.S. clinical trials for immediate-release DynaCirc® (isradipine) Capsules, volunteered or elicited, and considered by the investigator to be at least possibly drug related.

[See second table above]

In open-label, long-term studies of up to two years in duration with immediate-release DynaCirc® (isradipine) Capsules, the adverse experiences reported were generally the same as those reported in the short-term controlled trials. The overall frequencies of these adverse events were slightly higher in the long-term than in the controlled studies, but in the controlled studies most adverse reactions were mild and transient.

Continued on next page

DynaCirc CR—Cont.

OVERDOSAGE

Although there is no well documented experience with DynaCirc® (isradipine) overdosage, available data suggest that, as with other dihydropyridines, gross overdosage would result in excessive peripheral vasodilation with subsequent marked and probably prolonged systemic hypotension. Clinically significant hypotension overdosage calls for active cardiovascular support including monitoring of cardiac and respiratory function, elevation of lower extremities and attention to circulating fluid volume and urine output. A vasoconstrictor (such as epinephrine, norepinephrine, or levarterenol) may be helpful in restoring vascular tone and blood pressure, provided that there is no contraindication to its use. Since isradipine is highly protein bound, dialysis is not likely to be of benefit.

Significant lethality was observed in mice given oral doses of over 200 mg/kg and rabbits given about 50 mg/kg of isradipine. Rats tolerated doses of over 2000 mg/kg without effects on survival.

DOSAGE AND ADMINISTRATION

The dosage of DynaCirc CR® (isradipine) Controlled Release Tablets should be individualized. The recommended initial dose of DynaCirc CR® (isradipine) is 5 mg once-daily as monotherapy or in combination with a thiazide diuretic. An antihypertensive response usually occurs within 2 hours, with the peak antihypertensive response occurring 8–10 hours post-dose; blood pressure reduction is maintained for at least 24 hours following drug administration. If necessary, the dose may be adjusted in increments of 5 mg at 2–4 week intervals up to a maximum dose of 20 mg/day. Adverse experiences are increased in frequency above 10 mg/day.

DynaCirc CR® (isradipine) Controlled Release Tablets should be swallowed whole and should not be bitten or divided.

The bioavailability (increased AUC) of immediate-release DynaCirc® (isradipine) is increased in elderly patients (above 65 years of age), patients with hepatic functional impairment, and patients with mild renal impairment. Ordinarily, a starting dose of DynaCirc CR® (isradipine) 5 mg once-daily should be used in these patients.

HOW SUPPLIED

DynaCirc CR® (isradipine) Controlled Release Tablets

5 mg

A light pink, round, standard biconvex and film coated tablet. Printing is in red with "DynaCirc CR" in a semicircle with "5" centered within the semicircle.

Bottles of 100 controlled release tablets (NDC 65726-235-25)

Bottles of 30 controlled release tablets (NDC 65726-235-10)

10 mg

A beige, round, standard biconvex and film coated tablet. Printing is in red with "DynaCirc CR" in a semicircle with "10" centered within the semicircle.

Bottles of 100 controlled release tablets (NDC 65726-236-25)

Bottles of 30 controlled release tablets (NDC 65726-236-10)

Store and Dispense

Below 86°F (30°C) in a tight container, protected from moisture and humidity.

Jointly Manufactured for:
Novartis Pharmaceuticals Corporation
East Hanover, New Jersey 07936 *by*
Novartis Consumer Health Inc.
Lincoln, Nebraska 68517 *and* Alza Corporation
Vacaville, California 95638-94702
Distributed and Marketed by:
Reliant Pharmaceuticals, LLC
Liberty Corner, New Jersey 07938

T2000-48
89010601
REV: DECEMBER 2000 PRINTED IN USA 4078-42

Shown in Product Identification Guide, page 331

INNOPRAN XL™ ℞

[in-o-pran]
(propranolol hydrochloride)
Extended Release Capsules

DESCRIPTION

InnoPran XL (propranolol hydrochloride) is a nonselective, beta-adrenergic receptor-blocking agent for oral administration, available as an extended release product. Innopran XL is available as 80 mg and 120 mg capsules which contain sustained release beads. Each of the beads contains propranolol hydrochloride and is coated with dual membranes. These membranes are designed to retard release of propranolol hydrochloride for several hours after ingestion followed by the sustained release of propranolol.

The active ingredient in InnoPran XL is a synthetic beta-adrenergic receptor-blocking agent chemically described as 1-(Isopropylamino)-3-(1-naphthyloxy)-2-propanol hydrochloride. Its structural formula is:

[See chemical structure at top of next column]

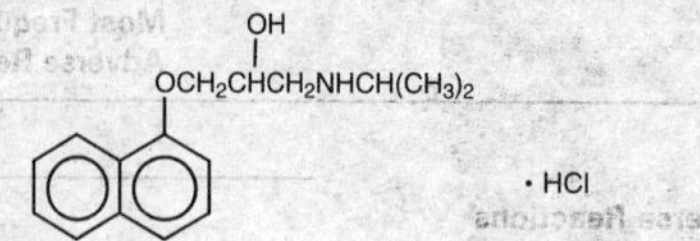

Propranolol hydrochloride is a stable, white, crystalline solid, which is readily soluble in water and ethanol. Its molecular weight is 295.81. Each capsule for oral administration contains sugar spheres, ethylcellulose, povidone, hypromellose phthalate, diethyl phthalate, hypromellose, polyethylene glycol, gelatin, titanium dioxide and black iron oxide. In addition, InnoPran XL 120 mg capsules contain yellow iron oxide.

CLINICAL PHARMACOLOGY

General

Propranolol is a nonselective, beta-adrenergic receptor-blocking agent possessing no other autonomic nervous system activity. It specifically competes with beta-adrenergic receptor-stimulating agents for available receptor sites. When access to beta-receptor sites is blocked by propranolol, chronotropic, inotropic, and vasodilator responses to beta-adrenergic stimulation are decreased proportionately. At dosages greater than required for beta blockade, propranolol also exerts a quinidine-like or anesthetic-like membrane action, which affects the cardiac action potential. The significance of the membrane action in the treatment of arrhythmias is uncertain.

Mechanism of Action

The mechanism of the antihypertensive effect of propranolol has not been established. Among factors that contribute to the antihypertensive action are: (1) decreased cardiac output, (2) inhibition of renin release by the kidneys, and (3) diminution of tonic sympathetic nerve outflow from vasomotor centers in the brain. Although total peripheral resistance may increase initially, it readjusts to or below the pretreatment level with chronic use of propranolol. Effects of propranolol on plasma volume appear to be minor and somewhat variable.

PHARMACOKINETICS AND DRUG METABOLISM

Absorption

Propranolol is highly lipophilic and is almost completely absorbed after oral administration. However, it undergoes high first-pass metabolism by the liver and on average, only about 25% of propranolol reaches the systemic circulation.

A single-dose, food-effect study in 36 healthy subjects showed that a high fat meal administered with InnoPran XL at 10 PM, increased the lag time from 3 to 5 hours and the time to reach the maximum concentration from 11.5 to 15.4 hours, under fed conditions, with no effect on the AUC. (See DOSAGE AND ADMINISTRATION).

Following multiple-dose administration of InnoPran XL at 10 PM under fasting conditions, the steady-state lag time was between 4-5 hours and propranolol peak plasma concentrations were reached approximately 12-14 hours after dosing. Propranolol trough levels were achieved 24-27 hours after dosing, and persisted for 3-5 hours after the next dose. The elimination half-life of propranolol was approximately 8 hours.

The plasma levels of propranolol showed dose proportional increases after single and multiple administration of 80, 120, and 160 mg of InnoPran XL.

At steady state, the bioavailability of 160-mg dose of InnoPran XL and propranolol hydrochloride long acting capsules did not differ significantly.

Distribution

Approximately 90% of circulating propranolol is bound to plasma proteins (albumin and alpha$_1$ acid glycoprotein). The binding is enantiomer-selective. The S-isomer is preferentially bound to alpha$_1$ glycoprotein and the R-isomer preferentially bound to albumin. The volume of distribution of propranolol is approximately 4 liters.

Metabolism and Elimination

Propranolol is extensively metabolized with most metabolites appearing in the urine. Propranolol is metabolized through three primary routes: aromatic hydroxylation (mainly 4-hydroxylation), N-dealkylation followed by further side-chain oxidation, and direct glucuronidation. It has been estimated that the percentage contributions of these routes to total metabolism are 42%, 41%, and 17%, respectively, but with considerable variability between individuals. The four major metabolites are propranolol glucuronide, naphthyloxylactic acid, and glucuronic acid and sulfate conjugates of 4-hydroxy propranolol.

In vitro studies have indicated that the aromatic hydroxylation of propranolol is catalyzed mainly by polymorphic CYP2D6. Side-chain oxidation is mediated mainly by CYP1A2 and to some extent by CYP2D6. 4-hydroxy propranolol is a weak inhibitor of CYP2D6.

Propranolol is also a substrate for CYP2C19 and a substrate for the intestinal efflux transporter, p-glycoprotein (p-gp). Studies suggest however that p-gp is not dose-limiting for intestinal absorption of propranolol in the usual therapeutic dose range.

In healthy subjects no difference was observed between CYP2D6 extensive metabolizers (EMs) and poor metabolizers (PMs) with respect to oral clearance or elimination half-life. Partial clearance to 4-hydroxy propranolol was significantly higher and to naphthyloxylactic acid was significantly lower in EMs than PMs.

Enantiomers

Of the two enantiomers of propranolol the S-enantiomer blocks beta-adrenergic receptors. In normal subjects receiving oral doses of racemic propranolol, S-enantiomer concentrations exceeded those of the R-enantiomer by 40-90% as a result of stereoselective hepatic metabolism.

Special Populations

Pediatric

The pharmacokinetics of InnoPran XL have not been investigated in patients under 18 years of age.

Geriatric

The pharmacokinetics of InnoPran XL have not been investigated in patients over 65 years of age. In a study of 12 elderly (62-79 years old) and 12 young (25-33 years old) healthy subjects, the clearance of S-enantiomer of propranolol was decreased in the elderly. Additionally, the half-life of both the R- and S-propranolol were prolonged in the elderly compared with the young (11 hours vs. 5 hours).

Gender

In a dose-proportionality study, the pharmacokinetics of InnoPran XL were evaluated in 22 male and 14 female healthy volunteers. Following single doses under fasting conditions, the mean AUC and C_{max} were about 49% and 16% higher for females across the dosage range. The mean elimination half-life was longer in females than in males (11 hours vs. 7.5 hours).

Race

A study conducted in 12 Caucasian and 13 African-American male subjects taking propranolol, showed that at steady state, the clearance of R- and S-propranolol were about 76% and 53% higher in African-Americans than in whites, respectively.

Renal Insufficiency

The pharmacokinetics of InnoPran XL have not been evaluated in patients with renal insufficiency. In a study conducted in 5 patients with chronic renal failure, 6 patients on regular dialysis, and 5 healthy subjects, who received a single oral dose of 40 mg of propranolol, the peak plasma concentrations (C_{max}) of propranolol in the chronic renal failure group were 2 to 3-fold higher (161±41 ng/ml) than those observed in the dialysis patients (47±9 ng/ml) and in the healthy subjects (26±1 ng/ml). Propranolol plasma clearance was also reduced in the patients with chronic renal failure.

Chronic renal failure has been associated with a decrease in drug metabolism via down regulation of hepatic cytochrome P450 activity.

Hepatic Insufficiency

The pharmacokinetics of InnoPran XL have not been evaluated in patients with hepatic impairment. However, propranolol is extensively metabolized by the liver. In a study conducted in 7 patients with cirrhosis and 9 healthy subjects receiving 80-mg oral propranolol every 8 hours for 7 doses, the steady-state unbound propranolol concentration in patients with cirrhosis was increased 3-fold in comparison to controls. In cirrhosis, the half-life increased to 11 hours compared to 4 hours (see PRECAUTIONS).

Drug Interactions

Interactions with Substrates, Inhibitors or Inducers of Cytochrome P-450 Enzymes

Because propranolol's metabolism involves multiple pathways in the cytochrome P-450 system (CYP2D6, 1A2, 2C19), administration of InnoPran XL with drugs that are metabolized by, or affect the activity (induction or inhibition) of one or more of these pathways may lead to clinically relevant drug interactions (see DRUG INTERACTIONS under PRECAUTIONS).

Substrates or Inhibitors of CYP2D6

Blood levels and/or toxicity of propranolol may be increased by administration of InnoPran XL with substrates or inhibitors of CYP2D6, such as amiodarone, cimetidine, delavudin, fluoxetine, paroxetine, quinidine, and ritonavir. No interactions were observed with either ranitidine or lansoprazole.

Substrates or Inhibitors of CYP1A2

Blood levels and/or toxicity of propranolol may be increased by administration of InnoPran XL with substrates or inhibitors of CYP1A2, such as imipramine, cimetidine, ciprofloxacin, fluvoxamine, isoniazid, ritonavir, theophylline, zileuton, zolmitriptan, and rizatriptan.

Substrates or Inhibitors of CYP2C19

Blood levels and/or toxicity of propranolol may be increased by administration of InnoPran XL with substrates or inhibitors of CYP2C19, such as fluconazole, cimetidine, fluoxetine, fluvoxamine, teniposide, and tolbutamide. No interaction was observed with omeprazole.

Inducers of Hepatic Drug Metabolism

Blood levels of propranolol may be decreased by administration of InnoPran XL with inducers such as rifampin and ethanol. Cigarette smoking also induces hepatic metabolism and has been shown to increase up to 100% the clearance of propranolol, resulting in decreased plasma concentrations.

Cardiovascular Drugs

Antiarrhythmics

The AUC of propafenone is increased by more than 200% by co-administration of propranolol.

The metabolism of propranolol is reduced by co-administration of quinidine, leading to a two-three fold increase in blood concentrations and greater degrees of clinical beta-blockade.

The metabolism of lidocaine is inhibited by co-administration of propranolol, resulting in a 25% increase in lidocaine concentrations.

Calcium channel blockers

The mean C_{max} and AUC of propranolol are increased respectively, by 50% and 30% by co-administration of nisoldipine and by 80% and 47%, by co-administration of nicardipine.

The mean C_{max} and AUC of nifedipine are increased by 64% and 79%, respectively, by co-administration of propranolol. Propranolol does not affect the pharmacokinetics of verapamil and norverapamil. Verapamil does not affect the pharmacokinetics of propranolol.

Non-Cardiovascular Drugs

Anti-Ulcer Drugs

Co-administration of propranolol with cimetidine, a non-specific CYP450 inhibitor, increased propranolol concentrations by about 40%. Co-administration with aluminum hydroxide gel (1200 mg) resulted in a 50% decrease in propranolol concentrations.

Co-administration of metoclopramide with propranolol did not have a significant effect on propranolol's pharmacokinetics.

Benzodiazepines

Propranolol can inhibit the metabolism of diazepam, resulting in increased concentrations of diazepam and its metabolites. Diazepam does not alter the pharmacokinetics of propranolol.

The pharmacokinetics of oxazepam, triazolam, lorazepam, and alprazolam are not affected by co-administration of propranolol.

Lipid Lowering Drugs

Co-administration of cholesteramine or colestipol with propranolol resulted in up to 50% decrease in propranolol concentrations.

Co-administration of propranolol with lovastatin or pravastatin decreased 20% to 25% the AUC of both, but did not alter their pharmacodynamics. Propranolol did not have an effect on the pharmacokinetics of fluvastatin.

Migraine Drugs

Administration of zolmitriptan or rizatriptan with propranolol resulted in increased concentrations of zolmitriptan (AUC increased by 56% and C_{max} by 37%) or rizatriptan (the AUC and C_{max} were increased by 67% and 75%, respectively).

Neuroleptic Drugs

Co-administration of propranolol at doses greater than or equal to 160 mg/day resulted in increased thioridazine plasma concentrations ranging from 50% to 370% and increased thioridazine metabolites concentrations ranging from 33% to 210%.

Co-administration of chlopromazine with propranolol resulted in increased plasma levels of both drugs (70% increase in propranolol concentrations).

Theophylline

Co-administration of theophylline with propranolol decreases theophylline oral clearance by 33% to 52%.

Warfarin

Concomitant administration of propranolol and warfarin has been shown to increase warfarin bioavailability and increase prothrombin time.

PHARMACODYNAMICS AND CLINICAL EFFECTS

Hypertension

In a double-blind, parallel, dose-response study in patients with mild-to-moderate hypertension (n=434), doses of InnoPran XL from 80 to 640 mg were taken once daily at approximately 10 PM. InnoPran XL significantly lowered sitting systolic and diastolic blood pressure when measurements were taken approximately 16 hours later. The placebo-subtracted diastolic blood pressure effect for the 80 and 120 mg doses were -3.0 and -4.0 mm Hg, respectively. Higher doses of InnoPran XL (160, 640 mg) had no additional blood pressure lowering effect when compared with 120 mg. The antihypertensive effects of InnoPran XL were seen in the elderly (greater than or equal to 65 years old) and men and women. There were too few non-caucasian patients to assess the efficacy of InnoPran XL in these patients.

INDICATIONS AND USAGE

Hypertension

InnoPran XL is indicated in the management of hypertension; it may be used alone or in combination with other antihypertensive agents.

CONTRAINDICATIONS

Propranolol is contraindicated in 1) cardiogenic shock; 2) sinus bradycardia and greater than first-degree block; 3) bronchial asthma; and 4) in patients with known hypersensitivity to propranolol hydrochloride.

WARNINGS

Cardiac Failure: Sympathetic stimulation may be a vital component supporting circulatory function in patients with congestive heart failure, and its inhibition by beta-blockade may precipitate more severe failure. Although beta-blockers should be avoided in overt congestive heart failure, some have been shown to be highly beneficial when used with close follow-up in patients with a history of failure who are well compensated and are receiving additional therapies, including diuretics as needed. Beta-adrenergic blocking agents do not abolish the inotropic action of digitalis on heart muscle.

Angina Pectoris: There have been reports of exacerbation of angina and, in some cases, myocardial infarction, following abrupt discontinuance of propranolol therapy. Therefore, when discontinuance of propranolol is planned, the dosage should be gradually reduced over at least a few weeks, and the patient should be cautioned against interruption or cessation of therapy without a physician's advice. If propranolol therapy is interrupted and exacerbation of angina occurs, it is usually advisable to reinstitute propranolol therapy and take other measures appropriate for the management of angina pectoris. Since coronary artery disease may be unrecognized, it may be prudent to follow the above advice in patients considered at risk of having occult atherosclerotic heart disease who are given propranolol for other indications.

Nonallergic Bronchospasm (e.g., Chronic Bronchitis, Emphysema): In general, patients with bronchospastic lung disease should not receive beta-blockers. Propranolol should be administered with caution in this setting since it may block bronchodilation produced by endogenous and exogenous catecholamine stimulation of beta-receptors.

Major Surgery: The necessity or desirability of withdrawal of beta-blocking therapy prior to major surgery is controversial. It should be noted, however, that the impaired ability of the heart to respond to reflex adrenergic stimuli in propranolol-treated patients may augment the risks of general anesthesia and surgical procedures.

Propranolol is a competitive inhibitor of beta-receptor agonists, and its effects can be reversed by administration of such agents, e.g., dobutamine or isoproterenol. However, such patients may be subject to protracted severe hypotension.

Diabetes and Hypoglycemia: Beta-adrenergic blockade may prevent the appearance of certain premonitory signs and symptoms (pulse rate and blood pressure changes) of acute hypoglycemia, especially in labile insulin-dependent diabetics. In these patients, it may be more difficult to adjust the dosage of insulin.

Propranolol therapy, particularly in infants and children, diabetic or not, has been associated with hypoglycemia especially during fasting, as in preparation for surgery. Hypoglycemia has been reported with propranolol use after prolonged physical exertion and in patients with renal insufficiency.

Thyrotoxicosis: Beta-adrenergic blockade may mask certain clinical signs of hyperthyroidism. Therefore, abrupt withdrawal of propranolol may be followed by an exacerbation of symptoms of hyperthyroidism, including thyroid storm. Propranolol may change thyroid-function tests, increasing T_4 and reversing T_3, and decreasing T_3.

Wolff-Parkinson-White Syndrome: Beta-adrenergic blockade in patients with Wolff-Parkinson-White syndrome and tachycardia has been associated with severe bradycardia requiring treatment with a pacemaker. In one case, this resulted after an initial dose of 5-mg propranolol.

PRECAUTIONS

General

Propranolol should be used with caution in patients with impaired hepatic or renal function. InnoPran XL is not indicated for the treatment of hypertensive emergencies.

Beta-adrenergic receptor blockade can cause reduction of intraocular pressure. Patients should be told that InnoPran XL may interfere with the glaucoma screening test. Withdrawal may lead to a return of intraocular pressure.

Risk of Anaphylactic Reaction. While taking beta-blockers, patients with a history of severe anaphylactic reaction to a variety of allergens may be more reactive to repeated challenge, either accidental, diagnostic, or therapeutic. Such patients may be unresponsive to the usual doses of epinephrine used to treat allergic reaction.

Clinical Laboratory Tests

In patients with hypertension, use of propranolol has been associated with elevated levels of serum potassium, and serum transaminases and alkaline phosphatase. In severe heart failure, the use of propranolol has been associated with increases in Blood Urea Nitrogen.

Drug Interactions

Caution should be exercised when InnoPran XL is administered with drugs that have an effect on CYP2D6, 1A2 or 2C19 metabolic pathways. Co-administration of such drugs with propranolol may lead to clinically relevant drug interactions and changes on its efficacy and/or toxicity (see DRUG INTERACTIONS in CLINICAL PHARMACOLOGY).

Cardiovascular Drugs

ACE Inhibitors

When combined with beta-blockers, ACE inhibitors can cause hypotension, particularly in the setting of acute myocardial infarction.

Certain ACE inhibitors have been reported to increase bronchial hyperreactivity when administered with propranolol.

The antihypertensive effects of clonidine may be antagonized by beta-blockers. InnoPran XL should be administered cautiously to patients withdrawing from clonidine.

Alpha Blockers

Prazosin has been associated with prolongation of first dose hypotension in the presence of beta-blockers.

Postural hypotension has been reported in patients taking both beta-blockers and terazosin or doxazosin.

Antiarrhythmics

Propafenone has negative inotropic and beta-blocking properties that can be additive to those of propranolol.

Quinidine increases the concentration of propranolol and produces greater degrees of clinical beta-blockade and may cause postural hypotension.

Disopyramide is a Type I antiarrhythmic drug with potent negative inotropic and chronotropic effects and has been associated with severe bradycardia, asystole and heart failure when administered with propranolol.

Amiodarone is an antiarrhythmic agent with negative chronotropic properties that may be additive to those seen with propranolol.

The clearance of lidocaine is reduced with administration of propranolol. Lidocaine toxicity has been reported following coadministration with propranolol.

Caution should be exercised when administering InnoPran XL with drugs that slow A-V nodal conduction, e.g., digitalis, lidocaine and calcium channel blockers.

Calcium Channel Blockers

Caution should be exercised when patients receiving a beta-blocker are administered a calcium-channel-blocking drug with negative inotropic and/or chronotropic effects. Both agents may depress myocardial contractility or atrioventricular conduction.

There have been reports of significant bradycardia, heart failure, and cardiovascular collapse with concurrent use of verapamil and beta-blockers.

Co-administration of propranolol and diltiazem in patients with cardiac disease has been associated with bradycardia, hypotension, high degree heart block, and heart failure.

Inotropic Agents

Patients on long-term therapy with propranolol may experience uncontrolled hypertension if administered epinephrine as a consequence of unopposed alpha-receptor stimulation. Epinephrine is therefore not indicated in the treatment of propranolol overdose (see OVERDOSAGE).

Isoproterenol and Dobutamine

Propranolol is a competitive inhibitor of beta-receptor agonists, and its effects can be reversed by administration of such agents, e.g., dobutamine or isoproterenol. Also, propranolol may reduce sensitivity to dobutamine stress echocardiography in patients undergoing evaluation for myocardial ischemia.

Reserpine

Patients receiving catecholamine-depleting drugs, such as reserpine and InnoPran XL, should be closely observed for excessive reduction of resting sympathetic nervous activity, which may result in hypotension, marked bradycardia, vertigo, syncopal attacks, or orthostatic hypotension. Administration of reserpine with propranolol may also potentiate depression.

Non-Cardiovascular Drugs

Anesthetic Agents

Methoxyflurane and trichloroethylene may depress myocardial contractility when administered with propranolol.

Antidepressants

The hypotensive effects of MAO inhibitors or tricyclic antidepressants may be exacerbated when administered with beta-blockers by interfering with the beta-blocking activity of propranolol.

Neuroleptic Drugs

Hypotension and cardiac arrest have been reported with the concomitant use of propranolol and haloperidol.

Non-Steroidal Anti-Inflammatory Drugs

Nonsteroidal anti-inflammatory drugs (NSAIDS) have been reported to blunt the antihypertensive effect of beta-adrenoreceptor blocking agents.

Administration of indomethacin with propranolol may reduce the efficacy of propranolol in reducing blood pressure and heart rate.

Thyroxine

Thyroxine may result in a lower than expected T_3 concentration when used concomitantly with propranolol.

Warfarin

Propranolol when administered with warfarin increases the concentration of warfarin. Prothrombin time, therefore, should be monitored.

Carcinogenesis, Mutagenesis, Impairment of Fertility

In dietary administration studies in which mice and rats were treated with propranolol for up to 18 months at doses of up to 150 mg/kg/day, there was no evidence of drug-related tumorigenesis. On a body surface area basis, this dose in the mouse and rat is, respectively, about equal to and about twice the maximum recommended human oral daily dose (MRHD) of 640 mg propranolol. In a study in which both male and female rats were exposed to propranolol in their diets at concentrations of up to 0.05% (about 50 mg/kg body weight and less than the MRHD), from 60 days prior to mating and throughout pregnancy and lactation for two generations, there were no effects on fertility. Based on differing results from Ames Tests performed by different laboratories, there is equivocal evidence for a genotoxic effect of propranolol in bacteria (S. typhimurium strain TA 1538).

Pregnancy: Pregnancy Category C

In a series of reproductive and developmental toxicology studies, propranolol was given to rats by gavage or in the diet throughout pregnancy and lactation. At doses of 150 mg/kg/day, but not at doses of 80 mg/kg/day (equivalent to the MRHD on a body surface area basis), treatment was associated with embryotoxicity (reduced litter size and increased resorption rates) as well as neonatal toxicity (deaths). Propranolol also was administered (in the feed) to rabbits (throughout pregnancy and lactation) at doses as high as 150 mg/kg/day (about 5 times the maximum recommended human oral daily dose). No evidence of embryo or neonatal toxicity was noted.

There are no adequate and well-controlled studies in pregnant women. Intrauterine growth retardation has been re-

Continued on next page

InnoPran XL—Cont.

ported for neonates whose mothers received propranolol during pregnancy. Neonates whose mothers received propranolol at parturition have exhibited bradycardia, hypoglycemia, and respiratory depression. Adequate facilities for monitoring such infants at birth should be available. InnoPran XL should be used during pregnancy only if the potential benefit justifies the potential risk to the fetus.

Nursing Mothers

Propranolol is excreted in human milk. Caution should be exercised when InnoPran XL is administered to a nursing mother.

Pediatric Use

Safety and effectiveness of propranolol in pediatric patients have not been established.

Geriatric Use

Clinical studies of InnoPran XL did not include sufficient numbers of subjects ages 65 and over to determine whether they respond differently from younger subjects. Other reported clinical experience has not identified differences in responses between the elderly and younger patients. In general, dose selection for an elderly patient should be cautious, usually starting at the low end of the dosing range, reflecting the greater frequency of decreased hepatic, renal, or cardiac function, and of concomitant disease or other drug therapy.

ADVERSE REACTIONS

Adverse events occurring at a rate of ≥3%, excluding those reported more commonly in placebo encountered in the InnoPran XL placebo-controlled hypertension trials and are plausibly related to treatment, are shown in Table 1.

Table 1. Treatment Emergent Adverse Events Reported In ≥ 3% of Subjects

		InnoPran XL	
Body System	**Placebo (N=88)**	**80 mg (N=89)**	**120 mg (N=85)**
Fatigue	3 (3.0%)	4 (5.0%)	6 (7.0%)
Dizziness (except vertigo)	2 (2.0%)	6 (7.0%)	3 (4.0%)
Constipation	0	3 (3.0%)	1 (1.0%)

The following adverse events were observed and have been reported with use of formulations of sustained- or immediate-release propranolol.

Cardiovascular: Bradycardia; congestive heart failure; intensification of AV block; hypotension; paresthesia of hands; thrombocytopenic purpura; arterial insufficiency, usually of the Raynaud type.

Central Nervous System: Light-headedness, mental depression manifested by insomnia, lassitude, weakness, fatigue; reversible mental depression progressing to catatonia; visual disturbances; hallucinations; vivid dreams; an acute reversible syndrome characterized by disorientation for time and place, short-term memory loss, emotional lability, slightly clouded sensorium, and decreased performance on neuropsychometrics. For immediate-release formulations, fatigue, lethargy, and vivid dreams appear dose related.

Gastrointestinal: Nausea, vomiting, epigastric distress, abdominal cramping, diarrhea, constipation, mesenteric arterial thrombosis, ischemic colitis.

Allergic: Pharyngitis and agranulocytosis; erythematous rash, fever combined with aching and sore throat; laryngospasm, and respiratory distress.

Respiratory: Bronchospasm.

Hematologic: Agranulocytosis, nonthrombocytopenic purpura, thrombocytopenic purpura.

Autoimmune: In extremely rare instances, systemic lupus erythematosus has been reported.

Miscellaneous: Alopecia, LE-like reactions, psoriasiform rashes, dry eyes, male impotence, and Peyronie's disease have been reported rarely. Oculomucocutaneous reactions involving the skin, serous membranes, and conjunctivae reported for a beta blocker (practolol) have not been associated with propranolol.

DOSAGE AND ADMINISTRATION

InnoPran XL should be administered once daily at bedtime (approximately 10 PM) and should be taken consistently either on an empty stomach or with food. The starting dose is 80 mg but dosage should be individualized and titration may be needed to a dose of 120 mg. In the clinical trial, doses of InnoPran XL above 120 mg had no additional effects on blood pressure (See PHARMACODYNAMICS AND CLINICAL EFFECTS). The time needed for full antihypertensive response is variable, but is usually achieved within 2-3 weeks.

OVERDOSAGE

Most overdoses of propranolol are mild and respond to supportive care.

Propranolol is not significantly dialyzable. In the event of overdose or exaggerated response, the following measures should be employed:

Decontamination: Gastric lavage

Supportive Therapy

Hypotension and bradycardia have been reported following propranolol overdose and should be treated appropriately. Glucagon can exert potent inotropic and chronotropic effects and may be particularly useful for the treatment of hypotension or depressed myocardial function after a propranolol overdose.

Glucagon should be administered as 50-150 mcg/kg intravenously followed by continuous drip of 1-5 mg/hour for positive chronotropic effect. Isoproterenol,dopamine or phosphodiesterase inhibitors may also be useful. Epinephrine, however, may provoke uncontrolled hypertension. Bradycardia can be treated with atropine or isoproterenol. Serious bradycardia may require temporary cardiac pacing.

The electrocardiogram, pulse, blood pressure, neurobehavioral status and intake and output balance must be monitored. Isoproterenol and aminophylline may be used for bronchospasm.

HOW SUPPLIED

InnoPran XL (propranolol hydrochloride) Extended Release Capsules

Each gray/white capsule, imprinted with "80", 2 segmented bands, "RD201", and Reliant logo contains 80 mg of propranolol hydrochloride in bottles of 30 (NDC 65726-250-10), bottles of 100 (NDC 65726-250-25), bottles of 500 (NDC 65726-250-35), and a Unit Dose package of 100 (NDC 65726-250-90).

Each gray/off-white capsule, imprinted with "120", 3 segmented bands "InnoPran XL" and Reliant logo contains 120 mg of propranolol hydrochloride in bottles of 30 (NDC 65726-251-10), bottles of 100 (NDC 65726-251-25), bottles of 500 (NDC 65726-251-35) , and a Unit Dose package of 100 (NDC 65726-251-90).

Store at 25°C (77°F); excursions permitted to 15-30°C (59-86°F) [see USP Controlled Room Temperature] in a tightly closed container. The unit dose packaging should be stored in the carton.

Rx only

April 2004

Reliant PHARMACEUTICALS LLC

Manufactured for:
Reliant Pharmaceuticals
Liberty Corner, NJ 07938
By:
Eurand America, Inc.
Vandalia, OH 45377

Address Medical Inquiries to:
Reliant Pharmaceuticals
Medical Affairs
110 Allen Road
Liberty Corner, NJ 07938 225R000

Shown in Product Identification Guide, page 331

LESCOL® ℞
(fluvastatin sodium)
Capsules
LESCOL® XL
(fluvastatin sodium)
Extended-Release Tablets
Rx only

Prescribing Information

DESCRIPTION

Lescol® (fluvastatin sodium), is a water-soluble cholesterol lowering agent which acts through the inhibition of 3-hydroxy-3-methylglutaryl-coenzyme A (HMG-CoA) reductase.

Fluvastatin sodium is [*R**, *S**-(*E*)]-(±)-7-[3-(4-fluorophenyl)-1-(1-methylethyl)-1*H*-indol-2-yl]-3,5-dihydroxy-6-heptenoic acid, monosodium salt. The empirical formula of fluvastatin sodium is $C_{24}H_{25}FNO_4$•Na, its molecular weight is 433.46 and its structural formula is:

$C_{24}H_{25}FNO_4$ • Na   Mol. wt. 433.46

This molecular entity is the first entirely synthetic HMG-CoA reductase inhibitor, and is in part structurally distinct from the fungal derivatives of this therapeutic class.

Fluvastatin sodium is a white to pale yellow, hygroscopic powder soluble in water, ethanol and methanol. Lescol is supplied as capsules containing fluvastatin sodium, equivalent to 20 mg or 40 mg of fluvastatin, for oral administration. Lescol® XL (fluvastatin sodium) is supplied as extended-release tablets containing fluvastatin sodium, equivalent to 80 mg of fluvastatin, for oral administration.

Active Ingredient: fluvastatin sodium

Inactive Ingredients in capsules: gelatin, magnesium stearate, microcrystalline cellulose, pregelatinized starch (corn), red iron oxide, sodium lauryl sulfate, talc, titanium dioxide, yellow iron oxide, and other ingredients.

Capsules may also include: benzyl alcohol, black iron oxide, butylparaben, carboxymethylcellulose sodium, edetate calcium disodium, methylparaben, propylparaben, silicon dioxide and sodium propionate.

Inactive Ingredients in extended-release tablets: microcrystalline cellulose, hydroxypropyl cellulose, hydroxypropyl methyl cellulose, potassium bicarbonate, povidone, magnesium stearate, iron oxide yellow, titanium dioxide and polyethylene glycol 8000.

CLINICAL PHARMACOLOGY

A variety of clinical studies have demonstrated that elevated levels of total cholesterol (Total-C), low density lipoprotein cholesterol (LDL-C), triglycerides (TG) and apolipoprotein B (a membrane transport complex for LDL-C) promote human atherosclerosis. Similarly, decreased levels of HDL-cholesterol (HDL-C) and its transport complex, apolipoprotein A, are associated with the development of atherosclerosis. Epidemiologic investigations have established that cardiovascular morbidity and mortality vary directly with the level of Total-C and LDL-C and inversely with the level of HDL-C.

Like LDL, cholesterol-enriched triglyceride-rich lipoproteins, including VLDL, IDL and remnants, can also promote atherosclerosis. Elevated plasma triglycerides are frequently found in a triad with low HDL-C levels and small LDL particles, as well as in association with non-lipid metabolic risk factors for coronary heart disease. As such, total plasma TG has not consistently been shown to be an independent risk factor for CHD. Furthermore, the independent effect of raising HDL or lowering TG on the risk of coronary and cardiovascular morbidity and mortality has not been determined.

In patients with hypercholesterolemia and mixed dyslipidemia, treatment with Lescol® (fluvastatin sodium) or Lescol® XL (fluvastatin sodium) reduced Total-C, LDL-C, apolipoprotein B, and triglycerides while producing an increase in HDL-C. Increases in HDL-C are greater in patients with low HDL-C (<35 mg/dL). Neither agent had a consistent effect on either Lp(a) or fibrinogen. The effect of Lescol or Lescol XL induced changes in lipoprotein levels, including reduction of serum cholesterol, on cardiovascular mortality has not been determined.

Mechanism of Action

Lescol is a competitive inhibitor of HMG-CoA reductase, which is responsible for the conversion of 3-hydroxy-3-methylglutaryl-coenzyme A (HMG-CoA) to mevalonate, a precursor of sterols, including cholesterol. The inhibition of cholesterol biosynthesis reduces the cholesterol in hepatic cells, which stimulates the synthesis of LDL receptors and thereby increases the uptake of LDL particles. The end result of these biochemical processes is a reduction of the plasma cholesterol concentration.

Pharmacokinetics/Metabolism

Oral Absorption

Fluvastatin is absorbed rapidly and completely following oral administration of the capsule, with peak concentrations reached in less than 1 hour. Following administration of a 10 mg dose, the absolute bioavailability is 24% (range 9%-50%). Administration with food reduces the rate but not the extent of absorption. At steady-state, administration of fluvastatin with the evening meal results in a two-fold decrease in C_{max} and more than two-fold increase in t_{max} as compared to administration 4 hours after the evening meal. No significant differences in extent of absorption or in the lipid-lowering effects were observed between the two administrations. After single or multiple doses above 20 mg, fluvastatin exhibits saturable first-pass metabolism resulting in higher-than-expected plasma fluvastatin concentrations.

Fluvastatin has two optical enantiomers, an active 3R, 5S and an inactive 3S,5R form. In vivo studies showed that stereo-selective hepatic binding of the active form occurs during the first pass resulting in a difference in the peak levels of the two enantiomers, with the active to inactive peak concentration ratio being about 0.7. The approximate ratio of the active to inactive approaches unity after the peak is seen and thereafter the two enantiomers decline with the same half-life. After an intravenous administration, bypassing the first-pass metabolism, the ratios of the enantiomers in plasma were similar throughout the concentration-time profiles.

Fluvastatin administered as Lescol XL 80 mg tablets reaches peak concentration in approximately 3 hours under fasting conditions, after a low-fat meal, or 2.5 hours after a low-fat meal. The mean relative bioavailability of the XL tablet is approximately 29% (range: 9%-66%) compared to that of the Lescol immediate release capsule administered under fasting conditions. Administration of a high fat meal delayed the absorption (T_{max}: 6H) and increased the bioavailability of the XL tablet by approximately 50%. Once Lescol XL begins to be absorbed, fluvastatin concentrations rise rapidly. The maximum concentration seen after a high fat meal is much less than the peak concentration following a single dose or twice daily dose of the 40 mg Lescol capsule. Overall variability in the pharmacokinetics of Lescol XL is large (42%-64% CV for C_{max} and AUC), and especially so after a high fat meal (63%-89% for C_{max} and AUC). Intrasubject variability in the pharmacokinetics of Lescol XL under fasting conditions (about 25% for C_{max} and AUC) tends to be much smaller as compared to the overall variability. Multiple peaks in plasma fluvastatin concentrations have been observed after Lescol XL administration.

Distribution

Fluvastatin is 98% bound to plasma proteins. The mean volume of distribution (VD_{ss}) is estimated at 0.35 L/kg. The parent drug is targeted to the liver and no active metabolites are present systemically. At therapeutic concentrations, the protein binding of fluvastatin is not affected by warfarin, salicylic acid and glyburide.

Metabolism

Fluvastatin is metabolized in the liver, primarily via hydroxylation of the indole ring at the 5- and 6-positions. N-dealkylation and beta-oxidation of the side-chain also occurs. The hydroxy metabolites have some pharmacologic activity, but do not circulate in the blood. Both enantiomers of fluvastatin are metabolized in a similar manner.

In vitro studies demonstrated that fluvastatin undergoes oxidative metabolism, predominantly via 2C9 isozyme systems (75%). Other isozymes that contribute to fluvastatin metabolism are 2C8 (~5%) and 3A4 (~20%). *(See PRECAUTIONS: Drug Interactions Section).*

Elimination

Fluvastatin is primarily (about 90%) eliminated in the feces as metabolites, with less than 2% present as unchanged drug. Urinary recovery is about 5%. After a radiolabeled dose of fluvastatin, the clearance was 0.8 L/h/kg. Following multiple oral doses of radiolabeled compound, there was no accumulation of fluvastatin; however, there was a 2.3 fold accumulation of total radioactivity.

Steady-state plasma concentrations show no evidence of accumulation of fluvastatin following immediate release capsule administration of up to 80 mg daily, as evidenced by a beta-elimination half-life of less than 3 hours. However, under conditions of maximum rate of absorption (i.e., fasting) systemic exposure to fluvastatin is increased 33% to 53% compared to a single 20 mg or 40 mg dose of the immediate release capsule. Following once daily administration of the 80 mg Lescol XL tablet for 7 days, systemic exposure to fluvastatin is increased (20%-30%) compared to a single dose of the 80 mg Lescol XL tablet. Terminal half-life of Lescol XL was about 9 hours as a result of the slow-release formulation.

Single-dose and steady-state pharmacokinetic parameters in 33 subjects with hypercholesterolemia for the capsules and in 35 healthy subjects for the extended-release tablets are summarized below:

[See table 1 above]

Special Populations

Renal Insufficiency: No significant (<6%) renal excretion of fluvastatin occurs in humans.

Hepatic Insufficiency: Fluvastatin is subject to saturable first-pass metabolism/sequestration by the liver and is eliminated primarily via the biliary route. Therefore, the potential exists for drug accumulation in patients with hepatic insufficiency. Caution should therefore be exercised when fluvastatin sodium is administered to patients with a history of liver disease or heavy alcohol ingestion *(see WARNINGS).*

Fluvastatin AUC and C_{max} values increased by about 2.5 fold in hepatic insufficiency patients. This result was attributed to the decreased presystemic metabolism due to hepatic dysfunction. The enantiomer ratios of the two isomers of fluvastatin in hepatic insufficiency patients were comparable to those observed in healthy subjects.

Age: Plasma levels of fluvastatin are not affected by age.

Gender: Women tend to have slightly higher (but statistically insignificant) fluvastatin concentrations than men for the immediate release capsule. This is most likely due to body weight differences, as adjusting for body weight decreases the magnitude of the differences seen. For Lescol XL, there are 67% and 77% increases in systemic availability for women over men under fasted and high fat meal conditions.

Pediatric: No data are available. Fluvastatin is not indicated for use in the pediatric population.

CLINICAL STUDIES

Hypercholesterolemia (heterozygous familial and non familial) and Mixed Dyslipidemia

In 12 placebo-controlled studies in patients with Type IIa or IIb hyperlipoproteinemia, Lescol® (fluvastatin sodium) alone was administered to 1621 patients in daily dose regimens of 20 mg, 40 mg, and 80 mg (40 mg twice daily) for at least 6 weeks duration. After 24 weeks of treatment, daily doses of 20 mg, 40 mg, and 80 mg (40 mg twice daily) resulted in median LDL-C reductions of 22% (n=747), 25% (n=748) and 36% (n=257), respectively. Lescol treatment produced dose-related reductions in Apo B and in triglycerides and increases in HDL-C. The median (25th, 75th percentile) percent changes from baseline in HDL-C after 12 weeks of treatment with Lescol at daily doses of 20 mg, 40 mg and 80 mg (40 mg twice daily) were +2 (-4,+10), +5 (-2,+12), and +4 (-3,+12), respectively. In a subgroup of patients with primary mixed dyslipidemia, defined as baseline TG levels ≥200 mg/dL, treatment with Lescol also produced significant decreases in Total-C, LDL-C, TG and Apo B and variable increases in HDL-C. The median (25th 75th percentile) percent changes from baseline in HDL-C after 12 weeks of treatment with Lescol at daily doses of 20 mg, 40 mg and 80 mg (40 mg twice daily) in this population were +4 (-2,+12), +8 (+1,+15), and +4 (-3,+13), respectively.

In a long-term open-label free titration study, after 96 weeks LDL-C decreases of 25% (20 mg, n=68), 31% (40 mg, n=298) and 34% (80 mg, n=209) were seen. No consistent effect on Lp(a) was observed.

Lescol® XL (fluvastatin sodium) Extended-Release Tablets have been studied in five controlled studies of patients with Type IIa or IIb hyperlipoproteinemia. Lescol XL was administered to over 900 patients in trials from 4 to 26 weeks in duration. In the three largest of these studies, Lescol XL given as a single daily dose of 80 mg significantly reduced Total-C, LDL-C, TG and Apo B. Therapeutic response is well established within two weeks, and a maximum response is achieved within four weeks. After four weeks of therapy, the median decrease in LDL-C was 38% and at week 24 endpoint the median LDL-C decrease was 35%. Significant increases in HDL-C were also observed. The median (25th and 75th percentile) percent changes from baseline in HDL-C for Lescol XL were +7(+0,+15) after 24 weeks of treatment.

[See table 2 above]

In patients with primary mixed dyslipidemia (Fredrickson Type IIb) as defined by baseline plasma triglycerides levels ≥200 mg/dL, Lescol XL 80 mg produced a median reduction in triglycerides of 25%. In these patients, Lescol XL 80 mg produced median (25th and 75th percentile) percent change from baseline in HDL-C of +11(+3,+20). Significant decreases in Total-C, LDL-C, and Apo B were also achieved. In these studies, patients with triglycerides >400 mg/dL were excluded.

Table 1
Single-Dose and Steady-State Pharmacokinetic Parameters

	C_{max} (ng/mL) mean±SD (range)	AUC (ng•h/mL) mean±SD (range)	t_{max} (hr) mean±SD (range)	CL/F (L/hr) mean±SD (range)	$t_{1/2}$ (hr) mean±SD (range)
Capsules					
20 mg single dose (n=17)	166±106 (48.9-517)	207±65 (111-288)	0.9±0.4 (0.5-2.0)	107±38.1 (69.5-181)	2.5±1.7 (0.5-6.6)
20 mg twice daily (n=17)	200±86 (71.8-366)	275±111 (91.6-467)	1.2±0.9 (0.5-4.0)	87.8±45 (42.8-218)	2.8±1.7 (0.9-6.0)
40 mg single dose (n=16)	273±189 (72.8-812)	456±259 (207-1221)	1,2±0.7 (0.75-3.0)	108±44.7 (32.8-193)	2.7±1.3 (0.8-5.9)
40 mg twice daily (n=16)	432±236 (119-990)	697±275 (359-1559)	1.2±0.6 (0.5-2.5)	64.2±21.1 (25.7-111)	2.7±1.3 (0.7-5.0)
Extended-Release Tablets 80 mg single dose (n=24)					
80 mg single dose, fasting (n=24)	126±53 (37-242)	579±341 (144-1760)	3.2±2.6 (1-12)		
80 mg single dose, fed-state high fat meal (n=24)	183±163 (21-733)	861±632 (199-3132)	6 (2-24)		
Extended-Release Tablets 80 mg following 7 days dosing (steady-state) (n=11)					
80 mg once daily, fasting (n=11)	102±42 (43.9-181)	630±326 (247-1406)	2.6±0.91 (1.5-4)		

Table 2
Median Percent Change in Lipid Parameters from Baseline to Week 24 Endpoint
All Placebo-Controlled Studies (Lescol®) and Active Controlled Trials (Lescol® XL)

Dose	Total Chol. N	Total Chol. % Δ	TG N	TG % Δ	LDL N	LDL % Δ	Apo B N	Apo B % Δ	HDL N	HDL % Δ
All Patients										
Lescol 20 mg[1]	747	-17	747	-12	747	-22	114	-19	747	+3
Lescol 40 mg[1]	748	-19	748	-14	748	-25	125	-18	748	+4
Lescol 40 mg twice daily[1]	257	-27	257	-18	257	-36	232	-28	257	+6
Lescol XL 80 mg[2]	750	-25	750	-19	748	-35	745	-27	750	+7
Baseline TG ≥200 mg/dL										
Lescol 20 mg[1]	148	-16	148	-17	148	-22	23	-19	148	+6
Lescol 40 mg[1]	179	-18	179	-20	179	-24	47	-18	179	+7
Lescol 40 mg twice daily[1]	76	-27	76	-23	76	-35	69	-28	76	+9
Lescol XL 80 mg[2]	239	-25	239	-25	237	-33	235	-27	239	+11

[1]Data for Lescol from 12 placebo controlled trials
[2]Data for Lescol XL 80 mg tablet from three 24 week controlled trials

Reduction in the Risk of Recurrent Cardiac Events

In the Lescol Intervention Prevention Study, the effect of Lescol 40 mg administered twice daily on the risk of recurrent cardiac events (time to first occurrence of cardiac death, nonfatal myocardial infarction, or revascularization) was assessed in 1677 patients with coronary heart disease who had undergone a percutaneous coronary intervention (PCI) procedure (mean time from PCI to randomization=3 days). In this multicenter, randomized, double-blind, placebo-controlled study, patients were treated with dietary/lifestyle counseling and either Lescol 40 mg (n=844) or placebo (n=833) given twice daily for a median of 3.9 years. The study population was 84% male, 98% Caucasian, with 37% >65 years of age. At baseline patients had total cholesterol between 100 and 367 mg/dL (mean 201 mg/dL), LDL-C between 42 and 243 mg/dL (mean 132 mg/dL), triglycerides between 15 and 270 mg/dL (mean 70 mg/dL) and HDL-C between 8 and 174 mg/dL (mean 39 mg/dL).

Lescol significantly reduced the risk of recurrent cardiac events (Figure 1) by 22% (p=0.013, 181 patients in the Lescol group vs. 222 patients in the placebo group). Revascularization procedures comprised the majority of the initial recurrent cardiac events (143 revascularization procedures in the Lescol group and 171 in the placebo group). Consistent trends in risk reduction were observed in patients >65 years of age.

[See figure 1 at top of next column]

Outcome data for the Lescol Intervention Prevention Study are shown in Figure 2. After exclusion of revascularization procedures (CABG and repeat PCI) occurring within the first 6 months of the initial procedure involving the originally instrumented site, treatment with Lescol was associated with a 32% (p=0.002) reduction in risk of late revascularization procedures (CABG or PCI occurring at the original site >6 months after the initial procedure, or at another site).

Figure 1. Primary Endpoint - Recurrent Cardiac Events (Cardiac Death, Nonfatal MI or Revascularization Procedure) (ITT Population)

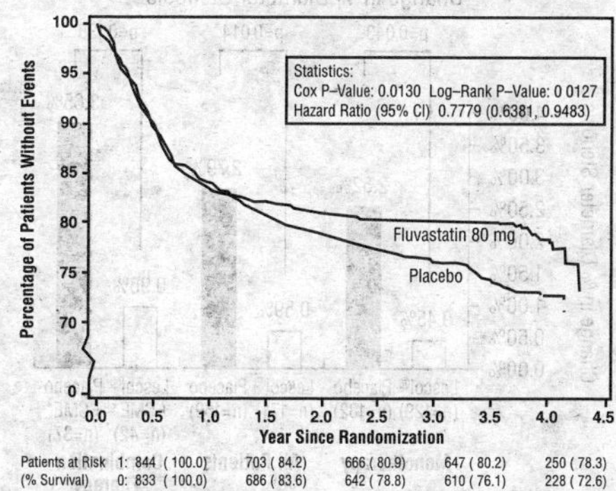

Figure 2. Lescol® Intervention Prevention Study - Primary and Secondary Endpoints

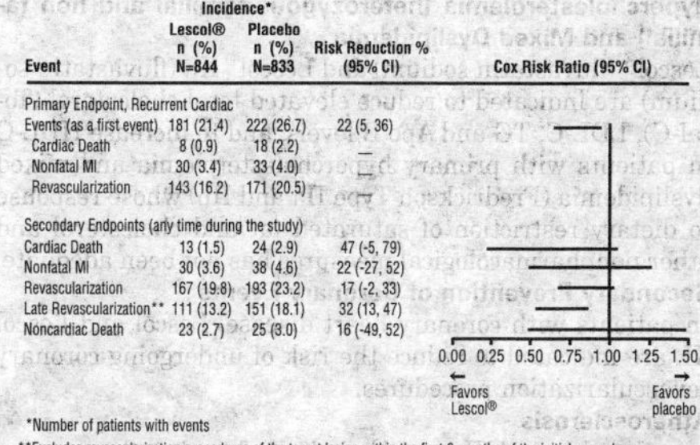

Event	Incidence* Lescol® n (%) N=844	Incidence* Placebo n (%) N=833	Risk Reduction % (95% CI)	Cox Risk Ratio (95% CI)
Primary Endpoint, Recurrent Cardiac Events (as a first event)	181 (21.4)	222 (26.7)	22 (5, 36)	
Cardiac Death	8 (0.9)	18 (2.2)		
Nonfatal MI	30 (3.4)	33 (4.0)		
Revascularization	143 (16.2)	171 (20.5)		
Secondary Endpoints (any time during the study)				
Cardiac Death	13 (1.5)	24 (2.9)	47 (-5, 79)	
Nonfatal MI	30 (3.6)	38 (4.6)	22 (-27, 52)	
Revascularization	167 (19.8)	193 (23.2)	17 (-2, 33)	
Late Revascularization**	111 (13.2)	151 (18.1)	32 (13, 47)	
Noncardiac Death	23 (2.7)	25 (3.0)	16 (-49, 52)	

*Number of patients with events
**Excludes revascularization procedurse of the target lesion within the first 6 months of the initial procedure

Atherosclerosis

In the Lipoprotein and Coronary Atherosclerosis Study (LCAS), the effect of Lescol therapy on coronary atherosclerosis was assessed by quantitative coronary angiography (QCA) in patients with coronary artery disease and mild to moderate hypercholesterolemia (baseline LDL-C range 115-

Continued on next page

Lescol—Cont.

190 mg/dL). In this randomized double-blind, placebo controlled trial, 429 patients were treated with conventional measures (Step 1 AHA Diet) and either Lescol 40 mg/day or placebo. In order to provide treatment to patients receiving placebo with LDL-C levels ≥160 mg/dL at baseline, adjunctive therapy with cholestyramine was added after week 12 to all patients in the study with baseline LDL-C values of ≥160 mg/dL. These baseline levels were present in 25% of the study population. Quantitative coronary angiograms were evaluated at baseline and 2.5 years in 340 (79%) angiographic evaluable patients.

Lescol significantly slowed the progression of coronary atherosclerosis. Compared to placebo, Lescol significantly slowed the progression of lesions as measured by within-patient per-lesion change in minimum lumen diameter (MLD), the primary endpoint (see Figure 3 below), percent diameter stenosis (Figure 4), and the formation of new lesions (13% of all fluvastatin patients versus 22% of all placebo patients). Additionally, a significant difference in favor of Lescol was found between all fluvastatin and all placebo patients in the distribution among the three categories of definite progression, definite regression, and mixed or no change. Beneficial angiographic results (change in MLD) were independent of patients' gender and consistent across a range of baseline LDL-C levels.

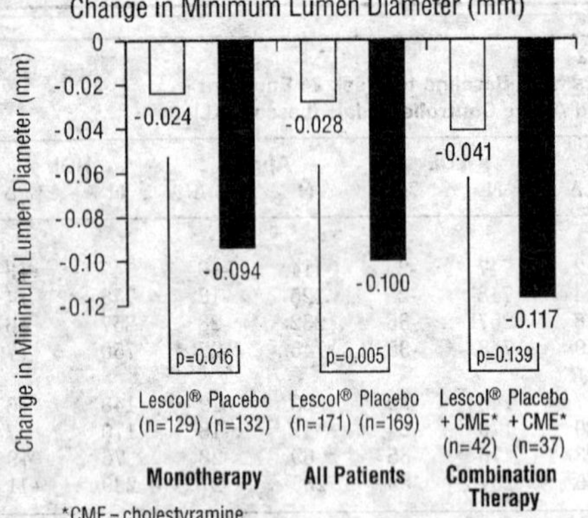

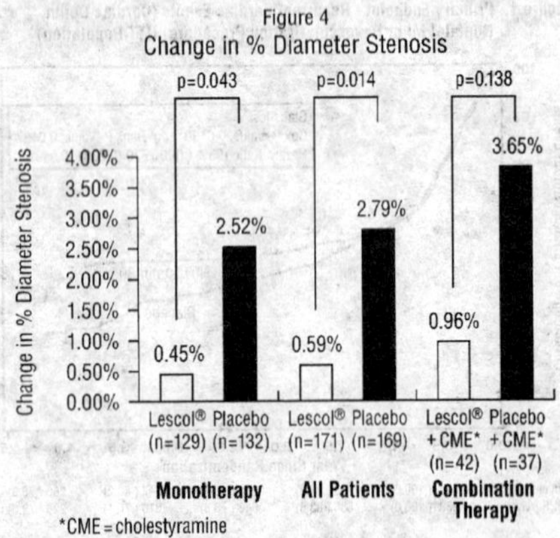

INDICATIONS AND USAGE

Therapy with lipid-altering agents should be used in addition to a diet restricted in saturated fat and cholesterol (see National Cholesterol Education Program (NCEP) Treatment Guidelines, below).

Hypercholesterolemia (heterozygous familial and non familial) and Mixed Dyslipidemia

Lescol® (fluvastatin sodium) and Lescol® XL (fluvastatin sodium) are indicated to reduce elevated total cholesterol (Total-C), LDL-C, TG and Apo B levels, and to increase HDL-C in patients with primary hypercholesterolemia and mixed dyslipidemia (Fredrickson Type IIa and IIb) whose response to dietary restriction of saturated fat and cholesterol and other nonpharmacological measures has not been adequate.

Secondary Prevention of Coronary Events

In patients with coronary heart disease, Lescol and Lescol XL are indicated to reduce the risk of undergoing coronary revascularization procedures.

Atherosclerosis

Lescol and Lescol XL are also indicated to slow the progression of coronary atherosclerosis in patients with coronary heart disease as part of a treatment strategy to lower total and LDL cholesterol to target levels.

Therapy with lipid-altering agents should be considered only after secondary causes for hyperlipidemia such as poorly controlled diabetes mellitus, hypothyroidism, nephrotic syndrome, dysproteinemias, obstructive liver disease, other medication, or alcoholism, have been excluded. Prior to initiation of fluvastatin sodium, a lipid profile

Table 3
NCEP Treatment Guidelines: LDL-C Goals and Cutpoints for Therapeutic Lifestyle Changes and Drug Therapy in Different Risk Categories

Risk Category	LDL Goal (mg/dL)	LDL Level at Which to Initiate Therapeutic Lifestyle Changes (mg/dL)	LDL Level at Which to Consider Drug Therapy (mg/dL)
CHD† or CHD risk equivalents (10-year risk >20%)	<100	≥100	≥130 (100-129: drug optional)††
2+ Risk factors (10-year risk ≤20%)	<130	≥130	10-year risk 10%-20%: ≥130 10-year risk <10%: ≥160
0–1 Risk factor†††	<160	≥160	≥190 (160–189: LDL-lowering drug optional)

†CHD, coronary heart disease

††Some authorities recommend use of LDL-lowering drugs in this category if an LDL-C level of <100mg/dL cannot be achieved by therapeutic lifestyle changes. Others prefer use of drugs that primarily modify triglycerides and HDL-C, e.g. nicotinic acid or fibrate. Clinical judgement also may call for deferring drug therapy in this subcategory.

†††Almost all people with 0-1 risk factor have 10-year risk <10%; thus, 10-year risk assessment in people with 0-1 risk factor is not necessary.

Table 4

Classification of Hyperlipoproteinemias

Type	Lipoproteins Elevated	Lipid Elevations: Major	Lipid Elevations: Minor
I (rare)	Chylomicrons	TG	↑ → C
IIa	LDL	C	–
IIb	LDL, VLDL	C	TG
III (rare)	IDL	C/TG	–
IV	VLDL	TG	↑ → C
V (rare)	Chylomicrons, VLDL	TG	↑ → C

C = cholesterol, TG = triglycerides, LDL = low density lipoprotein, VLDL = very low density lipoprotein, IDL = intermediate density lipoprotein

should be performed to measure Total-C, HDL-C and TG. For patients with TG <400 mg/dL (<4.5 mmol/L), LDL-C can be estimated using the following equation:

LDL-C = Total-C - HDL-C - 1/5 TG

For TG levels >400 mg/dL (>4.5 mmol/L), this equation is less accurate and LDL-C concentrations should be determined by ultracentrifugation. In many hypertriglyceridemic patients LDL-C may be low or normal despite elevated Total-C. In such cases, Lescol is not indicated.

Lipid determinations should be performed at intervals of no less than 4 weeks and dosage adjusted according to the patient's response to therapy.

The National Cholesterol Education Program (NCEP) Treatment Guidelines are summarized below:

[See table 3 above]

After the LDL-C goal has been achieved, if the TG is still ≥200 mg/dL, non-HDL-C (total-C minus HDL-C) becomes a secondary target of therapy. Non-HDL-C goals are set 30 mg/dL higher than LDL-C goals for each risk category.

At the time of hospitalization for an acute coronary event, consideration can be given to initiating drug therapy at discharge if the LDL-C level is ≥130 mg/dL (NCEP-ATP II).

Since the goal of treatment is to lower LDL-C, the NCEP recommends that the LDL-C levels be used to initiate and assess treatment response. Only if LDL-C levels are not available, should the Total-C be used to monitor therapy.

[See table 4 above]

Neither Lescol nor Lescol XL have been studied in conditions where the major abnormality is elevation of chylomicrons, VLDL, or IDL (i.e., hyperlipoproteinemia Types I, III, IV, or V).

CONTRAINDICATIONS

Hypersensitivity to any component of this medication. Lescol® (fluvastatin sodium) and Lescol® XL (fluvastatin sodium) are contraindicated in patients with active liver disease or unexplained, persistent elevations in serum transaminases *(see WARNINGS)*.

Pregnancy and Lactation

Atherosclerosis is a chronic process and discontinuation of lipid-lowering drugs during pregnancy should have little impact on the outcome of long-term therapy of primary hypercholesterolemia. Cholesterol and other products of cholesterol biosynthesis are essential components for fetal development (including synthesis of steroids and cell membranes). Since HMG-CoA reductase inhibitors decrease cholesterol synthesis and possibly the synthesis of other biologically active substances derived from cholesterol, they may cause fetal harm when administered to pregnant women. Therefore, HMG-CoA reductase inhibitors are contraindicated during pregnancy and in nursing mothers. **Fluvastatin sodium should be administered to women of childbearing age only when such patients are highly unlikely to conceive and have been informed of the potential hazards.** If the patient becomes pregnant while taking this class of drug, therapy should be discontinued and the patient apprised of the potential hazard to the fetus.

WARNINGS

Liver Enzymes

Biochemical abnormalities of liver function have been associated with HMG-CoA reductase inhibitors and other lipid-lowering agents. Approximately 1.1% of patients treated with Lescol® (fluvastatin sodium) capsules in worldwide trials developed dose-related, persistent elevations of transaminase levels to more than 3 times the upper limit of normal. Fourteen of these patients (0.6%) were discontinued from therapy. In all clinical trials, a total of 33/2969 patients (1.1%) had persistent transaminase elevations with an average fluvastatin exposure of approximately 71.2 weeks; 19 of these patients (0.6%) were discontinued. The majority of patients with these abnormal biochemical findings were asymptomatic.

In a pooled analysis of all placebo-controlled studies in which Lescol capsules were used, persistent transaminase elevations (>3 times the upper limit of normal [ULN] on two consecutive weekly measurements) occurred in 0.2%, 1.5%, and 2.7% of patients treated with 20, 40, and 80 mg (titrated to 40 mg twice daily) Lescol capsules, respectively. Ninety-one percent of the cases of persistent liver function test abnormalities (20 of 22 patients) occurred within 12 weeks of therapy and in all patients with persistent liver function test abnormalities there was an abnormal liver function test present at baseline or by week 8.

In the pooled analysis of the 24-week controlled trials, persistent transaminase elevation occurred in 1.9%, 1.8% and 4.9% of patients treated with Lescol® XL (fluvastatin sodium) 80 mg, Lescol 40 mg and Lescol 40 mg twice daily, respectively. In 13 of 16 patients treated with Lescol XL the abnormality occurred within 12 weeks of initiation of treatment with Lescol XL 80 mg.

It is recommended that liver function tests be performed before the initiation of therapy and at 12 weeks following initiation of treatment or elevation in dose. Patients who develop transaminase elevations or signs and symptoms of liver disease should be monitored to confirm the finding and should be followed thereafter with frequent liver function tests until the levels return to normal. Should an increase in AST or ALT of three times the upper limit of normal or greater persist (found on two consecutive occasions) withdrawal of fluvastatin sodium therapy is recommended.

Active liver disease or unexplained transaminase elevations are contraindications to the use of Lescol and Lescol XL *(see CONTRAINDICATIONS)*. Caution should be exercised when fluvastatin sodium is administered to patients with a history of liver disease or heavy alcohol ingestion *(see CLINICAL PHARMACOLOGY: Pharmacokinetics/Metabolism)*. Such patients should be closely monitored.

Skeletal Muscle

Rhabdomyolysis with renal dysfunction secondary to myoglobinuria has been reported with fluvastatin and with other drugs in this class. Myopathy, defined as muscle aching or muscle weakness in conjunction with increases in creatine phosphokinase (CPK) values to greater than 10 times the upper limit of normal, has been reported.

Myopathy should be considered in any patients with diffuse myalgias, muscle tenderness or weakness, and/or marked elevation of CPK. Patients should be advised to re-

port promptly unexplained muscle pain, tenderness or weakness, particularly if accompanied by malaise or fever. Fluvastatin sodium therapy should be discontinued if markedly elevated CPK levels occur or myopathy is diagnosed or suspected. Fluvastatin sodium therapy should also be temporarily withheld in any patient experiencing an acute or serious condition predisposing to the development of renal failure secondary to rhabdomyolysis, e.g., sepsis; hypotension; major surgery; trauma; severe metabolic, endocrine, or electrolyte disorders; or uncontrolled epilepsy.

The risk of myopathy and or rhabdomyolysis during treatment with HMG-CoA reductase inhibitors has been reported to be increased if therapy with either cyclosporine, gemfibrozil, erythromycin, or niacin is administered concurrently. Myopathy was not observed in a clinical trial in 74 patients involving patients who were treated with fluvastatin sodium together with niacin.

Uncomplicated myalgia has been observed infrequently in patients treated with Lescol at rates indistinguishable from placebo.

The use of fibrates alone may occasionally be associated with myopathy. The combined use of HMG-CoA reductase inhibitors and fibrates should generally be avoided.

PRECAUTIONS

General

Before instituting therapy with Lescol® (fluvastatin sodium) or Lescol® XL (fluvastatin sodium), an attempt should be made to control hypercholesterolemia with appropriate diet, exercise, and weight reduction in obese patients, and to treat other underlying medical problems *(see INDICATIONS AND USAGE)*.

The HMG-CoA reductase inhibitors may cause elevation of creatine phosphokinase and transaminase levels *(see WARNINGS and ADVERSE REACTIONS)*. This should be considered in the differential diagnosis of chest pain in a patient on therapy with fluvastatin sodium.

Homozygous Familial Hypercholesterolemia

HMG-CoA reductase inhibitors are reported to be less effective in patients with rare homozygous familial hypercholesterolemia, possibly because these patients have few functional LDL receptors.

Information for Patients

Patients should be advised to report promptly unexplained muscle pain, tenderness or weakness, particularly if accompanied by malaise or fever.

Women should be informed that if they become pregnant while receiving Lescol or Lescol XL the drug should be discontinued immediately to avoid possible harmful effects on a developing fetus from a relative deficit of cholesterol and biological products derived from cholesterol. In addition, Lescol or Lescol XL should not be taken during nursing. *(See CONTRAINDICATIONS.)*

Drug Interactions

The below listed drug interaction information is derived from studies using immediate release fluvastatin. Similar studies have not been conducted using the Lescol XL tablet.

***Immunosuppressive Drugs, Gemfibrozil, Niacin (Nicotinic Acid), Erythromycin** (See WARNINGS: Skeletal Muscle).*

In vitro data indicate that fluvastatin metabolism involves multiple Cytochrome P450 (CYP) isozymes. CYP2C9 isoenzyme is primarily involved in the metabolism of fluvastatin (~75%), while CYP2C8 and CYP3A4 isoenzymes are involved to a much less extent, i.e. ~5% and ~20%, respectively. If one pathway is inhibited in the elimination process of fluvastatin other pathways may compensate.

In vivo drug interaction studies with CYP3A4 inhibitors/substrates such as cyclosporine, erythromycin, and itraconazle result in minimal changes in the pharmacokinetics of fluvastatin, confirming less involvement of CYP3A4 isozyme. Concomitant administration of fluvastatin and phenytoin increased the levels of phenytoin and fluvastatin, suggesting predominant involvement of CYP2C9 in fluvastatin metabolism.

Niacin/Propranolol: Concomitant administration of immediate release fluvastatin sodium with niacin or propranolol has no effect on the bioavailability of fluvastatin sodium.

Cholestyramine: Administration of immediate release fluvastatin sodium concomitantly with, or up to 4 hours after cholestyramine, results in fluvastatin decreases of more than 50% for AUC and 50%-80% for C_{max}. However, administration of immediate release fluvastatin sodium 4 hours after cholestyramine resulted in a clinically significant additive effect compared with that achieved with either component drug.

Cyclosporine: Plasma cyclosporine levels remain unchanged when fluvastatin (20 mg daily) was administered concurrently in renal transplant recipients on stable cyclosporine regimens. Fluvastatin AUC increased 1.9 fold, and C_{max} increased 1.3 fold compared to historical controls.

Digoxin: In a crossover study involving 18 patients chronically receiving digoxin, a single 40 mg dose of immediate release fluvastatin had no effect on digoxin AUC, but had an 11% increase in digoxin C_{max} and small increase in digoxin urinary clearance.

Erythromycin: Erythromycin (500 mg, single dose) did not affect steady-state plasma levels of fluvastatin (40 mg daily).

Itraconazole: Concomitant administration of fluvastatin (40 mg) and itraconazole (100 mg daily × 4 days) does not affect plasma itraconazole or fluvastatin levels.

Gemfibrozil: There is no change in either fluvastatin (20 mg twice daily) or gemfibrozil (600 mg twice daily) plasma levels when these drugs are co-administered.

Phenytoin: Single morning dose administration of phenytoin (300 mg extended release) increased mean steady-state fluvastatin (40 mg) C_{max} by 27% and AUC by 40% whereas fluvastatin increased the mean phenytoin C_{max} by 5% and AUC by 20%. Patients on phenytoin should continue to be monitored appropriately when fluvastatin therapy is initiated or when the fluvastatin dosage is changed.

Diclofenac: Concurrent administration of fluvastatin (40 mg) increased the mean C_{max} and AUC of diclofenac by 60% and 25% respectively.

Tolbutamide: In healthy volunteers, concurrent administration of either single or multiple daily doses of fluvastatin sodium (40 mg) with tolbutamide (1 g) did not affect the plasma levels of either drug to a clinically significant extent.

Glibenclamide (Glyburide): In glibenclamide-treated NIDDM patients (n=32), administration of fluvastatin (40 mg twice daily for 14 days) increased the mean C_{max}, AUC, and $t_{1/2}$ of glibenclamide approximately 50%, 69% and 121%, respectively. Glibenclamide (5-20 mg daily) increased the mean C_{max} and AUC of fluvastatin by 44% and 51%, respectively. In this study there were no changes in glucose, insulin and C-peptide levels. However, patients on concomitant therapy with glibenclamide (glyburide) and fluvastatin should continue to be monitored appropriately when their fluvastatin dose is increased to 40 mg twice daily.

Losartan: Concomitant administration of fluvastatin with losartan has no effect on the bioavailability of either losartan or its active metabolite.

Cimetidine/Ranitidine/Omeprazole: Concomitant administration of immediate release fluvastatin sodium with cimetidine, ranitidine and omeprazole results in a significant increase in the fluvastatin C_{max} (43%, 70% and 50%, respectively) and AUC (24%-33%), with an 18%-23% decrease in plasma clearance.

Rifampicin: Administration of immediate release fluvastatin sodium to subjects pretreated with rifampicin results in significant reduction in C_{max} (59%) and AUC (51%), with a large increase (95%) in plasma clearance.

Warfarin: In vitro protein binding studies demonstrated no interaction at therapeutic concentrations. Concomitant administration of a single dose of warfarin (30 mg) in young healthy males receiving immediate release fluvastatin sodium (40 mg/day × 8 days) resulted in no elevation of racemic warfarin concentration. There was also no effect on prothrombin complex activity when compared to concomitant administration of placebo and warfarin. However, bleeding and/or increased prothrombin times have been reported in patients taking coumarin anticoagulants concomitantly with other HMG-CoA reductase inhibitors. Therefore, patients receiving warfarin-type anticoagulants should have their prothrombin times closely monitored when fluvastatin sodium is initiated or the dosage of fluvastatin sodium is changed.

Endocrine Function

HMG-CoA reductase inhibitors interfere with cholesterol synthesis and lower circulating cholesterol levels and, as such, might theoretically blunt adrenal or gonadal steroid hormone production.

Fluvastatin exhibited no effect upon non-stimulated cortisol levels and demonstrated no effect upon thyroid metabolism as assessed by TSH. Small declines in total testosterone have been noted in treated groups, but no commensurate elevation in LH occurred, suggesting that the observation was not due to a direct effect upon testosterone production. No effect upon FSH in males was noted. Due to the limited number of premenopausal females studied to date, no conclusions regarding the effect of fluvastatin upon female sex hormones may be made.

Two clinical studies in patients receiving fluvastatin at doses up to 80 mg daily for periods of 24 to 28 weeks demonstrated no effect of treatment upon the adrenal response to ACTH stimulation. A clinical study evaluated the effect of fluvastatin at doses up to 80 mg daily for 28 weeks upon the gonadal response to HCG stimulation. Although the mean total testosterone response was significantly reduced ($p<0.05$) relative to baseline in the 80 mg group, it was not significant in comparison to the changes noted in groups receiving either 40 mg of fluvastatin or placebo.

Patients treated with fluvastatin sodium who develop clinical evidence of endocrine dysfunction should be evaluated appropriately. Caution should be exercised if an HMG-CoA reductase inhibitor or other agent used to lower cholesterol levels is administered to patients receiving other drugs (e.g., ketoconazole, spironolactone, or cimetidine) that may decrease the levels of endogenous steroid hormones.

CNS Toxicity

CNS effects, as evidenced by decreased activity, ataxia, loss of righting reflex, and ptosis were seen in the following animal studies: the 18-month mouse carcinogenicity study at 50 mg/kg/day, the 6-month dog study at 36 mg/kg/day, the 6-month hamster study at 40 mg/kg/day, and in acute, high-dose studies in rats and hamsters (50 mg/kg), rabbits (300 mg/kg) and mice (1500 mg/kg). CNS toxicity in the acute high-dose studies was characterized (in mice) by conspicuous vacuolation in the ventral white columns of the spinal cord at a dose of 5000 mg/kg and (in rat) by edema with separation of myelinated fibers of the ventral spinal tracts and sciatic nerve at a dose of 1500 mg/kg. CNS toxicity, characterized by periaxonal vacuolation, was observed in the medulla of dogs that died after treatment for 5 weeks with 48 mg/kg/day; this finding was not observed in the remaining dogs when the dose level was lowered to 36 mg/kg/day. CNS vascular lesions, characterized by perivascular hemorrhages, edema, and mononuclear cell infiltration of perivascular spaces, have been observed in dogs treated with other members of this class. No CNS lesions have been observed after chronic treatment for up to 2 years with fluvastatin in the mouse (at doses up to 350 mg/kg/day), rat (up to 24 mg/kg/day), or dog (up to 16 mg/kg/day).

Prominent bilateral posterior Y suture lines in the ocular lens were seen in dogs after treatment with 1, 8, and 16 mg/kg/day for 2 years.

Carcinogenesis, Mutagenesis, Impairment of Fertility

A 2-year study was performed in rats at dose levels of 6, 9, and 18-24 (escalated after 1 year) mg/kg/day. These treatment levels represented plasma drug levels of approximately 9, 13, and 26-35 times the mean human plasma drug concentration after a 40 mg oral dose. A low incidence of forestomach squamous papillomas and 1 carcinoma of the forestomach at the 24 mg/kg/day dose level was considered to reflect the prolonged hyperplasia induced by direct contact exposure to fluvastatin sodium rather than to a systemic effect of the drug. In addition, an increased incidence of thyroid follicular cell adenomas and carcinomas was recorded for males treated with 18-24 mg/kg/day. The increased incidence of thyroid follicular cell neoplasm in male rats with fluvastatin sodium appears to be consistent with findings from other HMG-CoA reductase inhibitors. In contrast to other HMG-CoA reductase inhibitors, no hepatic adenomas or carcinomas were observed.

The carcinogenicity study conducted in mice at dose levels of 0.3, 15 and 30 mg/kg/day revealed, as in rats, a statistically significant increase in forestomach squamous cell papillomas in males and females at 30 mg/kg/day and in females at 15 mg/kg/day. These treatment levels represented plasma drug levels of approximately 0.05, 2, and 7 times the mean human plasma drug concentration after a 40 mg oral dose.

No evidence of mutagenicity was observed in vitro, with or without rat-liver metabolic activation, in the following studies: microbial mutagen tests using mutant strains of *Salmonella typhimurium* or *Escherichia coli;* malignant transformation assay in BALB/3T3 cells; unscheduled DNA synthesis in rat primary hepatocytes; chromosomal aberrations in V79 Chinese Hamster cells; HGPRT V79 Chinese Hamster cells. In addition, there was no evidence of mutagenicity in vivo in either a rat or mouse micronucleus test.

In a study in rats at dose levels for females of 0.6, 2 and 6 mg/kg/day and at dose levels for males of 2, 10 and 20 mg/kg/day, fluvastatin sodium had no adverse effects on the fertility or reproductive performance.

Seminal vesicles and testes were small in hamsters treated for 3 months at 20 mg/kg/day (approximately three times the 40 milligram human daily dose based on surface area, mg/m^2). There was tubular degeneration and aspermatogenesis in testes as well as vesiculitis of seminal vesicles. Vesiculitis of seminal vesicles and edema of the testes were also seen in rats treated for 2 years at 18 mg/kg/day (approximately 4 times the human C_{max} achieved with a 40 milligram daily dose).

Pregnancy

Pregnancy Category X

See CONTRAINDICATIONS.

Fluvastatin sodium produced delays in skeletal development in rats at doses of 12 mg/kg/day and in rabbits at doses of 10 mg/kg/day. Malaligned thoracic vertebrae were seen in rats at 36 mg/kg, a dose that produced maternal toxicity. These doses resulted in 2 times (rat at 12 mg/kg) or 5 times (rabbit at 10 mg/kg) the 40 mg human exposure based on mg/m^2 surface area. A study in which female rats were dosed during the third trimester at 12 and 24 mg/kg/day resulted in maternal mortality at or near term and postpartum. In addition, fetal and neonatal lethality were apparent. No effects on the dam or fetus occurred at 2 mg/kg/day. A second study at levels of 2, 6, 12 and 24 mg/kg/day confirmed the findings in the first study with neonatal mortality beginning at 6 mg/kg. A modified Segment III study was performed at dose levels of 12 or 24 mg/kg/day with or without the presence of concurrent supplementation with mevalonic acid, a product of HMG-CoA reductase which is essential for cholesterol biosynthesis. The concurrent administration of mevalonic acid completely prevented the maternal and neonatal mortality but did not prevent low body weights in pups at 24 mg/kg on days 0 and 7 postpartum. Therefore, the maternal and neonatal lethality observed with fluvastatin sodium reflect its exaggerated pharmacologic effect during pregnancy. There are no data with fluvastatin sodium in pregnant women. However, rare reports of congenital anomalies have been received following intrauterine exposure to other HMG-CoA reductase inhibitors. There has been one report of severe congenital bony deformity, tracheo-esophageal fistula, and anal atresia (VATER association) in a baby born to a woman who took another HMG-CoA reductase inhibitor with dextroamphetamine sulfate during the first trimester of pregnancy. **Lescol or Lescol XL should be administered to women of childbearing potential only when such patients are highly unlikely to conceive and have been informed of the potential hazards.** If a woman becomes pregnant while taking Lescol or Lescol XL, the drug should be discontinued and the patient advised again as to the potential hazards to the fetus.

Continued on next page

Lescol—Cont.

Nursing Mothers
Based on preclinical data, drug is present in breast milk in a 2:1 ratio (milk:plasma). Because of the potential for serious adverse reactions in nursing infants, nursing women should not take Lescol or Lescol XL *(see CONTRAINDICATIONS)*.
Pediatric Use
Safety and effectiveness in individuals less than 18 years old have not been established. Treatment in patients less than 18 years of age is not recommended at this time.
Geriatric Use
The effect of age on the pharmacokinetics of immediate release fluvastatin sodium was evaluated. Results indicate that for the general patient population plasma concentrations of fluvastatin sodium do not vary as a function of age. *(See also CLINICAL PHARMACOLOGY: Pharmacokinetics/Metabolism.)* Elderly patients (≥65 years of age) demonstrated a greater treatment response in respect to LDL-C, Total-C and LDL/HDL ratio than patients <65 years of age.

ADVERSE REACTIONS
In all clinical studies of Lescol® (fluvastatin sodium), 1.0% (32/2969) of fluvastatin-treated patients were discontinued due to adverse experiences attributed to study drug (mean exposure approximately 16 months ranging in duration from 1 to >36 months). This results in an exposure adjusted rate of 0.8% (32/4051) per patient year in fluvastatin patients in controlled studies compared to an incidence of 1.1% (4/355) in placebo patients. Adverse reactions have usually been of mild to moderate severity.
In controlled clinical studies, 3.9% (36/912) of patients treated with Lescol® XL (fluvastatin sodium) 80 mg discontinued due to adverse events (causality not determined).
Clinically relevant adverse experiences occurring in the Lescol and Lescol XL controlled studies with a frequency >2%, regardless of causality, include the following:

Table 5
Clinically Relevant Adverse Experiences Occurring in >2% Patients in Lescol® and Lescol XL® Controlled Studies

Adverse Event	Lescol®[1] (%) (N=2326)	Placebo[1] (%) (N=960)	Lescol® XL[2] (%) (N=912)
Musculoskeletal			
Myalgia	5.0	4.5	3.8
Arthritis	2.1	2.0	1.3
Arthropathy	NA	NA	3.2
Respiratory			
Sinusitis	2.6	1.9	3.5
Bronchitis	1.8	1.0	2.6
Gastrointestinal			
Dyspepsia	7.9	3.2	3.5
Diarrhea	4.9	4.2	3.3
Abdominal Pain	4.9	3.8	3.7
Nausea	3.2	2.0	2.5
Flatulence	2.6	2.5	1.4
Psychiatric Disorders			
Insomnia	2.7	1.4	0.8
Genitourinary			
Urinary Tract Infection	1.6	1.1	2.7
Miscellaneous			
Headache	8.9	7.8	4.7
Influenza-Like Symptoms	5.1	5.7	7.1
Accidental Trauma	5.1	4.8	4.2
Fatigue	2.7	2.3	1.6
Allergy	2.3	2.2	1.0

[1] Controlled trials with Lescol Capsules (20 and 40 mg daily and 40 mg twice daily)
[2] Controlled trials with Lescol XL 80 mg Tablets

The following effects have been reported with drugs in this class. Not all the effects listed below have necessarily been associated with fluvastatin sodium therapy.
Skeletal: muscle cramps, myalgia, myopathy, rhabdomyolysis, arthralgias.
Neurological: dysfunction of certain cranial nerves (including alteration of taste, impairment of extra-ocular movement, facial paresis), tremor, dizziness, vertigo, memory loss, paresthesia, peripheral neuropathy, peripheral nerve palsy, psychic disturbances, anxiety, insomnia, depression.
Hypersensitivity Reactions: An apparent hypersensitivity syndrome has been reported rarely which has included one or more of the following features: anaphylaxis, angioedema, lupus erythematosus-like syndrome, polymyalgia rheumatica, vasculitis, purpura, thrombocytopenia, leukopenia, hemolytic anemia, positive ANA, ESR increase, eosinophilia, arthritis, arthralgia, urticaria, asthenia, photosensitivity, fever, chills, flushing, malaise, dyspnea, toxic epidermal necrolysis, erythema multiforme, including Stevens-Johnson syndrome.
Gastrointestinal: pancreatitis, hepatitis, including chronic active hepatitis, cholestatic jaundice, fatty change in liver, and, rarely, cirrhosis, fulminant hepatic necrosis, and hepatoma; anorexia, vomiting.
Skin: alopecia, pruritus. A variety of skin changes (e.g., nodules, discoloration, dryness of skin/mucous membranes, changes to hair/nails) have been reported.
Reproductive: gynecomastia, loss of libido, erectile dysfunction.
Eye: progression of cataracts (lens opacities), ophthalmoplegia.
Laboratory Abnormalities: elevated transaminases, alkaline phosphatase, γ-glutamyl transpeptidase, and bilirubin; thyroid function abnormalities.
Concomitant Therapy
Fluvastatin sodium has been administered concurrently with cholestyramine and nicotinic acid. No adverse reactions unique to the combination or in addition to those previously reported for this class of drugs alone have been reported. Myopathy and rhabdomyolysis (with or without acute renal failure) have been reported when another HMG-CoA reductase inhibitor was used in combination with immunosuppressive drugs, gemfibrozil, erythromycin, or lipid-lowering doses of nicotinic acid. Concomitant therapy with HMG-CoA reductase inhibitors and these agents is generally not recommended. *(See WARNINGS: Skeletal Muscle.)*

OVERDOSAGE
The approximate oral LD_{50} is greater than 2 g/kg in mice and greater than 0.7 g/kg in rats.
The maximum single oral dose of Lescol® (fluvastatin sodium) capsules received by healthy volunteers was 80 mg. No clinically significant adverse experiences were seen at this dose. The maximum dose administered with an extended-release formulation was 640 mg for two weeks. This dose was not well tolerated and produced a variety of GI complaints and an increase in transaminase values (i.e., SGOT and SGPT).
There has been a single report of 2 children, one 2 years old and the other 3 years of age, either of whom may have possibly ingested fluvastatin sodium. The maximum amount of fluvastatin sodium that could have been ingested was 80 mg (4 × 20 mg capsules). Vomiting was induced by ipecac in both children and no capsules were noted in their emesis. Neither child experienced any adverse symptoms and both recovered from the incident without problems.
Should an accidental overdose occur, treat symptomatically and institute supportive measures as required. The dialyzability of fluvastatin sodium and of its metabolites in humans is not known at present.
Information about the treatment of overdose can often be obtained from a certified Regional Poison Control Center. Telephone numbers of certified Regional Poison Control Centers are listed in the Physicians' Desk Reference®.*

DOSAGE AND ADMINISTRATION
The patient should be placed on a standard cholesterol-lowering diet before receiving Lescol® (fluvastatin sodium) or Lescol® XL (fluvastatin sodium) and should continue on this diet during treatment with Lescol or Lescol XL. (See NCEP Treatment Guidelines for details on dietary therapy.)
For patients requiring LDL-C reduction to a goal of ≥25%, the recommended starting dose is 40 mg as one capsule, 80 mg as one Lescol XL tablet administered as a single dose in the evening or 80 mg in divided doses of the 40 mg capsule given twice daily. For patients requiring LDL-C reduction to a goal of <25% a starting dose of 20 mg may be used. The recommended dosing range is 20-80 mg/day. Lescol or Lescol XL may be taken without regard to meals, since there are no apparent differences in the lipid-lowering effects of fluvastatin sodium administered with the evening meal or 4 hours after the evening meal. Since the maximal reductions in LDL-C of a given dose are seen within 4 weeks, periodic lipid determinations should be performed and dosage adjustment made according to the patient's response to therapy and established treatment guidelines. The therapeutic effect of Lescol or Lescol XL is maintained with prolonged administration.
Concomitant Therapy
Lipid-lowering effects on total cholesterol and LDL cholesterol are additive when immediate release Lescol is combined with a bile-acid binding resin or niacin. When administering a bile-acid resin (e.g., cholestyramine) and fluvastatin sodium, Lescol should be administered at bedtime, at least 2 hours following the resin to avoid a significant interaction due to drug binding to resin. *(See also ADVERSE REACTIONS: Concomitant Therapy.)*
Dosage in Patients with Renal Insufficiency
Since fluvastatin sodium is cleared hepatically with less than 6% of the administered dose excreted into the urine, dose adjustments for mild to moderate renal impairment are not necessary. Fluvastatin has not been studied at doses greater than 40 mg in patients with severe renal impairment; therefore caution should be exercised when treating such patients at higher doses.

HOW SUPPLIED
Lescol® (fluvastatin sodium) Capsules
20 mg
Brown and light brown imprinted twice with "⚠" and "20" on one half and and the Lescol® (fluvastatin sodium) logo twice on the other half of the capsule.
Bottles of 30 capsules .... (NDC 0078-0176-15)
Bottles of 100 capsules .... (NDC 0078-0176-05)
40 mg
Brown and gold imprinted twice with "⚠" and "40" on one half and "LESCOL" and the Lescol® (fluvastatin sodium) logo twice on the other half of the capsule.
Bottles of 30 capsules .... (NDC 0078-0234-15)
Bottles of 100 capsules .... (NDC 0078-0234-05)
Lescol® XL (fluvastatin sodium) Extended-Release Tablets
80 mg
Yellow, round, slightly biconvex film-coated tablet with beveled edges debossed with "Lescol XL" on one side and "80" on the other.
Bottles of 30 tablets .... (NDC 0078-0354-15)
Bottle of 100 tablets .... (NDC 0078-0354-05)
Store and Dispense
Store at 25°C (77°F); excursions permitted to 15°C-30°C (59°F-86°F). [See USP Controlled Room Temperature]. Dispense in a tight container. Protect from light.

*Trademark of Medical Economics Company, Inc.
T2003-40
REV: MAY 2003 89011106
Shown in Product Identification Guide, page 331

RYTHMOL® SR ℞
[ryth-mul]
(propafenone hydrochloride) extended release CAPSULES

DESCRIPTION
RYTHMOL SR (propafenone hydrochloride) is an antiarrhythmic drug supplied in extended-release capsules of 225, 325 and 425 mg for oral administration.
The structural formula of propafenone HCl is given below:

$C_{21}H_{27}NO_3$•HCl M.W. = 377.92

2'-[2-Hydroxy-3-(propylamino)-propoxy]-3-phenylpropiophenone hydrochloride

Propafenone HCl has some structural similarities to beta-blocking agents. Propafenone HCl occurs as colorless crystals or white crystalline powder with a very bitter taste. It is slightly soluble in water (20°C), chloroform and ethanol. Rythmol SR are capsules filled with cylindrical-shaped 2 × 2 mm microtablets containing propafenone and the following inactive ingredients: antifoam, gelatin, hypromellose, red iron oxide, magnesium stearate, shellac, sodium lauryl sulfate, sodium dodecyl sulfate, soy lecithin and titanium dioxide.

CLINICAL PHARMACOLOGY
Mechanism of Action:
Propafenone is a Class 1C antiarrhythmic drug with local anesthetic effects, and a direct stabilizing action on myocardial membranes. The electrophysiological effect of propafenone manifests itself in a reduction of upstroke velocity (Phase 0) of the monophasic action potential. In Purkinje fibers, and to a lesser extent myocardial fibers, propafenone reduces the fast inward current carried by sodium ions. Diastolic excitability threshold is increased and effective refractory period prolonged. Propafenone reduces spontaneous automaticity and depresses triggered activity.
Studies in anesthetized dogs and isolated organ preparations show that propafenone has beta-sympatholytic activity at about 1/50 the potency of propranolol. Clinical studies employing isoproterenol challenge and exercise testing after single doses of propafenone indicate a beta-adrenergic blocking potency (per mg) about 1/40 that of propranolol in man. In clinical trials with the immediate release formulation, resting heart rate decreases of about 8% were noted at the higher end of the therapeutic plasma concentration range. At very high concentrations *in vitro*, propafenone can inhibit the slow inward current carried by calcium, but this calcium antagonist effect probably does not contribute to antiarrhythmic efficacy. Moreover, propafenone inhibits a variety of cardiac potassium currents in *in vitro* studies (i.e. the transient outward, the delayed rectifier, and the inward rectifier current). Propafenone has local anesthetic activity approximately equal to procaine. Compared to propafenone, the main metabolite, 5-hydroxypropafenone, has similar sodium and calcium channel activity, but about 10 times less beta-blocking activity (N-depropylpropafenone has weaker sodium channel activity but equivalent affinity for beta-receptors).
Electrophysiology:
Electrophysiology studies in patients with ventricular tachycardia (VT) have shown that propafenone prolongs atrioventricular (AV) conduction while having little or no effect on sinus node function. Both atrioventricular (AV) nodal conduction time (AH interval) and His-Purkinje conduction time (HV interval) are prolonged. Propafenone has little or no effect on the atrial functional refractory period, but AV nodal functional and effective refractory periods are prolonged. In patients with Wolff-Parkinson-White (WPW) syndrome, RYTHMOL immediate release tablets reduce conduction and increase the effective refractory period of the accessory pathway in both directions (see **ADVERSE REACTIONS/Electrocardiograms**).

Table 1: Analysis of tachycardia-free period (days) from Day 1 of randomization

	RYTHMOL SR Dose			
Parameter	225 mg BID (N = 126) n (%)	325 mg BID (N = 135) n (%)	425 mg BID (N = 136) n (%)	Placebo (N = 126) n (%)
Patients completing with terminating event†	66 (52)	56 (41)	41 (30)	87 (69)
Comparison of tachycardia-free periods				
Kaplan-Meier Median	112	291	*	41
Range	0 – 285	0 – 293	0 – 300	0 – 289
p-Value (Log-rank test)	0.014	< 0.0001	< 0.0001	--
Hazard Ratio compared to placebo	0.67	0.43	0.35	--
95% CI for Hazard Ratio	(0.49, 0.93)	(0.31, 0.61)	(0.24, 0.51)	--

*Fewer than 50% of the patients had events. The median time is not calculable.
†Terminating events comprised 91% atrial fibrillation, 5% atrial flutter, and 4% PSVT

Hemodynamics:
Studies in humans have shown that propafenone exerts a negative inotropic effect on the myocardium. Cardiac catheterization studies in patients with moderately impaired ventricular function (mean C.I.=2.61 L/min/m^2), utilizing intravenous propafenone infusions (loading dose of 2 mg/kg over 10 min+ followed by 2 mg/min for 30 min) that gave mean plasma concentrations of 3.0 μg/mL (a dose that produces plasma levels of propafenone greater than does recommended oral dosing), showed significant increases in pulmonary capillary wedge pressure, systemic and pulmonary vascular resistances and depression of cardiac output and cardiac index.

Pharmacokinetics and Metabolism:
Absorption/Bioavailability
Maximal plasma levels of propafenone are reached between three to eight hours following the administration of RYTHMOL SR. Propafenone is known to undergo extensive and saturable presystemic biotransformation which results in a dose and dosage form dependent absolute bioavailability; e.g., a 150 mg immediate release tablet had an absolute bioavailability of 3.4%, while a 300 mg immediate release tablet had an absolute bioavailability of 10.6%. Absorption from a 300 mg solution dose was rapid, with an absolute bioavailability of 21.4%. At still larger doses, above those recommended, bioavailability of propafenone from immediate release tablets increased still further.
Relative bioavailability assessments have been performed between RYTHMOL SR capsules and RYTHMOL immediate release tablets. In extensive metabolizers, the bioavailability of propafenone from the SR formulation was less than that of the immediate release formulation as the more gradual release of propafenone from the prolonged-release preparations resulted in an increase in overall first pass metabolism (see **Metabolism**). As a result of the increased first pass effect, higher daily doses of propafenone were required from the SR formulation relative to the immediate release formulation, to obtain similar exposure to propafenone. The relative bioavailability of propafenone from the 325 twice daily regimens of RYTHMOL SR approximates that of RYTHMOL immediate release 150 mg three times daily regimen. Mean exposure to 5-hydroxypropafenone was about 20-25% higher after SR capsule administration than after immediate-release tablet administration.
Food increased the exposure to propafenone 4-fold after single dose administration of 425 mg of RYTHMOL SR. However, in the multiple dose study (425 mg dose BID), the difference between the fed and fasted state was not significant.

Distribution
Following intravenous administration of propafenone, plasma levels decline in a bi-phasic manner consistent with a two compartment pharmacokinetic model. The average distribution half-life corresponding to the first phase was about five minutes. The volume of the central compartment was about 88 liters (1.1 L/kg) and the total volume of distribution about 252 liters.
In serum, propafenone is greater than 95% bound to proteins within the concentration range of 0.5 - 2 μg/mL. Protein binding decreases to about 88% in patients with severe hepatic dysfunction.

Metabolism
There are two genetically determined patterns of propafenone metabolism. In over 90% of patients, the drug is rapidly and extensively metabolized with an elimination half-life from 2-10 hours. These patients metabolize propafenone into two active metabolites: 5-hydroxypropafenone which is formed by CYP2D6 and N-depropylpropafenone (norpropafenone) which is formed by both CYP3A4 and CYP1A2. In less than 10% of patients, metabolism of propafenone is slower because the 5-hydroxy metabolite is not formed or is minimally formed. In these patients, the estimated propafenone elimination half-life ranges from 10-32 hours. Decreased ability to form the 5-hydroxy metabolite of propafenone is associated with a diminished ability to metabolize debrisoquine and a variety of other drugs such as encainide, metoprolol, and dextromethorphan whose metabolism is mediated by the CYP2D6 isozyme. In these patients, the N-depropylpropafenone metabolite occurs in quantities comparable to the levels occurring in extensive metabolizers.
As a consequence of the observed differences in metabolism, administration of RYTHMOL SR to slow and extensive metabolizers results in significant differences in plasma concentrations of propafenone, with slow metabolizers achieving concentrations about twice those of the extensive metabolizers at daily doses of 850 mg/day. At low doses the differences are greater, with slow metabolizers attaining concentrations about three to four times higher than extensive metabolizers. In extensive metabolizers, saturation of the hydroxylation pathway (CYP2D6) results in greater-than-linear increases in plasma levels following administration of RYTHMOL SR capsules. In slow metabolizers, propafenone pharmacokinetics are linear. Because the difference decreases at high doses and is mitigated by the lack of the active 5-hydroxy metabolite in the slow metabolizers, and because steady-state conditions are achieved after four to five days of dosing in all patients, the recommended dosing regimen of RYTHMOL SR is the same for all patients. The large intersubject variability in blood levels require that the dose of the drug be titrated carefully in patients with close attention paid to clinical and ECG evidence of toxicity (see **DOSAGE AND ADMINISTRATION**).
The 5-hydroxypropafenone and norpropafenone metabolites have electrophysiologic properties similar to propafenone *in vitro*. In man after administration of RYTHMOL SR, the 5-hydroxypropafenone metabolite is usually present in concentrations less than 40% of propafenone. The norpropafenone metabolite is usually present in concentrations less than 10% of propafenone.

Inter-Subject Variability:
With propafenone, there is a considerable degree of intersubject variability in pharmacokinetics which is due in large part to the first pass hepatic effect and non-linear pharmacokinetics in extensive metabolizers. A higher degree of inter-subject variability in pharmacokinetic parameters of propafenone was observed following both single and multiple dose administration of RYTHMOL SR capsules. Inter-subject variability appears to be substantially less in the poor metabolizer group than in the extensive metabolizer group, suggesting that a large portion of the variability is intrinsic to CYP2D6 polymorphism rather than to the formulation.
The clearance of propafenone is reduced and the elimination half-life increased in patients with significant hepatic dysfunction (see **PRECAUTIONS**). Decreased liver function also increases the bioavailability of propafenone. Absolute bioavailability assessments have not been determined for the RYTHMOL SR capsule formulation. Absolute bioavailability of RYTHMOL immediate release tablets has been demonstrated to be inversely related to indocyanine green clearance, reaching 60-70% at clearances of 7 mL/min and below.

Stereochemistry:
RYTHMOL is a racemic mixture. The R- and S-enantiomers of propafenone display stereoselective disposition characteristics. *In vitro* and *in vivo* studies have shown that the R-isomer of propafenone is cleared faster than the S-isomer via the 5-hydroxylation pathway (CYP2D6). This results in a higher ratio of S-propafenone to R-propafenone at steady state. Both enantiomers have equivalent potency to block sodium channels; however, the S-enantiomer is a more potent β-antagonist than the R-enantiomer. Following administration of RYTHMOL immediate release tablets or RYTHMOL SR capsules, the S/R ratio for the area under the plasma concentration-time curve was about 1.7. The S/R ratios of propafenone obtained after administration of 225, 325 and 425 mg RYTHMOL SR are independent of dose. In addition, no difference in the average values of the S/R ratios is evident between genotypes or over time.

Clinical Trials:
RYTHMOL SR has been evaluated in patients with a history of electrocardiographically documented recurrent episodes of symptomatic atrial fibrillation in two randomized, double-blind, placebo controlled trials.

RAFT
In one US multicenter study (Rythmol SR Atrial Fibrillation Trial, RAFT), three doses of RYTHMOL SR (225 mg BID, 325 mg BID and 425 mg BID) and placebo were compared in 523 patients with symptomatic, episodic atrial fibrillation. The patient population in this trial was 59% male with a mean age of 63 years, 91% White and 6% Black. The patients had a median history of atrial fibrillation of 13 months, and documented symptomatic atrial fibrillation within 12 months of study entry. Over 90% were NYHA Class I, and 21% had a prior electrical cardioversion. At baseline, 24% were treated with calcium channel blockers, 37% with beta blockers, and 38% with digoxin. Symptomatic arrhythmias after randomization were documented by transtelephonic electrocardiogram and centrally read and adjudicated by a blinded adverse event committee. RYTHMOL SR administered for up to 39 weeks was shown to prolong significantly the time to the first recurrence of symptomatic atrial arrhythmia, predominantly atrial fibrillation, from Day 1 of randomization (primary efficacy variable) compared to placebo, as shown in Table 1.
[See table 1 above]
There was a dose response for RYTHMOL SR for the tachycardia-free period as shown in the proportional hazard analysis and the Kaplan Meier curves presented in Figure 1.
[See figure 1 at top of next column]
In additional analyses, RYTHMOL SR (225 mg BID, 325 mg BID, and 425 mg BID) was also shown to prolong time to the first recurrence of symptomatic atrial fibrillation from Day 5 (steady-state pharmacokinetics were attained). The antiarrhythmic effect of RYTHMOL SR was not influenced by age, gender, history of cardioversion, duration of atrial fibrillation, frequency of atrial fibrillation or use of medication that lowers heart rate. Similarly, the antiarrhythmic effect of RYTHMOL SR was not influenced by the individual use of calcium channel blockers, beta-blockers or digoxin. Too few non-White patients were enrolled to assess the influence of race on effects of RYTHMOL SR (propafenone hydrochloride).
No difference in the average heart rate during the first recurrence of symptomatic arrhythmia between RYTHMOL SR and placebo was observed.

Figure 1: RAFT Kaplan-Meier Analysis for the Tachycardia-free period from Day 1 of randomization:

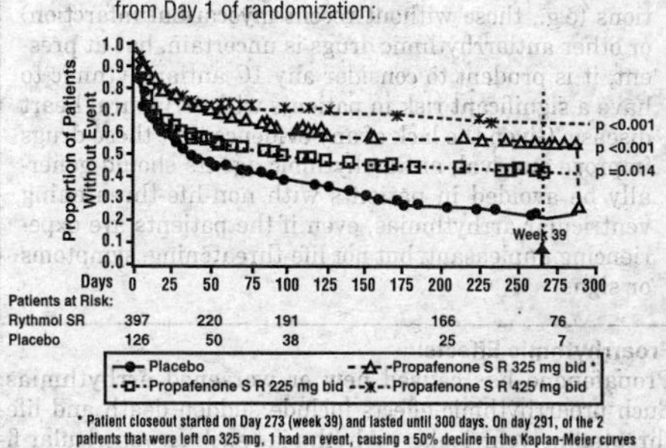

* Patient closeout started on Day 273 (week 39) and lasted until 300 days. On day 291, of the 2 patients that were left on 325 mg, 1 had an event, causing a 50% decline in the Kaplan-Meier curves

ERAFT
In a European multicenter trial [(European Rythmonorm SR Atrial Fibrillation Trial (ERAFT)], two doses of RYTHMOL SR (325 mg BID and 425 mg BID) and placebo were compared in 293 patients. The patient population in this trial was 61% male, 100% White with a mean age of 61 years. Patients had a median duration of atrial fibrillation of 3.3 years, and 61% were taking medications that lowered heart rate. At baseline, 15% of the patients were treated with calcium channel blockers (verapamil and diltiazem), 42% with beta-blockers and 8% with digoxin. During a qualifying period of up to 28 days, patients had to have one ECG-documented incident of symptomatic atrial fibrillation. The double-blind treatment phase consisted of a four day loading period followed by a 91-day efficacy period. Symptomatic arrhythmias were documented by electrocardiogram monitoring.
In ERAFT, RYTHMOL SR was shown to prolong the time to the first recurrence of symptomatic atrial arrhythmia from Day 5 of randomization (primary efficacy analysis). The proportional hazard analysis revealed that both RYTHMOL SR doses were superior to placebo. The antiarrhythmic effect of propafenone SR was not influenced by age, gender, duration of atrial fibrillation, frequency of atrial fibrillation or use of medication that lowers heart rate. It was also not influenced by the individual use of calcium channel blockers, beta-blockers or digoxin. Too few non-White patients were enrolled to assess the influence of race on the effects of RYTHMOL SR. There was a slight increase in the incidence of centrally diagnosed asymptomatic atrial fibrillation or atrial flutter in each of the two RYTHMOL SR treatment groups compared to placebo.

INDICATIONS AND USAGE

RYTHMOL SR is indicated to prolong the time to recurrence of symptomatic atrial fibrillation in patients without structural heart disease.
The use of RYTHMOL SR in patients with permanent atrial fibrillation or in patients exclusively with atrial flutter or PSVT has not been evaluated. RYTHMOL SR should not be used to control ventricular rate during atrial fibrillation.
The effect of RYTHMOL SR on mortality has not been determined (see black box **WARNINGS**).

Continued on next page

Rythmol SR—Cont.

CONTRAINDICATIONS

RYTHMOL SR is contraindicated in the presence of congestive heart failure, cardiogenic shock, sinoatrial, atrioventricular and intraventricular disorders of impulse generation or conduction (e.g., sick sinus node syndrome, atrioventricular block) in the absence of an artificial pacemaker, bradycardia, marked hypotension, bronchospastic disorders, electrolyte imbalance, or hypersensitivity to the drug.

WARNINGS

Mortality:
In the National Heart, Lung and Blood Institute's Cardiac Arrhythmia Suppression Trial (CAST), a long-term, multi-center, randomized, double-blind study in patients with asymptomatic non-life-threatening ventricular arrhythmias who had a myocardial infarction more than six days but less than two years previously, an increased rate of death or reversed cardiac arrest rate (7.7%; 56/730) was seen in patients treated with encainide or flecainide (Class 1C antiarrhythmics) compared with that seen in patients assigned to placebo (3.0%; 22/725). The average duration of treatment with encainide or flecainide in this study was ten months.
The applicability of the CAST results to other populations (e.g., those without recent myocardial infarction) or other antiarrhythmic drugs is uncertain, but at present, it is prudent to consider any 1C antiarrhythmic to have a significant risk in patients with structural heart disease. Given the lack of any evidence that these drugs improve survival, antiarrhythmic agents should generally be avoided in patients with non-life-threatening ventricular arrhythmias, even if the patients are experiencing unpleasant, but not life-threatening, symptoms or signs.

Proarrhythmic Effects:
Propafenone has caused new or worsened arrhythmias. Such proarrhythmic effects include sudden death and life-threatening ventricular arrhythmias such as ventricular fibrillation, ventricular tachycardia, asystole and Torsade de Pointes. It may also worsen premature ventricular contractions or supraventricular arrhythmias, and it may prolong the QT interval. It is therefore essential that each patient given RYTHMOL SR be evaluated electrocardiographically prior to and during therapy, to determine whether the response to RYTHMOL SR supports continued treatment. Because propafenone prolongs the QRS interval in the electrocardiogram, changes in the QT interval are difficult to interpret.
In a 474 patient U.S. uncontrolled, open label multicenter trial using the immediate release formulation in patients with symptomatic SVT, 1.9% (9/474) of these patients experienced ventricular tachycardia (VT) or ventricular fibrillation (VF) during the study. However, in four of the nine patients, the ventricular tachycardia was of atrial origin. Six of the nine patients that developed ventricular arrhythmias did so within 14 days of onset of therapy. About 2.3% (11/474) of all patients had recurrence of SVT during the study which could have been a change in the patients' arrhythmia behavior or could represent a proarrhythmic event. Case reports in patients treated with RYTHMOL for atrial fibrillation/flutter have included increased PVCs, VT, VF, Torsade de Pointes, asystole, and death.
In the RAFT study, there were five deaths, three in the pooled RYTHMOL SR group (0.8%) and two in the placebo group (1.6%). In the overall RYTHMOL SR and RYTHMOL immediate release database of eight studies, the mortality rate was 2.5% per year on RYTHMOL and 4.0% per year on placebo. Concurrent use of propafenone with other antiarrhythmic agents has not been well studied.

Use with Drugs that Prolong the QT Interval and Antiarrhythmic Agents:
The use of RYTHMOL SR (propafenone hydrochloride) in conjunction with other drugs that prolong the QT interval has not been extensively studied and is not recommended. Such drugs may include many antiarrhythmics, some phenothiazines, cisapride, bepridil, tricyclic antidepressants and oral macrolides. Class Ia and III antiarrhythmic agents should be withheld for at least five half-lives prior to dosing with RYTHMOL SR. The use of propafenone with Class Ia and III antiarrhythmic agents (including quinidine and amiodarone) is not recommended. There is only limited experience with the concomitant use of Class Ib or Ic antiarrhythmics.

Nonallergic Bronchospasm (e.g., chronic bronchitis, emphysema):
Patients with bronchospastic disease should not, in general, receive propafenone or other agents with beta-adrenergic-blocking activity.

Congestive Heart Failure:
Propafenone exerts a negative inotropic activity on the myocardium as well as beta blockade effects and may provoke overt congestive heart failure. In the U.S. trial (RAFT) in patients with symptomatic atrial fibrillation, congestive heart failure was reported in four (1.0%) patients receiving RYTHMOL SR (all doses), compared to one (0.8%) patient receiving placebo. Proarrhythmic effects are more likely to occur when propafenone is administered to patients with congestive heart failure (NYHA III and IV) or severe myocardial ischemia (see **CONTRAINDICATIONS**).

Conduction Disturbances:
Propafenone causes dose-related first degree AV block. Average PR interval prolongation and increases in QRS duration are also dose-related.
Propafenone should not be given to patients with atrioventricular and intraventricular conduction defects in the absence of a pacemaker (see **CONTRAINDICATIONS**).
In a U.S. trial (RAFT) in 523 patients with a history of symptomatic atrial fibrillation treated with RYTHMOL SR, electrocardiograms obtained in response to symptoms were associated with no patients having sinus rhythm with Mobitz Type I (Wenckenbach) second degree AV block, sinus rhythm with Mobitz Type II second degree AV block, or third degree AV block. Sinus bradycardia (rate <50 beats/min) was reported with the same frequency with RYTHMOL SR and placebo.

Effects on Pacemaker Threshold:
Propafenone may alter both pacing and sensing thresholds of artificial pacemakers. Pacemakers should be monitored and programmed accordingly during therapy.

Hematologic Disturbances:
Agranulocytosis (fever, chills, weakness, and neutropenia) has been reported in patients receiving propafenone. Generally, the agranulocytosis occurred within the first two months of propafenone therapy and upon discontinuation of therapy, the white count usually normalized by 14 days. Unexplained fever and/or decrease in white cell count, particularly during the initial three months of therapy, warrant consideration of possible agranulocytosis or granulocytopenia. Patients should be instructed to report promptly the development of any signs of infection such as fever, sore throat, or chills.

PRECAUTIONS

Hepatic Dysfunction:
Propafenone is highly metabolized by the liver and should, therefore, be administered cautiously to patients with impaired hepatic function. Severe liver dysfunction increases the bioavailability of propafenone to approximately 70% compared to 3-40% in patients with normal liver function when given RYTHMOL immediate release tablets. In eight patients with moderate to severe liver disease administered RYTHMOL immediate release tablets, the mean half-life was approximately nine hours. No studies are currently available comparing bioavailability of propafenone from RYTHMOL SR in patients with normal and impaired hepatic function. Increased bioavailability of propafenone in these patients may result in excessive accumulation. Careful monitoring for excessive pharmacological effects (see **OVERDOSAGE**) should be performed for patients with impaired hepatic function.

Renal Dysfunction:
Approximately 50% of propafenone metabolites are excreted in the urine following administration of RYTHMOL immediate release tablets. No studies have been performed to assess the percentage of metabolites eliminated in the urine following the administration of RYTHMOL SR capsules.
Until further data are available, RYTHMOL SR should be administered cautiously to patients with impaired renal function. These patients should be carefully monitored for signs of overdosage (see **OVERDOSAGE**).

Information for Patients:
Medications and Supplements:
Assessment of patients' medication history should include all over-the-counter, prescription and herbal/natural preparations with emphasis on preparations that may affect the pharmacodynamics or kinetics of RYTHMOL SR (see **WARNINGS/Use with Drugs that Prolong QT interval and Antiarrhythmic Agents**). Patients should be instructed to notify their health care providers of any change in over-the-counter, prescription and supplement use. If a patient is hospitalized or is prescribed new medication for any condition, the patient must inform the health care provider of ongoing RYTHMOL SR therapy. Patients should also check with their health care providers prior to taking a new over-the-counter medicine.
Electrolyte Imbalance:
If patients experience symptoms that may be associated with altered electrolyte balance, such as excessive or prolonged diarrhea, sweating, vomiting, or loss of appetite or thirst, these conditions should be immediately reported to their health care provider.
Dosing Schedule:
Patients should be instructed NOT to double the next dose if a dose is missed. The next dose should be taken at the usual time.

Elevated ANA Titers:
Positive ANA titers have been reported in patients receiving propafenone. They have been reversible upon cessation of treatment and may disappear even in the face of continued propafenone therapy. These laboratory findings were usually not associated with clinical symptoms, but there is one published case of drug-induced lupus erythematosus (positive rechallenge); it resolved completely upon discontinuation of therapy. Patients who develop an abnormal ANA test should be carefully evaluated and, if persistent or worsening elevation of ANA titers is detected, consideration should be given to discontinuing therapy.

Impaired Spermatogenesis:
Reversible disorders of spermatogenesis have been demonstrated in monkeys, dogs and rabbits after high dose intravenous administration of propafenone. Evaluation of the effects of short-term RYTHMOL administration on spermatogenesis in 11 normal subjects suggested that propafenone produced a reversible, short-term drop (within normal range) in sperm count. Subsequent evaluations in 11 patients receiving RYTHMOL chronically have found no effect of propafenone on sperm count.

Neuromuscular Dysfunction:
Exacerbation of myasthenia gravis has been reported during RYTHMOL immediate release tablet therapy.

Drug Interactions:
Drugs that inhibit CYP2D6, CYP1A2 and CYP3A4 might lead to increased plasma levels of propafenone. When propafenone is co-administered with inhibitors of these enzymes, the patients should be closely monitored and the dose adjusted accordingly.
Quinidine: Small doses of quinidine completely inhibit the hydroxylation metabolic pathway, making all patients, in effect, slow metabolizers (see **CLINICAL PHARMACOLOGY**). The use of quinidine with propafenone is not recommended.
Local Anesthetics: Concomitant use of local anesthetics (i.e., during pacemaker implantations, surgery, or dental use) may increase the risks of central nervous system side effects.
Digitalis: RYTHMOL immediate release tablets have been shown to produce dose-related increases in serum digoxin levels ranging from about 35% at 450 mg/day to 85% at 900 mg/day of RYTHMOL immediate release tablets without affecting digoxin renal clearance. Elevations of digoxin levels were maintained for up to 16 months during concomitant administration. Plasma digoxin levels of patients on concomitant therapy should be measured, and digoxin dosage should ordinarily be reduced when propafenone is started, especially if a relatively large digoxin dose is used or if plasma concentrations are relatively high.
Beta-Antagonists: In a study involving healthy subjects, concomitant administration of RYTHMOL immediate release tablets and propranolol resulted in substantial increases in propranolol plasma concentration and elimination half-life with no change in propafenone plasma levels from control values. Similar observations have been reported with metoprolol. Propafenone appears to inhibit the hydroxylation pathway for the two beta-antagonists (just as quinidine inhibits propafenone metabolism). Increased plasma concentrations of metoprolol could overcome its relative cardioselectivity. In RYTHMOL immediate release tablet clinical trials, patients who were receiving beta-blockers concurrently did not experience an increased incidence of side effects. While the therapeutic range for beta-blockers is wide, a reduction in dosage may be necessary during concomitant administration with propafenone.
Warfarin: In a study of eight healthy subjects receiving RYTHMOL immediate release tablets and warfarin concomitantly, mean steady-state warfarin plasma concentrations increased 39% with a corresponding increase in prothrombin times of approximately 25%. It is therefore recommended that prothrombin times be routinely monitored and the dose of warfarin be adjusted if necessary.
Cimetidine: Concomitant administration of RYTHMOL immediate release tablets and cimetidine in 12 healthy subjects resulted in a 20% increase in steady-state plasma concentrations of propafenone with no detectable changes in electrocardiographic parameters beyond that measured on propafenone alone.
Desipramine: Concomitant administration of propafenone and desipramine may result in elevated serum desipramine levels. Both desipramine, a tricyclic antidepressant, and propafenone are cleared by oxidative pathways of demethylation and hydroxylation carried out by the hepatic P-450 cytochrome.
Cyclosporin: Propafenone therapy may increase levels of cyclosporin.
Theophylline: Propafenone may increase theophylline concentration during concomitant therapy with the development of theophylline toxicity.
Rifampin: Rifampin may accelerate the metabolism and decrease the plasma levels and antiarrhythmic efficacy of propafenone.

Renal and Hepatic Toxicity in Animals:
Renal changes have been observed in the rat following six months of oral administration of propafenone HCl at doses of 180 and 360 mg/kg/day (about two and four times, respectively, the maximum recommended human daily dose [MRHD] on a mg/m^2 basis). Both inflammatory and non-inflammatory changes in the renal tubules, with accompanying interstitial nephritis, were observed. These changes were reversible, as they were not found in rats allowed to recover for six weeks. Fatty degenerative changes of the liver were found in rats following longer durations of administration of propafenone HCl at a dose of 270 mg/kg/day (about three times the MRHD on a mg/m^2 basis). There were no renal or hepatic changes at 90 mg/kg/day (equivalent to the MRHD on a mg/m^2 basis).

Carcinogenesis, Mutagenesis, Impairment of Fertility:
Lifetime maximally tolerated oral dose studies in mice (up to 360 mg/kg/day, about twice the maximum recommended human oral daily dose [MRHD] on a mg/m^2 basis) and rats (up to 270 mg/kg/day, about three times the MRHD on a mg/m^2 basis) provided no evidence of a carcinogenic potential for propafenone HCl.
Propafenone HCl tested negative for mutagenicity in the Ames (salmonella) test and in the *in vivo* mouse dominant lethal test. It tested negative for clastogenicity in the human lymphocyte chromosome aberration assay *in vitro* and in rat and Chinese hamster micronucleus tests, and other *in vivo* tests for chromosomal aberrations in rat bone marrow and Chinese hamster bone marrow and spermatogonia.

Table 2: Most common adverse events (≥2.0% in any RAFT propafenone SR treatment group and more common on propafenone than on placebo)

MedDRA Body System/Preferred Term	RYTHMOL SR 225 mg BID (N = 126) n (%)	RYTHMOL SR 325 mg BID (N = 135) n (%)	RYTHMOL SR 425 mg BID (N = 136) n (%)	Placebo (N = 126) n (%)
Mean exposure (days)	**124**	**149**	**141**	**91**
Cardiac disorders				
Angina pectoris	0 (0)	0 (0)	3 (2)	0 (0)
Atrial flutter	3 (2)	2 (1)	0 (0)	1 (1)
AV block first degree	3 (2)	3 (2)	4 (3)	0 (0)
Bradycardia	4 (3)	4 (3)	6 (4)	1 (1)
Cardiac failure congestive	0 (0)	1 (1)	3 (2)	1 (1)
Cardiac murmur	2 (2)	3 (2)	6 (4)	0 (0)
Edema	6 (5)	18 (13)	10 (7)	8 (6)
Eye disorders				
Vision blurred	1 (1)	1 (1)	5 (4)	0 (0)
Gastrointestinal disorders				
Constipation	10 (8)	19 (14)	16 (12)	3 (2)
Diarrhea	2 (2)	3 (2)	5 (4)	3 (2)
Dry mouth	1 (1)	1 (1)	5 (4)	1 (1)
Flatulence	3 (2)	3 (2)	1 (1)	0 (0)
Nausea	11 (9)	15 (11)	23 (17)	11 (9)
Vomiting	1 (1)	0 (0)	8 (6)	3 (2)
General disorder and administration site				
Fatigue	14 (11)	17 (13)	17 (13)	7 (6)
Weakness	4 (3)	6 (4)	6 (4)	3 (2)
Infections and infestations				
Upper respiratory tract infection	11 (9)	16 (12)	11 (8)	7 (6)
Investigations				
Blood alkaline phosphatase increased	0 (0)	0 (0)	4 (3)	0 (0)
Cardioactive drug level above therapeutic	1 (1)	1 (1)	3 (2)	1 (1)
Hematuria	2 (2)	2 (1)	4 (3)	3 (2)
Musculoskeletal, connective tissue and bone				
Muscle weakness	1 (1)	5 (4)	1 (1)	0 (0)
Nervous system disorders				
Dizziness (excluding vertigo)	29 (23)	28 (21)	29 (21)	18 (14)
Headache	8 (6)	12 (9)	14 (10)	11 (9)
Taste disturbance	7 (6)	18 (13)	30 (22)	1 (1)
Tremor	2 (2)	0 (0)	3 (2)	1 (1)
Somnolence	1 (1)	1 (1)	4 (3)	0 (0)
Psychiatric disorders				
Anxiety	12 (10)	17 (13)	16 (12)	13 (10)
Depression	1 (1)	4 (3)	0 (0)	2 (2)
Respiratory, thoracic and mediastinal disorder				
Dyspnea	16 (13)	23 (17)	17 (13)	9 (7)
Rales	2 (2)	1 (1)	3 (2)	0 (0)
Wheezing	0 (0)	0 (0)	3 (2)	0 (0)
Skin & subcutaneous tissue disorders				
Ecchymosis	2 (2)	3 (2)	5 (4)	0 (0)

Propafenone HCl, administered intravenously to rabbits, dogs, and monkeys, has been shown to decrease spermatogenesis. These effects were reversible, were not found following oral dosing of propafenone HCl, were seen at lethal or near lethal dose levels and were not seen in rats treated either orally or intravenously (see **PRECAUTIONS, Impaired Spermatogenesis**). Treatment of male rabbits for 10 weeks prior to mating at an oral dose of 120 mg/kg/day (about 2.4 times the MRHD on a mg/m^2 basis) or an intravenous dose of 3.5 mg/kg/day (a spermatogenesis-impairing dose) did not result in evidence of impaired fertility. Nor was there evidence of impaired fertility when propafenone HCl was administered orally to male and female rats at dose levels up to 270 mg/kg/day (about 3 times the MRHD on a mg/m^2 basis).

Pregnancy

Teratogenic Effects: *Pregnancy Category C.* Propafenone HCl has been shown to be embryotoxic (decreased survival) in rabbits and rats when given in oral maternally toxic doses of 150 mg/kg/day (about three times the maximum recommended human dose [MRHD] on a mg/m^2 basis) and 600 mg/kg/day (about six times the MRHD on a mg/m^2 basis), respectively. Although maternally tolerated doses (up to 270 mg/kg/day, about three times the MRHD on a mg/m^2 basis) produced no evidence of embryotoxicity in rats, post-implantation loss was elevated in all rabbit treatment groups (doses as low as 15 mg/kg/day, about 1/3 the MRHD on a mg/m^2 basis). There are no adequate and well-controlled studies in pregnant women. RYTHMOL SR (propafenone hydrochloride) should be used during pregnancy only if the potential benefit justifies the potential risk to the fetus.

Non-teratogenic Effects: In a study in which female rats received daily oral doses of propafenone HCl from mid-gestation through weaning of their offspring, doses as low as 90 mg/kg/day (equivalent to the MRHD on a mg/m^2 basis) produced increases in maternal deaths. Doses of 360 or more mg/kg/day (four or more times the MRHD on a mg/m^2 basis) resulted in reductions in neonatal survival, body weight gain and physiological development.

Labor and Delivery:

It is not known whether the use of propafenone during labor or delivery has immediate or delayed adverse effects on the fetus, or whether it prolongs the duration of labor or increases the need for forceps delivery or other obstetrical intervention.

Nursing Mothers:

Propafenone is excreted in human milk. Caution should be exercised when RYTHMOL SR is administered to a nursing mother.

Pediatric Use:

The safety and effectiveness of propafenone in pediatric patients have not been established.

Geriatric Use:

Of the total number of subjects in Phase III clinical studies of RYTHMOL SR (propafenone hydrochloride) 45.7 percent were 65 and over, while 15.7 percent were 75 and over. No overall differences in safety or effectiveness were observed between these subjects and younger subjects, but greater sensitivity of some older individuals at higher doses cannot be ruled out. The effect of age on the pharmacokinetics and pharmacodynamics of propafenone has not been studied.

ADVERSE REACTIONS

The data described below reflect exposure to RYTHMOL SR 225 mg BID in 126 patients, to RYTHMOL SR 325 mg BID in 135 patients, to RYTHMOL SR 425 mg BID in 136 patients, and to placebo in 126 patients for up to 39 weeks in a placebo-controlled trial (RAFT) conducted in the US. The most commonly reported adverse events in the trial included dizziness, chest pain, palpitations, taste disturbance, dyspnea, nausea, constipation, anxiety, fatigue, upper respiratory tract infection, influenza, first degree heart block and vomiting. The frequency of discontinuation due to adverse events was highest during the first 14 days of treatment. The majority of the patients with serious adverse events who withdrew or were discontinued recovered without sequelae.

Adverse events occurring in 2% or more of the patients in any of the RAFT propafenone SR treatment groups and more common with propafenone than with placebo, excluding those that are common in the population and those not plausibly related to drug therapy, are listed in Table 2.

[See table 2 at left]

No clinically important differences in incidence of adverse reactions were noted by age, or gender. Too few non-White patients were enrolled to assess adverse events according to race. Adverse events occurring in 2% or more of the patients in any of the ERAFT propafenone SR treatment groups and not listed in Table 2 include the following: bundle branch block left, bundle branch block right, conduction disorders, sinus bradycardia and hypotension.

Other adverse events reported with propafenone clinical trials not already listed in Table 3 include the following adverse events by body and preferred term.

Blood and lymphatic system disorders: anemia; lymphadenopathy; spleen disorder; thrombocytopenia; *Cardiac disorders:* angina unstable; arrhythmia; atrial hypertrophy; atrioventricular block; bundle branch block; bunch branch block left; bundle branch block right; cardiac arrest; cardiac disorder; conduction disorder; coronary artery disease; extrasystoles; myocardial infarction; nodal arrhythmia; palpitations; pericarditis; sinoatrial block; sinus arrest; sinus arrhythmia; sinus bradycardia; supraventricular extrasystoles; supraventricular tachycardia; ventricular arrhythmia; ventricular extrasystoles; ventricular hypertrophy; *Ear and labyrinth disorders:* hearing impaired; tinnitus; vertigo; *Eye disorders:* eye hemorrhage; eye inflammation; eyelid ptosis; miosis; retinal disorder; visual acuity reduced; *Gastrointestinal disorders:* abdominal distension; abdominal pain; dry throat; duodenitis; dyspepsia; dysphagia; eructation; gastritis; gastroesophageal reflux disease; gingival bleeding; glossitis; glossodynia; gum pain; halitosis; intestinal obstruction; melena; mouth ulceration; pancreatitis;

Continued on next page

Table 4: Number of patients according to the range of maximum QTc change compared to baseline over the study in each dose group (RAFT study)

Range of maximum QTc change	RYTHMOL SR			Placebo
	225 mg BID	325 mg BID	425 mg BID	
	N=119	N=129	N=123	N=120
	n (%)	n (%)	n (%)	n (%)
>20%	1 (1%)	6 (5%)	3 (2%)	5 (4%)
10-20%	19 (16%)	28 (22%)	32 (26%)	24 (20%)
≤10%	99 (83%)	95 (74%)	88 (72%)	91 (76%)

Rythmol SR—Cont.

peptic ulcer; rectal bleeding; sore throat; *General disorders and administration site conditions:* chest pain; feeling hot; hemorrhage; malaise; pain; pyrexia; *Hepato-biliary disorders:* hepatomegaly; *Investigations:* abnormal electrocardiogram; abnormal heart sounds; abnormal liver function tests; abnormal pulse; carotid bruit; decreased blood chloride; decreased blood pressure; decreased blood sodium; decreased hemoglobin; decreased neutrophil count; decreased platelet count; decreased prothrombin level; decreased red blood cell count; decreased weight; electrocardiogram QT prolonged; glycosuria present; heart rate irregular; increased alanine aminotransferase; increased aspartate aminotransferase; increased blood bilirubin; increased blood cholesterol; increased blood creatinine; increased blood glucose; increased blood lactate dehydrogenase; increased blood pressure; increased blood prolactin; increased blood triglycerides; increased blood urea; increased blood uric acid; increased eosinophil count; increased gamma-glutamyltransferase; increased monocyte count; increased prostatic specific antigen; increased prothrombin level; increased weight; increased white blood cell count; ketonuria present; proteinuria present; *Metabolism and nutrition disorders:* anorexia; dehydration; diabetes mellitus; gout; hypercholesterolemia; hyperglycemia; hyperlipidemia; hypokalemia; *Musculoskeletal, connective tissue and bone disorders:* arthritis; bursitis; collagen-vascular disease; costochondritis; joint disorder; muscle cramps; muscle spasms; myalgia; neck pain; pain in jaw; sciatica; tendonitis; *Nervous system disorders:* amnesia; ataxia; balance impaired; brain damage; cerebrovascular accident; dementia; gait abnormal; hypertonia; hypothesia; insomnia; paralysis; paresthesia; peripheral neuropathy; speech disorder; syncope; tongue hypoesthesia; *Psychiatric disorders:* decreased libido; emotional disturbance; mental disorder; neurosis; nightmare; sleep disorder; *Renal and urinary disorders:* dysuria; nocturia; oliguria; pyuria; renal failure; urinary casts; urinary frequency; urinary incontinence; urinary retention; urine abnormal; *Reproductive system and breast disorders:* breast pain; impotence; prostatism; *Respiratory, thoracic and mediastinal disorders:* atelectasis; breath sounds decreased; chronic obstructive airways disease; cough; epistaxis; hemoptysis; lung disorder; pleural effusion; pulmonary congestion; rales; respiratory failure; rhinitis; throat tightness; *Skin and subcutaneous tissue disorders:* alopecia; dermatitis; dry skin; erythema; nail abnormality; petechiae; pruritis; sweating increased; urticaria; *Vascular disorders:* arterial embolism limb; deep limb venous thrombosis; flushing; hematoma; hypertension; hypertensive crisis; hypotension; labile blood pressure; pallor; peripheral coldness; peripheral vascular disease; thrombosis.

Laboratory:

Electrocardiograms

Propafenone prolongs the PR and QRS intervals in patients with atrial and ventricular arrythmias. Prolongation of the QRS interval makes it difficult to interpret the effect of propafenone on the QT interval.

Table 3: Mean Change in 12-Lead Electrocardiogram Results (RAFT)

	RYTHMOL SR BID dosing			
	225 mg	325 mg	425 mg	Placebo
	n=126	n=135	n=136	n=126
PR (ms)	9±22	12±23	21±24	1±16
QRS (ms)	4±14	6±15	6±15	-2±12
QTc* (ms)	2±30	5±36	6±37	5±35

*Calculated using Bazett's correction factor

In RAFT, the distribution of the maximum changes in QTc compared to baseline over the study in each patient was similar in the RYTHMOL SR 225 mg BID, 325 mg BID, and 425 mg BID and placebo dose groups. Similar results were seen in the ERAFT study.

[See table 4 above]

OVERDOSAGE

The symptoms of overdosage may include hypotension, somnolence, bradycardia, intra-atrial and intraventricular conduction disturbances, and rarely convulsions and high grade ventricular arrhythmias. Defibrillation as well as infusion of dopamine and isoproterenol have been effective in controlling abnormal ventricular rhythm and blood pressure. Convulsions have been alleviated with intravenous diazepam. General supportive measures such as mechanical respiratory assistance and external cardiac massage may be necessary.

The hemodialysis of propafenone in patients with an overdose is expected to be of limited value in the removal of propafenone as a result of both its high protein binding (>95%) and large volume of distribution.

DOSAGE AND ADMINISTRATION

The dose of RYTHMOL SR must be individually titrated on the basis of response and tolerance. Therapy should be initiated with RYTHMOL SR 225 mg given every twelve hours. Dosage may be increased at a minimum of five day interval to 325 mg given every twelve hours. If additional therapeutic effect is needed, the dose of RYTHMOL SR may be increased to 425 mg given every twelve hours.

In patients with hepatic impairment or having significant widening of the QRS complex or second or third degree AV block, dose reduction should be considered.

RYTHMOL SR can be taken with or without food. Do not crush or further divide the contents of the capsule.

HOW SUPPLIED

RYTHMOL® SR (propafenone HCl) capsules are supplied as white, opaque, hard gelatin capsules containing either 225 mg, 325 mg, or 425 mg of propafenone HCl and imprinted in red with α and strength. The 325 mg strength is also imprinted with a single red band around ¾ of the circumference of the body; the 425 mg strength is imprinted with three bands around ¾ of the circumference of the body.

	NDC #65726-xxx-yy	
	Unit dose	Bottle of 100
225 mg	261-90	261-25
325 mg	262-90	262-25
425 mg	263-90	263-25

Storage: Store at 25°C (77°F); excursions permitted to 15-30°C (59-86°F) [see USP controlled room temperature]. Dispense in a tight container as defined in the USP.

℞ Only

RYTHMOL is a registered trademark of G. Petrik used under license by Abbott Laboratories

326F100

03-5323-R1

Revised: November, 2003

Distributed by:

Reliant Pharmaceuticals

Liberty Corner, New Jersey 07938 PRINTED IN U.S.A.

Shown in Product Identification Guide, page 331

IDENTIFICATION PROBLEM?
Turn to the **Product Identification Guide,** where you'll find more than 1600 products pictured in actual size and full color.

Roche Pharmaceuticals

Roche Laboratories Inc.
340 Kingsland Street
Nutley, NJ 07110-1199

For Medical Information:
(Including routine inquiries, adverse drug events and product complaints)
Call: (800) 526-6367
In Emergencies: 24-hour service
For the Medical Needs Program:
Call: (800) 285-4484
Write: Professional Product Information
Order Fulfillment
(800) 526-0625

ACCUTANE® ℞

[acc' u tane]

(isotretinoin)

CAPSULES

℞ only

CAUSES BIRTH DEFECTS

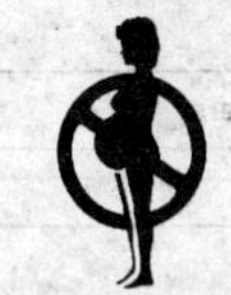

DO NOT GET PREGNANT

CONTRAINDICATIONS AND WARNINGS

Accutane must not be used by females who are pregnant. Although not every fetus exposed to Accutane has resulted in a deformed child, there is an extremely high risk that a deformed infant can result if pregnancy occurs while taking Accutane in any amount even for short periods of time. Potentially any fetus exposed during pregnancy can be affected. Presently, there are no accurate means of determining, after Accutane exposure, which fetus has been affected and which fetus has not been affected.

Major human fetal abnormalities related to Accutane administration in females have been documented. There is an increased risk of spontaneous abortion. In addition, premature births have been reported.

Documented external abnormalities include: skull abnormality; ear abnormalities (including anotia, micropinna, small or absent external auditory canals); eye abnormalities (including microphthalmia); facial dysmorphia; cleft palate. Documented internal abnormalities include: CNS abnormalities (including cerebral abnormalities, cerebellar malformation, hydrocephalus, microcephaly, cranial nerve deficit); cardiovascular abnormalities; thymus gland abnormality; parathyroid hormone deficiency. In some cases death has occurred with certain of the abnormalities previously noted.

Cases of IQ scores less than 85 with or without obvious CNS abnormalities have also been reported.

Accutane is contraindicated in females of childbearing potential unless the patient meets all of the following conditions:

- **Must NOT be pregnant or breast feeding.**
- **Must be capable of complying with the mandatory contraceptive measures required for Accutane therapy and understand behaviors associated with an increased risk of pregnancy.**
- **Must be reliable in understanding and carrying out instructions.**

Accutane must be prescribed under the *System to Manage Accutane Related Teratogenicity™* (S.M.A.R.T.™).

To prescribe Accutane, the prescriber must obtain a supply of yellow self-adhesive Accutane Qualification Stickers. To obtain these stickers:

1) **Read the booklet entitled *System to Manage Accutane Related Teratogenicity* (S.M.A.R.T.) *Guide to Best Practices.***
2) **Sign and return the completed S.M.A.R.T. *Letter of Understanding* containing the following Prescriber Checklist:**

- **I know the risk and severity of fetal injury/birth defects from Accutane**
- **I know how to diagnose and treat the various presentations of acne**
- **I know the risk factors for unplanned pregnancy and the effective measures for avoidance of unplanned pregnancy**
- **It is the informed patient's responsibility to avoid pregnancy during Accutane therapy and for 1 month after stopping Accutane. To help patients have the knowledge and tools to do so: Before beginning treatment of female patients with Accutane I will refer for expert, detailed pregnancy prevention counseling and prescribing, reimbursed by the manufacturer, OR I have the expertise to perform this function and elect to do so**

• I understand, and will properly use throughout the Accutane treatment course, the S.M.A.R.T. procedures for Accutane, including monthly pregnancy avoidance counseling, pregnancy testing and use of the yellow self-adhesive Accutane Qualification Stickers

3) To use the yellow self-adhesive Accutane Qualification Sticker: Accutane should not be prescribed or dispensed to any patient (male or female) without a yellow self-adhesive Accutane Qualification Sticker.

For female patients, the yellow self-adhesive Accutane Qualification Sticker signifies that she:

- **Must have had 2 negative urine or serum pregnancy tests with a sensitivity of at least 25 mIU/mL before receiving the initial Accutane prescription. The first test (a screening test) is obtained by the prescriber when the decision is made to pursue qualification of the patient for Accutane. The second pregnancy test (a confirmation test) should be done during the first 5 days of the menstrual period immediately preceding the beginning of Accutane therapy. For patients with amenorrhea, the second test should be done at least 11 days after the last act of unprotected sexual intercourse (without using 2 effective forms of contraception). Each month of therapy, the patient must have a negative result from a urine or serum pregnancy test. A pregnancy test must be repeated every month prior to the female patient receiving each prescription.**
- **Must have selected and have committed to use 2 forms of effective contraception simultaneously, at least 1 of which must be a primary form, unless absolute abstinence is the chosen method, or the patient has undergone a hysterectomy. Patients must use 2 forms of effective contraception for at least 1 month prior to initiation of Accutane therapy, during Accutane therapy, and for 1 month after discontinuing Accutane therapy. Counseling about contraception and behaviors associated with an increased risk of pregnancy must be repeated on a monthly basis.**

Effective forms of contraception include both primary and secondary forms of contraception. Primary forms of contraception include: tubal ligation, partner's vasectomy, intrauterine devices, birth control pills, and topical/injectable/implantable/insertable hormonal birth control products. Secondary forms of contraception include diaphragms, latex condoms, and cervical caps; each must be used with a spermicide.

Any birth control method can fail. Therefore, it is critically important that women of childbearing potential use 2 effective forms of contraception simultaneously. A drug interaction that decreases effectiveness of hormonal contraceptives has not been entirely ruled out for Accutane. Although hormonal contraceptives are highly effective, there have been reports of pregnancy from women who have used oral contraceptives, as well as topical/injectable/implantable/insertable hormonal birth control products. These reports occurred while these patients were taking Accutane. These reports are more frequent for women who use only a single method of contraception. Patients must receive written warnings about the rates of possible contraception failure (included in patient education kits).

Prescribers are advised to consult the package insert of any medication administered concomitantly with hormonal contraceptives, since some medications may decrease the effectiveness of these birth control products.

Patients should be prospectively cautioned not to self-medicate with the herbal supplement St. John's Wort because a possible interaction has been suggested with hormonal contraceptives based on reports of breakthrough bleeding on oral contraceptives shortly after starting St. John's Wort. Pregnancies have been reported by users of combined hormonal contraceptives who also used some form of St. John's Wort (see PRECAUTIONS).

- **Must have signed a Patient Information/Consent form that contains warnings about the risk of potential birth defects if the fetus is exposed to isotretinoin.**
- **Must have been informed of the purpose and importance of participating in the Accutane Survey and have been given the opportunity to enroll (see PRECAUTIONS).**

The yellow self-adhesive Accutane Qualification Sticker documents that the female patient is qualified, and includes the date of qualification, patient gender, cut-off date for filling the prescription, and up to a 30-day supply limit with no refills.

These yellow self-adhesive Accutane Qualification Stickers should also be used for male patients.

If a pregnancy does occur during treatment of a woman with Accutane, the prescriber and patient should discuss the desirability of continuing the pregnancy. Prescribers are strongly encouraged to report all cases of pregnancy to Roche @ 1-800-526-6367 where a Roche Pregnancy Prevention Program Specialist will be available to discuss Roche pregnancy information, or prescribers may contact the Food and Drug Administration MedWatch Program @ 1-800-FDA-1088.

Accutane should be prescribed only by prescribers who have demonstrated special competence in the diagnosis and treatment of severe recalcitrant nodular acne, are experienced in the use of systemic retinoids, have read the S.M.A.R.T. *Guide to Best Practices*, signed and returned the *completed* S.M.A.R.T. *Letter of Understanding*, and obtained yellow self-adhesive Accutane Qualification Stickers. Accutane should not be prescribed or dispensed without a yellow self-adhesive Accutane Qualification Sticker.

Table 1. Use of Pregnancy Tests and Accutane Qualification Stickers for Patients

Patient Type	Pregnancy Test Required	Qualification Date	Accutane Qualification Sticker Necessary	Dispense Within 7 Days of Qualification Date
All Males	No	Date Prescription Written	Yes	Yes
Females of Childbearing Potential	Yes	Date Sample Taken for Confirmatory Negative Pregnancy Test	Yes	Yes
Females* Not of Childbearing Potential	No	Date Prescription Written	Yes	Yes

***Females who have had a hysterectomy or who are postmenopausal are not considered to be of childbearing potential.**

INFORMATION FOR PHARMACISTS:

ACCUTANE MUST ONLY BE DISPENSED:

- **IN NO MORE THAN A 30-DAY SUPPLY**
- **ONLY ON PRESENTATION OF AN ACCUTANE PRESCRIPTION WITH A YELLOW SELF-ADHESIVE ACCUTANE QUALIFICATION STICKER**
- **WITHIN 7 DAYS OF THE QUALIFICATION DATE**
- **REFILLS REQUIRE A NEW PRESCRIPTION WITH A YELLOW SELF-ADHESIVE ACCUTANE QUALIFICATION STICKER**
- **NO TELEPHONE OR COMPUTERIZED PRESCRIPTIONS ARE PERMITTED.**

AN ACCUTANE MEDICATION GUIDE MUST BE GIVEN TO THE PATIENT EACH TIME ACCUTANE IS DISPENSED, AS REQUIRED BY LAW. THIS ACCUTANE MEDICATION GUIDE IS AN IMPORTANT PART OF THE RISK MANAGEMENT PROGRAM FOR THE PATIENT.

[See table 1 above]

DESCRIPTION

Isotretinoin, a retinoid, is available as Accutane in 10-mg, 20-mg and 40-mg soft gelatin capsules for oral administration. Each capsule contains beeswax, butylated hydroxyanisole, edetate disodium, hydrogenated soybean oil flakes, hydrogenated vegetable oil, and soybean oil. Gelatin capsules contain glycerin and parabens (methyl and propyl), with the following dye systems: 10 mg — iron oxide (red) and titanium dioxide; 20 mg — FD&C Red No. 3, FD&C Blue No. 1, and titanium dioxide; 40 mg — FD&C Yellow No. 6, D&C Yellow No. 10, and titanium dioxide.

Chemically, isotretinoin is 13-*cis*-retinoic acid and is related to both retinoic acid and retinol (vitamin A). It is a yellow to orange crystalline powder with a molecular weight of 300.44.

CLINICAL PHARMACOLOGY

Isotretinoin is a retinoid, which when administered in pharmacologic dosages of 0.5 to 1.0 mg/kg/day (see DOSAGE AND ADMINISTRATION), inhibits sebaceous gland function and keratinization. The exact mechanism of action of isotretinoin is unknown.

Nodular Acne

Clinical improvement in nodular acne patients occurs in association with a reduction in sebum secretion. The decrease in sebum secretion is temporary and is related to the dose and duration of treatment with Accutane, and reflects a reduction in sebaceous gland size and an inhibition of sebaceous gland differentiation.[1]

Pharmacokinetics

Absorption

Due to its high lipophilicity, oral absorption of isotretinoin is enhanced when given with a high-fat meal. In a crossover study, 74 healthy adult subjects received a single 80 mg oral dose (2 × 40 mg capsules) of Accutane under fasted and fed conditions. Both peak plasma concentration (C_{max}) and the total exposure (AUC) of isotretinoin were more than doubled following a standardized high-fat meal when compared with Accutane given under fasted conditions (see Table 2 below). The observed elimination half-life was unchanged. This lack of change in half-life suggests that food increases the bioavailability of isotretinoin without altering its disposition. The time to peak concentration (T_{max}) was also increased with food and may be related to a longer absorption phase. Therefore, Accutane capsules should always be taken with food (see DOSAGE AND ADMINISTRATION). Clinical studies have shown that there is no difference in the pharmacokinetics of isotretinoin between patients with nodular acne and healthy subjects with normal skin.

Table 2. Pharmacokinetic Parameters of Isotretinoin Mean (% CV), N=74

Accutane 2 × 40 mg Capsules	$AUC_{0-\infty}$ (ng·hr/mL)	C_{max} (ng/mL)	T_{max} (hr)	$t_{1/2}$ (hr)
Fed*	10,004 (22%)	862 (22%)	5.3 (77%)	21 (39%)
Fasted	3,703 (46%)	301 (63%)	3.2 (56%)	21 (30%)

*Eating a standardized high-fat meal

Distribution

Isotretinoin is more than 99.9% bound to plasma proteins, primarily albumin.

Metabolism

Following oral administration of isotretinoin, at least three metabolites have been identified in human plasma: 4-*oxo*-isotretinoin, retinoic acid (tretinoin), and 4-*oxo*-retinoic acid (4-*oxo*-tretinoin). Retinoic acid and 13-*cis*-retinoic acid are geometric isomers and show reversible interconversion. The administration of one isomer will give rise to the other. Isotretinoin is also irreversibly oxidized to 4-*oxo*-isotretinoin, which forms its geometric isomer 4-*oxo*-tretinoin.

After a single 80 mg oral dose of Accutane to 74 healthy adult subjects, concurrent administration of food increased the extent of formation of all metabolites in plasma when compared to the extent of formation under fasted conditions.

All of these metabolites possess retinoid activity that is in some in vitro models more than that of the parent isotretinoin. However, the clinical significance of these models is unknown. After multiple oral dose administration of isotretinoin to adult cystic acne patients (≥18 years), the exposure of patients to 4-*oxo*-isotretinoin at steady-state under fasted and fed conditions was approximately 3.4 times higher than that of isotretinoin.

In vitro studies indicate that the primary P450 isoforms involved in isotretinoin metabolism are 2C8, 2C9, 3A4, and 2B6. Isotretinoin and its metabolites are further metabolized into conjugates, which are then excreted in urine and feces.

Elimination

Following oral administration of an 80 mg dose of ^{14}C-isotretinoin as a liquid suspension, ^{14}C-activity in blood declined with a half-life of 90 hours. The metabolites of isotretinoin and any conjugates are ultimately excreted in the feces and urine in relatively equal amounts (total of 65% to 83%). After a single 80 mg oral dose of Accutane to 74 healthy adult subjects under fed conditions, the mean ± SD elimination half-lives ($t_{1/2}$) of isotretinoin and 4-*oxo*-isotretinoin were 21.0 ± 8.2 hours and 24.0 ± 5.3 hours, respectively. After both single and multiple doses, the observed accumulation ratios of isotretinoin ranged from 0.90 to 5.43 in patients with cystic acne.

Special Patient Populations

Pediatric Patients

The pharmacokinetics of isotretinoin were evaluated after single and multiple doses in 38 pediatric patients (12 to 15 years) and 19 adult patients (≥18 years) who received Accutane for the treatment of severe recalcitrant nodular acne. In both age groups, 4-*oxo*-isotretinoin was the major metabolite; tretinoin and 4-*oxo*-tretinoin were also observed. The dose-normalized pharmacokinetic parameters for isotretinoin following single and multiple doses are summarized in Table 3 for pediatric patients. There were no statistically significant differences in the pharmacokinetics of isotretinoin between pediatric and adult patients.

[See table 3 at top of next page]

In pediatric patients (12 to 15 years), the mean ± SD elimination half-lives ($t_{1/2}$) of isotretinoin and 4-*oxo*-isotretinoin were 15.7 ± 5.1 hours and 23.1 ± 5.7 hours, respectively. The accumulation ratios of isotretinoin ranged from 0.46 to 3.65 for pediatric patients.

INDICATIONS AND USAGE

Severe Recalcitrant Nodular Acne

Accutane is indicated for the treatment of severe recalcitrant nodular acne. Nodules are inflammatory lesions with a diameter of 5 mm or greater. The nodules may become suppurative or hemorrhagic. "Severe," by definition,[2] means "many" as opposed to "few or several" nodules. Because of significant adverse effects associated with its use, Accutane should be reserved for patients with severe nodular acne who are unresponsive to conventional therapy, including systemic antibiotics. In addition, Accutane is indicated only for those females who are not pregnant, because Accutane can cause severe birth defects (see boxed CONTRAINDICATIONS AND WARNINGS).

Continued on next page

Accutane—Cont.

A single course of therapy for 15 to 20 weeks has been shown to result in complete and prolonged remission of disease in many patients.[1,3,4] If a second course of therapy is needed, it should not be initiated until at least 8 weeks after completion of the first course, because experience has shown that patients may continue to improve while off Accutane. The optimal interval before retreatment has not been defined for patients who have not completed skeletal growth (see WARNINGS: Skeletal: Bone Mineral Density, Hyperostosis, and Premature Epiphyseal Closure).

CONTRAINDICATIONS

Pregnancy: Category X. See boxed CONTRAINDICATIONS AND WARNINGS.

Allergic Reactions

Accutane is contraindicated in patients who are hypersensitive to this medication or to any of its components. Accutane should not be given to patients who are sensitive to parabens, which are used as preservatives in the gelatin capsule (see PRECAUTIONS: Hypersensitivity).

WARNINGS

Psychiatric Disorders

Accutane may cause depression, psychosis and, rarely, suicidal ideation, suicide attempts, suicide, and aggressive and/or violent behaviors. Discontinuation of Accutane therapy may be insufficient; further evaluation may be necessary. No mechanism of action has been established for these events (see ADVERSE REACTIONS: Psychiatric). Prescribers should read the brochure, *Recognizing Psychiatric Disorders in Adolescents and Young Adults: A Guide for Prescribers of Accutane® (isotretinoin).*

Pseudotumor Cerebri

Accutane use has been associated with a number of cases of pseudotumor cerebri (benign intracranial hypertension), some of which involved concomitant use of tetracyclines. Concomitant treatment with tetracyclines should therefore be avoided. Early signs and symptoms of pseudotumor cerebri include papilledema, headache, nausea and vomiting, and visual disturbances. Patients with these symptoms should be screened for papilledema and, if present, they should be told to discontinue Accutane immediately and be referred to a neurologist for further diagnosis and care (see ADVERSE REACTIONS: Neurological).

Pancreatitis

Acute pancreatitis has been reported in patients with either elevated or normal serum triglyceride levels. **In rare instances, fatal hemorrhagic pancreatitis has been reported.** Accutane should be stopped if hypertriglyceridemia cannot be controlled at an acceptable level or if symptoms of pancreatitis occur.

Lipids

Elevations of serum triglycerides in excess of 800 mg/dL have been reported in patients treated with Accutane. Marked elevations of serum triglycerides were reported in approximately 25% of patients receiving Accutane in clinical trials. In addition, approximately 15% developed a decrease in high-density lipoproteins and about 7% showed an increase in cholesterol levels. In clinical trials, the effects on triglycerides, HDL, and cholesterol were reversible upon cessation of Accutane therapy. Some patients have been able to reverse triglyceride elevation by reduction in weight, restriction of dietary fat and alcohol, and reduction in dose while continuing Accutane.[5]

Blood lipid determinations should be performed before Accutane is given and then at intervals until the lipid response to Accutane is established, which usually occurs within 4 weeks. Especially careful consideration must be given to risk/benefit for patients who may be at high risk during Accutane therapy (patients with diabetes, obesity, increased alcohol intake, lipid metabolism disorder or familial history of lipid metabolism disorder). If Accutane therapy is instituted, more frequent checks of serum values for lipids and/or blood sugar are recommended (see PRECAUTIONS: Laboratory Tests).

The cardiovascular consequences of hypertriglyceridemia associated with Accutane are unknown. *Animal Studies:* In rats given 8 or 32 mg/kg/day of isotretinoin (1.3 to 5.3 times the recommended clinical dose of 1.0 mg/kg/day after normalization for total body surface area) for 18 months or longer, the incidences of focal calcification, fibrosis and inflammation of the myocardium, calcification of coronary, pulmonary and mesenteric arteries, and metastatic calcification of the gastric mucosa were greater than in control rats of similar age. Focal endocardial and myocardial calcifications associated with calcification of the coronary arteries were observed in two dogs after approximately 6 to 7 months of treatment with isotretinoin at a dosage of 60 to 120 mg/kg/day (30 to 60 times the recommended clinical dose of 1.0 mg/kg/day, respectively, after normalization for total body surface area).

Hearing Impairment

Impaired hearing has been reported in patients taking Accutane; in some cases, the hearing impairment has been reported to persist after therapy has been discontinued. Mechanism(s) and causality for this event have not been established. Patients who experience tinnitus or hearing impairment should discontinue Accutane treatment and be referred for specialized care for further evaluation (see ADVERSE REACTIONS: Special Senses).

Table 3. Pharmacokinetic Parameters of Isotretinoin Following Single and Multiple Dose Administration in Pediatric Patients, 12 to 15 Years of Age Mean (± SD), N=38*

Parameter	Isotretinoin (Single Dose)	Isotretinoin (Steady-State)
C_{max} (ng/mL)	573.25 (278.79)	731.98 (361.86)
$AUC_{(0-12)}$ (ng•hr/mL)	3033.37 (1394.17)	5082.00 (2184.23)
$AUC_{(0-24)}$ (ng•hr/mL)	6003.81 (2885.67)	–
T_{max} (hr)†	6.00 (1.00–24.60)	4.00 (0–12.00)
Css_{min} (ng/mL)	–	352.32 (184.44)
$T_{1/2}$ (hr)	–	15.69 (5.12)
CL/F (L/hr)	–	17.96 (6.27)

*The single and multiple dose data in this table were obtained following a non-standardized meal that is not comparable to the high-fat meal that was used in the study in Table 2.
†Median (range)

Hepatotoxicity

Clinical hepatitis considered to be possibly or probably related to Accutane therapy has been reported. Additionally, mild to moderate elevations of liver enzymes have been observed in approximately 15% of individuals treated during clinical trials, some of which normalized with dosage reduction or continued administration of the drug. If normalization does not readily occur or if hepatitis is suspected during treatment with Accutane, the drug should be discontinued and the etiology further investigated.

Inflammatory Bowel Disease

Accutane has been associated with inflammatory bowel disease (including regional ileitis) in patients without a prior history of intestinal disorders. In some instances, symptoms have been reported to persist after Accutane treatment has been stopped. Patients experiencing abdominal pain, rectal bleeding or severe diarrhea should discontinue Accutane immediately (see ADVERSE REACTIONS: Gastrointestinal).

Skeletal

Bone Mineral Density

Effects of multiple courses of Accutane on the developing musculoskeletal system are unknown. There is some evidence that long-term, high-dose, or multiple courses of therapy with isotretinoin have more of an effect than a single course of therapy on the musculoskeletal system. In an open-label clinical trial (N=217) of a single course of therapy with Accutane for severe recalcitrant nodular acne, bone density measurements at several skeletal sites were not significantly decreased (lumbar spine change >−4% and total hip change >−5%) or were increased in the majority of patients. One patient had a decrease in lumbar spine bone mineral density >4% based on unadjusted data. Sixteen (7.9%) patients had decreases in lumbar spine bone mineral density >4%, and all the other patients (92%) did not have significant decreases or had increases (adjusted for body mass index). Nine patients (4.5%) had a decrease in total hip bone mineral density >5% based on unadjusted data. Twenty-one (10.6%) patients had decreases in total hip bone mineral density >5%, and all the other patients (89%) did not have significant decreases or had increases (adjusted for body mass index). Follow-up studies performed in 8 of the patients with decreased bone mineral density for up to 11 months thereafter demonstrated increasing bone density in 5 patients at the lumbar spine, while the other 3 patients had lumbar spine bone density measurements below baseline values. Total hip bone mineral densities remained below baseline (range −1.6% to −7.6%) in 5 of 8 patients (62.5%).

In a separate open-label extension study of 10 patients, ages 13 to 18 years, who started a second course of Accutane 4 months after the first course, two patients showed a decrease in mean lumbar spine bone mineral density up to 3.25% (see PRECAUTIONS: Pediatric Use).

Spontaneous reports of osteoporosis, osteopenia, bone fractures, and delayed healing of bone fractures have been seen in the Accutane population. While causality to Accutane has not been established, an effect cannot be ruled out. Longer term effects have not been studied. It is important that Accutane be given at the recommended doses for no longer than the recommended duration.

Hyperostosis

A high prevalence of skeletal hyperostosis was noted in clinical trials for disorders of keratinization with a mean dose of 2.24 mg/kg/day. Additionally, skeletal hyperostosis was noted in 6 of 8 patients in a prospective study of disorders of keratinization.[6] Minimal skeletal hyperostosis and calcification of ligaments and tendons have also been observed by x-ray in prospective studies of nodular acne patients treated with a single course of therapy at recommended doses. The skeletal effects of multiple Accutane treatment courses for acne are unknown.

In a clinical study of 217 pediatric patients (12 to 17 years) with severe recalcitrant nodular acne, hyperostosis was not observed after 16 to 20 weeks of treatment with approximately 1 mg/kg/day of Accutane given in two divided doses. Hyperostosis may require a longer time frame to appear. The clinical course and significance remain unknown.

Premature Epiphyseal Closure

There are spontaneous reports of premature epiphyseal closure in acne patients receiving recommended doses of Accutane. The effect of multiple courses of Accutane on epiphyseal closure is unknown.

Vision Impairment

Visual problems should be carefully monitored. All Accutane patients experiencing visual difficulties should discontinue Accutane treatment and have an ophthalmological examination (see ADVERSE REACTIONS: Special Senses).

Corneal Opacities

Corneal opacities have occurred in patients receiving Accutane for acne and more frequently when higher drug dosages were used in patients with disorders of keratinization. The corneal opacities that have been observed in clinical trial patients treated with Accutane have either completely resolved or were resolving at follow-up 6 to 7 weeks after discontinuation of the drug (see ADVERSE REACTIONS: Special Senses).

Decreased Night Vision

Decreased night vision has been reported during Accutane therapy and in some instances the event has persisted after therapy was discontinued. Because the onset in some patients was sudden, patients should be advised of this potential problem and warned to be cautious when driving or operating any vehicle at night.

PRECAUTIONS

The Accutane Pregnancy Prevention and Risk Management Programs consist of the *System to Manage Accutane Related Teratogenicity* (S.M.A.R.T.) and the Accutane Pregnancy Prevention Program (PPP). S.M.A.R.T. should be followed for prescribing Accutane with the goal of preventing fetal exposure to isotretinoin. It consists of: 1) reading the booklet entitled *System to Manage Accutane Related Teratogenicity* (S.M.A.R.T.) *Guide to Best Practices,* 2) signing and returning the completed S.M.A.R.T. *Letter of Understanding* containing the Prescriber Checklist, 3) a yellow self-adhesive Accutane Qualification Sticker to be affixed to the prescription page. In addition, the patient educational material, *Be Smart, Be Safe, Be Sure,* should be used with each patient.

The following further describes each component:

1) The S.M.A.R.T. *Guide to Best Practices* includes: Accutane teratogenic potential, information on pregnancy testing, specific information about effective contraception, the limitations of contraceptive methods and behaviors associated with an increased risk of contraceptive failure and pregnancy, the methods to evaluate pregnancy risk, and the method to complete a qualified Accutane prescription.
2) The S.M.A.R.T. *Letter of Understanding* attests that Accutane prescribers understand that Accutane is a teratogen, have read the S.M.A.R.T. *Guide to Best Practices,* understand their responsibilities in preventing exposure of pregnant females to Accutane and the procedures for qualifying female patients as defined in the boxed CONTRAINDICATIONS AND WARNINGS.
   The Prescriber Checklist attests that Accutane prescribers know the risk and severity of injury/birth defects from Accutane; know how to diagnose and treat the various presentations of acne; know the risk factors for unplanned pregnancy and the effective measures for avoidance; will refer the patient for, or provide, detailed pregnancy prevention counseling to help the patient have knowledge and tools needed to fulfill their ultimate responsibility to avoid becoming pregnant; understand and properly use throughout the Accutane treatment course, the revised risk management procedures, including monthly pregnancy avoidance counseling, pregnancy testing, and use of qualified prescriptions with the yellow self-adhesive Accutane Qualification Sticker.
3) The yellow self-adhesive Accutane Qualification Sticker is used as documentation that the prescriber has qualified the female patient according to the qualification criteria (see boxed CONTRAINDICATIONS AND WARNINGS).
4) Accutane Pregnancy Prevention Program (PPP) is a systematic approach to comprehensive patient education about their responsibilities and includes education for contraception compliance and reinforcement of educational messages. The PPP includes information on the risks and benefits of Accutane which is linked to the Accutane Medication Guide dispensed by pharmacists with each prescription.
   Male and female patients are provided with separate booklets. Each booklet contains information on Accutane therapy, including precautions and warnings, an Informed Consent/Patient Agreement form, and a toll-free

line which provides Accutane information in 13 languages.

The booklet for male patients, *Be Smart, Be Safe, Be Sure, Accutane Risk Management Program for Men,* also includes information about male reproduction, a warning not to share Accutane with others or to donate blood during Accutane therapy and for 1 month following discontinuation of Accutane.

The booklet for female patients, *Be Smart, Be Safe, Be Sure, Accutane Pregnancy Prevention and Risk Management Program for Women,* also includes a referral program that offers females free contraception counseling, reimbursed by the manufacturer, by a reproductive specialist; a second Patient Information/Consent form concerning birth defects, obtaining her consent to be treated within this agreement; an enrollment form for the Accutane Survey; and a qualification checklist affirming the conditions under which female patients may receive Accutane. In addition, there is information on the types of contraceptive methods, the selection and use of appropriate, effective contraception, and the rates of possible contraceptive failure; a toll-free contraception counseling line; and patient education videos — the video "Be Prepared, Be Protected" and the video "Be Aware: The Risk of Pregnancy While on Accutane".

General

Although an effect of Accutane on bone loss is not established, physicians should use caution when prescribing Accutane to patients with a genetic predisposition for age-related osteoporosis, a history of childhood osteoporosis conditions, osteomalacia, or other disorders of bone metabolism. This would include patients diagnosed with anorexia nervosa and those who are on chronic drug therapy that causes drug-induced osteoporosis/osteomalacia and/or affects vitamin D metabolism, such as systemic corticosteroids and any anticonvulsant.

Patients may be at increased risk when participating in sports with repetitive impact where the risks of spondylolisthesis with and without pars fractures and hip growth plate injuries in early and late adolescence are known. There are spontaneous reports of fractures and/or delayed healing in patients while on treatment with Accutane or following cessation of treatment with Accutane while involved in these activities. While causality to Accutane has not been established, an effect cannot be ruled out.

Information for Patients and Prescribers

- Patients should be instructed to read the Medication Guide supplied as required by law when Accutane is dispensed. The complete text of the Medication Guide is reprinted at the end of this document. For additional information, patients should also read the *Patient Product Information, Important Information Concerning Your Treatment with Accutane® (isotretinoin).* All patients should sign the Informed Consent/Patient Agreement.
- Females of childbearing potential should be instructed that they must not be pregnant when Accutane therapy is initiated, and that they should use 2 forms of effective contraception 1 month before starting Accutane, while taking Accutane, and for 1 month after Accutane has been stopped. They should also sign a consent form prior to beginning Accutane therapy. They should be given an opportunity to enroll in the Accutane Survey and to review the patient videotapes provided by the manufacturer to the prescriber. The videos include information about contraception, the most common reasons that contraception fails, and the importance of using 2 forms of effective contraception when taking teratogenic drugs and comprehensive information about types of potential birth defects which could occur if a woman who is pregnant takes Accutane at any time during pregnancy. Female patients should be seen by their prescribers monthly and have a urine or serum pregnancy test performed each month during treatment to confirm negative pregnancy status before another Accutane prescription is written (see boxed CONTRAINDICATIONS AND WARNINGS).
- Accutane is found in the semen of male patients taking Accutane, but the amount delivered to a female partner would be about 1 million times lower than an oral dose of 40 mg. While the no-effect limit for isotretinoin-induced embryopathy is unknown, 20 years of postmarketing reports include 4 with isolated defects compatible with features of retinoid exposed fetuses. None of these cases had the combination of malformations characteristic of retinoid exposure, and all had other possible explanations for the defects observed.
- Patients may report mental health problems or family history of psychiatric disorders. These reports should be discussed with the patient and/or the patient's family. A referral to a mental health professional may be necessary. The physician should consider whether or not Accutane therapy is appropriate in this setting (see WARNINGS: Psychiatric Disorders).
- Patients should be informed that they must not share Accutane with anyone else because of the risk of birth defects and other serious adverse events.
- Patients should not donate blood during therapy and for 1 month following discontinuance of the drug because the blood might be given to a pregnant woman whose fetus must not be exposed to Accutane.
- Patients should be reminded to take Accutane with a meal (see DOSAGE AND ADMINISTRATION). To decrease the risk of esophageal irritation, patients should swallow the capsules with a full glass of liquid.
- Patients should be informed that transient exacerbation (flare) of acne has been seen, generally during the initial period of therapy.
- Wax epilation and skin resurfacing procedures (such as dermabrasion, laser) should be avoided during Accutane therapy and for at least 6 months thereafter due to the possibility of scarring (see ADVERSE REACTIONS: Skin and Appendages).
- Patients should be advised to avoid prolonged exposure to UV rays or sunlight.
- Patients should be informed that they may experience decreased tolerance to contact lenses during and after therapy.
- Patients should be informed that approximately 16% of patients treated with Accutane in a clinical trial developed musculoskeletal symptoms (including arthralgia) during treatment. In general, these symptoms were mild to moderate, but occasionally required discontinuation of the drug. Transient pain in the chest has been reported less frequently. In the clinical trial, these symptoms generally cleared rapidly after discontinuation of Accutane, but in some cases persisted (see ADVERSE REACTIONS: Musculoskeletal). There have been rare postmarketing reports of rhabdomyolysis, some associated with strenuous physical activity (see Laboratory Tests: CPK).
- Pediatric patients and their caregivers should be informed that approximately 29% (104/358) of pediatric patients treated with Accutane developed back pain. Back pain was severe in 13.5% (14/104) of the cases and occurred at a higher frequency in female than male patients. Arthralgias were experienced in 22% (79/358) of pediatric patients. Arthralgias were severe in 7.6% (6/79) of patients. Appropriate evaluation of the musculoskeletal system should be done in patients who present with these symptoms during or after a course of Accutane. Consideration should be given to discontinuation of Accutane if any significant abnormality is found.
- Neutropenia and rare cases of agranulocytosis have been reported. Accutane should be discontinued if clinically significant decreases in white cell counts occur.

Hypersensitivity

Anaphylactic reactions and other allergic reactions have been reported. Cutaneous allergic reactions and serious cases of allergic vasculitis, often with purpura (bruises and red patches) of the extremities and extracutaneous involvement (including renal) have been reported. Severe allergic reaction necessitates discontinuation of therapy and appropriate medical management.

Drug Interactions

- *Vitamin A:* Because of the relationship of Accutane to vitamin A, patients should be advised against taking vitamin supplements containing vitamin A to avoid additive toxic effects.
- *Tetracyclines:* Concomitant treatment with Accutane and tetracyclines should be avoided because Accutane use has been associated with a number of cases of pseudotumor cerebri (benign intracranial hypertension), some of which involved concomitant use of tetracyclines.
- *Micro-dosed Progesterone Preparations:* Micro-dosed progesterone preparations ("minipills" that do not contain an estrogen) may be an inadequate method of contraception during Accutane therapy. Although other hormonal contraceptives are highly effective, there have been reports of pregnancy from women who have used combined oral contraceptives, as well as topical/injectable/implantable/insertable hormonal birth control products. These reports are more frequent for women who use only a single method of contraception. It is not known if hormonal contraceptives differ in their effectiveness when used with Accutane. Therefore, it is critically important for women of childbearing potential to select and commit to use 2 forms of effective contraception simultaneously, at least 1 of which must be a primary form, unless absolute abstinence is the chosen method, or the patient has undergone a hysterectomy (see boxed CONTRAINDICATIONS AND WARNINGS).
- *Phenytoin:* Accutane has not been shown to alter the pharmacokinetics of phenytoin in a study in seven healthy volunteers. These results are consistent with the in vitro finding that neither isotretinoin nor its metabolites induce or inhibit the activity of the CYP 2C9 human hepatic P450 enzyme. Phenytoin is known to cause osteomalacia. No formal clinical studies have been conducted to assess if there is an interactive effect on bone loss between phenytoin and Accutane. Therefore, caution should be exercised when using these drugs together.
- *Systemic Corticosteroids:* Systemic corticosteroids are known to cause osteoporosis. No formal clinical studies have been conducted to assess if there is an interactive effect on bone loss between systemic corticosteroids and Accutane. Therefore, caution should be exercised when using these drugs together.

Prescribers are advised to consult the package insert of medication administered concomitantly with hormonal contraceptives, since some medications may decrease the effectiveness of these birth control products. **Accutane use is associated with depression in some patients (see WARNINGS: Psychiatric Disorders and ADVERSE REACTIONS: Psychiatric).** Patients should be prospectively cautioned not to self-medicate with the herbal supplement St. John's Wort because a possible interaction has been suggested with hormonal contraceptives based on reports of breakthrough bleeding on oral contraceptives shortly after starting St. John's Wort. Pregnancies have been reported by users of combined hormonal contraceptives who also used some form of St. John's Wort.

Laboratory Tests

Pregnancy Test

Female patients of childbearing potential must have negative results from 2 urine or serum pregnancy tests with a sensitivity of at least 25 mIU/mL before receiving the initial Accutane prescription. The first test is obtained by the prescriber when the decision is made to pursue qualification of the patient for Accutane (a screening test). The second pregnancy test (a confirmation test) should be done during the first 5 days of the menstrual period immediately preceding the beginning of Accutane therapy. For patients with amenorrhea, the second test should be done at least 11 days after the last act of unprotected sexual intercourse (without using 2 effective forms of contraception).

Each month of therapy, the patient must have a negative result from a urine or serum pregnancy test. A pregnancy test must be repeated each month prior to the female patient receiving each prescription.

- *Lipids:* Pretreatment and follow-up blood lipids should be obtained under fasting conditions. After consumption of alcohol, at least 36 hours should elapse before these determinations are made. It is recommended that these tests be performed at weekly or biweekly intervals until the lipid response to Accutane is established. The incidence of hypertriglyceridemia is 1 patient in 4 on Accutane therapy (see WARNINGS: Lipids).
- *Liver Function Tests:* Since elevations of liver enzymes have been observed during clinical trials, and hepatitis has been reported, pretreatment and follow-up liver function tests should be performed at weekly or biweekly intervals until the response to Accutane has been established (see WARNINGS: Hepatotoxicity).
- *Glucose:* Some patients receiving Accutane have experienced problems in the control of their blood sugar. In addition, new cases of diabetes have been diagnosed during Accutane therapy, although no causal relationship has been established.
- *CPK:* Some patients undergoing vigorous physical activity while on Accutane therapy have experienced elevated CPK levels; however, the clinical significance is unknown. There have been rare postmarketing reports of rhabdomyolysis, some associated with strenuous physical activity. In a clinical trial of 217 pediatric patients (12 to 17 years) with severe recalcitrant nodular acne, transient elevations in CPK were observed in 12% of patients, including those undergoing strenuous physical activity in association with reported musculoskeletal adverse events such as back pain, arthralgia, limb injury, or muscle sprain. In these patients, approximately half of the CPK elevations returned to normal within 2 weeks and half returned to normal within 4 weeks. No cases of rhabdomyolysis were reported in this trial.

Carcinogenesis, Mutagenesis and Impairment of Fertility

In male and female Fischer 344 rats given oral isotretinoin at dosages of 8 or 32 mg/kg/day (1.3 to 5.3 times the recommended clinical dose of 1.0 mg/kg/day, respectively, after normalization for total body surface area) for greater than 18 months, there was a dose-related increased incidence of pheochromocytoma relative to controls. The incidence of adrenal medullary hyperplasia was also increased at the higher dosage in both sexes. The relatively high level of spontaneous pheochromocytomas occurring in the male Fischer 344 rat makes it an equivocal model for study of this tumor; therefore, the relevance of this tumor to the human population is uncertain.

The Ames test was conducted with isotretinoin in two laboratories. The results of the tests in one laboratory were negative while in the second laboratory a weakly positive response (less than 1.6 × background) was noted in *S. typhimurium* TA100 when the assay was conducted with metabolic activation. No dose-response effect was seen and all other strains were negative. Additionally, other tests designed to assess genotoxicity (Chinese hamster cell assay, mouse micronucleus test, *S. cerevisiae* D7 assay, in vitro clastogenesis assay with human-derived lymphocytes, and unscheduled DNA synthesis assay) were all negative.

In rats, no adverse effects on gonadal function, fertility, conception rate, gestation or parturition were observed at oral dosages of isotretinoin of 2, 8, or 32 mg/kg/day (0.3, 1.3, or 5.3 times the recommended clinical dose of 1.0 mg/kg/day, respectively, after normalization for total body surface area).

In dogs, testicular atrophy was noted after treatment with oral isotretinoin for approximately 30 weeks at dosages of 20 or 60 mg/kg/day (10 or 30 times the recommended clinical dose of 1.0 mg/kg/day, respectively, after normalization for total body surface area). In general, there was microscopic evidence for appreciable depression of spermatogenesis but some sperm were observed in all testes examined and in no instance were completely atrophic tubules seen. In studies of 66 men, 30 of whom were patients with nodular acne under treatment with oral isotretinoin, no significant changes were noted in the count or motility of spermatozoa in the ejaculate. In a study of 50 men (ages 17 to 32 years) receiving Accutane (isotretinoin) therapy for nodular acne, no significant effects were seen on ejaculate volume, sperm count, total sperm motility, morphology or seminal plasma fructose.

Continued on next page

Accutane—Cont.

Pregnancy: Category X. See boxed CONTRAINDICATIONS AND WARNINGS.

Nursing Mothers

It is not known whether this drug is excreted in human milk. Because of the potential for adverse effects, nursing mothers should not receive Accutane.

Pediatric Use

The use of Accutane in pediatric patients less than 12 years of age has not been studied. The use of Accutane for the treatment of severe recalcitrant nodular acne in pediatric patients ages 12 to 17 years should be given careful consideration, especially for those patients where a known metabolic or structural bone disease exists (see PRECAUTIONS: General). Use of Accutane in this age group for severe recalcitrant nodular acne is supported by evidence from a clinical study comparing 103 pediatric patients (13 to 17 years) to 197 adult patients (≥18 years). Results from this study demonstrated that Accutane, at a dose of 1 mg/kg/day given in two divided doses, was equally effective in treating severe recalcitrant nodular acne in both pediatric and adult patients.

In studies with Accutane, adverse reactions reported in pediatric patients were similar to those described in adults except for the increased incidence of back pain and arthralgia (both of which were sometimes severe) and myalgia in pediatric patients (see ADVERSE REACTIONS).

In an open-label clinical trial (N=217) of a single course of therapy with Accutane for severe recalcitrant nodular acne, bone density measurements at several skeletal sites were not significantly decreased (lumbar spine change >−4% and total hip change >−5%) or were increased in the majority of patients. One patient had a decrease in lumbar spine bone mineral density >4% based on unadjusted data. Sixteen (7.9%) patients had decreases in lumbar spine bone mineral density >4%, and all the other patients (92%) did not have significant decreases or had increases (adjusted for body mass index). Nine patients (4.5%) had a decrease in total hip bone mineral density >5% based on unadjusted data. Twenty-one (10.6%) patients had decreases in total hip bone mineral density >5%, and all the other patients (89%) did not have significant decreases or had increases (adjusted for body mass index). Follow-up studies performed in 8 of the patients with decreased bone mineral density for up to 11 months thereafter demonstrated increasing bone density in 5 patients at the lumbar spine, while the other 3 patients had lumbar spine bone density measurements below baseline values. Total hip bone mineral densities remained below baseline (range −1.6% to −7.6%) in 5 of 8 patients (62.5%).

In a separate open-label extension study of 10 patients, ages 13 to 18 years, who started a second course of Accutane 4 months after the first course, two patients showed a decrease in mean lumbar spine bone mineral density up to 3.25% (see WARNINGS: Skeletal: Bone Mineral Density).

Geriatric Use

Clinical studies of isotretinoin did not include sufficient numbers of subjects aged 65 years and over to determine whether they respond differently from younger subjects. Although reported clinical experience has not identified differences in responses between elderly and younger patients, effects of aging might be expected to increase some risks associated with isotretinoin therapy (see WARNINGS and PRECAUTIONS).

ADVERSE REACTIONS

Clinical Trials and Postmarketing Surveillance

The adverse reactions listed below reflect the experience from investigational studies of Accutane, and the postmarketing experience. The relationship of some of these events to Accutane therapy is unknown. Many of the side effects and adverse reactions seen in patients receiving Accutane are similar to those described in patients taking very high doses of vitamin A (dryness of the skin and mucous membranes, eg, of the lips, nasal passage, and eyes).

Dose Relationship

Cheilitis and hypertriglyceridemia are usually dose related. Most adverse reactions reported in clinical trials were reversible when therapy was discontinued; however, some persisted after cessation of therapy (see WARNINGS and ADVERSE REACTIONS).

Body as a Whole

allergic reactions, including vasculitis, systemic hypersensitivity (see PRECAUTIONS: Hypersensitivity), edema, fatigue, lymphadenopathy, weight loss

Cardiovascular

palpitation, tachycardia, vascular thrombotic disease, stroke

Endocrine/Metabolic

hypertriglyceridemia (see WARNINGS: Lipids), alterations in blood sugar levels (see PRECAUTIONS: Laboratory Tests)

Gastrointestinal

inflammatory bowel disease (see WARNINGS: Inflammatory Bowel Disease), hepatitis (see WARNINGS: Hepatotoxicity), pancreatitis (see WARNINGS: Lipids), bleeding and inflammation of the gums, colitis, esophagitis/esophageal ulceration, ileitis, nausea, other nonspecific gastrointestinal symptoms

Hematologic

allergic reactions (see PRECAUTIONS: Hypersensitivity), anemia, thrombocytopenia, neutropenia, rare reports of agranulocytosis (see PRECAUTIONS: Information for Patients and Prescribers). See PRECAUTIONS: Laboratory Tests for other hematological parameters.

Musculoskeletal

skeletal hyperostosis, calcification of tendons and ligaments, premature epiphyseal closure, decreases in bone mineral density (see WARNINGS: Skeletal), musculoskeletal symptoms (sometimes severe) including back pain and arthralgia (see PRECAUTIONS: Information for Patients and Prescribers), transient pain in the chest (see PRECAUTIONS: Information for Patients and Prescribers), arthritis, tendonitis, other types of bone abnormalities, elevations of CPK/rare reports of rhabdomyolysis (see PRECAUTIONS: Laboratory Tests)

Neurological

pseudotumor cerebri (see WARNINGS: Pseudotumor Cerebri), dizziness, drowsiness, headache, insomnia, lethargy, malaise, nervousness, paresthesias, seizures, stroke, syncope, weakness

Psychiatric

suicidal ideation, suicide attempts, suicide, depression, psychosis, aggression, violent behaviors (see WARNINGS: Psychiatric Disorders), emotional instability

Of the patients reporting depression, some reported that the depression subsided with discontinuation of therapy and recurred with reinstitution of therapy.

Reproductive System

abnormal menses

Respiratory

bronchospasms (with or without a history of asthma), respiratory infection, voice alteration

Skin and Appendages

acne fulminans, alopecia (which in some cases persists), bruising, cheilitis (dry lips), dry mouth, dry nose, dry skin, epistaxis, eruptive xanthomas,[7] flushing, fragility of skin, hair abnormalities, hirsutism, hyperpigmentation and hypopigmentation, infections (including disseminated herpes simplex), nail dystrophy, paronychia, peeling of palms and soles, photoallergic/photosensitizing reactions, pruritus, pyogenic granuloma, rash (including facial erythema, seborrhea, and eczema), sunburn susceptibility increased, sweating, urticaria, vasculitis (including Wegener's granulomatosis; see PRECAUTIONS: Hypersensitivity), abnormal wound healing (delayed healing or exuberant granulation tissue with crusting; see PRECAUTIONS: Information for Patients and Prescribers)

Special Senses

Hearing

hearing impairment (see WARNINGS: Hearing Impairment), tinnitus.

Vision

corneal opacities (see WARNINGS: Corneal Opacities), decreased night vision which may persist (see WARNINGS: Decreased Night Vision), cataracts, color vision disorder, conjunctivitis, dry eyes, eyelid inflammation, keratitis, optic neuritis, photophobia, visual disturbances

Urinary System

glomerulonephritis (see PRECAUTIONS: Hypersensitivity), nonspecific urogenital findings (see PRECAUTIONS: Laboratory Tests for other urological parameters)

Laboratory

Elevation of plasma triglycerides (see WARNINGS: Lipids), decrease in serum high-density lipoprotein (HDL) levels, elevations of serum cholesterol during treatment

Increased alkaline phosphatase, SGOT (AST), SGPT (ALT), GGTP or LDH (see WARNINGS: Hepatotoxicity)

Elevation of fasting blood sugar, elevations of CPK (see PRECAUTIONS: Laboratory Tests), hyperuricemia

Decreases in red blood cell parameters, decreases in white blood cell counts (including severe neutropenia and rare reports of agranulocytosis; see PRECAUTIONS: Information for Patients and Prescribers), elevated sedimentation rates, elevated platelet counts, thrombocytopenia

White cells in the urine, proteinuria, microscopic or gross hematuria

Table 4. Accutane Dosing by Body Weight (Based on Administration With Food)

Body Weight		Total mg/day		
kilograms	pounds	0.5 mg/kg	1 mg/kg	2 mg/kg*
40	88	20	40	80
50	110	25	50	100
60	132	30	60	120
70	154	35	70	140
80	176	40	80	160
90	198	45	90	180
100	220	50	100	200

* See DOSAGE AND ADMINISTRATION: the recommended dosage range is 0.5 to 1.0 mg/kg/day.

OVERDOSAGE

The oral LD_{50} of isotretinoin is greater than 4000 mg/kg in rats and mice (>600 times the recommended clinical dose of 1.0 mg/kg/day after normalization of the rat dose for total body surface area and >300 times the recommended clinical dose of 1.0 mg/kg/day after normalization of the mouse dose for total body surface area) and is approximately 1960 mg/kg in rabbits (653 times the recommended clinical dose of 1.0 mg/kg/day after normalization for total body surface area). In humans, overdosage has been associated with vomiting, facial flushing, cheilosis, abdominal pain, headache, dizziness, and ataxia. All symptoms quickly resolved without apparent residual effects.

Accutane causes serious birth defects at any dosage (see boxed CONTRAINDICATIONS AND WARNINGS). Females of childbearing potential who present with isotretinoin overdose must be evaluated for pregnancy. Patients who are pregnant should receive counseling about the risks to the fetus, as described in the boxed CONTRAINDICATIONS AND WARNINGS. Non-pregnant patients must be warned to avoid pregnancy for at least one month and receive contraceptive counseling as described in the boxed CONTRAINDICATIONS AND WARNINGS. Educational materials for such patients can be obtained by calling the manufacturer. Because an overdose would be expected to result in higher levels of isotretinoin in semen than found during a normal treatment course, male patients should use a condom, or avoid reproductive sexual activity with a female who is or might become pregnant, for 30 days after the overdose. All patients with isotretinoin overdose should not donate blood for at least 30 days.

DOSAGE AND ADMINISTRATION

Accutane should be administered with a meal (see PRECAUTIONS: Information for Patients and Prescribers).

The recommended dosage range for Accutane is 0.5 to 1.0 mg/kg/day given in two divided doses with food for 15 to 20 weeks. In studies comparing 0.1, 0.5, and 1.0 mg/kg/day,[8] it was found that all dosages provided initial clearing of disease, but there was a greater need for retreatment with the lower dosages. During treatment, the dose may be adjusted according to response of the disease and/or the appearance of clinical side effects — some of which may be dose related. Adult patients whose disease is very severe with scarring or is primarily manifested on the trunk may require dose adjustments up to 2.0 mg/kg/day, as tolerated. Failure to take Accutane with food will significantly decrease absorption. Before upward dose adjustments are made, the patients should be questioned about their compliance with food instructions.

The safety of once daily dosing with Accutane has not been established. Once daily dosing is **not** recommended.

If the total nodule count has been reduced by more than 70% prior to completing 15 to 20 weeks of treatment, the drug may be discontinued. After a period of 2 months or more off therapy, and if warranted by persistent or recurring severe nodular acne, a second course of therapy may be initiated. The optimal interval before retreatment has not been defined for patients who have not completed skeletal growth. Long-term use of Accutane, even in low doses, has not been studied, and is not recommended. It is important that Accutane be given at the recommended doses for no longer than the recommended duration. The effect of long-term use of Accutane on bone loss is unknown (see WARNINGS: Skeletal: Bone Mineral Density, Hyperostosis, and Premature Epiphyseal Closure).

Contraceptive measures must be followed for any subsequent course of therapy (see boxed CONTRAINDICATIONS AND WARNINGS).

[See table 4 below]

Information for Pharmacists

Accutane must only be dispensed in no more than a 30-day supply and only on presentation of an Accutane prescription with a yellow self-adhesive Accutane Qualification Sticker within 7 days of the qualification date. **REFILLS REQUIRE A NEW WRITTEN PRESCRIPTION WITH A YELLOW SELF-ADHESIVE ACCUTANE QUALIFICATION STICKER WITHIN 7 DAYS OF THE QUALIFICATION DATE.** No telephone or computerized prescriptions are permitted.

An Accutane Medication Guide must be given to the patient each time Accutane is dispensed, as required by law. This Accutane Medication Guide is an important part of the risk management program for the patient.

HOW SUPPLIED

Soft gelatin capsules, 10 mg (light pink), imprinted ACCUTANE 10 ROCHE. Boxes of 100 containing 10 Prescription Paks of 10 capsules (NDC 0004-0155-49).

Soft gelatin capsules, 20 mg (maroon), imprinted ACCUTANE 20 ROCHE. Boxes of 100 containing 10 Prescription Paks of 10 capsules (NDC 0004-0169-49).

Soft gelatin capsules, 40 mg (yellow), imprinted ACCUTANE 40 ROCHE. Boxes of 100 containing 10 Prescription Paks of 10 capsules (NDC 0004-0156-49).

Storage

Store at controlled room temperature (59° to 86°F, 15° to 30°C). Protect from light.

REFERENCES

1. Peck GL, Olsen TG, Yoder FW, et al. Prolonged remissions of cystic and conglobate acne with 13-*cis*-retinoic acid. *N*

Engl J Med 300:329–333, 1979. 2. Pochi PE, Shalita AR, Strauss JS, Webster SB. Report of the consensus conference on acne classification. *J Am Acad Dermatol* 24:495–500, 1991. 3. Farrell LN, Strauss JS, Stranieri AM. The treatment of severe cystic acne with 13-*cis*-retinoic acid: evaluation of sebum production and the clinical response in a multiple-dose trial. *J Am Acad Dermatol* 3:602–611, 1980. 4. Jones H, Blanc D, Cunliffe WJ. 13-*cis*-retinoic acid and acne. *Lancet* 2:1048–1049, 1980. 5. Katz RA, Jorgensen H, Nigra TP. Elevation of serum triglyceride levels from oral isotretinoin in disorders of keratinization. *Arch Dermatol* 116:1369–1372, 1980. 6. Ellis CN, Madison KC, Pennes DR, Martel W, Voorhees JJ. Isotretinoin therapy is associated with early skeletal radiographic changes. *J Am Acad Dermatol* 10:1024–1029, 1984. 7. Dicken CH, Connolly SM. Eruptive xanthomas associated with isotretinoin (13-*cis*-retinoic acid). *Arch Dermatol* 116:951–952, 1980. 8. Strauss JS, Rapini RP, Shalita AR, et al. Isotretinoin therapy for acne: results of a multicenter dose-response study. *J Am Acad Dermatol* 10:490–496, 1984.

PATIENT INFORMATION/CONSENT (for female patients concerning birth defects)

To be completed by the patient, her parent/guardian* and signed by her prescriber.

Read each item below and initial in the space provided to show that you understand each item and agree to follow your prescriber's instructions. **Do not sign this consent and do not take Accutane if there is anything that you do not understand.**

*A parent or guardian of a minor patient (under age 18) must also read and initial each item before signing the consent.

____
(Patient's Name)

1. I understand that there is a very high risk that my unborn baby could have severe birth defects if I am pregnant or become pregnant while taking Accutane in any amount even for short periods of time. This is why I must not be pregnant while taking Accutane.
Initial: _____
2. I understand that I must not take Accutane (isotretinoin) if I am pregnant.
Initial: _____
3. I understand that I must not get pregnant during the entire time of my treatment and for 1 month after the end of my treatment with Accutane.
Initial: _____
4. I understand that I must avoid sexual intercourse completely, or I must use 2 separate, effective forms of birth control (contraception) **at the same time**. The only exception is if I have had surgery to remove the womb (a hysterectomy).
Initial: _____
5. I understand that birth control pills and topical/injectable/implantable/insertable hormonal birth control products are among the most effective forms of birth control. However, any form of birth control can fail. Therefore, I must use 2 different methods at the same time, every time I have sexual intercourse, even if 1 of the methods I choose is birth control pills or topical/injectable/implantable/insertable hormonal birth control.
Initial: _____
6. I will talk with my prescriber about any drugs or herbal products I plan to take during my Accutane treatment because hormonal birth control methods (for example, birth control pills) may not work if I am taking certain drugs or herbal products (for example, St. John's Wort).
Initial: _____
7. I understand that the following are considered effective forms of birth control:
Primary: Tubal ligation (tying my tubes), partner's vasectomy, birth control pills, topical/injectable/implantable/insertable hormonal birth control products, and an IUD (intrauterine device).
Secondary: Diaphragms, latex condoms, and cervical caps. Each must be used with a spermicide, which is a special cream or jelly that kills sperm.
I understand that at least 1 of my 2 methods of birth control must be a primary method.
Initial: _____
8. I understand that I may receive a free contraceptive (birth control) counseling session from a doctor or other family planning expert. My Accutane prescriber can give me an Accutane Patient Referral Form for this free consultation.
Initial: _____
9. I understand that I must begin using the birth control methods I have chosen as described above at least 1 month before I start taking Accutane.
Initial: _____
10. I understand that I cannot get a prescription for Accutane unless I have 2 negative pregnancy test results. The first pregnancy test should be done when my prescriber decides to prescribe Accutane. The second pregnancy test should be done during the first 5 days of my menstrual period right before starting Accutane therapy, or as instructed by my prescriber. I will then have 1 pregnancy test every month during my Accutane therapy.
Initial: _____
11. I understand that I should not start taking Accutane until I am sure that I am not pregnant and have negative results from 2 pregnancy tests.
Initial: _____
12. I have read and understand the materials my prescriber has given to me, including the *Patient Product Information, Important Information Concerning Your Treatment with Accutane® (isotretinoin)*. My prescriber gave me and asked me to watch the videos about contraception. I was told about a confidential counseling line that I may call for more information about birth control. I have received information on emergency contraception (birth control).
Initial: _____
13. I understand that I must stop taking Accutane right away and inform my prescriber if I get pregnant, miss my menstrual period, stop using birth control, or have sexual intercourse without using my 2 birth control methods at any time.
Initial: _____
14. My prescriber gave me information about the confidential Accutane Survey and explained to me how important it is to take part in the Accutane Survey.
Initial: _____
15. I understand that the yellow self-adhesive Accutane Qualification Sticker on my prescription for Accutane means that I am qualified to receive an Accutane prescription, because I:
   - have had 2 negative urine or serum pregnancy tests before receiving the initial Accutane prescription. I must have a negative result from a urine or serum pregnancy test repeated each month prior to my receiving each subsequent prescription.
   - have selected and committed to use 2 forms of effective contraception simultaneously, at least 1 of which must be a primary form, unless absolute abstinence is the chosen method, or I have undergone a hysterectomy. I must use 2 forms of contraception for at least 1 month prior to initiation of Accutane therapy, during therapy, and for 1 month after discontinuing therapy. I must receive counseling, repeated on a monthly basis, about contraception and behaviors associated with an increased risk of pregnancy.
   - have signed a Patient Information/Consent form that contains warnings about the risk of potential birth defects if I am pregnant or become pregnant and my unborn baby is exposed to isotretinoin.
   - have been informed of the purpose and importance of participating in the Accutane Survey and given the opportunity to enroll.

   Initial: _____

My prescriber has answered all my questions about Accutane and I understand that <u>it is my responsibility not to get pregnant during Accutane treatment or for 1 month after I stop taking Accutane</u>.
Initial: _____

I now authorize my prescriber ____________ to begin my treatment with Accutane.
Patient Signature:__________________Date:________
Parent/Guardian Signature (if under age 18): __________________Date: ________
Please print: Patient Name and Address________________
____________________Telephone ______________
I have fully explained to the patient, ______________, the nature and purpose of the treatment described above and the risks to females of childbearing potential. I have asked the patient if she has any questions regarding her treatment with Accutane and have answered those questions to the best of my ability.
Prescriber Signature: __________Date:__________

INFORMED CONSENT/PATIENT AGREEMENT (for all patients):

To be completed by patient (parent or guardian if patient is under age 18) and signed by the prescriber.

Read each item below and initial in the space provided if you understand each item and agree to follow your prescriber's instructions. A parent or guardian of a patient under age 18 must also read and understand each item before signing the agreement.

Do not sign this agreement and do not take Accutane if there is anything that you do not understand about all the information you have received about using Accutane.

1. I, ____,
(Patient's Name)
understand that Accutane is a medicine used to treat severe nodular acne that cannot be cleared up by any other acne treatments, including antibiotics. In severe nodular acne, many red, swollen, tender lumps form in the skin. If untreated, severe nodular acne can lead to permanent scars.
Initials: _____
2. My prescriber has told me about my choices for treating my acne.
Initials: _____
3. I understand that there are serious side effects that may happen while I am taking Accutane. These have been explained to me. These side effects include serious birth defects in babies of pregnant females. (Note: There is a second Informed Consent form for female patients concerning birth defects.)
Initials: _____
4. I understand that some patients, while taking Accutane or soon after stopping Accutane, have become depressed or developed other serious mental problems. Symptoms of these problems include sad, "anxious" or empty mood, irritability, anger, loss of pleasure or interest in social or sports activities, sleeping too much or too little, changes in weight or appetite, school or work performance going down, or trouble concentrating. Some patients taking Accutane have had thoughts about hurting themselves or putting an end to their own lives (suicidal thoughts). Some people tried to end their own lives. And some people have ended their own lives. There were reports that some of these people did not appear depressed. There have been reports of patients on Accutane becoming aggressive or violent. No one knows if Accutane caused these behaviors or if they would have happened even if the person did not take Accutane. Some people have had other signs of depression while taking Accutane (see #7 below).
Initials: _____
5. Before I start taking Accutane, I agree to tell my prescriber if, to the best of my knowledge, I have **ever** had symptoms of depression (see #7 below), been psychotic, attempted suicide, had any other mental problems, or take medicine for any of these problems. Being psychotic means having a loss of contact with reality, such as hearing voices or seeing things that are not there.
Initials: _____
6. Before I start taking Accutane, I agree to tell my prescriber if, to the best of my knowledge, anyone in my family has ever had symptoms of depression, been psychotic, attempted suicide, or had any other serious mental problems.
Initials: _____
7. Once I start taking Accutane, I agree to stop using Accutane and tell my prescriber right away if any of the following happen. I:
   - Start to feel sad or have crying spells
   - Lose interest in activities I once enjoyed
   - Sleep too much or have trouble sleeping
   - Become more irritable, angry, or aggressive than usual (for example, temper outbursts, thoughts of violence)
   - Have a change in my appetite or body weight
   - Have trouble concentrating
   - Withdraw from my friends or family
   - Feel like I have no energy
   - Have feelings of worthlessness or inappropriate guilt
   - Start having thoughts about hurting myself or taking my own life (suicidal thoughts)

   Initials: _____
8. **I agree to return to see my prescriber every month I take Accutane to get a new prescription for Accutane, to check my progress, and to check for signs of side effects.**
Initials: _____
9. Accutane will be prescribed just for me—I will not share Accutane with other people because it may cause serious side effects, including birth defects.
Initials: _____
10. I will not give blood while taking Accutane or for 1 month after I stop taking Accutane. I understand that if someone who is pregnant gets my donated blood, her baby may be exposed to Accutane and may be born with serious birth defects.
Initials: _____
11. I have read the *Patient Product Information, Important Information Concerning Your Treatment with Accutane® (isotretinoin)*, and other materials my provider gave me containing important safety information about Accutane. I understand all the information I received.
Initials: _____
12. My prescriber and I have decided I should take Accutane. I understand that each of my Accutane prescriptions must have a yellow self-adhesive Accutane Qualification Sticker on it. I understand that I can stop taking Accutane at any time. I agree to tell my prescriber if I stop taking Accutane.
Initials: _____

I now authorize my prescriber ________________________
to begin my treatment with Accutane.
Patient Signature: _______________Date:________
Parent/Guardian Signature (if under age 18): __________________Date: ________
Patient Name (print) _____________________________
Patient Address ________________________________
Telephone (___-___-___)
____

I have:
- fully explained to the patient, ______________, the nature and purpose of Accutane treatment, including its benefits and risks
- given the patient the appropriate educational materials, *Be Smart, Be Safe, Be Sure*, for Accutane and asked the patient if he/she has any questions regarding his/her treatment with Accutane
- answered those questions to the best of my ability
- placed the yellow self-adhesive Accutane Qualification Sticker on the prescription.

Prescriber Signature: ____________Date:_________

MEDICATION GUIDE

Read this Medication Guide every time you get a prescription or a refill for Accutane (ACK-u-tane). There may be new

Continued on next page

Accutane—Cont.

information. This information does not take the place of talking with your prescriber doctor or other health care provider).

What is the most important information I should know about Accutane?

Accutane is used to treat a type of severe acne (nodular acne) that has not been helped by other treatments, including antibiotics. However, Accutane can cause serious side effects. Before starting Accutane, discuss with your prescriber how bad your acne is, the possible benefits of Accutane, and its possible side effects, to decide if Accutane is right for you. Your prescriber will ask you to read and sign a form or forms indicating you understand some of the serious risks of Accutane.

Possible serious side effects of taking Accutane include *birth defects* and *mental disorders*.

1. **Birth defects. Accutane can cause birth defects (deformed babies) if taken by a pregnant woman.** It can also cause miscarriage (losing the baby before birth), premature (early) birth, or death of the baby. Do not take Accutane if you are pregnant or plan to become pregnant while you are taking Accutane. Do not get pregnant for 1 month after you stop taking Accutane. Also, if you get pregnant while taking Accutane, stop taking it right away and call your prescriber.
   All females should read the section in this Medication Guide "What are the important warnings for females taking Accutane?"
2. **Mental problems and suicide.** Some patients, while taking Accutane or soon after stopping Accutane, have become depressed or developed other serious mental problems. Symptoms of these problems include sad, "anxious" or empty mood, irritability, anger, loss of pleasure or interest in social or sports activities, sleeping too much or too little, changes in weight or appetite, school or work performance going down, or trouble concentrating. Some patients taking Accutane have had thoughts about hurting themselves or putting an end to their own lives (suicidal thoughts). Some people tried to end their own lives. And some people have ended their own lives. There were reports that some of these people did not appear depressed. There have been reports of patients on Accutane becoming aggressive or violent. No one knows if Accutane caused these behaviors or if they would have happened even if the person did not take Accutane.
   All patients should read the section in this Medication Guide "What are the signs of mental problems?"
   For other possible serious side effects of Accutane, see "What are the possible side effects of Accutane?" in this Medication Guide.

What are the important warnings for females taking Accutane?

You must not become pregnant while taking Accutane, or for 1 month after you stop taking Accutane. Accutane can cause severe birth defects in babies of women who take it while they are pregnant, even if they take Accutane for only a short time. **There is an extremely high risk that your baby will be deformed or will die** if you are pregnant while taking Accutane. Taking Accutane also increases the chance of miscarriage and premature births.

Female patients will not get their first prescription for Accutane unless there is proof they have had 2 negative pregnancy tests. The first test must be done when your prescriber decides to prescribe Accutane. The second pregnancy test must be done during the first 5 days of the menstrual period right before starting Accutane therapy, or as instructed by your prescriber. Each month of treatment, you must have a negative result from a urine or serum pregnancy test. Female patients cannot get another prescription for Accutane unless there is proof that they have had a negative pregnancy test.

A yellow self-adhesive Accutane Qualification Sticker on your prescription indicates to the pharmacist that you are qualified by your prescriber to get Accutane.

While you are taking Accutane, you **must** use effective birth control. **You must use 2 separate effective forms of birth control at the same time** for at least 1 month before starting Accutane, while you take it, and for 1 month after you stop taking it. You can either discuss effective birth control methods with your prescriber or go for a free visit to discuss birth control with another physician or family planning expert. Your prescriber can arrange this free visit, which will be paid for by the manufacturer.

You must use 2 separate forms of effective birth control because any method, including birth control pills and sterilization, can fail. There are only 2 reasons you would not need to use 2 separate methods of effective birth control:

1. You have had your womb removed by surgery (a hysterectomy).
2. You are absolutely certain you will not have genital-to-genital sexual contact with a male before, during, and for 1 month after Accutane treatment.

If you have sex at any time without using 2 forms of effective birth control, get pregnant, or miss your period, stop using Accutane and call your prescriber right away.

All patients should read the rest of this Medication Guide.

What are the signs of mental problems?

Tell your prescriber if, to the best of your knowledge, you or someone in your family has ever had any mental illness, including depression, suicidal behavior, or psychosis. Psychosis means a loss of contact with reality, such as hearing voices or seeing things that are not there. Also, tell your prescriber if you take medicines for any of these problems.

Stop using Accutane and tell your provider right away if you:

- Start to feel sad or have crying spells
- Lose interest in activities you once enjoyed
- Sleep too much or have trouble sleeping
- Become more irritable, angry, or aggressive than usual (for example, temper outbursts, thoughts of violence)
- Have a change in your appetite or body weight
- Have trouble concentrating
- Withdraw from your friends or family
- Feel like you have no energy
- Have feelings of worthlessness or inappropriate guilt
- Start having thoughts about hurting yourself or taking your own life (suicidal thoughts)

What is Accutane?

Accutane is used to treat the most severe form of acne (nodular acne) that cannot be cleared up by any other acne treatments, including antibiotics. In severe nodular acne, many red, swollen, tender lumps form in the skin. These can be the size of pencil erasers or larger. If untreated, nodular acne can lead to permanent scars. However, because Accutane can have serious side effects, you should talk with your prescriber about all of the possible treatments for your acne, and whether Accutane's possible benefits outweigh its possible risks.

Who should not take Accutane?

- **Do not take Accutane if you are pregnant, plan to become pregnant, or become pregnant during Accutane treatment.** Accutane causes severe birth defects. All females should read the section "What are the important warnings for females taking Accutane?" for more information and warnings about Accutane and pregnancy.
- Do not take Accutane unless you completely understand its possible risks and are willing to follow all of the instructions in this Medication Guide.

Tell your prescriber if you or someone in your family has had any kind of mental problems, asthma, liver disease, diabetes, heart disease, osteoporosis (bone loss), weak bones, anorexia nervosa (an eating disorder where people eat too little), or any other important health problems. Tell your prescriber about any food or drug allergies you have had in the past. These problems do not necessarily mean you cannot take Accutane, but your prescriber needs this information to discuss if Accutane is right for you.

How should I take Accutane?

- You will get no more than a 30-day supply of Accutane at a time, to be sure you check in with your prescriber each month to discuss side effects.
- Your prescription should have a special yellow self-adhesive sticker attached to it. The sticker is YELLOW. If your prescription does not have this yellow self-adhesive sticker, call your prescriber. The pharmacy should not fill your prescription unless it has the yellow self-adhesive sticker.
- The amount of Accutane you take has been specially chosen for you and may change during treatment.
- You will take Accutane 2 times a day with a meal, unless your prescriber tells you otherwise. Swallow your Accutane capsules with a full glass of liquid. This will help prevent the medication inside the capsule from irritating the lining of your esophagus (connection between mouth and stomach). For the same reason, do not chew or suck on the capsule.
- If you miss a dose, just skip that dose. Do **not** take 2 doses the next time.
- You should return to your prescriber as directed to make sure you don't have signs of serious side effects. Because some of Accutane's serious side effects show up in blood tests, some of these visits may involve blood tests (monthly visits for female patients should always include a urine or serum pregnancy test).

What should I avoid while taking Accutane?

- **Do not get pregnant** while taking Accutane. See "What is the most important information I should know about Accutane?" and "What are the important warnings for females taking Accutane?"
- **Do not breast feed** while taking Accutane and for 1 month after stopping Accutane. We do not know if Accutane can pass through your milk and harm the baby.
- **Do not give blood** while you take Accutane and for 1 month after stopping Accutane. If someone who is pregnant gets your donated blood, her baby may be exposed to Accutane and may be born with birth defects.
- **Do not take vitamin A** supplements. Vitamin A in high doses has many of the same side effects as Accutane. Taking both together may increase your chance of getting side effects.
- **Do not have cosmetic procedures to smooth your skin, including waxing, dermabrasion, or laser procedures, while you are using Accutane and for at least 6 months after you stop.** Accutane can increase your chance of scarring from these procedures. Check with your prescriber for advice about when you can have cosmetic procedures.
- **Avoid sunlight and ultraviolet lights** as much as possible. Tanning machines use ultraviolet lights. Accutane may make your skin more sensitive to light.
- **Do not use birth control pills that do not contain estrogen ("minipills").** They may not work while you take Accutane. Ask your prescriber or pharmacist if you are not sure what type you are using.
- **Talk with your doctor if you plan to take other drugs or herbal products.** This is especially important for patients using birth control pills and other hormonal types of birth control because the birth control may not work as effectively if you are taking certain drugs or herbal products. You should not take the herbal supplement St. John's Wort because this herbal supplement may make birth control pills not work as effectively.
- **Talk with your doctor if you are currently taking an oral or injected corticosteroid or anticonvulsant (seizure) medication prior to using Accutane.** These drugs may weaken your bones.
- **Do not share Accutane with other people.** It can cause birth defects and other serious health problems.
- **Do not take Accutane with antibiotics unless you talk to your prescriber.** For some antibiotics, you may have to stop taking Accutane until the antibiotic treatment is finished. Use of both drugs together can increase the chances of getting increased pressure in the brain.

What are the possible side effects of Accutane?

Accutane has possible serious side effects

- **Accutane can cause birth defects, premature births, and death in babies** whose mothers took Accutane while they were pregnant. See "What is the most important information I should know about Accutane?" and "What are the important warnings for females taking Accutane?"
- **Serious mental health problems.** See "What is the most important information I should know about Accutane?"
- **Serious brain problems.** Accutane can increase the pressure in your brain. This can lead to permanent loss of sight, or in rare cases, death. Stop taking Accutane and call your prescriber right away if you get any of these signs of increased brain pressure: bad headache, blurred vision, dizziness, nausea, or vomiting. Also, some patients taking Accutane have had seizures (convulsions) or stroke.
- **Abdomen (stomach area) problems.** Certain symptoms may mean that your internal organs are being damaged. These organs include the liver, pancreas, bowel (intestines), and esophagus (connection between mouth and stomach). If your organs are damaged, they may not get better even after you stop taking Accutane. Stop taking Accutane and call your prescriber if you get severe stomach, chest or bowel pain, trouble swallowing or painful swallowing, new or worsening heartburn, diarrhea, rectal bleeding, yellowing of your skin or eyes, or dark urine.
- **Bone and muscle problems.** Accutane may affect bones, muscles, and ligaments and cause pain in your joints or muscles. Tell your prescriber if you plan vigorous physical activity during treatment with Accutane. Tell your prescriber if you develop pain, particularly back pain or joint pain. There are reports that some patients have had stunted growth after taking Accutane for acne as directed. There are also some reports of broken bones or reduced healing of broken bones after taking Accutane for acne as directed. No one knows if taking Accutane for acne will affect your bones. If you have a broken bone, tell your provider that you are taking Accutane. Muscle weakness with or without pain can be a sign of serious muscle damage. If this happens, stop taking Accutane and call your prescriber right away.
- **Hearing problems.** Some people taking Accutane have developed hearing problems. It is possible that hearing loss can be permanent. Stop using Accutane and call your prescriber if your hearing gets worse or if you have ringing in your ears.
- **Vision problems.** While taking Accutane you may develop a sudden inability to see in the dark, so driving at night can be dangerous. This condition usually clears up after you stop taking Accutane, but it may be permanent. Other serious eye effects can occur. Stop taking Accutane and call your prescriber right away if you have any problems with your vision or dryness of the eyes that is painful or constant.
- **Lipid (fats and cholesterol in blood) problems.** Many people taking Accutane develop high levels of cholesterol and other fats in their blood. This can be a serious problem. Return to your prescriber for blood tests to check your lipids and to get any needed treatment. These problems generally go away when Accutane treatment is finished.
- **Allergic reactions.** In some people, Accutane can cause serious allergic reactions. Stop taking Accutane and get emergency care right away if you develop hives, a swollen face or mouth, or have trouble breathing. Stop taking Accutane and call your prescriber if you develop a fever, rash, or red patches or bruises on your legs.
- **Signs of other possibly serious problems.** Accutane may cause other problems. Tell your prescriber if you have trouble breathing (shortness of breath), are fainting, are very thirsty or urinate a lot, feel weak, have leg swelling, convulsions, slurred speech, problems moving, or any other serious or unusual problems. Frequent urination and thirst can be signs of blood sugar problems.

Serious permanent problems do not happen often. However, because the symptoms listed above may be signs of serious problems, if you get these symptoms, stop taking Accutane and call your prescriber. If not treated, they could lead to serious health problems. Even if these problems are treated, they may not clear up after you stop taking Accutane.

Accutane has less serious possible side effects

The common less serious side effects of Accutane are dry skin, chapped lips, dry eyes, and dry nose that may lead to nosebleeds. People who wear contact lenses may have trouble wearing them while taking Accutane and after therapy.

Sometimes, people's acne may get worse for a while. They should continue taking Accutane unless told to stop by their prescriber.
These are not all of Accutane's possible side effects. Your prescriber or pharmacist can give you more detailed information that is written for health care professionals.
This Medication Guide is only a summary of some important information about Accutane. Medicines are sometimes prescribed for purposes other than those listed in a Medication Guide. If you have any concerns or questions about Accutane, ask your prescriber. Do not use Accutane for a condition for which it was not prescribed.
Active Ingredient: Isotretinoin.
Inactive Ingredients: beeswax, butylated hydroxyanisole, edetate disodium, hydrogenated soybean oil flakes, hydrogenated vegetable oil, and soybean oil. Gelatin capsules contain glycerin and parabens (methyl and propyl), with the following dye systems: 10 mg — iron oxide (red) and titanium dioxide; 20 mg — FD&C Red No. 3, FD&C Blue No. 1, and titanium dioxide; 40 mg — FD&C Yellow No. 6, D&C Yellow No. 10, and titanium dioxide.
This Medication Guide has been approved by the U.S. Food and Drug Administration.

Revised: August 2003

Shown in Product Identification Guide, page 331

CELLCEPT® ℞

[*sĕl'sĕpt*]
(mycophenolate mofetil capsules)
(mycophenolate mofetil tablets)
CELLCEPT® ORAL SUSPENSION
(mycophenolate mofetil for oral suspension)
CELLCEPT® INTRAVENOUS
(mycophenolate mofetil hydrochloride for injection)

WARNING
Increased susceptibility to infection and the possible development of lymphoma may result from immunosuppression. Only physicians experienced in immunosuppressive therapy and management of renal, cardiac or hepatic transplant patients should use CellCept. Patients receiving the drug should be managed in facilities equipped and staffed with adequate laboratory and supportive medical resources. The physician responsible for maintenance therapy should have complete information requisite for the follow-up of the patient.

DESCRIPTION

CellCept (mycophenolate mofetil) is the 2-morpholinoethyl ester of mycophenolic acid (MPA), an immunosuppressive agent; inosine monophosphate dehydrogenase (IMPDH) inhibitor.
The chemical name for mycophenolate mofetil (MMF) is 2-morpholinoethyl (E)-6-(1,3-dihydro-4-hydroxy-6-methoxy-7-methyl-3-oxo-5-isobenzofuranyl)-4-methyl-4-hexenoate. It has an empirical formula of $C_{23}H_{31}NO_7$, a molecular weight of 433.50
Mycophenolate mofetil is a white to off-white crystalline powder. It is slightly soluble in water (43 µg/mL at pH 7.4); the solubility increases in acidic medium (4.27 mg/mL at pH 3.6). It is freely soluble in acetone, soluble in methanol, and sparingly soluble in ethanol. The apparent partition coefficient in 1-octanol/water (pH 7.4) buffer solution is 238. The pKa values for mycophenolate mofetil are 5.6 for the morpholino group and 8.5 for the phenolic group.
Mycophenolate mofetil hydrochloride has a solubility of 65.8 mg/mL in 5% Dextrose Injection USP (D5W). The pH of the reconstituted solution is 2.4 to 4.1.
CellCept is available for oral administration as capsules containing 250 mg of mycophenolate mofetil, tablets containing 500 mg of mycophenolate mofetil, and as a powder for oral suspension, which when constituted contains 200 mg/mL mycophenolate mofetil.
Inactive ingredients in CellCept 250 mg capsules include croscarmellose sodium, magnesium stearate, povidone (K-90) and pregelatinized starch. The capsule shells contain black iron oxide, FD&C blue #2, gelatin, red iron oxide, silicon dioxide, sodium lauryl sulfate, titanium dioxide, and yellow iron oxide.
Inactive ingredients in CellCept 500 mg tablets include black iron oxide, croscarmellose sodium, FD&C blue #2 aluminum lake, hydroxypropyl cellulose, hydroxypropyl methylcellulose, magnesium stearate, microcrystalline cellulose, polyethylene glycol 400, povidone (K-90), red iron oxide, talc, and titanium dioxide; may also contain ammonium hydroxide, ethyl alcohol, methyl alcohol, n-butyl alcohol, propylene glycol, and shellac.
Inactive ingredients in CellCept Oral Suspension include aspartame, citric acid anhydrous, colloidal silicon dioxide, methylparaben, mixed fruit flavor, sodium citrate dihydrate, sorbitol, soybean lecithin, and xanthan gum.
CellCept Intravenous is the hydrochloride salt of mycophenolate mofetil. The chemical name for the hydrochloride salt of mycophenolate mofetil is 2-morpholinoethyl (E)-6-(1,3-dihydro-4-hydroxy-6-methoxy-7-methyl-3-oxo-5-isobenzofuranyl)-4-methyl-4-hexenoate hydrochloride. It has an empirical formula of $C_{23}H_{31}NO_7$ HCl and a molecular weight of 469.96.
CellCept Intravenous is available as a sterile white to off-white lyophilized powder in vials containing mycophenolate mofetil hydrochloride for administration by intravenous infusion only. Each vial of CellCept Intravenous contains the equivalent of 500 mg mycophenolate mofetil as the hydrochloride salt. The inactive ingredients are polysorbate 80, 25 mg, and citric acid, 5 mg. Sodium hydroxide may have been used in the manufacture of CellCept Intravenous to adjust the pH. Reconstitution and dilution with 5% Dextrose Injection USP yields a slightly yellow solution of mycophenolate mofetil, 6 mg/mL. (For detailed method of preparation, see DOSAGE AND ADMINISTRATION.)

Pharmacokinetic Parameters for MPA [mean (±SD)] Following Administration of Mycophenolate Mofetil to Healthy Volunteers (Single Dose), Renal, Cardiac, and Hepatic Transplant Patients (Multiple Doses)

	Dose/Route	T_{max} (h)	C_{max} (µg/mL)	Total AUC (µg·h/mL)
Healthy Volunteers (single dose)	1 g/oral	0.80 (±0.36) (n=129)	24.5 (±9.5) (n=129)	63.9 (±16.2) (n=117)
Renal Transplant Patients (bid dosing) Time After Transplantation	**Dose/Route**	**T_{max} (h)**	**C_{max} (µg/mL)**	**Interdosing Interval AUC(0–12h) (µg·h/mL)**
5 days	1 g/iv	1.58 (±0.46) (n=31)	12.0 (±3.82) (n=31)	40.8 (±11.4) (n=31)
6 days	1 g/oral	1.33 (±1.05) (n=31)	10.7 (±4.83) (n=31)	32.9 (±15.0) (n=31)
Early (<40 days)	1 g/oral	1.31 (±0.76) (n=25)	8.16 (±4.50) (n=25)	27.3 (±10.9) (n=25)
Early (<40 days)	1.5 g/oral	1.21 (±0.81) (n=27)	13.5 (±8.18) (n=27)	38.4 (±15.4) (n=27)
Late (>3 months)	1.5 g/oral	0.90 (±0.24) (n=23)	24.1 (±12.1) (n=23)	65.3 (±35.4) (n=23)
Cardiac Transplant Patients (bid dosing) Time After Transplantation	**Dose/Route**	**T_{max} (h)**	**C_{max} (µg/mL)**	**Interdosing Interval AUC(0–12h) (µg·h/mL)**
Early (Day before discharge)	1.5 g/oral	1.8 (±1.3) (n=11)	11.5 (±6.8) (n=11)	43.3 (±20.8) (n=9)
Late (>6 months)	1.5 g/oral	1.1 (±0.7) (n=52)	20.0 (±9.4) (n=52)	54.1* (±20.4) (n=49)
Hepatic Transplant Patients (bid dosing) Time After Transplantation	**Dose/Route**	**T_{max} (h)**	**C_{max} (µg/mL)**	**Interdosing Interval AUC(0–12h) (µg·h/mL)**
4 to 9 days	1 g/iv	1.50 (±0.517) (n=22)	17.0 (±12.7) (n=22)	34.0 (±17.4) (n=22)
Early (5 to 8 days)	1.5 g/oral	1.15 (±0.432) (n=20)	13.1 (±6.76) (n=20)	29.2 (±11.9) (n=20)
Late (>6 months)	1.5 g/oral	1.54 (±0.51) (n=6)	19.3 (±11.7) (n=6)	49.3 (±14.8) (n=6)

**AUC(0–12h) values quoted are extrapolated from data from samples collected over 4 hours.*

CLINICAL PHARMACOLOGY

Mechanism of Action: Mycophenolate mofetil has been demonstrated in experimental animal models to prolong the survival of allogeneic transplants (kidney, heart, liver, intestine, limb, small bowel, pancreatic islets, and bone marrow). Mycophenolate mofetil has also been shown to reverse ongoing acute rejection in the canine renal and rat cardiac allograft models. Mycophenolate mofetil also inhibited proliferative arteriopathy in experimental models of aortic and cardiac allografts in rats, as well as in primate cardiac xenografts. Mycophenolate mofetil was used alone or in combination with other immunosuppressive agents in these studies. Mycophenolate mofetil has been demonstrated to inhibit immunologically mediated inflammatory responses in animal models and to inhibit tumor development and prolong survival in murine tumor transplant models.
Mycophenolate mofetil is rapidly absorbed following oral administration and hydrolyzed to form MPA, which is the active metabolite. MPA is a potent, selective, uncompetitive, and reversible inhibitor of inosine monophosphate dehydrogenase (IMPDH), and therefore inhibits the de novo pathway of guanosine nucleotide synthesis without incorporation into DNA. Because T- and B-lymphocytes are critically dependent for their proliferation on de novo synthesis of purines, whereas other cell types can utilize salvage pathways, MPA has potent cytostatic effects on lymphocytes. MPA inhibits proliferative responses of T- and B-lymphocytes to both mitogenic and allospecific stimulation. Addition of guanosine or deoxyguanosine reverses the cytostatic effects of MPA on lymphocytes. MPA also suppresses antibody formation by B-lymphocytes. MPA prevents the glycosylation of lymphocyte and monocyte glycoproteins that are involved in intercellular adhesion to endothelial cells and may inhibit recruitment of leukocytes into sites of inflammation and graft rejection. Mycophenolate mofetil did not inhibit early events in the activation of human peripheral blood mononuclear cells, such as the production of interleukin-1 (IL-1) and interleukin-2 (IL-2), but did block the coupling of these events to DNA synthesis and proliferation.
Pharmacokinetics: Following oral and intravenous administration, mycophenolate mofetil undergoes rapid and complete metabolism to MPA, the active metabolite. Oral absorption of the drug is rapid and essentially complete. MPA is metabolized to form the phenolic glucuronide of MPA (MPAG) which is not pharmacologically active. The parent drug, mycophenolate mofetil, can be measured systemically during the intravenous infusion; however, shortly (about 5 minutes) after the infusion is stopped or after oral administration, MMF concentration is below the limit of quantitation (0.4 µg/mL).
Absorption: In 12 healthy volunteers, the mean absolute bioavailability of oral mycophenolate mofetil relative to intravenous mycophenolate mofetil (based on MPA AUC) was 94%. The area under the plasma-concentration time curve (AUC) for MPA appears to increase in a dose-proportional fashion in renal transplant patients receiving multiple doses of mycophenolate mofetil up to a daily dose of 3 g (see table below on pharmacokinetic parameters).
Food (27 g fat, 650 calories) had no effect on the extent of absorption (MPA AUC) of mycophenolate mofetil when administered at doses of 1.5 g bid to renal transplant patients. However, MPA C_{max} was decreased by 40% in the presence of food (see DOSAGE AND ADMINISTRATION).

Continued on next page

CellCept—Cont.

Distribution: The mean (±SD) apparent volume of distribution of MPA in 12 healthy volunteers is approximately 3.6 (±1.5) and 4.0 (±1.2) L/kg following intravenous and oral administration, respectively. MPA, at clinically relevant concentrations, is 97% bound to plasma albumin. MPAG is 82% bound to plasma albumin at MPAG concentration ranges that are normally seen in stable renal transplant patients; however, at higher MPAG concentrations (observed in patients with renal impairment or delayed renal graft function), the binding of MPA may be reduced as a result of competition between MPAG and MPA for protein binding. Mean blood to plasma ratio of radioactivity concentrations was approximately 0.6 indicating that MPA and MPAG do not extensively distribute into the cellular fractions of blood.

In vitro studies to evaluate the effect of other agents on the binding of MPA to human serum albumin (HSA) or plasma proteins showed that salicylate (at 25 mg/dL with HSA) and MPAG (at ≥460 µg/mL with plasma proteins) increased the free fraction of MPA. At concentrations that exceeded what is encountered clinically, cyclosporine, digoxin, naproxen, prednisone, propranolol, tacrolimus, theophylline, tolbutamide, and warfarin did not increase the free fraction of MPA. MPA at concentrations as high as 100 µg/mL had little effect on the binding of warfarin, digoxin or propranolol, but decreased the binding of theophylline from 53% to 45% and phenytoin from 90% to 87%.

Metabolism: Following oral and intravenous dosing, mycophenolate mofetil undergoes complete metabolism to MPA, the active metabolite. Metabolism to MPA occurs presystemically after oral dosing. MPA is metabolized principally by glucuronyl transferase to form the phenolic glucuronide of MPA (MPAG) which is not pharmacologically active. In vivo, MPAG is converted to MPA via enterohepatic recirculation. The following metabolites of the 2-hydroxyethyl-morpholino moiety are also recovered in the urine following oral administration of mycophenolate mofetil to healthy subjects: N-(2-carboxymethyl)-morpholine, N-(2-hydroxyethyl)-morpholine, and the N-oxide of N-(2-hydroxyethyl)-morpholine.

Secondary peaks in the plasma MPA concentration-time profile are usually observed 6 to 12 hours postdose. The coadministration of cholestyramine (4 g tid) resulted in approximately a 40% decrease in the MPA AUC (largely as a consequence of lower concentrations in the terminal portion of the profile). These observations suggest that enterohepatic recirculation contributes to MPA plasma concentrations.

Increased plasma concentrations of mycophenolate mofetil metabolites (MPA 50% increase and MPAG about a 3-fold to 6-fold increase) are observed in patients with renal insufficiency (see CLINICAL PHARMACOLOGY: *Special Populations*).

Excretion: Negligible amount of drug is excreted as MPA (<1% of dose) in the urine. Orally administered radiolabeled mycophenolate mofetil resulted in complete recovery of the administered dose, with 93% of the administered dose recovered in the urine and 6% recovered in feces. Most (about 87%) of the administered dose is excreted in the urine as MPAG. At clinically encountered concentrations, MPA and MPAG are usually not removed by hemodialysis. However, at high MPAG plasma concentrations (>100 µg/mL), small amounts of MPAG are removed. Bile acid sequestrants, such as cholestyramine, reduce MPA AUC by interfering with enterohepatic circulation of the drug (see OVERDOSAGE).

Mean (±SD) apparent half-life and plasma clearance of MPA are 17.9 (±6.5) hours and 193 (±48) mL/min following oral administration and 16.6 (±5.8) hours and 177 (±31) mL/min following intravenous administration, respectively.

Pharmacokinetics in Healthy Volunteers, Renal, Cardiac, and Hepatic Transplant Patients: Shown below are the mean (±SD) pharmacokinetic parameters for MPA following the administration of mycophenolate mofetil given as single doses to healthy volunteers and multiple doses to renal, cardiac, and hepatic transplant patients. In the early posttransplant period (<40 days posttransplant), renal, cardiac, and hepatic transplant patients had mean MPA AUCs approximately 20% to 41% lower and mean C_{max} approximately 32% to 44% lower compared to the late transplant period (3 to 6 months posttransplant).

Mean MPA AUC values following administration of 1 g bid intravenous mycophenolate mofetil over 2 hours to renal transplant patients for 5 days were about 24% higher than those observed after oral administration of a similar dose in the immediate posttransplant phase. In hepatic transplant patients, administration of 1 g bid intravenous CellCept followed by 1.5 g bid oral CellCept resulted in mean MPA AUC values similar to those found in renal transplant patients administered 1 g CellCept bid.

[See table at top of previous page]

Two 500 mg tablets have been shown to be bioequivalent to four 250 mg capsules. Five mL of the 200 mg/mL constituted oral suspension have been shown to be bioequivalent to four 250 mg capsules.

Special Populations: Shown below are the mean (±SD) pharmacokinetic parameters for MPA following the administration of oral mycophenolate mofetil given as single doses to non-transplant subjects with renal or hepatic impairment.

[See first table above]

Pharmacokinetic Parameters for MPA [mean (±SD)] Following Single Doses of Mycophenolate Mofetil Capsules in Chronic Renal and Hepatic Impairment

Renal Impairment (no. of patients)	Dose	T_{max} (h)	C_{max} (µg/mL)	AUC(0–96h) (µg•h/mL)
Healthy Volunteers GFR >80 mL/min/1.73 m^2 (n=6)	1 g	0.75 (±0.27)	25.3 (±7.99)	45.0 (±22.6)
Mild Renal Impairment GFR 50 to 80 mL/min/1.73 m^2 (n=6)	1 g	0.75 (±0.27)	26.0 (±3.82)	59.9 (±12.9)
Moderate Renal Impairment GFR 25 to 49 mL/min/1.73 m^2 (n=6)	1 g	0.75 (±0.27)	19.0 (±13.2)	52.9 (±25.5)
Severe Renal Impairment GFR <25 mL/min/1.73 m^2 (n=7)	1 g	1.00 (±0.41)	16.3 (±10.8)	78.6 (±46.4)
Hepatic Impairment (no. of patients)	**Dose**	**T_{max} (h)**	**C_{max} (µg/mL)**	**AUC(0–48h) (µg•h/mL)**
Healthy Volunteers (n=6)	1 g	0.63 (±0.14)	24.3 (±5.73)	29.0 (±5.78)
Alcoholic Cirrhosis (n=18)	1 g	0.85 (±0.58)	22.4 (±10.1)	29.8 (±10.7)

Mean (±SD) Computed Pharmacokinetic Parameters for MPA by Age and Time After Allogeneic Renal Transplantation

Age Group	(n)	Time	T_{max} (h)		Dose Adjusted[a] C_{max} (µg/mL)		Dose Adjusted[a] AUC $_{0-12}$ (µg•h/mL)	
		Early (Day 7)						
1 to <2 yr	(6)[d]		3.03	(4.70)	10.3	(5.80)	22.5	(6.66)
1 to <6 yr	(17)		1.63	(2.85)	13.2	(7.16)	27.4	(9.54)
6 to <12 yr	(16)		0.940	(0.546)	13.1	(6.30)	33.2	(12.1)
12 to 18 yr	(21)		1.16	(0.830)	11.7	(10.7)	26.3	(9.14)[b]
		Late (Month 3)						
1 to <2 yr	(4)[d]		0.725	(0.276)	23.8	(13.4)	47.4	(14.7)
1 to <6 yr	(15)		0.989	(0.511)	22.7	(10.1)	49.7	(18.2)
6 to <12 yr	(14)		1.21	(0.532)	27.8	(14.3)	61.9	(19.6)
12 to 18 yr	(17)		0.978	(0.484)	17.9	(9.57)	53.6	(20.3)[c]
		Late (Month 9)						
1 to <2 yr	(4)[d]		0.604	(0.208)	25.6	(4.25)	55.8	(11.6)
1 to <6 yr	(12)		0.869	(0.479)	30.4	(9.16)	61.0	(10.7)
6 to <12 yr	(11)		1.12	(0.462)	29.2	(12.6)	66.8	(21.2)
12 to 18 yr	(14)		1.09	(0.518)	18.1	(7.29)	56.7	(14.0)

[a]adjusted to a dose of 600 mg/m^2
[b]n=20
[c]n=16
[d]a subset of 1 to <6 yr

Renal Insufficiency: In a single-dose study, MMF was administered as capsule or intravenous infusion over 40 minutes. Plasma MPA AUC observed after oral dosing to volunteers with severe chronic renal impairment [glomerular filtration rate (GFR) <25 mL/min/1.73 m^2] was about 75% higher relative to that observed in healthy volunteers (GFR >80 mL/min/1.73 m^2). In addition, the single-dose plasma MPAG AUC was 3-fold to 6-fold higher in volunteers with severe renal impairment than in volunteers with mild renal impairment or healthy volunteers, consistent with the known renal elimination of MPAG. No data are available on the safety of long-term exposure to this level of MPAG.

Plasma MPA AUC observed after single-dose (1 g) intravenous dosing to volunteers (n=4) with severe chronic renal impairment (GFR <25 mL/min/1.73 m^2) was 62.4 µg•h/mL (±19.3). Multiple dosing of mycophenolate mofetil in patients with severe chronic renal impairment has not been studied (see PRECAUTIONS: *General* and DOSAGE AND ADMINISTRATION).

In patients with delayed renal graft function posttransplant, mean MPA AUC(0–12h) was comparable to that seen in posttransplant patients without delayed renal graft function. There is a potential for a transient increase in the free fraction and concentration of plasma MPA in patients with delayed renal graft function. However, dose adjustment does not appear to be necessary in patients with delayed renal graft function. Mean plasma MPAG AUC(0–12h) was 2-fold to 3-fold higher than in posttransplant patients without delayed renal graft function (see PRECAUTIONS: *General* and DOSAGE AND ADMINISTRATION).

In 8 patients with primary graft non-function following renal transplantation, plasma concentrations of MPAG accumulated about 6-fold to 8-fold after multiple dosing for 28 days. Accumulation of MPA was about 1-fold to 2-fold.

The pharmacokinetics of mycophenolate mofetil are not altered by hemodialysis. Hemodialysis usually does not remove MPA or MPAG. At high concentrations of MPAG (>100 µg/mL), hemodialysis removes only small amounts of MPAG.

Hepatic Insufficiency: In a single-dose (1 g oral) study of 18 volunteers with alcoholic cirrhosis and 6 healthy volunteers, hepatic MPA glucuronidation processes appeared to be relatively unaffected by hepatic parenchymal disease when pharmacokinetic parameters of healthy volunteers and alcoholic cirrhosis patients within this study were compared. However, it should be noted that for unexplained reasons, the healthy volunteers in this study had about a 50% lower AUC as compared to healthy volunteers in other studies, thus making comparisons between volunteers with alcoholic cirrhosis and healthy volunteers difficult. Effects of hepatic disease on this process probably depend on the particular disease. Hepatic disease with other etiologies, such as primary biliary cirrhosis, may show a different effect. In a single-dose (1 g intravenous) study of 6 volunteers with severe hepatic impairment (aminopyrine breath test less than 0.2% of dose) due to alcoholic cirrhosis, MMF was rapidly converted to MPA. MPA AUC was 44.1 µg•h/mL (±15.5).

Pediatrics: The pharmacokinetic parameters of MPA and MPAG have been evaluated in 55 pediatric patients (ranging from 1 year to 18 years of age) receiving CellCept oral suspension at a dose of 600 mg/m^2 bid (up to a maximum of 1 g bid) after allogeneic renal transplantation. The pharmacokinetic data for MPA is provided in the following table:

[See second table above]

The CellCept oral suspension dose of 600 mg/m^2 bid (up to a maximum of 1 g bid) achieved mean MPA AUC values in pediatric patients similar to those seen in adult renal transplant patients receiving CellCept capsules at a dose of 1 g bid in the early posttransplant period. There was wide variability in the data. As observed in adults, early posttransplant MPA AUC values were approximately 45% to 53% lower than those observed in the later posttransplant period (>3 months). MPA AUC values were similar in the early and late posttransplant period across the 1 year to 18 year age range.

Gender: Data obtained from several studies were pooled to look at any gender-related differences in the pharmacokinetics of MPA (data were adjusted to 1 g oral dose). Mean (±SD) MPA AUC(0–12h) for males (n=79) was 32.0 (±14.5) and for females (n=41) was 36.5 (±18.8) µg•h/mL while mean (±SD) MPA C_{max} was 9.96 (±6.19) in the males and 10.6 (±5.64) µg/mL in the females. These differences are not of clinical significance.

Geriatrics: Pharmacokinetics in the elderly have not been studied.

CLINICAL STUDIES

The safety and efficacy of CellCept in combination with corticosteroids and cyclosporine for the prevention of organ rejection were assessed in randomized, double-blind, multicenter trials in renal (3 trials), in cardiac (1 trial), and in hepatic (1 trial) adult transplant patients.

Renal Transplant: The three renal studies compared two dose levels of oral CellCept (1 g bid and 1.5 g bid) with azathioprine (2 studies) or placebo (1 study) when administered in combination with cyclosporine (Sandimmune®*) and corticosteroids to prevent acute rejection episodes. One study also included antithymocyte globulin (ATGAM®†) induction therapy. These studies are described by geographic location of the investigational sites. One study was conducted in the USA at 14 sites, one study was conducted in Europe at 20 sites, and one study was conducted in Europe, Canada, and Australia at a total of 21 sites.

The primary efficacy endpoint was the proportion of patients in each treatment group who experienced treatment failure within the first 6 months after transplantation (defined as biopsy-proven acute rejection on treatment or the occurrence of death, graft loss or early termination from the study for any reason without prior biopsy-proven rejection). CellCept, when administered with antithymocyte globulin (ATGAM®) induction (one study) and with cyclosporine and corticosteroids (all three studies), was compared to the following three therapeutic regimens: (1) antithymocyte globulin (ATGAM®) induction/azathioprine/cyclosporine/corticosteroids, (2) azathioprine/cyclosporine/corticosteroids, and (3) cyclosporine/corticosteroids.

CellCept, in combination with corticosteroids and cyclosporine reduced (statistically significant at 0.05 level) the incidence of treatment failure within the first 6 months following transplantation. The following tables summarize the results of these studies. These tables show (1) the proportion of patients experiencing treatment failure, (2) the proportion of patients who experienced biopsy-proven acute rejection on treatment, and (3) early termination, for any reason other than graft loss or death, without a prior biopsy-proven acute rejection episode. Patients who prematurely discontinued treatment were followed for the occurrence of death or graft loss, and the cumulative incidence of graft loss and patient death are summarized separately. Patients who prematurely discontinued treatment were not followed for the occurrence of acute rejection after termination. More patients receiving CellCept discontinued without prior biopsy-proven rejection, death or graft loss than discontinued in the control groups, with the highest rate in the CellCept 3 g/day group. Therefore, the acute rejection rates may be underestimates, particularly in the CellCept 3 g/day group.

*Sandimmune is a registered trademark of Novartis Pharmaceuticals Corporation.
†ATGAM is a registered trademark of Pharmacia and Upjohn Company.

[See first table at right]

The cumulative incidence of 12-month graft loss or patient death is presented below. No advantage of CellCept with respect to graft loss or patient death was established. Numerically, patients receiving CellCept 2 g/day and 3 g/day experienced a better outcome than controls in all three studies; patients receiving CellCept 2 g/day experienced a better outcome than CellCept 3 g/day in two of the three studies. Patients in all treatment groups who terminated treatment early were found to have a poor outcome with respect to graft loss or patient death at 1 year.

[See second table at right]

Pediatrics: One open-label, safety and pharmacokinetic study of CellCept oral suspension 600 mg/m^2 bid (up to 1 g bid) in combination with cyclosporine and corticosteroids was performed at centers in the US (9), Europe (5) and Australia (1) in 100 pediatric patients (3 months to 18 years of age) for the prevention of renal allograft rejection. CellCept was well tolerated in pediatric patients (see ADVERSE REACTIONS), and the pharmacokinetics profile was similar to that seen in adult patients dosed with 1 g bid CellCept capsules (see CLINICAL PHARMACOLOGY: *Pharmacokinetics*). The rate of biopsy-proven rejection was similar across the age groups (3 months to <6 years, 6 years to <12 years, 12 years to 18 years). The overall biopsy-proven rejection rate at 6 months was comparable to adults. The combined incidence of graft loss (5%) and patient death (2%) at 12 months posttransplant was similar to that observed in adult renal transplant patients.

Cardiac Transplant: A double-blind, randomized, comparative, parallel-group, multicenter study in primary cardiac transplant recipients was performed at 20 centers in the United States, 1 in Canada, 5 in Europe and 2 in Australia. The total number of patients enrolled was 650; 72 never received study drug and 578 received study drug. Patients received CellCept 1.5 g bid (n=289) or azathioprine 1.5 to 3 mg/kg/day (n=289), in combination with cyclosporine (Sandimmune® or Neoral®*) and corticosteroids as maintenance immunosuppressive therapy. The two primary efficacy endpoints were: (1) the proportion of patients who, after transplantation, had at least one endomyocardial biopsy-proven rejection with hemodynamic compromise, or were retransplanted or died, within the first 6 months, and (2) the proportion of patients who died or were retransplanted during the first 12 months following transplantation. Patients who prematurely discontinued treatment were followed for the occurrence of allograft rejection for up to 6 months and for the occurrence of death for 1 year.

(1) Rejection: No difference was established between CellCept and azathioprine (AZA) with respect to biopsy-proven rejection with hemodynamic compromise.

*Neoral is a registered trademark of Novartis Pharmaceuticals Corporation.

(2) Survival: CellCept was shown to be at least as effective as AZA in preventing death or retransplantation at 1 year (see table below).

Renal Transplant Studies
Incidence of Treatment Failure
(Biopsy-proven Rejection or Early Termination for Any Reason)

USA Study† (N=499 patients)	**CellCept 2 g/day** (n=167 patients)	**CellCept 3 g/day** (n=166 patients)	**Azathioprine 1 to 2 mg/kg/day** (n=166 patients)
All treatment failures	31.1%	31.3%	47.6%
Early termination without prior acute rejection*	9.6%	12.7%	6.0%
Biopsy-proven rejection episode on treatment	19.8%	17.5%	38.0%
Europe/Canada/ Australia Study‡ (N=503 patients)	**CellCept 2 g/day (n=173 patients)**	**CellCept 3 g/day (n=164 patients)**	**Azathioprine 100 to 150 mg/day (n=166 patients)**
All treatment failures	38.2%	34.8%	50.0%
Early termination without prior acute rejection*	13.9%	15.2%	10.2%
Biopsy-proven rejection episode on treatment	19.7%	15.9%	35.5%
Europe Study§ (N=491 patients)	**CellCept 2 g/day (n=165 patients)**	**CellCept 3 g/day (n=160 patients)**	**Placebo (n=166 patients)**
All treatment failures	30.3%	38.8%	56.0%
Early termination without prior acute rejection*	11.5%	22.5%	7.2%
Biopsy-proven rejection episode on treatment	17.0%	13.8%	46.4%

*Does not include death and graft loss as reason for early termination.
†Antithymocyte globulin induction/MMF or azathioprine/cyclosporine/corticosteroids.
‡MMF or azathioprine/cyclosporine/corticosteroids.
§MMF or placebo/cyclosporine/corticosteroids.

Renal Transplant Studies
Cumulative Incidence of Combined Graft Loss or Patient Death at 12 Months

Study	CellCept 2 g/day	CellCept 3 g/day	Control (Azathioprine or Placebo)
USA	8.5%	11.5%	12.2%
Europe/Canada/Australia	11.7%	11.0%	13.6%
Europe	8.5%	10.0%	11.5%

Rejection at 6 Months/Death or Retransplantation at 1 Year

	All Patients		Treated Patients	
	AZA N = 323	CellCept N = 327	AZA N = 289	CellCept N = 289
Biopsy-proven rejection with hemodynamic compromise at 6 months*	121 (38%)	120 (37%)	100 (35%)	92 (32%)
Death or retransplantation at 1 year	49 (15.2%)	42 (12.8%)	33 (11.4%)	18 (6.2%)

*Hemodynamic compromise occurred if any of the following criteria were met: pulmonary capillary wedge pressure ≥20 mm or a 25% increase; cardiac index <2.0 L/min/m^2 or a 25% decrease; ejection fraction ≤30%; pulmonary artery oxygen saturation ≤60% or a 25% decrease; presence of new S_3 gallop; fractional shortening was ≤20% or a 25% decrease; inotropic support required to manage the clinical condition.

[See third table above]

Hepatic Transplant: A double-blind, randomized, comparative, parallel-group, multicenter study in primary hepatic transplant recipients was performed at 16 centers in the United States, 2 in Canada, 4 in Europe and 1 in Australia. The total number of patients enrolled was 565. Per protocol, patients received CellCept 1 g bid intravenously for up to 14 days followed by CellCept 1.5 g bid orally or azathioprine 1 to 2 mg/kg/day intravenously followed by azathioprine 1 to 2 mg/kg/day orally, in combination with cyclosporine (Neoral®) and corticosteroids as maintenance immunosuppressive therapy. The actual median oral dose of azathioprine on study was 1.5 mg/kg/day (range of 0.3 to 3.8 mg/kg/day) initially and 1.26 mg/kg/day (range of 0.3 to 3.8 mg/kg/day) at 12 months. The two primary endpoints were: (1) the proportion of patients who experienced, in the first 6 months posttransplantation, one or more episodes of biopsy-proven and treated rejection or death or retransplantation, and (2) the proportion of patients who experienced graft loss (death or retransplantation) during the first 12 months posttransplantation. Patients who prematurely discontinued treatment were followed for the occurrence of allograft rejection and for the occurrence of graft loss (death or retransplantation) for 1 year.

Results: In combination with corticosteroids and cyclosporine, CellCept obtained a lower rate of acute rejection at 6 months and a similar rate of death or retransplantation at 1 year compared to azathioprine.

Rejection at 6 Months/ Death or Retransplantation at 1 Year

	AZA N = 287	CellCept N = 278
Biopsy proven, treated rejection at 6 months (includes death or retransplantation)	137 (47.7%)	107 (38.5%)
Death or retransplantation at 1 year	42 (14.6%)	41 (14.7%)

INDICATIONS AND USAGE

Renal, Cardiac, and Hepatic Transplant: CellCept is indicated for the prophylaxis of organ rejection in patients receiving allogeneic renal, cardiac or hepatic transplants. CellCept should be used concomitantly with cyclosporine and corticosteroids.

Continued on next page

CellCept—Cont.

CellCept Intravenous is an alternative dosage form to CellCept capsules, tablets and oral suspension. CellCept Intravenous should be administered within 24 hours following transplantation. CellCept Intravenous can be administered for up to 14 days; patients should be switched to oral CellCept as soon as they can tolerate oral medication.

CONTRAINDICATIONS

Allergic reactions to CellCept have been observed; therefore, CellCept is contraindicated in patients with a hypersensitivity to mycophenolate mofetil, mycophenolic acid or any component of the drug product. CellCept Intravenous is contraindicated in patients who are allergic to Polysorbate 80 (TWEEN).

WARNINGS (see boxed WARNING)

Patients receiving immunosuppressive regimens involving combinations of drugs, including CellCept, as part of an immunosuppressive regimen are at increased risk of developing lymphomas and other malignancies, particularly of the skin (see ADVERSE REACTIONS). The risk appears to be related to the intensity and duration of immunosuppression rather than to the use of any specific agent. Oversuppression of the immune system can also increase susceptibility to infection, including opportunistic infections, fatal infections, and sepsis.

As usual for patients with increased risk for skin cancer, exposure to sunlight and UV light should be limited by wearing protective clothing and using a sunscreen with a high protection factor.

CellCept has been administered in combination with the following agents in clinical trials: antithymocyte globulin (ATGAM®), OKT3 (Orthoclone OKT® 3*), cyclosporine (Sandimmune®, Neoral®) and corticosteroids. The efficacy and safety of the use of CellCept in combination with other immunosuppressive agents have not been determined.

*Orthoclone OKT is a registered trademark of Ortho Biotech Inc.

Lymphoproliferative disease or lymphoma developed in 0.4% to 1% of patients receiving CellCept (2 g or 3 g) with other immunosuppressive agents in controlled clinical trials of renal, cardiac, and hepatic transplant patients (see ADVERSE REACTIONS).

In pediatric patients, no other malignancies besides lymphoproliferative disorder (2/148 patients) have been observed (see ADVERSE REACTIONS).

Adverse effects on fetal development (including malformations) occurred when pregnant rats and rabbits were dosed during organogenesis. These responses occurred at doses lower than those associated with maternal toxicity, and at doses below the recommended clinical dose for renal, cardiac or hepatic transplantation. There are no adequate and well-controlled studies in pregnant women. However, as CellCept has been shown to have teratogenic effects in animals, it may cause fetal harm when administered to a pregnant woman. Therefore, CellCept should not be used in pregnant women unless the potential benefit justifies the potential risk to the fetus.

Women of childbearing potential should have a negative serum or urine pregnancy test with a sensitivity of at least 50 mIU/mL within 1 week prior to beginning therapy. It is recommended that CellCept therapy should not be initiated by the physician until a report of a negative pregnancy test has been obtained.

Effective contraception must be used before beginning CellCept therapy, during therapy, and for 6 weeks following discontinuation of therapy, even where there has been a history of infertility, unless due to hysterectomy. Two reliable forms of contraception must be used simultaneously unless abstinence is the chosen method (see PRECAUTIONS: *Drug Interactions*). If pregnancy does occur during treatment, the physician and patient should discuss the desirability of continuing the pregnancy (see PRECAUTIONS: *Pregnancy* and *Information for Patients*).

In patients receiving CellCept (2 g or 3 g) in controlled studies for prevention of renal, cardiac or hepatic rejection, fatal infection/sepsis occurred in approximately 2% of renal and cardiac patients and in 5% of hepatic patients (see ADVERSE REACTIONS).

Severe neutropenia [absolute neutrophil count (ANC) <0.5 x $10^3/\mu L$] developed in up to 2.0% of renal, up to 2.8% of cardiac, and up to 3.6% of hepatic transplant patients receiving CellCept 3 g daily (see ADVERSE REACTIONS).

Patients receiving CellCept should be monitored for neutropenia (see PRECAUTIONS: *Laboratory Tests*). The development of neutropenia may be related to CellCept itself, concomitant medications, viral infections, or some combination of these causes. If neutropenia develops (ANC <1.3 x $10^3/\mu L$), dosing with CellCept should be interrupted or the dose reduced, appropriate diagnostic tests performed, and the patient managed appropriately (see DOSAGE AND ADMINISTRATION). Neutropenia has been observed most frequently in the period from 31 to 180 days posttransplant in patients treated for prevention of renal, cardiac, and hepatic rejection.

Patients receiving CellCept should be instructed to report immediately any evidence of infection, unexpected bruising, bleeding or any other manifestation of bone marrow depression.

Adverse Events in Controlled Studies in Prevention of Renal, Cardiac or Hepatic Allograft Rejection (Reported in ≥20% of Patients in the CellCept Group)

	Renal Studies			Cardiac Study		Hepatic Study	
	CellCept 2 g/day	CellCept 3 g/day	Azathioprine 1 to 2 mg/kg/day or 100 to 150 mg/day	CellCept 3 g/day	Azathioprine 1.5 to 3 mg/kg/day	CellCept 3 g/day	Azathioprine 1 to 2 mg/kg/day
	(n=336)	(n=330)	(n=326)	(n=289)	(n=289)	(n=277)	(n=287)
	%	%	%	%	%	%	%
Body as a Whole							
Pain	33.0	31.2	32.2	75.8	74.7	74.0	77.7
Abdominal pain	24.7	27.6	23.0	33.9	33.2	62.5	51.2
Fever	21.4	23.3	23.3	47.4	46.4	52.3	56.1
Headache	21.1	16.1	21.2	54.3	51.9	53.8	49.1
Infection	18.2	20.9	19.9	25.6	19.4	27.1	25.1
Sepsis	–	–	–	–	–	27.4	26.5
Asthenia	–	–	–	43.3	36.3	35.4	33.8
Chest pain	–	–	–	26.3	26.0	–	–
Back pain	–	–	–	34.6	28.4	46.6	47.4
Ascites	–	–	–	–	–	24.2	22.6
Hemic and Lymphatic							
Anemia	25.6	25.8	23.6	42.9	43.9	43.0	53.0
Leukopenia	23.2	34.5	24.8	30.4	39.1	45.8	39.0
Thrombocytopenia	–	–	–	23.5	27.0	38.3	42.2
Hypochromic anemia	–	–	–	24.6	23.5	–	–
Leukocytosis	–	–	–	40.5	35.6	22.4	21.3
Urogenital							
Urinary tract infection	37.2	37.0	33.7	–	–	–	–
Kidney function abnormal	–	–	–	21.8	26.3	25.6	28.9
Cardiovascular							
Hypertension	32.4	28.2	32.2	77.5	72.3	62.1	59.6
Hypotension	–	–	–	32.5	36.0	–	–
Cardiovascular disorder	–	–	–	25.6	24.2	–	–
Tachycardia	–	–	–	20.1	18.0	22.0	15.7
Metabolic and Nutritional							
Peripheral edema	28.6	27.0	28.2	64.0	53.3	48.4	47.7
Hypercholesteremia			–	41.2	38.4	–	–
Edema			–	26.6	25.6	28.2	28.2
Hypokalemia			–	31.8	25.6	37.2	41.1
Hyperkalemia	–	–	–	–	–	22.0	23.7
Hyperglycemia	–	–	–	46.7	52.6	43.7	48.8
Creatinine increased	–	–	–	39.4	36.0	–	–

(Table continued on next page)

CAUTION: CELLCEPT INTRAVENOUS SOLUTION SHOULD NEVER BE ADMINISTERED BY RAPID OR BOLUS INTRAVENOUS INJECTION.

PRECAUTIONS

General: Gastrointestinal bleeding (requiring hospitalization) has been observed in approximately 3% of renal, in 1.7% of cardiac, and in 5.4% of hepatic transplant patients treated with CellCept 3 g daily. In pediatric renal transplant patients, 5/148 cases of gastrointestinal bleeding (requiring hospitalization) were observed.

Gastrointestinal perforations have rarely been observed. Most patients receiving CellCept were also receiving other drugs known to be associated with these complications. Patients with active peptic ulcer disease were excluded from enrollment in studies with mycophenolate mofetil. Because CellCept has been associated with an increased incidence of digestive system adverse events, including infrequent cases of gastrointestinal tract ulceration, hemorrhage, and perforation, CellCept should be administered with caution in patients with active serious digestive system disease.

Subjects with severe chronic renal impairment (GFR <25 mL/min/1.73 m^2) who have received single doses of CellCept showed higher plasma MPA and MPAG AUCs relative to subjects with lesser degrees of renal impairment or normal healthy volunteers. No data are available on the safety of long-term exposure to these levels of MPAG. Doses of CellCept greater than 1 g administered twice a day to renal transplant patients should be avoided and they should be carefully observed (see CLINICAL PHARMACOLOGY: *Pharmacokinetics* and DOSAGE AND ADMINISTRATION). No data are available for cardiac or hepatic transplant patients with severe chronic renal impairment. CellCept may be used for cardiac or hepatic transplant patients with severe chronic renal impairment if the potential benefits outweigh the potential risks.

In patients with delayed renal graft function posttransplant, mean MPA AUC(0–12h) was comparable, but MPAG AUC(0–12h) was 2-fold to 3-fold higher, compared to that seen in posttransplant patients without delayed renal graft function. In the three controlled studies of prevention of renal rejection, there were 298 of 1483 patients (20%) with

Adverse Events in Controlled Studies in Prevention of Renal, Cardiac or Hepatic Allograft Rejection (Reported in ≥20% of Patients in the CellCept Group) *(cont.)*

	Renal Studies			Cardiac Study		Hepatic Study	
	CellCept 2 g/day	CellCept 3 g/day	Azathioprine 1 to 2 mg/kg/day or 100 to 150 mg/day	CellCept 3 g/day	Azathioprine 1.5 to 3 mg/kg/day	CellCept 3 g/day	Azathioprine 1 to 2 mg/kg/day
	(n=336)	(n=330)	(n=326)	(n=289)	(n=289)	(n=277)	(n=287)
	%	%	%	%	%	%	%
BUN increased	–	–	–	34.6	32.5	–	–
Lactic dehydrogenase increased	–	–	–	23.2	17.0	–	–
Hypomagnesemia	–	–	–	–	–	39.0	37.6
Hypocalcemia	–	–	–	–	–	30.0	30.0
Digestive							
Diarrhea	31.0	36.1	20.9	45.3	34.3	51.3	49.8
Constipation	22.9	18.5	22.4	41.2	37.7	37.9	38.3
Nausea	19.9	23.6	24.5	54.0	54.3	54.5	51.2
Dyspepsia	–	–	–	–	–	22.4	20.9
Vomiting	–	–	–	33.9	28.4	32.9	33.4
Anorexia	–	–	–	–	–	25.3	17.1
Liver function tests abnormal	–	–	–	–	–	24.9	19.2
Respiratory							
Infection	22.0	23.9	19.6	37.0	35.3	–	–
Dyspnea	–	–	–	36.7	36.3	31.0	30.3
Cough increased	–	–	–	31.1	25.6	–	–
Lung disorder	–	–	–	30.1	29.1	22.0	18.8
Sinusitis	–	–	–	26.0	19.0	–	–
Pleural effusion	–	–	–	–	–	34.3	35.9
Skin and Appendages							
Rash	–	–	–	22.1	18.0	–	–
Nervous System							
Tremor	–	–	–	24.2	23.9	33.9	35.5
Insomnia	–	–	–	40.8	37.7	52.3	47.0
Dizziness	–	–	–	28.7	27.7	–	–
Anxiety	–	–	–	28.4	23.9	–	–
Paresthesia	–	–	–	20.8	18.0	–	–

delayed graft function. Although patients with delayed graft function have a higher incidence of certain adverse events (anemia, thrombocytopenia, hyperkalemia) than patients without delayed graft function, these events were not more frequent in patients receiving CellCept than azathioprine or placebo. No dose adjustment is recommended for these patients; however, they should be carefully observed (see CLINICAL PHARMACOLOGY: *Pharmacokinetics* and DOSAGE AND ADMINISTRATION).

In cardiac transplant patients, the overall incidence of opportunistic infections was approximately 10% higher in patients treated with CellCept than in those receiving azathioprine therapy, but this difference was not associated with excess mortality due to infection/sepsis among patients treated with CellCept (see ADVERSE REACTIONS).

There were more herpes virus (H. simplex, H. zoster, and cytomegalovirus) infections in cardiac transplant patients treated with CellCept compared to those treated with azathioprine (see ADVERSE REACTIONS).

It is recommended that CellCept not be administered concomitantly with azathioprine because both have the potential to cause bone marrow suppression and such concomitant administration has not been studied clinically.

In view of the significant reduction in the AUC of MPA by cholestyramine, caution should be used in the concomitant administration of CellCept with drugs that interfere with enterohepatic recirculation because of the potential to reduce the efficacy of CellCept (see PRECAUTIONS: *Drug Interactions*).

On theoretical grounds, because CellCept is an IMPDH (inosine monophosphate dehydrogenase) inhibitor, it should be avoided in patients with rare hereditary deficiency of hypoxanthine-guanine phosphoribosyl-transferase (HGPRT) such as Lesch-Nyhan and Kelley-Seegmiller syndrome.

During treatment with CellCept, the use of live attenuated vaccines should be avoided and patients should be advised that vaccinations may be less effective (see PRECAUTIONS: *Drug Interactions: Live Vaccines*).

Phenylketonurics: CellCept Oral Suspension contains aspartame, a source of phenylalanine (0.56 mg phenylalanine/mL suspension). Therefore, care should be taken if CellCept Oral Suspension is administered to patients with phenylketonuria.

Information for Patients: Patients should be informed of the need for repeated appropriate laboratory tests while they are receiving CellCept. Patients should be given complete dosage instructions and informed of the increased risk of lymphoproliferative disease and certain other malignancies. Women of childbearing potential should be instructed of the potential risks during pregnancy, and that they should use effective contraception before beginning CellCept therapy, during therapy, and for 6 weeks after CellCept has been stopped (see WARNINGS and PRECAUTIONS: *Pregnancy*).

Laboratory Tests: Complete blood counts should be performed weekly during the first month, twice monthly for the second and third months of treatment, then monthly through the first year (see WARNINGS, ADVERSE REACTIONS and DOSAGE AND ADMINISTRATION).

Drug Interactions: Drug interaction studies with mycophenolate mofetil have been conducted with acyclovir, antacids, cholestyramine, cyclosporine, ganciclovir, oral contraceptives, and trimethoprim/sulfamethoxazole. Drug interaction studies have not been conducted with other drugs that may be commonly administered to renal, cardiac or hepatic transplant patients. CellCept has not been administered concomitantly with azathioprine.

Acyclovir: Coadministration of mycophenolate mofetil (1 g) and acyclovir (800 mg) to 12 healthy volunteers resulted in no significant change in MPA AUC and C_{max}. However, MPAG and acyclovir plasma AUCs were increased 10.6% and 21.9%, respectively. Because MPAG plasma concentrations are increased in the presence of renal impairment, as are acyclovir concentrations, the potential exists for the two drugs to compete for tubular secretion, further increasing the concentrations of both drugs.

Antacids With Magnesium and Aluminum Hydroxides: Absorption of a single dose of mycophenolate mofetil (2 g) was decreased when administered to ten rheumatoid arthritis patients also taking Maalox®* TC (10 mL qid). The C_{max} and AUC(0–24h) for MPA were 33% and 17% lower, respectively, than when mycophenolate mofetil was administered alone under fasting conditions. CellCept may be administered to patients who are also taking antacids containing magnesium and aluminum hydroxides; however, it is recommended that CellCept and the antacid not be administered simultaneously.

*Maalox is a registered trademark of Novartis Consumer Health, Inc.

Cholestyramine: Following single-dose administration of 1.5 g mycophenolate mofetil to 12 healthy volunteers pretreated with 4 g tid of cholestyramine for 4 days, MPA AUC decreased approximately 40%. This decrease is consistent with interruption of enterohepatic recirculation which may be due to binding of recirculating MPAG with cholestyramine in the intestine. Some degree of enterohepatic recirculation is also anticipated following intravenous administration of CellCept. Therefore, CellCept is not recommended to be given with cholestyramine or other agents that may interfere with enterohepatic recirculation.

Cyclosporine: Cyclosporine (Sandimmune®) pharmacokinetics (at doses of 275 to 415 mg/day) were unaffected by single and multiple doses of 1.5 g bid of mycophenolate mofetil in 10 stable renal transplant patients. The mean (±SD) AUC(0–12h) and C_{max} of cyclosporine after 14 days of multiple doses of mycophenolate mofetil were 3290 (±822) ng•h/mL and 753 (±161) ng/mL, respectively, compared to 3245 (±1088) ng•h/mL and 700 (±246) ng/mL, respectively, 1 week before administration of mycophenolate mofetil. The effect of cyclosporine on mycophenolate mofetil pharmacokinetics could not be evaluated in this study; however, plasma concentrations of MPA were similar to that for healthy volunteers.

Ganciclovir: Following single-dose administration to 12 stable renal transplant patients, no pharmacokinetic interaction was observed between mycophenolate mofetil (1.5 g) and intravenous ganciclovir (5 mg/kg). Mean (±SD) ganciclovir AUC and C_{max} (n=10) were 54.3 (±19.0) µg•h/mL and 11.5 (±1.8) µg/mL, respectively, after coadministration of the two drugs, compared to 51.0 (±17.0) µg•h/mL and 10.6 (±2.0) µg/mL, respectively, after administration of intravenous ganciclovir alone. The mean (±SD) AUC and C_{max} of MPA (n=12) after coadministration were 80.9 (±21.6) µg•h/mL and 27.8 (±13.9) µg/mL, respectively, compared to values of 80.3 (±16.4) µg•h/mL and 30.9 (±11.2) µg/mL, respectively, after administration of mycophenolate mofetil alone. Because MPAG plasma concentrations are increased in the presence of renal impairment, as are ganciclovir concentrations, the two drugs will compete for tubular secretion and thus further increases in concentrations of both drugs may occur. In patients with renal impairment in which MMF and ganciclovir are coadministered, patients should be monitored carefully.

Oral Contraceptives: A study of coadministration of CellCept (1 g bid) and combined oral contraceptives containing ethinylestradiol (0.02 mg to 0.04 mg) and levonorgestrel (0.05 mg to 0.20 mg), desogestrel (0.15 mg) or gestodene (0.05 mg to 0.10 mg) was conducted in 18 women with psoriasis over 3 consecutive menstrual cycles. Mean AUC(0–24h) was similar for ethinylestradiol and 3-keto desogestrel; however, mean levonorgestrel AUC(0–24h) significantly decreased by about 15%. There was large interpatient variability (%CV in the range of 60% to 70%) in the data, especially for ethinylestradiol. Mean serum levels of LH, FSH and progesterone were not significantly affected. CellCept may not have any influence on the ovulation-suppressing action of the studied oral contraceptives. However, it is recommended that oral contraceptives are coadministered with CellCept with caution and additional birth control methods be considered (see PRECAUTIONS: *Pregnancy*).

Trimethoprim/sulfamethoxazole: Following single-dose administration of mycophenolate mofetil (1.5 g) to 12 healthy male volunteers on day 8 of a 10 day course of Bactrim™* DS (trimethoprim 160 mg/sulfamethoxazole 800 mg) administered bid, no effect on the bioavailability of MPA was observed. The mean (±SD) AUC and C_{max} of MPA after concomitant administration were 75.2 (±19.8) µg•h/mL and 34.0 (±6.6) µg/mL, respectively, compared to 79.2 (±27.9) µg•h/mL and 34.2 (±10.7) µg/mL, respectively, after administration of mycophenolate mofetil alone.

*Bactrim is a trademark of Hoffmann-La Roche Inc.

Other Interactions: The measured value for renal clearance of MPAG indicates removal occurs by renal tubular secretion as well as glomerular filtration. Consistent with this, coadministration of probenecid, a known inhibitor of tubular secretion, with mycophenolate mofetil in monkeys results in a 3-fold increase in plasma MPAG AUC and a 2-fold increase in plasma MPA AUC. Thus, other drugs known to undergo renal tubular secretion may compete

Continued on next page

CellCept—Cont.

with MPAG and thereby raise plasma concentrations of MPAG or the other drug undergoing tubular secretion.

Drugs that alter the gastrointestinal flora may interact with mycophenolate mofetil by disrupting enterohepatic recirculation. Interference of MPAG hydrolysis may lead to less MPA available for absorption.

Live Vaccines: During treatment with CellCept, the use of live attenuated vaccines should be avoided and patients should be advised that vaccinations may be less effective (see PRECAUTIONS: *General*). Influenza vaccination may be of value. Prescribers should refer to national guidelines for influenza vaccination.

Carcinogenesis, Mutagenesis, Impairment of Fertility: In a 104-week oral carcinogenicity study in mice, mycophenolate mofetil in daily doses up to 180 mg/kg was not tumorigenic. The highest dose tested was 0.5 times the recommended clinical dose (2 g/day) in renal transplant patients and 0.3 times the recommended clinical dose (3 g/day) in cardiac transplant patients when corrected for differences in body surface area (BSA). In a 104-week oral carcinogenicity study in rats, mycophenolate mofetil in daily doses up to 15 mg/kg was not tumorigenic. The highest dose was 0.08 times the recommended clinical dose in renal transplant patients and 0.05 times the recommended clinical dose in cardiac transplant patients when corrected for BSA. While these animal doses were lower than those given to patients, they were maximal in those species and were considered adequate to evaluate the potential for human risk (see WARNINGS).

The genotoxic potential of mycophenolate mofetil was determined in five assays. Mycophenolate mofetil was genotoxic in the mouse lymphoma/thymidine kinase assay and the in vivo mouse micronucleus assay. Mycophenolate mofetil was not genotoxic in the bacterial mutation assay, the yeast mitotic gene conversion assay or the Chinese hamster ovary cell chromosomal aberration assay.

Mycophenolate mofetil had no effect on fertility of male rats at oral doses up to 20 mg/kg/day. This dose represents 0.1 times the recommended clinical dose in renal transplant patients and 0.07 times the recommended clinical dose in cardiac transplant patients when corrected for BSA. In a female fertility and reproduction study conducted in rats, oral doses of 4.5 mg/kg/day caused malformations (principally of the head and eyes) in the first generation offspring in the absence of maternal toxicity. This dose was 0.02 times the recommended clinical dose in renal transplant patients and 0.01 times the recommended clinical dose in cardiac transplant patients when corrected for BSA. No effects on fertility or reproductive parameters were evident in the dams or in the subsequent generation.

Pregnancy: *Category C.* In teratology studies in rats and rabbits, fetal resorptions and malformations occurred in rats at 6 mg/kg/day and in rabbits at 90 mg/kg/day, in the absence of maternal toxicity. These levels are equivalent to 0.03 to 0.92 times the recommended clinical dose in renal transplant patients and 0.02 to 0.61 times the recommended clinical dose in cardiac transplant patients on a BSA basis. In a female fertility and reproduction study conducted in rats, oral doses of 4.5 mg/kg/day caused malformations (principally of the head and eyes) in the first generation offspring in the absence of maternal toxicity. This dose was 0.02 times the recommended clinical dose in renal transplant patients and 0.01 times the recommended clinical dose in cardiac transplant patients when corrected for BSA.

There are no adequate and well-controlled studies in pregnant women. CellCept should not be used in pregnant women unless the potential benefit justifies the potential risk to the fetus. Effective contraception must be used before beginning CellCept therapy, during therapy and for 6 weeks after CellCept has been stopped (see WARNINGS and PRECAUTIONS: *Information for Patients*).

Nursing Mothers: Studies in rats treated with mycophenolate mofetil have shown mycophenolic acid to be excreted in milk. It is not known whether this drug is excreted in human milk. Because many drugs are excreted in human milk, and because of the potential for serious adverse reactions in nursing infants from mycophenolate mofetil, a decision should be made whether to discontinue nursing or to discontinue the drug, taking into account the importance of the drug to the mother.

Pediatric Use: Based on pharmacokinetic and safety data in pediatric patients after renal transplantation, the recommended dose of CellCept oral suspension is 600 mg/m^2 bid (up to a maximum of 1 g bid). Also see CLINICAL PHARMACOLOGY, CLINICAL STUDIES, ADVERSE REACTIONS, and DOSAGE AND ADMINISTRATION.

Safety and effectiveness in pediatric patients receiving allogeneic cardiac or hepatic transplants have not been established.

Geriatric Use: Clinical studies of CellCept did not include sufficient numbers of subjects aged 65 and over to determine whether they respond differently from younger subjects. Other reported clinical experience has not identified differences in responses between the elderly and younger patients. In general dose selection for an elderly patient should be cautious, reflecting the greater frequency of decreased hepatic, renal or cardiac function and of concomitant or other drug therapy. Elderly patients may be at an increased risk of adverse reactions compared with younger individuals (see ADVERSE REACTIONS).

ADVERSE REACTIONS

The principal adverse reactions associated with the administration of CellCept include diarrhea, leukopenia, sepsis, vomiting, and there is evidence of a higher frequency of certain types of infections eg, opportunistic infection (see WARNINGS). The adverse event profile associated with the administration of CellCept Intravenous has been shown to be similar to that observed after administration of oral dosage forms of CellCept.

CellCept Oral: The incidence of adverse events for CellCept was determined in randomized, comparative, double-blind trials in prevention of rejection in renal (2 active, 1 placebo-controlled trials), cardiac (1 active-controlled trial), and hepatic (1 active-controlled trial) transplant patients.

Elderly patients (≥65 years), particularly those who are receiving CellCept as part of a combination immunosuppressive regimen, may be at increased risk of certain infections (including cytomegalovirus [CMV] tissue invasive disease) and possibly gastrointestinal hemorrhage and pulmonary edema, compared to younger individuals (see PRECAUTIONS).

Safety data are summarized below for all active-controlled trials in renal (2 trials), cardiac (1 trial), and hepatic (1 trial) transplant patients. Approximately 53% of the renal patients, 65% of the cardiac patients, and 48% of the hepatic patients have been treated for more than 1 year. Adverse events reported in ≥20% of patients in the CellCept treatment groups are presented below.

[See table on pages 2858 and 2859]

The placebo-controlled renal transplant study generally showed fewer adverse events occurring in ≥20% of patients. In addition, those that occurred were not only qualitatively similar to the azathioprine-controlled renal transplant studies, but also occurred at lower rates, particularly for infection, leukopenia, hypertension, diarrhea and respiratory infection.

The above data demonstrate that in three controlled trials for prevention of renal rejection, patients receiving 2 g/day of CellCept had an overall better safety profile than did patients receiving 3 g/day of CellCept.

The above data demonstrate that the types of adverse events observed in multicenter controlled trials in renal, cardiac, and hepatic transplant patients are qualitatively similar except for those that are unique to the specific organ involved.

Sepsis, which was generally CMV viremia, was slightly more common in renal transplant patients treated with CellCept compared to patients treated with azathioprine. The incidence of sepsis was comparable in CellCept and in azathioprine-treated patients in cardiac and hepatic studies.

In the digestive system, diarrhea was increased in renal and cardiac transplant patients receiving CellCept compared to patients receiving azathioprine, but was comparable in hepatic transplant patients treated with CellCept or azathioprine.

Patients receiving CellCept alone or as part of an immunosuppressive regimen are at increased risk of developing lymphomas and other malignancies, particularly of the skin (see WARNINGS). The incidence of malignancies among the 1483 patients treated in controlled trials for the prevention of renal allograft rejection who were followed for ≥1 year was similar to the incidence reported in the literature for renal allograft recipients.

Lymphoproliferative disease or lymphoma developed in 0.4% to 1% of patients receiving CellCept (2 g or 3 g daily) with other immunosuppressive agents in controlled clinical trials of renal, cardiac, and hepatic transplant patients followed for at least 1 year (see WARNINGS). Non-melanoma skin carcinomas occurred in 1.6% to 4.2% of patients, other types of malignancy in 0.7% to 2.1% of patients. Three-year safety data in renal and cardiac transplant patients did not reveal any unexpected changes in incidence of malignancy compared to the 1-year data.

In pediatric patients, no other malignancies besides lymphoproliferative disorder (2/148 patients) have been observed.

Severe neutropenia (ANC <0.5 × 10^3/µL) developed in up to 2.0% of renal transplant patients, up to 2.8% of cardiac transplant patients and up to 3.6% of hepatic transplant patients receiving CellCept 3 g daily (see WARNINGS, PRECAUTIONS: *Laboratory Tests* and DOSAGE AND ADMINISTRATION).

All transplant patients are at increased risk of opportunistic infections. The risk increases with total immunosuppressive load (see WARNINGS). The following table shows the incidence of opportunistic infections that occurred in the renal, cardiac, and hepatic transplant populations in the azathioprine-controlled prevention trials:

[See table below]

The following other opportunistic infections occurred with an incidence of less than 4% in CellCept patients in the above azathioprine-controlled studies: Herpes zoster, visceral disease; Candida, urinary tract infection, fungemia/disseminated disease, tissue invasive disease; Cryptococcosis; Aspergillus/Mucor; Pneumocystis carinii.

In the placebo-controlled renal transplant study, the same pattern of opportunistic infection was observed compared to the azathioprine-controlled renal studies, with a notably lower incidence of the following: Herpes simplex and CMV tissue-invasive disease.

In patients receiving CellCept (2 g or 3 g) in controlled studies for prevention of renal, cardiac or hepatic rejection, fatal infection/sepsis occurred in approximately 2% of renal and cardiac patients and in 5% of hepatic patients (see WARNINGS).

In cardiac transplant patients, the overall incidence of opportunistic infections was approximately 10% higher in patients treated with CellCept than in those receiving azathioprine, but this difference was not associated with excess mortality due to infection/sepsis among patients treated with CellCept.

The following adverse events were reported with 3% to <20% incidence in renal, cardiac, and hepatic transplant patients treated with CellCept, in combination with cyclosporine and corticosteroids.

Viral and Fungal Infections in Controlled Studies in Prevention of Renal, Cardiac or Hepatic Transplant Rejection

	Renal Studies			Cardiac Study		Hepatic Study	
	CellCept 2 g/day	CellCept 3 g/day	Azathioprine 1 to 2 mg/kg/day or 100 to 150 mg/day	CellCept 3 g/day	Azathioprine 1.5 to 3 mg/kg/day	CellCept 3 g/day	Azathioprine 1 to 2 mg/kg/day
	(n=336)	(n=330)	(n=326)	(n=289)	(n=289)	(n=277)	(n=287)
	%	%	%	%	%	%	%
Herpes simplex	16.7	20.0	19.0	20.8	14.5	10.1	5.9
CMV							
–Viremia/syndrome	13.4	12.4	13.8	12.1	10.0	14.1	12.2
–Tissue invasive disease	8.3	11.5	6.1	11.4	8.7	5.8	8.0
Herpes zoster	6.0	7.6	5.8	10.7	5.9	4.3	4.9
–Cutaneous disease	6.0	7.3	5.5	10.0	5.5	4.3	4.9
Candida	17.0	17.3	18.1	18.7	17.6	22.4	24.4
–Mucocutaneous	15.5	16.4	15.3	18.0	17.3	18.4	17.4

Adverse Events Reported in 3% to <20% of Patients Treated With CellCept in Combination With Cyclosporine and Corticosteroids

Body System	
Body as a Whole	abdomen enlarged, abscess, accidental injury, cellulitis, chills occurring with fever, cyst, face edema, flu syndrome, hemorrhage, hernia, lab test abnormal, malaise, neck pain, pelvic pain, peritonitis
Hemic and Lymphatic	coagulation disorder, ecchymosis, pancytopenia, petechia, polycythemia, prothrombin time increased, thromboplastin time increased
Urogenital	acute kidney failure, albuminuria, dysuria, hydronephrosis, hematuria, impotence, kidney failure, kidney tubular necrosis, nocturia, oliguria, pain, prostatic disorder, pyelonephritis, scrotal edema, urine abnormality, urinary frequency, urinary incontinence, urinary retention, urinary tract disorder

Cardiovascular	angina pectoris, arrhythmia, arterial thrombosis, atrial fibrillation, atrial flutter, bradycardia, cardiovascular disorder, congestive heart failure, extrasystole, heart arrest, heart failure, hypotension, pallor, palpitation, pericardial effusion, peripheral vascular disorder, postural hypotension, pulmonary hypertension, supraventricular tachycardia, supraventricular extrasystoles, syncope, tachycardia, thrombosis, vasodilatation, vasospasm, ventricular extrasystole, ventricular tachycardia, venous pressure increased
Metabolic and Nutritional	abnormal healing, acidosis, alkaline phosphatase increased, alkalosis, bilirubinemia, creatinine increased, dehydration, gamma glutamyl transpeptidase increased, generalized edema, gout, hypercalcemia, hypercholesteremia, hyperlipemia, hyperphosphatemia, hyperuricemia, hypervolemia, hypocalcemia, hypochloremia, hypoglycemia, hyponatremia, hypophosphatemia, hypoproteinemia, hypovolemia, hypoxia, lactic dehydrogenase increased, respiratory acidosis, SGOT increased, SGPT increased, thirst, weight gain, weight loss
Digestive	anorexia, cholangitis, cholestatic jaundice, dysphagia, esophagitis, flatulence, gastritis, gastroenteritis, gastrointestinal disorder, gastrointestinal hemorrhage, gastrointestinal moniliasis, gingivitis, gum hyperplasia, hepatitis, ileus, infection, jaundice, liver damage, liver function tests abnormal, melena, mouth ulceration, nausea and vomiting, oral moniliasis, rectal disorder, stomach ulcer, stomatitis
Respiratory	apnea, asthma, atelectasis, bronchitis, epistaxis, hemoptysis, hiccup, hyperventilation, lung edema, lung disorder, neoplasm, pain, pharyngitis, pleural effusion, pneumonia, pneumothorax, respiratory disorder, respiratory moniliasis, rhinitis, sinusitis, sputum increased, voice alteration
Skin and Appendages	acne, alopecia, fungal dermatitis, hemorrhage, hirsutism, pruritus, rash, skin benign neoplasm, skin carcinoma, skin disorder, skin hypertrophy, skin ulcer, sweating, vesiculobullous rash
Nervous	agitation, anxiety, confusion, convulsion, delirium, depression, dry mouth, emotional lability, hallucinations, hypertonia, hypesthesia, nervousness, neuropathy, paresthesia, psychosis, somnolence, thinking abnormal, vertigo
Endocrine	Cushing's syndrome, diabetes mellitus, hypothyroidism, parathyroid disorder
Musculoskeletal	arthralgia, joint disorder, leg cramps, myalgia, myasthenia, osteoporosis
Special Senses	abnormal vision, amblyopia, cataract (not specified), conjunctivitis, deafness, ear disorder, ear pain, eye hemorrhage, tinnitus, lacrimation disorder

Pediatrics: The type and frequency of adverse events in a clinical study in 100 pediatric patients 3 months to 18 years of age dosed with CellCept oral suspension 600 mg/m^2 bid (up to 1 g bid) were generally similar to those observed in adult patients dosed with CellCept capsules at a dose of 1 g bid with the exception of abdominal pain, fever, infection, pain, sepsis, diarrhea, vomiting, pharyngitis, respiratory tract infection, hypertension, and anemia, which were observed in a higher proportion in pediatric patients.

CellCept Intravenous: The adverse event profile of CellCept Intravenous was determined from a single, double-blind, controlled comparative study of the safety of 2 g/day of intravenous and oral CellCept in renal transplant patients in the immediate posttransplant period (administered for the first 5 days). The potential venous irritation of CellCept Intravenous was evaluated by comparing the adverse events attributable to peripheral venous infusion of CellCept Intravenous with those observed in the intravenous placebo group; patients in this group received active medication by the oral route.

Adverse events attributable to peripheral venous infusion were phlebitis and thrombosis, both observed at 4% in patients treated with CellCept Intravenous.

In the active controlled study in hepatic transplant patients, 2 g/day of CellCept Intravenous were administered in the immediate posttransplant period (up to 14 days). The safety profile of intravenous CellCept was similar to that of intravenous azathioprine.

Postmarketing Experience

Digestive: colitis (sometimes caused by cytomegalovirus), pancreatitis, isolated cases of intestinal villous atrophy.

Resistance Mechanism Disorders: Serious life-threatening infections such as meningitis and infectious endocarditis have been reported occasionally and there is evidence of a higher frequency of certain types of serious infections such as tuberculosis and atypical mycobacterial infection.

Respiratory: Interstitial lung disorders, including fatal pulmonary fibrosis, have been reported rarely and should be considered in the differential diagnosis of pulmonary symptoms ranging from dyspnea to respiratory failure in posttransplant patients receiving CellCept.

OVERDOSAGE

There has been no reported experience of overdosage of mycophenolate mofetil in humans. The highest dose administered to renal transplant patients in clinical trials has been 4 g/day. In limited experience with cardiac and hepatic transplant patients in clinical trials, the highest doses used were 4 g/day or 5 g/day. At doses of 4 g/day or 5 g/day, there appears to be a higher rate, compared to the use of 3 g/day or less, of gastrointestinal intolerance (nausea, vomiting, and/or diarrhea), and occasional hematologic abnormalities, principally neutropenia, leading to a need to reduce or discontinue dosing.

In acute oral toxicity studies, no deaths occurred in adult mice at doses up to 4000 mg/kg or in adult monkeys at doses up to 1000 mg/kg; these were the highest doses of mycophenolate mofetil tested in these species. These doses represent 11 times the recommended clinical dose in renal transplant patients and approximately 7 times the recommended clinical dose in cardiac transplant patients when corrected for BSA. In adult rats, deaths occurred after single-oral doses of 500 mg/kg of mycophenolate mofetil. The dose represents approximately 3 times the recommended clinical dose in cardiac transplant patients when corrected for BSA.

MPA and MPAG are usually not removed by hemodialysis. However, at high MPAG plasma concentrations (>100 µg/mL), small amounts of MPAG are removed. By increasing excretion of the drug, MPA can be removed by bile acid sequestrants, such as cholestyramine (see CLINICAL PHARMACOLOGY: *Pharmacokinetics*).

DOSAGE AND ADMINISTRATION

RENAL TRANSPLANTATION:

Adults: A dose of 1 g administered orally or intravenously (over NO LESS THAN 2 HOURS) twice a day (daily dose of 2 g) is recommended for use in renal transplant patients. Although a dose of 1.5 g administered twice daily (daily dose of 3 g) was used in clinical trials and was shown to be safe and effective, no efficacy advantage could be established for renal transplant patients. Patients receiving 2 g/day of CellCept demonstrated an overall better safety profile than did patients receiving 3 g/day of CellCept.

Pediatrics: The recommended dose of CellCept oral suspension is 600 mg/m^2 administered twice daily (up to a maximum daily dose of 2 g/10 mL oral suspension). Patients with a body surface area of 1.25 m^2 to 1.5 m^2 may be dosed with CellCept capsules at a dose of 750 mg twice daily (1.5 g daily dose). Patients with a body surface area >1.5 m^2 may be dosed with CellCept capsules or tablets at a dose of 1 g twice daily (2 g daily dose).

CARDIAC TRANSPLANTATION: A dose of 1.5 g bid administered intravenously (over NO LESS THAN 2 HOURS) or 1.5 g bid oral (daily dose of 3 g) is recommended for use in adult cardiac transplant patients.

HEPATIC TRANSPLANTATION: A dose of 1 g bid administered intravenously (over NO LESS THAN 2 HOURS) or 1.5 g bid oral (daily dose of 3 g) is recommended for use in adult hepatic transplant patients.

CellCept Capsules, Tablets, and Oral Suspension: The initial oral dose of CellCept should be given as soon as possible following renal, cardiac or hepatic transplantation. Food had no effect on MPA AUC, but has been shown to decrease MPA C_{max} by 40%. Therefore, it is recommended that CellCept be administered on an empty stomach. However, in stable renal transplant patients, CellCept may be administered with food if necessary.

Note:

If required, CellCept Oral Suspension can be administered via a nasogastric tube with a minimum size of 8 French (minimum 1.7 mm interior diameter).

Patients With Hepatic Impairment: No dose adjustments are recommended for renal patients with severe hepatic parenchymal disease. However, it is not known whether dose adjustments are needed for hepatic disease with other etiologies (see CLINICAL PHARMACOLOGY: *Pharmacokinetics*).

No data are available for cardiac transplant patients with severe hepatic parenchymal disease.

Geriatrics: The recommended oral dose of 1 g bid for renal transplant patients, 1.5 g bid for cardiac transplant patients, and 1 g bid administered intravenously or 1.5 g bid administered orally in hepatic transplant patients is appropriate for elderly patients (see PRECAUTIONS: *Geriatric Use*).

Preparation of Oral Suspension

It is recommended that CellCept Oral Suspension be constituted by the pharmacist prior to dispensing to the patient. CellCept Oral Suspension should not be mixed with any other medication.

Mycophenolate mofetil has demonstrated teratogenic effects in rats and rabbits. There are no adequate and well-controlled studies in pregnant women. (See WARNINGS, PRECAUTIONS, ADVERSE REACTIONS, and HANDLING AND DISPOSAL.) Care should be taken to avoid inhalation or direct contact with skin or mucous membranes of the dry powder or the constituted suspension. If such contact occurs, wash thoroughly with soap and water; rinse eyes with water.

1. Tap the closed bottle several times to loosen the powder.
2. Measure 94 mL of water in a graduated cylinder.
3. Add approximately half the total amount of water for constitution to the bottle and shake the closed bottle well for about 1 minute.
4. Add the remainder of water and shake the closed bottle well for about 1 minute.
5. Remove the child-resistant cap and push bottle adapter into neck of bottle.
6. Close bottle with child-resistant cap tightly. This will assure the proper seating of the bottle adapter in the bottle and child-resistant status of the cap.

Dispense with patient instruction sheet and oral dispensers. It is recommended to write the date of expiration of the constituted suspension on the bottle label. (The shelf-life of the constituted suspension is 60 days.)

After constitution the oral suspension contains 200 mg/mL mycophenolate mofetil. Store constituted suspension at 25°C (77°F); excursions permitted to 15° to 30°C (59° to 86°F). Storage in a refrigerator at 2° to 8°C (36° to 46°F) is acceptable. Do not freeze. Discard any unused portion 60 days after constitution.

CellCept Intravenous: CellCept Intravenous is an alternative dosage form to CellCept capsules, tablets and oral suspension recommended for patients unable to take oral CellCept. CellCept Intravenous should be administered within 24 hours following transplantation. CellCept Intravenous can be administered for up to 14 days; patients should be switched to oral CellCept as soon as they can tolerate oral medication.

CellCept Intravenous must be reconstituted and diluted to a concentration of 6 mg/mL using 5% Dextrose Injection USP. CellCept Intravenous is incompatible with other intravenous infusion solutions. Following reconstitution, CellCept Intravenous must be administered by slow intravenous infusion over a period of NO LESS THAN 2 HOURS by either peripheral or central vein.

CAUTION: CELLCEPT INTRAVENOUS SOLUTION SHOULD NEVER BE ADMINISTERED BY RAPID OR BOLUS INTRAVENOUS INJECTION (see WARNINGS).

Preparation of Infusion Solution (6 mg/mL)

Caution should be exercised in the handling and preparation of solutions of CellCept Intravenous. Avoid direct contact of the prepared solution of CellCept Intravenous with skin or mucous membranes. If such contact occurs, wash thoroughly with soap and water; rinse eyes with plain water. (See WARNINGS, PRECAUTIONS, ADVERSE REACTIONS, and HANDLING AND DISPOSAL.)

CellCept Intravenous does not contain an antibacterial preservative; therefore, reconstitution and dilution of the product must be performed under aseptic conditions.

CellCept Intravenous infusion solution must be prepared in two steps: the first step is a reconstitution step with 5% Dextrose Injection USP, and the second step is a dilution step with 5% Dextrose Injection USP. A detailed description of the preparation is given below:

Step 1

a. Two (2) vials of CellCept Intravenous are used for preparing each 1 g dose, whereas three (3) vials are needed for each 1.5 g dose. Reconstitute the contents of each vial by injecting 14 mL of 5% Dextrose Injection USP.
b. Gently shake the vial to dissolve the drug.
c. Inspect the resulting slightly yellow solution for particulate matter and discoloration prior to further dilution. Discard the vials if particulate matter or discoloration is observed.

Step 2

a. To prepare a 1 g dose, further dilute the contents of the two reconstituted vials (approx. 2 × 15 mL) into 140 mL of 5% Dextrose Injection USP. To prepare a 1.5 g dose, further dilute the contents of the three reconstituted vials (approx. 3 × 15 mL) into 210 mL of 5% Dextrose Injection USP. The final concentration of both solutions is 6 mg mycophenolate mofetil per mL.
b. Inspect the infusion solution for particulate matter or discoloration. Discard the infusion solution if particulate matter or discoloration is observed.

If the infusion solution is not prepared immediately prior to administration, the commencement of administration of the infusion solution should be within 4 hours from reconstitution and dilution of the drug product. Keep solutions at 25°C (77°F); excursions permitted to 15° to 30°C (59° to 86°F).

CellCept Intravenous should not be mixed or administered concurrently via the same infusion catheter with other intravenous drugs or infusion admixtures.

Dosage Adjustments: In renal transplant patients with severe chronic renal impairment (GFR <25 mL/min/

Continued on next page

CellCept—Cont.

1.73 m^2) outside the immediate posttransplant period, doses of CellCept greater than 1 g administered twice a day should be avoided. These patients should also be carefully observed. No dose adjustments are needed in renal transplant patients experiencing delayed graft function postoperatively (see CLINICAL PHARMACOLOGY: *Pharmacokinetics* and PRECAUTIONS: *General*).

No data are available for cardiac or hepatic transplant patients with severe chronic renal impairment. CellCept may be used for cardiac or hepatic transplant patients with severe chronic renal impairment if the potential benefits outweigh the potential risks.

If neutropenia develops (ANC $<1.3 \times 10^3/\mu L$), dosing with CellCept should be interrupted or the dose reduced, appropriate diagnostic tests performed, and the patient managed appropriately (see WARNINGS, ADVERSE REACTIONS, and PRECAUTIONS: *Laboratory Tests*).

HANDLING AND DISPOSAL: Mycophenolate mofetil has demonstrated teratogenic effects in rats and rabbits (see PRECAUTIONS: Pregnancy). CellCept tablets should not be crushed and CellCept capsules should not be opened or crushed. Avoid inhalation or direct contact with skin or mucous membranes of the powder contained in CellCept capsules and CellCept Oral Suspension (before or after constitution). If such contact occurs, wash thoroughly with soap and water; rinse eyes with plain water. Should a spill occur, wipe up using paper towels wetted with water to remove spilled powder or suspension. Caution should be exercised in the handling and preparation of solutions of CellCept Intravenous. Avoid direct contact of the prepared solution of CellCept Intravenous with skin or mucous membranes. If such contact occurs, wash thoroughly with soap and water; rinse eyes with plain water.

HOW SUPPLIED

CellCept (mycophenolate mofetil capsules)
250 mg
Blue-brown, two-piece hard gelatin capsules, printed in black with "CellCept 250" on the blue cap and "Roche" on the brown body. Supplied in the following presentations:

NDC Number	Size
NDC 0004-0259-01	Bottle of 100
NDC 0004-0259-05	Package containing 12 bottles of 120
NDC 0004-0259-43	Bottle of 500

Storage: Store at 25°C (77°F); excursions permitted to 15° to 30°C (59° to 86°F).

CellCept (mycophenolate mofetil tablets)
500 mg
Lavender-colored, caplet-shaped, film-coated tablets printed in black with "CellCept 500" on one side and "Roche" on the other. Supplied in the following presentations:

NDC Number	Size
NDC 0004-0260-01	Bottle of 100
NDC 0004-0260-43	Bottle of 500

Storage and Dispensing Information: Store at 25°C (77°F); excursions permitted to 15° to 30°C (59° to 86°F). Dispense in light-resistant containers, such as the manufacturer's original containers.

CellCept Oral Suspension (mycophenolate mofetil for oral suspension)
Supplied as a white to off-white powder blend for constitution to a white to off-white mixed-fruit flavor suspension. Supplied in the following presentation:

NDC Number	Size
NDC 0004-0261-29	225 mL bottle with bottle adapter and 2 oral dispensers

Storage: Store dry powder at 25°C (77°F); excursions permitted to 15° to 30°C (59° to 86°F). Store constituted suspension at 25°C (77°F); excursions permitted to 15° to 30°C (59° to 86°F) for up to 60 days. Storage in a refrigerator at 2° to 8°C (36° to 46°F) is acceptable. Do not freeze.

CellCept Intravenous (mycophenolate mofetil hydrochloride for injection)
Supplied in a 20 mL, sterile vial containing the equivalent of 500 mg mycophenolate mofetil as the hydrochloride salt in cartons of 4 vials:

NDC Number
NDC 0004-0298-09

Storage: Store powder and reconstituted/infusion solutions at 25°C (77°F); excursions permitted to 15° to 30°C (59° to 86°F).

Revised: March 2003

Shown in Product Identification Guide, page 331

COPEGUS® ℞
[*cō pĕg' ŭs*]
(ribavirin, USP)
TABLETS

COPEGUS (ribavirin) monotherapy is not effective for the treatment of chronic hepatitis C virus infection and should not be used alone for this indication (see WARNINGS).

The primary clinical toxicity of ribavirin is hemolytic anemia. The anemia associated with ribavirin therapy may result in worsening of cardiac disease that has led to fatal and nonfatal myocardial infarctions. Patients with a history of significant or unstable cardiac disease should not be treated with ribavirin (see WARNINGS, ADVERSE REACTIONS, and DOSAGE AND ADMINISTRATION).

Significant teratogenic and/or embryocidal effects have been demonstrated in all animal species exposed to ribavirin. In addition, ribavirin has a multiple dose half-life of 12 days, and it may persist in non-plasma compartments for as long as 6 months. Ribavirin therapy is contraindicated in women who are pregnant and in the male partners of women who are pregnant. Extreme care must be taken to avoid pregnancy during therapy and for 6 months after completion of therapy in both female patients and in female partners of male patients who are taking ribavirin therapy. At least two reliable forms of effective contraception must be utilized during treatment and during the 6-month posttreatment follow-up period (see CONTRAINDICATIONS, WARNINGS, and PRECAUTIONS: Information for Patients, and Pregnancy: Category X).

DESCRIPTION

COPEGUS, the Hoffmann-La Roche brand name for ribavirin, is a nucleoside analogue with antiviral activity. The chemical name of ribavirin is 1-β-D-ribofuranosyl-1*H*-1,2,4-triazole-3-carboxamide and has the following structural formula:

CONH$_2$ N N N HOCH$_2$ O HO OH

The empirical formula of ribavirin is $C_8H_{12}N_4O_5$ and the molecular weight is 244.2. Ribavirin is a white to off-white powder. It is freely soluble in water and slightly soluble in anhydrous alcohol.

COPEGUS (ribavirin) is available as a light pink to pink colored, flat, oval-shaped, film-coated tablet for oral administration. Each tablet contains 200 mg of ribavirin and the following inactive ingredients: pregelatinized starch, microcrystalline cellulose, sodium starch glycolate, corn starch, and magnesium stearate. The coating of the tablet contains Chromatone-P® or Opadry® Pink (made by using hydroxypropyl methyl cellulose, talc, titanium dioxide, synthetic yellow iron oxide, and synthetic red iron oxide), ethyl cellulose (ECD-30), and triacetin.

Mechanism of Action
Ribavirin is a synthetic nucleoside analogue. The mechanism by which the combination of ribavirin and an interferon product exerts its effects against the hepatitis C virus has not been fully established.

CLINICAL PHARMACOLOGY

Pharmacokinetics
Multiple dose ribavirin pharmacokinetic data are available for HCV patients who received ribavirin in combination with peginterferon alfa-2a. Following administration of 1200 mg/day with food for 12 weeks mean±SD (n=39; body weight >75 kg) $AUC_{0\text{-}12hr}$ was 25,361±7110 ng•hr/mL and C_{max} was 2748±818 ng/mL. The average time to reach C_{max} was 2 hours. Trough ribavirin plasma concentrations following 12 weeks of dosing with food were 1662±545 ng/mL in HCV infected patients who received 800 mg/day (n=89), and 2112±810 ng/mL in patients who received 1200 mg/day (n=75; body weight >75 kg).

The terminal half-life of ribavirin following administration of a single oral dose of COPEGUS is about 120 to 170 hours. The total apparent clearance following administration of a single oral dose of COPEGUS is about 26 L/h. There is extensive accumulation of ribavirin after multiple dosing (twice daily) such that the C_{max} at steady state was four-fold higher than that of a single dose.

Effect of Food on Absorption of Ribavirin
Bioavailability of a single oral dose of ribavirin was increased by co-administration with a high-fat meal. The absorption was slowed (T_{max} was doubled) and the $AUC_{0\text{-}192h}$ and C_{max} increased by 42% and 66%, respectively, when COPEGUS was taken with a high-fat meal compared with fasting conditions (see **PRECAUTIONS** and **DOSAGE AND ADMINISTRATION**).

Elimination and Metabolism
The contribution of renal and hepatic pathways to ribavirin elimination after administration of COPEGUS is not known. In vitro studies indicate that ribavirin is not a substrate of CYP450 enzymes.

Special Populations
Race
There were insufficient numbers of non-Caucasian subjects studied to adequately determine potential pharmacokinetic differences between populations.

Renal Dysfunction
The pharmacokinetics of ribavirin following administration of COPEGUS have not been studied in patients with renal impairment and there are limited data from clinical trials on administration of COPEGUS in patients with creatinine clearance <50 mL/min. Therefore, patients with creatinine clearance <50 mL/min should not be treated with COPEGUS (see **WARNINGS** and **DOSAGE AND ADMINISTRATION**).

Hepatic Impairment
The effect of hepatic impairment on the pharmacokinetics of ribavirin following administration of COPEGUS has not been evaluated. The clinical trials of COPEGUS were restricted to patients with Child-Pugh class A disease.

Pediatric Patients
Pharmacokinetic evaluations in pediatric patients have not been performed.

Elderly Patients
Pharmacokinetic evaluations in elderly patients have not been performed.

Gender
Ribavirin pharmacokinetics, when corrected for weight, are similar in male and female patients.

Drug Interactions
In vitro studies indicate that ribavirin does not inhibit CYP450 enzymes.

Nucleoside Analogues
Ribavirin has been shown in vitro to inhibit phosphorylation of zidovudine and stavudine which could lead to decreased antiretroviral activity. Exposure to didanosine or its active metabolite (dideoxyadenosine 5'-triphosphate) is increased when didanosine is co-administered with ribavirin, which could cause or worsen clinical toxicities (see **PRECAUTIONS: Drug Interactions**).

Clinical Studies
The safety and effectiveness of PEGASYS® in combination with COPEGUS for the treatment of hepatitis C virus infection were assessed in two randomized controlled clinical trials. All patients were adults, had compensated liver disease, detectable hepatitis C virus, liver biopsy diagnosis of chronic hepatitis, and were previously untreated with interferon. Approximately 20% of patients in both studies had compensated cirrhosis (Child-Pugh class A).

In study NV15801 (described as study 4 in the PEGASYS Package Insert), patients were randomized to receive either PEGASYS 180 µg sc once weekly (qw) with an oral placebo, PEGASYS 180 µg qw with COPEGUS 1000 mg po (body weight <75 kg) or 1200 mg po (body weight ≥75 kg) or REBETRON® (interferon alfa-2b 3 MIU sc tiw plus ribavirin 1000 mg or 1200 mg po). All patients received 48 weeks of therapy followed by 24 weeks of treatment-free follow-up. COPEGUS or placebo treatment assignment was blinded. PEGASYS in combination with COPEGUS resulted in a higher SVR (defined as undetectable HCV RNA at the end of the 24-week treatment-free follow-up period) compared to PEGASYS alone or interferon alfa-2b and ribavirin (Table 1). In all treatment arms, patients with viral genotype 1, regardless of viral load, had a lower response rate to PEGASYS in combination with COPEGUS compared to patients with other viral genotypes.

Table 1 Sustained Virologic Response (SVR) to Combination Therapy (Study NV15801*)

	Interferon alfa-2b+ Ribavirin 1000 mg or 1200 mg	PEGASYS + placebo	PEGASYS + COPEGUS 1000 mg or 1200 mg
All patients	197/444 (44%)	65/224 (29%)	241/453 (53%)
Genotype 1	103/285 (36%)	29/145 (20%)	132/298 (44%)
Genotypes 2-6	94/159 (59%)	36/79 (46%)	109/155 (70%)

Difference in overall treatment response (PEGASYS/COPEGUS–Interferon alfa-2b/ribavirin) was 9% (95% CI 2.3, 15.3).
* Described as study 4 in the PEGASYS Package Insert.

In study NV15942 (described as study 5 in the PEGASYS Package Insert), all patients received PEGASYS 180 µg sc qw and were randomized to treatment for either 24 or 48 weeks and to a COPEGUS dose of either 800 mg or 1000 mg/1200 mg (for body weight <75 kg/≥75 kg). Assignment to the four treatment arms was stratified by viral genotype and baseline HCV viral titer. Patients with genotype 1 and high viral titer (defined as $>2 \times 10^6$ HCV RNA copies/mL serum) were preferentially assigned to treatment for 48 weeks.

Genotype 1
Irrespective of baseline viral titer, treatment for 48 weeks with PEGASYS and 1000 mg or 1200 mg of COPEGUS resulted in higher SVR (defined as undetectable HCV RNA at the end of the 24-week treatment-free follow-up period) compared to shorter treatment (24 weeks) and/or 800 mg COPEGUS.

Genotype non-1
Irrespective of baseline viral titer, treatment for 24 weeks with PEGASYS and 800 mg of COPEGUS resulted in a similar SVR compared to longer treatment (48 weeks) and/or 1000 mg or 1200 mg of COPEGUS (see Table 2).

[See table 2 at bottom of next page]

Among the 36 patients with genotype 4, response rates were similar to those observed in patients with genotype 1 (data not shown). The numbers of patients with genotype 5 and 6 were too few to allow for meaningful assessment.

Treatment Response in Patient Subgroups

Treatment response rates are lower in patients with poor prognostic factors receiving pegylated interferon alpha therapy. In studies NV15801 and NV15942, treatment response rates were lower in patients older than 40 years (50% vs 66%), in patients with cirrhosis (47% vs 59%), in patients weighing over 85 kg (49% vs 60%), and in patients with genotype 1 with high vs low viral load (43% vs 56%). African American patients had lower response rates compared to Caucasians.

Paired liver biopsies were performed on approximately 20% of patients in studies NV15801 and NV15942. Modest reductions in inflammation compared to baseline were seen in all treatment groups.

In studies NV15801 and NV15942, lack of early virologic response at 12 weeks (defined as HCV RNA undetectable or >2log10 lower than baseline) was grounds for discontinuation of treatment. Of patients who lacked an early viral response at 12 weeks and completed a recommended course of therapy despite a protocol-defined option to discontinue therapy, 5/39 (13%) achieved an SVR. Of patients who lacked an early viral response at 24 weeks, nineteen completed a full course of therapy and none achieved an SVR.

INDICATIONS AND USAGE

COPEGUS in combination with PEGASYS (peginterferon alfa-2a) is indicated for the treatment of adults with chronic hepatitis C virus infection who have compensated liver disease and have not been previously treated with interferon alpha. Patients in whom efficacy was demonstrated included patients with compensated liver disease and histological evidence of cirrhosis (Child-Pugh class A).

CONTRAINDICATIONS

COPEGUS (ribavirin) is contraindicated in:

- Patients with known hypersensitivity to COPEGUS or to any component of the tablet.
- Women who are pregnant.
- Men whose female partners are pregnant.
- Patients with hemoglobinopathies (eg, thalassemia major or sickle-cell anemia).

COPEGUS and PEGASYS combination therapy is contraindicated in patients with:

- Autoimmune hepatitis.
- Hepatic decompensation (Child-Pugh class B and C) before or during treatment.

WARNINGS

COPEGUS must not be used alone because ribavirin monotherapy is not effective for the treatment of chronic hepatitis C virus infection. The safety and efficacy of COPEGUS have only been established when used together with PEGASYS (pegylated interferon alfa-2a, recombinant).

COPEGUS and PEGASYS should be discontinued in patients who develop evidence of hepatic decompensation during treatment.

There are significant adverse events caused by COPEGUS/PEGASYS therapy, including severe depression and suicidal ideation, hemolytic anemia, suppression of bone marrow function, autoimmune and infectious disorders, pulmonary dysfunction, pancreatitis, and diabetes. The PEGASYS package insert and MEDICATION GUIDE should be reviewed in their entirety prior to initiation of combination treatment for additional safety information.

General

Treatment with COPEGUS and PEGASYS should be administered under the guidance of a qualified physician and may lead to moderate to severe adverse experiences requiring dose reduction, temporary dose cessation or discontinuation of therapy.

Pregnancy

Ribavirin may cause birth defects and/or death of the exposed fetus. Extreme care must be taken to avoid pregnancy in female patients and in female partners of male patients. Ribavirin has demonstrated significant teratogenic and/or embryocidal effects in all animal species in which adequate studies have been conducted. These effects occurred at doses as low as one twentieth of the recommended human dose of ribavirin. COPEGUS THERAPY SHOULD NOT BE STARTED UNLESS A REPORT OF A NEGATIVE PREGNANCY TEST HAS BEEN OBTAINED IMMEDIATELY PRIOR TO PLANNED INITIATION OF THERAPY. Patients should be instructed to use at least two forms of effective contraception during treatment and for 6 months after treatment has been stopped. Pregnancy testing should occur monthly during COPEGUS therapy and for 6 months after therapy has stopped (see CONTRAINDICATIONS and PRECAUTIONS: Information for Patients and Pregnancy: Category X).

Anemia

The primary toxicity of ribavirin is hemolytic anemia (hemoglobin <10 g/dL), which was observed in approximately 13% of COPEGUS and PEGASYS treated patients in clinical trials (see PRECAUTIONS: Laboratory Tests). The anemia associated with COPEGUS occurs within 1 to 2 weeks of initiation of therapy. BECAUSE THE INITIAL DROP IN HEMOGLOBIN MAY BE SIGNIFICANT, IT IS ADVISED THAT HEMOGLOBIN OR HEMATOCRIT BE OBTAINED PRETREATMENT AND AT WEEK 2 AND WEEK 4 OF THERAPY OR MORE FREQUENTLY IF CLINICALLY INDICATED. Patients should then be followed as clinically appropriate.

Fatal and nonfatal myocardial infarctions have been reported in patients with anemia caused by ribavirin. Patients should be assessed for underlying cardiac disease before initiation of ribavirin therapy. Patients with pre-existing cardiac disease should have electrocardiograms administered before treatment, and should be appropriately monitored during therapy. If there is any deterioration of cardiovascular status, therapy should be suspended or discontinued (see DOSAGE AND ADMINISTRATION: COPEGUS Dosage Modification Guidelines). Because cardiac disease may be worsened by drug induced anemia, patients with a history of significant or unstable cardiac disease should not use COPEGUS (see ADVERSE REACTIONS).

Pulmonary

Pulmonary symptoms, including dyspnea, pulmonary infiltrates, pneumonitis and occasional cases of fatal pneumonia, have been reported during therapy with ribavirin and interferon. In addition, sarcoidosis or the exacerbation of sarcoidosis has been reported. If there is evidence of pulmonary infiltrates or pulmonary function impairment, the patient should be closely monitored, and if appropriate, combination COPEGUS/PEGASYS treatment should be discontinued.

Other

COPEGUS and PEGASYS therapy should be suspended in patients with signs and symptoms of pancreatitis, and discontinued in patients with confirmed pancreatitis.

COPEGUS should not be used in patients with creatinine clearance <50 mL/min (see **CLINICAL PHARMACOLOGY: Special Populations**).

COPEGUS must be discontinued immediately and appropriate medical therapy instituted if an acute hypersensitivity reaction (eg, urticaria, angioedema, bronchoconstriction, anaphylaxis) develops. Transient rashes do not necessitate interruption of treatment.

PRECAUTIONS

The safety and efficacy of COPEGUS and PEGASYS therapy for the treatment of HIV infection, adenovirus, RSV, parainfluenza or influenza infections have not been established. COPEGUS should not be used for these indications. Ribavirin for inhalation has a separate package insert, which should be consulted if ribavirin inhalation therapy is being considered.

The safety and efficacy of COPEGUS and PEGASYS therapy have not been established in liver or other organ transplant patients, patients with decompensated liver disease due to hepatitis C virus infection, patients who are non-responders to interferon therapy or patients co-infected with HBV or HIV.

Information for Patients

Patients must be informed that ribavirin may cause birth defects and/or death of the exposed fetus. COPEGUS therapy must not be used by women who are pregnant or by men whose female partners are pregnant. Extreme care must be taken to avoid pregnancy in female patients and in female partners of male patients taking COPEGUS therapy and for 6 months posttherapy. COPEGUS therapy should not be initiated until a report of a negative pregnancy test has been obtained immediately prior to initiation of therapy. Patients must perform a pregnancy test monthly during therapy and for 6 months posttherapy.

Female patients of childbearing potential and male patients with female partners of childbearing potential must be advised of the teratogenic/embryocidal risks and must be instructed to practice effective contraception during COPEGUS therapy and for 6 months posttherapy. Patients should be advised to notify the healthcare provider immediately in the event of a pregnancy (see **CONTRAINDICATIONS** and **WARNINGS**).

The most common adverse event associated with ribavirin is anemia, which may be severe (see **ADVERSE REACTIONS**). Patients should be advised that laboratory evaluations are required prior to starting COPEGUS therapy and periodically thereafter (see **Laboratory Tests**). It is advised that patients be well hydrated, especially during the initial stages of treatment.

Patients who develop dizziness, confusion, somnolence, and fatigue should be cautioned to avoid driving or operating machinery.

Patients should be informed regarding the potential benefits and risks attendant to the use of COPEGUS. Instructions on appropriate use should be given, including review of the contents of the enclosed MEDICATION GUIDE, which is not a disclosure of all or possible adverse effects.

Patients should be advised to take COPEGUS with food.

Laboratory Tests

Before beginning COPEGUS therapy, standard hematological and biochemical laboratory tests must be conducted for all patients. Pregnancy screening for women of childbearing potential must be done.

After initiation of therapy, hematological tests should be performed at 2 weeks and 4 weeks and biochemical tests should be performed at 4 weeks. Additional testing should be performed periodically during therapy. Monthly pregnancy testing should be done during combination therapy and for 6 months after discontinuing therapy.

The entrance criteria used for the clinical studies of COPEGUS and PEGASYS combination therapy may be considered as a guideline to acceptable baseline values for initiation of treatment:

- Platelet count ≥90,000 cells/mm^3
- Absolute neutrophil count (ANC) ≥1500 cells/mm^3
- TSH and T_4 within normal limits or adequately controlled thyroid function
- ECG (see **WARNINGS**)

The maximum drop in hemoglobin usually occurred during the first 8 weeks of initiation of COPEGUS therapy. Because of this initial acute drop in hemoglobin, it is advised that a complete blood count should be obtained pretreatment and at week 2 and week 4 of therapy or more frequently if clinically indicated. Additional testing should be performed periodically during therapy. Patients should then be followed as clinically appropriate.

Drug Interactions

Results from a pharmacokinetic sub-study demonstrated no pharmacokinetic interaction between PEGASYS (peginterferon alfa-2a) and ribavirin.

Nucleoside Analogues

Didanosine

Co-administration of COPEGUS and didanosine is not recommended. Reports of fatal hepatic failure, as well as peripheral neuropathy, pancreatitis, and symptomatic hyperlactatemia/lactic acidosis have been reported in clinical trials (see **CLINICAL PHARMACOLOGY: Drug Interactions**).

Stavudine and Zidovudine

Ribavirin can antagonize the in vitro antiviral activity of stavudine and zidovudine against HIV. Therefore, concomitant use of ribavirin with either of these drugs should be avoided (see **CLINICAL PHARMACOLOGY: Drug Interactions**).

Carcinogenesis, Mutagenesis, Impairment of Fertility

Carcinogenesis

The carcinogenic potential of ribavirin has not been fully determined. In a p53 (+/−) mouse carcinogenicity study at doses up to the maximum tolerated dose of 100 mg/kg/day, ribavirin was not oncogenic. However, on a body surface area basis, this dose was 0.5 times the maximum recommended human 24-hour dose of ribavirin. A study to assess the carcinogenic potential of ribavirin in rats is ongoing.

Mutagenesis

Ribavirin demonstrated mutagenic activity in the in vitro mouse lymphoma assay. No clastogenic activity was observed in an in vivo mouse micronucleus assay at doses up to 2000 mg/kg. However, results from studies published in the literature show clastogenic activity in the in vivo mouse micronucleus assay at oral doses up to 2000 mg/kg. A dominant lethal assay in rats was negative, indicating that if mutations occurred in rats they were not transmitted through male gametes. However, potential carcinogenic risk to humans cannot be excluded.

Impairment of Fertility

In a fertility study in rats, ribavirin showed a marginal reduction in sperm counts at the dose of 100 mg/kg/day with no effect on fertility. Upon cessation of treatment, total recovery occurred after 1 spermatogenesis cycle. Abnormalities in sperm were observed in studies in mice designed to evaluate the time course and reversibility of ribavirin-induced testicular degeneration at doses of 15 to 150 mg/kg/day (approximately 0.1-0.8 times the maximum recommended human 24-hour dose of ribavirin) administered for 3 to 6 months. Upon cessation of treatment, essentially total recovery from ribavirin-induced testicular toxicity was apparent within 1 or 2 spermatogenic cycles.

Female patients of childbearing potential and male patients with female partners of childbearing potential should not receive COPEGUS unless the patient and his/her partner are using effective contraception (two reliable forms). Based on a multiple dose half-life ($t_{1/2}$) of ribavirin of 12 days, effective contraception must be utilized for 6 months posttherapy (ie, 15 half-lives of clearance for ribavirin).

No reproductive toxicology studies have been performed using PEGASYS in combination with COPEGUS. However, peginterferon alfa-2a and ribavirin when administered sep-

Table 2 Sustained Virologic Response as a Function of Genotype (Study NV15942*)

	24 Weeks Treatment		48 Weeks Treatment	
	PEGASYS + COPEGUS 800 mg (N=207)	PEGASYS + COPEGUS 1000 mg or 1200 mg** (N=280)	PEGASYS + COPEGUS 800 mg (N=361)	PEGASYS + COPEGUS 1000 mg or 1200 mg** (N=436)
Genotype 1	29/101 (29%)	48/118 (41%)	99/250 (40%)	138/271 (51%)
Gentoype 2-3	79/96 (82%)	116/144 (81%)	75/99 (76%)	117/153 (76%)

* Described as study 5 in the PEGASYS Package Insert.

**1000 mg for body weight <75 kg; 1200 mg for body weight ≥75 kg.

Continued on next page

Copegus—Cont.

arately, each has adverse effects on reproduction. It should be assumed that the effects produced by either agent alone would also be caused by the combination of the two agents.

Pregnancy

Pregnancy: Category X (see **CONTRAINDICATIONS**)
Ribavirin produced significant embryocidal and/or teratogenic effects in all animal species in which adequate studies have been conducted. Malformations of the skull, palate, eye, jaw, limbs, skeleton, and gastrointestinal tract were noted. The incidence and severity of teratogenic effects increased with escalation of the drug dose. Survival of fetuses and offspring was reduced.

In conventional embryotoxicity/teratogenicity studies in rats and rabbits, observed no-effect dose levels were well below those for proposed clinical use (0.3 mg/kg/day for both the rat and rabbit; approximately 0.06 times the recommended human 24-hour dose of ribavirin). No maternal toxicity or effects on offspring were observed in a peri/postnatal toxicity study in rats dosed orally at up to 1 mg/kg/day (approximately 0.01 times the maximum recommended human 24-hour dose of ribavirin).

Treatment and Posttreatment: Potential Risk to the Fetus
Ribavirin is known to accumulate in intracellular components from where it is cleared very slowly. It is not known whether ribavirin is contained in sperm, and if so, will exert a potential teratogenic effect upon fertilization of the ova. In a study in rats, it was concluded that dominant lethality was not induced by ribavirin at doses up to 200 mg/kg for 5 days (up to 1.7 times the maximum recommended human dose of ribavirin). However, because of the potential human teratogenic effects of ribavirin, male patients should be advised to take every precaution to avoid risk of pregnancy for their female partners.

COPEGUS should not be used by pregnant women or by men whose female partners are pregnant. Female patients of childbearing potential and male patients with female partners of childbearing potential should not receive COPEGUS unless the patient and his/her partner are using effective contraception (two reliable forms) during therapy and for 6 months posttherapy.

Ribavirin Pregnancy Registry
A Ribavirin Pregnancy Registry has been established to monitor maternal-fetal outcomes of of female patients and female partners of male patients exposed to ribavirin during treatment and for 6 months following cessation of treatment. Healthcare providers and patients are encouraged to report such cases by calling 1-800-593-2214.

Animal Toxicology
Long-term study in the mouse and rat (18-24 months; dose 20-75 and 10-40 mg/kg/day, respectively, approximately 0.1-0.4 times the maximum human daily dose of ribavirin) have demonstrated a relationship between chronic ribavirin exposure and an increased incidence of vascular lesions (microscopic hemorrhages) in mice. In rats, retinal degeneration occurred in controls, but the incidence was increased in ribavirin-treated rats.

Nursing Mothers

It is not known whether ribavirin is excreted in human milk. Because many drugs are excreted in human milk and to avoid any potential for serious adverse reactions in nursing infants from ribavirin, a decision should be made either to discontinue nursing or therapy with COPEGUS, based on the importance of the therapy to the mother.

Pediatric Use

Safety and effectiveness of COPEGUS have not been established in patients below the age of 18.

Geriatric Use

Clinical studies of COPEGUS and PEGASYS did not include sufficient numbers of subjects aged 65 or over to determine whether they respond differently from younger subjects. Specific pharmacokinetic evaluations for ribavirin in the elderly have not been performed. The risk of toxic reactions to this drug may be greater in patients with impaired renal function. COPEGUS should not be administered to patients with creatinine clearance <50 mL/min. (see **CLINICAL PHARMACOLOGY: Special Populations**).

Effect of Gender

No clinically significant differences in the pharmacokinetics of ribavirin were observed between male and female subjects.

ADVERSE REACTIONS

PEGASYS in combination with COPEGUS causes a broad variety of serious adverse reactions (see **BOXED WARNING** and **WARNINGS**). In all studies, one or more serious adverse reactions occurred in 10% of patients receiving PEGASYS in combination with COPEGUS.

The most common life-threatening or fatal events induced or aggravated by PEGASYS and COPEGUS were depression, suicide, relapse of drug abuse/overdose, and bacterial infections; each occurred at a frequency of <1%.

Nearly all patients in clinical trials experienced one or more adverse events. The most commonly reported adverse reactions were psychiatric reactions, including depression, irritability, anxiety, and flu-like symptoms such as fatigue, pyrexia, myalgia, headache and rigors.

Ten percent of patients receiving 48 weeks of therapy with PEGASYS in combination with COPEGUS discontinued therapy. The most common reasons for discontinuation of therapy were psychiatric, flu-like syndrome (eg, lethargy, fatigue, headache), dermatologic and gastrointestinal disorders.

The most common reason for dose modification in patients receiving combination therapy was for laboratory abnormalities; neutropenia (20%) and thrombocytopenia (4%) for PEGASYS and anemia (22%) for COPEGUS.

PEGASYS dose was reduced in 12% of patients receiving 1000 mg to 1200 mg COPEGUS for 48 weeks and in 7% of patients receiving 800 mg COPEGUS for 24 weeks. COPEGUS dose was reduced in 21% of patients receiving 1000 mg to 1200 mg COPEGUS for 48 weeks and 12% in patients receiving 800 mg COPEGUS for 24 weeks.

Because clinical trials are conducted under widely varying and controlled conditions, adverse reaction rates observed in clinical trials of a drug cannot be directly compared to rates in the clinical trials of another drug. Also, the adverse event rates listed here may not predict the rates observed in a broader patient population in clinical practice.

Table 3 Adverse Reactions Occurring in ≥5% of Patients in Hepatitis C Clinical Trials (Study NV15801*)

Body System	PEGASYS 180 µg + 1000 mg or 1200 mg COPEGUS 48 wk	Intron A + 1000 mg or 1200 mg REBETOL® 48 wk
	N=451	N=443
	%	%
Application Site Disorders		
Injection site reaction	23	16
Endocrine Disorders		
Hypothyroidism	4	5
Flu-like Symptoms and Signs		
Fatigue/Asthenia	65	68
Pyrexia	41	55
Rigors	25	37
Pain	10	9
Gastrointestinal		
Nausea/vomiting	25	29
Diarrhea	11	10
Abdominal pain	8	9
Dry mouth	4	7
Dyspepsia	6	5
Hematologic**		
Lymphopenia	14	12
Anemia	11	11
Neutropenia	27	8
Thrombocytopenia	5	<1
Metabolic and Nutritional		
Anorexia	24	26
Weight decrease	10	10
Musculoskeletal, Connective Tissue and Bone		
Myalgia	40	49
Arthralgia	22	23
Back pain	5	5
Neurological		
Headache	43	49
Dizziness (excluding vertigo)	14	14
Memory impairment	6	5
Psychiatric		
Irritability/Anxiety/ Nervousness	33	38
Insomnia	30	37
Depression	20	28
Concentration impairment	10	13
Mood alteration	5	6
Resistance Mechanism Disorders		
Overall	12	10
Respiratory, Thoracic and Mediastinal		
Dyspnea	13	14
Cough	10	7
Dyspnea exertional	4	7
Skin and Subcutaneous Tissue		
Alopecia	28	33
Pruritus	19	18
Dermatitis	16	13
Dry Skin	10	13
Rash	8	5
Sweating Increased	6	5
Eczema	5	4
Visual Disorders		
Vision Blurred	5	2

* Described as study 4 in the PEGASYS Package Insert.
** Severe hematologic abnormalities.

Patients treated for 24 weeks with PEGASYS and 800 mg COPEGUS were observed to have lower incidence of serious adverse events (3% vs 10%), hemoglobin <10g/dL (3% vs 15%), dose modification of PEGASYS (30% vs 36%) and COPEGUS (19% vs 38%) and of withdrawal from treatment (5% vs 15%) compared to patients treated for 48 weeks with PEGASYS and 1000 mg or 1200 mg COPEGUS. On the other hand the overall incidence of adverse events appeared to be similar in the two treatment groups.

The most common serious adverse event (3%) was bacterial infection (eg, sepsis, osteomyelitis, endocarditis, pyelonephritis, pneumonia). Other SAEs occurred at a frequency of <1% and included: suicide, suicidal ideation, psychosis, aggression, anxiety, drug abuse and drug overdose, angina, hepatic dysfunction, fatty liver, cholangitis, arrhythmia, diabetes mellitus, autoimmune phenomena (eg, hyperthyroidism, hypothyroidism, sarcoidosis, systemic lupus erythematosis, rheumatoid arthritis) peripheral neuropathy, aplastic anemia, peptic ulcer, gastrointestinal bleeding, pancreatitis, colitis, corneal ulcer, pulmonary embolism, coma, myositis, and cerebral hemorrhage.

Laboratory Test Values

Anemia due to hemolysis is the most significant toxicity of ribavirin therapy. Anemia (hemoglobin <10 g/dL) was observed in 13% of COPEGUS and PEGASYS combination-treated patients in clinical trials. The maximum drop in hemoglobin occurred during the first 8 weeks of initiation of ribavirin therapy (see **DOSAGE AND ADMINISTRATION: Dose Modifications**).

OVERDOSAGE

No cases of overdose with COPEGUS have been reported in clinical trials.

DOSAGE AND ADMINISTRATION

The recommended dose of COPEGUS tablets is provided in Table 4. The recommended duration of treatment for patients previously untreated with ribavirin and interferon is 24 to 48 weeks.

The daily dose of COPEGUS is 800 mg to 1200 mg administered orally in two divided doses. The dose should be individualized to the patient depending on baseline disease characteristics (eg, genotype), response to therapy, and tolerability of the regimen (see Table 4).

In the pivotal clinical trials, patients were instructed to take COPEGUS with food; therefore, patients are advised to take COPEGUS with food.

[See table 4 at left]

Table 4 PEGASYS and COPEGUS Dosing Recommendations

Genotype	PEGASYS Dose	COPEGUS Dose	Duration
Genotype 1, 4	180 µg	<75 kg = 1000 mg ≥75 kg = 1200 mg	48 weeks 48 weeks
Genotype 2, 3	180 µg	800 mg	24 weeks

Genotypes non-1 showed no increased response to treatment beyond 24 weeks (see Table 2).
Data on genotypes 5 and 6 are insufficient for dosing recommendations.

Dose Modifications

If severe adverse reactions or laboratory abnormalities develop during combination COPEGUS/PEGASYS therapy, the dose should be modified or discontinued, if appropriate, until the adverse reactions abate. If intolerance persists after dose adjustment, COPEGUS/PEGASYS therapy should be discontinued.

COPEGUS should be administered with caution to patients with pre-existing cardiac disease (see Table 5). Patients should be assessed before commencement of therapy and should be appropriately monitored during therapy. If there is any deterioration of cardiovascular status, therapy should be stopped (see **WARNINGS**).

Table 5 COPEGUS Dosage Modification Guidelines

Laboratory Values	Reduce Only COPEGUS Dose to 600 mg/day* if:	Discontinue COPEGUS if:
Hemoglobin in patients with no cardiac disease	<10 g/dL	<8.5 g/dL
Hemoglobin in patients with history of stable cardiac disease	≥2 g/dL decrease in hemoglobin during any 4 week period treatment	<12 g/dL despite 4 weeks at reduced dose

*One 200 mg tablet in the morning and two 200 mg tablets in the evening.

Once COPEGUS has been withheld due to either a laboratory abnormality or clinical manifestation, an attempt may be made to restart COPEGUS at 600 mg daily and further increase the dose to 800 mg daily depending upon the physician's judgment. However, it is not recommended that COPEGUS be increased to its original assigned dose (1000 mg to 1200 mg).

Renal Impairment

COPEGUS should not be used in patients with creatinine clearance <50 mL/min (see **WARNINGS** and **CLINICAL PHARMACOLOGY: Special Populations**).

HOW SUPPLIED

COPEGUS™ (ribavirin) is available as tablets for oral administration. Each tablet contains 200 mg of ribavirin and is light pink to pink colored, flat, oval-shaped, film-coated, and engraved with RIB 200 on one side and ROCHE on the other side. They are packaged as bottle of 168 tablets (NDC 0004-0086-94).

Storage Conditions

Store the COPEGUS Tablets bottle at 25°C (77°F); excursions are permitted between 15° and 30°C (59° and 86°F) [see USP Controlled Room Temperature]. Keep bottle tightly closed.

REBETRON® is a registered trademark of Schering Corporation.

MEDICATION GUIDE

Read this Medication Guide carefully before you start taking COPEGUS and read the Medication Guide each time you get more COPEGUS. There may be new information. This information does not take the place of talking to your healthcare provider about your medical condition or your treatment.

What is the most important information I should know about COPEGUS?

1. **COPEGUS, a form of ribavirin, may cause birth defects or death of an unborn child. Therefore, if you are pregnant or your partner is pregnant or plans to become pregnant, do not take COPEGUS.** Female patients and female partners of male patients being treated with COPEGUS must not become pregnant during treatment and for 6 months after treatment has stopped.
   During this time you must have pregnancy tests that show you are not pregnant. You must also use 2 effective forms of birth control during therapy and for 6 months after stopping therapy. Male patients should use a condom with spermicide as one of the two forms.
   If pregnancy occurs, report the pregnancy to your healthcare provider right away. (See **"What should I avoid while taking COPEGUS?"**)
   If you or a female sexual partner becomes pregnant, you should tell your healthcare provider. There is a Ribavirin Pregnancy Registry that collects information about pregnancy outcomes of female patients and female partners of male patients exposed to ribavirin. You or your healthcare provider are encouraged to contact the Registry at 1-800-593-2214
2. **COPEGUS can cause a dangerous drop in your red blood cell count.** COPEGUS can cause anemia, which is a decrease in the number of red blood cells. This can be dangerous, especially if you have heart or breathing problems. This may cause a worsening of heart (cardiovascular) or circulatory problems. Some patients may get chest pain and rarely, a heart attack. Patients with a history of heart disease have the highest chance of this. Tell your healthcare provider, before taking COPEGUS if you have or have ever had any heart or breathing problems. Your healthcare provider should check your red blood cell count before you start treatment with COPEGUS and often during the first 4 weeks of treatment. Your red blood cell count may be done more often if you have any heart or breathing problems.
3. **Do not take COPEGUS alone to treat hepatitis C virus infection.** COPEGUS does not treat hepatitis C virus infections by itself. COPEGUS should be used in combination with PEGASYS® (peginterferon alfa-2a) to treat continuing (chronic) hepatitis C virus infections. You should read the Medication Guide for PEGASYS because it has additional important information about treatment that is not covered in this Medication Guide. Your healthcare provider or pharmacist should give you a copy of the PEGASYS Medication Guide.

What is COPEGUS?

COPEGUS is the antiviral medicine ribavirin. It is used in combination with a medicine called PEGASYS (peginterferon alfa-2a) to treat some adults with chronic hepatitis C whose liver still works normally, and who have not been treated before with a medicine called an interferon alpha. It is not known how COPEGUS and PEGASYS work together to fight hepatitis C virus infections.

It is not known if treatment with COPEGUS and PEGASYS combination therapy can cure hepatitis C or if it can prevent liver damage (cirrhosis), liver failure or liver cancer that is caused by hepatitis C virus infections. It is not known if treatment with COPEGUS and PEGASYS combination therapy will prevent an infected person from spreading the hepatitis C virus to another person.

Treatment with COPEGUS has not been studied in children under 18 years of age.

Who should not take COPEGUS?

Do not use COPEGUS if:

- **You are a female and you are pregnant or plan to become pregnant** during treatment or during the 6 months after your treatment has ended. (See **"What is the most important information I should know about COPEGUS?"** and **"What should I avoid while taking COPEGUS?"**)
- **You are a male patient with a female sexual partner who is pregnant or plans to become pregnant** at any time while you are being treated with COPEGUS or during the 6 months after your treatment has ended. (See **"What is the most important information I should know about COPEGUS?"** and **"What should I avoid while taking COPEGUS?"**)
- **You are breast feeding. We do not know if COPEGUS can pass through your milk and if it can harm your baby. You will need to choose either to breast-feed or take COPEGUS, but not both.**
- **You have a liver disease called autoimmune hepatitis** (hepatitis caused by your immune system attacking your liver).
- **You have unstable or advanced liver disease.**
- **You are allergic to any of the ingredients in COPEGUS.** The active ingredient in COPEGUS is ribavirin. See the end of this Medication Guide for a list of all the ingredients in COPEGUS.

Tell your healthcare provider before starting treatment with COPEGUS in combination with PEGASYS (see also the PEGASYS Medication Guide) if you have any of the following medical conditions:

- **mental health problems, such as depression or anxiety:** COPEGUS and PEGASYS combination therapy may make them worse. Tell your healthcare provider if you are being treated or had treatment in the past for any mental problems, including depression, thoughts of ending your life (suicidal thoughts) or a feeling of loss of contact with reality, such as hearing voices or seeing things that are not there (psychosis). Tell your healthcare provider if you take any medicines for these problems.
- **high blood pressure, heart problems or have had a heart attack.** COPEGUS may worsen heart problems such as high blood pressure, increased heart rate, and chest pain. Tell your healthcare provider if you have or had a heart problem. Patients who have had certain heart problems should not take COPEGUS.
- **blood disorders,** including anemia (low red blood cell count), thalassemia (Mediterranean anemia) and sickle-cell anemia. COPEGUS can reduce the number of red blood cells you have. This may make you feel dizzy or weak and could worsen any heart problems you might have.
- **kidney problems.** If your kidneys do not work properly, you may have worse side effects from COPEGUS treatment and require a lower dose.
- **liver problems** (other than hepatitis C virus infection).
- **organ transplant,** and you are taking medicine that keeps your body from rejecting your transplant (suppresses your immune system).
- **thyroid disease.** COPEGUS and PEGASYS combination therapy may make your thyroid disease worse or harder to treat. COPEGUS and PEGASYS treatment may be stopped if you develop thyroid problems that cannot be controlled by medicine.
- **have or had drug or alcohol addiction or abuse.**
- **cancer.**
- **infection with hepatitis B virus and/or human immunodeficiency virus** (HIV, the virus that causes AIDS).
- **diabetes.** COPEGUS and PEGASYS combination therapy may make your diabetes worse or harder to treat.
- **past interferon treatment for hepatitis C virus infection that did not work for you.**

Tell your healthcare provider about all the medicines you take, including prescription and non-prescription medicines, vitamins or herbal supplements. Some medicines can cause serious side effects if taken while you also take COPEGUS. Some medicines may affect how COPEGUS works or COPEGUS may affect how your other medicines work. Be especially sure to tell your healthcare provider if you take any medicines to treat HIV.

For more information see the PEGASYS Medication Guide.

How should I take COPEGUS?

- Your healthcare provider will determine the right dose of COPEGUS based on your weight.
- Take COPEGUS 1 time in the morning and 1 time at night (2 times a day). Take COPEGUS the same 2 times each day.
- Take COPEGUS with food.
- It is very important to follow your dosing schedule and your healthcare provider's instructions on how to take your medicines.
- Take COPEGUS for as long as it is prescribed, and do not take more than your healthcare provider prescribes.
- If you miss a dose of COPEGUS and remember **the same day,** take the missed dose as soon as you remember. If **the whole day has passed,** ask your healthcare provider what to do. Do not take 2 doses at the same time.
- Your healthcare provider may adjust your dose of COPEGUS based on blood tests that show your response to treatment and side effects you may have.
- **Females taking COPEGUS or female sexual partners of male patients taking COPEGUS must have a pregnancy test:**
- before treatment begins
- every month during treatment
- for 6 months after treatment ends to make sure there is no pregnancy

It is also important not to use other ribavirin medicines without talking to your healthcare provider. Please see the PEGASYS Medication Guide for the proper use of PEGASYS injection.

What should I avoid while taking COPEGUS?

Avoid the following during COPEGUS treatment:

- **Do not get pregnant.** If you or your sexual partner get pregnant during treatment with COPEGUS or in the 6 months after treatment ends, tell your healthcare provider right away. (See **"What is the most important information I should know about treatment with COPEGUS?"**) Talk with your healthcare provider about birth control methods and how to avoid pregnancy. You must use extreme care to avoid pregnancy during and for 6 months after treatment in female and male patients.
- **Do not take COPEGUS alone to treat your hepatitis C virus infection.** COPEGUS should be used in combination with PEGASYS (peginterferon alfa-2a) to treat chronic hepatitis C virus infections. (See **"What is the most important information I should know about treatment with COPEGUS?"**)
- **Do not breast feed.** COPEGUS may pass through your milk and may harm your baby.
- **Do not drink alcohol,** including beer, wine, and liquor. This may make your liver disease worse.
- **Do not drive or operate machinery** if COPEGUS makes you feel tired, dizzy or confused.
- **Do not take other medicines unless your healthcare provider knows about them.** Take only medicines prescribed or approved by your healthcare provider. These include prescription and non-prescription medicines, vitamins or herbal supplements. Talk to your healthcare provider before starting any new medicine.

What are the possible side effects of COPEGUS?

The most serious possible side effects of COPEGUS are:

- **Harm to unborn children.** COPEGUS may cause birth defects or death of an unborn child. (For more details, see **"What is the most important information I should know about treatment with COPEGUS?"**)
- **Anemia.** Anemia is a reduction in the number of red blood cells you have. Anemia can be dangerous, especially if you have heart or breathing problems. Tell your healthcare provider right away if you feel tired, have chest pain or shortness of breath. These may be signs of low red blood cell counts.

Call your healthcare provider right away if you have any of the following symptoms. They may be signs of a serious side effect of COPEGUS and PEGASYS treatment.

- trouble breathing
- hives or swelling
- chest pain
- severe stomach pain or low back pain
- bloody diarrhea or bloody stools (bowel movements). These may look like black tar.
- bruising or unusual bleeding
- change in your vision
- high fever (temperature greater than 100.5°F)
- you have psoriasis (a skin disease) and it gets worse
- you become very depressed or think about suicide (ending your life)

The most common side effects of COPEGUS are likely to be the same as for other ribavirin products. These are:

- feeling tired
- nausea and appetite loss
- rash and itching
- cough

These are not all the possible side effects of COPEGUS treatment. For more information, ask your doctor or pharmacist and see the PEGASYS Medication Guide.

What should I know about hepatitis C infection?

Hepatitis C infection is a disease caused by a virus that infects the liver. Hepatitis C is more serious for some people than others. Most people who get hepatitis C carry the virus in their blood for the rest of their lives. Most of these people will have some liver damage, but many do not feel sick from the disease. In some people, the liver becomes badly dam-

Continued on next page

Copegus—Cont.

aged and scarred. This is called cirrhosis. Cirrhosis can cause the liver to stop working. Some people may get liver cancer or liver failure from the hepatitis C virus.

Hepatitis C virus is spread from one person to another by contact with an infected person's blood. You should talk to your healthcare provider about ways to prevent you from infecting others.

How should I store COPEGUS?

Store COPEGUS tablets at room temperature (77 °F).

Please refer to the PEGASYS Medication Guide for storage information about PEGASYS injection.

General information about the safe and effective use of COPEGUS

Medicines are sometimes prescribed for purposes other than those listed in a Medication Guide. Do not use COPEGUS for a condition for which it was not prescribed. Do not give COPEGUS to other people, even if they have the same symptoms that you have.

This Medication Guide summarizes the most important information about COPEGUS. If you would like more information, talk with your healthcare provider. You can ask your healthcare provider or pharmacist for information about COPEGUS that is written for healthcare professionals.

What are the ingredients in COPEGUS?

Active Ingredient: ribavirin

Inactive Ingredients: pregelatinized starch, sodium starch glycolate, cornstarch, microcrystalline cellulose, and magnesium stearate. The tablet is coated with aquacoat ECD-30, triacetin, and colored with a coating system composed of hydroxypropyl methyl cellulose, talc, titanium dioxide, synthetic yellow iron oxide, and synthetic red iron oxide.

This Medication Guide has been approved by the U.S. Food and Drug Administration.

CYTOVENE®-IV ℞

(ganciclovir sodium for injection)
FOR INTRAVENOUS INFUSION ONLY
CYTOVENE®
(ganciclovir capsules)
FOR ORAL ADMINISTRATION

The following text is complete prescribing information based on official labeling in effect June 2000.

WARNING: THE CLINICAL TOXICITY OF CYTOVENE AND CYTOVENE-IV INCLUDES GRANULOCYTOPENIA, ANEMIA AND THROMBOCYTOPENIA. IN ANIMAL STUDIES GANCICLOVIR WAS CARCINOGENIC, TERATOGENIC AND CAUSED ASPERMATOGENESIS.

CYTOVENE-IV IS INDICATED FOR USE *ONLY* IN THE TREATMENT OF CYTOMEGALOVIRUS (CMV) RETINITIS IN IMMUNOCOMPROMISED PATIENTS AND FOR THE PREVENTION OF CMV DISEASE IN TRANSPLANT PATIENTS AT RISK FOR CMV DISEASE.

CYTOVENE CAPSULES ARE INDICATED *ONLY* FOR PREVENTION OF CMV DISEASE IN PATIENTS WITH ADVANCED HIV INFECTION AT RISK FOR CMV DISEASE, FOR MAINTENANCE TREATMENT OF CMV RETINITIS IN IMMUNOCOMPROMISED PATIENTS, AND FOR PREVENTION OF CMV DISEASE IN SOLID ORGAN TRANSPLANT RECIPIENTS (see INDICATIONS AND USAGE).

BECAUSE CYTOVENE CAPSULES ARE ASSOCIATED WITH A RISK OF MORE RAPID RATE OF CMV RETINITIS PROGRESSION, THEY SHOULD BE USED AS MAINTENANCE TREATMENT ONLY IN THOSE PATIENTS FOR WHOM THIS RISK IS BALANCED BY THE BENEFIT ASSOCIATED WITH AVOIDING DAILY INTRAVENOUS INFUSIONS.

DESCRIPTION

Ganciclovir is a synthetic guanine derivative active against cytomegalovirus (CMV). CYTOVENE-IV and CYTOVENE are the brand names for ganciclovir sodium for injection and ganciclovir capsules, respectively.

CYTOVENE-IV is available as sterile lyophilized powder in strength of 500 mg per vial for intravenous administration only. Each vial of CYTOVENE-IV contains the equivalent of 500 mg ganciclovir as the sodium salt (46 mg sodium). Reconstitution with 10 mL of Sterile Water for Injection, USP, yields a solution with pH 11 and a ganciclovir concentration of approximately 50 mg/mL. Further dilution in an appropriate intravenous solution must be performed before infusion (see DOSAGE AND ADMINISTRATION).

CYTOVENE is available as 250 mg and 500 mg capsules. Each capsule contains 250 mg or 500 mg ganciclovir, respectively, and inactive ingredients croscarmellose sodium, magnesium stearate and povidone. Both hard gelatin shells consist of gelatin, titanium dioxide, yellow iron oxide and FD&C Blue No. 2.

Ganciclovir is a white to off-white crystalline powder with a molecular formula of $C_9H_{13}N_5O_4$ and a molecular weight of 255.23. The chemical name for ganciclovir is 9-[[2-hydroxy-1-(hydroxymethyl)ethoxy]methyl]guanine. Ganciclovir is a polar hydrophilic compound with a solubility of 2.6 mg/mL in water at 25°C and an n-octanol/water partition coefficient of 0.022. The pK_as for ganciclovir are 2.2 and 9.4.

Ganciclovir, when formulated as monosodium salt in the IV dosage form, is a white to off-white lyophilized powder with a molecular formula of $C_9H_{12}N_5NaO_4$, and a molecular weight of 277.22. The chemical name for ganciclovir sodium is 9-[[2-hydroxy-1-(hydroxymethyl) ethoxy]methyl]guanine, monosodium salt. The lyophilized powder has an aqueous solubility of greater than 50 mg/mL at 25°C. At physiological pH, ganciclovir sodium exists as the un-ionized form with a solubility of approximately 6 mg/mL at 37°C.

All doses in this insert are specified in terms of ganciclovir.

VIROLOGY

Mechanism of Action: Ganciclovir is an acyclic nucleoside analogue of 2′-deoxyguanosine that inhibits replication of herpes viruses. Ganciclovir has been shown to be active against cytomegalovirus (CMV) and herpes simplex virus (HSV) in human clinical studies.

To achieve anti-CMV activity, ganciclovir is phosphorylated first to the monophosphate form by a CMV-encoded (UL97 gene) protein kinase homologue, then to the di- and triphosphate forms by cellular kinases. Ganciclovir triphosphate concentrations may be 100-fold greater in CMV-infected than in uninfected cells, indicating preferential phosphorylation in infected cells. Ganciclovir triphosphate, once formed, persists for days in the CMV-infected cell. Ganciclovir triphosphate is believed to inhibit viral DNA synthesis by (1) competitive inhibition of viral DNA polymerases; and (2) incorporation into viral DNA, resulting in eventual termination of viral DNA elongation.

Antiviral Activity: The median concentration of ganciclovir that inhibits CMV replication (IC_{50}) in vitro (laboratory strains or clinical isolates) has ranged from 0.02 to 3.48 µg/mL. Ganciclovir inhibits mammalian cell proliferation (CIC_{50}) in vitro at higher concentrations ranging from 30 to 725 µg/mL. Bone marrow-derived colony-forming cells are more sensitive (CIC_{50} 0.028 to 0.7 µg/mL). The relationship of in vitro sensitivity of CMV to ganciclovir and clinical response has not been established.

Clinical Antiviral Effect of CYTOVENE-IV and CYTOVENE Capsules: *CYTOVENE-IV:* In a study of CYTOVENE-IV treatment of life- or sight-threatening CMV disease in immunocompromised patients, 121 of 314 patients had CMV cultured within 7 days prior to treatment and sequential posttreatment viral cultures of urine, blood, throat and/or semen. As judged by conversion to culture negativity, or a greater than 100-fold decrease in in vitro CMV titer, at least 83% of patients had a virologic response with a median response time of 7 to 15 days.

Antiviral activity of CYTOVENE-IV was demonstrated in two randomized studies for the prevention of CMV disease in transplant recipients (see table below).

[See table below]

CYTOVENE Capsules: In trials comparing CYTOVENE-IV with CYTOVENE capsules for the maintenance treatment of CMV retinitis in patients with AIDS, serial urine cultures and other available cultures (semen, biopsy specimens, blood and others) showed that a small proportion of patients remained culture-positive during maintenance therapy with no statistically significant differences in CMV isolation rates between treatment groups.

A study of CYTOVENE capsules (1000 mg q8h) for prevention of CMV disease in individuals with advanced HIV infection (ICM 1654) evaluated antiviral activity as measured by CMV isolation in culture; most cultures were from urine. At baseline, 40% (176/436) and 44% (92/210) of ganciclovir and placebo recipients, respectively, had positive cultures (urine or blood). After 2 months on treatment, 10% vs 44% of ganciclovir vs placebo recipients had positive cultures.

Viral Resistance: The current working definition of CMV resistance to ganciclovir in in vitro assays is IC_{50} >3.0 µg/mL (12.0 µM). CMV resistance to ganciclovir has been observed in individuals with AIDS and CMV retinitis who have never received ganciclovir therapy. Viral resistance has also been observed in patients receiving prolonged treatment for CMV retinitis with CYTOVENE-IV. In a controlled study of oral ganciclovir for prevention of AIDS-associated CMV disease, 364 individuals had one or more cultures performed after at least 90 days of ganciclovir treatment. Of these, 113 had at least one positive culture. The last available isolate from each subject was tested for reduced sensitivity, and 2 of 40 were found to be resistant to ganciclovir. These resistant isolates were associated with subsequent treatment failure for retinitis.

The possibility of viral resistance should be considered in patients who show poor clinical response or experience persistent viral excretion during therapy. The principal mechanism of resistance to ganciclovir in CMV is the decreased ability to form the active triphosphate moiety; resistant viruses have been described that contain mutations in the UL97 gene of CMV that controls phosphorylation of ganciclovir. Mutations in the viral DNA polymerase have also been reported to confer viral resistance to ganciclovir.

Patients With Positive CMV Cultures

Time	Heart Allograft* (n=147) CYTOVENE-IV†	Heart Allograft* (n=147) Placebo	Bone Marrow Allograft (n=72) CYTOVENE-IV‡	Bone Marrow Allograft (n=72) Placebo
Pretreatment	1/67 (2%)	5/64 (8%)	37/37 (100%)	35/35 (100%)
Week 2	2/75 (3%)	11/67 (16%)	2/31 (6%)	19/28 (68%)
Week 4	3/66 (5%)	28/66 (43%)	0/24 (0%)	16/20 (80%)

* CMV seropositive or receiving graft from seropositive donor
† 5 mg/kg bid for 14 days followed by 6 mg/kg qd for 5 days/week for 14 days
‡ 5 mg/kg bid for 7 days followed by 5 mg/kg qd until day 100 posttransplant

CLINICAL PHARMACOLOGY

Pharmacokinetics:

BECAUSE THE MAJOR ELIMINATION PATHWAY FOR GANCICLOVIR IS RENAL, DOSAGE REDUCTIONS ACCORDING TO CREATININE CLEARANCE ARE REQUIRED FOR CYTOVENE-IV AND SHOULD BE CONSIDERED FOR CYTOVENE CAPSULES. FOR DOSING INSTRUCTIONS IN PATIENTS WITH RENAL IMPAIRMENT, REFER TO DOSAGE AND ADMINISTRATION.

Absorption: The absolute bioavailability of oral ganciclovir under fasting conditions was approximately 5% (n=6) and following food was 6% to 9% (n=32). When ganciclovir was administered orally with food at a total daily dosage of 3 g/day (500 mg q3h, 6 times daily and 1000 mg tid), the steady-state absorption as measured by area under the serum concentration vs time curve (AUC) over 24 hours and maximum serum concentrations (C_{max}) were similar following both regimens with an AUC_{0-24} of 15.9 ± 4.2 (mean ± SD) and 15.4 ± 4.3 µg·hr/mL and C_{max} of 1.02 ± 0.24 and 1.18 ± 0.36 µg/mL, respectively (n=16).

At the end of a 1-hour intravenous infusion of 5 mg/kg ganciclovir, total AUC ranged between 22.1 ± 3.2 (n=16) and 26.8 ± 6.1 µg·hr/mL (n=16) and C_{max} ranged between 8.27 ± 1.02 (n=16) and 9.0 ± 1.4 µg/mL (n=16).

Food Effects: When CYTOVENE capsules were given with a meal containing 602 calories and 46.5% fat at a dosage of 1000 mg every 8 hours to 20 HIV-positive subjects, the steady-state AUC increased by 22 ± 22% (range: -6% to 68%) and there was a significant prolongation of time to peak serum concentrations (T_{max}) from 1.8 ± 0.8 to 3.0 ± 0.6 hours and a higher C_{max} (0.85 ± 0.25 vs 0.96 ± 0.27 µg/mL) (n=20).

Distribution: The steady-state volume of distribution of ganciclovir after intravenous administration was 0.74 ± 0.15 L/kg (n=98). For CYTOVENE capsules, no correlation was observed between AUC and reciprocal weight (range: 55 to 128 kg); oral dosing according to weight is not required. Cerebrospinal fluid concentrations obtained 0.25 to 5.67 hours postdose in 3 patients who received 2.5 mg/kg ganciclovir intravenously q8h or q12h ranged from 0.31 to 0.68 µg/mL representing 24% to 70% of the respective plasma concentrations. Binding to plasma proteins was 1% to 2% over ganciclovir concentrations of 0.5 and 51 µg/mL.

Metabolism: Following oral administration of a single 1000 mg dose of ^{14}C-labeled ganciclovir, 86 ± 3% of the administered dose was recovered in the feces and 5 ± 1% was recovered in the urine (n=4). No metabolite accounted for more than 1% to 2% of the radioactivity recovered in urine or feces.

Elimination: When administered intravenously, ganciclovir exhibits linear pharmacokinetics over the range of 1.6 to 5.0 mg/kg and when administered orally, it exhibits linear kinetics up to a total daily dose of 4 g/day. Renal excretion of unchanged drug by glomerular filtration and active tubular secretion is the major route of elimination of ganciclovir. In patients with normal renal function, 91.3 ± 5.0% (n=4) of intravenously administered ganciclovir was recovered unmetabolized in the urine. Systemic clearance of intravenously administered ganciclovir was 3.52 ± 0.80 mL/min/kg (n=98) while renal clearance was 3.20 ± 0.80 mL/min/kg (n=47), accounting for 91 ± 11% of the systemic clearance (n=47). After oral administration of ganciclovir, steady-state is achieved within 24 hours. Renal clearance following oral administration was 3.1 ± 1.2 mL/min/kg (n=22). Half-life was 3.5 ± 0.9 hours (n=98) following IV administration and 4.8 ± 0.9 hours (n=39) following oral administration.

Special Populations: *Renal Impairment:* The pharmacokinetics following intravenous administration of CYTOVENE-IV solution were evaluated in 10 immunocompromised patients with renal impairment who received doses ranging from 1.25 to 5.0 mg/kg.

[See first table at top of next page]

The pharmacokinetics of ganciclovir following oral administration of CYTOVENE capsules were evaluated in 44 patients, who were either solid organ transplant recipients or HIV positive. Apparent oral clearance of ganciclovir decreased and AUC_{0-24h} increased with diminishing renal function (as expressed by creatinine clearance). Based on these observations, it is necessary to modify the dosage of ganciclovir in patients with renal impairment (see DOSAGE AND ADMINISTRATION).

Hemodialysis reduces plasma concentrations of ganciclovir by about 50% after both intravenous and oral administration.

Race/Ethnicity and Gender: The effects of race/ethnicity and gender were studied in subjects receiving a dose regimen of 1000 mg every 8 hours. Although the numbers of blacks (16%) and Hispanics (20%) were small, there appeared to be a trend towards a lower steady-state C_{max} and

Estimated Creatinine Clearance (mL/min)	n	Dose	Clearance (mL/min) Mean ± SD	Half-life (hours) Mean ± SD
50–79	4	3.2 – 5 mg/kg	128 ± 63	4.6 ± 1.4
25–49	3	3 – 5 mg/kg	57 ± 8	4.4 ± 0.4
<25	3	1.25 – 5 mg/kg	30 ± 13	10.7 ± 5.7

Population Characteristics in Studies ICM 1653, ICM 1774 and AVI 034

		ICM 1653 (n=121)	ICM 1774 (n=225)	AVI 034 (n=159)
Median age (years) Range		38 24–62	37 22–56	39 23–62
Sex	Males	116 (96%)	222 (99%)	148 (93%)
	Females	5 (4%)	3 (1%)	10 (6%)
Ethnicity	Asian	3 (3%)	5 (2%)	7 (4%)
	Black	11 (9%)	9 (4%)	3 (2%)
	Caucasian	98 (81%)	186 (83%)	140 (88%)
	Other	9 (7%)	25 (11%)	8 (5%)
Median CD_4 Count Range		9.5 0 – 141	7.0 0 – 80	10.0 0 – 320
Mean (SD) Observation Time (days)		107.9 (43.0)	97.6 (42.5)	80.9 (47.0)

AUC_{0-8} in these subpopulations as compared to Caucasians. No definitive conclusions regarding gender differences could be made because of the small number of females (12%); however, no differences between males and females were observed.

Pediatrics: Ganciclovir pharmacokinetics were studied in 27 neonates, aged 2 to 49 days. At an intravenous dose of 4 mg/kg (n=14) or 6 mg/kg (n=13), the pharmacokinetic parameters were, respectively, C_{max} of 5.5 ± 1.6 and 7.0 ± 1.6 µg/mL, systemic clearance of 3.14 ± 1.75 and 3.56 ± 1.27 mL/min/kg, and $t_{½}$ of 2.4 hours (harmonic mean) for both.

Ganciclovir phrmacokinetics were also studied in 10 pediatric patients, aged 9 months to 12 years. The pharmacokinetic characteristics of ganciclovir were the same after single and multiple (q12h) intravenous doses (5 mg/kg). The steady-state volume of distribution was 0.64 ± 0.22 L/kg, C_{max} was 7.9 ± 3.9 µg/mL, systemic clearance was 4.7 ± 2.2 mL/min/kg, and $t_{½}$ was 2.4 ± 0.7 hours. The pharmacokinetics of intravenous ganciclovir in pediatric patients are similar to those observed in adults.

Elderly: No studies have been conducted in adults older than 65 years of age.

INDICATIONS AND USAGE

CYTOVENE-IV is indicated for the treatment of CMV retinitis in immunocompromised patients, including patients with acquired immunodeficiency syndrome (AIDS).

CYTOVENE-IV is also indicated for the prevention of CMV disease in transplant recipients at risk for CMV disease (see CLINICAL TRIALS).

CYTOVENE capsules are indicated for the prevention of CMV disease in solid organ transplant recipients and in individuals with advanced HIV infection at risk for developing CMV disease. CYTOVENE capsules are also indicated as an alternative to the intravenous formulation for maintenance treatment of CMV retinitis in immunocompromised patients, including patients with AIDS, in whom retinitis is stable following appropriate induction therapy and for whom the risk of more rapid progression is balanced by the benefit associated with avoiding daily IV infusions (see CLINICAL TRIALS).

SAFETY AND EFFICACY OF **CYTOVENE-IV** AND **CYTOVENE** HAVE NOT BEEN ESTABLISHED FOR CONGENITAL OR NEONATAL CMV DISEASE; NOR FOR THE TREATMENT OF ESTABLISHED CMV DISEASE OTHER THAN RETINITIS; NOR FOR USE IN NON-IMMUNOCOMPROMISED INDIVIDUALS. THE SAFETY AND EFFICACY OF **CYTOVENE** CAPSULES HAVE NOT BEEN ESTABLISHED FOR TREATING ANY MANIFESTATION OF CMV DISEASE OTHER THAN MAINTENANCE TREATMENT OF CMV RETINITIS.

CLINICAL TRIALS

1. *Treatment of CMV Retinitis*

The diagnosis of CMV retinitis should be made by indirect ophthalmoscopy. Other conditions in the differential diagnosis of CMV retinitis include candidiasis, toxoplasmosis, histoplasmosis, retinal scars and cotton wool spots, any of which may produce a retinal appearance similar to CMV. For this reason it is essential that the diagnosis of CMV be established by an ophthalmologist familiar with the retinal presentation of these conditions. The diagnosis of CMV retinitis may be supported by culture of CMV from urine, blood, throat or other sites, but a negative CMV culture does not rule out CMV retinitis.

Studies With CYTOVENE-IV: In a retrospective, non-randomized, single-center analysis of 41 patients with AIDS and CMV retinitis diagnosed by ophthalmologic examination between August 1983 and April 1988, treatment with CYTOVENE-IV solution resulted in a significant delay in mean (median) time to first retinitis progression compared to untreated controls [105 (71) days from diagnosis vs 35 (29) days from diagnosis]. Patients in this series received induction treatment of CYTOVENE-IV 5 mg/kg bid for 14 to 21 days followed by maintenance treatment with either 5 mg/kg once daily, 7 days per week or 6 mg/kg once daily, 5 days per week (see DOSAGE AND ADMINISTRATION).

In a controlled, randomized study conducted between February 1989 and December 1990,[1] immediate treatment with CYTOVENE-IV was compared to delayed treatment in 42 patients with AIDS and peripheral CMV retinitis; 35 of 42 patients (13 in the immediate-treatment group and 22 in the delayed-treatment group) were included in the analysis of time to retinitis progression. Based on masked assessment of fundus photographs, the mean [95% CI] and median [95% CI] times to progression of retinitis were 66 days [39, 94] and 50 days [40, 84], respectively, in the immediate-treatment group compared to 19 days [11, 27] and 13.5 days [8, 18], respectively, in the delayed-treatment group.

Studies Comparing CYTOVENE Capsules to CYTOVENE-IV: [See second table above]

ICM 1653: In this randomized, open-label, parallel group trial, conducted between March 1991 and November 1992, patients with AIDS and newly diagnosed CMV retinitis received a 3-week induction course of CYTOVENE-IV solution, 5 mg/kg bid for 14 days followed by 5 mg/kg once daily for 1 additional week.[2] Following the 21-day intravenous induction course, patients with stable CMV retinitis were randomized to receive 20 weeks of maintenance treatment with either CYTOVENE-IV solution, 5 mg/kg once daily, or CYTOVENE capsules, 500 mg 6 times daily (3000 mg/day). The study showed that the mean [95% CI] and median [95% CI] times to progression of CMV retinitis, as assessed by masked reading of fundus photographs, were 57 days [44, 70] and 29 days [28, 43], respectively, for patients on oral therapy compared to 62 days [50, 73] and 49 days [29, 61], respectively, for patients on intravenous therapy. The difference [95% CI] in the mean time to progression between the oral and intravenous therapies (oral - IV) was -5 days [-22, 12]. See Figure 1 for comparison of the proportion of patients remaining free of progression over time.

ICM 1774: In this three-arm, randomized, open-label, parallel group trial, conducted between June 1991 and August 1993, patients with AIDS and stable CMV retinitis following from 4 weeks to 4 months of treatment with CYTOVENE-IV solution were randomized to receive maintenance treatment with CYTOVENE-IV solution, 5 mg/kg once daily, CYTOVENE capsules, 500 mg 6 times daily, or CYTOVENE capsules, 1000 mg tid for 20 weeks. The study showed that the mean [95% CI] and median [95% CI] times to progression of CMV retinitis, as assessed by masked reading of fundus photographs, were 54 days [48, 60] and 42 days [31, 54], respectively, for patients on oral therapy compared to 66 days [56, 76] and 54 days [41, 69], respectively, for patients on intravenous therapy. The difference [95% CI] in the mean time to progression between the oral and intravenous therapies (oral - IV) was -12 days [-24, 0]. See Figure 2 for comparison of the proportion of patients remaining free of progression over time.

AVI 034: In this randomized, open-label, parallel group trial, conducted between June 1991 and February 1993, patients with AIDS and newly diagnosed (81%) or previously treated (19%) CMV retinitis who had tolerated 10 to 21 days of induction treatment with CYTOVENE-IV, 5 mg/kg twice daily, were randomized to receive 20 weeks of maintenance treatment with either CYTOVENE capsules, 500 mg 6 times daily or CYTOVENE-IV solution, 5 mg/kg/day.[3] The mean [95% CI] and median [95% CI] times to progression of CMV retinitis, as assessed by masked reading of fundus photographs, were 51 days [44, 57] and 41 days [31, 45], respectively, for patients on oral therapy compared to 62 days [52, 72] and 60 days [42, 83], respectively, for patients on intravenous therapy. The difference [95% CI] in the mean time to progression between the oral and intravenous therapies (oral - IV) was -11 days [-24, 1]. See Figure 3 for comparison of the proportion of patients remaining free of progression over time.

Comparison of other CMV retinitis outcomes between oral and IV formulations (development of bilateral retinitis, progression into Zone 1, and deterioration of visual acuity), while not definitive, showed no marked differences between treatment groups in these studies. Because of low event rates among these endpoints, these studies are underpowered to rule out significant differences in these endpoints.

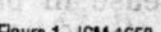
Figure 1 - ICM 1653

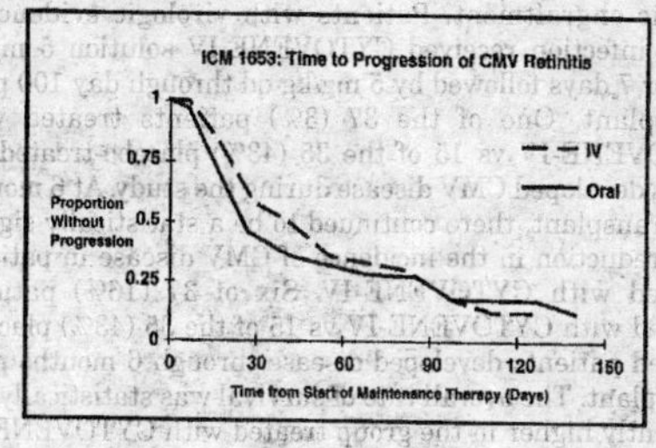

Figure 2 - ICM 1774

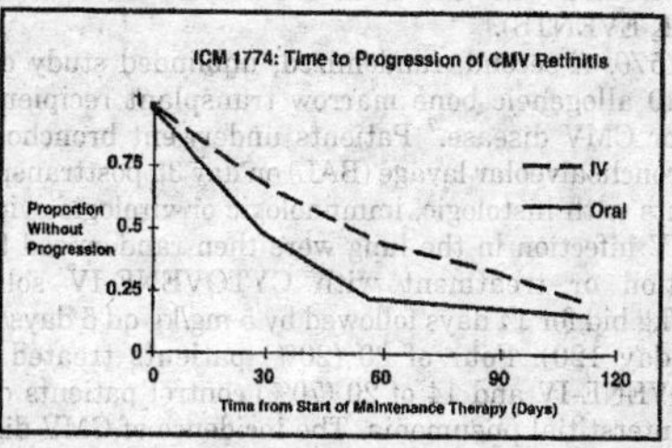

Figure 3 - AVI 034

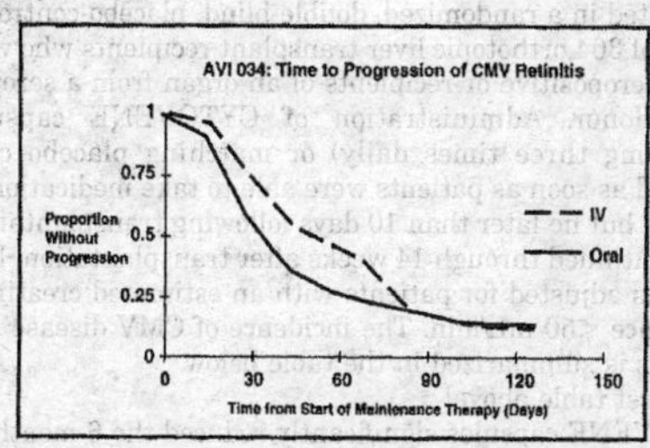

2. *Prevention of CMV Disease in Subjects With AIDS*

ICM 1654: In a double-blind study conducted between November 1992 and July 1994, 725 subjects with AIDS, who were CMV seropositive and/or culture positive, were randomized to receive CYTOVENE capsules, 1000 mg, every 8 hours, or placebo.[4] The study population had a median age of 38 years (range: 21 to 69); were 99% male; were 82% Caucasian, 10% Hispanic, 7% African-American and 1% Asian; and had a median CD_4 count of 21 (range: 0 to 100). The mean observation time was 351 days (range: 5 to 621). As shown in the following table, significantly more placebo recipients developed CMV disease.

Incidence of CMV Disease at 6, 12 and 18 Months After Enrollment (Kaplan-Meier Estimates)

	Incidence (Number Still At Risk) CMV Disease	
	Ganciclovir	Placebo
6 months	8% (397)	11% (190)
12 months	14% (225)	26% (92)
18 months	20% (27)	39% (9)

3. *Prevention of CMV Disease In Transplant Recipients*

CYTOVENE-IV: CYTOVENE-IV was evaluated in three randomized, controlled trials of prevention of CMV disease in organ transplant recipients.

ICM 1496: In a randomized, double-blind, placebo-controlled study of 149 heart transplant recipients[5] at risk for CMV infection (CMV seropositive or a seronegative recipient of an organ from a CMV seropositive donor), there was a statistically significant reduction in the overall incidence of

Continued on next page

Cytovene—Cont.

CMV disease in patients treated with CYTOVENE-IV. Immediately posttransplant, patients received CYTOVENE-IV solution 5 mg/kg bid for 14 days followed by 6 mg/kg qd for 5 days/week for an additional 14 days. Twelve of the 76 (16%) patients treated with CYTOVENE-IV vs 31 of the 73 (43%) placebo-treated patients developed CMV disease during the 120-day posttransplant observation period. No significant differences in hematologic toxicities were seen between the two treatment groups (refer to table in ADVERSE EVENTS).

ICM 1689: In a randomized, double-blind, placebo-controlled study of 72 bone marrow transplant recipients[6] with asymptomatic CMV infection (CMV positive culture of urine, throat or blood) there was a statistically significant reduction in the incidence of CMV disease in patients treated with CYTOVENE-IV following successful hematopoietic engraftment. Patients with virologic evidence of CMV infection received CYTOVENE-IV solution 5 mg/kg bid for 7 days followed by 5 mg/kg qd through day 100 posttransplant. One of the 37 (3%) patients treated with CYTOVENE-IV vs 15 of the 35 (43%) placebo-treated patients developed CMV disease during the study. At 6 months posttransplant, there continued to be a statistically significant reduction in the incidence of CMV disease in patients treated with CYTOVENE-IV. Six of 37 (16%) patients treated with CYTOVENE-IV vs 15 of the 35 (43%) placebo-treated patients developed disease through 6 months posttransplant. The overall rate of survival was statistically significantly higher in the group treated with CYTOVENE-IV, both at day 100 and day 180 posttransplant. Although the differences in hematologic toxicities were not statistically significant, the incidence of neutropenia was higher in the group treated with CYTOVENE-IV (refer to table in ADVERSE EVENTS).

ICM 1570: A second, randomized, unblinded study evaluated 40 allogeneic bone marrow transplant recipients at risk for CMV disease.[7] Patients underwent bronchoscopy and bronchoalveolar lavage (BAL) on day 35 posttransplant. Patients with histologic, immunologic or virologic evidence of CMV infection in the lung were then randomized to observation or treatment with CYTOVENE-IV solution (5 mg/kg bid for 14 days followed by 5 mg/kg qd 5 days/week until day 120). Four of 20 (20%) patients treated with CYTOVENE-IV and 14 of 20 (70%) control patients developed interstitial pneumonia. The incidence of CMV disease was significantly lower in the group treated with CYTOVENE-IV, consistent with the results observed in ICM 1689.

CYTOVENE Capsules: *GAN040:* CYTOVENE capsules were evaluated in a randomized, double-blind, placebo-controlled study of 304 orthotopic liver transplant recipients who were CMV seropositive or recipients of an organ from a seropositive donor. Administration of CYTOVENE capsules (1000 mg three times daily) or matching placebo commenced as soon as patients were able to take medication by mouth, but no later than 10 days following transplantation, and continued through 14 weeks after transplantation. Dosing was adjusted for patients with an estimated creatinine clearance <50 mL/min. The incidence of CMV disease at 6 months is summarized in the table below.

[See first table above]

CYTOVENE capsules significantly reduced the 6-month incidence of CMV disease in patients at increased risk of CMV disease, including seronegative recipients of organs from seropositive donors (15% [3/21] with CYTOVENE capsules vs 44% [11/25] with placebo), and patients receiving antilymphocyte antibodies (5% [2/44] with CYTOVENE capsules vs 33% [12/37] with placebo). The incidence of HSV infection at 6 months was 4% (5/150) in ganciclovir vs 24% (36/154) in placebo recipients (relative risk: 0.13; 95% CI: 0.05, 0.32).

Incidence of CMV Disease at 6 Months (Kaplan-Meier Estimates)

CMV Disease at 6 months	Ganciclovir (n=150)	Placebo (n=154)	Relative Risk (95% Cl)
CMV Disease,* N (%)	7 (4.8%)	29 (18.9%)	0.22 (0.10, 0.51)
CMV syndrome†	6 (4.1%)	19 (12.4%)	
CMV hepatitis	1 (0.7%)	9 (5.9%)	
CMV GI disease	0 (0.0%)	3 (2.0%)	
CMV lung disease	0 (0.0%)	4 (2.6%)	

* One or more CMV endpoints
† CMV syndrome: CMV viremia and unexplained fever, accompanied by malaise and/or neutropenia.

Laboratory Data:

Selected Laboratory Abnormalities in Trials for Treatment of CMV Retinitis and Prevention of CMV Diseases

	CMV Retinitis Treatment*		CMV Disease Prevention§	
Treatment	CYTOVENE Capsules† 3000 mg/day	CYTOVENE-IV‡ 5 mg/kg/day	CYTOVENE Capsules[ll] 3000 mg/day	Placebo¶
Subjects, number	320	175	478	234
Neutropenia:				
<500 ANC/μL	18%	25%	10%	6%
500 – <749	17%	14%	16%	7%
750 – <1000	19%	26%	22%	16%
Anemia: Hemoglobin:				
<6.5 g/dL	2%	5%	1%	<1%
6.5 – <8.0	10%	16%	5%	3%
8.0 – <9.5	25%	26%	15%	16%
Maximum Serum Creatinine:				
≥2.5 mg/dL	1%	2%	1%	2%
≥1.5 – <2.5	12%	14%	19%	11%

* Pooled data from Treatment Studies, ICM 1653. Study ICM 1774 and Study AVI 034
† Mean time on therapy = 91 days, including allowed reinduction treatment periods
‡ Mean time on therapy = 103 days, including allowed reinduction treatment periods
§ Data from Prevention Study, ICM 1654
ll Mean time on ganciclovir = 269 days
¶ Mean time on placebo = 240 days
(See discussion of clinical trials under INDICATIONS AND USAGE.)

CONTRAINDICATIONS

CYTOVENE-IV and CYTOVENE are contraindicated in patients with hypersensitivity to ganciclovir or acyclovir.

WARNINGS

Hematologic: **CYTOVENE-IV and CYTOVENE should not be administered if the absolute neutrophil count is less than 500 cells/μL or the platelet count is less than 25,000 cells/μL.** Granulocytopenia (neutropenia), anemia and thrombocytopenia have been observed in patients treated with CYTOVENE-IV and CYTOVENE. The frequency and severity of these events vary widely in different patient populations (see ADVERSE EVENTS).

CYTOVENE-IV and CYTOVENE should, therefore, be used with caution in patients with pre-existing cytopenias or with a history of cytopenic reactions to other drugs, chemicals or irradiation. Granulocytopenia usually occurs during the first or second week of treatment but may occur at any time during treatment. Cell counts usually begin to recover within 3 to 7 days of discontinuing drug. Colony-stimulating factors have been shown to increase neutrophil and white blood cell counts in patients receiving CYTOVENE-IV solution for treatment of CMV retinitis.

Impairment of Fertility: Animal data indicate that administration of ganciclovir causes inhibition of spermatogenesis and subsequent infertility. These effects were reversible at lower doses and irreversible at higher doses (see PRECAUTIONS: *Carcinogenesis, Mutagenesis* and *Impairment of Fertility*). Although data in humans have not been obtained regarding this effect, it is considered probable that ganciclovir at the recommended doses causes temporary or permanent inhibition of spermatogenesis. Animal data also indicate that suppression of fertility in females may occur.

Teratogenesis: Because of the mutagenic and teratogenic potential of ganciclovir, women of childbearing potential should be advised to use effective contraception during treatment. Similarly, men should be advised to practice barrier contraception during and for at least 90 days following treatment with CYTOVENE-IV or CYTOVENE (see *Pregnancy:* Category C).

PRECAUTIONS

General: In clinical studies with CYTOVENE-IV, the maximum single dose administered was 6 mg/kg by intravenous infusion over 1 hour. Larger doses have resulted in increased toxicity. It is likely that more rapid infusions would also result in increased toxicity (see OVERDOSAGE). Administration of CYTOVENE-IV solution should be accompanied by adequate hydration.

Initially reconstituted solutions of CYTOVENE-IV have a high pH (pH 11). Despite further dilution in intravenous fluids, phlebitis and/or pain may occur at the site of intravenous infusion. Care must be taken to infuse solutions containing CYTOVENE-IV only into veins with adequate blood flow to permit rapid dilution and distribution (see DOSAGE AND ADMINISTRATION).

Since ganciclovir is excreted by the kidneys, normal clearance depends on adequate renal function. IF RENAL FUNCTION IS IMPAIRED, DOSAGE ADJUSTMENTS ARE REQUIRED FOR CYTOVENE-IV AND SHOULD BE CONSIDERED FOR CYTOVENE CAPSULES. Such adjustments should be based on measured or estimated creatinine clearance values (see DOSAGE AND ADMINISTRATION).

Information for Patients: All patients should be informed that the major toxicities of ganciclovir are granulocytopenia (neutropenia), anemia and thrombocytopenia and that dose modifications may be required, including discontinuation. The importance of close monitoring of blood counts while on therapy should be emphasized. Patients should be informed that ganciclovir has been associated with elevations in serum creatinine.

Patients should be instructed to take CYTOVENE capsules with food to maximize bioavailability.

Patients should be advised that ganciclovir has caused decreased sperm production in animals and may cause infertility in humans. Women of childbearing potential should be advised that ganciclovir causes birth defects in animals and should not be used during pregnancy. Women of childbearing potential should be advised to use effective contraception during treatment with CYTOVENE-IV or CYTOVENE. Similarly, men should be advised to practice barrier contraception during and for at least 90 days following treatment with CYTOVENE-IV or CYTOVENE.

Patients should be advised that ganciclovir causes tumors in animals. Although there is no information from human studies, ganciclovir should be considered a potential carcinogen.

All HIV+ Patients: These patients may be receiving zidovudine (Retrovir®*). Patients should be counseled that treatment with both ganciclovir and zidovudine simultaneously may not be tolerated by some patients and may result in severe granulocytopenia (neutropenia). Patients with AIDS may be receiving didanosine (Videx®†). Patients should be counseled that concomitant treatment with both ganciclovir and didanosine can cause didanosine serum concentrations to be significantly increased.

HIV+ Patients With CMV Retinitis: Ganciclovir is not a cure for CMV retinitis, and immunocompromised patients may continue to experience progression of retinitis during or following treatment. Patients should be advised to have ophthalmologic follow-up examinations at a minimum of every 4 to 6 weeks while being treated with CYTOVENE-IV or CYTOVENE. Some patients will require more frequent follow-up.

Transplant Recipients: Transplant recipients should be counseled regarding the high frequency of impaired renal function in transplant recipients who received CYTOVENE-IV solution in controlled clinical trials, particularly in patients receiving concomitant administration of nephrotoxic agents such as cyclosporine and amphotericin B. Although the specific mechanism of this toxicity, which in most cases was reversible, has not been determined, the higher rate of renal impairment in patients receiving CYTOVENE-IV solution compared with those who received placebo in the same trials may indicate that CYTOVENE-IV played a significant role.

Laboratory Testing: Due to the frequency of neutropenia, anemia and thrombocytopenia in patients receiving CYTOVENE-IV and CYTOVENE (see ADVERSE EVENTS), it is recommended that complete blood counts and platelet counts be performed frequently, especially in patients in whom ganciclovir or other nucleoside analogues have previously resulted in leukopenia or in whom neutrophil counts are less than 1000 cells/μL at the beginning of treatment. Increased serum creatinine levels have been observed in trials evaluating both CYTOVENE-IV and CYTOVENE. Patients should have serum creatinine or creatinine clearance values monitored carefully to allow for dosage adjustments in renally impaired patients (see DOSAGE AND ADMINISTRATION).

Drug Interactions: *Didanosine:* At an oral dose of 1000 mg of CYTOVENE every 8 hours and didanosine, 200 mg every 12 hours, the steady-state didanosine AUC_{0-12} increased 111 ± 114% (range: 10% to 493%) when didanosine was administered either 2 hours prior to or concurrent with administration of CYTOVENE (n=12 patients, 23 observations). A decrease in steady-state ganciclovir AUC of 21 ± 17% (range: -44% to 5%) was observed when didanosine was administered 2 hours prior to administration of CYTOVENE, but ganciclovir AUC was not affected by the presence of didanosine when the two drugs were administered simultaneously (n=12). There were no significant changes in renal clearance for either drug.

When the standard intravenous ganciclovir induction dose (5 mg/kg infused over 1 hour every 12 hours) was coadministered with didanosine at a dose of 200 mg orally every 12 hours, the steady-state didanosine AUC_{0-12} increased 70 ± 40% (range: 3% to 121%, n=11) and C_{max} increased 49 ± 48% (range: -28% to 125%). In a separate study, when the standard intravenous ganciclovir maintenance dose (5 mg/kg infused over 1 hour every 24 hours) was coadministered with didanosine at a dose of 200 mg orally every 12 hours, didanosine AUC_{0-12} increased 50 ± 26% (range: 22% to 110%, n=11) and C_{max} increased 36 ± 36% (range: -27% to 94%) over the first didanosine dosing interval. Didanosine plasma concentrations (AUC_{12-24}) were unchanged during the dosing intervals when ganciclovir was not coadministered. Ganciclovir pharmacokinetics were not affected by didanosine. In neither study were there significant changes in the renal clearance of either drug.

Zidovudine: At an oral dose of 1000 mg of CYTOVENE every 8 hours, mean steady-state ganciclovir AUC_{0-8} decreased 17 ± 25% (range: -52% to 23%) in the presence of zidovudine, 100 mg every 4 hours (n=12). Steady-state zidovudine AUC_{0-4} increased 19 ± 27% (range: -11% to 74%) in the presence of ganciclovir.

Since both zidovudine and ganciclovir have the potential to cause neutropenia and anemia, some patients may not tolerate concomitant therapy with these drugs at full dosage.

Probenecid: At an oral dose of 1000 mg of CYTOVENE every 8 hours (n=10), ganciclovir AUC_{0-8} increased 53 ± 91% (range: -14% to 299%) in the presence of probenecid, 500 mg every 6 hours. Renal clearance of ganciclovir decreased 22 ± 20% (range: -54% to -4%), which is consistent with an interaction involving competition for renal tubular secretion.

Imipenem-cilastatin: Generalized seizures have been reported in patients who received ganciclovir and imipenem-cilastatin. These drugs should not be used concomitantly unless the potential benefits outweigh the risks.

Other Medications: It is possible that drugs that inhibit replication of rapidly dividing cell populations such as bone marrow, spermatogonia and germinal layers of skin and gastrointestinal mucosa may have additive toxicity when administered concomitantly with ganciclovir. Therefore, drugs such as dapsone, pentamidine, flucytosine, vincristine, vinblastine, adriamycin, amphotericin B, trimethoprim/sulfamethoxazole combinations or other nucleoside analogues, should be considered for concomitant use with ganciclovir only if the potential benefits are judged to outweigh the risks.

No formal drug interaction studies of CYTOVENE-IV or CYTOVENE and drugs commonly used in transplant recipients have been conducted. Increases in serum creatinine were observed in patients treated with CYTOVENE-IV plus either cyclosporine or amphotericin B, drugs with known potential for nephrotoxicity (see ADVERSE EVENTS). In a retrospective analysis of 93 liver allograft recipients receiving ganciclovir (5 mg/kg infused over 1 hour every 12 hours) and oral cyclosporine (at therapeutic doses), there was no evidence of an effect on cyclosporine whole blood concentrations.

Carcinogenesis, Mutagenesis‡: Ganciclovir was carcinogenic in the mouse at oral doses of 20 and 1000 mg/kg/day (approximately 0.1× and 1.4×, respectively, the mean drug exposure in humans following the recommended intravenous dose of 5 mg/kg, based on area under the plasma concentration curve [AUC] comparisons). At the dose of 1000 mg/kg/day there was a significant increase in the incidence of tumors of the preputial gland in males, forestomach (nonglandular mucosa) in males and females, and reproductive tissues (ovaries, uterus, mammary gland, clitoral gland and vagina) and liver in females. At the dose of 20 mg/kg/day, a slightly increased incidence of tumors was noted in the preputial and harderian glands in males, forestomach in males and females, and liver in females. No carcinogenic effect was observed in mice administered ganciclovir at 1 mg/kg/day (estimated as 0.01× the human dose based on AUC comparison). Except for histiocytic sarcoma of the liver, ganciclovir-induced tumors were generally of epithelial or vascular origin. Although the preputial and clitoral glands, forestomach and harderian glands of mice do not have human counterparts, ganciclovir should be considered a potential carcinogen in humans.

Ganciclovir increased mutations in mouse lymphoma cells and DNA damage in human lymphocytes in vitro at concentrations between 50 to 500 and 250 to 2000 µg/mL, respectively. In the mouse micronucleus assay, ganciclovir was clastogenic at doses of 150 and 500 mg/kg (IV) (2.8 to 10× human exposure based on AUC) but not 50 mg/kg (exposure approximately comparable to the human based on AUC). Ganciclovir was not mutagenic in the Ames Salmonella assay at concentrations of 500 to 5000 µg/mL.

Impairment of Fertility‡: Ganciclovir caused decreased mating behavior, decreased fertility, and an increased incidence of embryolethality in female mice following intravenous doses of 90 mg/kg/day (approximately 1.7× the mean drug exposure in humans following the dose of 5 mg/kg, based on AUC comparisons). Ganciclovir caused decreased fertility in male mice and hypospermatogenesis in mice and dogs following daily oral or intravenous administration of doses ranging from 0.2 to 10 mg/kg. Systemic drug exposure (AUC) at the lowest dose showing toxicity in each species ranged from 0.03 to 0.1× the AUC of the recommended human intravenous dose.

***Pregnancy:* Category C‡:** Ganciclovir has been shown to be embryotoxic in rabbits and mice following intravenous administration and teratogenic in rabbits. Fetal resorptions were present in at least 85% of rabbits and mice administered 60 mg/kg/day and 108 mg/kg/day (2× the human exposure based on AUC comparisons), respectively. Effects observed in rabbits included: fetal growth retardation, embryolethality, teratogenicity and/or maternal toxicity. Teratogenic changes included cleft palate, anophthalmia/microphthalmia, aplastic organs (kidney and pancreas), hydrocephaly and brachygnathia. In mice, effects observed were maternal/fetal toxicity and embryolethality.

Daily intravenous doses of 90 mg/kg administered to female mice prior to mating, during gestation, and during lactation caused hypoplasia of the testes and seminal vesicles in the month-old male offspring, as well as pathologic changes in the nonglandular region of the stomach (see *Carcinogenesis, Mutagenesis*). The drug exposure in mice as estimated by the AUC was approximately 1.7× the human AUC.

Ganciclovir may be teratogenic or embryotoxic at dose levels recommended for human use. There are no adequate and well-controlled studies in pregnant women. CYTOVENE-IV or CYTOVENE should be used during pregnancy only if the potential benefits justify the potential risk to the fetus.

‡Footnote: All dose comparisons presented in the *Carcinogenesis, Mutagenesis, Impairment of Fertility* and *Pregnancy* subsections are based on the human AUC following administration of a single 5 mg/kg intravenous infusion of CYTOVENE-IV as used during the maintenance phase of treatment. Compared with the single 5 mg/kg intravenous infusion, human exposure is doubled during the intravenous induction phase (5 mg/kg bid) and approximately halved during maintenance treatment with CYTOVENE capsules (1000 mg tid). The cross-species dose comparisons should be divided by 2 for intravenous induction treatment with CYTOVENE-IV and multiplied by 2 for CYTOVENE capsules.

Nursing Mothers: It is not known whether ganciclovir is excreted in human milk. However, many drugs are excreted in human milk and, because carcinogenic and teratogenic effects occurred in animals treated with ganciclovir, the possibility of serious adverse reactions from ganciclovir in nursing infants is considered likely (see *Pregnancy:* Category C). Mothers should be instructed to discontinue nursing if they are receiving CYTOVENE-IV or CYTOVENE. The minimum interval before nursing can safely be resumed after the last dose of CYTOVENE-IV or CYTOVENE is unknown.

Pediatric Use: **SAFETY AND EFFICACY OF CYTOVENE-IV AND CYTOVENE IN PEDIATRIC PATIENTS HAVE NOT BEEN ESTABLISHED. THE USE OF CYTOVENE-IV OR CYTOVENE IN THE PEDIATRIC POPULATION WARRANTS EXTREME CAUTION DUE TO THE PROBABILITY OF LONG-TERM CARCINOGENICITY AND REPRODUCTIVE TOXICITY. ADMINISTRATION TO PEDIATRIC PATIENTS SHOULD BE UNDERTAKEN ONLY AFTER CAREFUL EVALUATION AND ONLY IF THE POTENTIAL BENEFITS OF TREATMENT OUTWEIGH THE RISKS.**

The spectrum of adverse events reported in 120 immunocompromised pediatric clinical trial participants with serious CMV infections receiving CYTOVENE-IV solution were similar to those reported in adults. Granulocytopenia (17%) and thrombocytopenia (10%) were the most common adverse events reported.

Sixteen pediatric patients (8 months to 15 years of age) with life- or sight-threatening CMV infections were evaluated in an open-label, CYTOVENE-IV solution, pharmacokinetics study. Adverse events reported for more than one pediatric patient were as follows: hypokalemia (4/16, 25%), abnormal kidney function (3/16, 19%), sepsis (3/16, 19%), thrombocytopenia (3/16, 19%), leukopenia (2/16, 13%), coagulation disorder (2/16, 13%), hypertension (2/16, 13%), pneumonia (2/16, 13%) and immune system disorder (2/16, 13%).

There has been very limited clinical experience using CYTOVENE-IV for the treatment of CMV retinitis in patients under the age of 12 years. Two pediatric patients (ages 9 and 5 years) showed improvement or stabilization of retinitis for 23 and 9 months, respectively. These pediatric patients received induction treatment with 2.5 mg/kg tid followed by maintenance therapy with 6 to 6.5 mg/kg once per day, 5 to 7 days per week. When retinitis progressed during once-daily maintenance therapy, both pediatric patients were treated with the 5 mg/kg bid regimen. Two other pediatric patients (ages 2.5 and 4 years) who received similar induction regimens showed only partial or no response to treatment. Another pediatric patient, a 6-year-old with T-cell dysfunction, showed stabilization of retinitis for 3 months while receiving continuous infusions of CYTOVENE-IV at doses of 2 to 5 mg/kg/24 hours. Continuous infusion treatment was discontinued due to granulocytopenia.

Eleven of the 72 patients in the placebo-controlled trial in bone marrow transplant recipients were pediatric patients, ranging in age from 3 to 10 years (5 treated with CYTOVENE-IV and 6 with placebo). Five of the pediatric patients treated with CYTOVENE-IV received 5 mg/kg intravenously bid for up to 7 days; 4 patients went on to receive 5 mg/kg qd up to day 100 posttransplant. Results were similar to those observed in adult transplant recipients treated with CYTOVENE-IV. Two of the 6 placebo-treated pediatric patients developed CMV pneumonia vs none of the 5 patients treated with CYTOVENE-IV. The spectrum of adverse events in the pediatric group was similar to that observed in the adult patients.

CYTOVENE capsules have not been studied in pediatric patients under age 13.

Geriatric Use: The pharmacokinetic profiles of CYTOVENE-IV and CYTOVENE in elderly patients have not been established. Since elderly individuals frequently have a reduced glomerular filtration rate, particular attention should be paid to assessing renal function before and during administration of CYTOVENE-IV or CYTOVENE (see DOSAGE AND ADMINISTRATION).

Clinical studies of CYTOVENE-IV and CYTOVENE did not include sufficient numbers of subjects aged 65 and over to determine whether they respond differently from younger subjects. In general, dose selection for an elderly patient should be cautious, reflecting the greater frequency of decreased hepatic, renal, or cardiac function, and of concomitant disease or other drug therapy. CYTOVENE-IV and CYTOVENE are known to be substantially excreted by the kidney, and the risk of toxic reactions to this drug may be greater in patients with impaired renal function. Because elderly patients are more likely to have decreased renal function, care should be taken in dose selection. In addition, renal function should be monitored and dosage adjustments should be made accordingly (see *Use in Patients With Renal Impairment* and DOSAGE AND ADMINISTRATION).

Use in Patients With Renal Impairment: CYTOVENE-IV and CYTOVENE should be used with caution in patients with impaired renal function because the half-life and plasma/serum concentrations of ganciclovir will be increased due to reduced renal clearance (see DOSAGE AND ADMINISTRATION and ADVERSE EVENTS: *Renal Toxicity*).

Hemodialysis has been shown to reduce plasma levels of ganciclovir by approximately 50%.

ADVERSE EVENTS

Adverse events that occurred during clinical trials of CYTOVENE-IV solution and CYTOVENE capsules are summarized below, according to the participating study subject population.

Subjects With AIDS: Three controlled, randomized, phase 3 trials comparing CYTOVENE-IV and CYTOVENE capsules for maintenance treatment of CMV retinitis have been completed. During these trials, CYTOVENE-IV or CYTOVENE capsules were prematurely discontinued in 9% of subjects because of adverse events. In a placebo-controlled, randomized, phase 3 trial of CYTOVENE capsules for prevention of CMV disease in AIDS, treatment was prematurely discontinued because of adverse events, new or worsening intercurrent illness, or laboratory abnormalities in 19.5% of subjects treated with CYTOVENE capsules and 16% of subjects receiving placebo. Laboratory data and adverse events reported during the conduct of these controlled trials are summarized below.

[See second table at top of previous page]

Adverse Events: The following table shows selected adverse events reported in 5% or more of the subjects in three controlled clinical trials during treatment with either CYTOVENE-IV solution (5 mg/kg/day) or CYTOVENE capsules (3000 mg/day), and in one controlled clinical trial in which CYTOVENE capsules (3000 mg/day) were compared to placebo for the prevention of CMV disease.

[See first table at top of next page]

The following events were frequently observed in clinical trials but occurred with equal or greater frequency in placebo-treated subjects: abdominal pain, nausea, flatulence, pneumonia, paresthesia, rash.

Retinal Detachment: Retinal detachment has been observed in subjects with CMV retinitis both before and after initiation of therapy with ganciclovir. Its relationship to therapy with ganciclovir is unknown. Retinal detachment occurred in 11% of patients treated with CYTOVENE-IV solution and in 8% of patients treated with CYTOVENE capsules. Patients with CMV retinitis should have frequent ophthalmologic evaluations to monitor the status of their retinitis and to detect any other retinal pathology.

Transplant Recipients: There have been three controlled clinical trials of CYTOVENE-IV solution and one controlled clinical trial of CYTOVENE capsules for the prevention of CMV disease in transplant recipients. Laboratory data and adverse events reported during these trials are summarized below.

Laboratory Data: The following table shows the frequency of granulocytopenia (neutropenia) and thrombocytopenia observed:

[See second table at top of next page]

The following table shows the frequency of elevated serum creatinine values in these controlled clinical trials:

[See first table at top of page 2871]

In 3 out of 4 trials, patients receiving either CYTOVENE-IV solution or CYTOVENE capsules had elevated serum creatinine levels when compared to those receiving placebo. Most patients in these studies also received cyclosporine. The mechanism of impairment of renal function is not known.

Continued on next page

Cytovene—Cont.

However, careful monitoring of renal function during therapy with CYTOVENE-IV solution or CYTOVENE capsules is essential, especially for those patients receiving concomitant agents that may cause nephrotoxicity.

General: Other adverse events that were thought to be "probably" or "possibly" related to CYTOVENE-IV solution or CYTOVENE capsules in controlled clinical studies in either subjects with AIDS or transplant recipients are listed below. These events all occurred in at least 3 subjects.

Body as a Whole: abdomen enlarged, asthenia, chest pain, edema, headache, injection site inflammation, malaise, pain
Digestive System: abnormal liver function test, aphthous stomatitis, constipation, dyspepsia, eructation
Hemic and Lymphatic System: pancytopenia
Respiratory System: cough increased, dyspnea
Nervous System: abnormal dreams, anxiety, confusion, depression, dizziness, dry mouth, insomnia, seizures, somnolence, thinking abnormal, tremor
Skin and Appendages: alopecia, dry skin
Special Senses: abnormal vision, taste perversion, tinnitus, vitreous disorder
Metabolic and Nutritional Disorders: creatinine increased, SGOT increased, SGPT increased, weight loss
Cardiovascular System: hypertension, phlebitis, vasodilatation
Urogenital System: creatinine clearance decreased, kidney failure, kidney function abnormal, urinary frequency
Musculoskeletal System: arthralgia, leg cramps, myalgia, myasthenia

The following adverse events reported in patients receiving ganciclovir may be potentially fatal: gastrointestinal perforation, multiple organ failure, pancreatitis and sepsis.

Adverse Events Reported During Postmarketing Experience With CYTOVENE-IV and CYTOVENE Capsules: The following events have been identified during post-approval use of the drug. Because they are reported voluntarily from a population of unknown size, estimates of frequency cannot be made. These events have been chosen for inclusion due to either the seriousness, frequency of reporting, the apparent causal connection or a combination of these factors:
acidosis, allergic reaction, anaphylactic reaction, arthritis, bronchospasm, cardiac arrest, cardiac conduction abnormality, cataracts, cholelithiasis, cholestasis, congenital anomaly, dry eyes, dysesthesia, dysphasia, elevated triglyceride levels, encephalopathy, exfoliative dermatitis, extrapyramidal reaction, facial palsy, hallucinations, hemolytic anemia, hemolytic uremic syndrome, hepatic failure, hepatitis, hypercalcemia, hyponatremia, inappropriate serum ADH, infertility, intestinal ulceration, intracranial hypertension, irritability, loss of memory, loss of sense of smell, myelopathy, oculomotor nerve paralysis, peripheral ischemia, pulmonary fibrosis, renal tubular disorder, rhabdomyolysis, Stevens-Johnson syndrome, stroke, testicular hypotrophy, Torsades de Pointes, vasculitis, ventricular tachycardia

OVERDOSAGE

CYTOVENE-IV: Overdosage with CYTOVENE-IV has been reported in 17 patients (13 adults and 4 children under 2 years of age). Five patients experienced no adverse events following overdosage at the following doses: 7 doses of 11 mg/kg over a 3-day period (adult), single dose of 3500 mg (adult), single dose of 500 mg (72.5 mg/kg) followed by 48 hours of peritoneal dialysis (4-month-old), single dose of approximately 60 mg/kg followed by exchange transfusion (18-month-old), 2 doses of 500 mg instead of 31 mg (21-month-old).

Irreversible pancytopenia developed in 1 adult with AIDS and CMV colitis after receiving 3000 mg of CYTOVENE-IV solution on each of 2 consecutive days. He experienced worsening GI symptoms and acute renal failure that required short-term dialysis. Pancytopenia developed and persisted until his death from a malignancy several months later.

Other adverse events reported following overdosage included: persistent bone marrow suppression (1 adult with neutropenia and thrombocytopenia after a single dose of 6000 mg), reversible neutropenia or granulocytopenia (4 adults, overdoses ranging from 8 mg/kg daily for 4 days to a single dose of 25 mg/kg), hepatitis (1 adult receiving 10 mg/kg daily, and one 2 kg infant after a single 40 mg dose), renal toxicity (1 adult with transient worsening of hematuria after a single 500 mg dose, and 1 adult with elevated creatinine (5.2 mg/dL) after a single 5000 to 7000 mg dose), and seizure (1 adult with known seizure disorder after 3 days of 9 mg/kg). In addition, 1 adult received 0.4 mL (instead of 0.1 mL) CYTOVENE-IV solution by intravitreal injection, and experienced temporary loss of vision and central retinal artery occlusion secondary to increased intraocular pressure related to the injected fluid volume.

CYTOVENE Capsules: There have been no reports of overdosage with CYTOVENE capsules. Doses as high as 6000 mg/day, given either as 1000 mg 6 times daily or as 2000 mg tid, did not result in overt toxicity other than transient neutropenia. Daily doses of more than 6000 mg have not been studied.

Since ganciclovir is dialyzable, dialysis may be useful in reducing serum concentrations. Adequate hydration should be maintained. The use of hematopoietic growth factors should be considered.

DOSAGE AND ADMINISTRATION

CAUTION—DO NOT ADMINISTER CYTOVENE-IV SOLUTION BY RAPID OR BOLUS INTRAVENOUS INJECTION. THE TOXICITY OF CYTOVENE-IV MAY BE INCREASED AS A RESULT OF EXCESSIVE PLASMA LEVELS.

CAUTION—INTRAMUSCULAR OR SUBCUTANEOUS INJECTION OF RECONSTITUTED CYTOVENE-IV SOLUTION MAY RESULT IN SEVERE TISSUE IRRITATION DUE TO HIGH pH (11).

Dosage: THE RECOMMENDED DOSE FOR CYTOVENE-IV SOLUTION AND CYTOVENE CAPSULES SHOULD NOT BE EXCEEDED. THE RECOMMENDED INFUSION RATE FOR CYTOVENE-IV SOLUTION SHOULD NOT BE EXCEEDED.

For Treatment of CMV Retinitis in Patients With Normal Renal Function:

1. Induction Treatment

The recommended initial dosage for patients with normal renal function is 5 mg/kg (given intravenously at a constant rate over 1 hour) every 12 hours for 14 to 21 days. CYTOVENE capsules should not be used for induction treatment.

2. Maintenance Treatment

CYTOVENE-IV: Following induction treatment, the recommended maintenance dosage of CYTOVENE-IV solution is 5 mg/kg given as a constant-rate intravenous infusion over 1 hour once daily, 7 days per week or 6 mg/kg once daily, 5 days per week.

CYTOVENE Capsules: Following induction treatment, the recommended maintenance dosage of CYTOVENE capsules is 1000 mg tid with food. Alternatively, the dosing regimen of 500 mg 6 times daily every 3 hours with food, during waking hours, may be used.

For patients who experience progression of CMV retinitis while receiving maintenance treatment with either formulation of ganciclovir, reinduction treatment is recommended.

For the Prevention of CMV Disease in Patients With Advanced HIV Infection and Normal Renal Function:

CYTOVENE Capsules: The recommended prophylactic dose of CYTOVENE capsules is 1000 mg tid with food.

For the Prevention of CMV Disease in Transplant Recipients With Normal Renal Function:

CYTOVENE-IV: The recommended initial dosage of CYTOVENE-IV solution for patients with normal renal function is 5 mg/kg (given intravenously at a constant rate over 1 hour) every 12 hours for 7 to 14 days, followed by 5 mg/kg once daily, 7 days per week or 6 mg/kg once daily, 5 days per week.

CYTOVENE Capsules: The recommended prophylactic dosage of CYTOVENE capsules is 1000 mg tid with food.

The duration of treatment with CYTOVENE-IV solution and CYTOVENE capsules in transplant recipients is dependent upon the duration and degree of immunosuppression. In controlled clinical trials in bone marrow allograft recipients, treatment with CYTOVENE-IV was continued until day 100 to 120 posttransplantation. CMV disease occurred in several patients who discontinued treatment with CYTOVENE-IV solution prematurely. In heart allograft recipients, the onset of newly diagnosed CMV disease occurred after treatment with CYTOVENE-IV was stopped at day 28 posttransplant, suggesting that continued dosing may be necessary to prevent late occurrence of CMV disease in this patient population. In a controlled clinical trial of liver allograft recipients, treatment with CYTOVENE capsules was continued through week 14 posttransplantation (see INDICATIONS AND USAGE section for a more detailed discussion).

Renal Impairment:

CYTOVENE-IV: For patients with impairment of renal function, refer to the table below for recommended doses of CYTOVENE-IV solution and adjust the dosing interval as indicated:

Selected Adverse Events Reported ≥5% of Subjects in Three Randomized Phase 3 Studies Comparing CYTOVENE Capsules to CYTOVENE-IV Solution for Maintenance Treatment of CMV Retinitis and in One Phase 3 Randomized Study Comparing Cytovene Capsules to Placebo for Prevention of CMV Disease

		Maintenance Treatment Studies		Prevention Study	
Body System	Adverse Event	Capsules (n=326)	IV (n=179)	Capsules (n=478)	Placebo (n=234)
Body as a Whole	Fever	38%	48%	35%	33%
	Infection	9%	13%	8%	4%
	Chills	7%	10%	7%	4%
	Sepsis	4%	15%	3%	2%
Digestive System	Diarrhea	41%	44%	48%	42%
	Anorexia	15%	14%	19%	16%
	Vomiting	13%	13%	14%	11%
Hemic and Lymphatic System	Leukopenia	29%	41%	17%	9%
	Anemia	19%	25%	9%	7%
	Thrombocytopenia	6%	6%	3%	1%
Nervous System	Neuropathy	8%	9%	21%	15%
Other	Sweating	11%	12%	14%	12%
	Pruritus	6%	5%	10%	9%
Catheter Related*	Total Catheter Events	6%	22%	–	–
	Catheter Infection	4%	9%	–	–
	Catheter Sepsis	1%	8%	–	–

* Some of these events also appear under other body systems.

Controlled Trials – Transplant Recipients

	CYTOVENE-IV				CYTOVENE Capsules	
	Heart Allograft*		Bone Marrow Allograft†		Liver Allograft‡	
	CYTOVENE-IV (n=76)	Placebo (n=73)	CYTOVENE-IV (n=57)	Control (n=55)	CYTOVENE Capsules (n=150)	Placebo (n=154)
Neutropenia						
Minimum ANC <500/µL	4%	3%	12%	6%	3%	1%
Minimum ANC 500–1000/µL	3%	8%	29%	17%	3%	2%
TOTAL ANC ≤1000/µL	7%	11%	41%	23%	6%	3%
Thrombocytopenia						
Platelet count <25,000/µL	3%	1%	32%	28%	0%	3%
Platelet count 25,000–50,000/µL	5%	3%	25%	37%	5%	3%
TOTAL Platelet ≤50,000/µL	8%	4%	57%	65%	5%	6%

* Study ICM 1496. Mean duration of treatment = 28 days
† Study ICM 1570 and ICM 1689. Mean duration of treatment = 45 days
‡ Study GAN040. Mean duration of ganciclovir treatment = 82 days
(See discussion of clinical trials under INDICATIONS AND USAGE.)

Controlled Trials – Transplant Recipients

	CYTOVENE-IV						CYTOVENE Capsules	
	Heart Allograft ICM 1496		Bone Marrow Allograft ICM 1570		Bone Marrow Allograft ICM 1689		Liver Allograft Study 040	
Maximum Serum Creatinine Levels	CYTOVENE-IV (n=76)	Placebo (n=73)	CYTOVENE-IV (n=20)	Control (n=20)	CYTOVENE-IV (n=37)	Placebo (n=35)	CYTOVENE Capsules (n=150)	Placebo (n=154)
Serum Creatinine ≥2.5 mg/dL	18%	4%	20%	0%	0%	0%	16%	10%
Serum Creatinine ≥1.5 –<2.5 mg/dL	58%	69%	50%	35%	43%	44%	39%	42%

[See first table below]

Dosing for patients undergoing hemodialysis should not exceed 1.25 mg/kg 3 times per week, following each hemodialysis session. CYTOVENE-IV should be given shortly after completion of the hemodialysis session, since hemodialysis has been shown to reduce plasma levels by approximately 50%.

CYTOVENE Capsules: In patients with renal impairment, the dose of CYTOVENE capsules should be modified as shown below:

[See second table below]

Patient Monitoring: Due to the frequency of granulocytopenia, anemia and thrombocytopenia in patients receiving ganciclovir (see ADVERSE EVENTS), it is recommended that complete blood counts and platelet counts be performed frequently, especially in patients in whom ganciclovir or other nucleoside analogues have previously resulted in cytopenia, or in whom neutrophil counts are less than 1000 cells/µL at the beginning of treatment. Patients should have serum creatinine or creatinine clearance values followed carefully to allow for dosage adjustments in renally impaired patients (see DOSAGE AND ADMINISTRATION).

Reduction of Dose: Dosage reductions in renally impaired patients are required for CYTOVENE-IV and should be considered for CYTOVENE capsules (see *Renal Impairment*). Dosage reductions should also be considered for those with neutropenia, anemia and/or thrombocytopenia (see ADVERSE EVENTS). Ganciclovir should not be administered in patients with severe neutropenia (ANC less than 500/µL) or severe thrombocytopenia (platelets less than 25,000/µL).

Method of Preparation of CYTOVENE IV Solution: Each 10 mL clear glass vial contains ganciclovir sodium equivalent to 500 mg of ganciclovir and 46 mg of sodium. The contents of the vial should be prepared for administration in the following manner:

1. *Reconstituted Solution:*
   a. Reconstitute lyophilized CYTOVENE-IV by injecting 10 mL of Sterile Water for Injection, USP, into the vial. DO NOT USE BACTERIOSTATIC WATER FOR INJECTION CONTAINING PARABENS. IT IS INCOMPATIBLE WITH CYTOVENE-IV AND MAY CAUSE PRECIPITATION.
   b. Shake the vial to dissolve the drug.
   c. Visually inspect the reconstituted solution for particulate matter and discoloration prior to proceeding with infusion solution. Discard the vial if particulate matter or discoloration is observed.
   d. Reconstituted solution in the vial is stable at room temperature for 12 hours. It should not be refrigerated.
2. *Infusion Solution:*
   Based on patient weight, the appropriate volume of the reconstituted solution (ganciclovir concentration 50 mg/mL) should be removed from the vial and added to an acceptable (see below) infusion fluid (typically 100 mL) for delivery over the course of 1 hour. Infusion concentrations greater than 10 mg/mL are not recommended. The following infusion fluids have been determined to be chemically and physically compatible with CYTOVENE-IV solution: 0.9% Sodium Chloride, 5% Dextrose, Ringer's Injection and Lactated Ringer's Injection, USP.

CYTOVENE-IV, when reconstituted with sterile water for injection, further diluted with 0.9% sodium chloride injection, and stored refrigerated at 5°C in polyvinyl chloride (PVC) bags, remains physically and chemically stable for 14 days.

However, because CYTOVENE-IV is reconstituted with nonbacteriostatic sterile water, it is recommended that the infusion solution be used within 24 hours of dilution to reduce the risk of bacterial contamination. The infusion should be refrigerated. Freezing is not recommended.

Handling and Disposal: Caution should be exercised in the handling and preparation of solutions of CYTOVENE-IV and in the handling of CYTOVENE capsules. Solutions of CYTOVENE-IV are alkaline (pH 11). Avoid direct contact with the skin or mucous membranes of the powder contained in CYTOVENE capsules or of CYTOVENE-IV solutions. If such contact occurs, wash thoroughly with soap and water; rinse eyes thoroughly with plain water. CYTOVENE capsules should not be opened or crushed.

Because ganciclovir shares some of the properties of antitumor agents (ie, carcinogenicity and mutagenicity), consideration should be given to handling and disposal according to guidelines issued for antineoplastic drugs. Several guidelines on this subject have been published.[8–10]

There is no general agreement that all of the procedures recommended in the guidelines are necessary or appropriate.

HOW SUPPLIED

CYTOVENE®-IV (ganciclovir sodium for injection) is supplied in 10 mL sterile vials, each containing ganciclovir sodium equivalent to 500 mg of ganciclovir, in cartons of 25 (NDC 0004-6940-03).

Store vials at temperatures below 40°C (104°F).

CYTOVENE® (ganciclovir capsules) 250 mg are two-pieced, size No. 1, opaque green hard gelatin capsules with ROCHE and CYTOVENE 250 mg imprinted on the capsules in dark blue ink and with two blue lines partially encircling the capsule body. Each capsule contains 250 mg of ganciclovir as a white to off-white powder. CYTOVENE capsules are supplied as follows: Bottles of 180 capsules (NDC 0004-0269-48).

CYTOVENE® (ganciclovir capsules) 500 mg are two-pieced, size No. 0 elongated, opaque yellow/opaque green hard gelatin capsules with ROCHE and CYTOVENE 500 mg imprinted on the capsules in dark blue ink and with two blue lines partially encircling the capsule body. Each capsule contains 500 mg of ganciclovir as a white to off-white powder. CYTOVENE capsules are supplied as follows:

Bottles of 180 capsules (NDC 0004-0278-48).

Store between 5° and 25°C (41° and 77°F).

*Retrovir is a registered trademark of Glaxo Wellcome.

†Videx is a registered trademark of Bristol-Meyers Squibb.

REFERENCES

1. Spector SA, Weingeis T, Pollard R, et al. A randomized, controlled study of intravenous ganciclovir therapy for cytomegalovirus peripheral retinitis in patients with AIDS. *J Inf Dis.* 1993; 168:557–563. **2.** Drew WL, Ives D, Lalezari JP, et al. Oral ganciclovir as maintenance treatment for cytomegalovirus retinitis in patients with AIDS. *New Engl J Med.* 1995; 333:615–620. **3.** The Oral Ganciclovir European and Australian Cooperative Study Group. Intravenous vs oral ganciclovir: European/Australian comparative study of efficacy and safety in the prevention of cytomegalovirus retinitis recurrence in patients with AIDS. *AIDS.* 1995; 9:471–477. **4.** Spector SA, McKinley GF, Lalezari JP, Samo T, et al. Oral ganciclovir for the prevention of cytomegalovirus disease in persons with AIDS. *New Engl J Med.* 1996; 334: 1491–1497. **5.** Merigan TC, Renlund DG, Keay S, et al. A controlled trial of ganciclovir to prevent cytomegalovirus disease after heart transplantation. *New Engl J Med.* 1992; 326:1182–1186. **6.** Goodrich JM, Mori M, Gleaves CA, et al. Early treatment with ganciclovir to prevent cytomegalovirus disease after allogeneic bone marrow transplantation. *New Engl J Med.* 1991; 325:1601–1607. **7.** Schmidt GM, Horak DA, Niland JC, et al. The City of Hope-Stanford-Syntex CMV Study Group. A randomized, controlled trial of prophylactic ganciclovir for cytomegalovirus pulmonary infection in recipients of allogeneic bone marrow transplants. *New Engl J Med.* 1991; 15:1005–1011. **8.** Recommendations for the Safe Handling of Cytotoxic Drugs. US Department of Health and Human Services, National Institutes of Health, Bethesda, MD, September, 1992. NIH Publication No. 92–2621. **9.** American Society of Hospital Pharmacists technical assistance bulletin on handling cytotoxic and hazardous drugs. *Am J Hosp Pharm.* 1990; 47:1033–1049. **10.** Controlling Occupational Exposures to Hazardous Drugs. US Department of Labor. Occupational Health and Safety Administration. OSHA Technical Manual. Section V - Chapter 3, September 22, 1995.

Distributed by Roche Laboratories Inc., Nutley, NJ 07110

Revised: September 2000

Shown in Product Identification Guide, page 331

Creatinine Clearance* (mL/min)	CYTOVENE-IV Induction Dose (mg/kg)	Dosing Interval (hours)	CYTOVENE-IV Maintenance Dose (mg/kg)	Dosing Interval (hours)
≥70	5.0	12	5.0	24
50 – 69	2.5	12	2.5	24
25 – 49	2.5	24	1.25	24
10 – 24	1.25	24	0.625	24
<10	1.25	3 times per week, following hemodialysis	0.625	3 times per week, following hemodialysis

*Creatinine clearance can be related to serum creatinine by the formulas given below.

Creatinine Clearance* mL/min	CYTOVENE Capsule Dosages
≥70	1000 mg tid or 500 mg q3h, 6x/day
50 – 69	1500 mg qd or 500 mg tid
25 – 49	1000 mg qd or 500 mg bid
10 – 24	500 mg qd
<10	500 mg 3 times per week, following hemodialysis

* Creatinine clearance can be related to serum creatinine by the following formulas:

$$\text{Creatinine clearance for males} = \frac{(140 - \text{age [yrs]})\ (\text{body wt [kg]})}{(72)\ (\text{serum creatinine [mg/dL]})}$$

$$\text{Creatinine clearance for females} = 0.85 \times \text{male value}$$

DEMADEX® ℞

[*dĕ'mă-dĕks*]

(torsemide)

TABLETS

INJECTION

DESCRIPTION

DEMADEX (torsemide) is a diuretic of the pyridine-sulfonylurea class. Its chemical name is 1-isopropyl-3-[(4-*m*-toluidino-3-pyridyl) sulfonyl]urea.

Its empirical formula is $C_{16}H_{20}N_4O_3S$, its pKa is 7.1, and its molecular weight is 348.43.

Torsemide is a white to off-white crystalline powder. The tablets for oral administration also contain lactose NF, crospovidone NF, povidone USP, microcrystalline cellulose NF, and magnesium stearate NF. Torsemide ampuls for intravenous injection contain a sterile solution of torsemide (10 mg/mL), polyethylene glycol-400 NF, tromethamine USP, and sodium hydroxide NF (as needed to adjust pH) in water for injection USP.

CLINICAL PHARMACOLOGY

Mechanism of Action

Micropuncture studies in animals have shown that torsemide acts from within the lumen of the thick ascending portion of the loop of Henle, where it inhibits the $Na^+/K^+/2Cl^-$-carrier system. Clinical pharmacology studies have confirmed this site of action in humans, and effects in other segments of the nephron have not been demonstrated. Di-

Continued on next page

Demadex—Cont.

uretic activity thus correlates better with the rate of drug excretion in the urine than with the concentration in the blood.
Torsemide increases the urinary excretion of sodium, chloride, and water, but it does not significantly alter glomerular filtration rate, renal plasma flow, or acid-base balance.

Pharmacokinetics and Metabolism

The bioavailability of DEMADEX tablets is approximately 80%, with little intersubject variation; the 90% confidence interval is 75% to 89%. The drug is absorbed with little first-pass metabolism, and the serum concentration reaches its peak (C_{max}) within 1 hour after oral administration. C_{max} and area under the serum concentration-time curve (AUC) after oral administration are proportional to dose over the range of 2.5 mg to 200 mg. Simultaneous food intake delays the time to C_{max} by about 30 minutes, but overall bioavailability (AUC) and diuretic activity are unchanged. Absorption is essentially unaffected by renal or hepatic dysfunction.
The volume of distribution of torsemide is 12 liters to 15 liters in normal adults or in patients with mild to moderate renal failure or congestive heart failure. In patients with hepatic cirrhosis, the volume of distribution is approximately doubled.
In normal subjects the elimination half-life of torsemide is approximately 3.5 hours. Torsemide is cleared from the circulation by both hepatic metabolism (approximately 80% of total clearance) and excretion into the urine (approximately 20% of total clearance in patients with normal renal function). The major metabolite in humans is the carboxylic acid derivative, which is biologically inactive. Two of the lesser metabolites possess some diuretic activity, but for practical purposes metabolism terminates the action of the drug.
Because torsemide is extensively bound to plasma protein (>99%), very little enters tubular urine via glomerular filtration. Most renal clearance of torsemide occurs via active secretion of the drug by the proximal tubules into tubular urine.
In patients with decompensated congestive heart failure, hepatic and renal clearance are both reduced, probably because of hepatic congestion and decreased renal plasma flow, respectively. The total clearance of torsemide is approximately 50% of that seen in healthy volunteers, and the plasma half-life and AUC are correspondingly increased. Because of reduced renal clearance, a smaller fraction of any given dose is delivered to the intraluminal site of action, so at any given dose there is less natriuresis in patients with congestive heart failure than in normal subjects.
In patients with renal failure, renal clearance of torsemide is markedly decreased but total plasma clearance is not significantly altered. A smaller fraction of the administered dose is delivered to the intraluminal site of action, and the natriuretic action of any given dose of diuretic is reduced. A diuretic response in renal failure may still be achieved if patients are given higher doses. The total plasma clearance and elimination half-life of torsemide remain normal under the conditions of impaired renal function because metabolic elimination by the liver remains intact.
In patients with hepatic cirrhosis, the volume of distribution, plasma half-life, and renal clearance are all increased, but total clearance is unchanged.
The pharmacokinetic profile of torsemide in healthy elderly subjects is similar to that in young subjects except for a decrease in renal clearance related to the decline in renal function that commonly occurs with aging. However, total plasma clearance and elimination half-life remain unchanged.

Clinical Effects

The diuretic effects of DEMADEX begin within 10 minutes of intravenous dosing and peak within the first hour. With oral dosing, the onset of diuresis occurs within 1 hour and the peak effect occurs during the first or second hour. Independent of the route of administration, diuresis lasts about 6 to 8 hours. In healthy subjects given single doses, the dose-response relationship for sodium excretion is linear over the dose range of 2.5 mg to 20 mg. The increase in potassium excretion is negligible after a single dose of up to 10 mg and only slight (5 mEq to 15 mEq) after a single dose of 20 mg.

Congestive Heart Failure

DEMADEX has been studied in controlled trials in patients with New York Heart Association Class II to Class IV congestive heart failure. Patients who received 10 mg to 20 mg of daily DEMADEX in these studies achieved significantly greater reductions in weight and edema than did patients who received placebo.

Nonanuric Renal Failure

In single-dose studies in patients with nonanuric renal failure, high doses of DEMADEX (20 mg to 200 mg) caused marked increases in water and sodium excretion. In patients with nonanuric renal failure, severe enough to require hemodialysis, chronic treatment with up to 200 mg of daily DEMADEX has not been shown to change steady-state fluid retention. When patients in a study of acute renal failure received total daily doses of 520 mg to 1200 mg of DEMADEX, 19% experienced seizures. Ninety-six patients were treated in this study; 6/32 treated with torsemide experienced seizures, 6/32 treated with comparably high doses of furosemide experienced seizures, and 1/32 treated with placebo experienced a seizure.

Hepatic Cirrhosis

When given with aldosterone antagonists, DEMADEX also caused increases in sodium and fluid excretion in patients with edema or ascites due to hepatic cirrhosis. Urinary sodium excretion rate relative to the urinary excretion rate of DEMADEX is less in cirrhotic patients than in healthy subjects (possibly because of the hyperaldosteronism and resultant sodium retention that are characteristic of portal hypertension and ascites). However, because of the increased renal clearance of DEMADEX in patients with hepatic cirrhosis, these factors tend to balance each other, and the result is an overall natriuretic response that is similar to that seen in healthy subjects. Chronic use of any diuretic in hepatic disease has not been studied in adequate and well-controlled trials.

Essential Hypertension

In patients with essential hypertension, DEMADEX has been shown in controlled studies to lower blood pressure when administered once a day at doses of 5 mg to 10 mg. The antihypertensive effect is near maximal after 4 to 6 weeks of treatment, but it may continue to increase for up to 12 weeks. Systolic and diastolic supine and standing blood pressures are all reduced. There is no significant orthostatic effect, and there is only a minimal peak-trough difference in blood pressure reduction.
The antihypertensive effects of DEMADEX are, like those of other diuretics, on the average greater in black patients (a low-renin population) than in nonblack patients.
When DEMADEX is first administered, daily urinary sodium excretion increases for at least a week. With chronic administration, however, daily sodium loss comes into balance with dietary sodium intake. If the administration of DEMADEX is suddenly stopped, blood pressure returns to pretreatment levels over several days, without overshoot.
DEMADEX has been administered together with β-adrenergic blocking agents, ACE inhibitors, and calcium-channel blockers. Adverse drug interactions have not been observed, and special dosage adjustment has not been necessary.

INDICATIONS AND USAGE

DEMADEX is indicated for the treatment of edema associated with congestive heart failure, renal disease, or hepatic disease. Use of torsemide has been found to be effective for the treatment of edema associated with chronic renal failure. Chronic use of any diuretic in hepatic disease has not been studied in adequate and well-controlled trials.
DEMADEX intravenous injection is indicated when a rapid onset of diuresis is desired or when oral administration is impractical.
DEMADEX is indicated for the treatment of hypertension alone or in combination with other antihypertensive agents.

CONTRAINDICATIONS

DEMADEX is contraindicated in patients with known hypersensitivity to DEMADEX or to sulfonylureas.
DEMADEX is contraindicated in patients who are anuric.

WARNINGS

Hepatic Disease With Cirrhosis and Ascites

DEMADEX should be used with caution in patients with hepatic disease with cirrhosis and ascites, since sudden alterations of fluid and electrolyte balance may precipitate hepatic coma. In these patients, diuresis with DEMADEX (or any other diuretic) is best initiated in the hospital. To prevent hypokalemia and metabolic alkalosis, an aldosterone antagonist or potassium-sparing drug should be used concomitantly with DEMADEX.

Ototoxicity

Tinnitus and hearing loss (usually reversible) have been observed after rapid intravenous injection of other loop diuretics and have also been observed after oral DEMADEX. It is not certain that these events were attributable to DEMADEX. Ototoxicity has also been seen in animal studies when very high plasma levels of torsemide were induced. Administered intravenously, DEMADEX should be injected slowly over 2 minutes, and single doses should not exceed 200 mg.

Volume and Electrolyte Depletion

Patients receiving diuretics should be observed for clinical evidence of electrolyte imbalance, hypovolemia, or prerenal azotemia. Symptoms of these disturbances may include one or more of the following: dryness of the mouth, thirst, weakness, lethargy, drowsiness, restlessness, muscle pains or cramps, muscular fatigue, hypotension, oliguria, tachycardia, nausea, and vomiting. Excessive diuresis may cause dehydration, blood-volume reduction, and possibly thrombosis and embolism, especially in elderly patients. In patients who develop fluid and electrolyte imbalances, hypovolemia, or prerenal azotemia, the observed laboratory changes may include hyper- or hyponatremia, hyper- or hypochloremia, hyper- or hypokalemia, acid-base abnormalities, and increased blood urea nitrogen (BUN). If any of these occur, DEMADEX should be discontinued until the situation is corrected; DEMADEX may be restarted at a lower dose.
In controlled studies in the United States, DEMADEX was administered to hypertensive patients at doses of 5 mg or 10 mg daily. After 6 weeks at these doses, the mean decrease in serum potassium was approximately 0.1 mEq/L. The percentage of patients who had a serum potassium level below 3.5 mEq/L at any time during the studies was essentially the same in patients who received DEMADEX (1.5%) as in those who received placebo (3%). In patients followed for 1 year, there was no further change in mean serum potassium levels. In patients with congestive heart failure, hepatic cirrhosis, or renal disease treated with DEMADEX at doses higher than those studied in United States antihypertensive trials, hypokalemia was observed with greater frequency, in a dose-related manner.
In patients with cardiovascular disease, especially those receiving digitalis glycosides, diuretic-induced hypokalemia may be a risk factor for the development of arrhythmias. The risk of hypokalemia is greatest in patients with cirrhosis of the liver, in patients experiencing a brisk diuresis, in patients who are receiving inadequate oral intake of electrolytes, and in patients receiving concomitant therapy with corticosteroids or ACTH.
Periodic monitoring of serum potassium and other electrolytes is advised in patients treated with DEMADEX.

PRECAUTIONS

Laboratory Values

Potassium: See WARNINGS.

Calcium

Single doses of DEMADEX increased the urinary excretion of calcium by normal subjects, but serum calcium levels were slightly increased in 4- to 6-week hypertension trials. In a long-term study of patients with congestive heart failure, the average 1-year change in serum calcium was a decrease of 0.10 mg/dL (0.02 mmol/L). Among 426 patients treated with DEMADEX for an average of 11 months, hypocalcemia was not reported as an adverse event.

Magnesium

Single doses of DEMADEX caused healthy volunteers to increase their urinary excretion of magnesium, but serum magnesium levels were slightly increased in 4- to 6-week hypertension trials. In long-term hypertension studies, the average 1-year change in serum magnesium was an increase of 0.03 mg/dL (0.01 mmol/L). Among 426 patients treated with DEMADEX for an average of 11 months, one case of hypomagnesemia (1.3 mg/dL [0.53 mmol/L]) was reported as an adverse event.
In a long-term clinical study of DEMADEX in patients with congestive heart failure, the estimated annual change in serum magnesium was an increase of 0.2 mg/dL (0.08 mmol/L), but these data are confounded by the fact that many of these patients received magnesium supplements. In a 4-week study in which magnesium supplementation was not given, the rate of occurrence of serum magnesium levels below 1.7 mg/dL (0.70 mmol/L) was 6% and 9% in the groups receiving 5 mg and 10 mg of DEMADEX, respectively.

Blood Urea Nitrogen (BUN), Creatinine and Uric Acid

DEMADEX produces small dose-related increases in each of these laboratory values. In hypertensive patients who received 10 mg of DEMADEX daily for 6 weeks, the mean increase in blood urea nitrogen was 1.8 mg/dL (0.6 mmol/L), the mean increase in serum creatinine was 0.05 mg/dL (4 mmol/L), and the mean increase in serum uric acid was 1.2 mg/dL (70 mmol/L). Little further change occurred with long-term treatment, and all changes reversed when treatment was discontinued.
Symptomatic gout has been reported in patients receiving DEMADEX, but its incidence has been similar to that seen in patients receiving placebo.

Glucose

Hypertensive patients who received 10 mg of daily DEMADEX experienced a mean increase in serum glucose concentration of 5.5 mg/dL (0.3 mmol/L) after 6 weeks of therapy, with a further increase of 1.8 mg/dL (0.1 mmol/L) during the subsequent year. In long-term studies in diabetics, mean fasting glucose values were not significantly changed from baseline. Cases of hyperglycemia have been reported but are uncommon.

Serum Lipids

In the controlled short-term hypertension studies in the United States, daily doses of 5 mg, 10 mg, and 20 mg of DEMADEX were associated with increases in total plasma cholesterol of 4, 4, and 8 mg/dL (0.10 to 0.20 mmol/L), respectively. The changes subsided during chronic therapy.
In the same short-term hypertension studies, daily doses of 5 mg, 10 mg and 20 mg of DEMADEX were associated with mean increases in plasma triglycerides of 16, 13 and 71 mg/dL (0.15 to 0.80 mmol/L), respectively.
In long-term studies of 5 mg to 20 mg of DEMADEX daily, no clinically significant differences from baseline lipid values were observed after 1 year of therapy.

Other

In long-term studies in hypertensive patients, DEMADEX has been associated with small mean decreases in hemoglobin, hematocrit, and erythrocyte count and small mean increases in white blood cell count, platelet count, and serum alkaline phosphatase. Although statistically significant, all of these changes were medically inconsequential. No significant trends have been observed in any liver enzyme tests other than alkaline phosphatase.

Drug Interactions

In patients with essential hypertension, DEMADEX has been administered together with beta-blockers, ACE inhibitors, and calcium-channel blockers. In patients with congestive heart failure, DEMADEX has been administered together with digitalis glycosides, ACE inhibitors, and organic nitrates. None of these combined uses was associated with new or unexpected adverse events.
Torsemide does not affect the protein binding of glyburide or of warfarin, the anticoagulant effect of phenprocoumon (a related coumarin derivative), or the pharmacokinetics of digoxin or carvedilol (a vasodilator/beta-blocker). In healthy subjects, coadministration of DEMADEX was associated with significant reduction in the renal clearance of spirono-

lactone, with corresponding increases in the AUC. However, clinical experience indicates that dosage adjustment of either agent is not required.

Because DEMADEX and salicylates compete for secretion by renal tubules, patients receiving high doses of salicylates may experience salicylate toxicity when DEMADEX is concomitantly administered. Also, although possible interactions between torsemide and nonsteroidal anti-inflammatory agents (including aspirin) have not been studied, coadministration of these agents with another loop diuretic (furosemide) has occasionally been associated with renal dysfunction.

The natriuretic effect of DEMADEX (like that of many other diuretics) is partially inhibited by the concomitant administration of indomethacin. This effect has been demonstrated for DEMADEX under conditions of dietary sodium restriction (50 mEq/day) but not in the presence of normal sodium intake (150 mEq/day).

The pharmacokinetic profile and diuretic activity of torsemide are not altered by cimetidine or spironolactone. Coadministration of digoxin is reported to increase the area under the curve for torsemide by 50%, but dose adjustment of DEMADEX is not necessary.

Concomitant use of torsemide and cholestyramine has not been studied in humans but, in a study in animals, coadministration of cholestyramine decreased the absorption of orally administered torsemide. If DEMADEX and cholestyramine are used concomitantly, simultaneous administration is not recommended.

Coadministration of probenecid reduces secretion of DEMADEX into the proximal tubule and thereby decreases the diuretic activity of DEMADEX.

Other diuretics are known to reduce the renal clearance of lithium, inducing a high risk of lithium toxicity, so coadministration of lithium and diuretics should be undertaken with great caution, if at all. Coadministration of lithium and DEMADEX has not been studied.

Other diuretics have been reported to increase the ototoxic potential of aminoglycoside antibiotics and of ethacrynic acid, especially in the presence of impaired renal function. These potential interactions with DEMADEX have not been studied.

Carcinogenesis, Mutagenesis and Impairment of Fertility

No overall increase in tumor incidence was found when torsemide was given to rats and mice throughout their lives at doses up to 9 mg/kg/day (rats) and 32 mg/kg/day (mice). On a body-weight basis, these doses are 27 to 96 times a human dose of 20 mg; on a body-surface-area basis, they are 5 to 8 times this dose. In the rat study, the high-dose female group demonstrated renal tubular injury, interstitial inflammation, and a statistically significant increase in renal adenomas and carcinomas. The tumor incidence in this group was, however, not much higher than the incidence sometimes seen in historical controls. Similar signs of chronic non-neoplastic renal injury have been reported in high-dose animal studies of other diuretics such as furosemide and hydrochlorothiazide.

No mutagenic activity was detected in any of a variety of in vivo and in vitro tests of torsemide and its major human metabolite. The tests included the Ames test in bacteria (with and without metabolic activation), tests for chromosome aberrations and sister-chromatid exchanges in human lymphocytes, tests for various nuclear anomalies in cells found in hamster and murine bone marrow, tests for unscheduled DNA synthesis in mice and rats, and others.

In doses up to 25 mg/kg/day (75 times a human dose of 20 mg on a body-weight basis; 13 times this dose on a body-surface-area basis), torsemide had no adverse effect on the reproductive performance of male or female rats.

Pregnancy

Pregnancy Category B. There was no fetotoxicity or teratogenicity in rats treated with up to 5 mg/kg/day of torsemide (on a mg/kg basis, this is 15 times a human dose of 20 mg/day; on a mg/m^2 basis, the animal dose is 10 times the human dose), or in rabbits, treated with 1.6 mg/kg/day (on a mg/kg basis, 5 times the human dose of 20 mg/kg/day; on a mg/m^2 basis, 1.7 times this dose). Fetal and maternal toxicity (decrease in average body weight, increase in fetal resorption and delayed fetal ossification) occurred in rabbits and rats given doses 4 (rabbits) and 5 (rats) times larger. Adequate and well-controlled studies have not been carried out in pregnant women. Because animal reproduction studies are not always predictive of human response, this drug should be used during pregnancy only if clearly needed.

Labor and Delivery

The effect of DEMADEX on labor and delivery is unknown.

Nursing Mothers

It is not known whether DEMADEX is excreted in human milk. Because many drugs are excreted in human milk, caution should be exercised when DEMADEX is administered to a nursing woman.

Pediatric Use

Safety and effectiveness in pediatric patients have not been established.

Administration of another loop diuretic to severely premature infants with edema due to patent ductus arteriosus and hyaline membrane disease has occasionally been associated with renal calcifications, sometimes barely visible on X-ray but sometimes in staghorn form, filling the renal pelves. Some of these calculi have been dissolved, and hypercalciuria has been reported to have decreased, when chlorothiazide has been coadministered along with the loop diuretic. In other premature neonates with hyaline membrane disease, another loop diuretic has been reported to increase the risk of persistent patent ductus arteriosus, possibly through a prostaglandin-E-mediated process. The use of DEMADEX in such patients has not been studied.

Geriatric Use

Of the total number of patients who received DEMADEX in United States clinical studies, 24% were 65 or older while about 4% were 75 or older. No specific age-related differences in effectiveness or safety were observed between younger patients and elderly patients.

ADVERSE REACTIONS

At the time of approval, DEMADEX had been evaluated for safety in approximately 4000 subjects: over 800 of these subjects received DEMADEX for at least 6 months, and over 380 were treated for more than 1 year. Among these subjects were 564 who received DEMADEX during United States-based trials in which 274 other subjects received placebo.

The reported side effects of DEMADEX were generally transient, and there was no relationship between side effects and age, sex, race, or duration of therapy. Discontinuation of therapy due to side effects occurred in 3.5% of United States patients treated with DEMADEX and in 4.4% of patients treated with placebo. In studies conducted in the United States and Europe, discontinuation rates due to side effects were 3.0% (38/1250) with DEMADEX and 3.4% (13/380) with furosemide in patients with congestive heart failure, 2.0% (8/409) with DEMADEX and 4.8% (11/230) with furosemide in patients with renal insufficiency, and 7.6% (13/170) with DEMADEX and 0% (0/33) with furosemide in patients with cirrhosis.

The most common reasons for discontinuation of therapy with DEMADEX were (in descending order of frequency) dizziness, headache, nausea, weakness, vomiting, hyperglycemia, excessive urination, hyperuricemia, hypokalemia, excessive thirst, hypovolemia, impotence, esophageal hemorrhage, and dyspepsia. Dropout rates for these adverse events ranged from 0.1% to 0.5%.

The side effects considered possibly or probably related to study drug that occurred in United States placebo-controlled trials in more than 1% of patients treated with DEMADEX are shown in Table 1.

Table 1. Reactions Possibly or Probably Drug-Related United States Placebo-Controlled Studies Incidence (Percentages of Patients)

	DEMADEX (N=564)	Placebo (N=274)
Headache	7.3	9.1
Excessive Urination	6.7	2.2
Dizziness	3.2	4.0
Rhinitis	2.8	2.2
Asthenia	2.0	1.5
Diarrhea	2.0	1.1
ECG Abnormality	2.0	0.4
Cough Increase	2.0	1.5
Constipation	1.8	0.7
Nausea	1.8	0.4
Arthralgia	1.8	0.7
Dyspepsia	1.6	0.7
Sore Throat	1.6	0.7
Myalgia	1.6	1.5
Chest Pain	1.2	0.4
Insomnia	1.2	1.8
Edema	1.1	1.1
Nervousness	1.1	0.4

The daily doses of DEMADEX used in these trials ranged from 1.25 mg to 20 mg, with most patients receiving 5 mg to 10 mg; the duration of treatment ranged from 1 to 52 days, with a median of 41 days. Of the side effects listed in the table, only "excessive urination" occurred significantly more frequently in patients treated with DEMADEX than in patients treated with placebo. In the placebo-controlled hypertension studies whose design allowed side-effect rates to be attributed to dose, excessive urination was reported by 1% of patients receiving placebo, 4% of those treated with 5 mg of daily DEMADEX, and 15% of those treated with 10 mg. The complaint of excessive urination was generally not reported as an adverse event among patients who received DEMADEX for cardiac, renal, or hepatic failure.

Serious adverse events reported in the clinical studies for which a drug relationship could not be excluded were atrial fibrillation, chest pain, diarrhea, digitalis intoxication, gastrointestinal hemorrhage, hyperglycemia, hyperuricemia, hypokalemia, hypotension, hypovolemia, shunt thrombosis, rash, rectal bleeding, syncope, and ventricular tachycardia.

Angioedema has been reported in a patient exposed to DEMADEX who was later found to be allergic to sulfa drugs.

Of the adverse reactions during placebo-controlled trials listed without taking into account assessment of relatedness to drug therapy, arthritis and various other nonspecific musculoskeletal problems were more frequently reported in association with DEMADEX than with placebo, even though gout was somewhat more frequently associated with placebo. These reactions did not increase in frequency or severity with the dose of DEMADEX. One patient in the group treated with DEMADEX withdrew due to myalgia, and one in the placebo group withdrew due to gout.

Hypokalemia: See WARNINGS.

OVERDOSAGE

There is no human experience with overdoses of DEMADEX, but the signs and symptoms of overdosage can be anticipated to be those of excessive pharmacologic effect: dehydration, hypovolemia, hypotension, hyponatremia, hypokalemia, hypochloremic alkalosis, and hemoconcentration. Treatment of overdosage should consist of fluid and electrolyte replacement.

Laboratory determinations of serum levels of torsemide and its metabolites are not widely available.

No data are available to suggest physiological maneuvers (eg, maneuvers to change the pH of the urine) that might accelerate elimination of torsemide and its metabolites. Torsemide is not dialyzable, so hemodialysis will not accelerate elimination.

DOSAGE AND ADMINISTRATION

General

DEMADEX tablets may be given at any time in relation to a meal, as convenient. Special dosage adjustment in the elderly is not necessary.

Because of the high bioavailability of DEMADEX, oral and intravenous doses are therapeutically equivalent, so patients may be switched to and from the intravenous form with no change in dose. DEMADEX intravenous injection should be administered either slowly as a bolus over a period of 2 minutes or administered as a continuous infusion.

If DEMADEX is administered through an IV line, it is recommended that, as with other IV injections, the IV line be flushed with Normal Saline (Sodium Chloride Injection, USP) before and after administration. DEMADEX injection is formulated above pH 8.3. Flushing the line is recommended to avoid the potential for incompatibilities caused by differences in pH which could be indicated by color change, haziness or the formation of a precipitate in the solution.

If DEMADEX is administered as a continuous infusion, stability has been demonstrated through 24 hours at room temperature in plastic containers for the following fluids and concentrations:

200 mg DEMADEX (10 mg/mL) added to:
- 250 mL Dextrose 5% in water
- 250 mL 0.9% Sodium Chloride
- 500 mL 0.45% Sodium Chloride

50 mg DEMADEX (10 mg/mL) added to:
- 500 mL Dextrose 5% in water
- 500 mL 0.9% Sodium Chloride
- 500 mL 0.45% Sodium Chloride

Before administration, the solution of DEMADEX should be visually inspected for discoloration and particulate matter. If either is found, the ampul should not be used.

Congestive Heart Failure

The usual initial dose is 10 mg or 20 mg of once-daily oral or intravenous DEMADEX. If the diuretic response is inadequate, the dose should be titrated upward by approximately doubling until the desired diuretic response is obtained. Single doses higher than 200 mg have not been adequately studied.

Chronic Renal Failure

The usual initial dose of DEMADEX is 20 mg of once-daily oral or intravenous DEMADEX. If the diuretic response is inadequate, the dose should be titrated upward by approximately doubling until the desired diuretic response is obtained. Single doses higher than 200 mg have not been adequately studied.

Hepatic Cirrhosis

The usual initial dose is 5 mg or 10 mg of once-daily oral or intravenous DEMADEX, administered together with an aldosterone antagonist or a potassium-sparing diuretic. If the diuretic response is inadequate, the dose should be titrated upward by approximately doubling until the desired diuretic response is obtained. Single doses higher than 40 mg have not been adequately studied.

Chronic use of any diuretic in hepatic disease has not been studied in adequate and well-controlled trials.

Hypertension

The usual initial dose is 5 mg once daily. If the 5 mg dose does not provide adequate reduction in blood pressure within 4 to 6 weeks, the dose may be increased to 10 mg once daily. If the response to 10 mg is insufficient, an additional antihypertensive agent should be added to the treatment regimen.

HOW SUPPLIED

DEMADEX for oral administration is available as white, scored tablets containing 5 mg, 10 mg, 20 mg, or 100 mg of torsemide. The tablets are supplied in bottles and Tel-E-Dose®* packages of 100 as follows:

[See table above]

Dose	Shape	Bottle	Tel-E-Dose
5 mg	elliptical	NDC 0004-0262-01	NDC 0004-0262-49
10 mg	elliptical	NDC 0004-0263-01	NDC 0004-0263-49
20 mg	elliptical	NDC 0004-0264-01	NDC 0004-0264-49
100 mg	capsule shaped	NDC 0004-0265-01	NDC 0004-0265-49

Continued on next page

Demadex—Cont.

Each tablet is debossed on the scored side with the logo BM and 102, 103, 104, or 105 (for 5 mg, 10 mg, 20 mg, or 100 mg, respectively). On the opposite side, the tablet is debossed with 5, 10, 20, or 100 to indicate the dose.
DEMADEX for intravenous injection is supplied in clear ampuls containing 2 mL (20 mg, NDC 0004-0267-06) or 5 mL (50 mg, NDC 0004-0268-06) of a 10 mg/mL sterile solution. The ampuls are supplied in boxes of 10.

Storage

Store all dosage forms at 15° to 30°C (59° to 86°F). Do not freeze.

*Tel-E-Dose is a registered trademark of Hoffmann-La Roche Inc.

Revised: April 2003

Shown in Product Identification Guide, page 331

EC-NAPROSYN® ℞
(naproxen)
Delayed-Release Tablets

NAPROSYN® ℞
(naproxen)
Tablets

ANAPROX®/ANAPROX® DS ℞
(naproxen sodium)
Tablets

NAPROSYN® ℞
(naproxen)
Suspension
℞ only

DESCRIPTION

Naproxen is a member of the arylacetic acid group of nonsteroidal anti-inflammatory drugs.
The chemical names for naproxen and naproxen sodium are (S)-6-methoxy-α-methyl-2-naphthaleneacetic acid and (S)-6-methoxy-α-methyl-2-naphthaleneacetic acid, sodium salt, respectively.
Naproxen is an odorless, white to off-white crystalline substance. It is lipid-soluble, practically insoluble in water at low pH and freely soluble in water at high pH. The octanol/water partition coefficient of naproxen at pH 7.4 is 1.6 to 1.8. Naproxen sodium is a white to creamy white, crystalline solid, freely soluble in water at neutral pH.
NAPROSYN (naproxen) Tablets contain 250 mg, 375 mg or 500 mg of naproxen and croscarmellose sodium, iron oxides, povidone and magnesium stearate.
EC-NAPROSYN (naproxen) Delayed-Release Tablets are enteric-coated tablets containing 375 mg or 500 mg of naproxen and croscarmellose sodium, povidone and magnesium stearate. The enteric coating dispersion contains methacrylic acid copolymer, talc, triethyl citrate, sodium hydroxide and purified water. The dispersion may also contain simethicone emulsion. The dissolution of this enteric-coated naproxen tablet is pH dependent with rapid dissolution above pH 6. There is no dissolution below pH 4.
Each ANAPROX 275 mg and ANAPROX DS 550 mg tablet contains naproxen sodium, the active ingredient, with magnesium stearate, microcrystalline cellulose, povidone and talc. The coating suspension for the ANAPROX 275 mg tablet may contain hydroxypropyl methylcellulose 2910, Opaspray K-1-4210A, polyethylene glycol 8000 or Opadry YS-1-4215. The coating suspension for the ANAPROX DS 550 mg tablet may contain hydroxypropyl methylcellulose 2910, Opaspray K-1-4227, polyethylene glycol 8000 or Opadry YS-1-4216.
NAPROSYN (naproxen) Suspension for oral administration contains 125 mg/5 mL of naproxen in a vehicle containing sucrose, magnesium aluminum silicate, sorbitol solution and sodium chloride (30 mg/5 mL, 1.5 mEq), methylparaben, fumaric acid, FD&C Yellow No. 6, imitation pineapple flavor, imitation orange flavor and purified water. The pH of the suspension ranges from 2.2 to 3.7.

CLINICAL PHARMACOLOGY

Naproxen is a nonsteroidal anti-inflammatory drug (NSAID) with analgesic and antipyretic properties. The sodium salt of naproxen has been developed as a more rapidly absorbed formulation of naproxen for use as an analgesic. The naproxen anion inhibits prostaglandin synthesis but beyond this its mode of action is unknown.
Pharmacokinetics: Naproxen itself is rapidly and completely absorbed from the gastrointestinal tract with an in vivo bioavailability of 95%. The different dosage forms of NAPROSYN are bioequivalent in terms of extent of absorption (AUC) and peak concentration (C_{max}); however, the products do differ in their pattern of absorption. These differences between naproxen products are related to both the chemical form of naproxen used and its formulation. Even with the observed differences in pattern of absorption, the elimination half-life of naproxen is unchanged across products ranging from 12 to 17 hours. Steady-state levels of naproxen are reached in 4 to 5 days, and the degree of naproxen accumulation is consistent with this half-life. This suggests that the differences in pattern of release play only a negligible role in the attainment of steady-state plasma levels.
Absorption:
Immediate Release: After administration of NAPROSYN tablets, peak plasma levels are attained in 2 to 4 hours. After oral administration of ANAPROX, peak plasma levels are attained in 1 to 2 hours. The difference in rates between the two products is due to the increased aqueous solubility of the sodium salt of naproxen used in ANAPROX. Peak plasma levels of naproxen given as NAPROSYN Suspension are attained in 1 to 4 hours.
Delayed Release: EC-NAPROSYN is designed with a pH-sensitive coating to provide a barrier to disintegration in the acidic environment of the stomach and to lose integrity in the more neutral environment of the small intestine. The enteric polymer coating selected for EC-NAPROSYN dissolves above pH 6. When EC-NAPROSYN was given to fasted subjects, peak plasma levels were attained about 4 to 6 hours following the first dose (range: 2 to 12 hours). An in vivo study in man using radiolabeled EC-NAPROSYN tablets demonstrated that EC-NAPROSYN dissolves primarily in the small intestine rather than the stomach, so the absorption of the drug is delayed until the stomach is emptied.
When EC-NAPROSYN and NAPROSYN were given to fasted subjects (n=24) in a crossover study following 1 week of dosing, differences in time to peak plasma levels (T_{max}) were observed, but there were no differences in total absorption as measured by C_{max} and AUC:
[See table below]
Antacid Effects: When EC-NAPROSYN was given as a single dose with antacid (54 mEq buffering capacity), the peak plasma levels of naproxen were unchanged, but the time to peak was reduced (mean T_{max} fasted 5.6 hours, mean T_{max} with antacid 5 hours), although not significantly.
Food Effects: When EC-NAPROSYN was given as a single dose with food, peak plasma levels in most subjects were achieved in about 12 hours (range: 4 to 24 hours). Residence time in the small intestine until disintegration was independent of food intake. The presence of food prolonged the time the tablets remained in the stomach, time to first detectable serum naproxen levels, and time to maximal naproxen levels (T_{max}), but did not affect peak naproxen levels (C_{max}).
Distribution:
Naproxen has a volume of distribution of 0.16 L/kg. At therapeutic levels naproxen is greater than 99% albumin-bound. At doses of naproxen greater than 500 mg/day there is less than proportional increase in plasma levels due to an increase in clearance caused by saturation of plasma protein binding at higher doses (average trough C_{ss} 36.5, 49.2 and 56.4 mg/L with 500, 1000 and 1500 mg daily doses of naproxen). However, the concentration of unbound naproxen continues to increase proportionally to dose.
Metabolism:
Naproxen is extensively metabolized to 6-0-desmethyl naproxen, and both parent and metabolites do not induce metabolizing enzymes.
Elimination:
The clearance of naproxen is 0.13 mL/min/kg. Approximately 95% of the naproxen from any dose is excreted in the urine, primarily as naproxen (less than 1%), 6-0-desmethyl naproxen (less than 1%) or their conjugates (66% to 92%). The plasma half-life of the naproxen anion in humans ranges from 12 to 17 hours. The corresponding half-lives of both naproxen's metabolites and conjugates are shorter than 12 hours, and their rates of excretion have been found to coincide closely with the rate of naproxen disappearance from the plasma. In patients with renal failure metabolites may accumulate.
Special Populations:
Pediatric Patients: In pediatric patients aged 5 to 16 years with arthritis, plasma naproxen levels following a 5 mg/kg single dose of naproxen suspension (see DOSAGE AND ADMINISTRATION) were found to be similar to those found in normal adults following a 500 mg dose. The terminal half-life appears to be similar in pediatric and adult patients. Pharmacokinetic studies of naproxen were not performed in pediatric patients younger than 5 years of age. Pharmacokinetic parameters appear to be similar following administration of naproxen suspension or tablets in pediatric patients. EC-NAPROSYN has not been studied in subjects under the age of 18.
Renal Insufficiency: Naproxen pharmacokinetics has not been determined in subjects with renal insufficiency. Given that naproxen, its metabolites and conjugates are primarily excreted by the kidney, the potential exists for naproxen metabolites to accumulate in the presence of renal insufficiency.

	EC-NAPROSYN* 500 mg bid	NAPROSYN* 500 mg bid
C_{max} (μg/mL)	94.9 (18%)	97.4 (13%)
T_{max} (hours)	4 (39%)	1.9 (61%)
$AUC_{0-12\ hr}$ (μg•hr/mL)	845 (20%)	767 (15%)

* Mean value (coefficient of variation)

CLINICAL STUDIES

General Information: Naproxen has been studied in patients with rheumatoid arthritis, osteoarthritis, juvenile arthritis, ankylosing spondylitis, tendonitis and bursitis, and acute gout. Improvement in patients treated for rheumatoid arthritis was demonstrated by a reduction in joint swelling, a reduction in duration of morning stiffness, a reduction in disease activity as assessed by both the investigator and patient, and by increased mobility as demonstrated by a reduction in walking time. Generally, response to naproxen has not been found to be dependent on age, sex, severity or duration of rheumatoid arthritis.
In patients with osteoarthritis, the therapeutic action of naproxen has been shown by a reduction in joint pain or tenderness, an increase in range of motion in knee joints, increased mobility as demonstrated by a reduction in walking time, and improvement in capacity to perform activities of daily living impaired by the disease.
In a clinical trial comparing standard formulations of naproxen 375 mg bid (750 mg a day) vs 750 mg bid (1500 mg/day), 9 patients in the 750 mg group terminated prematurely because of adverse events. Nineteen patients in the 1500 mg group terminated prematurely because of adverse events. Most of these adverse events were gastrointestinal events.
In clinical studies in patients with rheumatoid arthritis, osteoarthritis, and juvenile arthritis, naproxen has been shown to be comparable to aspirin and indomethacin in controlling the aforementioned measures of disease activity, but the frequency and severity of the milder gastrointestinal adverse effects (nausea, dyspepsia, heartburn) and nervous system adverse effects (tinnitus, dizziness, lightheadedness) were less in naproxen-treated patients than in those treated with aspirin or indomethacin.
In patients with ankylosing spondylitis, naproxen has been shown to decrease night pain, morning stiffness and pain at rest. In double-blind studies the drug was shown to be as effective as aspirin, but with fewer side effects.
In patients with acute gout, a favorable response to naproxen was shown by significant clearing of inflammatory changes (eg, decrease in swelling, heat) within 24 to 48 hours, as well as by relief of pain and tenderness.
Naproxen has been studied in patients with mild to moderate pain secondary to postoperative, orthopedic, postpartum episiotomy and uterine contraction pain and dysmenorrhea. Onset of pain relief can begin within 1 hour in patients taking naproxen and within 30 minutes in patients taking naproxen sodium. Analgesic effect was shown by such measures as reduction of pain intensity scores, increase in pain relief scores, decrease in numbers of patients requiring additional analgesic medication, and delay in time to remedication. The analgesic effect has been found to last for up to 12 hours.
Naproxen may be used safely in combination with gold salts and/or corticosteroids; however, in controlled clinical trials, when added to the regimen of patients receiving corticosteroids, it did not appear to cause greater improvement over that seen with corticosteroids alone. Whether naproxen has a "steroid-sparing" effect has not been adequately studied. When added to the regimen of patients receiving gold salts, naproxen did result in greater improvement. Its use in combination with salicylates is not recommended because there is evidence that aspirin increases the rate of excretion of naproxen and data are inadequate to demonstrate that naproxen and aspirin produce greater improvement over that achieved with aspirin alone. In addition, as with other NSAIDs, the combination may result in higher frequency of adverse events than demonstrated for either product alone.
In ^{51}Cr blood loss and gastroscopy studies with normal volunteers, daily administration of 1000 mg of naproxen as 1000 mg of NAPROSYN (naproxen) or 1100 mg of ANAPROX (naproxen sodium) has been demonstrated to cause statistically significantly less gastric bleeding and erosion than 3250 mg of aspirin.
Three 6-week, double-blind, multicenter studies with EC-NAPROSYN (naproxen) (375 or 500 mg bid, n=385) and NAPROSYN (375 or 500 mg bid, n=279) were conducted comparing EC-NAPROSYN with NAPROSYN, including 355 rheumatoid arthritis and osteoarthritis patients who had a recent history of NSAID-related GI symptoms. These studies indicated that EC-NAPROSYN and NAPROSYN showed no significant differences in efficacy or safety and had similar prevalence of minor GI complaints. Individual patients, however, may find one formulation preferable to the other.
Five hundred and fifty-three patients received EC-NAPROSYN during long-term open-label trials (mean length of treatment was 159 days). The rates for clinically-diagnosed peptic ulcers and GI bleeds were similar to what has been historically reported for long-term NSAID use.

INDIVIDUALIZATION OF DOSAGE

Although NAPROSYN, NAPROSYN Suspension, EC-NAPROSYN, ANAPROX and ANAPROX DS all circulate in the plasma as naproxen, they have pharmacokinetic differences that may affect onset of action. Onset of pain relief can begin within 30 minutes in patients taking naproxen sodium and within 1 hour in patients taking naproxen. Because EC-NAPROSYN dissolves in the small intestine rather than in the stomach, the absorption of the drug is delayed compared to the other naproxen formulations (see CLINICAL PHARMACOLOGY).

The recommended strategy for initiating therapy is to choose a formulation and a starting dose likely to be effective for the patient and then adjust the dosage based on observation of benefit and/or adverse events. A lower dose should be considered in patients with renal or hepatic impairment or in elderly patients (see PRECAUTIONS).

Analgesia/Dysmenorrhea/Bursitis and Tendonitis: Because the sodium salt of naproxen is more rapidly absorbed, ANAPROX/ANAPROX DS is recommended for the management of acute painful conditions when prompt onset of pain relief is desired. The recommended starting dose is 550 mg followed by 550 mg every 12 hours or 275 mg every 6 to 8 hours, as required. The initial total daily dose should not exceed 1375 mg of naproxen sodium. Thereafter, the total daily dose should not exceed 1100 mg of naproxen sodium. NAPROSYN may also be used for treatment of acute pain and dysmenorrhea. EC-NAPROSYN is not recommended for initial treatment of acute pain because absorption of naproxen is delayed compared to other naproxen-containing products (see CLINICAL PHARMACOLOGY and INDICATIONS AND USAGE).

Acute Gout: The recommended starting dose is 750 mg of NAPROSYN followed by 250 mg every 8 hours until the attack has subsided. ANAPROX may also be used at a starting dose of 825 mg followed by 275 mg every 8 hours as needed. EC-NAPROSYN is not recommended because of the delay in absorption (see CLINICAL PHARMACOLOGY).

Osteoarthritis/Rheumatoid Arthritis/Ankylosing Spondylitis: The recommended dose of naproxen is NAPROSYN or NAPROSYN Suspension 250 mg, 375 mg or 500 mg taken twice daily (morning and evening) or EC-NAPROSYN 375 mg or 500 mg taken twice daily. Naproxen sodium may also be used (see DOSAGE AND ADMINISTRATION).

During long-term administration the dose of naproxen may be adjusted up or down depending on the clinical response of the patient. A lower daily dose may suffice for long-term administration. In patients who tolerate lower doses well, the dose may be increased to 1500 mg per day for up to 6 months when a higher level of anti-inflammatory/analgesic activity is required. When treating patients with naproxen 1500 mg/day (as NAPROSYN or 1650 mg of ANAPROX), the physician should observe sufficient increased clinical benefit to offset the potential increased risk. The morning and evening doses do not have to be equal in size and administration of the drug more frequently than twice daily does not generally make a difference in response (see CLINICAL PHARMACOLOGY).

Juvenile Arthritis: The use of NAPROSYN Suspension allows for more flexible dose titration. In pediatric patients, doses of 5 mg/kg/day produced plasma levels of naproxen similar to those seen in adults taking 500 mg of naproxen (see CLINICAL PHARMACOLOGY).

The recommended total daily dose is approximately 10 mg/kg given in two divided doses (ie, 5 mg/kg given twice a day) (see DOSAGE AND ADMINISTRATION).

INDICATIONS AND USAGE

Naproxen as NAPROSYN, EC-NAPROSYN, ANAPROX, ANAPROX DS or NAPROSYN Suspension are indicated for the treatment of rheumatoid arthritis, osteoarthritis, ankylosing spondylitis and juvenile arthritis.

Naproxen as NAPROSYN Suspension is recommended for juvenile rheumatoid arthritis in order to obtain the maximum dosage flexibility based on the patient's weight.

Naproxen as NAPROSYN, ANAPROX, ANAPROX DS and NAPROSYN Suspension are also indicated for the treatment of tendonitis, bursitis, acute gout, and for the management of pain and primary dysmenorrhea. EC-NAPROSYN is not recommended for initial treatment of acute pain because the absorption of naproxen is delayed compared to absorption from other naproxen-containing products (see CLINICAL PHARMACOLOGY and DOSAGE AND ADMINISTRATION).

CONTRAINDICATIONS

All naproxen products are contraindicated in patients who have had allergic reactions to prescription as well as to over-the-counter products containing naproxen. It is also contraindicated in patients in whom aspirin or other nonsteroidal anti-inflammatory/analgesic drugs induce the syndrome of asthma, rhinitis, and nasal polyps. Both types of reactions have the potential of being fatal. Anaphylactoid reactions to naproxen, whether of the true allergic type or the pharmacologic idiosyncratic (eg, aspirin hypersensitivity syndrome) type, usually but not always occur in patients with a known history of such reactions. Therefore, careful questioning of patients for such things as asthma, nasal polyps, urticaria, and hypotension associated with nonsteroidal anti-inflammatory drugs before starting therapy is important. In addition, if such symptoms occur during therapy, treatment should be discontinued.

WARNINGS

Risk of GI Ulceration, Bleeding and Perforation With NSAID Therapy: Serious gastrointestinal toxicity such as bleeding, ulceration and perforation can occur at any time, with or without warning symptoms, in patients treated chronically with NSAID therapy. Although minor upper gastrointestinal problems, such as dyspepsia, are common, usually developing early in therapy, physicians should remain alert for ulceration and bleeding in patients treated chronically with NSAIDs even in the absence of previous GI tract symptoms. In patients observed in clinical trials of several months to 2 years' duration, symptomatic upper GI ulcers, gross bleeding or perforation appear to occur in approximately 1% of patients treated for 3 to 6 months and in about 2% to 4% of patients treated for 1 year.

Physicians should inform patients about the signs and/or symptoms of serious GI toxicity and what steps to take if they occur.

Studies to date with all naproxen products have not identified any subset of patients not at risk of developing peptic ulceration and bleeding or any differences between different naproxen products in their propensity to cause peptic ulceration and bleeding. Except for a prior history of serious GI events and other risk factors known to be associated with peptic ulcer disease, such as alcoholism, smoking, etc., no risk factors (eg, age, sex) have been associated with increased risk. Elderly or debilitated patients seem to tolerate ulceration or bleeding less well than other individuals and most spontaneous reports of fatal GI events are in this population. Studies to date are inconclusive concerning the relative risk of various NSAIDs in causing such reactions. High doses of any NSAID probably carry a greater risk of these reactions, although controlled clinical trials showing this do not exist in most cases. In considering the use of relatively large doses (within the recommended dosage range), sufficient benefit should be anticipated to offset the potential increased risk of GI toxicity.

PRECAUTIONS

General: **NAPROXEN-CONTAINING PRODUCTS SUCH AS NAPROSYN, EC-NAPROSYN, ANAPROX, ANAPROX DS, NAPROSYN SUSPENSION, ALEVE®*, AND OTHER NAPROXEN PRODUCTS SHOULD NOT BE USED CONCOMITANTLY SINCE THEY ALL CIRCULATE IN THE PLASMA AS THE NAPROXEN ANION.**

If the steroid dose is reduced or eliminated during therapy, the steroid dosage should be reduced slowly and the patient should be observed closely for any evidence of adverse effects, including adrenal insufficiency and exacerbation of symptoms of arthritis.

Patients with initial hemoglobin values of 10 grams or less who are to receive long-term therapy should have hemoglobin values determined periodically.

The antipyretic and anti-inflammatory activities of the drug may reduce fever and inflammation, thus diminishing their utility as diagnostic signs in detecting complications of presumed noninfectious, noninflammatory painful conditions.

Because of adverse eye findings in animal studies with drugs of this class, it is recommended that ophthalmic studies be carried out if any change or disturbance in vision occurs.

Renal Effects: As with other nonsteroidal anti-inflammatory drugs, long-term administration of naproxen to animals has resulted in renal papillary necrosis and other abnormal renal pathology. In humans, there have been reports of acute interstitial nephritis, hematuria, proteinuria and occasionally nephrotic syndrome associated with naproxen-containing products and other NSAIDs since they have been marketed.

A second form of renal toxicity has been seen in patients taking naproxen as well as other nonsteroidal anti-inflammatory drugs. In patients with prerenal conditions leading to a reduction in renal blood flow or blood volume, where the renal prostaglandins have a supportive role in the maintenance of renal perfusion, administration of a nonsteroidal anti-inflammatory drug may cause a dose-dependent reduction in prostaglandin formation and precipitate overt renal decompensation. Patients at greatest risk of this reaction are those with impaired renal function, heart failure, liver dysfunction, those taking diuretics and the elderly. Discontinuation of nonsteroidal anti-inflammatory therapy is typically followed by recovery to the pretreatment state.

Naproxen and its metabolites are eliminated primarily by the kidneys; therefore, the drug should be used with caution in patients with significantly impaired renal function, and the monitoring of serum creatinine and/or creatinine clearance is advised in these patients. Caution should be used if the drug is given to patients with creatinine clearance of less than 20 mL/minute because accumulation of naproxen metabolites has been seen in such patients.

Chronic alcoholic liver disease and probably other diseases with decreased or abnormal plasma proteins (albumin) reduce the total plasma concentration of naproxen, but the plasma concentration of unbound naproxen is increased. Caution is advised when high doses are required and some adjustment of dosage may be required in these patients. It is prudent to use the lowest effective dose.

Studies indicate that although total plasma concentration of naproxen is unchanged, the unbound plasma fraction of naproxen is increased in the elderly. Caution is advised when high doses are required and some adjustment of dosage may be required in elderly patients. As with other drugs used in the elderly, it is prudent to use the lowest effective dose.

Hepatic Function: As with other nonsteroidal anti-inflammatory drugs, borderline elevations of one or more liver tests may occur in up to 15% of patients. These abnormalities may progress, may remain essentially unchanged, or may be transient with continued therapy. The SGPT (ALT) test is probably the most sensitive indicator of liver dysfunction. Meaningful (3 times the upper limit of normal) elevations of SGPT or SGOT (AST) occurred in controlled clinical trials in less than 1% of patients. A patient with symptoms and/or signs suggesting liver dysfunction or in whom an abnormal liver test has occurred, should be evaluated for evidence of the development of more severe hepatic reaction while on therapy with naproxen. Severe hepatic reactions, including jaundice and cases of fatal hepatitis, have been reported with naproxen as with other nonsteroidal anti-inflammatory drugs. Although such reactions are rare, if abnormal liver tests persist or worsen, if clinical signs and symptoms consistent with liver disease develop, or if systemic manifestations occur (eg, eosinophilia, rash, etc.), naproxen should be discontinued.

Fluid Retention and Edema: Peripheral edema has been observed in some patients receiving naproxen. Since each ANAPROX or ANAPROX DS tablet contains 25 mg or 50 mg of sodium (about 1 mEq per each 250 mg of naproxen), and each teaspoonful of NAPROSYN Suspension contains 39 mg (about 1.5 mEq per each 125 mg of naproxen) of sodium, this should be considered in patients whose overall intake of sodium must be severely restricted. For these reasons, ANAPROX, ANAPROX DS and NAPROSYN Suspension should be used with caution in patients with fluid retention, hypertension or heart failure.

Information for Patients: Naproxen, in NAPROSYN, EC-NAPROSYN, ANAPROX, ANAPROX DS and NAPROSYN Suspension, like other drugs of this class, is not free of side effects. The side effects of these formulations of naproxen can cause discomfort and, rarely, there are more serious side effects, such as gastrointestinal bleeding, which may result in hospitalization and even fatal outcomes.

NSAIDs (Nonsteroidal Anti-Inflammatory Drugs) are often essential agents in the management of arthritis and have a major role in the treatment of pain, but they also may be commonly employed for conditions that are less serious.

Physicians may wish to discuss with their patients the potential risks (see WARNINGS, PRECAUTIONS and ADVERSE REACTIONS) and likely benefits of naproxen treatment, particularly when it is used for less serious conditions where treatment without NSAIDs may represent an acceptable alternative to both the patient and physician.

Caution should be exercised by patients whose activities require alertness if they experience drowsiness, dizziness, vertigo or depression during therapy with naproxen.

Laboratory Tests: Because serious GI tract ulceration and bleeding can occur without warning symptoms, physicians should follow patients chronically treated with naproxen for signs and symptoms of ulceration and bleeding and should inform them of the importance of this follow-up and what they should do if certain signs and symptoms do appear (see WARNINGS: *Risk of GI Ulcerations, Bleeding and Perforation With NSAID Therapy*).

Drug Interactions: The use of NSAIDs in patients who are receiving ACE inhibitors may potentiate renal disease states (see PRECAUTIONS: *Renal Effects*).

In vitro studies have shown that naproxen anion, because of its affinity for protein, may displace from their binding sites other drugs that are also albumin-bound (see CLINICAL PHARMACOLOGY: *Pharmacokinetics*).

Theoretically, the naproxen anion itself could likewise be displaced. Short-term controlled studies failed to show that taking the drug significantly affects prothrombin times when administered to individuals on coumarin-type anticoagulants. Caution is advised nonetheless, since interactions have been seen with other nonsteroidal agents of this class. Similarly, patients receiving the drug and a hydantoin, sulfonamide or sulfonylurea should be observed for signs of toxicity to these drugs (see CLINICAL STUDIES: *General Information*).

Concomitant administration of naproxen and aspirin is not recommended because naproxen is displaced from its binding sites during the concomitant administration of aspirin, resulting in lower plasma concentrations and peak plasma levels.

The natriuretic effect of furosemide has been reported to be inhibited by some drugs of this class. Inhibition of renal lithium clearance leading to increases in plasma lithium concentrations has also been reported. Naproxen and other nonsteroidal anti-inflammatory drugs can reduce the antihypertensive effect of propranolol and other beta-blockers.

Probenecid given concurrently increases naproxen anion plasma levels and extends its plasma half-life significantly.

Caution should be used if naproxen is administered concomitantly with methotrexate. Naproxen, naproxen sodium and other nonsteroidal anti-inflammatory drugs have been reported to reduce the tubular secretion of methotrexate in an animal model, possibly increasing the toxicity of methotrexate.

Due to the gastric pH elevating effects of H_2-blockers, sucralfate and intensive antacid therapy, concomitant administration of EC-NAPROSYN is not recommended.

Drug/Laboratory Test Interactions: Naproxen may decrease platelet aggregation and prolong bleeding time. This effect should be kept in mind when bleeding times are determined.

The administration of naproxen may result in increased urinary values for 17-ketogenic steroids because of an interaction between the drug and/or its metabolites with m-di-nitrobenzene used in this assay. Although 17-hydroxycorticosteroid measurements (Porter-Silber test) do not appear to be artifactually altered, it is suggested that therapy with naproxen be temporarily discontinued 72 hours before adrenal function tests are performed if the Porter-Silber test is to be used.

Continued on next page

EC-Naprosyn/Anaprox—Cont.

Naproxen may interfere with some urinary assays of 5-hydroxy indoleacetic acid (5HIAA).

Carcinogenesis: A 2-year study was performed in rats to evaluate the carcinogenic potential of naproxen at rat doses of 8, 16, and 24 mg/kg/day (50, 100, and 150 mg/m^2). The maximum dose used was 0.28 times the systemic exposure to humans at the recommended dose. No evidence of tumorigenicity was found.

Pregnancy: *Teratogenic Effects:* Pregnancy Category B. Reproduction studies have been performed in rats at 20 mg/kg/day (125 mg/m^2/day, 0.23 times the human systemic exposure), rabbits at 20 mg/kg/day (220 mg/m^2/day, 0.27 times the human systemic exposure), and mice at 170 mg/kg/day (510 mg/m^2/day, 0.28 times the human systemic exposure) with no evidence of impaired fertility or harm to the fetus due to the drug. There are no adequate and well-controlled studies in pregnant women. Because animal reproduction studies are not always predictive of human response, naproxen should not be used during pregnancy unless clearly needed.

Nonteratogenic Effects: There is some evidence to suggest that when inhibitors of prostaglandin synthesis are used to delay preterm labor there is an increased risk of neonatal complications such as necrotizing enterocolitis, patent ductus arteriosus and intracranial hemorrhage. Naproxen treatment given in late pregnancy to delay parturition has been associated with persistent pulmonary hypertension, renal dysfunction and abnormal prostaglandin E levels in preterm infants. Because of the known effect of drugs of this class on the human fetal cardiovascular system (closure of ductus arteriosus), use during third trimester should be avoided.

Nursing Mothers: The naproxen anion has been found in the milk of lactating women at a concentration of approximately 1% of that found in plasma. Because of the possible adverse effects of prostaglandin-inhibiting drugs on neonates, use in nursing mothers should be avoided.

Pediatric Use: Safety and effectiveness in pediatric patients below the age of 2 years have not been established. Pediatric dosing recommendations for juvenile arthritis are based on well-controlled studies (see DOSAGE AND ADMINISTRATION). There are no adequate effectiveness or dose-response data for other pediatric conditions, but the experience in juvenile arthritis and other use experience have established that single doses of 2.5 to 5 mg/kg (as naproxen suspension, see DOSAGE AND ADMINISTRATION), with total daily dose not exceeding 15 mg/kg/day, are well tolerated in pediatric patients over 2 years of age.

ADVERSE REACTIONS

The following adverse reactions are divided into three parts based on frequency and whether or not the possibility exists of a causal relationship between naproxen and these adverse events. In those reactions listed as "Probable Causal Relationship" there is at least 1 case for each adverse reaction where there is evidence to suggest that there is a causal relationship between drug usage and the reported event.

Adverse reactions reported in controlled clinical trials in 960 patients treated for rheumatoid arthritis or osteoarthritis are listed below. In general, reactions in patients treated chronically were reported 2 to 10 times more frequently than they were in short-term studies in the 962 patients treated for mild to moderate pain or for dysmenorrhea. The most frequent complaints reported related to the gastrointestinal tract.

A clinical study found gastrointestinal reactions to be more frequent and more severe in rheumatoid arthritis patients taking daily doses of 1500 mg naproxen compared to those taking 750 mg naproxen (see CLINICAL PHARMACOLOGY).

In controlled clinical trials with about 80 pediatric patients and in well-monitored, open-label studies with about 400 pediatric patients with juvenile arthritis treated with naproxen, the incidence of rash and prolonged bleeding times were increased, the incidence of gastrointestinal and central nervous system reactions were about the same, and the incidence of other reactions were lower in pediatric patients than in adults.

The following adverse reactions are divided into three parts based on frequency and causal relationship.

Incidence greater than 1% (Probable Causal Relationship):

Gastrointestinal: constipation*, heartburn*, abdominal pain*, nausea*, dyspepsia, diarrhea, stomatitis

Central Nervous System: headache*, dizziness*, drowsiness*, lightheadedness, vertigo

Dermatologic: itching (pruritus)*, skin eruptions*, ecchymoses*, sweating, purpura

Special Senses: tinnitus*, hearing disturbances, visual disturbances

Cardiovascular: edema*, dyspnea*, palpitations

General: thirst

*Incidence of reported reaction between 3% and 9%. Those reactions occurring in less than 3% of the patients are unmarked.

Incidence less than 1% (Probable Causal Relationship):

The following adverse reactions were reported less frequently than 1% during controlled clinical trials and through voluntary reports since marketing. Those reactions observed through voluntary reporting since marketing are italicized.

Gastrointestinal: *abnormal liver function tests, colitis,* gastrointestinal bleeding and/or *perforation, hematemesis,* jaundice, pancreatitis, melena, vomiting

Renal: *glomerular nephritis, hematuria, hyperkalemia, interstitial nephritis, nephrotic syndrome, renal disease, renal failure, renal papillary necrosis*

Hematologic: agranulocytosis, *eosinophilia, granulocytopenia, leukopenia,* thrombocytopenia

Central Nervous System: *depression, dream abnormalities,* inability to concentrate, *insomnia, malaise, myalgia, muscle weakness*

Dermatologic: *alopecia, photosensitive dermatitis, urticaria,* skin rashes, *photosensitivity reactions resembling porphyria cutanea tarda, epidermolysis bullosa*

Special Senses: *hearing impairment*

Cardiovascular: *congestive heart failure*

Respiratory: *eosinophilic pneumonitis*

General: *anaphylactoid reactions, angioneurotic edema, menstrual disorders, pyrexia (chills and fever)*

Incidence less than 1% (Causal Relationship Unknown):

These observations are being listed to serve as alerting information to the physician.

Hematologic: *aplastic anemia, hemolytic anemia*

Central Nervous System: *aseptic meningitis, cognitive dysfunction*

Dermatologic: *epidermal necrolysis, erythema multiforme, Stevens-Johnson syndrome*

Gastrointestinal: *nonpeptic gastrointestinal ulceration, ulcerative stomatitis*

Cardiovascular: *vasculitis*

General: *hyperglycemia, hypoglycemia*

OVERDOSAGE

Significant naproxen overdosage may be characterized by drowsiness, heartburn, indigestion, nausea or vomiting. Because naproxen sodium may be rapidly absorbed, high and early blood levels should be anticipated. A few patients have experienced seizures, but it is not clear whether or not these were drug-related. It is not known what dose of the drug would be life-threatening. The oral LD_{50} of the drug is 543 mg/kg in rats, 1234 mg/kg in mice, 4110 mg/kg in hamsters, and greater than 1000 mg/kg in dogs.

Should a patient ingest a large number of tablets or a large volume of suspension, accidentally or purposefully, the stomach may be emptied and usual supportive measures employed. In animals 0.5 g/kg of activated charcoal was effective in reducing plasma levels of naproxen. Hemodialysis does not decrease the plasma concentration of naproxen because of the high degree of its protein binding.

DOSAGE AND ADMINISTRATION

[See table below]

To maintain the integrity of the enteric coating, the EC-NAPROSYN tablet should not be broken, crushed or chewed during ingestion.

During long-term administration, the dose of naproxen may be adjusted up or down depending on the clinical response of the patient. A lower daily dose may suffice for long-term administration. The morning and evening doses do not have to be equal in size and the administration of the drug more frequently than twice daily is not necessary.

In patients who tolerate lower doses well, the dose may be increased to naproxen 1500 mg per day for limited periods of up to 6 months when a higher level of anti-inflammatory/analgesic activity is required. When treating such patients with naproxen 1500 mg/day, the physician should observe sufficient increased clinical benefits to offset the potential increased risk (see CLINICAL PHARMACOLOGY and INDIVIDUALIZATION OF DOSAGE).

Juvenile Arthritis: The recommended total daily dose of naproxen is approximately 10 mg/kg given in 2 divided doses (ie, 5 mg/kg given twice a day). A measuring cup marked in 1/2 teaspoon and 2.5 milliliter increments is provided with the NAPROSYN Suspension. The following table may be used as a guide for dosing of NAPROSYN Suspension:

Patient's Weight	Dose	Administered as
13 kg (29 lb)	62.5 mg bid	2.5 mL (1/2 tsp) twice daily
25 kg (55 lb)	125 mg bid	5.0 mL (1 tsp) twice daily
38 kg (84 lb)	187.5 mg bid	7.5 mL (1 1/2 tsp) twice daily

Management of Pain, Primary Dysmenorrhea and Acute Tendonitis and Bursitis: The recommended starting dose is 550 mg of naproxen sodium as ANAPROX/ANAPROX DS followed by 550 mg every 12 hours or 275 mg every 6 to 8 hours as required. The initial total daily dose should not exceed 1375 mg of naproxen sodium. Thereafter, the total daily dose should not exceed 1100 mg of naproxen sodium. NAPROSYN may also be used but EC-NAPROSYN is not recommended for initial treatment of acute pain because absorption of naproxen is delayed compared to other naproxen-containing products (see CLINICAL PHARMACOLOGY, INDICATIONS AND USAGE and INDIVIDUALIZATION OF DOSAGE).

Acute Gout: The recommended starting dose is 750 mg of NAPROSYN followed by 250 mg every 8 hours until the attack has subsided. ANAPROX may also be used at a starting dose of 825 mg followed by 275 mg every 8 hours. EC-NAPROSYN is not recommended because of the delay in absorption (see CLINICAL PHARMACOLOGY).

HOW SUPPLIED

NAPROSYN Tablets: 250 mg: round, yellow, biconvex, engraved with NPR LE 250 on one side and scored on the other. Packaged in light-resistant bottles of 100.

100's (bottle): NDC 0004-6313-01.

375 mg: pink, biconvex oval, engraved with NPR LE 375 on one side. Packaged in light-resistant bottles of 100 and 500.

100's (bottle): NDC 0004-6314-01; 500's (bottle): NDC 0004-6314-14.

500 mg: yellow, capsule-shaped, engraved with NPR LE 500 on one side and scored on the other. Packaged in light-resistant bottles of 100 and 500.

100's (bottle): NDC 0004-6316-01; 500's (bottle): NDC 0004-6316-14.

Store at 15° to 30°C (59° to 86°F) in well-closed containers; dispense in light-resistant containers.

NAPROSYN Suspension: 125 mg/5 mL (contains 39 mg sodium, about 1.5 mEq/teaspoon): Available in 1 pint (473 mL) light-resistant bottles (NDC 0004-0028-28).

Store at 15° to 30°C (59° to 86°F); avoid excessive heat, above 40°C (104°F). Dispense in light-resistant containers.

EC-NAPROSYN Delayed-Release Tablets: 375 mg: white, capsule-shaped, imprinted with EC-NAPROSYN on one side and 375 on the other. Packaged in light-resistant bottles of 100.

100's (bottle): NDC 0004-6415-01.

500 mg: white, capsule-shaped, imprinted with EC-NAPROSYN on one side and 500 on the other. Packaged in light-resistant bottles of 100.

100's (bottle): NDC 0004-6416-01.

Store at 15° to 30°C (59° to 86°F) in well-closed containers; dispense in light-resistant containers.

ANAPROX Tablets: Naproxen sodium 275 mg: light blue, oval-shaped, engraved with NPS-275 on one side. Packaged in bottles of 100.

100's (bottle): NDC 0004-6202-01.

Store at 15° to 30°C (59° to 86°F) in well-closed containers.

ANAPROX DS Tablets: Naproxen sodium 550 mg: dark blue, oblong-shaped, engraved with NPS 550 on one side and scored on both sides. Packaged in bottles of 100 and 500.

100's (bottle): NDC 0004-6203-01; 500's (bottle): NDC 0004-6203-14.

Store at 15° to 30°C (59° to 86°F) in well-closed containers.

* ALEVE is a registered trademark of Bayer-Roche L.L.C.

Revised: May 2003

Shown in Product Identification Guide, page 331

Rheumatoid Arthritis, Osteoarthritis and Ankylosing Spondylitis:

NAPROSYN	250 mg or 375 mg or 500 mg	twice daily twice daily twice daily
ANAPROX	275 mg (naproxen 250 mg with 25 mg sodium)	twice daily
ANAPROX DS	550 mg (naproxen 500 mg with 50 mg sodium)	twice daily
NAPROSYN Suspension	250 mg (10 mL/2 tsp) or 375 mg (15 mL/3 tsp) or 500 mg (20 mL/4 tsp)	twice daily twice daily twice daily
EC-NAPROSYN	375 mg or 500 mg	twice daily twice daily

FORTOVASE® ℞

[fōr-tō-vās]

(saquinavir)

SOFT GELATIN CAPSULES

Product identification in this document includes: INVIRASE® in reference to saquinavir mesylate; FORTOVASE in reference to saquinavir, and saquinavir in reference to the active base.

DESCRIPTION

FORTOVASE brand of saquinavir is an inhibitor of the human immunodeficiency virus (HIV) protease. FORTOVASE is available as beige, opaque, soft gelatin capsules for oral administration in a 200-mg strength (as saquinavir free base). Each capsule also contains the inactive ingredients medium chain mono- and diglycerides, povidone and dl-alpha tocopherol. Each capsule shell contains gelatin and glycerol 85% with the following colorants: red iron oxide, yellow iron oxide, and titanium dioxide. The chemical name for saquinavir is N-tert-butyl-decahydro-2-[2(R)-hydroxy-4-phenyl-3(S)-[[N-(2-quinolylcarbonyl)-L-asparaginyl]amino]butyl]-(4aS,8aS)-isoquinoline-3(S)-carboxamide which has a molecular formula $C_{38}H_{50}N_6O_5$ and a molecular weight of 670.86.

Saquinavir is a white to off-white powder and is insoluble in aqueous medium at 25°C.

MICROBIOLOGY

Mechanism of Action

Saquinavir is an inhibitor of HIV protease. HIV protease is an enzyme required for the proteolytic cleavage of viral polyprotein precursors into individual functional proteins found in infectious HIV. Saquinavir is a peptide-like substrate analogue that binds to the protease active site and inhibits the activity of the enzyme. Saquinavir inhibition prevents cleavage of the viral polyproteins resulting in the formation of immature noninfectious virus particles.

Antiviral Activity

In vitro antiviral activity of saquinavir was assessed in lymphoblastoid and monocytic cell lines and in peripheral blood lymphocytes. Saquinavir inhibited HIV activity in both acutely and chronically infected cells. IC_{50} and IC_{90} values (50% and 90% inhibitory concentrations) were in the range of 1 to 30 nM and 5 to 80 nM, respectively. In the presence of 40% human serum, the mean IC_{50} of saquinavir against laboratory strain HIV-1 RF in MT4 cells was 37.7 ± 5 nM, representing a 4-fold increase in IC_{50} value. In cell culture, saquinavir demonstrated additive to synergistic effects against HIV-1 in combination with reverse transcriptase inhibitors (didanosine, lamivudine, nevirapine, stavudine, zalcitabine and zidovudine) without enhanced cytotoxicity. Saquinavir in combination with the protease inhibitors amprenavir, atazanavir, or lopinavir resulted in synergistic antiviral activity.

Drug Resistance

HIV-1 mutants with reduced susceptibility to saquinavir have been selected during in vitro passage. Genotypic analyses of these isolates showed several substitutions in the HIV protease gene. Only the G48V and L90M substitutions were associated with reduced susceptibility to saquinavir, and conferred an increase in the IC_{50}value of 8- and 3-fold, respectively.

HIV-1 isolates with reduced susceptibility (≥4-fold increase in the IC_{50} value) to saquinavir emerged in some patients treated with INVIRASE. Genotypic analysis of these isolates identified resistance conferring primary mutations in the protease gene G48V and L90M, and secondary mutations L10I/R/V, I54V/L, A71V/T, G73S, V77I, V82A and I84V that contributed additional resistance to saquinavir. Forty-one isolates from 37 patients failing therapy with INVIRASE had a median decrease in susceptibility to saquinavir of 4.3 fold.

The degree of reduction in in vitro susceptibility to saquinavir of clinical isolates bearing substitutions G48V and L90M depends on the number of secondary mutations present. In general, higher levels of resistance are associated with greater number of mutations only in association with either or both of the primary mutations G48V and L90M. No data are currently available to address the development of resistance in patients receiving saquinavir/ritonavir.

Cross-resistance

Among protease inhibitors, variable cross-resistance has been observed. In one clinical study, 22 HIV-1 isolates with reduced susceptibility (>4-fold increase in the IC_{50} value) to saquinavir following therapy with INVIRASE were evaluated for cross-resistance to amprenavir, indinavir, nelfinavir and ritonavir. Six of the 22 isolates (27%) remained susceptible to all 4 protease inhibitors, 12 of the 22 isolates (55%) retained susceptibility to at least one of the PIs and 4 out of the 22 isolates (18%) displayed broad cross-resistance to all PIs.

Sixteen (73%) and 11 (50%) of the 22 isolates remained susceptible (<4-fold) to amprenavir and indinavir, respectively. Four of 16 (25%) and 9 of 21 (43%) with available data remained susceptible to nelfinavir and ritonavir, respectively. After treatment failure with amprenavir, cross-resistance to saquinavir was evaluated. HIV-1 isolates from 22/22 patients failing treatment with amprenavir and containing one or more mutations M46L/I , I50V, I54L, V32I, I47V, and I84V were susceptible to saquinavir.

CLINICAL PHARMACOLOGY

Pharmacokinetics

The pharmacokinetic properties of saquinavir when administered as FORTOVASE have been evaluated in healthy volunteers (n=207) and HIV-infected patients (n=91) after single-oral doses (range: 300 mg to 1200 mg) and multiple-oral doses (range: 400 mg to 1200 mg tid). The disposition properties of saquinavir have been studied in healthy volunteers after intravenous doses of 6, 12, 36 or 72 mg (n=21).

HIV-infected patients administered FORTOVASE (1200 mg tid) had AUC and maximum plasma concentration (C_{max}) values approximately twice those observed in healthy volunteers receiving the same treatment regimen. The mean AUC values at week 1 were 4159 (CV 88%) and 8839 (CV 82%) ng•h/mL, and C_{max} values were 1420 (CV 81%) and 2477 (CV 76%) ng/mL for healthy volunteers and HIV-infected patients, respectively.

Absorption and Bioavailability in Adults

The absolute bioavailability of saquinavir administered as FORTOVASE has not been assessed. However, following single 600-mg doses, the relative bioavailability of saquinavir as FORTOVASE compared to saquinavir administered as INVIRASE was estimated as 331% (95% CI: 207% to 530%). The absolute bioavailability of saquinavir administered as INVIRASE averaged 4% (CV 73%, range: 1% to 9%) in 8 healthy volunteers who received a single 600-mg dose (3 x 200 mg) of INVIRASE following a high-fat breakfast (48 g protein, 60 g carbohydrate, 57 g fat; 1006 kcal). In healthy volunteers receiving single doses of FORTOVASE (300 mg to 1200 mg) and in HIV-infected patients receiving multiple doses of FORTOVASE (400 mg to 1200 mg tid), a greater than dose-proportional increase in saquinavir plasma concentrations has been observed.

Comparison of pharmacokinetic parameters between single- and multiple-dose studies shows that following multiple dosing of FORTOVASE (1200 mg tid) in healthy male volunteers (n=18), the steady-state AUC was 80% (95% CI: 22% to 176%) higher than that observed after a single 1200-mg dose (n=30).

Saquinavir plasma concentrations remained stable over a 60-week period of continued treatment in patients in a phase III substudy.

When administered as the sole protease inhibitor, it has been shown that FORTOVASE 1200 mg tid provides an 8-fold increase in AUC compared with INVIRASE 600 mg tid.

FORTOVASE in combination with ritonavir at doses of 400/400 mg bid, or 1000/100 mg bid provide saquinavir systemic exposures over a 24-hour period similar to or greater than those achieved with FORTOVASE 1200 mg tid.

[See table 1 above]

Table 1 Pharmacokinetic Parameters of Saquinavir at Steady-State After Administration of Different Regimens in HIV-Infected Patients

Dosing Regimen	n	$AUC_{0-\tau}$ (ng•h/mL)	AUC_{0-24h} (ng•h/mL)	C_{min} (ng/mL)
FORTOVASE 1200 mg tid (arithmetic mean)	31	7249	21747	216
INVIRASE 400 mg bid + ritonavir 400 mg bid (arithmetic mean± SD)	7	16000±8000	32000	480±360
INVIRASE 1000 mg bid + ritonavir 100 mg bid (geometric mean and 95% CI)	24	14607 (10218-20882)	29214	371 (245-561)
FORTOVASE 1000 mg bid + ritonavir 100 mg bid (geometric mean and 95% CI)	24	19085 (13943-26124)	38170	433 (301-622)

τ is the dosing interval (ie, 8h if tid and 12h if bid).

Table 2 Effect of FORTOVASE on the Pharmacokinetics of Coadministered Drugs

Coadministered Drug	FORTOVASE or FORTOVASE/ritonavir Dose	N	% Change for Coadministered Drug AUC (95%CI)	C_{max} (95%CI)
Clarithromycin 500 mg bid × 7 days	1200 mg tid × 7 days	12V		
Clarithromycin			↑45% (17-81%)	↑39% (10-76%)
14-OH clarithromycin metabolite			↓24% (5-40%)	↓34% (14-50%)
Midazolam 7.5–mg oral single dose	1200 mg tid × 5 days	6V	↑514%	↑235%
Nelfinavir 750-mg single dose	1200 mg tid × 4 days	14P	↑18% (5-33%)	↔
Rifabutin 300 mg once daily	1200 mg tid	14P	↑44%	↑45%
Ritonavir 400 mg bid × 14 days	400 mg bid × 14 days	8V	↔	↔
Sildenafil 100-mg single dose	1200 mg tid × 8 days	27V	↑210% (150-300%)	↑140% (80-230%)
Terfenadine[ϕ] 60 mg bid × 11 days*	1200 mg tid × 4 days	12V		
Terfenadine			↑368% (257-514%)	↑253% (164-373%)
Terfenadine acid metabolite			↑120% (89-156%)	↑93% (59-133%)
Efavirenz 600 mg	1200 mg tid	13V	↓12%	↓13%
Ketoconazole 400 mg once daily	1200 mg tid	12V	↔	↔
Enfuvirtide 90 mg SC q12h (bid) for 7 days	1000/100 mg bid	12 P	↔	↔

↑ Denotes an average increase in exposure by the percentage indicated.
↓ Denotes an average decrease in exposure by the percentage indicated.
↔Denotes no statistically significant change in exposure was observed.
* FORTOVASE should not be coadministered with terfenadine (see PRECAUTIONS: Drug Interactions).
P Patient
V Healthy Volunteers
ϕ No longer marketed in the US.

Food Effect

The mean 12-hour AUC after a single 800-mg oral dose of saquinavir in healthy volunteers (n=12) was increased from 167 ng•h/mL (CV 45%), under fasting conditions, to 1120 ng•h/mL (CV 54%) when FORTOVASE was given following a high-fat breakfast (45 g protein, 76 g carbohydrate, 55 g fat; 961 kcal). The effect of food with INVIRASE has been shown to persist for up to 2 hours. The mean 12-hour AUC after a single 1200-mg oral dose of FORTOVASE in healthy volunteers (n=12) was increased from 952 ng•h/mL, following a light meal (21 g protein, 50 g carbohydrate, 28 g fat; 524 kcal) to 1388 ng•h/mL when FORTOVASE was given following a high-fat breakfast (45 g protein, 76 g carbohydrate, 55 g fat; 961 kcal).

Saquinavir exposure was similar when FORTOVASE plus ritonavir (1000-mg/100-mg bid) was administered following a high-fat (45 g fat) or moderate-fat (20 g fat) breakfast.

Distribution in Adults

The mean steady-state volume of distribution following intravenous administration of a 12-mg dose of saquinavir (n=8) was 700 L (CV 39%), suggesting saquinavir partitions into tissues. It has been shown that saquinavir, up to 30 µg/mL, is approximately 97% bound to plasma proteins.

Metabolism and Elimination in Adults

In vitro studies using human liver microsomes have shown that the metabolism of saquinavir is cytochrome P450 mediated with the specific isoenzyme, CYP3A4, responsible for more than 90% of the hepatic metabolism. Based on in vitro studies, saquinavir is rapidly metabolized to a range of mono- and di-hydroxylated inactive compounds. In a mass balance study using 600 mg ^{14}C-saquinavir mesylate (n=8), 88% and 1% of the orally administered radioactivity was recovered in feces and urine, respectively, within 5 days of dosing. In an additional 4 subjects administered 10.5 mg ^{14}C-saquinavir intravenously, 81% and 3% of the intravenously administered radioactivity was recovered in feces and urine, respectively, within 5 days of dosing. In mass balance studies, 13% of circulating radioactivity in plasma was attributed to unchanged drug after oral administration and the remainder attributed to saquinavir metabolites. Following intravenous administration, 66% of circulating radioactivity was attributed to unchanged drug and the remainder attributed to saquinavir metabolites, suggesting that saquinavir undergoes extensive first-pass metabolism.

Systemic clearance of saquinavir was rapid, 1.14 L/h/kg (CV 12%) after intravenous doses of 6, 36, and 72 mg. The mean residence time of saquinavir was 7 hours (n=8).

Special Populations

Hepatic or Renal Impairment

Saquinavir pharmacokinetics in patients with hepatic or renal impairment has not been investigated (see PRECAUTIONS). Only 1% of saquinavir is excreted in the urine, so the impact of renal impairment on saquinavir elimination should be minimal.

Gender, Race and Age

The effect of gender was investigated in healthy volunteers receiving single 1200-mg doses of FORTOVASE (n=12 females, 18 males). No effect of gender was apparent on the pharmacokinetics of saquinavir in this study.

Continued on next page

Fortovase—Cont.

The effect of race on the pharmacokinetics of saquinavir has not been investigated.

Pediatric Patients

The pharmacokinetics of saquinavir in pediatric patients differs significantly from that in adults. Children have a markedly higher apparent clearance than adults and administration of saquinavir alone will not give consistently therapeutic plasma levels. The pharmacokinetics of saquinavir when coadministered with ritonavir to pediatric patients is under investigation.

Geriatric Patients

The pharmacokinetics of saquinavir when administered as FORTOVASE have not been sufficiently investigated in patients >65 years of age.

Drug Interactions (see PRECAUTIONS: Drug Interactions)

It is important to be aware that, when coadministered with ritonavir, the occurrence and magnitude of drug interactions may differ from those seen with FORTOVASE when administered as the sole protease inhibitor. When ritonavir is coadministered, prescribers should refer to the prescribing information for ritonavir regarding drug interactions associated with this drug.

Table 2 summarizes the effect of FORTOVASE on the geometric mean AUC and C_{max} of coadministered drugs. Table 3 summarizes the effect of coadministered drugs on the geometric mean AUC and C_{max} of saquinavir.

[See table 2 at top of previous page]

[See table 3 at right]

For information regarding clinical recommendations, see PRECAUTIONS: Drug Interactions, Table 6.

INDICATIONS AND USAGE

FORTOVASE is indicated for use in combination with other antiretroviral agents for the treatment of HIV infection. This indication is based on studies that showed increased saquinavir concentrations and improved antiviral activity for FORTOVASE 1200 mg tid compared to INVIRASE 600 mg tid.

In treatment-naive and treatment-experienced patients, the efficacy of FORTOVASE (with or without ritonavir coadministration) has not been compared against the efficacy of antiretroviral regimens currently considered standard of care.

Description of Clinical Studies

When used in combination with other antiretroviral agents, FORTOVASE and INVIRASE have been shown to decrease plasma HIV RNA levels and increase CD4 cell counts in an open-label randomized study (NV15355) in treatment-naive, HIV-infected patients. In addition, in a randomized, double-blind study (NV14256) in ZDV-experienced, HIV-infected patients, a combination regimen of FORTOVASE and HIVID was shown to be superior to either INVIRASE or HIVID monotherapy in decreasing the cumulative incidence of clinical disease progression to AIDS-defining events or death. It should be noted that HIV treatment regimens that were used in the initial clinical studies of INVIRASE are no longer considered standard of care.

FORTOVASE 1000 mg bid coadministered with ritonavir 100 mg bid was studied in a heterogeneous population of 148 HIV infected patients (MaxCmin 1 study). At baseline 42 were treatment naive and 106 were treatment experienced (of which 52 had an HIV RNA level <400 copies/mL at baseline). Results showed that 91/148 (61%) subjects achieved and/or sustained and HIV RNA level <400 copies/mL at the completion of 48 weeks.

Study NV15182 was an open-label safety study of FORTOVASE in combination with other antiretroviral agents in HIV-infected patients. The 48-week safety results from this study are displayed in the ADVERSE REACTIONS section.

CONTRAINDICATIONS

FORTOVASE is contraindicated in patients with clinically significant hypersensitivity to saquinavir or to any of the components contained in the capsule.

FORTOVASE should not be administered concurrently with terfenadine, cisapride, astemizole, pimozide, triazolam, midazolam, or ergot derivatives, because competition for CYP3A4 by saquinavir could result in inhibition of the metabolism of these drugs and create the potential for serious and/or life-threatening reactions, such as cardiac arrhythmias or prolonged sedation (see PRECAUTIONS: Drug Interactions).

FORTOVASE is contraindicated in patients with severe hepatic impairment (see PRECAUTIONS: Hepatic Effects).

FORTOVASE should not be administered concurrently with drugs listed in Table 4 (also see PRECAUTIONS: Drug Interactions, Table 5).

Table 3 Effect of Coadministered Drugs on FORTOVASE Pharmacokinetics

Coadministered Drug	FORTOVASE Dose	N	% Change for Saquinavir AUC (95%CI)	% Change for Saquinavir C_{max} (95%CI)
Clarithromycin 500 mg bid × 7 days	1200 mg tid × 7 days	12V	↑177% (108-269%)	↑187% (105-300%)
Efavirenz 600 mg	1200 mg tid	13V	↓62%	↓50%
Indinavir 800 mg q8h × 2 days	1200-mg single dose	6V	↑364% (190-644%)	↑299% (138-568%)
Ketoconazole 400 mg once daily	1200 mg tid	12V	↑190%	↑171%
Nelfinavir 750 mg × 4 days	1200-mg single dose	14P	↑392% (271-553%)	↑179% (105-280%)
Rifabutin 300 mg once daily	1200 mg tid	14P	↓47%	↓31%
Rifampin 600 mg once daily	1200 mg tid × 14 days	14V	↓70%	↓65%
Ritonavir 100 mg bid	1000 mg bid†	24P	↑176%	↑153%
Ritonavir 400 mg bid × 14 days*	400 mg tid × 14 days†	8V	↑121% (7–359%)	↑64%[§]
Lopinavir/ritonavir 400/100 mg bid, 15 days	800 mg bid, 10 days combo vs. 1200 mg tid, 5 days alone	14V	↑9.62-fold (8.05, 11.49)^	↑6.34-fold (5.32, 7.55)^
400/100 mg bid, 20 days	1200 mg bid, 5 days combo vs. 1200 mg tid 5 days alone	10V	↑9.91-fold (8.28, 11.86)^	↑6.44-fold (5.59, 7.41)^

↑ Denotes an average increase in exposure by the percentage indicated.
↓ Denotes an average decrease in exposure by the percentage indicated.
* When ritonavir was combined with the same dose of either INVIRASE or FORTOVASE, actual mean plasma exposures (AUC_{0-12}, 18200 ng•h/mL, 20000 ng•h/mL, respectively) were not significantly different.
^ 90% CI reported
† Compared to standard FORTOVASE 1200 mg tid regimen (n=33).
P Patient
V Healthy Volunteers

Table 5 Drugs That Should Not Be Coadministered With FORTOVASE

Drug Class: Drug Name	Clinical Comment
Antiarrhythmics: Amiodarone, bepridil, flecainide, propafenone, quinidine	CONTRAINDICATED due to potential for serious and/or life-threatening reactions.
Antihistamines: astemizole*, terfenadine*	CONTRAINDICATED due to potential for serious and/or life-threatening cardiac arrhythmias.
Ergot Derivatives: Dihydroergotamine, ergonovine, ergotamine, methylergonovine	CONTRAINDICATED due to potential for serious and life-threatening reactions such as acute ergot toxicity characterized by peripheral vasospasm and ischemia of the extremities and other tissues.
Antimycobacterial Agents: rifampin	WARNING coadministration with rifampin is not recommended because rifampin markedly decreases the concentration of saquinavir. The safety and efficacy of this combination have not been established.
Garlic Capsules	Garlic capsules should not be used while taking saquinavir (FORTOVASE) as the sole protease inhibitor due to the risk of decreased saquinavir plasma concentrations. No data are available for the coadministration of INVIRASE/ritonavir or FORTOVASE/ritonavir and garlic capsules.
GI Motility Agent: cisapride*	CONTRAINDICATED due to potential for serious and/or life-threatening reactions such as cardiac arrhythmias.
Herbal Products: St. John's wort (hypericum perforatum)	WARNING coadministration may lead to loss of virologic response and possible resistance to FORTOVASE or to the class of protease inhibitors.
HMG-CoA Reductase Inhibitors: lovastatin, simvastatin	WARNING potential for serious reactions such as risk of myopathy including rhabdomyolysis.
Sedatives/Hypnotics: triazolam, midazolam	CONTRAINDICATED due to potential for serious and/or life-threatening reactions such as prolonged or increased sedation or respiratory depression.

* No longer marketed in the US.

Table 4 Drugs That Are Contraindicated With FORTOVASE

Drug Class	Drugs Within Class That Are Contraindicated With FORTOVASE
Antiarrhythmics	Amiodarone, bepridil, flecainide, propafenone, quinidine
Antihistamines	Astemizole*, terfenadine*
Ergot Derivatives	Dihydroergotamine, ergonovine, ergotamine, methylergonovine
Antimycobacterial Agents	Rifampin
GI Motility Agent	Cisapride*
Neuroleptics	Pimozide
Sedative/Hypnotics	Triazolam, midazolam

*No longer marketed in the US.

If FORTOVASE is coadministered with ritonavir, the ritonavir label should be reviewed for additional contraindicated drugs.

WARNINGS

ALERT: Find out about medicines that should not be taken with FORTOVASE. This statement is included on the product's bottle label.

Interaction with HMG-CoA Reductase Inhibitors

Concomitant use of FORTOVASE with lovastatin or simvastatin is not recommended. Caution should be exercised if HIV protease inhibitors, including FORTOVASE, are used concurrently with other HMG-CoA reductase inhibitors that are also metabolized by the CYP3A4 pathway (eg, atorvastatin). Since increased concentrations of statins can, in rare cases, cause severe adverse events such as myopathy including rhabdomyolysis, this risk may be increased when HIV protease inhibitors, including saquinavir, are used in combination with these drugs.

Interaction with St. John's Wort (hypericum perforatum)

Concomitant use of FORTOVASE and St. John's wort (hypericum perforatum) or products containing St. John's wort is not recommended. Coadministration of protease inhibitors, including FORTOVASE, with St. John's wort is expected to substantially decrease protease inhibitor concentrations and may result in sub-optimal levels of FORTOVASE and lead to loss of virologic response and possible resistance to FORTOVASE or to the class of protease inhibitors.

Interaction with Garlic Capsules
Garlic capsules should not be used while taking saquinavir as the sole protease inhibitor due to the risk of decreased saquinavir plasma concentrations. No data are available for the coadministration of FORTOVASE/ritonavir or INVIRASE/ritonavir and garlic capsules.
Diabetes Mellitus and Hyperglycemia
New onset diabetes mellitus, exacerbation of pre-existing diabetes mellitus and hyperglycemia have been reported during postmarketing surveillance in HIV-infected patients receiving protease-inhibitor therapy. Some patients required either initiation or dose adjustments of insulin or oral hypoglycemic agents for the treatment of these events. In some cases diabetic ketoacidosis has occurred. In those patients who discontinued protease-inhibitor therapy, hyperglycemia persisted in some cases. Because these events have been reported voluntarily during clinical practice, estimates of frequency cannot be made and a causal relationship between protease-inhibitor therapy and these events has not been established.

PRECAUTIONS

General
FORTOVASE (saquinavir) soft gelatin capsules and INVIRASE (saquinavir mesylate) capsules are not bioequivalent and cannot be used interchangeably when used as the sole protease inhibitor. Only FORTOVASE should be used for the initiation of therapy that includes saquinavir as a sole protease inhibitor (see DOSAGE AND ADMINISTRATION) since FORTOVASE soft gelatin capsules provide greater bioavailability and efficacy than INVIRASE capsules.
If a serious or severe toxicity occurs during treatment with FORTOVASE, FORTOVASE should be interrupted until the etiology of the event is identified or the toxicity resolves. At that time, resumption of treatment with full-dose FORTOVASE may be considered. For antiretroviral agents used in combination with FORTOVASE, physicians should refer to the complete product information for these drugs for dose adjustment recommendations and for information regarding drug-associated adverse reactions.
Hepatic Effects
The use of FORTOVASE by patients with hepatic impairment has not been studied. In the absence of such studies, caution should be exercised, as increases in saquinavir levels and/or increases in liver enzymes may occur. In patients with underlying hepatitis B or C, cirrhosis, chronic alcoholism and/or other underlying liver abnormalities there have been reports of worsening liver disease.
Renal Effects
Renal clearance is only a minor elimination pathway; the principal route of metabolism and excretion for saquinavir is by the liver. Therefore, no dose adjustment is necessary for patients with renal impairment. However, patients with severe renal impairment have not been studied and caution should be exercised when prescribing saquinavir in this population.
Hemophilia
There have been reports of spontaneous bleeding in patients with hemophilia A and B treated with protease inhibitors. In some patients additional factor VIII was required. In the majority of reported cases treatment with protease inhibitors was continued or restarted. A causal relationship between protease-inhibitor therapy and these episodes has not been established.
Hyperlipidemia
Elevated cholesterol and/or triglyceride levels have been observed in some patients taking saquinavir in combination with ritonavir. Marked elevation in triglyceride levels is a risk factor for development of pancreatitis. Cholesterol and triglyceride levels should be monitored prior to initiating combination dosing regimen of FORTOVASE or INVIRASE with ritonavir, and at periodic intervals while on such therapy. In these patients, lipid disorders should be managed as clinically appropriate.
Fat Redistribution
Redistribution/accumulation of body fat including central obesity, dorsocervical fat enlargement (buffalo hump), facial wasting, peripheral wasting, breast enlargement, and "cushingoid appearance" have been observed in patients receiving antiretroviral therapy. A causal relationship between protease inhibitor therapy and these events has not been established and the long-term consequences are currently unknown.
Resistance/Cross-resistance
Varying degrees of cross-resistance among protease inhibitors have been observed. Continued administration of FORTOVASE therapy following loss of viral suppression may increase the likelihood of cross-resistance to other protease inhibitors (see MICROBIOLOGY).
Information for Patients
A statement to patients and health care providers is included on the product's bottle label: **ALERT: Find out about medicines that should NOT be taken with FORTOVASE.** A Patient Package Insert (PPI) for FORTOVASE is available for patient information.
Patients should be informed that any change from INVIRASE to FORTOVASE or FORTOVASE to INVIRASE coadministered with ritonavir should be made only under the supervision of a physician.
FORTOVASE may interact with some drugs; therefore, patients should be advised to report to their doctor the use of any other prescription, nonprescription medication, or herbal products, particularly St. John's wort.

Table 6 Established and Other Potentially Significant Drug Interactions: Alteration in Dose or Regimen May Be Recommended Based on Drug Interaction Studies or Predicted Interaction (Information in the table applies to FORTOVASE with or without ritonavir, unless otherwise indicated)

Concomitant Drug Class: Drug Name	Effect on Concentration of Saquinavir or Concomitant Drug	Clinical Comment
	HIV-Antiviral Agents	
Non-nucleoside reverse transcriptase inhibitor: Delavirdine	**FORTOVASE** ↑ Saquinavir Effect on delavirdine is not well established **FORTOVASE/ritonavir** Interaction has not been evaluated	Appropriate doses of the combination with respect to safety and efficacy have not been established.
Non-nucleoside reverse transcriptase inhibitor: Efavirenz*, nevirapine	**FORTOVASE** ↓ Saquinavir ↓ Efavirenz **FORTOVASE/ritonavir** Interaction has not been evaluated	FORTOVASE should not be given as the sole protease inhibitor to patients taking efavirenz or nevirapine. Appropriate doses of the combination of efavirenz or nevirapine and FORTOVASE/ritonavir with respect to safety and efficacy have not been established.
HIV protease inhibitor: Indinavir*	**FORTOVASE** ↑ Saquinavir Effect on indinavir is not well established **FORTOVASE/ritonavir** Interaction has not been evaluated	Appropriate doses of the combination with respect to safety and efficacy have not been established.
HIV protease inhibitor: Nelfinavir*	**FORTOVASE** ↑ Saquinavir ↑ Nelfinavir **FORTOVASE/ritonavir** Interaction has not been evaluated	Saquinavir 1200 mg bid with nelfinavir 1250 mg bid results in adequate plasma drug concentrations for both protease inhibitors.
HIV protease inhibitor: Ritonavir*	**FORTOVASE** ↑ Saquinavir ↔ Ritonavir	The recommended dose regimen when ritonavir is given to increase saquinavir concentrations is 1000 mg saquinavir plus ritonavir 100 mg twice daily.
HIV protease inhibitor: Lopinavir/ritonavir (coformulated capsule)*	**FORTOVASE** ↑ Saquinavir Effect on lopinavir is not well established	FORTOVASE (SQV) 800 mg bid + KALETRA produces ↑ AUC, ↑ C_{max}, and ↑ C_{min} relative to FORTOVASE 1200 mg tid (see CLINICAL PHARMACOLOGY: Table 3)
HIV fusion inhibitor: Enfuvirtide*	**FORTOVASE** Interaction has not been evaluated **FORTOVASE/ritonavir** ↔ Enfuvirtide	No clinically significant interaction was noted from a study in 12 HIV patients who received enfuvirtide concomitantly with FORTOVASE/ritonavir 1000/100 mg bid. No dose adjustments are required.
	Other Agents	
Antiarrhythmics: Lidocaine (systemic)	↑ Antiarrhythmics	Caution is warranted and therapeutic concentration monitoring, if available, is recommended for antiarrhythmics given with FORTOVASE or FORTOVASE/ritonavir
Anticoagulant: Warfarin		Concentrations of warfarin may be affected. It is recommended that INR (international normalized ratio) be monitored.
Anticonvulsants: Carbamazepine, phenobarbital, phenytoin	**FORTOVASE** ↓ Saquinavir Effect on carbamazepine, phenobarbital, and phenytoin is not well established **FORTOVASE/ritonavir** Interaction has not been evaluated	Use with caution, FORTOVASE may be less effective due to decreased saquinavir plasma concentrations in patients taking these agents concomitantly.
Anti-infective: Clarithromycin*	**FORTOVASE** ↑ Saquinavir ↑ Clarithromycin **FORTOVASE/ritonavir** Interaction has not been evaluated	No dose adjustment is required when the two drugs are coadministered for a limited time at the doses studied (clarithromycin 500 mg bid and FORTOVASE 1200 mg tid for 7 days). For patients with renal impairment, the following dosage adjustments should be considered: • For patients with CL_{CR} 30 to 60 mL/min the dose of clarithromycin should be reduced by 50%. • For patients with CL_{CR} <30 mL/min the dose of clarithromycin should be decreased by 75%. No dose adjustment for patients with normal renal function is necessary.

(Table continued on next page)

Patients should be informed that FORTOVASE is not a cure for HIV infection and that they may continue to acquire illnesses associated with advanced HIV infection, including opportunistic infections. Patients should be advised that FORTOVASE should be used only in combination with other active antiretroviral medications.
Patients should be informed that redistribution or accumulation of body fat may occur in patients receiving protease inhibitors and that the cause and long-term health effects of these conditions are not known at this time.
Patients should be told that the long-term effects of FORTOVASE are unknown at this time. They should be informed that FORTOVASE therapy has not been shown to reduce the risk of transmitting HIV to others through sexual contact or blood contamination.
Patients should be advised that FORTOVASE should be taken within 2 hours after a full meal. When FORTOVASE is coadministered with ritonavir a light meal is sufficient (see CLINICAL PHARMACOLOGY: Pharmacokinetics). Patients should be advised of the importance of taking their medication every day, as prescribed, to achieve maximum benefit. Patients should not alter the dose or discontinue therapy without consulting their physician. If a dose is missed, patients should take the next dose as soon as possible. However, the patient should not double the next dose. Patients should be informed that refrigerated (36° to 46°F, 2° to 8°C) capsules of FORTOVASE remain stable until the

Continued on next page

Fortovase—Cont.

expiration date printed on the label. Once brought to room temperature [at or below 77°F (25°C)], capsules should be used within 3 months.

Laboratory Tests

Clinical chemistry tests, viral load, and CD4 count should be performed prior to initiating FORTOVASE therapy and at appropriate intervals thereafter. Elevated nonfasting triglyceride levels have been observed in patients in saquinavir trials. Triglyceride levels should be periodically monitored during therapy. For comprehensive information concerning laboratory test alterations associated with use of other antiretroviral therapies, physicians should refer to the complete product information for these drugs.

Drug Interactions

Several drug interaction studies have been completed with both INVIRASE and FORTOVASE. Observations from drug interaction studies with FORTOVASE may not be predictive for INVIRASE. If ritonavir is coadministered, prescribers should also refer to the prescribing information for ritonavir regarding drug interactions associated with this agent.

The metabolism of saquinavir is mediated by cytochrome P450, with the specific isoenzyme CYP3A4 responsible for 90% of the hepatic metabolism. Additionally, saquinavir is a substrate for P-Glycoprotein (Pgp). Therefore, drugs that affect CYP3A4 and/or Pgp, may modify the pharmacokinetics of saquinavir. Similarly, saquinavir might also modify the pharmacokinetics of other drugs that are substrates for CYP3A4 or Pgp.

Drugs that are contraindicated specifically due to the expected magnitude of interaction and potential for serious adverse events are listed in Table 4 under CONTRAINDICATIONS. Additional drugs that are not recommended for coadministration with FORTOVASE are included in Table 5. These recommendations are based on either drug interaction studies or predicted interactions due to the expected magnitude of interaction and potential for serious events or loss of efficacy.

Drug interactions that have been established based on drug interaction studies are listed with the pharmacokinetic results in Table 2, which summarizes the effect of saquinavir, administered as FORTOVASE, on the geometric mean AUC and C_{max} of coadministered drugs and Table 3, which summarizes the effect of coadministered drugs on the geometric mean AUC and C_{max} of saquinavir. Clinical dose recommendations can be found in Table 6. The magnitude of interactions may be different when FORTOVASE is given with ritonavir.

[See table 5 on page 2878]

If FORTOVASE is coadministered with ritonavir, the ritonavir label should be reviewed for additional drugs that should not be coadministered.

[See table 6 on previous page and at right]

Drugs That Are Mainly Metabolized by CYP3A4

Although specific studies have not been performed, coadministration with drugs that are mainly metabolized by CYP3A4 (eg, calcium channel blockers, dapsone, disopyramide, quinine, amiodarone, quinidine, warfarin, tacrolimus, cyclosporine, ergot derivatives, pimozide, carbamazepine, fentanyl, alfentanyl, alprazolam, nefazodone and triazolam) may have elevated plasma concentrations when coadministered with saquinavir; therefore, these combinations should be used with caution. If FORTOVASE is coadministered with ritonavir, the ritonavir label should be reviewed for additional drugs that should not be coadministered.

Inducers of CYP3A4

Coadministration with compounds that are potent inducers of CYP3A4 (eg, phenobarbital, phenytoin, dexamethasone, carbamazepine) may result in decreased plasma levels of saquinavir.

Carcinogenesis, Mutagenesis and Impairment of Fertility

Carcinogenesis

Carcinogenicity studies found no indication of carcinogenic activity in rats and mice administered saquinavir for approximately 2 years. The plasma exposures (AUC values) in the respective species were up to approximately 60% of (using rat) and equivalent to (using mouse) those obtained in humans at the recommended clinical dose (FORTOVASE 1200 mg tid).

Mutagenesis

Mutagenicity and genotoxicity studies, with and without metabolic activation where appropriate, have shown that saquinavir has no mutagenic activity in vitro in either bacterial (Ames test) or mammalian cells (Chinese hamster lung V79/HPRT test). Saquinavir does not induce chromosomal damage in vivo in the mouse micronucleus assay or in vitro in human peripheral blood lymphocytes and does not induce primary DNA damage in vitro in the unscheduled DNA synthesis test.

Impairment of Fertility

Fertility and reproductive performance were not affected in rats at plasma exposures (AUC values) approximately 50% of those achieved in humans at the recommended dose.

Pregnancy

Teratogenic Effects

Category B. Reproduction studies conducted with saquinavir in rats have shown no embryotoxicity or teratogenicity at plasma exposures (AUC values) approximately 50% of those achieved in humans at the recommended dose or in rabbits at plasma exposures approximately 40% of those achieved at the recommended clinical dose of FORTOVASE. Distribution studies in these species showed that placental transfer of saquinavir is low (less than 5% of maternal plasma concentrations).

Studies in rats indicated that exposure to saquinavir from late pregnancy through lactation at plasma concentrations (AUC values) approximately 50% of those achieved in humans at the recommended dose of FORTOVASE had no effect on the survival, growth and development of offspring to weaning. Clinical experience in pregnant women is limited. Saquinavir should be used during pregnancy only if the potential benefit justifies the potential risk to the fetus.

Antiretroviral Pregnancy Registry

To monitor maternal-fetal outcomes of pregnant women exposed to antiretroviral medications, including FORTOVASE, an Antiretroviral Pregnancy Registry has

Table 6 *(cont.)* **Established and Other Potentially Significant Drug Interactions: Alteration in Dose or Regimen May Be Recommended Based on Drug Interaction Studies or Predicted Interaction (Information in the table applies to FORTOVASE with or without ritonavir, unless otherwise indicated)**

Concomitant Drug Class: Drug Name	Effect on Concentration of Saquinavir or Concomitant Drug	Clinical Comment
	Other Agents (continued)	
Antifungal: Ketoconazole*, itraconazole	**FORTOVASE** ↑ Saquinavir ↔ Ketoconazole **FORTOVASE/ritonavir** Interaction has not been evaluated	No dose adjustment is required when the two drugs are coadministered for a limited time at the doses studied (ketoconazole 400 mg qd and FORTOVASE 1200 mg tid). A similar increase in plasma concentrations of saquinavir could occur with itraconazole.
Antimycobacterial Rifabutin*	↓ Saquinavir ↑ Rifabutin	FORTOVASE should not be given as the sole protease inhibitor to patients taking rifabutin. Appropriate doses of the combination of rifabutin and FORTOVASE/ritonavir with respect to safety and efficacy have not been established.
Antimycobacterial Rifampin*	**FORTOVASE** ↓ Saquinavir **FORTOVASE/ritonavir** Interaction has not been evaluated	FORTOVASE should not be given as the sole protease inhibitor to patients taking rifampin. Appropriate doses of the combination of rifampin and FORTOVASE/ritonavir with respect to safety and efficacy have not been established.
Benzodiazepines: Alprazolam, clorazepate, diazepam, flurazepam	↑ Benzodiazepines	Clinical significance is unknown; however, a decrease in benzodiazepine dose may be needed.
Calcium channel blockers: Diltiazem, felodipine, nifedipine, nicardipine, nimodipine, verapamil, amlodipine, nisoldipine, isradipine	↑ Calcium channel blockers	Caution is warranted and clinical monitoring of patients is recommended.
Corticosteroid: Dexamethasone	**FORTOVASE** ↓ Saquinavir **FORTOVASE/ritonavir** Interaction has not been evaluated	Use with caution, FORTOVASE may be less effective due to decreased saquinavir plasma concentrations in patients taking these agents concomitantly.
Histamine H_2-receptor antagonist: Ranitidine	**FORTOVASE** ↑ Saquinavir **FORTOVASE/ritonavir** Interaction has not been evaluated	The increase is not thought to be clinically relevant and no dose adjustment of FORTOVASE is recommended. Appropriate doses of the combination of ranitidine and FORTOVASE/ritonavir with respect to safety and efficacy have not been established.
HMG-CoA reductase inhibitors: Simvastatin, lovastatin, atorvastatin	↑ HMG-CoA reductase inhibitors	The combination of FORTOVASE with simvastatin and lovastatin should be avoided. Use lowest possible dose of atorvastatin and with careful monitoring or consider other HMG-CoA reductase inhibitors such as pravastatin, fluvastatin and rosuvastatin.
Immunosuppressants: Cyclosporine, tacrolimus, rapamycin	↑ Immunosuppressants	Therapeutic concentration monitoring is recommended for immunosuppressant agents when coadministered with FORTOVASE or FORTOVASE/ritonavir.
Narcotic analgesic: Methadone	**FORTOVASE/ritonavir** ↓ Methadone	Dosage of methadone may need to be increased when coadministered with FORTOVASE/ritonavir.
Oral contraceptives: Ethinyl estradiol	**FORTOVASE/ritonavir** ↓ Ethinyl estradiol	Alternative or additional contraceptive measures should be used when estrogen-based oral contraceptives and FORTOVASE/ritonavir are coadministered.
PDE5 inhibitor (phosphodiesterase type 5 inhibitors): Sildenafil*, vardenafil, tadalafil	↑ Sildenafil ↔ Saquinavir ↑ Vardenafil ↑ Tadalafil **FORTOVASE/ritonavir** Interaction has not been evaluated, but expect increased concentrations of PDE5 inhibitors.	Use sildenafil with caution at reduced doses of 25 mg every 48 hours with increased monitoring of adverse events when administered concomitantly with FORTOVASE or FORTOVASE/ritonavir. Use vardenafil with caution at reduced doses of no more than 2.5 mg every 72 hours with increased monitoring of adverse events when administered concomitantly with FORTOVASE or FORTOVASE/ritonavir. Use tadalafil with caution at reduced doses of no more than 10 mg every 72 hours with increased monitoring of adverse events when administered concomitantly with FORTOVASE or FORTOVASE/ritonavir.
Tricyclic antidepressants: Amitriptyline, imipramine	↑ Tricyclics	Therapeutic concentration monitoring is recommended for tricyclic antidepressants when coadministered with FORTOVASE/ritonavir.

*See CLINICAL PHARMACOLOGY: Pharmacokinetics, Tables 2 and 3 for magnitude of interactions

been established. Physicians are encouraged to register patients by calling 1-800-258-4263.

Nursing Mothers

The Centers for Disease Control and Prevention recommend that HIV-infected mothers not breast-feed their infants to avoid risking postnatal transmission of HIV. It is not known whether saquinavir is excreted in human milk. Because of both the potential for HIV transmission and the potential for serious adverse reactions in nursing infants, **mothers should be instructed not to breast-feed if they are receiving antiretroviral medications, including FORTOVASE.**

Pediatric Use

FORTOVASE should not be administered as a sole protease inhibitor to pediatric patients ≤16 years of age due to the risk of reduced saquinavir plasma concentrations compared to adults.

Safety and effectiveness of saquinavir when coadministered with ritonavir to pediatric patients is under investigation.

Geriatric Use

Clinical studies of FORTOVASE did not include sufficient numbers of subjects aged 65 and over to determine whether they respond differently from younger subjects. In general, caution should be taken when dosing FORTOVASE in elderly patients due to the greater frequency of decreased hepatic, renal, or cardiac function, and of concomitant disease or other drug therapy.

ADVERSE REACTIONS (see PRECAUTIONS)

The safety of FORTOVASE was studied in more than 500 patients who received the drug either alone or in combination with other antiretroviral agents. The majority of treatment-related adverse events were of mild intensity. The most frequently reported treatment-emergent adverse events among patients receiving FORTOVASE in combination with other antiretroviral agents were diarrhea, nausea, abdominal discomfort, and dyspepsia.

Clinical adverse events of at least moderate intensity, which occurred in ≥2% of patients in studies NV15182 (an open-label, single-arm safety study) and NV15355 (an open-label randomized study comparing FORTOVASE and INVIRASE) are summarized in Table 7. The median duration of treatment in studies NV15182 and NV15355 were 52 and 18 weeks, respectively. In NV15182, more than 300 patients were on treatment for approximately 1 year.

FORTOVASE did not appear to alter the pattern, frequency or severity of known major toxicities associated with the use of nucleoside analogues. Physicians should refer to the complete product information for other antiretroviral agents as appropriate for drug-associated adverse reactions to these other agents.

Rare occurrences of the following serious adverse experiences have been reported during clinical trials of FORTOVASE and/or INVIRASE and were considered at least possibly related to use of study drugs: confusion, ataxia and weakness; seizures; headache; acute myeloblastic leukemia; hemolytic anemia; thrombocytopenia; thrombocytopenia and intracranial hemorrhage leading to death; attempted suicide; Stevens-Johnson syndrome; bullous skin eruption and polyarthritis; severe cutaneous reaction associated with increased liver function tests; isolated elevation of transaminases; exacerbation of chronic liver disease with Grade 4 elevated liver function tests, jaundice, ascites, and right and left upper quadrant abdominal pain; pancreatitis leading to death; intestinal obstruction; portal hypertension; thrombophlebitis; peripheral vasoconstriction; drug fever; nephrolithiasis; and acute renal insufficiency.

Table 7 Percentage of Patients With Treatment-Emergent Adverse Events* of at Least Moderate Intensity, Occurring in ≥2% of Patients

	NV15182 (48 weeks)	NV15355 (48 weeks) Naive Patients
ADVERSE EVENT	**FORTOVASE + TOC† N=442**	**FORTOVASE + 2 RTIs‡ N=90**
Gastrointestinal		
Diarrhea	19.9	15.6
Nausea	10.6	13.3
Abdominal Discomfort	8.6	10.0
Dyspepsia	8.4	7.8
Flatulence	5.7	10.0
Vomiting	2.9	4.4
Abdominal Pain	2.3	4.4
Constipation	–	3.3
Body as a Whole		
Fatigue	4.8	8.9
Appetite Decreased	–	2.2
Chest Pain	–	2.2
Central and Peripheral Nervous System		
Headaches	5.0	5.6
Psychiatric Disorders		
Depression	2.7	–
Insomnia	–	5.6
Anxiety	–	2.2
Libido Disorder	–	3.3
Special Senses Disorders		
Taste Alteration	–	4.4
Musculoskeletal Disorders		
Pain	–	3.3
Dermatological Disorders		
Eczema	–	–
Rash	–	–
Verruca	–	2.2

*Includes adverse events at least possibly related to study drug or of unknown intensity and/or relationship to treatment (corresponding to ACTG Grade 2, 3 and 4).
†Antiretroviral Treatment of Choice.
‡Reverse Transcriptase Inhibitor.

Table 9 Percentage of Patients with Marked Laboratory Abnormalities*

		NV15182 (48 weeks)	NV15355 (48 weeks) Naive Patients
BIOCHEMISTRY	**Limit**	**FORTOVASE + TOC† N=442**	**FORTOVASE + 2 RTIs‡ N=90**
Alkaline Phosphatase (high)	>5 x ULN§	0.5	0.0
Calcium (high)	>12.5 mg/dL	0.2	0.0
Creatine Kinase (high)	>4 x ULN§	7.8	6.0
Gamma GT (high)	>5 x ULN§	5.7	5.0
Glucose (low)	<40 mg/dL	6.4	3.5
Glucose (high)	>250 mg/dL	1.4	0.0
Phosphate (low)	<1.5 mg/dL	0.5	1.0
Potassium (high)	>6.5 mEq/L	2.7	3.5
Serum Amylase (high)	>2 x ULN§	1.9	ND
SGOT (AST) (high)	>5 x ULN§	4.1	0.0
SGPT (ALT) (high)	>5 x ULN§	5.7	1.0
Sodium (high)	>157 mEq/L	0.7	0.0
Sodium (low)	<123 mEq/L	0.0	1.0
Total Bilirubin (high)	>2.5 x ULN§	1.6	0.0
Triglycerides (high)	>750 mg/dL	0.0	2.0
HEMATOLOGY			
Hemoglobin (low)	<7.0 gm/dL	0.7	1.0
Absolute Neutrophil Count (low)	<750 mm^3	2.9	1.0
Platelets (low)	<50,000 mm^3	0.9	0.0

* ACTG Grade 3 or above.
† Antiretroviral Treatment of Choice.
‡ Reverse Transcriptase Inhibitor.
§ ULN = Upper limit of normal range.
ND Not done.

Concomitant Therapy with Ritonavir

Table 8 Grade 2, 3 and 4 Adverse Events (All Causality) Reported in ≥2% of Adult Patients in the MaxCmin 1 Study of FORTOVASE in Combination with Ritonavir 1000/100 mg bid

	FORTOVASE 1000 mg plus Ritonavir 100 mg bid (48 weeks) N=148 n(%=n/N)
Endocrine Disorders	
Diabetes mellitus/ hyperglycemia	4 (2.7)
Lipodystrophy	8 (5.4)
Gastrointestinal Disorders	
Nausea	16 (10.8)
Vomiting	11 (7.4)
Diarrhea	12 (8.1)
Abdominal Pain	9 (6.1)
Constipation	3 (2.0)
General Disorders and Administration Site Conditions	
Fatigue	9 (6.1)
Fever	5 (3.4)
Musculoskeletal Disorders	
Back Pain	3 (2.0)
Respiratory Disorders	
Pneumonia	8 (5.4)
Bronchitis	4 (2.7)
Influenza	4 (2.7)
Sinusitis	4 (2.7)
Dermatological Disorders	
Rash	5 (3.4)
Pruritus	5 (3.4)
Dry lips/skin	3 (2.0)
Eczema	3 (2.0)

Includes events with unknown relationship to study drug.

Laboratory Abnormalities

In the MaxCmin 1 study, Grade 3 and 4 thrombocytopenia (2.0% of patients) and anemia (2.0%) were observed with FORTOVASE in combination with ritonavir. At 48 weeks, other lab abnormalities included increased ALT, increased AST, increased GGT, hyperglycemia, hypertriglyceridemia, increased TSH, neutropenia, raised amylase, and increased LDH.

Table 9 summarizes the percentage of patients with marked laboratory abnormalities in study NV15182 and NV15355 (median duration of treatment was 52 and 18 weeks, respectively). In study NV15182, by 48 weeks <1% of patients discontinued treatment due to laboratory abnormalities.

In the safety study (NV15182), 27% to 33% of subjects experienced 1 grade shifts in ALT and AST during the 48-week study period. In 46% of such events, there was a single abnormal transaminase level with no evidence of persistently elevated enzyme values during the course of study. Only 3% to 4% of patients had ≥3 grade shifts in transaminase levels and less than 0.5% of patients had to discontinue the study for increased liver function test values.

[See table 9 above]

Additional marked lab abnormalities have been observed with INVIRASE. These include: calcium (low), phosphate (low), potassium (low), sodium (low).

Monotherapy and Combination Studies

Other clinical adverse experiences of any intensity, at least remotely related to FORTOVASE and INVIRASE, including those in <2% of patients, are listed below by body system.

Autonomic Nervous System

Mouth dry, night sweats, sweating increased

Body as a Whole

Allergic reaction, anorexia, appetite decreased, appetite disturbances, asthenia, chest pain, edema, fever, intoxication, malaise, olfactory disorder, pain body, pain pelvic, retrosternal pain, shivering, trauma, wasting syndrome, weakness generalized, weight decrease, redistribution/accumulation of body fat (see PRECAUTIONS: Fat Redistribution)

Cardiovascular/Cerebrovascular

Cyanosis, heart murmur, heart rate disorder, heart valve disorder, hypertension, hypotension, stroke, syncope, vein distended

Central and Peripheral Nervous System

Ataxia, cerebral hemorrhage, confusion, convulsions, dizziness, dysarthria, dysesthesia, hyperesthesia, hyperreflexia, hyporeflexia, light-headed feeling, myelopolyradiculoneuritis, neuropathy, numbness extremities, numbness face, paresis, paresthesia, peripheral neuropathy, poliomyelitis, prickly sensation, progressive multifocal leukoencephalopathy, spasms, tremor, unconsciousness

Dermatological

Acne, alopecia, chalazion, dermatitis, dermatitis seborrheic, erythema, folliculitis, furunculosis, hair changes, hot flushes, nail disorder, papillomatosis, papular rash, photosensitivity reaction, pigment changes skin, parasites external, pruritus, psoriasis, rash maculopapular, rash pruritic, red face, skin disorder, skin nodule, skin syndrome, skin ulceration, urticaria, verruca, xeroderma

Endocrine/Metabolic

Dehydration, diabetes mellitus, hyperglycemia, hypoglycemia, hypothyroidism, thirst, triglyceride increase, weight increase

Continued on next page

Fortovase—Cont.

Gastrointestinal
Abdominal distention, bowel movements frequent, buccal mucosa ulceration, canker sores oral, cheilitis, colic abdominal, dysphagia, esophageal ulceration, esophagitis, eructation, fecal incontinence, feces bloodstained, feces discolored, gastralgia, gastritis, gastroesophageal reflux, gastrointestinal inflammation, gingivitis, glossitis, hemorrhage rectum, hemorrhoids, infectious diarrhea, melena, painful defecation, parotid disorder, pruritus ani, pyrosis, salivary glands disorder, stomach upset, stomatitis, taste unpleasant, toothache, tooth disorder, ulcer gastrointestinal
Hematologic
Anemia, neutropenia, pancytopenia, splenomegaly
Liver and Biliary
Cholangitis sclerosing, cholelithiasis, hepatitis, hepatomegaly, hepatosplenomegaly, jaundice, liver enzyme disorder, pancreatitis
Musculoskeletal
Arthralgia, arthritis, back pain, cramps leg, cramps muscle, lumbago, musculoskeletal disorders, myalgia, myopathy, pain facial, pain jaw, pain leg, pain musculoskeletal, stiffness, tissue changes
Neoplasm
Kaposi's sarcoma, tumor
Platelet, Bleeding, Clotting
Bleeding dermal, hemorrhage, microhemorrhages, thrombocytopenia
Psychiatric
Agitation, amnesia, anxiety attack, behavior disturbances, dreaming excessive, euphoria, hallucination, intellectual ability reduced, irritability, lethargy, overdose effect, psychic disorder, psychosis, somnolence, speech disorder
Reproductive System
Epididymitis, erectile impotence, impotence, menstrual disorder, menstrual irregularity, penis disorder, prostate enlarged, vaginal discharge
Resistance Mechanism
Abscess, angina tonsillaris, candidiasis, cellulitis, herpes simplex, herpes zoster, infection bacterial, infection mycotic, infection staphylococcal, infestation parasitic, influenza, lymphadenopathy, molluscum contagiosum, moniliasis
Respiratory
Asthma bronchial, bronchitis, cough, dyspnea, epistaxis, hemoptysis, laryngitis, pharyngitis, pneumonia, pulmonary disease, respiratory disorder, rhinitis, rhinitis allergic atopic, sinusitis, upper respiratory tract infection
Special Senses
Blepharitis, conjunctivitis, cytomegalovirus retinitis, dry eye syndrome, earache, ear pressure, eye irritation, hearing decreased, otitis, taste unpleasant, tinnitus, visual disturbance, xerophthalmia
Urinary System
Micturition disorder, nocturia, renal calculus, renal colic, urinary tract bleeding, urinary tract infection

Postmarketing Experience with INVIRASE and FORTOVASE

Additional adverse events that have been observed during the postmarketing period are similar to those seen in clinical trials with INVIRASE and FORTOVASE and administration of INVIRASE and FORTOVASE in combination with ritonavir.

OVERDOSAGE

Two cases of FORTOVASE overdosage have been received (one case with unknown amount of FORTOVASE, the second case 3.6 to 4 grams at once). No adverse events have been reported in both cases. There were 2 patients who had overdoses with INVIRASE. No acute toxicities or sequelae were noted in the first patient after ingesting 8 grams of INVIRASE as a single dose. The patient was treated with induction of emesis within 2 to 4 hours after ingestion. The second patient ingested 2.4 grams of INVIRASE in combination with 600 mg of ritonavir and experienced pain in the throat that lasted for 6 hours and then resolved.

DOSAGE AND ADMINISTRATION

FORTOVASE (saquinavir) soft gelatin capsules and INVIRASE (saquinavir mesylate) capsules are not bioequivalent and cannot be used interchangeably When using saquinavir as the sole protease inhibitor in an antiviral regimen, FORTOVASE is the recommended formulation. INVIRASE may be considered only if it is combined with ritonavir, which significantly inhibits saquinavir's metabolism to provide plasma saquinavir levels at least equal to those achieved with FORTOVASE at the recommended dose of 1200 mg tid (see CLINICAL PHARMACOLOGY: Drug Interactions).

Adults (Over the Age of 16 Years)

FORTOVASE Administered Without Ritonavir:

- FORTOVASE 1200-mg tid (6 × 200-mg capsules)
- FORTOVASE should be taken with a meal or up to 2 hours after a meal

FORTOVASE Administered With Ritonavir:

- FORTOVASE 1000-mg bid (5 × 200-mg capsules) in combination with ritonavir 100-mg bid
- Ritonavir should be taken at the same time as FORTOVASE
- FORTOVASE and ritonavir should be taken within 2 hours after a meal

When used in combination with nucleoside analogues, the dosage of FORTOVASE should not be reduced as this will lead to greater than dose proportional decreases in saquinavir plasma levels.

Patients should be advised that FORTOVASE, like other protease inhibitors, is recommended for use in combination with active antiretroviral therapy. Greater activity has been observed when new antiretroviral therapies are begun at the same time as FORTOVASE. As with all protease inhibitors, adherence to the prescribed regimen is strongly recommended. Concomitant therapy should be based on a patient's prior drug exposure.

Monitoring of Patients

Clinical chemistry tests, viral load, and CD4 count should be performed prior to initiating FORTOVASE therapy and at appropriate intervals thereafter. For comprehensive patient monitoring recommendations for other antiretroviral therapies, physicians should refer to the complete product information for these drugs.

Dose Adjustment for Combination Therapy with FORTOVASE

For serious toxicities that may be associated with FORTOVASE, the drug should be interrupted. For recipients of combination therapy with FORTOVASE and other antiretroviral agents, dose adjustment of the other antiretroviral agents should be based on the known toxicity profile of the individual drug. FORTOVASE dose adjustments may be required with some other antiretroviral agents (see PRECAUTIONS: Drug Interactions). Physicians should refer to the complete product information for these drugs for comprehensive dose adjustment recommendations and drug-associated adverse reactions.

HOW SUPPLIED

FORTOVASE 200-mg capsules are beige, opaque, soft gelatin capsules with ROCHE and 0246 imprinted on the capsule shell — bottles of 180 (NDC 0004-0246-48).

The capsules should be refrigerated at 36° to 46°F (2° to 8°C) in tightly closed bottles until dispensed.

For patient use, refrigerated (36° to 46°F, 2° to 8°C) capsules of FORTOVASE remain stable until the expiration date printed on the label. Once brought to room temperature [at or below 77°F (25°C)], capsules should be used within 3 months.

HIVID and INVIRASE are registered trademarks of Hoffmann-La Roche Inc. KALETRA is a registered trademark of Abbott Laboratories.

Manufactured by:
F. Hoffmann-La Roche Ltd., Basel, Switzerland

Revised: December 2003

Shown in Product Identification Guide, page 331

FUZEON™ ℞

[fūe'zē-ŏn]
(enfuvirtide)
for Injection
℞ only

DESCRIPTION

FUZEON (enfuvirtide) is an inhibitor of the fusion of HIV-1 with CD4+ cells. Enfuvirtide is a linear 36-amino acid synthetic peptide with the N-terminus acetylated and the C-terminus is a carboxamide. It is composed of naturally occurring L-amino acid residues.

Enfuvirtide is a white to off-white amorphous solid. It has negligible solubility in pure water and the solubility increases in aqueous buffers (pH 7.5) to 85-142 g/100 mL. The empirical formula of enfuvirtide is $C_{204}H_{301}N_{51}O_{64}$, and the molecular weight is 4492. It has the following primary amino acid sequence:

CH_3CO-Tyr-Thr-Ser-Leu-Ile-His-Ser-Leu-Ile-Glu-Glu-Ser-Gln-Asn-Gln-Gln-Glu-Lys-Asn-Glu-Gln-Glu-Leu-Leu-Glu-Leu-Asp-Lys-Trp-Ala-Ser-Leu-Trp-Asn-Trp-Phe-NH_2.

The drug product, FUZEON (enfuvirtide) for Injection, is a white to off-white, sterile, lyophilized powder. Each single-use vial contains 108 mg of enfuvirtide for the delivery of 90 mg. Prior to subcutaneous administration, the contents of the vial are reconstituted with 1.1 mL of Sterile Water for Injection giving a volume of approximately 1.2 mL to provide the delivery of 1 mL of the solution. Each 1 mL of the reconstituted solution contains approximately 90 mg of enfuvirtide with approximate amounts of the following excipients: 22.55 mg of mannitol, 2.39 mg of sodium carbonate (anhydrous), and sodium hydroxide and hydrochloric acid for pH adjustment as needed. The reconstituted solution has an approximate pH of 9.0.

MICROBIOLOGY

Mechanism of Action

Enfuvirtide interferes with the entry of HIV-1 into cells by inhibiting fusion of viral and cellular membranes. Enfuvirtide binds to the first heptad-repeat (HR1) in the gp41 subunit of the viral envelope glycoprotein and prevents the conformational changes required for the fusion of viral and cellular membranes.

Antiviral Activity In Vitro

The in vitro antiviral activity of enfuvirtide was assessed by infecting different CD4+ cell types with laboratory and clinical isolates of HIV-1. The IC_{50} (50% inhibitory concentration) for enfuvirtide in laboratory and primary isolates representing HIV-1 clades A to G ranged from 4 to 280 nM (18 to 1260 ng/mL). The IC_{50} for baseline clinical isolates ranged from 0.089 to 107 nM (0.4 to 480 ng/mL) by the cMAGI assay (n=130) and from 1.56 to 1680 nM (7 to 7530 ng/mL) by a recombinant phenotypic entry assay (n=612). Enfuvirtide was similarly active in vitro against R5, X4, and dual tropic viruses. Enfuvirtide has no activity against HIV-2.

Enfuvirtide exhibited additive to synergistic effects in cell culture assays when combined with individual members of various antiretroviral classes, including zidovudine, lamivudine, nelfinavir, indinavir, and efavirenz.

Drug Resistance

HIV-1 isolates with reduced susceptibility to enfuvirtide have been selected in vitro. Genotypic analysis of the in vitro-selected resistant isolates showed mutations that resulted in amino acid substitutions at the enfuvirtide binding HR1 domain positions 36 to 38 of the HIV-1 envelope glycoprotein gp41. Phenotypic analysis of site-directed mutants in positions 36 to 38 in an HIV-1 molecular clone showed a 5-fold to 684-fold decrease in susceptibility to enfuvirtide.

In clinical trials, HIV-1 isolates with reduced susceptibility to enfuvirtide have been recovered from subjects treated with FUZEON in combination with other antiretroviral agents. Posttreatment HIV-1 virus from 185 subjects exhibited decreases in susceptibility to enfuvirtide ranging from 4-fold to 422-fold relative to their respective baseline virus and exhibited genotypic changes in gp41 amino acids 36 to 45. Substitutions in this region were observed with decreasing frequency at amino acid positions 38, 43, 36, 40, 42, and 45.

Cross-resistance

HIV-1 clinical isolates resistant to nucleoside analogue reverse transcriptase inhibitors (NRTI), non-nucleoside analogue reverse transcriptase inhibitors (NNRTI), and protease inhibitors (PI) were susceptible to enfuvirtide in cell culture.

CLINICAL PHARMACOLOGY

Pharmacokinetics

The pharmacokinetic properties of enfuvirtide were evaluated in HIV-1 infected adult and pediatric patients.

Absorption

Following a 90-mg single subcutaneous injection of FUZEON into the abdomen in 12 HIV-1 infected subjects, the mean (±SD) C_{max} was 4.59 ± 1.5 µg/mL, AUC was 55.8 ± 12.1 µg•h/mL and the median T_{max} was 8 hours (ranged from 3 to 12 h). The absolute bioavailability (using a 90-mg intravenous dose as a reference) was 84.3% ± 15.5%. Following 90-mg bid dosing of FUZEON subcutaneously in combination with other antiretroviral agents in 11 HIV-1 infected subjects, the mean (±SD) steady-state C_{max} was 5.0 ± 1.7 µg/mL, C_{trough} was 3.3 ± 1.6 µg/mL, $AUC_{0\text{-}12h}$ was 48.7 ± 19.1 µg•h/mL, and the median T_{max} was 4 hours (ranged from 4 to 8 h).

Absorption of the 90-mg dose was comparable when injected into the subcutaneous tissue of the abdomen, thigh or arm.

Distribution

The mean (±SD) steady-state volume of distribution after intravenous administration of a 90-mg dose of FUZEON (N=12) was 5.5 ± 1.1 L.

Enfuvirtide is approximately 92% bound to plasma proteins in HIV-infected plasma over a concentration range of 2 to 10 µg/mL. It is bound predominantly to albumin and to a lower extent to α-1 acid glycoprotein.

Metabolism/Elimination

As a peptide, enfuvirtide is expected to undergo catabolism to its constituent amino acids, with subsequent recycling of the amino acids in the body pool.

Mass balance studies to determine elimination pathway(s) of enfuvirtide have not been performed in humans.

In vitro studies with human microsomes and hepatocytes indicate that enfuvirtide undergoes hydrolysis to form a deamidated metabolite at the C-terminal phenylalanine residue, M3. The hydrolysis reaction is not NADPH dependent. The M3 metabolite is detected in human plasma following administration of enfuvirtide, with an AUC ranging from 2.4% to 15% of the enfuvirtide AUC.

Following a 90-mg single subcutaneous dose of enfuvirtide (N=12) the mean ±SD elimination half-life of enfuvirtide is 3.8 ± 0.6 h and the mean ±SD apparent clearance was 24.8 ± 4.1 mL/h/kg. Following 90-mg bid dosing of FUZEON subcutaneously in combination with other antiretroviral agents in 11 HIV-1 infected subjects, the mean ±SD apparent clearance was 30.6 ± 10.6 mL/h/kg.

Special Populations

Hepatic Insufficiency

Formal pharmacokinetic studies of enfuvirtide have not been conducted in patients with hepatic impairment.

Renal Insufficiency

Formal pharmacokinetic studies of enfuvirtide have not been conducted in patients with renal insufficiency. However, analysis of plasma concentration data from subjects in clinical trials indicated that the clearance of enfuvirtide is not affected in patients with creatinine clearance greater than 35 mL/min. The effect of creatinine clearance less than 35 mL/min on enfuvirtide clearance is unknown.

Gender and Weight

GENDER

Analysis of plasma concentration data from subjects in clinical trials indicated that the clearance of enfuvirtide is 20% lower in females than males after adjusting for body weight.

WEIGHT

Enfuvirtide clearance decreases with decreased body weight irrespective of gender. Relative to the clearance of a 70-kg male, a 40-kg male will have 20% lower clearance and a

110-kg male will have a 26% higher clearance. Relative to a 70-kg male, a 40-kg female will have a 36% lower clearance and a 110-kg female will have the same clearance.
No dose adjustment is recommended for weight or gender.
Race
Analysis of plasma concentration data from subjects in clinical trials indicated that the clearance of enfuvirtide was not different in Blacks compared to Caucasians. Other pharmacokinetic studies suggest no difference between Asians and Caucasians after adjusting for body weight.
Pediatric Patients
The pharmacokinetics of enfuvirtide have been studied in 18 pediatric subjects aged 6 through 16 years at a dose of 2 mg/kg. Enfuvirtide pharmacokinetics were determined in the presence of concomitant medications including antiretroviral agents. A dose of 2 mg/kg bid (maximum 90 mg bid) provided enfuvirtide plasma concentrations similar to those obtained in adult patients receiving 90 mg bid.
In the 18 pediatric subjects receiving the 2 mg/kg bid dose, the mean ±SD steady-state AUC was 53.6 ± 21.4 μg•h/mL, C_{max} was 5.9 ± 2.2 μg/mL, C_{trough} was 3.0 ± 1.5 μg/mL, and apparent clearance was 40 ± 14 mL/h/kg.
Geriatric Patients
The pharmacokinetics of enfuvirtide have not been studied in patients over 65 years of age.
Drug Interactions
Influence of FUZEON on the Metabolism of Concomitant Drugs
Based on the results from an in vitro human microsomal study, enfuvirtide is not an inhibitor of CYP450 enzymes. In an in vivo human metabolism study (N=12), FUZEON at the recommended dose of 90 mg bid did not alter the metabolism of CYP3A4, CYP2D6, CYP1A2, CYP2C19 or CYP2E1 substrates.
Influence of Concomitant Drugs on the Metabolism of Enfuvirtide
In separate pharmacokinetic interaction studies, coadministration of ritonavir (N=12), saquinavir/ritonavir (N=12), and rifampin (N=12) did not result in clinically significant pharmacokinetic interactions with FUZEON (see Table 1).
[See table 1 above]

Table 1 Effect of Ritonavir, Saquinavir/Ritonavir, and Rifampin on the Steady-State Pharmacokinetics of Enfuvirtide (90 mg bid)*

Coadministered Drug	Dose of Coadministered Drug	N	% Change of Enfuvirtide Pharmacokinetic Parameters† (90% CI)		
			C_{max}	AUC	C_{trough}
Ritonavir	200 mg, q12h, 4 days	12	↑24 (↑9 to ↑41)	↑22 (↑8 to ↑37)	↑14 (↑2 to ↑28)
Saquinavir/Ritonavir	1000/100 mg, q12h, 4 days	12	⇔	↑14 (↑5 to ↑24)	↑26 (↑17 to ↑35)
Rifampin	600 mg, qd, 10 days	12	⇔	⇔	↓15 (↓22 to ↓7)

*All studies were performed in HIV-1+ subjects using a sequential crossover design.
†↑ = Increase; ↓ = Decrease; ⇔ = No Effect (↑ or ↓ <10%)

INDICATIONS AND USAGE

FUZEON in combination with other antiretroviral agents is indicated for the treatment of HIV-1 infection in treatment-experienced patients with evidence of HIV-1 replication despite ongoing antiretroviral therapy.
This indication is based on analyses of plasma HIV-1 RNA levels and CD4 cell counts in controlled studies of FUZEON of 24 weeks duration. Subjects enrolled were treatment-experienced adults; many had advanced disease. There are no studies of FUZEON in antiretroviral naive patients. There are no results from controlled trials evaluating the effect of FUZEON on clinical progression of HIV-1.

Description of Clinical Studies
Studies in Antiretroviral Experienced Patients
Studies T20-301 and T20-302 are ongoing, randomized, controlled, open-label, multicenter trials in HIV-1 infected subjects. Subjects were required to have either (1) viremia despite 3 to 6 months prior therapy with a nucleoside reverse transcriptase inhibitor (NRTI), non-nucleoside reverse transcriptase inhibitor (NNRTI), and protease inhibitor (PI) or (2) viremia and documented resistance or intolerance to at least one member in each of the NRTI, NNRTI, and PI classes.
All subjects received an individualized background regimen consisting of 3 to 5 antiretroviral agents selected on the basis of the subject's prior treatment history and baseline genotypic and phenotypic viral resistance measurements. Subjects were then randomized at a 2:1 ratio to FUZEON 90 mg bid with background regimen or background regimen alone. Demographic characteristics for studies T20-301 and T20-302 are shown in Table 2. Subjects had prior exposure to a median of 12 antiretrovirals for a median of 7 years.

Table 2 T20-301 and T20-302 Pooled Subject Demographics

	FUZEON + Background Regimen	Background Regimen
	N=661	N=334
Sex		
Male	90%	90%
Female	10%	10%
Race		
White	89%	89%
Black	8%	7%
Mean Age (yr) (range)	43 (16-67)	43 (24-82)
Median Baseline HIV-1 RNA (log_{10} copies/mL)	5.2 (3.5-6.7)	5.1 (3.7-7.1)
Median Baseline CD4 Cell Count (cells/mm³)	88 (1-994)	97 (1-847)

The change in plasma HIV-1 RNA from baseline to week 24 was -1.52 log_{10} copies/mL for subjects receiving FUZEON plus background regimen compared to -0.73 log_{10} copies/mL for subjects receiving the background regimen only (see Table 3).
Subjects with two or more active drugs in their background regimen were more likely to achieve a HIV-1 RNA of <400 copies/mL.

Table 3 Outcomes of Randomized Treatment at Week 24 (Pooled Studies T20-301 and T20-302)

Outcomes	FUZEON + Background Regimen 90 mg bid	Background Regimen
	N=661	N=334
HIV-1 RNA Log Change from Baseline (log_{10} copies/mL)*	-1.52	-0.73
CD4+ cell count Change from Baseline (cells/mm³)#	+71	+35
HIV RNA ≥1 log below Baseline	342 (52%)	86 (26%)
HIV RNA <400 copies/mL	247 (37%)	54 (16%)
HIV RNA <50 copies/mL	151 (23%)	30 (9%)
Discontinued due to adverse reactions/labs †	40 (6%)	12 (4%)
Discontinued due to injection site reactions†	20 (3%)	N/A
Discontinued due to other reasons†ϕ§	36 (5%)	14 (4%)

* Based on results from pooled data of T20-301 and T20-302 on ITT population (week 24 viral load for subjects who were lost to follow-up, discontinued therapy, or switched from their original randomization, is replaced by their baseline value).
# Last value carried forward
† Percentages based on safety population FUZEON+background (N=663) and background (N=337).
ϕ As per the judgment of the investigator.
§ Includes discontinuations from loss to follow-up, treatment refusal, and other reasons.

CONTRAINDICATIONS

FUZEON is contraindicated in patients with known hypersensitivity to FUZEON or any of its components (see WARNINGS).

WARNINGS

Local Injection Site Reactions
The most common adverse events associated with FUZEON use are local injection site reactions. Manifestations may include pain and discomfort, induration, erythema, nodules and cysts, pruritus, and ecchymosis. Nine percent of patients had local reactions that required analgesics or limited usual activities (see ADVERSE REACTIONS). Reactions are often present at more than one injection site. Patients must be familiar with the FUZEON *Injection Instructions* in order to know how to inject FUZEON appropriately and how to monitor carefully for signs or symptoms of cellulitis or local infection.
Pneumonia
An increased rate of bacterial pneumonia was observed in subjects treated with FUZEON in the Phase 3 clinical trials compared to the control arm (see ADVERSE REACTIONS). It is unclear if the increased incidence of pneumonia is related to FUZEON use. However, because of this finding, patients with HIV infection should be carefully monitored for signs and symptoms of pneumonia, especially if they have underlying conditions which may predispose them to pneumonia. Risk factors for pneumonia included low initial CD4 cell count, high initial viral load, intravenous drug use, smoking, and a prior history of lung disease (see ADVERSE REACTIONS).
Hypersensitivity Reactions
Hypersensitivity reactions have been associated with FUZEON therapy and may recur on re-challenge. Hypersensitivity reactions have included individually and in combination: rash, fever, nausea and vomiting, chills, rigors, hypotension, and elevated serum liver transaminases. Other adverse events that may be immune mediated and have been reported in subjects receiving FUZEON include primary immune complex reaction, respiratory distress glomerulonephritis, and Guillain-Barre syndrome. Patients developing signs and symptoms suggestive of a systemic hypersensitivity reaction should discontinue FUZEON and should seek medical evaluation immediately. Therapy with FUZEON should not be restarted following systemic signs and symptoms consistent with a hypersensitivity reaction. Risk factors that may predict the occurrence or severity of hypersensitivity to FUZEON have not been identified (see ADVERSE REACTIONS).

PRECAUTIONS

Non-HIV Infected Individuals
There is a theoretical risk that FUZEON use may lead to the production of anti-enfuvirtide antibodies which cross react with HIV gp41. This could result in a false positive HIV test with an ELISA assay; a confirmatory western blot test would be expected to be negative. FUZEON has not been studied in non-HIV infected individuals.
Information for Patients
To assure safe and effective use of FUZEON, the following information and instructions should be given to patients:

- Patients should be informed that injection site reactions occur commonly. Patients must be familiar with the FUZEON *Injection Instructions* for instructions on how to appropriately inject FUZEON and how to carefully monitor for signs or symptoms of cellulitis or local infection. Patients should be instructed when to contact their healthcare provider about these reactions.
- Patients should be made aware that an increased rate of bacterial pneumonia was observed in subjects treated with FUZEON in Phase 3 clinical trials compared to the control arm. Patients should be advised to seek medical evaluation immediately if they develop signs or symptoms suggestive of pneumonia (cough with fever, rapid breathing, shortness of breath) (see WARNINGS).
- Patients should be advised of the possibility of a hypersensitivity reaction to FUZEON. Patients should be advised to discontinue therapy and immediately seek medical evaluation if they develop signs/symptoms of hypersensitivity (see WARNINGS).
- FUZEON is not a cure for HIV-1 infection and patients may continue to contract illnesses associated with HIV-1 infection. The long-term effects of FUZEON are unknown at this time. FUZEON therapy has not been shown to reduce the risk of transmitting HIV-1 to others through sexual contact or blood contamination.
- FUZEON must be taken as part of a combination antiretroviral regimen. Use of FUZEON alone may lead to rapid development of virus resistant to FUZEON and possibly other agents of the same class.
- Patients and caregivers must be instructed in the use of aseptic technique when administering FUZEON in order to avoid injection site infections. Appropriate training for FUZEON reconstitution and self-injection must be given by a healthcare provider, including a careful review of the FUZEON Patient Package Insert and FUZEON *Injection Instructions*. The first injection should be performed under the supervision of an appropriately qualified healthcare provider. It is recommended that the patient and/or caregiver's understanding and use of aseptic self-injection techniques and procedures be periodically re-evaluated.
- Patients should contact their healthcare provider for any questions regarding the administration of FUZEON. Patients should be told not to reuse needles or syringes, and be instructed in safe disposal procedures including the use of a puncture-resistant container for disposal of used needles and syringes. Patients must be instructed on the safe disposal of full containers as per local requirements. Caregivers who experience an accidental needlestick after patient injection should contact a healthcare provider immediately.
- Patients should inform their healthcare provider if they are pregnant, plan to become pregnant or become pregnant while taking this medication.
- Patients should inform their healthcare provider if they are breast-feeding.

Continued on next page

Fuzeon—Cont.

- Patients should not change the dose or dosing schedule of FUZEON or any antiretroviral medication without consulting their healthcare provider.
- Patients should contact their healthcare provider immediately if they stop taking FUZEON or any other drug in their antiretroviral regimen.
- Patients should be told that they can obtain more information on the self-administration of FUZEON at www.FUZEON.com or by calling 1-877-4-FUZEON (1-877-438-9366).

Patients should be advised that no studies have been conducted on the ability to drive or operate machinery while taking FUZEON. If patients experience dizziness while taking FUZEON, they should be advised to talk to their healthcare provider before driving or operating machinery.

Drug Interactions

CYP450 Metabolized Drugs

Results from in vitro and in vivo studies suggest that enfuvirtide is unlikely to have significant drug interactions with concomitantly administered drugs metabolized by CYP450 enzymes (see CLINICAL PHARMACOLOGY).

Antiretroviral Agents

No drug interactions with other antiretroviral medications have been identified that would warrant alteration of either the enfuvirtide dose or the dose of the other antiretroviral medication.

Carcinogenesis, Mutagenesis, Impairment of Fertility

Carcinogenesis

Long-term animal carcinogenicity studies of enfuvirtide have not been conducted.

Mutagenesis

Enfuvirtide was neither mutagenic nor clastogenic in a series of in vivo and in vitro assays including the Ames bacterial reverse mutation assay, a mammalian cell forward gene mutation assay in AS52 Chinese Hamster ovary cells or an in vivo mouse micronucleus assay.

Impairment of Fertility

Enfuvirtide produced no adverse effects on fertility in male or female rats at doses of up to 30 mg/kg/day administered by subcutaneous injection (1.6 times the maximum recommended adult human daily dose on a m^2 basis).

Pregnancy

Pregnancy Category B. Reproduction studies have been performed in rats and rabbits at doses up to 27 times and 3.2 times the adult human dose on a m^2 basis. The animal studies revealed no evidence of harm to the fetus from enfuvirtide. There are no adequate and well-controlled studies in pregnant women. Because animal reproduction studies are not always predictive of human response, this drug should be used during pregnancy only if clearly needed.

Antiretroviral Pregnancy Registry

To monitor maternal-fetal outcomes of pregnant women exposed to FUZEON and other antiretroviral drugs, an Antiretroviral Pregnancy Registry has been established. Physicians are encouraged to register patients by calling 1-800-258-4263.

Nursing Mothers

The Centers for Disease Control and Prevention recommends that HIV- infected mothers not breast-feed their infants to avoid the risk of postnatal transmission of HIV. It is not known whether enfuvirtide is excreted in human milk. Because of both the potential for HIV transmission and the potential for serious adverse reactions in nursing infants, **mothers should be instructed not to breast-feed if they are receiving FUZEON.**

Studies where radio-labeled ^{3}H-enfuvirtide was administered to lactating rats indicated that radioactivity was present in the milk. It is not known whether the radioactivity in the milk was from radio-labeled enfuvirtide or from radio-labeled metabolites of enfuvirtide (ie, amino acids and peptide fragments).

Pediatric Use

The safety and pharmacokinetics of FUZEON have not been established in pediatric subjects below 6 years of age. Limited efficacy data is available in pediatric subjects 6 years of age and older.

Thirty-five HIV-1 infected pediatric subjects ages 6 through 16 years have received FUZEON in two open-label, single-arm clinical trials. Adverse experiences were similar to those observed in adult patients.

Study T20-204 was an open-label, multicenter trial that evaluated the safety, and antiviral activity of FUZEON in treatment-experienced pediatric subjects. Eleven subjects from 6 to 12 years were enrolled (median age of 9 years). Median baseline CD4 cell count was 509 cells/µL and the median baseline HIV-1 RNA was 4.5 $\log_{10}$ copies/mL.

Ten of the 11 study subjects completed 48 weeks of chronic therapy. By week 48, 6/11 (55%) subjects had ≥1 $\log_{10}$ decline in HIV-1 RNA and 4/11 (36%) subjects were below 400 copies/mL of HIV-1 RNA. The median changes from baseline in HIV-1 RNA and CD4 cell count were -1.48 $\log_{10}$ copies/mL and 122 cells/µL, respectively.

Study T20-310 is an ongoing, open-label, multicenter trial evaluating the pharmacokinetics, safety, and antiviral activity of FUZEON in treatment-experienced pediatric subjects and adolescents. Twenty-four subjects from 6 through 16 years were enrolled (median age of 13 years). Median baseline CD4 cell count was 143 cells/µL and the median baseline HIV-1 RNA was 5.0 $\log_{10}$ copies/mL. The evaluation of the antiviral activity is ongoing.

Table 4 Summary of Individual Signs/Symptoms Characterizing Local Injection Site Reactions to Enfuvirtide in Studies T20-301 and T20-302 Combined (% of Subjects)

	N=663		
Event Category	**Any Severity Grade**	**% of Events Comprising Grade 3 Reactions**	**% of Events Comprising Grade 4 Reactions**
Pain/Discomfort[a]	95%	9%	0%
Induration[b]	89%	41%	16%
Erythema[c]	89%	22%	10%
Nodules and Cysts[d]	76%	26%	0%
Pruritus[e]	62%	4%	NA
Ecchymosis[f]	48%	8%	5%

[a] Grade 3 = severe pain requiring analgesics (or narcotic analgesics for ≤72 hours) and/or limiting usual activities; Grade 4 = severe pain requiring hospitalization or prolongation of hospitalization, resulting in death, or persistent or significant disability/incapacity, or life-threatening, or medically significant.
[b] Grade 3 = ≥25 mm but <50 mm; Grade 4 = ≥50 mm average diameter.
[c] Grade 3 = ≥50 mm but <85 mm average diameter; Grade 4 = ≥85 mm average diameter.
[d] Grade 3 = ≥3 cm; Grade 4 = if draining.
[e] Grade 3 = refractory to topical treatment or requiring oral or parenteral treatment; Grade 4 = not applicable.
[f] Grade 3 = >3 cm but ≤ 5 cm; Grade 4 = >5 cm.

Table 5 Percentage of Patients With Selected Treatment-Emergent Adverse Events* Reported in ≥2% of Adult Patients and Occurring More Frequently in Patients Treated With FUZEON (Pooled Studies T20-301/T20-302 at 24 Weeks)

Adverse Event (by System Organ Class)	**FUZEON+ Background Regimen**	**Background Regimen**
	N=663	**N=334**
Nervous System Disorders		
Peripheral Neuropathy	8.9%	6.3%
Taste Disturbance	2.4%	1.5%
Psychiatric Disorders		
Insomnia	11.3%	8.7%
Depression	8.6%	7.2%
Anxiety	5.7%	3.0%
Respiratory, Thoracic, and Mediastinal Disorders		
Cough	7.4%	5.4%
Infections		
Sinusitis	6.2%	2.1%
Herpes Simplex	5.0%	3.9%
Skin Papilloma	4.2%	1.5%
Influenza	3.9%	1.8%
General		
Weight Decreased	6.5%	5.1%
Appetite Decreased	6.3%	2.4%
Asthenia	5.7%	4.2%
Anorexia	2.6%	1.8%
Influenza-like Illness	2.3%	0.9%
Skin and Subcutaneous Tissue Disorders		
Pruritus Nos	5.1%	4.2%
Musculoskeletal, Connective, Tissue, and Bone Disorders		
Myalgia	5.0%	2.4%
Gastrointestinal Disorders		
Constipation	3.9%	2.7%
Abdominal Pain Upper	3.0%	2.7%
Pancreatitis	2.4%	0.9%
Eye Disorders		
Conjunctivitis	2.4%	0.9%
Blood and Lymphatic System Disorders		
Lymphadenopathy	2.3%	0.3%

*Excludes Injection Site Reactions

Geriatric Use

Clinical studies of FUZEON did not include sufficient numbers of subjects aged 65 and over to determine whether they respond differently from younger subjects.

ADVERSE REACTIONS

The overall safety profile of FUZEON is based on 1188 subjects who received at least 1 dose of FUZEON during various clinical trials. This includes 1153 adults, 608 of whom received the recommended dose for greater than 24 weeks, and 35 pediatric subjects.

Assessment of treatment-emergent adverse events is based on the pooled data from the two Phase 3 studies T20-301 and T20-302.

Local Injection Site Reactions

Local injection site reactions were the most frequent adverse events associated with the use of FUZEON. In Phase 3 clinical studies (T20-301 and T20-302), 98% of subjects had at least 1 local injection site reaction (ISR). Three percent of subjects discontinued treatment with FUZEON because of ISRs. Eighty-six percent of subjects experienced their first ISR during the initial week of treatment. The majority of ISRs were associated with mild to moderate pain at the injection site, erythema, induration, and the presence of nodules or cysts. For most subjects the severity of signs and symptoms associated with ISRs did not change during the 24 weeks of treatment. In 17% of subjects an individual ISR lasted for longer than 7 days. Because of the frequency and duration of individual ISRs, 23% of subjects had six or more ongoing ISRs at any given time. Individual signs and symptoms characterizing local ISRs are summarized in Table 4. Infection at the injection site (including abscess and cellulitis) was reported in 1% of subjects.

[See table 4 above]

Other Adverse Events

Hypersensitivity reactions have been attributed to FUZEON (≤ 1%) and in some cases have recurred upon rechallenge (see WARNINGS).

The events most frequently reported in subjects receiving FUZEON+background regimen, excluding injection site reactions, were diarrhea (26.8%), nausea (20.1%), and fatigue (16.1%). These events were also commonly observed in subjects that received background regimen alone: diarrhea (33.5%), nausea (23.7%), and fatigue (17.4%).

Treatment-emergent adverse events (% of subjects), excluding ISRs, from Phase 3 studies are summarized for adult subjects, regardless of severity and causality, in Table 5. Only events occurring in ≥2% of subjects and at a higher rate in subjects treated with FUZEON are summarized in Table 5; events that occurred at a higher rate in the control arms are not displayed.

[See table 5 at top of previous page]

An increased rate of bacterial pneumonia was observed in subjects treated with FUZEON in the Phase 3 clinical trials compared to the control arm (4.68 pneumonia events per 100 patient-years versus 0.61 events per 100 patient-years, respectively). Approximately half of the study subjects with pneumonia required hospitalization. One subject death in the FUZEON arm was attributed to pneumonia. Risk factors for pneumonia included low initial CD4 lymphocyte count, high initial viral load, intravenous drug use, smoking, and a prior history of lung disease. It is unclear if the increased incidence of pneumonia was related to FUZEON use. However, because of this finding patients with HIV infection should be carefully monitored for signs and symptoms of pneumonia, especially if they have underlying conditions which may predispose them to pneumonia (see WARNINGS).

Less Common Events

The following adverse events have been reported in 1 or more subjects; however, a causal relationship to FUZEON has not been established.

Immune System Disorders: worsening abacavir hypersensitivity reaction

Renal and Urinary Disorders: renal insufficiency (glomerulonephritis); renal failure

Blood and Lymphatic Disorders: thrombocytopenia; neutropenia, and fever

Endocrine and Metabolic: hyperglycemia

Infections and Infestations: pneumonia

Nervous System Disorders: Guillain-Barre syndrome (fatal); sixth nerve palsy

Laboratory Abnormalities

Table 6 shows the treatment-emergent laboratory abnormalities that occurred in at least 2% of subjects and more frequently in those receiving FUZEON+background regimen than background regimen alone from studies T20-301 and T20-302.

[See table 6 at right]

Adverse Events in Pediatric Patients

FUZEON has been studied in 35 pediatric subjects 6 through 16 years of age with duration of FUZEON exposure ranging from 1 dose to 48 weeks. Adverse experiences seen during clinical trials were similar to those observed in adult subjects.

OVERDOSAGE

There are no reports of human experience of acute overdose with FUZEON. The highest dose administered to 12 subjects in a clinical trial was 180 mg as a single dose subcutaneously. There is no specific antidote for overdose with FUZEON. Treatment of overdose should consist of general supportive measures.

DOSAGE AND ADMINISTRATION

Adults

The recommended dose of FUZEON is 90 mg (1 mL) twice daily injected subcutaneously into the upper arm, anterior thigh or abdomen. Each injection should be given at a site different from the preceding injection site, and only where there is no current injection site reaction from an earlier dose. FUZEON should not be injected into moles, scar tissue, bruises or the navel. Additional detailed information regarding the administration of FUZEON is described in the FUZEON *Injection Instructions*.

Pediatric Patients

No data are available to establish a dose recommendation of FUZEON in pediatric patients below the age of 6 years. In pediatric patients 6 years through 16 years of age, the recommended dosage of FUZEON is 2 mg/kg twice daily up to a maximum dose of 90 mg twice daily injected subcutaneously into the upper arm, anterior thigh or abdomen. Each injection should be given at a site different from the preceding injection site and only where there is no current injection site reaction from an earlier dose. FUZEON should not be injected into moles, scar tissue, bruises or the navel. Table 7 contains dosing guidelines for FUZEON based on body weight. Weight should be monitored periodically and the FUZEON dose adjusted accordingly.

[See table 7 at right]

Directions for Use

For more detailed instructions, see FUZEON *Injection Instructions*.

Subcutaneous Administration

FUZEON must only be reconstituted with 1.1 mL of Sterile Water for Injection. After adding sterile water, the vial should be gently tapped for 10 seconds and then gently rolled between the hands to avoid foaming and to ensure all particles of drug are in contact with the liquid and no drug remains on the vial wall. The vial should then be allowed to stand until the powder goes completely into solution, which could take up to 45 minutes. Reconstitution time can be reduced by gently rolling the vial between the hands until the product is completely dissolved. Before the solution is withdrawn for administration, the vial should be inspected visually to ensure that the contents are fully dissolved in solution, and that the solution is clear, colorless and without bubbles or particulate matter. If there is evidence of particulate matter, the vial must not be used and should be returned to the pharmacy.

FUZEON contains no preservatives. Once reconstituted, FUZEON should be injected immediately or kept refrigerated in the original vial until use. Reconstituted FUZEON must be used within 24 hours. The subsequent dose of FUZEON can be reconstituted in advance and must be stored in the refrigerator in the original vial and used within 24 hours. Refrigerated reconstituted solution should be brought to room temperature before injection and the vial should be inspected visually again to ensure that the contents are fully dissolved in solution and that the solution is clear, colorless, and without bubbles or particulate matter.

The reconstituted solution should be injected subcutaneously in the upper arm, abdomen or anterior thigh. The injection should be given at a site different from the preceding injection site and only where there is no current injection site reaction. Also, do not inject into moles, scar tissue, bruises or the navel. A vial is suitable for single use only; unused portions must be discarded (see FUZEON *Injection Instructions*).

Patients should contact their healthcare provider for any questions regarding the administration of FUZEON. Information about the self-administration of FUZEON may also be obtained by calling the toll-free number 1-877-4-FUZEON (1-877-438-9366) or at the FUZEON website, www.FUZEON.com. Patients should be taught to recognize the signs and symptoms of injection site reactions and instructed when to contact their healthcare provider about these reactions.

HOW SUPPLIED

FUZEON (enfuvirtide) for Injection is a white to off-white, sterile, lyophilized powder and it is packaged in a single-use

Continued on next page

Table 6 Percentage of Treatment-Emergent Laboratory Abnormalities That Occurred in ≥2% of Adult Patients and More Frequently in Patients Receiving FUZEON (Pooled Studies T20-301 and T20-302 at 24 Weeks)

Laboratory Parameters	Grading	FUZEON+ Background Regimen	Background Regimen
		N=663	N=334
Eosinophilia			
1-2 X ULN (0.7 × 10^9/L)	0.7-1.4 × 10^9/L)	8.3%	1.5%
>2 X ULN (0.7 × 10^9/L)	>1.4 × 10^9/L)	1.8%	0.9%
Amylase (U/L)			
Gr. 3	>2-5 × ULN	6.2%	3.6%
Gr. 4	>5 × ULN or clinical pancreatitis	0.9%	0.6%
Lipase (U/L)			
Gr. 3	>2-5 × ULN	5.9%	3.6%
Gr. 4	>5 × ULN	2.3%	1.8%
Triglycerides (mmol/L)			
Gr. 3	>1000 mg/dL	8.9%	7.2%
ALT			
Gr. 3	>5-10 × ULN	3.5%	2.1%
Gr. 4	>10 × ULN	0.9%	0.6%
AST			
Gr. 3	>5-10 × ULN	3.6%	3.0%
Gr. 4	>10 × ULN	1.2%	0.6%
Creatine Phosphokinase (U/L)			
Gr. 3	>5-10 × ULN	5.9%	3.6%
Gr. 4	>10 × ULN	2.3%	3.6%
GGT (U/L)			
Gr. 3	>5-10 × ULN	3.5%	3.3%
Gr. 4	>10 × ULN	2.4%	1.8%
Hemoglobin (g/dL)			
Gr. 3	6.5-7.9 g/dL	1.5%	0.9%
Gr. 4	<6.5 g/dL	0.6%	0.6%

Table 7 Pediatric Dosing Guidelines

Weight		Dose per bid Injection (mg/dose)	Injection Volume (90 mg enfuvirtide per mL)
Kilograms (kg)	Pounds (lbs)		
11.0 to 15.5	24 to 34	27	0.3 mL
15.6 to 20.0	>34 to 44	36	0.4 mL
20.1 to 24.5	>44 to 54	45	0.5 mL
24.6 to 29.0	>54 to 64	54	0.6 mL
29.1 to 33.5	>64 to 74	63	0.7 mL
33.6 to 38.0	>74 to 84	72	0.8 mL
38.1 to 42.5	>84 to 94	81	0.9 mL
≥42.6	>94	90	1.0 mL

Fuzeon—Cont.

clear glass vial containing 108 mg of enfuvirtide for the delivery of approximately 90 mg/1 mL when reconstituted with 1.1 mL of Sterile Water for Injection.
FUZEON is available in a Convenience Kit containing 60 single-use vials (2 cartons of 30 each) of FUZEON (90 mg strength), 60 vials (2 cartons of 30 each) of Sterile Water for Injection (1.1 mL per vial), 60 reconstitution syringes (3 cc), 60 administration syringes (1 cc), alcohol wipes, Package Insert, Patient Package Insert, and Injection Instruction Guide (NDC 0004-0380-39).

Storage Conditions
Store at 25°C (77°F); excursions permitted to 15° to 30°C (59° to 86°F) [See USP Controlled Room Temperature].
Reconstituted solution should be stored under refrigeration at 2° to 8°C (36° to 46°F) and used within 24 hours.
Roche and FUZEON are trademarks of Hoffmann-La Roche Inc.
FUZEON has been jointly developed by Trimeris, Inc. and Hoffmann-La Roche Inc. FUZEON is manufactured by Hoffmann-La Roche Inc.
Distributed by:
Roche Pharmaceuticals
Roche Laboratories Inc.
340 Kingsland Street
Nutley, New Jersey 07110-1199
www.rocheusa.com
Licensed from:
Trimeris, Inc.
4727 University Drive
Durham, North Carolina 27707
www.trimeris.com

Issued: March 2003

HIVID® ℞
[hī-vĭd]
(zalcitabine)
TABLETS

WARNING:
THE USE OF HIVID HAS BEEN ASSOCIATED WITH SIGNIFICANT CLINICAL ADVERSE REACTIONS, SOME OF WHICH ARE POTENTIALLY FATAL. HIVID CAN CAUSE SEVERE PERIPHERAL NEUROPATHY AND BECAUSE OF THIS SHOULD BE USED WITH EXTREME CAUTION IN PATIENTS WITH PREEXISTING NEUROPATHY. HIVID MAY ALSO RARELY CAUSE PANCREATITIS AND PATIENTS WHO DEVELOP ANY SYMPTOMS SUGGESTIVE OF PANCREATITIS WHILE USING HIVID SHOULD HAVE THERAPY SUSPENDED IMMEDIATELY UNTIL THIS DIAGNOSIS IS EXCLUDED.
LACTIC ACIDOSIS AND SEVERE HEPATOMEGALY WITH STEATOSIS, INCLUDING FATAL CASES, HAVE BEEN REPORTED WITH THE USE OF ANTIRETROVIRAL NUCLEOSIDE ANALOGUES ALONE OR IN COMBINATION, INCLUDING HIVID (SEE WARNINGS).
IN ADDITION, RARE CASES OF HEPATIC FAILURE AND DEATH CONSIDERED POSSIBLY RELATED TO UNDERLYING HEPATITIS B AND HIVID HAVE BEEN REPORTED (SEE WARNINGS AND PRECAUTIONS).

DESCRIPTION

HIVID is the Hoffmann-La Roche brand of zalcitabine [formerly called 2′,3′-dideoxycytidine (ddC)], a synthetic pyrimidine nucleoside analogue active against the human immunodeficiency virus (HIV). HIVID is available as film-coated tablets for oral administration in strengths of 0.375 mg and 0.750 mg. Each tablet also contains the inactive ingredients lactose, microcrystalline cellulose, croscarmellose sodium, magnesium stearate, hydroxypropyl methylcellulose, polyethylene glycol, and polysorbate 80 along with the following colorant system: 0.375 mg tablet — synthetic brown, black, red and yellow iron oxides, and titanium dioxide; 0.750 mg tablet — synthetic black iron oxide and titanium dioxide. The chemical name for zalcitabine is 4-amino-1-beta-D-2′,3′-dideoxyribofuranosyl-2-(1H)-pyrimidone or 2′,3′-dideoxycytidine with the molecular formula $C_9H_{13}N_3O_3$ and a molecular weight of 211.22.
Zalcitabine is a white to off-white crystalline powder with an aqueous solubility of 76.4 mg/mL at 25°C.

MICROBIOLOGY

Mechanism of Action: Zalcitabine is a synthetic nucleoside analogue of the naturally occurring nucleoside deoxycytidine, in which the 3′-hydroxyl group is replaced by hydrogen. Within cells, zalcitabine is converted to the active metabolite, dideoxycytidine 5′-triphosphate (ddCTP), by the sequential action of cellular enzymes. Dideoxycytidine 5′-triphosphate inhibits the activity of the HIV-reverse transcriptase both by competing for utilization of the natural substrate, deoxycytidine 5′-triphosphate (dCTP), and by its incorporation into viral DNA. The lack of a 3′-OH group in the incorporated nucleoside analogue prevents the formation of the 5′ to 3′ phosphodiester linkage essential for DNA chain elongation and, therefore, the viral DNA growth is terminated. The active metabolite, ddCTP, is also an inhibitor of cellular DNA polymerase-beta and mitochondrial DNA polymerase-gamma and has been reported to be incorporated into the DNA of cells in culture.

In Vitro HIV Susceptibility: The in vitro anti-HIV activity of zalcitabine was assessed by infecting cell lines of lymphoblastic and monocytic origin and peripheral blood lymphocytes with laboratory and clinical isolates of HIV. The IC_{50} and IC_{95} values (50% and 95% inhibitory concentration) were in the range of 30 to 500 nM and 100 to 1000 nM, respectively (1 nM = 0.21 ng/mL). Zalcitabine showed antiviral activity in all acute infections; however, activity was substantially less in chronically infected cells. In drug combination studies with zidovudine (ZDV) or saquinavir, zalcitabine showed additive to synergistic activity in cell culture. The relationship between the in vitro susceptibility of HIV to reverse-transcriptase inhibitors and the inhibition of HIV replication in humans has not been established.

Drug Resistance: HIV isolates with a reduction in sensitivity to zalcitabine (ddC) have been isolated from a small number of patients treated with HIVID by 1 year of therapy. Genetic analysis of these isolates showed point mutations (Lys 65 Arg or Asn, Thr 69 Asp, Leu 74 Val, Val 75 Thr or Ala, Met 184 Val or Tyr 215 Cys) in the pol gene that encodes for the reverse transcriptase. Combination therapy with HIVID and ZDV does not appear to prevent the emergence of zidovudine-resistant isolates.

Cross-resistance: The potential for cross-resistance between HIV-reverse transcriptase inhibitors and HIV-protease inhibitors is low because of the different enzyme targets involved. The point mutation at position 69 appears to be specific to ddC in its selection and effect. Additionally, the point mutations at positions 65, 74, 75, and 184 are associated with resistance to didanosine (ddI), that at position 75 with resistance to stavudine (d4T), and those at positions 65 (Lys to Arg), and 184 (Met to Val) with resistance to lamivudine (3TC). HIV isolates with multidrug resistance to ZDV, ddI, ddC, d4T, and 3TC were recovered from a small number of patients treated for 1 year with the combination of ZDV, ddI or ddC. The pattern of resistance mutations in the combination therapy was different (Ala 62 Val, Val 75 Ile, Phe 77 Leu, Phe 116 Tyr and Gln 151 Met) from monotherapy with mutation 151 being most significant for multidrug resistance.

CLINICAL PHARMACOLOGY

Pharmacokinetics: The pharmacokinetics of zalcitabine has been evaluated in studies in HIV-infected patients following 0.01 mg/kg, 0.03 mg/kg, and 1.5 mg oral doses, and a 1.5 mg intravenous dose administered as a 1-hour infusion.
Absorption and Bioavailability in Adults: Following oral administration to HIV-infected patients, the mean absolute bioavailability of zalcitabine was >80% (30% CV, range 23% to 124%, n=19). The absorption rate of a 1.5 mg oral dose of zalcitabine (n=20) was reduced when administered with food. This resulted in a 39% decrease in mean maximum plasma concentrations (C_{max}) from 25.2 ng/mL (35% CV, range 11.6 to 37.5 ng/mL) to 15.5 ng/mL (24% CV, range 9.1 to 23.7 ng/mL), and a twofold increase in time to achieve maximum plasma concentrations from a mean of 0.8 hours under fasting conditions to 1.6 hours when the drug was given with food. The extent of absorption (as reflected by AUC) was decreased by 14%, from 72 ng·hr/mL (28% CV, range 43 to 119 ng·hr/mL) to 62 ng·hr/mL (23% CV, range 42 to 91 ng·hr/mL). The clinical relevance of these decreases is unknown. Absorption of zalcitabine does not appear to be reduced in patients with diarrhea not caused by an identified pathogen.
Distribution in Adults: The steady-state volume of distribution following intravenous administration of a 1.5 mg dose of zalcitabine averaged 0.534 (± 0.127) L/kg (24% CV, range 0.304 to 0.734 L/kg, n=20). Cerebrospinal fluid obtained from 9 patients at 2 to 3.5 hours following 0.06 mg/kg or 0.09 mg/kg intravenous infusion showed measurable concentrations of zalcitabine. The CSF:plasma concentration ratio ranged from 9% to 37% (mean 20%), demonstrating penetration of the drug through the blood-brain barrier. The clinical relevance of these ratios has not been evaluated.
Metabolism and Elimination in Adults: Zalcitabine is phosphorylated intracellularly to zalcitabine triphosphate, the active substrate for HIV-reverse transcriptase. Concentrations of zalcitabine triphosphate are too low for quantitation following administration of therapeutic doses to humans.
Zalcitabine does not undergo a significant degree of metabolism by the liver. The primary metabolite of zalcitabine that has been identified is dideoxyuridine (ddU), which accounts for less than 15% of an oral dose in both urine and feces (n=4). Approximately 10% of an orally administered radiolabeled dose of zalcitabine appears in the feces (n=10), comprised primarily of unchanged drug and ddU. Renal excretion of unchanged drug appears to be the primary route of elimination, accounting for approximately 80% of an intravenous dose and 60% of an orally administered dose within 24 hours after dosing (n=19). The mean elimination half-life is 2 hours and generally ranges from 1 to 3 hours in individual patients. Total clearance following an intravenous dose averaged 285 mL/min (29% CV, range 165 to 447 mL/min, n=20). Renal clearance averaged approximately 235 mL/min or about 80% of total clearance (30% CV, range 129 to 348 mL/min, n=20). Renal clearance exceeds glomerular filtration rate suggesting renal tubular secretion contributes to the elimination of zalcitabine by the kidneys.
In patients with impaired kidney function, prolonged elimination of zalcitabine may be expected. Preliminary results from 7 patients with renal impairment (estimated creatinine clearance <55 mL/min) indicate that the half-life was prolonged (up to 8.5 hours) in these patients compared to those with normal renal function. Maximum plasma concentrations were higher in some patients after a single dose (see PRECAUTIONS).
In patients with normal renal function, the pharmacokinetics of zalcitabine was not altered during 3 times daily multiple dosing (n=9). Accumulation of drug in plasma during this regimen was negligible. The drug was <4% bound to plasma proteins, indicating that drug interactions involving binding-site displacement are unlikely (see *Drug Interactions*).

Drug Interactions: *Zidovudine:* There was no significant pharmacokinetic interaction between zidovudine and zalcitabine when single doses of zalcitabine (1.5 mg) and zidovudine (200 mg) were coadministered to 12 HIV-positive patients.
Probenecid: Following administration of a single oral 1.5 mg dose of zalcitabine alone during probenecid treatment (500 mg at 8 and 2 hours before and 4 hours after zalcitabine dosing) to 12 HIV-positive patients, mean renal clearance decreased from 310 mL/min (28% CV) to 180 mL/min (22% CV) and AUC increased from 59 ng•hr/mL (27% CV) to 91 ng•hr/mL (22% CV), indicating an increase in exposure of approximately 50% to zalcitabine. Mean half-life of zalcitabine increased from 1.7 to 2.5 hours (see PRECAUTIONS).
Cimetidine: Administration of a single dose of 1.5 mg zalcitabine with a single dose of 800 mg cimetidine to 12 HIV-positive patients resulted in a decrease in renal clearance from 224 mL/min (27% CV) to 171 mL/min (39% CV) and an increase in AUC from 75 ng•hr/mL (29% CV) to 102 ng•hr/mL (35% CV) (see PRECAUTIONS) indicating an increase in exposure of approximately 36% to zalcitabine.
Maalox: Concomitant administration of Maalox® TC (30 mL) with single dose of 1.5 mg zalcitabine to 12 HIV-positive patients resulted in a decrease in mean C_{max} from 25.2 ng/mL (28% CV) to 18.4 ng/mL (34% CV) and AUC from 75 ng•hr/mL (29% CV, n=10) to 58 ng•hr/mL (36% CV, n=10) indicating a decrease in bioavailability of approximately 25% to zalcitabine (see PRECAUTIONS).
Metoclopramide: Administration of a single dose of 1.5 mg zalcitabine with 20 mg metoclopramide (10 mg 1 hour before and 10 mg 4 hours after zalcitabine dose) to 12 HIV-positive patients resulted in a decrease in AUC from 69 ng•hr/mL (16% CV) to 62 ng•hr/mL (21% CV) indicating a decrease in bioavailability of approximately 10% (see PRECAUTIONS).
Loperamide: Administration of a single dose of 1.5 mg zalcitabine during loperamide treatment (4 mg 16 hours before zalcitabine, 2 mg at 10 hours and 4 hours before zalcitabine, and 2 mg 2 hours after the zalcitabine dose) to 12 HIV-positive patients with diarrhea resulted in no significant pharmacokinetic interaction between zalcitabine and loperamide.

Pharmacokinetics in Pediatric Patients: For pharmacokinetic properties in pediatric patients, see PRECAUTIONS: *Pediatric Use.* Limited pharmacokinetic data have been reported for 5 HIV-positive pediatric patients using doses of 0.03 and 0.04 mg/kg HIVID administered orally every 6 hours.[1] The mean bioavailability of zalcitabine in these pediatric patients was 54% and mean apparent systemic clearance was 150 mL/min/m^2. Due to the small number of subjects and different analytical techniques, it is difficult to make comparisons between pediatric and adult data.

INDICATIONS AND USAGE

HIVID is indicated in combination with antiretroviral agents for the treatment of HIV infection. This indication is based on study results showing a reduction in the rate of disease progression (AIDS-defining events or death) in patients with limited prior antiretroviral therapy who were treated with the combination of HIVID and zidovudine (see *Description of Clinical Studies*). This indication is also based on a study showing a reduction in both mortality and AIDS-defining clinical events for patients who received INVIRASE® (saquinavir mesylate) in combination with HIVID compared to patients who received either HIVID or INVIRASE alone.

Description of Clinical Studies: The use of HIVID in combination with zidovudine is based on the clinical results from study ACTG 175. ACTG 175 was a randomized, double-blind, controlled trial that compared zidovudine 200 mg three times daily; didanosine 200 mg twice daily; zidovudine+didanosine; and zidovudine+HIVID 0.750 mg three times daily. A total of 2467 HIV-infected adults (mean baseline CD_4 count = 352 cells/mm^3) with no prior AIDS-defining event enrolled with the following demographics: male (82%), Caucasian (70%), mean age of 35 years, asymptomatic HIV infection (81%) and prior antiretroviral use (57%, mean duration = 89.5 weeks). The overall mean duration of study treatment was 99 weeks. The incidence of AIDS-defining events or death is shown in Table 1.
[See table 1 at bottom of next page]
Although no antiretroviral agent should be used as monotherapy, a description of CPCRA 002 is included here as it provides a comparison of the safety and efficacy of HIVID compared to ddI.
CPCRA 002 was a randomized, multicenter, open-label study in which HIVID was compared to ddI as treatment for patients with advanced HIV infection (median CD_4 cell count = 37 cells/mm^3) who were clinically intolerant to ZDV, or who had met criteria for having disease progression while receiving ZDV.[2] Patients in this study had a mean of

17.5 months of prior ZDV use. The median duration of treatment for both HIVID and ddI was 34 weeks. The results demonstrate that HIVID was at least as efficacious as ddI in terms of time to an AIDS-defining event or death, while for survival alone the results favored HIVID. However, most of the patients (66%) in either group had disease progression over the median 16 months of follow-up. Overall rates of study drug intolerance, discontinuation and adverse events were similar for the two groups, although the types of events were different.

A clinical study (N3300/ACTG 114) has demonstrated ZDV to be superior to HIVID as monotherapy for advanced HIV disease (CD_4 cell count ≤200 cells/mm^3) in previously untreated patients.[3,4] The final analysis of this study indicated that 134 patients (42%) in the HIVID group with a median follow-up of 85 weeks and 120 patients (38%) in the ZDV group with a median follow-up of 96 weeks died with a relative risk for mortality of ZDV to HIVID of 0.54.

CONTRAINDICATIONS

HIVID is contraindicated in patients with clinically significant hypersensitivity to zalcitabine or to any of the excipients contained in the tablets.

WARNINGS

SIGNIFICANT CLINICAL ADVERSE REACTIONS, SOME OF WHICH ARE POTENTIALLY FATAL, HAVE BEEN REPORTED WITH HIVID. PATIENTS WITH DECREASED CD_4 CELL COUNTS APPEAR TO HAVE AN INCREASED INCIDENCE OF ADVERSE EVENTS.

1. Peripheral Neuropathy:

THE MAJOR CLINICAL TOXICITY OF HIVID IS PERIPHERAL NEUROPATHY, WHICH MAY OCCUR IN UP TO 1/3 OF PATIENTS WITH ADVANCED DISEASE TREATED WITH HIVID. The incidence in patients with less-advanced disease is lower.

HIVID-related peripheral neuropathy is a sensorimotor neuropathy characterized initially by numbness and burning dysesthesia involving the distal extremities. These symptoms may be followed by sharp shooting pains or severe continuous burning pain if the drug is not withdrawn. The neuropathy may progress to severe pain requiring narcotic analgesics and is potentially irreversible. In some patients, symptoms of neuropathy may initially progress despite discontinuation of HIVID. With prompt discontinuation of HIVID, the neuropathy is usually slowly reversible. There are no data regarding the use of HIVID in patients with preexisting peripheral neuropathy since these patients were excluded from clinical trials; therefore, HIVID should be used with extreme caution in these patients. Individuals with moderate or severe peripheral neuropathy, as evidenced by symptoms accompanied by objective findings, are advised to avoid HIVID.

HIVID should be used with caution in patients with a risk of developing peripheral neuropathy: patients with low CD_4 cell counts (CD_4 <50 cells/mm^3), diabetes, weight loss and/or patients receiving HIVID concomitantly with drugs that have the potential to cause peripheral neuropathy (see PRECAUTIONS: *Drug Interactions*). Careful monitoring is strongly recommended for these individuals.

HIVID should be stopped promptly if signs or symptoms of peripheral neuropathy occur, such as when moderate discomfort from numbness, tingling, burning or pain of the extremities progresses, or any related symptoms occur that are accompanied by an objective finding (see DOSAGE AND ADMINISTRATION).

2. Pancreatitis:

PANCREATITIS, WHICH HAS BEEN FATAL IN SOME CASES, HAS BEEN OBSERVED WITH THE ADMINISTRATION OF HIVID. Pancreatitis is an uncommon complication of HIVID occurring in up to 1.1% of patients.

Patients with a history of pancreatitis or known risk factors for the development of pancreatitis should be followed more closely while on HIVID therapy. Of 528 HIVID-treated patients enrolled in an expanded-access safety study (N3544), who had a history of prior pancreatitis or increased amylase, 28 (5.3%) developed pancreatitis and an additional 23 (4.4%) developed asymptomatic elevated serum amylase.

Treatment with HIVID should be stopped immediately if clinical signs or symptoms (nausea, vomiting, abdominal pain) or if abnormalities in laboratory values (hyperamylasemia associated with dysglycemia, rising triglyceride level, decreasing serum calcium) suggestive of pancreatitis should occur. If clinical pancreatitis develops during HIVID administration, it is recommended that HIVID be permanently discontinued. Treatment with HIVID should also be interrupted if treatment with another drug known to cause pancreatitis (eg, intravenous pentamidine) is required (see *Drug Interactions*).

3. Lactic Acidosis/Severe Hepatomegaly With Steatosis and Hepatic Toxicity:

Lactic acidosis and severe hepatomegaly with steatosis, including fatal cases, have been reported with the use of nucleoside analogues alone or in combination, including HIVID and other antiretrovirals.[5,6] A majority of these cases have been in women. Obesity and prolonged nucleoside exposure may be risk factors. Particular caution should be exercised when administering HIVID to any patient with known risk factors for liver disease; however, cases have also been reported in patients with no known risk factors. Treatment with HIVID should be suspended in any patient who develops clinical or laboratory findings suggestive of lactic acidosis or pronounced hepatotoxicity (which may include hepatomegaly and steatosis even in the absence of marked transaminase elevations).

IN ADDITION, RARE CASES OF HEPATIC FAILURE AND DEATH CONSIDERED POSSIBLY RELATED TO UNDERLYING HEPATITIS B AND HIVID HAVE BEEN REPORTED. Treatment with HIVID in patients with preexisting liver disease, liver enzyme abnormalities, a history of ethanol abuse or hepatitis should be approached with caution. Treatment with HIVID should be suspended in any patient who develops clinical or laboratory findings suggestive of pronounced hepatotoxicity. In clinical trials, drug interruption was recommended if liver function tests exceeded >5 times the upper limit of normal.

4. Other Serious Toxicities:

a) *Oral Ulcers:* Severe oral ulcers occurred in up to 3% of patients receiving HIVID in CPCRA 002 and ACTG 175; less severe oral ulcerations have occurred at higher frequencies in other clinical trials.

b) *Esophageal Ulcers:* Infrequent cases of esophageal ulcers have also been attributed to HIVID therapy. Interruption of HIVID should be considered in patients who develop esophageal ulcers that do not respond to specific treatment for opportunistic pathogens in order to assess a possible relationship to HIVID.

c) *Cardiomyopathy/Congestive Heart Failure:* Cardiomyopathy and congestive heart failure in patients with AIDS have been associated with the use of nucleoside analogues. Infrequent cases have been reported in patients receiving HIVID. Treatment with HIVID in patients with baseline cardiomyopathy or history of congestive heart failure should be approached with caution.

d) *Anaphylactoid Reaction:* An anaphylactoid reaction was reported in a patient receiving both HIVID and zidovudine. In addition, there have been several reports of hypersensitivity reactions (including anaphylactic reaction or urticaria without other signs of anaphylaxis).

PRECAUTIONS

General:

1. *Renal Impairment:* Patients with renal impairment (estimated creatinine clearance <55 mL/min) may be at a greater risk of toxicity from HIVID due to decreased drug clearance. Dosage adjustment is recommended in these patients (see DOSAGE AND ADMINISTRATION).
2. *Lymphoma:* High doses of zalcitabine, administered for 3 months to $B_6C_3F_1$ mice (resulting in plasma concentrations over 1000 times those seen in patients taking the recommended doses of HIVID) induced an increased incidence of thymic lymphoma.[7] Although the pathogenesis of the effect is uncertain, a predisposition to chemically induced thymic lymphoma and high rates of spontaneous lymphoreticular neoplasms have previously been noted in this strain of mice.[8]

   The incidence of lymphomas was reviewed in 13 comparative studies conducted by Roche, the NIAID and the NCI, as well as 7 Roche expanded-access studies that included HIVID. In one study, ACTG 155, a statistically significant increased rate of lymphomas was seen in patients receiving HIVID or combination HIVID and zidovudine compared to zidovudine alone (rates of 0, 1.3, and 2.3 per 100 person years for zidovudine, HIVID, and combination HIVID and zidovudine, respectively; log rank p-value=0.01, pooling HIVID, and combination HIVID and zidovudine vs zidovudine, p-value=0.003). Based on review of the literature, the incidence of lymphomas in HIV-infected patients with advanced disease on zidovudine monotherapy would be expected to be approximately 1 to 2 per 100 person years of follow-up.

   None of the other comparative studies evaluated showed a statistically significant difference in rates of lymphomas in patients receiving HIVID. In a large, controlled clinical trial (ACTG 175) HIVID in combination with zidovudine was not associated with an increase in the incidence of lymphoma over that seen with zidovudine monotherapy (6 of 615 and 9 of 619, respectively).

   Lymphoma has been identified as a consequence of HIV infection. This most likely represents a consequence of prolonged immunosuppression; however, an association between the occurrence of lymphoma and antiviral therapy cannot be excluded.
3. *Fat Redistribution:* Redistribution/accumulation of body fat including central obesity, dorsocervical fat enlargement (buffalo hump), peripheral wasting, facial wasting, breast enlargement, and "cushingoid appearance" have been observed in patients receiving antiretroviral therapy. The mechanism and long-term consequences of these events are currently unknown. A causal relationship has not been established.

Table 1. First AIDS-defining Event or Death and Death Only by Study Arm and Antiretroviral Experience in ACTG 175

Antiretroviral Experience	Event	Treatment			
		zidovudine	Zidovudine + didanosine	zidovudine + HIVID	didanosine
Overall	n	619	613	615	620
	AIDS/Death	96 (16%)	65 (11%)	76 (12%)	71 (11%)
	Death Only	54 (9%)	31 (5%)	40 (7%)	29 (5%)
Naive	n	269	263	267	268
	AIDS/Death	32 (12%)	20 (8%)	16 (6%)	23 (9%)
	Death Only	18 (7%)	11 (4%)	9 (3%)	11 (4%)
Experienced	n	350	350	348	352
	AIDS/Death	64 (18%)	45 (13%)	60 (17%)	48 (14%)
	Death Only	36 (10%)	20 (6%)	31 (9%)	18 (5%)

Patients receiving HIVID or any other antiretroviral therapy may continue to develop opportunistic infections and other complications of HIV infections, and therefore should remain under close clinical observation by physicians experienced in the treatment of patients with associated HIV diseases.

The duration of clinical benefit from antiretroviral therapy may be limited. Alterations in antiretroviral therapy should be considered in cases of disease progression, either clinical or as demonstrated by viral rebound (increase in HIV RNA after initial decline).

Information for Patients: Patients should be informed that HIVID is not a cure for HIV infection and that they may continue to acquire illnesses associated with advanced HIV infection, including opportunistic infections.

Patients should be told that there is currently no data demonstrating that HIVID therapy can reduce the risk of transmitting HIV to others through sexual contact or blood contamination.

Patients should be advised to take HIVID every day as prescribed. Patients should not alter the dose or discontinue therapy without consulting with their physician. If a dose is missed, patients should take the dose as soon as possible and then return to their normal schedule. However, if a dose is skipped, the patient should not double the next dose.

Patients should be instructed that the major toxicity of HIVID is peripheral neuropathy. Pancreatitis and hepatic toxicity are other serious potentially life-threatening toxicities that have been reported in patients treated with HIVID.

Patients should be advised of the early symptoms of these conditions and instructed to promptly report them to their physician. Since the development of peripheral neuropathy appears to be dose-related to HIVID, patients should be advised to follow their physicians' instructions regarding the prescribed dose.

Patients should be informed that redistribution or accumulation of body fat may occur in patients receiving antiretroviral therapy and that the cause and long-term health effects of these conditions are not known at this time.

Laboratory Tests: Complete blood counts and clinical chemistry tests should be performed prior to initiating HIVID therapy and at appropriate intervals thereafter. Baseline testing of serum amylase and triglyceride levels should be performed in individuals with a prior history of pancreatitis, increased amylase, those on parenteral nutrition or with a history of ethanol abuse.

Drug Interactions: *Zidovudine:* There is no significant pharmacokinetic interaction between ZDV and zalcitabine which has been confirmed clinically. Zalcitabine also has no significant effect on the intracellular phosphorylation of ZDV, as shown in vitro in peripheral blood mononuclear cells or in two other cell lines (U937 and Molt-4). In the same study it was shown that didanosine and stavudine had no significant effect on the intracellular phosphorylation of zalcitabine in peripheral blood mononuclear cells.

Lamivudine: In vitro studies in peripheral blood mononuclear cells, U937 and Molt-4 cells revealed that lamivudine significantly inhibited zalcitabine phosphorylation in a dose dependent manner. Effects were already seen with doses corresponding to relevant plasma levels in humans, and the intracellular phosphorylation of zalcitabine to its three metabolites (including the active zalcitabine triphosphate metabolite) was significantly inhibited. Zalcitabine inhibited lamivudine phosphorylation at high concentration ratios (10 and 100); however, it is considered to be unlikely that this decrease of phosphorylated lamivudine concentration is of clinical significance, as lamivudine is a more efficient substrate for deoxycytidine kinase than zalcitabine. These in vitro studies suggest that concomitant administration of zalcitabine and lamivudine in humans may result in sub-therapeutic concentrations of active phosphorylated zalcitabine, which may lead to a decreased antiretroviral effect of zalcitabine. It is unknown how the effect seen in these in vitro studies translates into clinical consequences. **Concomitant use of zalcitabine and lamivudine is not recommended.**

Saquinavir: The combination of HIVID, saquinavir, and ZDV has been studied (as triple combination) in adults.

Continued on next page

Hivid—Cont.

Pharmacokinetic data suggest that absorption, metabolism, and elimination of each of these drugs are unchanged when they are used together.
Drugs Associated With Peripheral Neuropathy: The concomitant use of HIVID with drugs that have the potential to cause peripheral neuropathy should be avoided where possible. Drugs that have been associated with peripheral neuropathy include antiretroviral nucleoside analogues, chloramphenicol, cisplatin, dapsone, disulfiram, ethionamide, glutethimide, gold, hydralazine, iodoquinol, isoniazid, metronidazole, nitrofurantoin, phenytoin, ribavirin, and vincristine. Concomitant use of HIVID with didanosine is not recommended.
Intravenous Pentamidine: Treatment with HIVID should be interrupted when the use of a drug that has the potential to cause pancreatitis is required. Death due to fulminant pancreatitis possibly related to intravenous pentamidine and HIVID has been reported. If intravenous pentamidine is required to treat *Pneumocystis carinii* pneumonia, treatment with HIVID should be interrupted (see WARNINGS).
Amphotericin, Foscarnet, and Aminoglycosides: Drugs such as amphotericin, foscarnet, and aminoglycosides may increase the risk of developing peripheral neuropathy (see WARNINGS: *Peripheral Neuropathy*) or other HIVID-associated adverse events by interfering with the renal clearance of zalcitabine (thereby raising systemic exposure). Patients who require the use of one of these drugs with HIVID should have frequent clinical and laboratory monitoring with dosage adjustment for any significant change in renal function.
Probenecid or Cimetidine: Concomitant administration of probenecid or cimetidine decreases the elimination of zalcitabine, most likely by inhibition of renal tubular secretion of zalcitabine. Patients receiving these drugs in combination with zalcitabine should be monitored for signs of toxicity and the dose of zalcitabine reduced if warranted.
Magnesium/Aluminum-containing Antacid Products: Absorption of zalcitabine is moderately reduced (approximately 25%) when coadministered with magnesium/aluminum-containing antacid products. The clinical significance of this reduction is not known, hence zalcitabine is not recommended to be ingested simultaneously with magnesium/aluminum-containing antacids.
Metoclopramide: Bioavailability is mildly reduced (approximately 10%) when zalcitabine and metoclopramide are coadministered (see CLINICAL PHARMACOLOGY: *Drug Interactions*).
Doxorubicin: Doxorubicin caused a decrease in zalcitabine phosphorylation (>50% inhibition of total phosphate formation) in U937/Molt 4 cells. Although there may be decreased zalcitabine activity because of lessened active metabolite formation, the clinical relevance of these in vitro results are not known.

Carcinogenesis, Mutagenesis and Impairment of Fertility:
Carcinogenesis: Zalcitabine was administered orally by dietary admixture to CRL:CD-1® (ICR) Br mice at dosages of 3, 83, or 250 mg/kg/day for 2 years. Plasma exposures (as measured by AUC) at these doses were 6-fold to 704-fold greater than the systemic exposure in humans with the therapeutic dose. Zalcitabine was administered orally by dietary admixture to CDF® (F-344)/Cr1BR/CdBR rats at dosages of 3, 28, 83, or 250 mg/kg/day. At the highest dose tested, the systemic exposure to zalcitabine was 833 times the systemic exposure in humans with the therapeutic dose. A significant increase in thymic lymphoma in all zalcitabine dose groups and Harderian gland (a gland of the eye of rodents) adenoma in the two highest dose groups was observed in female CD-1 mice after 2 years of dosing. No increase in tumor incidence was observed in rats or male mice treated with zalcitabine. In an independent study, administration of zalcitabine to $B_6C_3F_1$ mice at a dose of 1000 mg/kg/day for 3 months induced an increased incidence of thymic lymphoma. A high rate of spontaneous lymphoreticular neoplasms have previously been noted in this strain of mice.
Mutagenesis: Zalcitabine was positive in a cell transformation assay and induced chromosomal aberrations in vitro in human peripheral blood lymphocytes. Oral doses of zalcitabine at 2500 and 4500 mg/kg were clastogenic in the mouse micronucleus assay. Zalcitabine showed no evidence of mutagenicity in Ames tests, Chinese hamster lung cell assays and the mouse lymphoma assay. An unscheduled DNA synthesis assay in rat hepatocytes showed that zalcitabine had no effect on DNA repair.
Impairment of Fertility: Fertility and reproductive performance were assessed in rats at plasma concentrations up to 2142 times those achieved with the maximum recommended human dose (MRHD) based on AUC measurements. No adverse effects on rate of conception or general reproductive performance were observed. The highest dose was associated with embryolethality and evidence of teratogenicity. The next lower dose studied (plasma concentrations equivalent to 485 times the MRHD) was associated with a lower frequency of embryotoxicity but no teratogenicity. The fertility of F_1 males was significantly reduced at a calculated dose of 2142 (but not 485) times the MRHD (based on AUC measurements) in a teratology study in which rat mothers were dosed on gestation days 7 to 15. No adverse effects were observed on the fertility of parents or F_1 generation in the study of fertility and general reproductive performance or in the perinatal and postnatal reproduction study.

Table 2. Percentage of Patients With Clinical Adverse Experience ≥ Grade 3*† in ≥1% of Patients Receiving HIVID

	CPCRA 002* ZDV Intolerant or Failure		ACTG 175‡ ZDV Naive/Experienced	
	HIVID 0.750 mg q8h n=237	ddI 250 mg q12h n=230	ZDV 200 mg q8h n=619	HIVID+ZDV 0.750 mg q8h +200 mg q8h n=615
Body System/Adverse Event				
Systemic				
Fatigue	3.8	2.6	2.7	2.3
Headache	2.1	1.3	2.4	2.6
Fever	1.7	0.4	2.7	2.9
Gastrointestinal				
Abdominal Pain	3.0	7.0	2.3	1.8
Oral Lesions/Stomatitis§	3.0	0.0	0.6	1.5
Vomiting/Nausea§	3.4	7.0	4.9	2.1
Diarrhea/Constipation§	2.5	17.4	2.9	1.0
Hepatic				
Abnormal Hepatic Function	8.9	7.0	‖	‖
Neurological				
Convulsions	1.3	2.2		
Peripheral Neuropathy¶	28.3	13.0	3.1	3.3
Skin				
Rash/Pruritus/Urticaria	3.4	3.9	1.8	1.6
Metabolic and Nutrition				
Pancreatitis	0.0	1.7	0.2	0.5
Psychological				
Depression	0.4	0.0	1.1	1.8
Musculoskeletal				
Painful/Swollen Joints	0.4	0.0	0.3	1.0

* Grade 2 Adverse Events possibly or probably related to treatment or unassessable were included if study drug dosage was changed or interrupted.
† Grade 3 severity: event causing marked limitation in activity, requiring medical care and possible hospitalization. Grade 4 severity: completely disabling, unable to care for self, requiring active medical intervention, probable hospitalization or hospice care.
‡ All relationships.
§ Adverse experiences were combined to form this category.
‖ See Table 3.
¶ CPCRA 002 included patients who were dose-adjusted for Grade 2 events; ACTG 175 required dose adjustment for Grade 2 peripheral neuropathy but recorded only Grade 3 events.

Pregnancy: *Teratogenic Effects:* Pregnancy Category C. Zalcitabine has been shown to be teratogenic in mice at calculated exposure levels of 1365 and 2730 times that of the MRHD (based on AUC measurements). In rats, zalcitabine was teratogenic at a calculated exposure level of 2142 times the MRHD but not at an exposure level of 485 times the MRHD. In a perinatal and postnatal study in the rat, a high incidence of hydrocephalus was observed in the F_1 offspring derived from litters of dams treated with 1071 (but not 485) times the MRHD (based on AUC measurements). There are no adequate and well-controlled studies of zalcitabine in pregnant women. HIVID should be used during pregnancy only if the potential benefit justifies the potential risk to the fetus. Fertile women should not receive HIVID unless they are using effective contraception during therapy. If pregnancy occurs, physicians are encouraged to report such cases by calling (800) 526-6367.
Nonteratogenic Effects: Increased embryolethality was observed in pregnant mice at doses 2730 times the MRHD and in pregnant rats above 485 (but not 98) times the MRHD (based on AUC measurements). Average fetal body weight was significantly decreased in mice at doses of 1365 times the MRHD and in rats at 2142 times the MRHD (based on AUC measurements). In a perinatal and postnatal study, the learning and memory of a significant number of F_1 offspring were impaired, and they tended to stay hyperactive for a longer period of time. These effects, observed at a calculated exposure level of 1071 (but not 485) times the MRHD (based on AUC measurements), were considered to result from extensive damage to or gross underdevelopment of the brain of these F_1 offspring consistent with the finding of hydrocephalus.
Antiretroviral Pregnancy Registry: To monitor maternal-fetal outcomes of pregnant women exposed to HIVID, an Antiretroviral Pregnancy Registry has been established. Physicians are encouraged to register patients by calling 1-800-258-4263.
Nursing Mothers: **The Centers for Disease Control and Prevention recommend HIV-infected mothers not breast-feed their infants to avoid risking postnatal transmission of HIV.** It is not known whether zalcitabine is excreted in human milk. Because of both the potential for HIV transmission and the potential for serious adverse reactions in nursing infants, **mothers should be instructed not to breast-feed if they are receiving antiretroviral medications, including HIVID.**
Pediatric Use: *Pharmacokinetics in Pediatric Patients:* Limited pharmacokinetic data have been reported for 5 HIV-positive pediatric patients using doses of 0.03 and 0.04 mg/kg HIVID administered orally every 6 hours.[1] The mean bioavailability of zalcitabine in these pediatric patients was 54% and mean apparent systemic clearance was 150 mL/min/m^2. Due to the small number of subjects and different analytical techniques, it is difficult to make comparisons between pediatric and adult data.
Safety and effectiveness of HIVID in HIV-infected pediatric patients younger than 13 years of age have not been established.
Geriatric Use: Clinical studies of HIVID did not include sufficient numbers of subjects aged 65 and over to determine whether they respond differently from younger subjects. In general, dose selection for an elderly patient should be cautious, reflecting the greater frequency of decreased hepatic, renal, or cardiac function, and of concomitant disease or other drug therapy. HIVID is known to be substantially excreted by the kidney, and the risk of toxic reactions to this drug may be greater in patients with impaired renal function. Because elderly patients are more likely to have decreased renal function, care should be taken in dose selection. In addition, renal function should be monitored and dosage adjustments should be made accordingly (see PRECAUTIONS: *General: Renal Impairment* and DOSAGE AND ADMINISTRATION).

ADVERSE REACTIONS (See WARNINGS.)

Tables 2 and 3 summarize the clinical adverse events and laboratory abnormalities, respectively, that occurred in ≥1% of patients in the comparative monotherapy trial (CPCRA 002) of HIVID vs didanosine (ddI), and the comparative combination trial (ACTG 175) of zidovudine (ZDV) monotherapy vs HIVID and zidovudine combination therapy, respectively. Other studies have found a higher or lower incidence of adverse experiences depending upon disease status, generally being lower in patients with less advanced disease.
[See table 2 at left]
[See table 3 at bottom of next page]
Additional clinical adverse experiences associated with HIVID that occurred in <1% of patients in CPCRA 002 (at least possibly related, Grade 3 or higher), ACTG 175 (any relationship, Grade 3/4) or in other clinical studies are listed below by body system. Several of these events occurred in slightly higher rates in other studies. The incidence of adverse experiences varied in different studies, generally being lower in patients with less-advanced disease.
Body as a Whole: abnormal weight loss, asthenia, cachexia, chest tightness or pain, chills, cutaneous/allergic reaction, debilitation, difficulty moving, dry eyes/mouth, edema, facial pain or swelling, flank pain, flushing, increased sweating, lymphadenopathy, hypersensitivity reactions (see WARNINGS), malaise, night sweats, pain, pelvic/groin pain, rigors, redistribution/accumulation of body fat (see PRECAUTIONS: *Fat Redistribution*).

Cardiovascular: abnormal cardiac movement, arrhythmia, atrial fibrillation, cardiac failure, cardiac dysrhythmias, cardiomyopathy, heart racing, hypertension, palpitation, subarachnoid hemorrhage, syncope, tachycardia, ventricular ectopy.

Endocrine/Metabolic: abnormal triglycerides, abnormal lipase, altered serum glucose, decreased bicarbonate, diabetes mellitus, glycosuria, gout, hot flushes, hypercalcemia, hyperkalemia, hyperlipemia, hypernatremia, hyperuricemia, hypocalcemia, hypoglycemia, hypokalemia, hypomagnesemia, hyponatremia, hypophosphatemia, increased nonprotein nitrogen, lactic acidosis.

Gastrointestinal: abdominal bloating or cramps, acute pancreatitis, anal/rectal pain, anorexia, bleeding gums, bloody or black stools, colitis, dental abscess, dry mouth, dyspepsia, dysphagia, enlarged abdomen, epigastric pain, eructation, esophageal pain, esophageal ulcers, esophagitis, flatulence, gagging with pills, gastritis, gastrointestinal hemorrhage, gingivitis, glossitis, gum disorder, heartburn, hemorrhagic pancreatitis, hemorrhoids, increased saliva, left quadrant pain, melena, mouth lesion, odynophagia, painful sore gums, painful swallowing, pancreatitis, rectal hemorrhage, rectal mass, rectal ulcers, salivary gland enlargement, sore tongue, sore throat, tongue disorder, tongue ulcer, toothache, unformed/loose stools, vomiting.

Hematologic: absolute neutrophil count alteration, anemia, epistaxis, decreased hematocrit, granulocytosis, hemoglobinemia, leukopenia, neutrophilia, platelet alteration, purpura, thrombus, unspecified hematologic toxicity, white blood cell alteration.

Hepatic: abnormal lactate dehydrogenase, bilirubinemia, cholecystitis, decreased alkaline phosphatase, hepatitis, hepatocellular damage, hepatomegaly, increased alkaline phosphatase, jaundice.

Musculoskeletal: arthralgia, arthritis, arthropathy, arthrosis, back pain, backache, bone pains/aches, bursitis, cold extremities, extremity pain, joint inflammation, leg cramps, muscle aches, muscle weakness, muscle disorder, muscle stiffness, muscle cramps, myalgia, myopathy, myositis, neck pain, rib pain, stiff neck.

Neurological: abnormal coordination, aphasia, ataxia, Bell's palsy, confusion, decreased concentration, decreased neurological function, disequilibrium, dizziness, dysphonia, facial nerve palsy, focal motor seizures, grand mal seizure, hyperkinesia, hypertonia, hypokinesia, memory loss, migraine, neuralgia, neuritis, paralysis, seizures, speech disorder, status epilepticus, stupor, tremor, twitch, vertigo.

Psychological: acute psychotic disorder, acute stress reaction, agitation, amnesia, anxiety, confusion, decreased motivation, decreased sexual desire, depersonalization, emotional lability, euphoria, hallucination, impaired concentration, insomnia, manic reaction, mood swings, nervousness, paranoid state, somnolence, suicide attempt, dementia.

Respiratory: acute nasopharyngitis, chest congestion, coughing, cyanosis, difficulty breathing, dry nasal mucosa, dyspnea, flu-like symptoms, hemoptysis, nasal discharge, pharyngitis, rales/rhonchi, respiratory distress, sinus congestion, sinus pain, sinusitis, wheezing.

Skin: acne, alopecia, bullous eruptions, carbuncle/furuncle, cellulitis, cold sore, dermatitis, dry skin, dry rash desquamation, erythematous rash, exfoliative dermatitis, finger inflammation, follicular rash, impetigo, infection, itchy rash, lip blisters/lesions, macular/papular rash, maculopapular rash, moniliasis, mucocutaneous/skin disorder, nail disorder, photosensitivity reaction, pruritic disorder, pruritus, skin disorder, skin lesions, skin fissure, skin ulcer, urticaria.

Special Senses: abnormal vision, blurred vision, burning eyes, decreased taste, decreased vision, ear pain/problem, ear blockage, eye abnormality, eye inflammation, eye itching, eye pain, eye irritation, eye redness, eye hemorrhage, fluid in ears, hearing loss, increased tears, loss of taste, mucopurulent conjunctivitis, parosmia, photophobia, smell dysfunction, taste perversion, tinnitus, unequal-sized pupils, xerophthalmia, yellow sclera.

Urogenital: abnormal renal function, acute renal failure, albuminuria, bladder pain, dysuria, frequent urination, genital lesion/ulcer, increased blood urea nitrogen, increased creatinine, micturition frequency, nocturia, painful penis sore, pain on urination, penile edema, polyuria, renal cyst, renal calculus, testicular swelling, toxic nephropathy, urinary retention, vaginal itch, vaginal ulcer, vaginal pain, vaginal/cervix disorder, vaginal discharge.

OVERDOSAGE

Acute Overdosage: Inadvertent pediatric overdoses have occurred with doses up to 1.5 mg/kg HIVID. Pediatric patients had prompt gastric lavage and treatment with activated charcoal and had no sequelae. Mixed overdoses including HIVID and other drugs have led to drowsiness and vomiting (with HIVID or placebo, zidovudine and trimethoprim/sulfamethoxazole [TMP/SMX]), or increased GGT (with 18.75 mg HIVID with zidovudine and lormetazepam) or increased creatine phosphokinase (with HIVID or placebo, zidovudine, fluconazole, dapsone and wine). There is no experience with acute HIVID overdosage at higher doses and sequelae are unknown. There is no known antidote for HIVID overdosage. It is not known whether zalcitabine is dialyzable by peritoneal dialysis or hemodialysis.

Chronic Overdosage: In an initial dose-finding study in which zalcitabine was administered at doses 25 times (0.25 mg/kg every 8 hours) the currently recommended dose, one patient discontinued HIVID after 1½ weeks of treatment subsequent to the development of a rash and fever. In the early Phase 1 studies, all patients receiving zalcitabine at approximately 6 times the current total daily recommended dose experienced peripheral neuropathy by week 10. Eighty percent of patients who received approximately 2 times the current total daily recommended dose experienced peripheral neuropathy by week 12.

DOSAGE AND ADMINISTRATION

Patients should be advised that HIVID is recommended for use in combination with active antiretroviral therapy. Greater activity has been observed when new antiretroviral therapies are begun at the same time as HIVID. Concomitant therapy should be based on a patient's prior drug exposure. The recommended regimen is one 0.750 mg tablet of HIVID orally every 8 hours (2.25 mg HIVID total daily dose) in combination with other antiretroviral agents. Please refer to the complete product information for each of the other antiretroviral agents for the recommended doses of these agents. Based on preliminary data, the recommended HIVID dosage reduction for patients with impaired renal function is: creatinine clearance 10 to 40 mL/min: 0.750 mg of HIVID every 12 hours; creatinine clearance <10 mL/min: 0.750 mg of HIVID every 24 hours.

Monitoring of Patients: Complete blood counts and clinical chemistry tests should be performed prior to initiating HIVID therapy and at appropriate intervals thereafter. For comprehensive patient monitoring recommendations for other antiretroviral therapies, physicians should refer to the complete product information for these drugs. Serum amylase levels should be monitored in those individuals who have a history of elevated amylase, pancreatitis, ethanol abuse, who are on parenteral nutrition or who are otherwise at high risk of pancreatitis. Careful monitoring for signs or symptoms suggestive of peripheral neuropathy is recommended, particularly in individuals with a low CD_4 cell count or who are at a greater risk of developing peripheral neuropathy while on therapy (see WARNINGS).

Dose Adjustment for HIVID: For toxicities that are likely to be associated with HIVID (eg, peripheral neuropathy, severe oral ulcers, pancreatitis, elevated liver function tests especially in patients with chronic Hepatitis B), HIVID should be interrupted or dose reduced. FOR SEVERE TOXICITIES OR THOSE PERSISTING AFTER DOSE REDUCTION, HIVID SHOULD BE INTERRUPTED. For recipients of combination therapy with HIVID and other antiretroviral agents, dose adjustments or interruption for each drug should be based on the known toxicity profile of the individual drugs. SEE INFORMATION FOR EACH DRUG USED IN COMBINATION FOR A DESCRIPTION OF KNOWN DRUG-ASSOCIATED ADVERSE REACTIONS.

Patients developing moderate discomfort with signs or symptoms of peripheral neuropathy should stop HIVID. HIVID-associated peripheral neuropathy may continue to worsen despite interruption of HIVID. HIVID should be reintroduced at 50% dose — 0.375 mg every 8 hours only if all findings related to peripheral neuropathy have improved to mild symptoms. HIVID should be permanently discontinued if patients experience severe discomfort related to peripheral neuropathy or moderate discomfort that progresses. If other moderate to severe clinical adverse reactions or laboratory abnormalities (such as increased liver function tests) occur, then HIVID and/or the other potential causative agent(s) should be interrupted until the adverse reaction abates. HIVID and/or the other potential causative agent(s) should then be carefully reintroduced at lower doses if appropriate. If adverse reactions recur at the reduced dose, therapy should be discontinued. The minimum effective dose of HIVID in combination with zidovudine for the treatment of adult patients with advanced HIV infection has not been established.

In patients with poor bone marrow reserve, particularly those patients with advanced symptomatic HIV disease, frequent monitoring of hematologic indices is recommended to detect serious anemia or granulocytopenia. Significant toxicities, such as anemia (hemoglobin of <7.5 gm/dL or reduction of >25% of baseline) and/or granulocytopenia (granulocyte count of <750 cells/mm^3 or reduction of >50% from baseline), may require a treatment interruption of HIVID and zidovudine until evidence of marrow recovery is observed. For less severe anemia or granulocytopenia, a reduction in daily dose of zidovudine in those patients receiving combination therapy may be adequate. In patients who experience hematologic toxicity, reduction in hemoglobin may occur as early as 2 to 4 weeks after initiation of therapy, and granulocytopenia usually occurs after 6 to 8 weeks of therapy. In patients who develop significant anemia, dose modification does not necessarily eliminate the need for transfusion. If marrow recovery occurs following dose modification, gradual increases in dose may be appropriate depending on hematologic indices and patient tolerance. For more details, refer to the complete product information for zidovudine.

HOW SUPPLIED

HIVID 0.375 mg tablets are oval, beige, film-coated tablets with "HIVID 0.375" imprinted on one side and "ROCHE" on the other side — bottles of 100 (NDC 0004-0220-01). HIVID 0.750 mg tablets are oval, gray, film-coated tablets with "HIVID 0.750" imprinted on one side and "ROCHE" on the other side — bottles of 100 (NDC 0004-0221-01).

The tablets should be stored in tightly closed bottles at 59° to 86°F (15° to 30°C).

REFERENCES

1. Pizzo PA, Butler K, Balis F, et al. Dideoxycytidine alone and in an alternating schedule with zidovudine in children with symptomatic human immunodeficiency virus infection. *J Pediatr.* 1990;117(5): 799–808.
2. Abrams DI, Goldman AI, Launer C, et al. A comparative trial of didanosine or zalcitabine after treatment with zidovudine in patients with human immunodeficiency virus infection. *N Engl J Med.* 1994;330(10): 657–662.
3. Follansbee S, Drew L, Olson R, et al. The efficacy of zalcitabine (ddC, HIVID) versus zidovudine (ZDV) as monotherapy in ZDV-naive patients with advanced HIV disease; a randomized, double-blind, comparative trial (ACTG 114; N3300). IXth International Conference on AIDS/IV STD World Congress, Berlin, Germany, June 7–11, 1993. Poster PO-B26-2113.
4. Remick S, Follansbee S, Olson R, et al. Safety and tolerance of zalcitabine (ddC, HIVID) in a double-blind comparative trial (ACTG 114; N3300). IXth International Conference on AIDS/IV STD World Congress, Berlin, Germany, June 7–11, 1993. Poster PO-B26-2115.
5. "Dear Doctor" letter, Burroughs Wellcome Co., June 1, 1993.
6. Food and Drug Administration Antiviral Drugs Advisory Committee Meeting, "Mitochondrial Damage Associated with Nucleoside Analogues," Rockville, MD, September 21, 1993.
7. Sanders VM, Elwell MR, Heath JE, et al. Induction of Thymic Lymphoma in Mice Administered the Dideoxynucleoside ddC. *Fundamental and Applied Toxicology.* 1995;27: 263–269.
8. Irons RD, Le AT, Som DB, et al. 2′3′-Dideoxycytidine-induced Thymic Lymphoma Correlates with Species-specific Suppression of a Subpopulation of Primitive Hematopoietic Progenitor Cells in Mouse but Not Rat or Human Bone Marrow. *J Clin Invest.* 1995;95: 2777–2782.

Revised: September 2002

Shown in Product Identification Guide, page 331

Table 3. Percentage of Patients With Laboratory Abnormalities—Protocol Grade 3/4

	CPCRA 002* ZDV Intolerant or Failure		ACTG 175 ZDV Naive/Experienced	
	HIVID 0.750 mg q8h n=237	ddI 250 mg q12h n=230	ZDV 200 mg q8h n=619	HIVID+ZDV 0.750 mg q8h +200 mg q8h n=615
Laboratory Abnormality				
Anemia (<7.5 gm/dL)	8.4	7.4	1.8	3.1
Leukopenia (<1500 cells/mm^3)	13.1	9.6	N/A	N/A
Eosinophilia (>1000 cells/mm^3 or 25%)	2.5	1.7	N/A	N/A
Neutropenia (<750 cells/mm^3)	16.9	11.7	1.9	4.2
Thrombocytopenia (<50,000 cells/mm^3)	1.3	4.8	1.1	1.8
CPK Elevation* (>4 × ULN)	0.8	0.0	5.8	5.7
ALT (SGPT) (>5 × ULN)	N/A	N/A	3.6	5.0
AST (SGOT) (>5 × ULN)	7.6	5.7	2.9	4.1
Bilirubin (>2.5 × ULN)	0.8	0.9	0.5	1.0
GGT (>5 × ULN)	N/A	N/A	0.5	1.0
Amylase (>2 × ULN)	5.1	3.9	1.0	1.5
Hyperglycemia* (>250 mg/dL)	0.0	1.7	0.8	2.0

*Grade 3 or higher reported for CPCRA 002.
N/A Not available.

Continued on next page

INVIRASE® ℞

[ĭn-vər-ās]
(saquinavir mesylate)
CAPSULES

WARNING

INVIRASE® (saquinavir mesylate) capsules and FORTOVASE® (saquinavir) soft gelatin capsules are not bioequivalent and cannot be used interchangeably. INVIRASE may be used only if it is combined with ritonavir, which significantly inhibits saquinavir's metabolism to provide plasma saquinavir levels at least equal to those achieved with FORTOVASE. When using saquinavir as the sole protease inhibitor in an antiviral regimen, FORTOVASE is the recommended formulation (see CLINICAL PHARMACOLOGY: Drug Interactions).

Product identification in this document includes: INVIRASE in reference to saquinavir mesylate; FORTOVASE in reference to saquinavir soft gel formulation, and saquinavir in reference to the active base.

DESCRIPTION

INVIRASE brand of saquinavir mesylate is an inhibitor of the human immunodeficiency virus (HIV) protease. INVIRASE is available as light brown and green, opaque hard gelatin capsules for oral administration in a 200-mg strength (as saquinavir free base). Each capsule also contains the inactive ingredients lactose, microcrystalline cellulose, povidone K30, sodium starch glycolate, talc, and magnesium stearate. Each capsule shell contains gelatin and water with the following dye systems: red iron oxide, yellow iron oxide, black iron oxide, FD&C Blue #2, and titanium dioxide. The chemical name for saquinavir mesylate is N-tert-butyl-decahydro-2-[2(R)-hydroxy-4-phenyl-3(S)-[[N-(2-quinolylcarbonyl)-L-asparaginyl]amino]butyl]-(4aS, 8aS)-isoquinoline-3(S)-carboxamide methanesulfonate with a molecular formula $C_{38}H_{50}N_6O_5 \bullet CH_4O_3S$ and a molecular weight of 766.96. The molecular weight of the free base is 670.86.

Saquinavir mesylate is a white to off-white, very fine powder with an aqueous solubility of 2.22 mg/mL at 25°C.

MICROBIOLOGY

Mechanism of Action

Saquinavir is an inhibitor of HIV protease. HIV protease is an enzyme required for the proteolytic cleavage of viral polyprotein precursors into individual functional proteins found in infectious HIV. Saquinavir is a peptide-like substrate analogue that binds to the protease active site and inhibits the activity of the enzyme. Saquinavir inhibition prevents cleavage of the viral polyproteins resulting in the formation of immature noninfectious virus particles.

Antiviral Activity

In vitro antiviral activity of saquinavir was assessed in lymphoblastoid and monocytic cell lines and in peripheral blood lymphocytes. Saquinavir inhibited HIV activity in both acutely and chronically infected cells. IC_{50} and IC_{90} values (50% and 90% inhibitory concentrations) were in the range of 1 to 30 nM and 5 to 80 nM, respectively. In the presence of 40% human serum, the mean IC_{50} of saquinavir against laboratory strain HIV-1 RF in MT4 cells was 37.7± 5nM representing a 4-fold increase in the IC_{50} value. In cell culture, saquinavir demonstrated additive to synergistic effects against HIV-1 in combination with reverse transcriptase inhibitors (didanosine, lamivudine, nevirapine, stavudine, zalcitabine and zidovudine) without enhanced cytotoxicity. Saquinavir in combination with the protease inhibitors amprenavir, atazanavir, or lopinavir resulted in synergistic antiviral activity.

Drug Resistance

HIV-1 mutants with reduced susceptibility to saquinavir have been selected during in vitro passage. Genotypic analyses of these isolates showed several substitutions in the HIV protease gene. Only the G48V and L90M substitutions were associated with reduced susceptibility to saquinavir, and conferred an increase in the IC_{50} value of 8- and 3-fold, respectively.

HIV-1 isolates with reduced susceptibility (≥4-fold increase in the IC_{50} value) to saquinavir emerged in some patients treated with INVIRASE. Genotypic analysis of these isolates identified resistance conferring primary mutations in the protease gene G48V and L90M, and secondary mutations L10I/R/V, I54V/L, A71V/T, G73S, V77I, V82A and I84V that contributed additional resistance to saquinavir. Forty-one isolates from 37 patients failing therapy with INVIRASE had a median decrease in susceptibility to saquinavir of 4.3 fold.

The degree of reduction in in vitro susceptibility to saquinavir of clinical isolates bearing substitutions G48V and L90M depends on the number of secondary mutations present. In general, higher levels of resistance are associated with greater number of mutations only in association with either or both of the primary mutations G48V and L90M. No data are currently available to address the development of resistance in patients receiving saquinavir/ritonavir.

Cross-resistance

Among protease inhibitors, variable crossresistance has been observed. In one clinical study, 22 HIV-1 isolates with reduced susceptibility (>4-fold increase in the IC_{50} value) to saquinavir following therapy with INVIRASE were evaluated for cross-resistance to amprenavir, indinavir, nelfinavir and ritonavir. Six of the 22 isolates (27%) remained susceptible to all 4 protease inhibitors, 12 of the 22 isolates (55%) retained susceptibility to at least one of the PIs and 4 out of the 22 isolates (18%) displayed broad cross- resistance to all PIs. Sixteen (73%) and 11 (50%) of the 22 isolates remained susceptible (<4-fold) to amprenavir and indinavir, respectively. Four of 16 (25%) and nine of 21 (43%) with available data remained susceptible to nelfinavir and ritonavir, respectively.

After treatment failure with amprenavir, cross-resistance to saquinavir was evaluated. HIV-1 isolates from 22/22 patients failing treatment with amprenavir and containing one or more mutations M46L/I, I50V, I54L, V32I, I47V, and I84V were susceptible to saquinavir.

Table 1 Pharmacokinetic Parameters of Saquinavir at Steady-State After Administration of Different Regimens in HIV-Infected Patients

Dosing Regimen	N	AUC_τ (ng•h/mL)	AUC_{24h} (ng•h/mL)	C_{min} (ng/mL)
INVIRASE 600 mg tid (arithmetic mean, %CV)	10	866 (62)	2598	79
FORTOVASE 1200 mg tid (arithmetic mean)	31	7249	21747	216
INVIRASE 400 mg bid + ritonavir 400 mg bid (arithmetic mean ±SD)	7	16000±8000	32000	480±360
INVIRASE 1000 mg bid + ritonavir 100 mg bid (geometric mean and 95% CI)	24	14607 (10218-20882)	29214	371 (245-561)
FORTOVASE 1000 mg bid + ritonavir 100 mg bid (geometric mean and 95% CI)	24	19085 (13943-26124)	38170	433 (301-622)

τ is the dosing interval (ie, 8h if tid and 12h if bid)

Table 2 Effect of FORTOVASE or INVIRASE on the Pharmacokinetics of Coadministered Drugs

Coadministered Drug	FORTOVASE or FORTOVASE/ ritonavir Dose	N	% Change for Coadministered Drug	
			AUC (95%CI)	C_{max} (95%CI)
Clarithromycin 500 mg bid × 7 days Clarithromycin 14-OH clarithromycin metabolite	1200 mg tid × 7 days	12V	 ↑45% (17-81%) ↓24% (5-40%)	 ↑39% (10-76%) ↓34% (14-50%)
Midazolam 7.5-mg oral single dose	1200 mg tid ×5 days	6V	↑514%	↑235%
Ketoconazole 400 mg once daily	1200 mg tid	12V	↔	↔
Enfuvirtide 90 mg SCq 12h (bid) for 7 days	1000/100 mg bid	12P	↔	↔
Nelfinavir 750-mg single dose	1200 mg tid × 4 days	14P	↑18% (5-33%)	↔
Rifabutin 300 mg once daily	1200 mg tid	14P	↑44%	↑45%
Ritonavir 400 mg bid × 14 days	400 mg bid ×14 days	8V	↔	↔
Sildenafil 100-mg single dose	1200 mg tid ×8 days	27V	↑210% (150-300%)	↑140% (80-230%)
Terfenadine[ϕ] 60 mg bid × 11 days* Terfenadine Terfendadine acid metabolite	1200 mg tid × 4 days	12V	 ↑368% (257-514%) ↑120% (89-156%)	 ↑253% (164-373%) ↑93% (59-133%)
Efavirenz 600 mg	1200 mg tid	13V	↓12%	↓13%

↑ Denotes an average increase in exposure by the percentage indicated.
↓ Denotes an average decrease in exposure by the percentage indicated.
↔Denotes no statistically significant change in exposure was observed.
* FORTOVASE or INVIRASE/ritonavir should not be coadministered with terfenadine (see PRECAUTIONS: Drug Interactions).
P Patient
V Healthy Volunteers
ϕ No longer marketed in the US.

CLINICAL PHARMACOLOGY

Pharmacokinetics

The pharmacokinetic properties of INVIRASE have been evaluated in healthy volunteers (n=351) and HIV-infected patients (n=270) after single- and multiple-oral doses of 25, 75, 200, and 600 mg tid and in healthy volunteers after intravenous doses of 6, 12, 36 or 72 mg (n=21). The pharmacokinetics of INVIRASE/ritonavir 400/400 mg bid and INVIRASE/ritonavir 1000/100 mg bid have also been evaluated in HIV-infected patients.

HIV-infected patients administered INVIRASE (600-mg TID) had AUC and maximum plasma concentration (C_{max}) values approximately 2–2.5 times those observed in healthy volunteers receiving the same treatment regimen.

Absorption and Bioavailability in Adults

Absolute bioavailability of saquinavir administered as INVIRASE averaged 4% (CV 73%, range: 1% to 9%) in 8 healthy volunteers who received a single 600-mg dose (3 × 200 mg) of saquinavir mesylate following a high-fat breakfast (48 g protein, 60 g carbohydrate, 57 g fat; 1006 kcal). The low bioavailability is thought to be due to a combination of incomplete absorption and extensive first-pass metabolism. Following single 600-mg doses, the relative bioavailability of saquinavir as FORTOVASE compared to saquinavir administered as INVIRASE was estimated at 331% (95% CI 207% to 530%).

When administered as the sole protease inhibitor, it has been shown that FORTOVASE 1200 mg tid provides an 8-fold increase in AUC compared with INVIRASE 600 mg tid (see Table 1).

INVIRASE in combination with ritonavir at doses of 1000/100 mg bid or 400/400 mg bid provides saquinavir systemic exposures over a 24-hour period similar to or greater than those achieved with FORTOVASE 1200 mg tid (see Table 1).

[See table 1 above]

Food Effect

No food effect data are available for INVIRASE in combination with ritonavir.

The mean 24-hour AUC after a single 600-mg oral dose (6 × 100 mg) in healthy volunteers (n=6) was increased from 24 ng•h/mL (CV 33%), under fasting conditions, to 161 ng•h/mL (CV 35%) when INVIRASE was given following a high-fat breakfast (48 g protein, 60 g carbohydrate, 57 g fat; 1006 kcal). Saquinavir 24-hour AUC and C_{max} (n=6) following the administration of a higher calorie meal (943 kcal, 54 g fat) were on average 2 times higher than after a lower calorie, lower fat meal (355 kcal, 8 g fat). The effect of food has been shown to persist for up to 2 hours.

Saquinavir exposure was similar when FORTOVASE plus ritonavir (1000-mg/100-mg bid) were administered following a high-fat (45 g fat) or moderate-fat (20 g fat) breakfast.

Distribution in Adults

The mean steady-state volume of distribution following intravenous administration of a 12-mg dose of saquinavir (n=8) was 700 L (CV 39%), suggesting saquinavir partitions into tissues. Saquinavir was approximately 98% bound to plasma proteins over a concentration range of 15 to 700 ng/mL. In 2 patients receiving saquinavir mesylate 600 mg tid, cerebrospinal fluid concentrations were negligible when compared to concentrations from matching plasma samples.

Table 3 Effect of Coadministered Drugs on FORTOVASE or INVIRASE Pharmacokinetics

Coadministered Drug	FORTOVASE Dose	N	% Change for Saquinavir AUC (95%CI)	% Change for Saquinavir C_{max} (95%CI)
Clarithromycin 500 mg bid × 7 days	1200 mg tid × 7 days	12V	↑177% (108-269%)	↑187% (105-300%)
Efavirenz 600 mg	1200 mg tid	13V	↓62%	↓50%
Indinavir 800 mg q8h × 2 days	1200-mg single dose	6V	↑364% (190-644%)	↑299% (138-568%)
Ketoconazole 400 mg once daily	1200 mg tid	12V	↑190%	↑171%
Nelfinavir 750 mg × 4 days	1200-mg single dose	14P	↑392% (271-553%)	↑179% (105-280%)
Rifabutin 300 mg once daily	1200 mg tid	14P	↓47%	↓39%
Rifampin 600 mg once daily	1200 mg tid × 14 days	14V	↓70%	↓65%
Ritonavir 100 mg bid	1000 mg bid†	24P	↑176%	↑153%
Ritonavir 400 mg bid × 14 days*	400 mg bid × 14 days†	8V	↑121% (7-359%)	↑64%§
Lopinavir/ritonavir 400/100 mg bid, 15 days	800 mg bid, 10 day combo vs. 1200 mg tid, 5 days alone	14V	↑9.62-fold (8.05, 11.49)^	↑6.34-fold (5.32, 7.55)^
400/100 mg bid, 20 days	1200 mg bid, 10 day combo vs. 1200 mg tid, 5 days alone	10V	↑9.91-fold (8.28, 11.86)^	↑6.44-fold (5.59, 7.41)^
Coadministered Drug	**INVIRASE Dose**	**N**	**% Change for Saquinavir AUC (95%CI)**	**% Change for Saquinavir C_{max} (95%CI)**
Rifabutin 150 mg every 3 days or 300 mg every 7 days	400 mg bid + 400 mg ritonavir bid	24P	↑19%	↑39%
Ritonavir 400 mg bid steady state*	400 mg bid steady state‡	7P	↑1587% (808-3034%)	↑1277% (577-2702%)
Ritonavir 100 mg bid	1000 mg bid‡	24P	↑1124%	↑1325%

↑ Denotes an average increase in exposure by the percentage indicated.
↓ Denotes an average decrease in exposure by the percentage indicated.
↔Denotes no statistically significant change in exposure was observed.
* When ritonavir was combined with the same dose of either INVIRASE or FORTOVASE, actual mean plasma exposures (AUC_{12}, 18200 ng·h/mL, 20000 ng·h/mL, respectively) were not significantly different.
^ 90% CI reported
† Compared to standard FORTOVASE 1200 mg tid regimen (n=33).
‡ Compared to standard INVIRASE 600 mg tid regimen (n=114).
§ Did not reach statistical significance.
P Patient
V Healthy Volunteers

Metabolism and Elimination in Adults
In vitro studies using human liver microsomes have shown that the metabolism of saquinavir is cytochrome P450 mediated with the specific isoenzyme, CYP3A4, responsible for more than 90% of the hepatic metabolism. Based on in vitro studies, saquinavir is rapidly metabolized to a range of mono- and di-hydroxylated inactive compounds. In a mass balance study using 600 mg ^{14}C-saquinavir mesylate (n=8), 88% and 1% of the orally administered radioactivity was recovered in feces and urine, respectively, within 5 days of dosing. In an additional 4 subjects administered 10.5 mg ^{14}C-saquinavir intravenously, 81% and 3% of the intravenously administered radioactivity was recovered in feces and urine, respectively, within 5 days of dosing. In mass balance studies, 13% of circulating radioactivity in plasma was attributed to unchanged drug after oral administration and the remainder attributed to saquinavir metabolites. Following intravenous administration, 66% of circulating radioactivity was attributed to unchanged drug and the remainder attributed to saquinavir metabolites, suggesting that saquinavir undergoes extensive first-pass metabolism.
Systemic clearance of saquinavir was rapid, 1.14 L/h/kg (CV 12%) after intravenous doses of 6, 36, and 72 mg. The mean residence time of saquinavir was 7 hours (n=8).
Special Populations
Hepatic or Renal Impairment
Saquinavir pharmacokinetics in patients with hepatic or renal impairment has not been investigated (see PRECAUTIONS). Only 1% of saquinavir is excreted in the urine, so the impact of renal impairment on saquinavir elimination should be minimal.
Gender, Race, and Age
Pharmacokinetic data were available for 17 women in the Phase I/II studies. Pooled data did not reveal an apparent effect of gender on the pharmacokinetics of saquinavir.
The effect of race on the pharmacokinetics of saquinavir has not been investigated.
Pediatric Patients
The pharmacokinetics of saquinavir when administered as INVIRASE has not been sufficiently investigated in pediatric patients.
Geriatric Patients
The pharmacokinetics of saquinavir when administered as INVIRASE have not been sufficiently investigated in patients >65 years of age.
Drug Interactions (see PRECAUTIONS: Drug Interactions)
Several drug interaction studies have been completed with both INVIRASE and FORTOVASE. It is important to be aware that, when INVIRASE is coadministered with ritonavir, the occurrence and magnitude of drug interactions may differ from those seen with FORTOVASE when administered as the sole protease inhibitor. Because ritonavir is coadministered, prescribers should refer to the prescribing information for ritonavir regarding drug interactions associated with this drug.
Table 2 summarizes the effect of FORTOVASE on the geometric mean AUC and C_{max} of coadministered drugs. Table 3 summarizes the effect of coadministered drugs on the geometric mean AUC and C_{max} of saquinavir.
[See table 2 at top of previous page]
[See table 3 above]
For information regarding clinical recommendations, see PRECAUTIONS: Drug Interactions, Table 6.

INDICATIONS AND USAGE

INVIRASE in combination with ritonavir and other antiretroviral agents is indicated for the treatment of HIV infection. The twice daily administration of INVIRASE in combination with ritonavir is supported by safety data from the MaxCmin 1 study (see Table 7) and pharmacokinetic data (see Table 1). The efficacy of INVIRASE with ritonavir or FORTOVASE (with or without ritonavir coadministration) has not been compared against the efficacy of antiretroviral regimens currently considered standard of care.

Description of Clinical Studies

In a randomized, double-blind clinical study (NV14256) in ZDV-experienced, HIV-infected patients, INVIRASE in combination with HIVID was shown to be superior to either INVIRASE or HIVID monotherapy in decreasing the cumulative incidence of clinical disease progression to AIDS-defining events or death. Furthermore, in a randomized study (ACTG229/NV14255), patients with advanced HIV infection with history of prolonged ZDV treatment and who were given INVIRASE 600 mg tid + ZDV + HIVID experienced greater increases in CD4 cell counts as compared to those who received INVIRASE + ZDV or HIVID + ZDV. It should be noted that HIV treatment regimens that were used in these initial clinical studies of INVIRASE are no longer considered standard of care.
FORTOVASE 1000 mg bid coadministered with ritonavir 100 mg bid was studied in a heterogeneous population of 148 HIV-infected patients (MaxCmin 1 study). At baseline 42 were treatment naïve and 106 were treatment experienced (of which 52 had an HIV RNA level <400 copies/mL at baseline). Results showed that 91/148 (61%) subjects achieved and/or sustained an HIV RNA level <400 copies/mL at the completion of 48 weeks.

CONTRAINDICATIONS

INVIRASE may be used only if it is combined with ritonavir, which significantly inhibits saquinavir's metabolism and provides plasma saquinavir levels at least equal to those achieved with FORTOVASE.
INVIRASE is contraindicated in patients with clinically significant hypersensitivity to saquinavir or to any of the components contained in the capsule.
INVIRASE/ritonavir should not be administered concurrently with terfenadine, cisapride, astemizole, pimozide, triazolam, midazolam or ergot derivatives. Inhibition of CYP3A4 by saquinavir could result in elevated plasma concentrations of these drugs, potentially causing serious or life-threatening reactions, such as cardiac arrhythmias or prolonged sedation (see PRECAUTIONS: Drug Interactions).
INVIRASE when administered with ritonavir is contraindicated in patients with severe hepatic impairment.
INVIRASE should not be administered concurrently with drugs listed in Table 4 (also see PRECAUTIONS: Drug Interactions, Table 5).

Table 4 Drugs That Are Contraindicated With INVIRASE/Ritonavir

Drug Class	Drugs Within Class That Are Contraindicated With INVIRASE
Antiarrhythmics	Amiodarone, bepridil, flecainide, propafenone, quinidine
Antihistamines	Astemizole, terfenadine
Ergot Derivatives	Dihydroergotamine, ergonovine, ergotamine, methylergonovine
Antimycobacterial Agents	Rifampin*
GI Motility Agent	Cisapride
Neuroleptics	Pimozide
Sedative/Hypnotics	Triazolam, midazolam

*INVIRASE used as a sole protease inhibitor

WARNINGS

ALERT: Find out about medicines that should not be taken with INVIRASE. This statement is included on the product's bottle label.

Interaction with HMG-CoA Reductase Inhibitors

Concomitant use of INVIRASE with lovastatin or simvastatin is not recommended. Caution should be exercised if HIV protease inhibitors, including INVIRASE, are used concurrently with other HMG-CoA reductase inhibitors that are also metabolized by the CYP3A4 pathway (eg, atorvastatin). Since increased concentrations of statins can, in rare cases, cause severe adverse events such as myopathy including rhabdomyolysis, this risk may be increased when HIV protease inhibitors, including saquinavir, are used in combination with these drugs.

Interaction with St. John's Wort (hypericum perforatum)

Concomitant use of INVIRASE and St. John's wort (hypericum perforatum) or products containing St. John's wort is not recommended. Coadministration of protease inhibitors, including INVIRASE, with St. John's wort is expected to substantially decrease protease-inhibitor concentrations and may result in sub-optimal levels of INVIRASE and lead to loss of virologic response and possible resistance to INVIRASE or to the class of protease inhibitors.

Interaction with Garlic Capsules

Garlic capsules should not be used while taking saquinavir as the sole protease inhibitor due to the risk of decreased saquinavir plasma concentrations. No data are available for the coadministration of INVIRASE/ritonavir or FORTOVASE/ritonavir and garlic capsules.

Diabetes Mellitus and Hyperglycemia

New onset diabetes mellitus, exacerbation of preexisting diabetes mellitus and hyperglycemia have been reported during postmarketing surveillance in HIV-infected patients receiving protease-inhibitor therapy. Some patients required either initiation or dose adjustments of insulin or oral hypoglycemic agents for the treatment of these events. In

Continued on next page

Invirase—Cont.

some cases diabetic ketoacidosis has occurred. In those patients who discontinued protease-inhibitor therapy, hyperglycemia persisted in some cases. Because these events have been reported voluntarily during clinical practice, estimates of frequency cannot be made and a causal relationship between protease-inhibitor therapy and these events has not been established.

PRECAUTIONS

General

INVIRASE (saquinavir mesylate) capsules and FORTOVASE (saquinavir) soft gelatin capsules are not bioequivalent and cannot be used interchangeably when used as the sole protease inhibitor. Only FORTOVASE should be used for the initiation of therapy that includes saquinavir as a sole protease inhibitor (see DOSAGE AND ADMINISTRATION) since FORTOVASE soft gelatin capsules provide greater bioavailability and efficacy than INVIRASE capsules.

If a serious or severe toxicity occurs during treatment with INVIRASE, INVIRASE should be interrupted until the etiology of the event is identified or the toxicity resolves. At that time, resumption of treatment with full-dose INVIRASE may be considered. For antiretroviral agents used in combination with INVIRASE, physicians should refer to the complete product information for these drugs for dose adjustment recommendations and for information regarding drug-associated adverse reactions.

Hepatic Effects

The use of INVIRASE (in combination with ritonavir) by patients with hepatic impairment has not been studied. In the absence of such studies, caution should be exercised, as increases in saquinavir levels and/or increases in liver enzymes may occur.

In patients with underlying hepatitis B or C, cirrhosis, chronic alcoholism and/or other underlying liver abnormalities there have been reports of worsening liver disease.

Renal Effects

Renal clearance is only a minor elimination pathway; the principal route of metabolism and excretion for saquinavir is by the liver. Therefore, no initial dose adjustment is necessary for patients with renal impairment. However, patients with severe renal impairment have not been studied, and caution should be exercised when prescribing saquinavir in this population.

Hemophilia

There have been reports of spontaneous bleeding in patients with hemophilia A and B treated with protease inhibitors. In some patients additional factor VIII was required. In the majority of reported cases treatment with protease inhibitors was continued or restarted. A causal relationship between protease inhibitor therapy and these episodes has not been established.

Hyperlipidemia

Elevated cholesterol and/or triglyceride levels have been observed in some patients taking saquinavir in combination with ritonavir. Marked elevation in triglyceride levels is a risk factor for development of pancreatitis. Cholesterol and triglyceride levels should be monitored prior to initiating combination dosing regimen of FORTOVASE or INVIRASE with ritonavir, and at periodic intervals while on such therapy. In these patients, lipid disorders should be managed as clinically appropriate.

Lactose Intolerance

Each capsule contains lactose (anhydrous) 63.3 mg. This quantity should not induce specific symptoms of intolerance.

Fat Redistribution

Redistribution/accumulation of body fat including central obesity, dorsocervical fat enlargement (buffalo hump), facial wasting, peripheral wasting, breast enlargement, and "cushingoid appearance" have been observed in patients receiving antiretroviral therapy. A causal relationship between protease-inhibitor therapy and these events has not been established and the long-term consequences are currently unknown.

Resistance/Cross-resistance

Varying degrees of cross-resistance among protease inhibitors have been observed. Continued administration of INVIRASE therapy following loss of viral suppression may increase the likelihood of cross-resistance to other protease inhibitors (see MICROBIOLOGY).

Information for Patients

A statement to patients and health care providers is included on the product's bottle label: **ALERT: Find out about medicines that should NOT be taken with INVIRASE.**

Patients should be informed that any change from INVIRASE to FORTOVASE or FORTOVASE to INVIRASE coadministered with a drug which inhibits its metabolism, such as ritonavir, should be made only under the supervision of a physician.

INVIRASE may interact with some drugs; therefore, patients should be advised to report to their doctor the use of any other prescription, nonprescription medication, or herbal products, particularly St. John's wort.

Patients should be informed that INVIRASE is not a cure for HIV infection and that they may continue to acquire illnesses associated with advanced HIV infection, including opportunistic infections. Patients should be advised that **INVIRASE may be used only if it is combined with ritonavir, which significantly inhibits saquinavir's metabolism to provide plasma saquinavir levels at least equal to those achieved with FORTOVASE.**

Patients should be informed that redistribution or accumulation of body fat may occur in patients receiving protease inhibitors and that the cause and long-term health effects of these conditions are not known at this time.

Patients should be told that the long-term effects of INVIRASE are unknown at this time. They should be informed that INVIRASE therapy has not been shown to reduce the risk of transmitting HIV to others through sexual contact or blood contamination.

Patients should be advised that INVIRASE administered with ritonavir should be taken within 2 hours after a full meal (see CLINICAL PHARMACOLOGY: Pharmacokinetics). When INVIRASE is taken without food, concentrations of saquinavir in the blood are substantially reduced and may result in no antiviral activity. Patients should be advised of the importance of taking their medication every day, as prescribed, to achieve maximum benefit. Patients should not alter the dose or discontinue therapy without consulting their physician. If a dose is missed, patients should take the next dose as soon as possible. However, the patient should not double the next dose.

Laboratory Tests

Clinical chemistry tests, viral load, and CD4 count should be performed prior to initiating INVIRASE therapy and at appropriate intervals thereafter. Elevated nonfasting triglyceride levels have been observed in patients in saquinavir trials. Triglyceride levels should be periodically monitored during therapy. For comprehensive information concerning laboratory test alterations associated with use of other antiretroviral therapies, physicians should refer to the complete product information for these drugs.

Drug Interactions

Several drug interaction studies have been completed with both INVIRASE and FORTOVASE. Observations from drug interaction studies with FORTOVASE may not be predictive for INVIRASE. Because ritonavir is coadministered, prescribers should also refer to the prescribing information for ritonavir regarding drug interactions associated with this agent.

The metabolism of saquinavir is mediated by cytochrome P450, with the specific isoenzyme CYP3A4 responsible for 90% of the hepatic metabolism. Additionally, saquinavir is a substrate for P-Glycoprotein (Pgp). Therefore, drugs that affect CYP3A4 and/or Pgp, may modify the pharmacokinetics of saquinavir. Similarly, saquinavir might also modify the pharmacokinetics of other drugs that are substrates for CYP3A4 or Pgp.

Drugs that are contraindicated specifically due to the expected magnitude of interaction and potential for serious adverse events are listed in Table 4 under CONTRAINDICATIONS. Additional drugs that are not recommended for coadministration with INVIRASE and ritonavir are included in Table 5. These recommendations are based on either drug interaction studies or predicted interactions due to the expected magnitude of interaction and potential for serious events or loss of efficacy.

Drug interactions that have been established based on drug interaction studies are listed with the pharmacokinetic results in Table 2, which summarizes the effect of saquinavir, administered as FORTOVASE or INVIRASE, on the geometric mean AUC and C_{max} of coadministered drugs and Table 3, which summarizes the effect of coadministered drugs on the geometric mean AUC and C_{max} of saquinavir. Clinical dose recommendations can be found in Table 6. The magnitude of the interactions may be different when INVIRASE or FORTOVASE are given with ritonavir.

When coadministering INVIRASE/ritonavir with any agent having a narrow therapeutic margin, such as anticoagulants, anticonvulsants, and antiarrhythmics, special attention is warranted. With some agents, the metabolism may be induced, resulting in decreased concentrations. Examples and clinical dose recommendations can be found in Table 6.

Table 5 Drugs That Should Not Be Coadministered With INVIRASE/Ritonavir

Drug Class: Drug Name	Clinical Comment
Antiarrhythmics: Amiodarone, bepridil, flecainide, propafenone, quinidine	CONTRAINDICATED due to potential for serious and/or life-threatening reactions.
Antihistamines: astemizole*, terfenadine*	CONTRAINDICATED due to potential for serious and/or life-threatening cardiac arrhythmias.
Ergot Derivatives: Dihydroergotamine, ergonovine, ergotamine, methylergonovine	CONTRAINDICATED due to potential for serious and life-threatening reactions such as acute ergot toxicity characterized by peripheral vasospasm and ischemia of the extremities and other tissues.
Antimycobacterial Agents: rifampin	CONTRAINDICATED since the coadministration of this product with saquinavir in an antiretroviral regimen reduces the plasma concentrations of saquinavir.
Garlic Capsules	Garlic capsules should not be used while taking saquinavir (FORTOVASE) as the sole protease inhibitor due to the risk of decreased saquinavir plasma concentrations. No data are available for the coadministration of INVIRASE/ritonavir or FORTOVASE/ritonavir and garlic capsules.
GI Motility Agent: cisapride*	CONTRAINDICATED due to potential for serious and/or life-threatening reactions such as cardiac arrhythmias.
Herbal Products: St. John's wort (hypericum perforatum)	WARNING coadministration may lead to loss of virologic response and possible resistance to INVIRASE or to the class of protease inhibitors.
HMG-CoA Reductase Inhibitors: lovastatin, simvastatin	WARNING potential for serious reactions such as risk of myopathy including rhabdomyolysis.
Sedatives/Hypnotics: triazolam, midazolam	CONTRAINDICATED due to potential for serious and/or life-threatening reactions such as prolonged or increased sedation or respiratory depression.

*No longer marketed in the US.

[See table 6 on pages 2893 and 2894]

Drugs That Are Mainly Metabolized by CYP3A4

Although specific studies have not been performed, coadministration with drugs that are mainly metabolized by CYP3A4 (eg, calcium channel blockers, dapsone, disopyramide, quinine, amiodarone, quinidine, warfarin, tacrolimus, cyclosporine, ergot derivatives, pimozide, carbamazepine, fentanyl, alfentanyl, alprazolam, and triazolam) may have elevated plasma concentrations when coadministered with saquinavir; therefore, these combinations should be used with caution. Since INVIRASE is coadministered with ritonavir, the ritonavir label should be reviewed for additional drugs that should not be coadministered.

Inducers of CYP3A4

Coadministration with compounds that are potent inducers of CYP3A4 (eg, phenobarbital, phenytoin, dexamethasone, carbamazepine) may result in decreased plasma levels of saquinavir.

Carcinogenesis, Mutagenesis and Impairment of Fertility

Carcinogenesis

Carcinogenicity studies found no indication of carcinogenic activity in rats and mice administered saquinavir for approximately 2 years. The plasma exposures (AUC values) in the respective species were up to 6-fold (using rat) and 12-fold (using mouse) higher than those obtained in humans at the recommended clinical dose.

Mutagenesis

Mutagenicity and genotoxicity studies, with and without metabolic activation where appropriate, have shown that saquinavir has no mutagenic activity in vitro in either bacterial (Ames test) or mammalian cells (Chinese hamster lung V79/HPRT test). Saquinavir does not induce chromosomal damage in vivo in the mouse micronucleus assay or in vitro in human peripheral blood lymphocytes, and does not induce primary DNA damage in vitro in the unscheduled DNA synthesis test.

Impairment of Fertility

Fertility and reproductive performance were not affected in rats at plasma exposures (AUC values) up to 5 times those achieved in humans at the recommended dose.

Pregnancy

Teratogenic Effects: Category B

Reproduction studies conducted with saquinavir in rats have shown no embryotoxicity or teratogenicity at plasma exposures (AUC values) up to 5 times those achieved in humans at the recommended dose or in rabbits at plasma exposures 4 times those achieved at the recommended clinical dose. Studies in rats indicated that exposure to saquinavir from late pregnancy through lactation at plasma concentrations (AUC values) up to 5 times those achieved in humans at the recommended dose had no effect on the survival, growth, and development of offspring to weaning. Clinical experience in pregnant women is limited. Saquinavir should be used during pregnancy only if the potential benefit justifies the potential risk to the fetus.

Table 6 **Established and Other Potentially Significant Drug Interactions: Alteration in Dose or Regimen May Be Recommended Based on Drug Interaction Studies or Predicted Interaction (Information in the table applies to INVIRASE/ritonavir)**

Concomitant Drug Class: Drug Name	Effect on Concentration of Saquinavir or Concomitant Drug	Clinical Comment
	HIV-Antiviral Agents	
Non-nucleoside reverse transcriptase inhibitor: Delavirdine	↑ Saquinavir Effect on delavirdine is not well established **INVIRASE/ritonavir** Interaction has not been evaluated	Appropriate doses of the combination with respect to safety and efficacy have not been established.
Non-nucleoside reverse transcriptase inhibitor: Efavirenz*, nevirapine	↓ Saquinavir ↓ Efavirenz **INVIRASE/ritonavir** Interaction has not been evaluated	INVIRASE should not be given as the sole protease inhibitor to patients. Appropriate doses of the combination of efavirenz or nevirapine and INVIRASE/ritonavir with respect to safety and efficacy have not been established.
HIV protease inhibitor: Indinavir*	↑ Saquinavir Effect on indinavir is not well established **INVIRASE/ritonavir** Interaction has not been evaluated	Appropriate doses of the combination of indinavir and INVIRASE/ritonavir with respect to safety and efficacy have not been established.
HIV protease inhibitor: Nelfinavir*	↑ Saquinavir ↑ Nelfinavir **INVIRASE/ritonavir** Interaction has not been evaluated	Saquinavir 1200 mg bid with nelfinavir 1250 mg bid results in adequate plasma drug concentrations for both protease inhibitors.
HIV protease inhibitor: Ritonavir*	↑ Saquinavir ↔Ritonavir	The recommended dose regimen when ritonavir is given to increase saquinavir concentrations is 1000 mg saquinavir plus ritonavir 100 mg twice daily.
HIV protease inhibitor: Lopinavir/ritonavir (coformulated capsule)*	↑ Saquinavir Effect on lopinavir is not well established	FORTOVASE (SQV) 800 mg bid + KALETRA produces ↑ AUC, ↑ C_{max}, and ↑ C_{min} relative to FORTOVASE 1200 mg tid (see CLINICAL PHARMACOLOGY: Table 3)
HIV fusion inhibitor: Enfuvirtide*	FORTOVASE Interaction has not been evaluated FORTOVASE/ritonavir ↔enfuvirtide	No clinically significant interaction was noted from a study in 12 HIV patients who received enfuvirtide concomitantly with FORTOVASE/ritonavir 1000/100 mg bid. No dose adjustments are required.
	Other Agents	
Antiarrhythmics: Lidocaine (systemic)	↑ Antiarrhythmics	Caution is warranted and therapeutic concentration monitoring, if available, is recommended for antiarrhythmics given with INVIRASE/ritonavir
Anticoagulant: Warfarin		Concentrations of warfarin may be affected. It is recommended that INR (international normalized ratio) be monitored.
Anticonvulsants: Carbamazepine, phenobarbital, phenytoin	↓ Saquinavir Effect on carbamazepine, phenobarbital, and phenytoin is not well established **INVIRASE/ritonavir** Interaction has not been evaluated	Use with caution, saquinavir may be less effective due to decreased saquinavir plasma concentrations in patients taking these agents concomitantly.
Anti-infective: Clarithromycin*	↑ Saquinavir ↑ Clarithromycin **INVIRASE/ritonavir** Interaction has not been evaluated	No dose adjustment is required when the two drugs are coadministered for a limited time at the doses studied (clarithromycin 500 mg bid and FORTOVASE 1200 mg tid for 7 days). For patients with renal impairment, the following dosage adjustments should be considered: • For patients with CL_{CR} 30 to 60 mL/min the dose of clarithromycin should be reduced by 50%. • For patients with CL_{CR} <30 mL/min the dose of clarithromycin should be decreased by 75%. No dose adjustment for patients with normal renal function is necessary.
Antifungal: Ketoconazole*, itraconazole	↑ Saquinavir ↔Ketoconazole **INVIRASE/ritonavir** Interaction has not been evaluated	No dose adjustment is required when the two drugs are coadministered for a limited time at the doses studied (ketoconazole 400 mg qd and FORTOVASE 1200 mg tid). A similar increase in plasma concentrations of saquinavir could occur with itraconazole.

(Table continued on next page)

Antiretroviral Pregnancy Registry
To monitor maternal-fetal outcomes of pregnant women exposed to antiretroviral medications, including INVIRASE, an Antiretroviral Pregnancy Registry has been established. Physicians are encouraged to register patients by calling 1-800-258-4263.

Nursing Mothers
The Centers for Disease Control and Prevention recommend that HIV-infected mothers not breast-feed their infants to avoid risking postnatal transmission of HIV. It is not known whether saquinavir is excreted in human milk. Because of both the potential for HIV transmission and the potential for serious adverse reactions in nursing infants, **mothers should be instructed not to breast-feed if they are receiving antiretroviral medications, including INVIRASE.**

Pediatric Use
Safety and effectiveness of INVIRASE in HIV-infected pediatric patients younger than 16 years of age have not been established.

Geriatric Use
Clinical studies of INVIRASE did not include sufficient numbers of subjects aged 65 and over to determine whether they respond differently from younger subjects. In general, caution should be taken when dosing INVIRASE in elderly patients due to the greater frequency of decreased hepatic, renal or cardiac function, and of concomitant disease or other drug therapy.

ADVERSE REACTIONS (see PRECAUTIONS)
INVIRASE may be used only if it is combined with ritonavir, which significantly inhibits saquinavir's metabolism to provide plasma saquinavir levels at least equal to those achieved with FORTOVASE. See Concomitant Therapy with Ritonavir Adverse Reactions for safety information with the recommended dosage regimen.
The safety of INVIRASE was studied in patients who received the drug either alone or in combination with zidovudine and/or HIVID (zalcitabine, ddC). The majority of adverse events were of mild intensity. The most frequently reported adverse events among patients receiving INVIRASE in clinical trials (excluding those toxicities known to be associated with zidovudine and HIVID when used in combinations) were diarrhea, abdominal discomfort, and nausea.
The following grade 2 to grade 4 adverse events, (considered at least possibly related to study drug or of unknown relationship) occurred in ≥2% of patients receiving INVIRASE 600 mg tid alone or in combination with zidovudine and/or HIVID: abdominal discomfort, abdominal pain, appetite disturbances, asthenia, buccal mucosa ulceration, diarrhea, dizziness, dyspepsia, extremity numbness, headache, mucosa damage, musculoskeletal pain, myalgia, nausea, paresthesia, peripheral neuropathy, pruritus, and rash.
Rare occurrences of the following serious adverse experiences have been reported during clinical trials of INVIRASE and were considered at least possibly related to use of study drugs: confusion, ataxia, and weakness; acute myeloblastic leukemia; hemolytic anemia; attempted suicide; Stevens-Johnson syndrome; seizures; severe cutaneous reaction associated with increased liver function tests; isolated elevation of transaminases; thrombophlebitis; headache; thrombocytopenia; exacerbation of chronic liver disease with Grade 4 elevated liver function tests, jaundice, ascites, and right and left upper quadrant abdominal pain; drug fever; bullous skin eruption and polyarthritis; pancreatitis leading to death; nephrolithiasis; thrombocytopenia and intracranial hemorrhage leading to death; peripheral vasoconstriction; portal hypertension; intestinal obstruction. These events were reported from a database of >6000 patients. Over 100 patients on INVIRASE therapy have been followed for >2 years.

Concomitant Therapy with Ritonavir Adverse Reactions
In combination with ritonavir the recommended dose of INVIRASE is 1000 mg two times daily with ritonavir 100 mg two times daily in combination with other antiretroviral agents. Table 7 lists grades 2, 3 and 4 related adverse events that occurred in ≥2% of patients receiving FORTOVASE with ritonavir (1000/100 mg bid).

Table 7 **Grade 2, 3 and 4 Related Adverse Events* (All Causality) Reported in ≥2% of Adult Patients in the MaxCmin 1 Study of FORTOVASE in Combination with Ritonavir 1000/100 mg bid**

	FORTOVASE 1000 mg plus Ritonavir 100 mg bid (48 weeks) N=148 n(%=n/N)
Endocrine Disorders	
Diabetes mellitus/hyperglycemia	4 (2.7)
Lipodystrophy	8 (5.4)
Gastrointestinal Disorders	
Nausea	16 (10.8)
Vomiting	11 (7.4)

Continued on next page

Invirase—Cont.

Diarrhea	12 (8.1)
Abdominal Pain	9 (6.1)
Constipation	3 (2.0)
General Disorders and Administration Site Conditions	
Fatigue	9 (6.1)
Fever	5 (3.4)
Musculoskeletal Disorders	
Back Pain	3 (2.0)
Respiratory Disorders	
Pneumonia	8 (5.4)
Bronchitis	4 (2.7)
Influenza	4 (2.7)
Sinusitis	4 (2.7)
Dermatological Disorders	
Rash	5 (3.4)
Pruritus	5 (3.4)
Dry lips/skin	3 (2.0)
Eczema	3 (2.0)

*Includes events with unknown relationship to study drug

Additionally, adverse events that occurred in clinical trials with FORTOVASE, which are not listed above, are listed for completeness. However, due to the higher bioavailability of FORTOVASE, these adverse events might not be predictive of the safety profile of INVIRASE.

Experience from Clinical Trials with FORTOVASE

The safety of FORTOVASE was studied in more than 500 patients who received the drug either alone or in combination with other antiretroviral agents. The most frequently reported adverse events among patients receiving FORTOVASE in combination with other antiretroviral agents were diarrhea, nausea, abdominal discomfort, and dyspepsia. Clinical adverse events of at least moderate intensity, which occurred in ≥2% of patients in 2 studies with FORTOVASE, which are not listed above, are listed below by body system.

Gastrointestinal Disorders: constipation, flatulence, vomiting

Body as a Whole: appetite decreased, chest pain, fatigue

Psychological: depression, insomnia, anxiety, libido disorder

Special Senses: taste alteration

Skin and Appendages: verruca, eczema

Laboratory Abnormalities with INVIRASE

Grade 3 and 4 lab abnormalities have been observed with FORTOVASE in combination with ritonavir. At 48 weeks, lab abnormalities included increased ALT, anemia, increased AST, increased GGT, hyperglycemia, hypertriglyceridemia, increased TSH, neutropenia, raised amylase, raised LDH, and thrombocytopenia.

INVIRASE may be used only if it is combined with ritonavir, which significantly inhibits saquinavir's metabolism to provide plasma saquinavir levels at least equal to those achieved with FORTOVASE.

In studies NV14255/ACTG 229 and NV14256, the following grade 3 or grade 4 abnormalities in laboratory tests were reported among patients receiving INVIRASE 600 mg tid alone or in combination with ZDV and/or HIVID:

Biochemistry

- Incidence between <1% and 4%-hypoglycemia, hyper- or hypocalcemia, hypophosphatemia, hyper- or hypokalemia, hyper- or hyponatremia, raised serum amylase grade 3 or 4 elevations in transaminases (SGOT [AST] SGPT [ALT]), hyperbilirubinemia
- Incidence of ≤5%: hyperglycemia. Incidence of between 7% and 12%: elevated creatine phosphokinase.

Hematology

- Incidence of ≤2%: thrombocytopenia and anemia. Incidence of between 1% and 8%: leucopenia.

Additional marked lab abnormalities have been observed with FORTOVASE. These include: alkaline phosphatase (high), gamma GT (high), and triglycerides (high).

Monotherapy and Combination Studies

Other clinical adverse experiences of any intensity, at least remotely related to INVIRASE, including those in <2% of patients on arms containing INVIRASE in studies NV14255/ACTG229 and NV14256, and those in smaller clinical trials, are listed below by body system.

Body as a Whole: allergic reaction, anorexia, chest pain, edema, fatigue, fever, intoxication, parasites external, retrosternal pain, shivering, wasting syndrome, weakness generalized, weight decrease, redistribution/accumulation of body fat (see PRECAUTIONS: Fat Redistribution)

Table 6 *(cont.)* **Established and Other Potentially Significant Drug Interactions: Alteration in Dose or Regimen May Be Recommended Based on Drug Interaction Studies or Predicted Interaction (Information in the table applies to INVIRASE/ritonavir)**

Concomitant Drug Class: Drug Name	Effect on Concentration of Saquinavir or Concomitant Drug	Clinical Comment
	Other Agents (continued)	
Antimycobacterial Rifabutin*	↓ Saquinavir ↑ Rifabutin	INVIRASE should not be given as the sole protease inhibitor to patients. Appropriate doses of the combination of rifabutin and INVIRASE/ritonavir with respect to safety and efficacy have not been established.
Antimycobacterial Rifampin*	↓ Saquinavir ↑ Rifabutin **INVIRASE/ritonavir** Interaction has not been evaluated	INVIRASE should not be given as the sole protease inhibitor to patients. Appropriate doses of the combination of rifampin and INVIRASE/ritonavir with respect to safety and efficacy have not been established.
Benzodiazepines: Alprazolam, clorazepate, diazepam, flurazepam	↑ Benzodiazepines	Clinical significance is unknown; however, a decrease in benzodiazepine dose may be needed.
Calcium channel blockers: Diltiazem, felodipine, nifedipine, nicardipine, nimodipine, verapamil, amlodipine, nisoldipine, isradipine	↑ Calcium channel blockers	Caution is warranted and clinical monitoring of patients is recommended.
Corticosteroid: Dexamethasone	↓ Saquinavir **INVIRASE/ritonavir** Interaction has not been evaluated	Use with caution, saquinavir may be less effective due to decreased saquinavir plasma concentrations in patients taking these agents concomitantly.
Histamine H_2-receptor antagonist: Ranitidine	↑ Saquinavir **INVIRASE/ritonavir** Interaction has not been evaluated	The increase is not thought to be clinically relevant and no dose adjustment of FORTOVASE is recommended. Appropriate doses of the combination of ranitidine and INVIRASE/ritonavir with respect to safety and efficacy have not been established.
HMG-CoA reductase inhibitors: Simvastatin, lovastatin, atorvastatin	↑ HMG-CoA reductase inhibitors	The combination of INVIRASE/ritonavir with simvastatin and lovastatin should be avoided. Use lowest possible dose of atorvastatin and with careful monitoring or consider other HMG-CoA reductase inhibitors such as pravastatin, fluvastatin and rosuvastatin.
Immunosuppressants: Cyclosporine, tacrolimus, rapamycin	↑ Immunosuppressants	Therapeutic concentration monitoring is recommended for immunosuppressant agents when coadministered with INVIRASE/ritonavir.
Narcotic analgesic: Methadone	↓ Methadone	Dosage of methadone may need to be increased when coadministered with INVIRASE/ritonavir.
Oral contraceptives: Ethinyl estradiol	↓ Ethinyl estradiol	Alternative or additional contraceptive measures should be used when estrogen-based oral contraceptives and INVIRASE/ritonavir are coadministered.
PDE5 inhibitors (phosphodiesterase type 5 inhibitors): Sildenafil*, vardenafil, tadalafil	↑ Sildenafil ↔Saquinavir ↑ Vardenafil ↑ Tadalafil	**Use sildenafil with caution at** reduced doses of 25 mg every 48 hours with increased monitoring of adverse events when administered concomitantly with INVIRASE/ritonavir. Use vardenafil with caution at reduced doses of no more than 2.5 mg every 72 hours with increased monitoring of adverse events when administered concomitantly with INVIRASE/ritonavir. Use tadalafil with caution at reduced doses of no more than 10 mg every 72 hours with increased monitoring of adverse events when administered concomitantly with INVIRASE/ritonavir.
Tricyclic antidepressants: Amitriptyline, imipramine	↑ Tricyclics	Therapeutic concentration monitoring is recommended for tricyclic antidepressants when coadministered with INVIRASE/ritonavir.

*See CLINICAL PHARMACOLOGY: Pharmacokinetics, Tables 2 and 3 for magnitude of interactions

Cardiovascular: cyanosis, heart murmur, heart valve disorder, hypertension, hypotension, syncope, vein distended

Endocrine/Metabolic: dehydration, diabetes mellitus, dry eye syndrome, hyperglycemia, weight increase, xerophthalmia

Gastrointestinal: cheilitis, colic abdominal, constipation, dyspepsia, dysphagia, esophagitis, eructation, feces bloodstained, feces discolored, flatulence, gastralgia, gastritis, gastrointestinal inflammation, gingivitis, glossitis, hemorrhage rectum, hemorrhoids, hepatitis, hepatomegaly, hepa-

tosplenomegaly, infectious diarrhea, jaundice, liver enzyme disorder, melena, pain pelvic, painful defecation, pancreatitis, parotid disorder, salivary glands disorder, stomach upset, stomatitis, toothache, tooth disorder, vomiting
Hematologic: anemia, bleeding dermal, microhemorrhages, neutropenia, pancytopenia, splenomegaly, thrombocytopenia
Musculoskeletal: arthralgia, arthritis, back pain, cramps leg, cramps muscle, creatine phosphokinase increased, musculoskeletal disorders, stiffness, tissue changes, trauma
Neurological: ataxia, bowel movements frequent, confusion, convulsions, dysarthria, dysesthesia, heart rate disorder, hyperesthesia, hyperreflexia, hyporeflexia, light-headed feeling, mouth dry, myelopolyradiculoneuritis, numbness face, pain facial, paresis, poliomyelitis, prickly sensation, progressive multifocal leukoencephalopathy, spasms, tremor, unconsciousness
Psychological: agitation, amnesia, anxiety, anxiety attack, depression, dreaming excessive, euphoria, hallucination, insomnia, intellectual ability reduced, irritability, lethargy, libido disorder, overdose effect, psychic disorder, psychosis, somnolence, speech disorder, suicide attempt
Reproductive System: impotence, prostate enlarged, vaginal discharge
Resistance Mechanism: abscess, angina tonsillaris, candidiasis, cellulitis, herpes simplex, herpes zoster, infection bacterial, infection mycotic, infection staphylococcal, influenza, lymphadenopathy, moniliasis, tumor
Respiratory: bronchitis, cough, dyspnea, epistaxis, hemoptysis, laryngitis, pharyngitis, pneumonia, pulmonary disease, respiratory disorder, rhinitis, sinusitis, upper respiratory tract infection
Skin and Appendages: acne, alopecia, chalazion, dermatitis, dermatitis seborrheic, eczema, erythema, folliculitis, furunculosis, hair changes, hot flushes, nail disorder, night sweats, papillomatosis, photosensitivity reaction, pigment changes skin, rash maculopapular, skin disorder, skin nodule, skin ulceration, sweating increased, urticaria, verruca, xeroderma
Special Senses: blepharitis, earache, ear pressure, eye irritation, hearing decreased, otitis, taste alteration, tinnitus, visual disturbance
Urinary System: micturition disorder, renal calculus, urinary tract bleeding, urinary tract infection

Postmarketing Experience with INVIRASE and FORTOVASE

Additional adverse events that have been observed during the postmarketing period are similar to those seen in clinical trials with INVIRASE and FORTOVASE and administration of INVIRASE and FORTOVASE in combination with ritonavir.

OVERDOSAGE

No acute toxicities or sequelae were noted in 1 patient who ingested 8 grams of INVIRASE as a single dose. The patient was treated with induction of emesis within 2 to 4 hours after ingestion. A second patient ingested 2.4 grams of INVIRASE in combination with 600 mg of ritonavir and experienced pain in the throat that lasted for 6 hours and then resolved. In an exploratory Phase II study of oral dosing with INVIRASE at 7200 mg/day (1200 mg q4h), there were no serious toxicities reported through the first 25 weeks of treatment.

DOSAGE AND ADMINISTRATION

INVIRASE (saquinavir mesylate) capsules and FORTOVASE (saquinavir) soft gelatin capsules are not bioequivalent and cannot be used interchangeably. INVIRASE may be used only if it is combined with ritonavir, because it significantly inhibits saquinavir's metabolism to provide plasma saquinavir levels at least equal to those achieved with FORTOVASE at the recommended dose of 1200 mg tid. When using saquinavir as the sole protease inhibitor in an antiretroviral regimen, FORTOVASE is the recommended formulation (see CLINICAL PHARMACOLOGY: Drug Interactions).

Adults (Over the Age of 16 Years)

- INVIRASE 1000-mg bid (5 x 200-mg capsules) in combination with ritonavir 100-mg bid.
- Ritonavir should be taken at the same time as INVIRASE.
- INVIRASE and ritonavir should be taken within 2 hours after a meal.

Monitoring of Patients

Clinical chemistry tests, viral load, and CD4 count should be performed prior to initiating INVIRASE therapy and at appropriate intervals thereafter. For comprehensive patient monitoring recommendations for other nucleoside analogues, physicians should refer to the complete product information for these drugs.

Dose Adjustment for Combination Therapy with INVIRASE

For serious toxicities that may be associated with INVIRASE, the drug should be interrupted. INVIRASE at doses less than 1000 mg with 100 mg ritonavir bid are not recommended since lower doses have not shown antiviral activity. For recipients of combination therapy with INVIRASE and ritonavir, dose adjustments may be necessary. These adjustments should be based on the known toxicity profile of the individual agent and the pharmacokinetic interaction between saquinavir and the coadministered drug (see PRECAUTIONS: Drug Interactions). Physicians should refer to the complete product information for these drugs for comprehensive dose adjustment recommendations and drug-associated adverse reactions of nucleoside analogues.

HOW SUPPLIED

INVIRASE 200-mg capsules are light brown and green opaque capsules with ROCHE and 0245 imprinted on the capsule shell — bottles of 270 (NDC 0004-0245-15).
The capsules should be stored at 59° to 86°F (15° to 30°C) in tightly closed bottles.
HIVID, FORTOVASE and VERSED are registered trademarks of Hoffmann-La Roche Inc.
KALETRA is a registered trademark of Abbott Laboratories.
Manufactured by:
F. Hoffmann-La Roche Ltd., Basel, Switzerland
or Hoffmann-La Roche Inc., Nutley, New Jersey

Revised: December 2003

Shown in Product Identification Guide, page 331

KLONOPIN® TABLETS ℂ ℞

[klon'o-pin]
(clonazepam)

KLONOPIN® WAFERS

(clonazepam orally disintegrating tablets)

DESCRIPTION

Klonopin, a benzodiazepine, is available as scored tablets with a K-shaped perforation containing 0.5 mg of clonazepam and unscored tablets with a K-shaped perforation containing 1 mg or 2 mg of clonazepam. Each tablet also contains lactose, magnesium stearate, microcrystalline cellulose and corn starch, with the following colorants: 0.5 mg—FD&C Yellow No. 6 Lake; 1 mg—FD&C Blue No. 1 Lake and FD&C Blue No. 2 Lake.
Klonopin is also available as an orally disintegrating tablet containing 0.125 mg, 0.25 mg, 0.5 mg, 1 mg or 2 mg clonazepam. Each orally disintegrating tablet also contains gelatin, mannitol, methylparaben sodium, propylparaben sodium and xanthan gum.
Chemically, clonazepam is 5-(2-chlorophenyl)-1,3-dihydro-7-nitro-2*H*-1,4-benzodiazepin-2-one. It is a light yellow crystalline powder. It has a molecular weight of 315.72.

CLINICAL PHARMACOLOGY

Pharmacodynamics: The precise mechanism by which clonazepam exerts its antiseizure and antipanic effects is unknown, although it is believed to be related to its ability to enhance the activity of gamma aminobutyric acid (GABA), the major inhibitory neurotransmitter in the central nervous system. Convulsions produced in rodents by pentylenetetrazol or, to a lesser extent, electrical stimulation are antagonized, as are convulsions produced by photic stimulation in susceptible baboons. A taming effect in aggressive primates, muscle weakness and hypnosis are also produced. In humans, clonazepam is capable of suppressing the spike and wave discharge in absence seizures (petit mal) and decreasing the frequency, amplitude, duration and spread of discharge in minor motor seizures.
Pharmacokinetics: Clonazepam is rapidly and completely absorbed after oral administration. The absolute bioavailability of clonazepam is about 90%. Maximum plasma concentrations of clonazepam are reached within 1 to 4 hours after oral administration. Clonazepam is approximately 85% bound to plasma proteins. Clonazepam is highly metabolized, with less than 2% unchanged clonazepam being excreted in the urine. Biotransformation occurs mainly by reduction of the 7-nitro group to the 4-amino derivative. This derivative can be acetylated, hydroxylated and glucuronidated. Cytochrome P-450 including CYP3A, may play an important role in clonazepam reduction and oxidation. The elimination half-life of clonazepam is typically 30 to 40 hours. Clonazepam pharmacokinetics are dose-independent throughout the dosing range. There is no evidence that clonazepam induces its own metabolism or that of other drugs in humans.
Pharmacokinetics in Demographic Subpopulations and in Disease States: Controlled studies examining the influence of gender and age on clonazepam pharmacokinetics have not been conducted, nor have the effects of renal or liver disease on clonazepam pharmacokinetics been studied. Because clonazepam undergoes hepatic metabolism, it is possible that liver disease will impair clonazepam elimination. Thus, caution should be exercised when administering clonazepam to these patients.
Clinical Trials: *Panic Disorder:* The effectiveness of Klonopin in the treatment of panic disorder was demonstrated in two double-blind, placebo-controlled studies of adult outpatients who had a primary diagnosis of panic disorder (DSM-IIIR) with or without agoraphobia. In these studies, Klonopin was shown to be significantly more effective than placebo in treating panic disorder on change from baseline in panic attack frequency, the Clinician's Global Impression Severity of Illness Score and the Clinician's Global Impression Improvement Score.
Study 1 was a 9-week, fixed-dose study involving Klonopin doses of 0.5, 1, 2, 3 or 4 mg/day or placebo. This study was conducted in four phases: a 1-week placebo lead-in, a 3-week upward titration, a 6-week fixed dose and a 7-week discontinuance phase. A significant difference from placebo was observed consistently only for the 1 mg/day group. The difference between the 1 mg dose group and placebo in reduction from baseline in the number of full panic attacks was approximately 1 panic attack per week. At endpoint, 74% of patients receiving clonazepam 1 mg/day were free of full panic attacks, compared to 56% of placebo-treated patients.
Study 2 was a 6-week, flexible-dose study involving Klonopin in a dose range of 0.5 to 4 mg/day or placebo. This study was conducted in three phases: a 1-week placebo lead-in, a 6-week optimal-dose and a 6-week discontinuance phase. The mean clonazepam dose during the optimal dosing period was 2.3 mg/day. The difference between Klonopin and placebo in reduction from baseline in the number of full panic attacks was approximately 1 panic attack per week. At endpoint, 62% of patients receiving clonazepam were free of full panic attacks, compared to 37% of placebo-treated patients.
Subgroup analyses did not indicate that there were any differences in treatment outcomes as a function of race or gender.

INDICATIONS AND USAGE

Seizure Disorders: Klonopin is useful alone or as an adjunct in the treatment of the Lennox-Gastaut syndrome (petit mal variant), akinetic and myoclonic seizures. In patients with absence seizures (petit mal) who have failed to respond to succinimides, Klonopin may be useful.
In some studies, up to 30% of patients have shown a loss of anticonvulsant activity, often within 3 months of administration. In some cases, dosage adjustment may reestablish efficacy.
Panic Disorder: Klonopin is indicated for the treatment of panic disorder, with or without agoraphobia, as defined in DSM-IV. Panic disorder is characterized by the occurrence of unexpected panic attacks and associated concern about having additional attacks, worry about the implications or consequences of the attacks, and/or a significant change in behavior related to the attacks.
The efficacy of Klonopin was established in two 6- to 9-week trials in panic disorder patients whose diagnoses corresponded to the DSM-IIIR category of panic disorder (see CLINICAL PHARMACOLOGY: *Clinical Trials*).
Panic disorder (DSM-IV) is characterized by recurrent unexpected panic attacks, ie, a discrete period of intense fear or discomfort in which four (or more) of the following symptoms develop abruptly and reach a peak within 10 minutes: (1) palpitations, pounding heart or accelerated heart rate; (2) sweating; (3) trembling or shaking; (4) sensations of shortness of breath or smothering; (5) feeling of choking; (6) chest pain or discomfort; (7) nausea or abdominal distress; (8) feeling dizzy, unsteady, lightheaded or faint; (9) derealization (feelings of unreality) or depersonalization (being detached from oneself); (10) fear of losing control; (11) fear of dying; (12) paresthesias (numbness or tingling sensations); (13) chills or hot flushes.
The effectiveness of Klonopin in long-term use, that is, for more than 9 weeks, has not been systematically studied in controlled clinical trials. The physician who elects to use Klonopin for extended periods should periodically reevaluate the long-term usefulness of the drug for the individual patient (see DOSAGE AND ADMINISTRATION).

CONTRAINDICATIONS

Klonopin should not be used in patients with a history of sensitivity to benzodiazepines, nor in patients with clinical or biochemical evidence of significant liver disease. It may be used in patients with open angle glaucoma who are receiving appropriate therapy but is contraindicated in acute narrow angle glaucoma.

WARNINGS

Interference With Cognitive and Motor Performance: Since Klonopin produces CNS depression, patients receiving this drug should be cautioned against engaging in hazardous occupations requiring mental alertness, such as operating machinery or driving a motor vehicle. They should also be warned about the concomitant use of alcohol or other CNS-depressant drugs during Klonopin therapy (see PRECAUTIONS: *Drug Interactions* and *Information for Patients*).
Pregnancy Risks: Data from several sources raise concerns about the use of Klonopin during pregnancy.
Animal Findings: In three studies in which Klonopin was administered orally to pregnant rabbits at doses of 0.2, 1, 5 or 10 mg/kg/day (low dose approximately 0.2 times the maximum recommended human dose of 20 mg/day for seizure disorders and equivalent to the maximum dose of 4 mg/day for panic disorder, on a mg/m^2 basis) during the period of organogenesis, a similar pattern of malformations (cleft palate, open eyelid, fused sternebrae and limb defects) was observed in a low, non-dose-related incidence in exposed litters from all dosage groups. Reductions in maternal weight gain occurred at dosages of 5 mg/kg/day or greater and reduction in embryo-fetal growth occurred in one study at a dosage of 10 mg/kg/day. No adverse maternal or embryo-fetal effects were observed in mice and rats following administration during organogenesis of oral doses up to 15 mg/kg/day or 40 mg/kg/day, respectively (4 and 20 times the maximum recommended human dose of 20 mg/day for seizure disorders and 20 and 100 times the maximum dose of 4 mg/day for panic disorder, respectively, on a mg/m^2 basis).
General Concerns and Considerations About Anticonvulsants: Recent reports suggest an association between the use of anticonvulsant drugs by women with epilepsy and an elevated incidence of birth defects in children born to these

Continued on next page

Klonopin—Cont.

women. Data are more extensive with respect to diphenylhydantoin and phenobarbital, but these are also the most commonly prescribed anticonvulsants; less systematic or anecdotal reports suggest a possible similar association with the use of all known anticonvulsant drugs.

In children of women treated with drugs for epilepsy, reports suggesting an elevated incidence of birth defects cannot be regarded as adequate to prove a definite cause and effect relationship. There are intrinsic methodologic problems in obtaining adequate data on drug teratogenicity in humans; the possibility also exists that other factors (eg, genetic factors or the epileptic condition itself) may be more important than drug therapy in leading to birth defects. The great majority of mothers on anticonvulsant medication deliver normal infants. It is important to note that anticonvulsant drugs should not be discontinued in patients in whom the drug is administered to prevent seizures because of the strong possibility of precipitating status epilepticus with attendant hypoxia and threat to life. In individual cases where the severity and frequency of the seizure disorder are such that the removal of medication does not pose a serious threat to the patient, discontinuation of the drug may be considered prior to and during pregnancy; however, it cannot be said with any confidence that even mild seizures do not pose some hazards to the developing embryo or fetus.

General Concerns About Benzodiazepines: An increased risk of congenital malformations associated with the use of benzodiazepine drugs has been suggested in several studies. There may also be non-teratogenic risks associated with the use of benzodiazepines during pregnancy. There have been reports of neonatal flaccidity, respiratory and feeding difficulties, and hypothermia in children born to mothers who have been receiving benzodiazepines late in pregnancy. In addition, children born to mothers receiving benzodiazepines late in pregnancy may be at some risk of experiencing withdrawal symptoms during the postnatal period.

Advice Regarding the Use of Klonopin in Women of Childbearing Potential: In general, the use of Klonopin in women of childbearing potential, and more specifically during known pregnancy, should be considered only when the clinical situation warrants the risk to the fetus.

The specific considerations addressed above regarding the use of anticonvulsants for epilepsy in women of childbearing potential should be weighed in treating or counseling these women.

Because of experience with other members of the benzodiazepine class, Klonopin is assumed to be capable of causing an increased risk of congenital abnormalities when administered to a pregnant woman during the first trimester. Because use of these drugs is rarely a matter of urgency in the treatment of panic disorder, their use during the first trimester should almost always be avoided. The possibility that a woman of childbearing potential may be pregnant at the time of institution of therapy should be considered. If this drug is used during pregnancy, or if the patient becomes pregnant while taking this drug, the patient should be apprised of the potential hazard to the fetus. Patients should also be advised that if they become pregnant during therapy or intend to become pregnant, they should communicate with their physician about the desirability of discontinuing the drug.

Withdrawal Symptoms: Withdrawal symptoms of the barbiturate type have occurred after the discontinuation of benzodiazepines (see DRUG ABUSE AND DEPENDENCE).

PRECAUTIONS

General: *Worsening of Seizures:* When used in patients in whom several different types of seizure disorders coexist, Klonopin may increase the incidence or precipitate the onset of generalized tonic-clonic seizures (grand mal). This may require the addition of appropriate anticonvulsants or an increase in their dosages. The concomitant use of valproic acid and Klonopin may produce absence status.

Laboratory Testing During Long-Term Therapy: Periodic blood counts and liver function tests are advisable during long-term therapy with Klonopin.

Risks of Abrupt Withdrawal: The abrupt withdrawal of Klonopin, particularly in those patients on long-term, high-dose therapy, may precipitate status epilepticus. Therefore, when discontinuing Klonopin, gradual withdrawal is essential. While Klonopin is being gradually withdrawn, the simultaneous substitution of another anticonvulsant may be indicated.

Caution in Renally Impaired Patients: Metabolites of Klonopin are excreted by the kidneys; to avoid their excess accumulation, caution should be exercised in the administration of the drug to patients with impaired renal function.

Hypersalivation: Klonopin may produce an increase in salivation. This should be considered before giving the drug to patients who have difficulty handling secretions. Because of this and the possibility of respiratory depression, Klonopin should be used with caution in patients with chronic respiratory diseases.

Information for Patients: Physicians are advised to discuss the following issues with patients for whom they prescribe Klonopin:

Dose Changes: To assure the safe and effective use of benzodiazepines, patients should be informed that, since benzodiazepines may produce psychological and physical dependence, it is advisable that they consult with their physician before either increasing the dose or abruptly discontinuing this drug.

Interference With Cognitive and Motor Performance: Because benzodiazepines have the potential to impair judgment, thinking or motor skills, patients should be cautioned about operating hazardous machinery, including automobiles, until they are reasonably certain that Klonopin therapy does not affect them adversely.

Pregnancy: Patients should be advised to notify their physician if they become pregnant or intend to become pregnant during therapy with Klonopin (see WARNINGS).

Nursing: Patients should be advised not to breastfeed an infant if they are taking Klonopin.

Concomitant Medication: Patients should be advised to inform their physicians if they are taking, or plan to take, any prescription or over-the-counter drugs, since there is a potential for interactions.

Alcohol: Patients should be advised to avoid alcohol while taking Klonopin.

Drug Interactions: *Effect of Clonazepam on the Pharmacokinetics of Other Drugs:* Clonazepam does not appear to alter the pharmacokinetics of phenytoin, carbamazepine or phenobarbital. The effect of clonazepam on the metabolism of other drugs has not been investigated.

Effect of Other Drugs on the Pharmacokinetics of Clonazepam: Literature reports suggest that ranitidine, an agent that decreases stomach acidity, does not greatly alter clonazepam pharmacokinetics.

In a study in which the 2 mg clonazepam orally disintegrating tablet was administered with and without propantheline (an anticholinergic agent with multiple effects on the GI tract) to healthy volunteers, the AUC of clonazepam was 10% lower and the C_{max} of clonazepam was 20% lower when the orally disintegrating tablet was given with propantheline compared to when it was given alone.

Fluoxetine does not affect the pharmacokinetics of clonazepam. Cytochrome P-450 inducers, such as phenytoin, carbamazepine and phenobarbital, induce clonazepam metabolism, causing an approximately 30% decrease in plasma clonazepam levels. Although clinical studies have not been performed, based on the involvement of the cytochrome P-450 3A family in clonazepam metabolism, inhibitors of this enzyme system, notably oral antifungal agents, should be used cautiously in patients receiving clonazepam.

Pharmacodynamic Interactions: The CNS-depressant action of the benzodiazepine class of drugs may be potentiated by alcohol, narcotics, barbiturates, nonbarbiturate hypnotics, antianxiety agents, the phenothiazines, thioxanthene and butyrophenone classes of antipsychotic agents, monoamine oxidase inhibitors and the tricyclic antidepressants, and by other anticonvulsant drugs.

Carcinogenesis, Mutagenesis, Impairment of Fertility: Carcinogenicity studies have not been conducted with clonazepam.

The data currently available are not sufficient to determine the genotoxic potential of clonazepam.

In a two-generation fertility study in which clonazepam was given orally to rats at 10 and 100 mg/kg/day (low dose approximately 5 times and 24 times the maximum recommended human dose of 20 mg/day for seizure disorder and 4 mg/day for panic disorder, respectively, on a mg/m^2 basis), there was a decrease in the number of pregnancies and in the number of offspring surviving until weaning.

Pregnancy: *Teratogenic Effects:* Pregnancy Category D (see WARNINGS).

Labor and Delivery: The effect of Klonopin on labor and delivery in humans has not been specifically studied; however, perinatal complications have been reported in children born to mothers who have been receiving benzodiazepines late in pregnancy, including findings suggestive of either excess benzodiazepine exposure or of withdrawal phenomena (see WARNINGS: *Pregnancy Risks*).

Nursing Mothers: Mothers receiving Klonopin should not breastfeed their infants.

Pediatric Use: Because of the possibility that adverse effects on physical or mental development could become apparent only after many years, a benefit-risk consideration of the long-term use of Klonopin is important in pediatric patients being treated for seizure disorder (see INDICATIONS AND USAGE and DOSAGE AND ADMINISTRATION).

Safety and effectiveness in pediatric patients with panic disorder below the age of 18 have not been established.

Geriatric Use: Clinical studies of Klonopin did not include sufficient numbers of subjects aged 65 and over to determine whether they respond differently from younger subjects. Other reported clinical experience has not identified differences in responses between the elderly and younger patients. In general, dose selection for an elderly patient should be cautious, usually starting at the low end of the dosing range, reflecting the greater frequency of decreased hepatic, renal, or cardiac function, and of concomitant disease or other drug therapy.

Because clonazepam undergoes hepatic metabolism, it is possible that liver disease will impair clonazepam elimination. Metabolites of Klonopin are excreted by the kidneys; to avoid their excess accumulation, caution should be exercised in the administration of the drug to patients with impaired renal function. Because elderly patients are more likely to have decreased hepatic and/or renal function, care should be taken in dose selection, and it may be useful to assess hepatic and/or renal function at the time of dose selection.

Sedating drugs may cause confusion and over-sedation in the elderly; elderly patients generally should be started on low doses of Klonopin and observed closely.

ADVERSE REACTIONS

The adverse experiences for Klonopin are provided separately for patients with seizure disorders and with panic disorder.

Seizure Disorders: The most frequently occurring side effects of Klonopin are referable to CNS depression. Experience in treatment of seizures has shown that drowsiness has occurred in approximately 50% of patients and ataxia in approximately 30%. In some cases, these may diminish with time; behavior problems have been noted in approximately 25% of patients. Others, listed by system, are:

Neurologic: Abnormal eye movements, aphonia, choreiform movements, coma, diplopia, dysarthria, dysdiadochokinesis, "glassy-eyed" appearance, headache, hemiparesis, hypotonia, nystagmus, respiratory depression, slurred speech, tremor, vertigo

Psychiatric: Confusion, depression, amnesia, hallucinations, hysteria, increased libido, insomnia, psychosis, suicidal attempt (the behavior effects are more likely to occur in patients with a history of psychiatric disturbances). The following paradoxical reactions have been observed: excitability, irritability, aggressive behavior, agitation, nervousness, hostility, anxiety, sleep disturbances, nightmares and vivid dreams

Respiratory: Chest congestion, rhinorrhea, shortness of breath, hypersecretion in upper respiratory passages

Cardiovascular: Palpitations

Dermatologic: Hair loss, hirsutism, skin rash, ankle and facial edema

Gastrointestinal: Anorexia, coated tongue, constipation, diarrhea, dry mouth, encopresis, gastritis, increased appetite, nausea, sore gums

Genitourinary: Dysuria, enuresis, nocturia, urinary retention

Musculoskeletal: Muscle weakness, pains

Miscellaneous: Dehydration, general deterioration, fever, lymphadenopathy, weight loss or gain

Hematopoietic: Anemia, leukopenia, thrombocytopenia, eosinophilia

Hepatic: Hepatomegaly, transient elevations of serum transaminases and alkaline phosphatase

Panic Disorder: Adverse events during exposure to Klonopin were obtained by spontaneous report and recorded by clinical investigators using terminology of their own choosing. Consequently, it is not possible to provide a meaningful estimate of the proportion of individuals experiencing adverse events without first grouping similar types of events into a smaller number of standardized event categories. In the tables and tabulations that follow, CIGY dictionary terminology has been used to classify reported adverse events, except in certain cases in which redundant terms were collapsed into more meaningful terms, as noted below.

The stated frequencies of adverse events represent the proportion of individuals who experienced, at least once, a treatment-emergent adverse event of the type listed. An event was considered treatment-emergent if it occurred for the first time or worsened while receiving therapy following baseline evaluation.

Adverse Findings Observed in Short-Term, Placebo-Controlled Trials:

Adverse Events Associated With Discontinuation of Treatment:

Overall, the incidence of discontinuation due to adverse events was 17% in Klonopin compared to 9% for placebo in the combined data of two 6- to 9-week trials. The most common events (≥1%) associated with discontinuation and a dropout rate twice or greater for Klonopin than that of placebo included the following:

Adverse Event	Klonopin (N=574)	Placebo (N=294)
Somnolence	7%	1%
Depression	4%	1%
Dizziness	1%	<1%
Nervousness	1%	0%
Ataxia	1%	0%
Intellectual Ability Reduced	1%	0%

Adverse Events Occurring at an Incidence of 1% or More Among Klonopin-Treated Patients:

Table 1 enumerates the incidence, rounded to the nearest percent, of treatment-emergent adverse events that occurred during acute therapy of panic disorder from a pool of two 6- to 9-week trials. Events reported in 1% or more of patients treated with Klonopin (doses ranging from 0.5 to 4 mg/day) and for which the incidence was greater than that in placebo-treated patients are included.

The prescriber should be aware that the figures in Table 1 cannot be used to predict the incidence of side effects in the course of usual medical practice where patient characteristics and other factors differ from those that prevailed in the clinical trials. Similarly, the cited frequencies cannot be compared with figures obtained from other clinical investi-

gations involving different treatments, uses and investigators. The cited figures, however, do provide the prescribing physician with some basis for estimating the relative contribution of drug and nondrug factors to the side effect incidence in the population studied.
[See table 1 at right]

Commonly Observed Adverse Events:
Table 2. Incidence of Most Commonly Observed Adverse Events* in Acute Therapy in Pool of 6- to 9-Week Trials

Adverse Event (Roche Preferred Term)	Clonazepam (N=574)	Placebo (N=294)
Somnolence	37%	10%
Depression	7%	1%
Coordination Abnormal	6%	0%
Ataxia	5%	0%

* Treatment-emergent events for which the incidence in the clonazepam patients was ≥5% and at least twice that in the placebo patients.

Treatment-Emergent Depressive Symptoms:
In the pool of two short-term placebo-controlled trials, adverse events classified under the preferred term "depression" were reported in 7% of Klonopin-treated patients compared to 1% of placebo-treated patients, without any clear pattern of dose relatedness. In these same trials, adverse events classified under the preferred term "depression" were reported as leading to discontinuation in 4% of Klonopin-treated patients compared to 1% of placebo-treated patients. While these findings are noteworthy, Hamilton Depression Rating Scale (HAM-D) data collected in these trials revealed a larger decline in HAM-D scores in the clonazepam group than the placebo group suggesting that clonazepam-treated patients were not experiencing a worsening or emergence of clinical depression.
Other Adverse Events Observed During the Premarketing Evaluation of Klonopin in Panic Disorder:
Following is a list of modified CIGY terms that reflect treatment-emergent adverse events reported by patients treated with Klonopin at multiple doses during clinical trials. All reported events are included except those already listed in Table 1 or elsewhere in labeling, those events for which a drug cause was remote, those event terms which were so general as to be uninformative, and events reported only once and which did not have a substantial probability of being acutely life-threatening. It is important to emphasize that, although the events occurred during treatment with Klonopin, they were not necessarily caused by it.
Events are further categorized by body system and listed in order of decreasing frequency. These adverse events were reported infrequently, which is defined as occurring in 1/100 to 1/1000 patients.
Body as a Whole: weight increase, accident, weight decrease, wound, edema, fever, shivering, abrasions, ankle edema, edema foot, edema periorbital, injury, malaise, pain, cellulitis, inflammation localized
Cardiovascular Disorders: chest pain, hypotension postural
Central and Peripheral Nervous System Disorders: migraine, paresthesia, drunkenness, feeling of enuresis, paresis, tremor, burning skin, falling, head fullness, hoarseness, hyperactivity, hypoesthesia, tongue thick, twitching
Gastrointestinal System Disorders: abdominal discomfort, gastrointestinal inflammation, stomach upset, toothache, flatulence, pyrosis, saliva increased, tooth disorder, bowel movements frequent, pain pelvic, dyspepsia, hemorrhoids
Hearing and Vestibular Disorders: vertigo, otitis, earache, motion sickness
Heart Rate and Rhythm Disorders: palpitation
Metabolic and Nutritional Disorders: thirst, gout
Musculoskeletal System Disorders: back pain, fracture traumatic, sprains and strains, pain leg, pain nape, cramps muscle, cramps leg, pain ankle, pain shoulder, tendinitis, arthralgia, hypertonia, lumbago, pain feet, pain jaw, pain knee, swelling knee
Platelet, Bleeding and Clotting Disorders: bleeding dermal
Psychiatric Disorders: insomnia, organic disinhibition, anxiety, depersonalization, dreaming excessive, libido loss, appetite increased, libido increased, reactions decreased, aggressive reaction, apathy, attention lack, excitement, feeling mad, hunger abnormal, illusion, nightmares, sleep disorder, suicide ideation, yawning
Reproductive Disorders, Female: breast pain, menstrual irregularity
Reproductive Disorders, Male: ejaculation decreased
Resistance Mechanism Disorders: infection mycotic, infection viral, infection streptococcal, herpes simplex infection, infectious mononucleosis, moniliasis
Respiratory System Disorders: sneezing excessive, asthmatic attack, dyspnea, nosebleed, pneumonia, pleurisy
Skin and Appendages Disorders: acne flare, alopecia, xeroderma, dermatitis contact, flushing, pruritus, pustular reaction, skin burns, skin disorder
Special Senses Other, Disorders: taste loss
Urinary System Disorders: dysuria, cystitis, polyuria, urinary incontinence, bladder dysfunction, urinary retention, urinary tract bleeding, urine discoloration
Vascular (Extracardiac) Disorders: thrombophlebitis leg

Table 1. Treatment-Emergent Adverse Event Incidence in 6- to 9-Week Placebo-Controlled Clinical Trials*

Clonazepam Maximum Daily Dose						
Adverse Event by Body System	**<1mg n=96 %**	**1-<2mg n=129 %**	**2-<3mg n=113 %**	**≥3mg n=235 %**	**All Klonopin Groups N=574 %**	**Placebo N=294 %**
Central & Peripheral Nervous System						
Somnolence†	26	35	50	36	37	10
Dizziness	5	5	12	8	8	4
Coordination Abnormal†	1	2	7	9	6	0
Ataxia†	2	1	8	8	5	0
Dysarthria†	0	0	4	3	2	0
Psychiatric						
Depression	7	6	8	8	7	1
Memory Disturbance	2	5	2	5	4	2
Nervousness	1	4	3	4	3	2
Intellecutal Ability Reduced	0	2	4	3	2	0
Emotional Lability	0	1	2	2	1	1
Libido Decreased	0	1	3	1	1	0
Confusion	0	2	2	1	1	0
Respiratory System						
Upper Respiratory Tract Infection†	10	10	7	6	8	4
Sinusitis	4	2	8	4	4	3
Rhinitis	3	2	4	2	2	1
Coughing	2	2	4	0	2	0
Pharyngitis	1	1	3	2	2	1
Bronchitis	1	0	2	2	1	1
Gastrointestinal System						
Constipation†	0	1	5	3	2	2
Appetite Decreased	1	1	0	3	1	1
Abdominal Pain†	2	2	2	0	1	1
Body as a Whole						
Fatigue	9	6	7	7	7	4
Allergic Reaction	3	1	4	2	2	1
Musculoskeletal						
Myalgia	2	1	4	0	1	1
Resistance Mechanism Disorders						
Influenza	3	2	5	5	4	3
Urinary System						
Micturition Frequency	1	2	2	1	1	0
Urinary Tract Infection†	0	0	2	2	1	0
Vision Disorders						
Blurred Vision	1	2	3	0	1	1
Reproductive Disorders‡						
Female						
Dysmenorrhea	0	6	5	2	3	2
Colpitis	4	0	2	1	1	1
Male						
Ejaculation Delayed	0	0	2	2	1	0
Impotence	3	0	2	1	1	0

*Events reported by at least 1% of patients treated with Klonopin and for which the incidence was greater than that for placebo.
†Indicates that the p-value for the dose-trend test (Cochran-Mantel-Haenszel) for adverse event incidence was ≤0.10.
‡Denominators for events in gender-specific systems are: n=240 (clonazepam), 102 (placebo) for male, and 334 (clonazepam), 192 (placebo) for female.

Vision Disorders: eye irritation, visual disturbance, diplopia, eye twitching, styes, visual field defect, xerophthalmia

DRUG ABUSE AND DEPENDENCE

Controlled Substance Class: Clonazepam is a Schedule IV controlled substance.
Physical and Psychological Dependence: Withdrawal symptoms, similar in character to those noted with barbiturates and alcohol (eg, convulsions, psychosis, hallucinations, behavioral disorder, tremor, abdominal and muscle cramps) have occurred following abrupt discontinuance of clonazepam. The more severe withdrawal symptoms have usually been limited to those patients who received excessive doses over an extended period of time. Generally milder withdrawal symptoms (eg, dysphoria and insomnia) have been reported following abrupt discontinuance of benzodiazepines taken continuously at therapeutic levels for several months. Consequently, after extended therapy, abrupt discontinuation should generally be avoided and a gradual dosage tapering schedule followed (see DOSAGE AND ADMINISTRATION). Addiction-prone individuals (such as drug addicts or alcoholics) should be under careful surveillance when receiving clonazepam or other psychotropic agents because of the predisposition of such patients to habituation and dependence.
Following the short-term treatment of patients with panic disorder in Studies 1 and 2 (see CLINICAL PHARMACOLOGY: *Clinical Trials*), patients were gradually withdrawn during a 7-week downward-titration (discontinuance) period. Overall, the discontinuance period was associated with good tolerability and a very modest clinical deterioration, without evidence of a significant rebound phenomenon. However, there are not sufficient data from adequate and well-controlled long-term clonazepam studies in patients with panic disorder to accurately estimate the risks of withdrawal symptoms and dependence that may be associated with such use.

OVERDOSAGE

Human Experience: Symptoms of clonazepam overdosage, like those produced by other CNS depressants, include somnolence, confusion, coma and diminished reflexes.
Overdose Management: Treatment includes monitoring of respiration, pulse and blood pressure, general supportive measures and immediate gastric lavage. Intravenous fluids should be administered and an adequate airway maintained. Hypotension may be combated by the use of levarterenol or metaraminol. Dialysis is of no known value.
Flumazenil, a specific benzodiazepine-receptor antagonist, is indicated for the complete or partial reversal of the sedative effects of benzodiazepines and may be used in situations when an overdose with a benzodiazepine is known or suspected. Prior to the administration of flumazenil, necessary measures should be instituted to secure airway, ventilation and intravenous access. Flumazenil is intended as an adjunct to, not as a substitute for, proper management of benzodiazepine overdose. Patients treated with flumazenil should be monitored for resedation, respiratory depression and other residual benzodiazepine effects for an appropriate period after treatment. **The prescriber should be aware of a risk of seizure in association with flumazenil treatment, particularly in long-term benzodiazepine users and in cyclic antidepressant overdose.** The complete flumazenil package insert, including CONTRAINDICATIONS, WARNINGS and PRECAUTIONS, should be consulted prior to use.

Continued on next page

Klonopin—Cont.

Flumazenil is not indicated in patients with epilepsy who have been treated with benzodiazepines. Antagonism of the benzodiazepine effect in such patients may provoke seizures.

Serious sequelae are rare unless other drugs or alcohol have been taken concomitantly.

DOSAGE AND ADMINISTRATION

Clonazepam is available as a tablet or an orally disintegrating tablet (wafer). The tablets should be administered with water by swallowing the tablet whole. The orally disintegrating tablet should be administered as follows: After opening the pouch, peel back the foil on the blister. Do not push tablet through foil. Immediately upon opening the blister, using dry hands, remove the tablet and place it in the mouth. Tablet disintegration occurs rapidly in saliva so it can be easily swallowed with or without water.

Seizure Disorders: *Adults:* The initial dose for adults with seizure disorders should not exceed 1.5 mg/day divided into three doses. Dosage may be increased in increments of 0.5 to 1 mg every 3 days until seizures are adequately controlled or until side effects preclude any further increase. Maintenance dosage must be individualized for each patient depending upon response. Maximum recommended daily dose is 20 mg.

The use of multiple anticonvulsants may result in an increase of depressant adverse effects. This should be considered before adding Klonopin to an existing anticonvulsant regimen.

Pediatric Patients: Klonopin is administered orally. In order to minimize drowsiness, the initial dose for infants and children (up to 10 years of age or 30 kg of body weight) should be between 0.01 and 0.03 mg/kg/day but not to exceed 0.05 mg/kg/day given in two or three divided doses. Dosage should be increased by no more than 0.25 to 0.5 mg every third day until a daily maintenance dose of 0.1 to 0.2 mg/kg of body weight has been reached, unless seizures are controlled or side effects preclude further increase. Whenever possible, the daily dose should be divided into three equal doses. If doses are not equally divided, the largest dose should be given before retiring.

Geriatric Patients: There is no clinical trial experience with Klonopin in seizure disorder patients 65 years of age and older. In general, elderly patients should be started on low doses of Klonopin and observed closely (see PRECAUTIONS: *Geriatric Use*).

Panic Disorder: *Adults:* The initial dose for adults with panic disorder is 0.25 mg bid. An increase to the target dose for most patients of 1 mg/day may be made after 3 days. The recommended dose of 1 mg/day is based on the results from a fixed dose study in which the optimal effect was seen at 1 mg/day. Higher doses of 2, 3 and 4 mg/day in that study were less effective than the 1 mg/day dose and were associated with more adverse effects. Nevertheless, it is possible that some individual patients may benefit from doses of up to a maximum dose of 4 mg/day, and in those instances, the dose may be increased in increments of 0.125 to 0.25 mg bid every 3 days until panic disorder is controlled or until side effects make further increases undesired. To reduce the inconvenience of somnolence, administration of one dose at bedtime may be desirable.

Treatment should be discontinued gradually, with a decrease of 0.125 mg bid every 3 days, until the drug is completely withdrawn.

There is no body of evidence available to answer the question of how long the patient treated with clonazepam should remain on it. Therefore, the physician who elects to use Klonopin for extended periods should periodically reevaluate the long-term usefulness of the drug for the individual patient.

Pediatric Patients: There is no clinical trial experience with Klonopin in panic disorder patients under 18 years of age.

Geriatric Patients: There is no clinical trial experience with Klonopin in panic disorder patients 65 years of age and older. In general, elderly patients should be started on low doses of Klonopin and observed closely (see PRECAUTIONS: *Geriatric Use*).

HOW SUPPLIED

Klonopin tablets are available as scored tablets with a K-shaped perforation—0.5 mg, orange (NDC 0004-0068-01); and unscored tablets with a K-shaped perforation—1 mg, blue (NDC 0004-0058-01); 2 mg, white (NDC 0004-0098-01)—bottles of 100.

Imprint on tablets:

0.5 mg—1/2 KLONOPIN (front)
ROCHE (scored side)

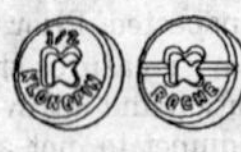

1 mg—1 KLONOPIN (front)
ROCHE (reverse side)

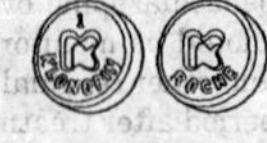

2 mg—2 KLONOPIN (front)
ROCHE (reverse side)

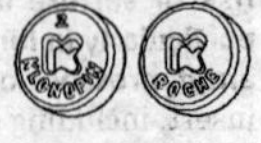

Klonopin Wafers (clonazepam orally disintegrating tablets) are white, round and debossed with the tablet strength expressed as a fraction or whole number (1/8, 1/4, 1/2, 1, or 2). The tablets are available in blister packages of 60 (10 pouches/carton) as follows:

0.125 mg	debossed 1/8, (NDC 0004-0279-22)
0.25 mg	debossed 1/4, (NDC 0004-0280-22)
0.5 mg	debossed 1/2, (NDC 0004-0281-22)
1 mg	debossed 1, (NDC 0004-0282-22)
2 mg	debossed 2, (NDC 0004-0283-22)

Store at 25°C (77°F); excursions permitted to 15° to 30°C (59° to 86°F).

Revised: July 2001

Shown in Product Identification Guide, page 331

KYTRIL ℞
(granisetron hydrochloride)
Injection

DESCRIPTION

KYTRIL (granisetron hydrochloride) Injection is an antinauseant and antiemetic agent. Chemically it is *endo*-N-(9-methyl-9-azabicyclo [3.3.1] non-3-yl)-1-methyl-1H-indazole-3-carboxamide hydrochloride with a molecular weight of 348.9 (312.4 free base). Its empirical formula is $C_{18}H_{24}N_4O \bullet HCl$.

Granisetron hydrochloride is a white to off-white solid that is readily soluble in water and normal saline at 20°C. KYTRIL Injection is a clear, colorless, sterile, nonpyrogenic, aqueous solution for intravenous administration.

KYTRIL is available in 1 mL single-dose and 4 mL multi-dose vials.

Single-Dose Vials

Each 1 mL of preservative-free aqueous solution contains 1.12 mg granisetron hydrochloride equivalent to granisetron, 1 mg and sodium chloride, 9 mg. The solution's pH ranges from 4.7 to 7.3.

Multi-Dose Vials

Each 1 mL contains 1.12 mg granisetron hydrochloride equivalent to granisetron, 1 mg; sodium chloride, 9 mg; citric acid, 2 mg; and benzyl alcohol, 10 mg, as a preservative. The solution's pH ranges from 4.0 to 6.0.

CLINICAL PHARMACOLOGY

Granisetron is a selective 5-hydroxytryptamine$_3$ (5-HT$_3$) receptor antagonist with little or no affinity for other serotonin receptors, including 5-HT$_1$; 5-HT$_{1A}$; 5-HT$_{1B/C}$; 5-HT$_2$; for alpha$_1$-, alpha$_2$- or beta-adrenoreceptors; for dopamine-D$_2$; or for histamine-H$_1$; benzodiazepine; picrotoxin or opioid receptors.

Serotonin receptors of the 5-HT$_3$ type are located peripherally on vagal nerve terminals and centrally in the chemoreceptor trigger zone of the area postrema. During chemotherapy-induced vomiting, mucosal enterochromaffin cells release serotonin, which stimulates 5-HT$_3$ receptors. This evokes vagal afferent discharge and may induce vomiting. Animal studies demonstrate that, in binding to 5-HT$_3$ receptors, granisetron blocks serotonin stimulation and subsequent vomiting after emetogenic stimuli such as cisplatin. In the ferret animal model, a single granisetron injection prevented vomiting due to high-dose cisplatin or arrested vomiting within 5 to 30 seconds.

In most human studies, granisetron has had little effect on blood pressure, heart rate or ECG. No evidence of an effect on plasma prolactin or aldosterone concentrations has been found in other studies.

KYTRIL Injection exhibited no effect on oro-cecal transit time in normal volunteers given a single intravenous infusion of 50 mcg/kg or 200 mcg/kg. Single and multiple oral doses slowed colonic transit in normal volunteers.

Pharmacokinetics

Chemotherapy-Induced Nausea and Vomiting

In adult cancer patients undergoing chemotherapy and in volunteers, mean pharmacokinetic data obtained from an infusion of a single 40 mcg/kg dose of KYTRIL Injection are shown in Table 1.

[See table 1 below]

Distribution

Plasma protein binding is approximately 65% and granisetron distributes freely between plasma and red blood cells.

Metabolism

Granisetron metabolism involves N-demethylation and aromatic ring oxidation followed by conjugation. In vitro liver microsomal studies show that granisetron's major route of metabolism is inhibited by ketoconazole, suggestive of metabolism mediated by the cytochrome P-450 3A subfamily. Animal studies suggest that some of the metabolites may also have 5-HT$_3$ receptor antagonist activity.

Elimination

Clearance is predominantly by hepatic metabolism. In normal volunteers, approximately 12% of the administered dose is eliminated unchanged in the urine in 48 hours. The remainder of the dose is excreted as metabolites, 49% in the urine, and 34% in the feces.

Subpopulations

Gender

There was high inter- and intra-subject variability noted in these studies. No difference in mean AUC was found between males and females, although males had a higher C_{max} generally.

Geriatrics

The ranges of the pharmacokinetic parameters in geriatric volunteers (mean age 71 years), given a single 40 mcg/kg intravenous dose of KYTRIL Injection, were generally similar to those in younger healthy volunteers; mean values were lower for clearance and longer for half-life in the geriatric patients (see Table 1).

Pediatric Patients

A pharmacokinetic study in pediatric cancer patients (2 to 16 years of age), given a single 40 mcg/kg intravenous dose of KYTRIL Injection, showed that volume of distribution and total clearance increased with age. No relationship with age was observed for peak plasma concentration or terminal phase plasma half-life. When volume of distribution and total clearance are adjusted for body weight, the pharmacokinetics of granisetron are similar in pediatric and adult cancer patients.

Renal Failure Patients

Total clearance of granisetron was not affected in patients with severe renal failure who received a single 40 mcg/kg intravenous dose of KYTRIL Injection.

Hepatically Impaired Patients

A pharmacokinetic study in patients with hepatic impairment due to neoplastic liver involvement showed that total clearance was approximately halved compared to patients without hepatic impairment. Given the wide variability in pharmacokinetic parameters noted in patients and the good tolerance of doses well above the recommended 10 mcg/kg dose, dosage adjustment in patients with possible hepatic functional impairment is not necessary.

Postoperative Nausea and Vomiting

In adult patients (age range, 18 to 64 years) recovering from elective surgery and receiving general balanced anesthesia, mean pharmacokinetic data obtained from a single 1 mg dose of KYTRIL Injection administered intravenously over 30 seconds are shown in Table 2.

[See table 2 at top of next page]

The pharmacokinetics of granisetron in patients undergoing surgery were similar to those seen in cancer patients undergoing chemotherapy.

CLINICAL TRIALS

Chemotherapy-Induced Nausea and Vomiting

Single-Day Chemotherapy

Cisplatin-Based Chemotherapy

In a double-blind, placebo-controlled study in 28 cancer patients, KYTRIL Injection, administered as a single intravenous infusion of 40 mcg/kg, was significantly more effective than placebo in preventing nausea and vomiting induced by cisplatin chemotherapy (see Table 3).

[See table 3 at top of next page]

KYTRIL Injection was also evaluated in a randomized dose response study of cancer patients receiving cisplatin ≥75 mg/m^2. Additional chemotherapeutic agents included: anthracyclines, carboplatin, cytostatic antibiotics, folic acid derivatives, methylhydrazine, nitrogen mustard analogs, podophyllotoxin derivatives, pyrimidine analogs, and vinca alkaloids. KYTRIL Injection doses of 10 and 40 mcg/kg were superior to 2 mcg/kg in preventing cisplatin-induced nausea and vomiting, but 40 mcg/kg was not significantly superior to 10 mcg/kg (see Table 4).

[See table 4 on next page]

Table 1. Pharmacokinetic Parameters in Adult Cancer Patients Undergoing Chemotherapy and in Volunteers, Following a Single Intravenous 40 mcg/kg Dose of KYTRIL Injection

	Peak Plasma Concentration (ng/mL)	Terminal Phase Plasma Half-Life (h)	Total Clearance (L/h/kg)	Volume of Distribution (L/kg)
Cancer Patients				
Mean	63.8*	8.95*	0.38*	3.07*
Range	18.0 to 176	0.90 to 31.1	0.14 to 1.54	0.85 to 10.4
Volunteers				
21 to 42 years				
Mean	64.3†	4.91†	0.79†	3.04†
Range	11.2 to 182	0.88 to 15.2	0.20 to 2.56	1.68 to 6.13
65 to 81 years				
Mean	57.0†	7.69†	0.44†	3.97†
Range	14.6 to 153	2.65 to 17.7	0.17 to 1.06	1.75 to 7.01

*5-minute infusion.
†3-minute infusion.

KYTRIL Injection was also evaluated in a double-blind, randomized dose response study of 353 patients stratified for high (≥80 to 120 mg/m^2) or low (50 to 79 mg/m^2) cisplatin dose. Response rates of patients for both cisplatin strata are given in Table 5.

[See table 5 at right]

For both the low and high cisplatin strata, the 10, 20, and 40 mcg/kg doses were more effective than the 5 mcg/kg dose in preventing nausea and vomiting within 24 hours of chemotherapy administration. The 10 mcg/kg dose was at least as effective as the higher doses.

Moderately Emetogenic Chemotherapy

KYTRIL Injection, 40 mcg/kg, was compared with the combination of chlorpromazine (50 to 200 mg/24 hours) and dexamethasone (12 mg) in patients treated with moderately emetogenic chemotherapy, including primarily carboplatin >300 mg/m^2, cisplatin 20 to 50 mg/m^2 and cyclophosphamide >600 mg/m^2. KYTRIL Injection was superior to the chlorpromazine regimen in preventing nausea and vomiting (see Table 6).

[See table 6 at right]

In other studies of moderately emetogenic chemotherapy, no significant difference in efficacy was found between KYTRIL doses of 40 mcg/kg and 160 mcg/kg.

Repeat-Cycle Chemotherapy

In an uncontrolled trial, 512 cancer patients received KYTRIL Injection, 40 mcg/kg, prophylactically, for two cycles of chemotherapy, 224 patients received it for at least four cycles, and 108 patients received it for at least six cycles. KYTRIL Injection efficacy remained relatively constant over the first six repeat cycles, with complete response rates (no vomiting and no moderate or severe nausea in 24 hours) of 60% to 69%. No patients were studied for more than 15 cycles.

Pediatric Studies

A randomized double-blind study evaluated the 24-hour response of 80 pediatric cancer patients (age 2 to 16 years) to KYTRIL Injection 10, 20 or 40 mcg/kg. Patients were treated with cisplatin ≥60 mg/m^2, cytarabine ≥3 g/m^2, cyclophosphamide ≥1 g/m^2 or nitrogen mustard ≥6 mg/m^2 (see Table 7).

[See table 7 at top of next page]

A second pediatric study compared KYTRIL Injection 20 mcg/kg to chlorpromazine plus dexamethasone in 88 patients treated with ifosfamide ≥3 g/m^2/day for two or three days. KYTRIL Injection was administered on each day of ifosfamide treatment. At 24 hours, 22% of KYTRIL Injection patients achieved complete response (no vomiting and no moderate or severe nausea in 24 hours) compared with 10% on the chlorpromazine regimen. The median number of vomiting episodes with KYTRIL Injection was 1.5; with chlorpromazine it was 7.0.

Postoperative Nausea and Vomiting

Prevention of Postoperative Nausea and Vomiting

The efficacy of KYTRIL Injection for prevention of postoperative nausea and vomiting was evaluated in 868 patients, of which 833 were women, 35 men, 484 Caucasians, 348 Asians, 18 Blacks, 18 Other, with 61 patients 65 years or older. KYTRIL was evaluated in two randomized, double-blind, placebo-controlled studies in patients who underwent elective gynecological surgery or cholecystectomy and received general anesthesia. Patients received a single intravenous dose of KYTRIL Injection (0.1 mg, 1 mg or 3 mg) or placebo either 5 minutes before induction of anesthesia or immediately before reversal of anesthesia. The primary endpoint was the proportion of patients with no vomiting for 24 hours after surgery. Episodes of nausea and vomiting and use of rescue antiemetic therapy were recorded for 24 hours after surgery. In both studies, KYTRIL Injection (1 mg) was more effective than placebo in preventing postoperative nausea and vomiting (see Table 8). No additional benefit was seen in patients who received the 3 mg dose.

[See table 8 at top of next page]

Gender/Race

There were too few male and Black patients to adequately assess differences in effect in either population.

Treatment of Postoperative Nausea and Vomiting

The efficacy of KYTRIL Injection for treatment of postoperative nausea and vomiting was evaluated in 844 patients, of which 731 were women, 113 men, 777 Caucasians, 6 Asians, 41 Blacks, 20 Other, with 107 patients 65 years or older. KYTRIL Injection was evaluated in two randomized, double-blind, placebo-controlled studies of adult surgical patients who received general anesthesia with no prophylactic antiemetic agent, and who experienced nausea or vomiting within 4 hours postoperatively. Patients received a single intravenous dose of KYTRIL Injection (0.1 mg, 1 mg or 3 mg) or placebo after experiencing postoperative nausea or vomiting. Episodes of nausea and vomiting and use of rescue antiemetic therapy were recorded for 24 hours after administration of study medication. KYTRIL Injection was more effective than placebo in treating postoperative nausea and vomiting (see Table 9). No additional benefit was seen in patients who received the 3 mg dose.

[See table 9 on next page]

Gender/Race

There were too few male and Black patients to adequately assess differences in effect in either population.

INDICATIONS AND USAGE

KYTRIL Injection is indicated for:

- The prevention of nausea and/or vomiting associated with initial and repeat courses of emetogenic cancer therapy, including high-dose cisplatin.

Table 2. Pharmacokinetic Parameters in 16 Adult Surgical Patients Following a Single Intravenous 1 mg Dose of KYTRIL Injection

	Terminal Phase Plasma Half-Life (h)	Total Clearance (L/h/kg)	Volume of Distribution (L/kg)
Mean	8.63	0.28	2.42
Range	1.77 to 17.73	0.07 to 0.71	0.71 to 4.13

Table 3. Prevention of Chemotherapy-Induced Nausea and Vomiting—Single-Day High-Dose Cisplatin Therapy[1]

	KYTRIL Injection	Placebo	*P*-Value
Number of Patients	14	14	
Response Over 24 Hours			
Complete Response[2]	93%	7%	<0.001
No Vomiting	93%	14%	<0.001
No More Than Mild Nausea	93%	7%	<0.001

[1] Cisplatin administration began within 10 minutes of KYTRIL Injection infusion and continued for 1.5 to 3.0 hours. Mean cisplatin dose was 86 mg/m^2 in the KYTRIL Injection group and 80 mg/m^2 in the placebo group.

[2] No vomiting and no moderate or severe nausea.

Table 4. Prevention of Chemotherapy-Induced Nausea and Vomiting—Single-Day High-Dose Cisplatin Therapy[1]

	KYTRIL Injection (mcg/kg)			*P*-Value (vs. 2 mcg/kg)	
	2	10	40	10	40
Number of Patients	52	52	53		
Response Over 24 Hours					
Complete Response[2]	31%	62%	68%	<0.002	<0.001
No Vomiting	38%	65%	74%	<0.001	<0.001
No More Than Mild Nausea	58%	75%	79%	NS	0.007

[1] Cisplatin administration began within 10 minutes of KYTRIL Injection infusion and continued for 2.6 hours (mean). Mean cisplatin doses were 96 to 99 mg/m^2.

[2] No vomiting and no moderate or severe nausea.

Table 5. Prevention of Chemotherapy-Induced Nausea and Vomiting—Single-Day High-Dose and Low-Dose Cisplatin Therapy[1]

	KYTRIL Injection (mcg/kg)				*P*-Value (vs. 5 mcg/kg)		
	5	10	20	40	10	20	40
High-Dose Cisplatin							
Number of Patients	40	49	48	47			
Response Over 24 Hours							
Complete Response[2]	18%	41%	40%	47%	0.018	0.025	0.004
No Vomiting	28%	47%	44%	53%	NS	NS	0.016
No Nausea	15%	35%	38%	43%	0.036	0.019	0.005
Low-Dose Cisplatin							
Number of Patients	42	41	40	46			
Response Over 24 Hours							
Complete Response[2]	29%	56%	58%	41%	0.012	0.009	NS
No Vomiting	36%	63%	65%	43%	0.012	0.008	NS
No Nausea	29%	56%	38%	33%	0.012	NS	NS

[1] Cisplatin administration began within 10 minutes of KYTRIL Injection infusion and continued for 2 hours (mean). Mean cisplatin doses were 64 and 98 mg/m^2 for low and high strata.

[2] No vomiting and no use of rescue antiemetic.

Table 6. Prevention of Chemotherapy-Induced Nausea and Vomiting—Single-Day Moderately Emetogenic Chemotherapy

	KYTRIL Injection	Chlorpromazine[1]	*P*-Value
Number of Patients	133	133	
Response Over 24 Hours			
Complete Response[2]	68%	47%	<0.001
No Vomiting	73%	53%	<0.001
No More Than Mild Nausea	77%	59%	<0.001

[1] Patients also received dexamethasone, 12 mg.

[2] No vomiting and no moderate or severe nausea.

- The prevention and treatment of postoperative nausea and vomiting. As with other antiemetics, routine prophylaxis is not recommended in patients in whom there is little expectation that nausea and/or vomiting will occur postoperatively. In patients where nausea and/or vomiting must be avoided during the postoperative period, KYTRIL Injection is recommended even where the incidence of postoperative nausea and/or vomiting is low.

CONTRAINDICATIONS

KYTRIL Injection is contraindicated in patients with known hypersensitivity to the drug or to any of its components.

WARNINGS

Hypersensitivity reactions may occur in patients who have exhibited hypersensitivity to other selective 5-HT$_3$ receptor antagonists.

PRECAUTIONS

KYTRIL is not a drug that stimulates gastric or intestinal peristalsis. It should not be used instead of nasogastric suction. The use of KYTRIL in patients following abdominal surgery or in patients with chemotherapy-induced nausea and vomiting may mask a progressive ileus and/or gastric distention.

Drug Interactions

Granisetron does not induce or inhibit the cytochrome P-450 drug-metabolizing enzyme system. There have been no definitive drug-drug interaction studies to examine pharmacokinetic or pharmacodynamic interaction with other drugs, but in humans, KYTRIL Injection has been safely administered with drugs representing benzodiazepines, neuroleptics and anti-ulcer medications commonly prescribed with antiemetic treatments. KYTRIL Injection also does not appear to interact with emetogenic cancer chemotherapies. Because granisetron is metabolized by hepatic cytochrome P-450 drug-metabolizing enzymes, inducers or inhibitors of these enzymes may change the clearance and, hence, the half-life of granisetron.

Continued on next page

Table 7. Prevention of Chemotherapy-Induced Nausea and Vomiting in Pediatric Patients

	KYTRIL Injection Dose (mcg/kg)		
	10	**20**	**40**
Number of Patients	29	26	25
Median Number of Vomiting Episodes	2	3	1
Complete Response Over 24 Hours[1]	21%	31%	32%

[1] No vomiting and no moderate or severe nausea.

Table 8. Prevention of Postoperative Nausea and Vomiting in Adult Patients

Study and Efficacy Endpoint	Placebo	KYTRIL 0.1 mg	KYTRIL 1 mg	KYTRIL 3 mg
Study 1				
Number of Patients	**133**	**132**	**134**	**128**
No Vomiting				
0 to 24 hours	34%	45%	63%**	62%**
No Nausea				
0 to 24 hours	22%	28%	50%**	42%**
No Nausea or Vomiting				
0 to 24 hours	18%	27%	49%**	42%**
No Use of Rescue Antiemetic Therapy				
0 to 24 hours	60%	67%	75%*	77%*
Study 2				
Number of Patients	**117**	**—**	**110**	**114**
No Vomiting				
0 to 24 hours	56%	—	77%**	75%*
No Nausea				
0 to 24 hours	37%	—	59%**	56%*

*P<0.05
**P<0.001 versus placebo
Note: No Vomiting = no vomiting and no use of rescue antiemetic therapy; No Nausea = no nausea and no use of rescue antiemetic therapy

Table 9. Treatment of Postoperative Nausea and Vomiting in Adult Patients

Study and Efficacy Endpoint	Placebo	KYTRIL 0.1 mg	KYTRIL 1 mg	KYTRIL 3 mg
Study 3				
Number of Patients	**133**	**128**	**133**	**125**
No Vomiting				
0 to 6 hours	26%	53%***	58%***	60%***
0 to 24 hours	20%	38%***	46%***	49%***
No Nausea				
0 to 6 hours	17%	40%***	41%***	42%***
0 to 24 hours	13%	27%**	30%**	37%***
No Use of Rescue Antiemetic Therapy				
0 to 6 hours	—	—	—	—
0 to 24 hours	33%	51%**	61%***	61%***
Study 4				
Number of Patients (All Patients)	**162**	**163**	**—**	**—**
No Vomiting				
0 to 6 hours	20%	32%*	—	—
0 to 24 hours	14%	23%*	—	—
No Nausea				
0 to 6 hours	13%	18%	—	—
0 to 24 hours	9%	14%	—	—
No Nausea to Vomiting				
0 to 6 hours	13%	18%	—	—
0 to 24 hours	9%	14%	—	—
No Use of Rescue Antiemetic Therapy				
0 to 6 hours	—	—	—	—
0 to 24 hours	24%	34%*	—	—
Number of Patients (Treated for Vomiting)[1]	**86**	**103**	**—**	**—**
No Vomiting				
0 to 6 hours	21%	27%	—	—
0 to 24 hours	14%	20%	—	—

*P<0.05
**P<0.01
***P<0.001 versus placebo
[1]Protocol Specified Analysis: Patients who had vomiting prior to treatment
Note: No vomiting = no vomiting and no use of rescue antiemetic therapy; No nausea = no nausea and no use of rescue antiemetic therapy

Kytril Injection—Cont.

Carcinogenesis, Mutagenesis, Impairment of Fertility
In a 24-month carcinogenicity study, rats were treated orally with granisetron 1, 5 or 50 mg/kg/day (6, 30 or 300 mg/m²/day). The 50 mg/kg/day dose was reduced to 25 mg/kg/day (150 mg/m²/day) during week 59 due to toxicity. For a 50 kg person of average height (1.46 m² body surface area), these doses represent 16, 81 and 405 times the recommended clinical dose (0.37 mg/m², iv) on a body surface area basis. There was a statistically significant increase in the incidence of hepatocellular carcinomas and adenomas in males treated with 5 mg/kg/day (30 mg/m²/day, 81 times the recommended human dose based on body surface area) and above, and in females treated with 25 mg/kg/day (150 mg/m²/day, 405 times the recommended human dose based on body surface area). No increase in liver tumors was observed at a dose of 1 mg/kg/day (6 mg/m²/day, 16 times the recommended human dose based on body surface area) in males and 5 mg/kg/day (30 mg/m²/day, 81 times the recommended human dose based on body surface area) in females. In a 12-month oral toxicity study, treatment with granisetron 100 mg/kg/day (600 mg/m²/day, 1622 times the recommended human dose based on body surface area) produced hepatocellular adenomas in male and female rats while no such tumors were found in the control rats. A 24-month mouse carcinogenicity study of granisetron did not show a statistically significant increase in tumor incidence, but the study was not conclusive.

Because of the tumor findings in rat studies, KYTRIL Injection should be prescribed only at the dose and for the indication recommended (see INDICATIONS AND USAGE and DOSAGE AND ADMINISTRATION).

Granisetron was not mutagenic in an in vitro Ames test and mouse lymphoma cell forward mutation assay, and in vivo mouse micronucleus test and in vitro and ex vivo rat hepatocyte UDS assays. It, however, produced a significant increase in UDS in HeLa cells in vitro and a significant increased incidence of cells with polyploidy in an in vitro human lymphocyte chromosomal aberration test.

Granisetron at subcutaneous doses up to 6 mg/kg/day (36 mg/m²/day, 97 times the recommended human dose based on body surface area) was found to have no effect on fertility and reproductive performance of male and female rats.

Pregnancy
Teratogenic Effects. *Pregnancy Category B.*
Reproduction studies have been performed in pregnant rats at intravenous doses up to 9 mg/kg/day (54 mg/m²/day, 146 times the recommended human dose based on body surface area) and pregnant rabbits at intravenous doses up to 3 mg/kg/day (35.4 mg/m²/day, 96 times the recommended human dose based on body surface area) and have revealed no evidence of impaired fertility or harm to the fetus due to granisetron. There are, however, no adequate and well-controlled studies in pregnant women. Because animal reproduction studies are not always predictive of human response, this drug should be used during pregnancy only if clearly needed.

Nursing Mothers
It is not known whether granisetron is excreted in human milk. Because many drugs are excreted in human milk, caution should be exercised when KYTRIL Injection is administered to a nursing woman.

Pediatric Use
See DOSAGE AND ADMINISTRATION for use in chemotherapy-induced nausea and vomiting in pediatric patients 2 to 16 years of age. Safety and effectiveness in pediatric patients under 2 years of age have not been established. Safety and effectiveness of KYTRIL Injection have not been established in pediatric patients for the prevention or treatment of postoperative nausea or vomiting.

Geriatric Use
During chemotherapy clinical trials, 713 patients 65 years of age or older received KYTRIL Injection. Effectiveness and safety were similar in patients of various ages.

During postoperative nausea and vomiting clinical trials, 168 patients 65 years of age or older, of which 47 were 75 years of age or older, received KYTRIL Injection. Clinical studies of KYTRIL Injection did not include sufficient numbers of subjects aged 65 years and over to determine whether they respond differently from younger subjects. Other reported clinical experience has not identified differences in responses between the elderly and younger patients.

ADVERSE REACTIONS

Chemotherapy-Induced Nausea and Vomiting
The following have been reported during controlled clinical trials or in the routine management of patients. The percentage figures are based on clinical trial experience only. Table 10 gives the comparative frequencies of the five most commonly reported adverse events (≥3%) in patients receiving KYTRIL Injection, in single-day chemotherapy trials. These patients received chemotherapy, primarily cisplatin, and intravenous fluids during the 24-hour period following KYTRIL Injection administration. Events were generally recorded over seven days post-KYTRIL Injection administration. In the absence of a placebo group, there is uncertainty as to how many of these events should be attributed to KYTRIL, except for headache, which was clearly more frequent than in comparison groups.

Table 10. Principal Adverse Events in Clinical Trials—Single-Day Chemotherapy

	Percent of Patients With Event	
	KYTRIL Injection 40 mcg/kg (n=1268)	**Comparator[1] (n=422)**
Headache	14%	6%
Asthenia	5%	6%
Somnolence	4%	15%
Diarrhea	4%	6%
Constipation	3%	3%

[1] Metoclopramide/dexamethasone and phenothiazines/dexamethasone.

In over 3,000 patients receiving KYTRIL Injection (2 to 160 mcg/kg) in single-day and multiple-day clinical trials with emetogenic cancer therapies, adverse events, other than those in Table 10, were observed; attribution of many of these events to KYTRIL is uncertain.

Hepatic: In comparative trials, mainly with cisplatin regimens, elevations of AST and ALT (>2 times the upper limit of normal) following administration of KYTRIL Injection occurred in 2.8% and 3.3% of patients, respectively. These frequencies were not significantly different from those seen with comparators (AST: 2.1%; ALT: 2.4%).

Cardiovascular: Hypertension (2%); hypotension, arrhythmias such as sinus bradycardia, atrial fibrillation, varying degrees of A-V block, ventricular ectopy including non-sustained tachycardia, and ECG abnormalities have been observed rarely.

Central Nervous System: Agitation, anxiety, CNS stimulation and insomnia were seen in less than 2% of patients. Extrapyramidal syndrome occurred rarely and only in the presence of other drugs associated with this syndrome.
Hypersensitivity: Rare cases of hypersensitivity reactions, sometimes severe (eg, anaphylaxis, shortness of breath, hypotension, urticaria) have been reported.
Other: Fever (3%), taste disorder (2%), skin rashes (1%). In multiple-day comparative studies, fever occurred more frequently with KYTRIL Injection (8.6%) than with comparative drugs (3.4%, $P<0.014$), which usually included dexamethasone.

Postoperative Nausea and Vomiting

The adverse events listed in Table 11 were reported in ≥2% of adults receiving KYTRIL Injection 1 mg during controlled clinical trials.

Table 11. Adverse Events ≥ 2%

	Percent of Patients With Event	
	KYTRIL Injection 1 mg (n=267)	Placebo (n=266)
Pain	10.1	8.3
Constipation	9.4	12.0
Anemia	9.4	10.2
Headache	8.6	7.1
Fever	7.9	4.5
Abdominal Pain	6.0	6.0
Hepatic Enzymes Increased	5.6	4.1
Insomnia	4.9	6.0
Bradycardia	4.5	5.3
Dizziness	4.1	3.4
Leukocytosis	3.7	4.1
Anxiety	3.4	3.8
Hypotension	3.4	3.8
Diarrhea	3.4	1.1
Flatulence	3.0	3.0
Infection	3.0	2.3
Dyspepsia	3.0	1.9
Hypertension	2.6	4.1
Urinary Tract Infection	2.6	3.4
Oliguria	2.2	1.5
Coughing	2.2	1.1

In a clinical study conducted in Japan, the types of adverse events differed notably from those reported above in Table 11. The adverse events in the Japanese study that occurred in ≥2% of patients and were more frequent with KYTRIL 1 mg than with placebo were: fever (56% to 50%), sputum increased (2.7% to 1.7%), and dermatitis (2.7% to 0%).

OVERDOSAGE

There is no specific antidote for KYTRIL Injection overdosage. In case of overdosage, symptomatic treatment should be given. Overdosage of up to 38.5 mg of granisetron hydrochloride injection has been reported without symptoms or only the occurrence of a slight headache.

DOSAGE AND ADMINISTRATION

Prevention of Chemotherapy-Induced Nausea and Vomiting

The recommended dosage for KYTRIL Injection is 10 mcg/kg administered intravenously within 30 minutes before initiation of chemotherapy, and only on the day(s) chemotherapy is given.
Infusion Preparation
KYTRIL Injection may be administered intravenously either undiluted over 30 seconds, or diluted with 0.9% Sodium Chloride or 5% Dextrose and infused over 5 minutes.
Stability
Intravenous infusion of KYTRIL Injection should be prepared at the time of administration. However, KYTRIL Injection has been shown to be stable for at least 24 hours when diluted in 0.9% Sodium Chloride or 5% Dextrose and stored at room temperature under normal lighting conditions.
As a general precaution, KYTRIL Injection should not be mixed in solution with other drugs. Parenteral drug products should be inspected visually for particulate matter and discoloration before administration whenever solution and container permit.
Pediatric Patients
The recommended dose in pediatric patients 2 to 16 years of age is 10 mcg/kg (see CLINICAL TRIALS). Pediatric patients under 2 years of age have not been studied.
Geriatric Patients, Renal Failure Patients or Hepatically Impaired Patients
No dosage adjustment is recommended (see CLINICAL PHARMACOLOGY: Pharmacokinetics).

Prevention and Treatment of Postoperative Nausea and Vomiting

The recommended dosage for prevention of postoperative nausea and vomiting is 1 mg of KYTRIL, undiluted, administered intravenously over 30 seconds, before induction of anesthesia or immediately before reversal of anesthesia.
The recommended dosage for the treatment of nausea and/or vomiting after surgery is 1 mg of KYTRIL, undiluted, administered intravenously over 30 seconds.
Pediatric Patients
Safety and effectiveness of KYTRIL Injection have not been established in pediatric patients for the prevention or treatment of postoperative nausea or vomiting.
Geriatric Patients, Renal Failure Patients or Hepatically Impaired Patients
No dosage adjustment is recommended (see CLINICAL PHARMACOLOGY: Pharmacokinetics).

HOW SUPPLIED

KYTRIL Injection, 1 mg/mL (free base), is supplied in 1 mL Single-Use Vials and 4 mL Multi-Dose Vials.
NDC 0004-0239-09 (package of 1 Single-Dose Vial)
NDC 0004-0240-09 (package of 1 Multi-Dose Vial)

Storage

Store single-dose vials and multi-dose vials at 25°C (77°F); excursions permitted to 15° to 30°C (59° to 86°F). [See USP Controlled Room Temperature]
Once the multi-dose vial is penetrated, its contents should be used within 30 days.
Do not freeze. Protect from light.

Revised: August 2002

KYTRIL® ℞
(granisetron hydrochloride)
TABLETS
ORAL SOLUTION

DESCRIPTION

KYTRIL Tablets and KYTRIL Oral Solution contain granisetron hydrochloride, an antinauseant and antiemetic agent. Chemically it is *endo*-N-(9-methyl-9-azabicyclo [3.3.1] non-3-yl)-1-methyl-1H-indazole-3-carboxamide hydrochloride with a molecular weight of 348.9 (312.4 free base). Its empirical formula is $C_{18}H_{24}N_4O \bullet HCl$.
Granisetron hydrochloride is a white to off-white solid that is readily soluble in water and normal saline at 20°C.
Tablets for Oral Administration: Each white, triangular, biconvex, film-coated KYTRIL Tablet contains 1.12 mg granisetron hydrochloride equivalent to granisetron, 1 mg. Inactive ingredients are: hydroxypropyl methylcellulose, lactose, magnesium stearate, microcrystalline cellulose, polyethylene glycol, polysorbate 80, sodium starch glycolate, and titanium dioxide.
Oral Solution: Each 10 mL of clear, orange-colored, orange-flavored KYTRIL Oral Solution contains 2.24 mg of granisetron hydrochloride equivalent to 2 mg granisetron. Inactive ingredients: citric acid anhydrous, FD&C Yellow No. 6, orange flavor, purified water, sodium benzoate, and sorbitol.

CLINICAL PHARMACOLOGY

Granisetron is a selective 5-hydroxytryptamine$_3$ (5-HT$_3$) receptor antagonist with little or no affinity for other serotonin receptors, including 5-HT$_1$; 5-HT$_{1A}$; 5-HT$_{1B/C}$; 5-HT$_2$; for alpha$_1$-, alpha$_2$-, or beta-adrenoreceptors; for dopamine-D$_2$; or for histamine-H$_1$; benzodiazepine; picrotoxin or opioid receptors.
Serotonin receptors of the 5-HT$_3$ type are located peripherally on vagal nerve terminals and centrally in the chemoreceptor trigger zone of the area postrema. During chemotherapy that induces vomiting, mucosal enterochromaffin cells release serotonin, which stimulates 5-HT$_3$ receptors. This evokes vagal afferent discharge, inducing vomiting. Animal studies demonstrate that, in binding to 5-HT$_3$ receptors, granisetron blocks serotonin stimulation and subsequent vomiting after emetogenic stimuli such as cisplatin. In the ferret animal model, a single granisetron injection prevented vomiting due to high-dose cisplatin or arrested vomiting within 5 to 30 seconds.
In most human studies, granisetron has had little effect on blood pressure, heart rate or ECG. No evidence of an effect on plasma prolactin or aldosterone concentrations has been found in other studies.
Following single and multiple oral doses, KYTRIL Tablets slowed colonic transit in normal volunteers. However, KYTRIL had no effect on oro-cecal transit time in normal volunteers when given as a single intravenous (IV) infusion of 50 mcg/kg or 200 mcg/kg.
Pharmacokinetics: In healthy volunteers and adult cancer patients undergoing chemotherapy, administration of KYTRIL Tablets produced mean pharmacokinetic data shown in Table 1.
[See table 1 below]
The effects of gender on the pharmacokinetics of KYTRIL Tablets have not been studied. However, after intravenous infusion of KYTRIL, no difference in mean AUC was found between males and females, although males had a higher C_{max} generally.
When KYTRIL Tablets were administered with food, AUC was decreased by 5% and C_{max} increased by 30% in non-fasted healthy volunteers who received a single dose of 10 mg.
Granisetron metabolism involves N-demethylation and aromatic ring oxidation followed by conjugation. Animal studies suggest that some of the metabolites may also have 5-HT$_3$ receptor antagonist activity.
Clearance is predominantly by hepatic metabolism. In normal volunteers, approximately 11% of the orally administered dose is eliminated unchanged in the urine in 48 hours. The remainder of the dose is excreted as metabolites, 48% in the urine and 38% in the feces.
In vitro liver microsomal studies show that granisetron's major route of metabolism is inhibited by ketoconazole, suggestive of metabolism mediated by the cytochrome P-450 3A subfamily.
Plasma protein binding is approximately 65% and granisetron distributes freely between plasma and red blood cells.
A 2 mg dose of KYTRIL Oral Solution is bioequivalent to the corresponding dose of KYTRIL Tablets (1 mg × 2) and may be used interchangeably.
In elderly and pediatric patients and in patients with renal failure or hepatic impairment, the pharmacokinetics of granisetron was determined following administration of intravenous KYTRIL:
Elderly: The ranges of the pharmacokinetic parameters in elderly volunteers (mean age 71 years), given a single 40 mcg/kg intravenous dose of KYTRIL Injection, were generally similar to those in younger healthy volunteers; mean values were lower for clearance and longer for half-life in the elderly.
Renal Failure Patients: Total clearance of granisetron was not affected in patients with severe renal failure who received a single 40 mcg/kg intravenous dose of KYTRIL Injection.
Hepatically Impaired Patients: A pharmacokinetic study with intravenous KYTRIL in patients with hepatic impairment due to neoplastic liver involvement showed that total clearance was approximately halved compared to patients without hepatic impairment. Given the wide variability in pharmacokinetic parameters noted in patients and the good tolerance of doses well above the recommended dose, dosage adjustment in patients with possible hepatic functional impairment is not necessary.
Pediatric Patients: A pharmacokinetic study in pediatric cancer patients (2 to 16 years of age), given a single 40 mcg/kg intravenous dose of KYTRIL Injection, showed that volume of distribution and total clearance increased with age. No relationship with age was observed for peak plasma concentration or terminal phase plasma half-life. When volume of distribution and total clearance are adjusted for body weight, the pharmacokinetics of granisetron are similar in pediatric and adult cancer patients.

CLINICAL TRIALS

Chemotherapy-Induced Nausea and Vomiting: KYTRIL Tablets prevent nausea and vomiting associated with initial and repeat courses of emetogenic cancer therapy, as shown by 24-hour efficacy data from studies using both moderately and highly-emetogenic chemotherapy.
Moderately Emetogenic Chemotherapy: The first trial compared KYTRIL Tablets doses of 0.25 mg to 2 mg bid, in 930 cancer patients receiving, principally, cyclophosphamide, carboplatin, and cisplatin (20 mg/m^2 to 50 mg/m^2). Efficacy was based on complete response (ie, no vomiting, no moderate or severe nausea, no rescue medication), no vomiting, and no nausea. Table 2 summarizes the results of this study.
[See table 2 at top of next page]
Results from a second double-blind, randomized trial evaluating KYTRIL Tablets 2 mg qd and KYTRIL Tablets 1 mg bid were compared to prochlorperazine 10 mg bid derived from a historical control. At 24 hours, there was no statistically significant difference in efficacy between the two KYTRIL Tablet regimens. Both regimens were statistically superior to the prochlorperazine control regimen (see Table 3).

Continued on next page

Table 1. Pharmacokinetic Parameters (Median [range]) Following KYTRIL Tablets (granisetron hydrochloride)

	Peak Plasma Concentration (ng/mL)	Terminal Phase Plasma Half-Life (h)	Volume of Distribution (L/kg)	Total Clearance (L/h/kg)
Cancer Patients 1 mg bid, 7 days (n=27)	5.99 [0.63 to 30.9]	N.D.*	N.D.	0.52 [0.09 to 7.37]
Volunteers single 1 mg dose (n=39)	3.63 [0.27 to 9.14]	6.23 [0.96 to 19.9]	3.94 [1.89 to 39.4]	0.41 [0.11 to 24.6]

* Not determined after oral administration; following a single intravenous dose of 40 mcg/kg, terminal phase half-life was determined to be 8.95 hours.
N.D. Not determined.

Kytril Tabs/Oral Solution—Cont.

[See table 3 at right]
Results from a KYTRIL Tablets 2 mg qd alone treatment arm in a third double-blind, randomized trial, were compared to prochlorperazine (PCPZ), 10 mg bid, derived from a historical control. The 24-hour results for KYTRIL Tablets 2 mg qd were statistically superior to PCPZ for all efficacy parameters: complete response (58%), no vomiting (79%), no nausea (51%), total control (49%). The PCPZ rates are shown in Table 3.

Cisplatin-Based Chemotherapy: The first double-blind trial compared KYTRIL Tablets 1 mg bid, relative to placebo (historical control), in 119 cancer patients receiving high-dose cisplatin (mean dose 80 mg/m^2). At 24 hours, KYTRIL Tablets 1 mg bid was significantly ($P<0.001$) superior to placebo (historical control) in all efficacy parameters: complete response (52%), no vomiting (56%) and no nausea (45%). The placebo rates were 7%, 14%, and 7%, respectively, for the three efficacy parameters.

Results from a KYTRIL Tablets 2 mg qd alone treatment arm in a second double-blind, randomized trial, were compared to both KYTRIL Tablets 1 mg bid and placebo historical controls. The 24-hour results for KYTRIL Tablets 2 mg qd were: complete response (44%), no vomiting (58%), no nausea (46%), total control (40%). The efficacy of KYTRIL Tablets 2 mg qd was comparable to KYTRIL Tablets 1 mg bid and statistically superior to placebo. The placebo rates were 7%, 14%, 7%, and 7%, respectively, for the four parameters.

No controlled study comparing granisetron injection with the oral formulation to prevent chemotherapy-induced nausea and vomiting has been performed.

Radiation-Induced Nausea and Vomiting: ***Total Body Irradiation:*** In a double-blind randomized study, 18 patients receiving KYTRIL Tablets, 2 mg daily, experienced significantly greater antiemetic protection compared to patients in a historical negative control group who received conventional (non-5-HT$_3$ antagonist) antiemetics. Total body irradiation consisted of 11 fractions of 120 cGy administered over 4 days, with three fractions on each of the first 3 days, and two fractions on the fourth day. KYTRIL Tablets were given one hour before the first radiation fraction of each day. Twenty-two percent (22%) of patients treated with KYTRIL Tablets did not experience vomiting or receive rescue antiemetics over the entire 4-day dosing period, compared to 0% of patients in the historical negative control group ($P<0.01$). In addition, patients who received KYTRIL Tablets also experienced significantly fewer emetic episodes during the first day of radiation and over the 4-day treatment period, compared to patients in the historical negative control group. The median time to the first emetic episode was 36 hours for patients who received KYTRIL Tablets.

Fractionated Abdominal Radiation: The efficacy of KYTRIL Tablets, 2 mg daily, was evaluated in a double-blind, placebo-controlled randomized trial of 260 patients. KYTRIL Tablets were given 1 hour before radiation, composed of up to 20 daily fractions of 180 to 300 cGy each. The exceptions were patients with seminoma or those receiving whole abdomen irradiation who initially received 150 cGy per fraction. Radiation was administered to the upper abdomen with a field size of at least 100 cm^2.

The proportion of patients without emesis and those without nausea for KYTRIL Tablets, compared to placebo, was statistically significant ($P<0.0001$) at 24 hours after radiation, irrespective of the radiation dose. KYTRIL was superior to placebo in patients receiving up to 10 daily fractions of radiation, but was not superior to placebo in patients receiving 20 fractions.

Patients treated with KYTRIL Tablets (n=134) had a significantly longer time to the first episode of vomiting (35 days vs. 9 days, $P<0.001$) relative to those patients who received placebo (n=126), and a significantly longer time to the first episode of nausea (11 days vs. 1 day, $P<0.001$). KYTRIL provided significantly greater protection from nausea and vomiting than placebo.

INDICATIONS AND USAGE

KYTRIL (granisetron hydrochloride) is indicated for the prevention of:

nausea and vomiting associated with initial and repeat courses of emetogenic cancer therapy, including high-dose cisplatin.

nausea and vomiting associated with radiation, including total body irradiation and fractionated abdominal radiation.

CONTRAINDICATIONS

KYTRIL is contraindicated in patients with known hypersensitivity to the drug or any of its components.

PRECAUTIONS

Drug Interactions: Granisetron does not induce or inhibit the cytochrome P-450 drug-metabolizing enzyme system. There have been no definitive drug-drug interaction studies to examine pharmacokinetic or pharmacodynamic interaction with other drugs but, in humans, KYTRIL Injection has been safely administered with drugs representing benzodiazepines, neuroleptics, and anti-ulcer medications commonly prescribed with antiemetic treatments. KYTRIL Injection also does not appear to interact with emetogenic cancer chemotherapies. Because granisetron is metabolized by hepatic cytochrome P-450 drug-metabolizing enzymes, inducers or inhibitors of these enzymes may change the clearance and, hence, the half-life of granisetron.

Table 2. Prevention of Nausea and Vomiting 24 Hours Post-Chemotherapy[1]

	Percentages of Patients KYTRIL Tablet Dose			
Efficacy Measures	0.25 mg bid (n=229) %	0.5 mg bid (n=235) %	1 mg bid (n=233) %	2 mg bid (n=233) %
Complete Response[2]	61	70*	81*†	72*
No Vomiting	66	77*	88*	79*
No Nausea	48	57	63*	54

1. Chemotherapy included oral and injectable cyclophosphamide, carboplatin, cisplatin (20 mg/m^2 to 50 mg/m^2), dacarbazine, doxorubicin, epirubicin.
2. No vomiting, no moderate or severe nausea, no rescue medication.
* Statistically significant ($P<0.01$) vs. 0.25 mg bid.
† Statistically significant ($P<0.01$) vs. 0.5 mg bid.

Table 3. Prevention of Nausea and Vomiting 24 Hours Post-Chemotherapy[1]

	Percentages of Patients		
Efficacy Measures	KYTRIL Tablets 1 mg bid (n=354) %	KYTRIL Tablets 2 mg qd (n=343) %	Prochlorperazine[2] 10 mg bid (n=111) %
Complete Response[3]	69*	64*	41
No Vomiting	82*	77*	48
No Nausea	51*	53*	35
Total Control[4]	51*	50*	33

1. Moderately emetogenic chemotherapeutic agents included cisplatin (20 mg/m^2 to 50 mg/m^2), oral and intravenous cyclophosphamide, carboplatin, dacarbazine, doxorubicin.
2. Historical control from a previous double-blind KYTRIL trial.
3. No vomiting, no moderate or severe nausea, no rescue medication.
4. No vomiting, no nausea, no rescue medication.
* Statistically significant ($P<0.05$) vs. prochlorperazine historical control.

Table 4. Principal Adverse Events in Clinical Trials

	Percent of Patients With Event			
	KYTRIL[1] Tablets 1 mg bid (n=978)	KYTRIL[1] Tablets 2 mg qd (n=1450)	Comparator[2] (n=599)	Placebo (n=185)
Headache[3]	21%	20%	13%	12%
Constipation	18%	14%	16%	8%
Asthenia	14%	18%	10%	4%
Diarrhea	8%	9%	10%	4%
Abdominal pain	6%	4%	6%	3%
Dyspepsia	4%	6%	5%	4%

1. Adverse events were recorded for 7 days when KYTRIL Tablets were given on a single day and for up to 28 days when KYTRIL Tablets were administered for 7 or 14 days.
2. Metoclopramide/dexamethasone; phenothiazines/dexamethasone; dexamethasone alone; prochlorperazine.
3. Usually mild to moderate in severity.

Carcinogenesis, Mutagenesis, Impairment of Fertility: In a 24-month carcinogenicity study, rats were treated orally with granisetron 1, 5 or 50 mg/kg/day (6, 30 or 300 mg/m^2/day). The 50 mg/kg/day dose was reduced to 25 mg/kg/day (150 mg/m^2/day) during week 59 due to toxicity. For a 50 kg person of average height (1.46 m^2 body surface area), these doses represent 4, 20, and 101 times the recommended clinical dose (1.48 mg/m^2, oral) on a body surface area basis. There was a statistically significant increase in the incidence of hepatocellular carcinomas and adenomas in males treated with 5 mg/kg/day (30 mg/m^2/day, 20 times the recommended human dose based on body surface area) and above, and in females treated with 25 mg/kg/day (150 mg/m^2/day, 101 times the recommended human dose based on body surface area). No increase in liver tumors was observed at a dose of 1 mg/kg/day (6 mg/m^2/day, 4 times the recommended human dose based on body surface area) in males and 5 mg/kg/day (30 mg/m^2/day, 20 times the recommended human dose based on body surface area) in females. In a 12-month oral toxicity study, treatment with granisetron 100 mg/kg/day (600 mg/m^2/day, 405 times the recommended human dose based on body surface area) produced hepatocellular adenomas in male and female rats while no such tumors were found in the control rats. A 24-month mouse carcinogenicity study of granisetron did not show a statistically significant increase in tumor incidence, but the study was not conclusive.

Because of the tumor findings in rat studies, KYTRIL (granisetron hydrochloride) should be prescribed only at the dose and for the indication recommended (see INDICATIONS AND USAGE, and DOSAGE AND ADMINISTRATION).

Granisetron was not mutagenic in in vitro Ames test and mouse lymphoma cell forward mutation assay, and in vivo mouse micronucleus test and in vitro and ex vivo rat hepatocyte UDS assays. It, however, produced a significant increase in UDS in HeLa cells in vitro and a significant increased incidence of cells with polyploidy in an in vitro human lymphocyte chromosomal aberration test.

Granisetron at oral doses up to 100 mg/kg/day (600 mg/m^2/day, 405 times the recommended human dose based on body surface area) was found to have no effect on fertility and reproductive performance of male and female rats.

Pregnancy: ***Teratogenic Effects:*** Pregnancy Category B. Reproduction studies have been performed in pregnant rats at oral doses up to 125 mg/kg/day (750 mg/m^2/day, 507 times the recommended human dose based on body surface area) and pregnant rabbits at oral doses up to 32 mg/kg/day (378 mg/m^2/day, 255 times the recommended human dose based on body surface area) and have revealed no evidence of impaired fertility or harm to the fetus due to granisetron. There are, however, no adequate and well-controlled studies in pregnant women. Because animal reproduction studies are not always predictive of human response, this drug should be used during pregnancy only if clearly needed.

Nursing Mothers: It is not known whether granisetron is excreted in human milk. Because many drugs are excreted in human milk, caution should be exercised when KYTRIL is administered to a nursing woman.

Pediatric Use: Safety and effectiveness in pediatric patients have not been established.

Geriatric Use: During clinical trials, 325 patients 65 years of age or older received KYTRIL Tablets; 298 were 65 to 74 years of age, and 27 were 75 years of age or older. Efficacy and safety were maintained with increasing age.

ADVERSE REACTIONS

Chemotherapy-Induced Nausea and Vomiting: Over 3700 patients have received KYTRIL Tablets in clinical trials with emetogenic cancer therapies consisting primarily of cyclophosphamide or cisplatin regimens.

In patients receiving KYTRIL Tablets 1 mg bid for 1, 7 or 14 days, or 2 mg qd for 1 day, adverse experiences reported in more than 5% of the patients with comparator and placebo incidences are listed in Table 4.

[See table 4 above]

Other adverse events reported in clinical trials were:

Gastrointestinal: In single-day dosing studies in which adverse events were collected for 7 days, nausea (20%) and vomiting (12%) were recorded as adverse events after the 24-hour efficacy assessment period.

Hepatic: In comparative trials, elevation of AST and ALT (>2 times the upper limit of normal) following the administration of KYTRIL Tablets occurred in 5% and 6% of patients, respectively. These frequencies were not significantly different from those seen with comparators (AST: 2%; ALT: 9%).

Cardiovascular: Hypertension (1%); hypotension, angina pectoris, atrial fibrillation, and syncope have been observed rarely.
Central Nervous System: Dizziness (5%), insomnia (5%), anxiety (2%), somnolence (1%). One case compatible with, but not diagnostic of, extrapyramidal symptoms has been reported in a patient treated with KYTRIL Tablets.
Hypersensitivity: Rare cases of hypersensitivity reactions, sometimes severe (eg, anaphylaxis, shortness of breath, hypotension, urticaria) have been reported.
Other: Fever (5%). Events often associated with chemotherapy also have been reported: leukopenia (9%), decreased appetite (6%), anemia (4%), alopecia (3%), thrombocytopenia (2%).
Over 5000 patients have received injectable KYTRIL in clinical trials.
Table 5 gives the comparative frequencies of the five commonly reported adverse events (≥ 3%) in patients receiving KYTRIL Injection, 40 mcg/kg, in single-day chemotherapy trials. These patients received chemotherapy, primarily cisplatin, and intravenous fluids during the 24-hour period following KYTRIL Injection administration.

Table 5. Principal Adverse Events in Clinical Trials—Single-Day Chemotherapy

	Percent of Patients with Event	
	KYTRIL Injection[1] 40 mcg/kg (n=1268)	Comparator[2] (n=422)
Headache	14%	6%
Asthenia	5%	6%
Somnolence	4%	15%
Diarrhea	4%	6%
Constipation	3%	3%

1. Adverse events were generally recorded over 7 days post-KYTRIL Injection administration.
2. Metoclopramide/dexamethasone and phenothiazines/dexamethasone.

In the absence of a placebo group, there is uncertainty as to how many of these events should be attributed to KYTRIL, except for headache, which was clearly more frequent than in comparison groups.
Radiation-Induced Nausea and Vomiting: In controlled clinical trials, the adverse events reported by patients receiving KYTRIL Tablets and concurrent radiation were similar to those reported by patients receiving KYTRIL Tablets prior to chemotherapy. The most frequently reported adverse events were diarrhea, asthenia, and constipation. Headache, however, was less prevalent in this patient population.

OVERDOSAGE

There is no specific treatment for granisetron hydrochloride overdosage. In case of overdosage, symptomatic treatment should be given. Overdosage of up to 38.5 mg of granisetron hydrochloride injection has been reported without symptoms or only the occurrence of a slight headache.

DOSAGE AND ADMINISTRATION

Emetogenic Chemotherapy: The recommended adult dosage of oral KYTRIL (granisetron hydrochloride) is 2 mg once daily or 1 mg twice daily. In the 2 mg once-daily regimen, two 1 mg tablets or 10 mL of KYTRIL Oral Solution (2 teaspoonfuls, equivalent to 2 mg of granisetron) are given up to 1 hour before chemotherapy. In the 1 mg twice-daily regimen, the first 1 mg tablet or one teaspoonful (5 mL) of KYTRIL Oral Solution is given up to 1 hour before chemotherapy, and the second tablet or second teaspoonful (5 mL) of KYTRIL Oral Solution, 12 hours after the first. Either regimen is administered only on the day(s) chemotherapy is given. Continued treatment, while not on chemotherapy, has not been found to be useful.
Use in the Elderly, Pediatric Patients, Renal Failure Patients or Hepatically Impaired Patients: No dosage adjustment is recommended (see CLINICAL PHARMACOLOGY: Pharmacokinetics).
Radiation (Either Total Body Irradiation or Fractionated Abdominal Radiation): The recommended adult dosage of oral KYTRIL is 2 mg once daily. Two 1 mg tablets or 10 mL of KYTRIL Oral Solution (2 teaspoonfuls, equivalent to 2 mg of granisetron) are taken within 1 hour of radiation.
Pediatric Use: There is no experience with oral KYTRIL in the prevention of radiation-induced nausea and vomiting in pediatric patients.
Use in the Elderly: No dosage adjustment is recommended.

HOW SUPPLIED

Tablets: White, triangular, biconvex, film-coated tablets; tablets are debossed K1 on one face.
1 mg Unit of Use 2's: NDC 0004-0241-33
1 mg SUP 20's: NDC 0004-0241-26 (intended for institutional use only)
Store between 15° and 30°C (59° and 86°F). Keep container closed tightly. Protect from light.
Oral Solution: Clear, orange-colored, orange-flavored, 2 mg/10 mL, in 30 mL amber glass bottles with child-resistant closures: NDC 0004-0237-09
Store at 25°C (77°F); excursions permitted to 15° to 30°C (59° to 86°F) [see USP Controlled Room Temperature]. Keep bottle closed tightly and stored in an upright position. Protect from light.

Distributed by Roche Laboratories Inc., Nutley, New Jersey 07110-1199

Revised: June 2001

Shown in Product Identification Guide, page 331

LARIAM®

℞

[lar-ē-um]
brand of
mefloquine hydrochloride
TABLETS
℞ only

DESCRIPTION

Lariam (mefloquine hydrochloride) is an antimalarial agent available as 250-mg tablets of mefloquine hydrochloride (equivalent to 228.0 mg of the free base) for oral administration.
Mefloquine hydrochloride is a 4-quinolinemethanol derivative with the specific chemical name of (R*, S*)-(±)-α-2-piperidinyl-2,8-bis (trifluoromethyl)-4-quinolinemethanol hydrochloride. It is a 2-aryl substituted chemical structural analog of quinine. The drug is a white to almost white crystalline compound, slightly soluble in water.
Mefloquine hydrochloride has a calculated molecular weight of 414.78.
The inactive ingredients are ammonium-calcium alginate, corn starch, crospovidone, lactose, magnesium stearate, microcrystalline cellulose, poloxamer #331, and talc.

CLINICAL PHARMACOLOGY

Pharmacokinetics
Absorption
The absolute oral bioavailability of mefloquine has not been determined since an intravenous formulation is not available. The bioavailability of the tablet formation compared with an oral solution was over 85%. The presence of food significantly enhances the rate and extent of absorption, leading to about a 40% increase in bioavailability. In healthy volunteers, plasma concentrations peak 6 to 24 hours (median, about 17 hours) after a single dose of Lariam. In a similar group of volunteers, maximum plasma concentrations in µg/L are roughly equivalent to the dose in milligrams (for example, a single 1000 mg dose produces a maximum concentration of about 1000 µg/L). In healthy volunteers, a dose of 250 mg once weekly produces maximum steady-state plasma concentrations of 1000 to 2000 µg/L, which are reached after 7 to 10 weeks.
Distribution
In healthy adults, the apparent volume of distribution is approximately 20 L/kg, indicating extensive tissue distribution. Mefloquine may accumulate in parasitized erythrocytes. Experiments conducted in vitro with human blood using concentrations between 50 and 1000 mg/mL showed a relatively constant erythrocyte-to-plasma concentration ratio of about 2 to 1. The equilibrium reached in less than 30 minutes was found to be reversible. Protein binding is about 98%.
Mefloquine crosses the placenta. Excretion into breast milk appears to be minimal (see **PRECAUTIONS: Nursing Mothers**).
Metabolism
Two metabolites have been identified in humans. The main metabolite, 2,8-*bis*-trifluoromethyl-4-quinoline carboxylic acid, is inactive in *Plasmodium falciparum*. In a study in healthy volunteers, the carboxylic acid metabolite appeared in plasma 2 to 4 hours after a single oral dose. Maximum plasma concentrations, which were about 50% higher than those of mefloquine, were reached after 2 weeks. Thereafter, plasma levels of the main metabolite and mefloquine declined at a similar rate. The area under the plasma concentration-time curve (AUC) of the main metabolite was 3 to 5 times larger than that of the parent drug. The other metabolite, an alcohol, was present in minute quantities only.
Elimination
In several studies in healthy adults, the mean elimination half-life of mefloquine varied between 2 and 4 weeks, with an average of about 3 weeks. Total clearance, which is essentially hepatic, is in the order of 30 mL/min. There is evidence that mefloquine is excreted mainly in the bile and feces. In volunteers, urinary excretion of unchanged mefloquine and its main metabolite under steady-state condition accounted for about 9% and 4% of the dose, respectively. Concentrations of other metabolites could not be measured in the urine.
Pharmacokinetics in Special Clinical Situations
Children and the Elderly
No relevant age-related changes have been observed in the pharmacokinetics of mefloquine. Therefore, the dosage for children has been extrapolated from the recommended adult dose.
No pharmacokinetic studies have been performed in patients with renal insufficiency since only a small proportion of the drug is eliminated renally. Mefloquine and its main metabolite are not appreciably removed by hemodialysis. No special chemoprophylactic dosage adjustments are indicated for dialysis patients to achieve concentrations in plasma similar to those in healthy persons.
Although clearance of mefloquine may increase in late pregnancy, in general, pregnancy has no clinically relevant effect on the pharmacokinetics of mefloquine.
The pharmacokinetics of mefloquine may be altered in acute malaria.
Pharmacokinetic differences have been observed between various ethnic populations. In practice, however, these are of minor importance compared with host immune status and sensitivity of the parasite.
During long-term prophylaxis (>2 years), the trough concentrations and the elimination half-life of mefloquine were similar to those obtained in the same population after 6 months of drug use, which is when they reached steady state.
In vitro and in vivo studies showed no hemolysis associated with glucose-6-phosphate dehydrogenase deficiency (see **ANIMAL TOXICOLOGY**).
Microbiology
Mechanism of Action
Mefloquine is an antimalarial agent which acts as a blood schizonticide. Its exact mechanism of action is not known.
Activity In Vitro and In Vivo
Mefloquine is active against the erythrocytic stages of *Plasmodium* species (see **INDICATIONS AND USAGE**). However, the drug has no effect against the exoerythrocytic (hepatic) stages of the parasite. Mefloquine is effective against malaria parasites resistant to chloroquine (see **INDICATIONS AND USAGE**).
Drug Resistance
Strains of *P. falciparum* with decreased susceptibility to mefloquine can be selected in vitro or in vivo. Resistance of *P. falciparum* to mefloquine has been reported in areas of multi-drug resistance in South East Asia. Increased incidences of resistance have also been reported in other parts of the world.
Cross-Resistance
Cross-resistance between mefloquine and halofantrine and cross-resistance between mefloquine and quinine have been observed in some regions.

INDICATIONS AND USAGE

Treatment of Acute Malaria Infections
Lariam is indicated for the treatment of mild to moderate acute malaria caused by mefloquine-susceptible strains of *P. falciparum* (both chloroquine-susceptible and resistant strains) or by *Plasmodium vivax*. There are insufficient clinical data to document the effect of mefloquine in malaria caused by *P. ovale* or *P. malariae*.
Note: Patients with acute *P. vivax* malaria, treated with Lariam, are at high risk of relapse because Lariam does not eliminate exoerythrocytic (hepatic phase) parasites. To avoid relapse, after initial treatment of the acute infection with Lariam, patients should subsequently be treated with an 8-aminoquinoline derivative (eg, primaquine).
Prevention of Malaria
Lariam is indicated for the prophylaxis of *P. falciparum* and *P. vivax* malaria infections, including prophylaxis of chloroquine-resistant strains of *P. falciparum*.

CONTRAINDICATIONS

Use of Lariam is contraindicated in patients with a known hypersensitivity to mefloquine or related compounds (eg, quinine and quinidine) or to any of the excipients contained in the formulation. Lariam should not be prescribed for prophylaxis in patients with active depression, a recent history of depression, generalized anxiety disorder, psychosis, or schizophrenia or other major psychiatric disorders, or with a history of convulsions.

WARNINGS

In case of life-threatening, serious or overwhelming malaria infections due to *P. falciparum*, patients should be treated with an intravenous antimalarial drug. Following completion of intravenous treatment, Lariam may be given to complete the course of therapy.
Data on the use of halofantrine subsequent to administration of Lariam suggest a significant, potentially fatal prolongation of the QTc interval of the ECG. Therefore, halofantrine must not be given simultaneously with or subsequent to Lariam. No data are available on the use of Lariam after halofantrine (see PRECAUTIONS: Drug Interactions).
Mefloquine may cause psychiatric symptoms in a number of patients, ranging from anxiety, paranoia, and depression to hallucinations and psychotic behavior. On occasions, these symptoms have been reported to continue long after mefloquine has been stopped. Rare cases of suicidal ideation and suicide have been reported though no relationship to drug administration has been confirmed. To minimize the chances of these adverse events, mefloquine should not be taken for prophylaxis in patients with active depression or with a recent history of depression, generalized anxiety disorder, psychosis, or schizophrenia or other major psychiatric disorders. Lariam should be used with caution in patients with a previous history of depression.
During prophylactic use, if psychiatric symptoms such as acute anxiety, depression, restlessness or confusion occur, these may be considered prodromal to a more serious event. In these cases, the drug must be discontinued and an alternative medication should be substituted.
Concomitant administration of Lariam and quinine or quinidine may produce electrocardiographic abnormalities.
Concomitant administration of Lariam and quinine or chloroquine may increase the risk of convulsions.

Continued on next page

Lariam—Cont.

PRECAUTIONS

General

Hypersensitivity reactions ranging from mild cutaneous events to anaphylaxis cannot be predicted.

In patients with epilepsy, Lariam may increase the risk of convulsions. The drug should therefore be prescribed only for curative treatment in such patients and only if there are compelling medical reasons for its use (see **PRECAUTIONS: Drug Interactions**).

Caution should be exercised with regard to activities requiring alertness and fine motor coordination such as driving, piloting aircraft, operating machinery, and deep-sea diving, as dizziness, a loss of balance, or other disorders of the central or peripheral nervous system have been reported during and following the use of Lariam. These effects may occur after therapy is discontinued due to the long half-life of the drug. Lariam should be used with caution in patients with psychiatric disturbances because mefloquine use has been associated with emotional disturbances (see **ADVERSE REACTIONS**).

In patients with impaired liver function the elimination of mefloquine may be prolonged, leading to higher plasma levels.

This drug has been administered for longer than 1 year. If the drug is to be administered for a prolonged period, periodic evaluations including liver function tests should be performed. Although retinal abnormalities seen in humans with long-term chloroquine use have not been observed with mefloquine use, long-term feeding of mefloquine to rats resulted in dose-related ocular lesions (retinal degeneration, retinal edema and lenticular opacity at 12.5 mg/kg/day and higher) (see **ANIMAL TOXICOLOGY**). Therefore, periodic ophthalmic examinations are recommended.

Parenteral studies in animals show that mefloquine, a myocardial depressant, possesses 20% of the antifibrillatory action of quinidine and produces 50% of the increase in the PR interval reported with quinine. The effect of mefloquine on the compromised cardiovascular system has not been evaluated. However, transitory and clinically silent ECG alterations have been reported during the use of mefloquine. Alterations included sinus bradycardia, sinus arrhythmia, first degree AV-block, prolongation of the QTc interval and abnormal T waves (see also cardiovascular effects under **PRECAUTIONS: Drug Interactions** and **ADVERSE REACTIONS**). The benefits of Lariam therapy should be weighed against the possibility of adverse effects in patients with cardiac disease.

Laboratory Tests

Periodic evaluation of hepatic function should be performed during prolonged prophylaxis.

Information for Patients

Medication Guide: As required by law, a Lariam Medication Guide is supplied to patients when Lariam is dispensed. An information wallet card is also supplied to patients when Lariam is dispensed. Patients should be instructed to read the Medication Guide when Lariam is received and to carry the information wallet card with them when they are taking Lariam. The complete texts of the Medication Guide and information wallet card are reprinted at the end of this document.

Patients should be advised:

- that malaria can be a life-threatening infection in the traveler;
- that Lariam is being prescribed to help prevent or treat this serious infection;
- that in a small percentage of cases, patients are unable to take this medication because of side effects, and it may be necessary to change medications;
- that when used as prophylaxis, the first dose of Lariam should be taken 1 week prior to arrival in an endemic area;
- that if the patients experience psychiatric symptoms such as acute anxiety, depression, restlessness or confusion, these may be considered prodromal to a more serious event. In these cases, the drug must be discontinued and an alternative medication should be substituted;
- that no chemoprophylactic regimen is 100% effective, and protective clothing, insect repellents, and bednets are important components of malaria prophylaxis;
- to seek medical attention for any febrile illness that occurs after return from a malarious area and to inform their physician that they may have been exposed to malaria.

Drug Interactions

Drug-drug interactions with Lariam have not been explored in detail. There is one report of cardiopulmonary arrest, with full recovery, in a patient who was taking a beta blocker (propranolol) (see **PRECAUTIONS: General**). The effects of mefloquine on the compromised cardiovascular system have not been evaluated. The benefits of Lariam therapy should be weighed against the possibility of adverse effects in patients with cardiac disease.

Because of the danger of a potentially fatal prolongation of the QTc interval, halofantrine must not be given simultaneously with or subsequent to Lariam (see **WARNINGS**).

Concomitant administration of Lariam and other related compounds (eg, quinine, quinidine and chloroquine) may produce electrocardiographic abnormalities and increase the risk of convulsions (see **WARNINGS**). If these drugs are to be used in the initial treatment of severe malaria, Lariam administration should be delayed at least 12 hours after the last dose. There is evidence that the use of halofantrine after mefloquine causes a significant lengthening of the QTc interval. Clinically significant QTc prolongation has not been found with mefloquine alone.

This appears to be the only clinically relevant interaction of this kind with Lariam, although theoretically, coadministration of other drugs known to alter cardiac conduction (eg, anti-arrhythmic or beta-adrenergic blocking agents, calcium channel blockers, antihistamines or H_1-blocking agents, tricyclic antidepressants and phenothiazines) might also contribute to a prolongation of the QTc interval. There are no data that conclusively establish whether the concomitant administration of mefloquine and the above listed agents has an effect on cardiac function.

In patients taking an anticonvulsant (eg, valproic acid, carbamazepine, phenobarbital or phenytoin), the concomitant use of Lariam may reduce seizure control by lowering the plasma levels of the anticonvulsant. Therefore, patients concurrently taking antiseizure medication and Lariam should have the blood level of their antiseizure medication monitored and the dosage adjusted appropriately (see **PRECAUTIONS: General**).

When Lariam is taken concurrently with oral live typhoid vaccines, attenuation of immunization cannot be excluded. Vaccinations with attenuated live bacteria should therefore be completed at least 3 days before the first dose of Lariam.

No other drug interactions are known. Nevertheless, the effects of Lariam on travelers receiving comedication, particularly diabetics or patients using anticoagulants, should be checked before departure.

In clinical trials, the concomitant administration of sulfadoxine and pyrimethamine did not alter the adverse reaction profile.

Carcinogenesis, Mutagenesis, Impairment of Fertility

Carcinogenesis

The carcinogenic potential of mefloquine was studied in rats and mice in 2-year feeding studies at doses of up to 30 mg/kg/day. No treatment-related increases in tumors of any type were noted.

Mutagenesis

The mutagenic potential of mefloquine was studied in a variety of assay systems including: Ames test, a host-mediated assay in mice, fluctuation tests and a mouse micronucleus assay. Several of these assays were performed with and without prior metabolic activation. In no instance was evidence obtained for the mutagenicity of mefloquine.

Impairment of Fertility

Fertility studies in rats at doses of 5, 20, and 50 mg/kg/day of mefloquine have demonstrated adverse effects on fertility in the male at the high dose of 50 mg/kg/day, and in the female at doses of 20 and 50 mg/kg/day. Histopathological lesions were noted in the epididymides from male rats at doses of 20 and 50 mg/kg/day. Administration of 250 mg/week of mefloquine (base) in adult males for 22 weeks failed to reveal any deleterious effects on human spermatozoa.

Pregnancy

Teratogenic Effects

Pregnancy Category C. Mefloquine has been demonstrated to be teratogenic in rats and mice at a dose of 100 mg/kg/day. In rabbits, a high dose of 160 mg/kg/day was embryotoxic and teratogenic, and a dose of 80 mg/kg/day was teratogenic but not embryotoxic. There are no adequate and well-controlled studies in pregnant women. However, clinical experience with Lariam has not revealed an embryotoxic or teratogenic effect. Mefloquine should be used during pregnancy only if the potential benefit justifies the potential risk to the fetus. Women of childbearing potential who are traveling to areas where malaria is endemic should be warned against becoming pregnant. Women of childbearing potential should also be advised to practice contraception during malaria prophylaxis with Lariam and for up to 3 months thereafter. However, in the case of unplanned pregnancy, malaria chemoprophylaxis with Lariam is not considered an indication for pregnancy termination.

Nursing Mothers

Mefloquine is excreted in human milk in small amounts, the activity of which is unknown. Based on a study in a few subjects, low concentrations (3% to 4%) of mefloquine were excreted in human milk following a dose equivalent to 250 mg of the free base. Because of the potential for serious adverse reactions in nursing infants from mefloquine, a decision should be made whether to discontinue the drug, taking into account the importance of the drug to the mother.

Pediatric Use

Use of Lariam to treat acute, uncomplicated *P. falciparum* malaria in pediatric patients is supported by evidence from adequate and well-controlled studies of Lariam in adults with additional data from published open-label and comparative trials using Lariam to treat malaria caused by *P. falciparum* in patients younger than 16 years of age. The safety and effectiveness of Lariam for the treatment of malaria in pediatric patients below the age of 6 months have not been established.

In several studies, the administration of Lariam for the treatment of malaria was associated with early vomiting in pediatric patients. Early vomiting was cited in some reports as a possible cause of treatment failure. If a second dose is not tolerated, the patient should be monitored closely and alternative malaria treatment considered if improvement is not observed within a reasonable period of time (see **DOSAGE AND ADMINISTRATION**).

Geriatric Use

Clinical studies of Lariam did not include sufficient numbers of subjects aged 65 and over to determine whether they respond differently from younger subjects. Other reported clinical experience has not identified differences in responses between the elderly and younger patients. Since electrocardiographic abnormalities have been observed in individuals treated with Lariam (see **PRECAUTIONS**) and underlying cardiac disease is more prevalent in elderly than in younger patients, the benefits of Lariam therapy should be weighed against the possibility of adverse cardiac effects in elderly patients.

ADVERSE REACTIONS

Clinical

At the doses used for treatment of acute malaria infections, the symptoms possibly attributable to drug administration cannot be distinguished from those symptoms usually attributable to the disease itself.

Among subjects who received mefloquine for prophylaxis of malaria, the most frequently observed adverse experience was vomiting (3%). Dizziness, syncope, extrasystoles and other complaints affecting less than 1% were also reported.

Among subjects who received mefloquine for treatment, the most frequently observed adverse experiences included: dizziness, myalgia, nausea, fever, headache, vomiting, chills, diarrhea, skin rash, abdominal pain, fatigue, loss of appetite, and tinnitus. Those side effects occurring in less than 1% included bradycardia, hair loss, emotional problems, pruritus, asthenia, transient emotional disturbances and telogen effluvium (loss of resting hair). Seizures have also been reported.

Two serious adverse reactions were cardiopulmonary arrest in one patient shortly after ingesting a single prophylactic dose of mefloquine while concomitantly using propranolol (see **PRECAUTIONS: Drug Interactions**), and encephalopathy of unknown etiology during prophylactic mefloquine administration. The relationship of encephalopathy to drug administration could not be clearly established.

Postmarketing

Postmarketing surveillance indicates that the same kind of adverse experiences are reported during prophylaxis, as well as acute treatment.

The most frequently reported adverse events are nausea, vomiting, loose stools or diarrhea, abdominal pain, dizziness or vertigo, loss of balance, and neuropsychiatric events such as headache, somnolence, and sleep disorders (insomnia, abnormal dreams). These are usually mild and may decrease despite continued use.

Occasionally, more severe neuropsychiatric disorders have been reported such as: sensory and motor neuropathies (including paresthesia, tremor and ataxia), convulsions, agitation or restlessness, anxiety, depression, mood changes, panic attacks, forgetfulness, confusion, hallucinations, aggression, psychotic or paranoid reactions and encephalopathy. Rare cases of suicidal ideation and suicide have been reported though no relationship to drug administration has been confirmed.

Other infrequent adverse events include:

Cardiovascular Disorders: circulatory disturbances (hypotension, hypertension, flushing, syncope), chest pain, tachycardia or palpitation, bradycardia, irregular pulse, extrasystoles, A-V block, and other transient cardiac conduction alterations

Skin Disorders: rash, exanthema, erythema, urticaria, pruritus, edema, hair loss, erythema multiforme, and Stevens-Johnson syndrome

Musculoskeletal Disorders: muscle weakness, muscle cramps, myalgia, and arthralgia

Other Symptoms: visual disturbances, vestibular disorders including tinnitus and hearing impairment, dyspnea, asthenia, malaise, fatigue, fever, sweating, chills, dyspepsia and loss of appetite

Laboratory

The most frequently observed laboratory alterations which could be possibly attributable to drug administration were decreased hematocrit, transient elevation of transaminases, leukopenia and thrombocytopenia. These alterations were observed in patients with acute malaria who received treatment doses of the drug and were attributed to the disease itself.

During prophylactic administration of mefloquine to indigenous populations in malaria-endemic areas, the following occasional alterations in laboratory values were observed: transient elevation of transaminases, leukocytosis or thrombocytopenia.

Because of the long half-life of mefloquine, adverse reactions to Lariam may occur or persist up to several weeks after the last dose.

OVERDOSAGE

In cases of overdosage with Lariam, the symptoms mentioned under **ADVERSE REACTIONS** may be more pronounced. The following procedure is recommended in case of overdosage: Induce vomiting or perform gastric lavage, as appropriate. Monitor cardiac function (if possible by ECG) and neuropsychiatric status for at least 24 hours. Provide symptomatic and intensive supportive treatment as required, particularly for cardiovascular disturbances.

DOSAGE AND ADMINISTRATION (see INDICATIONS AND USAGE)

Adult Patients

Treatment of mild to moderate malaria in adults caused by *P. vivax* or mefloquine-susceptible strains of *P. falciparum*.

Five tablets (1250 mg) mefloquine hydrochloride to be given as a single oral dose. The drug should not be taken on an empty stomach and should be administered with at least 8 oz (240 mL) of water.

If a full-treatment course with Lariam does not lead to improvement within 48 to 72 hours, Lariam should not be used for retreatment. An alternative therapy should be used. Similarly, if previous prophylaxis with mefloquine has failed, Lariam should not be used for curative treatment.

Note: Patients with acute *P. vivax* malaria, treated with Lariam, are at high risk of relapse because Lariam does not eliminate exoerythrocytic (hepatic phase) parasites. To avoid relapse after initial treatment of the acute infection with Lariam, patients should subsequently be treated with an 8-aminoquinoline derivative (eg, primaquine).

Malaria Prophylaxis

One 250 mg Lariam tablet once weekly.

Prophylactic drug administration should begin 1 week before arrival in an endemic area. Subsequent weekly doses should be taken regularly, always on the same day of each week, preferably after the main meal. To reduce the risk of malaria after leaving an endemic area, prophylaxis must be continued for 4 additional weeks to ensure suppressive blood levels of the drug when merozoites emerge from the liver. Tablets should not be taken on an empty stomach and should be administered with at least 8 oz (240 mL) of water.

In certain cases, eg, when a traveler is taking other medication, it may be desirable to start prophylaxis 2 to 3 weeks prior to departure, in order to ensure that the combination of drugs is well tolerated (see **PRECAUTIONS: Drug Interactions**).

When prophylaxis with Lariam fails, physicians should carefully evaluate which antimalarial to use for therapy.

Pediatric Patients

Treatment of mild to moderate malaria in pediatric patients caused by mefloquine-susceptible strains of *P. falciparum*.

Twenty (20) to 25 mg/kg body weight. Splitting the total therapeutic dose into 2 doses taken 6 to 8 hours apart may reduce the occurrence or severity of adverse effects. Experience with Lariam in infants less than 3 months old or weighing less than 5 kg is limited. The drug should not be taken on an empty stomach and should be administered with ample water. The tablets may be crushed and suspended in a small amount of water, milk or other beverage for administration to small children and other persons unable to swallow them whole.

If a full-treatment course with Lariam does not lead to improvement within 48 to 72 hours, Lariam should not be used for retreatment. An alternative therapy should be used. Similarly, if previous prophylaxis with mefloquine has failed, Lariam should not be used for curative treatment.

In pediatric patients, the administration of Lariam for the treatment of malaria has been associated with early vomiting. In some cases, early vomiting has been cited as a possible cause of treatment failure (see **PRECAUTIONS**). If a significant loss of drug product is observed or suspected because of vomiting, a second full dose of Lariam should be administered to patients who vomit less than 30 minutes after receiving the drug. If vomiting occurs 30 to 60 minutes after a dose, an additional half-dose should be given. If vomiting recurs, the patient should be monitored closely and alternative malaria treatment considered if improvement is not observed within a reasonable period of time.

The safety and effectiveness of Lariam to treat malaria in pediatric patients below the age of 6 months have not been established.

Malaria Prophylaxis

The following doses have been extrapolated from the recommended adult dose. Neither the pharmacokinetics, nor the clinical efficacy of these doses have been determined in children owing to the difficulty of acquiring this information in pediatric subjects. The recommended prophylactic dose of Lariam is approximately 5 mg/kg body weight once weekly. One 250 mg Lariam tablet should be taken once weekly in pediatric patients weighing over 45 kg. In pediatric patients weighing less than 45 kg, the weekly dose decreases in proportion to body weight:

30 to 45 kg:	3/4 tablet
20 to 30 kg:	1/2 tablet
10 to 20 kg:	1/4 tablet
5 to 10 kg:	1/8 tablet*

*Approximate tablet fraction based on a dosage of 5 mg/kg body weight. Exact doses for children weighing less than 10 kg may best be prepared and dispensed by pharmacists.

Experience with Lariam in infants less than 3 months old or weighing less than 5 kg is limited.

HOW SUPPLIED

Lariam is available as scored, white, round tablets, containing 250 mg of mefloquine hydrochloride in unit-dose packages of 25 (NDC 0004-0172-02). Imprint on tablets: LARIAM 250 ROCHE

Tablets should be stored at 25°C (77°F); excursions permitted to 15° to 30°C (59° to 86°F).

ANIMAL TOXICOLOGY

Ocular lesions were observed in rats fed mefloquine daily for 2 years. All surviving rats given 30 mg/kg/day had ocular lesions in both eyes characterized by retinal degeneration, opacity of the lens, and retinal edema. Similar but less severe lesions were observed in 80% of female and 22% of male rats fed 12.5 mg/kg/day for 2 years. At doses of 5 mg/kg/day, only corneal lesions were observed. They occurred in 9% of rats studied.

Revised: May 2004

MEDICATION GUIDE

This Medication Guide is intended only for travelers who are taking Lariam to prevent malaria. The information may not apply to patients who are sick with malaria and who are taking Lariam to treat malaria.

An information wallet card is provided with this Medication Guide. Carry it with you when you are taking Lariam.

This Medication Guide was revised in May 2004. Please read it before you start taking Lariam and each time you get a refill. There may be new information. This Medication Guide does not take the place of talking with your prescriber (doctor or other health care provider) about Lariam and malaria prevention. Only you and your prescriber can decide if Lariam is right for you. If you cannot take Lariam, you may be able to take a different medicine to prevent malaria.

What is the most important information I should know about Lariam?

1. **Take Lariam exactly as prescribed to prevent malaria.** Malaria is an infection that can cause death and is spread to humans through mosquito bites. If you travel to parts of the world where the mosquitoes carry the malaria parasite, you must take a malaria prevention medicine. Lariam is one of a small number of medications approved to prevent and to treat malaria. If taken correctly, Lariam is effective at preventing malaria but, like all medications, it may produce side effects in some patients.
2. **Lariam can rarely cause serious mental problems in some patients.** The most frequently reported side effects with Lariam, such as nausea, difficulty sleeping, and bad dreams are usually mild and do not cause people to stop taking the medicine. However, people taking Lariam occasionally experience severe anxiety, feelings that people are against them, hallucinations (seeing or hearing things that are not there, for example), depression, unusual behavior, or feeling disoriented. There have been reports that in some patients these side effects continue after Lariam is stopped. Some patients taking Lariam think about killing themselves, and there have been rare reports of suicides. It is not known whether Lariam was responsible for these suicides.
3. **You need to take malaria prevention medicine before you travel to a malaria area, while you are in a malaria area, and after you return from a malaria area.** Medicines approved in the United States for malaria prevention include Lariam, doxycycline, atovaquone/proguanil, hydroxychloroquine, and chloroquine. Not all of these drugs work equally as well in all areas of the world where there is malaria. The chloroquines, for example, do not work in areas where the malaria parasite has developed resistance to chloroquine. Lariam may be effective against malaria that is resistant to chloroquine or other drugs. All drugs to treat malaria have side effects that are different for each one. For example, some may make your skin more sensitive to sunlight (Lariam does not do this). However, if you use Lariam to prevent malaria and you develop a sudden onset of anxiety, depression, restlessness, confusion (possible signs of more serious mental problems), or you develop other serious side effects, contact a doctor or other health care provider. It may be necessary to stop taking Lariam and use another malaria prevention medicine instead. If you can't get another medicine, leave the malaria area. However, be aware that leaving the malaria area may not protect you from getting malaria. You still need to take a malaria prevention medicine.

Who should not take Lariam?

Do not take Lariam to **prevent** malaria if you

- **have depression or had depression recently**
- **have had recent mental illness or problems**, including anxiety disorder, schizophrenia (a severe type of mental illness), or psychosis (losing touch with reality)
- **have or had seizures (epilepsy or convulsions)**
- **are allergic to quinine or quinidine (medicines related to Lariam)**

Tell your prescriber about all your medical conditions. Lariam may not be right for you if you have certain conditions, especially the ones listed below:

- **Heart disease.** Lariam may not be right for you.
- **Pregnancy.** Tell your prescriber if you are pregnant or plan to become pregnant. It is dangerous for the mother and for the unborn baby (fetus) to get malaria during pregnancy. Therefore, ask your prescriber if you should take Lariam or another medicine to prevent malaria while you are pregnant.
- **Breast-feeding.** Lariam can pass through your milk and may harm the baby. Therefore, ask your prescriber whether you will need to stop breast-feeding or use another medicine.
- **Liver problems.**

Tell your prescriber about all the medicines you take, including prescription and non-prescription medicines, vitamins, and herbal supplements. Some medicines may give you a higher chance of having serious side effects from Lariam.

How should I take Lariam?

Take Lariam exactly as prescribed. If you are an adult or pediatric patient weighing 45 kg (99 pounds) or less, your prescriber will tell you the correct dose based on your weight.

To prevent malaria

- For adults and pediatric patients weighing over 45 kg, take 1 tablet of Lariam at least 1 week before you travel to a malaria area (or 2 to 3 weeks before you travel to a malaria area, if instructed by your prescriber). This starts the prevention and also helps you see how Lariam affects you and the other medicines you take. **Take 1 Lariam tablet once a week,** on the same day each week, while in a malaria area.
- **Continue taking Lariam for 4 weeks after returning from a malaria area.** If you cannot continue taking Lariam due to side effects or for other reasons, contact your prescriber.
- Take Lariam just after a meal and with at least 1 cup (8 ounces) of water.
- For children, Lariam can be given with water or crushed and mixed with water or sugar water. The prescriber will tell you the correct dose for children based on the child's weight.
- If you are told by a doctor or other health care provider to stop taking Lariam due to side effects or for other reasons, it will be necessary to take another malaria medicine. You must take **malaria prevention medicine before you travel to a malaria area, while you are in a malaria area, and after you return from a malaria area. If you don't have access to a doctor or other health care provider or to another medicine besides Lariam and have to stop taking it, leave the malaria area. However, be aware that leaving the malaria area may not protect you from getting malaria. You still need to take a malaria prevention medicine.**

What should I avoid while taking Lariam?

- **Halofantrine (marketed under various brand names),** a medicine used to treat malaria. Taking both of these medicines together can cause serious heart problems that can cause death.
- **Do not become pregnant.** Women should use effective birth control while taking Lariam.
- **Quinine, quinidine, or chloroquine (other medicines used to treat malaria).** Taking these medicines with Lariam could cause changes in your heart rate or increase the risk of seizures.

In addition:

- **Be careful driving or in other activities** needing alertness and careful movements (fine motor coordination). Lariam can cause dizziness or loss of balance, even after you stop taking it.
- **Be aware that certain vaccines may not work if given while you are taking Lariam.** Your prescriber may want you to finish taking your vaccines at least 3 days before starting Lariam.

What are the possible side effects of Lariam?

Lariam, like all medicines, may cause side effects in some patients. The most frequently reported side effects with Lariam when used for prevention of malaria include nausea, vomiting, diarrhea, dizziness, difficulty sleeping, and bad dreams. These are usually mild and do not cause people to stop taking the medicine.

Lariam may cause serious mental problems in some patients (see "What is the most important information I should know about Lariam?").

Lariam may affect your liver and your eyes if you take it for a long time. Your prescriber will tell you if you should have your eyes and liver checked while taking Lariam.

What else should I know about preventing malaria?

- **Find out whether you need malaria prevention.** Before you travel, talk with your prescriber about your travel plans to determine whether you need to take medicine to prevent malaria. Even in those countries where malaria is present, there may be areas of the country that are free of malaria. In general, malaria is more common in rural (country) areas than in big cities, and it is more common during rainy seasons, when mosquitoes are most common. You can get information about the areas of the world where malaria occurs from the Centers for Disease Control and Prevention (CDC) and from local authorities in the countries you visit. If possible, plan your travel to reduce the risk of malaria.
- **Take medicine to prevent malaria infection.** Without malaria prevention medicine, you have a higher risk of getting malaria. Malaria starts with flu-like symptoms, such as chills, fever, muscle pains, and headaches. However, malaria can make you very sick or cause death if you don't seek medical help immediately. These symptoms may disappear for a while, and you may think you are well. But, the symptoms return later and then it may be too late for successful treatment.

  Malaria can cause confusion, coma, and seizures. It can cause kidney failure, breathing problems, and severe damage to red blood cells. However, malaria can be easily diagnosed with a blood test, and if caught in time, can be effectively treated.

  If you get flu-like symptoms (chills, fever, muscle pains, or headaches) after you return from a malaria area, get medical help right away and tell your prescriber that you may have been exposed to malaria.

  People who have lived for many years in areas with malaria may have some immunity to malaria (they do not get it as easily) and may not take malaria prevention medicine. This does not mean that you don't need to take malaria prevention medicine.
- **Protect against mosquito bites.** Medicines do not always completely prevent your catching malaria from mosquito

Continued on next page

Lariam—Cont.

bites. So protect yourself very well against mosquitoes. Cover your skin with long sleeves and long pants, and use mosquito repellent and bednets while in malaria areas. If you are out in the bush, you may want to pre-wash your clothes with permethrin. This is a mosquito repellent that may be effective for weeks after use. Ask your prescriber for other ways to protect yourself.

General information about the safe and effective use of Lariam.

Medicines are sometimes prescribed for conditions not listed in Medication Guides. If you have any concerns about Lariam, ask your prescriber. This Medication Guide contains certain important information for travelers visiting areas with malaria. Your prescriber or pharmacist can give you information about Lariam that was written for health care professionals. Do not use Lariam for a condition for which it was not prescribed. Do not share Lariam with other people.

This Medication Guide has been approved by the U.S. Food and Drug Administration.

Reprint of information wallet card:

Roche

Lariam® (mefloquine hydrochloride) Tablets

Carry this information wallet card with you when you are taking Lariam.

You need to take malaria prevention medicine before you travel to a malaria area, while you are in a malaria area, and after you return from a malaria area.

If taken correctly, Lariam is effective at preventing malaria but, like all medications, it may produce side effects in some patients.

If you use Lariam to prevent malaria and you develop a sudden onset of anxiety, depression, restlessness, confusion (possible signs of more serious mental problems), or you develop other serious side effects, contact a doctor or other health care provider. It may be necessary to stop taking Lariam and use another malaria prevention medicine.

Other medicines approved in the United States for malaria prevention include: doxycycline, atovaquone/ proguanil, hydroxy-chloroquine, and chloroquine. Not all malaria medicines work equally well in malaria areas. The chloroquines, for example, do not work in many parts of the world. If you can't get another medicine, leave the malaria area. However, be aware that leaving the malaria area may not protect you from getting malaria. You still need to take a malaria prevention medicine.

Please read the Medication Guide for additional information on Lariam.

Card Revised: May 2004

Manufactured by:
F. Hoffmann-La Roche Ltd., Basel, Switzerland
Distributed by: Roche Pharmaceuticals Inc., Nutley, New Jersey 07110
Roche Laboratories Inc.

Medication Guide Revised: May 2004

Shown in Product Identification Guide, page 331

PEGASYS®
(peginterferon alfa-2a) ℞

Alpha interferons, including PEGASYS (peginterferon alfa-2a), may cause or aggravate fatal or life-threatening neuropsychiatric, autoimmune, ischemic, and infectious disorders. Patients should be monitored closely with periodic clinical and laboratory evaluations. Therapy should be withdrawn in patients with persistently severe or worsening signs or symptoms of these conditions. In many, but not all cases, these disorders resolve after stopping PEGASYS therapy (see WARNINGS and ADVERSE REACTIONS).

Use with Ribavirin. Ribavirin, including COPEGUS®, may cause birth defects and/or death of the fetus. Extreme care must be taken to avoid pregnancy in female patients and in female partners of male patients. Ribavirin causes hemolytic anemia. The anemia associated with ribavirin therapy may result in a worsening of cardiac disease. Ribavirin is genotoxic and mutagenic and should be considered a potential carcinogen (see COPEGUS Package Insert for additional information and other WARNINGS).

DESCRIPTION

PEGASYS, peginterferon alfa-2a, is a covalent conjugate of recombinant alfa-2a interferon (approximate molecular weight [MW] 20,000 daltons) with a single branched bis-monomethoxy polyethylene glycol (PEG) chain (approximate MW 40,000 daltons). The PEG moiety is linked at a single site to the interferon alfa moiety via a stable amide bond to lysine. Peginterferon alfa-2a has an approximate molecular weight of 60,000 daltons. Interferon alfa-2a is produced using recombinant DNA technology in which a cloned human leukocyte interferon gene is inserted into and expressed in *Escherichia coli*.

PEGASYS is supplied as an injectable solution in vials and prefilled syringes.

180 µg/1.0 mL Vial: A vial contains approximately 1.2 mL of solution to deliver 1.0 mL of drug product. Subcutaneous (sc) administration of 1.0 mL delivers 180 µg of drug product (expressed as the amount of interferon alfa-2a), 8.0 mg sodium chloride, 0.05 mg polysorbate 80, 10.0 mg benzyl alcohol, 2.62 mg sodium acetate trihydrate, and 0.05 mg acetic acid. The solution is colorless to light yellow and the pH is 6.0 ± 0.5.

180 µg/0.5 mL Prefilled Syringe: Each syringe contains 0.6 mL of solution to deliver 0.5 mL of drug product. Subcutaneous (sc) administration of 0.5 mL delivers 180 µg of drug product (expressed as the amount of interferon alfa-2a), 4.0 mg sodium chloride, 0.025 mg polysorbate 80, 5.0 mg benzyl alcohol, 1.3085 mg sodium acetate trihydrate, and 0.0231 mg acetic acid. The solution is colorless to light yellow and the pH is 6.0 ± 0.5.

CLINICAL PHARMACOLOGY

Pharmacodynamics

Interferons bind to specific receptors on the cell surface initiating intracellular signaling via a complex cascade of protein-protein interactions leading to rapid activation of gene transcription. Interferon-stimulated genes modulate many biological effects including the inhibition of viral replication in infected cells, inhibition of cell proliferation and immunomodulation. The clinical relevance of these in vitro activities is not known.

PEGASYS stimulates the production of effector proteins such as serum neopterin and 2', 5'-oligoadenylate synthetase.

Pharmacokinetics

Maximal serum concentrations (C_{max}) occur between 72 to 96 hours post-dose. The C_{max} and AUC measurements of PEGASYS increase in a dose-related manner. Week 48 mean trough concentrations (16 ng/mL; range 4 to 28) at 168 hours post-dose are approximately 2-fold higher than week 1 mean trough concentrations (8 ng/mL; range 0 to 15). Steady-state serum levels are reached within 5 to 8 weeks of once weekly dosing. The peak to trough ratio at week 48 is approximately 2.0.

The mean systemic clearance in healthy subjects given PEGASYS was 94 mL/h, which is approximately 100-fold lower than that for interferon alfa-2a (ROFERON®-A). The mean terminal half-life after sc dosing in patients with chronic hepatitis C was 80 hours (range 50 to 140 hours) compared to 5.1 hours (range 3.7 to 8.5 hours) for ROFERON®-A.

Special Populations

Gender and Age

PEGASYS administration yielded similar pharmacokinetics in male and female healthy subjects. The AUC was increased from 1295 to 1663 ng·h/mL in subjects older than 62 years taking 180 µg PEGASYS, but peak concentrations were similar (9 vs 10 ng/mL) in those older and younger than 62 years.

Pediatric Patients

The pharmacokinetics of PEGASYS have not been adequately studied in pediatric patients.

Renal Dysfunction

In patients with end stage renal disease undergoing hemodialysis, there is a 25% to 45% reduction in PEGASYS clearance (see **PRECAUTIONS: Renal Impairment**).

The pharmacokinetics of ribavirin following administration of COPEGUS have not been studied in patients with renal impairment and there are limited data from clinical trials on administration of COPEGUS in patients with creatinine clearance <50 mL/min. Therefore, patients with creatinine clearance <50 mL/min should not be treated with COPEGUS (see **WARNINGS** and **DOSAGE AND ADMINISTRATION**).

Effect of Food on Absorption of Ribavirin

Bioavailability of a single oral dose of ribavirin was increased by co-administration with a high-fat meal. The absorption was slowed (T_{max} was doubled) and the $AUC_{0\text{-}192h}$ and C_{max} increased by 42% and 66%, respectively, when COPEGUS was taken with a high-fat meal compared with fasting conditions (see **DOSAGE AND ADMINISTRATION**).

Drug Interactions

Nucleoside Analogues

Ribavirin has been shown in vitro to inhibit phosphorylation of zidovudine and stavudine, which could lead to decreased anti-retroviral activity. Exposure to didanosine or its active metabolite (dideoxyadenosine 5'-triphosphate) is increased when didanosine is co-administered with ribavirin (see **PRECAUTIONS: Drug Interactions**).

Methadone

The pharmacokinetics of concomitant administration of methadone and PEGASYS were evaluated in 24 PEGASYS naïve chronic hepatitis C patients (15 male, 9 female) who received 180 mg PEGASYS subcutaneously weekly. All patients were on stable methadone maintenance therapy (median dose 95 mg, range 30 mg to 150 mg) prior to receiving PEGASYS. Mean methadone PK parameters were 10% to 15% higher after 4 weeks of PEGASYS treatment as compared to baseline (see **PRECAUTIONS: Drug Interactions**). Methadone did not significantly alter the PK of PEGASYS as compared to a PK study of 6 chronic hepatitis C patients not receiving methadone.

CLINICAL STUDIES

PEGASYS Monotherapy (Studies 1, 2, and 3)

The safety and effectiveness of PEGASYS for the treatment of hepatitis C virus infection were assessed in three randomized, open-label, active-controlled clinical studies. All patients were adults, had compensated liver disease, detectable hepatitis C virus (HCV), liver biopsy diagnosis of chronic hepatitis, and were previously untreated with interferon. All patients received therapy by sc injection for 48 weeks, and were followed for an additional 24 weeks to assess the durability of response. In studies 1 and 2, approximately 20% of subjects had cirrhosis or bridging fibrosis. Study 3 enrolled patients with a histological diagnosis of cirrhosis (78%) or bridging fibrosis (22%).

In study 1 (n=630), patients received either ROFERON-A (interferon alfa-2a) 3 MIU three times/week (tiw), PEGASYS 135 µg once each week (qw) or PEGASYS 180 µg qw. In study 2 (n=526), patients received either ROFERON-A 6 MIU tiw for 12 weeks followed by 3 MIU tiw for 36 weeks or PEGASYS 180 µg qw. In study 3 (n=269), patients received ROFERON-A 3 MIU tiw, PEGASYS 90 µg qw or PEGASYS 180 µg once each week.

In all three studies, treatment with PEGASYS 180 µg resulted in significantly more patients who experienced a sustained response (defined as undetectable HCV RNA and normalization of ALT on or after study week 68) compared to treatment with ROFERON-A. In study 1, response to PEGASYS 135 µg was not different from response to 180 µg. In study 3, response to PEGASYS 90 µg was intermediate between PEGASYS 180 µg and ROFERON-A.

[See table 1 below]

Matched pre- and post-treatment liver biopsies were obtained in approximately 70% of patients. Similar modest reductions in inflammation compared to baseline were observed in all treatment groups.

Of the patients who did not demonstrate either undetectable HCV RNA or at least a 2log[10] drop in HCV RNA titer from baseline by 12 weeks of PEGASYS 180 µg therapy, 2% (3/156) achieved a sustained virologic response (see **DOSAGE AND ADMINISTRATION**).

Averaged over study 1, study 2, and study 3, response rates to PEGASYS were 23% among patients with viral genotype 1 and 48% in patients with other viral genotypes. The treatment response rates were similar in men and women.

PEGASYS/COPEGUS Combination Therapy (Studies 4 and 5)

The safety and effectiveness of PEGASYS in combination with COPEGUS for the treatment of hepatitis C virus infection were assessed in two randomized controlled clinical trials. All patients were adults, had compensated liver disease, detectable hepatitis C virus, liver biopsy diagnosis of chronic hepatitis, and were previously untreated with interferon. Approximately 20% of patients in both studies had compensated cirrhosis (Child-Pugh class A).

Table 1 Sustained Response to Monotherapy Treatment

	Study 1			Study 2			Study 3		
	ROFERON-A 3 MIU (N=207)	**PEGASYS 180 µg (N=208)**	**DIFF* (95% CI)**	**ROFERON-A 6/3 MIU (N=261)**	**PEGASYS 180 µg (N=265)**	**DIFF* (95% CI)**	**ROFERON-A 3 MIU (N=86)**	**PEGASYS 180 µg (N=87)**	**DIFF* (95% CI)**
Combined Virologic and Biologic Sustained Response	11%	24%	13 (6, 20)	17%	35%	18 (11, 25)	7%	23%	16 (6, 26)
Sustained Virologic Response**	11%	26%	15 (8, 23)	19%	38%	19 (11, 26)	8%	30%	22 (11, 33)

* Percent difference between PEGASYS and Roferon-A treatment
** COBAS AMPLICOR® HCV Test, version 2.0

In study 4, patients were randomized to receive either PEGASYS 180 μg sc once weekly (qw) with an oral placebo, PEGASYS 180 μg qw with COPEGUS 1000 mg po (body weight <75 kg) or 1200 mg po (body weight ≥75 kg) or REBETRON™ (interferon alfa-2b 3 MIU sc tiw plus ribavirin 1000 mg or 1200 mg po). All patients received 48 weeks of therapy followed by 24 weeks of treatment-free follow-up. COPEGUS or placebo treatment assignment was blinded. PEGASYS in combination with COPEGUS resulted in a higher SVR (defined as undetectable HCV RNA at the end of the 24-week treatment-free follow-up period) compared to PEGASYS alone or interferon alfa-2b and ribavirin. In all treatment arms, patients with viral genotype 1, regardless of viral load, had a lower response rate.

[See table 2 at right]

In study 5, all patients received PEGASYS 180 μg sc qw and were randomized to treatment for either 24 or 48 weeks and to a COPEGUS dose of either 800 mg or 1000 mg/1200 mg (for body weight <75 kg / ≥75 kg). Assignment to the four treatment arms was stratified by viral genotype and baseline HCV viral titer. Patients with genotype 1 and high viral titer (defined as $>2 \times 10^6$ HCV RNA copies/mL serum) were preferentially assigned to treatment for 48 weeks.

Genotype 1

Irrespective of baseline viral titer, treatment for 48 weeks with PEGASYS and 1000 mg or 1200 mg of COPEGUS resulted in higher SVR (defined as undetectable HCV RNA at the end of the 24-week treatment-free follow-up period) compared to shorter treatment (24 weeks) and/or 800 mg COPEGUS.

Genotype non-1

Irrespective of baseline viral titer, treatment for 24 weeks with PEGASYS and 800 mg of COPEGUS resulted in a similar SVR compared to longer treatment (48 weeks) and/or 1000 mg or 1200 mg of COPEGUS.

[See table 3 at right]

Among the 36 patients with genotype 4, response rates were similar to those observed in patients with genotype 1 (data not shown). The numbers of patients with genotype 5 and 6 were too few to allow for meaningful assessment.

Treatment Response in Patient Subgroups

Treatment response rates are lower in patients with poor prognostic factors receiving pegylated interferon alpha therapy. In studies 4 and 5, treatment response rates were lower in patients older than 40 years (50% vs 66%), in patients with cirrhosis (47% vs 59%), in patients weighing over 85 kg (49% vs 60%), and in patients with genotype 1 with high vs low viral load (43% vs 56%). African American patients had lower response rates compared to Caucasians.

Paired liver biopsies were performed on approximately 20% of patients in studies 4 and 5. Modest reductions in inflammation compared to baseline were seen in all treatment groups.

In studies 4 and 5, lack of early virologic response at 12 weeks (defined as HCV RNA undetectable or $>2\log^{10}$ lower than baseline) was grounds for discontinuation of treatment. Of patients who lacked an early viral response at 12 weeks and completed a recommended course of therapy despite a protocol-defined option to discontinue therapy, 5/39 (13%) achieved an SVR. Of patients who lacked an early viral response at 24 weeks, nineteen completed a full course of therapy and none achieved an SVR.

INDICATIONS AND USAGE

PEGASYS, peginterferon alfa-2a, alone or in combination with COPEGUS, is indicated for the treatment of adults with chronic hepatitis C virus infection who have compensated liver disease and have not been previously treated with interferon alpha. Patients in whom efficacy was demonstrated included patients with compensated liver disease and histological evidence of cirrhosis (Child-Pugh class A).

CONTRAINDICATIONS

PEGASYS is contraindicated in patients with:

- Hypersensitivity to PEGASYS or any of its components
- Autoimmune hepatitis
- Hepatic decompensation (Child-Pugh class B and C) before or during treatment

PEGASYS is contraindicated in neonates and infants because it contains benzyl alcohol. Benzyl alcohol is associated with an increased incidence of neurologic and other complications in neonates and infants, which are sometimes fatal.

PEGASYS and COPEGUS combination therapy is additionally contraindicated in:

- Patients with known hypersensitivity to COPEGUS or to any component of the tablet
- Women who are pregnant
- Men whose female partners are pregnant
- Patients with hemoglobinopathies (eg, thalassemia major, sickle-cell anemia)

WARNINGS

General

Patients should be monitored for the following serious conditions, some of which may become life threatening. Patients with persistently severe or worsening signs or symptoms should have their therapy withdrawn (see **BOXED WARNING**).

Neuropsychiatric

Life-threatening or fatal neuropsychiatric reactions may manifest in patients receiving therapy with PEGASYS and include suicide, suicidal ideation, depression, relapse of drug addiction, and drug overdose. These reactions may occur in patients with and without previous psychiatric illness.

Table 2 Sustained Virologic Response to Combination Therapy (Study 4)

	Interferon alfa-2b+ Ribavirin 1000 mg or 1200 mg	PEGASYS + Placebo	PEGASYS + COPEGUS 1000 mg or 1200 mg
All patients	197/444 (44%)	65/224 (29%)	241/453 (53%)
Genotype 1	103/285 (36%)	29/145 (20%)	132/298 (44%)
Genotypes 2-6	94/159 (59%)	36/79 (46%)	109/155 (70%)

Difference in overall treatment response (PEGASYS/COPEGUS – Interferon alfa-2b/ribavirin) was 9% (95% CI 2.3, 15.3).

Table 3 Sustained Virologic Response as a Function of Genotype (Study 5)

	24 Weeks Treatment		48 Weeks Treatment	
	PEGASYS + COPEGUS 800 mg (N=207)	**PEGASYS + COPEGUS 1000 mg or 1200 mg* (N=280)**	**PEGASYS + COPEGUS 800 mg (N=361)**	**PEGASYS + COPEGUS 1000 mg or 1200 mg* (N=436)**
Genotype 1	29/101 (29%)	48/118 (41%)	99/250 (40%)	138/271 (51%)
Genotype 2-3	79/96 (82%)	116/144 (81%)	75/99 (76%)	117/153 (76%)

*1000 mg for body weight <75 kg; 1200 mg for body weight ≥75 kg.

PEGASYS should be used with extreme caution in patients who report a history of depression. Neuropsychiatric adverse events observed with alpha interferon treatment include aggressive behavior, psychoses, hallucinations, bipolar disorders, and mania. Physicians should monitor all patients for evidence of depression and other psychiatric symptoms. Patients should be advised to report any sign or symptom of depression or suicidal ideation to their prescribing physicians. In severe cases, therapy should be stopped immediately and psychiatric intervention instituted (see **ADVERSE REACTIONS** and **DOSAGE AND ADMINISTRATION**).

Infections

Serious and severe bacterial infections, some fatal, have been observed in patients treated with alpha interferons including PEGASYS. Some of the infections have been associated with neutropenia. PEGASYS should be discontinued in patients who develop severe infections and appropriate antibiotic therapy instituted.

Bone Marrow Toxicity

PEGASYS suppresses bone marrow function and may result in severe cytopenias. Ribavirin may potentiate the neutropenia and lymphopenia induced by alpha interferons including PEGASYS. Very rarely alpha interferons may be associated with aplastic anemia. It is advised that complete blood counts (CBC) be obtained pre-treatment and monitored routinely during therapy (see **PRECAUTIONS: Laboratory Tests**).

PEGASYS and COPEGUS should be used with caution in patients with baseline neutrophil counts <1500 cells/mm³, with baseline platelet counts <90,000 cells/mm³ or baseline hemoglobin <10 g/dL. PEGASYS therapy should be discontinued, at least temporarily, in patients who develop severe decreases in neutrophil and/or platelet counts (see **DOSAGE AND ADMINISTRATION: Dose Modifications**).

Cardiovascular Disorders

Hypertension, supraventricular arrhythmias, chest pain, and myocardial infarction have been observed in patients treated with PEGASYS.

PEGASYS should be administered with caution to patients with pre-existing cardiac disease. Because cardiac disease may be worsened by ribavirin-induced anemia, patients with a history of significant or unstable cardiac disease should not use COPEGUS (see **WARNINGS: Anemia** and **COPEGUS Package Insert**).

Hypersensitivity

Severe acute hypersensitivity reactions (eg, urticaria, angioedema, bronchoconstriction, anaphylaxis) have been rarely observed during alpha interferon and ribavirin therapy. If such reaction occurs, therapy with PEGASYS and COPEGUS should be discontinued and appropriate medical therapy immediately instituted.

Endocrine Disorders

PEGASYS causes or aggravates hypothyroidism and hyperthyroidism. Hyperglycemia, hypoglycemia, and diabetes mellitus have been observed to develop in patients treated with PEGASYS. Patients with these conditions at baseline who cannot be effectively treated by medication should not begin PEGASYS therapy. Patients who develop these conditions during treatment and cannot be controlled with medication may require discontinuation of PEGASYS therapy.

Autoimmune Disorders

Development or exacerbation of autoimmune disorders including myositis, hepatitis, ITP, psoriasis, rheumatoid arthritis, interstitial nephritis, thyroiditis, and systemic lupus erythematosus have been reported in patients receiving alpha interferon. PEGASYS should be used with caution in patients with autoimmune disorders.

Pulmonary Disorders

Dyspnea, pulmonary infiltrates, pneumonia, bronchiolitis obliterans, interstitial pneumonitis and sarcoidosis, some resulting in respiratory failure and/or patient deaths, may be induced or aggravated by PEGASYS or alpha interferon therapy. Patients who develop persistent or unexplained pulmonary infiltrates or pulmonary function impairment should discontinue treatment with PEGASYS.

Colitis

Ulcerative, and hemorrhagic/ischemic colitis, sometimes fatal, have been observed within 12 weeks of starting alpha interferon treatment. Abdominal pain, bloody diarrhea, and fever are the typical manifestations of colitis. PEGASYS should be discontinued immediately if these symptoms develop. The colitis usually resolves within 1 to 3 weeks of discontinuation of alpha interferon.

Pancreatitis

Pancreatitis, sometimes fatal, has occurred during alpha interferon and ribavirin treatment. PEGASYS and COPEGUS should be suspended if symptoms or signs suggestive of pancreatitis are observed. PEGASYS and COPEGUS should be discontinued in patients diagnosed with pancreatitis.

Ophthalmologic Disorders

Decrease or loss of vision, retinopathy including macular edema, retinal artery or vein thrombosis, retinal hemorrhages and cotton wool spots, optic neuritis, and papilledema are induced or aggravated by treatment with PEGASYS or other alpha interferons. All patients should receive an eye examination at baseline. Patients with preexisting ophthalmologic disorders (eg, diabetic or hypertensive retinopathy) should receive periodic ophthalmologic exams during interferon alpha treatment. Any patient who develops ocular symptoms should receive a prompt and complete eye examination. PEGASYS treatment should be discontinued in patients who develop new or worsening ophthalmologic disorders.

Pregnancy: Use with Ribavirin (also, see COPEGUS Package Insert.)

Ribavirin may cause birth defects and/or death of the exposed fetus. Extreme care must be taken to avoid pregnancy in female patients and in female partners of male patients taking PEGASYS and COPEGUS combination therapy. COPEGUS THERAPY SHOULD NOT BE STARTED UNLESS A REPORT OF A NEGATIVE PREGNANCY TEST HAS BEEN OBTAINED IMMEDIATELY PRIOR TO INITIATION OF THERAPY. Women of childbearing potential and men must use two forms of effective contraception during treatment and for at least six months after treatment has concluded. Routine monthly pregnancy tests must be performed during this time (see BOXED WARNING, CONTRAINDICATIONS, PRECAUTIONS: Information for Patients, and COPEGUS Package Insert).

Anemia

The primary toxicity of ribavirin is hemolytic anemia. Hemoglobin <10 g/dL was observed in approximately 13% of COPEGUS and PEGASYS treated patients in clinical trials (see **PRECAUTIONS: Laboratory Tests**). The anemia associated with COPEGUS occurs within 1 to 2 weeks of initiation of therapy with maximum drop in hemoglobin observed during the first eight weeks. BECAUSE THE INITIAL DROP IN HEMOGLOBIN MAY BE SIGNIFICANT, IT IS ADVISED THAT HEMOGLOBIN OR HEMATOCRIT BE OBTAINED PRE-TREATMENT AND AT WEEK 2 AND WEEK 4 OF THERAPY OR MORE FREQUENTLY IF CLINICALLY INDICATED. Patients should then be followed as clinically appropriate.

Fatal and nonfatal myocardial infarctions have been reported in patients with anemia caused by ribavirin. Patients should be assessed for underlying cardiac disease before initiation of ribavirin therapy. Patients with preexisting cardiac disease should have electrocardiograms administered before treatment, and should be appropriately monitored during therapy. If there is any deterioration of cardiovascular status, therapy should be suspended or discontinued (see **DOSAGE AND ADMINISTRATION: COPEGUS Dosage Modification Guidelines**). Because cardiac disease may be worsened by drug-induced anemia, patients with a history of significant or unstable cardiac disease should not use COPEGUS (see **COPEGUS Package Insert**).

Continued on next page

Pegasys—Cont.

Renal

It is recommended that renal function be evaluated in all patients started on COPEGUS. COPEGUS should not be administered to patients with creatinine clearance <50 mL/min (see **CLINICAL PHARMACOLOGY: Special Populations**).

PRECAUTIONS

General

The safety and efficacy of PEGASYS alone or in combination with COPEGUS for the treatment of hepatitis C have not been established in:

- Patients who have failed other alpha interferon treatments
- Liver or other organ transplant recipients
- Patients co-infected with human immunodeficiency virus (HIV) or hepatitis B virus (HBV)

Renal Impairment

A 25% to 45% higher exposure to PEGASYS is seen in subjects undergoing hemodialysis. In patients with impaired renal function, signs and symptoms of interferon toxicity should be closely monitored. Doses of PEGASYS should be adjusted accordingly. PEGASYS should be used with caution in patients with creatinine clearance <50 mL/min (see **DOSAGE AND ADMINISTRATION: Dose Modifications**).

Information for Patients

Patients receiving PEGASYS alone or in combination with COPEGUS should be directed in its appropriate use, informed of the benefits and risks associated with treatment, and referred to the PEGASYS and, if applicable, COPEGUS (ribavirin) MEDICATION GUIDES.

PEGASYS and COPEGUS combination therapy must not be used by women who are pregnant or by men whose female partners are pregnant. COPEGUS therapy should not be initiated until a report of a negative pregnancy test has been obtained immediately before starting therapy. Female patients of childbearing potential and male patients with female partners of childbearing potential must be advised of the teratogenic/embryocidal risks and must be instructed to practice effective contraception during COPEGUS therapy and for 6 months post-therapy. Patients should be advised to notify the physician immediately in the event of a pregnancy (see **CONTRAINDICATIONS** and **WARNINGS**).

Women of childbearing potential and men must use two forms of effective contraception during treatment and during the 6 months after treatment has concluded; routine monthly pregnancy tests must be performed during this time (see **CONTRAINDICATIONS** and **COPEGUS Package Insert**).

If pregnancy does occur during treatment or during 6 months post-therapy, the patient must be advised of the significant teratogenic risk of COPEGUS therapy to the fetus. To monitor maternal-fetal outcomes of pregnant women exposed to COPEGUS, the COPEGUS Pregnancy Registry has been established. Physicians and patients are strongly encouraged to register by calling 1-800-526-6367.

Patients should be advised that laboratory evaluations are required before starting therapy and periodically thereafter (see **Laboratory Tests**). Patients should be instructed to remain well hydrated, especially during the initial stages of treatment. Patients should be advised to take COPEGUS with food.

Patients should be informed that it is not known if therapy with PEGASYS alone or in combination with COPEGUS will prevent transmission of HCV infection to others or prevent cirrhosis, liver failure or liver cancer that might result from HCV infection. Patients who develop dizziness, confusion, somnolence, and fatigue should be cautioned to avoid driving or operating machinery.

If home use is prescribed, a puncture-resistant container for the disposal of used needles and syringes should be supplied to the patients. Patients should be thoroughly instructed in the importance of proper disposal and cautioned against any reuse of any needles and syringes. The full container should be disposed of according to the directions provided by the physician (see **MEDICATION GUIDE**).

Laboratory Tests

Before beginning PEGASYS or PEGASYS and COPEGUS combination therapy, standard hematological and biochemical laboratory tests are recommended for all patients. Pregnancy screening for women of childbearing potential must be performed.

After initiation of therapy, hematological tests should be performed at 2 weeks and 4 weeks and biochemical tests should be performed at 4 weeks. Additional testing should be performed periodically during therapy. In the clinical studies, the CBC (including hemoglobin level and white blood cell and platelet counts) and chemistries (including liver function tests and uric acid) were measured at 1, 2, 4, 6, and 8, and then every 4 weeks or more frequently if abnormalities were found. Thyroid stimulating hormone (TSH) was measured every 12 weeks. Monthly pregnancy testing should be performed during combination therapy and for 6 months after discontinuing therapy.

The entrance criteria used for the clinical studies of PEGASYS may be considered as a guideline to acceptable baseline values for initiation of treatment:

- Platelet count ≥90,000 cells/mm^3 (as low as 75,000 cells/mm^3 in patients with cirrhosis)
- Caution should be exercised in initiating treatment in any patient with baseline risk of severe anemia (eg, spherocytosis, history of GI bleeding).
- Absolute neutrophil count (ANC) ≥1500 cells/mm^3
- Serum creatinine concentration <1.5 × upper limit of normal
- TSH and T_4 within normal limits or adequately controlled thyroid function

PEGASYS treatment was associated with decreases in WBC, ANC, lymphocytes, and platelet counts often starting within the first 2 weeks of treatment (see **ADVERSE REACTIONS**). Dose reduction is recommended in patients with hematologic abnormalities (see **DOSAGE AND ADMINISTRATION: Dose Modifications**).

While fever is commonly caused by PEGASYS therapy, other causes of persistent fever must be ruled out, particularly in patients with neutropenia (see **WARNINGS: Infections**).

Transient elevations in ALT (2-fold to 5-fold above baseline) were observed in some patients receiving PEGASYS, and were not associated with deterioration of other liver function tests. When the increase in ALT levels is progressive despite dose reduction or is accompanied by increased bilirubin, PEGASYS therapy should be discontinued (see **DOSAGE AND ADMINISTRATION: Dose Modifications**).

Drug Interactions

Treatment with PEGASYS once weekly for 4 weeks in healthy subjects was associated with an inhibition of P450 1A2 and a 25% increase in theophylline AUC. Theophylline serum levels should be monitored and appropriate dose adjustments considered for patients given both theophylline and PEGASYS (see **PRECAUTIONS**). There was no effect on the pharmacokinetics of representative drugs metabolized by CYP 2C9, CYP 2C19, CYP 2D6 or CYP 3A4.

In a PK study of HCV patients concomitantly receiving methadone, treatment with PEGASYS once weekly for 4 weeks was associated with methadone levels that were 10% to 15% higher than at baseline (see **CLINICAL PHARMACOLOGY: Drug Interactions**). The clinical significance of this finding is unknown; however, patients should be monitored for the signs and symptoms of methadone toxicity.

In patients with chronic hepatitis C treated with PEGASYS in combination with COPEGUS, PEGASYS treatment did not affect ribavirin distribution or clearance.

Nucleoside Analogues

Didanosine

Co-administration of COPEGUS and didanosine is not recommended. Reports of fatal hepatic failure, as well as peripheral neuropathy, pancreatitis, and symptomatic hyperlactatemia/lactic acidosis have been reported in clinical trials (see **CLINICAL PHARMACOLOGY: Drug Interactions**).

Stavudine and Zidovudine

Ribavirin can antagonize the in vitro antiviral activity of stavudine and zidovudine against HIV. Therefore, concomitant use of ribavirin with either of these drugs should be avoided.

Carcinogenesis, Mutagenesis, Impairment of Fertility

Carcinogenesis

PEGASYS has not been tested for its carcinogenic potential.

Mutagenesis

PEGASYS did not cause DNA damage when tested in the Ames bacterial mutagenicity assay and in the in vitro chromosomal aberration assay in human lymphocytes, either in the presence or absence of metabolic activation.

Use With Ribavirin

Ribavirin is genotoxic and mutagenic. The carcinogenic potential of ribavirin has not been fully determined. In a p53 (+/-) mouse carcinogenicity study at doses up to the maximum tolerated dose of 100 mg/kg/day ribavirin was not oncogenic. However, on a body surface area basis, this dose was 0.5 times maximum recommended human 24-hour dose of ribavirin. A study in rats to assess the carcinogenic potential of ribavirin is ongoing (see COPEGUS Package Insert).

Impairment of Fertility

PEGASYS may impair fertility in women. Prolonged menstrual cycles and/or amenorrhea were observed in female cynomolgus monkeys given sc injections of 600 µg/kg/dose (7200 µg/m^2/dose) of PEGASYS every other day for one month, at approximately 180 times the recommended weekly human dose for a 60 kg person (based on body surface area). Menstrual cycle irregularities were accompanied by both a decrease and delay in the peak 17β-estradiol and progesterone levels following administration of PEGASYS to female monkeys. A return to normal menstrual rhythm followed cessation of treatment. Every other day dosing with 100 µg/kg (1200 µg/m^2) PEGASYS (equivalent to approximately 30 times the recommended human dose) had no effects on cycle duration or reproductive hormone status.

The effects of PEGASYS on male fertility have not been studied. However, no adverse effects on fertility were observed in male Rhesus monkeys treated with non-pegylated interferon alfa-2a for 5 months at doses up to 25×10^6 IU/kg/day.

Use With Ribavirin

Ribavirin has shown reversible toxicity in animal studies of male fertility (see **COPEGUS Package Insert**).

Pregnancy

Pregnancy: Category C

PEGASYS has not been studied for its teratogenic effect. Non-pegylated interferon alfa-2a treatment of pregnant Rhesus monkeys at approximately 20 to 500 times the human weekly dose resulted in a statistically significant increase in abortions. No teratogenic effects were seen in the offspring delivered at term. PEGASYS should be assumed to have abortifacient potential. There are no adequate and well-controlled studies of PEGASYS in pregnant women. PEGASYS is to be used during pregnancy only if the potential benefit justifies the potential risk to the fetus. PEGASYS is recommended for use in women of childbearing potential only when they are using effective contraception during therapy.

Pregnancy: Category X: Use With Ribavirin (see CONTRAINDICATIONS)

Significant teratogenic and/or embryocidal effects have been demonstrated in all animal species exposed to ribavirin. COPEGUS therapy is contraindicated in women who are pregnant and in the male partners of women who are pregnant (see CONTRAINDICATIONS, WARNINGS, and COPEGUS Package Insert).

If pregnancy occurs in a patient or partner of a patient during treatment or during the 6 months after treatment cessation, such cases should be reported to the COPEGUS Pregnancy Registry at 1-800-526-6367.

Nursing Mothers

It is not known whether peginterferon or ribavirin or its components are excreted in human milk. The effect of orally ingested peginterferon or ribavirin from breast milk on the nursing infant has not been evaluated. Because of the potential for adverse reactions from the drugs in nursing infants, a decision must be made whether to discontinue nursing or discontinue PEGASYS and COPEGUS treatment.

Pediatric Use

The safety and effectiveness of PEGASYS, alone or in combination with COPEGUS in patients below the age of 18 years have not been established.

PEGASYS contains benzyl alcohol. Benzyl alcohol has been reported to be associated with an increased incidence of neurological and other complications in neonates and infants, which are sometimes fatal (see **CONTRAINDICATIONS**).

Geriatric Use

Younger patients have higher virologic response rates than older patients. Clinical studies of PEGASYS alone or in combination with COPEGUS did not include sufficient numbers of subjects aged 65 or over to determine whether they respond differently from younger subjects. Adverse reactions related to alpha interferons, such as CNS, cardiac, and systemic (eg, flu-like) effects may be more severe in the elderly and caution should be exercised in the use of PEGASYS in this population. PEGASYS and COPEGUS are excreted by the kidney, and the risk of toxic reactions to this therapy may be greater in patients with impaired renal function. Because elderly patients are more likely to have decreased renal function, care should be taken in dose selection and it may be useful to monitor renal function. PEGASYS should be used with caution in patients with creatinine clearance <50 mL/min and COPEGUS should not be administered to patients with creatinine clearance <50 mL/min.

ADVERSE REACTIONS

PEGASYS alone or in combination with COPEGUS causes a broad variety of serious adverse reactions (see **BOXED WARNING** and **WARNINGS**). In all studies, one or more serious adverse reactions occurred in 10% of patients receiving PEGASYS alone or in combination with COPEGUS.

The most common life-threatening or fatal events induced or aggravated by PEGASYS and COPEGUS were depression, suicide, relapse of drug abuse/overdose, and bacterial infections; each occurred at a frequency of <1%.

Nearly all patients in clinical trials experienced one or more adverse events. The most commonly reported adverse reactions were psychiatric reactions, including depression, irritability, anxiety, and flu-like symptoms such as fatigue, pyrexia, myalgia, headache, and rigors.

Overall 11% of patients receiving 48 weeks of therapy with PEGASYS either alone (7%) or in combination with COPEGUS (10%) discontinued therapy. The most common reasons for discontinuation of therapy were psychiatric, flu-like syndrome (eg, lethargy, fatigue, headache), dermatologic, and gastrointestinal disorders.

The most common reason for dose modification in patients receiving combination therapy was for laboratory abnormalities, neutropenia (20%) and thrombocytopenia (4%) for PEGASYS and anemia (22%) for COPEGUS.

PEGASYS dose was reduced in 12% of patients receiving 1000 mg to 1200 mg COPEGUS for 48 weeks and in 7% of patients receiving 800 mg COPEGUS for 24 weeks. COPEGUS dose was reduced in 21% of patients receiving 1000 mg to 1200 mg COPEGUS for 48 weeks and 12% in patients receiving 800 mg COPEGUS for 24 weeks.

Because clinical trials are conducted under widely varying and controlled conditions, adverse reaction rates observed in clinical trials of a drug cannot be directly compared to rates in the clinical trials of another drug. Also, the adverse event rates listed here may not predict the rates observed in a broader patient population in clinical practice.

[See table 4 at bottom of next page]

Patients treated for 24 weeks with PEGASYS and 800 mg COPEGUS were observed to have lower incidence of serious adverse events (3% vs 10%), Hgb <10 g/dL (3% vs 15%), dose modification of PEGASYS (30% vs 36%) and COPEGUS (19% vs 38%) and of withdrawal from treatment (5% vs 15%) compared to patients treated for 48 weeks with

PEGASYS and 1000 mg or 1200 mg COPEGUS. On the other hand the overall incidence of adverse events appeared to be similar in the two treatment groups.

The most common serious adverse event (3%) was bacterial infection (eg, sepsis, osteomyelitis, endocarditis, pyelonephritis, pneumonia). Other SAEs occurred at a frequency of <1% and included: suicide, suicidal ideation, psychosis, aggression, anxiety, drug abuse and drug overdose, angina, hepatic dysfunction, fatty liver, cholangitis, arrhythmia, diabetes mellitus, autoimmune phenomena (eg, hyperthyroidism, hypothyroidism, sarcoidosis, systemic lupus erythematosus, rheumatoid arthritis), peripheral neuropathy, aplastic anemia, peptic ulcer, gastrointestinal bleeding, pancreatitis, colitis, corneal ulcer, pulmonary embolism, coma, myositis, and cerebral hemorrhage.

Laboratory Test Values

Hemoglobin

The hemoglobin concentration decreased below 12 g/dL in 17% (median Hgb drop = 2.2 g/dL) of monotherapy and 52% (median Hgb drop = 3.7 g/dL) of combination therapy patients. Severe anemia (Hgb <10 g/dL) was encountered in 13% of patients receiving combination therapy and 2% of monotherapy recipients. Dose modification for anemia was required in 22% of ribavirin recipients treated for 48 weeks. Hemoglobin decreases in PEGASYS monotherapy were generally mild and did not require dose modification (see **DOSAGE AND ADMINISTRATION: Dose Modifications**).

Neutrophils

Decreases in neutrophil count below normal were observed in 95% of patients treated with PEGASYS either alone or in combination with COPEGUS. Severe potentially life-threatening neutropenia (ANC <0.5×10^9/L) occurred in approximately 5% of patients receiving PEGASYS either alone or in combination with COPEGUS. Seventeen percent of patients receiving PEGASYS monotherapy and 20% to 24% of patients receiving PEGASYS/COPEGUS combination therapy required modification of interferon dosage for neutropenia. Two percent of patients required permanent reductions of PEGASYS dosage and <1% required permanent discontinuation. Median neutrophil counts return to pre-treatment levels 4 weeks after cessation of therapy (see **DOSAGE AND ADMINISTRATION: Dose Modifications**).

Lymphocytes

Decreases in lymphocyte count are induced by interferon alpha therapy. Lymphopenia was observed during both monotherapy (86%) and combination therapy with PEGASYS and COPEGUS (94%). Severe lymphopenia (<0.5×10^9/L) occurred in approximately 5% of monotherapy patients and 14% of combination PEGASYS and COPEGUS therapy recipients. Dose adjustments were not required by protocol. Median lymphocyte counts return to pre-treatment levels after 4 to 12 weeks of the cessation of therapy. The clinical significance of the lymphopenia is not known.

Platelets

Platelet counts decreased in 52% of patients treated with PEGASYS alone (median drop 45% from baseline), 33% of patients receiving combination with COPEGUS (median drop 30% from baseline). Median platelet counts return to pre-treatment levels 4 weeks after the cessation of therapy.

Triglycerides

Triglyceride levels are elevated in patients receiving alfa interferon therapy and were elevated in the majority of patients participating in clinical studies receiving either PEGASYS alone or in combination with COPEGUS. Random levels higher ≥400 mg/dL were observed in about 20% of patients.

ALT Elevations

Less than 1% of patients experienced marked elevations (5- to 10-fold above baseline) in ALT levels during treatment. These transaminase elevations were on occasion associated with hyperbilirubinemia and were managed by dose reduction or discontinuation of study treatment. Liver function test abnormalities were generally transient. One case was attributed to autoimmune hepatitis, which persisted beyond study medication discontinuation (see **DOSAGE AND ADMINISTRATION: Dose Modifications**).

Thyroid Function

PEGASYS alone or in combination with COPEGUS was associated with the development of abnormalities in thyroid laboratory values, some with associated clinical manifestations. Hypothyroidism or hyperthyroidism requiring treatment, dose modification or discontinuation occurred in 4% and 1% of PEGASYS treated patients and 4% and 2% of PEGASYS and COPEGUS treated patients, respectively. Approximately half of the patients, who developed thyroid abnormalities during PEGASYS treatment, still had abnormalities during the follow-up period (see **PRECAUTIONS: Laboratory Tests**).

Immunogenicity

Nine percent (71/834) of patients treated with PEGASYS with or without COPEGUS developed binding antibodies to interferon alfa-2a, as assessed by an ELISA assay. Three percent of patients (25/835) receiving PEGASYS with or without COPEGUS, developed low-titer neutralizing antibodies (using an assay of a sensitivity of 100 INU/mL). The clinical and pathological significance of the appearance of serum neutralizing antibodies is unknown. No apparent correlation of antibody development to clinical response or adverse events was observed. The percentage of patients whose test results were considered positive for antibodies is highly dependent on the sensitivity and specificity of the assays.

Additionally, the observed incidence of antibody positivity in these assays may be influenced by several factors including sample timing and handling, concomitant medications, and underlying disease. For these reasons, comparison of the incidence of antibodies to PEGASYS with the incidence of antibodies to these products may be misleading.

OVERDOSAGE

There is limited experience with overdosage. The maximum dose received by any patient was 7 times the intended dose of PEGASYS (180 μg/day for 7 days). There were no serious reactions attributed to overdosages. Weekly doses of up to 630 μg have been administered to patients with cancer. Dose-limiting toxicities were fatigue, elevated liver enzymes, neutropenia, and thrombocytopenia. There is no specific antidote for PEGASYS. Hemodialysis and peritoneal dialysis are not effective.

DOSAGE AND ADMINISTRATION

There are no safety and efficacy data on treatment for longer than 48 weeks. Consideration should be given to discontinuing therapy after 12 to 24 weeks of therapy if the patient has failed to demonstrate an early virologic response (see **CLINICAL STUDIES**).

PEGASYS

The recommended dose of PEGASYS monotherapy is 180 μg (1.0 mL vial or 0.5 mL prefilled syringe) once weekly for 48 weeks by subcutaneous administration in the abdomen or thigh.

PEGASYS and COPEGUS Combination

The recommended dose of PEGASYS when used in combination with ribavirin is 180 μg (1.0 mL vial or 0.5 mL prefilled syringe) once weekly. The recommended dose of COPEGUS and duration for PEGASYS/COPEGUS therapy is based on viral genotype (see Table 5).

The daily dose of COPEGUS is 800 mg to 1200 mg administered orally in two divided doses. The dose should be indi-

Continued on next page

Table 4 Adverse Reactions Occurring in ≥5% of Patients in Hepatitis C Clinical Trials (Pooled Studies 1, 2, 3, and Study 4)

Body System	PEGASYS 180 μg 48 week†	ROFERON-A*†	PEGASYS 180 μg + 1000 mg or 1200 mg COPEGUS 48 week**	Intron A + 1000 mg or 1200 mg REBETOL® 48 week**
	N=559	N=554	N=451	N=443
	%	%	%	%
Application Site Disorders				
Injection site reaction	22	18	23	16
Endocrine Disorders				
Hypothyroidism	3	2	4	5
Flu-like Symptoms and Signs				
Fatigue/Asthenia	56	57	65	68
Pyrexia	37	41	41	55
Rigors	35	44	25	37
Pain	11	12	10	9
Gastrointestinal				
Nausea/Vomiting	24	33	25	29
Diarrhea	16	16	11	10
Abdominal pain	15	15	8	9
Dry mouth	6	3	4	7
Dyspepsia	<1	1	6	5
Hematologic‡				
Lymphopenia	3	5	14	12
Anemia	2	1	11	11
Neutropenia	21	8	27	8
Thrombocytopenia	5	2	5	<1
Metabolic and Nutritional				
Anorexia	17	17	24	26
Weight decrease	4	3	10	10
Musculoskeletal, Connective Tissue and Bone				
Myalgia	37	38	40	49
Arthralgia	28	29	22	23
Back pain	9	10	5	5
Neurological				
Headache	54	58	43	49
Dizziness (excluding vertigo)	16	12	14	14
Memory impairment	5	4	6	5
Psychiatric				
Irritability/Anxiety/Nervousness	19	22	33	38
Insomnia	19	23	30	37
Depression	18	19	20	28
Concentration impairment	8	10	10	13
Mood alteration	3	2	5	6
Resistance Mechanism Disorders				
Overall	10	6	12	10
Respiratory, Thoracic and Mediastinal				
Dyspnea	4	2	13	14
Cough	4	3	10	7
Dyspnea exertional	<1	<1	4	7
Skin and Subcutaneous Tissue				
Alopecia	23	30	28	33
Pruritus	12	8	19	18
Dermatitis	8	3	16	13
Dry skin	4	3	10	13
Rash	5	4	8	5
Sweating increased	6	7	6	5
Eczema	1	1	5	4
Visual Disorders				
Vision blurred	4	2	5	2

† Pooled studies 1, 2, and 3

* Either 3 MIU or 6/3 MIU of ROFERON-A

** Study 4

‡ Severe hematologic abnormalities

Pegasys—Cont.

vidualized to the patient depending on baseline disease characteristics (eg, genotype), response to therapy, and tolerability of the regimen.
Since COPEGUS absorption increases when administered with a meal, patients are advised to take COPEGUS with food.
[See table 5 at right]
A patient should self-inject PEGASYS only if the physician determines that it is appropriate and the patient agrees to medical follow-up as necessary and training in proper injection technique has been provided to him/her (see illustrated PEGASYS **MEDICATION GUIDE** for directions on injection site preparation and injection instructions).
PEGASYS should be inspected visually for particulate matter and discoloration before administration, and not used if particulate matter is visible or product is discolored. Vials and prefilled syringes with particulate matter or discoloration should be returned to the pharmacist.

Dose Modifications

If severe adverse reactions or laboratory abnormalities develop during combination COPEGUS/PEGASYS therapy, the dose should be modified or discontinued, if appropriate, until the adverse reactions abate. If intolerance persists after dose adjustment, COPEGUS/PEGASYS therapy should be discontinued.

PEGASYS

General

When dose modification is required for moderate to severe adverse reactions (clinical and/or laboratory), initial dose reduction to 135 µg (which is 0.75 mL for the vials or adjustment to the corresponding graduation mark for the syringes) is generally adequate. However, in some cases, dose reduction to 90 µg (which is 0.5 mL for the vials or adjustment to the corresponding graduation mark for the syringes) may be needed. Following improvement of the adverse reaction, re-escalation of the dose may be considered (see **WARNINGS, PRECAUTIONS**, and **ADVERSE REACTIONS**).

Hematological

[See table 6 at right]

Psychiatric: Depression

[See table 7 at right]

Renal Function

In patients with end-stage renal disease requiring hemodialysis, dose reduction to 135 µg PEGASYS is recommended. Signs and symptoms of interferon toxicity should be closely monitored.

Liver Function

In patients with progressive ALT increases above baseline values, the dose of PEGASYS should be reduced to 135 µg. If ALT increases are progressive despite dose reduction or accompanied by increased bilirubin or evidence of hepatic decompensation, therapy should be immediately discontinued.

COPEGUS

[See table 8 at right]

Once COPEGUS has been withheld due to a laboratory abnormality or clinical manifestation, an attempt may be made to restart COPEGUS at 600 mg daily and further increase the dose to 800 mg daily depending upon the physician's judgment. However, it is not recommended that COPEGUS be increased to the original dose (1000 mg or 1200 mg).

Renal Impairment

COPEGUS should not be used in patients with creatinine clearance <50 mL/min (see **WARNINGS** and **COPEGUS Package Insert**).

Table 5 PEGASYS and COPEGUS Dosing Recommendations

Genotype	PEGASYS Dose	COPEGUS Dose	Duration
Genotype 1, 4	180 µg	<75 kg = 1000 mg ≥75 kg = 1200 mg	48 weeks 48 weeks
Genotype 2, 3	180 µg	800 mg	24 weeks

Genotypes 2 & 3 showed no increased response to treatment beyond 24 weeks (see Table 3). Data on genotypes 5 and 6 are insufficient for dosing recommendations.

Table 6 PEGASYS Hematological Dose Modification Guidelines

Laboratory Values	PEGASYS Dose Reduction	Discontinue PEGASYS if:
ANC <750/mm^3	135 µg	ANC <500/mm^3, treatment should be suspended until ANC values return to more than 1000/mm^3. Reinstitute at 90 µg and monitor ANC
Platelet <50,000/mm^3	90 µg	Platelet count <25,000/mm^3

Table 7 Guidelines for Modification or Discontinuation of PEGASYS and for Scheduling Visits for Patients with Depression

Depression Severity	Initial Management (4-8 weeks)		Depression		
	Dose modification	Visit schedule	Remains stable	Improves	Worsens
Mild	No change	Evaluate once weekly by visit and/or phone	Continue weekly visit schedule	Resume normal visit schedule	(See moderate or severe depression)
Moderate	Decrease PEGASYS dose to 135 µg (in some cases dose reduction to 90 µg may be needed)	Evaluate once weekly (office visit at least every other week)	Consider psychiatric consultation. Continue reduced dosing	If symptoms improve and are stable for 4 weeks, may resume normal visit schedule. Continue reduced dosing or return to normal dose	(See severe depression)
Severe	Discontinue PEGASYS permanently	Obtain immediate psychiatric consultation	Psychiatric therapy necessary		

Table 8 COPEGUS Dosage Modification Guidelines

Laboratory Values	Reduce Only COPEGUS Dose to 600 mg/day* if:	Discontinue COPEGUS if:
Hemoglobin in patients with no cardiac disease	<10 g/dL	<8.5 g/dL
Hemoglobin in patients with history of stable cardiac disease	≥2 g/dL decrease in hemoglobin during any 4 week period treatment	<12 g/dL despite 4 weeks at reduced dose

* One 200 mg tablet in the morning and two 200 mg tablets in the evening.

HOW SUPPLIED

Single Dose Vial

Each PEGASYS (peginterferon alfa-2a) 180 µg single use, clear glass vial provides 1.0 mL containing 180 µg peginterferon alfa-2a for sc injection. Each package contains 1 vial (NDC 0004-0350-09).

Vials Monthly Convenience Pack

Four vials of PEGASYS (peginterferon alfa-2a), 180 µg single use, clear glass vials, in a box with 4 syringes and 8 alcohol swabs (NDC 0004-0350-39). Each syringe is a 1 mL (1 cc) volume syringe supplied with a 27 gauge, 1/2 inch needle with needle-stick protection device.

Prefilled Syringes Monthly Convenience Pack

Four prefilled syringes of PEGASYS (peginterferon alfa-2a), 180 µg single use, graduated, clear glass prefilled syringes, in a box with 4 needles and 4 alcohol swabs (NDC 0004-0352-39). Each syringe is a 0.5 mL (1/2 cc) volume syringe supplied with a 27 gauge, 1/2 inch needle with needle-stick protection device.

Storage

Store in the refrigerator at 2° to 8°C (36° to 46°F). Do not freeze or shake. Protect from light. Vials and prefilled syringes are for single use only. Discard any unused portion.
REBETRON™ is a trademark of Schering Corporation.

Revised: December 2003

MEDICATION GUIDE
PEGASYS®
(peginterferon alfa-2a)

Before you start taking PEGASYS (PEG-ah-sis), alone or in combination with COPEGUS® (Co-PEG-UHS), please read this Medication Guide carefully. Read this Medication Guide each time you refill your prescription in case new information has been added and make sure the pharmacist has given you the medicine your healthcare provider prescribed for you. Reading the information in this Medication Guide does not take the place of talking with your healthcare provider.

If you are taking PEGASYS in combination with COPEGUS, you should also read the Medication Guide for COPEGUS (ribavirin, USP) Tablets.

What is the most important information I should know about PEGASYS therapy?

PEGASYS, taken alone or in combination with COPEGUS, is a treatment for some people who are infected with hepatitis C virus. However, PEGASYS and COPEGUS can have serious side effects that may cause death in rare cases. Before starting PEGASYS therapy, you should talk with your healthcare provider about the possible benefits and the possible side effects of treatment, to decide if either of these treatments is right for you. If you begin treatment you will need to see your healthcare provider regularly for examinations and blood tests to make sure your treatment is working and to check for side effects.

The most serious possible side effects of PEGASYS taken alone or in combination with COPEGUS include:

Risks to Pregnancy:

Taking PEGASYS in combination with COPEGUS tablets can cause death, serious birth defects or other harm to your unborn child. If you are a woman of childbearing age, you must have negative pregnancy tests just before beginning treatment, during treatment, and for 6 months after you have stopped treatment. You must not become pregnant while either you or your partner are being treated with the PEGASYS/COPEGUS combination therapy or for 6 months after stopping therapy. Men and women should use two forms of birth control while taking the combination therapy and for the 6 months after treatment is completed. If you are a man, one of the two forms of birth control should be a condom. You must use birth control even if you believe that you are not fertile or that your fertility is low. You should talk to your healthcare provider about birth control for you and your partner.

If you are pregnant, you or your male partner must not take PEGASYS/COPEGUS combination therapy. If you or your partner are being treated and you become pregnant either during treatment or within 6 months of stopping treatment, call your healthcare provider right away.

Mental health problems:

PEGASYS may cause some patients to develop mood or behavioral problems. Signs of these problems include irritability (getting easily upset), depression (feeling low, feeling bad about yourself or feeling hopeless), and anxiety. Some patients may have aggressive behavior. Some patients may develop thoughts about ending their lives (suicidal thoughts) and may attempt to do so. A few patients have ever ended their lives. Former drug addicts may fall back into drug addiction or overdose. You must tell your healthcare provider if you are being treated for a mental illness or have a history of mental illness or if you are or have ever been addicted to drugs or alcohol. Call your healthcare provider immediately if you develop any of these problems while on PEGASYS treatment.

Blood problems:

Many patients taking PEGASYS have had a drop in the number of their white blood cells and their platelets. If the numbers of these blood cells are too low, you could be at risk for serious infections or bleeding.

COPEGUS causes a decrease in the number of your red blood cells (anemia). This can be dangerous, especially for patients who already have heart or circulatory (cardiovascular) problems. If you have or have ever had any cardiovascular problems, talk with your healthcare provider before taking the combination of PEGASYS and COPEGUS.

Infections:

Some patients taking interferon have had serious infections. Sometimes these infections have been fatal. If you develop a fever that does not go away or gets higher, call your healthcare provider right away. Your healthcare provider will need to examine you to rule out your having a serious infection.

Body organ problems:

Some patients may experience lung problems (such as difficulty breathing or pneumonia) and eye problems that can cause blurred vision or loss of your vision.

Call your healthcare provider immediately if you develop any of these conditions:

- **You become very depressed or think about suicide**
- **You have severe chest pain**
- **You have trouble breathing**
- **You have a change in your vision**
- **You become pregnant**
- **You notice unusual bleeding or bruising**
- **You have psoriasis (a skin disease) and it gets worse while taking PEGASYS**
- **High fever or a fever that does not go away**
- **You have severe stomach pain or lower back pain**
- **Bloody diarrhea**

For more information on possible side effects with PEGASYS therapy, alone or in combination with COPEGUS, please read the section on ***"What are the possible side effects of PEGASYS, and PEGASYS taken with COPEGUS?"*** *in this Medication Guide. You should also read the Medication Guide for COPEGUS tablets if you are taking that medicine with PEGASYS.*

What is PEGASYS?

PEGASYS is a drug used to treat adults who have a lasting (chronic) infection with hepatitis C virus and who show signs that the virus is damaging the liver. Patients with hepatitis C have the virus in their blood and in their liver. PEGASYS reduces the amount of virus in the body and helps the body's immune system fight the virus. The drug COPEGUS are tablets that may be taken with PEGASYS to help fight the virus infection. Do not take COPEGUS by itself.

In some patients that have received PEGASYS treatment for approximately one year, the amount of the hepatitis C virus in the body was decreased to a level so low that it could not be measured by blood tests. After 3 months of therapy, your healthcare provider may ask you to have a blood test to help determine how you are responding to your treatment.

It is not known if PEGASYS, used alone or in combination with COPEGUS, can cure hepatitis C (permanently eliminate the virus) or if it can prevent liver failure or liver cancer that is caused by hepatitis C infection.

It is also not known if PEGASYS, alone or in combination with COPEGUS, will prevent one infected person from infecting another person with hepatitis C.

Who should not take PEGASYS, or PEGASYS with COPEGUS?

Do not take PEGASYS or PEGASYS/COPEGUS therapy if you:

- are pregnant, planning to get pregnant during treatment or during the 6 months after treatment or breast-feeding
- are a male patient with a female sexual partner who is pregnant or plans to become pregnant at any time while you are being treated with COPEGUS or during the 6 months after your treatment has ended
- have hepatitis caused by your immune system attacking your liver (autoimmune hepatitis) or unstable liver disease
- had an allergic reaction to another alpha interferon or are allergic to any of the ingredients in PEGASYS or COPEGUS tablets
- Do not take PEGASYS, alone or in combination with COPEGUS, if you have abnormal red blood cells such as sickle-cell anemia or thalassemia major.

If you have ever had any of the following conditions or serious medical problems, tell your healthcare provider before you start taking PEGASYS:

- History of or current severe mental illness (such as depression or anxiety)
- History of drug or alcohol addiction or abuse
- History of heart disease or previous heart attack
- History of cancer
- Autoimmune disease (where the body's immune system attacks the body's own cells), such as psoriasis (a skin disease), systemic lupus erythematosus, rheumatoid arthritis
- Kidney problems
- Blood disorders
- You take a medicine called theophylline
- Diabetes (high blood sugar)
- Problems with the thyroid gland
- Liver problems, other than hepatitis C
- Hepatitis B infection
- HIV infection
- Colitis (an inflammation of the bowels)

You should tell your healthcare provider if you are taking or planning to take other prescription or nonprescription medicines or vitamin and mineral supplements or herbal medicines.

If you have any questions about your health condition or about taking PEGASYS alone or in combination with COPEGUS, you should talk to your healthcare provider.

How should I take PEGASYS, or PEGASYS with COPEGUS?

PEGASYS is given by injection under the skin (subcutaneous injection). PEGASYS comes in two different forms (a liquid in a single use vial and a liquid in a prefilled syringe). Your healthcare provider will determine which is best for you. Your healthcare provider will also decide whether you will take PEGASYS alone or with COPEGUS. Your dose of PEGASYS is given as a single injection once per week. At some point, your healthcare provider may change your dose of PEGASYS or COPEGUS. Do not change your dose unless your healthcare provider tells you to change it. It is important that you take PEGASYS and COPEGUS exactly as your healthcare provider tells you. Once you start treatment with PEGASYS, do not switch to another brand of interferon without talking to your healthcare provider. Other interferons may not have the same effect on the treatment of your disease. Switching brands will also require a change in your dose.

Take your prescribed dose of PEGASYS once a week, on the same day of each week and at approximately the same time. Your total dose of COPEGUS tablets should be divided so you take it twice a day with food (breakfast and dinner). Taking half your dose of COPEGUS in the morning and the other half at night will keep the medicine in your body at a steady level. Do not take more than your prescribed dose of PEGASYS or COPEGUS. **Be sure to read the Medication Guide for COPEGUS (ribavirin, USP) for complete instructions on how to take the COPEGUS tablets.**

Your healthcare provider will train you and/or the person that will be giving you the PEGASYS injections on the proper way to give injections. Whether you give yourself the injection or another person gives the injection to you, it is important that you are comfortable with preparing and injecting a dose of PEGASYS, and you understand the instructions in "How do I inject PEGASYS?" **At the end of this guide (see Appendix) there are detailed instructions on how to prepare and give yourself an injection of PEGASYS using the form your healthcare provider has prescribed for you.**

If you miss a dose and you remember **within 2 days** of when you should have taken PEGASYS, give yourself an injection of PEGASYS as soon as you remember. Take your next dose on the day you would usually take it. **If more than 2 days** have passed, ask your healthcare provider what you should do. If you miss a dose of COPEGUS, take the missed dose as soon as you remember during the same day. Do not take 2 doses too close together in time. If it is late in the day, wait until the next day and go back on schedule. **Do not double the next dose.**

If you take more than the prescribed amount of PEGASYS, call your healthcare provider right away. Your healthcare provider may want to examine you and take blood for testing.

You must get regular blood tests to help your healthcare provider check how the treatment is working and to check for side effects.

What should I avoid while taking PEGASYS, or PEGASYS with COPEGUS?

- If you are pregnant do not start taking or continue taking COPEGUS in combination with PEGASYS.
- Avoid becoming pregnant while taking PEGASYS, alone or in combination with COPEGUS. PEGASYS, alone or in combination with COPEGUS, may harm your unborn child (death or serious birth defects) or cause you to lose your baby (miscarry). **If you or your partner become pregnant during or within 6 months after treatment with COPEGUS, immediately report the pregnancy to your healthcare provider. You or your healthcare provider should call 1-800-526-6367.** When you call this number, you will be asked for information about you and/or your partner that will be added to a pregnancy registry. This information will be used to help you and your healthcare provider make decisions about your treatment for hepatitis in the future. You, your partner and/or your healthcare provider may also be asked follow-up information on the outcome of the pregnancy.
- Do not breast-feed your baby while on PEGASYS, alone or in combination with COPEGUS.

What are the possible side effects of PEGASYS, and PEGASYS taken with COPEGUS?

Possible, serious side effects include:

- **Risk to pregnancy, mental health problems including suicidal thoughts, blood problems, infections, and body organ problems:** *See "What is the most important information I should know about PEGASYS therapy?" in this Medication Guide.*
- **Autoimmune problems:** Some patients may develop a disease where the body's own immune system begins to attack itself (autoimmune disease) while on PEGASYS therapy. These diseases can include psoriasis or thyroid problems. In some patients who already have an autoimmune disease, the disease may worsen while on PEGASYS therapy.
- **Heart problems:** PEGASYS may cause some patients to experience chest pain, and very rarely a heart attack. Patients who already have heart disease could be at greatest risk. Tell your healthcare provider if you have or have had a heart problem in the past.

Common, but less serious, side effects include:

- **Flu-like symptoms:** Most patients who take PEGASYS have flu-like symptoms that usually lessen after the first few weeks of treatment. Flu-like symptoms may include fever, chills, muscle aches, joint pain, and headaches. Taking pain and fever reducers such as acetaminophen or ibuprofen before you take PEGASYS can help with these symptoms. You can also try taking PEGASYS at night. You may be able to sleep through the symptoms.
- **Extreme fatigue (tiredness):** Many patients may become extremely tired while on PEGASYS therapy.
- **Upset stomach:** Nausea, taste changes, diarrhea, and loss of appetite occur commonly.
- **Blood sugar problems:** Some patients may develop a problem with the way their body controls their blood sugar and may develop diabetes.
- **Skin reactions:** Some patients may develop rash, dry or itchy skin, and redness and swelling at the site of injection.
- **Hair thinning:** Temporary hair loss is not uncommon during treatment with PEGASYS.
- **Trouble sleeping**

These are not all of the side effects of PEGASYS, and PEGASYS taken with COPEGUS. Your healthcare provider or pharmacist can give you a more complete list.

Talk to your healthcare provider if you are worried about side effects or find them very bothersome.

General advice about prescription medicines

Medicines are sometimes prescribed for purposes other than those listed in a Medication Guide. If you have any concerns or questions about PEGASYS, contact your healthcare provider. Do not use PEGASYS for a condition or person other than that for which it is prescribed. If you want to know more about PEGASYS, your healthcare provider or pharmacist will be able to provide you with detailed information that is written for healthcare providers.

If you are taking COPEGUS (ribavirin, USP) in combination with PEGASYS, also read the Medication Guide supplied with that medicine.

Keep this and all drugs out of the reach of children.

This Medication Guide has been approved by the U.S. Food and Drug Administration.

Revised: December 2003

Medication Guide Appendix: Instructions for Preparing and Giving a Dose with a PEGASYS® Prefilled Syringe

How should I store PEGASYS Prefilled Syringes?

PEGASYS must be stored in the refrigerator at a temperature of 2°C to 8°C (36°F to 46°F). Do not leave PEGASYS outside of the refrigerator for more than 24 hours. Do not freeze PEGASYS. Keeping PEGASYS at temperatures outside the recommended range can destroy the medicine.

Each PEGASYS prefilled syringe can only be used once. Discard after use.

Do not shake the prefilled syringe of PEGASYS. If PEGASYS is shaken too hard, it will not work properly. Protect PEGASYS from light during storage.

Keep this and all other medicines out of the reach of children.

How do I prepare and inject PEGASYS?

You should read through all of these directions and ask your healthcare provider for help if you have any questions before trying to give yourself an injection. It is important to follow these directions carefully. Talk to your healthcare provider if you have any questions about PEGASYS.

Your healthcare provider may not want you to take all the medicine that comes in the prefilled syringe. To appropriately administer the dose that your healthcare provider tells you to take, you may have to get rid of some of the medicine before injecting the medicine.

If you ever switch between using prefilled syringes and vials, talk to your healthcare provider about how much PEGASYS to use. Equal volumes of liquid from the prefilled syringes and the vials DO NOT contain the same amount of PEGASYS. If you switch between prefilled syringes and vials, you will have to adjust the volume of liquid that you use to give your injection. If you do not adjust this, you could accidentally take too much or too little of your medicine.

If you are giving this injection to someone else, a healthcare provider must teach you how to avoid needle sticks. Being stuck by a used needle can pass diseases on to you.

The prefilled syringes are used for injecting PEGASYS under the surface of the skin (subcutaneous).

1. Collect all the materials you will need before you start to give the injection:
   - One PEGASYS prefilled syringe Monthly Convenience Pack containing an inner carton holding the PEGASYS prefilled syringe
   - A puncture-resistant container for cleaning up when you are finished
2. Open the convenience pack and look at the contents.
   - Each convenience pack has everything you need for the PEGASYS injection.
     - 4 single use syringes filled with medicine (should be colorless to light yellow)
     - four 27 gauge, 1/2 inch needles with needle stick protection device
     - 4 alcohol swabs
   - Do not use PEGASYS if:
     - the medicine is cloudy
     - the medicine has particles floating in it
     - the medicine is any color besides colorless to light yellow
     - the expiration date has passed
3. Warm the refrigerated medicine by gently rolling it in the palms of your hands for about one minute. Do not shake.
4. Wash your hands with soap and warm water to prevent infection.

Continued on next page

Pegasys—Cont.

5. Attachment of the needle to the PEGASYS prefilled syringe:
   - Remove the needle from its package. Do not remove the needle shield yet. Keep the needle covered until just before you give the injection.

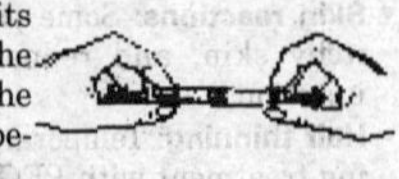

   - Remove and discard the rubber cap from the tip of the syringe barrel.
   - Put the needle onto the end of the syringe barrel so it fits tightly.
   - Here is a picture of the assembled syringe:
   - Keep the syringe in a horizontal position until ready for use.

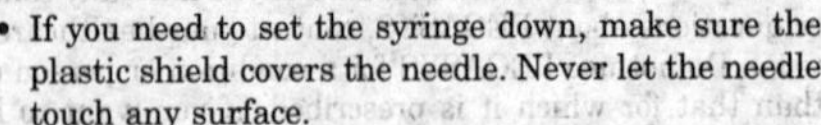

   - If you need to set the syringe down, make sure the plastic shield covers the needle. Never let the needle touch any surface.
6. Decide where you will give the injection.
   - Pick a place on your stomach or thigh (see the picture at right). Avoid your navel and waistline. You should use a different place each time you give yourself an injection.

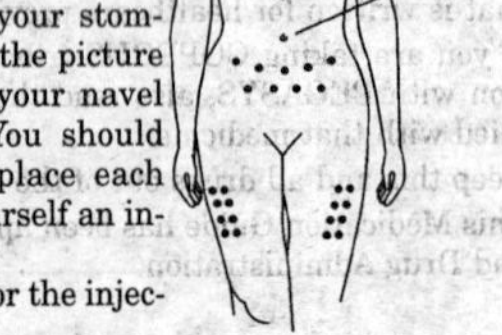

7. Prepare your skin for the injection.
   - To minimize the discomfort from injections, you may want to gently tap the area where you plan to give yourself an injection.
   - Clean the area using the alcohol pad. Let the skin dry for 10 seconds.
8. Uncover the needle.
   - Remove the plastic safety shield covering the needle. Do not remove the orange cap that is attached to the end of the syringe and above the needle that is the needle-stick protection device.

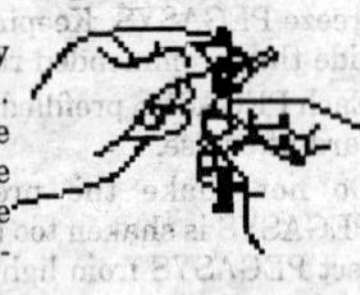

9. Remove air bubbles from the syringe.
   - Hold the syringe with the needle pointing up to the ceiling.
   - Using your thumb and finger, tap the syringe to bring air bubbles to the top.
   - Press the plunger in slightly to push air bubbles out of the syringe.
   - Your healthcare provider may not want you to take all the medicine that comes in the prefilled syringe.
   - To appropriately administer the dose that your healthcare provider tells you to take, you may have to get rid of some of the medicine before injecting the medicine.
   - The syringe has markings for 180 mcg, 135 mcg, and 90 mcg. Your healthcare provider will tell you which mark to use.
   - Once you know which mark to use, slowly and carefully press on the plunger rod of the syringe to push out medicine from the syringe. Keep pressing until the edge of the plunger stopper reaches the right mark on the side of the syringe.

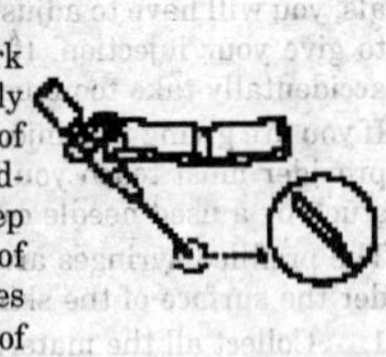

   - Do not decrease or increase your dose of PEGASYS unless your healthcare provider tells you to.
10. Give the injection of PEGASYS.
    - Position the point of the needle (the bevel) so it is facing up.
    - Pinch a fold of skin on your stomach or thigh firmly with your thumb and forefinger.
    - Hold the syringe like a pencil at a 45° to 90° angle to your skin. In one quick motion, insert the needle as far as it will go into the pinched area of skin. Pull the plunger of the syringe back very slightly. If blood comes into the syringe, the needle has entered a blood vessel. **Do not inject. Withdraw the needle and discard the syringe as outlined in step 11. Repeat the above steps with a new prefilled syringe and prepare a new site.**

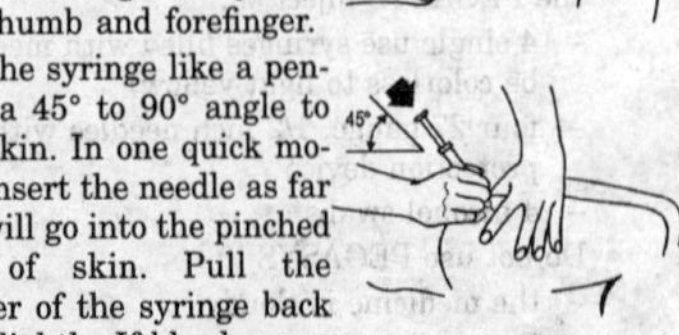

    - If no blood appears, release your skin and slowly push the plunger all the way down so that you get all of your medicine.
    - Pull out the needle at same angle you put it in.
    - Wipe the area with an alcohol swab.
11. For safety reasons, before you dispose of the syringe and needle, place the free end of the orange cap on a flat surface and push down on it until it clicks and covers over the needle. Always place used syringes and needles in a puncture-resistant container immediately after use and never reuse them. Keep your disposal container out of the reach of children.

How should I dispose of materials used to inject PEGASYS?

There may be special state and local laws for disposal of used needles and syringes. Your healthcare provider or pharmacist should provide you with instructions on how to properly dispose of your used syringes and needles. Always follow these instructions.

The instructions below should be used as a general guide for proper disposal:

- The needles and syringes should never be reused.
- Place all used needles and syringes in a puncture-proof disposable container that is available through your pharmacy or healthcare provider (Sharp's container).
- DO NOT use glass or clear plastic containers for disposal of needles and syringes.
- Dispose of the full container as instructed by your healthcare provider or pharmacist.

DO NOT throw the container in your household trash. DO NOT recycle. Keep the container out of the reach of children.

Appendix revision date: December 2003

Medication Guide Appendix: Instructions for Preparing and Giving a Dose with a PEGASYS® Vial

How should I store PEGASYS vials?

PEGASYS must be stored in the refrigerator at a temperature of 2°C to 8°C (36°F to 46°F). Do not leave PEGASYS outside of the refrigerator for more than 24 hours. Do not freeze PEGASYS. Keeping PEGASYS at temperatures outside the recommended range can destroy the medicine.

Each PEGASYS vial can only be used once. Discard after use.

Do not shake the vial of PEGASYS. If PEGASYS is shaken too hard, it will not work properly.

Protect PEGASYS from light during storage.

Keep this and all other medicines out of the reach of children.

How do I inject PEGASYS?

The following instructions will help you learn how to measure your dose and give yourself an injection of PEGASYS. You should read through all of these directions and ask your healthcare provider for help if you have any questions before trying to give yourself an injection. It is important to follow these directions carefully. Talk to your healthcare provider if you have any questions about PEGASYS.

If you are giving an injection to someone else, a healthcare provider must teach you how to avoid needle sticks. Being stuck by a used needle can pass diseases on to you.

1. Collect all the materials you will need before you start to give the injection:
   - One vial of PEGASYS
   - One syringe and needle
   - Several alcohol pads
   - A puncture-resistant container to dispose of the needle and syringe when you are finished

If you have received the PEGASYS Convenience Pack, it includes PEGASYS, safety syringes and needles with a needle-stick protection device attached, and alcohol swabs.

2. Check the date on the carton the PEGASYS comes in and make sure the expiration date has not passed, then remove a vial from the package and look at the medicine.
   - Do not use PEGASYS if:
     – the medicine is cloudy
     – the medicine has particles floating in it
     – the medicine is any color besides colorless to light yellow
     – the expiration date has passed
3. Warm the refrigerated medicine by gently rolling it in the palms of your hands for about one minute. Do not shake.
4. Wash your hands with soap and warm water to prevent infection.
5. Take the vial of PEGASYS and flip off the plastic top covering the vial opening, and clean the rubber stopper on the top of the vial with a different alcohol pad.

If you are not sure how much medicine to use or which mark to use, STOP and call your healthcare provider right away.

6. Remove the needle and syringe from their packaging and attach the needle to the end of the syringe.
   - If you are using a syringe and needle supplied with the PEGASYS Convenience Pack, the needle is already attached to the syringe and it will have a needle-stick protection device attached. Remove the clear protective cap from the end of the needle. Do not remove the orange cap that is attached to the end of the syringe and above the needle that is the needle-stick protection device.

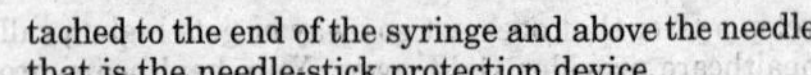

   - Pull the plunger back so the end of it is to the mark on the syringe barrel that matches the dose prescribed for you by your healthcare provider. This will pull air into the syringe barrel.
   - Push the needle through the center of the stopper on the vial.
   - Slowly inject all the air from the syringe into the air space above the solution. Do not inject air into the fluid.
   - Keep the needle inside the vial and turn both upside down. Hold the vial and syringe straight up. Slowly pull back on the plunger until the medicine is in the syringe up to the mark that matches your dose. Make sure the needle tip always stays in the medicine (not in the air space above it).
   - When the medicine is up to the right mark on the syringe barrel, take the syringe and needle out of the rubber stopper on the vial.
   - Keep the syringe pointing up until you are ready to use it.
   - If you need to set the syringe down, make sure that you never let the needle touch any surface.
7. Remove air bubbles from the syringe.
   - Hold the syringe with the needle pointing up to the ceiling.
   - Using your thumb and finger, tap the syringe to bring air bubbles to top.
   - Press the plunger in slightly to push air bubbles out of the syringe.

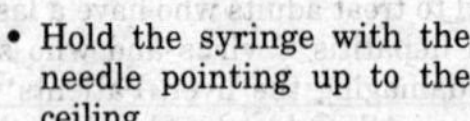

8. Decide where you will give the injection.
   - Pick a place on your stomach or thigh (see the picture below). Avoid your navel and waistline. You should use a different place each time you give yourself an injection.
9. Prepare your skin for the injection.
   - To minimize the discomfort from injections, you may want to gently tap the area where you plan to give yourself an injection.
   - Clean the area using an alcohol pad. Let the skin dry for 10 seconds.
10. Give the injection of PEGASYS.
    - Position the point of the needle (the bevel) so it is facing up.
    - Pinch a fold of skin on your stomach or thigh firmly between your thumb and forefinger.
    - Hold the syringe like a pencil at a 45° to 90° angle to your skin. In one quick motion, insert the needle as far as it will go into the pinched area of skin. Pull the plunger of the syringe back very slightly. If blood comes into the syringe, the needle has entered a blood vessel. **Do not inject. Withdraw the needle and discard the syringe as outlined in step 11. Repeat the above steps with a new vial and syringe and prepare a new site.**

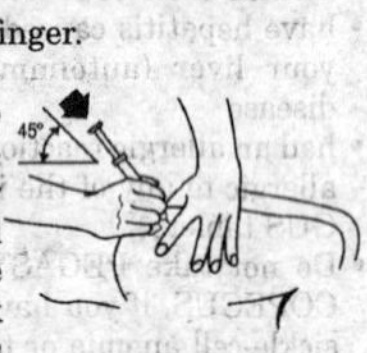

    - If no blood appears, release your skin and slowly push the plunger all the way down so that you get all of your medicine.
    - Pull out the needle at same angle you put it in. Wipe the area with an alcohol pad.
11. For safety reasons, always place used syringes and needles in a puncture-resistant container immediately after use and never reuse them.
    - If you are using a syringe with a needle-stick protection device, before you dispose of the syringe and needle, place the free end of the orange cap on a flat surface and push down on it until it clicks and covers over the needle.

How should I dispose of materials used to inject PEGASYS?

There may be special state and local laws for disposal of used needles and syringes. Your healthcare provider or pharmacist should provide you with instructions on how to properly dispose of your used syringes and needles. Always follow these instructions.

The instructions below should be used as a general guide for proper disposal:

- The needles and syringes should never be reused.
- Place all used needles and syringes in a puncture-proof disposable container that is available through your pharmacy or healthcare provider (Sharp's container).
- DO NOT use glass or clear plastic containers for disposal of needles and syringes.

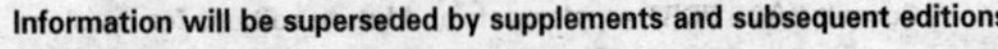

- Dispose of the full container as instructed by your health-care provider or pharmacist.

DO NOT throw the container in your household trash. DO NOT recycle. Keep the container out of the reach of children.

Appendix revision date: December 2003

Hoffmann-La Roche Inc., Nutley, New Jersey 07110-1199
U.S. Govt. Lic. No. 0136

ROCALTROL® ℞

brand of calcitriol
CAPSULES and ORAL SOLUTION

DESCRIPTION

Rocaltrol (calcitriol) is a synthetic vitamin D analog which is active in the regulation of the absorption of calcium from the gastrointestinal tract and its utilization in the body. Rocaltrol is available as capsules containing 0.25 mcg or 0.5 mcg calcitriol and as an oral solution containing 1 mcg/mL of calcitriol. All dosage forms contain butylated hydroxyanisole (BHA) and butylated hydroxytoluene (BHT) as antioxidants. The capsules contain a fractionated triglyceride of coconut oil, and the oral solution contains a fractionated triglyceride of palm seed oil. Gelatin capsule shells contain glycerin, parabens (methyl and propyl) and sorbitol, with the following dye systems: 0.25 mcg — FD&C Yellow No. 6 and titanium dioxide; 0.5 mcg — FD&C Red No. 3, FD&C Yellow No. 6 and titanium dioxide. The oral solution contains no additional adjuvants or coloring principles.

Calcitriol is a white, crystalline compound which occurs naturally in humans. It has a calculated molecular weight of 416.65 and is soluble in organic solvents but relatively insoluble in water. Chemically, calcitriol is 9,10-seco(5Z,7E)-5,7,10(19)-cholestatriene-1α, 3β, 25-triol.

The other names frequently used for calcitriol are 1α,25-dihydroxycholecalciferol, 1,25-dihydroxyvitamin D_3, 1,25-DHCC, 1,25$(OH)_2D_3$ and 1,25-diOHC.

CLINICAL PHARMACOLOGY

Man's natural supply of vitamin D depends mainly on exposure to the ultraviolet rays of the sun for conversion of 7-dehydrocholesterol in the skin to vitamin D_3 (cholecalciferol). Vitamin D_3 must be metabolically activated in the liver and the kidney before it is fully active as a regulator of calcium and phosphorus metabolism at target tissues. The initial transformation of vitamin D_3 is catalyzed by a vitamin D_3-25-hydroxylase enzyme (25-OHase) present in the liver, and the product of this reaction is 25-hydroxyvitamin D_3 [25-$(OH)D_3$]. Hydroxylation of 25-$(OH)D_3$ occurs in the mitochondria of kidney tissue, activated by the renal 25-hydroxyvitamin D_3-1 alpha-hydroxylase (alpha-OHase), to produce 1,25-$(OH)_2D_3$ (calcitriol), the active form of vitamin D_3. Endogenous synthesis and catabolism of calcitriol, as well as physiological control mechanisms affecting these processes, play a critical role regulating the serum level of calcitriol. Physiological daily production is normally 0.5 to 1.0 mcg and is somewhat higher during periods of increased bone synthesis (eg, growth or pregnancy).

Pharmacodynamics

The two known sites of action of calcitriol are intestine and bone. A calcitriol receptor-binding protein appears to exist in the mucosa of human intestine. Additional evidence suggests that calcitriol may also act on the kidney and the parathyroid glands. Calcitriol is the most active known form of vitamin D_3 in stimulating intestinal calcium transport. In acutely uremic rats calcitriol has been shown to stimulate intestinal calcium absorption.

The kidneys of uremic patients cannot adequately synthesize calcitriol, the active hormone formed from precursor vitamin D. Resultant hypocalcemia and secondary hyperparathyroidism are a major cause of the metabolic bone disease of renal failure. However, other bone-toxic substances which accumulate in uremia (eg, aluminum) may also contribute. The beneficial effect of Rocaltrol in renal osteodystrophy appears to result from correction of hypocalcemia and secondary hyperparathyroidism. It is uncertain whether Rocaltrol produces other independent beneficial effects. Rocaltrol treatment is not associated with an accelerated rate of renal function deterioration. No radiographic evidence of extraskeletal calcification has been found in predialysis patients following treatment. The duration of pharmacologic activity of a single dose of calcitriol is about 3 to 5 days.

Pharmacokinetics

Absorption

Calcitriol is rapidly absorbed from the intestine. Peak serum concentrations (above basal values) were reached within 3 to 6 hours following oral administration of single doses of 0.25 to 1.0 mcg of Rocaltrol. Following a single oral dose of 0.5 mcg, mean serum concentrations of calcitriol rose from a baseline value of 40.0±4.4 (SD) pg/mL to 60.0±4.4 pg/mL at 2 hours, and declined to 53.0±6.9 at 4 hours, 50±7.0 at 8 hours, 44±4.6 at 12 hours, and 41.5±5.1 at 24 hours.

Following multiple-dose administration, serum calcitriol levels reached steady-state within 7 days.

Distribution

Calcitriol is approximately 99.9% bound in blood. Calcitriol and other vitamin D metabolites are transported in blood, by an alpha-globulin vitamin D binding protein. There is evidence that maternal calcitriol may enter the fetal circulation. Calcitriol is transferred into human breast milk at low levels (ie, 2.2±0.1 pg/mL).

Metabolism

In vivo and in vitro studies indicate the presence of two pathways of metabolism for calcitriol. The first pathway involves the 24-hydroxylase as the first step in catabolism of calcitriol. There is definite evidence of 24-hydroxylase activity in the kidney; this enzyme is also present in many target tissues which possess the vitamin D receptor such as the intestine. The end product of this pathway is a side chain shortened metabolite, calcitroic acid. The second pathway involves the conversion of calcitriol via the stepwise hydroxylation of carbon-26 and carbon-23, and cyclization to yield ultimately 1α, 25R$(OH)_2$-26, 23S-lactone D_3. The lactone appears to be the major metabolite circulating in humans, with mean serum concentrations of 131±17 pg/mL. In addition, several other metabolites of calcitriol have been identified: 1α, 25$(OH)_2$-24-oxo-D_3; 1α, 23,25$(OH)_3$-24-oxo-D_3; 1α, 24R,25$(OH)_3D_3$; 1α, 25S,26$(OH)_3D_3$; 1α, 25$(OH)_2$-23-oxo-D_3; 1α, 25R,26$(OH)_3$-23-oxo-D_3; 1α, (OH)24,25,26,27-tetranor-COOH-D_3.

Excretion

Enterohepatic recycling and biliary excretion of calcitriol occur. The metabolites of calcitriol are excreted primarily in feces. Following intravenous administration of radiolabeled calcitriol in normal subjects, approximately 27% and 7% of the radioactivity appeared in the feces and urine, respectively, within 24 hours. When a 1-mcg oral dose of radiolabeled calcitriol was administered to normal subjects, approximately 10% of the total radioactivity appeared in urine within 24 hours. Cumulative excretion of radioactivity on the sixth day following intravenous administration of radiolabeled calcitriol averaged 16% in urine and 49% in feces. The elimination half-life of calcitriol in serum after single oral doses is about 5 to 8 hours in normal subjects.

Special Populations

Pediatric Pharmacokinetics

The steady-state pharmacokinetics of oral Rocaltrol were determined in a small group of pediatric patients (age range: 1.8 to 16 years) undergoing peritoneal dialysis. Rocaltrol was administered for 2 months at an average dose of 10.2 ng/kg (SD 5.5 ng/kg). In this pediatric population, mean C_{max} was 116 pmol/L, mean serum half-life was 27.4 hours, and mean clearance was 15.3 mL/hr/kg.[1]

Geriatric

No studies have examined the pharmacokinetics of calcitriol in geriatric patients.

Gender

Controlled studies examining the influence of gender on calcitriol have not been conducted.

Hepatic Insufficiency

Controlled studies examining the influence of hepatic disease on calcitriol have not been conducted.

Renal Insufficiency

Lower predose and peak calcitriol levels in serum were observed in patients with nephrotic syndrome and in patients undergoing hemodialysis compared with healthy subjects. The elimination half-life of calcitriol increased by at least twofold in chronic renal failure and hemodialysis patients compared with healthy subjects. Peak serum levels in patients with nephrotic syndrome were reached in 4 hours. For patients requiring hemodialysis peak serum levels were reached in 8 to 12 hours; half-lives were estimated to be 16.2 and 21.9 hours, respectively.

INDICATIONS AND USAGE

Predialysis Patients

Rocaltrol is indicated in the management of secondary hyperparathyroidism and resultant metabolic bone disease in patients with moderate to severe chronic renal failure (Ccr 15 to 55 mL/min) not yet on dialysis. In children, the creatinine clearance value must be corrected for a surface area of 1.73 square meters. A serum iPTH level of ≥ 100 pg/mL is strongly suggestive of secondary hyperparathyroidism.

Dialysis Patients

Rocaltrol is indicated in the management of hypocalcemia and the resultant metabolic bone disease in patients undergoing chronic renal dialysis. In these patients, Rocaltrol administration enhances calcium absorption, reduces serum alkaline phosphatase levels, and may reduce elevated parathyroid hormone levels and the histological manifestations of osteitis fibrosa cystica and defective mineralization.

Hypoparathyroidism Patients

Rocaltrol is also indicated in the management of hypocalcemia and its clinical manifestations in patients with postsurgical hypoparathyroidism, idiopathic hypoparathyroidism, and pseudohypoparathyroidism.

CONTRAINDICATIONS

Rocaltrol should not be given to patients with hypercalcemia or evidence of vitamin D toxicity. Use of Rocaltrol in patients with known hypersensitivity to Rocaltrol (or drugs of the same class) or any of the inactive ingredients is contraindicated.

WARNINGS

Overdosage of any form of vitamin D is dangerous (see **OVERDOSAGE**). Progressive hypercalcemia due to overdosage of vitamin D and its metabolites may be so severe as to require emergency attention. Chronic hypercalcemia can lead to generalized vascular calcification, nephrocalcinosis and other soft-tissue calcification. **The serum calcium times phosphate (Ca × P) product should not be allowed to exceed 70 mg^2/dL^2.** Radiographic evaluation of suspect anatomical regions may be useful in the early detection of this condition.

Rocaltrol is the most potent metabolite of vitamin D available. The administration of Rocaltrol to patients in excess of their daily requirements can cause hypercalcemia, hypercalciuria, and hyperphosphatemia. Therefore, pharmacologic doses of vitamin D and its derivatives should be withheld during Rocaltrol treatment to avoid possible additive effects and hypercalcemia. If treatment is switched from ergocalciferol (vitamin D_2) to calcitriol, it may take several months for the ergocalciferol level in the blood to return to the baseline value (see **OVERDOSAGE**).

Calcitriol increases inorganic phosphate levels in serum. While this is desirable in patients with hypophosphatemia, caution is called for in patients with renal failure because of the danger of ectopic calcification. A non-aluminum phosphate-binding compound and a low-phosphate diet should be used to control serum phosphorus levels in patients undergoing dialysis.

Magnesium-containing preparations (eg, antacids) and Rocaltrol should not be used concomitantly in patients on chronic renal dialysis because such use may lead to the development of hypermagnesemia.

Studies in dogs and rats given calcitriol for up to 26 weeks have shown that small increases of calcitriol above endogenous levels can lead to abnormalities of calcium metabolism with the potential for calcification of many tissues in the body.

PRECAUTIONS

General

Excessive dosage of Rocaltrol induces hypercalcemia and in some instances hypercalciuria; therefore, early in treatment during dosage adjustment, serum calcium should be determined twice weekly. In dialysis patients, a fall in serum alkaline phosphatase levels usually antedates the appearance of hypercalcemia and may be an indication of impending hypercalcemia. An abrupt increase in calcium intake as a result of changes in diet (eg, increased consumption of dairy products) or uncontrolled intake of calcium preparations may trigger hypercalcemia.

Should hypercalcemia develop, treatment with Rocaltrol should be stopped immediately. During periods of hypercalcemia, serum calcium and phosphate levels must be determined daily. When normal levels have been attained, treatment with Rocaltrol can be continued, at a daily dose 0.25 mcg lower than that previously used. An estimate of daily dietary calcium intake should be made and the intake adjusted when indicated. Rocaltrol should be given cautiously to patients on digitalis, because hypercalcemia in such patients may precipitate cardiac arrhythmias.

Immobilized patients, eg, those who have undergone surgery, are particularly exposed to the risk of hypercalcemia. In patients with normal renal function, chronic hypercalcemia may be associated with an increase in serum creatinine. While this is usually reversible, it is important in such patients to pay careful attention to those factors which may lead to hypercalcemia. Rocaltrol therapy should always be started at the lowest possible dose and should not be increased without careful monitoring of the serum calcium. An estimate of daily dietary calcium intake should be made and the intake adjusted when indicated.

Patients with normal renal function taking Rocaltrol should avoid dehydration. Adequate fluid intake should be maintained.

Information for Patients

The patient and his or her caregivers should be informed about compliance with dosage instructions, adherence to instructions about diet and calcium supplementation, and avoidance of the use of unapproved nonprescription drugs. Patients and their caregivers should also be carefully informed about the symptoms of hypercalcemia (see **ADVERSE REACTIONS**).

The effectiveness of Rocaltrol therapy is predicated on the assumption that each patient is receiving an adequate daily intake of calcium. Patients are advised to have a dietary intake of calcium at a minimum of 600 mg daily. The U.S. RDA for calcium in adults is 800 mg to 1200 mg.

Laboratory Tests

For dialysis patients, serum calcium, phosphorus, magnesium, and alkaline phosphatase should be determined periodically. For hypoparathyroid patients, serum calcium, phosphorus, and 24-hour urinary calcium should be determined periodically. For predialysis patients, serum calcium, phosphorus, alkaline phosphatase, creatinine, and intact PTH (iPTH) should be determined initially. Thereafter, serum calcium, phosphorus, alkaline phosphatase, and creatine should be determined monthly for a 6-month period and then determined periodically. Intact PTH (iPTH) should be determined periodically every 3 to 4 months at the time of visits. During the titration period of treatment with Rocaltrol, serum calcium levels should be checked at least twice weekly (see **DOSAGE AND ADMINISTRATION**).

Drug Interactions

Cholestyramine

Cholestyramine has been reported to reduce intestinal absorption of fat-soluble vitamins; as such it may impair intestinal absorption of Rocaltrol (see **WARNINGS** and **PRECAUTIONS: General**).

Phenytoin/Phenobarbital

The coadministration of phenytoin or phenobarbital will not affect plasma concentrations of calcitriol, but may reduce endogenous plasma levels of 25$(OH)D_3$ by accelerating metabolism. Since blood level of calcitriol will be reduced, higher doses of Rocaltrol may be necessary if these drugs are administered simultaneously.

Thiazides

Thiazides are known to induce hypercalcemia by the reduction of calcium excretion in urine. Some reports have shown that the concomitant administration of thiazides with Rocaltrol causes hypercalcemia. Therefore, precaution should be taken when coadministration is necessary.

Continued on next page

Rocaltrol—Cont.

Digitalis
Calcitriol dosage must be determined with care in patients undergoing treatment with digitalis, as hypercalcemia in such patients may precipitate cardiac arrhythmias (see **PRECAUTIONS: General**).
Ketoconazole
Ketoconazole may inhibit both synthetic and catabolic enzymes of calcitriol. Reductions in serum endogenous calcitriol concentrations have been observed following the administration of 300 mg/day to 1200 mg/day ketoconazole for a week to healthy men. However, in vivo drug interaction studies of ketoconazole with Rocaltrol have not been investigated.
Corticosteroids
A relationship of functional antagonism exists between vitamin D analogues, which promote calcium absorption, and corticosteroids, which inhibit calcium absorption.
Phosphate-Binding Agents
Since Rocaltrol also has an effect on phosphate transport in the intestine, kidneys and bones, the dosage of phosphate-binding agents must be adjusted in accordance with the serum phosphate concentration.
Vitamin D
Since calcitriol is the most potent active metabolite of vitamin D_3, pharmacological doses of vitamin D and its derivatives should be withheld during treatment with Rocaltrol to avoid possible additive effects and hypercalcemia (see **WARNINGS**).
Calcium Supplements
Uncontrolled intake of additional calcium-containing preparations should be avoided (see **PRECAUTIONS: General**).
Magnesium
Magnesium-containing preparations (eg, antacids) may cause hypermagnesemia and should therefore not be taken during therapy with Rocaltrol by patients on chronic renal dialysis.

Carcinogenesis, Mutagenesis and Impairment of Fertility
Long-term studies in animals have not been conducted to evaluate the carcinogenic potential of Rocaltrol. Rocaltrol is not mutagenic in vitro in the Ames Test, nor is it genotoxic in vivo in the Mouse Micronucleus Test. No significant effects of Rocaltrol on fertility and/or general reproductive performances were observed in a Segment I study in rats at doses of up to 0.3 mcg/kg (approximately 3 times the maximum recommended dose based on body surface area).

Pregnancy
Teratogenic Effects
Pregnancy Category C. Rocaltrol has been found to be teratogenic in rabbits when given at doses of 0.08 and 0.3 mcg/kg (approximately 2 and 6 times the maximum recommended dose based on mg/m^2). All 15 fetuses in 3 litters at these doses showed external and skeletal abnormalities. However, none of the other 23 litters (156 fetuses) showed external and skeletal abnormalities compared with controls.
Teratogenicity studies in rats at doses up to 0.45 mcg/kg (approximately 5 times maximum recommended dose based on mg/m^2) showed no evidence of teratogenic potential. There are no adequate and well-controlled studies in pregnant women. Rocaltrol should be used during pregnancy only if the potential benefit justifies the potential risk to the fetus.
Nonteratogenic Effects
In the rabbit, dosages of 0.3 mcg/kg/day (approximately 6 times maximum recommended dose based on surface area) administered on days 7 to 18 of gestation resulted in 19% maternal mortality, a decrease in mean fetal body weight and a reduced number of newborn surviving to 24 hours. A study of perinatal and postnatal development in rats resulted in hypercalcemia in the offspring of dams given Rocaltrol at doses of 0.08 or 0.3 mcg/kg/day (approximately 1 and 3 times the maximum recommended dose based on mg/m^2), hypercalcemia and hypophosphatemia in dams given Rocaltrol at a dose of 0.08 or 0.3 mcg/kg/day, and increased serum urea nitrogen in dams given Rocaltrol at a dose of 0.3 mcg/kg/day. In another study in rats, maternal weight gain was slightly reduced at a dose of 0.3 mcg/kg/day (approximately 3 times the maximum recommended dose based on mg/m^2) administered on days 7 to 15 of gestation. The offspring of a woman administered 17 mcg/day to 36 mcg/day of Rocaltrol (approximately 17 to 36 times the maximum recommended dose), during pregnancy manifested mild hypercalcemia in the first 2 days of life which returned to normal at day 3.

Nursing Mothers
Calcitriol from ingested Rocaltrol may be excreted in human milk. Because many drugs are excreted in human milk and because of the potential for serious adverse reactions from Rocaltrol in nursing infants, a mother should not nurse while taking Rocaltrol.

Pediatric Use
Safety and effectiveness of Rocaltrol in pediatric patients undergoing dialysis have not been established. The safety and effectiveness of Rocaltrol in pediatric predialysis patients is based on evidence from adequate and well-controlled studies of Rocaltrol in adults with predialysis chronic renal failure and additional supportive data from non-placebo controlled studies in pediatric patients. Dosing guidelines have not been established for pediatric patients under 1 year of age with hypoparathyroidism or for pediatric patients less than 6 years of age with pseudohypoparathyroidism (see **DOSAGE AND ADMINISTRATION: Hypoparathyroidism**).
Oral doses of Rocaltrol ranging from 10 to 55 ng/kg/day have been shown to improve calcium homeostasis and bone disease in pediatric patients with chronic renal failure for whom hemodialysis is not yet required (predialysis). Long-term calcitriol therapy is well tolerated by pediatric patients. The most common safety issues are mild, transient episodes of hypercalcemia, hyperphosphatemia, and increases in the serum calcium times phosphate (Ca × P) product which are managed effectively by dosage adjustment or temporary discontinuation of the vitamin D derivative.

Geriatric Use
Clinical studies of Rocaltrol did not include sufficient numbers of subjects aged 65 and over to determine whether they respond differently from younger subjects. Other reported clinical experience has not identified differences in responses between the elderly and younger patients. In general, dose selection for an elderly patient should be cautious, usually starting at the low end of the dosing range, reflecting the greater frequency of decreased hepatic, renal, or cardiac function, and of concomitant disease or other drug therapy.

ADVERSE REACTIONS

Since Rocaltrol is believed to be the active hormone which exerts vitamin D activity in the body, adverse effects are, in general, similar to those encountered with excessive vitamin D intake, ie, hypercalcemia syndrome or calcium intoxication (depending on the severity and duration of hypercalcemia) (see **WARNINGS**). Because of the short biological half-life of calcitriol, pharmacokinetic investigations have shown normalization of elevated serum calcium within a few days of treatment withdrawal, ie, much faster than in treatment with vitamin D_3 preparations.
The early and late signs and symptoms of vitamin D intoxication associated with hypercalcemia include:
Early: weakness, headache, somnolence, nausea, vomiting, dry mouth, constipation, muscle pain, bone pain, metallic taste, and anorexia, abdominal pain or stomach ache.
Late: polyuria, polydipsia, anorexia, weight loss, nocturia, conjunctivitis (calcific), pancreatitis, photophobia, rhinorrhea, pruritus, hyperthermia, decreased libido, elevated BUN, albuminuria, hypercholesterolemia, elevated SGOT (AST) and SGPT (ALT), ectopic calcification, nephrocalcinosis, hypertension, cardiac arrhythmias, dystrophy, sensory disturbances, dehydration, apathy, arrested growth, urinary tract infections, and, rarely, overt psychosis.
In clinical studies on hypoparathyroidism and pseudohypoparathyroidism, hypercalcemia was noted on at least one occasion in about 1 in 3 patients and hypercalciuria in about 1 in 7 patients. Elevated serum creatinine levels were observed in about 1 in 6 patients (approximately one half of whom had normal levels at baseline).
In concurrent hypercalcemia and hyperphosphatemia, soft-tissue calcification may occur; this can be seen radiographically (see **WARNINGS**).
In patients with normal renal function, chronic hypercalcemia may be associated with an increase in serum creatinine (see **PRECAUTIONS: General**).
Hypersensitivity reactions (pruritus, rash, urticaria, and very rarely severe erythematous skin disorders) may occur in susceptible individuals. One case of erythema multiforme and one case of allergic reaction (swelling of lips and hives all over the body) were confirmed by rechallenge.

OVERDOSAGE

Administration of Rocaltrol to patients in excess of their daily requirements can cause hypercalcemia, hypercalciuria, and hyperphosphatemia. Since calcitriol is a derivative of vitamin D, the signs and symptoms of overdose are the same as for an overdose of vitamin D (see **ADVERSE REACTIONS**). High intake of calcium and phosphate concomitant with Rocaltrol may lead to similar abnormalities. The serum calcium times phosphate (Ca × P) product should not be allowed to exceed 70 mg^2/dL^2. High levels of calcium in the dialysate bath may contribute to the hypercalcemia (see **WARNINGS**).

Treatment of Hypercalcemia and Overdosage in Dialysis Patients and Hypoparathyroidism Patients
General treatment of hypercalcemia (greater than 1 mg/dL above the upper limit of the normal range) consists of immediate discontinuation of Rocaltrol therapy, institution of a low-calcium diet and withdrawal of calcium supplements. Serum calcium levels should be determined daily until normocalcemia ensues. Hypercalcemia frequently resolves in 2 to 7 days. When serum calcium levels have returned to within normal limits, Rocaltrol therapy may be reinstituted at a dose of 0.25 mcg/day less than prior therapy. Serum calcium levels should be obtained at least twice weekly after all dosage changes and subsequent dosage titration. In dialysis patients, persistent or markedly elevated serum calcium levels may be corrected by dialysis against a calcium-free dialysate.

Treatment of Hypercalcemia and Overdosage in Predialysis Patients
If hypercalcemia ensues (greater than 1 mg/dL above the upper limit of the normal range), adjust dosage to achieve normocalcemia by reducing Rocaltrol therapy from 0.5 mcg to 0.25 mcg daily. If the patient is receiving a therapy of 0.25 mcg daily, discontinue Rocaltrol until patient becomes normocalcemic. Calcium supplements should also be reduced or discontinued. Serum calcium levels should be determined 1 week after withdrawal of calcium supplements. If serum calcium levels have returned to normal, Rocaltrol therapy may be reinstituted at a dosage of 0.25 mcg/day if previous therapy was at a dosage of 0.5 mcg/day. If Rocaltrol therapy was previously administered at a dosage of 0.25 mcg/day, Rocaltrol therapy may be reinstituted at a dosage of 0.25 mcg every other day. If hypercalcemia is persistent at the reduced dosage, serum PTH should be measured. If serum PTH is normal, discontinue Rocaltrol therapy and monitor patient in 3 months' time.

Treatment of Hyperphosphatemia in Predialysis Patients
If serum phosphorus levels exceed 5.0 mg/dL to 5.5 mg/dL, a calcium-containing phosphate-binding agent (ie, calcium carbonate or calcium acetate) should be taken with meals. Serum phosphorus levels should be determined as described earlier (see **PRECAUTIONS: Laboratory Tests**). Aluminum-containing gels should be used with caution as phosphate-binding agents because of the risk of slow aluminum accumulation.

Treatment of Accidental Overdosage of Rocaltrol
The treatment of acute accidental overdosage of Rocaltrol should consist of general supportive measures. If drug ingestion is discovered within a relatively short time, induction of emesis or gastric lavage may be of benefit in preventing further absorption. If the drug has passed through the stomach, the administration of mineral oil may promote its fecal elimination. Serial serum electrolyte determinations (especially calcium), rate of urinary calcium excretion, and assessment of electrocardiographic abnormalities due to hypercalcemia should be obtained. Such monitoring is critical in patients receiving digitalis. Discontinuation of supplemental calcium and a low-calcium diet are also indicated in accidental overdosage. Due to the relatively short duration of the pharmacological action of calcitriol, further measures are probably unnecessary. Should, however, persistent and markedly elevated serum calcium levels occur, there are a variety of therapeutic alternatives which may be considered, depending on the patient's underlying condition. These include the use of drugs such as phosphates and corticosteroids as well as measures to induce an appropriate forced diuresis. The use of peritoneal dialysis against a calcium-free dialysate has also been reported.

DOSAGE AND ADMINISTRATION

The optimal daily dose of Rocaltrol must be carefully determined for each patient. Rocaltrol can be administered orally either as a capsule (0.25 mcg or 0.50 mcg) or as an oral solution (1 mcg/mL). Rocaltrol therapy should always be started at the lowest possible dose and should not be increased without careful monitoring of serum calcium.
The effectiveness of Rocaltrol therapy is predicated on the assumption that each patient is receiving an adequate but not excessive daily intake of calcium. Patients are advised to have a dietary intake of calcium at a minimum of 600 mg daily. The U.S. RDA for calcium in adults is 800 mg to 1200 mg. To ensure that each patient receives an adequate daily intake of calcium, the physician should either prescribe a calcium supplement or instruct the patient in proper dietary measures.
Because of improved calcium absorption from the gastrointestinal tract, some patients on Rocaltrol may be maintained on a lower calcium intake. Patients who tend to develop hypercalcemia may require only low doses of calcium or no supplementation at all.
During the titration period of treatment with Rocaltrol, serum calcium levels should be checked at least twice weekly. When the optimal dosage of Rocaltrol has been determined, serum calcium levels should be checked every month (or as given below for individual indications). Samples for serum calcium estimation should be taken without a tourniquet.

Dialysis Patients
The recommended initial dose of Rocaltrol is 0.25 mcg/day. If a satisfactory response in the biochemical parameters and clinical manifestations of the disease state is not observed, dosage may be increased by 0.25 mcg/day at 4 to 8 week intervals. During this titration period, serum calcium levels should be obtained at least twice weekly, and if hypercalcemia is noted, the drug should be immediately discontinued until normocalcemia ensues (see **PRECAUTIONS: General**). Phosphorus, magnesium, and alkaline phosphatase should be determined periodically.
Patients with normal or only slightly reduced serum calcium levels may respond to Rocaltrol doses of 0.25 mcg every other day. Most patients undergoing hemodialysis respond to doses between 0.5 and 1 mcg/day.
Oral Rocaltrol may normalize plasma ionized calcium in some uremic patients, yet fail to suppress parathyroid hyperfunction. In these individuals with autonomous parathyroid hyperfunction, oral Rocaltrol may be useful to maintain normocalcemia, but has not been shown to be adequate treatment for hyperparathyroidism.

Hypoparathyroidism
The recommended initial dosage of Rocaltrol is 0.25 mcg/day given in the morning. If a satisfactory response in the biochemical parameters and clinical manifestations of the disease is not observed, the dose may be increased at 2- to 4-week intervals. During the dosage titration period, serum calcium levels should be obtained at least twice weekly and, if hypercalcemia is noted, Rocaltrol should be immediately discontinued until normocalcemia ensues (see **PRECAUTIONS: General**). Careful consideration should also be

given to lowering the dietary calcium intake. Serum calcium, phosphorus, and 24-hour urinary calcium should be determined periodically.

Most adult patients and pediatric patients age 6 years and older have responded to dosages in the range of 0.5 mcg to 2 mcg daily. Pediatric patients in the 1 to 5 year age group with hypoparathyroidism have usually been given 0.25 mcg to 0.75 mcg daily. The number of treated patients with pseudohypoparathyroidism less than 6 years of age is too small to make dosage recommendations.

Malabsorption is occasionally noted in patients with hypoparathyroidism; hence, larger doses of Rocaltrol may be needed.

Predialysis Patients

The recommended initial dosage of Rocaltrol is 0.25 mcg/day in adults and pediatric patients 3 years of age and older. This dosage may be increased if necessary to 0.5 mcg/day. For pediatric patients less than 3 years of age, the recommended initial dosage of Rocaltrol is 10 to 15 ng/kg/day.

HOW SUPPLIED

Capsules: 0.25 mcg calcitriol in soft gelatin, light orange, oval capsules, imprinted with ROCALTROL 0.25 ROCHE; bottles of 30 (NDC 0004-0143-23), and bottles of 100 (NDC 0004-0143-01).

Capsules: 0.5 mcg calcitriol in soft gelatin, dark orange, oblong capsules, imprinted with ROCALTROL 0.5 ROCHE; bottles of 100 (NDC 0004-0144-01).

Oral Solution: a clear, colorless to pale yellow oral solution containing 1 mcg/mL of calcitriol; each amber glass bottle of 15 mL of oral solution supplied with 20 single-use, graduated oral dispensers (NDC 0004-9115-00).

Rocaltrol Capsules and Oral Solution should be protected from light.

Store at 59° to 86°F (15° to 30°C).

REFERENCE

1. Jones CL, et al. Comparisons between oral and intraperitoneal 1,25-dihydroxyvitamin D_3 therapy in children treated with peritoneal dialysis. *Clin Nephrol.* 1994; 42: 44–49.

Revised: July 2004

Shown in Product Identification Guide, page 331

ROCEPHIN® ℞

[ro-sef ' in]

(ceftriaxone sodium)

FOR INJECTION

To reduce the development of drug-resistant bacteria and maintain the effectiveness of Rocephin and other antibacterial drugs, Rocephin should be used only to treat or prevent infections that are proven or strongly suspected to be caused by bacteria.

DESCRIPTION

Rocephin is a sterile, semisynthetic, broad-spectrum cephalosporin antibiotic for intravenous or intramuscular administration. Ceftriaxone sodium is (6*R*,7*R*)-7-[2-(2-Amino-4-thiazolyl)glyoxylamido]-8-oxo-3-[[(1,2,5,6-tetrahydro-2-methyl-5,6-dioxo-*as*-triazin-3-yl)thio]methyl]-5-thia-1-azabicyclo[4.2.0]oct-2-ene-2-carboxylic acid, 7^2-(*Z*)-(*O*-methyloxime), disodium salt, sesquaterhydrate.

The chemical formula of ceftriaxone sodium is $C_{18}H_{16}N_8Na_2O_7S_3 \cdot 3.5H_2O$. It has a calculated molecular weight of 661.59.

Rocephin is a white to yellowish-orange crystalline powder which is readily soluble in water, sparingly soluble in methanol and very slightly soluble in ethanol. The pH of a 1% aqueous solution is approximately 6.7. The color of Rocephin solutions ranges from light yellow to amber, depending on the length of storage, concentration and diluent used.

Rocephin contains approximately 83 mg (3.6 mEq) of sodium per gram of ceftriaxone activity.

CLINICAL PHARMACOLOGY

Average plasma concentrations of ceftriaxone following a single 30-minute intravenous (IV) infusion of a 0.5, 1 or 2 gm dose and intramuscular (IM) administration of a single 0.5 (250 mg/mL or 350 mg/mL concentrations) or 1 gm dose in healthy subjects are presented in Table 1.

[See table 1 above]

TABLE 1. Ceftriaxone Plasma Concentrations After Single Dose Administration

Dose/Route	Average Plasma Concentrations (µg/mL)								
	0.5 hr	1 hr	2 hr	4 hr	6 hr	8 hr	12 hr	16 hr	24 hr
0.5 gm IV*	82	59	48	37	29	23	15	10	5
0.5 gm IM 250 mg/mL	22	33	38	35	30	26	16	ND	5
0.5 gm IM 350 mg/mL	20	32	38	34	31	24	16	ND	5
1 gm IV*	151	111	88	67	53	43	28	18	9
1 gm IM	40	68	76	68	56	44	29	ND	ND
2 gm IV*	257	192	154	117	89	74	46	31	15

*IV doses were infused at a constant rate over 30 minutes.
ND = Not determined.

Ceftriaxone was completely absorbed following IM administration with mean maximum plasma concentrations occurring between 2 and 3 hours postdosing. Multiple IV or IM doses ranging from 0.5 to 2 gm at 12- to 24-hour intervals resulted in 15% to 36% accumulation of ceftriaxone above single dose values.

Ceftriaxone concentrations in urine are high, as shown in Table 2.

[See table 2 above]

TABLE 2. Urinary Concentrations of Ceftriaxone After Single Dose Administration

Dose/Route	Average Urinary Concentrations (µg/mL)					
	0-2 hr	2-4 hr	4-8 hr	8-12 hr	12-24 hr	24-48 hr
0.5 gm IV	526	366	142	87	70	15
0.5 gm IM	115	425	308	127	96	28
1 gm IV	995	855	293	147	132	32
1 gm IM	504	628	418	237	ND	ND
2 gm IV	2692	1976	757	274	198	40

ND = Not determined.

Thirty-three percent to 67% of a ceftriaxone dose was excreted in the urine as unchanged drug and the remainder was secreted in the bile and ultimately found in the feces as microbiologically inactive compounds. After a 1 gm IV dose, average concentrations of ceftriaxone, determined from 1 to 3 hours after dosing, were 581 µg/mL in the gallbladder bile, 788 µg/mL in the common duct bile, 898 µg/mL in the cystic duct bile, 78.2 µg/gm in the gallbladder wall and 62.1 µg/mL in the concurrent plasma.

Over a 0.15 to 3 gm dose range in healthy adult subjects, the values of elimination half-life ranged from 5.8 to 8.7 hours; apparent volume of distribution from 5.78 to 13.5 L; plasma clearance from 0.58 to 1.45 L/hour; and renal clearance from 0.32 to 0.73 L/hour. Ceftriaxone is reversibly bound to human plasma proteins, and the binding decreased from a value of 95% bound at plasma concentrations of <25 µg/mL to a value of 85% bound at 300 µg/mL. Ceftriaxone crosses the blood placenta barrier.

The average values of maximum plasma concentration, elimination half-life, plasma clearance and volume of distribution after a 50 mg/kg IV dose and after a 75 mg/kg IV dose in pediatric patients suffering from bacterial meningitis are shown in Table 3. Ceftriaxone penetrated the inflamed meninges of infants and pediatric patients; CSF concentrations after a 50 mg/kg IV dose and after a 75 mg/kg IV dose are also shown in Table 3.

[See table 3 above]

TABLE 3. Average Pharmacokinetic Parameters of Ceftriaxone in Pediatric Patients With Meningitis

	50 mg/kg IV	75 mg/kg IV
Maximum Plasma Concentrations (µg/mL)	216	275
Elimination Half-life (hr)	4.6	4.3
Plasma Clearance (mL/hr/kg)	49	60
Volume of Distribution (mL/kg)	338	373
CSF Concentration—inflamed meninges (µg/mL)	5.6	6.4
Range (µg/mL)	1.3-18.5	1.3-44
Time after dose (hr)	3.7 (± 1.6)	3.3 (± 1.4)

Compared to that in healthy adult subjects, the pharmacokinetics of ceftriaxone were only minimally altered in elderly subjects and in patients with renal impairment or hepatic dysfunction (Table 4); therefore, dosage adjustments are not necessary for these patients with ceftriaxone dosages up to 2 gm per day. Ceftriaxone was not removed to any significant extent from the plasma by hemodialysis. In 6 of 26 dialysis patients, the elimination rate of ceftriaxone was markedly reduced, suggesting that plasma concentrations of ceftriaxone should be monitored in these patients to determine if dosage adjustments are necessary.

[See table 4 above]

TABLE 4. Average Pharmacokinetic Parameters of Ceftriaxone in Humans

Subject Group	Elimination Half-Life (hr)	Plasma Clearance (L/hr)	Volume of Distribution (L)
Healthy Subjects	5.8-8.7	0.58-1.45	5.8-13.5
Elderly Subjects (mean age, 70.5 yr)	8.9	0.83	10.7
Patients With Renal Impairment			
Hemodialysis Patients (0-5 mL/min)*	14.7	0.65	13.7
Severe (5-15 mL/min)	15.7	0.56	12.5
Moderate (16-30 mL/min)	11.4	0.72	11.8
Mild (31-60 mL/min)	12.4	0.70	13.3
Patients With Liver Disease	8.8	1.1	13.6

*Creatinine clearance.

Pharmacokinetics in the Middle Ear Fluid: In one study, total ceftriaxone concentrations (bound and unbound) were measured in middle ear fluid obtained during the insertion of tympanostomy tubes in 42 pediatric patients with otitis media. Sampling times were from 1 to 50 hours after a single intramuscular injection of 50 mg/kg of ceftriaxone. Mean (± SD) ceftriaxone levels in the middle ear reached a peak of 35 (± 12) µg/mL at 24 hours, and remained at 19 (± 7) µg/mL at 48 hours. Based on middle ear fluid ceftriaxone concentrations in the 23 to 25 hour and the 46 to 50 hour sampling time intervals, a half-life of 25 hours was calculated. Ceftriaxone is highly bound to plasma proteins. The extent of binding to proteins in the middle ear fluid is unknown.

Microbiology: The bactericidal activity of ceftriaxone results from inhibition of cell wall synthesis. Ceftriaxone has a high degree of stability in the presence of beta-lactamases, both penicillinases and cephalosporinases, of gram-negative and gram-positive bacteria.

Ceftriaxone has been shown to be active against most strains of the following microorganisms, both in vitro and in clinical infections described in the INDICATIONS AND USAGE section.

Aerobic gram-negative microorganisms:

Acinetobacter calcoaceticus
Enterobacter aerogenes
Enterobacter cloacae
Escherichia coli
Haemophilus influenzae (including ampicillin-resistant and beta-lactamase producing strains)
Haemophilus parainfluenzae
Klebsiella oxytoca
Klebsiella pneumoniae
Moraxella catarrhalis (including beta-lactamase producing strains)
Morganella morganii
Neisseria gonorrhoeae (including penicillinase- and nonpenicillinase-producing strains)
Neisseria meningitidis
Proteus mirabilis
Proteus vulgaris
Serratia marcescens

Ceftriaxone is also active against many strains of *Pseudomonas aeruginosa*.

NOTE: Many strains of the above organisms that are multiply resistant to other antibiotics, eg, penicillins, cephalosporins, and aminoglycosides, are susceptible to ceftriaxone.

Aerobic gram-positive microorganisms:

Staphylococcus aureus (including penicillinase-producing strains)
Staphylococcus epidermidis
Streptococcus pneumoniae
Streptococcus pyogenes
Viridans group streptococci

Continued on next page

Rocephin—Cont.

NOTE: Methicillin-resistant staphylococci are resistant to cephalosporins, including ceftriaxone. Most strains of Group D streptococci and enterococci, eg, *Enterococcus (Streptococcus) faecalis*, are resistant.
Anaerobic microorganisms:
Bacteroides fragilis
Clostridium species
Peptostreptococcus species
NOTE: Most strains of *Clostridium difficile* are resistant.
The following in vitro data are available, **but their clinical significance is unknown**. Ceftriaxone exhibits in vitro minimal inhibitory concentrations (MICs) of ≤8 µg/mL or less against most strains of the following microorganisms, however, the safety and effectiveness of ceftriaxone in treating clinical infections due to these microorganisms have not been established in adequate and well-controlled clinical trials.
Aerobic gram-negative microorganisms:
Citrobacter diversus
Citrobacter freundii
Providencia species (including *Providencia rettgeri*)
Salmonella species (including *Salmonella typhi*)
Shigella species
Aerobic gram-positive microorganisms:
Streptococcus agalactiae
Anaerobic microorganisms:
Prevotella (Bacteroides) bivius
Porphyromonas (Bacteroides) melaninogenicus

Susceptibility Tests:
Dilution Techniques: Quantitative methods are used to determine antimicrobial minimal inhibitory concentrations (MICs). These MICs provide estimates of the susceptibility of bacteria to antimicrobial compounds. The MICs should be determined using a standardized procedure.[1] Standardized procedures are based on a dilution method (broth or agar) or equivalent with standardized inoculum concentrations and standardized concentrations of ceftriaxone powder. The MIC values should be interpreted according to the following criteria[2] for aerobic organisms other than *Haemophilus* spp, *Neisseria gonorrhoeae*, and *Streptococcus* spp, including *Streptococcus pneumoniae:*

MIC (µg/mL)	Interpretation
≤8	(S) Susceptible
16-32	(I) Intermediate
≥64	(R) Resistant

The following interpretive criteria[2] should be used when testing *Haemophilus* species using Haemophilus Test Media (HTM).

MIC (µg/mL)	Interpretation
≤2	(S) Susceptible

The absence of resistant strains precludes defining any categories other than "Susceptible". Strains yielding results suggestive of a "Nonsusceptible" category should be submitted to a reference laboratory for further testing.
The following interpretive criteria[2] should be used when testing *Neisseria gonorrhoeae* when using GC agar base and 1% defined growth supplement.

MIC (µg/mL)	Interpretation
≤0.25	(S) Susceptible

The absence of resistant strains precludes defining any categories other than "Susceptible". Strains yielding results suggestive of a "Nonsusceptible" category should be submitted to a reference laboratory for further testing.
The following interpretive criteria[2] should be used when testing *Streptococcus* spp including *Streptococcus pneumoniae* using cation-adjusted Mueller-Hinton broth with 2 to 5% lysed horse blood.

MIC (µg/mL)	Interpretation
≤0.5	(S) Susceptible
1	(I) Intermediate
≥2	(R) Resistant

A report of "Susceptible" indicates that the pathogen is likely to be inhibited if the antimicrobial compound in the blood reaches the concentrations usually achievable. A report of "Intermediate" indicates that the results should be considered equivocal, and if the microorganism is not fully susceptible to alternative, clinically feasible drugs, the test should be repeated. This category implies possible clinical applicability in body sites where the drug is physiologically concentrated or in situations where high dosage of the drug can be used. This category also provides a buffer zone which prevents small uncontrolled technical factors from causing major discrepancies in interpretation. A report of "Resistant" indicates that the pathogen is not likely to be inhibited if the antimicrobial compound in the blood reaches the concentrations usually achievable; other therapy should be selected.

Standardized susceptibility test procedures require the use of laboratory control microorganisms to control the technical aspects of the laboratory procedures. Standardized ceftriaxone powder should provide the following MIC values:[2]

Microorganism	ATCC® #	MIC (µg/mL)
Escherichia coli	25922	0.03-0.12
Staphylococcus aureus	29213	1-8*
Pseudomonas aeruginosa	27853	8-32
Haemophilus influenzae	49247	0.06-0.25
Neisseria gonorrhoeae	49226	0.004-0.015
Streptococcus pneumoniae	49619	0.03-0.12

*A bimodal distribution of MICs results at the extremes of the acceptable range should be suspect and control validity should be verified with data from other control strains.

Diffusion Techniques: Quantitative methods that require measurement of zone diameters also provide reproducible estimates of the susceptibility of bacteria to antimicrobial compounds. One such standardized procedure[3] requires the use of standardized inoculum concentrations. This procedure uses paper discs impregnated with 30 µg of ceftriaxone to test the susceptibility of microorganisms to ceftriaxone. Reports from the laboratory providing results of the standard single-disc susceptibility test with a 30 µg ceftriaxone disc should be interpreted according to the following criteria for aerobic organisms other than *Haemophilus* spp, *Neisseria gonorrhoeae* and *Streptococcus* spp:

Zone Diameter (mm)	Interpretation
≥21	(S) Susceptible
14-20	(I) Intermediate
≤13	(R) Resistant

The following interpretive criteria[3] should be used when testing *Haemophilus* species when using Haemophilus Test Media (HTM).

Zone Diameter (mm)	Interpretation
≥26	(S) Susceptible

The absence of resistant strains precludes defining any categories other than "Susceptible". Strains yielding results suggestive of a "Nonsusceptible" category should be submitted to a reference laboratory for further testing.
The following interpretive criteria[3] should be used when testing *Neisseria gonorrhoeae* when using GC agar base and 1% defined growth supplement.

Zone Diameter (mm)	Interpretation
≥35	(S) Susceptible

The absence of resistant strains precludes defining any categories other than "Susceptible". Strains yielding results suggestive of a "Nonsusceptible" category should be submitted to a reference laboratory for further testing.
The following interpretive criteria[3] should be used when testing *Streptococcus* spp other than *Streptococcus pneumoniae* when using Mueller-Hinton agar supplemented with 5% sheep blood incubated in 5% CO_2.

Zone Diameter (mm)	Interpretation
≥27	(S) Susceptible
25-26	(I) Intermediate
≤24	(R) Resistant

Interpretation should be as stated above for results using dilution techniques. Interpretation involves correlation of the diameter obtained in the disc test with the MIC for ceftriaxone.
Disc diffusion interpretive criteria for ceftriaxone discs against *Streptococcus pneumoniae* are not available, however, isolates of pneumococci with oxacillin zone diameters of >20 mm are susceptible (MIC ≤0.06 µg/mL) to penicillin and can be considered susceptible to ceftriaxone. *Streptococcus pneumoniae* isolates should not be reported as penicillin (ceftriaxone) resistant or intermediate based solely on an oxacillin zone diameter of ≤19 mm. The ceftriaxone MIC should be determined for those isolates with oxacillin zone diameters ≤19 mm.
As with standardized dilution techniques, diffusion methods require the use of laboratory control microorganisms that are used to control the technical aspects of the laboratory procedures. For the diffusion technique, the 30 µg ceftriaxone disc should provide the following zone diameters in these laboratory test quality control strains:[3]

Microorganism	ATCC® #	Zone Diameter Ranges (mm)
Escherichia coli	25922	29-35
Staphylococcus aureus	25923	22-28
Pseudomonas aeruginosa	27853	17-23
Haemophilus influenzae	49247	31-39
Neisseria gonorrhoeae	49226	39-51
Streptococcus pneumoniae	49619	30-35

Anaerobic Techniques: For anaerobic bacteria, the susceptibility to ceftriaxone as MICs can be determined by standardized test methods.[4] The MIC values obtained should be interpreted according to the following criteria:

MIC (µg/mL)	Interpretation
≤16	(S) Susceptible
32	(I) Intermediate
≥64	(R) Resistant

As with other susceptibility techniques, the use of laboratory control microorganisms is required to control the technical aspects of the laboratory standardized procedures. Standardized ceftriaxone powder should provide the following MIC values for the indicated standardized anaerobic dilution[4] testing method:
[See table below]

Method	Microorganism	ATCC® #	MIC (µg/mL)
Agar	*Bacteroides fragilis*	25285	32-128
	Bacteroides thetaiotaomicron	29741	64-256
Broth	*Bacteroides thetaiotaomicron*	29741	32-128

ATCC® is a registered trademark of the American Type Culture Collection.

INDICATIONS AND USAGE

Before instituting treatment with Rocephin, appropriate specimens should be obtained for isolation of the causative organism and for determination of its susceptibility to the drug. Therapy may be instituted prior to obtaining results of susceptibility testing.
To reduce the development of drug-resistant bacteria and maintain the effectiveness of Rocephin and other antibacterial drugs, Rocephin should be used only to treat or prevent infections that are proven or strongly suspected to be caused by susceptible bacteria. When culture and susceptibility information are available, they should be considered in selecting or modifying antibacterial therapy. In the absence of such data, local epidemiology and susceptibility patterns may contribute to the empiric selection of therapy.
Rocephin is indicated for the treatment of the following infections when caused by susceptible organisms:
LOWER RESPIRATORY TRACT INFECTIONS caused by *Streptococcus pneumoniae, Staphylococcus aureus, Haemophilus influenzae, Haemophilus parainfluenzae, Klebsiella pneumoniae, Escherichia coli, Enterobacter aerogenes, Proteus mirabilis* or *Serratia marcescens.*
ACUTE BACTERIAL OTITIS MEDIA caused by *Streptococcus pneumoniae, Haemophilus influenzae* (including beta-lactamase producing strains) or *Moraxella catarrhalis* (including beta-lactamase producing strains).
NOTE: In one study lower clinical cure rates were observed with a single dose of Rocephin compared to 10 days of oral therapy. In a second study comparable cure rates were observed between single dose Rocephin and the comparator. The potentially lower clinical cure rate of Rocephin should be balanced against the potential advantages of parenteral therapy (see CLINICAL STUDIES).
SKIN AND SKIN STRUCTURE INFECTIONS caused by *Staphylococcus aureus, Staphylococcus epidermidis, Streptococcus pyogenes,* Viridans group streptococci, *Escherichia coli, Enterobacter cloacae, Klebsiella oxytoca, Klebsiella pneumoniae, Proteus mirabilis, Morganella morganii,* * *Pseudomonas aeruginosa, Serratia marcescens, Acinetobacter calcoaceticus, Bacteroides fragilis** or *Peptostreptococcus* species.
URINARY TRACT INFECTIONS (complicated and uncomplicated) caused by *Escherichia coli, Proteus mirabilis, Proteus vulgaris, Morganella morganii* or *Klebsiella pneumoniae.*
UNCOMPLICATED GONORRHEA (cervical/urethral and rectal) caused by *Neisseria gonorrhoeae*, including both penicillinase- and nonpenicillinase-producing strains, and pharyngeal gonorrhea caused by nonpenicillinase-producing strains of *Neisseria gonorrhoeae.*
PELVIC INFLAMMATORY DISEASE caused by *Neisseria gonorrhoeae*. Rocephin, like other cephalosporins, has no activity against *Chlamydia trachomatis*. Therefore, when cephalosporins are used in the treatment of patients with pelvic inflammatory disease and *Chlamydia trachomatis* is one of the suspected pathogens, appropriate antichlamydial coverage should be added.
BACTERIAL SEPTICEMIA caused by *Staphylococcus aureus, Streptococcus pneumoniae, Escherichia coli, Haemophilus influenzae* or *Klebsiella pneumoniae.*
BONE AND JOINT INFECTIONS caused by *Staphylococcus aureus, Streptococcus pneumoniae, Escherichia coli, Proteus mirabilis, Klebsiella pneumoniae* or *Enterobacter* species.
INTRA-ABDOMINAL INFECTIONS caused by *Escherichia coli, Klebsiella pneumoniae, Bacteroides fragilis, Clostridium* species (Note: most strains of *Clostridium difficile* are resistant) or *Peptostreptococcus* species.
MENINGITIS caused by *Haemophilus influenzae, Neisseria meningitidis* or *Streptococcus pneumoniae*. Rocephin has also been used successfully in a limited number of cases of meningitis and shunt infection caused by *Staphylococcus epidermidis** and *Escherichia coli.**

*Efficacy for this organism in this organ system was studied in fewer than ten infections.

SURGICAL PROPHYLAXIS: The preoperative administration of a single 1 gm dose of Rocephin may reduce the incidence of postoperative infections in patients undergoing surgical procedures classified as contaminated or potentially contaminated (eg, vaginal or abdominal hysterectomy or cholecystectomy for chronic calculous cholecystitis in high-risk patients, such as those over 70 years of age, with acute cholecystitis not requiring therapeutic antimicrobials, obstructive jaundice or common duct bile stones) and in surgical patients for whom infection at the operative site would present serious risk (eg, during coronary artery bypass surgery). Although Rocephin has been shown to have been as effective as cefazolin in the prevention of infection following coronary artery bypass surgery, no placebo-controlled trials have been conducted to evaluate any cephalosporin antibiotic in the prevention of infection following coronary artery bypass surgery.

When administered prior to surgical procedures for which it is indicated, a single 1 gm dose of Rocephin provides protection from most infections due to susceptible organisms throughout the course of the procedure.

CONTRAINDICATIONS

Rocephin is contraindicated in patients with known allergy to the cephalosporin class of antibiotics.

WARNINGS

BEFORE THERAPY WITH ROCEPHIN IS INSTITUTED, CAREFUL INQUIRY SHOULD BE MADE TO DETERMINE WHETHER THE PATIENT HAS HAD PREVIOUS HYPERSENSITIVITY REACTIONS TO CEPHALOSPORINS, PENICILLINS OR OTHER DRUGS. THIS PRODUCT SHOULD BE GIVEN CAUTIOUSLY TO PENICILLIN-SENSITIVE PATIENTS. ANTIBIOTICS SHOULD BE ADMINISTERED WITH CAUTION TO ANY PATIENT WHO HAS DEMONSTRATED SOME FORM OF ALLERGY, PARTICULARLY TO DRUGS. SERIOUS ACUTE HYPERSENSITIVITY REACTIONS MAY REQUIRE THE USE OF SUBCUTANEOUS EPINEPHRINE AND OTHER EMERGENCY MEASURES.

Pseudomembranous colitis has been reported with nearly all antibacterial agents, including ceftriaxone, and may range in severity from mild to life-threatening. Therefore, it is important to consider this diagnosis in patients who present with diarrhea subsequent to the administration of antibacterial agents.

Treatment with antibacterial agents alters the normal flora of the colon and may permit overgrowth of clostridia. Studies indicate that a toxin produced by *Clostridium difficile* is one primary cause of "antibiotic-associated colitis".

After the diagnosis of pseudomembranous colitis has been established, appropriate therapeutic measures should be initiated. Mild cases of pseudomembranous colitis usually respond to drug discontinuation alone. In moderate to severe cases, consideration should be given to management with fluids and electrolytes, protein supplementation and treatment with an antibacterial drug clinically effective against *Clostridium difficile* colitis.

PRECAUTIONS

General: Prescribing Rocephin in the absence of a proven or strongly suspected bacterial infection or a prophylactic indication is unlikely to provide benefit to the patient and increases the risk of the development of drug-resistant bacteria.

Although transient elevations of BUN and serum creatinine have been observed, at the recommended dosages, the nephrotoxic potential of Rocephin is similar to that of other cephalosporins.

Ceftriaxone is excreted via both biliary and renal excretion (see CLINICAL PHARMACOLOGY). Therefore, patients with renal failure normally require no adjustment in dosage when usual doses of Rocephin are administered, but concentrations of drug in the serum should be monitored periodically. If evidence of accumulation exists, dosage should be decreased accordingly.

Dosage adjustments should not be necessary in patients with hepatic dysfunction; however, in patients with both hepatic dysfunction and significant renal disease, Rocephin dosage should not exceed 2 gm daily without close monitoring of serum concentrations.

Alterations in prothrombin times have occurred rarely in patients treated with Rocephin. Patients with impaired vitamin K synthesis or low vitamin K stores (eg, chronic hepatic disease and malnutrition) may require monitoring of prothrombin time during Rocephin treatment. Vitamin K administration (10 mg weekly) may be necessary if the prothrombin time is prolonged before or during therapy.

Prolonged use of Rocephin may result in overgrowth of nonsusceptible organisms. Careful observation of the patient is essential. If superinfection occurs during therapy, appropriate measures should be taken.

Rocephin should be prescribed with caution in individuals with a history of gastrointestinal disease, especially colitis. **There have been reports of sonographic abnormalities in the gallbladder of patients treated with Rocephin; some of these patients also had symptoms of gallbladder disease.** These abnormalities appear on sonography as an echo without acoustical shadowing suggesting sludge or as an echo with acoustical shadowing which may be misinterpreted as gallstones. The chemical nature of the sonographically detected material has been determined to be predominantly a ceftriaxone-calcium salt. **The condition appears to be transient and reversible upon discontinuation of Rocephin and institution of conservative management.** Therefore, Rocephin should be discontinued in patients who develop signs and symptoms suggestive of gallbladder disease and/or the sonographic findings described above.

Information for Patients: Patients should be counseled that antibacterial drugs including Rocephin should only be used to treat bacterial infections. They do not treat viral infections (eg, common cold). When Rocephin is prescribed to treat a bacterial infection, patients should be told that although it is common to feel better early in the course of therapy, the medication should be taken exactly as directed. Skipping doses or not completing the full course of therapy may (1) decrease the effectiveness of the immediate treatment and (2) increase the likelihood that bacteria will develop resistance and will not be treatable by Rocephin or other antibacterial drugs in the future.

Carcinogenesis, Mutagenesis, Impairment of Fertility: *Carcinogenesis:* Considering the maximum duration of treatment and the class of the compound, carcinogenicity studies with ceftriaxone in animals have not been performed. The maximum duration of animal toxicity studies was 6 months.

Mutagenesis: Genetic toxicology tests included the Ames test, a micronucleus test and a test for chromosomal aberrations in human lymphocytes cultured in vitro with ceftriaxone. Ceftriaxone showed no potential for mutagenic activity in these studies.

Impairment of Fertility: Ceftriaxone produced no impairment of fertility when given intravenously to rats at daily doses up to 586 mg/kg/day, approximately 20 times the recommended clinical dose of 2 gm/day.

Pregnancy: *Teratogenic Effects:* Pregnancy Category B. Reproductive studies have been performed in mice and rats at doses up to 20 times the usual human dose and have no evidence of embryotoxicity, fetotoxicity or teratogenicity. In primates, no embryotoxicity or teratogenicity was demonstrated at a dose approximately 3 times the human dose.

There are, however, no adequate and well-controlled studies in pregnant women. Because animal reproductive studies are not always predictive of human response, this drug should be used during pregnancy only if clearly needed.

Nonteratogenic Effects: In rats, in the Segment I (fertility and general reproduction) and Segment III (perinatal and postnatal) studies with intravenously administered ceftriaxone, no adverse effects were noted on various reproductive parameters during gestation and lactation, including postnatal growth, functional behavior and reproductive ability of the offspring, at doses of 586 mg/kg/day or less.

Nursing Mothers: Low concentrations of ceftriaxone are excreted in human milk. Caution should be exercised when Rocephin is administered to a nursing woman.

Pediatric Use: Safety and effectiveness of Rocephin in neonates, infants and pediatric patients have been established for the dosages described in the DOSAGE AND ADMINISTRATION section. In vitro studies have shown that ceftriaxone, like some other cephalosporins, can displace bilirubin from serum albumin. Rocephin should not be administered to hyperbilirubinemic neonates, especially prematures.

ADVERSE REACTIONS

Rocephin is generally well tolerated. In clinical trials, the following adverse reactions, which were considered to be related to Rocephin therapy or of uncertain etiology, were observed:

LOCAL REACTIONS— pain, induration and tenderness was 1% overall. Phlebitis was reported in <1% after IV administration. The incidence of warmth, tightness or induration was 17% (3/17) after IM administration of 350 mg/mL and 5% (1/20) after IM administration of 250 mg/mL.

HYPERSENSITIVITY—rash (1.7%). Less frequently reported (<1%) were pruritus, fever or chills.

HEMATOLOGIC—eosinophilia (6%), thrombocytosis (5.1%) and leukopenia (2.1%). Less frequently reported (<1%) were anemia, hemolytic anemia, neutropenia, lymphopenia, thrombocytopenia and prolongation of the prothrombin time.

GASTROINTESTINAL—diarrhea (2.7%). Less frequently reported (<1%) were nausea or vomiting, and dysgeusia. The onset of pseudomembranous colitis symptoms may occur during or after antibacterial treatment (see WARNINGS).

HEPATIC—elevations of SGOT (3.1%) or SGPT (3.3%). Less frequently reported (<1%) were elevations of alkaline phosphatase and bilirubin.

RENAL—elevations of the BUN (1.2%). Less frequently reported (<1%) were elevations of creatinine and the presence of casts in the urine.

CENTRAL NERVOUS SYSTEM—headache or dizziness were reported occasionally (<1%).

GENITOURINARY—moniliasis or vaginitis were reported occasionally (<1%).

MISCELLANEOUS—diaphoresis and flushing were reported occasionally (<1%).

Other rarely observed adverse reactions (<0.1%) include abdominal pain, agranulocytosis, allergic pneumonitis, anaphylaxis, basophilia, biliary lithiasis, bronchospasm, colitis, dyspepsia, epistaxis, flatulence, gallbladder sludge, glycosuria, hematuria, jaundice, leukocytosis, lymphocytosis, monocytosis, nephrolithiasis, palpitations, a decrease in the prothrombin time, renal precipitations, seizures, and serum sickness.

OVERDOSAGE

In the case of overdosage, drug concentration would not be reduced by hemodialysis or peritoneal dialysis. There is no specific antidote. Treatment of overdosage should be symptomatic.

DOSAGE AND ADMINISTRATION

Rocephin may be administered intravenously or intramuscularly.

ADULTS: The usual adult daily dose is 1 to 2 grams given once a day (or in equally divided doses twice a day) depending on the type and severity of infection. The total daily dose should not exceed 4 grams.

If *Chlamydia trachomatis* is a suspected pathogen, appropriate antichlamydial coverage should be added, because ceftriaxone sodium has no activity against this organism.

For the treatment of uncomplicated gonococcal infections, a single intramuscular dose of 250 mg is recommended.

For preoperative use (surgical prophylaxis), a single dose of 1 gram administered intravenously 1/2 to 2 hours before surgery is recommended.

PEDIATRIC PATIENTS: For the treatment of skin and skin structure infections, the recommended total daily dose is 50 to 75 mg/kg given once a day (or in equally divided doses twice a day). The total daily dose should not exceed 2 grams.

For the treatment of acute bacterial otitis media, a single intramuscular dose of 50 mg/kg (not to exceed 1 gram) is recommended (see INDICATIONS AND USAGE).

For the treatment of serious miscellaneous infections other than meningitis, the recommended total daily dose is 50 to 75 mg/kg, given in divided doses every 12 hours. The total daily dose should not exceed 2 grams.

In the treatment of meningitis, it is recommended that the initial therapeutic dose be 100 mg/kg (not to exceed 4 grams). Thereafter, a total daily dose of 100 mg/kg/day (not to exceed 4 grams daily) is recommended. The daily dose may be administered once a day (or in equally divided doses every 12 hours). The usual duration of therapy is 7 to 14 days.

Generally, Rocephin therapy should be continued for at least 2 days after the signs and symptoms of infection have disappeared. The usual duration of therapy is 4 to 14 days; in complicated infections, longer therapy may be required.

When treating infections caused by *Streptococcus pyogenes*, therapy should be continued for at least 10 days.

No dosage adjustment is necessary for patients with impairment of renal or hepatic function; however, blood levels should be monitored in patients with severe renal impairment (eg, dialysis patients) and in patients with both renal and hepatic dysfunctions.

DIRECTIONS FOR USE

Intramuscular Administration: Reconstitute Rocephin powder with the appropriate diluent (see COMPATIBILITY AND STABILITY).

Inject diluent into vial, shake vial thoroughly to form solution. Withdraw entire contents of vial into syringe to equal total labeled dose.

After reconstitution, each 1 mL of solution contains approximately 250 mg or 350 mg equivalent of ceftriaxone according to the amount of diluent indicated below. If required, more dilute solutions could be utilized. **A 350 mg/mL concentration is not recommended for the 250 mg vial since it may not be possible to withdraw the entire contents.**

As with all intramuscular preparations, Rocephin should be injected well within the body of a relatively large muscle; aspiration helps to avoid unintentional injection into a blood vessel.

Vial Dosage Size	Amount of Diluent to be Added	
	250 mg/mL	350 mg/mL
250 mg	0.9 mL	—
500 mg	1.8 mL	1.0 mL
1 gm	3.6 mL	2.1 mL
2 gm	7.2 mL	4.2 mL

Intravenous Administration: Rocephin should be administered intravenously by infusion over a period of 30 minutes. Concentrations between 10 mg/mL and 40 mg/mL are recommended; however, lower concentrations may be used if desired. Reconstitute vials or "piggyback" bottles with an appropriate IV diluent (see COMPATIBILITY AND STABILITY).

Vial Dosage Size	Amount of Diluent to be Added
250 mg	2.4 mL
500 mg	4.8 mL
1 gm	9.6 mL
2 gm	19.2 mL

After reconstitution, each 1 mL of solution contains approximately 100 mg equivalent of ceftriaxone. Withdraw entire contents and dilute to the desired concentration with the appropriate IV diluent.

Piggyback Bottle Dosage Size	Amount of Diluent to be Added
1 gm	10 mL
2 gm	20 mL

After reconstitution, further dilute to 50 mL or 100 mL volumes with the appropriate IV diluent.

COMPATIBILITY AND STABILITY: Rocephin sterile powder should be stored at room temperature—77°F (25°C)—or below and protected from light. After reconstitution, protection from normal light is not necessary. The color of solution ranges from light yellow to amber, depending on the length of storage, concentration and diluent used.

Rocephin *intramuscular* solutions remain stable (loss of potency less than 10%) for the following time periods:

[See first table at top of next page]

Continued on next page

Rocephin—Cont.

Rocephin *intravenous* solutions, at concentrations of 10, 20 and 40 mg/mL, remain stable (loss of potency less than 10%) for the following time periods stored in glass or PVC containers:
[See second table at right]
Similarly, Rocephin *intravenous* solutions, at concentrations of 100 mg/mL, remain stable in the IV piggyback glass containers for the above specified time periods.
The following *intravenous* Rocephin solutions are stable at room temperature (25°C) for 24 hours, at concentrations between 10 mg/mL and 40 mg/mL: Sodium Lactate (PVC container), 10% Invert Sugar (glass container), 5% Sodium Bicarbonate (glass container), Freamine III (glass container), Normosol-M in 5% Dextrose (glass and PVC containers), Ionosol-B in 5% Dextrose (glass container), 5% Mannitol (glass container), 10% Mannitol (glass container).
Ceftriaxone has been shown to be compatible with Flagyl®* IV (metronidazole hydrochloride). The concentration should not exceed 5 to 7.5 mg/mL metronidazole hydrochloride with ceftriaxone 10 mg/mL as an admixture. The admixture is stable for 24 hours at room temperature only in 0,9% sodium chloride injection or 5% dextrose in water (D5W). No compatibility studies have been conducted with the Flagyl® IV RTU® (metronidazole) formulation or using other diluents. Metronidazole at concentrations greater than 8 mg/mL will precipitate. Do not refrigerate the admixture as precipitation will occur.

* Registered trademark of SCS Pharmaceuticals.

Vancomycin and fluconazole are physically incompatible with ceftriaxone in admixtures. When either of these drugs is to be administered concomitantly with ceftriaxone by intermittent intravenous infusion, it is recommended that they be given sequentially, with thorough flushing of the intravenous lines (with one of the compatible fluids) between the administrations.
After the indicated stability time periods, unused portions of solutions should be discarded.
NOTE: Parenteral drug products should be inspected visually for particulate matter before administration.
Rocephin reconstituted with 5% Dextrose or 0.9% Sodium Chloride solution at concentrations between 10 mg/mL and 40 mg/mL, and then stored in frozen state (−20°C) in PVC or polyolefin containers, remains stable for 26 weeks. Reconstituted ADD-Vantage units, however, should not be stored in a frozen state (−20°C).
All frozen solutions of Rocephin, including those frozen following reconstitution and those supplied premixed as a frozen solution in Galaxy containers, should be thawed at room temperature before use. After thawing, unused portions should be discarded. **DO NOT REFREEZE**.
Rocephin solutions should *not* be physically mixed with or piggybacked into solutions containing other antimicrobial drugs or into diluent solutions other than those listed above, due to possible incompatibility.

ANIMAL PHARMACOLOGY

Concretions consisting of the precipitated calcium salt of ceftriaxone have been found in the gallbladder bile of dogs and baboons treated with ceftriaxone.
These appeared as a gritty sediment in dogs that received 100 mg/kg/day for 4 weeks. A similar phenomenon has been observed in baboons but only after a protracted dosing period (6 months) at higher dose levels (335 mg/kg/day or more). The likelihood of this occurrence in humans is considered to be low, since ceftriaxone has a greater plasma half-life in humans, the calcium salt of ceftriaxone is more soluble in human gallbladder bile and the calcium content of human gallbladder bile is relatively low.

HOW SUPPLIED

Rocephin is supplied as a sterile crystalline powder in glass vials and piggyback bottles. The following packages are available:
Vials containing 250 mg equivalent of ceftriaxone. Box of 1 (NDC 0004-1962-02) and box of 10 (NDC 0004-1962-01).
Vials containing 500 mg equivalent of ceftriaxone. Box of 1 (NDC 0004-1963-02) and box of 10 (NDC 0004-1963-01).
Vials containing 1 gm equivalent of ceftriaxone. Box of 1 (NDC 0004-1964-04) and box of 10 (NDC 0004-1964-01).
Piggyback bottles containing 1 gm equivalent of ceftriaxone. Box of 1 (NDC 0004-1964-02).
Vials containing 2 gm equivalent of ceftriaxone. Box of 10 (NDC 0004-1965-01).
Piggyback bottles containing 2 gm equivalent of ceftriaxone. Box of 1 (NDC 0004-1965-02).
Bulk pharmacy containers, containing 10 gm equivalent of ceftriaxone. Box of 1 (NDC 0004-1971-01). NOT FOR DIRECT ADMINISTRATION.
Rocephin is also supplied as a sterile crystalline powder in ADD-Vantage®* Vials as follows:
ADD-Vantage Vials containing 1 gm equivalent of ceftriaxone. Box of 10 (NDC 0004-1964-05).
ADD-Vantage Vials containing 2 gm equivalent of ceftriaxone. Box of 10 (NDC 0004-1965-05).
NOTE: Rocephin sterile powder should be stored at room temperature, 77°F (25°C) or below, and protected from light.
Rocephin is also supplied premixed as a frozen, iso-osmotic, sterile, nonpyreogenic solution of ceftriaxone sodium in 50 mL single dose Galaxy®† containers (PL 2040 plastic), is manufactured for Roche Laboratories Inc. by Baxter Healthcare Corporation, Deerfield, Illinois 60015. The following strengths are available:
1 gm equivalent of ceftriaxone, iso-osmotic with approximately 1.9 gm Dextrose Hydrous, USP, added (NDC 0004-2002-78).
2 gm equivalent of ceftriaxone, iso-osmotic with approximately 1.2 gm Dextrose Hydrous, USP, added (NDC 0004-2003-78).
NOTE: Frozen Rocephin should be stored at or below −20°C/−4°F.

*Registered trademark of Abbott Laboratories, Inc.
†Registered trademark of Baxter International Inc.

Diluent	Concentration mg/ml	Storage: Room Temp. (25°C)	Storage: Refrigerated (4°C)
Sterile Water for Injection	100	2 days	10 days
	250, 350	24 hours	3 days
0.9% Sodium Chloride Solution	100	2 days	10 days
	250, 350	24 hours	3 days
5% Dextrose Solution	100	2 days	10 days
	250, 350	24 hours	3 days
Bacteriostatic Water + 0.9% Benzyl Alcohol	100	24 hours	10 days
	250, 350	24 hours	3 days
1% Lidocaine Solution (without epinephrine)	100	24 hours	10 days
	250, 350	24 hours	3 days

Diluent	Storage: Room Temp. (25°C)	Storage: Refrigerated (4°C)
Sterile Water	2 days	10 days
0.9% Sodium Chloride Solution	2 days	10 days
5% Dextrose Solution	2 days	10 days
10% Dextrose Solution	2 days	10 days
5% Dextrose + 0.9% Sodium Chloride Solution*	2 days	Incompatible
5% Dextrose + 0.45% Sodium Chloride Solution	2 days	Incompatible

*Data available for 10 to 40 mg/mL concentrations in this diluent in PVC containers only.

Clinical Efficacy in Evaluable Population

Study Day	Ceftriaxone Single Dose	Comparator - 10 Days of Oral Therapy	95% Confidence Interval	Statistical Outcome
Study 1 - US		amoxicillin/clavulanate		
14	74% (220/296)	82% (247/302)	(−14.4%, −0.5%)	Ceftriaxone is lower than control at study day 14 and 28.
28	58% (167/288)	67% (200/297)	(−17.5%, −1.2%)	
Study 2 - US[5]		TMP-SMZ		
14	54% (113/210)	60% (124/206)	(−16.4%, 3.6%)	Ceftriaxone is equivalent to control at study day 14 and 28.
28	35% (73/206)	45% (93/205)	(−19.9%, 0.0%)	

Organism	Study Day 13-15: No. Analyzed	Study Day 13-15: No. Erad. (%)	Study Day 30+2: No. Analyzed	Study Day 30+2: No. Erad. (%)
Streptococcus pneumoniae	38	32 (84)	35	25 (71)
Haemophilus influenzae	33	28 (85)	31	22 (71)
Moraxella catarrhalis	15	12 (80)	15	9 (60)

CLINICAL STUDIES

Clinical Trials in Pediatric Patients With Acute Bacterial Otitis Media: In two adequate and well-controlled US clinical trials a single IM dose of ceftriaxone was compared with a 10 day course of oral antibiotic in pediatric patients between the ages of 3 months and 6 years. The clinical cure rates and statistical outcome appear in the table below:
[See third table above]
An open-label bacteriologic study of ceftriaxone without a comparator enrolled 108 pediatric patients, 79 of whom had positive baseline cultures for one or more of the common pathogens. The results of this study are tabulated as follows:
Week 2 and 4 Bacteriologic Eradication Rates in the Per Protocol Analysis in the Roche Bacteriologic Study by pathogen:
[See fourth table above]

REFERENCES

1. National Committee for Clinical Laboratory Standards, *Methods for Dilution Antimicrobial Susceptibility Tests for Bacteria that Grow Aerobically;* Approved Standard-Fifth Edition. NCCLS document M7-A5 (ISBN 1-56238-309-9). NCCLS, Wayne, PA 19087-1898, 2000.
2. National Committee for Clinical Laboratory Standards, Supplemental Tables. NCCLS document M100-S10(M7) (ISBN 1-56238-309-9). NCCLS, Wayne, PA 19087-1898, 2000.
3. National Committee for Clinical Laboratory Standards, *Performance Standards for Antimicrobial Disk Susceptibility Tests;* Approved Standard-Seventh Edition. NCCLS document M2-A7 (ISBN 1-56238-393-0). NCCLS, Wayne, PA 19087-1898, 2000.
4. National Committee for Clinical Laboratory Standards, *Methods for Antimicrobial Susceptibility Testing of Anaerobic Bacteria;* Approved Standard-Fourth Edition. NCCLS document M11-A4 (ISBN 1-56238-210-1). NCCLS, Wayne, PA 19087-1898, 1997.
5. Barnett ED, Teele DW, Klein JO, et al. *Comparison of Ceftriaxone and Trimethoprim-Sulfamethoxazole for Acute Otitis Media.* Pediatrics. Vol. 99, No. 1, January 1997.

Revised: May 2004

ROFERON®-A ℞

[ro-fear'on]
(Interferon alfa-2a, recombinant)

> Alpha interferons, including Interferon alfa-2a, cause or aggravate fatal or life-threatening neuropsychiatric, autoimmune, ischemic, and infectious disorders. Patients should be monitored closely with periodic clinical and laboratory evaluations. Patients with persistently severe or worsening signs or symptoms of these conditions should be withdrawn from therapy. In many, but not all cases, these disorders resolve after stopping Interferon alfa-2a therapy (see WARNINGS and ADVERSE REACTIONS).

DESCRIPTION

Roferon-A (Interferon alfa-2a, recombinant) is a sterile protein product for use by injection. Roferon-A is manufactured by recombinant DNA technology that employs a genetically engineered *Escherichia coli* bacterium containing DNA that codes for the human protein. Interferon alfa-2a, recombinant is a highly purified protein containing 165 amino acids, and it has an approximate molecular weight of 19,000 daltons. Fermentation is carried out in a defined nutrient medium containing the antibiotic tetracycline hydrochloride, 5 mg/L. However, the presence of the antibiotic is not detectable in the final product. Roferon-A is supplied in prefilled syringes. Each glass syringe barrel contains 0.5 mL of product. In addition, there is a needle, which is ½ inch in length.
Single Use Prefilled Syringes:
3 million IU (11.1 mcg/0.5 mL) Roferon-A per syringe—The solution is colorless and each 0.5 mL contains 3 MIU of Interferon alfa-2a, recombinant, 3.605 mg sodium chloride, 0.1 mg polysorbate 80, 5 mg benzyl alcohol as a preservative and 0.385 mg ammonium acetate.
6 million IU (22.2 mcg/0.5 mL) Roferon-A per syringe—The solution is colorless and each 0.5 mL contains 6 MIU of Interferon alfa-2a, recombinant, 3.605 mg sodium chloride, 0.1 mg polysorbate 80, 5 mg benzyl alcohol as a preservative and 0.385 mg ammonium acetate.

9 million IU (33.3 mcg/0.5 mL) Roferon-A per syringe—The solution is colorless and each 0.5 mL contains 9 MIU of Interferon alfa-2a, recombinant, 3.605 mg sodium chloride, 0.1 mg polysorbate 80, 5 mg benzyl alcohol as a preservative and 0.385 mg ammonium acetate.
The route of administration is by subcutaneous injection.

CLINICAL PHARMACOLOGY

The mechanism by which Interferon alfa-2a, recombinant, or any other interferon, exerts antitumor or antiviral activity is not clearly understood. However, it is believed that direct antiproliferative action against tumor cells, inhibition of virus replication and modulation of the host immune response play important roles in antitumor and antiviral activity.
The biological activities of Interferon alfa-2a, recombinant are species-restricted, ie, they are expressed in a very limited number of species other than humans. As a consequence, preclinical evaluation of Interferon alfa-2a, recombinant has involved in vitro experiments with human cells and some in vivo experiments.[1] Using human cells in culture, Interferon alfa-2a, recombinant has been shown to have antiproliferative and immunomodulatory activities that are very similar to those of the mixture of interferon alfa subtypes produced by human leukocytes. In vivo, Interferon alfa-2a, recombinant has been shown to inhibit the growth of several human tumors growing in immunocompromised (nude) mice. Because of its species-restricted activity, it has not been possible to demonstrate antitumor activity in immunologically intact syngeneic tumor model systems, where effects on the host immune system would be observable. However, such antitumor activity has been repeatedly demonstrated with, for example, mouse interferon-alfa in transplantable mouse tumor systems. The clinical significance of these findings is unknown.
The metabolism of Interferon alfa-2a, recombinant is consistent with that of alfa interferons in general. Alfa interferons are totally filtered through the glomeruli and undergo rapid proteolytic degradation during tubular reabsorption, rendering a negligible reappearance of intact alfa interferon in the systemic circulation. Small amounts of radiolabeled Interferon alfa-2a, recombinant appear in the urine of isolated rat kidneys, suggesting near complete reabsorption of Interferon alfa-2a, recombinant catabolites. Liver metabolism and subsequent biliary excretion are considered minor pathways of elimination for alfa interferons.
The serum concentrations of Interferon alfa-2a, recombinant reflected a large intersubject variation in both healthy volunteers and patients with disseminated cancer.
In healthy people, Interferon alfa-2a, recombinant exhibited an elimination half-life of 3.7 to 8.5 hours (mean 5.1 hours), volume of distribution at steady-state of 0.223 to 0.748 L/kg (mean 0.400 L/kg) and a total body clearance of 2.14 to 3.62 mL/min/kg (mean 2.79 mL/min/kg) after a 36 MIU (2.2×10^8pg) intravenous infusion. After intramuscular and subcutaneous administrations of 36 MIU, peak serum concentrations ranged from 1500 to 2580 pg/mL (mean 2020 pg/mL) at a mean time to peak of 3.8 hours and from 1250 to 2320 pg/mL (mean 1730 pg/mL) at a mean time to peak of 7.3 hours, respectively. The apparent fraction of the dose absorbed after intramuscular injection was greater than 80%.
The pharmacokinetics of Interferon alfa-2a, recombinant after single intramuscular doses to patients with disseminated cancer were similar to those found in healthy volunteers. Dose proportional increases in serum concentrations were observed after single doses up to 198 MIU. There were no changes in the distribution or elimination of Interferon alfa-2a, recombinant during twice daily (0.5 to 36 MIU), once daily (1 to 54 MIU), or three times weekly (1 to 136 MIU) dosing regimens up to 28 days of dosing. Multiple intramuscular doses of Interferon alfa-2a, recombinant resulted in an accumulation of two to four times the single dose serum concentrations. There is no pharmacokinetic information in patients with chronic hepatitis C, hairy cell leukemia, and chronic myelogenous leukemia.
Serum neutralizing activity, determined by a highly sensitive enzyme immunoassay, and a neutralization bioassay, was detected in approximately 25% of all patients who received Roferon-A.[2] Antibodies to human leukocyte interferon may occur spontaneously in certain clinical conditions (cancer, systemic lupus erythematosus, herpes zoster) in patients who have never received exogenous interferon.[3] The significance of the appearance of serum neutralizing activity is not known.
CLINICAL STUDIES: Studies have shown that Roferon-A can normalize serum ALT, improve liver histology and reduce viral load in patients with chronic hepatitis C. Other studies have shown that Roferon-A can produce clinically meaningful tumor regression or disease stabilization in patients with hairy cell leukemia.[4,5] In Ph-positive Chronic Myelogenous Leukemia, Roferon-A supplemented with intermittent chemotherapy has been shown to prolong overall survival and to delay disease progression compared to patients treated with chemotherapy alone.[6] In addition, Roferon-A has been shown to produce sustained complete cytogenetic responses in a small subset of patients with CML in chronic phase. The activity of Roferon-A in Ph-negative CML has not been determined.
EFFECTS ON CHRONIC HEPATITIS C: The safety and efficacy of Roferon-A was evaluated in multiple clinical trials involving over 2000 patients 18 years of age or older with hepatitis, with or without cirrhosis, who had elevated serum alanine aminotransferase (ALT) levels and tested positive for antibody to hepatitis C. Roferon-A was given three times a week (tiw) by subcutaneous (SC) or intramuscular (IM) injection in a variety of dosing regimens, including dose escalation and de-escalation regimens. Normalization of serum ALT was defined in all studies as two consecutive normal serum ALT values at least 21 days apart. A sustained response (SR) was defined as normalization of ALT both at the end of treatment and at the end of at least 6 months of treatment-free follow-up.

Table 1. — ALT Normalization in Patients Receiving Therapy With Roferon-A for 12 Months

Study No.	Dose (MIU)	N	End of Treatment [% (95% CI)]	End of Observation (Sustained Response SR) [% (95% CI)]*
1**	3	56	23	11
2	3	117	23	12
1 and 2 Combined	3	173	23 (17-30)	12 (7-17)
3	6-3	210	25 (19-31)	19 (14-25)

* All patients were followed for 6 months after end of treatment.
**EOT and SR rates for Placebo (study 1) were 0.

In trials in which Roferon-A was administered for 6 months, 6 MIU, 3 MIU, and 1 MIU were directly compared. Six MIU was associated with higher SR rates but greater toxicity (see ADVERSE REACTIONS). In studies in which the same dose of Roferon-A was administered for 6 or 12 months, the longer duration was associated with higher SR rates and adverse events were no more severe or frequent in the second 6 months than in the first 6 months. Based on these data, the recommended regimens are 3 MIU for 12 months or 6 MIU for the first 3 months followed by 3 MIU for the next 9 months (see Table 1 and DOSAGE AND ADMINISTRATION). There are no direct comparisons of these two regimens.
Younger patients (eg, less than 35 years of age) and patients without cirrhosis on liver biopsy were more likely to respond completely to Roferon-A than those patients greater than 35 years of age or patients with cirrhosis on liver biopsy.
In the two studies in which Roferon-A was administered subcutaneously three times weekly for 12 months, 20/173 (12%) patients experienced a sustained response to therapy (see Table 1). Of these patients, 15/173 (9%) maintained this sustained response during continuous follow-up for up to four years. Patients who have ALT normalization but who fail to have a sustained response following an initial course of therapy may benefit from retreatment with higher doses of Roferon-A (see DOSAGE AND ADMINISTRATION).
A subset of patients had liver biopsies performed both before and after treatment with Roferon-A. An improvement in liver histology as assessed by Knodell Histology Activity Index was generally observed.
A retrospective subgroup analysis of 317 patients from two studies suggested a correlation between improvement in liver histology, durable serum ALT response rates, and decreased viral load as measured by the polymerase chain reaction (PCR).
[See table 1 above]
EFFECTS ON Ph-POSITIVE CHRONIC MYELOGENOUS LEUKEMIA (CML): Roferon-A was evaluated in two trials of patients with chronic phase CML. Study DM84-38 was a single center phase II study conducted at the MD Anderson Cancer Center, which enrolled 91 patients, 81% were previously treated, 82% were Ph positive, and 63% received Roferon-A within 1 year of diagnosis. Study MI400 was a multicenter randomized phase III study conducted in Italy by the Italian Cooperative Study Group on CML in 335 patients; 226 Roferon-A and 109 chemotherapy. Patients with Ph-positive, newly diagnosed or minimally treated CML were randomized (ratio 2:1) to either Roferon-A or conventional chemotherapy with either hydroxyurea or busulfan.
In study DM84-38, patients started Roferon-A at 9 MIU/day, whereas in study MI400, it was progressively escalated from 3 to 9 MIU/day over the first month. In both trials, dose escalation for insufficient hematologic response, and dose attenuation or interruption for toxicity was permitted. No formal guidelines for dose attenuation were given in the chemotherapy arm of study MI400. In addition, in the Roferon-A arm, the MI400 protocol allowed the addition of intermittent single agent chemotherapy for insufficient hematologic response to Roferon-A alone. In this trial, 44% of the Roferon-A treated patients also received intermittent single agent chemotherapy at some time during the study.
The two studies were analyzed according to uniform response criteria. For hematologic response: complete response (WBC $<9\times10^9$/L, normalization of the differential with no immature forms in the peripheral blood, disappearance of splenomegaly), partial response (>50% decrease from baseline of WBC to $<20\%\times10^9$/L). For cytogenetic response: complete response (0% Ph-positive metaphases), partial response (1% to 34% Ph-positive metaphases).
In study DM84-38, the median survival from initiation of Roferon-A was 47 months. In study MI400, the median survival for the patients on the interferon arm was 69 months, which was significantly better than the 55 months seen in the chemotherapy control group (48 patients in study MI400 proceeded to BMT and in study DM84-38, 15 patients proceeded to BMT). Roferon-A treatment significantly delayed disease progression to blastic phase as evidenced by a median time to disease progression of 69 months to 46 months with chemotherapy.
By multivariate analysis of prognostic factors associated with all 335 patients entered into the randomized study, treatment with Roferon-A (with or without intermittent additional chemotherapy; p=0.006), Sokal index[7] (p=0.006) and WBC (p=0.023) were the three variables associated with an improved survival, independent of other baseline characteristics (Karnofsky performance status and hemoglobin being the other factors entered into the model).
In study MI400, overall hematologic responses, [complete responses (CR) and partial responses (PR)], were observed in approximately 60% of patients treated with Roferon-A (40% CR, 20% PR), compared to 70% with chemotherapy (30% CR, 40% PR). The median time to reach a complete hematologic response was 5 months in the Roferon-A arm and 4 months in the chemotherapy arm. The overall cytogenetic response rate (CR+PR), in patients receiving Roferon-A, was 10% and 12% in studies MI400 and DM84-38, respectively, according to the intent-to-treat principle. In contrast, only 2% of the patients in the chemotherapy arm of study MI400 achieved a cytogenetic response (with no complete responses). Cytogenetic responses were observed only in patients who had complete hematologic responses. In study DM84-38, hematologic and cytogenetic response rates were higher in the subset of patients treated with Roferon-A within 1 year of diagnosis (76% and 17%, respectively) compared to the subset initiating Roferon-A therapy more than 1 year from diagnosis (29% and 4%, respectively). In an exploratory analysis, patients who achieved a cytogenetic response lived longer than those who did not.
Severe adverse events were observed in 66% and 31% of patients on study DM84-38 and MI400, respectively. Dose reduction and temporary cessation of therapy was required frequently. Permanent cessation of Roferon-A, due to intolerable side effects, was required in 15% and 23% of patients on studies DM84-38 and MI400, respectively (see ADVERSE REACTIONS).
Limited data are available on the use of Roferon-A in children with Ph-positive, adult-type CML. A published report on 15 children with CML suggests a safety profile similar to that seen in adult CML; clinical responses were also observed[8] (see DOSAGE AND ADMINISTRATION).
EFFECTS ON HAIRY CELL LEUKEMIA: A multicenter US phase II study (N2752) enrolled 218 patients; 75 were evaluable for efficacy in a preliminary analysis; 218 patients were evaluable for safety. Patients were to receive a starting dose of Roferon-A up to 6 MIU/m²/day, for an induction period of 4 to 6 months. Responding patients were to receive 12 months maintenance therapy.
During the first 1 to 2 months of treatment of patients with hairy cell leukemia, significant depression of hematopoiesis was likely to occur. Subsequently, there was improvement in circulating blood cell counts. Of the 75 patients who were evaluable for efficacy following at least 16 weeks of therapy, 46 (61%) achieved complete or partial response. Twenty-one patients (28%) had a minor remission, 8 (11%) remained stable, and none had worsening of disease. All patients who achieved either a complete or partial response had complete or partial normalization of all peripheral blood elements including hemoglobin level, white blood cell, neutrophil, monocyte and platelet counts with a concomitant decrease in peripheral blood and bone marrow hairy cells. Responding patients also exhibited a marked reduction in red blood cell and platelet transfusion requirements, a decrease in infectious episodes and improvement in performance status. The probability of survival for 2 years in patients receiving Roferon-A (94%) was statistically increased compared to a historical control group (75%).

INDICATIONS AND USAGE

Roferon-A is indicated for the treatment of chronic hepatitis C and hairy cell leukemia in patients 18 years of age or older. In addition, it is indicated for chronic phase, Philadelphia chromosome (Ph) positive chronic myelogenous leukemia (CML) patients who are minimally pretreated (within 1 year of diagnosis).
FOR PATIENTS WITH CHRONIC HEPATITIS C: Roferon-A is indicated for use in patients with chronic hepatitis C diagnosed by HCV antibody and/or a history of exposure to hepatitis C who have compensated liver disease and are 18 years of age or older. A liver biopsy and a serum test for the presence of antibody to HCV should be performed to establish the diagnosis of chronic hepatitis C. Other causes of hepatitis, including hepatitis B, should be excluded prior to therapy with Roferon-A.

CONTRAINDICATIONS

Roferon-A is contraindicated in patients with known hypersensitivity to alfa interferon or any component of the product. The injectable solutions contain benzyl alcohol and are contraindicated in any individual with a known allergy to that preservative.

Continued on next page

Roferon-A—Cont.

WARNINGS

Roferon-A should be administered under the guidance of a qualified physician (see DOSAGE AND ADMINISTRATION). Appropriate management of the therapy and its complications is possible only when adequate facilities are readily available.

DEPRESSION AND SUICIDAL BEHAVIOR INCLUDING SUICIDAL IDEATION, SUICIDAL ATTEMPTS AND SUICIDES HAVE BEEN REPORTED IN ASSOCIATION WITH TREATMENT WITH ALFA INTERFERONS, INCLUDING ROFERON-A. Patients to be treated with Roferon-A should be informed that depression and suicidal ideation may be side effects of treatment and should be advised to report these side effects immediately to the prescribing physician. Patients receiving Roferon-A therapy should receive close monitoring for the occurrence of depressive symptomatology. Cessation of treatment should be considered for patients experiencing depression. Although dose reduction or treatment cessation may lead to resolution of the depressive symptomatology, depression may persist and suicides have occurred after withdrawing therapy (see PRECAUTIONS and ADVERSE REACTIONS).

Central nervous system adverse reactions have been reported in a number of patients. These reactions included decreased mental status, dizziness, impaired memory, agitation, manic behavior and psychotic reactions. More severe obtundation and coma have been rarely observed. Most of these abnormalities were mild and reversible within a few days to 3 weeks upon dose reduction or discontinuation of Roferon-A therapy. Careful periodic neuropsychiatric monitoring of all patients is recommended.

Roferon-A should be used with caution in patients with severe preexisting cardiac disease, severe renal or hepatic disease, seizure disorders and/or compromised central nervous system function.

Roferon-A should be administered with caution to patients with cardiac disease or with any history of cardiac illness. Acute, self-limited toxicities (ie, fever, chills) frequently associated with Roferon-A administration may exacerbate preexisting cardiac conditions. Rarely, myocardial infarction has occurred in patients receiving Roferon-A. Cases of cardiomyopathy have been observed on rare occasions in patients treated with alfa interferons.

Patients with a history of autoimmune hepatitis or a history of autoimmune disease and patients who are immunosuppressed transplant recipients should not be treated with Roferon-A. Controlled studies of Roferon-A therapy in patients with advanced cirrhosis and/or decompensated liver disease have not been performed. In chronic hepatitis C, initiation of alfa-interferon therapy, including Roferon-A, has been reported to cause transient liver abnormalities, which in patients with poorly compensated liver disease can result in increased ascites, hepatic failure or death.

Leukopenia and elevation of hepatic enzymes occurred frequently but were rarely dose-limiting. Thrombocytopenia occurred less frequently. Proteinuria and increased cells in urinary sediment were also seen infrequently. Dose-limiting hepatic or renal toxicities were unusual. Infrequently, severe renal toxicities, sometimes requiring renal dialysis, have been reported with alfa-interferon therapy alone or in combination with IL-2 (see PRECAUTIONS).

Infrequently, severe or fatal gastrointestinal hemorrhage has been reported in association with alfa-interferon therapy.

Alpha interferons suppress bone marrow function and may result in severe cytopenias including very rare events of aplastic anemia. It is advised that complete blood counts (CBC) be obtained pretreatment and monitored routinely during therapy. Alpha interferon therapy should be discontinued in patients who develop severe decreases in neutrophil ($<0.5 \times 10^9$/L) or platelet counts ($<25 \times 10^9$/L).

Caution should be exercised when administering Roferon-A to patients with myelosuppression or when Roferon-A is used in combination with other agents that are known to cause myelosuppression. Synergistic toxicity has been observed when Roferon-A is administered in combination with zidovudine (AZT).[9]

Hyperglycemia has been observed rarely in patients treated with Roferon-A. Symptomatic patients should have their blood glucose measured and followed-up accordingly. Patients with diabetes mellitus may require adjustment of their anti-diabetic regimen.

The injectable solutions contain benzyl alcohol and should not be used by patients with a known allergy to benzyl alcohol. This product is not indicated for use in neonates or infants and should not be used by patients in that age group. There have been rare reports of death in neonates and infants associated with excessive exposure to benzyl alcohol. There have been reports of permanent neuropsychiatric deficits and multiple system organ failure associated with benzyl alcohol in neonates and infants. The amount of benzyl alcohol at which toxicity or adverse effects may occur in neonates or infants is not known (see CONTRAINDICATIONS).

Ophthalmologic Disorders: Decrease or loss of vision, retinopathy including macular edema, retinal artery or vein thrombosis, retinal hemorrhages and cotton wool spots, optic neuritis, and papilledema are induced or aggravated by treatment with Interferon alfa-2a or other alpha interferons. All patients should receive an eye examination at baseline. Patients with preexisting ophthalmologic disorders (eg, diabetic or hypertensive retinopathy) should receive periodic ophthalmologic exams during interferon alpha treatment. Any patient who develops ocular symptoms should receive a prompt and complete eye examination. Interferon alfa-2a treatment should be discontinued in patients who develop new or worsening ophthalmologic disorders.

PRECAUTIONS

General: In all instances where the use of Roferon-A is considered for chemotherapy, the physician must evaluate the need and usefulness of the drug against the risk of adverse reactions. Most adverse reactions are reversible if detected early. If severe reactions occur, the drug should be reduced in dosage or discontinued and appropriate corrective measures should be taken according to the clinical judgment of the physician. Reinstitution of Roferon-A therapy should be carried out with caution and with adequate consideration of the further need for the drug and, alertness to possible recurrence of toxicity. The minimum effective doses of Roferon-A for treatment of hairy cell leukemia and chronic myelogenous leukemia have not been established.

Variations in dosage and adverse reactions exist among different brands of Interferon. Therefore, do not use different brands of Interferon in a single treatment regimen.

Rare cases of autoimmune diseases including thrombocytopenia, vasculitis, Raynaud's phenomenon, rheumatoid arthritis, lupus erythematosus, and rhabdomyolysis have been observed in patients treated with alpha interferons. Any patient developing an autoimmune disorder during treatment should be closely monitored and, if appropriate, treatment should be discontinued.

Information for Patient: Patients should be cautioned not to change brands of Interferon without medical consultation, as a change in dosage may result. Patients should be informed regarding the potential benefits and risks attendant to the use of Roferon-A. If home use is determined to be desirable by the physician, instructions on appropriate use should be given, including review of the contents of the enclosed Medication Guide. Patients should be well hydrated, especially during the initial stages of treatment.

Patients should be thoroughly instructed in the importance of proper disposal procedures and cautioned against reusing syringes and needles. If home use is prescribed, a puncture-resistant container for the disposal of used syringes and needles should be supplied to the patient. The full container should be disposed of according to directions provided by the physician (see Medication Guide).

Patients receiving high-dose alfa interferon should be cautioned against performing tasks that require complete mental alertness such as operating machinery or driving a motor vehicle. Patients to be treated with Roferon-A should be informed that depression and suicidal ideation may be side effects of treatment and should be advised to report these side effects immediately to the prescribing physician.

Laboratory Tests: Complete blood with differential platelet counts and clinical chemistry tests should be performed before initiation of Roferon-A therapy and at appropriate periods during therapy. Since responses of hairy cell leukemia, chronic hepatitis C and chronic myelogenous leukemia are not generally observed for 1 to 3 months after initiation of treatment, very careful monitoring for severe depression of blood cell counts is warranted during the initial phase of treatment.

Those patients who have preexisting cardiac abnormalities and/or are in advanced stages of cancer should have electrocardiograms taken before and during the course of treatment.

For patients being treated for chronic hepatitis C, serum ALT should be evaluated before therapy to establish baselines and repeated at week 2 and monthly thereafter following initiation of therapy for monitoring clinical response. Patients with neutrophil count $<1500/mm^3$, platelet count $<75{,}000/mm^3$, hemoglobin <10 g/dL and creatinine >1.5 mg/dL were excluded from several major chronic hepatitis C studies; patients with these laboratory abnormalities should be carefully monitored if treated with Roferon-A.

Patients with preexisting thyroid abnormalities may be treated if normal thyroid stimulating hormone (TSH) levels can be maintained by medication. Testing of TSH levels in these patients is recommended at baseline and every 3 months following initiation of therapy.

Triglyceride levels should be monitored periodically during treatment. Elevated triglyceride levels have been observed in chronic hepatitis C and chronic myelogenous leukemia patients treated with interferon alfa therapy, including Roferon-A.

Drug Interactions: Roferon-A has been reported to reduce the clearance of theophylline.[10,11] The clinical relevance of this interaction is presently unknown. Interactions between Roferon-A and other drugs have not been fully evaluated. Caution should be exercised when administering Roferon-A in combination with other potentially myelosuppressive agents (see WARNINGS).

Other Drug Interactions: Alfa interferons may affect the oxidative metabolic process by reducing the activity of hepatic microsomal cytochrome enzymes in the P450 group. Although the clinical relevance is still unclear, this should be taken into account when prescribing concomitant therapy with drugs metabolized by this route.

The neurotoxic, hematotoxic or cardiotoxic effects of previously or concurrently administered drugs may be increased by interferons. Interactions could occur following concurrent administration of centrally acting drugs. Use of Roferon-A in conjunction with interleukin-2 may potentiate risks of renal failure.

Carcinogenesis, Mutagenesis, Impairment of Fertility:

Carcinogenesis: Roferon-A has not been tested for its carcinogenic potential.

Mutagenesis: A. Internal Studies — Ames tests using six different tester strains, with and without metabolic activation, were performed with Roferon-A up to a concentration of 1920 µg/plate. There was no evidence of mutagenicity.

Human lymphocyte cultures were treated in vitro with Roferon-A at noncytotoxic concentrations. No increase in the incidence of chromosomal damage was noted.

B. Published Studies — There are no published studies on the mutagenic potential of Roferon-A. However, a number of studies on the genotoxicity of human leukocyte interferon have been reported.

A chromosomal defect following the addition of human leukocyte interferon to lymphocyte cultures from a patient suffering from a lymphoproliferative disorder has been reported.

In contrast, other studies have failed to detect chromosomal abnormalities following treatment of lymphocyte cultures from healthy volunteers with human leukocyte interferon.

It has also been shown that human leukocyte interferon protects primary chick embryo fibroblasts from chromosomal aberrations produced by gamma rays.

Impairment of Fertility: Roferon-A has been studied for its effect on fertility in Macaca mulatta (rhesus monkeys). Nonpregnant rhesus females treated with Roferon-A at doses of 5 and 25 MIU/kg/day have shown menstrual cycle irregularities, including prolonged or shortened menstrual periods and erratic bleeding; these cycles were considered to be anovulatory on the basis that reduced progesterone levels were noted and that expected increases in preovulatory estrogen and luteinizing hormones were not observed. These monkeys returned to a normal menstrual rhythm following discontinuation of treatment.

Pregnancy Category C: Roferon-A has been associated with statistically significant, dose-related increases in abortions in pregnant rhesus monkeys treated with 1, 5, or 25 MIU/kg/day (approximately 20 to 500 times the human weekly dose, when scaled by body surface area) during the early to midfetal period of organogenesis (gestation day 22 to 70). Abortifacient activity was also observed in 2/6 pregnant rhesus monkeys treated with 25 MIU/kg/day Roferon-A (500 times the human dose) during the period of late fetal development (days 79 to 100 of gestation). No teratogenic effects were seen in either study. However, the validity of extrapolating doses used in animal studies to human doses is not established. Therefore, no direct comparison of the doses that induced fetal death in monkeys to dose levels of Roferon-A used clinically can be made. There are no adequate and well-controlled studies of Roferon-A in pregnant women. Roferon-A is to be used during pregnancy only if the potential benefit justifies the potential risk to the fetus.

Roferon-A is recommended for use in women of childbearing potential only when they are using effective contraception during therapy.

The injectable solution contains benzyl alcohol. The excipient benzyl alcohol can be transmitted via the placenta. The possibility of toxicity should be taken into account in premature infants after the administration of Roferon-A solution for injection immediately prior to birth or Cesarean section.

Male fertility and teratologic evaluations have yielded no significant adverse effects to date.

Nursing Mothers: It is not known whether this drug is excreted in human milk. Because many drugs are excreted in human milk and because of the potential for serious adverse reactions in nursing infants from Roferon-A, a decision should be made whether to discontinue nursing or to discontinue the drug, taking into account the importance of the drug to the mother.

Pediatric Use: Use of Roferon-A in children with Ph-positive adult-type CML is supported by evidence from adequate and well-controlled studies of Roferon-A in adults with additional data from the literature on the use of alfa interferon in children with CML. A published report on 15 children with Ph-positive adult-type CML suggests a safety profile similar to that seen in adult CML; clinical responses were also observed[8] (see DOSAGE AND ADMINISTRATION).

For all other indications, safety and effectiveness have not been established in patients below the age of 18 years.

The injectable solutions are not indicated for use in neonates or infants and should not be used by patients in that age group. There have been rare reports of death in neonates and infants associated with excessive exposure to benzyl alcohol (see WARNINGS).

Geriatric Use: In clinical studies of Roferon-A in chronic hepatitis C, 101 patients were 65 years old or older. The numbers were insufficient to determine if antiviral responses differ from younger subjects. There were greater proportions of geriatric patients with serious adverse reactions (9% vs. 6%), withdrawals due to adverse reactions (11% vs. 6%), and WHO grade III neutropenia and thrombocytopenia.

Clinical studies of Roferon-A in chronic myelogenous leukemia or hairy cell leukemia did not include sufficient numbers of subjects aged 65 or older to determine whether they respond differently from younger subjects.

This drug is known to be excreted by the kidney, and the risk of toxic reactions to this drug may be greater in pa-

Table 2.—Significant Abnormal Laboratory Test Values

	Chronic Hepatitis C (n=203) 3 MIU tiw	Chronic Myelogenous Leukemia‡		Hairy Cell Leukemia (n=218)
		US Study (n=91)	Non-US Study (n=219)	
Leukopenia	1.5%	20%	3%	45%*
Neutropenia	10%	22%	0%	68%*
Thrombocytopenia	4.5%	27%	5%	62%*
Anemia (Hb)	0%	15%	4%	31%*
SGOT	NAP	5%	1%	9%
Alk. Phosphatase	0%	3%	1%	3%
LDH	NAP	NA	NA	<1%
Proteinuria	0%	NA	NA	10%†

*In the majority of patients, initial hematologic laboratory test values were abnormal due to their underlying disease.
†Ten percent of the patients experienced a proteinuria >1+ at least once.
‡Patients enrolled in the two clinical studies receiving at least one dose of Roferon-A.
NAP = Not applicable.
NA = Not assessed.

tients with impaired renal function. Because elderly patients are more likely to have decreased renal function, these patients should receive careful monitoring, including renal function.

ADVERSE REACTIONS

Depressive illness and suicidal behavior, including suicidal ideation and suicides, have been reported in association with the use of alfa-interferon products. The incidence of reported depression has varied substantially among trials, possibly related to the underlying disease, dose, duration of therapy and degree of monitoring, but has been reported to be 15% or higher (see WARNINGS).

FOR PATIENTS WITH CHRONIC HEPATITIS C: The most frequent adverse experiences were reported to be possibly or probably related to therapy with 3 MIU tiw Roferon-A, were mostly mild to moderate in severity and manageable without the need for discontinuation of therapy. A relative increase in the incidence, severity and seriousness of adverse events was observed in patients receiving doses above 3 MIU tiw.

Adverse reactions associated with the 3 MIU dose include:

Flu-like Symptoms: Fatigue (58%), myalgia/arthralgia (51%), flu-like symptoms (33%), fever (28%), chills (23%), asthenia (6%), sweating (5%), leg cramps (3%) and malaise (1%).

Central and Peripheral Nervous System: Headache (52%), dizziness (13%), paresthesia (7%), confusion (7%), concentration impaired (4%) and change in taste or smell (3%).

Gastrointestinal: Nausea/vomiting (33%), diarrhea (20%), anorexia (14%), abdominal pain (12%), flatulence (3%), liver pain (3%), digestion impaired (2%) and gingival bleeding (2%).

Psychiatric: Depression (16%), irritability (15%), insomnia (14%), anxiety (5%) and behavior disturbances (3%).

Pulmonary and Cardiovascular: Dryness or inflammation of oropharynx (6%), epistaxis (4%), rhinitis (3%), arrhythmia (1%) and sinusitis (<1%).

Skin: Injection site reaction (29%), partial alopecia (19%), rash (8%), dry skin or pruritus (7%), hematoma (1%), psoriasis (<1%), cutaneous eruptions (<1%), eczema (<1%) and seborrhea (<1%).

Other: Conjunctivitis (4%), menstrual irregularity (2%) and visual acuity decreased (<1%).

Patients receiving 6 MIU tiw experienced a higher incidence of severe psychiatric events (9%) than those receiving 3 MIU tiw (6%) in two large US studies. In addition, more patients withdrew from these studies when receiving 6 MIU tiw (11%) than when receiving 3 MIU tiw (7%). Up to half of patients receiving 3 MIU or 6 MIU tiw withdrawing from the study experienced depression or other psychiatric adverse events. At higher doses anxiety, sleep disorders, and irritability were observed more frequently. An increased incidence of fatigue, myalgia/arthralgia, headache, fever, chills, alopecia, sleep disturbances and dry skin or pruritus was also generally observed during treatment with higher doses of Roferon-A.

Generally there were fewer adverse events reported in the second 6 months of treatment than in the first 6 months for patients treated with 3 MIU tiw. Patients tolerant of initial therapy with Roferon-A generally tolerate re-treatment at the same dose, but tend to experience more adverse reactions at higher doses.

Infrequent adverse events (>1% but ≤3% incidence) included: cold feeling, cough, muscle cramps, diaphoresis, dyspnea, eye pain, reactivation of herpes simplex, lethargy, edema, sexual dysfunction, shaking, skin lesions, stomatitis, tooth disorder, urinary tract infection, weakness in extremities.

Triglyceride levels were not evaluated in the clinical trials. However, hypertriglyceridemia has been reported post marketing in patients receiving Roferon-A therapy for chronic hepatitis C.

FOR PATIENTS WITH CHRONIC MYELOGENOUS LEUKEMIA:

For patients with chronic myelogenous leukemia, the percentage of adverse events, whether related to drug therapy or not, experienced by patients treated with rIFNα-2a is given below. Severe adverse events were observed in 66% and 31% of patients on study DM84-38 and MI400, respectively. Dose reduction and temporary cessation of therapy were required frequently. Permanent cessation of Roferon-A, due to intolerable side effects, was required in 15% and 23% of patients on studies DM84-38 and MI400, respectively.

Flu-like Symptoms: Fever (92%), asthenia or fatigue (88%), myalgia (68%), chills (63%), arthralgia/bone pain (47%) and headache (44%).

Gastrointestinal: Anorexia (48%), nausea/vomiting (37%) and diarrhea (37%).

Central and Peripheral Nervous System: Headache (44%), depression (28%), decreased mental status (16%), dizziness (11%), sleep disturbances (11%), paresthesia (8%), involuntary movements (7%) and visual disturbance (6%).

Pulmonary and Cardiovascular: Coughing (19%), dyspnea (8%) and dysrhythmia (7%).

Skin: Hair changes (including alopecia) (18%), skin rash (18%), sweating (15%), dry skin (7%) and pruritus (7%).

Uncommon adverse events (<4%) reported in clinical studies included chest pain, syncope, hypotension, impotence, alterations in taste or hearing, confusion, seizures, memory loss, disturbances of libido, bruising and coagulopathy. Miscellaneous adverse events that were rarely observed included Coombs' positive hemolytic anemia, aplastic anemia, hypothyroidism, cardiomyopathy, hypertriglyceridemia and bronchospasm.

FOR PATIENTS WITH HAIRY CELL LEUKEMIA:

Constitutional (100%): Fever (92%), fatigue (86%), headache (64%), chills (64%), weight loss (33%), dizziness (21%) and flu-like symptoms (16%).

Integumentary (79%): Skin rash (44%), diaphoresis (22%), partial alopecia (17%), dry skin (17%) and pruritus (13%).

Musculoskeletal (73%): Myalgia (71%), joint or bone pain (25%) and arthritis or polyarthritis (5%).

Gastrointestinal (69%): Anorexia (43%), nausea/vomiting (39%) and diarrhea (34%).

Head and Neck (45%): Throat irritation (21%), rhinorrhea (12%) and sinusitis (11%).

Pulmonary (40%): Coughing (16%), dyspnea (12%) and pneumonia (11%).

Central Nervous System (39%): Dizziness (21%), depression (16%), sleep disturbance (10%), decreased mental status (10%), anxiety (6%), lethargy (6%), visual disturbance (6%) and confusion (5%).

Cardiovascular (39%): Chest pain (11%), edema (11%) and hypertension (11%).

Pain (34%): Pain (24%) and pain in back (16%).

Peripheral Nervous System (23%): Paresthesia (12%) and numbness (12%).

Rarely (<5%), central nervous system effects including gait disturbance, nervousness, syncope and vertigo, as well as cardiac adverse events including murmur, thrombophlebitis and hypotension were reported. Adverse experiences that occurred rarely, and may have been related to underlying disease, included ecchymosis, epistaxis, bleeding gums and petechiae. Urticaria and inflammation at the site of injection were also rarely observed.

IN OTHER INVESTIGATIONAL STUDIES OF ROFERON-A:

The following infrequent adverse events have been reported in one or more of the approved clinical indications as well as with the investigational use of Roferon-A (<5%): pancreatitis, colitis, gastrointestinal hemorrhage, stomatitis, thyroid dysfunction (including hypothyroidism and hyperthyroidism), diabetes (in some patients requiring insulin therapy), and pneumonitis (some cases responding to interferon cessation and corticosteroid therapy). In addition to the adverse experiences noted above, other adverse experiences that occurred included: abdominal fullness, hypermotility, hepatitis, gait disturbance, hallucinations, encephalopathy, psychomotor retardation, coma, stroke, transient ischemic attacks, dysphasia, sedation, apathy, irritability, hyperactivity, claustrophobia, loss of libido, congestive heart failure, myocardial infarction, Raynaud's phenomenon, hot flashes, tachypnea, ischemic retinopathy, excessive salivation and anaphylactic reactions. These adverse experiences occurred rarely (<1%).

The following events have been rarely observed (<3%) in some patients receiving Roferon-A: autoimmune diseases, ie, vasculitis, arthritis, hemolytic anemia and lupus erythematosus syndrome. The mechanism by which these events develop and their relationship to Roferon-A therapy are unclear. Similar events have been reported for other types of interferon.

ABNORMAL LABORATORY TEST VALUES: The percentage of patients with chronic hepatitis C, hairy cell leukemia, and with chronic myelogenous leukemia who experienced a significant abnormal laboratory test value (*NCI or WHO grades III or IV*) at least once during their treatment with Roferon-A is shown in Table 2:

[See table 2 above]

Elevated triglyceride levels have been observed in patients receiving interferon therapy, including Roferon-A.

CHRONIC HEPATITIS C: The incidence of neutropenia (*WHO grades III or IV*) was over twice as high in those treated with 6 MIU tiw (21%) as those treated with 3 MIU tiw (10%).

CHRONIC MYELOGENOUS LEUKEMIA: In the two clinical studies, a severe or life-threatening anemia was seen in up to 15% of patients. A severe or life-threatening leukopenia and thrombocytopenia were observed in up to 20% and 27% of patients, respectively. Changes were usually reversible when therapy was discontinued. One case of aplastic anemia and one case of Coombs' positive hemolytic anemia were seen in 310 patients treated with rIFNα-2a in clinical studies. Severe cytopenias led to discontinuation of therapy in 4% of all Roferon-A treated patients.

Transient increases in liver transaminases or alkaline phosphatase of any intensity were seen in up to 50% of patients during treatment with Roferon-A. Only 5% of patients had a severe or life-threatening increase in SGOT. In the clinical studies, such abnormalities required termination of therapy in less than 1% of patients.

HAIRY CELL LEUKEMIA: Increases in serum phosphorus (≥1.6 mmol/L) and serum uric acid (≥9.1 mg/dL) were observed in 9% and 10% of patients, respectively. The increase in serum uric acid is likely to be related to the underlying disease. Decreases in serum calcium (≤1.9 mmol/L) and serum phosphorus (≤0.9 mmol/L) were seen in 28% and 22% of patients, respectively.

OVERDOSAGE

There are no reports of overdosage, but repeated large doses of interferon can be associated with profound lethargy, fatigue, prostration, and coma. Such patients should be hospitalized for observation and appropriate supportive treatment given.

DOSAGE AND ADMINISTRATION

Roferon-A recommended dosing regimens are different for each of the following indications as described below.

Note: Parenteral drug products should be inspected visually for particulate matter and discoloration before administration, whenever solution and container permit.

Roferon-A is administered subcutaneously.

CHRONIC HEPATITIS C: The recommended dosage of Roferon-A for the treatment of chronic hepatitis C is 3 MIU three times a week (tiw) administered subcutaneously for 12 months (48 to 52 weeks). As an alternative, patients may be treated with an induction dose of 6 MIU tiw for the first 3 months (12 weeks) followed by 3 MIU tiw for 9 months (36 weeks). Normalization of serum ALT generally occurs within a few weeks after initiation of treatment in responders. Approximately 90% of patients who respond to Roferon-A do so within the first 3 months of treatment; however, patients responding to Roferon-A with a reduction in ALT should complete 12 months of treatment. Patients who have no response to Roferon-A within the first 3 months of therapy are not likely to respond with continued treatment; treatment discontinuation should be considered in these patients.

Patients who tolerate and partially or completely respond to therapy with Roferon-A but relapse following its discontinuation may be re-treated. Re-treatment with either 3 MIU tiw or with 6 MIU tiw for 6 to 12 months may be considered. Please see ADVERSE REACTIONS regarding the increased frequency of adverse reactions associated with treatment with higher doses.

Temporary dose reduction by 50% is recommended in patients who do not tolerate the prescribed dose. If adverse events resolve, treatment with the original prescribed dose can be re-initiated. In patients who cannot tolerate the reduced dose, cessation of therapy, at least temporarily, is recommended.

CHRONIC MYELOGENOUS LEUKEMIA: For patients with Ph-positive CML in chronic phase: Prior to initiation of therapy, a diagnosis of Philadelphia chromosome positive CML in chronic phase by the appropriate peripheral blood, bone marrow and other diagnostic testing should be made. Monitoring of hematologic parameters should be done regularly (eg, monthly). Since significant cytogenetic changes are not readily apparent until after hematologic response has occurred, and usually not until several months of therapy have elapsed, cytogenetic monitoring may be performed at less frequent intervals. Achievement of complete cytogenetic response has been observed up to 2 years following the start of Roferon-A treatment.

The recommended initial dose of Roferon-A is 9 MIU daily administered as a subcutaneous injection. Based on clinical experience,[3] short-term tolerance may be improved by gradually increasing the dose of Roferon-A over the first week of administration from 3 MIU daily for 3 days to 6 MIU daily for 3 days to the target dose of 9 MIU daily for the duration of the treatment period.

Continued on next page

Roferon-A—Cont.

The optimal dose and duration of therapy have not yet been determined. Even though the median time to achieve a complete hematologic response was 5 months in study MI400, hematologic responses have been observed up to 18 months after treatment start. Treatment should be continued until disease progression. If severe side effects occur, a treatment interruption or a reduction in either the dose or the frequency of injections may be necessary to achieve the individual maximally tolerated dose (see PRECAUTIONS).
Limited data are available on the use of Roferon-A in children with CML. In one report of 15 children with Ph-positive, adult-type CML doses between 2.5 to 5 MIU/m²/day given intramuscularly were tolerated.[8] In another study, severe adverse effects including deaths were noted in children with previously untreated, Ph-negative, juvenile CML, who received interferon doses of 30 MIU/m²/day.[12]
HAIRY CELL LEUKEMIA: Prior to initiation of therapy, tests should be performed to quantitate peripheral blood hemoglobin, platelets, granulocytes and hairy cells and bone marrow hairy cells. These parameters should be monitored periodically (eg, monthly) during treatment to determine whether response to treatment has occurred. If a patient does not respond within 6 months, treatment should be discontinued. If a response to treatment does occur, treatment should be continued until no further improvement is observed and these laboratory parameters have been stable for about 3 months. Patients with hairy cell leukemia have been treated for up to 24 consecutive months. The optimal duration of treatment for this disease has not been determined.
The induction dose of Roferon-A is 3 MIU daily for 16 to 24 weeks, administered as a subcutaneous injection. The recommended maintenance dose is 3 MIU, tiw. Dose reduction by one-half or withholding of individual doses may be needed when severe adverse reactions occur. The use of doses higher than 3 MIU is not recommended in hairy cell leukemia.

HOW SUPPLIED

Single Use Prefilled Syringes: (for subcutaneous administration)

3 million IU Roferon-A per syringe — Each 0.5 mL contains 3 MIU of Interferon alfa-2a, recombinant, 3.605 mg sodium chloride, 0.1 mg polysorbate 80, 5 mg benzyl alcohol as a preservative and 0.385 mg ammonium acetate. Boxes of 1 (NDC 0004-2015-09); Boxes of 6 (NDC 0004-2015-07).

6 million IU Roferon-A per syringe — Each 0.5 mL contains 6 MIU of Interferon alfa-2a, recombinant, 3.605 mg sodium chloride, 0.1 mg polysorbate 80, 5 mg benzyl alcohol as a preservative and 0.385 mg ammonium acetate. Boxes of 1 (NDC 0004-2016-09); Boxes of 6 (NDC 0004-2016-07).

9 million IU Roferon-A per syringe — Each 0.5 mL contains 9 MIU of Interferon alfa-2a, recombinant, 3.605 mg sodium chloride, 0.1 mg polysorbate 80, 5 mg benzyl alcohol as a preservative and 0.385 mg ammonium acetate. Boxes of 1 (NDC 0004-2017-09); Boxes of 6 (NDC 0004-2017-07).

Storage: The prefilled syringe should be stored in the refrigerator at 36° to 46°F (2° to 8°C) Do *not* freeze or shake. Protect Roferon-A from light during storage.

REFERENCES

1. Trown PW, et al. *Cancer.* 1986; 57(suppl):1648-1656.
2. Itri LM, et al. *Cancer.* 1987; 59:668-674.
3. Jones GJ, Itri LM. *Cancer.* 1986; 57(suppl):1709-1715.
4. Foon KA, et al. *Blood.* 1984; 64(suppl 1):164a.
5. Quesada Jr, et al. *Cancer.* 1986; 57(suppl):1678-1680.
6. The Italian Cooperative Study Group on CML. *N Engl J Med.* 1994; 330:820-825.
7. Sokal JE, et al. *Blood.* 1984; 63(4):789-799.
8. Dow LW, et al. *Cancer.* 1991; 68:1678-1684.
9. Krown SE, et al. *Proc Am Soc Clin Oncol.* 1988; 7:1.
10. Williams SJ, et al. *Lancet.* 1987; 2:939-941.
11. Jonkman JHG, et al. *Br J Clin Pharmacol.* 1989; 2(27): 795-802.
12. Maybee D, et al. *Proc Annu Meet Am Soc Clin Oncol.* 1992; 11:A950.

Revised: October 2003

MEDICATION GUIDE

Roferon®-A
(Interferon alfa-2a, recombinant)
Solution for Injection – Prefilled Syringes

Before you start taking Roferon-A (ro-FER-on), please read this Medication Guide carefully. Read this Medication Guide each time you refill your prescription in case new information has been added. This information does not take the place of talking with your healthcare provider.

What is the most important information I should know about Roferon-A?

Roferon is used to treat people with hepatitis C, hairy cell leukemia and Philadelphia chromosome positive chronic myelogenous leukemia (CML). However, Roferon-A can cause some serious side effects that may cause death in rare cases. Before starting Roferon-A, you should talk with your healthcare provider about the possible benefits and the possible side effects of treatment, to decide if Roferon-A is right for you. While taking Roferon-A, you will need to see your healthcare provider regularly for medical examinations and blood tests to make sure your treatment is working and to check for side effects.
The most serious possible side effects of Roferon-A treatment include:

1. **Mental health problems:** Roferon-A may cause some patients to develop mood or behavioral problems. Signs of these problems include irritability (getting easily upset), depression (feeling low, feeling bad about yourself or feeling hopeless), and anxiety. Some patients may have aggressive behavior and think about hurting others. Some patients may develop thoughts about ending their lives (suicidal thoughts) and may attempt to do so. A few patients have even ended their lives. Former drug addicts may fall back into drug addiction or overdose. You must tell your healthcare provider if you are being treated for a mental illness or have a history of mental illness or if you are or have ever been addicted to drugs or alcohol. Call your healthcare provider immediately if you develop any of these problems while on Roferon-A treatment.
2. **Heart problems:** Roferon-A may cause some patients to experience high blood pressure, a fast heartbeat, chest pain, and very rarely a heart attack. Tell your healthcare provider if you have or have had any heart problems in the past.
3. **Blood problems:** Many patients taking Roferon-A have had a drop in the number of their white blood cells and their platelets. If the numbers of these blood cells are too low, you could be at risk for infections or bleeding.

Stop taking Roferon-A and call your healthcare provider immediately if you develop any of these symptoms:

- **You become very depressed or think about suicide**
- **You have severe chest pain**
- **You have trouble breathing**
- **You have a change in your vision**
- **You notice unusual bleeding or bruising**
- **High fever**
- **Severe stomach pain. If the pain is in the lower part of your stomach area it could mean that your bowels are inflamed (colitis)**

For more information on possible side effects with Roferon-A therapy, please read the section on "What are the possible side effects of Roferon-A?" in this Medication Guide.

What is Roferon-A?

Roferon-A is a treatment that is used for some people who are infected with the hepatitis C virus, hairy cell leukemia, and Philadelphia chromosome positive chronic myelogenous leukemia (CML). Patients with hepatitis C have the virus that causes hepatitis in their blood and liver. Patients with hairy cell leukemia produce abnormal white blood cells that travel to the spleen where they trap and destroy normal blood cells. In CML, your body produces too many of certain blood cells. Roferon-A works in these conditions by reducing the amount of virus in the body, destroying cells that may be harmful to your body and keeping the body from producing too many cells.

Who should not take Roferon-A?

Do not use Roferon-A if:

- You are pregnant or breast-feeding or are planning to become pregnant.
- You are allergic to alpha interferons, *Escherichia coli*-derived products or any component of Roferon-A.
- You have autoimmune hepatitis (hepatitis caused by your immune system attacking your liver).

If you have or have had any of the following conditions or serious medical problems, discuss them with your doctor before taking Roferon-A:

- History of or current severe mental illness (such as depression or anxiety)
- Previous heart attack or heart problems
- Sleep problems
- High blood pressure
- Autoimmune disease (where the body's immune system attacks the body's own cells), such as vasculitis, psoriasis, systemic lupus erythematosus, rheumatoid arthritis
- Kidney problems
- Blood disorders-Low blood counts or bleeding problems
- You take a medicine called theophylline
- Diabetes (high blood sugar)
- Thyroid problems
- Liver problems, other than hepatitis C
- Hepatitis B infection
- HIV infection (the virus that causes AIDS)
- Problems with your vision
- Colitis
- Body organ transplant and are taking medicine that keeps your body from rejecting your transplant (suppresses your immune system)
- Alcoholism
- Drug abuse or addiction

If you have any doubts about your health condition or about taking Roferon-A, talk to your healthcare provider.

What should I avoid while taking Roferon-A?

- Avoid becoming pregnant while taking Roferon-A. Roferon-A may harm your unborn child or cause you to lose your baby (miscarry).
- You should not breast-feed your baby while taking Roferon-A.

How should I take Roferon-A?

To get the most benefit from this medicine, it is important to take Roferon-A exactly as your healthcare provider tells you.
Your healthcare provider will tell you how much medicine to take and how often to take it. Once you start treatment with Roferon-A, do not switch to another brand of interferon without talking to your doctor. Other interferons may not have the same effect on the treatment of your disease. Switching brands will also require a change in your dose. Your healthcare provider will tell you how long you need to use Roferon-A.
Over time, your healthcare provider may change your dose of Roferon-A. Do not change your dose unless your doctor tells you to change it.
Roferon-A is supplied in prefilled syringes. Whether you give yourself the injection or another person gives the injection to you, it is important to follow the instructions in this Medication Guide (see the appendix "Instructions for Preparing and Giving a Dose with a Roferon-A Prefilled Syringe").
If you miss a dose of Roferon-A, take the missed dose as soon as possible during the same day or the next day, then continue on your regular dosing schedule. If several days go by after you miss a dose, check with your doctor about what to do. Do not double the next dose or take more than one dose a day unless your doctor tells you to. Call your doctor right away if you take more than your prescribed Roferon-A dose. Your doctor may wish to examine you more closely and take blood for testing.
You must get regular blood tests to help your healthcare provider check how the treatment is working and to check for side effects.
Tell your doctor if you are taking or planning to take other prescription or non-prescription medicines, including vitamins and mineral supplements and herbal medicines.

What are the possible side effects of Roferon-A?

Possible, serious side effects include:

- **Mental health problems including suicide, suicidal thoughts, heart problems, and blood problems:** See the section "What is the most important information I should know about Roferon-A?".
- **Other body organ problems:** Some patients may experience lung problems (such as difficulty breathing or pneumonia) and vision problems.
- **New or worsening autoimmune disease:** Some patients may develop an autoimmune disease (a disease where the body's own immune system begins to attack itself) while on Roferon-A therapy. These diseases can include vasculitis (an inflammation of your blood vessels), rheumatoid arthritis or lupus erythematosus, psoriasis or thyroid problems. In some patients who already have an autoimmune disease, the disease may worsen while on Roferon-A therapy.

Common, but less serious, side effects include:

- **Flu-like symptoms:** Most patients who take Roferon-A have flu-like symptoms that usually lessen after the first few weeks of treatment. Flu-like symptoms may include unusual tiredness, fever, chills, muscle aches, and joint pain. Taking acetaminophen or ibuprofen before you take Roferon-A can help with these symptoms. You can also try taking Roferon-A at night. You may be able to sleep through the symptoms.
- **Extreme fatigue (tiredness):** Many patients may become extremely tired while on Roferon-A therapy.
- **Upset stomach:** Nausea, taste changes, diarrhea, and loss of appetite occur commonly.
- **Blood sugar problems:** Some patients may develop a problem with the way their body controls their blood sugar and may develop diabetes.
- **Thyroid problems:** Some patients may develop changes in their thyroid function. Symptoms of these changes may include feeling hot or cold all the time, trouble concentrating, changes in your skin (your skin may become very dry), and changes in your weight.
- **Skin reactions:** Some patients may develop a rash, dry or itchy skin, and redness and swelling at the site of injection.
- **Sleep disturbances and headache:** Trouble sleeping and headaches may also occur during Roferon-A therapy.
- **Hair thinning:** Hair loss is not uncommon while using Roferon-A. This hair loss is temporary and hair growth should return after you stop taking Roferon-A.

These are not all of the side effects of Roferon-A. Your doctor or pharmacist can give you a more complete list.
Talk to your healthcare provider if you are worried about side effects or find them very bothersome.

General advice about prescription medicines

Medicines are sometimes prescribed for purposes other than those listed in a Medication Guide. If you have any concerns or questions about Roferon-A, contact your healthcare provider. Do not use Roferon-A for a condition or person other than that for which it is prescribed. If you want to know more about Roferon-A, your healthcare provider or pharmacist will be able to provide you with detailed information that is written for healthcare providers.
This Medication Guide has been approved by the U.S. Food and Drug Administration.
Keep this and all other medications out of the reach of children.
Revised: September 2003

Medication Guide Appendix: Instructions for Preparing and Giving a Dose with a Roferon-A Prefilled Syringe

How should I store Roferon-A?

Roferon-A must be stored in the refrigerator at a temperature of 36°F to 46°F (2°C to 8°C). Do not leave Roferon-A outside of the refrigerator for more than 24 hours. Do not freeze Roferon-A. Keeping Roferon-A at temperatures outside the recommended range can destroy the medicine. Do not shake Roferon-A. Shaking can destroy Roferon-A so that it will not work. Protect Roferon-A from light during storage.

How do I inject Roferon-A?

The instructions that follow will help you learn how to use Roferon-A prefilled syringes. Please read all of these directions before trying to take your medicine. It is important to follow these directions carefully. Talk to your healthcare provider if you have any concerns about how to use Roferon-A. Whether you are giving yourself an injection or if you are giving this injection to someone else, a healthcare provider must teach you how to inject.

The prefilled syringes are used for injecting Roferon-A under the surface of the skin (subcutaneous).

1. Collect all the materials you will need before you start to give the injection:
   - one sterile Roferon-A prefilled syringe with needle
   - alcohol swabs
   - puncture-resistant disposable container
2. Check the expiration date on the package to make sure that it has not passed and check the solution in the syringe. The solution in the syringe should be clear or colorless to light yellow in color.
   - Do not use Roferon-A if:
     – the medicine is cloudy
     – the medicine has particles floating in it
     – the medicine is any color besides clear or colorless to light yellow
     – it has passed the expiration date
3. Warm the refrigerated medicine by gently rolling the syringe in the palms of your hands for about one minute.
4. Wash your hands with soap and warm water. This step is very important to help prevent infection.
5. Roferon-A prefilled syringe:

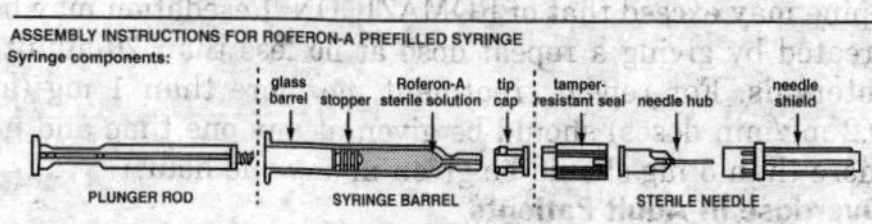

6. Assemble syringe:
   - Place the plunger rod into the open end of the syringe barrel.
   - Gently screw the rod into the plunger stopper until snug. DO NOT USE FORCE.

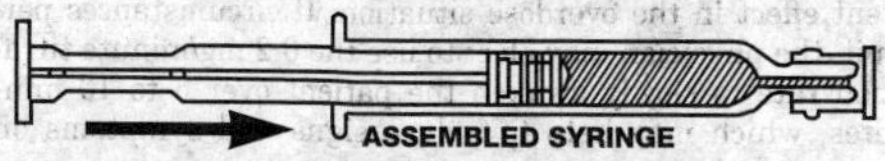

7. Prepare the needle:
   - Turn and pull off the bright yellow tamper-resistant seal from needle. A "click" sound means that the needle is OK to use.

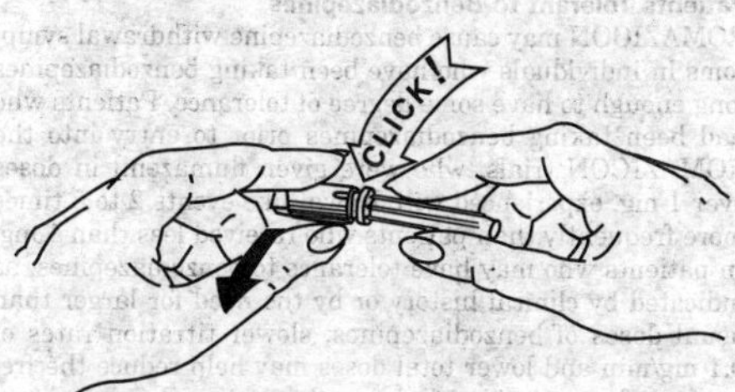

IF YOU DO NOT HEAR A "CLICK", DO NOT USE THE NEEDLE AND DO NOT REMOVE THE CLEAR NEEDLE SHIELD. DISCARD THE NEEDLE IN THE PUNCTURE-PROOF CONTAINER.

If you have another needle, proceed again with Step 7. If no alternate needle is available, contact your healthcare provider to make arrangements for a replacement needle.

8. To attach the needle to the prefilled syringe:

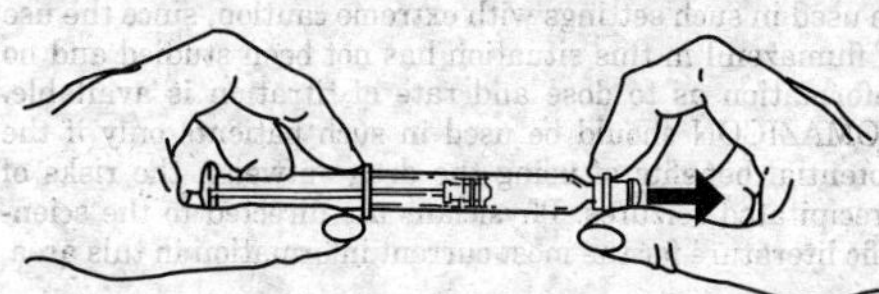

   - Remove the grey tip cap from syringe barrel.

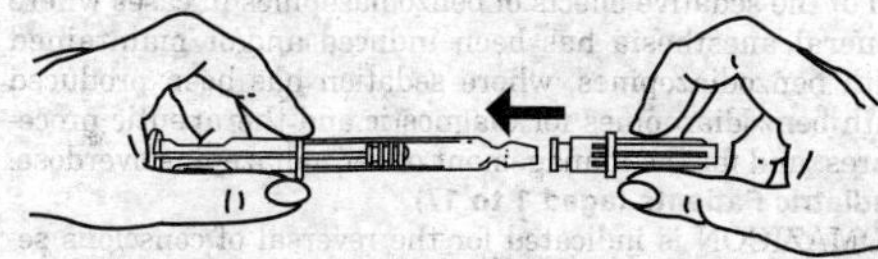

   - Place the needle onto the end of the syringe barrel so it fits snugly. Do not remove the clear needle shield.
9. Choose an injection site:
   - You should choose a different spot each time you give or receive an injection. The common sites to use are:
   - abdomen, avoiding the navel and waistline area
   - thigh
     [See first figure at top of next column]
   - If someone else is giving you the injection, then the upper, outer arm can be used as an injection site.
     [See second figure at top of next column]
10. Preparing the injection site:
    - Clean the skin where the injection will be given with an alcohol swab and allow the site to dry for 10 seconds.
11. Injecting Roferon-A:
    - Hold the pale yellow hub between your thumb and forefinger and carefully (to avoid a needle-stick) remove the clear needle shield with your other hand. The syringe is ready for injection.

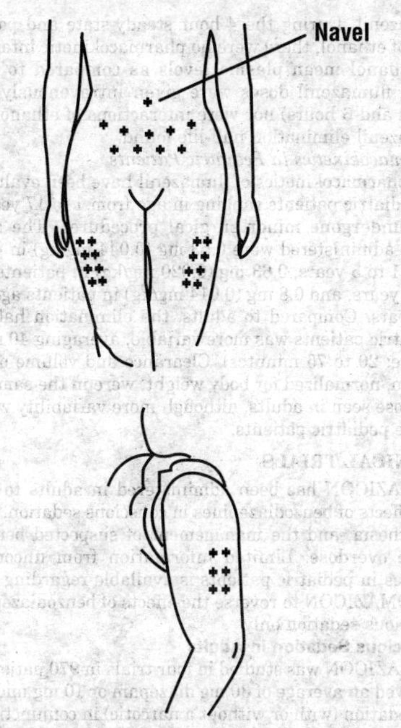

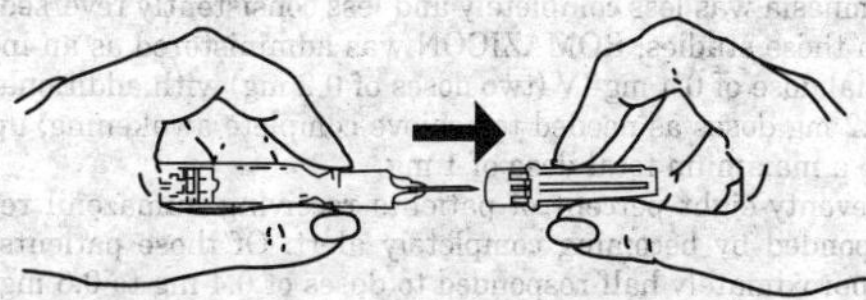

   - Keep the syringe in a horizontal position until ready for use.

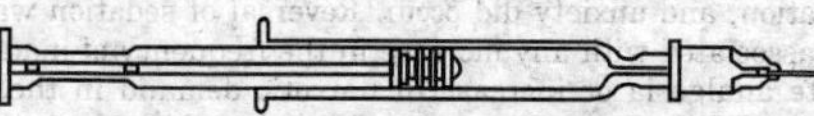

   - Holding the syringe with the needle facing up, tap the syringe barrel to bring air bubbles to the top.
   - Press the plunger slightly to push the air bubbles out through the needle.
   - Hold the syringe horizontally, and position the bevel of the needle so the point of the needle is facing up.

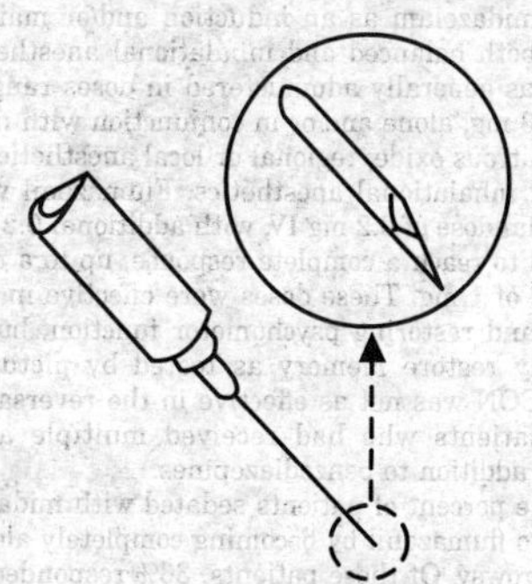

   - Pinch an area of skin firmly between your thumb and forefinger.

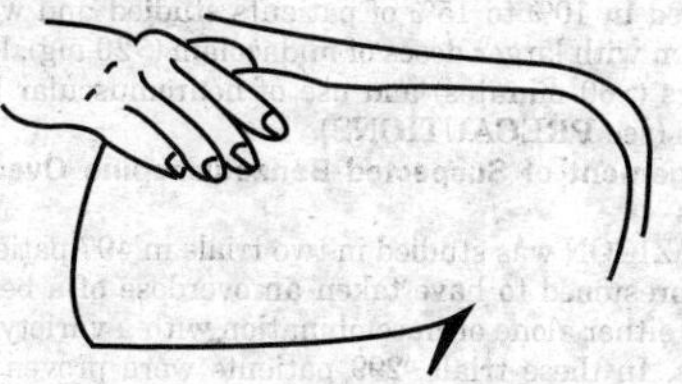

   - Hold the needle like a pencil at a 45° to 90° angle to skin and using a quick dart-like motion, insert the needle as far as it will go.

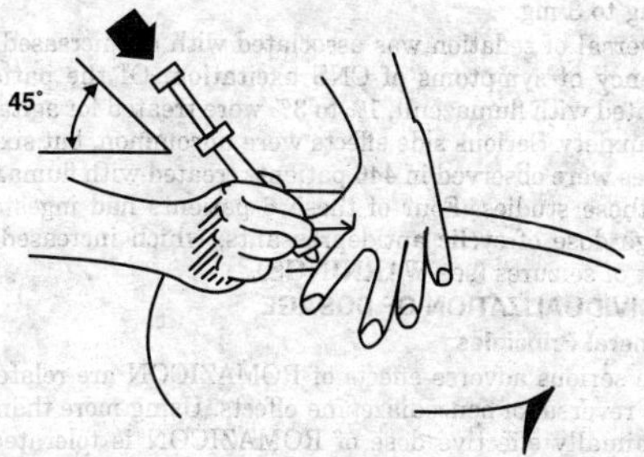

   - Once inserted, draw back slowly on the syringe. If blood appears in the syringe, the needle has entered a blood vessel.

Do not inject Roferon-A at that site and discard the syringe. Use a new syringe for the injection and use at a different injection site.

   - If blood does not appear in the syringe then slowly push the plunger all the way down so that you get all of your medicine.
   - Withdraw the needle at same angle it was inserted. See instructions for disposal of the needle and syringe in the section "How should I dispose of materials used to inject Roferon-A?".
   - When you are finished, place an alcohol swab over the injection site and press slightly.

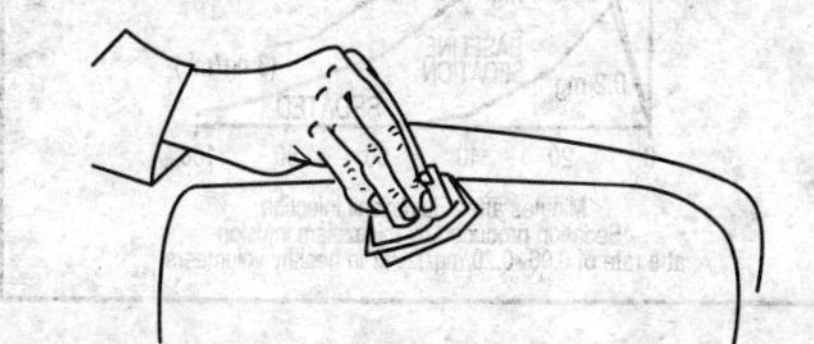

   - Do not reuse syringes and needles. Use a new prefilled syringe and needle for each injection.

How should I dispose of materials used to inject Roferon-A?

- Do not recap the needle.
- Place the entire syringe and needle in a puncture-resistant container. A home "Sharps Container" may be purchased at your pharmacy or you can use a hard plastic container with a screw top or a coffee can with a plastic lid. You should talk to your healthcare provider about how to properly dispose of a full container of used syringes. There may be special state or local laws about disposing used syringes and needles, so please check with your physician, nurse or pharmacist for instructions. DO NOT throw the filled container in the household trash and DO NOT recycle.
- The needle cover and alcohol swabs can be thrown in the regular trash. You should always keep your syringes and disposal container out of the reach of children.

Appendix revision date: September 2003

U.S. Govt. Lic. No. 0136

ROMAZICON® ℞

[ro-măs´ĕ-kŏn]

(flumazenil)

INJECTION

DESCRIPTION

ROMAZICON® (flumazenil) is a benzodiazepine receptor antagonist. Chemically, flumazenil is ethyl 8-fluoro-5,6-dihydro-5-methyl-6-oxo-4H-imidazo [1,5-a](1,4) benzodiazepine-3-carboxylate. Flumazenil has an imidazobenzodiazepine structure, a calculated molecular weight of 303.3. Flumazenil is a white to off-white crystalline compound with an octanol:buffer partition coefficient of 14 to 1 at pH 7.4. It is insoluble in water but slightly soluble in acidic aqueous solutions. ROMAZICON is available as a sterile parenteral dosage form for intravenous administration. Each mL contains 0.1 mg of flumazenil compounded with 1.8 mg of methylparaben, 0.2 mg of propylparaben, 0.9% sodium chloride, 0.01% edetate disodium, and 0.01% acetic acid; the pH is adjusted to approximately 4 with hydrochloric acid and/or, if necessary, sodium hydroxide.

CLINICAL PHARMACOLOGY

Flumazenil, an imidazobenzodiazepine derivative, antagonizes the actions of benzodiazepines on the central nervous system. Flumazenil competitively inhibits the activity at the benzodiazepine recognition site on the GABA/benzodiazepine receptor complex. Flumazenil is a weak partial agonist in some animal models of activity, but has little or no agonist activity in man.

Flumazenil does not antagonize the central nervous system effects of drugs affecting GABA-ergic neurons by means other than the benzodiazepine receptor (including ethanol, barbiturates, or general anesthetics) and does not reverse the effects of opioids.

In animals pretreated with high doses of benzodiazepines over several weeks, ROMAZICON elicited symptoms of benzodiazepine withdrawal, including seizures. A similar effect was seen in adult human subjects.

Pharmacodynamics:

Intravenous ROMAZICON has been shown to antagonize sedation, impairment of recall, psychomotor impairment and ventilatory depression produced by benzodiazepines in healthy human volunteers.

The duration and degree of reversal of sedative benzodiazepine effects are related to the dose and plasma concentrations of flumazenil as shown in the following data from a study in normal volunteers.

[See figure at top of next column]

Generally, doses of approximately 0.1 mg to 0.2 mg (corresponding to peak plasma levels of 3 to 6 ng/mL) produce partial antagonism, whereas higher doses of 0.4 to 1 mg (peak plasma levels of 12 to 28 ng/mL) usually produce complete antagonism in patients who have received the usual

Continued on next page

Romazicon—Cont.

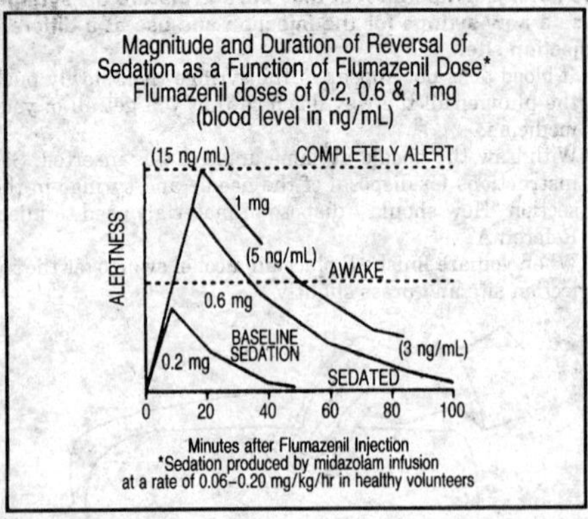

sedating doses of benzodiazepines. The onset of reversal is usually evident within 1 to 2 minutes after the injection is completed. Eighty percent response will be reached within 3 minutes, with the peak effect occurring at 6 to 10 minutes. The duration and degree of reversal are related to the plasma concentration of the sedating benzodiazepine as well as the dose of ROMAZICON given.

In healthy volunteers, ROMAZICON did not alter intraocular pressure when given alone and reversed the decrease in intraocular pressure seen after administration of midazolam.

Pharmacokinetics

After IV administration, plasma concentrations of flumazenil follow a two-exponential decay model. The pharmacokinetics of flumazenil are dose-proportional up to 100 mg.

Distribution

Flumazenil is extensively distributed in the extravascular space with an initial distribution half-life of 4 to 11 minutes and a terminal half-life of 40 to 80 minutes. Peak concentrations of flumazenil are proportional to dose, with an apparent initial volume of distribution of 0.5 L/kg. The volume of distribution at steady-state is 0.9 to 1.1 L/kg. Flumazenil is a weak lipophilic base. Protein binding is approximately 50% and the drug shows no preferential partitioning into red blood cells. Albumin accounts for two thirds of plasma protein binding.

Metabolism

Flumazenil is completely (99%) metabolized. Very little unchanged flumazenil (≤1%) is found in the urine. The major metabolites of flumazenil identified in urine are the deethylated free acid and its glucuronide conjugate. In preclinical studies there was no evidence of pharmacologic activity exhibited by the de-ethylated free acid.

Elimination

Elimination of radiolabeled drug is essentially complete within 72 hours, with 90% to 95% of the radioactivity appearing in urine and 5% to 10% in the feces. Clearance of flumazenil occurs primarily by hepatic metabolism and is dependent on hepatic blood flow. In pharmacokinetic studies of normal volunteers, total clearance ranged from 0.8 to 1.0 L/hr/kg.

Pharmacokinetic parameters following a 5-minute infusion of a total of 1 mg of ROMAZICON mean (coefficient of variation, range):

C_{max}(ng/mL)	24 (38%, 11-43)
AUC (ng·hr/mL)	15 (22%, 10-22)
V_{ss}(L/kg)	1 (24%, 0.8-1.6)
Cl (L/hr/kg)	1 (20%, 0.7-1.4)
Half-life (min)	54 (21%, 41-79)

Food Effects:

Ingestion of food during an intravenous infusion of the drug results in a 50% increase in clearance, most likely due to the increased hepatic blood flow that accompanies a meal.

Special Populations

The Elderly

The pharmacokinetics of flumazenil are not significantly altered in the elderly.

Gender

The pharmacokinetics of flumazenil are not different in male and female subjects.

Renal Failure (creatinine clearance <10 mL/min) and Hemodialysis

The pharmacokinetics of flumazenil are not significantly affected.

Patients With Liver Dysfunction

For patients with moderate liver dysfunction, their mean total clearance is decreased to 40% to 60% and in patients with severe liver dysfunction, it is decreased to 25% of normal value, compared with age-matched healthy subjects. This results in a prolongation of the half-life to 1.3 hours in patients with moderate hepatic impairment and 2.4 hours in severely impaired patients. Caution should be exercised with initial and/or repeated dosing to patients with liver disease.

Drug-Drug Interaction:

The pharmacokinetic profile of flumazenil is unaltered in the presence of benzodiazepine agonists and the kinetic profiles of those benzodiazepines studied (ie, diazepam, flunitrazepam, lormetazepam, and midazolam) are unaltered by flumazenil. During the 4-hour steady-state and post infusion of ethanol, there were no pharmacokinetic interactions on ethanol mean plasma levels as compared to placebo when flumazenil doses were given intravenously (at 2.5 hours and 6 hours) nor were interactions of ethanol on the flumazenil elimination half-life found.

Pharmacokinetics in Pediatric Patients

The pharmacokinetics of flumazenil have been evaluated in 29 pediatric patients ranging in age from 1 to 17 years who had undergone minor surgical procedures. The average doses administered were 0.53 mg (0.044 mg/kg) in patients aged 1 to 5 years, 0.63 mg (0.020 mg/kg) in patients aged 6 to 12 years, and 0.8 mg (0.014 mg/kg) in patients aged 13 to 17 years. Compared to adults, the elimination half-life in pediatric patients was more variable, averaging 40 minutes (range: 20 to 75 minutes). Clearance and volume of distribution, normalized for body weight, were in the same range as those seen in adults, although more variability was seen in the pediatric patients.

CLINICAL TRIALS

ROMAZICON has been administered in adults to reverse the effects of benzodiazepines in conscious sedation, general anesthesia, and the management of suspected benzodiazepine overdose. Limited information from uncontrolled studies in pediatric patients is available regarding the use of ROMAZICON to reverse the effects of benzodiazepines in conscious sedation only.

Conscious Sedation in Adults

ROMAZICON was studied in four trials in 970 patients who received an average of 30 mg diazepam or 10 mg midazolam for sedation (with or without a narcotic) in conjunction with both inpatient and outpatient diagnostic or surgical procedures. ROMAZICON was effective in reversing the sedating and psychomotor effects of the benzodiazepine; however, amnesia was less completely and less consistently reversed. In these studies, ROMAZICON was administered as an initial dose of 0.4 mg IV (two doses of 0.2 mg) with additional 0.2 mg doses as needed to achieve complete awakening, up to a maximum total dose of 1 mg.

Seventy-eight percent of patients receiving flumazenil responded by becoming completely alert. Of those patients, approximately half responded to doses of 0.4 mg to 0.6 mg, while the other half responded to doses of 0.8 mg to 1 mg. Adverse effects were infrequent in patients who received 1 mg of ROMAZICON or less, although injection site pain, agitation, and anxiety did occur. Reversal of sedation was not associated with any increase in the frequency of inadequate analgesia or increase in narcotic demand in these studies. While most patients remained alert throughout the 3-hour postprocedure observation period, resedation was observed to occur in 3% to 9% of the patients, and was most common in patients who had received high doses of benzodiazepines (see **PRECAUTIONS**).

General Anesthesia in Adults

ROMAZICON was studied in four trials in 644 patients who received midazolam as an induction and/or maintenance agent in both balanced and inhalational anesthesia. Midazolam was generally administered in doses ranging from 5 mg to 80 mg, alone and/or in conjunction with muscle relaxants, nitrous oxide, regional or local anesthetics, narcotics and/or inhalational anesthetics. Flumazenil was given as an initial dose of 0.2 mg IV, with additional 0.2 mg doses as needed to reach a complete response, up to a maximum total dose of 1 mg. These doses were effective in reversing sedation and restoring psychomotor function, but did not completely restore memory as tested by picture recall. ROMAZICON was not as effective in the reversal of sedation in patients who had received multiple anesthetic agents in addition to benzodiazepines.

Eighty-one percent of patients sedated with midazolam responded to flumazenil by becoming completely alert or just slightly drowsy. Of those patients, 36% responded to doses of 0.4 mg to 0.6 mg, while 64% responded to doses of 0.8 mg to 1 mg.

Resedation in patients who responded to ROMAZICON occurred in 10% to 15% of patients studied and was more common with larger doses of midazolam (>20 mg), long procedures (>60 minutes) and use of neuromuscular blocking agents (see **PRECAUTIONS**).

Management of Suspected Benzodiazepine Overdose in Adults

ROMAZICON was studied in two trials in 497 patients who were presumed to have taken an overdose of a benzodiazepine, either alone or in combination with a variety of other agents. In these trials, 299 patients were proven to have taken a benzodiazepine as part of the overdose, and 80% of the 148 who received ROMAZICON responded by an improvement in level of consciousness. Of the patients who responded to flumazenil, 75% responded to a total dose of 1 mg to 3 mg.

Reversal of sedation was associated with an increased frequency of symptoms of CNS excitation. Of the patients treated with flumazenil, 1% to 3% were treated for agitation or anxiety. Serious side effects were uncommon, but six seizures were observed in 446 patients treated with flumazenil in these studies. Four of these 6 patients had ingested a large dose of cyclic antidepressants, which increased the risk of seizures (see **WARNINGS**).

INDIVIDUALIZATION OF DOSAGE

General Principles

The serious adverse effects of ROMAZICON are related to the reversal of benzodiazepine effects. Using more than the minimally effective dose of ROMAZICON is tolerated by most patients but may complicate the management of patients who are physically dependent on benzodiazepines or patients who are depending on benzodiazepines for therapeutic effect (such as suppression of seizures in cyclic antidepressant overdose).

In high-risk patients, it is important to administer the smallest amount of ROMAZICON that is effective. The 1-minute wait between individual doses in the dose-titration recommended for general clinical populations may be too short for high-risk patients. This is because it takes 6 to 10 minutes for any single dose of flumazenil to reach full effects. Practitioners should slow the rate of administration of ROMAZICON administered to high-risk patients as recommended below.

Anesthesia and Conscious Sedation in Adult Patients

ROMAZICON is well tolerated at the recommended doses in individuals who have no tolerance to (or dependence on) benzodiazepines. The recommended doses and titration rates in anesthesia and conscious sedation (0.2 mg to 1 mg given at 0.2 mg/min) are well tolerated in patients receiving the drug for reversal of a single benzodiazepine exposure in most clinical settings (see **ADVERSE REACTIONS**). The major risk will be resedation because the duration of effect of a long-acting (or large dose of a short-acting) benzodiazepine may exceed that of ROMAZICON. Resedation may be treated by giving a repeat dose at no less than 20-minute intervals. For repeat treatment, no more than 1 mg (at 0.2 mg/min doses) should be given at any one time and no more than 3 mg should be given in any one hour.

Overdose in Adult Patients

The risk of confusion, agitation, emotional lability, and perceptual distortion with the doses recommended in patients with benzodiazepine overdose (3 mg to 5 mg administered as 0.5 mg/min) may be greater than that expected with lower doses and slower administration. The recommended doses represent a compromise between a desirable slow awakening and the need for prompt response and a persistent effect in the overdose situation. If circumstances permit, the physician may elect to use the 0.2 mg/minute titration rate to slowly awaken the patient over 5 to 10 minutes, which may help to reduce signs and symptoms on emergence.

ROMAZICON has no effect in cases where benzodiazepines are not responsible for sedation. Once doses of 3 mg to 5 mg have been reached without clinical response, additional ROMAZICON is likely to have no effect.

Patients Tolerant to Benzodiazepines

ROMAZICON may cause benzodiazepine withdrawal symptoms in individuals who have been taking benzodiazepines long enough to have some degree of tolerance. Patients who had been taking benzodiazepines prior to entry into the ROMAZICON trials, who were given flumazenil in doses over 1 mg, experienced withdrawal-like events 2 to 5 times more frequently than patients who received less than 1 mg.

In patients who may have tolerance to benzodiazepines, as indicated by clinical history or by the need for larger than usual doses of benzodiazepines, slower titration rates of 0.1 mg/min and lower total doses may help reduce the frequency of emergent confusion and agitation. In such cases, special care must be taken to monitor the patients for resedation because of the lower doses of ROMAZICON used.

Patients Physically Dependent on Benzodiazepines

ROMAZICON is known to precipitate withdrawal seizures in patients who are physically dependent on benzodiazepines, even if such dependence was established in a relatively few days of high-dose sedation in Intensive Care Unit (ICU) environments. The risk of either seizures or resedation in such cases is high and patients have experienced seizures before regaining consciousness. ROMAZICON should be used in such settings with extreme caution, since the use of flumazenil in this situation has not been studied and no information as to dose and rate of titration is available. ROMAZICON should be used in such patients only if the potential benefits of using the drug outweigh the risks of precipitated seizures. Physicians are directed to the scientific literature for the most current information in this area.

INDICATIONS AND USAGE

Adult Patients

ROMAZICON is indicated for the complete or partial reversal of the sedative effects of benzodiazepines in cases where general anesthesia has been induced and/or maintained with benzodiazepines, where sedation has been produced with benzodiazepines for diagnostic and therapeutic procedures, and for the management of benzodiazepine overdose.

Pediatric Patients (aged 1 to 17)

ROMAZICON is indicated for the reversal of conscious sedation induced with benzodiazepines (see **PRECAUTIONS: Pediatric Use**).

CONTRAINDICATIONS

ROMAZICON is contraindicated:

- in patients with a known hypersensitivity to flumazenil or benzodiazepines.
- in patients who have been given a benzodiazepine for control of a potentially life-threatening condition (eg, control of intracranial pressure or status epilepticus).
- in patients who are showing signs of serious cyclic antidepressant overdose (see **WARNINGS**).

WARNINGS

THE USE OF ROMAZICON HAS BEEN ASSOCIATED WITH THE OCCURRENCE OF SEIZURES.

THESE ARE MOST FREQUENT IN PATIENTS WHO HAVE BEEN ON BENZODIAZEPINES FOR LONG-TERM SEDATION OR IN OVERDOSE CASES WHERE PA-

TIENTS ARE SHOWING SIGNS OF SERIOUS CYCLIC ANTIDEPRESSANT OVERDOSE. PRACTITIONERS SHOULD INDIVIDUALIZE THE DOSAGE OF ROMAZICON AND BE PREPARED TO MANAGE SEIZURES.

Risk of Seizures

The reversal of benzodiazepine effects may be associated with the onset of seizures in certain high-risk populations. Possible risk factors for seizures include: concurrent major sedative-hypnotic drug withdrawal, recent therapy with repeated doses of parenteral benzodiazepines, myoclonic jerking or seizure activity prior to flumazenil administration in overdose cases, or concurrent cyclic antidepressant poisoning.

ROMAZICON is not recommended in cases of serious cyclic antidepressant poisoning, as manifested by motor abnormalities (twitching, rigidity, focal seizure), dysrhythmia (wide QRS, ventricular dysrhythmia, heart block), anticholinergic signs (mydriasis, dry mucosa, hypoperistalsis), and cardiovascular collapse at presentation. In such cases ROMAZICON should be withheld and the patient should be allowed to remain sedated (with ventilatory and circulatory support as needed) until the signs of antidepressant toxicity have subsided. Treatment with ROMAZICON has no known benefit to the seriously ill mixed-overdose patient other than reversing sedation and should not be used in cases where seizures (from any cause) are likely.

Most convulsions associated with flumazenil administration require treatment and have been successfully managed with benzodiazepines, phenytoin or barbiturates. Because of the presence of flumazenil, higher than usual doses of benzodiazepines may be required.

Hypoventilation

Patients who have received ROMAZICON for the reversal of benzodiazepine effects (after conscious sedation or general anesthesia) should be monitored for resedation, respiratory depression, or other residual benzodiazepine effects for an appropriate period (up to 120 minutes) based on the dose and duration of effect of the benzodiazepine employed.

This is because ROMAZICON has not been established in patients as an effective treatment for hypoventilation due to benzodiazepine administration. In healthy male volunteers, ROMAZICON is capable of reversing benzodiazepine-induced depression of the ventilatory responses to hypercapnia and hypoxia after a benzodiazepine alone. However, such depression may recur because the ventilatory effects of typical doses of ROMAZICON (1 mg or less) may wear off before the effects of many benzodiazepines. The effects of ROMAZICON on ventilatory response following sedation with a benzodiazepine in combination with an opioid are inconsistent and have not been adequately studied. The availability of flumazenil does not diminish the need for prompt detection of hypoventilation and the ability to effectively intervene by establishing an airway and assisting ventilation.

Overdose cases should always be monitored for resedation until the patients are stable and resedation is unlikely.

PRECAUTIONS

Return of Sedation

ROMAZICON may be expected to improve the alertness of patients recovering from a procedure involving sedation or anesthesia with benzodiazepines, but should not be substituted for an adequate period of postprocedure monitoring. The availability of ROMAZICON does not reduce the risks associated with the use of large doses of benzodiazepines for sedation.

Patients should be monitored for resedation, respiratory depression (see **WARNINGS**), or other persistent or recurrent agonist effects for an adequate period of time after administration of ROMAZICON.

Resedation is least likely in cases where ROMAZICON is administered to reverse a low dose of a short-acting benzodiazepine (<10 mg midazolam). It is most likely in cases where a large single or cumulative dose of a benzodiazepine has been given in the course of a long procedure along with neuromuscular blocking agents and multiple anesthetic agents.

Profound resedation was observed in 1% to 3% of adult patients in the clinical studies. In clinical situations where resedation must be prevented in adult patients, physicians may wish to repeat the initial dose (up to 1 mg of ROMAZICON given at 0.2 mg/min) at 30 minutes and possibly again at 60 minutes. This dosage schedule, although not studied in clinical trials, was effective in preventing resedation in a pharmacologic study in normal volunteers.

The use of ROMAZICON to reverse the effects of benzodiazepines used for conscious sedation has been evaluated in one open-label clinical trial involving 107 pediatric patients between the ages of 1 and 17 years. This study suggested that pediatric patients who have become fully awake following treatment with flumazenil may experience a recurrence of sedation, especially younger patients (ages 1 to 5). Resedation was experienced in 7 of 60 patients who were fully alert 10 minutes after the start of ROMAZICON administration. No patient experienced a return to the baseline level of sedation. Mean time to resedation was 25 minutes (range: 19 to 50 minutes) (see **PRECAUTIONS: Pediatric Use**). The safety and effectiveness of repeated flumazenil administration in pediatric patients experiencing resedation have not been established.

Use in the ICU

ROMAZICON should be used with caution in the ICU because of the increased risk of unrecognized benzodiazepine dependence in such settings. ROMAZICON may produce convulsions in patients physically dependent on benzodiazepines (see **INDIVIDUALIZATION OF DOSAGE** and **WARNINGS**).

Administration of ROMAZICON to diagnose benzodiazepine-induced sedation in the ICU is not recommended due to the risk of adverse events as described above. In addition, the prognostic significance of a patient's failure to respond to flumazenil in cases confounded by metabolic disorder, traumatic injury, drugs other than benzodiazepines, or any other reasons not associated with benzodiazepine receptor occupancy is unknown.

Use in Overdosage

ROMAZICON is intended as an adjunct to, not as a substitute for, proper management of airway, assisted breathing, circulatory access and support, internal decontamination by lavage and charcoal, and adequate clinical evaluation.

Necessary measures should be instituted to secure airway, ventilation and intravenous access prior to administering flumazenil. Upon arousal, patients may attempt to withdraw endotracheal tubes and/or intravenous lines as the result of confusion and agitation following awakening.

Head Injury

ROMAZICON should be used with caution in patients with head injury as it may be capable of precipitating convulsions or altering cerebral blood flow in patients receiving benzodiazepines. It should be used only by practitioners prepared to manage such complications should they occur.

Use With Neuromuscular Blocking Agents

ROMAZICON should not be used until the effects of neuromuscular blockade have been fully reversed.

Use in Psychiatric Patients

ROMAZICON has been reported to provoke panic attacks in patients with a history of panic disorder.

Pain on Injection

To minimize the likelihood of pain or inflammation at the injection site, ROMAZICON should be administered through a freely flowing intravenous infusion into a large vein. Local irritation may occur following extravasation into perivascular tissues.

Use in Respiratory Disease

The primary treatment of patients with serious lung disease who experience serious respiratory depression due to benzodiazepines should be appropriate ventilatory support (see **PRECAUTIONS**) rather than the administration of ROMAZICON. Flumazenil is capable of partially reversing benzodiazepine-induced alterations in ventilatory drive in healthy volunteers, but has not been shown to be clinically effective.

Use in Cardiovascular Disease

ROMAZICON did not increase the work of the heart when used to reverse benzodiazepines in cardiac patients when given at a rate of 0.1 mg/min in total doses of less than 0.5 mg in studies reported in the clinical literature. Flumazenil alone had no significant effects on cardiovascular parameters when administered to patients with stable ischemic heart disease.

Use in Liver Disease

The clearance of ROMAZICON is reduced to 40% to 60% of normal in patients with mild to moderate hepatic disease and to 25% of normal in patients with severe hepatic dysfunction (see **CLINICAL PHARMACOLOGY: Pharmacokinetics**). While the dose of flumazenil used for initial reversal of benzodiazepine effects is not affected, repeat doses of the drug in liver disease should be reduced in size or frequency.

Use in Drug- and Alcohol-Dependent Patients

ROMAZICON should be used with caution in patients with alcoholism and other drug dependencies due to the increased frequency of benzodiazepine tolerance and dependence observed in these patient populations.

ROMAZICON is not recommended either as a treatment for benzodiazepine dependence or for the management of protracted benzodiazepine abstinence syndromes, as such use has not been studied.

The administration of flumazenil can precipitate benzodiazepine withdrawal in animals and man. This has been seen in healthy volunteers treated with therapeutic doses of oral lorazepam for up to 2 weeks who exhibited effects such as hot flushes, agitation and tremor when treated with cumulative doses of up to 3 mg doses of flumazenil.

Similar adverse experiences suggestive of flumazenil precipitation of benzodiazepine withdrawal have occurred in some adult patients in clinical trials. Such patients had a short-lived syndrome characterized by dizziness, mild confusion, emotional lability, agitation (with signs and symptoms of anxiety), and mild sensory distortions. This response was dose-related, most common at doses above 1 mg, rarely required treatment other than reassurance and was usually short lived. When required, these patients (5 to 10 cases) were successfully treated with usual doses of a barbiturate, a benzodiazepine, or other sedative drug.

Practitioners should assume that flumazenil administration may trigger dose-dependent withdrawal syndromes in patients with established physical dependence on benzodiazepines and may complicate the management of withdrawal syndromes for alcohol, barbiturates and cross-tolerant sedatives.

Drug Interactions

Interaction with central nervous system depressants other than benzodiazepines has not been specifically studied; however, no deleterious interactions were seen when ROMAZICON was administered after narcotics, inhalational anesthetics, muscle relaxants and muscle relaxant antagonists administered in conjunction with sedation or anesthesia.

Particular caution is necessary when using ROMAZICON in cases of mixed drug overdosage since the toxic effects (such as convulsions and cardiac dysrhythmias) of other drugs taken in overdose (especially cyclic antidepressants) may emerge with the reversal of the benzodiazepine effect by flumazenil (see **WARNINGS**).

The use of ROMAZICON is not recommended in epileptic patients who have been receiving benzodiazepine treatment for a prolonged period. Although ROMAZICON exerts a slight intrinsic anticonvulsant effect, its abrupt suppression of the protective effect of a benzodiazepine agonist can give rise to convulsions in epileptic patients.

ROMAZICON blocks the central effects of benzodiazepines by competitive interaction at the receptor level. The effects of nonbenzodiazepine agonists at benzodiazepine receptors, such as zopiclone, triazolopyridazines and others, are also blocked by ROMAZICON.

The pharmacokinetics of benzodiazepines are unaltered in the presence of flumazeniland vice versa.

There is no pharmacokinetic interaction between ethanol and flumazenil.

Use in Ambulatory Patients

The effects of ROMAZICON may wear off before a long-acting benzodiazepine is completely cleared from the body. In general, if a patient shows no signs of sedation within 2 hours after a 1-mg dose of flumazenil, serious resedation at a later time is unlikely. An adequate period of observation must be provided for any patient in whom either long-acting benzodiazepines (such as diazepam) or large doses of short-acting benzodiazepines (such as >10 mg of midazolam) have been used (see **INDIVIDUALIZATION OF DOSAGE**).

Because of the increased risk of adverse reactions in patients who have been taking benzodiazepines on a regular basis, it is particularly important that physicians query patients or their guardians carefully about benzodiazepine, alcohol and sedative use as part of the history prior to any procedure in which the use of ROMAZICON is planned (see **PRECAUTIONS: Use in Drug- and Alcohol-Dependent Patients**).

Information for Patients

ROMAZICON does not consistently reverse amnesia. Patients cannot be expected to remember information told to them in the postprocedure period and instructions given to patients should be reinforced in writing or given to a responsible family member. Physicians are advised to discuss with patients or their guardians, both before surgery and at discharge, that although the patient may feel alert at the time of discharge, the effects of the benzodiazepine (eg, sedation) may recur. As a result, the patient should be instructed, preferably in writing, that their memory and judgment may be impaired and specifically advised:

1. Not to engage in any activities requiring complete alertness, and not to operate hazardous machinery or a motor vehicle during the first 24 hours after discharge, and it is certain no residual sedative effects of the benzodiazepine remain.
2. Not to take any alcohol or non-prescription drugs during the first 24 hours after flumazenil administration or if the effects of the benzodiazepine persist.

Laboratory Tests

No specific laboratory tests are recommended to follow the patient's response or to identify possible adverse reactions.

Drug/Laboratory Test Interactions

The possible interaction of flumazenil with commonly used laboratory tests has not been evaluated.

Carcinogenesis, Mutagenesis, Impairment of Fertility

Carcinogenesis

No studies in animals to evaluate the carcinogenic potential of flumazenil have been conducted.

Mutagenesis

No evidence for mutagenicity was noted in the Ames test using five different tester strains. Assays for mutagenic potential in *S. cerevisiae* D7 and in Chinese hamster cells were considered to be negative as were blastogenesis assays in vitro in peripheral human lymphocytes and in vivo in a mouse micronucleus assay. Flumazenil caused a slight increase in unscheduled DNA synthesis in rat hepatocyte culture at concentrations which were also cytotoxic; no increase in DNA repair was observed in male mouse germ cells in an in vivo DNA repair assay.

Impairment of Fertility

A reproduction study in male and female rats did not show any impairment of fertility at oral dosages of 125 mg/kg/day. From the available data on the area under the curve (AUC) in animals and man the dose represented 120× the human exposure from a maximum recommended intravenous dose of 5 mg.

Pregnancy

Pregnancy Category C

There are no adequate and well-controlled studies of the use of flumazenil in pregnant women. Flumazenil should be used during pregnancy only if the potential benefit justifies the potential risk to the fetus.

Teratogenic Effects

Flumazenil has been studied for teratogenicity in rats and rabbits following oral treatments of up to 150 mg/kg/day.

Continued on next page

Romazicon—Cont.

The treatments during the major organogenesis were on days 6 to 15 of gestation in the rat and days 6 to 18 of gestation in the rabbit. No teratogenic effects were observed in rats or rabbits at 150 mg/kg; the dose, based on the available data on the area under the plasma concentration-time curve (AUC) represented 120× to 600× the human exposure from a maximum recommended intravenous dose of 5 mg in humans. In rabbits, embryocidal effects (as evidenced by increased preimplantation and postimplantation losses) were observed at 50 mg/kg or 200× the human exposure from a maximum recommended intravenous dose of 5 mg. The no-effect dose of 15 mg/kg in rabbits represents 60× the human exposure.

Nonteratogenic Effects

An animal reproduction study was conducted in rats at oral dosages of 5, 25, and 125 mg/kg/day of flumazenil. Pup survival was decreased during the lactating period, pup liver weight at weaning was increased for the high-dose group (125 mg/kg/day) and incisor eruption and ear opening in the offspring were delayed; the delay in ear opening was associated with a delay in the appearance of the auditory startle response. No treatment-related adverse effects were noted for the other dose groups. Based on the available data from AUC, the effect level (125 mg/kg) represents 120× the human exposure from 5 mg, the maximum recommended intravenous dose in humans. The no-effect level represents 24× the human exposure from an intravenous dose of 5 mg.

Labor and Delivery

The use of ROMAZICON to reverse the effects of benzodiazepines used during labor and delivery is not recommended because the effects of the drug in the newborn are unknown.

Nursing Mothers

Caution should be exercised when deciding to administer ROMAZICON to a nursing woman because it is not known whether flumazenil is excreted in human milk.

Pediatric Use

The safety and effectiveness of ROMAZICON have been established in pediatric patients 1 year of age and older. Use of ROMAZICON in this age group is supported by evidence from adequate and well-controlled studies of ROMAZICON in adults with additional data from uncontrolled pediatric studies including one open-label trial.

The use of ROMAZICON to reverse the effects of benzodiazepines used for conscious sedation was evaluated in one uncontrolled clinical trial involving 107 pediatric patients between the ages of 1 and 17 years. At the doses used, ROMAZICON's safety was established in this population. Patients received up to 5 injections of 0.01 mg/kg flumazenil up to a maximum total dose of 1.0 mg at a rate not exceeding 0.2 mg/min.

Of 60 patients who were fully alert at 10 minutes, 7 experienced resedation. Resedation occurred between 19 and 50 minutes after the start of ROMAZICON administration. None of the patients experienced a return to the baseline level of sedation. All 7 patients were between the ages of 1 and 5 years. The types and frequency of adverse events noted in these pediatric patients were similar to those previously documented in clinical trials with ROMAZICON to reverse conscious sedation in adults. No patient experienced a serious adverse event attributable to flumazenil.

The safety and efficacy of ROMAZICON in the reversal of conscious sedation in pediatric patients below the age of 1 year have not been established (see **CLINICAL PHARMACOLOGY: Pharmacokinetics in Pediatric Patients**).

The safety and efficacy of ROMAZICON have not been established in pediatric patients for reversal of the sedative effects of benzodiazepines used for induction of general anesthesia, for the management of overdose, or for the resuscitation of the newborn, as no well-controlled clinical studies have been performed to determine the risks, benefits and dosages to be used. However, published anecdotal reports discussing the use of ROMAZICON in pediatric patients for these indications have reported similar safety profiles and dosing guidelines to those described for the reversal of conscious sedation.

The risks identified in the adult population with ROMAZICON use also apply to pediatric patients. Therefore, consult the **CONTRAINDICATIONS, WARNINGS, PRECAUTIONS**, and **ADVERSE REACTIONS** sections when using ROMAZICON in pediatric patients.

Geriatric Use

Of the total number of subjects in clinical studies of flumazenil, 248 were 65 and over. No overall differences in safety or effectiveness were observed between these subjects and younger subjects. Other reported clinical experience has not identified differences in responses between the elderly and younger patients, but greater sensitivity of some older individuals cannot be ruled out.

The pharmacokinetics of flumazenil have been studied in the elderly and are not significantly different from younger patients. Several studies of ROMAZICON in subjects over the age of 65 and one study in subjects over the age of 80 suggest that while the doses of benzodiazepine used to induce sedation should be reduced, ordinary doses of ROMAZICON may be used for reversal.

ADVERSE REACTIONS

Serious Adverse Reactions

Deaths have occurred in patients who received ROMAZICON in a variety of clinical settings. The majority of deaths occurred in patients with serious underlying disease or in patients who had ingested large amounts of non-benzodiazepine drugs (usually cyclic antidepressants), as part of an overdose.

Serious adverse events have occurred in all clinical settings, and convulsions are the most common serious adverse events reported. ROMAZICON administration has been associated with the onset of convulsions in patients with severe hepatic impairment and in patients who are relying on benzodiazepine effects to control seizures, are physically dependent on benzodiazepines, or who have ingested large doses of other drugs (mixed-drug overdose) (see **WARNINGS**).

Two of the 446 patients who received ROMAZICON in controlled clinical trials for the management of a benzodiazepine overdose had cardiac dysrhythmias (1 ventricular tachycardia, 1 junctional tachycardia).

Adverse Events in Clinical Studies

The following adverse reactions were considered to be related to ROMAZICON administration (both alone and for the reversal of benzodiazepine effects) and were reported in studies involving 1875 individuals who received flumazenil in controlled trials. Adverse events most frequently associated with flumazenil alone were limited to dizziness, injection site pain, increased sweating, headache, and abnormal or blurred vision (3% to 9%).

Body as a Whole: fatigue (asthenia, malaise), headache, injection site pain*, injection site reaction (thrombophlebitis, skin abnormality, rash)

Cardiovascular System: cutaneous vasodilation (sweating, flushing, hot flushes)

Digestive System: nausea, vomiting (11%)

Nervous System: agitation (anxiety, nervousness, dry mouth, tremor, palpitations, insomnia, dyspnea, hyperventilation)*, dizziness (vertigo, ataxia) (10%), emotional lability (crying abnormal, depersonalization, euphoria, increased tears, depression, dysphoria, paranoia)

Special Senses: abnormal vision (visual field defect, diplopia), paresthesia (sensation abnormal, hypoesthesia)

All adverse reactions occurred in 1% to 3% of cases unless otherwise marked.

*indicates reaction in 3% to 9% of cases.

Observed percentage reported if greater than 9%.

The following adverse events were observed infrequently (less than 1%) in the clinical studies, but were judged as probably related to ROMAZICON administration and/or reversal of benzodiazepine effects:

Nervous System: confusion (difficulty concentrating, delirium), convulsions (see **WARNINGS**), somnolence (stupor)

Special Senses: abnormal hearing (transient hearing impairment, hyperacusis, tinnitus)

The following adverse events occurred with frequencies less than 1% in the clinical trials. Their relationship to ROMAZICON administration is unknown, but they are included as alerting information for the physician.

Body as a Whole: rigors, shivering

Cardiovascular System: arrhythmia (atrial, nodal, ventricular extrasystoles), bradycardia, tachycardia, hypertension, chest pain

Digestive System: hiccup

Nervous System: speech disorder (dysphonia, thick tongue)

Not included in this list is operative site pain that occurred with the same frequency in patients receiving placebo as in patients receiving flumazenil for reversal of sedation following a surgical procedure.

Additional Adverse Reactions Reported During Postmarketing Experience

The following events have been reported during postapproval use of ROMAZICON.

Nervous System: Fear, panic attacks in patients with a history of panic disorders.

Withdrawal symptoms may occur following rapid injection of ROMAZICON in patients with long-term exposure to benzodiazepines.

DRUG ABUSE AND DEPENDENCE

ROMAZICON acts as a benzodiazepine antagonist, blocks the effects of benzodiazepines in animals and man, antagonizes benzodiazepine reinforcement in animal models, produces dysphoria in normal subjects, and has had no reported abuse in foreign marketing.

Although ROMAZICON has a benzodiazepine-like structure it does not act as a benzodiazepine agonist in man and is not a controlled substance.

OVERDOSAGE

Large intravenous doses (exceeding those recommended) of ROMAZICON, when administered to healthy normal volunteers in the absence of a benzodiazepine agonist, produced no serious adverse reactions, severe signs or symptoms, or clinically significant laboratory test abnormalities. In clinical studies, most adverse reactions to flumazenil were an extension of the pharmacologic effects of the drug in reversing benzodiazepine effects.

Reversal with an excessively high dose of ROMAZICON may produce anxiety, agitation, increased muscle tone, hyperesthesia and possibly convulsions. Convulsions have been treated with barbiturates, benzodiazepines and phenytoin, generally with prompt resolution of the seizures (see **WARNINGS**).

DOSAGE AND ADMINISTRATION

ROMAZICON is recommended for intravenous use only. It is compatible with 5% dextrose in water, lactated Ringer's and normal saline solutions. If ROMAZICON is drawn into a syringe or mixed with any of these solutions, it should be discarded after 24 hours. For optimum sterility, ROMAZICON should remain in the vial until just before use. As with all parenteral drug products, ROMAZICON should be inspected visually for particulate matter and discoloration prior to administration, whenever solution and container permit.

To minimize the likelihood of pain at the injection site, ROMAZICON should be administered through a freely running intravenous infusion into a large vein.

Reversal of Conscious Sedation

Adult Patients

For the reversal of the sedative effects of benzodiazepines administered for conscious sedation, the recommended initial dose of ROMAZICON is 0.2 mg (2 mL) administered intravenously over 15 seconds. If the desired level of consciousness is not obtained after waiting an additional 45 seconds, a second dose of 0.2 mg (2 mL) can be injected and repeated at 60-second intervals where necessary (up to a maximum of 4 additional times) to a maximum total dose of 1 mg (10 mL). The dosage should be individualized based on the patient's response, with most patients responding to doses of 0.6 mg to 1 mg (see **INDIVIDUALIZATION OF DOSAGE**).

In the event of resedation, repeated doses may be administered at 20-minute intervals as needed. For repeat treatment, no more than 1 mg (given as 0.2 mg/min) should be administered at any one time, and no more than 3 mg should be given in any one hour.

It is recommended that ROMAZICON be administered as the series of small injections described (not as a single bolus injection) to allow the practitioner to control the reversal of sedation to the approximate endpoint desired and to minimize the possibility of adverse effects (see **INDIVIDUALIZATION OF DOSAGE**).

Pediatric Patients

For the reversal of the sedative effects of benzodiazepines administered for conscious sedation in pediatric patients greater than 1 year of age, the recommended initial dose is 0.01 mg/kg (up to 0.2 mg) administered intravenously over 15 seconds. If the desired level of consciousness is not obtained after waiting an additional 45 seconds, further injections of 0.01 mg/kg (up to 0.2 mg) can be administered and repeated at 60-second intervals where necessary (up to a maximum of 4 additional times) to a maximum total dose of 0.05 mg/kg or 1 mg, whichever is lower. The dose should be individualized based on the patient's response. The mean total dose administered in the pediatric clinical trial of flumazenil was 0.65 mg (range: 0.08 mg to 1.00 mg). Approximately one-half of patients required the maximum of five injections.

Resedation occurred in 7 of 60 pediatric patients who were fully alert 10 minutes after the start of ROMAZICON administration (see **PRECAUTIONS: Pediatric Use**). The safety and efficacy of repeated flumazenil administration in pediatric patients experiencing resedation have not been established.

It is recommended that ROMAZICON be administered as the series of small injections described (not as a single bolus injection) to allow the practitioner to control the reversal of sedation to the approximate endpoint desired and to minimize the possibility of adverse effects (see **INDIVIDUALIZATION OF DOSAGE**).

The safety and efficacy of ROMAZICON in the reversal of conscious sedation in pediatric patients below the age of 1 year have not been established.

Reversal of General Anesthesia in Adult Patients

For the reversal of the sedative effects of benzodiazepines administered for general anesthesia, the recommended initial dose of ROMAZICON is 0.2 mg (2 mL) administered intravenously over 15 seconds. If the desired level of consciousness is not obtained after waiting an additional 45 seconds, a further dose of 0.2 mg (2 mL) can be injected and repeated at 60-second intervals where necessary (up to a maximum of 4 additional times) to a maximum total dose of 1 mg (10 mL). The dosage should be individualized based on the patient's response, with most patients responding to doses of 0.6 mg to 1 mg (see **INDIVIDUALIZATION OF DOSAGE**).

In the event of resedation, repeated doses may be administered at 20-minute intervals as needed. For repeat treatment, no more than 1 mg (given as 0.2 mg/min) should be administered at any one time, and no more than 3 mg should be given in any one hour.

It is recommended that ROMAZICON be administered as the series of small injections described (not as a single bolus injection) to allow the practitioner to control the reversal of sedation to the approximate endpoint desired and to minimize the possibility of adverse effects (see **INDIVIDUALIZATION OF DOSAGE**).

Management of Suspected Benzodiazepine Overdose in Adult Patients

For initial management of a known or suspected benzodiazepine overdose, the recommended initial dose of ROMAZICON is 0.2 mg (2 mL) administered intravenously over 30 seconds. If the desired level of consciousness is not obtained after waiting 30 seconds, a further dose of 0.3 mg (3 mL) can be administered over another 30 seconds. Further doses of 0.5 mg (5 mL) can be administered over 30 seconds at 1-minute intervals up to a cumulative dose of 3 mg.

Do not rush the administration of ROMAZICON. Patients should have a secure airway and intravenous access before administration of the drug and be awakened gradually (see **PRECAUTIONS**).

Most patients with a benzodiazepine overdose will respond to a cumulative dose of 1 mg to 3 mg of ROMAZICON, and doses beyond 3 mg do not reliably produce additional effects. On rare occasions, patients with a partial response at 3 mg may require additional titration up to a total dose of 5 mg (administered slowly in the same manner).

If a patient has not responded 5 minutes after receiving a cumulative dose of 5 mg of ROMAZICON, the major cause of sedation is likely not to be due to benzodiazepines, and additional ROMAZICON is likely to have no effect.

In the event of resedation, repeated doses may be given at 20-minute intervals if needed. For repeat treatment, no more than 1 mg (given as 0.5 mg/min) should be given at any one time and no more than 3 mg should be given in any one hour.

Safety and Handling

ROMAZICON is supplied in sealed dosage forms and poses no known risk to the healthcare provider. Routine care should be taken to avoid aerosol generation when preparing syringes for injection, and spilled medication should be rinsed from the skin with cool water.

HOW SUPPLIED

5 mL multiple-use vials containing 0.1 mg/mL flumazenil — boxes of 10 (NDC 0004-6911-06); 10 mL multiple-use vials containing 0.1 mg/mL flumazenil — boxes of 10 (NDC 0004-6912-06).

Storage

Store at 25° (77°F); excursions permitted to 15° to 30°C (59° to 86°F) [See USP Controlled Room Temperature].

Revised: December 2003

TAMIFLU® ℞

[*tă-mĭ-flew*]

(oseltamivir phosphate)
CAPSULES
AND FOR ORAL SUSPENSION

DESCRIPTION

TAMIFLU (oseltamivir phosphate) is available as a capsule containing 75 mg oseltamivir for oral use, in the form of oseltamivir phosphate, and as a powder for oral suspension, which when constituted with water as directed contains 12 mg/mL oseltamivir base. In addition to the active ingredient, each capsule contains pregelatinized starch, talc, povidone K 30, croscarmellose sodium, and sodium stearyl fumarate. The capsule shell contains gelatin, titanium dioxide, yellow iron oxide, black iron oxide, and red iron oxide. Each capsule is printed with blue ink, which includes FD&C Blue No. 2 as the colorant. In addition to the active ingredient, the powder for oral suspension contains xanthan gum, monosodium citrate, sodium benzoate, sorbitol, saccharin sodium, titanium dioxide, and tutti-frutti flavoring.

Oseltamivir phosphate is a white crystalline solid with the chemical name (3R,4R,5S)-4-acetylamino-5-amino-3(1-ethylpropoxy)-1-cyclohexene-1-carboxylic acid, ethyl ester, phosphate (1:1). The chemical formula is $C_{16}H_{28}N_2O_4$ (free base). The molecular weight is 312.4 for oseltamivir free base and 410.4 for oseltamivir phosphate salt.

MICROBIOLOGY

Mechanism of Action

Oseltamivir is an ethyl ester prodrug requiring ester hydrolysis for conversion to the active form, oseltamivir carboxylate. The proposed mechanism of action of oseltamivir is inhibition of influenza virus neuraminidase with the possibility of alteration of virus particle aggregation and release.

Antiviral Activity In Vitro

The antiviral activity of oseltamivir carboxylate against laboratory strains and clinical isolates of influenza virus was determined in cell culture assays. The concentrations of oseltamivir carboxylate required for inhibition of influenza virus were highly variable depending on the assay method used and the virus tested. The 50% and 90% inhibitory concentrations (IC_{50} and IC_{90}) were in the range of 0.0008 μM to >35 μM and 0.004 μM to >100 μM, respectively (1 μM=0.284 μg/mL). The relationship between the in vitro antiviral activity in cell culture and the inhibition of influenza virus replication in humans has not been established.

Resistance

Influenza A virus isolates with reduced susceptibility to oseltamivir carboxylate have been recovered in vitro by passage of virus in the presence of increasing concentrations of oseltamivir carboxylate. Genetic analysis of these isolates showed that reduced susceptibility to oseltamivir carboxylate is associated with mutations that result in amino acid changes in the viral neuraminidase or viral hemagglutinin or both. Resistance mutations selected in vitro in neuraminidase are I222T and H274Y in influenza A N1 and I222T and R292K in influenza A N2. Mutations E119V, R292K and R305Q have been selected in avian influenza A neuraminidase N9. Mutations A28T and R124M have been selected in the hemagglutinin of influenza A H3N2 and mutation H154Q in the hemagglutinin of a reassortant human/avian virus H1N9.

In clinical studies in the treatment of naturally acquired infection with influenza virus, 1.3% (4/301) of posttreatment isolates in adult patients and adolescents, and 8.6% (9/105) in pediatric patients aged 1 to 12 years showed emergence of influenza variants with decreased neuraminidase susceptibility in vitro to oseltamivir carboxylate. Mutations in influenza A resulting in decreased susceptibility were H274Y in neuraminidase N1 and E119V and R292K in neuraminidase N2. Insufficient information is available to fully characterize the risk of emergence of TAMIFLU resistance in clinical use.

In clinical studies of postexposure and seasonal prophylaxis, determination of resistance was limited by the low overall incidence rate of influenza infection and prophylactic effect of TAMIFLU.

Cross-resistance

Cross-resistance between zanamivir-resistant influenza mutants and oseltamivir-resistant influenza mutants has been observed in vitro. Due to limitations in the assays available to detect drug-induced shifts in virus susceptibility, an estimate of the incidence of oseltamivir resistance and possible cross-resistance to zanamivir in clinical isolates cannot be made. However, two of the three oseltamivir-induced mutations (E119V, H274Y and R292K) in the viral neuraminidase from clinical isolates occur at the same amino acid residues as two of the three mutations (E119G/A/D, R152K and R292K) observed in zanamivir-resistant virus.

Immune Response

No influenza vaccine interaction study has been conducted. In studies of naturally acquired and experimental influenza, treatment with TAMIFLU did not impair normal humoral antibody response to infection.

CLINICAL PHARMACOLOGY

Pharmacokinetics

Absorption and Bioavailability

Oseltamivir is readily absorbed from the gastrointestinal tract after oral administration of oseltamivir phosphate and is extensively converted predominantly by hepatic esterases to oseltamivir carboxylate. At least 75% of an oral dose reaches the systemic circulation as oseltamivir carboxylate. Exposure to oseltamivir is less than 5% of the total exposure after oral dosing (Table 1).

[See table 1 above]

Table 1. Mean (% CV) Pharmacokinetic Parameters of Oseltamivir and Oseltamivir Carboxylate After a Multiple 75 mg Capsule Twice Daily Oral Dose (n=20)

Parameter	Oseltamivir	Oseltamivir Carboxylate
C_{max} (ng/mL)	65.2 (26)	348 (18)
AUC_{0-12h} (ng•h/mL)	112 (25)	2719 (20)

Plasma concentrations of oseltamivir carboxylate are proportional to doses up to 500 mg given twice daily (see **DOSAGE AND ADMINISTRATION**).

Coadministration with food has no significant effect on the peak plasma concentration (551 ng/mL under fasted conditions and 441 ng/mL under fed conditions) and the area under the plasma concentration time curve (6218 ng•h/mL under fasted conditions and 6069 ng•h/mL under fed conditions) of oseltamivir carboxylate.

Distribution

The volume of distribution (V_{ss}) of oseltamivir carboxylate, following intravenous administration in 24 subjects, ranged between 23 and 26 liters.

The binding of oseltamivir carboxylate to human plasma protein is low (3%). The binding of oseltamivir to human plasma protein is 42%, which is insufficient to cause significant displacement-based drug interactions.

Metabolism

Oseltamivir is extensively converted to oseltamivir carboxylate by esterases located predominantly in the liver. Neither oseltamivir nor oseltamivir carboxylate is a substrate for, or inhibitor of, cytochrome P450 isoforms.

Elimination

Absorbed oseltamivir is primarily (>90%) eliminated by conversion to oseltamivir carboxylate. Plasma concentrations of oseltamivir declined with a half-life of 1 to 3 hours in most subjects after oral administration. Oseltamivir carboxylate is not further metabolized and is eliminated in the urine. Plasma concentrations of oseltamivir carboxylate declined with a half-life of 6 to 10 hours in most subjects after oral administration. Oseltamivir carboxylate is eliminated entirely (>99%) by renal excretion. Renal clearance (18.8 L/h) exceeds glomerular filtration rate (7.5 L/h) indicating that tubular secretion occurs, in addition to glomerular filtration. Less than 20% of an oral radiolabeled dose is eliminated in feces.

Special Populations

Renal Impairment

Administration of 100 mg of oseltamivir phosphate twice daily for 5 days to patients with various degrees of renal impairment showed that exposure to oseltamivir carboxylate is inversely proportional to declining renal function. Oseltamivir carboxylate exposures in patients with normal and abnormal renal function administered various dose regimens of oseltamivir are described in Table 2.

[See table 2 above]

Table 2. Oseltamivir Carboxylate Exposures in Patients With Normal and Reduced Serum Creatinine Clearance

Parameter	Normal Renal Function			Impaired Renal Function				
	75 mg qd	75 mg bid	150 mg bid	Creatinine Clearance <10 mL/min		Creatinine Clearance >10 and <30 mL/min		
				CAPD	Hemodialysis			
				30 mg weekly	30 mg alternate HD cycle	75 mg daily	75 mg alternate days	30 mg daily
C_{max}	259*	348*	705*	766	850	1638	1175	655
C_{min}	39*	138*	288*	62	48	864	209	346
AUC_{48}	7476*	10876*	21864*	17381	12429	62636	21999	25054

*Observed values. All other values are predicted.
AUC normalized to 48 hours.

Pediatric Patients

The pharmacokinetics of oseltamivir and oseltamivir carboxylate have been evaluated in a single dose pharmacokinetic study in pediatric patients aged 5 to 16 years (n=18) and in a small number of pediatric patients aged 3 to 12 years (n=5) enrolled in a clinical trial. Younger pediatric patients cleared both the prodrug and the active metabolite faster than adult patients resulting in a lower exposure for a given mg/kg dose. For oseltamivir carboxylate, apparent total clearance decreases linearly with increasing age (up to 12 years). The pharmacokinetics of oseltamivir in pediatric patients over 12 years of age are similar to those in adult patients.

Geriatric Patients

Exposure to oseltamivir carboxylate at steady-state was 25% to 35% higher in geriatric patients (age range 65 to 78 years) compared to young adults given comparable doses of oseltamivir. Half-lives observed in the geriatric patients were similar to those seen in young adults. Based on drug exposure and tolerability, dose adjustments are not required for geriatric patients for either treatment or prophylaxis (see **DOSAGE AND ADMINISTRATION: Special Dosage Instructions**).

INDICATIONS AND USAGE

Treatment of Influenza

TAMIFLU is indicated for the treatment of uncomplicated acute illness due to influenza infection in patients 1 year and older who have been symptomatic for no more than 2 days.

Prophylaxis of Influenza

TAMIFLU is indicated for the prophylaxis of influenza in adult patients and adolescents 13 years and older.

TAMIFLU is not a substitute for early vaccination on an annual basis as recommended by the Centers for Disease Control's Immunization Practices Advisory Committee.

Description of Clinical Studies: Studies in Naturally Occurring Influenza

Treatment of Influenza

Adult Patients

Two phase III placebo-controlled and double-blind clinical trials were conducted: one in the USA and one outside the USA. Patients were eligible for these trials if they had fever >100°F, accompanied by at least one respiratory symptom (cough, nasal symptoms or sore throat) and at least one systemic symptom (myalgia, chills/sweats, malaise, fatigue or headache) and influenza virus was known to be circulating in the community. In addition, all patients enrolled in the trials were allowed to take fever-reducing medications.

Of 1355 patients enrolled in these two trials, 849 (63%) patients were influenza-infected (age range 18 to 65 years; median age 34 years; 52% male; 90% Caucasian; 31% smokers). Of the 849 influenza-infected patients, 95% were infected with influenza A, 3% with influenza B, and 2% with influenza of unknown type.

TAMIFLU was started within 40 hours of onset of symptoms. Subjects participating in the trials were required to self-assess the influenza-associated symptoms as "none", "mild", "moderate" or "severe". Time to improvement was calculated from the time of treatment initiation to the time

Continued on next page

Tamiflu—Cont.

when all symptoms (nasal congestion, sore throat, cough, aches, fatigue, headaches, and chills/sweats) were assessed as "none" or "mild". In both studies, at the recommended dose of TAMIFLU 75 mg twice daily for 5 days, there was a 1.3 day reduction in the median time to improvement in influenza-infected subjects receiving TAMIFLU compared to subjects receiving placebo. Subgroup analyses of these studies by gender showed no differences in the treatment effect of TAMIFLU in men and women.

In the treatment of influenza, no increased efficacy was demonstrated in subjects receiving treatment of 150 mg TAMIFLU twice daily for 5 days.

Geriatric Patients

Three double-blind placebo-controlled treatment trials were conducted in patients ≥65 years of age in three consecutive seasons. The enrollment criteria were similar to that of adult trials with the exception of fever being defined as >97.5°F. Of 741 patients enrolled, 476 (65%) patients were influenza-infected. Of the 476 influenza-infected patients, 95% were infected with influenza type A and 5% with influenza type B.

In the pooled analysis, at the recommended dose of TAMIFLU 75 mg twice daily for 5 days, there was a 1 day reduction in the median time to improvement in influenza-infected subjects receiving TAMIFLU compared to those receiving placebo (p=NS). However, the magnitude of treatment effect varied between studies.

Pediatric Patients

One double-blind placebo-controlled treatment trial was conducted in pediatric patients aged 1 to 12 years (median age 5 years), who had fever (>100°F) plus one respiratory symptom (cough or coryza) when influenza virus was known to be circulating in the community. Of 698 patients enrolled in this trial, 452 (65%) were influenza-infected (50% male; 68% Caucasian). Of the 452 influenza-infected patients, 67% were infected with influenza A and 33% with influenza B.

The primary endpoint in this study was the time to freedom from illness, a composite endpoint which required 4 individual conditions to be met. These were: alleviation of cough, alleviation of coryza, resolution of fever, and parental opinion of a return to normal health and activity. TAMIFLU treatment of 2 mg/kg twice daily, started within 48 hours of onset of symptoms, significantly reduced the total composite time to freedom from illness by 1.5 days compared to placebo. Subgroup analyses of this study by gender showed no differences in the treatment effect of TAMIFLU in males and females.

Prophylaxis of Influenza

The efficacy of TAMIFLU in preventing naturally occurring influenza illness has been demonstrated in three seasonal prophylaxis studies and a postexposure prophylaxis study in households. The primary efficacy parameter for all these studies was the incidence of laboratory confirmed clinical influenza. Laboratory confirmed clinical influenza was defined as oral temperature ≥99.0°F/37.2°C plus at least one respiratory symptom (cough, sore throat, nasal congestion) and at least one constitutional symptom (aches and pain, fatigue, headache, chills/sweats), all recorded within 24 hours, plus either a positive virus isolation or a fourfold increase in virus antibody titers from baseline.

In a pooled analysis of two seasonal prophylaxis studies in healthy unvaccinated adults (aged 13 to 65 years), TAMIFLU 75 mg once daily taken for 42 days during a community outbreak reduced the incidence of laboratory confirmed clinical influenza from 4.8% (25/519) for the placebo group to 1.2% (6/520) for the TAMIFLU group.

In a seasonal prophylaxis study in elderly residents of skilled nursing homes, TAMIFLU 75 mg once daily taken for 42 days reduced the incidence of laboratory confirmed clinical influenza from 4.4% (12/272) for the placebo group to 0.4% (1/276) for the TAMIFLU group. About 80% of this elderly population were vaccinated, 14% of subjects had chronic airway obstructive disorders, and 43% had cardiac disorders.

In a study of postexposure prophylaxis in household contacts (aged ≥13 years) of an index case, TAMIFLU 75 mg once daily administered within 2 days of onset of symptoms in the index case and continued for 7 days reduced the incidence of laboratory confirmed clinical influenza from 12% (24/200) in the placebo group to 1% (2/205) for the TAMIFLU group. Index cases did not receive TAMIFLU in the study.

CONTRAINDICATIONS

TAMIFLU is contraindicated in patients with known hypersensitivity to any of the components of the product.

PRECAUTIONS

General

There is no evidence for efficacy of TAMIFLU in any illness caused by agents other than influenza viruses Types A and B.

Use of TAMIFLU should not affect the evaluation of individuals for annual influenza vaccination in accordance with guidelines of the Centers for Disease Control and Prevention Advisory Committee on Immunization Practices.

Efficacy of TAMIFLU in patients who begin treatment after 40 hours of symptoms has not been established.

Efficacy of TAMIFLU in the treatment of subjects with chronic cardiac disease and/or respiratory disease has not been established. No difference in the incidence of complications was observed between the treatment and placebo groups in this population. No information is available regarding treatment of influenza in patients with any medical condition sufficiently severe or unstable to be considered at imminent risk of requiring hospitalization.

Safety and efficacy of repeated treatment or prophylaxis courses have not been studied.

Efficacy of TAMIFLU for treatment or prophylaxis has not been established in immunocompromised patients.

Serious bacterial infections may begin with influenza-like symptoms or may coexist with or occur as complications during the course of influenza. TAMIFLU has not been shown to prevent such complications.

Hepatic Impairment

The safety and pharmacokinetics in patients with hepatic impairment have not been evaluated.

Renal Impairment

Dose adjustment is recommended for patients with a serum creatinine clearance <30 mL/min (see **DOSAGE AND ADMINISTRATION**).

Information for Patients

Patients should be instructed to begin treatment with TAMIFLU as soon as possible from the first appearance of flu symptoms. Similarly, prevention should begin as soon as possible after exposure, at the recommendation of a physician.

Patients should be instructed to take any missed doses as soon as they remember, except if it is near the next scheduled dose (within 2 hours), and then continue to take TAMIFLU at the usual times.

TAMIFLU is not a substitute for a flu vaccination. Patients should continue receiving an annual flu vaccination according to guidelines on immunization practices.

Drug Interactions

Information derived from pharmacology and pharmacokinetic studies of oseltamivir suggests that clinically significant drug interactions are unlikely.

Oseltamivir is extensively converted to oseltamivir carboxylate by esterases, located predominantly in the liver. Drug interactions involving competition for esterases have not been extensively reported in literature. Low protein binding of oseltamivir and oseltamivir carboxylate suggests that the probability of drug displacement interactions is low.

In vitro studies demonstrate that neither oseltamivir nor oseltamivir carboxylate is a good substrate for P450 mixed-function oxidases or for glucuronyl transferases.

Cimetidine, a non-specific inhibitor of cytochrome P450 isoforms and competitor for renal tubular secretion of basic or cationic drugs, has no effect on plasma levels of oseltamivir or oseltamivir carboxylate.

Clinically important drug interactions involving competition for renal tubular secretion are unlikely due to the known safety margin for most of these drugs, the elimination characteristics of oseltamivir carboxylate (glomerular filtration and anionic tubular secretion) and the excretion capacity of these pathways. Coadministration of probenecid results in an approximate twofold increase in exposure to oseltamivir carboxylate due to a decrease in active anionic tubular secretion in the kidney. However, due to the safety margin of oseltamivir carboxylate, no dose adjustments are required when coadministering with probenecid.

Coadministration with amoxicillin does not alter plasma levels of either compound, indicating that competition for the anionic secretion pathway is weak.

In six subjects, multiple doses of oseltamivir did not affect the single-dose pharmacokinetics of acetaminophen.

Carcinogenesis, Mutagenesis, and Impairment of Fertility

Long-term carcinogenicity tests with oseltamivir are underway but have not been completed. However, a 26-week dermal carcinogenicity study of oseltamivir carboxylate in FVB/Tg.AC transgenic mice was negative. The animals were dosed at 40, 140, 400 or 780 mg/kg/day in two divided doses. The highest dose represents the maximum feasible dose based on the solubility of the compound in the control vehicle. A positive control, tetradecanoyl phorbol-13-acetate administered at 2.5 µg per dose three times per week gave a positive response.

Oseltamivir was found to be non-mutagenic in the Ames test and the human lymphocyte chromosome assay with and without enzymatic activation and negative in the mouse micronucleus test. It was found to be positive in a Syrian Hamster Embryo (SHE) cell transformation test. Oseltamivir carboxylate was non-mutagenic in the Ames test and the L5178Y mouse lymphoma assay with and without enzymatic activation and negative in the SHE cell transformation test.

In a fertility and early embryonic development study in rats, doses of oseltamivir at 50, 250, and 1500 mg/kg/day were administered to females for 2 weeks before mating, during mating and until day 6 of pregnancy. Males were dosed for 4 weeks before mating, during and for 2 weeks after mating. There were no effects on fertility, mating performance or early embryonic development at any dose level. The highest dose was approximately 100 times the human systemic exposure (AUC_{0-24h}) of oseltamivir carboxylate.

Pregnancy

Pregnancy Category C: There are insufficient human data upon which to base an evaluation of risk of TAMIFLU to the pregnant woman or developing fetus. Studies for effects on embryo-fetal development were conducted in rats (50, 250, and 1500 mg/kg/day) and rabbits (50, 150, and 500 mg/kg/day) by the oral route. Relative exposures at these doses were, respectively, 2, 13, and 100 times human exposure in the rat and 4, 8, and 50 times human exposure in the rabbit. Pharmacokinetic studies indicated that fetal exposure was seen in both species. In the rat study, minimal maternal toxicity was reported in the 1500 mg/kg/day group. In the rabbit study, slight and marked maternal toxicities were observed, respectively, in the 150 and 500 mg/kg/day groups. There was a dose-dependent increase in the incidence rates of a variety of minor skeletal abnormalities and variants in the exposed offspring in these studies. However, the individual incidence rate of each skeletal abnormality or variant remained within the background rates of occurrence in the species studied.

Because animal reproductive studies may not be predictive of human response and there are no adequate and well-controlled studies in pregnant women, TAMIFLU should be used during pregnancy only if the potential benefit justifies the potential risk to the fetus.

Nursing Mothers

In lactating rats, oseltamivir and oseltamivir carboxylate are excreted in the milk. It is not known whether oseltamivir or oseltamivir carboxylate is excreted in human milk. TAMIFLU should, therefore, be used only if the potential benefit for the lactating mother justifies the potential risk to the breast-fed infant.

Geriatric Use

The safety of TAMIFLU has been established in clinical studies which enrolled 741 subjects (374 received placebo and 362 received TAMIFLU). Some seasonal variability was noted in the clinical efficacy outcomes (see **Description of Clinical Studies: Studies in Naturally Occurring Influenza: Treatment of Influenza:** Geriatric Patients).

Safety and efficacy have been demonstrated in elderly residents of nursing homes who took TAMIFLU for up to 42 days for the prevention of influenza. Many of these individuals had cardiac and/or respiratory disease, and most had received vaccine that season (see **Description of Clinical Studies: Studies in Naturally Occurring Influenza: Prophylaxis of Influenza**).

Pediatric Use

The safety and efficacy of TAMIFLU in pediatric patients younger than 1 year of age have not been studied. TAMIFLU is not indicated for either treatment or prophylaxis of influenza in pediatric patients younger than 1 year of age because of uncertainties regarding the rate of development of the human blood-brain barrier and the unknown clinical significance of non-clinical animal toxicology data for human infants (see **ANIMAL TOXICOLOGY**).

ANIMAL TOXICOLOGY

In a 2-week study in unweaned rats, administration of a single dose of 1000 mg/kg oseltamivir phosphate to 7-day-old rats resulted in deaths associated with unusually high exposure to the prodrug. However, at 2000 mg/kg, there were no deaths or other significant effects in 14-day-old unweaned rats. Further follow-up investigations of the unexpected deaths of 7-day-old rats at 1000 mg/kg revealed that the concentrations of the prodrug in the brains were approximately 1500-fold those of the brains of adult rats administered the same oral dose of 1000 mg/kg, and those of the active metabolite were approximately 3-fold higher. Plasma levels of the prodrug were 10-fold higher in 7-day-old rats as compared with adult rats. These observations suggest that the levels of oseltamivir in the brains of rats decrease with increasing age and most likely reflect the maturation stage of the blood-brain barrier. No adverse effects occurred at 500 mg/kg/day administered to 7- to 21-day-old rats. At this dosage, the exposure to prodrug was approximately 800-fold the exposure expected in a 1-year-old child.

ADVERSE REACTIONS

Treatment Studies in Adult Patients

A total of 1171 patients who participated in adult phase III controlled clinical trials for the treatment of influenza were treated with TAMIFLU. The most frequently reported adverse events in these studies were nausea and vomiting. These events were generally of mild to moderate degree and usually occurred on the first 2 days of administration. Less than 1% of subjects discontinued prematurely from clinical trials due to nausea and vomiting.

Adverse events that occurred with an incidence of ≥1% in 1440 patients taking placebo or TAMIFLU 75 mg twice daily in adult phase III treatment studies are shown in Table 3. This summary includes 945 healthy young adults and 495 "at risk" patients (elderly patients and patients with chronic cardiac or respiratory disease). Those events reported numerically more frequently in patients taking TAMIFLU compared with placebo were nausea, vomiting, bronchitis, insomnia, and vertigo.

[See table 3 at top of next page]

Adverse events included are: all events reported in the treatment studies with frequency ≥1% in the oseltamivir 75 mg bid group.

Additional adverse events occurring in <1% of patients receiving TAMIFLU for treatment included unstable angina, anemia, pseudomembranous colitis, humerus fracture, pneumonia, pyrexia, and peritonsillar abscess.

Prophylaxis Studies

A total of 3434 subjects (adolescents, healthy adults and elderly) participated in phase III prophylaxis studies, of whom 1480 received the recommended dose of 75 mg once daily for up to 6 weeks. Adverse events were qualitatively very similar to those seen in the treatment studies, despite a longer duration of dosing (Table 3). Events reported more frequently in subjects receiving TAMIFLU compared to subjects receiving placebo in prophylaxis studies, and more commonly than in treatment studies, were aches and pains, rhinorrhea, dyspepsia and upper respiratory tract infections. However, the difference in incidence between TAMIFLU and placebo for these events was less than 1%. There were no clinically relevant differences in the safety profile of the 942 elderly subjects who received TAMIFLU or placebo, compared with the younger population.

Treatment Studies in Pediatric Patients

A total of 1032 pediatric patients aged 1 to 12 years (including 698 otherwise healthy pediatric patients aged 1 to 12 years and 334 asthmatic pediatric patients aged 6 to 12 years) participated in phase III studies of TAMIFLU given for the treatment of influenza. A total of 515 pediatric patients received treatment with TAMIFLU oral suspension. Adverse events occurring in >1% of pediatric patients receiving TAMIFLU treatment are listed in Table 4. The most frequently reported adverse event was vomiting. Other events reported more frequently by pediatric patients treated with TAMIFLU included abdominal pain, epistaxis, ear disorder, and conjunctivitis. These events generally occurred once and resolved despite continued dosing. They did not cause discontinuation of drug in the vast majority of cases.

The adverse event profile in adolescents is similar to that described for adult patients and pediatric patients aged 1 to 12 years.

[See table 4 at right]

Observed During Clinical Practice for Treatment

The following adverse reactions have been identified during postmarketing use of TAMIFLU. Because these reactions are reported voluntarily from a population of uncertain size, it is not possible to reliably estimate their frequency or establish a causal relationship to TAMIFLU exposure.

General: Rash, swelling of the face or tongue, toxic epidermal necrolysis

Digestive: Hepatitis, liver function tests abnormal

Cardiac: Arrhythmia

Neurologic: Seizure, confusion

Metabolic: Aggravation of diabetes

Table 3. Most Frequent Adverse Events in Studies in Naturally Acquired Influenza

Adverse Event	Treatment: Placebo N=716	Treatment: Oseltamivir 75 mg bid N=724	Prophylaxis: Placebo N=1434	Prophylaxis: Oseltamivir 75 mg qd N=1480
Nausea (without vomiting)	40 (5.6%)	72 (9.9%)	56 (3.9%)	104 (7.0%)
Vomiting	21 (2.9%)	68 (9.4%)	15 (1.0%)	31 (2.1%)
Diarrhea	70 (9.8%)	48 (6.6%)	38 (2.6%)	48 (3.2%)
Bronchitis	15 (2.1%)	17 (2.3%)	17 (1.2%)	11 (0.7%)
Abdominal pain	16 (2.2%)	16 (2.2%)	23 (1.6%)	30 (2.0%)
Dizziness	25 (3.5%)	15 (2.1%)	21 (1.5%)	24 (1.6%)
Headache	14 (2.0%)	13 (1.8%)	251 (17.5%)	298 (20.1%)
Cough	12 (1.7%)	9 (1.2%)	86 (6.0%)	83 (5.6%)
Insomnia	6 (0.8%)	8 (1.1%)	14 (1.0%)	18 (1.2%)
Vertigo	4 (0.6%)	7 (1.0%)	3 (0.2%)	4 (0.3%)
Fatigue	7 (1.0%)	7 (1.0%)	107 (7.5%)	117 (7.9%)

Table 4. Adverse Events Occurring On Treatment in >1% of Pediatric Patients Enrolled in Phase III Trials of TAMIFLU Treatment of Naturally Acquired Influenza

Adverse Event	Placebo N=517	TAMIFLU 2 mg/kg twice daily N=515
Vomiting	48 (9.3%)	77 (15.0%)
Diarrhea	55 (10.6%)	49 (9.5%)
Otitis media	58 (11.2%)	45 (8.7%)
Abdominal pain	20 (3.9%)	24 (4.7%)
Asthma (including aggravated)	19 (3.7%)	18 (3.5%)
Nausea	22 (4.3%)	17 (3.3%)
Epistaxis	13 (2.5%)	16 (3.1%)
Pneumonia	17 (3.3%)	10 (1.9%)
Ear disorder	6 (1.2%)	9 (1.7%)
Sinusitis	13 (2.5%)	9 (1.7%)
Bronchitis	11 (2.1%)	8 (1.6%)
Conjunctivitis	2 (0.4%)	5 (1.0%)
Dermatitis	10 (1.9%)	5 (1.0%)
Lymphadenopathy	8 (1.5%)	5 (1.0%)
Tympanic membrane disorder	6 (1.2%)	5 (1.0%)

OVERDOSAGE

At present, there has been no experience with overdose. Single doses of up to 1000 mg of TAMIFLU have been associated with nausea and/or vomiting.

DOSAGE AND ADMINISTRATION

TAMIFLU may be taken with or without food (see **CLINICAL PHARMACOLOGY: Pharmacokinetics**). However, when taken with food, tolerability may be enhanced in some patients.

Standard Dosage – Treatment of Influenza:

Adults and Adolescents

The recommended oral dose of TAMIFLU for treatment of influenza in adults and adolescents 13 years and older is 75 mg twice daily for 5 days. Treatment should begin within 2 days of onset of symptoms of influenza.

Pediatric Patients

TAMIFLU is not indicated for treatment of influenza in pediatric patients younger than 1 year.

The recommended oral dose of TAMIFLU oral suspension for pediatric patients 1 year and older or adult patients who cannot swallow a capsule is:

[See third table at right]

Body Weight in kg	Body Weight in lbs	Recommended Dose for 5 Days	Number of Bottles Needed to Obtain the Recommended Dose
≤15 kg	≤33 lbs	30 mg twice daily	1
>15 kg to 23 kg	>33 lbs to 51 lbs	45 mg twice daily	2
>23 kg to 40 kg	>51 lbs to 88 lbs	60 mg twice daily	2
>40 kg	>88 lbs	75 mg twice daily	3

An oral dosing dispenser with 30 mg, 45 mg, and 60 mg graduations is provided with the oral suspension; the 75 mg dose can be measured using a combination of 30 mg and 45 mg. It is recommended that patients use this dispenser. In the event that the dispenser provided is lost or damaged, another dosing syringe or other device may be used to deliver the following volumes: 2.5 mL (1/2 tsp) for children ≤15 kg, 3.8 mL (3/4 tsp) for >15 to 23 kg, 5.0 mL (1 tsp) for >23 to 40 kg, and 6.2 mL (1 1/4 tsp) for >40 kg.

Standard Dosage – Prophylaxis of Influenza:

The safety and efficacy of TAMIFLU for prophylaxis of influenza in pediatric patients younger than 13 years of age have not been established.

The recommended oral dose of TAMIFLU for prophylaxis of influenza in adults and adolescents 13 years and older following close contact with an infected individual is 75 mg once daily for at least 7 days. Therapy should begin within 2 days of exposure. The recommended dose for prophylaxis during a community outbreak of influenza is 75 mg once daily. Safety and efficacy have been demonstrated for up to 6 weeks. The duration of protection lasts for as long as dosing is continued.

Special Dosage Instructions

Hepatic Impairment

The safety and pharmacokinetics in patients with hepatic impairment have not been evaluated.

Renal Impairment

For plasma concentrations of oseltamivir carboxylate predicted to occur following various dosing schedules in patients with renal impairment, see **CLINICAL PHARMACOLOGY: Pharmacokinetics:** Special Populations.

Treatment of Influenza

Dose adjustment is recommended for patients with creatinine clearance between 10 and 30 mL/min receiving TAMIFLU for the treatment of influenza. In these patients it is recommended that the dose be reduced to 75 mg of TAMIFLU once daily for 5 days. No recommended dosing regimens are available for patients undergoing routine hemodialysis and continuous peritoneal dialysis treatment with end-stage renal disease.

Prophylaxis of Influenza

For the prophylaxis of influenza, dose adjustment is recommended for patients with creatinine clearance between 10 and 30 mL/min receiving TAMIFLU. In these patients it is recommended that the dose be reduced to 75 mg of TAMIFLU every other day or 30 mg TAMIFLU oral suspension every day. No recommended dosing regimens are available for patients undergoing routine hemodialysis and continuous peritoneal dialysis treatment with end-stage renal disease.

Geriatric Patients

No dose adjustment is required for geriatric patients (see **CLINICAL PHARMACOLOGY: Pharmacokinetics:** Special Populations and **PRECAUTIONS**).

Preparation of TAMIFLU Oral Suspension

It is recommended that TAMIFLU oral suspension be constituted by the pharmacist prior to dispensing to the patient:

1. Tap the closed bottle several times to loosen the powder.
2. Measure **23 mL** of water in a graduated cylinder.
3. Add the total amount of water for constitution to the bottle and shake the closed bottle well for 15 seconds.
4. Remove the child-resistant cap and push bottle adapter into the neck of the bottle.
5. Close bottle with child-resistant cap tightly. This will assure the proper seating of the bottle adapter in the bottle and child-resistant status of the cap.

NOTE: SHAKE THE TAMIFLU ORAL SUSPENSION WELL BEFORE EACH USE.

The constituted oral suspension should be used within 10 days of preparation; the pharmacist should write the date of expiration of the constituted suspension on a pharmacy label. The patient package insert and oral dispenser should be dispensed to the patient.

HOW SUPPLIED

TAMIFLU Capsules

Supplied as 75-mg (75 mg free base equivalent of the phosphate salt) grey/light yellow hard gelatin capsules. "ROCHE" is printed in blue ink on the grey body and "75 mg" is printed in blue ink on the light yellow cap. Available in blister packages of 10 (NDC 0004-0800-85).

Storage

Store the capsules at 25°C (77°F); excursions permitted to 15° to 30°C (59° to 86°F). [See USP Controlled Room Temperature]

TAMIFLU for Oral Suspension

Supplied as a white powder blend for constitution to a white tutti-frutti–flavored suspension. Available in glass bottles containing 25 mL of suspension after constitution equivalent to 300 mg oseltamivir base. Each bottle is supplied with a bottle adapter and 1 oral dispenser (NDC 0004-0810-95).

Storage

Store dry powder at 25°C (77°F); excursions permitted to 15° to 30°C (59° to 86°F). [See USP Controlled Room Temperature]

Store constituted suspension under refrigeration at 2° to 8°C (36° to 46°F). Do not freeze.

Manufactured by F. Hoffmann-La Roche Ltd., Basel, Switzerland

Distributed by Roche Laboratories Inc., Nutley, New Jersey 07110-1199

Licensor: Gilead Sciences, Inc., Foster City, California 94404

Revised: June 2004

Shown in Product Identification Guide, page 331

TICLID® ℞

[tye' klid]

(ticlopidine hydrochloride)

Tablets

WARNING: TICLID can cause life-threatening hematological adverse reactions, including neutropenia/agranulocytosis, thrombotic thrombocytopenic purpura (TTP) and aplastic anemia.

Neutropenia/Agranulocytosis: **Among 2048 patients in clinical trials in stroke patients, there were 50 cases (2.4%) of neutropenia (less than 1200 neutrophils/mm³), and the neutrophil count was below 450/mm³ in 17 of these patients (0.8% of the total population).**

TTP: **One case of thrombotic thrombocytopenic purpura was reported during clinical trials in stroke patients. Based on postmarketing data, US physicians reported about 100 cases between 1992 and 1997. Based**

Continued on next page

Ticlid—Cont.

on an estimated patient exposure of 2 million to 4 million, and assuming an event reporting rate of 10% (the true rate is not known), the incidence of ticlopidine-associated TTP may be as high as one case in every 2000 to 4000 patients exposed.

Aplastic Anemia: **Aplastic anemia was not seen during clinical trials in stroke patients, but US physicians reported about 50 cases between 1992 and 1998. Based on an estimated patient exposure of 2 million to 4 million, and assuming an event reporting rate of 10% (the true rate is not known), the incidence of ticlopidine-associated aplastic anemia may be as high as one case in every 4000 to 8000 patients exposed.**

Monitoring of Clinical and Hematologic Status: **Severe hematological adverse reactions may occur within a few days of the start of therapy. The incidence of TTP peaks after about 3 to 4 weeks of therapy and neutropenia peaks at approximately 4 to 6 weeks. The incidence of aplastic anemia peaks after about 4 to 8 weeks of therapy. The incidence of the hematologic adverse reactions declines thereafter. Only a few cases of neutropenia, TTP, or aplastic anemia have arisen after more than 3 months of therapy.**

Hematological adverse reactions cannot be reliably predicted by any identified demographic or clinical characteristics. During the first 3 months of treatment, patients receiving TICLID must, therefore, be hematologically and clinically monitored for evidence of neutropenia or TTP. If any such evidence is seen, TICLID should be immediately discontinued.

The detection and treatment of ticlopidine-associated hematological adverse reactions are further described under WARNINGS.

DESCRIPTION

TICLID (ticlopidine hydrochloride) is a platelet aggregation inhibitor. Chemically it is 5-[(2-chlorophenyl)methyl]-4,5,6,7-tetrahydrothieno [3,2-c] pyridine hydrochloride.

Ticlopidine hydrochloride is a white crystalline solid. It is freely soluble in water and self-buffers to a pH of 3.6. It also dissolves freely in methanol, is sparingly soluble in methylene chloride and ethanol, slightly soluble in acetone and insoluble in a buffer solution of pH 6.3. It has a molecular weight of 300.25.

TICLID tablets for oral administration are provided as white, oval, film-coated, blue-imprinted tablets containing 250 mg of ticlopidine hydrochloride. Each tablet also contains citric acid, magnesium stearate, microcrystalline cellulose, povidone, starch and stearic acid as inactive ingredients. The white film-coating contains hydroxypropylmethyl cellulose, polyethylene glycol and titanium dioxide. Each tablet is printed with blue ink, which includes FD&C Blue #1 aluminum lake as the colorant. The tablets are identified with Ticlid on one side and 250 on the reverse side.

CLINICAL PHARMACOLOGY

Mechanism of Action: When taken orally, ticlopidine hydrochloride causes a time- and dose-dependent inhibition of both platelet aggregation and release of platelet granule constituents, as well as a prolongation of bleeding time. The intact drug has no significant in vitro activity at the concentrations attained in vivo; and, although analysis of urine and plasma indicates at least 20 metabolites, no metabolite which accounts for the activity of ticlopidine has been isolated.

Ticlopidine hydrochloride, after oral ingestion, interferes with platelet membrane function by inhibiting ADP-induced platelet-fibrinogen binding and subsequent platelet-platelet interactions. The effect on platelet function is irreversible for the life of the platelet, as shown both by persistent inhibition of fibrinogen binding after washing platelets ex vivo and by inhibition of platelet aggregation after resuspension of platelets in buffered medium.

Pharmacokinetics and Metabolism: After oral administration of a single 250-mg dose, ticlopidine hydrochloride is rapidly absorbed with peak plasma levels occurring at approximately 2 hours after dosing and is extensively metabolized. Absorption is greater than 80%. Administration after meals results in a 20% increase in the AUC of ticlopidine.

Ticlopidine hydrochloride displays nonlinear pharmacokinetics and clearance decreases markedly on repeated dosing. In older volunteers the apparent half-life of ticlopidine after a single 250-mg dose is about 12.6 hours; with repeat dosing at 250 mg bid, the terminal elimination half-life rises to 4 to 5 days and steady-state levels of ticlopidine hydrochloride in plasma are obtained after approximately 14 to 21 days.

Ticlopidine hydrochloride binds reversibly (98%) to plasma proteins, mainly to serum albumin and lipoproteins. The binding to albumin and lipoproteins is nonsaturable over a wide concentration range. Ticlopidine also binds to alpha-1 acid glycoprotein. At concentrations attained with the recommended dose, only 15% or less ticlopidine in plasma is bound to this protein.

Ticlopidine hydrochloride is metabolized extensively by the liver; only trace amounts of intact drug are detected in the urine. Following an oral dose of radioactive ticlopidine hydrochloride administered in solution, 60% of the radioactivity is recovered in the urine and 23% in the feces. Approximately $^{1}/_{3}$ of the dose excreted in the feces is intact ticlopidine hydrochloride, possibly excreted in the bile. Ticlopidine hydrochloride is a minor component in plasma (5%) after a single dose, but at steady-state is the major component (15%). Approximately 40% to 50% of the radioactive metabolites circulating in plasma are covalently bound to plasma proteins, probably by acylation.

Clearance of ticlopidine decreases with age. Steady-state trough values in elderly patients (mean age 70 years) are about twice those in younger volunteer populations.

Hepatically Impaired Patients: The effect of decreased hepatic function on the pharmacokinetics of TICLID was studied in 17 patients with advanced cirrhosis. The average plasma concentration of ticlopidine in these subjects was slightly higher than that seen in older subjects in a separate trial (see CONTRAINDICATIONS).

Renally Impaired Patients: Patients with mildly (Ccr 50 to 80 mL/min) or moderately (Ccr 20 to 50 mL/min) impaired renal function were compared to normal subjects (Ccr 80 to 150 mL/min) in a study of the pharmacokinetic and platelet pharmacodynamic effects of TICLID (250 mg bid) for 11 days. Concentrations of unchanged TICLID were measured after a single 250-mg dose and after the final 250-mg dose on Day 11.

AUC values of ticlopidine increased by 28% and 60% in mild and moderately impaired patients, respectively, and plasma clearance decreased by 37% and 52%, respectively, but there were no statistically significant differences in ADP-induced platelet aggregation. In this small study (26 patients), bleeding times showed significant prolongation only in the moderately impaired patients.

Pharmacodynamics: In healthy volunteers over the age of 50, substantial inhibition (over 50%) of ADP-induced platelet aggregation is detected within 4 days after administration of ticlopidine hydrochloride 250 mg bid, and maximum platelet aggregation inhibition (60% to 70%) is achieved after 8 to 11 days. Lower doses cause less, and more delayed, platelet aggregation inhibition, while doses above 250 mg bid give little additional effect on platelet aggregation but an increased rate of adverse effects. The dose of 250 mg bid is the only dose that has been evaluated in controlled clinical trials.

After discontinuation of ticlopidine hydrochloride, bleeding time and other platelet function tests return to normal within 2 weeks, in the majority of patients.

At the recommended therapeutic dose (250 mg bid), ticlopidine hydrochloride has no known significant pharmacological actions in man other than inhibition of platelet function and prolongation of the bleeding time.

CLINICAL TRIALS: *Stroke Patients*

The effect of ticlopidine on the risk of stroke and cardiovascular events was studied in two multicenter, randomized, double-blind trials.

1. Study in Patients Experiencing Stroke Precursors: In a trial comparing ticlopidine and aspirin (The Ticlopidine Aspirin Stroke Study or TASS), 3069 patients (1987 men, 1082 women) who had experienced such stroke precursors as transient ischemic attack (TIA), transient monocular blindness (amaurosis fugax), reversible ischemic neurological deficit or minor stroke, were randomized to ticlopidine 250 mg bid or aspirin 650 mg bid. The study was designed to follow patients for at least 2 years and up to 5 years.

Over the duration of the study, TICLID significantly reduced the risk of fatal and nonfatal stroke by 24% (p = .011) from 18.1 to 13.8 per 100 patients followed for 5 years, compared to aspirin. During the first year, when the risk of stroke is greatest, the reduction in risk of stroke (fatal and nonfatal) compared to aspirin was 48%; the reduction was similar in men and women.

2. Study in Patients Who Had a Completed Atherothrombotic Stroke: In a trial comparing ticlopidine with placebo (The Canadian American Ticlopidine Study or CATS) 1073 patients who had experienced a previous atherothrombotic stroke were treated with TICLID 250 mg bid or placebo for up to 3 years.

TICLID significantly reduced the overall risk of stroke by 24% (p = .017) from 24.6 to 18.6 per 100 patients followed for 3 years, compared to placebo. During the first year the reduction in risk of fatal and nonfatal stroke over placebo was 33%.

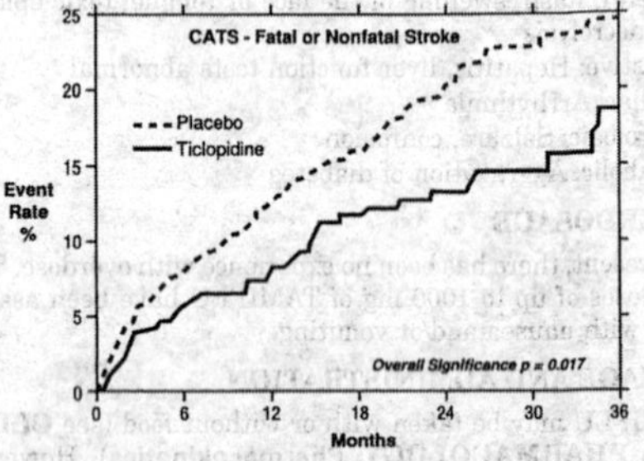

Stent Patients: The ability of TICLID to reduce the rate of thrombotic events after the placement of coronary artery stents has been studied in five randomized trials, one of substantial size (Stent Anticoagulation Restenosis Study or STARS) described below, and four smaller studies. In these trials, ticlopidine 250 mg bid with ASA (dose range from 100 mg bid to 325 mg qd) was compared to aspirin alone or to anticoagulant therapy plus aspirin. The trials enrolled patients undergoing both planned (elective) and unplanned coronary stent placement. The types of stents used, the use of intravascular ultrasound, and the use of high-pressure stent deployment varied among the trials, although all patients in STARS received a Palmaz-Schatz stent. The primary efficacy endpoints of the trials were similar, and included death, myocardial infarction and the need for repeat coronary angioplasty or CABG. All trials followed patients for at least 30 days.

In STARS, patients were randomized to receive one of three regimens for 4 weeks: aspirin alone, aspirin plus coumadin, or aspirin plus ticlopidine. Therapy was initiated following successful coronary stent placement. The primary endpoint was the incidence of stent thrombosis, defined as death, Q-Wave MI, or angiographic thrombus within the stented vessel demonstrated at the time of documented ischemia requiring emergent revascularization. The incidence rates for the primary endpoint and its components at 30 days are shown in the table below.

[See table below]

The use of ticlopidine plus aspirin did not affect the rate of non-Q-wave MIs when compared with aspirin alone or aspirin plus anticoagulants in STARS.

The use of ticlopidine plus aspirin was associated with a lower rate of recurrent cardiovascular events when compared with aspirin alone or aspirin plus anticoagulants in the other four randomized trials.

The rate of serious bleeding complications and neutropenia in STARS are shown in the table below. There were no cases of thrombotic thrombocytopenic purpura (TTP) or aplastic anemia reported in 1346 patients who received ticlopidine plus aspirin in the five randomized trials.

[See table at top of next page]

INDICATIONS AND USAGE: TICLID is indicated:

- to reduce the risk of thrombotic stroke (fatal or nonfatal) in patients who have experienced stroke precursors, and in patients who have had a completed thrombotic stroke. Because TICLID is associated with a risk of life-threatening blood dyscrasias including thrombotic thrombocytopenic purpura (TTP), neutropenia/agranulocytosis and aplastic anemia (see BOXED WARNING and WARNINGS), TICLID should be reserved for patients who are intolerant or allergic to aspirin therapy or who have failed aspirin therapy.
- as adjunctive therapy with aspirin to reduce the incidence of subacute stent thrombosis in patients undergoing successful coronary stent implantation (see CLINICAL TRIALS).

TICLID® (ticlopidine hydrochloride)

STARS	TICLID + Aspirin N=546	Aspirin N=557	Coumadin + Aspirin N=550	Odds Ratio (95% C.I.)*	p-Value*
Primary Endpoint	3 (0.5%)	20 (3.6%)	15 (2.7%)	0.15 (0.03, 0.51)	<0.001
Deaths	0 (0%)	1 (0.2%)	0 (0%)	=	=
Q-Wave MI (Recurrent and Procedure Related)	1 (0.2%)	12 (2.2%)	8 (1.5%)	0.08 (0.002, 0.57)	0.004
Angiographically Evident Thrombosis	3 (0.5%)	16 (2.9%)	15 (2.7%)	0.19 (0.03, 0.66)	0.005

* Comparison of TICLID plus aspirin to aspirin alone.

CONTRAINDICATIONS

The use of TICLID is contraindicated in the following conditions:

- Hypersensitivity to the drug
- Presence of hematopoietic disorders such as neutropenia and thrombocytopenia or a past history of either TTP or aplastic anemia
- Presence of a hemostatic disorder or active pathological bleeding (such as bleeding peptic ulcer or intracranial bleeding)
- Patients with severe liver impairment

WARNINGS

Hematological Adverse Reactions: *Neutropenia:* Neutropenia may occur suddenly. Bone-marrow examination typically shows a reduction in white blood cell precursors. After withdrawal of ticlopidine, the neutrophil count usually rises to >1200/mm^3 within 1 to 3 weeks.

Thrombocytopenia: Rarely, thrombocytopenia may occur in isolation or together with neutropenia.

Thrombotic Thrombocytopenic Purpura (TTP): TTP is characterized by thrombocytopenia, microangiopathic hemolytic anemia (schistocytes [fragmented RBCs] seen on peripheral smear), neurological findings, renal dysfunction, and fever. The signs and symptoms can occur in any order, in particular, clinical symptoms may precede laboratory findings by hours or days. With **prompt** treatment (often including plasmapheresis), 70% to 80% of patients will survive with minimal or no sequelae. Because platelet transfusions may accelerate thrombosis in patients with TTP on ticlopidine, they should, if possible, be avoided.

Aplastic Anemia: Aplastic anemia is characterized by anemia, thrombocytopenia and neutropenia together with a bone marrow examination that shows decreases in the precursor cells for red blood cells, white blood cells, and platelets. Patients may present with signs or symptoms suggestive of infection, in association with low white blood cell and platelet counts. **Prompt** treatment, which may include the use of drugs to stimulate the bone marrow, can minimize the mortality associated with aplastic anemia.

Monitoring for Hematologic Adverse Reactions: Starting just before initiating treatment and continuing through the third month of therapy, patients receiving TICLID must be monitored every 2 weeks. Because of ticlopidine's long plasma half-life, patients who discontinue ticlopidine during this 3-month period should continue to be monitored for 2 weeks after discontinuation. More frequent monitoring, and monitoring after the first 3 months of therapy, is necessary only in patients with clinical signs (eg, signs or symptoms suggestive of infection) or laboratory signs (eg, neutrophil count less than 70% of the baseline count, decrease in hematocrit or platelet count) that suggest incipient hematological adverse reactions.

Clinically, fever might suggest neutropenia, TTP, or aplastic anemia; TTP might also be suggested by weakness, pallor, petechiae or purpura, dark urine (due to blood, bile pigments, or hemoglobin) or jaundice, or neurological changes. Patients should be told to discontinue TICLID and to contact the physician immediately upon the occurrence of any of these findings.

Laboratory monitoring should include a complete blood count, with special attention to the absolute neutrophil count (WBC × % neutrophils), platelet count, and the appearance of the peripheral smear. Ticlopidine is occasionally associated with thrombocytopenia unrelated to TTP or aplastic anemia. Any acute, unexplained reduction in **hemoglobin** or platelet count should prompt further investigation for a diagnosis of TTP, and the appearance of **schistocytes** (fragmented RBCs) on the smear should be treated as presumptive evidence of TTP. A simultaneous decrease in platelet count and WBC count should prompt further investigation for a diagnosis of aplastic anemia. If there are laboratory signs of TTP or aplastic anemia, or if the neutrophil count is confirmed to be <1200/mm^3, then TICLID should be discontinued immediately.

Other Hematological Effects: Rare cases of agranulocytosis, pancytopenia, or leukemia have been reported in postmarketing experience, some of which have been fatal. All forms of hematological adverse reactions are potentially fatal.

Cholesterol Elevation: TICLID therapy causes increased serum cholesterol and triglycerides. Serum total cholesterol levels are increased 8% to 10% within 1 month of therapy and persist at that level. The ratios of the lipoprotein subfractions are unchanged.

Anticoagulant Drugs: The tolerance and long-term safety of coadministration of TICLID with heparin, oral anticoagulants or fibrinolytic agents have not been established. In trials for cardiac stenting, patients received heparin and TICLID concomitantly for approximately 12 hours. If a patient is switched from an anticoagulant or fibrinolytic drug to TICLID, the former drug should be discontinued prior to TICLID administration.

PRECAUTIONS

General: TICLID should be used with caution in patients who may be at risk of increased bleeding from trauma, surgery or pathological conditions. If it is desired to eliminate the antiplatelet effects of TICLID prior to elective surgery, the drug should be discontinued 10 to 14 days prior to surgery. Several controlled clinical studies have found increased surgical blood loss in patients undergoing surgery during treatment with ticlopidine. In TASS and CATS it

STARS	TICLID + Aspirin N=546	Aspirin N=557	Coumadin + Aspirin N=550
Hemorrhagic Complications	30 (5.5%)	10 (1.8%)	34 (6.2%)
Cerebrovascular Accident	0 (0%)	2 (0.4%)	1 (0.2%)
Neutropenia (≤1200/mm^3)	3 (0.5%)	0 (0%)	1 (0.2%)

was recommended that patients have ticlopidine discontinued prior to elective surgery. Several hundred patients underwent surgery during the trials, and no excessive surgical bleeding was reported.

Prolonged bleeding time is normalized within 2 hours after administration of 20 mg methylprednisolone IV. Platelet transfusions may also be used to reverse the effect of TICLID on bleeding. Because platelet transfusions may accelerate thrombosis in patients with TTP on ticlopidine, they should, if possible, be avoided.

GI Bleeding: TICLID prolongs template bleeding time. The drug should be used with caution in patients who have lesions with a propensity to bleed (such as ulcers). Drugs that might induce such lesions should be used with caution in patients on TICLID (see CONTRAINDICATIONS).

Use in Hepatically Impaired Patients: Since ticlopidine is metabolized by the liver, dosing of TICLID or other drugs metabolized in the liver may require adjustment upon starting or stopping concomitant therapy. Because of limited experience in patients with severe hepatic disease, who may have bleeding diatheses, the use of TICLID is not recommended in this population (see CLINICAL PHARMACOLOGY and CONTRAINDICATIONS).

Use in Renally Impaired Patients: There is limited experience in patients with renal impairment. Decreased plasma clearance, increased AUC values and prolonged bleeding times can occur in renally impaired patients. In controlled clinical trials no unexpected problems have been encountered in patients having mild renal impairment, and there is no experience with dosage adjustment in patients with greater degrees of renal impairment. Nevertheless, for renally impaired patients, it may be necessary to reduce the dosage of ticlopidine or discontinue it altogether if hemorrhagic or hematopoietic problems are encountered (see CLINICAL PHARMACOLOGY).

***Information for the Patient* (see Patient Leaflet):** Patients should be told that a decrease in the number of white blood cells (neutropenia) or platelets (thrombocytopenia) can occur with TICLID, especially during the first 3 months of treatment and that neutropenia, if it is severe, can result in an increased risk of infection. They should be told it is critically important to obtain the scheduled blood tests to detect neutropenia or thrombocytopenia. Patients should also be reminded to contact their physicians if they experience any indication of infection such as fever, chills, or sore throat, any of which might be a consequence of neutropenia. Thrombocytopenia may be part of a syndrome called TTP. Symptoms and signs of TTP, such as fever, weakness, difficulty speaking, seizures, yellowing of skin or eyes, dark or bloody urine, pallor or petechiae (pinpoint hemorrhagic spots on the skin), should be reported immediately.

All patients should be told that it may take them longer than usual to stop bleeding when they take TICLID and that they should report any unusual bleeding to their physician. Patients should tell physicians and dentists that they are taking TICLID before any surgery is scheduled and before any new drug is prescribed.

Patients should be told to promptly report side effects of TICLID such as severe or persistent diarrhea, skin rashes or subcutaneous bleeding or any signs of cholestasis, such as yellow skin or sclera, dark urine, or light-colored stools. Patients should be told to take TICLID with food or just after eating in order to minimize gastrointestinal discomfort.

Laboratory Tests: *Liver Function:* TICLID therapy has been associated with elevations of alkaline phosphatase, bilirubin, and transaminases, which generally occurred within 1 to 4 months of therapy initiation. In controlled clinical trials in stroke patients the incidence of elevated alkaline phosphatase (greater than two times upper limit of normal) was 7.6% in ticlopidine patients, 6% in placebo patients and 2.5% in aspirin patients. The incidence of elevated AST (SGOT) (greater than two times upper limit of normal) was 3.1% in ticlopidine patients, 4% in placebo patients and 2.1% in aspirin patients. No progressive increases were observed in closely monitored clinical trials (eg, no transaminase greater than 10 times the upper limit of normal was seen), but most patients with these abnormalities had therapy discontinued. Occasionally patients had developed minor elevations in bilirubin.

Postmarketing experience includes rare individuals with elevations in their transaminases and bilirubin to >10× above the upper limits of normal. Based on postmarketing and clinical trial experience, liver function testing, including ALT, AST, and GGT, should be considered whenever liver dysfunction is suspected, particularly during the first 4 months of treatment.

Drug Interactions: Therapeutic doses of TICLID caused a 30% increase in the plasma half-life of antipyrine and may cause analogous effects on similarly metabolized drugs. Therefore, the dose of drugs metabolized by hepatic microsomal enzymes with low therapeutic ratios or being given to patients with hepatic impairment may require adjustment to maintain optimal therapeutic blood levels when starting or stopping concomitant therapy with ticlopidine. Studies of specific drug interactions yielded the following results:

Aspirin and Other NSAIDs: Ticlopidine potentiates the effect of aspirin or other NSAIDs on platelet aggregation. The safety of concomitant use of ticlopidine and NSAIDs has not been established. The safety of concomitant use of ticlopidine and aspirin beyond 30 days has not been established (see CLINICAL TRIALS: *Stent Patients*). Aspirin did not modify the ticlopidine-mediated inhibition of ADP-induced platelet aggregation, but ticlopidine potentiated the effect of aspirin on collagen-induced platelet aggregation. Caution should be exercised in patients who have lesions with a propensity to bleed, such as ulcers. Long-term concomitant use of aspirin and ticlopidine is not recommended (see PRECAUTIONS: *GI Bleeding*).

Antacids: Administration of TICLID after antacids resulted in an 18% decrease in plasma levels of ticlopidine.

Cimetidine: Chronic administration of cimetidine reduced the clearance of a single dose of TICLID by 50%.

Digoxin: Coadministration of TICLID with digoxin resulted in a slight decrease (approximately 15%) in digoxin plasma levels. Little or no change in therapeutic efficacy of digoxin would be expected.

Theophylline: In normal volunteers, concomitant administration of TICLID resulted in a significant increase in the theophylline elimination half-life from 8.6 to 12.2 hours and a comparable reduction in total plasma clearance of theophylline.

Phenobarbital: In 6 normal volunteers, the inhibitory effects of TICLID on platelet aggregation were not altered by chronic administration of phenobarbital.

Phenytoin: In vitro studies demonstrated that ticlopidine does not alter the plasma protein binding of phenytoin. However, the protein binding interactions of ticlopidine and its metabolites have not been studied in vivo. Several cases of elevated phenytoin plasma levels with associated somnolence and lethargy have been reported following coadministration with TICLID. Caution should be exercised in coadministering this drug with TICLID, and it may be useful to remeasure phenytoin blood concentrations.

Propranolol: In vitro studies demonstrated that ticlopidine does not alter the plasma protein binding of propranolol. However, the protein binding interactions of ticlopidine and its metabolites have not been studied in vivo. Caution should be exercised in coadministering this drug with TICLID.

Other Concomitant Therapy: Although specific interaction studies were not performed, in clinical studies TICLID was used concomitantly with beta blockers, calcium channel blockers and diuretics without evidence of clinically significant adverse interactions (see PRECAUTIONS).

Food Interaction: The oral bioavailability of ticlopidine is increased by 20% when taken after a meal. Administration of TICLID with food is recommended to maximize gastrointestinal tolerance. In controlled trials in stroke patients TICLID was taken with meals.

Carcinogenesis, Mutagenesis, Impairment of Fertility: In a 2-year oral carcinogenicity study in rats, ticlopidine at daily doses of up to 100 mg/kg (610 mg/m^2) was not tumorigenic. For a 70-kg person (1.73 m^2 body surface area) the dose represents 14 times the recommended clinical dose on a mg/kg basis and two times the clinical dose on body surface area basis. In a 78-week oral carcinogenicity study in mice, ticlopidine at daily doses up to 275 mg/kg (1180 mg/m^2) was not tumorigenic. The dose represents 40 times the recommended clinical dose on a mg/kg basis and four times the clinical dose on body surface area basis.

Ticlopidine was not mutagenic in vitro in the Ames test, the rat hepatocyte DNA-repair assay, or the Chinese-hamster fibroblast chromosomal aberration test; or in vivo in the mouse spermatozoid morphology test, the Chinese-hamster micronucleus test, or the Chinese-hamster bone-marrow-cell sister-chromatid exchange test. Ticlopidine was found to have no effect on fertility of male and female rats at oral doses up to 400 mg/kg/day.

Pregnancy: *Teratogenic Effects:* Pregnancy: Category B. Teratology studies have been conducted in mice (doses up to 200 mg/kg/day), rats (doses up to 400 mg/kg/day) and rabbits (doses up to 200 mg/kg/day). Doses of 400 mg/kg in rats, 200 mg/kg/day in mice and 100 mg/kg in rabbits produced maternal toxicity, as well as fetal toxicity, but there was no evidence of a teratogenic potential of ticlopidine. There are, however, no adequate and well-controlled studies in pregnant women. Because animal reproduction studies are not always predictive of a human response, this drug should be used during pregnancy only if clearly needed.

Nursing Mothers: Studies in rats have shown ticlopidine is excreted in the milk. It is not known whether this drug is excreted in human milk. Because many drugs are excreted in human milk and because of the potential for serious adverse reactions in nursing infants from ticlopidine, a deci-

Continued on next page

Ticlid—Cont.

sion should be made whether to discontinue nursing or to discontinue the drug, taking into account the importance of the drug to the mother.

Pediatric Use: Safety and effectiveness in pediatric patients have not been established.

Geriatric Use: Clearance of ticlopidine is somewhat lower in elderly patients and trough levels are increased. The major clinical trials with TICLID in stroke patients were conducted in an elderly population with an average age of 64 years. Of the total number of patients in the therapeutic trials, 45% of patients were over 65 years old and 12% were over 75 years old. No overall differences in effectiveness or safety were observed between these patients and younger patients, and other reported clinical experience has not identified differences in responses between the elderly and younger patients, but greater sensitivity of some older individuals cannot be ruled out.

ADVERSE REACTIONS

Adverse reactions in stroke patients were relatively frequent with over 50% of patients reporting at least one. Most (30% to 40%) involved the gastrointestinal tract. Most adverse effects are mild, but 21% of patients discontinued therapy because of an adverse event, principally diarrhea, rash, nausea, vomiting, GI pain and neutropenia. Most adverse effects occur early in the course of treatment, but a new onset of adverse effects can occur after several months.

The incidence rates of adverse events listed in the following table were derived from multicenter, controlled clinical trials in stroke patients described above comparing TICLID, placebo and aspirin over study periods of up to 5.8 years. Adverse events considered by the investigator to be probably drug-related that occurred in at least 1% of patients treated with TICLID are shown in the following table:

[See table below]

Incidence of discontinuation, regardless of relationship to therapy, is shown in parentheses.

Hematological: Neutropenia/thrombocytopenia, TTP, aplastic anemia (see BOXED WARNING and WARNINGS), leukemia, agranulocytosis, eosinophilia, pancytopenia, thrombocytosis and bone-marrow depression have been reported.

Gastrointestinal: TICLID therapy has been associated with a variety of gastrointestinal complaints including diarrhea and nausea. The majority of cases are mild, but about 13% of patients discontinued therapy because of these. They usually occur within 3 months of initiation of therapy and typically are resolved within 1 to 2 weeks without discontinuation of therapy. If the effect is severe or persistent, therapy should be discontinued. In some cases of severe or bloody diarrhea, colitis was later diagnosed.

Hemorrhagic: TICLID has been associated with increased bleeding, spontaneous posttraumatic bleeding and perioperative bleeding including, but not limited to, gastrointestinal bleeding. It has also been associated with a number of bleeding complications such as ecchymosis, epistaxis, hematuria and conjunctival hemorrhage.

Intracerebral bleeding was rare in clinical trials in stroke patients with TICLID, with an incidence no greater than that seen with comparator agents (ticlopidine 0.5%, aspirin 0.6%, placebo 0.75%). It has also been reported postmarketing.

Rash: Ticlopidine has been associated with a maculopapular or urticarial rash (often with pruritus). Rash usually occurs within 3 months of initiation of therapy with a mean onset time of 11 days. If drug is discontinued, recovery occurs within several days. Many rashes do not recur on drug rechallenge. There have been rare reports of severe rashes, including Stevens-Johnson syndrome, erythema multiforme and exfoliative dermatitis.

Less Frequent Adverse Reactions (Probably Related): Clinical adverse experiences occurring in 0.5% to 1.0% of stroke patients in controlled trials include:

Digestive System: GI fullness
Skin and Appendages: urticaria
Nervous System: headache
Body as a Whole: asthenia, pain
Hemostatic System: epistaxis
Special Senses: tinnitus

In addition, rarer, relatively serious and potentially fatal events associated with the use of TICLID have also been reported from postmarketing experience: Hemolytic anemia with reticulocytosis, immune thrombocytopenia, hepatitis, hepatocellular jaundice, cholestatic jaundice, hepatic necrosis, hepatic failure, peptic ulcer, renal failure, nephrotic syndrome, hyponatremia, vasculitis, sepsis, allergic reactions (including angioedema, allergic pneumonitis, and anaphylaxis), systemic lupus (positive ANA), peripheral neuropathy, serum sickness, arthropathy and myositis.

OVERDOSAGE

One case of deliberate overdosage with TICLID has been reported by a foreign postmarketing surveillance program. A 38-year-old male took a single 6000-mg dose of TICLID (equivalent to 24 standard 250-mg tablets). The only abnormalities reported were increased bleeding time and increased SGPT. No special therapy was instituted and the patient recovered without sequelae.

Single oral doses of ticlopidine at 1600 mg/kg and 500 mg/kg were lethal to rats and mice, respectively. Symptoms of acute toxicity were GI hemorrhage, convulsions, hypothermia, dyspnea, loss of equilibrium and abnormal gait.

DOSAGE AND ADMINISTRATION

Stroke:

The recommended dose of TICLID is 250 mg bid taken with food. Other doses have not been studied in controlled trials for these indications.

Coronary Artery Stenting: The recommended dose of TICLID is 250 mg bid taken with food together with antiplatelet doses of aspirin for up to 30 days of therapy following successful stent implantation.

HOW SUPPLIED

TICLID is available in white, oval, film-coated 250-mg tablets, printed in blue with Ticlid on one side and 250 on the other. They are provided in unit of use bottles of 30 tablets (NDC 0004-0018-23) and 60 tablets (NDC 0004-0018-22) and 500 tablets (NDC 0004-0018-14).

Store at 15° to 30°C (59° to 86°F).

IMPORTANT INFORMATION ABOUT TICLID (ticlopidine HCl) TABLETS

The information in this leaflet is intended to help you use TICLID safely. Please read the leaflet carefully. Although it does not contain all the detailed medical information that is provided to your doctor, it provides facts about TICLID that are important for you to know. If you still have questions after reading this leaflet or if you have questions at any time during your treatment with TICLID, check with your doctor.

Why TICLID was Prescribed by Your Doctor:

Stroke Patients: TICLID is recommended to help reduce your risk of having a stroke, but only for patients who have had a stroke or early stroke warning symptoms while on aspirin, or for those who have these symptoms but are intolerant or allergic to aspirin.

Stent Patients: TICLID is recommended with aspirin for up to 30 days in patients who have had a stent implanted in their coronary arteries to reduce the risk of blood clots forming inside the stent.

Special Warning for Users of TICLID/Necessary Blood Tests:

TICLID is not prescribed for those who can take aspirin to reduce the risk of stroke because TICLID can cause life-threatening blood problems. **Getting your blood tests done and reporting symptoms to your doctor as soon as possible can avoid serious complications.**

The white cells of the blood that fight infection may drop to dangerous levels (a condition called neutropenia). This occurs in about 2.4% (1 in 40) of people on ticlopidine. You should be on the lookout for signs of infection such as fever, chills or sore throat. If this problem is caught early, it can almost always be reversed, but if undetected it can be fatal.

Another problem that has occurred in some patients taking ticlopidine is a decrease in cells called platelets (a condition called thrombocytopenia). This may occur as part of a syndrome that includes injury to red blood cells, causing anemia, kidney abnormalities, neurologic changes and fever. This condition is called TTP and can be fatal.

Things you should watch for as possible early signs of TTP are yellow skin or eye color, pinpoint dots (rash) on the skin, pale color, fever, weakness on a side of the body, or dark urine. **If any of these occur, contact your doctor immediately.**

Both complications occur most frequently in the first 90 days after TICLID is started. To make sure you don't develop either of these problems, your doctor will arrange for you to have your blood tested before you start taking TICLID and then every 2 weeks for the first 3 months you are on TICLID. If detected, neutropenia and thrombocytopenia can almost always be reversed. It is essential that you keep your appointments for the blood tests and that you call your doctor immediately if you have any indication that you may have TTP or neutropenia. If you stop taking TICLID for any reason within the first 3 months, you will still need to have your blood tested for an additional 2 weeks after you have stopped taking TICLID.

Rarely, decreases in the white blood cells, red blood cells and platelets can occur together. This condition is called aplastic anemia and can be fatal.

Things you should watch for as possible early signs of aplastic anemia are feeling of excessive weakness and tiredness, paleness, bruising, and bleeding from areas such as your nose or gums. You may also develop signs of infection such as fever. **If any of these occur, contact your doctor immediately.**

Other Warnings and Precautions: A few people may develop jaundice while being treated with TICLID. The signs of jaundice are yellowing of the skin or the whites of the eyes or consistent darkening of the urine or lightening in the color of the stools. These symptoms should be reported to your physician promptly.

If any of the symptoms described above for neutropenia, TTP, aplastic anemia or jaundice occur, contact your doctor immediately.

TICLID should be used only as directed by your doctor. Do not give TICLID to anyone else. **Keep TICLID out of reach of children!**

Some people may have such side effects as diarrhea, skin rash, stomach or intestinal discomfort. If any of these problems are persistent, or if you are concerned about them, bring them to your doctor's attention.

It may take longer than usual to stop bleeding when taking TICLID. Tell your doctor if you have any more bleeding or bruising than usual, and, if you have emergency surgery, be sure to let your doctor or dentist know that you are taking TICLID. Also, tell your doctor well in advance of any planned surgery (including tooth extraction), because he or she may recommend that you stop taking TICLID temporarily.

How TICLID Works: *Stroke Patients:* A stroke occurs when a clot (or thrombus) forms in a blood vessel in the brain or forms in another part of the body and breaks off, then travels to the brain (an embolus). In both cases the blood supply to part of the brain is blocked and that part of the brain is damaged. TICLID works by making the blood less likely to clot, although not so much less that it causes you to become likely to bleed, unless you have a bleeding disorder or some injury (such as a bleeding ulcer of the stomach or intestine) that is especially likely to bleed.

Stent Patients: A heart attack or angina (chest pain) can occur when fatty deposits block the arteries that carry oxygen and nutrient-rich blood to your heart. To decrease the chance of fatty deposits building up over time, your doctor may recommend the placement of a coronary stent. TICLID may be given to you with aspirin to make blood clots less likely to form inside the stent so that the artery remains open.

Who Should Not Take TICLID? Contact your doctor immediately and do not take TICLID if:

- you have an allergic reaction to TICLID
- you have a blood disorder or a serious bleeding problem, such as a bleeding stomach ulcer
- you have previously been told you had TTP or aplastic anemia
- you have severe liver disease or other liver problems
- you are pregnant or you are planning to become pregnant
- you are breastfeeding

Distributed by Roche Laboratories Inc., Nutley, NJ 07110

Revised: March 2001

Shown in Product Identification Guide, page 331

Percent of Patients With Adverse Events in Controlled Studies (TASS and CATS)

Event	TICLID (n= 2048) Incidence	Aspirin (n = 1527) Incidence	Placebo (n = 536) Incidence
Any Events	*60.0 (20.9)*	*53.2 (14.5)*	*34.3 (6.1)*
Diarrhea	12.5 (6.3)	5.2 (1.8)	4.5 (1.7)
Nausea	7.0 (2.6)	6.2 (1.9)	1.7 (0.9)
Dyspepsia	7.0 (1.1)	9.0 (2.0)	0.9 (0.2)
Rash	5.1 (3.4)	1.5 (0.8)	0.6 (0.9)
GI Pain	3.7 (1.9)	5.6 (2.7)	1.3 (0.4)
Neutropenia	2.4 (1.3)	0.8 (0.1)	1.1 (0.4)
Purpura	2.2 (0.2)	1.6 (0.1)	0.0 (0.0)
Vomiting	1.9 (1.4)	1.4 (0.9)	0.9 (0.4)
Flatulence	1.5 (0.1)	1.4 (0.3)	0.0 (0.0)
Pruritus	1.3 (0.8)	0.3 (0.1)	0.0 (0.0)
Dizziness	1.1 (0.4)	0.5 (0.4)	0.0 (0.0)
Anorexia	1.0 (0.4)	0.5 (0.3)	0.0 (0.0)
Abnormal Liver Function Test	1.0 (0.7)	0.3 (0.3)	0.0 (0.0)

TORADOL® IV/IM ℞

[tōr-ă-dŏl]

(ketorolac tromethamine injection)

TORADOL® ORAL

(ketorolac tromethamine tablets)

WARNING

TORADOL, a nonsteroidal anti-inflammatory drug (NSAID), is indicated for the short-term (up to 5 days in adults) management of moderately severe acute pain that requires analgesia at the opioid level. It is NOT indicated for minor or chronic painful conditions. TORADOL is a potent NSAID analgesic, and its administration carries many risks. The resulting NSAID-related adverse events can be serious in certain patients for whom TORADOL is indicated, especially when the drug is used inappropriately. Increasing the dose of TORADOL beyond the label recommendations will not provide better efficacy but will result in increasing the risk of developing serious adverse events.

GASTROINTESTINAL EFFECTS

- TORADOL can cause peptic ulcers, gastrointestinal bleeding and/or perforation. Therefore, TORADOL is CONTRAINDICATED in patients with active peptic ulcer disease, in patients with recent gastrointestinal bleeding or perforation, and in patients with a history of peptic ulcer disease or gastrointestinal bleeding.

RENAL EFFECTS

- TORADOL is CONTRAINDICATED in patients with advanced renal impairment and in patients at risk for renal failure due to volume depletion (see WARNINGS).

RISK OF BLEEDING

- TORADOL inhibits platelet function and is, therefore, CONTRAINDICATED in patients with suspected or confirmed cerebrovascular bleeding, patients with hemorrhagic diathesis, incomplete hemostasis and those at high risk of bleeding (see WARNINGS and PRECAUTIONS).
- TORADOL is CONTRAINDICATED as prophylactic analgesic before any major surgery and is CONTRAINDICATED intraoperatively when hemostasis is critical because of the increased risk of bleeding.

HYPERSENSITIVITY

- Hypersensitivity reactions, ranging from bronchospasm to anaphylactic shock, have occurred and appropriate counteractive measures must be available when administering the first dose of TORADOL$^{IV/IM}$ (see CONTRAINDICATIONS and WARNINGS). TORADOL is CONTRAINDICATED in patients with previously demonstrated hypersensitivity to ketorolac tromethamine or allergic manifestations to aspirin or other nonsteroidal anti-inflammatory drugs (NSAIDs).

INTRATHECAL OR EPIDURAL ADMINISTRATION

- TORADOL is CONTRAINDICATED for intrathecal or epidural administration due to its alcohol content.

LABOR, DELIVERY AND NURSING

- The use of TORADOL in labor and delivery is CONTRAINDICATED because it may adversely affect fetal circulation and inhibit uterine contractions.
- The use of TORADOL is CONTRAINDICATED in nursing mothers because of the potential adverse effects of prostaglandin-inhibiting drugs on neonates.

CONCOMITANT USE WITH NSAIDs

- TORADOL is CONTRAINDICATED in patients currently receiving ASA or NSAIDs because of the cumulative risk of inducing serious NSAID-related side effects.

DOSAGE AND ADMINISTRATION

TORADOL^{ORAL}

- TORADOL^{ORAL} is indicated only as continuation therapy to TORADOL$^{IV/IM}$, and the combined duration of use of TORADOL$^{IV/IM}$ and TORADOL^{ORAL} is not to exceed 5 days because of the increased risk of serious adverse events.
- The recommended total daily dose of TORADOL^{ORAL} (maximum 40 mg) is significantly lower than for TORADOL$^{IV/IM}$ (maximum 120 mg) (see DOSAGE AND ADMINISTRATION and *Transition from TORADOL$^{IV/IM}$ to TORADOL^{ORAL}*).

SPECIAL POPULATIONS

- Dosage should be adjusted for patients 65 years or older, for patients under 50 kg (110 lbs) of body weight (see DOSAGE AND ADMINISTRATION) and for patients with moderately elevated serum creatinine (see WARNINGS). Doses of TORADOL$^{IV/IM}$ are not to exceed 60 mg (total dose per day) in these patients. TORADOL$^{IV/IM}$ is indicated as a single dose therapy in pediatric patients (see DOSAGE AND ADMINISTRATION); not to exceed 30 mg for IM administration and 15 mg for IV administration.

DESCRIPTION

TORADOL (ketorolac tromethamine) is a member of the pyrrolo-pyrrole group of nonsteroidal anti-inflammatory drugs (NSAIDs). The chemical name for ketorolac tromethamine is (±)-5-benzoyl-2,3-dihydro-1H-pyrrolizine-1-carboxylic acid, compound with 2-amino-2-(hydroxymethyl)-1,3-propanediol (1:1).

TORADOL is a racemix mixture of [−]S and [+]R ketorolac tromethamine. Ketorolac tromethamine may exist in three crystal forms. All forms are equally soluble in water. Ketorolac tromethamine has a pKa of 3.5 and an n-octanol/water partition coefficient of 0.26. The molecular weight of ketorolac tromethamine is 376.41. Its molecular formula is $C_{19}H_{24}N_2O_6$.

TORADOL is available for intravenous (IV) or intramuscular (IM) administration as: 15 mg in 1 mL (1.5%) and 30 mg in 1 mL (3%) in sterile solution; 60 mg in 2 mL (3%) of ketorolac tromethamine in sterile solution is available for IM administration only. The solutions contain 0.1% citric acid, 10% (w/v) alcohol, USP, and 6.68 mg, 4.35 mg and 8.70 mg, respectively, of sodium chloride in sterile water. The pH is adjusted with sodium hydroxide or hydrochloric acid, and the solutions are packaged with nitrogen. The sterile solutions are clear and slightly yellow in color.

TORADOL^{ORAL} is available as round, white, film-coated, red-printed tablets. Each tablet contains 10 mg ketorolac tromethamine, the active ingredient, with added lactose, magnesium stearate and microcrystalline cellulose. The white film-coating contains hydroxypropyl methylcellulose, polyethylene glycol and titanium dioxide.

The tables are printed with red ink that includes FD&C Red #40 Aluminum lake as the colorant. There is a large T printed on both sides of the tablet, as well as the word TORADOL on one side, and the word ROCHE on the other.

Table 1. Table of Approximate Average Pharmacokinetic Parameters (Mean ± SD) Following Oral, Intramuscular and Intravenous Doses of TORADOL

Pharmacokinetic Parameters (units)	Oral*		Intramuscular†		Intravenous Bolus‡	
	10 mg	15 mg	30 mg	60 mg	15 mg	30 mg
Bioavailability (extent)	100%					
T_{max}[1] (min)	44 ± 34	33 ± 21[§]	44 ± 29	33 ± 21[§]	1.1 ± 0.7[§]	2.9 ± 1.8
C_{max}[2] (μg/mL) [single-dose]	0.87 ± 0.22	1.14 ± 0.32[§]	2.42 ± 0.68	4.55 ± 1.27[§]	2.47 ± 0.51[§]	4.65 ± 0.96
C_{max} (μg/mL) [steady state qid]	1.05 ± 0.26[§]	1.56 ± 0.44[§]	3.11 ± 0.87[§]	N/A[‖]	3.09 ± 1.17[§]	6.85 ± 2.61
C_{min}[3] (μg/mL) [steady state qid]	0.29 ± 0.07[§]	0.47 ± 0.13[§]	0.93 ± 0.26[§]	N/A	0.61 ± 0.21[§]	1.04 ± 0.35
C_{avg}[4] (μg/mL) [steady state qid]	0.59 ± 0.20[§]	0.94 ± 0.29[§]	1.88 ± 0.59[§]	N/A	1.09 ± 0.30[§]	2.17 ± 0.59
Vβ[5] (L/kg)	0.175 ± 0.039				0.210 ± 0.044	

% Dose metabolized = <50 % Dose excreted in feces = 6

% Dose excreted in urine = 91 % Plasma protein binding = 99

* Derived from PO pharmacokinetic studies in 77 normal fasted volunteers

† Derived from IM pharmacokinetic studies in 54 normal volunteers

‡ Derived from IV pharmacokinetic studies in 24 normal volunteers

§ Mean value was simulated from observed plasma concentration data and standard deviation was simulated from percent coefficient of variation for observed C_{max} and T_{max} data

‖ Not applicable because 60 mg is only recommended as a single dose

1 Time-to-peak plasma concentration

2 Peak plasma concentration

3 Trough plasma concentration

4 Average plasma concentration

5 Volume of distribution

CLINICAL PHARMACOLOGY

Pharmacodynamics: Ketorolac tromethamine is a nonsteroidal anti-inflammatory drug (NSAID) that exhibits analgesic activity in animal models. Ketorolac tromethamine inhibits synthesis of prostaglandins and may be considered a peripherally acting analgesic. The biological activity of ketorolac tromethamine is associated with the S-form. Ketorolac tromethamine possesses no sedative or anxiolytic properties.

The peak analgesic effect of TORADOL occurs within 2 to 3 hours and is not statistically significantly different over the recommended dosage range of TORADOL. The greatest difference between large and small doses of TORADOL by either route is in the duration of analgesia.

Pharmacokinetics: Ketorolac tromethamine is a racemic mixture of [−]S- and [+]R-enantiomeric forms, with the S-form having analgesic activity.

Comparison of IV, IM and Oral Pharmacokinetics: The pharmacokinetics of ketorolac tromethamine, following IV, IM and oral doses of TORADOL, are compared in Table 1. In adults, the extent of bioavailability following administration of the ORAL and IM forms of TORADOL was equal to that following an IV bolus.

Linear Kinetics: In adults, following administration of single ORAL, IM or IV doses of TORADOL in the recommended dosage ranges, the clearance of the racemate does not change. This implies that the pharmacokinetics of ketorolac tromethamine in adults, following single or multiple IM, IV or recommended oral doses of TORADOL, are linear. At the higher recommended doses, there is a proportional increase in the concentrations of free and bound racemate.

Absorption: TORADOL is 100% absorbed after oral administration (see Table 1). Oral administration of TORADOL after a high-fat meal resulted in decreased peak and delayed time-to-peak concentrations of ketorolac tromethamine by about 1 hour. Antacids did not affect the extent of absorption.

Distribution: The mean apparent volume (Vβ) of ketorolac tromethamine following complete distribution was approximately 13 liters. This parameter was determined from single-dose data. The ketorolac tromethamine racemate has been shown to be highly protein bound (99%). Nevertheless, even plasma concentrations as high as 10 μg/mL will only occupy approximately 5% of the albumin binding sites. Thus, the unbound fraction for each enantiomer will be constant over the therapeutic range. A decrease in serum albumin, however, will result in increased free drug concentrations.

Ketorolac tromethamine is excreted in human milk (see PRECAUTIONS: *Lactation and Nursing*).

Metabolism: Ketorolac tromethamine is largely metabolized in the liver. The metabolic products are hydroxylated and conjugated forms of the parent drug. The products of metabolism, and some unchanged drug, are excreted in the urine.

Excretion: The principal route of elimination of ketorolac and its metabolites is renal. About 92% of a given dose is found in the urine, approximately 40% as metabolites and 60% as unchanged ketorolac. Approximately 6% of a dose is excreted in the feces. A single-dose study with 10 mg TORADOL (n=9) demonstrated that the S-enantiomer is cleared approximately two times faster than the R-enantiomer and that the clearance was independent of the route of administration. This means that the ratio of S/R plasma concentrations decreases with time after each dose. There is little or no inversion of the R- to S- form in humans. The clearance of the racemate in normal subjects, elderly individuals and in hepatically and renally impaired patients is outlined in Table 2 (see CLINICAL PHARMACOLOGY: *Kinetics in Special Populations*).

The half-life of the ketorolac tromethamine S-enantiomer was approximately 2.5 hours (SD ± 0.4) compared with 5 hours (SD ± 1.7) for the R-enantiomer. In other studies, the half-life for the racemate has been reported to lie within the range of 5 to 6 hours.

Accumulation: TORADOL administered as an IV bolus every 6 hours for 5 days to healthy subjects (n=13), showed no significant difference in C_{max} on Day 1 and Day 5. Trough levels averaged 0.29 μg/mL (SD ± 0.13) on Day 1 and 0.55 μg/mL (SD ± 0.23) on Day 6. Steady state was approached after the fourth dose.

Accumulation of ketorolac tromethamine has not been studied in special populations (geriatric, pediatric, renal failure or hepatic disease patients).

Kinetics in Special Populations

Geriatric Patients: Based on single-dose data only, the half-life of the ketorolac tromethamine racemate increased from 5 to 7 hours in the elderly (65 to 78 years) compared with young healthy volunteers (24 to 35 years) (see Table 2). There was little difference in the C_{max} for the two groups (elderly, 2.52 μg/mL ± 0.77; young, 2.99 μg/mL ± 1.03) (see PRECAUTIONS: *Geriatric Use*).

Pediatric Patients: Following a single intravenous bolus dose of 0.5 mg/kg in 10 children 4 to 8 years old, the half-life was 6 hours (range: 3.5 to 10 h), the average clearance was 0.042 L/hr/kg and the Vd was 0.26 L/kg (range: 0.19 to 0.44 L/kg). In a second study, following a single intravenous dose of 0.6 mg/kg in 24 children 3 to 18 years old, C_{max} was 4.3 ± 1.7 mcg/mL, T_{max} was 10.25 ± 1.15 minutes, half-life was 3.8 ± 2.6 hours, Cl was 0.0678 L/hr/kg and Vd was 0.25 L/kg. The volume of distribution and clearance of ketorolac in pediatric patients was twice that observed in adult subjects (see Tables 1 and 2). There are no pharmacokinetic data available for TORADOL administration by the IM route in pediatric patients.

Renal Insufficiency: Based on single-dose data only, the mean half-life of ketorolac tromethamine in renally impaired patients is between 6 and 19 hours and is dependent on the extent of the impairment. There is poor correlation between creatinine clearance and total ketorolac tromethamine clearance in the elderly and populations with renal impairment (r=0.5).

In patients with renal disease, the AUC_∞ of each enantiomer increased by approximately 100% compared with healthy volunteers. The volume of distribution doubles for the S-enantiomer and increases by 1/5th for the R-enantiomer. The increase in volume of distribution of ketorolac tromethamine implies an increase in unbound fraction.

The AUC_∞-ratio of the ketorolac tromethamine each enantiomers in healthy subjects and patients remained similar, indicating there was no selective excretion of either enantiomer in patients compared to healthy subjects (see WARNINGS: *Renal Effects* and Table 2).

Hepatic Insufficiency: There was no significant difference in estimates of half-life, AUC_∞ and C_{max} in 7 patients with liver disease compared to healthy volunteers (see PRECAUTIONS: *Hepatic Effects* and Table 2).

Race: Pharmacokinetic differences due to race have not been identified.

[See table 1 above]

[See table 2 at bottom of next page]

IV Administration: In normal adult subjects (n=37), the total clearance of 30 mg IV-administered TORADOL was 0.030 (0.0.17-0.051) L/h/kg. The terminal half-life was 5.6 (4.0-7.9) hours. (See *Kinetics in Special Populations* for use of TORADOL^{IV} in pediatric patients.)

Continued on next page

Toradol—Cont.

Clinical Studies

Adult Patients: The analgesic efficacy of intramuscularly, intravenously and orally administered TORADOL was investigated in two postoperative pain models: general surgery (orthopedic, gynecologic and abdominal) and oral surgery (removal of impacted third molars). The studies were double-blind, single- and multiple-dose, parallel trial designs in patients with moderate to severe pain at baseline. TORADOL$^{IV/IM}$ was compared as follows: IM to meperidine or morphine administered intramuscularly and IV to morphine administered either directly IV or through a PCA (Patient-Controlled Analgesia) pump.

Short-Term Use (up to 5 days) Studies: In adults, the comparisons of intramuscular administration during the first hour, the onset of analgesic action was similar for TORADOL and the narcotics, but the duration of analgesia was longer with TORADOL than with the opioid comparators meperidine or morphine.

In a multidose, postoperative (general surgery) double-blind trial of TORADOL^{IM} 30 mg versus morphine 6 and 12 mg IM, each drug given on an as needed basis for up to 5 days, the overall analgesic effect of TORADOL^{IM} 30 mg was between that of morphine 6 and 12 mg. The majority of patients treated with either TORADOL or morphine were dosed for up to 3 days; a small percentage of patients received 5 days of dosing.

In clinical settings where perioperative morphine was allowed, TORADOL^{IV} 30 mg, given once or twice as needed, provided analgesia comparable to morphine 4 mg IV once or twice as needed.

There was relatively limited experience with 5 consecutive days of TORADOL^{IV} use in controlled clinical trials, as most patients were given the drug for 3 days or less. The adverse events seen with IV-administered TORADOL were similar to those observed with IM-administered TORADOL, as would be expected based on the similar pharmacokinetics and bioequivalence (AUC, clearance, plasma half-life) of IV and IM routes of TORADOL administration.

Pediatric Patients: The analgesic efficacy of single doses of TORADOL$^{IV/IM}$ has been demonstrated by showing a decrease in the need for supplemental narcotic in pediatric patients receiving ketorolac as compared to placebo. See discussion of these results under *Clinical Studies With Concomitant Use of Opioids* below.

Clinical Studies With Concomitant Use of Opioids

Adults Patients: Clinical studies in postoperative pain management have demonstrated that TORADOL$^{IV/IM}$, when used in combination with opioids, significantly reduced opioid consumption. This combination may be useful in the subpopulation of patients especially prone to opioid-related complications. TORADOL and narcotics should not be administered in the same syringe.

In a postoperative study, where all patients received morphine by a PCA device, patients treated with TORADOL^{IV} as fixed intermittent boluses (eg, 30 mg initial dose followed by 15 mg q3h), required significantly less morphine (26%) than the placebo group. Analgesia was significantly superior, at various postdosing pain assessment times, in the patients receiving TORADOL^{IV} plus PCA morphine as compared to patients receiving PCA-administered morphine alone.

Pediatric Patients: TORADOL^{IM} injection reduced the need for supplemental opioid (fentanyl) when a 1 mg/kg dose was administered immediately following tonsillectomy compared to saline controls (see WARNINGS: *Hemorrhage*). In another study, when a single bolus dose of 0.9 mg/kg of TORADOL^{IV} was given to pediatric patients ages 5 to 12 years, compared to saline, a reduction in supplemental opioid was needed following various surgical procedures. In a third study less supplemental morphine was needed in pediatric patients ages 8 to 16 years, who received a 0.8 mg/kg IV injection of TORADOL in conjunction with morphine following orthopedic surgical procedures, compared to morphine alone. In a study in pediatric patients ages 3 to 12 years, TORADOL^{IV} demonstrated a slower onset of analgesia, but a longer duration of action compared to morphine. There is limited data available to support the use of multiple doses of TORADOL$^{IV/IM}$ in pediatric patients. There are also insufficient data available to support the use of TORADOL^{ORAL} in pediatric patients.

Postmarketing Surveillance Study: A large postmarketing observational, nonrandomized study, involving approximately 10,000 patients receiving TORADOL, demonstrated that the risk of clinically serious gastrointestinal (GI) bleeding was dose-dependent (see Tables 3A and 3B). This was particularly true in elderly patients who received an average daily dose greater than 60 mg/day of TORADOL (see Table 3A).

Table 3. Incidence of Clinically Serious GI Bleeding as Related to Age, Total Daily Dose, and History of GI Perforation, Ulcer, Bleeding (PUB) After up to 5 Days of Treatment With TORADOL$^{IV/IM}$

A. Adult Patients Without History of PUB

Age of Patients	Total Daily Dose of TORADOL$^{IV/IM}$			
	≤60 mg	>60 to 90 mg	>90 to 120 mg	>120 mg
<65 years of age	0.4%	0.4%	0.9%	4.6%
≥65 years of age	1.2%	2.8%	2.2%	7.7%

B. Adult Patients With History of PUB

Age of Patients	Total Daily Dose of TORADOL$^{IV/IM}$			
	≤60 mg	>60 to 90 mg	>90 to 120 mg	>120 mg
<65 years of age	2.1%	4.6%	7.8%	15.4%
≥65 years of age	4.7%	3.7%	2.8%	25.0%

INDICATIONS AND USAGE

Adult Patients: TORADOL is indicated for the short-term (≤5 days) management of moderately severe acute pain that requires analgesia at the opioid level, usually in a postoperative setting. Therapy should always be initiated with TORADOL$^{IV/IM}$, and TORADOL^{ORAL} is to be used only as continuation treatment, if necessary. Combined use of TORADOL$^{IV/IM}$ and TORADOL^{ORAL} is not to exceed 5 days of use because of the potential of increasing the frequency and severity of adverse reactions associated with the recommended doses (see WARNINGS, PRECAUTIONS, DOSAGE AND ADMINISTRATION, and ADVERSE REACTIONS). Patients should be switched to alternative analgesics as soon as possible, but TORADOL therapy is not to exceed 5 days.

Pediatric Patients: The safety and effectiveness of single doses of TORADOL$^{IV/IM}$ have been established in pediatric patients between the ages of 2 and 16 years. TORADOL, as a single injectable dose, has been shown to be effective in the management of moderately severe acute pain that requires analgesia at the opioid level, usually in the postoperative setting. There is limited data available to support the use of multiple doses of TORADOL in pediatric patients. Safety and effectiveness have not been established in pediatric patients below the age of 2 years. Use of TORADOL in pediatric patients is supported by evidence from adequate and well-controlled studies of TORADOL in adults with additional pharmacokinetic, efficacy and safety data on its use in pediatric patients available in the published literature (see CLINICAL PHARMACOLOGY: *Clinical Studies*, WARNINGS, and PRECAUTIONS).

TORADOL$^{IV/IM}$ has been used concomitantly with morphine and meperidine and has shown an opioid-sparing effect. For breakthrough pain, it is recommended to supplement the lower end of the TORADOL$^{IV/IM}$ dosage range with low doses of narcotics prn, unless otherwise contraindicated. TORADOL$^{IV/IM}$ and narcotics should not be administered in the same syringe (see DOSAGE AND ADMINISTRATION: *Pharmaceutical Information for TORADOL$^{IV/IM}$*).

CONTRAINDICATIONS (see also Boxed WARNING):

- TORADOL is CONTRAINDICATED in patients with active peptic ulcer disease, in patients with recent gastrointestinal bleeding or perforation and in patients with a history of peptic ulcer disease or gastrointestinal bleeding.
- TORADOL is CONTRAINDICATED in patients with advanced renal impairment or in patients at risk for renal failure due to volume depletion (see WARNINGS for correction of volume depletion).
- TORADOL is CONTRAINDICATED in labor and delivery because, through its prostaglandin synthesis inhibitory effect, it may adversely affect fetal circulation and inhibit uterine contractions, thus increasing the risk of uterine hemorrhage.
- The use of TORADOL is CONTRAINDICATED in nursing mothers because of the potential adverse events of prostaglandin-inhibiting drugs on neonates.
- TORADOL is CONTRAINDICATED in patients with previously demonstrated hypersensitivity to ketorolac tromethamine, allergic manifestations to aspirin or other nonsteroidal anti-inflammatory drugs (NSAIDs).
- TORADOL is CONTRAINDICATED as prophylactic analgesic before any major surgery and is CONTRAINDICATED intraoperatively when hemostasis is critical because of the increased risk of bleeding.
- TORADOL inhibits platelet function and is, therefore, CONTRAINDICATED in patients with suspected or confirmed cerebrovascular bleeding, hemorrhagic diathesis, incomplete hemostasis and those at high risk of bleeding (see WARNINGS and PRECAUTIONS).
- TORADOL is CONTRAINDICATED in patients currently receiving ASA or NSAIDs because of the cumulative risks of inducing serious NSAID-related adverse events.
- TORADOL$^{IV/IM}$ is CONTRAINDICATED for neuraxial (epidural or intrathecal) administration due to its alcohol content.
- The concomitant use of TORADOL and probenecid is CONTRAINDICATED.

WARNINGS (see also Boxed WARNING):

The combined use of TORADOL$^{IV/IM}$ and TORADOL^{ORAL} is not to exceed 5 days in adults. Only single doses of TORADOL$^{IV/IM}$ are recommended for use in pediatric patients.

The most serious risks associated with TORADOL are:

- ***Gastrointestinal (GI) Effects – Risk of GI Ulceration, Bleeding, and Perforation:*** TORADOL is CONTRAINDICATED in patients with previously documented peptic ulcers and/or GI bleeding. Serious gastrointestinal toxicity, such as bleeding, ulceration and perforation, can occur at any time, with or without warning symptoms, in patients treated with TORADOL. Studies to date with NSAIDs have not identified any subset of patients not at risk of developing peptic ulceration and bleeding. Elderly or debilitated patients seem to tolerate ulceration or bleeding less well than other individuals, and most spontaneous reports of fatal GI events are in this population. Postmarketing experience with parenterally administered TORADOL suggests that there may be a greater risk of gastrointestinal ulcerations, bleeding and perforation in the elderly.

The incidence and severity of gastrointestinal complications increases with increasing dose of, and duration of treatment with, TORADOL. In a nonrandomized, in-hospital postmarketing surveillance study comparing parenteral TORADOL to parenteral opioids, higher rates of clinically serious GI bleeding were seen in adult patients <65 years of age who received an average total daily dose of more than 90 mg of TORADOL$^{IV/IM}$ per day (see CLINICAL PHARMACOLOGY: *Postmarketing Surveillance Study*).

The same study showed that elderly (≥65 years of age) and debilitated patients are more susceptible to gastrointestinal complications. A history of peptic ulcer disease was revealed as another risk factor that increases the pos-

Table 2. The Influence of Age, Liver, and Kidney Function on the Clearance and Terminal Half-life of TORADOL (IM[1] and ORAL[2]) in Adult Populations

Type of Subjects	Total Clearance [in L/h/kg][3] IM Mean (range)	Total Clearance [in L/h/kg][3] ORAL Mean (range)	Terminal Half-life [in hours] IM Mean (range)	Terminal Half-life [in hours] ORAL Mean (range)
Normal Subjects IM (n=54) mean age=32, range=18–60 Oral (n=77) mean age=32, range=20–60	0.023 (0.010–0.046)	0.025 (0.013–0.050)	5.3 (3.5–9.2)	5.3 (2.4–9.0)
Healthy Elderly Subjects IM (n=13), Oral (n=12) mean age=72, range=65–78	0.019 (0.013–0.034)	0.024 (0.018–0.034)	7.0 (4.7–8.6)	6.1 (4.3–7.6)
Patients with Hepatic Dysfunction IM and Oral (n=7) mean age=51, range=43–64	0.029 (0.013–0.066)	0.033 (0.019–0.051)	5.4 (2.2–6.9)	4.5 (1.6–7.6)
Patients with Renal Impairment IM (n=25), Oral (n=9) serum creatinine=1.9–5.0 mg/dL, mean age (IM)=54, range=35–71 mean age (Oral)=57, range=39–70	0.015 (0.005–0.043)	0.016 (0.007–0.052)	10.3 (5.9–19.2)	10.8 (3.4–18.9)
Renal Dialysis Patients IM and Oral (n=9) mean age=40, range=27–63	0.016 (0.003–0.036)	—	13.6 (8.0–39.1)	—

[1] Estimated from 30 mg single IM doses of ketorolac tromethamine
[2] Estimated from 10 mg single oral doses of ketorolac tromethamine
[3] Liters/hour/kilogram

sibility of developing serious gastrointestinal complications during TORADOL therapy (see Tables 3A and 3B).

- ***Hemorrhage:*** Because prostaglandins play an important role in hemostasis and NSAIDs affect platelet aggregation as well, use of TORADOL in patients who have coagulation disorders should be undertaken very cautiously, and those patients should be carefully monitored. Patients on therapeutic doses of anticoagulants (eg, heparin or dicumarol derivatives) have an increased risk of bleeding complications if given TORADOL concurrently; therefore, physicians should administer such concomitant therapy only extremely cautiously. The concurrent use of TORADOL and prophylactic low-dose heparin (2500 to 5000 units q12h), warfarin and dextrans have not been studied extensively, but may also be associated with an increased risk of bleeding. Until data from such studies are available, physicians should carefully weigh the benefits against the risks and use such concomitant therapy in these patients only extremely cautiously. In patients who receive anticoagulants for any reason, there is an increased risk of intramuscular hematoma formation from administered TORADOL$^{\underline{IM}}$ (see PRECAUTIONS: *Drug Interactions*). Patients receiving therapy that affects hemostasis should be monitored closely.

  In postmarketing experience, postoperative hematomas and other signs of wound bleeding have been reported in association with the perioperative use of TORADOL$^{\underline{IV/IM}}$. Therefore, perioperative use of TORADOL should be avoided and postoperative use be undertaken with caution when hemostasis is critical (see WARNINGS and PRECAUTIONS).
- ***Pediatrics and Tonsillectomy:*** Physicians should consider the increased risk of bleeding before deciding to administer TORADOL in patients following tonsillectomy. TORADOL$^{\underline{IV/IM}}$ is not recommended for use in pediatric patients below the age of 2 years. In a retrospective analysis of patients having undergone tonsillectomy with or without adenoidectomy, the risk of bleeding was 10.1% in patients administered TORADOL$^{\underline{IV/IM}}$ compared to 2.2% in those receiving opioids. The postoperative hemorrhage rate in patients 12 years and younger was 6.5% and 3.3% with and without TORADOL, respectively. In a prospective study of TORADOL in pediatric patients (ages 3 to 9 years) undergoing tonsillectomy with or without adenoidectomy, the overall incidence of bleeding was similar between the patients receiving TORADOL and morphine (16.3% versus 17%, respectively). However, during the first 24 hours after surgery, a higher incidence of bleeding was observed in the TORADOL$^{\underline{IV/IM}}$ group (14.3%) versus the morphine group (4.2%).
- ***Anaphylactoid Reactions:*** Anaphylactoid reactions may occur in patients without a known previous exposure or hypersensitivity to aspirin, TORADOL or other NSAIDs, or in individuals with a history of angioedema, bronchospastic reactivity (eg, asthma) and nasal polyps. Anaphylactoid reactions, like anaphylaxis, may have a fatal outcome.
- ***Impaired Renal Function: TORADOL should be used with caution in patients with impaired renal function or a history of kidney disease because it is a potent inhibitor of prostaglandin synthesis.*** Renal toxicity with TORADOL has been seen in patients with conditions leading to a reduction in blood volume and/or renal blood flow where renal prostaglandins have a supportive role in the maintenance of renal perfusion. In these patients administration of TORADOL may cause a dose-dependent reduction in renal prostaglandin formation and may precipitate acute renal failure. Patients at greatest risk of this reaction are those with impaired renal function, dehydration, heart failure, liver dysfunction, those taking diuretics and the elderly. Discontinuation of TORADOL therapy is usually followed by recovery to the pretreatment state.

  Renal Effects: TORADOL and its metabolites are eliminated primarily by the kidneys, which, in patients with reduced creatinine clearance, will result in diminished clearance of the drug (see CLINICAL PHARMACOLOGY). Therefore, TORADOL should be used with caution in patients with impaired renal function (see DOSAGE AND ADMINISTRATION) and such patients should be followed closely. With the use of TORADOL, there have been reports of acute renal failure, interstitial nephritis and nephrotic syndrome.

  Because patients with underlying renal insufficiency are at increased risk of developing acute renal failure, the risks and benefits should be assessed prior to giving TORADOL to these patients. Hence, in patients with moderately elevated serum creatinine, it is recommended that the daily dose of TORADOL$^{\underline{IV/IM}}$ be reduced by half, not to exceed 60 mg/day. **TORADOL IS CONTRAINDICATED IN PATIENTS WITH SERUM CREATININE CONCENTRATIONS INDICATING ADVANCED RENAL IMPAIRMENT (see CONTRAINDICATIONS).**

  Hypovolemia should be corrected before treatment with TORADOL is initiated.
- ***Fluid Retention and Edema:*** Fluid retention, edema, retention of NaCl, oliguria, elevations of serum urea nitrogen and creatinine have been reported in clinical trials with TORADOL. Therefore, TORADOL should be used only very cautiously in patients with cardiac decompensation, hypertension or similar conditions.
- ***Pregnancy:*** In late pregnancy, as with other NSAIDs, TORADOL should be avoided because it may cause premature closure of the ductus arteriosus.

PRECAUTIONS: *General:*

- *Hepatic Effects: TORADOL should be used with caution in patients with impaired hepatic function or a history of liver disease.* Treatment with TORADOL may cause elevations of liver enzymes, and, in patients with pre-existing liver dysfunction, it may lead to the development of a more severe hepatic reaction. The administration of TORADOL should be discontinued in patients in whom an abnormal liver test has occurred as a result of TORADOL therapy.
- *Hematologic Effects:* TORADOL inhibits platelet aggregation and may prolong bleeding time; therefore, it is contraindicated as a preoperative medication, and caution should be used when hemostasis is critical. Unlike aspirin, the inhibition of platelet function by TORADOL disappears within 24 to 48 hours after the drug is discontinued. TORADOL does not appear to affect platelet count, prothrombin time (PT) or partial thromboplastin time (PTT). In controlled clinical studies, where TORADOL was administered intramuscularly or intravenously postoperatively, the incidence of clinically significant postoperative bleeding was 0.4% for TORADOL compared to 0.2% in the control groups receiving narcotic analgesics.

Information for Patients: TORADOL is a potent NSAID and may cause serious side effects such as gastrointestinal bleeding or kidney failure, which may result in hospitalization and even fatal outcome.

Physicians, when prescribing TORADOL, should inform their patients or their guardians of the potential risk of TORADOL treatment (see Boxed WARNING, WARNINGS, PRECAUTIONS, and ADVERSE REACTIONS sections).

Advise patients not to given TORADOL$^{\underline{ORAL}}$ to other family members and to discard any unused drug.

Remember that the total duration of TORADOL therapy is not to exceed 5 days in adults or a single dose in pediatric patients ages 2 to 16 years.

Drug Interactions: Ketorolac is highly bound to human plasma protein (mean 99.2%).

Warfarin, Digoxin, Salicylate, and Heparin

The in vitro binding of ***warfarin*** to plasma proteins is only slightly reduced by ketorolac tromethamine (99.5% control vs 99.3%) when ketorolac plasma concentrations reach 5 to 10 µg/mL. Ketorolac does not alter ***digoxin*** protein binding. In vitro studies indicate that, at therapeutic concentrations of ***salicylate*** (300 µg/mL), the binding of ketorolac was reduced from approximately 99.2% to 97.5%, representing a potential twofold increase in unbound ketorolac plasma levels. Therapeutic concentrations of ***digoxin, warfarin, ibuprofen, naproxen, piroxicam, acetaminophen, phenytoin*** and ***tolbutamide*** did not alter ketorolac tromethamine protein binding.

In a study involving 12 adult volunteers, TORADOL$^{\underline{ORAL}}$ was coadministered with a single dose of 25 mg ***warfarin***, causing no significant changes in pharmacokinetics or pharmacodynamics of warfarin. In another study, TORADOL$^{\underline{IV/IM}}$ was given with two doses of 5000 U of ***heparin*** to 11 healthy volunteers, resulting in a mean template bleeding time of 6.4 minutes (3.2 to 11.4 min) compared to a mean of 6.0 minutes (3.4 to 7.5 min) for heparin alone and 5.1 minutes (3.5 to 8.5 min) for placebo. Although these results do not indicate a significant interaction between TORADOL and warfarin or heparin, the administration of TORADOL to patients taking anticoagulants should be done extremely cautiously, and patients should be closely monitored (see WARNINGS and PRECAUTIONS).

Furosemide

TORADOL$^{\underline{IV/IM}}$ reduced the diuretic response to ***furosemide*** in normovolemic healthy subjects by approximately 20% (mean sodium and urinary output decreased 17%).

Probenecid

Concomitant administration of TORADOL$^{\underline{ORAL}}$ and ***probenecid*** resulted in decreased clearance of ketorolac and significant increases in ketorolac plasma levels (total AUC increased approximately threefold from 5.4 to 17.8 µg/h/mL) and terminal half-life increased approximately twofold from 6.6 to 15.1 hours. Therefore, concomitant use of TORADOL and probenecid is contraindicated.

Lithium

Inhibition of renal ***lithium*** clearance, leading to an increase in plasma lithium concentration, has been reported with some prostaglandin synthesis-inhibiting drugs. The effect of TORADOL on plasma lithium has not been studied, but cases of increased lithium plasma levels during TORADOL therapy have been reported.

Methotrexate

Concomitant administration of ***methotrexate*** and some NSAIDs has been reported to reduce the clearance of methotrexate, enhancing the toxicity of methotrexate. The effect of TORADOL on methotrexate clearance has not been studied.

Nondepolarizing Muscle Relaxants

In postmarketing experience there have been reports of a possible interaction between TORADOL$^{\underline{IV/IM}}$ and ***nondepolarizing muscle relaxants*** that resulted in apnea. The concurrent use of TORADOL with muscle relaxants has not been formally studied.

ACE Inhibitors

Concomitant use of ***ACE inhibitors*** may increase the risk of renal impairment, particularly in volume-depleted patients.

Antiepileptic Drugs

Sporadic cases of seizures have been reported during concomitant use of TORADOL and ***antiepileptic drugs*** (phenytoin, carbamazepine).

Psychoactive Drugs

Hallucinations have been reported when TORADOL was used in patients taking ***psychoactive drugs*** (fluoxetine, thiothixene, alprazolam).

Morphine

TORADOL$^{\underline{IV/IM}}$ has been administered concurrently with ***morphine*** in several clinical trials of postoperative pain without evidence of adverse interactions. Do not mix TORADOL and morphine in the same syringe.

There is no evidence in animal or human studies that TORADOL induces or inhibits hepatic enzymes capable of metabolizing itself or other drugs.

Carcinogenesis, Mutagenesis and Impairment of Fertility:

An 18-month study in mice with oral doses of ketorolac tromethamine at 2 mg/kg/day (0.9 times of human systemic exposure at the recommended IM or IV dose of 30 mg qid, based on area-under-the-plasma-concentration curve [AUC]), and a 24-month study in rats at 5 mg/kg/day (0.5 times the human AUC) showed no evidence of tumorigenicity.

Ketorolac tromethamine was not mutagenic in the Ames test, unscheduled DNA synthesis and repair, and in forward mutation assays. Ketorolac tromethamine did not cause chromosome breakage in the in vivo mouse micronucleus assay. At 1590 µg/mL and at higher concentrations, ketorolac tromethamine increased the incidence of chromosomal aberrations in Chinese hamster ovarian cells.

Impairment of fertility did not occur in male or female rats at oral doses of 9 mg/kg (0.9 times the human AUC) and 16 mg/kg (1.6 times the human AUC) of ketorolac tromethamine, respectively.

Pregnancy: Pregnancy Category C. Reproduction studies have been performed during organogenesis using daily oral doses of ketorolac tromethamine at 3.6 mg/kg (0.37 times the human AUC) in rabbits and at 10 mg/kg (1.0 times the human AUC) in rats. Results of these studies did not reveal evidence of teratogenicity to the fetus. Oral doses of ketorolac tromethamine at 1.5 mg/kg (0.14 times the human AUC), administered after gestation Day 17, caused dystocia and higher pup mortality in rats. There are no adequate and well-controlled studies of TORADOL in pregnant women. TORADOL should be used during pregnancy only if the potential benefit justifies the potential risk to the fetus.

Labor and Delivery: The use of TORADOL is contraindicated in labor and delivery because, through its prostaglandin synthesis inhibitory effect, it may adversely affect fetal circulation and inhibit uterine contractions, thus increasing the risk of uterine hemorrhage (see CONTRAINDICATIONS).

Lactation and Nursing: After a single administration of 10 mg of TORADOL$^{\underline{ORAL}}$ to humans, the maximum milk concentration observed was 7.3 ng/mL, and the maximum milk-to-plasma ratio was 0.037. After 1 day of dosing (qid), the maximum milk concentration was 7.9 ng/mL, and the maximum milk-to-plasma ratio was 0.025. Because of the possible adverse effects of prostaglandin-inhibiting drugs on neonates, use in nursing mothers is contraindicated.

Pediatric Use: The safety and effectiveness of single doses of TORADOL$^{\underline{IV/IM}}$ have been established in pediatric patients between the ages of 2 and 16 years. TORADOL$^{\underline{IV/IM}}$ has been shown to be effective in the management of moderately severe acute pain that requires analgesia at the opioid level, usually in a postoperative setting. Safety and efficacy in pediatric patients below the age of 2 have not been established. Therefore, TORADOL$^{\underline{IV/IM}}$ is not recommended in pediatric patients below the age of 2. The risk of bleeding was greater in those patients administered TORADOL$^{\underline{IV/IM}}$ following tonsillectomy. Physicians should consider the increased risk of bleeding before deciding to administer TORADOL$^{\underline{IV/IM}}$ in patients following tonsillectomy (see WARNINGS: *Hemorrhage* and *Pediatrics and Tonsillectomy*).

The risks identified in the adult population with TORADOL$^{\underline{IV/IM}}$ use also apply to pediatric patients. Therefore, consult the CONTRAINDICATIONS, WARNINGS, PRECAUTIONS, and ADVERSE REACTIONS sections when prescribing TORADOL$^{\underline{IV/IM}}$ to pediatric patients.

Geriatric Use (≥65 years of age): Because ketorolac tromethamine may be cleared more slowly by the elderly (see CLINICAL PHARMACOLOGY) who are also more sensitive to the adverse effects of NSAIDs (see WARNINGS: *Renal Effects*), extra caution and reduced dosages (see DOSAGE AND ADMINISTRATION) must be used when treating the elderly with TORADOL$^{\underline{IV/IM}}$. The lower end of the TORADOL$^{\underline{IV/IM}}$ dosage range is recommended for patients over 65 years of age, and total daily dose is not to exceed 60 mg. The incidence and severity of gastrointestinal complications increases with increasing dose of, and duration of treatment with, TORADOL.

ADVERSE REACTIONS

Adverse reaction rates increase with higher doses of TORADOL. Practitioners should be alert for the severe complications of treatment with TORADOL, such as GI ulceration, bleeding and perforation, postoperative bleeding, acute renal failure, anaphylactic and anaphylactoid reactions and liver failure (see Boxed WARNING, WARNINGS, PRECAUTIONS, and DOSAGE AND ADMINISTRATION). These NSAID-related complications can be serious in certain patients for whom TORADOL is indicated, especially when the drug is used inappropriately.

Continued on next page

Toradol—Cont.

The Adverse Reactions Listed Below Were Reported in Clinical Trials as Probably Related to TORADOL:

• Incidence Greater Than 1%

Percentage of incidence in parentheses for those events reported in 3% or more patients.

Body as a Whole: edema (4%)
Cardiovascular: hypertension
Dermatologic: pruritus, rash
Gastrointestinal: nausea (12%), dyspepsia (12%), gastrointestinal pain (13%), diarrhea (7%), constipation, flatulence, gastrointestinal fullness, vomiting, stomatitis
Hemic and Lymphatic: purpura
Nervous System: headache (17%), drowsiness (6%), dizziness (7%), sweating
Injection-site pain was reported by 2% of patients in multi-dose studies.

• Incidence 1% or Less

Body as a Whole: weight gain, fever, infections, asthenia
Cardiovascular: palpitation, pallor, syncope
Dermatologic: urticaria
Gastrointestinal: gastritis, rectal bleeding, eructation, anorexia, increased appetite
Hemic and Lymphatic: epistaxis, anemia, eosinophilia
Nervous System: tremors, abnormal dreams, hallucinations, euphoria, extrapyramidal symptoms, vertigo, paresthesia, depression, insomnia, nervousness, excessive thirst, dry mouth, abnormal thinking, inability to concentrate, hyperkinesis, stupor
Respiratory: dyspnea, pulmonary edema, rhinitis, cough
Special Senses: abnormal taste, abnormal vision, blurred vision, tinnitus, hearing loss
Urogenital: hematuria, proteinuria, oliguria, urinary retention, polyuria, increased urinary frequency

The Following Adverse Events Were Reported From Post-marketing Experience:

Body as a Whole: hypersensitivity reactions such as anaphylaxis, anaphylactoid reaction, laryngeal edema, tongue edema (see Boxed WARNING and WARNINGS), angioedema, myalgia
Cardiovascular: hypotension, flushing
Dermatologic: Lyell's syndrome, Stevens-Johnson syndrome, exfoliative dermatitis, maculopapular rash, urticaria
Gastrointestinal: peptic ulceration, GI hemorrhage, GI perforation (see Boxed WARNING and WARNINGS), melena, acute pancreatitis, hematemesis, esophagitis
Hemic and Lymphatic: postoperative wound hemorrhage (rarely requiring blood transfusion — see Boxed WARNING, WARNINGS, and PRECAUTIONS), thrombocytopenia, leukopenia
Hepatic: hepatitis, liver failure, cholestatic jaundice
Nervous System: convulsions, psychosis, aseptic meningitis
Respiratory: asthma, bronchospasm
Urogenital: acute renal failure (see Boxed WARNING and WARNINGS), flank pain with or without hematuria and/or azotemia, interstitial nephritis, hyponatremia, hyperkalemia, hemolytic uremic syndrome

OVERDOSAGE

Symptoms following acute NSAIDs overdoses are usually limited to lethargy, drowsiness, nausea, vomiting, and epigastric pain, which are generally reversible with supportive care. Gastrointestinal bleeding can occur. Hypertension, acute renal failure, respiratory depression and coma may occur, but are rare. Anaphylactoid reactions have been reported with therapeutic ingestion of NSAIDs, and may occur following an overdose.

Patients should be managed by symptomatic and supportive care following a NSAIDs overdose. There are no specific antidotes. Emesis and/or activated charcoal (60 g to 100 g in adults, 1 g/kg to 2 g/kg in children) and/or osmotic cathartic may be indicated in patients seen within 4 hours of ingestion with symptoms or following a large oral overdose (5 to 10 times the usual dose).

In controlled overdosage, daily doses of 360 mg of TORADOL$^{IV/IM}$ given for 5 days (three times the highest recommended dose), caused abdominal pain and peptic ulcers which healed after discontinuation of dosing. Metabolic acidosis has been reported following intentional overdosage. Single overdoses of TORADOL have been variously associated with abdominal pain, nausea, vomiting, hyperventilation, peptic ulcers and/or erosive gastritis and renal dysfunction which have resolved after discontinuation of dosing. Dialysis does not significantly clear ketorolac tromethamine from the blood stream.

DOSAGE AND ADMINISTRATION

IN ADULTS, THE COMBINED DURATION OF USE OF TORADOL$^{IV/IM}$ AND TORADOL^{ORAL} IS NOT TO EXCEED 5 DAYS. IN ADULTS, THE USE OF TORADOL^{ORAL} IS ONLY INDICATED AS CONTINUATION THERAPY TO TORADOL$^{IV/IM}$.

TORADOL$^{IV/IM}$

Adults Patients: TORADOL$^{IV/IM}$ may be used as a single or multiple dose on a regular or prn schedule for the management of moderately severe acute pain that requires analgesia at the opioid level, usually in a postoperative setting. Hypovolemia should be corrected prior to the administration of TORADOL (see WARNINGS: *Renal Effects*). Patients should be switched to alternative analgesics as soon as possible, but TORADOL therapy is not to exceed 5 days.

When administering TORADOL$^{IV/IM}$, the IV bolus must be given over no less than 15 seconds. The IM administration should be given slowly and deeply into the muscle. The analgesic effect begins in ~30 minutes with maximum effect in 1 to 2 hours after dosing IV or IM, Duration of analgesic effect is usually 4 to 6 hours.

Single-Dose Treatment: The Following Regimen Should Be Limited to Single Administration Use Only

Adult Patients:

IM Dosing:

- *Patients <65 years of age:* One dose of 60 mg.
- *Patients ≥65 years of age, renally impaired and/or less than 50 kg (110 lbs) of body weight:* One dose of 30 mg.

IV Dosing:

- *Patients <65 years of age:* One dose of 30 mg.
- *Patients ≥65 years of age, renally impaired and/or less than 50 kg (110 lbs) of body weight:* One dose of 15 mg.

Pediatric Patients (2 to 16 years of age): The pediatric population should receive only a single dose of TORADOL injection, as follows:

IM Dosing:

- One dose of 1 mg/kg up to a maximum of 30 mg.

IV Dosing:

- One dose of 0.5 mg/kg up to a maximum of 15 mg.

Multiple-Dose Treatment (IV or IM) in Adults

- *Patients <65 years of age:* The recommended dose is 30 mg TORADOL$^{IV/IM}$ every 6 hours. The maximum daily dose should not exceed 120 mg.
- *For Patients ≥65 years of age, renally impaired patients (see WARNINGS) and patients less than 50 kg (110 lbs):* The recommended dose is 15 mg TORADOL$^{IV/IM}$ every 6 hours. The maximum daily dose for these populations should not exceed 60 mg.

For breakthrough pain do not increase the dose or the frequency of TORADOL. Consideration should be given to supplementing these regimens with low doses of opioids prn unless otherwise contraindicated.

Pharmaceutical Information for TORADOL$^{IV/IM}$: Parenteral drug products should be inspected visually for particulate matter and discoloration prior to administration whenever solution and container permit.

TORADOL$^{IV/IM}$ should not be mixed in a small volume (eg, in a syringe) with morphine sulfate, meperidine hydrochloride, promethazine hydrochloride or hydroxyzine hydrochloride; this will result in precipitation of ketorolac from solution.

TORADOL^{ORAL} is indicated ONLY as continuation therapy to TORADOL$^{IV/IM}$ for the management of moderately severe acute pain that requires analgesia at the opioid level (see also PRECAUTIONS: *Information for Patients*).

Transition From TORADOL$^{IV/IM}$ to TORADOL^{ORAL} in Adults: The recommended TORADOL^{ORAL} dose is as follows:

- *Adult Patients <65 years of age:* 2 tablets as a first oral dose for patients who received **60 mg IM single dose, 30 mg IV single dose or 30 multiple dose.** TORADOL$^{IV/IM}$ followed by 1 tablet TORADOL^{ORAL} every 4 to 6 hours, not to exceed 40 mg/24 h of TORADOL^{ORAL}.
- *Patients ≥65 years of age, renally impaired and/or less than 50 kg (110 lbs) of body weight:* 1 tablet as a first oral dose for patients who received **30 mg IM single dose, 15 mg IV single dose or 15 mg multiple dose.** TORADOL$^{IV/IM}$ followed by 1 tablet TORADOL^{ORAL} every 4 to 6 hours, not to exceed 40 mg/24 h of TORADOL^{ORAL}.

Shortening the recommended dosing intervals may result in increased frequency and severity of adverse reactions.

In adults, the maximum combined duration of use (parenteral and oral TORADOL is limited to 5 days.

HOW SUPPLIED

TORADOL$^{IV/IM}$ for intramuscular or intravenous use is available in a sterile vial:

15 mg: 15 mg/mL, 1 mL fill per 2 mL single use vial, box of 10 (NDC 0004-6925-06).

30 mg: 30 mg/mL, 1 mL fill per 2 mL single use vial, box of 10 (NDC 0004-6926-06).

For IM Single-Dose Use Only; Not Intended for IV Use — 60 mg: 30 mg/mL, 2 mL fill per 2 mL single use vial, box of 1 (NDC 0004-6927-09).

Store vials at 15° to 30°C (59° to 86°F) with protection from light.

TORADOL^{ORAL} 10 mg tablets are round, white, film-coated, red printed tablets. There is a large T printed on both sides of the tablet, with TORADOL on one side, and ROCHE on the other, available in bottles of 100 tablets (NDC 0004-0273-01).

Store bottles at 15° to 30°C (59° to 86°F).

Revised: September 2002

Shown in Product Identification Guide, page 331

VALCYTE® ℞

(valganciclovir hydrochloride tablets)

> **WARNING**
> **THE CLINICAL TOXICITY OF VALCYTE, WHICH IS METABOLIZED TO GANCICLOVIR, INCLUDES GRANULOCYTOPENIA, ANEMIA AND THROMBOCYTOPENIA. IN ANIMAL STUDIES GANCICLOVIR WAS CARCINOGENIC, TERATOGENIC AND CAUSED ASPERMATOGENESIS.**

DESCRIPTION

Valcyte (valganciclovir HCl tablets) contains valganciclovir hydrochloride (valganciclovir HCl), a hydrochloride salt of the L-valyl ester of ganciclovir that exists as a mixture of two diastereomers. Ganciclovir is a synthetic guanine derivative active against cytomegalovirus (CMV).

Valcyte is available as a 450 mg tablet for oral administration. Each tablet contains 496.3 mg of valganciclovir HCl (corresponding to 450 mg of valganciclovir), and the inactive ingredients microcrystalline cellulose, povidone K-30, crospovidone and stearic acid. The film-coat applied to the tablets contains Opadry Pink®.

Valganciclovir HCl is a white to off-white crystalline powder with a molecular formula of $C_{14}H_{22}N_6O_5 \cdot HCl$ and a molecular weight of 390.83. The chemical name for valganciclovir HCl is L-Valine, 2-[(2-amino-1,6-dihydro-6-oxo-9H-purin-9-yl)methoxy]-3-hydroxypropyl ester, monohydrochloride. Valganciclovir HCl is a polar hydrophilic compound with a solubility of 70 mg/mL in water at 25°C at a pH of 7.0 and an n-octanol/water partition coefficient of 0.0095 at pH 7.0. The pKa for valganciclovir HCl is 7.6.

All doses in this insert are specified in terms of valganciclovir.

VIROLOGY

Mechanism of Action

Valganciclovir is an L-valyl ester (prodrug) of ganciclovir that exists as a mixture of two diastereomers. After oral administration, both diastereomers are rapidly converted to ganciclovir by intestinal and hepatic esterases. Ganciclovir is a synthetic analogue of 2′-deoxyguanosine, which inhibits replication of human cytomegalovirus in vitro and in vivo. In CMV-infected cells ganciclovir is initially phosphorylated to ganciclovir monophosphate by the viral protein kinase, pUL97. Further phosphorylation occurs by cellular kinases to produce ganciclovir triphosphate, which is then slowly metabolized intracellularly (half-life 18 hours). As the phosphorylation is largely dependent on the viral kinase, phosphorylation of ganciclovir occurs preferentially in virus-infected cells. The virustatic activity of ganciclovir is due to inhibition of viral DNA synthesis by ganciclovir triphosphate.

Antiviral Activity

The quantitative relationship between the in vitro susceptibility of human herpesviruses to antivirals and clinical response to antiviral therapy has not been established, and virus sensitivity testing has not been standardized. Sensitivity test results, expressed as the concentration of drug required to inhibit the growth of virus in cell culture by 50% (IC_{50}), vary greatly depending upon a number of factors. Thus the IC_{50} of ganciclovir that inhibits human CMV replication in vitro (laboratory and clinical isolates) has ranged from 0.02 to 5.75 μg/mL (0.08 to 22.94 μM). Ganciclovir inhibits mammalian cell proliferation (IC_{50}) in vitro at higher concentrations ranging from 10.21 to >250 μg/mL (40 to >1000 μM). Bone marrow-derived colony-forming cells are more sensitive (IC_{50} = 0.69 to 3.06 μg/mL: 2.7 to 12 μM).

Viral Resistance

Viruses resistant to ganciclovir can arise after prolonged treatment with valganciclovir by selection of mutations in either the viral protein kinase gene (UL97) responsible for ganciclovir monophosphorylation and/or in the viral DNA polymerase gene (UL54). Virus with mutations in the UL97 gene is resistant to ganciclovir alone, whereas virus with mutations in the UL54 gene may show cross-resistance to other antivirals that target the same sites on viral DNA polymerase.

The current working definition of CMV resistance to ganciclovir in in vitro assays is $IC_{50} \geq 1.5$ μg/mL (≥ 6.0 μM). CMV resistance to ganciclovir has been observed in individuals with AIDS and CMV retinitis who have never received ganciclovir therapy. Viral resistance has also been observed in patients receiving prolonged treatment for CMV retinitis with ganciclovir. The possibility of viral resistance should be considered in patients who show poor clinical response or experience persistent viral excretion during therapy.

CLINICAL PHARMACOLOGY

Pharmacokinetics

BECAUSE THE MAJOR ELIMINATION PATHWAY FOR GANCICLOVIR IS RENAL, DOSAGE REDUCTIONS ACCORDING TO CREATININE CLEARANCE ARE REQUIRED FOR VALCYTE TABLETS. FOR DOSING INSTRUCTIONS IN PATIENTS WITH RENAL IMPAIRMENT, REFER TO DOSAGE AND ADMINISTRATION.

The pharmacokinetic properties of valganciclovir have been evaluated in HIV- and CMV-seropositive patients, patients with AIDS and CMV retinitis and in solid organ transplant patients.

The ganciclovir pharmacokinetic measures following administration of 900 mg Valcyte and 5 mg/kg intravenous ganciclovir and 1000 mg three times daily oral ganciclovir in HIV-positive/CMV-positive patients are summarized in Table 1.

[See table 1 at top of next page]

The area under the plasma concentration-time curve (AUC) for ganciclovir administered as Valcyte tablets is comparable to the ganciclovir AUC for intravenous ganciclovir. Ganciclovir C_{max} following Valcyte administration is 40% lower than following intravenous ganciclovir administration. During maintenance dosing, ganciclovir $AUC_{0\text{-}24\ hr}$ and C_{max} following oral ganciclovir administration (1000 mg three times daily) are lower relative to Valcyte and intravenous ganciclovir. The ganciclovir C_{min} following intravenous ganciclovir and Valcyte administration are less than the ganciclovir C_{min} following oral ganciclovir administration. The clinical significance of the differences in ganciclovir pharmacokinetics for these three ganciclovir delivery systems is unknown.

Figure 1. Ganciclovir Plasma Concentration Time Profiles in HIV-positive/CMV-positive Patients*

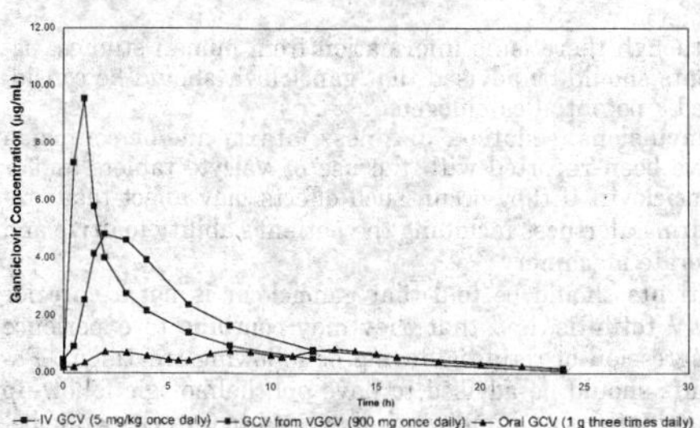

*Plasma concentration-time profiles for ganciclovir (GCV) from Valcyte (VGCV) and intravenous ganciclovir were obtained from a multiple dose study (study WV15376 n=21 and n=18, respectively) in HIV-positive/CMV-positive patients with CMV retinitis. The plasma concentration-time profile for oral ganciclovir was obtained from a multiple dose study (GAN2230 n=24) in HIV-positive/CMV-positive patients without CMV retinitis.

In solid organ transplant recipients, the mean systemic exposure to ganciclovir was 1.7 × higher following administration of 900 mg Valcyte tablets once daily versus 1000 mg ganciclovir capsules three times daily, when both drugs were administered according to their renal function dosing algorithms. The systemic ganciclovir exposures attained were comparable across kidney, heart and liver transplant recipients based on a population pharmacokinetics evaluation (see Table 2).

[See table 2 at right]

In a pharmacokinetic study in liver transplant patients, the ganciclovir $AUC_{0\text{-}24\ hr}$ achieved with 900 mg valganciclovir was 41.7 ± 9.9 µg•h/mL (n=28) and the $AUC_{0\text{-}24\ hr}$ achieved with the approved dosage of 5 mg/kg intravenous ganciclovir was 48.2 ± 17.3 µg•h/mL (n=27).

Absorption

Valganciclovir, a prodrug of ganciclovir, is well absorbed from the gastrointestinal tract and rapidly metabolized in the intestinal wall and liver to ganciclovir. The absolute bioavailability of ganciclovir from Valcyte tablets following administration with food was approximately 60% (3 studies, n=18; n=16; n=28). Ganciclovir median T_{max} following administration of 450 mg to 2625 mg Valcyte tablets ranged from 1 to 3 hours. Dose proportionality with respect to ganciclovir AUC following administration of Valcyte tablets was demonstrated only under fed conditions. Systemic exposure to the prodrug, valganciclovir, is transient and low, and the AUC_{24} and C_{max} values are approximately 1% and 3% of those of ganciclovir, respectively.

Food Effects

When Valcyte tablets were administered with a high fat meal containing approximately 600 total calories (31.1 g fat, 51.6 g carbohydrates and 22.2 g protein) at a dose of 875 mg once daily to 16 HIV-positive subjects, the steady-state ganciclovir AUC increased by 30% (95% CI 12% to 51%), and the C_{max} increased by 14% (95% CI -5% to 36%), without any prolongation in time to peak plasma concentrations (T_{max}). Valcyte tablets should be administered with food (see DOSAGE AND ADMINISTRATION).

Distribution

Due to the rapid conversion of valganciclovir to ganciclovir, plasma protein binding of valganciclovir was not determined. Plasma protein binding of ganciclovir is 1% to 2% over concentrations of 0.5 and 51 µg/mL. When ganciclovir was administered intravenously, the steady-state volume of distribution of ganciclovir was 0.703 ± 0.134 L/kg (n=69).

After administration of Valcyte tablets, no correlation was observed between ganciclovir AUC and reciprocal weight; oral dosing of Valcyte tablets according to weight is not required.

Metabolism

Valganciclovir is rapidly hydrolyzed to ganciclovir; no other metabolites have been detected. No metabolite of orally administered radiolabeled ganciclovir (1000 mg single dose) accounted for more than 1% to 2% of the radioactivity recovered in the feces or urine.

Elimination

The major route of elimination of valganciclovir is by renal excretion as ganciclovir through glomerular filtration and active tubular secretion. Systemic clearance of intravenously administered ganciclovir was 3.07 ± 0.64 mL/min/kg (n=68) while renal clearance was 2.99 ± 0.67 mL/min/kg (n=16).

The terminal half-life ($t_{1/2}$) of ganciclovir following oral administration of Valcyte tablets to either healthy or HIV-positive/CMV-positive subjects was 4.08 ± 0.76 hours (n=73), and that following administration of intravenous ganciclovir was 3.81 ± 0.71 hours (n=69). In heart, kidney, kidney-pancreas, and liver transplant patients, the terminal elimination half-life of ganciclovir following oral administration of Valcyte was 6.48 ± 1.38 hours, and following oral administration of Cytovene was 8.56 ± 3.62.

Table 1 Mean Ganciclovir Pharmacokinetic* Measures in Healthy Volunteers and HIV-positive/CMV-positive Adults at Maintenance Dosage

Formulation	Valcyte Tablets	Cytovene®-IV	Cytovene®
Dosage	900 mg once daily with food	5 mg/kg once daily	1000 mg three times daily with food
$AUC_{0\text{-}24\ hr}$ (µg•h/mL)	29.1 ± 9.7 (3 studies, n=57)	26.5 ± 5.9 (4 studies, n=68)	Range of means 12.3 to 19.2 (6 studies, n=94)
C_{max} (µg/mL)	5.61 ± 1.52 (3 studies, n=58)	9.46 ± 2.02 (4 studies, n=68)	Range of means 0.955 to 1.40 (6 studies, n=94)
Absolute oral bioavailability (%)	59.4 ± 6.1 (2 studies, n=32)	Not Applicable	Range of means 6.22± 1.29 to 8.53 ± 1.53 (2 studies, n=32)
Elimination half-life (hr)	4.08 ± 0.76 (4 studies, n=73)	3.81 ± 0.71 (4 studies, n=69)	Range of means 3.86 to 5.03 (4 studies, n=61)
Renal clearance (mL/min/kg)	3.21 ± 0.75 (1 study, n=20)	2.99 ± 0.67 (1 study, n=16)	Range of means 2.67 to 3.98 (3 studies, n=30)

*Data were obtained from single and multiple dose studies in healthy volunteers, HIV-positive patients, and HIV-positive/CMV-positive patients with and without retinitis. Patients with CMV retinitis tended to have higher ganciclovir plasma concentrations than patients without CMV retinitis.

Table 2 Mean Ganciclovir Pharmacokinetic Measures by Organ Type (Study PV 16000)

Parameter	Cytovene Capsules	Valcyte Tablets
Dosage	1000 mg three times daily with food	900 mg once daily with food
Heart Transplant Recipients	N=13	N=17
$AUC_{0\text{-}24\ hr}$ (µg•h/mL)	26.6 ± 11.6	40.2 ± 11.8
C_{max} (µg/ml)	1.4 ± 0.5	4.9 ± 1.1
Elimination half-life (hr)	8.47 ± 2.84	6.58 ± 1.50
Liver Transplant Recipients	N=33	N=75
$AUC_{0\text{-}24\ hr}$ (µg•h/mL)	24.9 ± 10.2	46.0 ± 16.1
C_{max} (µg/ml)	1.3 ± 0.4	5.4 ± 1.5
Elimination half-life (hr)	7.68 ± 2.74	6.18 ± 1.42
Kidney Transplant Recipients	N=36	N=68
$AUC_{0\text{-}24\ hr}$ (µg•h/mL)	31.3 ± 10.3	48.2 ± 14.6
C_{max} (µg/ml)	1.5 ± 0.5	5.3 ± 1.5
Elimination half-life (hr)	9.44 ± 4.37	6.77 ± 1.25

* Includes kidney-pancreas

Table 3 Pharmacokinetics of Ganciclovir From a Single Oral Dose of 900 mg Valcyte Tablets

Estimated Creatinine Clearance (mL/min)	N	Apparent Clearance (mL/min) Mean ± SD	AUC_{last} (µg•h/mL) Mean± SD	Half-life (hours) Mean± SD
51-70	6	249 ± 99	49.5 ± 22.4	4.85 ± 1.4
21-50	6	136 ± 64	91.9 ± 43.9	10.2 ± 4.4
11-20	6	45 ± 11	223 ± 46	21.8 ± 5.2
≤10	6	12.8 ± 8	366 ± 66	67.5 ± 34

Special Populations

Renal Impairment

The pharmacokinetics of ganciclovir from a single oral dose of 900 mg Valcyte tablets were evaluated in 24 otherwise healthy individuals with renal impairment.

[See table 3 at right]

Decreased renal function results in decreased clearance of ganciclovir from valganciclovir, and a corresponding increase in terminal half-life. Therefore, dosage adjustment is required for patients with impaired renal function (see PRECAUTIONS: General).

Hemodialysis

Hemodialysis reduces plasma concentrations of ganciclovir by about 50% following Valcyte administration. Patients receiving hemodialysis (CrCl <10 mL/min) cannot use Valcyte tablets because the daily dose of Valcyte tablets required for these patients is less than 450 mg (see PRECAUTIONS: General and DOSAGE AND ADMINISTRATION: Hemodialysis Patients).

Patients with Hepatic Impairment

The safety and efficacy of Valcyte tablets have not been studied in patients with hepatic impairment.

Race/Ethnicity and Gender

Insufficient data are available to demonstrate any effect of race or gender on the pharmacokinetics of valganciclovir.

Pediatrics

Valcyte tablets have not been studied in pediatric patients; the pharmacokinetic characteristics of Valcyte tablets in these patients have not been established (see PRECAUTIONS: Pediatric Use).

Geriatrics

No studies of Valcyte tablets have been conducted in adults older than 65 years of age (see PRECAUTIONS: Geriatric Use).

INDICATIONS AND USAGE

Valcyte tablets are indicated for the treatment of cytomegalovirus (CMV) retinitis in patients with acquired immunodeficiency syndrome (AIDS) (see CLINICAL TRIALS).

Valcyte is indicated for the prevention of cytomegalovirus (CMV) disease in kidney, heart, and kidney-pancreas transplant patients at high risk (Donor CMV seropositive/Recipient CMV seronegative [(D+/R-)]).

Valcyte is not indicated for use in liver transplant patients (see CLINICAL TRIALS and WARNINGS).

The safety and efficacy of Valcyte for the prevention of CMV disease in other solid organ transplant patients such as lung transplant patients have not been established.

CLINICAL TRIALS

Induction Therapy of CMV Retinitis

Study WV15376

In a randomized, open-label controlled study, 160 patients with AIDS and newly diagnosed CMV retinitis were randomized to receive treatment with either Valcyte tablets (900 mg twice daily for 21 days, then 900 mg once daily for 7 days) or with intravenous ganciclovir solution (5 mg/kg twice daily for 21 days, then 5 mg/kg once daily for 7 days). Study participants were: male (91%), White (53%), Hispanic (31%), and Black (11%). The median age was 39 years, the median baseline HIV-1 RNA was 4.9 $\log_{10}$, and the median CD_4 cell count was 23 cells/mm^3. A determination of CMV retinitis progression by the masked review of retinal photographs taken at baseline and week 4 was the primary outcome measurement of the 3-week induction therapy. Table 4 provides the outcomes at 4 weeks.

Continued on next page

Valcyte—Cont.

Table 4 Week 4 Masked Review of Retinal Photographs in Study WV15376

	Cytovene-IV	Valcyte
Determination of CMV retinitis progression at Week 4	N=80	N=80
Progressor	7	7
Non-progressor	63	64
Death	2	1
Discontinuations due to Adverse Events	1	2
Failed to return	1	1
CMV not confirmed at baseline or no interpretable baseline photos	6	5

Maintenance Therapy of CMV Retinitis
No comparative clinical data are available on the efficacy of Valcyte for the maintenance therapy of CMV retinitis because all patients in study WV15376 received open-label Valcyte after week 4. However, the AUC for ganciclovir is similar following administration of 900 mg Valcyte tablets once daily and 5 mg/kg intravenous ganciclovir once daily. Although the ganciclovir C_{max} is lower following Valcyte administration compared to intravenous ganciclovir, it is higher than the C_{max} obtained following oral ganciclovir administration (see Figure 1 in CLINICAL PHARMACOLOGY). Therefore, use of Valcyte as maintenance therapy is supported by a plasma concentration-time profile similar to that of two approved products for maintenance therapy of CMV retinitis.

Prevention of CMV Disease in Heart, Kidney, Kidney-Pancreas, and Liver Transplantation
A double-blind, double-dummy active comparator study was conducted in 372 heart, liver, kidney, and kidney-pancreas transplant patients at high-risk for CMV disease (D+/R-). Patients were randomized (2 Valcyte: 1 oral ganciclovir) to receive either Valcyte (900 mg once daily) or oral ganciclovir (1000 mg three times a day) starting within 10 days of transplantation until Day 100 posttransplant. The proportion of patients who developed CMV disease, including CMV syndrome and/or tissue-invasive disease during the first 6 months posttransplant was similar between the Valcyte arm (12.1%, N=239) and the oral ganciclovir arm (15.2%, N=125). However, in liver transplant patients, the incidence of tissue-invasive CMV disease was significantly higher in the Valcyte group compared with the ganciclovir group. These results are summarized in Table 5.
Mortality at six months was 3.7% (9/244) in the Valcyte group and 1.6% (2/126) in the oral ganciclovir group.
[See table 5 below]

CONTRAINDICATIONS
Valcyte tablets are contraindicated in patients with hypersensitivity to valganciclovir or ganciclovir.

WARNINGS
THE CLINICAL TOXICITY OF VALCYTE, WHICH IS METABOLIZED TO GANCICLOVIR, INCLUDES GRANULOCYTOPENIA, ANEMIA AND THROMBOCYTOPENIA. IN ANIMAL STUDIES GANCICLOVIR WAS CARCINOGENIC, TERATOGENIC AND CAUSED ASPERMATOGENESIS.

Hematologic
Valcyte tablets should not be administered if the absolute neutrophil count is less than 500 cells/µL, the platelet count is less than 25,000/µL, or the hemoglobin is less than 8 g/dL. Severe leukopenia, neutropenia, anemia, thrombocytopenia, pancytopenia, bone marrow depression and aplastic anemia have been observed in patients treated with Valcyte tablets (and ganciclovir) (see PRECAUTIONS: Laboratory Testing and ADVERSE EVENTS).
Valcyte tablets should, therefore, be used with caution in patients with pre-existing cytopenias, or who have received or who are receiving myelosuppressive drugs or irradiation. Cytopenia may occur at any time during treatment and may increase with continued dosing. Cell counts usually begin to recover within 3 to 7 days of discontinuing drug.

Impairment of Fertility
Animal data indicate that administration of ganciclovir causes inhibition of spermatogenesis and subsequent infertility. These effects were reversible at lower doses and irreversible at higher doses (see PRECAUTIONS: Carcinogenesis, Mutagenesis and Impairment of Fertility). It is considered probable that in humans, Valcyte at the recommended doses may cause temporary or permanent inhibition of spermatogenesis. Animal data also indicate that suppression of fertility in females may occur.

Teratogenesis, Carcinogenesis and Mutagenesis
Because of the mutagenic and teratogenic potential of ganciclovir, women of childbearing potential should be advised to use effective contraception during treatment. Similarly, men should be advised to practice barrier contraception during, and for at least 90 days following, treatment with Valcyte tablets (see PRECAUTIONS: Carcinogenesis, Mutagenesis and Impairment of Fertility, and Pregnancy: Category C).
In animal studies, ganciclovir was found to be mutagenic and carcinogenic. Valcyte should, therefore, be considered a potential teratogen and carcinogen in humans with the potential to cause birth defects and cancers (see DOSAGE AND ADMINISTRATION: Handling and Disposal).

Tissue Invasive CMV Disease in Liver Transplant Patients
In liver transplant patients, there was a significantly higher incidence of tissue-invasive CMV disease in the Valcyte-treated group compared with the oral ganciclovir group (see CLINICAL TRIALS).

PRECAUTIONS
General
Strict adherence to dosage recommendations is essential to avoid overdose.
The bioavailability of ganciclovir from Valcyte tablets is significantly higher than from ganciclovir capsules. Patients switching from ganciclovir capsules should be advised of the risk of overdosage if they take more than the prescribed number of Valcyte tablets. Valcyte tablets cannot be substituted for Cytovene capsules on a one-to-one basis (see DOSAGE AND ADMINISTRATION).
Since ganciclovir is excreted by the kidneys, normal clearance depends on adequate renal function. IF RENAL FUNCTION IS IMPAIRED, DOSAGE ADJUSTMENTS ARE REQUIRED FOR VALCYTE TABLETS. Such adjustments should be based on measured or estimated creatinine clearance values (see DOSAGE AND ADMINISTRATION: Renal Impairment).
For patients on hemodialysis (CrCl <10 mL/min) it is recommended that ganciclovir be used (in accordance with the dose-reduction algorithm cited in the Cytovene®-IV and Cytovene® Capsules complete product information section on DOSAGE AND ADMINISTRATION: Renal Impairment) rather than Valcyte tablets (see DOSAGE AND ADMINISTRATION: Hemodialysis and CLINICAL PHARMACOLOGY: Special Populations: Hemodialysis).

Information for Patients (see Patient Information)
Valcyte tablets cannot be substituted for ganciclovir capsules on a one-to-one basis. Patients switching from ganciclovir capsules should be advised of the risk of overdosage if they take more than the prescribed number of Valcyte tablets (see OVERDOSAGE and DOSAGE AND ADMINISTRATION).
Valcyte is changed to ganciclovir once it is absorbed into the body. All patients should be informed that the major toxicities of ganciclovir include granulocytopenia (neutropenia), anemia and thrombocytopenia and that dose modifications may be required, including discontinuation. The importance of close monitoring of blood counts while on therapy should be emphasized. Patients should be informed that ganciclovir has been associated with elevations in serum creatinine. Patients should be instructed to take Valcyte tablets with food to maximize bioavailability.
Patients should be advised that ganciclovir has caused decreased sperm production in animals and may cause decreased fertility in humans. Women of childbearing potential should be advised that ganciclovir causes birth defects in animals and should not be used during pregnancy. Because of the potential for serious adverse events in nursing infants, mothers should be instructed not to breast-feed if they are receiving Valcyte tablets. Women of childbearing potential should be advised to use effective contraception during treatment with Valcyte tablets. Similarly, men should be advised to practice barrier contraception during and for at least 90 days following treatment with Valcyte tablets.
Although there is no information from human studies, patients should be advised that ganciclovir should be considered a potential carcinogen.
Convulsions, sedation, dizziness, ataxia and/or confusion have been reported with the use of Valcyte tablets and/or ganciclovir. If they occur, such effects may affect tasks requiring alertness including the patient's ability to drive and operate machinery.
Patients should be told that ganciclovir is not a cure for CMV retinitis, and that they may continue to experience progression of retinitis during or following treatment. Patients should be advised to have ophthalmologic follow-up examinations at a minimum of every 4 to 6 weeks while being treated with Valcyte tablets. Some patients will require more frequent follow-up.

Laboratory Testing
Due to the frequency of neutropenia, anemia and thrombocytopenia in patients receiving Valcyte tablets (see ADVERSE EVENTS), it is recommended that complete blood counts and platelet counts be performed frequently, especially in patients in whom ganciclovir or other nucleoside analogues have previously resulted in leukopenia, or in whom neutrophil counts are less than 1000 cells/µL at the beginning of treatment. Increased monitoring for cytopenias may be warranted if therapy with oral ganciclovir is changed to Valcyte, because of increased plasma concentrations of ganciclovir after Valcyte administration (see CLINICAL PHARMACOLOGY).
Increased serum creatinine levels have been observed in trials evaluating Valcyte tablets. Patients should have serum creatinine or creatinine clearance values monitored carefully to allow for dosage adjustments in renally impaired patients (see DOSAGE AND ADMINISTRATION: Renal Impairment). The mechanism of impairment of renal function is not known.

Drug Interactions
Drug Interaction Studies Conducted With Valcyte
No in vivo drug-drug interaction studies were conducted with valganciclovir. However, because valganciclovir is rapidly and extensively converted to ganciclovir, interactions associated with ganciclovir will be expected for Valcyte tablets.
Drug Interaction Studies Conducted With Ganciclovir
Binding of ganciclovir to plasma proteins is only about 1% to 2%, and drug interactions involving binding site displacement are not anticipated.
Drug-drug interaction studies were conducted in patients with normal renal function. Patients with impaired renal function may have increased concentrations of ganciclovir and the coadministered drug following concomitant administration of Valcyte tablets and drugs excreted by the same pathway as ganciclovir. Therefore, these patients should be closely monitored for toxicity of ganciclovir and the coadministered drug.
[See table 6 on next page]
[See table 7 at bottom of next page]

Carcinogenesis, Mutagenesis and Impairment of Fertility[‡]
No long-term carcinogenicity studies have been conducted with Valcyte. However, upon oral administration, valganciclovir is rapidly and extensively converted to ganciclovir. Therefore, like ganciclovir, valganciclovir is a potential carcinogen.
Ganciclovir was carcinogenic in the mouse at oral doses that produced exposures approximately 0.1× and 1.4×, respectively, the mean drug exposure in humans following the recommended intravenous dose of 5 mg/kg, based on area under the plasma concentration curve (AUC) comparisons. At the higher dose there was a significant increase in the incidence of tumors of the preputial gland in males, forestomach (nonglandular mucosa) in males and females, and reproductive tissues (ovaries, uterus, mammary gland, clitoral gland and vagina) and liver in females. At the lower dose, a slightly increased incidence of tumors was noted in the preputial and harderian glands in males, forestomach in males and females, and liver in females. Ganciclovir should be considered a potential carcinogen in humans.
Valganciclovir increases mutations in mouse lymphoma cells. In the mouse micronucleus assay, valganciclovir was clastogenic. Valganciclovir was not mutagenic in the Ames Salmonella assay. Ganciclovir increased mutations in mouse lymphoma cells and DNA damage in human lymphocytes in vitro. In the mouse micronucleus assay, ganciclovir was clastogenic. Ganciclovir was not mutagenic in the Ames Salmonella assay.
Valganciclovir is converted to ganciclovir and therefore is expected to have similar reproductive toxicity effects as ganciclovir (see WARNINGS: Impairment of Fertility). Ganciclovir caused decreased mating behavior, decreased fertility, and an increased incidence of embryolethality in female mice following intravenous doses that produced an exposure approximately 1.7× the mean drug exposure in humans following the dose of 5 mg/kg, based on AUC comparisons. Ganciclovir caused decreased fertility in male mice and hypospermatogenesis in mice and dogs following daily oral or intravenous administration. Systemic drug exposure (AUC) at the lowest dose showing toxicity in each species ranged

Table 5 Percentage of Patrients with CMV Disease and Tissue-Invasive CMV Disease by Organ Type: Endpoint Committee, 6 Month ITT Population

Organ	CMV Disease[1]		Tissue-Invasive CMV Disease		CMV Syndrome	
	VGCV (N=239)	GCV (N=125)	VGCV (N=239)	GCV (N=125)	VGCV (N=239)	GCV (N=125)
Liver (n=177)	19% (22/118)	12% (7/59)	14% (16/118)	3% (2/59)	5% (6/118)	9% (5/59)
Kidney (n=120)	6% (5/81)	23% (9/39)	1% (1/81)	5% (2/39)	5% (4/81)	18% (7/39)
Heart (n=56)	6% (2/35)	10% (2/21)	0% (0/35)	5% (1/21)	6% (2/35)	5% (1/21)
Kidney/Pancreas (n=11)	0% (0/5)	17% (1/6)	0% (0/5)	17% (1/6)	0% (0/5)	0% (0/6)

GCV = oral ganciclovir; VGCV = Valcyte
[1] Number of Patients with CMV Disease = Number of Patients with Tissue-Invasive CMV Disease + Number of Patients with CMV Syndrome.

from 0.03 to 0.1× the AUC of the recommended human intravenous dose. Valganciclovir caused similar effects on spermatogenesis in mice, rats, and dogs. It is considered likely that ganciclovir (and valganciclovir) could cause inhibition of human spermatogenesis.

Pregnancy

Category C‡

Valganciclovir is converted to ganciclovir and therefore is expected to have reproductive toxicity effects similar to ganciclovir. Ganciclovir has been shown to be embryotoxic in rabbits and mice following intravenous administration, and teratogenic in rabbits. Fetal resorptions were present in at least 85% of rabbits and mice administered doses that produced 2× the human exposure based on AUC comparisons. Effects observed in rabbits included: fetal growth retardation, embryolethality, teratogenicity and/or maternal toxicity. Teratogenic changes included cleft palate, anophthalmia/microphthalmia, aplastic organs (kidney and pancreas), hydrocephaly and brachygnathia. In mice, effects observed were maternal/fetal toxicity and embryolethality.

Daily intravenous doses administered to female mice prior to mating, during gestation, and during lactation caused hypoplasia of the testes and seminal vesicles in the month-old male offspring, as well as pathologic changes in the nonglandular region of the stomach (see WARNINGS: Teratogenesis, Carcinogenesis and Mutagenesis). The drug exposure in mice as estimated by the AUC was approximately 1.7× the human AUC.

Data obtained using an ex vivo human placental model show that ganciclovir crosses the placenta and that simple diffusion is the most likely mechanism of transfer. The transfer was not saturable over a concentration range of 1 to 10 mg/mL and occurred by passive diffusion.

Valganciclovir may be teratogenic or embryotoxic at dose levels recommended for human use. There are no adequate and well-controlled studies in pregnant women. Valcyte tablets should be used during pregnancy only if the potential benefit justifies the potential risk to the fetus.

‡**Footnote:** All dose comparisons presented in the Carcinogenesis, Mutagenesis and Impairment of Fertility, and Pregnancy subsections are based on the human AUC following administration of a single 5 mg/kg infusion of intravenous ganciclovir.

Table 6 Results of Drug Interaction Studies with Ganciclovir: Effects of Coadministered Drug on Ganciclovir Plasma AUC and C_{max} Values

Coadministered Drug	Ganciclovir Dosage	n	Ganciclovir Pharmacokinetic (PK) Parameter	Clinical Comment
Zidovudine 100 mg every 4 hours	1000 mg every 8 hours	12	AUC ↓ 17 ± 25% (range: -52% to 23%)	Zidovudine and Valcyte each have the potential to cause neutropenia and anemia. Some patients may not tolerate concomitant therapy at full dosage.
Didanosine 200 mg every 12 hours administered 2 hours before ganciclovir	1000 mg every 8 hours	12	AUC ↓ 21 ± 17% (range: -44% to 5%)	Effect not likely to be clinically significant.
Didanosine 200 mg every 12 hours stimultaneously administered with ganciclovir	1000 mg every 8 hours	12	No effect on ganciclovir PK parameters observed	No effect expected.
	IV ganciclovir 5 mg/kg twice daily	11	No effect on ganciclovir PK parameters observed	No effect expected.
	IV ganciclovir 5 mg/kg once daily	11	No effect on ganciclovir PK parameters observed	No effect expected.
Probenecid 500 mg every 6 hours	1000 mg every 8 hours	10	AUC ↑ 53 ± 91% (range: -14% to 299%) Ganciclovir renal clearance ↓ 22 ± 20% (Range: -54% to -4%)	Patients taking probenecid and Valcyte should be monitored for evidence of ganciclovir toxicity.
Zalcitabine 0.75 mg every 8 hours administered 2 hours before ganciclovir	1000 mg every 8 hours	10	AUC ↑ 13%	Effect not likely to be clinically significant.
Trimethoprim 200 mg once daily	1000 mg every 8 hours	12	Ganciclovir renal clearance ↓ 16.3% Half-life ↑ 15%	Effect not likely to be clinically significant.
Mycophenolate Mofetil 1.5 g single dose	IV ganciclovir 5 mg/kg single dose	12	No effect on ganciclovir PK parameters observed (patients with normal renal function)	Patients with renal impairment should be monitored carefully as levels of metabolites of both drugs may increase.

Table 7 Results of Drug Interaction Studies With Ganciclovir: Effects of Ganciclovir on Plasma AUC and C_{max} Values of Coadministered Drug

Coadministered Drug	Ganciclovir Dosage	N	Coadministered Drug Pharmacokinetic (PK) Parameter	Clinical Comment
Zidovudine 100 mg every 4 hours	1000 mg every 8 hours	12	AUC_{0-4} ↑ 19 ± 27% (range: -11% to 74%)	Zidovudine and Valcyte each have the potential to cause neutropenia and anemia. Some patients may not tolerate concomitant therapy at full dosage.
Didanosine 200 mg every 12 hours when administered 2 hours prior to or concurrent with ganciclovir	1000 mg every 8 hours	12	AUC_{0-12} ↑ 111 ± 114% (range: 10% to 493%)	Patients should be closely monitored for didanosine toxicity.
Didanosine 200 mg every 12 hours	IV ganciclovir 5 mg/kg twice daily	11	AUC_{0-12} ↑ 70 ± 40% (range: 3% to 121%) C_{max} ↑ 49 ± 48% (range: -28% to 125%)	Patients should be closely monitored for didanosine toxicity.
Didanosine 200 mg every 12 hours	IV ganciclovir 5 mg/kg once daily	11	AUC_{0-12} ↑ 50 ± 26% (range: 22% to 110%) C_{max} ↑ 36 ± 36% (range: -27% to 94%)	Patients should be closely monitored for didanosine toxicity.
Zalcitabine 0.75 mg every 8 hours administered 2 hours before ganciclovir	1000 mg every 8 hours	10	No clinically relevant PK parameter changes	No effect expected.
Trimethoprim 200 mg once daily	1000 mg every 8 hours	12	Increase (12%) in C_{min}	Effect not likely to be clinically significant.
Mycophenolate Mofetil (MMF) 1.5 g single dose	IV ganciclovir 5 mg/kg single dose	12	No PK interaction observed (patients with normal renal function)	Patients with renal impairment should be monitored carefully as levels of metabolites of both drugs may increase.

Nursing Mothers

It is not known whether ganciclovir or valganciclovir is excreted in human milk. Because valganciclovir caused granulocytopenia, anemia and thrombocytopenia in clinical trials and ganciclovir was mutagenic and carcinogenic in animal studies, the possibility of serious adverse events from ganciclovir in nursing infants is possible (see WARNINGS). Because of potential for serious adverse events in nursing infants, **mothers should be instructed not to breast-feed if they are receiving Valcyte tablets.** In addition, the Centers for Disease Control and Prevention recommend that HIV-infected mothers not breast-feed their infants to avoid risking postnatal transmission of HIV.

Pediatric Use

Safety and effectiveness of Valcyte tablets in pediatric patients have not been established.

Geriatric Use

The pharmacokinetic characteristics of Valcyte in elderly patients have not been established. Since elderly individuals frequently have a reduced glomerular filtration rate, particular attention should be paid to assessing renal function before and during administration of Valcyte (see DOSAGE AND ADMINISTRATION).

Clinical studies of Valcyte did not include sufficient numbers of subjects aged 65 and over to determine whether they respond differently from younger subjects. In general, dose selection for an elderly patient should be cautious, reflecting the greater frequency of decreased hepatic, renal, or cardiac function, and of concomitant disease or other drug therapy. Valcyte is known to be substantially excreted by the kidney, and the risk of toxic reactions to this drug may be greater in patients with impaired renal function. Because elderly patients are more likely to have decreased renal function, care should be taken in dose selection. In addition, renal function should be monitored and dosage adjustments should be made accordingly (see PRECAUTIONS: General, CLINICAL PHARMACOLOGY: Special Populations: Renal Impairment, and DOSAGE AND ADMINISTRATION: Renal Impairment).

ADVERSE EVENTS

Experience With Valcyte Tablets

Valganciclovir, a prodrug of ganciclovir, is rapidly converted to ganciclovir after oral administration. Adverse events known to be associated with ganciclovir usage can therefore be expected to occur with Valcyte tablets.

Treatment of CMV Retinitis in AIDS Patients

As shown in Table 8, the safety profiles of Valcyte tablets and intravenous ganciclovir during 28 days of randomized therapy (21 days induction dose and 7 days maintenance dose) in 158 patients were comparable, with the exception of catheter-related infection, which occurred with greater frequency in patients randomized to receive IV ganciclovir.

Table 8 Percentage of Selected Adverse Events Occurring During the Randomized Phase of Study WV15376

Adverse Event	Valcyte Arm N=79	Intravenous Ganciclovir Arm N=79
Diarrhea	16%	10%
Neutropenia	11%	13%
Nausea	8%	14%
Headache	9%	5%
Anemia	8%	8%
Catheter-related infection	3%	11%

Tables 9 and 10 show the pooled adverse event data and abnormal laboratory values from two single arm, open-label clinical trials, study WV15376 and WV15705. A total of 370

Continued on next page

Valcyte—Cont.

patients received maintenance therapy with Valcyte tablets 900 mg once daily. Approximately 252 (68%) of these patients received Valcyte tablets for more than nine months (maximum duration was 36 months).

Table 9 Pooled Selected Adverse Events Reported in ≥5% of Patients in Two Clinical Studies in CMV Retinitis

Adverse Events According to Body System	Patients with CMV Retinitis (Studies WV15376 and WV15705) Valcyte (N=370) (%)
Gastrointestinal system	
Diarrhea	41
Nausea	30
Vomiting	21
Abdominal pain	15
Body as a whole	
Pyrexia	31
Headache	22
Hemic and lymphatic system	
Neutropenia	27
Anemia	26
Thrombocytopenia	6
Central and peripheral nervous system	
Insomnia	16
Peripheral neuropathy	9
Paresthesia	8
Special senses	
Retinal detachment	15

Table 10 Pooled Laboratory Abnormalities Reported in Two Clinical Studies in the Treatment of CMV Retinitis

Laboratory Abnormalities	CMV Retinitis Patients (Studies WV15376 and WV15705) Valcyte (N=370) (%)
Neutropenia: AUC /μL	
<500	19
500 – <750	17
750 – <1000	17
Anemia: Hemoglobin g/dL	
<6.5	7
6.5 – <8.0	13
8.0 – <9.5	16
Thrombocytopenia: Platelets/μL	
<25000	4
25000 – <50000	6
50000 – <100000	22
Serum Creatinine: mg/dL	
>2.5	3
>1.5 – 2.5	12

Prevention of CMV Disease in Selected Solid Organ Transplantation

Table 11 shows selected adverse events regardless of severity and drug relationship with an incidence of ≥5% from a clinical trial, PV16000 (up to 28 days after study treatment) where heart, kidney, kidney-pancreas and liver transplant patients received Valcyte (N=244) or oral ganciclovir (N=126). The majority of the adverse events were of mild or moderate intensity.

Table 11 Percentage of Selected Grades 1-4 Adverse Events Reported in ≥5% of Selected Solid Organ Transplant Patients in Study PV16000

Adverse Event	Valcyte (N=244) %	Oral Ganciclovir (N=126) %
Diarrhea	30	29
Tremors	28	25
Graft rejection	24	30
Nausea	23	23
Headache	22	27
Insomnia	20	16
Hypertension	18	15
Vomiting	16	14
Leukopenia	14	7
Pyrexia	13	14

Table 13 Dose Modifications for Patients With Impaired Renal Function

CrCl* (mL/min)	Induction Dose	Maintenance Prevention Dose
≥ 60	900 mg twice daily	900 mg once daily
40 – 59	450 mg twice daily	450 mg once daily
25 – 39	450 mg once daily	450 mg every 2 days
10 – 24	450 mg every 2 days	450 mg twice weekly

*An estimated creatinine clearance can be related to serum creatinine by the following formulas:

For males = $\frac{(140 - \text{age [years]}) \times (\text{body weight [kg]})}{(72) \times (\text{serum creatinine [mg/dL]})}$

For females = 0.85 × male value

Laboratory adverse events are those reported by investigators.

Adverse events not included in Table 11, which either occurred at a frequency of ≥5% in clinical study PV16000, or were selected serious adverse events reported in studies WV15376, WV15705, or PV16000 with a frequency of <5% are listed below.

Allergic reactions: valganciclovir hypersensitivity
Bleeding complications: potentially life-threatening bleeding associated with thrombocytopenia
Central and peripheral nervous system: paresthesia, dizziness (excluding vertigo), convulsion
Gastrointestinal disorders: abdominal pain, constipation, dyspepsia, abdominal distention, ascites
General disorders and administration site disorders: fatigue, pain, edema, peripheral edema, weakness
Hemic system: anemia, neutropenia, thrombocytopenia, pancytopenia, bone marrow depression, aplastic anemia
Hepatobiliary disorders: abnormal hepatic function
Infections and infestations: pharyngitis/nasopharyngitis, upper respiratory tract infection, urinary tract infection, local and systemic infections and sepsis, postoperative wound infection
Injury, poisoning and procedural complications: postoperative complications, postoperative pain, increased wound drainage, wound dehiscence
Metabolism and nutrition disorders: hyperkalemia, hypokalemia, hypomagnesemia, hyperglycemia, appetite decreased, dehydration, hypophosphatemia, hypocalcemia
Musculoskeletal and connective tissue disorders: back pain, arthralgia, muscle cramps, limb pain
Psychiatric disorders: depression, psychosis, hallucinations, confusion, agitation
Renal and urinary disorders: renal impairment, dysuria, decreased creatinine clearance
Respiratory, thoracic and mediastinal disorders: cough, dyspnea, rhinorrhea, pleural effusion
Skin and subcutaneous tissue disorders: dermatitis, pruritus, acne
Vascular disorders: hypotension

Laboratory abnormalities reported with Valcyte tablets in one study in solid organ transplant patients are listed in Table 12.

Table 12 Laboratory Abnormalities Reported in Selected Solid Organ Transplant Patients in Study PV16000

Laboratory Abnormalities	Valcyte (N=244) %	Oral Cytovene (N=126) %
Neutropenia: ANC/μL		
<500	5	3
500 – <750	3	2
750 – <1000	5	2
Anemia: Hemoglobin g/dL		
<6.5	1	2
6.5 – <8.0	5	7
8.0 – <9.5	31	25
Thrombocytopenia: Platelets/μL		
<25000	0	2
25000 – <50000	1	3
50000 – <100000	18	21
Serum Creatinine: mg/dL		
>2.5	14	21
>1.5 – 2.5	45	47

Experience With Ganciclovir

Valganciclovir is rapidly converted to ganciclovir upon oral administration. Adverse events reported with Valcyte in general were similar to those reported with ganciclovir (Cytovene). Please refer to the Cytovene product information for more information on postmarketing adverse events associated with ganciclovir.

OVERDOSAGE

Overdose Experience With Valcyte Tablets

One adult developed fatal bone marrow depression (medullary aplasia) after several days of dosing that was at least 10-fold greater than recommended for the patient's estimated degree of renal impairment.

It is expected that an overdose of Valcyte tablets could also possibly result in increased renal toxicity (see PRECAUTIONS: General and DOSAGE AND ADMINISTRATION: Renal Impairment).

Since ganciclovir is dialyzable, dialysis may be useful in reducing serum concentrations in patients who have received an overdose of Valcyte tablets (see CLINICAL PHARMACOLOGY: Special Populations: *Hemodialysis*). Adequate hydration should be maintained. The use of hematopoietic growth factors should be considered (see CLINICAL PHARMACOLOGY: Special Populations: *Hemodialysis*).

Overdose Experience With Intravenous Ganciclovir

Reports of overdoses with intravenous ganciclovir have been received from clinical trials and during postmarketing experience. The majority of patients experienced one or more of the following adverse events:

Hematological toxicity: pancytopenia, bone marrow depression, medullary aplasia, leukopenia, neutropenia, granulocytopenia
Hepatotoxicity: hepatitis, liver function disorder
Renal toxicity: worsening of hematuria in a patient with pre-existing renal impairment, acute renal failure, elevated creatinine
Gastrointestinal toxicity: abdominal pain, diarrhea, vomiting
Neurotoxicity: generalized tremor, convulsion

DOSAGE AND ADMINISTRATION

Strict adherence to dosage recommendations is essential to avoid overdose. Valcyte tablets cannot be substituted for Cytovene capsules on a one-to-one basis.

Valcyte tablets are administered orally, and should be taken with food (see CLINICAL PHARMACOLOGY: Absorption). After oral administration, valganciclovir is rapidly and extensively converted into ganciclovir. The bioavailability of ganciclovir from Valcyte tablets is significantly higher than from ganciclovir capsules. Therefore the dosage and administration of Valcyte tablets as described below should be closely followed (see PRECAUTIONS: General and OVERDOSAGE).

For the Treatment of CMV Retinitis in Patients With Normal Renal Function

Induction:
For patients with active CMV retinitis, the recommended dosage is 900 mg (two 450 mg tablets) twice a day for 21 days with food.
Maintenance:
Following induction treatment, or in patients with inactive CMV retinitis, the recommended dosage is 900 mg (two 450 mg tablets) once daily with food.

For the Prevention of CMV Disease in Heart, Kidney, and Kidney-Pancreas Transplantation

For patients who have received a kidney, heart, or kidney-pancreas transplant, the recommended dose is 900 mg (two 450 mg tablets) once daily with food starting within 10 days of transplantation until 100 days posttransplantation.

Renal Impairment

Serum creatinine or creatinine clearance levels should be monitored carefully. Dosage adjustment is required according to creatinine clearance as shown in Table 13 (see PRECAUTIONS: General and CLINICAL PHARMACOLOGY: Special Populations: Renal Impairment). Increased monitoring for cytopenias may be warranted in patients with renal impairment (see PRECAUTIONS: Laboratory Testing). [See table 13 above]

Hemodialysis Patients

Valcyte should not be prescribed to patients receiving hemodialysis (see CLINICAL PHARMACOLOGY: Special Populations: Hemodialysis and PRECAUTIONS: General).

For patients on hemodialysis (CrCl <10 mL/min) a dose recommendation cannot be given (see CLINICAL PHARMACOLOGY: Special Populations: Hemodialysis).

Handling and Disposal

Caution should be exercised in the handling of Valcyte tablets. Tablets should not be broken or crushed. Since valganciclovir is considered a potential teratogen and carcinogen in humans, caution should be observed in handling broken tablets (see WARNINGS: Teratogenesis, Carcinogenesis and Mutagenesis). Avoid direct contact of broken or crushed tablets with skin or mucous membranes. If such contact occurs, wash thoroughly with soap and water, and rinse eyes thoroughly with plain water.

Because ganciclovir shares some of the properties of antitumor agents (ie, carcinogenicity and mutagenicity), consideration should be given to handling and disposal according to guidelines issued for antineoplastic drugs. Several guidelines on this subject have been published (see REFERENCES).

There is no general agreement that all of the procedures recommended in the guidelines are necessary or appropriate.

HOW SUPPLIED

Valcyte (valganciclovir HCl tablets) is available as 450 mg pink convex oval tablets with "VGC" on one side and "450" on the other side. Each tablet contains valganciclovir HCl equivalent to 450 mg valganciclovir. Valcyte is supplied in bottles of 60 tablets (NDC 0004-0038-22).

Storage

Store at 25°C (77°F); excursions permitted to 15°C to 30°C (59°F to 86°F) [See USP controlled room temperature].

REFERENCES

1. Recommendations for the Safe Handling of Cytotoxic Drugs. US Department of Health and Human Services, National Institutes of Health, Bethesda, MD, September 1992. NIH Publication No. 92-2621
2. American Society of Hospital Pharmacists technical assistance bulletin on handling cytotoxic and hazardous drugs. Am J Hosp Pharm. 1990; 47:1033-1049
3. Controlling Occupational Exposures to Hazardous Drugs. US Department of Labor. Occupational Health and Safety Administration. OSHA Technical Manual. Section VI - Chapter 2, January 20, 1999

PATIENT INFORMATION

Read the Patient Information that comes with Valcyte before you start using it and each time you get a refill. There may be new information. This information does not take the place of talking with your healthcare provider.

What is the most important information I should know about Valcyte?

- **Valcyte can affect your blood cells and bone marrow causing serious and life-threatening problems.** Valcyte can lower the amount of your white blood cells, red blood cells, and platelets. Your doctor may do regular blood tests to check your blood cells while you are taking Valcyte. Based on these tests, your doctor may change your dose or tell you to stop taking Valcyte.
- **Valcyte may cause cancer.** Valcyte causes cancer in animals. It is not known if Valcyte causes cancer in people.
- **Valcyte may cause birth defects.** Valcyte causes birth defects in animals. It is not known if Valcyte causes birth defects in people. Valcyte should not be used during pregnancy. **Tell your doctor right away if you get pregnant while taking Valcyte. If you can get pregnant, you should use effective birth control during treatment with Valcyte. Men should use a condom during treatment with Valcyte, and for 90 days after treatment, if their partner can get pregnant.** Talk to your doctor if you have questions about birth control. Valcyte may lower the amount of sperm in a man's body and cause fertility problems.
- **Valcyte changes into the medicine ganciclovir once it is in your body.** Ganciclovir is also the active ingredient in Cytovene® Capsules and Cytovene-IV®. Do not take Valcyte and Cytovene at the same time. The dose of medicine in Valcyte Tablets and Cytovene Capsules is different. **One tablet of Valcyte has more medicine than one capsule of Cytovene. This means that one Valcyte tablet cannot be substituted for one Cytovene Capsule. You could overdose and become very sick.** Talk to your doctor or pharmacist if you have questions about your medicine.

What is Valcyte?

Valcyte is an "antiviral" medicine used:

- to treat cytomegalovirus (CMV) retinitis in people who have acquired immunodeficiency syndrome (AIDS). When CMV virus infects the eyes, it is called CMV retinitis.
- to prevent cytomegalovirus (CMV) disease in people who have received a **heart, kidney, or kidney-pancreas** transplant and who have a chance for getting CMV disease.

Valcyte may:

- slow the growth of CMV virus in your body. CMV is an infection caused by a herpesvirus called cytomegalovirus. If CMV retinitis isn't treated, it can cause blindness. Valcyte may protect your eyesight from damage due to CMV disease. CMV can also infect other parts of the body.
- prevent CMV disease for up to 6 months after **heart, kidney, or kidney-pancreas** transplant. Valcyte may prevent CMV virus from spreading into healthy cells.

Valcyte does not cure CMV retinitis. You may still get retinitis or worsening of retinitis during or after treatment with Valcyte. Therefore, it is important to stay under a doctor's care and have your eyes checked regularly. Valcyte has not been studied in children or in adults older than age 65.

Who should not take Valcyte?

Do not take Valcyte if you:

- **are receiving hemodialysis.** The use of ganciclovir (Cytovene Capsules) rather than Valcyte tablets is recommended. Valcyte does not come in the right dose for people on hemodialysis.
- **are allergic to any of its ingredients or if you have ever had a serious reaction to ganciclovir (Cytovene Capsules or Cytovene-IV).** See the end of this leaflet for a list of the ingredients in Valcyte.

In addition, Valcyte is not for use in prevention of CMV disease in patients who have received a liver transplant.

More research is needed before Valcyte can be recommended for use in the prevention of CMV disease in other organ transplant patients such as liver or lung transplant patients.

Before taking Valcyte, tell your doctor:

- **if you are pregnant or plan to become pregnant.** Valcyte may cause birth defects. (See "What is the most important information I should know about Valcyte?")
- **if you are breast-feeding.** It is not known if Valcyte passes into your milk and if it may harm your baby. You should not breast-feed if you are HIV-positive because of the chance of passing the HIV virus to your baby through your milk.
- **if you have kidney problems.** Your doctor may give you a lower dose of Valcyte, or check you more often if you are taking Valcyte.
- **if you have blood cell problems**
- **if you are having radiation treatment**
- **about all the medicines you take,** including prescription and non-prescription medicines, vitamins and herbal supplements. **Do not take Cytovene Capsules if you are taking Valcyte tablets.** Valcyte and other medicines may affect each other. These interactions may cause serious problems. The following medicines may need dose changes if you are also taking Valcyte:
  - Videx® (didanosine, ddI)
  - Retrovir® (zidovudine, ZDV, AZT)
  - Probenecid

  Tell your doctor if you take medicines such as chemotherapy medicines that can lower your bone marrow function.

How should I take Valcyte?

- Take Valcyte exactly as your doctor prescribes it. Your dose of Valcyte will depend on your medical condition. If you have kidney problems or are over age 65, your doctor may give you a lower dose of Valcyte.
  - the usual dose for adults to get active CMV retinitis under control (induction therapy) is two 450 mg tablets twice a day for 21 days.
  - the usual dose for adults to help keep CMV retinitis under control (maintenance therapy) is two 450 mg tablets once a day.
  - the usual dose to prevent CMV in adults who have had a **heart, kidney, or kidney-pancreas** transplant is two 450 mg tablets once a day starting within 10 days of transplant and continuing until 100 days after the transplant.
- Take Valcyte with food.
- Do not break or crush Valcyte tablets.
- If you miss a dose of Valcyte, take the missed dose as soon as you remember. Then, take the next dose at the usual scheduled time. However, if it is almost time for your next dose, **do not take the missed dose.**
- Do not let your Valcyte run out. The amount of virus in your blood may increase if your medicine is stopped, even for a short time.
- If you take too much Valcyte, call your local poison control center or emergency room right away. You may need treatment in a hospital.
- Do not substitute Valcyte tablets for Cytovene capsules. Talk to your doctor, nurse or pharmacist if you have questions about your medicine.

What should I avoid while taking Valcyte?

- **Do not get pregnant.** Valcyte causes birth defects in animals. It is not known if Valcyte causes birth defects in people. Valcyte should not be used during pregnancy. **Tell your doctor right away if you get pregnant while taking Valcyte. If you can get pregnant, you should use effective birth control during treatment with Valcyte. Men should use a condom during treatment with Valcyte, and for 90 days after treatment, if their partner can get pregnant.** Talk to your doctor if you have questions about birth control. Valcyte may lower the amount of sperm in a man's body and cause fertility problems.
- **Do not breast-feed.** Valcyte may harm your baby. You should not breast-feed if you are HIV-positive because of the chance of passing the HIV virus to your baby through your milk.
- **Do not drive a car or operate other dangerous machinery until you know how Valcyte affects you.** Valcyte can cause seizures, sleepiness, dizziness, unsteady movements, and confusion.
- **Do not break or crush Valcyte tablets.** Avoid contact with broken Valcyte tablets on your skin, mucous membranes or eyes. If contact occurs, wash your skin well with soap and water or rinse your eyes well with plain water.

What are the possible side effects of Valcyte?

See "What is the most important information I should know about Valcyte?" for details on the most serious side effects.

Valcyte can also cause the following serious side effects:

- **kidney problems.** Valcyte may affect your kidney function. Your doctor may do regular blood tests called serum creatinine levels to check your kidney function while you are taking Valcyte.
- **brain and nerve problems.** Valcyte may cause seizures, sleepiness, dizziness, unsteady movements, and confusion.

Common side effects of Valcyte include diarrhea, nausea, vomiting, stomach pain, fever, headache, shaky movements (tremors), graft rejection, swelling of the legs, constipation, back pain, trouble sleeping, and high blood pressure.

Common changes in blood tests for people taking Valcyte include low white blood cells (neutropenia or leukopenia), low red blood cells (anemia), increased blood creatinine levels, increased calcium in the blood, and abnormal liver function. Talk to your doctor about side effects that bother you or that won't go away.

These are not all the side effects of Valcyte. For more information, ask your doctor or pharmacist.

How do I store Valcyte?

- Store Valcyte at room temperature, 59° to 86° F (15° to 30° C.)
- **Keep Valcyte and all medicines out of the reach of children.**

General information about Valcyte.

Medicines are sometimes prescribed for conditions that are not mentioned in patient information leaflets. Do not use Valcyte for a condition for which it was not prescribed. Do not give Valcyte to other people, even if they have the same symptoms you have. It may harm them.

This leaflet summarizes the most important information about Valcyte. If you would like more information, talk with your doctor. You can ask your doctor or pharmacist for information about Valcyte that is written for health professionals. Information about Valcyte is also available at 1-800-526-6367 (toll-free).

What are the ingredients in Valcyte?

Active Ingredient: Valganciclovir HCl

Inactive Ingredients: microcrystalline cellulose, povidone K-30, crospovidone, and stearic acid. The film-coated applied to the tablets contains Opadry Pink®.

Cytovene is a registered trademark of Hoffmann-LaRoche Inc.

Videx is a registered trademark of Bristol-Myers Squibb Company.

Retrovir is a registered trademark of GlaxoSmithKline.

Valcyte tablets are manufactured by Patheon Inc., Mississauga, Ontario, Canada L5N 7K9

Revised: September 2003

Shown in Product Identification Guide, page 332

VESANOID®

℞

[ves'ă noid]
(tretinoin)
Capsules

WARNINGS

1. Experienced Physician and Institution

Patients with acute promyelocytic leukemia (APL) are at high risk in general and can have severe adverse reactions to VESANOID (tretinoin). VESANOID should therefore be administered under the supervision of a physician who is experienced in the management of patients with acute leukemia and in a facility with laboratory and supportive services sufficient to monitor drug tolerance and protect and maintain a patient compromised by drug toxicity, including respiratory compromise. Use of VESANOID requires that the physician concludes that the possible benefit to the patient outweighs the following known adverse effects of the therapy.

2. Retinoic Acid-APL Syndrome

About 25% of patients with APL treated with VESANOID have experienced a syndrome called the retinoic-acid-APL (RA-APL) syndrome characterized by fever, dyspnea, weight gain, radiographic pulmonary infiltrates and pleural or pericardial effusions. This syndrome has occasionally been accompanied by impaired myocardial contractility and episodic hypotension. It has been observed with or without concomitant leukocytosis. Endotracheal intubation and mechanical ventilation have been required in some cases due to progressive hypoxemia, and several patients have expired with multiorgan failure. The syndrome generally occurs during the first month of treatment, with some cases reported following the first dose of VESANOID.

The management of the syndrome has not been defined rigorously, but high-dose steroids given at the first suspicion of the RA-APL syndrome appear to reduce morbidity and mortality. At the first signs suggestive of the syndrome (unexplained fever, dyspnea and/or weight gain, abnormal chest auscultatory findings or radiographic abnormalities), high-dose steroids (dexamethasone 10 mg intravenously administered every 12 hours for 3 days or until the resolution of symptoms) should be immediately initiated, irrespective of the leukocyte count. The majority of patients do not require termination of VESANOID therapy during treatment of the RA-APL syndrome.

3. Leukocytosis at Presentation and Rapidly Evolving Leukocytosis During VESANOID Treatment

During VESANOID treatment about 40% of patients will develop rapidly evolving leukocytosis. Patients who

Continued on next page

Vesanoid—Cont.

present with high WBC at diagnosis (>5×10⁹/L) have an increased risk of a further rapid increase in WBC counts. Rapidly evolving leukocytosis is associated with a higher risk of life-threatening complications.
If signs and symptoms of the RA-APL syndrome are present together with leukocytosis, treatment with high-dose steroids should be initiated immediately. Some investigators routinely add chemotherapy to VESANOID treatment in the case of patients presenting with a WBC count of >5×10⁹/L or in the case of a rapid increase in WBC count for patients leukopenic at start of treatment, and have reported a lower incidence of the RA-APL syndrome. Consideration could be given to adding full-dose chemotherapy (including an anthracycline if not contraindicated) to the VESANOID therapy on day 1 or 2 for patients presenting with a WBC count of >5×10⁹/L, or immediately, for patients presenting with a WBC count of <5×10⁹/L, if the WBC count reaches ≥6×10⁹/L by day 5, or ≥10×10⁹/L by day 10, or ≥15×10⁹/L by day 28.

4. Teratogenic Effects. Pregnancy Category D – see WARNINGS
There is a high risk that a severely deformed infant will result if VESANOID is administered during pregnancy. If, nonetheless, it is determined that VESANOID represents the best available treatment for a pregnant woman or a woman of childbearing potential, it must be assured that the patient has received full information and warnings of the risk to the fetus if she were to be pregnant and of the risk of possible contraception failure and has been instructed in the need to use two reliable forms of contraception simultaneously during therapy and for 1 month following discontinuation of therapy, and has acknowledged her understanding of the need for using dual contraception, unless abstinence is the chosen method.
Within 1 week prior to the institution of VESANOID therapy, the patient should have blood or urine collected for a serum or urine pregnancy test with a sensitivity of at least 50 mIU/mL. When possible, VESANOID therapy should be delayed until a negative result from this test is obtained. When a delay is not possible, the patient should be placed on two reliable forms of contraception. Pregnancy testing and contraception counseling should be repeated monthly throughout the period of VESANOID treatment.

DESCRIPTION

VESANOID (tretinoin) is a retinoid that induces maturation of acute promyelocytic leukemia (APL) cells in culture. It is available in a 10 mg soft gelatin capsule for oral administration. Each capsule also contains beeswax, butylated hydroxyanisole, edetate disodium, hydrogenated soybean oil flakes, hydrogenated vegetable oils and soybean oil. The gelatin capsule shell contains glycerin, yellow iron oxide, red iron oxide, titanium dioxide, methylparaben and propylparaben.
Chemically, tretinoin is all-*trans* retinoic acid and is related to retinol (Vitamin A). It is a yellow to light orange crystalline powder with a molecular weight of 300.44.

CLINICAL PHARMACOLOGY

Mechanism of Action
Tretinoin is not a cytolytic agent but instead induces cytodifferentiation and decreased proliferation of APL cells in culture and in vivo. In APL patients, tretinoin treatment produces an initial maturation of the primitive promyelocytes derived from the leukemic clone, followed by a repopulation of the bone marrow and peripheral blood by normal, polyclonal hematopoietic cells in patients achieving complete remission (CR). The exact mechanism of action of tretinoin in APL is unknown.

Pharmacokinetics
Tretinoin activity is primarily due to the parent drug. In human pharmacokinetics studies, orally administered drug was well absorbed into the systemic circulation, with approximately two-thirds of the administered radiolabel recovered in the urine. The terminal elimination half-life of tretinoin following initial dosing is 0.5 to 2 hours in patients with APL. There is evidence that tretinoin induces its own metabolism. Plasma tretinoin concentrations decrease on average to one-third of their day 1 values during 1 week of continuous therapy. Mean ± SD peak tretinoin concentrations decreased from 394 ± 89 to 138 ± 139 ng/mL, while area under the curve (AUC) values decreased from 537 ± 191 ng·h/mL to 249 ± 185 ng·h/mL during 45 mg/m² daily dosing in 7 APL patients. Increasing the dose to "correct" for this change has not increased response.
Absorption
A single 45 mg/m² (~80 mg) oral dose to APL patients resulted in a mean ± SD peak tretinoin concentration of 347 ± 266 ng/mL. Time to reach peak concentration was between 1 and 2 hours.
Distribution
The apparent volume of distribution of tretinoin has not been determined. Tretinoin is greater than 95% bound in plasma, predominately to albumin. Plasma protein binding remains constant over the concentration range of 10 to 500 ng/mL.
Metabolism
Tretinoin metabolites have been identified in plasma and urine. Cytochrome P450 enzymes have been implicated in the oxidative metabolism of tretinoin. Metabolites include 13-*cis* retinoic acid, 4-oxo *trans* retinoic acid, 4-oxo *cis* retinoic acid, and 4-oxo *trans* retinoic acid glucuronide. In APL patients, daily administration of a 45 mg/m² dose of tretinoin resulted in an approximately tenfold increase in the urinary excretion of 4-oxo *trans* retinoic acid glucuronide after 2 to 6 weeks of continuous dosing, when compared to baseline values.
Excretion
Studies with radiolabeled drug have demonstrated that after the oral administration of 2.75 and 50 mg doses of tretinoin, greater than 90% of the radioactivity was recovered in the urine and feces. Based upon data from 3 subjects, approximately 63% of radioactivity was recovered in the urine within 72 hours and 31% appeared in the feces within 6 days.
Special Populations
The pharmacokinetics of tretinoin have not been separately evaluated in women, in members of different ethnic groups, or in individuals with renal or hepatic insufficiency.
Drug-Drug Interactions
In 13 patients who had received daily doses of tretinoin for 4 consecutive weeks, administration of ketoconazole (400 to 1200 mg oral dose) 1 hour prior to the administration of the tretinoin dose on day 29 led to a 72% increase (218 ± 224 vs 375 ± 285 ng·h/mL) in tretinoin mean plasma AUC. The precise cytochrome P450 enzymes involved in these interactions have not been specified; *CYP* 3A4, 2C8 and 2E have been implicated in various preliminary reports.

Clinical Studies
VESANOID has been investigated in 114 previously treated APL patients and in 67 previously untreated ("de novo") patients in one open-label, uncontrolled single investigator clinical study (Memorial Sloan-Kettering Cancer Center [MSKCC]) and in two cohorts of compassionate cases treated by multiple investigators under the auspices of the National Cancer Institute (NCI). All patients received 45 mg/m²/day as a divided oral dose for up to 90 days or 30 days beyond the day that CR was reached. Results are shown in the following table:
[See table below]
The median time to CR was between 40 and 50 days (range: 2 to 120 days). Most patients in these studies received cytotoxic chemotherapy during the remission phase. These results compare to the 30% to 50% CR rate and ≤6 month median survival reported for cytotoxic chemotherapy of APL in the treatment of relapse.
Ten of 15 pediatric cases achieved CR (8 of 10 males and 2 of 5 females). There were insufficient patients of black, Hispanic or Asian derivation to estimate relative response rates in these groups, but responses were seen in each category. Responses were seen in 3 of 4 patients for whom cytogenetic analysis failed to detect the t(15;17) translocation typically seen in APL. The t(15;17) translocation results in the PML/RARα gene, which appears necessary for this disease. Molecular genetic studies were not conducted in these cases, but it is likely they represent cases with a masked translocation giving rise to PML/RARα. Responses to tretinoin have not been observed in cases in which PML/RARα fusion has been shown to be absent.

INDICATIONS AND USAGE

VESANOID (tretinoin) capsules are indicated for the induction of remission in patients with acute promyelocytic leukemia (APL), French-American-British (FAB) classification M3 (including the M3 variant), characterized by the presence of the t(15;17) translocation and/or the presence of the PML/RARα gene who are refractory to, or who have relapsed from, anthracycline chemotherapy, or for whom anthracycline-based chemotherapy is contraindicated. VESANOID is for the induction of remission only. The optimal consolidation or maintenance regimens have not been defined, but all patients should receive an accepted form of remission consolidation and/or maintenance therapy for APL after completion of induction therapy with VESANOID.

CONTRAINDICATIONS

VESANOID is contraindicated in patients with a known hypersensitivity to retinoids. VESANOID should not be given to patients who are sensitive to parabens, which are used as preservatives in the gelatin capsule.

WARNINGS

Pregnancy Category D – See Boxed WARNINGS
Tretinoin has teratogenic and embryotoxic effects in mice, rats, hamsters, rabbits and pigtail monkeys, and may be expected to cause fetal harm when administered to a pregnant woman. Tretinoin causes fetal resorptions and a decrease in live fetuses in all animals studied. Gross external, soft tissue and skeletal alterations occurred at doses higher than 0.7 mg/kg/day in mice, 2 mg/kg/day in rats, 7 mg/kg/day in hamsters, and at a dose of 10 mg/kg/day, the only dose tested, in pigtail monkeys (about 1/20, 1/4, and 1/2 and 4 times the human dose, respectively, on a mg/m² basis).
There are no adequate and well-controlled studies in pregnant women. Although experience with humans administered VESANOID is extremely limited, increased spontaneous abortions and major human fetal abnormalities related to the use of other retinoids have been documented in humans. Reported defects include abnormalities of the CNS, musculoskeletal system, external ear, eye, thymus and great vessels; and facial dysmorphia, cleft palate, and parathyroid hormone deficiency. Some of these abnormalities were fatal. Cases of IQ scores less than 85, with or without obvious CNS abnormalities, have also been reported. All fetuses exposed during pregnancy can be affected and at the present time there is no antepartum means of determining which fetuses are and are not affected.
Effective contraception must be used by all females during VESANOID therapy and for 1 month following discontinuation of therapy. Contraception must be used even when there is a history of infertility or menopause, unless a hysterectomy has been performed. Whenever contraception is required, it is recommended that two reliable forms of contraception be used simultaneously, unless abstinence is the chosen method. If pregnancy does occur during treatment, the physician and patient should discuss the desirability of continuing or terminating the pregnancy.

Patients Without the t(15;17) Translocation
Initiation of therapy with VESANOID may be based on the morphological diagnosis of acute promyelocytic leukemia. Confirmation of the diagnosis of APL should be sought by detection of the t(15;17) genetic marker by cytogenetic studies. If these are negative, PML/RARα fusion should be sought using molecular diagnostic techniques. The response rate of other AML subtypes to VESANOID has not been demonstrated; therefore, patients who lack the genetic marker should be considered for alternative treatment.

Retinoic Acid-APL (RA-APL) Syndrome
In up to 25% of patients with APL treated with VESANOID, a syndrome occurs which can be fatal (see boxed WARNINGS and ADVERSE REACTIONS).

Leukocytosis at Presentation and Rapidly Evolving Leukocytosis During VESANOID Treatment
See boxed WARNINGS.

Pseudotumor Cerebri
Retinoids, including VESANOID, have been associated with pseudotumor cerebri (benign intracranial hypertension), especially in pediatric patients. Early signs and symptoms of pseudotumor cerebri include papilledema, headache, nausea and vomiting, and visual disturbances. Patients with these symptoms should be evaluated for pseudotumor cerebri, and, if present, appropriate care should be instituted in concert with neurological assessment.

Lipids
Up to 60% of patients experienced hypercholesterolemia and/or hypertriglyceridemia, which were reversible upon completion of treatment. The clinical consequences of temporary elevation of triglycerides and cholesterol are unknown, but venous thrombosis and myocardial infarction have been reported in patients who ordinarily are at low risk for such complications.

Elevated Liver Function Test Results
Elevated liver function test results occur in 50% to 60% of patients during treatment. Liver function test results should be carefully monitored during treatment and consideration be given to a temporary withdrawal of VESANOID if test results reach >5 times the upper limit of normal values. However, the majority of these abnormalities resolve without interruption of VESANOID or after completion of treatment.

PRECAUTIONS

General
VESANOID has potentially significant toxic side effects in APL patients. Patients undergoing therapy should be closely observed for signs of respiratory compromise and/or leukocytosis (see boxed WARNINGS). Supportive care appropriate for APL patients, eg, prophylaxis for bleeding, prompt therapy for infection, should be maintained during therapy with VESANOID.

Laboratory Tests
The patient's hematologic profile, coagulation profile, liver function test results, and triglyceride and cholesterol levels should be monitored frequently.

	MSKCC		NCI Cohort 1		NCI Cohort 2	
	Relapsed n=20	De Novo n=15	Relapsed* n=48	De Novo n=14	Relapsed n=46	De Novo† n=38
Complete Remission	16 (80%)	11 (73%)	24 (50%)	5 (36%)	24 (52%)	26 (68%)
Median Survival (Mo)	10.8	NR	5.8	0.5	8.8	NR
Median Follow-up (Mo)	9.9	42.9	5.6	1.2	8.0	13.1
RA-APL Syndrome	4 (20%)	5 (33%)	10 (21%)	6 (43%)	NA	NA

NR = Not Reached
NA = Not Available
*Including 9 chemorefractory patients
†Including 8 patients who received chemotherapy but failed to enter remission

Drug Interactions
Limited clinical data on potential drug interactions are available. As VESANOID is metabolized by the hepatic P450 system, there is a potential for alteration of pharmacokinetics parameters in patients administered concomitant medications that are also inducers or inhibitors of this system. Medications that generally induce hepatic P450 enzymes include rifampicin, glucocorticoids, phenobarbital and pentobarbital. Medications that generally inhibit hepatic P450 enzymes include ketoconazole, cimetidine, erythromycin, verapamil, diltiazem and cyclosporine. To date there are no data to suggest that co-use with these medications increases or decreases either efficacy or toxicity of VESANOID.

Effect of Food
No data on the effect of food on the absorption of VESANOID are available. The absorption of retinoids as a class has been shown to be enhanced when taken together with food.

Carcinogenesis, Mutagenesis and Impairment of Fertility
No long-term carcinogenicity studies with tretinoin have been conducted. In short-term carcinogenicity studies, tretinoin at a dose of 30 mg/kg/day (about 2 times the human dose on a mg/m^2 basis) was shown to increase the rate of diethylnitrosamine (DEN)-induced mouse liver adenomas and carcinomas. Tretinoin was negative when tested in the Ames and Chinese hamster V79 cell HGPRT assays for mutagenicity. A twofold increase in the sister chromatid exchange (SCE) has been demonstrated in human diploid fibroblasts, but other chromosome aberration assays, including an in vitro assay in human peripheral lymphocytes and an in vivo mouse micronucleus assay, did not show a clastogenic or aneuploidogenic effect. Adverse effects on fertility and reproductive performance were not observed in studies conducted in rats at doses up to 5 mg/kg/day (about 2/3 the human dose on a mg/m^2 basis). In a 6-week toxicology study in dogs, minimal to marked testicular degeneration, with increased numbers of immature spermatozoa, were observed at 10 mg/kg/day (about 4 times the equivalent human dose in mg/m^2).

Nursing Mothers
It is not known whether this drug is excreted in human milk. Because many drugs are excreted in human milk, and because of the potential for serious adverse reactions from VESANOID in nursing infants, mothers should discontinue nursing prior to taking this drug.

Pediatric Use
There are limited clinical data on the pediatric use of VESANOID. Of 15 pediatric patients (age range: 1 to 16 years) treated with VESANOID, the incidence of complete remission was 67%. Safety and effectiveness in pediatric patients below the age of 1 year have not been established. Some pediatric patients experience severe headache and pseudotumor cerebri, requiring analgesic treatment and lumbar puncture for relief. Increased caution is recommended in the treatment of pediatric patients. Dose reduction may be considered for pediatric patients experiencing serious and/or intolerable toxicity; however, the efficacy and safety of VESANOID at doses lower than 45 mg/m^2/day have not been evaluated in the pediatric population.

Geriatric Use
Of the total number of subjects in clinical studies of VESANOID, 21.4% were 60 and over. No overall differences in safety or effectiveness were observed between these subjects and younger subjects, and other reported clinical experience has not identified differences in responses between the elderly and younger patients, but greater sensitivity of some older individuals cannot be ruled out.

ADVERSE REACTIONS

Virtually all patients experience some drug-related toxicity, especially headache, fever, weakness, and fatigue. These adverse effects are seldom permanent or irreversible nor do they usually require interruption of therapy. Some of the adverse events are common in patients with APL, including hemorrhage, infections, gastrointestinal hemorrhage, disseminated intravascular coagulation, pneumonia, septicemia, and cerebral hemorrhage. The following describes the adverse events, regardless of drug relationship, that were observed in patients treated with VESANOID.

Typical Retinoid Toxicity
The most frequently reported adverse events were similar to those described in patients taking high doses of vitamin A and included headache (86%), fever (83%), skin/mucous membrane dryness (77%), bone pain (77%), nausea/vomiting (57%), rash (54%), mucositis (26%), pruritus (20%), increased sweating (20%), visual disturbances (17%), ocular disorders (17%), alopecia (14%), skin changes (14%), changed visual acuity (6%), bone inflammation (3%), visual field defects (3%).

RA-APL Syndrome
APL patients treated with VESANOID have experienced a syndrome characterized by fever, dyspnea, weight gain, radiographic pulmonary infiltrates and pleural or pericardial effusions. This syndrome has occasionally been accompanied by impaired myocardial contractility and episodic hypotension and has been observed with or without concomitant leukocytosis. Some patients have expired due to progressive hypoxemia and multiorgan failure. The syndrome generally occurs during the first month of treatment, with some cases reported following the first dose of VESANOID. The management of the syndrome has not been defined rigorously, but high-dose steroids given at the first signs of the syndrome appear to reduce morbidity and mortality. Treatment with dexamethasone, 10 mg intravenously administered every 12 hours for 3 days or until resolution of symptoms, should be initiated without delay at the first suspicion of symptoms (one or more of the following: fever, dyspnea, weight gain, abnormal chest auscultatory findings or radiographic abnormalities). Sixty percent or more of patients treated with VESANOID may require high-dose steroids because of these symptoms. The majority of patients do not require termination of VESANOID therapy during treatment of the syndrome.

Body as a Whole
General disorders related to VESANOID administration and/or associated with APL included malaise (66%), shivering (63%), hemorrhage (60%), infections (58%), peripheral edema (52%), pain (37%), chest discomfort (32%), edema (29%), disseminated intravascular coagulation (26%), weight increase (23%), injection site reactions (17%), anorexia (17%), weight decrease (17%), myalgia (14%), flank pain (9%), cellulitis (8%), face edema (6%), fluid imbalance (6%), pallor (6%), lymph disorders (6%), acidosis (3%), hypothermia (3%), ascites (3%).

Respiratory System Disorders
Respiratory system disorders were commonly reported in APL patients administered VESANOID. The majority of these events are symptoms of the RA-APL syndrome (see boxed WARNINGS). Respiratory system adverse events included upper respiratory tract disorders (63%), dyspnea (60%), respiratory insufficiency (26%), pleural effusion (20%), pneumonia (14%), rales (14%), expiratory wheezing (14%), lower respiratory tract disorders (9%), pulmonary infiltration (6%), bronchial asthma (3%), pulmonary edema (3%), larynx edema (3%), unspecified pulmonary disease (3%).

Ear Disorders
Ear disorders were consistently reported, with earache or feeling of fullness in the ears reported by 23% of the patients. Hearing loss and other unspecified auricular disorders were observed in 6% of patients, with infrequent (<1%) reports of irreversible hearing loss.

Gastrointestinal Disorders
GI disorders included GI hemorrhage (34%), abdominal pain (31%), other gastrointestinal disorders (26%), diarrhea (23%), constipation (17%), dyspepsia (14%), abdominal distention (11%), hepatosplenomegaly (9%), hepatitis (3%), ulcer (3%), unspecified liver disorder (3%).

Cardiovascular and Heart Rate and Rhythm Disorders
Arrhythmias (23%), flushing (23%), hypotension (14%), hypertension (11%), phlebitis (11%), cardiac failure (6%) and for 3% of patients: cardiac arrest, myocardial infarction, enlarged heart, heart murmur, ischemia, stroke, myocarditis, pericarditis, pulmonary hypertension, secondary cardiomyopathy.

Central and Peripheral Nervous System Disorders and Psychiatric
Dizziness (20%), paresthesias (17%), anxiety (17%), insomnia (14%), depression (14%), confusion (11%), cerebral hemorrhage (9%), intracranial hypertension (9%), agitation (9%), hallucination (6%) and for 3% of patients: abnormal gait, agnosia, aphasia, asterixis, cerebellar edema, cerebellar disorders, convulsions, coma, CNS depression, dysarthria, encephalopathy, facial paralysis, hemiplegia, hyporeflexia, hypotaxia, no light reflex, neurologic reaction, spinal cord disorder, tremor, leg weakness, unconsciousness, dementia, forgetfulness, somnolence, slow speech.

Urinary System Disorders
Renal insufficiency (11%), dysuria (9%), acute renal failure (3%), micturition frequency (3%), renal tubular necrosis (3%), enlarged prostate (3%).

Miscellaneous Adverse Events
Isolated cases of erythema nodosum, basophilia and hyperhistaminemia, Sweet's syndrome, organomegaly, hypercalcemia, pancreatitis and myositis have been reported.

OVERDOSAGE

There has been no experience with acute overdosage in humans. The maximal tolerated dose in patients with myelodysplastic syndrome or solid tumors was 195 mg/m^2/day. The maximal tolerated dose in pediatric patients was lower at 60 mg/m^2/day. Overdosage with other retinoids has been associated with transient headache, facial flushing, cheilosis, abdominal pain, dizziness and ataxia. These symptoms have quickly resolved without apparent residual effects.

DOSAGE AND ADMINISTRATION

The recommended dose is 45 mg/m^2/day administered as two evenly divided doses until complete remission is documented. Therapy should be discontinued 30 days after achievement of complete remission or after 90 days of treatment, whichever occurs first.

If after initiation of treatment of VESANOID the presence of the t(15;17) translocation is not confirmed by cytogenetics and/or by polymerase chain reaction studies and the patient has not responded to VESANOID, alternative therapy appropriate for acute myelogenous leukemia should be considered.

VESANOID is for the induction of remission only. Optimal consolidation or maintenance regimens have not been determined. All patients should, therefore, receive a standard consolidation and/or maintenance chemotherapy regimen for APL after induction therapy with VESANOID, unless otherwise contraindicated.

HOW SUPPLIED

VESANOID is supplied as 10 mg capsules, two-tone (lengthwise), orange-yellow and reddish-brown and imprinted VESANOID 10 ROCHE. Supplied in high-density polyethylene, opaque bottles of 100 capsules with child-resistant closure (NDC 0004-0250-01).

Store at 15° to 30°C (59° to 86°F). Protect from light.

27898475

Revised: March 2003

Shown in Product Identification Guide, page 332

XELODA® ℞

[*zē'lōdă*]
(capecitabine)
TABLETS

> **WARNING**
> XELODA Warfarin Interaction: Patients receiving concomitant capecitabine and oral coumarin-derivative anticoagulant therapy should have their anticoagulant response (INR or prothrombin time) monitored frequently in order to adjust the anticoagulant dose accordingly. A clinically important XELODA-Warfarin drug interaction was demonstrated in a clinical pharmacology trial (see CLINICAL PHARMACOLOGY and PRECAUTIONS). Altered coagulation parameters and/or bleeding, including death, have been reported in patients taking XELODA concomitantly with coumarin-derivative anticoagulants such as warfarin and phenprocoumon. Postmarketing reports have shown clinically significant increases in prothrombin time (PT) and INR in patients who were stabilized on anticoagulants at the time XELODA was introduced. These events occurred within several days and up to several months after initiating XELODA therapy and, in a few cases, within 1 month after stopping XELODA. These events occurred in patients with and without liver metastases. Age greater than 60 and a diagnosis of cancer independently predispose patients to an increased risk of coagulopathy.

DESCRIPTION

XELODA (capecitabine) is a fluoropyrimidine carbamate with antineoplastic activity. It is an orally administered systemic prodrug of 5'-deoxy-5-fluorouridine (5'-DFUR) which is converted to 5-fluorouracil.

The chemical name for capecitabine is 5'-deoxy-5-fluoro-N-[(pentyloxy) carbonyl]-cytidine and has a molecular weight of 359.35.

Capecitabine is a white to off-white crystalline powder with an aqueous solubility of 26 mg/mL at 20°C.

XELODA is supplied as biconvex, oblong film-coated tablets for oral administration. Each light peach-colored tablet contains 150 mg capecitabine and each peach-colored tablet contains 500 mg capecitabine. The inactive ingredients in XELODA include: anhydrous lactose, croscarmellose sodium, hydroxypropyl methylcellulose, microcrystalline cellulose, magnesium stearate and purified water. The peach or light peach film coating contains hydroxypropyl methylcellulose, talc, titanium dioxide, and synthetic yellow and red iron oxides.

CLINICAL PHARMACOLOGY

XELODA is relatively non-cytotoxic in vitro. This drug is enzymatically converted to 5-fluorouracil (5-FU) in vivo.

Bioactivation: Capecitabine is readily absorbed from the gastrointestinal tract. In the liver, a 60 kDa carboxylesterase hydrolyzes much of the compound to 5'-deoxy-5-fluorocytidine (5'- DFCR). Cytidine deaminase, an enzyme found in most tissues, including tumors, subsequently converts 5'-DFCR to 5'-deoxy-5-fluorouridine (5'-DFUR). The enzyme, thymidine phosphorylase (dThdPase), then hydrolyzes 5'-DFUR to the active drug 5-FU. Many tissues throughout the body express thymidine phosphorylase. Some human carcinomas express this enzyme in higher concentrations than surrounding normal tissues.

Metabolic Pathway of Capecitabine to 5-FU

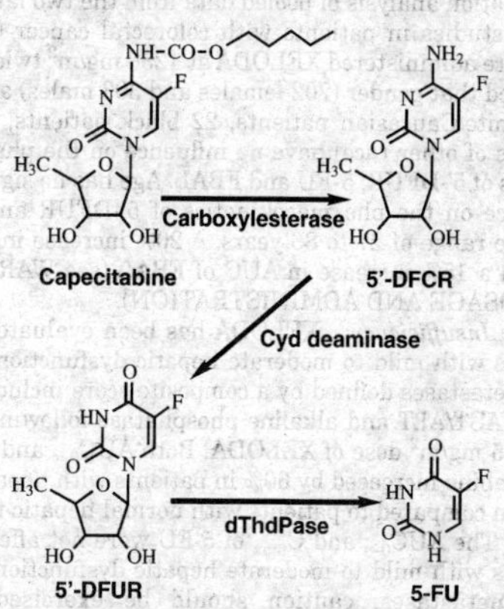

Mechanism of Action: Both normal and tumor cells metabolize 5-FU to 5-fluoro-2'-deoxyuridine monophosphate (FdUMP) and 5-fluorouridine triphosphate (FUTP). These metabolites cause cell injury by two different mechanisms.

Continued on next page

Xeloda—Cont.

First, FdUMP and the folate cofactor, N^{5-10}-methylenetetrahydrofolate, bind to thymidylate synthase (TS) to form a covalently bound ternary complex. This binding inhibits the formation of thymidylate from 2'-deoxyuridylate. Thymidylate is the necessary precursor of thymidine triphosphate, which is essential for the synthesis of DNA, so that a deficiency of this compound can inhibit cell division. Second, nuclear transcriptional enzymes can mistakenly incorporate FUTP in place of uridine triphosphate (UTP) during the synthesis of RNA. This metabolic error can interfere with RNA processing and protein synthesis.

Pharmacokinetics in Colorectal Tumors and Adjacent Healthy Tissue: Following oral administration of XELODA 7 days before surgery in patients with colorectal cancer, the median ratio of 5-FU concentration in colorectal tumors to adjacent tissues was 2.9 (range from 0.9 to 8.0). These ratios have not been evaluated in breast cancer patients or compared to 5-FU infusion.

Human Pharmacokinetics: The pharmacokinetics of XELODA and its metabolites have been evaluated in about 200 cancer patients over a dosage range of 500 to 3500 mg/m^2/day. Over this range, the pharmacokinetics of XELODA and its metabolite, 5'-DFCR were dose proportional and did not change over time. The increases in the AUCs of 5'-DFUR and 5-FU, however, were greater than proportional to the increase in dose and the AUC of 5-FU was 34% higher on day 14 than on day 1. The elimination half-life of both parent capecitabine and 5-FU was about ¾ of an hour. The inter-patient variability in the C_{max} and AUC of 5-FU was greater than 85%.

Following oral administration of 825 mg/m^2 capecitabine twice daily for 14 days, Japanese patients (n=18) had about 36% lower C_{max} and 24% lower AUC for capecitabine than the Caucasian patients (n=22). Japanese patients had also about 25% lower C_{max} and 34% lower AUC for FBAL than the Caucasian patients. The clinical significance of these differences is unknown. No significant differences occurred in the exposure to other metabolites (5'-DFCR, 5'- DFUR, and 5-FU).

Absorption, Distribution, Metabolism and Excretion: Capecitabine reached peak blood levels in about 1.5 hours (T_{max}) with peak 5-FU levels occurring slightly later, at 2 hours. Food reduced both the rate and extent of absorption of capecitabine with mean C_{max} and $AUC_{0-\infty}$ decreased by 60% and 35%, respectively. The C_{max} and $AUC_{0-\infty}$ of 5-FU were also reduced by food by 43% and 21%, respectively. Food delayed T_{max} of both parent and 5-FU by 1.5 hours (see PRECAUTIONS and DOSAGE AND ADMINISTRATION).

Plasma protein binding of capecitabine and its metabolites is less than 60% and is not concentration-dependent. Capecitabine was primarily bound to human albumin (approximately 35%).

Capecitabine is extensively metabolized enzymatically to 5-FU. The enzyme dihydropyrimidine dehydrogenase hydrogenates 5-FU, the product of capecitabine metabolism, to the much less toxic 5-fluoro-5, 6-dihydro-fluorouracil (FUH_2). Dihydropyrimidinase cleaves the pyrimidine ring to yield 5-fluoro-ureido-propionic acid (FUPA). Finally, β-ureido-propionase cleaves FUPA to α-fluoro-β-alanine (FBAL) which is cleared in the urine.

Capecitabine and its metabolites are predominantly excreted in urine; 95.5% of administered capecitabine dose is recovered in urine. Fecal excretion is minimal (2.6%). The major metabolite excreted in urine is FBAL which represents 57% of the administered dose. About 3% of the administered dose is excreted in urine as unchanged drug.

A clinical phase 1 study evaluating the effect of XELODA on the pharmacokinetics of docetaxel (Taxotere®) and the effect of docetaxel on the pharmacokinetics of XELODA was conducted in 26 patients with solid tumors. XELODA was found to have no effect on the pharmacokinetics of docetaxel (C_{max} and AUC) and docetaxel has no effect on the pharmacokinetics of capecitabine and the 5-FU precursor 5'-DFUR.

Special Populations:

A population analysis of pooled data from the two large controlled studies in patients with colorectal cancer (n=505) who were administered XELODA at 1250 mg/m^2 twice a day indicated that gender (202 females and 303 males) and race (455 white/Caucasian patients, 22 black patients, and 28 patients of other race) have no influence on the pharmacokinetics of 5'-DFUR, 5-FU and FBAL. Age has no significant influence on the pharmacokinetics of 5'-DFUR and 5-FU over the range of 27 to 86 years. A 20% increase in age results in a 15% increase in AUC of FBAL (see WARNINGS and DOSAGE AND ADMINISTRATION).

Hepatic Insufficiency: XELODA has been evaluated in 13 patients with mild to moderate hepatic dysfunction due to liver metastases defined by a composite score including bilirubin, AST/ALT and alkaline phosphatase following a single 1255 mg/m^2 dose of XELODA. Both $AUC_{0-\infty}$ and C_{max} of capecitabine increased by 60% in patients with hepatic dysfunction compared to patients with normal hepatic function (n=14). The $AUC_{0-\infty}$ and C_{max} of 5-FU were not affected. In patients with mild to moderate hepatic dysfunction due to liver metastases, caution should be exercised when XELODA is administered. The effect of severe hepatic dysfunction on XELODA is not known (see PRECAUTIONS and DOSAGE AND ADMINISTRATION).

Renal Insufficiency: Following oral administration of 1250 mg/m^2 capecitabine twice a day to cancer patients with varying degrees of renal impairment, patients with moderate (creatinine clearance = 30 to 50 mL/min) and severe (creatinine clearance <30 mL/min) renal impairment showed 85% and 258% higher systemic exposure to FBAL on day 1 compared to normal renal function patients (creatinine clearance >80 mL/min). Systemic exposure to 5'-DFUR was 42% and 71% greater in moderately and severely renal impaired patients, respectively, than in normal patients. Systemic exposure to capecitabine was about 25% greater in both moderately and severely renal impaired patients (see CONTRAINDICATIONS, WARNINGS, and DOSAGE AND ADMINISTRATION).

Drug-Drug Interactions:

Anticoagulants: In four patients with cancer, chronic administration of capecitabine (1250 mg/m^2 bid) with a single 20 mg dose of warfarin increased the mean AUC of S-warfarin by 57% and decreased its clearance by 37%. Baseline corrected AUC of INR in these 4 patients increased by 2.8-fold, and the maximum observed mean INR value was increased by 91% (see Boxed WARNING and PRECAUTIONS: *Drug-Drug Interactions*).

Drugs Metabolized by Cytochrome P450 Enzymes: In vitro enzymatic studies with human liver microsomes indicated that capecitabine and its metabolites (5'-DFUR, 5'-DFCR, 5-FU, and FBAL) had no inhibitory effects on substrates of cytochrome P450 for the major isoenzymes such as 1A2, 2A6, 3A4, 2C9, 2C19, 2D6, and 2E1.

Antacid: When Maalox® (20 mL), an aluminum hydroxide- and magnesium hydroxide-containing antacid, was administered immediately after XELODA (1250 mg/m^2, n=12 cancer patients), AUC and C_{max} increased by 16% and 35%, respectively, for capecitabine and by 18% and 22%, respectively, for 5'-DFCR. No effect was observed on the other three major metabolites (5'-DFUR, 5-FU, FBAL) of XELODA.

XELODA has a low potential for pharmacokinetic interactions related to plasma protein binding.

CLINICAL STUDIES

Colorectal Carcinoma: The recommended dose of XELODA was determined in an open-label, randomized clinical study, exploring the efficacy and safety of continuous therapy with capecitabine (1331 mg/m^2/day in two divided doses, n=39), intermittent therapy with capecitabine (2510 mg/m^2/day in two divided doses, n=34), and intermittent therapy with capecitabine in combination with oral leucovorin (LV) (capecitabine 1657 mg/m^2/day in two divided doses, n=35; leucovorin 60 mg/day) in patients with advanced and/or metastatic colorectal carcinoma in the first-line metastatic setting. There was no apparent advantage in response rate to adding leucovorin to XELODA; however, toxicity was increased. XELODA, 1250 mg/m^2 twice daily for 14 days followed by a 1-week rest, was selected for further clinical development based on the overall safety and efficacy profile of the three schedules studied.

Data from two open-label, multicenter, randomized, controlled clinical trials involving 1207 patients support the use of XELODA in the first-line treatment of patients with metastatic colorectal carcinoma. The two clinical studies were identical in design and were conducted in 120 centers in different countries. Study 1 was conducted in the US, Canada, Mexico, and Brazil; Study 2 was conducted in Europe, Israel, Australia, New Zealand, and Taiwan. Altogether, in both trials, 603 patients were randomized to treatment with XELODA at a dose of 1250 mg/m^2 twice daily for 2 weeks followed by a 1-week rest period and given as 3-week cycles; 604 patients were randomized to treatment with 5-FU and leucovorin (20 mg/m^2 leucovorin IV followed by 425 mg/m^2 IV bolus 5-FU, on days 1 to 5, every 28 days).

In both trials, overall survival, time to progression and response rate (complete plus partial responses) were assessed. Responses were defined by the World Health Organization criteria and submitted to a blinded independent review committee (IRC). Differences in assessments between the investigator and IRC were reconciled by the sponsor, blinded to treatment arm, according to a specified algorithm. Survival was assessed based on a non-inferiority analysis.

The baseline demographics for XELODA and 5-FU/LV patients are shown in Table 1.

[See table 1 above]

The efficacy endpoints for the two phase 3 trials are shown in Tables 2 and 3.

[See table 2 above]

[See table 3 above]

Table 1. Baseline Demographics of Controlled Colorectal Trials

	Study 1		Study 2	
	XELODA (n=302)	**5-FU/LV (n=303)**	**XELODA (n=301)**	**5-FU/LV (n=301)**
Age (median, years) Range	64 (23-86)	63 (24-87)	64 (29-84)	64 (36-86)
Gender Male (%) Female (%)	 181 (60) 121 (40)	 197 (65) 106 (35)	 172 (57) 129 (43)	 173 (57) 128 (43)
Karnofsky PS (median) Range	90 (70-100)	90 (70-100)	90 (70-100)	90 (70-100)
Colon (%) Rectum (%)	222 (74) 79 (26)	232 (77) 70 (23)	199 (66) 101 (34)	196 (65) 105 (35)
Prior radiation therapy (%)	52 (17)	62 (21)	42 (14)	42 (14)
Prior adjuvant 5-FU (%)	84 (28)	110 (36)	56 (19)	41 (14)

Table 2. Efficacy of XELODA vs 5-FU/LV in Colorectal Cancer (Study 1)

	XELODA (n=302)	**5-FU/LV (n=303)**
Overall Response Rate (%, 95% C.I.)	21 (16-26)	11 (8-15)
(*p*-value)	0.0014	
Time to Progression (Median, days, 95% C.I.)	128 (120-136)	131 (105-153)
Hazard Ratio (XELODA/5-FU/LV) 95% C.I. for Hazard Ratio	0.99 (0.84-1.17)	
Survival (Median, days, 95% C.I.)	380 (321-434)	407 (366-446)
Hazard Ratio (XELODA/5-FU/LV) 95% C.I. for Hazard Ratio	1.00 0.84-1.18	

Table 3. Efficacy of XELODA vs 5-FU/LV in Colorectal Cancer (Study 2)

	XELODA (n=301)	**5-FU/LV (n=301)**
Overall Response Rate (%, 95% C.I.)	21 (16–26)	14 (10–18)
(*p*-value)	0.027	
Time to Progression (Median, days, 95% C.I.)	137 (128–165)	131 (102–156)
Hazard Ratio (XELODA/5-FU/LV) 95% C.I. for Hazard Ratio	0.97 0.82–1.14	
Survival (Median, days, 95% C.I.)	404 (367–452)	369 (338–430)
Hazard Ratio (XELODA/5-FU/LV) 95% C.I. for Hazard Ratio	0.92 0.78–1.09	

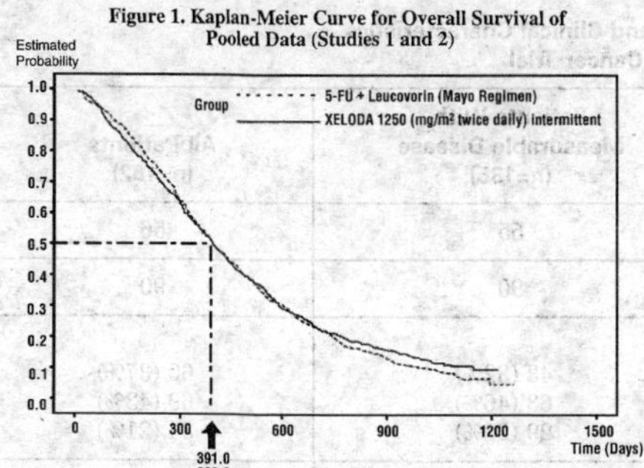

Figure 1. Kaplan-Meier Curve for Overall Survival of Pooled Data (Studies 1 and 2)

XELODA was superior to 5-FU/LV for objective response rate in Study 1 and Study 2. The similarity of XELODA and 5-FU/LV in these studies was assessed by examining the potential difference between the two treatments. In order to assure that XELODA has a clinically meaningful survival effect, statistical analyses were performed to determine the percent of the survival effect of 5-FU/LV that was retained by XELODA. The estimate of the survival effect of 5-FU/LV was derived from a meta-analysis of ten randomized studies from the published literature comparing 5-FU to regimens of 5-FU/LV that were similar to the control arms used in these Studies 1 and 2. The method for comparing the treatments was to examine the worst case (95% confidence upper bound) for the difference between 5-FU/LV and XELODA, and to show that loss of more than 50% of the 5-FU/LV survival effect was ruled out. It was demonstrated that the percent of the survival effect of 5-FU/LV maintained was at least 61% for Study 2 and 10% for Study 1. The pooled result is consistent with a retention of at least 50% of the effect of 5-FU/LV. It should be noted that these values for preserved effect are based on the upper bound of the 5-FU/LV vs XELODA difference. These results do not exclude the possibility of true equivalence of XELODA to 5-FU/LV (see Tables 2 and 3 and Figure 1).

Breast Carcinoma: XELODA has been evaluated in clinical trials in combination with docetaxel (Taxotere®) and as monotherapy.

Breast Cancer Combination Therapy: The dose of XELODA used in the phase 3 clinical trial in combination with docetaxel was based on the results of a phase 1 study, where a range of doses of docetaxel administered in 3-week cycles in combination with an intermittent regimen of XELODA (14 days of treatment, followed by a 7-day rest period) were evaluated. The combination dose regimen was selected based on the tolerability profile of the 75 mg/m² administered in 3-week cycles of docetaxel in combination with 1250 mg/m² twice daily for 14 days of XELODA administered in 3-week cycles. The approved dose of 100 mg/m² of docetaxel administered in 3-week cycles was the control arm of the phase 3 study.

XELODA in combination with docetaxel was assessed in an open-label, multicenter, randomized trial in 75 centers in Europe, North America, South America, Asia, and Australia. A total of 511 patients with metastatic breast cancer resistant to, or recurring during or after an anthracycline-containing therapy, or relapsing during or recurring within 2 years of completing an anthracycline-containing adjuvant therapy were enrolled. Two hundred and fifty-five (255) patients were randomized to receive XELODA 1250 mg/m² twice daily for 14 days followed by 1 week without treatment and docetaxel 75 mg/m² as a 1-hour intravenous infusion administered in 3-week cycles. In the monotherapy arm, 256 patients received docetaxel 100 mg/m² as a 1-hour intravenous infusion administered in 3-week cycles. Patient demographics are provided in Table 4.

[See table 4 above]

XELODA in combination with docetaxel resulted in statistically significant improvement in time to disease progression, overall survival and objective response rate compared to monotherapy with docetaxel as shown in Table 5 and Figures 2 and 3.

[See table 5 above]

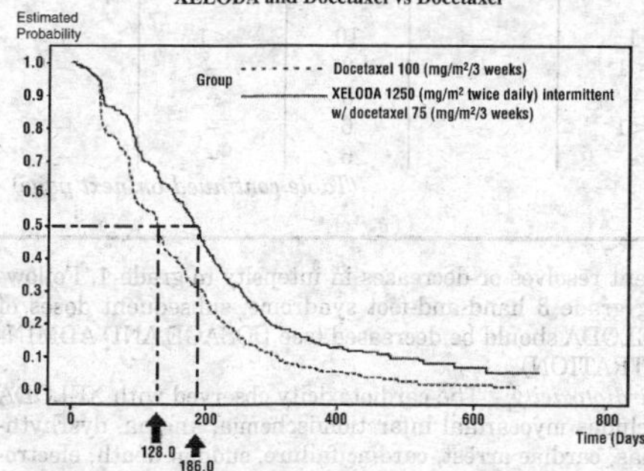

Figure 2. Kaplan-Meier Estimates for Time to Disease Progression – XELODA and Docetaxel vs Docetaxel

[See figure 3 at top of next column]

Breast Cancer Monotherapy: The antitumor activity of XELODA as a monotherapy was evaluated in an open-label single-arm trial conducted in 24 centers in the US and Canada. A total of 162 patients with stage IV breast cancer were enrolled. The primary endpoint was tumor response rate in

Table 4. Baseline Demographics and Clinical Characteristics XELODA and Docetaxel Combination vs Docetaxel in Breast Cancer Trial

	XELODA + Docetaxel (n=255)	Docetaxel (n=256)
Age (median, years)	52	51
Karnofsky PS (median)	90	90
Site of Disease		
Lymph nodes	121 (47%)	125 (49%)
Liver	116 (45%)	122 (48%)
Bone	107 (42%)	119 (46%)
Lung	95 (37%)	99 (39%)
Skin	73 (29%)	73 (29%)
Prior Chemotherapy		
Anthracycline[1]	255 (100%)	256 (100%)
5-FU	196 (77%)	189 (74%)
Paclitaxel	25 (10%)	22 (9%)
Resistance to an Anthracycline		
No resistance	19 (7%)	19 (7%)
Progression on anthracycline therapy	65 (26%)	73 (29%)
Stable disease after 4 cycles of anthracycline therapy	41 (16%)	40 (16%)
Relapsed within 2 years of completion of anthracycline-adjuvant therapy	78 (31%)	74 (29%)
Experienced a brief response to anthracycline therapy, with subsequent progression while on therapy or within 12 months after last dose	51 (20%)	50 (20%)
No. of Prior Chemotherapy Regimens for Treatment of Metastatic Disease		
0	89 (35%)	80 (31%)
1	123 (48%)	135 (53%)
2	43 (17%)	39 (15%)
3	0 (0%)	2 (1%)

[1]Includes 10 patients in combination and 18 patients in monotherapy arms treated with an anthracenedione

Table 5. Efficacy of XELODA and Docetaxel Combination vs Docetaxel Monotherapy

Efficacy Parameter	Combination Therapy	Monotherapy	p-value	Hazard Ratio
Time to Disease Progression				
Median Days	186	128	0.0001	0.643
95% C.I.	(165-198)	(105-136)		
Overall Survival				
Median Days	442	352	0.0126	0.775
95% C.I.	(375-497)	(298-387)		
Response Rate[1]	32%	22%	0.009	NA[2]

[1] The response rate reported represents a reconciliation of the investigator and IRC assessments performed by the sponsor according to a predefined algorithm.
[2] NA = Not Applicable

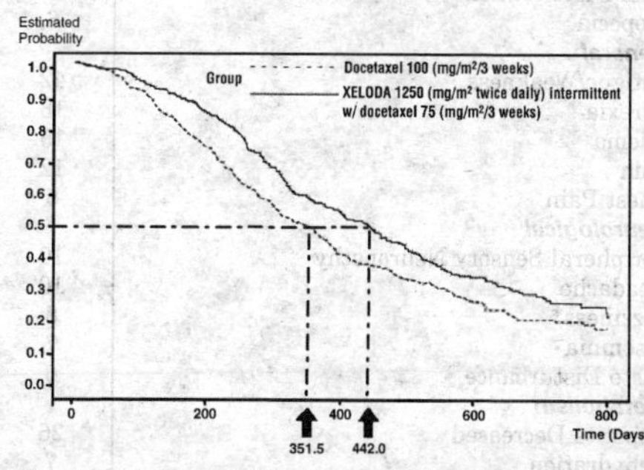

Figure 3. Kaplan-Meier Estimates of Survival – XELODA and Docetaxel vs Docetaxel

patients with measurable disease, with response defined as a ≥50% decrease in sum of the products of the perpendicular diameters of bidimensionally measurable disease for at least 1 month. XELODA was administered at a dose of 1255 mg/m² twice daily for 2 weeks followed by a 1-week rest period and given as 3-week cycles. The baseline demographics and clinical characteristics for all patients (n=162) and those with measurable disease (n=135) are shown in Table 6. Resistance was defined as progressive disease while on treatment, with or without an initial response, or relapse within 6 months of completing treatment with an anthracycline-containing adjuvant chemotherapy regimen.

[See table 6 at top of next page]

Antitumor responses for patients with disease resistant to both paclitaxel and an anthracycline are shown in Table 7.

Table 7. Response Rates in Doubly-Resistant Patients Single-Arm Breast Cancer Trial

	Resistance to Both Paclitaxel and an Anthracycline (n=43)
CR	0
PR[1]	11
CR + PR[1]	11
Response Rate[1] (95% C.I.)	25.6% (13.5, 41.2)
Duration of Response,[1] Median in days[2] (Range)	154 (63-233)

[1]Includes 2 patients treated with an anthracenedione
[2]From date of first response

For the subgroup of 43 patients who were doubly resistant, the median time to progression was 102 days and the median survival was 255 days. The objective response rate in this population was supported by a response rate of 18.5% (1 CR, 24 PRs) in the overall population of 135 patients with measurable disease, who were less resistant to chemotherapy (see Table 6). The median time to progression was 90 days and the median survival was 306 days.

INDICATIONS AND USAGE

Colorectal Cancer: XELODA is indicated as first-line treatment of patients with metastatic colorectal carcinoma when treatment with fluoropyrimidine therapy alone is preferred. Combination chemotherapy has shown a survival benefit compared to 5-FU/LV alone. A survival benefit over 5-FU/LV has not been demonstrated with XELODA monotherapy. Use of XELODA instead of 5-FU/LV in combinations has not been adequately studied to assure safety or preservation of the survival advantage.

Breast Cancer Combination Therapy: XELODA in combination with docetaxel is indicated for the treatment of patients with metastatic breast cancer after failure of prior anthracycline-containing chemotherapy.

Breast Cancer Monotherapy: XELODA monotherapy is also indicated for the treatment of patients with metastatic breast cancer resistant to both paclitaxel and an anthracycline-containing chemotherapy regimen or resistant to paclitaxel and for whom further anthracycline therapy is not indicated, eg, patients who have received cumulative doses

Continued on next page

Xeloda—Cont.

of 400 mg/m² of doxorubicin or doxorubicin equivalents. Resistance is defined as progressive disease while on treatment, with or without an initial response, or relapse within 6 months of completing treatment with an anthracycline-containing adjuvant regimen.

CONTRAINDICATIONS

XELODA is contraindicated in patients with known hypersensitivity to capecitabine or to any of its components. XELODA is contraindicated in patients who have a known hypersensitivity to 5-fluorouracil. XELODA is contraindicated in patients with known dihydropyrimidine dehydrogenase (DPD) deficiency. XELODA is also contraindicated in patients with severe renal impairment (creatinine clearance below 30 mL/min [Cockroft and Gault]) (see CLINICAL PHARMACOLOGY: *Special Populations*).

WARNINGS

Renal Insufficiency: Patients with moderate renal impairment at baseline require dose reduction (see DOSAGE AND ADMINISTRATION). Patients with mild and moderate renal impairment at baseline should be carefully monitored for adverse events. Prompt interruption of therapy with subsequent dose adjustments is recommended if a patient develops a grade 2 to 4 adverse event as outlined in Table 14 in DOSAGE AND ADMINISTRATION.

Coagulopathy: See Boxed WARNING.

Diarrhea: XELODA can induce diarrhea, sometimes severe. Patients with severe diarrhea should be carefully monitored and given fluid and electrolyte replacement if they become dehydrated. In the overall clinical trial safety database of XELODA monotherapy (N=875), the median time to first occurrence of grade 2 to 4 diarrhea was 34 days (range from 1 to 369 days). The median duration of grade 3 to 4 diarrhea was 5 days. National Cancer Institute of Canada (NCIC) grade 2 diarrhea is defined as an increase of 4 to 6 stools/day or nocturnal stools, grade 3 diarrhea as an increase of 7 to 9 stools/day or incontinence and malabsorption, and grade 4 diarrhea as an increase of ≥10 stools/day or grossly bloody diarrhea or the need for parenteral support. If grade 2, 3 or 4 diarrhea occurs, administration of XELODA should be immediately interrupted until the diarrhea resolves or decreases in intensity to grade 1. Following a reoccurrence of grade 2 diarrhea or occurrence of any grade 3 or 4 diarrhea, subsequent doses of XELODA should be decreased (see DOSAGE AND ADMINISTRATION). Standard antidiarrheal treatments (eg, loperamide) are recommended.

Necrotizing enterocolitis (typhlitis) has been reported.

Geriatric Patients: Patients ≥80 years old may experience a greater incidence of grade 3 or 4 adverse events (see PRECAUTIONS: *Geriatric Use*). In the overall clinical trial safety database of XELODA monotherapy (N=875), 62% of the 21 patients ≥80 years of age treated with XELODA experienced a treatment-related grade 3 or 4 adverse event: diarrhea in 6 (28.6%), nausea in 3 (14.3%), hand-and-foot syndrome in 3 (14.3%), and vomiting in 2 (9.5%) patients. Among the 10 patients 70 years of age and greater (no patients were >80 years of age) treated with XELODA in combination with docetaxel, 30% (3 out of 10) of patients experienced grade 3 or 4 diarrhea and stomatitis, and 40% (4 out of 10) experienced grade 3 hand-and-foot syndrome.

Among the 67 patients ≥60 years of age receiving XELODA in combination with docetaxel, the incidence of grade 3 or 4 treatment-related adverse events, treatment-related serious adverse events, withdrawals due to adverse events, treatment discontinuations due to adverse events and treatment discontinuations within the first two treatment cycles was higher than in the <60 years of age patient group.

Pregnancy: XELODA may cause fetal harm when given to a pregnant woman. Capecitabine at doses of 198 mg/kg/day during organogenesis caused malformations and embryo death in mice. In separate pharmacokinetic studies, this dose in mice produced 5'-DFUR AUC values about 0.2 times the corresponding values in patients administered the recommended daily dose. Malformations in mice included cleft palate, anophthalmia, microphthalmia, oligodactyly, polydactyly, syndactyly, kinky tail and dilation of cerebral ventricles. At doses of 90 mg/kg/day, capecitabine given to pregnant monkeys during organogenesis caused fetal death. This dose produced 5'-DFUR AUC values about 0.6 times the corresponding values in patients administered the recommended daily dose. There are no adequate and well-controlled studies in pregnant women using XELODA. If the drug is used during pregnancy, or if the patient becomes pregnant while receiving this drug, the patient should be apprised of the potential hazard to the fetus. Women of childbearing potential should be advised to avoid becoming pregnant while receiving treatment with XELODA.

PRECAUTIONS

General: Patients receiving therapy with XELODA should be monitored by a physician experienced in the use of cancer chemotherapeutic agents. Most adverse events are reversible and do not need to result in discontinuation, although doses may need to be withheld or reduced (see DOSAGE AND ADMINISTRATION).

Combination With Other Drugs: Use of XELODA in combination with irinotecan has not been adequately studied.

Hand-and-Foot Syndrome: Hand-and-foot syndrome (palmar-plantar erythrodysesthesia or chemotherapy-induced acral erythema) is a cutaneous toxicity (median time to onset of 79 days, range from 11 to 360 days) with a severity range of grades 1 to 3. Grade 1 is characterized by any of the following: numbness, dysesthesia/paresthesia, tingling, painless swelling or erythema of the hands and/or feet and/or discomfort which does not disrupt normal activities. Grade 2 hand-and-foot syndrome is defined as painful erythema and swelling of the hands and/or feet and/or discomfort affecting the patient's activities of daily living. Grade 3 hand-and-foot syndrome is defined as moist desquamation, ulceration, blistering or severe pain of the hands and/or feet and/or severe discomfort that causes the patient to be unable to work or perform activities of daily living. If grade 2 or 3 hand-and-foot syndrome occurs, administration of XELODA should be interrupted until the event resolves or decreases in intensity to grade 1. Following grade 3 hand-and-foot syndrome, subsequent doses of XELODA should be decreased (see DOSAGE AND ADMINISTRATION).

Cardiotoxicity: The cardiotoxicity observed with XELODA includes myocardial infarction/ischemia, angina, dysrhythmias, cardiac arrest, cardiac failure, sudden death, electrocardiographic changes, and cardiomyopathy. These adverse events may be more common in patients with a prior history of coronary artery disease.

Dihydropyrimidine Dehydrogenase Deficiency: Rarely, unexpected, severe toxicity (eg, stomatitis, diarrhea, neutropenia and neurotoxicity) associated with 5-fluorouracil has been attributed to a deficiency of dihydropyrimidine dehy-

Table 6. Baseline Demographics and Clinical Characteristics
Single Arm Breast Cancer Trial

	Patients With Measurable Disease (n=135)	All Patients (n=162)
Age (median, years)	55	56
Karnofsky PS	90	90
No. Disease Sites		
1-2	43 (32%)	60 (37%)
3-4	63 (46%)	69 (43%)
>5	29 (22%)	34 (21%)
Dominant Site of Disease		
Visceral[1]	101 (75%)	110 (68%)
Soft Tissue	30 (22%)	35 (22%)
Bone	4 (3%)	17 (10%)
Prior Chemotherapy		
Paclitaxel	135 (100%)	162 (100%)
Anthracycline[2]	122 (90%)	147 (91%)
5-FU	110 (81%)	133 (82%)
Resistance to Paclitaxel	103 (76%)	124 (77%)
Resistance to an Anthracycline[2]	55 (41%)	67 (41%)
Resistance to both Paclitaxel and an Anthracycline[2]	43 (32%)	51 (31%)

[1]Lung, pleura, liver, peritoneum
[2]Includes 2 patients treated with an anthracenedione

Table 8. Pooled Phase 3 Colorectal Trials:
Percent Incidence of Adverse Events Related or Unrelated to Treatment in ≥5% of Patients

Adverse Event	XELODA (n=596)			5-FU/LV (n=593)		
	Total %	Grade 3 %	Grade 4 %	Total %	Grade 3 %	Grade 4 %
Number of Patients With > One Adverse Event	96	52	9	94	45	9
Body System/Adverse Event						
GI						
Diarrhea	55	13	2	61	10	2
Nausea	43	4	–	51	3	<1
Vomiting	27	4	<1	30	4	<1
Stomatitis	25	2	<1	62	14	1
Abdominal Pain	35	9	<1	31	5	–
Gastrointestinal Motility Disorder	10	<1	–	7	<1	–
Constipation	14	1	<1	17	1	–
Oral Discomfort	10	–	–	10	–	–
Upper GI Inflammatory Disorders	8	<1	–	10	1	–
Gastrointestinal Hemorrhage	6	1	<1	3	1	–
Ileus	6	4	1	5	2	1
Skin and Subcutaneous						
Hand-and-Foot Syndrome	54	17	NA	6	1	NA
Dermatitis	27	1	–	26	1	–
Skin Discoloration	7	<1	–	5	–	–
Alopecia	6	–	–	21	<1	–
General						
Fatigue/Weakness	42	4	–	46	4	–
Pyrexia	18	1	–	21	2	–
Edema	15	1	–	9	1	–
Pain	12	1	–	10	1	–
Chest Pain	6	1	–	6	1	<1
Neurological						
Peripheral Sensory Neuropathy	10	–	–	4	–	–
Headache	10	1	–	7	–	–
Dizziness*	8	<1	–	8	<1	–
Insomnia	7	–	–	7	–	–
Taste Disturbance	6	1	–	11	<1	1
Metabolism						
Appetite Decreased	26	3	<1	31	2	<1
Dehydration	7	2	<1	8	3	1
Eye						
Eye Irritation	13	–	–	10	<1	–
Vision Abnormal	5	–	–	2	–	–
Respiratory						
Dyspnea	14	1	–	10	<1	1
Cough	7	<1	1	8	–	–
Pharyngeal Disorder	5	–	–	5	–	–
Epistaxis	3	<1	–	6	–	–
Sore Throat	2	–	–	6	–	–

(Table continued on next page)

drogenase (DPD) activity. A link between decreased levels of DPD and increased, potentially fatal toxic effects of 5-fluorouracil therefore cannot be excluded.

Hepatic Insufficiency: Patients with mild to moderate hepatic dysfunction due to liver metastases should be carefully monitored when XELODA is administered. The effect of severe hepatic dysfunction on the disposition of XELODA is not known (see CLINICAL PHARMACOLOGY and DOSAGE AND ADMINISTRATION).

Hyperbilirubinemia: In the overall clinical trial safety database of XELODA monotherapy (N=875), grade 3 (1.5-3 × ULN) hyperbilirubinemia occurred in 15.2% (n=133) and grade 4 (>3 × ULN) hyperbilirubinemia occurred in 3.9% (n=34) of 875 patients with either metastatic breast or colorectal cancer who received at least one dose of XELODA 1250 mg/m^2 twice daily as monotherapy for 2 weeks followed by a 1-week rest period. Of 566 patients who had hepatic metastases at baseline and 309 patients without hepatic metastases at baseline, grade 3 or 4 hyperbilirubinemia occurred in 22.8% and 12.3%, respectively. Of the 167 patients with grade 3 or 4 hyperbilirubinemia, 18.6% (n=31) also had postbaseline elevations (grades 1 to 4, without elevations at baseline) in alkaline phosphatase and 27.5% (n=46) had postbaseline elevations in transaminases at any time (not necessarily concurrent). The majority of these patients, 64.5% (n=20) and 71.7% (n=33), had liver metastases at baseline. In addition, 57.5% (n=96) and 35.3% (n=59) of the 167 patients had elevations (grades 1 to 4) at both prebaseline and postbaseline in alkaline phosphatase or transaminases, respectively. Only 7.8% (n=13) and 3.0% (n=5) had grade 3 or 4 elevations in alkaline phosphatase or transaminases.

In the 596 patients treated with XELODA as first-line therapy for metastatic colorectal cancer, the incidence of grade 3 or 4 hyperbilirubinemia was similar to the overall clinical trial safety database of XELODA monotherapy. The median time to onset for grade 3 or 4 hyperbilirubinemia in the colorectal cancer population was 64 days and median total bilirubin increased from 8 μm/L at baseline to 13 μm/L during treatment with XELODA. Of the 136 colorectal cancer patients with grade 3 or 4 hyperbilirubinemia, 49 patients had grade 3 or 4 hyperbilirubinemia as their last measured value, of which 46 had liver metastases at baseline.

In 251 patients with metastatic breast cancer who received a combination of XELODA and docetaxel, grade 3 (1.5 to 3 × ULN) hyperbilirubinemia occurred in 7% (n=17) and grade 4 (>3 × ULN) hyperbilirubinemia occurred in 2% (n=5).

If drug-related grade 2 to 4 elevations in bilirubin occur, administration of XELODA should be immediately interrupted until the hyperbilirubinemia resolves or decreases in intensity to grade 1. NCIC grade 2 hyperbilirubinemia is defined as 1.5 × normal, grade 3 hyperbilirubinemia as 1.5 to 3 × normal and grade 4 hyperbilirubinemia as >3 × normal. (See recommended dose modifications under DOSAGE AND ADMINISTRATION.)

Hematologic: In 875 patients with either metastatic breast or colorectal cancer who received a dose of 1250 mg/m^2 administered twice daily as monotherapy for 2 weeks followed by a 1-week rest period, 3.2%, 1.7%, and 2.4% of patients had grade 3 or 4 neutropenia, thrombocytopenia or decreases in hemoglobin, respectively. In 251 patients with metastatic breast cancer who received a dose of XELODA in combination with docetaxel, 68% had grade 3 or 4 neutropenia, 2.8% had grade 3 or 4 thrombocytopenia, and 9.6% had grade 3 or 4 anemia.

Carcinogenesis, Mutagenesis and Impairment of Fertility: Adequate studies investigating the carcinogenic potential of XELODA have not been conducted. Capecitabine was not mutagenic in vitro to bacteria (Ames test) or mammalian cells (Chinese hamster V79/HPRT gene mutation assay). Capecitabine was clastogenic in vitro to human peripheral blood lymphocytes but not clastogenic in vivo to mouse bone marrow (micronucleus test). Fluorouracil causes mutations in bacteria and yeast. Fluorouracil also causes chromosomal abnormalities in the mouse micronucleus test in vivo.

Impairment of Fertility: In studies of fertility and general reproductive performance in mice, oral capecitabine doses of 760 mg/kg/day disturbed estrus and consequently caused a decrease in fertility. In mice that became pregnant, no fetuses survived this dose. The disturbance in estrus was reversible. In males, this dose caused degenerative changes in the testes, including decreases in the number of spermatocytes and spermatids. In separate pharmacokinetic studies, this dose in mice produced 5'-DFUR AUC values about 0.7 times the corresponding values in patients administered the recommended daily dose.

Information for Patients (see Patient Package Insert): Patients and patients' caregivers should be informed of the expected adverse effects of XELODA, particularly nausea, vomiting, diarrhea, and hand-and-foot syndrome, and should be made aware that patient-specific dose adaptations during therapy are expected and necessary (see DOSAGE AND ADMINISTRATION). Patients should be encouraged to recognize the common grade 2 toxicities associated with XELODA treatment.

Diarrhea: Patients experiencing grade 2 diarrhea (an increase of 4 to 6 stools/day or nocturnal stools) or greater should be instructed to stop taking XELODA immediately. Standard antidiarrheal treatments (eg, loperamide) are recommended.

Nausea: Patients experiencing grade 2 nausea (food intake significantly decreased but able to eat intermittently) or greater should be instructed to stop taking XELODA immediately. Initiation of symptomatic treatment is recommended.

Table 8 *(cont.)*. Pooled Phase 3 Colorectal Trials: Percent Incidence of Adverse Events Related or Unrelated to Treatment in ≥5% of Patients

Adverse Event	**XELODA (n=596)**			**5-FU/LV (n=593)**		
	Total %	**Grade 3 %**	**Grade 4 %**	**Total %**	**Grade 3 %**	**Grade 4 %**
Number of Patients With > One Adverse Event	96	52	9	94	45	9
Body System/Adverse Event						
Musculoskeletal						
Back Pain	10	2	—	9	<1	–
Arthralgia	8	1	—	6	1	–
Vascular						
Venous Thrombosis	8	3	<1	6	2	–
Psychiatric						
Mood Alteration	5	–	–	6	<1	–
Depression	5	–	–	4	<1	–
Infections						
Viral	5	<1	–	5	<1	–
Blood and Lymphatic						
Anemia	80	2	<1	79	1	<1
Neutropenia	13	1	2	46	8	13
Hepatobiliary						
Hyperbilirubinemia	48	18	5	17	3	3

– Not observed
* Excluding vertigo
NA = Not Applicable

Vomiting: Patients experiencing grade 2 vomiting (2 to 5 episodes in a 24-hour period) or greater should be instructed to stop taking XELODA immediately. Initiation of symptomatic treatment is recommended.

Hand-and-Foot Syndrome: Patients experiencing grade 2 hand-and-foot syndrome (painful erythema and swelling of the hands and/or feet and/or discomfort affecting the patients' activities of daily living) or greater should be instructed to stop taking XELODA immediately.

Stomatitis: Patients experiencing grade 2 stomatitis (painful erythema, edema or ulcers of the mouth or tongue, but able to eat) or greater should be instructed to stop taking XELODA immediately. Initiation of symptomatic treatment is recommended (see DOSAGE AND ADMINISTRATION).

Fever and Neutropenia: Patients who develop a fever of 100.5°F or greater or other evidence of potential infection should be instructed to call their physician.

Drug-Food Interaction: In all clinical trials, patients were instructed to administer XELODA within 30 minutes after a meal. Since current safety and efficacy data are based upon administration with food, it is recommended that XELODA be administered with food (see DOSAGE AND ADMINISTRATION).

Drug-Drug Interactions:

Antacid: The effect of an aluminum hydroxide- and magnesium hydroxide-containing antacid (Maalox) on the pharmacokinetics of XELODA was investigated in 12 cancer patients. There was a small increase in plasma concentrations of XELODA and one metabolite (5'-DFCR); there was no effect on the 3 major metabolites (5'-DFUR, 5-FU and FBAL).

Anticoagulants: Patients receiving concomitant capecitabine and oral coumarin-derivative anticoagulant therapy should have their anticoagulant response (INR or prothrombin time) monitored closely with great frequency and the anticoagulant dose should be adjusted accordingly (see Boxed WARNING and CLINICAL PHARMACOLOGY). Altered coagulation parameters and/or bleeding have been reported in patients taking XELODA concomitantly with coumarin-derivative anticoagulants such as warfarin and phenprocoumon. These events occurred within several days and up to several months after initiating XELODA therapy and, in a few cases, within 1 month after stopping XELODA. These events occurred in patients with and without liver metastases. In a drug interaction study with single-dose warfarin administration, there was a significant increase in the mean AUC of S-warfarin. The maximum observed INR value increased by 91%. This interaction is probably due to an inhibition of cytochrome P450 2C9 by capecitabine and/or its metabolites (see CLINICAL PHARMACOLOGY).

CYP2C9 substrates: Other than warfarin, no formal drug-drug interaction studies between XELODA and other CYP2C9 substrates have been conducted. Care should be exercised when XELODA is coadministered with CYP2C9 substrates.

Phenytoin: The level of phenytoin should be carefully monitored in patients taking XELODA and phenytoin dose may need to be reduced (see DOSAGE AND ADMINISTRATION: *Dose Modification Guidelines*). Postmarketing reports indicate that some patients receiving XELODA and phenytoin had toxicity associated with elevated phenytoin levels. Formal drug-drug interaction studies with phenytoin have not been conducted, but the mechanism of interaction is presumed to be inhibition of the CYP2C9 isoenzyme by capecitabine and/or its metabolites (see PRECAUTIONS: *Drug-Drug Interactions: Anticoagulants*).

Leucovorin: The concentration of 5-fluorouracil is increased and its toxicity may be enhanced by leucovorin. Deaths from severe enterocolitis, diarrhea, and dehydration have been reported in elderly patients receiving weekly leucovorin and fluorouracil.

Pregnancy: *Teratogenic Effects:* Category D (see WARNINGS). Women of childbearing potential should be advised to avoid becoming pregnant while receiving treatment with XELODA.

Nursing Women: Lactating mice given a single oral dose of capecitabine excreted significant amounts of capecitabine metabolites into the milk. Because of the potential for serious adverse reactions in nursing infants from capecitabine, it is recommended that nursing be discontinued when receiving XELODA therapy.

Pediatric Use: The safety and effectiveness of XELODA in persons <18 years of age have not been established.

Geriatric Use: Physicians should pay particular attention to monitoring the adverse effects of XELODA in the elderly (see WARNINGS: *Geriatric Patients*).

ADVERSE REACTIONS

Colorectal Cancer: Table 8 shows the adverse events occurring in ≥5% of patients from pooling the two phase 3 trials in colorectal cancer. Rates are rounded to the nearest whole number. A total of 596 patients with metastatic colorectal cancer were treated with 1250 mg/m^2 twice a day of XELODA administered for 2 weeks followed by a 1-week rest period, and 593 patients were administered 5-FU and leucovorin in the Mayo regimen (20 mg/m^2 leucovorin IV followed by 425 mg/m^2 IV bolus 5-FU, on days 1-5, every 28 days). In the pooled colorectal database the median duration of treatment was 139 days for capecitabine-treated patients and 140 days for 5-FU/LV-treated patients. A total of 78 (13%) and 63 (11%) capecitabine and 5-FU/LV-treated patients, respectively, discontinued treatment because of adverse events/intercurrent illness. A total of 82 deaths due to all causes occurred either on study or within 28 days of receiving study drug: 50 (8.4%) patients randomized to XELODA and 32 (5.4%) randomized to 5-FU/LV.

[See table 8 on previous page and above]

Breast Cancer Combination: The following data are shown for the combination study with XELODA and docetaxel in patients with metastatic breast cancer in Table 9. In the XELODA and docetaxel combination arm the treatment was XELODA administered orally 1250 mg/m^2 twice daily as intermittent therapy (2 weeks of treatment followed by 1 week without treatment) for at least 6 weeks and docetaxel administered as a 1-hour intravenous infusion at a dose of 75 mg/m^2 on the first day of each 3-week cycle for at least 6 weeks. In the monotherapy arm docetaxel was administered as a 1-hour intravenous infusion at a dose of 100 mg/m^2 on the first day of each 3-week cycle for at least 6 weeks. The mean duration of treatment was 129 days in the combination arm and 98 days in the monotherapy arm. A total of 66 patients (26%) in the combination arm and 49 (19%) in the monotherapy arm withdrew from the study because of adverse events. The percentage of patients requiring dose reductions due to adverse events was 65% in the combination arm and 36% in the monotherapy arm. The percentage of patients requiring treatment interruptions due to adverse events in the combination arm was 79%. Treatment interruptions were part of the dose modification scheme for the combination therapy arm but not for the docetaxel monotherapy-treated patients.

[See table 9 at top of next page]

[See table 10 on page 2949]

Breast Cancer XELODA Monotherapy: The following data are shown for the study in stage IV breast cancer patients who received a dose of 1250 mg/m^2 administered twice daily for 2 weeks followed by a 1-week rest period. The mean duration of treatment was 114 days. A total of 13 out of 162

Continued on next page

Xeloda—Cont.

patients (8%) discontinued treatment because of adverse events/intercurrent illness.
[See table 11 on next page]

OTHER ADVERSE EVENTS:

XELODA and Docetaxel in Combination: Shown below by body system are the clinically relevant adverse events in <5% of patients in the overall clinical trial safety database of 251 patients (Study Details) reported as related to the administration of XELODA in combination with docetaxel and that were clinically at least remotely relevant. In parentheses is the incidence of grade 3 and 4 occurrences of each adverse event.

It is anticipated that the same types of adverse events observed in the XELODA monotherapy studies may be observed in patients treated with the combination of XELODA plus docetaxel.

Gastrointestinal: ileus (0.39), necrotizing enterocolitis (0.39), esophageal ulcer (0.39), hemorrhagic diarrhea (0.80)
Neurological: ataxia (0.39), syncope (1.20), taste loss (0.80), polyneuropathy (0.39), migraine (0.39)
Cardiac: supraventricular tachycardia (0.39)
Infection: neutropenic sepsis (2.39), sepsis (0.39), bronchopneumonia (0.39)
Blood and Lymphatic: agranulocytosis (0.39), prothrombin decreased (0.39)
Vascular: hypotension (1.20), venous phlebitis and thrombophlebitis (0.39), postural hypotension (0.80)
Renal: renal failure (0.39)
Hepatobiliary: jaundice (0.39), abnormal liver function tests (0.39), hepatic failure (0.39), hepatic coma (0.39), hepatotoxicity (0.39)
Immune System: hypersensitivity (1.20)

XELODA Monotherapy: Shown below by body system are the clinically relevant adverse events in <5% of patients in the overall clinical trial safety database of 875 patients (phase 3 colorectal studies — 596 patients, phase 2 colorectal study — 34 patients, phase 2 breast cancer studies — 245 patients) reported as related to the administration of XELODA and that were clinically at least remotely relevant. In parentheses is the incidence of grade 3 or 4 occurrences of each adverse event.

Gastrointestinal: abdominal distension, dysphagia, proctalgia, ascites (0.1), gastric ulcer (0.1), ileus (0.3), toxic dilation of intestine, gastroenteritis (0.1)
Skin and Subcutaneous: nail disorder (0.1), sweating increased (0.1), photosensitivity reaction (0.1), skin ulceration, pruritus, radiation recall syndrome (0.2)
General: chest pain (0.2), influenza-like illness, hot flushes, pain (0.1), hoarseness, irritability, difficulty in walking, thirst, chest mass, collapse, fibrosis (0.1), hemorrhage, edema, sedation
Neurological: insomnia, ataxia (0.5), tremor, dysphasia, encephalopathy (0.1), abnormal coordination, dysarthria, loss of consciousness (0.2), impaired balance
Metabolism: increased weight, cachexia (0.4), hypertriglyceridemia (0.1), hypokalemia, hypomagnesemia
Eye: conjunctivitis
Respiratory: cough (0.1), epistaxis (0.1), asthma (0.2), hemoptysis, respiratory distress (0.1), dyspnea
Cardiac: tachycardia (0.1), bradycardia, atrial fibrillation, ventricular extrasystoles, extrasystoles, myocarditis (0.1), pericardial effusion
Infections: laryngitis (1.0), bronchitis (0.2), pneumonia (0.2), bronchopneumonia (0.2), keratoconjunctivitis, sepsis (0.3), fungal infections (including candidiasis) (0.2)
Musculoskeletal: myalgia, bone pain (0.1), arthritis (0.1), muscle weakness
Blood and Lymphatic: leukopenia (0.2), coagulation disorder (0.1), bone marrow depression (0.1), idiopathic thrombocytopenia purpura (1.0), pancytopenia (0.1)
Vascular: hypotension (0.2), hypertension (0.1), lymphoedema (0.1), pulmonary embolism (0.2), cerebrovascular accident (0.1)
Psychiatric: depression, confusion (0.1)
Renal: renal impairment (0.6)
Ear: vertigo
Hepatobiliary: hepatic fibrosis (0.1), hepatitis (0.1), cholestatic hepatitis (0.1), abnormal liver function tests
Immune System: drug hypersensitivity (0.1)
Postmarketing: hepatic failure

Table 9. Percent Incidence of Adverse Events Considered Related or Unrelated to Treatment in ≥5% of Patients Participating in the XELODA and Docetaxel Combination vs Docetaxel Monotherapy Study

Adverse Event	XELODA 1250 mg/m²/bid With Docetaxel 75 mg/m²/3 weeks (n=251)			Docetaxel 100 mg/m²/3 weeks (n=255)		
	Total %	Grade 3 %	Grade 4 %	Total %	Grade 3 %	Grade 4 %
Number of Patients With at Least one Adverse Event	99	76.5	29.1	97	57.6	31.8
Body System/Adverse Event						
GI						
Diarrhea	67	14	<1	48	5	<1
Stomatitis	67	17	<1	43	5	–
Nausea	45	7	–	36	2	–
Vomiting	35	4	1	24	2	–
Constipation	20	2	–	18	–	–
Abdominal Pain	30	<3	<1	24	2	–
Dyspepsia	14	–	–	8	1	–
Dry Mouth	6	<1	–	5	–	–
Skin and Subcutaneous						
Hand-and-Foot Syndrome	63	24	NA	8	1	NA
Alopecia	41	6	–	42	7	–
Nail Disorder	14	2	–	15	–	–
Dermatitis	8	–	–	11	1	–
Rash Erythematous	9	<1	–	5	–	–
Nail Discoloration	6	–	–	4	<1	–
Onycholysis	5	1	–	5	1	–
Pruritus	4	–	–	5	–	–
General						
Pyrexia	28	2	–	34	2	–
Asthenia	26	4	<1	25	6	–
Fatigue	22	4	–	27	6	–
Weakness	16	2	–	11	2	–
Pain in Limb	13	<1	–	13	2	–
Lethargy	7	–	–	6	2	–
Pain	7	<1	–	5	1	–
Chest Pain (non-cardiac)	4	<1	–	6	2	–
Influenza-like Illness	5	–	–	5	–	–
Neurological						
Taste Disturbance	16	<1	–	14	<1	–
Headache	15	3	–	15	2	–
Paresthesia	12	<1	–	16	1	–
Dizziness	12	–	–	8	<1	–
Insomnia	8	–	–	10	<1	–
Peripheral Neuropathy	6	–	–	10	1	–
Hypoaesthesia	4	<1	–	8	<1	–
Metabolism						
Anorexia	13	1	–	11	<1	–
Appetite Decreased	10	–	–	5	–	–
Weight Decreased	7	–	–	5	–	–
Dehydration	10	2	–	7	<1	<1
Eye						
Lacrimation Increased	12	–	–	7	<1	–
Conjunctivitis	5	–	–	4	–	–
Eye Irritation	5	–	–	1	–	–
Musculoskeletal						
Arthralgia	15	2	–	24	3	–
Myalgia	15	2	–	25	2	–
Back Pain	12	<1	–	11	3	–
Bone Pain	8	<1	–	10	2	–
Cardiac						
Edema	33	<2	–	34	<3	1
Blood						
Neutropenic Fever	16	3	13	21	5	16
Respiratory						
Dyspnea	14	2	<1	16	2	–
Cough	13	1	–	22	<1	–
Sore Throat	12	2	–	11	<1	–
Epistaxis	7	<1	–	6	–	–
Rhinorrhea	5	–	–	3	–	–
Pleural Effusion	2	1	–	7	4	–
Infection						
Oral Candidiasis	7	<1	–	8	<1	–
Urinary Tract Infection	6	<1	–	4	–	–
Upper Respiratory Tract	4	–	–	5	1	–
Vascular						
Flushing	5	–	–	5	–	–
Lymphoedema	3	<1	–	5	1	–
Psychiatric						
Depression	5	–	–	5	1	–

–Not observed
NA = Not Applicable

OVERDOSAGE

The manifestations of acute overdose would include nausea, vomiting, diarrhea, gastrointestinal irritation and bleeding, and bone marrow depression. Medical management of overdose should include customary supportive medical interventions aimed at correcting the presenting clinical manifestations. Although no clinical experience using dialysis as a treatment for XELODA overdose has been reported, dialysis may be of benefit in reducing circulating concentrations of 5'-DFUR, a low–molecular-weight metabolite of the parent compound.

Single doses of XELODA were not lethal to mice, rats, and monkeys at doses up to 2000 mg/kg (2.4, 4.8, and 9.6 times the recommended human daily dose on a mg/m² basis).

DOSAGE AND ADMINISTRATION

The recommended dose of XELODA is 1250 mg/m² administered orally twice daily (morning and evening; equivalent to 2500 mg/m² total daily dose) for 2 weeks followed by a 1-week rest period given as 3-week cycles. XELODA tablets should be swallowed with water within 30 minutes after a meal. In combination with docetaxel, the recommended dose of XELODA is 1250 mg/m² twice daily for 2 weeks followed by a 1-week rest period, combined with docetaxel at 75 mg/m² as a 1-hour intravenous infusion every 3 weeks. Pre-medication, according to the docetaxel labeling, should be started prior to docetaxel administration for patients receiving the XELODA plus docetaxel combination. Table 12 displays the total daily dose by body surface area and the number of tablets to be taken at each dose.
[See table 12 at bottom of next page]

Dose Modification Guidelines: Patients should be carefully monitored for toxicity. Toxicity due to XELODA administration may be managed by symptomatic treatment, dose interruptions and adjustment of XELODA dose. Once the dose has been reduced it should not be increased at a later time.

The dose of phenytoin and the dose of a coumarin-derivative anticoagulants may need to be reduced when either drug is administered concomitantly with XELODA (see PRECAUTIONS: *Drug-Drug Interactions*).

Dose modification for the use of XELODA and docetaxel in combination is shown in Table 13.
[See table 13 at top of page 2950]

Dose modification for the use of XELODA as monotherapy is shown in Table 14.
[See table 14 at top of page 2951]

Dosage modifications are not recommended for grade 1 events. Therapy with XELODA should be interrupted upon the occurrence of a grade 2 or 3 adverse experience. Once the adverse event has resolved or decreased in intensity to grade 1, then XELODA therapy may be restarted at full dose or as adjusted according to Table 14. If a grade 4 experience occurs, therapy should be discontinued or interrupted until resolved or decreased to grade 1, and therapy should be restarted at 50% of the original dose. Doses of XELODA omitted for toxicity are not replaced or restored; instead the patient should resume the planned treatment cycles.

Adjustment of Starting Dose in Special Populations:

Hepatic Impairment: In patients with mild to moderate hepatic dysfunction due to liver metastases, no starting dose adjustment is necessary; however, patients should be carefully monitored. Patients with severe hepatic dysfunction have not been studied.

Renal Impairment: No adjustment to the starting dose of XELODA is recommended in patients with mild renal impairment (creatinine clearance = 51 to 80 mL/min [Cockroft and Gault, as shown below]). In patients with moderate renal impairment (baseline creatinine clearance = 30 to 50 mL/min), a dose reduction to 75% of the XELODA starting dose when used as monotherapy or in combination with docetaxel (from 1250 mg/m^2 to 950 mg/m^2 twice daily) is recommended (see CLINICAL PHARMACOLOGY: *Special Populations*). Subsequent dose adjustment is recommended as outlined in Table 14 if a patient develops a grade 2 to 4 adverse event (see WARNINGS).

[See second table at top of page 2951]

Geriatrics: Physicians should exercise caution in monitoring the effects of XELODA in the elderly. Insufficient data are available to provide a dosage recommendation.

Table 10. Percent of Patients With Laboratory Abnormalities Participating in the XELODA and Docetaxel Combination vs Docetaxel Monotherapy Study

Adverse Event	XELODA 1250 mg/m^2/bid With Docetaxel 75 mg/m^2/3 weeks (n=251)			Docetaxel 100 mg/m^2/3 weeks (n=255)		
Body System/Adverse Event	**Total %**	**Grade 3 %**	**Grade 4 %**	**Total %**	**Grade 3 %**	**Grade 4 %**
Hematologic						
Leukopenia	91	37	24	88	42	33
Neutropenia/Granulocytopenia	86	20	49	87	10	66
Thrombocytopenia	41	2	1	23	1	2
Anemia	80	7	3	83	5	<1
Lymphocytopenia	99	48	41	98	44	40
Hepatobiliary						
Hyperbilirubinemia	20	7	2	6	2	2

Table 11. Percent Incidence of Adverse Events Considered Remotely, Possibly or Probably Related to Treatment in ≥5% of Patients Participating in the Single Arm Trial in Stage IV Breast Cancer

Adverse Event	Phase 2 Trial in Stage IV Breast Cancer (n=162)		
Body System/Adverse Event	**Total %**	**Grade 3 %**	**Grade 4 %**
GI			
Diarrhea	57	12	3
Nausea	53	4	–
Vomiting	37	4	–
Stomatitis	24	7	–
Abdominal Pain	20	4	–
Constipation	15	1	–
Dyspepsia	8	–	–
Skin and Subcutaneous			
Hand-and-Foot Syndrome	57	11	N/A
Dermatitis	37	1	–
Nail Disorder	7		–
General			
Fatigue	41	8	–
Pyrexia	12	1	–
Pain in Limb	6	1	–
Neurological			
Paresthesia	21	1	–
Headache	9	1	–
Dizziness	8		–
Insomnia	8	–	–
Metabolism			
Anorexia	23	3	–
Dehydration	7	4	1
Eye			
Eye Irritation	15	–	–
Musculoskeletal			
Myalgia	9		–
Cardiac			
Edema	9	1	–
Blood			
Neutropenia	26	2	2
Thrombocytopenia	24	3	1
Anemia	72	3	1
Lymphopenia	94	44	15
Hepatobiliary			
Hyperbilirubinemia	22	9	2

–Not observed or applicable
NA = Not Applicable

Table 12. XELODA Dose Calculation According to Body Surface Area

Dose Level 1250 mg/m^2 Twice a Day		Number of Tablets to be Taken at Each Dose (Morning and Evening)	
Surface Area (m^2)	**Total Daily* Dose (mg)**	**150 mg**	**500 mg**
≤ 1.25	3000	0	3
1.26-1.37	3300	1	3
1.38-1.51	3600	2	3
1.52-1.65	4000	0	4
1.66-1.77	4300	1	4
1.78-1.91	4600	2	4
1.92-2.05	5000	0	5
2.06-2.17	5300	1	5
≥ 2.18	5600	2	5

*Total Daily Dose divided by 2 to allow equal morning and evening doses

HOW SUPPLIED

XELODA is supplied as biconvex, oblong film-coated tablets, available in bottles as follows:

150 mg
color: light peach
engraving: XELODA on one side, 150 on the other
150 mg tablets are packaged in bottles of 60 (NDC 0004-1100-20) and 120 (NDC 0004-1100-51).

500 mg
color: peach
engraving: XELODA on one side, 500 on the other
500 mg tablets are packaged in bottles of 120 (NDC 0004-1101-50) and 240 (NDC 0004-1101-16).

Storage Conditions: Store at 25°C (77°F); excursions permitted to 15° to 30°C (59° to 86°F). [See USP Controlled Room Temperature]. KEEP TIGHTLY CLOSED.

Maalox is a registered trademark of Novartis.
Taxotere is a registered trademark of Aventis Pharmaceuticals Products Inc.
For full Taxotere prescribing information, please refer to Taxotere Package Insert.

PATIENT PACKAGE INSERT (text only):

Patient Information
XELODA® (capecitabine) Tablets

Read this leaflet before you start taking XELODA® [zeh-LOE-duh] and each time you renew your prescription. It contains important information. However, this information does not take the place of talking with your doctor. This information cannot cover all possible risks and benefits of XELODA. Your doctor should always be your first choice for detailed information about your medical condition and this medicine.

What is XELODA?

XELODA is a medicine you take by mouth (orally) that is used to treat:

- cancer of the colon or rectum that has spread to other parts of the body (metastatic colorectal cancer) when fluoropyrimidine therapy alone is preferred. Patients and physicians should note that combination chemotherapy has shown a survival benefit compared to 5-FU/LV alone. A survival benefit over 5-FU/LV has not been demonstrated with XELODA monotherapy.
- breast cancer that has spread to other parts of the body and has not responded to treatment with certain other medicines. These medicines include paclitaxel (Taxol®) and anthracycline-containing therapy such as Adriamycin® and doxorubicin.

XELODA is changed in the body to the substance 5-fluorouracil. In some patients with colon, rectum or breast cancer, this substance stops cancer cells from growing and decreases the size of the tumor.

Who should not take XELODA?

1. DO NOT TAKE XELODA IF YOU

- are nursing a baby. Tell your doctor if you are nursing. XELODA may pass to the baby in your milk and harm the baby.
- are allergic to 5-fluorouracil.
- are allergic to capecitabine or to any of its ingredients.
- have a known lack of the enzyme DPD (dihydropyrimidine dehydrogenase).

2. TELL YOUR DOCTOR IF YOU

- **take a blood thinner such as warfarin (Coumadin®). This is very important because XELODA may increase the effect of the blood thinner. If you are taking blood thinners and XELODA, your doctor needs to check how fast your blood clots more frequently and adjust the dose of the blood thinner, if needed.**
- take phenytoin (Dilantin®). Your doctor needs to test the levels of phenytoin in your blood more often or change your dose of phenytoin.
- are pregnant. XELODA may not be right for you.
- have kidney problems. Your doctor may prescribe a different medicine or reduce the XELODA dose.
- have liver problems. You may need to be checked for liver problems while you take XELODA.
- take the vitamin folic acid. It may affect how XELODA works.

How should I take XELODA?

Your doctor will prescribe a dose and treatment plan that is right for *you*. Your doctor may want you to take a combination of 150 mg and 500 mg tablets for each dose. If a com-

Continued on next page

Xeloda—Cont.

bination of tablets is prescribed, you must correctly identify the tablets. Taking the wrong tablets could cause an overdose (too much medicine) or underdose (too little medicine). The 150 mg tablets are light peach in color and have 150 engraved on one side. The 500 mg tablets are peach in color and have 500 engraved on one side. Your doctor may change the amount of medicine you take during your treatment. Your doctor may prescribe XELODA Tablets in combination with Taxotere® or docetaxel injection.

- Take the tablets in the combination prescribed by your doctor for your **morning and evening** doses.
- Take the tablets **within 30 minutes after the end of a meal** (breakfast and dinner).
- **Swallow XELODA with water.**
- If you miss a dose of XELODA, do not take the missed dose at all and do not double the next one. Instead, continue your regular dosing schedule and check with your doctor.
- It is recommended that XELODA be taken for 14 days followed by a 7-day rest period (no drug), given as a 21-day cycle. Your doctor will tell you how many cycles of treatment you will need.
- In case of accidental swallowing, or if you suspect that too much medicine has been taken, contact your doctor or local poison control center or emergency room **right away**.

What should I avoid while taking XELODA?

- Women should not become pregnant while taking XELODA. XELODA may harm your unborn child. Use effective birth control while taking XELODA. Tell your doctor if you become pregnant.
- Men should practice birth control measures while taking XELODA.
- Do not breast-feed. XELODA may pass through your milk and harm the baby.

What are the most common side effects of XELODA?

The most common side effects of XELODA are:

- diarrhea, nausea, vomiting, stomatitis (sores in mouth and throat), abdominal (stomach area) pain, upset stomach, constipation, loss of appetite, and dehydration (too much water loss from the body). These side effects are more common in patients age 80 and older.
- hand-and-foot syndrome (palms of the hands or soles of the feet tingle, become numb, painful, swollen or red), rash, dry, itchy or discolored skin, nail problems, and hair loss.
- tiredness, weakness, dizziness, headache, fever, pain (including chest, back, joint, and muscle pain), trouble sleeping, and taste problems.

These side effects may differ when taking XELODA in combination with Taxotere. Please consult your doctor for possible side effects that may be caused by taking XELODA with Taxotere.

If you are concerned about these or any other side effects while taking XELODA, talk to your doctor.

Do not continue to take XELODA until you have talked to your doctor if you have the side effects listed below, or other side effects that concern you. Your doctor can help reduce the chance that the side effects will continue or become serious. Your doctor may tell you to decrease the dose or stop XELODA treatment for a while.

Contact your doctor right away if you have:

- ***Diarrhea:*** if you have more than 4 bowel movements each day or any diarrhea at night
- ***Vomiting:*** if you vomit more than once in a 24-hour time period
- ***Nausea:*** if you lose your appetite, and the amount of food you eat each day is much less than usual
- ***Stomatitis:*** if you have pain, redness, swelling or sores in your mouth
- ***Hand-and-Foot Syndrome:*** if you have pain and swelling or redness of your hands or feet that prevents normal activity
- ***Fever or Infection:*** if you have a temperature of 100.5°F or greater, or other signs of infection

If caught early, most of these side effects usually improve after you stop taking XELODA. If they do not improve within 2 to 3 days, call your doctor again. After side effects have improved, your doctor will tell you whether to start taking XELODA again and what dose to use.

How should I store and use XELODA?

- **Never share XELODA with anyone.**
- **XELODA should be stored at normal room temperature (about 65° to 85°F).**
- **Keep this and all other medications out of the reach of children.**
- **In case of accidental ingestion or if you suspect that more than the prescribed dose of this medication has been taken, contact your doctor or local poison control center or emergency room IMMEDIATELY.**

General advice about prescription medicines:

Medicines are sometimes prescribed for conditions that are not mentioned in patient information leaflets. Do not use XELODA for a condition for which it was not prescribed. Do not give XELODA to other people, even if they have the same symptoms you have. It may harm them.

This leaflet summarizes the most important information about XELODA. If you would like more information, talk with your doctor. You can ask your pharmacist or doctor for information about XELODA that is written for health professionals.

Table 13. XELODA in Combination With Docetaxel Dose Reduction Schedule

Toxicity NCIC Grades*	Grade 2	Grade 3	Grade 4
1st appearance	Grade 2 occurring during the 14 days of XELODA treatment: interrupt XELODA treatment until resolved to grade 0-1. Treatment may be resumed during the cycle at the same dose of XELODA. Doses of XELODA missed during a treatment cycle are not to be replaced. Prophylaxis for toxicities should be implemented where possible. Grade 2 persisting at the time the next XELODA/docetaxel treatment is due: delay treatment until resolved to grade 0-1, then continue at 100% of the original XELODA and docetaxel dose. Prophylaxis for toxicities should be implemented where possible.	Grade 3 occurring during the 14 days of XELODA treatment: interrupt the XELODA treatment until resolved to grade 0-1. Treatment may be resumed during the cycle at 75% of the XELODA dose. Doses of XELODA missed during a treatment cycle are not to be replaced. Prophylaxis for toxicities should be implemented where possible. Grade 3 persisting at the time the next XELODA/docetaxel treatment is due: delay treatment until resolved to grade 0-1. For patients developing grade 3 toxicity at any time during the treatment cycle, upon resolution to grade 0-1, subsequent treatment cycles should be continued at 75% of the original XELODA dose and at 55 mg/m^2 of docetaxel. Prophylaxis for toxicities should be implemented where possible.	Discontinue treatment unless treating physician considers it to be in the best interest of the patient to continue with XELODA at 50% of original dose.
2nd appearance of same toxicity	Grade 2 occurring during the 14 days of XELODA treatment: interrupt XELODA treatment until resolved to grade 0-1. Treatment may be resumed during the cycle at 75% of original XELODA dose. Doses of XELODA missed during a treatment cycle are not to be replaced. Prophylaxis for toxicities should be implemented where possible. Grade 2 persisting at the time the next XELODA/docetaxel treatment is due: delay treatment until resolved to grade 0-1. For patients developing 2nd occurrence of grade 2 toxicity at any time during the treatment cycle, upon resolution to grade 0-1, subsequent treatment cycles should be continued at 75% of the original XELODA dose and at 55 mg/m^{2}of docetaxel. Prophylaxis for toxicities should be implemented where possible.	Grade 3 occurring during the 14 days of XELODA treatment: interrupt the XELODA treatment until resolved to grade 0-1. Treatment may be resumed during the cycle at 50% of the XELODA dose. Doses of XELODA missed during a treatment cycle are not to be replaced. Prophylaxis for toxicities should be implemented where possible. Grade 3 persisting at the time the next XELODA/docetaxel treatment is due: delay treatment until resolved to grade 0-1. For patients developing grade 3 toxicity at any time during the treatment cycle, upon resolution to grade 0-1, subsequent treatment cycles should be continued at 50% of the original XELODA dose and the docetaxel discontinued. Prophylaxis for toxicities should be implemented where possible.	Discontinue treatment.
3rd appearance of same toxicity	Grade 2 occurring during the 14 days of XELODA treatment: interrupt XELODA treatment until resolved to grade 0-1. Treatment may be resumed during the cycle at 50% of the original XELODA dose. Doses of XELODA missed during a treatment cycle are not to be replaced. Prophylaxis for toxicities should be implemented where possible. Grade 2 persisting at the time the next XELODA/docetaxel treatment is due: delay treatment until resolved to grade 0-1. For patients developing 3rd occurrence of grade 2 toxicity at any time during the treatment cycle, upon resolution to grade 0-1, subsequent treatment cycles should be continued at 50% of the original XELODA dose and the docetaxel discontinued. Prophylaxis for toxicities should be implemented where possible.	Discontinue treatment.	
4th appearance of same toxicity	Discontinue treatment.		

*National Cancer Institute of Canada Common Toxicity Criteria were used except for hand-and-foot syndrome (see PRECAUTIONS).

Adriamycin is a registered trademark of Pharmacia & Upjohn Company.

Coumadin is a registered trademark of DuPont Pharma.

Dilantin is a registered trademark of Parke-Davis.

Taxol is a registered trademark of Bristol-Myers Squibb Company.

Table 14. Recommended Dose Modifications

Toxicity NCIC Grades*	During a Course of Therapy	Dose Adjustment for Next Treatment (% of starting dose)
• *Grade 1*	Maintain dose level	Maintain dose level
• *Grade 2*		
-1st appearance	Interrupt until resolved to grade 0-1	100%
-2nd appearance	Interrupt until resolved to grade 0-1	75%
-3rd appearance	Interrupt until resolved to grade 0-1	50%
-4th appearance	Discontinue treatment permanently	
• *Grade 3*		
-1st appearance	Interrupt until resolved to grade 0-1	75%
-2nd appearance	Interrupt until resolved to grade 0-1	50%
-3rd appearance	Discontinue treatment permanently	
• *Grade 4*		
-1st appearance	Discontinue permanently *OR* If physician deems it to be in the patient's best interest to continue, interrupt until resolved to grade 0-1	50%

*National Cancer Institute of Canada Common Toxicity Criteria were used except for the hand-and-foot syndrome (see PRECAUTIONS).

Cockroft and Gault Equation:

$$\text{Creatinine clearance for males} = \frac{(140 - \text{age [yrs]})\ (\text{body wt [kg]})}{(72)\ (\text{serum creatinine [mg/dL]})}$$

Creatinine clearance for females = 0.85 × male value

Taxotere is a registered trademark of Aventis Pharmaceuticals Products Inc.

Revised: April 2003

Shown in Product Identification Guide, page 332

XENICAL®

℞

[zen'ĭ-cal]
(orlistat)
CAPSULES

DESCRIPTION

XENICAL (orlistat) is a lipase inhibitor for obesity management that acts by inhibiting the absorption of dietary fats. Orlistat is (S)-2-formylamino-4-methyl-pentanoic acid (S)-1-[[(2S, 3S)-3-hexyl-4-oxo-2-oxetanyl] methyl]-dodecyl ester. Its empirical formula is $C_{29}H_{53}NO_5$, and its molecular weight is 495.7. It is a single diastereomeric molecule that contains four chiral centers, with a negative optical rotation in ethanol at 529 nm.
Orlistat is a white to off-white crystalline powder. Orlistat is practically insoluble in water, freely soluble in chloroform, and very soluble in methanol and ethanol. Orlistat has no pK_a within the physiological pH range.
XENICAL is available for oral administration in dark-blue, hard-gelatin capsules, with light-blue imprinting. Each capsule contains 120 mg of the active ingredient, orlistat. The capsules also contain the inactive ingredients microcrystalline cellulose, sodium starch glycolate, sodium lauryl sulfate, povidone, and talc. Each capsule shell contains gelatin, titanium dioxide, and FD&C Blue No.1, with printing of pharmaceutical glaze NF, titanium dioxide, and FD&C Blue No.1 aluminum lake.

CLINICAL PHARMACOLOGY

Mechanism of Action
Orlistat is a reversible inhibitor of lipases. It exerts its therapeutic activity in the lumen of the stomach and small intestine by forming a covalent bond with the active serine residue site of gastric and pancreatic lipases. The inactivated enzymes are thus unavailable to hydrolyze dietary fat in the form of triglycerides into absorbable free fatty acids and monoglycerides. As undigested triglycerides are not absorbed, the resulting caloric deficit may have a positive effect on weight control. Systemic absorption of the drug is therefore not needed for activity. At the recommended therapeutic dose of 120 mg three times a day, orlistat inhibits dietary fat absorption by approximately 30%.
Pharmacokinetics
Absorption
Systemic exposure to orlistat is minimal. Following oral dosing with 360 mg ^{14}C-orlistat, plasma radioactivity peaked at approximately 8 hours; plasma concentrations of intact orlistat were near the limits of detection (<5 ng/mL). In therapeutic studies involving monitoring of plasma samples, detection of intact orlistat in plasma was sporadic and concentrations were low (<10 ng/mL or 0.02 µM), without evidence of accumulation, and consistent with minimal absorption.
The average absolute bioavailability of intact orlistat was assessed in studies with male rats at oral doses of 150 and 1000 mg/kg/day and in male dogs at oral doses of 100 and 1000 mg/kg/day and found to be 0.12%, 0.59% in rats and 0.7%, 1.9% in dogs, respectively.
Distribution
In vitro orlistat was >99% bound to plasma proteins (lipoproteins and albumin were major binding proteins). Orlistat minimally partitioned into erythrocytes.
Metabolism
Based on animal data, it is likely that the metabolism of orlistat occurs mainly within the gastrointestinal wall. Based on an oral ^{14}C-orlistat mass balance study in obese patients, two metabolites, M1 (4-member lactone ring hydrolyzed) and M3 (M1 with N-formyl leucine moiety cleaved), accounted for approximately 42% of total radioactivity in plasma. M1 and M3 have an open β-lactone ring and extremely weak lipase inhibitory activity (1000- and 2500-fold less than orlistat, respectively). In view of this low inhibitory activity and the low plasma levels at the therapeutic dose (average of 26 ng/mL and 108 ng/mL for M1 and M3, respectively, 2 to 4 hours after a dose), these metabolites are considered pharmacologically inconsequential. The primary metabolite M1 had a short half-life (approximately 3 hours) whereas the secondary metabolite M3 disappeared at a slower rate (half-life approximately 13.5 hours). In obese patients, steady-state plasma levels of M1, but not M3, increased in proportion to orlistat doses.
Elimination
Following a single oral dose of 360 mg ^{14}C-orlistat in both normal weight and obese subjects, fecal excretion of the unabsorbed drug was found to be the major route of elimination. Orlistat and its M1 and M3 metabolites were also subject to biliary excretion. Approximately 97% of the administered radioactivity was excreted in feces; 83% of that was found to be unchanged orlistat. The cumulative renal excretion of total radioactivity was <2% of the given dose of 360 mg ^{14}C-orlistat. The time to reach complete excretion (fecal plus urinary) was 3 to 5 days. The disposition of orlistat appeared to be similar between normal weight and obese subjects. Based on limited data, the half-life of the absorbed orlistat is in the range of 1 to 2 hours.
Special Populations
Because the drug is minimally absorbed, studies in special populations (geriatric, different races, patients with renal and hepatic insufficiency) were not conducted.
Pediatrics
Plasma concentrations of orlistat and its metabolites M1 and M3 were similar to those found in adults at the same dose level. Daily fecal fat excretions were 27% and 7% of dietary intake in orlistat and placebo treatment groups, respectively.
Drug-Drug Interactions
Drug-drug interaction studies indicate that XENICAL had no effect on pharmacokinetics and/or pharmacodynamics of alcohol, digoxin, glyburide, nifedipine (extended-release tablets), oral contraceptives, phenytoin, pravastatin, or warfarin. Alcohol did not affect the pharmacodynamics of orlistat.
Other Short-term Studies
Adults
In several studies of up to 6-weeks duration, the effects of therapeutic doses of XENICAL on gastrointestinal and systemic physiological processes were assessed in normal-weight and obese subjects. Postprandial cholecystokinin plasma concentrations were lowered after multiple doses of XENICAL in two studies but not significantly different from placebo in two other experiments. There were no clinically significant changes observed in gallbladder motility, bile composition or lithogenicity, or colonic cell proliferation rate, and no clinically significant reduction of gastric emptying time or gastric acidity. In addition, no effects on plasma triglyceride levels or systemic lipases were observed with the administration of XENICAL in these studies. In a 3-week study of 28 healthy male volunteers, XENICAL (120 mg three times a day) did not significantly affect the balance of calcium, magnesium, phosphorus, zinc, copper, and iron.
Pediatrics
In a 3-week study of 32 obese adolescents aged 12 to 16 years, XENICAL (120 mg three times a day) did not significantly affect the balance of calcium, magnesium, phosphorus, zinc, or copper. The iron balance was decreased by 64.7 µmole/24 hours and 40.4 µmole/24 hours in orlistat and placebo treatment groups, respectively.
Dose-response Relationship
A simple maximum effect (E_{max}) model was used to define the dose-response curve of the relationship between XENICAL daily dose and fecal fat excretion as representative of gastrointestinal lipase inhibition. The dose-response curve demonstrated a steep portion for doses up to approximately 400 mg daily, followed by a plateau for higher doses. At doses greater than 120 mg three times a day, the percentage increase in effect was minimal.

CLINICAL STUDIES

Observational epidemiologic studies have established a relationship between obesity and visceral fat and the risks for cardiovascular disease, type 2 diabetes, certain forms of cancer, gallstones, certain respiratory disorders, and an increase in overall mortality. These studies suggest that weight loss, if maintained, may produce health benefits for obese patients who have or are at risk of developing weight-related comorbidities. The long-term effects of orlistat on morbidity and mortality associated with obesity have not been established.
The effects of XENICAL on weight loss, weight maintenance, and weight regain and on a number of comorbidities (eg, type 2 diabetes, lipids, blood pressure) were assessed in seven long-term (1- to 2-years duration) multicenter, double-blind, placebo-controlled clinical trials. During the first year of therapy, weight loss and weight maintenance were assessed. During the second year of therapy, some studies assessed continued weight loss and weight maintenance and others assessed the effect of orlistat on weight regain. These studies included over 2800 patients treated with XENICAL and 1400 patients treated with placebo. The majority of these patients had obesity-related risk factors and comorbidities. In these 7 studies, treatment with XENICAL and placebo designates treatment with XENICAL plus diet and placebo plus diet, respectively.
During the weight loss and weight maintenance period, a well-balanced, reduced-calorie diet that was intended to result in an approximate 20% decrease in caloric intake and provide 30% of calories from fat was recommended to all patients. In addition, all patients were offered nutritional counseling.
One-year Results: Weight Loss, Weight Maintenance, and Risk Factors
Weight loss was observed within 2 weeks of initiation of therapy and continued for 6 to 12 months.
Pooled data from five clinical trials indicated that the overall mean weight loss from randomization to the end of 6 months and 1 year of treatment in the intent-to-treat population were 12.4 lbs and 13.4 lbs in the patients treated with XENICAL and 6.2 lbs and 5.8 lbs in the placebo-treated patients, respectively. During the 4-week placebo lead-in period of the studies, an additional 5 to 6 lb weight loss was also observed in the same patients. Of the patients who completed 1 year of treatment, 57% of the patients treated with XENICAL (120 mg three times a day) and 31% of the placebo-treated patients lost at least 5% of their baseline body weight.
The percentages of patients achieving ≥5% and ≥10% weight loss after 1 year in five large multicenter studies for the intent-to-treat populations are presented in Table 1.
[See table 1 at top of next page]
The relative changes in risk factors associated with obesity following 1 year of therapy with XENICAL and placebo are presented for the population as a whole and for the population with abnormal values at randomization.
Population as a Whole
The changes in metabolic, cardiovascular and anthropometric risk factors associated with obesity based on pooled data for five clinical studies, regardless of the patient's risk factor status at randomization, are presented in Table 2. One year of therapy with XENICAL resulted in relative improvement in several risk factors.

Continued on next page

Table 1 Percentage of Patients Losing ≥5% and ≥10% of Body Weight From Randomization After 1-Year Treatment*

	Intent-to-Treat Population†									
	≥5% Weight Loss					≥10% Weight Loss				
Study No.	XENICAL	n	Placebo	n	p-value	XENICAL	n	Placebo	n	p-value
14119B	35.5%	110	21.3%	108	0.021	16.4%	110	6.5%	108	0.022
14119C	54.8%	343	27.4%	340	<0.001	24.8%	343	8.2%	340	<0.001
14149	50.6%	241	26.3%	236	<0.001	22.8%	241	11.9%	236	0.02
14161‡	37.1%	210	16.0%	212	<0.001	19.5%	210	3.8%	212	<0.001
14185	42.6%	657	22.4%	223	<0.001	17.7%	657	9.9%	223	0.006

The diet utilized during year 1 was a reduced-calorie diet.

* Treatment designates XENICAL 120 mg three times a day plus diet or placebo plus diet
† Last observation carried forward
‡ All studies, with the exception of 14161, were conducted at centers specialized in treating obesity and complications of obesity. Study 14161 was conducted with primary care physicians.

Table 3 Percentage of Patients Losing ≥5% and ≥10% of Body Weight From Randomization After 2-Year Treatment*

	Intent-to-Treat Population†									
	≥5% Weight Loss					≥10% Weight Loss				
Study No.	XENICAL	n	Placebo	n	p-value	XENICAL	n	Placebo	n	p-value
14119C	45.1%	133	23.6%	123	<0.001	24.8%	133	6.5%	123	<0.001
14149	43.3%	178	27.2%	158	0.002	18.0%	178	9.5%	158	0.025
14161‡	25.0%	148	15.0%	113	0.049	16.9%	148	3.5%	113	0.001
14185	34.0%	147	27.9%	122	0.279	17.7%	147	11.5%	122	0.154

The diet utilized during year 2 was designed for weight maintenance and not weight loss.

* Treatment designates XENICAL 120 mg three times a day plus diet or placebo plus diet
† Last observation carried forward
‡ All studies, with the exception of 14161 were conducted at centers specializing in treating obesity or complictions of obesity. Study 14161 was conducted with primary care physicians.

Xenical—Cont.

Table 2 Mean Change in Risk Factors From Randomization Following 1-Year Treatment* Population as a Whole

Risk Factor	XENICAL 120 mg†	Placebo†
Metabolic:		
Total Cholesterol	-2.0%	+5.0%
LDL-Cholesterol	-4.0%	+5.0%
HDL-Cholesterol	+9.3%	+12.8%
LDL/HDL	-0.37	-0.20
Triglycerides	+1.34%	+2.9%
Fasting Glucose, mmol/L	-0.04	+0.0
Fasting Insulin, pmol/L	-6.7	+5.2
Cardiovascular:		
Systolic Blood Pressure, mm Hg	-1.01	+0.58
Diastolic Blood Pressure, mm Hg	-1.19	+0.46
Anthropometric:		
Waist Circumference, cm	-6.45	-4.04
Hip Circumference, cm	-5.31	-2.96

* Treatment designates XENICAL 120 mg three times a day plus diet or placebo plus diet
† Intent-to-treat population at week 52, observed data based on pooled data from 5 studies

Population With Abnormal Risk Factors at Randomization
The changes from randomization following 1-year treatment in the population with abnormal lipid levels (LDL ≥ 130 mg/dL, LDL/HDL ≥ 3.5, HDL <35 mg/dL) were greater for XENICAL compared to placebo with respect to LDL-cholesterol (-7.83% vs +1.14%) and the LDL/HDL ratio (-0.64 vs -0.46). HDL increased in the placebo group by 20.1% and in the XENICAL group by 18.8%. In the population with abnormal blood pressure at baseline (systolic BP ≥ 140 mm Hg), the change in SBP from randomization to 1 year was greater for XENICAL (-10.89 mm Hg) than placebo (-5.07 mm Hg). For patients with a diastolic blood pressure ≥90 mm Hg, XENICAL patients decreased by -7.9 mm Hg while the placebo patients decreased by -5.5 mm Hg. Fasting insulin decreased more for XENICAL than placebo (-39 vs -16 pmol/L) from randomization to 1 year in the population with abnormal baseline values (≥120 pmol/L). A greater reduction in waist circumference for XENICAL vs placebo (-7.29 vs -4.53 cm) was observed in the population with abnormal baseline values (≥100 cm).

Effect on Weight Regain
Three studies were designed to evaluate the effects of XENICAL compared to placebo in reducing weight regain after a previous weight loss achieved following either diet alone (one study, 14302) or prior treatment with XENICAL (two studies, 14119C and 14185). The diet utilized during the 1- year weight regain portion of the studies was a weight-maintenance diet, rather than a weight-loss diet, and patients received less nutritional counseling than patients in weight-loss studies. For studies 14119C and 14185, patients' previous weight loss was due to 1 year of treatment with XENICAL in conjunction with a mildly hypocaloric diet. Study 14302 was conducted to evaluate the effects of 1 year of treatment with XENICAL on weight regain in patients who had lost 8% or more of their body weight in the previous 6 months on diet alone.
In study 14119C, patients treated with placebo regained 52% of the weight they had previously lost while the patients treated with XENICAL regained 26% of the weight they had previously lost (p<0.001). In study 14185, patients treated with placebo regained 63% of the weight they had previously lost while the patients treated with XENICAL regained 35% of the weight they had lost (p<0.001). In study 14302, patients treated with placebo regained 53% of the weight they had previously lost while the patients treated with XENICAL regained 32% of the weight that they had lost (p<0.001).

Two-year Results: Long-term Weight Control and Risk Factors
The treatment effects of XENICAL were examined for 2 years in four of the five 1-year weight management clinical studies previously discussed (see Table 1). At the end of year 1, the patients' diets were reviewed and changed where necessary. The diet prescribed in the second year was designed to maintain patient's current weight. XENICAL was shown to be more effective than placebo in long-term weight control in four large, multicenter, 2-year double-blind, placebo-controlled studies.
Pooled data from four clinical studies indicate that 40% of all patients treated with 120 mg three times a day of XENICAL and 24% of patients treated with placebo who completed 2 years of the same therapy had ≥5% loss of body weight from randomization. Pooled data from four clinical studies indicate that the relative weight loss advantage between XENICAL 120 mg three times a day and placebo treatment groups was the same after 2 years as for 1 year, indicating that the pharmacologic advantage of XENICAL was maintained over 2 years. In the same studies cited in the **One-year Results** (see Table 1), the percentages of patients achieving a ≥5% and ≥10% weight loss after 2 years are shown in Table 3.
[See table 3 at left]
The relative changes in risk factors associated with obesity following 2 years of therapy were also assessed in the population as a whole and the population with abnormal risk factors at randomization.

Population as a Whole
The relative differences in risk factors between treatment with XENICAL and placebo were similar to the results following 1 year of therapy for total cholesterol, LDL-cholesterol, LDL/HDL ratio, triglycerides, fasting glucose, fasting insulin, diastolic blood pressure, waist circumference, and hip circumference. The relative differences between treatment groups for HDL cholesterol and systolic blood pressure were less than that observed in the year one results.

Population With Abnormal Risk Factors at Randomization
The relative differences in risk factors between treatment with XENICAL and placebo were similar to the results following 1 year of therapy for LDL- and HDL-cholesterol, triglycerides, fasting insulin, diastolic blood pressure, and waist circumference. The relative differences between treatment groups for LDL/HDL ratio and isolated systolic blood pressure were less than that observed in the year one results.

Study of Patients With Type 2 Diabetes
A 1-year double-blind, placebo-controlled study in type 2 diabetics (N=321) stabilized on sulfonylureas was conducted. Thirty percent of patients treated with XENICAL achieved at least a 5% or greater reduction in body weight from randomization compared to 13% of the placebo-treated patients (p<0.001). Table 4 describes the changes over 1 year of treatment with XENICAL compared to placebo, in sulfonylurea usage and dose reduction as well as in hemoglobin HbA1c, fasting glucose, and insulin.

Table 4 Mean Changes in Body Weight and Glycemic Control From Randomization Following 1-Year Treatment in Patients With Type 2 Diabetes

	XENICAL 120 mg* (n=162)	Placebo* (n=159)	Statistical Significance
% patients who discontinued dose of oral sulfonylurea	11.7%	7.5%	†
% patients who decreased dose of oral sulfonylurea	31.5%	21.4%	
Average reduction in sulfonylurea medication dose	-22.8%	-9.1%	†
Body weight change (lbs)	-8.9	-4.2	†
HbA1c	-0.18%	+0.28%	†
Fasting glucose, mmol/L	-0.02	+0.54	†
Fasting insulin, pmol/L	-19.68	-18.02	ns

Statistical significance based on intent-to-treat population, last observation carried forward.
* Treatment designates XENICAL 120 mg three times a day plus diet or placebo plus diet
† Statistically significant (p ≤ 0.05) based on intent-to-treat, last observation carried forward
ns nonsignificant, p>0.05

In addition, XENICAL (n=162) compared to placebo (n=159) was associated with significant lowering for total cholesterol (-1.0% vs +9.0%, p≤0.05), LDL-cholesterol (-3.0% vs +10.0%, p≤0.05), LDL/HDL ratio (-0.26 vs -0.02, p≤0.05) and triglycerides (+2.54% vs +16.2%, p≤0.05), respectively. For HDL cholesterol, there was a +6.49% increase on XENICAL and +8.6% increase on placebo, p>0.05. Systolic blood pressure increased by +0.61 mm Hg on XENICAL and increased by +4.33 mm Hg on placebo, p>0.05. Diastolic blood pressure decreased by -0.47 mm Hg for XENICAL and by -0.5 mm Hg for placebo, p>0.05.

Glucose Tolerance in Obese Patients
Two-year studies that included oral glucose tolerance tests were conducted in obese patients not previously diagnosed or treated for type 2 diabetes and whose baseline oral glucose tolerance test (OGTT) status at randomization was either normal, impaired, or diabetic.
The progression from a normal OGTT at randomization to a diabetic or impaired OGTT following 2 years of treatment with XENICAL (n=251) or placebo (n=207) were compared. Following treatment with XENICAL, 0.0% and 7.2% of the patients progressed from normal to diabetic and normal to impaired, respectively, compared to 1.9% and 12.6% of the placebo treatment group, respectively.
In patients found to have an impaired OGTT at randomization, the percent of patients improving to normal or deteriorating to diabetic status following 1 and 2 years of treat-

ment with XENICAL compared to placebo are presented. After 1 year of treatment, 45.8% of the placebo patients and 73% of the XENICAL patients had a normal oral glucose tolerance test while 10.4% of the placebo patients and 2.6% of the XENICAL patients became diabetic. After 2 years of treatment, 50% of the placebo patients and 71.7% of the XENICAL patients had a normal oral glucose tolerance test while 7.5% of placebo patients were found to be diabetic and 1.7% of XENICAL patients were found to be diabetic after treatment.

Pediatric Clinical Studies

The effects of XENICAL on body mass index (BMI) and weight loss were assessed in a 54-week multicenter, double-blind, placebo-controlled study in 539 obese adolescents (357 receiving XENICAL 120 mg three times a day, 182 receiving placebo), aged 12 to 16 years. All study participants had a baseline BMI that was 2 units greater than the US weighted mean for the 95th percentile based on age and gender. Body mass index was the primary efficacy parameter because it takes into account changes in height and body weight, which occur in growing children.

During the study, all patients were instructed to take a multivitamin containing fat-soluble vitamins at least 2 hours before or after ingestion of XENICAL. Patients were also maintained on a well-balanced, reduced-calorie diet that was intended to provide 30% of calories from fat. In addition, all patients were placed on a behavior modification program and offered exercise counseling.

Approximately 65% of patients in each treatment group completed the study.

Following one year of treatment, BMI decreased by an average of 0.55 kg/m^2 in the XENICAL-treated patients and increased by an average of 0.31 kg/m^2 in the placebo-treated patients (p=0.001).

The percentages of patients achieving ≥5% and ≥10% reduction in BMI and body weight after 52 weeks of treatment for the intent-to-treat population are presented in Table 5.

[See table 5 at right]

Table 5 Percentages of Patients with ≥5% and ≥10% Decrease in Body Mass Index and Body Weight After 1-Year Treatment* (Protocol NM16189)

	Intent-to-Treat Population‡							
	≥5% Decrease				≥10% Decrease			
	XENICAL	n	Placebo	n	XENICAL	n	Placebo	n
BMI	26.5%	347	15.7%	178	13.3%	347	4.5%	178
Body Weight	19.0%	348	11.7%	180	9.5%	348	3.3%	180

* Treatment designates XENICAL 120 mg three times a day plus diet or placebo plus diet

‡ Last observation carried forward

INDICATIONS AND USAGE

XENICAL is indicated for obesity management including weight loss and weight maintenance when used in conjunction with a reduced-calorie diet. XENICAL is also indicated to reduce the risk for weight regain after prior weight loss. XENICAL is indicated for obese patients with an initial body mass index (BMI) ≥30 kg/m^2 or ≥27 kg/m^2 in the presence of other risk factors (eg, hypertension, diabetes, dyslipidemia).

Table 6 illustrates body mass index (BMI) according to a variety of weights and heights. The BMI is calculated by dividing weight in kilograms by height in meters squared. For example, a person who weighs 180 lbs and is 5′5″ would have a BMI of 30.

[See table 6 at right]

Table 6 Body Mass Index (BMI), kg/m^2*

WEIGHT (lb)

HEIGHT (ft/in)	120	130	140	150	160	170	180	190	200	210	220	230	240	250	260	270	280	290	300	310	320
4'10"	25	27	29	31	34	36	38	40	42	44	46	48	50	52	54	57	59	61	63	65	67
4'11"	24	26	28	30	32	34	36	38	40	43	45	47	49	51	53	55	57	59	61	63	65
5'0"	23	25	27	29	31	33	35	37	39	41	43	45	47	49	51	53	55	57	59	61	63
5'1"	23	25	27	28	30	32	34	36	38	40	42	44	45	47	49	51	53	55	57	59	61
5'2"	22	24	26	27	29	31	33	35	37	38	40	42	44	46	48	49	51	53	55	57	59
5'3"	21	23	25	27	28	30	32	34	36	37	39	41	43	44	46	48	50	51	53	55	57
5'4"	21	22	24	26	28	29	31	33	34	36	38	40	41	43	45	46	48	50	52	53	55
5'5"	20	22	23	25	27	28	30	32	33	35	37	38	40	42	43	45	47	48	50	52	53
5'6"	19	21	23	24	26	27	29	31	32	34	36	37	39	40	42	44	45	47	49	50	52
5'7"	19	20	22	24	25	27	28	30	31	33	35	36	38	39	41	42	44	46	47	49	50
5'8"	18	20	21	23	24	26	27	29	30	32	34	35	37	38	40	41	43	44	46	47	49
5'9"	18	19	21	22	24	25	27	28	30	31	33	34	36	37	38	40	41	43	44	46	47
5'10"	17	19	20	22	23	24	26	27	29	30	32	33	35	36	37	39	40	42	43	45	46
5'11"	17	18	20	21	22	24	25	27	28	29	31	32	34	35	36	38	39	41	42	43	45
6'0"	16	18	19	20	22	23	24	26	27	29	30	31	33	34	35	37	38	39	41	42	43
6'1"	16	17	19	20	21	22	24	25	26	28	29	30	32	33	34	36	37	38	40	41	42
6'2"	15	17	18	19	21	22	23	24	26	27	28	30	31	32	33	35	36	37	39	40	41

* Conversion Factors:

Weight in lbs ÷ 2.2 = weight in kilograms (kg)

Height in inches x 0.0254 = height in meters (m)

1 foot = 12 inches

CONTRAINDICATIONS

XENICAL is contraindicated in patients with chronic malabsorption syndrome or cholestasis, and in patients with known hypersensitivity to XENICAL or to any component of this product.

WARNINGS

Miscellaneous

Organic causes of obesity (eg, hypothyroidism) should be excluded before prescribing XENICAL.

Preliminary data from a XENICAL and cyclosporine drug interaction study indicate a reduction in cyclosporine plasma levels when XENICAL was coadministered with cyclosporine. Therefore, XENICAL and cyclosporine should not be coadministered. To reduce the chance of a drug-drug interaction, cyclosporine should be taken at least 2 hours before or after XENICAL in patients taking both drugs. In addition, in those patients whose cyclosporine levels are being measured, more frequent monitoring should be considered.

PRECAUTIONS

General

Patients should be advised to adhere to dietary guidelines (see DOSAGE AND ADMINISTRATION). Gastrointestinal events (see ADVERSE REACTIONS) may increase when XENICAL is taken with a diet high in fat (>30% total daily calories from fat). The daily intake of fat should be distributed over three main meals. If XENICAL is taken with any one meal very high in fat, the possibility of gastrointestinal effects increases.

Patients should be strongly encouraged to take a multivitamin supplement that contains fat-soluble vitamins to ensure adequate nutrition because XENICAL has been shown to reduce the absorption of some fat-soluble vitamins and beta-carotene (see DOSAGE AND ADMINISTRATION). In addition, the levels of vitamin D and beta-carotene may be low in obese patients compared with non-obese subjects. The supplement should be taken once a day at least 2 hours before or after the administration of XENICAL, such as at bedtime.

Table 7 illustrates the percentage of adult patients on XENICAL and placebo who developed a low vitamin level on two or more consecutive visits during 1 and 2 years of therapy in studies in which patients were not previously receiving vitamin supplementation.

Table 7 Incidence of Low Vitamin Values on Two or More Consecutive Visits (Nonsupplemented Adult Patients With Normal Baseline Values - First and Second Year)

	Placebo*	XENICAL*
Vitamin A	1.0%	2.2%
Vitamin D	6.6%	12.0%
Vitamin E	1.0%	5.8%
Beta-carotene	1.7%	6.1%

* Treatment designates placebo plus diet or XENICAL plus diet

Table 8 illustrates the percentage of adolescent patients on XENICAL and placebo who developed a low vitamin level on two or more consecutive visits during the 1-year study.

Table 8 Incidence of Low Vitamin Values on Two or More Consecutive Visits (Pediatric Patients With Normal Baseline Values*)

	Placebo**	XENICAL**
Vitamin A	0.0%	0.0%
Vitamin D	0.7%	1.4%
Vitamin E	0.0%	0.0%
Beta-carotene	0.8%	1.5%

*All patients were treated with vitamin supplementation throughout the course of the study

** Treatment designates placebo plus diet or XENICAL plus diet

Some patients may develop increased levels of urinary oxalate following treatment with XENICAL. Caution should be exercised when prescribing XENICAL to patients with a history of hyperoxaluria or calcium oxalate nephrolithiasis.

Weight-loss induction by XENICAL may be accompanied by improved metabolic control in diabetics, which might require a reduction in dose of oral hypoglycemic medication (eg, sulfonylureas, metformin) or insulin (see CLINICAL STUDIES).

Misuse Potential

As with any weight-loss agent, the potential exists for misuse of XENICAL in inappropriate patient populations (eg, patients with anorexia nervosa or bulimia). See INDICATIONS AND USAGE for recommended prescribing guidelines.

Information for Patients

Patients should read the Patient Information before starting treatment with XENICAL and each time their prescription is renewed.

Drug Interactions

Alcohol

In a multiple-dose study in 30 normal-weight subjects, coadministration of XENICAL and 40 grams of alcohol (eg, approximately 3 glasses of wine) did not result in alteration of alcohol pharmacokinetics, orlistat pharmacodynamics (fecal fat excretion), or systemic exposure to orlistat.

Cyclosporine

Preliminary data from a XENICAL and cyclosporine drug interaction study indicate a reduction in cyclosporine plasma levels when XENICAL was coadministered with cyclosporine (see WARNINGS).

Digoxin

In 12 normal-weight subjects receiving XENICAL 120 mg three times a day for 6 days, XENICAL did not alter the pharmacokinetics of a single dose of digoxin.

Fat-soluble Vitamin Supplements and Analogues

A pharmacokinetic interaction study showed a 30% reduction in beta-carotene supplement absorption when concomitantly administered with XENICAL. XENICAL inhibited absorption of a vitamin E acetate supplement by approximately 60%. The effect of orlistat on the absorption of supplemental vitamin D, vitamin A, and nutritionally-derived vitamin K is not known at this time.

Glyburide

In 12 normal-weight subjects receiving orlistat 80 mg three times a day for 5 days, orlistat did not alter the pharmacokinetics or pharmacodynamics (blood glucose-lowering) of glyburide.

Nifedipine (extended-release tablets)

In 17 normal-weight subjects receiving XENICAL 120 mg three times a day for 6 days, XENICAL did not alter the bioavailability of nifedipine (extended-release tablets).

Oral Contraceptives

In 20 normal-weight female subjects, the treatment of XENICAL 120 mg three times a day for 23 days resulted in no changes in the ovulation-suppressing action of oral contraceptives.

Phenytoin

In 12 normal-weight subjects receiving XENICAL 120 mg three times a day for 7 days, XENICAL did not alter the pharmacokinetics of a single 300-mg dose of phenytoin.

Pravastatin

In a 2-way crossover study of 24 normal-weight, mildly hypercholesterolemic patients receiving XENICAL 120 mg three times a day for 6 days, XENICAL did not affect the pharmacokinetics of pravastatin.

Warfarin

In 12 normal-weight subjects, administration of XENICAL 120 mg three times a day for 16 days did not result in any change in either warfarin pharmacokinetics (both R- and S-enantiomers) or pharmacodynamics (prothrombin time and serum Factor VII). Although undercarboxylated osteocalcin, a marker of vitamin K nutritional status, was unaltered with XENICAL administration, vitamin K levels tended to decline in subjects taking XENICAL. Therefore, as vitamin K absorption may be decreased with XENICAL, patients on chronic stable doses of warfarin who are prescribed XENICAL should be monitored closely for changes in coagulation parameters.

Carcinogenesis, Mutagenesis, Impairment of Fertility

Carcinogenicity studies in rats and mice did not show a carcinogenic potential for orlistat at doses up to 1000 mg/kg/day and 1500 mg/kg/day, respectively. For mice and rats,

Continued on next page

Xenical—Cont.

these doses are 38 and 46 times the daily human dose calculated on an area under concentration vs time curve basis of total drug-related material.

Orlistat had no detectable mutagenic or genotoxic activity as determined by the Ames test, a mammalian forward mutation assay (V79/HPRT), an in vitro clastogenesis assay in peripheral human lymphocytes, an unscheduled DNA synthesis assay (UDS) in rat hepatocytes in culture, and an in vivo mouse micronucleus test.

When given to rats at a dose of 400 mg/kg/day in a fertility and reproduction study, orlistat had no observable adverse effects. This dose is 12 times the daily human dose calculated on a body surface area (mg/m^2) basis.

Pregnancy

Teratogenic Effects: Pregnancy Category B.

Teratogenicity studies were conducted in rats and rabbits at doses up to 800 mg/kg/day. Neither study showed embryotoxicity or teratogenicity. This dose is 23 and 47 times the daily human dose calculated on a body surface area (mg/m^2) basis for rats and rabbits, respectively.

The incidence of dilated cerebral ventricles was increased in the mid- and high-dose groups of the rat teratology study. These doses were 6 and 23 times the daily human dose calculated on a body surface area (mg/m^2) basis for the mid- and high-dose levels, respectively. This finding was not reproduced in two additional rat teratology studies at similar doses.

There are no adequate and well-controlled studies of XENICAL in pregnant women. Because animal reproductive studies are not always predictive of human response, XENICAL is not recommended for use during pregnancy.

Nursing Mothers

It is not known if orlistat is secreted in human milk. Therefore, XENICAL should not be taken by nursing women.

Pediatric Use

The safety and efficacy of XENICAL have been evaluated in obese adolescent patients aged 12 to 16 years. Use of XENICAL in this age group is supported by evidence from adequate and well-controlled studies of XENICAL in adults with additional data from a 54-week efficacy and safety study and a 21-day mineral balance study in obese adolescent patients aged 12 to 16 years. Patients treated with XENICAL had a mean reduction in BMI of 0.55 kg/m^2 compared with an average increase of 0.31 kg/m^2 in placebo-treated patients (p=0.001). In both adolescent studies, adverse effects were generally similar to those described in adults and included fatty/oily stool, oily spotting, and oily evacuation. In a subgroup of 152 orlistat and 77 placebo patients from the 54-week study, changes in body composition measured by DEXA were similar in both treatment groups with the exception of fat mass, which was significantly reduced in patients treated with XENICAL compared to patients treated with placebo (-2.5 kg vs -0.6 kg, p=0.033). Because XENICAL can interfere with the absorption of fat-soluble vitamins, all patients should take a daily multivitamin that contains vitamins A, D, E, K, and beta-carotene. The supplement should be taken at least 2 hours before or after XENICAL (see CLINICAL PHARMACOLOGY: Other Short-term Studies; CLINICAL STUDIES: Pediatric Clinical Studies; ADVERSE REACTIONS: Pediatric Patients). XENICAL has not been studied in pediatric patients below the age of 12 years.

Geriatric Use

Clinical studies of XENICAL did not include sufficient numbers of patients aged 65 years and older to determine whether they respond differently from younger patients.

ADVERSE REACTIONS

Commonly Observed (based on first year and second year data - XENICAL 120 mg three times a day versus placebo): Gastrointestinal (GI) symptoms were the most commonly observed treatment-emergent adverse events associated with the use of XENICAL in double-blind, placebo-controlled clinical trials and are primarily a manifestation of the mechanism of action. (Commonly observed is defined as an incidence of ≥5% and an incidence in the XENICAL 120 mg group that is at least twice that of placebo.)

[See table 9 above]

Table 9 Commonly Observed Adverse Events

Adverse Event	Year 1 XENICAL* % Patients (N=1913)	Year 1 Placebo* % Patients (N=1466)	Year 2 XENICAL* % Patients (N=613)	Year 2 Placebo* % Patients (N=524)
Oily Spotting	26.6	1.3	4.4	0.2
Flatus with Discharge	23.9	1.4	2.1	0.2
Fecal Urgency	22.1	6.7	2.8	1.7
Fatty/Oily Stool	20.0	2.9	5.5	0.6
Oily Evacuation	11.9	0.8	2.3	0.2
Increased Defecation	10.8	4.1	2.6	0.8
Fecal Incontinence	7.7	0.9	1.8	0.2

* Treatment designates XENICAL three times a day plus diet or placebo plus diet

These and other commonly observed adverse reactions were generally mild and transient, and they decreased during the second year of treatment. In general, the first occurrence of these events was within 3 months of starting therapy. Overall, approximately 50% of all episodes of GI adverse events associated with orlistat treatment lasted for less than 1 week, and a majority lasted for no more than 4 weeks. However, GI adverse events may occur in some individuals over a period of 6 months or longer.

Discontinuation of Treatment

In controlled clinical trials, 8.8% of patients treated with XENICAL discontinued treatment due to adverse events, compared with 5.0% of placebo-treated patients. For XENICAL, the most common adverse events resulting in discontinuation of treatment were gastrointestinal.

Incidence in Controlled Clinical Trials

The following table lists other treatment-emergent adverse events from seven multicenter, double-blind, placebo-controlled clinical trials that occurred at a frequency of ≥2% among patients treated with XENICAL 120 mg three times a day and with an incidence that was greater than placebo during year 1 and year 2, regardless of relationship to study medication.

Table 10 Other Treatment-Emergent Adverse Events From Seven Placebo-Controlled Clinical Trials

Body System/Adverse Event	Year 1 XENICAL* % Patients (N=1913)	Year 1 Placebo* % Patients (N=1466)	Year 2 XENICAL* % Patients (N=613)	Year 2 Placebo* % Patients (N=524)
Gastrointestinal System				
Abdominal Pain/Discomfort	25.5	21.4	–	–
Nausea	8.1	7.3	3.6	2.7
Infectious Diarrhea	5.3	4.4	–	–
Rectal Pain/Discomfort	5.2	4.0	3.3	1.9
Tooth Disorder	4.3	3.1	2.9	2.3
Gingival Disorder	4.1	2.9	2.0	1.5
Vomiting	3.8	3.5	–	–
Respiratory System				
Influenza	39.7	36.2	–	–
Upper Respiratory Infection	38.1	32.8	26.1	25.8
Lower Respiratory Infection	7.8	6.6	–	–
Ear, Nose & Throat Symptoms	2.0	1.6	–	–
Musculoskeletal System				
Back Pain	13.9	12.1	–	–
Pain Lower Extremities	–	–	10.8	10.3
Arthritis	5.4	4.8	–	–
Myalgia	4.2	3.3	–	–
Joint Disorder	2.3	2.2	–	–
Tendonitis	–	–	2.0	1.9
Central Nervous System				
Headache	30.6	27.6	–	–
Dizziness	5.2	5.0	–	–
Body as a Whole				
Fatigue	7.2	6.4	3.1	1.7
Sleep Disorder	3.9	3.3	–	–
Skin & Appendages				
Rash	4.3	4.0	–	–
Dry Skin	2.1	1.4	–	–
Reproductive, Female				
Menstrual Irregularity	9.8	7.5	–	–
Vaginitis	3.8	3.6	2.6	1.9
Urinary System				
Urinary Tract Infection	7.5	7.3	5.9	4.8
Psychiatric Disorder				
Psychiatric Anxiety	4.7	2.9	2.8	2.1
Depression	–	–	3.4	2.5
Hearing & Vestibular Disorders				
Otitis	4.3	3.4	2.9	2.5
Cardiovascular Disorders				
Pedal Edema	–	–	2.8	1.9

* Treatment designates XENICAL 120 mg three times a day plus diet or placebo plus diet
– None reported at a frequency ≥2% and greater than placebo

[See table 10 above]

Other Clinical Studies or Postmarketing Surveillance

Rare cases of hypersensitivity have been reported with the use of XENICAL. Signs and symptoms have included pruritus, rash, urticaria, angioedema, and anaphylaxis.

Preliminary data from a XENICAL and cyclosporine drug interaction study indicate a reduction in cyclosporine plasma levels when XENICAL was coadministered with cyclosporine (see WARNINGS).

Pediatric Patients

In clinical trials with XENICAL in adolescent patients ages 12 to 16 years, the profile of adverse reactions was generally similar to that observed in adults.

OVERDOSAGE

Single doses of 800 mg XENICAL and multiple doses of up to 400 mg three times a day for 15 days have been studied in normal weight and obese subjects without significant adverse findings.

Should a significant overdose of XENICAL occur, it is recommended that the patient be observed for 24 hours. Based on human and animal studies, systemic effects attributable to the lipase-inhibiting properties of orlistat should be rapidly reversible.

DOSAGE AND ADMINISTRATION

The recommended dose of XENICAL is one 120-mg capsule three times a day with each main meal containing fat (during or up to 1 hour after the meal).

The patient should be on a nutritionally balanced, reduced-calorie diet that contains approximately 30% of calories from fat. The daily intake of fat, carbohydrate, and protein should be distributed over three main meals. If a meal is occasionally missed or contains no fat, the dose of XENICAL can be omitted.

Because XENICAL has been shown to reduce the absorption of some fat-soluble vitamins and beta-carotene, patients should be counseled to take a multivitamin containing fat-

soluble vitamins to ensure adequate nutrition (see PRECAUTIONS: General). The supplement should be taken at least 2 hours before or after the administration of XENICAL, such as at bedtime.
Doses above 120 mg three times a day have not been shown to provide additional benefit.
Based on fecal fat measurements, the effect of XENICAL is seen as soon as 24 to 48 hours after dosing. Upon discontinuation of therapy, fecal fat content usually returns to pretreatment levels within 48 to 72 hours.
The safety and effectiveness of XENICAL beyond 2 years have not been determined at this time.

HOW SUPPLIED

XENICAL is a dark-blue, hard-gelatin capsule containing pellets of powder.
XENICAL 120 mg Capsules: Dark-blue, two-piece, No. 1 opaque hard-gelatin capsule imprinted with Roche and XENICAL 120 in light-blue ink — bottle of 90 (NDC 0004-0256-52).

Storage Conditions

Store at 25°C (77°F); excursions permitted to 15° to 30°C (59° to 86°F) [see USP Controlled Room Temperature]. **Keep bottle tightly closed.**
XENICAL should not be used after the given expiration date.

Revised: December 2003

Shown in Product Identification Guide, page 332

ZENAPAX® ℞

[*zĕn-ă-păks*]
(daclizumab)
STERILE CONCENTRATE FOR INJECTION

> WARNING
> **Only physicians experienced in immunosuppressive therapy and management of organ transplant patients should prescribe ZENAPAX® (daclizumab). The physician responsible for ZENAPAX administration should have complete information requisite for the follow-up of the patient. ZENAPAX should only be administered by healthcare personnel trained in the administration of the drug who have available adequate laboratory and supportive medical resources.**

DESCRIPTION

ZENAPAX® (Daclizumab) is an immunosuppressive, humanized IgG1 monoclonal antibody produced by recombinant DNA technology that binds specifically to the alpha subunit (p55 alpha, CD25, or Tac subunit) of the human high-affinity interleukin-2 (IL-2) receptor that is expressed on the surface of activated lymphocytes.
Daclizumab is a composite of human (90%) and murine (10%) antibody sequences. The human sequences were derived from the constant domains of human IgG1 and the variable framework regions of the Eu myeloma antibody. The murine sequences were derived from the complementarity-determining regions of a murine anti-Tac antibody. The molecular weight predicted from the DNA sequence is 144 kilodaltons.
ZENAPAX 25 mg/5 mL is supplied as a clear, sterile, colorless concentrate for further dilution and intravenous administration. Each milliliter of ZENAPAX contains 5 mg of daclizumab and 3.6 mg sodium phosphate monobasic monohydrate, 11 mg sodium phosphate dibasic heptahydrate, 4.6 mg sodium chloride, 0.2 mg polysorbate 80, and may contain hydrochloric acid or sodium hydroxide to adjust the pH to 6.9. No preservatives are added.

CLINICAL PHARMACOLOGY

General

Mechanism of Action
Daclizumab functions as an IL-2 receptor antagonist that binds with high-affinity to the Tac subunit of the high-affinity IL-2 receptor complex and inhibits IL-2 binding. Daclizumab binding is highly specific for Tac, which is expressed on activated but not resting lymphocytes. Administration of ZENAPAX inhibits IL-2-mediated activation of lymphocytes, a critical pathway in the cellular immune response involved in allograft rejection.
While in the circulation, ZENAPAX impairs the response of the immune system to antigenic challenges. Whether the ability to respond to repeated or ongoing challenges with those antigens returns to normal after ZENAPAX is cleared is unknown (see **PRECAUTIONS**).

Pharmacokinetics

Adults
In clinical trials involving renal allograft patients treated with a 1 mg/kg IV dose of ZENAPAX every 14 days for a total of five doses, peak serum concentration (mean ± SD) rose between the first dose (21 ± 14 µg/mL) and fifth dose (32 ± 22 µg/mL). The mean trough serum concentration before the fifth dose was 7.6 ± 4.0 µg/mL. Population pharmacokinetic analysis of the data using a two-compartment open model gave the following values for a reference patient (45-year-old male Caucasian patient with a body weight of 80 kg and no proteinuria): systemic clearance = 15 mL/hour, volume of central compartment = 2.5 liter, volume of peripheral compartment = 3.4 liter. The estimated terminal elimination half-life for the reference patient was 20 days (480 hours), which is similar to the terminal elimination half-life for human IgG (18 to 23 days). Bayesian estimates of terminal elimination half-life ranged from 11 to 38 days for the 123 patients included in the population analysis. The influence of body weight on systemic clearance supports the dosing of ZENAPAX on a milligram per kilogram (mg/kg) basis. For patients studied, this dosing maintained drug exposure within 30% of the reference exposure. Covariate analyses showed that no dosage adjustments based on age, race, gender or degree of proteinuria, are required for renal allograft patients. The estimated interpatient variability (percent coefficient of variation) in systemic clearance and central volume of distribution were 15% and 27%, respectively.
Pediatrics
Pharmacokinetic parameters were evaluated in 61 pediatric patients treated with a 1 mg/kg IV dose of ZENAPAX every 14 days for a total of five doses. Peak serum concentration (mean ± SD) rose between the first dose (16 ± 12 µg/mL) and fifth dose (21 ± 14 µg/mL). The mean trough serum concentration before the fifth dose was 5.0 ± 2.7 µg/mL. Population pharmacokinetic analysis of the data using a two-compartment open model gave the following values for a reference patient (Caucasian patient with a body weight of 29.7 kg): systemic clearance = 10 mL/hour, volume of central compartment = 2.0 liter, volume of peripheral compartment = 1.4 liter. The estimated terminal elimination half-life for the reference patient was 13 days (317 hours). For the patients studied, this dosing maintained drug exposure within 50% of the reference exposure. Covariate analyses suggested that disposition parameters were not influenced to a clinically relevant extent by race, gender or degree of proteinuria. The estimated interpatient variability (percent coefficient of variation) in systemic clearance and central volume of distribution were 30% and 40%, respectively.

Pharmacodynamics

In vitro and in vivo data suggest that serum levels of 5 to 10 µg/mL are necessary for saturation of the Tac subunit of the IL-2 receptors to block the responses of activated T lymphocytes. At the recommended dosage regimen, daclizumab saturates the Tac subunit of the IL-2 receptor for approximately 90 and 120 days posttransplant, respectively in pediatric and adult patients. The duration of clinically significant IL-2 receptor blockade after the recommended course of ZENAPAX is not known. No significant changes to circulating lymphocyte numbers or cell phenotypes were observed by flow cytometry. Cytokine release syndrome has not been observed after ZENAPAX administration.

CLINICAL STUDIES

The safety and efficacy of ZENAPAX for the prophylaxis of acute organ rejection in adult patients receiving their first cadaveric kidney transplant were assessed in two randomized, double-blind, placebo-controlled, multicenter trials. These trials compared a dose of 1.0 mg/kg of ZENAPAX with placebo when each was administered as part of standard immunosuppressive regimens containing either cyclosporine and corticosteroids (double-therapy trial, no US sites) or cyclosporine, corticosteroids, and azathioprine (triple-therapy trial, predominantly US sites) to prevent acute renal allograft rejection. ZENAPAX dosing was initiated within 24 hours pretransplant, with subsequent doses given every 14 days for a total of five doses.
The primary efficacy endpoint of both trials was the proportion of patients who developed a biopsy-proven acute rejection episode within the first 6 months following transplantation. As shown in Table 1, this incidence was significantly lower in the group treated with ZENAPAX in both the double-therapy and triple-therapy trials.

Table 1. Efficacy Parameters

	Triple-therapy Regimen (cyclosporine, corticosteroids, and azathioprine)			Double-therapy Regimen (cyclosporine and corticosteroids)		
	Placebo (N=134)	ZENAPAX (N=126)	p-value	Placebo (N=134)	ZENAPAX (N=141)	p-value
Incidence of biopsy-proven acute rejection at 6 months						
No. of patients	47 (35%)	28 (22%)	0.03	63 (47%)	39 (28%)	0.001
Incidence of biopsy-proven acute rejection at 1 year						
No. of patients	51 (38%)	35 (28%)	n.s.	65 (49%)	39 (28%)	<0.001
Graft survival at 3 years posttransplant						
No. of patients with functioning graft	111 (83%)	106 (84%)	n.s.	105 (78%)	116 (82%)	n.s.
Patient survival at 3 years posttransplant						
No. of patients	126 (94%)	116 (92%)	n.s.	118 (88%)	135 (96%)	0.02

n.s. = not significant

[See table 1 above]
Treatment with ZENAPAX was associated with better patient survival up to 3 years posttransplant in the double-therapy study. No difference in patient survival was observed in the triple-therapy study between patients treated with ZENAPAX or placebo up to 3 years posttransplant. No difference was observed for graft survival between treatment groups in both studies at 3 years posttransplant.
The incidence of delayed graft function was not different between patients treated with placebo or ZENAPAX in either study. No difference in graft function was observed 1 year and 3 years posttransplant in either study between patients treated with placebo or ZENAPAX.
In a randomized, double-blind study to assess tolerability, pharmacokinetics, and drug interactions in renal allograft recipients, ZENAPAX (50 patients) or placebo (25 patients) was added to an immunosuppressive regimen of cyclosporine, mycophenolate mofetil, and corticosteroids. In this study, the addition of ZENAPAX did not result in an increased incidence of adverse events or a change in the types of adverse events reported. The incidence of the combined endpoint of biopsy-proven or clinically presumptive acute rejection was 20% (5 of 25 patients) in the placebo group and 12% (6 of 50 patients) in the ZENAPAX group. Although numerically lower, the difference in acute rejection was not significant. However, in a randomized, double-blind, placebo-controlled trial of ZENAPAX in cardiac transplant recipients (n=434) receiving concomitant cyclosporine, mycophenolate mofetil, and corticosteroids, mortality was increased in patients randomized to receive ZENAPAX compared with those randomized to receive placebo (see **WARNINGS** and **ADVERSE REACTIONS**).

INDICATION AND USAGE

ZENAPAX is indicated for the prophylaxis of acute organ rejection in patients receiving renal transplants. It is used as part of an immunosuppressive regimen that includes cyclosporine and corticosteroids.
The efficacy of ZENAPAX for the prophylaxis of acute rejection in recipients of other solid organ allografts has not been demonstrated.

CONTRAINDICATION

ZENAPAX is contraindicated in patients with known hypersensitivity to daclizumab or to any components of this product.

WARNINGS: See Boxed WARNING.

The use of ZENAPAX as part of an immunosuppressive regimen including cyclosporine, mycophenolate mofetil, and corticosteroids may be associated with an increase in mortality. In a randomized, double-blind, placebo-controlled trial of ZENAPAX for the prevention of allograft rejection in 434 cardiac transplant recipients receiving concomitant cyclosporine, mycophenolate mofetil, and corticosteroids, mortality at 6 and 12 months was increased in those patients receiving ZENAPAX compared to those receiving placebo (7% vs 5%, respectively at 6 months; 10% vs 6% respectively at 12 months). Some, but not all, of the increase in mortality appeared related to a higher incidence of severe infections. Concomitant use of anti-lymphocyte antibody therapy may also be a factor in some of the fatal infections.
ZENAPAX should be administered under qualified medical supervision. Patients should be informed of the potential benefits of therapy and the risks associated with administration of immunosuppressive therapy.
While the incidence of lymphoproliferative disorders and opportunistic infections in the limited clinical trial experience was no higher in patients treated with ZENAPAX compared with placebo-treated patients, patients on immunosuppressive therapy are at increased risk for developing lymphoproliferative disorders and opportunistic infections and should be monitored accordingly.

Hypersensitivity

Severe, acute (onset within 24 hours) hypersensitivity reactions including anaphylaxis have been observed both on initial exposure to ZENAPAX and following re-exposure. These reactions may include hypotension, bronchospasm, wheezing, laryngeal edema, pulmonary edema, cyanosis, hypoxia, respiratory arrest, cardiac arrhythmia, cardiac arrest, peripheral edema, loss of consciousness, fever, rash, urticaria, diaphoresis, pruritus, and/or injection site reactions. If a severe hypersensitivity reaction occurs, therapy with ZENAPAX should be permanently discontinued. Medications for the treatment of severe hypersensitivity reactions including anaphylaxis should be available for immediate use. Patients previously administered ZENAPAX should only be re-exposed to a subsequent course of therapy with caution. The potential risks of such re-administration, specifically those associated with immunosuppression, are not known.

PRECAUTIONS

General

It is not known whether ZENAPAX use will have a long-term effect on the ability of the immune system to respond to antigens first encountered during ZENAPAX-induced immunosuppression.
Re-administration of ZENAPAX after an initial course of therapy has not been studied in humans. The potential

Continued on next page

Zenapax—Cont.

risks of such re-administration, specifically those associated with immunosuppression and/or the occurrence of anaphylaxis/anaphylactoid reactions, are not known.

Drug Interactions

The following medications have been administered with ZENAPAX in clinical trials in renal allograft patients with no incremental increase in adverse reactions: cyclosporine, mycophenolate mofetil, ganciclovir, acyclovir, azathioprine, and corticosteroids. Very limited experience exists in these patients with the use of ZENAPAX concomitantly with tacrolimus, muromonab-CD3, antithymocyte globulin, and anti-lymphocyte globulin.

In renal allograft recipients (n=50) treated with ZENAPAX and mycophenolate mofetil, no pharmacokinetic interaction between ZENAPAX and mycophenolic acid, the active metabolite of mycophenolate mofetil, was observed.

However, in a large clinical study in cardiac transplant recipients (n=434), the use of ZENAPAX as part of an immunosuppression regimen including cyclosporine, mycophenolate mofetil, and corticosteroids was associated with an increase in mortality, particularly in patients receiving concomitant anti-lymphocyte antibody therapy and in patients who developed severe infections (see **WARNINGS** and **ADVERSE REACTIONS**: **Incidence of Infectious Episodes**).

Carcinogenesis, Mutagenesis and Impairment of Fertility

Long-term studies to evaluate the carcinogenic potential of ZENAPAX have not been performed. ZENAPAX was not genotoxic in the Ames or the V79 chromosomal aberration assays, with or without metabolic activation. The effect of ZENAPAX on fertility is not known, because animal reproduction studies have not been conducted with ZENAPAX (see **WARNINGS** and **ADVERSE REACTIONS**).

Pregnancy

Pregnancy Category C: Animal reproduction studies have not been conducted with ZENAPAX. Therefore, it is not known whether ZENAPAX can cause fetal harm when administered to pregnant women or can affect reproductive capacity. In general, IgG molecules are known to cross the placental barrier. ZENAPAX should not be used in pregnant women unless the potential benefit justifies the potential risk to the fetus. Women of childbearing potential should use effective contraception before beginning ZENAPAX therapy, during therapy, and for 4 months after completion of ZENAPAX therapy.

Nursing Mothers

It is not known whether ZENAPAX is excreted in human milk. Because many drugs are excreted in human milk, including human antibodies, and because of the potential for adverse reactions, a decision should be made to discontinue nursing or to discontinue the drug, taking into account the importance of the drug to the mother.

Pediatric Use

The safety and effectiveness of ZENAPAX have been established in pediatric patients from 11 months to 17 years of age. Use of ZENAPAX in this age group is supported by evidence from adequate and well-controlled studies of ZENAPAX in adults with additional pediatric pharmacokinetic data (see **CLINICAL PHARMACOLOGY**). Data from the pediatric pharmacokinetic study were also analyzed for efficacy, immunogenicity and safety. In an open-label study, 60 pediatric renal transplant recipients [median age of 10 years] received standard immunosuppressive agents in addition to a regimen of ZENAPAX administered at a dose of 1.0 mg/kg at intervals of 14 days for a total of 5 doses, starting immediately before transplantation. In this study, the combined incidence of biopsy-proven and clinically presumptive acute rejection at 1 year posttransplant was 17% (10/60). Patient and graft survival at 1 year posttransplant were 100% and 96.7%, respectively. The incidence of anti-daclizumab antibodies (34%) observed in the first 3 months posttransplant was higher than the incidence previously observed in adult patients (14%) (see **ADVERSE REACTIONS**: **Immunogenicity**).

The safety profile of ZENAPAX in pediatric transplant patients was shown to be comparable with that in adult transplant patients with the exception of the following adverse events, which occurred more frequently in pediatric patients (>15% difference in incidence): diarrhea, post-operative pain, fever, vomiting, aggravated hypertension, pruritus, and infections of the upper respiratory tract and urinary tract.

It is not known whether the immune response to vaccines, infection, and other antigenic stimuli administered or encountered during ZENAPAX therapy is impaired or whether such response will remain impaired after ZENAPAX therapy.

Also see **CLINICAL PHARMACOLOGY** and **DOSAGE AND ADMINISTRATION**.

Geriatric Use

Clinical studies of ZENAPAX did not include sufficient numbers of subjects age 65 and older to determine whether they respond differently from younger subjects. Caution must be used in giving immunosuppressive drugs to elderly patients.

ADVERSE REACTIONS

Because clinical trials are conducted under widely varying conditions, adverse reactions rates observed in the clinical trials of a drug cannot be directly compared to rates in the clinical trials of another drug. Rates observed in clinical studies may not reflect those observed in clinical practice. Adverse reaction information obtained in clinical trials does, however, provide a basis for identifying adverse events that appear to be related to drug use and for approximating the rate of occurrence.

The safety of ZENAPAX was determined in four clinical studies of renal allograft rejection, three of which were randomized controlled clinical trials, in 629 patients receiving renal allografts of whom 336 received ZENAPAX and 293 received placebo. All patients received concomitant cyclosporine and corticosteroids. In these clinical trials, ZENAPAX did not appear to alter the pattern, frequency or severity of known major toxicities associated with the use of immunosuppressive drugs.

The use of ZENAPAX was associated with a higher incidence of mortality when compared to placebo in a large (n=434) randomized controlled study of patients receiving cardiac transplants (see **WARNINGS** and **Incidence of Infectious Episodes**).

Adverse events were reported by 95% of the patients in the placebo-treated group and 96% of the patients in the group treated with ZENAPAX. The proportion of patients prematurely withdrawn from the combined studies because of adverse events was 8.5% in the placebo-treated group and 8.6% in the group treated with ZENAPAX.

ZENAPAX did not increase the number of serious adverse events observed compared with placebo. The most frequently reported adverse events were gastrointestinal disorders, which were reported with equal frequency in ZENAPAX- (67%) and placebo-treated (68%) patient groups.

The incidence and types of adverse events were similar in both placebo-treated patients and patients treated with ZENAPAX. The following adverse events occurred in ≥5% of patients treated with ZENAPAX. These events included: *Gastrointestinal System:* constipation, nausea, diarrhea, vomiting, abdominal pain, pyrosis, dyspepsia, abdominal distention, epigastric pain not food-related; *Metabolic and Nutritional:* edema extremities, edema; *Central and Peripheral Nervous System:* tremor, headache, dizziness; *Urinary System:* oliguria, dysuria, renal tubular necrosis; *Body as a Whole—General:* posttraumatic pain, chest pain, fever, pain, fatigue; *Autonomic Nervous System:* hypertension, hypotension, aggravated hypertension; *Respiratory System:* dyspnea, pulmonary edema, coughing; *Skin and Appendages:* impaired wound healing without infection, acne; *Psychiatric:* insomnia; *Musculoskeletal System:* musculoskeletal pain, back pain; *Heart Rate and Rhythm:* tachycardia; *Vascular Extracardiac:* thrombosis; *Platelet, Bleeding and Clotting Disorders:* bleeding; *Hemic and Lymphatic:* lymphocele.

The following adverse events occurred in <5% and ≥2% of patients treated with ZENAPAX. These included: *Gastrointestinal System:* flatulence, gastritis, hemorrhoids; *Metabolic and Nutritional:* fluid overload, diabetes mellitus, dehydration; *Urinary System:* renal damage, hydronephrosis, urinary tract bleeding, urinary tract disorder, renal insufficiency; *Body as a Whole—General:* shivering, generalized weakness; *Central and Peripheral Nervous System:* urinary retention, leg cramps, prickly sensation; *Respiratory System:* atelectasis, congestion, pharyngitis, rhinitis, hypoxia, rales, abnormal breath sounds, pleural effusion; *Skin and Appendages:* pruritus, hirsutism, rash, night sweats, increased sweating; *Psychiatric:* depression, anxiety; *Musculoskeletal System:* arthralgia, myalgia; *Vision:* vision blurred; *Application Site:* application site reaction.

Incidence of Malignancies

One and 3 years posttransplant, the incidence of malignancies was 2.7% and 7.8%, respectively, in the placebo group compared with 1.5% and 6.4%, respectively, in the ZENAPAX group. Addition of ZENAPAX did not increase the number of posttransplant lymphomas up to 3 years posttransplant. Lymphomas occurred at a frequency of ≤1.5% in both placebo-treated and ZENAPAX-treated groups.

Hyperglycemia

No differences in abnormal hematologic or chemical laboratory test results were seen between groups treated with placebo or ZENAPAX with the exception of fasting blood glucose. Fasting blood glucose was measured in a small number of patients treated with placebo or ZENAPAX. A total of 16% (10 of 64 patients) of placebo-treated and 32% (28 of 88 patients) of patients treated with ZENAPAX had high fasting blood glucose values. Most of these high values occurred either on the first day posttransplant when patients received high doses of corticosteroids or in patients with diabetes.

Incidence of Infectious Episodes

The overall incidence of infectious episodes, including viral infections, fungal infections, bacteremia and septicemia, and pneumonia, was not higher in patients treated with ZENAPAX than in placebo-treated patients in trials of renal transplantation. In a large randomized study of ZENAPAX used for the prevention of allograft rejection in patients receiving cardiac allografts, more patients receiving ZENAPAX experienced severe or fatal infections after 12 months of therapy when compared to those receiving placebo (10% vs 7%, respectively). The risks of infection or death may be increased in patients receiving concomitant anti-lymphocyte antibody therapy (see **WARNINGS**).

The types of infections reported in trials of renal transplantation were similar in both the ZENAPAX-treated and the placebo-treated groups. Cytomegalovirus infection was reported in 16% of the patients in the placebo group and 13% of the patients in the ZENAPAX group. One exception was cellulitis and wound infections, which occurred in 4.1% of placebo-treated patients and 8.4% of patients treated with ZENAPAX. At 1 year posttransplant, 7 placebo patients and 1 patient treated with ZENAPAX had died of an infection. At 3 years posttransplant, 8 placebo patients and 4 patients treated with ZENAPAX had died of infection.

Immunogenicity

Low titers of anti-idiotype antibodies to daclizumab were detected in the adult patients treated with ZENAPAX with an overall incidence of 14%. The incidence of anti-daclizumab antibodies observed in the pediatric patients was 34%. No antibodies that affected efficacy, safety, serum levels or any other clinically relevant parameter examined were detected. The data reflect the percentage of patients whose test results were considered positive for antibodies to daclizumab in an ELISA assay and are highly dependent on the sensitivity and specificity of the assay. Additionally, the observed incidence of antibody positivity in the assay may be influenced by several factors including sample handling, timing of sample collection, concomitant medications and underlying disease. For these reasons, comparison of the incidence of antibodies to daclizumab with the incidence of antibodies to other products may be misleading.

Post-Marketing Experience

The following adverse reactions have been identified and reported during post-approval use of ZENAPAX (daclizumab). Because the reports of these reactions are voluntary and the population is of uncertain size, it is not always possible to reliably estimate the frequency of the reaction or establish a causal relationship to drug exposure.

Severe acute hypersensitivity reactions including anaphylaxis characterized by hypotension, bronchospasm, wheezing, laryngeal edema, pulmonary edema, cyanosis, hypoxia, respiratory arrest, cardiac arrhythmia, cardiac arrest, peripheral edema, loss of consciousness, fever, rash, urticaria, diaphoresis, pruritus, and/or injection site reactions, as well as cytokine release syndrome, have been reported during post-marketing experience with ZENAPAX. The relationship between these reactions and the development of antibodies to ZENAPAX is unknown.

OVERDOSAGE

There have not been any reports of overdoses with ZENAPAX. A maximum tolerated dose has not been determined in patients. A dose of 1.5 mg/kg has been administered to bone marrow transplant recipients without any associated adverse events.

DOSAGE AND ADMINISTRATION

ZENAPAX is used as part of an immunosuppressive regimen that includes cyclosporine and corticosteroids. The recommended dose for ZENAPAX in adult and pediatric patients is 1.0 mg/kg (see **PRECAUTIONS**: **Pediatric Use**). The calculated volume of ZENAPAX should be mixed with 50 mL of sterile 0.9% sodium chloride solution and administered via a peripheral or central vein over a 15-minute period.

Based on the clinical trials, the standard course of ZENAPAX therapy is five doses. The first dose should be given no more than 24 hours before transplantation. The four remaining doses should be given at intervals of 14 days.

No dosage adjustment is necessary for patients with severe renal impairment. No dosage adjustments based on other identified covariates (age, gender, proteinuria, race) are required for renal allograft patients. No data are available for administration in patients with severe hepatic impairment.

Instructions for Administration:

- ZENAPAX IS NOT FOR DIRECT INJECTION. The calculated volume should be diluted in 50 mL of sterile 0.9% sodium chloride solution before intravenous administration to patients. When mixing the solution, gently invert the bag in order to avoid foaming; DO NOT SHAKE.
- Parenteral drug products should be inspected visually for particulate matter and discoloration before administration. If particulate matter is present or the solution colored, do not use.
- Care must be taken to assure sterility of the prepared solution, since the drug product does not contain any antimicrobial preservative or bacteriostatic agents.
- ZENAPAX is a colorless solution provided as a single-use vial; any unused portion of the drug should be discarded.
- Once the infusion is prepared, it should be administered intravenously within 4 hours. If it must be held longer, it should be refrigerated between 2° to 8°C (36° to 46°F) for up to 24 hours. After 24 hours, the prepared solution should be discarded.
- No incompatibility between ZENAPAX and polyvinyl chloride or polyethylene bags or infusion sets has been observed. No data are available concerning the incompatibility of ZENAPAX with other drug substances. Other drug substances should not be added or infused simultaneously through the same intravenous line.
- ZENAPAX should only be administered by healthcare personnel trained in the administration of the drug who have available adequate laboratory and supportive medical resources.

HOW SUPPLIED

ZENAPAX is supplied in single-use glass vials. Each vial contains 25 mg of daclizumab in 5 mL of solution (NDC 0004-0501-09). Vials should be stored between the temperatures of 2° to 8°C (36° to 46°F); do not shake or freeze. Protect undiluted solution against direct light. Diluted medication is stable for 24 hours at 4°C or for 4 hours at room temperature.

US Govt. Lic. No. 0136

Revised: July 2003

EDUCATIONAL MATERIAL

Please contact your Roche representative concerning availability of educational programs and material.

Roche Pharmaceuticals

Roche Products Inc.
Manati, Puerto Rico 00674

For Medical Information Contact:
Roche Laboratories Inc
(800) 526-6367
Order Fulfillment:
Roche Laboratories Inc
(800) 526-0625

VALIUM® ©ꝶ

[val 'ee-um]
brand of diazepam
TABLETS

The following text is complete prescribing information based on official labeling in effect June 2001.

DESCRIPTION

Valium (diazepam) is a benzodiazepine derivative. The chemical name of diazepam is 7-chloro-1,3-dihydro-1-methyl -5- phenyl-2H-1,4-benzodiazepin-2-one. It is a colorless crystalline compound, insoluble in water. The empirical formula is $C_{16}H_{13}ClN_2O$ and the molecular weight is 284.75. Valium is available for oral administration as tablets containing 2 mg, 5 mg or 10 mg diazepam. In addition to the active ingredient diazepam, each tablet contains the following inactive ingredients: anhydrous lactose, corn starch, pregelatinized starch and calcium stearate with the following dyes: 5-mg tablets contain FD&C Yellow No. 6 and D&C Yellow No. 10; 10-mg tablets contain FD&C Blue No. 1. Valium 2-mg tablets contain no dye.

PHARMACOLOGY

In animals, Valium appears to act on parts of the limbic system, the thalamus and hypothalamus, and induces calming effects. Valium, unlike chlorpromazine and reserpine, has no demonstrable peripheral autonomic blocking action, nor does it produce extrapyramidal side effects; however, animals treated with Valium do have a transient ataxia at higher doses. Valium was found to have transient cardiovascular depressor effects in dogs. Long-term experiments in rats revealed no disturbances of endocrine function.

Oral LD_{50} of diazepam is 720 mg/kg in mice and 1240 mg/kg in rats. Intraperitoneal administration of 400 mg/kg to a monkey resulted in death on the sixth day.

Reproduction Studies: A series of rat reproduction studies was performed with diazepam in oral doses of 1, 10, 80 and 100 mg/kg. At 100 mg/kg there was a decrease in the number of pregnancies and surviving offspring in these rats. Neonatal survival of rats at doses lower than 100 mg/kg was within normal limits. Several neonates in these rat reproduction studies showed skeletal or other defects. Further studies in rats at doses up to and including 80 mg/kg/day did not reveal teratological effects on the offspring.

In humans, measurable blood levels of Valium were obtained in maternal and cord blood, indicating placental transfer of the drug.

INDICATIONS

Valium is indicated for the management of anxiety disorders or for the short-term relief of the symptoms of anxiety. Anxiety or tension associated with the stress of everyday life usually does not require treatment with an anxiolytic.

In acute alcohol withdrawal, Valium may be useful in the symptomatic relief of acute agitation, tremor, impending or acute delirium tremens and hallucinosis.

Valium is a useful adjunct for the relief of skeletal muscle spasm due to reflex spasm to local pathology (such as inflammation of the muscles or joints, or secondary to trauma); spasticity caused by upper motor neuron disorders (such as cerebral palsy and paraplegia); athetosis; and stiff-man syndrome.

Oral Valium may be used adjunctively in convulsive disorders, although it has not proved useful as the sole therapy.

The effectiveness of Valium in long-term use, that is, more than 4 months, has not been assessed by systematic clinical studies. The physician should periodically reassess the usefulness of the drug for the individual patient.

CONTRAINDICATIONS

Valium is contraindicated in patients with a known hypersensitivity to this drug and, because of lack of sufficient clinical experience, in pediatric patients under 6 months of age. It may be used in patients with open angle glaucoma who are receiving appropriate therapy, but is contraindicated in acute narrow angle glaucoma.

WARNINGS

Valium is not of value in the treatment of psychotic patients and should not be employed in lieu of appropriate treatment. As is true of most preparations containing CNS-acting drugs, patients receiving Valium should be cautioned against engaging in hazardous occupations requiring complete mental alertness such as operating machinery or driving a motor vehicle.

As with other agents which have anticonvulsant activity, when Valium is used as an adjunct in treating convulsive disorders, the possibility of an increase in the frequency and/or severity of grand mal seizures may require an increase in the dosage of standard anticonvulsant medication. Abrupt withdrawal of Valium in such cases may also be associated with a temporary increase in the frequency and/or severity of seizures.

Since Valium has a central nervous system depressant effect, patients should be advised against the simultaneous ingestion of alcohol and other CNS-depressant drugs during Valium therapy.

Usage in Pregnancy: **An increased risk of congenital malformations associated with the use of minor tranquilizers (diazepam, meprobamate and chlordiazepoxide) during the first trimester of pregnancy has been suggested in several studies. Because use of these drugs is rarely a matter of urgency, their use during this period should almost always be avoided. The possibility that a woman of childbearing potential may be pregnant at the time of institution of therapy should be considered. Patients should be advised that if they become pregnant during therapy or intend to become pregnant they should communicate with their physicians about the desirability of discontinuing the drug.**

Management of Overdosage: Manifestations of Valium overdosage include somnolence, confusion, coma and diminished reflexes. Respiration, pulse and blood pressure should be monitored, as in all cases of drug overdosage, although, in general, these effects have been minimal following overdosage. General supportive measures should be employed, along with immediate gastric lavage. Intravenous fluids should be administered and an adequate airway maintained. Hypotension may be combated by the use of Levophed® (levarterenol) or Aramine (metaraminol). Dialysis is of limited value. As with the management of intentional overdosage with any drug, it should be borne in mind that multiple agents may have been ingested.

Flumazenil, a specific benzodiazepine-receptor antagonist, is indicated for the complete or partial reversal of the sedative effects of benzodiazepines and may be used in situations when an overdose with a benzodiazepine is known or suspected. Prior to the administration of flumazenil, necessary measures should be instituted to secure airway, ventilation, and intravenous access. Flumazenil is intended as an adjunct to, not as a substitute for, proper management of benzodiazepine overdose. Patients treated with flumazenil should be monitored for resedation, respiratory depression and other residual benzodiazepine effects for an appropriate period after treatment. **The prescriber should be aware of a risk of seizure in association with flumazenil treatment, particularly in long-term benzodiazepine users and in cyclic antidepressant overdose.** The complete flumazenil package insert, including CONTRAINDICATIONS, WARNINGS and PRECAUTIONS, should be consulted prior to use.

Withdrawal symptoms of the barbiturate type have occurred after the discontinuation of benzodiazepines. (See DRUG ABUSE AND DEPENDENCE section.)

PRECAUTIONS

If Valium is to be combined with other psychotropic agents or anticonvulsant drugs, careful consideration should be given to the pharmacology of the agents to be employed—particularly with known compounds which may potentiate the action of Valium, such as phenothiazines, narcotics, barbiturates, MAO inhibitors and other antidepressants. The usual precautions are indicated for severely depressed patients or those in whom there is any evidence of latent depression; particularly the recognition that suicidal tendencies may be present and protective measures may be necessary. The usual precautions in treating patients with impaired renal or hepatic function should be observed.

In elderly and debilitated patients, it is recommended that the dosage be limited to the smallest effective amount to preclude the development of ataxia or oversedation (2 mg to $2^1/_2$ mg once or twice daily, initially, to be increased gradually as needed and tolerated).

The clearance of Valium and certain other benzodiazepines can be delayed in association with Tagamet (cimetidine) administration. The clinical significance of this is unclear.

Information for Patients: To assure the safe and effective use of benzodiazepines, patients should be informed that, since benzodiazepines may produce psychological and physical dependence, it is advisable that they consult with their physician before either increasing the dose or abruptly discontinuing this drug.

Pediatric Use: Safety and effectiveness in pediatric patients below the age of 6 months have not been established.

ADVERSE REACTIONS

Side effects most commonly reported were drowsiness, fatigue and ataxia. Infrequently encountered were confusion, constipation, depression, diplopia, dysarthria, headache, hypotension, incontinence, jaundice, changes in libido, nausea, changes in salivation, skin rash, slurred speech, tremor, urinary retention, vertigo and blurred vision. Paradoxical reactions such as acute hyperexcited states, anxiety, hallucinations, increased muscle spasticity, insomnia, rage, sleep disturbances and stimulation have been reported; should these occur, use of the drug should be discontinued.

Because of isolated reports of neutropenia and jaundice, periodic blood counts and liver function tests are advisable during long-term therapy. Minor changes in EEG patterns, usually low-voltage fast activity, have been observed in patients during and after Valium therapy and are of no known significance.

DRUG ABUSE AND DEPENDENCE

Withdrawal symptoms, similar in character to those noted with barbiturates and alcohol (convulsions, tremor, abdominal and muscle cramps, vomiting and sweating), have occurred following abrupt discontinuance of diazepam. The more severe withdrawal symptoms have usually been limited to those patients who had received excessive doses over an extended period of time. Generally milder withdrawal symptoms (eg, dysphoria and insomnia) have been reported following abrupt discontinuance of benzodiazepines taken continuously at therapeutic levels for several months. Consequently, after extended therapy, abrupt discontinuation should generally be avoided and a gradual dosage tapering schedule followed. Addiction-prone individuals (such as drug addicts or alcoholics) should be under careful surveillance when receiving diazepam or other psychotropic agents because of the predisposition of such patients to habituation and dependence.

DOSAGE AND ADMINISTRATION

Dosage should be individualized for maximum beneficial effect. While the usual daily dosages given below will meet the needs of most patients, there will be some who may require higher doses. In such cases dosage should be increased cautiously to avoid adverse effects.

	USUAL DAILY DOSE
ADULTS:	
Management of Anxiety Disorders and Relief of Symptoms of Anxiety.	Depending upon severity of symptoms—2 mg to 10 mg, 2 to 4 times daily
Symptomatic Relief in Acute Alcohol Withdrawal.	10 mg, 3 or 4 times during the first 24 hours, reducing to 5 mg, 3 or 4 times daily as needed
Adjunctively for Relief of Skeletal Muscle Spasm.	2 mg to 10 mg, 3 or 4 times daily
Adjunctively in Convulsive Disorders.	2 mg to 10 mg, 2 to 4 times daily
Geriatric Patients, or in the presence of debilitating disease.	2 mg to $2^1/_2$ mg, 1 or 2 times daily initially; increase gradually as needed and tolerated
PEDIATRIC PATIENTS:	
Because of varied responses to CNS-acting drugs, initiate therapy with lowest dose and increase as required. Not for use in pediatric patients under 6 months.	1 mg to $2^1/_2$ mg, 3 or 4 times daily initially; increase gradually as needed and tolerated

HOW SUPPLIED

For oral administration, Valium is supplied as round, flat-faced scored tablets with V-shaped perforation and beveled edges. Valium is available as follows: 2 mg, white—bottles of 100 (NDC 0140-0004-01) and 500 (NDC 0140-0004-14); 5 mg, yellow—bottles of 100 (NDC 0140-0005-01) and 500 (NDC 0140-0005-14); 10 mg, blue—bottles of 100 (NDC 0140-0006-01) and 500 (NDC 0140-0006-14).

Engraved on tablets:

2 mg—2 VALIUM® (front)
ROCHE (twice on scored side)

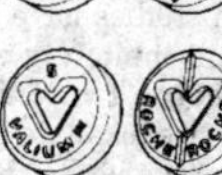

5 mg—5 VALIUM® (front)
ROCHE (twice on scored side)

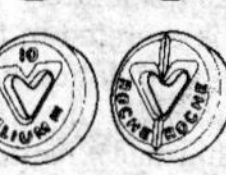

10 mg—10 VALIUM® (front)
ROCHE (twice on scored side)

*Levophed is a registered trademark of Abbott Laboratories.
†Aramine is a registered trademark of MERCK & CO., INC.

Storage: Store at room temperature 59° to 86°F (15° to 30°C). Dispense in tight, light-resistant containers as defined in USP/NF.

Revised: March 2000

Shown in Product Identification Guide, page 332

Romark Pharmaceuticals A Division of Romark Laboratories L.C.
3000 BAYPORT DRIVE
SUITE 200
TAMPA, FL 33607

For Medical Information:
Telephone: (877) 925-4642
Fax: (813) 282-9055

ALINIA® ℞

[ă-lĭ-nē-ă]
(nitazoxanide) Tablets
(nitazoxanide) for Oral Suspension

DESCRIPTION

Alinia Tablets and Alinia for Oral Suspension contain the active ingredient, nitazoxanide, a synthetic antiprotozoal agent for oral administration. Nitazoxanide is a light yellow crystalline powder. It is poorly soluble in ethanol and practically insoluble in water. Chemically, nitazoxanide is 2-acetyloxy-*N*-(5-nitro-2-thiazolyl)benzamide. The molecular formula is $C_{12}H_9N_3O_5S$ and the molecular weight is 307.3. The structural formula is:

Alinia Tablets contain 500 mg of nitazoxanide and the following inactive ingredients: maize starch, pregelatinized corn starch, hydroxypropyl methylcellulose, sucrose, sodium starch glycollate, talc, magnesium stearate, soy lecithin, polyvinyl alcohol, xanthan gum, titanium dioxide, talc, FD&C Yellow No. 10 Aluminum Lake, FD&C Yellow No. 6 Aluminum Lake, and FD&C Blue No. 2 Aluminum Lake.

Alinia for Oral Suspension, after reconstitution, contains 100 mg nitazoxanide per 5 mL and the following inactive ingredients: sodium benzoate, sucrose, xanthan gum, microcrystalline cellulose and carboxymethylcellulose sodium, anhydrous citric acid, sodium citrate dihydrate, acacia gum, sugar syrup, FD&C Red #40 and natural strawberry flavoring.

CLINICAL PHARMACOLOGY

Absorption: Following oral administration of Alinia Tablets or Oral Suspension, maximum plasma concentrations of the active metabolites tizoxanide and tizoxanide glucuronide are observed within 1-4 hours. The parent nitazoxanide is not detected in plasma. Pharmacokinetic parameters of tizoxanide and tizoxanide glucuronide are shown in Tables 1 and 2 below.

[See table 1 above]
[See table 2 above]

Table 1. Mean (±SD) plasma pharmacokinetic parameter values following administration of a single dose of one 500 mg Alinia Tablet with food to subjects ≥12 years of age

	Tizoxanide			Tizoxanide glucuronide		
Age	C_{max} (µg/mL)	T_{max}* (hr)	AUC_τ (µg•hr/mL)	C_{max} (µg/mL)	T_{max}* (hr)	AUC_τ (µg•hr/mL)
12-17 years	9.1 (6.1)	4.0 (1-4)	39.5 (24.2)	7.3 (1.9)	4.0 (2-8)	46.5 (18.2)
≥18 years	10.6 (2.0)	3.0 (2-4)	41.9 (6.0)	10.5 (1.4)	4.5 (4-6)	63.0 (12.3)

* T_{max} is given as a Mean (Range)

Table 2. Mean (± SD) plasma pharmacokinetic parameter values following administration of a single dose of Alinia for Oral Suspension with food to subjects 1 through 11 years of age

		Tizoxanide			Tizoxanide glucuronide		
Age	Dose	C_{max} (µg/mL)	T_{max}* (hr)	AUC_{inf} (µg•hr/mL)	C_{max} (µg/mL)	T_{max}* (hr)	AUC_{inf} (µg•hr/mL)
1-3 years	100mg	3.11 (2.0)	3.5 (2-4)	11.7 (4.46)	3.64 (1.16)	4.0 (3-4)	19.0 (5.03)
4-11 years	200mg	3.00 (0.99)	2.0 (1-4)	13.5 (3.3)	2.84 (0.97)	4.0 (2-4)	16.9 (5.00)

* T_{max} is given as a Mean (Range)

Alinia for Oral Suspension is not bioequivalent to Alinia Tablets. The relative bioavailability of the suspension compared to the tablet was 70%.

Effect of Food: When Alinia Tablets are administered with food, the AUC_τ of tizoxanide and tizoxanide glucuronide in plasma is increased almost two-fold and the C_{max} is increased by almost 50%.

When Alinia for Oral Suspension was administered with food, the AUC_τ of tizoxanide and tizoxanide glucuronide increased by about 45-50% and the C_{max} increased by ≤10%.

Alinia Tablets and for Oral Suspension were administered with food in clinical trials and hence they are recommended to be administered with food (see **DOSAGE AND ADMINISTRATION**).

Multiple dosing: Following oral administration of a single Alinia Tablet every 12 hours for 7 consecutive days, there was no significant accumulation of nitazoxanide metabolites tizoxanide or tizoxanide glucuronide detected in plasma.

Distribution: In plasma, more than 99% of tizoxanide is bound to proteins.

Metabolism: Following oral administration in humans, nitazoxanide is rapidly hydrolyzed to an active metabolite, tizoxanide (desacetyl-nitazoxanide). Tizoxanide then undergoes conjugation, primarily by glucuronidation. *In vitro* metabolism studies have demonstrated that tizoxanide has no significant inhibitory effect on cytochrome P450 enzymes.

Elimination: Tizoxanide is excreted in the urine, bile and feces, and tizoxanide glucuronide is excreted in urine and bile. Approximately two-thirds of the oral dose of nitazoxanide is excreted in the feces and one-third in the urine.

Special Populations

Patients with Impaired Hepatic and/or Renal Function: The pharmacokinetics of nitazoxanide in patients with impaired hepatic and/or renal function has not been studied.

Geriatric Patients: The pharmacokinetics of nitazoxanide in geriatric patients has not been studied.

Pediatric Patients: The pharmacokinetics of nitazoxanide following administration of Alinia Tablets in pediatric patients less than 12 years of age has not been studied. The pharmacokinetics of nitazoxanide following administration of Alinia for Oral Suspension in pediatric patients less than one year of age has not been studied.

MICROBIOLOGY

Mechanism of action

The antiprotozoal activity of nitazoxanide is believed to be due to interference with the pyruvate:ferredoxin oxido-reductase (PFOR) enzyme-dependent electron transfer reaction which is essential to anaerobic energy metabolism. Studies have shown that the PFOR enzyme from *Giardia lamblia* directly reduces nitazoxanide by transfer of electrons in the absence of ferredoxin. The DNA-derived PFOR protein sequence of *Cryptosporidium parvum* appears to be similar to that of *Giardia lamblia*. Interference with the PFOR enzyme-dependent electron transfer reaction may not be the only pathway by which nitazoxanide exhibits antiprotozoal activity.

Activity *in vitro*

Nitazoxanide and its metabolite, tizoxanide, are active *in vitro* in inhibiting the growth of (i) sporozoites and oocysts of *Cryptosporidium parvum* and (ii) trophozoites of *Giardia lamblia*.

Drug Resistance

A potential for development of resistance by *Cryptosporidium parvum* or *Giardia lamblia* to nitazoxanide has not been examined.

Susceptibility Tests:

For protozoa such as *Cryptosporidium parvum* and *Giardia lamblia*, standardized tests for use in clinical microbiology laboratories are not available.

INDICATIONS AND USAGE

Diarrhea caused by *Giardia lamblia*:

Alinia for Oral Suspension (patients 1 year of age and older) and Alinia Tablets (patients 12 years and older) are indicated for the treatment of diarrhea caused by *Giardia lamblia*.

Diarrhea caused by *Cryptosporidium parvum*:

Alinia for Oral Suspension is indicated for patients 1 through 11 years of age for the treatment of diarrhea caused by *Cryptosporidium parvum*.

Alinia for Oral Suspension and Alinia Tablets have not been shown to be superior to placebo for the treatment of diarrhea caused by *Cryptosporidium parvum* in HIV- infected or immunodeficient patients (see **CLINICAL STUDIES**).

The safety and effectiveness of Alinia for Oral Suspension or Alinia Tablets for the treatment of diarrhea caused by *Cryptosporidium parvum* in patients 12 years of age and older have not been established.

CONTRAINDICATIONS

Alinia Tablets and Alinia for Oral Suspension are contraindicated in patients with a prior hypersensitivity to nitazoxanide or any other ingredient in the formulations.

PRECAUTIONS

General: The pharmacokinetics of nitazoxanide in patients with compromised renal or hepatic function have not been studied. Therefore, nitazoxanide must be administered with caution to patients with hepatic and biliary disease, to patients with renal disease and to patients with combined renal and hepatic disease.

Information for Patients

Alinia Tablets and Alinia for Oral Suspension should be taken with food.

Diabetic patients and caregivers should be aware that the oral suspension contains 1.48 grams of sucrose per 5 mL.

Drug Interactions

Tizoxanide is highly bound to plasma protein (>99.9%). Therefore, caution should be used when administering nitazoxanide concurrently with other highly plasma protein-bound drugs with narrow therapeutic indices, as competition for binding sites may occur (e.g., warfarin). *In vitro* metabolism studies have demonstrated that tizoxanide has no significant inhibitory effect on cytochrome P450 enzymes. Although no drug-drug interaction studies have been conducted *in vivo*, it is expected that no significant interaction would occur when nitazoxanide is co-administered with drugs that either are metabolized by or inhibit cytochrome P450 enzymes.

Carcinogenesis, Mutagenesis, Impairment of Fertility

Long-term carcinogenicity studies have not been conducted. Nitazoxanide was not genotoxic in the Chinese hamster ovary (CHO) cell chromosomal aberration assay or the mouse micronucleus assay. Nitazoxanide was genotoxic in one tester strain (TA 100) in the Ames bacterial mutation assay.

Nitazoxanide did not adversely affect male or female fertility in the rat at 2400 mg/kg/day (approximately 20 times the clinical adult dose adjusted for body surface area).

Pregnancy: Teratogenic Effects

Pregnancy Category B: Reproduction studies have been performed at doses up to 3200 mg/kg/day in rats (approximately 26 times the clinical adult dose adjusted for body surface area) and 100 mg/kg/day in rabbits (approximately 2 times the clinical adult dose adjusted for surface area) and have revealed no evidence of impaired fertility or harm to the fetus due to nitazoxanide. There are, however, no adequate and well-controlled studies in pregnant women.

Nursing Mothers

It is not known whether nitazoxanide is excreted in human milk. Because many drugs are excreted in human milk, caution should be exercised when nitazoxanide is administered to a nursing woman.

Pediatric Use

A single Alinia Tablet contains a greater amount of nitazoxanide than is recommended for pediatric dosing and should therefore not be used in pediatric patients 11 years or younger. Alinia for Oral Suspension should be used for dosing nitazoxanide in pediatric patients. (See **DOSAGE AND ADMINISTRATION**)

Safety and effectiveness of Alinia for Oral Suspension in pediatric patients less than one year of age have not been studied.

Geriatrics

Clinical studies of Alinia Tablets and Alinia for Oral Suspension did not include sufficient numbers of subjects aged 65 and over to determine whether they respond differently from younger subjects. In general, the greater frequency of decreased hepatic, renal, or cardiac function, and of concomitant disease or other drug therapy in elderly patients should be considered when prescribing Alinia Tablets and Alinia for Oral Suspension. As stated in the **PRECAUTIONS** section, this therapy must be administered with caution to patients with renal and or hepatic impairment.

HIV-Infected or Immunodeficient Patients

Alinia Tablets and Alinia for Oral Suspension have not been studied for the treatment of diarrhea caused by *Giardia lamblia* in HIV-infected or immunodeficient patients. Alinia Tablets and Alinia for Oral Suspension have not been shown to be superior to placebo for the treatment of diarrhea caused by *Cryptosporidium parvum* in HIV-infected or immunodeficient patients (see **CLINICAL STUDIES**).

ADVERSE REACTIONS

Alinia Tablets: In controlled and uncontrolled clinical studies of 1,628 HIV-uninfected patients age 12 years and older who received various dosage regimens of Alinia Tablets, the most common adverse events reported regardless of causality assessment were: abdominal pain (6.7%), diarrhea (4.3%), headache (3.1%) and nausea (3.1%). In placebo-controlled clinical trials using the recommended dose, the rates of occurrence of these events did not differ significantly from those of the placebo. In placebo-controlled trials of HIV-uninfected patients age 12 years and older who received Alinia Tablets for the treatment of diarrhea caused by *Giardia lamblia*, approximately 1% of patients discontinued therapy because of an adverse event.

Adverse events occurring in less than 1% of the patients age 12 years and older participating in clinical trials of Alinia Tablets are listed below:

Body as a Whole: asthenia, fever, pain, allergic reaction, pelvic pain, chills, chills and fever, flu syndrome.

Nervous System: dizziness, somnolence, insomnia, tremor, hypesthesia.

Indication	Age	Dosage	Duration
Treatment of diarrhea caused by *Giardia lamblia*	1-3 years	5 mL of Alinia for Oral Suspension (100 mg nitazoxanide) every 12 hours with food	3 days
	4-11 years	10 mL of Alinia for Oral Suspension (200 mg nitazoxanide) every 12 hours with food	
	≥12 years	1 Alinia Tablet (500 mg nitazoxanide) every 12 hours with food or 25 mL of Alinia for Oral Suspension (500 mg nitazoxanide) every 12 hours with food	
Treatment of diarrhea caused by *Cryptosporidium parvum*	1-3 years	5 mL of Alinia for Oral Suspension (100 mg nitazoxanide) every 12 hours with food	3 days
	4-11 years	10 mL of Alinia for Oral Suspension (200 mg nitazoxanide) every 12 hours with food	

Adult and Adolescent Patients with Diarrhea Caused by *Giardia lamblia*
Clinical Response Rates* 4 to 7 Days Post-therapy % (Number of Successes/Total)

	Alinia Tablets	Alinia for Oral Suspension	Placebo Tablets
Study 1	85% (46/54)¶ §	83% (45/54)¶ §	44% (12/27)
Study 2	100% (8/8)	-	30% (3/10)

*Includes all patients randomized with *Giardia lamblia* as the sole pathogen. Patients failing to complete the studies were treated as failures.
¶Clinical response rates statistically significantly higher when compared to placebo.
§The 95% confidence interval of the difference in response rates for the tablet and suspension is (-14%, 17%).

Pediatric Patients with Diarrhea Caused by *Giardia lamblia*
Clinical Response Rates 7 to 10 Days Following Initiation of Therapy
Intent-to-Treat and Per Protocol Analyses
% (Number of Successes/Total), [95% Confidence Interval]

Population	Nitazoxanide (3 days)	Metronidazole (5 days)	95% CI Diff§
Intent-to-treat analysis†	85% (47/55)	80% (44/55)	[-9%, 20%]
Per protocol analysis¶	90% (43/48)	83% (39/47)	[-8%, 21%]

†Intent-to-treat analysis includes all patients randomized with patients not completing the study treated as failures.
¶Per protocol analysis includes only patients who took all of their medication and completed the study. Seven patients in each treatment group missed at least one dose of medication and one in the metronidazole treatment group was lost to follow-up.
§95% Confidence Interval on the difference in response rates (nitazoxanide-metronidazole).

Pediatric Patients with Diarrhea Caused by *Cryptosporidium parvum* Clinical Response Rates 3 to 7 Days Post-therapy, Intent-to-Treat Analyses % (Number of Successes/Total)

Population	Nitazoxanide*	Placebo
Outpatient Study, age 1 – 11 years	88% (21/24)	38% (9/24)
Inpatient Study, Malnourished¶, age 12–35 months	56% (14/25)	23% (5/22)

*Clinical response rates statistically significantly higher compared to placebo.
¶ 60% considered severely underweight, 19% moderately underweight, 17% mild underweight.

Digestive System: vomiting, dyspepsia, anorexia, flatulence, constipation, dry mouth, thirst.
Urogenital System: discolored urine, dysuria, amenorrhea, metrorrhagia, kidney pain, edema labia.
Metabolic & Nutrition: increased SGPT.
Hemic & Lymphatic Systems: anemia, leukocytosis.
Skin: rash, pruritus.
Special Senses: eye discoloration, ear ache.
Respiratory System: epistaxis, lung disease, pharyngitis.
Cardiovascular System: tachycardia, syncope, hypertension.
Muscular System: myalgia, leg cramps, spontaneous bone fracture.

Alinia for Oral Suspension: In controlled and uncontrolled clinical studies of 613 HIV-uninfected pediatric patients who received Alinia for Oral Suspension, the most frequent adverse events reported regardless of causality assessment were: abdominal pain (7.8%), diarrhea (2.1%), vomiting (1.1%) and headache (1.1%). These were typically mild and transient in nature. In placebo-controlled clinical trials, the rates of occurrence of these events did not differ significantly from those of the placebo. None of the 613 pediatric patients discontinued therapy because of adverse events.

Adverse events occurring in less than 1% of the pediatric patients participating in clinical trials of Alinia for Oral Suspension are listed below:
Digestive System: nausea, anorexia, flatulence, appetite increase, enlarged salivary glands.
Body as a Whole: fever, infection, malaise.
Metabolic & Nutrition: increased creatinine, increased SGPT.
Skin: pruritus, sweat.
Special Senses: eye discoloration (pale yellow).
Respiratory System: rhinitis.
Nervous System: dizziness.
Urogenital System: discolored urine.

The adverse events seen in adult patients treated with Alinia for Oral Suspension were similar to those observed in adult patients treated with Alinia Tablets.

OVERDOSAGE

Information on nitazoxanide overdosage is not available. In acute studies in rodents and dogs, the oral LD_{50} was higher than 10,000 mg/kg. Single oral doses of up to 4000 mg nitazoxanide have been administered to healthy adult volunteers without significant adverse effects. In the event of overdose, gastric lavage may be appropriate soon after oral administration. Patients should be carefully observed and given symptomatic and supportive treatment.

DOSAGE AND ADMINISTRATION

[See first table above]
Safety and effectiveness of Alinia for Oral Suspension and Alinia Tablets for the treatment of diarrhea caused by *Cryptosporidium parvum* in patients 12 years and older have not been established.
A single Alinia tablet contains a greater amount of nitazoxanide than is recommended for pediatric dosing and should therefore not be used in pediatric patients 11 years or younger.
Alinia Tablets and Alinia for Oral Suspension have not been studied for the treatment of *Giardia lamblia* in HIV-infected or immunodeficient patients. Alinia Tablets and Alinia for Oral Suspension have not been shown to be superior to placebo for the treatment of diarrhea caused by *Cryptosporidium parvum* in HIV-infected or immunodeficient patients (see **CLINICAL STUDIES**).

DIRECTIONS FOR MIXING ALINIA FOR ORAL SUSPENSION
Prepare a suspension at time of dispensing as follows: The amount of water required for preparation of the suspension is 48 mL. Tap bottle until all powder flows freely. Add approximately one-half of the total amount of water required for reconstitution and shake vigorously to suspend powder. Add remainder of water and again shake vigorously.
The container should be kept tightly closed, and the suspension should be shaken well before each administration. The suspension may be stored for 7 days, after which any unused portion must be discarded.

HOW SUPPLIED

Alinia Tablets are round, yellow, film-coated tablets debossed with ALINIA on one side and 500 on the other side. Each tablet contains 500 mg of nitazoxanide. The tablets are packaged in HDPE bottles of 60 tablets and blister cards of 6 tablets.
Bottles of 60 NDC 67546-111-11
Boxes of 3 blister cards NDC 67546-111-32
(Alinia 3-Day Therapy Packs™)

Alinia for Oral Suspension is a pink-colored powder formulation that, when reconstituted as directed, contains 100 mg nitazoxanide/5 mL. The reconstituted suspension has a pink color and strawberry flavor. Alinia for Oral Suspension is available as:
Bottles of 60 mL NDC 67546-212-21

Storage and Stability: Store the tablets, unsuspended powder, and the reconstituted oral suspension at 25°C (77°F); excursions permitted to 15-30°C (59-86°F). [See USP Controlled Room Temperature]

CLINICAL STUDIES

Diarrhea caused by *Giardia lamblia* in adults and adolescents 12 years of age or older:
In a double-blind, controlled study (Study 1) conducted in Peru and Egypt in adults and adolescents with diarrhea caused by *Giardia lamblia*, a three-day course of treatment with Alinia Tablets administered 500 mg BID was compared with a placebo tablet and Alinia for Oral Suspension administered 500 mg/25 mL of suspension BID for 3 days. A second double-blind, controlled study (Study 2) conducted in Egypt in adults and adolescents with diarrhea caused by *Giardia lamblia* compared Alinia Tablets administered 500 mg BID for 3 days to a placebo. For both of these studies, clinical response was evaluated 4 to 7 days following the end of treatment. A clinical response of 'well' was defined as 'no symptoms, no watery stools and no more than 2 soft stools with no hematochezia within the past 24 hours' or 'no symptoms and no unformed stools within the past 48 hours.' The following clinical response rates were obtained:
[See second table at left]
Some of the patients with 'well' clinical responses had *Giardia lamblia* cysts in their stool samples 4 to 7 days following the end of treatment. The relevance of stool examination results in these patients is unknown. Patients should be managed based upon clinical response to treatment.

Diarrhea caused by *Giardia lamblia* in pediatric patients 1 through 11 years of age:
In a randomized, controlled study conducted in Peru in 110 pediatric patients with diarrhea caused by *Giardia lamblia*, a three-day course of treatment with nitazoxanide (100 mg BID in pediatric patients ages 24-47 months, 200 mg BID in pediatric patients ages 4 through 11 years) was compared to a five-day course of treatment with metronidazole (125 mg BID in pediatric patients ages 2 through 5 years, 250 mg BID in pediatric patients ages 6 through 11 years). Clinical response was evaluated 7 to 10 days following initiation of treatment with a 'well' response defined as 'no symptoms, no watery stools and no more than 2 soft stools with no hematochezia within the past 24 hours' or 'no symptoms and no unformed stools within the past 48 hours.' The following clinical cure rates were obtained:
[See third table at left]
Some of the patients with 'well' clinical responses had *Giardia lamblia* cysts in their stool samples 4 to 7 days following the end of treatment. The relevance of stool examination results in these patients is unknown. Patients should be managed based upon clinical response to treatment.

Diarrhea caused by *Cryptosporidium parvum* in pediatric patients 1 through 11 years of age:
In two double-blind, controlled studies in pediatric patients with diarrhea caused by *Cryptosporidium parvum*, a three-day course of treatment with nitazoxanide (100 mg BID in pediatric patients ages 12-47 months, 200 mg BID in pediatric patients ages 4 through 11 years) was compared with a placebo. One study was conducted in Egypt in outpatients ages 1 through 11 years with diarrhea caused by *C. parvum*. Another study was conducted in Zambia in malnourished pediatric patients admitted to the hospital with diarrhea caused by *C. parvum*. Clinical response was evaluated 3 to 7 days post-therapy with a 'well' response defined as 'no symptoms, no watery stools and no more than 2 soft stools with no hematochezia within the past 24 hours' or 'no symptoms and no unformed stools within the past 48 hours.' The following clinical response rates were obtained:
[See fourth table above]
Some of the patients with 'well' clinical responses had *Cryptosporidium* oocysts in their stool samples 3 to 7 days following the end of treatment. The relevance of stool examination results in these patients is unknown. Patients should be managed based upon clinical response to treatment.
Another double-blind, placebo-controlled study was conducted in hospitalized, severely malnourished pediatric patients with acquired immune deficiency syndrome (AIDS) in Zambia. In this study, a three day course of nitazoxanide suspension (100 mg BID in pediatric patients ages 12-47 months, 200 mg BID in pediatric patients ages 4 through 11 years) did not produce clinical cure rates that were significantly different from the placebo control.

Rx Only
US Patents No. 5,578,621; 6,020,353; 5,968,961; 5,387,598; 6,117,894; 5,965,590.
DATE OF ISSUANCE: July, 2004

Romark Pharmaceuticals
A division of Romark Laboratories, L.C.
3000 Bayport Drive, Suite 200
Tampa FL 33607
Telephone: 813-282-8544, Fax: 813-282-4910
E-mail: customer.service@romark.com
Web site: www.romark.com

Ross Products Division

ABBOTT LABORATORIES
COLUMBUS, OH 43215-1724 USA

Direct Inquiries to:
1-800-227-5767

PEDIALYTE® OTC

[*pē 'dē-ah-līt"*]
Oral Electrolyte Maintenance Solution

USAGE

To quickly replace fluids and electrolytes lost during diarrhea and vomiting to help prevent dehydration in infants and children; for maintenance of water and electrolytes following corrective parenteral therapy for severe diarrhea. Pedialyte is designed to promote fluid absorption more effectively than common household beverages.

Features:

- Ready To Use—no mixing or dilution necessary.
- Balanced electrolytes to replace diarrheal stool losses and provide maintenance requirements.
- Provides glucose to promote sodium and water absorption.
- Unflavored liquid form available for young infants; fruit-flavored, bubble gum-flavored and grape-flavored liquids formulated with improved taste to enhance compliance in older infants and children.
- Plastic liter bottles are resealable and allow easy measuring and pouring.
- 8-fl-oz cherry and apple flavors; single-serving size is easy for children to hold and drink.
- Freezer Pops (2.1 fl oz Pedialyte per sleeve) are available in multiple flavors to encourage compliance with fluid intake recommendations for children 1 year of age and older.
- Widely available in grocery, drug and discount stores.
- Low osmolality; 270 mOsm/kg water for flavored; 250 mOsm/kg water for unflavored.

AVAILABILITY

Ready To Use:

1-liter (33.8-fl-oz) plastic bottles; 8 per case; Unflavored, No. 00336; Fruit Flavor, No. 00365; Bubble Gum Flavor, No. 51752; Grape Flavor, No. 00240.
8-fl-oz glass bottles; 4 six-packs per case; Unflavored, No. 00160.
2.1-fl-oz sleeve Freezer Pops; 8 sixteen-sleeve boxes per case; Grape, Cherry, Orange and Blue Raspberry, No. 00245.
8-fl-oz plastic bottles; 8 four-packs per case; Cherry, No. 54981; Apple, No. 57425.

DOSAGE

Refer to Administration Guide to restore fluid and minerals lost in diarrhea and vomiting.
Pedialyte should be offered frequently in amounts tolerated. Total daily intake should be adjusted to meet individual needs, based on thirst and response to therapy. The suggested intakes for maintenance are based on water requirements for ordinary energy expenditure.[1]
[See table below]

INGREDIENTS:

Unflavored: (Pareve, Ⓤ) Water, dextrose; Less than 2% of: potassium citrate, sodium chloride, sodium citrate, and citric acid.
Fruit Flavor: (Pareve, Ⓤ) Water, dextrose; Less than 2% of: fructose, citric acid, natural and artificial fruit flavors, potassium citrate, sodium chloride, sodium citrate, sucralose, acesulfame potassium and Yellow 6.
Grape Flavor: (Pareve, Ⓤ) Water, dextrose; Less than 2% of: fructose, citric acid, potassium citrate, sodium chloride, artificial grape flavor, sodium citrate, sucralose, acesulfame potassium, Red 40 and Blue 1.
Bubble Gum Flavor: (Pareve, Ⓤ) Water, dextrose; Less than 2% of: fructose, citric acid, potassium citrate, sodium chloride, sodium citrate, artificial bubble gum flavor, sucralose, acesulfame potassium and Red 40.
Freezer Pops: (Pareve,Ⓤ) Water, dextrose; Less than 2% of: citric acid, sodium chloride, sodium carboxymethylcellulose, potassium citrate, potassium sorbate, sodium benzoate, sucralose and acesulfame potassium; **Grape** also contains: Natural and artificial grape flavor, Red 40 and Blue 1; **Cherry** also contains: Natural and artificial cherry flavor and Red 40; **Orange** also contains: Natural and artificial orange flavor, Yellow 6 and Red 40; **Blue Raspberry** also contains: Natural and artificial blue raspberry flavor and Blue 1.
Cherry Singles: (Pareve, Ⓤ) Water, dextrose; Less than 2% of: fructose, citric acid, sodium chloride, potassium citrate, sodium citrate, artificial cherry flavor, potassium sorbate, sodium benzoate, sucralose, acesulfame potassium and Red 40.
Apple Singles: (Pareve, Ⓤ) Water, dextrose; Less than 2% of: fructose, citric acid, sodium chloride, potassium citrate, sodium citrate, potassium sorbate, sodium benzoate, artificial apple flavor, caramel color, acesulfame potassium and sucralose.

UNFLAVORED PEDIALYTE LIQUID PROVIDES (per liter):
Sodium, 45 mEq; potassium, 20 mEq; chloride, 35 mEq; dextrose, 25 g; Calories, 100.
(FAN 9003)

FLAVORED PEDIALYTE LIQUID PROVIDES (per liter):
Sodium, 45 mEq; potassium, 20 mEq; chloride, 35 mEq; dextrose, 20 g; fructose, 5 g; Calories, 100.
(FAN 9003)

PEDIALYTE FREEZER POPS PROVIDE (per liter):
Sodium, 45 mEq; potassium, 20 mEq; chloride, 35 mEq; dextrose, 25 g; Calories, 100.

PEDIALYTE SINGLES PROVIDE (8 fl oz):
Sodium, 10.6 mEq; potassium, 4.7 mEq; chloride, 8.3 mEq; dextrose, 4.7 g; fructose, 1.2 g; Calories 24.
(FAN 9003)

PEDIAZOLE® ℞

(8030)
erythromycin ethylsuccinate
and sulfisoxazole acetyl
for oral suspension

Rx only

To reduce the development of drug-resistant bacteria and maintain the effectiveness of Pediazole and other antibacterial drugs, Pediazole should be used only to treat or prevent infections that are proven or strongly suspected to be caused by bacteria.

DESCRIPTION

Pediazole is a combination of erythromycin ethylsuccinate, USP, and sulfisoxazole acetyl, USP. When reconstituted with water as directed on the label, the granules form a white, strawberry-banana flavor suspension that provides the equivalent of 200 mg erythromycin activity and the equivalent of 600 mg of sulfisoxazole activity per teaspoonful (5 mL).
Erythromycin is produced by a strain of *Saccaropolyspora erythraea* and belongs to the macrolide group of antibiotics. It is basic and readily forms salts and esters. Erythromycin ethylsuccinate is the 2′-ethylsuccinyl ester of erythromycin. It is essentially a tasteless form of the antibiotic suitable for oral administration, particularly in suspension dosage forms. The chemical name is erythromycin 2′-(ethyl succinate). Erythromycin ethylsuccinate has the following structural formula:

Sulfisoxazole acetyl or N[1]-acetyl sulfisoxazole is an ester of sulfisoxazole. Chemically, sulfisoxazole is N-(3,4-Dimethyl-5-isoxazolyl)-N-sulfanilylacetamide. Sulfisoxazole acetyl has the following structural formula:

Inactive Ingredients: Citric acid, magnesium aluminum silicate, poloxamer, sodium carboxymethylcellulose, sodium citrate, sucrose and artificial flavoring.

CLINICAL PHARMACOLOGY

Orally administered erythromycin ethylsuccinate suspensions are readily and reliably absorbed. Erythromycin ethylsuccinate products have demonstrated rapid and consistent absorption in both fasting and nonfasting conditions. However, higher serum concentrations are obtained when these products are given with food. Bioavailability data are available from Ross Products Division. Erythromycin is largely bound to plasma proteins. After absorption, erythromycin diffuses readily into most body fluids. In the absence of meningeal inflammation, low concentrations are normally achieved in the spinal fluid, but the passage of the drug across the blood-brain barrier increases in meningitis. Erythromycin crosses the placental barrier and is excreted in human milk. Erythromycin is not removed by peritoneal dialysis or hemodialysis.
In the presence of normal hepatic function, erythromycin is concentrated in the liver and is excreted in the bile; the effect of hepatic dysfunction on biliary excretion of erythromycin is not known. After oral administration, less than 5% of the administered dose can be recovered in the active form in the urine.
Wide variation in blood levels may result following identical doses of a sulfonamide. Blood levels should be measured in patients receiving these drugs for serious infections. Free sulfonamide blood levels of 50 to 150 mcg/mL may be considered therapeutically effective for most infections, with blood levels of 120 to 150 mcg/mL being optimal for serious infections. The maximum sulfonamide level should be 200 mcg/mL, because adverse reactions occur more frequently above this concentration.
Following oral administration, sulfisoxazole is rapidly and completely absorbed; the small intestine is the major site of absorption, but some of the drug is absorbed from the stomach. Sulfonamides are present in the blood as free, conjugated (acetylated and possibly other forms), and protein-bound forms. The amount present as "free" drug is considered to be the therapeutically active form. Approximately 85% of a dose of sulfisoxazole is bound to plasma proteins, primarily to albumin; 65% to 72% of the unbound portion is in the nonacetylated form.
Maximum plasma concentrations of intact sulfisoxazole following a single 2-g oral dose of sulfisoxazole to healthy adult volunteers ranged from 127 to 211 mcg/mL (mean, 169 mcg/mL), and the time of peak plasma concentration ranged from 1 to 4 hours (mean, 2.5 hours). The elimination half-life of sulfisoxazole ranged from 4.6 to 7.8 hours after oral administration. The elimination of sulfisoxazole has been shown to be slower in elderly subjects (63 to 75 years) with diminished renal function (creatinine clearance 37 to 68 mL/min).[1] After multiple-dose oral administration of 500 mg q.i.d. to healthy volunteers, the average steady-state plasma concentrations of intact sulfisoxazole ranged from 49.9 to 88.8 mcg/mL (mean, 63.4 mcg/mL).[2]
Sulfisoxazole and its acetylated metabolites are excreted primarily by the kidneys through glomerular filtration. Concentrations of sulfisoxazole are considerably higher in the urine than in the blood. The mean urinary recovery following oral administration of sulfisoxazole is 97% within 48 hours; 52% of this is intact drug, and the remainder is the N[4]-acetylated metabolite.
Sulfisoxazole is distributed only in extracellular body fluids. It is excreted in human milk. It readily crosses the placental barrier. In healthy subjects, cerebrospinal fluid concentrations of sulfisoxazole vary; in patients with meningitis, however, concentrations of free drug in cerebrospinal fluid as high as 94 mcg/mL have been reported.

Microbiology:

Pediazole has been formulated to contain sulfisoxazole for concomitant use with erythromycin.
Erythromycin acts by inhibition of protein synthesis by binding 50 S ribosomal subunits of susceptible organisms. It

Pedialyte Administration Guide for Infants and Young Children*

Age	2 Weeks	3 Months	6	9	1 Years	1½	2	2½	3	3½	4
Approximate Weight† (lb)	9	14	18	21	23	26	28	30	32	34	36
(kg)	4.0	6.4	8.2	9.5	10.5	11.8	12.7	13.6	14.4	15.3	16.3
PEDIALYTE fl oz/day for Maintenance**	16 to 20	30 to 34	36 to 42	39 to 45	42 to 47	47 to 52	48 to 53	51 to 56	53 to 57	54 to 57	55 to 59

* Administration Guide does not apply to infants less than 1 week of age. For children over 4 years, maintenance intakes may exceed 2 liters daily. If there is vomiting or fever, or if diarrhea continues beyond 24 hours, consult the child's physician.
** Fluid intake is total fluid requirement from oral electrolyte solution, formula or other fluids, but does not take into account ongoing stool losses. Fluid loss in the stool should be replaced by consumption of an extra amount of Pedialyte equal to stool losses, in addition to fluid maintenance requirement in this Administration Guide. Pedialyte Freezer Pops are to be used with Pedialyte Oral Electrolyte Maintenance Solution or other appropriate fluids to help prevent dehydration.
† Weight based on the 50th percentile of weight for age for boys from the National Center for Health Statistics (NCHS) Centers for Disease Control and Prevention (CDC) growth charts. Kuczmarski RJ, Ogden CL, Grummer-Strawn LM, et al: CDC Growth Charts: United States. Data from Vital and Health Statistics of the Centers for Disease Control and Prevention/National Center for Health Statistics. *Advance Data*, no. 314, December 4, 2000.

1. Extrapolated from Barness L, Curran JS: Nutrition, in Nelson WE, Behrman RE, Kliegman RM, Arvin AM: *Nelson Textbook of Pediatrics*, ed 15. Philadelphia: WB Saunders Co, 1996, pp 141-143.

does not affect nucleic acid synthesis. Antagonism has been demonstrated *in vitro* between erythromycin and clindamycin, lincomycin, and chloramphenicol.
The sulfonamides are bacteriostatic agents, and the spectrum of activity is similar for all. Sulfonamides inhibit bacterial synthesis of dihydrofolic acid by preventing the condensation of the pteridine with *para*-aminobenzoic acid through competitive inhibition of the enzyme dihydropteroate synthetase. Resistant strains have altered dihydropteroate synthetase with reduced affinity for sulfonamides or produce increased quantities of *para*-aminobenzoic acid.

Susceptibility Testing:

Diffusion Techniques: Quantitative methods that require measurement of zone diameters provide reproducible estimates of the susceptibility of bacteria to antimicrobial compounds. One such standardized procedure[3] that has been recommended for use with disks to test the susceptibility of microorganisms to the combination erythromycin ethylsuccinate and sulfisoxazole acetyl uses the 15 mcg erythromycin disk and the 250 (300) mcg sulfisoxazole disk. Interpretation involves correlation of the diameter obtained in the disk tests with the respective MIC for erythromycin and sulfisoxazole.
Reports from the laboratory providing results of standard single-disk susceptibility tests should be interpreted according to the following criteria.[3-5]

With a 15 mcg erythromycin disk:

Zone Diameter	Interpretation
≥23	Susceptible (S)
14–22	Intermediate (I)
≤13	Resistant (R)

With a 250 (or 300) mcg sulfisoxazole disk:

Zone Diameter	Interpretation
≥17	Susceptible (S)
13–16	Intermediate (I)
≤12	Resistant (R)

A report of "Susceptible" indicates that the pathogen is likely to be inhibited by usually achievable concentrations of the antimicrobial compound in blood. A report of "Intermediate" indicates that the result should be considered equivocal, and, if the microorganism is not fully susceptible to alternative, clinically feasible drugs, the test should be repeated. This category implies possible clinical applicability in body sites where the drug is physiologically concentrated or in situations where high dosage of drug can be used. This category also provides a buffer zone that prevents small uncontrolled technical factors from causing major discrepancies in interpretation. A report of "Resistant" indicates that usually achievable concentrations of the antimicrobial compound in the blood are unlikely to be inhibitory and that other therapy should be selected.
Measurement of MIC or MBC and achieved antimicrobial compound concentrations may be appropriate to guide therapy in some infections. (See CLINICAL PHARMACOLOGY section for further information on drug concentrations and other pharmacokinetic properties of this antimicrobial drug product.)
Standardized susceptibility test procedures require the use of laboratory control microorganisms. The 15 mcg erythromycin disk and the 250 (or 300) mcg sulfisoxazole disk should provide the following zone diameters in these laboratory test quality control strains:

Microorganism	Zone Diameter (mm)
15 mcg Erythromycin Disk:	
S. aureus ATCC 25923	22–30
250 (or 300) mcg Sulfisoxazole Disk:	
E. coli ATCC 25922	18–26
S. aureus ATCC 25923	24–34

Dilution Techniques: Quantitative methods that are used to determine minimum inhibitory concentrations provide reproducible estimates of the susceptibility of bacteria to antimicrobial compounds. One such standardized procedure uses a standardized dilution method (broth, agar, or microdilution) or equivalent with erythromycin or sulfisoxazole powder. The MIC values obtained should be intrepreted according to the following criteria:

MIC (mcg/mL)	Interpretation
With Erythromycin Powder:	
≤0.5	Susceptible (S)
1–4	Intermediate (I)
≥8	Resistant (R)
With Sulfisoxazole Powder:	
≤256	Susceptible (S)
≥512	Resistant (R)

Interpretation should be as stated above for results using diffusion techniques.

As with standard diffusion techniques, dilution methods require the use of laboratory control microorganisms. Standard erythromycin and sulfisoxazole powders should provide the following MIC values:

Microorganism	MIC (mcg/mL)
With Erythromycin Powder:	
S. aureus ATCC 25923	0.12–0.5
E. faecalis ATCC 29212	1–4
With Sulfisoxazole Powder:	
S. aureus ATCC 29213	32–128
E. faecalis ATCC 29212	32–128
E. coli ATCC 25922	8–32

INDICATIONS AND USAGE

For treatment of ACUTE OTITIS MEDIA in children that is caused by susceptible strains of *Haemophilus influenzae*.
To reduce the development of drug-resistant bacteria and maintain the effectiveness of Pediazole, USP, and other antibacterial drugs, Pediazole should be used only to treat or prevent infections that are proven or strongly suspected to be caused by susceptible bacteria. When culture and susceptibility information are available, they should be considered in selecting or modifying antibacterial therapy. In the absence of such data, local epidemiology and susceptibility patterns may contribute to the empiric selection of therapy.

CONTRAINDICATIONS

Pediazole is contraindicated in the following patient populations:

Patients with a known hypersensitivity to either of its components, children younger than 2 months, pregnant women *at term*, and mothers nursing infants less than 2 months of age.

Use in pregnant women at term, in children less than 2 months of age, and in mothers nursing infants less than 2 months of age is contraindicated because sulfonamides may promote kernicterus in the newborn by displacing bilirubin from plasma proteins.
Erythromycin is contraindicated in patients taking terfenadine, astemizole or cisapride. **(See PRECAUTIONS—Drug Interactions.)**

WARNINGS

FATALITIES ASSOCIATED WITH THE ADMINISTRATION OF SULFONAMIDES, ALTHOUGH RARE, HAVE OCCURRED DUE TO SEVERE REACTIONS INCLUDING STEVENS-JOHNSON SYNDROME, TOXIC EPIDERMAL NECROLYSIS, FULMINANT HEPATIC NECROSIS, AGRANULOCYTOSIS, APLASTIC ANEMIA, AND OTHER BLOOD DYSCRASIAS.
SULFONAMIDES, INCLUDING SULFONAMIDE-CONTAINING PRODUCTS SUCH AS PEDIAZOLE, SHOULD BE DISCONTINUED AT THE FIRST APPEARANCE OF SKIN RASH OR ANY SIGN OF ADVERSE REACTION. In rare instances, a skin rash may be followed by a more severe reaction, such as Stevens-Johnson syndrome, toxic epidermal necrolysis, hepatic necrosis, and serious blood disorders. **(See PRECAUTIONS.)**
Clinical signs such as sore throat, fever, arthralgia, pallor, rash, purpura, or jaundice may be early indications of serious reactions.
There have been reports of hepatic dysfunction including increased liver enzymes, and hepatocellular and/or cholestatic hepatitis, with or without jaundice, occurring in patients receiving oral erythromycin products.
Cough, shortness of breath, and pulmonary infiltrates are hypersensitivity reactions of the respiratory tract that have been reported in association with sulfonamide treatment.
The sulfonamides should not be used for the treatment of group A beta-hemolytic streptococcal infections. In an established infection, they will not eradicate the streptococcus and, therefore, will not prevent sequelae such as rheumatic fever.
Pseudomembranous colitis has been reported with nearly all antibacterial agents, including Pediazole, and may range in severity from mild to life-threatening. Therefore, it is important to consider this diagnosis in patients who present with diarrhea subsequent to the administration of antibacterial agents.
Treatment with antibacterial agents alters the normal flora of the colon and may permit overgrowth of clostridia. Studies indicate that a toxin produced by *Clostridium difficile* is one primary cause of "antibiotic-associated colitis."
After diagnosis of pseudomembranous colitis has been established, therapeutic measures should be initiated. Mild cases of pseudomembranous colitis usually respond to drug discontinuation alone. In moderate to severe cases, consideration should be given to management with fluids and electrolytes, protein supplementation, and treatment with an antibacterial drug clinically effective against *Clostridium difficile* colitis.
There have been reports suggesting that erythromycin does not reach the fetus in adequate concentration to prevent congenital syphilis. Infants born to women treated during pregnancy with erythromycin for early syphilis should be treated with an appropriate penicillin regimen.
Rhabdomyolysis with or without renal impairment has been reported in seriously ill patients receiving erythromycin concomitantly with lovastatin. Therefore, patients receiving concomitant lovastatin and erythromycin should be carefully monitored for creatine kinase (CK) and serum transaminase levels. (See package insert for lovastatin.)

PRECAUTIONS

General: Prescribing Pediazole in the absence of a proven or strongly suspected bacterial infection or a prophylactic indication is unlikely to provide benefit to the patient and increases the risk of the development of drug-resistant bacteria.
Erythromycin is principally excreted by the liver. Caution should be exercised when erythromycin is administered to patients with impaired hepatic function. **(See CLINICAL PHARMACOLOGY and WARNINGS sections.)**
Prolonged or repeated use of erythromycin may result in an overgrowth of nonsusceptible bacteria or fungi. If superinfection occurs, erythromycin should be discontinued and appropriate therapy instituted.
There have been reports that erythromycin may aggravate the weakness of patients with myasthenia gravis.
When indicated, incision and drainage or other surgical procedures should be performed in conjunction with antibiotic therapy.
Sulfonamides should be given with caution to patients with impaired renal or hepatic function and to those with severe allergy or bronchial asthma. In glucose-6-phosphate dehydrogenase-deficient individuals, hemolysis may occur; this reaction is frequently dose-related.
Information for Patients: Patients should be counseled that antibacterial drugs including Pediazole should only be used to treat bacterial infections. They do not treat viral infections (eg, the common cold). When Pediazole is prescribed to treat a bacterial infection, patients should be told that although it is common to feel better early in the course of therapy, the medication should be taken exactly as directed. Skipping doses or not completing the full course of therapy may (1) decrease the effectiveness of the immediate treatment and (2) increase the likelihood that bacteria will develop resistance and will not be treatable by Pediazole or other antibacterial drugs in the future.
Patients should maintain an adequate fluid intake to prevent crystalluria and stone formation.
Laboratory Tests: Complete blood counts should be done frequently in patients receiving sulfonamides. If a significant reduction in the count of any formed blood element is noted, Pediazole should be discontinued. Urinalysis with careful microscopic examination and renal function tests should be performed during therapy, particularly for those patients with impaired renal function. Blood levels should be measured in patients receiving a sulfonamide for serious infections. **(See INDICATIONS AND USAGE.)**
Drug/Laboratory Test Interactions: Erythromycin interferes with the fluorometric determination of urinary catecholamines.
Drug Interactions: Erythromycin use in patients who are receiving high doses of theophylline may be associated with an increase in serum theophylline levels and potential theophylline toxicity. In case of theophylline toxicity and/or elevated serum theophylline levels, the dose of theophylline should be reduced while the patient is receiving concomitant erythromycin therapy.
Concomitant administration of erythromycin and digoxin has been reported to result in elevated digoxin serum levels.
There have been reports of increased anticoagulant effects when erythromycin and oral anticoagulants were used concomitantly. Increased anticoagulation effects due to this drug may be more pronounced in the elderly.
Concurrent use of erythromycin and ergotamine or dihydroergotamine has been associated in some patients with acute ergot toxicity characterized by severe peripheral vasospasm and dysesthesia.
Triazolobenzodiazepines (such as triazolam and alprazolam) and related benzodiazepines: Erythromycin has been reported to decrease the clearance of triazolam and midazolam and thus may increase the pharmacologic effect of these benzodiazepines.
HMG-CoA Reductase Inhibitors: Erythromycin has been reported to increase concentrations of HMG-CoA Reductase Inhibitors (eg, lovastatin and simvastatin). Rare reports of rhabdomyolysis have been reported in patients taking these drugs concomitantly.
The use of erythromycin in patients concurrently taking drugs metabolized by the cytochrome P450 system may be associated with elevations in serum levels of these other drugs. There have been reports of interactions of erythromycin with carbamazepine, cyclosporine, tacrolimus, hexobarbital, phenytoin, alfentanil, cisapride, disopyramide, quinidine, methylprednisolone, cilostazol, vinblastine, sildenafil, lovastatin, and bromocriptine, valproate, terfenadine, and astemizole. Serum concentrations of drugs metabolized by the cytochrome P450 system should be monitored closely in patients concurrently receiving erythromycin.
Erythromycin has been reported to significantly alter the metabolism of the nonsedating antihistamines terfenadine and astemizole when taken concomitantly. Rare cases of serious cardiovascular adverse events, including electrocardiographic QT/QTc interval prolongation, cardiac arrest, torsades de pointes, and other ventricular arrhythmias, have been observed. **(See CONTRAINDICATIONS.)** In addition, deaths have been reported rarely with concomitant administration of terfenadine and erythromycin.

Continued on next page

Pediazole—Cont.

It has been reported that sulfisoxazole may prolong the prothrombin time in patients who are receiving the anticoagulants including warfarin. This interaction should be kept in mind when Pediazole is given to patients already on anticoagulant therapy, and the prothrombin time or other suitable coagulation test should be monitored.
It has been proposed that sulfisoxazole competes with thiopental for plasma protein binding. In one study involving 48 patients, intravenous sulfisoxazole resulted in a decrease in the amount of thiopental required for anesthesia and in a shortening of the awakening time. It is not known whether chronic oral doses of sulfisoxazole have a similar effect. Until more is known about this interaction, physicians should be aware that patients receiving sulfisoxazole might require less thiopental for anesthesia.
Sulfonamides can displace methotrexate from plasma protein binding sites, thus increasing free methotrexate concentrations. Studies in man have shown sulfisoxazole infusions to decrease plasma protein-bound methotrexate by one fourth.
Sulfisoxazole can also potentiate the blood-sugar-lowering activity of sulfonylureas, as well as cause hypoglycemia by itself.
Carcinogenesis, Mutagenesis, Impairment of Fertility:
Carcinogenesis: Pediazole has not undergone adequate trials relating to carcinogenicity; each component, however, has been evaluated separately. Long-term (2-year) oral studies conducted in rats with erythromycin ethylsuccinate did not provide evidence of tumorigenicity. Sulfisoxazole was not carcinogenic in either sex when administered to mice by gavage for 103 weeks at dosages up to approximately 18 times the highest recommended human dose or to rats at 4 times the highest recommended human daily dose. Rats appear to be especially susceptible to the goitrogenic effects of sulfonamides, and long-term administration of sulfonamides has resulted in thyroid malignancies in this species.
Mutagenesis: There are no studies available that adequately evaluate the mutagenic potential of Pediazole or either of its components. Ames mutagenic assays have not been performed with sulfisoxazole. However, sulfisoxazole was not observed to be mutagenic in *E. coli* Sd-4-73 when tested in the absence of a metabolic activating system. There was no apparent effect on male or female fertility in rats fed erythromycin (base) at levels up to 0.25% of diet.
Impairment of Fertility: Pediazole has not undergone adequate trials relating to impairment of fertility. In a reproduction study in rats given 7 times the highest recommended human dose per day of sulfisoxazole, no effects were observed regarding mating behavior, conception rate or fertility index (percent pregnant).
Pregnancy: Teratogenic Effects. Pregnancy Category C. At dosages 7 times the highest recommended human daily dose, sulfisoxazole was not teratogenic in either rats or rabbits. However, in two other teratogenicity studies, cleft palates developed in both rats and mice, and skeletal defects were also observed in rats after administration of 9 times the human therapeutic dose of sulfisoxazole.
There is no evidence of teratogenicity or any other adverse effect on reproduction in female rats fed erythromycin base (up to 0.25% of diet) prior to and during mating, during gestation, and through weaning of two successive litters. There are, however, no adequate and well-controlled studies in pregnant women. Because animal reproduction studies are not always predictive of human response, this drug should be used during pregnancy only if clearly needed. Erythromycin has been reported to cross the placental barrier in humans, but fetal plasma levels are generally low.
There are no adequate or well-controlled studies of Pediazole in either laboratory animals or in pregnant women. It is not known whether Pediazole can cause fetal harm when administered to a pregnant woman prior to term or can affect reproduction capacity. Pediazole should be used during pregnancy only if the potential benefit justifies the potential risk to the fetus.
Nonteratogenic Effects: Kernicterus may occur in the newborn as a result of treatment of a pregnant woman *at term* with sulfonamides. **(See CONTRAINDICATIONS.)**
Labor and Delivery: The effects of erythromycin and sulfisoxazole on labor and delivery are unknown.
Nursing Mothers: Both erythromycin and sulfisoxazole are excreted in human milk. **Because of the potential for the development of kernicterus in neonates due to the displacement of bilirubin from plasma proteins by sulfisoxazole, a decision should be made whether to discontinue nursing or discontinue the drug, taking into account the importance of the drug to the mother. (See CONTRAINDICATIONS.)**
Pediatric Use: **See INDICATIONS AND USAGE** and **DOSAGE AND ADMINISTRATION** sections. Not for use in children under 2 months of age. **(See CONTRAINDICATIONS.)**
Geriatric Use: Clinical studies of Pediazole did not include adult or geriatric populations. **See INDICATIONS AND USAGE** and **DOSAGE AND ADMINISTRATION** sections.

ADVERSE REACTIONS

Erythromycin ethylsuccinate: The most frequent side effects of oral erythromycin preparations are gastrointestinal and are dose-related. They include nausea, vomiting, abdominal pain, diarrhea and anorexia. Symptoms of hepatitis, hepatic dysfunction and/or abnormal liver-function test results may occur. **(See WARNINGS section.)** Pseudomembranous colitis has been rarely reported in association with erythromycin therapy.
Allergic reactions ranging from urticaria to anaphylaxis have occurred. Skin reactions ranging from mild eruptions to erythema multiforme, Stevens-Johnson Syndrome, and toxic epidermal necrolysis have been reported rarely.
There have been isolated reports of reversible hearing loss occurring chiefly in patients with renal insufficiency and in patients receiving high doses of erythromycin.
Onset of pseudomembranous colitis symptoms may occur during or after antibiotic treatment. **(See WARNINGS.)**
Sulfisoxazole acetyl: Included in the listing that follows are adverse reactions that have been reported with other sulfonamide products: Pharmacologic similarities require that each of the reactions be considered with Pediazole administration.
Allergic/Dermatologic: Anaphylaxis, erythema multiforme (Stevens-Johnson syndrome), toxic epidermal necrolysis (Lyell's syndrome), exfoliative dermatitis, angioedema, arteritis, vasculitis, allergic myocarditis, serum sickness, rash, urticaria, pruritus, photosensitivity, and conjunctival and scleral injection, generalized allergic reactions and generalized skin eruptions. In addition, periarteritis nodosa and systemic lupus erythematosus have been reported. **(See WARNINGS.)**
Cardiovascular: Tachycardia, palpitations, syncope, and cyanosis.
Rarely, erythromycin has been associated with the production of ventricular arrhythmias, including ventricular tachycardia and torsade de pointes, in individuals with prolonged QT intervals.
Endocrine: The sulfonamides bear certain chemical similarities to some goitrogens, diuretics (acetazolamide and the thiazides) and oral hypoglycemic agents. Cross-sensitivity may exist with these agents. Developments of goiter, diuresis, and hypoglycemia have occurred rarely in patients receiving sulfonamides.
Gastrointestinal: Hepatitis, hepatocellular necrosis, jaundice, pseudomembranous colitis, nausea, emesis, anorexia, abdominal pain, diarrhea, gastrointestinal hemorrhage, melena, flatulence, glossitis, stomatitis, salivary gland enlargement, and pancreatitis. Onset of pseudomembranous colitis symptoms may occur during or after treatment with sulfisoxazole, a component of Pediazole. **(See WARNINGS.)**
The sulfisoxazole acetyl component of Pediazole has been reported to cause increased elevation of liver-associated enzymes in patients with hepatitis.
Genitourinary: Crystalluria, hematuria, BUN and creatinine elevations, nephritis, and toxic nephrosis with oliguria and anuria. Acute renal failure and urinary retention have also been reported.
The frequency of renal complications, commonly associated with some sulfonamides, is lower in patients receiving the more soluble sulfonamides such as sulfisoxazole.
Hematologic: Leukopenia, agranulocytosis, aplastic anemia, thrombocytopenia, purpura, hemolytic anemia, anemia, eosinophilia, clotting disorders including hypoprothrombinemia and hypofibrinogenemia, sulfhemoglobinemia, and methemoglobinemia.
Musculoskeletal: Arthralgia, myalgia.
Neurologic: Headache, dizziness, peripheral neuritis, paresthesia, convulsions, tinnitus, vertigo, ataxia, and intracranial hypertension.
Psychiatric: Psychosis, hallucination, disorientation, depression, anxiety and apathy.
Respiratory: Cough, shortness of breath, and pulmonary infiltrates. **(See WARNINGS.)**
Vascular: Angioedema, arteritis, and vasculitis.
Miscellaneous: Edema (including periorbital), pyrexia, drowsiness, weakness, fatigue, lassitude, rigors, flushing, hearing loss, insomnia, pneumonitis and chills.

OVERDOSAGE

No information is available on a specific result of overdose with Pediazole. Overdosage of erythromycin should be handled with the prompt elimination of unabsorbed drug and all other appropriate measures should be instituted. Erythromycin is not removed by peritoneal dialysis or hemodialysis.
The amount of a single dose of sulfisoxazole that is either associated with symptoms of overdosage or is likely to be life-threatening has not been reported. Signs and symptoms of overdosage reported with sulfonamides include anorexia, colic, nausea, vomiting, dizziness, headache, drowsiness and unconsciousness. Pyrexia, hematuria and crystalluria may be noted. Blood dyscrasias and jaundice are potential late manifestations of overdosage.
General principles of treatment include the immediate discontinuation of the drug, instituting gastric lavage or emesis, forcing oral fluids, and administering intravenous fluids if urine output is low and renal function is normal. The patient should be monitored with blood counts and appropriate blood chemistries, including electrolytes. If the patient becomes cyanotic, the possibility of methemoglobinemia should be considered and, if present, the condition should be treated appropriately with intravenous 1% methylene blue. If a significant blood dyscrasia or jaundice occurs, specific therapy should be instituted for these complications. Peritoneal dialysis is not effective, and hemodialysis is only moderately effective in removing sulfonamides.
The acute toxicity of sulfisoxazole in animals is as follows:

Species	LD_{50} ± S.E. · (mg/kg)
mouse	5700 ± 235
rats	>10,000
rabbits	>2000

DOSAGE AND ADMINISTRATION

PEDIAZOLE SHOULD NOT BE ADMINISTERED TO INFANTS LESS THAN 2 MONTHS OF AGE BECAUSE OF CONTRAINDICATIONS OF SYSTEMIC SULFONAMIDES IN THIS AGE GROUP.
For Acute Otitis Media in Children: The dose of Pediazole can be calculated based on the erythromycin component (50 mg/kg/day) or the sulfisoxazole component (150 mg/kg/day to a maximum of 6 g/day). The total daily dose of Pediazole should be administered in equally divided doses three or four times a day for 10 days. Pediazole may be administered without regard to meals.
The following approximate dosage schedules are recommended for using Pediazole:
Children: Two months of age or older

FOUR-TIMES-A-DAY SCHEDULE

Weight	Dose—every 6 hours
Less than 8 kg (<18 lb)	Adjust dosage by body weight
8 kg (18 lb)	1/2 teaspoonful (2.5 mL)
16 kg (35 lb)	1 teaspoonful (5 mL)
24 kg (53 lb)	1 1/2 teaspoonfuls (7.5 mL)
Over 32 kg (over 70 lb)	2 teaspoonfuls (10 mL)

THREE-TIMES-A-DAY SCHEDULE

Weight	Dose—every 8 hours
Less than 6 kg (<13 lb)	Adjust dosage by body weight
6 kg (13 lb)	1/2 teaspoonful (2.5 mL)
12 kg (26 lb)	1 teaspoonful (5 mL)
18 kg (40 lb)	1 1/2 teaspoonfuls (7.5 mL)
24 kg (53 lb)	2 teaspoonfuls (10 mL)
Over 30 kg (over 66 lb)	2 1/2 teaspoonfuls (12.5 mL)

TO PATIENT: Shake before using. Oversize bottle provides shake space. Keep tightly closed. Store in the refrigerator. Use within 14 days. Unused portion should be discarded after 14 days.

HOW SUPPLIED

Pediazole Suspension is available for teaspoon dosage in 100-mL (**NDC** 0074-8030-13), 150-mL (**NDC** 0074-8030-43), 200-mL (**NDC** 0074-8030-53) and 250-mL (**NDC** 0074-8030-73) bottles, in the form of granules to be reconstituted with water. The suspension provides erythromycin ethylsuccinate equivalent to 200 mg erythromycin activity and sulfisoxazole acetyl equivalent to 600 mg sulfisoxazole per teaspoonful (5 mL).
Before mixing, store below 86°F (30°C).

REFERENCES

1. Boisvert A, Barbeau G, Belanger PM: Pharmacokinetics of sulfisoxazole in young and elderly subjects. *Gerontology* 1984;30:125-131.
2. Oie S, Gambertoglio JG, Fleckenstein L: Comparison of the disposition of total and unbound sulfisoxazole after single and multiple dosing. *J Pharmacokinet Biopharm* 1982;10:157-172.
3. National Committee for Clinical Laboratory Standards: *Performance Standards for Antimicrobial Disk Susceptibility Tests, Fifth Edition.* Approved Standard NCCLS Document M2-A5, Vol 13, No. 24. Villanova, Pa: NCCLS, 1993.
4. National Committee for Clinical Laboratory Standards: *Methods for Dilution Antimicrobial Susceptibility Tests for Bacteria that Grow Aerobically, Third Edition.* Approved Standard NCCLS Document M7-A3, Vol 13, No. 25. Villanova, Pa: NCCLS, 1993.
5. National Committee for Clinical Laboratory Standards: *Performance Standard for Antimicrobial Susceptibility Testing, Third Edition.* Supplement, NCCLS Document M100-S3 (ISBN 1-56238-136-9). Villanova, Pa: NCCLS, 1993.

Revised: March, 2004

PEDIASURE® and PEDIASURE® ENTERAL FORMULA OTC

[*pē 'dē-ah-shur "*]
Complete, Balanced Nutrition®

PediaSure Enteral Formula and PediaSure Enteral Formula With Fiber

USAGE

Nutritionally complete, balanced, enteral formulas especially designed for tube feeding of children 1–13 years of age. May be used as the sole source of nutrition or as a sup-

plement. PediaSure Enteral contains 1000 calories and 30 grams of protein per liter. Meets or exceeds 100% of the Dietary Reference Intakes (DRIs) for protein, vitamins, and minerals for children 1–8 years of age in 1000 mL and for children 9–13 years of age in 1500 mL. Meets DRIs for children ages 4–13 with less volume than other pediatric tube-feeding products, and PediaSure Enteral Formulas are the only pediatric products to meet the nutrient needs of children up to age 13.* The fat content is 35% of total calories. The fatty acid profile complies with American Academy of Pediatrics' (AAP) recommendation for less than 10% of calories from saturated fat and less than 300 mg per day of dietary cholesterol and the National Academy of Sciences' recommendation of an n6:n3 fatty acid ratio of less than 10:1. Calcium:phosphorus ratio of 1.2:1 meets recommendations by the AAP for growing children.
PediaSure Enteral Formula with Fiber contains 8 grams of dietary fiber per liter. Fiber blend provides soluble (53%) and insoluble (47%) fiber and FOS (fructooligosaccharides). FOS is a prebiotic that stimulates the growth and activity of beneficial bacteria (e.g., bifidobacteria) in the colon; helps create an environment unfavorable to the growth of pathogenic bacteria in at-risk patients; is fermented to short-chain fatty acids, a preferred energy source for cells of the colon, helping to maintain GI tract integrity; and acts as a functional fiber representing the type of fiber found in fruits and vegetables.

*As compared with the standard and fiber-containing versions of Kindercal® TF, Nutren Junior®, and Resource® Just For Kids. Kindercal, Nutren Junior and Resource are not trademarks of Abbott Laboratories.

Not for parenteral use.
Not intended for infants under 1 year of age unless specified by a physician.

AVAILABILITY

Ready to Use
8-fl-oz (237-mL) cans: 24 per case; PediaSure Enteral Formula, Vanilla, No. 51804; PediaSure Enteral Formula With Fiber, Vanilla, No. 51806.

INGREDIENTS (enteral)

Ⓤ-D Water, corn maltodextrin, milk protein concentrate, sugar (sucrose), high oleic safflower oil, soy oil, medium chain triglycerides; Less than 0.5% of: natural and artificial flavor, dextrose, potassium citrate, magnesium phosphate, cellulose gel, salt (sodium chloride), potassium chloride, calcium phosphate, potassium phosphate, choline chloride, soy lecithin, mono- and diglycerides, carrageenan, ascorbic acid, cellulose gum, m-inositol, taurine, ferrous sulfate, dl-alpha-tocopheryl acetate, L-carnitine, zinc sulfate, calcium pantothenate, niacinamide, manganese sulfate, thiamine chloride hydrochloride, pyridoxine hydrochloride, riboflavin, cupric sulfate, vitamin A palmitate, folic acid, biotin, chromium chloride, potassium iodide, sodium selenate, sodium molybdate, phylloquinone, vitamin D_3, and cyanocobalamin.
(FAN 7818-01)

INGREDIENTS (enteral with fiber)

Ⓤ-D Water, corn maltodextrin, milk protein concentrate, sugar (sucrose), high oleic safflower oil, soy oil, medium chain triglycerides; Less than 0.5% of: fructooligosaccharides, natural and artificial flavor, oat fiber, dextrose, soy fiber, potassium citrate, magnesium phosphate, gum arabic, salt (sodium chloride), potassium chloride, calcium phosphate, potassium phosphate, cellulose gum, choline chloride, soy lecithin, mono- and diglycerides, ascorbic acid, carrageenan, m-inositol, taurine, ferrous sulfate, dl-alpha-tocopheryl acetate, L-carnitine, zinc sulfate, calcium pantothenate, niacinamide, manganese sulfate, thiamine chloride hydrochloride, pyridoxine hydrochloride, riboflavin, cupric sulfate, vitamin A palmitate, folic acid, biotin, chromium chloride, potassium iodide, sodium selenate, sodium molybdate, phylloquinone, vitamin D_3, and cyanocobalamin.
(FAN 7818-01)

NUTRITION INFORMATION	***Per 8 fl oz***
Calories	237
Protein, g	7.1
Carbohydrate, g	31.4 (32.7*)
Dietary Fiber, g	1.9†
Fat, g	9.4
Water, g	202 (201*)
Vitamin A, IU	380
Vitamin D, IU	120
Vitamin E, IU	5.4
Vitamin K, mcg	14
Vitamin C, mg	24
Folic Acid, mcg	71
Thiamine (Vitamin B_1), mg	0.64
Riboflavin (Vitamin B_2), mg	0.50
Vitamin B_6, mg	0.62
Vitamin B_{12}, mcg	1.4
Niacin, mg	2.4
Choline, mg	71
Biotin, mcg	76
Pantothenic Acid, mg	2.4
Inositol, mg	19
Sodium, mg	90
Potassium, mg	310
Chloride, mg	240
Calcium, mg	230
Phosphorus, mg	200
Magnesium, mg	47
Iodine, mcg	23
Manganese, mg	0.36
Copper, mg	0.24
Zinc, mg	1.4
Iron, mg	3.3
Chromium, mcg	7.1
Molybdenum, mcg	8.5
Selenium, mcg	7.6
L-Carnitine, mg	4
Taurine, mg	17

*Enteral with Fiber
†1.2g of total dietary fiber from a patented fiber blend and 0.7g of fructooligosaccarides.

PediaSure and PediaSure with Fiber

USAGE

Nutritionally complete, balanced formulas especially designed for oral feeding of children 1–10 years of age. May be used as the sole source of nutrition or as a supplement. PediaSure meets or exceeds 100% of the NAS/NRC RDAs for children 1–6 years of age in 1000 mL (approx. 34 fl oz) and for children 7–10 years of age in 1300 mL (approx. 44 fl oz). Calcium:phosphorus ratio of 1.2:1 meets recommendations by the American Academy of Pediatrics Committee on Nutrition (AAPCON) for growing children. PediaSure is ideal for children whose nutrient needs are increased or who may be undernourished due to illness or poor appetite. PediaSure is formulated to support catch-up growth in children with failure to thrive and is well tolerated. "Kid Approved" vanilla, chocolate, strawberry, banana cream, and orange cream flavors encourage compliance (retail and institutional PediaSure). Also available with fiber.

Not for parenteral use.
Not intended for infants under 1 year of age unless specified by a physician.

AVAILABILITY

Ready to Use
8-fl-oz (237 mL) cans: 24 per case; Vanilla, No. 00373 (retail), Vanilla, No. 55897 (institution); Chocolate, No. 51812 (retail), Chocolate, No. 51882 (institution); Strawberry, No. 51810 (retail), Strawberry, No. 51880 (institution); Banana Cream, No. 51808 (retail), Banana Cream, No. 51884 (institution); Orange Cream, No. 57014 (retail), Orange Cream, No. 57841 (institution), PediaSure With Fiber, Vanilla, No. 50652 (retail).

COMPOSITION

Ready to Use PediaSure Vanilla (other flavors have similar composition and nutrient values. PediaSure With Fiber also contains 8 grams soy fiber per liter. For specific information, see product labels).

INGREDIENTS (institutional)

Ⓤ-D Water, sugar (sucrose), corn maltodextrin, sodium caseinate, high oleic safflower oil, soy oil, medium chain triglycerides, whey protein concentrate; Less than 0.5% of: calcium phosphate, natural and artificial flavor, potassium citrate, magnesium chloride, cellulose gel, potassium phosphate, potassium chloride, soy lecithin, mono- and diglycerides, choline chloride, carrageenan, ascorbic acid, cellulose gum, m-inositol, taurine, ferrous sulfate, zinc sulfate, salt (sodium chloride), niacinamide, dl-alpha-tocopheryl acetate, L-carnitine, calcium pantothenate, thiamine chloride hydrochloride, pyridoxine hydrochloride, riboflavin, manganese sulfate, cupric sulfate, vitamin A palmitate, folic acid, biotin, potassium iodide, sodium selenate, sodium molybdate, phylloquinone, vitamin D_3, and cyanocobalamin.
(FAN 7842-02)

INGREDIENTS (retail)

Ⓤ-D Water, sugar (sucrose), maltodextrin (corn), sodium caseinate, high-oleic safflower oil, soy oil, fractionated coconut oil (medium-chain triglycerides), whey protein concentrate; Less than 0.5% of: calcium phosphate tribasic, natural and artificial flavor, potassium citrate, magnesium chloride, cellulose gel, potassium phosphate dibasic, potassium chloride, soy lecithin, mono- and diglycerides, choline chloride, carrageenan, ascorbic acid, cellulose gum, m-inositol, taurine, ferrous sulfate, zinc sulfate, sodium chloride, niacinamide, alpha-tocopheryl acetate, L-carnitine, calcium pantothenate, thiamine chloride hydrochloride, pyridoxine hydrochloride, riboflavin, manganese sulfate, cupric sulfate, vitamin A palmitate, folic acid, biotin, potassium iodide, sodium selenate, sodium molybdate, phylloquinone, vitamin D_3 and cyanocobalamin.
(FAN 9060-02)

INGREDIENTS (retail with fiber)

Ⓤ-D Water, sugar (sucrose), maltodextrin (corn), sodium caseinate, high-oleic safflower oil, soy oil, fractionated coconut oil (medium-chain triglycerides), whey protein concentrate, soy fiber; Less than 0.5% of: calcium phosphate tribasic, natural and artificial flavor, potassium citrate, magnesium chloride, potassium phosphate dibasic, potassium chloride, soy lecithin, mono- and diglycerides, choline chloride, carrageenan, ascorbic acid, m-inositol, taurine, ferrous sulfate, zinc sulfate, sodium chloride, niacinamide, alpha- tocopheryl acetate, L-carnitine, calcium pantothenate, thiamine chloride hydrochloride, pyridoxine hydrochloride, riboflavin, manganese sulfate, cupric sulfate, vitamin A palmitate, folic acid, biotin, phylloquinone, potassium iodide, sodium selenate, sodium molybdate, phylloquinone, vitamin D_3 and cyanocobalamin.
(FAN 9060-02)

NUTRITION INFORMATION	***Per 8 fl oz***
Calories	237
Protein, g	7.1
Carbohydrate, g	26 (26.9)*
Fat, g	11.8
Water, g	200
Vitamin A, IU	610
Vitamin D, IU	120
Vitamin E, IU	5.4
Vitamin K, mcg	9.0
Vitamin C, mg	24
Folic Acid, mcg	88
Thiamine (Vitamin B_1), mg	0.64
Riboflavin (Vitamin B_2), mg	0.50
Vitamin B_6, mg	0.62
Vitamin B_{12}, mcg	1.4
Niacin, mg	4.0
Choline, mg	71
Biotin, mcg	76
Pantothenic Acid, mg	2.4
Inositol, mg	19
Sodium, mg	90
Potassium, mg	310
Chloride, mg	240
Calcium, mg	230
Phosphorus, mg	190
Magnesium, mg	47
Iodine, mcg	23
Manganese, mg	0.24
Copper, mg	0.24
Zinc, mg	2.8
Iron, mg	3.3
Chromium, mcg	7.1
Molybdenum, mcg	8.5
Selenium, mcg	5.4
L-Carnitine, mg	4
Taurine, mg	17

*PediaSure With Fiber includes soy fiber (a source of dietary fiber that provides 1.2 calories and 1.2 g of total dietary fiber).

SURVANTA® ℞
(beractant)
intratracheal suspension

Sterile Suspension
For Intratracheal Administration Only

DESCRIPTION

SURVANTA® (beractant) Intratracheal Suspension is a sterile, non-pyrogenic pulmonary surfactant intended for intratracheal use only. It is a natural bovine lung extract containing phospholipids, neutral lipids, fatty acids, and surfactant-associated proteins to which colfosceril palmitate (dipalmitoylphosphatidylcholine), palmitic acid, and tripalmitin are added to standardize the composition and to mimic surface-tension lowering properties of natural lung surfactant. The resulting composition provides 25 mg/mL phospholipids (including 11.0-15.5 mg/mL disaturated phosphatidylcholine), 0.5-1.75 mg/mL triglycerides, 1.4-3.5 mg/mL free fatty acids, and less than 1.0 mg/mL protein. It is suspended in 0.9% sodium chloride solution, and heat-sterilized. SURVANTA contains no preservatives. Its protein content consists of two hydrophobic, low molecular weight, surfactant-associated proteins commonly known as SP-B and SP-C. It does not contain the hydrophilic, large molecular weight surfactant-associated protein known as SP-A.
Each mL of SURVANTA contains 25 mg of phospholipids. It is an off-white to light brown liquid supplied in single-use glass vials containing 4 mL (100 mg phospholipids) or 8 mL (200 mg phospholipids).

CLINICAL PHARMACOLOGY

Endogenous pulmonary surfactant lowers surface tension on alveolar surfaces during respiration and stabilizes the alveoli against collapse at resting transpulmonary pressures. Deficiency of pulmonary surfactant causes Respiratory Distress Syndrome (RDS) in premature infants. SURVANTA replenishes surfactant and restores surface activity to the lungs of these infants.

Activity

In vitro, SURVANTA reproducibly lowers minimum surface tension to less than 8 dynes/cm as measured by the pulsating bubble surfactometer and Wilhelmy Surface Balance. *In situ,* SURVANTA restores pulmonary compliance to excised rat lungs artificially made surfactant-deficient. *In vivo,* single SURVANTA doses improve lung pressure-volume measurements, lung compliance, and oxygenation in premature rabbits and sheep.

Continued on next page

Survanta—Cont.

Animal Metabolism

SURVANTA is administered directly to the target organ, the lungs, where biophysical effects occur at the alveolar surface. In surfactant-deficient premature rabbits and lambs, alveolar clearance of radio-labelled lipid components of SURVANTA is rapid. Most of the dose becomes lung-associated within hours of administration, and the lipids enter endogenous surfactant pathways of reutilization and recycling. In surfactant-sufficient adult animals, SURVANTA clearance is more rapid than in premature and young animals. There is less reutilization and recycling of surfactant in adult animals.

Limited animal experiments have not found effects of SURVANTA on endogenous surfactant metabolism. Precursor incorporation and subsequent secretion of saturated phosphatidylcholine in premature sheep are not changed by SURVANTA treatments.

No information is available about the metabolic fate of the surfactant-associated proteins in SURVANTA. The metabolic disposition in humans has not been studied.

Clinical Studies

Clinical effects of SURVANTA were demonstrated in six single-dose and four multiple-dose randomized, multicenter, controlled clinical trials involving approximately 1700 infants. Three open trials, including a Treatment IND, involved more than 8500 infants. Each dose of SURVANTA in all studies was 100 mg phospholipids/kg birth weight and was based on published experience with Surfactant TA, a lyophilized powder dosage form of SURVANTA having the same composition.

Prevention Studies

Infants of 600-1250 g birth weight and 23 to 29 weeks estimated gestational age were enrolled in two *multiple-dose* studies. A dose of SURVANTA was given within 15 minutes of birth to prevent the development of RDS. Up to three additional doses in the first 48 hours, as often as every 6 hours, were given if RDS subsequently developed and infants required mechanical ventilation with an $FiO_2 \geq 0.30$. Results of the studies at 28 days of age are shown in Table 1.

TABLE 1

Study 1

	SURVANTA	Control	P-Value
Number infants studied	119	124	
Incidence of RDS (%)	27.6	63.5	<0.001
Death due to RDS (%)	2.5	19.5	<0.001
Death or BPD due to RDS (%)	48.7	52.8	0.536
Death due to any cause (%)	7.6	22.8	0.001
Air Leaks[a](%)	5.9	21.7	0.001
Pulmonary interstitial emphysema (%)	20.8	40.0	0.001

Study 2[b]

	SURVANTA	Control	P-Value
Number infants studied	91	96	
Incidence of RDS (%)	28.6	48.3	0.007
Death due to RDS (%)	1.1	10.5	0.006
Death or BPD due to RDS (%)	27.5	44.2	0.018
Death due to any cause[c](%)	16.5	13.7	0.633
Air Leaks[a](%)	14.5	19.6	0.374
Pulmonary interstitial emphysema (%)	26.5	33.2	0.298

[a] Pneumothorax or pneumopericardium

[b] Study discontinued when Treatment IND initiated

[c] No cause of death in the SURVANTA group was significantly increased; the higher number of deaths in this group was due to the sum of all causes.

Rescue Studies

Infants of 600-1750 g birth weight with RDS requiring mechanical ventilation and an $FiO_2 \geq 0.40$ were enrolled in two *multiple-dose* rescue studies. The initial dose of SURVANTA was given after RDS developed and before 8 hours of age. Infants could receive up to three additional doses in the first 48 hours, as often as every 6 hours, if they required mechanical ventilation and an $FiO_2 \geq 0.30$. Results of the studies at 28 days of age are shown in Table 2.

TABLE 2

Study 3[a]

	SURVANTA	Control	P-Value
Number infants studied	198	193	
Death due to RDS (%)	11.6	18.1	0.071
Death or BPD due to RDS (%)	59.1	66.8	0.102
Death due to any cause (%)	21.7	26.4	0.285
Air Leaks[b](%)	11.8	29.5	<0.001
Pulmonary interstitial emphysema (%)	16.3	34.0	<0.001

Study 4

	SURVANTA	Control	P-Value
Number infants studied	204	203	
Death due to RDS (%)	6.4	22.3	<0.001
Death or BPD due to RDS (%)	43.6	63.4	<0.001
Death due to any cause (%)	15.2	28.2	0.001
Air Leaks[b] (%)	11.2	22.2	0.005
Pulmonary interstitial emphysema (%)	20.8	44.4	<0.001

[a] Study discontinued when Treatment IND initiated

[b] Pneumothorax or pneumopericardium

Acute Clinical Effects

Marked improvements in oxygenation may occur within minutes of administration of SURVANTA.

All controlled clinical studies with SURVANTA provided information regarding the acute effects of SURVANTA on the arterial-alveolar oxygen ratio (a/APO_2), FiO_2, and mean airway pressure (MAP) during the first 48 to 72 hours of life. Significant improvements in these variables were sustained for 48-72 hours in SURVANTA-treated infants in four single-dose and two multiple-dose rescue studies and in two multiple-dose prevention studies. In the single-dose prevention studies, FiO_2 improved significantly.

INDICATIONS AND USAGE

SURVANTA is indicated for prevention and treatment ("rescue") of Respiratory Distress Syndrome (RDS) (hyaline membrane disease) in premature infants. SURVANTA significantly reduces the incidence of RDS, mortality due to RDS and air leak complications.

Prevention

In premature infants less than 1250 g birth weight or with evidence of surfactant deficiency, give SURVANTA as soon as possible, preferably within 15 minutes of birth.

Rescue

To treat infants with RDS confirmed by x-ray and requiring mechanical ventilation, give SURVANTA as soon as possible, preferably by 8 hours of age.

CONTRAINDICATIONS

None known.

WARNINGS

SURVANTA is intended for intratracheal use only.

SURVANTA CAN RAPIDLY AFFECT OXYGENATION AND LUNG COMPLIANCE. Therefore, its use should be restricted to a highly supervised clinical setting with immediate availability of clinicians experienced with intubation, ventilator management, and general care of premature infants. Infants receiving SURVANTA should be frequently monitored with arterial or transcutaneous measurement of systemic oxygen and carbon dioxide.

DURING THE DOSING PROCEDURE, TRANSIENT EPISODES OF BRADYCARDIA AND DECREASED OXYGEN SATURATION HAVE BEEN REPORTED. If these occur, stop the dosing procedure and initiate appropriate measures to alleviate the condition. After stabilization, resume the dosing procedure.

PRECAUTIONS

General

Rales and moist breath sounds can occur transiently after administration. Endotracheal suctioning or other remedial action is not necessary unless clear-cut signs of airway obstruction are present.

Increased probability of post-treatment nosocomial sepsis in SURVANTA-treated infants was observed in the controlled clinical trials (Table 3). The increased risk for sepsis among SURVANTA-treated infants was not associated with increased mortality among these infants. The causative organisms were similar in treated and control infants. There was no significant difference between groups in the rate of post-treatment infections other than sepsis.

Use of SURVANTA in infants less than 600 g birth weight or greater than 1750 g birth weight has not been evaluated in controlled trials. There is no controlled experience with use of SURVANTA in conjunction with experimental therapies for RDS (eg, high-frequency ventilation or extracorporeal membrane oxygenation).

No information is available on the effects of doses other than 100 mg phospholipids/kg, more than four doses, dosing more frequently than every 6 hours, or administration after 48 hours of age.

Carcinogenesis, Mutagenesis, Impairment of Fertility

Carcinogenicity studies have not been performed with SURVANTA. SURVANTA was negative when tested in the Ames test for mutagenicity. Using the maximum feasible dose volume, SURVANTA up to 500 mg phospholipids/kg/day (approximately one-third the premature infant dose based on $mg/m^2/day$) was administered subcutaneously to newborn rats for 5 days. The rats reproduced normally and there were no observable adverse effects in their offspring.

ADVERSE REACTIONS

The most commonly reported adverse experiences were associated with the dosing procedure. In the multiple-dose controlled clinical trials, each dose of SURVANTA was divided into four quarter-doses which were instilled through a catheter inserted into the endotracheal tube by briefly disconnecting the endotracheal tube from the ventilator. Transient bradycardia occurred with 11.9% of *doses*. Oxygen desaturation occurred with 9.8% of *doses*.

Other reactions during the dosing procedure occurred with fewer than 1% of doses and included endotracheal tube reflux, pallor, vasoconstriction, hypotension, endotracheal tube blockage, hypertension, hypocarbia, hypercarbia, and apnea. No deaths occurred during the dosing procedure, and all reactions resolved with symptomatic treatment.

The occurrence of concurrent illnesses common in premature infants was evaluated in the controlled trials. The rates in all controlled studies are in Table 3.

TABLE 3

	All Controlled Studies		
	SURVANTA	Control	
Concurrent Event	(%)	(%)	P-Value[a]
Patent ductus arteriosus	46.9	47.1	0.814
Intracranial hemorrhage	48.1	45.2	0.241
Severe intracranial hemorrhage	24.1	23.3	0.693
Pulmonary air leaks	10.9	24.7	<0.001
Pulmonary interstitial emphysema	20.2	38.4	<0.001
Necrotizing enterocolitis	6.1	5.3	0.427
Apnea	65.4	59.6	0.283
Severe apnea	46.1	42.5	0.114
Post-treatment sepsis	20.7	16.1	0.019
Post-treatment infection	10.2	9.1	0.345
Pulmonary hemorrhage	7.2	5.3	0.166

[a]*P*-value comparing groups in controlled studies

When all controlled studies were pooled, there was no difference in intracranial hemorrhage. However, in one of the single-dose rescue studies and one of the multiple-dose prevention studies, the rate of intracranial hemorrhage was significantly higher in SURVANTA patients than control patients (63.3% *v* 30.8%, *P*=0.001; and 48.8% *v* 34.2%, *P*=0.047, respectively). The rate in a Treatment IND involving approximately 8100 infants was lower than in the controlled trials.

In the controlled clinical trials, there was no effect of SURVANTA on results of common laboratory tests: white blood cell count and serum sodium, potassium, bilirubin, creatinine.

More than 4300 pretreatment and posttreatment serum samples from approximately 1500 patients were tested by Western Blot Immunoassay for antibodies to surfactant-associated proteins SP-B and SP-C. No IgG or IgM antibodies were detected.

Several other complications are known to occur in premature infants. The following conditions were reported in the controlled clinical studies. The rates of the complications were not different in treated and control infants, and none of the complications were attributed to SURVANTA.

Respiratory: lung consolidation, blood from the endotracheal tube, deterioration after weaning, respiratory decompensation, subglottic stenosis, paralyzed diaphragm, respiratory failure.

Cardiovascular: hypotension, hypertension, tachycardia, ventricular tachycardia, aortic thrombosis, cardiac failure, cardio-respiratory arrest, increased apical pulse, persistent fetal circulation, air embolism, total anomalous pulmonary venous return.

Gastrointestinal: abdominal distention, hemorrhage, intestinal perforations, volvulus, bowel infarct, feeding intolerance, hepatic failure, stress ulcer.

Renal: renal failure, hematuria.

Hematologic: coagulopathy, thrombocytopenia, disseminated intravascular coagulation.

Central Nervous System: seizures.

Endocrine/Metabolic: adrenal hemorrhage, inappropriate ADH secretion, hyperphosphatemia.

Musculoskeletal: inguinal hernia.

Systemic: fever, deterioration.

Follow-Up Evaluations

To date, no long-term complications or sequelae of SURVANTA therapy have been found.

Single-Dose Studies

Six-month adjusted-age follow-up evaluations of 232 infants (115 treated) demonstrated no clinically important differences between treatment groups in pulmonary and neurologic sequelae, incidence or severity of retinopathy of prematurity, rehospitalizations, growth, or allergic manifestations.

Multiple-Dose Studies

Six-month adjusted-age follow-up evaluations have been completed in 631 (345 treated) of 916 surviving infants. There were significantly less cerebral palsy and need for supplemental oxygen in SURVANTA infants than controls. Wheezing at the time of examination was significantly more frequent among SURVANTA infants, although there was no difference in bronchodilator therapy.

Final twelve-month follow-up data from the multiple-dose studies are available from 521 (272 treated) of 909 surviving infants. There was significantly less wheezing in SURVANTA infants than controls, in contrast to the six-month results. There was no difference in the incidence of cerebral palsy at twelve months.

Twenty-four month adjusted-age evaluations were completed in 429 (226 treated) of 906 surviving infants. There were significantly fewer SURVANTA infants with rhonchi, wheezing, and tachypnea at the time of examination. No other differences were found.

OVERDOSAGE

Overdosage with SURVANTA has not been reported. Based on animal data, overdosage might result in acute airway obstruction. Treatment should be symptomatic and supportive.

Rales and moist breath sounds can transiently occur after SURVANTA is given, and do not indicate overdosage. Endotracheal suctioning or other remedial action is not required unless clear-cut signs of airway obstruction are present.

DOSAGE AND ADMINISTRATION

FOR INTRATRACHEAL ADMINISTRATION ONLY.

SURVANTA should be administered by or under the supervision of clinicians experienced in intubation, ventilator management, and general care of premature infants.

Marked improvements in oxygenation may occur within minutes of administration of SURVANTA. Therefore, frequent and careful clinical observation and monitoring of systemic oxygenation are essential to avoid hyperoxia.

Review of audiovisual instructional materials describing dosage and administration procedures is recommended before using SURVANTA. Materials are available upon request from Ross Products Division, Abbott Laboratories Inc.

Dosage

Each dose of SURVANTA is 100 mg of phospholipids/kg birth weight (4 mL/kg). The SURVANTA DOSING CHART shows the total dosage for a range of birth weights.

SURVANTA DOSING CHART

WEIGHT (grams)	TOTAL DOSE (mL)	WEIGHT (grams)	TOTAL DOSE (mL)
600- 650	2.6	1301-1350	5.4
651- 700	2.8	1351-1400	5.6
701- 750	3.0	1401-1450	5.8
751- 800	3.2	1451-1500	6.0
801- 850	3.4	1501-1550	6.2
851- 900	3.6	1551-1600	6.4
901- 950	3.8	1601-1650	6.6
951-1000	4.0	1651-1700	6.8
1001-1050	4.2	1701-1750	7.0
1051-1100	4.4	1751-1800	7.2
1101-1150	4.6	1801-1850	7.4
1151-1200	4.8	1851-1900	7.6
1201-1250	5.0	1901-1950	7.8
1251-1300	5.2	1951-2000	8.0

Four doses of SURVANTA can be administered in the first 48 hours of life. Doses should be given no more frequently than every 6 hours.

Directions for Use

SURVANTA should be inspected visually for discoloration prior to administration. The color of SURVANTA is off-white to light brown. If settling occurs during storage, swirl the vial gently (DO NOT SHAKE) to redisperse. Some foaming at the surface may occur during handling and is inherent in the nature of the product.

SURVANTA is stored refrigerated (2–8°C). Date and time need to be recorded in the box on front of the carton or vial, whenever SURVANTA is removed from the refrigerator. Before administration, SURVANTA should be warmed by standing at room temperature for at least 20 minutes or warmed in the hand for at least 8 minutes. ARTIFICIAL WARMING METHODS SHOULD NOT BE USED. If a prevention dose is to be given, preparation of SURVANTA should begin before the infant's birth.

Unopened, unused vials of SURVANTA that have been warmed to room temperature may be returned to the refrigerator within 24 hours of warming, and stored for future use. SURVANTA SHOULD NOT BE REMOVED FROM THE REFRIGERATOR FOR MORE THAN 24 HOURS. SURVANTA SHOULD NOT BE WARMED AND RETURNED TO THE REFRIGERATOR MORE THAN ONCE.

Each single-use vial of SURVANTA should be entered only once. Used vials with residual drug should be discarded.

SURVANTA DOES NOT REQUIRE RECONSTITUTION OR SONICATION BEFORE USE.

Dosing Procedures

General

SURVANTA is administered intratracheally by instillation through a 5 French end-hole catheter. The catheter can be inserted into the infant's endotracheal tube without interrupting ventilation by passing the catheter through a neonatal suction valve attached to the endotracheal tube. Alternatively, SURVANTA can be instilled through the catheter by briefly disconnecting the endotracheal tube from the ventilator.

The neonatal suction valve used for administering SURVANTA should be a type that allows entry of the catheter into the endotracheal tube without interrupting ventilation and also maintains a closed airway circuit system by sealing the valve around the catheter.

If the neonatal suction valve is used, the catheter should be rigid enough to pass easily into the endotracheal tube. A very soft and pliable catheter may twist or curl within the neonatal suction valve. The length of the catheter should be shortened so that the tip of the catheter protrudes just beyond the end of the endotracheal tube above the infant's carina. SURVANTA should not be instilled into a mainstem bronchus.

To ensure homogenous distribution of SURVANTA throughout the lungs, each dose is divided into *four quarter-doses.* Each quarter-dose is administered with the infant in a different position. The recommended positions are:

- Head and body inclined 5–10° down, head turned to the right
- Head and body inclined 5–10° down, head turned to the left
- Head and body inclined 5–10° up, head turned to the right
- Head and body inclined 5–10° up, head turned to the left

The dosing procedure is facilitated if one person administers the dose while another person positions and monitors the infant.

First Dose

Determine the total dose of SURVANTA from the SURVANTA DOSING CHART based on the infant's birth weight. Slowly withdraw the entire contents of the vial into a plastic syringe through a large-gauge needle (eg, at least 20 gauge). DO NOT FILTER SURVANTA AND AVOID SHAKING.

Attach the premeasured 5 French end-hole catheter to the syringe. Fill the catheter with SURVANTA. Discard excess SURVANTA through the catheter so that only the total dose to be given remains in the syringe.

BEFORE ADMINISTERING SURVANTA, assure proper placement and patency of the endotracheal tube. At the discretion of the clinician, the endotracheal tube may be suctioned before administering SURVANTA. The infant should be allowed to stabilize before proceeding with dosing.

In the prevention strategy, weigh, intubate and stabilize the infant. Administer the dose as soon as possible after birth, preferably within 15 minutes. Position the infant appropriately and gently inject the first quarter-dose through the catheter over 2-3 seconds.

After administration of the first quarter-dose, remove the catheter from the endotracheal tube. Manually ventilate with a hand-bag with sufficient oxygen to prevent cyanosis, at a rate of 60 breaths/minute, and sufficient positive pressure to provide adequate air exchange and chest wall excursion.

In the rescue strategy, the first dose should be given as soon as possible after the infant is placed on a ventilator for management of RDS. In the clinical trials, immediately before instilling the first quarter-dose, the infant's ventilator settings were changed to rate 60/minute, inspiratory time 0.5 second, and FiO_2 1.0.

Position the infant appropriately and gently inject the first quarter-dose through the catheter over 2–3 seconds. After administration of the first quarter-dose, remove the catheter from the endotracheal tube and continue mechanical ventilation.

In both strategies, ventilate the infant for at least 30 seconds or until stable. Reposition the infant for instillation of the next quarter-dose.

Instill the remaining quarter-doses using the same procedures. After instillation of each quarter-dose, remove the catheter and ventilate for at least 30 seconds or until the infant is stabilized. After instillation of the final quarter-dose, remove the catheter without flushing it. Do not suction the infant for 1 hour after dosing unless signs of significant airway obstruction occur.

AFTER COMPLETION OF THE DOSING PROCEDURE, RESUME USUAL VENTILATOR MANAGEMENT AND CLINICAL CARE.

Repeat Doses

The dosage of SURVANTA for repeat doses is also 100 mg phospholipids/kg and is based on the infant's birth weight. The infant should not be reweighed for determination of the SURVANTA dosage. Use the SURVANTA DOSING CHART to determine the total dosage.

The need for additional doses of SURVANTA is determined by evidence of continuing respiratory distress. Using the following criteria for redosing, significant reductions in mortality due to RDS were observed in the multiple-dose clinical trials with SURVANTA.

Dose no sooner than 6 hours after the preceding dose if the infant remains intubated and requires at least 30% inspired oxygen to maintain a PaO_2 less than or equal to 80 torr.

Radiographic confirmation of RDS should be obtained before administering additional doses to those who received a prevention dose.

Prepare SURVANTA and position the infant for administration of each quarter-dose as previously described. After instillation of each quarter-dose, remove the dosing catheter from the endotracheal tube and ventilate the infant for at least 30 seconds or until stable.

In the clinical studies, ventilator settings used to administer repeat doses were different than those used for the first dose. For repeat doses, the FiO_2 was increased by 0.20 or an amount sufficient to prevent cyanosis. The ventilator delivered a rate of 30/minute with an inspiratory time less than 1.0 second. If the infant's pretreatment rate was 30 or greater, it was left unchanged during SURVANTA instillation.

Manual hand-bag ventilation should not be used to administer repeat doses. DURING THE DOSING PROCEDURE, VENTILATOR SETTINGS MAY BE ADJUSTED AT THE DISCRETION OF THE CLINICIAN TO MAINTAIN APPROPRIATE OXYGENATION AND VENTILATION.

AFTER COMPLETION OF THE DOSING PROCEDURE, RESUME USUAL VENTILATOR MANAGEMENT AND CLINICAL CARE.

Dosing Precautions

If an infant experiences bradycardia or oxygen desaturation during the dosing procedure, stop the dosing procedure and initiate appropriate measures to alleviate the condition. After the infant has stabilized, resume the dosing procedure.

Rales and moist breath sounds can occur transiently after administration of SURVANTA. Endotracheal suctioning or other remedial action is unnecessary unless clear-cut signs of airway obstruction are present.

HOW SUPPLIED

SURVANTA (beractant) Intratracheal Suspension is supplied in single-use glass vials containing 4 mL (NDC 0074-1040-04) or 8 mL (NDC 0074-1040-08) of SURVANTA. Each milliliter contains 25 mg of phospholipids suspended in 0.9% sodium chloride solution. The color is off-white to light brown.

Store unopened vials at refrigeration temperature (2-8°C). Protect from light. Store vials in carton until ready for use. Vials are for single use only. Upon opening, discard unused drug.

October, 1999

Shown in Product Identification Guide, page 332

PEDIAFLOR® Drops ℞
Sodium Fluoride Oral Solution, USP
1.7 fl oz (50 mL) bottles, calibrated dropper

VI-DAYLIN® ADC VITAMINS Drops OTC
Dietary Supplement of Vitamins A, D, and C
50 mL Spil-gard® bottles, calibrated dropper

VI-DAYLIN® ADC VITAMINS + IRON Drops OTC
Dietary Supplement of Vitamins A, D, and C with Iron
50 mL Spil-gard® bottles, calibrated dropper

VI-DAYLIN® MULTIVITAMIN Drops OTC
Multivitamin Supplement
50 mL Spil-gard® bottles, calibrated dropper

VI-DAYLIN® MULTIVITAMIN + IRON Drops OTC
Multivitamin/Iron Supplement
50 mL Spil-gard® bottles, calibrated dropper

VI-DAYLIN®/F ADC VITAMINS Drops With Fluoride ℞
ADC Vitamins/Fluoride
50 mL Spil-gard® bottles, calibrated dropper

VI-DAYLIN®/F ADC VITAMINS + IRON Drops With Fluoride ℞
ADC Vitamins/Fluoride/Iron Supplement
50 mL Spil-gard® bottles, calibrated dropper

VI-DAYLIN®/F MULTIVITAMIN Drops With Fluoride ℞
Multivitamins/Fluoride
50 mL Spil-gard® bottles, calibrated dropper

VI-DAYLIN®/F MULTIVITAMIN + IRON Drops With Fluoride ℞
Multivitamins/Fluoride/Iron Supplement
50 mL Spil-gard® bottles, calibrated dropper

VI-DAYLIN® MULTIVITAMIN Liquid OTC
Multivitamin Supplement
16-fl-oz (473 mL) bottles
8-fl-oz (237 mL) bottles

VI-DAYLIN® MULTIVITAMIN + IRON Liquid OTC
Multivitamin/Iron Supplement
16-fl-oz (473 mL) bottles
8-fl-oz (237 mL) bottles

EDUCATIONAL MATERIAL

A complete program of educational services for health care professionals and patients is available.
Contact your local Ross representative.

For information on over-the-counter drugs, consult PDR For Nonprescription Drugs and Dietary Supplements.

Roxane Laboratories, Inc.

P.O. BOX 16532
COLUMBUS, OH 43216-6532

Direct Inquiries to:
Technical Product Information
P.O. Box 16532
Columbus, OH 43216-6532
1-800-962-8364

ROXANE LABORATORIES, INC PRODUCT LIST

Acetylcysteine Solution USP 10%, 20%
Alprazolam Intensol™ Oral Solution (Concentrate) CIV 1mg/mL
Azathioprine Tablets USP 50mg
Butorphanol Tartrate Nasal Spray CIV 10mg/mL
Calcitriol Oral Solution 1 mcg/mL
Calcium Carbonate Tablets USP 1250mg
Calcium Carbonate Oral Suspension (not USP) 1250mg/5mL
Calcium Gluconate Tablets USP 500mg
Clotrimazole Troche 10 mg
Cocaine Hydrochloride Topical Solution CII 4%,10%
Codeine Sulfate Tablets USP CII 15mg, 30mg, 60mg
Cromolyn Sodium Inhalation Solution USP 20mg/2mL
Cyclophosphamide Tablets USP 25mg, 50mg
Dexamethasone Intensol™ Oral Solution (Concentrate) 1 mg per mL
Dexamethasone Oral Solution 0.5mg/5mL
Dexamethasone Tablets USP 0.5 mg, 0.75mg, 1mg, 1.5mg, 2mg, 4mg, 6mg
Diazepam Intensol™ Oral Solution (Concentrate) CIV 5 mg/mL
Diazepam Oral Solution USP CIV 5 mg/5 mL
Diclofenac Sodium Delayed-Release Tablets USP 50mg, 75mg
Digoxin Elixir USP 0.05mg/mL
DHT™ Dihydrotachysterol Tablets USP 0.125mg, 0.4mg
DHT™ Intensol™ Oral Solution (Concentrate) 0.2 mg/mL
Diphenoxylate Hydrochloride and Atropine Sulfate Oral Solution USP CV 2mg/0.02mg/4mL, 2.5mg/0.025mg/5mL, 5mg/0.05mg/10mL
Dolophine® Hydrochloride Tablets (Methadone Hydrochloride Tablets USP) CII 5mg, 10mg
Flecainide Acetate Tablets USP 50mg, 100mg, 150mg
Fluconazole Tablets, 100mg, 150mg, 200mg
Furosemide Oral Solution USP 10mg/mL, 40mg/5mL
Furosemide Tablets USP 20mg, 40mg, 80mg
Hydromorphone Hydrochloride Tablets USP CII 2mg, 4mg, 8 mg
Ipratropium Bromide Nasal Spray 0.03% (21mcg/spray), 0.06% (42mcg/spray)
Lactulose Solution USP 10g/15mL
Leucovorin Calcium Tablets USP 5mg, 10mg, 15mg, 25mg
Levorphanol Tartrate Tablets USP CII 2 mg
Lidocaine Viscous 2% (Lidocaine Hydrochloride Oral Topical Solution USP 2%)
Lidocaine Hydrochloride Topical Solution USP 4%
Lithium Carbonate Capsules USP 150mg, 300mg, 600mg
Lithium Carbonate Tablets USP 300mg
Lithium Carbonate Extended Release Tablets USP 450mg
Lithium Citrate Syrup USP 8mEq per 5mL, 16mEq per 10mL
Loperamide Hydrochloride Oral Solution 1mg/5mL
Lorazepam Intensol™ Oral Concentrate USP CIV 2mg/mL
Megestrol Acetate Oral Suspension USP 40mg/mL
Megestrol Acetate Tablets USP 20mg, 40mg
Meperidine Hydrochloride Tablets USP CII 100mg
Meperidine Hydrochloride Syrup USP CII 50mg/5mL
Mercaptopurine Tablets USP, 50mg
Methadone Hydrochloride Intensol™ Oral Concentrate USP CII 10mg/mL
Methadone Hydrochloride Tablets USP CII 5mg, 10mg
Methadone Hydrochloride Oral Solution USP CII 5mg/5mL, 10mg/5mL
Methotrexate Tablets USP 2.5mg
Mexiletine Hydrochloride Capsules USP 150mg, 200mg, 250mg
Midazolam Hydrochloride Syrup CIV 2mg/mL
Milk of Magnesia Concentrated (Lemon Flavored) 100mL, 400mL
Mirtazapine Tablets 15 mg, 30 mg, 45 mg
Morphine Sulfate (Immediate Release) Tablets CII 15mg, 30mg
Morphine Sulfate (Immediate Release) Oral Solution CII 10mg/5mL, 20mg/10mL, 20mg/5mL
Naproxen Oral Suspension USP 125mg/5mL
Oxycodone and Acetaminophen Capsules USP CII 5mg/500mg
PredniSONE Intensol™ Oral Solution (Concentrate) 5mg/mL
PredniSONE Oral Solution USP 5mg/5mL
PredniSONE Tablets USP 1mg, 2.5mg, 5mg, 10mg, 20mg, 50mg
Propantheline Bromide Tablets USP 15mg
Propranolol Hydrochloride Oral Solution 20mg/5mL and 40mg/5 mL
Pseudoephedrine Hydrochloride Tablets USP 30mg, 60mg
Roxicet™ Oral Solution (Oxycodone Hydrochloride 5mg and Acetaminophen 325mg/5mL) CII
Roxicet™ Tablets (Oxycodone 5mg and Acetaminophen 325mg Tablets USP) CII
Roxicet 5/500™ Caplets (Oxycodone HCl 5mg and Acetaminophen Tablets 500mg USP) CII
Saliva Substitute
Sodium Polystyrene Sulfonate Suspension USP 15g/60mL; 30g/120mL and 50g/200mL
Tamoxifen Citrate Tablets USP 10mg, 20mg
Triazolam Tablets USP CIV 0.125mg, 0.25mg

Salix Pharmaceuticals, Inc.

8540 COLONNADE CENTER DR.
SUITE 501
RALEIGH, NC 27615

Direct Inquiries to:
(866) 669-7597 Phone
(919) 862-1095 Fax
www.salix.com

For adverse events, product quality complaints and patient information requests:
Product Information Center
(800) 508-0024 Phone
(510) 595-8183 Fax
E-mail: medical.affairs@salix.com

AZASAN® ℞

[*ayz-uh-san*]
Azathioprine Tablets, USP
25 mg Scored Tablets
75 mg Scored Tablets
100 mg Scored Tablets

> **WARNING:** Chronic immunosuppression with this purine antimetabolite increases *risk of neoplasia* in humans. Physicians using this drug should be very familiar with this risk as well as with the mutagenic potential to both men and women and with possible hematologic toxicities. See WARNINGS.

DESCRIPTION

AZASAN®, an immunosuppressive antimetabolite, is available in tablet form for oral administration. Each scored tablet contains 25 mg, 75 mg or 100 mg azathioprine and the inactive ingredients lactose monohydrate, pregelatinized starch, povidone, corn starch, magnesium stearate, and stearic acid.

Azathioprine is chemically 1*H*-purine, 6-[(1-methyl-4-nitro-1*H*-imidazol-5-yl)thio]-. The structural formula of azathioprine is:

$C_9H_7N_7O_2S$ M.W.277.27

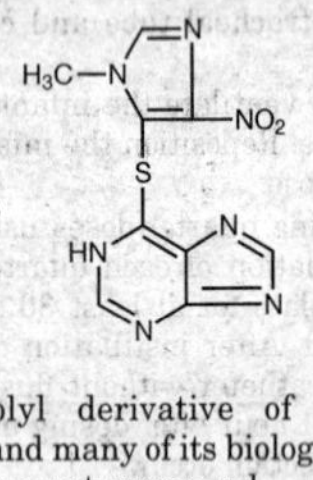

It is an imidazolyl derivative of 6-mercaptopurine (PURINETHOL®) and many of its biological effects are similar to those of the parent compound.

Azathioprine is insoluble in water, but may be dissolved with addition of one molar equivalent of alkali. The sodium salt of azathioprine is sufficiently soluble to make a 10 mg/mL water solution which is stable for 24 hours at 59° to 77°F (15° to 25°C). Azathioprine is stable in solution at neutral or acid pH but hydrolysis to mercaptopurine occurs in excess sodium hydroxide (0.1N), especially on warming. Conversion to mercaptopurine also occurs in the presence of sulfhydryl compounds such as cysteine, glutathione, and hydrogen sulfide.

CLINICAL PHARMACOLOGY

Metabolism: Azathioprine is well absorbed following oral administration. Maximum serum radioactivity occurs at 1 to 2 hours after oral ^{35}S-azathioprine and decays with a half-life of 5 hours. This is not an estimate of the half-life of azathioprine itself but is the decay rate for all ^{35}S-containing metabolites of the drug. Because of extensive metabolism, only a fraction of the radioactivity is present as azathioprine. Usual doses produce blood levels of azathioprine, and of mercaptopurine derived from it, which are low (<1 mcg/mL). Blood levels are of little predictive value for therapy since the magnitude and duration of clinical effects correlate with thiopurine nucleotide levels in tissues rather than with plasma drug levels. Azathioprine and mercaptopurine are moderately bound to serum proteins (30%) and are partially dialyzable.

Azathioprine is cleaved in vivo to mercaptopurine. Both compounds are rapidly eliminated from blood and are oxidized or methylated in erythrocytes and liver; no azathioprine or mercaptopurine is detectable in urine after 8 hours. Conversion to inactive 6-thiouric acid by xanthine oxidase is an important degradative pathway, and the inhibition of this pathway in patients receiving allopurinol is the basis for the azathioprine dosage reduction required in these patients (see PRECAUTIONS: Drug Interactions). Proportions of metabolites are different in individual patients, and this presumably accounts for variable magnitude and duration of drug effects. Renal clearance is probably not important in predicting biological effectiveness or toxicities, although dose reduction is practiced in patients with poor renal function.

Homograft Survival: Summary information from transplant centers and registries indicates relatively universal use of AZASAN® with or without other immunosuppressive agents. Although the use of azathioprine for inhibition of renal homograft rejection is well established, the mechanism(s) for this action are somewhat obscure. The drug suppresses hypersensitivities of the cell-mediated type and causes variable alterations in antibody production. Suppression of T-cell effects, including ablation of T-cell suppression, is dependent on the temporal relationship to antigenic stimulus or engraftment. This agent has little effect on established graft rejections or secondary responses.

Alterations in specific immune responses or immunologic functions in transplant recipients are difficult to relate specifically to immunosuppression by azathioprine. These patients have subnormal responses to vaccines, low numbers of T-cells, and abnormal phagocytosis by peripheral blood cells, but their mitogenic responses, serum immunoglobulins, and secondary antibody responses are usually normal.

Immunoinflammatory Response: Azathioprine suppresses disease manifestations as well as underlying pathology in animal models of autoimmune disease. For example, the severity of adjuvant arthritis is reduced by azathioprine.

The mechanisms whereby azathioprine affects autoimmune diseases are not known. Azathioprine is immunosuppressive, delayed hypersensitivity and cellular cytotoxicity tests being suppressed to a greater degree than are antibody responses. In the rat model of adjuvant arthritis, azathioprine has been shown to inhibit the lymph node hyperplasia which precedes the onset of the signs of the disease. Both the immunosuppressive and therapeutic effects in animal models are dose-related. Azathioprine is considered a slow-acting drug and effects may persist after the drug has been discontinued.

INDICATIONS AND USAGE

AZASAN® is indicated as an adjunct for the prevention of rejection in renal homotransplantation. It is also indicated for the management of severe, active rheumatoid arthritis unresponsive to rest, aspirin, or other nonsteroidal anti-inflammatory drugs, or to agents in the class of which gold is an example.

Renal Homotransplantation: AZASAN® is indicated as an adjunct for the prevention of rejection in renal homotransplantation. Experience with over 16,000 transplants shows a 5-year patient survival of 35% to 55%, but this is dependent on donor, match for HLA antigens, anti-donor and anti B-cell alloantigen antibody, and other variables. The effect of azathioprine on these variables has not been tested in controlled trials.

Rheumatoid Arthritis: AZASAN® is indicated only in adult patients meeting criteria for classic or definite rheumatoid arthritis as specified by the American Rheumatism Association. AZASAN® should be restricted to patients with severe, active and erosive disease not responsive to conventional management including rest, aspirin, or other nonsteroidal drugs or to agents in the class of which gold is an example. Rest, physiotherapy, and salicylates should be continued while AZASAN® is given, but it may be possible to reduce the dose of corticosteroids in patients on AZASAN®. The combined use of AZASAN® with gold, antimalarials, or penicillamine has not been studied for either added benefit or unexpected adverse effects. The use of AZASAN® with these agents cannot be recommended.

CONTRAINDICATIONS

AZASAN® should not be given to patients who have shown hypersensitivity to the drug.

AZASAN® should not be used for treating rheumatoid arthritis in pregnant women.

Patients with rheumatoid arthritis previously treated with alkylating agents (cyclophosphamide, chlorambucil, melphalan, or others) may have a prohibitive risk of neoplasia if treated with AZASAN®.

WARNINGS

Severe *leukopenia, thrombocytopenia, macrocytic anemia,* and/or *pancytopenia* may occur in patients on AZASAN®. Severe bone marrow depression may also occur. Individuals with inherited low or absent thiopurine methyltransferase (TPMT) activity may be at increased risk of developing severe, life-threatening myelotoxicity from AZASAN®. Prospective TPMT genotyping or phenotyping may help identify such patients.

Hematologic toxicities are dose related and may be more severe in renal transplant patients whose homograft is undergoing rejection. It is suggested that patients on AZASAN® have complete blood counts, including platelet counts, weekly during the first month, twice monthly for the second and third months of treatment, then monthly or more frequently if dosage alterations or other therapy changes are necessary. Delayed hematologic suppression may occur. Prompt reduction in dosage or temporary withdrawal of the drug may be necessary if there is a rapid fall in, or persistently low leukocyte count, or other evidence of bone marrow depression. Leukopenia does not correlate with therapeutic effect; therefore, the dose should not be increased intentionally to lower the white blood cell count.

Serious infections are a constant hazard for patients receiving chronic immunosuppression, especially for homograft recipients. Fungal, viral, bacterial, and protozoal infections may be fatal and should be treated vigorously. Reduction of azathioprine dosage and/or use of other drugs should be considered.

AZASAN® is mutagenic in animals and humans, carcinogenic in animals, and may increase the patient's *risk of neoplasia*. Renal transplant patients are known to have an increased risk of malignancy, predominantly skin cancer and reticulum cell or lymphomatous tumors. The risk of post-transplant lymphomas may be increased in patients who receive aggressive treatment with immunosuppressive drugs. The degree of immunosuppression is determined not only by the immunosuppressive regimen but also by a number of other patient factors. The number of immunosuppressive agents may not necessarily increase the risk of post-transplant lymphomas. However, transplant patients who receive multiple immunosuppressive agents may be at risk for over-immunosuppression; therefore, immunosuppressive drug therapy should be maintained at the lowest effective levels. Information is available on the spontaneous neoplasia risk in rheumatoid arthritis, and on neoplasia following immunosuppressive therapy of other autoimmune disease. It has not been possible to define the precise *risk of neoplasia* due to AZASAN®. The data suggest the risk may be elevated in patients with rheumatoid arthritis, though lower than for renal transplant patients. However, acute myelogenous leukemia as well as solid tumors have been reported in patients with rheumatoid arthritis who have received azathioprine. Data on neoplasia in patients receiving AZASAN® can be found under ADVERSE REACTIONS.

AZASAN® has been reported to cause temporary depression in spermatogenesis and reduction in sperm viability and sperm count in mice at doses 10 times the human therapeutic dose; a reduced percentage of fertile matings occurred when animals received 5 mg/kg.

Pregnancy: Pregnancy Category D. AZASAN® can cause fetal harm when administered to a pregnant woman. AZASAN® should not be given during pregnancy without careful weighing of risk versus benefit. Whenever possible, use of AZASAN® in pregnant patients should be avoided. This drug should not be used for treating rheumatoid arthritis in pregnant women.

AZASAN® is teratogenic in rabbits and mice when given in doses equivalent to the human dose (5 mg/kg daily). Abnormalities included skeletal malformations and visceral anomalies.

Limited immunologic and other abnormalities have occurred in a few infants born of renal allograft recipients on AZASAN®. In a detailed case report, documented lymphopenia, diminished IgG and IgM levels, CMV infection, and a decreased thymic shadow were noted in an infant born to a mother receiving 150 mg azathioprine and 30 mg prednisone daily throughout pregnancy. At 10 weeks most features were normalized. DeWitte et al reported pancytopenia and severe immune deficiency in a preterm infant whose mother received 125 mg azathioprine and 12.5 mg prednisone daily. There have been two published reports of abnormal physical findings. Williamson and Karp described an infant born with preaxial polydactyly whose mother received azathioprine 200 mg daily and prednisone 20 mg every other day during pregnancy. Tallent et al described an infant with a large myelomeningocele in the upper lumbar region, bilateral dislocated hips, and bilateral talipes equinovarus. The father was on long-term azathioprine therapy.

Benefit versus risk must be weighed carefully before use of AZASAN® in patients of reproductive potential. There are no adequate and well-controlled studies in pregnant women. If this drug is used during pregnancy or if the patient becomes pregnant while taking this drug, the patient should be apprised of the potential hazard to the fetus. Women of childbearing age should be advised to avoid becoming pregnant.

PRECAUTIONS

General: A gastrointestinal hypersensitivity reaction characterized by severe nausea and vomiting has been reported. These symptoms may also be accompanied by diarrhea, rash, fever, malaise, myalgias, elevations in liver enzymes, and occasionally, hypotension. Symptoms of gastrointestinal toxicity most often develop within the first several weeks of AZASAN® therapy and are reversible upon discontinuation of the drug. The reaction can recur within hours after rechallenge with a single dose of AZASAN®.

Information for Patients: Patients being started on AZASAN® should be informed of the necessity of periodic blood counts while they are receiving the drug and should be encouraged to report any unusual bleeding or bruising to their physician. They should be informed of the danger of infection while receiving AZASAN® and asked to report signs and symptoms of infection to their physician. Careful dosage instructions should be given to the patient, especially when AZASAN® is being administered in the presence of impaired renal function or concomitantly with allopurinol (see PRECAUTIONS - Drug Interactions subsection and DOSAGE AND ADMINISTRATION). Patients should be advised of the potential risks of the use of AZASAN® during pregnancy and during the nursing period. The increased risk of neoplasia following therapy with AZASAN® should be explained to the patient.

Laboratory Tests: See WARNINGS and ADVERSE REACTIONS sections.

Drug Interactions:

Use with Allopurinol: The principal pathway for detoxification of AZASAN® is inhibited by allopurinol. Patients receiving AZASAN® and allopurinol concomitantly should have a dose reduction of AZASAN®, to approximately 1/3 to 1/4 the usual dose.

Use with Other Agents Affecting Myelopoiesis: Drugs which may affect leukocyte production, including co-trimoxazole, may lead to exaggerated leukopenia, especially in renal transplant recipients.

Use with Angiotensin-Converting Enzyme Inhibitors: The use of angiotensin-converting enzyme inhibitors to control hypertension in patients on azathioprine has been reported to induce severe leukopenia.

Carcinogenesis, Mutagenesis, Impairment of Fertility: See WARNINGS section.

Pregnancy: ***Teratogenic Effects:*** Pregnancy Category D. See WARNINGS section.

Nursing Mothers: The use of AZASAN® in nursing mothers is not recommended. Azathioprine or its metabolites are transferred at low levels both transplacentally and in breast milk. Because of the potential for tumorgenicity shown for azathioprine, a decision should be made whether to discontinue nursing or discontinue the drug, taking into account the importance of the drug to the mother.

Pediatric Use: Safety and efficacy of azathioprine in pediatric patients have not been established.

ADVERSE REACTIONS

The principal and potentially serious toxic effects of AZASAN® are hematologic and gastrointestinal. The risks of secondary infection and neoplasia are also significant (see WARNINGS). The frequency and severity of adverse reactions depend on the dose and duration of AZASAN® as well as on the patient's underlying disease or concomitant therapies. The incidence of hematologic toxicities and neoplasia encountered in groups of renal homograft recipients is significantly higher than that in studies employing AZASAN® for rheumatoid arthritis. The relative incidences in clinical studies are summarized below:

Toxicity	Renal Homograft	Rheumatoid Arthritis
Leukopenia		
Any Degree	>50%	28%
<2500/mm^3	16%	5.3%
Infections	20%	<1%
Neoplasia		*
Lymphoma	0.5%	
Others	2.8%	

*Data on the rate and risk of neoplasia among persons with rheumatoid arthritis treated with azathioprine are limited. The incidence of lymphoproliferative disease in patients with RA appears to be significantly higher than that in the general population. In one completed study, the rate of lymphoproliferative disease in RA patients receiving higher than recommended doses of azathioprine (5 mg/kg/day) was 1.8 cases per 1000 patient years of follow-up, compared with 0.8 cases per 1000 patient years of follow-up in those not receiving azathioprine. However, the proportion of the increased risk attributable to the azathioprine dosage or to other therapies (i.e., alkylating agents) received by azathioprine-treated patients cannot be determined.

Hematologic: Leukopenia and/or thrombocytopenia are dose dependent and may occur late in the course of therapy with AZASAN®. Dose reduction or temporary withdrawal allows reversal of these toxicities. Infection may occur as a secondary manifestation of bone marrow suppression or leukopenia, but the incidence of infection in renal homotransplantation is 30 to 60 times that in rheumatoid arthritis. Macrocytic anemia and/or bleeding have been reported in two patients on azathioprine.

Gastrointestinal: Nausea and vomiting may occur within the first few months of AZASAN® therapy, and occurred in approximately 12% of 676 rheumatoid arthritis patients. The frequency of gastric disturbance often can be reduced by administration of the drug in divided doses and/or after meals. However, in some patients, nausea and vomiting may be severe and may be accompanied by symptoms such as diarrhea, fever, malaise, and myalgias (see PRECAUTIONS). Vomiting with abdominal pain may occur rarely with a hypersensitivity pancreatitis. Hepatotoxicity manifest by elevation of serum alkaline phosphatase, bilirubin, and/or serum transaminases is known to occur following azathioprine use, primarily in allograft recipients. Hepatotoxicity has been uncommon (less than 1%) in rheumatoid arthritis patients. Hepatotoxicity following transplantation most often occurs within 6 months of transplantation and is generally reversible after interruption of AZASAN®. A rare, but life-threatening hepatic veno-occlusive disease associated with chronic administration of azathioprine has been described in transplant patients and in one patient receiving azathioprine for panuveitis. Periodic measurement of serum transaminases, alkaline phosphatase, and bilirubin is indicated for early detection of hepatotoxicity. If hepatic veno-occlusive disease is clinically suspected, AZASAN® should be permanently withdrawn.

Others: Additional side effects of low frequency have been reported. These include skin rashes (approximately 2%), alopecia, fever, arthralgias, diarrhea, steatorrhea and negative nitrogen balance (all less than 1%).

OVERDOSAGE

The oral LD_{50}s for single doses of AZASAN® in mice and rats are 2500 mg/kg and 400 mg/kg, respectively. Very large doses of this antimetabolite may lead to marrow hypoplasia, bleeding, infection, and death. About 30% of AZASAN® is bound to serum proteins, but approximately 45% is removed during an 8-hour hemodialysis. A single case has been reported of a renal transplant patient who ingested a single dose of 7500 mg azathioprine. The immediate toxic reactions were nausea, vomiting, and diarrhea, followed by mild leukopenia and mild abnormalities in liver function. The white blood cell count, SGOT, and bilirubin returned to normal 6 days after the overdose.

DOSAGE AND ADMINISTRATION

Renal Homotransplantation: The dose of AZASAN® required to prevent rejection and minimize toxicity will vary with individual patients; this necessitates careful management. The initial dose is usually 3 to 5 mg/kg daily, beginning at the time of transplant. AZASAN® is usually given as a single daily dose on the day of, and in a minority of cases 1 to 3 days before, transplantation. AZASAN® is often initiated with the intravenous administration of the sodium salt, with subsequent use of tablets (at the same dose level) after the postoperative period. Intravenous administration of the sodium salt is indicated only in patients unable to tolerate oral medications. Dose reduction to maintenance levels of 1 to 3 mg/kg daily is usually possible. The dose of AZASAN® should not be increased to toxic levels because of threatened rejection. Discontinuation may be necessary for severe hematologic or other toxicity, even if rejection of the homograft may be a consequence of drug withdrawal.

Rheumatoid Arthritis: AZASAN® is usually given on a daily basis. The initial dose should be approximately 1 mg/kg (50 to 100 mg) given as a single dose or on a twice daily schedule. The dose may be increased, beginning at 6 to 8 weeks and thereafter by steps at 4-week intervals, if there are no serious toxicities and if initial response is unsatisfactory. Dose increments should be 0.5 mg/kg daily, up to a maximum dose of 2.5 mg/kg/day. Therapeutic response occurs after several weeks of treatment, usually 6 to 8; an adequate trial should be a minimum of 12 weeks. Patients not improved after 12 weeks can be considered refractory. AZASAN® may be continued long-term in patients with clinical response, but patients should be monitored carefully, and gradual dosage reduction should be attempted to reduce risk of toxicities.

Maintenance therapy should be at the lowest effective dose, and the dose given can be lowered decrementally with changes of 0.5 mg/kg or approximately 25 mg daily every 4 weeks while other therapy is kept constant. The optimum duration of maintenance AZASAN® has not been determined. AZASAN® can be discontinued abruptly, but delayed effects are possible.

Use in Renal Dysfunction: Relatively oliguric patients, especially those with tubular necrosis in the immediate post-cadaveric transplant period, may have delayed clearance of AZASAN® or its metabolites, may be particularly sensitive to this drug, and are usually given lower doses.

Procedures for proper handling and disposal of this immunosuppressive antimetabolite drug should be considered. Several guidelines on this subject have been published.[1-7] There is no general agreement that all of the procedures recommended in the guideline are necessary or appropriate.

HOW SUPPLIED

AZASAN® Tablets, USP are available in:

25 mg, oval-shaped, yellow, scored tablets,
- 100 count bottles (NDC 65649-251-41)
- 15 count samples (NDC 65649-251-51)

75 mg, triangle-shaped, yellow, scored tablets,
- 100 count bottles (NDC 65649-231-41)
- 15 count samples (NDC 65649-231-51)

100 mg, diamond-shaped, yellow, scored tablets,
- 100 count bottles (NDC 65649-241-41)
- 15 count samples (NDC 65649-241-51)

Rx only.

Store at 20° to 25°C (68° to 77° F) [See USP Controlled Room Temperature]

Store in a dry place and protect from light.

Dispense in a tight, light-resistant container as defined in the USP.

REFERENCES

1. Recommendations for the Safe Handling of Parenteral Antineoplastic Drugs, NIH Publication No. 83-2621. For sale by the Superintendent of Documents, U.S. Government Printing Office, Washington, DC 20402.
2. AMA Council Report, Guidelines for Handling Parenteral Antineoplastics. *JAMA*, 1985;253(11):1590-1592.
3. National Study Commission on Cytotoxic Exposure - Recommendations for Handling Cytotoxic Agents. Available from Louis P. Jeffrey, ScD., Chairman, National Study Commission on Cytotoxic Exposure, Massachusetts College of Pharmacy and Allied Health Sciences, 179 Longwood Avenue, Boston, Massachusetts 02115.

Continued on next page

Azasan—Cont.

4. Clinical Oncological Society of Australia, Guidelines and Recommendations for Safe Handling of Antineoplastic Agents. Med J Australia, 1983;1:426-428.
5. Jones RB, et al: Safe Handling of Chemotherapeutic Agents: A Report from the Mount Sinai Medical Center. *CA-A Cancer Journal for Clinicians*, 1983;(Sept/Oct) 258-263.
6. American Society of Hospital Pharmacists Technical Assistance Bulletin on Handling Cytotoxic and Hazardous Drugs. *Am J Hosp Pharm*, 1990;47:1033-1049.
7. OSHA Work-Practice Guidelines for Personnel Dealing with Cytotoxic (Antineoplastic) Drugs. *Am J Hosp Pharm*, 1986; 43:1193-1204.

Manufactured by:
AAI Development Services
An aaiPharma® Company
Wilmington, NC 28405
Manufactured for:
Salix
Pharmaceuticals, Inc.
Raleigh, NC 27615
PC 3290B
Rev 12/2003

Shown in Product Identification Guide, page 332

COLAZAL® ℞

[kôl a zal]
(balsalazide disodium)
Capsules

PRODUCT OVERVIEW

KEY FACTS

COLAZAL® (balsalazide disodium) is an oral prodrug containing mesalamine (5-aminosalicylic acid) and is indicated for the treatment of mildly to moderately active ulcerative colitis. Each *COLAZAL®* capsule contains 750mg of balsalazide disodium. The approved dosage is three capsules, three times per day. Ninety-nine percent of the balsalazide travels intact to the colon where the enzyme, azoreductase, produced by colonic bacteria, cleaves the molecule and releases the mesalamine for anti-inflammatory activity.

MAJOR USES

Two double-masked, clinical studies (N=259) have shown *COLAZAL®* to be effective in the treatment of the signs and symptoms of active ulcerative colitis. In one study, the indicated dose of *COLAZAL®* showed superior effectiveness to a lower dose of *COLAZAL®*. The percentage of patients improved in measures of stool blood, stool frequency and sigmoidoscopic score after eight weeks of treatment. A second study, conducted in Europe, confirmed these findings of symptomatic improvement.

SAFETY INFORMATION

The most frequently reported adverse events in clinical trials (N=259) included headache (8%), abdominal pain (6%) and nausea (5%). The overall reporting of adverse events was similar to those reported by patients receiving placebo. *COLAZAL®* is contraindicated in patients with hypersensitivity to salicylates or to any components of the *COLAZAL®* capsules or balsalazide metabolites. *COLAZAL®* capsules are sulfa-free and do not contain lactose.

PRODUCT ILLUSTRATION

COLAZAL® capsules are available as 750mg gelatin capsules, 280 capsules per bottle. The usual course of therapy is eight to twelve weeks.

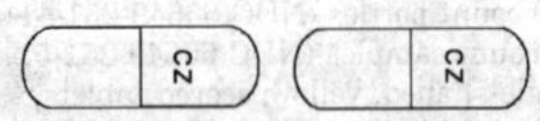

750mg Capsules

DESCRIPTION

Each *COLAZAL®* capsule contains 750 mg of balsalazide disodium, a prodrug that is enzymatically cleaved in the colon to produce mesalamine (5–aminosalicylic acid), an anti inflammatory drug. Each daily dose of *COLAZAL®* (6.75 grams) is equivalent to 2.4 grams of mesalamine. Balsalazide disodium has the chemical name (E)-5-[[-4-[[(2-carboxyethyl) amino]carbonyl] phenyl]azo]-2-hydroxybenzoic acid, disodium salt, dihydrate. Its structural formula is:

NaOOC / HO–C₆H₃–N=N–C₆H₄–C(=O)–NH–CH₂–CH₂–COONa • 2 H₂O

Molecular Weight: 437.32
Molecular Formula: $C_{17}H_{13}N_3O_6Na_2 \cdot 2H_2O$

Balsalazide disodium is a stable, odorless orange to yellow microcrystalline powder. It is freely soluble in water and isotonic saline, sparingly soluble in methanol and ethanol, and practically insoluble in all other organic solvents.

Inactive Ingredients: Each hard gelatin capsule contains colloidal silicon dioxide and magnesium stearate. The sodium content of each capsule is approximately 86 mg.

CLINICAL PHARMACOLOGY

Balsalazide disodium is delivered intact to the colon where it is cleaved by bacterial azoreduction to release equimolar quantities of mesalamine, which is the therapeutically active portion of the molecule, and 4-aminobenzoyl-β-alanine. The recommended dose of 6.75 grams/day, for the treatment of active disease, provides 2.4 grams of free 5-aminosalicylic acid to the colon.

The 4-aminobenzoyl-β-alanine carrier moiety released when balsalazide disodium is cleaved is only minimally absorbed and largely inert. The mechanism of action of 5-aminosalicylic acid is unknown, but appears to be topical rather than systemic. Mucosal production of arachidonic acid metabolites, both through the cyclooxygenase pathways, i.e., prostanoids, and through the lipoxygenase pathways, i.e., leukotrienes and hydroxyeicosatetraenoic acids, is increased in patients with chronic inflammatory bowel disease, and it is possible that 5-aminosalicylic acid diminishes inflammation by blocking production of arachidonic acid metabolites in the colon.

Pharmacokinetics: *COLAZAL®* capsules contain granules of balsalazide disodium which are insoluble in acid and designed to be delivered to the colon intact. Upon reaching the colon, bacterial azoreductases cleave the compound to release 5-aminosalicylic acid the therapeutically active portion of the molecule, and 4-aminobenzoyl-β-alanine.

Absorption: In healthy individuals, the systemic absorption of intact balsalazide was very low and variable. The mean C_{max} occurs approximately 1–2 hours after single oral doses of 1.5 grams or 2.25 grams. The absolute bioavailability of this compound was not determined. In a study of ulcerative colitis patients receiving balsalazide, 1.5 grams twice daily, for over one year, systemic drug exposure, based on mean AUC values, was up to 60 times greater (8 ng*hr/mL to 480 ng*hr/mL) to after equivalent multiple doses of 1.5 grams twice daily when compared to healthy subjects who received the same dose. There was a large intersubject variability in the plasma concentration of balsalazide versus time profiles in all studies, thus its half-life could not be determined. The effect of food intake on the absorption of this compound was not studied.

Distribution: The binding of balsalazide to human plasma proteins was ≥ 99%.

Metabolism: The products of the azoreduction of this compound, 5-aminosalicylic acid and 4-aminobenzoyl-β-alanine, and their N-acetylated metabolites have been identified in plasma, urine and feces.

Elimination: Less than 1% of an oral dose was recovered as parent compound, 5-aminosalicylic acid or 4-aminobenzoyl-β-alanine in the urine of healthy subjects after single and multiple doses of *COLAZAL®*, while up to 25% of the dose was recovered as the N-acetylated metabolites. In a study with 10 healthy volunteers, 65% of a single 2.25 gram dose of *COLAZAL®* was recovered as 5-aminosalicylic acid, 4–aminobenzoyl-β-alanine, and the N-acetylated metabolites in feces, while <1% of the dose was recovered as parent compound.

In a study that examined the disposition of balsalazide in patients who were taking 3–6 grams of *COLAZAL®* daily for more than one year and who were in remission from ulcerative colitis, less than 1% of an oral dose was recovered as intact balsalazide in the urine. Less than 4% of the dose was recovered as 5-aminosalicylic acid, while virtually no 4-aminobenzoyl-β-alanine was detected in urine. The urinary recovery of the N-acetylated metabolites comprised 20–25% of the balsalazide dose. No fecal recovery studies were performed in this population.

Special Populations

Geriatric: No information is available for the geriatric population.

Pediatric: The safety and effectiveness of balsalazide in the pediatric population have not been established.

Gender: No adequate and well-controlled studies which examine balsalazide in males versus females are available.

Renal Insufficiency: No adequate and well-controlled studies which examine balsalazide disposition in patients with mild, moderate, and severe renal impairment are available.

Hepatic Insufficiency: No information is available for patients with hepatic impairment.

Race: No information is available which examines balsalazide in different races.

Pharmacodynamic/Pharmacokinetic Relationship: No information is available.

Drug-Drug Interactions: Neither in vitro nor in vivo drug-drug interaction studies have been performed with balsalazide.

CLINICAL TRIALS

Two randomized, double-blind studies were conducted.

In the first trial, 103 patients with active mild to moderate ulcerative colitis with sigmoidoscopy findings of friable or spontaneously bleeding mucosa were randomized and treated with balsalazide 6.75 grams/day or balsalazide 2.25 grams/day. The primary efficacy endpoint was reduction of rectal bleeding and improvement of at least one of the other assessed symptoms (stool frequency, patient functional assessment, abdominal pain, sigmoidoscopic grade, and physician's global assessment (PGA)). Outcome assessment for rectal bleeding at each interim period (week 2, 4, and 8) encompassed a 4 day period (96 hours). Results demonstrated a statistically significant difference between high and low doses of *COLAZAL®* (Figure 1).

Figure 1: Percentage of Patients Improved at 8 Weeks

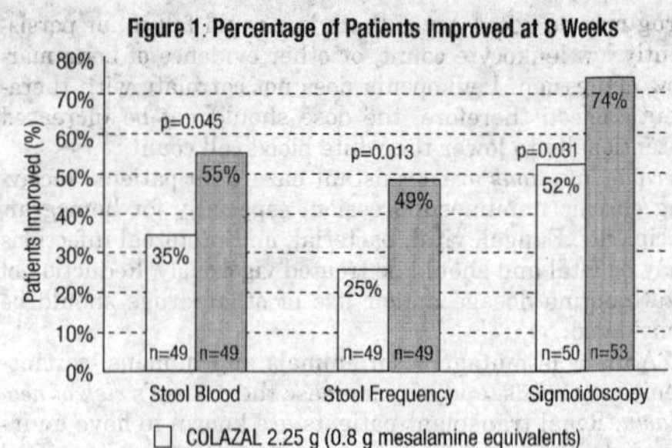

A second study, conducted in Europe, confirmed findings of symptomatic improvement.

INDICATIONS AND USAGE

COLAZAL® is indicated for the treatment of mildly to moderately active ulcerative colitis. Safety and effectiveness of *COLAZAL®* beyond 12 weeks has not been established.

CONTRAINDICATIONS

COLAZAL® is contraindicated in patients with hypersensitivity to salicylates or to any of the components of *COLAZAL®* capsules or balsalazide metabolites.

PRECAUTIONS

Of the 259 patients treated with *COLAZAL®* 6.75 grams/day in controlled clinical trials of active disease, exacerbation of the symptoms of colitis, possibly related to drug use, has been reported by 3 patients.

General: Patients with pyloric stenosis may have prolonged gastric retention of *COLAZAL®* capsules.

Renal: At doses up to 2000 mg/kg (approximately 21 times the recommended 6.75 grams/day dose on a mg/kg basis for a 70 kg person), *COLAZAL®* had no nephrotoxic effects in rats or dogs. Renal toxicity has been observed in animals and patients given other mesalamine products. Therefore, caution should be exercised when administering *COLAZAL®* to patients with known renal dysfunction or a history of renal disease.

Drug Interactions: No drug interaction studies have been conducted for *COLAZAL®*, however the use of orally administered antibiotics could, theoretically, interfere with the release of mesalamine in the colon.

Carcinogenesis, Mutagenesis, Impairment of Fertility: In a 24 month rat (Sprague Dawley) carcinogenicity study, oral (dietary) balsalazide disodium at doses up to 2 grams/kg/day was not tumorigenic. For a 50 kg person of average height this dose represents 2.4 times the recommended human dose on a body surface area basis.

Balsalazide disodium was not genotoxic in the following in vitro or in vivo tests: Ames test, human lymphocyte chromosomal aberration test, and mouse lymphoma cell (L5178Y/TK+/−) forward mutation test, or mouse micronucleus test. However, it was genotoxic in the in vitro Chinese hamster lung cell (CH V79/HGPRT) forward mutation test.

4-aminobenzoyl-β-alanine, a metabolite of balsalazide disodium, was not genotoxic in the Ames test and the mouse lymphoma cell (L5178Y/TK+/−) forward mutation test but was positive in the human lymphocyte chromosomal aberration test. N-acetyl-4-aminobenzoyl-β-alanine, a conjugated metabolite of balsalazide disodium, was not genotoxic in Ames test, the mouse lymphoma cell (L5178Y/TK+/−) forward mutation test, or the human lymphocyte chromosomal aberration test. Balsalazide disodium at oral doses up to 2 grams/kg/day, 2.4 times the recommended human dose based on body surface area, was found to have no effect on fertility and reproductive performance in rats.

Pregnancy—Teratogenic Effects: Pregnancy Category B. Reproduction studies were performed in rats and rabbits at oral doses up to 2 grams/kg/day, 2.4 and 4.7 times the recommended human dose based on body surface area for the rat and rabbit, respectively, and revealed no evidence of impaired fertility or harm to the fetus due to balsalazide disodium. There are, however, no adequate and well-controlled studies in pregnant women. Because animal reproduction studies are not always predictive of human response, this drug should be used during pregnancy only if clearly needed.

Nursing Mothers: It is not known whether balsalazide disodium is excreted in human milk. Because many drugs are excreted in human milk, caution should be exercised when *COLAZAL®* is administered to a nursing woman.

Pediatric Use: Safety and effectiveness of *COLAZAL®* in pediatric patients have not been established.

ADVERSE REACTIONS

Over 1000 patients received treatment with *COLAZAL®* in domestic and foreign clinical trials. In four controlled clinical trials patients receiving a *COLAZAL®* dose of 6.75 grams/day most frequently reported the following events (reporting frequency ≥3%), headache (8%), abdominal pain (6%), diarrhea (5%), nausea (5%), vomiting (4%), respiratory infection (4%), and arthralgia (4%). Withdrawal from therapy due to adverse events was comparable among patients on *COLAZAL®* and placebo.

Adverse events reported by 1% or more of patients who participated in the four well-controlled, Phase 3 trials are presented by treatment group (Table 1).

Table 1. Adverse Events Occurring in at Least 1% of *COLAZAL®* and Ulcerative Colitis Patients in Controlled Trials

Adverse Event	*COLAZAL®* 6.75 grams/day [N = 259]	Placebo [N = 35]
Headache	22 (8%)	3 (9%)
Abdominal pain	16 (6%)	1 (3%)
Nausea	14 (5%)	2 (6%)
Diarrhea	14 (5%)	1 (3%)
Vomiting	11 (4%)	2 (6%)
Respiratory	9 (4%)	5 (14%)
Arthralgia	9 (4%)	–
Rhinitis	6 (2%)	–
Insomnia	6 (2%)	–
Fatigue	6 (2%)	–
Rectal bleeding	5 (2%)	1 (3%)
Flatulence	5 (2%)	–
Fever	5 (2%)	–
Dyspepsia	5 (2%)	–
Pharyngitis	4 (2%)	–
Pain	4 (2%)	1 (3%)
Coughing	4 (2%)	–
Back pain	4 (2%)	1 (3%)
Anorexia	4 (2%)	–
Urinary tract infection	3 (1%)	–
Sinusitis	3 (1%)	1 (3%)
Myalgia	3 (1%)	–
Frequent stools	3 (1%)	1 (3%)
Flu-like disorder	3 (1%)	–
Dry mouth	3 (1%)	–
Dizziness	3 (1%)	2 (6%)
Cramps	3 (1%)	–
Constipation	3 (1%)	–

The number of placebo patients is too small for valid comparisons. Some adverse events, such as abdominal pain, fatigue, and nausea were reported more frequently in women subjects than in men. Abdominal pain, rectal bleeding, and anemia can be part of the clinical presentation of ulcerative colitis.

The following adverse events, presented by body system, have also been infrequently reported by patients taking *COLAZAL®* during clinical trials (n = 513) for the treatment of active acute ulcerative colitis or from foreign post-marketing reports. In most cases no relationship to *COLAZAL®* has been established.

Body as a Whole: abdomen enlarged, asthenia, chest pain, chills, edema, hot flushes, malaise

Cardiovascular and vascular: bradycardia, deep venous thrombosis, hypertension, leg ulcer, palpitations, pericarditis

Gastrointestinal: amylase increased, bowel irregularity, ulcerative colitis aggravated, diarrhea with blood, diverticulosis, epigastric pain, eructation, fecal incontinence, feces abnormal, gastroenteritis, giardiasis, glossitis, hemorrhoids, melena, neoplasm benign, pancreatitis, ulcerative stomatitis, stools frequent, tenesmus, tongue discoloration

Hematologic: anemia, epistaxis, fibrinogen plasma increase, hemorrhage, prothrombin decrease, prothrombin increase, thrombocythemia

Liver and biliary: bilirubin increase, hepatic function abnormal, SGOT increase, SGPT increase

Lymphatic: eosinophilia, granulocytopenia, leukocytosis, leukopenia, lymphadenopathy, lymphoma-like disorder, lymphopenia

Metabolic and nutritional: creatine phosphokinase increased, hypocalcemia, hypokalemia, hypoproteinemia, LDH increase, weight decrease, weight increase

Musculoskeletal: arthritis, arthropathy, stiffness in legs

Nervous: aphasia, dysphonia, gait abnormal, hypertonia, hypoesthesia, paresis, spasm generalized, tremor

Psychiatric: anxiety, depression, nervousness, somnolence

Reproductive: menstrual disorder

Resistance Mechanism: abscess, immunoglobulins decrease, infection, moniliasis, viral infection

Respiratory: bronchospasm, dyspnea, hemoptysis

Skin: alopecia, angioedema, dermatitis, dry skin, erythema nodosum, erythematous rash, pruritus, pruritus ani, psoriasis, skin ulceration

Special Senses: conjunctivitis, earache, ear infection, iritis, parosmia, taste perversion, tinnitus, vision abnormal

Urinary: hematuria, interstitial nephritis, micturition frequency, polyuria, pyuria

Post Marketing Reports:

The following events have been identified during post-approval use in clinical practice, of products which contain (or are metabolized to) mesalamine. Because they are reported voluntarily from a population of unknown size, estimates of frequency cannot be made. These events have been chosen for inclusion due to a combination of seriousness, frequency of reporting, or potential causal connection to mesalamine.

Gastrointestinal: Reports of hepatotoxicity, including elevated liver function tests (SGOT/AST, SGPT/ALT, GGT, LDH, alkaline phosphatase, bilirubin), jaundice, cholestatic jaundice, cirrhosis, hepatocellular damage including liver necrosis and liver failure. Some of these cases were fatal, however, no fatalities associated with these events were reported in *COLAZAL®* clinical trials. One case of Kawasaki-like syndrome which included hepatic function changes was also reported, however, this event was not reported in *COLAZAL®* clinical trials.

DRUG ABUSE AND DEPENDENCY

Abuse: None reported

Dependency: Drug dependence has not been reported with chronic administration of mesalamine.

OVERDOSAGE

No case of overdose has occurred with *COLAZAL®*. A 3–year-old boy is reported to have ingested 2 grams of another mesalamine product. He was treated with ipecac and activated charcoal with no adverse reactions.

If an overdose occurs with *COLAZAL®* use, treatment should be supportive, with particular attention to correction of electrolyte abnormalities.

A single oral dose of balsalazide disodium at 5 grams/kg or 4-aminobenzoyl-β-alanine, a metabolite of balsalazide disodium, at 1 gram/kg was non-lethal in mice and rats. No symptoms of acute toxicity were seen at these doses.

DOSAGE AND ADMINISTRATION

For Treatment of Active Ulcerative Colitis the usual dose in adults is three 750 mg *COLAZAL®* capsules to be taken three times a day for a total daily dose of 6.75 grams for a duration of 8 weeks. Some patients in the clinical trials required treatment for up to 12 weeks.

HOW SUPPLIED

COLAZAL® is available as beige capsules containing 750 mg balsalazide and CZ imprinted in black.

NDC 65649-101-02 Bottles of 280 capsules

Store at 25°C (77°F); excursions permitted to 15–30°C (59–86°F). See USP Controlled Room Temperature.

℞ only

Manufactured for Salix Pharmaceuticals, Inc., Raleigh, N.C. 27615

* *COLAZAL®* is a registered trademark of Salix Pharmaceuticals, Inc.

(6075.02/August 2002)

Shown in Product Identification Guide, page 332

XIFAXAN™ ℞

[zuh fax in]

(rifaximin)

Tablets 200 mg

DESCRIPTION

XIFAXAN™ Tablets contain rifaximin, a semi-synthetic, non-systemic antibiotic. The chemical name for rifaximin is (2*S*,16*Z*,18*E*,20*S*,21*S*,22*R*,23*R*,24*R*,25*S*,26*S*,27*S*,28*E*)-5,6,21,23,25-pentahydroxy-27-methoxy-2,4,11,16,20,22,24,26-octamethyl-2,7-(epoxypentadeca-[1,11,13]trienimino) benzofuro[4,5-e]pyrido[1,2-α]-benzimida-zole-1,15(2*H*)-dione,25-acetate. The empirical formula is $C_{43}H_{51}N_3O_{11}$ and its molecular weight is 785.9. The chemical structure is represented below:

XIFAXAN™ Tablets for oral administration are film-coated and contain 200 mg of rifaximin. Inactive ingredients are colloidal silicon dioxide, disodium edetate, glycerol palmitostearate, hypromellose, microcrystalline cellulose, propylene glycol, red iron oxide, sodium starch glycolate, talc, and titanium dioxide.

CLINICAL PHARMACOLOGY

Pharmacokinetics

Absorption: The mean pharmacokinetic parameters of rifaximin in 14 healthy subjects after a single oral 400-mg dose given as 2 × 200 mg doses under fed and fasting conditions are summarized in Table 1.

Table 1. Effect of Food on the Mean ± S.D. Pharmacokinetic Parameters Following a Single 400-mg Dose of Rifaximin (N = 14)

Parameter	Fasting	Fed
C_{max} (ng/mL)	3.80 ± 1.32	9.63 ± 5.93
T_{max} (h)	1.21 ± 0.47	1.90 ± 1.52
Half-Life (h)	5.85 ± 4.34	5.95 ± 1.88
AUC (ng•h/mL)	18.35 ± 9.48	34.70 ± 9.23
% Excreted in Urine	0.023 ± 0.009	0.051 ± 0.017

Rifaximin can be administered with or without food. Systemic absorption of rifaximin was low in both the fasting state and when administered within 30 minutes of a high-fat breakfast.

^{14}C-Rifaximin was administered as a single dose to 4 healthy male subjects. The mean overall recovery of radioactivity in the urine and feces of 3 subjects during the 168 hours after administration was 96.94 ± 5.64% of the dose. Radioactivity was excreted almost exclusively in the feces (96.62 ± 5.67% of the dose), with only a small proportion of the dose (mean 0.32% of the dose) excreted in urine. Analysis of fecal extracts indicated that rifaximin was being excreted as unchanged drug. The amount of radioactivity in urine (<0.4% of the dose) suggests that rifaximin is poorly absorbed from the gastrointestinal tract and is almost exclusively and completely excreted in feces as unchanged drug. Mean rifaximin pharmacokinetic parameters were C_{max} 4.3 ± 2.8 ng/mL and AUC_t 19.5 ± 16.5 ng•h/mL with a median T_{max} of 1.25 hours.

Systemic absorption of rifaximin (200 mg three times daily) was also evaluated in 13 subjects with shigellosis on Days 1 and 3 of a three-day course of treatment. Rifaximin concentrations and exposures were low and variable. There was no evidence of accumulation of rifaximin following repeated administration for 3 days (9 doses). Peak plasma rifaximin concentrations after 3 and 9 consecutive doses ranged from 0.81 to 3.4 ng/mL on Day 1 and 0.68 to 2.26 ng/mL on Day 3. Similarly, $AUC_{0\text{-}last}$ estimates were 6.95 ± 5.15 ng•h/mL on Day 1 and 7.83 ± 4.94 ng•h/mL on Day 3. Rifaximin is not suitable for treating systemic bacterial infections because less than 0.4% of the drug is absorbed after oral administration (see **WARNINGS**).

Distribution: Animal pharmacokinetic studies have demonstrated that 80% to 90% of orally administered rifaximin is concentrated in the gut with less than 0.2% in the liver and kidney, and less than 0.01% in other tissues. In adults with infectious diarrhea treated with rifaximin 800 mg daily for three days, concentrations of rifaximin in stools averaged ~8000 μg/g the day after treatment ended.

Metabolism: *In vitro* drug interactions studies have shown that rifaximin, at concentrations ranging from 2 to 200 ng/mL, did not inhibit human hepatic cytochrome P450 isoenzymes: 1A2, 2A6, 2B6, 2C9, 2C19, 2D6, 2E1, and 3A4. In an *in vitro* hepatocyte induction model, rifaximin was shown to induce cytochrome P450 3A4 (CYP3A4), an isoenzyme which rifampin is known to induce. Two clinical drug-drug interaction studies using midazolam and an oral contraceptive containing ethinyl estradiol and norgestimate demonstrated that rifaximin did not alter the pharmacokinetics of these drugs (see **Drug-Drug Interactions**).

Excretion: Rifaximin is excreted primarily in the feces. After oral administration of 400 mg ^{14}C-rifaximin to healthy volunteers, approximately 97% of the dose was recovered in feces, almost entirely as unchanged drug, and 0.32% was recovered in the urine.

Special Populations

Geriatric: The pharmacokinetics of rifaximin in patients ≥65 years of age has not been studied.

Pediatric: The pharmacokinetics of rifaximin has not been studied in pediatric patients of any age.

Gender: The effect of gender on the pharmacokinetics of rifaximin has not been studied.

Renal Insufficiency: The pharmacokinetics of rifaximin in patients with impaired renal function has not been studied.

Hepatic Insufficiency: Mean peak rifaximin plasma concentrations of 13.5 ng/mL were detected in hepatic encephalopathy patients administered rifaximin 800 mg three times daily for 7 days. Less than 0.1% of the administered dose was recovered after 7 days. Because of the limited systemic absorption of rifaximin, no specific dosing adjustments are recommended for patients with hepatic insufficiency.

Drug-Drug Interactions

In an *in vitro* hepatocyte induction model, rifaximin was shown to induce cytochrome P450 3A4 (CYP3A4), an isoenzyme which rifampin is known to induce. Two clinical drug-drug interaction studies were conducted using midazolam and an oral contraceptive containing ethinyl estradiol and norgestimate to assess the effect of rifaximin on the pharmacokinetics of these drugs.

The midazolam study was an open-label, randomized, crossover, drug-interaction trial designed to assess the effect of rifaximin 200 mg administered orally (PO) every 8 hours (Q8H) for 3 days and every 8 hours for 7 days, on the pharmacokinetics of a single dose of either midazolam 2 mg intravenous (IV) or midazolam 6 mg PO. No significant difference was observed in the metrics of systemic exposure or elimination of IV or PO midazolam or its major metabolite, 1′-hydroxymidazolam, between midazolam alone or together with rifaximin. Therefore, rifaximin was not shown to significantly affect intestinal or hepatic CYP3A4 activity.

The oral contraceptive study utilized an open-label, crossover design in 28 healthy female subjects to determine if rifaximin 200 mg PO administered Q8H for 3 days altered the pharmacokinetics of a single dose of an oral contraceptive containing 0.07 mg ethinyl estradiol and 0.50 mg norgestimate. Results showed that the pharmacokinetics of single doses of ethinyl estradiol and norgestimate were not altered by rifaximin.

Microbiology

Rifaximin acts by binding to the beta-subunit of bacterial DNA-dependent RNA polymerase resulting in inhibition of bacterial RNA synthesis.

Escherichia coli has been shown to develop resistance to rifaximin *in vitro*. However, the clinical significance of such an effect has not been studied.

Continued on next page

Xifaxan—Cont.

Rifaximin is a structural analog of rifampin. Organisms with high rifaximin minimum inhibitory concentration (MIC) values also have elevated MIC values against rifampin. Cross-resistance between rifaximin and other classes of antimicrobials has not been studied.
Rifaximin has been shown to be active against the following pathogen in clinical studies of infectious diarrhea as described in the **INDICATIONS AND USAGE** section: *Escherichia coli* (enterotoxigenic and enteroaggregative strains).

Susceptibility Tests

In vitro susceptibility testing was performed according to the National Committee for Clinical Laboratory Standards (NCCLS) agar dilution method M7-A6[1]. However, the correlation between susceptibility testing and clinical outcome has not been determined.

INDICATIONS AND USAGE

XIFAXAN™ Tablets are indicated for the treatment of patients (≥12 years of age) with travelers' diarrhea caused by noninvasive strains of *Escherichia coli* (see **WARNINGS, Microbiology**, and **CLINICAL STUDIES**).
XIFAXAN™ Tablets should not be used in patients with diarrhea complicated by fever or blood in the stool or diarrhea due to pathogens other than *Escherichia coli*.

CONTRAINDICATIONS

XIFAXAN™ Tablets are contraindicated in patients with a hypersensitivity to rifaximin, any of the rifamycin antimicrobial agents, or any of the components in XIFAXAN™ Tablets.

WARNINGS

XIFAXAN™ Tablets were not found to be effective in patients with diarrhea complicated by fever and/or blood in the stool or diarrhea due to pathogens other than *Escherichia coli*. XIFAXAN™ Tablets are not effective in cases of travelers' diarrhea due to *Campylobacter jejuni*. The effectiveness of XIFAXAN™ Tablets in travelers' diarrhea caused by *Shigella* spp. and *Salmonella* spp. has not been proven. XIFAXAN™ Tablets should not be used in patients where *Campylobacter jejuni, Shigella* spp., or *Salmonella* spp. may be suspected as causative pathogens.
XIFAXAN™ Tablets should be discontinued if diarrhea symptoms get worse or persist more than 24-48 hours and alternative antibiotic therapy should be considered.
Pseudomembranous colitis has been reported with nearly all antibacterial agents and may range in severity from mild to life-threatening. Therefore, it is important to consider this diagnosis in patients who present with diarrhea subsequent to the administration of antibacterial agents.
Treatment with antibacterial agents alters the normal flora of the colon and may permit overgrowth of clostridia. Studies indicate that a toxin produced by *Clostridium difficile* is the primary cause of "antibiotic-associated colitis."
After the diagnosis of pseudomembranous colitis has been established, therapeutic measures should be initiated. Mild cases of pseudomembranous colitis usually respond to drug discontinuation alone. In moderate to severe cases, consideration should be given to management with fluids and electrolytes, protein supplementation, and treatment with an antibacterial drug clinically effective against *Clostridium difficile*.

PRECAUTIONS

General

The use of antibiotics may promote the overgrowth of nonsusceptible organisms. Should superinfection occur during therapy, appropriate measures should be taken.

Information for Patients

Patients should be advised that XIFAXAN™ Tablets may be taken with or without food. Patients should be advised that XIFAXAN™ Tablets should be discontinued if their diarrhea persists **more than 24-48 hours** or worsens, or if they have fever and/or blood in the stool that they should seek medical care (see **Patient Information**).

Drug-Drug Interactions

Although *in vitro* studies demonstrated the potential of rifaximin to interact with cytochrome P450 3A4 (CYP3A4), a clinical drug-drug interaction study demonstrated that rifaximin did not significantly affect the pharmacokinetics of midazolam either presystemically or systemically. An additional clinical drug-drug interaction study showed no effect of rifaximin on the presystemic metabolism of an oral contraceptive containing ethinyl estradiol and norgestimate. Therefore, clinical interactions with drugs metabolized by human cytochrome P450 isoenzymes are not expected (see **Pharmacokinetics** and **Drug-Drug Interactions**).

Carcinogenesis, Mutagenesis, Impairment of Fertility

Carcinogenicity studies were not conducted. Rifaximin was not genotoxic in the bacterial reverse mutation assay, chromosomal aberration assay, rat bone marrow micronucleus assay, and the CHO/HGPRT mutation assay. There was no effect on fertility in male or female rats following the administration of rifaximin at doses up to 300 mg/kg (approximately 5 times the clinical dose, adjusted for body surface area).

Pregnancy—Teratogenic Effects (Pregnancy Category C)

Pregnancy

Pregnancy category C: Rifaximin was teratogenic in rats at doses of 150 to 300 mg/kg (approximately 2.5 to 5 times the clinical dose, adjusted for body surface area) and in rabbits at doses of 62.5 to 1000 mg/kg (approximately 2 to 33 times the clinical dose, adjusted for body surface area). These effects include cleft palate, agnatha, jaw shorterning, hemorrhage, eye partially open, small eyes, brachygnathia, incomplete ossification, and increased thoracolumbar vertebrae. There are no adequate and well controlled studies in pregnant women. XIFAXAN™ Tablets should be used during pregnancy only if the potential benefit outweighs the potential risk to the fetus.

Use during lactation

It is not known whether rifaximin is excreted in human milk. Because many drugs are excreted in human milk and because of the potential for adverse reactions in nursing infants from XIFAXAN™ Tablets, a decision should be made whether to discontinue nursing or to discontinue the drug, taking into account the importance of the drug to the mother.

Pediatric Use

The safety and effectiveness of XIFAXAN™ Tablets in pediatric patients less than 12 years of age have not been established.

Geriatric Use

Clinical studies of XIFAXAN™ Tablets did not include sufficient numbers of subjects aged 65 and over to determine whether they respond differently than younger subjects.

ADVERSE REACTIONS

The safety of XIFAXAN™ Tablets 200 mg taken three times a day (TID) was evaluated in 320 patients in two placebo-controlled clinical trials with 95% of patients receiving at least three days of treatment with XIFAXAN™ Tablets. All adverse events for XIFAXAN™ Tablets 200 mg TID that occurred at a frequency ≥2% in the two placebo-controlled trials combined are provided in Table 2. (These include adverse events that may be attributable to the underlying disease.)

Table 2. All Adverse Events With an Incidence ≥2% Among Patients Receiving XIFAXAN™ Tablets, 600 mg/day, in Placebo-Controlled Studies

MedDRA Preferred Term	Number (%) of Patients	
	XIFAXAN™ Tablets, 600 mg/day (N = 320)	Placebo N = 228
Flatulence	36 (11.3%)	45 (19.7%)
Headache	31 (9.7%)	21 (9.2%)
Abdominal Pain NOS	23 (7.2%)	23 (10.1%)
Rectal Tenesmus	23 (7.2%)	20 (8.8%)
Defecation Urgency	19 (5.9%)	21 (9.2%)
Nausea	17 (5.3%)	19 (8.3%)
Constipation	12 (3.8%)	8 (3.5%)
Pyrexia	10 (3.1%)	10 (4.4%)
Vomiting NOS	7 (2.2%)	4 (1.8%)

The following adverse events, presented by body system, have also been reported in <2% of patients taking XIFAXAN™ Tablets in the two placebo-controlled clinical trials where the 200 mg taken three times a day dose was used. The following includes adverse events regardless of causal relationship to drug exposure.
Blood and Lymphatic System Disorders: lymphocytosis, monocytosis, neutropenia
Ear and Labyrinth Disorders: ear pain, motion sickness, tinnitus
Gastrointestinal Disorders: abdominal distension, diarrhea NOS, dry throat, fecal abnormality NOS, gingival disorder NOS, inguinal hernia NOS, dry lips, stomach discomfort
General Disorders and Administration Site Conditions: chest pain, fatigue, malaise, pain NOS, weakness
Infections and Infestations: dysentery NOS, respiratory tract infection NOS, upper respiratory tract infection NOS
Injury and Poisoning: sunburn
Investigations: aspartate aminotransferase increased, blood in stool, blood in urine, weight decreased
Metabolic and Nutritional Disorders: anorexia, dehydration
Musculoskeletal, Connective Tissue, and Bone Disorders: arthralgia, muscle spasms, myalgia, neck pain
Nervous System Disorders: abnormal dreams, dizziness, migraine NOS, syncope, loss of taste
Psychiatric Disorders: insomnia
Renal and Urinary Disorders: choluria, dysuria, hematuria, polyuria, proteinuria, urinary frequency
Respiratory, Thoracic, and Mediastinal Disorders: dyspnea NOS, nasal passage irritation, nasopharyngitis, pharyngitis, pharyngolaryngeal pain, rhinitis NOS, rhinorrhea
Skin and Subcutaneous Tissue Disorders: clamminess, rash NOS, sweating increased
Vascular Disorders: hot flashes NOS

Postmarketing Experience

The following events: hypersensitivity reactions, including allergic dermatitis, rash, angioneurotic edema, urticaria, and pruritus; have been identified during foreign post-approval use of XIFAXAN™ Tablets. Because these events are reported voluntarily from a population of uncertain size, it is not always possible to estimate their frequency or establish a causal relationship to drug exposure.

DRUG ABUSE AND DEPENDENCY

Abuse

None reported.

Dependency

None reported.

OVERDOSAGE

No specific information is available on the treatment of overdosage with XIFAXAN™ Tablets. In clinical studies at doses higher than the recommended dose (> 600 mg/day), adverse events were similar to the recommended dose (200 mg taken three times a day) and to placebo. In the case of overdosage, discontinue XIFAXAN™ Tablets, treat symptomatically, and institute supportive measures as required.

DOSAGE AND ADMINISTRATION

XIFAXAN™ Tablets can be administered orally with or without food. For travelers' diarrhea, the recommended dose is one 200 mg tablet taken three times a day for 3 days.

HOW SUPPLIED

XIFAXAN™ Tablets are available as circular, pink-colored, biconvex tablets containing 200 mg rifaximin, debossed with "Sx" on one side.
NDC 65649-301-03 Bottles of 30 tablets
Store XIFAXAN™ Tablets at 20–25°C (68–77°F); excursions permitted to 15–30°C (59–86°F). See USP Controlled Room Temperature.

CLINICAL STUDIES

The efficacy of rifaximin (200 mg orally taken three times a day for 3 days) was evaluated in two-randomized, multi-center, double-blind, placebo controlled studies in adult subjects with travelers' diarrhea. One study was conducted at clinical sites in Mexico, Guatemala, and Kenya (Study 1). The other study was conducted in Mexico, Guatemala, Peru, and India (Study 2). Stool specimens were collected before treatment and 1 to 3 days following the end of treatment to identify enteric pathogens. The predominant pathogen in both studies was *Escherichia coli*.
The clinical efficacy of rifaximin was assessed by the time to return to normal, formed stools and resolution of symptoms. The primary efficacy endpoint was time to last unformed stool (TLUS) which is defined as the time to the last unformed stool passed, after which clinical cure was declared. Table 3 displays the median TLUS and the number of patients who achieved clinical cure for the intent to treat population (ITT) of Study 1. The duration of diarrhea was significantly shorter in patients treated with rifaximin than in the placebo group. More rifaximin-treated patients were classified as clinical cures than were those in the placebo group.

Table 3. Clinical Response in Study 1 (ITT population)

	Rifaximin (n=125)	Placebo (n=129)	Estimate (97.5% CI)	P-Value
Median TLUS (hours)	32.5	58.6	1.78[a] (1.26, 2.50)	0.0002
Clinical cure, n (%)	99 (79.2)	78 (60.5)	18.7[b] (5.3, 32.1)	0.001

a Hazard Ratio
b Difference in rates

Microbiological eradication (defined as the absence of a baseline pathogen in culture of stool after 72 hours of therapy) rates for Study 1 are presented in Table 4 for patients with any pathogen at baseline and for the subset of patients with *Escherichia coli* at baseline. *Escherichia coli* was the only pathogen with sufficient numbers to allow comparisons between treatment groups.
Even though rifaximin had microbiologic activity similar to placebo, it demonstrated a clinically significant reduction in duration of diarrhea and a higher clinical cure rate than placebo. Therefore, patients should be managed based on clinical response to therapy rather than microbiologic response.

Table 4. Microbiologic Eradication Rates in Study 1 Subjects with a Baseline Pathogen

	Rifaximin	Placebo
Overall	48/70 (68.6)	41/61 (67.2)
E. coli	38/53 (71.7)	40/54 (74.1)

Study 2 provided additional information to support the results presented for Study 1. This study also provided evidence that rifaximin-treated subjects with fever and/or blood in the stool at baseline had prolonged TLUS. These subjects had lower clinical cure rates than those without fever or blood in the stool at baseline. Many of the patients with fever and/or blood in the stool (dysentery-like diarrheal syndromes) had invasive pathogens, primarily *Campylobacter jejuni*, isolated in the baseline stool.
Also in this study, the majority of the rifaximin-treated subjects who had *Campylobacter jejuni* isolated as a sole pathogen at baseline failed treatment and the resulting clinical cure rate for these patients was 23.5% (4/17). In addition to not being different from placebo, the microbiologic eradication rates for subjects with *Campylobacter jejuni* isolated at baseline were much lower than the eradication rates seen for *Escherichia coli*.
In an unrelated Phase 1, open-label, pharmacokinetic study of oral XIFAXAN™ Tablets 200 mg taken every 8 hours for 3 days, 15 adult subjects were challenged with *Shigella flex-*

neri 2a, of whom 13 developed diarrhea or dysentery and were treated with rifaximin. Although this open-label challenge trial was not adequate to assess the effectiveness of rifaximin in the treatment of shigellosis, the following observations were noted. Eight subjects received rescue treatment with ciprofloxacin either because of lack of response to rifaximin treatment within 24 hours (2), or because they developed severe dysentery (5), or because of recurrence of *Shigella flexneri* in the stool (1). Five of the 13 subjects received ciprofloxacin although they did not have evidence of severe disease or relapse.

REFERENCES

1. Methods for dilution antimicrobial susceptibility tests for bacteria that grow aerobically. National Committee for Clinical Laboratory Standards, Sixth Edition, Wayne PA. *Approved Standard NCCLS Document M7-A6* January 2003; 23 (2).

Rx Only

Manufactured for Salix Pharmaceuticals, Inc., Raleigh, NC 27615,
under license from Alfa Wassermann S.p.A.

XIFAXAN™ is a trademark of Salix Pharmaceuticals, Inc., under license from Alfa Wassermann S.p.A.

6255.00/June 2004
2316-25-04A

Shown in Product Identification Guide, page 332

Sandoz Pharmaceuticals Corporation

PLEASE NOTE:
Due to the merger of CibaGeneva Pharmaceuticals and Sandoz Pharmaceuticals Corporation, please refer to **Novartis Pharmaceuticals Corporation** for branded product information and Geneva Pharmaceuticals, Inc. for branded generic product information.

SangStat Medical Corporation

6300 DUMBARTON CIRCLE
FREMONT, CA 94555

Direct Inquiries to:
Medical and Scientific Information
(877) 264-7828
Customer Service
(888) 764-7828

THYMOGLOBULIN® ℞

Anti-thymocyte Globulin (Rabbit)
Sterile Lyophilized Preparation
For Intravenous Use Only
Rx only

> **WARNING**
> Thymoglobulin® should only be used by physicians experienced in immunosuppressive therapy for the management of renal transplant patients.

DESCRIPTION

Thymoglobulin® [Anti-thymocyte Globulin (Rabbit)] is a purified, pasteurized, gamma immune globulin, obtained by immunization of rabbits with human thymocytes. This immunosuppressive product contains cytotoxic antibodies directed against antigens expressed on human T-lymphocytes. Thymoglobulin is a sterile, freeze-dried product for intravenous administration after reconstitution with sterile Water for Injection, USP (WFI).

Each package contains two 7 mL vials:

Vial 1: Freeze-Dried Thymoglobulin Formulation	
Active Ingredient: Anti-thymocyte Globulin (Rabbit)	25 mg
Inactive ingredients: Glycine (50 mg), mannitol (50 mg), sodium chloride (10 mg)	
Vial 2: Diluent	
Sterile Water for Injection, USP	5 mL

The reconstituted preparation contains approximately 5 mg/mL of Thymoglobulin, of which >90% is rabbit gamma immune globulin (IgG). The reconstituted solution has a pH of 7.0 ± 0.4. Human red blood cells are used in the manufacturing process to deplete cross-reactive antibodies to non-T-cell antigens. The manufacturing process is validated to remove or inactivate potential exogenous viruses. All human red blood cells are from US registered or FDA licensed blood banks. A viral inactivation step (pasteurization, i.e., heat treatment of active ingredient at 60°C/10 hr) is performed for each lot. Each Thymoglobulin lot is released following potency testing (lymphocytotoxicity and E-rosette inhibition assays), and cross-reactive antibody testing (hemagglutination, platelet agglutination, anti-human serum protein antibody, antiglomerular basement membrane antibody, and fibroblast toxicity assays on every fifth lot).

Table 1. Response to Study Treatment by Rejection Severity and Study Half

	Total		First Half		Second Half	
	Thymoglobulin	Atgam	Thymoglobulin	Atgam	Thymoglobulin	Atgam
Baseline Rejection Severity:	**Success/n (%)**		**Success/n (%)**		**Success/n (%)**	
Mild	9/10 (90.0%)	5/8 (62.5%)	5/5 (100%)	1/3 (33.3%)	4/5 (80.0%)	4/5 (80.0%)
Moderate	44/58 (75.5%)	41/58 (70.7%)	22/26 (84.6%)	22/32 (68.8%)	22/32 (68.8%)	19/26 (73.1%)
Severe	11/14 (71.6%)	8/14 (57.1%)	6/8 (75.0%)	3/8 (37.5%)	5/6 (83.3%)	5/6 (83.3%)
Overall	64/82 (78.0%)	54/80 (67.5%)	33/39 (84.6%)	26/43 (60.5%)	31/43 (72.1%)	28/37 (75.7%)
Weighted estimate of difference (Thymoglobulin—Atgam)	11.1%[a]		19.3%		−3.2%	
Lower one-sided 95% confidence bound	0.07%		4.6%		−19.7%	
p-value[b]	0.061[c]		0.008[d]		0.625[d]	

a. across rejection severity and study half
b. under null hypothesis of equivalence (Cochran-Mantel-Haenszel test)
c. one-sided stratified on rejection severity and study half
d. one-sided stratified on rejection severity

PHARMACOLOGY

Mechanism of Action

The mechanism of action by which polyclonal antilymphocyte preparations suppress immune responses is not fully understood. Possible mechanisms by which Thymoglobulin may induce immunosuppression *in vivo* include: T-cell clearance from the circulation and modulation of T-cell activation, homing, and cytotoxic activities. Thymoglobulin includes antibodies against T-cell markers such as CD2, CD3, CD4, CD8, CD11a, CD18, CD25, CD44, CD45, HLA-DR, HLA Class I heavy chains, and β2 microglobulin.[1,2,3,4,5] *In vitro,* Thymoglobulin (concentrations >0.1 mg/mL) mediates T-cell suppressive effects via inhibition of proliferative responses to several mitogens.[2,3,4] In patients, T-cell depletion is usually observed within a day from initiating Thymoglobulin therapy.[7,9,10] Thymoglobulin has not been shown to be effective for treating antibody (humoral) mediated rejections.

Pharmacokinetics and Immunogenicity

After an intravenous dose of 1.25 to 1.5 mg/kg/day (over 4 hours for 7–11 days) 4–8 hours post-infusion, Thymoglobulin levels were on average 21.5 μg/mL (10–40 μg/mL) with a half-life of 2–3 days after the first dose, and 87 μg/mL (23–170 μg/mL) after the last dose.[9] During the Thymoglobulin* Phase III randomized trial, of the 108 of 163 patients evaluated, anti-rabbit antibodies developed in 68% of the Thymoglobulin-treated patients, and anti-horse antibodies developed in 78% of the Atgam®**-treated patients (p=n.s.). No controlled studies have been conducted to study the effect of anti-rabbit antibodies on repeat use of Thymoglobulin. However, monitoring the lymphocyte count to ensure that T-cell depletion is achieved upon retreatment with Thymoglobulin is recommended.[8] Based on data collected from a limited number of patients (Clinical study Phase III, n=12), T-cell counts are presented in the chart below. These data were collected using flow cytometry (FACSCAN, Becton-Dickinson).

Mean T-Cell Counts Following Initiation of Thymoglobulin Therapy

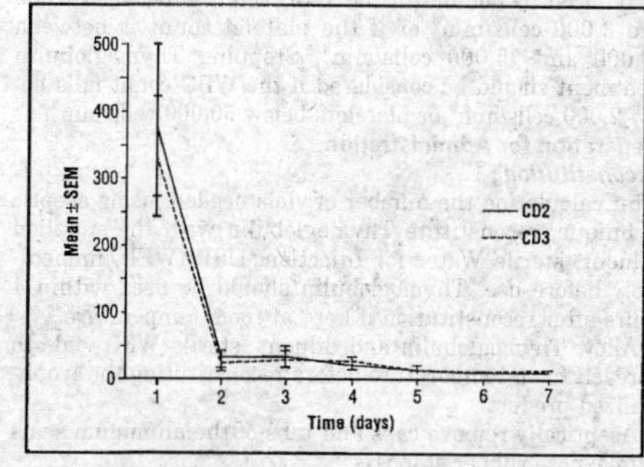

Clinical Trials

US Phase III Study

A controlled, double-blind, multicenter, randomized clinical trial comparing Thymoglobulin and Atgam was conducted at 28 US transplant centers in renal transplant patients (n=163) with biopsy-proven Banff Grade II (moderate), Grade III (severe), or steroid-resistant Grade I (mild) acute graft rejection. This clinical trial rejected the null hypothesis that Thymoglobulin was more than 20% less effective in reversing acute rejection than Atgam. The overall weighted estimate of the treatment difference (Thymoglobulin-Atgam success rate) was 11.1% with a lower 95% confidence bound of 0.07%. Therefore, Thymoglobulin was at least as effective as Atgam in reversing acute rejection episodes.[8]

*Thymoglobulin is a registered trademark of SangStat Medical Corporation, Fremont, CA, USA
** Atgam is a registered trademark of Pharmacia & Upjohn, Kalamazoo, MI, USA

In the study, patients were randomized to receive 7 to 14 days of Thymoglobulin (1.5 mg/kg/day) or Atgam (15 mg/kg/day). For the entire study, the two treatment groups were comparable with respect to donor and recipient characteristics. During the trial, the FDA approved new maintenance immunosuppressive agents (tacrolimus and mycophenolate). Off-protocol use of these agents occurred during the second half of the study in some patients without affecting the overall conclusions (Thymoglobulin 22/43, Atgam 20/37; p=0.826). The results however are presented for the first and second halves of the study (Table 1). In Table 1, successful treatment is presented as those patients whose serum creatinine levels (14 days from the diagnosis of rejection) returned to baseline and whose graft was functioning on day 30 after the end of therapy.

[See table 1 above]

There were no significant differences between the two treatments with respect to (i) day 30 serum creatinine levels relative to baseline, (ii) improvement rate in post-treatment histology, (iii) one-year post-rejection Kaplan-Meier patient survival (Thymoglobulin 93%, n=82 and Atgam 96%, n=80), (iv) day 30 and (v) one-year post-rejection graft survival (Thymoglobulin 83%, n=82; Atgam 75%, n=80).

INDICATIONS AND USAGE

Thymoglobulin is indicated for the treatment of renal transplant acute rejection in conjunction with concomitant immunosuppression.

CONTRAINDICATIONS

Thymoglobulin is contraindicated in patients with history of allergy or anaphylaxis to rabbit proteins, or who have an acute viral illness.

WARNINGS

Thymoglobulin should only be used by physicians experienced in immunosuppressive therapy for the treatment of renal transplant patients. Medical surveillance is required during Thymoglobulin infusion. In rare instances, anaphylaxis has been reported with Thymoglobulin use. In such cases, the infusion should be terminated immediately. Medical personnel should be available to treat patients who experience anaphylaxis. Emergency treatment such as 0.3 mL to 0.5 mL aqueous epinephrine (1:1000 dilution) subcutaneously and other resuscitative measures including oxygen, intravenous fluids, antihistamines, corticosteroids, pressor amines, and airway management, as clinically indicated, should be provided. Thymoglobulin or other rabbit immunoglobulins should not be administered again for such patients. Thrombocytopenia or neutropenia may result from cross-reactive antibodies and is reversible following dose adjustments.

PRECAUTIONS

General

Thymoglobulin infusion may produce fever and chills. To minimize these, the first dose should be infused over a min-

Continued on next page

Thymoglobulin—Cont.

imum of 6 hours into a high-flow vein. Also, premedication with corticosteroids, acetaminophen, and/or an antihistamine and/or slowing the infusion rate may reduce reaction incidence and intensity (see **DOSAGE AND ADMINISTRATION**).

Prolonged use or overdosage of Thymoglobulin in association with other immunosuppressive agents may cause over-immunosuppression resulting in severe infections and may increase the incidence of lymphoma or post-transplant lymphoproliferative disease (PTLD) or other malignancies. Appropriate antiviral, antibacterial, antiprotozoal, and/or antifungal prophylaxis is recommended.

Laboratory Tests

During Thymoglobulin therapy, monitoring the lymphocyte count (i.e., total lymphocyte and/or T-cell subset) may help assess the degree of T-cell depletion (see **Pharmacokinetics and Immunogenicity**). For safety, WBC and platelet counts should also be monitored (see **DOSAGE AND ADMINISTRATION**).

Drug Interactions

- Because Thymoglobulin is administered to patients receiving a standard immunosuppressive regimen, this may predispose patients to over-immunosuppression. Many transplant centers decrease maintenance immunosuppression therapy during the period of antibody therapy.
- Thymoglobulin can stimulate the production of antibodies which cross-react with rabbit immune globulins (see **Pharmacokinetics and Immunogenicity**).

Drug/Laboratory Test Interactions

Thymoglobulin has not been shown to interfere with any routine clinical laboratory tests which do not use immunoglobulins. Thymoglobulin may interfere with rabbit antibody-based immunoassays and with cross-match or panel-reactive antibody cytotoxicity assays.

Carcinogenesis, Mutagenesis, Impairment of Fertility

The carcinogenic and mutagenic potential of Thymoglobulin and its potential to impair fertility have not been studied.

Pregnancy: Pregnancy Category C

Animal reproduction studies have not been conducted with Thymoglobulin. It is also not known whether Thymoglobulin can cause fetal harm or can affect reproduction capacity. Thymoglobulin should be given to a pregnant woman only if clearly needed.

Nursing Mothers

Thymoglobulin has not been studied in nursing women. It is not known whether this drug is excreted in human milk. Because many drugs are excreted in human milk, caution should be exercised when Thymoglobulin is administered to a nursing woman.

Pediatric Use

The safety and effectiveness of Thymoglobulin in pediatric patients has not been established in controlled trials. However, the dose, efficacy, and adverse event profile are not thought to be different from adults based on limited European studies and US compassionate use.[6]

ADVERSE REACTIONS

Thymoglobulin adverse events are generally manageable or reversible. In the US Phase III controlled clinical trial (n = 163) comparing the efficacy and safety of Thymoglobulin and Atgam, there were no significant differences in clinically significant adverse events between the two treatment groups (Table 2). Malignancies were reported in 3 patients who received Thymoglobulin and in 3 patients who received Atgam during the one-year follow-up period. These included two PTLDs in the Thymoglobulin group and two PTLDs in the Atgam group. Infections occurring in both treatment groups during the 3-month follow-up are summarized in Table 3. No significant differences were seen between the Thymoglobulin and Atgam groups for all types of infections, and the incidence of cytomegalovirus (CMV) infection was equivalent in both groups. (Viral prophylaxis was by the center's discretion during antibody treatment, but all centers used gancyclovir infusion during treatment.)

[See table 2 above]
[See table 3 at left]

Table 2. Frequently Reported and Significant Adverse Events*

	Thymoglobulin n = 82		Atgam n = 81		
Preferred Term	**No. of Patients**	**(%)**	**No. of Patients**	**(%)**	**p Value†**
Frequently Reported Events					
Fever	52	(63.4)	51	(63.0)	1.0
Chills	47	(57.3)	35	(43.2)	0.086
Leukopenia	47	(57.3)	24	(29.6)	<0.001
Pain	38	(46.3)	35	(43.2)	0.753
Headache	33	(40.2)	28	(34.6)	0.518
Abdominal pain	31	(37.8)	22	(27.2)	0.181
Diarrhea	30	(36.6)	26	(32.1)	0.622
Hypertension	30	(36.6)	23	(28.4)	0.316
Nausea	30	(36.6)	23	(28.4)	0.316
Thrombocytopenia	30	(36.6)	36	(44.4)	0.341
Peripheral edema	28	(34.1)	28	(34.6)	1.0
Dyspnea	23	(28.0)	16	(19.8)	0.271
Asthenia	22	(26.8)	26	(32.1)	0.495
Hyperkalemia	22	(26.8)	15	(18.5)	0.262
Tachycardia	22	(26.8)	19	(23.5)	0.719
Significant Events§					
Leukopenia	47	(57.3)	24	(29.6)	<0.001
Malaise	11	(13.4)	3	(3.7)	0.047
Dizziness	7	(8.5)	20	(24.7)	0.006

*Treatment Emergent Adverse Events (TEAE) are summarized. Frequently reported adverse events are those reported by more than 25% of patients in a treatment group; significant adverse events are those where the incidence rate differed between treatment groups by a significance level of ≤0.05.
†p value comparing treatment groups using Fisher's exact test.
§statistically significant differences in the AEs

Table 3. Infections

	Thymoglobulin n=82			Atgam n=81			
BODY SYSTEM Preferred Term	**No. of Patients**	**(%)**	**Total Reports**	**No. of Patients**	**(%)**	**Total Reports**	**p Value†**
BODY AS A WHOLE	30	(36.6)	36	22	(27.2)	29	0.240
Infection	25	(30.5)	26	19	(23.5)	21	0.378
Other	14	(17.1)	15	11	(13.6)	12	0.665
CMV	11	(13.4)	11	9	(11.1)	9	0.812
Sepsis	10	(12.2)	10	7	(9.6)	7	0.610
Moniliasis	0	(0.0)	0	1	(1.2)	1	0.497
DIGESTIVE	5	(6.1)	5	3	(3.7)	3	0.720
Gastrointestinal moniliasis	4	(4.9)	4	1	(1.2)	1	0.367
Oral moniliasis	3	(3.7)	0	2	(2.5)	1	0.497
Gastritis	1	(1.2)	1	0	(0.0)	0	1.000
RESPIRATORY	0	(0.0)	0	1	(1.2)	1	0.497
Pneumonia	0	(0.0)	0	1	(1.2)	1	0.497
SKIN	4	(4.9)	4	0	(0.0)	0	0.120
Herpes simplex	4	(4.9)	4	0	(0.0)	0	0.120
UROGENITAL	15	(18.3)	15	22	(29.2)	22	0.195
Urinary tract infection	15	(18.3)	15	21	(25.9)	21	0.262
Vaginitis	0	(0.0)	0	1	(1.2)	1	0.497
NOT SPECIFIED	0	(0.0)	0	2	(2.5)	2	0.245

†p value comparing treatment groups using Fisher's exact test.

OVERDOSAGE

Thymoglobulin overdosage may result in leukopenia or thrombocytopenia, which can be managed with dose reduction (see **DOSAGE AND ADMINISTRATION**).

DOSAGE AND ADMINISTRATION

The recommended dosage of Thymoglobulin for treatment of acute renal graft rejection is 1.5 mg/kg of body weight administered daily for 7 to 14 days. The recommended route of administration is intravenous infusion using a high-flow vein. Thymoglobulin should be infused over a minimum of 6 hours for the first infusion and over at least 4 hours on subsequent days of therapy. Thymoglobulin should be administered through an in-line 0.22 µm filter.

Thymoglobulin is supplied as two vials: one vial contains lyophilized (solid) Thymoglobulin (25 mg) and the second vial contains 5 mL sterile Water for Injection, USP (WFI) labeled as "Diluent". For vial reconstitution, dilution in infusion solution and infusion procedure, see **Preparation for Administration**. Investigations indicate that Thymoglobulin is well tolerated and less likely to produce side effects when administered at the recommended rate. Administration of antiviral prophylactic therapy is recommended. Premedication with corticosteroids, acetaminophen, and/or an antihistamine 1 hour prior to the infusion is recommended and may reduce the incidence and intensity of side effects during the infusion (see **PRECAUTIONS: General**). Medical personnel should monitor patients for adverse events during and after infusion. Monitoring T-cell counts (absolute and/or subsets) to assess the level of T-cell depletion is recommended. Total white blood cell and platelet counts should be monitored.

Overdosage of Thymoglobulin may result in leukopenia and/or thrombocytopenia. The Thymoglobulin dose should be reduced by one-half if the WBC count is between 2,000 and 3,000 cells/mm^3 or if the platelet count is between 50,000 and 75,000 cells/mm^3. Stopping Thymoglobulin treatment should be considered if the WBC count falls below 2,000 cells/mm^3 or platelets below 50,000 cells/mm^3.

Preparation for Administration

Reconstitution

After calculating the number of vials needed, using aseptic technique, reconstitute Thymoglobulin with the supplied Diluent, sterile Water for Injection, USP (WFI), immediately before use. Thymoglobulin should be used within 4 hours after reconstitution if kept at room temperature.

1. Allow Thymoglobulin and diluent (sterile WFI) vials to reach room temperature before reconstituting the lyophilized product.
2. Aseptically remove caps and tabs of the aluminum seals to expose rubber stoppers.
3. Clean stoppers with germicidal or alcohol swab.
4. Aseptically remove 5 mL of diluent (sterile WFI) using a sterile, single-use syringe and inject it slowly into the vial containing Thymoglobulin lyophilized powder.
5. Reconstitute each vial of Thymoglobulin lyophilized powder with 5 mL of sterile diluent.
6. Rotate vial gently until powder is completely dissolved. Each reconstituted vial contains 25 mg or 5 mg/mL of Thymoglobulin.
7. Inspect solution for particulate matter after reconstitution. Should some particulate matter remain, continue to gently rotate the vial until no particulate matter is visible. If particulate matter persists, discard this vial.

Dilution

1. Transfer the contents of the calculated number of Thymoglobulin vials into the bag of infusion solution (saline or dextrose). Recommended volume: per one vial of Thymoglobulin use 50 mL of infusion solution (total volume usually between 50 to 500 mL).
2. Mix the solution by inverting the bag gently only once or twice.

Infusion

1. Follow the manufacturer's instructions for the infusion administration set. Infuse through a 0.22-micron filter into a high-flow vein.
2. Set the flow rate to deliver the dose over a minimum of 6 hours for the first dose and over at least 4 hours for subsequent doses.

HOW SUPPLIED

Thymoglobulin is available as sterile, lyophilized powder to be reconstituted with sterile diluent. Each package contains two 7 mL vials:

Vial 1:
Freeze-Dried Thymoglobulin Formulation (25 mg)

NDC# 62053-534-25
Vial 2:
Diluent (sterile Water for Injection, USP) (>5 mL)
NDC# 62053-535-05

Storage

- Store in refrigerator between +2°C to +8°C (36°F to 46°F).
- Protect from light.
- Do not freeze.
- Do not use after the expiration date indicated on the label.
- Reconstituted vials of Thymoglobulin should be used within 4 hours.
- Infusion solutions of Thymoglobulin must be used immediately.
- Any unused drug remaining after infusion must be discarded.

REFERENCES

1. Bonnefoy-Bérard N, et al. Antibodies against functional leukocyte surface molecules in polyclonal antilymphocyte and antithymocyte globulins. *Transplantation* (1991)**51**:669–673.
2. Bonnefoy-Bérard N, et al. Inhibition of CD25 (IL-2Rα) expression and T-cell proliferation by polyclonal antithymocyte globulins. *Immunology* (1992)**77**:61–67.
3. Bonnefoy-Bérard N, et al. Antiproliferative effect of anti-lymphocyte globulins on B cells and B-cell lines. *Blood* (1992)**79**:2164–2170.
4. Bonnefoy-Bérard N, Revillard J-P. Mechanisms of immunosuppression induced by antithymocyte globulins and OKT3. *J Heart Lung Transplant* (1996)**15**:435–442.
5. Bourdage J, et al. Comparative polyclonal antithymocyte globulin and anti-lymphocyte/antilymphoblast globulin anti-CD antigen analysis by flow cytometry. *Transplantation* (1995)**59**:1194–1200.
6. Broyer M, et al. Triple therapy including cyclosporine A versus conventional regimen—a randomized prospective study in pediatric kidney transplantation. *Transplant Proc* (1987)**19**:3582–3585.
7. Clark KR, et al. Administration of ATG according to the absolute T lymphocyte count during therapy for steroid-resistant rejection. *Transpl Int* (1993)**6**:18–21.
8. Gaber AO, et al. Results of the double-blind, randomized, multicenter, phase III clinical trial of Thymoglobulin versus Atgam in the treatment of acute graft rejection episodes after renal transplantation. *Transplantation* (1998)**66**:29–37.
9. Guttmann RD, et al. Pharmacokinetics, foreign protein immune response, cytokine release, and lymphocyte subsets in patients receiving Thymoglobuline and immunosuppression. *Transplant Proc* (1997)**29**(suppl 7A): 24S–26S.
10. Ippoliti G, et al. Prophylactic use of rabbit ATG vs horse ALG in heart-transplanted patients under Sandimmun (CyA) therapy: clinical and immunological effects. *Clin Transplantation* (1989)**3**:204–208.

License Holder and Manufacturer:
IMTIX-SANGSTAT
Lyon, France
US License No. 1271
Distributed by:
SangStat Medical Corporation
Fremont, CA 94555

SANGSTAT
SangStat Medical Corporation 90152102-0198 Rev. 0402

SANKYO Pharma Inc.

TWO HILTON COURT
PARSIPPANY, NJ 07054

Direct Inquiries to:
1-877-4SANKYO
www.sankyopharma.com

BENICAR® TABLETS ℞
(olmesartan medoxomil)

USE IN PREGNANCY
When used in pregnancy during the second and third trimesters, drugs that act directly on the renin-angiotensin system can cause injury and even death to the developing fetus. When pregnancy is detected, BENICAR® should be discontinued as soon as possible. See **WARNINGS, Fetal/Neonatal Morbidity and Mortality.**

DESCRIPTION

BENICAR® (olmesartan medoxomil), a prodrug, is hydrolyzed to olmesartan during absorption from the gastrointestinal tract. Olmesartan is a selective AT_1 subtype angiotensin II receptor antagonist.
Olmesartan medoxomil is described chemically as 2,3-dihydroxy-2-butenyl 4-(1-hydroxy-1-methylethyl)-2-propyl-1-[*p*-(*o*-1*H*-tetrazol-5-ylphenyl)benzyl]imidazole-5-carboxylate, cyclic 2,3-carbonate.
Its empirical formula is $C_{29}H_{30}N_6O_6$ and its structural formula is:

Olmesartan medoxomil is a white to light yellowish-white powder or crystalline powder with a molecular weight of 558.59. It is practically insoluble in water and sparingly soluble in methanol. BENICAR® is available for oral use as film-coated tablets containing 5 mg, 20 mg, or 40 mg of olmesartan medoxomil and the following inactive ingredients: hydroxypropylcellulose, lactose, low-substituted hydroxypropylcellulose, magnesium stearate, microcrystalline cellulose, talc, titanium dioxide, and (5 mg only) yellow iron oxide.

CLINICAL PHARMACOLOGY

Mechanism of Action

Angiotensin II is formed from angiotensin I in a reaction catalyzed by angiotensin converting enzyme (ACE, kininase II). Angiotensin II is the principal pressor agent of the renin-angiotensin system, with effects that include vasoconstriction, stimulation of synthesis and release of aldosterone, cardiac stimulation and renal reabsorption of sodium. Olmesartan blocks the vasoconstrictor effects of angiotensin II by selectively blocking the binding of angiotensin II to the AT_1 receptor in vascular smooth muscle. Its action is, therefore, independent of the pathways for angiotensin II synthesis.
An AT_2 receptor is found also in many tissues, but this receptor is not known to be associated with cardiovascular homeostasis. Olmesartan has more than a 12,500-fold greater affinity for the AT_1 receptor than for the AT_2 receptor.
Blockade of the renin-angiotensin system with ACE inhibitors, which inhibit the biosynthesis of angiotensin II from angiotensin I, is a mechanism of many drugs used to treat hypertension. ACE inhibitors also inhibit the degradation of bradykinin, a reaction also catalyzed by ACE. Because olmesartan medoxomil does not inhibit ACE (kininase II), it does not affect the response to bradykinin. Whether this difference has clinical relevance is not yet known.
Blockade of the angiotensin II receptor inhibits the negative regulatory feedback of angiotensin II on renin secretion, but the resulting increased plasma renin activity and circulating angiotensin II levels do not overcome the effect of olmesartan on blood pressure.

Pharmacokinetics

General
Olmesartan medoxomil is rapidly and completely bioactivated by ester hydrolysis to olmesartan during absorption from the gastrointestinal tract. Olmesartan appears to be eliminated in a biphasic manner with a terminal elimination half-life of approximately 13 hours. Olmesartan shows linear pharmacokinetics following single oral doses of up to 320 mg and multiple oral doses of up to 80 mg. Steady-state levels of olmesartan are achieved within 3 to 5 days and no accumulation in plasma occurs with once-daily dosing.
The absolute bioavailability of olmesartan is approximately 26%. After oral administration, the peak plasma concentration (C_{max}) of olmesartan is reached after 1 to 2 hours. Food does not affect the bioavailability of olmesartan.
Metabolism and Excretion
Following the rapid and complete conversion of olmesartan medoxomil to olmesartan during absorption, there is virtually no further metabolism of olmesartan. Total plasma clearance of olmesartan is 1.3 L/h, with a renal clearance of 0.6 L/h. Approximately 35% to 50% of the absorbed dose is recovered in urine while the remainder is eliminated in feces via the bile.
Distribution
The volume of distribution of olmesartan is approximately 17 L. Olmesartan is highly bound to plasma proteins (99%) and does not penetrate red blood cells. The protein binding is constant at plasma olmesartan concentrations well above the range achieved with recommended doses.
In rats, olmesartan crossed the blood-brain barrier poorly, if at all. Olmesartan passed across the placental barrier in rats and was distributed to the fetus. Olmesartan was distributed to milk at low levels in rats.

Special Populations

Pediatric: The pharmacokinetics of olmesartan have not been investigated in patients <18 years of age.
Geriatrics: The pharmacokinetics of olmesartan were studied in the elderly (≥65 years). Overall, maximum plasma concentrations of olmesartan were similar in young adults and the elderly. Modest accumulation of olmesartan was observed in the elderly with repeated dosing; $AUC_{ss,\tau}$ was 33% higher in elderly patients, corresponding to an approximate 30% reduction in CL_R.
Gender: Minor differences were observed in the pharmacokinetics of olmesartan in women compared to men. AUC and C_{max} were 10-15% higher in women than in men.
Renal Insufficiency: In patients with renal insufficiency, serum concentrations of olmesartan were elevated compared to subjects with normal renal function. After repeated dosing, the AUC was approximately tripled in patients with severe renal impairment (creatinine clearance <20 mL/min). The pharmacokinetics of olmesartan in patients undergoing hemodialysis has not been studied.
Hepatic Insufficiency: Increases in $AUC_{0-\infty}$ and C_{max} were observed in patients with moderate hepatic impairment compared to those in matched controls, with an increase in AUC of about 60%.

Drug Interactions: See PRECAUTIONS, Drug Interactions.

Pharmacodynamics

Olmesartan medoxomil doses of 2.5 to 40 mg inhibit the pressor effects of angiotensin I infusion. The duration of the inhibitory effect was related to dose, with doses of olmesartan medoxomil >40 mg giving >90% inhibition at 24 hours.
Plasma concentrations of angiotensin I and angiotensin II and plasma renin activity (PRA) increase after single and repeated administration of olmesartan medoxomil to healthy subjects and hypertensive patients. Repeated administration of up to 80 mg olmesartan medoxomil had minimal influence on aldosterone levels and no effect on serum potassium.

Clinical Trials

The antihypertensive effects of BENICAR® have been demonstrated in seven placebo-controlled studies at doses ranging from 2.5 to 80 mg for 6 to 12 weeks, each showing statistically significant reductions in peak and trough blood pressure. A total of 2693 patients (2145 BENICAR®; 548 placebo) with essential hypertension were studied. BENICAR® once daily (QD) lowered diastolic and systolic blood pressure. The response was dose-related, as shown in the following graph. An olmesartan medoxomil dose of 20 mg daily produces a trough sitting BP reduction over placebo of about 10/6 mm Hg and a dose of 40 mg daily produces a trough sitting BP reduction over placebo of about 12/7 mm Hg. Olmesartan medoxomil doses greater than 40 mg had little additional effect. The onset of the antihypertensive effect occurred within 1 week and was largely manifest after 2 weeks.

BENICAR® Dose Response
Placebo-Adjusted Reduction
in Blood Pressure (mm Hg)

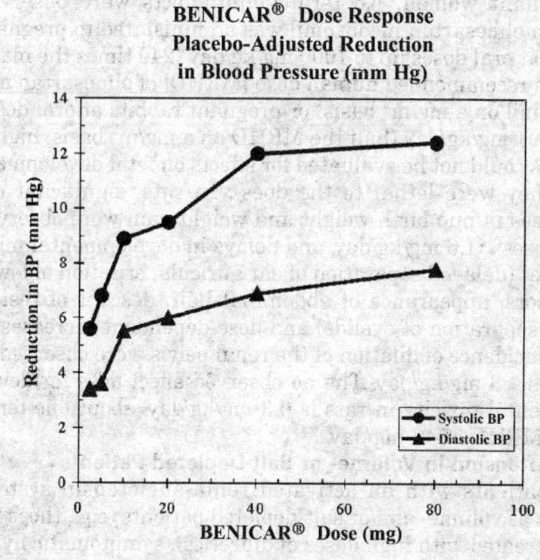

Data above are from seven placebo-controlled studies (2145 BENICAR® patients, 548 placebo patients). The blood pressure lowering effect was maintained throughout the 24-hour period with BENICAR® once daily, with trough-to-peak ratios for systolic and diastolic response between 60 and 80%. The blood pressure lowering effect of BENICAR®, with and without hydrochlorothiazide, was maintained in patients treated for up to 1 year. There was no evidence of tachyphylaxis during long-term treatment with BENICAR® or rebound effect following abrupt withdrawal of olmesartan medoxomil after 1 year of treatment.
The antihypertensive effect of BENICAR® was similar in men and women and in patients older and younger than 65 years. The effect was smaller in black patients (usually a low-renin population), as has been seen with other ACE inhibitors, angiotensin receptor blockers and beta-blockers. BENICAR® had an additional blood pressure lowering effect when added to hydrochlorothiazide.

INDICATIONS AND USAGE

BENICAR® is indicated for the treatment of hypertension. It may be used alone or in combination with other antihypertensive agents.

CONTRAINDICATIONS

BENICAR® is contraindicated in patients who are hypersensitive to any component of this product.

WARNINGS

Fetal/Neonatal Morbidity and Mortality

Drugs that act directly on the renin-angiotensin system can cause fetal and neonatal morbidity and death when administered to pregnant women. Several dozen cases have been reported in the world literature of patients who were taking angiotensin converting enzyme inhibitors. When pregnancy is detected, BENICAR® should be discontinued as soon as possible.

Continued on next page

Benicar—Cont.

The use of drugs that act directly on the renin-angiotensin system during the second and third trimesters of pregnancy has been associated with fetal and neonatal injury, including hypotension, neonatal skull hypoplasia, anuria, reversible or irreversible renal failure and death. Oligohydramnios has also been reported, presumably resulting from decreased fetal function; oligohydramnios in this setting has been associated with fetal limb contractures, craniofacial deformation and hypoplastic lung development. Prematurity, intrauterine growth retardation and patent ductus arteriosus have also been reported, although it is not clear whether these occurrences were due to exposure to the drug.

These adverse effects do not appear to have resulted from intrauterine drug exposure that has been limited to the first trimester. Mothers whose embryos and fetuses are exposed to an angiotensin II receptor antagonist only during the first trimester should be so informed. Nonetheless, when patients become pregnant, physicians should have the patient discontinue the use of BENICAR® as soon as possible. Rarely (probably less often than once in every thousand pregnancies), no alternative to a drug acting on the renin-angiotensin system will be found. In these rare cases, the mothers should be apprised of the potential hazards to their fetuses and serial ultrasound examinations should be performed to assess the intra-amniotic environment.

If oligohydramnios is observed, BENICAR® should be discontinued unless it is considered life-saving for the mother. Contraction stress testing (CST), a nonstress test (NST) or biophysical profiling (BPP) may be appropriate, depending upon the week of pregnancy. Patients and physicians should be aware, however, that oligohydramnios may not appear until after the fetus has sustained irreversible injury.

Infants with histories of *in utero* exposure to an angiotensin II receptor antagonist should be closely observed for hypotension, oliguria and hyperkalemia. If oliguria occurs, attention should be directed toward support of blood pressure and renal perfusion. Exchange transfusion or dialysis may be required as means of reversing hypotension and/or substituting for disordered renal function.

There is no clinical experience with the use of BENICAR® in pregnant women. No teratogenic effects were observed when olmesartan medoxomil was administered to pregnant rats at oral doses up to 1000 mg/kg/day (240 times the maximum recommended human dose [MRHD] of olmesartan medoxomil on a mg/m^2 basis) or pregnant rabbits at oral doses up to 1 mg/kg/day (half the MRHD on a mg/m^2 basis; higher doses could not be evaluated for effects on fetal development as they were lethal to the does). In rats, significant decreases in pup birth weight and weight gain were observed at doses ≥1.6 mg/kg/day, and delays in developmental milestones (delayed separation of ear auricula, eruption of lower incisors, appearance of abdominal hair, descent of testes, and separation of eyelids) and dose-dependent increases in the incidence of dilation of the renal pelvis were observed at doses ≥8 mg/kg/day. The no observed effect dose for developmental toxicity in rats is 0.3 mg/kg/day, about one-tenth the MRHD of 40 mg/day.

Hypotension in Volume- or Salt-Depleted Patients

In patients with an activated renin-angiotensin system, such as volume- and/or salt-depleted patients (e.g., those being treated with high doses of diuretics), symptomatic hypotension may occur after initiation of treatment with BENICAR®. Treatment should start under close medical supervision. If hypotension does occur, the patient should be placed in the supine position and, if necessary, given an intravenous infusion of normal saline (See **DOSAGE AND ADMINISTRATION**). A transient hypotensive response is not a contraindication to further treatment, which usually can be continued without difficulty once the blood pressure has stabilized.

PRECAUTIONS

General

Impaired Renal Function: As a consequence of inhibiting the renin-angiotensin-aldosterone system, changes in renal function may be anticipated in susceptible individuals treated with olmesartan medoxomil. In patients whose renal function may depend upon the activity of the renin-angiotensin-aldosterone system (e.g. patients with severe congestive heart failure), treatment with angiotensin converting enzyme inhibitors and angiotensin receptor antagonists has been associated with oliguria and/or progressive azotemia and (rarely) with acute renal failure and/or death. Similar results may be anticipated in patients treated with olmesartan medoxomil. (See **CLINICAL PHARMACOLOGY, Special Populations.**)

In studies of ACE inhibitors in patients with unilateral or bilateral renal artery stenosis, increases in serum creatinine or blood urea nitrogen (BUN) have been reported. There has been no long-term use of olmesartan medoxomil in patients with unilateral or bilateral renal artery stenosis, but similar results may be expected.

Information for Patients

Pregnancy: Female patients of childbearing age should be told about the consequences of second and third trimester exposure to drugs that act on the renin-angiotensin system and they should be told also that these consequences do not appear to have resulted from intrauterine drug exposure that has been limited to the first trimester. These patients should be asked to report pregnancies to their physicians as soon as possible.

Drug Interactions

No significant drug interactions were reported in studies in which olmesartan medoxomil was co-administered with digoxin or warfarin in healthy volunteers. The bioavailability of olmesartan was not significantly altered by the co-administration of antacids [$Al(OH)_3/Mg(OH)_2$]. Olmesartan medoxomil is not metabolized by the cytochrome P450 system and has no effects on P450 enzymes; thus, interactions with drugs that inhibit, induce or are metabolized by those enzymes are not expected.

Carcinogenesis, Mutagenesis, Impairment of Fertility

Olmesartan medoxomil was not carcinogenic when administered by dietary administration to rats for up to 2 years. The highest dose tested (2000 mg/kg/day) was, on a mg/m^2 basis, about 480 times the maximum recommended human dose (MRHD) of 40 mg/day. Two carcinogenicity studies conducted in mice, a 6-month gavage study in the p53 knockout mouse and a 6-month dietary administration study in the Hras2 transgenic mouse, at doses of up to 1000 mg/kg/day (about 120 times the MRHD), revealed no evidence of a carcinogenic effect of olmesartan medoxomil.

Both olmesartan medoxomil and olmesartan tested negative in the *in vitro* Syrian hamster embryo cell transformation assay and showed no evidence of genetic toxicity in the Ames (bacterial mutagenicity) test. However, both were shown to induce chromosomal aberrations in cultured cells *in vitro* (Chinese hamster lung) and tested positive for thymidine kinase mutations in the *in vitro* mouse lymphoma assay. Olmesartan medoxomil tested negative *in vivo* for mutations in the MutaMouse intestine and kidney and for clastogenicity in mouse bone marrow (micronucleus test) at oral doses of up to 2000 mg/kg (olmesartan not tested).

Fertility of rats was unaffected by administration of olmesartan medoxomil at dose levels as high as 1000 mg/kg/day (240 times the MRHD) in a study in which dosing was begun 2 (female) or 9 (male) weeks prior to mating.

Pregnancy

Pregnancy Categories C (first trimester) and D (second and third trimesters). See **WARNINGS, Fetal/Neonatal Morbidity and Mortality.**

Nursing Mothers

It is not known whether olmesartan is excreted in human milk, but olmesartan is secreted at low concentration in the milk of lactating rats. Because of the potential for adverse effects on the nursing infant, a decision should be made whether to discontinue nursing or discontinue the drug, taking into account the importance of the drug to the mother.

Pediatric Use

Safety and effectiveness in pediatric patients have not been established.

Geriatric Use

Of the total number of hypertensive patients receiving BENICAR® in clinical studies, more than 20% were 65 years of age and over, while more than 5% were 75 years of age and older. No overall differences in effectiveness or safety were observed between elderly patients and younger patients. Other reported clinical experience has not identified differences in responses between the elderly and younger patients, but greater sensitivity of some older individuals cannot be ruled out.

ADVERSE REACTIONS

BENICAR® has been evaluated for safety in more than 3825 patients/subjects, including more than 3275 patients treated for hypertension in controlled trials. This experience included about 900 patients treated for at least 6 months and more than 525 for at least 1 year. Treatment with BENICAR® was well tolerated, with an incidence of adverse events similar to placebo. Events generally were mild, transient and had no relationship to the dose of olmesartan medoxomil.

The overall frequency of adverse events was not dose-related. Analysis of gender, age and race groups demonstrated no differences between olmesartan medoxomil and placebo-treated patients. The rate of withdrawals due to adverse events in all trials of hypertensive patients was 2.4% (i.e. 79/3278) of patients treated with olmesartan medoxomil and 2.7% (i.e. 32/1179) of control patients. In placebo-controlled trials, the only adverse event that occurred in more than 1% of patients treated with olmesartan medoxomil and at a higher incidence versus placebo was dizziness (3% vs. 1%).

The following adverse events occurred in placebo-controlled clinical trials at an incidence of more than 1% of patients treated with olmesartan medoxomil, but also occurred at about the same or greater incidence in patients receiving placebo: back pain, bronchitis, creatine phosphokinase increased, diarrhea, headache, hematuria, hyperglycemia, hypertriglyceridemia, influenza-like symptoms, pharyngitis, rhinitis and sinusitis.

The incidence of cough was similar in placebo (0.7%) and BENICAR® (0.9%) patients.

Other (potentially important) adverse events that have been reported with an incidence of greater than 0.5%, whether or not attributed to treatment, in the more than 3100 hypertensive patients treated with olmesartan medoxomil monotherapy in controlled or open-label trials are listed below.

Body as a Whole: chest pain, peripheral edema
Central and Peripheral Nervous System: vertigo
Gastrointestinal: abdominal pain, dyspepsia, gastroenteritis, nausea
Heart Rate and Rhythm Disorders: tachycardia
Metabolic and Nutritional Disorders: hypercholesterolemia, hyperlipemia, hyperuricemia
Musculoskeletal: arthralgia, arthritis, myalgia
Skin and Appendages: rash

Facial edema was reported in 5 patients receiving olmesartan medoxomil. Angioedema has been reported with angiotensin II antagonists.

Laboratory Test Findings: In controlled clinical trials, clinically important changes in standard laboratory parameters were rarely associated with administration of olmesartan medoxomil.

Hemoglobin and Hematocrit: Small decreases in hemoglobin and hematocrit (mean decreases of approximately 0.3 g/dL and 0.3 volume percent, respectively) were observed.

Liver Function Tests: Elevations of liver enzymes and/or serum bilirubin were observed infrequently. Five patients (0.1%) assigned to olmesartan medoxomil and one patient (0.2%) assigned to placebo in clinical trials were withdrawn because of abnormal liver chemistries (transaminases or total bilirubin). Of the five olmesartan medoxomil patients, three had elevated transaminases, which were attributed to alcohol use, and one had a single elevated bilirubin value, which normalized while treatment continued.

Post-Marketing Experience: Rare cases of angioedema and rhabdomyolysis have been reported in patients receiving olmesartan medoxomil.

OVERDOSAGE

Limited data are available related to overdosage in humans. The most likely manifestations of overdosage would be hypotension and tachycardia; bradycardia could be encountered if parasympathetic (vagal) stimulation occurs. If symptomatic hypotension should occur, supportive treatment should be initiated. The dialyzability of olmesartan is unknown.

DOSAGE AND ADMINISTRATION

Dosage must be individualized. The usual recommended starting dose of BENICAR® is 20 mg once daily when used as monotherapy in patients who are not volume-contracted. For patients requiring further reduction in blood pressure after 2 weeks of therapy, the dose of BENICAR® may be increased to 40 mg. Doses above 40 mg do not appear to have greater effect. Twice-daily dosing offers no advantage over the same total dose given once daily.

No initial dosage adjustment is recommended for elderly patients, for patients with moderate to marked renal impairment (creatinine clearance <40mL/min) or with moderate to marked hepatic dysfunction (see CLINICAL PHARMACOLOGY, Special Populations). For patients with possible depletion of intravascular volume (e.g., patients treated with diuretics, particularly those with impaired renal function), BENICAR® should be initiated under close medical supervision and consideration should be given to use of a lower starting dose (see WARNINGS, Hypotension in Volume- and Salt-Depleted Patients).

BENICAR® may be administered with or without food.

If blood pressure is not controlled by BENICAR® alone, a diuretic may be added. BENICAR® may be administered with other antihypertensive agents.

HOW SUPPLIED

BENICAR® is supplied as yellow, round, film-coated tablets containing 5 mg of olmesartan medoxomil, as white, round, film-coated tablets containing 20 mg of olmesartan medoxomil, and as white, oval-shaped, film-coated tablets containing 40 mg of olmesartan medoxomil. Tablets are debossed with Sankyo on one side and C12, C14, or C15 on the other side of the 5, 20, and 40 mg tablets, respectively.

Tablets are supplied as follows:

[See table below]

Storage

Store at 20-25°C (68-77°F) [See USP Controlled Room Temperature].

Manufactured by Sankyo Pharma GmbH, Munich, Germany

Manufactured for Sankyo Pharma Inc., Parsippany, New Jersey 07054

Rx Only

Revised May 2004

SANKYO

	5 mg	20 mg	40 mg
Bottle of 30	NDC 65597-101-30	NDC 65597-103-30	NDC 65597-104-30
Bottle of 90	Not available	NDC 65597-103-90	NDC 65597-104-90
Blister 10 cards X 10		NDC 65597-103-10	NDC 65597-104-10

BENICAR HCT™ Tablets ℞
(OLMESARTAN MEDOXOMIL-HYDROCHLOROTHIAZIDE)

USE IN PREGNANCY
When used in pregnancy during the second and third trimesters, drugs that act directly on the renin-angiotensin system can cause injury and even death to the developing fetus. When pregnancy is detected, BENICAR HCT™ should be discontinued as soon as possible. See **WARNINGS, Fetal/Neonatal Morbidity and Mortality.**

DESCRIPTION
BENICAR HCT™ (olmesartan medoxomil-hydrochlorothiazide) is a combination of an angiotensin II receptor antagonist (AT_1 subtype), olmesartan medoxomil, and a thiazide diuretic, hydrochlorothiazide (HCTZ).
Olmesartan medoxomil, a prodrug, is hydrolyzed to olmesartan during absorption from the gastrointestinal tract.
Olmesartan medoxomil is 2,3-dihydroxy-2-butenyl 4-(1-hydroxy-1-methylethyl)-2-propyl-1-[*p*-(*o*-1*H*-tetrazol-5-ylphenyl)benzyl]imidazole-5-carboxylate, cyclic 2, 3-carbonate.
Its empirical formula is $C_{29}H_{30}N_6O_6$ and its structural formula is:

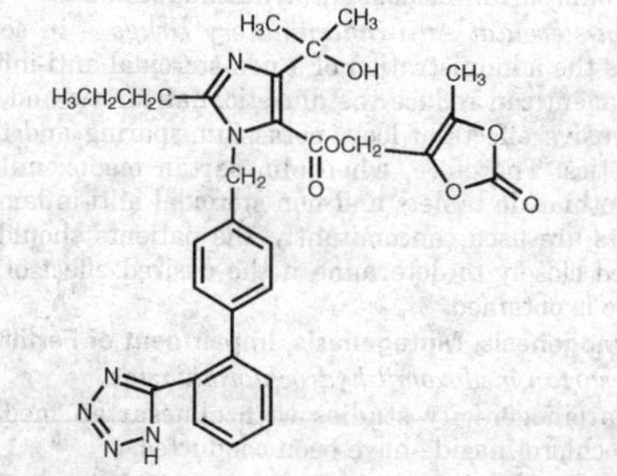

Olmesartan medoxomil is a white to light yellowish-white powder or crystalline powder with a molecular weight of 558.6. It is practically insoluble in water and sparingly soluble in methanol.
Hydrochlorothiazide is 6-chloro-3,4-dihydro-2*H*-1,2,4-benzo-thiadiazine-7-sulfonamide 1,1-dioxide. Its empirical formula is $C_7H_8ClN_3O_4S_2$ and its structural formula is:

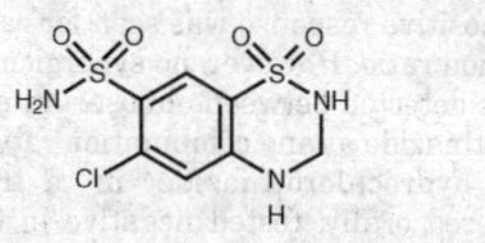

Hydrochlorothiazide is a white, or practically white, crystalline powder with a molecular weight of 297.7. Hydrochlorothiazide is slightly soluble in water but freely soluble in sodium hydroxide solution.
BENICAR HCT™ is available for oral administration in tablets containing 20 mg or 40 mg of olmesartan medoxomil combined with 12.5 mg of hydrochlorothiazide, or 40 mg of olmesartan medoxomil combined with 25 mg of hydrochlorothiazide. Inactive ingredients include: hydroxypropylcellulose, hypromellose, lactose, low-substituted hydroxypropylcellulose, magnesium stearate, microcrystalline cellulose, red iron oxide, talc, titanium dioxide and yellow iron oxide.

CLINICAL PHARMACOLOGY
Mechanism of Action
Olmesartan medoxomil
Angiotensin II is formed from angiotensin I in a reaction catalyzed by angiotensin converting enzyme (ACE, kininase II). Angiotensin II is the principal pressor agent of the renin-angiotensin system, with effects that include vasoconstriction, stimulation of synthesis and release of aldosterone, cardiac stimulation and renal reabsorption of sodium. Olmesartan blocks the vasoconstrictor effects of angiotensin II by selectively blocking the binding of angiotensin II to the AT_1 receptor in vascular smooth muscle. Its action is, therefore, independent of the pathways for angiotensin II synthesis.
An AT_2 receptor is found also in many tissues, but this receptor is not known to be associated with cardiovascular homeostasis. Olmesartan has more than a 12,500-fold greater affinity for the AT_1 receptor than for the AT_2 receptor.
Blockade of the renin-angiotensin system with ACE inhibitors, which inhibit the biosynthesis of angiotensin II from angiotensin I, is a mechanism of many drugs used to treat hypertension. ACE inhibitors also inhibit the degradation of bradykinin, a reaction also catalyzed by ACE. Because olmesartan medoxomil does not inhibit ACE (kininase II), it does not affect the response to bradykinin. Whether this difference has clinical relevance is not yet known.
Blockade of the angiotensin II receptor inhibits the negative regulatory feedback of angiotensin II on renin secretion, but the resulting increased plasma renin activity and circulating angiotensin II levels do not overcome the effect of olmesartan on blood pressure.
Hydrochlorothiazide
Hydrochlorothiazide is a thiazide diuretic. Thiazides affect the renal tubular mechanisms of electrolyte reabsorption, directly increasing excretion of sodium and chloride in approximately equivalent amounts. Indirectly, the diuretic action of hydrochlorothiazide reduces plasma volume, with consequent increases in plasma renin activity, increases in aldosterone secretion, increases in urinary potassium loss, and decreases in serum potassium. The renin-aldosterone link is mediated by angiotensin II, so co-administration of an angiotensin II receptor antagonist tends to reverse the potassium loss associated with these diuretics.
The mechanism of the antihypertensive effect of thiazides is not fully understood.

Pharmacokinetics
General
Olmesartan medoxomil
Olmesartan medoxomil is rapidly and completely bioactivated by ester hydrolysis to olmesartan during absorption from the gastrointestinal tract. Olmesartan appears to be eliminated in a biphasic manner with a terminal elimination half-life of approximately 13 hours. Olmesartan shows linear pharmacokinetics following single oral doses of up to 320 mg and multiple oral doses of up to 80 mg. Steady-state levels of olmesartan are achieved within 3 to 5 days and no accumulation in plasma occurs with once-daily dosing.
The absolute bioavailability of olmesartan is approximately 26%. After oral administration, the peak plasma concentration (C_{max}) of olmesartan is reached after 1 to 2 hours. Food does not affect the bioavailability of olmesartan.
Hydrochlorothiazide
When plasma levels have been followed for at least 24 hours, the plasma half-life has been observed to vary between 5.6 and 14.8 hours.
Metabolism and Excretion
Olmesartan medoxomil
Following the rapid and complete conversion of olmesartan medoxomil to olmesartan during absorption, there is virtually no further metabolism of olmesartan. Total plasma clearance of olmesartan is 1.3 L/h, with a renal clearance of 0.6 L/h. Approximately 35% to 50% of the absorbed dose is recovered in urine while the remainder is eliminated in feces via the bile.
Hydrochlorothiazide
Hydrochlorothiazide is not metabolized but is eliminated rapidly by the kidney. At least 61% of the oral dose is eliminated unchanged within 24 hours.
Distribution
Olmesartan
The volume of distribution of olmesartan is approximately 17 L. Olmesartan is highly bound to plasma proteins (99%) and does not penetrate red blood cells. The protein binding is constant at plasma olmesartan concentrations well above the range achieved with recommended doses.
In rats, olmesartan crossed the blood-brain barrier poorly, if at all. Olmesartan passed across the placental barrier in rats and was distributed to the fetus. Olmesartan was distributed to milk at low levels in rats.
Hydrochlorothiazide
Hydrochlorothiazide crosses the placental but not the blood-brain barrier and is excreted in breast milk.
Special Populations
Pediatric: The pharmacokinetics of olmesartan have not been investigated in patients <18 years of age.
Geriatric: The pharmacokinetics of olmesartan were studied in the elderly (≥65 years). Overall, maximum plasma concentrations of olmesartan were similar in young adults and the elderly. Modest accumulation of olmesartan was observed in the elderly with repeated dosing; $AUC_{ss,\tau}$ was 33% higher in elderly patients, corresponding to an approximate 30% reduction in CL_R.
Gender: Minor differences were observed in the pharmacokinetics of olmesartan in women compared to men. AUC and C_{max} were 10-15% higher in women than in men.
Renal Insufficiency: In patients with renal insufficiency, serum concentrations of olmesartan were elevated compared to subjects with normal renal function. After repeated dosing, the AUC was approximately tripled in patients with severe renal impairment (creatinine clearance <20 mL/min). The pharmacokinetics of olmesartan in patients undergoing hemodialysis has not been studied.
Hepatic Insufficiency: Increases in $AUC_{0-\infty}$ and C_{max} for olmesartan were observed in patients with moderate hepatic impairment compared to those in matched controls, with an increase in AUC of about 60%.
Drug Interactions: See **PRECAUTIONS, Drug Interactions.**

Pharmacodynamics
Olmesartan medoxomil
Olmesartan medoxomil doses of 2.5 to 40 mg inhibit the pressor effects of angiotensin I infusion. The duration of the inhibitory effect was related to dose, with doses of olmesartan medoxomil >40 mg giving >90% inhibition at 24 hours.
Plasma concentrations of angiotensin I and angiotensin II and plasma renin activity (PRA) increase after single and repeated administration of olmesartan medoxomil to healthy subjects and hypertensive patients. Repeated administration of up to 80 mg olmesartan medoxomil had minimal influence on aldosterone levels and no effect on serum potassium.
Hydrochlorothiazide
After oral administration of hydrochlorothiazide, diuresis begins within 2 hours, peaks in about 4 hours and lasts about 6 to 12 hours.

Clinical Trials
Olmesartan medoxomil
The antihypertensive effects of olmesartan medoxomil have been demonstrated in seven placebo-controlled studies at doses ranging from 2.5 to 80 mg for 6 to 12 weeks, each showing statistically significant reductions in peak and trough blood pressure. A total of 2693 patients (2145 olmesartan medoxomil; 548 placebo) with essential hypertension were studied. Olmesartan medoxomil once daily (QD) lowered diastolic and systolic blood pressure. The response was dose-related. An olmesartan medoxomil dose of 20 mg daily produces a trough sitting BP reduction over placebo of about 10/6 mm Hg and a dose of 40 mg daily produces a trough sitting BP reduction over placebo of about 12/7 mm Hg. Olmesartan medoxomil doses greater than 40 mg had little additional effect. The onset of the antihypertensive effect occurred within 1 week and was largely manifest after 2 weeks.
The blood pressure lowering effect was maintained throughout the 24-hour period with olmesartan medoxomil once daily, with trough-to-peak ratios for systolic and diastolic response between 60 and 80%.
The blood pressure lowering effect of olmesartan medoxomil, with and without hydrochlorothiazide, was maintained in patients treated for up to 1 year. There was no evidence of tachyphylaxis during long-term treatment with olmesartan medoxomil or rebound effect following abrupt withdrawal of olmesartan medoxomil after 1 year of treatment.
The antihypertensive effect of olmesartan medoxomil was similar in men and women and in patients older and younger than 65 years. The effect was smaller in black patients (usually a low-renin population), as has been seen with other ACE inhibitors, angiotensin receptor blockers and beta-blockers. Olmesartan medoxomil had an additional blood pressure lowering effect when added to hydrochlorothiazide.
Olmesartan medoxomil-hydrochlorothiazide
In clinical trials 1230 patients were exposed to the combination of olmesartan medoxomil (2.5 mg to 40 mg) and hydrochlorothiazide (12.5 mg to 25 mg). These trials included one placebo-controlled factorial trial (n=502) in mild-moderate hypertensives with combinations of olmesartan medoxomil (10 mg, 20 mg, 40 mg or placebo) and hydrochlorothiazide (12.5 mg, 25 mg or placebo). The antihypertensive effect of the combination on trough blood pressure was related to the dose of each component (see table below).

Placebo-Adjusted Changes in Sitting Systolic/Diastolic Blood Pressure (mmHg)

	Olmesartan Medoxomil dose			
HCTZ dose	0 mg	10 mg	20 mg	40 mg
0 mg	–	7/5	12/5	13/7
12.5 mg	5/1	17/8	17/8	16/10
25 mg	14/5	19/11	22/11	24/14

Once-daily dosing with 20 mg olmesartan medoxomil and 12.5 mg hydrochlorothiazide, 40 mg olmesartan medoxomil and 12.5 mg hydrochlorothiazide or 40 mg olmesartan medoxomil and 25 mg hydrochlorothiazide produced mean placebo-adjusted blood pressure reductions at trough (24 hours post-dosing) ranging from 17/8 to 24/14 mm Hg.
The onset of the antihypertensive effect occurred within 1 week and was near maximal at 4 weeks. The antihypertensive effect was independent of gender, but there were too few subjects to identify response differences based on race or age greater than or less than 65 years. No appreciable changes in trough heart rate were observed with combination therapy in the placebo-controlled trial.

INDICATIONS AND USAGE
BENICAR HCT™ is indicated for the treatment of hypertension. This fixed dose combination is not indicated for initial therapy (see **DOSAGE AND ADMINISTRATION**).

CONTRAINDICATIONS
BENICAR HCT™ is contraindicated in patients who are hypersensitive to any component of this product.
Because of the hydrochlorothiazide component, this product is contraindicated in patients with anuria or hypersensitivity to other sulfonamide-derived drugs.

WARNINGS
Fetal/Neonatal Morbidity and Mortality
Drugs that act directly on the renin-angiotensin system can cause fetal and neonatal morbidity and death when administered to pregnant women. Several dozen cases have been reported in the world literature of patients who were taking angiotensin converting enzyme inhibitors. When pregnancy is detected, BENICAR HCT™ should be discontinued as soon as possible.
The use of drugs that act directly on the renin-angiotensin system during the second and third trimesters of pregnancy has been associated with fetal and neonatal injury, including hypotension, neonatal skull hypoplasia, anuria, reversible or irreversible renal failure and death. Oligohydramnios has also been reported, presumably resulting from

Continued on next page

Benicar HCT—Cont.

decreased fetal function; oligohydramnios in this setting has been associated with fetal limb contractures, craniofacial deformation and hypoplastic lung development. Prematurity, intrauterine growth retardation and patent ductus arteriosus have also been reported, although it is not clear whether these occurrences were due to exposure to the drug.

These adverse effects do not appear to have resulted from intrauterine drug exposure that has been limited to the first trimester. Mothers whose embryos and fetuses are exposed to an angiotensin II receptor antagonist only during the first trimester should be so informed. Nonetheless, when patients become pregnant, physicians should have the patient discontinue the use of BENICAR HCT™ as soon as possible.

Rarely (probably less often than once in every thousand pregnancies), no alternative to a drug acting on the renin-angiotensin system will be found. In these rare cases, the mothers should be apprised of the potential hazards to their fetuses and serial ultrasound examinations should be performed to assess the intra-amniotic environment.

If oligohydramnios is observed, BENICAR HCT™ should be discontinued unless it is considered life-saving for the mother. Contraction stress testing (CST), a non-stress test (NST) or biophysical profiling (BPP) may be appropriate, depending upon the week of pregnancy. Patients and physicians should be aware, however, that oligohydramnios may not appear until after the fetus has sustained irreversible injury.

Infants with histories of *in utero* exposure to an angiotensin II receptor antagonist should be closely observed for hypotension, oliguria and hyperkalemia. If oliguria occurs, attention should be directed toward support of blood pressure and renal perfusion. Exchange transfusion or dialysis may be required as means of reversing hypotension and/or substituting for disordered renal function.

There is no clinical experience with the use of BENICAR HCT™ in pregnant women. No teratogenic effects were observed when 1.6:1 combinations of olmesartan medoxomil and hydrochlorothiazide were administered to pregnant mice at oral doses up to 1625 mg/kg/day (122 times the maximum recommended human dose [MRHD] on a mg/m^2 basis) or pregnant rats at oral doses up to 1625 mg/kg/day (280 times the MRHD on a mg/m^2 basis). In rats, however, fetal body weights at 1625 mg/kg/day (a toxic, sometimes lethal dose in the dams) were significantly lower than control. The no observed effect dose for developmental toxicity in rats, 162.5 mg/kg/day, is about 28 times, on a mg/m^2 basis, the MRHD of BENICAR HCT™ (40 mg olmesartan medoxomil/25 mg hydrochlorothiazide/day).

Thiazides cross the placental barrier and appear in cord blood. There is a risk of fetal or neonatal jaundice, thrombocytopenia and possibly other adverse reactions that have occurred in adults.

Hypotension in Volume- or Salt-Depleted Patients

In patients with an activated renin-angiotensin system, such as volume- or salt-depleted patients (*e.g.*, those being treated with high doses of diuretics), symptomatic hypotension may occur after initiation of treatment with BENICAR HCT™, as with any angiotensin receptor blocker. Treatment should start under close medical supervision. If hypotension does occur, the patient should be placed in the supine position and, if necessary, given an intravenous infusion of normal saline (See **DOSAGE AND ADMINISTRATION**). When electrolyte and fluid imbalances have been corrected, therapy usually can be continued without difficulty. A transient hypotensive response is not a contraindication to further treatment.

Hydrochlorothiazide

Hepatic Impairment

Thiazides should be used with caution in patients with impaired hepatic function or progressive liver disease, since minor alterations of fluid and electrolyte balance may precipitate hepatic coma.

Hypersensitivity Reaction

Hypersensitivity reactions to hydrochlorothiazide may occur in patients with or without a history of allergy or bronchial asthma, but are more likely in patients with such a history.

Systemic Lupus Erythematosus

Thiazide diuretics have been reported to cause exacerbation or activation of systemic lupus erythematosus.

Lithium Interaction

Lithium generally should not be given with thiazides (see **PRECAUTIONS: Drug Interactions**; *Hydrochlorothiazide, Lithium*).

PRECAUTIONS

General

Olmesartan medoxomil-hydrochlorothiazide

In a double-blind clinical trial of various doses of olmesartan medoxomil and hydrochlorothiazide, the incidence of hypertensive patients who developed hypokalemia (serum potassium <3.4 mEq/L) was 2.1%; the incidence of hyperkalemia (serum potassium >5.7 mEq/L) was 0.4%. In this trial, no patient discontinued due to increases or decreases in serum potassium.

Hydrochlorothiazide

Periodic determinations of serum electrolytes to detect possible electrolyte imbalance should be performed at appropriate intervals. All patients receiving thiazide therapy should be observed for clinical signs of fluid or electrolyte imbalance: hyponatremia, hypochloremic alkalosis and hypokalemia. Serum and urine electrolyte determinations are important when the patient is vomiting excessively or receiving parenteral fluids. Warning signs or symptoms of fluid and electrolyte imbalance, irrespective of cause, include dryness of mouth, thirst, weakness, lethargy, drowsiness, restlessness, confusion, seizures, muscle pains or cramps, muscular fatigue, hypotension, oliguria, tachycardia and gastrointestinal disturbances such as nausea and vomiting.

Hypokalemia may develop, especially with brisk diuresis, when severe cirrhosis is present, or after prolonged therapy. Interference with adequate oral electrolyte intake will also contribute to hypokalemia. Hypokalemia may cause cardiac arrhythmia and may also sensitize or exaggerate the response of the heart to the toxic effects of digitalis (e.g., increased ventricular irritability).

Although any chloride deficit is generally mild and usually does not require specific treatment except under extraordinary circumstances (as in liver disease or renal disease), chloride replacement may be required in the treatment of metabolic alkalosis.

Dilutional hyponatremia may occur in edematous patients in hot weather; appropriate therapy is water restriction, rather than administration of salt except in rare instances when the hyponatremia is life-threatening. In actual salt depletion, appropriate replacement is the therapy of choice.

Hyperuricemia may occur or frank gout may be precipitated in certain patients receiving thiazide therapy.

In diabetic patients dosage adjustments of insulin or oral hypoglycemic agents may be required. Hyperglycemia may occur with thiazide diuretics. Thus latent diabetes mellitus may become manifest during thiazide therapy.

The antihypertensive effects of the drug may be enhanced in the post-sympathectomy patient.

If progressive renal impairment becomes evident consider withholding or discontinuing diuretic therapy.

Thiazides have been shown to increase the urinary excretion of magnesium; this may result in hypomagnesemia.

Thiazides may decrease urinary calcium excretion. Thiazides may cause intermittent and slight elevation of serum calcium in the absence of known disorders of calcium metabolism. Marked hypercalcemia may be evidence of hyperparathyroidism. Thiazides should be discontinued before carrying out tests for parathyroid function.

Increases in cholesterol and triglyceride levels may be associated with thiazide diuretic therapy.

Impaired Renal Function

As a consequence of inhibiting the renin-angiotensin-aldosterone system, changes in renal function may be anticipated in susceptible individuals treated with olmesartan medoxomil. In patients whose renal function may depend upon the activity of the renin-angiotensin-aldosterone system (e.g. patients with severe congestive heart failure), treatment with angiotensin converting enzyme inhibitors and angiotensin receptor antagonists has been associated with oliguria and/or progressive azotemia and (rarely) with acute renal failure and/or death. Similar results may be anticipated in patients treated with olmesartan medoxomil. (See **CLINICAL PHARMACOLOGY, *Special Populations***)

In studies of ACE inhibitors in patients with unilateral or bilateral renal artery stenosis, increases in serum creatinine or blood urea nitrogen (BUN) have been reported. There has been no long-term use of olmesartan medoxomil in patients with unilateral or bilateral renal artery stenosis, but similar results may be expected.

Thiazides should be used with caution in severe renal disease. In patients with renal disease, thiazides may precipitate azotemia. Cumulative effects of the drug may develop in patients with impaired renal function.

Information for Patients

Pregnancy: Female patients of childbearing age should be told about the consequences of second and third trimester exposure to drugs that act on the renin-angiotensin system and they should be told also that these consequences do not appear to have resulted from intrauterine drug exposure that has been limited to the first trimester. These patients should be asked to report pregnancies to their physicians as soon as possible.

Symptomatic Hypotension: A patient receiving BENICAR HCT™ should be cautioned that lightheadedness can occur, especially during the first days of therapy, and that it should be reported to the prescribing physician. The patients should be told that if syncope occurs, BENICAR HCT™ should be discontinued until the physician has been consulted.

All patients should be cautioned that inadequate fluid intake, excessive perspiration, diarrhea or vomiting can lead to an excessive fall in blood pressure, with the same consequences of light-headedness and possible syncope.

Drug Interactions

Olmesartan medoxomil

No significant drug interactions were reported in studies in which olmesartan medoxomil was co-administered with hydrochlorothiazide, digoxin or warfarin in healthy volunteers. The bioavailability of olmesartan was not significantly altered by the co-administration of antacids [$Al(OH)_3/Mg(OH)_2$]. Olmesartan medoxomil is not metabolized by the cytochrome P450 system and has no effects on P450 enzymes; thus, interactions with drugs that inhibit, induce or are metabolized by those enzymes are not expected.

Hydrochlorothiazide

When administered concurrently the following drugs may interact with thiazide diuretics:

Alcohol, Barbiturates, Or Narcotics – potentiation of orthostatic hypotension may occur.

Antidiabetic Drugs (oral agents and insulin) – dosage adjustment of the antidiabetic drug may be required.

Other Antihypertensive Drugs – additive effect or potentiation.

Cholestyramine and Colestipol Resins – absorption of hydrochlorothiazide is impaired in the presence of anionic exchange resins. Single doses of either cholestyramine or colestipol resins bind the hydrochlorothiazide and reduce its absorption from the gastrointestinal tract by up to 85 and 43 percent, respectively.

Corticosteriods, ACTH – intensified electrolyte depletion, particularly hypokalemia.

Pressor Amines (e.g. Norepinephrine) – possible decreased response to pressor amines but not sufficient to preclude their use.

Skeletal Muscle Relaxants, Non depolarizing (e.g. Tubocurarine) – possible increased responsiveness to the muscle relaxant.

Lithium – should not generally be given with diuretics. Diuretic agents reduce the renal clearance of lithium and add a high risk of lithium toxicity. Refer to the package insert for lithium preparations before use of such preparation with olmesartan medoxomil-hydrochlorothiazide.

Non-steroidal Anti-inflammatory Drugs – in some patients the administration of a non-steroidal anti-inflammatory agent can reduce the diuretic, natriuretic and antihypertensive effects of loop, potassium-sparing and thiazide diuretics. Therefore, when olmesartan medoxomil-hydrochlorothiazide tablets and non-steroidal anti-inflammatory agents are used concomitantly, the patients should be observed closely to determine if the desired effect of the diuretic is obtained.

Carcinogenesis, Mutagenesis, Impairment of Fertility

Olmesartan medoxomil-hydrochlorothiazide

No carcinogenicity studies with olmesartan medoxomil-hydrochlorothiazide have been conducted.

Olmesartan medoxomil-hydrochlorothiazide in a ratio of 20:12.5 was negative in the *Salmonella-Escherichia coli*/mammalian microsome reverse mutation test up to the maximum recommended plate concentration for the standard assays. Olmesartan medoxomil and hydrochlorothiazide were tested individually and in combination ratios of 40:12.5, 20:12.5 and 10:12.5, for clastogenic activity in the *in vitro* Chinese hamster lung (CHL) chromosomal aberration assay. A positive response was seen for each component and combination ratio. However, no synergism in clastogenic activity was detected between olmesartan medoxomil and hydrochlorothiazide at any combination ratio. Olmesartan medoxomil hydrochlorothiazide in a ratio of 20:12.5, administered orally, tested negative in the *in vivo* mouse bone marrow erythrocyte micronucleus assay at administered doses of up to 3144 mg/kg.

No studies of impairment of fertility with olmesartan medoxomil-hydrochlorothiazide have been conducted.

Olmesartan medoxomil

Olmesartan medoxomil was not carcinogenic when administered by dietary administration to rats for up to 2 years. The highest dose tested (2000 mg/kg/day) was, on a mg/m^2 basis, about 480 times the maximum recommended human dose (MRHD) of 40 mg/day. Two carcinogenicity studies conducted in mice, a 6-month gavage study in the p53 knockout mouse and a 6-month dietary administration study in the Hras2 transgenic mouse, at doses of up to 1000 mg/kg/day (about 120 times the MRHD), revealed no evidence of a carcinogenic effect of olmesartan medoxomil.

Both olmesartan medoxomil and olmesartan tested negative in the *in vitro* Syrian hamster embryo cell transformation assay and showed no evidence of genetic toxicity in the Ames (bacterial mutagenicity) test. However, both were shown to induce chromosomal aberrations in cultured cells *in vitro* (Chinese hamster lung) and both tested positive for thymidine kinase mutations in the *in vitro* mouse lymphoma assay. Olmesartan medoxomil tested negative *in vivo* for mutations in the MutaMouse intestine and kidney, and for clastogenicity in mouse bone marrow (micronucleus test) at oral doses of up to 2000 mg/kg (olmesartan not tested).

Fertility of rats was unaffected by administration of olmesartan medoxomil at dose levels as high as 1000 mg/kg/day (240 times the MRHD) in a study in which dosing was begun 2 (female) or 9 (male) weeks prior to mating.

Hydrochlorothiazide

Two-year feeding studies in mice and rats conducted under the auspices of the National Toxicology Program (NTP) uncovered no evidence of a carcinogenic potential of hydrochlorothiazide in female mice (at doses of up to approximately 600 mg/kg/day) or in male and female rats (at doses of up to approximately 100 mg/kg/day). The NTP, however, found equivocal evidence for hepatocarcinogenicity in male mice.

Hydrochlorothiazide was not genotoxic *in vitro* in the Ames mutagenicity assay of *Salmonella typhimurium* strains TA 98, TA 100, TA 1535, TA 1537 and TA 1538, or in the Chinese Hamster Ovary (CHO) test for chromosomal aberrations. It was also not genotoxic *in vivo* in assays using mouse germinal cell chromosomes, Chinese hamster bone marrow chromosomes, or the *Drosophila* sex-linked recessive lethal trait gene. Positive test results were obtained in the *in vitro* CHO Sister Chromatid Exchange (clastogenicity) assay, the Mouse Lymphoma Cell (mutagenicity) assay and the *Aspergillus nidulans* non-disjunction assay.

Hydrochlorothiazide had no adverse effects on the fertility of mice and rats of either sex in studies wherein these species were exposed, via their diet, to doses of up to 100 and 4 mg/kg, respectively, prior to mating and throughout gestation.

Pregnancy

Pregnancy Categories C (first trimester) and D (second and third trimesters)

(See **WARNINGS: Fetal/Neonatal Morbidity and Mortality**)

Nursing Mothers

It is not known whether olmesartan is excreted in human milk, but olmesartan is secreted at low concentration in the milk of lactating rats. Because of the potential for adverse effects on the nursing infant, a decision should be made whether to discontinue nursing or discontinue the drug, taking into account the importance of the drug to the mother.

Thiazides appear in human milk. Because of the potential for adverse effects on the nursing infant, a decision should be made whether to discontinue nursing or discontinue the drug, taking into account the importance of the drug to the mother.

Pediatric Use

Safety and effectiveness in pediatric patients have not been established.

Geriatric Use

Clinical studies of BENICAR HCT™ did not include sufficient numbers of subjects aged 65 and over to determine whether they respond differently from younger subjects. Other reported clinical experience has not identified differences in responses between the elderly and younger patients. In general, dose selection for an elderly patient should be cautious, usually starting at the low end of the dosing range, reflecting the greater frequency of decreased hepatic, renal or cardiac function and of concomitant diseases or other drug therapy.

Olmesartan and hydrochlorothiazide are substantially excreted by the kidney, and the risk of toxic reactions to this drug may be greater in patients with impaired renal function.

ADVERSE REACTIONS

Olmesartan medoxomil-hydrochlorothiazide

Olmesartan medoxomil-hydrochlorothiazide has been evaluated for safety in 1243 hypertensive patients. Treatment with olmesartan medoxomil-hydrochlorothiazide was well tolerated, with an incidence of adverse events similar to placebo. Events generally were mild, transient and had no relationship to the dose of olmesartan medoxomil-hydrochlorothiazide.

In the clinical trials, the overall frequency of adverse events was not dose-related. Analysis of gender, age and race groups demonstrated no differences between olmesartan medoxomil-hydrochlorothiazide and placebo-treated patients. The rate of withdrawals due to adverse events in all trials of hypertensive patients was 2.0% (25/1243) of patients treated with olmesartan medoxomil-hydrochlorothiazide and 2.0% (7/342) of patients treated with placebo.

In a placebo-controlled clinical trial, the following adverse events reported with olmesartan medoxomil-hydrochlorothiazide occurred in >2% of patients, and more often on the olmesartan medoxomil-hydrochlorothiazide combination than on placebo, regardless of drug relationship:

[See first table above]

	Olmesartan/HCTZ (N=247) (%)	Placebo (N=42) (%)	Olmesartan (N=125) (%)	HCTZ (N=88) (%)
Gastrointestinal				
Nausea	3	0	2	1
Metabolic				
Hyperuricemia	4	2	0	2
Nervous System				
Dizziness	9	2	1	8
Respiratory				
Upper Respiratory Tract Infection	7	0	6	7

The following adverse events were also reported at a rate of >2%, but were as, or more, common in the placebo group: headache and urinary tract infection.

Other adverse events that have been reported with an incidence of greater than 1.0%, whether or not attributed to treatment, in the more than 1200 hypertensive patients treated with olmesartan medoxomil-hydrochlorothiazide in controlled or open-label trials are listed below.

Body as a Whole: chest pain, back pain, peripheral edema

Central and Peripheral Nervous System: vertigo

Gastrointestinal: abdominal pain, dyspepsia, gastroenteritis, diarrhea

Liver and Biliary System: SGOT increased, GGT increased, SGPT increased

Metabolic and Nutritional: hyperlipemia, creatine phosphokinase increased, hyperglycemia

Musculoskeletal: arthritis, arthralgia, myalgia

Respiratory System: coughing

Skin and Appendages Disorders: rash

Urinary System: hematuria

Facial edema was reported in 2/1243 patients receiving olmesartan medoxomil-hydrochlorothiazide. Angioedema has been reported with angiotensin II receptor antagonists.

Olmesartan medoxomil

Other adverse events that have been reported with an incidence of greater than 0.5%, whether or not attributed to treatment, in more than 3100 hypertensive patients treated with olmesartan medoxomil monotherapy in controlled or open-label trials are tachycardia and hypercholesterolemia.

Hydrochlorothiazide

Other adverse experiences that have been reported with hydrochlorothiazide, without regard to causality, are listed below:

Body as a Whole: weakness

Digestive: pancreatitis, jaundice (intrahepatic cholestatic jaundice), sialadenitis, cramping, gastric irritation

Hematologic: aplastic anemia, agranulocytosis, leukopenia, hemolytic anemia, thrombocytopenia

Hypersensitivity: purpura, photosensitivity, urticaria, necrotizing angiitis (vasculitis and cutaneous vasculitis), fever, respiratory distress including pneumonitis and pulmonary edema, anaphylactic reactions

Metabolic: hyperglycemia, glycosuria, hyperuricemia

Musculoskeletal: muscle spasm

Nervous System/Psychiatric: restlessness

Renal: renal failure, renal dysfunction, interstitial nephritis

Skin: erythema multiforme including Stevens-Johnson syndrome, exfoliative dermatitis including toxic epidermal necrolysis

Special Senses: transient blurred vision, xanthopsia

Laboratory Test Findings

In controlled clinical trials, clinically important changes in standard laboratory parameters were rarely associated with administration of olmesartan medoxomil-hydrochlorothiazide.

Creatinine, Blood Urea Nitrogen: Increases in blood urea nitrogen (BUN) and serum creatinine of >50% were observed in 1.3% of patients. No patients were discontinued from clinical trials of olmesartan medoxomil-hydrochlorothiazide due to increased BUN or creatinine.

Hemoglobin and Hematocrit: A greater than 20% decrease in hemoglobin and hematocrit was observed in 0.0% and 0.4% (one patient), respectively, of olmesartan medoxomil-hydrochlorothiazide patients, compared with 0.0% and 0.0%, respectively, in placebo-treated patients. No patients were discontinued due to anemia.

Post-Marketing Experience: Rare cases of angioedema and rhabdomyolysis have been reported in patients receiving olmesartan medoxomil.

OVERDOSAGE

Olmesartan medoxomil

Limited data are available related to overdosage in humans. The most likely manifestations of overdosage would be hypotension and tachycardia; bradycardia could be encountered if parasympathetic (vagal) stimulation occurs. If symptomatic hypotension should occur, supportive treatment should be initiated. The dialyzability of olmesartan is unknown.

No lethality was observed in acute toxicity studies in mice and rats given single oral doses up to 2000 mg/kg olmesartan medoxomil. The minimum lethal oral dose of olmesartan medoxomil in dogs was greater than 1500 mg/kg.

Hydrochlorothiazide

The most common signs and symptoms of overdose observed in humans are those caused by electrolyte depletion (hypokalemia, hypochloremia, hyponatremia) and dehydration resulting from excessive diuresis. If digitalis has also been administered, hypokalemia may accentuate cardiac arrhythmias. The degree to which hydrochlorothiazide is removed by hemodialysis has not been established. The oral LD_{50} of hydrochlorothiazide is greater than 10 g/kg in both mice and rats.

DOSAGE AND ADMINISTRATION

The usual recommended starting dose of BENICAR® (olmesartan medoxomil) is 20 mg once daily when used as monotherapy in patients who are not volume-contracted. For patients requiring further reduction in blood pressure after 2 weeks of therapy, the dose may be increased to 40 mg. Doses above 40 mg do not appear to have greater effect. Twice-daily dosing offers no advantage over the same total dose given once daily. No initial dosage adjustment is recommended for elderly patients, for patients with moderate to marked renal impairment (creatinine clearance <40mL/min) or with moderate to marked hepatic dysfunction (see **CLINICAL PHARMACOLOGY, *Special Populations***). For patients with possible depletion of intravascular volume (e.g., patients treated with diuretics, particularly those with impaired renal function), BENICAR® should be initiated under close medical supervision and consideration should be given to use of a lower starting dose (see **WARNINGS, Hypotension in Volume- or Salt-Depleted Patients**).

Hydrochlorothiazide is effective in doses between 12.5 mg and 50 mg once daily.

The side effects (see **WARNINGS**) of BENICAR® are generally rare and independent of dose; those of hydrochlorothiazide are most typically dose-dependent (primarily hypokalemia). Some dose-independent phenomena (e.g., pancreatitis) do occur with hydrochlorothiazide. Therapy with any combination of olmesartan medoxomil and hydrochlorothiazide will be associated with both sets of dose-independent side effects.

To minimize dose-independent side effects, it is usually appropriate to begin combination therapy only after a patient has failed to achieve the desired effect with monotherapy.

Replacement Therapy

BENICAR HCT™ (olmesartan medoxomil-hydrochlorothiazide) may be substituted for its titrated components.

Dose Titration by Clinical Effect

BENICAR HCT™ is available in strengths of 20 mg/12.5 mg, 40 mg/12.5 mg and 40 mg/25 mg. A patient whose blood pressure is inadequately controlled by BENICAR® or hydrochlorothiazide alone may be switched to once daily BENICAR HCT™ (olmesartan medoxomil-hydrochlorothiazide).

Dosing should be individualized. Depending on the blood pressure response, the dose may be titrated at intervals of 2-4 weeks.

If blood pressure is not controlled by BENICAR® alone, hydrochlorothiazide may be added starting with a dose of 12.5 mg and later titrated to 25 mg once daily.

If a patient is taking hydrochlorothiazide, BENICAR® may be added starting with a dose of 20 mg once daily and titrated to 40 mg, for inadequate blood pressure control. If large doses of hydrochlorothiazide have been used as monotherapy and volume depletion or hyponatremia is present, caution should be used when adding BENICAR® or switching to BENICAR HCT™ as marked decreases in blood pressure may occur (see **WARNINGS, Hypotension in Volume- or Salt-Depleted Patients**). Consideration should be given to reducing the dose of hydrochlorothiazide to 12.5 mg before adding BENICAR®. The antihypertensive effect of BENICAR HCT™ is related to the dose of both components over the range of 10 mg/12.5 mg to 40 mg/25 mg (see **CLINICAL PHARMACOLOGY, Clinical Trials**). The dose of BENICAR HCT™ is one tablet once daily. More than one tablet daily is not recommended.

BENICAR HCT™ may be administered with other antihypertensive agents.

Patients with Renal Impairment

The usual regimens of therapy with BENICAR HCT™ may be followed provided the patient's creatinine clearance is >30 mL/min. In patients with more severe renal impairment, loop diuretics are preferred to thiazides, so BENICAR HCT™ is not recommended.

Patients with Hepatic Impairment

No dosage adjustment is necessary with hepatic impairment (see **CLINICAL PHARMACOLOGY, *Special Populations***).

	20 mg/12.5 mg	40 mg/12.5 mg	40 mg/25 mg
Bottle of 30 tablets	NDC 65597-105-30	NDC 65597-106-30	NDC 65597-107-30
Bottle of 90 tablets	NDC 65597-105-90	NDC 65597-106-90	NDC 65597-107-90
10 Blister cards of 10 tablets	NDC 65597-105-10	NDC 65597-106-10	NDC 65597-107-10
Bottle of 1000 tablets	NDC 65597-105-11	NDC 65597-106-11	NDC 65597-107-11

Continued on next page

Benicar HCT—Cont.

HOW SUPPLIED

BENICAR HCT™ is supplied as 20 mg/12.5 mg: reddish-yellow, circular, film-coated tablets, approximately 8.5 mm in diameter, with "Sankyo" debossed on one side and "C22" on the other side. Each tablet contains 20 mg of olmesartan medoxomil and 12.5 mg of hydrochlorothiazide.
40 mg/12.5 mg: reddish-yellow, oval, film-coated tablets, approximately 15 x 7 mm, with "Sankyo" debossed on one side and "C23" on the other side. Each tablet contains 40 mg of olmesartan medoxomil and 12.5 mg of hydrochlorothiazide.
40 mg/25 mg: pink, oval, film-coated tablets, approximately 15 x 7 mm, with "Sankyo" debossed on one side and "C25" on the other side. Each tablet contains 40 mg of olmesartan medoxomil and 25 mg of hydrochlorothiazide.
Tablets are supplied as follows:
[See second table at top of previous page]

Storage
Store at 20-25°(68-77°F) [See USP Controlled Room Temperature].
Manufactured for Sankyo Pharma Inc., Parsippany, NJ 07054
Manufactured by Sankyo Pharma GmbH, Munich, Germany
Rx Only
May 2004
SANKYO

WELCHOL® Tablets ℞

[wĕl-chōl]
(colesevelam hydrochloride)
[koe le sev' e lam]

DESCRIPTION

WelChol® contains colesevelam hydrochloride (hereafter referred to as colesevelam), a non-absorbed, polymeric, lipid-lowering agent intended for oral administration. Colesevelam is a high capacity bile acid binding molecule. Colesevelam is poly (allylamine hydrochloride) cross-linked with epichlorohydrin and alkylated with 1-bromodecane and (6-bromohexyl)-trimethylammonium bromide. Colesevelam is hydrophilic, and insoluble in water.
WelChol® is an off-white, film-coated, solid tablet containing 625 mg colesevelam. In addition, each tablet contains the following inactive ingredients: magnesium stearate, microcrystalline cellulose, silicon dioxide, HPMC (hydroxypropyl methylcellulose), and acetylated monoglyceride. The tablets are imprinted using a water-soluble black ink.

CLINICAL PHARMACOLOGY

Mechanism of Action
The mechanism of action for the lipid-lowering activity of colesevelam, the active pharmaceutical ingredient in WelChol®, has been evaluated in various *in vitro* and *in vivo* studies. These studies have demonstrated that colesevelam binds bile acids, including glycocholic acid, the major bile acid in humans.
Cholesterol is the sole precursor of bile acids. During normal digestion, bile acids are secreted into the intestine. A major portion of bile acids are then absorbed from the intestinal tract and returned to the liver via the enterohepatic circulation.
Colesevelam is a non-absorbed, lipid-lowering polymer that binds bile acids in the intestine, impeding their reabsorption. As the bile acid pool becomes depleted, the hepatic enzyme, cholesterol 7-α-hydroxylase, is upregulated, which increases the conversion of cholesterol to bile acids. This causes an increased demand for cholesterol in the liver cells, resulting in the dual effect of increasing transcription and activity of the cholesterol biosynthetic enzyme, hydroxymethyl-glutaryl-coenzyme A (HMG-CoA) reductase, and increasing the number of hepatic low-density lipoprotein (LDL) receptors. These compensatory effects result in increased clearance of LDL cholesterol (LDL-C) from the blood, resulting in decreased serum LDL-C levels.[1, 2] Serum triglyceride levels may increase or remain unchanged.
Clinical studies have demonstrated that elevated levels of total cholesterol (total-C), LDL-C, and apolipoprotein B (Apo B, a protein associated with LDL-C) are associated with an increased risk of atherosclerosis in humans. Similarly, decreased levels of high-density lipoprotein cholesterol (HDL-C) are associated with the development of atherosclerosis[1]. Epidemiological investigations have established that cardiovascular morbidity and mortality vary directly with the levels of total-C and LDL-C, and inversely with the level of HDL-C.
The combination of colesevelam and an HMG-CoA reductase inhibitor is effective in further lowering serum total-C and LDL-C levels beyond that achieved by either agent alone. The effects of colesevelam either alone or with an HMG-CoA reductase inhibitor on cardiovascular morbidity and mortality have not been determined.

Pharmacokinetics
Colesevelam is a hydrophilic, water-insoluble polymer that is not hydrolyzed by digestive enzymes and is not absorbed. In 16 healthy volunteers, an average of 0.05% of a single ^{14}C-labeled colesevelam dose was excreted in the urine when given following 28 days of chronic dosing of 1.9 grams of colesevelam twice per day.

Table 1: WelChol® 24 Week Trial - Percentage Change in Lipid Parameters From Baseline

GRAMS/DAY	N	TOTAL-C	LDL-C	APO B	HDL-C	NON-HDL-C	TG
Placebo	88	+1	0	0	−1	+1	+5
3.8 g (6 tablets)	95	−7*	−15*	−12*	+3*	−10*	+10
4.5 g (7 tablets)	94	−10*	−18*	−12*	+3	−13*	+9

*p<0.05 for lipid parameters compared to placebo, for Apo B compared to baseline LDL-C, total-C, and Apo B are mean values; HDL-C and TG are median values.

Table 2: WelChol® in Combination with Atorvastatin, Simvastatin, and Lovastatin – Percentage Change in Lipid Parameters

DOSE/DAY	N	TOTAL-C	LDL-C	APO B	HDL-C	NON-HDL-C	TG
Atorvastatin Trial (4-week)							
Placebo	19	+4	+3	−3	+4	+4	+10
Atorvastatin 10 mg	18	−27*	−38*	−32*	+8	−35*	−24*
WelChol® 3.8 g/ Atorvastatin 10 mg	18	−31*	−48*	−38*	+11	−40*	−1
Atorvastatin 80 mg	20	−39*	−53*	−46*	+6	−50*	−33*
Simvastatin Trial (6-week)							
Placebo	33	−2	−4	−4*	−3	−2	+6
Simvastatin 10 mg	35	−19*	−26*	−20*	+3*	−24*	−17*
WelChol® 3.8 g/ Simvastatin 10 mg	34	−28*	−42*	−33*	+10*	−37*	−12*
Simvastatin 20 mg	39	−23*	−34*	−26*	+7*	−30*	−12*
WelChol® 2.3 g/ Simvastatin 20 mg	37	−29*	−42*	−32*	+4*	−37*	−12*
Lovastatin Trial (4-week)							
Placebo	26	+1	0	0	+1	+1	+1
Lovastatin 10 mg	26	−14*	−22*	−16*	+5	−19*	0
WelChol® 2.3 g/ Lovastatin 10 mg together	27	−21*	−34*	−24*	+4	−27*	−1
WelChol® 2.3 g/ Lovastatin 10 mg apart	23	−21*	−32*	−24*	+2	−28*	−2

*p<0.05 for lipid parameters compared to placebo, for Apo B compared to baseline LDL-C, total-C and Apo B are mean values; HDL-C and TG are median values.

Clinical Trials
WelChol® reduces total-C, LDL-C, and Apo B, and increases HDL-C when administered either alone or in combination with an HMG-CoA reductase inhibitor in patients with primary hypercholesterolemia.
Approximately 1400 patients were studied in eight clinical trials with treatment durations ranging from 4 to 50 weeks. With the exception of one long-term study, all studies were multicenter, randomized, double-blind, and placebo-controlled. A maximum therapeutic response to WelChol® was achieved within 2 weeks and was maintained during long-term therapy.
In a study in patients with LDL-C between 130 and 220 mg/dL (mean 158 mg/dL), WelChol® was given for 24 weeks in divided doses with the morning and evening meals. As shown in Table 1 below, the mean LDL-C reductions were 15% and 18% at the 3.8 g and 4.5 g doses. The respective mean total-C reductions were 7% and 10%. The mean Apo B reductions were 12% in both treatment groups. WelChol® at both doses increased HDL-C by 3%. There were small increases in triglycerides (TG) at both WelChol® doses that were not statistically different from placebo.
[See table 1 above]
In a study in 98 patients with LDL-C between 145 and 250 mg/dL (mean 169 mg/dL), WelChol® 3.8 g was given for 6 weeks as a single dose with breakfast, a single dose with dinner, or as divided doses with breakfast and dinner. The mean LDL-C reductions were 18%, 15%, and 18% for the three dosing regimens, respectively. The reductions with these three regimens were not statistically different from one another.
Co-administration of WelChol® and an HMG-CoA reductase inhibitor (atorvastatin, lovastatin, or simvastatin) demonstrated an additive reduction of LDL-C in three clinical studies. As demonstrated in Table 2 below, WelChol® doses of 2.3 g to 3.8 g resulted in additional 8% to 16% reductions in LDL-C above that seen with the HMG-CoA reductase inhibitor alone.
[See table 2 above]
In all three studies, the LDL-C reduction achieved with the combination of WelChol® and any given dose of HMG-CoA reductase inhibitor therapy was statistically superior to that achieved with WelChol® or that dose of the HMG-CoA reductase inhibitor alone.
The LDL-C reduction with atorvastatin 80 mg was not statistically significantly different from the combination of WelChol® 3.8 g and atorvastatin 10 mg.

INDICATIONS AND USAGE

WelChol®, administered alone or in combination with an HMG-CoA reductase inhibitor, is indicated as adjunctive therapy to diet and exercise for the reduction of elevated LDL cholesterol in patients with primary hypercholesterolemia (Fredrickson Type IIa).
Therapy with lipid lowering agents should be a component of multiple risk-factor intervention in patients at significant increased risk for atherosclerotic vascular disease due to hypercholesterolemia. Lipid altering agents should be used in addition to a diet restricted in saturated fat and cholesterol and when the response to diet and other non-pharmacological means has been inadequate.
Prior to initiating therapy with WelChol®, secondary causes of hypercholesterolemia (i.e., poorly controlled diabetes mellitus, hypothyroidism, nephrotic syndrome, dysproteinemias, obstructive liver disease, other drug therapy, alcoholism) should be excluded, and a lipid profile obtained to assess total-C, HDL-C, and TG. For individuals with TG less than 400 mg/dL, LDL-C can be estimated using the following equation.[3]

LDL-C = Total-C – [(TG/5) + HDL-C]

Periodic determination of serum cholesterol levels in patients as outlined in the National Cholesterol Education Program (NCEP) guidelines should be done to confirm a favorable initial and long-term response. The NCEP treatment guidelines are presented in Table 3.
[See table 3 at bottom of next page]

Major Risk Factors (Exclusive of LDL Cholesterol) That Modify LDL Goals*

- Cigarette smoking
- Hypertension (BP ≥140/90 mmHg or on anti-hypertensive medication)
- Low HDL cholesterol (<40 mg/dL) †

- Family history of premature CHD (CHD in male first degree relative <55 years; CHD in female first degree relative <65 years)
- Age (men ≥45 years; women ≥55 years)

* In ATP III, diabetes is regarded as a CHD risk equivalent.
† HDL cholesterol ≥60 mg/dL counts as a "negative" risk factor; its presence removes one risk factor from the total count.

After the LDL-C goal has been achieved, if the TG is still ≥200mg/dL, non HDL-C (total-C minus HDL-C) becomes a secondary target of therapy. Non-HDL-C goals are set 30 mg/dL higher than LDL-C goals for each risk category.

CONTRAINDICATIONS

WelChol® is contraindicated in individuals with bowel obstruction and in individuals who have shown hypersensitivity to any of the components of WelChol®.

PRECAUTIONS

General

Patients with TG levels greater than 300 mg/dL were excluded from WelChol® clinical trials. Caution should be exercised when treating patients with TG levels greater than 300 mg/dL.

In non-clinical safety studies, rats administered colesevelam at doses greater than 30-fold the projected human clinical dose experienced hemorrhage from vitamin K deficiency. WelChol® did not induce any clinically significant reduction in the absorption of vitamins A, D, E, or K during clinical trials of up to one year. However, caution should be exercised when treating patients with a susceptibility to vitamin K or fat soluble vitamin deficiencies.

The safety and efficacy of WelChol® in patients with dysphagia, swallowing disorders, severe gastrointestinal motility disorders, or major gastrointestinal tract surgery have not been established. Consequently, caution should be exercised when WelChol® is used in patients with these gastrointestinal disorders.

Information for the Patient

WelChol® may be taken once per day with a meal, or taken twice per day in divided doses with meals. Patients should be directed to take WelChol® with a liquid and a meal, and adhere to their NCEP-recommended diet. Patients should tell their physicians if they are pregnant, are intending to become pregnant, or are breastfeeding.

Laboratory Tests

Serum total-C, LDL-C and TG levels should be determined periodically based on NCEP guidelines to confirm favorable initial and adequate long-term responses.

Drug Interactions

WelChol® has been studied in several human drug interaction studies in which it was administered with a meal and the test drug. WelChol® was found to have no significant effect on the bioavailability of digoxin, fenofibrate, lovastatin, metoprolol, quinidine, valproic acid, and warfarin. WelChol® decreased the Cmax and AUC of sustained-release verapamil (Calan SR®) by approximately 31% and 11%, respectively. Since there is a high degree of variability in the bioavailability of verapamil, the clinical significance of this finding is unclear. In clinical studies, co-administration of WelChol® with atorvastatin, lovastatin, or simvastatin did not interfere with the lipid-lowering activity of the HMG-CoA reductase inhibitor. Other drugs have not been studied. When administering other drugs for which alterations in blood levels could have a clinically significant effect on safety or efficacy, physicians should consider monitoring drug levels or effects.

Carcinogenesis, Mutagenesis, Impairment of Fertility

A 104-week carcinogenicity study with colesevelam (WelChol®) was conducted in CD-1 mice, at oral dietary doses up to 3 g/kg/day. This dose was approximately 50 times the maximum recommended human dose of 4.5 g/day, based on body weight, mg/kg. There were no significant drug-induced tumor findings in male or female mice. In a 104-week carcinogenicity study with colesevelam (WelChol®) in Harlan Sprague-Dawley rats, a statistically significant increase in the incidence of pancreatic acinar cell adenoma was seen in male rats at doses >1.2 g/kg/day (approximately 20 times the maximum human dose, based on body weight, mg/kg) (trend test only). A statistically significant increase in thyroid C-cell adenoma was seen in female rats at 2.4 g/kg/day (approximately 40 times the maximum human dose, based on body weight, mg/kg).

Colesevelam and four degradants present in the drug substance have been evaluated for mutagenicity in the Ames test and a mammalian chromosomal aberration test. The four degradants and an extract of the parent compound did not exhibit genetic toxicity in an *in vitro* bacterial mutagenesis assay in *S. typhimurium* and *E. coli* (Ames assay) with or without rat liver metabolic activation. An extract of the parent compound was positive in the Chinese Hamster Ovary (CHO) cell chromosomal aberration assay in the presence of metabolic activation and negative in the absence of metabolic activation. The results of the CHO cell chromosomal aberration assay with two of the four degradants, decylamine HCl and aminohexyltrimethyl ammonium chloride HCl, were equivocal in the absence of metabolic activation and negative in the presence of metabolic activation. The other two degradants, didecylamine HCl and 6-decylamino-hexyltrimethyl ammonium chloride HCl, were negative in the presence and absence of metabolic activation.

Colesevelam did not impair fertility in rats at doses of up to 3 g/kg/day (approximately 50 times the maximum human dose, based on body weight, mg/kg).

PREGNANCY

Pregnancy Category B

Reproduction studies have been performed in rats and rabbits at doses up to 3 g/kg/day and 1 g/kg/day, respectively (approximately 50 and 17 times the maximum human dose, based on body weight, mg/kg) and have revealed no evidence of harm to the fetus due to colesevelam. There are, however, no adequate and well-controlled studies in pregnant women. Because animal reproduction studies are not always predictive of human response, this drug should be used during pregnancy only if clearly needed. Requirements for vitamins and other nutrients are increased in pregnancy. The effect of WelChol® on the absorption of vitamins has not been studied in pregnant women.

Pediatric Use

The safety and efficacy of colesevelam (WelChol®) have not been established in pediatric patients.

Geriatric Use

There is no evidence for special considerations when colesevelam (WelChol®) is administered to elderly patients.

ADVERSE REACTIONS

WelChol® treatment-emergent adverse events that occurred in greater than 2% of patients in an integrated safety analysis are presented in Table 4.

Table 4: Frequent (>2%) Treatment-Emergent Adverse Events By Treatment Category

BODY SYSTEM/ ADVERSE EVENT	PLACEBO (N=258) %	WELCHOL® ONLY (N=807) %
Body as a Whole		
Infection	13	10
Headache	8	6
Pain	7	5
Back Pain	6	3
Abdominal Pain	5	5
Flu Syndrome	3	3
Accidental Injury	3	4
Asthenia	2	4
Digestive System		
Flatulence	14	12
Constipation	7	11
Diarrhea	7	5
Nausea	4	4
Dyspepsia	3	8
Respiratory System		
Sinusitis	4	2
Rhinitis	3	3
Cough Increased	2	2
Pharyngitis	2	3
Musculoskeletal System		
Myalgia	0	2

Table 3: NCEP Guidelines

RISK CATEGORY	LCL-C GOAL	LDL LEVEL AT WHICH TO INITIATE THERAPEUTIC LIFESTYLE CHANGES (TLC)	LDL LEVEL AT WHICH TO CONSIDER DRUG THERAPY
CHD or CHD Risk Equivalents (10-year risk >20%)	<100 mg/dL	≥100 mg/dL	≥130 mg/dL (100-129 mg/dL: drug optional)*
2+ Risk Factors (10-year risk ≤20%)	<130 mg/dL	≥130 mg/dL	10-year risk 10-20%: ≥130 mg/dL
			10-year risk <10%: ≥160 mg/dL
0-1 Risk Factor†	<160 mg/dL	≥160 mg/dL	≥190 mg/dL (160-189 mg/dL: LDL-lowering drug optional)

* Some authorities recommended use of LDL cholesterol-lowering drugs in the category if LDL cholesterol <100 mg/dL cannot be achieved by therapeutic lifestyle changes. Other prefer use of drugs that primarily modify triglycerides and HDL cholesterol e.g., nicotinic acid or fibrate. Clinical judgment also may call for deferring drug therapy in this subcategory.
† Almost all people with 0-1 risk factor have a 10-year risk <10%, thus 10-year risk assessment in people with 0-1 risk factor is not necessary.

OVERDOSAGE

Because WelChol® is not absorbed, the risk of systemic toxicity is low. Doses in excess of 4.5 g per day have not been tested.

DOSAGE AND ADMINISTRATION

Monotherapy

The recommended starting dose of WelChol® is 3 tablets taken twice per day with meals or 6 tablets once per day with a meal. The WelChol® dose can be increased to 7 tablets, depending upon the desired therapeutic effect. WelChol® should be taken with a liquid.

Combination Therapy

WelChol®, at doses of 4 to 6 tablets per day, has been shown to be safe and effective when dosed at the same time (i.e., co-administered) as an HMG-CoA reductase inhibitor or when the two drugs are dosed apart. [**CLINICAL PHARMACOLOGY, Clinical Trials**]. WelChol® should be taken with a liquid. For maximal therapeutic effect in combination with an HMG-CoA reductase inhibitor, the recommended dose of WelChol® is 3 tablets taken twice per day with meals or 6 tablets taken once per day with a meal.

HOW SUPPLIED

WelChol® (colesevelam hydrocholoride), 625 mg, is supplied as an off-white, solid tablet imprinted with the word "Sankyo" over "C01".

WelChol® Tablets are available as follows:
Bottles of 540 – NDC 65597-701-54
Bottles of 180—NDC 65597-701-18

Storage

Store at 25°C (77°F); excursions permitted to 15-30°C (59-86°F) [see USP Controlled Room Temperature]. Brief exposure to 40°C does not adversely affect the product. Protect from moisture.

References

1. Grundy SM, Ahrens EH, Salen G. Interruption of the enterohepatic circulation of bile acids in man: comparative effects of cholestyramine and ileal exclusion on cholesterol metabolism. J Lab Clin Med 1971; 78: 94-121.
2. Shepherd J, Packard CJ, Bicker S, Veitch LTD, Gemmell MH. Cholestyramine promotes receptor-mediated low-density-lipoprotein catabolism. N Engl J Med 1980; 302: 1219-22.
3. Friedewald WT, Levy RI, Fredrickson DS: Estimation of the concentration of LDL cholesterol in plasma without use of a preparative ultracentrifuge. Clin. Chem. 1972; 18(6): 499.

Manufactured for: Sankyo Pharma Inc.
Parsippany, New Jersey 07054
by: Patheon YM Inc.
Toronto, Ontario M3B 1Y5
Active Ingredient: Product of Austria
Licensed From: GelTex Pharmaceuticals, Inc.
Rx Only
Issued: October 2003
Version: 8

For EMERGENCY telephone numbers, consult the **Manufacturers' Index.**

Sanofi-Synthelabo Inc.
90 PARK AVENUE
NEW YORK, NY 10016

Direct Inquiries to:
(212) 551-4000

For Medical Information Contact:
Product Information Services
(800) 446-6267

Sales and Ordering:
East Coast: (800) 223-1062
West Coast: (800) 223-5511

AMBIEN® ©IV ℞
[am' bē-ĕn]
(zolpidem tartrate)

DESCRIPTION

Ambien (zolpidem tartrate), is a non-benzodiazepine hypnotic of the imidazopyridine class and is available in 5-mg and 10-mg strength tablets for oral administration.

Chemically, zolpidem is N,N,6-trimethyl-2-p-tolylimidazo[1,2-a] pyridine-3-acetamide L-(+)-tartrate (2:1). It has the following structure:

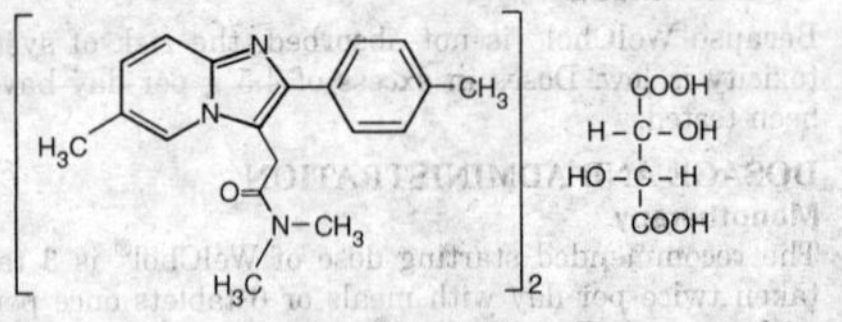

Zolpidem tartrate is a white to off-white crystalline powder that is sparingly soluble in water, alcohol, and propylene glycol. It has a molecular weight of 764.88.

Each Ambien tablet includes the following inactive ingredients: hydroxypropyl methylcellulose, lactose, magnesium stearate, microcrystalline cellulose, polyethylene glycol, sodium starch glycolate, and titanium dioxide; the 5-mg tablet also contains FD&C Red No. 40, iron oxide colorant, and polysorbate 80.

CLINICAL PHARMACOLOGY

Pharmacodynamics: Subunit modulation of the $GABA_A$ receptor chloride channel macromolecular complex is hypothesized to be responsible for sedative, anticonvulsant, anxiolytic, and myorelaxant drug properties. The major modulatory site of the $GABA_A$ receptor complex is located on its alpha (α) subunit and is referred to as the benzodiazepine (BZ) or omega (ω) receptor. At least three subtypes of the (ω) receptor have been identified.

While zolpidem is a hypnotic agent with a chemical structure unrelated to benzodiazepines, barbiturates, or other drugs with known hypnotic properties, it interacts with a GABA-BZ receptor complex and shares some of the pharmacological properties of the benzodiazepines. In contrast to the benzodiazepines, which nonselectively bind to and activate all omega receptor subtypes, zolpidem in vitro binds the (ω_1) receptor preferentially with a high affinity ratio of the $alpha_1/alpha_5$ subunits. The (ω_1) receptor is found primarily on the Lamina IV of the sensorimotor cortical regions, substantia nigra (parsreticulata), cerebellum molecular layer, olfactory bulb, ventral thalamic complex, pons, inferior colliculus, and globus pallidus. This selective binding of zolpidem on the (ω_1) receptor is not absolute, but it may explain the relative absence of myorelaxant and anticonvulsant effects in animal studies as well as the preservation of deep sleep (stages 3 and 4) in human studies of zolpidem at hypnotic doses.

Pharmacokinetics: The pharmacokinetic profile of Ambien is characterized by rapid absorption from the GI tract and a short elimination half-life ($T_{1/2}$) in healthy subjects. In a single-dose crossover study in 45 healthy subjects administered 5- and 10-mg zolpidem tartrate tablets, the mean peak concentrations (C_{max}) were 59 (range: 29 to 113) and 121 (range: 58 to 272) ng/mL, respectively, occurring at a mean time (T_{max}) of 1.6 hours for both. The mean Ambien elimination half-life was 2.6 (range: 1.4 to 4.5) and 2.5 (range: 1.4 to 3.8) hours, for the 5- and 10-mg tablets, respectively. Ambien is converted to inactive metabolites that are eliminated primarily by renal excretion. Ambien demonstrated linear kinetics in the dose range of 5 to 20 mg. Total protein binding was found to be 92.5 ± 0.1% and remained constant, independent of concentration between 40 and 790 ng/mL. Zolpidem did not accumulate in young adults following nightly dosing with 20-mg zolpidem tartrate tablets for 2 weeks.

A food-effect study in 30 healthy male volunteers compared the pharmacokinetics of Ambien 10 mg when administered while fasting or 20 minutes after a meal. Results demonstrated that with food, mean AUC and C_{max} were decreased by 15% and 25%, respectively, while mean T_{max} was prolonged by 60% (from 1.4 to 2.2 hr). The half-life remained unchanged. These results suggest that, for faster sleep onset, Ambien should not be administered with or immediately after a meal.

In the elderly, the dose for Ambien should be 5 mg (see *Precautions and Dosage and Administration*). This recommendation is based on several studies in which the mean C_{max}, $T_{1/2}$, and AUC were significantly increased when compared to results in young adults. In one study of eight elderly subjects (>70 years), the means for C_{max}, $T_{1/2}$, and AUC significantly increased by 50% (255 vs 384 ng/mL), 32% (2.2 vs 2.9 hr), and 64% (955 vs 1,562 ng hr/mL), respectively, as compared to younger adults (20 to 40 years) following a single 20-mg oral zolpidem dose. Ambien did not accumulate in elderly subjects following nightly oral dosing of 10 mg for 1 week.

The pharmacokinetics of Ambien in eight patients with chronic hepatic insufficiency were compared to results in healthy subjects. Following a single 20-mg oral zolpidem dose, mean C_{max} and AUC were found to be two times (250 vs 499 ng/mL) and five times (788 vs 4,203 ng hr/mL) higher, respectively, in hepatically compromised patients. T_{max} did not change. The mean half-life in cirrhotic patients of 9.9 hr (range: 4.1 to 25.8 hr) was greater than that observed in normals of 2.2 hr (range: 1.6 to 2.4 hr). Dosing should be modified accordingly in patients with hepatic insufficiency (see *Precautions and Dosage and Administration*).

The pharmacokinetics of zolpidem tartrate were studied in 11 patients with end-stage renal failure (mean Cl_{Cr} = 6.5 ± 1.5 mL/min) undergoing hemodialysis three times a week, who were dosed with zolpidem 10 mg orally each day for 14 or 21 days. No statistically significant differences were observed for C_{max}, T_{max}, half-life, and AUC between the first and last day of drug administration when baseline concentration adjustments were made. On day 1, C_{max} was 172 ± 29 ng/mL (range: 46 to 344 ng/mL). After repeated dosing for 14 or 21 days, C_{max} was 203 ± 32 ng/mL (range: 28 to 316 ng/mL). On day 1, T_{max} was 1.7 ± 0.3 hr (range: 0.5 to 3.0 hr); after repeated dosing T_{max} was 0.8 ± 0.2 hr (range: 0.5 to 2.0 hr). This variation is accounted for by noting that last-day serum sampling began 10 hours after the previous dose, rather than after 24 hours. This resulted in residual drug concentration and a shorter period to reach maximal serum concentration. On day 1, $T_{1/2}$ was 2.4 ± 0.4 hr (range: 0.4 to 5.1 hr). After repeated dosing, $T_{1/2}$ was 2.5 ± 0.4 hr (range: 0.7 to 4.2 hr). AUC was 796 ± 159 ng hr/mL after the first dose and 818 ± 170 ng• hr/mL after repeated dosing. Zolpidem was not hemodialyzable. No accumulation of unchanged drug appeared after 14 or 21 days. Ambien (zolpidem tartrate) pharmacokinetics were not significantly different in renally impaired patients. No dosage adjustment is necessary in patients with compromised renal function. As a general precaution, these patients should be closely monitored.

Postulated relationship between elimination rate of hypnotics and their profile of common untoward effects: The type and duration of hypnotic effects and the profile of unwanted effects during administration of hypnotic drugs may be influenced by the biologic half-life of administered drug and any active metabolites formed. When half-lives are long, drug or metabolites may accumulate during periods of nightly administration and be associated with impairment of cognitive and/or motor performance during waking hours; the possibility of interaction with other psychoactive drugs or alcohol will be enhanced. In contrast, if half-lives, including half-lives of active metabolites, are short, drug and metabolites will be cleared before the next dose is ingested, and carryover effects related to excessive sedation or CNS depression should be minimal or absent. Ambien has a short half-life and no active metabolites. During nightly use for an extended period, pharmacodynamic tolerance or adaptation to some effects of hypnotics may develop. If the drug has a short elimination half-life, it is possible that a relative deficiency of the drug or its active metabolites (ie, in relationship to the receptor site) may occur at some point in the interval between each night's use. This sequence of events may account for two clinical findings reported to occur after several weeks of nightly use of other rapidly eliminated hypnotics, namely, increased wakefulness during the last third of the night, and the appearance of increased signs of daytime anxiety. Increased wakefulness during the last third of the night as measured by polysomnography has not been observed in clinical trials with Ambien.

Controlled trials supporting safety and efficacy

Transient insomnia: Normal adults experiencing transient insomnia (n=462) during the first night in a sleep laboratory were evaluated in a double-blind, parallel group, single-night trial comparing two doses of zolpidem (7.5 and 10 mg) and placebo. Both zolpidem doses were superior to placebo on objective (polysomnographic) measures of sleep latency, sleep duration, and number of awakenings.

Normal elderly adults (mean age 68) experiencing transient insomnia (n=35) during the first two nights in a sleep laboratory were evaluated in a double-blind, crossover, 2-night trial comparing four doses of zolpidem (5, 10, 15 and 20 mg) and placebo. All zolpidem doses were superior to placebo on the two primary PSG parameters (sleep latency and efficiency) and all four subjective outcome measures (sleep duration, sleep latency, number of awakenings, and sleep quality).

Chronic insomnia: Zolpidem was evaluated in two controlled studies for the treatment of patients with chronic insomnia (most closely resembling primary insomnia, as defined in the APA Diagnostic and Statistical Manual of Mental Disorders, DSM-IV™). Adult outpatients with chronic insomnia (n=75) were evaluated in a double-blind, parallel group, 5-week trial comparing two doses of zolpidem tartrate (10 and 15 mg) and placebo. On objective (polysomnographic) measures of sleep latency and sleep efficiency, zolpidem 15 mg was superior to placebo for all 5 weeks; zolpidem 10 mg was superior to placebo on sleep latency for the first 4 weeks and on sleep efficiency for weeks 2 and 4. Zolpidem was comparable to placebo on number of awakenings at both doses studied.

Adult outpatients (n=141) with chronic insomnia were also evaluated in a double-blind, parallel group, 4-week trial comparing two doses of zolpidem (10 and 15 mg) and placebo. Zolpidem 10 mg was superior to placebo on a subjective measure of sleep latency for all 4 weeks, and on subjective measures of total sleep time, number of awakenings, and sleep quality for the first treatment week. Zolpidem 15 mg was superior to placebo on a subjective measure of sleep latency for the first 3 weeks, on a subjective measure of total sleep time for the first week, and on number of awakenings and sleep quality for the first 2 weeks.

Next-day residual effects: Next-day residual effects of Ambien were evaluated in seven studies involving normal volunteers. In three studies in adults (including one study in a phase advance model of transient insomnia) and in one study in elderly subjects, a small but statistically significant decrease in performance was observed in the Digit Symbol Substitution Test (DSST) when compared to placebo. Studies of Ambien in non-elderly patients with insomnia did not detect evidence of next-day residual effects using the DSST, the Multiple Sleep Latency Test (MSLT), and patient ratings of alertness.

Rebound effects: There was no objective (polysomnographic) evidence of rebound insomnia at recommended doses seen in studies evaluating sleep on the nights following discontinuation of Ambien (zolpidem tartrate). There was subjective evidence of impaired sleep in the elderly on the first post-treatment night at doses above the recommended elderly dose of 5 mg.

Memory impairment: Controlled studies in adults utilizing objective measures of memory yielded no consistent evidence of next-day memory impairment following the administration of Ambien. However, in one study involving zolpidem doses of 10 and 20 mg, there was a significant decrease in next-morning recall of information presented to subjects during peak drug effect (90 minutes post-dose), ie, these subjects experienced anterograde amnesia. There was also subjective evidence from adverse event data for anterograde amnesia occurring in association with the administration of Ambien, predominantly at doses above 10 mg.

Effects on sleep stages: In studies that measured the percentage of sleep time spent in each sleep stage, Ambien has generally been shown to preserve sleep stages. Sleep time spent in stages 3 and 4 (deep sleep) was found comparable to placebo with only inconsistent, minor changes in REM (paradoxical) sleep at the recommended dose.

INDICATIONS AND USAGE

Ambien (zolpidem tartrate) is indicated for the short-term treatment of insomnia. Ambien has been shown to decrease sleep latency and increase the duration of sleep for up to 35 days in controlled clinical studies (see *Clinical Pharmacology: Controlled trials supporting safety and efficacy*).

Hypnotics should generally be limited to 7 to 10 days of use, and reevaluation of the patient is recommended if they are to be taken for more than 2 to 3 weeks. Ambien should not be prescribed in quantities exceeding a 1-month supply (see *Warnings*).

CONTRAINDICATIONS

None known.

WARNINGS

Since sleep disturbances may be the presenting manifestation of a physical and/or psychiatric disorder, symptomatic treatment of insomnia should be initiated only after a careful evaluation of the patient. The failure of insomnia to remit after 7 to 10 days of treatment may indicate the presence of a primary psychiatric and/or medical illness which should be evaluated. Worsening of insomnia or the emergence of new thinking or behavior abnormalities may be the consequence of an unrecognized psychiatric or physical disorder. Such findings have emerged during the course of treatment with sedative/hypnotic drugs, including Ambien. Because some of the important adverse effects of Ambien appear to be dose related (see *Precautions* and *Dosage and Administration*), it is important to use the smallest possible effective dose, especially in the elderly.

A variety of abnormal thinking and behavior changes have been reported to occur in association with the use of sedative/hypnotics. Some of these changes may be characterized by decreased inhibition (eg, aggressiveness and extroversion that seemed out of character), similar to effects produced by alcohol and other CNS depressants. Other reported behavioral changes have included bizarre behavior, agitation, hallucinations, and depersonalization. Amnesia and other neuro-psychiatric symptoms may occur unpredictably. In primarily depressed patients, worsening of depression, including suicidal thinking, has been reported in association with the use of sedative/hypnotics.

It can rarely be determined with certainty whether a particular instance of the abnormal behaviors listed above is drug induced, spontaneous in origin, or a result of an underlying psychiatric or physical disorder. Nonetheless, the emergence of any new behavioral sign or symptom of concern requires careful and immediate evaluation.

Following the rapid dose decrease or abrupt discontinuation of sedative/hypnotics, there have been reports of signs and symptoms similar to those associated with withdrawal from other CNS-depressant drugs (see *Drug Abuse and Dependence*).

Ambien, like other sedative/hypnotic drugs, has CNS-depressant effects. Due to the rapid onset of action, Ambien should only be ingested immediately prior to going to bed. Patients should be cautioned against engaging in hazardous occupations requiring complete mental alertness or motor coordination such as operating machinery or driving a motor vehicle after ingesting the drug, including potential impairment of the performance of such activities that may occur the day following ingestion of Ambien. Ambien showed additive effects when combined with alcohol and should not be taken with alcohol. Patients should also be cautioned about possible combined effects with other CNS-depressant drugs. Dosage adjustments may be necessary when Ambien is administered with such agents because of the potentially additive effects.

PRECAUTIONS

General

Use in the elderly and/or debilitated patients: Impaired motor and/or cognitive performance after repeated exposure or unusual sensitivity to sedative/hypnotic drugs is a concern in the treatment of elderly and/or debilitated patients. Therefore, the recommended Ambien dosage is 5 mg in such patients (see *Dosage and Administration*) to decrease the possibility of side effects. These patients should be closely monitored.

Use in patients with concomitant illness: Clinical experience with Ambien (zolpidem tartrate) in patients with concomitant systemic illness is limited. Caution is advisable in using Ambien in patients with diseases or conditions that could affect metabolism or hemodynamic responses. Although studies did not reveal respiratory depressant effects at hypnotic doses of Ambien in normals or in patients with mild to moderate chronic obstructive pulmonary disease (COPD), a reduction in the Total Arousal Index together with a reduction in lowest oxygen saturation and increase in the times of oxygen desaturation below 80% and 90% was observed in patients with mild-to-moderate sleep apnea when treated with Ambien (10 mg) when compared to placebo. However, precautions should be observed if Ambien is prescribed to patients with compromised respiratory function, since sedative/hypnotics have the capacity to depress respiratory drive. Post-marketing reports of respiratory insufficiency, most of which involved patients with pre-existing respiratory impairment, have been received. Data in end-stage renal failure patients repeatedly treated with Ambien did not demonstrate drug accumulation or alterations in pharmacokinetic parameters. No dosage adjustment in renally impaired patients is required; however, these patients should be closely monitored (see *Pharmacokinetics*). A study in subjects with hepatic impairment did reveal prolonged elimination in this group; therefore, treatment should be initiated with 5 mg in patients with hepatic compromise, and they should be closely monitored.

Use in depression: As with other sedative/hypnotic drugs, Ambien should be administered with caution to patients exhibiting signs or symptoms of depression. Suicidal tendencies may be present in such patients and protective measures may be required. Intentional over-dosage is more common in this group of patients; therefore, the least amount of drug that is feasible should be prescribed for the patient at any one time.

Information for patients: Patient information is printed at the end of this insert. To assure safe and effective use of Ambien, this information and instructions provided in the patient information section should be discussed with patients.

Laboratory tests: There are no specific laboratory tests recommended.

Drug interactions

CNS-active drugs: Ambien was evaluated in healthy volunteers in single-dose interaction studies for several CNS drugs. A study involving haloperidol and zolpidem revealed no effect of haloperidol on the pharmacokinetics or pharmacodynamics of zolpidem. Imipramine in combination with zolpidem produced no pharmacokinetic interaction other than a 20% decrease in peak levels of imipramine, but there was an additive effect of decreased alertness. Similarly, chlorpromazine in combination with zolpidem produced no pharmacokinetic interaction, but there was an additive effect of decreased alertness and psychomotor performance. The lack of a drug interaction following single-dose administration does not predict a lack following chronic administration.

An additive effect on psychomotor performance between alcohol and zolpidem was demonstrated.

A single-dose interaction study with zolpidem 10 mg and fluoxetine 20 mg at steady-state levels in male volunteers did not demonstrate any clinically significant pharmacokinetic or pharmacodynamic interactions. When multiple doses of zolpidem and fluoxetine at steady-state concentrations were evaluated in healthy females, the only significant change was a 17% increase in the zolpidem half-life. There was no evidence of an additive effect in psychomotor performance.

Following five consecutive nightly doses of zolpidem 10 mg in the presence of sertraline 50 mg (17 consecutive daily doses, at 7:00 am, in healthy female volunteers), zolpidem C_{max} was significantly higher (43%) and T_{max} was significantly decreased (53%). Pharmacokinetics of sertraline and N-desmethylsertraline were unaffected by zolpidem.

Since the systematic evaluations of Ambien (zolpidem tartrate) in combination with other CNS-active drugs have been limited, careful consideration should be given to the pharmacology of any CNS-active drug to be used with zolpidem. Any drug with CNS-depressant effects could potentially enhance the CNS-depressant effects of zolpidem.

Drugs that affect drug metabolism via cytochrome P450: A randomized, double-blind, crossover interaction study in ten healthy volunteers between itraconazole (200 mg once daily for 4 days) and a single dose of zolpidem (10 mg) given 5 hours after the last dose of itraconazole resulted in a 34% increase in $AUC_{0-\infty}$ of zolpidem. There were no significant pharmacodynamic effects of zolpidem on subjective drowsiness, postural sway, or psychomotor performance.

A randomized, placebo-controlled, crossover interaction study in eight healthy female volunteers between 5 consecutive daily doses of rifampin (600 mg) and a single dose of zolpidem (20 mg) given 17 hours after the last dose of rifampin showed significant reductions of the AUC (−73%), C_{max} (−58%), and $T_{1/2}$ (−36%) of zolpidem together with significant reductions in the pharmacodynamic effects of zolpidem.

Other drugs: A study involving cimetidine/zolpidem and ranitidine/zolpidem combinations revealed no effect of either drug on the pharmacokinetics or pharmacodynamics of zolpidem. Zolpidem had no effect on digoxin kinetics and did not affect prothrombin time when given with warfarin in normal subjects. Zolpidem's sedative/hypnotic effect was reversed by flumazenil; however, no significant alterations in zolpidem pharmacokinetics were found.

Drug/Laboratory test interactions: Zolpidem is not known to interfere with commonly employed clinical laboratory tests. In addition, clinical data indicate that zolpidem does not cross-react with benzodiazepines, opiates, barbiturates, cocaine, cannabinoids, or amphetamines in two standard urine drug screens.

Carcinogenesis, mutagenesis, impairment of fertility

Carcinogenesis: Zolpidem was administered to rats and mice for 2 years at dietary dosages of 4, 18, and 80 mg/kg/day. In mice, these dosages are 26 to 520 times or 2 to 35 times the maximum 10-mg human dose on a mg/kg or mg/m^2 basis, respectively. In rats these doses are 43 to 876 times or 6 to 115 times the maximum 10-mg human dose on a mg/kg or mg/m^2 basis, respectively. No evidence of carcinogenic potential was observed in mice. Renal liposarcomas were seen in 4/100 rats (3 males, 1 female) receiving 80 mg/kg/day and a renal lipoma was observed in one male rat at the 18 mg/kg/ day dose. Incidence rates of lipoma and liposarcoma for zolpidem were comparable to those seen in historical controls and the tumor findings are thought to be a spontaneous occurrence.

Mutagenesis: Zolpidem did not have mutagenic activity in several tests including the Ames test, genotoxicity in mouse lymphoma cells in vitro, chromosomal aberrations in cultured human lymphocytes, unscheduled DNA synthesis in rat hepatocytes in vitro, and the micronucleus test in mice.

Impairment of fertility: In a rat reproduction study, the high dose (100 mg base/kg) of zolpidem resulted in irregular estrus cycles and prolonged precoital intervals, but there was no effect on male or female fertility after daily oral doses of 4 to 100 mg base/kg or 5 to 130 times the recommended human dose in mg/m^2. No effects on any other fertility parameters were noted.

Pregnancy

Teratogenic effects: Pregnancy Category B. Studies to assess the effects of zolpidem on human reproduction and development have not been conducted.

Teratology studies were conducted in rats and rabbits.

In rats, adverse maternal and fetal effects occurred at 20 and 100 mg base/kg and included dose-related maternal lethargy and ataxia and a dose-related trend to incomplete ossification of fetal skull bones. Underossification of various fetal bones indicates a delay in maturation and is often seen in rats treated with sedative/hypnotic drugs. There were no teratogenic effects after zolpidem administration. The no-effect dose for maternal or fetal toxicity was 4 mg base/kg or 5 times the maximum human dose on a mg/m^2 basis.

In rabbits, dose-related maternal sedation and decreased weight gain occurred at all doses tested. At the high dose, 16 mg base/kg, there was an increase in postimplantation fetal loss and underossification of sternebrae in viable fetuses. These fetal findings in rabbits are often secondary to reductions in maternal weight gain. There were no frank teratogenic effects. The no-effect dose for fetal toxicity was 4 mg base/kg or 7 times the maximum human dose on a mg/m^2 basis.

Because animal reproduction studies are not always predictive of human response, this drug should be used during pregnancy only if clearly needed.

Nonteratogenic effects: Studies to assess the effects on children whose mothers took zolpidem during pregnancy have not been conducted. However, children born of mothers taking sedative/hypnotic drugs may be at some risk for withdrawal symptoms from the drug during the postnatal period. In addition, neonatal flaccidity has been reported in infants born of mothers who received sedative/hypnotic drugs during pregnancy.

Labor and delivery: Ambien (zolpidem tartrate) has no established use in labor and delivery.

Nursing mothers: Studies in lactating mothers indicate that the half-life of zolpidem is similar to that in young normal volunteers (2.6 ± 0.3 hr). Between 0.004 and 0.019% of the total administered dose is excreted into milk, but the effect of zolpidem on the infant is unknown.

In addition, in a rat study, zolpidem inhibited the secretion of milk. The no-effect dose was 4 mg base/kg or 6 times the recommended human dose in mg/m^2.

The use of Ambien in nursing mothers is not recommended.

Pediatric use: Safety and effectiveness in pediatric patients below the age of 18 have not been established.

Geriatric use: A total of 154 patients in U.S. controlled clinical trials and 897 patients in non-U.S. clinical trials who received zolpidem were ≥60 years of age. For a pool of U.S. patients receiving zolpidem at doses of ≤10 mg or placebo, there were three adverse events occurring at an incidence of at least 3% for zolpidem and for which the zolpidem incidence was at least twice the placebo incidence (ie, they could be considered drug related).

Adverse Event	Zolpidem	Placebo
Dizziness	3%	0%
Drowsiness	5%	2%
Diarrhea	3%	1%

A total of 30/1,959 (1.5%) non-U.S. patients receiving zolpidem reported falls, including 28/30 (93%) who were ≥70 years of age. Of these 28 patients, 23 (82%) were receiving zolpidem doses >10 mg. A total of 24/1,959 (1.2%) non-U.S. patients receiving zolpidem reported confusion, including 18/24 (75%) who were ≥70 years of age. Of these 18 patients, 14 (78%) were receiving zolpidem doses >10 mg.

ADVERSE REACTIONS

Associated with discontinuation of treatment: Approximately 4% of 1,701 patients who received zolpidem at all doses (1.25 to 90 mg) in U.S. premarketing clinical trials discontinued treatment because of an adverse clinical event. Events most commonly associated with discontinuation from U.S. trials were daytime drowsiness (0.5%), dizziness (0.4%), headache (0.5%), nausea (0.6%), and vomiting (0.5%).

Approximately 4% of 1,959 patients who received zolpidem at all doses (1 to 50 mg) in similar foreign trials discontinued treatment because of an adverse event. Events most commonly associated with discontinuation from these trials were daytime drowsiness (1.1%), dizziness/vertigo (0.8%), amnesia (0.5%), nausea (0.5%), headache (0.4%), and falls (0.4%).

Data from a clinical study in which selective serotonin reuptake inhibitor- (SSRI) treated patients were given zolpidem revealed that four of the seven discontinuations during double-blind treatment with zolpidem (n=95) were associated with impaired concentration, continuing or aggravated depression, and manic reaction; one patient treated with placebo (n=97) was discontinued after an attempted suicide.

Incidence in controlled clinical trials

Most commonly observed adverse events in controlled trials: During short-term treatment (up to 10 nights) with Ambien at doses up to 10 mg, the most commonly observed adverse events associated with the use of zolpidem and seen at statistically significant differences from placebo-treated patients were drowsiness (reported by 2% of zolpidem patients), dizziness (1%), and diarrhea (1%). During longer-term treatment (28 to 35 nights) with zolpidem at doses up to 10 mg, the most commonly observed adverse events associated with the use of zolpidem and seen at statistically significant differences from placebo-treated patients were dizziness (5%) and drugged feelings (3%).

Adverse events observed at an incidence of ≥1% in controlled trials: The following tables enumerate treatment-emergent adverse event frequencies that were observed at an incidence equal to 1% or greater among patients with insomnia who received Ambien in U.S. placebo-controlled trials. Events reported by investigators were classified utilizing a modified World Health Organization (WHO) dictionary of preferred terms for the purpose of establishing event frequencies. The prescriber should be aware that these figures cannot be used to predict the incidence of side effects in the course of usual medical practice, in which patient characteristics and other factors differ from those that prevailed in these clinical trials. Similarly, the cited frequencies cannot be compared with figures obtained from other clinical investigators involving related drug products and uses, since each group of drug trials is conducted under a different set of conditions. However, the cited figures provide the physician with a basis for estimating the relative contribution of drug and nondrug factors to the incidence of side effects in the population studied.

The following table was derived from a pool of 11 placebo-controlled short-term U.S. efficacy trials involving zolpidem in doses ranging from 1.25 to 20 mg. The table is limited to data from doses up to and including 10 mg, the highest dose recommended for use.

[See first table at top of next page]

Continued on next page

This product information was prepared in September 2004. On these and other products of Sanofi-Synthelabo Inc., detailed information may be obtained on a current basis by direct inquiry to Product Information Services, 90 Park Avenue, New York, NY 10016 (toll free 1-800-446-6267).

Ambien—Cont.

The following table was derived from a pool of three placebo-controlled long-term efficacy trials involving Ambien (zolpidem tartrate). These trials involved patients with chronic insomnia who were treated for 28 to 35 nights with zolpidem at doses of 5, 10, or 15 mg. The table is limited to data from doses up to and including 10 mg, the highest dose recommended for use. The table includes only adverse events occurring at an incidence of at least 1% for zolpidem patients.

[See second table at right]

Dose relationship for adverse events: There is evidence from dose comparison trials suggesting a dose relationship for many of the adverse events associated with zolpidem use, particularly for certain CNS and gastrointestinal adverse events.

Adverse event incidence across the entire preapproval database: Ambien (zolpidem tartrate) was administered to 3,660 subjects in clinical trials throughout the U.S., Canada, and Europe. Treatment-emergent adverse events associated with clinical trial participation were recorded by clinical investigators using terminology of their own choosing. To provide a meaningful estimate of the proportion of individuals experiencing treatment-emergent adverse events, similar types of untoward events were grouped into a smaller number of standardized event categories and classified utilizing a modified World Health Organization (WHO) dictionary of preferred terms. The frequencies presented, therefore, represent the proportions of the 3,660 individuals exposed to zolpidem, at all doses, who experienced an event of the type cited on at least one occasion while receiving zolpidem. All reported treatment-emergent adverse events are included, except those already listed in the table above of adverse events in placebo-controlled studies, those coding terms that are so general as to be uninformative, and those events where a drug cause was remote. It is important to emphasize that, although the events reported did occur during treatment with Ambien, they were not necessarily caused by it.

Adverse events are further classified within body system categories and enumerated in order of decreasing frequency using the following definitions: frequent adverse events are defined as those occurring in greater than 1/100 subjects; infrequent adverse events are those occurring in 1/100 to 1/1,000 patients; rare events are those occurring in less than 1/1,000 patients.

Autonomic nervous system: Infrequent: increased sweating, pallor, postural hypotension, syncope. Rare: abnormal accommodation, altered saliva, flushing, glaucoma, hypotension, impotence, increased saliva, tenesmus.

Body as a whole: Frequent: asthenia. Infrequent: edema, falling, fever, malaise, trauma. Rare: allergic reaction, allergy aggravated, abdominal body sensation, anaphylactic shock, face edema, hot flashes, increased ESR, pain, restless legs, rigors, tolerance increased, weight decrease.

Cardiovascular system: Infrequent: cerebrovascular disorder, hypertension, tachycardia. Rare: angina pectoris, arrhythmia, arteritis, circulatory failure, extrasystoles, hypertension aggravated, myocardial infarction, phlebitis, pulmonary embolism, pulmonary edema, varicose veins, ventricular tachycardia.

Central and peripheral nervous system: Frequent: ataxia, confusion, euphoria, insomnia, vertigo. Infrequent: agitation, decreased cognition, detached, difficulty concentrating, dysarthria, emotional lability, hallucination, hypoesthesia, illusion, leg cramps, migraine, paresthesia, sleeping (after daytime dosing), speech disorder, stupor, tremor. Rare: abnormal gait, abnormal thinking, aggressive reaction, apathy, appetite increased, decreased libido, delusion, dementia, depersonalization, dysphasia, feeling strange, hypokinesia, hypotonia, hysteria, intoxicated feeling, manic reaction, neuralgia, neuritis, neuropathy, neurosis, panic attacks, paresis, personality disorder, somnambulism, suicide attempts, tetany, yawning.

Gastrointestinal system: Frequent: hiccup. Infrequent: constipation, dysphagia, flatulence, gastroenteritis. Rare: enteritis, eructation, esophagospasm, gastritis, hemorrhoids, intestinal obstruction, rectal hemorrhage, tooth caries.

Hematologic and lymphatic system: Rare: anemia, hyperhemoglobinemia, leukopenia, lymphadenopathy, macrocytic anemia, purpura, thrombosis.

Immunologic system: Rare: abscess, herpes simplex, herpes zoster, otitis externa, otitis media.

Liver and biliary system: Infrequent: abnormal hepatic function, increased SGPT. Rare: bilirubinemia, increased SGOT.

Metabolic and nutritional: Infrequent: hyperglycemia, thirst. Rare: gout, hypercholesteremia, hyperlipidemia, increased alkaline phosphatase, increased BUN, periorbital edema.

Musculoskeletal system: Infrequent: arthritis. Rare: arthrosis, muscle weakness, sciatica, tendinitis.

Reproductive system: Infrequent: menstrual disorder, vaginitis. Rare: breast fibroadenosis, breast neoplasm, breast pain.

Respiratory system: Infrequent: bronchitis, coughing, dyspnea. Rare: bronchospasm, epistaxis, hypoxia, laryngitis, pneumonia.

Skin and appendages: Infrequent: pruritus. Rare: acne, bullous eruption, dermatitis, furunculosis, injection-site inflammation, photosensitivity reaction, urticaria.

Incidence of Treatment-Emergent Adverse Experiences in Short-term Placebo-Controlled Clinical Trials

(Percentage of patients reporting)

Body System/ Adverse Event*	Zolpidem (≤10 mg) (N=685)	Placebo (N=473)
Central and Peripheral Nervous System		
Headache	7	6
Drowsiness	2	–
Dizziness	1	–
Gastrointestinal System		
Nausea	2	3
Diarrhea	1	–
Musculoskeletal System		
Myalgia	1	2

*Events reported by at least 1% of Ambien patients are included.

Incidence of Treatment-Emergent Adverse Experiences in Long-term Placebo-Controlled Clinical Trials

(Percentage of patients reporting)

Body System/ Adverse Event*	Zolpidem (≤10 mg) (N=152)	Placebo (N=161)
Autonomic Nervous System		
Dry mouth	3	1
Body as a Whole		
Allergy	4	1
Back pain	3	2
Influenza-like symptoms	2	–
Chest pain	1	–
Fatigue	1	2
Cardiovascular System		
Palpitation	2	–
Central and Peripheral Nervous System		
Headache	19	22
Drowsiness	8	5
Dizziness	5	1
Lethargy	3	1
Drugged feeling	3	–
Lightheadedness	2	1
Depression	2	1
Abnormal dreams	1	–
Amnesia	1	–
Anxiety	1	1
Nervousness	1	3
Sleep disorder	1	–
Gastrointestinal System		
Nausea	6	6
Dyspepsia	5	6
Diarrhea	3	2
Abdominal pain	2	2
Constipation	2	1
Anorexia	1	1
Vomiting	1	1
Immunologic System		
Infection	1	1
Musculoskeletal System		
Myalgia	7	7
Arthralgia	4	4
Respiratory System		
Upper respiratory infection	5	6
Sinusitis	4	2
Pharyngitis	3	1
Rhinitis	1	3
Skin and Appendages		
Rash	2	1
Urogenital System		
Urinary tract infection	2	2

*Events reported by at least 1% of patients treated with Ambien.

Special senses: Frequent: diplopia, vision abnormal. Infrequent: eye irritation, eye pain, scleritis, taste perversion, tinnitus. Rare: conjunctivitis, corneal ulceration, lacrimation abnormal, parosmia, photopsia.

Urogenital system: Infrequent: cystitis, urinary incontinence. Rare: acute renal failure, dysuria, micturition frequency, nocturia, polyuria, pyelonephritis, renal pain, urinary retention.

DRUG ABUSE AND DEPENDENCE

Controlled substance: Zolpidem tartrate is classified as a Schedule IV controlled substance by federal regulation.

Abuse and dependence: Studies of abuse potential in former drug abusers found that the effects of single doses of Ambien (zolpidem tartrate) 40 mg were similar, but not identical, to diazepam 20 mg, while zolpidem tartrate 10 mg was difficult to distinguish from placebo.

Sedative/hypnotics have produced withdrawal signs and symptoms following abrupt discontinuation. These reported symptoms range from mild dysphoria and insomnia to a withdrawal syndrome that may include abdominal and muscle cramps, vomiting, sweating, tremors, and convulsions. The U.S. clinical trial experience from zolpidem does not reveal any clear evidence for withdrawal syndrome. Nevertheless, the following adverse events included in DSM-III-R criteria for uncomplicated sedative/hypnotic withdrawal were reported during U.S. clinical trials following placebo substitution occurring within 48 hours following last zolpidem treatment: fatigue, nausea, flushing, lightheadedness, uncontrolled crying, emesis, stomach cramps, panic attack, nervousness, and abdominal discomfort. These reported adverse events occurred at an incidence of 1% or less. However, available data cannot provide a reliable estimate of the incidence, if any, of dependence during treatment at recommended doses. Rare post-marketing reports of abuse, dependence and withdrawal have been received.

Because persons with a history of addiction to, or abuse of, drugs or alcohol are at increased risk of habituation and dependence, they should be under careful surveillance when receiving zolpidem or any other hypnotic.

OVERDOSAGE

Signs and symptoms: In European postmarketing reports of overdose with zolpidem alone, impairment of consciousness has ranged from somnolence to light coma. There was one case each of cardiovascular and respiratory compromise. Individuals have fully recovered from zolpidem tartrate overdoses up to 400 mg (40 times the maximum recommended dose). Overdose cases involving multiple CNS-depressant agents, including zolpidem, have resulted in more severe symptomatology, including fatal outcomes.

Recommended treatment: General symptomatic and supportive measures should be used along with immediate gastric lavage where appropriate. Intravenous fluids should be administered as needed. Flumazenil may be useful. As in all cases of drug overdose, respiration, pulse, blood pressure, and other appropriate signs should be monitored and general supportive measures employed. Hypotension and CNS depression should be monitored and treated by appropriate medical intervention. Sedating drugs should be withheld following zolpidem overdosage, even if excitation occurs. The value of dialysis in the treatment of overdosage has not been determined, although hemodialysis studies in patients with renal failure receiving therapeutic doses have demonstrated that zolpidem is not dialyzable.

Poison control center: As with the management of all overdosage, the possibility of multiple drug ingestion should be considered. The physician may wish to consider contacting a poison control center for up-to-date information on the management of hypnotic drug product overdosage.

DOSAGE AND ADMINISTRATION

The dose of Ambien should be individualized.

The recommended dose for adults is 10 mg immediately before bedtime.

Downward dosage adjustment may be necessary when Ambien is administered with agents having known CNS-depressant effects because of the potentially additive effects. Elderly or debilitated patients may be especially sensitive to the effects of Ambien (zolpidem tartrate). Patients with hepatic insufficiency do not clear the drug as rapidly as normals. An initial 5-mg dose is recommended in these patients (see *Precautions*).

The total Ambien dose should not exceed 10 mg.

HOW SUPPLIED

Ambien 5-mg tablets are capsule-shaped, pink, film coated, with, AMB 5 debossed on one side and 5401 on the other and supplied as:

NDC Number	Size
0024-5401-31	bottle of 100
0024-5401-34	carton of 100 unit dose
0024-5401-50	bottle of 500
0024-5401-10	Ambien PAK™ of 30 unit dose

Ambien 10-mg tablets are capsule-shaped, white, film coated, with AMB 10 debossed on one side and 5421 on the other and supplied as:

NDC Number	Size
0024-5421-31	bottle of 100
0024-5421-34	carton of 100 unit dose
0024-5421-50	bottle of 500
0024-5421-10	Ambien PAK™ of 30 unit dose

Store at controlled room temperature 20°–25° C (68°–77°F).

Rx only

INFORMATION FOR PATIENTS TAKING AMBIEN

Your doctor has prescribed Ambien to help you sleep. The following information is intended to guide you in the safe use of this medicine.

It is not meant to take the place of your doctor's instructions. If you have any questions about Ambien tablets be sure to ask your doctor or pharmacist.

Ambien is used to treat different types of sleep problems, such as:

- trouble falling asleep
- waking up too early in the morning
- waking up often during the night

Some people may have more than one of these problems.

Ambien belongs to a group of medicines known as the "sedative/hypnotics," or simply, sleep medicines. There are many different sleep medicines available to help people sleep better. Sleep problems are usually temporary, requiring treatment for only a short time, usually 1 or 2 days up to 1 or 2 weeks. Some people have chronic sleep problems that may require more prolonged use of sleep medicine. However, you should not use these medicines for long periods without talking with your doctor about the risks and benefits of prolonged use.

SIDE EFFECTS

Most common side effects: All medicines have side effects. Most common side effects of sleep medicines include:

- drowsiness
- dizziness
- lightheadedness
- difficulty with coordination

You may find that these medicines make you sleepy during the day. How drowsy you feel depends upon how your body reacts to the medicine, which sleep medicine you are taking, and how large a dose your doctor has prescribed. Daytime drowsiness is best avoided by taking the lowest dose possible that will still help you sleep at night. Your doctor will work with you to find the dose of Ambien that is best for you.

To manage these side effects while you are taking this medicine:

- When you first start taking Ambien or any other sleep medicine until you know whether the medicine will still have some carryover effect in you the next day, use extreme care while doing anything that requires complete alertness, such as driving a car, operating machinery, or piloting an aircraft.
- NEVER drink alcohol while you are being treated with Ambien or any sleep medicine. Alcohol can increase the side effects of Ambien or any other sleep medicine.
- Do not take any other medicines without asking your doctor first. This includes medicines you can buy without a prescription. Some medicines can cause drowsiness and are best avoided while taking Ambien.
- Always take the exact dose of Ambien prescribed by your doctor. Never change your dose without talking to your doctor first.

SPECIAL CONCERNS

There are some special problems that may occur while taking sleep medicines.

Memory problems: Sleep medicines may cause a special type of memory loss or "amnesia." When this occurs, a person may not remember what has happened for several hours after taking the medicine. This is usually not a problem since most people fall asleep after taking the medicine. Memory loss can be a problem, however, when sleep medicines are taken while traveling, such as during an airplane flight and the person wakes up before the effect of the medicine is gone. This has been called "traveler's amnesia."

Memory problems are not common while taking Ambien. In most instances memory problems can be avoided if you take Ambien only when you are able to get a full night's sleep (7 to 8 hours) before you need to be active again. Be sure to talk to your doctor if you think you are having memory problems.

Tolerance: When sleep medicines are used every night for more than a few weeks, they may lose their effectiveness to help you sleep. This is known as "tolerance." Sleep medicines should, in most cases, be used only for short periods of time, such as 1 or 2 days and generally no longer than 1 or 2 weeks. If your sleep problems continue, consult your doctor, who will determine whether other measures are needed to overcome your sleep problems.

Dependence: Sleep medicines can cause dependence, especially when these medicines are used regularly for longer than a few weeks or at high doses. Some people develop a need to continue taking their medicines. This is known as dependence or "addiction."

When people develop dependence, they may have difficulty stopping the sleep medicine. If the medicine is suddenly stopped, the body is not able to function normally and unpleasant symptoms (see *Withdrawal*) may occur. They may find they have to keep taking the medicine either at the prescribed dose or at increasing doses just to avoid withdrawal symptoms.

All people taking sleep medicines have some risk of becoming dependent on the medicine. However, people who have been dependent on alcohol or other drugs in the past may have a higher chance of becoming addicted to sleep medicines. This possibility must be considered before using these medicines for more than a few weeks.

If you have been addicted to alcohol or drugs in the past, it is important to tell your doctor before starting Ambien or any sleep medicine.

Withdrawal: Withdrawal symptoms may occur when sleep medicines are stopped suddenly after being used daily for a long time. In some cases, these symptoms can occur even if the medicine has been used for only a week or two.

In mild cases, withdrawal symptoms may include unpleasant feelings. In more severe cases, abdominal and muscle cramps, vomiting, sweating, shakiness, and rarely, seizures may occur. These more severe withdrawal symptoms are very uncommon.

Another problem that may occur when sleep medicines are stopped is known as "rebound insomnia." This means that a person may have more trouble sleeping the first few nights after the medicine is stopped than before starting the medicine. If you should experience rebound insomnia, do not get discouraged. This problem usually goes away on its own after 1 or 2 nights.

If you have been taking Ambien or any other sleep medicine for more than 1 or 2 weeks, do not stop taking it on your own. Always follow your doctor's directions.

Changes in behavior and thinking: Some people using sleep medicines have experienced unusual changes in their thinking and/or behavior. These effects are not common. However, they have included:

- more outgoing or aggressive behavior than normal
- loss of personal identity
- confusion
- strange behavior
- agitation
- hallucinations
- worsening of depression
- suicidal thoughts

How often these effects occur depends on several factors, such as a person's general health, the use of other medicines, and which sleep medicine is being used. Clinical experience with Ambien suggests that it is uncommonly associated with these behavior changes.

It is also important to realize that it is rarely clear whether these behavior changes are caused by the medicine, an illness, or occur on their own. In fact, sleep problems that do not improve may be due to illnesses that were present before the medicine was used. If you or your family notice any changes in your behavior, or if you have any unusual or disturbing thoughts, call your doctor immediately.

Pregnancy: Sleep medicines may cause sedation of the unborn baby when used during the last weeks of pregnancy.

Be sure to tell your doctor if you are pregnant, if you are planning to become pregnant, or if you become pregnant while taking Ambien.

SAFE USE OF SLEEPING MEDICINES

To ensure the safe and effective use of Ambien or any other sleep medicine, you should observe the following cautions:

1. Ambien is a prescription medicine and should be used ONLY as directed by your doctor. Follow your doctor's instructions about how to take, when to take, and how long to take Ambien.
2. Never use Ambien or any other sleep medicine for longer than directed by your doctor.
3. If you notice any unusual and/or disturbing thoughts or behavior during treatment with Ambien or any other sleep medicine, contact your doctor.
4. Tell your doctor about any medicines you may be taking, including medicines you may buy without a prescription. You should also tell your doctor if you drink alcohol. DO NOT use alcohol while taking Ambien or any other sleep medicine.
5. Do not take Ambien unless you are able to get a full night's sleep before you must be active again. For example, Ambien should not be taken on an overnight airplane flight of less than 7 to 8 hours since "traveler's amnesia" may occur.
6. Do not increase the prescribed dose of Ambien or any other sleep medicine unless instructed by your doctor.
7. When you first start taking Ambien or any other sleep medicine until you know whether the medicine will still have some carryover effect in you the next day, use extreme care while doing anything that requires complete alertness, such as driving a car, operating machinery, or piloting an aircraft.
8. Be aware that you may have more sleeping problems the first night or two after stopping Ambien or any other sleep medicine.
9. Be sure to tell your doctor if you are pregnant, if you are planning to become pregnant, or if you become pregnant while taking Ambien.
10. As with all prescription medicines, never share Ambien or any other sleep medicine with anyone else. Always store Ambien or any other sleep medicine in the original container out of reach of children.
11. Ambien works very quickly. You should only take Ambien right before going to bed and are ready to go to sleep.

sanofi~synthelabo

Distributed by:
Sanofi-Synthelabo Inc.
New York, NY 10016

Ambien® Ⓒ
(zolpidem tartrate)

Revised March 2004

ZSS-5C

Shown in Product Identification Guide, page 332

ARALEN® ℞

[*ă-ră-lĕn*]

(chloroquine phosphate, USP)

For Malaria and Extraintestinal Amebiasis

DESCRIPTION

ARALEN, chloroquine phosphate, USP, is a 4-aminoquinoline compound for oral administration. It is a white, odorless, bitter tasting, crystalline substance, freely soluble in water.

ARALEN is an antimalarial and amebicidal drug.

Chemically, it is 7-chloro-4-[[4- (diethylamino)-1-methylbutyl]amino] quinoline phosphate (1:2) and has the following structural formula:

Each tablet contains 500 mg of chloroquine phosphate USP, equivalent to 300 mg chloroquine base.

Inactive Ingredients: Carnauba Wax, Colloidal Silicon Dioxide, Dibasic Calcium Phosphate, Hydroxypropyl Methylcellulose, Magnesium Stearate, Microcrystalline Cellulose, Polyethylene Glycol, Polysorbate 80, Pregelatinized Starch, Sodium Starch Glycolate, Stearic Acid, Titanium Dioxide.

CLINICAL PHARMACOLOGY

Chloroquine is rapidly and almost completely absorbed from the gastrointestinal tract, and only a small proportion of the administered dose is found in the stools. Approximately 55% of the drug in the plasma is bound to nondiffusible plasma constituents. Excretion of chloroquine is quite slow, but is increased by acidification of the urine. Chloroquine is deposited in the tissues in considerable amounts. In animals, from 200 to 700 times the plasma concentration may be found in the liver, spleen, kidney, and lung; leukocytes also concentrates the drug. The brain and spinal cord, in contrast, contain only 10 to 30 times the amount present in plasma.

Continued on next page

This product information was prepared in September 2004. On these and other products of Sanofi-Synthelabo Inc., detailed information may be obtained on a current basis by direct inquiry to Product Information Services, 90 Park Avenue, New York, NY 10016 (toll free 1-800-446-6267).

Aralen—Cont.

Chloroquine undergoes appreciable degradation in the body. The main metabolite is desethylchloroquine, which accounts for one fourth of the total material appearing in the urine; bisdesethylchloroquine, a carboxylic acid derivative, and other metabolic products as yet uncharacterized are found in small amounts. Slightly more than half of the urinary drug products can be accounted for as unchanged chloroquine.

Microbiology

Mechanism of Action: Chloroquine is an antimalarial agent. While the drug can inhibit certain enzymes, its effect is believed to result, at least in part, from its interaction with DNA. However, the mechanism of plasmodicidal action of chloroquine is not completely certain.

Activity *in vitro* and *in vivo*: Chloroquine is active against the erythrocytic forms of *Plasmodium vivax, Plasmodium malariae*, and susceptible strains of *Plasmodium falciparum* (but not the gametocytes of *P. falciparum*). It is not effective against exoerythrocytic forms of the parasite.

In vitro studies with trophozoites of *Entamoeba histolytica* have demonstrated that chloroquine also possess amebicidal activity comparable to that of emetine.

Drug Resistance: Resistance of *Plasmodium falciparum* to chloroquine is widespread and cases of *Plasmodium vivax* resistance have been reported.

INDICATIONS AND USAGE

ARALEN is indicated for the suppressive treatment and for acute attacks of malaria due to *P. vivax, P. malariae, P. ovale*, and susceptible strains of *P. falciparum*. The drug is also indicated for the treatment of extraintestinal amebiasis.

ARALEN does not prevent relapses in patients with vivax or malariae malaria because it is not effective against exoerythrocytic forms of the parasite, nor will it prevent vivax or malariae infection when administered as a prophylactic. It is highly effective as a suppressive agent in patients with vivax or malariae malaria, in terminating acute attacks, and significantly lengthening the interval between treatment and relapse. In patients with falciparum malaria it abolishes the acute attack and effects complete cure of the infection, unless due to a resistant strain of *P. falciparum*.

CONTRAINDICATIONS

Use of this drug is contraindicated in the presence of retinal or visual field changes either attributable to 4-aminoquinoline compounds or to any other etiology, and in patients with known hypersensitivity to 4-aminoquinoline compounds. However, in the treatment of acute attacks of malaria caused by susceptible strains of plasmodia, the physician may elect to use this drug after carefully weighing the possible benefits and risks to the patient.

WARNINGS

It has been found that certain strains of *P. falciparum* have become resistant to 4-aminoquinoline compounds (including chloroquine and hydroxychloroquine). Chloroquine resistance is widespread and, at present, is particularly prominent in various parts of the world including sub-Saharan Africa, Southeast Asia, the Indian subcontinent, and over large portions of South America, including the Amazon basin[1].

Before using chloroquine for prophylaxis, it should be ascertained whether chloroquine is appropriate for use in the region to be visited by the traveler.

Chloroquine should not be used for treatment of *P. falciparum* infections acquired in areas of chloroquine resistance or malaria occuring in patients where chloroquine prophylaxis has failed.

Patients infected with a resistant strain of plasmodia as shown by the fact that normally adequate doses have failed to prevent or cure clinical malaria or parasitemia should be treated with another form of antimalarial therapy.

Irreversible retinal damage has been observed in some patients who had received long-term or high-dosage 4-aminoquinoline therapy. Retinopathy has been reported to be dose related.

When prolonged therapy with any anti-malarial compound is contemplated, initial (base line) and periodic ophthalmologic examinations (including visual acuity, expert slit-lamp, funduscopic, and visual field tests) should be performed.

If there is any indication (past or present) of abnormality in the visual acuity, visual field, or retinal macular areas (such as pigmentary changes, loss of foveal reflex), or any visual symptoms (such as light flashes and streaks) which are not fully explainable by difficulties of accommodation or corneal opacities, the drug should be discontinued immediately and the patient closely observed for possible progression. Retinal changes (and visual disturbances) may progress even after cessation of therapy.

All patients on long-term therapy with this preparation should be questioned and examined periodically, including testing knee and ankle reflexes, to detect any evidence of muscular weakness. If weakness occurs, discontinue the drug.

A number of fatalities have been reported following the accidental ingestion of chloroquine, sometimes in relatively small doses (0.75 g or 1 g chloroquine phosphate in one 3-year-old child). Patients should be strongly warned to keep this drug out of the reach of children because they are especially sensitive to the 4-aminoquinoline compounds.

Use of ARALEN in patients with psoriasis may precipitate a severe attack of psoriasis.When used in patients with porphyria the condition may be exacerbated. The drug should not be used in these conditions unless in the judgment of the physician the benefit to the patient outweighs the potential risks.

Usage in Pregnancy: Radioactively tagged chloroquine administered intraveneously to pregnant pigmented CBA mice passed rapidly across the placenta and accumulated selectively in the melanin structures of the fetal eyes. It was retained in the ocular tissues for five months after the drug had been eliminated from the rest of the body[2]. There are no adequate and well-controlled studies evaluating the safety and efficacy of chloroquine in pregnant women. Usage of chloroquine during pregnancy should be avoided except in the suppression or treatment of malaria when in the judgment of the physician the benefit outweighs the potential risk to the fetus.

PRECAUTIONS

Hematological

Effects/Laboratory Tests

Complete blood cell counts should be made periodically if patients are given prolonged therapy. If any severe blood disorder appears which is not attributable to the disease under treatment, discontinuance of the drug should be considered.

The drug should be administered with caution to patients having G-6-PD (glucose-6 phosphate dehydrogenase) deficiency.

Auditory Effects

In patients with preexisting auditory damage, chloroquine should be administered with caution. In case of any defects in hearing, chloroquine should be immediately discontinued, and the patient closely observed (see ADVERSE REACTIONS).

Hepatic Effects

Since this drug is known to concentrate in the liver, it should be used with caution in patients with hepatic disease or alcoholism or in conjunction with known hepatotoxic drugs.

Central Nervous System Effects

Patients with history of epilepsy should be advised about the risk of chloroquine provoking seizures.

Drug Interactions

Antacids and kaolin: Antacids and kaolin can reduce absorption of chloroquine; an interval of at least 4 hours between intake of these agents and chloroquine should be observed.

Cimetidine: Cimetidine can inhibit the metabolism of chloroquine, increasing its plasma level. Concomitant use of cimetidine should be avoided.

Ampicillin: In a study of healthy volunteers, chloroquine significantly reduced the bioavailability of ampicillin. An interval of at least two hours between intake of this agent and chloroquine should be observed.

Cyclosporin: After introduction of chloroquine (oral form), a sudden increase in serum cyclosporin level has been reported. Therefore, close monitoring of serum cyclosporin level is recommended and, if necessary, chloroquine should be discontinued.

Pregnancy

See WARNINGS, Usage in Pregnancy.

Nursing Mothers

Because of the potential for serious adverse reactions in nursing infants from chloroquine, a decision should be made whether to discontinue nursing or to discontinue the drug, taking into account the potential clinical benefit of the drug to the mother.

Pediatric Use

See WARNINGS and DOSAGE AND ADMINISTRATION.

Geriatric Use

Clinical studies of Aralen did not include sufficient numbers of subjects aged 65 and over to determine whether they respond differently from younger subjects. However, this drug is known to be substantially excreted by the kidney, and the risk of toxic reactions to this drug may be greater in patients with impaired renal function. Because elderly patients are more likely to have decreased renal function, care should be taken in dose selection and it may be useful to monitor renal function.

ADVERSE REACTIONS

Special Senses: Ocular: Irreversible retinal damage in patients receiving long-term or high-dosage 4-aminoquinoline therapy; visual disturbances (blurring of vision and difficulty of focusing or accommodation); nyctalopia; scotomatous vision with field defects of paracentral, pericentral ring types, and typically temporal scotomas, e.g., difficulty in reading with words tending to disappear, seeing half an object, misty vision, and fog before the eyes.

Auditory: Nerve type deafness; tinnitus, reduced hearing in patients with pre-existing auditory damage.

Musculoskeletal system: Skeletal muscle myopathy or neuromyopathy leading to progressive weakness and atrophy of proximal muscle groups, which may be associated with mild sensory changes, depression of tendon reflexes and abnormal nerve conduction, have been noted.

Gastrointestinal system: Anorexia, nausea, vomiting, diarrhea, abdominal cramps.

Skin and appendages: Pleomorphic skin eruptions, skin and mucosal pigmentary changes; lichen planus-like eruptions, pruritus, photosensitivity and hair loss and bleaching of hair pigment.

Hematologic system: Rarely, aplastic anemia, reversible agranulocytosis, thrombocytopenia and neutropenia.

Central Nervous system: Convulsive seizures. Mild and transient headache. Neuropsychiatric changes including psychosis, delirium, personality changes and depression.

Cardiovascular system: Rarely, hypotension, electrocardiographic change (particularly, inversion or depression of the T-wave with widening of the QRS complex), and cardiomyopathy.

OVERDOSAGE

Symptoms: Chloroquine is very rapidly and completely absorbed after ingestion. Toxic doses of chloroquine can be fatal. As little as 1 g may be fatal in children. Toxic symptoms can occur within minutes. These consist of headache, drowsiness, visual disturbances, nausea and vomiting, cardiovascular collapse, shock and convulsions followed by sudden and early respiratory and cardiac arrest. The electrocardiogram may reveal atrial standstill, nodal rhythm, prolonged intraventricular conduction time, and progressive bradycardia leading to ventricular fibrillation and/or arrest.

Treatment: Treatment is symptomatic and must be prompt with immediate evacuation of the stomach by emesis (at home, before transportation to the hospital) or gastric lavage until the stomach is completely emptied. If finely powdered, activated charcoal is introduced by stomach tube, after lavage, and within 30 minutes after ingestion of the antimalarial, it may inhibit further intestinal absorption of the drug. To be effective, the dose of activated charcoal should be at least five times the estimated dose of chloroquine ingested.

Convulsions, if present, should be controlled before attempting gastric lavage. If due to cerebral stimulation, cautious administration of an ultra short-acting barbiturate may be tried but, if due to anoxia, it should be corrected by oxygen administration and artificial respiration. Monitor ECG. In shock with hypotension, a potent vasopressor should be administered. Replace fluids and electrolytes as needed. Cardiac compressing or pacing may be indicated to sustain the circulation. Because of the importance of supporting respiration, tracheal intubation or tracheostomy, followed by gastric lavage, may also be necessary. Peritoneal dialysis and exchange transfusions have also been suggested to reduce the level of the drug in the blood.

A patient who survives the acute phase and is asymptomatic should be closely observed for at least six hours. Fluids may be forced, and sufficient ammonium chloride (8 g daily in divided doses for adults) may be administered for a few days to acidify the urine to help promote urinary excretion in cases of both overdosage or sensitivity.

DOSAGE AND ADMINISTRATION

The dosage of chloroquine phosphate is often expressed in terms of equivalent chloroquine base. Each 500 mg tablet of ARALEN contains the equivalent of 300 mg chloroquine base. In infants and children the dosage is preferably calculated by body weight.

Malaria: Suppression—**Adult Dose:** 500 mg (= 300 mg base) on exactly the same day of each week.

Pediatric Dose: The weekly suppressive dosage is 5 mg calculated as base, per kg of body weight, but should not exceed the adult dose regardless of weight.

If circumstances permit, suppressive therapy should begin two weeks prior to exposure. However, failing this in adults, an initial double (loading) dose of 1 g (= 600 mg base), or in children 10 mg base/kg may be taken in two divided doses, six hours apart. The suppressive therapy should be continued for eight weeks after leaving the endemic area.

For Treatment of Acute Attack.

Adults: An initial dose of 1 g (= 600 mg base) followed by an additional 500 mg (= 300 mg base) after six to eight hours and a single dose of 500 mg (= 300 mg base) on each of two consecutive days. This represents a total dose of 2.5 g chloroquine phosphate or 1.5 g base in three days.

The dosage for adults of low body weight and for infants and children should be determined as follows:

First dose: 10 mg base per kg (but not exceeding a single dose of 600 mg base).

Second dose: (6 hours after first dose) 5 mg base per kg (but not exceeding a single dose of 300 mg base).

Third dose: (24 hours after first dose) 5 mg base per kg.

Fourth dose: (36 hours after first dose) 5 mg base per kg.

For radical cure of vivax and malariae malaria concomitant therapy with an 8-aminoquinoline compound is necessary.

Extraintestinal Amebiasis: Adults, 1 g (600 mg base) daily for two days, followed by 500 mg (300 mg base) daily for at least two to three weeks. Treatment is usually combined with an effective intestinal amebicide.

Geriatric Use

See PRECAUTIONS, Geriatric Use.

HOW SUPPLIED

Tablets containing 500 mg chloroquine phosphate USP, equivalent to 300 mg of chloroquine base, bottles of 25 (NDC 0024-0084-01).

White, film-coated convex, discoid tablet, 1/2 inch in diameter with an uncoated core, printed in black ink with a stylized "W" on one side and an "A77" on the other side.

Dispense in tight, light-resistant container as defined in the USP/NF.

Store at 25° C (77° F); excursions permitted to 15° - 30° C (59° - 86° F) [see USP Controlled Room Temperature]

REFERENCES
1. Malaria Deaths Following Inappropriate Malaria Chemoprophylaxis–United States, 2001. MMWR Weekly, 2001; 50(28): 597-599.
2. Ullberg S, Lindquist N G, Sjostrand S E: Accumulation of chorioretinotoxic drugs in the foetal eye. Nature 1970; 227: 1257.

sanofi~synthelabo
Manufactured for
Sanofi-Synthelabo Inc.
New York, NY 10016
by Bayer Corporation
Myerstown, PA 17067
Printed In USA
Revised June 2003

ASW-2G

AVAPRO® ℞
(irbesartan) Tablets

USE IN PREGNANCY
When used in pregnancy during the second and third trimesters, drugs that act directly on the renin-angiotensin system can cause injury and even death to the developing fetus. When pregnancy is detected, AVAPRO should be discontinued as soon as possible. See **WARNINGS: Fetal/Neonatal Morbidity and Mortality.**

DESCRIPTION

AVAPRO* (irbesartan) is an angiotensin II receptor (AT_1 subtype) antagonist.
Irbesartan is a non-peptide compound, chemically described as a 2-butyl-3-[*p*-(*o*-1*H*-tetrazol-5-ylphenyl)benzyl]-1,3-diazaspiro[4,4]non-1-en-4-one.
Its empirical formula is $C_{25}H_{28}N_6O$, and the structural formula:

[structural formula: O, N, N, (CH₂)₃CH₃, N, N, N, N, H]

Irbesartan is a white to off-white crystalline powder with a molecular weight of 428.5. It is a nonpolar compound with a partition coefficient (octanol/water) of 10.1 at pH of 7.4. Irbesartan is slightly soluble in alcohol and methylene chloride and practically insoluble in water.
AVAPRO is available for oral administration in unscored tablets containing 75 mg, 150 mg, or 300 mg of irbesartan. Inactive ingredients include: lactose, microcrystalline cellulose, pregelatinized starch, croscarmellose sodium, poloxamer 188, silicon dioxide and magnesium stearate.

CLINICAL PHARMACOLOGY

Mechanism of Action
Angiotensin II is a potent vasoconstrictor formed from angiotensin I in a reaction catalyzed by angiotensin-converting enzyme (ACE, kininase II). Angiotensin II is the principal pressor agent of the renin-angiotensin system (RAS) and also stimulates aldosterone synthesis and secretion by adrenal cortex, cardiac contraction, renal resorption of sodium, activity of sympathetic nervous system, and smooth muscle cell growth. Irbesartan blocks the vasoconstrictor and aldosterone-secreting effects of angiotensin II by selectively binding to the AT_1 angiotensin II receptor. There is also an AT_2 receptor in many tissues, but it is not involved in cardiovascular homeostasis.
Irbesartan is a specific competitive antagonist of AT_1 receptors with a much greater affinity (more than 8500-fold) for the AT_1 receptor than for the AT_2 receptor and no agonist activity.
Blockade of the AT_1 receptor removes the negative feedback of angiotensin II on renin secretion, but the resulting increased plasma renin activity and circulating angiotensin II do not overcome the effects of irbesartan on blood pressure.
Irbesartan does not inhibit ACE or renin or affect other hormone receptors or ion channels known to be involved in the cardiovascular regulation of blood pressure and sodium homeostasis. Because irbesartan does not inhibit ACE, it does not affect the response to bradykinin; whether this has clinical relevance is not known.

Pharmacokinetics
Irbesartan is an orally active agent that does not require biotransformation into an active form. The oral absorption of irbesartan is rapid and complete with an average absolute bioavailability of 60–80%. Following oral administration of AVAPRO, peak plasma concentrations of irbesartan are attained at 1.5–2 hours after dosing. Food does not affect the bioavailability of AVAPRO.
Irbesartan exhibits linear pharmacokinetics over the therapeutic dose range.
The terminal elimination half-life of irbesartan averaged 11–15 hours. Steady-state concentrations are achieved within 3 days. Limited accumulation of irbesartan (<20%) is observed in plasma upon repeated once-daily dosing.

Metabolism and Elimination
Irbesartan is metabolized via glucuronide conjugation and oxidation. Following oral or intravenous administration of ^{14}C-labeled irbesartan, more than 80% of the circulating plasma radioactivity is attributable to unchanged irbesartan. The primary circulating metabolite is the inactive irbesartan glucuronide conjugate (approximately 6%). The remaining oxidative metabolites do not add appreciably to irbesartan's pharmacologic activity.
Irbesartan and its metabolites are excreted by both biliary and renal routes. Following either oral or intravenous administration of ^{14}C-labeled irbesartan, about 20% of radioactivity is recovered in the urine and the remainder in the feces, as irbesartan or irbesartan glucuronide.
In vitro studies of irbesartan oxidation by cytochrome P450 isoenzymes indicated irbesartan was oxidized primarily by 2C9; metabolism by 3A4 was negligible. Irbesartan was neither metabolized by, nor did it substantially induce or inhibit, isoenzymes commonly associated with drug metabolism (1A1, 1A2, 2A6, 2B6, 2D6, 2E1). There was no induction or inhibition of 3A4.

Distribution
Irbesartan is 90% bound to serum proteins (primarily albumin and α_1-acid glycoprotein) with negligible binding to cellular components of blood. The average volume of distribution is 53–93 liters. Total plasma and renal clearances are in the range of 157–176 and 3.0–3.5 mL/min, respectively. With repetitive dosing, irbesartan accumulates to no clinically relevant extent.
Studies in animals indicate that radiolabeled irbesartan weakly crosses the blood brain barrier and placenta. Irbesartan is excreted in the milk of lactating rats.
* Registered trademark of Sanofi

Special Populations
Pediatric: Irbesartan pharmacokinetics have not been investigated in patients <18 years of age.
Gender: No gender related differences in pharmacokinetics were observed in healthy elderly (age 65–80 years) or in healthy young (age 18–40 years) subjects. In studies of hypertensive patients, there was no gender difference in half-life or accumulation, but somewhat higher plasma concentrations of irbesartan were observed in females (11–44%). No gender-related dosage adjustment is necessary.
Geriatric: In elderly subjects (age 65–80 years), irbesartan elimination half-life was not significantly altered, but AUC and C_{max} values were about 20–50% greater than those of young subjects (age 18–40 years). No dosage adjustment is necessary in the elderly.
Race: In healthy black subjects, irbesartan AUC values were approximately 25% greater than whites; there was no difference in C_{max} values.
Renal Insufficiency: The pharmacokinetics of irbesartan were not altered in patients with renal impairment or in patients on hemodialysis. Irbesartan is not removed by hemodialysis. No dosage adjustment is necessary in patients with mild to severe renal impairment unless a patient with renal impairment is also volume depleted. (See **WARNINGS: Hypotension in Volume- or Salt-depleted Patients** and **DOSAGE AND ADMINISTRATION.)**
Hepatic Insufficiency: The pharmacokinetics of irbesartan following repeated oral administration were not significantly affected in patients with mild to moderate cirrhosis of the liver. No dosage adjustment is necessary in patients with hepatic insufficiency.
Drug Interactions: (See **PRECAUTIONS: Drug Interactions.)**

Pharmacodynamics
In healthy subjects, single oral irbesartan doses of up to 300 mg produced dose-dependent inhibition of the pressor effect of angiotensin II infusions. Inhibition was complete (100%) 4 hours following oral doses of 150 mg or 300 mg and partial inhibition was sustained for 24 hours (60% and 40% at 300 mg and 150 mg, respectively).
In hypertensive patients, angiotensin II receptor inhibition following chronic administration of irbesartan causes a 1.5–2 fold rise in angiotensin II plasma concentration and a 2–3 fold increase in plasma renin levels. Aldosterone plasma concentrations generally decline following irbesartan administration, but serum potassium levels are not significantly affected at recommended doses.
In hypertensive patients, chronic oral doses of irbesartan (up to 300 mg) had no effect on glomerular filtration rate, renal plasma flow or filtration rate, renal plasma flow or filtration fraction. In multiple dose studies in hypertensive patients, there were no clinically important effects on fasting triglycerides, total cholesterol, HDL-cholesterol, or fasting glucose concentrations. There was no effect on serum uric acid during chronic oral administration, and no uricosuric effect.

Clinical Studies
The antihypertensive effects of AVAPRO (irbesartan) were examined in seven (7) major placebo-controlled 8–12 week trials in patients with baseline diastolic blood pressures of 95–110 mmHg. Doses of 1–900 mg were included in these trials in order to fully explore the dose-range of irbesartan. These studies allowed comparison of once- or twice-daily regimens at 150 mg/day, comparisons of peak and trough effects, and comparisons of response by gender, age, and race. Two of the seven placebo-controlled trials identified above examined the antihypertensive effects of irbesartan and hydrochlorothiazide in combination.
The seven (7) studies of irbesartan monotherapy included a total of 1915 patients randomized to irbesartan (1–900 mg) and 611 patients randomized to placebo. Once-daily doses of 150 and 300 mg provided statistically and clinically significant decreases in systolic and diastolic blood pressure with trough (24 hours post-dose) effects after 6–12 weeks of treatment compared to placebo, of about 8–10/5–6 and 8–12/5–8 mmHg, respectively. No further increase in effect was seen at dosages greater than 300 mg. The dose-response relationships for effects on systolic and diastolic pressure are shown in Figures 1 and 2.

Figure 1.
Placebo-subtracted reduction in trough SeSBP; integrated analysis

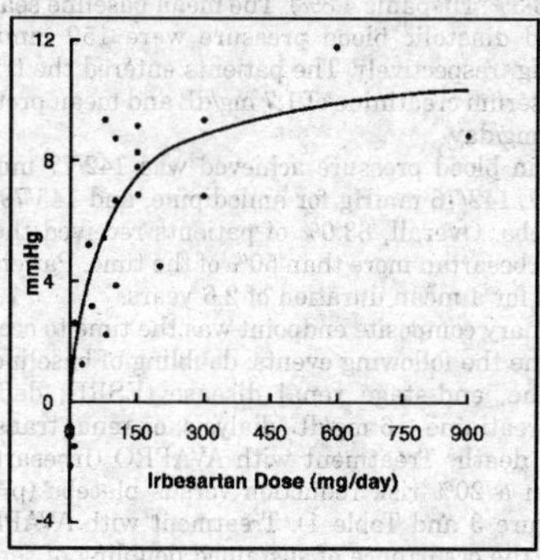

Figure 2.
Placebo-subtracted reduction in trough SeDBP; integrated analysis

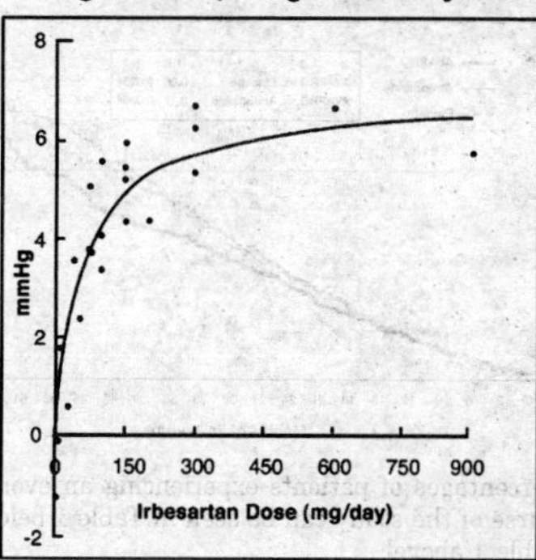

Once-daily administration of therapeutic doses of irbesartan gave peak effects at around 3–6 hours and, in one ambulatory blood pressure monitoring study, again around 14 hours. This was seen with both once-daily and twice-daily dosing. Trough-to-peak ratios by systolic and diastolic response were generally between 60–70%. In a continuous blood pressure monitoring study, once-daily dosing with 150 mg gave trough and mean 24-hour responses similar to those observed in patients receiving twice-daily dosing at the same total daily dose.
In controlled trials, the addition of irbesartan to hydrochlorothiazide doses of 6.25, 12.5, or 25 mg produced further dose-related reductions in blood pressure similar to those achieved with the same monotherapy dose of irbesartan. HCTZ aldo had an approximately additive effect.
Analysis of age, gender, and race subgroups of patients showed that men and women, and patients over and under 65 years of age, had generally similar responses. Irbesartan was effective in reducing blood pressure regardless of race, although the effect was somewhat less in blacks (usually a low-renin population).
The effect of irbesartan is apparent after the first dose and it is close to its full observed effect at 2 weeks. At the end of an 8-week exposure, about 2/3 of the antihypertensive effect was still present one week after the last dose. Rebound hypertension was not observed. There was essentially no change in average heart rate in irbesartan-treated patients in controlled trials.

Nephropathy in Type 2 Diabetic Patients
The Irbesartan Diabetic Nephropathy Trial (IDNT) was a randomized, placebo- and active-controlled, double-blind multicenter study, conducted worldwide in 1715 patients

Continued on next page

This product information was prepared in September 2004. On these and other products of Sanofi-Synthelabo Inc., detailed information may be obtained on a current basis by direct inquiry to Product Information Services, 90 Park Avenue, New York, NY 10016 (toll free 1-800-446-6267).

Avapro—Cont.

with type 2 diabetes, hypertension (SeSBP >135 mmHg or SeDBP >85 mmHg), and nephropathy (serum creatinine 1.0 to 3.0 mg/dL in females or 1.2 to 3.0 mg/dL in males and proteinuria ≥900 mg/day). Patients were randomized to receive AVAPRO 75 mg, amlodipine 2.5 mg, or matching placebo once-daily. Patients were titrated to a maintenance dose of AVAPRO 300 mg, or amlodipine 10 mg, as tolerated. Additional antihypertensive agents (excluding ACE inhibitors, angiotensin II receptor antagonists and calcium channel blockers) were added as needed to achieve blood pressure goal (≤135/85 or 10 mmHg reduction in systolic blood pressure if higher than 160 mmHg) for patients in all groups.

The study population was 66.5% male, 72.9% below 65 years of age and 72% White, (Asian/Pacific Islander 5.0%, Black 13.3%, Hispanic 4.8%). The mean baseline seated systolic and diastolic blood pressure were 159 mmHg and 87 mmHg, respectively. The patients entered the trial with a mean serum creatinine of 1.7 mg/dL and mean proteinuria of 4144 mg/day.

The mean blood pressure achieved was 142/77 mmHg for AVAPRO, 142/76 mmHg for amlodipine, and 145/79 mmHg for placebo. Overall, 83.0% of patients received the target dose of irbesartan more than 50% of the time. Patients were followed for a mean duration of 2.6 years.

The primary composite endpoint was the time to occurrence of any one the following events: doubling of baseline serum creatinine, end-stage renal disease (ESRD; defined by serum creatinine ≥6 mg/dL, dialysis, or renal transplantation) or death. Treatment with AVAPRO (irbesartan) resulted in a 20% risk reduction versus placebo (p=0.0234) (see Figure 3 and Table 1). Treatment with AVAPRO also reduced the occurrence of sustained doubling of serum creatinine as a separate end point (33%), but had no significant effect on ESRD alone and no effect on overall mortality (see Table 1).

Figure 3.
IDNT: Kaplan-Meier Estimates Of Primary Endpoint
(Doubling of Serum Creatinine, End-Stage Renal Disease or All-Cause Mortality)

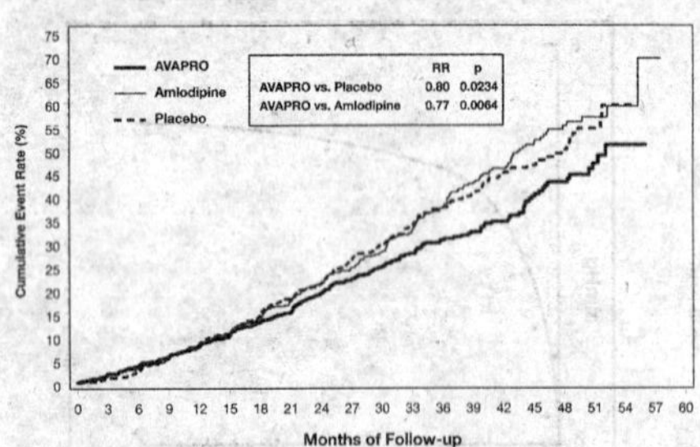

Table 1: IDNT: Components of Primary Composite Endpoint

	Comparison with placebo				Comparison with amlodipine		
	AVAPRO N=579 (%)	Placebo N=569 (%)	Hazard Ratio	95% CI	Amlodipine N=567 (%)	Hazard Ratio	95% CI
Primary Composite Endpoint	32.6	39.0	0.80	0.66–0.97 (p=0.0234)	41.1	0.77	0.63–0.93
Breakdown of first occurring event contributing to primary endpoint							
2× creatinine	14.2	19.5	—	—	22.8	—	—
ESRD	7.4	8.3	—	—	8.8	—	—
Death	11.1	11.2	—	—	9.5	—	—
Incidence of total events over entire period of follow-up							
2× creatinine	16.9	23.7	0.67	0.52–0.87	25.4	0.63	0.49–0.81
ESRD	14.2	17.8	0.77	0.57–1.03	18.3	0.77	0.57–1.03
Death	15.0	16.3	0.92	0.69–1.23	14.6	1.04	0.77–1.40

Table 2: IDNT: Primary Efficacy Outcome Within Subgroups

Baseline Factors	AVAPRO N=579 (%)	Comparison with placebo: Placebo N=569 (%)	Hazard Ratio	95% CI
Gender				
Male	27.5	36.7	0.68	0.53–0.88
Female	42.3	44.6	0.98	0.72–1.34
Race				
White	29.5	37.3	0.75	0.60–0.95
Non-White	42.6	43.5	0.95	0.67–1.34
Age (years)				
< 65	31.8	39.9	0.77	0.62–0.97
≥ 65	35.1	36.8	0.88	0.61–1.29

The percentages of patients experiencing an event during the course of the study can be seen in Table 1 below:

[See table 1 above]

The secondary endpoint of the study was a composite of cardiovascular mortality and morbidity (myocardial infarction, hospitalization for heart failure, stroke with permanent neurological deficit, amputation). There were no statistically significant differences among treatment groups in these endpoints. Compared with placebo, AVAPRO significantly reduced proteinuria by about 27%, an effect that was evident within 3 months of starting therapy. AVAPRO (irbesartan) significantly reduced the rate of loss of renal function (glomerular filtration rate), as measured by the reciprocal of the serum creatinine concentration, by 18.2%.

Table 2 presents results for demographic subgroups. Subgroup analyses are difficult to interpret and it is not known whether these observations represent true differences or chance effects. For the primary endpoint, AVAPRO's favorable effects were seen in patients also taking other antihypertensive medications (angiotensin II receptor antagonists, angiotensin converting enzyme inhibitors and calcium channel blockers were not allowed), oral hypoglycemic agents, and lipid-lowering agents.

[See table 2 above]

INDICATIONS AND USAGE

AVAPRO (irbesartan) is indicated for the treatment of hypertension. It may be used alone or in combination with other antihypertensive agents.

Nephropathy in Type 2 Diabetic Patients

AVAPRO (irbesartan) is indicated for the treatment of diabetic nephropathy with an elevated serum creatinine and proteinuria (>300 mg/day) in patients with type 2 diabetes and hypertension. In this population, AVAPRO reduces the rate of progression of nephropathy as measured by the occurrence of doubling of serum creatinine or end-stage renal disease (need for dialysis or renal transplantation) (see **CLINICAL PHARMACOLOGY: Clinical Studies**).

CONTRAINDICATIONS

AVAPRO is contraindicated in patients who are hypersensitive to any component of this product.

WARNINGS

Fetal/Neonatal Morbidity and Mortality

Drugs that act directly on the renin-angiotensin system can cause fetal and neonatal morbidity and death when administered to pregnant women. Several dozen cases have been reported in the world literature in patients who were taking angiotensin-converting-enzyme inhibitors. When pregnancy is detected, AVAPRO should be discontinued as soon as possible.

The use of drugs that act directly on the renin-angiotensin system during the second and third trimesters of pregnancy has been associated with fetal and neonatal injury, including hypotension, neonatal skull hypoplasia, anuria, reversible or irreversible renal failure, and death. Oligohydramnios has also been reported, presumably resulting from decreased fetal renal function; oligohydramnios in this setting has been associated with fetal limb contractures, craniofacial deformation and hypoplastic lung development. Prematurity, intrauterine growth retardation, and patent ductus arteriosus have also been reported, although it is not clear whether these occurrences were due to exposure to the drug.

These adverse effects do not appear to have resulted from intrauterine drug exposure that has been limited to the first trimester.

Mothers whose embryos and fetuses are exposed to an angiotensin II receptor antagonist only during the first trimester should be so informed. Nonetheless, when patients become pregnant, physicians should have the patient discontinue the use of AVAPRO as soon as possible.

Rarely (probably less often than once in every thousand pregnancies), no alternative to a drug acting on the renin-angiotensin system will be found. In these rare cases, the mothers should be apprised of the potential hazards to their fetuses, and serial ultrasound examinations should be performed to assess the intraamniotic environment.

If oligohydramnios is observed, AVAPRO should be discontinued unless it is considered life-saving for the mother. Contraction stress testing (CST), a non-stress test (NST), or biophysical profiling (BPP) may be appropriate depending upon the week of pregnancy. Patients and physicians should be aware, however, that oligohydramnios may not appear until after the fetus has sustained irreversible injury.

Infants with histories of *in utero* exposure to an angiotensin II receptor antagonist should be closely observed for hypotension, oliguria, and hyperkalemia. If oliguria occurs, attention should be directed toward support of blood pressure and renal perfusion. Exchange transfusion or dialysis may be required as means of reversing hypotension and/or substituting for disordered renal function.

When pregnant rats were treated with irbesartan from day 0 to day 20 of gestation (oral doses of 50, 180, and 650 mg/kg/day), increased incidences of renal pelvic cavitation, hydroureter and/or absence of renal papilla were observed in fetuses at doses ≥50 mg/kg/day [approximately equivalent to the maximum recommended human dose (MRHD), 300 mg/day, on a body surface area basis]. Subcutaneous edema was observed in fetuses at doses ≥180 mg/kg/day (about 4 times the MRHD on a body surface area basis). As these anomalies were not observed in rats in which irbesartan exposure (oral doses of 50, 150 and 450 mg/kg/day) was limited to gestation days 6–15, they appear to reflect late gestational effects of the drug. In pregnant rabbits, oral doses of 30 mg irbesartan/kg/day were associated with maternal mortality and abortion. Surviving females receiving this dose (about 1.5 times the MRHD of a body surface area basis) had a slight increase in early resorptions and a corresponding decrease in live fetuses. Irbesartan was found to cross the placental barrier in rats and rabbits.

Radioactivity was present in the rat and rabbit fetus during late gestation and in rat milk following oral doses of radiolabeled irbesartan.

Hypotension in Volume- or Salt-depleted Patients

Excessive reduction of blood pressure was rarely seen (<0.1%) in patients with uncomplicated hypertension. Initiation of antihypertensive therapy may cause symptomatic hypotension in patients with intravascular volume- or sodium-depletion, e.g., in patients treated virgorously with diuretics or in patients on dialysis. Such volume depletion should be corrected prior to administration of AVAPRO (irbesartan), or a low starting dose should be used (see **DOSAGE AND ADMINISTRATION**).

If hypotension occurs, the patient should be placed in the supine position and, if necessary, given an intravenous infusion of normal saline. A transient hypotensive response is not a contraindication to further treatment, which usually can be continued without difficulty once the blood pressure has stabilized.

PRECAUTIONS

Impaired Renal Function

As a consequence of inhibiting the renin-angiotensin-aldosterone system, changes in renal function may be anticipated in susceptible individuals. In patients whose renal function may depend on the activity of the renin-angiotensin-aldosterone system (e.g., patients with severe congestive heart failure), treatment with angiotensin-converting-enzyme inhibitors has been associated with oliguria and/or progressive azotemia and (rarely) with acute renal failure and/or death. AVAPRO would be expected to behave similarly. In studies of ACE inhibitors in patients with unilateral or bilateral renal artery stenosis, increases in serum creatinine or BUN have been reported. There has been no known use of AVAPRO in patients with unilateral or bilateral renal artery stenosis, but a similar effect should be anticipated.

Information for Patients

Pregnancy: Female patients of childbearing age should be told about the consequences of second- and third-trimester exposure to drugs that act on the remin-angiotensin system, and they should also be told that these consequences do not appear to have resulted from intrauterine drug exposure that has been limited to the first trimester. These patients should be asked to report pregnancies to their physicians as soon as possible.

Drug Interactions

No significant drug-drug pharmacokinetic (or pharmacodynamic) interactions have been found in interaction studies with hydrochlorothiazide, digoxin, warfarin, and nifedipine. *In vitro* studies show significant inhibition of the formation of oxidized irbesartan metabolites with the known cytochrome CYP 2C9 substrates/inhibitors sulphenazole, tolbutamide and nifedipine. However, in clinical studies the consequences of concomitant irbesartan on the pharmacodynamics of warfarin were negligible. Based on *in vitro* data, no interaction would be expected with drugs whose metabolism is dependent upon cytochrome P450 isozymes 1A1, 1A2, 2A6, 2B6, 2D6, 2E1, or 3A4.

In separate studies of patients receiving maintenance doses of warfarin, hydrochlorothiazide, or digoxin, irbesartan administration for 7 days had no effect on the pharmacodynamics of warfarin (prothrombin time) or pharmacokinetics of digoxin. The pharmacokinetics of irbesartan were not affected by coadministration of nifedipine or hydrochlorothiazide.

Carcinogenesis, Mutagenesis, Impairment of Fertility

No evidence of carcinogenicity was observed when irbesartan was administered at doses of up to 500/1000 mg/kg/day (males/females, respectively) in rats and 1000 mg/kg/day in mice for up to two years. For male and female rats, 500 mg/kg/day provided an average systemic exposure to irbesartan (AUC_{0-24h}, bound plus unbound) about 3 and 11 times, respectively, the average systemic exposure in humans receiving the maximum recommended dose (MRD) of 300 mg irbesartan/day, whereas 1000 mg/kg/day (administered to females only) provided an average systemic exposure about 21 times that reported for humans at the MRD. For male and female mice, 1000 mg/kg/day provided an exposure to irbesartan about 3 and 5 times, respectively, the human exposure at 300 mg/day.

Irbesartan was not mutagenic in a battery of *in vitro* tests (Ames microbial test, rat hepatocyte DNA repair test, V79 mammalian-cell forward gene-mutation assay). Irbesartan was negative in several tests for induction of chromosomal aberrations (*in vitro*—human lymphocyte assay; *in vivo*—mouse micronucleus study).

Irbesartan had no adverse effects on fertility or mating of male or female rats at oral doses ≤650 mg/kg/day, the highest dose providing a systemic exposure to irbesartan (AUC_{0-24h}, bound plus unbound) about 5 times that found in humans receiving the maximum recommended dose of 300 mg/day.

Pregnancy

Pregnancy Categories C (first trimester) and D (second and third trimester).

See **WARNINGS: Fetal/Neonatal Morbidity and Mortality.**

Nursing Mothers

It is not known whether irbesartan is excreted in human milk, but irbesartan or some metabolite of irbesartan is secreted at low concentration in the milk of lactating rats. Because of the potential for adverse effects on the nursing infant, a decision should be made whether to discontinue nursing or discontinue the drug, taking into account the importance of the drug to the mother.

Pediatric Use

Safety and effectiveness in pediatric patients have not been established.

Geriatric Use

Of the 1965 subjects in controlled clinical studies of Avapro (irbesartan) for hypertension, 15% were age 65 and over, but few were over age 75. No striking differences in antihypertensive effect or in adverse events appear to be present in this database, but there were insufficient numbers of aged subjects to enable detection of less than striking differences. Greater or lesser sensitivity of some older individuals cannot be ruled out. (See **Pharmacokinetics, Special Populations,** and **Clinical Studies.**)

ADVERSE REACTIONS

Hypertension

AVAPRO has been evaluated for safety in more than 4300 patients with hypertension and about 5000 subjects overall. This experience includes 1303 patients treated for over 6 months and 407 patients for 1 year or more. Treatment with AVAPRO was well-tolerated, with an incidence of adverse events similar to placebo. These events generally were mild and transient with no relationship to the doses of AVAPRO.

In placebo-controlled clinical trials, discontinuation of therapy due to a clinical adverse event was required in 3.3 percent of patients treated with AVAPRO, versus 4.5 percent of patients given placebo.

In placebo-controlled clinical trials, the adverse event experiences that occurred in at least 1% of patients treated with AVAPRO (n=1965) and at a higher incidence versus placebo (n=641) included diarrhea (3% vs. 2%), dyspepsia/heartburn (2% vs. 1%), musculoskeletal trauma (2% vs. 1%), fatigue (4% vs. 3%), and upper respiratory infection (9% vs. 6%). None of these differences were significant.

The following adverse events occurred at an incidence of 1% or greater in patients treated with irbesartan, but were at least as frequent or more frequent in patients recieving placebo: abdominal pain, anxiety/nervousness, chest pain, dizziness, edema, headache, influenza, musculoskeletal pain, pharyngitis, nausea/vomiting, rash, rhinitis, sinus abnormailty, tachycardia and urinary tract infection.

Irbesartan use was not associated with an increased incidence of dry cough, as is typically associated with ACE inhibitor use. In placebo controlled studies, the incidence of cough in irbesartan treated patients was 2.8% versus 2.7% in patients receiving placebo.

The incidence of hypotension or orthostatic hypotension was low in irbesartan treated patients (0.4%), unrelated to dosage, and similar to the incidence among placebo treated patients (0.2%). Dizziness, syncope, and vertigo were reported with equal or less frequency in patients receiving irbesartan compared with placebo.

In addition, the following potentially important events occurred in less than 1% of the 1965 patients and at least 5 patients (0.3%) receiving irbesartan in clinical studies, and those less frequent, clinically significant events (listed by body system). It cannot be determined whether these events were causally related to irbesartan:

Body as a Whole: fever, chills, facial edema, upper extremity edema;

Cardiovascular: flushing, hypertension, cardiac murmur, myocardial infarction, angina pectoris, arrhythmic/conduction disorder, cardio-respiratory arrest, heart failure, hypertensive crisis;

Dermatologic: pruritus, dermatitis, ecchymosis, erythema face, urticaria;

Endocrine/Metabolic/Electrolyte Imbalances: sexual dysfunction, libido change, gout;

Gastrointestinal: constipation, oral lesion, gastroenteritis, flatulence, abdominal distention;

Musculoskeletal/Connective Tissue: extremity swelling, muscle cramp, arthritis, muscle ache, musculoskeletal chest pain, joint stiffness, bursitis, muscle weakness;

Nervous System: sleep disturbance, numbness, somnolence, emotional disturbance, depression, paresthesia, tremor, transient ischemic attack, cerebrovascular accident;

Renal/Genitourinary: abnormal urination, prostate disorder;

Respiratory: epistaxis, tracheobronchitis, congestion, pulmonary congestion, dyspnea, wheezing;

Special Senses: vision disturbance, hearing abnormality, ear infection, ear pain, conjunctivitis, other eye disturbance, eyelid abnormality, ear abnormality.

Nephropathy in Type 2 Diabetic Patients

In clinical studies in patients with hypertension and type 2 diabetic renal disease, the adverse drug experiences were similar to those seen in patients with hypertension with the exception of an increased incidence of orthostatic symptoms (dizziness, orthostatic dizziness, and orthostatic hypotension) observed in IDNT (proteinuria ≥900 mg/day, and serum creatinine ranging from 1.0–3.0 mg/dL). In this trial, orthostatic symptoms occurred more frequently in the AVAPRO group (dizziness 10.2%, orthostatic dizziness, 5.4%, orthostatic hypotension 5.4%) than in the placebo group (dizziness 6.0%, orthostatic dizziness 2.7%, orthostatic hypotension 3.2%).

Post-Marketing Experience: The following have been very rarely reported in post-marketing experience: urticaria; angioedema (involving swelling of the face, lips, pharynx, and/or tongue); increased liver function tests; jaundice. Hyperkalemia has been rarely reported.

Laboratory Test Findings

In controlled clinical trials, clincally important differences in laboratory tests were rarely associated with administration of AVAPRO.

Creatinine, Blood Urea Nitrogen: Minor increases in blood urea nitrogen (BUN) or serum creatinine were observed in less than 0.7% of patients with essential hypertension treated with AVAPRO alone versus 0.9% on placebo. (See **PRECAUTIONS: Impaired Renal Function.**)

Hematologic: Mean decreases in hemoglobin of 0.2 g/dL were observed in 0.2% of patients receiving AVAPRO compared to 0.3% of placebo treated patients. Neutropenia (<1000 cells/mm^3) occurred at similar frequencies among patients receiving AVAPRO (0.3%) and placebo treated patients (0.5%).

Nephropathy in Type 2 Diabetic Patients

Hyperkalemia: In IDNT (proteinuria ≥900 mg/day, and serum creatinine ranging from 1.0–3.0 mg/dL), the percent of patients with hyperkalemia (>6 mEq/L) was 18.6% in the AVAPRO group vs. 6.0% in the placebo group. Discontinuations due to hyperkalemia in the AVAPRO group were 2.1% vs. 0.4% in the placebo group.

OVERDOSAGE

No data are available in regard to overdosage in humans. However, daily doses of 900 mg for 8 weeks were well-tolerated. The most likely manifestations of overdosage are expected to be hypotension and tachycardia; bradycardia might also occur from overdose. Irbesartan is not removed by hemodialysis.

To obtain up-to-date information about the treatment of overdosage, a good resource is a certified Regional Poison-Control Center. Telephone numbers of certified poison-control centers are listed in the *Physicians' Desk Reference* (PDR). In managing overdose, consider the possibilities of multiple-drug interactions, drug-drug interactions, and unusual drug kinetics in the patient.

Laboratory determinations of serum levels of irbesartan are not widely available, and such determinations have, in any event, no known established role in the management of irbesartan overdose.

Acute oral toxicity studies with irbesartan in mice and rats indicated acute lethal doses were in excess of 2000 mg/kg, about 25- and 50-fold the maximum recommended human dose (300 mg) on a mg/m^2 basis, respectively.

DOSAGE AND ADMINISTRATION

AVAPRO may be administered with other antihypertensive agents and with or without food.

Hypertension

The recommended initial dose of AVAPRO is 150 mg once daily. Patients requiring further reduction in blood pressure should be titrated to 300 mg once daily.

A low dose of a diuretic may be added, if blood pressure is not controlled by AVAPRO alone. Hydrochlorothiazide has been shown to have an additive effect (see **CLINICAL PHARMACOLOGY: Clinical Studies**). Patients not adequately treated by the maximum dose of 300 mg once daily are unlikely to derive additional benefit from a higher dose or twice-daily dosing.

No dosage adjustment is necessary in elderly patients, or in patients with hepatic impairment or mild to severe renal impairment.

Nephropathy in Type 2 Diabetic Patients

The recommended target maintenance dose is 300 mg once daily. There are no data on the clinical effects of lower doses of AVAPRO on diabetic nephropathy (see **CLINICAL PHARMACOLOGY: Clinical Studies**).

Pediatric Patients

Children (<6 years): Safety and effectiveness have not been established.

Children (6–12 years): An initial dose of 75 mg once daily is reasonable. Patients requiring further reduction in blood pressure should be titrated to 150 mg once daily (see **PRECAUTIONS: Pediatric Use**).

Adolescent patients (13–16 years): An initial dose of 150 mg once daily is reasonable. Patients requiring further reduction in blood pressure should be titrated to 300 mg once daily. Higher doses are not recommended (see **PRECAUTIONS: Pediatric Use**).

Volume- and Salt-depleted Patients

A lower initial dose or AVAPRO (75 mg) is recommended in patients with depletion of intravascular volume or salt (e.g., patients treated vigorously with diuretics or on hemodialysis) (see **WARNINGS: Hypotension in Volume- of Salt-depleted Patients**).

HOW SUPPLIED

AVAPRO® (irbesartan) is available as white to off-white biconvex oval tablets, debossed with a heart shape on one side and a portion of the NDC code on the other. Unit-of-use bottles contain 30, 90, or 500 tablets and blister packs contain 100 tablets, as follows:

	75 mg	150 mg	300 mg
Debossing	2771	2772	2773
Bottle of 30	0087-2771-31	0087-2772-31	0087-2773-31
Bottle of 90	0087-2771-32	0087-2772-32	0087-2773-32
Bottle of 500		0087-2772-15	0087-2773-15
Blister of 100	0087-2771-35	0087-2772-35	

[See table above]

Storage

Store at a temperature between 15° C and 30° C (59° F and 85° F) [USP].

Distributed by:

Bristol-Myers Squibb Sanofi-Synthelabo Partnership

New York, NY 10016

Revised September 2002 J4641H 1092944A6

Shown in Product Identification Guide, page 332

DEMEROL® ℞

[dĕ-mər-ŏl]

(meperidine hydrochloride, USP)

WARNING: May be habit forming

DESCRIPTION

Meperidine hydrochloride, a white crystalline substance with a melting point of 186° C to 189° C. It is readily soluble

Continued on next page

This product information was prepared in September 2004. On these and other products of Sanofi-Synthelabo Inc., detailed information may be obtained on a current basis by direct inquiry to Product Information Services, 90 Park Avenue, New York, NY 10016 (toll free 1-800-446-6267).

Demerol—Cont.

in water and has a neutral reaction and a slightly bitter taste. The solution is not decomposed by a short period of boiling.

The syrup is a pleasant-tasting, nonalcoholic, banana-flavored solution containing 50 mg of DEMEROL, brand of meperidine hydrochloride, per 5 mL teaspoon (25 drops contain 13 mg of DEMEROL). The tablets contain 50 mg or 100 mg of the analgesic.

Inactive Ingredients—TABLETS: Calcium Sulfate, Dibasic Calcium Phosphate, Starch, Stearic Acid, Talc. SYRUP: Benzoic Acid, Flavor, Liquid Glucose, Purified Water, Saccharin Sodium.

Chemically, DEMEROL is 4-Piperidinecarboxylic acid, 1-methyl-4-phenyl-, ethyl ester, hydrochloride and has the following structure:

H_3C—N ... O ... CH_3 • HCl

CLINICAL PHARMACOLOGY

Meperidine hydrochloride is a narcotic analgesic with multiple actions qualitatively similar to those of morphine; the most prominent of these involve the central nervous system and organs composed of smooth muscle. The principal actions of therapeutic value are analgesia and sedation.

There is some evidence which suggests that meperidine may produce less smooth muscle spasm, constipation, and depression of the cough reflex than equianalgesic doses of morphine. Meperidine, in 60 mg to 80 mg parenteral doses, is approximately equivalent in analgesic effect to 10 mg of morphine. The onset of action is slightly more rapid than with morphine, and the duration of action is slightly shorter. Meperidine is significantly less effective by the oral than by the parenteral route, but the exact ratio of oral to parenteral effectiveness is unknown.

INDICATIONS AND USAGE

DEMEROL is indicated for the relief of moderate to severe pain.

CONTRAINDICATIONS

DEMEROL is contraindicated in patients with hypersensitivity to meperidine.

Meperidine is contraindicated in patients who are receiving monoamine oxidase (MAO) inhibitors or those who have recently received such agents. Therapeutic doses of meperidine have occasionally precipitated unpredictable, severe, and occasionally fatal reactions in patients who have received such agents within 14 days. The mechanism of these reactions is unclear, but may be related to a preexisting hyperphenylalaninemia. Some have been characterized by coma, severe respiratory depression, cyanosis, and hypotension, and have resembled the syndrome of acute narcotic overdose. In other reactions the predominant manifestations have been hyperexcitability, convulsions, tachycardia, hyperpyrexia, and hypertension. Although it is not known that other narcotics are free of the risk of such reactions, virtually all of the reported reactions have occurred with meperidine. If a narcotic is needed in such patients, a sensitivity test should be performed in which repeated, small, incremental doses of morphine are administered over the course of several hours while the patient's condition and vital signs are under careful observation. (Intravenous hydrocortisone or prednisolone have been used to treat severe reactions, with the addition of intravenous chlorpromazine in those cases exhibiting hypertension and hyperpyrexia. The usefulness and safety of narcotic antagonists in the treatment of these reactions is unknown.)

WARNINGS

DEMEROL is an opioid agonist and a Schedule II controlled substance with an abuse liability similar to morphine.

DEMEROL can be abused in a manner similar to other opioid agonists, legal or illicit. This should be considered when prescribing or dispensing DEMEROL in situations where the physician or pharmacist is concerned about an increased risk of misuse, abuse, or diversion.

Misuse, Abuse, and Diversion of Opioids

Meperidine is an opioid agonist of the morphine-type. Such drugs are sought by drug abusers and people with addiction disorders and are subject to criminal diversion.

Meperidine can be abused in a manner similar to other opioid agonists, legal or illicit. This should be considered when prescribing or dispensing DEMEROL in situations where the physician or pharmacist is concerned about an increased risk of misuse, abuse, or diversion.

DEMEROL has been reported as being abused by crushing, chewing, snorting, or injecting the dissolved product. These practices will result in the uncontrolled delivery of the opioid and pose a significant risk to the abuser that could result in overdose or death (see **WARNINGS** and **DRUG ABUSE AND ADDICTION**).

Concerns about abuse, addiction, and diversion should not prevent the proper management of pain.

Healthcare professionals should contact their State Professional Licensing Board or State Controlled Substances Authority for information on how to prevent and detect abuse or diversion of this product.

Interactions with Alcohol and Drugs of Abuse

Meperidine may be expected to have additive effects when used in conjunction with alcohol, other opioids, or illicit drugs that cause central nervous system depression.

Head Injury and Increased Intracranial Pressure: The respiratory depressant effects of meperidine and its capacity to elevate cerebrospinal fluid pressure may be markedly exaggerated in the presence of head injury, other intracranial lesions, or a preexisting increase in intracranial pressure. Furthermore, narcotics produce adverse reactions which may obscure the clinical course of patients with head injuries. In such patients, meperidine must be used with extreme caution and only if its use is deemed essential.

Asthma and Other Respiratory Conditions: Meperidine should be used with extreme caution in patients having an acute asthmatic attack, patients with chronic obstructive pulmonary disease or cor pulmonale, patients having a substantially decreased respiratory reserve, and patients with preexisting respiratory depression, hypoxia, or hypercapnia. In such patients, even usual therapeutic doses of narcotics may decrease respiratory drive while simultaneously increasing airway resistance to the point of apnea.

Hypotensive Effect: The administration of meperidine may result in severe hypotension in the postoperative patient or any individual whose ability to maintain blood pressure has been compromised by a depleted blood volume or the administration of drugs such as the phenothiazines or certain anesthetics.

Usage in Ambulatory Patients: Meperidine may impair the mental and/or physical abilities required for the performance of potentially hazardous tasks such as driving a car or operating machinery. The patient should be cautioned accordingly.

Meperidine, like other narcotics, may produce orthostatic hypotension in ambulatory patients.

Usage in Pregnancy: Meperidine should not be used in pregnant women prior to the labor period, unless in the judgment of the physician the potential benefits outweigh the possible risks, because safe use in pregnancy prior to labor has not been established relative to possible adverse effects on fetal development.

Labor and Delivery: Meperidine crosses the placental barrier and can produce depression of respiration and psychophysiologic functions in the newborn. Resuscitation may be required (See OVERDOSAGE).

Nursing Mothers: Meperidine appears in the milk of nursing mothers receiving the drug. Due to the potential for serious adverse reactions in nursing infants, a decision should be made whether to discontinue nursing or to discontinue the drug, taking into account the potential benefits of the drug to the nursing woman.

PRECAUTIONS

General

Opioid analgesics can have a narrow therapeutic index in certain patient populations, particularly when combined with CNS depressant drugs. The use of these products should be reserved for cases where the benefits of opioid analgesia outweigh the known risks of respiratory depression, altered mental state, and postural hypotension.

Use of DEMEROL may be associated with increased potential risks and should be used with caution in the following conditions: sickle cell anemia, pheochromocytoma, acute alcoholism; adrenocortical insufficiency (e.g., Addison's disease); CNS depression or coma; delirium tremens; debilitated patients; kyphoscoliosis associated with respiratory depression; myxedema or hypothyroidism; prostatic hypertrophy or urethral stricture; severe impairment of hepatic, pulmonary, or renal function; and toxic psychosis.

The administration of meperidine may obscure the diagnosis or clinical course in patients with acute abdominal conditions. All opioids may induce or aggravate seizures in some clinical settings.

Interactions with other CNS Depressants

DEMEROL should be used with caution and consideration should be given to starting with a reduced dosage in patients who are concurrently receiving other central nervous system depressants including sedatives or hypnotics, general anesthetics, phenothiazines, other tranquilizers, and alcohol. Drug-drug interactions may result in respiratory depression, hypotension, profound sedation, or coma if these drugs are taken in combination with the usual doses of DEMEROL.

Interactions with Mixed Agonist/Antagonist Opioid Analgesics

Agonist/antagonist analgesics (i.e., pentazocine, nalbuphine, butorphanol, and buprenorphine) should be administered with caution to a patient who has received or is receiving a course of therapy with a pure opioid agonist analgesic such as meperidine. In this situation, mixed agonist/antagonist analgesics may reduce the analgesic effect of medperidine and/or may precipitate withdrawal symptoms in these patients.

Supraventricular Tachycardias: Meperidine should be used with caution in patients with atrial flutter and other supraventricular tachycardias because of a possible vagolytic action which may produce a significant increase in the ventricular response rate.

Convulsions: Meperidine may aggravate preexisting convulsions in patients with convulsive disorders. If dosage is escalated substantially above recommended levels because of tolerance development, convulsions may occur in individuals without a history of convulsive disorders.

Acute Abdominal Conditions: The administration of meperidine or other narcotics may obscure the diagnosis or clinical course in patients with acute abdominal conditions.

Tolerance and Physical Dependence

Tolerance is the need for increasing doses of opioids to maintain a defined effect such as analgesia (in the absence of disease progression or other external factors). Physical dependence is manifested by withdrawal symptoms after abrupt discontinuation of a drug or upon administration of an antagonist. Physical dependence and tolerance are not unusual during chronic opioid therapy.

The opioid abstinence or withdrawal syndrome is characterized by some or all of the following: restlessness, lacrimation, rhinorrhea, yawning, perspiration, chills, myalgia, mydriasis. Other symptoms also may develop, including: irritability, anxiety, backache, joint pain, weakness, abdominal cramps, insomnia, nausea, anorexia, vomiting, diarrhea, or increased blood pressure, respiratory rate, or heart rate.

In general, opioids used regularly should not be abruptly discontinued.

Use in Drug and Alcohol Addiction

DEMEROL is an opioid with no approved use in the management of addictive disorders. Its proper usage in individuals with drug or alcohol dependence, either active or in remission, is for the management of pain requiring opioid analgesia. Demerol should be used with caution in patients with alcoholism and other drug dependencies due to the increased frequency of narcotic tolerance, dependence, and the risk of addiction observed in these patient populations. Abuse of DEMEROL in combination with other CNS depressant drugs can result in serious risk to the patient.

Information for Patients/Caregivers

If clinically advisable, patients receiving DEMEROL (meperidine hydrochloride) tablets or their caregivers should be given the following information by the physician, nurse, pharmacist, or caregiver:

1. Patients should be aware that DEMEROL tablets contain meperidine, which is a morphine-like substance.
2. Patients should be advised to report pain and adverse experiences occurring during therapy. Individualization of dosage is essential to make optimal use of this medication.
3. Patients should be advised not to adjust the dose of DEMEROL without consulting the prescribing professional.
4. Patients should be advised that DEMEROL may impair mental and/or physical ability required for the performance of potentially hazardous tasks (e.g., driving, operating heavy machinery).
5. Patients should not combine DEMEROL with alcohol or other central nervous system depressants (sleep aids, tranquilizers) except by the orders of the prescribing physician, because dangerous additive effects may occur, resulting in serious injury or death.
6. Women of childbearing potential who become, or are planning to become pregnant should be advised to consult their physician regarding the effects of analgesics and other drug use during pregnancy on themselves and their unborn child.
7. Patients should be advised that DEMEROL is a potential drug of abuse. They should protect it from theft, and it should never be given to anyone other than the individual for whom it was prescribed.
8. Patients should be advised that if they have been receiving treatment with DEMEROL for more than a few weeks and cessation of therapy is indicated, it may be appropriate to taper the DEMEROL dose, rather than abruptly discontinue it, due to the risk of precipitating withdrawal symptoms. Their physician can provide a dose schedule to accomplish a gradual discontinuation of the medication.
9. Patients should be instructed to keep DEMEROL in a secure place out of the reach of children. When DEMEROL is no longer needed, the unused tablets should be destroyed by flushing down the toilet.

Drug Interactions: Also see WARNINGS.

Acyclovir: Plasma concentrations of meperidine and its metabolite, normeperidine, may be increased by acyclovir; thus caution should be used with concomitant administration.

Cimetidine: Cimetidine reduced the clearance and volume of distribution of meperidine and also the formation of the metabolite, normeperidine, in healthy subjects; thus, caution should be used with concomitant administration.

Phenytoin: The hepatic metabolism of meperidine may be enhanced by phenytoin. Concomitant administration resulted in reduced half-life and bioavailability with increased clearance of meperidine in healthy subjects; however, blood concentrations of normeperidine were increased.

Ritonavir: Plasma concentrations of the active metabolite normeperidine may be increased by ritonavir; thus concomitant administration should be avoided.

Opioid analgesics, including DEMEROL, may enhance the neuromuscular blocking action of skeletal muscle relaxants and produce an increased degree of respiratory depression.

Special Risk Patients: Meperidine should be given with caution and the initial dose should be reduced in certain patients such as the elderly or debilitated, and those with severe impairment of hepatic or renal function, Sickle Cell Anemia, hypothyroidism, Addison's disease, Pheochromocytoma and prostatic hypertrophy or urethral stricture. In patients with pheochromocytoma, meperidine has been reported to provoke hypertension.

Usage in Hepatically Impaired Patients: Accumulation of meperidine and/or its active metabolite, normeperidine, can

occur in patients with hepatic impairment. Meperidine should therefore be used with caution in patients with hepatic impairment.
Usage in Renally Impaired Patients: Accumulation of meperidine and/or its active metabolite, normeperidine, can also occur in patients with renal impairment. Meperidine should therefore be used with caution in patients with renal impairment.
Carcinogenesis, mutagenesis, impairment of fertility: Studies to assess the carcinogenic or mutagenic potential of meperidine have not been conducted. Studies to determine the effect of meperidine on fertility have not been conducted.
Pregnancy: Teratogenic effects. Pregnancy Category C: Animal reproduction studies have not been conducted with meperidine. It is also not known whether DEMEROL can cause fetal harm when administered to a pregnant woman or can affect reproduction capacity. DEMEROL should be given to a pregnant woman only if clearly needed.
Labor and Delivery: See WARNINGS.
Nursing Mothers: See WARNINGS.
Pediatric Use: Literature reports indicate that meperidine has a slower elimination rate in neonates and young infants compared to older children and adults. Neonates and young infants may also be more susceptible to the effects, especially the respiratory depressant effects. Meperidine should therefore be used with caution in neonates and young infants, and any potential benefits of the drug weighed against the relative risk to a pediatric patient.
Geriatric Use: Clinical studies of DEMEROL during product development did not include sufficient numbers of subjects aged 65 and over to evaluate age-related differences in safety or efficacy. Literature reports indicate that geriatric patients have a slower elimination rate compared to young patients and they may be more susceptible to the effects of meperidine. A reduction in the total daily dose of meperidine may be required in elderly patients, and the potential benefits of the drug weighed against the relative risk to a geriatric patient.

ADVERSE REACTIONS

The major hazards of meperidine, as with other narcotic analgesics, are respiratory depression and, to a lesser degree, circulatory depression; respiratory arrest, shock, and cardiac arrest have occurred.
The most frequently observed adverse reactions include lightheadedness, dizziness, sedation, nausea, vomiting, and sweating. These effects seem to be more prominent in ambulatory patients and in those who are not experiencing severe pain. In such individuals, lower doses are advisable. Some adverse reactions in ambulatory patients may be alleviated if the patient lies down.
Other adverse reactions include:
Nervous System: Euphoria, dysphoria, weakness, headache, agitation, tremor, uncoordinated muscle movements, (e.g. muscle twitches, myoclonus), severe convulsions, transient hallucinations and disorientation, visual disturbances.
Gastrointestinal: Dry mouth, constipation, biliary tract spasm.
Cardiovascular: Flushing of the face, tachycardia, bradycardia, palpitation, hypotension (see WARNINGS), syncope.
Genitourinary: Urinary retention.
Allergic: Pruritus, urticaria, other skin rashes, wheal and flare over the vein with intravenous injection.

DOSAGE AND ADMINISTRATION

For Relief of Pain

Dosage should be adjusted according to the severity of the pain and the response of the patient. Meperidine is less effective orally than on parenteral administration. The dose of DEMEROL should be proportionately reduced (usually by 25 to 50 percent) when administered concomitantly with phenothiazines and many other tranquilizers since they potentiate the action of DEMEROL.
Adults: The usual dosage is 50 mg to 150 mg orally, every 3 or 4 hours as necessary.
Pediatric Patients: The usual dosage is 1.1 mg/kg to 1.8 mg/kg orally, up to the adult dose, every 3 or 4 hours as necessary.
Each dose of the syrup should be taken in one-half glass of water, since if taken undiluted, it may exert a slight topical anesthetic effect on mucous membranes.

DRUG ABUSE AND ADDICTION

DEMEROL contains meperidine, a mu-agonist opioid with an abuse liability similar to morphine and is a Schedule II controlled substance. Meperidine, like morphine and other opioids used in analgesia, can be abused and is subject to criminal diversion.

Drug addiction is characterized by compulsive use, use for non-medical purposes, and continued use despite harm or risk of harm. Drug addiction is a treatable disease, utilizing a multi-disciplinary approach, but relapse is common.
"Drug seeking" behavior is very common in addicts and drug abusers. Drug-seeking tactics include emergency calls or visits near the end of office hours, refusal to undergo appropriate examination, testing or referral, repeated "loss" of prescriptions, tampering with prescriptions and reluctance to provide prior medical records or contact information for other treating physician(s). "Doctor shopping" to obtain additional prescriptions is common among drug abusers and people suffering from untreated addiction.
Abuse and addiction are separate and distinct from physical dependence and tolerance. Physicians should be aware that addiction may not be accompanied by concurrent tolerance and symptoms of physical dependence in all addicts. In addition, abuse of opioids can occur in the absence of true addiction and is characterized by misuse for non-medical purposes, often in combination with other psychoactive substances. DEMEROL, like other opioids, has been diverted for non-medical use. Careful record-keeping of prescribing information, including quantity, frequency, and renewal requests is strongly advised.
Abuse of DEMEROL poses a risk of overdose and death. This risk is increased with concurrent abuse of DEMEROL with alcohol and other substances. Due to the presence of talc as one of the excipients in tablets, parenteral abuse of crushed tablets can be expected to result in local tissue necrosis, infection, pulmonary granulomas, and increased risk of endocarditis and valvular heart disease. In addition, parenteral drug abuse is commonly associated with transmission of infectious diseases such as hepatitis and HIV.
Proper assessment of the patient, proper prescribing practices, periodic re-evaluation of therapy, and proper dispensing and storage are appropriate measures that help to limit abuse of opioid drugs.

OVERDOSAGE

Symptoms: Serious overdosage with meperidine is characterized by respiratory depression (a decrease in respiratory rate and/or tidal volume, Cheyne-Stokes respiration, cyanosis), extreme somnolence progressing to stupor or coma, skeletal muscle flaccidity, cold and clammy skin, and sometimes bradycardia and hypotension. In severe overdosage, particularly by the intravenous route, apnea, circulatory collapse, cardiac arrest, and death may occur.
Treatment: Primary attention should be given to the reestablishment of adequate respiratory exchange through provision of a patent airway and institution of assisted or controlled ventilation. The narcotic antagonist, naloxone hydrochloride, is a specific antidote against respiratory depression which may result from overdosage or unusual sensitivity to narcotics, including meperidine. Therefore, an appropriate dose of this antagonist should be administered, preferably by the intravenous route, simultaneously with efforts at respiratory resuscitation.
An antagonist should not be administered in the absence of clinically significant respiratory or cardiovascular depression.
Oxygen, intravenous fluids, vasopressors, and other supportive measures should be employed as indicated.
In cases of overdosage with DEMEROL tablets, the stomach should be evacuated by emesis or gastric lavage.
NOTE: In an individual physically dependent on narcotics, the administration of the usual dose of a narcotic antagonist will precipitate an acute withdrawal syndrome. The severity of this syndrome will depend on the degree of physical dependence and the dose of antagonist administered. The use of narcotic antagonists in such individuals should be avoided if possible. If a narcotic antagonist must be used to treat serious respiratory depression in the physically dependent patient, the antagonist should be administered with extreme care and only one-fifth to one-tenth the usual initial dose administered.

SAFETY AND HANDLING

Demerol® (meperidine HCl) tablets and syrup are dosage forms that contain meperidine hydrochloride which is a controlled substance. Like morphine, meperidine is controlled under Schedule II of the Controlled Substances Act. Meperidine, like all opioids, is liable to diversion and misuse and should be handled accordingly. Patients and their families should be instructed to flush any DEMEROL syrup or DEMEROL tablets that are no longer needed.
DEMEROL has been targeted for theft and diversion by criminals. Healthcare professionals should contact their State Professional Licensing Board or State Controlled Substance Authority for information on how to prevent and detect abuse or diversion of this product.

HOW SUPPLIED

For Oral Use

Tablets are white, round and convex: the 50 mg tablet is scored.
Tablets of 50 mg, bottles of 100 (NDC 0024-0335-04), bottles of 500 (NDC 0024-0335-06), Hospital Blister Pak of 25 (NDC 0024-0335-02), **100 mg**, bottles of 100 (NDC 0024-0337-04).
SYRUP, nonalcoholic, banana-flavored 50 mg per 5 mL teaspoon, bottles of 16 fl oz (NDC 0024-0332-06).
Store at 25° C (77° F); excursions permitted to 15°-30° C (59°-86° F) [See USP Controlled Room Temperature].
sanofi~synthelabo
Manufactured for Sanofi-Synthelabo Inc.
New York, NY 10016
by Bayer Corporation
Myerstown, PA 17067

Revised July 2003
DSW 3L(O)

Shown in Product Identification Guide, page 332

ELIGARD® 7.5 mg ℞
[ĕl'-ə gärd]
(leuprolide acetate for injectable suspension)

DESCRIPTION

ELIGARD® 7.5 mg is a sterile polymeric matrix formulation of leuprolide acetate for subcutaneous injection. It is designed to deliver 7.5 mg of leuprolide acetate at a controlled rate over a one month therapeutic period.
Leuprolide acetate is a synthetic nonapeptide analog of naturally occurring gonadotropin releasing hormone (GnRH or LH-RH) that, when given continuously, inhibits pituitary gonadotropin secretion and suppresses testicular and ovarian steroidogenesis. The analog possesses greater potency than the natural hormone. The chemical name is 5-oxo-L-prolyl-L-histidyl-L-tryptophyl-L-seryl-L-tyrosyl-D-leucyl-L-leucyl-L-arginyl-N-ethyl-L-prolinamide acetate (salt) with the following structural formula:

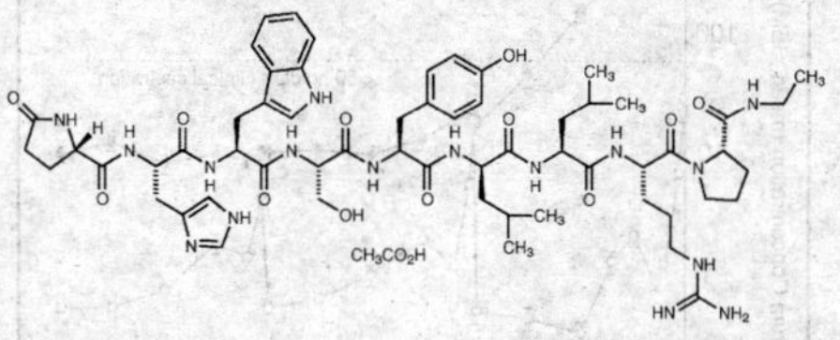

ELIGARD® 7.5 mg is prefilled and supplied in two separate, sterile syringes whose contents are mixed immediately prior to administration. The two syringes are joined and the single dose product is mixed until it is homogenous. ELIGARD® 7.5 mg is administered subcutaneously where it forms a solid drug delivery depot.
One syringe contains the ATRIGEL® Delivery System and the other contains leuprolide acetate. The ATRIGEL® Delivery System is a polymeric (non-gelatin containing) delivery system consisting of a biodegradable poly(DL-lactide-co-glycolide) (PLGH) polymer formulation dissolved in a biocompatible solvent, *N*-methyl-2-pyrrolidone (NMP). PLGH is a co-polymer with a 50:50 molar ratio of DL-lactide to glycolide containing carboxyl end groups. The second syringe contains leuprolide acetate and the constituted product is designed to deliver 7.5 mg of leuprolide acetate at the time of subcutaneous injection.
ELIGARD® 7.5 mg delivers 7.5 mg of leuprolide acetate (equivalent to approximately 7.0 mg leuprolide free base) dissolved in 160 mg *N*-methyl-2-pyrrolidone and 82.5 mg poly(DL-lactide-co-glycolide). The approximate weight of the administered formulation is 250 mg.

CLINICAL PHARMACOLOGY

Leuprolide acetate, an LH-RH agonist, acts as a potent inhibitor of gonadotropin secretion when given continuously in therapeutic doses. Animal and human studies indicate that after an initial stimulation, chronic administration of leuprolide acetate results in suppression of ovarian and testicular steroidogenesis. This effect is reversible upon discontinuation of drug therapy.
In humans, administration of leuprolide acetate results in an initial increase in circulating levels of luteinizing hormone (LH) and follicle stimulating hormone (FSH), leading to a transient increase in levels of the gonadal steroids (testosterone and dihydrotestosterone in males, and estrone and estradiol in premenopausal females). However, continuous administration of leuprolide acetate results in decreased levels of LH and FSH. In males, testosterone is reduced to below castrate threshold ($\leq$ 50 ng/dL). These decreases occur within two to four weeks after initiation of treatment. Long-term studies have shown that continuation of therapy with leuprolide acetate maintains testosterone below the castrate level for up to seven years.

PHARMACODYNAMICS

Following the first dose of ELIGARD® 7.5 mg, mean serum testosterone concentrations transiently increased, then fell to below castrate threshold ($\leq$ 50 ng/dL) within three weeks (Figure 1). Continued monthly treatment maintained castrate testosterone suppression throughout the study. No breakthrough of testosterone concentrations above castrate threshold (> 50 ng/dL) occurred at any time during the study once castrate suppression was achieved.
Leuprolide acetate is not active when given orally.

PHARMACOKINETICS

Absorption: The pharmacokinetics/pharmacodynamics observed during three once monthly injections (ELIGARD® 7.5 mg) in 20 patients with advanced carcinoma of the prostate is shown in Figure 1. Mean serum leuprolide concentrations following the initial injection rose to 25.3 ng/mL (C_{max}) at approximately 5 hours after injection. After the initial increase following each injection, serum concentrations remained relatively constant (0.28 – 2.00 ng/mL). There was no evidence of significant accumulation during repeated dosing. Nondetectable leuprolide plasma concentrations have been observed during chronic ELIGARD® 7.5 mg administration, but testosterone levels were maintained at castrate levels.
[See figure 1 at top of next column]
Distribution: The mean steady-state volume of distribution of leuprolide following intravenous bolus administration to healthy male volunteers was 27 L.[1] *In vitro* binding to human plasma proteins ranged from 43% to 49%.
Metabolism: In healthy male volunteers, a 1 mg bolus of leuprolide administered intravenously revealed that the

Continued on next page

This product information was prepared in September 2004. On these and other products of Sanofi-Synthelabo Inc., detailed information may be obtained on a current basis by direct inquiry to Product Information Services, 90 Park Avenue, New York, NY 10016 (toll free 1-800-446-6267).

Eligard 7.5 mg—Cont.

Figure 1-Pharmacokinetic/Pharmacodynamic Response (N=20) to ELIGARD® 7.5 mg - Patients dosed initially and at Months 1 and 2

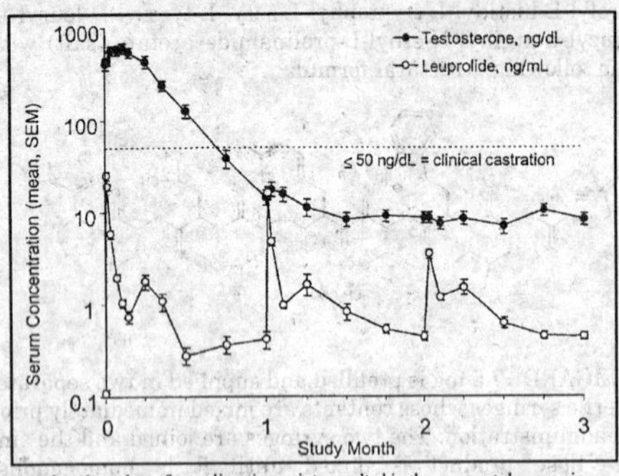

A reduced number of sampling timepoints resulted in the apparent decrease in C_{max} values with the second and third doses of ELIGARD® 7.5 mg (Figure 1).

mean systemic clearance was 8.34 L/h, with a terminal elimination half-life of approximately 3 hours based on a two compartment model.[1]

No drug metabolism study was conducted with ELIGARD® 7.5 mg. Upon administration with different leuprolide acetate formulations, the major metabolite of leuprolide acetate is a pentapeptide (M-1) metabolite.

Excretion: No drug excretion study was conducted with ELIGARD® 7.5 mg.

Special Populations:

Geriatrics: The majority (70%) of the 128 patients studied in these clinical trials were age 70 and older.

Pediatrics: The safety and effectiveness of ELIGARD® 7.5 mg in pediatric patients have not been established (see **CONTRAINDICATIONS**).

Race: In patients studied (26 White, 2 Hispanic), mean serum leuprolide concentrations were similar.

Renal and Hepatic Insufficiency: The pharmacokinetics of ELIGARD® 7.5 mg in hepatically and renally impaired patients have not been determined.

Drug-Drug Interactions: No pharmacokinetic drug-drug interaction studies were conducted with ELIGARD® 7.5 mg.

CLINICAL STUDIES

In one open-label, multicenter study (AGL9904), 120 patients with advanced prostate cancer were treated with six monthly injections of ELIGARD® 7.5 mg. Eighty-nine patients had stage C disease and 31 patients had stage D disease. This study evaluated the achievement and maintenance of serum testosterone suppression over six months of therapy.

The mean testosterone concentration increased from 361.3 ng/dL at Baseline to 574.6 ng/dL at Day 3 following the initial subcutaneous injection. The mean serum testosterone concentration then decreased to below Baseline by Day 10 and was 21.8 ng/dL on Day 28. At the conclusion of the study (Month 6), mean testosterone concentration was 6.1 ng/dL (Figure 2).

Serum testosterone was suppressed to below the castrate threshold (≤ 50 ng/dL) by Day 28 (Week 4) in 112 of 119 (94.1%) patients remaining in the study. The remaining seven patients all attained the castrate threshold by Day 42. Once testosterone suppression at or below serum concentrations of 50 ng/dL was achieved, no patients (0%) demonstrated breakthrough (concentration above 50 ng/dL) at any time in the study. All 117 evaluable patients in the study at Month 6 (two patients withdrew for reasons unrelated to drug) had testosterone concentrations of ≤ 50 ng/dL.

Figure 2. ELIGARD® 7.5 mg Mean Serum Testosterone Concentrations (n=117)

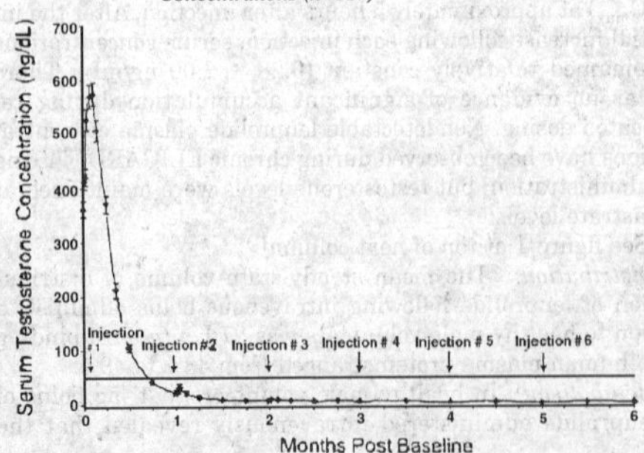

Serum PSA decreased in all patients whose Baseline values were elevated above the normal limit. Mean values were reduced 94% from Baseline to Month 6. At Month 6, PSA levels had decreased to within normal limits in 94% of patients who presented with elevated levels at Baseline.

Other secondary efficacy endpoints evaluated included WHO performance status, bone pain, urinary pain and urinary signs and symptoms. At Baseline, 88% of patients were classified as "fully active" by the WHO performance status scale (Status=0) and 11% as "restricted in strenuous activity but ambulatory and able to carry out work of a light or sedentary nature" (Status=1). These percentages were unchanged at Month 6. At Baseline, patients experienced little bone pain, with a mean score of 1.22 (range 1–9) on a scale of 1 (no pain) to 10 (worst pain possible). At Month 6, the mean bone pain score was essentially unchanged at 1.26 (range 1–7). Urinary pain, scored on the same scale, was similarly low, with a mean of 1.12 at Baseline (range 1–5) and 1.07 at Month 6 (range 1–8). Urinary signs and symptoms were similarly low at Baseline and decreased modestly at Month 6. In addition, there was a reduction in patients with prostate abnormalities detected during physical exam from 102 (85%) at Screening to 77 (64%) at Month 6.

INDICATIONS AND USAGE

ELIGARD® 7.5 mg is indicated for the palliative treatment of advanced prostate cancer.

CONTRAINDICATIONS

1. ELIGARD® 7.5 mg is contraindicated in patients with hypersensitivity to GnRH, GnRH agonist analogs or any of the components of ELIGARD® 7.5 mg. Anaphylactic reactions to synthetic GnRH or GnRH agonist analogs have been reported in the literature.[2]
2. ELIGARD® 7.5 mg is contraindicated in women and in pediatric patients and was not studied in women or children. Moreover, leuprolide acetate can cause fetal harm when administered to a pregnant woman. Major fetal abnormalities were observed in rabbits but not in rats after administration of leuprolide acetate throughout gestation. There were increased fetal mortality and decreased fetal weights in rats and rabbits. The effects on fetal mortality are expected consequences of the alterations in hormonal levels brought about by this drug. The possibility exists that spontaneous abortion may occur.

WARNINGS

ELIGARD® 7.5 mg, like other LH-RH agonists, causes a transient increase in serum concentrations of testosterone during the first week of treatment. Patients may experience worsening of symptoms or onset of new signs and symptoms during the first few weeks of treatment, including bone pain, neuropathy, hematuria, or bladder outlet obstruction. Isolated cases of ureteral obstruction and/or spinal cord compression, which may contribute to paralysis with or without fatal complications, have been observed in the palliative treatment of advanced prostate cancer using LH-RH agonists. (see **PRECAUTIONS**).

If spinal cord compression or renal impairment develops, standard treatment of these complications should be instituted.

PRECAUTIONS

General: Patients with metastatic vertebral lesions and/or with urinary tract obstruction should be closely observed during the first few weeks of therapy (see **WARNINGS** section).

Laboratory tests: Response to ELIGARD® 7.5 mg should be monitored by measuring serum concentrations of testosterone and prostate-specific antigen periodically.

In the majority of patients, testosterone levels increased above Baseline during the first week, declining thereafter to Baseline levels or below by the end of the second week. Castrate levels were generally reached within two to four weeks and once achieved were maintained for the duration of treatment. No increases to above the castrate level occurred in any of the patients.

Results of testosterone determinations are dependent on assay methodology. It is advisable to be aware of the type and precision of the assay methodology to make appropriate clinical and therapeutic decisions.

Drug Interactions: See **PHARMACOKINETICS**

Drug/Laboratory Test Interactions: Therapy with leuprolide results in suppression of the pituitary-gonadal system. Results of diagnostic tests of pituitary gonadotropic and gonadal functions conducted during and after leuprolide therapy may be affected.

Carcinogenesis, Mutagenesis, Impairment of Fertility: Two-year carcinogenicity studies were conducted with leuprolide acetate in rats and mice. In rats, a dose-related increase of benign pituitary hyperplasia and benign pituitary adenomas was noted at 24 months when the drug was administered subcutaneously at high daily doses (0.6 to 4 mg/kg). There was a significant but not dose-related increase of pancreatic islet-cell adenomas in females and of testicular interstitial cell adenomas in males (highest incidence in the low dose group). In mice, no leuprolide acetate-induced tumors or pituitary abnormalities were observed at a dose as high as 60 mg/kg for two years. Patients have been treated with leuprolide acetate for up to three years with doses as high as 10 mg/day and for two years with doses as high as 20 mg/day without demonstrable pituitary abnormalities. No carcinogenicity studies have been conducted with ELIGARD® 7.5 mg.

Mutagenicity studies have been performed with leuprolide acetate using bacterial and mammalian systems and with ELIGARD® 7.5 mg in bacterial systems. These studies provided no evidence of a mutagenic potential.

Pregnancy, Teratogenic Effects: Pregnancy category X. (See **CONTRAINDICATIONS**).

Pediatric Use: ELIGARD® 7.5 mg is contraindicated in pediatric patients and was not studied in children (see **CONTRAINDICATIONS**).

ADVERSE REACTIONS

The safety of ELIGARD® 7.5 mg was evaluated in eight surgically castrated males and 120 patients with advanced prostate cancer in two clinical trials. ELIGARD® 7.5 mg, like other LH-RH analogs, caused a transient increase in serum testosterone concentrations during the first week of treatment. Therefore, potential exacerbations of signs and symptoms of the disease during the first few weeks of treatment are of concern in patients with vertebral metastases and/or urinary obstruction or hematuria. If these conditions are aggravated, it may lead to neurological problems such as weakness and/or paresthesia of the lower limbs or worsening of urinary symptoms (see **WARNINGS** and **PRECAUTIONS**).

In Study AGL9904, 120 patients were dosed with ELIGARD® 7.5 mg for up to six months and injection sites were closely monitored. In all, 716 injections of ELIGARD® 7.5 mg were administered. Transient burning/stinging was reported following 248 (34.6%) injections, with the majority (84%) of these events reported as mild. Pain was reported following 4.3% of study injections (18.3% of patients) and was generally reported as brief in duration and mild in intensity.

Erythema was reported following 2.6% of injections (12.5% of patients). These events were all reported as mild and generally resolved within a few days post-injection. Mild bruising was reported following 2.5% of injections (11.7% of patients). Pruritis, induration, and ulceration was reported following 1.4% (11 patients), 0.4% (3 patients), and 0.1% (1 patient) of study injections, respectively.

These localized adverse events were non-recurrent over time. No patient discontinued therapy due to an injection site adverse event.

The following possibly or probably related systemic adverse events occurred during clinical trials of up to six months of treatment with ELIGARD® 7.5 mg, and were reported in ≥ 2% of patients (Tables 1 and 2). Often, causality is difficult to assess in patients with metastatic prostate cancer. Reactions considered not drug-related are excluded.

[See table 1 above]

Table 1: Incidence (%) of Possibly or Probably Related Systemic Adverse Events Reported by ≥ 2% of Patients (n = 120) Treated with ELIGARD® 7.5 mg for up to Six Months in Study AGL9904

Body System	Adverse Event	Number	Percent
Body as a Whole	Malaise and Fatigue	21	17.5%
	Dizziness	4	3.3%
Cardiovascular	Hot flashes/sweats*	68	56.7%
Genitourinary	Atrophy of Testes*	6	5.0%
Digestive	Gastroenteritis/Colitis	3	2.5%

[See table 2 above]

Table 2: Incidence (%) of Possibly or Probably-Related Systemic Adverse Events Reported by ≥ 2% of Surgically Castrated Patients (n = 8) Treated with a Single-Dose of ELIGARD® 7.5 mg in Study AGL9802

Body System	Adverse Event	Number	Percent
Cardiovascular	Hot flashes/sweats*	2	25.0%

In addition, the following possibly or probably related systemic adverse events were reported by < 2% of the patients using ELIGARD® 7.5 mg in clinical studies.

General: Sweating, insomnia, syncope
Gastrointestinal: Flatulence, constipation
Hematologic: Decreased red blood cell count, hematocrit and hemoglobin
Metabolic: Weight gain
Musculoskeletal: Tremor, backache, joint pain
Nervous: Disturbance of smell and taste, depression, vertigo
Skin: Alopecia
Urogenital: Testicular soreness, impotence*, decreased libido*, gynecomastia, breast soreness

*Expected pharmacological consequences of testosterone suppression. In the patient populations studied, a total of 86 hot flash/sweats adverse events were reported in 70 patients. Of these, 71 events (83%) were mild; 14 (16%) were moderate; 1 (1%) was severe.

Changes in Bone Density: Decreased bone density has been reported in the medical literature in men who have had orchiectomy or who have been treated with an LH-RH agonist analog.[3] It can be anticipated that long periods of medical castration in men will have effects on bone density.

OVERDOSAGE

In clinical trials using daily subcutaneous leuprolide acetate in patients with prostate cancer, doses as high as 20 mg/day for up to two years caused no adverse effects differing from those observed with the 1 mg/day dose.

DOSAGE AND ADMINISTRATION

The recommended dose of ELIGARD® 7.5 mg is one injection every month. The injection delivers 7.5 mg of leuprolide acetate, incorporated in a polymer formulation. It is administered subcutaneously and provides continuous release of leuprolide for one month.

Once mixed, ELIGARD® 7.5 mg should be discarded if not administered within 30 minutes.

As with other drugs administered by subcutaneous injection, the injection site should vary periodically. The specific injection location chosen should be an area with sufficient soft or loose subcutaneous tissue. In clinical trials, the injection was administered in the upper- or mid-abdominal area. Avoid areas with brawny or fibrous subcutaneous tissue or locations that could be rubbed or compressed (i.e., with a belt or clothing waistband).

Mixing and Administration Procedure

IMPORTANT: Allow the product to reach room temperature before using. **Once mixed, the product must be administered within 30 minutes.**

Follow the instructions as directed to ensure proper preparation of ELIGARD® 7.5 mg prior to administration:

ELIGARD® 7.5 mg is packaged in a pouch that contains two smaller pouches (Figure 3), a needle cartridge and a desiccant pack (Figure 4). Syringe A pouch contains the sterile Syringe A pre-filled with the ATRIGEL® polymer system and a long white replacement plunger rod (Figure 5). Syringe B pouch contains the sterile Syringe B pre-filled with leuprolide acetate powder (Figure 6).

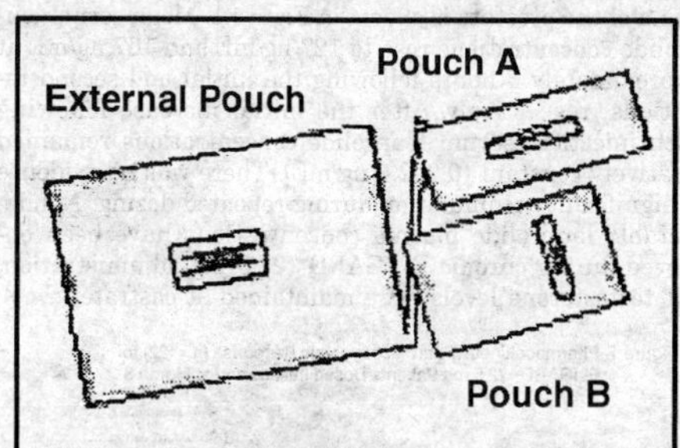

Figure 3

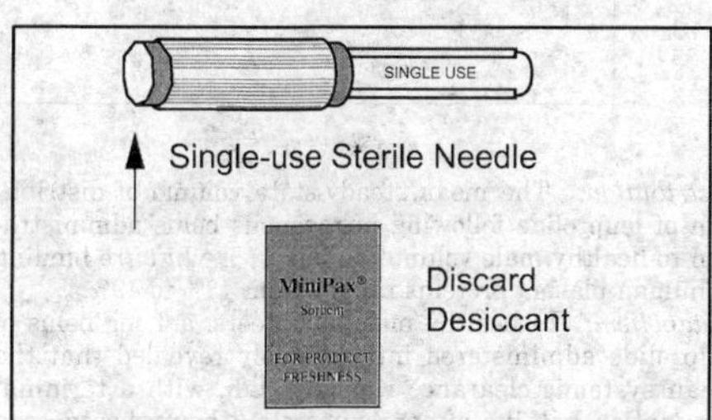

Figure 4

Syringe A Pouch

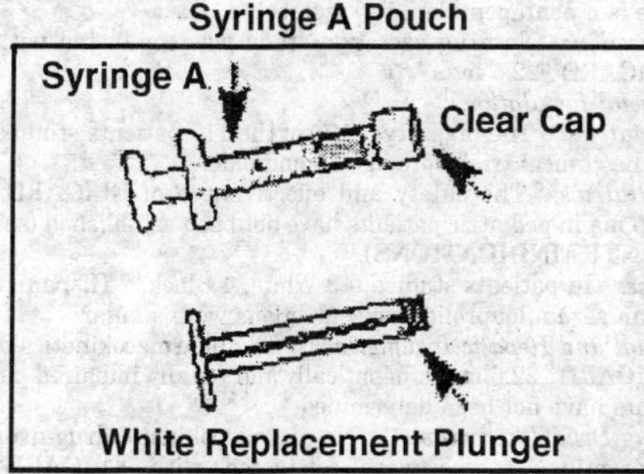

Figure 5

[See figure 6 at top of next column]

1. On a clean field, open all of the pouches and remove the contents. Discard the desiccant pack.

[See figure 7 at top of next column]
[See figure 8 in next column]

2. Pull out the blue-tipped short plunger rod and attached stopper from Syringe B and discard (Figure 7). Gently insert the long, white replacement plunger rod into the gray primary stopper remaining in Syringe B by twisting it in place (Figure 8).

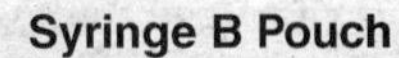

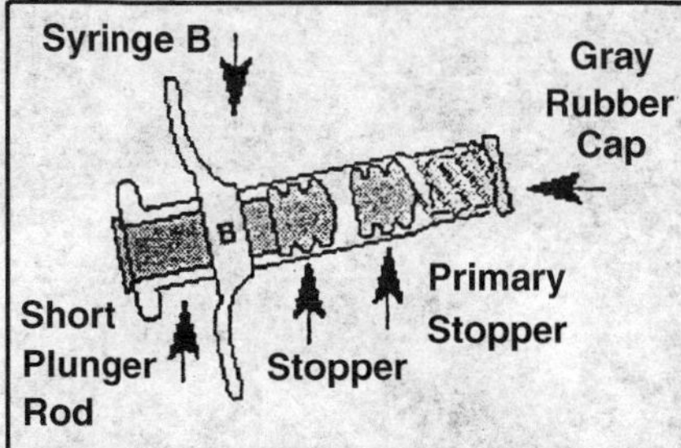

Figure 6

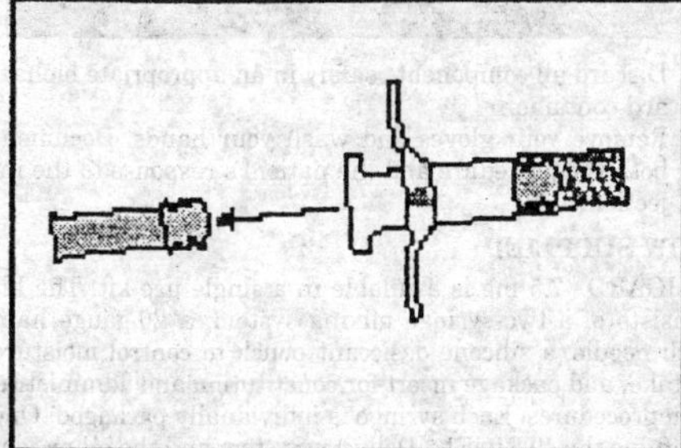

Figure 7

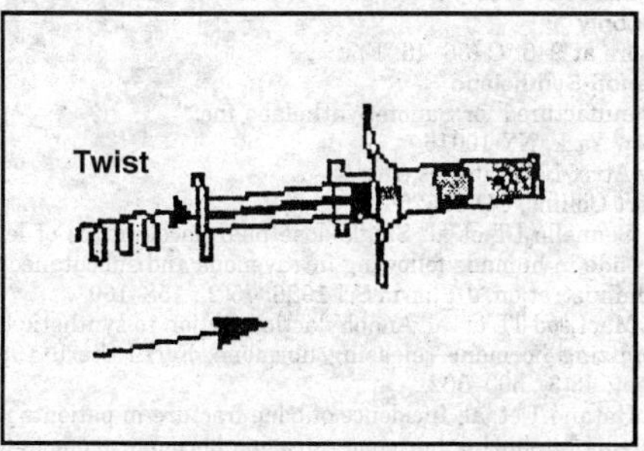

Figure 8

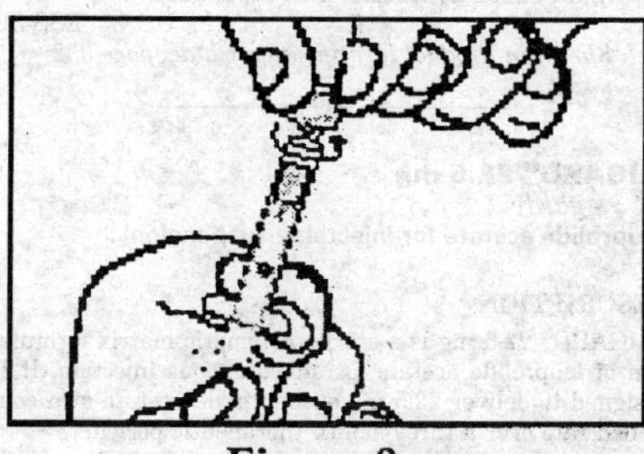

Figure 9

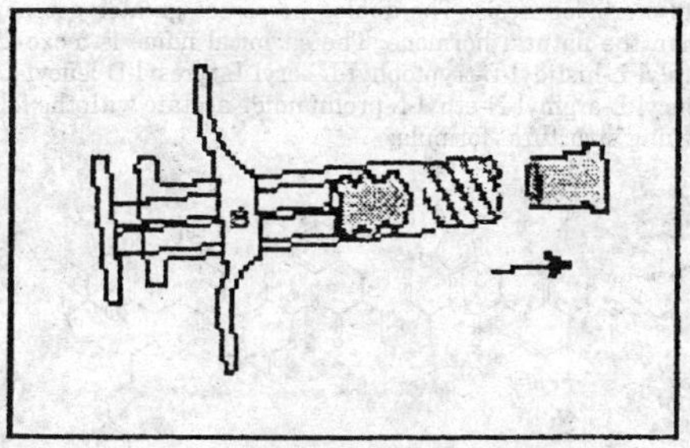

Figure 10

3. Unscrew the clear cap from Syringe A (Figure 9). Remove the gray rubber cap from Syringe B (Figure 10).

[See figure 11 at top of next column]

4. Join the two syringes together by pushing in and twisting until secure (Figure 11).

[See figure 12 at top of next column]

5. Inject the liquid contents of Syringe A into Syringe B containing the leuprolide acetate. Thoroughly mix the product by pushing the contents of both syringes back and forth between syringes (approximately 45 seconds) to obtain a uniform suspension (Figure 12). When thoroughly mixed, the suspension will appear a light tan to tan color. **Please note: Product must be mixed as described; shaking will not provide adequate mixing of the product.**

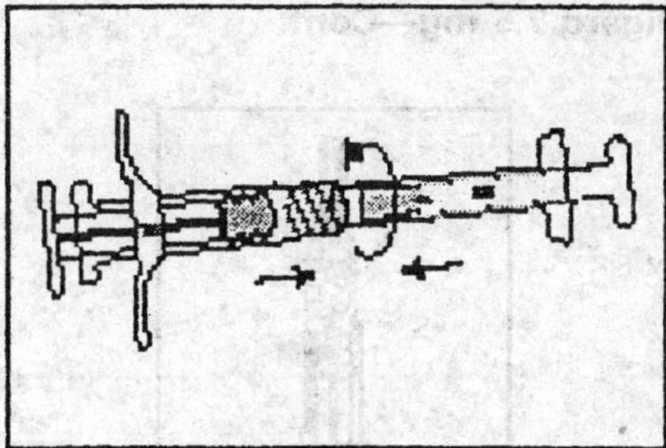

Figure 11

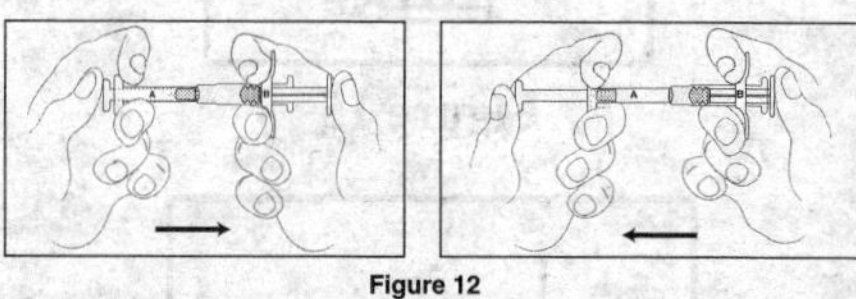

Figure 12

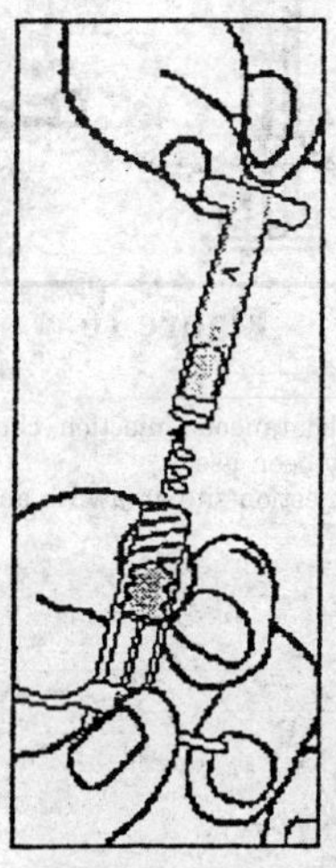

Figure 13

6. Hold the syringes vertically with Syringe B on the bottom. The syringes should remain securely coupled. Draw the entire mixed product into Syringe B (short, wide syringe) by depressing the Syringe A plunger and slightly withdrawing the Syringe B plunger. Uncouple Syringe A while continuing to push down on the Syringe A plunger (Figure 13). **Please note: Small air bubbles will remain in the formulation—this is acceptable.**

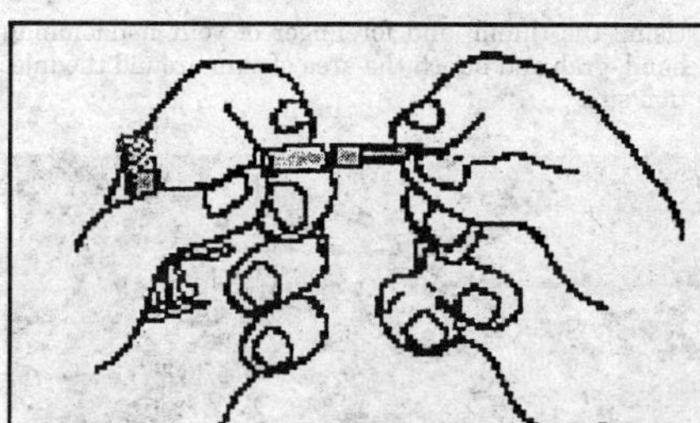

Figure 14

[See figure 15 at top of next column]
[See figure 16 at top of next column]

7. Hold Syringe B upright. Remove the pink cap on the bottom of the sterile needle cartridge by twisting it (Figure 14). Attach the needle cartridge to the end of Syringe B (Figure 15) by pushing in and turning the needle until it is firmly seated. Do not twist the needle onto the syringe until it is stripped. Pull off the clear needle cartridge cover prior to administration (Figure 16).
8. Choose an injection site on the abdomen, upper buttocks, or anywhere with adequate amounts of subcutaneous tissue that does not have excessive pigment, nodules, lesions, or hair. Since you can vary the injection

Continued on next page

This product information was prepared in September 2004. On these and other products of Sanofi-Synthelabo Inc., detailed information may be obtained on a current basis by direct inquiry to Product Information Services, 90 Park Avenue, New York, NY 10016 (toll free 1-800-446-6267).

Eligard 7.5 mg—Cont.

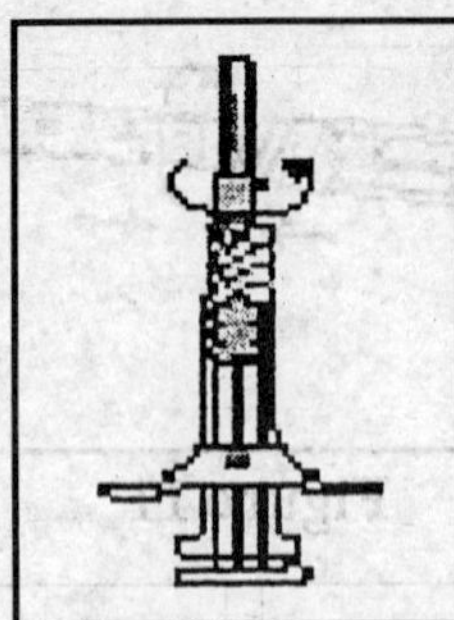

Figure 15

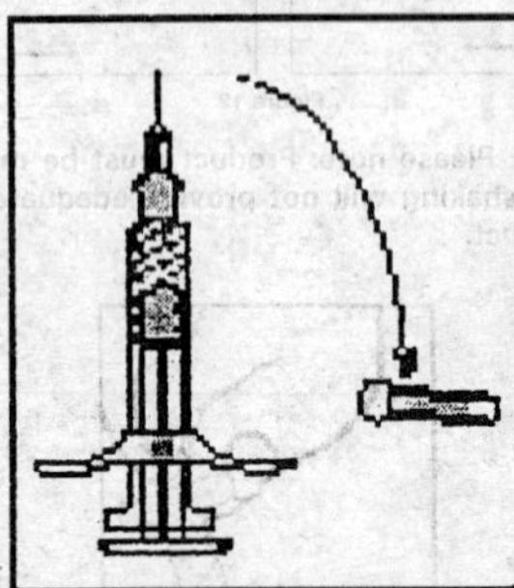

Figure 16

site with a subcutaneous injection, choose an area that hasn't recently been used.

9. Cleanse the injection-site area with an alcohol swab.[4]

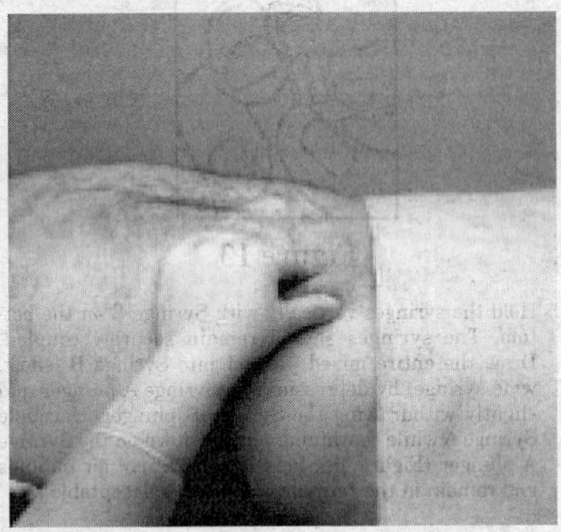

10. Using the thumb and forefinger of your nondominant hand, grab and bunch the area of skin around the injection site.[4]

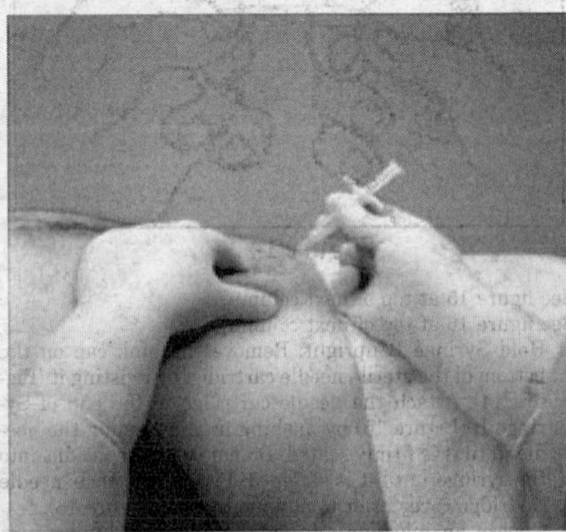

11. Using your dominant hand, insert the needle quickly. The approximate angle you use will depend on the amount and fullness of the subcutaneous tissue and the length of the needle. [4]

[See figure at top of next column]

12. After the needle is inserted, release the skin with your nondominant hand.[4]
13. Inject the drug using a slow, steady push. Press down on the plunger until the syringe is empty.[4]
14. Withdraw the needle quickly at the same angle used for insertion.[4]
15. Gently massage the injection area with a cotton ball or gauze pad.[4]

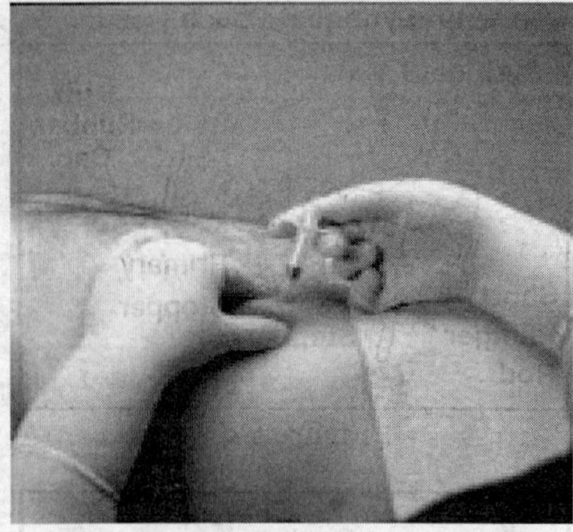

16. Discard all components safely in an appropriate biohazard container.
17. Remove your gloves and wash your hands. Document both the procedure and the patient's response to the injection.

HOW SUPPLIED

ELIGARD® 7.5 mg is available in a single use kit. The kit consists of a two-syringe mixing system, a 20-gauge half-inch needle, a silicone desiccant pouch to control moisture uptake, and package insert for constitution and administration procedures. Each syringe is individually packaged. One contains the ATRIGEL® Delivery System and the other contains leuprolide acetate. When constituted, ELIGARD® 7.5 mg is administered as a single dose.
(NDC 0024-0793-75)

Rx only

Store at 2–8 °C (36–46 °F)

Sanofi-Synthelabo

Manufactured for Sanofi-Synthelabo Inc.
New York, NY 10016
by Atrix Laboratories, Inc.
Fort Collins, CO 80525

1. Sennello LT et al. Single-dose pharmacokinetics of leuprolide in humans following intravenous and subcutaneous administration. J Pharm Sci 1986; 75(2): 158–160.
2. MacLeod TL et. al. Anaphylactic reaction to synthetic luteinizing hormone releasing hormone. Fertil Steril 1987 Sept; 48(3): 500–502.
3. Hatano T et. al. Incidence of bone fracture in patients receiving luteinizing hormone-releasing hormone agonists for prostate cancer. BJU International 2000 86: 449–452.
4. National Institutes of Health. Giving a subcutaneous injection. Bethesda, MD; 2002.

04295 Rev 5 7/03 Revised July 2003

ESS-3D

Shown in Product Identification Guide, page 332

ELIGARD® 22.5 mg ℞

[el' ə - gärd]

(leuprolide acetate for injectable suspension)

DESCRIPTION

ELIGARD® 22.5 mg is a sterile polymeric matrix formulation of leuprolide acetate for subcutaneous injection. It is designed to deliver 22.5 mg of leuprolide acetate at a controlled rate over a three-month therapeutic period.

Leuprolide acetate is a synthetic nonapeptide analog of naturally occurring gonadotropin releasing hormone (GnRH or LH-RH) that, when given continuously, inhibits pituitary gonadotropin secretion and suppresses testicular and ovarian steroidogenesis. The analog possesses greater potency than the natural hormone. The chemical name is 5-oxo-L-prolyl-L-histidyl-L-tryptophyl-L-seryl-L-tyrosyl-D-leucyl-L-leucyl-L-arginyl-N-ethyl-L-prolinamide acetate with the following structural formula:

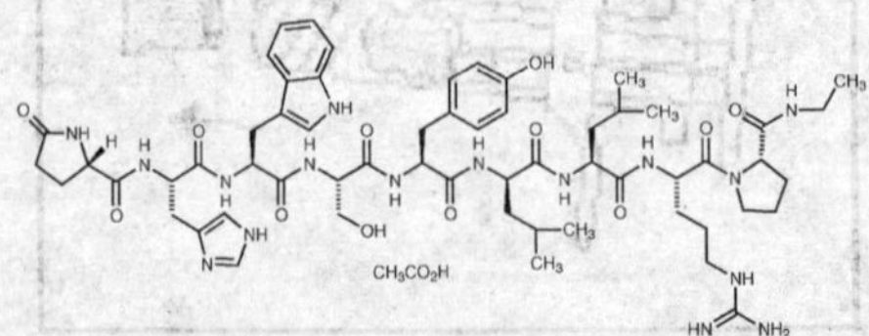

ELIGARD® 22.5 mg is prefilled and supplied in two separate, sterile syringes whose contents are mixed immediately prior to administration. The two syringes are joined and the single dose product is mixed until it is homogenous. ELIGARD® 22.5 mg is administered once every three months subcutaneously where it forms a solid drug delivery depot.

One syringe contains the ATRIGEL® Delivery System, and the other contains leuprolide acetate. ATRIGEL® is a polymeric (non-gelatin containing) delivery system consisting of a biodegradable, poly (DL-lactide-co-glycolide) (PLG) polymer formulation dissolved in a biocompatible solvent, *N*-methyl-2-pyrrolidone (NMP). PLG is a co-polymer with a 75:25 molar ratio of DL-lactide to glycolide with hexanediol. The second syringe contains leuprolide acetate and the constituted product is designed to deliver 22.5 mg of leuprolide acetate at the time of subcutaneous injection.

ELIGARD® 22.5 mg delivers 22.5 mg of leuprolide acetate (equivalent to approximately 21 mg leuprolide free base) dissolved in 193.9 mg *N*-methyl-2-pyrrolidone and 158.6 mg poly (DL-lactide-co-glycolide). The approximate weight of the administered formulation is 375 mg.

CLINICAL PHARMACOLOGY

Leuprolide acetate, an LH-RH agonist, acts as a potent inhibitor of gonadotropin secretion when given continuously in therapeutic doses. Animal and human studies indicate that after an initial stimulation, chronic administration of leuprolide acetate results in suppression of testicular and ovarian steroidogenesis. This effect is reversible upon discontinuation of drug therapy.

In humans, administration of leuprolide acetate results in an initial increase in circulating levels of luteinizing hormone (LH) and follicle stimulating hormone (FSH), leading to a transient increase in the levels of gonadal steroids (testosterone and dihydrotestosterone in males, and estrone and estradiol in premenopausal females). However, continuous administration of leuprolide acetate results in decreased levels of LH and FSH. In males, testosterone is reduced to below castrate threshold (≤ 50 ng/dL). These decreases occur within two to four weeks after initiation of treatment. Long-term studies have shown that continuation of therapy with leuprolide acetate maintains testosterone below the castrate level for up to seven years.

PHARMACODYNAMICS

Following the first dose of ELIGARD® 22.5 mg, mean serum testosterone concentrations transiently increased, then fell to below castrate threshold (≤ 50 ng/dL) within three weeks (Figure 1). Continued treatment maintained castrate testosterone suppression throughout the study. No breakthrough of testosterone concentrations above castrate threshold (> 50 ng/dL) occurred at any time during the study once castrate suppression was achieved in a subset of 22 patients.

Leuprolide acetate is not active when given orally.

PHARMACOKINETICS

Absorption: The pharmacokinetics/pharmacodynamics observed during two injections every three months (ELIGARD® 22.5 mg) in 22 patients with advanced carcinoma of the prostate is shown in Figure 1. Mean serum leuprolide concentrations rose to 127 ng/mL and 107 ng/mL at approximately 5 hours following the initial and second injections, respectively. After the initial increase following each injection, serum leuprolide concentrations remained relatively constant (0.2–2.0 ng/mL). There was no evidence of significant accumulation during repeated dosing. Nondetectable leuprolide plasma concentrations have been observed during chronic ELIGARD® 22.5 mg administration, but testosterone levels were maintained at castrate levels.

Figure 1. Pharmacokinetic/Pharmacodynamic Response (n = 22) to ELIGARD® 22.5 mg Patients Dosed Initially and at Month 3

Testosterone (ng/dL)
Leuprolide (ng/mL)
≤ 50 ng/dL = clinical castration
Serum Concentration (mean, SEM)
Study Month

Distribution: The mean steady-state volume of distribution of leuprolide following intravenous bolus administration to healthy male volunteers was 27 L.[1] *In vitro* binding to human plasma proteins ranged from 43% to 49%.

Metabolism: In healthy male volunteers, a 1 mg bolus of leuprolide administered intravenously revealed that the mean systemic clearance was 8.34 L/h, with a terminal elimination half-life of approximately 3 hours based on a two compartment model.[1]

No drug metabolism study was conducted with ELIGARD® 22.5 mg. Upon administration with different leuprolide acetate formulations, the major metabolite of leuprolide acetate is a pentapeptide (M-1) metabolite.

Excretion: No drug excretion study was conducted with ELIGARD® 22.5 mg.

Special Populations:

Geriatrics: The majority (71%) of the 117 patients studied in the clinical trial were age 70 and older.

Pediatrics: The safety and effectiveness of ELIGARD® 22.5 mg in pediatric patients have not been established (see **CONTRAINDICATIONS**).

Race: In patients studied (19 White, 4 Black, 2 Hispanic), mean serum leuprolide concentrations were similar.

Renal and Hepatic Insufficiency: The pharmacokinetics of ELIGARD® 22.5 mg in hepatically and renally impaired patients have not been determined.

Drug-Drug Interactions: No pharmacokinetic drug-drug interaction studies were conducted with ELIGARD® 22.5 mg.

CLINICAL STUDIES

In one open-label, multicenter study (AGL9909), 117 patients with advanced prostate cancer were treated with at least a single injection of study drug. Of these, 113 patients received a total of two injections of ELIGARD® 22.5 mg, given once every three months. Two patients had stage A disease, 19 patients had stage B, 60 patients had stage C, and 36 patients had stage D. This study evaluated the achievement and maintenance of castrate serum testoster-

one suppression over six months of therapy. A total of 111 patients completed the study.
The mean testosterone concentration increased from 367.1 ng/dL at Baseline to 588.0 ng/dL at Day 2 following the initial subcutaneous injection. The mean serum testosterone concentration then decreased to below Baseline by Day 14 and was 27.7 ng/dL on Day 21. At the conclusion of the study (Month 6), mean testosterone concentration was 10.1 ng/dL (Figure 2).
Of the original 117 patients, one received less than a full dose of ELIGARD® 22.5 mg at Baseline, never suppressed, and was withdrawn at Day 73 and given an alternate treatment. In the remaining 116 patients who did receive the full dose at Baseline, serum testosterone was suppressed to below the castrate threshold (≤ 50 ng/dL) by Day 28 (Week 4) in 115 of 116 patients (99%). By Day 35, all 116 patients (100%) who received a full dose at Baseline attained the castrate threshold. Once testosterone suppression at or below serum concentrations of 50 ng/dL was achieved, only one patient (< 1%) demonstrated breakthrough (concentrations above 50 ng/dL) following the initial injection; that patient remained below the castrate threshold following the second injection. All 111 evaluable patients in the study at Month 6 had testosterone concentrations of ≤ 50 ng/dL.
All non-evaluable patients who attained castration by Day 28 maintained castration at each timepoint up to and including the time of withdrawal.

Figure 2. ELIGARD® 22.5 mg Mean Serum Testosterone Concentrations (n = 111)

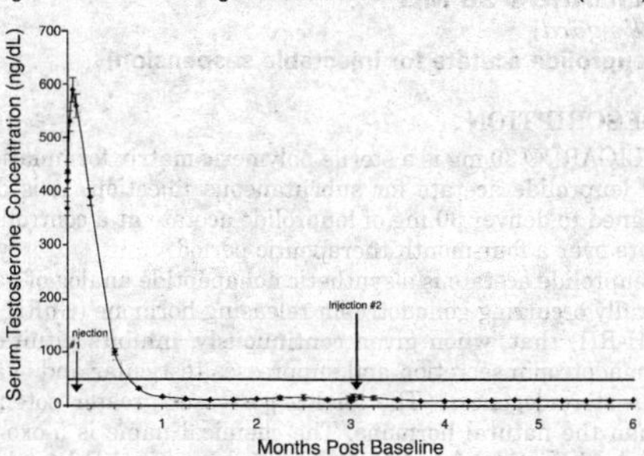

Serum PSA decreased in all patients whose Baseline values were elevated above the normal limit. Mean values were reduced 98% from Baseline to Month 6. At Month 6, PSA levels had decreased to within normal limits in 91% of patients who presented with elevated levels at Baseline.
Other secondary efficacy endpoints evaluated included WHO performance status, bone pain, urinary pain, and urinary signs and symptoms. At Baseline, 94% of patients were classified as "fully active" by the WHO performance status scale (Status=0) and 6% as "restricted in strenuous activity but ambulatory and able to carry out work of a light or sedentary nature" (Status=1). At Month 6, these percentages were changed to 96% (Status=0) and 4% (Status=1). At Baseline, patients experienced little bone pain, with a mean score of 1.20 (range 1-9) on a scale of 1 (no pain) to 10 (worst pain possible). At Month 6, the mean bone pain score was essentially unchanged at 1.22 (range 1-5). Urinary pain, scored on the same scale, was similarly low, with a mean of 1.02 at Baseline (range 1-2) and 1.10 at Month 6 (range 1-8). Urinary signs and symptoms demonstrated a mean score of 1.09 at Baseline (range 1-4) and increased to 1.18 at Month 6 (range 1-7). In addition, there was a reduction in patients with prostate abnormalities detected during physical exam from 96 (82%) at Screening to 76 (65%) at Month 6.

INDICATIONS AND USAGE

ELIGARD® 22.5 mg is indicated for the palliative treatment of advanced prostate cancer.

CONTRAINDICATIONS

1. ELIGARD® 22.5 mg is contraindicated in patients with hypersensitivity to GnRH, GnRH agonist analogs or any of the components of ELIGARD® 22.5 mg. Anaphylactic reactions to synthetic GnRH or GnRH agonist analogs have been reported in the literature.[2]
2. ELIGARD® 22.5 mg is contraindicated in women and in pediatric patients and was not studied in women or children. Moreover, leuprolide acetate can cause fetal harm when administered to a pregnant woman. Major fetal abnormalities were observed in rabbits but not in rats after administration of leuprolide acetate throughout gestation. There were increased fetal mortality and decreased fetal weights in rats and rabbits. The effects on fetal mortality are expected consequences of the alterations in hormonal levels brought about by this drug. The possibility exists that spontaneous abortion may occur.

WARNINGS

ELIGARD® 22.5 mg, like other LH-RH agonists, causes a transient increase in serum concentrations of testosterone during the first week of treatment. Patients may experience worsening of symptoms or onset of new signs and symptoms during the first few weeks of treatment, including bone pain, neuropathy, hematuria, or bladder outlet obstruction. Isolated cases of ureteral obstruction and/or spinal cord compression, which may contribute to paralysis with or without fatal complications, have been observed in the palliative treatment of advanced prostate cancer using LH-RH agonists (see **PRECAUTIONS**).

Table 1: Incidence (%) of Possibly or Probably Related Systemic Adverse Events Reported by ≥ 2% of Patients (n = 117) Treated with ELIGARD® 22.5 mg for up to Six Months; Study AGL9909

Body System	Adverse Event	Number	Percent
Vascular Disorders	Hot flashes/sweats*	66	56.4%
Body as a Whole	Fatigue	7	6.0%
Genitourinary	Urinary frequency	3	2.6%
Gastrointestinal	Nausea	4	3.4%
Skin and Subcutaneous Tissue	Pruritis	3	2.6%
Musculoskeletal	Arthralgia	4	3.4%

If spinal cord compression or renal impairment develops, standard treatment of these complications should be instituted.

PRECAUTIONS

General: Patients with metastatic vertebral lesions and/or with urinary tract obstruction should be closely observed during the first few weeks of therapy (see **WARNINGS** section).
Laboratory tests: Response to ELIGARD® 22.5 mg should be monitored by measuring serum concentrations of testosterone and prostate specific antigen periodically.
In the majority of patients, testosterone levels increased above Baseline during the first week, declining thereafter to Baseline levels or below by the end of the second week. Castrate levels were generally reached within two to four weeks and once achieved were maintained for the duration of treatment.
Results of testosterone determinations are dependent on assay methodology. It is advisable to be aware of the type and precision of the assay methodology to make appropriate clinical and therapeutic decisions.
Drug Interactions: See **PHARMACOKINETICS**
Drug/Laboratory Test Interactions: Therapy with leuprolide acetate results in suppression of the pituitary-gonadal system. Results of diagnostic tests of pituitary gonadotropic and gonadal functions conducted during and after leuprolide therapy may be affected.
Carcinogenesis, Mutagenesis, Impairment of Fertility: Two-year carcinogenicity studies were conducted with leuprolide acetate in rats and mice. In rats, a dose-related increase of benign pituitary hyperplasia and benign pituitary adenomas was noted at 24 months when the drug was administered subcutaneously at high daily doses (0.6 to 4 mg/kg). There was a significant but not dose-related increase of pancreatic islet-cell adenomas in females and of testicular interstitial cell adenomas in males (highest incidence in the low dose group). In mice, no leuprolide acetate-induced tumors or pituitary abnormalities were observed at a dose as high as 60 mg/kg for two years. Patients have been treated with leuprolide acetate for up to three years with doses as high as 10 mg/day and for two years with doses as high as 20 mg/day without demonstrable pituitary abnormalities. No carcinogenicity studies have been conducted with ELIGARD® 22.5 mg.
Mutagenicity studies were performed with leuprolide acetate using bacterial and mammalian systems and with ELIGARD® 7.5 mg in bacterial systems. These studies provided no evidence of a mutagenic potential.
Pregnancy, Teratogenic Effects: Pregnancy category X (see **CONTRAINDICATIONS**).
Pediatric Use: ELIGARD® 22.5 mg is contraindicated in pediatric patients and was not studied in children (see **CONTRAINDICATIONS**).

ADVERSE REACTIONS

The safety of ELIGARD® 22.5 mg was evaluated in 117 patients with advanced prostate cancer. ELIGARD® 22.5 mg, like other LH-RH analogs, caused a transient increase in serum testosterone concentrations during the first two weeks of treatment. Therefore, potential exacerbations of signs and symptoms of the disease during the first weeks of treatment are of concern in patients with vertebral metastases and/or urinary obstruction or hematuria. If these conditions are aggravated, it may lead to neurological problems such as weakness and/or paresthesia of the lower limbs or worsening of urinary symptoms (see **WARNINGS** and **PRECAUTIONS**).
In Study AGL9909, 117 patients were dosed with ELIGARD® 22.5 mg every three months for up to six months and injection sites were closely monitored. In all, 230 injections of ELIGARD® 22.5 mg were administered. Transient burning/stinging was reported following 50 injections (21.7%), with the majority (86%) of these events reported as mild. Pain was reported following 3.5% of study injections (6.0% of patients) and was generally reported as brief in duration and mild in intensity.
Erythema was reported following 2 injections (0.9% of study injections, 1.7% of patients). One of the reports characterized the erythema as mild and resolved within 7 days. The other was moderate and resolved within 15 days. Neither patient experienced erythema at multiple injections. Mild bruising was reported following 4 injections (1.7% of study injections, 3.4% of patients). Mild pruritis was reported following 1 injection (0.4% of study injections, 0.9% of patients).
These localized adverse events were nonrecurrent over time. No patient discontinued therapy due to an injection site adverse event.
The following possibly or probably related systemic adverse events occurred during clinical trials of up to six months of treatment with ELIGARD® 22.5 mg, and were reported in ≥2% of patients (Table 1). Often, causality is difficult to assess in patients with metastatic prostate cancer. Reactions considered not drug-related are excluded.
[See table 1 above]
In addition, the following possibly or probably related systemic adverse events were reported by < 2% of the patients using ELIGARD® 22.5 mg in the clinical study.
Gastrointestinal: Dyspepsia
General: Rigors, weakness, lethargy
Renal: Difficulties with urination, pain on urination, scanty urination, bladder spasm, blood in urine and urinary retention
Reproductive: Breast tenderness*, testicular atrophy*, testicular pain, gynecomastia*, impotence*
Skin: Clamminess, night sweats*, sweating increased*
Vascular: Hypertension, hypotension

* Expected pharmacological consequence of testosterone suppression. In the patient population studied, a total of 84 hot flash/sweats events were reported in 66 patients. Of these, 73 events (87%) were described as mild; 11 (13%) as moderate; none were severe.

Changes in Bone Density: Decreased bone density has been reported in the medical literature in men who have had orchiectomy or who have been treated with an LH-RH agonist analog.[3] It can be anticipated that long periods of medical castration in men will have effects on bone density.

OVERDOSAGE

In clinical trials using daily subcutaneous injections of leuprolide acetate in patients with prostate cancer, doses as high as 20 mg/day for up to two years caused no adverse effects differing from those observed with the 1 mg/day dose.

DOSAGE AND ADMINISTRATION

The recommended dose of ELIGARD® 22.5 mg is one injection every three months. The injection delivers 22.5 mg of leuprolide acetate, incorporated in a polymer formulation. It is administered subcutaneously and provides continuous release of leuprolide for three months.
Once mixed, ELIGARD® 22.5 mg should be discarded if not administered within 30 minutes.
As with other drugs administered by subcutaneous injection, the injection site should vary periodically. The specific injection location chosen should be an area with sufficient soft or loose subcutaneous tissue. In clinical trials, the injection was administered in the upper- or mid-abdominal area. Avoid areas with brawny or fibrous subcutaneous tissue or locations that could be rubbed or compressed (i.e., with a belt or clothing waistband).

Mixing and Administration Procedure

IMPORTANT:
Allow the product to reach room temperature before using.
Once mixed, the product must be administered within 30 minutes.
Follow the instructions as directed to ensure proper preparation of ELIGARD® 22.5 mg prior to administration:
ELIGARD® 22.5 mg is packaged in a pouch that contains two smaller pouches (Figure 3), a needle cartridge and a desiccant pack (Figure 4). Syringe A pouch contains the sterile Syringe A pre-filled with the ATRIGEL® polymer system and a long white replacement plunger rod (Figure 5). Syringe B pouch contains the sterile Syringe B pre-filled with leuprolide acetate powder (Figure 6).

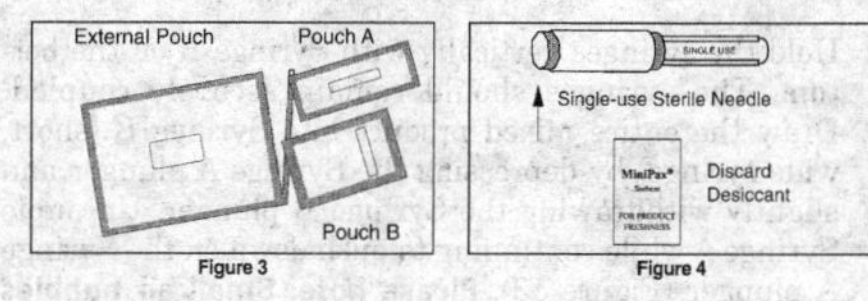

Figure 3 Figure 4

Continued on next page

This product information was prepared in September 2004. On these and other products of Sanofi-Synthelabo Inc., detailed information may be obtained on a current basis by direct inquiry to Product Information Services, 90 Park Avenue, New York, NY 10016 (toll free 1-800-446-6267).

Eligard 22.5 mg—Cont.

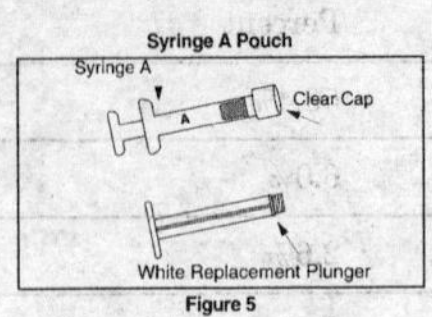

Figure 5

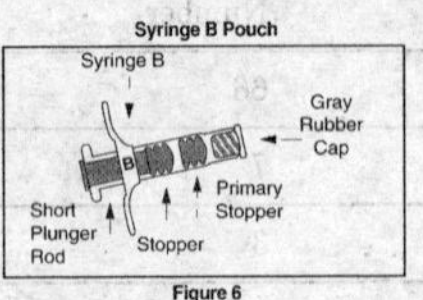

Figure 6

1. On a clean field, open all of the pouches and remove the contents. Discard the desiccant pack.

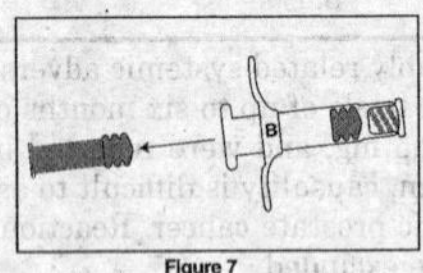
Figure 7

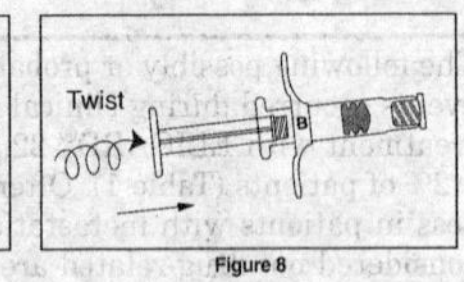

Figure 8

2. Pull out the blue-tipped short plunger rod and attached stopper from Syringe B and discard (Figure 7). Gently insert the long, white replacement plunger rod into the gray primary stopper remaining in Syringe B by twisting it in place (Figure 8).

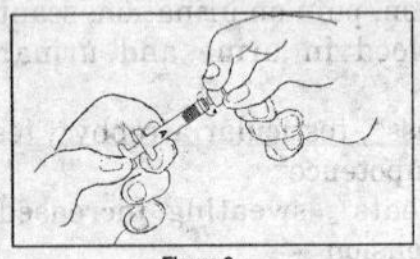
Figure 9

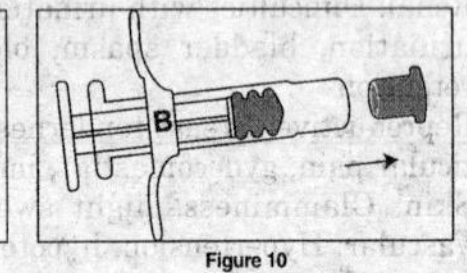
Figure 10

3. Unscrew the clear cap from Syringe A (Figure 9). Remove the gray rubber cap from Syringe B (Figure 10).

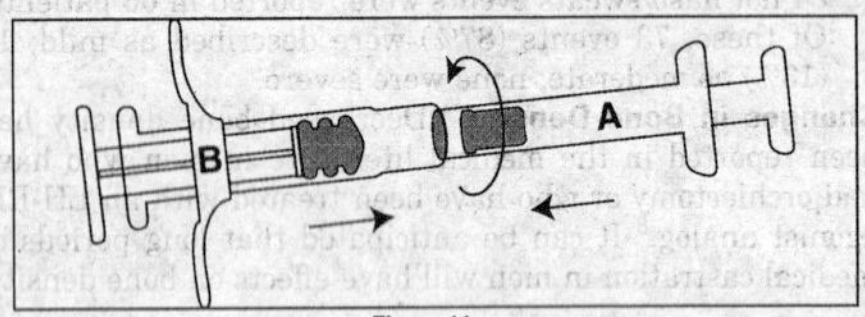
Figure 11

4. Join the two syringes together by pushing in and twisting until secure (Figure 11).

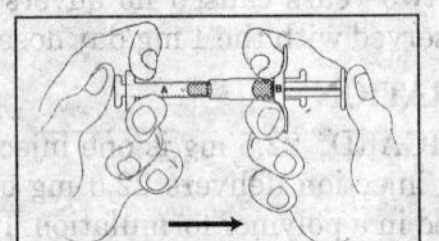

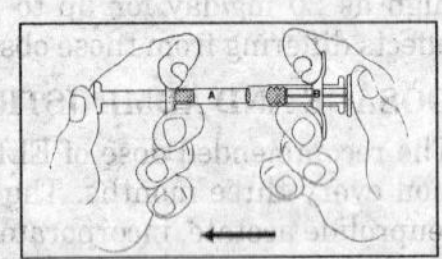
Figure 12

5. Inject the liquid contents of Syringe A into Syringe B containing the leuprolide acetate. Thoroughly mix the product by pushing the contents of both syringes back and forth between syringes (approximately 45 seconds) to obtain a uniform suspension (Figure 12). When thoroughly mixed, the suspension will appear colorless to pale yellow in color. **Please note: Product must be mixed as described; shaking will not provide adequate mixing of the product.**

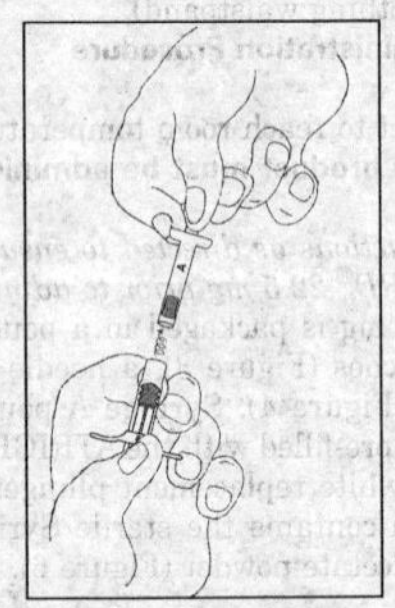
Figure 13

6. Hold the syringes vertically with Syringe B on the bottom. The syringes should remain securely coupled. Draw the entire mixed product into Syringe B (short, wide syringe) by depressing the Syringe A plunger and slightly withdrawing the Syringe B plunger. Uncouple Syringe A while continuing to push down on the Syringe A plunger (Figure 13). **Please note: Small air bubbles will remain in the formulation – this is acceptable.**

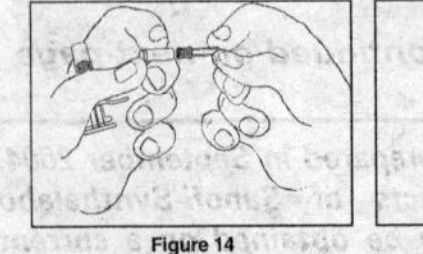
Figure 14

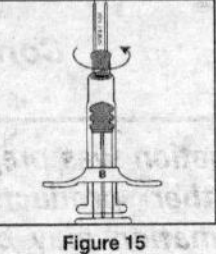
Figure 15

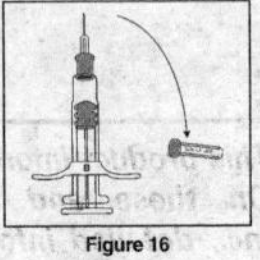
Figure 16

7. Hold Syringe B upright. Remove the pink cap on the bottom of the sterile needle cartridge by twisting it (Figure 14). Attach the needle cartridge to the end of Syringe B (Figure 15) by pushing in and turning the needle until it is firmly seated. Do not twist the needle onto the syringe until it is stripped. Pull off the clear needle cartridge cover prior to administration (Figure 16).
8. Choose an injection site on the abdomen, upper buttocks, or anywhere with adequate amounts of subcutaneous tissue that does not have excessive pigment, nodules, lesions, or hair. Since you can vary the injection site with a subcutaneous injection, choose an area that hasn't recently been used.
9. Cleanse the injection-site area with an alcohol swab.[4]

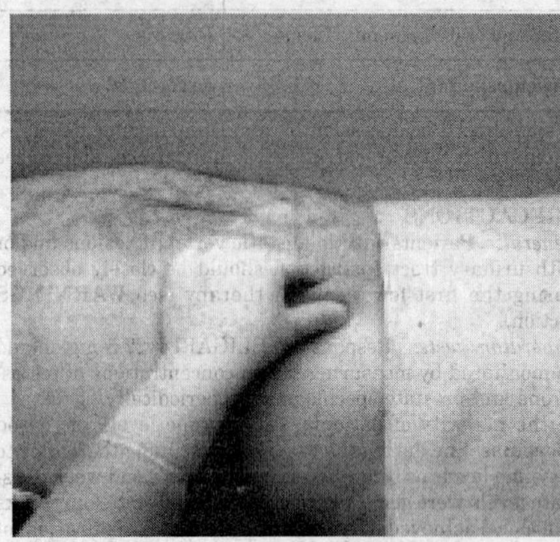

10. Using the thumb and forefinger of your nondominant hand, grab and bunch the area of skin around the injection site.[4]

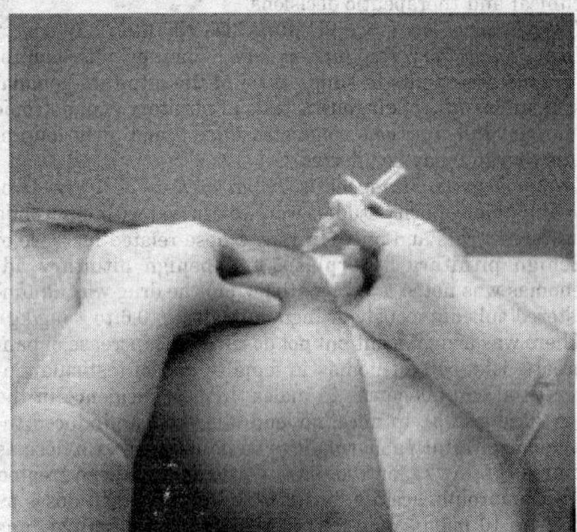

11. Using your dominant hand, insert the needle quickly. The approximate angle you use will depend on the amount and fullness of the subcutaneous tissue and the length of the needle.[4]

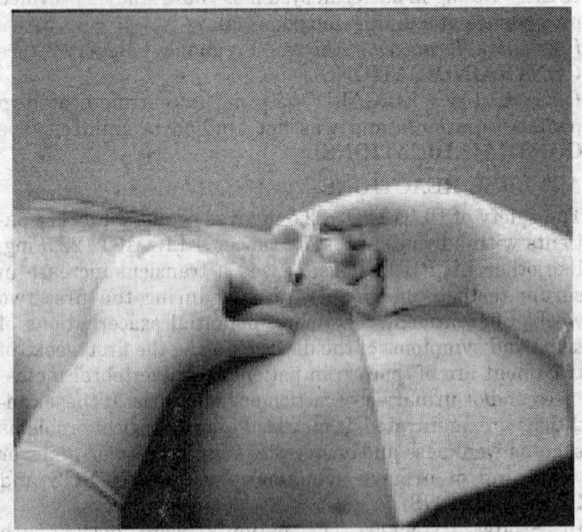

12. After the needle is inserted, release the skin with your nondominant hand.[4]
13. Inject the drug using a slow, steady push. Press down on the plunger until the syringe is empty.[4]
14. Withdraw the needle quickly at the same angle used for insertion.[4]
15. Gently massage the injection area with a cotton ball or gauze pad.[4]
16. Discard all componennts safely in an appropriate biohazard container.
17. Remove your gloves and wash your hands. Document both the procedure and the patient's response to the injection.

HOW SUPPLIED

ELIGARD® 22.5 mg is available in a single use kit. The kit consists of a two-syringe mixing system, a 20-gauge half-inch needle, a silicone desiccant pouch to control moisture uptake, and a package insert for constitution and administration procedures. Each syringe is individually packaged. One contains the ATRIGEL® Delivery System and the other contains leuprolide acetate. When constituted, ELIGARD® 22.5 mg is administered as a single dose.
(NDC 0024-0222-05)
Rx only
Store at 2-8 °C (35.6–46.4 °F)
sanofi-synthelabo
Manufactured for Sanofi-Synthelabo Inc.
New York, NY 10016
by Atrix Laboratories, Inc.
Fort Collins, CO 80525

1. Sennello LT et al. Single-dose pharmacokinetics of leuprolide in humans following intravenous and subcutaneous administration. J Pharm Sci 1986; 75(2): 158-160.
2. MacLeod TL et al. Anaphylactic reaction to synthetic luteinizing hormone releasing hormone. Fertil Steril 1987 Sept; 48(3): 500-502.
3. Hatano T et al. Incidence of bone fracture in patients receiving luteinizing hormone-releasing hormone agonists for prostate cancer. BJU International 2000 86: 449-452.
4. National Institutes of Health. Giving a subcutaneous injection, Bethesda, MD; 2002.

04109 Rev 5 8/04 Revised August 2004
ESS-6E

Shown in Product Identification Guide, page 332

ELIGARD® 30 MG ℞

[*el' ə-gärd*]
(leuprolide acetate for injectable suspension)

DESCRIPTION

ELIGARD® 30 mg is a sterile polymeric matrix formulation of leuprolide acetate for subcutaneous injection. It is designed to deliver 30 mg of leuprolide acetate at a controlled rate over a four-month therapeutic period.

Leuprolide acetate is a synthetic nonapeptide analog of naturally occurring gonadotropin releasing hormone (GnRH or LH-RH) that, when given continuously, inhibits pituitary gonadotropin secretion and suppresses testicular and ovarian steroidogenesis. The analog possesses greater potency than the natural hormone. The chemical name is 5-oxo-L-prolyl-L-histidyl-L-tryptophyl-L-seryl-L-tyrosyl-D-leucyl-L-leucyl-L-arginyl-N-ethyl-L-prolinamide acetate (salt) with the following structural formula:

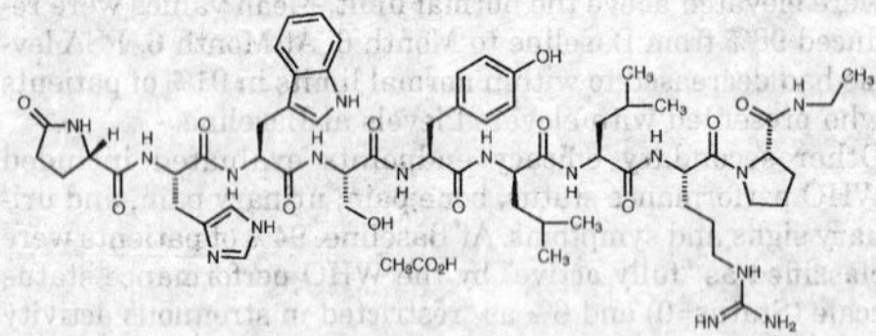

ELIGARD® 30 mg is prefilled and supplied in two separate, sterile syringes whose contents are mixed immediately prior to administration. The two syringes are joined and the single dose product is mixed until it is homogenous. ELIGARD® 30 mg is administered once every four months subcutaneously, where it forms a solid drug delivery depot. One syringe contains the ATRIGEL® Delivery System and the other contains leuprolide acetate. ATRIGEL® is a polymeric (non-gelatin containing) delivery system consisting of a biodegradable poly(DL-lactide-co-glycolide) (PLG) polymer formulation dissolved in a biocompatible solvent, *N*-methyl-2-pyrrolidone (NMP). PLG is a co-polymer with a 75:25 molar ratio of DL-lactide to glycolide with hexanediol. The second syringe contains leuprolide acetate and the constituted product is designed to deliver 30 mg of leuprolide acetate at the time of subcutaneous injection.

ELIGARD® 30 mg delivers 30 mg of leuprolide acetate (equivalent to approximately 28 mg leuprolide free base) dissolved in 258.5 mg *N*-methyl-2-pyrrolidone and 211.5 mg poly(DL-lactide-co-glycolide). The approximate weight of the administered formulation is 500 mg.

CLINICAL PHARMACOLOGY

Leuprolide acetate, an LH-RH agonist, acts as a potent inhibitor of gonadotropin secretion when given continuously in therapeutic doses. Animal and human studies indicate that after an initial stimulation, chronic administration of leuprolide acetate results in suppression of testicular and ovarian steroidogenesis. This effect is reversible upon discontinuation of drug therapy.

In humans, administration of leuprolide acetate results in an initial increase in circulating levels of luteinizing hormone (LH) and follicle stimulating hormone (FSH), leading to a transient increase in levels of the gonadal steroids (testosterone and dihydrotestosterone in males, and estrone and estradiol in premenopausal females). However, continuous administration of leuprolide acetate results in decreased levels of LH and FSH. In males, testosterone is reduced to below castrate threshold (≤ 50 ng/dL). These decreases occur within two to four weeks after initiation of treatment. Long-term studies have shown that continuation of therapy with leuprolide acetate maintains testosterone below the castrate level for up to seven years.

PHARMACODYNAMICS

Following the first dose of ELIGARD® 30 mg, mean serum testosterone concentrations transiently increased, then fell to below castrate threshold (≤ 50 ng/dL) within three weeks (Figure 1). One patient withdrew from the study at Day 14.

Of the 89 patients remaining in the study, 85 (96%) had serum testosterone below the castrate threshold by Month 1 (Day 28). By Day 42, 89 (100%) of patients attained castrate testosterone suppression. Once castrate testosterone suppression was achieved, 3 patients (3%) demonstrated breakthrough (concentrations above 50 ng/dL after achieving castrate levels).

Leuprolide acetate is not active when given orally.

PHARMACOKINETICS

Absorption: The pharmacokinetics/pharmacodynamics observed during injections administered initially and at four months (ELIGARD® 30 mg) in 24 patients with advanced carcinoma of the prostate is shown in Figure 1. Mean serum leuprolide concentrations following the initial injection rose rapidly to 150 ng/mL (C_{max}) at approximately 3.3 hours after injection. After the initial increase following each injection, mean serum concentrations remained relatively constant (0.1–1.0 ng/mL). There was no evidence of significant accumulation during repeated dosing. Nondetectable leuprolide plasma concentrations have been occasionally observed during ELIGARD® 30 mg administration, but testosterone levels were maintained at castrate levels.

Figure 1. Pharmacokinetic/Pharmacodynamic Response (N = 24) to ELIGARD® 30 mg-Patients dosed initially and at Month 4

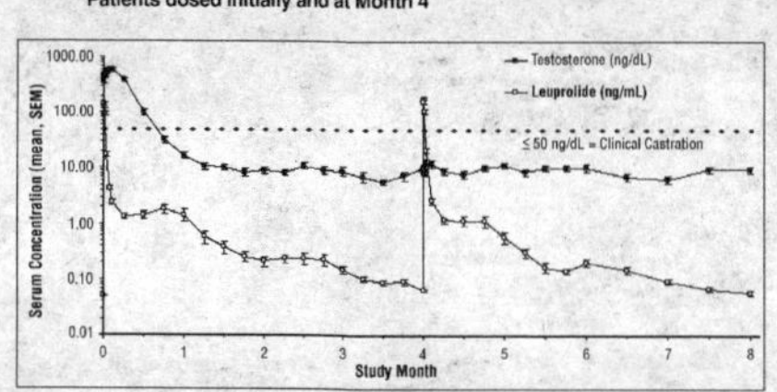

Distribution: The mean steady-state volume of distribution of leuprolide following intravenous bolus administration to healthy male volunteers was 27 L.[1] *In vitro* binding to human plasma proteins ranged from 43% to 49%.

Metabolism: In healthy male volunteers, a 1 mg bolus of leuprolide administered intravenously revealed that the mean systemic clearance was 8.34 L/h, with a terminal elimination half-life of approximately 3 hours based on a two compartment model.[1]

No drug metabolism study was conducted with ELIGARD® 30 mg. Upon administration with different leuprolide acetate formulations, the major metabolite of leuprolide acetate is a pentapeptide (M-1) metabolite.

Excretion: No drug excretion study was conducted with ELIGARD® 30 mg.

Special Populations:

Geriatrics: The majority (71%) of the 90 patients studied in the clinical trial were age 70 and older.

Pediatrics: The safety and effectiveness of ELIGARD® 30 mg in pediatric patients have not been established (see **CONTRAINDICATIONS**).

Race: In patients studied (18 White, 4 Black, 2 Hispanic), mean serum leuprolide concentrations were similar.

Renal and Hepatic Insufficiency: The pharmacokinetics of ELIGARD® 30 mg in hepatically and renally impaired patients have not been determined.

Drug-Drug Interactions: No pharmacokinetic drug-drug interaction studies were conducted with ELIGARD® 30 mg.

CLINICAL STUDIES

In one open-label, multicenter study (AGL0001), 90 patients with prostate cancer were treated with at least a single injection of study drug. Of these, 85 patients received a total of two injections of ELIGARD® 30 mg given once every four months. Two patients had Jewett stage A disease, 38 had stage B disease, 16 had stage C disease and 34 patients had stage D disease. This study evaluated the achievement and maintenance of castrate serum testosterone suppression over eight months of therapy. A total of 82 patients completed the study.

The mean testosterone concentration increased from 385.5 ng/dL at Baseline to 610.0 ng/dL at Day 2 following the initial subcutaneous injection. The mean serum testosterone concentration then decreased to below Baseline by Day 14 and was 17.2 ng/dL on Day 28. At the conclusion of the study (Month 8), mean testosterone concentration was 12.4 ng/dL (Figure 2).

Of the original 90 patients, one patient withdrew on Day 14. Serum testosterone was suppressed to below the castrate threshold (≤ 50 ng/dL) by Day 28 in 85 of 89 (96%) patients remaining in the study. All 89 (100%) of patients remaining in the study attained the castrate threshold by Day 42. Once testosterone suppression at or below serum concentrations of 50 ng/dL was achieved, three patients (3%) demonstrated breakthrough (concentration above 50 ng/dL) during the study. In the first of these patients, a single serum testosterone concentration of 53 ng/dL was reported on the day after the second injection. In this patient, castrate suppression was reported for all other timepoints. In the second patient, a serum testosterone concentration of 66 ng/dL was reported immediately prior to the second injection. This rose to a maximum concentration of 147 ng/dL on the second day after the second injection. In this patient, castrate suppression was again reached on the seventh day after the second injection and was maintained thereafter. In the final patient, serum testosterone concentrations above 50 ng/dL were reported at 2 and at 8 hours after the second injection. Serum testosterone concentration rose to a maximum of 110 ng/dL on the third day after the second injection. In this patient, castrate suppression was again reached eighteen days after the second injection and was maintained until the final day of the study, when a single serum testosterone concentration of 55 ng/dL was reported. Of 82 evaluable patients in the study at Month 8, 81 had testosterone concentrations of ≤ 50 ng/dL.

Table 1: Incidence (%) of Possibly or Probably Related Systemic Adverse Events Reported by ≥ 2% of Patients (n = 90) Treated with ELIGARD® 30 mg for up to Eight Months in Study AGL0001

Body System	Adverse Event	Number	Percent
Vascular	Hot flashes*	66	73.3%
General Disorders	Fatigue	12	13.3%
Reproductive	Testicular atrophy*	4	4.4%
	Gynecomastia*	2	2.2%
	Testicular pain	2	2.2%
Skin	Clamminess*	4	4.4%
	Night sweats*	3	3.3%
	Alopecia	2	2.2%
Renal/Urinary	Nocturia	2	2.2%
	Urinary frequency	2	2.2%
Nervous system	Dizziness	4	4.4%
Psychiatric	Decreased libido*	3	3.3%
Musculoskeletal	Myalgia	2	2.2%
Gastrointestinal	Nausea	2	2.2%

In addition, the following possibly or probably related systemic adverse events were reported by 1.1% of patients using ELIGARD® 30 mg in the clinical study.

General: Lethargy

Reproductive: Breast enlargement*, erectile dysfunction*, reduced penis size

Renal/Urinary: Urinary urgency, incontinence

Psychiatric: Insomnia, depression

Musculoskeletal: Muscle atrophy, limb pain

* Expected pharmacological consequences of testosterone suppression. In the patient population studied, a total of 75 hot flash adverse events were reported in 66 patients. Of these, 57 events (76%) were mild; 16 (21%) were moderate; 2 (3%) were severe.

All seven non-evaluable patients who had achieved castration by Day 28 maintained castration at each timepoint, up to and including the time of withdrawal.

Figure 2. ELIGARD® 30 mg Mean Serum Testosterone Concentrations (n = 90)

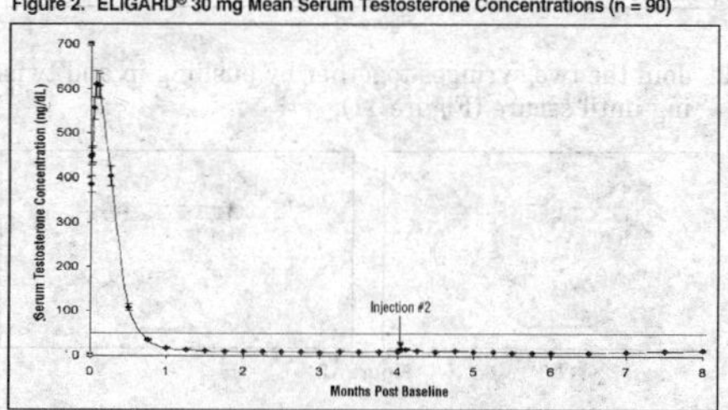

Serum PSA decreased in all patients whose Baseline values were elevated above the normal limit. Mean values were reduced 86% from Baseline to Month 8. At Month 8, PSA levels had decreased to within normal limits in 93% of patients who presented with elevated levels at Baseline.

Other secondary efficacy endpoints evaluated included WHO performance status, bone pain, urinary pain and urinary signs and symptoms. At Baseline, 90% of patients were classified as "fully active" by the WHO performance status scale (Status=0) and 10% as "restricted in strenuous activity but ambulatory and able to carry out work of a light or sedentary nature" (Status=1). At Month 8, the percentage of fully active men decreased slightly to 87%, the percentage of men classified as restricted increased slightly to 12%, and one patient (1%) was classified as unable to carry out work activities (Status=2). At Baseline, patients experienced little bone pain, with a mean score of 1.20 (range 1-7) on a scale of 1 (no pain) to 10 (worst pain possible). At Month 8, the mean bone pain score was essentially unchanged at 1.19 (range 1-8). Urinary pain, scored on the same scale, was similarly low, with a mean of 1.01 at Baseline (range 1-2) and all patients had a score of 1 by Month 8. Urinary signs and symptoms were similarly low at Baseline and decreased modestly at Month 8. In addition, there was a reduction in patients with prostate abnormalities detected during physical exam from 66 (73%) at Screening to 54 (60%) at Month 8.

INDICATIONS AND USAGE

ELIGARD® 30 mg is indicated for the palliative treatment of advanced prostate cancer.

CONTRAINDICATIONS

1. ELIGARD® 30 mg is contraindicated in patients with hypersensitivity to GnRH, GnRH agonist analogs or any of the components of ELIGARD® 30 mg. Anaphylactic reactions to synthetic GnRH or GnRH agonist analogs have been reported in the literature.[2]
2. ELIGARD® 30 mg is contraindicated in women and in pediatric patients and was not studied in women or children. Moreover, leuprolide acetate can cause fetal harm when administered to a pregnant woman. Major fetal abnormalities were observed in rabbits but not in rats after administration of leuprolide acetate throughout gestation. There were increased fetal mortality and decreased fetal weights in rats and rabbits. The effects on fetal mortality are expected consequences of the alterations in hormonal levels brought about by this drug. The possibility exists that spontaneous abortion may occur.

WARNINGS

ELIGARD® 30 mg, like other LH-RH agonists, causes a transient increase in serum concentrations of testosterone during the first week of treatment. Patients may experience worsening of symptoms or onset of new signs and symptoms during the first few weeks of treatment, including bone pain, neuropathy, hematuria, or bladder outlet obstruction. Isolated cases of ureteral obstruction and/or spinal cord compression, which may contribute to paralysis with or without fatal complications, have been observed in the palliative treatment of advanced prostate cancer using LH-RH agonists (see **PRECAUTIONS**).

If spinal cord compression or ureteral obstruction develops, standard treatment of these complications should be instituted.

PRECAUTIONS

General: Patients with metastatic vertebral lesions and/or with urinary tract obstruction should be closely observed during the first few weeks of therapy (see **WARNINGS** section).

Laboratory Tests: Response to ELIGARD® 30 mg should be monitored by measuring serum concentrations of testosterone and prostate specific antigen periodically.

In the majority of patients, testosterone levels increased above Baseline during the first week, declining thereafter to Baseline levels or below by the end of the third week. Castrate levels were generally reached within two to four weeks, with most (86/89) patients remaining suppressed throughout the study.

Results of testosterone determinations are dependent on assay methodology. It is advisable to be aware of the type and precision of the assay methodology to make appropriate clinical and therapeutic decisions.

Drug Interactions: See **PHARMACOKINETICS**

Drug/Laboratory Test Interactions: Therapy with leuprolide acetate results in suppression of the pituitary-gonadal system. Results of diagnostic tests of pituitary gonadotropic

Continued on next page

This product information was prepared in September 2004. On these and other products of Sanofi-Synthelabo Inc., detailed information may be obtained on a current basis by direct inquiry to Product Information Services, 90 Park Avenue, New York, NY 10016 (toll free 1-800-446-6267).

Eligard 30 mg—Cont.

and gonadal functions conducted during and after leuprolide therapy may be affected.

Carcinogenesis, Mutagenesis, Impairment of Fertility: Two-year carcinogenicity studies were conducted with leuprolide acetate in rats and mice. In rats, a dose-related increase of benign pituitary hyperplasia and benign pituitary adenomas was noted at 24 months when the drug was administered subcutaneously at high daily doses (0.6 to 4 mg/kg). There was a significant but not dose-related increase of pancreatic islet-cell adenomas in females and of testicular interstitial cell adenomas in males (highest incidence in the low dose group). In mice, no leuprolide acetate-induced tumors or pituitary abnormalities were observed at a dose as high as 60 mg/kg for two years. Patients have been treated with leuprolide acetate for up to three years with doses as high as 10 mg/day and for two years with doses as high as 20 mg/day without demonstrable pituitary abnormalities. No carcinogenicity studies have been conducted with ELIGARD® 30 mg.

Mutagenicity studies have been performed with leuprolide acetate using bacterial and mammalian systems and with ELIGARD® 7.5 mg in bacterial systems. These studies provided no evidence of a mutagenic potential.

Pregnancy, Teratogenic Effects: Pregnancy category X (see **CONTRAINDICATIONS**).

Pediatric Use: ELIGARD® 30 mg is contraindicated in pediatric patients and was not studied in children (see **CONTRAINDICATIONS**).

ADVERSE REACTIONS

The safety of ELIGARD® 30 mg was evaluated in 90 patients with advanced prostate cancer. ELIGARD® 30 mg, like other LH-RH analogs, caused a transient increase in serum testosterone concentrations during the first week of treatment. Therefore, potential exacerbations of signs and symptoms of the disease during the first weeks of treatment are of concern in patients with vertebral metastases and/or urinary obstruction or hematuria. If these conditions are aggravated, it may lead to neurological problems such as weakness and/or paresthesia of the lower limbs or worsening of urinary symptoms (see **WARNINGS** and **PRECAUTIONS**).

In Study AGL0001, 90 patients were dosed with ELIGARD® 30 mg every four months for up to eight months and injection sites were closely monitored. In all, 175 injections of ELIGARD® 30 mg were administered. Transient burning/stinging was reported at the injection site following 35 (20%) injections, with all (100%) of these events reported as mild. Pain was reported following 2.3% of study injections (3.3% of patients) and was generally reported as mild in intensity. A single event reported as moderate pain resolved within two minutes and all 3 mild pain events resolved within several days. Erythema was reported following 1.1% of injections (2.2% of patients). These events were all reported as mild and generally resolved within a few days post-injection.

These localized adverse events were non-recurrent over time. No patient discontinued therapy due to an injection site adverse event.

The following possibly or probably related systemic adverse events occurred during clinical trials of up to eight months of treatment with ELIGARD® 30 mg, and were reported in ≥ 2% of patients (Table 1). Often, causality is difficult to assess in patients with metastatic prostate cancer. Reactions considered not drug-related are excluded.

[See table 1 at top of previous page]

Changes in Bone Density: Decreased bone density has been reported in the medical literature in men who have had orchiectomy or who have been treated with an LH-RH agonist analog.[3] It can be anticipated that long periods of medical castration in men will have effects on bone density.

OVERDOSAGE

In clinical trials using daily subcutaneous injections of leuprolide acetate in patients with prostate cancer, doses as high as 20 mg/day for up to two years caused no adverse effects differing from those observed with the 1 mg/day dose.

DOSAGE AND ADMINISTRATION

The recommended dose of ELIGARD® 30 mg is one injection every four months. The injection delivers 30 mg of leuprolide acetate, incorporated in a polymer formulation. It is administered subcutaneously and provides continuous release of leuprolide for four months.

Once mixed, ELIGARD® 30 mg should be discarded if not administered within 30 minutes.

As with other drugs administered by subcutaneous injection, the injection site should vary periodically.

Mixing and Administration Procedure

IMPORTANT: Allow the product to reach room temperature before using. **Once mixed, the product must be administered within 30 minutes.**

Follow the instructions as directed to ensure proper preparation of ELIGARD® 30 mg prior to administration:

ELIGARD® 30 mg is packaged in a pouch that contains two smaller pouches (Figure 3), a needle cartridge and a desiccant pack (Figure 4). Syringe A pouch contains the sterile Syringe A pre-filled with the ATRIGEL® polymer system and a long white replacement plunger rod (Figure 5). Syringe B pouch contains the sterile Syringe B pre-filled with leuprolide acetate powder (Figure 6).

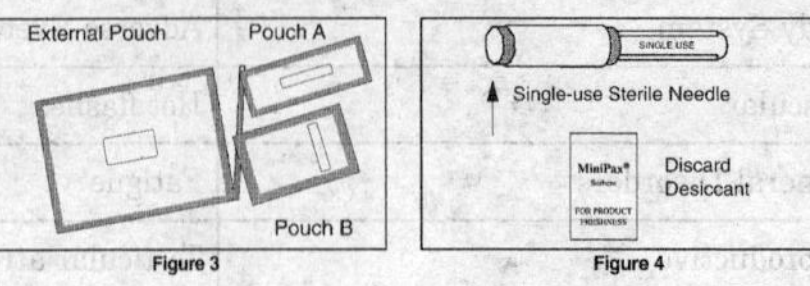

Figure 3 Figure 4

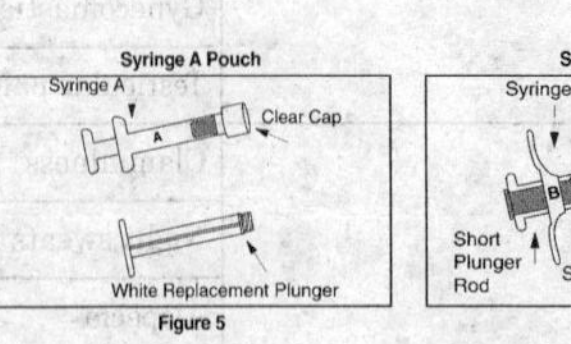

Figure 5 Figure 6

1. On a clean field, open all of the pouches and remove the contents. Discard the desiccant pack.

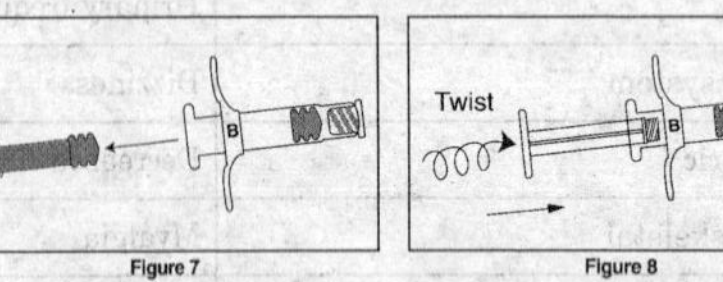

Figure 7 Figure 8

2. Pull out the blue-tipped short plunger rod and attached stopper from Syringe B and discard (Figure 7). Gently insert the long, white replacement plunger rod into the gray primary stopper remaining in Syringe B by twisting it in place (Figure 8).

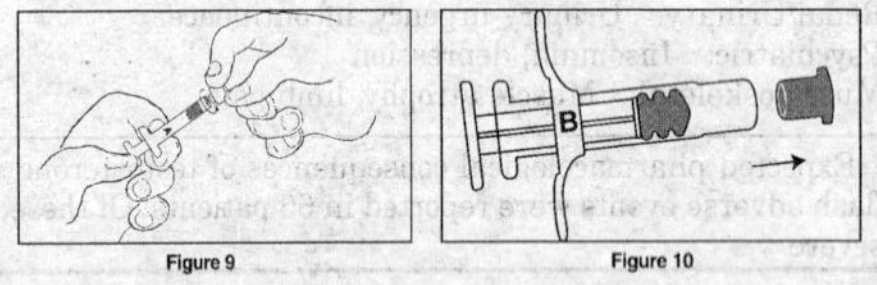
Figure 9 Figure 10

3. Unscrew the clear cap from Syringe A (Figure 9). Remove the gray rubber cap from Syringe B (Figure 10).

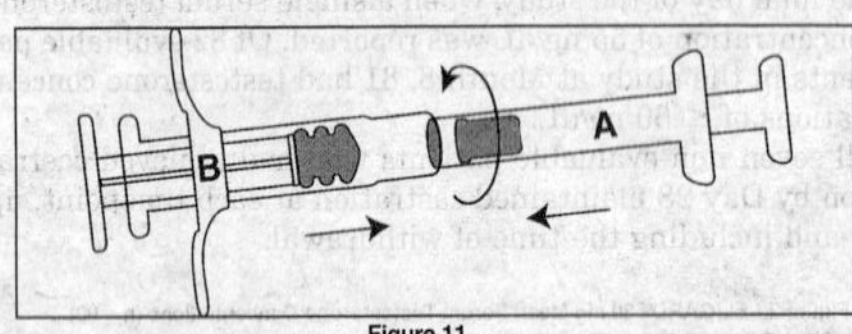
Figure 11

4. Join the two syringes together by pushing in and twisting until secure (Figure 11).

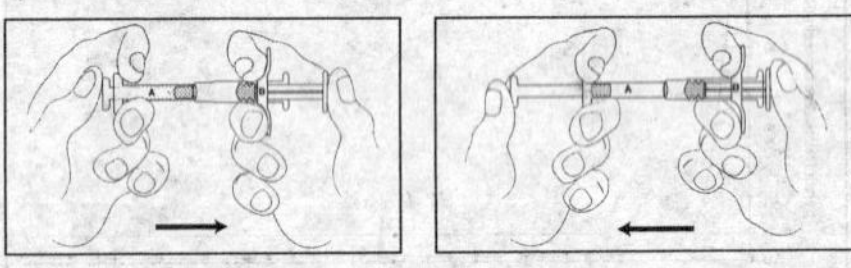
Figure 12

5. Inject the liquid contents of Syringe A into Syringe B containing the leuprolide acetate. Thoroughly mix the product by pushing the contents of both syringes back and forth between syringes (approximately 45 seconds) to obtain a uniform suspension (Figure 12). When thoroughly mixed, the suspension will appear colorless to pale yellow in color. **Please note: Product must be mixed as described; shaking will not provide adequate mixing of the product.**

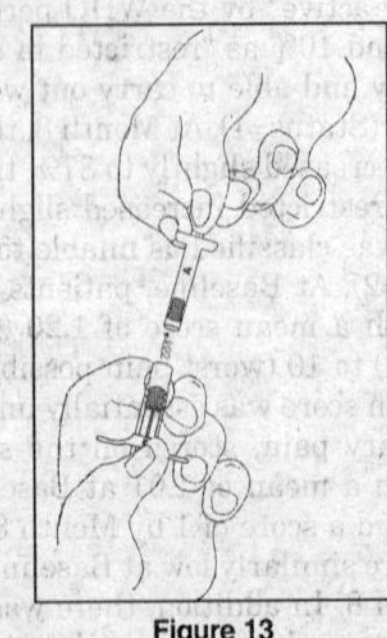
Figure 13

6. Hold the syringes vertically with Syringe B on the bottom. The syringes should remain securely coupled. Draw the entire mixed product into Syringe B (short, wide syringe) by depressing the Syringe A plunger and slightly withdrawing the Syringe B plunger. Uncouple Syringe A while continuing to push down on the Syringe A plunger (Figure 13). **Please note: Small air bubbles will remain in the formulation – this is acceptable.**

[See figures 14, 15, and 16 at top of next column]

7. Hold Syringe B upright. Remove the pink cap on the bottom of the sterile needle cartridge by twisting it (Figure 14). Attach the needle cartridge to the end of Syringe B (Figure 15) by pushing in and turning the needle until it is firmly seated. Do not twist the needle onto the syringe until it is stripped. Pull off the clear needle cartridge cover prior to administration (Figure 16).

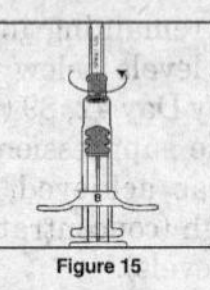
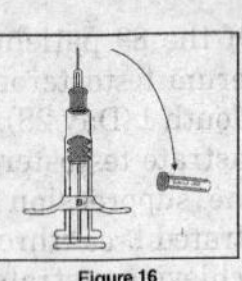
Figure 14 Figure 15 Figure 16

8. Choose an injection site on the abdomen, upper buttocks, or anywhere with adequate amounts of subcutaneous tissue that does not have excessive pigment, nodules, lesions, or hair. Since you can vary the injection site with a subcutaneous injection, choose an area that hasn't recently been used.
9. Cleanse the injection site area with an alcohol swab.[4]

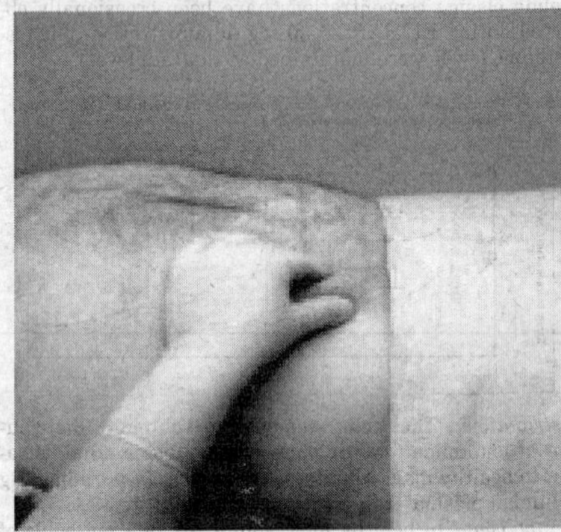

10. Using the thumb and forefinger of your nondominant hand, grab and bunch the area of skin around the injection site.[4]

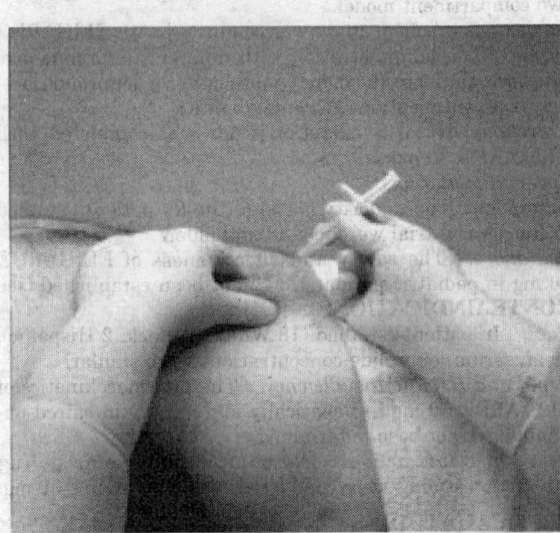

11. Using your dominant hand, insert the needle quickly. The approximate angle you use will depend on the amount and fullness of the subcutaneous tissue and the length of the needle.[4]

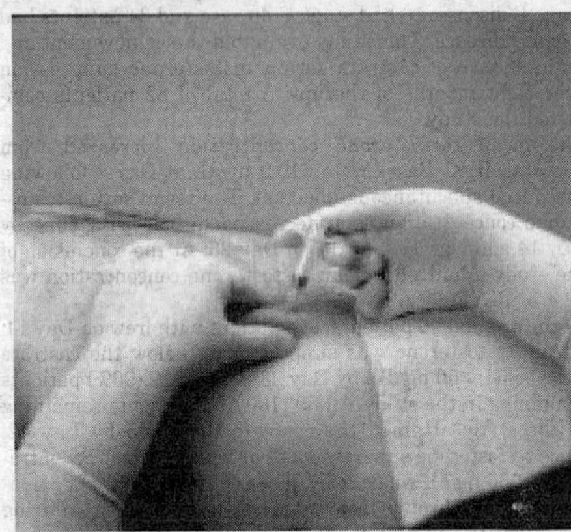

12. After the needle is inserted, release the skin with your nondominant hand.[4]
13. Inject the drug using a slow, steady push. Press down on the plunger until the syringe is empty.[4]
14. Withdraw the needle quickly at the same angle used for insertion.[4]
15. Gently massage the injection area with a cotton ball or gauze pad.[4]
16. Discard all componennts safely in an appropriate bio-hazard container.
17. Remove your gloves and wash your hands. Document both the procedure and the patient's response to the injection.

HOW SUPPLIED

ELIGARD® 30 mg is available in a single use kit. The kit consists of a two-syringe mixing system, a 20-gauge 5/8-inch needle, a silicone desiccant pouch to control moisture uptake, and a package insert for constitution and administration procedures. Each syringe is individually packaged. One contains the ATRIGEL® Delivery System and the other contains leuprolide acetate. When constituted, ELIGARD® 30 mg is administered as a single dose.
(NDC 0024-0610-30)

Rx only

Store at 2–8 °C (35.6–46.4 °F)

sanofi~synthelabo
Manufactured for Sanofi-Synthelabo Inc.
New York, NY 10016
by Atrix Laboratories, Inc.
Fort Collins, CO 80525

1 Sennello LT et al. Single-dose pharmacokinetics of leuprolide in humans following intravenous and subcutaneous administration. J Pharm Sci 1986; 75(2): 158-160.
2 MacLeod TL et. al. Anaphylactic reaction to synthetic luteinizing hormone releasing hormone. Fertil Steril 1987 Sept; 48(3): 500-502.
3 Hatano T et. al. Incidence of bone fracture in patients receiving luteinizing hormone-releasing hormone agonists for prostate cancer. BJU International 2000 86: 449-452.
4 National Instituites of Health. Giving a subcutaneous injection, Bethesda, Md; 2002.

04305 Rev 4 8/04 Revised August 2004

Shown in Product Identification Guide, page 332

ELITEK™ ℞
(rasburicase)

BOXED WARNINGS

Anaphylaxis
ELITEK may cause severe hypersensitivity reactions including anaphylaxis. ELITEK should be immediately and permanently discontinued in any patient developing clinical evidence of a serious hypersensitivity reaction (see **WARNINGS, Anaphylaxis** and **ADVERSE REACTIONS, Immunogenicity**).

Hemolysis
ELITEK administered to patients with glucose-6-phosphate dehydrogenase (G6PD) deficiency can cause severe hemolysis. ELITEK administration should be immediately and permanently discontinued in any patient developing hemolysis. It is recommended that patients at higher risk for G6PD deficiency (e.g., patients of African or Mediterranean ancestry) be screened prior to starting ELITEK therapy (see **CONTRAINDICATIONS** and **WARNINGS, Hemolysis**).

Methemoglobinemia
ELITEK use has been associated with methemoglobinemia. ELITEK administration should be immediately and permanently discontinued in any patient identified as having developed methemoglobinemia (see **WARNINGS, Methemoglobinemia**).

Interference with Uric Acid Measurements
ELITEK will cause enzymatic degradation of the uric acid within blood samples left at room temperature, resulting in spuriously low uric acid levels. To ensure accurate measurements, blood must be collected into prechilled tubes containing heparin anticoagulant and immediately immersed and maintained in an ice water bath; plasma samples must be assayed within 4 hours of sample collection (see **PRECAUTIONS, Laboratory Test Interactions**).

DESCRIPTION

ELITEK (rasburicase) is a recombinant urate-oxidase enzyme produced by a genetically modified *Saccharomyces cerevisiae* strain. The cDNA coding for rasburicase was cloned from a strain of *Aspergillus flavus*.
Rasburicase is a tetrameric protein with identical subunits of a molecular mass of about 34kDa. The molecular formula of the monomer is $C_{1523}H_{2383}N_{417}O_{462}S_7$. The monomer, made up of a single 301 amino acid polypeptide chain, has no intra- or inter-disulfide bridges and is N-terminal acetylated. The drug product is a sterile, white to off-white, lyophilized powder intended for intravenous administration following reconstitution. ELITEK is supplied in 3-mL colorless, glass vials containing 1.5 mg rasburicase, 10.6 mg mannitol, 15.9 mg L-alanine, and between 12.6 and 14.3 mg of dibasic sodium phosphate.
The diluent solution for reconstitution, supplied in a 2 mL clear, glass ampule, is composed of 1.0 mL sterile Water for Injection, USP, and 1.0 mg Poloxamer 188. The product reconstituted with diluent is a clear, colorless solution.

CLINICAL PHARMACOLOGY

In humans, uric acid is the final step in the catabolic pathway of purines. Rasburicase catalyzes enzymatic oxidation of uric acid into an inactive and soluble metabolite (allantoin). Rasburicase is only active at the end of the purine catabolic pathway.
Pharmacokinetics of rasburicase were evaluated in two studies that enrolled patients with lymphoid leukemia (B and T cell), non-Hodgkin's lymphoma (including Burkitt's lymphoma) or acute myelogenous leukemia. ELITEK exposure, as measured by $AUC_{0-24\ hr}$ and C_{max}, tended to increase linearly with doses over a limited dose range (0.15 to 0.20mg/kg). The overall elimination half-life was 18 hours. No accumulation of rasburicase was observed between days 1 and 5 of dosing. ELITEK mean volume of distribution was 110 to 127 mL/kg in pediatric patients. There are insufficient data to characterize pharmacokinetics in adult patients.

CLINICAL STUDIES

ELITEK was administered in three studies to 265 patients with acute leukemia or non-Hodgkin's lymphoma. The clinical studies were largely limited to pediatric patients (246 of 265). ELITEK was administered as a 30-minute infusion once (n=251) or twice (n=14) daily at a dose of 0.15 or 0.20 mg/kg/dose (total daily dose 0.20–0.40 mg/kg/day). ELITEK was administered prior to and concurrent with anti-tumor therapy, which consisted of either systemic chemotherapy (n=196) or steroids (n=69).

Study 1
Study 1 was a randomized, open-label, controlled study conducted at six institutions, in which 52 pediatric patients were randomized to receive either ELITEK (n=27) or allopurinol (n=25).[1] The dose of allopurinol varied according to local institutional practice. ELITEK was administered as an intravenous infusion over 30 minutes once (n=26) or twice (n=1) daily at a dose of 0.20 mg/kg/dose (total daily dose 0.20–0.40 mg/kg/day). Initiation of dosing was permitted at any time between 4 to 48 hours before the start of anti-tumor therapy and could be continued for 5 to 7 days after initiation of anti-tumor therapy. Patients were stratified at randomization on the basis of underlying malignant disease (leukemia or lymphoma) and baseline serum or plasma uric acid levels (<8.0 mg/dL and ≥8.0 mg/dL). The primary study objective was to demonstrate a greater reduction in uric acid concentration over 96 hours ($AUC_{0-96\ hr}$) in the ELITEK group as compared to the allopurinol group. Uric acid $AUC_{0-96\ hr}$ was defined as the area under the curve for plasma uric acid levels (mg•hr/dL), measured from the last value prior to the first dose of ELITEK until 96 hours after that first dose. Plasma uric acid levels were used for all uric acid $AUC_{0-96\ hr}$ calculations (see **PRECAUTIONS, Laboratory Test Interactions**).
The demographics of the two study arms (ELITEK vs. allopurinol) were as follows: age <13 years (82% vs. 76%), males (59% vs. 72%), Caucasian (59% vs. 72%), ECOG performance status 0 (89% vs. 84%), and leukemia (74% vs. 76%). The median interval, in hours, between initiation of ELITEK and of anti-tumor treatment was 20 hours, with a range of 70 hours before to 10 hours after the initiation of anti-tumor treatment (n=24, data not reported for 3 patients).
The uric acid $AUC_{0-96\ hr}$ was significantly lower in the ELITEK group (128 ± s.e. 14 mg•hr/dL) as compared to the allopurinol group (328 ± s.e. 26 mg•hr/dL). All but one patient in the ELITEK arm had reduction and maintenance of uric acid levels to within or below the normal range during the treatment. The incidence of renal dysfunction was similar in the two study arms; one patient in the allopurinol arm developed acute renal failure.

Study 2
Study 2 was a multi-institutional, single-arm study conducted in 89 pediatric and 18 adult patients with hematologic malignancies. Patients received ELITEK at a dose of 0.15 mg/kg/day. The primary efficacy objective was determination of the proportion of patients with maintained plasma uric acid concentration at 48 hours where maintenance of uric acid concentration was defined as: 1) achievement of uric acid concentration ≤6.5 mg/dL (patients <13 years) or ≤7.5 mg/dL (patients ≥13 years) within a designated time point (48 hours) from initiation of ELITEK and maintained until 24 hours after the last administration of study drug; and 2) control of uric acid level without the need for allopurinol or other agents.
The study population demographics were: age <13 years (76%), males (61%), Caucasian (91%), ECOG performance status = 0 (92%), and leukemia (89%).
The proportion of patients with maintenance of uric acid concentration at 48 hours in Study 2 was 99% (106/107).

Study 3
Study 3 was a multi-institutional, single-arm study conducted in 130 pediatric patients and 1 adult patient with hematologic malignancies.[2] Patients received ELITEK at either a dose of 0.15 mg/kg/day (n=12) or 0.20 mg/kg/day (n=119). The primary efficacy objective was determination of the proportion of patients with maintained plasma uric acid concentration at 48 hours as defined for Study 2 above. The study population demographics were: age <13 years (76%), Caucasian (83%), males (67%), ECOG = 0 (67%), and leukemia (88%).
The proportion of patients with maintenance of uric acid concentration at 48 hours in Study 3 was 92% in the 0.15 mg/kg group (n=12) and 95% in the 0.20 mg/kg group (n=119).

Pooled Analyses
Dosing
For the pooled data set of the 3 clinical studies (n=265), total daily dosing for ELITEK ranged from 0.15 to 0.40 mg/kg/day with the majority receiving 0.20 mg/kg/day. The maximum daily doses received were 0.15 mg/kg/day in 116 patients, 0.20 mg/kg/day in 135 patients, 0.30 mg/kg/day (divided doses) in 3 patients, and 0.40 mg/kg/day (divided doses) in 11 patients. The safety and effectiveness of twice-daily dosing with ELITEK have not been established due to insufficient data (see **DOSAGE AND ADMINISTRATION**).
Reduction of Uric Acid Levels
Data from the 3 studies (n=265) were pooled and analyzed according to the plasma uric acid levels over time. The pretreatment plasma uric acid concentration was ≥8 mg/dL in 61 patients and was <8 mg/dL in 200 patients. The median uric acid concentration at baseline, at 4 hours following the first dose of ELITEK, and the per patient fall in plasma uric acid concentration from baseline to 4 hours were calculated in those patients with both pre-treatment and 4-hour post-treatment values. Among patients with pre-treatment uric acid ≥8.0 mg/dL [baseline median 10.6 mg/dL (range 8.1–36.4)], the median per-patient change in plasma uric acid concentration by 4 hours after the first dose was a decrease of 9.1 mg/dL (0.3–19.3 mg/dL). Among the patients with a pre-treatment plasma uric acid level < 8 mg/dL [baseline median 4.6 mg/dL (range 0.2–7.9 mg/dL)], the median per-patient change in plasma uric acid concentration by 4 hours after the first dose was a decrease of 4.1 mg/dL (0.1–7.6 mg/dL).

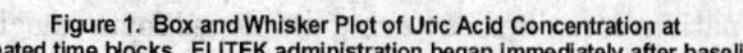
Figure 1. Box and Whisker Plot of Uric Acid Concentration at designated time blocks. ELITEK administration began immediately after baseline.

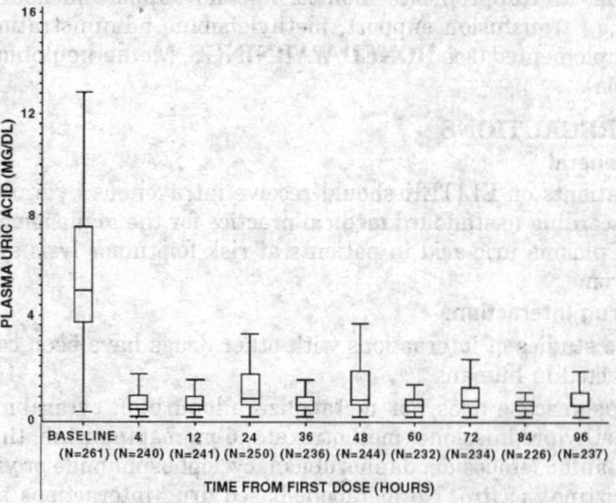

Figure 1 is a box and whisker plot of plasma uric acid levels inclusive of 261 of the 265 ELITEK treated patients from Studies 1, 2, and 3. Of the 261 evaluable patients, plasma uric acid concentration was maintained (see **CLINICAL STUDIES, Study 2**, for the definition of uric acid concentration maintenance) by 4 hours for 92% of patients (240/261), by 24 hours for 93% of patients (245/261), by 48 hours for 97% of patients (254/261), by 72 hours for 99% of patients (260/261), and by 96 hours for 100% of patients (261/261). Of the subset of 61 patients whose plasma uric acid level was elevated at baseline (≥8 mg/dL), plasma uric acid concentration was maintained by 4 hours for 72% of patients (44/61), by 24 hours for 80% of patients (49/61), by 48 hours for 92% of patients (56/61), by 72 hours for 98% of patients (60/61), and by 96 hours for 100% (61/61).

INDICATIONS AND USAGE

ELITEK (rasburicase) is indicated for the initial management of plasma uric acid levels in pediatric patients with leukemia, lymphoma, and solid tumor malignancies who are receiving anti-cancer therapy expected to result in tumor lysis and subsequent elevation of plasma uric acid.

CONTRAINDICATIONS

ELITEK is contraindicated in individuals deficient in glucose-6-phosphate dehydrogenase (G6PD) (see **BOXED WARNINGS, Hemolysis** and **WARNINGS, Hemolysis**).
ELITEK is contraindicated in patients with a known history of anaphylaxis or hypersensitivity reactions, hemolytic reactions or methemoglobinemia reactions to ELITEK or any of the excipients (see **BOXED WARNINGS** and **WARNINGS**).

WARNINGS

Anaphylaxis
The safety and efficacy of ELITEK have been established only for a single course of treatment [once daily for 5 days (see **DOSAGE AND ADMINISTRATION**)].
ELITEK may cause severe allergic reactions including anaphylaxis. Signs and symptoms of these reactions include anaphylactic shock, bronchospasm, chest pain, dyspnea, hypotension and/or urticaria. ELITEK administration should be immediately and permanently discontinued in any patient developing clinical evidence of a serious hypersensitivity reaction (see **BOXED WARNINGS, Anaphylaxis** and **ADVERSE REACTIONS, Immunogenicity**).

Hemolysis
ELITEK is contraindicated in patients with G6PD deficiency because hydrogen peroxide is one of the major by-products of the conversion of uric acid to allantoin. In clinical studies, two patients developed severe hemolytic

Continued on next page

This product information was prepared in September 2004. On these and other products of Sanofi-Synthelabo Inc., detailed information may be obtained on a current basis by direct inquiry to Product Information Services, 90 Park Avenue, New York, NY 10016 (toll free 1-800-446-6267).

Elitek—Cont.

reactions [National Cancer Institute Common Toxicity Criteria[3] (NCI CTC) grade 3 and 4] within 2–4 days of the start of ELITEK. G6PD deficiency was subsequently identified in one of these patients. ELITEK administration should be immediately and permanently discontinued in any patient developing hemolysis, and appropriate patient monitoring and support measures initiated (e.g., transfusion support). It is recommended that patients at higher risk for G6PD deficiency (e.g., patients of African or Mediterranean ancestry) be screened prior to starting ELITEK therapy (see **BOXED WARNINGS, Hemolysis** and **CONTRAINDICATIONS**).

Methemoglobinemia

In clinical studies, methemoglobinemia has been reported in 2 patients receiving ELITEK. Both patients developed serious hypoxemia requiring intervention with the appropriate medical support measures. It is not known whether patients with deficiency of cytochrome b_5 reductase (formerly known as methemoglobin reductase) or of other enzymes with antioxidant activity are at increased risk for methemoglobinemia or hemolytic anemia. ELITEK administration should be immediately and permanently discontinued in any patient identified as having developed methemoglobinemia, and appropriate monitoring and support measures (e.g., transfusion support, methyleneblue administration) implemented (see **BOXED WARNINGS, Methemoglobinemia**).

PRECAUTIONS

General

Patients on ELITEK should receive intravenous hydration according to standard medical practice for the management of plasma uric acid in patients at risk for tumor lysis syndrome.

Drug Interactions

No studies of interactions with other drugs have been conducted in humans.

Rasburicase does not metabolize allopurinol, cytarabine, methylprednisolone, methotrexate, 6-mercaptopurine, thioguanine, etoposide, daunorubicin, cyclophosphamide or vincristine *in vitro*. No metabolic-based drug interactions are therefore anticipated with these agents in patients.

In preclinical *in vivo* studies, rasburicase did not affect the activity of isoenzymes CYP1A, CYP2A, CYP2B, CYP2C, CYP2E, and CYP3A, suggesting no induction nor inhibition potential. Clinically relevant P450-mediated drug-drug interactions are therefore not anticipated in patients treated with the recommended ELITEK dose and dosing schedule.

Laboratory Test Interactions

At room temperature, ELITEK causes enzymatic degradation of the uric acid in blood/plasma/serum samples potentially resulting in spuriously low plasma uric acid assay readings. The following special sample handling procedure must be followed to avoid *ex vivo* uric acid degradation.

Uric acid must be analyzed in plasma. Blood must be collected into prechilled tubes containing heparin anticoagulant. Samples must be **immediately immersed in an ice water bath**. Plasma samples must be prepared by centrifugation in a pre-cooled centrifuge (4°C). Finally, the plasma must be maintained in an ice water bath and analyzed for uric acid within four hours of collection (see **BOXED WARNINGS, Interference with Uric Acid Measurement**).

Carcinogenesis, Mutagenesis, Impairment of Fertility

Long-term studies in animals to evaluate carcinogenic potential have not been performed.

ELITEK was non-genotoxic in the Ames, unscheduled DNA synthesis, chromosome analysis, mouse lymphoma, and micronucleus tests.

ELITEK did not affect reproductive performance or fertility in male or female rats at doses 8-fold higher than the human dose when corrected for differences in body surface area.

Pregnancy Category C

Animal reproduction studies have not been conducted with ELITEK. It is also not known whether ELITEK can cause fetal harm when administered to a pregnant woman or can affect reproduction capacity. ELITEK should be given to a pregnant woman only if clearly needed.

Nursing Mothers

It is not known whether this drug is excreted in human milk. Because many drugs are excreted in human milk and because of the potential for serious adverse reactions in nursing infants, a decision should be made whether to discontinue nursing or to discontinue ELITEK, taking into account the importance of the drug to the mother.

Pediatric Use

The efficacy and safety of ELITEK was studied in 246 pediatric patients ranging in age from 1 month to 17 years. There were an insufficient number of patients in the 0–6 months age group (n=7) to determine whether they respond differently from older children. These patients were pooled into the <2 years of age group (n=24). Children <2 years of age had a higher mean uric acid $AUC_{0-96\ hr}$ than those age 2–17 years (150 ± s.e. 16 mg•hr/dL vs. 108 ± s.e. 4 mg•hr/dL, respectively). In addition, the data suggest that children <2 years of age had a lower rate of success at achieving maintenance uric acid concentration by 48 hours [83% (95% CI of 62 to 95) vs. 93% (95% CI of 89 to 95), respectively]. Children <2 years old also experienced more toxicity. The following adverse events were observed more frequently in children less than 2 years of age compared to those age 2–17 years respectively: vomiting (75% vs. 55%), diarrhea (63% vs. 20%), fever (50% vs. 38%), and rash (38% vs. 10%).

Geriatric Use

Five of the 19 adults among the 265 patients enrolled in clinical studies of ELITEK, were age 65 or greater. Therefore, there are insufficient data to determine whether geriatric subjects, or adults in general, respond differently from pediatric subjects.

ADVERSE REACTIONS

Because clinical trials are conducted under widely varying conditions, adverse reaction rates observed in the clinical trials of a drug cannot be directly compared to rates in the clinical trials of another drug and may not reflect the rates observed in practice. The adverse reaction information from clinical trials does, however, provide a basis for identifying the adverse events that appear to be related to drug use and for approximating rates.

The data described below reflect exposure to ELITEK in 703 patients [63% male, 37% female; median age 10 years (range 10 days to 88 years); 73% Caucasian, 9% African, 4% Asian, 14% other/unknown]. ELITEK was studied for adverse reactions, regardless of severity, in 347 patients (265 pediatric and 82 adults) enrolled in one active-controlled trial (Study 1), two uncontrolled trials (Studies 2 and 3), and one uncontrolled safety trial (n=82). Additionally, an expanded access experience enrolled 356 patients, for whom reliably collected data were limited to serious adverse reactions.

Among the 703 patients for whom serious adverse reactions were assessed, the most serious adverse reactions caused by ELITEK were allergic reactions including anaphylaxis (<1%), rash (1%), hemolysis (<1%), and methemoglobinemia (<1%) (see **BOXED WARNINGS** and **WARNINGS**). The commonly observed serious adverse reactions were fever (5%), neutropenia with fever (4%), respiratory distress (3%), sepsis (3%), neutropenia (2%), and mucositis (2%). The following additional serious adverse reactions were observed in ≤1% of patients regardless of causality: acute renal failure, arrhythmia, cardiac failure, cardiac arrest, cellulitis, cerebrovascular disorder, chest pain, convulsions, cyanosis, diarrhea, dehydration, hot flushes, ileus, infection, intestinal obstruction, hemorrhage, myocardial infarction, paresthesia, pancytopenia, pneumonia, pulmonary edema, pulmonary hypertension, retinal hemorrhage, rigors, thrombosis, and thrombophlebitis.

Among the 347 patients for whom all adverse reactions regardless of severity were assessed, the most frequently observed adverse reactions (incidence ≥10%) were vomiting (50%), fever (46%), nausea (27%), headache (26%), abdominal pain (20%), constipation (20%), diarrhea (20%), mucositis (15%), and rash (13%). In Study 1, an active control study, the following adverse events occurred more frequently in ELITEK-treated subjects than allopurinol-treated subjects: vomiting, fever, nausea, diarrhea, and headache. Although the incidence of rash was similar in the two arms, severe rash (NCI CTC[3], Grade 3 or 4) was reported only in one ELITEK-treated patient.

Immunogenicity

ELITEK is immunogenic in healthy volunteers, and can elicit antibodies that inhibit the activity of rasburicase *in vitro* (see **BOXED WARNINGS, Anaphylaxis** and **WARNINGS, Anaphylaxis**).

In a study of 28 healthy volunteers, the incidence of antibody responses to either a single dose or to 5 daily doses was assessed. Binding antibodies to rasburicase were detected by ELISA in 17/28 (61%) volunteers and neutralizing antibodies were detected in 18/28 (64%) volunteers. Time to detection of antibodies ranged from 1 to 6 weeks after ELITEK exposure. In two subjects with extended follow-up, antibodies persisted for 333 and 494 days.

The incidence of antibody responses in patients with hematologic malignancy has not been adequately assessed. In clinical trials of patients with hematologic malignancies, 24 of the 218 patients tested (11%) developed antibodies by day 28 following ELITEK administration. However, this is not a reliable estimate of the true incidence of antibody responses in patients with hematologic malignancies, because the data from the healthy volunteer study indicate that antibody may not be detectable until some time point beyond day 28.

The incidence of antibody responses detected is highly dependent on the sensitivity and specificity of the assay, which have not been fully evaluated. Additionally, the observed incidence of antibody positivity in an assay may be influenced by several factors, including serum sampling, timing and methodology, concomitant medications, and underlying disease. For these reasons, comparison of the incidence of antibodies to ELITEK with the incidence of antibodies to other products may be misleading.

OVERDOSAGE

No cases of overdosage with ELITEK have been reported. The maximum dose of ELITEK that has been administered as a single dose is 0.20 mg/kg; the maximum daily dose that has been administered is 0.40 mg/kg/day. According to the mechanism of action of ELITEK, an overdose will lead to low or undetectable plasma uric acid concentration, which has no known clinical consequences. Patients suspected of receiving an overdose should be monitored, and general supportive measures should be initiated as no specific antidote for ELITEK has been identified.

DOSAGE AND ADMINISTRATION

The recommended dose and schedule of ELITEK is 0.15 or 0.20 mg/kg as a single daily dose for 5 days. Because the safety and effectiveness of other schedules have not been established, dosing beyond 5 days or administration of more than one course of ELITEK is not recommended. Chemotherapy should be initiated 4 to 24 hours after the first dose of ELITEK. **DO NOT ADMINISTER AS A BOLUS INFUSION.** ELITEK should be administered as an intravenous infusion over 30 minutes.

Reconstitution Procedure

Determine the number of vials of ELITEK needed to achieve the proper dosage, based on the individual patient's weight and the dose per kilogram. ELITEK must be reconstituted in the diluent provided. Add 1 mL of the provided reconstitution solution (diluent) to each vial of ELITEK and mix by swirling very gently. **Do not shake or vortex.** Parenteral drug products should be inspected visually for particulate matter and discoloration prior to administration, and discarded if particulate matter is visible or if product is discolored.

Further Dilution and Administration

Using aseptic technique and syringes of appropriate volume, remove the predetermined dose of ELITEK from the reconstituted vials and inject into an infusion bag containing the appropriate volume of 0.9% sterile sodium chloride, to achieve a final total volume of 50 mL. This final solution for injection is to be infused over 30 minutes. **No filters should be used for the infusion.**

The reconstituted ELITEK contains no preservatives and must be administered within 24 hours of reconstitution. The reconstituted or diluted solution can be stored up to 24 hours at 2–8°C. Discard any unused product.

ELITEK should be infused through a different line than that used for the infusion of other concomitant medications. If use of a separate line is not possible, the line should be flushed with at least 15 mL of saline solution prior to and after infusion with ELITEK.

HOW SUPPLIED

NDC 0024-5150-10: One carton containing 3 single-use vials each containing 1.5 mg of rasburicase and 3 ampules each containing 1.0 mL diluent.

Storage and Handling

The lyophilized drug product and the diluent for reconstitution should be stored at 2–8°C (36–46°F). Do not freeze. Protect from light.

REFERENCES

1. Goldman SC, Holcenberg JS, Finklestein JZ. A randomized comparison between rasburicase and allopurinol in children with lymphoma or leukemia at high risk for tumor lysis. *Blood.* 2001;97:2998–3003.

2. Pui C-H, Mahmoud HH, Wiley JM et al. Recombinant urate oxidase for the prophylaxis or treatment of hyperuricemia in patients with leukemia or lymphoma. *J Clin Oncol.* 2001;19:697–704.

3. National Cancer Institute Common Toxicity Criteria, Version 2.0 (http://ctep.cancer.gov/reporting/ctc.html).

sanofi~synthelabo
Manufactured and distributed by Sanofi-Synthelabo Inc.
New York, NY 10016
U.S. License No. 1294
Printed in USA
Revised March 2004
ESS-4B

ELOXATIN™ ℞

[ē-lŏks-ă-tĭn]

(oxaliplatin for injection)

> **WARNING**
>
> ELOXATIN (oxaliplatin for injection) should be administered under the supervision of a qualified physician experienced in the use of cancer chemotherapeutic agents. Appropriate management of therapy and complications is possible only when adequate diagnostic and treatment facilities are readily available.
>
> Anaphylactic-like reactions to ELOXATIN have been reported, and may occur within minutes of ELOXATIN administration. Epinephrine, corticosteroids, and antihistamines have been employed to alleviate symptoms (see WARNINGS and ADVERSE REACTIONS).

DESCRIPTION

ELOXATIN™ (oxaliplatin for injection) is an antineoplastic agent with the molecular formula $C_8H_{14}N_2O_4Pt$ and the chemical name of *cis*-[(1*R*,2*R*)-1,2-cyclohexanediamine-*N*,*N*'] [oxalato(2-)-*O*,*O*'] platinum. Oxaliplatin is an organoplatinum complex in which the platinum atom is complexed with 1,2-diaminocyclohexane (DACH) and with an oxalate ligand as a leaving group.

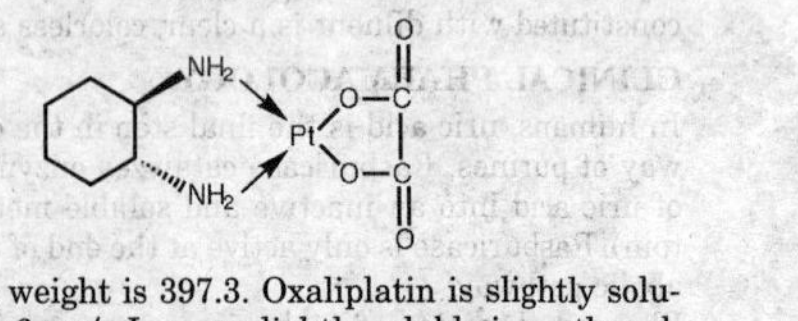

The molecular weight is 397.3. Oxaliplatin is slightly soluble in water at 6 mg/mL, very slightly soluble in methanol, and practically insoluble in ethanol and acetone.

ELOXATIN is supplied in vials containing 50 mg or 100 mg of oxaliplatin as a sterile, preservative-free lyophilized powder for reconstitution. Lactose monohydrate is present as an inactive ingredient at 450 mg and 900 mg in the 50 mg and 100 mg dosage strengths, respectively.

CLINICAL PHARMACOLOGY

Mechanism of Action

Oxaliplatin undergoes nonenzymatic conversion in physiologic solutions to active derivatives via displacement of the labile oxalate ligand. Several transient reactive species are formed, including monoaquo and diaquo DACH platinum, which covalently bind with macromolecules. Both inter- and intrastrand Pt-DNA crosslinks are formed. Crosslinks are formed between the *N7* positions of two adjacent guanines (GG), adjacent adenine-guanines (AG), and guanines separated by an intervening nucleotide (GNG). These crosslinks inhibit DNA replication and transcription. Cytotoxicity is cell-cycle nonspecific.

Pharmacology

In vivo studies have shown antitumor activity of oxaliplatin against colon carcinoma. In combination with 5-fluorouracil (5-FU), oxaliplatin exhibits *in vitro* and *in vivo* antiproliferative activity greater than either compound alone in several tumor models [HT29 (colon), GR (mammary), and L1210 (leukemia)].

Human Pharmacokinetics

The reactive oxaliplatin derivatives are present as a fraction of the unbound platinum in plasma ultrafiltrate. The decline of ultrafilterable platinum levels following oxaliplatin administration is triphasic, characterized by two relatively short distribution phases ($t_{1/2\alpha}$; 0.43 hours and $t_{1/2\beta}$; 16.8 hours) and a long terminal elimination phase ($t_{1/2\gamma}$; 391 hours). Pharmacokinetic parameters obtained after a single 2-hour IV infusion of ELOXATIN at a dose of 85 mg/m^2 expressed as ultrafilterable platinum were C_{max} of 0.814 µg/mL and volume of distribution of 440 L.

Interpatient and intrapatient variability in ultrafilterable platinum exposure (AUC_{0-48}) assessed over 3 cycles was moderate to low (23% and 6%, respectively). A pharmacodynamic relationship between platinum ultrafiltrate levels and clinical safety and effectiveness has not been established.

Distribution

At the end of a 2-hour infusion of ELOXATIN, approximately 15% of the administered platinum is present in the systemic circulation. The remaining 85% is rapidly distributed into tissues or eliminated in the urine. In patients, plasma protein binding of platinum is irreversible and is greater than 90%. The main binding proteins are albumin and gammaglobulins. Platinum also binds irreversibly and accumulates (approximately 2-fold) in erythrocytes, where it appears to have no relevant activity. No platinum accumulation was observed in plasma ultrafiltrate following 85 mg/m^2 every two weeks.

Metabolism

Oxaliplatin undergoes rapid and extensive nonenzymatic biotransformation. There is no evidence of cytochrome P450-mediated metabolism *in vitro*.

Up to 17 platinum-containing derivatives have been observed in plasma ultrafiltrate samples from patients, including several cytotoxic species (monochloro DACH platinum, dichloro DACH platinum, and monoaquo and diaquo DACH platinum) and a number of noncytotoxic, conjugated species.

Elimination

The major route of platinum elimination is renal excretion. At five days after a single 2-hour infusion of ELOXATIN, urinary elimination accounted for about 54% of the platinum eliminated, with fecal excretion accounting for only about 2%. Platinum was cleared from plasma at a rate (10–17 L/h) that was similar to or exceeded the average human glomerular filtration rate (GFR; 7.5 L/h). There was no significant effect of gender on the clearance of ultrafilterable platinum. The renal clearance of ultrafilterable platinum is significantly correlated with GFR (see ADVERSE REACTIONS).

Pharmacokinetics in Special Populations

Renal Impairment

The AUC_{0-48hr} of platinum in the plasma ultrafiltrate increases as renal function decreases. The AUC_{0-48hr} of platinum in patients with mild (creatinine clearance, CL_{cr} 50 to 80 mL/min), moderate (CL_{cr} 30 to <50 mL/min) and severe renal (CL_{cr} <30 mL/min) impairment is increased by about 60, 140 and 190%, respectively, compared to patients with normal renal function (CL_{cr} >80 mL/min)] (see PRECAUTIONS and ADVERSE REACTIONS).

Drug - Drug Interactions

No pharmacokinetic interaction between 85 mg/m^2 of ELOXATIN and 5-FU has been observed in patients treated every 2 weeks, but increases of 5-FU plasma concentrations by approximately 20% have been observed with doses of 130 mg/m^2 of ELOXATIN administered every 3 weeks. *In vitro*, platinum was not displaced from plasma proteins by the following medications: erythromycin, salicylate, sodium valproate, granisetron, and paclitaxel. *In vitro*, oxaliplatin is not metabolized by, nor does it inhibit, human cytochrome P450 isoenzymes. No P450-mediated drug-drug interactions are therefore anticipated in patients.

Since platinum containing species are eliminated primarily through the kidney, clearance of these products may be decreased by co-administration of potentially nephrotoxic compounds, although this has not been specifically studied.

Table 1 – Dosing Regimens in Patients Previously Untreated for Advanced Colorectal Cancer Clinical Trial

Treatment Arm	Dose	Regimen
ELOXATIN + 5-FU/LV FOLFOX4 (N=267)	**Day 1: ELOXATIN: 85 mg/m^2 (2-hour infusion) + LV 200 mg/m^2 (2-hour infusion), followed by 5-FU: 400 mg/m^2 (bolus), 600 mg/m^2 (22-hour infusion) Day 2: LV 200 mg/m^2 (2-hour infusion), followed by 5-FU: 400 mg/m^2 (bolus), 600 mg/m^2 (22-hour infusion)**	q2w
irinotecan + 5-FU/LV IFL (N=264)	Day 1: irinotecan 125 mg/m^2 as a 90-min infusion + LV 20 mg/m^2 as a 15-min infusion or IV push, followed by 5-FU 500 mg/m^2 IV bolus weekly × 4	q6w
ELOXATIN + irinotecan IROX (N=264)	Day 1: ELOXATIN: 85 mg/m^2 IV (2-hour infusion) + irinotecan 200 mg/m^2 IV over 30 minutes	q3w

Table 2 – Patient Demographics and Dosing in Patients Previously Untreated for Advanced Colorectal Cancer Clinical Trial

	ELOXATIN + 5-FU/LV N=267	irinotecan + 5-FU/LV N=264	ELOXATIN + irinotecan N=264
Sex: Male (%)	58.8	65.2	61.0
Female (%)	41.2	34.8	39.0
Median age (years)	61.0	61.0	61.0
<65 years of age (%)	61	62	63
≥65 years of age (%)	39	38	37
ECOG (%)			
0,1	94.4	95.5	94.7
2	5.6	4.5	5.3
Involved organs (%)			
Colon only	0.7	0.8	0.4
Liver only	39.3	44.3	39.0
Liver + other	41.2	38.6	40.9
Lung only	6.4	3.8	5.3
Other (including lymph nodes)	11.6	11.0	12.9
Not reported	0.7	1.5	1.5
Prior radiation (%)	3.0	1.5	3.0
Prior surgery (%)	74.5	79.2	81.8
Prior adjuvant (%)	15.7	14.8	15.2

CLINICAL STUDIES

Combination Therapy with ELOXATIN and 5-FU/LV in Patients Previously Untreated for Advanced Colorectal Cancer

A North American, multicenter, open-label, randomized controlled study was sponsored by the National Cancer Institute (NCI) as an intergroup study led by the North Central Cancer Treatment Group (NCCTG). The study had 7 arms at different times during its conduct, four of which were closed due to either changes in the standard of care, toxicity, or simplification. During the study, the control arm was changed to irinotecan plus 5-FU/LV. The results reported below compared the efficacy and safety of two experimental regimens, ELOXATIN in combination with infusional 5-FU/LV and a combination of ELOXATIN plus irinotecan, to an approved control regimen of irinotecan plus 5-FU/LV in 795 concurrently randomized patients previously untreated for locally advanced or metastatic colorectal cancer. After completion of enrollment, the dose of irinotecan plus 5-FU/LV was decreased due to toxicity. Patients had to be at least 18 years of age, have known locally advanced, locally recurrent, or metastatic colorectal adenocarcinoma not curable by surgery or amenable to radiation therapy with curative intent, histologically proven colorectal adenocarcinoma, measurable or evaluable disease, with an ECOG performance status 0,1, or 2. Patients had to have granulocyte count ≥ 1.5 x 10^9/L, platelets ≥ 100 x 10^9/L, hemoglobin ≥9.0 gm/dL, creatinine ≤ 1.5 x ULN, total bilirubin ≤ 1.5 mg/dL, AST ≤ 5 x ULN, and alkaline phosphatase ≤ 5 x ULN. Patients may have received adjuvant therapy for resected Stage II or III disease without recurrence within 12 months. The patients were stratified for ECOG performance status (0, 1 vs. 2), prior adjuvant chemotherapy (yes vs. no), prior immunotherapy (yes vs. no), and age (<65 vs.≥65 years). Although no post study treatment was specified in the protocol, 65 to 72% of patients received additional post study chemotherapy after study treatment discontinuation on all arms. Fifty eight percent of patients on the ELOXATIN plus 5-FU/LV arm received an irinotecan-containing regimen and 23% of patients on the irinotecan plus 5-FU/LV arm received oxaliplatin-containing regimens. Oxaliplatin was not commercially available during the trial.

The following table presents the dosing regimens of the three arms of the study.

[See table 1 above]

The following table presents the demographics and dosing of the patient population entered into this study.

[See table 2 above]

The length of a treatment cycle was 2 weeks for the ELOXATIN and 5-FU/LV regimen; 6 weeks for the irinotecan plus 5-FU/LV regimen; and 3 weeks for the ELOXATIN plus irinotecan regimen. The median number of cycles administered per patient was 10 (23.9 weeks) for the ELOXATIN and 5-FU/LV regimen, 4 (23.6 weeks) for the irinotecan plus 5-FU/LV regimen, and 7 (21.0 weeks) for the ELOXATIN plus irinotecan regimen.

Patients treated with the ELOXATIN and 5-FU/LV combination had a significantly longer time to tumor progression based on investigator assessment, longer overall survival, and a significantly higher confirmed response rate based on investigator assessment compared to patients given irinotecan plus 5-FU/LV. The following table summarizes the efficacy results.

[See table 3 at top of next page]

The numbers in the response rate and TTP analysis are based on unblinded investigator assessment.

Figure 1 illustrates the Kaplan-Meier survival curves for the comparison of ELOXATIN and 5-FU/LV combination and ELOXATIN plus irinotecan to irinotecan plus 5-FU/LV.

Continued on next page

This product information was prepared in September 2004. On these and other products of Sanofi-Synthelabo Inc., detailed information may be obtained on a current basis by direct inquiry to Product Information Services, 90 Park Avenue, New York, NY 10016 (toll free 1-800-446-6267).

Eloxatin—Cont.

Figure 1 illustrates the Kaplan-Meier survival curves for the comparison of ELOXATIN and 5-FU/LV combination and ELOXATIN plus irinotecan to irinotecan plus 5-FU/LV.

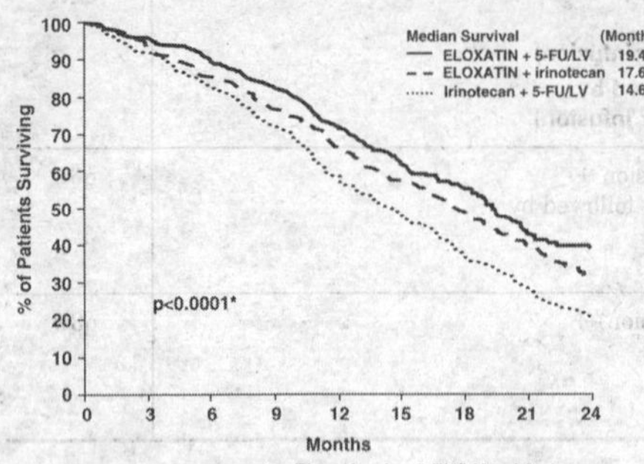

*Log rank test comparing Eloxatin plus 5-FU/LV to irinotecan plus 5-FU/LV.

A descriptive subgroup analysis demonstrated that the improvement in survival for ELOXATIN plus 5-FU/LV compared to irinotecan plus 5-FU/LV appeared to be maintained across age groups, prior adjuvant therapy, and number of organs involved. An estimated survival advantage in ELOXATIN plus 5-FU/LV versus irinotecan plus 5-FU/LV was seen in both genders; however it was greater among women than men. Insufficient subgroup sizes prevented analysis by race.

Combination Therapy with ELOXATIN and 5-FU/LV in Previously Treated Patients with Advanced Colorectal Cancer

A multicenter, open-label, randomized, three arm controlled study was conducted in the US and Canada comparing the efficacy and safety of ELOXATIN in combination with an infusional schedule of 5-FU/LV to the same dose and schedule of 5-FU/LV alone and to single agent oxaliplatin in patients with advanced colorectal cancer who had relapsed/progressed during or within 6 months of first line therapy with bolus 5-FU/LV and irinotecan. The study was intended to be analyzed for response rate after 450 patients were enrolled. Survival will be subsequently assessed in all patients enrolled in the completed study. Accrual to this study is complete, with 821 patients enrolled. Patients in the study had to be at least 18 years of age, have unresectable, measurable, histologically proven colorectal adenocarcinoma, with a Karnofsky performance status >50%. Patients had to have SGOT(AST) and SGPT(ALT) ≤ 2x the institution's upper limit of normal (ULN), unless liver metastases were present and documented at baseline by CT or MRI scan, in which case ≤ 5x ULN was permitted. Patients had to have alkaline phosphatase ≤ 2x the institution's ULN, unless liver metastases were present and documented at baseline by CT or MRI scan, in which cases ≤ 5x ULN was permitted. Prior radiotherapy was permitted if it had been completed at least 3 weeks before randomization.

The dosing regimens of the three arms of the study are presented in the table below.

[See table 4 at right]

Patients entered into the study for evaluation of response must have had at least one unidimensional lesion measuring ≥20mm using conventional CT or MRI scans, ≥10mm using a spiral CT scan. Tumor response and progression were assessed every 3 cycles (6 weeks) using the Response Evaluation Criteria in Solid Tumors (RECIST) until radiological documentation of progression or for 13 months following the first dose of study drug(s), whichever came first. Confirmed responses were based on two tumor assessments separated by at least 4 weeks.

The demographics of the patient population entered into this study are shown in the table below.

[See table 5 at right and on next page]

The median number of cycles administered per patient was 6 for the ELOXATIN and 5-FU/LV combination and 3 each for 5-FU/LV alone and ELOXATIN alone.

Patients treated with the combination of ELOXATIN and 5-FU/LV had an increased response rate compared to patients given 5-FU/LV or oxaliplatin alone. The efficacy results are summarized in the tables below.

[See table 6 at top of next page]
[See table 7 on next page]

At the time of the interim analysis 49% of the radiographic progression events had occurred. In this interim analysis an estimated 2-month increase in median time to radiographic progression was observed compared to 5-FU/LV alone.

Of the 13 patients who had tumor response to the combination of ELOXATIN and 5-FU/LV, 5 were female and 8 were male, and responders included patients <65 years old and ≥65 years old. The small number of non-Caucasian participants made efficacy analyses in these populations uninterpretable.

INDICATIONS AND USAGE

ELOXATIN, used in combination with infusional 5-FU/LV, is indicated for the treatment of advanced carcinoma of the colon or rectum.

CONTRAINDICATIONS

ELOXATIN should not be administered to patients with a history of known allergy to ELOXATIN or other platinum compounds.

Table 3 – Summary of Efficacy

	ELOXATIN + 5-FU/LV N=267	irinotecan + 5-FU/LV N=264	ELOXATIN + irinotecan N=264
Survival (ITT)			
Number of deaths N (%)	155 (58.1)	192 (72.7)	175 (66.3)
Median survival (months)	19.4	14.6	17.6
Hazard Ratio and (95% confidence interval)	0.65 (0.53–0.80)*		
P-value	<0.0001*	–	–
TTP (ITT, investigator assessment)			
Percentage of progressors	82.8	81.8	89.4
Median TTP (months)	8.7	6.9	6.5
Hazard Ratio and (95% confidence interval)	0.74 (0.61–0.89)*		
P-value	0.0014*	–	–
Response Rate (investigator assessment)**			
Patients with measurable disease	210	212	215
Complete response N (%)	13 (6.2)	5 (2.4)	7 (3.3)
Partial response N (%)	82 (39.0)	64 (30.2)	67 (31.2)
Complete and partial response N (%)	95 (45.2)	69 (32.5)	74 (34.4)
95% confidence interval	(38.5–52.0)	(26.2–38.9)	(28.1–40.8)
P-value	0.0080*	–	–

*Compared to irinotecan plus 5-FU/LV (IFL) arm
**Based on all patients with measurable disease at baseline

Table 4 – Dosing Regimens in Refractory and Relapsed Colorectal Cancer Clinical Trial

Treatment Arm	Dose	Regimen
ELOXATIN + 5-FU/LV (N=152)	**Day 1: ELOXATIN: 85 mg/m² (2-hour infusion) + LV 200 mg/m² (2-hour infusion), followed by 5-FU: 400 mg/m² (bolus), 600 mg/m² (22-hour infusion)** **Day 2: LV 200 mg/m² (2-hour infusion), followed by 5-FU: 400 mg/m² (bolus), 600 mg/m² (22-hour infusion)**	**q2w**
5-FU/LV (N=151)	Day 1: LV 200 mg/m² (2-hour infusion), followed by 5-FU: 400 mg/m² (bolus), 600 mg/m² (22-hour infusion) Day 2: LV 200 mg/m² (2-hour infusion), followed by 5-FU: 400 mg/m² (bolus), 600 mg/m² (22-hour infusion)	q2w
ELOXATIN (N=156)	Day 1: ELOXATIN 85 mg/m²(2-hour infusion)	q2w

Table 5 – Patient Demographics in Refractory and Relapsed Colorectal Cancer Clinical Trial

	5-FU/LV (N=151)	ELOXATIN (N=156)	ELOXATIN + 5-FU/LV (N=152)
Sex: Male (%)	54.3	60.9	57.2
Female (%)	45.7	39.1	42.8
Median age (years)	60.0	61.0	59.0
Range	21-80	27-79	22-88
Race (%)			
Caucasian	87.4	84.6	88.8
Black	7.9	7.1	5.9
Asian	1.3	2.6	2.6
Other	3.3	5.8	2.6
KPS (%)			
70–100	94.7	92.3	95.4
50–60	2.6	4.5	2.0
Not reported	2.6	3.2	2.6

(Table continued on next page)

WARNINGS

As in the case for other platinum compounds, hypersensitivity and anaphylactic/anaphylactoid reactions to ELOXATIN have been reported (see ADVERSE REACTIONS). These allergic reactions were similar in nature and severity to those reported with other platinum-containing compounds, i.e., rash, urticaria, erythema, pruritus, and, rarely, bronchospasm and hypotension. These reactions occur within minutes of administration and should be managed with appropriate supportive therapy. Drug-related deaths associated with platinum compounds from this reaction have been reported.

Pregnancy Category D

ELOXATIN may cause fetal harm when administered to a pregnant woman. Pregnant rats were administered 1 mg/kg/day oxaliplatin (less than one-tenth the recommended human dose based on body surface area) during gestation days 1-5 (pre-implantation), 6-10, or 11-16 (during organogenesis). Oxaliplatin caused developmental mortality (increased early resorptions) when administered on days 6-10 and 11-16 and adversely affected fetal growth (decreased fetal weight, delayed ossification) when administered on days 6-10. If this drug is used during pregnancy or if the patient becomes pregnant while taking this drug, the patient should be apprised of the potential hazard to the fetus. Women of childbearing potential should be advised to avoid becoming pregnant while receiving treatment with ELOXATIN.

PRECAUTIONS

General

ELOXATIN should be administered under the supervision of a qualified physician experienced in the use of cancer chemotherapeutic agents. Appropriate management of therapy and complications is possible only when adequate diagnostic and treatment facilities are readily available.

Neuropathy

Neuropathy was graded using a study-specific neurotoxicity scale, which was different than the National Cancer Institute Common Toxicity Criteria, Version 2.0 (NCI CTC) (see below).

In the previously treated study, neuropathy information was collected to establish that ELOXATIN is associated with two types of neuropathy:

- **An acute, reversible, primarily peripheral, sensory neuropathy that is of early onset, occurring within hours or one to two days of dosing, that resolves within 14 days, and that frequently recurs with further dosing.** The symptoms may be precipitated or exacerbated by exposure to cold temperature or cold objects and they usually present as transient paresthesia, dysesthesia and hypoesthesia in the hands, feet, perioral area, or throat. Jaw spasm, abnormal tongue sensation, dysarthria, eye pain, and a feeling of chest pressure have also been observed. The acute, reversible pattern of sensory neuropathy was observed in about 56% of study patients who received ELOXATIN with 5-FU/LV. In any individual cycle acute neurotoxicity was observed in approximately 30% of patients. Ice (mucositis prophylaxis) should be avoided during the infusion of ELOXATIN because cold temperature can exacerbate acute neurological symptoms (see DOSAGE AND ADMINISTRATION: Dose Modifications).

  An acute syndrome of pharyngolaryngeal dysesthesia seen in 1-2% (grade 3/4) of patients previously untreated for advanced colorectal cancer, and the previously treated patients is characterized by subjective sensations of dysphagia or dyspnea, without any laryngospasm or bronchospasm (no stridor or wheezing).
- **A persistent (>14 days), primarily peripheral, sensory neuropathy that is usually characterized by paresthesias, dysesthesias, hypoesthesias, but may also include deficits in proprioception that can interfere with daily activities (e.g. writing, buttoning, swallowing, and difficulty walking from impaired proprioception).** These forms of neuropathy occurred in 48% of the study patients receiving ELOXATIN with 5-FU/LV. Persistent neuropathy can occur without any prior acute neuropathy event. The majority of the patients (80%) who developed grade 3 persistent neuropathy progressed from prior Grade 1 or 2 events. These symptoms may improve in some patients upon discontinuation of ELOXATIN.

Overall, neuropathy was reported in patients previously untreated for advanced colorectal cancer in 82% (all grades) and 19% (grade 3/4), and in the previously treated patients in 74% (all grades) and 7% (grade 3/4) events. Information regarding reversibility of neuropathy was not available from the trial for patients who had not been previously treated for colorectal cancer.

Neurotoxicity scale:

The grading scale for paresthesias/dysesthesias was: Grade 1, resolved and did not interfere with functioning; Grade 2, interfered with function but not daily activities; Grade 3, pain or functional impairment that interfered with daily activities; Grade 4, persistent impairment that is disabling or life-threatening.

Pulmonary Toxicity

ELOXATIN has been associated with pulmonary fibrosis (<1% of study patients), which may be fatal. The combined incidence of cough, dyspnea and hypoxia was 43% (any grade) and 7% (grade 3 and 4) in the ELOXATIN plus 5-FU/LV arm compared to 32% (any grade) and 5% (grade 3 and 4) in the irinotecan plus 5-FU/LV arm of unknown duration for patients with previously untreated colorectal cancer. In case of unexplained respiratory symptoms such as non-productive cough, dyspnea, crackles, or radiological pulmonary infiltrates, ELOXATIN should be discontinued until further pulmonary investigation excludes interstitial lung disease or pulmonary fibrosis.

Information for Patients

Patients and patients' caregivers should be informed of the expected side effects of ELOXATIN, particularly its neurologic effects, both the acute, reversible effects, and the persistent neurosensory toxicity. Patients should be informed that the acute neurosensory toxicity may be precipitated or exacerbated by exposure to cold or cold objects. Patients should be instructed to avoid cold drinks, use of ice, and should cover exposed skin prior to exposure to cold temperature or cold objects.

Table 5 *(cont.)* – Patient Demographics in Refractory and Relapsed Colorectal Cancer Clinical Trial

	5-FU/LV (N=151)	ELOXATIN (N=156)	ELOXATIN + 5-FU/LV (N=152)
Prior radiotherapy (%)	25.2	19.2	25.0
Prior pelvic radiation (%)	18.5	13.5	21.1
Number of metastatic sites (%)			
1	27.2	31.4	25.7
≥2	72.2	67.9	74.3
Liver involvement (%)			
Liver only	22.5	25.6	18.4
Liver + other	60.3	59.0	53.3

Table 6 - Response Rates (ITT Analysis)

Best Response	5-FU/LV (N=151)	ELOXATIN (N=156)	ELOXATIN + 5-FU/LV (N=152)
CR	0	0	0
PR	0	2 (1%)	13 (9%)
p-value	0.0002 for 5-FU/LV vs. ELOXATIN + 5-FU/LV		
95% CI	0-2.4%	0.2-4.6%	4.6-14.2%

Table 7 - Summary of Radiographic Time to Progression*

Arm	5-FU/LV (N=151)	ELOXATIN (N=156)	ELOXATIN + 5-FU/LV (N=152)
No. of Progressors	74	101	50
No. of patients with no radiological evaluation beyond baseline	22 (15%)	16 (10%)	17 (11%)
Median TTP (months)	2.7	1.6	4.6
95% CI	1.8-3.0	1.4-2.7	4.2-6.1

*This is not an ITT analysis. Events were limited to radiographic disease progression documented by independent review of radiographs. Clinical progression was not included in this analysis, and 18% of patients were excluded from the analysis based on unavailability of the radiographs for independent review.

Table 8 – Adverse Experience Reported in Patients Previously Untreated for Advanced Colorectal Cancer Clinical Trial (≥5% of all patients and with ≥1% NCI Grade 3/4 events)

	ELOXATIN + 5-FU/LV N=259		irinotecan + 5-FU/LV N=256		ELOXATIN + irinotecan N=258	
Adverse Event (WHO/Pref)	**All Grades (%)**	**Grade 3/4 (%)**	**All Grades (%)**	**Grade 3/4 (%)**	**All Grades (%)**	**Grade 3/4 (%)**
Any Event	99	82	98	70	99	76
Allergy/Immunology						
Hypersensitivity	12	2	5	0	6	1
Cardiovascular						
Thrombosis	6	5	6	6	3	3
Hypotension	5	3	6	3	4	3

(Table continued on next page)

Patients must be adequately informed of the risk of low blood cell counts and instructed to contact their physician immediately should fever, particularly if associated with persistent diarrhea, or evidence of infection develop.

Patients should be instructed to contact their physician if persistent vomiting, diarrhea, signs of dehydration, cough or breathing difficulties occur, or signs of allergic reaction appear.

Laboratory Tests

Standard monitoring of the white blood cell count with differential, hemoglobin, platelet count, and blood chemistries (including ALT, AST, bilirubin and creatinine) is recommended before each ELOXATIN cycle (see DOSAGE AND ADMINISTRATION).

Laboratory Test Interactions

None known.

Carcinogenesis, Mutagenesis, Impairment of Fertility

Long-term animal studies have not been performed to evaluate the carcinogenic potential of oxaliplatin. Oxaliplatin was not mutagenic to bacteria (Ames test) but was mutagenic to mammalian cells *in vitro* (L5178Y mouse lymphoma assay). Oxaliplatin was clastogenic both *in vitro* (chromosome aberration in human lymphocytes) and *in vivo* (mouse bone marrow micronucleus assay).

In a fertility study, male rats were given oxaliplatin at 0, 0.5, 1, or 2 mg/kg/day for five days every 21 days for a total of three cycles prior to mating with females that received two cycles of oxaliplatin on the same schedule. A dose of 2 mg/kg/day (less than one-seventh the recommended human dose on a body surface area basis) did not affect pregnancy rate, but caused developmental mortality (increased early resorptions, decreased live fetuses, decreased live births) and delayed growth (decreased fetal weight). Testicular damage, characterized by degeneration, hypoplasia, and atrophy, was observed in dogs administered oxaliplatin at 0.75 mg/kg/day x 5 days every 28 days for three cycles. A no

Continued on next page

This product information was prepared in September 2004. On these and other products of Sanofi-Synthelabo Inc., detailed information may be obtained on a current basis by direct inquiry to Product Information Services, 90 Park Avenue, New York, NY 10016 (toll free 1-800-446-6267).

Table 8 *(cont.)* – Adverse Experience Reported in Patients Previously Untreated for Advanced Colorectal Cancer Clinical Trial (≥5% of all patients and with ≥1% NCI Grade 3/4 events)

	ELOXATIN + 5-FU/LV N=259		irinotecan + 5-FU/LV N=256		ELOXATIN + irinotecan N=258	
Adverse Event (WHO/Pref)	**All Grades (%)**	**Grade 3/4 (%)**	**All Grades (%)**	**Grade 3/4 (%)**	**All Grades (%)**	**Grade 3/4 (%)**
Constitutional Symptoms/Pain/Ocular/Visual						
Fatigue	70	7	58	11	66	16
Abdominal Pain	29	8	31	7	39	10
Myalgia	14	2	6	0	9	2
Pain	7	1	5	1	6	1
Vision abnormal	5	0	2	1	6	1
Neuralgia	5	0	0	0	2	1
Dermatology/Skin						
Skin reaction–hand/foot	7	1	2	1	1	0
Injection site reaction	6	0	1	0	4	1
Gastrointestinal						
Nausea	71	6	67	15	83	19
Diarrhea	56	12	65	29	76	25
Vomiting	41	4	43	13	64	23
Stomatitis	38	0	25	1	19	1
Anorexia	35	2	25	4	27	5
Constipation	32	4	27	2	21	2
Diarrhea-colostomy	13	2	16	7	16	3
Gastrointestinal NOS	5	2	4	2	3	2
Hematology/Infection						
Infection no ANC	10	4	5	1	7	2
Infection—ANC	8	8	12	11	9	8
Lymphopenia	6	2	4	1	5	2
Febrile neutropenia	4	4	15	14	12	11
Hepatic/Metabolic/Laboratory/Renal						
Hyperglycemia	14	2	11	3	12	3
Hypokalemia	11	3	7	4	6	2
Dehydration	9	5	16	11	14	7
Hypoalbuminemia	8	0	5	2	9	1
Hyponatremia	8	2	7	4	4	1
Urinary frequency	5	1	2	1	3	1
Neurology						
Overall Neuropathy	82	19	18	2	69	7
Paresthesias	77	18	16	2	62	6
Pharyngo-laryngeal dysesthesias	38	2	1	0	28	1
Neuro-sensory	12	1	2	0	9	1
Neuro NOS	1	0	1	0	1	0
Pulmonary						
Cough	35	1	25	2	17	1
Dyspnea	18	7	14	3	11	2
Hiccups	5	1	2	0	3	2

Eloxatin—Cont.

effect level was not identified. This daily dose is approximately one-sixth of the recommended human dose on a body surface area basis.

Pregnancy Category D-See WARNINGS

Nursing Mothers - It is not known whether ELOXATIN or its derivatives are excreted in human milk. Because many drugs are excreted in human milk and because of the potential for serious adverse reactions in nursing infants from ELOXATIN, a decision should be made whether to discontinue nursing or delay the use of the drug, taking into account the importance of the drug to the mother.

Pediatric Use - The safety and effectiveness of ELOXATIN in pediatric patients have not been established.

Patients with Renal Impairment - The safety and effectiveness of the combination of ELOXATIN and 5-FU/LV in patients with renal impairment have not been evaluated. The combination of ELOXATIN and 5-FU/LV should be used with caution in patients with preexisting renal impairment since the primary route of platinum elimination is renal. Clearance of ultrafilterable platinum is decreased in patients with mild, moderate, and severe renal impairment. A pharmacodynamic relationship between platinum ultrafiltrate levels and clinical safety and effectiveness has not been established (see CLINICAL PHARMACOLOGY and ADVERSE REACTIONS).

Geriatric Use - No significant effect of age on the clearance of ultrafilterable platinum has been observed. In the previously untreated for advanced colorectal cancer randomized clinical trial (see CLINICAL STUDIES) of ELOXATIN, 160 patients treated with ELOXATIN and 5-FU/LV were < 65 years and 99 patients were ≥ 65 years. The same efficacy improvements in response rate, time to tumor progression, and overall survival were observed in the ≥ 65 year old patients as in the overall study population. In the previously treated randomized clinical trial (see CLINICAL STUDIES) of ELOXATIN, 95 patients treated with ELOXATIN and 5-FU/LV were < 65 years and 55 patients were ≥ 65 years. The rates of overall adverse events, including grade 3 and 4 events, were similar across and within arms in the different age groups in both studies. The incidence of diarrhea, dehydration, hypokalemia, leukopenia, fatigue and syncope were higher in patients ≥ 65 years old. No adjustment to starting dose was required in patients ≥ 65 years old.

Drug Interactions - No specific cytochrome P-450-based drug interaction studies have been conducted. No pharmacokinetic interaction between 85 mg/m^2 ELOXATIN and 5-FU/LV has been observed in patients treated every 2 weeks. Increases of 5-FU plasma concentrations by approximately 20% have been observed with doses of 130 mg/m^2 ELOXATIN dosed every 3 weeks. Since platinum containing species are eliminated primarily through the kidney, clearance of these products may be decreased by co-administration of potentially nephrotoxic compounds; although, this has not been specifically studied (see CLINICAL PHARMACOLOGY).

ADVERSE REACTIONS

More than 4,000 patients with advanced colorectal cancer have been treated in clinical studies with ELOXATIN either as a single agent or in combination with other medications. The most common adverse reactions were peripheral sensory neuropathies, fatigue, neutropenia, nausea, emesis, and diarrhea (see PRECAUTIONS).

Patients Previously Untreated for Advanced Colorectal Cancer

Two-hundred and fifty nine patients were treated in the ELOXATIN and 5-FU/LV combination arm of the randomized trial in patients previously untreated for advanced colorectal cancer (see CLINICAL STUDIES). The adverse event profile in this study was similar to that seen in other studies and the adverse reactions in this trial are shown in the tables below.

Both 5-FU and ELOXATIN are associated with gastrointestinal and hematologic adverse events. When ELOXATIN is administered in combination with 5-FU, the incidence of these events is increased.

The incidence of death within 30 days of treatment in the previously untreated for advanced colorectal cancer study, regardless of causality, was 3% with the ELOXATIN and 5-FU/LV combination, 5% with irinotecan plus 5-FU/LV, and 3% with ELOXATIN plus irinotecan. Deaths within 60 days from initiation of therapy were 2.3% with the ELOXATIN and 5-FU/LV combination, 5.1% with irinotecan plus 5-FU/LV, and 3.1% with ELOXATIN plus irinotecan.

The following table provides adverse events reported in the previously untreated for advanced colorectal cancer study (see CLINICAL STUDIES) by body system and decreasing order of frequency in the ELOXATIN and 5-FU/LV combination arm for events with overall incidences ≥5% and for grade 3/4 events with incidences ≥ 1%. This table does not include hematologic and blood chemistry abnormalities; these are shown separately below.

[See table 8 on previous page and at left]

The following table provides adverse events reported in the previously untreated for advanced colorectal cancer study (see CLINICAL STUDIES) by body system and decreasing order of frequency in the ELOXATIN and 5-FU/LV combination arm for events with overall incidences ≥5% but with incidences < 1% NCI Grade 3/4 events.

Table 9 - Adverse Experience Reported in Patients Previously Untreated for Advanced Colorectal Cancer Clinical Trial (≥5% of all patients but with < 1% NCI Grade 3/4 events)

	ELOXATIN + 5-FU/LV N=259	irinotecan + 5-FU/ LV N=256	ELOXATIN + irinotecan N=258
Adverse Event (WHO/Pref)	**All Grades (%)**	**All Grades (%)**	**All Grades (%)**
Allergy/Immunology			
Rash	11	4	7
Rhinitis allergic	10	6	6
Cardiovascular			
Edema	15	13	10

Constitutional Symptoms/Pain/Ocular/Visual			
Headache	13	6	9
Weight loss	11	9	11
Epistaxis	10	2	2
Tearing	9	1	2
Rigors	8	2	7
Dysphasia	5	3	3
Sweating	5	6	12
Arthralgia	5	5	8
Dermatology/Skin			
Alopecia	38	44	67
Flushing	7	2	5
Pruritus	6	4	2
Dry Skin	6	2	5
Gastrointestinal			
Taste perversion	14	6	8
Dyspepsia	12	7	5
Flatulence	9	6	5
Mouth Dryness	5	2	3
Hematology/Infection			
Fever no ANC	16	9	9
Hepatic/Metabolic/Laboratory/Renal			
Hypocalcemia	7	5	4
Elevated Creatinine	4	4	5
Neurology			
Insomnia	13	9	11
Depression	9	5	7
Dizziness	8	6	10
Anxiety	5	2	6

Adverse events were similar in men and women and in patients <65 and ≥65 years, but older patients may have been more susceptible to diarrhea, dehydration, hypokalemia, leukopenia, fatigue and syncope. The following additional adverse events, at least possibly related to treatment and potentially important, were reported in ≥2% and <5% of the patients in the ELOXATIN and 5-FU/LV combination arm (listed in decreasing order of frequency): metabolic, pneumonitis, catheter infection, vertigo, prothrombin time, pulmonary, rectal bleeding, dysuria, nail changes, chest pain, rectal pain, syncope, hypertension, hypoxia, unknown infection, bone pain, pigmentation changes, and urticaria.

Previously Treated Patients with Advanced Colorectal Cancer

Four hundred and fifty patients (about 150 receiving the combination of ELOXATIN and 5-FU/LV) were studied in a randomized trial in patients with refractory and relapsed colorectal cancer (see CLINICAL STUDIES). The adverse event profile in this study was similar to that seen in other studies and the adverse reactions in this trial are shown in the tables below.

Thirteen percent of patients in the ELOXATIN and 5-FU/LV combination arm and 18% in the 5-FU/LV arm of the previously treated study had to discontinue treatment because of adverse effects related to gastrointestinal, or hematologic adverse events, or neuropathies. Both 5-FU and ELOXATIN are associated with gastrointestinal and hematologic adverse events. When ELOXATIN is administered in combination with 5-FU, the incidence of these events is increased.

The incidence of death within 30 days of treatment in the previously treated study, regardless of causality, was 5% with the ELOXATIN and 5-FU/LV combination, 8% with ELOXATIN alone, and 7% with 5-FU/LV. Of the 7 deaths that occurred on the ELOXATIN and 5-FU/LV combination arm within 30 days of stopping treatment, 3 may have been treatment related, associated with gastrointestinal bleeding or dehydration.

The following table provides adverse events reported in the previously treated study (see CLINICAL STUDIES) by body system and in decreasing order of frequency in the ELOXATIN and 5-FU/LV combination arm for events with overall incidences ≥5% and for grade 3/4 events with incidences ≥ 1%. This table does not include hematologic and blood chemistry abnormalities; these are shown separately below.

[See table 10 above]

Table 10 – Adverse Experience Reported in Previously Treated Colorectal Cancer Clinical Trial (≥5% of all patients and with ≥1% NCI Grade 3/4 events)

	5-FU/LV (N=142)		ELOXATIN (N=153)		ELOXATIN + 5-FU/LV (N=150)	
Adverse Event (WHO/Pref)	**All Grades (%)**	**Grade 3/4 (%)**	**All Grades (%)**	**Grade 3/4 (%)**	**All Grades (%)**	**Grade 3/4 (%)**
Any Event	98	41	100	46	99	73
Cardiovascular						
Dyspnea	11	2	13	7	20	4
Coughing	9	0	11	0	19	1
Edema	13	1	10	1	15	1
Thromboembolism	4	2	2	1	9	8
Chest Pain	4	1	5	1	8	1
Constitutional Symptoms/Pain						
Fatigue	52	6	61	9	68	7
Back Pain	16	4	11	0	19	3
Pain	9	3	14	3	15	2
Dermatology/Skin						
Injection Site Reaction	5	1	9	0	10	3
Gastrointestinal						
Diarrhea	44	3	46	4	67	11
Nausea	59	4	64	4	65	11
Vomiting	27	4	37	4	40	9
Stomatitis	32	3	14	0	37	3
Abdominal Pain	31	5	31	7	33	4
Anorexia	20	1	20	2	29	3
Gastroesophageal Reflux	3	0	1	0	5	2
Hematology/Infection						
Fever	23	1	25	1	29	1
Febrile Neutropenia	1	1	0	0	6	6
Hepatic/Metabolic/Laboratory/Renal						
Hypokalemia	3	1	3	2	9	4
Dehydration	6	4	5	3	8	3
Neurology						
Neuropathy	17	0	76	7	74	7
Acute	10	0	65	5	56	2
Persistent	9	0	43	3	48	6

The following table provides adverse events reported in the previously treated study (see CLINICAL STUDIES) by body system and in decreasing order of frequency in the ELOXATIN and 5-FU/LV combination arm for events with overall incidences ≥5% but with incidences <1% NCI Grade 3/4 events.

Table 11 - Adverse Experience Reported in Previously Treated Colorectal Cancer Clinical Trial (≥5% of all patients but with < 1% NCI Grade 3/4 events)

	5-FU/LV (N = 142)	ELOXATIN (N = 153)	ELOXATIN +5-FU/LV (N = 150)
Adverse Event (WHO/Pref)	**All Grades (%)**	**All Grades (%)**	**All Grades (%)**
Allergy/Immunology			
Rhinitis	4	6	15
Allergic Reaction	1	3	10
Rash	5	5	9
Cardiovascular			
Peripheral Edema	11	5	10
Constitutional Symptoms/Pain/Ocular/Visual			
Headache	8	13	17
Arthralgia	10	7	10
Epistaxis	1	2	9
Abnormal Lacrimation	6	1	7
Rigors	6	9	7
Dermatology/Skin			
Hand-Foot Syndrome	13	1	11
Flushing	2	3	10
Alopecia	3	3	7
Gastrointestinal			
Constipation	23	31	32
Dyspepsia	10	7	14
Taste Perversion	1	5	13
Mucositis	10	2	7

Continued on next page

This product information was prepared in September 2004. On these and other products of Sanofi-Synthelabo Inc., detailed information may be obtained on a current basis by direct inquiry to Product Information Services, 90 Park Avenue, New York, NY 10016 (toll free 1-800-446-6267).

Eloxatin—Cont.

Flatulence	6	3	5
Hepatic/Metabolic/Laboratory/Renal			
Hematuria	4	0	6
Dysuria	1	1	6
Neurology			
Dizziness	8	7	13
Insomnia	4	11	9
Pulmonary			
Upper Resp Tract Infection	4	7	10
Pharyngitis	10	2	9
Hiccup	0	2	5

Adverse events were similar in men and women and in patients <65 and ≥65 years, but older patients may have been more susceptible to dehydration, diarrhea, hypokalemia and fatigue. The following additional adverse events, at least possibly related to treatment and potentially important, were reported in ≥2% and <5% of the patients in the ELOXATIN and 5-FU/LV combination arm (listed in decreasing order of frequency): anxiety, myalgia, erythematous rash, increased sweating, conjunctivitis, weight decrease, dry mouth, rectal hemorrhage, depression, ataxia, ascites, hemorrhoids, muscle weakness, nervousness, tachycardia, abnormal micturition frequency, dry skin, pruritus, hemoptysis, purpura, vaginal hemorrhage, melena, somnolence, pneumonia, proctitis, involuntary muscle contractions, intestinal obstruction, gingivitis, tenesmus, hot flashes, enlarged abdomen, urinary incontinence.

Hematologic

The following tables list the hematologic changes occurring in ≥5% of patients, based on laboratory values and NCI grade, with the exception of anemia in the patients previously untreated for advanced colorectal cancer, which is based on AE reporting and NCI grade alone.

[See table 12 above]
[See table 13 at right]

Thrombocytopenia

Thrombocytopenia was frequently reported with the combination of ELOXATIN and 5-FU/LV. The incidence of Grade 3/4 thrombocytopenia in the patients previously untreated for advanced colorectal cancer and the previously treated patients was 3-5%. Grade 3/4 hemorrhagic events in both patient populations were reported at low frequency and the incidence of these events was greater for the combination of ELOXATIN and 5-FU/LV over the irinotecan plus 5-FU/LV or 5-FU/LV control groups. In the previously untreated patients, the incidence of epistaxis was 10% in the ELOXATIN and 5-FU/LV arm, and 2% and 1% respectively in the irinotecan plus 5-FU/LV or irinotecan plus ELOXATIN arms. The requirement for platelet transfusion was not increased in the ELOXATIN and 5-FU/LV arm. The incidence of all hemorrhagic events in the previously treated patients was also higher on the ELOXATIN combination arm compared to the 5-FU/LV arm. These events included gastrointestinal bleeding, hematuria and epistaxis.

Neutropenia

Neutropenia was frequently observed with the combination of ELOXATIN and 5-FU/LV, with Grade 3 and 4 events reported in 35% and 18% of the patients previously untreated for advanced colorectal cancer, respectively. Grade 3 and 4 events were reported in 27% and 17% of previously treated patients, respectively. The incidence of febrile neutropenia in the patients previously untreated for advanced colorectal cancer was 15% (3% of cycles) in the irinotecan plus 5-FU/LV arm and 4% (less than 1% of cycles) in the ELOXATIN and 5-FU/LV combination arm. Additionally, in this same population, infection with grade 3 or 4 neutropenia was 12% in the irinotecan plus 5-FU/LV, and 8% in the ELOXATIN and 5-FU/LV combination. The incidence of febrile neutropenia in the previously treated patients was 1% in the 5-FU/LV arm and 6% (less than 1% of cycles) in the ELOXATIN and 5-FU/LV combination arm.

Gastrointestinal

In patients previously untreated for advanced colorectal cancer receiving the combination of ELOXATIN and 5-FU/LV, the incidence of Grade 3 and 4 vomiting and diarrhea was less compared to irinotecan plus 5-FU/LV controls (see table). In previously treated patients receiving the combination of ELOXATIN and 5-FU/LV, the incidence of Grade 3 and 4 nausea, vomiting, diarrhea, and mucositis/stomatitis increased compared to 5-FU/LV controls (see table).

The incidence of gastrointestinal adverse events in the previously untreated and previously treated patients appears to be similar across cycles. Premedication with antiemetics, including 5-HT_3 blockers, is recommended. Diarrhea and mucositis may be exacerbated by the addition of ELOXATIN to 5-FU/LV, and should be managed with appropriate supportive care. Since cold temperature can exacerbate acute neurological symptoms, ice (mucositis prophylaxis) should be avoided during the infusion of ELOXATIN.

Table 12 – Adverse Hematologic Experiences in Patients Previously Untreated for Advanced Colorectal Cancer (≥5% of patients)

	ELOXATIN + 5-FU/LV N=259		irinotecan + 5-FU/LV N=256		ELOXATIN + irinotecan N=258	
Hematology Parameter	**All Grades (%)**	**Grade 3/4 (%)**	**All Grades (%)**	**Grade 3/4 (%)**	**All Grades (%)**	**Grade 3/4 (%)**
Anemia	27	3	28	4	25	3
Leukopenia	85	20	84	23	76	24
Neutropenia	81	53	77	44	71	36
Thrombocytopenia	71	5	26	2	44	4

Table 13 – Adverse Hematologic Experiences in Previously Treated Patients (≥5% of patients)

	5-FU/LV (N=142)		ELOXATIN (N=153)		ELOXATIN + 5-FU/LV (N=150)	
Hematology Parameter	**All Grades (%)**	**Grade 3/4 (%)**	**All Grades (%)**	**Grade 3/4 (%)**	**All Grades (%)**	**Grade 3/4 (%)**
Anemia	68	2	64	1	81	2
Leukopenia	34	1	13	0	76	19
Neutropenia	25	5	7	0	73	44
Thrombocytopenia	20	0	30	3	64	4

Table 14 – Adverse Hepatic – Clinical Chemistry Experience in Patients Previously Untreated for Advanced Colorectal Cancer (≥5% of patients)

	ELOXATIN +5-FU/LV N=259		irinotecan + 5-FU/LV N=256		ELOXATIN + irinotecan N=258	
Clinical Chemistry	**All Grades (%)**	**Grade 3/4 (%)**	**All Grades (%)**	**Grade 3/4 (%)**	**All Grades (%)**	**Grade 3/4 (%)**
ALT (SGPT-ALAT)	6	1	2	0	5	2
AST (SGOT-ASAT)	17	1	2	1	11	1
Alkaline Phosphatase	16	0	8	0	14	2
Total Bilirubin	6	1	3	1	3	2

Table 15 – Adverse Hepatic – Clinical Chemistry Experience in Previously Treated Patients (≥5% of patients)

	5-FU/LV (N=142)		ELOXATIN (N=153)		ELOXATIN + 5-FU/LV (N=150)	
Clinical Chemistry	**All Grades (%)**	**Grade 3/4 (%)**	**All Grades (%)**	**Grade 3/4 (%)**	**All Grades (%)**	**Grade 3/4 (%)**
ALT (SGPT-ALAT)	28	3	36	1	31	0
AST (SGOT-ASAT)	39	2	54	4	47	0
Total Bilirubin	22	6	13	5	13	1

Dermatologic

ELOXATIN did not increase the incidence of alopecia compared to 5-FU/LV alone. No complete alopecia was reported. The incidence of hand-foot syndrome in patients previously untreated for advanced colorectal cancer was 2% in the irinotecan plus 5-FU/LV arm and 7% in the ELOXATIN and 5-FU/LV combination arm. The incidence of hand-foot syndrome in previously treated patients was 13% in the 5-FU/LV arm and 11% in the ELOXATIN and 5-FU/LV combination arm.

Care of Intravenous Site:

Extravasation may result in local pain and inflammation that may be severe and lead to complications, including necrosis. Injection site reaction, including redness, swelling, and pain, has been reported.

Neurologic

Overall, neuropathy was reported in patients previously untreated for advanced colorectal cancer in 82% (all grades) and 19% (grade 3/4), and in the previously treated patients in 74% (all grades) and 7% (grade 3/4) events. ELOXATIN is consistently associated with two types of peripheral neuropathy (see PRECAUTIONS, Neuropathy). In the previously treated patients, the incidence of overall and Grade 3/4 persistent peripheral neuropathy was 48% and 6%, respectively. The majority of the patients (80%) that developed grade 3 persistent neuropathy progressed from prior Grade 1 or 2 events. The median number of cycles administered on the ELOXATIN with 5-FU/LV combination arm in the previously treated patients was 6.

Pulmonary

ELOXATIN has been associated with pulmonary fibrosis (see PRECAUTIONS, Pulmonary Toxicity).

Allergic Reactions

Hypersensitivity to ELOXATIN has been observed (<2% Grade 3/4) in clinical studies. These allergic reactions which can be fatal, can occur at any cycle, and were similar in nature and severity to those reported with other platinum-containing compounds such as, rash, urticaria, erythema, pruritus, and, rarely, bronchospasm and hypotension. The symptoms associated with hypersensitivity reactions reported in the previously untreated patients were urticaria, pruritus, flushing of the face, diarrhea associated with oxaliplatin infusion, shortness of breath, bronchospasm, diaphoresis, chest pains, hypotension, disorientation and syncope. These reactions are usually managed with standard epinephrine, corticosteroid, antihistamine therapy, and may require discontinuation of therapy (see WARNINGS for anaphylactic/anaphylactoid reactions).

Anticoagulation and Hemorrhage

There have been reports while on study and from post-marketing surveillance of prolonged prothrombin time and INR occasionally associated with hemorrhage in patients who received ELOXATIN plus 5-FU/LV while on anticoagulants. Patients receiving ELOXATIN plus 5-FU/LV and requiring oral anticoagulants may require closer monitoring.

Renal

About 5-10% of patients in all groups had some degree of elevation of serum creatinine. The incidence of Grade 3/4 elevations in serum creatinine in the ELOXATIN and 5-FU/LV combination arm was 1% in the previously treated patients.

Hepatic

The following tables list the clinical chemistry changes associated with hepatic toxicity occurring in ≥5% of patients, based on adverse events reported and NCI CTC grade for patients previously untreated for advanced colorectal cancer, laboratory values and NCI CTC grade for previously treated patients.

[See table 14 above]
[See table 15 above]

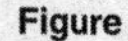

Thromboembolism

The incidence of thromboembolic events was 6 and 9% of the patients previously untreated for advanced colorectal cancer and previously treated patients in the ELOXATIN and 5-FU/LV combination arm, respectively.

Postmarketing Experience

The following events have been reported from worldwide postmarketing experience.

Body as a whole:

-angioedema, anaphylactic shock

Central and peripheral nervous system disorders:

-loss of deep tendon reflexes, dysarthria, Lhermitte's sign, cranial nerve palsies, fasciculations

Gastrointestinal system disorders:

-severe diarrhea/vomiting resulting in hypokalemia, metabolic acidosis; ileus; intestinal obstruction, pancreatitis

Hearing and vestibular system disorders:

-deafness

Platelet, bleeding, and clotting disorders:

-immuno-allergic thrombocytopenia

-prolongation of prothrombin time and of INR in patients receiving anticoagulants

Red Blood Cell disorders:

-hemolytic uremic syndrome

Respiratory system disorders:

-pulmonary fibrosis, and other interstitial lung diseases

Vision disorders:

-decrease of visual acuity, visual field disturbance, optic neuritis

OVERDOSAGE

There have been five ELOXATIN overdoses reported. One patient received two 130 mg/m^2 doses of ELOXATIN (cumulative dose of 260 mg/m^2) within a 24 hour period. The patient experienced Grade 4 thrombocytopenia (<25,000/mm^3) without any bleeding, which resolved. Two other patients were mistakenly administered ELOXATIN instead of carboplatin. One patient received a total ELOXATIN dose of 500 mg and the other received 650 mg. The first patient experienced dyspnea, wheezing, paresthesia, profuse vomiting and chest pain on the day of administration. She developed respiratory failure and severe bradycardia, and subsequently did not respond to resuscitation efforts. The other patient also experienced dyspnea, wheezing, paresthesia, and vomiting. Her symptoms resolved with supportive care. Another patient who was mistakenly administered a 700 mg dose experienced rapid onset of dysesthesia. Inpatient supportive care was given, including hydration, electrolyte support, and platelet transfusion. Recovery occurred 15 days after the overdose. The last patient received an overdose of oxaliplatin at 360 mg instead of 120 mg over a 1-hour infusion by mistake. At the end of the infusion, the patient experienced 2 episodes of vomiting, laryngospasm, and paresthesia. The patient fully recovered from the laryngospasm within half an hour. At the time of reporting, 1 hour after onset of the event, the patient was recovering from paresthesia. There is no known antidote for ELOXATIN overdose. In addition to thrombocytopenia, the anticipated complications of an ELOXATIN overdose include myelosuppression, nausea and vomiting, diarrhea, and neurotoxicity. Patients suspected of receiving an overdose should be monitored, and supportive treatment should be administered.

DOSAGE AND ADMINISTRATION

The recommended dose schedule given every two weeks is as follows:

Day 1: ELOXATIN 85 mg/m^2 IV infusion in 250-500 mL D5W and leucovorin 200 mg/m^2 IV infusion in D5W both given over 120 minutes at the same time in separate bags using a Y-line, followed by 5-FU 400 mg/m^2 IV bolus given over 2-4 minutes, followed by 5-FU 600 mg/m^2 IV infusion in 500 mL D5W (recommended) as a 22-hour continuous infusion.

Day 2: Leucovorin 200 mg/m^2 IV infusion over 120 minutes, followed by 5-FU 400 mg/m^2 IV bolus given over 2-4 minutes, followed by 5-FU 600 mg/m^2 IV infusion in 500 mL D5W (recommended) as a 22-hour continuous infusion.

[See figure 2 above]

Repeat cycle every 2 weeks.

The administration of ELOXATIN does not require prehydration.

Premedication with antiemetics, including 5-HT_3 blockers with or without dexamethasone, is recommended.

For information on 5-fluorouracil and leucovorin, see the respective package inserts.

Dose Modification Recommendations

Prior to subsequent therapy cycles, patients should be evaluated for clinical toxicities and laboratory tests (see Laboratory Tests). Neuropathy was graded using a study-specific neurotoxicity scale (see PRECAUTIONS, Neuropathy). Other toxicities were graded by the NCI CTC, Version 2.0.

Prolongation of infusion time for ELOXATIN from 2 hours to 6 hours decreases the C_{max} by an estimated 32% and may mitigate acute toxicities. The infusion times for 5-FU and leucovorin do not need to be changed.

For patients who experience persistent Grade 2 neurosensory events that do not resolve, a dose reduction of ELOXATIN to 65 mg/m^2 should be considered. For patients with persistent Grade 3 neurosensory events, discontinuing therapy should be considered. The 5-FU/LV regimen need not be altered.

Figure 2

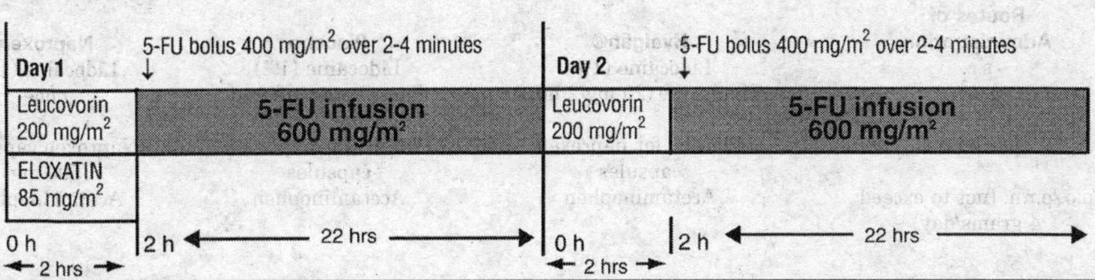

A dose reduction of ELOXATIN to 65 mg/m^2 and 5-FU by 20% (300 mg/m^2 bolus and 500 mg/m^2 22 hour infusion) is recommended for patients after recovery from grade 3/4 gastrointestinal (despite prophylactic treatment) or grade 4 neutropenia or grade 3/4 thrombocytopenia. The next dose should be delayed until: neutrophils ≥1.5 x 10^9/L, and platelets ≥75 x 10^9/L.

Preparation of Infusion Solution

RECONSTITUTION OR FINAL DILUTION MUST NEVER BE PERFORMED WITH A SODIUM CHLORIDE SOLUTION OR OTHER CHLORIDE-CONTAINING SOLUTIONS.

The lyophilized powder is reconstituted by adding 10 mL (for the 50 mg vial) or 20 mL (for the 100 mg vial) of Water for Injection, USP or 5% Dextrose Injection, USP. **Do not administer the reconstituted solution without further dilution.** The reconstituted solution must be further diluted in an infusion solution of 250-500 mL of 5% Dextrose Injection, USP.

After reconstitution in the original vial, the solution may be stored up to 24 hours under refrigeration [2-8°C (36-46°F)]. After final dilution with 250-500 mL of 5% Dextrose Injection, USP, the shelf life is **6 hours at room temperature [20-25°C (68-77°F)] or up to 24 hours under refrigeration [2-8°C (36-46°F)].** ELOXATIN is not light sensitive.

ELOXATIN is incompatible in solution with alkaline medications or media (such as basic solutions of 5-FU) and must not be mixed with these or administered simultaneously through the same infusion line. **The infusion line should be flushed with D5W prior to administration of any concomitant medication.**

Parenteral drug products should be inspected visually for particulate matter and discoloration prior to administration and discarded if present.

Needles or intravenous administration sets containing aluminum parts that may come in contact with ELOXATIN should not be used for the preparation or mixing of the drug. Aluminum has been reported to cause degradation of platinum compounds.

HOW SUPPLIED

ELOXATIN is supplied in clear, glass, single-use vials with gray elastomeric stoppers and aluminum flip-off seals containing 50 mg or 100 mg of oxaliplatin as a sterile, preservative-free lyophilized powder for reconstitution. Lactose monohydrate is also present as an inactive ingredient.

NDC 0024-0596-02: 50 mg single-use vial with green flip-off seal individually packaged in a carton.

NDC 0024-0597-04: 100 mg single-use vial with dark blue flip-off seal individually packaged in a carton.

Storage

Store under normal lighting conditions at 25°C (77°F); excursions permitted to 15-30°C (59-86°F) [see USP controlled room temperature].

Handling and Disposal

As with other potentially toxic anticancer agents, care should be exercised in the handling and preparation of infusion solutions prepared from ELOXATIN. The use of gloves is recommended. If a solution of ELOXATIN contacts the skin, wash the skin immediately and thoroughly with soap and water. If ELOXATIN contacts the mucous membranes, flush thoroughly with water.

Procedures for the handling and disposal of anticancer drugs should be considered. Several guidelines on the subject have been published [1–8]. There is no general agreement that all of the procedures recommended in the guidelines are necessary or appropriate.

REFERENCES

1. ONS Clinical Practice Committee. Cancer Chemotherapy Guidelines and Recommendations for Practice. Pittsburgh, Pa: Oncology Nursing Society; 1999:32-41.
2. Recommendations for the safe handling of parenteral antineoplastic drugs. NIH Publication No. 83-2621. For sale by the Superintendent of Documents, U.S. Government Printing Office, Washington, D.C. 20402.
3. AMA Council Report. Guidelines for handling parenteral antineoplastics. *JAMA* 1985;253(11):1590-1592.
4. National Study Commission on Cytotoxic Exposure. Recommendations for handling cytotoxic agents. Available from Louis P. Jeffrey, Sc.D., Chairman, National Study Commission on Cytotoxic Exposure, Massachusetts College of Pharmacy and Allied Health Sciences, 179 Longwood Avenue, Boston, MA 02115.
5. Clinical Oncological Society of Australia. Guidelines and recommendations for safe handling of antineoplastic agents. *Med J Australia* 1983;1:426-428.
6. Jones RB, et al. Safe handling of chemotherapeutic agents: a report from the Mount Sinai Medical Center. *Ca - A Cancer Journal for Clinicians.* Sept./Oct. 1983: 258-263.
7. American Society of Hospital Pharmacists. ASHP Technical Assistance Bulletin on handling cytotoxic and hazardous drugs. *Am J Hosp Pharm* 1990;47:1033-1049.
8. Controlling Occupational Exposure to Hazardous Drugs. (OSHA Work-Practice Guidelines). *Am J Hosp Pharm* 1996;53:1669-1685.

sanofi~synthelabo

Distributed by Sanofi-Synthelabo Inc.
New York, NY 10016
Manufactured for Sanofi-Synthelabo Inc. by Ben Venue Laboratories
Bedford, OH 44146-0568
ESS-5A Rev. 01/04

HYALGAN® ℞
sodium hyaluronate

LABELING

CAUTION

Federal law restricts this device to sale by or on the order of a physician.

DESCRIPTION

Hyalgan® is a viscous solution consisting of a high molecular weight (500,000–730,000 daltons) fraction of purified natural sodium hyaluronate in buffered physiological sodium chloride, having a pH of 6.8–7.5. The sodium hyaluronate is extracted from rooster combs. Hyaluronic acid is a natural complex sugar of the glycosaminoglycan family and is a long-chain polymer containing repeating disaccharide units of Na-glucuronate-N-acetylglucosamine.

INDICATIONS

Hyalgan® is indicated for the treatment of pain in osteoarthritis (OA) of the knee in patients who have failed to respond adequately to conservative nonpharmacologic therapy, and to simple analgesics, e.g., acetaminophen.

CONTRAINDICATIONS

- Do not administer to patients with known hypersensitivity to hyaluronate preparations.
- Intra-articular injections are contraindicated in cases of past and present infections or skin diseases in the area of the injection site.

WARNINGS

- Do not concomitantly use disinfectants containing quaternary ammonium salts for skin preparation because hyaluronic acid can precipitate in their presence.
- Anaphylactoid and allergic reactions have been reported with this product. See Adverse Events Section for more detail.
- Transient increases in inflammation in the injected knee following Hyalgan® injection in some patients with inflammatory arthritis such as rheumatoid arthritis or gouty arthritis have been reported.

PRECAUTIONS

General

- The effectiveness of a single treatment cycle of less than 3 injections has not been established.
- The safety and effectiveness of the use of Hyalgan® in joints other than the knee have not been established.
- The safety and effectiveness of the use of Hyalgan® concomitantly with other intra-articular injectables have not been established.
- Use caution when injecting Hyalgan® into patients who are allergic to avian proteins, feathers, and egg products.
- Strict aseptic administration technique must be followed.
- **STERILE CONTENTS.** The vial/syringe is intended for single use. The contents of the vial must be used immediately once the container has been opened. Discard any unused Hyalgan®.
- Do not use Hyalgan® if the package is opened or damaged. Store in the original packaging (protected from light) below 77° F (25° C). DO NOT FREEZE.
- Remove joint effusion, if present, before injecting Hyalgan®.

Continued on next page

This product information was prepared in September 2004. On these and other products of Sanofi-Synthelabo Inc., detailed information may be obtained on a current basis by direct inquiry to Product Information Services, 90 Park Avenue, New York, NY 10016 (toll free 1-800-446-6267).

TABLE 2. STUDY DESIGN

Routes of Administration	Hyalgan®	Placebo	Naproxen
s.c.	Lidocaine (1%)	Lidocaine (1%)	Lidocaine (1%)
i.a.*	Hyalgan® (20 mg/2 mL)	Phosphate-Buffered Saline (2 mL)	none
p.o./b.i.d.	Placebo for naproxen capsules	Placebo for naproxen capsules	Naproxen capsules (500 mg)
p.o./p.r.n. (not to exceed 4 grams/day)	Acetaminophen	Acetaminophen	Acetaminophen

Legend: s.c. = subcutaneous; i.a. = intra-articular; p.o. = by mouth; b.i.d. = twice a day; p.r.n. = as needed
* Synovial fluid was aspirated (when present) in the Hyalgan® and placebo groups.

TABLE 3
Demographic Characteristics of All Randomized Subjects

DEMOGRAPHIC VARIABLE	TREATMENT			
	Hyalgan® N = 164	Placebo N = 168	Naproxen N = 163	TOTAL N = 495
AGE (years):				
Mean	63.5	64.3	63.2	63.7
SD	10.1	10.0	9.2	9.8
Range	41–90	44–85	40–80	40–90
Gender [N (%)]:				
Female	99 (60.3)	91 (54.1)	99 (60.7)	289 (58.4)
Male	65 (39.6)	77 (45.8)	64 (39.3)	206 (41.6)
Race [N (%)]:				
Caucasian	137 (83.6)	135 (80.4)	133 (81.6)	405 (81.8)
Black	23 (14.0)	32 (19.0)	25 (15.3)	80 (16.2)
Other	4 (4.2)	1 (1.0)	5 (3.1)	10 (2.0)
Height (cm):				
Mean	167.8	168.6	167.6	168.0
SD	8.8	10.7	11.9	10.5
Range	145–190	142–193	102–198	102–198
Weight (kg):				
Mean	88.4	88.1	89.7	88.7
SD	18.0	18.2	18.4	18.2
Range	46–139	49–170	45–150	45–170
NSAIDs Use (N, %)	107 (65.2)	117 (69.6)	113 (69.3)	337 (68.1)
Use of Assistive Devices (N, %)	35 (21.3)	34 (20.2)	32 (19.6)	101 (20.4)
Physical Therapy (N, %)	20 (12.2)	17 (10.1)	25 (15.3)	62 (12.5)

Legend: cm = centimeters; kg = kilograms; SD = standard deviation

TABLE 4
Clinical Results

Evaluation	Success Criteria	Results
100 mm VAS for pain during 50- foot walk.	A statistically significant (alpha = 0.05) reduction on mean VAS for Hyalgan® when compared to placebo at Week 26. This difference was also to exceed one fourth of the Standard Deviation of the mean change from baseline.	At Week 26, the difference between the Hyalgan®-treated group and the placebo-treated group adjusted means was 8.85 mm (p = 0.0043), which is a difference of approximately one-third of a standard deviation (Table 5).
Masked Evaluator Categorical Assessment of subject pain (0=none to 5=disabled) during the 48 hours preceding visits.	The number of Hyalgan®-treated subjects showing improvement at Week 26 was to be concordant with the VAS results; however, not required to be independently statistically significant.	At Week 26 the masked evaluator's categorical assessment of pain indicated that the Hyalgan®-treated subjects experienced less pain than the placebo-treated subjects (Table 6).

(Table continued on next page)

Hyalgan—Cont.

Information for Patients

- Provide patients with a copy of the Patient Information prior to use.
- Transient pain and/or swelling of the injected joint may occur after intra-articular injection of Hyalgan®.
- As with any invasive joint procedure, it is recommended that the patient avoid any strenuous activities or prolonged (i.e., more than 1 hour) weight-bearing activities such as jogging or tennis within 48 hours following the intra-articular injection.

Use in Specific Populations

- **Pregnancy:** *Teratogenic Effects*—Reproductive toxicity studies, including multigeneration studies, have been performed in rats and rabbits at doses up to 11 times the anticipated human dose (1.43 mg/kg per treatment cycle) and have revealed no evidence of impaired fertility or harm to the experimental animal fetus due to intra-articular injections of Hyalgan®. Animal reproduction studies are not always predictive of human response. The safety and effectiveness of Hyalgan® have not been established in pregnant women.
- **Nursing Mothers:** It is not known if Hyalgan® is excreted in human milk. The safety and effectiveness of Hyalgan® have not been established in lactating women.
- **Pediatrics:** The safety and effectiveness of Hyalgan® have not been demonstrated in children.

ADVERSE EVENTS

Hyalgan® was investigated in a pivotal clinical investigation conducted in the United States in which there were three arms (164 subjects treated with Hyalgan®; 168 with placebo; and 163 with naproxen) (refer to Table 1). Common adverse events reported for the Hyalgan®-treated subjects were gastrointestinal complaints, injection site pain, knee swelling/effusion, local skin reactions (rash, ecchymosis), pruritus, and headache. Swelling and effusion, local skin reactions (ecchymosis and rash), and headache occurred at equal frequency in the Hyalgan®- and placebo-treated groups. Hyalgan®-treated subjects had 48/164 (29%) incidents of gastrointestinal complaints that were not statistically different from the placebo-treated group. A statistically significant difference in the occurrence of pain at the injection site was noted in the Hyalgan®-treated subjects: 38/164 (23%) in comparison to 22/168 (13%) in the placebo-treated subjects (p = 0.022). There were 6/164 (4%) premature discontinuations in Hyalgan®-treated subjects due to injection site pain in comparison to 1/168 (<1%) in the placebo-treated subjects. These differences were not statistically significant.

Two (2/164, 1.2%) Hyalgan®-treated subjects and 3/168 (1.8%) placebo-treated subjects were reported to have positive bacterial cultures of effusion aspirated from the treated knee. The two Hyalgan®-treated subjects and two of the placebo-treated subjects did not exhibit evidence of infection clinically or subsequently and were not treated with antibiotics. One of the placebo-treated subjects was hospitalized and received presumptive treatment for septic arthritis.

Hyalgan® has been in clinical use in Europe since 1987. Analysis of the adverse events that have been reported with the use of Hyalgan® in Europe reveals that most of the events are related to local symptoms such as pain, swelling/effusion, and warmth or redness at the injection site. In the two events reported as anaphylactoid reactions, Hyalgan® treatment was discontinued and both had favorable outcomes. Three cases of allergic reactions were reported in which the patients were discontinued from Hyalgan® treatment and the incidents resolved. Seven cases of fever were reported in which three of the cases were reported to be associated with local reactions; pyogenic arthritis was reported to be ruled out in these three cases. All the fever patients were discontinued from Hyalgan® treatment and all incidents resolved. One incident of shock (which was described as a "hypotensive crisis") was reported. The incident resolved and Hyalgan® treatment was continued.

Adverse experience data from the literature contain no evidence of increased risk relating to retreatment with Hyalgan®. The frequency and severity of adverse events occurring during repeat treatment cycles did not increase over that reported for a single treatment cycle. (Carrabba et al., 1995; Carrabba et al., 1991; Kotz and Kolarz, 1999; Scali, 1995).

TABLE 1
Incidence[1] of Adverse Events Occurring in More Than 5% of All Subjects

Adverse Event	Hyalgan® N = 164	Placebo N = 168
Gastrointestinal Complaints[2]	48 (29%)	59 (36%)
Injection site pain[3]	38 (23%)[4]	22 (13%)
Headache	30 (18%)	29 (17%)
Local skin[5]	23 (14%)	17 (10%)
Local joint pain and swelling[6]	21 (13%)	22 (13%)
Pruritus (local)	12 (7%)	7 (4%)

Notes: [1] Number and % of subjects
[2] Severe in 4 Hyalgan®-treated subjects and 4 placebo-treated subjects
[3] Severe in 5 Hyalgan®-treated subjects and 2 placebo-treated subjects
[4] Statistically significant (p=0.02)
[5] Includes ecchymosis and rash
[6] Severe in 2 Hyalgan®-treated subjects (1.2%) and 1 placebo-treated subjects

CLINICAL STUDY

The use of Hyalgan® as a treatment for pain in OA of the knee was investigated in a multicenter clinical trial conducted in the United States.

Study Design

This study was a double-masked, placebo and naproxen-controlled, multicenter prospective clinical trial with three treatment arms, as summarized in Table 2. A total of 495 subjects with moderate to severe pain was randomized (at baseline evaluation) into three treatment groups in a ratio of 1:1:1 Hyalgan®, placebo, or naproxen.

[See table 2 above]

Patient Population and Demographics

The demographics of trial participants were comparable across treatment groups with regard to age, sex, race, height, weight, history of osteoarthritis, prior use of NSAIDs, prior physical therapy, and use of assistive devices (refer to Table 3).

[See table 3 above]

Evaluation Schedule

After meeting initial screening requirements NSAID therapy was discontinued. After 2 weeks, all subjects returned for baseline evaluations. The baseline evaluation included assessment of three primary effectiveness criteria; measurement of pain during a 50-foot walk test using a 100 mm Visual Analog Scale (VAS), a categorical assessment (0 = none to 5 = disabled) of pain, as assessed by a masked evaluator, during the 48 hours preceding the visit, and a categorical assessment (0 = none to 5 = disabled) of pain, as assessed by the subject, during the 48 hours preceding the visit.

All subjects who completed the NSAID washout period and met all entry requirements received their first injection after randomization. All subjects received subcutaneous lidocaine injections. Intra-articular injections (Hyalgan®, placebo) were administered weekly for a total of 5 injections (Weeks 0–4). The naproxen group received 500 mg of naproxen to be taken b.i.d. for 26 weeks.

Subsequent visits and evaluations took place at Weeks 5, 9, 12, 16, 21, and 26. Safety and effectiveness criteria were assessed and recorded at these time periods.

Clinical Results

For this trial, overall success for effectiveness was defined as meeting all four of the success criteria listed in Table 4 using scores from week 26. The criteria were met (refer to Tables 4 through 8).

[See table 4 on previous page and above]
[See table 5 above]
[See table 6 above]
[See table 7 at top of next page]
[See table 8 at top of next page]

Additional Analyses

a. An analysis of study completers was performed as follows: Success was defined as 1) achieving a 20 mm decrease in the VAS for the 50-foot walk test by Week 5, and 2) maintaining this improvement through Week 26. In this analysis greater proportions of Hyalgan®-treated subjects (59/105, 56%) than either placebo- (47/115, 41%) or naproxen-treated subjects (51/113, 45%) were successful under this definition. The Hyalgan®-placebo comparison was statistically significant ($p = 0.031$, Fisher's Exact Test).

Since patients were not followed beyond Week 26, it is unknown how long pain relief continued. There are reports in the literature of some patients experiencing benefit beyond 26 weeks.

b. *Categorical Assessment of Pain—Subjects:* A longitudinal analysis of categorical assessment of pain by the subject, which analyzed the percentage of subjects who attained success revealed that a significantly higher percentage of Hyalgan®-treated subjects as compared to the placebo-treated subjects (55/105, 52% vs 43/115, 37%, $p = 0.030$, Fisher's Exact Test) achieved success (an improvement of greater than or equal to one point on the five-point scale) and maintained this success from Week 5 until Week 26.

Supplementary Clinical Information

Three randomized, controlled clinical investigations were performed that provide information about a three-injection treatment course of Hyalgan®. In all of the studies the patients were followed for 60 days.

Two studies provided a comparison to placebo. One of the placebo-controlled studies evaluated two treatment doses of Hyalgan®, 20 mg/2 ml and 40 mg/2 ml. The 20 mg/2 ml treatment arm included 19 knees, the 40 mg/2 ml included 20 knees, and the placebo arm included 18 knees. The other placebo study included 20 knees in the treatment group and 18 knees in the placebo-treatment group. The third study provided a comparison between patients treated with three weekly injections of Hyalgan® followed by 2 weekly treatments with arthrocentesis with patients treated with arthrocentesis for five weeks, and arthrocentesis and placebo injections for five weeks. Additional arms of this study assessed additional treatment regimens. Statistical evaluation of the data was performed at day 60. In this study only patients considered to be a success were followed beyond day 60. These patients were followed for 180 days, however, due to the number of dropouts, statistical evaluation was not performed on data gathered at time points beyond day 60. The results of these investigations reported that the three-injection Hyalgan® treated patients experienced pain relief beginning at day 21 and continuing throughout the remaining 60-day observation period.

Safety

In order for the product to be considered safe, the incidence of severe swelling and pain consequent to intra-articular injection should be less than 5%. This criterion was met as indicated in Table 1. See the Adverse Events Section.

DETAILED DEVICE DESCRIPTION

Each vial or syringe contains:

Sodium Hyaluronate	20.0 mg
Sodium chloride	17.0 mg
Monobasic sodium phosphate • $2H_2O$	0.1 mg
Dibasic sodium phosphate • $12H_2O$	1.2 mg
Water for injection	q.s.* to 2.0 mL

*q.s. = up to

HOW SUPPLIED

Hyalgan® is supplied as a sterile, non-pyrogenic solution in 2 mL vials or 2 mL pre-filled syringes.

DIRECTIONS FOR USE

Hyalgan® is administered by intra-articular injection. A treatment cycle consists of five injections given at weekly intervals. Some patients may experience benefit with three injections given at weekly intervals. This has been noted in studies reported in the literature in which patients treated with three injections were followed for 60 days.

Precaution: Do not use Hyalgan® if the package is opened or damaged. Store in the original packaging (protected from light) below 77° F (25° C). DO NOT FREEZE.

TABLE 4 *(cont.)*
Clinical Results

Evaluation	Success Criteria	Results
Subjects' Categorical Assessment of pain (0=none to 5=disabled) during the 48 hours preceding visits.	The number of Hyalgan®-treated subjects showing improvement at Week 26 was to be concordant with the VAS results; however, not required to be independently statistically significant.	At Week 26 the subjects' categorical assessment of pain indicated that the Hyalgan®-treated subjects experienced less pain than the placebo-treated subjects (Table 7).
Magnitude of the observed effect for Hyalgan® versus placebo on both the VAS and the categorical pain assessments.	At Week 26 the magnitude of the observed effect for Hyalgan® versus placebo on both the VAS and the categorical pain assessments were to be at least 50% of those observed for the naproxen group.	The improvement in pain on the VAS exhibited by the Hyalgan®-treated group relative to the placebo-treated group were at least 50% of the benefits exhibited by the naproxen-treated group relative to the placebo-treated group. The results of the categorical assessments by the masked evaluator and the subject indicated that improvement of the Hyalgan®-treated group relative to the placebo-treated group was at least 50% of the benefits exhibited by the naproxen-treated group relative to the placebo-treated group (Table 8).

TABLE 5
ANCOVA of 50-Foot Walk Test (mm) VAS by Week for All Completed Subjects

	Week							
	3	4	5	9	12	16	21	26
Adjusted Means Hyalgan®	27.23	21.54	19.29	20.04	20.26	20.83	18.44	17.88
Placebo	32.35	28.57	25.67	24.28	26.66	25.44	24.77	26.73
Hyalgan® versus Placebo	5.13	7.03	6.39	4.24	6.40	4.61	6.33	8.846
p-value	0.06	0.01	0.01	0.1	0.03	0.1	0.02	0.004

TABLE 6
Masked Evaluators' Categorical Assessments of Pain for Completed Subjects in Prior 48 Hours: Level of Pain by Treatment Group at Baseline and Week 26

	NUMBER (%) OF SUBJECTS IN CATEGORY					
	Hyalgan®		Placebo		Naproxen	
	Baseline	Week 26	Baseline	Week 26	Baseline	Week 26
None (0)	0 (0.0)	27 (25.7)	0 (0.0)	15 (13.0)	0 (0.0)	17 (15.0)
Slight (1)	1 (1.0)	23 (21.9)	0 (0.0)	27 (23.5)	0 (0.0)	32 (28.3)
Mild (2)	2 (1.9)	24 (22.9)	2 (1.7)	29 (25.2)	2 (1.8)	27 (23.9)
Moderate (3)	69 (65.7)	26 (24.8)	85 (73.9)	34 (29.6)	79 (70.5)	28 (24.8)
Marked (4)	33 (31.4)	5 (4.8)	28 (24.3)	10 (8.7)	31 (27.7)	9 (8.0)
TOTAL	105 (100)	105 (100)	115 (100)	115 (100)	112* (100)	113 (100)

*One Naproxen treated subject was missing a Baseline assessment.

Precaution: Strict aseptic administration technique must be followed.

Warning: Do not concomitantly use disinfectants containing quaternary ammonium salts for skin preparation because hyaluronic acid can precipitate in their presence.

Inject subcutaneous lidocaine or similar local anesthetic prior to injection of Hyalgan®.

Precaution: Remove joint effusion, if present, before injection of Hyalgan®.

Do not use the same syringe for removing joint effusion and for injecting Hyalgan®.

Take care to remove the tip cap of the syringe and needle aseptically.

Inject Hyalgan® into the joint through a 20-gauge needle.

Precaution: The vial/syringe is intended for single use. The contents of the vial must be used immediately once the container has been opened. Discard any unused Hyalgan®. Inject the full 2 mL in one knee only. If treatment is bilateral, a separate vial should be used for each knee.

MANUFACTURED BY
Fidia Farmaceutici S.p.A.
Via Ponte della Fabbrica 3/A
35031 Abano Terme, Padua (PD), Italy

DISTRIBUTED BY
Sanofi-Synthelabo Inc.
90 Park Avenue
New York, NY 10016

REFERENCES

1. M. Carrabba et al., 1991 Hyaluronic acid sodium salt (Hyalgan®) in the treatment of patients with osteoarthritis of the knee: a controlled trial versus Orgotein, Final Report, April 1991. Data on file.
2. M. Carrabba et al., 1995. Effectiveness and safety of 1, 3 and 5 injections of 20 mg/2 ml Hyalgan® in comparison with a placebo and with arthrocentesis only, in the treatment of knee osteoarthritis. European Journal of Rheumatology and Inflammation 15:25–31.
3. M. Dougados et al., 1993. High molecular weight sodium hyaluronate (hyalectin) in osteoarthritis of the knee: a one-year placebo-controlled trial. Osteoarthritis and Cartilage 1:97–103.
4. R. Kotz and G. Kolarz, 1997 pulished as R. Kotz and G. Kolarz, 1999. Intra-articular hyaluronic acid: duration of effect and results of repeated treatment cycles. The American Journal of Orthopedics, 28:5–7.

Continued on next page

This product information was prepared in September 2004. On these and other products of Sanofi-Synthelabo Inc., detailed information may be obtained on a current basis by direct inquiry to Product Information Services, 90 Park Avenue, New York, NY 10016 (toll free 1-800-446-6267).

TABLE 7
Subjects' Categorical Assessments of Pain for Completed Subjects in Prior 48 Hours: Level of Pain by Treatment Group at Baseline and Week 26

	NUMBER (%) OF SUBJECTS IN CATEGORY					
	Hyalgan®		Placebo		Naproxen	
	Baseline	Week 26	Baseline	Week 26	Baseline	Week 26
None (0)	1 (1.0)	23 (21.9)	0 (0.0)	14 (12.2)	0 (0.0)	13 (11.5)
Slight (1)	2 (1.9)	27 (25.7)	0 (0.0)	24 (20.9)	1 (0.9)	31 (27.4)
Mild (2)	6 (5.7)	19 (18.1)	8 (7.0)	24 (20.9)	7 (6.2)	26 (23.0)
Moderate (3)	62 (59.0)	26 (24.8)	78 (67.8)	40 (34.8)	72 (63.7)	31 (27.4)
Marked (4)	34 (32.4)	10 (9.5)	29 (25.2)	13 (11.3)	33 (29.2)	12 (10.6)
TOTAL	105 (100)	105 (100)	115 (100)	115 (100)	113 (100)	113 (100)

TABLE 8
Hyalgan® Effect as a Percentage of the Naproxen-Placebo Difference

Assessment	Hyalgan® (HYL)	Placebo (PLA)	Naproxen (NAP)	HYL-PLA	NAP-HYL	NAP-PLA	(HYL-PLA) % of (NAP-PLA)
VAS for 50 foot Walk Baseline Adjusted Mean Effect Sizes From ANCOVA				−8.85 mm on a 100 mm VAS	4.12 mm on a 100 mm VAS	−4.73* mm on a 100 mm VAS	187%
% of Subjects Improved by Masked Evaluators	78.1	69.6	73.2	8.5	−4.9	3.6	236%
% of Subjects Improved by Subjects	73.3	62.6	67.3	10.7	−6.0	4.7	228%

*Imputed as (NAP-HYL)+(HYL-PLA).
Note that Effectiveness Success Criterion D is satisfied since ((HYL-PLA) % of (NAP-PLA))>50% for all three of the above pain assessments.

Hyalgan—Cont.

5. G. Leardini et al., 1987. Intra-articular sodium hyaluronate (Hyalgan®) in gonarthrosis. Clinical Trials Journal 24(4):341–350.
6. J.J. Scali, 1995. Intra-articular hyaluronic acid in the treatment of osteoarthritis of the knee: a long term study 15(1):57–62.

07241191
Revised July 2001

Shown in Product Identification Guide, page 332

PLAQUENIL® ℞
HYDROXYCHLOROQUINE SULFATE, USP

WARNING
PHYSICIANS SHOULD COMPLETELY FAMILIARIZE THEMSELVES WITH THE COMPLETE CONTENTS OF THIS LEAFLET BEFORE PRESCRIBING HYDROXYCHLOROQUINE.

DESCRIPTION

Hydroxychloroquine sulfate is a colorless crystalline solid, soluble in water to at least 20 percent; chemically the drug is 2-[[4-[(7-Chloro-4- quinolyl) amino] pentyl] ethylamino] ethanol sulfate (1:1).

Plaquenil (hydroxychloroquine sulfate) tablets contain 200 mg hydroxychloroquine sulfate, equivalent to 155 mg base, and are for oral administration.

Inactive Ingredients: Dibasic Calcium Phosphate, Hydroxypropyl Methylcellulose, Magnesium Stearate, Polyethylene glycol 400, Polysorbate 80, Starch, Titanium Dioxide.

ACTIONS

The drug possesses antimalarial actions and also exerts a beneficial effect in lupus erythematosus (chronic discoid or systemic) and acute or chronic rheumatoid arthritis. The precise mechanism of action is not known.

INDICATIONS

PLAQUENIL is indicated for the suppressive treatment and treatment of acute attacks of malaria due to *Plasmodium vivax, P. malariae, P. ovale,* and susceptible strains of *P. falciparum.* It is also indicated for the treatment of discoid and systemic lupus erythematosus, and rheumatoid arthritis.

CONTRAINDICATIONS

Use of this drug is contraindicated (1) in the presence of retinal or visual field changes attributable to any 4-aminoquinoline compound, (2) in patients with known hypersensitivity to 4-aminoquinoline compounds, and (3) for long-term therapy in children.

WARNINGS, General

PLAQUENIL is not effective against chloroquine-resistant strains of *P. falciparum.*

Children are especially sensitive to the 4-aminoquinoline compounds. A number of fatalities have been reported following the accidental ingestion of chloroquine, sometimes in relatively small doses (0.75 g or 1 g in one 3- year-old child). Patients should be strongly warned to keep these drugs out of the reach of children.

Use of PLAQUENIL in patients with psoriasis may precipitate a severe attack of psoriasis. When used in patients with porphyria the condition may be exacerbated. The preparation should not be used in these conditions unless in the judgment of the physician the benefit to the patient outweighs the possible hazard.

Usage in Pregnancy—Usage of this drug during pregnancy should be avoided except in the suppression or treatment of malaria when in the judgment of the physician the benefit outweighs the possible hazard. It should be noted that radioactively-tagged chloroquine administered intravenously to pregnant, pigmented CBA mice passed rapidly across the placenta. It accumulated selectively in the melanin structures of the fetal eyes and was retained in the ocular tissues for five months after the drug had been eliminated from the rest of the body.

PRECAUTIONS, General

Antimalarial compounds should be used with caution in patients with hepatic disease or alcoholism or in conjunction with known hepatotoxic drugs.

Periodic blood cell counts should be made if patients are given prolonged therapy. If any severe blood disorder appears which is not attributable to the disease under treatment, discontinuation of the drug should be considered. The drug should be administered with caution in patients having G-6-PD (glucose-6-phosphate dehydrogenase) deficiency.

OVERDOSAGE

The 4-aminoquinoline compounds are very rapidly and completely absorbed after ingestion, and in accidental overdosage, or rarely with lower doses in hypersensitive patients, toxic symptoms may occur within 30 minutes. These consist of headache, drowsiness, visual disturbances, cardiovascular collapse, and convulsions, followed by sudden and early respiratory and cardiac arrest. The electrocardiogram may reveal atrial standstill, nodal rhythm, prolonged intraventricular conduction time, and progressive bradycardia leading to ventricular fibrillation and/or arrest. Treatment is symptomatic and must be prompt with immediate evacuation of the stomach by emesis (at home, before transportation to the hospital) or gastric lavage until the stomach is completely emptied. If finely powdered, activated charcoal is introduced by the stomach tube, after lavage, and within 30 minutes after ingestion of the tablets, it may inhibit further intestinal absorption of the drug. To be effective, the dose of activated charcoal should be at least five times the estimated dose of hydroxychloroquine ingested. Convulsions, if present, should be controlled before attempting gastric lavage. If due to cerebral stimulation, cautious administration of an ultrashort-acting barbiturate may be tried but, if due to anoxia, it should be corrected by oxygen administration, artificial respiration or, in shock with hypotension, by vasopressor therapy. Because of the importance of supporting respiration, tracheal intubation or tracheostomy, followed by gastric lavage, may also be necessary. Exchange transfusions have been used to reduce the level of 4-aminoquinoline drug in the blood.

A patient who survives the acute phase and is asymptomatic should be closely observed for at least six hours. Fluids may be forced, and sufficient ammonium chloride (8 g daily in divided doses for adults) may be administered for a few days to acidify the urine to help promote urinary excretion in cases of both overdosage and sensitivity.

MALARIA

ACTIONS

Like chloroquine phosphate, USP, PLAQUENIL is highly active against the erythrocytic forms of *P. vivax* and *malariae* and most strains of *P. falciparum* (but not the gametocytes of *P. falciparum*).

PLAQUENIL does not prevent relapses in patients with *vivax* or *malariae* malaria because it is not effective against exo-erythrocytic forms of the parasite, nor will it prevent *vivax* or *malariae* infection when administered as a prophylactic. It is highly effective as a suppressive agent in patients with *vivax* or *malariae* malaria, in terminating acute attacks, and significantly lengthening the interval between treatment and relapse. In patients with *falciparum* malaria, it abolishes the acute attack and effects complete cure of the infection, unless due to a resistant strain of *P. falciparum.*

INDICATIONS

PLAQUENIL is indicated for the treatment of acute attacks and suppression of malaria.

WARNING

In recent years, it has been found that certain strains of *P. falciparum* have become resistant to 4-aminoquinoline compounds (including hydroxychloroquine) as shown by the fact that normally adequate doses have failed to prevent or cure clinical malaria or parasitemia. Treatment with quinine or other specific forms of therapy is therefore advised for patients infected with a resistant strain of parasites.

ADVERSE REACTIONS

Following the administration in doses adequate for the treatment of an acute malarial attack, mild and transient headache, dizziness, and gastrointestinal complaints (diarrhea, anorexia, nausea, abdominal cramps and, on rare occasions, vomiting) may occur. Cardiomyopathy has been rarely reported with high daily dosages of hydroxychloroquine.

DOSAGE AND ADMINISTRATION

One tablet of 200 mg of hydroxychloroquine sulfate is equivalent to 155 mg base.

Malaria: Suppression—*In adults,* 400 mg (=310 mg base) on exactly the same day of each week. *In infants and children,* the weekly suppressive dosage is 5 mg, calculated as base, per kg of body weight, but should not exceed the adult dose regardless of weight.

If circumstances permit, suppressive therapy should begin two weeks prior to exposure. However, failing this, in adults an initial double (loading) dose of 800 mg (= 620 mg base), or in children 10 mg base/kg may be taken in two divided doses, six hours apart. The suppressive therapy should be continued for eight weeks after leaving the endemic area.

Treatment of the acute attack—*In adults,* an initial dose of 800 mg (= 620 mg base) followed by 400 mg (= 310 mg base) in six to eight hours and 400 mg (= 310 mg base) on each of two consecutive days (total 2 g hydroxychloroquine sulfate or 1.55 g base). An alternative method, employing a single dose of 800 mg (= 620 mg base), has also proved effective.

The dosage for adults may also be calculated on the basis of body weight; this method is preferred for infants and children. A total dose representing 25 mg of base per kg of body weight is administered in three days, as follows:

First dose: 10 mg base per kg (but not exceeding a single dose of 620 mg base).
Second dose: 5 mg base per kg (but not exceeding a single dose of 310 mg base) 6 hours after first dose.
Third dose: 5 mg base per kg 18 hours after second dose.
Fourth dose: 5 mg base per kg 24 hours after third dose.

For radical cure of *vivax* and *malariae* malaria concomitant therapy with an 8-aminoquinoline compound is necessary.

LUPUS ERYTHEMATOSUS AND RHEUMATOID ARTHRITIS

INDICATIONS

PLAQUENIL is useful in patients with the following disorders who have not responded satisfactorily to drugs with less potential for serious side effects: lupus erythematosus (chronic discoid and systemic) and acute or chronic rheumatoid arthritis.

WARNINGS

PHYSICIANS SHOULD COMPLETELY FAMILIARIZE THEMSELVES WITH THE COMPLETE CONTENTS OF THIS LEAFLET BEFORE PRESCRIBING PLAQUENIL.

Irreversible retinal damage has been observed in some patients who had received long-term or high-dosage 4-aminoquinoline therapy for discoid and systemic lupus erythematosus, or rheumatoid arthritis. Retinopathy has been reported to be dose related.

When prolonged therapy with any antimalarial compound is contemplated, initial (base line) and periodic (every three months) ophthalmologic examinations (including visual acuity, expert slit-lamp, funduscopic, and visual field tests) should be performed.

If there is any indication of abnormality in the visual acuity, visual field, or retinal macular areas (such as pigmentary changes, loss of foveal reflex), or any visual symptoms (such as light flashes and streaks) which are not fully explainable by difficulties of accommodation or corneal opacities, the drug should be discontinued immediately and the patient closely observed for possible progression. Retinal changes (and visual disturbances) may progress even after cessation of therapy.

All patients on long-term therapy with this preparation should be questioned and examined periodically, including the testing of knee and ankle reflexes, to detect any evidence of muscular weakness. If weakness occurs, discontinue the drug.

In the treatment of rheumatoid arthritis, if objective improvement (such as reduced joint swelling, increased mobility) does not occur within six months, the drug should be discontinued. Safe use of the drug in the treatment of juvenile arthritis has not been established.

PRECAUTIONS

Dermatologic reactions to PLAQUENIL may occur and, therefore, proper care should be exercised when it is administered to any patient receiving a drug with a significant tendency to produce dermatitis.

The methods recommended for early diagnosis of "chloroquine retinopathy" consist of (1) funduscopic examination of the macula for fine pigmentary disturbances or loss of the foveal reflex and (2) examination of the central visual field with a small red test object for pericentral or paracentral scotoma or determination of retinal thresholds to red. Any unexplained visual symptoms, such as light flashes or streaks should also be regarded with suspicion as possible manifestations of retinopathy.

If serious toxic symptoms occur from overdosage or sensitivity, it has been suggested that ammonium chloride (8 g daily in divided doses for adults) be administered orally three or four days a week for several months after therapy has been stopped, as acidification of the urine increases renal excretion of the 4-aminoquinoline compounds by 20 to 90 percent. However, caution must be exercised in patients with impaired renal function and/or metabolic acidosis.

ADVERSE REACTIONS

Not all of the following reactions have been observed with every 4-aminoquinoline compound during long-term therapy, but they have been reported with one or more and should be borne in mind when drugs of this class are administered. Adverse effects with different compounds vary in type and frequency.

CNS Reactions: Irritability, nervousness, emotional changes, nightmares, psychosis, headache, dizziness, vertigo, tinnitus, nystagmus, nerve deafness, convulsions, ataxia.

Neuromuscular Reactions: Skeletal muscle palsies or skeletal muscle myopathy or neuromyopathy leading to progressive weakness and atrophy of proximal muscle groups which may be associated with mild sensory changes, depression of tendon reflexes and abnormal nerve conduction.

Ocular Reactions:

A. *Ciliary body:* Disturbance of accommodation with symptoms of blurred vision. This reaction is dose related and reversible with cessation of therapy.

B. *Cornea:* Transient edema, punctate to lineal opacities, decreased corneal sensitivity. The corneal changes, with or without accompanying symptoms (blurred vision, halos around lights, photophobia), are fairly common, but reversible. Corneal deposits may appear as early as three weeks following initiation of therapy.

The incidence of corneal changes and visual side effects appears to be considerably lower with hydroxychloroquine than with chloroquine.

C. *Retina:*

Macula: Edema, atrophy, abnormal pigmentation (mild pigment stippling to a "bull's-eye" appearance), loss of foveal reflex, increased macular recovery time following exposure to a bright light (photo-stress test), elevated retinal threshold to red light in macular, paramacular, and peripheral retinal areas.

Other fundus changes include optic disc pallor and atrophy, attenuation of retinal arterioles, fine granular pigmentary disturbances in the peripheral retina and prominent choroidal patterns in advanced stage.

D. *Visual field defects:* pericentral or paracentral scotoma, central scotoma with decreased visual acuity, rarely field constriction.

The most common visual symptoms attributed to the retinopathy are: reading and seeing difficulties (words, letters, or parts of objects missing), photophobia, blurred distance vision, missing or blacked out areas in the central or peripheral visual field, light flashes and streaks.

Retinopathy appears to be dose related and has occurred within several months (rarely) to several years of daily therapy; a small number of cases have been reported several years after antimalarial drug therapy was discontinued. It has not been noted during prolonged use of weekly doses of the 4-aminoquinoline compounds for suppression of malaria.

Patients with retinal changes may have visual symptoms or may be asymptomatic (with or without visual field changes). Rarely scotomatous vision or field defects may occur without obvious retinal change.

Retinopathy may progress even after the drug is discontinued. In a number of patients, early retinopathy (macular pigmentation sometimes with central field defects) diminished or regressed completely after therapy was discontinued. Paracentral scotoma to red targets (sometimes called "premaculopathy") is indicative of early retinal dysfunction which is usually reversible with cessation of therapy.

A small number of cases of retinal changes have been reported as occurring in patients who received only hydroxychloroquine. These usually consisted of alteration in retinal pigmentation which was detected on periodic ophthalmologic examination; visual field defects were also present in some instances. A case of delayed retinopathy has been reported with loss of vision starting one year after administration of hydroxychloroquine had been discontinued.

Dermatologic Reactions: Bleaching of hair, alopecia, pruritus, skin and mucosal pigmentation, photosensitivity, and skin eruptions (urticarial, morbilliform, lichenoid, maculopapular, purpuric, erythema annulare centrifugum, Stevens Johnsons syndrome, acute generalized exanthematous pustulosis, and exfoliative dermatitis).

Hematologic Reactions: Various blood dyscrasias such as aplastic anemia, agranulocytosis, leukopenia, thrombocytopenia (hemolysis in individuals with glucose-6-phosphate dehydrogenase (G-6-PD) deficiency).

Gastrointestinal Reactions: Anorexia, nausea, vomiting, diarrhea, and abdominal cramps.

Isolated cases of abnormal liver function and fulminant hepatic failure.

Miscellaneous Reactions: Weight loss, lassitude, exacerbation or precipitation of porphyria and nonlight-sensitive psoriasis.

Cardiomyopathy has been rarely reported with high daily dosages of hydroxychloroquine.

DOSAGE AND ADMINISTRATION

One tablet of hydroxychloroquine sulfate, 200 mg, is equivalent to 155 mg base.

Lupus erythematosus —Initially, the average *adult* dose is 400 mg (=310 mg base) once or twice daily. This may be continued for several weeks or months, depending on the response of the patient. For prolonged maintenance therapy, a smaller dose, from 200 mg to 400 mg (= 155 mg to 310 mg base) daily will frequently suffice.

The incidence of retinopathy has been reported to be higher when this maintenance dose is exceeded.

Rheumatoid arthritis —The compound is cumulative in action and will require several weeks to exert its beneficial therapeutic effects, whereas minor side effects may occur relatively early. Several months of therapy may be required before maximum effects can be obtained. If objective improvement (such as reduced joint swelling, increased mobility) does not occur within six months, the drug should be discontinued. Safe use of the drug in the treatment of juvenile rheumatoid arthritis has not been established.

Initial dosage —In ***adults,*** from 400 mg to 600 mg (=310 mg to 465 mg base) daily, each dose to be taken with a meal or a glass of milk. In a small percentage of patients, troublesome side effects may require temporary reduction of the initial dosage. Later (usually from five to ten days), the dose may gradually be increased to the optimum response level, often without return of side effects.

Maintenance dosage —When a good response is obtained (usually in four to twelve weeks), the dosage is reduced by 50 percent and continued at a usual maintenance level of 200 mg to 400 mg (=155 mg to 310 mg base) daily, each dose to be taken with a meal or a glass of milk. The incidence of retinopathy has been reported to be higher when this maintenance dose is exceeded.

Should a relapse occur after medication is withdrawn, therapy may be resumed or continued on an intermittent schedule if there are no ocular contraindications.

Corticosteroids and salicylates may be used in conjunction with this compound, and they can generally be decreased gradually in dosage or eliminated after the drug has been used for several weeks. When gradual reduction of steroid dosage is indicated, it may be done by reducing every four to five days the dose of cortisone by no more than from 5 mg to 15 mg; of hydrocortisone from 5 mg to 10 mg; of prednisolone and prednisone from 1 mg to 2.5 mg; of methylprednisolone and triamcinolone from 1 mg to 2 mg; and of dexamethasone from 0.25 mg to 0.5 mg.

HOW SUPPLIED

Plaquenil tablets are white, to off-white, film coated tablets imprinted "PLAQUENIL" on one face in black ink. Each tablet contains 200 mg hydroxychloroquine sulfate (equivalent to 155 mg base). Bottles of 100 tablets (NDC 0024-1562-10).

Dispense in a tight, light-resistant container as defined in the USP/NF.

Store at room temperature up to 30°C (86°F).

PSW-5H (A)

Revised April 2002

Shown in Product Identification Guide, page 332

PLAVIX® ℞

[plā-vĭcks]

(clopidogrel bisulfate tablets)

DESCRIPTION

PLAVIX (clopidogrel bisulfate) is an inhibitor of ADP -induced platelet aggregation acting by direct inhibition of adenosine diphosphate (ADP) binding to its receptor and of the subsequent ADP-mediated activation of the glycoprotein GPIIb/IIIa complex. Chemically it is methyl (+)-(*S*)-α-(2-chlorophenyl)-6,7-dihydrothieno[3,2-c]pyridine-5(4*H*)-acetate sulfate (1:1). The empirical formula of clopidogrel bisulfate is $C_{16}H_{16}ClNO_2S \bullet H_2SO_4$ and its molecular weight is 419.9.

The structural formula is as follows:

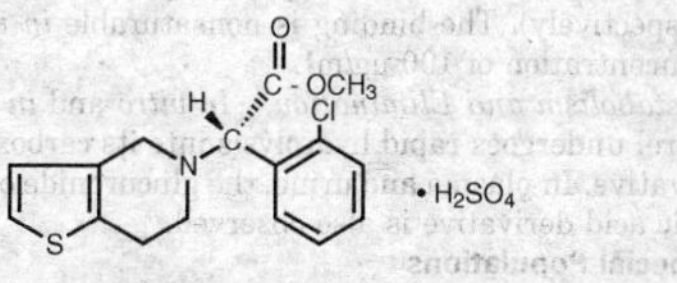

Clopidogrel bisulfate is a white to off-white powder. It is practically insoluble in water at neutral pH but freely soluble at pH 1. It also dissolves freely in methanol, dissolves sparingly in methylene chloride, and is practically insoluble in ethyl ether. It has a specific optical rotation of about +56°.

PLAVIX for oral administration is provided as pink, round, biconvex, debossed film-coated tablets containing 97.875 mg of clopidogrel bisulfate which is the molar equivalent of 75 mg of clopidogrel base.

Each tablet contains hydrogenated castor oil, hydroxypropylcellulose, mannitol, microcrystalline cellulose and polyethylene glycol 6000 as inactive ingredients. The pink film coating contains ferric oxide, hydroxypropyl methylcellulose 2910, lactose monohydrate, titanium dioxide and triacetin. The tablets are polished with Carnauba wax.

CLINICAL PHARMACOLOGY

Mechanism of Action

Clopidogrel is an inhibitor of platelet aggregation. A variety of drugs that inhibit platelet function have been shown to decrease morbid events in people with established cardiovascular atherosclerotic disease as evidenced by stroke or transient ischemic attacks, myocardial infarction, unstable angina or the need for vascular bypass or angioplasty. This indicates that platelets participate in the initiation and/or evolution of these events and that inhibiting them can reduce the event rate.

Pharmacodynamic Properties

Clopidogrel selectively inhibits the binding of adenosine diphosphate (ADP) to its platelet receptor and the subsequent ADP-mediated activation of the glycoprotein GPIIb/IIIa complex, thereby inhibiting platelet aggregation. Biotransformation of clopidogrel is necessary to produce inhibition of platelet aggregation, but an active metabolite responsible for the activity of the drug has not been isolated. Clopidogrel also inhibits platelet aggregation induced by agonists other than ADP by blocking the amplification of platelet activation by released ADP. Clopidogrel does not inhibit phosphodiesterase activity.

Clopidogrel acts by irreversibly modifying the platelet ADP receptor. Consequently, platelets exposed to clopidogrel are affected for the remainder of their lifespan.

Dose dependent inhibition of platelet aggregation can be seen 2 hours after single oral doses of PLAVIX. Repeated doses of 75 mg PLAVIX per day inhibit ADP-induced platelet aggregation on the first day, and inhibition reaches steady state between Day 3 and Day 7. At steady state, the average inhibition level observed with a dose of 75 mg PLAVIX per day was between 40% and 60%. Platelet aggregation and bleeding time gradually return to baseline values after treatment is discontinued, generally in about 5 days.

Pharmacokinetics and Metabolism

After repeated 75-mg oral doses of clopidogrel (base), plasma concentrations of the parent compound, which has no platelet inhibiting effect, are very low and are generally below the quantification limit (0.00025 mg/L) beyond 2 hours after dosing. Clopidogrel is extensively metabolized by the liver. The main circulating metabolite is the carbox-

Continued on next page

This product information was prepared in September 2004. On these and other products of Sanofi-Synthelabo Inc., detailed information may be obtained on a current basis by direct inquiry to Product Information Services, 90 Park Avenue, New York, NY 10016 (toll free 1-800-446-6267).

Plavix—Cont.

ylic acid derivative, and it too has no effect on platelet aggregation. It represents about 85% of the circulating drug-related compounds in plasma.
Following an oral dose of ^{14}C-labeled clopidogrel in humans, approximately 50% was excreted in the urine and approximately 46% in the feces in the 5 days after dosing. The elimination half-life of the main circulating metabolite was 8 hours after single and repeated administration. Covalent binding to platelets accounted for 2% of radiolabel with a half-life of 11 days.
Effect of Food: Administration of PLAVIX (clopidogrel bisulfate) with meals did not significantly modify the bioavailability of clopidogrel as assessed by the pharmacokinetics of the main circulating metabolite.
Absorption and Distribution: Clopidogrel is rapidly absorbed after oral administration of repeated doses of 75 mg clopidogrel (base), with peak plasma levels (≅3 mg/L) of the main circulating metabolite occurring approximately 1 hour after dosing. The pharmacokinetics of the main circulating metabolite are linear (plasma concentrations increased in proportion to dose) in the dose range of 50 to 150 mg of clopidogrel. Absorption is at least 50% based on urinary excretion of clopidogrel-related metabolites.
Clopidogrel and the main circulating metabolite bind reversibly *in vitro* to human plasma proteins (98% and 94%, respectively). The binding is nonsaturable *in vitro* up to a concentration of 100 µg/mL.
Metabolism and Elimination: *In vitro* and *in vivo*, clopidogrel undergoes rapid hydrolysis into its carboxylic acid derivative. In plasma and urine, the glucuronide of the carboxylic acid derivative is also observed.

Special Populations

Geriatric Patients: Plasma concentrations of the main circulating metabolite are significantly higher in elderly (≥75 years) compared to young healthy volunteers but these higher plasma levels were not associated with differences in platelet aggregation and bleeding time. No dosage adjustment is needed for the elderly.
Renally Impaired Patients: After repeated doses of 75 mg PLAVIX per day, plasma levels of the main circulating metabolite were lower in patients with severe renal impairment (creatinine clearance from 5 to 15 mL/min) compared to subjects with moderate renal impairment (creatinine clearance 30 to 60 mL/min) or healthy subjects. Although inhibition of ADP-induced platelet aggregation was lower (25%) than that observed in healthy volunteers, the prolongation of bleeding time was similar to healthy volunteers receiving 75 mg of PLAVIX per day.
Gender: No significant difference was observed in the plasma levels of the main circulating metabolite between males and females. In a small study comparing men and women, less inhibition of ADP-induced platelet aggregation was observed in women, but there was no difference in prolongation of bleeding time. In the large, controlled clinical study (Clopidogrel vs. Aspirin in Patients at Risk of Ischemic Events; CAPRIE), the incidence of clinical outcome events, other adverse clinical events, and abnormal clinical laboratory parameters was similar in men and women.
Race: Pharmacokinetic differences due to race have not been studied.

CLINICAL STUDIES

The clinical evidence for the efficacy of PLAVIX is derived from two double-blind trials: the CAPRIE study (Clopidogrel vs. Aspirin in Patients at Risk of Ischemic Events), a comparison of PLAVIX to aspirin, and the CURE study (Clopidogrel in Unstable Angina to Prevent Recurrent Ischemic Events), a comparison of PLAVIX to placebo, both given in combination with aspirin and other standard therapy.
The CAPRIE trial was a 19,185-patient, 304-center, international, randomized, double-blind, parallel-group study comparing PLAVIX (75 mg daily) to aspirin (325 mg daily). The patients randomized had: 1) recent histories of myocardial infarction (within 35 days); 2) recent histories of ischemic stroke (within 6 months) with at least a week of residual neurological signs; or 3) objectively established peripheral arterial disease. Patients received randomized treatment for an average of 1.6 years (maximum of 3 years). The trial's primary outcome was the time to first occurrence of new ischemic stroke (fatal or not), new myocardial infarction (fatal or not), or other vascular death. Deaths not easily attributable to nonvascular causes were all classified as vascular.

Table 1: Outcome Events in the CAPRIE Primary Analysis

Patients	PLAVIX 9599	aspirin 9586
IS (fatal or not)	438 (4.6%)	461 (4.8%)
MI (fatal or not)	275 (2.9%)	333 (3.5%)
Other vascular death	226 (2.4%)	226 (2.4%)
Total	939 (9.8%)	1020 (10.6%)

As shown in the table, PLAVIX (clopidogrel bisulfate) was associated with a lower incidence of outcome events of every kind. The overall risk reduction (9.8% vs. 10.6%) was 8.7%, P=0.045. Similar results were obtained when all-cause mortality and all-cause strokes were counted instead of vascular mortality and ischemic strokes (risk reduction 6.9%). In patients who survived an on-study stroke or myocardial infarction, the incidence of subsequent events was again lower in the PLAVIX group.
The curves showing the overall event rate are shown in Figure 1. The event curves separated early and continued to diverge over the 3-year follow-up period.

Figure 1: Fatal or Non-Fatal Vascular Events in the CAPRIE Study

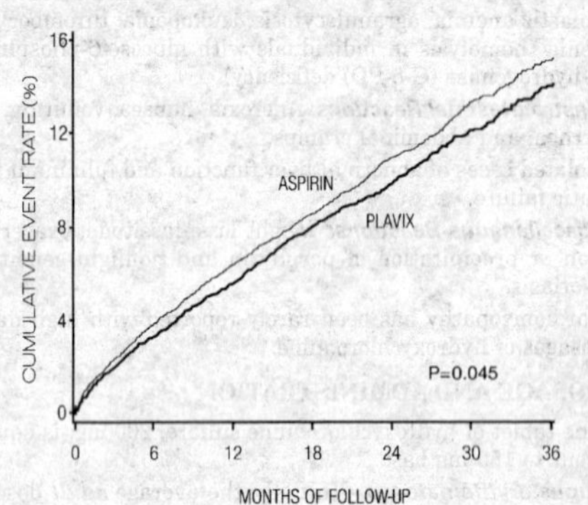

Although the statistical significance favoring PLAVIX over aspirin was marginal (P=0.045), and represents the result of a single trial that has not been replicated, the comparator drug, aspirin, is itself effective (vs. placebo) in reducing cardiovascular events in patients with recent myocardial infarction or stroke. Thus, the difference between PLAVIX and placebo, although not measured directly, is substantial.
The CAPRIE trial included a population that was randomized on the basis of 3 entry criteria. The efficacy of PLAVIX relative to aspirin was heterogeneous across these randomized subgroups (P=0.043). It is not clear whether this difference is real or a chance occurrence. Although the CAPRIE trial was not designed to evaluate the relative benefit of PLAVIX over aspirin in the individual patient subgroups, the benefit appeared to be strongest in patients who were enrolled because of peripheral vascular disease (especially those who also had a history of myocardial infarction) and weaker in stroke patients. In patients who were enrolled in the trial on the sole basis of a recent myocardial infarction, PLAVIX was not numerically superior to aspirin.
In the meta-analyses of studies of aspirin vs. placebo in patients similar to those in CAPRIE, aspirin was associated with a reduced incidence of thrombotic events. There was a suggestion of heterogeneity in these studies too, with the effect strongest in patients with a history of myocardial infarction, weaker in patients with a history of stroke, and not discernible in patients with a history of peripheral vascular disease. With respect to the inferred comparison of PLAVIX to placebo, there is no indication of heterogeneity.
The CURE study included 12,562 patients with acute coronary syndrome without ST segment elevation (unstable angina or non-Q-wave myocardial infarction) and presenting within 24 hours of onset of the most recent episode of chest pain or symptoms consistent with ischemia. Patients were required to have either ECG changes compatible with new ischemia (without ST segment elevation) or elevated cardiac enzymes or troponin I or T to at least twice the upper limit of normal. The patient population was largely Caucasian (82%) and included 38% women, and 52% patients ≥65 years of age.
Patients were randomized to receive PLAVIX (300 mg loading dose followed by 75 mg/day) or placebo, and were treated for up to one year. Patients also received aspirin (75–325 mg once daily) and other standard therapies such as heparin. The use of GPIIb/IIIa inhibitors was not permitted for three days prior to randomization.
The number of patients experiencing the primary outcome (CV death, MI, or stroke) was 582 (9.30%) in the PLAVIX-treated group and 719 (11.41%) in the placebo-treated group, a 20% relative risk reduction (95% CI of 10%-28%; p=0.00009) for the PLAVIX-treated group (see Table 2).
At the end of 12 months, the number of patients experiencing the co-primary outcome (CV death, MI, stroke or refractory ischemia) was 1035 (16.54%) in the PLAVIX-treated group and 1187 (18.83%) in the placebo-treated group, a 14% relative risk reduction (95% CI of 6%-21%, p=0.0005) for the PLAVIX-treated group (see Table 2).
In the PLAVIX-treated group, each component of the two primary endpoints (CV death, MI, stroke, refractory ischemia) occurred less frequently than in the placebo-treated group.
[See table 2 below]
The benefits of PLAVIX were maintained throughout the course of the trial (up to 12 months).

Figure 2: Cardiovascular Death, Myocardial Infarction, and Stroke in the CURE Study

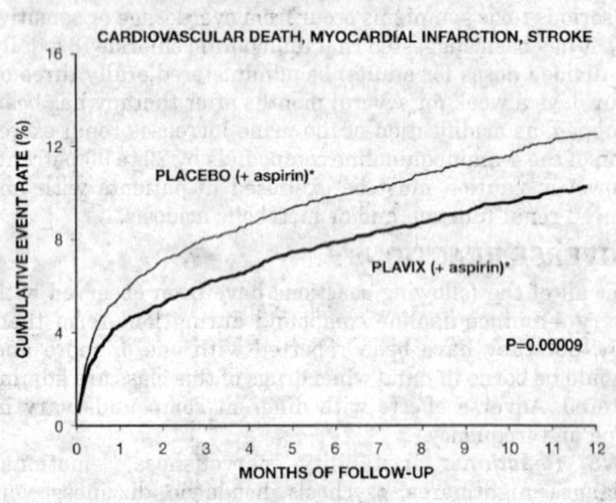

*Other standard therapies were used as appropriate

In CURE, the use of PLAVIX was associated with a lower incidence of CV death, MI or stroke in patient populations with different characteristics, as shown in Figure 3. The benefits associated with PLAVIX (clopidogrel bisulfate tablets) were independent of the use of other acute and long-term cardiovascular therapies, including heparin/LMWH (low molecular weight heparin), IV glycoprotein IIb/IIIa (GPIIb/IIIa) inhibitors, lipid-lowering drugs, beta-blockers, and ACE-inhibitors. The efficacy of PLAVIX was observed independently of the dose of aspirin (75-325 mg once daily). The use of oral anticoagulants, non-study anti-platelet drugs and chronic NSAIDs was not allowed in CURE.
[See figure 3 at top of next column]
The use of PLAVIX in CURE was associated with a decrease in the use of thrombolytic therapy (71 patients [1.1%] in the PLAVIX group, 126 patients [2.0%] in the placebo group; relative risk reduction of 43%, P=0.0001), and GPIIb/IIIa inhibitors (369 patients [5.9%] in the PLAVIX group, 454 patients [7.2%] in the placebo group; relative risk reduction of 18%, P=0.003). The use of PLAVIX in CURE did not impact the number of patients treated with CABG or PCI (with or without stenting), (2253 patients [36.0%] in the PLAVIX group, 2324 patients [36.9%] in the placebo group; relative risk reduction of 4.0%, P=0.1658).

INDICATIONS AND USAGE

PLAVIX (clopidogrel bisulfate) is indicated for the reduction of thrombotic events as follows:

- **Recent MI, Recent Stroke or Established Peripheral Arterial Disease**
  For patients with a history of recent myocardial infarction (MI), recent stroke, or established peripheral arterial disease, PLAVIX has been shown to reduce the rate

Table 2: Outcome Events in the CURE Primary Analysis

Outcome	PLAVIX (+ aspirin)* (n=6259)		Placebo (+ aspirin)* (n=6303)		Relative Risk Reduction (%) (95% CI)
Primary outcome (Cardiovascular death, MI, Stroke)	582	(9.3%)	719	(11.4%)	20% (10.3, 27.9) P=0.00009
Co-primary outcome (Cardiovascular death, MI, Stroke, Refractory Ischemia)	1035	(16.5%)	1187	(18.8%)	14% (6.2, 20.6) P=0.00052)
All Individual Outcome Events:†					
CV death	318	(5.1%)	345	(5.5%)	7% (-7.7, 20.6)
MI	324	(5.2%)	419	(6.6%)	23% (11.0, 33.4)
Stroke	75	(1.2%)	87	(1.4%)	14% (-17.7, 36.6)
Refractory ischemia	544	(8.7%)	587	(9.3%)	7% (-4.0, 18.0)

* Other standard therapies were used as appropriate.
† The individual components do not represent a breakdown of the primary and co-primary outcomes, but rather the total number of subjects experiencing an event during the course of the study.

Figure 3: Hazard Ratio for Patient Baseline Characteristics and On-Study Concomitant Medications/Interventions for the CURE Study

Baseline Characteristics		N	Percent Events PLAVIX (+aspirin)*	Placebo (+aspirin)*
Overall		12562	9.3	11.4
Diagnosis	Non-Q-W	3295	12.7	15.5
	Unst Ang	8298	7.3	8.7
	Other	968	15.1	19.7
Elev Card Enzy	No	9381	8.8	10.9
	Yes	3176	10.7	13.0
ST Depr >1.0mm	No	7273	7.5	8.9
	Yes	5288	11.8	14.8
Diabetes	No	9721	7.9	9.9
	Yes	2840	14.2	16.7
Previous MI	No	8517	7.8	9.5
	Yes	4044	12.5	15.4
Previous Stroke	No	12055	8.9	11.0
	Yes	506	17.9	22.4
Concomitant Medication / Therapy				
Heparin/LMWH	No	951	4.9	7.7
	Yes	11611	9.7	11.7
Aspirin	<100mg	1927	8.5	9.7
	100-200mg	7428	9.2	10.9
	>200mg	3201	9.9	13.7
GPIIb/IIIa Antag	No	11739	8.9	10.8
	Yes	823	15.7	19.2
Beta-Blocker	No	2032	9.9	12.0
	Yes	10530	9.2	11.3
ACEI	No	4813	6.3	8.1
	Yes	7749	11.2	13.5
Lipid-Lowering	No	4461	10.9	13.1
	Yes	8101	8.4	10.5
PTCA/CABG	No	7977	8.1	10.0
	Yes	4585	11.4	13.8

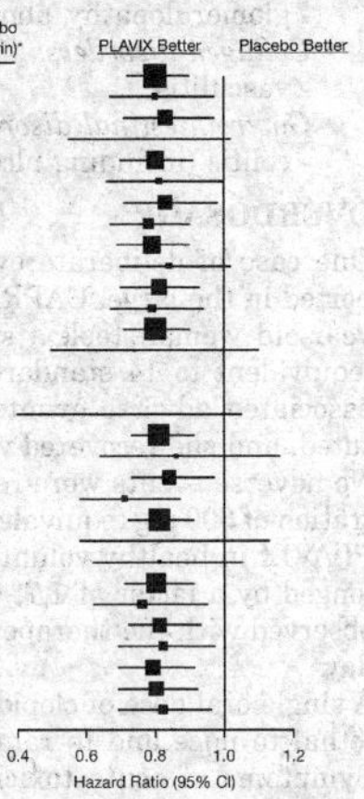

PLAVIX Better | Placebo Better

0.4 0.6 0.8 1.0 1.2

Hazard Ratio (95% CI)

*Other standard therapies were used as appropriate

of a combined endpoint of new ischemic stroke (fatal or not), new MI (fatal or not), and other vascular death.

- **Acute Coronary Syndrome**

  For patients with acute coronary syndrome (unstable angina/non-Q-wave MI) including patients who are to be managed medically and those who are to be managed with percutaneous coronary intervention (with or without stent) or CABG, PLAVIX has been shown to decrease the rate of a combined endpoint of cardiovascular death, MI, or stroke as well as the rate of a combined endpoint of cardiovascular death, MI, stroke, or refractory ischemia.

CONTRAINDICATIONS

The use of PLAVIX is contraindicated in the following conditions:

- Hypersensitivity to the drug substance or any component of the product.
- Active pathological bleeding such as peptic ulcer or intracranial hemorrhage.

WARNINGS

Thrombotic thrombocytopenic purpura (TTP): TTP has been reported rarely following use of PLAVIX, sometimes after a short exposure (<2 weeks). TTP is a serious condition requiring prompt treatment. It is characterized by thrombocytopenia, microangiopathic hemolytic anemia (schistocytes [fragmented RBCs] seen on peripheral smear), neurological findings, renal dysfunction, and fever. TTP was not seen during clopidogrel's clinical trials, which included over 17,500 clopidogrel-treated patients. In world-wide postmarketing experience, however, TTP has been reported at a rate of about four cases per million patients exposed, or about 11 cases per million patient-years. The background rate is thought to be about four cases per million person-years.

PRECAUTIONS

General

As with other antiplatelet agents, PLAVIX prolongs the bleeding time and therefore should be used with caution in patients who may be at risk of increased bleeding from trauma, surgery, or other pathological conditions (particularly gastrointestinal and intraocular). If a patient is to undergo elective surgery and an antiplatelet effect is not desired, PLAVIX should be discontinued 5 days prior to surgery.

Due to the risk of bleeding and undesirable hematological effects, blood cell count determination and/or other appropriate testing should be promptly considered, whenever such suspected clinical symptoms arise during the course of treatment (see **ADVERSE REACTIONS**).

GI Bleeding: In CAPRIE, PLAVIX was associated with a rate of gastrointestinal bleeding of 2.0%, vs. 2.7% on aspirin. In CURE, the incidence of major gastrointestinal bleeding was 1.3% vs. 0.7% (PLAVIX + aspirin vs. placebo + aspirin, respectively). PLAVIX should be used with caution in patients who have lesions with a propensity to bleed (such as ulcers). Drugs that might induce such lesions should be used with caution in patients taking PLAVIX.

Use in Hepatically Impaired Patients: Experience is limited in patients with severe hepatic disease, who may have bleeding diatheses. PLAVIX should be used with caution in this population.

Use in Renally-impaired Patients: Experience is limited in patients with severe renal impairment. PLAVIX should be used with caution in this population.

Information for Patients

Patients should be told that it may take them longer than usual to stop bleeding when they take PLAVIX, and that they should report any unusual bleeding to their physician. Patients should inform physicians and dentists that they are taking PLAVIX before any surgery is scheduled and before any new drug is taken.

Drug Interactions

Study of specific drug interactions yielded the following results:

Aspirin: Aspirin did not modify the clopidogrel-mediated inhibition of ADP-induced platelet aggregation. Concomitant administration of 500 mg of aspirin twice a day for 1 day did not significantly increase the prolongation of bleeding time induced by PLAVIX. PLAVIX potentiated the effect of aspirin on collagen-induced platelet aggregation. PLAVIX and aspirin have been administered together for up to one year.

Table 3: CURE Incidence of Bleeding Complications (% Patients)

Event	PLAVIX (+ aspirin)* (n=6259)	Placebo (+ aspirin)* (n=6303)	P-value
Major bleeding†	3.7‡	2.7§	0.001
Life-threatening bleeding	2.2	1.8	0.13
Fatal	0.2	0.2	
5 g/dL hemoglobin drop	0.9	0.9	
Requiring surgical intervention	0.7	0.7	
Hemorrhagic strokes	0.1	0.1	
Requiring inotropes	0.5	0.5	
Requiring transfusion (≥4 units)	1.2	1.0	
Other major bleeding	1.6	1.0	0.005
Significantly disabling	0.4	0.3	
Intraocular bleeding with significant loss of vision	0.05	0.03	
Requiring 2-3 units of blood	1.3	0.9	
Minor bleeding¶	5.1	2.4	<0.001

* Other standard therapies were used as appropriate.
† Life threatening and other major bleeding.
‡ Major bleeding event rate for PLAVIX + aspirin was dose-dependent on aspirin: <100 mg=2.6%; 100-200 mg=3.5%; >200 mg=4.9%
§ Major bleeding event rate for placebo + aspirin was dose-dependent on aspirin: <100 mg=2.0%; 100-200 mg=2.3%; >200 mg=4.0%
¶ Led to interruption of study medication.

Heparin: In a study in healthy volunteers, PLAVIX did not necessitate modification of the heparin dose or alter the effect of heparin on coagulation. Coadministration of heparin had no effect on inhibition of platelet aggregation induced by PLAVIX.

Nonsteroidal Anti-Inflammatory Drugs (NSAIDs): In healthy volunteers receiving naproxen, concomitant administration of PLAVIX was associated with increased occult gastrointestinal blood loss. NSAIDs and PLAVIX should be coadministered with caution.

Warfarin: Because of the increased risk of bleeding, the concomitant administration of warfarin with PLAVIX should be undertaken with caution. (See **Precautions–General.**)

Other Concomitant Therapy: No clinically significant pharmacodynamic interactions were observed when PLAVIX was coadministered with **atenolol, nifedipine,** or both atenolol and nifedipine. The pharmacodynamic activity of PLAVIX was also not significantly influenced by the coadministration of **phenobarbital, cimetidine** or **estrogen**.

The pharmacokinetics of **digoxin** or **theophylline** were not modified by the coadministration of PLAVIX (clopidogrel bisulfate).

At high concentrations *in vitro*, clopidogrel inhibits P_{450} (2C9). Accordingly, PLAVIX may interfere with the metabolism of **phenytoin, tamoxifen, tolbutamide, warfarin, torsemide, fluvastatin,** and many **non-steroidal anti-inflammatory agents**, but there are no data with which to predict the magnitude of these interactions. Caution should be used when any of these drugs is coadministered with PLAVIX.

In addition to the above specific interaction studies, patients entered into clinical trials with PLAVIX received a variety of concomitant medications including **diuretics, beta-blocking agents, angiotensin converting enzyme inhibitors, calcium antagonists, cholesterol lowering agents, coronary vasodilators, antidiabetic agents** (including **insulin**), **antiepileptic agents, hormone replacement therapy, heparins** (unfractionated and LMWH) and **GPIIb/IIIa antagonists** without evidence of clinically significant adverse interactions. The use of oral anticoagulants, non-study antiplatelet drug and chronic NSAIDs was not allowed in CURE and there are no data on their concomitant use with clopidogrel.

Drug/Laboratory Test Interactions

None known.

Carcinogenesis, Mutagenesis, Impairment of Fertility

There was no evidence of tumorigenicity when clopidogrel was administered for 78 weeks to mice and 104 weeks to rats at dosages up to 77 mg/kg per day, which afforded plasma exposures >25 times that in humans at the recommended daily dose of 75 mg.

Clopidogrel was not genotoxic in four *in vitro* tests (Ames test, DNA-repair test in rat hepatocytes, gene mutation assay in Chinese hamster fibroblasts, and metaphase chromosome analysis of human lymphocytes) and in one *in vivo* test (micronucleus test by oral route in mice).

Clopidogrel was found to have no effect on fertility of male and female rats at oral doses up to 400 mg/kg per day (52 times the recommended human dose on a mg/m^2 basis).

Pregnancy

Pregnancy Category B. Reproduction studies performed in rats and rabbits at doses up to 500 and 300 mg/kg/day (respectively, 65 and 78 times the recommended daily human dose on a mg/m^2 basis), revealed no evidence of impaired fertility or fetotoxicity due to clopidogrel. There are, however, no adequate and well-controlled studies in pregnant women. Because animal reproduction studies are not always predictive of a human response, PLAVIX should be used during pregnancy only if clearly needed.

Nursing Mothers

Studies in rats have shown that clopidogrel and/or its metabolites are excreted in the milk. It is not known whether this drug is excreted in human milk. Because many drugs are excreted in human milk and because of the potential for serious adverse reactions in nursing infants, a decision should be made whether to discontinue nursing or to discontinue the drug, taking into account the importance of the drug to the nursing woman.

Pediatric Use

Safety and effectiveness in the pediatric population have not been established.

ADVERSE REACTIONS

PLAVIX has been evaluated for safety in more than 17,500 patients, including over 9,000 patients treated for 1 year or more. The overall tolerability of PLAVIX in CAPRIE was similar to that of aspirin regardless of age, gender and race, with an approximately equal incidence (13%) of patients withdrawing from treatment because of adverse reactions. The clinically important adverse events observed in CAPRIE and CURE are discussed below.

Hemorrhagic: In CAPRIE patients receiving PLAVIX, gastrointestinal hemorrhage occurred at a rate of 2.0%, and required hospitalization in 0.7%. In patients receiving aspirin, the corresponding rates were 2.7% and 1.1%, respectively. The incidence of intracranial hemorrhage was 0.4% for PLAVIX compared to 0.5% for aspirin.

In CURE, PLAVIX use with aspirin was associated with an increase in bleeding compared to placebo with aspirin (see Table 3). There was an excess in major bleeding in patients receiving PLAVIX plus aspirin compared with placebo plus aspirin, primarily gastrointestinal and at puncture sites. The incidence of intracranial hemorrhage (0.1%), and fatal bleeding (0.2%), was the same in both groups.

In patients receiving both PLAVIX and aspirin in CURE, the incidence of bleeding is described in Table 3.

[See table 3 above]

Ninety-two percent (92%) of the patients in the CURE study received heparin/LMWH, and the rate of bleeding in these patients was similar to the overall results.

There was no excess in major bleeds within seven days after coronary bypass graft surgery in patients who stopped therapy more than five days prior to surgery (event rate 4.4% PLAVIX + aspirin; 5.3% placebo + aspirin). In patients who remained on therapy within five days of bypass graft surgery, the event rate was 9.6% for PLAVIX + aspirin, and 6.3% for placebo + aspirin.

Neutropenia/agranulocytosis: Ticlopidine, a drug chemically similar to PLAVIX, is associated with a 0.8% rate of severe neutropenia (less than 450 neutrophils/µL). In CAPRIE severe neutropenia was observed in six patients, four on PLAVIX and two on aspirin. Two of the 9599 patients who received PLAVIX and none of the 9586 patients who received aspirin had neutrophil counts of zero. One of the four PLAVIX patients in CAPRIE was receiving cytotoxic chemotherapy, and another recovered and returned to the trial after only temporarily interrupting treatment with PLAVIX (clopidogrel bisulfate). In CURE, the numbers of patients with thrombocytopenia (19 PLAVIX + aspirin vs. 24 placebo + aspirin) or neutropenia (3 vs. 3) were similar. Although the risk of myelotoxicity with PLAVIX thus appears to be quite low, this possibility should be considered when a patient receiving PLAVIX demonstrates fever or other sign of infection.

Continued on next page

This product information was prepared in September 2004. On these and other products of Sanofi-Synthelabo Inc., detailed information may be obtained on a current basis by direct inquiry to Product Information Services, 90 Park Avenue, New York, NY 10016 (toll free 1-800-446-6267).

Plavix—Cont.

Gastrointestinal: Overall, the incidence of gastrointestinal events (e.g. abdominal pain, dyspepsia, gastritis and constipation) in patients receiving PLAVIX (clopidogrel bisulfate) was 27.1%, compared to 29.8% in those receiving aspirin in the CAPRIE trial. In the CURE trial the incidence of these gastrointestinal events for patients receiving PLAVIX + aspirin was 11.7% compared to 12.5% for those receiving placebo + aspirin.

In the CAPRIE trial, the incidence of peptic, gastric or duodenal ulcers was 0.7% for PLAVIX and 1.2% for aspirin. In the CURE trial the incidence of peptic, gastric or duodenal ulcers was 0.4% for PLAVIX + aspirin and 0.3% for placebo + aspirin.

Cases of diarrhea were reported in the CAPRIE trial in 4.5% of patients in the PLAVIX group compared to 3.4% in the aspirin group. However, these were rarely severe (PLAVIX=0.2% and aspirin=0.1%). In the CURE trial, the incidence of diarrhea for patients receiving PLAVIX + aspirin was 2.1% compared to 2.2% for those receiving placebo + aspirin.

In the CAPRIE trial, the incidence of patients withdrawing from treatment because of gastrointestinal adverse reactions was 3.2% for PLAVIX and 4.0% for aspirin. In the CURE trial, the incidence of patients withdrawing from treatment because of gastrointestinal adverse reactions was 0.9% for PLAVIX + aspirin compared with 0.8% for placebo + aspirin.

Rash and Other Skin Disorders: In the CAPRIE trial, the incidence of skin and appendage disorders in patients receiving PLAVIX was 15.8% (0.7% serious); the corresponding rate in aspirin patients was 13.1% (0.5% serious). In the CURE trial the incidence of rash or other skin disorders in patients receiving PLAVIX + aspirin was 4.0% compared to 3.5% for those receiving placebo + aspirin.

In the CAPRIE trial, the overall incidence of patients withdrawing from treatment because of skin and appendage disorders adverse reactions was 1.5% for PLAVIX and 0.8% for aspirin. In the CURE trial, the incidence of patients withdrawing because of skin and appendage disorders adverse reactions was 0.7% for PLAVIX + aspirin compared with 0.3% for placebo + aspirin.

Adverse events occurring in ≥2.5% of patients on PLAVIX in the CAPRIE controlled clinical trial are shown below regardless of relationship to PLAVIX. The median duration of therapy was 20 months, with a maximum of 3 years.

Table 4: Adverse Events Occurring in ≥2.5% of PLAVIX Patients in CAPRIE

Body System Event	% Incidence (% Discontinuation) PLAVIX [n=9599]	Aspirin [n=9586]
Body as a Whole–general disorders		
Chest Pain	8.3 (0.2)	8.3 (0.3)
Accidental/Inflicted Injury	7.9 (0.1)	7.3 (0.1)
Influenza-like symptoms	7.5 (<0.1)	7.0 (<0.1)
Pain	6.4 (0.1)	6.3 (0.1)
Fatigue	3.3 (0.1)	3.4 (0.1)
Cardiovascular disorders, general		
Edema	4.1 (<0.1)	4.5 (<0.1)
Hypertension	4.3 (<0.1)	5.1 (<0.1)
Central & peripheral nervous system disorders		
Headache	7.6 (0.3)	7.2 (0.2)
Dizziness	6.2 (0.2)	6.7 (0.3)
Gastrointestinal system disorders		
Abdominal pain	5.6 (0.7)	7.1 (1.0)
Dyspepsia	5.2 (0.6)	6.1 (0.7)
Diarrhea	4.5 (0.4)	3.4 (0.3)
Nausea	3.4 (0.5)	3.8 (0.4)
Metabolic & nutritional disorders		
Hypercholesterolemia	4.0 (0)	4.4 (<0.1)
Musculo-skeletal system disorders		
Arthralgia	6.3 (0.1)	6.2 (0.1)
Back Pain	5.8 (0.1)	5.3 (<0.1)
Platelet, bleeding, & clotting disorders		
Purpura/Bruise	5.3 (0.3)	3.7 (0.1)
Epistaxis	2.9 (0.2)	2.5 (0.1)
Psychiatric disorders		
Depression	3.6 (0.1)	3.9 (0.2)
Respiratory system disorders		
Upper resp tract infection	8.7 (<0.1)	8.3 (<0.1)
Dyspnea	4.5 (0.1)	4.7 (0.1)
Rhinitis	4.2 (0.1)	4.2 (<0.1)
Bronchitis	3.7 (0.1)	3.7 (0)
Coughing	3.1 (<0.1)	2.7 (<0.1)
Skin & appendage disorders		
Rash	4.2 (0.5)	3.5 (0.2)
Pruritus	3.3 (0.3)	1.6 (0.1)
Urinary system disorders		
Urinary tract infection	3.1 (0)	3.5 (0.1)

Incidence of discontinuation, regardless of relationship to therapy, is shown in parentheses.

Adverse events occurring in ≥2.0% of patients on PLAVIX in the CURE controlled clinical trial are shown below regardless of relationship to PLAVIX.

Table 5: Adverse Events Occurring in ≥2.0% of PLAVIX Patients in CURE

Body System Event	% Incidence (% Discontinuation) PLAVIX (+ aspirin)* [n=6259]	Placebo (+ aspirin)* [n=6303]
Body as a Whole–general disorders		
Chest Pain	2.7 (<0.1)	2.8 (0.0)
Central & peripheral nervous system disorders		
Headache	3.1 (0.1)	3.2 (0.1)
Dizziness	2.4 (0.1)	2.0 (<0.1)
Gastrointestinal system disorders		
Abdominal pain	2.3 (0.3)	2.8 (0.3)
Dyspepsia	2.0 (0.1)	1.9 (<0.1)
Diarrhea	2.1 (0.1)	2.2 (0.1)

* Other standard therapies were used as appropriate.

Other adverse experiences of potential importance occurring in 1% to 2.5% of patients receiving PLAVIX (clopidogrel bisulfate) in the CAPRIE or CURE controlled clinical trials are listed below regardless of relationship to PLAVIX. In general, the incidence of these events was similar to that in patients receiving aspirin (in CAPRIE) or placebo + aspirin (in CURE).

Autonomic Nervous System Disorders: Syncope, Palpitation. *Body as a Whole-general disorders:* Asthenia, Fever, Hernia. *Cardiovascular disorders:* Cardiac failure. *Central and peripheral nervous system disorders:* Cramps legs, Hypoaesthesia, Neuralgia, Paraesthesia, Vertigo. *Gastrointestinal system disorders:* Constipation, Vomiting. *Heart rate and rhythm disorders:* Fibrillation atrial. *Liver and biliary system disorders:* Hepatic enzymes increased. *Metabolic and nutritional disorders:* Gout, hyperuricemia, non-protein nitrogen (NPN) increased. *Musculo-skeletal system disorders:* Arthritis, Arthrosis. *Platelet, bleeding & clotting disorders:* GI hemorrhage, hematoma, platelets decreased. *Psychiatric disorders:* Anxiety, Insomnia. *Red blood cell disorders:* Anemia. *Respiratory system disorders:* Pneumonia, Sinusitis. *Skin and appendage disorders:* Eczema, Skin ulceration. *Urinary system disorders:* Cystitis. *Vision disorders:* Cataract, Conjunctivitis.

Other potentially serious adverse events which may be of clinical interest but were rarely reported (<1%) in patients who received PLAVIX in the CAPRIE or CURE controlled clinical trials are listed below regardless of relationship to PLAVIX. In general, the incidence of these events was similar to that in patients receiving aspirin (in CAPRIE) or placebo + aspirin (in CURE).

Body as a whole: Allergic reaction, necrosis ischemic. *Cardiovascular disorders:* Edema generalized. *Gastrointestinal system disorders:* Gastric ulcer perforated, gastritis hemorrhagic, upper GI ulcer hemorrhagic. *Liver and Biliary system disorders:* Bilirubinemia, hepatitis infectious, liver fatty. *Platelet, bleeding and clotting disorders:* hemarthrosis, hematuria, hemoptysis, hemorrhage intracranial, hemorrhage retroperitoneal, hemorrhage of operative wound, ocular hemorrhage, pulmonary hemorrhage, purpura allergic, thrombocytopenia. *Red blood cell disorders:* Anemia aplastic, anemia hypochromic. *Reproductive disorders, female:* Menorrhagia. *Respiratory system disorders:* Hemothorax. *Skin and appendage disorders:* Bullous eruption, rash erythematous, rash maculopapular, urticaria. *Urinary system disorders:* Abnormal renal function, acute renal failure. *White cell and reticuloendothelial system disorders:* Agranulocytosis, granulocytopenia, leukemia, leukopenia, neutrophils decreased.

Postmarketing Experience

The following events have been reported spontaneously from worldwide postmarketing experience:

- *Body as a whole:*
  - hypersensitivity reactions, anaphylactoid reactions
- *Central and Peripheral Nervous System disorders:*
  - confusion, hallucinations, taste disorders
- *Liver and Biliary system disorders:*
  - abnormal liver function test, hepatitis (non-infectious)
- *Platelet, Bleeding and Clotting disorders:*
  - cases of bleeding with fatal outcome (especially intracranial, gastrointestinal and retroperitoneal hemorrhage)
  - agranulocytosis, aplastic anemia/pancytopenia, thrombotic thrombocytopenic purpura (TTP) — see **WARNINGS**.
  - conjunctival, ocular and retinal bleeding
- *Respiratory system disorders:*
  - bronchospasm
- *Skin and Appendage disorders:*
  - angioedema, erythema multiforme
- *Urinary system disorders:*
  - glomerulopathy, abnormal creatinine levels
- *Collagen disorders:*
  - vasculitis
- *Gastrointestinal disorders:*
  - colitis (including ulcerative or lymphocytic colitis)

OVERDOSAGE

One case of deliberate overdosage with PLAVIX was reported in the large, CAPRIE controlled clinical study. A 34-year-old woman took a single 1,050-mg dose of PLAVIX (equivalent to 14 standard 75-mg tablets). There were no associated adverse events. No special therapy was instituted, and she recovered without sequelae.

No adverse events were reported after single oral administration of 600 mg (equivalent to 8 standard 75-mg tablets) of PLAVIX in healthy volunteers. The bleeding time was prolonged by a factor of 1.7, which is similar to that typically observed with the therapeutic dose of 75 mg of PLAVIX per day.

A single oral dose of clopidogrel at 1500 or 2000 mg/kg was lethal to mice and to rats and at 3000 mg/kg to baboons. Symptoms of acute toxicity were vomiting (in baboons), prostration, difficult breathing, and gastrointestinal hemorrhage in all species.

Recommendations About Specific Treatment:

Based on biological plausibility, platelet transfusion may be appropriate to reverse the pharmacological effects of PLAVIX if quick reversal is required.

DOSAGE AND ADMINISTRATION

Recent MI, Recent Stroke, or Established Peripheral Arterial Disease

The recommended daily dose of PLAVIX is 75 mg once daily.

Acute Coronary Syndrome

For patients with acute coronary syndrome (unstable angina/non-Q-wave MI), PLAVIX should be initiated with a single 300 mg loading dose and then continued at 75 mg once daily. Aspirin (75 mg-325 mg once daily) should be initiated and continued in combination with PLAVIX. In CURE, most patients with Acute Coronary Syndrome also received heparin acutely (see **CLINICAL STUDIES**).

PLAVIX can be administered with or without food.

No dosage adjustment is necessary for elderly patients or patients with renal disease. (See **Clinical Pharmacology: Special Populations.**)

HOW SUPPLIED

PLAVIX (clopidogrel bisulfate) is available as a pink, round, biconvex, film-coated tablet debossed with "75" on one side and "1171" on the other. Tablets are provided as follows:

NDC 63653-1171-6 bottles of 30
NDC 63653-1171-1 bottles of 90
NDC 63653-1171-5 bottles of 500
NDC 63653-1171-3 blisters of 100

Storage

Store at 25° C (77° F); excursions permitted to 15°–30° C (59°–86° F) [See USP Controlled Room Temperature]

Distributed by:
Bristol-Myers Squibb/Sanofi Pharmaceuticals Partnership
New York, NY 10016
sanofi~synthelabo
Bristol-Myers Squibb Company
PLAVIX® is a registered trademark of Sanofi-Synthelabo.
51-021345-04
Revised July 2003

Shown in Product Identification Guide, page 332

UROXATRAL® ℞

[ur-ŏks-ă-trăl]
(alfuzosin HCl extended-release tablets)

DESCRIPTION

Each UROXATRAL (alfuzosin HCl extended-release tablets) tablet contains 10 mg alfuzosin hydrochloride as the active ingredient. Alfuzosin hydrochloride is a white to off-white crystalline powder that melts at approximately 240°C. It is freely soluble in water, sparingly soluble in alcohol, and practically insoluble in dichloromethane.

Alfuzosin hydrochloride is (R,S)-N-[3-[(4-amino-6,7-dimethoxy-2-quinazolinyl) methylamino] propyl] tetrahydro-2-furancarboxamide hydrochloride. The empirical formula of alfuzosin hydrochloride is $C_{19}H_{27}N_5O_4$•HCl. The molecular weight of alfuzosin hydrochloride is 425.9. Its structural formula is:

The tablet also contains the following inactive ingredients: colloidal silicon dioxide (NF), ethylcellulose (NF), hydrogenated castor oil (NF), hydroxypropyl methylcellulose (USP), magnesium stearate (NF), mannitol (USP), microcrystalline cellulose (NF), povidone (USP), and yellow ferric oxide (NF).

CLINICAL PHARMACOLOGY

The symptoms associated with benign prostatic hyperplasia (BPH) such as urinary frequency, nocturia, weak stream, hesitancy and incomplete emptying are related to two components, anatomical (static) and functional (dynamic). The static component is related to the prostate size. Prostate size alone does not correlate with symptom severity. The dynamic component is a function of the smooth muscle tone in the prostate and its capsule, the bladder neck, and the bladder base as well as the prostatic urethra. The smooth muscle tone is regulated by alpha-adrenergic receptors. Alfuzosin exhibits selectivity for alpha$_1$-adrenergic receptors in the lower urinary tract. Blockade of these adrenoreceptors can cause smooth muscle in the bladder neck and prostate to relax, resulting in an improvement in urine flow and a reduction in symptoms of BPH.

UROXATRAL (alfuzosin HCl extended-release) is a selective antagonist of post-synaptic alpha$_1$-adrenoreceptors, which are located in the prostate, bladder base, bladder neck, prostatic capsule, and prostatic urethra.

Pharmacokinetics

The pharmacokinetics of UROXATRAL have been evaluated in adult healthy male volunteers after single and/or multiple administration with daily doses ranging from 7.5 mg to 30 mg, and in patients with BPH at doses from 7.5 mg to 15 mg.

Absorption: The absolute bioavailability of UROXATRAL 10 mg tablets under fed conditions is 49%. Following multiple dosing of 10 mg UROXATRAL under fed conditions, the time to maximum concentration is 8 hours. C_{max} and AUC_{0-24} are 13.6 (SD = 5.6) ng/mL and 194 (SD = 75) ng.h/mL, respectively. UROXATRAL exhibits linear kinetics following single and multiple dosing up to 30 mg. Steady-state plasma levels are reached with the second dose of UROXATRAL administration. Steady-state alfuzosin plasma concentrations are 1.2- to 1.6-fold higher than those observed after a single administration.

Effect of Food: As illustrated in Figure 1, the extent of absorption is 50% lower under fasting conditions. Therefore, UROXATRAL should be taken immediately following a meal. (See DOSAGE AND ADMINISTRATION.)

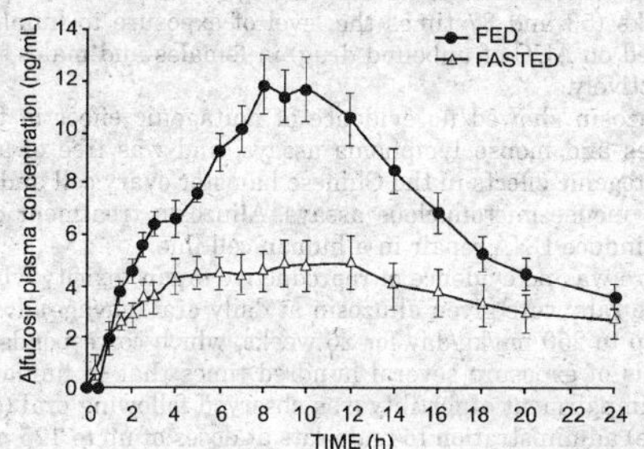

Figure 1 – Mean (SEM) Alfuzosin Plasma Concentration-Time Profiles after a Single Administration of UROXATRAL 10 mg tablets to 8 Healthy Middle-Aged Male Volunteers in Fed and Fasted States

Distribution: The volume of distribution following intravenous administration in healthy male middle-aged volunteers was 3.2 L/kg. Results of *in vitro* studies indicate that alfuzosin is moderately bound to human plasma proteins (82% to 90%), with linear binding over a wide concentration range (5 to 5,000 ng/mL).

Metabolism: Alfuzosin undergoes extensive metabolism by the liver, with only 11% of the administered dose excreted unchanged in the urine. Alfuzosin is metabolized by three metabolic pathways: oxidation, O-demethylation, and N-dealkylation. The metabolites are not pharmacologically active. CYP3A4 is the principal hepatic enzyme isoform involved in its metabolism.

Excretion and Elimination: Following oral administration of ^{14}C-labeled alfuzosin solution, the recovery of radioactivity after 7 days (expressed as a percentage of the administered dose) was 69% in feces and 24% in urine. Following oral administration of UROXATRAL 10 mg tablets, the apparent elimination half-life is 10 hours.

Special Populations

Elderly: In a pharmacokinetic assessment during phase 3 clinical studies in patients with BPH, there was no relationship between peak plasma concentrations of alfuzosin and age. However, trough levels were positively correlated with age. The concentrations in subjects ≥75 years of age were approximately 35% greater than in those below 65 years of age.

Patients with Renal Impairment: The pharmacokinetic profiles of UROXATRAL 10 mg tablets in subjects with normal renal function (CL_{CR}>80 mL/min), mild impairment (CL_{CR} 60 to 80 mL/min), moderate impairment (CL_{CR} 30 to 59 mL/min), and severe impairment (CL_{CR} <30 mL/min) were compared. These clearances were calculated by the Cockcroft-Gault formula. Relative to subjects with normal renal function, the mean C_{max} and AUC values were increased by approximately 50% in patients with mild, moderate, or severe renal impairment. (See PRECAUTIONS, Special Populations).

Patients with Hepatic Insufficiency: In patients with moderate or severe hepatic insufficiency (Child-Pugh categories B and C), the plasma apparent clearance (CL/F) was reduced to approximately one-third to one-fourth that observed in healthy subjects. This reduction in clearance results in three to four-fold higher plasma concentrations of alfuzosin in these patients compared to healthy subjects. Therefore, UROXATRAL is contraindicated in patients with moderate to severe hepatic impairment (See **CONTRAINDICATIONS**). The pharmacokinetics of UROXATRAL have not been studied in patients with mild hepatic insufficiency. (See PRECAUTIONS, Special Populations).

Table 1. Mean QT and QTc changes in msec (95% CI) from baseline at T_{max} (relative to placebo) with different methodologies to correct for effect of heart rate.

Drug/Dose	QT	Fridericia method	Population-specific method	Subject-specific method
Alfuzosin 10 mg	-5.8 (-10.2, -1.4)	4.9 (0.9, 8.8)	1.8 (-1.4, 5.0)	1.8 (-1.3, 5.0)
Alfuzosin 40 mg	-4.2 (-8.5, 0.2)	7.7 (1.9, 13.5)	4.2 (-0.6, 9.0)	4.3 (-0.5, 9.2)
Moxifloxacin *400 mg	6.9 (2.3, 11.5)	12.7 (8.6, 16.8)	11.0 (7.0, 15.0)	11.1 (7.2, 15.0)

* Active control

Drug-Drug Interactions

Metabolic interactions

CYP3A4 is the principal hepatic enzyme isoform involved in the metabolism of alfuzosin.

Potent CYP3A4 inhibitors

Repeated administration of 400 mg of ketoconazole, a potent inhibitor of CYP3A4, increased alfuzosin C_{max} 2.3-fold and AUC_{last} 3.2-fold following a single 10 mg dose of alfuzosin. Therefore, UROXATRAL should not be co-administered with potent inhibitors of CYP3A4 because exposure is increased, (e.g., ketoconazole, itraconazole, or ritonavir). (See **CONTRAINDICATIONS**).

Moderate CYP3A4 inhibitors

Diltiazem: Repeated co-administration of 240 mg/day of diltiazem, a moderately-potent inhibitor of CYP3A4, with 7.5 mg/day (2.5 mg three times daily) alfuzosin (equivalent to the exposure with UROXATRAL) increased the C_{max} and AUC_{0-24} of alfuzosin 1.5- and 1.3-fold, respectively. Alfuzosin increased the C_{max} and AUC_{0-12} of diltiazem 1.4-fold. Although no changes in blood pressure were observed in this study, diltiazem is an antihypertensive medication and the combination of UROXATRAL and anti-hypertensive medications has the potential to cause hypotension in some patients. (See **WARNINGS**).

In human liver microsomes, at concentrations that are achieved at the therapeutic dose, alfuzosin did not inhibit CYP1A2, 2A6, 2C9, 2C19, 2D6 or 3A4 isoenzymes. In primary culture of human hepatocytes, alfuzosin did not induce CYP1A, 2A6 or 3A4 isoenzymes.

Other interactions

Warfarin: Multiple dose administration of an immediate release tablet formulation of alfuzosin 5 mg twice daily for six days to six healthy male volunteers did not affect the pharmacological response to a single 25 mg oral dose of warfarin.

Digoxin: Repeated co-administration of UROXATRAL 10 mg tablets and digoxin 0.25 mg/day for 7 days did not influence the steady-state pharmacokinetics of either drug.

Cimetidine: Repeated administration of 1 g/day cimetidine increased both alfuzosin C_{max} and AUC values by 20%.

Atenolol: Single administration of 100 mg atenolol with a single dose of 2.5 mg of an immediate release alfuzosin tablet in eight healthy young male volunteers increased alfuzosin C_{max} and AUC values by 28% and 21%, respectively. Alfuzosin increased atenolol C_{max} and AUC values by 26% and 14%, respectively. In this study, the combination of alfuzosin with atenolol caused significant reductions in mean blood pressure and in mean heart rate. (See **WARNINGS**.)

Hydrochlorothiazide: Single administration of 25 mg hydrochlorothiazide did not modify the pharmacokinetic parameters of alfuzosin. There was no evidence of pharmacodynamic interaction between alfuzosin and hydrochlorothiazide in the 8 patients in this study.

Electrophysiology

The effect of 10 mg and 40 mg alfuzosin on QT interval was evaluated in a double-blind, randomized, placebo and active-controlled (moxifloxacin 400 mg), 4-way crossover single dose study in 45 healthy white male subjects aged 19 to 45 years. The QT interval was measured at the time of peak alfuzosin plasma concentrations. The 40 mg dose of alfuzosin was chosen because this dose achieves higher blood levels than those achieved with the co-administration of UROXATRAL and ketoconazole 400 mg. Table 1 summarizes the effect on uncorrected QT and mean corrected QT interval (QTc) with different methods of correction (Fridericia, population-specific, and subject-specific correction methods) at the time of peak alfuzosin plasma concentrations. No single one of these correction methodologies is known to be more valid. The mean change of heart rate associated with a 10 mg dose of alfuzosin in this study was 5.2 beats/minute and 5.8 beats/minute with 40 mg alfuzosin. The change in heart rate with moxifloxacin was 2.8 beats/minute.

[See table 1 above]

The QT effect appeared greater for 40 mg compared to 10 mg alfuzosin. The effect of the highest alfuzosin dose (four times the therapeutic dose) studied did not appear as large as that of the active control moxifloxacin at its therapeutic dose. This study, however, was not designed to make direct statistical comparisons between the drugs or the dose levels. There has been no signal of Torsade de Pointes in the extensive post-marketing experience with alfuzosin outside the United States.

Clinical Studies

Three randomized placebo-controlled, double-blind, parallel-arm, 12-week studies were conducted with the 10 mg daily dose of alfuzosin. In these three studies, 1,608 patients [mean age 64.2 years, range 49-92 years; Caucasian (96.1%), Black (1.6%), Asian (1.1%), Other (1.2) were randomized and 473 patients received UROXATRAL 10 mg daily. Table 1 provides the results of the three studies that evaluated the 10 mg dose.

There were two primary efficacy variables in these three studies. The International Prostate Symptom Score (IPSS, or AUA Symptom Score) consists of seven questions that assess the severity of both irritative (frequency, urgency, nocturia) and obstructive (incomplete emptying, stopping and starting, weak stream, and pushing or straining) symptoms, with possible scores ranging from 0 to 35. The second efficacy variable was peak urinary flow rate. The peak flow rate was measured just prior to the next dose in study 2 and on average at 16 hours post-dosing in studies 1 and 3.

There was a statistically significant reduction from baseline to last assessment (Week 12) in the IPSS versus placebo in all three studies, indicating a reduction in symptom severity (Table 2 and Figures 2, 3, and 4).

[See table 2 at top of next page]

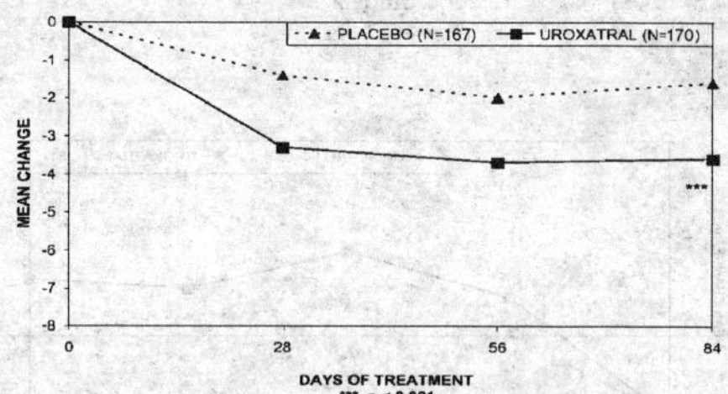

Figure 2 — Mean Change from Baseline in Total Symptom Score, by Visit: Study 1

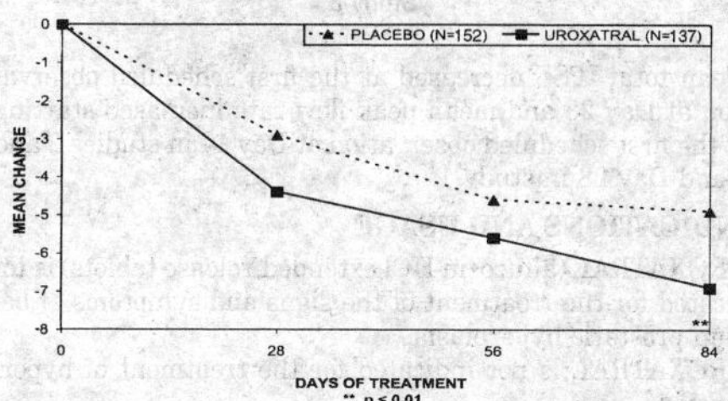

Figure 3 — Mean Change from Baseline in Total Symptom Score, by Visit: Study 2

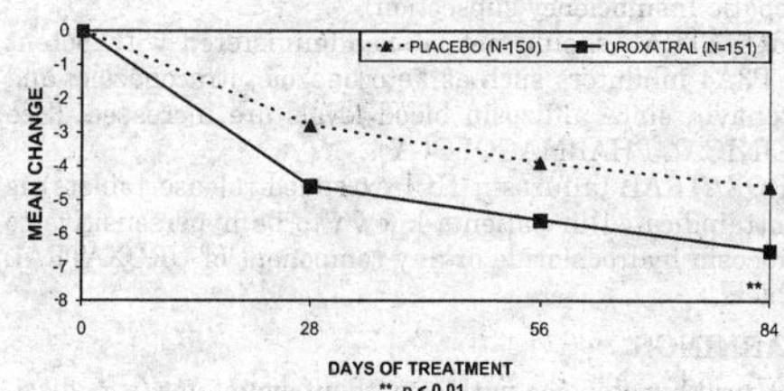

Figure 4 — Mean Change from Baseline in Total Symptom Score, by Visit: Study 3

Peak urinary flow rate was increased statistically significantly from baseline to last assessment (Week 12) versus placebo in studies 1 and 2 (Table 3 and Figures 5, 6, and 7).

Continued on next page

This product information was prepared in September 2004. On these and other products of Sanofi-Synthelabo Inc., detailed information may be obtained on a current basis by direct inquiry to Product Information Services, 90 Park Avenue, New York, NY 10016 (toll free 1-800-446-6267).

Uroxatral—Cont.

[See table 3 at right]

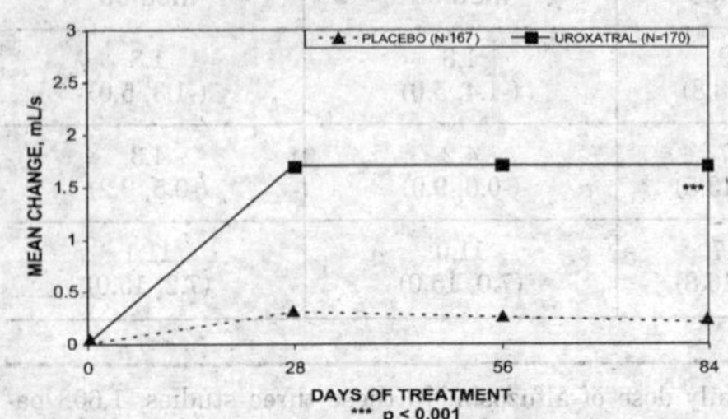

Figure 5 — Mean Change from Baseline in Peak Urine Flow Rate (mL/s), by Visit: Study 1

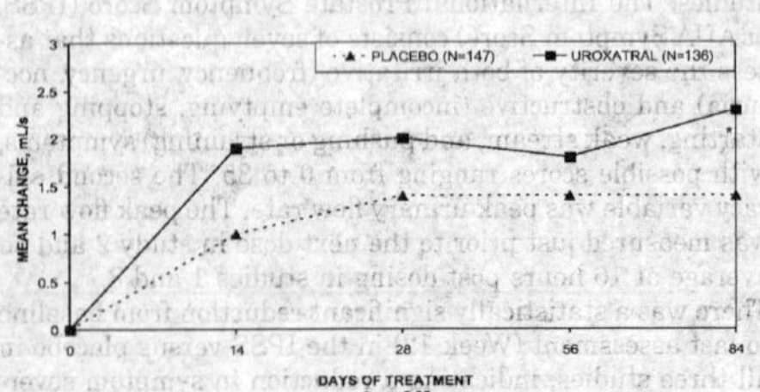

Figure 6 — Mean Change from Baseline in Peak Urine Flow Rate (mL/s), by Visit: Study 2

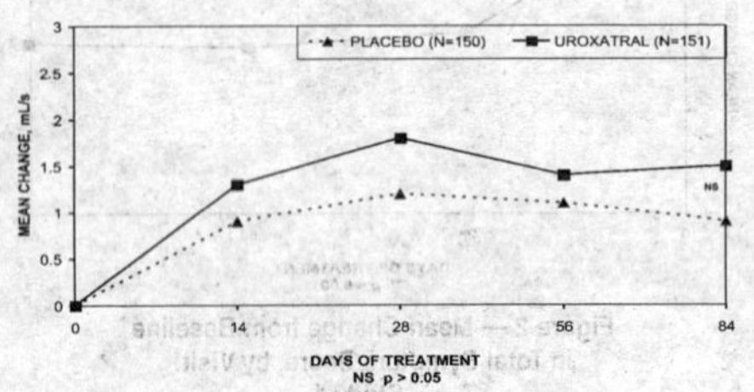

Figure 7 — Mean Change from Baseline in Peak Urine Flow Rate (mL/s), by Visit: Study 3

Mean total IPSS decreased at the first scheduled observation at Day 28 and mean peak flow rate increased starting at the first scheduled observation at Day 14 in studies 2 and 3 and Day 28 in study 1.

INDICATIONS AND USAGE

UROXATRAL (alfuzosin HCl extended-release tablets) is indicated for the treatment of the signs and symptoms of benign prostatic hyperplasia.

UROXATRAL is not indicated for the treatment of hypertension.

CONTRAINDICATIONS

UROXATRAL should not be used in patients with moderate or severe hepatic insufficiency, (Childs-Pugh categories B and C) since alfuzosin blood levels are increased in these patients. (See CLINICAL PHARMACOLOGY, Patients with Hepatic Insufficiency subsection).

UROXATRAL should not be co-administered with potent CYP3A4 inhibitors such as ketoconazole, itraconazole, and ritonavir, since alfuzosin blood levels are increased. (See CLINICAL PHARMACOLOGY).

UROXATRAL (alfuzosin HCl extended-release tablets) is contraindicated in patients known to be hypersensitive to alfuzosin hydrochloride or any component of UROXATRAL tablets.

WARNINGS

Postural hypotension with or without symptoms (e.g., dizziness) may develop within a few hours following administration of UROXATRAL (alfuzosin HCl extended-release tablets). As with other alpha-blockers, there is a potential for syncope. Patients should be warned of the possible occurrence of such events and should avoid situations where injury could result should syncope occur. Care should be taken when UROXATRAL is administered to patients with symptomatic hypotension or patients who have had a hypotensive response to other medications.

PRECAUTIONS

General

Prostatic Carcinoma: Carcinoma of the prostate and BPH cause many of the same symptoms. These two diseases frequently coexist. Therefore, patients thought to have BPH should be examined prior to starting therapy with UROXATRAL (alfuzosin HCl extended-release tablets) to rule out the presence of carcinoma of the prostate.

Table 2 — Mean Change (SD) from Baseline to week 12 in International Prostate Symptom Score in Three Randomized, Controlled, Double Blind Studies

	Study 1		Study 2		Study 3	
Symptom Score	**Placebo (n=167)**	**UROXATRAL 10 mg (n=170)**	**Placebo (n=152)**	**UROXATRAL 10 mg (n=137)**	**Placebo (n=150)**	**UROXATRAL 10 mg (n=151)**
Total symptom score						
Baseline	18.2 (6.4)	18.2 (6.3)	17.7 (4.1)	17.3 (3.5)	17.7 (5.0)	18.0 (5.4)
Change[a]	-1.6 (5.8)	-3.6 (4.8)	-4.9 (5.9)	-6.9 (4.9)	-4.6 (5.8)	-6.5 (5.2)
p-value	0.001		0.002		0.007	

[a]Difference between baseline value and last value

Table 3 — Mean (SD) from Baseline in Peak Urine Flow Rate (mL/sec) in Three Randomized, Controlled, Double-Blind Studies

	Study 1		Study 2		Study 3	
	Placebo (n=167)	**UROXATRAL 10 mg (n=170)**	**Placebo (n=147)**	**UROXATRAL 10 mg (n=136)**	**Placebo (n=150)**	**UROXATRAL 10 mg (n=136)**
Mean Peak flow rate						
Baseline	10.2 (4.0)	9.9 (3.9)	9.2 (2.0)	9.4 (1.9)	9.3 (2.6)	9.5 (3.0)
Change[a]	0.2 (3.5)	1.7 (4.2)	1.4 (3.2)	2.3 (3.6)	0.9 (3.0)	1.5 (3.3)
p-value	0.0004		0.03		0.22	

[a]Difference between baseline value and last value

Drug-Drug Interactions: The pharmacokinetic and pharmacodynamic interactions between UROXATRAL and other alpha-blockers have not been determined. However, interactions may be expected, and UROXATRAL should NOT be used in combination with other alpha-blockers.

Coronary Insufficiency: If symptoms of angina pectoris should newly appear or worsen, UROXATRAL should be discontinued.

Hepatic Insufficiency: UROXATRAL should not be given to patients with moderate or severe hepatic insufficiency. (See **CONTRAINDICATIONS**). The pharmacokinetics of UROXATRAL have not been studied in patients with mild hepatic insufficiency (See CLINICAL PHARMACOLOGY, Patients with Hepatic Insufficiency).

Renal Insufficiency: Systemic exposure was increased by approximately 50% in pharmacokinetic studies of patients with mild, moderate, and severe renal insufficiency (See CLINICAL PHARMACOLOGY, Special Populations). In phase 3 studies, the safety profile of patients with mild (n=172) or moderate (n=56) renal impairment was similar to the patients with normal renal function in those studies. Safety data are available in only a limited number of patients (n=6) with creatinine clearance below 30 mL/min; therefore, caution should be exercised when UROXATRAL is administered in patients with severe renal insufficiency.

Patients with Congenital or Acquired QT Prolongation: In a study of QT effect in 45 healthy males (See CLINICAL PHARMACOLOGY, Electrophysiology), the QT effect appeared less with alfuzosin 10 mg than with 40 mg, and the effect of alfuzosin 40 mg did not appear as large as that of the active control moxifloxacin at its therapeutic dose. This observation should be considered in clinical decisions to prescribe UROXATRAL for patients with a known history of QT prolongation or patients who are taking medications known to prolong QT, although there has been no signal of Torsades de Pointe in the extensive post-marketing experience with alfuzosin outside the United States. There are no known PK/PD studies of the effects of other alpha blockers on cardiac repolarization.

Information for Patients

Patients should be told about the possible occurrence of symptoms related to postural hypotension, such as dizziness, when beginning UROXATRAL, and they should be cautioned about driving, operating machinery, or performing hazardous tasks during this period.

UROXATRAL should be taken with food and with the same meal each day.

Patients should be advised not to crush or chew UROXATRAL tablets.

Laboratory Tests

No laboratory test interactions with UROXATRAL tablets are known.

Pediatric Use

UROXATRAL is not indicated for use in children.

Geriatric Use

Of the total number of subjects in clinical studies of UROXATRAL, 48% were 65 years of age and over, whereas 11% were 75 and over. No overall differences in safety or effectiveness were observed between these subjects and younger subjects. (See CLINICAL PHARMACOLOGY, Elderly subsection.)

Carcinogenesis, Mutagenesis, and Impairment of Fertility

There was no evidence of a drug-related increase in the incidence of tumors in mice following dietary administration of 100 mg/kg/day alfuzosin for 98 weeks (13 and 15 times the level of exposure to humans based on AUC of unbound drug) in females and males, respectively. The highest dose tested in female mice may not have constituted a maximally tolerated dose. Likewise, there was no evidence of a drug-related increase in the incidence of tumors in rats following dietary administration of 100 mg/kg/day alfuzosin for 104 weeks (53 and 37 times the level of exposure to humans based on AUC of unbound drug) in females and males, respectively.

Alfuzosin showed no evidence of mutagenic effect in the Ames and mouse lymphoma assays, and was free of any clastogenic effects in the Chinese hamster ovary cell and *in vivo* mouse micronucleus assays. Alfuzosin treatment did not induce DNA repair in a human cell line.

There was no evidence of reproductive organ toxicity when male rats were given alfuzosin at daily oral (gavage) doses of up to 250 mg/kg/day for 26 weeks, which corresponds to levels of exposure several hundred times that in humans. No impairment of fertility was observed following oral (gavage) administration to male rats at doses of up to 125 mg/kg/day for 70 days. Estrous cycling was inhibited in rats and dogs at doses of 25 mg/kg and 20 mg/kg, respectively, corresponding to levels of systemic exposure (based on AUC of unbound drug) 12- and 18-fold higher, respectively, than in humans, although this did not result in impaired fertility in rats.

Pregnancy

Teratogenic Effects, Pregnancy and Lactation Category B. UROXATRAL is not indicated for use in women.

There was no evidence of teratogenicity or embryotoxicity in rats at maternal (oral gavage) doses up to 250 mg/kg/day, corresponding to systemic exposure levels 1,200-fold higher than in humans. In rabbits, up to the dose of 100 mg/kg/day (approximately 3 times the clinical dose by body surface area) given orally (via gavage), no evidence of fetal toxicity or teratogenicity was seen.

Gestation was slightly prolonged in rats with a maternal dose >5 mg/kg/day (oral gavage), which corresponds to systemic exposure levels (based on AUC of unbound drug) 12 times higher than human exposure levels, but there were no difficulties with parturition.

Nursing Mothers

UROXATRAL is not indicated for use in women.

ADVERSE REACTIONS

The incidence of treatment-emergent adverse events has been ascertained from 3 placebo-controlled clinical trials involving 1,608 men in which daily doses of 10 and 15 mg alfuzosin were evaluated. In these 3 trials, 473 men received UROXATRAL (alfuzosin HCl 10 mg extended-release tablets). In these studies, 4% of patients taking UROXATRAL (alfuzosin HCl extended-release tablets) 10 mg tablets withdrew from the study due to adverse events, compared with 3% in the placebo group.

Table 4 summarizes the treatment-emergent adverse events that occurred in ≥2% of patients receiving UROXATRAL, and at an incidence numerically higher than that of the placebo group. In general, the adverse events seen in long-term use were similar in type and frequency to the events described below for the 3-month trials.

Table 4 — Treatment-Emergent Adverse Events Occurring in ≥2% of UROXATRAL-Treated Patients and More Frequently than with Placebo in 3-Month Placebo-Controlled Clinical Studies

Adverse Event	Placebo (n=678)	UROXATRAL (n=473)
Dizziness	19 (2.8%)	27 (5.7%)
Upper respiratory tract infection	4 (0.6%)	14 (3.0%)

Headache	12 (1.8%)	14 (3.0%)
Fatigue	12 (1.8%)	13 (2.7%)

The following adverse events, reported by between 1% and 2% of patients receiving UROXATRAL and occurring more frequently than with placebo, are listed alphabetically by body system and by decreasing frequency within body system: Gastrointestinal system:
Body as a whole: pain
Gastrointestinal system: abdominal pain, dyspepsia, constipation, nausea
Reproductive system: impotence
Respiratory system: bronchitis, sinusitis, pharyngitis
The following adverse events have also been reported in postmarketing experience: rash, tachycardia, chest pain, priapism.
Signs and Symptoms of Orthostasis in Clinical Studies: The adverse events related to orthostasis that occurred in the double-blind phase 3 studies with alfuzosin 10 mg are summarized in Table 5. Approximately 20% to 30% of patients in these studies were taking antihypertensive medication.

Table 5 — Number (%) of Patients with Symptoms Possibly Associated with Orthostasis in 3-Month Placebo-Controlled Clinical Studies

Symptoms	Placebo (n=678)	UROXATRAL (n=473)
Dizziness	19 (2.8%)	27 (5.7%)
Hypotension or postural hypotension	0	2 (0.4%)
Syncope	0	1 (0.2%)

Multiple testing for blood pressure changes or orthostatic hypotension was conducted in the three controlled studies at each scheduled clinic visit (Days 14, 28, 56, and 84). Patients with a decrease in systolic blood pressure of >20 mm Hg after 2 minutes standing following being supine were excluded from the three trials. These tests were considered positive for blood pressure decrease if (1) supine systolic blood pressure was ≤90 mm Hg, with a decrease ≥20 mm Hg versus baseline, and/or (2) supine diastolic blood pressure was ≤50 mm Hg, with a decrease ≥15 mm Hg versus baseline. The tests were considered positive for orthostatic hypotension if there was a decrease in systolic blood pressure of ≥20 mm Hg upon standing from the supine position during the orthostatic tests. According to these definitions, decreased systolic blood pressure was observed in none of the 674 placebo patients and 1 (0.2%) of the 469 UROXATRAL patients. Decreased diastolic blood pressure was observed in 3 (0.4%) of the placebo patients and in 4 (0.9%) of the UROXATRAL patients. A positive orthostatic test was seen in 52 (7.7%) of placebo patients and in 31 (6.6%) of the UROXATRAL patients.
No vital sign measurements were obtained following first dose administration in the phase 3 studies, except for a subset of patients in study 1 who had blood pressure measurements 12 to 16 hours after the first dose to assess the potential to produce orthostatic hypotension. None of these 35 UROXATRAL treated patients showed a positive test for systolic, diastolic or orthostatic blood pressure change.

OVERDOSAGE

Should overdose of UROXATRAL (alfuzosin HCl extended-release tablets) lead to hypotension, support of the cardiovascular system is of first importance. Restoration of blood pressure and normalization of heart rate may be accomplished by keeping the patient in the supine position. If this measure is inadequate, then the administration of intravenous fluids should be considered. If necessary, vasopressors should then be used, and the renal function should be monitored and supported as needed. Alfuzosin is 82% to 90% protein-bound; therefore, dialysis may not be of benefit.

DOSAGE AND ADMINISTRATION

The recommended dosage is one 10 mg UROXATRAL (alfuzosin HCl extended-release tablets) tablet daily to be taken immediately after the same meal each day. The tablets should not be chewed or crushed.

HOW SUPPLIED

UROXATRAL (alfuzosin HCl extended-release tablets) 10 mg is available as a round, three-layer tablet: one white layer between two yellow layers, debossed with X10. UROXATRAL is supplied as follows:

Package	NDC Number
Bottles of 30	0024-4200-30
Bottles of 100	0024-4200-10
Hospital Unit Dose (blister packs containing 10 cards of 10 tablets each)	0024-4200-20

Rx only.
Store at 25°C (77°F); excursions permitted to 15° to 30°C (59° to 86°F) [see USP Controlled Room Temperature].
Protect from light and moisture.
Keep UROXATRAL out of reach of children.
42003790
HPG13824-01
Distributed by:
sanofi-synthelabo
Sanofi-Synthelabo Inc., New York, NY 10016

UROXATRAL® is a registered trademark of Sanofi-Synthelabo.
USS-1 Revised June 2003

Santen Inc.

for further product information see
VISTAKON® Pharmaceuticals, LLC

Santarus, Inc

10590 WEST OCEAN AIR DRIVE
SUITE 200
SAN DIEGO, CA 92130

Direct Inquiries to:
PH# (888) 778-0887
FAX# 858-314-5701
E-MAIL-CONTACT@SANTARUS.COM

ZEGERID™ ℞
[zĕ-gər-īd]
(omeprazole)
Powder for Oral Suspension
Rx only

DESCRIPTION

The active ingredient in ZEGERID™ (omeprazole) powder for oral suspension, is a substituted benzimidazole, 5-methoxy-2-[[(4-methoxy-3, 5-dimethyl-2-pyridinyl) methyl]sulfinyl]-1*H*-benzimidazole, a racemic mixture of two enantiomers that inhibits gastric acid secretion. Its empirical formula is $C_{17}H_{19}N_3O_3S$, with a molecular weight of 345.42. The structural formula is:

Omeprazole is a white to off-white crystalline powder which melts with decomposition at about 155°C. It is a weak base, freely soluble in ethanol and methanol, and slightly soluble in acetone and isopropanol and very slightly soluble in water. The stability of omeprazole is a function of pH; it is rapidly degraded in acid media, but has acceptable stability under alkaline conditions.
ZEGERID™ Powder for Oral Suspension is supplied in unit dose packets as an immediate-release formulation to be constituted with water for oral administration. Each packet contains 20 mg of omeprazole and the following excipients: sodium bicarbonate, sucrose, sucralose, xanthan gum, xylitol, and flavorings.

CLINICAL PHARMACOLOGY

Omeprazole is acid labile and thus rapidly degraded by gastric acid. ZEGERID™ Powder for Oral Suspension is an immediate-release formulation that contains sodium bicarbonate to protect omeprazole from acid degradation.

Pharmacokinetics

Absorption

When ZEGERID™ is administered on an empty stomach 1 hour prior to a meal, absorption of omeprazole is rapid, with mean peak plasma levels of omeprazole occurring at around 30 minutes (range 10 to 90 minutes) after a single dose or repeated once-daily administration (see figures below).

Mean Plasma Omeprazole Concentrations (Days 1 and 7)

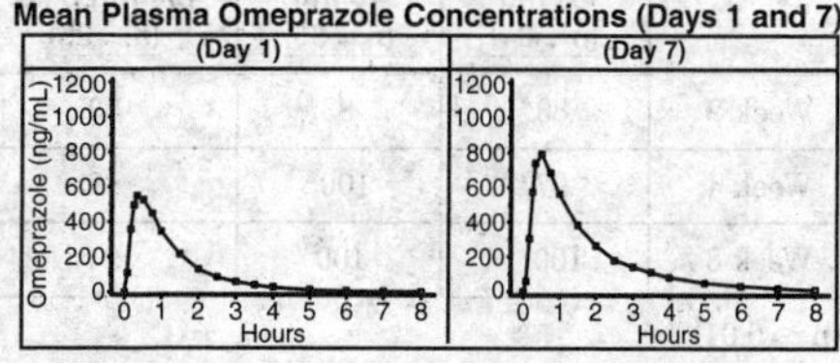

The AUC(0-inf)(ng*hr/mL) was 1446 after 7 days of 20 mg daily doses and the Tmax was approximately 30 minutes. Following single or repeated once daily dosing, peak plasma concentrations of omeprazole from ZEGERID™ are approximately proportional from 20 to 40 mg doses, but a greater than linear mean AUC (three-fold increase) is observed when doubling the dose to 40 mg. The bioavailability of omeprazole from ZEGERID™ Powder for Oral Suspension increases upon repeated administration of ZEGERID™.

Pharmacokinetic Parameters of ZEGERID™ Following Oral 20 mg Once-Daily Dosing for 1 and 7 Days

Parameter	Day 1
AUC(0-inf) (ng*hr/mL)	825
Coefficient of variation	72%
Cmax (ng/mL)	672
Coefficient of variation	44%
Tmax (min)	29.8
T½ (hr)	0.86

Values represent arithmetic means.

Parameter	Day 7
AUC(0-inf) (ng*hr/mL)	1446
Coefficient of variation	61%
Cmax (ng/mL)	902
Coefficient of variation	40%
Tmax (min)	28.3
T½ (hr)	1.08

Values represent arithmetic means.

When ZEGERID™ is administered 1 hour after a meal, Cmax and AUC are reduced by 63% and 24%, respectively, relative to administration prior to a meal.

Distribution

Omeprazole is bound to plasma proteins. Protein binding is approximately 95%.

Metabolism

Absolute bioavailability (compared to intravenous administration) is about 30-40% at doses of 20-40 mg, due in large part to pre-systemic metabolism.

Excretion

In healthy subjects, the mean plasma half-life is 1 hour (range 0.4 to 3.2 hours), and the total body clearance is 500-600 mL/min.
Following single dose oral administration of omeprazole, little if any unchanged drug is excreted in urine. The majority of the dose (about 77%) is eliminated in urine as at least six metabolites. Two metabolites have been identified as hydroxyomeprazole and the corresponding carboxylic acid. The remainder of the dose was recoverable in feces. This implies a significant biliary excretion of the metabolites of omeprazole. Three metabolites have been identified in plasma — the sulfide and sulfone derivatives of omeprazole, and hydroxyomeprazole. These metabolites have very little or no antisecretory activity.

Special Populations

Geriatric

The elimination rate of omeprazole was somewhat decreased in the elderly, and bioavailability was increased. Omeprazole was 76% bioavailable when a single 40 mg oral dose of omeprazole (buffered solution) was administered to healthy elderly subjects, versus 58% in young subjects given the same dose. Nearly 70% of the dose was recovered in urine as metabolites of omeprazole and no unchanged drug was detected. The plasma clearance of omeprazole was 250 mL/min (about half that of young subjects) and its plasma half-life averaged one hour, similar to that of young healthy subjects.

Pediatric

The pharmacokinetics of ZEGERID™ have not been studied in patients < 18 years of age.

Gender

There are no known differences in the absorption or excretion of omeprazole between males and females.

Hepatic insufficiency

In patients with chronic hepatic disease, the bioavailability of omeprazole increased to approximately 100% compared to an I.V. dose, reflecting decreased first-pass effect, and the mean plasma half-life of the drug increased to nearly 3 hours compared to the mean half-life of 1 hour in healthy subjects. Plasma clearance averaged 70 mL/min, compared to a value of 500-600 mL/min in normal subjects.

Renal insufficiency

In patients with chronic renal impairment, whose creatinine clearance ranged between 10 and 62 mL/min/1.73m^2, the disposition of omeprazole was very similar to that in healthy volunteers, although there was a slight increase in bioavailability. Because urinary excretion is a primary route of excretion of omeprazole metabolites, their elimination slowed in proportion to the decreased creatinine clearance.

Asians

In pharmacokinetic studies of single 20 mg omeprazole doses, an increase in AUC of approximately four fold was noted in Asian subjects compared to Caucasians.
Dose adjustment, particularly where maintenance of healing of erosive esophagitis is indicated, for the hepatically impaired and Asian subjects should be considered.

Drug-Drug Interactions

When omeprazole 40 mg once daily was given in combination with clarithromycin 500 mg every 8 hours to healthy adult male subjects, the steady-state plasma concentrations of omeprazole were increased by the concomitant administration of clarithromycin (Cmax, AUC(0–24) and T1/2 increased 30%, 89%, and 34%, respectively).

Pharmacodynamics

Mechanism of Action

Omeprazole belongs to a class of antisecretory compounds, the substituted benzimidazoles, that do not exhibit anticho-

Continued on next page

Zegerid—Cont.

linergic or H2 histamine antagonistic properties, but that suppress gastric acid secretion by specific inhibition of the H+/K+ ATPase enzyme system at the secretory surface of the gastric parietal cell. Because this enzyme system is regarded as the acid (proton) pump within the gastric mucosa, omeprazole has been characterized as a gastric acid-pump inhibitor, in that it blocks the final step of acid production. This effect is dose-related and leads to inhibition of both basal and stimulated acid secretion irrespective of the stimulus. Animal studies indicate that after rapid disappearance from plasma, omeprazole can be found within the gastric mucosa for a day or more.

Antisecretory Activity

Results from a study of the antisecretory effect of repeated once-daily dosing of 20 mg of ZEGERID™ in healthy subjects (n = 28) is shown below.

Effect of ZEGERID™ 20 mg on Intragastric pH on Day 7

Parameter	
% Decrease from Baseline for Integrated Intragastric Acidity (mmol*hr/L)	82%/(24%)*
% Time Gastric pH > 4 (hours)	51% (12.2 h) /(43%)*
Median pH	4.2/(37%)*

Values represent medians. All parameters were measured over a 24-hour period.

*Coefficient of variation

The antisecretory effect thus lasts far longer than would be expected from the very short plasma half-life (1 hour) apparently due to irreversible binding to the parietal H+/K+ ATPase enzyme. Repeated single daily oral doses of ZEGERID™ 20 mg have produced nearly 100% inhibition of 24-hour integrated intragastric acidity in some subjects.

Enterochromaffin-like (ECL) Cell Effects

In 24 month carcinogenicity studies in rats, a dose-related significant increase in gastric carcinoid tumors and ECL cell hyperplasia was observed in both male and female animals (see PRECAUTIONS, Carcinogenesis, Mutagenesis, Impairment of Fertility). Carcinoid tumors have also been observed in rats subjected to fundectomy or long-term treatment with other proton pump inhibitors or high doses of H2-receptor antagonists.

Human gastric biopsy specimens have been obtained from more than 3000 patients treated with omeprazole in long-term clinical trials. The incidence of ECL cell hyperplasia in these studies increased with time; however, no case of ECL cell carcinoids, dysplasia, or neoplasia has been found in these patients. (See also CLINICAL PHARMACOLOGY, Pathological Hypersecretory Conditions.)

However, these studies are of insufficient duration and size to rule out the possible influence of long-term administration of omeprazole on the development of any premalignant or malignant conditions.

Serum Gastrin Effects

In studies involving more than 200 patients, serum gastrin levels increased during the first 1 to 2 weeks of once-daily administration of therapeutic doses of omeprazole in parallel with inhibition of acid secretion. No further increase in serum gastrin occurred with continued treatment. In comparison with histamine H2-receptor antagonists, the median increases produced by 20 mg doses of omeprazole were higher (1.3 to 3.6 fold vs. 1.1 to 1.8 fold increase). Gastrin values returned to pretreatment levels, usually within 1 to 2 weeks after discontinuation of therapy.

Other Effects

Systemic effects of omeprazole in the CNS, cardiovascular and respiratory systems have not been found to date. Omeprazole, given in oral doses of 30 or 40 mg for 2 to 4 weeks, had no effect on thyroid function, carbohydrate metabolism, or circulating levels of parathyroid hormone, cortisol, estradiol, testosterone, prolactin, cholecystokinin or secretin.

No effect on gastric emptying of the solid and liquid components of a test meal was demonstrated after a single dose of omeprazole 90 mg. In healthy subjects, a single I.V. dose of omeprazole (0.35 mg/kg) had no effect on intrinsic factor secretion. No systematic dose-dependent effect has been observed on basal or stimulated pepsin output in humans. However, when intragastric pH is maintained at 4.0 or above, basal pepsin output is low, and pepsin activity is decreased.

As do other agents that elevate intragastric pH, omeprazole administered for 14 days in healthy subjects produced a significant increase in the intragastric concentrations of viable bacteria. The pattern of the bacterial species was unchanged from that commonly found in saliva. All changes resolved within three days of stopping treatment.

The course of Barrett's esophagus in 106 patients was evaluated in a U.S. double-blind controlled study of omeprazole 40 mg b.i.d. for 12 months followed by 20 mg b.i.d. for 12 months or ranitidine 300 mg b.i.d. for 24 months. No clinically significant impact on Barrett's mucosa by antisecretory therapy was observed. Although neosquamous epithelium developed during antisecretory therapy, complete elimination of Barrett's mucosa was not achieved. No significant difference was observed between treatment groups in development of dysplasia in Barrett's mucosa and no patient developed esophageal carcinoma during treatment. No significant differences between treatment groups were observed in development of ECL cell hyperplasia, corpus atrophic gastritis, corpus intestinal metaplasia, or colon polyps exceeding 3 mm in diameter (see also CLINICAL PHARMACOLOGY, Enterochromaffin-like (ECL) Cell Effects).

Clinical Studies

Duodenal Ulcer Disease

Active Duodenal Ulcer—In a multicenter, double-blind, placebo controlled study of 147 patients with endoscopically documented duodenal ulcer, the percentage of patients healed (per protocol) at 2 and 4 weeks was significantly higher with omeprazole 20 mg once a day than with placebo ($p \leq 0.01$).

Treatment of Active Duodenal Ulcer
% of Patients Healed

	Omeprazole 20 mg a.m. (n = 99)	Placebo a.m. (n = 48)
Week 2	41*	13
Week 4	75*	27

*($p \leq 0.01$)

Complete daytime and nighttime pain relief occurred significantly faster ($p \leq 0.01$) in patients treated with omeprazole 20 mg than in patients treated with placebo. At the end of the study, significantly more patients who had received omeprazole had complete relief of daytime pain ($p \leq 0.05$) and nighttime pain ($p \leq 0.01$).

In a multicenter, double-blind study of 293 patients with endoscopically documented duodenal ulcer, the percentage of patients healed (per protocol) at 4 weeks was significantly higher with omeprazole 20 mg once a day than with ranitidine 150 mg b.i.d. ($p < 0.01$).

Treatment of Active Duodenal Ulcer
% of Patients Healed

	Omeprazole 20 mg a.m. (n = 145)	Ranitidine 150 mg b.i.d. (n = 148)
Week 2	42	34
Week 4	82*	63

*($p < 0.01$)

Healing occurred significantly faster in patients treated with omeprazole than in those treated with ranitidine 150 mg b.i.d. ($p < 0.01$).

In a foreign multinational randomized, double-blind study of 105 patients with endoscopically documented duodenal ulcer, 20 mg and 40 mg of omeprazole were compared to 150 mg b.i.d. of ranitidine at 2, 4 and 8 weeks. At 2 and 4 weeks both doses of omeprazole were statistically superior (per protocol) to ranitidine, but 40 mg was not superior to 20 mg of omeprazole, and at 8 weeks there was no significant difference between any of the active drugs.

Treatment of Active Duodenal Ulcer
% of Patients Healed

	Omeprazole		Ranitidine
	20 mg (n = 34)	40 mg (n = 36)	150 mg b.i.d. (n = 35)
Week 2	83*	83*	53
Week 4	97*	100*	82
Week 8	100	100	94

*($p \leq 0.01$)

Gastroesophageal Reflux Disease (GERD)

Symptomatic GERD

A placebo controlled study was conducted in Scandinavia to compare the efficacy of omeprazole 20 mg or 10 mg once daily for up to 4 weeks in the treatment of heartburn and other symptoms in GERD patients without erosive esophagitis. Results are shown below.

% Successful Symptomatic Outcome[a]

	Omeprazole 20 mg a.m.	Omeprazole 10 mg a.m.	Placebo a.m.
All patients	46*,† (n = 205)	31† (n = 199)	13 (n = 105)
Patients with confirmed GERD	56*,† (n = 115)	36† (n = 109)	14 (n = 59)

[a]Defined as complete resolution of heartburn

*($p < 0.005$) versus 10 mg

†($p < 0.005$) versus placebo

Erosive Esophagitis

In a U.S. multicenter double-blind placebo controlled study of 20 mg or 40 mg of omeprazole in patients with symptoms of GERD and endoscopically diagnosed erosive esophagitis of grade 2 or above, the percentage healing rates (per protocol) were as follows:

Week	20 mg Omeprazole (n = 83)	40 mg Omeprazole (n = 87)	Placebo (n = 43)
4	39*	45*	7
8	74*	75*	14

*($p < 0.01$) Omeprazole versus placebo.

In this study, the 40 mg dose was not superior to the 20 mg dose of omeprazole in the percentage healing rate. Other controlled clinical trials have also shown that omeprazole is effective in severe GERD. In comparisons with histamine H2-receptor antagonists in patients with erosive esophagitis, grade 2 or above, omeprazole in a dose of 20 mg was significantly more effective than the active controls. Complete daytime and nighttime heartburn relief occurred significantly faster ($p < 0.01$) in patients treated with omeprazole than in those taking placebo or histamine H2-receptor antagonists.

In this and five other controlled GERD studies, significantly more patients taking 20 mg omeprazole (84%) reported complete relief of GERD symptoms than patients receiving placebo (12%).

Long Term Maintenance Treatment of Erosive Esophagitis

In a U.S. double-blind, randomized, multicenter, placebo controlled study, two dose regimens of omeprazole were studied in patients with endoscopically confirmed healed esophagitis. Results to determine maintenance of healing of erosive esophagitis are shown below.

Life Table Analysis

	Omeprazole 20 mg q.d. (n = 138)	Omeprazole 20 mg 3 days per week (n = 137)	Placebo (n = 131)
Percent in endoscopic remission at 6 months	70*	34	11

*($p < 0.01$) Omeprazole 20 mg q.d. versus Omeprazole 20 mg 3 consecutive days per week or placebo.

In an international multicenter double-blind study, omeprazole 20 mg daily and 10 mg daily were compared to ranitidine 150 mg twice daily in patients with endoscopically confirmed healed esophagitis. The table below provides the results of this study for maintenance of healing of erosive esophagitis.

Life Table Analysis

	Omeprazole 20 mg q.d. (n = 131)	Omeprazole 10 mg q.d. (n = 133)	Ranitidine 150 mg b.i.d. (n = 128)
Percent in endoscopic remission at 12 months	77*	58‡	46

*($p = 0.01$) Omeprazole 20 mg q.d. versus Omeprazole 10 mg q.d. or Ranitidine.

‡($p = 0.03$) Omeprazole 10 mg q.d. versus Ranitidine.

In patients who initially had grades 3 or 4 erosive esophagitis, for maintenance after healing 20 mg daily of omeprazole was effective, while 10 mg did not demonstrate effectiveness.

INDICATIONS AND USAGE

Duodenal Ulcer

ZEGERID™ is indicated for short-term treatment of active duodenal ulcer. Most patients heal within four weeks. Some patients may require an additional four weeks of therapy.

Treatment of Gastroesophageal Reflux Disease (GERD)

Symptomatic GERD

ZEGERID™, is indicated for the treatment of heartburn and other symptoms associated with GERD.

Erosive Esophagitis
ZEGERID™, is indicated for the short-term treatment (4-8 weeks) of erosive esophagitis which has been diagnosed by endoscopy. (See CLINICAL PHARMACOLOGY, Clinical Studies.)
The efficacy of ZEGERID™ used for longer than 8 weeks in these patients has not been established. In the rare instance of a patient not responding to 8 weeks of treatment, it may be helpful to give up to an additional 4 weeks of treatment. If there is recurrence of erosive esophagitis or GERD symptoms (e.g. heartburn), additional 4-8 week courses of omeprazole may be considered.

Maintenance of Healing of Erosive Esophagitis
ZEGERID™ Powder for Oral Suspension is indicated to maintain healing of erosive esophagitis.
Controlled studies do not extend beyond 12 months.

CONTRAINDICATIONS

ZEGERID™ is contraindicated in patients with known hypersensitivity to any components of the formulation.

PRECAUTIONS

General
Symptomatic response to therapy with omeprazole does not preclude the presence of gastric malignancy.
Atrophic gastritis has been noted occasionally in gastric corpus biopsies from patients treated long-term with omeprazole.
ZEGERID™ contains 460 mg sodium per dose in the form of sodium bicarbonate. This should be taken into consideration for patients on a sodium-restricted diet.
ZEGERID™ contains 1680 mg (20 mEq) of sodium bicarbonate. Sodium bicarbonate is contraindicated in patients with metabolic alkalosis and hypocalcemia. Sodium bicarbonate should be used with caution in patients with Bartter's syndrome, hypokalemia, and respiratory alkalosis. Long-term administration of bicarbonate with calcium or milk can cause milk-alkali syndrome.

Information for Patients
ZEGERID™ is supplied as a powder for oral suspension. It should be taken on an empty stomach at least 1 hour prior to a meal.
ZEGERID™ is available as 20 mg single-dose packets. Directions for use: Empty packet contents into a small cup containing 2 tablespoons of water. DO NOT USE OTHER LIQUIDS OR FOODS. Stir well and drink immediately. Refill cup with water and drink.

Drug Interactions
Other
Omeprazole can prolong the elimination of diazepam, warfarin and phenytoin, drugs that are metabolized by oxidation in the liver. There have been reports of increased INR and prothrombin time in patients receiving proton pump inhibitors, including omeprazole, and warfarin concomitantly. Increases in INR and prothrombin time may lead to abnormal bleeding and even death. Patients treated with proton pump inhibitors and warfarin may need to be monitored for increases in INR and prothrombin time. Although in healthy subjects no interaction with theophylline or propranolol was found, there have been clinical reports of interaction with other drugs metabolized via the cytochrome P-450 system (e.g., cyclosporine, disulfiram, benzodiazepines). Patients should be monitored to determine if it is necessary to adjust the dosage of these drugs when taken concomitantly with ZEGERID™.
Because of its profound and long-lasting inhibition of gastric acid secretion, it is theoretically possible that omeprazole may interfere with absorption of drugs where gastric pH is an important determinant of their bioavailability (e.g., ketoconazole, ampicillin esters, and iron salts). In the clinical trials, antacids were used concomitantly with the administration of omeprazole.
Co-administration of omeprazole and clarithromycin have resulted in increases of plasma levels of omeprazole, clarithromycin, and 14-hydroxy-clarithromycin (see also **CLINICAL PHARMACOLOGY, Pharmacokinetics**).

Carcinogenesis, Mutagenesis, Impairment of Fertility
In two 24-month carcinogenicity studies in rats, omeprazole at daily doses of 1.7, 3.4, 13.8, 44.0 and 140.8 mg/kg/day (about 0.7 to 57 times the human dose of 20 mg per day, based on body surface area) produced gastric ECL cell carcinoids in a dose-related manner in both male and female rats; the incidence of this effect was markedly higher in female rats, which had higher blood levels of omeprazole. Gastric carcinoids seldom occur in the untreated rat. In addition, ECL cell hyperplasia was present in all treated groups of both sexes. In one of these studies, female rats were treated with 13.8 mg omeprazole/kg/day (about 5.7 times the human dose of 20 mg per day, based on body surface area) for one year, then followed for an additional year without the drug. No carcinoids were seen in these rats. An increased incidence of treatment-related ECL cell hyperplasia was observed at the end of one year (94% treated vs 10% controls). By the second year the difference between treated and control rats was much smaller (46% vs 26%) but still showed more hyperplasia in the treated group. Gastric adenocarcinoma was seen in one rat (2%). No similar tumor was seen in male or female rats treated for two years. For this strain of rat no similar tumor has been noted historically, but a finding involving only one tumor is difficult to interpret. In a 52-week toxicity study in Sprague-Dawley rats, brain astrocytomas were found in a small number of males that received omeprazole at dose levels of 0.4, 2, and 16 mg/kg/day (about 0.2 to 6.5 times the human dose of 20 mg/day, based on body surface area). No astrocytomas were observed in female rats in this study. In a 2-year carcinogenicity study in Sprague-Dawley rats, no astrocytomas were found in males and females at the high dose of 140.8 mg/kg/day (about 57 times the human dose of 20 mg per day, based on body surface area). A 78-week mouse carcinogenicity study of omeprazole did not show increased tumor occurrence, but the study was not conclusive. A 26-week p53 (+/−) transgenic mouse carcinogenicity study was not positive.
Omeprazole was positive for clastogenic effects in an *in vitro* human lymphocyte chromosomal aberration assay, in one of two *in vivo* mouse micronucleus tests, and in an in vivo bone marrow cell chromosomal aberration assay. Omeprazole was negative in the *in vitro* Ames *Salmonella typhimurium* assay, an *in vitro* mouse lymphoma cell forward mutation assay and an *in vivo* rat liver DNA damage assay.
Omeprazole at oral doses up to 138.0 mg/kg/day (about 56 times the human dose of 20 mg per day, based on body surface area) was found to have no effect on fertility and reproductive performance.

Pregnancy
Pregnancy Category C
There are no adequate and well-controlled studies on the use of omeprazole in pregnant women. The vast majority of reported experience with omeprazole during human pregnancy is first trimester exposure and the duration of use is rarely specified, e.g., intermittent vs. chronic. An expert review of published data on experiences with omeprazole use during pregnancy by TERIS – the Teratogen Information System – concluded that therapeutic doses during pregnancy are unlikely to pose a substantial teratogenic risk (the quantity and quality of data were assessed as fair).
Three epidemiological studies compared the frequency of congenital abnormalities among infants born to women who used omeprazole during pregnancy to the frequency of abnormalities among infants of women exposed to H2-receptor antagonists or other controls. A population-based prospective cohort epidemiological study from the Swedish Medical Birth Registry, covering approximately 99% of pregnancies, reported on 955 infants (824 exposed during the first trimester with 39 of these exposed beyond first trimester, and 131 exposed after the first trimester) whose mothers used omeprazole during pregnancy. In utero exposure to omeprazole was not associated with increased risk of any malformation (odds ratio 0.82, 95% CI 0.50-1.34), low birth weight or low Apgar score. The number of infants born with ventricular septal defects and the number of stillborn infants was slightly higher in the omeprazole exposed infants than the expected number in the normal population. The author concluded that both effects may be random.
A retrospective cohort study reported on 689 pregnant women exposed to either H2-blockers or omeprazole in the first trimester (134 exposed to omeprazole). The overall malformation rate was 4.4% (95% CI 3.6-5.3) and the malformation rate for first trimester exposure to omeprazole was 3.6% (95% CI 1.5-8.1). The relative risk of malformations associated with first trimester exposure to omeprazole compared with nonexposed women was 0.9 (95% CI 0.3-2.2). The study could effectively rule out a relative risk greater than 2.5 for all malformations. Rates of preterm delivery or growth retardation did not differ between the groups.
A controlled prospective observational study followed 113 women exposed to omeprazole during pregnancy (89% first trimester exposures). The reported rates of major congenital malformations was 4% for the omeprazole group, 2% for controls exposed to nonteratogens, and 2.8% in disease-paired controls (background incidence of major malformations 1-5%). Rates of spontaneous and elective abortions, preterm deliveries gestational age at delivery, and mean birth weight did not differ between the groups. The sample size in this study has 80% power to detect a 5-fold increase in the rate of major malformation.
Several studies have reported no apparent adverse short term effects on the infant when single dose oral or intravenous omeprazole was administered to over 200 pregnant women as premedication for cesarean section under general anesthesia.
Teratology studies conducted in pregnant rats at omeprazole doses up to 138 mg/kg/day (about 56 times the human dose of 20 mg/day, based on body surface area) and in pregnant rabbits at doses up to 69 mg/kg/day (about 56 times the human dose of 20 mg per day, based on body surface area) did not disclose any evidence for a teratogenic potential of omeprazole.
In rabbits, omeprazole in a dose range of 6.9 to 69.1 mg/kg/day (about 5.6 to 56 times the human dose of 20 mg per day, based on body surface area) produced dose-related increases in embryo-lethality, fetal resorptions and pregnancy disruptions. In rats, dose-related embryo/fetal toxicity and postnatal developmental toxicity were observed in offspring resulting from parents treated with omeprazole at 13.8 to 138.0 mg/kg/day (about 5.6 to 56 times the human dose of 20 mg per day, based on body surface area).
Chronic use of sodium bicarbonate may lead to systemic alkalosis and increased sodium intake can produce edema and weight increase. There are no adequate and well-controlled studies in pregnant women. Because animal studies and studies in humans cannot rule out the possibility of harm, omeprazole should be used during pregnancy only if the potential benefit to pregnant women justifies the potential risk to the fetus.

Nursing Mothers
Omeprazole concentrations have been measured in breast milk of a woman following oral administration of 20 mg. The peak concentration of omeprazole in breast milk was less than 7% of the peak serum concentration. The concentration will correspond to 0.004 mg of omeprazole in 200 mL of milk. In rats, omeprazole administration during late gestation and lactation at doses of 13.8 to 138 mg/kg/day (about 5.6 to 56 times the human dose of 20 mg per day, based on body surface area) resulted in decreased weight gain in pups. Because omeprazole is excreted in human milk, because of the potential for serious adverse reactions in nursing infants from omeprazole, and because of the potential for tumorigenicity shown for omeprazole in rat carcinogenicity studies, a decision should be made whether to discontinue nursing or to discontinue the drug, taking into account the importance of the drug to the mother. In addition, sodium bicarbonate should be used with caution in nursing mothers.

Pediatric Use
There are no adequate and well-controlled studies in pediatric patients with ZEGERID™.

Geriatric Use
Omeprazole was administered to over 2000 elderly individuals (≥ 65 years of age) in clinical trials in the U.S. and Europe. There were no differences in safety and effectiveness between the elderly and younger subjects. Other reported clinical experience has not identified differences in response between the elderly and younger subjects, but greater sensitivity of some older individuals cannot be ruled out.
Pharmacokinetic studies with omeprazole have shown the elimination rate was somewhat decreased in the elderly and bioavailability was increased. The plasma clearance of omeprazole was 250 mL/min (about half that of young subjects). The plasma half-life averaged one hour, about the same as that in nonelderly, healthy subjects taking ZEGERID™. However, no dosage adjustment is necessary in the elderly. (See CLINICAL PHARMACOLOGY.)

ADVERSE REACTIONS

Omeprazole was generally well tolerated during domestic and international clinical trials in 3096 patients.
In the U.S. clinical trial population of 465 patients, the following adverse experiences were reported to occur in 1% or more of patients on therapy with omeprazole. Numbers in parentheses indicate percentages of the adverse experiences considered by investigators as possibly, probably or definitely related to the drug.

	Omeprazole (n = 465)	Placebo (n = 64)	Ranitidine (n = 195)
Headache	6.9 (2.4)	6.3	7.7 (2.6)
Diarrhea	3.0 (1.9)	3.1 (1.6)	2.1 (0.5)
Abdominal Pain	2.4 (0.4)	3.1	2.1
Nausea	2.2 (0.9)	3.1	4.1 (0.5)
URI	1.9	1.6	2.6
Dizziness	1.5 (0.6)	0.0	2.6 (1.0)
Vomiting	1.5 (0.4)	4.7	1.5 (0.5)
Rash	1.5 (1.1)	0.0	0.0
Constipation	1.1 (0.9)	0.0	0.0
Cough	1.1	0.0	1.5
Asthenia	1.1 (0.2)	1.6 (1.6)	1.5 (1.0)
Back Pain	1.1	0.0	0.5

The following adverse reactions which occurred in 1% or more of omeprazole-treated patients have been reported in international double-blind, and open-label, clinical trials in which 2,631 patients and subjects received omeprazole.

Incidence of Adverse Experiences ≥ 1%
Causal Relationship not Assessed

	Omeprazole (n = 2631)	Placebo (n = 120)
Body as a Whole, site unspecified		
Abdominal pain	5.2	3.3
Asthenia	1.3	0.8
Digestive System		
Constipation	1.5	0.8
Diarrhea	3.7	2.5
Flatulence	2.7	5.8
Nausea	4.0	6.7

Continued on next page

Zegerid—Cont.

Vomiting	3.2	10.0
Acid regurgitation	1.9	3.3
Nervious System / Psychiatric		
Headache	2.9	2.5

Additional adverse reactions occurring in < 1% of patients or subjects in domestic and/or international trials conducted with omeprazole, or occurring since the drug was marketed, are shown below within each body system. In many instances, the relationship to omeprazole was unclear.

Body as a Whole
Allergic reactions, including, rarely, anaphylaxis (see also *Skin* below), fever, pain, fatigue, malaise, abdominal swelling.

Cardiovascular
Chest pain or angina, tachycardia, bradycardia, palpitation, elevated blood pressure, and peripheral edema.

Gastrointestinal
Pancreatitis (some fatal), anorexia, irritable colon, flatulence, fecal discoloration, esophageal candidiasis, mucosal atrophy of the tongue, dry mouth. During treatment with omeprazole, gastric fundic gland polyps have been noted rarely. These polyps are benign and appear to be reversible when treatment is discontinued.
Gastroduodenal carcinoids have been reported in patients with ZE syndrome on long-term treatment with omeprazole. This finding is believed to be a manifestation of the underlying condition, which is known to be associated with such tumors.

Hepatic
Mild and, rarely, marked elevations of liver function tests [ALT (SGPT), AST (SGOT), γ-glutamyl transpeptidase, alkaline phosphatase, and bilirubin (jaundice)]. In rare instances, overt liver disease has occurred, including hepatocellular, cholestatic, or mixed hepatitis, liver necrosis (some fatal), hepatic failure (some fatal), and hepatic encephalopathy.

Metabolic / Nutritional
Hyponatremia, hypoglycemia, and weight gain.

Musculoskeletal
Muscle cramps, myalgia, muscle weakness, joint pain, and leg pain.

Nervous System / Psychiatric
Psychic disturbances including depression, aggression, hallucinations, confusion, insomnia, nervousness, tremors, apathy, somnolence, anxiety, dream abnormalities; vertigo; paresthesia; and hemifacial dysesthesia.

Respiratory
Epistaxis, pharyngeal pain

Skin
Rash and rarely, cases of severe generalized skin reactions including toxic epidermal necrolysis (TEN; some fatal), Stevens-Johnson syndrome, and erythema multiforme (some severe); purpura and/or petechiae (some with rechallenge); skin inflammation, urticaria, angioedema, pruritus, alopecia, dry skin, and hyperhidrosis.

Special Senses
Tinnitus, taste perversion

Ocular
Blurred vision, ocular irritation, dry eye syndrome, optic atrophy, anterior ischemic optic neuropathy, optic neuritis and double vision.

Urogenital
Interstitial nephritis (some with positive rechallenge), urinary tract infection, microscopic pyuria, urinary frequency, elevated serum creatinine, proteinuria, hematuria, glycosuria, testicular pain, and gynecomastia.

Hematologic
Rare instances of pancytopenia, agranulocytosis (some fatal), thrombocytopenia, neutropenia, anemia, leucocytosis, and hemolytic anemia have been reported.
The incidence of clinical adverse experiences in patients greater than 65 years of age was similar to that in patients 65 years of age or less.
Additional adverse reactions that could be caused by sodium bicarbonate, include metabolic alkalosis, seizures, and tetany.

OVERDOSAGE

Reports have been received of overdosage with omeprazole in humans. Doses ranged up to 2400 mg (120 times the usual recommended clinical dose). Manifestations were variable, but included confusion, drowsiness, blurred vision, tachycardia, nausea, vomiting, diaphoresis, flushing, headache, dry mouth, and other adverse reactions similar to those seen in normal clinical experience. (See ADVERSE REACTIONS.) Symptoms were transient, and no serious clinical outcome has been reported when omeprazole was taken alone. No specific antidote for omeprazole overdosage is known. Omeprazole is extensively protein bound and is, therefore, not readily dialyzable. In the event of overdosage, treatment should be symptomatic and supportive.
As with the management of any overdose, the possibility of multiple drug ingestion should be considered. For current information on treatment of any drug overdose, a certified Regional Poison Control Center should be contacted. Telephone numbers are listed in the Physicians' Desk Reference (PDR) or local telephone book.
Single oral doses of omeprazole at 1350, 1339, and 1200 mg/kg were lethal to mice, rats, and dogs, respectively. Animals given these doses showed sedation, ptosis, tremors, convulsions, and decreased activity, body temperature, and respiratory rate and increased depth of respiration.
In addition, a sodium bicarbonate overdose may cause hypocalcemia, hypokalemia, hypernatremia, and seizures.

DOSAGE AND ADMINISTRATION

Short-Term Treatment of Active Duodenal Ulcer
The recommended adult oral dose of omeprazole, is 20 mg once daily. Most patients heal within four weeks. Some patients may require an additional four weeks of therapy. (See INDICATIONS AND USAGE.)

Gastroesophageal Reflux Disease (GERD)
The recommended adult oral dose for the treatment of patients with symptomatic GERD and no esophageal lesions is 20 mg daily for up to 4 weeks. The recommended adult oral dose for the treatment of patients with erosive esophagitis and accompanying symptoms due to GERD is 20 mg daily for 4 to 8 weeks. (See INDICATIONS AND USAGE.)

Maintenance of Healing of Erosive Esophagitis
The recommended adult oral dose is 20 mg daily. (See CLINICAL PHARMACOLOGY, Clinical Studies.)

Preparation and Administration of Suspension
ZEGERID™ should be taken on an empty stomach 1 hour before a meal.
ZEGERID™ is supplied as unit dose packets containing an immediate-release formulation of omeprazole 20 mg.
Directions for use: Empty packet contents into a small cup containing 2 tablespoons of WATER. DO NOT USE OTHER LIQUIDS OR FOODS. Stir well and drink immediately. Refill cup with water and drink.

HOW SUPPLIED

ZEGERID™ is a white, flavored powder packaged in individual 20 mg dose packets. It is supplied as follows:
NDC 68012-052-30 Cartons of 30: 20 mg unit dose packets

Storage
Store ZEGERID™ in its original individual packets. Store at 25°C (68 - 77°F): excursions permitted to 15 - 30°C (59 - 86°F). **[see USP Controlled Room Temperature]**
ZEGERID™ is a trademark of Santarus, Inc.
Manufactured for: Santarus, Inc., San Diego, CA 92130
By: Patheon Inc., Whitby, Ontario L1N 5Z5
Shown in Product Identification Guide, page 332

Savient Pharmaceuticals, Inc.

ONE TOWER CENTER
FOURTEENTH FLOOR
EAST BRUNSWICK, NJ 08816

For Medical or Reimbursement Information Contact:
886-OXANDRIN or visit
http:\\www.oxandrin.com
For Product Ordering please call: (800) 741-2698
Fax: (800) 741-2696

DELATESTRYL® Ⓒ℞

[dē-lăt-'strĭl]
Testosterone Enanthate Injection USP
Multiple Dose Vial
Rx only

DESCRIPTION

DELATESTRYL (Testosterone Enanthate Injection) provides testosterone enanthate, a derivative of the primary endogenous androgen testosterone, for intramuscular administration. In their active form, androgens have a 17-beta-hydroxy group. Esterification of the 17-beta-hyroxy group increases the duration of action of testosterone; hydrolysis to free testosterone occurs in vivo. Each mL of sterile, colorless to pale yellow solution provides 200 mg testosterone enanthate in sesame oil with 5 mg chlorobutanol (chloral derivative) as a preservative.
Testosterone enanthate is designated chemically as androst-4-en-3-one, 17-[(1-oxoheptyl)-oxy]-, (17β)-. Structural formula:

$OCO(CH_2)_5CH_3$ CH3 H

$C_{26}H_{40}O_3$ MW 400.60

CLINICAL PHARMACOLOGY

Endogenous androgens are responsible for the normal growth and development of the male sex organs and for maintenance of secondary sex characteristics. These effects include growth and maturation of prostate, seminal vesicles, penis, and scrotum; development of male hair distribution, such as beard, pubic, chest, and axillary hair; laryngeal enlargement; vocal chord thickening; alterations in body musculature; and fat distribution.
Androgens also cause retention of nitrogen, sodium, potassium, and phosphorus, and decreased urinary excretion of calcium. Androgens have been reported to increase protein anabolism and decrease protein catabolism. Nitrogen balance is improved only when there is sufficient intake of calories and protein.
Androgens are responsible for the growth spurt of adolescence and for the eventual termination of linear growth, which is brought about by fusion of the epiphyseal growth centers. In children, exogenous androgens accelerate linear growth rates but may cause a disproportionate advancement in bone maturation. Use over long periods may result in fusion of the epiphyseal growth centers and termination of growth process. Androgens have been reported to stimulate the production of red blood cells by enhancing the production of erythropoietic stimulating factor.
During exogenous administration of androgens, endogenous testosterone release is inhibited through feedback inhibition of pituitary luteinizing hormone (LH). At large doses of exogenous androgens, spermatogenesis may also be suppressed through feedback inhibition of pituitary follicle stimulating hormone (FSH).
There is a lack of substantial evidence that androgens are effective in fractures, surgery, convalescence, and functional uterine bleeding.

PHARMACOKINETICS
Testosterone esters are less polar than free testosterone. Testosterone esters in oil injected intramuscularly are absorbed slowly from the lipid phase; thus testosterone enanthate can be given at intervals of two to four weeks.
Testosterone in plasma is 98 percent bound to a specific testosterone-estradiol binding globulin, and about two percent is free. Generally, the amount of this sex-hormone binding globulin in the plasma will determine the distribution of testosterone between free and bound forms, and the free testosterone concentration will determine its half-life.
About 90 percent of a dose of testosterone is excreted in the urine as glucuronic and sulfuric acid conjugates of testosterone and its metabolites; about six percent of a dose is excreted in the feces, mostly in the unconjugated form. Inactivation of testosterone occurs primarily in the liver. Testosterone is metabolized to various 17-keto steroids through two different pathways. There are considerable variations of the half-life of testosterone as reported in the literature, ranging from 10 to 100 minutes.
In responsive tissues, the activity of testosterone appears to depend on reduction to dihydrotestosterone, which binds to cytosol receptor proteins. The steroid-receptor complex is transported to the nucleus where it initiates transcription events and cellular changes related to androgen action.

INDICATIONS AND USAGE

Males
DELATESTRYL (Testosterone Enanthate Injection) is indicated for replacement therapy in conditions associated with a deficiency or absence of endogenous testosterone.
Primary hypogonadism (congenital or acquired)—Testicular failure due to cryptorchidism, bilateral torsion, orchitis, vanishing testis syndrome, or orchidectomy.
Hypogonadotropic hypogonadism (congenital or acquired)—Idiopathic gonadotropin or luteinizing hormone-releasing hormone (LHRH) deficiency, or pituitary-hypothalamic injury from tumors, trauma, or radiation. (Appropriate adrenal cortical and thyroid hormone replacement therapy are still necessary, however, and are actually of primary importance.)
If the above conditions occur prior to puberty, androgen replacement therapy will be needed during the adolescent years for development of secondary sexual characteristics. Prolonged androgen treatment will be required to maintain sexual characteristics in these and other males who develop testosterone deficiency after puberty.
Delayed puberty—DELATESTRYL (Testosterone Enanthate Injection) may be used to stimulate puberty in carefully selected males with clearly delayed puberty. These patients usually have a familial pattern of delayed puberty that is not secondary to a pathological disorder; puberty is expected to occur spontaneously at a relatively late date. Brief treatment with conservative doses may occasionally be justified in these patients if they do not respond to psychological support. The potential adverse effect on bone maturation should be discussed with the patient and parents prior to androgen administration. An X-ray of the hand and wrist to determine bone age should be obtained every six months to assess the effect of treatment on the epiphyseal centers (see WARNINGS).

Females
Metastatic mammary cancer—DELATESTRYL (Testosterone Enanthate Injection) may be used secondarily in women with advancing inoperable metastatic (skeletal) mammary cancer who are one to five years postmenopausal. Primary goals of therapy in these women include ablation of the ovaries. Other methods of counteracting estrogen activity are adrenalectomy, hypophysectomy, and/or antiestrogen therapy. This treatment has also been used in premenopausal women with breast cancer who have benefited from oophorectomy and are considered to have a hormone-responsive tumor. Judgment concerning androgen therapy should be made by an oncologist with expertise in this field.

CONTRAINDICATIONS

Androgens are contraindicated in men with carcinomas of the breast or with known or suspected carcinomas of the prostate and in women who are or may become pregnant. When administered to pregnant women, androgens cause

virilization of the external genitalia of the female fetus. This virilization includes clitoromegaly, abnormal vaginal development, and fusion of genital folds to form a scrotal-like structure. The degree of masculinization is related to the amount of drug given and the age of the fetus and is most likely to occur in the female fetus when the drugs are given in the first trimester. If the patient becomes pregnant while taking androgens, she should be apprised of the potential hazard to the fetus.
This preparation is also contraindicated in patients with a history of hypersensitivity to any of its components.

WARNINGS

In patients with breast cancer and in immobilized patients, androgen therapy may cause hypercalcemia by stimulating osteolysis. In patients with cancer, hypercalcemia may indicate progression of bony metastasis. If hypercalcemia occurs, the drug should be discontinued and appropriate measures instituted.
Prolonged use of high doses of androgens has been associated with the development of peliosis hepatis and hepatic neoplasms including hepatocellular carcinoma (see PRECAUTIONS, Carcinogenesis). Peliosis hepatis can be a life-threatening or fatal complication.
If cholestatic hepatitis with jaundice appears or if liver function tests become abnormal, the androgen should be discontinued and the etiology should be determined. Drug-induced jaundice is reversible when the medication is discontinued.
Geriatric patients treated with androgens may be at an increased risk for the development of prostatic hypertrophy and prostatic carcinoma.
Due to sodium and water retention, edema with or without congestive heart failure may be a serious complication in patients with preexisting cardiac, renal, or hepatic disease. In addition to discontinuation of the drug, diuretic therapy may be required. If the administration of testosterone enanthate is restarted, a lower dose should be used.
Gynecomastia frequently develops and occasionally persists in patients being treated for hypogonadism.
Androgen therapy should be used cautiously in healthy males with delayed puberty. The effect on bone maturation should be monitored by assessing bone age of the wrist and hand every six months. In children, androgen treatment may accelerate bone maturation without producing compensatory gain in linear growth. This adverse effect may result in compromised adult stature. The younger the child the greater the risk of compromising final mature height.

PRECAUTIONS

General
Women should be observed for signs of virilization (deepening of the voice, hirsutism, acne, clitoromegaly, and menstrual irregularities). Discontinuation of drug therapy at the time of evidence of mild virilism is necessary to prevent irreversible virilization. Such virilization is usual following androgen use at high doses and is not prevented by concomitant use of estrogens. A decision may be made by the patient and the physician that some virilization will be tolerated during treatment for breast carcinoma.
Because androgens may alter serum cholesterol concentration, caution should be used when administering these drugs to patients with a history of myocardial infarction or coronary artery disease. Serial determinations of serum cholesterol should be made and therapy adjusted accordingly. A causal relationship between myocardial infarction and hypercholesterolemia has not been established.
Information for Patients
Male adolescent patients receiving androgens for delayed puberty should have bone development checked every six months.
The physician should instruct patients to report any of the following side effects of androgens:
Adult or adolescent males—too frequent or persistent erections of the penis.
Women—hoarseness, acne, changes in menstrual periods, or more facial hair.
All patients—Any nausea, vomiting, changes in skin color, or ankle swelling.
Laboratory Tests
Women with disseminated breast carcinoma should have frequent determination of urine and serum calcium levels during the course of androgen therapy (see WARNINGS).
Periodic (every six months) X-ray examinations of bone age should be made during treatment of pre-pubertal males to determine the rate of bone maturation and the effects of androgen therapy on the epiphyseal centers.
Hemoglobin and hematocrit should be checked periodically for polycythemia in patients who are receiving high doses of androgens.
Drug Interactions
When administered concurrently, the following drugs may interact with androgens:
Anticoagulants, oral—C-17 substituted derivatives of testosterone, such as methandrostenolone, have been reported to decrease the anticoagulant requirement. Patients receiving oral anticoagulant therapy require close monitoring especially when androgens are started or stopped.
Antidiabetic drugs and insulin—In diabetic patients, the metabolic effects of androgens may decrease blood glucose and insulin requirements.
ACTH and corticosteroids—Enhanced tendency toward edema. Use caution when giving these drugs together, especially in patients with hepatic or cardiac disease.
Oxyphenbutazone—Elevated serum levels of oxyphenbutazone may result.
Drug/Laboratory Test Interferences
Androgens may decrease levels of thyroxine-binding globulin, resulting in decreased total T_4 serum levels and increased resin uptake of T_3 and T_4. Free thyroid hormone levels remain unchanged, however, and there is no clinical evidence of thyroid dysfunction.
Carcinogenesis
Testosterone has been tested by subcutaneous injection and implantation in mice and rats. The implant induced cervical-uterine tumors in mice, which metastasized in some cases. There is suggestive evidence that injection of testosterone into some strains of female mice increases their susceptibility to hepatoma. Testosterone is also known to increase the number of tumors and decrease the degree of differentiation of chemically induced carcinomas of the liver in rats.
There are rare reports of hepatocellular carcinoma in patients receiving long-term therapy with androgens in high doses. Withdrawal of the drugs did not lead to regression of the tumors in all cases.
Geriatric patients treated with androgens may be at an increased risk for the development of prostatic hypertrophy and prostatic carcinoma.
Pregnancy: Teratogenic Effects
Category X (see CONTRAINDICATIONS).
Nursing Mothers
It is not known whether androgens are excreted in human milk. Because many drugs are excreted in human milk and because of the potential for serious adverse reactions in nursing infants from androgens, a decision should be made whether to discontinue nursing or to discontinue the drug, taking into account the importance of the drug to the mother.
Pediatric Use
Androgen therapy should be used very cautiously in pediatric patients and only by specialists who are aware of the adverse effects on bone maturation. Skeletal maturation must be monitored every six months by an X-ray of the hand and wrist (see INDICATIONS AND USAGE, and WARNINGS).

ADVERSE REACTIONS

Endocrine and Urogenital, Female—The most common side effects of androgen therapy are amenorrhea and other menstrual irregularities, inhibition of gonadotropin secretion, and virilization, including deepening of the voice and clitoral enlargement. The latter usually is not reversible after androgens are discontinued. When administered to a pregnant woman, androgens cause virilization of the external genitalia of the female fetus. *Male*—Gynecomastia, and excessive frequency and duration of penile erections. Oligospermia may occur at high dosages (see CLINICAL PHARMACOLOGY).
Skin and Appendages—Hirsutism, male pattern baldness, and acne.
Fluid and Electrolyte Disturbances—Retention of sodium, chloride, water, potassium, calcium (see WARNINGS), and inorganic phosphates.
Gastrointestinal—Nausea, cholestatic jaundice, alterations in liver function tests; rarely, hepatocellular neoplasms, peliosis hepatis (see WARNINGS).
Hematologic—Suppression of clotting factors II, V, VII, and X; bleeding in patients on concomitant anticoagulant therapy; polycythemia.
Nervous System—Increased or decreased libido, headache, anxiety, depression, and generalized paresthesia.
Metabolic—Increased serum cholesterol.
Miscellaneous—Rarely, anaphylactoid reactions; inflammation and pain at injection site.

DRUG ABUSE AND DEPENDENCE

DELATESTRYL is classified as a controlled substance under the Anabolic Steroids Control Act of 1990 and has been assigned to Schedule III.

OVERDOSAGE

There have been no reports of acute overdosage with androgens.

DOSAGE AND ADMINISTRATION

Dosage and duration of therapy with DELATESTRYL (Testosterone Enanthate Injection) will depend on age, sex, diagnosis, patient's response to treatment, and appearance of adverse effects. When properly given, injections of DELATESTRYL are well tolerated. Care should be taken to inject the preparation deeply into the gluteal muscle following the usual precautions for intramuscular administration. In general, total doses above 400 mg per month are not required because of the prolonged action of the preparation. Injections more frequently than every two weeks are rarely indicated. NOTE: Use of a wet needle or wet syringe may cause the solution to become cloudy; however this does not affect the potency of the material. Parenteral drug products should be inspected visually for particulate matter and discoloration prior to administration, whenever solution and container permit. DELATESTRYL is a clear, colorless to pale yellow solution.
Male hypogonadism: As replacement therapy, i.e., for eunuchism, the suggested dosage is 50 to 400 mg every 2 to 4 weeks.
In males with delayed puberty: Various dosage regimens have been used; some call for lower dosages initially with gradual increases as puberty progresses, with or without a decrease to maintenance levels. Other regimens call for higher dosage to induce pubertal changes and lower dosage for maintenance after puberty. The chronological and skeletal ages must be taken into consideration, both in determining the initial dose and in adjusting the dose. Dosage is within the range of 50 to 200 mg every 2 to 4 weeks for a limited duration, for example, 4 to 6 months. X-rays should be taken at appropriate intervals to determine the amount of bone maturation and skeletal development (see INDICATIONS AND USAGE, and WARNINGS).
Palliation of inoperable mammary cancer in women: A dosage of 200 to 400 mg every 2 to 4 weeks is recommended. Women with metastatic breast carcinoma must be followed closely because androgen therapy occasionally appears to accelerate the disease.

HOW SUPPLIED

DELATESTRYL (Testosterone Enanthate Injection) is available in a 5 mL (200 mg/mL) multiple dose vial (NDC 54396-328-40).
Storage
DELATESTRYL (Testosterone Enanthate Injection) should be stored at room temperature. Warming and rotating the syringe unit or vial between the palms of the hands will redissolve any crystals that may have formed during storage at low temperatures.
Manufactured for:
Savient Pharmaceuticals, Inc.
East Brunswick, NJ 08816
Manufactured by:
SAB-Pharma Inc.
Boucherville, QC, Canada J4B 7K8
Made in Canada
Revised: July 2003
100216B
Shown in Product Identification Guide, page 332

OXANDRIN® CIII ℞

[ŏks-ăn-drĭn]
(oxandrolone tablets, USP)

DESCRIPTION

OXANDRIN® oral tablets contain 2.5 mg or 10 mg of the anabolic steroid oxandrolone.
Oxandrolone is 17β-hydroxy-17α-methyl-2-oxa-5α-androstan-3-one with the following structural formula:

Inactive ingredients include cornstarch, lactose, magnesium stearate, and hypromellose.

CLINICAL PHARMACOLOGY

Anabolic steroids are synthetic derivatives of testosterone. Certain clinical effects and adverse reactions demonstrate the androgenic properties of this class of drugs. Complete dissociation of anabolic and androgenic effects has not been achieved. The actions of anabolic steroids are therefore similar to those of male sex hormones with the possibility of causing serious disturbances of growth and sexual development if given to young children. Anabolic steroids suppress the gonadotropic functions of the pituitary and may exert a direct effect upon the testes.
During exogenous administration of anabolic androgens, endogenous testosterone release is inhibited through inhibition of pituitary luteinizing hormone (LH). At large doses, spermatogenesis may be suppressed through feedback inhibition of pituitary follicle-stimulating hormone (FSH).
Anabolic steroids have been reported to increase low-density lipoproteins and decrease high-density lipoproteins. These levels revert to normal on discontinuation of treatment.

INDICATIONS AND USAGE

Oxandrin is indicated as adjunctive therapy to promote weight gain after weight loss following extensive surgery, chronic infections, or severe trauma, and in some patients who without definite pathophysiologic reasons fail to gain or to maintain normal weight, to offset the protein catabolism associated with prolonged administration of corticosteroids, and for the relief of the bone pain frequently accompanying osteoporosis (See **DOSAGE AND ADMINISTRATION**).

DRUG ABUSE AND DEPENDENCE

Oxandrolone is classified as a controlled substance under the Anabolic Steroids Control Act of 1990 and has been assigned to Schedule III (non-narcotic).

CONTRAINDICATIONS

1. Known or suspected carcinoma of the prostate or the male breast.
2. Carcinoma of the breast in females with hypercalcemia (androgenic anabolic steroids may stimulate osteolytic bone resorption).

Continued on next page

Oxandrin—Cont.

3. Pregnancy, because of possible masculinization of the fetus. Oxandrin has been shown to cause embryotoxicity, fetotoxicity, infertility, and masculinization of female animal offspring when given in doses 9 times the human dose.
4. Nephrosis, the nephrotic phase of nephritis.
5. Hypercalcemia.

WARNINGS

PELIOSIS HEPATIS, A CONDITION IN WHICH LIVER AND SOMETIMES SPLENIC TISSUE IS REPLACED WITH BLOOD-FILLED CYSTS, HAS BEEN REPORTED IN PATIENTS RECEIVING ANDROGENIC ANABOLIC STEROID THERAPY. THESE CYSTS ARE SOMETIMES PRESENT WITH MINIMAL HEPATIC DYSFUNCTION, BUT AT OTHER TIMES THEY HAVE BEEN ASSOCIATED WITH LIVER FAILURE. THEY ARE OFTEN NOT RECOGNIZED UNTIL LIFE-THREATENING LIVER FAILURE OR INTRA-ABDOMINAL HEMORRHAGE DEVELOPS. WITHDRAWAL OF DRUG USUALLY RESULTS IN COMPLETE DISAPPEARANCE OF LESIONS.

LIVER CELL TUMORS ARE ALSO REPORTED. MOST OFTEN THESE TUMORS ARE BENIGN AND ANDROGEN-DEPENDENT, BUT FATAL MALIGNANT TUMORS HAVE BEEN REPORTED. WITHDRAWAL OF DRUG OFTEN RESULTS IN REGRESSION OR CESSATION OF PROGRESSION OF THE TUMOR. HOWEVER, HEPATIC TUMORS ASSOCIATED WITH ANDROGENS OR ANABOLIC STEROIDS ARE MUCH MORE VASCULAR THAN OTHER HEPATIC TUMORS AND MAY BE SILENT UNTIL LIFE-THREATENING INTRA-ABDOMINAL HEMORRHAGE DEVELOPS. BLOOD LIPID CHANGES THAT ARE KNOWN TO BE ASSOCIATED WITH INCREASED RISK OF ATHEROSCLEROSIS ARE SEEN IN PATIENTS TREATED WITH ANDROGENS OR ANABOLIC STEROIDS. THESE CHANGES INCLUDE DECREASED HIGH-DENSITY LIPOPROTEINS AND SOMETIMES INCREASED LOW-DENSITY LIPOPROTEINS. THE CHANGES MAY BE VERY MARKED AND COULD HAVE A SERIOUS IMPACT ON THE RISK OF ATHEROSCLEROSIS AND CORONARY ARTERY DISEASE.

Cholestatic hepatitis and jaundice may occur with 17-alpha-alkylated androgens at a relatively low dose. If cholestatic hepatitis with jaundice appears or if liver function tests become abnormal, oxandrolone should be discontinued and the etiology should be determined. Drug-induced jaundice is reversible when the medication is discontinued.

In patients with breast cancer, anabolic steroid therapy may cause hypercalcemia by stimulating osteolysis. Oxandrolone therapy should be discontinued if hypercalcemia occurs.

Edema with or without congestive heart failure may be a serious complication in patients with pre-existing cardiac, renal, or hepatic disease. Concomitant administration of adrenal cortical steroid or ACTH may increase the edema.

In children, androgen therapy may accelerate bone maturation without producing compensatory gain in linear growth. This adverse effect results in compromised adult height. The younger the child, the greater the risk of compromising final mature height. The effect on bone maturation should be monitored by assessing bone age of the left wrist and hand every 6 months (See **PRECAUTIONS: Laboratory Tests**).

Geriatric patients treated with androgenic anabolic steroids may be at an increased risk for the development of prostatic hypertrophy and prostatic carcinoma.

ANABOLIC STEROIDS HAVE NOT BEEN SHOWN TO ENHANCE ATHLETIC ABILITY.

PRECAUTIONS

Concurrent dosing of oxandrolone and warfarin may result in unexpectedly large increases in the INR or prothrombin time (PT). When oxandrolone is prescribed to patients being treated with warfarin, doses of warfarin may need to be decreased significantly to maintain the desirable INR level and diminish the risk of potentially serious bleeding (See PRECAUTIONS: Drug Interactions).

General:

Women should be observed for signs of virilization (deepening of the voice, hirsutism, acne, clitoromegaly). Discontinuation of drug therapy at the time of evidence of mild virilism is necessary to prevent irreversible virilization. Some virilizing changes in women are irreversible even after prompt discontinuance of therapy and are not prevented by concomitant use of estrogens. Menstrual irregularities may also occur.

Anabolic steroids may cause suppression of clotting factors II, V, VII, and X, and an increase in prothrombin time.

Information for patients:

The physician should instruct patients to report immediately any use of warfarin and any bleeding.

The physician should instruct patients to report any of the following side effects of androgens:

Males: Too frequent or persistent erections of the penis, appearance or aggravation of acne.

Females: Hoarseness, acne, changes in menstrual periods, or more facial hair.

All patients: Nausea, vomiting, changes in skin color, or ankle swelling.

Laboratory Tests:

Women with disseminated breast carcinoma should have frequent determination of urine and serum calcium levels during the course of therapy (See **WARNINGS**).

Because of the hepatotoxicity associated with the use of 17-alpha-alkylated androgens, liver function tests should be obtained periodically.

Periodic (every 6 months) x-ray examinations of bone age should be made during treatment of children to determine the rate of bone maturation and the effects of androgen therapy on the epiphyseal centers.

Serum lipids and high-density lipoprotein cholesterol determinations should be done periodically as androgenic anabolic steroids have been reported to increase low-density lipoproteins. Serum cholesterol levels may increase during therapy. Therefore, caution is required when administering these agents to patients with a history of myocardial infarction or coronary artery disease. Serial determinations of serum cholesterol should be made and therapy adjusted accordingly.

Hemoglobin and hematocrit should be checked periodically for polycythemia in patients who are receiving high doses of anabolic steroids.

Drug interactions

Anticoagulants:

Anabolic steroids may increase sensitivity to oral anticoagulants. Dosage of the anticoagulant may have to be decreased in order to maintain desired prothrombin time. Patients receiving oral anticoagulant therapy require close monitoring, especially when anabolic steroids are started or stopped.

Warfarin:

A multidose study of oxandrolone, given as 5 or 10 mg BID in 15 healthy subjects concurrently treated with warfarin, resulted in a mean increase in S-warfarin half-life from 26 to 48 hours and AUC from 4.55 to 12.08 ng*hr/mL: similar increases in R-warfarin half-life and AUC were also detected. Microscopic hematuria (9/15) and gingival bleeding (1/15) were also observed. A 5.5-fold decrease in the mean warfarin dose from 6.13 mg/day to 1.13 mg/day (approximately 80-85% reduction of warfarin dose), was necessary to maintain a target INR of 1.5. When oxandrolone therapy is initiated in a patient already receiving treatment with warfarin, the INR or prothrombin time (PT) should be monitored closely and the dose of warfarin adjusted as necessary until a stable target INR or PT has been achieved. Furthermore, in patients receiving both drugs, careful monitoring of the INR or PT, and adjustment of the warfarin dosage if indicated are recommended when the oxandrolone dose is changed or discontinued. Patients should be closely monitored for signs and symptoms of occult bleeding.

Oral hypoglycemic agents:

Oxandrolone may inhibit the metabolism of oral hypoglycemic agents.

Adrenal steroids or ACTH:

In patients with edema, concomitant administration with adrenal cortical steroids or ACTH may increase the edema.

Drug/Laboratory test interactions:

Anabolic steroids may decrease levels of thyroxine-binding globulin, resulting in decreased total T_4 serum levels and increased resin uptake of T_3 and T_4.

Free thyroid hormone levels remain unchanged. In addition, a decrease in PBI and radioactive iodine uptake may occur.

Carcinogenesis, mutagenesis, impairment of fertility

Animal data:

Oxandrolone has not been tested in laboratory animals for carcinogenic or mutagenic effects. In 2-year chronic oral rat studies, a dose-related reduction of spermatogenesis and decreased organ weights (testes, prostate, seminal vesicles, ovaries, uterus, adrenals, and pituitary) were shown.

Human data:

Liver cell tumors have been reported in patients receiving long-term therapy with androgenic anabolic steroids in high doses (See **WARNINGS**). Withdrawal of the drugs did not lead to regression of the tumors in all cases.

Geriatric patients treated with androgenic anabolic steroids may be at an increased risk for the development of prostatic hypertrophy and prostatic carcinoma.

Pregnancy:

Teratogenic effects-Pregnancy Category X (See **CONTRAINDICATIONS**).

Nursing mothers:

It is not known whether anabolic steroids are excreted in human milk. Because of the potential of serious adverse reactions in nursing infants from oxandrolone, a decision should be made whether to discontinue nursing or to discontinue the drug, taking into account the importance of the drug to the mother.

Pediatric use:

Anabolic agents may accelerate epiphyseal maturation more rapidly than linear growth in children and the effect may continue for 6 months after the drug has been stopped. Therefore, therapy should be monitored by x-ray studies at 6-month intervals in order to avoid the risk of compromising adult height. Androgenic anabolic steroid therapy should be used very cautiously in children and only by specialists who are aware of the effects on bone maturation (See **WARNINGS**).

ADVERSE REACTIONS

The following adverse reactions have been associated with use of anabolic steroids:

Hepatic: Cholestatic jaundice with, rarely, hepatic necrosis and death. Hepatocellular neoplasms and peliosis hepatis with long-term therapy (See **WARNINGS**). Reversible changes in liver function tests also occur including increased bromsulfophthalein (BSP) retention, and increases in serum bilirubin, aspartate aminotransferase (AST, SGOT) and alkaline phosphatase.

In males:

Prepubertal: Phallic enlargement and increased frequency or persistence of erections.

Postpubertal: Inhibition of testicular function, testicular atrophy and oligospermia, impotence, chronic priapism, epididymitis, and bladder irritability.

In females:

Clitoral enlargement, menstrual irregularities.

CNS: Habituation, excitation, insomnia, depression, and changes in libido.

Hematologic: Bleeding in patients on concomitant oral anticoagulant therapy.

Breast: Gynecomastia.

Larynx: Deepening of the voice in females.

Hair: Hirsutism and male pattern baldness in females.

Skin: Acne (especially in females and prepubertal males).

Skeletal: Premature closure of epiphyses in children (See **PRECAUTIONS: Pediatric use**).

Fluid and electrolytes: Edema, retention of serum electrolytes (sodium chloride, potassium, phosphate, calcium).

Metabolic/Endocrine: Decreased glucose tolerance (See **PRECAUTIONS: Laboratory Tests**), increased creatinine excretion, increased serum levels of creatinine phosphokinase (CPK). Masculinization of the fetus. Inhibition of gonadotropin secretion.

OVERDOSAGE

No symptoms or signs associated with overdosage have been reported. It is possible that sodium and water retention may occur.

The oral LD_{50} of oxandrolone in mice and dogs is greater than 5,000 mg/kg. No specific antidote is known, but gastric lavage may be used.

DOSAGE AND ADMINISTRATION

Therapy with anabolic steroids is adjunctive to and not a replacement for conventional therapy. The duration of therapy with Oxandrin (oxandrolone) will depend on the response of the patient and the possible appearance of adverse reactions. Therapy should be intermittent.

Adults: The response of individuals to anabolic steroids varies. The daily adult dosage is 2.5 mg to 20 mg given in 2 to 4 divided doses. The desired response may be achieved with as little as 2.5 mg or as much as 20 mg daily. A course of therapy of 2 to 4 weeks is usually adequate. This may be repeated intermittently as indicated.

Children: For children the total daily dosage of Oxandrin is ≤ 0.1 mg per kilogram body weight or ≤ 0.045 mg per pound of body weight. This may be repeated intermittently as indicated.

HOW SUPPLIED

Oxandrin 2.5 mg tablets are oval, white, and scored with BTG on one side and "11" on each side of the scoreline on the other side; bottles of 100 (NDC 54396-111-11).

Oxandrin 10 mg tablets are capsule shaped, white, with BTG on one side and "10" on the other side; bottles of 60 (NDC 54396-110-60).

℞ only

Issued: August 2003

Manufactured for
Savient Pharmaceuticals, Inc. by:
DSM Pharmaceuticals, Inc.
Greenville, NC 27834
Pfizer Co.,
New York, NY, 10017
Address medical inquiries to:
Savient Pharmaceuticals, Inc.
Medical Affairs
1 Tower Center
Fourteenth Floor
East Brunswick, NJ 08816

Shown in Product Identification Guide, page 332

IDENTIFICATION PROBLEM?
Turn to the **Product Identification Guide**, where you'll find more than 1600 products pictured in actual size and full color.

Scandipharm, Inc.

22 INVERNESS CENTER PARKWAY
BIRMINGHAM, AL 35242

(For prescribing information, see listing under AXCAN SCANDIPHARM INC.)

Schering Corporation

a wholly-owned subsidiary of Schering-Plough Corporation
GALLOPING HILL ROAD
KENILWORTH, NJ 07033

Direct Inquiries to:
(908) 298-4000
CUSTOMER SERVICE:
(800) 222-7579
FAX: (908) 595-3729

For Medical Information Contact:
Schering Laboratories
Drug Information Services
2000 Galloping Hill Road
Kenilworth, NJ 07033
(800) 526-4099
FAX: (973) 921-7228

Product Identification Codes

To provide quick and positive identification of Schering Products, we have imprinted the product identification number of the National Drug Code on most tablets and capsules. In some cases, identification letters also appear. Additionally, the following telephone number is provided for inquiries:

Drug Information Services
1-800-526-4099

CLARINEX® ℞

[klă-rĭ-nĕks]
(desloratadine)
TABLETS, REDITABS® TABLETS

DESCRIPTION

CLARINEX (desloratadine) Tablets are light blue, round, film coated tablets containing 5 mg desloratadine, an antihistamine, to be administered orally. It also contains the following excipients: dibasic calcium phosphate dihydrate USP, microcrystalline cellulose NF, corn starch NF, talc USP, carnauba wax NF, white wax NF, coating material consisting of lactose monohydrate, hydroxypropyl methylcellulose, titanium dioxide, polyethylene glycol, and FD&C Blue # 2 Aluminum Lake.

The CLARINEX RediTabs® brand of desloratadine orally-disintegrating tablets is a pink colored, round, tablet shaped unit with a "C" debossed on one side. Each RediTabs unit contains 5 mg of desloratadine. It also contains the following inactive ingredients: gelatin Type B NF, mannitol USP, aspartame NF, polarcrillin potassium NF, citric acid USP, red dye and tutti frutti flavoring.

Desloratadine is a white to off-white powder that is slightly soluble in water, but very soluble in ethanol and propylene glycol. It has an empirical formula: $C_{19}H_{19}ClN_2$ and a molecular weight of 310.8. The chemical name is 8-chloro-6,11-dihydro-11-(4-piperdinylidene)-5*H*-benzo[5,6]cyclohepta[1,2-*b*]pyridine and has the following structure:

CLINICAL PHARMACOLOGY

Mechanism of Action: Desloratadine is a long-acting tricyclic histamine antagonist with selective H_1-receptor histamine antagonist activity. Receptor binding data indicates that at a concentration of 2-3 ng/mL (7 nanomolar), desloratadine shows significant interaction with the human histamine H_1-receptor. Desloratadine inhibited histamine release from human mast cells *in vitro*.

Results of a radiolabeled tissue distribution study in rats and a radioligand H_1-receptor binding study in guinea pigs showed that desloratadine did not readily cross the blood brain barrier.

Pharmacokinetics: Absorption: Following oral administration of desloratadine 5 mg once daily for 10 days to normal healthy volunteers, the mean time to maximum plasma concentrations (T_{max}) occurred at approximately 3 hours post dose and mean steady state peak plasma concentrations (C_{max}) and area under the concentration-time curve (AUC) of 4 ng/mL and 56.9 ng.hr/mL were observed, respectively. Neither food nor grapefruit juice had an effect on the bioavailability (C_{max} and AUC) of desloratadine.

Table 1
Changes in Desloratadine and 3-Hydroxydesloratadine Pharmacokinetics in Healthy Male and Female Volunteers

	Desloratadine		3-Hydroxydesloratadine	
	C_{max}	AUC 0-24 hrs	C_{max}	AUC 0-24 hrs
Erythromycin (500 mg Q8h)	+24%	+14%	+43%	+40%
Ketoconazole (200 mg Q12h)	+45%	+39%	+43%	+72%
Azithromycin (500 mg day 1, 250 mg QD × 4 days)	+15%	+5%	+15%	+4%
Fluoxetine (20 mg QD)	+15%	+0%	+17%	+13%
Cimetidine (600 mg Q12h)	+12%	+19%	-11%	-3%

The pharmacokinetic profile of CLARINEX RediTabs Tablets was evaluated in a three-way crossover study in 30 adult volunteers. A single CLARINEX RediTabs Tablet containing 5 mg of desloratadine was bioequivalent to a single 5 mg CLARINEX Tablet and was bioequivalent to 10 mL of CLARINEX Syrup containing 5 mg of desloratadine for both desloratadine and 3-hydroxydesloratadine. In a separate study with 30 adult volunteers, food or water had no effect on the bioavailability (AUC and C_{max}) of CLARINEX RediTabs Tablets, however, food shifted the desloratadine median T_{max} value from 2.5 to 4 hr.

Distribution: Desloratadine and 3-hydroxydesloratadine are approximately 82% to 87% and 85% to 89%, bound to plasma proteins, respectively. Protein binding of desloratadine and 3-hydroxydesloratadine was unaltered in subjects with impaired renal function.

Metabolism: Desloratadine (a major metabolite of loratadine) is extensively metabolized to 3-hydroxydesloratadine, an active metabolite, which is subsequently glucuronidated. The enzyme(s) responsible for the formation of 3-hydroxydesloratadine have not been identified. Data from clinical trials indicate that a subset of the general patient population has a decreased ability to form 3-hydroxydesloratadine, and are slow metabolizers of desloratadine. In pharmacokinetic studies (n=1087), approximately 7% of subjects were slow metabolizers of desloratadine (defined as a subject with an AUC ratio of 3-hydroxydesloratadine to desloratadine less than 0.1, or a subject with a desloratadine half-life exceeding 50 hours). The frequency of slow metabolizers is higher in Blacks (approximately 20% of Blacks were slow metabolizers in pharmacokinetic studies, n=276). The median exposure (AUC) to desloratadine in the slow metabolizers was approximately 6-fold greater than the subjects who are not slow metabolizers. Subjects who are slow metabolizers of desloratadine cannot be prospectively identified and will be exposed to higher levels of desloratadine following dosing with the recommended dose of desloratadine. Although not seen in these pharmacokinetic studies, patients who are slow metabolizers may be more susceptible to dose-related adverse events.

Elimination: The mean elimination half-life of desloratadine was 27 hours. C_{max} and AUC values increased in a dose proportional manner following single oral doses between 5 and 20 mg. The degree of accumulation after 14 days of dosing was consistent with the half-life and dosing frequency. A human mass balance study documented a recovery of approximately 87% of the ^{14}C-desloratadine dose, which was equally distributed in urine and feces as metabolic products. Analysis of plasma 3-hydroxydesloratadine showed similar T_{max} and half-life values compared to desloratadine.

Special Populations: Geriatric: In older subjects (≥ 65 years old; n=17) following multiple-dose administration of CLARINEX Tablets, the mean C_{max} and AUC values for desloratadine were 20% greater than in younger subjects (< 65 years old). The oral total body clearance (CL/F) when normalized for body weight was similar between the two age groups. The mean plasma elimination half-life of desloratadine was 33.7 hr in subjects ≥ 65 years old. The pharmacokinetics for 3-hydroxydesloratadine appeared unchanged in older versus younger subjects. These age-related differences are unlikely to be clinically relevant and no dosage adjustment is recommended in elderly subjects.

Renally Impaired: Desloratadine pharmacokinetics following a single dose of 7.5 mg were characterized in patients with mild (n=7; creatinine clearance 51–69 mL/min/1.73 m^2), moderate (n=6; creatinine clearance 34–43 mL/min/1.73 m^2), and severe (n=6; creatinine clearance 5–29 mL/min/1.73 m^2) renal impairment or hemodialysis dependent (n=6) patients. In patients with mild and moderate renal impairment, median C_{max} and AUC values increased by approximately 1.2- and 1.9-fold, respectively, relative to subjects with normal renal function. In patients with severe renal impairment or who were hemodialysis dependent, C_{max} and AUC values increased by approximately 1.7- and 2.5-fold, respectively. Minimal changes in 3-hydroxydesloratadine concentrations were observed. Desloratadine and 3-hydroxydesloratadine were poorly removed by hemodialysis. Plasma protein binding of desloratadine and 3-hydroxydesloratadine was unaltered by renal impairment. Dosage adjustment for patients with renal impairment is recommended (see **DOSAGE AND ADMINISTRATION** section).

Hepatically Impaired: Desloratadine pharmacokinetics were characterized following a single oral dose in patients with mild (n=4), moderate (n=4), and severe (n=4) hepatic impairment as defined by the Child-Pugh classification of hepatic function and 8 subjects with normal hepatic function. Patients with hepatic impairment, regardless of severity, had approximately a 2.4-fold increase in AUC as compared with normal subjects. The apparent oral clearance of desloratadine in patients with mild, moderate, and severe hepatic impairment was 37%, 36%, and 28% of that in normal subjects, respectively. An increase in the mean elimination half-life of desloratadine in patients with hepatic impairment was observed. For 3-hydroxydesloratadine, the mean C_{max} and AUC values for patients with hepatic impairment were not statistically significantly different from subjects with normal hepatic function. Dosage adjustment for patients with hepatic impairment is recommended (see **DOSAGE AND ADMINISTRATION** section).

Gender: Female subjects treated for 14 days with CLARINEX Tablets had 10% and 3% higher desloratadine C_{max} and AUC values, respectively, compared with male subjects. The 3-hydroxydesloratadine C_{max} and AUC values were also increased by 45% and 48%, respectively, in females compared with males. However, these apparent differences are not likely to be clinically relevant and therefore no dosage adjustment is recommended.

Race: Following 14 days of treatment with CLARINEX Tablets, the C_{max} and AUC values for desloratadine were 18% and 32% higher, respectively, in Blacks compared with Caucasians. For 3-hydroxydesloratadine there was a corresponding 10% reduction in C_{max} and AUC values in Blacks compared to Caucasians. These differences are not likely to be clinically relevant and therefore no dose adjustment is recommended.

Drug Interactions: In two controlled crossover clinical pharmacology studies in healthy male (n=12 in each study) and female (n=12 in each study) volunteers, desloratadine 7.5 mg (1.5 times the daily dose) once daily was coadministered with erythromycin 500 mg every 8 hours or ketoconazole 200 mg every 12 hours for 10 days. In 3 separate controlled, parallel group clinical pharmacology studies, desloratadine at the clinical dose of 5 mg has been coadministered with azithromycin 500 mg followed by 250 mg once daily for 4 days (n=18) or with fluoxetine 20 mg once daily for 7 days after a 23 day pretreatment period with fluoxetine (n=18) or with cimetidine 600 mg every 12 hours for 14 days (n=18) under steady state conditions to normal healthy male and female volunteers. Although increased plasma concentrations (C_{max} and AUC 0-24 hrs) of desloratadine and 3-hydroxydesloratadine were observed (see Table 1), there were no clinically relevant changes in the safety profile of desloratadine, as assessed by electrocardiographic parameters (including the corrected QT interval), clinical laboratory tests, vital signs, and adverse events.

[See table 1 above]

Pharmacodynamics: Wheal and Flare: Human histamine skin wheal studies following single and repeated 5 mg doses of desloratadine have shown that the drug exhibits an antihistaminic effect by 1 hour; this activity may persist for as long as 24 hours. There was no evidence of histamine-induced skin wheal tachyphylaxis within the desloratadine 5 mg group over the 28 day treatment period. The clinical relevance of histamine wheal skin testing is unknown.

Effects on QT_c: Single dose administration of desloratadine did not alter the corrected QT interval (QT_c) in rats (up to 12 mg/kg, oral), or guinea pigs (25 mg/kg, intravenous). Repeated oral administration at doses up to 24 mg/kg for durations up to 3 months in monkeys did not alter the QT_c at an estimated desloratadine exposure (AUC) that was approximately 955 times the mean AUC in humans at the recommended daily oral dose. See **OVERDOSAGE** section for information on human QT_c experience.

Clinical Trials: Seasonal Allergic Rhinitis: The clinical efficacy and safety of CLARINEX Tablets were evaluated in over 2,300 patients 12 to 75 years of age with seasonal allergic rhinitis. A total of 1,838 patients received 2.5–20 mg/day of CLARINEX in 4 double-blind, randomized, placebo-controlled clinical trials of 2 to 4 weeks' duration conducted in the United States. The results of these studies demonstrated the efficacy and safety of CLARINEX 5 mg in the treatment of adult and adolescent patients with seasonal allergic rhinitis. In a dose ranging trial, CLARINEX 2.5-

Continued on next page

Information on Schering products appearing on these pages is effective as of June 2003.

Clarinex—Cont.

20 mg/day was studied. Doses of 5, 7.5, 10, and 20 mg/day were superior to placebo; and no additional benefit was seen at doses above 5.0 mg. In the same study, an increase in the incidence of somnolence was observed at doses of 10 mg/day and 20 mg/day (5.2% and 7.6%, respectively), compared to placebo (2.3%).

In 2 four-week studies of 924 patients (aged 15 to 75 years) with seasonal allergic rhinitis and concomitant asthma, CLARINEX Tablets 5 mg once daily improved rhinitis symptoms, with no decrease in pulmonary function. This supports the safety of administering CLARINEX Tablets to adult patients with seasonal allergic rhinitis with mild to moderate asthma.

CLARINEX Tablets 5 mg once daily significantly reduced the Total Symptom Scores (the sum of individual scores of nasal and non-nasal symptoms) in patients with seasonal allergic rhinitis. See Table 2.

[See table 2 at right]

There were no significant differences in the effectiveness of CLARINEX Tablets 5 mg across subgroups of patients defined by gender, age, or race.

Perennial Allergic Rhinitis: The clinical efficacy and safety of CLARINEX Tablets 5 mg were evaluated in over 1,300 patients 12 to 80 years of age with perennial allergic rhinitis. A total of 685 patients received 5 mg/day of CLARINEX in 2 double-blind, randomized, placebo-controlled clinical trials of 4 weeks' duration conducted in the United States and internationally. In one of these studies CLARINEX Tablets 5 mg once daily was shown to significantly reduce symptoms of perennial allergic rhinitis (Table 3).

[See table 3 at right]

Chronic Idiopathic Urticaria: The efficacy and safety of CLARINEX Tablets 5 mg once daily was studied in 416 chronic idiopathic urticaria patients 12 to 84 years of age, of whom 211 received CLARINEX. In two double-blind, placebo-controlled, randomized clinical trials of six weeks' duration, at the pre-specified one-week primary time point evaluation, CLARINEX Tablets significantly reduced the severity of pruritus when compared to placebo (Table 4). Secondary endpoints were also evaluated and during the first week of therapy CLARINEX Tablets 5 mg reduced the secondary endpoints, "Number of Hives" and the "Size of the Largest Hive," when compared to placebo.

[See table 4 at right]

INDICATIONS AND USAGE

Allergic Rhinitis: CLARINEX Tablets 5 mg are indicated for the relief of the nasal and non-nasal symptoms of allergic rhinitis (seasonal and perennial) in patients 12 years of age and older.

Chronic Idiopathic Urticaria: CLARINEX Tablets are indicated for the symptomatic relief of pruritus, reduction in the number of hives, and size of hives, in patients with chronic idiopathic urticaria 12 years of age and older.

CONTRAINDICATIONS

CLARINEX Tablets 5 mg are contraindicated in patients who are hypersensitive to this medication or to any of its ingredients, or to loratadine.

PRECAUTIONS

Carcinogenesis, Mutagenesis, Impairment of Fertility: The carcinogenic potential of desloratadine was assessed using loratadine studies. In an 18-month study in mice and a 2-year study in rats, loratadine was administered in the diet at doses up to 40 mg/kg/day in mice (estimated desloratadine and desloratadine metabolite exposures were approximately 3 times the AUC in humans at the recommended daily oral dose) and 25 mg/kg/day in rats (estimated desloratadine and desloratadine metabolite exposures were approximately 30 times the AUC in humans at the recommended daily oral dose). Male mice given 40 mg/kg/day loratadine had a significantly higher incidence of hepatocellular tumors (combined adenomas and carcinomas) than concurrent controls. In rats, a significantly higher incidence of hepatocellular tumors (combined adenomas and carcinomas) was observed in males given 10 mg/kg/day and in males and females given 25 mg/kg/day. The estimated desloratadine and desloratadine metabolite exposures of rats given 10 mg/kg of loratadine were approximately 7 times the AUC in humans at the recommended daily oral dose. The clinical significance of these findings during long-term use of desloratadine is not known.

In genotoxicity studies with desloratadine, there was no evidence of genotoxic potential in a reverse mutation assay (*Salmonella/E. coli* mammalian microsome bacterial mutagenicity assay) or in two assays for chromosomal aberrations (human peripheral blood lymphocyte clastogenicity assay and mouse bone marrow micronucleus assay).

There was no effect on female fertility in rats at desloratadine doses up to 24 mg/kg/day (estimated desloratadine and desloratadine metabolite exposures were approximately 130 times the AUC in humans at the recommended daily oral dose). A male specific decrease in fertility, demonstrated by reduced female conception rates, decreased sperm numbers and motility, and histopathologic testicular changes, occurred at an oral desloratadine dose of 12 mg/kg in rats (estimated desloratadine exposures were approximately 45 times the AUC in humans at the recommended daily oral dose). Desloratadine had no effect on fertility in rats at an oral dose of 3 mg/kg/day (estimated desloratadine and desloratadine metabolite exposures were approximately 8 times the AUC in humans at the recommended daily oral dose).

Table 2
TOTAL SYMPTOM SCORE (TSS)
Changes in a 2 Week Clinical Trial in Patients with Seasonal Allergic Rhinitis

Treatment Group (n)	Mean Baseline* (sem)	Change from Baseline** (sem)	Placebo Comparison (P-value)
CLARINEX 5.0 mg (171)	14.2 (0.3)	-4.3 (0.3)	P<0.01
Placebo (173)	13.7 (0.3)	-2.5 (0.3)	

* At baseline, a total nasal symptom score (sum of 4 individual symptoms) of at least 6 and a total non-nasal symptom score (sum of 4 individual symptoms) of at least 5 (each symptom scored 0 to 3 where 0=no symptom and 3=severe symptoms) was required for trial eligibility. TSS ranges from 0=no symptoms to 24=maximal symptoms.
**Mean reduction in TSS averaged over the 2-week treatment period.

Table 3
TOTAL SYMPTOM SCORE (TSS)
Changes in a 4 Week Clinical Trial in Patients with Perennial Allergic Rhinitis

Treatment Group (n)	Mean Baseline* (sem)	Change from Baseline** (sem)	Placebo Comparison (P-value)
CLARINEX 5.0 mg (337)	12.37 (0.18)	-4.06 (0.21)	P=0.01
Placebo (337)	12.30 (0.18)	-3.27 (0.21)	

* At baseline, average of total symptom score (sum of 5 individual nasal symptoms and 3 non-nasal symptoms, each symptom scored 0 to 3 where 0=no symptom and 3=severe symptoms) of at least 10 was required for trial eligibility. TSS ranges from 0=no symptoms to 24=maximal symptoms.
**Mean reduction in TSS averaged over the 4-week treatment period.

Table 4
PRURITUS SYMPTOM SCORE
Changes in the First Week of a Clinical Trial in Patients with Chronic Idiopathic Urticaria

Treatment Group (n)	Mean Baseline (sem)	Change from Baseline* (sem)	Placebo Comparison (P-value)
CLARINEX 5.0 mg (115)	2.19 (0.04)	-1.05 (0.07)	P<0.01
Placebo (110)	2.21 (0.04)	-0.52 (0.07)	

Pruritus scored 0 to 3 where 0=no symptom to 3=maximal symptom
*Mean reduction in pruritus averaged over the first week of treatment.

Pregnancy Category C: Desloratadine was not teratogenic in rats at doses up to 48 mg/kg/day (estimated desloratadine and desloratadine metabolite exposures were approximately 210 times the AUC in humans at the recommended daily oral dose) or in rabbits at doses up to 60 mg/kg/day (estimated desloratadine exposures were approximately 230 times the AUC in humans at the recommended daily oral dose). In a separate study, an increase in pre-implantation loss and a decreased number of implantations and fetuses were noted in female rats at 24 mg/kg (estimated desloratadine and desloratadine metabolite exposures were approximately 120 times the AUC in humans at the recommended daily oral dose). Reduced body weight and slow righting reflex were reported in pups at doses of 9 mg/kg/day or greater (estimated desloratadine and desloratadine metabolite exposures were approximately 50 times or greater than the AUC in humans at the recommended daily oral dose). Desloratadine had no effect on pup development at an oral dose of 3 mg/kg/day (estimated desloratadine and desloratadine metabolite exposures were approximately 7 times the AUC in humans at the recommended daily oral dose). There are, however, no adequate and well-controlled studies in pregnant women. Because animal reproduction studies are not always predictive of human response, desloratadine should be used during pregnancy only if clearly needed.

Nursing Mothers: Desloratadine passes into breast milk, therefore a decision should be made whether to discontinue nursing or to discontinue desloratadine, taking into account the importance of the drug to the mother.

Pediatric Use: The safety and effectiveness of CLARINEX Tablets in pediatric patients under 12 years of age have not been established.

Geriatric Use: Clinical studies of desloratadine did not include sufficient numbers of subjects aged 65 and over to determine whether they respond differently from younger subjects. Other reported clinical experience has not identified differences between the elderly and younger patients. In general, dose selection for an elderly patient should be cautious, reflecting the greater frequency of decreased hepatic, renal, or cardiac function, and of concomitant disease or other drug therapy. (see **CLINICAL PHARMACOLOGY – Special Populations**).

Information for Patients: Patients should be instructed to use CLARINEX Tablets as directed. As there are no food effects on bioavailability, patients can be instructed that CLARINEX Tablets may be taken without regard to meals. Patients should be advised not to increase the dose or dosing frequency as studies have not demonstrated increased effectiveness at higher doses and somnolence may occur.

Phenylketonurics: CLARINEX RediTabs Tablets contain phenylalanine 1.75 mg per tablet.

ADVERSE REACTIONS

Allergic Rhinitis: In multiple-dose placebo-controlled trials, 2,834 patients received CLARINEX Tablets at doses of 2.5 mg to 20 mg daily, of whom 1,655 patients received the recommended daily dose of 5 mg. In patients receiving 5 mg daily, the rate of adverse events was similar between CLARINEX and placebo-treated patients. The percent of patients who withdrew prematurely due to adverse events was 2.4% in the CLARINEX group and 2.6% in the placebo group. There were no serious adverse events in these trials in patients receiving desloratadine. All adverse events that were reported by greater than or equal to 2% of patients who received the recommended daily dose of CLARINEX Tablets (5.0 mg once-daily), and that were more common with CLARINEX Tablet than placebo, are listed in Table 5.

Table 5
Incidence of Adverse Events Reported by ≥ 2%
of Allergic Rhinitis Patients in Placebo-Controlled,
Multiple-Dose Clinical Trials

Adverse Experience	CLARINEX Tablets 5 mg (n=1,655)	Placebo (n=1,652)
Pharyngitis	4.1%	2.0%
Dry Mouth	3.0%	1.9%
Myalgia	2.1%	1.8%
Fatigue	2.1%	1.2%
Somnolence	2.1%	1.8%
Dysmenorrhea	2.1%	1.6%

The frequency and magnitude of laboratory and electrocardiographic abnormalities were similar in CLARINEX and placebo-treated patients.

There were no differences in adverse events for subgroups of patients as defined by gender, age, or race.

Chronic Idiopathic Urticaria: In multiple-dose, placebo-controlled trials of chronic idiopathic urticaria, 211 patients received CLARINEX Tablets and 205 received placebo. Adverse events that were reported by greater than or equal to 2% of patients who received CLARINEX Tablets and that were more common with CLARINEX than placebo were (rates for CLARINEX and placebo, respectively): headache (14%, 13%), nausea (5%, 2%), fatigue (5%, 1%), dizziness (4%, 3%), pharyngitis (3%, 2%), dyspepsia (3%, 1%), and myalgia (3%, 1%).

The following spontaneous adverse events have been reported during the marketing of desloratadine: tachycardia, palpitations and rarely hypersensitivity reactions (such as rash, pruritus, urticaria, edema, dyspnea, and anaphylaxis), and elevated liver enzymes including bilirubin.

DRUG ABUSE AND DEPENDENCE

There is no information to indicate that abuse or dependency occurs with CLARINEX Tablets.

OVERDOSAGE

Information regarding acute overdosage is limited to experience from clinical trials conducted during the development of the CLARINEX product. In a dose ranging trial, at doses of 10 mg and 20 mg/day somnolence was reported.

Single daily doses of 45 mg were given to normal male and female volunteers for 10 days. All ECGs obtained in this study were manually read in a blinded fashion by a cardiologist. In CLARINEX-treated subjects, there was an increase in mean heart rate of 9.2 bpm relative to placebo. The QT interval was corrected for heart rate (QT_c) by both the Bazett and Fridericia methods. Using the QT_c (Bazett) there was a mean increase of 8.1 msec in CLARINEX-treated subjects relative to placebo. Using QT_c (Fridericia) there was a mean increase of 0.4 msec in CLARINEX-treated subjects relative to placebo. No clinically relevant adverse events were reported.

In the event of overdose, consider standard measures to remove any unabsorbed drug. Symptomatic and supportive treatment is recommended. Desloratadine and 3-hydroxydesloratadine are not eliminated by hemodialysis.

Lethality occurred in rats at oral doses of 250 mg/kg or greater (estimated desloratadine and desloratadine metabolite exposures were approximately 120 times the AUC in humans at the recommended daily oral dose). The oral median lethal dose in mice was 353 mg/kg (estimated desloratadine exposures were approximately 290 times the human daily oral dose on a mg/m^2 basis). No deaths occurred at oral doses up to 250 mg/kg in monkeys (estimated desloratadine exposures were approximately 810 times the human daily oral dose on a mg/m^2 basis).

DOSAGE AND ADMINISTRATION

In adults and children 12 years of age and over, the recommended dose of CLARINEX Tablets is 5 mg once daily. In patients with liver or renal impairment, a starting dose of one 5 mg tablet every other day is recommended based on pharmacokinetic data.

Administration of CLARINEX RediTabs Tablets: Place CLARINEX RediTabs Tablet on the tongue. Tablet disintegration occurs rapidly. Administer with or without water. Take tablet immediately after opening the blister.

HOW SUPPLIED

CLARINEX Tablets: Embossed "C5", light blue film coated tablets; that are packaged in high-density polyethylene plastic bottles of 100 (NDC 0085-1264-01) and 500 (NDC 0085-1264-02). Also available, CLARINEX Unit-of-Use package of 30 tablets (3 × 10; 10 blisters per card) (NDC 0085-1264-04); and Unit Dose-Hospital Pack of 100 Tablets (10 × 10; 10 blisters per card) (NDC 0085-1264-03).

Protect Unit-of-Use packaging and Unit Dose-Hospital Pack from excessive moisture.

Store at 25°C (77°F); excursions permitted to 15–30°C (59–86°F) [see USP Controlled Room Temperature]

Heat Sensitive. Avoid exposure at or above 30°C (86°F).

CLARINEX REDITABS (desloratadine orally-disintegrating tablets) 5 mg: "C" debossed, pink tablets in foil/foil blisters.

Packs of 30 tablets (containing 3 x 10's) NDC 0085-1280-01.

Store at 25°C (77°F); excursions permitted to 15–30°C (59–86°F) [see USP Controlled Room Temperature]

Schering®

Schering Corporation
Kenilworth, NJ 07033 USA

Rev. 7/03 **23882159T**

CLARINEX REDITABS brand of desloratadine orally-disintegrating tablets are manufactured for Schering Corporation by Cardinal Health UK. 416 Limited, England.

DIPROLENE® AF ℞

[*dĭp-rō-lēn*]

(brand of augmented betamethasone dipropionate)*

Cream, 0.05%

(potency expressed as betamethasone)

*Vehicle augments the penetration of the steroid.

For Dermatologic Use Only – Not for Ophthalmic Use

PRODUCT INFORMATION

DESCRIPTION

DIPROLENE® AF Cream 0.05% contains betamethasone dipropionate, USP, a synthetic adrenocorticosteroid, for dermatologic use in an emollient base. Betamethasone, an analog of prednisolone, has a high degree of corticosteroid activity and a slight degree of mineralocorticoid activity. Betamethasone dipropionate is the 17, 21-dipropionate ester of betamethasone.

Chemically, betamethasone dipropionate is 9-fluoro-11β,17,21-trihydroxy-16β-methylpregna-1,4-diene-3,20-dione 17,21-dipropionate, with the empirical formula $C_{28}H_{37}FO_7$, a molecular weight of 504.6, and the following structural formula:

[See chemical structure at top of next column]

Betamethasone dipropionate is a white to creamy white, odorless crystalline powder, insoluble in water.

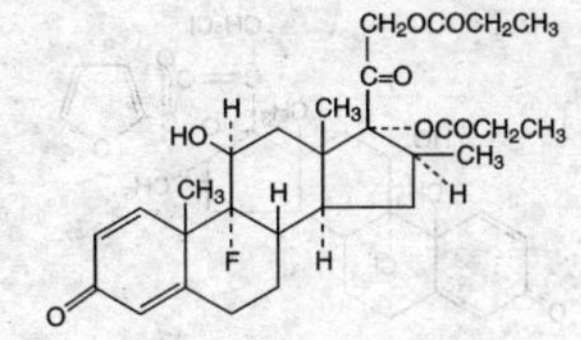

Each gram of DIPROLENE AF Cream 0.05% contains: 0.643 mg betamethasone dipropionate, USP (equivalent to 0.5 mg betamethasone) in an emollient cream base of purified water, USP; chlorocresol; propylene glycol, USP; white petrolatum, USP; white wax, NF; cyclomethicone; sorbitol solution, USP; glyceryl oleate/propylene glycol; ceteareth-30; carbomer 940, NF; and sodium hydroxide R.

CLINICAL PHARMACOLOGY

The corticosteroids are a class of compounds comprising steroid hormones secreted by the adrenal cortex and their synthetic analogs. In pharmacologic doses, corticosteroids are used primarily for their anti-inflammatory and/or immunosuppressive effects.

Topical corticosteroids, such as betamethasone dipropionate, are effective in the treatment of corticosteroid-responsive dermatoses primarily because of their anti-inflammatory, antipruritic, and vasoconstrictive actions. However, while the physiologic, pharmacologic, and clinical effects of the corticosteroids are well known, the exact mechanisms of their actions in each disease are uncertain. Betamethasone dipropionate, a corticosteroid, has been shown to have topical (dermatologic) and systemic pharmacologic and metabolic effects characteristic of this class of drugs.

Pharmacokinetics: The extent of percutaneous absorption of topical corticosteroids is determined by many factors including the vehicle, the integrity of the epidermal barrier, and the use of occlusive dressings. (See **DOSAGE AND ADMINISTRATION** section.)

Topical corticosteroids can be absorbed through normal intact skin. Inflammation and/or other disease processes in the skin may increase percutaneous absorption. Occlusive dressings substantially increase the percutaneous absorption of topical corticosteroids. (See **DOSAGE AND ADMINISTRATION** section.)

Once absorbed through the skin, topical corticosteroids enter pharmacokinetic pathways similar to systemically administered corticosteroids. Corticosteroids are bound to plasma proteins in varying degrees, are metabolized primarily in the liver and excreted by the kidneys. Some of the topical corticosteroids and their metabolites are also excreted into the bile.

DIPROLENE AF Cream 0.05% was applied once daily at 7 grams per day for 1 week to diseased skin, in adult patients with psoriasis or atopic dermatitis, to study its effects on the hypothalamic-pituitary-adrenal (HPA) axis. The results suggested that the drug caused a slight lowering of adrenal corticosteroid secretion, although in no case did plasma cortisol levels go below the lower limit of the normal range.

Sixty-seven pediatric patients ages 1 to 12 years, with atopic dermatitis, were enrolled in an open-label, hypothalamic-pituitary-adrenal (HPA) axis safety study. DIPROLENE AF Cream 0.05% was applied twice daily for 2 to 3 weeks over a mean body surface area of 58% (range 35% to 95%). In 19 of 60 (32%) evaluable patients, adrenal suppression was indicated by either a $\leq$ 5 mcg/dL pre-stimulation cortisol, or a cosyntropin post-stimulation cortisol $\leq$ 18 mcg/dL and/or an increase of $<$ 7 mcg/dL from the baseline cortisol. Studies performed with DIPROLENE AF Cream 0.05% indicate that it is in the high range of potency as compared with other topical corticosteroids.

INDICATIONS AND USAGE

DIPROLENE AF Cream 0.05% is a high-potency corticosteroid indicated for relief of the inflammatory and pruritic manifestations of corticosteroid-responsive dermatoses in patients 13 years and older.

CONTRAINDICATIONS

DIPROLENE AF Cream 0.05% is contraindicated in patients who are hypersensitive to betamethasone dipropionate, to other corticosteroids, or to any ingredient in this preparation.

PRECAUTIONS

General: Systemic absorption of topical corticosteroids has produced reversible HPA axis suppression, manifestations of Cushing's syndrome, hyperglycemia, and glucosuria in some patients.

Conditions which augment systemic absorption include the application of the more potent corticosteroids, use over large surface areas, prolonged use, and the addition of occlusive dressings. Use of more than one corticosteroid-containing product at the same time may increase total systemic glucocorticoid exposure. (See **DOSAGE AND ADMINISTRATION** section.)

Therefore, patients receiving a large dose of a potent topical steroid applied to a large surface area should be evaluated periodically for evidence of HPA axis suppression by using the urinary free cortisol and ACTH stimulation tests. If HPA axis suppression is noted, an attempt should be made to withdraw the drug, to reduce the frequency of application, or to substitute a less potent steroid.

Recovery of HPA axis function is generally prompt and complete upon discontinuation of the drug. In an open-label pediatric study of 60 evaluable patients, of the 19 who showed evidence of suppression, 4 patients were tested 2 weeks after discontinuation of DIPROLENE AF Cream 0.05%, and 3 of the 4 (75%) had complete recovery of HPA axis function. Infrequently, signs and symptoms of steroid withdrawal may occur, requiring supplemental systemic corticosteroids. Children may absorb proportionally larger amounts of topical corticosteroids and thus be more susceptible to systemic toxicity. (See **PRECAUTIONS – Pediatric Use.**)

If irritation develops, topical corticosteroids should be discontinued and appropriate therapy instituted.

In the presence of dermatological infections, the use of an appropriate antifungal or antibacterial agent should be instituted. If a favorable response does not occur promptly, the corticosteroid should be discontinued until the infection has been adequately controlled.

Information for Patients: Patients using topical corticosteroids should receive the following information and instructions. This information is intended to aid in the safe and effective use of this medication. It is not a disclosure of all possible adverse or intended effects.

1. This medication is to be used as directed by the physician and should not be used longer than the prescribed time period. It is for external use only. Avoid contact with the eyes.
2. Patients should be advised not to use this medication for any disorder other than that for which it was prescribed.
3. The treated skin area should not be bandaged or otherwise covered or wrapped as to be occlusive. (See **DOSAGE AND ADMINISTRATION** section.)
4. Patients should report any signs of local adverse reactions.
5. Other corticosteroid-containing products should not be used with DIPROLENE AF Cream 0.05% without first talking to your physician.

Laboratory Tests: The following tests may be helpful in evaluating HPA axis suppression:

Urinary free cortisol test
ACTH stimulation test

Carcinogenesis, Mutagenesis, and Impairment of Fertility: Long-term animal studies have not been performed to evaluate the carcinogenic potential of betamethasone dipropionate.

Betamethasone was negative in the bacterial mutagenicity assay (*Salmonella typhimurium* and *Escherichia coli*), and in the mammalian cell mutagenicity assay (CHO/HGPRT). It was positive in the *in vitro* human lymphocyte chromosome aberration assay, and equivocal in the *in vivo* mouse bone marrow micronucleus assay. This pattern of response is similar to that of dexamethasone and hydrocortisone.

Reproductive studies with betamethasone dipropionate carried out in rabbits at doses of 1.0 mg/kg by the intramuscular route and in mice up to 33 mg/kg by the intramuscular route indicated no impairment of fertility except for dose-related increases in fetal resorption rates in both species. These doses are approximately 5- and 38-fold the human dose based on a mg/m^2 comparison, respectively.

Pregnancy: Teratogenic Effects: Pregnancy Category C: Corticosteroids are generally teratogenic in laboratory animals when administered systemically at relatively low dosage levels.

Betamethasone dipropionate has been shown to be teratogenic in rabbits when given by the intramuscular route at doses of 0.05 mg/kg. This dose is approximately 0.2-fold the maximum human dose based on a mg/m^2 comparison. The abnormalities observed included umbilical hernias, cephalocele and cleft palates.

Some corticosteroids have been shown to be teratogenic after dermal application in laboratory animals. There are no adequate and well-controlled studies in pregnant women on teratogenic effects from topically applied corticosteroids. Therefore, topical corticosteroids should be used during pregnancy only if the potential benefit justifies the potential risk to the fetus. Drugs of this class should not be used extensively on pregnant patients, in large amounts, or for prolonged periods of time.

Nursing Mothers: It is not known whether topical administration of corticosteroids can result in sufficient systemic absorption to produce detectable quantities in breast milk. Systemically administered corticosteroids are secreted into breast milk in quantities not likely to have a deleterious effect on the infant. Nevertheless, a decision should be made whether to discontinue nursing or to discontinue the drug, taking into account the importance of the drug to the mother.

Pediatric Use: Use of DIPROLENE AF Cream 0.05% in pediatric patients 12 years of age and younger is not recommended. (See **CLINICAL PHARMACOLOGY** and **ADVERSE REACTIONS** sections.) In an open-label study, 19 of 60 (32%) evaluable pediatric patients (aged 3 months-12 years old) using DIPROLENE AF Cream 0.05% for treatment of atopic dermatitis demonstrated HPA axis suppres-

Continued on next page

Information on Schering products appearing on these pages is effective as of June 2003.

Diprolene AF—Cont.

sion. The proportion of patients with adrenal suppression in this study was progressively greater, the younger the age group. (See **CLINICAL PHARMACOLOGY Pharmacokinetics.**)

Pediatric patients may demonstrate greater susceptibility to topical corticosteroid-induced HPA axis suppression and Cushing's syndrome than mature patients because of a larger skin surface area to body weight ratio. The study described above supports this premise, as adrenal suppression in 9-12 year olds, 6-8 year olds, 2-5 year olds, and 3 months-1 year old was 17%, 32%, 38% and 50% respectively. Hypothalamic-pituitary-adrenal (HPA) axis suppression, Cushing's syndrome, and intracranial hypertension have been reported in children receiving topical corticosteroids. Manifestations of adrenal suppression in children include linear growth retardation, delayed weight gain, low plasma cortisol levels, and absence of response to ACTH stimulation. Manifestations of intracranial hypertension include bulging fontanelles, headaches, and bilateral papilledema. Chronic corticosteroid therapy may interfere with the growth and development of children.

ADVERSE REACTIONS

The only local adverse reaction reported to be possibly or probably related to treatment with DIPROLENE AF Cream 0.05% during adult, controlled clinical studies was stinging. It occurred in 1 patient, 0.4%, of the 242 patients or subjects involved in the studies.

Adverse reactions reported to be possibly or probably related to treatment with DIPROLENE AF Cream 0.05% during a pediatric clinical study include signs of skin atrophy (telangiectasia, bruising, shininess). Skin atrophy occurred in 7 of 67 (10%) patients, involving all age groups from 3 months-12 years of age.

The following local adverse reactions are reported infrequently when topical corticosteroids are used as recommended. These reactions are listed in an approximate decreasing order of occurrence: burning, itching, irritation, dryness, folliculitis, hypertrichosis, acneiform eruptions, hypopigmentation, perioral dermatitis, allergic contact dermatitis, maceration of the skin, secondary infection, skin atrophy, striae, miliaria.

Systemic absorption of topical corticosteroids has produced reversible hypothalamic-pituitary-adrenal (HPA) axis suppression, manifestations of Cushing's syndrome, hyperglycemia, and glucosuria in some patients.

OVERDOSAGE

Topically applied corticosteroids can be absorbed in sufficient amounts to produce systemic effects. (See **PRECAUTIONS.**)

DOSAGE AND ADMINISTRATION

Apply a thin film of DIPROLENE AF Cream to the affected skin areas once or twice daily. Treatment with DIPROLENE AF Cream 0.05% should be limited to 45 g per week.

DIPROLENE AF Cream 0.05% is not to be used with occlusive dressings.

HOW SUPPLIED

DIPROLENE AF Cream 0.05% is supplied in 15-g (NDC 0085-0517-01) and 50-g (NDC 0085-0517-04) tubes; boxes of one.

Store between 2° and 30°C (36° and 86°F).

Schering®

Schering Corporation
Kenilworth, NJ 07033 USA
Rev. 10/01 17968645
18670330T

ELOCON® ℞

[ĕl'ō-cŏn]

brand of mometasone furoate cream, USP
Cream 0.1%
For Dermatologic Use Only
Not for Ophthalmic Use

DESCRIPTION

ELOCON® (mometasone furoate cream, USP) Cream 0.1% contains mometasone furoate, USP for dermatologic use. Mometasone furoate is a synthetic corticosteroid with anti-inflammatory activity.

Chemically, mometasone furoate is 9α,21-Dichloro-11β,17-dihydroxy-16α-methylpregna-1,4-diene-3,20-dione 17-(2-furoate), with the empirical formula $C_{27}H_{30}Cl_2O_6$, a molecular weight of 521.4 and the following structural formula:

[See chemical structure at top of next column]

Mometasone furoate is a white to off-white powder practically insoluble in water, slightly soluble in octanol, and moderately soluble in ethyl alcohol.

Each gram of ELOCON Cream 0.1% contains: 1 mg mometasone furoate, USP in a cream base of hexylene glycol, NF; phosphoric acid, NF; propylene glycol stearate (55% monoester); stearyl alcohol and ceteareth-20; titanium dioxide, USP; aluminum starch octenylsuccinate (Gamma Irradiated); white wax, NF; white petrolatum, USP; and purified water, USP.

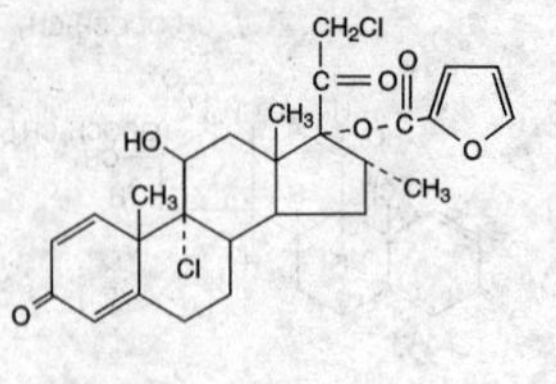

CH₂Cl C=O CH₃ -O-C HO CH₃ CH₃ Cl O

CLINICAL PHARMACOLOGY

Like other topical corticosteroids, mometasone furoate has anti-inflammatory, antipruritic, and vasoconstrictive properties. The mechanism of the anti-inflammatory activity of the topical steroids, in general, is unclear. However, corticosteroids are thought to act by the induction of phospholipase A_2 inhibitory proteins, collectively called lipocortins. It is postulated that these proteins control the biosynthesis of potent mediators of inflammation such as prostaglandins and leukotrienes by inhibiting the release of their common precursor arachidonic acid. Arachidonic acid is released from membrane phospholipids by phospholipase A_2.

Pharmacokinetics:

The extent of percutaneous absorption of topical corticosteroids is determined by many factors including the vehicle and the integrity of the epidermal barrier. Occlusive dressings with hydrocortisone for up to 24 hours have not been demonstrated to increase penetration; however, occlusion of hydrocortisone for 96 hours markedly enhances penetration. Studies in humans indicate that approximately 0.4% of the applied dose of ELOCON Cream 0.1% enters the circulation after 8 hours of contact on normal skin without occlusion. Inflammation and/or other disease processes in the skin may increase percutaneous absorption.

Studies performed with ELOCON Cream 0.1% indicate that it is in the medium range of potency as compared with other topical corticosteroids.

In a study evaluating the effects of mometasone furoate cream on the hypothalamic-pituitary-adrenal (HPA) axis, 15 grams were applied twice daily for 7 days to six adult patients with psoriasis or atopic dermatitis. The cream was applied without occlusion to at least 30% of the body surface. The results show that the drug caused a slight lowering of adrenal corticosteroid secretion.

In a pediatric trial, 24 atopic dermatitis patients, of which 19 patients were age 2 to 12 years, were treated with ELOCON Cream 0.1% once daily. The majority of patients cleared within 3 weeks.

Ninety-seven pediatric patients ages 6 to 23 months with atopic dermatitis were enrolled in an open-label, hypothalamic-pituitary-adrenal (HPA) axis safety study. ELOCON Cream 0.1% was applied once daily for approximately 3 weeks over a mean body surface area of 41% (range 15% to 94%). In approximately 16% of patients who showed normal adrenal function by Cortrosyn test before starting treatment, adrenal suppression was observed at the end of treatment with ELOCON Cream 0.1%. The criteria for suppression were: basal cortisol level of ≤5 mcg/dL, 30-minute post-stimulation level of ≤18 mcg/dL, or an increase of <7 mcg/dL. Follow-up testing 2 to 4 weeks after stopping treatment, available for 5 of the patients, demonstrated suppressed HPA axis function in one patient, using these same criteria.

INDICATIONS AND USAGE

ELOCON Cream 0.1% is a medium potency corticosteroid indicated for the relief of the inflammatory and pruritic manifestations of corticosteroid-responsive dermatoses.

ELOCON (mometasone furoate cream, USP) Cream 0.1% may be used in pediatric patients 2 years of age or older, although the safety and efficacy of drug use for longer than 3 weeks have not been established (see **PRECAUTIONS**–**Pediatric Use** section). Since safety and efficacy of ELOCON Cream 0.1% have not been established in pediatric patients below 2 years of age, its use in this age group is not recommended.

CONTRAINDICATIONS

ELOCON Cream 0.1% is contraindicated in those patients with a history of hypersensitivity to any of the components in the preparation.

PRECAUTIONS

General:

Systemic absorption of topical corticosteroids can produce reversible hypothalamic-pituitary-adrenal (HPA) axis suppression with the potential for glucocorticosteroid insufficiency after withdrawal of treatment. Manifestations of Cushing's syndrome, hyperglycemia, and glucosuria can also be produced in some patients by systemic absorption of topical corticosteroids while on treatment.

Patients applying a topical steroid to a large surface area or to areas under occlusion should be evaluated periodically for evidence of HPA axis suppression. This may be done by using the ACTH stimulation, A.M. plasma cortisol, and urinary free cortisol tests.

In a study evaluating the effects of mometasone furoate cream on the hypothalamic-pituitary-adrenal (HPA) axis, 15 grams were applied twice daily for 7 days to six adult patients with psoriasis or atopic dermatitis. The cream was applied without occlusion to at least 30% of the body surface. The results show that the drug caused a slight lowering of adrenal corticosteroid secretion.

If HPA axis suppression is noted, an attempt should be made to withdraw the drug, to reduce the frequency of application, or to substitute a less potent corticosteroid. Recovery of HPA axis function is generally prompt upon discontinuation of topical corticosteroids. Infrequently, signs and symptoms of glucocorticosteroid insufficiency may occur requiring supplemental systemic corticosteroids. For information on systemic supplementation, see Prescribing Information for those products.

Pediatric patients may be more susceptible to systemic toxicity from equivalent doses due to their larger skin surface to body mass ratios (see **PRECAUTIONS — Pediatric Use**).

If irritation develops, ELOCON Cream 0.1% should be discontinued and appropriate therapy instituted. Allergic contact dermatitis with corticosteroids is usually diagnosed by observing a failure to heal rather than noting a clinical exacerbation as with most topical products not containing corticosteroids. Such an observation should be corroborated with appropriate diagnostic patch testing.

If concomitant skin infections are present or develop, an appropriate antifungal or antibacterial agent should be used. If a favorable response does not occur promptly, use of ELOCON Cream 0.1% should be discontinued until the infection has been adequately controlled.

Information for Patients:

Patients using topical corticosteroids should receive the following information and instructions:

1. This medication is to be used as directed by the physician. It is for external use only. Avoid contact with the eyes.
2. This medication should not be used for any disorder other than that for which it was prescribed.
3. The treated skin area should not be bandaged or otherwise covered or wrapped so as to be occlusive, unless directed by the physician.
4. Patients should report to their physician any signs of local adverse reactions.
5. Parents of pediatric patients should be advised not to use ELOCON Cream 0.1% in the treatment of diaper dermatitis. ELOCON Cream 0.1% should not be applied in the diaper area as diapers or plastic pants may constitute occlusive dressing (see **DOSAGE AND ADMINISTRATION**).
6. This medication should not be used on the face, underarms, or groin areas unless directed by the physician.
7. As with other corticosteroids, therapy should be discontinued when control is achieved. If no improvement is seen within 2 weeks, contact the physician.
8. Other corticosteroid-containing products should not be used with ELOCON Cream 0.1% without first consulting with the physician.

Laboratory Tests: The following tests may be helpful in evaluating patients for HPA axis suppression:

ACTH stimulation test
A.M. plasma cortisol test
Urinary free cortisol test

Carcinogenesis, Mutagenesis, Impairment of Fertility:

Long-term animal studies have not been performed to evaluate the carcinogenic potential of ELOCON (mometasone furoate cream, USP) Cream 0.1%. Long-term carcinogenicity studies of mometasone furoate were conducted by the inhalation route in rats and mice. In a 2-year carcinogenicity study in Sprague-Dawley rats, mometasone furoate demonstrated no statistically significant increase of tumors at inhalation doses up to 67 mcg/kg (approximately 0.04 times the estimated maximum clinical topical dose from ELOCON Cream 0.1% on a mcg/m² basis). In a 19-month carcinogenicity study in Swiss CD-1 mice, mometasone furoate demonstrated no statistically significant increase in the incidence of tumors at inhalation doses up to 160 mcg/kg (approximately 0.05 times the estimated maximum clinical topical dose from ELOCON Cream 0.1% on a mcg/m² basis).

Mometasone furoate increased chromosomal aberrations in an *in vitro* Chinese hamster ovary cell assay, but did not increase chromosomal aberrations in an *in vitro* Chinese hamster lung cell assay. Mometasone furoate was not mutagenic in the Ames test or mouse lymphoma assay, and was not clastogenic in an *in vivo* mouse micronucleus assay, a rat bone marrow chromosomal aberration assay, or a mouse male germ-cell chromosomal aberration assay. Mometasone furoate also did not induce unscheduled DNA synthesis *in vivo* in rat hepatocytes.

In reproductive studies in rats, impairment of fertility was not produced in male or female rats by subcutaneous doses up to 15 mcg/kg (approximately 0.01 times the estimated maximum clinical topical dose from ELOCON Cream 0.1% on a mcg/m² basis).

Pregnancy *Teratogenic Effects: Pregnancy Category C:*

Corticosteroids have been shown to be teratogenic in laboratory animals when administered systemically at relatively low dosage levels. Some corticosteroids have been shown to be teratogenic after dermal application in laboratory animals.

When administered to pregnant rats, rabbits, and mice, mometasone furoate increased fetal malformations. The doses that produced malformations also decreased fetal growth, as measured by lower fetal weights and/or delayed ossification. Mometasone furoate also caused dystocia and related complications when administered to rats during the end of pregnancy.

In mice, mometasone furoate caused cleft palate at subcutaneous doses of 60 mcg/kg and above. Fetal survival was reduced at 180 mcg/kg. No toxicity was observed at 20 mcg/kg. (Doses of 20, 60, and 180 mcg/kg in the mouse are approximately 0.01, 0.02, and 0.05 times the estimated maximum clinical topical dose from ELOCON Cream 0.1% on a mcg/m^2 basis).

In rats, mometasone furoate produced umbilical hernias at topical doses of 600 mcg/kg and above. A dose of 300 mcg/kg produced delays in ossification, but no malformations. (Doses of 300 and 600 mcg/kg in the rat are approximately 0.2 and 0.4 times the estimated maximum clinical topical dose from ELOCON Cream 0.1% on a mcg/m^2 basis).

In rabbits, mometasone furoate caused multiple malformations (eg, flexed front paws, gallbladder agenesis, umbilical hernia, hydrocephaly) at topical doses of 150 mcg/kg and above (approximately 0.2 times the estimated maximum clinical topical dose from ELOCON Cream 0.1% on a mcg/m^2 basis). In an oral study, mometasone furoate increased resorptions and caused cleft palate and/or head malformations (hydrocephaly and domed head) at 700 mcg/kg. At 2800 mcg/kg most litters were aborted or resorbed. No toxicity was observed at 140 mcg/kg. (Doses at 140, 700, and 2800 mcg/kg in the rabbit are approximately 0.2, 0.9, and 3.6 times the estimated maximum clinical topical dose from ELOCON Cream 0.1% on a mcg/m^2 basis).

When rats received subcutaneous doses of mometasone furoate throughout pregnancy or during the later stages of pregnancy, 15 mcg/kg caused prolonged and difficult labor and reduced the number of live births, birth weight, and early pup survival. Similar effects were not observed at 7.5 mcg/kg. (Doses of 7.5 and 15 mcg/kg in the rat are approximately 0.005 and 0.01 times the estimated maximum clinical topical dose from ELOCON Cream 0.1% on a mcg/m^2 basis).

There are no adequate and well-controlled studies of teratogenic effects from topically applied corticosteroids in pregnant women. Therefore, topical corticosteroids should be used during pregnancy only if the potential benefit justifies the potential risk to the fetus.

Nursing Mothers:

Systemically administered corticosteroids appear in human milk and could suppress growth, interfere with endogenous corticosteroid production, or cause other untoward effects. It is not known whether topical administration of corticosteroids could result in sufficient systemic absorption to produce detectable quantities in human milk. Because many drugs are excreted in human milk, caution should be exercised when ELOCON Cream 0.1% is administered to a nursing woman.

Pediatric Use:

ELOCON Cream 0.1% may be used with caution in pediatric patients 2 years of age or older, although the safety and efficacy of drug use for longer than 3 weeks have not been established. Use of ELOCON Cream 0.1% is supported by results from adequate and well-controlled studies in pediatric patients with corticosteroid-responsive dermatoses. Since safety and efficacy of ELOCON Cream 0.1% have not been established in pediatric patients below 2 years of age, its use in this age group is not recommended.

ELOCON Cream 0.1% caused HPA axis suppression in approximately 16% of pediatric patients ages 6 to 23 months, who showed normal adrenal function by Cortrosyn test before starting treatment, and were treated for approximately 3 weeks over a mean body surface area of 41% (range 15% to 94%). The criteria for suppression were: basal cortisol level of ≤5 mcg/dL, 30-minute post-stimulation level of ≤18 mcg/dL, or an increase of <7 mcg/dL. Follow-up testing 2 to 4 weeks after study completion, available for 5 of the patients, demonstrated suppressed HPA axis function in one patient, using these same criteria. Long-term use of topical corticosteroids has not been studied in this population (see **CLINICAL PHARMACOLOGY – Pharmacokinetics** section).

Because of a higher ratio of skin surface area to body mass, pediatric patients are at a greater risk than adults of HPA axis suppression and Cushing's syndrome when they are treated with topical corticosteroids. They are, therefore, also at greater risk of adrenal insufficiency during and/or after withdrawal of treatment. Pediatric patients may be more susceptible than adults to skin atrophy, including striae, when they are treated with topical corticosteroids. Pediatric patients applying topical corticosteroids to greater than 20% of body surface are at higher risk of HPA axis suppression.

HPA axis suppression, Cushing's syndrome, linear growth retardation, delayed weight gain, and intracranial hypertension have been reported in pediatric patients receiving topical corticosteroids. Manifestations of adrenal suppression in children include low plasma cortisol levels, and an absence of response to ACTH stimulation. Manifestations of intracranial hypertension include bulging fontanelles, headaches, and bilateral papilledema.

ELOCON (mometasone furoate cream, USP) Cream 0.1% should not be used in the treatment of diaper dermatitis.

Geriatric Use:

Clinical studies of ELOCON Cream 0.1% included 190 subjects who were 65 years of age and over and 39 subjects who were 75 years of age and over. No overall differences in safety or effectiveness were observed between these subjects and younger subjects, and other reported clinical experience has not identified differences in responses between the elderly and younger patients. However, greater sensitivity of some older individuals cannot be ruled out.

ADVERSE REACTIONS

In controlled clinical studies involving 319 patients, the incidence of adverse reactions associated with the use of ELOCON Cream 0.1% was 1.6%. Reported reactions included burning, pruritus, and skin atrophy. Reports of rosacea associated with the use of ELOCON Cream 0.1% have also been received. In controlled clinical studies (n=74) involving pediatric patients 2 to 12 years of age, the incidence of adverse experiences associated with the use of ELOCON Cream 0.1% was approximately 7%. Reported reactions included stinging, pruritus, and furunculosis.

The following adverse reactions were reported to be possibly or probably related to treatment with ELOCON Cream 0.1% during clinical studies in 4% of 182 pediatric patients 6 months to 2 years of age: decreased glucocorticoid levels, 2; paresthesia, 2; folliculitis,1; moniliasis, 1; bacterial infection, 1; skin depigmentation, 1. The following signs of skin atrophy were also observed among 97 patients treated with ELOCON Cream 0.1% in a clinical study: shininess 4, telangiectasia 1, loss of elasticity 4, loss of normal skin markings 4, thinness 1, and bruising 1. Striae were not observed in this study.

The following additional local adverse reactions have been reported infrequently with topical corticosteroids, but may occur more frequently with the use of occlusive dressings. These reactions are listed in an approximate decreasing order of occurrence: irritation, dryness, folliculitis, hypertrichosis, acneiform eruptions, hypopigmentation, perioral dermatitis, allergic contact dermatitis, secondary infection, striae, and miliaria.

OVERDOSAGE

Topically applied ELOCON Cream 0.1% can be absorbed in sufficient amounts to produce systemic effects (see **PRECAUTIONS** section).

DOSAGE AND ADMINISTRATION

Apply a thin film of ELOCON Cream 0.1% to the affected skin areas once daily. ELOCON Cream 0.1% may be used in pediatric patients 2 years of age or older. Since safety and efficacy of ELOCON Cream 0.1% have not been adequately established in pediatric patients below 2 years of age, its use in this age group is not recommended (see **PRECAUTIONS – Pediatric Use** section).

As with other corticosteroids, therapy should be discontinued when control is achieved. If no improvement is seen within 2 weeks, reassessment of diagnosis may be necessary. Safety and efficacy of ELOCON Cream 0.1% in pediatric patients for more than 3 weeks of use have not been established.

ELOCON Cream 0.1% should not be used with occlusive dressings unless directed by a physician. ELOCON Cream 0.1% should not be applied in the diaper area if the child still requires diapers or plastic pants as these garments may constitute occlusive dressing.

HOW SUPPLIED

ELOCON Cream 0.1% is supplied in 15-g (NDC 0085-0567-01) and 45-g (NDC 0085-0567-02) tubes; boxes of one.

Store ELOCON Cream 0.1% between 2° and 25°C (36° and 77°F).

ELOCON®
brand of mometasone furoate cream, USP
Cream 0.1%
For Dermatologic Use Only
Not for Ophthalmic Use

Schering Corporation
Kenilworth, NJ 07033 USA
Rev. 12/02 17969366
18724332T

Shown in Product Identification Guide, page 332

ELOCON® ℞
[el'ō-cŏn]
brand of mometasone furoate ointment, USP
Ointment 0.1%
For Dermatologic Use Only
Not for Ophthalmic Use

DESCRIPTION

ELOCON® (mometasone furoate ointment, USP) Ointment 0.1% contains mometasone furoate, USP for dermatologic use. Mometasone furoate is a synthetic corticosteroid with anti-inflammatory activity.

Chemically, mometasone furoate is 9α,21-Dichloro-11β,17-dihydroxy-16α-methylpregna-1,4-diene-3,20-dione 17-(2-furoate), with the empirical formula $C_{27}H_{30}Cl_2O_6$, a molecular weight of 521.4 and the following structural formula:

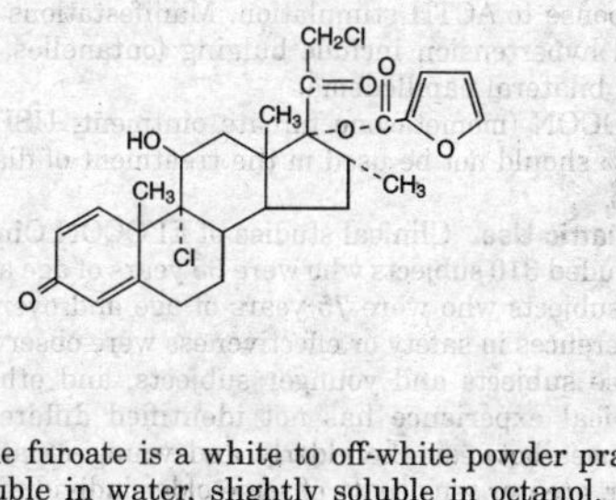

Mometasone furoate is a white to off-white powder practically insoluble in water, slightly soluble in octanol, and moderately soluble in ethyl alcohol.

Each gram contains: 1 mg mometasone furoate, USP in an ointment base of hexylene glycol; phosphoric acid; propylene glycol stearate (55% monoester); white wax; white petrolatum; and purified water.

CLINICAL PHARMACOLOGY

Like other topical corticosteroids, mometasone furoate has anti-inflammatory, anti-pruritic, and vasoconstrictive properties. The mechanism of the anti-inflammatory activity of the topical steroids, in general, is unclear. However, corticosteroids are thought to act by the induction of phospholipase A_2 inhibitory proteins, collectively called lipocortins. It is postulated that these proteins control the biosynthesis of potent mediators of inflammation such as prostaglandins and leukotrienes by inhibiting the release of their common precursor arachidonic acid. Arachidonic acid is released from membrane phospholipids by phospholipase A_2.

Pharmacokinetics The extent of percutaneous absorption of topical corticosteroids is determined by many factors including the vehicle and the integrity of the epidermal barrier. Occlusive dressings with hydrocortisone for up to 24 hours have not been demonstrated to increase penetration; however, occlusion of hydrocortisone for 96 hours markedly enhances penetration. Studies in humans indicate that approximately 0.7% of the applied dose of ELOCON Ointment 0.1% enters the circulation after 8 hours of contact on normal skin without occlusion. Inflammation and/or other disease processes in the skin may increase percutaneous absorption.

Studies performed with ELOCON Ointment 0.1% indicate that it is in the medium range of potency as compared with other topical corticosteroids.

In a study evaluating the effects of mometasone furoate ointment on the hypothalamic-pituitary-adrenal (HPA) axis, 15 grams were applied twice daily for 7 days to six adult patients with psoriasis or atopic dermatitis. The ointment was applied without occlusion to at least 30% of the body surface. The results show that the drug caused a slight lowering of adrenal corticosteroid secretion.

In a pediatric trial, 24 atopic dermatitis patients, of which 19 patients were age 2 to 12 years, were treated with ELOCON Cream 0.1% once daily. The majority of patients cleared within 3 weeks.

Sixty-three pediatric patients ages 6 to 23 months, with atopic dermatitis, were enrolled in an open-label, hypothalamic-pituitary-adrenal (HPA) axis safety study. ELOCON Ointment 0.1% was applied once daily for approximately 3 weeks over a mean body surface area of 39% (range 15% to 99%). In approximately 27% of patients who showed normal adrenal fuction by Cortrosyn test before starting treatment, adrenal suppression was observed at the end of treatment with ELOCON Ointment 0.1%. The criteria for suppression were: basal cortisol level of ≤5 mcg/dL, 30-minute post-stimulation level of ≤18 mcg/dL, or an increase of <7 mcg/dL. Follow-up testing 2 to 4 weeks after stopping treatment, available for 8 of the patients, demonstrated suppressed HPA axis function in 3 patients, using these same criteria.

INDICATIONS AND USAGE

ELOCON Ointment 0.1% is a medium potency corticosteroid indicated for the relief of the inflammatory and pruritic manifestations of corticosteroid-responsive dermatoses.

ELOCON (mometasone furoate ointment, USP) Ointment 0.1% may be used in pediatric patients 2 years of age or older, although the safety and efficacy of drug use for longer than 3 weeks have not been established (see **PRECAUTIONS – Pediatric Use**). Since safety and efficacy of ELOCON Ointment 0.1% have not been adequately established in pediatric patients below 2 years of age, its use in this age group is not recommended.

CONTRAINDICATIONS

ELOCON Ointment 0.1% is contraindicated in those patients with a history of hypersensitivity to any of the components in the preparation.

PRECAUTIONS

General: Systemic absorption of topical corticosteroids can produce reversible hypothalamic-pituitary-adrenal (HPA) axis suppression with the potential for glucocorticosteroid insufficiency after withdrawal of treatment. Manifestations of Cushing's syndrome, hyperglycemia, and glucosuria can also be produced in some patients by systemic absorption of topical corticosteroids while on treatment.

Patients applying a topical steroid to a large surface area or areas under occlusion should be evaluated periodically for evidence of HPA axis suppression. This may be done by using the ACTH stimulation, A.M. plasma cortisol, and urinary free cortisol tests.

In a study evaluating the effects of mometasone furoate ointment on the hypothalamic-pituitary-adrenal (HPA) axis, 15 grams were applied twice daily for 7 days to six adult patients with psoriasis or atopic dermatitis. The ointment was applied without occlusion to at least 30% of the body surface. The results show that the drug caused a slight lowering of adrenal corticosteroid secretion.

If HPA axis suppression is noted, an attempt should be made to withdraw the drug, to reduce the frequency of ap-

Continued on next page

Information on Schering products appearing on these pages is effective as of June 2003.

Elocon Ointment—Cont.

plication, or to substitute a less potent corticosteroid. Recovery of HPA axis function is generally prompt upon discontinuation of topical corticosteroids. Infrequently, signs and symptoms of glucocorticosteroid insufficiency may occur requiring supplemental systemic corticosteroids. For information on systemic supplementation, see Prescribing Information for those products.
Pediatric patients may be more susceptible to systemic toxicity from equivalent doses due to their larger skin surface to body mass ratios (see **PRECAUTIONS – Pediatric Use**).
If irritation develops, ELOCON Ointment 0.1% should be discontinued and appropriate therapy instituted. Allergic contact dermatitis with corticosteroids is usually diagnosed by observing failure to heal rather than noting a clinical exacerbation as with most topical products not containing corticosteroids. Such an observation should be corroborated with appropriate diagnostic patch testing.
If concomitant skin infections are present or develop, an appropriate antifungal or antibacterial agent should be used. If a favorable response does not occur promptly, use of ELOCON Ointment 0.1% should be discontinued until the infection has been adequately controlled.
Information for Patients Patients using topical corticosteroids should receive the following information and instructions:

1. This medication is to be used as directed by the physician. It is for external use only. Avoid contact with the eyes.
2. This medication should not be used for any disorder other than that for which it was prescribed.
3. The treated skin area should not be bandaged or otherwise covered or wrapped so as to be occlusive, unless directed by the physician.
4. Patients should report to their physician any signs of local adverse reactions.
5. Parents of pediatric patients should be advised not to use ELOCON Ointment 0.1% in the treatment of diaper dermatitis. ELOCON Ointment 0.1% should not be applied in the diaper area as diapers or plastic pants may constitute occlusive dressing (see **DOSAGE AND ADMINISTRATION**).
6. This medication should not be used on the face, underarms, or groin areas unless directed by the physician.
7. As with other corticosteroids, therapy should be discontinued when control is achieved. If no improvement is seen within 2 weeks, contact the physician.
8. Other corticosteroid-containing products should not be used with ELOCON Ointment 0.1% without first consulting with the physician.

Laboratory Tests The following tests may be helpful in evaluating patients for HPA axis suppression:
ACTH stimulation test
A.M. plasma cortisol test
Urinary free cortisol test
Carcinogenesis, Mutagenesis, Impairment of Fertility Long-term animal studies have not been performed to evaluate the carcinogenic potential of ELOCON (mometasone furoate ointment, USP) Ointment 0.1%. Long-term carcinogenicity studies of mometasone furoate were conducted by the inhalation route in rats and mice. In a 2-year carcinogenicity study in Sprague-Dawley rats, mometasone furoate demonstrated no statistically significant increase of tumors at inhalation doses up to 67 mcg/kg (approximately 0.04 times the estimated maximum clinical topical dose from ELOCON Ointment 0.1% on a mcg/m^2 basis). In a 19-month carcinogenicity study in Swiss CD-1 mice, mometasone furoate demonstrated no statistically significant increase in the incidence of tumors at inhalation doses up to 160 mcg/kg (approximately 0.05 times the estimated maximum clinical topical dose from ELOCON Ointment 0.1% on a mcg/m^2 basis).
Mometasone furoate increased chromosomal aberrations in an *in vitro* Chinese hamster ovary cell assay, but did not increase chromosomal aberrations in an *in vitro* Chinese hamster lung cell assay. Mometasone furoate was not mutagenic in the Ames test or mouse lymphoma assay, and was not clastogenic in an *in vivo* mouse micronucleus assay, a rat bone marrow chromosomal aberration assay, or a mouse male germ-cell chromosomal aberration assay. Mometasone furoate also did not induce unscheduled DNA synthesis *in vivo* in rat hepatocytes.
In reproductive studies in rats, impairment of fertility was not produced in male or female rats by subcutaneous doses up to 15 mcg/kg (approximately 0.01 times the estimated maximum clinical topical dose from ELOCON Ointment 0.1% on a mcg/m^2 basis).
Pregnancy *Teratogenic Effects: Pregnancy Category C:* Corticosteroids have been shown to be teratogenic in laboratory animals when administered systemically at relatively low dosage levels. Some corticosteroids have been shown to be teratogenic after dermal application in laboratory animals.
When administered to pregnant rats, rabbits, and mice, mometasone furoate increased fetal malformations. The doses that produced malformations also decreased fetal growth, as measured by lower fetal weights and/or delayed ossification. Mometasone furoate also caused dystocia and related complications when administered to rats during the end of pregnancy.
In mice, mometasone furoate caused cleft palate at subcutaneous doses of 60 mcg/kg and above. Fetal survival was reduced at 180 mcg/kg. No toxicity was observed at 20 mcg/kg. (Doses of 20, 60, and 180 mcg/kg in the mouse are approximately 0.01, 0.02, and 0.05 times the estimated maximum clinical topical dose from ELOCON Ointment 0.1% on a mcg/m^2 basis).
In rats, mometasone furoate produced umbilical hernias at topical doses of 600 mcg/kg and above. A dose of 300 mcg/kg produced delays in ossification, but no malformations. (Doses of 300 and 600 mcg/kg in the rat are approximately 0.2 and 0.4 times the estimated maximum clinical topical dose from ELOCON Ointment 0.1% on a mcg/m^2 basis).
In rabbits, mometasone furoate caused multiple malformations (eg, flexed front paws, gallbladder agenesis, umbilical hernia, hydrocephaly) at topical doses of 150 mcg/kg and above (approximately 0.2 times the estimated maximum clinical topical dose from ELOCON Ointment 0.1% on a mcg/m^2 basis). In an oral study, mometasone furoate increased resorptions and caused cleft palate and/or head malformations (hydrocephaly and domed head) at 700 mcg/kg. At 2800 mcg/kg most litters were aborted or resorbed. No toxicity was observed at 140 mcg/kg. (Doses of 140, 700, and 2800 mcg/kg in the rabbit are approximately 0.2, 0.9, and 3.6 times the estimated maximum clinical topical dose from ELOCON Ointment 0.1% on a mcg/m^2 basis).
When rats received subcutaneous doses of mometasone furoate throughout pregnancy or during the later stages of pregnancy, 15 mcg/kg caused prolonged and difficult labor and reduced the number of live births, birth weight, and early pup survival. Similar effects were not observed at 7.5 mcg/kg. (Doses of 7.5 and 15 mcg/kg in the rat are approximately 0.005 and 0.01 times the estimated maximum clinical topical dose from ELOCON Ointment 0.1% on a mcg/m^2 basis).
There are no adequate and well-controlled studies of teratogenic effects from topically applied corticosteroids in pregnant women. Therefore, topical corticosteroids should be used during pregnancy only if the potential benefit justifies the potential risk to the fetus.
Nursing Mothers Systemically administered corticosteroids appear in human milk and could suppress growth, interfere with endogenous corticosteroid production, or cause other untoward effects. It is not known whether topical administration of corticosteroids could result in sufficient systemic absorption to produce detectable quantities in human milk. Because many drugs are excreted in human milk, caution should be exercised when ELOCON Ointment 0.1% is administered to a nursing woman.
Pediatric Use ELOCON Ointment 0.1% may be used with caution in pediatric patients 2 years of age or older, although the safety and efficacy of drug use for longer than 3 weeks have not been established. Use of ELOCON Ointment 0.1% is supported by results from adequate and well-controlled studies in pediatric patients with corticosteroid-responsive dermatoses. Since safety and efficacy of ELOCON Ointment 0.1% have not been adequately established in pediatric patients below 2 years of age, its use in this age group is not recommended.
ELOCON Ointment 0.1% caused HPA axis suppression in approximately 27% of pediatric patients ages 6 to 23 months, who showed normal adrenal function by Cortrosyn test before starting treatment, and were treated for approximately 3 weeks over a mean body surface area of 39% (range 15% to 99%). The criteria for suppression were: basal cortisol level of ≤5 mcg/dL, 30-minute post-stimulation level of ≤18 mcg/dL, or an increase of <7 mcg/dL. Follow-up testing 2 to 4 weeks after stopping treatment, available for 8 of the patients, demonstrated suppressed HPA axis function in 3 patients, using these same criteria. Long-term use of topical corticosteroids has not been studied in this population (see **CLINICAL PHARMACOLOGY – Pharmacokinetics**).
Because of a higher ratio of skin surface area to body mass, pediatric patients are at a greater risk than adults of HPA axis suppression and Cushing's syndrome when they are treated with topical corticosteroids. They are, therefore, also at greater risk of glucocorticosteroid insufficiency during and/or after withdrawal of treatment. Pediatric patients may be more susceptible than adults to skin atrophy, including striae, when they are treated with topical corticosteroids. Pediatric patients applying topical corticosteroids to greater than 20% of body surface are at higher risk of HPA axis suppression.
HPA axis suppression, Cushing's syndrome, linear growth retardation, delayed weight gain, and intracranial hypertension have been reported in children receiving topical corticosteroids. Manifestations of adrenal suppression in children include low plasma cortisol levels, and absence of response to ACTH stimulation. Manifestations of intracranial hypertension include bulging fontanelles, headaches, and bilateral papilledema.
ELOCON (mometasone furoate ointment, USP) Ointment 0.1% should not be used in the treatment of diaper dermatitis.
Geriatric Use Clinical studies of ELOCON Ointment 0.1% included 310 subjects who were 65 years of age and over and 57 subjects who were 75 years of age and over. No overall differences in safety or effectiveness were observed between these subjects and younger subjects, and other reported clinical experience has not identified differences in responses between the elderly and younger patients. However, greater sensitivity of some older individuals cannot be ruled out.

ADVERSE REACTIONS

In controlled clinical studies involving 812 patients, the incidence of adverse reactions associated with the use of ELOCON Ointment 0.1% was 4.8%. Reported reactions included burning, pruritus, skin atrophy, tingling/stinging, and furunculosis. Reports of rosacea associated with the use of ELOCON Ointment 0.1% have been received. In controlled clinical studies (n=74) involving pediatric patients 2 to 12 years of age, the incidence of adverse experiences associated with the use of ELOCON Cream is approximately 7%. Reported reactions included stinging, pruritus, and furunculosis.
The following adverse reactions were reported to be possibly or probably related to treatment with ELOCON Ointment 0.1% during a clinical study, in 5% of 63 pediatric patients 6 months to 2 years of age: decreased glucocorticoid levels, 1; an unspecified skin disorder, 1; and a bacterial skin infection, 1. The following signs of skin atrophy were also observed among 63 patients treated with ELOCON Ointment 0.1% in a clinical study: shininess 4, telangiectasia 1, loss of elasticity 4, loss of normal skin markings 4, thinness 1. Striae and bruising were not observed in this study.
The following additional local adverse reactions have been reported infrequently with topical corticosteroids, but may occur more frequently with the use of occlusive dressings. These reactions are listed in an approximate decreasing order of occurrence: irritation, dryness, folliculitis, hypertrichosis, acneiform eruptions, hypopigmentation, perioral dermatitis, allergic contact dermatitis, secondary infection, striae, and miliaria.

OVERDOSAGE

Topically applied ELOCON Ointment 0.1% can be absorbed in sufficient amounts to produce systemic effects (see **PRECAUTIONS**).

DOSAGE AND ADMINISTRATION

Apply a thin film of ELOCON Ointment 0.1% to the affected skin areas once daily. ELOCON Ointment 0.1% may be used in pediatric patients 2 years of age or older. Since safety and efficacy of ELOCON Ointment 0.1% have not been adequately established in pediatric patients below 2 years of age, its use in this age group is not recommended (see **PRECAUTIONS – Pediatric Use**).
As with other corticosteroids, therapy should be discontinued when control is achieved. If no improvement is seen within 2 weeks, reassessment of diagnosis may be necessary. Safety and efficacy of ELOCON Ointment 0.1% in pediatric patients for more than 3 weeks have not been established.
ELOCON Ointment 0.1% should not be used with occlusive dressings unless directed by a physician. ELOCON Ointment 0.1% should not be applied in the diaper area if the child still requires diapers or plastic pants as these garments may constitute occlusive dressing.

HOW SUPPLIED

ELOCON Ointment 0.1% is supplied in 15 g (NDC 0085-0370-01) and 45 g (NDC 0085-0370-02) tubes; boxes of one.
Store at 25°C (77°F); excursions permitted to 15–30°C (59–86°F).
[See USP Controlled Room Temperature]
Schering Corporation
Kenilworth, NJ 07033 USA
Rev. 11/02 17969544
18724235T

Shown in Product Identification Guide, page 332

FORADIL® AEROLIZER® ℞

[fōr-ă-dĭl]
(formoterol fumarate inhalation powder)
Rx only

Prescribing Information

DESCRIPTION

FORADIL® AEROLIZER® consists of a capsule dosage form containing a dry powder formulation of FORADIL (formoterol fumarate) intended for oral inhalation only with the AEROLIZER® Inhaler.
Each clear, hard gelatin capsule contains a dry powder blend of 12 mcg of formoterol fumarate and 25 mg of lactose as a carrier.
The active component of FORADIL is formoterol fumarate, a racemate. Formoterol fumarate is a selective beta$_2$-adrenergic bronchodilator. Its chemical name is (±)-2-hydroxy-5-[(1RS)-1-hydroxy-2-[[(1RS)-2-(4-methoxyphenyl)-1-methylethyl]-amino]ethyl]formanilide fumarate dihydrate; its structural formula is

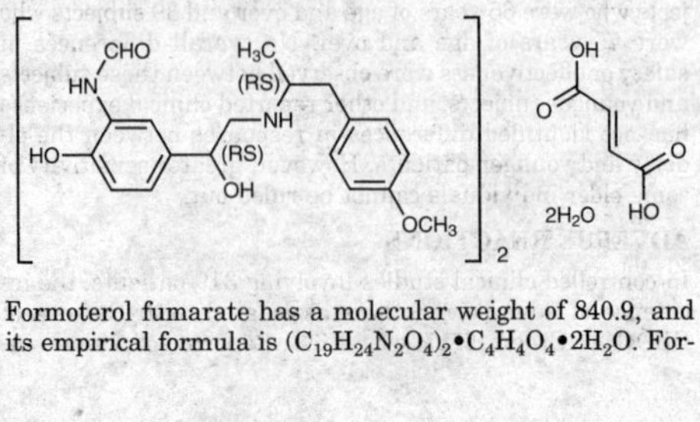

Formoterol fumarate has a molecular weight of 840.9, and its empirical formula is $(C_{19}H_{24}N_2O_4)_2 \bullet C_4H_4O_4 \bullet 2H_2O$. Formoterol fumarate is a white to yellowish crystalline powder, which is freely soluble in glacial acetic acid, soluble in methanol, sparingly soluble in ethanol and isopropanol, slightly soluble in water, and practically insoluble in acetone, ethyl acetate, and diethyl ether.

The AEROLIZER Inhaler is a plastic device used for inhaling FORADIL. The amount of drug delivered to the lung will depend on patient factors, such as inspiratory flow rate and inspiratory time. Under standardized in vitro testing at a fixed flow rate of 60 L/min for 2 seconds, the AEROLIZER Inhaler delivered 10 mcg of formoterol fumarate from the mouthpiece. Peak inspiratory flow rates (PIFR) achievable through the AEROLIZER Inhaler were evaluated in 33 adult and adolescent patients and 32 pediatric patients with mild-to-moderate asthma. Mean PIFR was 117.82 L/min (range 34-188 L/min) for adult and adolescent patients, and 99.66 L/min (range 43-187 L/min) for pediatric patients. Approximately ninety percent of each population studied generated a PIFR through the device exceeding 60 L/min.

To use the delivery system, a FORADIL capsule is placed in the well of the AEROLIZER Inhaler, and the capsule is pierced by pressing and releasing the buttons on the side of the device. The formoterol fumarate formulation is dispersed into the air stream when the patient inhales rapidly and deeply through the mouthpiece.

CLINICAL PHARMACOLOGY

Mechanism of Action

Formoterol fumarate is a long-acting selective beta$_2$-adrenergic receptor agonist (beta$_2$-agonist). Inhaled formoterol fumarate acts locally in the lung as a bronchodilator. In vitro studies have shown that formoterol has more than 200-fold greater agonist activity at beta$_2$-receptors than at beta$_1$-receptors. Although beta$_2$-receptors are the predominant adrenergic receptors in bronchial smooth muscle and beta$_1$-receptors are the predominant receptors in the heart, there are also beta$_2$-receptors in the human heart comprising 10%-50% of the total beta-adrenergic receptors. The precise function of these receptors has not been established, but they raise the possibility that even highly selective beta$_2$-agonists may have cardiac effects.

The pharmacologic effects of beta$_2$-adrenoceptor agonist drugs, including formoterol, are at least in part attributable to stimulation of intracellular adenyl cyclase, the enzyme that catalyzes the conversion of adenosine triphosphate (ATP) to cyclic-3′, 5′-adenosine monophosphate (cyclic AMP). Increased cyclic AMP levels cause relaxation of bronchial smooth muscle and inhibition of release of mediators of immediate hypersensitivity from cells, especially from mast cells.

In vitro tests show that formoterol is an inhibitor of the release of mast cell mediators, such as histamine and leukotrienes, from the human lung. Formoterol also inhibits histamine-induced plasma albumin extravasation in anesthetized guinea pigs and inhibits allergen-induced eosinophil influx in dogs with airway hyper-responsiveness. The relevance of these in vitro and animal findings to humans is unknown.

Animal Pharmacology

Studies in laboratory animals (minipigs, rodents, and dogs) have demonstrated the occurrence of cardiac arrhythmias and sudden death (with histologic evidence of myocardial necrosis) when beta-agonists and methylxanthines are administered concurrently. The clinical significance of these findings is unknown.

Pharmacokinetics

Information on the pharmacokinetics of formoterol in plasma has been obtained in healthy subjects by oral inhalation of doses higher than the recommended range and in Chronic Obstructive Pulmonary Disease (COPD) patients after oral inhalation of doses at and above the therapeutic dose. Urinary excretion of unchanged formoterol was used as an indirect measure of systemic exposure. Plasma drug disposition data parallel urinary excretion, and the elimination half-lives calculated for urine and plasma are similar.

Absorption

Following inhalation of a single 120 mcg dose of formoterol fumarate by 12 healthy subjects, formoterol was rapidly absorbed into plasma, reaching a maximum drug concentration of 92 pg/mL within 5 minutes of dosing. In COPD patients treated for 12 weeks with formoterol fumarate 12 or 24 mcg b.i.d., the mean plasma concentrations of formoterol ranged between 4.0 and 8.8 pg/mL and 8.0 and 17.3 pg/mL, respectively, at 10 min, 2 h and 6 h post inhalation.

Following inhalation of 12 to 96 mcg of formoterol fumarate by 10 healthy males, urinary excretion of both (R,R)- and (S,S)-enantiomers of formoterol increased proportionally to the dose. Thus, absorption of formoterol following inhalation appeared linear over the dose range studied.

In a study in patients with asthma, when formoterol 12 or 24 mcg twice daily was given by oral inhalation for 4 weeks or 12 weeks, the accumulation index, based on the urinary excretion of unchanged formoterol ranged from 1.63 to 2.08 in comparison with the first dose. For COPD patients, when formoterol 12 or 24 mcg twice daily was given by oral inhalation for 12 weeks, the accumulation index, based on the urinary excretion of unchanged formoterol was 1.19-1.38. This suggests some accumulation of formoterol in plasma with multiple dosing. The excreted amounts of formoterol at steady-state were close to those predicted based on single-dose kinetics. As with many drug products for oral inhalation, it is likely that the majority of the inhaled formoterol fumarate delivered is swallowed and then absorbed from the gastrointestinal tract.

Distribution

The binding of formoterol to human plasma proteins in vitro was 61%-64% at concentrations from 0.1 to 100 ng/mL. Binding to human serum albumin in vitro was 31%-38% over a range of 5 to 500 ng/mL. The concentrations of formoterol used to assess the plasma protein binding were higher than those achieved in plasma following inhalation of a single 120 mcg dose.

Metabolism

Formoterol is metabolized primarily by direct glucuronidation at either the phenolic or aliphatic hydroxyl group and O-demethylation followed by glucuronide conjugation at either phenolic hydroxyl groups. Minor pathways involve sulfate conjugation of formoterol and deformylation followed by sulfate conjugation. The most prominent pathway involves direct conjugation at the phenolic hydroxyl group. The second major pathway involves O-demethylation followed by conjugation at the phenolic 2′-hydroxyl group. Four cytochrome P450 isozymes (CYP2D6, CYP2C19, CYP2C9 and CYP2A6) are involved in the O-demethylation of formoterol. Formoterol did not inhibit CYP450 enzymes at therapeutically relevant concentrations. Some patients may be deficient in CYP2D6 or 2C19 or both. Whether a deficiency in one or both of these isozymes results in elevated systemic exposure to formoterol or systemic adverse effects has not been adequately explored.

Excretion

Following oral administration of 80 mcg of radiolabeled formoterol fumarate to 2 healthy subjects, 59%-62% of the radioactivity was eliminated in the urine and 32%-34% in the feces over a period of 104 hours. Renal clearance of formoterol from blood in these subjects was about 150 mL/min. Following inhalation of a 12 mcg or 24 mcg dose by 16 patients with asthma, about 10% and 15%-18% of the total dose was excreted in the urine as unchanged formoterol and direct conjugates of formoterol, respectively. Following inhalation of 12 mcg or 24 mcg dose by 18 patients with COPD the corresponding values were 7% and 6-9% of the dose, respectively.

Based on plasma concentrations measured following inhalation of a single 120 mcg dose by 12 healthy subjects, the mean terminal elimination half-life was determined to be 10 hours. From urinary excretion rates measured in these subjects, the mean terminal elimination half-lives for the (R,R)- and (S,S)-enantiomers were determined to be 13.9 and 12.3 hours, respectively. The (R,R)- and (S,S)-enantiomers represented about 40% and 60% of unchanged drug excreted in the urine, respectively, following single inhaled doses between 12 and 120 mcg in healthy volunteers and single and repeated doses of 12 and 24 mcg in patients with asthma. Thus, the relative proportion of the two enantiomers remained constant over the dose range studied and there was no evidence of relative accumulation of one enantiomer over the other after repeated dosing.

Special Populations

Gender: After correction for body weight, formoterol pharmacokinetics did not differ significantly between males and females.

Geriatric and Pediatric: The pharmacokinetics of formoterol have not been studied in the elderly population, and limited data are available in pediatric patients.

In a study of children with asthma who were 5 to 12 years of age, when formoterol fumarate 12 or 24 mcg was given twice daily by oral inhalation for 12 weeks, the accumulation index ranged from 1.18 to 1.84 based on urinary excretion of unchanged formoterol. Hence, the accumulation in children did not exceed that in adults, where the accumulation index ranged from 1.63 to 2.08 (see above). Approximately 6% and 6.5% to 9% of the dose was recovered in the urine of the children as unchanged and conjugated formoterol, respectively.

Hepatic/Renal Impairment: The pharmacokinetics of formoterol have not been studied in subjects with hepatic or renal impairment.

Pharmacodynamics

Systemic Safety and Pharmacokinetic/Pharmacodynamic Relationships

The major adverse effects of inhaled beta$_2$-agonists occur as a result of excessive activation of the systemic beta-adrenergic receptors. The most common adverse effects in adults and adolescents include skeletal muscle tremor and cramps, insomnia, tachycardia, decreases in plasma potassium, and increases in plasma glucose.

Pharmacokinetic/pharmacodynamic (PK/PD) relationships between heart rate, ECG parameters, and serum potassium levels and the urinary excretion of formoterol were evaluated in 10 healthy male volunteers (25 to 45 years of age) following inhalation of single doses containing 12, 24, 48, or 96 mcg of formoterol fumarate. There was a linear relationship between urinary formoterol excretion and decreases in serum potassium, increases in plasma glucose, and increases in heart rate.

In a second study, PK/PD relationships between plasma formoterol levels and pulse rate, ECG parameters, and plasma potassium levels were evaluated in 12 healthy volunteers following inhalation of a single 120 mcg dose of formoterol fumarate (10 times the recommended clinical dose). Reductions of plasma potassium concentration were observed in all subjects. Maximum reductions from baseline ranged from 0.55 to 1.52 mmol/L with a median maximum reduction of 1.01 mmol/L. The formoterol plasma concentration was highly correlated with the reduction in plasma potassium concentration. Generally, the maximum effect on plasma potassium was noted 1 to 3 hours after peak formoterol plasma concentrations were achieved. A mean maximum increase of pulse rate of 26 bpm was observed 6 hours post dose. The maximum increase of mean corrected QT interval (QTc) was 25 msec when calculated using Bazett's correction and was 8 msec when calculated using Fredericia's correction. The QTc returned to baseline within 12-24 hours post-dose. Formoterol plasma concentrations were weakly correlated with pulse rate and increase of QTc duration. The effects on plasma potassium, pulse rate, and QTc interval are known pharmacological effects of this class of study drug and were not unexpected at the very high formoterol dose (120 mcg single dose, 10 times the recommended single dose) tested in this study. These effects were well-tolerated by the healthy volunteers.

The electrocardiographic and cardiovascular effects of FORADIL AEROLIZER were compared with those of albuterol and placebo in two pivotal 12-week double-blind studies of patients with asthma. A subset of patients underwent continuous electrocardiographic monitoring during three 24-hour periods. No important differences in ventricular or supraventricular ectopy between treatment groups were observed. In these two studies, the total number of patients with asthma exposed to any dose of FORADIL AEROLIZER who had continuous electrocardiographic monitoring was about 200.

Continuous electrocardiographic monitoring was not included in the clinical studies of FORADIL AEROLIZER that were performed in COPD patients. The electrocardiographic effects of FORADIL AEROLIZER were evaluated versus placebo in a 12-month pivotal double-blind study of patients with COPD. An analysis of ECG intervals was performed for patients who participated at study sites in the United States, including 46 patients treated with FORADIL AEROLIZER 12 mcg twice daily, and 50 patients treated with FORADIL AEROLIZER 24 mcg twice daily. ECGs were performed pre-dose, and at 5-15 minutes and 2 hours post-dose at study baseline and after 3, 6 and 12 months of treatment. The results showed that there was no clinically meaningful acute or chronic effect on ECG intervals, including QTc, resulting from treatment with FORADIL AEROLIZER.

Tachyphylaxis/Tolerance

In a clinical study in 19 adult patients with mild asthma, the bronchoprotective effect of formoterol, as assessed by methacholine challenge, was studied following an initial dose of 24 mcg (twice the recommended dose) and after 2 weeks of 24 mcg twice daily. Tolerance to the bronchoprotective effects of formoterol was observed as evidenced by a diminished bronchoprotective effect on FEV$_1$ after 2 weeks of dosing, with loss of protection at the end of the 12 hour dosing period.

Rebound bronchial hyper-responsiveness after cessation of chronic formoterol therapy has not been observed.

In three large clinical trials in patients with asthma, while efficacy of formoterol versus placebo was maintained, a slightly reduced bronchodilatory response (as measured by 12-hour FEV$_1$ AUC) was observed within the formoterol arms over time, particularly with the 24 mcg twice daily dose (twice the daily recommended dose). A similarly reduced FEV$_1$ AUC over time was also noted in the albuterol treatment arms (180 mcg four times daily by metered-dose inhaler).

CLINICAL TRIALS

Adolescent and Adult Asthma Trials

In a placebo-controlled, single-dose clinical trial, the onset of bronchodilation (defined as a 15% or greater increase from baseline in FEV$_1$) was similar for FORADIL AEROLIZER and albuterol 180 mcg by metered-dose inhaler.

In single-dose and multiple-dose clinical trials, the maximum improvement in FEV$_1$ for FORADIL AEROLIZER 12 mcg generally occurred within 1 to 3 hours, and an increase in FEV$_1$ above baseline was observed for 12 hours in most patients.

FORADIL AEROLIZER was compared to albuterol 180 mcg four times daily by metered-dose inhaler, and placebo in a total of 1095 adult and adolescent patients 12 years of age and above with mild-to-moderate asthma (defined as FEV$_1$ 40%–80% of the patient's predicted normal value) who participated in two pivotal, 12-week, multi-center, randomized, double-blind, parallel group studies.

The results of both studies showed that FORADIL AEROLIZER 12 mcg twice daily resulted in significantly greater post-dose bronchodilation (as measured by serial FEV$_1$ for 12 hours post-dose) throughout the 12-week treatment period. Mean FEV$_1$ measurements from both studies are shown below for the first and last treatment days (see Figures 1 and 2).

Continued on next page

Information on Schering products appearing on these pages is effective as of June 2003.

Foradil—Cont.

Figure 1a
Mean FEV_1 from Clinical Trial A
First Treatment Day

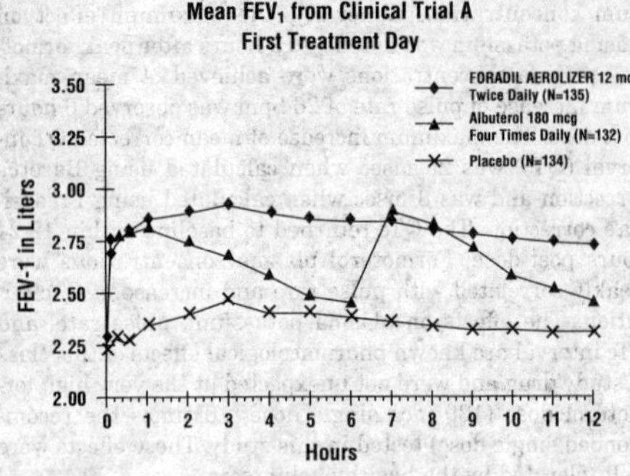

Figure 1b
Mean FEV_1 from Clinical Trial A
Last Treatment Day

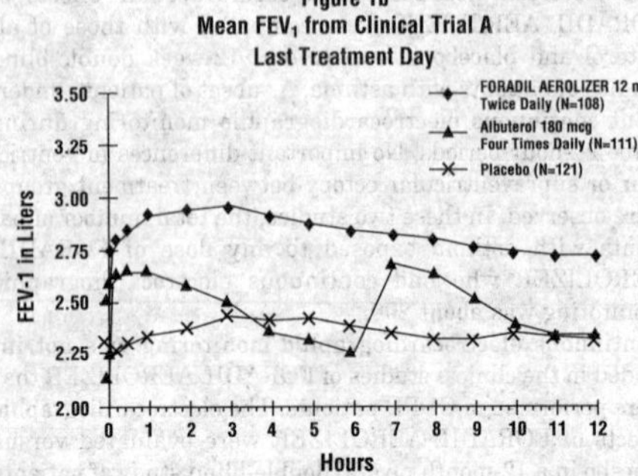

Figure 2a
Mean FEV_1 from Clinical Trial B
First Treatment Day

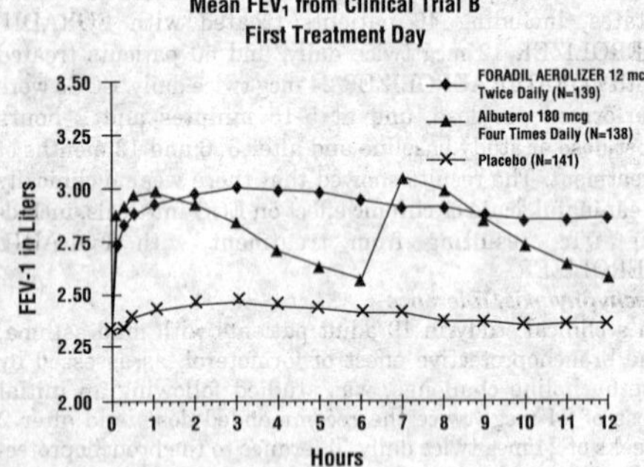

Figure 2b
Mean FEV_1 from Clinical Trial B
Last Treatment Day

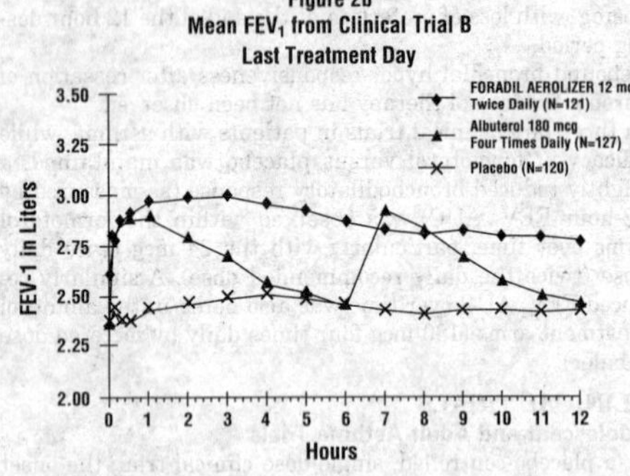

Compared with placebo and albuterol, patients treated with FORADIL AEROLIZER 12 mcg demonstrated improvement in many secondary efficacy endpoints, including improved combined and nocturnal asthma symptom scores, fewer nighttime awakenings, fewer nights in which patients used rescue medication, and higher morning and evening peak flow rates.

Pediatric Asthma Trial

A 12-month, multi-center, randomized, double-blind, parallel-group, study compared FORADIL AEROLIZER and placebo in a total of 518 children with asthma (ages 5-12 years) who required daily bronchodilators and anti-inflammatory treatment. Efficacy was evaluated on the first day of treatment, at Week 12, and at the end of treatment.

FORADIL AEROLIZER 12 mcg twice daily demonstrated a greater 12-hour FEV_1 AUC compared to placebo on the first day of treatment, after twelve weeks of treatment, and after one year of treatment.

Exercise-Induced Bronchospasm Trials

The effect of FORADIL AEROLIZER on exercise-induced bronchospasm (defined as >20% fall in FEV_1) was examined in four randomized, single-dose, double-blind, crossover studies in a total of 77 patients 4 to 41 years of age with exercise-induced bronchospasm. Exercise challenge testing was conducted 15 minutes, and 4, 8, and 12 hours following administration of a single dose of study drug (FORADIL AEROLIZER 12 mcg, albuterol 180 mcg by metered-dose inhaler, or placebo) on separate test days. FORADIL AEROLIZER 12 mcg and albuterol 180 mcg were each superior to placebo for FEV_1 measurements obtained 15 minutes after study drug administration. FORADIL AEROLIZER 12 mcg maintained superiority over placebo at 4, 8, and 12 hours after administration. Most subjects were protected from exercise-induced bronchospasm for up to 12 hours following administration of FORADIL AEROLIZER; however, some were not. The efficacy of FORADIL AEROLIZER in the prevention of exercise-induced bronchospasm when dosed on a regular twice daily regimen has not been studied.

Adult COPD Trials

In multiple-dose clinical trials in patients with COPD, FORADIL AEROLIZER 12 mcg was shown to provide onset of significant bronchodilation (defined as 15% or greater increase from baseline in FEV_1) within 5 minutes of oral inhalation after the first dose. Bronchodilation was maintained for at least 12 hours.

FORADIL AEROLIZER was studied in two pivotal, double-blind, placebo-controlled, randomized, multi-center, parallel-group trials in a total of 1634 adult patients (age range: 34-88 years; mean age: 63 years) with COPD who had a mean FEV_1 that was 46% of predicted. The diagnosis of COPD was based upon a prior clinical diagnosis of COPD, a smoking history (greater than 10 pack-years), age (at least 40 years), spirometry results (prebronchodilator baseline FEV_1 less than 70% of the predicted value, and at least 0.75 liters, with the FEV_1/VC being less than 88% for men and less than 89% for women), and symptom score (greater than zero on at least four of the seven days prior to randomization). These studies included approximately equal numbers of patients with and without baseline bronchodilator reversibility, defined as a 15% or greater increase FEV_1 after inhalation of 200 mcg of albuterol sulfate. A total of 405 patients received FORADIL AEROLIZER 12 mcg, administered twice daily. Each trial compared FORADIL AEROLIZER 12 mcg twice daily and FORADIL AEROLIZER 24 mcg twice daily with placebo and an active control drug. The active control drug was ipratropium bromide in COPD Trial A, and slow-release theophylline in COPD Trial B (the theophylline arm in this study was open-label). The treatment period was 12 weeks in COPD Trial A, and 12 months in COPD Trial B.

The results showed that FORADIL AEROLIZER 12 mcg twice daily resulted in significantly greater post-dose bronchodilation (as measured by serial FEV_1 for 12 hours post-dose; the primary efficacy analysis) compared to placebo when evaluated after 12 weeks of treatment in both trials, and after 12 months of treatment in the 12-month trial (COPD Trial B). Compared to FORADIL AEROLIZER 12 mcg twice daily, FORADIL AEROLIZER 24 mcg twice daily did not provide any additional benefit on a variety of endpoints including FEV_1.

Mean FEV_1 measurements after 12 weeks of treatment for one of the two major efficacy studies are shown in the figure below.

Figure 3
Mean FEV_1 after 12 Weeks of treatment
from COPD Trial A

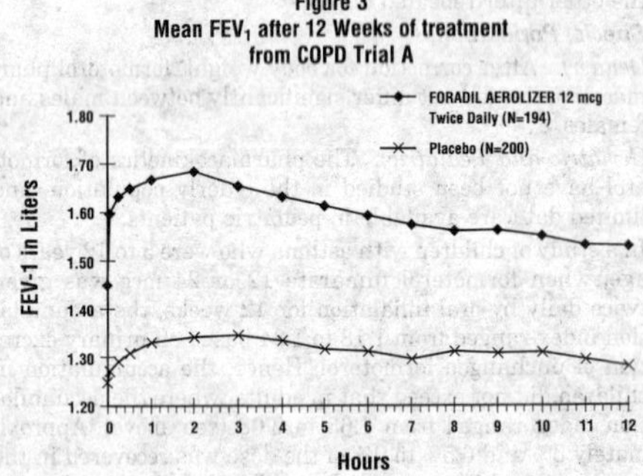

FORADIL AEROLIZER 12 mcg twice daily was statistically superior to placebo at all post-dose timepoints tested (from 5 minutes to 12 hours post-dose) throughout the 12-week (COPD Trial A) and 12-month (COPD Trial B) treatment periods.

In both pivotal trials compared with placebo, patients treated with FORADIL AEROLIZER 12 mcg demonstrated improved morning pre-medication peak expiratory flow rates and took fewer puffs of rescue albuterol.

INDICATIONS AND USAGE

FORADIL AEROLIZER is indicated for long-term, twice-daily (morning and evening) administration in the maintenance treatment of asthma and in the prevention of bronchospasm in adults and children 5 years of age and older with reversible obstructive airways disease, including patients with symptoms of nocturnal asthma, who require regular treatment with inhaled, short-acting, beta$_2$-agonists. It is not indicated for patients whose asthma can be managed by occasional use of inhaled, short-acting, beta$_2$-agonists.

FORADIL AEROLIZER is also indicated for the acute prevention of exercise-induced bronchospasm (EIB) in adults and children 5 years of age and older, when administered on an occasional, as-needed basis.

FORADIL AEROLIZER can be used to treat asthma concomitantly with short-acting beta$_2$-agonists, inhaled or systemic corticosteroids, and theophylline therapy (see PRECAUTIONS, Drug Interactions). A satisfactory clinical response to FORADIL AEROLIZER does not eliminate the need for continued treatment with an anti-inflammatory agent.

FORADIL AEROLIZER is indicated for the long-term, twice daily (morning and evening) administration in the maintenance treatment of bronchoconstriction in patients with Chronic Obstructive Pulmonary Disease including chronic bronchitis and emphysema.

CONTRAINDICATIONS

FORADIL (formoterol fumarate) is contraindicated in patients with a history of hypersensitivity to formoterol fumarate or to any components of this product.

WARNINGS

IMPORTANT INFORMATION: FORADIL AEROLIZER SHOULD NOT BE INITIATED IN PATIENTS WITH SIGNIFICANTLY WORSENING OR ACUTELY DETERIORATING ASTHMA, WHICH MAY BE A LIFE-THREATENING CONDITION. The use of FORADIL AEROLIZER in this setting is inappropriate.

FORADIL AEROLIZER IS NOT A SUBSTITUTE FOR INHALED OR ORAL CORTICOSTEROIDS. Corticosteroids should not be stopped or reduced at the time FORADIL AEROLIZER is initiated. (See PRECAUTIONS, Information for Patients and the accompanying Patient Instructions For Use.)

When beginning treatment with FORADIL AEROLIZER, patients who have been taking inhaled, short-acting beta$_2$-agonists on a regular basis (e.g., four times a day) should be instructed to discontinue the regular use of these drugs and use them only for symptomatic relief of acute asthma symptoms (see PRECAUTIONS, Information for Patients).

Paradoxical Bronchospasm

As with other inhaled beta$_2$-agonists, formoterol can produce paradoxical bronchospasm, that may be life-threatening. If paradoxical bronchospasm occurs, FORADIL AEROLIZER should be discontinued immediately and alternative therapy instituted.

Deterioration of Asthma

Asthma may deteriorate acutely over a period of hours or chronically over several days or longer. If the usual dose of FORADIL AEROLIZER no longer controls the symptoms of bronchoconstriction, and the patient's inhaled, short-acting beta$_2$-agonist becomes less effective or the patient needs more inhalation of short-acting beta$_2$-agonist than usual, these may be markers of deterioration of asthma. In this setting, a re-evaluation of the patient and the asthma treatment regimen should be undertaken at once, giving special consideration to the possible need for anti-inflammatory treatment, e.g., corticosteroids. Increasing the daily dosage of FORADIL AEROLIZER beyond the recommended dose in this situation is not appropriate. FORADIL AEROLIZER should not be used more frequently than twice daily (morning and evening) at the recommended dose.

Use of Anti-inflammatory Agents

The use of beta$_2$-agonists alone may not be adequate to control asthma in many patients. Early consideration should be given to adding anti-inflammatory agents, e.g., corticosteroids. There are no data demonstrating that FORADIL has any clinical anti-inflammatory effect and therefore it cannot be expected to take the place of corticosteroids. Patients who already require oral or inhaled corticosteroids for treatment of asthma should be continued on this type of treatment even if they feel better as a result of initiating or increasing the dose of FORADIL AEROLIZER. Any change in corticosteroid dosage, in particular a reduction, should be made ONLY after clinical evaluation (see PRECAUTIONS, Information for Patients).

Cardiovascular Effects

Formoterol fumarate, like other beta$_2$-agonists, can produce a clinically significant cardiovascular effect in some patients as measured by increases in pulse rate, blood pressure, and/or symptoms. Although such effects are uncommon after administration of FORADIL AEROLIZER at recommended doses, if they occur, the drug may need to be discontinued. In addition, beta-agonists have been reported to produce ECG changes, such as flattening of the T wave, prolongation of the QTc interval, and ST segment depression. The clinical significance of these findings is unknown. Therefore, formoterol fumarate, like other sympathomimetic amines, should be used with caution in patients with cardiovascular disorders, especially coronary insufficiency, cardiac arrhythmias, and hypertension (see PRECAUTIONS, General).

Immediate Hypersensitivity Reactions

Immediate hypersensitivity reactions may occur after administration of FORADIL AEROLIZER, as demonstrated by cases of anaphylactic reactions, urticaria, angioedema, rash, and bronchospasm.

Do Not Exceed Recommended Dose

Fatalities have been reported in association with excessive use of inhaled sympathomimetic drugs in patients with asthma. The exact cause of death is unknown, but cardiac arrest following an unexpected development of a severe acute asthmatic crisis and subsequent hypoxia is suspected.

PRECAUTIONS

General

FORADIL AEROLIZER should not be used to treat acute symptoms of asthma. FORADIL AEROLIZER has not been studied in the relief of acute asthma symptoms and extra doses should not be used for that purpose. When prescribing FORADIL AEROLIZER, the physician should also provide the patient with an inhaled, short-acting beta$_2$-agonist for treatment of symptoms that occur acutely, despite regular twice-daily (morning and evening) use of FORADIL AEROLIZER. Patients should also be cautioned that increasing inhaled beta$_2$-agonist use is a signal of deteriorating asthma. (See Information for Patients and the accompanying Patient Instructions For Use.)

Formoterol fumarate, like other sympathomimetic amines, should be used with caution in patients with cardiovascular disorders, especially coronary insufficiency, cardiac arrhythmias, and hypertension; in patients with convulsive disorders or thyrotoxicosis; and in patients who are unusually responsive to sympathomimetic amines. Clinically significant changes in systolic and/or diastolic blood pressure, pulse rate and electrocardiograms have been seen infrequently in individual patients in controlled clinical studies with formoterol. Doses of the related beta$_2$-agonist albuterol, when administered intravenously, have been reported to aggravate preexisting diabetes mellitus and ketoacidosis.

Beta-agonist medications may produce significant hypokalemia in some patients, possibly through intracellular shunting, which has the potential to produce adverse cardiovascular effects. The decrease in serum potassium is usually transient, not requiring supplementation.

Clinically significant changes in blood glucose and/or serum potassium were infrequent during clinical studies with long-term administration of FORADIL AEROLIZER at the recommended dose.

FORADIL® capsules should ONLY be used with the AEROLIZER® Inhaler and SHOULD NOT be taken orally. FORADIL® capsules should always be stored in the blister, and only removed IMMEDIATELY before use.

Information for Patients

It is important that patients understand how to use the AEROLIZER Inhaler appropriately and how it should be used in relation to other asthma medications they are taking (see the accompanying Patient Instructions For Use).

The active ingredient of FORADIL (formoterol fumarate) is a long-acting, bronchodilator used for the treatment of asthma, including nocturnal asthma, and for the prevention of exercise-induced bronchospasm. FORADIL AEROLIZER provides bronchodilation for up to 12 hours. Patients should be advised not to increase the dose or frequency of FORADIL AEROLIZER without consulting the prescribing physician. Patients should be warned not to stop or reduce concomitant asthma therapy without medical advice.

FORADIL AEROLIZER is not indicated to relieve acute asthma symptoms and extra doses should not be used for that purpose. Acute symptoms should be treated with an inhaled, short-acting, beta$_2$-agonist (the health-care provider should prescribe the patient with such medication and instruct the patient in how it should be used). Patients should be instructed to seek medical attention if their symptoms worsen, if FORADIL AEROLIZER treatment becomes less effective, or if they need more inhalations of a short-acting beta$_2$-agonist than usual. Patients should not inhale more than the contents of the prescribed number of capsules at any one time. The daily dosage of FORADIL AEROLIZER should not exceed one capsule twice daily (24 mcg total daily dose).

When FORADIL AEROLIZER is used for the prevention of EIB, the contents of one capsule should be taken at least 15 minutes prior to exercise. Additional doses of FORADIL AEROLIZER should not be used for 12 hours. Prevention of EIB has not been studied in patients who are receiving chronic FORADIL AEROLIZER administration twice daily and these patients should not use additional FORADIL AEROLIZER for prevention of EIB.

FORADIL AEROLIZER should not be used as a substitute for oral or inhaled corticosteroids. The dosage of these medications should not be changed and they should not be stopped without consulting the physician, even if the patient feels better after initiating treatment with FORADIL AEROLIZER.

Patients should be informed that treatment with beta$_2$-agonists may lead to adverse events which include palpitations, chest pain, rapid heart rate, tremor or nervousness.

Patients should be informed never to use FORADIL AEROLIZER with a spacer and never to exhale into the device.

Patients should avoid exposing the FORADIL capsules to moisture and should handle the capsules with dry hands. The AEROLIZER® Inhaler should never be washed and should be kept dry. The patient should always use the new AEROLIZER Inhaler that comes with each refill.

Women should be advised to contact their physician if they become pregnant or if they are nursing.

Patients should be told that in rare cases, the gelatin capsule might break into small pieces. These pieces should be retained by the screen built into the AEROLIZER Inhaler. However, it remains possible that rarely, tiny pieces of gelatin might reach the mouth or throat after inhalation. The capsule is less likely to shatter when pierced if: storage conditions are strictly followed, capsules are removed from the blister immediately before use, and the capsules are only pierced once.

Drug Interactions

If additional adrenergic drugs are to be administered by any route, they should be used with caution because the pharmacologically predictable sympathetic effects of formoterol may be potentiated.

Concomitant treatment with xanthine derivatives, steroids, or diuretics may potentiate any hypokalemic effect of adrenergic agonists.

The ECG changes and/or hypokalemia that may result from the administration of non-potassium sparing diuretics (such as loop or thiazide diuretics) can be acutely worsened by beta-agonists, especially when the recommended dose of the beta-agonist is exceeded. Although the clinical significance of these effects is not known, caution is advised in the coadministration of beta-agonist with non-potassium sparing diuretics.

Formoterol, as with other beta$_2$-agonists, should be administered with extreme caution to patients being treated with monamine oxidase inhibitors, tricyclic antidepressants, or drugs known to prolong the QTc interval because the action of adrenergic agonists on the cardiovascular system may be potentiated by these agents. Drugs that are known to prolong the QTc interval have an increased risk of ventricular arrhythmias.

Beta-adrenergic receptor antagonists (beta-blockers) and formoterol may inhibit the effect of each other when administered concurrently. Beta-blockers not only block the therapeutic effects of beta-agonists, such as formoterol, but may produce severe bronchospasm in asthmatic patients. Therefore, patients with asthma should not normally be treated with beta-blockers. However, under certain circumstances, e.g., as prophylaxis after myocardial infarction, there may be no acceptable alternatives to the use of beta-blockers in patients with asthma. In this setting, cardioselective beta-blockers could be considered, although they should be administered with caution.

Carcinogenesis, Mutagenesis, Impairment of Fertility

The carcinogenic potential of formoterol fumarate has been evaluated in 2-year drinking water and dietary studies in both rats and mice. In rats, the incidence of ovarian leiomyomas was increased at doses of 15 mg/kg and above in the drinking water study and at 20 mg/kg in the dietary study, but not at dietary doses up to 5 mg/kg (AUC exposure approximately 450 times human exposure at the maximum recommended daily inhalation dose). In the dietary study, the incidence of benign ovarian thecacell tumors was increased at doses of 0.5 mg/kg and above (AUC exposure at the low dose of 0.5 mg/kg was approximately 45 times human exposure at the maximum recommended daily inhalation dose). This finding was not observed in the drinking water study, nor was it seen in mice (see below).

In mice, the incidence of adrenal subcapsular adenomas and carcinomas was increased in males at doses of 69 mg/kg and above in the drinking water study, but not at doses up to 50 mg/kg (AUC exposure approximately 590 times human exposure at the maximum recommended daily inhalation dose) in the dietary study. The incidence of hepatocarcinomas was increased in the dietary study at doses of 20 and 50 mg/kg in females and 50 mg/kg in males, but not at doses up to 5 mg/kg in either males or females (AUC exposure approximately 60 times human exposure at the maximum recommended daily inhalation dose). Also in the dietary study, the incidence of uterine leiomyomas and leiomyosarcomas was increased at doses of 2 mg/kg and above (AUC exposure at the low dose of 2 mg/kg was approximately 25 times human exposure at the maximum recommended daily inhalation dose). Increases in leiomyomas of the rodent female genital tract have been similarly demonstrated with other beta-agonist drugs.

Formoterol fumarate was not mutagenic or clastogenic in the following tests: mutagenicity tests in bacterial and mammalian cells, chromosomal analyses in mammalian cells, unscheduled DNA synthesis repair tests in rat hepatocytes and human fibroblasts, transformation assay in mammalian fibroblasts and micronucleus tests in mice and rats.

Reproduction studies in rats revealed no impairment of fertility at oral doses up to 3 mg/kg (approximately 1000 times the maximum recommended daily inhalation dose in humans on a mg/m^2 basis).

Pregnancy, Teratogenic Effects, Pregnancy Category C

Formoterol fumarate has been shown to cause stillbirth and neonatal mortality at oral doses of 6 mg/kg (approximately 2000 times the maximum recommended daily inhalation dose in humans on a mg/m^2 basis) and above in rats receiving the drug during the late stage of pregnancy. These effects, however, were not produced at a dose of 0.2 mg/kg (approximately 70 times the maximum recommended daily inhalation dose in humans on a mg/m^2 basis). When given to rats throughout organogenesis, oral doses of 0.2 mg/kg and above delayed ossification of the fetus, and doses of 6 mg/kg and above decreased fetal weight. Formoterol fumarate did not cause malformations in rats or rabbits following oral administration. Because there are no adequate and well-controlled studies in pregnant women, FORADIL AEROLIZER should be used during pregnancy only if the potential benefit justifies the potential risk to the fetus.

Use in Labor and Delivery

Formoterol fumarate has been shown to cause stillbirth and neonatal mortality at oral doses of 6 mg/kg (approximately 2000 times the maximum recommended daily inhalation dose in humans on a mg/m^2 basis) and above in rats receiving the drug for several days at the end of pregnancy. These effects were not produced at a dose of 0.2 mg/kg (approximately 70 times the maximum recommended daily inhalation dose in humans on a mg/m^2 basis). There are no adequate and well-controlled human studies that have investigated the effects of FORADIL AEROLIZER during labor and delivery.

Because beta-agonists may potentially interfere with uterine contractility, FORADIL AEROLIZER should be used during labor only if the potential benefit justifies the potential risk.

Nursing Mothers

In reproductive studies in rats, formoterol was excreted in the milk. It is not known whether formoterol is excreted in human milk, but because many drugs are excreted in human milk, caution should be exercised if FORADIL AEROLIZER is administered to nursing women. There are no well-controlled human studies of the use of FORADIL AEROLIZER in nursing mothers.

Pediatric Use

Asthma

A total of 776 children 5 years of age and older with asthma were studied in three multiple-dose controlled clinical trials. Of the 512 children who received formoterol, 508 were 5-12 years of age, and approximately one third were 5-8 years of age.

Exercise-Induced Bronchospasm

A total of 25 pediatric patients, 4–11 years of age, were studied in two well-controlled single-dose clinical trials.

The safety and effectiveness of FORADIL AEROLIZER in pediatric patients below 5 years of age has not been established. (See CLINICAL TRIALS, Pediatric Asthma Trial, and ADVERSE REACTIONS, Experience in Pediatric, Adolescent and Adult Patients.)

Geriatric Use

Of the total number of patients who received FORADIL AEROLIZER in adolescent and adult chronic dosing asthma clinical trials, 318 were 65 years of age or older and 39 were 75 years of age and older. Of the 811 patients who received FORADIL AEROLIZER in two pivotal multiple-dose controlled clinical studies in patients with COPD, 395 (48.7%) were 65 years of age or older while 62 (7.6%) were 75 years of age or older. No overall differences in safety or effectiveness were observed between these subjects and younger subjects. A slightly higher frequency of chest infection was reported in the 39 asthma patients 75 years of age and older, although a causal relationship with FORADIL has not been established. Other reported clinical experience has not identified differences in responses between the elderly and younger adult patients, but greater sensitivity of some older individuals cannot be ruled out. (See PRECAUTIONS, Drug Interactions.)

ADVERSE REACTIONS

Adverse reactions to FORADIL are similar in nature to other selective beta$_2$-adrenoceptor agonists; e.g., angina, hypertension or hypotension, tachycardia, arrhythmias, nervousness, headache, tremor, dry mouth, palpitation, muscle cramps, nausea, dizziness, fatigue, malaise, hypokalemia, hyperglycemia, metabolic acidosis and insomnia.

Experience in Pediatric, Adolescent and Adult Patients with Asthma

Of the 5,824 patients in multiple-dose controlled clinical trials, 1,985 were treated with FORADIL AEROLIZER at the recommended dose of 12 mcg twice daily. The following table shows adverse events where the frequency was greater than or equal to 1% in the FORADIL twice daily group and where the rates in the FORADIL group exceeded placebo. Three adverse events showed dose ordering among tested doses of 6, 12 and 24 mcg administered twice daily; tremor, dizziness and dysphonia.

NUMBER AND FREQUENCY OF ADVERSE EXPERIENCES IN PATIENTS 5 YEARS OF AGE AND OLDER FROM MULTIPLE-DOSE CONTROLLED CLINICAL TRIALS

Adverse Event	FORADIL AEROLIZER 12 mcg twice daily		Placebo	
	n	(%)	n	(%)
Total Patients	1985	(100)	969	(100)
Infection viral	341	(17.2)	166	(17.1)
Bronchitis	92	(4.6)	42	(4.3)
Chest infection	54	(2.7)	4	(0.4)
Dyspnea	42	(2.1)	16	(1.7)
Chest pain	37	(1.9)	13	(1.3)
Tremor	37	(1.9)	4	(0.4)
Dizziness	31	(1.6)	15	(1.5)
Insomnia	29	(1.5)	8	(0.8)
Tonsillitis	23	(1.2)	7	(0.7)
Rash	22	(1.1)	7	(0.7)
Dysphonia	19	(1.0)	9	(0.9)

Experience in Children with Asthma

The safety of FORADIL AEROLIZER compared to placebo was investigated in one large, multicenter, randomized, double-blind clinical trial in 518 children with asthma (ages 5–12 years) in need of daily bronchodilators and anti-inflammatory treatment. The numbers and percent of patients who reported adverse events were comparable in the 12 mcg twice daily and placebo groups. In general, the pattern of the adverse events observed in children differed from the usual pattern seen in adults. The adverse events that were more frequent in the formoterol group than in the placebo group reflected infection/inflammation (viral infection, rhinitis, tonsillitis, gastroenteritis) or abdominal complaints (abdominal pain, nausea, dyspepsia).

Continued on next page

Information on Schering products appearing on these pages is effective as of June 2003.

Foradil—Cont.

Experience in Adult Patients with COPD

Of the 1634 patients in two pivotal multiple-dose Chronic Obstructive Pulmonary Disease (COPD) controlled trials, 405 were treated with FORADIL AEROLIZER 12 mcg twice daily. The numbers and percent of patients who reported adverse events were comparable in the 12 mcg twice daily and placebo groups. Adverse events (AE's) experienced were similar to those seen in asthmatic patients, but with a higher incidence of COPD-related AE's in both placebo and formoterol treated patients.

The following table shows adverse events where the frequency was greater than or equal to 1% in the FORADIL AEROLIZER group and where the rates in the FORADIL AEROLIZER group exceeded placebo. The two clinical trials included doses of 12 mcg and 24 mcg, administered twice daily. Seven adverse events showed dose ordering among tested doses of 12 and 24 mcg administered twice daily; pharyngitis, fever, muscle cramps, increased sputum, dysphonia, myalgia, and tremor.

NUMBER AND FREQUENCY OF ADVERSE EXPERIENCES IN ADULT COPD PATIENTS TREATED IN MULTIPLE-DOSE CONTROLLED CLINICAL TRIALS

Adverse Event	FORADIL AEROLIZER 12 mcg twice daily		Placebo	
	n	(%)	n	(%)
Total Patients	405	(100)	420	(100)
Upper respiratory tract infection	30	(7.4)	24	(5.7)
Pain back	17	(4.2)	17	(4.0)
Pharyngitis	14	(3.5)	10	(2.4)
Pain chest	13	(3.2)	9	(2.1)
Sinusitis	11	(2.7)	7	(1.7)
Fever	9	(2.2)	6	(1.4)
Cramps leg	7	(1.7)	2	(0.5)
Cramps muscle	7	(1.7)	0	
Anxiety	6	(1.5)	5	(1.2)
Pruritus	6	(1.5)	4	(1.0)
Sputum increased	6	(1.5)	5	(1.2)
Mouth dry	5	(1.2)	4	(1.0)
Trauma	5	(1.2)	0	

Overall, the frequency of all cardiovascular adverse events in the two pivotal studies was low and comparable to placebo (6.4% for FORADIL AEROLIZER 12 mcg twice daily, and 6.0% for placebo). There were no frequently-occurring specific cardiovascular adverse events for FORADIL AEROLIZER (frequency greater than or equal to 1% and greater than placebo).

Post Marketing Experience

In extensive worldwide marketing experience with FORADIL, serious exacerbations of asthma, including some that have been fatal, have been reported. While most of these cases have been in patients with severe or acutely deteriorating asthma (see WARNINGS), a few have occurred in patients with less severe asthma. The contribution of FORADIL to these cases could not be determined.

Rare reports of anaphylactic reactions, including severe hypotension and angioedema, have also been received in association with the use of formoterol fumarate inhalation powder.

DRUG ABUSE AND DEPENDENCE

There was no evidence in clinical trials of drug dependence with the use of FORADIL.

OVERDOSAGE

The expected signs and symptoms with overdosage of FORADIL AEROLIZER are those of excessive beta-adrenergic stimulation and/or occurrence or exaggeration of any of the signs and symptoms listed under ADVERSE REACTIONS, e.g., angina, hypertension or hypotension, tachycardia, with rates up to 200 beats/min., arrhythmias, nervousness, headache, tremor, seizures, muscle cramps, dry mouth, palpitation, nausea, dizziness, fatigue, malaise, hypokalemia, hyperglycemia, and insomnia. Metabolic acidosis may also occur. As with all inhaled sympathomimetic medications, cardiac arrest and even death may be associated with an overdose of FORADIL AEROLIZER.

Treatment of overdosage consists of discontinuation of FORADIL AEROLIZER together with institution of appropriate symptomatic and/or supportive therapy. The judicious use of a cardioselective beta-receptor blocker may be considered, bearing in mind that such medication can produce bronchospasm. There is insufficient evidence to determine if dialysis is beneficial for overdosage of FORADIL AEROLIZER. Cardiac monitoring is recommended in cases of overdosage.

The minimum acute lethal inhalation dose of formoterol fumarate in rats is 156 mg/kg (approximately 53,000 and 25,000 times the maximum recommended daily inhalation dose in adults and children, respectively, on a mg/m^2 basis). The median lethal oral doses in Chinese hamsters, rats, and mice provide even higher multiples of the maximum recommended daily inhalation dose in humans.

DOSAGE AND ADMINISTRATION

FORADIL capsules should be administered only by the oral inhalation route (see the accompanying Patient Instructions for Use) and only using the AEROLIZER Inhaler. FORADIL capsules should not be ingested (i.e., swallowed) orally. FORADIL capsules should always be stored in the blister, and only removed IMMEDIATELY BEFORE USE.

For Maintenance Treatment of Asthma

For adults and children 5 years of age and older, the usual dosage is the inhalation of the contents of one 12-mcg FORADIL capsule every 12 hours using the AEROLIZER® Inhaler. The patient must not exhale into the device. The total daily dose of FORADIL should not exceed one capsule twice daily (24 mcg total daily dose). More frequent administration or administration of a larger number of inhalations is not recommended. If symptoms arise between doses, an inhaled short-acting beta$_2$-agonist should be taken for immediate relief.

If a previously effective dosage regimen fails to provide the usual response, medical advice should be sought immediately as this is often a sign of destabilization of asthma. Under these circumstances, the therapeutic regimen should be re-evaluated and additional therapeutic options, such as inhaled or systemic corticosteroids, should be considered.

For Prevention of Exercise-Induced Bronchospasm (EIB)

For adults and children 5 years of age or older, the usual dosage is the inhalation of the contents of one 12-mcg FORADIL capsule at least 15 minutes before exercise administered on an occasional as-needed basis. When used intermittently as needed for prevention, protection may last up to 12 hours.

Additional doses of FORADIL AEROLIZER should not be used for 12 hours after the administration of this drug. Regular, twice-daily dosing has not been studied in preventing EIB. Patients who are receiving FORADIL AEROLIZER twice daily for maintenance treatment of their asthma should not use additional doses for prevention of EIB and may require a short-acting bronchodilator.

For Maintenance Treatment of Chronic Obstructive Pulmonary Disease (COPD)

The usual dosage is the inhalation of the contents of one 12 mcg FORADIL capsule every 12 hours using the AEROLIZER® inhaler.

A total daily dose of greater than 24 mcg is not recommended.

If a previously effective dosage regimen fails to provide the usual response, medical advice should be sought immediately as this is often a sign of destabilization of COPD. Under these circumstances, the therapeutic regimen should be re-evaluated and additional therapeutic options should be considered.

HOW SUPPLIED

FORADIL® AEROLIZER® contains: aluminum blister-packaged 12-mcg FORADIL (formoterol fumarate) clear gelatin capsules with "CG" printed on one end and "FXF" printed on the opposite end; one AEROLIZER® Inhaler; and Patient Instructions for Use

Unit Dose (blister pack)
Box of 12 (strips of 6) .... NDC 0085-1402-01

Unit Dose (blister pack)
Box of 60 (strips of 6) .... NDC 0085-1401-01

FORADIL® capsules should be used with the AEROLIZER® Inhaler only. The AEROLIZER® Inhaler should not be used with any other capsules.

Prior to dispensing: Store in a refrigerator, 2°C-8°C (36°F-46°F)

After dispensing to patient: Store at 20°C to 25°C (68°F to 77°F) [see USP Controlled Room Temperature]. Protect from heat and moisture. CAPSULES SHOULD ALWAYS BE STORED IN THE BLISTER AND ONLY REMOVED FROM THE BLISTER IMMEDIATELY BEFORE USE.

Always discard the FORADIL® capsules and AEROLIZER® Inhaler by the "Use by" date and always use the new AEROLIZER Inhaler provided with each new prescription.

Keep out of the reach of children.

REV: JUNE 2003 Printed in U.S.A. 89018802
26762910 Rev. 6/03

SCHERING CORPORATION
Manufactured by:
Novartis Pharma AG, Basle, Switzerland
for
Schering Corporation, Kenilworth, NJ 07033

GUANIDINE HYDROCHLORIDE ℞

[guă-nĭ-dīn]
Tablets

DESCRIPTION

Chemically, guanidine (amino-methanamidine) hydrochloride is a crystalline powder freely soluble in water and alcohol. The aqueous solution is neutral.

The structural formula is:

$$HN = C < \begin{matrix} NH_2 \\ NH_2 \end{matrix} \cdot HCl$$

Each tablet contains 125 mg of guanidine hydrochloride with no color additive in the base. It also contains the following inactive ingredients: colloidal silicon dioxide, magnesium stearate, mannitol, and microcrystalline cellulose.

CLINICAL PHARMACOLOGY

Guanidine apparently acts by enhancing the release of acetylcholine following a nerve impulse. It also appears to slow the rates of depolarization and repolarization of muscle cell membranes.

INDICATIONS AND USAGE

Guanidine is indicated for the reduction of the symptoms of muscle weakness and easy fatigability associated with the myasthenic syndrome of Eaton-Lambert. It is not indicated for treating myasthenia gravis. The Eaton-Lambert syndrome is ordinarily differentiated from myasthenia gravis by the usual association of the syndrome with small cell carcinoma of the lung, but myography may be necessary to make the diagnosis.

CONTRAINDICATIONS

Guanidine is contraindicated in individuals with a history of intolerance or allergy to this drug.

WARNINGS

Fatal bone-marrow suppression, apparently dose related, can occur with guanidine.

Safe use of guanidine hydrochloride in pregnancy has not been established. Therefore, the benefits of therapy must be weighed against the potential hazards. Because guanidine is excreted in milk, patients on this drug should discontinue breast-feeding.

Since there is inadequate experience in children who have received this drug, safety and efficacy in children have not been established.

PRECAUTIONS

Baseline blood studies should be followed by frequent red and white blood cell and differential counts. The drug should be discontinued upon appearance of bone-marrow suppression. Concurrent therapy with other drugs that may cause bone-marrow suppression should be avoided.

Renal function may be affected in some patients receiving guanidine. Patients should therefore have regular urine examinations and serum creatinine determinations while taking this drug.

Physicians should be given adequate precautions pertaining to the gastrointestinal side effects and the possibility of induced behavior disorders.

Treatment should not be continued longer than necessary.

ADVERSE REACTIONS

Anemia, leukopenia, and thrombocytopenia resulting from bone-marrow suppression attributable to guanidine have been reported. Other adverse reactions that have been observed are:

General: sore throat, rash, fever.

Neurologic: paresthesia of lips, face, hands, feet; cold sensations in hands and feet; nervousness, light-headedness, jitteriness, increased irritability; tremor, trembling sensation; ataxia; emotional lability; psychotic state; confusion; mood changes, and hallucinations.

Gastrointestinal: dry mouth; gastric irritation; anorexia; nausea; diarrhea; abdominal cramping. Gastrointestinal side effects may preclude the use of guanidine as a desired form of therapy.

Dermatologic: rash, flushing or pink complexion; folliculitis; petechiae, purpura, ecchymoses; sweating; skin eruptions; dryness and scaling of the skin.

Renal: elevation of blood creatinine, uremia; chronic interstitial nephritis, acute interstitial nephritis, and renal tubular necrosis.

Hepatic: abnormal liver function tests.

Cardiac: palpitation, tachycardia, atrial fibrillation, hypotension.

DOSAGE AND ADMINISTRATION

Initial dosage is usually between 10 and 15 mg/kg (5 to 7 mg/pound) of body weight per day in 3 or 4 divided doses. This dosage may be gradually increased to a total daily dosage of 35 mg/kg (16 mg/pound) of body weight per day or up to the development of side effects. As individual tolerance is highly variable, the dosage must be carefully titrated. Once a tolerable dose has been established, it should be continued. Occasionally removal of the primary neoplastic lesion may result in improvement of symptoms, permitting the discontinuance of guanidine.

OVERDOSAGE

Mild gastrointestinal disorders, such as anorexia, increased peristalsis, or diarrhea are early warnings that tolerance is being exceeded. These symptoms may be relieved by atropine, but nevertheless note should be taken of these symptoms and dosage reductions considered. Slight numbness or tingling of the lips and fingertips shortly after taking a dose of guanidine has been reported. This per se is not an indication to discontinue treatment and/or reduce dosage.

Severe guanidine intoxication is characterized by nervous hyperirritability, fibrillary tremors and convulsive contractions of muscle, salivation, vomiting, diarrhea, hypoglycemia, and circulatory disturbances. Administration of intravenous calcium gluconate may control the neuromuscular and convulsive symptoms and provide some relief of other toxic manifestations.

Atropine is more effective than calcium in relieving the G.I. symptoms, circulatory disturbances, and changes in blood sugar.

HOW SUPPLIED

Guanidine hydrochloride tablets: 125 mg, white, round tablet; impressed with the product identification number "KEY 74" on one side. Guanidine hydrochloride tablets are available in bottles of 100 (NDC 0085-0492-01).

Store at 25°C (77°F); excursions permitted to 15-30°C (59-86°F) [see USP Controlled Room Temperature].

Manufactured by
Schering Canada, Inc.
Pointe Claire, Quebec, Canada
for
Key Pharmaceuticals, Inc.
Kenilworth, NJ 07033 USA
Revised 5/03
27051812
81-483544

INTEGRILIN® ℞

[*ĭn-tĕg'-rĭl-in*]
(eptifibatide)
Injection

For Intravenous Administration

DESCRIPTION

Eptifibatide is a cyclic heptapeptide containing six amino acids and one mercaptopropionyl (des-amino cysteinyl) residue. An interchain disulfide bridge is formed between the cysteine amide and the mercaptopropionyl moieties. Chemically it is N^6-(aminoiminomethyl)-N^2-(3-mercapto-1-oxopropyl-L-lysylglycyl-L-α-aspartyl-L-tryptophyl-L-prolyl-L-cysteinamide, cyclic (1→6)-disulfide. Eptifibatide binds to the platelet receptor glycoprotein (GP) IIb/IIIa of human platelets and inhibits platelet aggregation.
The eptifibatide peptide is produced by solution-phase peptide synthesis, and is purified by preparative reverse-phase liquid chromatography and lyophilized. The structural formula is:

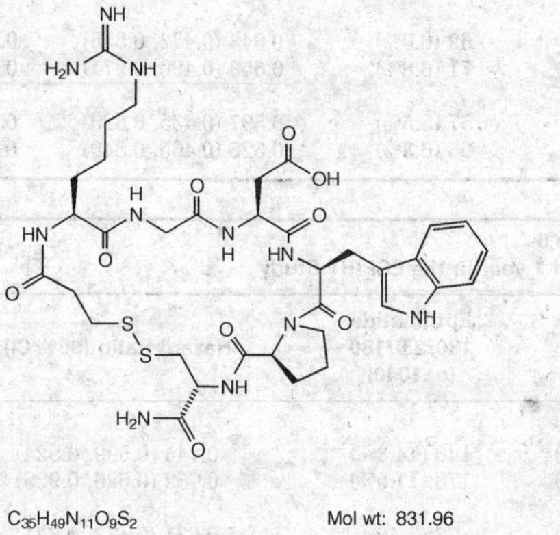

$C_{35}H_{49}N_{11}O_9S_2$ Mol wt: 831.96

INTEGRILIN (eptifibatide) Injection is a clear, colorless, sterile, non-pyrogenic solution for intravenous (IV) use. Each 10-mL vial contains 2 mg/mL of eptifibatide and each 100-mL vial contains either 0.75 mg/mL or 2 mg/mL of eptifibatide. Each vial of either size also contains 5.25 mg/mL citric acid and sodium hydroxide to adjust the pH to 5.35.

CLINICAL PHARMACOLOGY

Mechanism of Action. Eptifibatide reversibly inhibits platelet aggregation by preventing the binding of fibrinogen, von Willebrand factor, and other adhesive ligands to GP IIb/IIIa. When administered intravenously, eptifibatide inhibits *ex vivo* platelet aggregation in a dose- and concentration-dependent manner. Platelet aggregation inhibition is reversible following cessation of the eptifibatide infusion; this is thought to result from dissociation of eptifibatide from the platelet.
Pharmacodynamics. Infusion of eptifibatide into baboons caused a dose-dependent inhibition of *ex vivo* platelet aggregation, with complete inhibition of aggregation achieved at infusion rates greater than 5.0 µg/kg/min. In a baboon model that is refractory to aspirin and heparin, doses of eptifibatide that inhibit aggregation prevented acute thrombosis with only a modest prolongation (2- to 3-fold) of the bleeding time. Platelet aggregation in dogs was also inhibited by infusions of eptifibatide, with complete inhibition at 2.0 µg/kg/min. This infusion dose completely inhibited canine coronary thrombosis induced by coronary artery injury (Folts model).
Human pharmacodynamic data were obtained in healthy subjects and in patients presenting with unstable angina (UA) or non-ST-segment elevation myocardial infarction (NSTEMI) and/or undergoing percutaneous coronary interventions. Studies in healthy subjects enrolled only males; patient studies enrolled approximately one third women. In these studies, eptifibatide inhibited *ex vivo* platelet aggregation induced by adenosine diphosphate (ADP) and other agonists in a dose- and concentration-dependent manner. The effect of eptifibatide was observed immediately after administration of a 180 µg/kg intravenous bolus. Table 1 shows the effects of dosing regimens of eptifibatide used in the IMPACT II and PURSUIT studies on *ex vivo* platelet aggregation induced by 20 µM ADP in PPACK-anticoagulated platelet-rich plasma and on bleeding time. The effects of the dosing regimen used in ESPRIT on platelet aggregation have not been studied.

Table 2
Clinical Events in The PURSUIT Study

Death or MI	Placebo (n = 4739) n (%)	Eptifibatide (180/2.0) (n = 4722) n (%)	p-value
3 days	359 (7.6%)	279 (5.9%)	0.001
7 days	552 (11.6%)	477 (10.1%)	0.016
30 days			
Death or MI (Primary Endpoint)	745 (15.7%)	672 (14.2%)	0.042
Death	177 (3.7%)	165 (3.5%)	
Nonfatal MI	568 (12.0%)	507 (10.7%)	

Table 1
Platelet Inhibition and Bleeding Time

	IMPACT II 135/0.5*	PURSUIT 180/2.0**
Inhibition of platelet aggregation 15 min. after bolus	69%	84%
Inhibition of platelet aggregation at steady state	40–50%	>90%
Bleeding-time prolongation at steady state	<5×	<5×
Inhibition of platelet aggregation 4h after infusion discontinuation	<30%	<50%
Bleeding-time prolongation 6h after infusion discontinuation	1×	1.4×

*135 µg/kg bolus followed by a continuous infusion of 0.5 µg/kg/min
**180 µg/kg bolus followed by a continuous infusion of 2.0 µg/kg/min

The eptifibatide dosing regimen used in the ESPRIT study included two 180 µg/kg bolus doses given ten minutes apart combined with a continuous 2.0 µg/kg/min infusion.
When administered alone, eptifibatide has no measurable effect on prothrombin time (PT) or activated partial thromboplastin time (aPTT). (See also PRECAUTIONS: Drug Interactions).
There were no important differences between men and women or between age groups in the pharmacodynamic properties of eptifibatide. Differences among ethnic groups have not been assessed.
Pharmacokinetics. The pharmacokinetics of eptifibatide are linear and dose-proportional for bolus doses ranging from 90 to 250 µg/kg and infusion rates from 0.5 to 3.0 µg/kg/min. Plasma elimination half-life is approximately 2.5 hours. Administration of a single 180 µg/kg bolus combined with an infusion produces an early peak level, followed by a small decline prior to attaining steady state (within 4–6 hours). This decline can be prevented by administering a second 180 µg/kg bolus ten minutes after the first. The extent of eptifibatide binding to human plasma protein is about 25%. Clearance in patients with coronary artery disease is about 55–58 mL/kg/h. In healthy subjects, renal clearance accounts for approximately 50% of total body clearance, with the majority of the drug excreted in the urine as eptifibatide, deamidated eptifibatide, and other, more polar metabolites. No major metabolites have been detected in human plasma. In patients with moderate to severe renal insufficiency (creatinine clearance <50 mL/min using the Cockroft-Gault equation), the clearance of eptifibatide is reduced by approximately 50% and steady-state plasma levels approximately doubled (see WARNINGS, DOSAGE AND ADMINISTRATION).
Special Populations. Patients in clinical studies were older (range 20 to 94 years) than those in the clinical pharmacology studies. Elderly patients with coronary artery disease demonstrated higher plasma levels and lower total body clearance of eptifibatide when given the same dose as younger patients. Limited data are available on lighter weight (<50 kg) patients over 75 years of age.
No studies have been conducted in patients with hepatic impairment.
Males and females have not demonstrated any clinically significant differences in the pharmacokinetics of eptifibatide.

CLINICAL STUDIES

Eptifibatide was studied in three placebo-controlled, randomized studies. PURSUIT evaluated patients with acute coronary syndromes: unstable angina (UA) or non-ST-segment myocardial infarction (NSTEMI). Two other studies, ESPRIT and IMPACT II, evaluated patients about to undergo a percutaneous coronary intervention (PCI). Patients underwent primarily balloon angioplasty in IMPACT II and intracoronary stent placement, with or without angioplasty, in ESPRIT.
Non-ST-segment Elevation Acute Coronary Syndrome
Non-ST-segment elevation acute coronary syndrome is defined as prolonged (≥10 minutes) symptoms of cardiac ischemia within the previous 24 hours associated with either ST-segment changes (elevation between 0.6 mm and 1 mm or depression >0.5 mm), T-wave inversion (>1 mm), or positive CK-MB. This definition includes "unstable angina" and "NSTEMI" but excludes myocardial infarction that is associated with Q waves or greater degrees of ST-segment elevation.
PURSUIT (Platelet Glycoprotein IIb/IIIa in Unstable Angina: Receptor Suppression Using INTEGRILIN Therapy)
PURSUIT was a 726-center, 27-country, double-blind, randomized, placebo-controlled study in 10,948 patients presenting with UA or NSTEMI. Patients could be enrolled only if they had experienced cardiac ischemia at rest (≥10 minutes) within the previous 24 hours and had either ST-segment changes (elevations between 0.6 mm and 1 mm or depression >0.5 mm), T-wave inversion (>1 mm), or increased CK-MB. Important exclusion criteria included a history of bleeding diathesis, evidence of abnormal bleeding within the previous 30 days, uncontrolled hypertension, major surgery within the previous 6 weeks, stroke within the previous 30 days, any history of hemorrhagic stroke, serum creatinine >2.0 mg/dL, dependency on renal dialysis, or platelet count <100,000/mm^3.
Patients were randomized to either placebo, eptifibatide 180 µg/kg bolus followed by a 2.0 µg/kg/min infusion (180/2.0), or eptifibatide 180 µg/kg bolus followed by a 1.3 µg/kg/min infusion (180/1.3). The infusion was continued for 72 hours, until hospital discharge, or until the time of coronary artery bypass grafting (CABG), whichever occurred first, except that if PCI was performed, the eptifibatide infusion was continued for 24 hours after the procedure, allowing for a duration of infusion up to 96 hours.
The lower-infusion-rate arm was stopped after the first interim analysis when the two active-treatment arms appeared to have the same incidence of bleeding.
Patient age ranged from 20 to 94 (mean 63) years, and 65% were male. The patients were 89% Caucasian, 6% Hispanic, and 5% Black, recruited in the United States and Canada (40%), Western Europe (39%), Eastern Europe (16%), and Latin America (5%).
This was a "real world" study; each patient was managed according to the usual standards of the investigational site; frequencies of angiography, PCI, and CABG therefore differed widely from site to site and from country to country. Of the patients in PURSUIT, 13% were managed with PCI during drug infusion, of whom 50% received intracoronary stents; 87% were managed medically (without PCI during drug infusion).
The majority of patients received aspirin (75–325 mg once daily). Heparin was administered intravenously or subcutaneously, at the physician's discretion, most commonly as an intravenous bolus of 5000 U followed by a continuous infusion of 1000 U/h. For patients weighing less than 70 kg, the recommended heparin bolus dose was 60 U/kg followed by a continuous infusion of 12 U/kg/h. A target aPTT of 50–70 seconds was recommended. A total of 1250 patients underwent PCI within 72 hours after randomization, in which case they received intravenous heparin to maintain an activated clotting time (ACT) of 300–350 seconds.
The primary endpoint of the study was the occurrence of death from any cause or new myocardial infarction (MI) (evaluated by a blinded Clinical Endpoints Committee) within 30 days of randomization.
Compared to placebo, eptifibatide administered as a 180 µg/kg bolus followed by a 2.0 µg/kg/min infusion significantly (p=0.042) reduced the incidence of endpoint events (see Table 2). The reduction in the incidence of endpoint events in patients receiving eptifibatide was evident early during treatment, and this reduction was maintained through at least 30 days (see Figure 1). Table 2 also shows the incidence of the components of the primary endpoint, death (whether or not preceded by an MI) and new MI in surviving patients at 30 days.
[See table 2 above]
[See figure 1 at top of next column]
Treatment with eptifibatide prior to determination of patient management strategy reduced clinical events regardless of whether patients ultimately underwent diagnostic catheterization, revascularization (i.e., PCI or CABG surgery) or continued to receive medical management alone. Table 3 shows the incidence of death or MI within 72 hours.

Continued on next page

Information on Schering products appearing on these pages is effective as of June 2003.

Integrilin—Cont.

Figure 1
Kaplan-Meier Plot of Time to Death or Myocardial Infarction Within 30 Days of Randomization

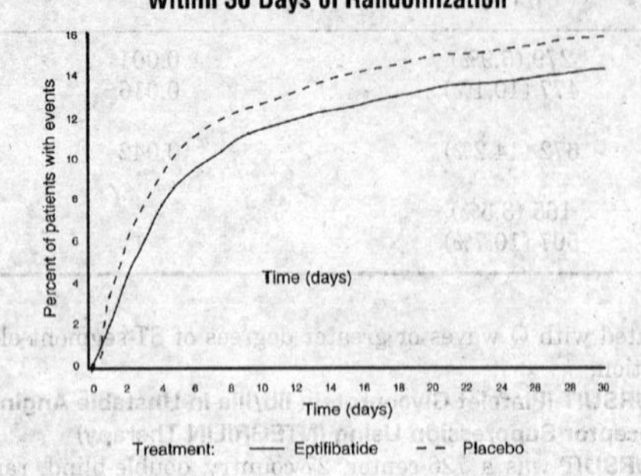

Table 3
Clinical Events (Death or MI) in the PURSUIT Study Within 72 Hours of Randomization

	Placebo	Eptifibatide 180/2.0
Overall Patient Population	n=4739	n=4722
- At 72 hours	7.6%	5.9%
Patients undergoing early PCI	n=631	n=619
- Pre-procedure (nonfatal MI only)	5.5%	1.8%
- At 72 hours	14.4%	9.0%
Patients not undergoing early PCI	n=4108	n=4103
- At 72 hours	6.5%	5.4%

All of the effect of eptifibatide was established within 72 hours (during the period of drug infusion), regardless of management strategy. Moreover, for patients undergoing early PCI, a reduction in events was evident prior to the procedure.

Follow-up data were available through 165 days for 10,611 patients enrolled in the PURSUIT trial (96.9 percent of the initial enrollment). This follow-up included 4,566 patients who received eptifibatide at the 180/2.0 dose. As reported by the investigators, the occurrence of death from any cause or new myocardial infarction for patients followed for at least 165 days was reduced from 13.6 percent with placebo to 12.1 percent with eptifibatide 180/2.0.

Percutaneous Coronary Intervention

IMPACT II (INTEGRILIN to Minimize Platelet Aggregation and Prevent Coronary Thrombosis II)

IMPACT II was a multi-center, double-blind, randomized, placebo-controlled study conducted in the United States in 4010 patients undergoing PCI. Major exclusion criteria included a history of bleeding diathesis, major surgery within 6 weeks of treatment, gastrointestinal bleeding within 30 days, any stroke or structural CNS abnormality, uncontrolled hypertension, PT >1.2 times control, hematocrit <30%, platelet count <100,000/mm^3, and pregnancy.

Patient age ranged from 24 to 89 (mean 60) years, and 75% were male. The patients were 92% Caucasian, 5% Black, and 3% Hispanic. Forty-one percent of the patients underwent PCI for ongoing ACS. Patients were randomly assigned to one of three treatment regimens, each incorporating a bolus dose initiated immediately prior to PCI followed by a continuous infusion lasting 20–24 hours: 1) 135 μg/kg bolus followed by a continuous infusion of 0.5 μg/kg/min of eptifibatide (135/0.5); 2) 135 μg/kg bolus followed by a continuous infusion of 0.75 μg/kg/min of eptifibatide (135/0.75); or 3) a matching placebo bolus followed by a matching placebo continuous infusion. Each patient received aspirin and an intravenous heparin bolus of 100 U/kg, with additional bolus infusions of up to 2000 additional units of heparin every 15 minutes to maintain an activated clotting time (ACT) of 300–350 seconds.

The primary endpoint was the composite of death, MI, or urgent revascularization, analyzed at 30 days after randomization in all patients who received at least one dose of study drug.

As shown in Table 4, each eptifibatide regimen reduced the rate of death, MI, or urgent intervention, although at 30 days, this finding was statistically significant only in the lower-dose eptifibatide group. As in the PURSUIT study, the effects of eptifibatide were seen early and persisted throughout the 30-day period.

[See table 4 above]

ESPRIT (Enhanced Suppression of the Platelet IIb/IIIa Receptor with INTEGRILIN Therapy)

The ESPRIT study was a multi-center, double-blind, randomized, placebo-controlled study conducted in the United States and Canada that enrolled 2064 patients undergoing elective or urgent PCI with intended intracoronary stent placement. Exclusion criteria included MI within the previous 24 hours, ongoing chest pain, administration of any oral anti-platelet or oral anticoagulant other than aspirin within 30 days of PCI (although loading doses of thienopyridine on the day of PCI were encouraged), planned PCI of a saphenous vein graft or subsequent "staged" PCI, prior stent placement in the target lesion, PCI within the previous 90 days, a history of bleeding diathesis, major surgery within 6 weeks of treatment, gastrointestinal bleeding within 30 days, any stroke or structural CNS abnormality, uncontrolled hypertension, PT >1.2 times control, hematocrit <30%, platelet count <100,000/mm^3, and pregnancy.

Patient age ranged from 24 to 93 (mean 62) years and 73% of patients were male. The study enrolled 90% Caucasian, 5% African American, 2% Hispanic and 1% Asian patients. Patients received a wide variety of stents. Patients were randomized either to placebo or eptifibatide administered as an intravenous bolus of 180 μg/kg followed immediately by a continuous infusion of 2.0 μg/kg/min, and a second bolus of 180 μg/kg administered 10 minutes later (180/2.0/180). Eptifibatide infusion was continued for 18–24 hours after PCI or until hospital discharge, whichever came first. Each patient received at least one dose of aspirin (162–325 mg) and 60 U/kg of heparin as a bolus (not to exceed 6000 Units) if not already receiving a heparin infusion. Additional boluses of heparin (10–40 U/kg) could be administered in order to reach a target ACT between 200 and 300 seconds.

The primary endpoint of the ESPRIT study was the composite of death, MI, urgent target vessel revascularization (UTVR) and "bailout" to open label eptifibatide due to a thrombotic complication of PCI (TBO) (e.g., visible thrombus, "no reflow", or abrupt closure) at 48 hours. MI, UTVR and TBO were evaluated by a blinded Clinical Events Committee.

As shown in Table 5, the incidence of the primary endpoint and selected secondary endpoints was significantly reduced in patients who received eptifibatide. A treatment benefit in patients who received eptifibatide was seen by 48 hours and at the end of the 30-day observation period.

[See table 5 above]

The need for thrombotic "bailout" was significantly reduced with eptifibatide at 48 hours (2.1% for placebo, 1.0% for eptifibatide; p=0.029). Consistent with previous studies of GP IIb/IIIa inhibitors, most of the benefit achieved acutely with eptifibatide was in the reduction of MI. Eptifibatide reduced the occurrence of MI at 48 hours from 9.0% for placebo to 5.4% (p=0.0015) and maintained that effect with significance at 30 days.

Follow-up (12 month) mortality data were available for 2024 patients (1017 on eptifibatide) enrolled in the ESPRIT trial (98.1% of the initial enrollment). Twelve-month clinical event data were available for 1964 patients (988 on eptifibatide) representing 95.2% of the initial enrollment. As shown in Table 6, the treatment effect of eptifibatide seen at 48 hours and 30 days appeared preserved at 6 months and 1 year. Most of the benefit was in reduction of MI.

[See table 6 above]

Table 4
Clinical Events in the IMPACT II Study

	Placebo n (%)	Eptifibatide (135/0.5) n (%)	Eptifibatide (135/0.75) n (%)
Patients	1285	1300	1286
Abrupt Closure	65 (5.1%)	36 (2.8%)	43 (3.3%)
p-value vs. placebo		0.003	0.030
Death, MI, or Urgent Intervention			
24 hours	123 (9.6%)	86 (6.6%)	89 (6.9%)
p-value vs. placebo		0.006	0.014
48 hours	131 (10.2%)	99 (7.6%)	102 (7.9%)
p-value vs. placebo		0.021	0.045
30 days (primary endpoint)	149 (11.6%)	118 (9.1%)	128 (10.0%)
p-value vs. placebo		0.035	0.179
Death or MI			
30 days	110 (8.6%)	89 (6.8%)	95 (7.4%)
p-value vs. placebo		0.102	0.272
6 months	151 (11.9%)*	136 (10.6%)*	130 (10.3%)*
p-value vs. placebo		0.297	0.182

*Kaplan-Meier estimate of event rate.

Table 5
Clinical Events in the ESPRIT Study

	Placebo (n=1024)	Eptifibatide 180/2.0/180 (n=1040)	Relative Risk (95% CI)	p-Value
Death, MI, Urgent Target Vessel Revascularization, or Thrombotic "Bailout"				
48 Hours (primary endpoint)	108 (10.5%)	69 (6.6%)	0.629 (0.471, 0.840)	0.0015
30 Days	120 (11.7%)	78 (7.5%)	0.640 (0.488, 0.840)	0.0011
Death, MI, Urgent Target Vessel Revascularization				
48 Hours	95 (9.3%)	62 (6.0%)	0.643 (0.472, 0.875)	0.0045
30 Days (key secondary endpoint)	107 (10.4%)	71 (6.8%)	0.653 (0.490, 0.871)	0.0034
Death or MI				
48 Hours	94 (9.2%)	57 (5.5%)	0.597 (0.435, 0.820)	0.0013
30 Days	104 (10.2%)	66 (6.3%)	0.625 (0.465, 0.840)	0.0016

Table 6
Clinical Events at 6 months and 1 year in the ESPRIT Study

	Placebo (n=1024)	Eptifibatide 180/2.0/180 (n=1040)	Hazard Ratio (95% CI)
Death, MI, or Target Vessel Revascularization			
6 Months	187 (18.5%)	146 (14.3%)	0.744 (0.599, 0.924)
1 Year	222 (22.1%)	178 (17.5%)	0.762 (0.626, 0.929)
Death, MI			
6 Months	117 (11.5%)	77 (7.4%)	0.631 (0.473, 0.841)
1 Year	126 (12.4%)	83 (8.0%)	0.630 (0.478, 0.832)

Percentages are Kaplan-Meier event rates.

INDICATIONS AND USAGE

INTEGRILIN is indicated:

- For the treatment of patients with acute coronary syndrome (unstable angina/non-ST-segment elevation myocardial infarction) including patients who are to be managed medically and those undergoing percutaneous coronary intervention (PCI). In this setting, INTEGRILIN has been shown to decrease the rate of a combined endpoint of death or new myocardial infarction.
- For the treatment of patients undergoing PCI, including those undergoing intracoronary stenting. In this setting, INTEGRILIN has been shown to decrease the rate of a combined endpoint of death, new myocardial infarction, or need for urgent intervention.

In the IMPACT II, PURSUIT and ESPRIT studies of eptifibatide, most patients received heparin and aspirin, as described in CLINICAL TRIALS.

CONTRAINDICATIONS

Treatment with eptifibatide is contraindicated in patients with:

- A history of bleeding diathesis, or evidence of active abnormal bleeding within the previous 30 days.
- Severe hypertension (systolic blood pressure >200 mm Hg or diastolic blood pressure >110 mm Hg) not adequately controlled on antihypertensive therapy.
- Major surgery within the preceding 6 weeks.

- History of stroke within 30 days or any history of hemorrhagic stroke.
- Current or planned administration of another parenteral GP IIb/IIIa inhibitor.
- Dependency on renal dialysis.
- Known hypersensitivity to any component of the product.

WARNINGS

Bleeding. Bleeding is the most common complication encountered during eptifibatide therapy. Administration of eptifibatide is associated with an increase in major and minor bleeding, as classified by the criteria of the Thrombolysis in Myocardial Infarction Study group (TIMI), (see ADVERSE REACTIONS). Most major bleeding associated with eptifibatide has been at the arterial access site for cardiac catheterization or from the gastrointestinal or genitourinary tract.

In patients undergoing percutaneous coronary interventions, patients receiving eptifibatide experience an increased incidence of major bleeding compared to those receiving placebo without a significant increase in transfusion requirement. Special care should be employed to minimize the risk of bleeding among these patients (see PRECAUTIONS). If bleeding cannot be controlled with pressure, infusion of eptifibatide and concomitant heparin should be stopped immediately.

Renal Insufficiency. Approximately 50% of eptifibatide is cleared by the kidney in patients with normal renal function. Total drug clearance is decreased by approximately 50% and steady-state plasma eptifibatide concentrations are doubled in patients with an estimated creatinine clearance <50 mL/min (using the Cockroft-Gault equation). Therefore, the infusion dose should be reduced to 1 µg/kg-min in such patients. If an estimated creatinine clearance is not available, the infusion dose should be reduced in patients with a serum creatinine >2 mg/dL (see DOSAGE AND ADMINISTRATION section). There has been no clinical experience in patients dependent on dialysis.

Platelet Count <100,000/mm^3. Because it is an inhibitor of platelet aggregation, caution should be exercised when administering eptifibatide to patients with a platelet count <100,000/mm^3; there has been no clinical experience with eptifibatide initiated in patients with a platelet count <100,000/mm^3.

PRECAUTIONS

Bleeding Precautions

Care of the Femoral Artery Access Site in Patients Undergoing Percutaneous Coronary Intervention (PCI). In patients undergoing PCI, treatment with eptifibatide is associated with an increase in major and minor bleeding at the site of arterial sheath placement. After PCI, eptifibatide infusion should be continued until hospital discharge or up to 18–24 hours, whichever comes first. Heparin use is discouraged after the PCI procedure. Early sheath removal is encouraged while eptifibatide is being infused. Prior to removing the sheath, it is recommended that heparin be discontinued for 3–4 hours and an aPTT of <45 seconds or ACT <150 seconds be achieved. In any case, both heparin and eptifibatide should be discontinued and sheath hemostasis should be achieved at least 2–4 hours before hospital discharge.

Use of Thrombolytics, Anticoagulants, and Other Antiplatelet Agents. In the IMPACT II, PURSUIT and ESPRIT studies, eptifibatide was used concomitantly with unfractionated heparin and aspirin (see CLINICAL STUDIES). In the ESPRIT study, clopidogrel or ticlopidine were used routinely starting the day of PCI. Because eptifibatide inhibits platelet aggregation, caution should be employed when it is used with other drugs that affect hemostasis, including **thrombolytics, oral anticoagulants, non-steroidal anti-inflammatory drugs,** and **dipyridamole**. To avoid potentially additive pharmacologic effects, concomitant treatment with **other inhibitors of platelet receptor GP IIb/IIIa** should be avoided.

There is only a small experience with concomitant use of eptifibatide and **thrombolytics**. In a study of 180 patients with acute myocardial infarction (AMI), eptifibatide (in regimens up to a bolus of 180 µg/kg followed by a continuous infusion of 0.75 µg/kg/min for 24 hours) was administered concomitantly with the approved "accelerated" regimen of alteplase, a thrombolytic agent. The studied regimens of eptifibatide did not increase the incidence of major bleeding or transfusion compared to the incidence seen when alteplase was given alone.

In the IMPACT II study, 15 patients received a thrombolytic agent in conjunction with the 135/0.5 dosing regimen, 2 of whom experienced a major bleed. In the PURSUIT study, 40 patients who received eptifibatide at the 180/2.0 dosing regimen received a thrombolytic agent, 10 of whom experienced a major bleed.

In another AMI study involving 181 patients, eptifibatide (in regimens up to a bolus of 180 µg/kg followed by a continuous infusion of up to 2.0 µg/kg/min for up to 72 hours) was administered concomitantly with streptokinase (1.5 million units over 60 minutes), another thrombolytic agent. At the highest studied infusion rates (1.3 µg/kg/min and 2.0 µg/kg/min), eptifibatide was associated with an increase in the incidence of bleeding and transfusions compared to the incidence seen when streptokinase was given alone.

These limited data on the use of eptifibatide in patients receiving thrombolytic agents do not allow an estimate of the bleeding risk associated with concomitant use of thrombolytics. Systemic thrombolytic therapy should be used with caution in patients who have received eptifibatide.

Table 7
Major Bleeding by Maximal aPTT Within 72 Hours in the PURSUIT Study

	Placebo n (%)	Eptifibatide 180/1.3* n (%)	Eptifibatide 180/2.0 n (%)
Maximum aPTT (seconds)			
<50	44/721(6.1%)	21/244(8.6%)	44/743(5.9%)
50–70 (recommended)	92/908(10.1%)	28/259(10.8%)	99/883(11.2%)
>70	281/2786(10.1%)	99/891(11.1%)	345/2811(12.3%)

*Administered only until the first interim analysis

Table 8
Bleeding Events and Transfusions in the PURSUIT, ESPRIT and IMPACT II Studies

PURSUIT	Placebo n (%)	Eptifibatide 180/1.3* n (%)	Eptifibatide 180/2.0 n (%)
Patients	4696	1472	4679
Major bleeding[a]	425 (9.3%)	152 (10.5%)	498 (10.8%)
Minor bleeding[a]	347 (7.6%)	152 (10.5%)	604 (13.1%)
Requiring Transfusions[b]	490 (10.4%)	188 (12.8%)	601 (12.8%)
ESPRIT	**Placebo n (%)**	**Eptifibatide 180/2.0/180 n (%)**	
Patients	1024	1040	
Major bleeding[a]	4 (0.4%)	13 (1.3%)	
Minor bleeding[a]	18 (2.0%)	29 (3.0%)	
Requiring Transfusions[b]	11 (1.1%)	16 (1.5%)	
IMPACT II	**Placebo n (%)**	**Eptifibatide 135/0.5 n (%)**	**Eptifibatide 135/0.75 n (%)**
Patients	1285	1300	1286
Major bleeding[a]	55 (4.5%)	55 (4.4%)	58 (4.7%)
Minor bleeding[a]	115 (9.3%)	146 (11.7%)	177 (14.2%)
Requiring Transfusions[b]	66 (5.1%)	71 (5.5%)	74 (5.8%)

Note: denominator is based on patients for whom data are available
* Administered only until the first interim analysis
[a] For major and minor bleeding, patients are counted only once according to the most severe classification.
[b] Includes transfusions of whole blood, packed red blood cells, fresh frozen plasma, cryoprecipitate, platelets, and autotransfusion during the initial hospitalization.

Minimization of Vascular and Other Trauma. Arterial and venous punctures, intramuscular injections, and the use of urinary catheters, nasotracheal intubation, and nasogastric tubes should be minimized. When obtaining intravenous access, non-compressible sites (e.g., subclavian or jugular veins) should be avoided.

Laboratory Tests. Before infusion of eptifibatide, the following laboratory tests should be performed to identify preexisting hemostatic abnormalities: hematocrit or hemoglobin, platelet count, serum creatinine, and PT/aPTT. In patients undergoing PCI, the activated clotting time (ACT) should also be measured.

Maintaining Target aPTT and ACT. The aPTT should be maintained between 50 and 70 seconds unless PCI is to be performed. In patients treated with heparin, bleeding can be minimized by close monitoring of the aPTT. Table 7 displays the risk of major bleeding according to the maximum aPTT attained within 72 hours in the PURSUIT study.

[See table 7 above]

The ESPRIT study stipulated a target ACT of 200 to 300 seconds during PCI. Patients receiving eptifibatide 180/2.0/180 (mean ACT 284 seconds) experienced an increased incidence of bleeding relative to placebo (mean ACT 276 seconds), primarily at the femoral artery access site. At these lower ACTs, bleeding was less than previously reported with eptifibatide in the PURSUIT and IMPACT II studies.

The aPTT or ACT should be checked prior to arterial sheath removal. The sheath should not be removed unless the aPTT is <45 seconds or the ACT is <150 seconds.

Thrombocytopenia. If the patient experiences a confirmed platelet decrease to <100,000/mm^3, INTEGRILIN and heparin should be discontinued and the condition appropriately monitored and treated.

Drug Interactions. Enoxaparin dosed as a 1.0 mg/kg subcutaneous injection q12h for four doses did not alter the pharmacokinetics of eptifibatide or the level of platelet aggregation in healthy adults.

Geriatric Use. The PURSUIT and IMPACT II clinical studies enrolled patients up to the age of 94 years (45% were age 65 and over; 12% were age 75 and older). There was no apparent difference in efficacy between older and younger patients treated with eptifibatide. The incidence of bleeding complications was higher in the elderly in both placebo and eptifibatide groups, and the incremental risk of eptifibatide-associated bleeding was greater in the older patients. No dose adjustment was made for elderly patients, but patients over 75 years of age had to weigh at least 50 kg to be enrolled in the PURSUIT study; no such limitation was stipulated in the ESPRIT study (see also ADVERSE REACTIONS).

Carcinogenesis, Mutagenesis, Impairment of Fertility. No long-term studies in animals have been performed to evaluate the carcinogenic potential of eptifibatide. Eptifibatide was not genotoxic in the Ames test, the mouse lymphoma cell (L 5178Y, TK$^{+/-}$) forward mutation test, the human lymphocyte chromosome aberration test, or the mouse micronucleus test. Administered by continuous intravenous infusion at total daily doses up to 72 mg/kg/day (about 4 times the recommended maximum daily human dose on a body surface area basis), eptifibatide had no effect on fertility and reproductive performance of male and female rats.

Pregnancy. Pregnancy Category B. Teratology studies have been performed by continuous intravenous infusion of eptifibatide in pregnant rats at total daily doses of up to 72 mg/kg/day (about 4 times the recommended maximum daily human dose on a body surface area basis) and in pregnant rabbits at total daily doses of up to 36 mg/kg/day (also about 4 times the recommended maximum daily human dose on a body surface area basis). These studies revealed no evidence of harm to the fetus due to eptifibatide. There are, however, no adequate and well-controlled studies in pregnant women with eptifibatide. Because animal reproduction studies are not always predictive of human response, eptifibatide should be used during pregnancy only if clearly needed.

Pediatric Use. Safety and effectiveness of eptifibatide in pediatric patients have not been studied.

Nursing Mothers. It is not known whether eptifibatide is excreted in human milk. Because many drugs are excreted in human milk, caution should be exercised when eptifibatide is administered to a nursing mother.

ADVERSE REACTIONS

A total of 16,782 patients were treated in the Phase III clinical trials (PURSUIT, ESPRIT and IMPACT II). These 16,782 patients had a mean age of 62 years (range 20 to 94 years). Eighty-nine percent of the patients were Caucasian, with the remainder being predominantly Black (5%) and Hispanic (5%). Sixty-eight percent were men. Because of the different regimens used in PURSUIT, IMPACT II and ESPRIT, data from the three studies were not pooled.

Continued on next page

Information on Schering products appearing on these pages is effective as of June 2003.

Integrilin—Cont.

Bleeding. The incidences of bleeding events and transfusions in the PURSUIT, IMPACT II and ESPRIT studies are shown in Table 8. Bleeding was classified as major or minor by the criteria of the TIMI study group. Major bleeding events consisted of intracranial hemorrhage and other bleeding that led to decreases in hemoglobin greater than 5 g/dL. Minor bleeding events included spontaneous gross hematuria, spontaneous hematemesis, other observed blood loss with a hemoglobin decrease of more than 3 g/dL, and other hemoglobin decreases that were greater than 4 g/dL but less than 5 g/dL. In patients who received transfusions, the corresponding loss in hemoglobin was estimated through an adaptation period of the method of Landefeld *et al.*

[See table 8 at top of previous page]

The majority of major bleeding events in the ESPRIT study occurred at the vascular access site (1 and 8 patients, or 0.1% and 0.8% in the placebo and eptifibatide groups, respectively). Bleeding at "other" locations occurred in 0.2% and 0.4% of patients, respectively.

In the PURSUIT study, the greatest increase in major bleeding in eptifibatide-treated patients compared to placebo was also associated with bleeding at the femoral artery access site (2.8% versus 1.3%). Oropharyngeal (primarily gingival), genito-urinary, gastrointestinal, and retroperitoneal bleeding were also seen more commonly in eptifibatide-treated patients compared to placebo-treated patients. Among patients experiencing a major bleed in the IMPACT II study, an increase in bleeding on eptifibatide versus placebo was observed only for the femoral artery access site (3.2% versus 2.8%).

Table 9 displays the incidence of TIMI major bleeding according to the cardiac procedures carried out in the PURSUIT study. The most common bleeding complications were related to cardiac revascularization (CABG-related or femoral artery access site bleeding). A corresponding table for ESPRIT is not presented as every patient underwent PCI in the ESPRIT study and only 11 patients underwent CABG.

[See table 9 above]

In the PURSUIT and ESPRIT studies, the risk of major bleeding with eptifibatide increased as patient weight decreased. This relationship was most apparent for patients weighing less than 70 kg.

Bleeding adverse events resulting in discontinuation of study drug were more frequent among patients receiving eptifibatide than placebo (4.6% versus 0.9% in ESPRIT, 8% versus 1% in PURSUIT, 3.5% versus 1.9% in IMPACT II).

Intracranial Hemorrhage and Stroke. Intracranial hemorrhage was rare in the PURSUIT, IMPACT II and ESPRIT clinical studies. In the PURSUIT study, 3 patients in the placebo group, 1 patient in the group treated with eptifibatide 180/1.3 and 5 patients in the group treated with eptifibatide 180/2.0 experienced a hemorrhagic stroke. The overall incidence of stroke was 0.5% in patients receiving eptifibatide 180/1.3, 0.7% in patients receiving eptifibatide 180/2.0, and 0.8% in placebo patients.

In the IMPACT II study, intracranial hemorrhage was experienced by 1 patient treated with eptifibatide 135/0.5, 2 patients treated with eptifibatide 135/0.75 and 2 patients in the placebo group. The overall incidence of stroke was 0.5% in patients receiving eptifibatide 135/0.5, 0.7% in patients receiving eptifibatide 135/0.75 and 0.7% in the placebo group.

In the ESPRIT study, there were 3 hemorrhagic strokes, 1 in the placebo group and 2 in the eptifibatide group. In addition there was 1 case of cerebral infarction in the eptifibatide group.

Thrombocytopenia. In the PURSUIT and IMPACT II studies, the incidence of thrombocytopenia (<100,000/mm^3 or ≥50% reduction from baseline) and the incidence of platelet transfusions were similar between patients treated with eptifibatide and placebo. In the ESPRIT study, the incidence was 0.6% in the placebo group and 1.2% in the eptifibatide group.

Allergic Reactions. In the PURSUIT study, anaphylaxis was reported in 7 patients receiving placebo (0.15%) and 7 patients receiving eptifibatide 180/2.0 (0.16%). In the IMPACT II study, anaphylaxis was reported in 1 patient (0.08%) on placebo and in no patients on eptifibatide. In the IMPACT II study, 2 patients (1 patient (0.04%) receiving eptifibatide and 1 patient (0.08%) receiving placebo) discontinued study drug because of allergic reactions. In the ESPRIT study, there were no cases of anaphylaxis reported. There were 3 patients who suffered an allergic reaction, 1 on placebo and 2 on eptifibatide. In addition, 1 patient in the placebo group was diagnosed with urticaria.

The potential for development of antibodies to eptifibatide has been studied in 433 subjects. Eptifibatide was non-antigenic in 412 patients receiving a single administration of eptifibatide (135 μg/kg bolus followed by a continuous infusion of either 0.5 μg/kg/min or 0.75 μg/kg/min), and in 21 subjects to whom eptifibatide (135 μg/kg bolus followed by a continuous infusion of 0.75 μg/kg/min) was administered twice, 28 days apart. In both cases, plasma for antibody detection was collected approximately 30 days after each dose. The development of antibodies to eptifibatide at higher doses has not been evaluated.

Other Adverse Reactions. In the PURSUIT and ESPRIT studies, the incidence of serious non-bleeding adverse events was similar in patients receiving placebo or eptifibatide (19% and 19%, respectively in PURSUIT; 6% and 7%, respectively in ESPRIT). In PURSUIT, the only serious non-bleeding adverse event that occurred at a rate of at least 1% and was more common with eptifibatide than placebo (7% versus 6%) was hypotension. Most of the serious non-bleeding events consisted of cardiovascular events typical of an unstable angina population. In the IMPACT II study, serious non-bleeding events that occurred in greater than 1% of patients were uncommon and similar in incidence between placebo- and eptifibatide-treated patients.

Discontinuation of study drug due to adverse events other than bleeding was uncommon in the PURSUIT, IMPACT II and ESPRIT studies, with no single event occurring in >0.5% of the study population (except for "other" in the ESPRIT study). In the PURSUIT study, non-bleeding adverse events leading to discontinuation occurred in the eptifibatide and placebo groups in the following body systems with an incidence of ≥0.1%: cardiovascular system (0.3% and 0.3%), digestive system (0.1% and 0.1%), hemic/lymphatic system (0.1% and 0.1%), nervous system (0.3% and 0.4%), urogenital system (0.1% and 0.1%), and whole body system (0.2% and 0.2%). In the ESPRIT study, the following non-bleeding adverse events leading to discontinuation occurred in the eptifibatide and placebo groups with an incidence of ≥0.1%: "other" (1.2% and 1.1%). In the IMPACT II study, non-bleeding adverse events leading to discontinuation occurred in the 135/0.5 eptifibatide and placebo groups in the following body systems with an incidence of ≥0.1%: whole body (0.3% and 0.1%), cardiovascular system (1.4% and 1.4%), digestive system (0.2% and 0%), hemic/lymphatic system (0.2% and 0%), nervous system (0.3% and 0.2%), and respiratory system (0.1% and 0.1%).

Post-Marketing Experience. The following adverse events have been reported in post-marketing experience, primarily with eptifibatide in combination with heparin and aspirin: cerebral, GI and pulmonary hemorrhage. Fatal bleeding events have been reported.

Table 9
Major Bleeding by Procedures in the PURSUIT Study

	Placebo n (%)	Eptifibatide 180/1.3* n (%)	Eptifibatide 180/2.0 n (%)
Patients	4577	1451	4604
Overall Incidence of Major Bleeding	425 (9.3%)	152 (10.5%)	498 (10.8%)
Breakdown by Procedure:			
CABG	375 (8.2%)	123 (8.5%)	377 (8.2%)
Angioplasty without CABG	27 (0.6%)	16 (1.1%)	64 (1.4%)
Angiography without angioplasty or CABG	11 (0.2%)	7 (0.5%)	29 (0.6%)
Medical Therapy Only	12 (0.3%)	6 (0.4%)	28 (0.6%)

Denominators are based on the total number of patients whose TIMI classification was resolved.
*Administered only until the first interim analysis

INTEGRILIN Dosing Charts by Weight

Patient Weight (kg)	Patient Weight (lb)	180 μg/kg Bolus Volume (from 2 mg/mL vial)	2.0 μg/kg/min Infusion Volume (from 2 mg/mL 100-mL vial)	2.0 μg/kg/min Infusion Volume (from 0.75 mg/mL 100-mL vial)	1.0 μg/kg/min Infusion Volume (from 2 mg/mL 100-mL vial)	1.0 μg/kg/min Infusion Volume (from 0.75 mg/mL 100-mL vial)
37–41	81–91	3.4 mL	2.0 mL/h	6.0 mL/h	1.0 mL/h	3.0 mL/h
42–46	92–102	4.0 mL	2.5 mL/h	7.0 mL/h	1.3 mL/h	3.5 mL/h
47–53	103–117	4.5 mL	3.0 mL/h	8.0 mL/h	1.5 mL/h	4.0 mL/h
54–59	118–130	5.0 mL	3.5 mL/h	9.0 mL/h	1.8 mL/h	4.5 mL/h
60–65	131–143	5.6 mL	3.8 mL/h	10.0 mL/h	1.9 mL/h	5.0 mL/h
66–71	144–157	6.2 mL	4.0 mL/h	11.0 mL/h	2.0 mL/h	5.5 mL/h
72–78	158–172	6.8 mL	4.5 mL/h	12.0 mL/h	2.3 mL/h	6.0 mL/h
79–84	173–185	7.3 mL	5.0 mL/h	13.0 mL/h	2.5 mL/h	6.5 mL/h
85–90	186–198	7.9 mL	5.3 mL/h	14.0 mL/h	2.7 mL/h	7.0 mL/h
91–96	199–212	8.5 mL	5.6 mL/h	15.0 mL/h	2.8 mL/h	7.5 mL/h
97–103	213–227	9.0 mL	6.0 mL/h	16.0 mL/h	3.0 mL/h	8.0 mL/h
104–109	228–240	9.5 mL	6.4 mL/h	17.0 mL/h	3.2 mL/h	8.5 mL/h
110–115	241–253	10.2 mL	6.8 mL/h	18.0 mL/h	3.4 mL/h	9.0 mL/h
116–121	254–267	10.7 mL	7.0 mL/h	19.0 mL/h	3.5 mL/h	9.5 mL/h
>121	>267	11.3 mL	7.5 mL/h	20.0 mL/h	3.7 mL/h	10.0 mL/h

OVERDOSAGE

There has been only limited experience with overdosage of eptifibatide. There were 8 patients in the IMPACT II study, 9 patients in the PURSUIT study and no patient in the ESPRIT study who received bolus doses and/or infusion doses more than double those called for in the protocols. None of these patients experienced an intracranial bleed or other major bleeding.

Eptifibatide was not lethal to rats, rabbits, or monkeys when administered by continuous intravenous infusion for 90 minutes at a total dose of 45 mg/kg (about 2 to 5 times the recommended maximum daily human dose on a body surface area basis). Symptoms of acute toxicity were loss of righting reflex, dyspnea, ptosis, and decreased muscle tone in rabbits and petechial hemorrhages in the femoral and abdominal areas of monkeys.

From *in vitro* studies, eptifibatide is not extensively bound to plasma proteins and thus may be cleared from plasma by dialysis.

DOSAGE AND ADMINISTRATION

The safety and efficacy of eptifibatide has been established in clinical studies that employed concomitant use of heparin and aspirin. Different dose regimens of eptifibatide were used in the major clinical studies. (See CLINICAL STUDIES.)

Acute Coronary Syndrome

The recommended adult dosage of eptifibatide in patients with acute coronary syndrome and normal renal function is an intravenous bolus of 180 μg/kg as soon as possible following diagnosis, followed by a continuous infusion of 2.0 μg/kg/min until hospital discharge or initiation of CABG surgery, up to 72 hours. If a patient is to undergo a percutaneous coronary intervention (PCI) while receiving eptifibatide, the infusion should be continued up to hospital discharge, or for up to 18–24 hours after the procedure, whichever comes first, allowing for up to 96 hours of therapy.

The recommended adult dosage of eptifibatide in patients with acute coronary syndrome with an estimated creatinine clearance (using the Cockroft-Gault equation)* < 50 mL/min or, if creatinine clearance is not available, a serum creatinine > 2.0 mg/dL, is an intravenous bolus of 180 μg/kg as soon as possible following diagnosis, immediately followed by a continuous infusion of 1.0 μg/kg-min.

Percutaneous Coronary Intervention (PCI)

The recommended adult dosage of eptifibatide in patients with normal renal function is an intravenous bolus of 180 μg/kg administered immediately before the initiation of PCI followed by a continuous infusion of 2.0 μg/kg/min and a second 180 μg/kg bolus 10 minutes after the first bolus. Infusion should be continued until hospital discharge, or for up to 18 to 24 hours, whichever comes first. A minimum of 12 hours of infusion is recommended.

The recommended adult dose of eptifibatide in patients with an estimated clearance (using the Cockroft-Gault equation)* <50 mL/min or, if creatinine clearance is not available, a serum creatinine >2.0 mg/dL, is an intravenous bolus of 180 μg/kg administered immediately before the initiation of the procedure, immediately followed by a continuous infusion of 1.0 μg/kg-min and a second 180 μg/kg bolus administered 10 minutes after the first.

In patients who undergo coronary artery bypass graft surgery, eptifibatide infusion should be discontinued prior to surgery.

*Using the Cockroft-Gault equation, creatinine clearance is calculated as:

Males: $\frac{(140-\text{age})\ (\text{body wt in kg})}{72\ (\text{serum creatinine})}$

Females: $\frac{(140-\text{age})\ (\text{body wt in kg})\ (0.85)}{72\ (\text{serum creatinine})}$

Aspirin and Heparin Dosing Recommendations

In the clinical trials that showed eptifibatide to be effective, most patients received concomitant aspirin and heparin. The recommended aspirin and heparin doses to be used are as follows:

Acute Coronary Syndrome
Aspirin:
160–325 mg po initially and daily thereafter
Heparin:
Target aPTT 50–70 seconds during medical management
- If weight ≥70 kg, 5000 U bolus followed by infusion of 1000 U/hr.
- If weight <70 kg, 60 U/kg bolus followed by infusion of 12 U/kg/hr.

Target ACT 200–300 seconds during PCI
- If heparin is initiated prior to PCI, additional boluses during PCI to maintain an ACT target of 200–300 seconds.
- Heparin infusion after the PCI is discouraged.

PCI
Aspirin:
160–325 mg po 1–24 hours prior to PCI and daily thereafter
Heparin:
Target ACT 200–300 seconds
- 60 U/kg bolus initially in patients not treated with heparin within 6 hours prior to PCI.
- Additional boluses during PCI to maintain ACT within target.
- Heparin infusion after the PCI is strongly discouraged.

Patients requiring thrombolytic therapy should have eptifibatide infusions stopped.
Instructions for Administration
1. Like other parenteral drug products, INTEGRILIN solutions should be inspected visually for particulate matter and discoloration prior to administration, whenever solution and container permit.
2. INTEGRILIN may be administered in the same intravenous line as alteplase, atropine, dobutamine, heparin, lidocaine, meperidine, metoprolol, midazolam, morphine, nitroglycerin, or verapamil. INTEGRILIN should not be administered through the same intravenous line as furosemide.
3. INTEGRILIN may be administered in the same IV line with 0.9% NaCl or 0.9% NaCl/5% dextrose. With either vehicle, the infusion may also contain up to 60 mEq/L of potassium chloride. No incompatibilities have been observed with intravenous administration sets. No compatibility studies have been performed with PVC bags.
4. The bolus dose(s) of INTEGRILIN should be withdrawn from the 10-mL vial into a syringe. The bolus dose(s) should be administered by IV push.
5. Immediately following the bolus dose administration, a continuous infusion of INTEGRILIN should be initiated. When using an intravenous infusion pump, INTEGRILIN should be administered undiluted directly from the 100-mL vial. The 100-mL vial should be spiked with a vented infusion set. Care should be taken to center the spike within the circle on the stopper top.

INTEGRILIN is to be administered by volume according to patient weight. Patients should receive INTEGRILIN according to the following table:
[See second table at top of previous page]

HOW SUPPLIED
INTEGRILIN (eptifibatide) Injection is supplied as a sterile solution in 10-mL vials containing 20 mg of eptifibatide (NDC 0085-1177-01) and 100-mL vials containing either 75 mg of eptifibatide (NDC 0085-1136-01) or 200 mg of eptifibatide (NDC 0085-1177-02).
Vials should be stored refrigerated at 2–8°C (36–46°F). Vials may be transferred to room temperature storage* for a period not to exceed 2 months. Upon transfer, vial cartons must be marked by the dispensing pharmacist with a "DISCARD BY" date (2 months from the transfer date or the labeled expiration date, whichever comes first).
Do not use beyond the labeled expiration date. Protect from light until administration. Discard any unused portion left in the vial.

* USP controlled Room Temperature: 25°C (77°F) with excursions permitted between 15–30°C (59–86°F).
Rx only
INTEGRILIN is a registered trademark of Millennium Pharmaceuticals, Inc.
Marketed By:
Millennium Pharmaceuticals, Inc.
Cambridge, MA 02139
and
Schering Corporation
Kenilworth, NJ 07033
Distributed By:
Schering Corporation
Kenilworth, NJ 07033

Issued June 2003
Rev 9

INTRON® A ℞
[*ĭn'tr-ŏn*]
Interferon alfa-2b, recombinant
For Injection

WARNING
Alpha interferons, including INTRON® A, cause or aggravate fatal or life-threatening neuropsychiatric, autoimmune, ischemic, and infectious disorders. Patients should be monitored closely with periodic clinical and laboratory evaluations. Patients with persistently severe or worsening signs or symptoms of these conditions should be withdrawn from therapy. In many but not all cases these disorders resolve after stopping INTRON A therapy. See **WARNINGS** and **ADVERSE REACTIONS**.

Powder for Injection

Vial Strength	mL Diluent	Final Concentration after Reconstitution million IU/mL*	mg INTRON A† Interferon alfa-2b, recombinant	Route of Administration
5 MIU	1	5	0.019	IM, SC, IV
10 MIU	2	5	0.038	IM, SC, IV, IL++
18 MIU	1	18	0.069	IM, SC, IV
25 MIU	5	5	0.096	IM, SC, IV
50 MIU	1	50	0.192	IM, SC, IV

*Each mL also contains 20 mg glycine, 2.3 mg sodium phosphate dibasic, 0.55 mg sodium phosphate monobasic, and 1.0 mg human albumin.
†Based on the specific activity of approximately 2.6×10^8 IU/mg protein, as measured by HPLC assay.
++The 10 MIU vial for intralesional use should be reconstituted with 1 mL of the provided diluent.

Solution Vials for Injection

Vial Strength	Final Concentration*	mg INTRON A† Interferon alfa-2b, recombinant	Route of Administration
3 MIU	3 million IU/0.5 mL	0.012	IM, SC
5 MIU	5 million IU/0.5 mL	0.019	IM, SC, IL
10 MIU	10 million IU/1.0 mL	0.038	IM, SC, IL
18‡ MIU multidose	3 million IU/0.5 mL	0.088	IM, SC
25¶ MIU multidose	5 million IU/0.5 mL	0.123	IM, SC, IL

*Each mL contains 7.5 mg sodium chloride, 1.8 mg sodium phosphate dibasic, 1.3 mg sodium phosphate monobasic, 0.1 mg edetate disodium, 0.1 mg polysorbate 80, and 1.5 mg m-cresol as a preservative.
† Based on the specific activity of approximately 2.6×10^8 IU/mg protein as measured by HPLC assay.
‡ This is a multidose vial which contains a total of 22.8 million IU of interferon alfa-2b, recombinant per 3.8 mL in order to provide the delivery of six 0.5-mL doses, each containing 3 million IU of INTRON A Interferon alfa-2b, recombinant for Injection (for a label strength of 18 million IU).
¶ This is a multidose vial which contains a total of 32.0 million IU of interferon alfa-2b, recombinant per 3.2 mL in order to provide the delivery of five 0.5-mL doses, each containing 5 million IU of INTRON A Interferon alfa-2b, recombinant for Injection (for a label strength of 25 million IU).

Solution in Multidose Pens for Injection

Pen Strength	Final Concentration*	INTRON A Dose Delivered (6 doses, 0.2 mL each)	mg INTRON A†	Route of Administration
18 MIU	22.5 MIU/1.5 mL	3 MIU/dose	0.087	SC
30 MIU	37.5 MIU/1.5 mL	5 MIU/dose	0.144	SC
60 MIU	75 MIU/1.5 mL	10 MIU/dose	0.288	SC

*Each mL also contains 7.5 mg sodium chloride, 1.8 mg sodium phosphate dibasic, 1.3 mg sodium phosphate monobasic, 0.1 mg edetate disodium, 0.1 mg polysorbate 80, and 1.5 mg m-cresol as a preservative.
† Based on the specific activity of approximately 2.6×10^8 IU/mg protein as measured by HPLC assay.

DESCRIPTION
INTRON A Interferon alfa-2b, recombinant for intramuscular, subcutaneous, intralesional, or intravenous Injection is a purified sterile recombinant interferon product.
Interferon alfa-2b, recombinant for Injection has been classified as an alfa interferon and is a water-soluble protein with a molecular weight of 19,271 daltons produced by recombinant DNA techniques. It is obtained from the bacterial fermentation of a strain of *Escherichia coli* bearing a genetically engineered plasmid containing an interferon alfa-2b gene from human leukocytes. The fermentation is carried out in a defined nutrient medium containing the antibiotic tetracycline hydrochloride at a concentration of 5 to 10 mg/L; the presence of this antibiotic is not detectable in the final product. The specific activity of Interferon alfa-2b, recombinant is approximately 2.6×10^8 IU/mg protein as measured by the HPLC assay.
[See first table above]
Prior to administration, the INTRON A Powder for Injection is to be reconstituted with the provided Diluent for INTRON A Interferon alfa-2b, recombinant for Injection (bacteriostatic water for injection) containing 0.9% benzyl alcohol as a preservative (see **DOSAGE AND ADMINISTRATION**) INTRON A Powder for Injection is a white to cream-colored powder.
[See second table above]
[See third table above]
These packages do not require reconstitution prior to administration (see **DOSAGE AND ADMINISTRATION**) INTRON A Solution for Injection is a clear, colorless solution.

CLINICAL PHARMACOLOGY
General The interferons are a family of naturally occurring small proteins and glycoproteins with molecular weights of approximately 15,000 to 27,600 daltons produced and secreted by cells in response to viral infections and to synthetic or biological inducers.
Preclinical Pharmacology Interferons exert their cellular activities by binding to specific membrane receptors on the cell surface. Once bound to the cell membrane, interferons initiate a complex sequence of intracellular events. *In vitro* studies demonstrated that these include the induction of certain enzymes, suppression of cell proliferation, immunomodulating activities such as enhancement of the phagocytic activity of macrophages and augmentation of the specific cytotoxicity of lymphocytes for target cells, and inhibition of virus replication in virus-infected cells.
In a study using human hepatoblastoma cell line, HB 611, the *in vitro* antiviral activity of alfa interferon was demonstrated by its inhibition of hepatitis B virus (HBV) replication.
The correlation between these *in vitro* data and the clinical results is unknown. Any of these activities might contribute to interferon's therapeutic effects.
Pharmacokinetics The pharmacokinetics of INTRON A Interferon alfa-2b, recombinant for Injection were studied in 12 healthy male volunteers following single doses of 5 million IU/m² administered intramuscularly, subcutaneously, and as a 30-minute intravenous infusion in a crossover design.
The mean serum INTRON A concentrations following intramuscular and subcutaneous injections were comparable. The maximum serum concentrations obtained via these routes were approximately 18 to 116 IU/mL and occurred 3 to 12 hours after administration. The elimination half-life of INTRON A Interferon alfa-2b, recombinant for Injection following both intramuscular and subcutaneous injections was approximately 2 to 3 hours. Serum concentrations were undetectable by 16 hours after the injections.
After intravenous administration, serum INTRON A concentrations peaked (135 to 273 IU/mL) by the end of the 30-

Continued on next page

Information on Schering products appearing on these pages is effective as of June 2003.

Intron A—Cont.

minute infusion, then declined at a slightly more rapid rate than after intramuscular or subcutaneous drug administration, becoming undetectable 4 hours after the infusion. The elimination half-life was approximately 2 hours.
Urine INTRON A concentrations following a single dose (5 million IU/m^2) were not detectable after any of the parenteral routes of administration. This result was expected since preliminary studies with isolated and perfused rabbit kidneys have shown that the kidney may be the main site of interferon catabolism.
There are no pharmacokinetic data available for the intralesional route of administration.
Serum Neutralizing Antibodies In INTRON A treated patients tested for antibody activity in clinical trials, serum anti-interferon neutralizing antibodies were detected in 0% (0/90) of patients with hairy cell leukemia, 0.8% (2/260) of patients treated intralesionally for condylomata acuminata, and 4% (1/24) of patients with AIDS-Related Kaposi's Sarcoma. Serum neutralizing antibodies have been detected in <3% of patients treated with higher INTRON A doses in malignancies other than hairy cell leukemia or AIDS-Related Kaposi's Sarcoma. The clinical significance of the appearance of serum anti-interferon neutralizing activity in these indications is not known.
Serum anti-interferon neutralizing antibodies were detected in 7% (12/168) of patients either during treatment or after completing 12 to 48 weeks of treatment with 3 million IU TIW of INTRON A therapy for chronic hepatitis C and in 13% (6/48) of patients who received INTRON A therapy for chronic hepatitis B at 5 million IU QD for 4 months, and in 3% (1/33) of patients treated at 10 million IU TIW. Serum anti-interferon neutralizing antibodies were detected in 9% (5/53) of pediatric patients who received INTRON A therapy for chronic hepatitis B at 6 million IU/m^2 TIW. Among all chronic hepatitis B or C patients, pediatric and adults with detectable serum neutralizing antibodies, the titers detected were low (22/24 with titers ≤1:40 and 2/24 with titers ≤ 1:160). The appearance of serum anti-interferon neutralizing activity did not appear to affect safety or efficacy.
Hairy Cell Leukemia In clinical trials in patients with hairy cell leukemia, there was depression of hematopoiesis during the first 1 to 2 months of INTRON A treatment, resulting in reduced numbers of circulating red and white blood cells, and platelets. Subsequently, both splenectomized and non-splenectomized patients achieved substantial and sustained improvements in granulocytes, platelets, and hemoglobin levels in 75% of treated patients and at least some improvement (minor responses) occurred in 90%. INTRON A treatment resulted in a decrease in bone marrow hypercellularity and hairy cell infiltrates. The hairy cell index (HCI), which represents the percent of bone marrow cellularity times the percent of hairy cell infiltrate, was ≥50% at the beginning of the study in 87% of patients. The percentage of patients with such an HCI decreased to 25% after 6 months and to 14% after 1 year. These results indicate that even though hematologic improvement had occurred earlier, prolonged INTRON A treatment may be required to obtain maximal reduction in tumor cell infiltrates in the bone marrow.
The percentage of patients with hairy cell leukemia who required red blood cell or platelet transfusions decreased significantly during treatment and the percentage of patients with confirmed and serious infections declined as granulocyte counts improved. Reversal of splenomegaly and of clinically significant hypersplenism was demonstrated in some patients.
A study was conducted to assess the effects of extended INTRON A treatment on duration of response for patients who responded to initial therapy. In this study, 126 responding patients were randomized to receive additional INTRON A treatment for 6 months or observation for a comparable period, after 12 months of initial INTRON A therapy. During this 6-month period, 3% (2/66) of INTRON A treated patients relapsed compared with 18% (11/60) who were not treated. This represents a significant difference in time to relapse in favor of continued INTRON A treatment (p=0.006/0.01, Log Rank/ Wilcoxon). Since a small proportion of the total population had relapsed, median time to relapse could not be estimated in either group. A similar pattern in relapses was seen when all randomized treatment, including that beyond 6 months, and available follow-up data were assessed. The 15% (10/66) relapses among INTRON A patients occurred over a significantly longer period of time than the 40% (24/60) with observation (p=0.0002/0.0001, Log Rank/Wilcoxon). Median time to relapse was estimated, using the Kaplan-Meier method, to be 6.8 months in the observation group but could not be estimated in the INTRON A group.
Subsequent follow-up with a median time of approximately 40 months demonstrated an overall survival of 87.8%. In a comparable historical control group followed for 24 months, overall median survival was approximately 40%.
Malignant Melanoma The safety and efficacy of INTRON A Interferon alfa-2b, recombinant for Injection was evaluated as adjuvant to surgical treatment in patients with melanoma who were free of disease (postsurgery) but at high risk for systemic recurrence. These included patients with lesions of Breslow thickness >4 mm, or patients with lesions of any Breslow thickness with primary or recurrent nodal involvement. In a randomized, controlled trial in 280 patients, 143 patients received INTRON A therapy at 20 million IU/m^2 intravenously five times per week for 4 weeks (induction phase) followed by 10 million IU/m^2 subcutaneously three times per week for 48 weeks (maintenance phase). INTRON A therapy was begun ≤56 days after surgical resection. The remaining 137 patients were observed. INTRON A therapy produced a significant increase in relapse-free and overall survival. Median time to relapse for the INTRON A treated patients vs observation patients was 1.72 years vs 0.98 years (p<0.01, stratified Log Rank). The estimated 5-year relapse-free survival rate, using the Kaplan-Meier method, was 37% for INTRON A treated patients vs 26% for observation patients. Median overall survival time for INTRON A treated patients vs observation patients was 3.82 years vs 2.78 years (p=0.047, stratified Log Rank). The estimated 5-year overall survival rate, using the Kaplan-Meier method, was 46% for INTRON A treated patients vs 37% for observation patients.
In a second study of 642 resected high-risk melanoma patients, subjects were randomized equally to one of three groups: high-dose INTRON A therapy for 1 year (same schedule as above), low-dose INTRON A therapy for 2 years (3 MU/d TIW SC), and observation. Consistent with the earlier trial, high-dose INTRON A therapy demonstrated an improvement in relapse-free survival (3-year estimated RFS 48% vs 41%; median RFS 2.4 vs 1.6 years, p=not significant). Relapse-free survival in the low-dose INTRON A arm was similar to that seen in the observation arm. Neither high-dose nor low-dose INTRON A therapy showed a benefit in overall survival as compared to observation in this study.
Follicular Lymphoma The safety and efficacy of INTRON A in conjunction with CHVP, a combination chemotherapy regimen, was evaluated as initial treatment in patients with clinically aggressive, large tumor burden, Stage III/IV follicular Non-Hodgkin's Lymphoma. Large tumor burden was defined by the presence of any one of the following: a nodal or extranodal tumor mass with a diameter of >7 cm; involvement of at least three nodal sites (each with a diameter of >3 cm); systemic symptoms; splenomegaly; serous effusion, orbital or epidural involvement; ureteral compression; or leukemia.
In a randomized, controlled trial, 130 patients received CHVP therapy and 135 patients received CHVP therapy plus INTRON A therapy at 5 million IU subcutaneously three times weekly for the duration of 18 months. CHVP chemotherapy consisted of cyclophosphamide 600 mg/m^2, doxorubicin 25 mg/m^2, and teniposide (VM-26) 60 mg/m^2, administered intravenously on Day 1 and prednisone at a daily dose of 40 mg/m^2 given orally on Days 1 to 5. Treatment consisted of six CHVP cycles administered monthly, followed by an additional six cycles administered every 2 months for 1 year. Patients in both treatment groups received a total of 12 CHVP cycles over 18 months.
The group receiving the combination of INTRON A therapy plus CHVP had a significantly longer progression-free survival (2.9 years vs 1.5 years, p=0.0001, Log Rank test). After a median follow-up of 6.1 years, the median survival for patients treated with CHVP alone was 5.5 years while median survival for patients treated with CHVP plus INTRON A therapy had not been reached (p=0.004, Log Rank test). In three additional published, randomized, controlled studies of the addition of interferon alfa to anthracycline-containing combination chemotherapy regimens,[1–3] the addition of interferon alfa was associated with significantly prolonged progression-free survival. Differences in overall survival were not consistently observed.
Condylomata Acuminata Condylomata acuminata (venereal or genital warts) are associated with infections of the human papilloma virus (HPV). The safety and efficacy of INTRON A Interferon alfa-2b, recombinant for Injection in the treatment of condylomata acuminata were evaluated in three controlled double-blind clinical trials. In these studies, INTRON A doses of 1 million IU per lesion were administered intralesionally three times a week (TIW), in ≤5 lesions per patient for 3 weeks. The patients were observed for up to 16 weeks after completion of the full treatment course.
INTRON A treatment of condylomata was significantly more effective than placebo, as measured by disappearance of lesions, decreases in lesion size, and by an overall change in disease status. Of 192 INTRON A treated patients and 206 placebo treated patients who were evaluable for efficacy at the time of best response during the course of the study, 42% of INTRON A patients vs 17% of placebo patients experienced clearing of all treated lesions. Likewise, 24% of INTRON A patients vs 8% of placebo patients experienced marked (≥75% to <100%) reduction in lesion size, 18% vs 9% experienced moderate (≥50% to ≤75%) reduction in lesion size, 10% vs 42% had a slight (<50%) reduction in lesion size, 5% vs 24% had no change in lesion size, and 0% vs 1% experienced exacerbation (p<0.001).
In one of these studies, 43% (54/125) of patients in whom multiple (≤3) lesions were treated, experienced complete clearing of all treated lesions during the course of the study. Of these patients, 81% remained cleared 16 weeks after treatment was initiated.
Patients who did not achieve total clearing of all their treated lesions had these same lesions treated with a second course of therapy. During this second course of treatment, 38% to 67% of patients had clearing of all treated lesions. The overall percentage of patients who had cleared all their treated lesions after two courses of treatment ranged from 57% to 85%.
INTRON A treated lesions showed improvement within 2 to 4 weeks after the start of treatment in the above study; maximal response to INTRON A therapy was noted 4 to 8 weeks after initiation of treatment.
The response to INTRON A therapy was better in patients who had condylomata for shorter durations than in patients with lesions for a longer duration.
Another study involved 97 patients in whom three lesions were treated with either an intralesional injection of 1.5 million IU of INTRON A Interferon alfa-2b, recombinant for Injection per lesion followed by a topical application of 25% podophyllin, or a topical application of 25% podophyllin alone. Treatment was given once a week for 3 weeks. The combined treatment of INTRON A Interferon alfa-2b, recombinant for Injection and podophyllin was shown to be significantly more effective than podophyllin alone, as determined by the number of patients whose lesions cleared. This significant difference in response was evident after the second treatment (Week 3) and continued through 8 weeks posttreatment. At the time of the patient's best response, 67% (33/49) of the INTRON A Interferon alfa-2b, recombinant for Injection and podophyllin treated patients had all three treated lesions clear while 42% (20/48) of the podophyllin treated patients had all three clear (p=0.003).
AIDS-Related Kaposi's Sarcoma The safety and efficacy of INTRON A Interferon alfa-2b, recombinant for Injection in the treatment of Kaposi's Sarcoma (KS), a common manifestation of the Acquired Immune Deficiency Syndrome (AIDS), were evaluated in clinical trials in 144 patients.
In one study, INTRON A doses of 30 million IU/m^2 were administered subcutaneously three times per week (TIW), to patients with AIDS-Related KS. Doses were adjusted for patient tolerance. The average weekly dose delivered in the first 4 weeks was 150 million IU; at the end of 12 weeks this averaged 110 million IU/week; and by 24 weeks averaged 75 million IU/week.
Forty-four percent of asymptomatic patients responded vs 7% of symptomatic patients. The median time to response was approximately 2 months and 1 month, respectively, for asymptomatic and symptomatic patients. The median duration of response was approximately 3 months and 1 month, respectively, for the asymptomatic and symptomatic patients. Baseline T4/T8 ratios were 0.46 for responders vs 0.33 for nonresponders.
In another study, INTRON A doses of 35 million IU were administered subcutaneously, daily (QD), for 12 weeks. Maintenance treatment, with every other day dosing (QOD), was continued for up to 1 year in patients achieving antitumor and antiviral responses. The median time to response was 2 months and the median duration of response was 5 months in the asymptomatic patients.
In all studies, the likelihood of response was greatest in patients with relatively intact immune systems as assessed by baseline CD4 counts (interchangeable with T4 counts). Results at doses of 30 million IU/m^2 TIW and 35 million IU/QD were subcutaneously similar and are provided together in TABLE 1. This table demonstrates the relationship of response to baseline CD4 count in both asymptomatic and symptomatic patients in the 30 million IU/m^2 TIW and the 35 million IU/QD treatment groups.
In the 30 million IU study group, 7% (5/72) of patients were complete responders and 22% (16/72) of the patients were partial responders. The 35 million IU study had 13% (3/23 patients) complete responders and 17% (4/23) partial responders.
For patients who received 30 million IU TIW, the median survival time was longer in patients with CD4 >200 (30.7 months) than in patients with CD4 ≤200 (8.9 months). Among responders, the median survival time was 22.6 months vs 9.7 months in nonresponders.

TABLE 1
*RESPONSE BY BASELINE CD4 COUNT**
IN AIDS-RELATED KS PATIENTS
30 million IU/m^2
TIW, SC and 35 million IU QD, SC

	Asymptomatic			*Symptomatic*	
CD4<200	4/14	(29%)		0/19	(0%)
200≤CD4≤400	6/12	(50%)	} 58%	0/5	(0%)
CD4>400	5/7	(71%)		0/0	(0%)

*Data for CD4, and asymptomatic and symptomatic classification were not available for all patients.

Chronic Hepatitis C The safety and efficacy of INTRON A Interferon alfa-2b, recombinant for Injection in the treatment of chronic hepatitis C was evaluated in 5 randomized clinical studies in which an INTRON A dose of 3 million IU three times a week (TIW) was assessed. The initial three studies were placebo-controlled trials that evaluated a 6-month (24 week) course of therapy. In each of the three studies, INTRON A therapy resulted in a reduction in serum alanine aminotransferase (ALT) in a greater proportion of patients vs control patients at the end of 6 months of dosing. During the 6 months of follow-up, approximately 50% of the patients who responded maintained their ALT response. A combined analysis comparing pretreatment and posttreatment liver biopsies revealed histological improvement in a statistically significantly greater proportion of INTRON A treated patients compared to controls.
Two additional studies have investigated longer treatment durations (up to 24 months).[5,6] Patients in the two studies to evaluate longer duration of treatment had hepatitis with or without cirrhosis in the absence of decompensated liver disease. Complete response to treatment was defined as normalization of the final two serum ALT levels during the treatment period. A sustained response was defined as a

complete response at the end of the treatment period with sustained normal ALT values lasting at least 6 months following discontinuation of therapy.

In Study 1, all patients were initially treated with INTRON A 3 million IU TIW subcutaneously for 24 weeks (run-in-period). Patients who completed the initial 24-week treatment period were then randomly assigned to receive no further treatment, or to receive 3 million IU TIW for an additional 48 weeks. In Study 2, patients who met the entry criteria were randomly assigned to receive INTRON A 3 million IU TIW subcutaneously for 24 weeks or to receive INTRON A 3 million IU TIW subcutaneously for 96 weeks. In both studies, patient follow-up was variable and some data collection was retrospective.

Results show that longer durations of INTRON A therapy improved the sustained response rate (see TABLE 2). In patients with complete responses (CR) to INTRON A therapy after 6 months of treatment (149/352 [42%]), responses were less often sustained if drug was discontinued (21/70 [30%]) than if it was continued for 18 to 24 months (44/79 [56%]). Of all patients randomized, the sustained response rate in the patients receiving 18 or 24 months of therapy was 22% and 26%, respectively, in the two trials. In patients who did not have a CR by 6 months, additional therapy did not result in significantly more responses, since almost all patients who responded to therapy did so within the first 16 weeks of treatment.

A subset (<50%) of patients from the combined extended dosing studies had liver biopsies performed both before and after INTRON A treatment. Improvement in necroinflammatory activity as assessed retrospectively by the Knodell (Study 1) and Scheuer (Study 2) Histology Activity Indices was observed in both studies. A higher number of patients (58%, 45/78) improved with extended therapy than with shorter (6 months) therapy (38%, 34/89) in this subset.

REBETRON® Combination Therapy containing INTRON A and REBETOL® (ribavirin, USP) Capsules has been shown to provide a significant reduction in virologic load and improved histologic response in patients with compensated liver disease who have relapsed following therapy with alfa interferon alone and in patients previously untreated with alfa interferon. See REBETRON Combination Therapy package insert for additional information.

[See table 2 above]

TABLE 2

SUSTAINED ALT RESPONSE RATE VS DURATION OF THERAPY

*IN **CHRONIC HEPATITIS C** PATIENTS*

INTRON A 3 Million IU TIW

Treatment Group—Number of Patients (%)*

Study Number	*INTRON A 3 million IU 24 weeks of treatment*		*INTRON A 3 million IU 72 or 96 weeks of treatment*†		*Difference (Extended– 24 weeks) (95% CI)*‡	
	ALT response at the end of follow-up					
1	12/101	(12%)	23/104	(22%)	10%	(-3, 24)
2	9/67	(13%)	21/80	(26%)	13%	(-4, 30)
Combined Studies	**21/168**	**(12.5%)**	**44/184**	**(24%)**	**11.4%**	**(2, 21)**
	ALT response at the end of treatment					
1	40/101	(40%)	51/104	(49%)	—	
2	32/67	(48%)	35/80	(44%)	—	

*Intent to treat groups.

† Study 1: 72 weeks of treatment; Study 2: 96 weeks of treatment.

‡ Confidence intervals adjusted for multiple comparisons due to 3 treatment arms in the study.

Chronic Hepatitis B ***Adults*** The safety and efficacy of INTRON A Interferon alfa-2b, recombinant for Injection in the treatment of chronic hepatitis B were evaluated in three clinical trials in which INTRON A doses of 30 to 35 million IU per week were administered subcutaneously (SC), as either 5 million IU daily (QD), or 10 million IU three times a week (TIW) for 16 weeks vs no treatment. All patients were 18 years of age or older with compensated liver disease, and had chronic hepatitis B virus (HBV) infection (serum HBsAg positive for at least 6 months) and HBV replication (serum HBeAg positive). Patients were also serum HBV-DNA positive, an additional indicator of HBV replication, as measured by a research assay.[7,8] All patients had elevated serum alanine aminotransferase (ALT) and liver biopsy findings compatible with the diagnosis of chronic hepatitis. Patients with the presence of antibody to human immunodeficiency virus (anti-HIV) or antibody to hepatitis delta virus (anti-HDV) in the serum were excluded from the studies.

Virologic response to treatment was defined in these studies as a loss of serum markers of HBV replication (HBeAg and HBV DNA). Secondary parameters of response included loss of serum HBsAg, decreases in serum ALT, and improvement in liver histology.

In each of two randomized controlled studies, a significantly greater proportion of INTRON A treated patients exhibited a virologic response compared with untreated control patients (see TABLE 3). In a third study without a concurrent control group, a similar response rate to INTRON A therapy was observed. Pretreatment with prednisone, evaluated in two of the studies, did not improve the response rate and provided no additional benefit.

The response to INTRON A therapy was durable. No patient responding to INTRON A therapy at a dose of 5 million IU QD or 10 million IU TIW, relapsed during the follow-up period which ranged from 2 to 6 months after treatment ended. The loss of serum HBeAg and HBV DNA was maintained in 100% of 19 responding patients followed for 3.5 to 36 months after the end of therapy.

In a proportion of responding patients, loss of HBeAg was followed by the loss of HBsAg. HBsAg was lost in 27% (4/15) of patients who responded to INTRON A therapy at a dose of 5 million IU QD, and 35% (8/23) of patients who responded to 10 million IU TIW. No untreated control patient lost HBsAg in these studies.

[See table 3 above]

TABLE 3

*VIROLOGIC RESPONSE**

*IN **CHRONIC HEPATITIS B** PATIENTS*

Treatment Group†—Number of Patients (%)

Study Number	*INTRON A 5 million IU QD*		*INTRON A 10 million IU TIW*		*Untreated Controls*		*P‡ Value*
1[7]	15/38	(39%)	—	—	3/42	(7%)	0.0009
2	—	—	10/24	(42%)	1/22	(5%)	0.005
3[8]	—	—	13/24§	(54%)	2/27	(7%)§	NA§
All Studies	**15/38**	**(39%)**	**23/48**	**(48%)**	**6/91**	**(7%)**	—

*Loss of HBeAg and HBV DNA by 6 months posttherapy.

† Patients pretreated with prednisone not shown.

‡ INTRON A treatment group vs untreated control.

§ Untreated control patients evaluated after 24-week observation period. A subgroup subsequently received INTRON A therapy. A direct comparison is not applicable (NA).

In an ongoing study to assess the long-term durability of virologic response, 64 patients responding to INTRON A therapy have been followed for 1.1 to 6.6 years after treatment; 95% (61/64) remain serum HBeAg negative and 49% (30/61) have lost serum HBsAg.

INTRON A therapy resulted in normalization of serum ALT in a significantly greater proportion of treated patients compared to untreated patients in each of two controlled studies (see TABLE 4). In a third study without a concurrent control group, normalization of serum ALT was observed in 50% (12/24) of patients receiving INTRON A therapy.

TABLE 4

*ALT RESPONSES**

*IN **CHRONIC HEPATITIS B** PATIENTS*

Treatment Group—Number of Patients (%)

Study Number	*INTRON A 5 million IU QD*		*INTRON A 10 million IU TIW*		*Untreated Controls*		*P† Value*
1	16/38	(42%)	—	—	8/42	(19%)	0.03
2	—	—	10/24	(42%)	1/22	(5%)	0.0034
3	—	—	12/24‡	(50%)	2/27	(7%)‡	NA‡
All Studies	**16/38**	**(42%)**	**22/48**	**(46%)**	**11/91**	**(12%)**	—

*Reduction in serum ALT to normal by 6 months posttherapy.

† INTRON A treatment group vs untreated control.

‡ Untreated control patients evaluated after 24-week observation period. A subgroup subsequently received INTRON A therapy. A direct comparison is not applicable (NA).

Virologic response was associated with a reduction in serum ALT to normal or near normal (≤1.5 × the upper limit of normal) in 87% (13/15) of patients responding to INTRON A therapy at 5 million IU QD, and 100% (23/23) of patients responding to 10 million IU TIW.

Improvement in liver histology was evaluated in Studies 1 and 3 by comparison of pretreatment and 6-month post-treatment liver biopsies using the semiquantitative Knodell Histology Activity Index.[9] No statistically significant difference in liver histology was observed in treated patients compared to control patients in Study 1. Although statistically significant histological improvement from baseline was observed in treated patients in Study 3 ($p \leq 0.01$), there was no control group for comparison. Of those patients exhibiting a virologic response following treatment with 5 million IU QD or 10 million IU TIW, histological improvement was observed in 85% (17/20) compared to 36% (9/25) of patients who were not virologic responders. The histological improvement was due primarily to decreases in severity of necrosis, degeneration, and inflammation in the periportal, lobular, and portal regions of the liver (Knodell Categories I + II + III). Continued histological improvement was observed in four responding patients who lost serum HBsAg and were followed 2 to 4 years after the end of INTRON A therapy.[10]

Pediatrics The safety and efficacy of INTRON A Interferon alfa-2b, recombinant for Injection in the treatment of chronic hepatitis B was evaluated in one randomized controlled trial of 149 patients ranging from 1 year to 17 years of age. Seventy-two patients were treated with 3 million IU/m² of INTRON A therapy administered subcutaneously three times a week (TIW) for 1 week; the dose was then escalated to 6 million IU/m² TIW for a minimum of 16 weeks up to 24 weeks. The maxiumum weekly dosage was 10 million IU TIW. Seventy-seven patients were untreated controls. Study entry and response criteria were identical to those described in the adult patient population.

Patients treated with INTRON A therapy had a better response (loss of HBV DNA and HBeAg at 24 weeks of follow up) compared to the untreated controls (24% [17/72] vs 10% [8/77] p=0.05). Sixteen of the 17 responders treated with INTRON A therapy remained HBV DNA and HBeAg negative and had a normal serum ALT 12 to 24 months after completion of treatment. Serum HBsAg became negative in 7 out of 17 patients who responded to INTRON A therapy. None of the control patients who had an HBV DNA and HBeAg response became HBsAg negative. At 24 weeks of follow up, normalization of serum ALT was similar in patients treated with INTRON A therapy (17%, 12/72) and in untreated control patients (16%, 12/77). Patients with a baseline HBV DNA <100 pg/mL were more likely to respond to INTRON A therapy than were patients with a baseline HBV DNA >100 pg/mL (35% vs 9%, respectively). Patients who contracted hepatitis B through maternal vertical transmission had lower response rates than those who contracted the disease by other means (5% vs 31%, respectively). There was no evidence that the effects on HBV DNA and HBeAg were limited to specific subpopulations based on age, gender, or race.

[See table 4 above]

INDICATIONS AND USAGE

Hairy Cell Leukemia INTRON A Interferon alfa-2b, recombinant for Injection is indicated for the treatment of patients 18 years of age or older with hairy cell leukemia.

Malignant Melanoma INTRON A Interferon alfa-2b, recombinant for Injection is indicated as adjuvant to surgical treatment in patients 18 years of age or older with malignant melanoma who are free of disease but at high risk for systemic recurrence, within 56 days of surgery.

Follicular Lymphoma INTRON A Interferon alfa-2b, recombinant for Injection is indicated for the initial treatment of clinically aggressive (see **Clinical Experience**) follicular Non-Hodgkin's Lymphoma in conjunction with anthracycline-containing combination chemotherapy in patients 18 years of age or older. Efficacy of INTRON A therapy in patients with low-grade, low-tumor burden follicular Non-Hodgkin's Lymphoma has not been demonstrated.

Condylomata Acuminata INTRON A Interferon alfa-2b, recombinant for Injection is indicated for intralesional treatment of selected patients 18 years of age or older with condylomata acuminata involving external surfaces of the genital and perianal areas (see **DOSAGE AND ADMINISTRATION**).

The use of this product in adolescents has not been studied.

AIDS-Related Kaposi's Sarcoma INTRON A Interferon alfa-2b, recombinant for Injection is indicated for the treatment of selected patients 18 years of age or older with AIDS-

Continued on next page

Information on Schering products appearing on these pages is effective as of June 2003.

Intron A—Cont.

Related Kaposi's Sarcoma. The likelihood of response to INTRON A therapy is greater in patients who are without systemic symptoms, who have limited lymphadenopathy and who have a relatively intact immune system as indicated by total CD4 count.

Chronic Hepatitis C INTRON A Interferon alfa-2b, recombinant for Injection is indicated for the treatment of chronic hepatitis C in patients 18 years of age or older with compensated liver disease who have a history of blood or blood-product exposure and/or are HCV antibody positive. Studies in these patients demonstrated that INTRON A therapy can produce meaningful effects on this disease, manifested by normalization of serum alanine aminotransferase (ALT) and reduction in liver necrosis and degeneration.

A liver biopsy should be performed to establish the diagnosis of chronic hepatitis. Patients should be tested for the presence of antibody to HCV. Patients with other causes of chronic hepatitis, including autoimmune hepatitis, should be excluded. Prior to initiation of INTRON A therapy, the physician should establish that the patient has compensated liver disease. The following patient entrance criteria for compensated liver disease were used in the clinical studies and should be considered before INTRON A treatment of patients with chronic hepatitis C:

- No history of hepatic encephalopathy, variceal bleeding, ascites, or other clinical signs of decompensation
- Bilirubin $\leq$2 mg/dL
- Albumin Stable and within normal limits
- Prothrombin Time <3 seconds prolonged
- WBC $\geq$3000/mm^3
- Platelets $\geq$70,000/mm^3

Serum creatinine should be normal or near normal.

Prior to initiation of INTRON A therapy, CBC and platelet counts should be evaluated in order to establish baselines for monitoring potential toxicity. These tests should be repeated at weeks 1 and 2 following initiation of INTRON A therapy, and monthly thereafter. Serum ALT should be evaluated at approximately 3-month intervals to assess response to treatment (see **DOSAGE AND ADMINISTRATION**).

Patients with preexisting thyroid abnormalities may be treated if thyroid-stimulating hormone (TSH) levels can be maintained in the normal range by medication. TSH levels must be within normal limits upon initiation of INTRON A treatment and TSH testing should be repeated at 3 and 6 months (see **PRECAUTIONS – Laboratory Tests**).

INTRON A in combination with REBETOL (ribavirin, USP) Capsules is indicated for the treatment of chronic hepatitis C in patients with compensated liver disease previously untreated with alfa interferon therapy or who have relapsed following alfa interferon therapy. See REBETRON Combination Therapy package insert for additional information.

Chronic Hepatitis B INTRON A Interferon alfa-2b, recombinant for Injection is indicated for the treatment of chronic hepatitis B in patients 1 year of age or older with compensated liver disease. Patients who have been serum HBsAg positive for at least 6 months and have evidence of HBV replication (serum HBeAg positive) with elevated serum ALT are candidates for treatment. Studies in these patients demonstrated that INTRON A therapy can produce virologic remission of this disease (loss of serum HBeAg), and normalization of serum aminotransferases. INTRON A therapy resulted in the loss of serum HBsAg in some responding patients.

Prior to initiation of INTRON A therapy, it is recommended that a liver biopsy be performed to establish the presence of chronic hepatitis and the extent of liver damage. The physician should establish that the patient has compensated liver disease. The following patient entrance criteria for compensated liver disease were used in the clinical studies and should be considered before INTRON A treatment of patients with chronic hepatitis B:

- No history of hepatic encephalopathy, variceal bleeding, ascites, or other signs of clinical decompensation
- Bilirubin Normal
- Albumin Stable and within normal limits
- Prothrombin Time *Adults* <3 seconds prolonged *Pediatrics* $\leq$2 seconds prolonged
- WBC $\geq$4000/mm^3
- Platelets *Adults* $\geq$100,000/mm^3 *Pediatrics* $\geq$150,000/mm^3

Patients with causes of chronic hepatitis other than chronic hepatitis B or chronic hepatitis C should not be treated with INTRON A Interferon alfa-2b, recombinant for Injection. CBC and platelet counts should be evaluated prior to initiation of INTRON A therapy in order to establish baselines for monitoring potential toxicity. These tests should be repeated at treatment weeks 1, 2, 4, 8, 12, and 16. Liver function tests, including serum ALT, albumin, and bilirubin, should be evaluated at treatment weeks 1, 2, 4, 8, 12, and 16. HBeAg, HBsAg, and ALT should be evaluated at the end of therapy, as well as 3- and 6-months posttherapy, since patients may become virologic responders during the 6-month period following the end of treatment. In clinical studies in adults, 39% (15/38) of responding patients lost HBeAg 1 to 6 months following the end of INTRON A therapy. Of responding patients who lost HBsAg, 58% (7/12) did so 1- to 6-months posttreatment.

A transient increase in ALT $\geq$2 × baseline value (flare) can occur during INTRON A therapy for chronic hepatitis B. In clinical trials in adults and pediatrics, this flare generally occurred 8 to 12 weeks after initiation of therapy and was more frequent in INTRON A responders (*adults* 63%, 24/38; *pediatrics* 59%, 10/17) than in nonresponders (*adults* 27%, 13/48; *pediatrics* 35%, 19/55). However, in adults and pediatrics, elevations in bilirubin $\geq$3 mg/dL ($\geq$2 times ULN) occurred infrequently (*adults* 2%, 2/86; *pediatrics* 3%, 2/72) during therapy. When ALT flare occurs, in general, INTRON A therapy should be continued unless signs and symptoms of liver failure are observed. During ALT flare, clinical symptomatology and liver function tests including ALT, prothrombin time, alkaline phosphatase, albumin, and bilirubin, should be monitored at approximately 2-week intervals (see **WARNINGS**).

DOSAGE AND ADMINISTRATION

IMPORTANT: INTRON A Interferon alfa-2b, is packaged as 1) powder for reconstitution/injection; 2) solution for injection; and 3) solution in prefilled, multidose cartridges in a multidose pen device for subcutaneous injection. Not all dosage forms and strengths are appropriate for some indications. It is important that you carefully read the instructions below for the indication you are treating to ensure you are using an appropriate dosage form and strength.

INTRON A SOLUTION FOR INJECTION IS NOT RECOMMENDED FOR INTRAVENOUS ADMINISTRATION.

Hairy Cell Leukemia The recommended dosage of INTRON A Interferon alfa-2b, recombinant for Injection for the treatment of hairy cell leukemia is 2 million IU/m^2 administered intramuscularly (see **WARNINGS**) or subcutaneously 3 times a week for up to 6 months. Responding patients may benefit from continued treatment. **NOTE: The 50 million IU strength of the INTRON A Powder for Injection is NOT to be used for the treatment of hairy cell leukemia.** Higher doses are not recommended.

If severe adverse reactions develop, the dosage should be modified (50% reduction) or therapy should be temporarily discontinued until the adverse reactions abate. If persistent or recurrent intolerance develops following adequate dosage adjustment, or disease progresses, INTRON A treatment should be discontinued. The minimum effective INTRON A dose has not been established.

Malignant Melanoma The recommended INTRON A treatment regimen includes induction treatment 5 consecutive days per week for 4 weeks as an intravenous (IV) infusion at a dose of 20 million IU/m^2, followed by maintenance treatment three times per week for 48 weeks as a subcutaneous (SC) injection, at a dose of 10 million IU/m^2.

In the clinical trial, the median daily INTRON A doses administered to patients were 19.1 million IU/m^2 during the induction phase and 9.1 million IU/m^2 during the maintenance phase. **NOTE: INTRON A Solution for Injection is NOT recommended for intravenous administration and should not be used for the induction phase of malignant melanoma.**

Regular laboratory testing should be performed to monitor laboratory abnormalities for the purposes of dose modification (see **PRECAUTIONS – Laboratory Tests**). If adverse reactions develop during INTRON A treatment, particularly if granulocytes decrease to <500/mm^3 or SGPT/SGOT rises to >5 × upper limit of normal, treatment should be temporarily discontinued until the adverse reactions abate. INTRON A treatment should be restarted at 50% of the previous dose. If intolerance persists after dose adjustments or if granulocytes decrease to <250/mm^3 or SGPT/SGOT rises to >10 × upper limit of normal, INTRON A therapy should be discontinued.

Follicular Lymphoma The recommended dosage of INTRON A Interferon alfa-2b, recombinant for Injection is 5 million IU subcutaneously three times per week for up to 18 months in conjunction with an anthracycline-containing chemotherapy regimen.

In published reports, the doses of myelosuppressive drugs were reduced by 25% from those utilized in a full-dose CHOP regimen, and cycle length increased by 33% (eg, from 21 to 28 days) when an alfa interferon was added to the regimen.[1,4] The dosing regimen should be modified for evidence of serious toxicity. The following dose modification guidelines for hematologic toxicity were used in the clinical trial: the chemotherapy regimen was delayed if either the neutrophil count was <1500/mm^3 or the platelet count was <75,000/mm^3. Administration of INTRON A therapy was temporarily interrupted for a neutrophil count <1000/mm^3, or a platelet count <50,000/mm^3, or reduced by 50% to 2.5 MIU TIW for a neutrophil count >1000/mm^3 but <1500/mm^3.

Reinstitution of the initial INTRON A dose (5 million IU TIW) was tolerated after resolution of hematologic toxicity ($\geq$1500/mm^3).

INTRON A therapy should be discontinued if SGOT exceeds >5 × the upper limit of normal or serum creatinine >2.0 mg/dL (see **WARNINGS**).

Condylomata Acuminata The 10 million IU vial of INTRON A Powder for Injection must be reconstituted with 1 mL of Diluent for INTRON A Interferon alfa-2b, recombinant for Injection (bacteriostatic water for injection). Do not reconstitute the 10 million IU vial of INTRON A Powder for Injection with more than 1 mL of diluent since the injection would be subpotent. Do not use the 5 million, 18 million, 25 million, or 50 million IU vials of INTRON A Powder for Injection for the treatment of condylomata acuminata since the resulting reconstituted solution would be either hypertonic or an inappropriate concentration. Do not use the 3 million IU vial or the 18 million IU multidose vial of INTRON A Solution for Injection for the intralesional treatment of condylomata acuminata since the concentrations are inappropriate for such use.

Inject 1.0 million IU of INTRON A Interferon alfa-2b, recombinant for Injection (either 0.1 mL of reconstituted 10 million IU INTRON A Powder for Injection or 0.1 mL of the 5 million IU, 10 million IU, or 25 million IU strengths of INTRON A Solution for Injection, each having a final concentration of 10 million IU/mL) into each lesion three times per week on alternate days, for 3 weeks. The injection should be administered intralesionally using a Tuberculin or similar syringe and a 25- to 30-gauge needle. The needle should be directed at the center of the base of the wart and at an angle almost parallel to the plane of the skin (approximating that in the commonly used PPD test). This will deliver the interferon to the dermal core of the lesion, infiltrating the lesion and causing a small wheal. Care should be taken not to go beneath the lesion too deeply; subcutaneous injection should be avoided, since this area is below the base of the lesion. Do not inject too superficially since this will result in possible leakage, infiltrating only the keratinized layer, and not the dermal core. As many as five lesions can be treated at one time. To reduce side effects, INTRON A injections may be administered in the evening, when possible. Additionally, acetaminophen may be administered at the time of injection to alleviate some of the potential side effects.

The maximum response usually occurs 4 to 8 weeks after initiation of the first treatment course. If results at 12 to 16 weeks after the initial treatment course has concluded are not satisfactory, a second course of treatment using the above dosage schedule may be instituted providing that clinical symptoms and signs, or changes in laboratory parameters (liver function tests, WBC, and platelets) do not preclude such a course of action.

Patients with 6 to 10 condylomata may receive a second (sequential) course of treatment at the above dosage schedule, to treat up to five additional condylomata per course of treatment. Patients with greater than 10 condylomata may receive additional sequences depending on how large a number of condylomata are present.

AIDS-Related Kaposi's Sarcoma The recommended INTRON A dosage is 30 million IU/m^2 three times a week administered subcutaneously or intramuscularly. **NOTE: INTRON A Solution for Injection should NOT be used for AIDS-Related Kaposi's Sarcoma since the concentrations are inappropriate.** The 18 million and 25 million IU multidose strengths of the INTRON A Solution for Injection should not be used for the treatment of AIDS-Related Kaposi's Sarcoma since the concentrations are inappropriate. The selected dosage regimen should be maintained unless the disease progresses rapidly or severe intolerance is manifested. If severe adverse reactions develop, the dosage should be modified (50% reduction) or therapy should be temporarily discontinued until the adverse reactions abate. When patients initiate therapy at 30 million IU/m^2 TIW, the average dose tolerated at the end of 12 weeks of therapy is 110 million IU/week and 75 million IU/week at the end of 24 weeks of therapy.

When disease stabilization or a response to treatment occurs, treatment should continue until there is no further evidence of tumor or until discontinuation is required by evidence of a severe opportunistic infection or adverse effect.

Chronic Hepatitis C The recommended dosage of INTRON A Interferon alfa-2b, recombinant for Injection for the treatment of chronic hepatitis C is 3 million IU three times a week (TIW) administered subcutaneously or intramuscularly. **NOTE: The 10 million IU vial of INTRON A Solution for Injection should NOT be used for chronic hepatitis C.** In patients tolerating therapy with normalization of ALT at 16 weeks of treatment, INTRON A therapy should be extended to 18 to 24 months (72 to 96 weeks) at 3 million IU TIW to improve the sustained response rate (see **CLINICAL PHARMACOLOGY – Chronic Hepatitis C**). Patients who do not normalize their ALTs after 16 weeks of therapy rarely achieve a sustained response with extension of treatment. Consideration should be given to discontinuing these patients from therapy.

If severe adverse reactions develop during INTRON A treatment, the dose should be modified (50% reduction) or therapy should be discontinued as indicated below. If intolerance persists after dose adjustment, INTRON A therapy should be discontinued.

See REBETRON Combination Therapy package insert for dosing when used in combination with REBETOL (ribavirin, USP) Capsules.

Chronic Hepatitis B ***Adults*** The recommended dosage of INTRON A Interferon alfa-2b, recombinant for Injection for the treatment of chronic hepatitis B is 30 to 35 million IU per week, administered subcutaneously or intramuscularly, either as 5 million IU daily (QD) or as 10 million IU three times a week (TIW) for 16 weeks.

Pediatrics The recommended dosage of INTRON A Interferon alfa-2b, recombinant for Injection for the treatment of chronic hepatitis B is 3 million IU/m^2 three times a week (TIW) for the first week of therapy followed by dose escalation to 6 million IU/m^2 TIW (maximum of 10 million IU TIW) administered subcutaneously for a total therapy duration of 16 to 24 weeks. **NOTE: The 3 million IU single-use vial and the 18 million IU multidose vial of INTRON A Solution for Injection should NOT be used for chronic hepatitis B.**

If severe adverse reactions or laboratory abnormalities develop during INTRON A therapy, the dose should be modified (50% reduction), or discontinued if appropriate, until the adverse reactions abate. If intolerance persists after dose adjustment, INTRON A therapy should be discontinued.

For patients with decreases in white blood cell, granulocyte, or platelet counts, the following guidelines for dose modification should be followed:

INTRON A Dose	*White Blood Cell Count*	*Granulocyte Count*	*Platelet Count*
Reduce 50%	$<1.5 \times 10^9$/L	$<0.75 \times 10^9$/L	$<50 \times 10^9$/L
Permanently Discontinue	$<1.0 \times 10^9$/L	$<0.5 \times 10^9$/L	$<25 \times 10^9$/L

INTRON A therapy was resumed at up to 100% of the initial dose when white blood cell, granulocyte, and/or platelet counts returned to normal or baseline values.

At the discretion of the physician, the patient may self-administer the medication. (see illustrated **PATIENT INFORMATION SHEET** for instructions).

Preparation and Administration of INTRON A Interferon alfa-2b, recombinant Powder for Injection for Intramuscular, Subcutaneous, or Intralesional Administration

Reconstitution of INTRON A Powder for Injection Inject the amount of Diluent for INTRON A Interferon alfa-2b, recombinant for Injection (bacteriostatic water for injection) stated in the chart below into the INTRON A vial. Swirl gently to hasten complete dissolution of the powder. The appropriate INTRON A dose should then be withdrawn and injected intramuscularly, subcutaneously, or intralesionally (see **PATIENT INFORMATION SHEET** for detailed instructions). After preparation and administration of the INTRON A injection, it is essential to follow the procedure for proper disposal of syringes and needles (see **PATIENT INFORMATION SHEET** for detailed instructions).

INTRON A Powder for Injection is not indicated for use in infants and should not be used in pediatric patients in this age group because when reconstituted with the provided diluent it contains benzyl alcohol (see **WARNINGS Chronic Hepatitis B**).

Preparation and Administration of INTRON A Interferon alfa-2b, recombinant Powder for Injection for Intravenous Infusion

The infusion solution should be prepared immediately prior to use. Based on the desired dose, the appropriate vial strength(s) of INTRON A Interferon alfa-2b, recombinant Powder for Injection should be reconstituted with the diluent provided. The appropriate INTRON A dose should then be withdrawn and injected into a 100-mL bag of 0.9% Sodium Chloride Injection, USP. The final concentration of INTRON A Interferon alfa-2b, recombinant for Injection should be not less than 10 million IU/100 mL. The prepared solution should be infused over a 20-minute period.

[See first table above]

Please refer to the **Patient Information Sheet** for detailed, step-by-step instructions on how to inject the INTRON A dose. After administration of INTRON A, it is essential to follow the procedure for proper disposal of syringes and needles.

Parenteral drug products should be inspected visually for particulate matter and discoloration prior to administration, whenever solution and container permit. INTRON A Interferon alfa-2b, recombinant for Injection may be administered using either sterilized glass or plastic disposable syringes.

Stability INTRON A Interferon alfa-2b, recombinant Powder for Injection provided in vials ranging from 5 to 50 million IU per vial, is stable at 45°C (113°F) for up to 7 days. After reconstitution with Diluent for INTRON A Interferon alfa-2b, recombinant for Injection (bacteriostatic water for injection) the solution is stable for 1 month at 2° to 8°C (36° to 46°F). The reconstituted solution is clear and colorless to light yellow.

Preparation and Administration of INTRON A Interferon alfa-2b, recombinant Solution for Injection

INTRON A Solution for Injection is supplied in single-use vials, multidose vials, and multidose pens. These Solutions for Injection do not require reconstitution prior to administration; the solution is clear and colorless. INTRON A Solution for Injection is not recommended for intravenous infusion.

Solution for Injection in Vials

For INTRON A Solution for Injection vials, the appropriate dose should be withdrawn from the vial and injected intramuscularly, subcutaneously, or intralesionally (5 million IU and 10 million IU single-use vials, and 25 million IU multidose vials only). The single-use 3, 5, and 10 million IU vials are supplied with B-D Safey-Lok* syringes. The Safety-Lok* syringe contains a plastic safety sleeve to be pulled over the needle after use. The syringe locks with an audible click when the green stripe on the safety sleeve covers the red stripe on the needle.

[See second table above]

Solution for Injection in Multidose Pens

The INTRON A Solution for Injection multidose pen contains a prefilled, multidose cartridge for subcutaneous administration. It is designed to deliver individual doses using a simple dial mechanism. The needles provided in the packaging should be used for the INTRON A Solution for Injection multidose pen only. A new needle is to be used each time a dose is delivered using the pen. To avoid the possible transmission of disease, each INTRON A Solution for Injection multidose pen is for single patient use only.

INTRON A Interferon alfa-2b, recombinant Powder for Injection

	5 million IU	10 million IU	18 million IU	25 million IU	50 million IU‡
Chronic Hepatitis B	1 mL	1 mL			
Chronic Hepatitis C					
Hairy Cell Leukemia	1 mL	2 mL		5 mL	
AIDS-Related Kaposi's Sarcoma					1 mL
Condylomata Acuminata		1 mL*			
Malignant Melanoma induction phase†	1 mL	1 mL	1 mL	5 mL	1 mL
maintenance phase	1 mL	1 mL	1 mL		1 mL
Follicular Lymphoma	1 mL	1 mL		5 mL	

*IMPORTANT: For patients with condylomata acuminata, reconstitute the 10 million IU vial with only 1 mL of the diluent provided to reach a final concentration of 10 million IU/mL to be administered intralesionally.
† Based on the desired dose, the appropriate vial strengths should be reconstituted and administered intravenously.
‡ This vial strength should be used only for the treatment of patients with AIDS-Related Kaposi's Sarcoma or malignant melanoma since the concentration is inappropriate for all other indications.

INTRON A Interferon alfa-2b, recombinant Solution for Injection

	3 million IU	5 million IU	10 million IU	18 million IU multidose*	25 million IU multidose†
Chronic Hepatitis B		✓	✓		✓§
Chronic Hepatitis C	✓			✓	
Hairy Cell Leukemia	✓	✓	✓	✓	✓
Condylomata Acuminata		✓			✓
Malignant Melanoma	✓‡	✓	✓	✓‡	✓¶
Follicular Lymphoma		✓			✓

*This is a multidose vial which contains a total of 22.8 million IU of interferon alfa-2b, recombinant per 3.8 mL in order to provide the delivery of six 0.5-mL doses, each containing 3 million IU of INTRON A Interferon alfa-2b, recombinant for Injection (for a label strength of 18 million IU).
† This is a multidose vial which contains a total of 32 million IU of interferon alfa-2b, recombinant per 3.2 mL in order to provide the delivery of five 0.5-mL doses, each containing 5 million IU of INTRON A Interferon alfa-2b, recombinant for Injection (for a label strength of 25 million IU).
‡ Use only for dose reduction.
§ Use only for the 5 MIU daily regimen.
¶ Use only for maintenance treatment.

INTRON A Interferon alfa-2b, recombinant Solution in Multidose Pens

	3 million IU/0.2 mL*	5 million IU/0.2 mL**	10 million IU/0.2 mL***
Chronic Hepatitis B		✓	✓
Chronic Hepatitis C	✓		
Hairy Cell Leukemia	✓	✓	
Malignant Melanoma			✓
Follicular Lymphoma		✓	

* The 3 million IU multidose pen contains a total of 22.5 million IU of interferon alfa-2b, recombinant per 1.5 mL in order to provide delivery of six 0.2-mL doses each containing 3 million IU of interferon alfa-2b, recombinant Solution for Injection (for a label strength of 18 million IU).

** The 5 million IU multidose pen contains a total of 37.5 million IU of interferon alfa-2b, recombinant per 1.5 mL in order to provide delivery of six 0.2-mL doses each containing 5 million IU of interferon alfa-2b, recombinant Solution for Injection (for a label strength of 30 million IU).

*** The 10 million IU multidose pen contains a total of 75 million IU of interferon alfa-2b, recombinant per 1.5 mL in order to provide delivery of six 0.2-mL doses each containing 10 million IU of interferon alfa-2b, recombinant Solution for Injection (for a label strength of 60 million IU).

Please refer to the **Patient Information Sheet** for detailed, step-by-step instructions on how to inject the INTRON A dose. After administration of INTRON A, it is essential to follow the procedure for proper disposal of syringes and needles.

Parenteral drug products should be inspected visually for particulate matter and discoloration prior to administration, whenever solution and container permit. INTRON A Interferon alfa-2b, recombinant for Injection may be administered using either sterilized glass or plastic disposable syringes.

Stability INTRON A Interferon alfa-2b, recombinant Solution for Injection multidose pens provided in strengths ranging from 18 to 60 million IU per pen is stable at 30°C (86°F) for up to 2 days. INTRON A Interferon alfa-2b, recombinant Solution for Injection provided in vials ranging from 3 to 25 million IU per vial, is stable at 35°C (95°F) for up to 7 days and at 30°C (86°F) for up to 14 days. The solution is clear and colorless.

CONTRAINDICATIONS

INTRON A Interferon alfa-2b, recombinant for Injection is contraindicated in patients with a history of hypersensitivity to interferon alfa or any component of the injection. REBETRON Combination Therapy containing INTRON A and REBETOL (ribavirin, USP) Capsules must not be used by women who are pregnant or by men whose female partners are pregnant. Extreme care must be taken to avoid pregnancy in female patients and in female partners of patients taking combination INTRON A/REBETOL therapy. Patients with autoimmune hepatitis must not be treated with combination INTRON A/REBETOL therapy. See REBETRON Combination Therapy package insert for additional information.

WARNINGS

General Moderate to severe adverse experiences may require modification of the patient's dosage regimen, or in some cases termination of INTRON A therapy. Because of the fever and other "flu-like" symptoms associated with INTRON A administration, it should be used cautiously in patients with debilitating medical conditions, such as those with a history of pulmonary disease (eg, chronic obstructive pulmonary disease), or diabetes mellitus prone to ketoacidosis. Caution should also be observed in patients with coagulation disorders (eg, thrombophlebitis, pulmonary embolism) or severe myelosuppression.

Patients with platelet counts of less than 50,000/mm^3 should not be administered INTRON A Interferon alfa-2b, recombinant for Injection intramuscularly, but instead by subcutaneous administration.

INTRON A therapy should be used cautiously in patients with a history of cardiovascular disease. Those patients with a history of myocardial infarction and/or previous or current arrhythmic disorder who require INTRON A therapy should be closely monitored (see **Laboratory Tests**). Cardiovascular adverse experiences, which include hypo-

Continued on next page

Information on Schering products appearing on these pages is effective as of June 2003.

Intron A—Cont.

tension, arrhythmia, or tachycardia of 150 beats per minute or greater, and rarely, cardiomyopathy and myocardial infarction have been observed in some INTRON A treated patients. Some patients with these adverse events had no history of cardiovascular disease. Transient cardiomyopathy was reported in approximately 2% of the AIDS-Related Kaposi's Sarcoma patients treated with INTRON A Interferon alfa-2b, recombinant for Injection. Hypotension may occur during INTRON A administration, or up to 2 days post-therapy, and may require supportive therapy including fluid replacement to maintain intravascular volume.

Supraventricular arrhythmias occurred rarely and appeared to be correlated with preexisting conditions and prior therapy with cardiotoxic agents. These adverse experiences were controlled by modifying the dose or discontinuing treatment, but may require specific additional therapy.

DEPRESSION AND SUICIDAL BEHAVIOR INCLUDING SUICIDAL IDEATION, SUICIDAL ATTEMPTS, AND COMPLETED SUICIDES HAVE BEEN REPORTED IN ASSOCIATION WITH TREATMENT WITH ALFA INTERFERONS, INCLUDING INTRON A THERAPY. Patients with a preexisting psychiatric condition, especially depression, or a history of severe psychiatric disorder should not be treated with INTRON A Interferon alfa-2b, recombinant for Injection.[11] INTRON A therapy should be discontinued for any patient developing severe depression or other psychiatric disorder during treatment. Obtundation and coma have also been observed in some patients, usually elderly, treated at higher doses. While these effects are usually rapidly reversible upon discontinuation of therapy, full resolution of symptoms has taken up to 3 weeks in a few severe episodes. Narcotics, hypnotics, or sedatives may be used concurrently with caution and patients should be closely monitored until the adverse effects have resolved.

Bone marrow toxicity INTRON A therapy suppresses bone marrow function and may result in severe cytopenias including very rare events of aplastic anemia. It is advised that complete blood counts (CBC) be obtained pretreatment and monitored routinely during therapy (see **PRECAUTIONS: Laboratory Tests**). INTRON A therapy should be discontinued in patients who develop severe decreases in neutrophil ($<0.5 \times 10^9$/L) or platelet counts ($<25 \times 10^9$/L) (see **DOSAGE AND ADMINISTRATION**: Guidelines for Dose Modification).

Ophthalmologic Disorders Decrease or loss of vision, retinopathy including macular edema, retinal artery or vein thrombosis, retinal hemorrhages and cotton wool spots; optic neuritis and papilledema may be induced or aggravated by treatment with Interferon alfa-2b or other alpha interferons. All patients should receive an eye examination at baseline. Patients with pre-existing ophthalmologic disorders (eg, diabetic or hypertensive retinopathy) should receive periodic ophthalmologic exams during interferon alpha treatment. Any patient who develops ocular symptoms should receive a prompt and complete eye examination. Interferon alfa-2b treatment should be discontinued in patients who develop new or worsening ophthalmologic disorders.

Infrequently, patients receiving INTRON A therapy developed thyroid abnormalities, either hypothyroid or hyperthyroid. The mechanism by which INTRON A Interferon alfa-2b, recombinant for Injection may alter thyroid status is unknown. Patients with preexisting thyroid abnormalities whose thyroid function cannot be maintained in the normal range by medication should not be treated with INTRON A Interferon alfa-2b, recombinant for Injection. Prior to initiation of INTRON A therapy, serum TSH should be evaluated. Patients developing symptoms consistent with possible thyroid dysfunction during the course of INTRON A therapy should have their thyroid function evaluated and appropriate treatment instituted. Therapy should be discontinued for patients developing thyroid abnormalities during treatment whose thyroid function cannot be normalized by medication. Discontinuation of INTRON A therapy has not always reversed thyroid dysfunction occurring during treatment.

Hepatotoxicity, including fatality, has been observed in interferon alfa treated patients, including those treated with INTRON A Interferon alfa-2b, recombinant for Injection. Any patient developing liver function abnormalities during treatment should be monitored closely and if appropriate, treatment should be discontinued.

Pulmonary infiltrates, pneumonitis and pneumonia, including fatality, have been observed in interferon alfa treated patients, including those treated with INTRON A Interferon alfa-2b, recombinant for Injection. The etiologic explanation for these pulmonary findings has yet to be established. Any patient developing fever, cough, dyspnea, or other respiratory symptoms should have a chest x-ray taken. If the chest x-ray shows pulmonary infiltrates or there is evidence of pulmonary function impairment, the patient should be closely monitored, and, if appropriate, interferon alfa treatment should be discontinued. While this has been reported more often in patients with chronic hepatitis C treated with interferon alfa, it has also been reported in patients with oncologic diseases treated with interferon alfa.

Rare cases of autoimmune diseases including thrombocytopenia, vasculitis, Raynaud's phenomenon, rheumatoid arthritis, lupus erythematosus, and rhabdomyolysis have been observed in patients treated with alfa interferons, including patients treated with INTRON A Interferon alfa-2b, recombinant for Injection. In very rare cases the event resulted in fatality. The mechanism by which these events develop and their relationship to interferon alfa therapy is not clear. Any patient developing an autoimmune disorder during treatment should be closely monitored and, if appropriate, treatment should be discontinued.

Diabetes mellitus and hyperglycemia have been observed rarely in patients treated with INTRON A Interferon alfa-2b, recombinant for Injection. Symptomatic patients should have their blood glucose measured and followed up accordingly. Patients with diabetes mellitus may require adjustment of their antidiabetic regimen.

The 50 million IU strength of the INTRON A Powder for Injection is not to be used for the treatment of hairy cell leukemia, condylomata acuminata, follicular lymphoma, chronic hepatitis C, or chronic hepatitis B. The 5 million, 18 million, and 25 million IU strengths of the INTRON A Powder for Injection are not to be used for the intralesional treatment of condylomata acuminata since the dilution required for the intralesional use would result in a hypertonic solution.

The INTRON A multidose pens, the 3 million IU vial, and the 18 million IU multidose vial of INTRON A Solution for Injection are not to be used for the treatment of condylomata acuminata. The INTRON A multidose pens and the 18 million and 25 million IU multidose vials of INTRON A Solution for Injection are not to be used for the treatment of AIDS-Related Kaposi's Sarcoma. INTRON A Solution for Injection is not recommended for the intravenous treatment of malignant melanoma.

The powder formulations of this product contain albumin, a derivative of human blood. Based on effective donor screening and product manufacturing processes, it carries an extremely remote risk for transmission of viral diseases. A theoretical risk for transmission of Creutzfeldt-Jakob disease (CJD) also is considered extremely remote. No cases of transmission of viral diseases or CJD have ever been identified for albumin.

AIDS-Related Kaposi's Sarcoma INTRON A therapy should not be used for patients with rapidly progressive visceral disease (see **CLINICAL PHARMACOLOGY**). Also of note, there may be synergistic adverse effects between INTRON A Interferon alfa-2b, recombinant for Injection and zidovudine. Patients receiving concomitant zidovudine have had a higher incidence of neutropenia than that expected with zidovudine alone. Careful monitoring of the WBC count is indicated in all patients who are myelosuppressed and in all patients receiving other myelosuppressive medications. The effects of INTRON A Interferon alfa-2b, recombinant for Injection when combined with other drugs used in the treatment of AIDS-Related disease are unknown.

Chronic Hepatitis C and Chronic Hepatitis B Patients with decompensated liver disease, autoimmune hepatitis or a history of autoimmune disease, and patients who are immunosuppressed transplant recipients should not be treated with INTRON A Interferon alfa-2b, recombinant for Injection. There are reports of worsening liver disease, including jaundice, hepatic encephalopathy, hepatic failure, and death following INTRON A therapy in such patients. Therapy should be discontinued for any patient developing signs and symptoms of liver failure.

Chronic hepatitis B patients with evidence of decreasing hepatic synthetic functions, such as decreasing albumin levels or prolongation of prothrombin time, who nevertheless meet the entry criteria to start therapy, may be at increased risk of clinical decompensation if a flare of aminotransferases occurs during INTRON A treatment. In such patients, if increases in ALT occur during INTRON A therapy for chronic hepatitis B, they should be followed carefully including close monitoring of clinical symptomatology and liver function tests, including ALT, prothrombin time, alkaline phosphatase, albumin, and bilirubin. In considering these patients for INTRON A therapy, the potential risks must be evaluated against the potential benefits of treatment.

INTRON A Interferon alfa-2b, recombinant Powder for Injection when reconstituted with the provided Diluent for INTRON A Interferon alfa-2b, recombinant for Injection (bacteriostatic water for injection) contains benzyl alcohol. There have been rare reports of death in infants associated with excessive exposure to benzyl alcohol. The amount of benzyl alcohol at which toxicity or adverse effects may occur in infants is not known. INTRON A **Powder for Injection** is not indicated for use in infants and should not be used in pediatric patients in this age group.

REBETRON Combination Therapy containing INTRON A and REBETOL (ribavirin, USP) Capsules was associated with hemolytic anemia. Hemoglobin <10 g/dL was observed in approximately 10% of patients in clinical trials. Anemia occurred within 1 to 2 weeks of initiation of ribavirin therapy. REBETRON Combination Therapy containing INTRON A and REBETOL is not recommended in patients with severe renal impairment and should be used with caution in patients with moderate renal impairment. See REBETRON Combination Therapy package insert for additional information.

PRECAUTIONS

General Acute serious hypersensitivity reactions (eg, urticaria, angioedema, bronchoconstriction, anaphylaxis) have been observed rarely in INTRON A treated patients; if such an acute reaction develops, the drug should be discontinued immediately and appropriate medical therapy instituted. Transient rashes have occurred in some patients following injection, but have not necessitated treatment interruption. While fever may be related to the flu-like syndrome reported commonly in patients treated with interferon, other causes of persistent fever should be ruled out.

There have been reports of interferon, including INTRON A Interferon alfa-2b, recombinant for Injection, exacerbating preexisting psoriasis and sarcoidosis as well as development of new sarcoidosis. Therefore, INTRON A therapy should be used in these patients only if the potential benefit justifies the potential risk.

Variations in dosage, routes of administration, and adverse reactions exist among different brands of interferon. Therefore, do not use different brands of interferon in any single treatment regimen.

Triglycerides Elevated triglyceride levels have been observed in patients treated with interferons including INTRON A therapy. Elevated triglyceride levels should be managed as clinically appropriate. Hypertriglyceridemia may result in pancreatitis. Discontinuation of INTRON A therapy should be considered for patients with persistently elevated triglycerides (eg, triglycerides > 1000 mg/dL) associated with symptoms of potential pancreatitis, such as abdominal pain, nausea, or vomiting.

Drug Interactions Interactions between INTRON A Interferon alfa-2b, recombinant for Injection and other drugs have not been fully evaluated. Caution should be exercised when administering INTRON A therapy in combination with other potentially myelosuppressive agents such as zidovudine. Concomitant use of alfa interferon and theophylline decreases theophylline clearance, resulting in a 100% increase in serum theophylline levels.

Information for Patients Patients receiving INTRON A treatment should be directed in its appropriate use, informed of benefits and risks associated with treatment, and referred to the **PATIENT INFORMATION SHEET**. This information is intended to aid in the safe and effective use of this medication. It is not a disclosure of all possible adverse or intended effects.

If home use is prescribed, a puncture-resistant container for the disposal of used syringes and needles should be supplied to the patient. Patients should be thoroughly instructed in the importance of proper disposal and cautioned against any reuse of needles and syringes. The full container should be disposed of according to the directions provided by the physician (see **PATIENT INFORMATION SHEET**).

Patients should be cautioned not to change brands of interferon without medical consultation as a change in dosage may result.

Patients receiving high INTRON A doses should be cautioned against performing tasks that would require complete mental alertness, such as operating machinery or driving a motor vehicle.

The most common adverse experiences occurring with INTRON A therapy are "flu-like" symptoms, such as fever, headache, fatigue, anorexia, nausea, or vomiting (see **ADVERSE REACTIONS**) and appear to decrease in severity as treatment continues. Some of these "flu-like" symptoms may be minimized by bedtime administration. Antipyretics may be used to prevent or partially alleviate the fever and headache. Another common adverse experience is thinning of the hair.

It is advised that patients be well hydrated, especially during the initial stages of treatment.

INTRON A in combination with REBETOL (ribavirin, USP) Capsules therapy must not be used by women who are pregnant or by men whose female partners are pregnant. Extreme care must be taken to avoid pregnancy in female patients and in female partners of patients taking INTRON A/REBETOL therapy. Combination INTRON A/REBETOL therapy should not be initiated until a report of a negative pregnancy test has been obtained immediately prior to initiation of therapy. See REBETRON Combination Therapy package insert for additional information.

Laboratory Tests In addition to those tests normally required for monitoring patients, the following laboratory tests are recommended for all patients on INTRON A therapy, prior to beginning treatment and then periodically thereafter.

- Standard hematologic tests – including hemoglobin, complete and differential white blood cell counts, and platelet count.
- Blood chemistries – electrolytes, liver function tests, and TSH.

Those patients who have preexisting cardiac abnormalities and/or are in advanced stages of cancer should have electrocardiograms taken prior to and during the course of treatment.

Mild-to-moderate leukopenia and elevated serum liver enzyme (SGOT) levels have been reported with intralesional administration of INTRON A Interferon alfa-2b, recombinant for Injection (see **ADVERSE REACTIONS**); therefore, the monitoring of these laboratory parameters should be considered.

Baseline chest x-rays are suggested and should be repeated if clinically indicated.

For malignant melanoma patients, differential WBC count and liver function tests should be monitored weekly during the induction phase of therapy and monthly during the maintenance phase of therapy.

For specific recommendations in chronic hepatitis C and chronic hepatitis B, see **INDICATIONS AND USAGE**.

TREATMENT-RELATED ADVERSE EXPERIENCES BY INDICATION
Dosing Regimens
*Percentage (%) of Patients**

	Malignant Melanoma	Follicular Lymphoma	Hairy Cell Leukemia	Condylomata Acuminata	AIDS-Related Kaposi's Sarcoma		Chronic Hepatitis C‖		Chronic Hepatitis B Adults	Chronic Hepatitis B Pediatrics
	20 MIU/m² Induction (IV) 10 MIU/m² Maintenance (SC)	5 MIU TIW/SC	2 MIU/m² TIW/SC	1 MIU/ lesion	30 MIU/m² TIW/SC	35 MIU QD/SC	3 MIU TIW	5 MIU QD	10 MIU TIW	6 MIU/m² TIW
ADVERSE EXPERIENCE	N=143	N=135	N=145	N=352	N=74	N=29	N=183	N=101	N=78	N=116
Application-Site Disorders			20							
injection site inflammation	—	1	—	—	—	—	5	3	—	—
other (≤5%)	burning, injection site bleeding, injection site pain, injection site reaction (5% in chronic hepatitis B pediatrics), itching									
Blood Disorders (<5%)	anemia, anemia hypochromic, granulocytopenia, hemolytic anemia, leukopenia, lymphocytosis, neutropenia (9% in chronic hepatitis C, 14% in chronic hepatitis B pediatrics), thrombocytopenia (10% in chronic hepatitis C) (bleeding 8% in malignant melanoma), thrombocytopenic purpura									
Body as a Whole										
facial edema	—	1	—	<1	—	10	<1	3	1	<1
weight decrease	3	13	<1	<1	5	3	10	2	5	3
other (≤5%)	allergic reaction, cachexia, dehydration, earache, hernia, edema, hypercalcemia, hyperglycemia, hypothermia, inflammation nonspecific, lymphadenitis, lymphadenopathy, mastitis, periorbital edema, poor peripheral circulation, peripheral edema (6% in follicular lymphoma), phlebitis superficial, scrotal/penile edema, thirst, weakness, weight increase									
Cardiovascular System Disorders (<5%)	angina, arrhythmia, atrial fibrillation, bradycardia, cardiac failure, cardiomegaly, cardiomyopathy, coronary artery disorder, extrasystoles, heart valve disorder, hematoma, hypertension (9% in chronic hepatitis C), hypotension, palpitations, phlebitis, postural hypotension, pulmonary embolism, Raynaud's disease, tachycardia, thrombosis, varicose vein									
Endocrine System Disorders (<5%)	aggravation of diabetes mellitus, goiter, gynecomastia, hyperglycemia, hyperthyroidism, hypertriglyceridemia, hypothyroidism, virilism									
Flu-like Symptoms										
fever	81	56	68	56	47	55	34	66	86	94
headache	62	21	39	47	36	21	43	61	44	57
chills	54	—	46	45	—	—	—	—	—	—
myalgia	75	16	39	44	34	28	43	59	40	27
fatigue	96	8	61	18	84	48	23	75	69	71
increased sweating	6	13	8	2	4	21	4	1	1	3
asthenia	—	63	7	—	11	—	40	5	15	5
rigors	2	7	—	—	30	14	16	38	42	30
arthralgia	6	8	8	9	—	3	16	19	8	15
dizziness	23	—	12	9	7	24	9	13	10	8
influenza-like symptoms	10	18	37	—	45	79	26	5	—	<1
back pain	—	15	19	6	1	3	—	—	—	—
dry mouth	1	2	19	—	22	28	5	6	5	—
chest pain	2	8	<1	<1	1	28	4	4	—	—
malaise	6	—	—	14	5	—	13	9	6	3
pain (unspecified)	15	9	18	3	3	3	—	—	—	—
other (<5%)	chest pain substernal, hyperthermia, rhinitis, rhinorrhea									
Gastrointestinal System Disorders										
diarrhea	35	19	18	2	18	45	13	19	8	12
anorexia	69	21	19	1	38	41	14	43	53	43
nausea	66	24	21	17	28	21	19	50	33	18
taste alteration	24	2	13	<1	5	7	2	10	—	—
abdominal pain	2	20	<5	1	5	21	16	5	4	23
loose stools	—	1	—	<1	—	10	2	2	—	2
vomiting	†	32	6	2	11	14	8	7	10	27
constipation	1	14	<1	—	1	10	4	5	—	2
gingivitis	2‡	7‡	—	—	—	14	—	1	—	—
dyspepsia	—	2	—	2	4	—	7	3	8	3
other (<5%)	abdominal ascites, abdominal distension, colitis, dysphagia, eructation, esophagitis, flatulence, gallstones, gastric ulcer, gastritis, gastroenteritis, gastrointestinal disorder (7% in follicular lymphoma), gastrointestinal hemorrhage, gastrointestinal mucosal discoloration, gingival bleeding, gum hyperplasia, halitosis, hemorrhoids, increased appetite, increased saliva, intestinal disorder, melena, mouth ulceration, mucositis, oral hemorrhage, oral leukoplakia, rectal bleeding after stool, rectal hemorrhage, stomatitis, stomatitis ulcerative, taste loss, tongue disorder, tooth disorder									
Liver and Biliary System Disorders (<5%)	abnormal hepatic function tests, biliary pain, bilirubinemia, hepatitis, increased lactate dehydrogenase, increased transaminases (SGOT/SGPT) (elevated SGOT 63% in malignant melanoma and 24% in follicular lymphoma), jaundice, right upper quadrant pain (15% in chronic hepatitis C), and very rarely, hepatic encephalopathy, hepatic failure, and death									
Musculoskeletal System Disorders										
musculoskeletal pain	—	18	—	—	—	—	21	9	1	10
other (<5%)	arteritis, arthritis, arthritis aggravated, arthrosis, bone disorder, bone pain, carpal tunnel syndrome, hyporeflexia, leg cramps, muscle atrophy, muscle weakness, polyarteritis nodosa, tendinitis, rheumatoid arthritis, spondylitis									
Nervous System and Psychiatric Disorders										
depression	40	9	6	3	9	28	19	17	6	4
paresthesia	13	13	6	1	3	21	5	6	3	<1
impaired concentration	—	1	—	<1	3	14	3	8	5	3
amnesia	§	1	<5	—	—	14	—	—	—	—
confusion	8	2	<5	4	12	10	1	—	—	2
hypoesthesia	—	1	<5	1	—	10	—	—	—	—
irritability	1	1	—	—	—	—	13	16	12	22

(Table continued on next page)

Carcinogenesis, Mutagenesis, Impairment of Fertility
Studies with INTRON A Interferon alfa-2b, recombinant for Injection have not been performed to determine carcinogenicity.

Interferon may impair fertility. In studies of interferon administration in nonhuman primates, menstrual cycle abnormalities have been observed. Decreases in serum estradiol and progesterone concentrations have been reported in women treated with human leukocyte interferon.[12] Therefore, fertile women should not receive INTRON A therapy unless they are using effective contraception during the therapy period. INTRON A therapy should be used with caution in fertile men.

Mutagenicity studies have demonstrated that INTRON A Interferon alfa-2b, recombinant for Injection is not mutagenic.

Studies in mice (0.1, 1.0 million IU/day), rats (4, 20, 100 million IU/kg/day), and cynomolgus monkeys (1.1 million IU/kg/day; 0.25, 0.75, 2.5 million IU/kg/day) injected with INTRON A Interferon alfa-2b, recombinant for Injection for up to 9 days, 3 months, and 1 month, respectively, have revealed no evidence of toxicity. However, in cynomolgus monkeys (4, 20, 100 million IU/kg/day) injected daily for 3 months with INTRON A Interferon alfa-2b, recombinant for Injection toxicity was observed at the mid and high doses and mortality was observed at the high dose.

However, due to the known species-specificity of interferon, the effects in animals are unlikely to be predictive of those in man.

INTRON A in combination with REBETOL (ribavirin, USP) Capsules should be used with caution in fertile men. See the REBETRON Combination Therapy package insert for additional information.

Continued on next page

Information on Schering products appearing on these pages is effective as of June 2003.

Intron A—Cont.

Pregnancy Category C INTRON A Interferon alfa-2b, recombinant for Injection has been shown to have abortifacient effects in *Macaca mulatta* (rhesus monkeys) at 15 and 30 million IU/kg (estimated human equivalent of 5 and 10 million IU/kg, based on body surface area adjustment for a 60 kg adult). There are no adequate and well-controlled studies in pregnant women. INTRON A therapy should be used during pregnancy only if the potential benefit justifies the potential risk to the fetus.

Pregnancy Category X applies to the REBETRON Combination Therapy containing INTRON A and REBETOL (ribavirin, USP) Capsules (see **CONTRAINDICATIONS**). See REBETRON Combination Therapy package insert for additional information.

Nursing Mothers It is not known whether this drug is excreted in human milk. However, studies in mice have shown that mouse interferons are excreted into the milk. Because of the potential for serious adverse reactions from the drug in nursing infants, a decision should be made whether to discontinue nursing or to discontinue INTRON A therapy, taking into account the importance of the drug to the mother.

Pediatric Use *General* Safety and effectiveness in pediatric patients below the age of 18 years have not been established for indications other than chronic hepatitis B.

Chronic Hepatitis B Safety and effectiveness in pediatric patients ranging in age from 1 to 17 years have been established based upon one controlled clinical trial (see **CLINICAL PHARMACOLOGY, INDICATIONS AND USAGE, DOSAGE AND ADMINISTRATION; Chronic Hepatitis B**). Safety and effectiveness in pediatric patients below the age of 1 year have not been established.

INTRON A Interferon alfa-2b, recombinant **Powder for Injection** when reconstituted with the provided Diluent for INTRON A Interferon alfa-2b, recombinant for Injection (bacteriostatic water for injection) contains benzyl alcohol and is not indicated for use in infants. There have been rare reports of death in infants associated with excessive exposure to benzyl alcohol. The amount of benzyl alcohol at which toxicity or adverse effects may occur in infants is not known (see **WARNINGS Chronic Hepatitis B**).

Geriatric Use In all clinical studies of INTRON A (interferon alfa-2b, recombinant), including studies as monotherapy and in combination with REBETOL (ribavirin, USP) Capsules, only a small percentage of the subjects were aged 65 and over. These numbers were too few to determine if they respond differently from younger subjects except for the clinical trials of INTRON A in combination with REBETOL, where elderly subjects had a higher frequency of anemia (67%) than did younger patients (28%).

In a database consisting of clinical study and postmarketing reports for various indications, cardiovascular adverse events and confusion were reported more frequently in elderly patients receiving INTRON A therapy compared to younger patients.

In general, INTRON A therapy should be administered to elderly patients cautiously, reflecting the greater frequency of decreased hepatic, renal, bone marrow, and/or cardiac function and concomitant disease or other drug therapy. INTRON A is known to be substantially excreted by the kidney, and the risk of adverse reactions to INTRON A may be greater in patients with impaired renal function. Because elderly patients often have decreased renal function, patients should be carefully monitored during treatment, and dose adjustments made based on symptoms and/or laboratory abnormalities (see **CLINICAL PHARMACOLOGY**, and **DOSAGE AND ADMINISTRATION**).

ADVERSE REACTIONS

General The adverse experiences listed below were reported to be possibly or probably related to INTRON A therapy during clinical trials. Most of these adverse reactions were mild to moderate in severity and were manageable. Some were transient and most diminished with continued therapy.

The most frequently reported adverse reactions were "flu-like" symptoms, particularly fever, headache, chills, myalgia, and fatigue. More severe toxicities are observed generally at higher doses and may be difficult for patients to tolerate. In addition, the following spontaneous adverse experiences have been reported during the marketing surveillance of INTRON A Interferon alfa-2b, recombinant for Injection: nephrotic syndrome, pancreatitis, psychosis, including hallucinations, renal failure, and renal insufficiency. Very rarely, INTRON A used alone or in combination with REBETOL (ribavirin, USP) Capsules may be associated with aplastic anemia. Rarely sarcoidosis or exacerbation of sarcoidosis has been reported.

[See table on previous page and below]

Hairy Cell Leukemia The adverse reactions most frequently reported during clinical trials in 145 patients with hairy cell leukemia were the "flu-like" symptoms of fever (68%), fatigue, (61%), and chills (46%).

Malignant Melanoma The INTRON A dose was modified because of adverse events in 65% (n=93) of the patients. INTRON A therapy was discontinued because of adverse events in 8% of the patients during induction and 18% of the patients during maintenance. The most frequently reported adverse reaction was fatigue which was observed in 96% of patients. Other adverse reactions that were recorded in >20% of INTRON A treated patients included neutropenia (92%), fever (81%), myalgia (75%), anorexia (69%), vomiting/nausea (66%), increased SGOT (63%), headache (62%),

TREATMENT-RELATED ADVERSE EXPERIENCES BY INDICATION (cont.)
Dosing Regimens
*Percentage (%) of Patients**

	MALIGNANT MELANOMA	FOLLICULAR LYMPHOMA	HAIRY CELL LEUKEMIA	CONDYLOMATA ACUMINATA	AIDS-RELATED KAPOSI'S SARCOMA		CHRONIC HEPATITIS C‖	CHRONIC HEPATITIS B		
								Adults		Pediatrics
	20 MIU/m² Induction (IV) 10 MIU/m² Maintenance (SC)	5 MIU TIW/SC	2 MIU/m² TIW/SC	1 MIU/ lesion	30 MIU/m² TIW/SC	35 MIU QD/SC	3 MIU TIW	5 MIU QD	10 MIU TIW	6 MIU/m² TIW
ADVERSE EXPERIENCE	N=143	N=135	N=145	N=352	N=74	N=29	N=183	N=101	N=78	N=116
somnolence	1	2	<5	3	3	—	33¶	14	9	5
anxiety	1	9	5	<1	1	3	5	2	—	3
insomnia	5	4	—	<1	3	3	12	11	6	8
nervousness	1	1	—	1	—	3	2	3	—	3
decreased libido	1	1	<5	—	—	—	1	5	1	—
other (<5%)	abnormal coordination, abnormal dreaming, abnormal gait, abnormal thinking, aggravated depression, aggressive reaction, agitation (7% in chronic hepatitis B pediatrics) alcohol intolerance, apathy, aphasia, ataxia, Bell's palsy, CNS dysfunction, coma, convulsions, delirium, dysphonia, emotional lability, extrapyramidal disorder, feeling of ebriety, flushing, hearing disorder, hearing impairment, hot flashes, hyperesthesia, hyperkinesia, hypertonia, hypokinesia, impaired consciousness, labyrinthine disorder, loss of consciousness, manic depression, manic reaction, migraine, neuralgia, neuritis, neuropathy, neurosis, paresis, paroniria, parosmia, personality disorder, polyneuropathy, psychosis, speech disorder, stroke, suicidal ideation, suicide attempt, syncope, tinnitus, tremor, twitching, vertigo (8% in follicular lymphoma)									
Reproduction System Disorders (<5%)	amenorrhea (12% in follicular lymphoma), dysmenorrhea, impotence, leukorrhea, menorrhagia, menstrual irregularity, pelvic pain, penis disorder, sexual dysfunction, uterine bleeding, vaginal dryness									
Resistance Mechanism Disorders										
moniliasis	—	1	—	<1	—	17	—	—	—	—
herpes simplex	1	2	—	1	—	3	1	5	—	—
other (<5%)	abscess, conjunctivitis, fungal infection, hemophilus, herpes zoster, infection, infection bacterial, infection nonspecific (7% in follicular lymphoma), infection parasitic, otitis media, sepsis, stye, trichomonas, upper respiratory tract infection, viral infection (7% in chronic hepatitis C)									
Respiratory System Disorders										
dyspnea	15	14	<1	—	1	34	3	5	—	—
coughing	6	13	<1	—	—	31	1	4	—	5
pharyngitis	2	8	<5	1	1	31	3	7	1	7
sinusitis	1	4	—	—	—	21	2	—	—	—
nonproductive coughing	2	7	—	—	—	14	0	1	—	—
nasal congestion	1	7	—	1	—	10	<1	4	—	—
other (≤5%)	asthma, bronchitis (10% in follicular lymphoma), bronchospasm, cyanosis, epistaxis (7% in chronic hepatitis B pediatrics), hemoptysis, hypoventilation, laryngitis, lung fibrosis, pleural effusion, orthopnea, pleural pain, pneumonia, pneumonitis, pneumothorax, rales, respiratory disorder, respiratory insufficiency, sneezing, tonsillitis, tracheitis, wheezing									
Skin and Appendages Disorders										
dermatitis	1	—	8	—	—	—	2	1	—	—
alopecia	29	23	8	—	12	31	28	26	38	17
pruritus	—	10	11	1	7	—	9	6	4	3
rash	19	13	25	—	9	10	5	8	1	5
dry skin	1	3	9	—	9	10	4	3	—	<1
other (<5%)	abnormal hair texture, acne, cellulitis, cyanosis of the hand, cold and clammy skin, dermatitis lichenoides, eczema, epidermal necrolysis, erythema, erythema nodosum, folliculitis, furunculosis, increased hair growth, lacrimal gland disorder, lacrimation, lipoma, maculopapular rash, melanosis, nail disorders, nonherpetic cold sores, pallor, peripheral ischemia, photosensitivity, pruritus genital, psoriasis, psoriasis aggravated, purpura (5% in chronic hepatitis C), rash erythematous, sebaceous cyst, skin depigmentation, skin discoloration, skin nodule, urticaria, vitiligo									
Urinary System Disorders (<5%)	albumin/protein in urine, cystitis, dysuria, hematuria, incontinence, increased BUN, micturition disorder, micturition frequency, nocturia, polyuria (10% in follicular lymphoma), renal insufficiency, urinary tract infection (5% in chronic hepatitis C)									
Vision Disorders (<5%)	abnormal vision, blurred vision, diplopia, dry eyes, eye pain, nystagmus, photophobia									

*Dash (—) indicates not reported
† Vomiting was reported with nausea as a single term
‡ Includes stomatitis/mucositis
§ Amnesia was reported with confusion as a single term
‖ Percentages based upon a summary of all adverse events during 18 to 24 months of treatment
¶ Predominantly lethargy

ABNORMAL LABORATORY TEST VALUES BY INDICATION
Dosing Regimens
Percentage (%) of Patients

	Malignant Melanoma	Follicular Lymphoma	Hairy Cell Leukemia	Condylomata Acuminata	AIDS-Related Kaposi's Sarcoma		Chronic Hepatitis C	Chronic Hepatitis B		
								Adults		Pediatrics
	20 MIU/m² Induction (IV) 10 MIU/m² Maintenance (SC)	5 MIU TIW/SC	2 MIU/m² TIW/SC	1 MIU/ lesion	30 MIU/m² TIW/SC	35 MIU QD/SC	3 MIU TIW	5 MIU QD	10 MIU TIW	6 MIU/m² TIW
Laboratory Tests	N=143	N=135	N=145	N=352	N=69–73	N=26–28	N=140–171	N=96–101	N=75–103	N=113–115
Hemoglobin	22	8	NA	—	1	15	26¶	32*	23*	17**
White Blood Cell Count	‖	—	NA	17	10	22	26†	68†	34†	9†
Platelet Count	15	13	NA	—	0	8	15‡	12‡	5‡	1‡
Serum Creatinine	3	2	0	—	—	—	6	3	0	3
Alkaline Phosphatase	13	—	4	—	—	—	—	8	4	0
Lactate Dehydrogenase	1	—	0	—	—	—	—	—	—	—
Serum Urea Nitrogen	12	4	0	—	—	—	—	2	0	2
SGOT	63	24	4	12	11	41	—	—	—	—
SGPT	2	—	13	—	10	15	—	—	—	—
Granulocyte Count										
• Total	92	36	NA		31	39	45§	75§	61§	70§
• 1000 –<1500/mm³	66						32	30	32	43
• 750 –<1000/mm³	—	21	—	—	—	—	10	24	18	18
• 500 –<750/mm³	25	—			—	—	1	17	9	7
• <500/mm³	1	13			—	—	2	4	2	2

NA—Not Applicable—Patients' initial hematologic laboratory test values were abnormal due to their condition.
* Decrease of ≥2 g/dL
**Decrease of ≥2 g/dL; 14% 2–<3 g/dL; 3%≥3g/dL
† Decrease to <3000/mm³
‡ Decrease to <70,000/mm³
§ Neutrophils plus bands
‖ White Blood Cell Count was reported as neutropenia
¶ Decrease of ≥2 g/dL; 20% 2–<3 g/dL; 6% ≥3 g/dL

chills (54%), depression (40%), diarrhea (35%), alopecia (29%), altered taste sensation (24%), dizziness/vertigo (23%), and anemia (22%).

Adverse reactions classified as severe or life threatening (ECOG Toxicity Criteria grade 3 or 4) were recorded in 66% and 14% of INTRON A treated patients, respectively. Severe adverse reactions recorded in >10% of INTRON A treated patients included neutropenia/leukopenia (26%), fatigue (23%), fever (18%), myalgia (17%), headache (17%), chills (16%), and increased SGOT (14%). Grade 4 fatigue was recorded in 4% and grade 4 depression was recorded in 2% of INTRON A treated patients. No other grade 4 AE was reported in more than 2 INTRON A treated patients. Lethal hepatotoxicity occurred in 2 INTRON A treated patients early in the clinical trial. No subsequent lethal hepatotoxicities were observed in the clinical trial. No subsequent lethal hepatotoxicities were observed with adequate monitoring of liver function tests (see **PRECAUTIONS—Laboratory Tests**).

Follicular Lymphoma Ninety-six percent of patients treated with CHVP plus INTRON A therapy and 91% of patients treated with CHVP alone reported an adverse event of any severity. Asthenia, fever, neutropenia, increased hepatic enzymes, alopecia, headache, anorexia, "flu-like" symptoms, myalgia, dyspnea, thrombocytopenia, paresthesia, and polyuria occurred more frequently in the CHVP plus INTRON A treated patients than in patients treated with CHVP alone. Adverse reactions classified as severe or life threatening (World Health Organization grade 3 or 4) recorded in >5% of CHVP plus INTRON A treated patients included neutropenia (34%), asthenia (10%) and vomiting (10%). The incidence of neutropenic infection was 6% in CHVP plus INTRON A vs 2% in CHVP alone. One patient in each treatment group required hospitalization.

Twenty-eight percent of CHVP plus INTRON A treated patients had a temporary modification/interruption of their INTRON A therapy, but only 13 patients (10%) permanently stopped INTRON A therapy because of toxicity. There were four deaths on study; two patients committed suicide in the CHVP plus INTRON A arm and two patients in the CHVP arm had unwitnessed sudden death. Three patients with hepaitis B (one of whom also had alcoholic cirrhosis) developed hepatotoxicity leading to discontinuation of INTRON A. Other reasons for discontinuation included intolerable asthenia (5/135), severe flu symptoms (2/135), and one patient each with exacerbation of ankylosing spondylitis, psychosis, and decreased ejection fraction.

Condylomata Acuminata Eighty-eight percent (311/352) of patients treated with INTRON A Interferon alfa-2b recombinant for injection for condylomata acuminata who were evaluable for safety, reported an adverse reaction during treatment. The incidence of the adverse reactions reported increased when the nuber of treated lesions increased from one to five. All 40 patients who had five warts treated, reported some type of adverse reaction during treatment.

Adverse reactions and abnormal laboratory test values reported by patients who were retreated were qualitatively and quantitatively similar to those reported during the initial INTRON A treatment period.

AIDS-Related Kaposi's Sarcoma In patients with AIDS-Related Kaposi's Sarcoma, some type of adverse reaction occurred in 100% of the 74 patients treated with 30 million IU/m² three times a week and in 97% of the 29 patients treated with 35 million IU per day.

Of these adverse reactions, those classified as severe (World Health Organization grade 3 or 4) were reported in 27% to 55% of patients. Severe adverse reactions in the 30 million IU/m² TIW study included: fatigue (20%), influenza-like symptoms (15%), anorexia (12%), dry mouth (4%), headache (4%), confusion (3%), fever (3%), myalgia (3%), and nausea and vomiting (1% each). Severe adverse reactions for patients who received the 35 million IU QD included: fever (24%), fatigue (17%), influenza-like symptoms (14%), dyspnea (14%), headache (10%), pharyngitis (7%), and ataxia, confusion, dysphagia, GI hemorrhage, abnormal hepatic function, increased SGOT, myalgia, cardiomyopathy, face edema, depression, emotional lability, suicide attempt, chest pain, and coughing (1 patient each). Overall, the incidence of severe toxicity was higher among patients who received the 35 million IU per day dose.

Chronic Hepatitis C Two studies of extended treatment (18 to 24 months) with INTRON A Interferon alfa-2b, recombinant for injection show that approximately 95% of all patients treated experience some type of adverse event and that patients treated for extended duration continue to experience adverse events throughout treatment. Most adverse events reported are mild to moderate in severity. However, 29/152 (19%) of patients treated for 18 to 24 months experienced a serious adverse event compared to 11/163 (7%) of those treated for 6 months. Adverse events which occur or persist during extended treatment are similar in type and severity to those occurring during short-course therapy.

Of the patients achieving a complete response after 6 months of therapy, 12/79 (15%) subsequently discontinued INTRON A treatment during extended therapy because of adverse events, and 23/79 (29%) experienced severe adverse events (WHO grade 3 or 4) during extended therapy.

In patients using REBETRON Combination Therapy containing INTRON A and REBETOL (ribavirin, USP) Capsules, the primary toxicity observed was hemolytic anemia. Reductions in hemoglobin levels occurred within the first 1 to 2 weeks of therapy. Cardiac and pulmonary events associated with anemia occurred in approximately 10% of patients treated with INTRON A/REBETOL therapy. See REBETRON Combination Therapy package insert for additional information.

Chronic Hepatitis B ***Adults*** In patients with chronic hepatitis B, some type of adverse reaction occurred in 98% of the 101 patients treated at 5 million IU QD and 90% of the 78 patients treated at 10 million IU TIW. Most of these adverse reactions were mild to moderate in severity, were manageable, and were reversible following the end of therapy.

Adverse reactions classified as severe (causing a significant interference with normal daily activities or clinical state) were reported in 21% to 44% of patients. The severe adverse reactions reported most frequently were the "flu-like" symptoms of fever (28), fatigue (15%), headache (5%), myalgia (4%), rigors (4%), and other severe "flu-like" symptoms which occurred in 1% to 3% of patients. Other severe adverse reactions occurring in more than one patient were alopecia (8%), anorexia (6%), depression (3%), nausea (3%), and vomiting (2%).

To manage side effects, the dose was reduced, or INTRON A therapy was interrupted in 25% to 38% of patients. Five percent of patients discontinued treatment due to adverse experiences.

Pediatrics In pediatric patients, the most frequently reported adverse events were those commonly associated with interferon treatment; flu-like symptoms (100%), gastrointestinal system disorders (46%), and nausea and vomiting (40%). Neutropenia (13%) and thrombocytopenia (3%) were also reported. None of the adverse events were life threatening. The majority were moderate to severe and resolved upon dose reduction or drug discontinuation.

[See table above]

OVERDOSAGE

There is limited experience with overdosage. Postmarketing surveillance includes reports of patients receiving a single dose as great as 10 times the recommended dose. In general, the primary effects of an overdosage are consistent with the effects seen with therapeutic doses of interferon alfa-2b. Hepatic enzyme abnormalities, renal failure, hemorrhage, and myocardial infarction have been reported with single administration overdoses and/or with longer durations of treatment than prescribed (see **ADVERSE REACTIONS**). Toxic effects after ingestion of interferon alfa-2b are not expected because interferons are poorly absorbed orally. Consultation with a poison center is recommended.

Treatment. There is no specific antidote for interferon alfa-2b. Hemodialysis and peritoneal dialysis are not considered effective for treatment of overdose.

HOW SUPPLIED

INTRON A Interferon alfa-2b, recombinant Powder for Injection INTRON A Interferon alfa-2b, recombinant Powder for Injection, 5 million IU per vial and Diluent for INTRON A Interferon alfa-2b, recombinant for Injection (bacteriostatic water for injection) 1 mL per vial; boxes containing 1 INTRON A vial and 1 vial of INTRON A Diluent (NDC 0085-0120-02).

INTRON A Interferon alfa-2b, recombinant Powder for Injection, 10 million IU per vial and Diluent for INTRON A Interferon alfa-2b, recombinant for Injection (bacteriostatic water for injection) 2 mL per vial; boxes containing 1 INTRON A vial and 1 vial of INTRON A Diluent (NDC 0085-0571-02).

INTRON A Interferon alfa-2b, recombinant Powder for Injection, 18 million IU per vial and Diluent for INTRON A Interferon alfa-2b, recombinant for Injection (bacteriostatic water for injection) 1 mL per vial; boxes containing 1 vial of INTRON A and 1 vial of INTRON A Diluent (NDC 0085-1110-01).

INTRON A Interferon alfa-2b, recombinant Powder for Injection, 25 million IU per vial and Diluent for INTRON A Interferon alfa-2b, recombinant for Injection (bacteriostatic water for injection) 5 mL per vial; boxes containing 1 INTRON A vial and 1 vial of INTRON A Diluent (NDC 0085-0285-02).

INTRON A Interferon alfa-2b, recombinant Powder for Injection, 50 million IU per vial and Diluent for INTRON A Interferon alfa-2b, recombinant for Injection (bacteriostatic water for injection) 1 mL per vial; boxes containing 1 INTRON A vial and 1 vial of INTRON A Diluent (NDC 0085-0539-01).

Store INTRON A Interferon alfa-2b, recombinant Powder for Injection both before and after reconstitution between 2° and 8°C (36° and 46°F).

Continued on next page

Information on Schering products appearing on these pages is effective as of June 2003.

Intron A—Cont.

INTRON A Interferon alfa-2b, recombinant Solution for Injection INTRON A Interferon alfa-2b, recombinant Solution for Injection, 6 doses of 3 million IU (18 million IU) multidose pen (22.5 million IU per 1.5 mL per pen); boxes containing 1 INTRON A multidose pen, six disposable needles and alcohol swabs (NDC 0085-1242-01).
INTRON A Interferon alfa-2b, recombinant Solution for Injection, 6 doses of 5 million IU (30 million IU) multidose pen (37.5 million IU per 1.5 mL per pen); boxes containing 1 INTRON A multidose pen, six disposable needles and alcohol swabs (NDC 0085-1235-01).
INTRON A Interferon alfa-2b, recombinant Solution for Injection, 6 doses of 10 million IU (60 million IU) multidose pen (75 million IU per 1.5 mL per pen); boxes containing 1 INTRON A multidose pen, six disposable needles and alcohol swabs (NDC 0085-1254-01).
INTRON A Interferon alfa-2b, recombinant Solution for Injection INTRON A, Pak-3, containing 6 INTRON A vials, 3 million IU per vial; 6 B-D Safety-Lok* syringes with a safety sleeve; and 6 alcohol swabs (NDC 0085-1184-02).
INTRON A Interferon alfa-2b, recombinant Solution for Injection INTRON A, Pak-5, containing 6 INTRON A vials, 5 million IU per vial; 6 B-D Safety-Lok* syringes with a safety sleeve; and 6 alcohol swabs (NDC 0085-1191-02).
INTRON A Interferon alfa-2b, recombinant Solution for Injection INTRON A, Pak-10, containing 6 INTRON A vials, 10 million IU per vial; 6 B-D Safety-Lok* syringes with a safety sleeve; and 6 alcohol swabs (NDC 0085-1179-02).
INTRON A Interferon alfa-2b, recombinant Solution for Injection, 18 million IU multidose vial (22.8 million IU per 3.8 mL per vial); boxes containing 1 vial of INTRON A Solution for Injection (NDC 0085-1168-01).
INTRON A Interferon alfa-2b, recombinant Solution for Injection, 25 million IU multidose vial (32 million IU per 3.2 mL per vial); boxes containing 1 vial of INTRON A Solution for Injection (NDC 0085-1133-01).
Store INTRON A Interferon alfa-2b, recombinant Solution for Injection between 2° and 8°C (36° and 46°F).
Rev. 6/02

*Safety-Lok is a registered trademark of Becton Dickinson and Company.
Schering Corporation
Kenilworth, NJ 07033 USA
B-24937623

REFERENCES

1. Smalley R, et al. *N Engl J Med.* 1992;327:1336-1341.
2. Aviles A, et al. *Leukemia and Lymphoma.* 1996;20:495-499.
3. Unterhalt M, et al. *Blood.* 1996;88 (10Suppl 1):1744A.
4. Schiller J, et al. *J Biol Response Mod.* 1989;8:252-261.
5. Poynard T, et al. *N Engl J Med.* 1995;332:(22)1457-1462.
6. Lin R, et al. *J Hepatol.* 1995;23:487-496.
7. Perrillo R, et al. *N Engl J Med.* 1990;323:295-301.
8. Perez V, et al. *J Hepatol.* 1990;11:S113-S117.
9. Knodell R, et al. *Hepatology.* 1981;1:431-435.
10. Perrillo R, et al. *Ann Intern Med.* 1991;115:113-115.
11. Renault P, et al. *Arch Intern Med.* 1987;147:1577-1580.
12. Kauppila A, et al. *Int J Cancer.* 1982;29:291-294.

NASONEX® ℞

[nā-sō-nĕks]
(mometasone furoate monohydrate)
Nasal Spray, 50 mcg*
FOR INTRANASAL USE ONLY
*calculated on the anhydrous basis

DESCRIPTION

Mometasone furoate monohydrate, the active component of NASONEX Nasal Spray, 50 mcg, is an anti-inflammatory corticosteroid having the chemical name, 9,21-Dichloro-11β,17-dihydroxy-16α-methylpregna-1,4-diene-3,20-dione 17-(2 furoate) monohydrate, and the following chemical structure:

Mometasone furoate monohydrate is a white powder, with an empirical formula of $C_{27}H_{30}Cl_2O_6 \cdot H_2O$, and a molecular weight of 539.45. It is practically insoluble in water; slightly soluble in methanol, ethanol, and isopropanol; soluble in acetone and chloroform; and freely soluble in tetrahydrofuran. Its partition coefficient between octanol and water is greater than 5000.
NASONEX Nasal Spray, 50 mcg is a metered-dose, manual pump spray unit containing an aqueous suspension of mometasone furoate monohydrate equivalent to 0.05% w/w mometasone furoate calculated on the anhydrous basis; in an aqueous medium containing glycerin, microcrystalline cellulose and carboxymethylcellulose sodium, sodium citrate, 0.25% w/w phenylethyl alcohol, citric acid, benzalkonium chloride, and polysorbate 80. The pH is between 4.3 and 4.9.
After initial priming (10 actuations), each actuation of the pump delivers a metered spray containing 100 mg of suspension containing mometasone furoate monohydrate equivalent to 50 mcg of mometasone furoate calculated on the anhydrous basis. Each bottle of NASONEX Nasal Spray, 50 mcg provides 120 sprays.

CLINICAL PHARMACOLOGY

NASONEX Nasal Spray, 50 mcg is a corticosteroid demonstrating anti-inflammatory properties. The precise mechanism of corticosteroid action on allergic rhinitis is not known. Corticosteroids have been shown to have a wide range of effects on multiple cell types (eg, mast cells, eosinophils, neutrophils, macrophages, and lymphocytes) and mediators (eg, histamine, eicosanoids, leukotrienes, and cytokines) involved in inflammation.
In two clinical studies utilizing nasal antigen challenge, NASONEX Nasal Spray, 50 mcg decreased some markers of the early- and late-phase allergic response. These observations included decreases (vs placebo) in histamine and eosinophil cationic protein levels, and reductions (vs baseline) in eosinophils, neutrophils, and epithelial cell adhesion proteins. The clinical significance of these findings is not known.
The effect of NASONEX Nasal Spray, 50 mcg on nasal mucosa following 12 months of treatment was examined in 46 patients with allergic rhinitis. There was no evidence of atrophy and there was a marked reduction in intraepithelial eosinophilia and inflammatory cell infiltration (eg, eosinophils, lymphocytes, monocytes, neutrophils, and plasma cells).
Pharmacokinetics: ***Absorption:*** Mometasone furoate monohydrate administered as a nasal spray is virtually undetectable in plasma from adult and pediatric subjects despite the use of a sensitive assay with a lower quantitation limit (LOQ) of 50 pcg/mL.
Distribution: The *in vitro* protein binding for mometasone furoate was reported to be 98% to 99% in concentration range of 5 to 500 ng/mL.
Metabolism: Studies have shown that any portion of a mometasone furoate dose which is swallowed and absorbed undergoes extensive metabolism to multiple metabolites. There are no major metabolites detectable in plasma. Upon *in vitro* incubation, one of the minor metabolites formed is 6β-hydroxy-mometasone furoate. In human liver microsomes, the formation of the metabolite is regulated by cytochrome P-450 3A4 (CYP3A4).
Elimination: Following intravenous administration, the effective plasma elimination half-life of mometasone furoate is 5.8 hours. Any absorbed drug is excreted as metabolites mostly via the bile, and to a limited extent, into the urine.
Special Populations: The effects of renal impairment, hepatic impairment, age, or gender on mometasone furoate pharmacokinetics have not been adequately investigated.
Pharmacodynamics: Three clinical pharmacology studies have been conducted in humans to assess the effect of NASONEX Nasal Spray, 50 mcg at various doses on adrenal function. In one study, daily doses of 200 and 400 mcg of NASONEX Nasal Spray, 50 mcg and 10 mg of prednisone were compared to placebo in 64 patients with allergic rhinitis. Adrenal function before and after 36 consecutive days of treatment was assessed by measuring plasma cortisol levels following a 6-hour Cortrosyn (ACTH) infusion and by measuring 24-hour urinary-free cortisol levels. NASONEX Nasal Spray, 50 mcg, at both the 200- and 400-mcg dose, was not associated with a statistically significant decrease in mean plasma cortisol levels post-Cortrosyn infusion or a statistically significant decrease in the 24-hour urinary-free cortisol levels compared to placebo. A statistically significant decrease in the mean plasma cortisol levels post-Cortrosyn infusion and 24-hour urinary-free cortisol levels was detected in the prednisone treatment group compared to placebo.
A second study assessed adrenal response to NASONEX Nasal Spray, 50 mcg (400 and 1600 mcg/day), prednisone (10 mg/day), and placebo, administered for 29 days in 48 male volunteers. The 24-hour plasma cortisol area under the curve (AUC_{0-24}), during and after an 8-hour Cortrosyn infusion and 24-hour urinary-free cortisol levels were determined at baseline and after 29 days of treatment. No statistically significant differences of adrenal function were observed with NASONEX Nasal Spray, 50 mcg compared to placebo.
A third study evaluated single, rising doses of NASONEX Nasal Spray, 50 mcg (1000, 2000, and 4000 mcg/day), orally administered mometasone furoate (2000, 4000, and 8000 mcg/day), orally administered dexamethasone (200, 400, and 800 mcg/day), and placebo (administered at the end of each series of doses) in 24 male volunteers. Dose administrations were separated by at least 72 hours. Determination of serial plasma cortisol levels at 8 AM and for the 24-hour period following each treatment were used to calculate the plasma cortisol area under the curve (AUC_{0-24}). In addition, 24-hour urinary-free cortisol levels were collected prior to initial treatment administration and during the period immediately following each dose. No statistically significant decreases in the plasma cortisol AUC, 8 AM cortisol levels, or 24-hour urinary-free cortisol levels were observed in volunteers treated with either NASONEX Nasal Spray, 50 mcg or oral mometasone, as compared with placebo treatment. Conversely, nearly all volunteers treated with the three doses of dexamethasone demonstrated abnormal 8 AM cortisol levels (defined as a cortisol level <10 mcg/dL), reduced 24-hour plasma AUC values, and decreased 24-hour urinary-free cortisol levels, as compared to placebo treatment.
Three clinical pharmacology studies have been conducted in pediatric patients to assess the effect of mometasone furoate nasal spray, on the adrenal function at daily doses of 50, 100, and 200 mcg vs placebo. In one study, adrenal function before and after 7 consecutive days of treatment was assessed in 48 pediatric patients with allergic rhinitis (ages 6 to 11 years) by measuring morning plasma cortisol and 24-hour urinary-free cortisol levels. Mometasone furoate nasal spray, at all three doses, was not associated with a statistically significant decrease in mean plasma cortisol levels or a statistically significant decrease in the 24-hour urinary-free cortisol levels compared to placebo. In the second study, adrenal function before and after 14 consecutive days of treatment was assessed in 48 pediatric patients (ages 3 to 5 years) with allergic rhinitis by measuring plasma cortisol levels following a 30-minute Cortrosyn infusion. Mometasone furoate nasal spray, 50 mcg, at all three doses (50, 100, and 200 mcg/day), was not associated with a statistically significant decrease in mean plasma cortisol levels post-Cortrosyn infusion compared to placebo. All patients had a normal response to Cortrosyn. In the third study, adrenal function before and after up to 42 consecutive days of once-daily treatment was assessed in 52 patients with allergic rhinitis (ages 2 to 5 years), 28 of whom received mometasone furoate nasal spray, 50 mcg per nostril (total daily dose 100 mcg), by measuring morning plasma cortisol and 24-hour urinary-free cortisol levels. Mometasone furoate nasal spray was not associated with a statistically significant decrease in mean plasma cortisol levels or a statistically significant decrease in the 24-hour urinary-free cortisol levels compared to placebo.
Clinical Studies: The efficacy and safety of NASONEX Nasal Spray, 50 mcg in the prophylaxis and treatment of seasonal allergic rhinitis and the treatment of perennial allergic rhinitis have been evaluated in 18 controlled trials, and one uncontrolled clinical trial, in approximately 3000 adults (ages 17 to 85 years) and adolescents (ages 12 to 16 years). This included 1757 males and 1453 females, including a total of 283 adolescents (182 boys and 101 girls) with seasonal allergic or perennial allergic rhinitis, treated with NASONEX Nasal Spray, 50 mcg at doses ranging from 50 to 800 mcg/day. The majority of patients were treated with 200 mcg/day. These trials evaluated the total nasal symptom scores that included stuffiness, rhinorrhea, itching, and sneezing. Patients treated with NASONEX Nasal Spray, 50 mcg, 200 mcg/day had a significant decrease in total nasal symptom scores compared to placebo-treated patients. No additional benefit was observed for mometasone furoate doses greater than 200 mcg/day. A total of 350 patients have been treated with NASONEX Nasal Spray, 50 mcg for 1 year or longer.
The efficacy and safety of NASONEX Nasal Spray, 50 mcg in the treatment of seasonal allergic and perennial allergic rhinitis in pediatric patients (ages 3 to 11 years) have been evaluated in four controlled trials. This included approximately 990 pediatric patients ages 3 to 11 years (606 males and 384 females) with seasonal allergic or perennial allergic rhinitis treated with mometasone furoate nasal spray at doses ranging from 25 to 200 mcg/day. Pediatric patients treated with NASONEX Nasal Spray, 50 mcg (100 mcg total daily dose, 374 patients) had a significant decrease in total nasal symptom (congestion, rhinorrhea, itching, and sneezing) scores, compared to placebo-treated patients. No additional benefit was observed for the 200-mcg mometasone furoate total daily dose in pediatric patients (ages 3 to 11 years). A total of 163 pediatric patients have been treated for 1 year.
In patients with seasonal allergic rhinitis, NASONEX Nasal Spray, 50 mcg, demonstrated improvement in nasal symptoms (vs placebo) within 11 hours after the first dose based on one single-dose, parallel-group study of patients in an outdoor "park" setting (park study) and one environmental exposure unit (EEU) study, and within 2 days in two randomized, double-blind, placebo-controlled, parallel-group seasonal allergic rhinitis studies. Maximum benefit is usually achieved within 1 to 2 weeks after initiation of dosing.
Prophylaxis of seasonal allergic rhinitis for patients 12 years of age and older with NASONEX Nasal Spray, 50 mcg, given at a dose of 200 mcg/day, was evaluated in two clinical studies in 284 patients. These studies were designed such that patients received 4 weeks of prophylaxis with NASONEX Nasal Spray, 50 mcg prior to the anticipated onset of the pollen season; however, some patients received only 2 to 3 weeks of prophylaxis. Patients receiving 2 to 4 weeks of prophylaxis with NASONEX Nasal Spray, 50 mcg demonstrated a statistically significantly smaller mean increase in total nasal symptom scores with onset of the pollen season as compared to placebo patients.

INDICATIONS AND USAGE

NASONEX Nasal Spray, 50 mcg is indicated for the treatment of the nasal symptoms of seasonal allergic and perennial allergic rhinitis, in adults and pediatric patients 2 years of age and older. NASONEX Nasal Spray, 50 mcg is indicated for the prophylaxis of the nasal symptoms of seasonal allergic rhinitis in adult and adolescent patients 12 years and older. In patients with a known seasonal allergen that precipitates nasal symptoms of seasonal allergic rhinitis, initiation of prophylaxis with NASONEX Nasal Spray, 50 mcg is recommended 2 to 4 weeks prior to the anticipated start of the pollen season. Safety and effectiveness of NASONEX Nasal Spray, 50 mcg in pediatric patients less than 2 years of age have not been established.

CONTRAINDICATIONS

Hypersensitivity to any of the ingredients of this preparation contraindicates its use.

WARNINGS

The replacement of a systemic corticosteroid with a topical corticosteroid can be accompanied by signs of adrenal insufficiency and, in addition, some patients may experience symptoms of withdrawal; ie, joint and/or muscular pain, lassitude, and depression. Careful attention must be given when patients previously treated for prolonged periods with systemic corticosteroids are transferred to topical corticosteroids, with careful monitoring for acute adrenal insufficiency in response to stress. This is particularly important in those patients who have associated asthma or other clinical conditions where too rapid a decrease in systemic corticosteroid dosing may cause a severe exacerbation of their symptoms.

If recommended doses of intranasal corticosteroids are exceeded or if individuals are particularly sensitive or predisposed by virtue of recent systemic steroid therapy, symptoms of hypercorticism may occur, including very rare cases of menstrual irregularities, acneiform lesions, and cushingoid features. If such changes occur, topical corticosteroids should be discontinued slowly, consistent with accepted procedures for discontinuing oral steroid therapy.

Persons who are on drugs which suppress the immune system are more susceptible to infections than healthy individuals. Chickenpox and measles, for example, can have a more serious or even fatal course in nonimmune children or adults on corticosteroids. In such children or adults who have not had these diseases, particular care should be taken to avoid exposure. How the dose, route, and duration of corticosteroid administration affects the risk of developing a disseminated infection is not known. The contribution of the underlying disease and/or prior corticosteroid treatment to the risk is also not known. If exposed to chickenpox, prophylaxis with varicella zoster immune globin (VZIG) may be indicated. If exposed to measles, prophylaxis with pooled intramuscular immunoglobulin (IG) may be indicated. (See the respective package inserts for complete VZIG and IG prescribing information.) If chickenpox develops, treatment with antiviral agents may be considered.

PRECAUTIONS

General: Intranasal corticosteroids may cause a reduction in growth velocity when administered to pediatric patients (see **PRECAUTIONS, Pediatric Use** section). In clinical studies with NASONEX Nasal Spray, 50 mcg, the development of localized infections of the nose and pharynx with *Candida albicans* has occurred only rarely. When such an infection develops, use of NASONEX Nasal Spray, 50 mcg should be discontinued and appropriate local or systemic therapy instituted, if needed.

Nasal corticosteroids should be used with caution, if at all, in patients with active or quiescent tuberculous infection of the respiratory tract, or in untreated fungal, bacterial, systemic viral infections, or ocular herpes simplex.

Rarely, immediate hypersensitivity reactions may occur after the intranasal administration of mometasone furoate monohydrate. Extremely rare instances of wheezing have been reported.

Rare instances of nasal septum perforation and increased intraocular pressure have also been reported following the intranasal application of aerosolized corticosteroids. As with any long-term topical treatment of the nasal cavity, patients using NASONEX Nasal Spray, 50 mcg over several months or longer should be examined periodically for possible changes in the nasal mucosa.

Because of the inhibitory effect of corticosteroids on wound healing, patients who have experienced recent nasal septum ulcers, nasal surgery, or nasal trauma should not use a nasal corticosteroid until healing has occurred.

Glaucoma and cataract formation was evaluated in one controlled study of 12 weeks' duration and one uncontrolled study of 12 months' duration in patients treated with NASONEX Nasal Spray, 50 mcg at 200 mcg/day, using intraocular pressure measurements and slit lamp examination. No significant change from baseline was noted in the mean intraocular pressure measurements for the 141 NASONEX-treated patients in the 12-week study, as compared with 141 placebo-treated patients. No individual NASONEX-treated patient was noted to have developed a significant elevation in intraocular pressure or cataracts in this 12-week study. Likewise, no significant change from baseline was noted in the mean intraocular pressure measurements for the 139 NASONEX-treated patients in the 12-month study and again, no cataracts were detected in these patients. Nonetheless, nasal and inhaled corticosteroids have been associated with the development of glaucoma and/or cataracts. Therefore, close follow-up is warranted in patients with a change in vision and with a history of glaucoma and/or cataracts.

When nasal corticosteroids are used at excessive doses, systemic corticosteroid effects such as hypercorticism and adrenal suppression may appear. If such changes occur, NASONEX Nasal Spray, 50 mcg should be discontinued slowly, consistent with accepted procedures for discontinuing oral steroid therapy.

Information for Patients: Patients being treated with NASONEX Nasal Spray, 50 mcg should be given the following information and instructions. This information is intended to aid in the safe and effective use of this medication. It is not a disclosure of all intended or possible adverse effects. Patients should use NASONEX Nasal Spray, 50 mcg at regular intervals (once daily) since its effectiveness depends on regular use. Improvement in nasal symptoms of allergic rhinitis has been shown to occur within 11 hours after the first dose based on one single-dose, parallel-group study of patients in an outdoor "park" setting (park study) and one environmental exposure unit (EEU) study and within 2 days after the first dose in two randomized, double-blind, placebo-controlled, parallel-group seasonal allergic rhinitis studies. Maximum benefit is usually achieved within 1 to 2 weeks after initiation of dosing. Patients should take the medication as directed and should not increase the prescribed dosage by using it more than once a day in an attempt to increase its effectiveness. Patients should contact their physician if symptoms do not improve, or if the condition worsens. To assure proper use of this nasal spray, and to attain maximum benefit, patients should read and follow the accompanying Patient's Instructions for Use carefully. Administration to young children should be aided by an adult.

Patients should be cautioned not to spray NASONEX Nasal Spray, 50 mcg into the eyes or directly onto the nasal septum.

Persons who are on immunosuppressant doses of corticosteroids should be warned to avoid exposure to chickenpox or measles, and patients should also be advised that if they are exposed, medical advice should be sought without delay.

Carcinogenesis, Mutagenesis, Impairment of Fertility: In a 2-year carcinogenicity study in Sprague Dawley rats, mometasone furoate demonstrated no statistically significant increase in the incidence of tumors at inhalation doses up to 67 mcg/kg (approximately 3 and 2 times the maximum recommended daily intranasal dose in adults and children, respectively, on a mcg/m^2 basis). In a 19-month carcinogenicity study in Swiss CD-1 mice, mometasone furoate demonstrated no statistically significant increase in the incidence of tumors at inhalation doses up to 160 mcg/kg (approximately 3 and 2 times the maximum recommended daily intranasal dose in adults and children, respectively, on a mcg/m^2 basis).

Mometasone furoate increased chromosomal aberrations in an *in vitro* Chinese hamster ovary-cell assay, but did not increase chromosomal aberrations in an *in vitro* Chinese hamster lung cell assay. Mometasone furoate was not mutagenic in the Ames test or mouse-lymphoma assay, and was not clastogenic in an *in vivo* mouse micronucleus assay and a rat bone marrow chromosomal aberration assay or a mouse male germ-cell chromosomal aberration assay. Mometasone furoate also did not induce unscheduled DNA synthesis *in vivo* in rat hepatocytes.

In reproductive studies in rats, impairment of fertility was not produced by subcutaneous doses up to 15 mcg/kg (less than the maximum recommended daily intranasal dose in adults on a mcg/m^2 basis).

Pregnancy: ***Teratogenic Effects: Pregnancy Category C:*** When administered to pregnant mice, rats, and rabbits, mometasone furoate increased fetal malformations. The doses that produced malformations also decreased fetal growth, as measured by lower fetal weights and/or delayed ossification. Mometasone furoate also caused dystocia and related complications when administered to rats during the end of pregnancy.

In mice, mometasone furoate caused cleft palate at subcutaneous doses of 60 mcg/kg and above (approximately equivalent to the maximum recommended daily intranasal dose in adults on a mcg/m^2 basis). Fetal survival was reduced at 180 mcg/kg (approximately 4 times the maximum recommended daily intranasal dose in adults on a mcg/m^2 basis). No toxicity was observed at 20 mcg/kg (less than the maximum recommended daily intranasal dose in adults on a mcg/m^2 basis).

In rats, mometasone furoate produced umbilical hernia at topical dermal doses of 600 mcg/kg and above (approximately 25 times the maximum recommended daily intranasal dose in adults on a mcg/m^2 basis). A dose of 300 mcg/kg (approximately 10 times the maximum recommended daily intranasal dose in adults on a mcg/m^2 basis) produced delays in ossification, but no malformations.

In rabbits, mometasone furoate caused multiple malformations (eg, flexed front paws, gallbladder agenesis, umbilical hernia, hydrocephaly) at topical dermal doses of 150 mcg/kg and above (approximately 10 times the maximum recommended daily intranasal dose in adults on a mcg/m^2 basis). In an oral study, mometasone furoate increased resorptions and caused cleft palate and/or head malformations (hydrocephaly or domed head) at 700 mcg/kg (approximately 55 times the maximum recommended daily intranasal dose in adults on a mcg/m^2 basis). At 2800 mcg/kg (approximately 230 times the maximum recommended daily intranasal dose in adults on a mcg/m^2 basis), most litters were aborted or resorbed. No toxicity was observed at 140 mcg/kg (approximately 10 times the maximum recommended daily intranasal dose in adults on a mcg/m^2 basis).

When rats received subcutaneous doses of mometasone furoate throughout pregnancy or during the later stages of pregnancy, 15 mcg/kg (less than the maximum recommended daily intranasal dose in adults on a mcg/m^2 basis) caused prolonged and difficult labor and reduced the number of live births, birth weight, and early pup survival. Similar effects were not observed at 7.5 mcg/kg (less than the maximum recommended daily intranasal dose in adults on a mcg/m^2 basis).

There are no adequate and well-controlled studies in pregnant women. NASONEX Nasal Spray, 50 mcg, like other corticosteroids, should be used during pregnancy only if the potential benefits justify the potential risk to the fetus. Experience with oral corticosteroids since their introduction in pharmacologic, as opposed to physiologic, doses suggests that rodents are more prone to teratogenic effects from corticosteroids than humans. In addition, because there is a natural increase in corticosteroid production during pregnancy, most women will require a lower exogenous corticosteroid dose and many will not need corticosteroid treatment during pregnancy.

Nonteratogenic Effects: Hypoadrenalism may occur in infants born to women receiving corticosteroids during pregnancy. Such infants should be carefully monitored.

Nursing Mothers: It is not known if mometasone furoate is excreted in human milk. Because other corticosteroids are excreted in human milk, caution should be used when NASONEX Nasal Spray, 50 mcg is administered to nursing women.

Pediatric Use: Controlled clinical studies have shown intranasal corticosteroids may cause a reduction in growth velocity in pediatric patients. This effect has been observed in the absence of laboratory evidence of hypothalamic-pituitary-adrenal (HPA) axis suppression, suggesting that growth velocity is a more sensitive indicator of systemic corticosteroid exposure in pediatric patients than some commonly used tests of HPA axis function. The long-term effects of this reduction in growth velocity associated with intranasal corticosteroids, including the impact on final adult height, are unknown. The potential for "catch up" growth following discontinuation of treatment with intranasal corticosteroids has not been adequately studied. The growth of pediatric patients receiving intranasal corticosteroids, including NASONEX Nasal Spray, 50 mcg should be monitored routinely (eg, via stadiometry). The potential growth effects of prolonged treatment should be weighed against clinical benefits obtained and the availability of safe and effective noncorticosteroid treatment alternatives. To minimize the systemic effects of intranasal corticosteroids, including NASONEX Nasal Spray, 50 mcg, each patient should be titrated to his/her lowest effective dose.

Seven hundred and twenty (720) patients 3 to 11 years of age were treated with mometasone furoate nasal spray, 50 mcg (100 mcg total daily dose) in controlled clinical trials (see **CLINICAL PHARMACOLOGY, Clinical Studies** section). Twenty-eight (28) patients 2 to 5 years of age were treated with mometasone furoate nasal spray, 50 mcg (100 mcg total daily dose) in a controlled trial to evaluate safety (see **CLINICAL PHARMACOLOGY, Pharmacokinetics** section). Safety and effectiveness in children less than 2 years of age have not been established.

A clinical study has been conducted for 1 year in pediatric patients (ages 3 to 9 years) to assess the effect of NASONEX Nasal Spray, 50 mcg (100 mcg total daily dose) on growth velocity. No statistically significant effect on growth velocity was observed for NASONEX Nasal Spray, 50 mcg compared to placebo. No evidence of clinically relevant HPA axis suppression was observed following a 30-minute cosyntropin infusion.

The potential of NASONEX Nasal Spray, 50 mcg to cause growth suppression in susceptible patients or when given at higher doses cannot be ruled out.

Geriatric Use: A total of 203 patients above 64 years of age (age range 64 to 85 years) have been treated with NASONEX Nasal Spray, 50 mcg for up to 3 months. The adverse reactions reported in this population were similar in type and incidence to those reported by younger patients.

ADVERSE REACTIONS

In controlled US and international clinical studies, a total of 3210 adult and adolescent patients ages 12 years and older received treatment with NASONEX Nasal Spray, 50 mcg at doses of 50 to 800 mcg/day. The majority of patients (n = 2103) were treated with 200 mcg/day. In controlled US and international studies, a total of 990 pediatric patients (ages 3 to 11 years) received treatment with NASONEX Nasal Spray, 50 mcg, at doses of 25 to 200 mcg/day. The majority of pediatric patients (720) were treated with 100 mcg/day. A total of 513 adult, adolescent, and pediatric patients have been treated for 1 year or longer. The overall incidence of adverse events for patients treated with NASONEX Nasal Spray, 50 mcg was comparable to patients treated with the vehicle placebo. Also, adverse events did not differ significantly based on age, sex, or race. Three percent or less of patients in clinical trials discontinued treatment because of adverse events; this rate was similar for the vehicle and active comparators.

All adverse events (regardless of relationship to treatment) reported by 5% or more of adult and adolescent patients ages 12 years and older who received NASONEX Nasal Spray, 50 mcg, 200 mcg/day and by pediatric patients ages 3 to 11 years who received NASONEX Nasal Spray, 50 mcg, 100 mcg/day in clinical trials vs placebo and that were more common with NASONEX Nasal Spray, 50 mcg than placebo, are displayed in the table below.

Continued on next page

Information on Schering products appearing on these pages is effective as of June 2003.

ADVERSE EVENTS FROM CONTROLLED CLINICAL TRIALS IN SEASONAL ALLERGIC AND PERENNIAL ALLERGIC RHINITIS (PERCENT OF PATIENTS REPORTING)

	Adult and Adolescent Patients 12 years and older		Pediatric Patients Ages 3 to 11 years	
	NASONEX 200 mcg (n = 2103)	VEHICLE PLACEBO (n = 1671)	NASONEX 100 mcg (n = 374)	VEHICLE PLACEBO (n = 376)
Headache	26	22	17	18
Viral Infection	14	11	8	9
Pharyngitis	12	10	10	10
Epistaxis/Blood-Tinged Mucus	11	6	8	9
Coughing	7	6	13	15
Upper Respiratory Tract Infection	6	2	5	4
Dysmenorrhea	5	3	1	0
Musculoskeletal Pain	5	3	1	1
Sinusitis	5	3	4	4
Vomiting	1	1	5	4

Nasonex—Cont.

[See table above]

Other adverse events which occurred in less than 5% but greater than or equal to 2% of mometasone furoate adult and adolescent patients (ages 12 years and older) treated with 200-mcg doses (regardless of relationship to treatment), and more frequently than in the placebo group included: arthralgia, asthma, bronchitis, chest pain, conjunctivitis, diarrhea, dyspepsia, earache, flu-like symptoms, myalgia, nausea, and rhinitis.

Other adverse events which occurred in less than 5% but greater than or equal to 2% of mometasone furoate pediatric patients ages 3 to 11 years treated with 100-mcg doses vs placebo (regardless of relationship to treatment) and more frequently than in the placebo group included: diarrhea, nasal irritation, otitis media, and wheezing.

The adverse event (regardless of relationship to treatment) reported by 5% of pediatric patients ages 2 to 5 years who received NASONEX Nasal Spray, 50 mcg, 100 mcg/day in a clinical trial vs placebo including 56 subjects (28 each NASONEX Nasal Spray, 50 mcg and placebo) and that was more common with NASONEX Nasal Spray, 50 mcg than placebo, included: upper respiratory tract infection (7% vs 0%, respectively). The other adverse event which occurred in less than 5% but greater than or equal to 2% of mometasone furoate pediatric patients ages 2 to 5 years treated with 100-mcg doses vs placebo (regardless of relationship to treatment) and more frequently than in the placebo group included: skin trauma.

Rare cases of nasal ulcers and nasal and oral candidiasis were also reported in patients treated with NASONEX Nasal Spray, 50 mcg, primarily in patients treated for longer than 4 weeks.

In postmarketing surveillance of this product, cases of nasal burning and irritation, anaphylaxis and angioedema, and rare cases of nasal septal perforation have been reported. Disturbances of taste and smell have been reported very rarely.

OVERDOSAGE

There are no data available on the effects of acute or chronic overdosage with NASONEX Nasal Spray, 50 mcg. Because of low systemic bioavailability, and an absence of acute drug-related systemic findings in clinical studies, overdose is unlikely to require any therapy other than observation. Intranasal administration of 1600 mcg (8 times the recommended dose of NASONEX Nasal Spray, 50 mcg) daily for 29 days, to healthy human volunteers, was well tolerated with no increased incidence of adverse events. Single intranasal doses up to 4000 mcg have been studied in human volunteers with no adverse effects reported. Single oral doses up to 8000 mcg have been studied in human volunteers with no adverse effects reported. Chronic overdosage with any corticosteroid may result in signs or symptoms of hypercorticism (see **PRECAUTIONS**). Acute overdosage with this dosage form is unlikely since one bottle of NASONEX Nasal Spray, 50 mcg contains approximately 8500 mcg of mometasone furoate.

DOSAGE AND ADMINISTRATION

Adults and Children 12 Years of Age and Older: The usual recommended dose for prophylaxis and treatment of the nasal symptoms of seasonal allergic rhinitis and treatment of the nasal symptoms of perennial allergic rhinitis is two sprays (50 mcg of mometasone furoate in each spray) in each nostril once daily (total daily dose of 200 mcg).

In patients with a known seasonal allergen that precipitates nasal symptoms of seasonal allergic rhinitis, prophylaxis with NASONEX Nasal Spray, 50 mcg (200 mcg/day) is recommended 2 to 4 weeks prior to the anticipated start of the pollen season.

Children 2 to 11 Years of Age: The usual recommended dose for treatment of the nasal symptoms of seasonal allergic and perennial allergic rhinitis is one spray (50 mcg of mometasone furoate in each spray) in each nostril once daily (total daily dose of 100 mcg).

Improvement in nasal symptoms of allergic rhinitis has been shown to occur within 11 hours after the first dose based on one single-dose, parallel-group study of patients in an outdoor "park" setting (park study) and one environmental exposure unit (EEU) study and within 2 days after the first dose in two randomized, double-blind, placebo-controlled, parallel-group seasonal allergic rhinitis studies. Maximum benefit is usually achieved within 1 to 2 weeks. Patients should use NASONEX Nasal Spray, 50 mcg only once daily at a regular interval.

Prior to initial use of NASONEX Nasal Spray, 50 mcg, the pump must be primed by actuating ten times or until a fine spray appears. The pump may be stored unused for up to 1 week without repriming. If unused for more than 1 week, reprime by actuating two times, or until a fine spray appears.

Directions for Use: Illustrated Patient's Instructions for Use accompany each package of NASONEX Nasal Spray, 50 mcg.

Directions for Cleaning: Illustrated Applicator Cleaning Instructions accompany each package of NASONEX Nasal Spray, 50 mcg.

HOW SUPPLIED

NASONEX (mometasone furoate monohydrate) Nasal Spray, 50 mcg is supplied in a white, high-density, polyethylene bottle fitted with a white metered-dose, manual spray pump, and teal-green cap. It contains 17 g of product formulation, 120 sprays, each delivering 50 mcg of mometasone furoate per actuation. Supplied with Patient's Instructions for Use (NDC 0085-1197-01).

Store at 25°C (77°F); excursions permitted to 15-30°C (59-86°F) [see USP Controlled Room Temperature]. Protect from light.

When NASONEX Nasal Spray, 50 mcg is removed from its cardboard container, prolonged exposure of the product to direct light should be avoided. Brief exposure to light, as with normal use, is acceptable.

SHAKE WELL BEFORE EACH USE.

Schering Corporation
Kenilworth, NJ 07033 USA

 Rev. 6/03

U.S. Patent No. D355,844

26405246T

PEG-INTRON® ℞

[pĕg ĭn-trŏn]

(Peginterferon alfa-2b)
Powder for Injection

Alpha interferons, including PEG-Intron, may cause or aggravate fatal or life-threatening neuropsychiatric, autoimmune, ischemic, and infectious disorders. Patients should be monitored closely with periodic clinical and laboratory evaluations. Patients with persistently severe or worsening signs or symptoms of these conditions should be withdrawn from therapy. In many but not all cases these disorders resolve after stopping PEG-Intron therapy. See WARNINGS, ADVERSE REACTIONS.

Use with Ribavirin. Ribavirin may cause birth defects and/or death of the unborn child. Extreme care must be taken to avoid pregnancy in female patients and in female partners of male patients. Ribavirin causes hemolytic anemia. The anemia associated with REBETOL therapy may result in a worsening of cardiac disease. Ribavirin is genotoxic and mutagenic and should be considered a potential carcinogen. (See REBETOL package insert for additional information and other warnings).

DESCRIPTION

PEG-Intron®, peginterferon alfa-2b, Powder for Injection is a covalent conjugate of recombinant alfa-2b interferon with monomethoxypolyethylene glycol (PEG). The average molecular weight of the PEG portion of the molecule is 12,000 daltons. The average molecular weight of the PEG-Intron molecule is approximately 31,000 daltons. The specific activity of peginterferon alfa-2b is approximately 0.7×10^8 IU/mg protein.

Interferon alfa-2b, is a water-soluble protein with a molecular weight of 19,271 daltons produced by recombinant DNA techniques. It is obtained from the bacterial fermentation of a strain of *Escherichia coli* bearing a genetically engineered plasmid containing an interferon gene from human leukocytes.

PEG-Intron is supplied in both vials and the Redipen™ for subcutaneous use.

Vials

Each vial contains either 74 µg, 118.4 µg, 177.6 µg, or 222 µg of PEG-Intron as a white to off-white tablet-like solid, that is whole/in pieces or as a loose powder, and 1.11 mg dibasic sodium phosphate anhydrous, 1.11 mg monobasic sodium phosphate dihydrate, 59.2 mg sucrose and 0.074 mg polysorbate 80. Following reconstitution with 0.7 mL of the supplied Sterile Water for Injection, USP, each vial contains PEG-Intron at strengths of either 50 µg per 0.5 mL, 80 µg per 0.5 mL, 120 µg per 0.5 mL, or 150 µg per 0.5 mL.

Redipen™

Redipen™ is a dual-chamber glass cartridge containing lyophilized PEG-Intron as a white to off-white tablet or powder that is whole or in pieces in the sterile active chamber and a second chamber containing Sterile Water for Injection, USP. Each PEG-Intron Redipen™ contains either 67.5 µg, 108 µg, 162 µg, or 202.5 µg of PEG-Intron, and 1.013 mg dibasic sodium phosphate anhydrous, 1.013 mg monobasic sodium phosphate dihydrate, 54 mg sucrose and 0.0675 mg polysorbate 80. Each cartridge is reconstituted to allow for the administration of up to 0.5 mL of solution. Following reconstitution, each Redipen™ contains PEG-Intron at strengths of either 50 µg per 0.5 mL, 80 µg per 0.5 mL, 120 µg per 0.5 mL, or 150 µg per 0.5 mL for a single use. Because a small volume of reconstituted solution is lost during preparation of PEG-Intron, each Redipen™ contains an excess amount of PEG-Intron powder and diluent to ensure delivery of the labeled dose.

CLINICAL PHARMACOLOGY

General: The biological activity of PEG-Intron is derived from its interferon alfa-2b moiety. Interferons exert their cellular activities by binding to specific membrane receptors on the cell surface and initiate a complex sequence of intracellular events. These include the induction of certain enzymes, suppression of cell proliferation, immunomodulating activities such as enhancement of the phagocytic activity of macrophages and augmentation of the specific cytotoxicity of lymphocytes for target cells, and inhibition of virus replication in virus-infected cells. Interferon alfa upregulates the Th1 T-helper cell subset in *in vitro* studies. The clinical relevance of these findings is not known.

Pharmacodynamics: PEG-Intron raises concentrations of effector proteins such as serum neopterin and 2′5′ oligoadenylate synthetase, raises body temperature, and causes reversible decreases in leukocyte and platelet counts. The correlation between the *in vitro* and *in vivo* pharmacologic and pharmacodynamic and clinical effects is unknown.

Pharmacokinetics: Following a single subcutaneous (SC) dose of PEG-Intron, the mean absorption half-life (t ½ k_a) was 4.6 hours. Maximal serum concentrations (C_{max}) occur between 15–44 hours post-dose, and are sustained for up to 48–72 hours. The C_{max} and AUC measurements of PEG-Intron increase in a dose-related manner. After multiple dosing, there is an increase in bioavailability of PEG-Intron. Week 48 mean trough concentrations (320 pg/mL; range 0, 2960) are approximately 3-fold higher than Week 4 mean trough concentrations (94 pg/mL; range 0, 416). The mean PEG-Intron elimination half-life is approximately 40 hours (range 22 to 60 hours) in patients with HCV infection. The apparent clearance of PEG-Intron is estimated to be approximately 22.0 mL/hr•kg. Renal elimination accounts for 30% of the clearance. Single dose peginterferon alfa-2b pharmacokinetics following a subcutaneous 1.0 µg/kg dose suggest the clearance of peginterferon alfa-2b is reduced by approximately half in subjects with impaired renal function (creatinine clearance <50 mL/minute).

Pegylation of interferon alfa-2b produces a product (PEG-Intron) whose clearance is lower than that of non-pegylated interferon alfa-2b. When compared to INTRON A, PEG-Intron (1.0 µg/kg) has approximately a seven-fold lower mean apparent clearance and a five-fold greater mean half-life permitting a reduced dosing frequency. At effective therapeutic doses, PEG-Intron has approximately ten-fold greater C_{max} and 50-fold greater AUC than interferon alfa-2b.

The pharmacokinetics of geriatric subjects (>65 years of age) treated with a single subcutaneous dose of 1.0 µg/kg of PEG-Intron were similar in C_{max}, AUC, clearance, or elimination half-life as compared to younger subjects (28 to 44 years of age).

During the 48 week treatment period with PEG-Intron, no differences in the pharmacokinetic profiles were observed between male and female patients with chronic hepatitis C infection.

Effect of Food on Absorption of Ribavirin Both AUC_{tf} and C_{max} increased by 70% when REBETOL Capsules were administered with a high-fat meal (841 kcal, 53.8 g fat, 31.6 g protein, and 57.4 g carbohydrate) in a single-dose pharmacokinetic study. (See **DOSAGE AND ADMINISTRATION**).

Drug Interactions: It is not known if PEG-Intron therapy causes clinically significant drug-drug interactions with drugs metabolized by the liver in patients with hepatitis C. In 12 healthy subjects known to be CYP2D6 extensive metabolizers, a single subcutaneous dose of 1 μg/kg PEG-Intron did not inhibit CYP1A2, 2C8/9, 2D6, hepatic 3A4 or N-acetyltransferase; the effects of PEG-Intron on CYP2C19 were not assessed.

CLINICAL STUDIES

PEG-Intron Monotherapy-Study 1

A randomized study compared treatment with PEG-Intron (0.5, 1.0, or 1.5 μg/kg once weekly SC) to treatment with INTRON A, (3 million units three times weekly SC) in 1219 adults with chronic hepatitis from HCV infection. The patients were not previously treated with interferon alfa, had compensated liver disease, detectable HCV RNA, elevated ALT, and liver histopathology consistent with chronic hepatitis. Patients were treated for 48 weeks and were followed for 24 weeks post-treatment. Seventy percent of all patients were infected with HCV genotype 1, and 74 percent of all patients had high baseline levels of HCV RNA (more than 2 million copies per mL of serum), two factors known to predict poor response to treatment.

Response to treatment was defined as undetectable HCV RNA and normalization of ALT at 24 weeks posttreatment. The response rates to the 1.0 and 1.5 μg/kg PEG-Intron doses were similar (approximately 24%) to each other and were both higher than the response rate to INTRON A (12%). (See **Table 1**)

[See table 1 above]

TABLE 1. Rates of Response to Treatment-Study 1

	A PEG-Intron 0.5 μg/kg (N=315)	B PEG-Intron 1.0 μg/kg (N=298)	C INTRON A 3 MIU TIW (N=307)	B-C (95% CI) Difference between PEG-Intron 1.0 μg/kg and INTRON A
Treatment Response (Combined Virologic Response and ALT Normalization)	17%	24%	12%	11 (5, 18)
Virologic Response[a]	18%	25%	12%	12 (6, 19)
ALT Normalization	24%	29%	18%	11 (5, 18)

[a]Serum HCV is measured by a research-based quantitative polymerase chain reaction assay by a central laboratory.

Patients with both viral genotype 1 and high serum levels of HCV RNA at baseline were less likely to respond to treatment with PEG-Intron. Among patients with the two unfavorable prognostic variables, 8% (12/157) responded to PEG-Intron treatment and 2% (4/169) responded to INTRON A. Doses of PEG-Intron higher than the recommended dose did not result in higher response rates in these patients.

Patients receiving PEG-Intron with viral genotype 1 had a response rate of 14% (28/199) while patients with other viral genotypes had a 45% (43/96) response rate.

Ninety-six percent of the responders in the PEG-Intron groups and 100% of responders in the INTRON A group first cleared their viral RNA by week-24 of treatment. See **DOSAGE AND ADMINISTRATION**.

The treatment response rates were similar in men and women. Response rates were lower in African American and Hispanic patients and higher in Asians compared to Caucasians. Although African Americans had a higher proportion of poor prognostic factors compared to Caucasians the number of non-Caucasians studied (9% of the total) was insufficient to allow meaningful conclusions about differences in response rates after adjusting for prognostic factors.

Liver biopsies were obtained before and after treatment in 60% of patients. A modest reduction in inflammation compared to baseline that was similar in all four treatment groups was observed.

PEG-Intron/REBETOL Combination Therapy-Study 2

A randomized study compared treatment with two PEG-Intron/REBETOL regimens [PEG-Intron 1.5 μg/kg SC once weekly (QW)/REBETOL 800 mg PO daily (in divided doses); PEG-Intron 1.5 μg/kg SC QW for 4 weeks then 0.5 μg/kg SC QW for 44 weeks/REBETOL 1000/1200 mg PO daily (in divided doses)] with INTRON A [3 MIU SC thrice weekly (TIW)/REBETOL 1000/1200 mg PO daily (in divided doses)] in 1530 adults with chronic hepatitis C. Interferon naïve patients were treated for 48 weeks and followed for 24 weeks posttreatment. Eligible patients had compensated liver disease, detectable HCV RNA, elevated ALT, and liver histopathology consistent with chronic hepatitis.

Response to treatment was defined as undetectable HCV RNA at 24 weeks posttreatment. The response rate to the PEG-Intron 1.5 μg/kg plus ribavirin 800 mg dose was higher than the response rate to INTRON A/REBETOL (See **Table 2**). The response rate to PEG-Intron 1.5 → 0.5 μg/kg/REBETOL was essentially the same as the response to INTRON A/REBETOL (data not shown).

[See table 2 above]

TABLE 2. Rates of Response to Treatment-Study 2

	PEG-Intron 1.5 μg/kg QW REBETOL 800 mg QD	INTRON A 3 MIU TIW REBETOL 1000/1200 mg QD
Overall[1,2] response	52% (264/511)	46% (231/505)
Genotype 1	41% (141/348)	33% (112/343)
Genotype 2-6	75% (123/163)	73% (119/162)

[1]Serum HCV RNA is measured with a research-based quantitative polymerase chain reaction assay by a central laboratory.
[2]Difference in overall treatment response (PEG-Intron/REBETOL vs. INTRON A/REBETOL) is 6% with 95% confidence interval of (0.18, 11.63) adjusted for viral genotype and presence of cirrhosis at baseline.

Patients with viral genotype 1, regardless of viral load, had a lower response rate to PEG-Intron (1.5 μg/kg)/REBETOL compared to patients with other viral genotypes. Patients with both poor prognostic factors (genotype 1 and high viral load) had a response rate of 30% (78/256) compared to a response rate of 29% (71/247) with INTRON A/REBETOL.

Patients with lower body weight tended to have higher adverse event rates (see **ADVERSE REACTIONS**) and higher response rates than patients with higher body weights. Differences in response rates between treatment arms did not substantially vary with body weight.

Treatment response rates with PEG-Intron/REBETOL were 49% in men and 56% in women. Response rates were lower in African American and Hispanic patients and higher in Asians compared to Caucasians. Although African Americans had a higher proportion of poor prognostic factors compared to Caucasians the number of non-Caucasians studied (11% of the total) was insufficient to allow meaningful conclusions about differences in response rates after adjusting for prognostic factors.

Liver biopsies were obtained before and after treatment in 68% of patients. Compared to baseline approximately 2/3 of patients in all treatment groups were observed to have a modest reduction in inflammation.

INDICATIONS AND USAGE

PEG-Intron, peginterferon alfa-2b, is indicated for use alone or in combination with REBETOL (ribavirin, USP) for the treatment of chronic hepatitis C in patients with compensated liver disease who have not been previously treated with interferon alpha and are at least 18 years of age.

CONTRAINDICATIONS

PEG-Intron is contraindicated in patients with:

- hypersensitivity to PEG-Intron or any other component of the product
- autoimmune hepatitis
- decompensated liver disease

PEG-Intron/REBETOL combination therapy is additionally contraindicated in:

- patients with hypersensitivity to ribavirin or any other component of the product
- women who are pregnant
- men whose female partners are pregnant
- patients with hemoglobinopathies (e.g., thalassemia major, sickle-cell anemia)

WARNINGS

Patients should be monitored for the following serious conditions, some of which may become life threatening. Patients with persistently severe or worsening signs or symptoms should be withdrawn from therapy.

Neuropsychiatric events

Life-threatening or fatal neuropsychiatric events, including suicide, suicidal and homicidal ideation, depression, relapse of drug addiction/overdose, and aggressive behavior have occurred in patients with and without a previous psychiatric disorder during PEG-Intron treatment and follow-up. Psychoses, hallucinations, bipolar disorders, and mania have been observed in patients treated with alpha interferons. PEG-Intron should be used with extreme caution in patients with a history of psychiatric disorders. Patients should be advised to report immediately any symptoms of depression and/or suicidal ideation to their prescribing physicians. Physicians should monitor all patients for evidence of depression and other psychiatric symptoms. In severe cases, PEG-Intron should be stopped immediately and psychiatric intervention instituted. (See **DOSAGE AND ADMINISTRATION: Dose Reduction.**)

Bone marrow toxicity

PEG-Intron suppresses bone marrow function, sometimes resulting in severe cytopenias. PEG-Intron should be discontinued in patients who develop severe decreases in neutrophil or platelet counts. (See **DOSAGE AND ADMINISTRATION: Dose Reduction**). Ribavirin may potentiate the neutropenia induced by interferon alpha. Very rarely alpha interferons may be associated with aplastic anemia.

Endocrine disorders

PEG-Intron causes or aggravates hypothyroidism and hyperthyroidism. Hyperglycemia has been observed in patients treated with PEG-Intron. Diabetes mellitus has been observed in patients treated with alpha interferons. Patients with these conditions who cannot be effectively treated by medication should not begin PEG-Intron therapy. Patients who develop these conditions during treatment and cannot be controlled with medication should not continue PEG-Intron therapy.

Cardiovascular events

Cardiovascular events, which include hypotension, arrhythmia, tachycardia, cardiomyopathy, angina pectoris, and myocardial infarction, have been observed in patients treated with PEG-Intron. PEG-Intron should be used cautiously in patients with cardiovascular disease. Patients with a history of myocardial infarction and arrhythmic disorder who require PEG-Intron therapy should be closely monitored (see **Laboratory Tests**). Patients with a history of significant or unstable cardiac disease should not be treated with PEG-Intron/REBETOL combination therapy. [See **REBETOL package insert.**]

Pulmonary disorders

Dyspnea, pulmonary infiltrates, pneumonia, bronchiolitis obliterans, interstitial pneumonitis and sarcoidosis some resulting in respiratory failure and/or patient deaths, may be induced or aggravated by PEG-Intron or alpha interferon therapy. Recurrence of respiratory failure has been observed with interferon rechallenge. PEG-Intron combination treatment should be suspended in patients who develop pulmonary infiltrates or pulmonary function impairment. Patients who resume interferon treatment should be closely monitored.

Colitis

Fatal and nonfatal ulcerative or hemorrhagic/ischemic colitis have been observed within 12 weeks of the start of alpha interferon treatment. Abdominal pain, bloody diarrhea, and fever are the typical manifestations. PEG-Intron treatment should be discontinued immediately in patients who develop these symptoms and signs. The colitis usually resolves within 1–3 weeks of discontinuation of alpha interferons.

Pancreatitis

Fatal and nonfatal pancreatitis have been observed in patients treated with alpha interferon. PEG-Intron therapy should be suspended in patients with signs and symptoms suggestive of pancreatitis and discontinued in patients diagnosed with pancreatitis.

Autoimmune disorders

Development or exacerbation of autoimmune disorders (e.g. thyroiditis, thrombocytopenia, rheumatoid arthritis, interstitial nephritis, systemic lupus erythematosus, psoriasis) have been observed in patients receiving PEG-Intron. PEG-Intron should be used with caution in patients with autoimmune disorders.

Ophthalmologic disorders

Decrease or loss of vision, retinopathy including macular edema, retinal artery or vein thrombosis, retinal hemorrhages and cotton wool spots, optic neuritis, and papilledema may be induced or aggravated by treatment with peginterferon alfa-2b or other alpha interferons. All patients should receive an eye examination at baseline. Patients with preexisting ophthalmologic disorders (e.g. diabetic or hypertensive retinopathy) should receive periodic ophthalmologic exams during interferon alpha treatment. Any patient who develops ocular symptoms should receive a prompt and complete eye examination. Peginterferon alfa-2b treatment should be discontinued in patients who develop new or worsening ophthalmologic disorders.

Hypersensitivity

Serious, acute hypersensitivity reactions (e.g., urticaria, angioedema, bronchoconstriction, anaphylaxis) have been rarely observed during alpha interferon therapy. If such a reaction develops during treatment with PEG-Intron, dis-

Continued on next page

Information on Schering products appearing on these pages is effective as of June 2003.

PEG-Intron—Cont.

continue treatment and institute appropriate medical therapy immediately. Transient rashes do not necessitate interruption of treatment.

Use with Ribavirin-(See also REBETOL Package Insert)

REBETOL may cause birth defects and/or death of the unborn child. REBETOL therapy should not be started until a report of a negative pregnancy test has been obtained immediately prior to planned initiation of therapy. Patients should use at least two forms of contraception and have monthly pregnancy tests (See BOXED WARNING, CONTRAINDICATIONS and PRECAUTIONS: Information for Patients and REBETOL package insert).

Anemia

Ribavirin caused hemolytic anemia in 10% of PEG-Intron/REBETOL treated patients within 1–4 weeks of initiation of therapy. Complete blood counts should be obtained pretreatment and at week 2 and week 4 of therapy or more frequently if clinically indicated. Anemia associated with REBETOL therapy may result in a worsening of cardiac disease. Decrease in dosage or discontinuation of REBETOL may be necessary. (See **DOSAGE AND ADMINISTRATION: Dose Reduction.**)

PRECAUTIONS

- PEG-Intron alone or in combination with REBETOL has not been studied in patients who have failed other alpha interferon treatments.
- The safety and efficacy of PEG-Intron alone or in combination with REBETOL for the treatment of hepatitis C in liver or other organ transplant recipients have not been studied. Preliminary data indicates that interferon alpha therapy may be associated with an increased rate of kidney graft rejection. Liver graft rejection has also been reported but a causal association to interferon alpha therapy has not been established.
- The safety and efficacy of PEG-Intron/REBETOL for the treatment of patients with HCV co-infected with HIV or HBV have not been established.

Triglycerides: Elevated triglyceride levels have been observed in patients treated with interferons including PEG-Intron therapy. Elevated triglyceride levels should be managed as clinically appropriate. Hypertriglyceridemia may result in pancreatitis. Discontinuation of PEG-Intron therapy should be considered for patients with persistently elevated triglycerides (eg, triglycerides >1000 mg/dL) associated with symptoms of potential pancreatitis, such as abdominal pain, nausea, or vomiting.

Patients with renal failure: Increases in serum creatinine levels have been observed in patients with renal insufficiency treated with interferons, including PEG-Intron. Patients with impairment of renal function should be closely monitored for signs and symptoms of interferon toxicity, including increases in serum creatinine, and doses of PEG-Intron should be adjusted accordingly. PEG-Intron should be used with caution in patients with creatinine clearance <50 mL/min; in considering these patients for PEG-Intron therapy, the potential risks must be evaluated against the potential benefits of treatment. REBETOL must not be used in patients with creatinine clearance <50 mL/min. (See **DOSAGE AND ADMINISTRATION: Dose Reduction**).

Information for Patients: Patients receiving PEG-Intron alone or in combination with REBETOL should be directed in its appropriate use, informed of the benefits and risks associated with treatment, and referred to the **MEDICATION GUIDES for PEG-Intron and, if applicable, REBETOL (ribavirin, USP).**

Patients must be informed that REBETOL may cause birth defects and/or death of the unborn child. Extreme care must be taken to avoid pregnancy in female patients and in female partners of male patients during treatment with combination PEG-Intron/REBETOL therapy and for 6 months post-therapy. Combination PEG-Intron/REBETOL therapy should not be initiated until a report of a negative pregnancy test has been obtained immediately prior to initiation of therapy. It is recommended that patients undergo monthly pregnancy tests during therapy and for 6 months post-therapy. **(See CONTRAINDICATIONS and REBETOL package insert).**

Patients should be informed that there are no data regarding whether PEG-Intron therapy will prevent transmission of HCV infection to others. Also, it is not known if treatment with PEG-Intron will cure hepatitis C or prevent cirrhosis, liver failure, or liver cancer that may be the result of infection with the hepatitis C virus.

Patients should be advised that laboratory evaluations are required before starting therapy and periodically thereafter (see **Laboratory Tests**). It is advised that patients be well hydrated, especially during the initial stages of treatment. "Flu-like" symptoms associated with administration of PEG-Intron may be minimized by bedtime administration of PEG-Intron or by use of antipyretics.

Patients should be advised to use a puncture-resistant container for the disposal of used syringes, needles, and the Redipen™. The full container should be disposed of in accordance with state and local laws. Patients should be thoroughly instructed in the importance of proper disposal. Patients should also be cautioned against reusing or sharing needles, syringes, or the Redipen™.

Laboratory Tests: PEG-Intron alone or in combination with ribavirin may cause severe decreases in neutrophil and platelet counts, and hematologic, endocrine (e.g. TSH) and hepatic abnormalities. Transient elevations in ALT (2–5 fold above baseline) were observed in 10% of patients treated with PEG-Intron, and was not associated with deterioration of other liver functions.

Patients on PEG-Intron or PEG-Intron/REBETOL combination therapy should have hematology and blood chemistry testing before the start of treatment and then periodically thereafter. In the clinical trial CBC (including hemoglobin, neutrophil and platelet counts) and chemistries (including AST, ALT, bilirubin, and uric acid) were measured during the treatment period at weeks 2, 4, 8, 12, and then at 6-week intervals or more frequently if abnormalities developed. TSH levels were measured every 12 weeks during the treatment period.

HCV RNA should be measured at 6 months of treatment. PEG-Intron or PEG-Intron/REBETOL combination therapy should be discontinued in patients with persistent high viral levels.

Patients who have pre-existing cardiac abnormalities should have electrocardiograms administered before treatment with PEG-Intron/REBETOL.

Carcinogenesis, Mutagenesis, and Impairment of Fertility

Carcinogenesis and Mutagenesis: PEG-Intron has not been tested for its carcinogenic potential. Neither PEG-Intron, nor its components interferon or methoxypolyethylene glycol caused damage to DNA when tested in the standard battery of mutagenesis assays, in the presence and absence of metabolic activation.

Use with Ribavirin: Ribavirin is genotoxic and mutagenic and should be considered a potential carcinogen. See REBETOL package insert for additional warnings relevant to PEG-Intron therapy in combination with ribavirin.

Impairment of Fertility: PEG-Intron may impair human fertility. Irregular menstrual cycles were observed in female cynomolgus monkeys given subcutaneous injections of 4239 µg/m^2 PEG-Intron alone every other day for one month, (approximately 345 times the recommended weekly human dose based upon body surface area). These effects included transiently decreased serum levels of estradiol and progesterone, suggestive of anovulation. Normal menstrual cycles and serum hormone levels resumed in these animals 2 to 3 months following cessation of PEG-Intron treatment. Every other day dosing with 262 µg/m^2 (approximately 21 times the weekly human dose) had no effects on cycle duration or reproductive hormone status. The effects of PEG-Intron on male fertility have not been studied.

Pregnancy Category C: PEG-Intron monotherapy: Non-pegylated Interferon alfa-2b, has been shown to have abortifacient effects in *Macaca mulatta* (rhesus monkeys) at 15 and 30 million IU/kg (estimated human equivalent of 5 and 10 million IU/kg, based on body surface area adjustment for a 60 kg adult). PEG-Intron should be assumed to also have abortifacient potential. There are no adequate and well-controlled studies in pregnant women. PEG-Intron therapy is to be used during pregnancy only if the potential benefit justifies the potential risk to the fetus. Therefore, PEG-Intron is recommended for use in fertile women only when they are using effective contraception during the treatment period.

Nursing Mothers: It is not known whether the components of PEG-Intron are excreted in human milk. Because of the potential for adverse reactions from the drug in nursing infants, a decision must be made whether to discontinue nursing or discontinue the treatment, taking into account the importance of the product to the mother.

Pregnancy Category X: Use with Ribavirin

Significant teratogenic and/or embryocidal effects have been demonstrated in all animal species exposed to ribavirin. REBETOL therapy is contraindicated in women who are pregnant and in the male partners of women who are pregnant. See CONTRAINDICATIONS and the REBETOL Package Insert.

If pregnancy occurs in a patient or partner of a patient during treatment with PEG-Intron and REBETOL during the 6 months after treatment cessation, physicians should report such cases by calling (800) 727-7064.

Pediatric. Safety and effectiveness in pediatric patients below the age of 18 years have not been established.

Geriatric. In general, younger patients tend to respond better than older patients to interferon-based therapies. Clinical studies of PEG-Intron alone or in combination with REBETOL did not include sufficient numbers of subjects aged 65 and over, however, to determine whether they respond differently than younger subjects. Treatment with alpha interferons, including PEG-Intron, is associated with neuropsychiatric, cardiac, pulmonary, GI and systemic (flu-like) adverse effects. Because these adverse reactions may be more severe in the elderly, caution should be exercised in use of PEG-Intron in this population. This drug is known to be substantially excreted by the kidney. Because elderly patients are more likely to have decreased renal function, the risk of toxic reactions to this drug may be greater in patients with impaired renal function. REBETOL should not be used in patients with creatinine clearance <50 mL/min. When using PEG-Intron/REBETOL therapy, refer also to the REBETOL Medication Guide.

ADVERSE REACTIONS

Nearly all study patients in clinical trials experienced one or more adverse events. In the PEG monotherapy trial the incidence of serious adverse events was similar (about 12%) in all treatment groups. In the PEG-Intron/REBETOL combination trial the incidence of serious adverse events was 17% in the PEG-Intron/REBETOL groups compared to 14% in the INTRON A/REBETOL group.

In many but not all cases, adverse events resolved after dose reduction or discontinuation of therapy. Some patients experienced ongoing or new serious adverse events during the 6-month follow-up period. In the PEG-Intron/REBETOL trial 13 patients experienced life-threatening psychiatric events (suicidal ideation or attempt) and one patient accomplished suicide.

There have been five patient deaths which occurred in clinical trials: one suicide in a patient receiving PEG-Intron monotherapy and one suicide in a patient receiving PEG-Intron/REBETOL combination therapy; two deaths among patients receiving INTRON A monotherapy (1 murder/suicide and 1 sudden death) and one patient death in the INTRON A/REBETOL group (motor vehicle accident).

Overall 10–14% of patients receiving PEG-Intron, alone or in combination with REBETOL, discontinued therapy compared with 6% treated with INTRON A alone and 13% treated with INTRON A in combination with REBETOL. The most common reasons for discontinuation of therapy were related to psychiatric, systemic (e.g. fatigue, headache), or gastrointestinal adverse events.

In the combination therapy trial, dose reductions due to adverse reactions occurred in 42% of patients receiving PEG-Intron (1.5 µg/kg)/REBETOL and in 34% of those receiving INTRON A/REBETOL. The majority of patients (57%) weighing 60 kg or less receiving PEG-Intron (1.5 µg/kg)/REBETOL required dose reduction. Reduction of interferon was dose related (PEG-Intron 1.5 µg/kg >PEG-Intron 0.5 µg/kg or INTRON A), 40%, 27%, 28%, respectively. Dose reduction for REBETOL was similar across all three groups, 33–35%. The most common reasons for dose modifications were neutropenia (18%), or anemia (9%). (see **Laboratory Values**). Other common reasons included depression, fatigue, nausea, and thrombocytopenia.

In the PEG-Intron/REBETOL combination trial the most common adverse events were psychiatric which occurred among 77% of patients and included most commonly depression, irritability, and insomnia, each reported by approximately 30-40% of subjects in all treatment groups. Suicidal behavior (ideation, attempts, and suicides) occurred in 2% of all patients during treatment or during follow-up after treatment cessation (see **WARNINGS**).

PEG-Intron induced fatigue or headache in approximately two-thirds of patients, and induced fever or rigors in approximately half of the patients. The severity of some of these systemic symptoms (e.g. fever and headache) tended to decrease as treatment continues. The incidence tends to be higher with PEG-Intron than with INTRON A therapy alone or in combination with REBETOL.

Application site inflammation and reaction (e.g. bruise, itchiness, irritation) occurred at approximately twice the incidence with PEG-Intron therapies (in up to 75% of patients) compared with INTRON A. However injection site pain was infrequent (2–3%) in all groups.

Other common adverse events in the PEG-Intron/REBETOL group included myalgia (56%), arthralgia (34%), nausea (43%), anorexia (32%), weight loss (29%), alopecia (36%), and pruritus (29%).

In the PEG-Intron monotherapy trial the incidence of severe adverse events was 13% in the INTRON A group and 17% in the PEG-Intron groups. In the PEG-Intron/REBETOL combination therapy trial the incidence of severe adverse events was 23% in the INTRON A/REBETOL group and 31–34% in the PEG-Intron/REBETOL groups. The incidence of life-threatening adverse events was ≤1% across all groups in the monotherapy and combination therapy trials.

Adverse events that occurred in the clinical trial at >5% incidence are provided in **Table 3** by treatment group. Due to potential differences in ascertainment procedures, adverse event rate comparisons across studies should not be made.

[See table 3 on next page]

Many patients continued to experience adverse events several months after discontinuation of therapy. By the end of the 6-month follow-up period the incidence of ongoing adverse events by body class in the PEG-Intron 1.5/REBETOL group was 33% (psychiatric), 20% (musculoskeletal), and 10% (for endocrine and for GI). In approximately 10–15% of patients weight loss, fatigue and headache had not resolved.

Individual serious adverse events occurred at a frequency ≤1% and included suicide attempt, suicidal ideation, severe depression; psychosis, aggressive reaction, relapse of drug addiction/overdose; nerve palsy (facial, oculomotor); cardiomyopathy, myocardial infarction, angina, pericardial effusion, retinal ischemia, retinal artery or vein thrombosis, blindness, decreased visual acuity, optic neuritis, transient ischemic attack, supraventricular arrhythmias, loss of consciousness; neutropenia, infection (sepsis, pneumonia, abscess, cellulitis); emphysema, bronchiolitis obliterans, pleural effusion, gastroenteritis, pancreatitis, gout, hyperglycemia, hyperthyroidism and hypothyroidism, autoimmune thrombocytopenia with or without purpura, rheumatoid arthritis, interstitial nephritis, lupus-like syndrome, sarcoidosis, aggravated psoriasis; urticaria, injection-site necrosis, vasculitis, phototoxicity.

Laboratory Values

Changes in selected laboratory values during treatment with PEG-Intron alone or in combination with REBETOL treatment are described below. **Decreases in hemoglobin, neutrophils, and platelets may require dose reduction or permanent discontinuation from therapy. (See DOSAGE AND ADMINISTRATION-Dose Reduction)**

Hemoglobin. REBETOL induced a decrease in hemoglobin levels in approximately two thirds of patients. Hemoglobin levels decreased to <11 g/dL in about 30% of patients. Severe anemia (<8 g/dL) occurred in <1% of patients. Dose modification was required in 9 and 13% of patients in the PEG-Intron/REBETOL and INTRON A/REBETOL groups. Hemoglobin levels become stable by treatment week 4–6 on average. Hemoglobin levels return to baseline between 4 and 12 weeks posttreatment. In the PEG-Intron monotherapy trial hemoglobin decreases were generally mild and dose modifications were rarely necessary. **(See DOSAGE AND ADMINISTRATION: Dose Reduction).**

Neutrophils. Decreases in neutrophil counts were observed in a majority of patients treated with PEG-Intron alone (70%) or as combination therapy with REBETOL (85%) and INTRON A/REBETOL (60%). Severe potentially life-threatening neutropenia (<0.5 × 10^9/L) occurred in 1% of patients treated with PEG-Intron monotherapy, 2% of patients treated with INTRON A/REBETOL and in 4% of patients treated with PEG-Intron/REBETOL. Two percent of patients receiving PEG-Intron monotherapy and 18% of patients receiving PEG-Intron/REBETOL required modification of interferon dosage. Few patients (≤1%) required permanent discontinuation of treatment. Neutrophil counts generally return to pre-treatment levels within 4 weeks of cessation of therapy. **(See DOSAGE AND ADMINISTRATION: Dose Reduction).**

Platelets. Platelet counts decrease in approximately 20% of patients treated with PEG-Intron alone or with REBETOL and in 6% of patients treated with INTRON A/REBETOL. Severe decreases in platelet counts (<50,000/mm^3) occur in <1% of patients. Patients may require discontinuation or dose modification as a result of platelet decreases. **(See DOSAGE AND ADMINISTRATION: Dose Reduction).** In the PEG-Intron/REBETOL combination therapy trial 1% or 3% of patients required dose modification of INTRON A or PEG-Intron respectively. Platelet counts generally returned to pretreatment levels within 4 weeks of the cessation of therapy.

Thyroid Function. Development of TSH abnormalities, with and without clinical manifestations, are associated with interferon therapies. Clinically apparent thyroid disorders occur among patients treated with either INTRON A or PEG-Intron (with or without REBETOL) at a similar incidence (5% for hypothyroidism and 3% for hyperthyroidism). Subjects developed new onset TSH abnormalities while on treatment and during the follow-up period. At the end of the follow-up period 7% of subjects still had abnormal TSH values.

Bilirubin and uric acid. In the PEG-Intron/REBETOL trial 10–14% of patients developed hyperbilirubinemia and 33–38% developed hyperuricemia in association with hemolysis. Six patients developed mild to moderate gout.

Postmarketing Experience

The following adverse reactions have been identified and reported during post-approval use of PEG-Intron therapy: seizures, hearing impairment, hearing loss, and peripheral neuropathy, cardiac ischemia, rhabdomyolysis, stomatitis, vertigo, renal insufficiency, renal failure, Stevens Johnson Syndrome, toxic epidermal necrolysis, and erythema multiforme. Because the reports of these reactions are voluntary and the population of uncertain size, it is not always possible to reliably estimate the frequency of the reaction or establish a causal relationship to drug exposure.

Immunogenicity: Approximately 2% of patients receiving PEG-Intron (32/1759) or INTRON A (11/728) with or without REBETOL developed low-titer (≤160) neutralizing antibodies to PEG-Intron or INTRON A. The clinical and pathological significance of the appearance of serum neutralizing antibodies is unknown. No apparent correlation of antibody development to clinical response or adverse events was observed. The incidence of post-treatment binding antibody ranged from 8 to 15 percent. The data reflect the percentage of patients whose test results were considered positive for antibodies to PEG-Intron in a Biacore assay that is used to measure binding antibodies, and in an antiviral neutralization assay, which measures serum-neutralizing antibodies. The percentage of patients whose test results were considered positive for antibodies is highly dependent on the sensitivity and specificity of the assays. Additionally the observed incidence of antibody positivity in these assays may be influenced by several factors including sample timing and handling, concomitant medications, and underlying disease. For these reasons, comparison of the incidence of antibodies to PEG-Intron with the incidence of antibodies to other products may be misleading.

TABLE 3. Adverse Events Occurring in >5% of Patients

	*Percentage of Patients Reporting Adverse Events**			
	Study 1		Study 2	
Adverse Events	**PEG-Intron 1.0 µg/kg (n=297)**	**INTRON A 3 MIU (n=303)**	**PEG-Intron 1.5 µg/kg/ REBETOL (n=511)**	**INTRON A/ REBETOL (n=505)**
Application Site				
Injection Site Inflammation/Reaction	47	20	75	49
Autonomic Nervous Sys.				
Mouth Dry	6	7	12	8
Sweating Increased	6	7	11	7
Flushing	6	3	4	3
Body as a Whole				
Fatigue/Asthenia	52	54	66	63
Headache	56	52	62	58
Rigors	23	19	48	41
Fever	22	12	46	33
Weight Decrease	11	13	29	20
RUQ Pain	8	8	12	6
Chest Pain	6	4	8	7
Malaise	7	6	4	6
Central/Periph. Nerv. Sys.				
Dizziness	12	10	21	17
Endocrine Disorders				
Hypothyroidism	5	3	5	4
Gastrointestinal				
Nausea	26	20	43	33
Anorexia	20	17	32	27
Diarrhea	18	16	22	17
Vomiting	7	6	14	12
Abdominal Pain	15	11	13	13
Dyspepsia	6	7	9	8
Constipation	1	3	5	5
Hematologic Disorders				
Neutropenia	6	2	26	14
Anemia	0	0	12	17
Leukopenia	<1	0	6	5
Thrombocytopenia	7	<1	5	2
Liver and Biliary System				
Hepatomegaly	6	5	4	4
Musculoskeletal				
Myalgia	54	53	56	50
Arthralgia	23	27	34	28
Musculoskeletal Pain	28	22	21	19
Psychiatric				
Insomnia	23	23	40	41
Depression	29	25	31	34
Anxiety/Emotional Lability/Irritability	28	34	47	47
Concentration Impaired	10	8	17	21
Agitation	2	2	8	5
Nervousness	4	3	6	6
Reproductive, Female				
Menstrual Disorder	4	3	7	6
Resistance Mechanism				
Infection Viral	11	10	12	12
Infection Fungal	<1	3	6	1
Respiratory System				
Dyspnea	4	2	26	24
Coughing	8	5	23	16
Pharyngitis	10	7	12	13
Rhinitis	2	2	8	6
Sinusitis	7	7	6	5
Skin and Appendages				
Alopecia	22	22	36	32
Pruritus	12	8	29	28
Rash	6	7	24	23
Skin Dry	11	9	24	23
Special Senses Other,				
Taste Perversion	<1	2	9	4
Vision Disorders				
Vision blurred	2	3	5	6
Conjunctivitis	4	2	4	5

* Patients reporting one or more adverse events. A patient may have reported more than one adverse event within a body system/organ class category.

OVERDOSAGE

There is limited experience with overdosage. In the clinical studies, a few patients accidentally received a dose greater than that prescribed. There were no instances in which a participant in the monotherapy or combination therapy trials received more than 10.5 times the intended dose of PEG-Intron. The maximum dose received by any patient was 3.45 µg/kg weekly over a period of approximately 12 weeks. The maximum known overdosage of REBETOL was an intentional ingestion of 10 g (fifty 200 mg capsules). There were no serious reactions attributed to these overdosages. In cases of overdosing, symptomatic treatment and close observation of the patient are recommended.

DOSAGE AND ADMINISTRATION

There are no safety and efficacy data on treatment for longer than one year. A patient should self-inject PEG-Intron only if the physician determines that it is appropriate and the patient agrees to medical follow-up as necessary and training in proper injection technique has been given to him/her. (See illustrated **MEDICATION GUIDE** for instructions.)

Continued on next page

Information on Schering products appearing on these pages is effective as of June 2003.

PEG-Intron—Cont.

It is recommended that patients receiving PEG-Intron, alone or in combination with ribavirin, be discontinued from therapy if HCV viral levels remain high after 6 months of therapy.

PEG-Intron Monotherapy

The recommended dose of PEG-Intron regimen is 1.0 µg/kg/week subcutaneously for one year. The dose should be administered on the same day of the week.

The volume of PEG-Intron to be injected depends on the patient weight (see **Table 4** below).

[See table 4 at right]

PEG-Intron/REBETOL Combination Therapy

When administered in combination with REBETOL, the recommended dose of PEG-Intron is 1.5 micrograms/kg/week. The volume of PEG-Intron to be injected depends on the strength of PEG-Intron and patient's body weight. (See **Table 5** below).

[See table 5 at right]

The recommended dose of REBETOL is 800 mg/day in 2 divided doses: two capsules (400 mg) with breakfast and two capsules (400 mg) with dinner. REBETOL should not be used in patients with creatinine clearance <50 mL/min.

Dose Reduction

If a serious adverse reaction develops during the course of treatment (See **WARNINGS**) discontinue or modify the dosage of PEG-Intron and/or REBETOL until the adverse event abates or decreases in severity. If persistent or recurrent serious adverse events develop despite adequate dosage adjustment, discontinue treatment. For guidelines for dose modifications and discontinuation based on laboratory parameters, see **Tables 6 and 7**. In the combination therapy trial dose reductions occurred among 42% of patients receiving PEG-Intron 1.5 µg/kg/REBETOL 800 mg daily including 57% of those patients weighing 60 kg or less (see **ADVERSE REACTIONS**).

[See table 6 at right]
[See table 7 at right]

Preparation and Administration

PEG-Intron Redipen™

PEG-Intron Redipen™ consists of a dual-chamber glass cartridge with sterile, lyophilized peginterferon alfa-2b in the active chamber and Sterile Water for Injection, USP in the diluent chamber. The PEG-Intron in the glass cartridge should appear as a white to off-white tablet shaped solid that is whole or in pieces, or powder. To reconstitute the lyophilized peginterferon alfa-2b in the Redipen™, hold the Redipen™ upright (dose button down) and press the two halves of the pen together until there is an audible click. Gently invert the pen to mix the solution. DO NOT SHAKE. The reconstituted solution has a concentration of either 50 µg per 0.5 mL, 80 µg per 0.5 mL, 120 µg per 0.5 mL, or 150 µg per 0.5 mL for a single subcutaneous injection. Visually inspect the solution for particulate matter and discoloration prior to administration. The reconstituted solution should be clear and colorless. Do not use if the solution is discolored or cloudy, or if particulates are present.

Keeping the pen upright, attach the supplied needle and select the appropriate PEG-Intron dose by pulling back on the dosing button until the dark bands are visible and turning the button until the dark band is aligned with the correct dose. The prepared PEG-Intron solution is to be injected subcutaneously.

The PEG-Intron Redipen™ is a single use pen and does not contain a preservative. The reconstituted solution should be used immediately and cannot be stored for more than 24 hours at 2°–8°C (See **Storage**). **DO NOT REUSE THE REDIPEN™.** The sterility of any remaining product can no longer be guaranteed. **DISCARD THE UNUSED PORTION.** Pooling of unused portions of some medications has been linked to bacterial contamination and morbidity.

PEG-Intron Vials

Two B-D Safety-Lok™ syringes are provided in the package; one syringe is for the reconstitution steps and one for the patient injection. There is a plastic safety sleeve to be pulled over the needle after use. The syringe locks with an audible click when the green stripe on the safety sleeve covers the red stripe on the needle. Instructions for the preparation and administration of PEG-Intron Powder for Injection are provided below.

Reconstitute the PEG-Intron lyophilized product with only 0.7 mL of 1 mL of supplied diluent (Sterile Water for Injection, USP). **The diluent vial is for single use only. The remaining diluent should be discarded.** No other medications should be added to solutions containing PEG-Intron, and PEG-Intron should not be reconstituted with other diluents. Swirl gently to hasten complete dissolution of the powder. The reconstituted solution should be clear and colorless. Visually inspect the solution for particulate matter and discoloration prior to administration. The solution should not be used if discolored or cloudy, or if particulates are present.

The appropriate PEG-Intron dose should be withdrawn and injected subcutaneously. PEG-Intron vials are for single use only and do not contain a preservative. The reconstituted solution should be used immediately and cannot be stored for more than 24 hours at 2°–8°C (See **Storage**). **DO NOT REUSE THE VIAL.** The sterility of any remaining product can no longer be guaranteed. **DISCARD THE UNUSED PORTION.** Pooling of unused portions of some medications has been linked to bacterial contamination and morbidity.

After preparation and administration of the PEG-Intron for injection, it is essential to follow the state and or local procedures for proper disposal of syringes, needles, and the Redipen™. A puncture-resistant container should be used for disposal. Patients should be instructed in how to properly dispose of used syringes, needles, or the Redipen™ and be cautioned against the reuse of these items.

Storage

PEG-Intron Redipen™

PEG-Intron Redipen™ should be stored at 2° to 8°C (36° to 46°F). After reconstitution, the solution should be used immediately, but may be stored up to 24 hours at 2° to 8°C (36° to 46°F). The reconstituted solution contains no preservative, and is clear and colorless. **DO NOT FREEZE.**

PEG-Intron Vials

PEG-Intron should be stored at 25°C (77°F); excursions permitted to 15–30°C (59–86°F) [see USP Controlled Room Temperature]. After reconstitution with supplied Diluent the solution should be used immediately, but may be stored up to 24 hours at 2° to 8°C (36° to 46°F). The reconstituted solution contains no preservative, is clear and colorless. **DO NOT FREEZE.**

HOW SUPPLIED

PEG-Intron Redipen™

PEG-Intron Redipen™ contains a dual-chamber glass cartridge with a white to off-white lyophilized powder active

TABLE 4. Recommended PEG-Intron Monotherapy Dosing

Body weight (kg)	PEG-Intron Redipen™ or Vial Strength to Use	Amount of PEG-Intron (µg) to Administer	Volume (mL)* of PEG-Intron to Administer
≤45 46–56	50 µg per 0.5 mL	40 50	0.4 0.5
57–72 73–88	80 µg per 0.5 mL	64 80	0.4 0.5
89–106 107–136	120 µg per 0.5 mL	96 120	0.4 0.5
137–160	150 µg per 0.5 mL	150	0.5

* When reconstituted as directed

TABLE 5. Recommended PEG-Intron Combination Therapy Dosing

Body weight (kg)	PEG-Intron Redipen™ or Vial Strength to Use	Amount of PEG-Intron (µg) to Administer	Volume (mL)* of PEG-Intron to Administer
<40	50 µg per 0.5 mL	50	0.5
40–50 51–60	80 µg per 0.5 mL	64 80	0.4 0.5
61–75 76–85	120 µg per 0.5 mL	96 120	0.4 0.5
>85	150 µg per 0.5 mL	150	0.5

* When reconstituted as directed

TABLE 6. Guidelines for Modification or Discontinuation of PEG-Intron or PEG-Intron/REBETOL and for Scheduling Visits for Patients with Depression

Depression Severity[1]	Initial Management (4–8 wks)		Depression		
	Dose modification	Visit schedule	Remains stable	Improves	Worsens
Mild	No change	Evaluate once weekly by visit and/or phone.	Continue weekly visit schedule.	Resume normal visit schedule.	(See moderate or severe depression)
Moderate	Decrease IFN dose 50%	Evaluate once weekly (office visit at least every other week).	Consider psychiatric consultation. Continue reduced dosing.	If symptoms improve and are stable for 4 wks, may resume normal visit schedule. Continue reducing dosing or return to normal dose.	(See severe depression)
Severe	Discontinue IFN/R permanently.	Obtain immediate psychiatric consultation.	Psychiatric therapy necessary		

[1]See DSM-IV for definitions

TABLE 7. Guidelines for Dose Modification and Discontinuation of PEG-Intron or PEG-Intron/REBETOL for Hematologic Toxicity

Laboratory Values		PEG-Intron	REBETOL
Hgb*	<10.0 g/dL <8.5 g/dL	------------------------- Permanently discontinue	Decrease by 200 mg/day Permanently discontinue
WBC	$<1.5 \times 10^9$/L $<1.0 \times 10^9$/L	Reduce dose by 50% Permanently discontinue	------------------------- Permanently discontinue
Neutrophils	$<0.75 \times 10^9$/L $<0.5 \times 10^9$/L	Reduce dose by 50% Permanently discontinue	------------------------- Permanently discontinue
Platelets	$<80 \times 10^9$/L $<50 \times 10^9$/L	Reduce dose by 50% Permanently discontinue	------------------------- Permanently discontinue

* For patients with a history of stable cardiac disease receiving PEG-Intron in combination with ribavirin, the PEG-Intron dose should be reduced by half and the ribavirin dose by 200 mg/day if a >2g/dL decrease in hemoglobin is observed during any 4 week period. Both PEG-Intron and ribavirin should be permanently discontinued if patients have hemoglobin levels <12 g/dL after this ribavirin dose reduction.

chamber and a sterile diluent chamber with Sterile Water for Injection, USP for subcutaneous use.

Each PEG-Intron Redipen™ Package Contains:	
A box containing one 50 µg per 0.5 mL PEG-Intron Redipen™ and 1 B-D needle and 2 alcohol swabs.	(NDC 0085-1323-01)
A box containing one 80 µg per 0.5 mL PEG-Intron Redipen™ and 1 B-D needle and 2 alcohol swabs.	(NDC 0085-1316-01)
A box containing one 120 µg per 0.5 mL PEG-Intron Redipen™ and 1 B-D needle and 2 alcohol swabs.	(NDC 0085-1297-01)
A box containing one 150 µg per 0.5 mL PEG-Intron Redipen™ and 1 B-D needle and 2 alcohol swabs.	(NDC 0085-1370-01)

PEG-Intron Vials

PEG-Intron is a white to off-white lyophilized powder supplied in 2-mL vials. The PEG-Intron Powder for Injection should be reconstituted with 0.7 mL of the supplied Diluent (Sterile Water for Injection, USP) prior to use.

Each PEG-Intron Package Contains:	
A box containing one 50 µg per 0.5 mL vial of PEG-Intron Powder for Injection and one 1 mL vial of Diluent (Sterile Water for Injection, USP), 2 B-D Safety-Lok™* syringes with a safety sleeve and 2 alcohol swabs.	(NDC 0085-1368-01)
A box containing one 80 µg per 0.5 mL vial of PEG-Intron Powder for Injection and one 1 mL vial of Diluent (Sterile Water for Injection, USP), 2 B-D Safety-Lok™* syringes with a safety sleeve and 2 alcohol swabs.	(NDC 0085-1291-01)
A box containing one 120 µg per 0.5 mL vial of PEG-Intron Powder for Injection and one 1 mL vial of Diluent (Sterile Water for Injection, USP), 2 B-D Safety-Lok™*syringes with a safety sleeve and 2 alcohol swabs.	(NDC 0085-1304-01)
A box containing one 150 µg per 0.5 mL vial of PEG-Intron Powder for Injection and one 1 mL vial of Diluent (Sterile Water for Injection, USP), 2 B-D Safety-Lok™*syringes with a safety sleeve and 2 alcohol swabs.	(NDC 0085-1279-01)

Schering Corporation
Kenilworth, NJ 07033 USA

Rev. 10/03 27664407T

*Safety-Lok is a trademark of Becton Dickinson and Company.

MEDICATION GUIDE
PEG-Intron® Redipen™

Single-dose
Delivery System
(Peginterferon alfa-2b)
Including appendix with instructions for using PEG-Intron® Redipen™ Single-dose Delivery System

Read this Medication Guide carefully before you start taking PEG-Intron (**Peg In-tron**) or PEG-Intron/REBETOL (**REB-eh-tole**) combination therapy. Read the Medication Guide each time you refill your prescription because there may be new information. The information in this Medication Guide does not take the place of talking with your doctor.

If you are taking PEG-Intron/REBETOL combination therapy, also read the Medication Guide for REBETOL (ribavirin, USP) Capsules.

What is the most important information I should know about PEG-Intron and PEG-Intron/REBETOL combination therapy?

PEG-Intron (peginterferon) is a treatment for some people who are infected with hepatitis C virus. However, PEG-Intron and PEG-Intron/ REBETOL combination therapy can have serious side effects that may cause death in rare cases. Before you decide to start treatment, you should talk to your doctor about the possible benefits and side effects of PEG-Intron or PEG-Intron/REBETOL combination therapy. If you begin treatment you will need to see your doctor regularly for medical examinations and lab tests to make sure your treatment is working and to check for side effects.

REBETOL capsules may cause birth defects and/or death of an unborn child. If you are pregnant, you or your male partner must not take PEG-Intron/ REBETOL combination therapy. You must not become pregnant while either you or your partner are being treated with the combination PEG-Intron/ REBETOL therapy, or for 6 months after stopping therapy. Men and women should use birth control while taking the combination therapy and for 6 months afterwards. If you or your partner are being treated and you become pregnant either during treatment or within 6 months of stopping treatment, call your doctor right away.

If you are taking PEG-Intron or PEG-Intron/REBETOL therapy you should call your doctor immediately if you develop any of these symptoms:

New or worsening mental health problems such as thoughts about killing or hurting yourself or others, trouble breathing, chest pain, severe stomach or lower back pain, bloody diarrhea or bloody bowel movements, high fever, bruising, bleeding, or decreased vision.

The most serious possible side effects of PEG-Intron and PEG-Intron/REBETOL therapy include:

Problems with Pregnancy. Combination PEG-Intron/ REBETOL therapy can cause death, serious birth defects, or other harm to your unborn child. If you are a woman of childbearing age you must not become pregnant during treatment and for 6 months after you have stopped therapy. You must have a negative pregnancy test immediately before beginning treatment, during treatment, and for 6 months after you have stopped therapy. Both male and female patients must use effective forms of birth control during treatment and for the 6 months after treatment is completed. Male patients should use a condom. If you are a female, you must use birth control even if you believe that you are not fertile or that your fertility is low. You should talk to your doctor about birth control for you and your partner.

Mental health problems and suicide. PEG-Intron and PEG-Intron/REBETOL therapies may cause patients to develop mood or behavioral problems. These can include irritability (getting easily upset) and depression (feeling low, feeling bad about yourself, or feeling hopeless). Some patients may have aggressive behavior. Former drug addicts may fall back into drug addiction or overdose. Some patients think about hurting or killing themselves or other people and some have killed (suicide) or hurt themselves or others. You must tell your doctor if you are being treated for a mental illness or had treatment in the past for any mental illness, including depression and suicidal behavior. You should tell your doctor if you have ever been addicted to drugs or alcohol.

Heart problems. Some patients taking PEG-Intron or PEG-Intron/REBETOL therapy may develop problems with their heart, including low blood pressure, fast heart rate, and very rarely, heart attacks. Tell your doctor if you have had any heart problems in the past.

Blood problems. PEG-Intron and PEG-Intron/REBETOL therapies commonly lower two types of blood cells (white blood cells and platelets). In some patients, these blood counts may fall to dangerously low levels. If your blood counts become very low, this could lead to infections or bleeding.

REBETOL therapy causes a decrease in the number of red blood cells you have (anemia). This can be dangerous, especially for patients who already have heart or circulatory (cardiovascular) problems. Talk with your doctor before taking combination PEG-Intron/REBETOL therapy if you have or have ever had any cardiovascular problems.

Body organ problems. Certain symptoms like severe stomach pain may mean that your internal organs are being damaged.

For other possible side effects, see "What are the possible side effects of PEG-Intron and PEG-Intron/REBETOL" in this Medication Guide.

What is PEG-Intron and PEG-Intron/REBETOL combination therapy?

The PEG-Intron product is a drug used to treat adults who have a lasting (chronic) infection with hepatitis C virus and who show signs that the virus is damaging the liver.

PEG-Intron/REBETOL combination therapy consists of two medications also used to treat hepatitis C infection. Patients with hepatitis C have the virus in their blood and in their liver. PEG-Intron reduces the amount of virus in the body and helps the body's immune system fight the virus. REBETOL (ribavirin) is a drug that helps to fight the viral infection but does not work when used by itself to treat chronic hepatitis C.

It is not known if PEG-Intron or PEG-Intron/REBETOL therapies can cure hepatitis C (permanently eliminate the virus) or if it can prevent liver failure or liver cancer that is caused by hepatitis C infection.

It is also not known if PEG-Intron or PEG-Intron/ REBETOL combination therapy will prevent one infected person from infecting another person with hepatitis C.

Who should not take PEG-Intron or PEG-Intron/REBETOL therapy?

Do not take PEG-Intron or PEG-Intron/REBETOL therapy if you:

- are pregnant, planning to get pregnant during treatment or during the 6 months after treatment, or breast-feeding.
- are a male patient with a female sexual partner who is pregnant or plans to become pregnant at any time while you are being treated with REBETOL or during the 6 months after your treatment has ended.
- have hepatitis caused by your immune system attacking your liver (autoimmune hepatitis) or unstable liver disease.
- had an allergic reaction to another alpha interferon or are allergic to any of the ingredients in PEG-Intron or REBETOL Capsules. If you have any doubts, ask your doctor.
- Do not take PEG-Intron/REBETOL combination therapy if you have abnormal red blood cells such as sickle-cell anemia or thalassemia major.

If you have any of the following conditions or serious medical problems, discuss them with your doctor before taking PEG-Intron or PEG-Intron/REBETOL therapy:

- depression or anxiety
- sleep problems
- high blood pressure
- previous heart attack, or other heart problems
- liver problems (other than hepatitis C infection)
- any kind of autoimmune disease (where the body's immune system attacks the body's own cells), such as psoriasis, systemic lupus erythematosus, rheumatoid arthritis
- thyroid problems
- diabetes
- colitis (inflammation of the bowels)
- cancer
- hepatitis B infection
- HIV infection
- kidney problems
- bleeding problems
- alcoholism
- drug abuse or addiction
- body organ transplant and are taking medicine that keeps your body from rejecting your transplant (suppresses your immune system).

How should I take PEG-Intron or PEG-Intron/REBETOL?

Your doctor will decide whether you will take PEG-Intron therapy alone or the combination of PEG-Intron/REBETOL, as well as the correct dose (based on your weight). PEG-Intron and PEG-Intron/REBETOL are given for one year. Take your prescribed dose of PEG-Intron once a week, on the same day of each week and at approximately the same time. Take the medicine for the full year and do not take more than the prescribed dose. REBETOL Capsules should be taken with food. When you take REBETOL with food, more of the medicine (70% more on average) is taken up by your body. You should take REBETOL the same way every day (twice a day with food) to keep the medicine in your body at a steady level. This will help your doctor to decide how your treatment is working and how to change the number of REBETOL capsules you take if you have side effects from REBETOL. **Be sure to read the Medication Guide for REBETOL (ribavirin, USP) for complete instructions on how to take the REBETOL capsules.**

You should be completely comfortable with how to prepare PEG-Intron; how to set the dose you take; and how to inject yourself before you use PEG-Intron for the first time. PEG-Intron comes in two different forms, a powder in a single-use vial and a Redipen™ single-use delivery system. See the attached appendix for detailed instructions for preparing and giving a dose of PEG-Intron.

If you miss a dose of the PEG-Intron product, take the missed dose as soon as possible during the same day or the next day, then continue on your regular dosing schedule. If several days go by after you miss a dose, check with your doctor about what to do. Do not double the next dose or take more than one dose a week without talking to your doctor. Call your doctor right away if you take more than your prescribed PEG-Intron dose. Your doctor may wish to examine you more closely, and take blood for testing.

If you miss a dose of REBETOL capsules, take the missed dose as soon as possible during the same day. If an entire day has gone by, check with your doctor about what to do. Do not double the next dose.

You must get regular blood tests to help your doctor check how the treatment is working and to check for side effects. Tell your doctor if you are taking or planning to take other prescription or non-prescription medicines, including vitamin and mineral supplements and herbal medicines.

What should I avoid while taking PEG-Intron or PEG-Intron/REBETOL therapies?

- If you are pregnant do not start taking PEG-Intron/ REBETOL combination therapy.
- Avoid becoming pregnant while taking PEG-Intron or PEG-Intron/REBETOL.

PEG-Intron and PEG-Intron/REBETOL may harm your unborn child (death or serious birth defects) or cause you to lose your baby (miscarry). **If you or your partner become pregnant during treatment or during the 6 months after treatment with PEG-Intron/REBETOL combination therapy, immediately report the pregnancy to your doctor. You or your doctor should call (800) 727-7064.** By calling this number, information about you and/or your partner will be added to a pregnancy registry that will be used to help you and your doctor make decisions about your treatment for

Continued on next page

Information on Schering products appearing on these pages is effective as of June 2003.

PEG-Intron—Cont.

hepatitis in the future. You, your partner and/or your physician will be asked to provide follow-up information on the outcome of the pregnancy.

- Do not breast-feed your baby while taking PEG-Intron.

What are the possible side effects of PEG-Intron and PEG-Intron/REBETOL combination therapy?

Possible, serious side effects include:

Mental health problems including suicide, blood problems, heart problems, body organ problems. See "What is the most important information I should know about PEG-Intron and PEG-Intron/REBETOL combination therapy?"

Other body organ problems. A few patients have lung problems (such as pneumonia or inflammation of the lung tissue), inflammation of the kidney, and eye disorders.

New or worsening autoimmune disease. Some patients taking PEG-Intron or PEG-Intron/REBETOL develop autoimmune diseases (a condition where the body's immune cells attack other cells or organs in the body), including rheumatoid arthritis, systemic lupus erythematosus, and psoriasis. In some patients who already have an autoimmune disease, the disease worsens on PEG-Intron and PEG-Intron/REBETOL combination therapy.

Common but less serious side effects include:

Flu-like symptoms. Most patients who take PEG-Intron or PEG-Intron/REBETOL therapy have "flu-like" symptoms (headache, muscle aches, tiredness and fever). Some of these symptoms (fever, headache) usually lessen after the first few weeks of therapy. You can reduce some of these symptoms by injecting your PEG-Intron dose at bedtime. Over-the-counter pain and fever reducers, such as acetaminophen or ibuprofen, can be used to prevent or reduce the fever and headache.

Extreme fatigue (tiredness). Many patients become extremely tired while on PEG-Intron or PEG-Intron/REBETOL combination therapy.

Appetite problems. Nausea, loss of appetite, and weight loss, occur commonly.

Thyroid problems. Some patients develop changes in the function of their thyroid. Symptoms of thyroid changes include the inability to concentrate, feeling cold or hot all the time, a change in your weight and changes to your skin.

Blood sugar problems. Some patients develop problems with the way their body controls their blood sugar and may develop high blood sugar or diabetes.

Skin reactions. Redness, swelling, and itching are common at the site of injection. If after several days these symptoms do not disappear contact your doctor. You may get a rash during therapy. If this occurs, your doctor may recommend medicine to treat the rash.

Hair thinning. Hair thinning is common during PEG-Intron and PEG-Intron/ REBETOL treatment. Hair loss stops and hair growth returns after therapy is stopped.

These are not all of the side effects of PEG-Intron or PEG-Intron/REBETOL combination therapy. Your doctor or pharmacist can give you a more complete list.

General advice about prescription medicines:

Medicines are sometimes prescribed for purposes other than those listed in a Medication Guide. If you have any concerns about PEG-Intron, ask your doctor. Your doctor or pharmacist can give you information about PEG-Intron that was written for health care professionals. Do not use PEG-Intron for a condition for which it was not prescribed. Do not share this medication with other people.

If you are taking PEG-Intron/REBETOL combination therapy, also read the Medication Guide for REBETOL (ribavirin, USP) Capsules.

This Medication Guide has been approved by the U.S. Food and Drug Administration.

How do I prepare and inject the PEG-Intron Redipen™ Dose?

The PEG-Intron Redipen™ system is for a single use, by one person only. The Redipen™ must not be shared. Use only the injection needle provided in the packaging for the PEG-Intron Redipen™ system. If you have problems with the Redipen™ system or the PEG-Intron solution, you should contact your nurse, doctor, or pharmacist.

The following instructions explain how to prepare and inject yourself with the PEG-Intron Redipen™ system. Please read the instructions carefully and follow them step by step. Your health care provider will instruct you on how to self-inject with the PEG-Intron Redipen™. Do not attempt to inject yourself unless you are sure you understand the procedure and requirements for self-injection.

How to use the PEG-Intron Redipen™ single-dose delivery system.

[See figure at top of next column]

Storing PEG-Intron

PEG-Intron Redipen™ should be stored in the refrigerator at 2° to 8°C (36° to 46°F); avoid exposure to heat. After mixing, the PEG-Intron solution should be used immediately but may be stored in the refrigerator up to 24 hours at 2° to 8°C (36° to 46°F). The solution contains no preservatives. DO NOT FREEZE.

I: Preparation

1. Find a clean, well-lit, non-slip flat working surface and assemble all of the supplies you will need for an injection. All of the supplies you will need are in the PEG-Intron Redipen™ package. The package contains:
   - a PEG-Intron Redipen™ single-dose delivery system
   - one disposable needle

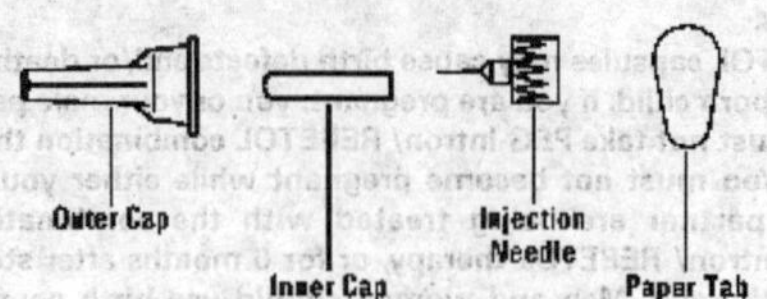

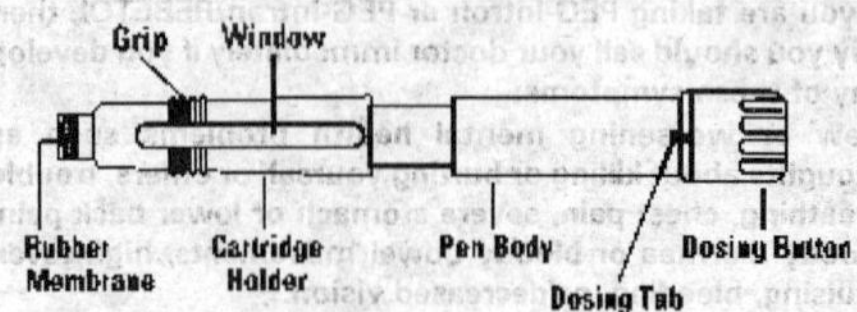

   - alcohol swabs, and
   - dose tray (the dose tray is the bottom half of the Redipen™ package)
2. Take the PEG-Intron Redipen™ system out of the refrigerator to allow the medicine to come to room temperature. Before removing the Redipen™ from the carton, check the expiration date printed on the PEG-Intron Redipen™ carton to make sure that the expiration date has not passed. Do not use if the expiration date has passed.
3. After taking the PEG-Intron Redipen™ system out of the carton, look in the window of the Redipen™ and make sure the PEG-Intron in the cartridge holder chamber is a white, to off-white tablet that is whole or in pieces or powder.
4. Wash your hands thoroughly with soap and water, rinse and towel dry. It is important to keep your work area, your hands, and injection site clean to minimize the risk of infection.

II: Mixing

Key points:

Before you mix the PEG-Intron, make sure it is at room temperature. It is important that you keep the PEG-Intron Redipen™ system UPRIGHT (dosing button down) as shown in Figure 1.

5. Hold the PEG-Intron Redipen™ system **UPRIGHT (Figure 1)** in the dose tray or on a flat non-slip surface with the dosing button down. You may want to hold the Redipen™ using the grip.
   - To mix the powder and the liquid, press the two halves of the pen together firmly until you hear the click.
   - Wait several seconds for the powder to completely dissolve.

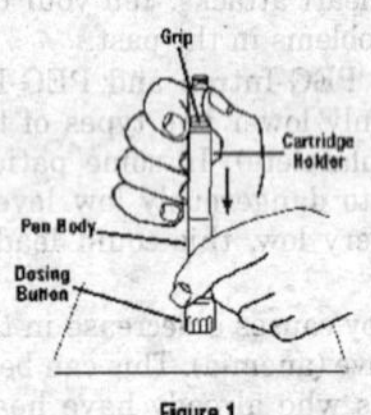

Figure 1

6. **Gently turn the PEG-Intron Redipen™ system upside down twice (Figure 2). To avoid excessive foaming, DO NOT SHAKE.**
   - Keeping the PEG-Intron Redipen™ system UPRIGHT, check through the Redipen™ window to see if the mixed PEG-Intron solution is completely dissolved. If there is still foam, wait until it settles. The solution should be clear, colorless, and without particles **before use**. It is normal to see some small bubbles near the top of the solution. Do not use if the solution is not clear, or if you see particles.

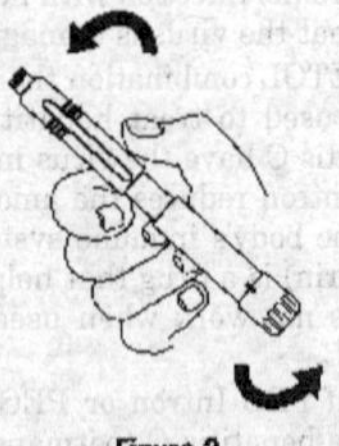

Figure 2

7. **Place the PEG-Intron Redipen™ system into the dose tray provided in the packaging (Figure 3). The dosing button will be on the bottom.**
   - Wipe the rubber membrane of the PEG-Intron Redipen™ system with one alcohol swab.
   - Remove the protective paper tab from the injection needle. Keeping the PEG-Intron Redipen™ system **UPRIGHT** in the dose tray, gently push the injection needle straight onto the Redipen™ system and screw it securely in place.
   - Keep the PEG-Intron Redipen™ system pointed up and keep the outer needle cap on.
   - You may see some liquid trickle out from under the cap for a few seconds after screwing the injection needle onto the Redipen™. Wait until this stops before going to the next step.

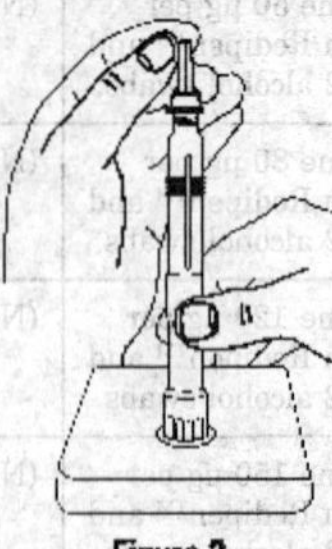

Figure 3

III: Setting the Dose

8. **Remove the PEG-Intron Redipen™ system from the dose tray (Figure 4).** Holding the PEG-Intron Redipen™ system firmly, pull the dosing button out as far as it will go, until you see the dark bands below the dosing button.

   Do not push the dosing button in until you are ready to self-inject the PEG-Intron dose.

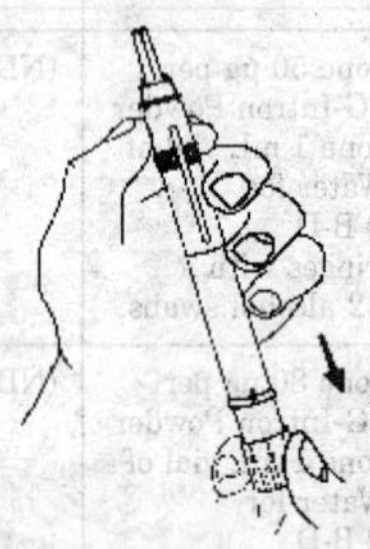

Figure 4

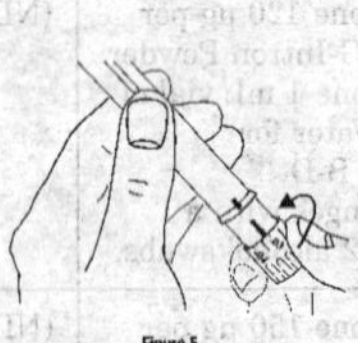

Figure 5

9. Turn the dosing button until your prescribed dose is lined up with the dosing tab (**Figure 5**).

IV: Injecting the PEG-Intron Dose

Choosing an Injection Site

The best sites for giving yourself an injection are those areas with a layer of fat between the skin and muscle, like your thigh, the outer surface of your upper arm, and abdomen. Do not inject yourself in the area near your navel or waistline. If you are very thin, you should only use the thigh or outer surface of the arm for injection.

You should use a different site each time you inject PEG-Intron to avoid soreness at any one site. Do not inject PEG-Intron into an area where the skin is irritated, red, bruised, infected, or has scars, stretch marks, or lumps.

10. Clean the skin where the injection is to be given with an alcohol swab, and wait for the area to dry.
11. Remove the outer cap from the needle (**Figure 6**). There may be some liquid around the inner needle cap. This is normal. Once the injection site is dry pull off the inner needle cap.

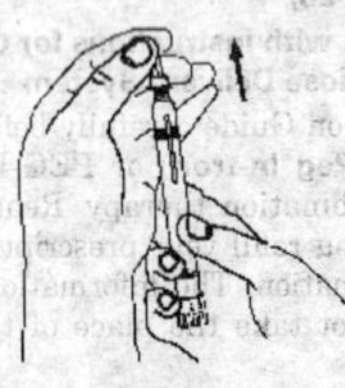

Figure 6

12. **Hold the PEG-Intron Redipen™ system with your fingers wrapped around the pen body barrel and your thumb on the dosing button (Figure 7).**
    - With your other hand, pinch the skin in the area you have cleaned for injection.
    - Insert the needle into the pinched skin at an angle of 45° to 90°.
    - Press the dosing button down slowly and firmly until you can't push it any further.
    - Keep your thumb pressed down on the dosing button for an additional 5 seconds to ensure that you get the complete dose.

• Remove the needle from your skin.

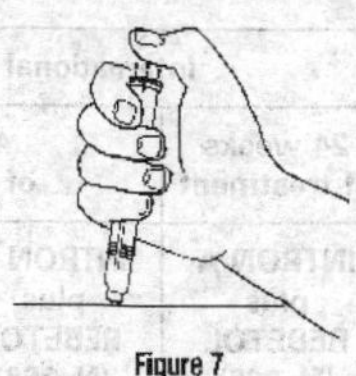
Figure 7

13. **Gently press the injection site with a small bandage or sterile gauze if necessary for a few seconds but** do not massage the injection site. If there is bleeding, cover with an adhesive bandage. Discard the PEG-Intron Redipen™ system with the needle still attached. DO NOT RECAP THE NEEDLE and DO NOT REUSE the Redipen™.
   • After 2 hours, check the injection site for redness, swelling, or tenderness. If you have a skin reaction and it doesn't clear up in a few days, contact your health care provider.

How do I dispose of the Redipen™?

Discard the Redipen™ system and needle and any solution remaining in the Redipen™ in a Sharps container or other puncture-proof container like a coffee can. DO NOT use glass or clear plastic containers. Your doctor or nurse will tell you how to dispose of a full container. Always keep the container out of reach of children.

Manufactured by:
Schering Corporation
Kenilworth, NJ 07033 USA
10/03 **27662404T**

REBETOL® ℞

[rē'bə-tōl]
(ribavirin, USP)
Capsules and Oral Solution

- **REBETOL monotherapy is not effective for the treatment of chronic hepatitis C virus infection and should not be used alone for this indication. (See WARNINGS).**
- **The primary toxicity of ribavirin is hemolytic anemia. The anemia associated with REBETOL therapy may result in worsening of cardiac disease that has led to fatal and nonfatal myocardial infarctions. Patients with a history of significant or unstable cardiac disease should not be treated with REBETOL. (See WARNINGS, ADVERSE REACTIONS and DOSAGE AND ADMINISTRATION).**
- **Significant teratogenic and/or embryocidal effects have been demonstrated in all animal species exposed to ribavirin. In addition, ribavirin has a multiple-dose half-life of 12 days, and so it may persist in nonplasma compartments for as long as 6 months. Therefore, REBETOL therapy is contraindicated in women who are pregnant and in the male partners of women who are pregnant. Extreme care must be taken to avoid pregnancy during therapy and for 6 months after completion of treatment in both female patients and in female partners of male patients who are taking REBETOL therapy. At least two reliable forms of effective contraception must be utilized during treatment and during the 6-month posttreatment follow-up-period. (See CONTRAINDICATIONS, WARNINGS, PRECAUTIONS—Information for Patients and Pregnancy Category X).**

DESCRIPTION

REBETOL®

REBETOL is Schering Corporation's brand name for ribavirin, a nucleoside analog. The chemical name of ribavirin is 1-β-D-ribofuranosyl-1*H*-1,2,4-triazole-3-carboxamide and has the following structural formula:

[structural formula: O, NH2, N, HO, O, OH, OH]

Ribavirin is a white, crystalline powder. It is freely soluble in water and slightly soluble in anhydrous alcohol. The empirical formula is $C_8H_{12}N_4O_5$ and the molecular weight is 244.21.

REBETOL Capsules consist of a white powder in a white, opaque, gelatin capsule. Each capsule contains 200 mg ribavirin and the inactive ingredients microcrystalline cellulose, lactose monohydrate, croscarmellose sodium, and magnesium stearate. The capsule shell consists of gelatin, sodium lauryl sulfate, silicon dioxide, and titanium dioxide. The capsule is printed with edible blue pharmaceutical ink which is made of shellac, anhydrous ethyl alcohol, isopropyl alcohol, n-butyl alcohol, propylene glycol, ammonium hydroxide, and FD&C Blue #2 aluminum lake.

REBETOL Oral Solution is a clear, colorless to pale or light yellow bubble gum-flavored liquid. Each milliliter of the solution contains 40 mg of ribavirin and the inactive ingredients sucrose, glycerin, sorbitol, propylene glycol, sodium citrate, citric acid, sodium benzoate, natural and artificial flavor for bubble gum #15864, and water.

Mechanism of Action

The mechanism of inhibition of hepatitis C virus (HCV) RNA by combination therapy with ribavirin and interferon products has not been established.

CLINICAL PHARMACOLOGY

Pharmacokinetics

Ribavirin Single- and multiple-dose pharmacokinetic properties in adults with chronic hepatitis C are summarized in **TABLE 1**. Ribavirin was rapidly and extensively absorbed following oral administration. However, due to first-pass metabolism, the absolute bioavailability averaged 64% (44%). There was a linear relationship between dose and AUC_{tf} (AUC from time zero to last measurable concentration) following single doses of 200–1200 mg ribavirin. The relationship between dose and C_{max} was curvilinear, tending to asymptote above single doses of 400–600 mg.

Upon multiple oral dosing, based on $AUC12_{hr}$, a sixfold accumulation of ribavirin was observed in plasma. Following oral dosing with 600 mg BID, steady-state was reached by approximately 4 weeks, with mean steady-state plasma concentrations of 2200 (37%) ng/mL. Upon discontinuation of dosing, the mean half-life was 298 (30%) hours, which probably reflects slow elimination from nonplasma compartments.

Effect of Food on Absorption of Ribavirin Both AUC_{tf} and C_{max} increased by 70% when REBETOL Capsules were administered with a high-fat meal (841 kcal, 53.8 g fat, 31.6 g protein, and 57.4 g carbohydrate) in a single-dose pharmacokinetic study. There are insufficient data to address the clinical relevance of these results. Clinical efficacy studies with REBETOL/INTRON A were conducted without instructions with respect to food consumption. During clinical studies with REBETOL/PEG-INTRON, all subjects were instructed to take REBETOL Capsules with food. (See **DOSAGE AND ADMINISTRATION**.)

Effect of Antacid on Absorption of Ribavirin Coadministration with an antacid containing magnesium, aluminum, and simethicone (Mylanta®[1]) resulted in a 14% decrease in mean ribavirin AUC_{tf}. The clinical relevance of results from this single-dose study is unknown.

TABLE 1. Mean (% CV) Pharmacokinetic Parameters for REBETOL When Administered Individually to Adults

Parameter	REBETOL		
	Single Dose 600 mg Oral Solution (N=14)	Single Dose 600 mg Capsules (N=12)	Multiple Dose 600 mg BID Capsules (N=12)
T_{max} (hr)	1.00(34)	1.7 (46)***	3 (60)
C_{max}*	872 (42)	782 (37)	3680 (85)
AUC_{tf}**	14098 (38)	13400 (48)	228000 (25)
$T_{1/2}$ (hr)		43.6 (47)	298 (30)
Apparent Volume of Distribution (L)		2825 (9)†	
Apparent Clearance (L/hr)		38.2 (40)	
Absolute Bioavailability		64% (44)††	

* ng/mL
** ng.hr/mL
*** N = 11
† data obtained from a single-dose pharmacokinetic study using ^{14}C labeled ribavirin; N = 5
†† N = 6

Ribavirin transport into nonplasma compartments has been most extensively studied in red blood cells, and has been identified to be primarily via an e_s-type equilibrative nucleoside transporter. This type of transporter is present on virtually all cell types and may account for the extensive volume of distribution. Ribavirin does not bind to plasma proteins.

Ribavirin has two pathways of metabolism: (i) a reversible phosphorylation pathway in nucleated cells; and (ii) a degradative pathway involving deribosylation and amide hydrolysis to yield a triazole carboxylic acid metabolite. Ribavirin and its triazole carboxamide and triazole carboxylic acid metabolites are excreted renally. After oral administration of 600 mg of ^{14}C-ribavirin, approximately 61% and 12% of the radioactivity was eliminated in the urine and feces, respectively, in 336 hours. Unchanged ribavirin accounted for 17% of the administered dose.

Results of *in vitro* studies using both human and rat liver microsome preparations indicated little or no cytochrome P450 enzyme-mediated metabolism of ribavirin, with minimal potential for P450 enzyme-based drug interactions.

No pharmacokinetic interactions were noted between INTRON A Injection and REBETOL Capsules in a multiple-dose pharmacokinetic study.

Drug Interactions Ribavirin has been shown *in vitro* to inhibit phosphorylation of zidovudine and stavudine which could lead to decreased antiretroviral activity. Exposure to didanosine or its active metabolite (dideoxyadenosine 5'-triphosphate) is increased when didanosine is co-administered with ribavirin, which could cause or worsen clinical toxicities (see **PRECAUTIONS: Drug Interactions**).

1. Trademark of Johnson & Johnson-Merck Consumer Pharmaceuticals Co.

Special Populations

Renal Dysfunction The pharmacokinetics of ribavirin were assessed after administration of a single oral dose (400 mg) of ribavirin to non HCV-infected subjects with varying degrees of renal dysfunction. The mean AUC_{tf} value was threefold greater in subjects with creatinine clearance values between 10 to 30 mL/min when compared to control subjects (creatinine clearance >90 mL/min). In subjects with creatinine clearance values between 30 to 60 mL/min, AUC_{tf} was twofold greater when compared to control subjects. The increased AUC_{tf} appears to be due to reduction of renal and non-renal clearance in these patients. Phase III efficacy trials included subjects with creatinine clearance values >50 mL/min. The multiple dose pharmacokinetics of ribavirin cannot be accurately predicted in patients with renal dysfunction. Ribavirin is not effectively removed by hemodialysis. Patients with creatinine clearance <50 mL/min should not be treated with REBETOL (See **WARNINGS**.)

Hepatic Dysfunction The effect of hepatic dysfunction was assessed after a single oral dose of ribavirin (600 mg). The mean AUC_{tf} values were not significantly different in subjects with mild, moderate, or severe hepatic dysfunction (Child-Pugh Classification A, B, or C) when compared to control subjects. However, the mean C_{max} values increased with severity of hepatic dysfunction and was twofold greater in subjects with severe hepatic dysfunction when compared to control subjects.

Elderly Patients Pharmacokinetic evaluations in elderly subjects have not been performed.

Gender There were no clinically significant pharmacokinetic differences noted in a single-dose study of eighteen male and eighteen female subjects.

Pediatric Patients Multiple-dose pharmacokinetic properties for REBETOL Capsules and INTRON A in pediatric patients with chronic hepatitis C between 5 and 16 years of age are summarized in **TABLE 2**. The pharmacokinetics of REBETOL and INTRON A (dose-normalized) are similar in adults and pediatric patients.

Complete pharmacokinetic characteristics of REBETOL Oral Solution have not been determined in pediatric patients. Ribavirin C_{min} values were similar following administration of REBETOL Oral Solution or REBETOL Capsules during 48 weeks of therapy in pediatric patients (3 to 16 years of age).

TABLE 2. Mean (% CV) Multiple-Dose Pharmacokinetic Parameters for INTRON A and REBETOL Capsules When Administered to Pediatric Patients With Chronic Hepatitis C

Parameter	REBETOL 15 mg/kg/day as 2 divided doses (n=17)	INTRON A 3 MIU/m² TIW (n=54)
T_{max} (hr)	1.9 (83)	5.9 (36)
C_{max} (ng/mL)	3275 (25)	51 (48)
AUC*	29774 (26)	622 (48)
Apparent clearance L/hr/kg	0.27 (27)	ND

*AUC_{12} (ng/hr/mL) for REBETOL; $AUC_{0\text{-}24}$ (IU hr/mL) for INTRON A
ND=not done
In this section of the label, numbers in parenthesis indicate % coefficient of variation.

INDICATIONS AND USAGE

REBETOL (ribavirin, USP) Capsules and Oral Solution are indicated in combination with INTRON A (interferon alfa-2b, recombinant) Injection for the treatment of chronic hepatitis C in patients 3 years of age and older with compensated liver disease previously untreated with alpha interferon or in patients 18 years of age and older who have relapsed following alpha interferon therapy.

REBETOL Capsules are indicated in combination with PEG-INTRON (peginterferon alfa-2b, recombinant) Injection for the treatment of chronic hepatitis C in patients with compensated liver disease who have not been previously treated with interferon alpha and are at least 18 years of age.

The safety and efficacy of REBETOL Capsules or Oral Solution with interferons other than INTRON A or PEG-INTRON products have not been established.

Continued on next page

Information on Schering products appearing on these pages is effective as of June 2003.

Rebetol—Cont.

Pediatric Use

Evidence of disease progression, such as hepatic inflammation and fibrosis, as well as prognostic factors for response, HCV genotype and viral load, should be considered when deciding to treat a pediatric patient. The benefits of treatment should be weighed against the safety findings observed (see **PRECAUTIONS Pediatric Use**) for pediatric subjects in the clinical trials.

Description of Clinical Studies

REBETOL/INTRON A Combination Therapy

Adult Patients

Previously Untreated Patients

Adults with compensated chronic hepatitis C and detectable HCV RNA (assessed by a central laboratory using a research-based RT-PCR assay) who were previously untreated with alpha interferon therapy were enrolled into two multicenter, double-blind trials (US and International) and randomized to receive REBETOL Capsules 1200 mg/day (1000 mg/day for patients weighing ≤75 kg) plus INTRON A Injection 3 MIU TIW or INTRON A Injection plus placebo for 24 or 48 weeks followed by 24 weeks of off-therapy follow-up. The International study did not contain a 24-week INTRON A plus placebo treatment arm. The US study enrolled 912 patients who, at baseline, were 67% male, 89% Caucasian with a mean Knodell HAI score (I+II+III) of 7.5, and 72% genotype 1. The International study, conducted in Europe, Israel, Canada, and Australia, enrolled 799 patients (65% male, 95% Caucasian, mean Knodell score 6.8, and 58% genotype 1).

Study results are summarized in **TABLE 3**.

[See table 3 at right]

Of patients who had not achieved HCV RNA below the limit of detection of the research based assay by week 24 of REBETOL/INTRON A treatment, less than 5% responded to an additional 24 weeks of combination treatment.

Among patients with HCV Genotype 1 treated with REBETOL/INTRON A therapy who achieved HCV RNA below the detection limit of the research-based assay by 24 weeks, those randomized to 48 weeks of treatment had higher virologic responses compared to those in the 24 week treatment group. There was no observed increase in response rates for patients with HCV nongenotype 1 randomized to REBETOL/INTRON A therapy for 48 weeks compared to 24 weeks.

Relapse Patients

Patients with compensated chronic hepatitis C and detectable HCV RNA (assessed by a central laboratory using a research-based RT-PCR assay) who had relapsed following one or two courses of interferon therapy (defined as abnormal serum ALT levels) were enrolled into two multicenter, double-blind trials (US and International) and randomized to receive REBETOL 1200 mg/day (1000 mg/day for patients weighing ≤75 kg) plus INTRON A 3 MIU TIW or INTRON A plus placebo for 24 weeks followed by 24 weeks of off-therapy follow-up. The US study enrolled 153 patients who, at baseline, were 67% male, 92% Caucasian with a mean Knodell HAI score (I+II+III) of 6.8, and 58% genotype 1. The International study, conducted in Europe, Israel, Canada, and Australia, enrolled 192 patients (64% male, 95% Caucasian, mean Knodell score 6.6, and 56% genotype 1).

Study results are summarized in **TABLE 4**.

[See table 4 at right]

Virologic and histologic responses were similar among male and female patients in both the previously untreated and relapse studies.

Pediatric Patients

Pediatric patients 3 to 16 years of age with compensated chronic hepatitis C and detectable HCV RNA (assessed by a central laboratory using a research-based RT-PCR assay) were treated with REBETOL 15 mg/kg per day plus INTRON A 3 MIU/m² TIW for 48 weeks followed by 24 weeks of off-therapy follow-up. A total of 118 patients received treatment who were 57% male, 80% Caucasian, and 78% genotype 1. Patients <5 years of age received REBETOL Oral Solution and those ≥5 years of age received either REBETOL Oral Solution or Capsules.

Study results are summarized in **TABLE 5**.

TABLE 5. Virologic Response: Previously Untreated Pediatric Patients*

	INTRON A 3 MIU/m² TIW Plus REBETOL 15 mg/kg/day
Overall Response[1] (n=118)	54 (46)
Genotype 1 (n=92)	33 (36)
Genotype non-1 (n=26)	21 (81)

*Number (%) of patients.

1. Defined as HCV RNA below limit of detection using a research-based RT-PCR assay at end of treatment and during follow-up.

Patients with viral genotype 1, regardless of viral load, had a lower response rate to INTRON A/REBETOL combination therapy compared to patients with genotype non-1, 36% versus 81%. Patients with both poor prognostic factors (genotype 1 and high viral load) had a response rate of 26% (13/50).

TABLE 3. Virologic and Histologic Responses: Previously Untreated Patients*

	US Study				International Study		
	24 weeks of treatment		48 weeks of treatment		24 weeks of treatment	48 weeks of treatment	
	INTRON A plus REBETOL (N=228)	INTRON A plus Placebo (N=231)	INTRON A plus REBETOL (N=228)	INTRON A plus Placebo (N=225)	INTRON A plus REBETOL (N=265)	INTRON A plus REBETOL (N=268)	INTRON A plus Placebo (N=266)
Virologic Response							
-Responder[1]	65 (29)	13 (6)	85 (37)	27 (12)	86 (32)	113 (42)	46 (17)
-Nonresponder	147 (64)	194 (84)	110 (48)	168 (75)	158 (60)	120 (45)	196 (74)
-Missing Data	16 (7)	24 (10)	33 (14)	30 (13)	21 (8)	35 (13)	24 (9)
Histologic Response							
-Improvement[1]	102 (45)	77 (33)	96 (42)	65 (29)	103 (39)	102 (38)	69 (26)
-No improvement	77 (34)	99 (43)	61 (27)	93 (41)	85 (32)	58 (22)	111 (41)
-Missing Data	49 (21)	55 (24)	71 (31)	67 (30)	77 (29)	108 (40)	86 (32)

*Number (%) of patients.

1. Defined as HCV RNA below limit of detection using a research-based RT-PCR assay at end of treatment and during follow-up period.
2. Defined as posttreatment (end of follow-up) minus pretreatment liver biopsy Knodell HAI score (I+II+III) improvement of ≥2 points.

TABLE 4. Virologic and Histologic Responses: Relapse Patients*

	US Study		International Study	
	INTRON A plus REBETOL (N=77)	INTRON A plus Placebo (N=76)	INTRON A plus REBETOL (N=96)	INTRON A plus Placebo (N=96)
Virologic Response				
-Responder[1]	33 (43)	3 (4)	46 (48)	5 (5)
-Nonresponder	36 (47)	66 (87)	45 (47)	91 (95)
-Missing Data	8 (10)	7 (9)	5 (5)	0 (0)
Histologic Response				
-Improvement[2]	38 (49)	27 (36)	49 (51)	30 (31)
-No improvement	23 (30)	37 (49)	29 (30)	44 (46)
-Missing Data	16 (21)	12 (16)	18 (19)	22 (23)

* Number (%) of patients.

1. Defined as HCV RNA below limit of detection using a research-based RT-PCR assay at end of treatment and during follow-up period.
2. Defined as posttreatment (end of follow-up) minus pretreatment liver biopsy Knodell HAI score (I+II+III) improvement of ≥2 points.

REBETOL/PEG-INTRON Combination Therapy

A randomized study compared treatment with two PEG-INTRON/ REBETOL regimens [PEG-INTRON 1.5 μg/kg SC once weekly (QW)/ REBETOL 800 mg PO daily (in divided doses); PEG-INTRON 1.5 μg/kg SC QW for 4 weeks then 0.5 μg/kg SC QW for 44 weeks/ REBETOL 1000/1200 mg PO daily (in divided doses)] with INTRON A [3 MIU SC thrice weekly (TIW)/REBETOL 1000/1200 mg PO daily (in divided doses)] in 1530 adults with chronic hepatitis C. Interferon naïve patients were treated for 48 weeks and followed for 24 weeks posttreatment. Eligible patients had compensated liver disease, detectable HCV RNA, elevated ALT, and liver histopathology consistent with chronic hepatitis.

Response to treatment was defined as undetectable HCV RNA at 24 weeks posttreatment (see **Table 6**).

TABLE 6. Rates of Response to Combination Treatment

	PEG-INTRON 1.5 μg/kg QW REBETOL 800 mg QD	INTRON A 3 MIU TIW REBETOL 1000/1200 mg QD
Overall[1,2] response	52% (264/511)	46% (231/505)
Genotype 1	41% (141/348)	33% (112/343)
Genotype 2-6	75% (123/163)	73% (119/162)

1. Serum HCV RNA was measured with a research-based quantitative polymerase chain reaction assay by a central laboratory.
2. Difference in overall treatment response (PEG-INTRON/REBETOL vs. INTRON A/REBETOL) is 6% with 95% confidence interval of (0.18, 11.63) adjusted for viral genotype and presence of cirrhosis at baseline.

The response rate to PEG-INTRON 1.5→0.5μg/kg/REBETOL was essentially the same as the response to INTRON A/REBETOL (data not shown).

Patients with viral genotype 1, regardless of viral load, had a lower response rate to PEG-INTRON (1.5 μg/kg)/REBETOL combination therapy compared to patients with other viral genotypes. Patients with both poor prognostic factors (genotype 1 and high viral load) had a response rate of 30% (78/256) compared to a response rate of 29% (71/247) with INTRON A/ REBETOL combination therapy.

Patients with lower body weight tended to have higher adverse event rates (see **ADVERSE REACTIONS**) and higher response rates than patients with higher body weights. Differences in response rates between treatment arms did not substantially vary with body weight.

Treatment response rates with PEG-INTRON/REBETOL combination therapy were 49% in men and 56% in women. Response rates were lower in African American and Hispanic patients and higher in Asians compared to Caucasians. Although African Americans had a higher proportion of poor prognostic factors compared to Caucasians the number of non-Caucasians studied (11% of the total) was insufficient to allow meaningful conclusions about differences in response rates after adjusting for prognostic factors.

Liver biopsies were obtained before and after treatment in 68% of patients. Compared to baseline approximately $^2/_3$ of patients in all treatment groups were observed to have a modest reduction in inflammation.

CONTRAINDICATIONS

Pregnancy

REBETOL Capsules and Oral Solution may cause birth defects and/or death of the exposed fetus. REBETOL therapy is contraindicated for use in women who are pregnant or in men whose female partners are pregnant. (See **WARNINGS, PRECAUTIONS–Information for Patients and Pregnancy Category X.**)

REBETOL Capsules and Oral Solution are contraindicated in patients with a history of hypersensitivity to ribavirin or any component of the capsule.

Patients with autoimmune hepatitis must not be treated with combination REBETOL/INTRON A therapy because using these medicines can make the hepatitis worse.

Patients with hemoglobinopathies (eg, thalassemia major, sickle-cell anemia) should not be treated with REBETOL Capsules or Oral Solution.

WARNINGS

Based on results of clinical trials ribavirin monotherapy is not effective for the treatment of chronic hepatitis C virus infection; therefore, REBETOL Capsules or Oral Solution must not be used alone. The safety and efficacy of REBETOL Capsules and Oral Solution have only been es-

tablished when used together with INTRON A (interferon alfa-2b, recombinant) as REBETRON Combination Therapy or with PEG-INTRON Injection.

There are significant adverse events caused by REBETOL/ INTRON A or PEG-INTRON therapy, including severe depression and suicidal ideation, hemolytic anemia, suppression of bone marrow function, autoimmune and infectious disorders, pulmonary dysfunction, pancreatitis, and diabetes. Suicidal ideation or attempts occurred more frequently among pediatric patients, primarily adolescents, compared to adult patients (2.4% versus 1%) during treatment and off-therapy follow-up. The REBETRON Combination Therapy and PEG-INTRON package inserts should be reviewed in their entirety prior to initiation of combination treatment for additional safety information.

Pregnancy

REBETOL Capsules and Oral Solution may cause birth defects and/or death of the exposed fetus. Extreme care must be taken to avoid pregnancy in female patients and in female partners of male patients. REBETOL has demonstrated significant teratogenic and/or embryocidal effects in all animal species in which adequate studies have been conducted. These effects occurred at doses as low as one twentieth of the recommended human dose of ribavirin. REBETOL THERAPY SHOULD NOT BE STARTED UNTIL A REPORT OF A NEGATIVE PREGNANCY TEST HAS BEEN OBTAINED IMMEDIATELY PRIOR TO PLANNED INITIATION OF THERAPY. Patients should be instructed to use at least two forms of effective contraception during treatment and during the six month period after treatment has been stopped based on multiple dose half-life of ribavirin of 12 days. Pregnancy testing should occur monthly during REBETOL therapy and for six months after therapy has stopped (see CONTRAINDICATIONS and PRECAUTIONS: Information for Patients and Pregnancy Category X).

Anemia

The primary toxicity of ribavirin is hemolytic anemia, which was observed in approximately 10% of REBETOL/ INTRON A-treated patients in clinical trials (see adverse reactions laboratory values—*hemoglobin*). The anemia associated with REBETOL capsules occurs within 1–2 weeks of initiation of therapy. BECAUSE THE INITIAL DROP IN HEMOGLOBIN MAY BE SIGNIFICANT, IT IS ADVISED THAT HEMOGLOBIN OR HEMATOCRIT BE OBTAINED PRETREATMENT AND AT WEEK 2 AND WEEK 4 OF THERAPY, OR MORE FREQUENTLY IF CLINICALLY INDICATED. Patients should then be followed as clinically appropriate.

Fatal and nonfatal myocardial infarctions have been reported in patients with anemia caused by REBETOL. Patients should be assessed for underlying cardiac disease before initiation of ribavirin therapy. Patients with preexisting cardiac disease should have electrocardiograms administered before treatment, and should be appropriately monitored during therapy. If there is any deterioration of cardiovascular status, therapy should be suspended or discontinued. (See DOSAGE AND ADMINISTRATION: Guidelines for Dose Modification.) Because cardiac disease may be worsened by drug induced anemia, patients with a history of significant or unstable cardiac disease should not use REBETOL. (See ADVERSE REACTIONS.)

REBETOL and INTRON A or PEG-INTRON therapy should be suspended in patients with signs and symptoms of pancreatitis and discontinued in patients with confirmed pancreatitis.

REBETOL should not be used in patients with creatinine clearance <50 mL/min. (See **Clinical Pharmacology, Special populations.**)

Pulmonary

Pulmonary symptoms, including dyspnea, pulmonary infiltrates, pneumonitis and pneumonia, have been reported during therapy with REBETOL/ INTRON A; occasional cases of fatal pneumonia have occurred. In addition, sarcoidosis or the exacerbation of sarcoidosis has been reported. If there is evidence of pulmonary infiltrates or pulmonary function impairment, the patient should be closely monitored, and if appropriate, combination REBETOL/ INTRON A treatment should be discontinued.

TABLE 7. Selected Treatment-Emergent Adverse Events: Previously Untreated and Relapse Adult Patients and Previously Untreated Pediatric Patients

	Percentage of Patients						
	US Previously Untreated Study				US Relapse Study		Pediatric Patients
	24 weeks of treatment		48 weeks of treatment		24 weeks of treatment		48 weeks of treatment
Patients Reporting Adverse Events*	**INTRON A plus REBETOL (N=228)**	**INTRON A plus Placebo (N=231)**	**INTRON A plus REBETOL (N=228)**	**INTRON A plus Placebo (N=225)**	**INTRON A plus REBETOL (N=77)**	**INTRON A plus Placebo (N=76)**	**INTRON A plus REBETOL (N=118)**
Application Site Disorders							
Injection site inflammation	13	10	12	14	6	8	14
Injection site reaction	7	9	8	9	5	3	19
Body as a Whole - General Disorders							
Headache	63	63	66	67	66	68	69
Fatigue	68	62	70	72	60	53	58
Rigors	40	32	42	39	43	37	25
Fever	37	35	41	40	32	36	61
Influenza-like symptoms	14	18	18	20	13	13	31
Asthenia	9	4	9	9	10	4	5
Chest pain	5	4	9	8	6	7	5
Central & Peripheral Nervous System Disorders							
Dizziness	17	15	23	19	26	21	20
Gastrointestinal System Disorders							
Nausea	38	35	46	33	47	33	33
Anorexia	27	16	25	19	21	14	51
Dyspepsia	14	6	16	9	16	9	<1
Vomiting	11	10	9	13	12	8	42
Musculoskeletal System Disorders							
Myalgia	61	57	64	63	61	58	32
Arthralgia	30	27	33	36	29	29	15
Musculoskeletal pain	20	26	28	32	22	28	21
Psyciatric Disorders							
Insomnia	39	27	39	30	26	25	14
Irritability	23	19	32	27	25	20	10
Depression	32	25	36	37	23	14	13
Emotional lability	7	6	11	8	12	8	16
Concentration impaired	11	14	14	14	10	12	5
Nervousness	4	2	4	4	5	4	3
Respiratory System Disorders							
Dyspnea	19	9	18	10	17	12	5
Sinusitis	9	7	10	14	12	7	<1
Skin and Appendages Disorders							
Alopecia	28	27	32	28	27	26	23
Rash	20	9	28	8	21	5	17
Pruritus	21	9	19	8	13	4	12
Special Senses, Other Disorders							
Taste perversion	7	4	8	4	6	5	<1

*Patients reporting one or more adverse events. A patient may have reported more than one adverse event within a body system/organ class category.

PRECAUTIONS

The safety and efficacy of REBETOL/INTRON A and PEG-INTRON therapy for the treatment of HIV infection, adenovirus, RSV, parainfluenza, or influenza infections have not been established. REBETOL Capsules should not be used for these indications. Ribavirin for inhalation has a separate package insert, which should be consulted if ribavirin inhalation therapy is being considered.

The safety and efficacy of REBETOL/INTRON A therapy has not been established in liver or other organ transplant patients, patients with decompensated liver disease due to hepatitis C infection, patients who are nonresponders to interferon therapy, or patients coinfected with HBV or HIV.

Information for Patients

Patients must be informed that REBETOL Capsules and Oral Solution may cause birth defects and/or death of the exposed fetus. REBETOL must not be used by women who are pregnant or by men whose female partners are pregnant. Extreme care must be taken to avoid pregnancy in female patients and in female partners of male patients taking REBETOL. REBETOL should not be initiated until a report of a negative pregnancy test has been obtained immediately prior to initiation of therapy. Patients must perform a pregnancy test monthly during therapy and for 6 months posttherapy. Women of childbearing potential must be counseled about use of effective contraception (two reliable forms) prior to initiating therapy. Patients (male and female) must be advised of the teratogenic/embryocidal risks and must be instructed to practice effective contraception during REBETOL and for 6 months posttherapy. Patients (male and female) should be advised to notify the physician immediately in the event of a pregnancy. (See **CONTRAINDICATIONS** and **WARNINGS.**)

If pregnancy does occur during treatment or during 6 months posttherapy, the patient must be advised of the teratogenic risk of REBETOL therapy to the fetus. Patients, or partners of patients, should immediately report any pregnancy that occurs during treatment or within 6 months after treatment cessation to their physician. Physicians should report such cases by calling 1-800-727-7064.

Patients receiving REBETOL Capsules should be informed of the benefits and risks associated with treatment, directed in its appropriate use, and referred to the patient **MEDICATION GUIDE**. Patients should be informed that the effect of treatment of hepatitis C infection on transmission is not known, and that appropriate precautions to prevent transmission of the hepatitis C virus should be taken.

The most common adverse experience occurring with REBETOL Capsules is anemia, which may be severe. (See **ADVERSE REACTIONS.**) Patients should be advised that laboratory evaluations are required prior to starting therapy and periodically thereafter. (See **Laboratory Tests.**) It is advised that patients be well hydrated, especially during the initial stages of treatment.

Laboratory Tests The following laboratory tests are recommended for all patients treated with REBETOL Capsules, prior to beginning treatment and then periodically thereafter.

- Standard hematologic tests—including hemoglobin (pretreatment, week 2 and week 4 of therapy, and as clinically appropriate [see **WARNINGS**]), complete and differential white blood cell counts, and platelet count.
- Blood chemistries—liver function tests and TSH.
- Pregnancy—including monthly monitoring for women of childbearing potential.
- ECG (See **WARNINGS.**)

Continued on next page

Information on Schering products appearing on these pages is effective as of June 2003.

Rebetol—Cont.

Carcinogenesis and Mutagenesis Ribavirin did not cause an increase in any tumor type when administered for 6 months in the transgenic p53 deficient mouse model at doses up to 300 mg/kg (estimated human equivalent of 25 mg/kg based on body surface area adjustment for a 60 kg adult; approximately 1.9 times the maximum recommended human daily dose). Ribavirin was non-carcinogenic when administered for 2 years to rats at doses up to 40 mg/kg (estimated human equivalent of 5.71 mg/kg based on body surface area adjustment for a 60 kg adult). However, this dose was less than the maximum tolerated dose, and therefore the study was not adequate to fully characterize the carcinogenic potential of ribavirin.

Ribavirin demonstrated increased incidences of mutation and cell transformation in multiple genotoxicity assays. Ribavirin was active in the Balb/3T3 *In Vitro* Cell Transformation Assay. Mutagenic activity was observed in the mouse lymphoma assay, and at doses of 20–200 mg/kg (estimated human equivalent of 1.67–16.7 mg/kg, based on body surface area adjustment for a 60 kg adult; 0.1–1 X the maximum recommended human 24-hour dose of ribavirin) in a mouse micronucleus assay. A dominant lethal assay in rats was negative, indicating that if mutations occurred in rats they were not transmitted through male gametes.

Impairment of Fertility Ribavirin demonstrated significant embryocidal and/or teratogenic effects at doses well below the recommended human dose in all animal species in which adequate studies have been conducted.

Fertile women and partners of fertile women should not receive REBETOL unless the patient and his/her partner are using effective contraception (two reliable forms). Based on a multiple dose half-life ($t_{1/2}$) of ribavirin of 12 days, effective contraception must be utilized for 6 months post-therapy (eg, 15 half-lives of clearance for ribavirin).

REBETOL should be used with caution in fertile men. In studies in mice to evaluate the time course and reversibility of ribavirin-induced testicular degeneration at doses of 15 to 150 mg/kg/day (estimated human equivalent of 1.25–12.5 mg/kg/day, based on body surface area adjustment for a 60 kg adult; 0.1–0.8 X the maximum human 24-hour dose of ribavirin) administered for 3 or 6 months, abnormalities in sperm occurred. Upon cessation of treatment, essentially total recovery from ribavirin-induced testicular toxicity was apparent within 1 or 2 spermatogenesis cycles.

Animal Toxicology Long-term studies in the mouse and rat (18–24 months; doses of 20–75 and 10–40 mg/kg/day, respectively [estimated human equivalent doses of 1.67–6.25 and 1.43–5.71 mg/kg/day, respectively, based on body surface area adjustment for a 60 kg adult; approximately 0.1–0.4 X the maximum human 24-hour dose of ribavirin]) have demonstrated a relationship between chronic ribavirin exposure and increased incidences of vascular lesions (microscopic hemorrhages) in mice. In rats, retinal degeneration occurred in controls, but the incidence was increased in ribavirin-treated rats.

Pregnancy Category X (see **CONTRAINDICATIONS**)

Ribavirin produced significant embryocidal and/or teratogenic effects in all animal species in which adequate studies have been conducted. Malformations of the skull, palate, eye, jaw, limbs, skeleton, and gastrointestinal tract were noted. The incidence and severity of teratogenic effects increased with escalation of the drug dose. Survival of fetuses and offspring was reduced. In conventional embryotoxicity/teratogenicity studies in rats and rabbits, observed no effect dose levels were well below those for proposed clinical use (0.3 mg/kg/day for both the rat and rabbit; approximately 0.06 X the recommended human 24-hour dose of ribavirin). No maternal toxicity or effects on offspring were observed in a peri/postnatal toxicity study in rats dosed orally at up to 1 mg/kg/day (estimated human equivalent dose of 0.17 mg/kg based on body surface area adjustment for a 60 kg adult; approximately 0.01 X the maximum recommended human 24-hour dose of ribavirin).

Treatment and Posttreatment: Potential Risk to the Fetus Ribavirin is known to accumulate in intracellular components from where it is cleared very slowly. It is not known whether ribavirin contained in sperm will exert a potential teratogenic effect upon fertilization of the ova. In a study in rats, it was concluded that dominant lethality was not induced by ribavirin at doses up to 200 mg/kg for 5 days (estimated human equivalent doses of 7.14–28.6 mg/kg, based on body surface area adjustment for a 60 kg adult; up to 1.7 X the maximum recommended human dose of ribavirin). However, because of the potential human teratogenic effects of ribavirin, male patients should be advised to take every precaution to avoid risk of pregnancy for their female partners.

Women of childbearing potential should not receive REBETOL unless they are using effective contraception (two reliable forms) during the therapy period. In addition, effective contraception should be utilized for 6 months post-therapy based on a multiple-dose half-life ($t_{1/2}$) of ribavirin of 12 days.

Male patients and their female partners must practice effective contraception (two reliable forms) during treatment with REBETOL and for the 6-month posttherapy period (eg, 15 half-lives for ribavirin clearance from the body).

If pregnancy occurs in a patient or partner of a patient during treatment or during the 6 months after treatment cessation, physicians should report such cases by calling 1-800-727-7064.

Nursing Mothers It is not known whether the REBETOL product is excreted in human milk. Because of the potential for serious adverse reactions from the drug in nursing infants, a decision should be made whether to discontinue nursing or to delay or discontinue REBETOL.

Geriatric Use Clinical studies of REBETOL/INTRON A or PEG-INTRON therapy did not include sufficient numbers of subjects aged 65 and over to determine if they respond differently from younger subjects.

REBETOL is known to be substantially excreted by the kidney, and the risk of toxic reactions to this drug may be greater in patients with impaired renal function. Because elderly patients often have decreased renal function, care should be taken in dose selection. Renal function should be monitored and dosage adjustments should be made accordingly. REBETOL should not be used in patients with creatinine clearance <50 mL/min. (See **WARNINGS**.)

In general, REBETOL Capsules should be administered to elderly patients cautiously, starting at the lower end of the dosing range, reflecting the greater frequency of decreased hepatic and/or cardiac function, and of concomitant disease or other drug therapy. In clinical trials, elderly subjects had a higher frequency of anemia (67%) than did younger patients (28%). (See **WARNINGS**.)

Pediatric Use Suicidal ideation or attempts occurred more frequently among pediatric patients, primarily adolescents, compared to adult patients (2.4% versus 1%) during treatment and off-therapy follow-up (see WARNINGS). As in adult patients, pediatric patients experienced other psychiatric adverse events (eg, depression, emotional lability, somnolence), anemia, and neutropenia (see **WARNINGS**). During a 48-week course of therapy there was a decrease in the rate of linear growth (mean percentile assignment decrease of 9%) and a decrease in the rate of weight gain (mean percentile assignment decrease of 13%). A general reversal of these trends was noted during the 24-week posttreatment period.

Drug Interactions

Didanosine: Co-administration of REBETOL Capsules or Oral Solution and didanosine is not recommended. Reports of fatal hepatic failure, as well as peripheral neuropathy, pancreatitis, and symptomatic hyperlactactemia/ lactic acidosis have been reported in clinical trials (see **CLINICAL PHARMACOLOGY: Drug Interactions**).

Stavudine and Zidovudine: Ribavirin may antagonize the in vitro antiviral activity of stavudine and zidovudine against HIV. Therefore, concomitant use of ribavirin with either of these drugs should be used with caution (see **CLINICAL PHARMACOLOGY: Drug Interactions**).

ADVERSE REACTIONS

The primary toxicity of ribavirin is hemolytic anemia. Reductions in hemoglobin levels occurred within the first 1–2 weeks of oral therapy. (See WARNINGS.) Cardiac and pulmonary events associated with anemia occurred in approximately 10% of patients. (See WARNINGS.)

REBETOL/INTRON A Combination Therapy

In clinical trials, 19% and 6% of previously untreated and relapse patients, respectively, discontinued therapy due to adverse events in the combination arms compared to 13% and 3% in the interferon arms. Selected treatment-emergent adverse events that occurred in the US studies with ≥5% incidence are provided in **TABLE 7** by treatment group. In general, the selected treatment-emergent adverse events were reported with lower incidence in the international studies as compared to the US studies with the exception of asthenia, influenza-like symptoms, nervousness, and pruritus.

Pediatric Patients

In clinical trials of 118 pediatric patients 3 to 16 years of age, 6% discontinued therapy due to adverse events. Dose modifications were required in 30% of patients, most commonly for anemia and neutropenia. In general, the adverse event profile in the pediatric population was similar to that observed in adults. Injection site disorders, fever, anorexia, vomiting, and emotional lability occurred more frequently in pediatric patients compared to adult patients. Conversely, pediatric patients experienced less fatigue, dyspepsia, arthralgia, insomnia, irritability, impaired concentration, dyspnea, and pruritus compared to adult patients. Selected treatment-emergent adverse events that occurred with ≥5% incidence among all pediatric patients who received the recommended dose of REBETOL/INTRON A combination therapy are provided in **Table 7**.

[See table at top of previous page]

In addition, the following spontaneous adverse events have been reported during the marketing surveillance of REBETOL/INTRON A therapy: hearing disorder and vertigo.

REBETOL/PEG-INTRON Combination Therapy

Overall, in clinical trials, 14% of patients receiving REBETOL in combination with PEG-INTRON, discontinued therapy compared with 13% treated with REBETOL in combination with INTRON A. The most common reasons for discontinuation of therapy were related to psychiatric, systemic (eg, fatigue, headache), or gastrointestinal adverse events. Adverse events that occurred in clinical trial at >5% incidence are provided in **Table 8** by treatment group. Safety and effectiveness of REBETOL in combination with PEG-INTRON has not been established in pediatric patients.

TABLE 8. Adverse Events Occurring in > 5% of Patients

Adverse Events	*Percentage of Patients Reporting Adverse Events**	
	PEG-INTRON 1.5 µg/kg/ REBETOL (N=511)	**INTRON A/ REBETOL (N=505)**
Application Site		
Injection Site Inflammation	25	18
Injection Site Reaction	58	36
Autonomic Nervous System		
Mouth Dry	12	8
Sweating Increased	11	7
Flushing	4	3
Body as a Whole		
Fatigue/Asthenia	66	63
Headache	62	58
Rigors	48	41
Fever	46	33
Weight Decrease	29	20
RUQ Pain	12	6
Chest Pain	8	7
Malaise	4	6
Central & Peripheral Nervous System		
Dizziness	21	17
Endocrine		
Hypothyroidism	5	4
Gastrointestinal		
Nausea	43	33
Anorexia	32	27
Diarrhea	22	17
Vomiting	14	12
Abdominal Pain	13	13
Dyspepsia	9	8
Constipation	5	5
Hematologic Disorders		
Neutropenia	26	14
Anemia	12	17
Leukopenia	6	5
Thrombocytopenia	5	2
Liver and Biliary System		
Hepatomegaly	4	4
Musculoskeletal		
Myalgia	56	50
Arthralgia	34	28
Musculoskeletal Pain	21	19
Psychiatric		
Insomnia	40	41
Depression	31	34
Anxiety/Emotional Lability/Irritability	47	47
Concentration Impaired	17	21
Agitation	8	5
Nervousness	6	6
Reproductive, Female		
Menstrual Disorder	7	6
Resistance Mechanism		
Infection Viral	12	12
Infection Fungal	6	1
Respiratory System		
Dyspnea	26	24
Coughing	23	16
Pharyngitis	12	13
Rhinitis	8	6
Sinusitis	6	5
Skin and Appendages		
Alopecia	36	32
Pruritus	29	28
Rash	24	23
Skin Dry	24	23
Special Senses, Other		
Taste Perversion	9	4

Vision Disorders		
Vision Blurred	5	6
Conjunctivitis	4	5

***Patients reporting one or more adverse events. A patient may have reported more than one adverse event within a body system/organ class category.**

Laboratory Values

REBETOL/INTRON A Combination Therapy

Changes in selected hematologic values (hemoglobin, white blood cells, neutrophils, and platelets) during therapy are described below. (See **TABLE 9**.)

Hemoglobin Hemoglobin decreases among patients receiving REBETOL therapy began at Week 1, with stabilization by Week 4. In previously untreated patients treated for 48 weeks the mean maximum decrease from baseline was 3.1 g/dL in the US study and 2.9 g/dL in the International study. In relapse patients the mean maximum decrease from baseline was 2.8 g/dL in the US study and 2.6 g/dL in the International study. Hemoglobin values returned to pretreatment levels within 4–8 weeks of cessation of therapy in most patients.

Bilirubin and Uric Acid Increases in both bilirubin and uric acid, associated with hemolysis, were noted in clinical trials. Most were moderate biochemical changes and were reversed within 4 weeks after treatment discontinuation. This observation occurs most frequently in patients with a previous diagnosis of Gilbert's syndrome. This has not been associated with hepatic dysfunction or clinical morbidity.

[See table 9 at right]

REBETOL/PEG-INTRON Combination Therapy

Changes in selected hematologic values (hemoglobin, white blood cells, neutrophils, and platelets) during therapy are described below. (See **TABLE 10**.)

Hemoglobin

REBETOL induced a decrease in hemoglobin levels in approximately two thirds of patients. Hemoglobin levels decreased to <11g/dL in about 30% of patients. Severe anemia (<8 g/dL) occurred in <1% of patients. Dose modification was required in 9 and 13% of patients in the PEG-INTRON/REBETOL and INTRON A/REBETOL groups.

Bilirubin and Uric Acid

In the REBETOL/PEG-INTRON combination trial 10–14% of patients developed hyperbilirubinemia and 33-38% developed hyperuricemia in association with hemolysis. Six patients developed mild to moderate gout.

TABLE 10. Selected Hematologic Values During Treatment with REBETOL plus PEG-INTRON

	Number (%) of Subjects	
	PEG-INTRON plus REBETOL (N=511)	**INTRON A plus REBETOL (N=505)**
Hemoglobin (g/dL)		
9.5–10.9	26	27
8.0–9.4	3	3
6.5–7.9	0.2	0.2
<6.5	0	0
Leukocytes ($\times 10^9$/L)		
2.0–2.9	46	41
1.5–1.9	24	8
1.0–1.4	5	1
<1.0	0	0
Neutrophils ($\times 10^9$/L)		
1.0–1.49	33	37
0.75–0.99	25	13
0.5–0.74	18	7
<0.5	4	2
Platelets ($\times 10^9$/L)		
70–99	15	5
50–69	3	0.8
30–49	0.2	0.2
<30	0	0
Total Bilirubin (mg/dL)		
1.5–3.0	10	13
3.1–6.0	0.6	0.2
6.1–12.0	0	0.2
>12.0	0	0
ALT (SGPT)		
2 × Baseline	0.6	0.2
2.1–5 × Baseline	3	1
5.1–10 × Baseline	0	0
>10 × Baseline	0	0

OVERDOSAGE

There is limited experience with overdosage. Acute ingestion of up to 20 grams of REBETOL Capsules, INTRON A ingestion of up to 120 million units, and subcutaneous doses of INTRON A up to 10 times the recommended doses have been reported. Primary effects that have been observed are increased incidence and severity of the adverse events related to the therapeutic use of INTRON A and REBETOL.

TABLE 9. Selected Hematologic Values During Treatment with REBETOL plus INTRON A: Previously Untreated and Relapse Adult Patients and Previously Untreated Pediatric Patients

	Percentage of Patients						
	US Previously Untreated Study				US Relapse Study		Pediatric Patients
	24 weeks of treatment		48 weeks of treatment		24 weeks of treatment		48 weeks of treatment
	INTRON A plus REBETOL (N=228)	**INTRON A plus Placebo (N=231)**	**INTRON A plus REBETOL (N=228)**	**INTRON A plus Placebo (N=225)**	**INTRON A plus REBETOL (N=77)**	**INTRON A plus Placebo (N=76)**	**INTRON A plus REBETOL (N=118)**
Hemoglobin (g/dL)							
9.5–10.9	24	1	32	1	21	3	24
8.0–9.4	5	0	4	0	4	0	3
6.5–7.9	0	0	0	0.4	0	0	0
<6.5	0	0	0	0	0	0	0
Leukocytes ($\times 10^9$/L)							
2.0–2.9	40	20	38	23	45	26	35
1.5–1.9	4	1	9	2	5	3	8
1.0–1.4	0.9	0	2	0	0	0	0
<1.0	0	0	0	0	0	0	0
Neutrophils ($\times 10^9$/L)							
1.0–1.49	30	32	31	44	42	34	37
0.75–0.99	14	15	14	11	16	18	15
0.5–0.74	9	9	14	7	8	4	16
<0.5	11	8	11	5	5	8	3
Platelets ($\times 10^9$/L)							
70–99	9	11	11	14	6	12	0.8
50–69	2	3	2	3	0	5	2
30–49	0	0.4	0	0.4	0	0	0
<30	0.9	0	1	0.9	0	0	0
Total Bilirubin (mg/dL)							
1.5–3.0	27	13	32	13	21	7	2
3.1–6.0	0.9	0.4	2	0	3	0	0
6.1–12.0	0	0	0.4	0	0	0	0
>12.0	0	0	0	0	0	0	0

However, hepatic enzyme abnormalities, renal failure, hemorrhage, and myocardial infarction have been reported with administration of single subcutaneous doses of INTRON A that exceed dosing recommendations.

There is no specific antidote for INTRON A or REBETOL overdose, and hemodialysis and peritoneal dialysis are not effective for treatment of overdose of either agent.

DOSAGE AND ADMINISTRATION

(see **CLINICAL PHARMACOLOGY, Special Populations**; see **WARNINGS**)

REBETOL/INTRON A Combination Therapy

Adults The recommended dose of REBETOL Capsules depends on the patient's body weight. The recommended dose of REBETOL is provided in **TABLE 11**.

The recommended duration of treatment for patients previously untreated with interferon is 24 to 48 weeks. The duration of treatment should be individualized to the patient depending on baseline disease characteristics, response to therapy, and tolerability of the regimen. (See **Description of Clinical Studies** and **ADVERSE REACTIONS**.) After 24 weeks of treatment virologic response should be assessed. Treatment discontinuation should be considered in any patient who has not achieved an HCV RNA below the limit of detection of the assay by 24 weeks. There are no safety and efficacy data on treatment for longer than 48 weeks in the previously untreated patient population.

In patients who relapse following non-pegylated interferon monotherapy, the recommended duration of treatment is 24 weeks. There are no safety and efficacy data on treatment for longer than 24 weeks in the relapse patient population.

TABLE 11. Recommended Dosing

Body weight	REBETOL Capsules
≤ 75 kg	2 × 200-mg capsules AM, 3 × 200-mg capsules PM daily p.o.
> 75 kg	3 × 200 mg capsules AM, 3 × 200 mg capsules PM daily p.o.

Pediatrics The recommended dose of REBETOL is 15 mg/kg per day orally (divided dose AM and PM). For children weighing ≤25 kg or who cannot swallow capsules, REBETOL Oral Solution is supplied in a concentration of 40 mg/mL. For children weighing >25 kg, either the Oral Solution or 200-mg capsule may be administered. Refer to **TABLE 12** for dosing recommendations for the 200-mg capsule to achieve the recommended dose.

The recommended duration of treatment is 48 weeks for pediatric patients with genotype 1. After 24 weeks of treatment virologic response should be assessed. Treatment discontinuation should be considered in any patient who has not achieved an HCV RNA below the limit of detection of the assay by this time. The recommended duration of treatment for pediatric patients with genotype 2/3 is 24 weeks. There are no safety and efficacy data on treatment for longer than 48 weeks in pediatrics.

TABLE 12. Pediatric Dosing

Body weight	REBETOL Capsules	INTRON A Injection
25–36 kg	1 × 200-mg capsules AM, 1 × 200-mg capsules PM daily p.o.	3 million IU/m² 3 times weekly s.c.
37–49 kg	1 × 200-mg capsules AM, 2 × 200-mg capsules PM daily p.o.	3 million IU/m² 3 times weekly s.c.
50–61 kg	2 × 200-mg capsules AM, 2 × 200-mg capsules PM daily p.o.	3 million IU/m² 3 times weekly s.c.
>61 kg	Refer to adult dosing table.	Refer to adult dosing table

REBETOL may be administered without regard to food, but should be administered in a consistent manner with respect to food intake. (See **CLINICAL PHARMACOLOGY**.)

REBETOL/PEG-INTRON Combination Therapy

The recommended dose of REBETOL Capsules is 800 mg/day in 2 divided doses: two capsules (400 mg) in the morning with food and two capsules (400 mg) in the evening with food.

***Dose Modifications* (TABLE 13)**

If severe adverse reactions or laboratory abnormalities develop during combination REBETOL/INTRON A therapy the dose should be modified, or discontinued if appropriate, until the adverse reactions abate. If intolerance persists after dose adjustment, REBETOL/INTRON A therapy should be discontinued.

REBETOL should not be used in patients with creatinine clearance <50 mL/min. (See **WARNINGS** and **CLINICAL PHARMACOLOGY, Special Populations**.)

Continued on next page

Information on Schering products appearing on these pages is effective as of June 2003.

Rebetol—Cont.

REBETOL should be administered with caution to patients with preexisting cardiac disease. Patients should be assessed before commencement of therapy and should be appropriately monitored during therapy. If there is any deterioration of cardiovascular status, therapy should be stopped. (See **WARNINGS**.)

For patients with a history of stable cardiovascular disease, a permanent dose reduction is required if the hemoglobin decreases by ≥2 g/dL during any 4-week period. In addition, for these cardiac history patients, if the hemoglobin remains <12 g/dL after 4 weeks on a reduced dose, the patient should discontinue combination REBETOL/INTRON A therapy.

It is recommended that a patient whose hemoglobin level falls below 10 g/dL have his/her REBETOL dose reduced to 600 mg daily (1 × 200-mg capsule AM, 2 × 200-mg capsules PM) for adults and 7.5 mg/kg per day (divided dose AM and PM) for pediatric patients. A patient whose hemoglobin level falls below 8.5 g/dL should be permanently discontinued from REBETOL therapy. (See **WARNINGS**.)

TABLE 13. Guidelines for Dose Modifications and Discontinuation for Anemia

Hemoglobin	Dose Reduction* REBETOL-600 mg daily adults 7.5 mg/kg daily for pediatrics	Permanent Discontinuation of REBETOL Treatment
No Cardiac History	**<10 g/dL**	**<8.5 g/dL**
Cardiac History Patients	**≥2 g/dL decrease during any 4-week period during treatment**	**<12 g/dL after 4 weeks of dose reduction**

HOW SUPPLIED

REBETOL 200-mg Capsules are white, opaque capsules with REBETOL, 200 mg, and the Schering Corporation logo imprinted on the capsule shell; the capsules are packaged in a bottle containing 42 capsules (NDC 0085-1327-04), 56 capsules (NDC 0085-1351-05), 70 capsules (NDC 0085-1385-07), and 84 capsules (NDC 0085-1194-03).

REBETOL Oral Solution 40 mg/mL is a clear, colorless to pale or light yellow bubble gum-flavored liquid and it is packaged in 4-oz. amber glass bottles (100 mL/bottle) with child-resistant closures (NDC 0085-1318-01).

Storage Conditions

The bottle of REBETOL Capsules should be stored at 25°C (77°F); excursions permitted to 15°–30°C (59°–86°F) [see USP Controlled Room Temperature].

REBETOL Oral Solution should be stored between 2° and 8°C (36° and 46°F) or at 25°C (77°F); excursions permitted to 15°–30°C (59°–86°F) [see USP Controlled Room Temperature].

Schering Corporation
Kenilworth, NJ 07033 USA
U.S. Patents 4,530,901 & 4,211,771

Rev. 9/03 27002404T

REBETRON® ℞

[rĕb-ĕ-trŏn]

Combination Therapy *containing* REBETOL® (ribavirin, USP) Capsules *and* INTRON® A (interferon alfa-2b, recombinant) Injection

CONTRAINDICATIONS AND WARNINGS

Combination REBETOL/INTRON A therapy is contraindicated in females who are pregnant and in the male partners of females who are pregnant. Extreme care must be taken to avoid pregnancy during therapy and for 6 months after completion of treatment in female patients, and in female partners of male patients who are taking combination REBETOL/INTRON A therapy. Females of childbearing potential and males must use two reliable forms of effective contraception during treatment and during the 6-month posttreatment follow-up period. Significant teratogenic and/or embryocidal effects have been demonstrated for ribavirin in all animal species studied. See CONTRAINDICATIONS and WARNINGS. REBETOL monotherapy is not effective for the treatment of chronic hepatitis C and should not be used for this indication. See WARNINGS.

Alpha interferons, including INTRON® A, cause or aggravate fatal or life-threatening neuropsychiatric, autoimmune, ischemic, and infectious disorders. Patients should be monitored closely with periodic clinical and laboratory evaluations. Patients with persistently severe or worsening signs or symptoms of these conditions should be withdrawn from therapy. In many but not all cases these disorders resolve after stopping INTRON A therapy. See **WARNINGS**, and **ADVERSE REACTIONS**.

DESCRIPTION

REBETOL®

REBETOL is Schering Corporation's brand name for ribavirin, a nucleoside analog with antiviral activity. The chemical name of ribavirin is 1-β-D-ribofuranosyl-1*H*-1,2,4-triazole-3-carboxamide and has the following structural formula:

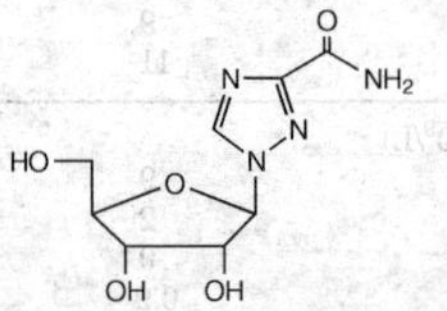

Ribavirin is a white, crystalline powder. It is freely soluble in water and slightly soluble in anhydrous alcohol. The empirical formula is $C_8H_{12}N_4O_5$ and the molecular weight is 244.21.

REBETOL Capsules consist of a white powder in a white, opaque, gelatin capsule. Each capsule contains 200 mg ribavirin and the inactive ingredients microcrystalline cellulose, lactose monohydrate, croscarmellose sodium, and magnesium stearate. The capsule shell consists of gelatin and titanium dioxide. The capsule is printed with edible blue pharmaceutical ink which is made of shellac, anhydrous ethyl alcohol, isopropyl alcohol, n-butyl alcohol, propylene glycol, ammonium hydroxide, and FD&C Blue #2 aluminum lake.

INTRON® A

INTRON A is Schering Corporation's brand name for interferon alfa-2b, recombinant, a purified, sterile, recombinant interferon product.

Interferon alfa-2b, recombinant has been classified as an alpha interferon and is a water-soluble protein composed of 165 amino acids with a molecular weight of 19,271 daltons produced by recombinant DNA techniques. It is obtained from the bacterial fermentation of a strain of *Escherichia coli* bearing a genetically engineered plasmid containing an interferon alfa-2b gene from human leukocytes. The fermentation is carried out in a defined nutrient medium containing the antibiotic tetracycline hydrochloride at a concentration of 5 to 10 mg/L; the presence of this antibiotic is not detectable in the final product.

INTRON A Injection is a clear, colorless solution. The 3 million IU vial of INTRON A Injection contains 3 million IU of interferon alfa-2b, recombinant per 0.5 mL. The 18 million IU multidose vial of INTRON A Injection contains a total of 22.8 million IU of interferon alfa-2b, recombinant per 3.8 mL (3 million IU/0.5 mL) in order to provide the delivery of six 0.5-mL doses, each containing 3 million IU of INTRON A (for a label strength of 18 million IU). The 18 million IU INTRON A Injection multidose pen contains a total of 22.5 million IU of interferon alfa-2b, recombinant per 1.5 mL (3 million IU/0.2 mL) in order to provide the delivery of six 0.2-mL doses, each containing 3 million IU of INTRON A (for a label strength of 18 million IU). Each mL also contains 7.5 mg sodium chloride, 1.8 mg sodium phosphate dibasic, 1.3 mg sodium phosphate monobasic, 0.1 mg edetate disodium, 0.1 mg polysorbate 80, and 1.5 mg m-cresol as a preservative.

Based on the specific activity of approximately 2.6×10^8 IU/mg protein as measured by HPLC assay, the corresponding quantities of interferon alfa-2b, recombinant in the vials and pen described above are approximately 0.012 mg, 0.088 mg, and 0.087 mg protein, respectively.

Mechanism of Action

Ribavirin/Interferon alfa-2b, recombinant The mechanism of inhibition of hepatitis C virus (HCV) RNA by combination therapy with REBETOL and INTRON A has not been established.

CLINICAL PHARMACOLOGY

Pharmacokinetics

Interferon alfa-2b, recombinant Single- and multiple-dose pharmacokinetic properties of INTRON A (interferon alfa-2b, recombinant) are summarized in **TABLE 1**. Following a single 3 million IU (MIU) subcutaneous dose in 12 patients with chronic hepatitis C, mean (% CV*) serum concentrations peaked at 7 (44%) hours. Following 4 weeks of subcutaneous dosing with 3 MIU three times a week (TIW), interferon serum concentrations were undetectable predose. However, a twofold increase in bioavailability was noted upon multiple dosing of interferon; the reason for this is unknown. Mean half-life values following single- and multiple-dose administrations were 6.8 (24%) hours and 6.5 (29%) hours, respectively.

Ribavirin Single- and multiple-dose pharmacokinetic properties in adults with chronic hepatitis C are summarized in **TABLE 1**. Ribavirin was rapidly and extensively absorbed following oral administration. However, due to first-pass metabolism, the absolute bioavailability averaged 64% (44%). There was a linear relationship between dose and AUC_{tf} (AUC from time zero to last measurable concentration) following single doses of 200-1200 mg ribavirin. The relationship between dose and C_{max} was curvilinear, tending to asymptote above single doses of 400-600 mg.

Upon multiple oral dosing, based on $AUC12_{hr}$, a sixfold accumulation of ribavirin was observed in plasma. Following oral dosing with 600 mg BID, steady-state was reached by approximately 4 weeks, with mean steady-state plasma concentrations of 2200 (37%) ng/mL. Upon discontinuation of dosing, the mean half-life was 298 (30%) hours, which probably reflects slow elimination from nonplasma compartments.

Effect of Food on Absorption of Ribavirin Both AUC_{tf} and C_{max} increased by 70% when REBETOL Capsules were administered with a high-fat meal (841 kcal, 53.8 g fat, 31.6 g protein, and 57.4 g carbohydrate) in a single-dose pharmacokinetic study. There are insufficient data to address the clinical relevance of these results. Clinical efficacy studies were conducted without instructions with respect to food consumption. (See **DOSAGE AND ADMINISTRATION**.)

Effect of Antacid on Absorption of Ribavirin Coadministration with an antacid containing magnesium, aluminum, and simethicone (Mylanta®) resulted in a 14% decrease in mean ribavirin AUC_{tf}. The clinical relevance of results from this single-dose study is unknown.

[See table 1 below]

Ribavirin transport into nonplasma compartments has been most extensively studied in red blood cells, and has been identified to be primarily via an e_s-type equilibrative nucleoside transporter. This type of transporter is present on virtually all cell types and may account for the extensive volume of distribution. Ribavirin does not bind to plasma proteins.

Ribavirin has two pathways of metabolism: (i) a reversible phosphorylation pathway in nucleated cells; and (ii) a degradative pathway involving deribosylation and amide hydrolysis to yield a triazole carboxylic acid metabolite. Ribavirin and its triazole carboxamide and triazole carboxylic acid metabolites are excreted renally. After oral administration of 600 mg of ^{14}C-ribavirin, approximately 61% and 12% of the radioactivity was eliminated in the urine and feces, respectively, in 336 hours. Unchanged ribavirin accounted for 17% of the administered dose.

Results of *in vitro* studies using both human and rat liver microsome preparations indicated little or no cytochrome P450 enzyme-mediated metabolism of ribavirin, with minimal potential for P450 enzyme-based drug interactions.

No pharmacokinetic interactions were noted between INTRON A Injection and REBETOL Capsules in a multiple-dose pharmacokinetic study.

Special Populations

Renal Dysfunction The pharmacokinetics of ribavirin were assessed after administration of a single oral dose (400 mg) of ribavirin to subjects with varying degrees of renal dysfunction. The mean AUC_{tf} value was threefold greater in subjects with creatinine clearance values between 10 to 30 mL/min when compared to control subjects (creatinine clearance >90 mL/min). This appears to be due to reduction of apparent clearance in these patients. Ribavirin was not removed by hemodialysis. Patients with creatinine clearance <50 mL/min should not be treated with REBETOL (see **WARNINGS**).

Hepatic Dysfunction The effect of hepatic dysfunction was assessed after a single oral dose of ribavirin (600 mg). The mean AUC_{tf} values were not significantly different in subjects with mild, moderate, or severe hepatic dysfunction (Child-Pugh Classification A, B, or C) when compared to control subjects. However, the mean C_{max} values increased with severity of hepatic dysfunction and was twofold

TABLE 1. Mean (% CV) Pharmacokinetic Parameters for INTRON A and REBETOL When Administered Individually to Adults with Chronic Hepatitis C

Parameter	INTRON A (N=12)		REBETOL (N=12)	
	Single Dose 3 MIU	Multiple Dose 3 MIU TIW	Single Dose 600 mg	Multiple Dose 600 mg BID
T_{max} (hr)	7 (44)	5 (37)	1.7 (46)***	3 (60)
C_{max}*	13.9 (32)	29.7 (33)	782 (37)	3680 (85)
AUC_{tf}**	142 (43)	333 (39)	13400 (48)	228000 (25)
$T_{1/2}$ (hr)	6.8 (24)	6.5 (29)	43.6 (47)	298 (30)
Apparent Volume of Distribution (L)			2825 (9)†	
Apparent Clearance (L/hr)	14.3 (17)		38.2 (40)	
Absolute Bioavailability			64% (44)††	

* IU/mL for INTRON A and ng/mL for REBETOL
** IU.hr/mL for INTRON A and ng.hr/mL for REBETOL
† Data obtained from a single-dose pharmacokinetic study using ^{14}C labeled ribavirin; N=5
†† N=6
*** N=11

greater in subjects with severe hepatic dysfunction when compared to control subjects.

Pediatric Patients Multiple-dose pharmacokinetic properties for ribavirin in pediatric patients with chronic hepatitis C between 5 and 16 years of age are summarized in **TABLE 2**.

TABLE 2. Mean (% CV) Pharmacokinetic Parameters for REBETOL When Administered to Pediatric Patients with Chronic Hepatitis C

Parameter	12 mg/kg/day as 2 divided doses (n=19)	15 mg/kg/day as 2 divided doses (n=19)
T_{max} (hr)	1.4 (60)	1.9 (81)
C_{max} (ng/mL)	2705 (17)	3243 (24)
AUC_{12} (ng*hr/mL)	25049 (16)	29620 (25)
Apparent Clearance (L/hr/kg)	0.25 (16)	0.27 (25)

Elderly Patients Pharmacokinetic evaluations for elderly subjects have not been performed.

Gender There were no clinically significant pharmacokinetic differences noted in a single-dose study of eighteen male and eighteen female subjects.

In this section of the label, numbers in parenthesis indicate % coefficient of variation.

INDICATIONS AND USAGE

REBETOL (ribavirin, USP) Capsules is indicated in combination with INTRON A (interferon alfa-2b, recombinant) Injection for the treatment of chronic hepatitis C in patients with compensated liver disease previously untreated with alpha interferon or who have relapsed following alpha interferon therapy.

Description of Clinical Studies

Previously Untreated Patients Adults with compensated chronic hepatitis C and detectable HCV RNA (assessed by a central laboratory using a research-based RT-PCR assay) who were previously untreated with alpha interferon therapy were enrolled into two multicenter, double-blind trials (US and International) and randomized to receive REBETOL Capsules 1200 mg/day (1000 mg/day for patients weighing ≤75 kg) plus INTRON A Injection 3 MIU TIW or INTRON A Injection plus placebo for 24 or 48 weeks followed by 24 weeks of off-therapy follow-up. The International study did not contain a 24-week INTRON A plus placebo treatment arm. The US study enrolled 912 patients who, at baseline, were 67% male, 89% caucasian with a mean Knodell HAI score (I+II+III) of 7.5, and 72% genotype 1. The International study, conducted in Europe, Israel, Canada, and Australia, enrolled 799 patients (65% male, 95% caucasian, mean Knodell score 6.8, and 58% genotype 1).

Study results are summarized in **TABLE 3**.

[See table 3 above]

TABLE 3. Virologic and Histologic Responses: Previously Untreated Patients*

	US Study				International Study		
	24 weeks of treatment		48 weeks of treatment		24 weeks of treatment	48 weeks of treatment	
	INTRON A plus REBETOL (N=228)	**INTRON A plus Placebo (N=231)**	**INTRON A plus REBETOL (N=228)**	**INTRON A plus Placebo (N=225)**	**INTRON A plus REBETOL (N=265)**	**INTRON A plus REBETOL (N=268)**	**INTRON A plus Placebo (N=266)**
Virologic Response							
–Responder[1]	65 (29)	13 (6)	85 (37)	27 (12)	86 (32)	113 (42)	46 (17)
–Nonresponder	147 (64)	194 (84)	110 (48)	168 (75)	158 (60)	120 (45)	196 (74)
–Missing data	16 (7)	24 (10)	33 (14)	30 (13)	21 (8)	35 (13)	24 (9)
Histologic Response							
–Improvement[2]	102 (45)	77 (33)	96 (42)	65 (29)	103 (39)	102 (38)	69 (26)
–No improvement	77 (34)	99 (43)	61 (27)	93 (41)	85 (32)	58 (22)	111 (41)
–Missing data	49 (21)	55 (24)	71 (31)	67 (30)	77 (29)	108 (40)	86 (32)

*Number (%) of patients

[1] Defined as HCV RNA below limit of detection using a research-based RT-PCR assay at end of treatment and during follow-up period.

[2] Defined as posttreatment (end of follow-up) minus pretreatment liver biopsy Knodell HAI score (I+II+III) improvement of ≥2 points.

Of patients who had not achieved HCV RNA below the limit of detection of the research-based assay by week 24 of REBETOL/INTRON A treatment, less than 5% responded to an additional 24 weeks of combination treatment.

Among patients with HCV genotype 1 treated with REBETOL/INTRON A therapy who achieved HCV RNA below the detection limit of the research-based assay by 24 weeks, those randomized to 48 weeks of treatment had higher virologic responses compared to those in the 24-week treatment group. There was no observed increase in response rates for patients with HCV nongenotype 1 randomized to REBETOL/INTRON A therapy for 48 weeks compared to 24 weeks.

Relapse Patients Patients with compensated chronic hepatitis C and detectable HCV RNA (assessed by a central laboratory using a research-based RT-PCR assay) who had relapsed following one or two courses of interferon therapy (defined as abnormal serum ALT levels) were enrolled into two multicenter, double-blind trials (US and International) and randomized to receive REBETOL 1200 mg/day (1000 mg/day for patients weighing ≤75 kg) plus INTRON A 3 MIU TIW or INTRON A plus placebo for 24 weeks followed by 24 weeks of off-therapy follow-up. The US study enrolled 153 patients who, at baseline, were 67% male, 92% caucasian with a mean Knodell HAI score (I+II+III) of 6.8, and 58% genotype 1. The International study, conducted in Europe, Israel, Canada, and Australia, enrolled 192 patients (64% male, 95% caucasian, mean Knodell score 6.6, and 56% genotype 1).

Study results are summarized in **TABLE 4**.

[See table 4 above]

TABLE 4. Virologic and Histologic Responses: Relapse Patients*

	US Study		International Study	
	INTRON A plus REBETOL (N=77)	**INTRON A plus Placebo (N=76)**	**INTRON A plus REBETOL (N=96)**	**INTRON A plus Placebo (N=96)**
Virologic Response				
–Responder[1]	33 (43)	3 (4)	46 (48)	5 (5)
–Nonresponder	36 (47)	66 (87)	45 (47)	91 (95)
–Missing data	8 (10)	7 (9)	5 (5)	0 (0)
Histologic Response				
–Improvement[2]	38 (49)	27 (36)	49 (51)	30 (31)
–No improvement	23 (30)	37 (49)	29 (30)	44 (46)
–Missing data	16 (21)	12 (16)	18 (19)	22 (23)

*Number (%) of patients

[1] Defined as HCV RNA below limit of detection using a research-based RT-PCR assay at end of treatment and during follow-up period.

[2] Defined as posttreatment (end of follow-up) minus pretreatment liver biopsy Knodell HAI score (I+II+III) improvement of ≥2 points.

Virologic and histologic responses were similar among male and female patients in both the previously untreated and relapse studies.

CONTRAINDICATIONS

Combination REBETOL/INTRON A therapy must not be used by females who are pregnant or by males whose female partners are pregnant. Extreme care must be taken to avoid pregnancy in female patients and in female partners of male patients taking combination REBETOL/INTRON A therapy. Combination REBETOL/INTRON A therapy should not be initiated until a report of a negative pregnancy test has been obtained immediately prior to initiation of therapy. Females of childbearing potential and males must use two forms of effective contraception during treatment and during the 6 months after treatment has been concluded. Significant teratogenic and/or embryocidal effects have been demonstrated for ribavirin in all animal species in which adequate studies have been conducted. These effects occurred at doses as low as one twentieth of the recommended human dose of REBETOL Capsules. If pregnancy occurs in a patient or partner of a patient during treatment or during the 6 months after treatment stops, physicians are encouraged to report such cases by calling (800) 727-7064. **See boxed CONTRAINDICATIONS AND WARNINGS. See WARNINGS.**

REBETOL Capsules in combination with INTRON A Injection is contraindicated in patients with a history of hypersensitivity to ribavirin and/or alpha interferon or any component of the capsule and/or injection.

Patients with autoimmune hepatitis must not be treated with combination REBETOL/INTRON A therapy.

WARNINGS

Pregnancy

Category X, may cause birth defects. See boxed CONTRAINDICATIONS AND WARNINGS. See CONTRAINDICATIONS.

Anemia

HEMOLYTIC ANEMIA (HEMOGLOBIN <10 G/DL) WAS OBSERVED IN APPROXIMATELY 10% OF REBETOL/INTRON A-TREATED PATIENTS IN CLINICAL TRIALS (SEE ADVERSE REACTIONS LABORATORY VALUES – *HEMOGLOBIN*). ANEMIA OCCURRED WITHIN 1–2 WEEKS OF INITIATION OF RIBAVIRIN THERAPY. BECAUSE OF THIS INITIAL ACUTE DROP IN HEMOGLOBIN, IT IS ADVISED THAT COMPLETE BLOOD COUNTS (CBC) SHOULD BE OBTAINED PRETREATMENT AND AT WEEK 2 AND WEEK 4 OF THERAPY OR MORE FREQUENTLY IF CLINICALLY INDICATED. PATIENTS SHOULD THEN BE FOLLOWED AS CLINICALLY APPROPRIATE.

The anemia associated with REBETOL/INTRON A therapy may result in deterioration of cardiac function and/or exacerbation of the symptoms of coronary disease. Patients should be assessed before initiation of therapy and should be appropriately monitored during therapy. If there is any deterioration of cardiovascular status, therapy should be suspended or discontinued. (See **DOSAGE AND ADMINISTRATION**.) Because cardiac disease may be worsened by drug induced anemia, patients with a history of significant or unstable cardiac disease should not use combination REBETOL/INTRON A therapy. (See **ADVERSE REACTIONS**.)

Similarly, patients with hemoglobinopathies (eg, thalassemia, sickle-cell anemia) should not be treated with combination REBETOL/INTRON A therapy.

Psychiatric

Severe psychiatric adverse events, including depression, psychoses, aggressive behavior, hallucinations, violent behavior (suicidal ideation, suicidal attempts, suicides), and rare instances of homicidal ideation have occurred during combination REBETOL/INTRON A therapy, both in patients with and without a previous psychiatric disorder. REBETOL/INTRON A therapy should be used with extreme caution in patients with a history of pre-existing psychiatric disorders, and all patients should be carefully monitored for evidence of depression and other psychiatric symptoms. Suspension of REBETOL/INTRON A therapy should be considered if psychiatric intervention and/or dose reduction is unsuccessful in controlling psychiatric symptoms. In severe cases, therapy should be stopped immediately and psychiatric intervention sought. (See ADVERSE REACTIONS.)

Bone Marrow Toxicity

INTRON A therapy suppresses bone marrow function and may result in severe cytopenias including very rare events of aplastic anemia. It is advised that complete blood counts (CBC) be obtained pre-treatment and monitored routinely during therapy (see **PRECAUTIONS: Laboratory Tests**). INTRON A therapy should be discontinued in patients who develop severe decreases in neutrophil ($<0.5 \times 10^9$/L) or platelet counts ($<25 \times 10^9$/L) (See **DOSAGE AND ADMINISTRATION: Guidelines for Dose Modifications**).

Pulmonary

Pulmonary symptoms, including dyspnea, pulmonary infiltrates, pneumonitis and pneumonia, have been reported during therapy with REBETOL/INTRON A; occasional cases of fatal pneumonia have occurred. In addition, sarcoidosis or the exacerbation of sarcoidosis has been reported. If there is evidence of pulmonary infiltrates or pulmonary function impairment, the patient should be closely monitored, and if appropriate, combination REBETOL/INTRON A treatment should be discontinued.

Other

- REBETOL Capsule monotherapy is not effective for the treatment of chronic hepatitis C and should not be used for this indication.

Continued on next page

Information on Schering products appearing on these pages is effective as of June 2003.

Rebetron—Cont.

- Fatal and nonfatal pancreatitis has been observed in patients treated with REBETOL/INTRON A therapy. REBETOL/INTRON A therapy should be suspended in patients with signs and symptoms of pancreatitis and discontinued in patients with confirmed pancreatitis.
- Combination REBETOL/INTRON A therapy should not be used in patients with creatinine clearance <50 mL/min.
- Diabetes mellitus and hyperglycemia have been observed in patients treated with INTRON A.
- Ophthalmologic disorders have been reported with treatment with alpha interferons (including INTRON A therapy). Investigators using alpha interferons have reported the occurrence of retinal hemorrhages, cotton wool spots, and retinal artery or vein obstruction in rare instances. Any patient complaining of loss of visual acuity or visual field should have an eye examination. Because these ocular events may occur in conjunction with other disease states, a visual exam prior to initiation of combination REBETOL/INTRON A therapy is recommended in patients with diabetes mellitus or hypertension.
- Acute serious hypersensitivity reactions (eg, urticaria, angioedema, bronchoconstriction, anaphylaxis) have been observed in INTRON A-treated patients; if such an acute reaction develops, combination REBETOL/INTRON A therapy should be discontinued immediately and appropriate medical therapy instituted.
- Combination REBETOL/INTRON A therapy should be discontinued for patients developing thyroid abnormalities during treatment whose thyroid function cannot be controlled by medication.

PRECAUTIONS

Exacerbation of autoimmune disease has been reported in patients receiving alpha interferon therapy (including INTRON A therapy). REBETOL/INTRON A therapy should be used with caution in patients with other autoimmune disorders.

There have been reports of interferon, including INTRON A (interferon alfa-2b, recombinant) exacerbating pre-existing psoriasis; therefore, combination REBETOL/INTRON A therapy should be used in these patients only if the potential benefit justifies the potential risk.

The safety and efficacy of REBETOL/INTRON A therapy has not been established in liver or other organ transplant patients, decompensated hepatitis C patients, patients who are nonresponders to interferon therapy, or patients coinfected with HBV or HIV.

The safety and efficacy of REBETOL Capsule monotherapy for the treatment of HIV infection, adenovirus, early RSV infection, parainfluenza, or influenza have not been established and REBETOL Capsules should not be used for these indications.

There is no information regarding the use of REBETOL Capsules with other interferons.

Triglycerides Elevated triglyceride levels have been observed in patients treated with interferon including REBETOL/INTRON A therapy. Elevated triglyceride levels should be managed as clinically appropriate. Severe hypertriglyceridemia (triglycerides >1000 mg/dL) may result in pancreatitis. Discontinuation of REBETOL/INTRON A therapy should be considered for patients with persistently elevated triglycerides (triglycerides >1000 mg/dL) associated with symptoms of potential pancreatitis, such as abdominal pain, nausea, or vomiting (see **WARNINGS - Other**).

Drug Interactions Nucleoside Analogues: Administration of nucleoside analogues has resulted in fatal and nonfatal lactic acidosis. Coadministration of ribavirin and nucleoside analogues should be undertaken with caution and only if the potential benefit outweighs the potential risks.

Information for Patients Combination REBETOL/INTRON A therapy must not be used by females who are pregnant or by males whose female partners are pregnant. Extreme care must be taken to avoid pregnancy in female patients and in female partners of male patients taking combination REBETOL/INTRON A therapy. Combination REBETOL/INTRON A therapy should not be initiated until a report of a negative pregnancy test has been obtained immediately prior to initiation of therapy. Patients must perform a pregnancy test monthly during therapy and for 6 months posttherapy. Females of childbearing potential must be counseled about use of effective contraception (two reliable forms) prior to initiating therapy. Patients (male and female) must be advised of the teratogenic/embryocidal risks and must be instructed to practice effective contraception during combination REBETOL/INTRON A therapy and for 6 months posttherapy. Patients (male and female) should be advised to notify the physician immediately in the event of a pregnancy. (See **CONTRAINDICATIONS**.)

If pregnancy does occur during treatment or during 6 months posttherapy, the patient must be advised of the significant teratogenic risk of REBETOL therapy to the fetus. Patients, or partners of patients, should immediately report any pregnancy that occurs during treatment or within 6 months after treatment cessation to their physician. Physicians are encouraged to report such cases by calling (800) 727-7064.

Patients receiving combination REBETOL/INTRON A treatment should be directed in its appropriate use, informed of the benefits and risks associated with treatment, and referred to the patient **MEDICATION GUIDE**. There are no data evaluating whether REBETOL/INTRON A therapy will prevent transmission of infection to others. Also, it is not known if treatment with REBETOL/INTRON A therapy will cure hepatitis C or prevent cirrhosis, liver failure, or liver cancer that may be the result of infection with the hepatitis C virus.

TABLE 5. Selected Treatment-Emergent Adverse Events: Previously Untreated and Relapse Patients

	Percentage of Patients					
	US Previously Untreated Study				US Relapse Study	
	24 weeks of treatment		48 weeks of treatment		24 weeks of treatment	
Patients Reporting Adverse Events*	**INTRON A plus REBETOL (N=228)**	**INTRON A plus Placebo (N=231)**	**INTRON A plus REBETOL (N=228)**	**INTRON A plus Placebo (N=225)**	**INTRON A plus REBETOL (N=77)**	**INTRON A plus Placebo (N=76)**
Application Site Disorders						
injection site inflammation	13	10	12	14	6	8
injection site reaction	7	9	8	9	5	3
Body as a Whole - General Disorders						
headache	63	63	66	67	66	68
fatigue	68	62	70	72	60	53
rigors	40	32	42	39	43	37
fever	37	35	41	40	32	36
influenza-like symptoms	14	18	18	20	13	13
asthenia	9	4	9	9	10	4
chest pain	5	4	9	8	6	7
Central & Peripheral Nervous System Disorders						
dizziness	17	15	23	19	26	21
Gastrointestinal System Disorders						
nausea	38	35	46	33	47	33
anorexia	27	16	25	19	21	14
dyspepsia	14	6	16	9	16	9
vomiting	11	10	9	13	12	8
Musculoskeletal System Disorders						
myalgia	61	57	64	63	61	58
arthralgia	30	27	33	36	29	29
musculoskeletal pain	20	26	28	32	22	28
Psychiatric Disorders						
insomnia	39	27	39	30	26	25
irritability	23	19	32	27	25	20
depression	32	25	36	37	23	14
emotional lability	7	6	11	8	12	8
concentration impaired	11	14	14	14	10	12
nervousness	4	2	4	4	5	4
Respiratory System Disorders						
dyspnea	19	9	18	10	17	12
sinusitis	9	7	10	14	12	7
Skin and Appendages Disorders						
alopecia	28	27	32	28	27	26
rash	20	9	28	8	21	5
pruritus	21	9	19	8	13	4
Special Senses, Other Disorders						
taste perversion	7	4	8	4	6	5

* Patients reporting one or more adverse events. A patient may have reported more than one adverse event within a body system/organ class category.

If home use is prescribed, a puncture-resistant container for the disposal of used syringes and needles should be supplied to the patient. Patients should be thoroughly instructed in the importance of proper disposal and cautioned against any reuse of needles and syringes. The full container should be disposed of according to the directions provided by the physician (see **MEDICATION GUIDE**). To avoid possible transmission of disease, do not share your multidose pen with anyone; it is for you and you alone.

The most common adverse experiences occurring with combination REBETOL/INTRON A therapy are "flu-like" symptoms, such as headache, fatigue, myalgia, and fever (see **ADVERSE REACTIONS**) and appear to decrease in severity as treatment continues. Some of these "flu-like" symptoms may be minimized by bedtime administration of INTRON A therapy. Antipyretics should be considered to prevent or partially alleviate the fever and headache. Another common adverse experience associated with INTRON A therapy is thinning of the hair.

Patients should be advised that laboratory evaluations are required prior to starting therapy and periodically thereafter (see **Laboratory Tests**). It is advised that patients be well hydrated, especially during the initial stages of treatment.

Laboratory Tests The following laboratory tests are recommended for all patients on combination REBETOL/INTRON A therapy, prior to beginning treatment and then periodically thereafter.

- Standard hematologic tests – including hemoglobin (pretreatment, week 2 and week 4 of therapy, and as clinically appropriate [see **WARNINGS**]), complete and differential white blood cell counts, and platelet count.
- Blood chemistries – liver function tests and TSH.
- Pregnancy – including monthly monitoring for females of childbearing potential.

Carcinogenesis and Mutagenesis Carcinogenicity studies with interferon alfa-2b, recombinant have not been performed because neutralizing activity appears in the serum after multiple dosing in all of the animal species tested. Adequate studies to assess the carcinogenic potential of ribavirin in animals have not been conducted. However, ribavirin is a nucleoside analog that has produced positive findings in multiple *in vitro* and animal *in vivo* genotoxicity assays, and should be considered a potential carcinogen. Further studies to assess the carcinogenic potential of ribavirin in animals are ongoing.

Mutagenicity studies have demonstrated that interferon alfa-2b, recombinant is not mutagenic. Ribavirin demonstrated increased incidences of mutation and cell transformation in multiple genotoxicity assays. Ribavirin was active in the Balb/3T3 *In Vitro* Cell Transformation Assay. Mutagenic activity was observed in the mouse lymphoma assay, and at doses of 20-200 mg/kg (estimated human equivalent of 1.67-16.7 mg/kg, based on body surface area adjustment for a 60 kg adult; 0.1-1 × the maximum recommended human 24-hour dose of ribavirin) in a mouse micronucleus assay. A dominant lethal assay in rats was negative, indicating that if mutations occurred in rats they were not transmitted through male gametes.

Impairment of Fertility No reproductive toxicology studies have been performed using interferon alfa-2b, recombinant in combination with ribavirin. However, evidence provided below for interferon alfa-2b, recombinant and ribavirin when administered alone indicate that both agents have adverse effects on reproduction. It should be assumed that the effects produced by either agent alone will also be caused by the combination of the two agents. Interferons may impair human fertility. In studies of interferon alfa-2b, recombinant administration in nonhuman primates, menstrual cycle abnormalities have been observed. Decreases in serum estradiol and progesterone concentrations have been reported in females treated with human leukocyte interferon. In addition, ribavirin demonstrated significant embryocidal and/or teratogenic effects at doses well below the recommended human dose in all animal species in which adequate studies have been conducted.

Fertile females and partners of fertile females should not receive combination REBETOL/INTRON A therapy unless the patient and his/her partner are using effective contraception (two reliable forms). Based on a multiple dose half-life ($t_{1/2}$) of ribavirin of 12 days, effective contraception must be utilized for 6 months posttherapy (eg, 15 half-lives of clearance for ribavirin).

Combination REBETOL/INTRON A therapy should be used with caution in fertile males. In studies in mice to evaluate the time course and reversibility of ribavirin-induced testicular degeneration at doses of 15 to 150 mg/kg/day (estimated human equivalent of 1.25-12.5 mg/kg/day, based on body surface area adjustment for a 60 kg adult; 0.1-0.8 × the maximum human 24-hour dose of ribavirin) administered for 3 or 6 months, abnormalities in sperm occurred. Upon cessation of treatment, essentially total recovery from ribavirin-induced testicular toxicity was apparent within 1 or 2 spermatogenesis cycles.

Animal Toxicology Long-term studies in the mouse and rat (18-24 months; doses of 20-75 and 10-40 mg/kg/day, respectively [estimated human equivalent doses of 1.67-6.25 and 1.43-5.71 mg/kg/day, respectively, based on body surface area adjustment for a 60 kg adult; approximately 0.1-0.4 × the maximum human 24-hour dose of ribavirin]) have demonstrated a relationship between chronic ribavirin exposure and increased incidences of vascular lesions (microscopic hemorrhages) in mice. In rats, retinal degeneration occurred in controls, but the incidence was increased in ribavirin-treated rats.

Pregnancy Category X (see **CONTRAINDICATIONS**) Interferon alfa-2b, recombinant has been shown to have abortifacient effects in *Macaca mulatta* (rhesus monkeys) at 15 and 30 million IU/kg (estimated human equivalent of 5 and 10 million IU/kg, based on body surface area adjustment for a 60 kg adult). There are no adequate and well-controlled studies in pregnant females.

Ribavirin produced significant embryocidal and/or teratogenic effects in all animal species in which adequate studies have been conducted. Malformations of the skull, palate, eye, jaw, limbs, skeleton, and gastrointestinal tract were noted. The incidence and severity of teratogenic effects increased with escalation of the drug dose. Survival of fetuses and offspring was reduced. In conventional embryotoxicity/teratogenicity studies in rats and rabbits, observed no effect dose levels were well below those for proposed clinical use (0.3 mg/kg/day for both the rat and rabbit; approximately 0.06 × the recommended human 24-hour dose of ribavirin). No maternal toxicity or effects on offspring were observed in a peri/postnatal toxicity study in rats dosed orally at up to 1 mg/kg/day (estimated human equivalent dose of 0.17 mg/kg based on body surface area adjustment for a 60 kg adult; approximately 0.01 × the maximum recommended human 24-hour dose of ribavirin).

Treatment and Posttreatment: Potential Risk to the Fetus

Ribavirin is known to accumulate in intracellular components from where it is cleared very slowly. It is not known whether ribavirin contained in sperm will exert a potential teratogenic effect upon fertilization of the ova. In a study in rats, it was concluded that dominant lethality was not induced by ribavirin at doses up to 200 mg/kg for 5 days (estimated human equivalent doses of 7.14–28.6 mg/kg, based on body surface area adjustment for a 60 kg adult; up to 1.7 × the maximum recommended human dose of ribavirin). However, because of the potential human teratogenic effects of ribavirin, male patients should be advised to take every precaution to avoid risk of pregnancy for their female partners.

Females of childbearing potential should not receive combination REBETOL/INTRON A therapy unless they are using effective contraception (two reliable forms) during the therapy period. In addition, effective contraception should be utilized for 6 months posttherapy based on a multiple dose half-life ($t_{1/2}$) of ribavirin of 12 days.

Male patients and their female partners must practice effective contraception (two reliable forms) during treatment with combination REBETOL/INTRON A therapy and for the 6-month posttherapy period (eg, 15 half-lives for ribavirin clearance from the body).

If pregnancy occurs in a patient or partner of a patient during treatment or during the 6 months after treatment cessation, physicians are encouraged to report such cases by calling (800) 727-7064.

Nursing Mothers It is not known whether REBETOL and INTRON A are excreted in human milk. However, studies in mice have shown that mouse interferons are excreted into the milk. Because of the potential for serious adverse reactions from the drugs in nursing infants, a decision should be made whether to discontinue nursing or to discontinue combination REBETOL/INTRON A therapy, taking into account the importance of the therapy to the mother.

Pediatric Use One hundred twenty-five pediatric patients between three and sixteen years of age with chronic hepatitis C virus infection (median duration 10.7 years) received REBETOL Capsules with INTRON A for up to 48 weeks. The overall sustained response rate cannot be calculated since all patients have not yet completed 24-weeks of off-therapy follow-up.

Suicidal ideation or attempts occurred more frequently among pediatric patients compared to adult patients (2.4% versus 1%) during treatment and off-therapy follow-up (see WARNINGS). As in adult patients, pediatric patients experienced other psychiatric adverse events (eg, depression, emotional lability, somnolence), anemia, and neutropenia (see **WARNINGS**). During a 48-week course of therapy

TABLE 6. Selected Hematologic Values During Treatment with REBETOL plus INTRON A: Previously Untreated and Relapse Patients

	Percentage of Patients					
	US Previously Untreated Study				US Relapse Study	
	24 weeks of treatment		48 weeks of treatment		24 weeks of treatment	
	INTRON A plus REBETOL (N=228)	**INTRON A plus Placebo (N=231)**	**INTRON A plus REBETOL (N=228)**	**INTRON A plus Placebo (N=225)**	**INTRON A plus REBETOL (N=77)**	**INTRON A plus Placebo (N=76)**
Hemoglobin (g/dL)						
9.5-10.9	24	1	32	1	21	3
8.0-9.4	5	0	4	0	4	0
6.5-7.9	0	0	0	0.4	0	0
<6.5	0	0	0	0	0	0
Leukocytes (× 10^9/L)						
2.0-2.9	40	20	38	23	45	26
1.5-1.9	4	1	9	2	5	3
1.0-1.4	0.9	0	2	0	0	0
<1.0	0	0	0	0	0	0
Neutrophils (× 10^9/L)						
1.0-1.49	30	32	31	44	42	34
0.75-0.99	14	15	14	11	16	18
0.5-0.74	9	9	14	7	8	4
<0.5	11	8	11	5	5	8
Platelets (× 10^9/L)						
70-99	9	11	11	14	6	12
50-69	2	3	2	3	0	5
30-49	0	0.4	0	0.4	0	0
<30	0.9	0	1	0.9	0	0
Total Bilirubin (mg/dL)						
1.5-3.0	27	13	32	13	21	7
3.1-6.0	0.9	0.4	2	0	3	0
6.1-12.0	0	0	0.4	0	0	0
>12.0	0	0	0	0	0	0

TABLE 7. Recommended Adult Dosing

Body weight	REBETOL Capsules	INTRON A Injection
≤75 kg	2 × 200-mg capsules AM, 3 × 200-mg capsules PM daily p.o.	3 million IU 3 times weekly s.c.
>75 kg	3 × 200-mg capsules AM, 3 × 200-mg capsules PM daily p.o.	3 million IU 3 times weekly s.c.

there was a decrease in the rate of linear growth (mean percentile assignment decrease of 7%) and a decrease in the rate of weight gain (mean percentile assignment decrease of 9%). A general reversal of these trends was noted during the 24-week posttreatment period.

Injection site disorders, fever, anorexia, vomiting, and emotional lability occurred more frequently in pediatric patients compared to adult patients. Conversely, pediatric patients experienced less fatigue, dyspepsia, arthralgia, insomnia, irritability, impaired concentration, dyspnea, and pruritus compared to adult patients.

Geriatric Use Clinical studies of REBETRON Combination Therapy did not include sufficient numbers of subjects aged 65 and over to determine if they respond differently from younger subjects. In clinical trials, elderly subjects had a higher frequency of anemia (67%) than did younger patients (28%) (see **WARNINGS**).

In general, REBETOL (ribavirin) should be administered to elderly patients cautiously, starting at the lower end of the dosing range, reflecting the greater frequency of decreased renal, hepatic and/or cardiac function, and of concomitant disease or other drug therapy.

REBETOL (ribavirin) is known to be substantially excreted by the kidney, and the risk of adverse reactions to ribavirin may be greater in patients with impaired renal function. Because elderly patients often have decreased renal function, care should be taken in dose selection. Renal function should be monitored and dosage adjustments of ribavirin should be made accordingly (see **DOSAGE AND ADMINISTRATION: Guidelines for Dose Modifications**). REBETOL should not be used in elderly patients with creatinine clearance <50mL/min (see **WARNINGS**).

REBETRON Combination Therapy should be used very cautiously in elderly patients with a history of psychiatric disorders (see **WARNINGS**).

ADVERSE REACTIONS

The safety of combination REBETOL/INTRON A therapy was evaluated in controlled trials of 1010 HCV-infected adults who were previously untreated with interferon therapy and were subsequently treated for 24 or 48 weeks with combination REBETOL/INTRON A therapy and in 173 HCV-infected patients who had relapsed after interferon therapy and were subsequently treated for 24 weeks with combination REBETOL/INTRON A therapy. (See **Description of Clinical Studies.**) Overall, 19% and 6% of previously untreated and relapse patients, respectively, discontinued therapy due to adverse events in the combination arms compared to 13% and 3% in the interferon arms.

The primary toxicity of ribavirin is hemolytic anemia. Reductions in hemoglobin levels occurred within the first 1–2 weeks of therapy (see WARNINGS). Cardiac and pulmonary events associated with anemia occurred in approximately 10% of patients treated with REBETOL/INTRON A therapy. (See WARNINGS.)

The most common psychiatric events occurring in US studies of previously untreated and relapse patients treated with REBETOL/INTRON A therapy, respectively, were insomnia (39%, 26%), depression (34%, 23%), and irritability (27%, 25%). Suicidal behavior (ideation, attempts, and suicides) occurred in 1% of patients. (See **WARNINGS.**) In addition, hearing disorders (tinnitus and hearing loss) and vertigo have occurred in patients treated with combination REBETOL/INTRON A therapy.

Selected treatment-emergent adverse events that occurred in the US studies with ≥5% incidence are provided in **TABLE 5** by treatment group. In general, the selected treatment-emergent adverse events reported with lower incidence in the international studies as compared to the US studies with the exception of asthenia, influenza-like symptoms, nervousness, and pruritus.

[See table 5 at top of previous page]

Laboratory Values

Changes in selected hematologic values (hemoglobin, white blood cells, neutrophils, and platelets) during combination REBETOL/INTRON A treatment are described below (see **TABLE 6**).

Hemoglobin Hemoglobin decreases among patients on combination therapy began at Week 1, with stabilization by Week 4. In previously untreated patients treated for 48 weeks, the mean maximum decrease from baseline was 3.1 g/dL in the US study and 2.9 g/dL in the International study. In relapse patients, the mean maximum decrease from baseline was 2.8 g/dL in the US study and 2.6 g/dL in the International study. Hemoglobin values returned to pretreatment levels within 4 to 8 weeks of cessation of therapy in most patients.

Neutrophils There were decreases in neutrophil counts in both the combination REBETOL/INTRON A and INTRON A plus placebo dose groups. In previously untreated patients treated for 48 weeks, the mean maximum

Continued on next page

Information on Schering products appearing on these pages is effective as of June 2003.

Rebetron—Cont.

decrease in neutrophil count in the US study was 1.3 × 10^9/L and in the International study was 1.5 × 10^9/L. In relapse patients the mean maximum decrease in neutrophil count in the US study was 1.3 × 10^9/L and in the International study was 1.6 × 10^9/L. Neutrophil counts returned to pretreatment levels within 4 weeks of cessation of therapy in most patients.

Platelets In both previously untreated and relapse patients mean platelet counts generally remained in the normal range in all treatment groups; however, mean platelet counts were 10% to 15% lower in the INTRON A plus placebo group than the REBETOL/INTRON A group. Mean platelet counts returned to baseline levels within 4 weeks after treatment discontinuation.

Thyroid Function Of patients who entered the previously untreated (24 and 48 week treatments) and relapse (24 week treatment) studies without thyroid abnormalities, approximately 3% to 6% and 1% to 2%, respectively, developed thyroid abnormalities requiring clinical intervention.

Bilirubin and Uric Acid Increases in both bilirubin and uric acid, associated with hemolysis, were noted in clinical trials. Most were moderate biochemical changes and were reversed within 4 weeks after treatment discontinuation. This observation occurs most frequently in patients with a previous diagnosis of Gilbert's syndrome. This has not been associated with hepatic dysfunction or clinical morbidity.

[See table 6 at top of previous page]

OVERDOSAGE

There is limited experience with overdosage. Acute ingestion of up to 20 grams of REBETOL Capsules, INTRON A ingestion of up to 120 million units, and subcutaneous doses of INTRON A up to 10 times the recommended doses have been reported. Primary effects that have been observed are increased incidence and severity of the adverse events related to the therapeutic use of INTRON A and REBETOL. However, hepatic enzyme abnormalities, renal failure, hemorrhage, and myocardial infarction have been reported with administration of single subcutaneous doses of INTRON A that exceed dosing recommendations.

There is no specific antidote for INTRON A or REBETOL, and hemodialysis and peritoneal dialysis are not effective for treatment of overdose of either agent.

DOSAGE AND ADMINISTRATION

INTRON A Injection should be administered subcutaneously and REBETOL Capsules should be administered orally. REBETOL may be administered without regard to food, but should be administered in a consistent manner. (See **CLINICAL PHARMACOLOGY**.)

Adults

The recommended dose of REBETOL Capsules depends on the patient's body weight. The recommended doses of REBETOL and INTRON A are given in **TABLE 7**.

The recommended duration of treatment for patients previously untreated with interferon is 24 to 48 weeks. The duration of treatment should be individualized to the patient depending on baseline disease characteristics, response to therapy, and tolerability of the regimen (see **Description of Clinical Studies** and **ADVERSE REACTIONS**). After 24 weeks of treatment virologic response should be assessed. Treatment discontinuation should be considered in any patient who has not achieved an HCV RNA below the limit of detection of the assay by 24 weeks. There are no safety and efficacy data on treatment for longer than 48 weeks in the previously untreated patient population.

In patients who relapse following interferon therapy, the recommended duration of treatment is 24 weeks. There are no safety and efficacy data on treatment for longer than 24 weeks in the relapse patient population.

[See table 7 on previous page]

Pediatrics

Efficacy of REBETOL and INTRON A for pediatric patients has not been established. Based on pharmacokinetic data, the following doses of REBETOL and INTRON A provide similar exposures in pediatric patients as observed in adult patients treated with the approved doses of REBETOL and INTRON A (see **TABLE 8**).

[See table 8 above]

Under no circumstances should REBETOL Capsules be opened, crushed, or broken (See **CONTRAINDICATIONS** and **WARNINGS**).

Dose Modifications (**TABLE 9**)

In clinical trials, approximately 26% of patients required modification of their dose of REBETOL Capsules, INTRON A Injection, or both agents. If severe adverse reactions or laboratory abnormalities develop during combination REBETOL/INTRON A therapy, the dose should be modified, or discontinued if appropriate, until the adverse reactions abate. If intolerance persists after dose adjustment, REBETOL/INTRON A therapy should be discontinued.

REBETOL/INTRON A therapy should be administered with caution to patients with pre-existing cardiac disease. Patients should be assessed before commencement of therapy and should be appropriately monitored during therapy. If there is any deterioration of cardiovascular status, therapy should be stopped. (See **WARNINGS**.)

For patients with a history of stable cardiovascular disease, a permanent dose reduction is required if the hemoglobin decreases by ≥2 g/dL during any 4-week period. In addition, for these cardiac history patients, if the hemoglobin remains <12 g/dL after 4 weeks on a reduced dose, the patient should discontinue combination REBETOL/INTRON A therapy.

It is recommended that a patient whose hemoglobin level falls below 10 g/dL have his/her REBETOL dose reduced to 600 mg daily (1 × 200-mg capsule AM, 2 × 200-mg capsules PM). A patient whose hemoglobin level falls below 8.5 g/dL should be permanently discontinued from REBETOL/ INTRON A therapy. (See **WARNINGS**.)

It is recommended that a patient who experiences moderate depression (persistent low mood, loss of interest, poor self image, and/or hopelessness) have his/her INTRON A dose temporarily reduced and/or be considered for medical ther-

Table 8. Pediatric Dosing

Body weight	REBETOL Capsules	INTRON A Injection
25-36 kg	1 × 200-mg capsule AM 1 × 200-mg capsule PM daily p.o.	3 million IU/m² 3 times weekly s.c.
37-49 kg	1 × 200-mg capsule AM 2 × 200-mg capsules PM daily p.o.	3 million IU/m² 3 times weekly s.c.
50-61 kg	2 × 200-mg capsules AM 2 × 200-mg capsules PM daily p.o.	3 million IU/m² 3 times weekly s.c.
>61 kg	Refer to adult dosing table	Refer to adult dosing table

TABLE 9. Guidelines for Dose Modifications

	Dose Reduction* REBETOL - Adults: 600 mg daily Pediatrics: half the dose INTRON A - Adults: 1.5 million IU TIW Pediatrics: 1.5 million IU/m² TIW	Permanent Discontinuation of Treatment REBETOL and INTRON A
Hemoglobin	<10 g/dL (REBETOL) **Cardiac History Patients Only.** **≥2 g/dL decrease during any 4-week period during treatment (REBETOL/INTRON A)**	<8.5 g/dL **Cardiac History Patients Only.** **<12 g/dL after 4 weeks of dose reduction**
White blood count	<1.5 × 10^9/L (INTRON A)	<1.0 × 10^9/L
Neutrophil count	<0.75 × 10^9/L (INTRON A)	<0.5 × 10^9/L
Platelet count	Adults: <50 × 10^9/L (INTRON A) Pediatrics: <80 × 10^9/L (INTRON A)	Adults: <25 × 10^9/L Pediatrics: <50 × 10^9/L

*Study medication to be dose reduced is shown in parenthesis.

Vial/Pen Label Strength	Fill Volume	Concentration
3 million IU vial	0.5 mL	3 million IU/0.5 mL
18 million IU multidose vial†	3.8 mL	3 million IU/0.5 mL
18 million IU multidose pen††	1.5 mL	3 million IU/0.2 mL

† This is a multidose vial which contains a total of 22.8 million IU of interferon alfa-2b, recombinant per 3.8 mL in order to provide the delivery of six 0.5-mL doses, each containing 3 million IU of interferon alfa-2b, recombinant (for a label strength of 18 million IU).

†† This is a multidose pen which contains a total of 22.5 million IU of interferon alfa-2b, recombinant per 1.5 mL in order to provide the delivery of six 0.2-mL doses, each containing 3 million IU of interferon alfa-2b, recombinant (for a label strength of 18 million IU).

	Each REBETRON Combination Package Consists of:	
For Patients ≤75 kg	A box containing 6 vials of INTRON A Injection (3 million IU in 0.5 mL per vial), 6 B-D Safety-Lok™ syringes with a safety sleeve, alcohol swabs, and one bottle containing 70 REBETOL Capsules.	(NDC 0085-1241-02)
	One 18 million IU multidose vial of INTRON A Injection (22.8 million IU per 3.8 mL; 3 million IU/0.5 mL), 6 B-D Safety Lok™ syringes with a safety sleeve, alcohol swabs, and one bottle containing 70 REBETOL Capsules.	(NDC 0085-1236-02)
	One 18 million IU INTRON A Injection multidose pen (22.5 million IU per 1.5 mL; 3 million IU/0.2 mL), 6 disposable needles, alcohol swabs, and one bottle containing 70 REBETOL Capsules.	(NDC 0085-1258-02)
For Patients >75 kg	A box containing 6 vials of INTRON A Injection (3 million IU in 0.5 mL per vial), 6 B-D Safety-Lok™ syringes with a safety sleeve, alcohol swabs, and one bottle containing 84 REBETOL Capsules.	(NDC 0085-1241-01)
	One 18 million IU multidose vial of INTRON A Injection (22.8 million IU per 3.8 mL; 3 million IU/0.5 mL), 6 B-D Safety Lok™ syringes with a safety sleeve, alcohol swabs, and one bottle containing 84 REBETOL Capsules.	(NDC 0085-1236-01)
	One 18 million IU INTRON A Injection multidose pen (22.5 million IU per 1.5 mL; 3 million IU/0.2 mL), 6 disposable needles, alcohol swabs, and one bottle containing 84 REBETOL Capsules.	(NDC 0085-1258-01)
For REBETOL Dose Reduction	A box containing 6 vials of INTRON A Injection (3 million IU in 0.5 mL per vial), 6 B-D Safety-Lok™ syringes with a safety sleeve, alcohol swabs, and one bottle containing 42 REBETOL Capsules.	(NDC 0085-1241-03)
	One 18 million IU multidose vial of INTRON A Injection (22.8 million IU per 3.8 mL; 3 million IU/0.5 mL), 6 B-D Safety Lok™ syringes with a safety sleeve, alcohol swabs, and one bottle containing 42 REBETOL Capsules.	(NDC 0085-1236-03)
	One 18 million IU INTRON A Injection multidose pen (22.5 million IU per 1.5 mL; 3 million IU/0.2 mL), 6 disposable needles, alcohol swabs, and one bottle containing 42 REBETOL Capsules.	(NDC 0085-1258-03)

apy. A patient experiencing severe depression or suicidal ideation/attempt should be discontinued from REBETOL/INTRON A therapy and followed closely with appropriate medical management. (See **WARNINGS**.)

[See table 9 on previous page]

Administration of INTRON A Injection

At the discretion of the physician, the patient may self-administer the INTRON A. (See illustrated **MEDICATION GUIDE** for instructions.)

The INTRON A Injection is supplied as a clear and colorless solution. The appropriate INTRON A dose should be withdrawn from the vial or set on the multidose pen and injected subcutaneously. The INTRON A Injection supplied with the B-D Safety Lok™ syringes contain a plastic sleeve to be pulled over the needle after use. The syringe locks with an audible click when the green stripe on the safety sleeve covers the red stripe on the needle. After administration of INTRON A Injection, it is essential to follow the procedure for proper disposal of syringes and needles. (See **MEDICATION GUIDE** for detailed instructions.)

[See third table at top of previous page]

Parenteral drug products should be inspected visually for particulate matter and discoloration prior to administration, whenever solution and container permit. INTRON A Injection may be administered using either sterilized glass or plastic disposable syringes.

Stability INTRON A Injection provided in vials is stable at 35°C (95°F) for up to 7 days and at 30°C (86°F) for up to 14 days. INTRON A Injection provided in a multidose pen is stable at 30°C (86°F) for up to 2 days. The solution is clear and colorless.

HOW SUPPLIED

REBETOL 200-mg Capsules are white, opaque capsules with REBETOL, 200 mg, and the Schering Corporation logo imprinted on the capsule shell; the capsules are packaged in a bottle.

INTRON A Injection is a clear, colorless solution packaged in single-dose and multidose vials, and a multidose pen.

INTRON A Injection and REBETOL Capsules are available in the following combination package presentations:

[See fourth table on previous page]

STORAGE CONDITIONS

Store the REBETOL Capsules plus INTRON A Injection combination package refrigerated between 2° and 8°C (36° and 46°F).

When separated, the individual bottle of REBETOL Capsules should be stored refrigerated between 2° and 8°C (36° and 46°F) or at 25°C (77°F); excursions are permitted between 15° and 30°C (59° and 86°F).

When separated, the individual vials of INTRON A Injection and the INTRON A multidose pen should be stored refrigerated between 2° and 8°C (36°and 46°F).

Schering Corporation
Kenilworth, NJ 07033 USA

B-25930614 Rev. 9/02
25272927T

RIBAVIRIN, USP CAPSULES ℞

[rī-bə-vī-rĭn]

- **Ribavirin monotherapy is not effective for the treatment of chronic hepatitis C virus infection and should not be used alone for this indication. (See WARNINGS.)**
- **The primary toxicity of ribavirin is hemolytic anemia. The anemia associated with ribavirin therapy may result in worsening of cardiac disease that has led to fatal and nonfatal myocardial infarctions. Patients with a history of significant or unstable cardiac disease should not be treated with ribavirin. (See WARNINGS, ADVERSE REACTIONS, and DOSAGE AND ADMINISTRATION.)**
- **Significant teratogenic and/or embryocidal effects have been demonstrated in all animal species exposed to ribavirin. In addition, ribavirin has a multiple-dose half-life of 12 days, and so it may persist in nonplasma compartments for as long as 6 months. Therefore, ribavirin therapy is contraindicated in women who are pregnant and in the male partners of women who are pregnant. Extreme care must be taken to avoid pregnancy during therapy and for 6 months after completion of treatment in both female patients and in female partners of male patients who are taking ribavirin therapy. At least two reliable forms of effective contraception must be utilized during treatment and during the 6-month posttreatment follow-up period. (See CONTRAINDICATIONS, WARNINGS, PRECAUTIONS–Information for Patients and Pregnancy Category X.)**

DESCRIPTION

Ribavirin is a nucleoside analog. The chemical name of ribavirin is 1-β-D-ribofuranosyl-1*H*-1,2,4-triazole-3-carboxamide and has the following structural formula:

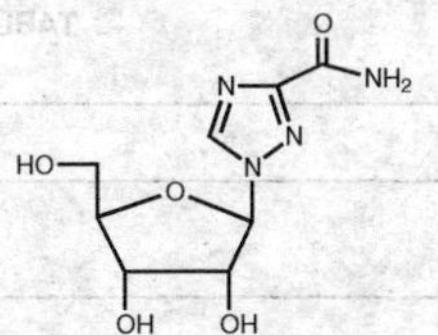

Ribavirin is a white, crystalline powder. It is freely soluble in water and slightly soluble in anhydrous alcohol. The empirical formula is $C_8H_{12}N_4O_5$ and the molecular weight is 244.21.

Ribavirin Capsules consist of a white powder in a white, opaque, gelatin capsule. Each capsule contains 200 mg ribavirin and the inactive ingredients microcrystalline cellulose, lactose monohydrate, croscarmellose sodium, and magnesium stearate. The capsule shell consists of gelatin, sodium lauryl sulfate, silicon dioxide, and titanium dioxide. The capsule is printed with edible blue pharmaceutical ink which is made of shellac, anhydrous ethyl alcohol, isopropyl alcohol, n-butyl alcohol, propylene glycol, ammonium hydroxide, and FD&C Blue #2 aluminum lake.

Mechanism of Action

The mechanism of inhibition of hepatitis C virus (HCV) RNA by combination therapy with interferon products has not been established.

CLINICAL PHARMACOLOGY

Pharmacokinetics

Ribavirin Single- and multiple-dose pharmacokinetic properties in adults with chronic hepatitis C are summarized in **TABLE 1**. Ribavirin was rapidly and extensively absorbed following oral administration. However, due to first-pass metabolism, the absolute bioavailability averaged 64% (44%). There was a linear relationship between dose and AUC_{tf} (AUC from time zero to last measurable concentration) following single doses of 200-1200 mg ribavirin. The relationship between dose and C_{max} was curvilinear, tending to asymptote above single doses of 400-600 mg.

Upon multiple oral dosing, based on $AUC12_{hr}$, a sixfold accumulation of ribavirin was observed in plasma. Following oral dosing with 600 mg BID, steady-state was reached by approximately 4 weeks, with mean steady-state plasma concentrations of 2200 (37%) ng/mL. Upon discontinuation of dosing, the mean half-life was 298 (30%) hours, which probably reflects slow elimination from nonplasma compartments.

Effect of Food on Absorption of Ribavirin Both AUC_{tf} and C_{max} increased by 70% when Ribavirin Capsules were administered with a high-fat meal (841 kcal, 53.8 g fat, 31.6 g protein, and 57.4 g carbohydrate) in a single-dose pharmacokinetic study. There are insufficient data to address the clinical relevance of these results. Clinical efficacy studies with Ribavirin/INTRON A were conducted without instructions with respect to food consumption. During clinical studies with Ribavirin/PEG-INTRON, all subjects were instructed to take Ribavirin Capsules with food. (See **DOSAGE AND ADMINISTRATION**.)

Effect of Antacid on Absorption of Ribavirin Coadministration with an antacid containing magnesium, aluminum, and simethicone (Mylanta®[1]) resulted in a 14% decrease in mean ribavirin AUC_{tf}. The clinical relevance of results from this single-dose study is unknown.

TABLE 1. Mean (% CV) Pharmacokinetic Parameters for Ribavirin When Administered Individually to Adults with Chronic Hepatitis C

Parameter	Ribavirin (N=12)	
	Single Dose 600 mg	Multiple Dose 600 mg BID
T_{max} (hr)	1.7 (46)***	3 (60)
C_{max}*	782 (37)	3680 (85)
AUC_{tf}**	13400 (48)	228000 (25)
$T_{1/2}$ (hr)	43.6 (47)	298 (30)
Apparent Volume of Distribution (L)	2825 (9)†	
Apparent Clearance (L/hr)	38.2 (40)	
Absolute Bioavailability	64% (44)††	

* ng/mL
** ng.hr/mL
*** N = 11
† data obtained from a single-dose pharmacokinetic study using ^{14}C labeled ribavirin; N = 5
†† N = 6

Ribavirin transport into nonplasma compartments has been most extensively studied in red blood cells, and has been identified to be primarily via an e_s-type equilibrative nucleoside transporter. This type of transporter is present on virtually all cell types and may account for the extensive volume of distribution. Ribavirin does not bind to plasma proteins.

Ribavirin has two pathways of metabolism: (i) a reversible phosphorylation pathway in nucleated cells; and (ii) a degradative pathway involving deribosylation and amide hydrolysis to yield a triazole carboxylic acid metabolite. Ribavirin and its triazole carboxamide and triazole carboxylic acid metabolites are excreted renally. After oral administration of 600 mg of ^{14}C-ribavirin, approximately 61% and 12% of the radioactivity was eliminated in the urine and feces, respectively, in 336 hours. Unchanged ribavirin accounted for 17% of the administered dose.

Results of *in vitro* studies using both human and rat liver microsome preparations indicated little or no cytochrome P450 enzyme-mediated metabolism of ribavirin, with minimal potential for P450 enzyme-based drug interactions.

No pharmacokinetic interactions were noted between INTRON A Injection and Ribavirin Capsules in a multiple-dose pharmacokinetic study.

1. Trademark of Johnson & Johnson-Merck Consumer Pharmaceuticals Co.

Special Populations

Renal Dysfunction The pharmacokinetics of ribavirin were assessed after administration of a single oral dose (400 mg) of ribavirin to non HCV-infected subjects with varying degrees of renal dysfunction. The mean AUC_{tf} value was threefold greater in subjects with creatinine clearance values between 10 to 30 mL/min when compared to control subjects (creatinine clearance >90 mL/min). In subjects with creatinine clearance values between 30 to 60 mL/min, AUC_{tf} was twofold greater when compared to control subjects. The increased AUC_{tf} appears to be due to reduction of renal and non-renal clearance in these patients. Phase III efficacy trials included subjects with creatinine clearance values >50 mL/min. The multiple dose pharmacokinetics of ribavirin cannot be accurately predicted in patients with renal dysfunction. Ribavirin is not effectively removed by hemodialysis. Patients with creatinine clearance <50 mL/min should not be treated with ribavirin (See **WARNINGS**.)

Hepatic Dysfunction The effect of hepatic dysfunction was assessed after a single oral dose of ribavirin (600 mg). The mean AUC_{tf} values were not significantly different in subjects with mild, moderate, or severe hepatic dysfunction (Child-Pugh Classification A, B, or C) when compared to control subjects. However, the mean C_{max} values increased with severity of hepatic dysfunction and was twofold greater in subjects with severe hepatic dysfunction when compared to control subjects.

Pediatric Patients Pharmacokinetic evaluations in pediatric subjects have not been performed.

Elderly Patients Pharmacokinetic evaluations in elderly subjects have not been performed.

Gender There were no clinically significant pharmacokinetic differences noted in a single-dose study of eighteen male and eighteen female subjects.

In this section of the label, numbers in parenthesis indicate % coefficient of variation.

INDICATIONS AND USAGE

Ribavirin, USP Capsules are indicated in combination with INTRON A (interferon alfa-2b, recombinant) Injection for the treatment of chronic hepatitis C in patients with compensated liver disease previously untreated with alpha interferon or who have relapsed following alpha interferon therapy.

Ribavirin Capsules are indicated in combination with PEG-INTRON (peg-interferon alfa-2b, recombinant) Injection for the treatment of chronic hepatitis C in patients with compensated liver disease who have not been previously treated with interferon alpha and are at least 18 years of age.

The safety and efficacy of Ribavirin Capsules with interferons other than INTRON A or PEG-INTRON products have not been established.

Description of Clinical Studies

Ribavirin/INTRON A Combination Therapy

Previously Untreated Patients

Adults with compensated chronic hepatitis C and detectable HCV RNA (assessed by a central laboratory using a research-based RT-PCR assay) who were previously untreated with alpha interferon therapy were enrolled into two multicenter, double-blind trials (US and International) and randomized to receive Ribavirin Capsules 1200 mg/day (1000 mg/day for patients weighing ≤75 kg) plus INTRON A Injection 3 MIU TIW or INTRON A Injection plus placebo for 24 or 48 weeks followed by 24 weeks of off-therapy follow-up. The International study did not contain a 24-week INTRON A plus placebo treatment arm. The US study enrolled 912 patients who, at baseline, were 67% male, 89% Caucasian with a mean Knodell HAI score (I+II+III) of 7.5, and 72% genotype 1. The International study, conducted in Europe, Israel, Canada, and Australia, enrolled 799 patients (65% male, 95% Caucasian, mean Knodell score 6.8, and 58% genotype 1).

Study results are summarized in **TABLE 2**.

[See table 2 at top of next page]

Of patients who had not achieved HCV RNA below the limit of detection of the research based assay by week 24 of Ribavirin/INTRON A treatment, less than 5% responded to an additional 24 weeks of combination treatment.

Among patients with HCV Genotype 1 treated with Ribavirin/INTRON A therapy who achieved HCV RNA below the detection limit of the research-based assay by 24 weeks, those randomized to 48 weeks of treatment had higher virologic responses compared to those in the 24 week

Continued on next page

Information on Schering products appearing on these pages is effective as of June 2003.

Ribavirin—Cont.

treatment group. There was no observed increase in response rates for patients with HCV nongenotype 1 randomized to Ribavirin/INTRON A therapy for 48 weeks compared to 24 weeks.

Relapse Patients

Patients with compensated chronic hepatitis C and detectable HCV RNA (assessed by a central laboratory using a research-based RT-PCR assay) who had relapsed following one or two courses of interferon therapy (defined as abnormal serum ALT levels) were enrolled into two multicenter, double-blind trials (US and International) and randomized to receive ribavirin 1200 mg/day (1000 mg/day for patients weighing ≤75 kg) plus INTRON A 3 MIU TIW or INTRON A plus placebo for 24 weeks followed by 24 weeks of off-therapy follow-up. The US study enrolled 153 patients who, at baseline, were 67% male, 92% Caucasian with a mean Knodell HAI score (I+II+III) of 6.8, and 58% genotype 1. The International study, conducted in Europe, Israel, Canada, and Australia, enrolled 192 patients (64% male, 95% Caucasian, mean Knodell score 6.6, and 56% genotype 1).

Study results are summarized in **TABLE 3.**

[See table 3 at right]

Virologic and histologic responses were similar among male and female patients in both the previously untreated and relapse studies.

Ribavirin/PEG-INTRON Combination Therapy

A randomized study compared treatment with two PEG-INTRON/Ribavirin regimens [PEG-INTRON 1.5 µg/kg SC once weekly (QW)/Ribavirin 800 mg PO daily (in divided doses); PEG-INTRON 1.5 µg/kg SC QW for 4 weeks then 0.5 µg/kg SC QW for 44 weeks/ Ribavirin 1000/1200 mg PO daily (in divided doses)] with INTRON A [3 MIU SC thrice weekly (TIW)/Ribavirin 1000/1200 mg PO daily (in divided doses)] in 1530 adults with chronic hepatitis C. Interferon naïve patients were treated for 48 weeks and followed for 24 weeks post-treatment. Eligible patients had compensated liver disease, detectable HCV RNA, elevated ALT, and liver histopathology consistent with chronic hepatitis.

Response to treatment was defined as undetectable HCV RNA at 24 weeks posttreatment (See **Table 4**).

TABLE 4. Rates of Response to Combination Treatment

	PEG-INTRON 1.5µg/kg QW Ribavirin 800 mg QD	INTRON A 3 MIU TIW Ribavirin 1000/1200 mg QD
Overall[1,2] response	52% (264/511)	46% (231/505)
Genotype 1	41% (141/348)	33% (112/343)
Genotype 2-6	75% (123/163)	73% (119/162)

1. Serum HCV RNA was measured with a research-based quantitative polymerase chain reaction assay by a central laboratory.
2. Difference in overall treatment response (PEG-INTRON/Ribavirin vs. INTRON A/Ribavirin) is 6% with 95% confidence interval of (0.18, 11.63) adjusted for viral genotype and presence of cirrhosis at baseline.

The response rate to PEG-INTRON 1.5→0.5µg/kg/Ribavirin was essentially the same as the response to INTRON A/Ribavirin (data not shown).

Patients with viral genotype 1, regardless of viral load, had a lower response rate to PEG-INTRON (1.5 µg/kg)/Ribavirin combination therapy compared to patients with other viral genotypes. Patients with both poor prognostic factors (genotype 1 and high viral load) had a response rate of 30% (78/256) compared to a response rate of 29% (71/247) with INTRON A/Ribavirin combination therapy.

Patients with lower body weight tended to have higher adverse event rates (see **ADVERSE REACTIONS**) and higher response rates than patients with higher body weights. Differences in response rates between treatment arms did not substantially vary with body weight.

Treatment response rates with PEG-INTRON/Ribavirin combination therapy were 49% in men and 56% in women. Response rates were lower in African American and Hispanic patients and higher in Asians compared to Caucasians. Although African Americans had a higher proportion of poor prognostic factors compared to Caucasians the number of non-Caucasians studied (11% of the total) was insufficient to allow meaningful conclusions about differences in response rates after adjusting for prognostic factors.

Liver biopsies were obtained before and after treatment in 68% of patients. Compared to baseline approximately $^2/_3$ of patients in all treatment groups were observed to have a modest reduction in inflammation.

CONTRAINDICATIONS

Pregnancy

Ribavirin Capsules may cause birth defects and/or death of the exposed fetus. Ribavirin therapy is contraindicated for use in women who are pregnant or in men whose female partners are pregnant. (See **WARNINGS, PRECAUTIONS-Information for Patients and Pregnancy Category**

TABLE 2. Virologic and Histologic Responses: Previously Untreated Patients*

	US Study			
	24 weeks of treatment		48 weeks of treatment	
	INTRON A plus Ribavirin (N=228)	INTRON A plus Placebo (N=231)	INTRON A plus Ribavirin (N=228)	INTRON A plus Placebo (N=225)
Virologic Response				
-Responder[1]	65 (29)	13 (6)	85 (37)	27 (12)
-Nonresponder	147 (64)	194 (84)	110 (48)	168 (75)
-Missing Data	16 (7)	24 (10)	33 (14)	30 (13)
Histologic Response				
-Improvement[2]	102 (45)	77 (33)	96 (42)	65 (29)
-No improvement	77 (34)	99 (43)	61 (27)	93 (41)
-Missing Data	49 (21)	55 (24)	71 (31)	67 (30)

	International Study		
	24 weeks of treatment	48 weeks of treatment	
	INTRON A plus Ribavirin (N=265)	INTRON A plus Ribavirin (N=268)	INTRON A plus Placebo (N=266)
Virologic Response			
-Responder[1]	86 (32)	113 (42)	46 (17)
-Nonresponder	158 (60)	120 (45)	196 (74)
-Missing Data	21 (8)	35 (13)	24 (9)
Histologic Response			
-Improvement[2]	103 (39)	102 (38)	69 (26)
-No improvement	85 (32)	58 (22)	111 (41)
-Missing Data	77 (29)	108 (40)	86 (32)

* Number (%) of patients.
1. Defined as HCV RNA below limit of detection using a research based RT-PCR assay at end of treatment and during follow-up period.
2. Defined as posttreatment (end of follow-up) minus pretreatment liver biopsy Knodell HAI score (I+II+III) improvement of ≥2 points.

TABLE 3. Virologic and Histologic Responses: Relapse Patients*

	US Study		International Study	
	INTRON A plus Ribavirin (N=77)	INTRON A plus Placebo (N=76)	INTRON A plus Ribavirin (N=96)	INTRON A plus Placebo (N=96)
Virologic Response				
-Responder[1]	33 (43)	3 (4)	46 (48)	5 (5)
-Nonresponder	36 (47)	66 (87)	45 (47)	91 (95)
-Missing Data	8 (10)	7 (9)	5 (5)	0 (0)
Histologic Response				
-Improvement[2]	38 (49)	27 (36)	49 (51)	30 (31)
-No improvement	23 (30)	37 (49)	29 (30)	44 (46)
-Missing Data	16 (21)	12 (16)	18 (19)	22 (23)

* Number (%) of patients.
1. Defined as HCV RNA below limit of detection using a research based RT-PCR assay at end of treatment and during follow-up period.
2. Defined as posttreatment (end of follow-up) minus pretreatment liver biopsy Knodell HAI score (I+II+III) improvement of ≥2 points.

X.) Ribavirin Capsules are contraindicated in patients with a history of hypersensitivity to ribavirin or any component of the capsule.

Patients with autoimmune hepatitis must not be treated with combination Ribavirin/INTRON A therapy because using these medicines can make the hepatitis worse.

Patients with hemoglobinopathies (eg, thalassemia major, sickle-cell anemia) should not be treated with Ribavirin Capsules.

WARNINGS

Based on results of clinical trials ribavirin monotherapy is not effective for the treatment of chronic hepatitis C virus infection; therefore, Ribavirin Capsules must not be used alone. The safety and efficacy of Ribavirin Capsules have only been established when used together with INTRON A (interferon alfa-2b, recombinant) as REBETRON Combination Therapy or with PEG-INTRON Injection.

There are significant adverse events caused by Ribavirin/INTRON A or PEG-INTRON therapy, including severe depression and suicidal ideation, hemolytic anemia, suppression of bone marrow function, autoimmune and infectious disorders, pulmonary dysfunction, pancreatitis, and diabetes. The REBETRON Combination Therapy and PEG-INTRON package inserts should be reviewed in their entirety prior to initiation of combination treatment for additional safety information.

Pregnancy

Ribavirin Capsules may cause birth defects and/or death of the exposed fetus. Extreme care must be taken to avoid pregnancy in female patients and in female partners of male patients. Ribavirin has demonstrated significant teratogenic and/or embryocidal effects in all animal species in which adequate studies have been conducted. These effects occurred at doses as low as one twentieth of the recommended human dose of ribavirin. RIBAVIRIN THERAPY SHOULD NOT BE STARTED UNTIL A REPORT OF A NEGATIVE PREGNANCY TEST HAS BEEN OBTAINED IMMEDIATELY PRIOR TO PLANNED INITIATION OF THERAPY. Patients should be instructed to use at least two forms of effective contraception during treatment and during the six month period after treatment has been stopped based on multiple dose half-life of ribavirin of 12 days. Pregnancy testing should occur monthly during ribavirin therapy and for six months after therapy has stopped (see CONTRAINDICATIONS and PRECAUTIONS: Information for Patients and Pregnancy Category X).

Anemia

The primary toxicity of ribavirin is hemolytic anemia, which was observed in approximately 10% of Ribavirin/INTRON A-treated patients in clinical trials (See ADVERSE REACTIONS: Laboratory Values - *Hemoglobin*). The anemia associated with ribavirin capsules occurs within 1–2 weeks of initiation of therapy. BECAUSE THE INITIAL DROP IN HEMOGLOBIN MAY BE SIGNIFICANT, IT IS ADVISED THAT HEMOGLOBIN OR HEMATOCRIT BE OBTAINED PRETREATMENT AND AT WEEK 2 AND WEEK 4 OF THERAPY, OR MORE FREQUENTLY IF CLINICALLY INDICATED. Patients should then be followed as clinically appropriate.

Fatal and nonfatal myocardial infarctions have been reported in patients with anemia caused by Ribavirin. Patients should be assessed for underlying cardiac disease before initiation of ribavirin therapy. Patients with preexisting cardiac disease should have electrocardiograms administered before treatment, and should be appropriately monitored during therapy. If there is any deterioration of cardiovascular status, therapy should be suspended or discontinued. (See DOSAGE AND ADMINISTRATION: Guidelines for Dose Modification.) Because cardiac disease may be worsened by drug induced anemia, patients with a history of significant or unstable cardiac disease should not use ribavirin. (See ADVERSE REACTIONS.)

Ribavirin and INTRON A or PEG-INTRON therapy should be suspended in patients with signs and symptoms of pancreatitis and discontinued in patients with confirmed pancreatitis.

Ribavirin should not be used in patients with creatinine clearance <50 mL/min. (See **Clinical Pharmacology, Special Populations.**)

Pulmonary

Pulmonary symptoms, including dyspnea, pulmonary infiltrates, pneumonitis and pneumonia, have been reported during therapy with Ribavirin/INTRON A; occasional cases of fatal pneumonia have occurred. In addition, sarcoidosis or the exacerbation of sarcoidosis has been reported. If there is evidence of pulmonary infiltrates or pulmonary function impairment, the patient should be closely monitored, and if appropriate, combination Ribavirin/INTRON A treatment should be discontinued.

PRECAUTIONS

The safety and efficacy of Ribavirin/INTRON A and PEG-INTRON therapy for the treatment of HIV infection, adenovirus, RSV, parainfluenza, or influenza infections have not been established. Ribavirin Capsules should not be used for these indications. Ribavirin for inhalation has a separate package insert, which should be consulted if ribavirin inhalation therapy is being considered.

The safety and efficacy of Ribavirin/INTRON A therapy has not been established in liver or other organ transplant patients, patients with decompensated liver disease due to hepatitis C infection, patients who are nonresponders to interferon therapy, or patients coinfected with HBV or HIV.

Information for Patients

Patients must be informed that Ribavirin Capsules may cause birth defects and/or death of the exposed fetus. Ribavirin must not be used by women who are pregnant or by men whose female partners are pregnant. Extreme care must be taken to avoid pregnancy in female patients and in female partners of male patients taking ribavirin. Ribavirin should not be initiated until a report of a negative pregnancy test has been obtained immediately prior to initiation of therapy. Patients must perform a pregnancy test monthly during therapy and for 6 months posttherapy. Women of childbearing potential must be counseled about use of effective contraception (two reliable forms) prior to initiating therapy. Patients (male and female) must be advised of the teratogenic/embryocidal risks and must be instructed to practice effective contraception during ribavirin and for 6 months posttherapy. Patients (male and female) should be advised to notify the physician immediately in the event of a pregnancy. (See **CONTRAINDICATIONS** and **WARNINGS**.)

If pregnancy does occur during treatment or during 6 months post-therapy, the patient must be advised of the teratogenic risk of ribavirin therapy to the fetus. Patients, or partners of patients, should immediately report any pregnancy that occurs during treatment or within 6 months after treatment cessation to their physician. Physicians should report such cases by calling 1-800-727-7064.

Patients receiving Ribavirin Capsules should be informed of the benefits and risks associated with treatment, directed in its appropriate use, and referred to the patient **MEDICATION GUIDE**. Patients should be informed that the effect of treatment of hepatitis C infection on transmission is not known, and that appropriate precautions to prevent transmission of the hepatitis C virus should be taken.

The most common adverse experience occurring with Ribavirin Capsules is anemia, which may be severe. (See **ADVERSE REACTIONS**.) Patients should be advised that laboratory evaluations are required prior to starting therapy and periodically thereafter. (See **Laboratory Tests**.) It is advised that patients be well hydrated, especially during the initial stages of treatment.

Laboratory Tests The following laboratory tests are recommended for all patients treated with Ribavirin Capsules, prior to beginning treatment and then periodically thereafter.

- Standard hematologic tests - including hemoglobin (pretreatment, week 2 and week 4 of therapy, and as clinically appropriate [see **WARNINGS**]), complete and differential white blood cell counts, and platelet count.
- Blood chemistries - liver function tests and TSH.
- Pregnancy - including monthly monitoring for women of childbearing potential.
- ECG (See **WARNINGS**)

Carcinogenesis and Mutagenesis Adequate studies to assess the carcinogenic potential of ribavirin in animals have not been conducted. However, ribavirin is a nucleoside analogue that has produced positive findings in multiple *in vitro* and animal *in vivo* genotoxicity assays, and should be considered a potential carcinogen. Further studies to assess the carcinogenic potential of ribavirin in animals are ongoing.

TABLE 5. Selected Treatment-Emergent Adverse Events: Previously Untreated and Relapse Patients

	Percentage of Patients					
	US Previously Untreated Study				US Relapse Study	
	24 weeks of treatment		48 weeks of treatment		24 weeks of treatment	
Patients Reporting Adverse Events*	INTRON A plus Ribavirin (N=228)	INTRON A plus Placebo (N=231)	INTRON A plus Ribavirin (N=228)	INTRON A plus Placebo (N=225)	INTRON A plus Ribavirin (N=77)	INTRON A plus Placebo (N=76)
Application Site Disorders						
injection site inflammation	13	10	12	14	6	8
injection site reaction	7	9	8	9	5	3
Body as a Whole – General Disorders						
Headache	63	63	66	67	66	68
Fatigue	68	62	70	72	60	53
Rigors	40	32	42	39	43	37
Fever	37	35	41	40	32	36
influenza-like symptoms	14	18	18	20	13	13
Asthenia	9	4	9	9	10	4
chest pain	5	4	9	8	6	7
Central & Peripheral Nervous System Disorders						
Dizziness	17	15	23	19	26	21
Gastrointestinal System Disorders						
Nausea	38	35	46	33	47	33
Anorexia	27	16	25	19	21	14
Dyspepsia	14	6	16	9	16	9
Vomiting	11	10	9	13	12	8
Musculoskeletal System Disorders						
Myalgia	61	57	64	63	61	58
Arthralgia	30	27	33	36	29	29
musculoskeletal pain	20	26	28	32	22	28
Psychiatric Disorders						
Insomnia	39	27	39	30	26	25
Irritability	23	19	32	27	25	20
Depression	32	25	36	37	23	14
emotional lability	7	6	11	8	12	8
concentration impaired	11	14	14	14	10	12
nervousness	4	2	4	4	5	4
Respiratory System Disorders						
Dyspnea	19	9	18	10	17	12
Sinusitis	9	7	10	14	12	7
Skin and Appendages Disorders						
Alopecia	28	27	32	28	27	26
Rash	20	9	28	8	21	5
Pruritus	21	9	19	8	13	4
Special Senses, Other Disorders						
taste perversion	7	4	8	4	6	5

*Patients reporting one or more adverse events. A patient may have reported more than one adverse event within a body system/organ class category.

Ribavirin demonstrated increased incidences of mutation and cell transformation in multiple genotoxicity assays. Ribavirin was active in the Balb/3T3 *In Vitro* Cell Transformation Assay. Mutagenic activity was observed in the mouse lymphoma assay, and at doses of 20-200 mg/kg (estimated human equivalent of 1.67-16.7 mg/kg, based on body surface area adjustment for a 60 kg adult; 0.1-1 × the maximum recommended human 24-hour dose of ribavirin) in a mouse micronucleus assay. A dominant lethal assay in rats was negative, indicating that if mutations occurred in rats they were not transmitted through male gametes.

Impairment of Fertility Ribavirin demonstrated significant embryocidal and/or teratogenic effects at doses well below the recommended human dose in all animal species in which adequate studies have been conducted.

Fertile women and partners of fertile women should not receive ribavirin unless the patient and his/her partner are using effective contraception (two reliable forms). Based on a multiple dose half-life ($t_{1/2}$) of ribavirin of 12 days, effective contraception must be utilized for 6 months posttherapy (eg, 15 half-lives of clearance for ribavirin).

Ribavirin should be used with caution in fertile men. In studies in mice to evaluate the time course and reversibility of ribavirin-induced testicular degeneration at doses of 15 to 150 mg/kg/day (estimated human equivalent of 1.25-12.5 mg/kg/day, based on body surface area adjustment for a 60 kg adult; 0.1-0.8 × the maximum human 24-hour dose of ribavirin) administered for 3 or 6 months, abnormalities in sperm occurred. Upon cessation of treatment, essentially total recovery from ribavirin-induced testicular toxicity was apparent within 1 or 2 spermatogenesis cycles.

Animal Toxicology Long-term studies in the mouse and rat (18-24 months; doses of 20-75 and 10-40 mg/kg/day, respectively [estimated human equivalent doses of 1.67-6.25 and 1.43-5.71 mg/ kg/day, respectively, based on body surface area adjustment for a 60 kg adult; approximately 0.1-0.4 × the maximum human 24-hour dose of ribavirin]) have demonstrated a relationship between chronic ribavirin exposure and increased incidences of vascular lesions (microscopic hemorrhages) in mice. In rats, retinal degeneration occurred in controls, but the incidence was increased in ribavirin-treated rats.

Pregnancy Category X (see **CONTRAINDICATIONS**)

Ribavirin produced significant embryocidal and/or teratogenic effects in all animal species in which adequate studies have been conducted. Malformations of the skull, palate, eye, jaw, limbs, skeleton, and gastrointestinal tract were noted. The incidence and severity of teratogenic effects increased with escalation of the drug dose. Survival of fetuses and offspring was reduced. In conventional embryotoxicity/teratogenicity studies in rats and rabbits, observed no effect dose levels were well below those for proposed clinical use (0.3 mg/kg/day for both the rat and rabbit; approximately 0.06 × the recommended human 24-hour dose of ribavirin). No maternal toxicity or effects on offspring were observed in a peri/postnatal toxicity study in rats dosed orally at up to 1 mg/kg/day (estimated human equivalent dose of 0.17 mg/kg based on body surface area adjustment for a 60 kg adult; approximately 0.01 × the maximum recommended human 24-hour dose of ribavirin).

Treatment and Posttreatment: Potential Risk to the Fetus

Ribavirin is known to accumulate in intracellular components from where it is cleared very slowly. It is not known whether ribavirin contained in sperm will exert a potential teratogenic effect upon fertilization of the ova. In a study in rats, it was concluded that dominant lethality was not induced by ribavirin at doses up to 200 mg/kg for 5 days (estimated human equivalent doses of 7.14-28.6 mg/kg, based on body surface area adjustment for a 60 kg adult; up to 1.7 × the maximum recommended human dose of ribavirin).

Continued on next page

Information on Schering products appearing on these pages is effective as of June 2003.

TABLE 7. Selected Hematologic Values During Treatment with Ribavirin plus INTRON A: Previously Untreated and Relapse Patients

	Percentage of Patients					
	US Previously Untreated Study				US Relapse Study	
	24 weeks of treatment		48 weeks of treatment		24 weeks of treatment	
	INTRON A plus Ribavirin (N=228)	INTRON A plus Placebo (N=231)	INTRON A plus Ribavirin (N=228)	INTRON A plus Placebo (N=225)	INTRON A plus Ribavirin (N=77)	INTRON A plus Placebo (N=76)
Hemoglobin (g/dL)						
9.5-10.9	24	1	32	1	21	3
8.0-9.4	5	0	4	0	4	0
6.5-7.9	0	0	0	0.4	0	0
<6.5	0	0	0	0	0	0
Leukocytes ($\times 10^9$/L)						
2.0-2.9	40	20	38	23	45	26
1.5-1.9	4	1	9	2	5	3
1.0-1.4	0.9	0	2	0	0	0
<1.0	0	0	0	0	0	0
Neutrophils ($\times 10^9$/L)						
1.0-1.49	30	32	31	44	42	34
0.75-0.99	14	15	14	11	16	18
0.5-0.74	9	9	14	7	8	4
<0.5	11	8	11	5	5	8
Platelets ($\times 10^9$/L)						
70-99	9	11	11	14	6	12
50-69	2	3	2	3	0	5
30-49	0	0.4	0	0.4	0	0
<30	0.9	0	1	0.9	0	0
Total Bilirubin (mg/dL)						
1.5-3.0	27	13	32	13	21	7
3.1-6.0	0.9	0.4	2	0	3	0
6.1-12.0	0	0	0.4	0	0	0
>12.0	0	0	0	0	0	0

Ribavirin—Cont.

However, because of the potential human teratogenic effects of ribavirin, male patients should be advised to take every precaution to avoid risk of pregnancy for their female partners.

Women of childbearing potential should not receive ribavirin unless they are using effective contraception (two reliable forms) during the therapy period. In addition, effective contraception should be utilized for 6 months post-therapy based on a multiple-dose half-life ($t_{1/2}$) of ribavirin of 12 days. Male patients and their female partners must practice effective contraception (two reliable forms) during treatment with ribavirin and for the 6-month posttherapy period (eg, 15 half-lives for ribavirin clearance from the body).

If pregnancy occurs in a patient or partner of a patient during treatment or during the 6 months after treatment cessation, physicians should report such cases by calling 1-800-727-7064.

Nursing Mothers It is not known whether the ribavirin product is excreted in human milk. Because of the potential for serious adverse reactions from the drug in nursing infants, a decision should be made whether to discontinue nursing or to delay or discontinue ribavirin.

Geriatric Use Clinical studies of Ribavirin/INTRON A or PEG-INTRON therapy did not include sufficient numbers of subjects aged 65 and over to determine if they respond differently from younger subjects.

Ribavirin is known to be substantially excreted by the kidney, and the risk of toxic reactions to this drug may be greater in patients with impaired renal function. Because elderly patients often have decreased renal function, care should be taken in dose selection. Renal function should be monitored and dosage adjustments should be made accordingly. Ribavirin should not be used in patients with creatinine clearance <50 mL/min. (See **WARNINGS.**)

In general, Ribavirin Capsules should be administered to elderly patients cautiously, starting at the lower end of the dosing range, reflecting the greater frequency of decreased hepatic and/or cardiac function, and of concomitant disease or other drug therapy. In clinical trials, elderly subjects had a higher frequency of anemia (67%) than did younger patients (28%). (See **WARNINGS.**)

Pediatric Use Safety and effectiveness in pediatric patients have not been established.

ADVERSE REACTIONS

The primary toxicity of ribavirin is hemolytic anemia. Reductions in hemoglobin levels occurred within the first 1–2 weeks of oral therapy. (See WARNINGS.) Cardiac and pulmonary events associated with anemia occurred in approximately 10% of patients. (See WARNINGS.)

Ribavirin/INTRON A Combination Therapy

In clinical trials, 19% and 6% of previously untreated and relapse patients, respectively, discontinued therapy due to adverse events in the combination arms compared to 13% and 3% in the interferon arms. Selected treatment-emergent adverse events that occurred in the US studies with ≥5% incidence are provided in **TABLE 5** by treatment group. In general, the selected treatment-emergent adverse events reported with lower incidence in the international studies as compared to the US studies with the exception of asthenia, influenza-like symptoms, nervousness, and pruritus.

[See table 5 at top of previous page]

In addition, the following spontaneous adverse events have been reported during the marketing surveillance of Ribavirin/INTRON A therapy: hearing disorder and vertigo.

Ribavirin/PEG-INTRON Combination Therapy

Overall, in clinical trials, 14% of patients receiving ribavirin in combination with PEG-INTRON, discontinued therapy compared with 13% treated with ribavirin in combination with INTRON A. The most common reasons for discontinuation of therapy were related to psychiatric, systemic (eg, fatigue, headache), or gastrointestinal adverse events. Adverse events that occurred in clinical trial at >5% incidence are provided in **Table 6** by treatment group.

TABLE 6. Adverse Events Occurring in > 5% of Patients

	*Percentage of Patients Reporting Adverse Events**	
Adverse Events	**PEG-INTRON 1.5 µg/kg/ Ribavirin (N=511)**	**INTRON A/ Ribavirin (N=505)**
Application Site		
Injection Site Inflammation	25	18
Injection Site Reaction	58	36
Autonomic Nervous System		
Mouth Dry	12	8
Sweating Increased	11	7
Flushing	4	3
Body as a Whole		
Fatigue/Asthenia	66	63
Headache	62	58
Rigors	48	41
Fever	46	33
Weight Decrease	29	20
RUO Pain	12	6
Chest Pain	8	7
Malaise	4	6
Central/Peripheral Nervous System		
Dizziness	21	17
Endocrine		
Hypothyroidism	5	4
Gastrointestinal		
Nausea	43	33
Anorexia	32	27
Diarrhea	22	17
Vomiting	14	12
Abdominal Pain	13	13
Dyspepsia	9	8
Constipation	5	5
Hematologic Disorders		
Neutropenia	26	14
Anemia	12	17
Leukopenia	6	5
Thrombocytopenia	5	2
Liver and Biliary System		
Hepatomegaly	4	4
Musculoskeletal		
Myalgia	56	50
Arthralgia	34	28
Musculoskeletal Pain	21	19
Psychiatric		
Insomnia	40	41
Depression	31	34
Anxiety/Emotional Lability/Irritability	47	47
Concentration Impaired	17	21
Agitation	8	5
Nervousness	6	6
Reproductive, Female		
Menstrual Disorder	7	6
Resistance Mechanism		
Infection Viral	12	12
Infection Fungal	6	1
Respiratory System		
Dyspnea	26	24
Coughing	23	16
Pharyngitis	12	13
Rhinitis	8	6
Sinusitis	6	5
Skin and Appendages		
Alopecia	36	32
Pruritus	29	28
Rash	24	23
Skin Dry	24	23
Special Senses, Other		
Taste Perversion	9	4
Vision Disorders		
Vision Blurred	5	6
Conjunctivitis	4	5

***Patients reporting one or more adverse events. A patient may have reported more than one adverse event within a body system/organ class category.**

Laboratory Values

Ribavirin/INTRON A Combination Therapy

Changes in selected hematologic values (hemoglobin, white blood cells, neutrophils, and platelets) during therapy are described below. (See **TABLE 7.**)

Hemoglobin Hemoglobin decreases among patients receiving ribavirin therapy began at Week 1, with stabilization by Week 4. In previously untreated patients treated for 48 weeks the mean maximum decrease from baseline was 3.1 g/dL in the US study and 2.9 g/dL in the International study. In relapse patients the mean maximum decrease from baseline was 2.8 g/dL in the US study and 2.6 g/dL in the International study. Hemoglobin values returned to pretreatment levels within 4-8 weeks of cessation of therapy in most patients.

Bilirubin and Uric Acid Increases in both bilirubin and uric acid, associated with hemolysis, were noted in clinical trials. Most were moderate biochemical changes and were reversed within 4 weeks after treatment discontinuation. This observation occurs most frequently in patients with a previous diagnosis of Gilbert's syndrome. This has not been associated with hepatic dysfunction or clinical morbidity.

[See table 7 above]

Ribavirin/PEG-INTRON Combination Therapy

Changes in selected hematologic values (hemoglobin, white blood cells, neutrophils, and platelets) during therapy are described below. (See **TABLE 8.**)

Hemoglobin

Ribavirin induced a decrease in hemoglobin levels in approximately two thirds of patients. Hemoglobin levels decreased to <11g/dL in about 30% of patients. Severe anemia (<8 g/dL) occurred in <1% of patients. Dose modification was required in 9 and 13% of patients in the PEG-INTRON/Ribavirin and INTRON A/Ribavirin groups.

Bilirubin and Uric

In the Ribavirin/PEG-INTRON combination trial 10-14% of patients developed hyperbilirubenemia and 33-38% developed hyperuricemia in association with hemolysis. Six patients developed mild to moderate gout.

TABLE 8. Selected Hematologic Values During Treatment with Ribavirin plus PEG-INTRON

	Number (%) of Subjects	
	PEG-INTRON plus Ribavirin (N=511)	INTRON A plus Ribavirin (N=505)
Hemoglobin (g/dL)		
9.5-10.9	26	27
8.0-9.4	3	3
6.5-7.9	0.2	0.2
<6.5	0	0
Leukocytes ($\times 10^9$/L)		
2.0-2.9	46	41
1.5-1.9	24	8
1.0-1.4	5	1
<1.0	0	0
Neutrophils ($\times 10^9$/L)		
1.0-1.49	33	37
0.75-0.99	25	13
0.5-0.74	18	7
<0.5	4	2
Platelets ($\times 10^9$/L)		
70-99	15	5
50-69	3	0.8
30-49	0.2	0.2
<30	0	0
Total Bilirubin (mg/dL)		
1.5-3.0	10	13
3.1-6.0	0.6	0.2
6.1-12.0	0	0.2
>12.0	0	0
ALT (SGPT)		
2 × Baseline	0.6	0.2
2.1-5 × Baseline	3	1
5.1-10 × Baseline	0	0
>10 × Baseline	0	0

OVERDOSAGE

There is limited experience with overdosage. Acute ingestion of up to 20 grams of Ribavirin Capsules, INTRON A ingestion of up to 120 million units, and subcutaneous doses of INTRON A up to 10 times the recommended doses have been reported. Primary effects that have been observed are increased incidence and severity of the adverse events related to the therapeutic use of INTRON A and ribavirin. However, hepatic enzyme abnormalities, renal failure, hemorrhage, and myocardial infarction have been reported with administration of single subcutaneous doses of INTRON A that exceed dosing recommendations.
There is no specific antidote for INTRON A or ribavirin, and hemodialysis and peritoneal dialysis are not effective for treatment of overdose of either agent.

DOSAGE AND ADMINISTRATION (see CLINICAL PHARMACOLOGY, Special Populations; see WARNINGS)

Ribavirin/INTRON A Combination Therapy
The recommended dose of Ribavirin Capsules depends on the patient's body weight. The recommended dose of ribavirin is provided in **TABLE 9**.
The recommended duration of treatment for patients previously untreated with interferon is 24 to 48 weeks. The duration of treatment should be individualized to the patient depending on baseline disease characteristics, response to therapy, and tolerability of the regimen. (See **Description of Clinical Studies** and **ADVERSE REACTIONS**.) After 24 weeks of treatment virologic response should be assessed. Treatment discontinuation should be considered in any patient who has not achieved an HCV RNA below the limit of detection of the assay by 24 weeks. There are no safety and efficacy data on treatment for longer than 48 weeks in the previously untreated patient population.
In patients who relapse following interferon therapy, the recommended duration of treatment is 24 weeks. There are no safety and efficacy data on treatment for longer than 24 weeks in the relapse patient population.

TABLE 9. Recommended Dosing

Body weight	Ribavirin Capsules
≤ 75 kg	2 × 200-mg capsules AM, 3 × 200-mg capsules PM daily p.o.
> 75 kg	3 × 200-mg capsules AM, 3 × 200-mg capsules PM daily p.o.

Ribavirin may be administered without regard to food, but should be administered in a consistent manner with respect to food intake. (See **CLINICAL PHARMACOLOGY**.)

Ribavirin/PEG-INTRON Combination Therapy
The recommended dose of Ribavirin Capsules is 800 mg/day in 2 divided doses: two capsules (400 mg) in the morning with food and two capsules (400 mg) in the evening with food.
***Dose Modifications* (TABLE 10)**
If severe adverse reactions or laboratory abnormalities develop during combination Ribavirin/INTRON A therapy the dose should be modified, or discontinued if appropriate, until the adverse reactions abate. If intolerance persists after dose adjustment, Ribavirin/INTRON A therapy should be discontinued.
Ribavirin should not be used in patients with creatinine clearance <50 mL/min. (See **WARNINGS** and **CLINICAL PHARMACOLOGY, Special Populations.**)
Ribavirin should be administered with caution to patients with preexisting cardiac disease. Patients should be assessed before commencement of therapy and should be appropriately monitored during therapy. If there is any deterioration of cardiovascular status, therapy should be stopped. (See **WARNINGS.**)
For patients with a history of stable cardiovascular disease, a permanent dose reduction is required if the hemoglobin decreases by ≥2 g/dL during any 4-week period. In addition, for these cardiac history patients, if the hemoglobin remains <12 g/dL after 4 weeks on a reduced dose, the patient should discontinue combination Ribavirin/INTRON A therapy.
It is recommended that a patient whose hemoglobin level falls below 10 g/dL have his/her ribavirin dose reduced to 600 mg daily (1 × 200-mg capsule AM, 2 × 200 mg capsules PM). A patient whose hemoglobin level falls below 8.5 g/dL should be permanently discontinued from ribavirin therapy. (See **WARNINGS.**)

TABLE 10. Guidelines for Dose Modifications and Discontinuation for Anemia

Hemoglobin	Dose Reduction* Ribavirin-600 mg daily	Permanent Discontinuation of Ribavirin Treatment
No Cardiac History	**<10 g/dL**	**<8.5 g/dL**
Cardiac History Patients	**≥2 g/dL decrease during any 4-week period during treatment**	**<12 g/dL after 4 weeks of dose reduction**

HOW SUPPLIED

Ribavirin 200-mg Capsules are white, opaque capsules with 200 mg and W-1523 imprinted on the capsule shell; the capsules are packaged in a bottle containing 42 capsules (NDC-59930-1523-4), 56 capsules (NDC 59930-1523-3), 70 capsules (NDC 59930-1523-2), and 84 capsules (NDC 59930-1523-1).
Storage Conditions
The bottle of Ribavirin Capsules should be stored at 25°C (77°F); excursions are permitted between 15° and 30°C (59° and 86°F).
Warrick Pharmaceuticals Corporation
Reno, NV 89506 USA
B-26964210 3/03

TEMODAR® ℞

[*tĕm-ō-dăr*]
(temozolomide)
Capsules

DESCRIPTION

TEMODAR Capsules for oral administration contain temozolomide, an imidazotetrazine derivative. The chemical name of temozolomide is 3,4-dihydro-3-methyl-4-oxoimidazo[5,1-d]-*as*-tetrazine-8-carboxamide. The structural formula is:

$CONH_2$ N N N N N CH_3 O

The material is a white to light tan/light pink powder with a molecular formula of $C_6H_6N_6O_2$ and a molecular weight of 194.15. The molecule is stable at acidic pH (<5), and labile at pH >7, hence can be administered orally. The prodrug, temozolomide, is rapidly hydrolyzed to the active 5-(3-methyltriazen-1-yl)imidazole-4-carboxamide (MTIC) at neutral and alkaline pH values, with hydrolysis taking place even faster at alkaline pH.
Each capsule contains either 5 mg, 20 mg, 100 mg, or 250 mg of temozolomide. The inactive ingredients for TEMODAR Capsules are lactose anhydrous, colloidal silicon dioxide, sodium starch glycolate, tartaric acid, and stearic acid. Gelatin capsule shells contain titanium dioxide. The capsules are imprinted with pharmaceutical ink.
TEMODAR 5 mg: green imprint contains pharmaceutical grade shellac, anhydrous ethyl alcohol, isopropyl alcohol, n-butyl alcohol, propylene glycol, ammonium hydroxide, titanium dioxide, yellow iron oxide, and FD&C Blue #2 aluminum lake.
TEMODAR 20 mg: brown imprint also contains pharmaceutical grade shellac, anhydrous ethyl alcohol, isopropyl alcohol, n-butyl alcohol, propylene glycol, purified water, ammonium hydroxide, potassium hydroxide, titanium dioxide, black iron oxide, yellow iron oxide, brown iron oxide, and red iron oxide.
TEMODAR 100 mg: blue imprint contains pharmaceutical glaze (modified) in an ethanol/shellac mixture, isopropyl alcohol, n-butyl alcohol, propylene glycol, titanium dioxide, and FD&C Blue #2 aluminum lake.
TEMODAR 250 mg: black imprint contains pharmaceutical grade shellac, anhydrous ethyl alcohol, isopropyl alcohol, n-butyl alcohol, propylene glycol, purified water, ammonium hydroxide, potassium hydroxide, and black iron oxide.

CLINICAL PHARMACOLOGY

Mechanism of Action: Temozolomide is not directly active but undergoes rapid nonenzymatic conversion at physiologic pH to the reactive compound MTIC. The cytotoxicity of MTIC is thought to be primarily due to alkylation of DNA. Alkylation (methylation) occurs mainly at the O^6 and N^7 positions of guanine.
Pharmacokinetics: Temozolomide is rapidly and completely absorbed after oral administration; peak plasma concentrations occur in 1 hour. Food reduces the rate and extent of temozolomide absorption. Mean peak plasma concentration and AUC decreased by 32% and 9%, respectively, and T_{max} increased 2-fold (from 1.1 to 2.25 hours) when temozolomide was administered after a modified high-fat breakfast. Temozolomide is rapidly eliminated with a mean elimination half-life of 1.8 hours and exhibits linear kinetics over the therapeutic dosing range. Temozolomide has a mean apparent volume of distribution of 0.4 L/kg (%CV=13%). It is weakly bound to human plasma proteins; the mean percent bound of drug-related total radioactivity is 15%.
Metabolism and Elimination: Temozolomide is spontaneously hydrolyzed at physiologic pH to the active species, 3-methyl-(triazen-1-yl)imidazole-4-carboxamide (MTIC) and to temozolomide acid metabolite. MTIC is further hydrolyzed to 5-amino-imidazole-4-carboxamide (AIC) which is known to be an intermediate in purine and nucleic acid biosynthesis and to methylhydrazine, which is believed to be the active alkylating species. Cytochrome P450 enzymes play only a minor role in the metabolism of temozolomide and MTIC. Relative to the AUC of temozolomide, the exposure to MTIC and AIC is 2.4% and 23%, respectively. About 38% of the administered temozolomide total radioactive dose is recovered over 7 days; 37.7% in urine and 0.8% in feces. The majority of the recovery of radioactivity in urine is as unchanged temozolomide (5.6%), AIC (12%), temozolomide acid metabolite (2.3%), and unidentified polar metabolite(s) (17%). Overall clearance of temozolomide is about 5.5 L/hr/m^2.
Special Populations: *Age* Population pharmacokinetic analysis indicates that age (range 19 to 78 years) has no influence on the pharmacokinetics of temozolomide. In the anaplastic astrocytoma study population, patients 70 years of age or older had a higher incidence of Grade 4 neutropenia and Grade 4 thrombocytopenia in the first cycle of therapy than patients under 70 years of age (see **PRECAUTIONS**). In the entire safety database, however, there did not appear to be a higher incidence in patients 70 years of age or older (see **ADVERSE REACTIONS**).
Gender Population pharmacokinetic analysis indicates that women have an approximately 5% lower clearance (adjusted for body surface area) for temozolomide than men. Women have higher incidences of Grade 4 neutropenia and thrombocytopenia in the first cycle of therapy than men (see **ADVERSE REACTIONS**).
Race The effect of race on the pharmacokinetics of temozolomide has not been studied.
Tobacco Use Population pharmacokinetic analysis indicates that the oral clearance of temozolomide is similar in smokers and nonsmokers.
Creatinine Clearance Population pharmacokinetic analysis indicates that creatinine clearance over the range of 36-130 mL/min/m^2 has no effect on the clearance of temozolomide after oral administration. The pharmacokinetics of temozolomide have not been studied in patients with severely impaired renal function (CLcr <36 mL/min/m^2). Caution should be exercised when TEMODAR is administered to patients with severe renal impairment. TEMODAR has not been studied in patients on dialysis.
Hepatically Impaired Patients In a pharmacokinetic study, the pharmacokinetics of temozolomide in patients with mild-to-moderate hepatic impairment (Child's-Pugh Class I–II) were similar to those observed in patients with normal hepatic function. Caution should be exercised when temozolomide is administered to patients with severe hepatic impairment.

Continued on next page

Information on Schering products appearing on these pages is effective as of June 2003.

Temodar—Cont.

Pediatrics Pediatric patients (3 to 17 years of age) and adult patients have similar clearance and half-life values for temozolomide. There is no clinical experience with the use of TEMODAR in children under the age of 3 years.

Drug-Drug Interactions In a multiple-dose study, administration of TEMODAR with ranitidine did not change the C_{max} or AUC values for temozolomide or MTIC.

Population analysis indicates that administration of valproic acid decreases the clearance of temozolomide by about 5% (see **PRECAUTIONS**).

Population analysis failed to demonstrate any influence of coadministered dexamethasone, prochlorperazine, phenytoin, carbamazepine, ondansetron, H_2-receptor antagonists, or phenobarbital on the clearance of orally administered temozolomide.

Clinical Studies A single-arm, multicenter study was conducted in 162 patients who had anaplastic astrocytoma at first relapse and who had a baseline Karnofsky performance status of 70 or greater. Patients had previously received radiation therapy and may also have previously received a nitrosourea with or without other chemotherapy. Fifty-four patients had disease progression on prior therapy with both a nitrosourea and procarbazine and their malignancy was considered refractory to chemotherapy (refractory anaplastic astrocytoma population). Median age of this subgroup of 54 patients was 42 years (19 to 76). Sixty-five percent were male. Seventy-two percent of patients had a KPS of ≥80. Sixty-three percent of patients had surgery other than a biopsy at the time of initial diagnosis. Of those patients undergoing resection, 73% underwent a subtotal resection and 27% underwent a gross total resection. Eighteen percent of patients had surgery at the time of first relapse. The median time from initial diagnosis to first relapse was 13.8 months (4.2 to 75.4).

TEMODAR was given for the first 5 consecutive days of a 28-day cycle at a starting dose of 150 mg/m²/day. If the nadir and day of dosing (Day 29, Day 1 of next cycle) absolute neutrophil count was ≥1.5 × 10⁹/L (1,500/μL) and the nadir and Day 29, Day 1 of next cycle, platelet count was ≥100 × 10⁹/L (100,000/μL), the TEMODAR dose was increased to 200 mg/m²/day for the first 5 consecutive days of a 28-day cycle.

In the refractory anaplastic astrocytoma population the overall tumor response rate (CR + PR) was 22% (12/54 patients) and the complete response rate was 9% (5/54 patients). The median duration of all responses was 50 weeks (range of 16 to 114 weeks) and the median duration of complete responses was 64 weeks (range of 52 to 114 weeks). In this population, progression-free survival at 6 months was 45% (95% confidence interval 31% to 58%) and progression-free survival at 12 months was 29% (95% confidence interval 16% to 42%). Median progression-free survival was 4.4 months. Overall survival at 6 months was 74% (95% confidence interval 62% to 86%) and 12-month overall survival was 65% (95% confidence interval 52% to 78%). Median overall survival was 15.9 months.

INDICATIONS AND USAGE

TEMODAR (temozolomide) Capsules are indicated for the treatment of adult patients with refractory anaplastic astrocytoma, ie, patients at first relapse who have experienced disease progression on a drug regimen containing a nitrosourea and procarbazine.

This indication is based on the response rate in the indicated population. No results are available from randomized controlled trials in recurrent anaplastic astrocytoma that demonstrate a clinical benefit resulting from treatment, such as improvement in disease-related symptoms, delayed disease progression, or improved survival.

CONTRAINDICATIONS

TEMODAR (temozolomide) Capsules are contraindicated in patients who have a history of hypersensitivity reaction to any of its components. TEMODAR is also contraindicated in patients who have a history of hypersensitivity to DTIC, since both drugs are metabolized to MTIC.

WARNINGS

Patients treated with TEMODAR may experience myelosuppression. Prior to dosing, patients must have an absolute neutrophil count (ANC) ≥1.5 × 10⁹/L and a platelet count ≥100 × 10⁹/L. A complete blood count should be obtained on Day 22 (21 days after the first dose) or within 48 hours of that day, and weekly until the ANC is above 1.5 × 10⁹/L and platelet count exceeds 100 × 10⁹/L. In the clinical trials, if the ANC fell to <1.0 × 10⁹/L or the platelet count was <50 × 10⁹/L during any cycle, the next cycle was reduced by 50 mg/m², but not below 100 mg/m². Patients who do not tolerate 100 mg/m² should not receive TEMODAR. Geriatric patients and women have been shown in clinical trials to have a higher risk of developing myelosuppression. Myelosuppression generally occurred late in the treatment cycle. The median nadirs occurred at 26 days for platelets (range 21 to 40 days) and 28 days for neutrophils (range 1 to 44 days). Only 14% (22/158) of patients had a neutrophil nadir and 20% (32/158) of patients had a platelet nadir which may have delayed the start of the next cycle. Neutrophil and platelet counts returned to normal, on average, within 14 days of nadir counts (see **PRECAUTIONS**).

Pregnancy: Temozolomide may cause fetal harm when administered to a pregnant woman. Five consecutive days of oral administration of 75 mg/m²/day in rats and 150 mg/m²/day in rabbits during the period of organogenesis (3/8 and 3/4 the maximum recommended human dose, respectively) caused numerous malformations of the external organs, soft tissues, and skeleton in both species. Doses of 150 mg/m²/day in rats and rabbits also caused embryolethality as indicated by increased resorptions. There are no adequate and well-controlled studies in pregnant women. If this drug is used during pregnancy, or if the patient becomes pregnant while taking this drug, the patient should be apprised of the potential hazard to the fetus. Women of childbearing potential should be advised to avoid becoming pregnant during therapy with TEMODAR.

PRECAUTIONS

Information for Patients: In clinical trials, the most frequently occurring adverse effects were nausea and vomiting. These were usually either self-limiting or readily controlled with standard antiemetic therapy. Capsules should not be opened. If capsules are accidentally opened or damaged, rigorous precautions should be taken with the capsule contents to avoid inhalation or contact with the skin or mucous membranes. The medication should be kept away from children and pets.

Drug Interaction: Administration of valproic acid decreases oral clearance of temozolomide by about 5%. The clinical implication of this effect is not known.

Patients with Severe Hepatic or Renal Impairment: Caution should be exercised when TEMODAR is administered to patients with severe hepatic or renal impairment (see **Special Populations**).

Geriatrics: Clinical studies of temozolomide did not include sufficient numbers of subjects aged 65 and over to determine whether they responded differently from younger subjects. Other reported clinical experience has not identified differences in responses between the elderly and younger patients. Caution should be exercised when treating elderly patients.

In the anaplastic astrocytoma study population, patients 70 years of age or older had a higher incidence of Grade 4 neutropenia and Grade 4 thrombocytopenia (2/8; 25%, p=.31 and 2/10; 20%, p=.09, respectively) in the first cycle of therapy than patients under 70 years of age (see **ADVERSE REACTIONS**).

Laboratory Tests: A complete blood count should be obtained on Day 22 (21 days after the first dose). Blood counts should be performed weekly until recovery if the ANC falls below 1.5 × 10⁹/L and the platelet count falls below 100 × 10⁹/L.

Carcinogenesis, Mutagenesis, and Impairment of Fertility: Standard carcinogenicity studies were not conducted with temozolomide. In rats treated with 200 mg/m² temozolomide (equivalent to the maximum recommended daily human dose) on 5 consecutive days every 28 days for 3 cycles, mammary carcinomas were found in both males and females. With 6 cycles of treatment at 25, 50, and 125 mg/m² (about 1/8 to 1/2 the maximum recommended daily human dose), mammary carcinomas were observed at all doses and fibrosarcomas of the heart, eye, seminal vesicles, salivary glands, abdominal cavity, uterus, and prostate; carcinoma of the seminal vesicles, schwannoma of the heart, optic nerve, and harderian gland; and adenomas of the skin, lung, pituitary, and thyroid were observed at the high dose.

Temozolomide was mutagenic *in vitro* in bacteria (Ames assay) and clastogenic in mammalian cells (human peripheral blood lymphocyte assays).

Reproductive function studies have not been conducted with temozolomide. However, multicycle toxicology studies in rats and dogs have demonstrated testicular toxicity (syncytial cells/immature sperm, testicular atrophy) at doses of 50 mg/m² in rats and 125 mg/m² in dogs (1/4 and 5/8, respectively, of the maximum recommended human dose on a body surface area basis).

Pregnancy Category D: See **WARNINGS** section.

Nursing Mothers: It is not known whether this drug is excreted in human milk. Because many drugs are excreted in human milk and because of the potential for serious adverse reactions in nursing infants from TEMODAR, patients receiving TEMODAR should discontinue nursing.

Pediatric Use: TEMODOR effectiveness in children has not been demonstrated. TEMODAR Capsules have been studied in 2 open label Phase 2 studies in pediatric patients (age 3-18 years) at a dose of 160-200 mg/m² daily for 5 days every 28 days. In one trial conducted by the Schering Corporation, 29 patients with recurrent brain stem glioma and 34 patients with recurrent high grade astrocytoma were enrolled. All patients had failed surgery and radiation therapy, while 31% also failed chemotherapy. In a second Phase 2 open label study conducted by the Children's Oncology Group (COG), 122 patients were enrolled, including medulloblastoma/PNET (29), high grade astrocytoma (23), low grade astrocytoma (22), brain stem glioma (16), ependymoma (14), other CNS tumors (9) and non-CNS tumors (9). The TEMODAR toxicity profile in children is similar to adults. Table 1 shows the adverse events in 122 children in the COG Phase 2 study.

[See table 1 below]

Table 1

Adverse Events Reported in Pediatric Cooperative Group Trial (≥10%)

Body System/Organ Class Adverse Event	No. (%) of TEMODAR Patients (N=122)[a] All Events	Gr 3/4
Subjects Reporting an AE	**107 (88)**	**69 (57)**
Body as a Whole		
Central and Peripheral Nervous System		
Central cerebral CNS cortex	22 (18)	13 (11)
Gastrointestinal System		
Nausea	56 (46)	5 (4)
Vomiting	62 (51)	4 (3)
Platelet, Bleeding and Clotting		
Thrombocytopenia	71 (58)	31 (25)
Red Blood Cell Disorders		
Decreased Hemoglobin	62 (51)	7 (6)
White Cell and RES Disorders		
Decreased WBC	71 (58)	21 (17)
Lymphopenia	73 (60)	48 (39)
Neutropenia	62 (51)	24 (20)

[a] These various tumors included the following: PNET-medulloblastoma, glioblastoma, low grade astrocytoma, brain stem tumor, ependymoma, mixed glioma, oligodendroglioma, neuroblastoma, Ewing's sarcoma, pineoblastoma, alveolar soft part sarcoma, neurofibrosarcoma, optic glioma, and osteosarcoma.

ADVERSE REACTIONS

Tables 2 and 3 show the incidence of adverse events in the 158 patients in the anaplastic astrocytoma study for whom data are available. In the absence of a control group, it is not clear in many cases whether these events should be attributed to temozolomide or the patients' underlying conditions, but nausea, vomiting, fatigue, and hematologic effects appear to be clearly drug related. The most frequently occurring side effects were nausea, vomiting, headache, and fatigue. The adverse events were usually NCI Common Toxicity Criteria (CTC) Grade 1 or 2 (mild to moderate in severity) and were self-limiting, with nausea and vomiting readily controlled with antiemetics. The incidence of severe nausea and vomiting (CTC Grade 3 or 4) was 10% and 6%, respectively. Myelosuppression (thrombocytopenia and neutropenia) was the dose-limiting adverse event. It usually occurred within the first few cycles of therapy and was not cumulative.

Myelosuppression occurred late in the treatment cycle and returned to normal, on average, within 14 days of nadir counts. The median nadirs occurred at 26 days for platelets (range 21 to 40 days) and 28 days for neutrophils (range 1 to 44 days). Only 14% (22/158) of patients had a neutrophil nadir and 20% (32/158) of patients had a platelet nadir which may have delayed the start of the next cycle (see **WARNINGS**). Less than 10% of patients required hospitalization, blood transfusion, or discontinuation of therapy due to myelosuppression.

In clinical trial experience with 110 to 111 women and 169 to 174 men (depending on measurements), there were higher rates of Grade 4 neutropenia (ANC <500 cells/μL) and thrombocytopenia (<20,000 cells/μL) in women than men in the first cycle of therapy: (12% versus 5% and 9% versus 3%, respectively).

In the entire safety database for which hematologic data exist (N=932), 7% (4/61) and 9.5% (6/63) of patients over age 70 experienced Grade 4 neutropenia or thrombocytopenia in the first cycle, respectively. For patients less than or equal to age 70, 7% (62/871) and 5.5% (48/879) experienced Grade 4 neutropenia or thrombocytopenia in the first cycle, respectively. Pancytopenia, leukopenia, and anemia have also been reported.

In addition, the following spontaneous adverse experiences have been reported during the marketing surveillance of TEMODAR Capsules: allergic reactions including rare cases of anaphylaxis. Rare cases of erythema multiforme have been reported which resolved after discontinuation of TEMODAR and, in some cases, recurred upon rechallenge. Rare cases of opportunistic infections including *Pneumocystis carinii* pneumonia (PCP) have also been reported.

Table 2

Adverse Events in the Anaplastic Astrocytoma Trial (≥5%)

	No. (%) of TEMODAR Patients (N=158)	
	All Events	**Grade 3/4**
Any Adverse Event	**153 (97)**	**79 (50)**
Body as a Whole		
Headache	65 (41)	10 (6)
Fatigue	54 (34)	7 (4)
Asthenia	20 (13)	9 (6)
Fever	21 (13)	3 (2)
Back pain	12 (8)	4 (3)
Cardiovascular		
Edema peripheral	17 (11)	1 (1)
Central and Peripheral Nervous System		
Convulsions	36 (23)	8 (5)
Hemiparesis	29 (18)	10 (6)
Dizziness	19 (12)	1 (1)
Coordination abnormal	17 (11)	2 (1)
Amnesia	16 (10)	6 (4)
Insomnia	16 (10)	0
Paresthesia	15 (9)	1 (1)
Somnolence	15 (9)	5 (3)
Paresis	13 (8)	4 (3)
Urinary incontinence	13 (8)	3 (2)
Ataxia	12 (8)	3 (2)
Dysphasia	11 (7)	1 (1)
Convulsions local	9 (6)	0
Gait abnormal	9 (6)	1 (1)
Confusion	8 (5)	0
Endocrine		
Adrenal hypercorticism	13 (8)	0
Gastrointestinal System		
Nausea	84 (53)	16 (10)
Vomiting	66 (42)	10 (6)
Constipation	52 (33)	1 (1)
Diarrhea	25 (16)	3 (2)
Abdominal pain	14 (9)	2 (1)
Anorexia	14 (9)	1 (1)
Metabolic		
Weight increase	8 (5)	0
Musculoskeletal System		
Myalgia	8 (5)	0
Psychiatric Disorders		
Anxiety	11 (7)	1 (1)
Depression	10 (6)	0
Reproductive Disorders		
Breast pain, female	4 (6)	0
Resistance Mechanism Disorders		
Infection viral	17 (11)	0
Respiratory System		
Upper respiratory tract infection	13 (8)	0
Pharyngitis	12 (8)	0
Sinusitis	10 (6)	0
Coughing	8 (5)	0
Skin and Appendages		
Rash	13 (8)	0
Pruritus	12 (8)	2 (1)
Urinary System		
Urinary tract infection	12 (8)	0
Micturition increased frequency	9 (6)	0
Vision		
Diplopia	8 (5)	0
Vision Abnormal*	8 (5)	0

*Blurred vision, visual deficit, vision changes, vision troubles.

Table 3

Adverse Hematologic Effects (Grade 3 to 4) in the Anaplastic Astrocytoma Trial

	TEMODAR[a]
Hemoglobin	7/158 (4%)
Lymphopenia	83/152 (55%)
Neutrophils	20/142 (14%)
Platelets	29/156 (19%)
WBC	18/158 (11%)

[a]Change from Grade 0 to 2 at baseline to Grade 3 or 4 during treatment.

OVERDOSAGE

Doses of 500, 750, 1,000, and 1,250 mg/m^2 (total dose per cycle over 5 days) have been evaluated clinically in patients. Dose-limiting toxicity was hematologic and was reported at 1,000 mg/m^2 and at 1,250 mg/m^2. Up to 1,000 mg/m^2 has been taken as a single dose, with only the expected effects of neutropenia and thrombocytopenia resulting. In the event of an overdose, hematologic evaluation is needed. Supportive measures should be provided as necessary.

DOSAGE AND ADMINISTRATION

Dosage of TEMODAR must be adjusted according to nadir neutrophil and platelet counts in the previous cycle and neutrophil and platelet counts at the time of initiating the next cycle. The initial dose is 150 mg/m^2 orally once daily for 5 consecutive days per 28-day treatment cycle. If both the nadir and day of dosing (Day 29, Day 1 of next cycle) absolute neutrophil counts (ANC) are ≥1.5 × 10^9/L (1,500/μL) and both the nadir and Day 29, Day 1 of next cycle platelet counts are ≥100 × 10^9/L (100,000/μL), the TEMODAR dose may be increased to 200 mg/m^2/day for 5 consecutive days per 28-day treatment cycle. During treatment, a complete blood count should be obtained on Day 22 (21 days after the first dose) or within 48 hours of that day, and weekly until the ANC is above 1.5 × 10^9/L (1,500/μL) and the platelet count exceeds 100 × 10^9/L (100,000/μL). The next cycle of TEMODAR should not be started until the ANC and platelet count exceed these levels. If the ANC falls to <1.0 × 10^9/L (1,000/μL) or the platelet count is <50 × 10^9/L (50,000/μL) during any cycle, the next cycle should be reduced by 50 mg/m^2, but not below 100 mg/m^2, the lowest recommended dose (see **Table 4**) (see **WARNINGS**). TEMODAR therapy can be continued until disease progression. In the clinical trial, treatment could be continued for a maximum of 2 years; but the optimum duration of therapy is not known. For TEMODAR dosage calculations based on body surface area (BSA), see **Table 5**. For suggested capsule combinations based on daily dose, see **Table 6**.

Table 4 Dosing Modification Table

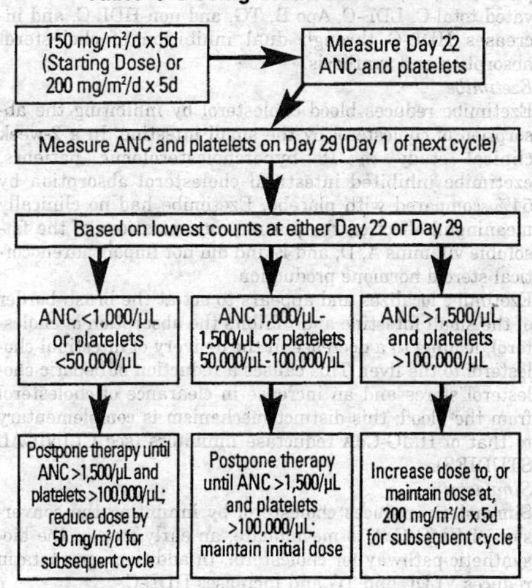

Table 5

Daily Dose Calculations by Body Surface Area (BSA) for 5 consecutive days per 28-day treatment cycle for the initial chemotherapy cycle (150 mg/m^2) and for subsequent chemotherapy cycles (200 mg/m^2) for patients whose nadir and day of dosing (Day 29, Day 1 of next cycle) absolute neutrophil count (ANC) is >1.5 × 10^9/L (1,500/μL) and whose nadir and Day 29, Day 1 of next cycle platelet count is >100 × 10^9/L (100,000/μL).

Total BSA (m^2)	150 mg/m^2 (mg daily)	200 mg/m^2 (mg daily)
0.5	75	100
0.6	90	120
0.7	105	140
0.8	120	160
0.9	135	180
1.0	150	200
1.1	165	220
1.2	180	240
1.3	195	260
1.4	210	280
1.5	225	300
1.6	240	320
1.7	255	340
1.8	270	360
1.9	285	380
2.0	300	400
2.1	315	420
2.2	330	440
2.3	345	460
2.4	360	480
2.5	375	500

Table 6

Suggested Capsule Combinations Based on Daily Dose

	Number of Daily Capsules by Strength (mg)			
Total Daily Dose (mg)	**250**	**100**	**20**	**5**
200	0	2	0	0
205	0	2	0	1
210	0	2	0	2
215	0	2	0	3
220	0	2	1	0
225	0	2	1	1
230	0	2	1	2
235	0	2	1	3
240	0	2	2	0
245	0	2	2	1
250	1	0	0	0
255	1	0	0	1
260	1	0	0	2
265	1	0	0	3
270	1	0	1	0
275	1	0	1	1
280	1	0	1	2
285	1	0	1	3
290	1	0	2	0
295	1	0	2	1
300	0	3	0	0
305	0	3	0	1
310	0	3	0	2
315	0	3	0	3
320	0	3	1	0
325	0	3	1	1
330	1	0	4	0
335	1	0	4	1
340	0	3	2	0
345	0	3	2	1
350	1	1	0	0
355	1	1	0	1
360	1	1	0	2
365	1	1	0	3
370	1	1	1	0
375	1	1	1	1
380	1	1	1	2
385	1	1	1	3
390	1	1	2	0
395	1	1	2	1
400	0	4	0	0
405	0	4	0	1
410	0	4	0	2
415	0	4	0	3
420	0	4	1	0
425	0	4	1	1
430	1	1	4	0
435	0	4	1	3
440	0	4	2	0
445	0	4	2	1
450	1	2	0	0
455	1	2	0	1
460	1	2	0	2
465	1	2	0	3
470	1	2	1	0
475	1	2	1	1
480	1	2	1	2
485	1	2	1	3
490	1	2	2	0
495	1	2	2	1
500	2	0	0	0

In the clinical trial, TEMODAR was administered under both fasting and nonfasting conditions; however, absorption is affected by food (see **CLINICAL PHARMACOLOGY**) and consistency of administration with respect to food is recommended. There are no dietary restrictions with temozolomide. To reduce nausea and vomiting, temozolomide should be taken on an empty stomach. Bedtime administra-

Continued on next page

Information on Schering products appearing on these pages is effective as of June 2003.

Temodar—Cont.

tion may be advised. Antiemetic therapy may be administered prior to and/or following administration of TEMODAR.

TEMODAR (temozolomide) Capsules should not be opened or chewed. They should be swallowed whole with a glass of water.

Handling and Disposal: Temozolomide causes the rapid appearance of malignant tumors in rats. Capsules should not be opened. If capsules are accidentally opened or damaged, rigorous precautions should be taken with the capsule contents to avoid inhalation or contact with the skin or mucous membranes. Procedures for proper handling and disposal of anticancer drugs should be considered.[1–7] Several guidelines on this subject have been published. There is no general agreement that all of the procedures recommended in the guidelines are necessary or appropriate.

HOW SUPPLIED

TEMODAR (temozolomide) Capsules are supplied in amber glass bottles with child-resistant polypropylene caps containing the following capsule strengths:

TEMODAR (temozolomide) Capsules 5 mg: 5 and 20 capsule bottles.

5 count—NDC 0085-1248-01
20 count—NDC 0085-1248-02

TEMODAR (temozolomide) Capsules 20 mg: 5 and 20 capsule bottles.

5 count—NDC 0085-1244-01
20 count—NDC 0085-1244-02

TEMODAR (temozolomide) Capsules 100 mg: 5 and 20 capsule bottles.

5 count—NDC 0085-1259-01
20 count—NDC 0085-1259-02

TEMODAR (temozolomide) Capsules 250 mg: 5 and 20 capsule bottles.

5 count—NDC 0085-1252-01
20 count—NDC 0085-1252-02

Store at 25°C (77°F); excursions permitted to 15°–30°C (59°–86°F).

[See USP Controlled Room Temperature]

REFERENCES

1. Recommendations for the Safe Handling of Parenteral Antineoplastic Drugs, NIH Publication No. 83-2621. For sale by the Superintendent of Documents, U.S. Government Printing Office, Washington, DC 20402.
2. AMA Council Report, Guidelines for Handling Parenteral Antineoplastics. *JAMA.* 1985;2.53(11):1590-1592.
3. National Study Commission on Cytotoxic Exposure—Recommendations for Handling Cytotoxic Agents. Available from Louis P. Jeffrey, ScD., Chairman, National Study Commission on Cytotoxic Exposure, Massachusetts College of Pharmacy and Allied Health Sciences, 179 Longwood Avenue, Boston, Massachusetts 02115.
4. Clinical Oncological Society of Australia, Guidelines and Recommendations for Safe Handling of Antineoplastic Agents. *Med J Australia.* 1983;1:426-428.
5. Jones RB, et al. Safe Handling Of Chemotherapeutic Agents: A Report from the Mount Sinai Medical Center. *CA—A Cancer Journal for Clinicians.* 1983;(Sept/Oct):258-263.
6. American Society of Hospital Pharmacists Technical Assistance Bulletin on Handling Cytotoxic and Hazardous Drugs. *Am J Hosp Pharm.* 1990;47:1033-1049.
7. Controlling Occupational Exposure to Hazardous Drugs. (OSHA Work-Practice Guidelines), *Am J Health-Syst Pharm.* 1996;53:1669-1685.

Schering Corporation
Kenilworth, NJ 07033 USA
Rev. 2/04 22487841

VYTORIN™ 10/10 ℞
(EZETIMIBE 10 MG/SIMVASTATIN 10 MG TABLETS)
VYTORIN™ 10/20 ℞
(EZETIMIBE 10 MG/SIMVASTATIN 20 MG TABLETS)
VYTORIN™ 10/40 ℞
(EZETIMIBE 10 MG/SIMVASTATIN 40 MG TABLETS)
VYTORIN™ 10/80 ℞
(EZETIMIBE 10 MG/SIMVASTATIN 80 MG TABLETS)

[*vī-tŏr-in*]

DESCRIPTION

VYTORIN contains ezetimibe, a selective inhibitor of intestinal cholesterol and related phytosterol absorption, and simvastatin, a 3-hydroxy-3-methylglutaryl-coenzyme A (HMG-CoA) reductase inhibitor.

The chemical name of ezetimibe is 1-(4-fluorophenyl)-3(R)-[3-(4-fluorophenyl)-3(S)-hydroxypropyl]- 4(S)-(4-hydroxyphenyl)-2-azetidinone. The empirical formula is $C_{24}H_{21}F_2NO_3$ and its molecular weight is 409.4.

Ezetimibe is a white, crystalline powder that is freely to very soluble in ethanol, methanol, and acetone and practically insoluble in water. Its structural formula is:

[See chemical structure at top of next column]

Simvastatin, an inactive lactone, is hydrolyzed to the corresponding β-hydroxyacid form, which is an inhibitor of HMG-CoA reductase. Simvastatin is butanoic acid, 2,2-dimethyl,

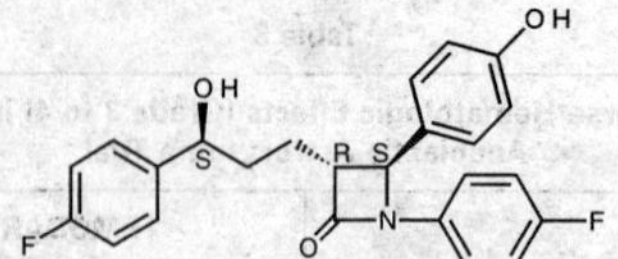

1,2,3,7,8,8a-hexahydro-3,7- dimethyl-8-[2-(tetrahydro-4-hydroxy-6-oxo-2*H*-pyran-2-yl)-ethyl]-1-naphthalenyl ester, [1*S*- [1α,3α,7β,8β(2*S**,4*S**),-8aβ]]. The empirical formula of simvastatin is $C_{25}H_{38}O_5$ and its molecular weight is 418.57. Simvastatin is a white to off-white, nonhygroscopic, crystalline powder that is practically insoluble in water, and freely soluble in chloroform, methanol and ethanol. Its structural formula is:

VYTORIN is available for oral use as tablets containing 10 mg of ezetimibe, and 10 mg of simvastatin (VYTORIN 10/10), 20 mg of simvastatin (VYTORIN 10/20), 40 mg of simvastatin (VYTORIN 10/40), or 80 mg of simvastatin (VYTORIN 10/80). Each tablet contains the following inactive ingredients: butylated hydroxyanisole NF, citric acid monohydrate USP, croscarmellose sodium NF, hydroxypropyl methylcellulose USP, lactose monohydrate NF, magnesium stearate NF, microcrystalline cellulose NF, and propyl gallate NF.

CLINICAL PHARMACOLOGY

Background

Clinical studies have demonstrated that elevated levels of total cholesterol (total-C), low-density lipoprotein cholesterol (LDL-C) and apolipoprotein B (Apo B), the major protein constituent of LDL, promote human atherosclerosis. In addition, decreased levels of high-density lipoprotein cholesterol (HDL-C) are associated with the development of atherosclerosis. Epidemiologic studies have established that cardiovascular morbidity and mortality vary directly with the level of total-C and LDL-C and inversely with the level of HDL-C. Like LDL, cholesterol-enriched triglyceride-rich lipoproteins, including very-low-density lipoproteins (VLDL), intermediate-density lipoproteins (IDL), and remnants, can also promote atherosclerosis. The independent effect of raising HDL-C or lowering triglycerides (TG) on the risk of coronary and cardiovascular morbidity and mortality has not been determined.

Mode of Action

VYTORIN

Plasma cholesterol is derived from intestinal absorption and endogenous synthesis. VYTORIN contains ezetimibe and simvastatin, two lipid-lowering compounds with complementary mechanisms of action. VYTORIN reduces elevated total-C, LDL-C, Apo B, TG, and non-HDL-C, and increases HDL-C through dual inhibition of cholesterol absorption and synthesis.

Ezetimibe

Ezetimibe reduces blood cholesterol by inhibiting the absorption of cholesterol by the small intestine. In a 2-week clinical study in 18 hypercholesterolemic patients, ezetimibe inhibited intestinal cholesterol absorption by 54%, compared with placebo. Ezetimibe had no clinically meaningful effect on the plasma concentrations of the fat-soluble vitamins A, D, and E and did not impair adrenocortical steroid hormone production.

Ezetimibe localizes and appears to act at the brush border of the small intestine and inhibits the absorption of cholesterol, leading to a decrease in the delivery of intestinal cholesterol to the liver. This causes a reduction of hepatic cholesterol stores and an increase in clearance of cholesterol from the blood; this distinct mechanism is complementary to that of HMG-CoA reductase inhibitors (see CLINICAL STUDIES).

Simvastatin

Simvastatin reduces cholesterol by inhibiting the conversion of HMG-CoA to mevalonate, an early step in the biosynthetic pathway for cholesterol. In addition, simvastatin reduces VLDL and TG and increases HDL-C.

Pharmacokinetics

Absorption

VYTORIN

VYTORIN is bioequivalent to coadministered ezetimibe and simvastatin.

Ezetimibe

After oral administration, ezetimibe is absorbed and extensively conjugated to a pharmacologically active phenolic glucuronide (ezetimibe-glucuronide).

Effect of Food on Oral Absorption

Ezetimibe

Concomitant food administration (high-fat or non-fat meals) had no effect on the extent of absorption of ezetimibe when administered as 10-mg tablets. The C_{max} value of ezetimibe was increased by 38% with consumption of high-fat meals.

Simvastatin

Relative to the fasting state, the plasma profiles of both active and total inhibitors of HMG-CoA reductase were not affected when simvastatin was administered immediately before an American Heart Association recommended low-fat meal.

Distribution

Ezetimibe

Ezetimibe and ezetimibe-glucuronide are highly bound (>90%) to human plasma proteins.

Simvastatin

Both simvastatin and its β-hydroxyacid metabolite are highly bound (approximately 95%) to human plasma proteins. When radiolabeled simvastatin was administered to rats, simvastatin-derived radioactivity crossed the blood-brain barrier.

Metabolism and Excretion

Ezetimibe

Ezetimibe is primarily metabolized in the small intestine and liver via glucuronide conjugation with subsequent biliary and renal excretion. Minimal oxidative metabolism has been observed in all species evaluated.

In humans, ezetimibe is rapidly metabolized to ezetimibe-glucuronide. Ezetimibe and ezetimibe-glucuronide are the major drug-derived compounds detected in plasma, constituting approximately 10 to 20% and 80 to 90% of the total drug in plasma, respectively. Both ezetimibe and ezetimibe-glucuronide are slowly eliminated from plasma with a half-life of approximately 22 hours for both ezetimibe and ezetimibe-glucuronide. Plasma concentration-time profiles exhibit multiple peaks, suggesting enterohepatic recycling. Following oral administration of ^{14}C-ezetimibe (20 mg) to human subjects, total ezetimibe (ezetimibe + ezetimibe-glucuronide) accounted for approximately 93% of the total radioactivity in plasma. After 48 hours, there were no detectable levels of radioactivity in the plasma.

Approximately 78% and 11% of the administered radioactivity were recovered in the feces and urine, respectively, over a 10-day collection period. Ezetimibe was the major component in feces and accounted for 69% of the administered dose, while ezetimibe-glucuronide was the major component in urine and accounted for 9% of the administered dose.

Simvastatin

Simvastatin is a lactone that is readily hydrolyzed *in vivo* to the corresponding β-hydroxyacid, a potent inhibitor of HMG-CoA reductase. Inhibition of HMG-CoA reductase is a basis for an assay in pharmacokinetic studies of the β-hydroxyacid metabolites (active inhibitors) and, following base hydrolysis, active plus latent inhibitors (total inhibitors) in plasma following administration of simvastatin. The major active metabolites of simvastatin present in human plasma are the β-hydroxyacid of simvastatin and its 6′- hydroxy, 6′-hydroxymethyl, and 6′-exomethylene derivatives.

Plasma concentrations of total radioactivity (simvastatin plus ^{14}C-metabolites) peaked at 4 hours and declined rapidly to about 10% of peak by 12 hours postdose. Simvastatin undergoes extensive first-pass extraction in the liver, its primary site of action, with subsequent excretion of drug equivalents in the bile. As a consequence of extensive hepatic extraction of simvastatin (estimated to be >60% in man), the availability of drug to the general circulation is low.

Following an oral dose of ^{14}C-labeled simvastatin in man, 13% of the dose was excreted in urine and 60% in feces. The latter represents absorbed drug equivalents excreted in bile, as well as any unabsorbed drug.

In a single-dose study in nine healthy subjects, it was estimated that less than 5% of an oral dose of simvastatin reaches the general circulation as active inhibitors.

Special Populations

Geriatric Patients

Ezetimibe

In a multiple-dose study with ezetimibe given 10 mg once daily for 10 days, plasma concentrations for total ezetimibe were about 2-fold higher in older (≥65 years) healthy subjects compared to younger subjects.

Simvastatin

In a study including 16 elderly patients between 70 and 78 years of age who received simvastatin 40 mg/day, the mean plasma level of HMG-CoA reductase inhibitory activity was increased approximately 45% compared with 18 patients between 18–30 years of age.

Pediatric Patients

Ezetimibe

In a multiple-dose study with ezetimibe given 10 mg once daily for 7 days, the absorption and metabolism of ezetimibe were similar in adolescents (10 to 18 years) and adults. Based on total ezetimibe, there are no pharmacokinetic differences between adolescents and adults. Pharmacokinetic data in the pediatric population <10 years of age are not available.

Gender

Ezetimibe

In a multiple-dose study with ezetimibe given 10 mg once daily for 10 days, plasma concentrations for total ezetimibe were slightly higher (<20%) in women than in men.

Race

Ezetimibe

Based on a meta-analysis of multiple-dose pharmacokinetic studies, there were no pharmacokinetic differences between Blacks and Caucasians. There were too few patients in other racial or ethnic groups to permit further pharmacokinetic comparisons.

Hepatic Insufficiency

Ezetimibe

After a single 10-mg dose of ezetimibe, the mean exposure (based on area under the curve [AUC]) to total ezetimibe was increased approximately 1.7-fold in patients with mild hepatic insufficiency (Child-Pugh score 5 to 6), compared to healthy subjects. The mean AUC values for total ezetimibe and ezetimibe increased approximately 3- to 4-fold and 5- to 6-fold, respectively, in patients with moderate (Child-Pugh score 7 to 9) or severe hepatic impairment (Child-Pugh score 10 to 15). In a 14-day, multiple-dose study (10 mg daily) in patients with moderate hepatic insufficiency, the mean AUC for total ezetimibe and ezetimibe increased approximately 4-fold compared to healthy subjects.

Renal Insufficiency

Ezetimibe

After a single 10-mg dose of ezetimibe in patients with severe renal disease (n=8; mean CrCl ≤30 mL/min/1.73 m^2), the mean AUC for total ezetimibe and ezetimibe increased approximately 1.5-fold, compared to healthy subjects (n=9).

Simvastatin

Pharmacokinetic studies with another statin having a similar principal route of elimination to that of simvastatin have suggested that for a given dose level higher systemic exposure may be achieved in patients with severe renal insufficiency (as measured by creatinine clearance).

***Drug Interactions* (See also PRECAUTIONS, *Drug Interactions*)**

No clinically significant pharmacokinetic interaction was seen when ezetimibe was coadministered with simvastatin. Specific pharmacokinetic drug interaction studies with VYTORIN have not been performed.

Cytochrome P450: Ezetimibe had no significant effect on a series of probe drugs (caffeine, dextromethorphan, tolbutamide, and IV midazolam) known to be metabolized by cytochrome P450 (1A2, 2D6, 2C8/9 and 3A4) in a "cocktail" study of twelve healthy adult males. This indicates that ezetimibe is neither an inhibitor nor an inducer of these cytochrome P450 isozymes, and it is unlikely that ezetimibe will affect the metabolism of drugs that are metabolized by these enzymes.

In a study of 12 healthy volunteers, simvastatin at the 80-mg dose had no effect on the metabolism of the probe cytochrome P450 isoform 3A4 (CYP3A4) substrates midazolam and erythromycin. This indicates that simvastatin is not an inhibitor of CYP3A4, and, therefore, is not expected to affect the plasma levels of other drugs metabolized by CYP3A4.

Simvastatin is a substrate for CYP3A4. Potent inhibitors of CYP3A4 can raise the plasma levels of HMG-CoA reductase inhibitory activity and increase the risk of myopathy. (See WARNINGS, *Myopathy/Rhabdomyolysis* and PRECAUTIONS, *Drug Interactions.*)

Antacids: In a study of twelve healthy adults, a single dose of antacid (Supralox™ 20 mL) administration had no significant effect on the oral bioavailability of total ezetimibe, ezetimibe-glucuronide, or ezetimibe based on AUC values. The C_{max} value of total ezetimibe was decreased by 30%.

Cholestyramine: In a study of forty healthy hypercholesterolemic (LDL-C ≥130 mg/dL) adult subjects, concomitant cholestyramine (4 g twice daily) administration decreased the mean AUC of total ezetimibe and ezetimibe approximately 55% and 80%, respectively.

Cyclosporine: In a study of eight post-renal transplant patients with mildly impaired or normal renal function (creatinine clearance of >50 mL/min), stable doses of cyclosporine (75 to 150 mg twice daily) increased the mean AUC and C_{max} values of total ezetimibe 3.4-fold (range 2.3- to 7.9-fold) and 3.9-fold (range 3.0- to 4.4-fold), respectively, compared to a historical healthy control population (n=17). In a different study, a renal transplant patient with severe renal insufficiency (creatinine clearance of 13.2 mL/min/1.73 m^2) who was receiving multiple medications, including cyclosporine, demonstrated a 12-fold greater exposure to total ezetimibe compared to healthy subjects.

Fenofibrate: In a study of thirty-two healthy hypercholesterolemic (LDL-C ≥130 mg/dL) adult subjects, concomitant fenofibrate (200 mg once daily) administration increased the mean C_{max} and AUC values of total ezetimibe approximately 64% and 48%, respectively. Pharmacokinetics of fenofibrate were not significantly affected by ezetimibe (10 mg once daily).

Gemfibrozil: In a study of twelve healthy adult males, concomitant administration of gemfibrozil (600 mg twice daily) significantly increased the oral bioavailability of total ezetimibe by a factor of 1.7. Ezetimibe (10 mg once daily) did not significantly affect the bioavailability of gemfibrozil.

Grapefruit Juice: Grapefruit juice contains one or more components that inhibit CYP3A4 and can increase the plasma concentrations of drugs metabolized by CYP3A4. In one study[1], 10 subjects consumed 200 mL of double-strength grapefruit juice (one can of frozen concentrate diluted with one rather than 3 cans of water) three times daily for 2 days and an additional 200 mL double-strength grapefruit juice together with, and 30 and 90 minutes following, a single dose of 60 mg simvastatin on the third day. This regimen of grapefruit juice resulted in mean increases in the concentration (as measured by the area under the concentration-time curve) of active and total HMG-CoA reductase inhibitory activity [measured using a radioenzyme inhibition assay both before (for active inhibitors) and after (for total inhibitors) base hydrolysis] of 2.4-fold and 3.6-fold, respectively, and of simvastatin and its β-hydroxyacid metabolite [measured using a chemical assay — liquid chromatography/tandem mass spectrometry] of 16-fold and 7-fold, respectively. In a second study, 16 subjects consumed one 8 oz glass of single-strength grapefruit juice (one can of frozen concentrate diluted with 3 cans of water) with breakfast for 3 consecutive days and a single dose of 20 mg simvastatin in the evening of the third day. This regimen of grapefruit juice resulted in a mean increase in the plasma concentration (as measured by the area under the concentration-time curve) of active and total HMG-CoA reductase inhibitory activity [using a validated enzyme inhibition assay different from that used in the first[1] study, both before (for active inhibitors) and after (for total inhibitors) base hydrolysis] of 1.13-fold and 1.18-fold, respectively, and of simvastatin and its β-hydroxyacid metabolite [measured using a chemical assay — liquid chromatography/tandem mass spectrometry] of 1.88-fold and 1.31-fold, respectively. The effect of amounts of grapefruit juice between those used in these two studies on simvastatin pharmacokinetics has not been studied.

Table 1
Response to VYTORIN in Patients with Primary Hypercholesterolemia
(Mean[a] % Change from Untreated Baseline[b])

Treatment (Daily Dose)	N	Total-C	LDL-C	Apo B	HDL-C	TG[a]	Non-HDL-C
Pooled data (All VYTORIN doses)[c]	609	−38	−53	−42	+7	−24	−49
Pooled data (All simvastatin doses)[c]	622	−28	−39	−32	+7	−21	−36
Ezetimibe 10 mg	149	−13	−19	−15	+5	−11	−18
Placebo	148	−1	−2	0	0	−2	−2
VYTORIN by dose							
10/10	152	−31	−45	−35	+8	−23	−41
10/20	156	−36	−52	−41	+10	−24	−47
10/40	147	−39	−55	−44	+6	−23	−51
10/80	154	−43	−60	−49	+6	−31	−56
Simvastatin by dose							
10 mg	158	−23	−33	−26	+5	−17	−30
20 mg	150	−24	−34	−28	+7	−18	−32
40 mg	156	−29	−41	−33	+8	−21	−38
80 mg	158	−35	−49	−39	+7	−27	−45

[a] For triglycerides, median % change from baseline
[b] Baseline - on no lipid-lowering drug
[c] VYTORIN doses pooled (10/10-10/80) significantly reduced total-C, LDL-C, Apo B, TG, and non-HDL-C compared to simvastatin, and significantly increased HDL-C compared to placebo.

[1] Lilja JJ, Kivisto KT, Neuvonen PJ. Clin Pharmacol Ther 1998;64(5):477-83.

ANIMAL PHARMACOLOGY

Ezetimibe

The hypocholesterolemic effect of ezetimibe was evaluated in cholesterol-fed Rhesus monkeys, dogs, rats, and mouse models of human cholesterol metabolism. Ezetimibe was found to have an ED_{50} value of 0.5 µg/kg/day for inhibiting the rise in plasma cholesterol levels in monkeys. The ED_{50} values in dogs, rats, and mice were 7, 30, and 700 µg/kg/day, respectively. These results are consistent with ezetimibe being a potent cholesterol absorption inhibitor.

In a rat model, where the glucuronide metabolite of ezetimibe (ezetimibe-glucuronide) was administered intraduodenally, the metabolite was as potent as ezetimibe in inhibiting the absorption of cholesterol, suggesting that the glucuronide metabolite had activity similar to the parent drug.

In 1-month studies in dogs given ezetimibe (0.03-300 mg/kg/day), the concentration of cholesterol in gallbladder bile increased ~2- to 4-fold. However, a dose of 300 mg/kg/day administered to dogs for one year did not result in gallstone formation or any other adverse hepatobiliary effects. In a 14-day study in mice given ezetimibe (0.3-5 mg/kg/day) and fed a low-fat or cholesterol-rich diet, the concentration of cholesterol in gallbladder bile was either unaffected or reduced to normal levels, respectively.

A series of acute preclinical studies was performed to determine the selectivity of ezetimibe for inhibiting cholesterol absorption. Ezetimibe inhibited the absorption of ^{14}C-cholesterol with no effect on the absorption of triglycerides, fatty acids, bile acids, progesterone, ethyl estradiol, or the fat-soluble vitamins A and D.

In 4- to 12-week toxicity studies in mice, ezetimibe did not induce cytochrome P450 drug metabolizing enzymes. In toxicity studies, a pharmacokinetic interaction of ezetimibe with HMG-CoA reductase inhibitors (parents or their active hydroxy acid metabolites) was seen in rats, dogs, and rabbits.

CLINICAL STUDIES

Primary Hypercholesterolemia

VYTORIN

VYTORIN reduces total-C, LDL-C, Apo B, TG, and non-HDL-C, and increases HDL-C in patients with hypercholesterolemia. Maximal to near maximal response is generally achieved within 2 weeks and maintained during chronic therapy.

VYTORIN is effective in men and women with hypercholesterolemia. Experience in non-Caucasians is limited and does not permit a precise estimate of the magnitude of the effects of VYTORIN.

In a multicenter, double-blind, placebo-controlled, 12-week trial, 1528 hypercholesterolemic patients were randomized to one of ten treatment groups: placebo, ezetimibe (10 mg), simvastatin (10 mg, 20 mg, 40 mg, or 80 mg), or VYTORIN (10/10, 10/20, 10/40, or 10/80).

When patients receiving VYTORIN were compared to those receiving all doses of simvastatin, VYTORIN significantly lowered total-C, LDL-C, Apo B, TG, and non-HDL-C. The effects of VYTORIN on HDL-C were similar to the effects seen with simvastatin. Further analysis showed VYTORIN significantly increased HDL-C compared with placebo. (See Table 1.) The lipid response to VYTORIN was similar in patients with TG levels greater than or less than 200 mg/dL.

[See table 1 above]

In a multicenter, double-blind, controlled, 23-week study, 710 patients with known CHD or CHD risk equivalents, as defined by the NCEP ATP III guidelines, and an LDL-C ≥130 mg/dL were randomized to one of four treatment groups: coadministered ezetimibe and simvastatin equivalent to VYTORIN (10/10, 10/20, and 10/40), or simvastatin 20 mg. Patients not reaching an LDL-C <100 mg/dL had their simvastatin dose titrated at 6-week intervals to a maximal dose of 80 mg.

At Week 5, the LDL-C reductions with VYTORIN 10/10, 10/20, or 10/40 were significantly larger than with simvastatin 20 mg (see Table 2).

Table 2
Response to VYTORIN after 5 Weeks in Patients with CHD or CHD Risk Equivalents and an LDL-C ≥130 mg/dL

	Simvastatin 20 mg	VYTORIN 10/10	VYTORIN 10/20	VYTORIN 10/40
N	253	251	109	97
Mean baseline LDL-C	174	165	167	171
Percent change LDL-C	−38	−47	−53	−59

In a multicenter, double-blind, 24-week, forced titration study, 788 patients with primary hypercholesterolemia, who had not met their NCEP ATP III target LDL-C goal, were randomized to receive coadministered ezetimibe and simvastatin equivalent to VYTORIN (10/10 and 10/20) or atorvastatin 10 mg. For all three treatment groups, the dose of the statin was titrated at 6-week intervals to 80 mg. At each pre-specified dose comparison, VYTORIN lowered LDL-C to a greater degree than atorvastatin (see Table 3).

[See table 3 at top of next page]

In a multicenter, double-blind, 24-week trial, 214 patients with type 2 diabetes mellitus treated with thiazolidinedi-

Continued on next page

Information on Schering products appearing on these pages is effective as of June 2003.

Vytorin—Cont.

ones (rosiglitazone or pioglitazone) for a minimum of 3 months and simvastatin 20 mg for a minimum of 6 weeks, were randomized to receive either simvastatin 40 mg or the coadministered active ingredients equivalent to VYTORIN 10/20. The median LDL-C and HbA1c levels at baseline were 89 mg/dL and 7.1%, respectively.

VYTORIN 10/20 was significantly more effective than doubling the dose of simvastatin to 40 mg. The median percent changes from baseline for VYTORIN vs simvastatin were: LDL-C -25% and -5%; total-C -16% and -5%; Apo B -19% and -5%; and non-HDL-C -23% and -5%. Results for HDL-C and TG between the two treatment groups were not significantly different.

Ezetimibe

In two multicenter, double-blind, placebo-controlled, 12-week studies in 1719 patients with primary hypercholesterolemia, ezetimibe significantly lowered total-C (-13%), LDL-C (-19%), Apo B (-14%), and TG (-8%), and increased HDL-C (+3%) compared to placebo. Reduction in LDL-C was consistent across age, sex, and baseline LDL-C.

Simvastatin

In two large, placebo-controlled clinical trials, the Scandinavian Simvastatin Survival Study (N=4,444 patients) and the Heart Protection Study (N=20,536 patients), the effects of treatment with simvastatin were assessed in patients at high risk of coronary events because of existing coronary heart disease, diabetes, peripheral vessel disease, history of stroke or other cerebrovascular disease. Simvastatin was proven to reduce: the risk of total mortality by reducing CHD deaths; the risk of non-fatal myocardial infarction and stroke; and the need for coronary and non-coronary revascularization procedures.

No incremental benefit of VYTORIN on cardiovascular morbidity and mortality over and above that demonstrated for simvastatin has been established.

Homozygous Familial Hypercholesterolemia (HoFH)

A double-blind, randomized, 12-week study was performed in patients with a clinical and/or genotypic diagnosis of HoFH. Data were analyzed from a subgroup of patients (n=14) receiving simvastatin 40 mg at baseline. Increasing the dose of simvastatin from 40 to 80 mg (n=5) produced a reduction of LDL-C of 13% from baseline on simvastatin 40 mg. Coadministered ezetimibe and simvastatin equivalent to VYTORIN (10/40 and 10/80 pooled, n=9), produced a reduction of LDL-C of 23% from baseline on simvastatin 40 mg. In those patients coadministered ezetimibe and simvastatin equivalent to VYTORIN (10/80, n=5), a reduction of LDL-C of 29% from baseline on simvastatin 40 mg was produced.

Table 3
Response to VYTORIN and Atorvastatin in Patients with Primary Hypercholesterolemia
(Mean[a] % Change from Untreated Baseline[b])

Treatment	N	Total-C	LDL-C	Apo B	HDL-C	TG[a]	Non-HDL-C
Week 6							
Atorvastatin 10 mg[c]	262	−28	−37	−32	+5	−23	−35
VYTORIN 10/10[d]	263	−34[f]	−46[f]	−38[f]	+8[f]	−26	−43[f]
VYTORIN 10/20[e]	263	−36[f]	−50[f]	−41[f]	+10[f]	−25	−46[f]
Week 12							
Atorvastatin 20 mg	246	−33	−44	−38	+7	−28	−42
VYTORIN 10/20	250	−37[f]	−50[f]	−41[f]	+9	−28	−46[f]
VYTORIN 10/40	252	−39[f]	−54[f]	−45[f]	+12[f]	−31	−50[f]
Week 18							
Atorvastatin 40 mg	237	−37	−49	−42	+8	−31	−47
VYTORIN 10/40[g]	482	−40[f]	−56[f]	−45[f]	+11[f]	−32	−52[f]
Week 24							
Atorvastatin 80 mg	228	−40	−53	−45	+6	−35	−50
VYTORIN 10/80[g]	459	−43[f]	−59[f]	−49[f]	+12[f]	−35	−55[f]

[a] For triglycerides, median % change from baseline
[b] Baseline - on no lipid-lowering drug
[c] Atorvastatin: 10 mg start dose titrated to 20 mg, 40 mg, and 80 mg through Weeks 6, 12, 18, and 24
[d] VYTORIN: 10/10 start dose titrated to 10/20, 10/40, and 10/80 through Weeks 6, 12, 18, and 24
[e] VYTORIN: 10/20 start dose titrated to 10/40, 10/40, and 10/80 through Weeks 6, 12, 18, and 24
[f] p≤0.05 for difference with atorvastatin in the specified week
[g] Data pooled for common doses of VYTORIN at Weeks 18 and 24.

Table 4
Summary of NCEP ATP III Guidelines

Risk Category	LDL Goal (mg/dL)	LDL Level at Which to Initiate Therapeutic Lifestyle Changes[a] (mg/dL)	LDL level at Which to Consider Drug Therapy (mg/dL)
CHD or CHD risk equivalents[b] (10-year risk >20%)[c]	<100	≥100	≥130 (100-129: drug optional)[d]
2+ Risk factors[e] (10-year risk ≤20%)[c]	<130	≥130	10-year risk 10–20%: ≥130[c] 10-year risk <10%: ≥160[c]
0–1 Risk factor[f]	<160	≥160	≥190 (160–189: LDL-lowering drug optional)

[a] Therapeutic lifestyle changes include: 1) dietary changes: reduced intake of saturated fats (<7% of total calories) and cholesterol (<200 mg per day), and enhancing LDL lowering with plant stanols/sterols (2 g/d) and increased viscous (soluble) fiber (10–25 g/d), 2) weight reduction, and 3) increased physical activity.
[b] CHD risk equivalents comprise: diabetes, multiple risk factors that confer a 10-year risk for CHD >20%, and other clinical forms of atherosclerotic disease (peripheral arterial disease, abdominal aortic aneurysm and symptomatic carotid artery disease).
[c] Risk assessment for determining the 10-year risk for developing CHD is carried out using the Framingham risk scoring. Refer to JAMA, May 16, 2001; 285 (19): 2486–2497, or the NCEP website (http://www.nhlbi.nih.gov) for more details.
[d] Some authorities recommend use of LDL-lowering drugs in this category if an LDL cholesterol <100 mg/dL cannot be achieved by therapeutic lifestyle changes. Others prefer use of drugs that primarily modify triglycerides and HDL, e.g., nicotinic acid or fibrate. Clinical judgment also may call for deferring drug therapy in this subcategory.
[e] Major risk factors (exclusive of LDL cholesterol) that modify LDL goals include cigarette smoking, hypertension (BP ≥140/90 mm Hg or on anti-hypertensive medication), low HDL cholesterol (<40 mg/dL), family history of premature CHD (CHD in male first-degree relative <55 years; CHD in female first-degree relative <65 years), age (men ≥45 years; women ≥55 years). HDL cholesterol ≥60 mg/dL counts as a "negative" risk factor; its presence removes one risk factor from the total count.
[f] Almost all people with 0-1 risk factor have a 10-year risk <10%; thus, 10-year risk assessment in people with 0-1 risk factor is not necessary.

INDICATIONS AND USAGE

Primary Hypercholesterolemia

VYTORIN is indicated as adjunctive therapy to diet for the reduction of elevated total-C, LDL-C, Apo B, TG, and non-HDL-C, and to increase HDL-C in patients with primary (heterozygous familial and non- familial) hypercholesterolemia or mixed hyperlipidemia.

Homozygous Familial Hypercholesterolemia (HoFH)

VYTORIN is indicated for the reduction of elevated total-C and LDL-C in patients with homozygous familial hypercholesterolemia, as an adjunct to other lipid-lowering treatments (e.g., LDL apheresis) or if such treatments are unavailable.

Therapy with lipid-altering agents should be a component of multiple risk-factor intervention in individuals at increased risk for atherosclerotic vascular disease due to hypercholesterolemia. Lipid- altering agents should be used in addition to an appropriate diet (including restriction of saturated fat and cholesterol) and when the response to diet and other non-pharmacological measures has been inadequate. (See NCEP Adult Treatment Panel (ATP) III Guidelines, summarized in Table 4.)

[See table 4 above]

Prior to initiating therapy with VYTORIN, secondary causes for dyslipidemia (i.e., diabetes, hypothyroidism, obstructive liver disease, chronic renal failure, and drugs that increase LDL-C and decrease HDL-C [progestins, anabolic steroids, and corticosteroids]), should be excluded or, if appropriate, treated. A lipid profile should be performed to measure total-C, LDL-C, HDL-C and TG. For TG levels >400 mg/dL (>4.5 mmol/L), LDL-C concentrations should be determined by ultracentrifugation.

At the time of hospitalization for an acute coronary event, lipid measures should be taken on admission or within 24 hours. These values can guide the physician on initiation of LDL-lowering therapy before or at discharge.

CONTRAINDICATIONS

Hypersensitivity to any component of this medication.

Active liver disease or unexplained persistent elevations in serum transaminases (see WARNINGS, *Liver Enzymes*).

Pregnancy and lactation. Atherosclerosis is a chronic process and the discontinuation of lipid-lowering drugs during pregnancy should have little impact on the outcome of long-term therapy of primary hypercholesterolemia. Moreover, cholesterol and other products of the cholesterol biosynthesis pathway are essential components for fetal development, including synthesis of steroids and cell membranes. Because of the ability of inhibitors of HMG-CoA reductase such as simvastatin to decrease the synthesis of cholesterol and possibly other products of the cholesterol biosynthesis pathway, VYTORIN is contraindicated during pregnancy and in nursing mothers. **VYTORIN should be administered to women of childbearing age only when such patients are highly unlikely to conceive.** If the patient becomes pregnant while taking this drug, VYTORIN should be discontinued immediately and the patient should be apprised of the potential hazard to the fetus (see PRECAUTIONS, *Pregnancy*).

WARNINGS

Myopathy/Rhabdomyolysis

In clinical trials, there was no excess of myopathy or rhabdomyolysis associated with ezetimibe compared with the relevant control arm (placebo or HMG-CoA reductase inhibitor alone). However, myopathy and rhabdomyolysis are known adverse reactions to HMG-CoA reductase inhibitors and other lipid-lowering drugs. In clinical trials, the incidence of CK >10 X the upper limit of normal [ULN] was 0.2% for VYTORIN.

Simvastatin, like other inhibitors of HMG-CoA reductase, occasionally causes myopathy manifested as muscle pain, tenderness or weakness with creatine kinase above 10 X ULN. Myopathy sometimes takes the form of rhabdomyolysis with or without acute renal failure secondary to myoglobinuria, and rare fatalities have occurred. The risk of myopathy is increased by high levels of HMG-CoA reductase inhibitory activity in plasma.

- **Because VYTORIN contains simvastatin, the risk of myopathy/rhabdomyolysis is increased by concomitant use of VYTORIN with the following:**

Potent inhibitors of CYP3A4: Cyclosporine, itraconazole, ketoconazole, erythromycin, clarithromycin, HIV protease inhibitors, nefazodone, or large quantities of grapefruit juice (>1 quart daily), particularly with higher doses of VYTORIN (see CLINICAL PHARMACOLOGY, *Pharmacokinetics*; PRECAUTIONS, *Drug Interactions, CYP3A4 Interactions*).

Other drugs:

Gemfibrozil, particularly with higher doses of VYTORIN (see CLINICAL PHARMACOLOGY, *Pharmacokinetics*; PRECAUTIONS, *Drug Interactions, Interactions with lipid-lowering drugs that can cause myopathy when given alone*).

Other lipid-lowering drugs (other fibrates or ≥1 g/day of niacin) that can cause myopathy when given alone (see PRECAUTIONS, *Drug Interactions, Interactions with lipid-lowering drugs that can cause myopathy when given alone*).

Amiodarone or verapamil with higher doses of VYTORIN (see PRECAUTIONS, *Drug Interactions, Other drug interactions*). In an ongoing clinical trial, myopathy has been reported in 6% of patients receiving simvastatin 80 mg and amiodarone. In an analysis of clinical trials involving 25,248 patients treated with simvastatin 20 to 80 mg, the incidence of myopathy was higher in patients receiving verapamil and simvastatin (4/635; 0.63%) than in patients taking simvastatin without a calcium channel blocker (13/21,224; 0.061%).

• **The risk of myopathy/rhabdomyolysis is dose related for simvastatin.** The incidence in clinical trials, in which patients were carefully monitored and some interacting drugs were excluded, has been approximately 0.02% at 20 mg, 0.07% at 40 mg and 0.3% at 80 mg.

Consequently:

1. Use of VYTORIN concomitantly with itraconazole, ketoconazole, erythromycin, clarithromycin, HIV protease inhibitors, nefazodone, or large quantities of grapefruit juice (>1 quart daily) should be avoided. If treatment with itraconazole, ketoconazole, erythromycin, or clarithromycin is unavoidable, therapy with VYTORIN should be suspended during the course of treatment. Concomitant use with other medicines labeled as having a potent inhibitory effect on CYP3A4 at therapeutic doses should be avoided unless the benefits of combined therapy outweigh the increased risk.

2. There is an increased risk of myopathy when simvastatin is used concomitantly with gemfibrozil or other fibrates; the safety and effectiveness of ezetimibe administered with fibrates have not been established. **Therefore, the concomitant use of VYTORIN and fibrates should be avoided.** (See PRECAUTIONS, *Drug Interactions, Other Drug Interactions, Fibrates.*)

3. Caution should be used when prescribing lipid-lowering doses (≥1 g/day) of niacin with VYTORIN, as niacin can cause myopathy when given alone. **The benefit of further alterations in lipid levels by the combined use of VYTORIN with niacin should be carefully weighed against the potential risks of this drug combination.**

4. The dose of VYTORIN should not exceed 10/10 mg daily in patients receiving concomitant medication with cyclosporine. The benefits of the use of VYTORIN in patients receiving cyclosporine should be carefully weighed against the risks of this combination. **(See PRECAUTIONS, *Drug Interactions, Other Drug Interactions, Cyclosporine.*)**

5. The dose of VYTORIN should not exceed 10/20 mg daily in patients receiving concomitant medication with amiodarone or verapamil. The combined use of VYTORIN at doses higher than 10/20 mg daily with amiodarone or verapamil should be avoided unless the clinical benefit is likely to outweigh the increased risk of myopathy.

6. All patients starting therapy with VYTORIN, or whose dose of VYTORIN is being increased, should be advised of the risk of myopathy and told to report promptly any unexplained muscle pain, tenderness or weakness. VYTORIN therapy should be discontinued immediately if myopathy is diagnosed or suspected. The presence of these symptoms, and/or a CK level >10 times the ULN indicates myopathy. In most cases, when patients were promptly discontinued from simvastatin treatment, muscle symptoms and CK increases resolved. Periodic CK determinations may be considered in patients starting therapy with VYTORIN or whose dose is being increased, but there is no assurance that such monitoring will prevent myopathy.

7. Many of the patients who have developed rhabdomyolysis on therapy with simvastatin have had complicated medical histories, including renal insufficiency usually as a consequence of long-standing diabetes mellitus. Such patients taking VYTORIN merit closer monitoring. Therapy with VYTORIN should be temporarily stopped a few days prior to elective major surgery and when any major medical or surgical condition supervenes.

Liver Enzymes

In three placebo-controlled, 12-week trials, the incidence of consecutive elevations (≥3 X ULN) in serum transaminases was 1.7% overall for patients treated with VYTORIN and appeared to be dose-related with an incidence of 2.6% for patients treated with VYTORIN 10/80. In controlled long-term (48-week) extensions, which included both newly-treated and previously-treated patients, the incidence of consecutive elevations (≥3 X ULN) in serum transaminases was 1.8% overall and 3.6% for patients treated with VYTORIN 10/80. These elevations in transaminases were generally asymptomatic, not associated with cholestasis, and returned to baseline after discontinuation of therapy or with continued treatment.

It is recommended that liver function tests be performed before the initiation of treatment with VYTORIN, and thereafter when clinically indicated. Patients titrated to the 10/80-mg dose should receive an additional test prior to titration, 3 months after titration to the 10/80-mg dose, and periodically thereafter (e.g., semiannually) for the first year of treatment. Patients who develop increased transaminase levels should be monitored with a second liver function evaluation to confirm the finding and be followed thereafter with frequent liver function tests until the abnormality(ies) return to normal. Should an increase in AST or ALT of 3 X ULN or greater persist, withdrawal of therapy with VYTORIN is recommended.

VYTORIN should be used with caution in patients who consume substantial quantities of alcohol and/or have a past history of liver disease. Active liver diseases or unexplained persistent transaminase elevations are contraindications to the use of VYTORIN.

PRECAUTIONS

Information for Patients

Patients should be advised about substances they should not take concomitantly with VYTORIN and be advised to report promptly unexplained muscle pain, tenderness, or weakness (see list below and WARNINGS, *Myopathy/Rhabdomyolysis*). Patients should also be advised to inform other physicians prescribing a new medication that they are taking VYTORIN.

Hepatic Insufficiency

Due to the unknown effects of the increased exposure to ezetimibe in patients with moderate or severe hepatic insufficiency, VYTORIN is not recommended in these patients. (See CLINICAL PHARMACOLOGY, *Pharmacokinetics, Special Populations.*)

***Drug Interactions* (See also CLINICAL PHARMACOLOGY, Drug Interactions)**

VYTORIN

CYP3A4 Interactions

Potent inhibitors of CYP3A4 (below) increase the risk of myopathy by reducing the elimination of the simvastatin component of VYTORIN.

See WARNINGS, *Myopathy/Rhabdomyolysis,* and CLINICAL PHARMACOLOGY, *Pharmacokinetics, Drug Interactions.*

Itraconazole
Ketoconazole
Erythromycin
Clarithromycin
HIV protease inhibitors
Nefazodone
Cyclosporine
Large quantities of grapefruit juice (>1 quart daily)

Interactions with lipid-lowering drugs that can cause myopathy when given alone

See WARNINGS, *Myopathy/Rhabdomyolysis.*

The risk of myopathy is increased by gemfibrozil and to a lesser extent by other fibrates and niacin (nicotinic acid) (≥1 g/day).

Other drug interactions

Amiodarone or Verapamil: The risk of myopathy/rhabdomyolysis is increased by concomitant administration of amiodarone or verapamil (see WARNINGS, *Myopathy/Rhabdomyolysis*).

Cholestyramine: Concomitant cholestyramine administration decreased the mean AUC of total ezetimibe approximately 55%. The incremental LDL-C reduction due to adding VYTORIN to cholestyramine may be reduced by this interaction.

Cyclosporine: Caution should be exercised when initiating VYTORIN in patients treated with cyclosporine due to increased exposure to ezetimibe. This exposure may be greater in patients with severe renal insufficiency. In patients treated with cyclosporine, the potential effects of the increased exposure to ezetimibe from concomitant use should be carefully weighed against the benefits of alterations in lipid levels provided by ezetimibe. In a pharmacokinetic study in post-renal transplant patients with mildly impaired or normal renal function (creatinine clearance of >50 mL/min), concomitant cyclosporine administration increased the mean AUC and C_{max} of total ezetimibe 3.4-fold (range 2.3- to 7.9-fold) and 3.9-fold (range 3.0- to 4.4-fold), respectively. In a separate study, the total ezetimibe exposure increased 12-fold in one renal transplant patient with severe renal insufficiency receiving multiple medications, including cyclosporine. (See CLINICAL PHARMACOLOGY, *Drug Interactions* and WARNINGS, *Myopathy/Rhabdomyolysis.*)

Digoxin: Concomitant administration of a single dose of digoxin in healthy male volunteers receiving simvastatin resulted in a slight elevation (less than 0.3 ng/mL) in plasma digoxin concentrations compared to concomitant administration of placebo and digoxin. Patients taking digoxin should be monitored appropriately when VYTORIN is initiated.

Fibrates: The safety and effectiveness of VYTORIN administered with fibrates have not been established.

Fibrates may increase cholesterol excretion into the bile, leading to cholelithiasis. In a preclinical study in dogs, ezetimibe increased cholesterol in the gallbladder bile (see ANIMAL PHARMACOLOGY). Coadministration of VYTORIN with fibrates is not recommended until use in patients is studied. (See WARNINGS, *Myopathy/Rhabdomyolysis.*)

Warfarin: Simvastatin 20-40 mg/day modestly potentiated the effect of coumarin anticoagulants: the prothrombin time, reported as International Normalized Ratio (INR), increased from a baseline of 1.7 to 1.8 and from 2.6 to 3.4 in a normal volunteer study and in a hypercholesterolemic patient study, respectively. With other statins, clinically evident bleeding and/or increased prothrombin time has been reported in a few patients taking coumarin anticoagulants concomitantly. In such patients, prothrombin time should be determined before starting VYTORIN and frequently enough during early therapy to insure that no significant alteration of prothrombin time occurs. Once a stable prothrombin time has been documented, prothrombin times can be monitored at the intervals usually recommended for patients on coumarin anticoagulants. If the dose of VYTORIN is changed or discontinued, the same procedure should be repeated. Simvastatin therapy has not been associated with bleeding or with changes in prothrombin time in patients not taking anticoagulants.

Ezetimibe

Fenofibrate: In a pharmacokinetic study, concomitant fenofibrate administration increased total ezetimibe concentrations approximately 1.5-fold.

Gemfibrozil: In a pharmacokinetic study, concomitant gemfibrozil administration increased total ezetimibe concentrations approximately 1.7-fold.

Simvastatin

Propranolol: In healthy male volunteers there was a significant decrease in mean C_{max}, but no change in AUC, for simvastatin total and active inhibitors with concomitant administration of single doses of simvastatin and propranolol. The clinical relevance of this finding is unclear. The pharmacokinetics of the enantiomers of propranolol were not affected.

CNS Toxicity

Optic nerve degeneration was seen in clinically normal dogs treated with simvastatin for 14 weeks at 180 mg/kg/day, a dose that produced mean plasma drug levels about 12 times higher than the mean plasma drug level in humans taking 80 mg/day.

A chemically similar drug in this class also produced optic nerve degeneration (Wallerian degeneration of retinogeniculate fibers) in clinically normal dogs in a dose-dependent fashion starting at 60 mg/kg/day, a dose that produced mean plasma drug levels about 30 times higher than the mean plasma drug level in humans taking the highest recommended dose (as measured by total enzyme inhibitory activity). This same drug also produced vestibulocochlear Wallerian-like degeneration and retinal ganglion cell chromatolysis in dogs treated for 14 weeks at 180 mg/kg/day, a dose that resulted in a mean plasma drug level similar to that seen with the 60 mg/kg/day dose.

CNS vascular lesions, characterized by perivascular hemorrhage and edema, mononuclear cell infiltration of perivascular spaces, perivascular fibrin deposits and necrosis of small vessels were seen in dogs treated with simvastatin at a dose of 360 mg/kg/day, a dose that produced mean plasma drug levels that were about 14 times higher than the mean plasma drug levels in humans taking 80 mg/day. Similar CNS vascular lesions have been observed with several other drugs of this class.

There were cataracts in female rats after two years of treatment with 50 and 100 mg/kg/day (22 and 25 times the human AUC at 80 mg/day, respectively) and in dogs after three months at 90 mg/kg/day (19 times) and at two years at 50 mg/kg/day (5 times).

Carcinogenesis, Mutagenesis, Impairment of Fertility

VYTORIN

No animal carcinogenicity or fertility studies have been conducted with the combination of ezetimibe and simvastatin. The combination of ezetimibe with simvastatin did not show evidence of mutagenicity *in vitro* in a microbial mutagenicity (Ames) test with *Salmonella typhimurium* and *Escherichia coli* with or without metabolic activation. No evidence of clastogenicity was observed *in vitro* in a chromosomal aberration assay in human peripheral blood lymphocytes with ezetimibe and simvastatin with or without metabolic activation. There was no evidence of genotoxicity at doses up to 600 mg/kg with the combination of ezetimibe and simvastatin (1:1) in the *in vivo* mouse micronucleus test.

Ezetimibe

A 104-week dietary carcinogenicity study with ezetimibe was conducted in rats at doses up to 1500 mg/kg/day (males) and 500 mg/kg/day (females) (~20 times the human exposure at 10 mg daily based on $AUC_{0\text{-}24hr}$ for total ezetimibe). A 104-week dietary carcinogenicity study with ezetimibe was also conducted in mice at doses up to 500 mg/kg/day (>150 times the human exposure at 10 mg daily based on $AUC_{0\text{-}24hr}$ for total ezetimibe). There were no statistically significant increases in tumor incidences in drug-treated rats or mice.

No evidence of mutagenicity was observed *in vitro* in a microbial mutagenicity (Ames) test with *Salmonella typhimurium* and *Escherichia coli* with or without metabolic activation. No evidence of clastogenicity was observed *in vitro* in a chromosomal aberration assay in human peripheral blood lymphocytes with or without metabolic activation. In addition, there was no evidence of genotoxicity in the *in vivo* mouse micronucleus test.

In oral (gavage) fertility studies of ezetimibe conducted in rats, there was no evidence of reproductive toxicity at doses up to 1000 mg/kg/day in male or female rats (~7 times the human exposure at 10 mg daily based on $AUC_{0\text{-}24hr}$ for total ezetimibe).

Simvastatin

In a 72-week carcinogenicity study, mice were administered daily doses of simvastatin of 25, 100, and 400 mg/kg body weight, which resulted in mean plasma drug levels approximately 1, 4, and 8 times higher than the mean human plasma drug level, respectively (as total inhibitory activity based on AUC) after an 80-mg oral dose. Liver carcinomas were significantly increased in high-dose females and mid- and high-dose males with a maximum incidence of 90% in males. The incidence of adenomas of the liver was significantly increased in mid- and high-dose females. Drug treatment also significantly increased the incidence of lung adenomas in mid- and high-dose males and females. Adenomas of the Harderian gland (a gland of the eye of rodents) were significantly higher in high-dose mice than in controls. No evidence of a tumorigenic effect was observed at 25 mg/kg/day.

In a separate 92-week carcinogenicity study in mice at doses up to 25 mg/kg/day, no evidence of a tumorigenic effect was observed (mean plasma drug levels were 1 times higher than humans given 80 mg simvastatin as measured by AUC).

In a two-year study in rats at 25 mg/kg/day, there was a statistically significant increase in the incidence of thyroid

Continued on next page

Information on Schering products appearing on these pages is effective as of June 2003.

Vytorin—Cont.

follicular adenomas in female rats exposed to approximately 11 times higher levels of simvastatin than in humans given 80 mg simvastatin (as measured by AUC).

A second two-year rat carcinogenicity study with doses of 50 and 100 mg/kg/day produced hepatocellular adenomas and carcinomas (in female rats at both doses and in males at 100 mg/kg/day). Thyroid follicular cell adenomas were increased in males and females at both doses; thyroid follicular cell carcinomas were increased in females at 100 mg/kg/day. The increased incidence of thyroid neoplasms appears to be consistent with findings from other HMG-CoA reductase inhibitors. These treatment levels represented plasma drug levels (AUC) of approximately 7 and 15 times (males) and 22 and 25 times (females) the mean human plasma drug exposure after an 80 milligram daily dose.

No evidence of mutagenicity was observed in a microbial mutagenicity (Ames) test with or without rat or mouse liver metabolic activation. In addition, no evidence of damage to genetic material was noted in an *in vitro* alkaline elution assay using rat hepatocytes, a V-79 mammalian cell forward mutation study, an *in vitro* chromosome aberration study in CHO cells, or an *in vivo* chromosomal aberration assay in mouse bone marrow.

There was decreased fertility in male rats treated with simvastatin for 34 weeks at 25 mg/kg body weight (4 times the maximum human exposure level, based on AUC, in patients receiving 80 mg/day); however, this effect was not observed during a subsequent fertility study in which simvastatin was administered at this same dose level to male rats for 11 weeks (the entire cycle of spermatogenesis including epididymal maturation). No microscopic changes were observed in the testes of rats from either study. At 180 mg/kg/day, (which produces exposure levels 22 times higher than those in humans taking 80 mg/day based on surface area, mg/m^2), seminiferous tubule degeneration (necrosis and loss of spermatogenic epithelium) was observed. In dogs, there was drug-related testicular atrophy, decreased spermatogenesis, spermatocytic degeneration and giant cell formation at 10 mg/kg/day, (approximately 2 times the human exposure, based on AUC, at 80 mg/day). The clinical significance of these findings is unclear.

Pregnancy

Pregnancy Category: X

See CONTRAINDICATIONS.

VYTORIN

As safety in pregnant women has not been established, treatment should be immediately discontinued as soon as pregnancy is recognized. VYTORIN should be administered to women of child-bearing potential only when such patients are highly unlikely to conceive and have been informed of the potential hazards.

Ezetimibe

In oral (gavage) embryo-fetal development studies of ezetimibe conducted in rats and rabbits during organogenesis, there was no evidence of embryolethal effects at the doses tested (250, 500, 1000 mg/kg/day). In rats, increased incidences of common fetal skeletal findings (extra pair of thoracic ribs, unossified cervical vertebral centra, shortened ribs) were observed at 1000 mg/kg/day (~10 times the human exposure at 10 mg daily based on $AUC_{0\text{-}24hr}$ for total ezetimibe). In rabbits treated with ezetimibe, an increased incidence of extra thoracic ribs was observed at 1000 mg/kg/day (150 times the human exposure at 10 mg daily based on $AUC_{0\text{-}24hr}$ for total ezetimibe). Ezetimibe crossed the placenta when pregnant rats and rabbits were given multiple oral doses.

Multiple-dose studies of ezetimibe coadministered with HMG-CoA reductase inhibitors (statins) in rats and rabbits during organogenesis result in higher ezetimibe and statin exposures. Reproductive findings occur at lower doses in coadministration therapy compared to monotherapy.

Simvastatin

Simvastatin was not teratogenic in rats at doses of 25 mg/kg/day or in rabbits at doses up to 10 mg/kg daily. These doses resulted in 3 times (rat) or 3 times (rabbit) the human exposure based on mg/m^2 surface area. However, in studies with another structurally-related HMG-CoA reductase inhibitor, skeletal malformations were observed in rats and mice.

Rare reports of congenital anomalies have been received following intrauterine exposure to HMG-CoA reductase inhibitors. In a review[2] of approximately 100 prospectively followed pregnancies in women exposed to simvastatin or another structurally related HMG-CoA reductase inhibitor, the incidences of congenital anomalies, spontaneous abortions and fetal deaths/stillbirths did not exceed what would be expected in the general population. The number of cases is adequate only to exclude a 3- to 4-fold increase in congenital anomalies over the background incidence. In 89% of the prospectively followed pregnancies, drug treatment was initiated prior to pregnancy and was discontinued at some point in the first trimester when pregnancy was identified.

Labor and Delivery

The effects of VYTORIN on labor and delivery in pregnant women are unknown.

Nursing Mothers

In rat studies, exposure to ezetimibe in nursing pups was up to half of that observed in maternal plasma. It is not known whether ezetimibe or simvastatin are excreted into human breast milk. Because a small amount of another drug in the same class as simvastatin is excreted in human milk and because of the potential for serious adverse reactions in nursing infants, women who are nursing should not take VYTORIN (see CONTRAINDICATIONS).

Pediatric Use

VYTORIN

There are insufficient data for the safe and effective use of VYTORIN in pediatric patients. (See *Ezetimibe* and *Simvastatin* below.)

Ezetimibe

The pharmacokinetics of ezetimibe in adolescents (10 to 18 years) have been shown to be similar to that in adults. Treatment experience with ezetimibe in the pediatric population is limited to 4 patients (9 to 17 years) with homozygous sitosterolemia and 5 patients (11 to 17 years) with HoFH. Treatment with ezetimibe in children (<10 years) is not recommended.

Simvastatin

Safety and effectiveness of simvastatin in patients 10–17 years of age with heterozygous familial hypercholesterolemia have been evaluated in a controlled clinical trial in adolescent boys and in girls who were at least 1 year post-menarche. Patients treated with simvastatin had an adverse experience profile generally similar to that of patients treated with placebo. **Doses greater than 40 mg have not been studied in this population.** In this limited controlled study, there was no detectable effect on growth or sexual maturation in the adolescent boys or girls, or any effect on menstrual cycle length in girls. Adolescent females should be counseled on appropriate contraceptive methods while on therapy with simvastatin (see CONTRAINDICATIONS and PRECAUTIONS, *Pregnancy*). Simvastatin has not been studied in patients younger than 10 years of age, nor in pre-menarchal girls.

Geriatric Use

Of the patients who received VYTORIN in clinical studies, 792 were 65 and older (this included 176 who were 75 and older). The safety of VYTORIN was similar between these patients and younger patients. Greater sensitivity of some older individuals cannot be ruled out. (See CLINICAL PHARMACOLOGY, *Special Populations* and ADVERSE REACTIONS.)

[2] Manson, J.M., Freyssinges, C., Ducrocq, M.B., Stephenson, W.P., Postmarketing Surveillance of Lovastatin and Simvastatin Exposure During Pregnancy, *Reproductive Toxicology*, 10(6):439–446, 1996.

ADVERSE REACTIONS

VYTORIN has been evaluated for safety in more than 3800 patients in clinical trials. VYTORIN was generally well tolerated.

Table 5 summarizes the frequency of clinical adverse experiences reported in ≥2% of patients treated with VYTORIN (n=1236) and at an incidence greater than placebo regardless of causality assessment from three similarly designed, placebo-controlled trials.

[See table 5 below]

Table 5*
Clinical Adverse Events Occurring in ≥2% of Patients Treated with VYTORIN and at an Incidence Greater than Placebo, Regardless of Causality

Body System/Organ Class Adverse Event	Placebo (%) n=311	Ezetimibe 10 mg (%) n=302	Simvastatin** (%) n=1234	VYTORIN** (%) n=1236
Body as a whole – general disorders				
Headache	6.4	6.0	5.9	6.8
Infection and infestations				
Influenza	1.0	1.0	1.9	2.6
Upper respiratory tract infection	2.6	5.0	5.0	3.9
Musculoskeletal and connective tissue disorders				
Myalgia	2.9	2.3	2.6	3.5
Pain in extremity	1.3	3.0	2.0	2.3

*Includes two placebo-controlled combination studies in which the active ingredients equivalent to VYTORIN were coadministered and one placebo-controlled study in which VYTORIN was administered.
**All doses.

Ezetimibe

Other adverse experiences reported with ezetimibe in placebo-controlled studies, regardless of causality assessment: *Body as a whole – general disorders:* fatigue; *Gastrointestinal system disorders:* abdominal pain, diarrhea; *Infection and infestations:* infection viral, pharyngitis, sinusitis; *Musculoskeletal system disorders:* arthralgia, back pain; *Respiratory system disorders:* coughing.

Post-marketing Experience

The following adverse reactions have been reported in post-marketing experience, regardless of causality assessment: Hypersensitivity reactions, including angioedema and rash; pancreatitis; nausea; cholelithiasis; cholecystitis.

Simvastatin

Other adverse experiences reported with simvastatin in placebo-controlled clinical studies, regardless of causality assessment: *Body as a whole – general disorders:* asthenia; *Eye disorders:* cataract; *Gastrointestinal system disorders:* abdominal pain, constipation, diarrhea, dyspepsia, flatulence, nausea; *Skin and subcutaneous tissue disorders:* eczema, pruritus, rash.

The following effects have been reported with other HMG-CoA reductase inhibitors. Not all the effects listed below have necessarily been associated with simvastatin therapy.

Musculoskeletal system disorders: muscle cramps, myalgia, myopathy, rhabdomyolysis, arthralgias.

Nervous system disorders: dysfunction of certain cranial nerves (including alteration of taste, impairment of extra-ocular movement, facial paresis), tremor, dizziness, memory loss, paresthesia, peripheral neuropathy, peripheral nerve palsy, psychic disturbances.

Ear and labyrinth disorders: vertigo.

Psychiatric disorders: anxiety, insomnia, depression, loss of libido.

Hypersensitivity Reactions: An apparent hypersensitivity syndrome has been reported rarely which has included one or more of the following features: anaphylaxis, angioedema, lupus erythematous-like syndrome, polymyalgia rheumatica, dermatomyositis, vasculitis, purpura, thrombocytopenia, leukopenia, hemolytic anemia, positive ANA, ESR increase, eosinophilia, arthritis, arthralgia, urticaria, asthenia, photosensitivity, fever, chills, flushing, malaise, dyspnea, toxic epidermal necrolysis, erythema multiforme, including Stevens-Johnson syndrome.

Gastrointestinal system disorders: pancreatitis, vomiting.

Hepatobiliary disorders: hepatitis, including chronic active hepatitis, cholestatic jaundice, fatty change in liver, and, rarely, cirrhosis, fulminant hepatic necrosis, and hepatoma.

Metabolism and nutrition disorders: anorexia.

Skin and subcutaneous tissue disorders: alopecia, pruritus. A variety of skin changes (e.g., nodules, discoloration, dryness of skin/mucous membranes, changes to hair/nails) have been reported.

Reproductive system and breast disorders: gynecomastia, erectile dysfunction.

Eye disorders: progression of cataracts (lens opacities), ophthalmoplegia.

Laboratory Abnormalities: elevated transaminases, alkaline phosphatase, γ-glutamyl transpeptidase, and bilirubin; thyroid function abnormalities.

Laboratory Tests

Marked persistent increases of serum transaminases have been noted (see WARNINGS, *Liver Enzymes*). About 5% of patients taking simvastatin had elevations of CK levels of 3 or more times the normal value on one or more occasions. This was attributable to the noncardiac fraction of CK. Muscle pain or dysfunction usually was not reported (see WARNINGS, *Myopathy/Rhabdomyolysis*).

Concomitant Lipid-Lowering Therapy

In controlled clinical studies in which simvastatin was administered concomitantly with cholestyramine, no adverse reactions peculiar to this concomitant treatment were observed. The adverse reactions that occurred were limited to those reported previously with simvastatin or cholestyramine.

Adolescent Patients (ages 10–17 years)

In a 48-week controlled study in adolescent boys and girls who were at least 1 year post-menarche, 10–17 years of age with heterozygous familial hypercholesterolemia (n=175), the safety and tolerability profile of the group treated with simvastatin (10–40 mg daily) was generally similar to that of the group treated with placebo, with the most common adverse experiences observed in both groups being upper respiratory infection, headache, abdominal pain, and nausea (see CLINICAL PHARMACOLOGY, *Special Populations* and PRECAUTIONS, *Pediatric Use*).

OVERDOSAGE

VYTORIN

No specific treatment of overdosage with VYTORIN can be recommended. In the event of an overdose, symptomatic and supportive measures should be employed.

Ezetimibe

In clinical studies, administration of ezetimibe, 50 mg/day to 15 healthy subjects for up to 14 days, or 40 mg/day to 18 patients with primary hypercholesterolemia for up to 56 days, was generally well tolerated.

A few cases of overdosage have been reported; most have not been associated with adverse experiences. Reported adverse experiences have not been serious.

Simvastatin
A few cases of overdosage with simvastatin have been reported; the maximum dose taken was 3.6 g. All patients recovered without sequelae.
The dialyzability of simvastatin and its metabolites in man is not known at present.

DOSAGE AND ADMINISTRATION

The patient should be placed on a standard cholesterol-lowering diet before receiving VYTORIN and should continue on this diet during treatment with VYTORIN. The dosage should be individualized according to the baseline LDL-C level, the recommended goal of therapy, and the patient's response. (See NCEP Adult Treatment Panel (ATP) III Guidelines, summarized in Table 4.) VYTORIN should be taken as a single daily dose in the evening, with or without food.
The dosage range is 10/10 mg/day through 10/80 mg/day. The recommended usual starting dose is 10/20 mg/day. Initiation of therapy with 10/10 mg/day may be considered for patients requiring less aggressive LDL-C reductions. Patients who require a larger reduction in LDL-C (greater than 55%) may be started at 10/40 mg/day. After initiation or titration of VYTORIN, lipid levels may be analyzed after 2 or more weeks and dosage adjusted, if needed. See below for dosage recommendations for patients receiving certain concomitant therapies and for those with renal insufficiency.

Patients with Homozygous Familial Hypercholesterolemia
The recommended dosage for patients with homozygous familial hypercholesterolemia is VYTORIN 10/40 mg/day or 10/80 mg/day in the evening. VYTORIN should be used as an adjunct to other lipid-lowering treatments (e.g., LDL apheresis) in these patients or if such treatments are unavailable.

Patients with Hepatic Insufficiency
No dosage adjustment is necessary in patients with mild hepatic insufficiency (see PRECAUTIONS, *Hepatic Insufficiency*).

Patients with Renal Insufficiency
No dosage adjustment is necessary in patients with mild or moderate renal insufficiency. However, for patients with severe renal insufficiency, VYTORIN should not be started unless the patient has already tolerated treatment with simvastatin at a dose of 5 mg or higher. Caution should be exercised when VYTORIN is administered to these patients and they should be closely monitored (see CLINICAL PHARMACOLOGY, *Pharmacokinetics* and WARNINGS, *Myopathy/Rhabdomyolysis*).

Geriatric Patients
No dosage adjustment is necessary in geriatric patients (see CLINICAL PHARMACOLOGY, *Special Populations*).

Coadministration with Bile Acid Sequestrants
Dosing of VYTORIN should occur either ≥2 hours before or ≥4 hours after administration of a bile acid sequestrant (see PRECAUTIONS, *Drug Interactions*).

Patients taking Cyclosporine
Caution should be exercised when initiating VYTORIN in the setting of cyclosporine. In patients taking cyclosporine, VYTORIN should not be started unless the patient has already tolerated treatment with simvastatin at a dose of 5 mg or higher. The dose of VYTORIN should not exceed 10/10 mg/day.

Patients taking Amiodarone or Verapamil
In patients taking amiodarone or verapamil concomitantly with VYTORIN, the dose should not exceed 10/20 mg/day (see WARNINGS, *Myopathy/Rhabdomyolysis* and PRECAUTIONS, *Drug Interactions, Other drug interactions*).

HOW SUPPLIED

No. 3873 — Tablets VYTORIN 10/10 are white to off-white capsule-shaped tablets with code "311" on one side.
They are supplied as follows:
NDC 66582-311-31 bottles of 30
NDC 66582-311-54 bottles of 90
NDC 66582-311-82 bottles of 1000 (If repackaged in blisters, then opaque or light-resistant blisters should be used.)
NDC 66582-311-28 unit dose packages of 100.
No. 3874 — Tablets VYTORIN 10/20 are white to off-white capsule-shaped tablets with code "312" on one side.
They are supplied as follows:
NDC 66582-312-31 bottles of 30
NDC 66582-312-54 bottles of 90
NDC 66582-312-82 bottles of 1000 (If repackaged in blisters, then opaque or light-resistant blisters should be used.)
NDC 66582-312-28 unit dose packages of 100.
No. 3875 — Tablets VYTORIN 10/40 are white to off-white capsule-shaped tablets with code "313" on one side.
They are supplied as follows:
NDC 66582-313-31 bottles of 30
NDC 66582-313-54 bottles of 90
NDC 66582-313-74 bottles of 500 (If repackaged in blisters, then opaque or light-resistant blisters should be used.)
NDC 66582-313-52 unit dose packages of 50.
No. 3876 — Tablets VYTORIN 10/80 are white to off-white capsule-shaped tablets with code "315" on one side.
They are supplied as follows:
NDC 66582-315-31 bottles of 30
NDC 66582-315-54 bottles of 90
NDC 66582-315-74 bottles of 500 (If repackaged in blisters, then opaque or light-resistant blisters should be used.)
NDC 66582-315-52 unit dose packages of 50.
Storage
Store at 20–25°C (68–77°F). [See USP Controlled Room Temperature.] Keep container tightly closed.

9619600
Issued July 2004
Printed in USA
MERCK/Schering-Plough Pharmaceuticals
Manufactured for:
MERCK/Schering-Plough Pharmaceuticals
North Wales, PA 19454, USA
By:
MSD Technology Singapore Pte. Ltd.
Singapore 637766

VYTORIN™ (ezetimibe/simvastatin) Tablets

Patient Information about VYTORIN (VI-tor-in)
Generic name: ezetimibe/simvastatin tablets
Read this information carefully before you start taking VYTORIN. Review this information each time you refill your prescription for VYTORIN as there may be new information. This information does not take the place of talking with your doctor about your medical condition or your treatment. If you have any questions about VYTORIN, ask your doctor. Only your doctor can determine if VYTORIN is right for you.

What is VYTORIN?
VYTORIN contains two cholesterol-lowering medications, ezetimibe and simvastatin, available as a tablet in four strengths:
— VYTORIN 10/10 (ezetimibe 10 mg/simvastatin 10 mg)
— VYTORIN 10/20 (ezetimibe 10 mg/simvastatin 20 mg)
— VYTORIN 10/40 (ezetimibe 10 mg/simvastatin 40 mg)
— VYTORIN 10/80 (ezetimibe 10 mg/simvastatin 80 mg)
VYTORIN is a medicine used to lower levels of total cholesterol, LDL (bad) cholesterol, and fatty substances called triglycerides in the blood. In addition, VYTORIN raises levels of HDL (good) cholesterol. It is used for patients who cannot control their cholesterol levels by diet alone. You should stay on a cholesterol-lowering diet while taking this medicine.
VYTORIN works to reduce your cholesterol in two ways. It reduces the cholesterol absorbed in your digestive tract, as well as the cholesterol your body makes by itself. VYTORIN does not help you lose weight.
For more information about cholesterol, see the section called "What should I know about high cholesterol?"

Who should not take VYTORIN?
Do not take VYTORIN:
- If you are allergic to ezetimibe or simvastatin, the active ingredients in VYTORIN, or to the inactive ingredients. For a list of inactive ingredients, see the "Inactive ingredients" section at the end of this information sheet.
- If you have active liver disease or repeated blood tests indicating possible liver problems.
- If you are pregnant, or think you may be pregnant, or planning to become pregnant or breast-feeding.

VYTORIN is not recommended for use in children under 10 years of age.

What should I tell my doctor before and while taking VYTORIN?
Tell your doctor right away if you experience unexplained muscle pain, tenderness, or weakness. This is because on rare occasions, muscle problems can be serious, including muscle breakdown resulting in kidney damage.
The risk of muscle breakdown is greater at higher doses of VYTORIN.
The risk of muscle breakdown is greater in patients with kidney problems.
Taking VYTORIN with certain substances can increase the risk of muscle problems. It is particularly important to tell your doctor if you are taking any of the following:
- cyclosporine
- antifungal agents (such as itraconazole or ketoconazole)
- fibric acid derivatives (such as gemfibrozil, bezafibrate, or fenofibrate)
- the antibiotics erythromycin and clarithromycin
- HIV protease inhibitors (such as indinavir, nelfinavir, ritonavir, and saquinavir)
- the antidepressant nefazodone
- amiodarone (a drug used to treat an irregular heartbeat)
- verapamil (a drug used to treat high blood pressure, chest pain associated with heart disease, or other heart conditions)
- large doses (≥1 g/day) of niacin or nicotinic acid
- large quantities of grapefruit juice (>1 quart daily)

It is also important to tell your doctor if you are taking coumarin anticoagulants (drugs that prevent blood clots, such as warfarin).
Tell your doctor about any prescription and nonprescription medicines you are taking or plan to take, including natural or herbal remedies.
Tell your doctor about all your medical conditions including allergies.
Tell your doctor if you:
- drink substantial quantities of alcohol or ever had liver problems. VYTORIN may not be right for you.
- are pregnant or plan to become pregnant. Do not use VYTORIN if you are pregnant, trying to become pregnant or suspect that you are pregnant. If you become pregnant while taking VYTORIN, stop taking it and contact your doctor immediately.
- are breast-feeding. Do not use VYTORIN if you are breast-feeding.

Tell other doctors prescribing a new medication that you are taking VYTORIN.

How should I take VYTORIN?
Your doctor has prescribed your dose of VYTORIN. The available doses of VYTORIN are 10/10, 10/20, 10/40, and 10/80. The usual daily starting dose is VYTORIN 10/20.
- Take VYTORIN once a day, in the evening, with or without food.
- Try to take VYTORIN as prescribed. If you miss a dose, do not take an extra dose. Just resume your usual schedule.
- Continue to follow a cholesterol-lowering diet while taking VYTORIN. Ask your doctor if you need diet information.
- Keep taking VYTORIN unless your doctor tells you to stop. If you stop taking VYTORIN, your cholesterol may rise again.

What should I do in case of an overdose?
Contact your doctor immediately.

What are the possible side effects of VYTORIN?
See your doctor regularly to check your cholesterol level and to check for side effects. Your doctor may do blood tests to check your liver before you start taking VYTORIN and during treatment.
In clinical studies patients reported the following common side effects while taking VYTORIN: headache and muscle pain (see What should I tell my doctor before and while taking VYTORIN?).
The following side effects have been reported in general use with either ezetimibe or simvastatin tablets (tablets that contain the active ingredients of VYTORIN):
- allergic reactions including swelling of the face, lips, tongue, and/or throat that may cause difficulty in breathing or swallowing (which may require treatment right away), and rash; inflammation of the pancreas; nausea; gallstones; inflammation of the gallbladder.

Tell your doctor if you are having these or any other medical problems while on VYTORIN. This is not a complete list of side effects. For a complete list, ask your doctor or pharmacist.

What should I know about high cholesterol?
Cholesterol is a type of fat found in your blood. Cholesterol comes from two sources. It is produced by your body and it comes from the food you eat. Your total cholesterol is made up of both LDL and HDL cholesterol.
LDL cholesterol is called "bad" cholesterol because it can build up in the wall of your arteries and form plaque. Over time, plaque build-up can cause a narrowing of the arteries. This narrowing can slow or block blood flow to your heart, brain, and other organs. High LDL cholesterol is a major cause of heart disease and stroke.
HDL cholesterol is called "good" cholesterol because it keeps the bad cholesterol from building up in the arteries.
Triglycerides also are fats found in your body.

General Information about VYTORIN
Medicines are sometimes prescribed for conditions that are not mentioned in patient information leaflets. Do not use VYTORIN for a condition for which it was not prescribed. Do not give VYTORIN to other people, even if they have the same condition you have. It may harm them.
This summarizes the most important information about VYTORIN. If you would like more information, talk with your doctor. You can ask your pharmacist or doctor for information about VYTORIN that is written for health professionals. For additional information, visit the following web site: vytorin.com.

Inactive ingredients:
Butylated hydroxyanisole NF, citric acid monohydrate USP, croscarmellose sodium NF, hydroxypropyl methylcellulose USP, lactose monohydrate NF, magnesium stearate NF, microcrystalline cellulose NF, and propyl gallate NF.

9621000 Issued July 2004
Manufactured for:
Merck/Schering-Plough Pharmaceuticals
North Wales, PA 19454, USA
By:
MSD Technology Singapore Pte. Ltd.
Singapore 637766

ZETIA® ℞
[zĕt' ē ă]
(ezetimibe)
TABLETS

DESCRIPTION

ZETIA (ezetimibe) is in a class of lipid-lowering compounds that selectively inhibits the intestinal absorption of cholesterol and related phytosterols. The chemical name of ezetimibe is 1-(4-fluorophenyl)-3(R)-[3-(4-fluorophenyl)-3(S)-hydroxypropyl]-4(S)-(4-hydroxyphenyl)-2-azetidinone.

Continued on next page

Information on Schering products appearing on these pages is effective as of June 2003.

Zetia—Cont.

The empirical formula is $C_{24}H_{21}F_2NO_3$. Its molecular weight is 409.4 and its structural formula is:

Ezetimibe is a white, crystalline powder that is freely to very soluble in ethanol, methanol, and acetone and practically insoluble in water. Ezetimibe has a melting point of about 163°C and is stable at ambient temperature. ZETIA is available as a tablet for oral administration containing 10 mg of ezetimibe and the following inactive ingredients: croscarmellose sodium NF, lactose monohydrate NF, magnesium stearate NF, microcrystalline cellulose NF, povidone USP, and sodium lauryl sulfate NF.

CLINICAL PHARMACOLOGY

Background

Clinical studies have demonstrated that elevated levels of total cholesterol (total-C), low density lipoprotein cholesterol (LDL-C) and apolipoprotein B (Apo B), the major protein constituent of LDL, promote human atherosclerosis. In addition, decreased levels of high density lipoprotein cholesterol (HDL-C) are associated with the development of atherosclerosis. Epidemiologic studies have established that cardiovascular morbidity and mortality vary directly with the level of total-C and LDL-C and inversely with the level of HDL-C. Like LDL, cholesterol-enriched triglyceride-rich lipoproteins, including very-low-density lipoproteins (VLDL), intermediate-density lipoproteins (IDL), and remnants, can also promote atherosclerosis. The independent effect of raising HDL-C or lowering triglycerides (TG) on the risk of coronary and cardiovascular morbidity and mortality has not been determined.

ZETIA reduces total-C, LDL-C, Apo B, and TG, and increases HDL-C in patients with hypercholesterolemia. Administration of ZETIA with an HMG-CoA reductase inhibitor is effective in improving serum total-C, LDL-C, Apo B, TG, and HDL-C beyond either treatment alone. The effects of ezetimibe given either alone or in addition to an HMG-CoA reductase inhibitor on cardiovascular morbidity and mortality have not been established.

Mode of Action

Ezetimibe reduces blood cholesterol by inhibiting the absorption of cholesterol by the small intestine. In a 2-week clinical study in 18 hypercholesterolemic patients, ZETIA inhibited intestinal cholesterol absorption by 54%, compared with placebo. ZETIA had no clinically meaningful effect on the plasma concentrations of the fat-soluble vitamins A, D, and E (in a study of 113 patients), and did not impair adrenocortical steroid hormone production (in a study of 118 patients).

The cholesterol content of the liver is derived predominantly from three sources. The liver can synthesize cholesterol, take up cholesterol from the blood from circulating lipoproteins, or take up cholesterol absorbed by the small intestine. Intestinal cholesterol is derived primarily from cholesterol secreted in the bile and from dietary cholesterol.

Ezetimibe has a mechanism of action that differs from those of other classes of cholesterol-reducing compounds (HMG-CoA reductase inhibitors, bile acid sequestrants [resins], fibric acid derivatives, and plant stanols).

Ezetimibe does not inhibit cholesterol synthesis in the liver, or increase bile acid excretion. Instead, ezetimibe localizes and appears to act at the brush border of the small intestine and inhibits the absorption of cholesterol, leading to a decrease in the delivery of intestinal cholesterol to the liver. This causes a reduction of hepatic cholesterol stores and an increase in clearance of cholesterol from the blood; this distinct mechanism is complementary to that of HMG-CoA reductase inhibitors (see CLINICAL STUDIES).

Pharmacokinetics

Absorption

After oral administration, ezetimibe is absorbed and extensively conjugated to a pharmacologically active phenolic glucuronide (ezetimibe-glucuronide). After a single 10-mg dose of ZETIA to fasted adults, mean ezetimibe peak plasma concentrations (C_{max}) of 3.4 to 5.5 ng/mL were attained within 4 to 12 hours (T_{max}). Ezetimibe-glucuronide mean C_{max} values of 45 to 71 ng/mL were achieved between 1 and 2 hours (T_{max}). There was no substantial deviation from dose proportionality between 5 and 20 mg. The absolute bioavailability of ezetimibe cannot be determined, as the compound is virtually insoluble in aqueous media suitable for injection. Ezetimibe has variable bioavailability; the coefficient of variation, based on inter-subject variability, was 35 to 60% for AUC values.

Effect of Food on Oral Absorption

Concomitant food administration (high fat or non-fat meals) had no effect on the extent of absorption of ezetimibe when administered as ZETIA 10-mg tablets. The C_{max} value of ezetimibe was increased by 38% with consumption of high fat meals. ZETIA can be administered with or without food.

Distribution

Ezetimibe and ezetimibe-glucuronide are highly bound (>90%) to human plasma proteins.

Table 1
Response to ZETIA in Patients with Primary Hypercholesterolemia (Mean[a] % Change from Untreated Baseline[b])

Treatment group		N	Total-C	LDL-C	Apo B	TG[a]	HDL-C
Study 1[c]	Placebo	205	+1	+1	-1	-1	-1
	Ezetimibe	622	-12	-18	-15	-7	+1
Study 2[c]	Placebo	226	+1	+1	-1	+2	-2
	Ezetimibe	666	-12	-18	-16	-9	+1
Pooled Data[c] (Studies 1 & 2)	Placebo	431	0	+1	-2	0	-2
	Ezetimibe	1288	-13	-18	-16	-8	+1

[a] For triglycerides, median % change from baseline
[b] Baseline - on no lipid-lowering drug
[c] ZETIA significantly reduced total-C, LDL-C, Apo B, and TG, and increased HDL-C compared to placebo.

Table 2
Response to Addition of ZETIA to On-going HMG-CoA Reductase Inhibitor Therapy[a] in Patients with Hypercholesterolemia (Mean[b] % Change from Treated Baseline[c])

Treatment (Daily Dose)	N	Total-C	LDL-C	Apo B	TG[b]	HDL-C
On-going HMG-CoA reductase inhibitor +Placebo[d]	390	-2	-4	-3	-3	+1
On-going HMG-CoA reductase inhibitor +ZETIA[d]	379	-17	-25	-19	-14	+3

[a] Patients receiving each HMG-CoA reductase inhibitor: 40% atorvastatin, 31% simvastatin, 29% others (pravastatin, fluvastatin, cerivastatin, lovastatin)
[b] For triglycerides, median % change from baseline
[c] Baseline - on an HMG-CoA reductase inhibitor alone.
[d] ZETIA + HMG-CoA reductase inhibitor significantly reduced total-C, LDL-C, Apo B, and TG, and increased HDL-C compared to HMG-CoA reductase inhibitor alone.

Metabolism and Excretion

Ezetimibe is primarily metabolized in the small intestine and liver via glucuronide conjugation (a phase II reaction) with subsequent biliary and renal excretion. Minimal oxidative metabolism (a phase I reaction) has been observed in all species evaluated.

In humans, ezetimibe is rapidly metabolized to ezetimibe-glucuronide. Ezetimibe and ezetimibe-glucuronide are the major drug-derived compounds detected in plasma, constituting approximately 10 to 20% and 80 to 90% of the total drug in plasma, respectively. Both ezetimibe and ezetimibe-glucuronide are slowly eliminated from plasma with a half-life of approximately 22 hours for both ezetimibe and ezetimibe-glucuronide. Plasma concentration-time profiles exhibit multiple peaks, suggesting enterohepatic recycling.

Following oral administration of ^{14}C-ezetimibe (20 mg) to human subjects, total ezetimibe (ezetimibe + ezetimibe-glucuronide) accounted for approximately 93% of the total radioactivity in plasma. After 48 hours, there were no detectable levels of radioactivity in the plasma.

Approximately 78% and 11% of the administered radioactivity were recovered in the feces and urine, respectively, over a 10-day collection period. Ezetimibe was the major component in feces and accounted for 69% of the administered dose, while ezetimibe-glucuronide was the major component in urine and accounted for 9% of the administered dose.

Special Populations

Geriatric Patients

In a multiple dose study with ezetimibe given 10 mg once daily for 10 days, plasma concentrations for total ezetimibe were about 2-fold higher in older (≥65 years) healthy subjects compared to younger subjects.

Pediatric Patients

In a multiple dose study with ezetimibe given 10 mg once daily for 7 days, the absorption and metabolism of ezetimibe were similar in adolescents (10 to 18 years) and adults. Based on total ezetimibe, there are no pharmacokinetic differences between adolescents and adults. Pharmacokinetic data in the pediatric population <10 years of age are not available.

Gender

In a multiple dose study with ezetimibe given 10 mg once daily for 10 days, plasma concentrations for total ezetimibe were slightly higher (<20%) in women than in men.

Race

Based on a meta-analysis of multiple-dose pharmacokinetic studies, there were no pharmacokinetic differences between Blacks and Caucasians. There were too few patients in other racial or ethnic groups to permit further pharmacokinetic comparisons.

Hepatic Insufficiency

After a single 10-mg dose of ezetimibe, the mean area under the curve (AUC) for total ezetimibe was increased approximately 1.7-fold in patients with mild hepatic insufficiency (Child-Pugh score 5 to 6), compared to healthy subjects. The mean AUC values for total ezetimibe and ezetimibe were increased approximately 3- to 4-fold and 5- to 6-fold, respectively, in patients with moderate (Child-Pugh score 7 to 9) or severe hepatic impairment (Child-Pugh score 10 to 15). In a 14-day, multiple-dose study (10 mg daily) in patients with moderate hepatic insufficiency, the mean AUC values for total ezetimibe and ezetimibe were increased approximately 4-fold on Day 1 and Day 14 compared to healthy subjects. Due to the unknown effects of the increased exposure to ezetimibe in patients with moderate or severe hepatic insufficiency, ZETIA is not recommended in these patients (see CONTRAINDICATIONS and PRECAUTIONS, *Hepatic Insufficiency*).

Renal Insufficiency

After a single 10-mg dose of ezetimibe in patients with severe renal disease (n=8; mean CrCl ≤30 mL/min/1.73 m^2), the mean AUC values for total ezetimibe, ezetimibe-glucuronide, and ezetimibe were increased approximately 1.5-fold, compared to healthy subjects (n=9).

Drug Interactions (See also PRECAUTIONS, *Drug Interactions*)

ZETIA had no significant effect on a series of probe drugs (caffeine, dextromethorphan, tolbutamide, and IV midazolam) known to be metabolized by cytochrome P450 (1A2, 2D6, 2C8/9 and 3A4) in a "cocktail" study of twelve healthy adult males. This indicates that ezetimibe is neither an inhibitor nor an inducer of these cytochrome P450 isozymes, and it is unlikely that ezetimibe will affect the metabolism of drugs that are metabolized by these enzymes.

Warfarin: Concomitant administration of ezetimibe (10 mg once daily) had no significant effect on bioavailability of warfarin and prothrombin time in a study of twelve healthy adult males.

Digoxin: Concomitant administration of ezetimibe (10 mg once daily) had no significant effect on the bioavailability of digoxin and the ECG parameters (HR, PR, QT, and QTc intervals) in a study of twelve healthy adult males.

Gemfibrozil: In a study of twelve healthy adult males, concomitant administration of gemfibrozil (600 mg twice daily) significantly increased the oral bioavailability of total ezetimibe by a factor of 1.7. Ezetimibe (10 mg once daily) did not significantly affect the bioavailability of gemfibrozil.

Oral Contraceptives: Co-administration of ezetimibe (10 mg once daily) with oral contraceptives had no significant effect on the bioavailability of ethinyl estradiol or levonorgestrel in a study of eighteen healthy adult females.

Cimetidine: Multiple doses of cimetidine (400 mg twice daily) had no significant effect on the oral bioavailability of ezetimibe and total ezetimibe in a study of twelve healthy adults.

Antacids: In a study of twelve healthy adults, a single dose of antacid (Supralox™ 20 mL) administration had no significant effect on the oral bioavailability of total ezetimibe, ezetimibe-glucuronide, or ezetimibe based on AUC values. The C_{max} value of total ezetimibe was decreased by 30%.

Glipizide: In a study of twelve healthy adult males, steady-state levels of ezetimibe (10 mg once daily) had no significant effect on the pharmacokinetics and pharmacodynamics of glipizide. A single dose of glipizide (10 mg) had no significant effect on the exposure to total ezetimibe or ezetimibe.

HMG-CoA Reductase Inhibitors: In studies of healthy hypercholesterolemic (LDL-C ≥130 mg/dL) adult subjects, concomitant administration of ezetimibe (10 mg once daily) had no significant effect on the bioavailability of either lovastatin, simvastatin, pravastatin, atorvastatin, or fluvastatin. No significant effect on the bioavailability of total ezetimibe and ezetimibe was demonstrated by either lovastatin (20 mg once daily), pravastatin (20 mg once daily), atorvastatin (10 mg once daily), or fluvastatin (20 mg once daily).

Fenofibrate: In a study of thirty-two healthy hypercholesterolemic (LDL-C ≥130 mg/dL) adult subjects, concomitant fenofibrate (200 mg once daily) administration increased the mean C_{max} and AUC values of total ezetimibe approximately 64% and 48%, respectively. Pharmacokinetics of fenofibrate were not significantly affected by ezetimibe (10 mg once daily).

Cholestyramine: In a study of forty healthy hypercholesterolemic (LDL-C ≥130 mg/dL) adult subjects, concomitant cholestyramine (4 g twice daily) administration decreased the mean AUC values of total ezetimibe and ezetimibe approximately 55% and 80%, respectively.

Cyclosporine: In a study of eight post-renal transplant patients with mildly impaired or normal renal function (creatinine clearance of >50 mL/min), stable doses of cyclosporine (75 to 150 mg twice daily) increased the mean AUC and C_{max} values of total ezetimibe 3.4-fold (range 2.3- to 7.9-fold) and 3.9-fold (range 3.0- to 4.4-fold), respectively, compared to a historical healthy control population (n=17). In a different study, a renal transplant patient with severe renal insufficiency (creatinine clearance of 13.2 mL/min/1.73 m^2) who was receiving multiple medications, including cyclosporine, demonstrated a 12-fold greater exposure to total ezetimibe compared to healthy subjects.

ANIMAL PHARMACOLOGY

The hypocholesterolemic effect of ezetimibe was evaluated in cholesterol-fed Rhesus monkeys, dogs, rats, and mouse models of human cholesterol metabolism. Ezetimibe was found to have an ED_{50} value of 0.5 µg/kg/day for inhibiting the rise in plasma cholesterol levels in monkeys. The ED_{50} values in dogs, rats, and mice were 7, 30, and 700 µg/kg/day, respectively. These results are consistent with ZETIA being a potent cholesterol absorption inhibitor.

In a rat model, where the glucuronide metabolite of ezetimibe (SCH 60663) was administered intraduodenally, the metabolite was as potent as the parent compound (SCH 58235) in inhibiting the absorption of cholesterol, suggesting that the glucuronide metabolite had activity similar to the parent drug.

In 1-month studies in dogs given ezetimibe (0.03-300 mg/kg/day), the concentration of cholesterol in gallbladder bile increased ~2- to 4-fold. However, a dose of 300 mg/kg/day administered to dogs for one year did not result in gallstone formation or any other adverse hepatobiliary effects. In a 14-day study in mice given ezetimibe (0.3-5 mg/kg/day) and fed a low-fat or cholesterol-rich diet, the concentration of cholesterol in gallbladder bile was either unaffected or reduced to normal levels, respectively.

A series of acute preclinical studies was performed to determine the selectivity of ZETIA for inhibiting cholesterol absorption. Ezetimibe inhibited the absorption of ^{14}C-cholesterol with no effect on the absorption of triglycerides, fatty acids, bile acids, progesterone, ethyl estradiol, or the fat-soluble vitamins A and D.

In 4- to 12-week toxicity studies in mice, ezetimibe did not induce cytochrome P450 drug metabolizing enzymes. In toxicity studies, a pharmacokinetic interaction of ezetimibe with HMG-CoA reductase inhibitors (parents or their active hydroxy acid metabolites) was seen in rats, dogs, and rabbits.

CLINICAL STUDIES

Primary Hypercholesterolemia

ZETIA reduces total-C, LDL-C, Apo B, and TG, and increases HDL-C in patients with hypercholesterolemia. Maximal to near maximal response is generally achieved within 2 weeks and maintained during chronic therapy.

ZETIA is effective in patients with hypercholesterolemia, in men and women, in younger and older patients, alone or administered with an HMG-CoA reductase inhibitor. Experience in pediatric and adolescent patients (ages 9 to 17) has been limited to patients with homozygous familial hypercholesterolemia (HoFH) or sitosterolemia.

Experience in non-Caucasians is limited and does not permit a precise estimate of the magnitude of the effects of ZETIA.

Monotherapy

In two, multicenter, double-blind, placebo-controlled, 12-week studies in 1719 patients with primary hypercholesterolemia, ZETIA significantly lowered total-C, LDL-C, Apo B, and TG, and increased HDL-C compared to placebo (see Table 1). Reduction in LDL-C was consistent across age, sex, and baseline LDL-C.

[See table 1 at top of previous page]

Combination with HMG-CoA Reductase Inhibitors

ZETIA Added to On-going HMG-CoA Reductase Inhibitor Therapy

In a multicenter, double-blind, placebo-controlled, 8-week study, 769 patients with primary hypercholesterolemia, known coronary heart disease or multiple cardiovascular risk factors who were already receiving HMG-CoA reductase inhibitor monotherapy, but who had not met their NCEP ATP II target LDL-C goal were randomized to receive either ZETIA or placebo in addition to their on-going HMG-CoA reductase inhibitor therapy.

ZETIA, added to on-going HMG-CoA reductase inhibitor therapy, significantly lowered total-C, LDL-C, Apo B, and TG, and increased HDL-C compared with an HMG-CoA reductase inhibitor administered alone (see Table 2). LDL-C reductions induced by ZETIA were generally consistent across all HMG-CoA reductase inhibitors.

[See table 2 at top of previous page]

ZETIA Initiated Concurrently with an HMG-CoA Reductase Inhibitor

In four, multicenter, double-blind, placebo-controlled, 12-week trials, in 2382 hypercholesterolemic patients, ZETIA or placebo was administered alone or with various doses of atorvastatin, simvastatin, pravastatin, or lovastatin.

When all patients receiving ZETIA with an HMG-CoA reductase inhibitor were compared to all those receiving the corresponding HMG-CoA reductase inhibitor alone, ZETIA significantly lowered total-C, LDL-C, Apo B, and TG, and, with the exception of pravastatin, increased HDL-C compared to the HMG-CoA reductase inhibitor administered alone. LDL-C reductions induced by ZETIA were generally consistent across all HMG-CoA reductase inhibitors. (See footnote c, Tables 3 to 6.)

[See table 3 above]

[See table 4 above]

[See table 5 at top of next page]

[See table 6 on next page]

Table 3
Response to ZETIA and Atorvastatin Initiated Concurrently in Patients with Primary Hypercholesterolemia (Mean[a] % Change from Untreated Baseline[b])

Treatment (Daily Dose)	N	Total-C	LDL-C	Apo B	TG[a]	HDL-C
Placebo	60	+4	+4	+3	-6	+4
ZETIA	65	-14	-20	-15	-5	+4
Atorvastatin 10 mg	60	-26	-37	-28	-21	+6
ZETIA + Atorvastatin 10 mg	65	-38	-53	-43	-31	+9
Atorvastatin 20 mg	60	-30	-42	-34	-23	+4
ZETIA + Atorvastatin 20 mg	62	-39	-54	-44	-30	+9
Atorvastatin 40 mg	66	-32	-45	-37	-24	+4
ZETIA + Atorvastatin 40 mg	65	-42	-56	-45	-34	+5
Atorvastatin 80 mg	62	-40	-54	-46	-31	+3
ZETIA + Atorvastatin 80 mg	63	-46	-61	-50	-40	+7
Pooled data (All Atorvastatin Doses)[c]	248	-32	-44	-36	-24	+4
Pooled data (All ZETIA + Atorvastatin Doses)[c]	255	-41	-56	-45	-33	+7

[a] For triglycerides, median % change from baseline
[b] Baseline - on no lipid-lowering drug
[c] ZETIA + all doses of atorvastatin pooled (10-80 mg) significantly reduced total-C, LDL-C, Apo B, and TG, and increased HDL-C compared to all doses of atorvastatin pooled (10-80 mg).

Table 4
Response to ZETIA and Simvastatin Initiated Concurrently in Patients with Primary Hypercholesterolemia (Mean[a] % Change from Untreated Baseline[b])

Treatment (Daily Dose)	N	Total-C	LDL-C	Apo B	TG[a]	HDL-C
Placebo	70	-1	-1	0	+2	+1
ZETIA	61	-13	-19	-14	-11	+5
Simvastatin 10 mg	70	-18	-27	-21	-14	+8
ZETIA + Simvastatin 10 mg	67	-32	-46	-35	-26	+9
Simvastatin 20 mg	61	-26	-36	-29	-18	+6
ZETIA + Simvastatin 20 mg	69	-33	-46	-36	-25	+9
Simvastatin 40 mg	65	-27	-38	-32	-24	+6
ZETIA + Simvastatin 40 mg	73	-40	-56	-45	-32	+11
Simvastatin 80 mg	67	-32	-45	-37	-23	+8
ZETIA + Simvastatin 80 mg	65	-41	-58	-47	-31	+8
Pooled data (All Simvastatin Doses)[c]	263	-26	-36	-30	-20	+7
Pooled data (All ZETIA + Simvastatin Doses)[c]	274	-37	-51	-41	-29	+9

[a] For triglycerides, median % change from baseline
[b] Baseline - on no lipid-lowering drug
[c] ZETIA + all doses of simvastatin pooled (10-80 mg) significantly reduced total-C, LDL-C, Apo B, and TG, and increased HDL-C compared to all doses of simvastatin pooled (10-80 mg).

Continued on next page

Information on Schering products appearing on these pages is effective as of June 2003.

Zetia—Cont.

Homozygous Familial Hypercholesterolemia (HoFH)
A study was conducted to assess the efficacy of ZETIA in the treatment of HoFH. This double-blind, randomized, 12-week study enrolled 50 patients with a clinical and/or genotypic diagnosis of HoFH, with or without concomitant LDL apheresis, already receiving atorvastatin or simvastatin (40 mg). Patients were randomized to one of three treatment groups, atorvastatin or simvastatin (80 mg), ZETIA administered with atorvastatin or simvastatin (40 mg), or ZETIA administered with atorvastatin or simvastatin (80 mg). Due to decreased bioavailability of ezetimibe in patients concomitantly receiving cholestyramine (see PRECAUTIONS), ezetimibe was dosed at least 4 hours before or after administration of resins. Mean baseline LDL-C was 341 mg/dL in those patients randomized to atorvastatin 80 mg or simvastatin 80 mg alone and 316 mg/dL in the group randomized to ZETIA plus atorvastatin 40 or 80 mg or simvastatin 40 or 80 mg. ZETIA, administered with atorvastatin or simvastatin (40 and 80 mg statin groups, pooled), significantly reduced LDL-C (21%) compared with increasing the dose of simvastatin or atorvastatin monotherapy from 40 to 80 mg (7%). In those treated with ZETIA plus 80 mg atorvastatin or with ZETIA plus 80 mg simvastatin, LDL-C was reduced by 27%.
Homozygous Sitosterolemia (Phytosterolemia)
A study was conducted to assess the efficacy of ZETIA in the treatment of homozygous sitosterolemia. In this multicenter, double-blind, placebo-controlled, 8-week trial, 37 patients with homozygous sitosterolemia with elevated plasma sitosterol levels (>5 mg/dL) on their current therapeutic regimen (diet, bile-acid-binding resins, HMG-CoA reductase inhibitors, ileal bypass surgery and/or LDL apheresis), were randomized to receive ZETIA (n=30) or placebo (n=7). Due to decreased bioavailability of ezetimibe in patients concomitantly receiving cholestyramine (see PRECAUTIONS), ezetimibe was dosed at least 2 hours before or 4 hours after resins were administered. Excluding the one subject receiving LDL apheresis, ZETIA significantly lowered plasma sitosterol and campesterol, by 21% and 24% from baseline, respectively. In contrast, patients who received placebo had increases in sitosterol and campesterol of 4% and 3% from baseline, respectively. For patients treated with ZETIA, mean plasma levels of plant sterols were reduced progressively over the course of the study. The effects of reducing plasma sitosterol and campesterol on reducing the risks of cardiovascular morbidity and mortality have not been established.
Reductions in sitosterol and campesterol were consistent between patients taking ZETIA concomitantly with bile acid sequestrants (n=8) and patients not on concomitant bile acid sequestrant therapy (n=21).

INDICATIONS AND USAGE

Primary Hypercholesterolemia
Monotherapy
ZETIA, administered alone, is indicated as adjunctive therapy to diet for the reduction of elevated total-C, LDL-C, and Apo B in patients with primary (heterozygous familial and non-familial) hypercholesterolemia.
Combination therapy with HMG-CoA reductase inhibitors
ZETIA, administered in combination with an HMG-CoA reductase inhibitor, is indicated as adjunctive therapy to diet for the reduction of elevated total-C, LDL-C, and Apo B in patients with primary (heterozygous familial and non-familial) hypercholesterolemia.
Homozygous Familial Hypercholesterolemia (HoFH)
The combination of ZETIA and atorvastatin or simvastatin, is indicated for the reduction of elevated total-C and LDL-C levels in patients with HoFH, as an adjunct to other lipid-lowering treatments (e.g., LDL apheresis) or if such treatments are unavailable.
Homozygous Sitosterolemia
ZETIA is indicated as adjunctive therapy to diet for the reduction of elevated sitosterol and campesterol levels in patients with homozygous familial sitosterolemia.
Therapy with lipid-altering agents should be a component of multiple risk-factor intervention in individuals at increased risk for atherosclerotic vascular disease due to hypercholesterolemia. Lipid-altering agents should be used in addition to an appropriate diet (including restriction of saturated fat and cholesterol) and when the response to diet and other non-pharmacological measures has been inadequate. (See NCEP Adult Treatment Panel (ATP) III Guidelines, summarized in Table 7.)
[See table 7 at bottom of next page]
Prior to initiating therapy with ZETIA, secondary causes for dyslipidemia (i.e., diabetes, hypothyroidism, obstructive liver disease, chronic renal failure, and drugs that increase LDL-C and decrease HDL-C [progestins, anabolic steroids, and corticosteroids]), should be excluded or, if appropriate, treated. A lipid profile should be performed to measure total-C, LDL-C, HDL-C and TG. For TG levels >400 mg/dL (>4.5 mmol/L), LDL-C concentrations should be determined by ultracentrifugation.
At the time of hospitalization for an acute coronary event, lipid measures should be taken on admission or within 24 hours. These values can guide the physician on initiation of LDL-lowering therapy before or at discharge.

Table 5
Response to ZETIA and Pravastatin Initiated Concurrently in Patients with Primary Hypercholesterolemia (Mean[a] % Change from Untreated Baseline[b])

Treatment (Daily Dose)	N	Total-C	LDL-C	Apo B	TG[a]	HDL-C
Placebo	65	0	-1	-2	-1	+2
ZETIA	64	-13	-20	-15	-5	+4
Pravastatin 10 mg	66	-15	-21	-16	-14	+6
ZETIA + Pravastatin 10 mg	71	-24	-34	-27	-23	+8
Pravastatin 20 mg	69	-15	-23	-18	-8	+8
ZETIA + Pravastatin 20 mg	66	-27	-40	-31	-21	+8
Pravastatin 40 mg	70	-22	-31	-26	-19	+6
ZETIA + Pravastatin 40 mg	67	-30	-42	-32	-21	+8
Pooled data (All Pravastatin Doses)[c]	205	-17	-25	-20	-14	+7
Pooled data (All ZETIA + Pravastatin Doses)[c]	204	-27	-39	-30	-21	+8

[a] For triglycerides, median % change from baseline
[b] Baseline - on no lipid-lowering drug
[c] ZETIA + all doses of pravastatin pooled (10-40 mg) significantly reduced total-C, LDL-C, Apo B, and TG compared to all doses of pravastatin pooled (10-40 mg).

Table 6
Response to ZETIA and Lovastatin Initiated Concurrently in Patients with Primary Hypercholesterolemia (Mean[a] % Change from Untreated Baseline[b])

Treatment (Daily Dose)	N	Total-C	LDL-C	Apo B	TG[a]	HDL-C
Placebo	64	+1	0	+1	+6	0
ZETIA	72	-13	-19	-14	-5	+3
Lovastatin 10 mg	73	-15	-20	-17	-11	+5
ZETIA + Lovastatin 10 mg	65	-24	-34	-27	-19	+8
Lovastatin 20 mg	74	-19	-26	-21	-12	+3
ZETIA + Lovastatin 20 mg	62	-29	-41	-34	-27	+9
Lovastatin 40 mg	73	-21	-30	-25	-15	+5
ZETIA + Lovastatin 40 mg	65	-33	-46	-38	-27	+9
Pooled data (All Lovastatin Doses)[c]	220	-18	-25	-21	-12	+4
Pooled data (All ZETIA + Lovastatin Doses)[c]	192	-29	-40	-33	-25	+9

[a] For triglycerides, median % change from baseline
[b] Baseline - on no lipid-lowering drug
[c] ZETIA + all doses of lovastatin pooled (10-40 mg) significantly reduced total-C, LDL-C, Apo B, and TG, and increased HDL-C compared to all doses of lovastatin pooled (10-40 mg).

CONTRAINDICATIONS

Hypersensitivity to any component of this medication.
The combination of ZETIA with an HMG-CoA reductase inhibitor is contraindicated in patients with active liver disease or unexplained persistent elevations in serum transaminases.
All HMG-CoA reductase inhibitors are contraindicated in pregnant and nursing women. When ZETIA is administered with an HMG-CoA reductase inhibitor in a woman of childbearing potential, refer to the pregnancy category and product labeling for the HMG-CoA reductase inhibitor. (See PRECAUTIONS, *Pregnancy*.)

PRECAUTIONS

Concurrent administration of ZETIA with a specific HMG-CoA reductase inhibitor should be in accordance with the product labeling for that HMG-CoA reductase inhibitor.
Liver Enzymes
In controlled clinical monotherapy studies, the incidence of consecutive elevations (≥3 × the upper limit of normal [ULN]) in serum transaminases was similar between ZETIA (0.5%) and placebo (0.3%).
In controlled clinical combination studies of ZETIA initiated concurrently with an HMG-CoA reductase inhibitor, the incidence of consecutive elevations (≥3 × ULN) in serum transaminases was 1.3% for patients treated with ZETIA administered with HMG-CoA reductase inhibitors and 0.4% for patients treated with HMG-CoA reductase inhibitors alone. These elevations in transaminases were generally asymptomatic, not associated with cholestasis, and returned to baseline after discontinuation of therapy or with continued treatment. When ZETIA is co-administered with an HMG-CoA reductase inhibitor, liver function tests should be performed at initiation of therapy and according to the recommendations of the HMG-CoA reductase inhibitor.
Skeletal Muscle
In clinical trials, there was no excess of myopathy or rhabdomyolysis associated with ZETIA compared with the relevant control arm (placebo or HMG-CoA reductase inhibitor alone). However, myopathy and rhabdomyolysis are known adverse reactions to HMG-CoA reductase inhibitors and other lipid-lowering drugs. In clinical trials, the incidence of CPK >10 X ULN was 0.2% for ZETIA vs 0.1% for placebo, and 0.1% for ZETIA co-administered with an HMG-CoA reductase inhibitor vs 0.4% for HMG-CoA reductase inhibitors alone.
Hepatic Insufficiency
Due to the unknown effects of the increased exposure to ezetimibe in patients with moderate or severe hepatic insufficiency, ZETIA is not recommended in these patients. (See CLINICAL PHARMACOLOGY, *Special Populations*.)
Drug Interactions (See also CLINICAL PHARMACOLOGY, *Drug Interactions*)

Cholestyramine: Concomitant cholestyramine administration decreased the mean AUC of total ezetimibe approximately 55%. The incremental LDL-C reduction due to adding ezetimibe to cholestyramine may be reduced by this interaction.
Fibrates: The safety and effectiveness of ezetimibe administered with fibrates have not been established.
Fibrates may increase cholesterol excretion into the bile, leading to cholelithiasis. In a preclinical study in dogs, ezetimibe increased cholesterol in the gallbladder bile (see ANIMAL PHARMACOLOGY). Co-administration of ZETIA with fibrates is not recommended until use in patients is studied.
Fenofibrate: In a pharmacokinetic study, concomitant fenofibrate administration increased total ezetimibe concentrations approximately 1.5-fold.
Gemfibrozil: In a pharmacokinetic study, concomitant gemfibrozil administration increased total ezetimibe concentrations approximately 1.7-fold.
HMG-CoA Reductase Inhibitors: No clinically significant pharmacokinetic interactions were seen when ezetimibe was co-administered with atorvastatin, simvastatin, pravastatin, lovastatin, or fluvastatin.
Cyclosporine: Caution should be exercised when initiating ezetimibe in patients treated with cyclosporine due to increased exposure to ezetimibe. This exposure may be greater in patients with severe renal insufficiency. In patients treated with cyclosporine, the potential effects of the increased exposure to ezetimibe from concomitant use should be carefully weighed against the benefits of alterations in lipid levels provided by ezetimibe. In a pharmacokinetic study in post-renal transplant patients with mildly impaired or normal renal function (creatinine clearance of >50 mL/min), concomitant cyclosporine administration increased the mean AUC and C_{max} of total ezetimibe 3.4-fold (range 2.3- to 7.9-fold) and 3.9-fold (range 3.0- to 4.4-fold), respectively. In a separate study, the total ezetimibe exposure increased 12-fold in one renal transplant patient with severe renal insufficiency receiving multiple medications, including cyclosporine (see CLINICAL PHARMACOLOGY, *Drug Interactions*).
Carcinogenesis, Mutagenesis, Impairment of Fertility
A 104-week dietary carcinogenicity study with ezetimibe was conducted in rats at doses up to 1500 mg/kg/day (males) and 500 mg/kg/day (females) (~20 times the human exposure at 10 mg daily based on $AUC_{0\text{-}24hr}$ for total ezetimibe). A 104-week dietary carcinogenicity study with ezetimibe was also conducted in mice at doses up to 500 mg/kg/day (>150 times the human exposure at 10 mg daily based on $AUC_{0\text{-}24hr}$ for total ezetimibe). There were no statistically significant increases in tumor incidences in drug-treated rats or mice.
No evidence of mutagenicity was observed *in vitro* in a microbial mutagenicity (Ames) test with *Salmonella typhimurium* and *Escherichia coli* with or without metabolic activation. No evidence of clastogenicity was observed *in vitro* in a chromosomal aberration assay in human peripheral blood lymphocytes with or without metabolic activation. In addition, there was no evidence of genotoxicity in the *in vivo* mouse micronucleus test.
In oral (gavage) fertility studies of ezetimibe conducted in rats, there was no evidence of reproductive toxicity at doses up to 1000 mg/kg/day in male or female rats (~7 times the human exposure at 10 mg daily based on $AUC_{0\text{-}24hr}$ for total ezetimibe).

Pregnancy
Pregnancy Category: C
There are no adequate and well-controlled studies of ezetimibe in pregnant women. Ezetimibe should be used during pregnancy only if the potential benefit justifies the risk to the fetus.
In oral (gavage) embryo-fetal development studies of ezetimibe conducted in rats and rabbits during organogenesis, there was no evidence of embryolethal effects at the doses tested (250, 500, 1000 mg/kg/day). In rats, increased incidences of common fetal skeletal findings (extra pair of thoracic ribs, unossified cervical vertebral centra, shortened ribs) were observed at 1000 mg/kg/day (~10 times the human exposure at 10 mg daily based on $AUC_{0\text{-}24hr}$ for total ezetimibe). In rabbits treated with ezetimibe, an increased incidence of extra thoracic ribs was observed at 1000 mg/kg/day (150 times the human exposure at 10 mg daily based on $AUC_{0\text{-}24hr}$ for total ezetimibe). Ezetimibe crossed the placenta when pregnant rats and rabbits were given multiple oral doses.
Multiple dose studies of ezetimibe given in combination with HMG-CoA reductase inhibitors (statins) in rats and rabbits during organogenesis result in higher ezetimibe and statin exposures. Reproductive findings occur at lower doses in combination therapy compared to monotherapy.
All HMG-CoA reductase inhibitors are contraindicated in pregnant and nursing women. When ZETIA is administered with an HMG-CoA reductase inhibitor in a woman of childbearing potential, refer to the pregnancy category and product labeling for the HMG-CoA reductase inhibitor. (See CONTRAINDICATIONS.)
Labor and Delivery
The effects of ZETIA on labor and delivery in pregnant women are unknown.
Nursing Mothers
In rat studies, exposure to total ezetimibe in nursing pups was up to half of that observed in maternal plasma. It is not known whether ezetimibe is excreted into human breast milk; therefore, ZETIA should not be used in nursing mothers unless the potential benefit justifies the potential risk to the infant.
Pediatric Use
The pharmacokinetics of ZETIA in adolescents (10 to 18 years) have been shown to be similar to that in adults. Treatment experience with ZETIA in the pediatric population is limited to 4 patients (9 to 17 years) in the sitosterolemia study and 5 patients (11 to 17 years) in the HoFH study. Treatment with ZETIA in children (<10 years) is not recommended. (See CLINICAL PHARMACOLOGY, *Special Populations.*)
Geriatric Use
Of the patients who received ZETIA in clinical studies, 948 were 65 and older (this included 206 who were 75 and older). The effectiveness and safety of ZETIA were similar between these patients and younger subjects. Greater sensitivity of some older individuals cannot be ruled out. (See CLINICAL PHARMACOLOGY, *Special Populations*, and ADVERSE REACTIONS.)

ADVERSE REACTIONS

ZETIA has been evaluated for safety in more than 4700 patients in clinical trials. Clinical studies of ZETIA (administered alone or with an HMG-CoA reductase inhibitor) demonstrated that ZETIA was generally well tolerated. The overall incidence of adverse events reported with ZETIA was similar to that reported with placebo, and the discontinuation rate due to adverse events was also similar for ZETIA and placebo.
Monotherapy
Adverse experiences reported in ≥2% of patients treated with ZETIA and at an incidence greater than placebo in placebo-controlled studies of ZETIA, regardless of causality assessment, are shown in Table 8.

Table 8*
Clinical Adverse Events Occurring in ≥2% of Patients Treated with ZETIA and at an Incidence Greater than Placebo, Regardless of Causality

Body System/Organ Class Adverse Event	Placebo (%) n = 795	ZETIA 10 mg (%) n = 1691
Body as a whole – general disorders		
Fatigue	1.8	2.2
Gastro-intestinal system disorders		
Abdominal pain	2.8	3.0
Diarrhea	3.0	3.7
Infection and infestations		
Infection viral	1.8	2.2
Pharyngitis	2.1	2.3
Sinusitis	2.8	3.6
Musculo-skeletal system disorders		
Arthralgia	3.4	3.8
Back pain	3.9	4.1
Respiratory system disorders		
Coughing	2.1	2.3

*Includes patients who received placebo or ZETIA alone reported in Table 9.

The frequency of less common adverse events was comparable between ZETIA and placebo.
Combination with an HMG-CoA Reductase Inhibitor
ZETIA has been evaluated for safety in combination studies in more than 2000 patients.
In general, adverse experiences were similar between ZETIA administered with HMG-CoA reductase inhibitors and HMG-CoA reductase inhibitors alone. However, the frequency of increased transaminases was slightly higher in patients receiving ZETIA administered with HMG-CoA reductase inhibitors than in patients treated with HMG-CoA reductase inhibitors alone. (See PRECAUTIONS, *Liver Enzymes.*)
Clinical adverse experiences reported in ≥2% of patients and at an incidence greater than placebo in four placebo-controlled trials where ZETIA was administered alone or initiated concurrently with various HMG-CoA reductase inhibitors, regardless of causality assessment, are shown in Table 9.
[See table 9 at top of next page]
Post-marketing Experience
The following adverse reactions have been reported in post-marketing experience, regardless of causality assessment: Hypersensitivity reactions, including angioedema and rash; pancreatitis; nausea; cholelithiasis; cholecystitis.

OVERDOSAGE

In clinical studies, administration of ezetimibe, 50 mg/day to 15 healthy subjects for up to 14 days, or 40 mg/day to 18 patients with primary hypercholesterolemia for up to 56 days, was generally well tolerated.
A few cases of overdosage with ZETIA have been reported; most have not been associated with adverse experiences. Reported adverse experiences have not been serious. In the event of an overdose, symptomatic and supportive measures should be employed.

DOSAGE AND ADMINISTRATION

The patient should be placed on a standard cholesterol-lowering diet before receiving ZETIA and should continue on this diet during treatment with ZETIA.
The recommended dose of ZETIA is 10 mg once daily. ZETIA can be administered with or without food.
ZETIA may be administered with an HMG-CoA reductase inhibitor for incremental effect. For convenience, the daily dose of ZETIA may be taken at the same time as the HMG-CoA reductase inhibitor, according to the dosing recommendations for the HMG-CoA reductase inhibitor.
Patients with Hepatic Insufficiency
No dosage adjustment is necessary in patients with mild hepatic insufficiency (see PRECAUTIONS, *Hepatic Insufficiency*).
Patients with Renal Insufficiency
No dosage adjustment is necessary in patients with renal insufficiency (see CLINICAL PHARMACOLOGY, *Special Populations*).
Geriatric Patients
No dosage adjustment is necessary in geriatric patients (see CLINICAL PHARMACOLOGY, *Special Populations*).
Co-administration with Bile Acid Sequestrants
Dosing of ZETIA should occur either ≥2 hours before or ≥4 hours after administration of a bile acid sequestrant (see PRECAUTIONS, *Drug Interactions*).

Continued on next page

Table 7
Summary of NCEP ATP III Guidelines

Risk Category	LDL Goal (mg/dL)	LDL Level at Which to Initiate Therapeutic Lifestyle Changes[a] (mg/dL)	LDL level at Which to Consider Drug Therapy (mg/dL)
CHD or CHD risk equivalents[b] (10-year risk >20%)[c]	<100	≥100	≥130 (100-129: drug optional)[d]
2+ Risk factors[e] (10-year risk ≤20%)[c]	<130	≥130	10-year risk 10-20%: ≥130[c] 10-year risk <10%: ≥160[c]
0-1 Risk factor[f]	<160	≥160	≥190 (160-189: LDL-lowering drug optional)

[a] Therapeutic lifestyle changes include: 1) dietary changes: reduced intake of saturated fats (<7% of total calories) and cholesterol (<200 mg per day), and enhancing LDL lowering with plant stanols/sterols (2 g/d) and increased viscous (soluble) fiber (10-25 g/d), 2) weight reduction, and 3) increased physical activity.
[b] CHD risk equivalents comprise: diabetes, multiple risk factors that confer a 10-year risk for CHD >20%, and other clinical forms of atherosclerotic disease (peripheral arterial disease, abdominal aortic aneurysm and symptomatic carotid artery disease).
[c] Risk assessment for determining the 10-year risk for developing CHD is carried out using the Framingham risk scoring. Refer to JAMA, May 16, 2001; 285 (19): 2486-2497, or the NCEP website (http://www.nhlbi.nih.gov) for more details.
[d] Some authorities recommend use of LDL-lowering drugs in this category if an LDL cholesterol <100 mg/dL cannot be achieved by therapeutic lifestyle changes. Others prefer use of drugs that primarily modify triglycerides and HDL, e.g., nicotinic acid or fibrate. Clinical judgment also may call for deferring drug therapy in this subcategory.
[e] Major risk factors (exclusive of LDL cholesterol) that modify LDL goals include cigarette smoking, hypertension (BP ≥140/90 mm Hg or on anti-hypertensive medication), low HDL cholesterol (<40 mg/dL), family history of premature CHD (CHD in male first-degree relative <55 years; CHD in female first-degree relative <65 years), age (men ≥45 years; women ≥55 years). HDL cholesterol ≥60 mg/dL counts as a "negative" risk factor; its presence removes one risk factor from the total count.
[f] Almost all people with 0-1 risk factor have a 10-year risk <10%; thus, 10-year risk assessment in people with 0-1 risk factor is not necessary.

Information on Schering products appearing on these pages is effective as of June 2003.

Table 9*
Clinical Adverse Events occurring in ≥2% of Patients and at an Incidence Greater than Placebo, Regardless of Causality, in ZETIA/Statin Combination Studies

Body System/Organ Class Adverse Event	Placebo (%) n=259	ZETIA 10 mg (%) n=262	All Statins** (%) n=936	ZETIA + All Statins** (%) n=925
Body as a whole – general disorders				
Chest pain	1.2	3.4	2.0	1.8
Dizziness	1.2	2.7	1.4	1.8
Fatigue	1.9	1.9	1.4	2.8
Headache	5.4	8.0	7.3	6.3
Gastro-intestinal system disorders				
Abdominal pain	2.3	2.7	3.1	3.5
Diarrhea	1.5	3.4	2.9	2.8
Infection and infestations				
Pharyngitis	1.9	3.1	2.5	2.3
Sinusitis	1.9	4.6	3.6	3.5
Upper respiratory tract infection	10.8	13.0	13.6	11.8
Musculo-skeletal system disorders				
Arthralgia	2.3	3.8	4.3	3.4
Back pain	3.5	3.4	3.7	4.3
Myalgia	4.6	5.0	4.1	4.5

*Includes four placebo-controlled combination studies in which ZETIA was initiated concurrently with an HMG-CoA reductase inhibitor.
**All Statins = all doses of all HMG-CoA reductase inhibitors.

Zetia—Cont.

HOW SUPPLIED

No. 3861 - Tablets ZETIA, 10 mg, are white to off-white, capsule-shaped tablets debossed with "414" on one side. They are supplied as follows:
NDC 66582-414-31 bottles of 30
NDC 66582-414-54 bottles of 90
NDC 66582-414-74 bottles of 500
NDC 66582-414-28 unit dose packages of 100.

Storage

Store at 25°C (77°F); excursions permitted to 15-30°C (59-86°F). [See USP Controlled Room Temperature.] Protect from moisture.
25751868T
REV 04
Issued August 2004
Printed in USA.
Manufactured for:
Merck/Schering-Plough Pharmaceuticals
North Wales, PA 19454, USA
By:
Schering Corporation
Kenilworth, NJ 07033, USA
or
Merck & Co., Inc.
Whitehouse Station, NJ 08889, USA

ZETIA® (ezetimibe) Tablets

Patient Information about ZETIA (zĕt'-ē-ă)

Generic name: ezetimibe (ĕ-zĕt'-ĕ-mīb)

Read this information carefully before you start taking ZETIA and each time you get more ZETIA. There may be new information. This information does not take the place of talking with your doctor about your medical condition or your treatment. If you have any questions about ZETIA, ask your doctor. Only your doctor can determine if ZETIA is right for you.

What is ZETIA?

ZETIA is a medicine used to lower levels of total cholesterol and LDL (bad) cholesterol in the blood. It is used for patients who cannot control their cholesterol levels by diet alone. It can be used by itself or with other medicines to treat high cholesterol. You should stay on a cholesterol-lowering diet while taking this medicine.

ZETIA works to reduce the amount of cholesterol your body absorbs. ZETIA does not help you lose weight.

For more information about cholesterol, see the "What should I know about high cholesterol?" section that follows.

Who should not take ZETIA?

- Do not take ZETIA if you are allergic to ezetimibe, the active ingredient in ZETIA, or to the inactive ingredients. For a list of inactive ingredients, see the "Inactive ingredients" section that follows.
- If you have active liver disease, do not take ZETIA while taking cholesterol-lowering medicines called statins.
- If you are pregnant or breast-feeding, do not take ZETIA while taking a statin.

What should I tell my doctor before and while taking ZETIA?

Tell your doctor about any prescription and non-prescription medicines you are taking or plan to take, including natural or herbal remedies.

Tell your doctor about all your medical conditions including allergies.

Tell your doctor if you:

- ever had liver problems. ZETIA may not be right for you.
- are pregnant or plan to become pregnant. Your doctor will decide if ZETIA is right for you.
- are breast-feeding. We do not know if ZETIA can pass to your baby through your milk. Your doctor will decide if ZETIA is right for you.
- experience unexplained muscle pain, tenderness, or weakness.

How should I take ZETIA?

- Take ZETIA once a day, with or without food. It may be easier to remember to take your dose if you do it at the same time every day, such as with breakfast, dinner, or at bedtime. If you also take another medicine to reduce your cholesterol, ask your doctor if you can take them at the same time.
- If you forget to take ZETIA, take it as soon as you remember. However, do not take more than one dose of ZETIA a day.
- Continue to follow a cholesterol-lowering diet while taking ZETIA. Ask your doctor if you need diet information.
- Keep taking ZETIA unless your doctor tells you to stop. It is important that you keep taking ZETIA even if you do not feel sick.

See your doctor regularly to check your cholesterol level and to check for side effects. Your doctor may do blood tests to check your liver before you start taking ZETIA with a statin and during treatment.

What are the possible side effects of ZETIA?

In clinical studies patients reported few side effects while taking ZETIA. These included stomach pain and feeling tired.

Additionally, the following side effects have been reported in general use: allergic reactions (which may require treatment right away) including swelling of the face, lips, tongue, and/or throat that may cause difficulty in breathing or swallowing, and rash; inflammation of the pancreas; nausea; gallstones; inflammation of the gallbladder.

Tell your doctor if you are have these or any other medical problems while on ZETIA. For a complete list of side effects, ask your doctor or pharmacist.

What should I know about high cholesterol?

Cholesterol is a type of fat found in your blood. Your total cholesterol is made up of LDL and HDL cholesterol.

LDL cholesterol is called "bad" cholesterol because it can build up in the wall of your arteries and form plaque. Over time, plaque build-up can cause a narrowing of the arteries. This narrowing can slow or block blood flow to your heart, brain, and other organs. High LDL cholesterol is a major cause of heart disease and stroke.

HDL cholesterol is called "good" cholesterol because it keeps the bad cholesterol from building up in the arteries.

Triglycerides also are fats found in your blood.

General Information about ZETIA

Medicines are sometimes prescribed for conditions that are not mentioned in patient information leaflets. Do not use ZETIA for a condition for which it was not prescribed. Do not give ZETIA to other people, even if they have the same condition you have. It may harm them.

This summarizes the most important information about ZETIA. If you would like more information, talk with your doctor. You can ask your pharmacist or doctor for information about ZETIA that is written for health professionals.

Inactive ingredients:

Croscarmellose sodium, lactose monohydrate, magnesium stearate, microcrystalline cellulose, povidone, and sodium lauryl sulfate.
25751760T
REV 04
Issued August 2004
Manufactured for:
Merck/Schering-Plough Pharmaceuticals
North Wales, PA 19454, USA
By:
Schering Corporation
Kenilworth, NJ 07033, USA
or
Merck & Co., Inc.
Whitehouse Station, NJ 08889, USA

Schwarz Pharma, Inc.

6140 W. EXECUTIVE DRIVE
MEQUON, WI 53092

For Medical Information Contact:
Schwarz Pharma, Inc.
Medical and Drug Information
(262) 238-9994
(800) 558-5114

COLYTE® ℞

(PEG-3350 & ELECTROLYTES for Oral Solution)
For Gastrointestinal Lavage
℞ Only

DESCRIPTION

colyte® is a colon lavage preparation provided as water-soluble components for solution. In solution each colyte® preparation delivers the following, in grams per liter.

Polyethylene glycol 3350	60.00
Sodium chloride	1.46
Potassium chloride	0.745
Sodium bicarbonate	1.68
Sodium sulfate	5.68

When dissolved in sufficient water to make 4 liters, the final solution contains 125 mEq/L sodium, 10 mEq/L potassium, 20 mEq/L bicarbonate, 80 mEq/L sulfate, 35 mEq/L chloride and 18 mEq/L polyethylene glycol 3350. The reconstituted solution is isosmotic and has a mildly salty taste. colyte® is administered orally or via nasogastric tube.

HOW SUPPLIED

colyte® is supplied in 4 liter and 18 oz. bottles. Each 4 liter bottle contains polyethylene glycol 3350 240 g, sodium chloride 5.84 g, potassium chloride 2.98 g, sodium bicarbonate 6.72 g, sodium sulfate (anhydrous) 22.72 g. Each 18 oz. bottle contains polyethylene glycol 3350 227.10 g, sodium chloride 5.53 g, potassium chloride 2.82 g, sodium bicarbonate 6.36 g, sodium sulfate (anhydrous) 21.50 g. Each preparation is supplied in powdered form, for oral administration as a solution.

colyte®	4 liter	NDC 0091-4401-23
	18 oz.	NDC 0091-4401-49

Store powder at controlled room temperature 15°–30°C (59°–86°F).
KEEP RECONSTITUTED SOLUTION REFRIGERATED. USE WITHIN 48 HOURS. DISCARD UNUSED PORTION.
Also available as:

colyte®-flavored	4 liter	NDC 0091-4403-05
	18 oz.	NDC 0091-4403-13
colyte® with flavor packs	4 liter	NDC 0091-7036-23

PCL2109F Rev. 05/03

COLYTE® WITH FLAVOR PACKS ℞

(PEG-3350 & ELECTROLYTES for oral solution)
For Gastrointestinal Lavage
℞ Only

DESCRIPTION

colyte® with flavor packs is a colon lavage preparation provided as water-soluble components for solution. In solution this preparation with one flavor pack added delivers the following, in grams per liter.

Polyethylene glycol 3350	60.00
Sodium chloride	1.46
Potassium chloride	0.745
Sodium bicarbonate	1.68
Sodium sulfate	5.68
Flavor ingredients	0.805

When dissolved in sufficient water to make 4 liters, the final solution contains 125 mEq/L sodium, 10 mEq/L potassium, 20 mEq/L bicarbonate, 80 mEq/L sulfate, 35 mEq/L chloride and 18 mEq/L polyethylene glycol 3350. The reconstituted solution is isosmotic and has a mild salty taste. This preparation can be used without the flavor packs and is administered orally or via nasogastric tube.

Each orange flavor pack (3.22 g) contains hypromellose, natural and artificial orange powder, saccharin sodium, colloidal silicon dioxide. Each citrus berry flavor pack (3.22 g) contains hypromellose, artificial citrus berry powder, saccharin sodium, colloidal silicon dioxide. Each lemon lime flavor pack (3.22 g) contains, hypromellose, natural and artificial lemon lime powder, Prosweet® Powder Natural, saccharin sodium, colloidal silicon dioxide. Each cherry flavor pack (3.22 g) contains hypromellose, artificial cherry powder, saccharin sodium, colloidal silicon dioxide. Each pineapple flavor pack (3.22 g) contains hypromellose, artificial pineapple flavor powder, Magna Sweet™, saccharin sodium, colloidal silicon dioxide.

CLINICAL PHARMACOLOGY

colyte® with flavor packs cleanses the bowel by induction of diarrhea. The osmotic activity of polyethylene glycol 3350, in combination with the electrolyte concentration, results in virtually no net absorption or excretion of ions or water. Accordingly, large volumes may be administered without significant changes in fluid and electrolyte balance.

INDICATIONS AND USAGE

colyte® with flavor packs is indicated for bowel cleansing prior to colonoscopy or barium enema X-ray examination.

CONTRAINDICATIONS

colyte® with flavor packs is contraindicated in patients known to be hypersensitive to any of the components.
colyte® with flavor packs is contraindicated in patients with ileus, gastrointestinal obstruction, gastric retention, bowel perforation, toxic colitis or toxic megacolon.

WARNINGS

Flavor packs are for use only in combination with the contents of the accompanying 4 liter container. No other additional ingredients (e.g., flavorings) should be added to the solution. colyte® with flavor packs should be used with caution in patients with severe ulcerative colitis.

PRECAUTIONS

General: Patients with impaired gag reflex, unconscious or semiconscious patients and patients prone to regurgitation or aspiration should be observed during the administration of colyte® with flavor packs, especially if it is administered via nasogastric tube.
If gastrointestinal obstruction or perforation is suspected appropriate studies should be performed to rule out these conditions before administration of colyte® with flavor packs.

INFORMATION FOR PATIENTS

colyte® with flavor packs produces a watery stool which cleanses the bowel prior to examination.
For best results, no solid food should be ingested during the 3–4 hour period prior to the initiation of colyte® with flavor packs administration. In no case should solid foods be eaten within 2 hours of drinking colyte® with flavor packs.
The rate of administration is 240 mL (8 fl. oz.) every 10 minutes. Rapid drinking of each portion is preferred rather than drinking small amounts continuously.
The first bowel movement should occur approximately one hour after the start of colyte® with flavor packs administration.
Administration of colyte® with flavor packs should be continued until the watery stool is clear and free of solid matter. This normally requires the consumption of approximately 3–4 liters (3–4 quarts), although more or less may be required in some patients. The unused portion should be discarded.

DRUG INTERACTIONS

Oral medication administered within one hour of the start of administration of colyte® with flavor packs may be flushed from the gastrointestinal tract and not absorbed.

CARCINOGENESIS, MUTAGENESIS, IMPAIRMENT OF FERTILITY

Studies to evaluate carcinogenic or mutagenic potential or potential to adversely affect male or female fertility have not been performed.

PREGNANCY

Category C. Animal reproduction studies have not been conducted with colyte® with flavor packs, and it is not known whether colyte® with flavor packs can affect reproductive capacity or harm the fetus when administered to a pregnant patient. colyte® with flavor packs should be given to a pregnant patient only if clearly needed.

PEDIATRIC USE

Safety and effectiveness in pediatric patients have not been established.

GERIATRIC USE

Published literature contains isolated reports of serious adverse reactions following the administration of PEG-ELS products in patients over 60 years of age. These adverse events include upper GI bleeding from Mallory-Weiss Tear, esophageal perforation, asystole, sudden dyspnea with pulmonary edema, and "butterfly-like" infiltrate on chest x-ray after vomiting and aspirating PEG.

ADVERSE REACTIONS

Nausea, abdominal fullness and bloating are the most frequent adverse reactions, occurring in up to 50% of patients. Abdominal cramps, vomiting and anal irritation occur less frequently. These adverse reactions are transient. Isolated cases of urticaria, rhinorrhea, dermatitis, and rarely anaphylaxis, angioedema, tongue edema, and face edema have been reported which may represent allergic reactions.

DOSAGE AND ADMINISTRATION

colyte® with flavor packs can be administered orally or by nasogastric tube. Patients should fast at least 3 hours prior to administration. A one hour waiting period after the appearance of clear liquid stool should be allowed prior to examination to complete bowel evacuation. No foods except clear liquids should be permitted prior to examination after colyte® with flavor packs administration.
ORAL: The recommended adult oral dose is 240 mL (8 fl. oz.) every 10 minutes (see INFORMATION FOR PATIENTS). Lavage is complete when fecal discharge is clear. Lavage is usually complete after the ingestion of 3–4 liters.
NASOGASTRIC TUBE: colyte® with flavor packs is administered at a rate of 20–30 mL per minute (1.2–1.8 L/hour).
PREPARATION OF colyte® with flavor packs SOLUTION:
This preparation can be used with or without the flavor packs.

1. To add flavor, tear open one flavor pack at the indicated marking and pour contents into the bottle BEFORE reconstitution. Discard unused flavor packs.
2. SHAKE WELL to incorporate flavoring into the powder.
3. Add tap water to FILL line. Replace cap tightly and mix or shake well until all ingredients have dissolved. (No other additional ingredients, e.g. flavorings, should be added to the solution.)

Note: If not using flavor packs, omit steps one and two, above.

HOW SUPPLIED

colyte® with flavor packs is supplied in 4 liter bottles with an attached package containing flavor packs. Each 4 liter bottle contains polyethylene glycol 3350 240 g, sodium chloride 5.84 g, potassium chloride 2.98 g, sodium bicarbonate 6.72 g, sodium sulfate (anhydrous) 22.72 g. This preparation is supplied in powdered form, for oral administration as a solution.

colyte® with flavor packs 4 liter NDC 0091-7036-23

Store powder at controlled room temperature 15°–30°C (59°–86°F).
KEEP RECONSTITUTED SOLUTION REFRIGERATED. USE WITHIN 48 HOURS. DISCARD UNUSED PORTION.
Also available as:

colyte®	4 liter	NDC 0091-4401-23
	18 oz.	NDC 0091-4401-49
colyte® -flavored	4 liter	NDC 0091-4403-05
	18 oz.	NDC 0091-4403-13

PCL3827F Rev. 09/03

Shown in Product Identification Guide, page 332

CORTIFOAM® ℞
(hydrocortisone acetate rectal aerosol) 10%
Rectal Foam
℞ Only

DESCRIPTION

Cortifoam® (hydrocortisone acetate rectal aerosol) 10% Rectal Foam contains hydrocortisone acetate 10% in a base containing propylene glycol, emulsifying wax, polyoxyethylene-10-stearyl ether, cetyl alcohol, methylparaben, propylparaben, trolamine, purified water and inert propellants: isobutane and propane.
Each application delivers approximately 900 mg of foam containing 80 mg of hydrocortisone (90 mg of hydrocortisone acetate).
The molecular weight of hydrocortisone acetate is 404.50. It is designated chemically as pregn-4-ene-3,20-dione, 21-(acetyloxy)-11, 17-dihydroxy-, (11β)-. The empirical formula is $C_{23}H_{32}O_6$ and the structural formula is:

Hydrocortisone acetate, a synthetic adrenocortical steroid, is a white to practically white, odorless, crystalline powder. It is insoluble in water (1 mg/100 mL) and slightly soluble in alcohol and chloroform.

HOW SUPPLIED

Cortifoam® is supplied in an aerosol container with a special rectal applicator. Each applicator delivers approximately 900 mg of foam containing approximately 80 mg of hydrocortisone as 90 mg of hydrocortisone acetate. When used correctly, the aerosol container will deliver a minimum of 14 applications.

NDC 0091-0695-20 15 g

Store at controlled room temperature, 20°–25°C (68°–77°F).
DO NOT REFRIGERATE.
Rx Only
PC2080D Rev. 06/02

Shown in Product Identification Guide, page 332

DILATRATE®-SR ℞
[*dī 'lă-trāt*]
(isosorbide dinitrate)
sustained release capsules
40 mg
℞ Only

DESCRIPTION

Isosorbide dinitrate (ISDN) is 1,4:3,6-dianhydro-D-glucitol 2,5 dinitrate, an organic nitrate whose structural formula is

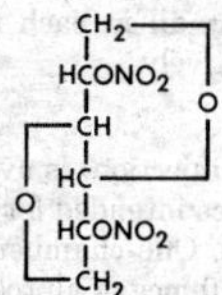

and whose molecular weight is 236.14. The organic nitrates are vasodilators, active on both arteries and veins. Each Dilatrate-SR sustained release capsule contains 40 mg of isosorbide dinitrate, in a microdialysis delivery system that causes the active drug to be released over an extended period. Each capsule also contains ethylcellulose, lactose, pharmaceutical glaze, starch, sucrose and talc. The capsule shells contain D&C Red 33, D&C Yellow 10, gelatin and titanium dioxide.

HOW SUPPLIED

Dilatrate®-SR (isosorbide dinitrate) 40 mg sustained release capsules are opaque pink and colorless capsules with white beadlets and are imprinted "Schwarz" and "0920". They are supplied as follows:
Bottles of 100 NDC 0091-0920-01
Store at controlled room temperature 15°–30°C (59°–86°F) in a dry place.
PC2088G Rev. 11/02

EDEX® ℞
[*ē-'deks*]
(alprostadil for injection)
For Intracavernous Use Only
Sterile Powder and Diluent
(sterile 0.9% sodium chloride) in Cartridges
℞ Only

DESCRIPTION

EDEX (alprostadil for injection) is a sterile, pyrogen-free powder containing alprostadil in an alfadex (α-cyclodextrin) inclusion complex. Alprostadil is an endogenous substance known as prostaglandin E_1 (PGE_1). EDEX is supplied in single-dose, dual-chamber cartridges.
EDEX is lyophilized in single-dose, dual-chamber cartridges intended for use with the reusable EDEX injection device. One chamber of the cartridge contains alprostadil, alfadex and lactose as a sterile, pyrogen-free powder. The other chamber contains 1.075 mL of sterile 0.9% sodium chloride. The EDEX cartridges are supplied in three strengths: 10 mcg cartridge (10.75 mcg alprostadil, 347.55 mcg α-cyclodextrin, 51.06 mg lactose); 20 mcg cartridge (21.5 mcg alprostadil, 695.2 mcg α-cyclodextrin, 51.06 mg lactose); 40 mcg cartridge (43.0 mcg alprostadil, 1,390.3 mcg α-cyclodextrin, 51.06 mg lactose). The EDEX injection device is used to reconstitute the sterile powder in one chamber with the sterile 0.9% sodium chloride in the other chamber. After reconstitution, the EDEX injection device is used to administer the intracavernous injection of alprostadil.
The chemical name for alprostadil is (1R,2R,3R)-3-Hydroxy-2-[(E)-(3S)-3-hydroxy-1-octenyl]-5-oxocyclopentane heptanoic acid. The empirical formula is $C_{20}H_{34}O_5$ and the molecular weight is 354.49. The chemical structure is:

The α-cyclodextrin inclusion complex improves the water solubility of alprostadil. The empirical formula of α-cyclodextrin is $C_{36}H_{60}O_{30}$ and the molecular weight is 972.85. The chemical structure is:

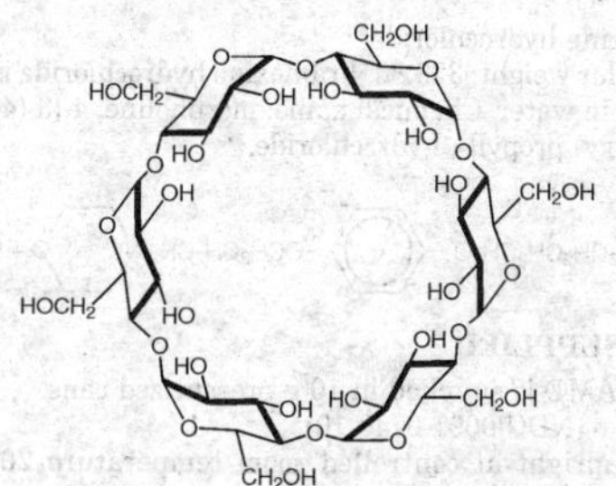

Continued on next page

Edex—Cont.

Alprostadil alfadex is a white, odorless, hygroscopic powder. It is freely soluble in water and practically insoluble in ethanol, ethyl acetate and ether. After reconstitution, the active ingredient, alprostadil, immediately dissociates from the α-cyclodextrin inclusion complex. The reconstituted solution is clear and colorless and has a pH between 4.0 and 8.0. When the single-dose, dual-chamber cartridge containing either 10.75, 21.5 or 43.0 mcg of alprostadil is placed into the EDEX injection device and reconstituted, the deliverable amount of alprostadil in each milliliter is 10, 20 or 40 micrograms, respectively.

HOW SUPPLIED

EDEX (alprostadil for injection) is available in single-dose, dual-chamber cartridges intended for use with the reusable EDEX injection device. One chamber of the cartridge contains 10.75, 21.5 or 43.0 mcg of alprostadil as a white, sterile, lyophilized powder. The other chamber contains 1.075 mL of sterile 0.9% sodium chloride. When the cartridge is placed into the EDEX injection device and reconstituted, the deliverable amount of alprostadil in each milliliter is 10, 20 or 40 micrograms, respectively. EDEX Cartridge 2 Pack contains one reusable EDEX injection device, two single-dose, dual-chamber cartridges, two 1/2 inch, 29 gauge (0.33 mm x 12.7 mm) needles, and four alcohol swabs. EDEX Cartridge 6 Pack contains one reusable EDEX injection device, six single-dose, dual-chamber cartridges, six 1/2 inch, 29 gauge (0.33 mm x 12.7 mm) needles, and twelve alcohol swabs.

The EDEX cartridges are supplied in the following packages:

EDEX Cartridge 2 Pack (includes one injection device, two cartridges, two needles and four alcohol swabs)

10 mcg	1 × 2 Pack	NDC 0091-1110-16
20 mcg	1 × 2 Pack	NDC 0091-1120-16
40 mcg	1 × 2 Pack	NDC 0091-1140-16

EDEX Cartridge 6 Pack (includes one injection device, 6 cartridges, 6 needles and twelve alcohol swabs)

10 mcg	1 × 6 Pack	NDC 0091-1110-20
20 mcg	1 × 6 Pack	NDC 0091-1120-20
40 mcg	1 × 6 Pack	NDC 0091-1140-20

Store at 25°C (77°F); excursions permitted between 15°–30°C (59°–86°F).

PC4766 Rev. 02/04

EPIFOAM® ℞

topical aerosol
(hydrocortisone acetate 1% and pramoxine hydrochloride 1%)
Rx Only

DESCRIPTION

Epifoam® (hydrocortisone acetate 1% and pramoxine hydrochloride 1%) is a topical aerosol foam containing: hydrocortisone acetate 1% and pramoxine hydrochloride 1% in a base containing: propylene glycol, cetyl alcohol, glyceryl monostearate and PEG 100 stearate blend, laureth-23, polyoxyl-40 stearate, methylparaben, propylparaben, trolamine, purified water, and inert propellants: isobutane and propane.

EPIFOAM® contains a synthetic steroid used as an anti-inflammatory/antipruritic agent, and a local anesthetic.

Hydrocortisone acetate

Molecular weight: 404.50. Solubility of hydrocortisone acetate in water: 1 mg/100 mL. Chemical name: Pregn-4-ene-3,20-dione, 21-(acetyloxy)-11, 17-dihydroxy- (11β)-.

Pramoxine hydrochloride

Molecular weight: 329.86. Pramoxine hydrochloride is freely soluble in water. Chemical name: morpholine, 4-[3-(4-butoxyphenoxy) propyl]-, hydrochloride.

HOW SUPPLIED

EPIFOAM® is supplied in 10 g pressurized cans.

10 g (NDC 0091-0740-10)

Store upright at controlled room temperature 20°–25°C (68°–77°F). Do not refrigerate.

PC2202E Rev. 06/03

Shown in Product Identification Guide, page 332

KUTRASE® Capsules ℞

[kū 'trās]
℞ **Only**

DESCRIPTION

kutrase® capsules contain three standardized digestive enzymes: lipase, amylase and protease. The source of the enzymes is pancreatin and they are designed for oral digestive enzyme supplement therapy. Each capsule provides the following enzymatic activity:

lipase	2,400 USP Units
amylase	30,000 USP Units
protease	30,000 USP Units

Each capsule also contains as inactive ingredients: colloidal silicon dioxide, D&C yellow #10, FD&C green #3, FD&C yellow #6, gelatin, sodium lauryl sulfate and titanium dioxide.

HOW SUPPLIED

kutrase® capsules are green and white capsules and are imprinted "SCHWARZ" and "4175".

Bottles of 100 capsules NDC 0091-4175-01

Store at controlled room temperature 15°–30°C (59°–86°F). Protect from high humidity.

PC4164B Rev. 08/03

KU-ZYME® CAPSULES ℞

[kū ' zīm]
℞ **Only**

DESCRIPTION

ku-zyme® capsules contain three standardized digestive enzymes: lipase, amylase and protease. The source of the enzymes is pancreatin and they are designed for oral digestive enzyme supplement therapy. Each capsule provides the following enzymatic activity:

lipase	1,200 USP Units
amylase	15,000 USP Units
protease	15,000 USP Units

Each capsule also contains as inactive ingredients: colloidal silicon dioxide, D&C yellow #10, FD&C yellow #6, gelatin, sodium lauryl sulfate and titanium dioxide.

HOW SUPPLIED

ku-zyme® capsules are yellow and white capsules and are imprinted "SCHWARZ" and "4122".

Bottles of 100 capsules NDC 0091-4122-01

Store at controlled room temperature 15°–30°C (59°–86°F). Protect from high humidity.

PC4166B Rev. 08/03

KU-ZYME® HP CAPSULES ℞

[kū ' zīm]
(pancrelipase capsules USP)
Rx Only

DESCRIPTION

KU-ZYME® HP Capsules (pancrelipase capsules USP) contain standardized lipase, amylase and protease obtained from hog pancreas and are designed for oral digestive enzyme replacement therapy. Each capsule contains:

lipase	8,000 USP Units
protease	30,000 USP Units
amylase	30,000 USP Units

Each capsule also contains as inactive ingredients: gelatin, lactose, magnesium stearate, titanium dioxide and other ingredients.

HOW SUPPLIED

KU-ZYME® HP Capsules (pancrelipase capsules USP) are white opaque capsules and are imprinted "SCHWARZ" and "525."

Bottles of 100 capsules NDC 0091-3525-01

Store at a temperature not exceeding 25°C (77°F). Protect from high humidity.

PC 3752B Rev. 08/03

LEVATOL® Tablets ℞

[lev 'a-tol]
(penbutolol sulfate) 20 mg

℞ **Only**

DESCRIPTION

levatol® (penbutolol sulfate) is a synthetic β-receptor antagonist for oral administration. The chemical name of penbutolol sulfate is (S)-1-tert-butylamino-3-(o-cyclopentylphenoxy)-2-propanol sulfate. It is provided as the levorotatory isomer. The empirical formula for penbutolol sulfate is $C_{36}H_{60}N_2O_8S$. Its molecular weight is 680.94. A dose of 20 mg is equivalent to 29.4 μmol. The structural formula is as follows:

[See chemical structure at top of next column]

Penbutolol is a white, odorless, crystalline powder. levatol is available as tablets for oral administration. Each tablet contains 20 mg of penbutolol sulfate. It also contains corn starch, D&C Yellow No. 10, lactose, magnesium stearate, povidone, silicon dioxide, talc, titanium dioxide, and other inactive ingredients.

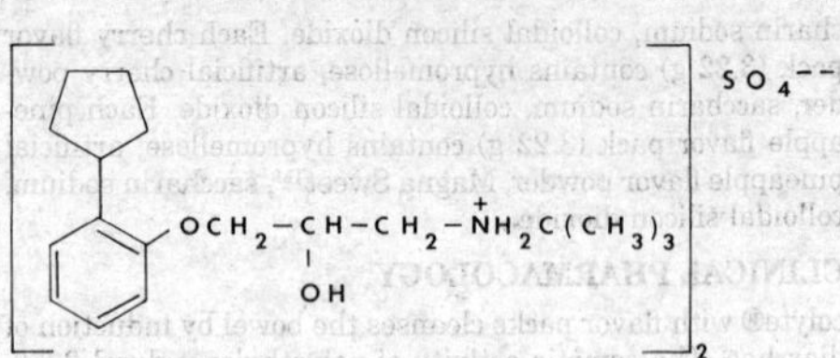

HOW SUPPLIED

levatol® (penbutolol sulfate) 20 mg tablets are yellow, scored, capsule-shaped and engraved "SP22". They are supplied as follows:

Bottles of 100 NDC 0091-4500-15

Store at controlled room temperature 20°–25°C (68°–77°F). Keep tightly closed and protect from light.

PC2077C Rev. 09/01

LEVSIN® PRODUCTS ℞

[lev 'sin]
(hyoscyamine sulfate USP)

LEVBID® Extended-Release Tablets
LEVSIN®/SL Tablets
LEVSIN® Tablets
LEVSIN® Elixir
LEVSIN® Drops (Oral Solution)
LEVSIN® Injection
LEVSINEX® TIMECAPS™
℞ **Only**

DESCRIPTION

levsin® (hyoscyamine sulfate USP) is one of the principal anticholinergic/antispasmodic components of belladonna alkaloids. The empirical formula is $(C_{17}H_{23}NO_3)_2 \cdot H_2SO_4 \cdot 2H_2O$ and the molecular weight is 712.85. Chemically, it is benzeneacetic acid, α-(hydroxymethyl)-,8-methyl-8-azabicyclo [3.2.1.] oct-3-yl ester, [3(S)-endo]-, sulfate (2:1), dihydrate.

levbid® extended-release tablets contain 0.375 mg of hyoscyamine sulfate in a formulation designed for oral b.i.d. dosage. Each levbid® extended-release tablet also contains as inactive ingredients: lactose, magnesium stearate, FD&C yellow #6 and other ingredients.

levsin®/SL tablets contain 0.125 mg hyoscyamine sulfate formulated for sublingual administration. However, the tablets may be chewed or taken orally. Each tablet also contains as inactive ingredients: colloidal silicon dioxide, dextrates, flavor, mannitol, and stearic acid.

levsin® tablets contain 0.125 mg hyoscyamine sulfate formulated for oral administration. Each tablet also contains as inactive ingredients: acacia, confectioner's sugar, corn starch, lactose, powdered cellulose and stearic acid.

levsin® elixir contains 0.125 mg hyoscyamine sulfate per 5 mL with 20% alcohol for oral administration. levsin® elixir also contains as inactive ingredients: FD&C red #40, FD&C yellow #6, flavor, glycerin, purified water, sorbitol solution and sucrose.

levsin® drops contain 0.125 mg hyoscyamine sulfate per mL with 5% alcohol for oral administration. levsin® drops also contain as inactive ingredients: FD&C red #40, FD&C yellow #6, flavor, glycerin, purified water, sodium citrate, sorbitol solution, and sucrose.

levsin® injection is a sterile solution containing 0.5 mg hyoscyamine sulfate per mL. The 1 mL ampuls contain as inactive ingredients: water for injection, pH is adjusted with hydrochloric acid when necessary.

levsinex® timecaps™ contain 0.375 mg hyoscyamine sulfate in an extended-release formulation designed for oral b.i.d. dosage. Each capsule also contains as inactive ingredients: FD&C blue #1, D&C red #28, FD&C red #40, FD&C yellow #6, gelatin, lactose monohydrate, sodium lauryl sulfate, magnesium stearate, silicon dioxide, titanium dioxide and other ingredients.

HOW SUPPLIED

levbid® (hyoscyamine sulfate, 0.375 mg) **extended-release tablets** are light orange, capsule-shaped, scored tablets. They are coded SP538.

Bottles of 100 tablets	NDC 0091-3538-01
Bottles of 500 tablets	NDC 0091-3538-05

levsin®/SL tablets (hyoscyamine sulfate tablets USP, 0.125 mg) are white, peppermint-flavored, octagonal shaped, scored, and imprinted with "SCHWARZ" on one side and "532" on the other.

Bottles of 100 tablets	NDC 0091-3532-01
Bottles of 500 tablets	NDC 0091-3532-05

levsin® tablets (hyoscyamine sulfate tablets USP, 0.125 mg) are white, scored and imprinted with "SCHWARZ" on one side and "531" on the other.

Bottles of 100 tablets	NDC 0091-3531-01
Bottles of 500 tablets	NDC 0091-3531-05

levsin® elixir (hyoscyamine sulfate elixir USP, 0.125 mg/5 mL) is orange colored and flavored and contains 20% alcohol.

Pints (473 mL) NDC 0091-4532-16

levsin® drops (hyoscyamine sulfate oral solution USP, 0.125 mg/mL) is orange colored and flavored.

15 mL dropper bottle NDC 0091-4538-15

levsin® injection (hyoscyamine sulfate injection USP, 0.5 mg/mL) is a clear, colorless and sterile solution.
1 mL ampuls-box of 5 NDC 0091-1536-05
levsinex® timecaps™ (hyoscyamine sulfate, 0.375 mg) Extended-Release Capsules are brown and white capsules imprinted "SCHWARZ" and "537."
Bottles of 100 capsules NDC 0091-3537-01
Bottles of 500 capsules NDC 0091-3537-05
Store at controlled room temperature 15°–30°C (59°–86°F).

MONOKET® TABLETS ℞
[män'-o-ket]
(isosorbide mononitrate)
℞ Only

DESCRIPTION
monoket®, an organic nitrate, is a vasodilator with effects on both arteries and veins. The empirical formula is $C_6H_9NO_6$ and the molecular weight is 191.14. The chemical name for Monoket® is 1,4:3,6-Dianhydro-D-glucitol 5-nitrate and the compound has the following structural formula:

[structural formula: H, OH, H, O, O, H, H, ONO_2]

monoket® is available in 10 mg and 20 mg tablets. Each tablet also contains as inactive ingredients: lactose, talc, colloidal silicon dioxide, starch, microcrystalline cellulose and aluminum stearate.

HOW SUPPLIED
monoket® (isosorbide mononitrate) 10 mg tablets are white, round, scored and engraved "10" on one side and engraved "SCHWARZ 610" on the other. They are supplied as follows:
Bottles of 100 NDC 0091-3610-01
monoket® (isosorbide mononitrate) 20 mg tablets are white, round, scored and engraved "20" on one side and engraved "SCHWARZ 620" on the other. They are supplied as follows:
Bottles of 100 NDC 0091-3620-01
Bottles of 180 NDC 0091-3620-18
Unit Dose Packages of 100 NDC 0091-3620-11
Store at controlled room temperature 15°–30°C (59°–86°F).
Keep tightly closed.
PC3734C Rev. 07/03

NULEV® ℞
[nū' lĕv]
(hyoscyamine sulfate orally disintegrating tablets)
0.125 mg
℞ Only

DESCRIPTION
NuLev® (hyoscyamine sulfate orally disintegrating tablets) 0.125 mg is formulated for oral administration using patented DuraSolv® technology. NuLev disintegrates within seconds after placement on the tongue, allowing it to be swallowed with or without water.
Hyoscyamine sulfate is one of the principal anticholinergic/antispasmodic components of belladonna alkaloids. The empirical formula is $(C_{17}H_{23}NO_3)_2 \bullet H_2SO_4 \bullet 2H_2O$ and the molecular weight is 712.85. Chemically, it is benzeneacetic acid, α-(hydroxymethyl)-, 8-methyl-8-azabicyclo [3.2.1.] oct-3-yl ester, [3(S)-endo]-, sulfate (2:1), dihydrate with the following structure:

[structural formula: N–CH_3; CH_2OH · H_2SO_4 · $2H_2O$; OOCCH; C_6H_5;]$_2$]

Each tablet also contains as inactive ingredients: aspartame, colloidal silicon dioxide, crospovidone, flavor, magnesium stearate, mannitol, microcrystalline cellulose.

HOW SUPPLIED
NuLev® (hyoscyamine sulfate orally disintegrating tablets) 0.125 mg are white, mint-flavored, round and imprinted with SP and 111.
Bottles of 100 tablets NDC 0091-3111-01
Store at 25°C (77°F); excursions permitted to 15–30°C (59–86°F).
Protect from moisture.
Dispense in tight, light-resistant container as defined in USP.
Manufactured For:
SCHWARZ
PHARMA
Milwaukee, Wisconsin 53201, USA
By:
CIMA™
Eden Prairie, MN 55344
NuLev® uses CIMA's DuraSolv® technology.
U.S. Patent Nos. 6,024,981 and 6,221,392.
PC4205A Rev. 03/03

PARCOPA™ ℞
(carbidopa-levodopa orally disintegrating tablets)

Rx only

DESCRIPTION
PARCOPA™ (carbidopa-levodopa orally disintegrating tablets) is a combination of carbidopa and levodopa for the treatment of Parkinson's disease and syndrome.
PARCOPA™ is an orally administered formulation of carbidopa-levodopa which rapidly disintegrates on the tongue and does not require water to aid dissolution or swallowing.
Carbidopa, an inhibitor of aromatic amino acid decarboxylation, is a white, crystalline compound, slightly soluble in water, with a molecular weight of 244.24. It is designated chemically as (–)-L-α-hydrazino-α-methyl-β-(3,4-dihydroxybenzene) propanoic acid monohydrate. Its empirical formula is $C_{10}H_{14}N_2O_4 \bullet H_2O$, and its structural formula is:

[structural formula: OH, HO, CH_3, CH_2CCOOH, $NHNH_2$, $\bullet H_2O$]

Tablet content is expressed in terms of anhydrous carbidopa which has a molecular weight of 226.23.
Levodopa, an aromatic amino acid, is a white, crystalline compound, slightly soluble in water, with a molecular weight of 197.2. It is designated chemically as (–)-L-α-amino-β-(3,4-dihydroxybenzene) propanoic acid. Its empirical formula is $C_9H_{11}NO_4$, and its structural formula is:

[structural formula: OH, HO, $CH_2CHCOOH$, NH_2]

PARCOPA™ is supplied as tablets in three strengths:
PARCOPA™ 25/100, containing 25 mg of carbidopa and 100 mg of levodopa.
PARCOPA™ 10/100, containing 10 mg of carbidopa and 100 mg of levodopa.
PARCOPA™ 25/250, containing 25 mg of carbidopa and 250 mg of levodopa.
Inactive ingredients are aspartame, citric acid, crospovidone, magnesium stearate, mannitol, microcrystalline cellulose, natural and artificial mint flavor and sodium bicarbonate. PARCOPA™ 10/100 and 25/250 also contain FD&C blue #2 HT aluminum lake. PARCOPA™ 25/100 also contains yellow 10 iron oxide.

CLINICAL PHARMACOLOGY
Parkinson's disease is a progressive, neurodegenerative disorder of the extrapyramidal nervous system affecting the mobility and control of the skeletal muscular system. Its characteristic features include resting tremor, rigidity, and bradykinetic movements. Symptomatic treatments, such as levodopa therapies, may permit the patient better mobility.

Mechanism of Action
Current evidence indicates that symptoms of Parkinson's disease are related to depletion of dopamine in the corpus striatum. Administration of dopamine is ineffective in the treatment of Parkinson's disease apparently because it does not cross the blood-brain barrier. However, levodopa, the metabolic precursor of dopamine, does cross the blood-brain barrier, and presumably is converted to dopamine in the brain. This is thought to be the mechanism whereby levodopa relieves symptoms of Parkinson's disease.

Pharmacodynamics
When levodopa is administered orally it is rapidly decarboxylated to dopamine in extracerebral tissues so that only a small portion of a given dose is transported unchanged to the central nervous system. For this reason, large doses of levodopa are required for adequate therapeutic effect and these may often be accompanied by nausea and other adverse reactions, some of which are attributable to dopamine formed in extracerebral tissues.
Since levodopa competes with certain amino acids for transport across the gut wall, the absorption of levodopa may be impaired in some patients on a high protein diet.
Carbidopa inhibits decarboxylation of peripheral levodopa. It does not cross the blood-brain barrier and does not affect the metabolism of levodopa within the central nervous system.
The incidence of levodopa-induced nausea and vomiting is less with carbidopa-levodopa than with levodopa. In many patients, this reduction in nausea and vomiting will permit more rapid dosage titration.
Since its decarboxylase inhibiting activity is limited to extracerebral tissues, administration of carbidopa with levodopa makes more levodopa available for transport to the brain.

Pharmacokinetics
Carbidopa reduces the amount of levodopa required to produce a given response by about 75 percent and, when administered with levodopa, increases both plasma levels and the plasma half-life of levodopa, and decreases plasma and urinary dopamine and homovanillic acid.
The plasma half-life of levodopa is about 50 minutes, without carbidopa. When carbidopa and levodopa are administered together, the half-life of levodopa is increased to about 1.5 hours. At steady state, the bioavailability of carbidopa from carbidopa-levodopa tablets is approximately 99% relative to the concomitant administration of carbidopa and levodopa.
In clinical pharmacologic studies, simultaneous administration of carbidopa and levodopa produced greater urinary excretion of levodopa in proportion to the excretion of dopamine than administration of the two drugs at separate times.
Pyridoxine hydrochloride (vitamin B_6), in oral doses of 10 mg to 25 mg, may reverse the effects of levodopa by increasing the rate of aromatic amino acid decarboxylation. Carbidopa inhibits this action of pyridoxine; therefore, PARCOPA™ can be given to patients receiving supplemental pyridoxine (vitamin B_6).

INDICATIONS AND USAGE
PARCOPA™ is indicated in the treatment of the symptoms of idiopathic Parkinson's disease (paralysis agitans), postencephalitic parkinsonism, and symptomatic parkinsonism which may follow injury to the nervous system by carbon monoxide intoxication and/or manganese intoxication.
PARCOPA™ is indicated in these conditions to permit the administration of lower doses of levodopa with reduced nausea and vomiting, with more rapid dosage titration, with a somewhat smoother response, and with supplemental pyridoxine (vitamin B_6).
In some patients, a somewhat smoother antiparkinsonian effect results from therapy with carbidopa-levodopa than with levodopa. However, patients with markedly irregular ("on-off") responses to levodopa have not been shown to benefit from carbidopa-levodopa therapy.
Although the administration of carbidopa permits control of parkinsonism and Parkinson's disease with much lower doses of levodopa, there is no conclusive evidence at present that this is beneficial other than in reducing nausea and vomiting, permitting more rapid titration, and providing a somewhat smoother response to levodopa.
Certain patients who responded poorly to levodopa have improved when carbidopa-levodopa was substituted. This is most likely due to decreased peripheral decarboxylation of levodopa which results from administration of carbidopa rather than to a primary effect of carbidopa on the nervous system. Carbidopa has not been shown to enhance the intrinsic efficacy of levodopa in parkinsonian syndromes.
In considering whether to give PARCOPA™ to patients already on levodopa who have nausea and/or vomiting, the practitioner should be aware that, while many patients may be expected to improve, some do not. Since one cannot predict which patients are likely to improve, this can only be determined by a trial of therapy. It should be further noted that in controlled trials comparing carbidopa-levodopa with levodopa, about half of the patients with nausea and/or vomiting on levodopa improved spontaneously despite being retained on the same dose of levodopa during the controlled portion of the trial.

CONTRAINDICATIONS
Nonselective monoamine oxidase (MAO) inhibitors are contraindicated for use with PARCOPA™. These inhibitors must be discontinued at least two weeks prior to initiating therapy with PARCOPA™. PARCOPA™ may be administered concomitantly with the manufacturer's recommended dose of an MAO inhibitor with selectivity for MAO type B (e.g., selegiline HCl) (See PRECAUTIONS, *Drug Interactions*).
PARCOPA™ is contraindicated in patients with known hypersensitivity to any component of this drug, and in patients with narrow-angle glaucoma.
Because levodopa may activate a malignant melanoma, PARCOPA™ should not be used in patients with suspicious, undiagnosed skin lesions or a history of melanoma.

WARNINGS
When PARCOPA™ (carbidopa-levodopa orally disintegrating tablets) is to be given to patients who are being treated with levodopa, levodopa must be discontinued at least twelve hours before therapy with PARCOPA™ (carbidopa-levodopa orally disintegrating tablets) is started. In order to reduce adverse reactions, it is necessary to individualize therapy. See DOSAGE AND ADMINISTRATION section before initiating therapy.
The addition of carbidopa with levodopa in the form of PARCOPA™ reduces the peripheral effects (nausea, vomiting) due to decarboxylation of levodopa; however, carbidopa does not decrease the adverse reactions due to the central effects of levodopa. Because carbidopa permits more levodopa to reach the brain and more dopamine to be formed, certain adverse CNS effects, e.g., dyskinesias (involuntary movements), may occur at lower dosages and sooner with PARCOPA™ than with levodopa alone.
Levodopa alone, as well as PARCOPA™, is associated with dyskinesias. The occurrence of dyskinesias may require dosage reduction.
As with levodopa, PARCOPA™ may cause mental disturbances. These reactions are thought to be due to increased brain dopamine following administration of levodopa. All

Continued on next page

Parcopa—Cont.

patients should be observed carefully for the development of depression with concomitant suicidal tendencies. Patients with past or current psychoses should be treated with caution.

PARCOPA™ should be administered cautiously to patients with severe cardiovascular or pulmonary disease, bronchial asthma, renal, hepatic or endocrine disease.

As with levodopa, care should be exercised in administering PARCOPA™ to patients with a history of myocardial infarction who have residual atrial, nodal, or ventricular arrhythmias. In such patients, cardiac function should be monitored with particular care during the period of initial dosage adjustment, in a facility with provisions for intensive cardiac care.

As with levodopa, treatment with PARCOPA™ may increase the possibility of upper gastrointestinal hemorrhage in patients with a history of peptic ulcer.

Neuroleptic Malignant Syndrome (NMS): Sporadic cases of a symptom complex resembling NMS have been reported in association with dose reductions or withdrawal of therapy with carbidopa-levodopa. Therefore, patients should be observed carefully when the dosage of PARCOPA™ is reduced abruptly or discontinued, especially if the patient is receiving neuroleptics.

NMS is an uncommon but life-threatening syndrome characterized by fever or hyperthermia. Neurological findings, including muscle rigidity, involuntary movements, altered consciousness, mental status changes; other disturbances, such as autonomic dysfunction, tachycardia, tachypnea, sweating, hyper- or hypotension; laboratory findings, such as creatine phosphokinase elevation, leukocytosis, myoglobinuria, and increased serum myoglobin have been reported.

The early diagnosis of this condition is important for the appropriate management of these patients. Considering NMS as a possible diagnosis and ruling out other acute illnesses (e.g., pneumonia, systemic infection, etc.) is essential. This may be especially complex if the clinical presentation includes both serious medical illness and untreated or inadequately treated extrapyramidal signs and symptoms (EPS). Other important considerations in the differential diagnosis include central anticholinergic toxicity, heat stroke, drug fever, and primary central nervous system (CNS) pathology.

The management of NMS should include: 1) intensive symptomatic treatment and medical monitoring and 2) treatment of any concomitant serious medical problems for which specific treatments are available. Dopamine agonists, such as bromocriptine, and muscle relaxants, such as dantrolene, are often used in the treatment of NMS, however, their effectiveness has not been demonstrated in controlled studies.

PRECAUTIONS

General

As with levodopa, periodic evaluations of hepatic, hematopoietic, cardiovascular, and renal function are recommended during extended therapy.

Patients with chronic wide-angle glaucoma may be treated cautiously with PARCOPA™ provided the intraocular pressure is well controlled and the patient is monitored carefully for changes in intraocular pressure during therapy.

Information for Patients

Phenylketonurics

Phenylketonuric patients should be informed that PARCOPA™ contains phenylalanine 3.4 mg per 25/100 orally disintegrating tablet, 3.4 mg per 10/100 orally disintegrating tablet, and 8.4 mg per 25/250 orally disintegrating tablet.

Patients should be instructed not to remove PARCOPA™ Tablets from the bottle until just prior to dosing. With dry hands, the tablet should be gently removed and immediately placed on the tongue to dissolve and be swallowed with the saliva.

The patient should be informed that PARCOPA™ is an immediate-release formulation of carbidopa-levodopa that is designed to begin release of ingredients within 30 minutes. It is important that PARCOPA™ be taken at regular intervals according to the schedule outlined by the physician. The patient should be cautioned not to change the prescribed dosage regimen and not to add any additional antiparkinson medications, including other carbidopa-levodopa preparations, without first consulting the physician.

Patients should be advised that sometimes a "wearing-off" effect may occur at the end of the dosing interval. The physician should be notified if such response poses a problem to lifestyle.

Patients should be advised that occasionally, dark color (red, brown, or black) may appear in saliva, urine, or sweat after ingestion of PARCOPA™. Although the color appears to be clinically insignificant, garments may become discolored.

The patient should be advised that a change in diet to foods that are high in protein may delay the absorption of levodopa and may reduce the amount taken up in the circulation. Excessive acidity also delays stomach emptying, thus delaying the absorption of levodopa. Iron salts (such as in multi-vitamin tablets) may also reduce the amount of levodopa available to the body. The above factors may reduce the clinical effectiveness of the levodopa or carbidopa-levodopa therapy.

NOTE: The suggested advice to patients being treated with PARCOPA™ is intended to aid in the safe and effective use of this medication. It is not a disclosure of all possible adverse or intended effects.

Laboratory Tests

Abnormalities in laboratory tests may include elevations of liver function tests such as alkaline phosphatase, SGOT (AST), SGPT (ALT), lactic dehydrogenase, and bilirubin. Abnormalities in blood urea nitrogen and positive Coombs test have also been reported. Commonly, levels of blood urea nitrogen, creatinine, and uric acid are lower during administration of carbidopa-levodopa than with levodopa.

Carbidopa-levodopa may cause a false-positive reaction for urinary ketone bodies when a test tape is used for determination of ketonuria. This reaction will not be altered by boiling the urine specimen. False-negative tests may result with the use of glucose-oxidase methods of testing for glucosuria.

Cases of falsely diagnosed pheochromocytoma in patients on carbidopa-levodopa therapy have been reported very rarely. Caution should be exercised when interpreting the plasma and urine levels of catecholamines and their metabolites in patients on levodopa or carbidopa-levodopa therapy.

Drug Interactions

Caution should be exercised when the following drugs are administered concomitantly with PARCOPA™ (carbidopa-levodopa orally disintegrating tablets).

Symptomatic postural hypotension has occurred when carbidopa-levodopa was added to the treatment of a patient receiving antihypertensive drugs. Therefore, when therapy with PARCOPA™ is started, dosage adjustment of the antihypertensive drug may be required.

For patients receiving MAO inhibitors (Type A or B), see CONTRAINDICATIONS. Concomitant therapy with selegiline and carbidopa-levodopa may be associated with severe orthostatic hypotension not attributable to carbidopa-levodopa alone (see CONTRAINDICATIONS).

There have been rare reports of adverse reactions, including hypertension and dyskinesia, resulting from the concomitant use of tricyclic antidepressants and carbidopa-levodopa.

Dopamine D_2 receptor antagonists (e.g., phenothiazines, butyrophenones, risperidone) and isoniazid may reduce the therapeutic effects of levodopa. In addition, the beneficial effects of levodopa in Parkinson's disease have been reported to be reversed by phenytoin and papaverine. Patients taking these drugs with PARCOPA™ should be carefully observed for loss of therapeutic response.

Iron salts may reduce the bioavailability of levodopa and carbidopa. The clinical relevance is unclear.

Although metoclopramide may increase the bioavailability of levodopa by increasing gastric emptying, metoclopramide may also adversely affect disease control by its dopamine receptor antagonistic properties.

Carcinogenesis, Mutagenesis, Impairment of Fertility

In a two-year bioassay of carbidopa and levodopa, no evidence of carcinogenicity was found in rats receiving doses of approximately two times the maximum daily human dose of carbidopa and four times the maximum daily human dose of levodopa.

In reproduction studies with carbidopa and levodopa, no effects on fertility were found in rats receiving doses of approximately two times the maximum daily human dose of carbidopa and four times the maximum daily human dose of levodopa.

Pregnancy

Pregnancy Category C. No teratogenic effects were observed in a study in mice receiving up to 20 times the maximum recommended human dose of carbidopa and levodopa. There was a decrease in the number of live pups delivered by rats receiving approximately two times the maximum recommended human dose of carbidopa and approximately five times the maximum recommended human dose of levodopa during organogenesis. Carbidopa and levodopa caused both visceral and skeletal malformations in rabbits at all doses and ratios of carbidopa/levodopa tested, which ranged from 10 times/5 times the maximum recommended human dose of carbidopa/levodopa to 20 times/10 times the maximum recommended human dose of carbidopa/levodopa.

There are no adequate or well-controlled studies in pregnant women. It has been reported from individual cases that levodopa crosses the human placental barrier, enters the fetus, and is metabolized. Carbidopa concentrations in fetal tissue appeared to be minimal. Use of PARCOPA™ in women of childbearing potential requires that the anticipated benefits of the drug be weighed against possible hazards to mother and child.

Nursing Mothers

It is not known whether this drug is excreted in human milk. Because many drugs are excreted in human milk, caution should be exercised when PARCOPA™ is administered to a nursing woman.

Pediatric Use

Safety and effectiveness in pediatric patients have not been established. Use of the drug in patients below the age of 18 is not recommended.

ADVERSE REACTIONS

The most common adverse reactions reported with carbidopa-levodopa therapy have included dyskinesias, such as choreiform, dystonic, and other involuntary movements and nausea.

The following other adverse reactions have been reported with carbidopa-levodopa:

Body as a Whole: chest pain, asthenia.

Cardiovascular: cardiac irregularities, hypotension, orthostatic effects including orthostatic hypotension, hypertension, syncope, phlebitis, palpitation.

Gastrointestinal: dark saliva, gastrointestinal bleeding, development of duodenal ulcer, anorexia, vomiting, diarrhea, constipation, dyspepsia, dry mouth, taste alterations.

Hematologic: agranulocytosis, hemolytic and non-hemolytic anemia, thrombocytopenia, leukopenia.

Hypersensitivity: angioedema, urticaria, pruritus, Henoch-Schonlein purpura, bullous lesions (including pemphigus-like reactions).

Musculoskeletal: back pain, shoulder pain, muscle cramps.

Nervous System/Psychiatric: psychotic episodes including delusions, hallucinations, and paranoid ideation, neuroleptic malignant syndrome (see WARNINGS), bradykinetic episodes ("on-off" phenomenon), confusion, agitation, dizziness, somnolence, dream abnormalities including nightmares, insomnia, paresthesia, headache, depression with or without development of suicidal tendencies, dementia, increased libido. Convulsions also have occurred; however, a causal relationship with carbidopa-levodopa has not been established.

Respiratory: dyspnea, upper respiratory infection.

Skin: rash, increased sweating, alopecia, dark sweat.

Urogenital: urinary tract infection, urinary frequency, dark urine.

Laboratory Tests: decreased hemoglobin and hematocrit; abnormalities in alkaline phosphatase, SGOT (AST), SGPT (ALT), lactic dehydrogenase, bilirubin, blood urea nitrogen (BUN), Coombs test; elevated serum glucose; white blood cells, bacteria, and blood in the urine.

Other adverse reactions that have been reported with levodopa alone and with various carbidopa-levodopa formulations, and may occur with PARCOPA™ are:

Body as a Whole: abdominal pain and distress, fatigue.

Cardiovascular: myocardial infarction.

Gastrointestinal: gastrointestinal pain, dysphagia, sialorrhea, flatulence, bruxism, burning sensation of the tongue, heartburn, hiccups.

Metabolic: edema, weight gain, weight loss.

Musculoskeletal: leg pain.

Nervous System/Psychiatric: ataxia, extrapyramidal disorder, falling, anxiety, gait abnormalities, nervousness, decreased mental acuity, memory impairment, disorientation, euphoria, blepharospasm (which may be taken as an early sign of excess dosage; consideration of dosage reduction may be made at this time), trismus, increased tremor, numbness, muscle twitching, activation of latent Horner's syndrome, peripheral neuropathy.

Respiratory: pharyngeal pain, cough.

Skin: malignant melanoma (see also CONTRAINDICATIONS), flushing.

Special Senses: oculogyric crises, diplopia, blurred vision, dilated pupils.

Urogenital: urinary retention, urinary incontinence, priapism.

Miscellaneous: bizarre breathing patterns, faintness, hoarseness, malaise, hot flashes, sense of stimulation.

Laboratory Tests: decreased white blood cell count and serum potassium; increased serum creatinine and uric acid; protein and glucose in urine.

OVERDOSAGE

Management of acute overdosage with PARCOPA™ is the same as management of acute overdosage with levodopa. Pyridoxine is not effective in reversing the actions of PARCOPA™.

General supportive measures should be employed, along with immediate gastric lavage. Intravenous fluids should be administered judiciously and an adequate airway maintained. Electrocardiographic monitoring should be instituted and the patient carefully observed for the development of arrhythmias; if required, appropriate antiarrhythmic therapy should be given. The possibility that the patient may have taken other drugs as well as PARCOPA™ should be taken into consideration. To date, no experience has been reported with dialysis; hence, its value in overdosage is not known.

Based on studies in which high doses of levodopa and/or carbidopa were administered, a significant proportion of rats and mice given single oral doses of levodopa of approximately 1500-2000 mg/kg are expected to die. A significant proportion of infant rats of both sexes are expected to die at a dose of 800 mg/kg. A significant proportion of rats are expected to die after treatment with similar doses of carbidopa. The addition of carbidopa in a 1:10 ratio with levodopa increases the dose at which a significant proportion of mice are expected to die to 3360 mg/kg.

DOSAGE AND ADMINISTRATION

Instructions for Use/Handling PARCOPA™ Tablets

Just prior to administration, GENTLY remove the tablet from the bottle with dry hands. IMMEDIATELY place the PARCOPA™ Tablet on top of the tongue where it will dissolve in seconds, then swallow with saliva. Administration with liquid is not necessary.

The optimum daily dosage of PARCOPA™ must be determined by careful titration in each patient. PARCOPA™ is available in a 1:4 ratio of carbidopa to levodopa (PARCOPA™ 25/100) as well as 1:10 ratio (PARCOPA™ 25/250 and PARCOPA™ 10/100). Tablets of the two ratios may be given separately or combined as needed to provide the optimum dosage.

Studies show that peripheral dopa decarboxylase is saturated by carbidopa at approximately 70 to 100 mg a day. Patients receiving less than this amount of carbidopa are more likely to experience nausea and vomiting.

Usual Initial Dosage

Dosage is best initiated with one tablet of PARCOPA™ 25/100 three times a day. This dosage schedule provides 75 mg of carbidopa per day. Dosage may be increased by one tablet every day or every other day, as necessary, until a dosage of eight tablets of PARCOPA™ 25/100 a day is reached.

If PARCOPA™ 10/100 is used, dosage may be initiated with one tablet three or four times a day. However, this will not provide an adequate amount of carbidopa for many patients. Dosage may be increased by one tablet every day or every other day until a total of eight tablets (2 tablets q.i.d.) is reached.

How to Transfer Patients from Levodopa

Levodopa must be discontinued at least twelve hours before starting PARCOPA™ (carbidopa-levodopa orally disintegrating tablets). A daily dosage of PARCOPA™ should be chosen that will provide approximately 25 percent of the previous levodopa dosage. Patients who are taking less than 1500 mg of levodopa a day should be started on one tablet of PARCOPA™ 25/100 three or four times a day. The suggested starting dosage for most patients taking more than 1500 mg of levodopa is one tablet of PARCOPA™ 25/250 three or four times a day.

Maintenance

Therapy should be individualized and adjusted according to the desired therapeutic response. At least 70 to 100 mg of carbidopa per day should be provided. When a greater proportion of carbidopa is required, one tablet of PARCOPA™ 25/100 may be substituted for each tablet of PARCOPA™ 10/100. When more levodopa is required, PARCOPA™ 25/250 should be substituted for PARCOPA™ 25/100 or PARCOPA™ 10/100. If necessary, the dosage of PARCOPA™ 25/250 may be increased by one-half or one tablet every day or every other day to a maximum of eight tablets a day. Experience with total daily dosages of carbidopa greater than 200 mg is limited.

Because both therapeutic and adverse responses occur more rapidly with PARCOPA™ than with levodopa alone, patients should be monitored closely during the dose adjustment period. Specifically, involuntary movements will occur more rapidly with PARCOPA™ than with levodopa. The occurrence of involuntary movements may require dosage reduction. Blepharospasm may be a useful early sign of excess dosage in some patients.

Addition of Other Antiparkinsonian Medications

Standard drugs for Parkinson's disease, other than levodopa without a decarboxylase inhibitor, may be used concomitantly while PARCOPA™ is being administered, although dosage adjustments may be required.

Interruption of Therapy

Sporadic cases of a symptom complex resembling Neuroleptic Malignant Syndrome (NMS) have been associated with dose reductions and withdrawal of carbidopa-levodopa. Patients should be observed carefully if abrupt reduction or discontinuation of PARCOPA™ is required, especially if the patient is receiving neuroleptics. (See WARNINGS.)

If general anesthesia is required, PARCOPA™ may be continued as long as the patient is permitted to take fluids and medication by mouth. If therapy is interrupted temporarily, the patient should be observed for symptoms resembling NMS, and the usual daily dosage may be administered as soon as the patient is able to take oral medication.

HOW SUPPLIED

PARCOPA™ (carbidopa-levodopa orally disintegrating tablets) 25/100 are yellow, round, flat-faced, mint-flavored, scored and engraved "25/100" on the unscored side and "SP" above and "342" below the score on the other side. They are supplied as follows:

Bottles of 100 NDC 0091-3342-01

PARCOPA™ (carbidopa-levodopa orally disintegrating tablets) 10/100 are blue, round, flat-faced, mint-flavored, scored and engraved "10/100" on the unscored side and "SP" above and "341" below the score on the other side. They are supplied as follows:

Bottles of 100 NDC 0091-3341-01

PARCOPA™ (carbidopa-levodopa orally disintegrating tablets) 25/250 are blue, round, flat-faced, mint-flavored, scored, and engraved "25/250" on the unscored side and "SP" above and "343" below the score on the other side. They are supplied as follows:

Bottles of 100 NDC 0091-3343-01

Storage

Store at 20° to 25°C (68° to 77°F); excursions permitted between 15° to 30°C (59° to 86°F) [See USP Controlled Room Temperature]. Protect from moisture and light.

Dispense in a tight, light-resistant container as defined in the USP/NF.

Manufactured for:
SCHWARZ PHARMA
Milwaukee, WI 53201, USA
By:
CIMA LABS INC.®
Eden Prairie, MN 55344, USA
PARCOPA™ uses CIMA® U.S. Patent Nos. 6,024,981 and 6,221,392.
PC4578
Rev. 01/03

PROCTOCREAM®•HC 2.5% ℞

(hydrocortisone cream USP, 2.5%)
[topical]
℞ Only

DESCRIPTION

proctoCream®•HC 2.5% contains Hydrocortisone [Pregn-4-ene-3, 20-dione, 11, 17,21-trihydroxy-, (11β)-] with the molecular formula $C_{21}H_{30}O_5$ and a molecular weight of 362.47, CAS 50-23-7. Each gram for topical administration contains: 25 mg of hydrocortisone in a base of glyceryl monostearate, polyoxyl 40 stearate, glycerin, paraffin, stearyl alcohol, isopropyl palmitate, sorbitan monostearate, benzyl alcohol, potassium sorbate, lactic acid, and purified water.

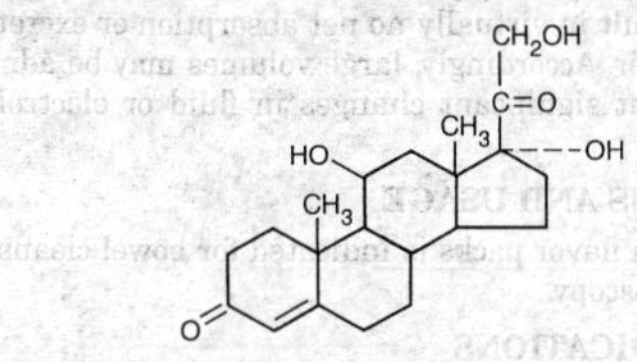

CH2OH C=O CH3 OH HO CH3 O

HOW SUPPLIED

proctoCream®•HC 2.5% (hydrocortisone cream USP, 2.5%) is supplied in 30 gram tubes.

30 g NDC 0091-4640-24

Store at controlled room temperature 15°-30°C (59°-86°F).

PC2178B Rev. 01/02

PROCTOFOAM®-HC ℞

(hydrocortisone acetate 1%
and pramoxine hydrochloride 1%)
topical aerosol
℞ Only

DESCRIPTION

Proctofoam®-HC (hydrocortisone acetate 1% and pramoxine hydrochloride 1%) is a topical aerosol foam for anal use containing hydrocortisone acetate 1% and pramoxine hydrochloride 1% in a hydrophilic base containing cetyl alcohol, emulsifying wax, methylparaben, polyoxyethylene-10 stearyl ether, propylene glycol, propylparaben, purified water, trolamine, and inert propellants: isobutane and propane.

Proctofoam®-HC contains a synthetic corticosteroid used as an anti-inflammatory/antipruritic agent and a local anesthetic.

Hydrocortisone acetate

Molecular weight: 404.50. Solubility of hydrocortisone acetate in water: 1 mg/100 mL.

Chemical name: pregn-4-ene-3,20-dione, 21-(acetyloxy)-11, 17-dihydroxy-,(11β)-.

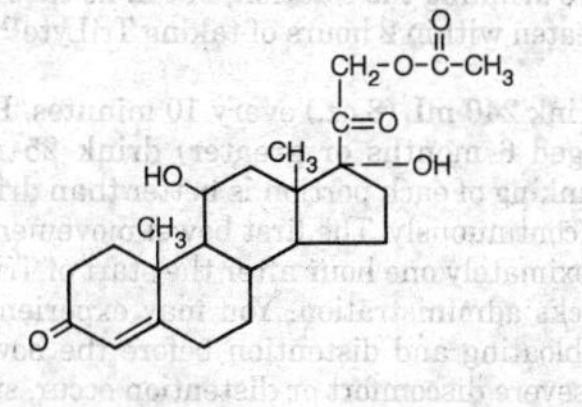

CH2-O-C-CH3 O C=O CH3 OH HO CH3 O

Pramoxine hydrochloride

Molecular weight: 329.86. Pramoxine hydrochloride is freely soluble in water.

Chemical name: morpholine, 4-[3-(4-butoxyphenoxy) propyl]-, hydrochloride.

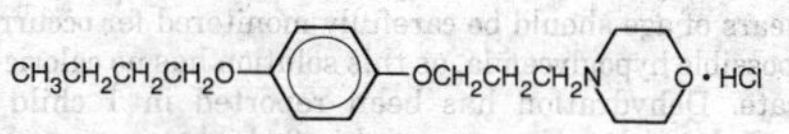

CH3CH2CH2CH2O— —OCH2CH2CH2N O • HCl

CLINICAL PHARMACOLOGY

Topical corticosteroids share anti-inflammatory, antipruritic and vasoconstrictive actions.

The mechanism of anti-inflammatory activity of the topical corticosteroids is unclear. Various laboratory methods, including vasoconstrictor assays, are used to compare and predict potencies and/or clinical efficacies of the topical corticosteroids. There is some evidence to suggest that a recognizable correlation exists between vasoconstrictor potency and therapeutic efficacy in man.

Pramoxine hydrochloride is a surface or local anesthetic which is not chemically related to the "caine" types of local anesthetics. Its unique chemical structure is likely to minimize the danger of cross-sensitivity reactions in patients allergic to other local anesthetics.

Pharmacokinetics: The extent of percutaneous absorption of topical corticosteroids is determined by many factors including the vehicle, the integrity of the epidermal barrier, and the use of occlusive dressings.

Topical corticosteroids can be absorbed through normal intact skin. Inflammation and/or other disease processes in the skin increase the percutaneous absorption of topical corticosteroids. Occlusive dressings substantially increase the percutaneous absorption of topical corticosteroids. Thus, occlusive dressings may be a valuable therapeutic adjunct for treatment of resistant dermatoses. (See DOSAGE AND ADMINISTRATION.)

Once absorbed through the skin, topical corticosteroids are handled through pharmacokinetic pathways similar to systemically administered corticosteroids. Corticosteroids are bound to plasma proteins in varying degrees. Corticosteroids are metabolized primarily in the liver and are then excreted by the kidneys. Some of the topical corticosteroids and their metabolites are also excreted into the bile.

INDICATIONS AND USAGE

Proctofoam®-HC is indicated for the relief of the inflammatory and pruritic manifestations of corticosteroid-responsive dermatoses of the anal region.

CONTRAINDICATIONS

Topical corticosteroid products are contraindicated in those patients with a history of hypersensitivity to any of the components of the preparation.

WARNINGS

Do not insert any part of the aerosol container directly into the anus. Avoid contact with the eyes. Contents of the container are under pressure. Do not burn or puncture the aerosol container. Do not store at temperature above 120°F (49°C). If there is no evidence of clinical improvement within two or three weeks after starting Proctofoam®-HC therapy, or if the patient's condition worsens, discontinue the drug. Keep this and all medicines out of the reach of children.

PRECAUTIONS

General: Systemic absorption of topical corticosteroids has produced reversible hypothalamic-pituitary-adrenal (HPA) axis suppression, manifestations of Cushing's syndrome, hyperglycemia, and glucosuria in some patients.

Conditions which augment systemic absorption include the application of the more potent steroids, use over large surface areas, prolonged use, and the addition of occlusive dressings. Therefore, patients receiving a large dose of a potent topical steroid applied to a large surface area or under an occlusive dressing should be evaluated periodically for evidence of HPA axis suppression by using the urinary free cortisol and ACTH stimulation tests. If HPA axis suppression is noted, an attempt should be made to withdraw the drug, to reduce the frequency of application, or to substitute a less potent steroid.

Recovery of HPA axis function is generally prompt and complete upon discontinuation of the drug. Infrequently, signs and symptoms of steroid withdrawal may occur, requiring supplemental systemic corticosteroids.

Pediatric patients may absorb proportionally larger amounts of topical corticosteroids and thus be more susceptible to systemic toxicity. (see PRECAUTIONS – *Pediatric Use.*)

If irritation develops, topical corticosteroids should be discontinued and appropriate therapy instituted.

In the presence of dermatological infections, the use of an appropriate antifungal or antibacterial agent should be instituted. If a favorable response does not occur promptly, the corticosteroid should be discontinued until the infection has been adequately controlled.

Information for the Patient: Patients using topical corticosteroids should receive the following information and instructions:

1. This medication is to be used as directed by the physician. It is for anal or perianal use only. Avoid contact with eyes.
2. Be advised not to use this medication for any disorder other than for which it has been prescribed.
3. Report any signs of adverse reactions.

Laboratory Tests: The following tests may be helpful in evaluating the HPA axis suppression:

Urinary free cortisol test
ACTH stimulation test

Carcinogenesis, Mutagenesis, Impairment of Fertility: Long-term animal studies have not been performed to evaluate the carcinogenic potential or the effect on fertility of topical corticosteroids.

Studies to determine mutagenicity with prednisolone and hydrocortisone have revealed negative results.

Pregnancy: Teratogenic Effects. Pregnancy Category C. Corticosteroids are generally teratogenic in laboratory animals when administered systemically at relatively low dosage levels. The more potent corticosteroids have been shown to be teratogenic after dermal application in laboratory animals. There are no adequate, well-controlled studies of teratogenic effects from topically applied corticosteroids in pregnant women. Therefore, topical corticosteroids should be used during pregnancy only if the potential benefit justifies the potential risk to the fetus. Drugs of this class should not be used extensively on pregnant patients, in large amounts, or for prolonged periods of time.

Nursing Mothers: It is not known whether topical administration of corticosteroids could result in sufficient systemic absorption to produce detectable quantities in breast milk. Systemically administered corticosteroids are secreted into breast milk in quantities *not* likely to have a deleterious effect on the infant. Nevertheless, caution should be exercised when topical corticosteroids are administered to a nursing woman.

Continued on next page

Proctofoam-HC—Cont.

Pediatric Use: Pediatric patients may demonstrate greater susceptibility to topical corticosteroid-induced HPA axis suppression and Cushing's syndrome than mature patients because of a larger skin surface area to body weight ratio.
Hypothalamic-pituitary-adrenal (HPA) axis suppression, Cushing's syndrome, and intracranial hypertension have been reported in pediatric patients receiving topical corticosteroids. Manifestations of adrenal suppression in pediatric patients include linear growth retardation, delayed weight gain, low plasma cortisol levels, and absense of response to ACTH stimulation. Manifestations of intracranial hypertension include bulging fontanelles, headaches, and bilateral papilledema.
Administration of topical corticosteroids to pediatric patients should be limited to the least amount compatible with an effective therapeutic regimen. Chronic corticosteroid therapy may interfere with the growth and development of pediatric patients.

ADVERSE REACTIONS

The following local adverse reactions are reported infrequently with topical corticosteroids, but may occur more frequently with the use of occlusive dressings. These reactions are listed in an approximate decreasing order of occurrence: burning, itching, irritation, dryness, folliculitis, hypertrichosis, acneiform eruptions, hypopigmentation, perioral dermatitis, allergic contact dermatitis, maceration of the skin, secondary infection, skin atrophy, striae and miliaria.

OVERDOSAGE

Topically applied corticosteroids can be absorbed in sufficient amounts to produce systemic effects. (See PRECAUTIONS.)

DOSAGE AND ADMINISTRATION

Apply to affected area 3 to 4 times daily. Use the applicator supplied for anal administration. For perianal use, transfer a small quantity to a tissue and rub in gently.
Directions for Use.

1. Place cap on top of container. Shake foam container vigorously for 5–10 seconds before each use. **Do not remove container cap during use of the product.**
2. Hold container upright on a level surface and gently place the tip of the applicator onto the nose of the container cap. **CONTAINER MUST BE HELD UPRIGHT TO OBTAIN PROPER FLOW OF MEDICATION.**
3. Pull plunger past the fill line on the applicator barrel.
4. Hold the container and applicator at eye level. Place the index and middle fingers on the container cap flanges and the thumb beneath the container. Support the applicator with your other hand. Prime the container by pressing down firmly on flanges and then release. With initial priming, a burst of air may come out of the container. It usually requires 1–2 pumps for foam to appear.
5. To fill applicator barrel, **press down firmly** on cap flanges, hold for 1–2 seconds, and release. **Wait 5–10 seconds to allow foam to expand in applicator barrel. Repeat until foam reaches fill line.** It usually requires **3–4 pumps** for foam to reach fill line. Remove applicator from container cap. **Note:** If foam goes beyond fill line, it will continue to expand and flow backwards resulting in foam build-up under cap.
6. Hold applicator firmly by barrel, making sure thumb and middle finger are positioned securely underneath and resting against barrel wings. Place index finger over the plunger. Gently insert tip into anus. Once in place, push plunger to expel foam, then withdraw applicator. **CAUTION:** Do not insert any part of the aerosol container directly into the anus. Apply to anus only with enclosed applicator. Do not insert any part of applicator past the anus into rectum.
7. After each use, applicator parts should be pulled apart for thorough cleaning with warm water. Since some foam will appear under the cap, the cap and underlying tip should be pulled apart and rinsed to help prevent build-up of foam and possible blockage.

HOW SUPPLIED

Proctofoam®-HC is supplied in an aerosol container with a special anal applicator. When used correctly, the aerosol container will deliver a minimum of 14 applications. **Store upright at controlled room temperature 20°–25°C (68°–77°F). DO NOT REFRIGERATE.**

NDC 0091-0690-10 10g

Marketed by:
Blansett Pharmacal
No. Little Rock, AR 72115
For:
SCHWARZ
PHARMA
Milwaukee, WI 53201, USA
PC2585H Rev. 06/03

Shown in Product Identification Guide, page 332

TRILYTE™ with flavor packs ℞

[*trī-līt*]
(PEG-3350, sodium chloride, sodium bicarbonate and potassium chloride for oral solution)
Rx Only

DESCRIPTION

TriLyte is a white powder for reconstitution containing 420 g polyethylene glycol 3350, 5.72 g sodium bicarbonate, 11.2 g sodium chloride, 1.48 g potassium chloride. Flavor packs, each containing 3.22 g of flavoring ingredients, are attached to the 4 liter bottle. See individual flavor packs for complete listing of ingredients. When dissolved in water to a volume of 4 liters, TriLyte™ with flavor packs (PEG-3350, sodium chloride, sodium bicarbonate and potassium chloride for oral solution) is an isosmotic solution, for oral administration, having a pleasant mineral water taste. One flavor pack can be added before reconstitution to flavor the solution. TriLyte™ with flavor packs is administered orally or via nasogastric tube as a gastrointestinal lavage.

CLINICAL PHARMACOLOGY

TriLyte™ with flavor packs induces a diarrhea which rapidly cleanses the bowel, usually within 4 hours. The osmotic activity of polyethylene glycol 3350 and the electrolyte concentration result in virtually no net absorption or excretion of ions or water. Accordingly, large volumes may be administered without significant changes in fluid or electrolyte balance.

INDICATIONS AND USAGE

TriLyte™ with flavor packs is indicated for bowel cleansing prior to colonoscopy.

CONTRAINDICATIONS

TriLyte™ with flavor packs is contraindicated in patients known to be hypersensitive to any of the components. TriLyte™ with flavor packs is contraindicated in patients with ileus, gastrointestinal obstruction, gastric retention, bowel perforation, toxic colitis or toxic megacolon.

WARNINGS

The flavor packs are for use only with the accompanying 4 liter bottle. No additional ingredients, e.g. flavorings, should be added to the solution. TriLyte™ with flavor packs should be used with caution in patients with severe ulcerative colitis. Use of TriLyte™ with flavor packs in children younger than 2 years of age should be carefully monitored for occurrence of possible hypoglycemia, as this solution has no caloric substrate. Dehydration has been reported in 1 child and hypokalemia has been reported in 3 children.

PRECAUTIONS

General: Patients with impaired gag reflex, unconscious, or semiconscious patients, and patients prone to regurgitation or aspiration should be observed during the administration of TriLyte™ with flavor packs, especially if it is administered via nasogastric tube. If a patient experiences severe bloating, distention or abdominal pain, administration should be slowed or temporarily discontinued until the symptoms abate. If gastrointestinal obstruction or perforation is suspected, appropriate studies should be performed to rule out these conditions before administration of TriLyte™ with flavor packs.
Information for Patients: TriLyte™ with flavor packs produces a watery stool which cleanses the bowel before examination. Prepare the solution according to the instructions on the bottle. It is more palatable if chilled. For best results, no solid food should be consumed during the 3 to 4 hour period before drinking the solution, but in no case should solid foods be eaten within 2 hours of taking TriLyte™ with flavor packs.
Adults drink 240 mL (8 oz.) every 10 minutes. Pediatric patients (aged 6 months or greater) drink 25 mL/kg/hour. Rapid drinking of each portion is better than drinking small amounts continuously. The first bowel movement should occur approximately one hour after the start of TriLyte™ with flavor packs administration. You may experience some abdominal bloating and distention before the bowels start to move. If severe discomfort or distention occur, stop drinking temporarily or drink each portion at longer intervals until these symptoms disappear. Continue drinking until the watery stool is clear and free of solid matter. This usually requires at least 3 liters. Any unused portion should be discarded.
Use of TriLyte™ with flavor packs in children younger than 2 years of age should be carefully monitored for occurrence of possible hypoglycemia, as this solution has no caloric substrate. Dehydration has been reported in 1 child and hypokalemia has been reported in 3 children.
Drug Interactions: Oral medication administered within one hour of the start of administration of TriLyte™ with flavor packs may be flushed from the gastrointestinal tract and not absorbed.
Carcinogenesis, Mutagenesis, Impairment of Fertility: Carcinogenic and reproductive studies with animals have not been performed.
Pregnancy: Category C. Animal reproduction studies have not been conducted with TriLyte™ with flavor packs. It is also not known whether TriLyte™ with flavor packs can cause fetal harm when administered to a pregnant woman or can affect reproductive capacity. TriLyte™ with flavor packs should be given to a pregnant woman only if clearly needed.
Pediatric Use: Safety and effectiveness of TriLyte™ with flavor packs in pediatric patients aged 6 months and older is supported by evidence from adequate and well-controlled clinical trials of a similar product in adults with additional safety and efficacy data from published studies of similar formulations.

ADVERSE REACTIONS

Nausea, abdominal fullness and bloating are the most common adverse reactions (occurring in up to 50% of patients) to administration of TriLyte™ with flavor packs. Abdominal cramps, vomiting and anal irritation occur less frequently. These adverse reactions are transient and subside rapidly. Isolated cases of urticaria, rhinorrhea, dermatitis and (rarely) anaphylactic reaction have been reported which may represent allergic reactions.
Published literature contains isolated reports of serious adverse reactions following the administration of PEG-ELS products in patients over 60 years of age. These adverse events include upper GI bleeding from Mallory-Weiss Tear, esophageal perforation, asystole, sudden dyspnea with pulmonary edema, and "butterfly-like" infiltrate on chest X-ray after vomiting and aspirating PEG.

DOSAGE AND ADMINISTRATION

TriLyte™ with flavor packs is usually administered orally, but may be given via nasogastric tube to patients who are unwilling or unable to drink the solution. Ideally, the patient should fast for approximately three or four hours prior to TriLyte™ with flavor packs administration, but in no case should solid food be given for at least two hours before the solution is given.
Oral Administration: Adults: At a rate of 240 mL (8 oz.) every 10 minutes, until the rectal effluent is clear or 4 liters are consumed. **Pediatric Patients (aged 6 months or greater):** At a rate of 25 mL/kg/hour, until the rectal effluent is clear or 4 liters are consumed. Rapid drinking of each portion is preferred to drinking small amounts continuously.
Nasogastric Tube Administration: Adults: At a rate of 20-30 mL per minute (1.2-1.8 liters per hour). **Pediatric Patients (aged 6 months or greater):** At a rate of 25 mL/kg/hour, until the rectal effluent is clear or 4 liters are consumed.
The first bowel movement should occur approximately one hour after the start of TriLyte™ with flavor packs administration. Ingestion of 4 liters of TriLyte™ with flavor packs solution prior to gastrointestinal examination produces satisfactory preparation in over 95% of patients.
Various regimens have been used. One method is to schedule patients for examination in midmorning or later, allowing the patients 3 hours for drinking and an additional 1 hour period for complete bowel evacuation. Another method is to administer TriLyte™ with flavor packs on the evening before the examination.
Preparation of the Solution: This preparation can be used with or without the flavor packs. The pharmacist should dispense the bottle and the attached flavor packs to the patient.

1. To add flavor, tear open one flavor pack at the indicated marking and pour contents into the bottle BEFORE reconstitution. Discard unused flavor packs.
2. SHAKE WELL to incorporate flavoring into the powder.
3. Add tap water to the top of the FILL line marked 4 liters. Replace cap tightly and SHAKE WELL until all ingredients have dissolved. No additional ingredients, e.g. flavorings, should be added to the solution.

Note: If not using a flavor pack, omit steps 1 and 2 above. Dissolution is facilitated by using lukewarm water. The solution is more palatable if chilled before administration. However, chilled solution is not recommended for infants. The reconstituted solution should be refrigerated and used within 48 hours. Discard any unused portion.

HOW SUPPLIED

TriLyte™ with flavor packs (PEG-3350, sodium chloride, sodium bicarbonate and potassium chloride for oral solution) is supplied in a 4 liter bottle with an attached package containing flavor packs. This preparation is supplied in powdered form (white to off-white powder) for oral administration as a solution following reconstitution. Each 4 liter bottle contains polyethylene glycol 3350 420 g, sodium bicarbonate 5.72 g, sodium chloride 11.2 g, potassium chloride 1.48 g. Each flavor pack contains 3.22 g of flavoring ingredients. When made up to 4 liters volume with water, the solution contains PEG-3350 31.3 mmol/L, sodium 65 mmol/L, chloride 53 mmol/L, bicarbonate 17 mmol/L and potassium 5 mmol/L.

TriLyte™ with flavor packs 4 liter NDC 0091-0447-23
Rx Only
STORAGE: Store in sealed container at 25°C (77°F); excursions permitted between 15° - 30° C (59° - 86°F). When reconstituted, keep solution refrigerated. Use within 48 hours. Discard unused portion.
SCHWARZ PHARMA, Inc.
Milwaukee, WI 53201, USA

Shown in Product Identification Guide, page 333

UNIRETIC® TABLETS ℞

(moexipril HCl/hydrochlorothiazide)
7.5 mg / 12.5 mg
15 mg / 12.5 mg
15 mg / 25 mg
℞ Only

USE IN PREGNANCY
When used in pregnancy during the second and third trimesters, ACE inhibitors can cause injury and even death to the developing fetus. When pregnancy is detected, uniretic® should be discontinued as soon as possible. **See WARNINGS, Fetal/Neonatal Morbidity and Mortality.**

DESCRIPTION

uniretic® (moexipril hydrochloride/hydrochlorothiazide) is a combination of an angiotensin-converting enzyme (ACE) inhibitor, moexipril hydrochloride, and a diuretic, hydrochlorothiazide. Moexipril hydrochloride is a fine white to off-white powder. It is soluble (about 10% weight-to-volume) in distilled water at room temperature. It has the empirical formula $C_{27}H_{34}N_2O_7$•HCl and a molecular weight of 535.04. It is chemically described as [3S-[2[R*(R*)],3R*]]-2-[2-[[1-(Ethoxycarbonyl)-3-phenyl-propyl]amino]-1-oxopropyl]-1,2,3,4-tetrahydro-6,7-dimethoxy-3-isoquinolinecarboxylic acid, monohydrochloride. Moexipril hydrochloride is a non-sulfhydryl containing precursor of the active ACE inhibitor moexiprilat and its structural formula is:

OCH3 COOH CH3 COOC2H5 N NH O OCH3 • HCl

Hydrochlorothiazide is a white, or practically white, crystalline powder. It is slightly soluble in water, freely soluble in sodium hydroxide solution, in n-butylamine and in dimethylformamide. Hydrochlorothiazide has the empirical formula $C_7H_8ClN_3O_4S_2$ and a molecular weight of 297.75. It is chemically described as *2H*-1,2,4-Benzothiadiazine-7-sulfonamide,6-chloro-3,4-dihydro-,1,1-dioxide. Hydrochlorothiazide is a thiazide diuretic and its structural formula is:

O O S H2N O O S NH Cl N H

uniretic® is available for oral administration in three tablet strengths. The inactive ingredients in all strengths are lactose, magnesium oxide, crospovidone, magnesium stearate and gelatin. The film coating in all strengths contains hypromellose, hydroxypropyl cellulose, polyethylene glycol 6000, magnesium stearate and titanium dioxide. In addition, the film coating for uniretic® 7.5 mg / 12.5 mg and uniretic® 15 mg / 25 mg contains ferric oxide.

CLINICAL PHARMACOLOGY

Mechanism of Action

Moexipril Hydrochloride

Moexipril hydrochloride is a prodrug for moexiprilat, which inhibits ACE in humans and animals. The mechanism through which moexiprilat lowers blood pressure is believed to be primarily inhibition of ACE activity. ACE is a peptidyl dipeptidase that catalyzes the conversion of the inactive decapeptide angiotensin I to the vasoconstrictor substance angiotensin II. Angiotensin II is a potent peripheral vasoconstrictor that also stimulates aldosterone secretion by the adrenal cortex and provides negative feedback on renin secretion. ACE is identical to kininase II, an enzyme that degrades bradykinin, an endothelium-dependent vasodilator. Moexiprilat is about 1000 times as potent as moexipril in inhibiting ACE and kininase II. Inhibition of ACE results in decreased angiotensin II formation, leading to decreased vasoconstriction, increased plasma renin activity, and decreased aldosterone secretion. The latter results in diuresis and natriuresis and a small increase in serum potassium concentration (mean increases of about 0.25 mEq/L were seen when moexipril was used alone).

Whether increased levels of bradykinin, a potent vasodepressor peptide, play a role in the therapeutic effects of moexipril remains to be elucidated. Although the principal mechanism of moexipril in blood pressure reduction is believed to be through the renin-angiotensin-aldosterone system, ACE inhibitors have some effect on blood pressure even in apparent low-renin hypertension. As is the case with other ACE inhibitors, however, the antihypertensive effect of moexipril is smaller in black patients, a predominantly low-renin population, than in nonblack hypertensive patients. Although moexipril monotherapy is less effective in blacks than in nonblacks, the efficacy of combination therapy appears to be independent of race.

Hydrochlorothiazide

Hydrochlorothiazide is a thiazide diuretic and antihypertensive. Thiazides affect the distal renal tubular mechanisms of electrolyte reabsorption, directly increasing excretion of sodium and chloride in approximately equivalent amounts. Indirectly, the diuretic action of hydrochlorothiazide reduces plasma volume, with consequent increases in plasma renin activity, increases in aldosterone secretion, increases in urinary potassium loss, and decreases in serum potassium. The renin-aldosterone link is mediated by angiotensin, so coadministration of an ACE inhibitor tends to reverse the potassium loss associated with these diuretics. The mechanism of the antihypertensive effect of thiazides is unknown.

Pharmacokinetics

Moexipril-Hydrochlorothiazide

Following oral administration of uniretic®, the moexipril peak plasma concentration was reached within 0.8 hour and the peak plasma concentration of moexiprilat occurred 1.6 hours after administration. After reaching the peak plasma level (C_{max}), moexiprilat plasma concentrations decreased biphasically. After administration of uniretic®, renal excretion of unchanged hydrochlorothiazide is about 60% in 24 hours. The pharmacokinetics of moexipril and hydrochlorothiazide after administration of uniretic® are not different, respectively, from the pharmacokinetics of moexipril and hydrochlorothiazide from immediate-release monotherapy formulations.

Moexipril Hydrochloride

Moexipril's antihypertensive activity is almost entirely due to its deesterified metabolite, moexiprilat. Bioavailability of oral moexipril is about 13% compared to intravenous (I.V.) moexipril (both measuring the metabolite moexiprilat), and is markedly affected by food, which reduces C_{max} and AUC (see Absorption). Moexipril should therefore be taken in a fasting state. The time of peak plasma concentration (T_{max}) of moexiprilat is about 1 ½ hours and elimination half-life ($t_{½}$) is estimated at 2 to 9 hours in various studies, the variability reflecting a complex elimination pattern that is not simply exponential. Like all ACE inhibitors, moexiprilat has a prolonged terminal elimination phase, presumably reflecting slow release of drug bound to the ACE. Accumulation of moexiprilat with repeated dosing is minimal, about 30%, compatible with a functional elimination $t_{½}$ of about 12 hours. Over the dose range of 7.5 to 30 mg, pharmacokinetics are approximately dose proportional.

Absorption: Moexipril is incompletely absorbed, with bioavailability as moexiprilat of about 13%. Bioavailability varies with formulation and food intake which reduces C_{max} and AUC of moexiprilat by about 70% and 40% respectively after the ingestion of a low-fat breakfast or by 80% and 50% respectively after the ingestion of a high-fat breakfast.

Distribution: The clearance (CL) for moexipril is 441 mL/min and for moexiprilat 232 mL/min with a $t_{½}$ of 1.3 and 9.8 hours, respectively. Moexiprilat is about 50% protein bound. The volume of distribution of moexiprilat is about 2.8 L/kg.

Metabolism and Excretion: Moexipril is relatively rapidly converted to its active metabolite moexiprilat, but persists longer than some other ACE inhibitor prodrugs, such that its $t_{½}$ is over one hour and it has a significant AUC. Both moexipril and moexiprilat are converted to diketopiperazine derivatives and unidentified metabolites. After I.V. administration of moexipril, about 40% of the dose appears in urine as moexiprilat, about 26% as moexipril, with small amounts of the metabolites; about 20% of the I.V. dose appears in feces, principally as moexiprilat. After oral administration, only about 7% of the dose appears in urine as moexiprilat, about 1% as moexipril, with about 5% as other metabolites. Fifty-two percent of the dose is recovered in feces as moexiprilat and 1% as moexipril.

Special Populations:

Decreased Renal Function: The effective elimination $t_{½}$ and AUC of both moexipril and moexiprilat are increased with decreasing renal function. There is insufficient information available to characterize this relationship fully, but at creatinine clearances in the range of 10 to 40 mL/min, the $t_{½}$ of moexiprilat is increased by a factor of 3 to 4.

Decreased Hepatic Function: In patients with mild to moderate cirrhosis given single 15 mg doses of moexipril, the C_{max} of moexipril was increased by about 50% and the AUC increased by about 120%, while the C_{max} for moexiprilat was decreased by about 50% and the AUC increased by almost 300%.

Elderly Patients: In elderly male subjects (65–80 years old) with clinically normal renal and hepatic function, the AUC and C_{max} of moexiprilat are about 30% greater than in younger subjects (19–42 years old).

Pharmacokinetic Interactions With Other Drugs: No clinically important pharmacokinetic interactions occurred when moexipril was administered concomitantly with hydrochlorothiazide, digoxin, or cimetidine.

Hydrochlorothiazide

Absorption: After oral administration, 60–80% of a single dose of hydrochlorothiazide is absorbed. The reported studies of food effects on hydrochlorothiazide absorption have been inconclusive. The absorption of hydrochlorothiazide is reported to be reduced by 50% in patients with congestive heart failure. Hydrochlorothiazide exhibits dose proportionality over the dose range of 12.5 to 75 mg.

Distribution: The apparent volume of distribution has been observed to vary between 1.5–4.2 L/kg. Hydrochlorothiazide accumulates in red blood cells, so that whole blood levels are higher than those measured in plasma. Equilibrium between whole blood levels and plasma levels is reached 4 hours after oral administration. Hydrochlorothiazide crosses the placental barrier. Hydrochlorothiazide has a protein binding of 21–24%.

Metabolism and Excretion: Hydrochlorothiazide is not metabolized. Hydrochlorothiazide is eliminated rapidly by the kidney. More than 60 percent of the oral dose is eliminated unchanged within 24 hours. When plasma levels have been followed for at least 24 hours, the plasma half-life has been observed to vary between 5.6 and 14.8 hours. The renal clearance has been observed to vary between 3.1–5.5 mL/min/kg.

Special Populations:

Decreased Renal Function: In a study of patients with impaired renal function (mean creatinine clearance of 19 mL/min), the elimination half-life of hydrochlorothiazide was increased to 21 hours.

Pharmacokinetic Interactions With Other Drugs: Coadministration of propantheline or guanabenz increased the absorption of hydrochlorothiazide and coadministration of cholestyramine or colestipol decreased the absorption of hydrochlorothiazide.

Pharmacodynamics and Clinical Effect

Moexipril—Hydrochlorothiazide

In uniretic® clinical trials using moexipril doses of 3.75–30 mg and hydrochlorothiazide doses of 3.125–50 mg, the antihypertensive effects were sustained for at least 24 hours and they increased with increasing dose of either component. The extent of blood pressure reduction seen with uniretic® was approximately additive as compared to monotherapy of each component. The antihypertensive effects of uniretic® continue during therapy for up to 24 months. The effectiveness of uniretic® was not significantly influenced by patient age or gender. Although moexipril monotherapy is less effective in blacks than in nonblacks, the efficacy of uniretic® appears to be independent of race. By blocking the renin-angiotensin-aldosterone axis, administration of moexipril tends to reduce the potassium loss associated with hydrochlorothiazide. In uniretic® controlled clinical trials, the average change in serum potassium was near zero in subjects who received 3.75 mg / 6.25 mg or 7.5 mg / 12.5 mg, but subjects who received 15 mg / 12.5 mg or 15 mg / 25 mg experienced a mild decrease in serum potassium, similar to that experienced by subjects who received the same dose of hydrochlorothiazide monotherapy.

Moexipril Hydrochloride

Single and multiple doses of 15 mg or more of moexipril give sustained inhibition of plasma ACE activity of 80–90%, beginning within 2 hours and lasting 24 hours (80%).

In controlled trials, the peak effects of orally administered moexipril increased with the dose administered over a dose range of 7.5 to 60 mg, given once a day. Antihypertensive effects were first detectable about 1 hour after dosing, with a peak effect between 3 and 6 hours after dosing. Just before dosing (i.e., at trough), the antihypertensive effects were less prominently related to dose and the antihypertensive effect tended to diminish during the 24-hour dosing interval when the drug was administered once a day.

In multiple-dose studies in the dose range of 7.5 to 30 mg once daily, moexipril lowered sitting blood pressure at trough by 4–11/3–6 mmHg more than placebo, a tendency toward increased response with higher doses. These effects are typical of ACE inhibitors; there are no trials of adequate size comparing moexipril with other antihypertensive agents.

Higher doses of moexipril generally leave a greater fraction of the peak blood pressure effect still present at trough. During dose titration, any decision as to the adequacy of a dosing regimen should be based on trough blood pressure measurements. If diastolic blood pressure control is not adequate at the end of the dosing interval, the dose can be increased or given as a divided (BID) regimen.

During chronic therapy, the antihypertensive effect of any dose of moexipril is generally evident within 2 weeks of treatment, with maximal reduction after 4 weeks. The antihypertensive effects of moexipril have been proven to continue during therapy for up to 24 months.

Moexipril, like other ACE inhibitors, is less effective in decreasing trough blood pressures in blacks than in nonblacks. Placebo-corrected trough group diastolic blood pressure effects in blacks in the proposed dose range were +1 to −3 mmHg compared with responses in nonblacks of −4 to −6 mmHg.

The effectiveness of moexipril was not significantly influenced by patient age, gender, or weight. Moexipril has been shown to have antihypertensive activity in both pre- and postmenopausal women who have participated in placebo-controlled clinical trials.

INDICATIONS AND USAGE

uniretic® is indicated for treatment of patients with hypertension. **This fixed combination is not indicated for the initial therapy of hypertension (see DOSAGE AND ADMINISTRATION).**

In using uniretic®, consideration should be given to the fact that another ACE inhibitor, captopril, has caused agranulocytosis, particularly in patients with renal impairment or collagen-vascular disease. Available data are insufficient to show that uniretic® does not have a similar risk (see WARNINGS, Neutropenia/Agranulocytosis). In addition, ACE inhibitors, for which adequate data are available, cause a higher rate of angioedema in black than in nonblack patients (see WARNINGS, Angioedema).

CONTRAINDICATIONS

uniretic® is contraindicated in patients who are hypersensitive to any component of this product and in patients with a history of angioedema related to previous treatment with an ACE inhibitor. Because of the hydrochlorothiazide component, this product is contraindicated in patients with anuria or hypersensitivity to other sulfonamide-derived drugs. Hypersensitivity reactions are more likely to occur in patients with a history of allergy or bronchial asthma.

WARNINGS

Anaphylactoid and Possibly Related Reactions

Presumably because angiotensin-converting enzyme inhibitors affect the metabolism of eicosanoids and polypeptides, including endogenous bradykinin, patients receiving ACE inhibitors, including uniretic®, may be subject to a variety of adverse reactions, some of them serious.

Head and Neck Angioedema: Angioedema involving the face, extremities, lips, tongue, glottis, and/or larynx has been reported in patients treated with ACE inhibitors, including moexipril. Symptoms suggestive of angioedema or facial edema occurred in <0.5% of moexipril-treated patients in placebo-controlled trials. None of the cases were considered life-threatening and all resolved either without treatment or with medication (antihistamines or glucocorti-

Continued on next page

Uniretic—Cont.

coids). One patient treated with hydrochlorothiazide alone experienced laryngeal edema. No instances of angioedema were reported in placebo-treated patients.

In cases of angioedema, treatment with uniretic® should be promptly discontinued and the patient carefully observed until the swelling disappears. In instances where swelling has been confined to the face and lips, the condition has generally resolved without treatment, although antihistamines have been useful in relieving symptoms.

Angioedema associated with involvement of the tongue, glottis, or larynx may be fatal due to airway obstruction. Appropriate therapy, e.g., subcutaneous epinephrine solution 1:1000 (0.3 to 0.5 mL) and/or measures to ensure a patent airway, should be promptly provided (see ADVERSE REACTIONS).

Intestinal Angioedema: Intestinal angioedema has been reported in patients treated with ACE inhibitors. These patients presented with abdominal pain (with or without nausea or vomiting); in some cases there was no prior history of facial angioedema and C-1 esterase levels were normal. The angioedema was diagnosed by procedures including abdominal CT scan or ultrasound, or at surgery, and symptoms resolved after stopping the ACE inhibitor. Intestinal angioedema should be included in the differential diagnosis of patients on ACE inhibitors presenting with abdominal pain.

Anaphylactoid Reactions During Desensitization: Two patients undergoing desensitizing treatment with hymenoptera venom while receiving ACE inhibitors sustained life-threatening anaphylactoid reactions. In the same patients, these reactions did not occur when ACE inhibitors were temporarily withheld, but they reappeared when the ACE inhibitors were inadvertently readministered.

Anaphylactoid Reactions During Membrane Exposure: Anaphylactoid reactions have been reported in patients dialyzed with high-flux membranes and treated concomitantly with an ACE inhibitor. Anaphylactoid reactions have also been reported in patients undergoing low-density lipoprotein apheresis with dextran sulfate absorption.

Hypotension

uniretic® can cause symptomatic hypotension, although, as with other ACE inhibitors, this is unusual in uncomplicated hypertensive patients treated with uniretic® alone. Symptomatic hypotension is most likely to occur in patients who have been salt- and/or volume-depleted as a result of prolonged diuretic therapy, dietary salt restriction, dialysis, diarrhea, or vomiting. Volume- and/or salt-depletion should be corrected before initiating therapy with uniretic® (see ADVERSE REACTIONS).

The thiazide component of uniretic® may potentiate the action of other antihypertensive drugs, especially ganglionic or peripheral adrenergic-blocking drugs. The antihypertensive effects of the thiazide component may also be enhanced in the postsympathectomy patient.

In patients with congestive heart failure, with or without associated renal insufficiency, ACE inhibitor therapy may cause excessive hypotension, which may be associated with oliguria or progressive azotemia, and rarely, with acute renal failure and death. In these patients, uniretic® therapy should be started under close medical supervision, and patients should be followed closely for the first two weeks of treatment and whenever the dose of uniretic® is increased. Care in avoiding hypotension should also be taken in patients with ischemic heart disease, aortic stenosis, or cerebrovascular disease, in whom an excessive decrease in blood pressure could result in a myocardial infarction or a cerebrovascular accident.

If hypotension occurs, the patient should be placed in a supine position and, if necessary, treated with an intravenous infusion of normal saline. uniretic® treatment usually can be continued following restoration of blood pressure and volume.

Impaired Renal Function

uniretic® should be used with caution in patients with severe renal disease. Thiazide diuretics may precipitate azotemia in such patients and the effects of repeated dosing may be cumulative.

As a consequence of inhibition of the renin-angiotensin-aldosterone system, changes in renal function may be anticipated in susceptible individuals. There is no clinical experience of uniretic® in the treatment of hypertension in patients with renal failure.

Some hypertensive patients with no apparent preexisting renal vascular disease have developed increases in blood urea nitrogen and serum creatinine, usually minor and transient, especially when moexipril has been given concomitantly with a thiazide diuretic. This is more likely to occur in patients with preexisting renal impairment. There may be a need for dose adjustment of uniretic®. **Evaluation of hypertensive patients should always include assessment of renal function** (see DOSAGE AND ADMINISTRATION).

In hypertensive patients with severe congestive heart failure, whose renal function may depend on the activity of the renin-angiotensin-aldosterone system, treatment with ACE inhibitors, including moexipril, may be associated with oliguria and/or progressive azotemia and, rarely, acute renal failure and/or death.

In hypertensive patients with unilateral or bilateral renal artery stenosis, increases in blood urea nitrogen and serum creatinine have been observed in some patients following ACE inhibitor therapy. These increases were almost always reversible upon discontinuation of the ACE inhibitor and/or diuretic therapy. In such patients, renal function should be monitored during the first few weeks of therapy.

Neutropenia/Agranulocytosis

Another ACE inhibitor, captopril, has been shown to cause agranulocytosis and bone marrow depression, rarely in patients with uncomplicated hypertension, but more frequently in hypertensive patients with renal impairment, especially if they also have a collagen-vascular disease such as systemic lupus erythematosus or scleroderma. Although there were no instances of severe neutropenia (absolute neutrophil count <500/mm^3) among patients given moexipril, as with other ACE inhibitors, monitoring of white blood cell counts should be considered for patients who have collagen-vascular disease, especially if the disease is associated with impaired renal function. Available data from clinical trials of moexipril are insufficient to show that moexipril does not cause agranulocytosis at rates similar to captopril.

Fetal/Neonatal Morbidity and Mortality

ACE inhibitors can cause fetal and neonatal morbidity and death when administered to pregnant women. Several dozen cases have been reported in the world literature. When pregnancy is detected, ACE inhibitors should be discontinued as soon as possible.

The use of ACE inhibitors during the second and third trimesters of pregnancy has been associated with fetal and neonatal injury, including hypotension, neonatal skull hypoplasia, anuria, reversible or irreversible renal failure, and death. Oligohydramnios has also been reported, presumably resulting from decreased fetal renal function; oligohydramnios in this setting has been associated with fetal limb contractures, craniofacial deformation, and hypoplastic lung development. Prematurity, intrauterine growth retardation, and patent ductus arteriosus have also been reported, although it is not clear whether these were caused by the ACE inhibitor exposure.

Fetal and neonatal morbidity do not appear to have resulted from intrauterine ACE inhibitor exposure limited to the first trimester. Mothers who have used ACE inhibitors only during the first trimester should be informed of this. Nonetheless, when patients become pregnant, physicians should make every effort to discontinue the use of uniretic® as soon as possible.

Rarely (probably less often than once in every thousand pregnancies), no alternative to ACE inhibitors will be found. In these rare cases, the mothers should be apprised of the potential hazards to their fetuses, and serial ultrasound examinations should be performed to assess the intraamniotic environment.

If oligohydramnios is observed, uniretic® should be discontinued unless it is considered life-saving for the mother. Contraction stress testing (CST), a non-stress test (NST), or biophysical profiling (BPP) may be appropriate, depending upon the week of pregnancy. Patients and physicians should be aware, however, that oligohydramnios may not be detected until after the fetus has sustained irreversible injury. Infants with histories of *in utero* exposure to ACE inhibitors should be closely observed for hypotension, oliguria, and hyperkalemia. If oliguria occurs, attention should be directed toward support of blood pressure and renal perfusion. Exchange transfusion or peritoneal dialysis may be required as means of reversing hypotension and/or substituting for disordered renal function. Theoretically, the ACE inhibitor could be removed from the neonatal circulation by exchange transfusion, but no experience with this procedure has been reported.

Intrauterine exposure to thiazide diuretics is associated with fetal or neonatal jaundice, thrombocytopenia, and possibly other adverse reactions that have occurred in adults. Reproduction studies with the combination of moexipril hydrochloride and hydrochlorothiazide (ratio 7.5:12.5) indicated that the combination possessed no teratogenic properties up to the lethal dose of 800 mg/kg/day in rats and up to the maternotoxic dose of 160 mg/kg/day in rabbits.

Hepatic Failure

Rarely, ACE inhibitors have been associated with a syndrome that starts with cholestatic jaundice and progresses to fulminant hepatic necrosis and sometimes death. The mechanism of this syndrome is not understood. Patients receiving ACE inhibitors who develop jaundice or marked elevations of hepatic enzymes should discontinue the ACE Inhibitor and receive appropriate medical follow-up.

Impaired Hepatic Function

uniretic® should be used with caution in patients with impaired hepatic function or progressive liver disease, since minor alterations of fluid and electrolyte balance may precipitate hepatic coma. In patients with mild to moderate cirrhosis given single 15 mg doses of moexipril, the C_{max} of moexipril was increased by about 50% and the AUC increased by about 120%, while the C_{max} for moexiprilat was decreased by about 50% and the AUC increased by almost 300%. No formal pharmacokinetic studies have been carried out with uniretic® in hypertensive patients with impaired liver function.

Systemic Lupus Erythematosus

Thiazide diuretics have been reported to cause exacerbation or activation of systemic lupus erythematosus.

PRECAUTIONS

General

Serum Electrolyte Imbalances: In clinical trials with moexipril monotherapy, persistent hyperkalemia (serum potassium above 5.4 mEq/L) occurred in approximately 1.3% of hypertensive patients receiving moexipril. Risk factors for the development of hyperkalemia with ACE inhibitors include renal insufficiency, diabetes mellitus, and the concomitant use of potassium-sparing diuretics, potassium supplements, and/or potassium-containing salt substitutes. Treatment with thiazide diuretics has been associated with hypokalemia, hyponatremia, and hypochloremic alkalosis. These disturbances sometimes manifest as one or more of the following: dryness of mouth, thirst, weakness, lethargy, drowsiness, restlessness, muscle pains or cramps, muscular fatigue, hypotension, oliguria, tachycardia, nausea, and vomiting. Hypokalemia has also been reported to sensitize or exaggerate the response of the heart to the toxic effects of digitalis. The risk of hypokalemia is greatest in patients with cirrhosis of the liver, in patients experiencing a brisk diuresis, in patients who are receiving inadequate oral intake of electrolytes, and in patients receiving concomitant therapy with corticosteroids or ACTH.

The opposite effects of moexipril and hydrochlorothiazide on serum potassium will approximately counterbalance each other in many patients, so that little net effect upon serum potassium will be seen. Initial and periodic determinations of serum electrolytes to detect possible electrolyte imbalance should be performed at appropriate intervals.

Chloride deficits generally are mild and require specific treatment only under extraordinary circumstances (e.g., in liver disease or renal disease). Dilutional hyponatremia may occur in edematous patients; appropriate therapy is water restriction rather than administration of salt, except in rare instances when the hyponatremia is life-threatening. In actual salt depletion, appropriate replacement is the therapy of choice.

Calcium excretion is reduced by thiazides. In a few patients on prolonged thiazide therapy, pathological changes in the parathyroid gland have been seen, with hypercalcemia and hypophosphatemia. More serious complications of hyperparathyroidism (renal lithiasis, bone resorption, and peptic ulceration) have not been seen. Thiazides enhance urinary excretion of magnesium and hypomagnesemia may result.

Other Metabolic Disturbances: Thiazide diuretics may reduce glucose tolerance and may raise serum levels of cholesterol, triglycerides, and uric acid. These effects are usually minor, but frank gout or overt diabetes may be precipitated in susceptible patients.

Surgery/Anesthesia: In patients undergoing major surgery or during anesthesia with agents that produce hypotension, moexipril may block the effects of compensatory renin release. If hypotension occurs in this setting and is considered to be due to this mechanism, it can be corrected by volume expansion.

Cough: Presumably due to the inhibition of the degradation of endogenous bradykinin, persistent nonproductive cough has been reported with all ACE inhibitors, always resolving after discontinuation of therapy. ACE inhibitor-induced cough should be considered in the differential diagnosis of cough. In placebo-controlled trials with uniretic®, cough was present in 3% of uniretic® patients and 1% of patients given placebo.

Information for Patients

Food: Patients should be advised to take uniretic® one hour before a meal (see CLINICAL PHARMACOLOGY and DOSAGE AND ADMINISTRATION).

Angioedema: Angioedema, including laryngeal edema, may occur with treatment with ACE inhibitors, usually occurring early in therapy (within the first month). Patients should be so advised and told to report immediately any signs or symptoms suggesting angioedema (swelling of the face, extremities, eyes, lips, tongue, difficulty in breathing) and to take no more drug until they have consulted with the prescribing physician.

Symptomatic Hypotension: Patients should be cautioned that lightheadedness can occur with uniretic®, especially during the first few days of therapy. If fainting occurs, the patient should stop taking uniretic® and consult the prescribing physician.

All patients should be cautioned that excessive perspiration and dehydration may lead to an excessive fall in blood pressure because of reduction in fluid volume. Other causes of volume depletion such as vomiting or diarrhea may also lead to a fall in blood pressure; patients should be advised to consult their physician if they develop these conditions.

Hyperkalemia: Patients should be told not to use potassium supplements or salt substitutes containing potassium without consulting their physician.

Neutropenia: Patients should be told to report promptly any indication of infection (e.g., sore throat, fever) that could be a sign of neutropenia.

Pregnancy: Female patients of childbearing age should be told about the consequences of second- and third-trimester exposure to ACE inhibitors and should also be told that these consequences do not appear to have resulted from intrauterine ACE inhibitor exposure that has been limited to the first trimester. Patients should be asked to report pregnancies to their physicians as soon as possible.

Drug Interactions

Potassium Supplements and Potassium-Sparing Diuretics: As noted above (*Serum Electrolyte Imbalances*), the net effect of uniretic® may be to elevate a patient's serum potassium, to reduce it, or to leave it unchanged. Potassium-sparing diuretics (spironolactone, amiloride, triamterene) or potassium supplements can increase the risk of hyperkalemia. If concomitant use of such agents is indicated, they should be given with caution, and the patient's serum potassium should be monitored.

Oral Anticoagulants: Interaction studies with warfarin failed to identify any clinically important effect of moexipril monotherapy on the serum concentrations of the anticoagulant or on its anticoagulant effect.
Lithium: Increased serum lithium levels and symptoms of lithium toxicity have been reported in patients receiving ACE inhibitors during therapy with lithium. Because renal clearance of lithium is reduced by thiazides, the risk of lithium toxicity is presumably raised further when, as in therapy with uniretic®, a thiazide diuretic is coadministered with the ACE inhibitor. These drugs should be coadministered with caution, and frequent monitoring of serum lithium levels is recommended.
Alcohol, Barbiturates, or Narcotics: Potentiation of orthostatic hypotension may occur in patients on thiazide diuretic therapy with concomitant use of alcohol, barbiturates, or narcotics.
Antidiabetic Agents: Use of thiazide diuretics concomitantly with antidiabetic agents (oral agents and insulin) may require dosage adjustment of the antidiabetic agent. Moexipril has been used in clinical trials concomitantly with oral hypoglycemic agents and there was no evidence of any clinically important adverse interactions.
Cholestyramine and Colestipol Resins: Absorption of hydrochlorothiazide is impaired in the presence of anionic exchange resins. Single doses of either cholestyramine or colestipol resins bind the hydrochlorothiazide and reduce its absorption from the gastrointestinal tract by up to 85% and 43%, respectively.
Corticosteroids, ACTH: Use of thiazide diuretics concomitantly with corticosteroids or ACTH may intensify electrolyte depletion, particularly hypokalemia.
Pressor Amines: Thiazide diuretics may decrease arterial responsiveness to pressor amines (e.g. norepinephrine), but not enough to preclude effectiveness of the pressor agent for therapeutic use.
Skeletal Muscle Relaxants, Nondepolarizing: Thiazide diuretics may increase the responsiveness to tubocurarine.
Non-steroidal Anti-inflammatory Drugs: In some patients, the administration of a non-steroidal anti-inflammatory agent can reduce the diuretic, natriuretic, and antihypertensive effects of loop, potassium-sparing and thiazide diuretics. Thus, when uniretic® and non-steroidal anti-inflammatory agents are used concomitantly, the patient should be observed closely to determine if the desired effect of the diuretic is obtained.
Other Agents: No clinically important pharmacokinetic interactions occurred when moexipril was administered concomitantly with digoxin or cimetidine.
Moexipril has been used in clinical trials concomitantly with calcium-channel-blocking agents, diuretics, H_2 blockers, digoxin, and cholesterol-lowering agents. There was no evidence of clinically important adverse interactions. In general, ACE inhibitors have less than additive effects with beta-adrenergic blockers, presumably because both work by inhibiting the renin-angiotensin system.
Coadministration of propantheline or guanabenz increased the absorption of hydrochlorothiazide.

Carcinogenesis, Mutagenesis, Impairment of Fertility

Moexipril Hydrochloride

No evidence of carcinogenicity was detected in long-term studies when moexipril was administered to mice and rats at doses up to 14 or 27.3 times the Maximum Recommended Human Dose (MRHD) on a mg/m^2 basis. No mutagenicity was detected in the Ames test and microbial reverse mutation assay, with and without metabolic activation, or in an *in vivo* nucleus anomaly test. However, increased chromosomal aberration frequency in Chinese hamster ovary (CHO) cells was detected under metabolic activation conditions at a 20-hour harvest time. Reproduction studies have been performed in rabbits at oral doses up to 0.7 times the MRHD on a mg/m^2 basis, and in rats up to 90.9 times the MRHD on a mg/m^2 basis. No indication of impaired fertility, reproductive toxicity, or teratogenicity was observed.

Hydrochlorothiazide

Under the auspices of the National Toxicology Program, rats and mice received hydrochlorothiazide in their feed for two years, at doses up to 600 mg/kg/day in mice and up to 100 mg/kg/day in rats. These studies uncovered no evidence of a carcinogenic potential of hydrochlorothiazide in rats or female mice, but there was equivocal evidence of hepatocarcinogenicity in male mice. Hydrochlorothiazide was not genotoxic in *in vitro* assays using strains TA 98, TA 100, TA 1535, TA 1537, and TA 1538 of *Salmonella typhimurium* (the Ames test); in the CHO test for chromosomal aberrations; or in *in vivo* assays using mouse germinal cell chromosomes, Chinese hamster bone marrow chromosomes; and the *Drosophila* sex-linked recessive lethal trait gene. Positive test results were obtained in the *in vitro* CHO Sister Chromatid Exchange (clastogenicity) test and in the Mouse Lymphoma Cell (mutagenicity) assays, using concentrations of hydrochlorothiazide of 43–1300 mcg/mL. Positive test results were also obtained in the *Aspergillus nidulans* nondisjunction assay, using an unspecified concentration of hydrochlorothiazide.
Hydrochlorothiazide had no adverse effects on the fertility of mice and rats of either sex in studies wherein these species were exposed, via their diets, to doses up to 100 and 4 mg/kg/day, respectively, prior to mating and throughout gestation.

Pregnancy

Pregnancy Categories C (first trimester) and D (second and third trimesters). See WARNINGS, Fetal/Neonatal Morbidity and Mortality.

Nursing Mothers

It is not known whether moexipril or moexiprilat is excreted in human milk. Thiazides are excreted in human milk. Because of the potential for serious adverse reactions in nursing infants from hydrochlorothiazide and the unknown effects of moexipril or moexiprilat in infants, a decision should be made whether to discontinue nursing or to discontinue uniretic®, taking into account the importance of the drug to the mother.

Pediatric Use

Safety and effectiveness of uniretic® in pediatric patients have not been established.

Geriatric Use

Of the patients who received uniretic® in controlled clinical studies, 24% were 65 years of age or older. No overall differences in effectiveness or safety were observed between these patients and younger patients. In elderly patients receiving moexipril, plasma levels of drug are slightly higher and renal clearance is reduced when compared to younger patients, but these effects did not have detectable consequences. Hydrochlorothiazide is known to be substantially excreted by the kidney, and the risk of toxic reactions to this drug may be greater in patients with impaired renal function. Because elderly patients are more likely to have decreased renal function, care should be taken in dose selection, and it may be useful to monitor renal function.

ADVERSE REACTIONS

uniretic® has been evaluated for safety in more than 1140 patients with hypertension with more than 120 treated for more than one year. uniretic® has not demonstrated a potential for causing adverse experiences different from those previously associated with other ACE inhibitor/diuretic combinations. The overall incidence of reported adverse events was slightly less in patients treated with uniretic® than patients treated with placebo.
Adverse experiences were usually mild and transient, and there was no relationship between adverse experiences and gender, race, age, or total daily dosage (except for serum potassium decreases at 50 mg hydrochlorothiazide) within the moexipril/ hydrochlorothiazide dosage range of 3.75 mg / 3.125 mg to 30 mg / 50 mg. Discontinuation of therapy due to adverse experiences was required in 5.3% of patients treated with uniretic® and in 8.4% of patients treated with placebo. The most common reasons for discontinuation of therapy with uniretic® were cough (0.5%) and dizziness (0.5%).
All adverse experiences considered at least possibly related to treatment that occurred at any dose in placebo-controlled trials of once-daily dosing in more than 1% of patients treated with uniretic® and that were at least as frequent in the uniretic® group as in the placebo group are shown in the following table.

Adverse Events in Placebo-Controlled Trials

ADVERSE EVENT	UNIRETIC (N=506 N (%)	PLACEBO (N=202) N (%)
Cough	15 (3)	2 (1)
Dizziness	7 (1.4)	2 (1)
Fatigue	5 (1)	1 (0.5)

Other adverse experiences occurring in more than 1% of patients treated with uniretic® in controlled or uncontrolled trials, some of which were of uncertain drug relationship, listed in decreasing frequency include: upper respiratory infection, headache, pain, flu syndrome, pharyngitis, hyperuricemia, diarrhea, back pain, rhinitis, sinusitis, abnormal ECG, infection, abdominal pain, chest pain, dyspepsia, hyperglycemia, hypokalemia, rash, vertigo, nausea, hypertonia, increased SGPT, urinary tract infection, impotence, peripheral edema, pyuria, bronchitis, and fever. See WARNINGS and PRECAUTIONS for discussion of anaphylactoid reactions, angioedema, hypotension, neutropenia/agranulocytosis, fetal/neonatal morbidity and mortality, serum electrolyte imbalances, and cough.
The following adverse experiences, some of which are of uncertain drug relationship, were reported in uniretic® controlled or uncontrolled clinical trials in less than 1% of patients or have been attributed to other ACE inhibitors. Within each organ system, adverse experiences are listed in decreasing frequency.
Cardiovascular: palpitation, flushing, syncope, tachycardia, myocardial infarct, hypotension, postural hypotension, arrhythmia, first degree AV block, ventricular extrasystoles, atrial fibrillation, migraine, hemorrhage, sinus bradycardia, bigeminy, bradycardia, bundle branch block, heart arrest, myocardial ischemia, peripheral vascular disorder, prolonged QT interval, inverted T wave, ventricular fibrillation
Dermatologic: eczema, pruritus, sweating, acne, dry skin, herpes simplex, contact dermatitis, herpes zoster, psoriasis, alopecia, angioedema, erythema nodosum, fungal dermatitis, furunculosis, maculopapular rash, purpuric rash, skin carcinoma, subcutaneous nodule, urticaria, pemphigus
Gastrointestinal: vomiting, constipation, gastroenteritis, periodontal abscess, cholelithiasis, gastritis, gingivitis, esophagitis, flatulence, anorexia, colitis, dysphagia, tooth caries, cheilitis, enteritis, eructation, gastrointestinal carcinoma, gastrointestinal hemorrhage, glossitis, increased appetite, jaundice, melena, rectal hemorrhage, stomatitis, tongue discoloration, tongue edema
Hematologic: anemia, hypochromic anemia, leukopenia, abnormal erythrocytes, ecchymosis, lymphocytosis, hemolysis, lymphadenopathy, eosinophilia, petechia, abnormal WBC, hemolytic anemia
Metabolic: hyperlipemia, increased SGOT, gout, bilirubinemia, increased creatinine, hypercholesterolemia, increased BUN, increased CPK, diabetes mellitus, hyponatremia, thirst, edema, increased alkaline phosphatase, increased amylase, dehydration, decreased glucose tolerance, goiter, hypercalcemia, hyperkalemia, hypocalcemia, hypochloremia, hypoproteinemia, weight gain
Neurologic/Psychiatric: insomnia, postural dizziness, somnolence, dry mouth, anxiety, nervousness, paresthesia, depression, neuritis, hypesthesia, decreased libido, neuralgia, amnesia, ataxia, cerebral infarct, emotional lability, facial paralysis, hypokinesia, neurosis, vocal cord paralysis
Renal: albuminuria, urinary frequency, hematuria, glycosuria, cystitis, dysuria, nocturia, polyuria, kidney calculus, pyelonephritis, urate crystalluria, urinary casts, urinary retention
Respiratory: epistaxis, pneumonia, dyspnea, asthma, lung carcinoma, hemoptysis, laryngitis, voice alteration, eosinophilic pneumonitis
Urogenital: vaginal hemorrhage, breast carcinoma, scrotal edema, vaginitis, breast enlargement, breast pain, dysmenorrhea, leukorrhea
Other: asthenia, conjunctivitis, myalgia, arthralgia, arthrosis, hernia, neck pain, cyst, tenosynovitis, abnormal vision, allergic reaction, arthritis, cataract, cellulitis, moniliasis, otitis media, eye hemorrhage, chills, abscess, bursitis, deafness, ear pain, glaucoma, iritis, neck rigidity, photosensitivity, retinal degeneration, tinnitus
Monotherapy with moexipril has been evaluated for safety in over 3000 patients. In clinical trials, the observed adverse experiences with moexipril were similar to those seen in the uniretic® trials.
Hydrochlorothiazide: The following adverse reactions have been reported with hydrochlorothiazide and, within each organ system, are listed by decreasing severity.
Cardiovascular: orthostatic hypotension (may be potentiated by alcohol, barbiturates, or narcotics)
Gastrointestinal: pancreatitis, jaundice (intrahepatic cholestatic, see WARNINGS), sialadenitis, vomiting, diarrhea, cramping, nausea, gastric irritation, constipation, anorexia
Neurologic/Psychiatric: vertigo, dizziness, transient blurred vision, headache, paresthesia, xanthopsia, weakness, restlessness
Musculoskeletal: muscle spasm
Hematologic: aplastic anemia, agranulocytosis, leukopenia, thrombocytopenia
Metabolic: hyperglycemia, glycosuria, hyperuricemia
Hypersensitivity: necrotizing angiitis, Stevens-Johnson syndrome, respiratory distress including pneumonitis and pulmonary edema, purpura, urticaria, rash, photosensitivity

Clinical Laboratory Test Findings

Serum Electrolytes: See PRECAUTIONS, General.
Creatinine and Blood Urea Nitrogen: As with other ACE inhibitors, minor increases in blood urea nitrogen or serum creatinine, reversible upon discontinuation of therapy, were observed in less than 1% of patients with essential hypertension who were treated with uniretic®. Increases are more likely to occur in patients with compromised renal function (see PRECAUTIONS, General).
Other (causal relationship unknown): Clinically important changes in standard laboratory tests were rarely associated with uniretic® administration.

OVERDOSAGE

No specific information is available on the treatment of overdosage with uniretic®. Treatment should be symptomatic and supportive. Therapy with uniretic® should be discontinued and the patient observed closely. Suggested measures include induction of emesis and/or gastric lavage and correction of dehydration, electrolyte imbalance and hypotension by established procedures.
Single oral doses of 2 g/kg moexipril were associated with significant lethality in mice. Rats, however, tolerated single oral doses of up to 3 g/kg. The oral LD_{50} of hydrochlorothiazide is greater than 10 g/kg in mice and rats. For the combination of moexipril hydrochloride and hydrochlorothiazide (ratio 7.5:12.5), the approximate LD_{50} was around 10 g/kg for mice and above 10 g/kg for rats. Addition of hydrochlorothiazide to moexipril hydrochloride did not increase the acute toxicity due to moexipril hydrochloride.
Human overdoses of moexipril have not been reported. In case reports of overdoses with other ACE inhibitors, hypotension has been the principal adverse effect noted. The most common signs and symptoms observed with an overdose of hydrochlorothiazide have been those of dehydration and electrolyte depletion (hypokalemia, hypochloremia, hyponatremia). If digitalis has also been administered, hypokalemia may accentuate cardiac arrhythmias.
No data are available to suggest that physiological maneuvers (e.g., maneuvers to change the pH of the urine) would accelerate elimination of moexipril and its metabolites. The dialyzability of moexipril is not known.
Angiotensin II could presumably serve as a specific antagonist-antidote in the setting of moexipril overdose, but angiotensin II is essentially unavailable outside of research facilities. Because the hypotensive effect of moexipril is achieved through vasodilation and effective hypovolemia, it is reason-

Continued on next page

Uniretic—Cont.

able to treat moexipril overdose by infusion of normal saline solution. In addition, renal function and serum potassium should be monitored.

DOSAGE AND ADMINISTRATION

Moexipril and hydrochlorothiazide are effective treatments for hypertension. The recommended dosage range of moexipril is 7.5 to 30 mg daily, administered in a single or two divided doses one hour before meals, while hydrochlorothiazide is effective in a dosage of 12.5 to 50 mg daily.

The side effects (see WARNINGS) of moexipril are generally rare and apparently independent of dose; those of hydrochlorothiazide are a mixture of dose-dependent phenomena (primarily hypokalemia) and dose-independent phenomena (e.g., pancreatitis), the former much more common than the latter. Therapy with any combination of moexipril and hydrochlorothiazide will be associated with both sets of dose-independent side effects, but regimens in which moexipril is combined with low doses of hydrochlorothiazide produce minimal effects on serum potassium. In uniretic® controlled clinical trials, the average change in serum potassium was near zero in subjects who received 3.75 mg / 6.25 mg or 7.5 mg / 12.5 mg, but subjects who received 15 mg / 12.5 mg or 15 mg / 25 mg experienced a mild decrease in serum potassium, similar to that experienced by subjects who received the same dose of hydrochlorothiazide monotherapy. To minimize dose-independent side effects, it is usually appropriate to begin combination therapy only after a patient has failed to achieve the desired effect with monotherapy.

Dose Titration Guided by Clinical Effect: A patient whose blood pressure is not adequately controlled with either moexipril or hydrochlorothiazide monotherapy may be given uniretic® 7.5 mg / 12.5 mg, uniretic® 15 mg / 12.5 mg or uniretic® 15 mg / 25 mg one hour before a meal. Further increases of moexipril, hydrochlorothiazide or both depend on clinical response. The hydrochlorothiazide dose should generally not be increased until 2–3 weeks have elapsed.

Total daily doses above 30 mg / 50 mg a day have not been studied in hypertensive patients. Patients whose blood pressures are adequately controlled with 25 mg of hydrochlorothiazide daily, but who experience significant potassium loss with this regimen, may achieve blood pressure control without electrolyte disturbance if they are switched to moexipril 3.75 mg/hydrochlorothiazide 6.25 mg (one-half of the uniretic® 7.5 mg / 12.5 mg tablet). For patients who experience an excessive reduction in blood pressure with uniretic® 7.5 mg / 12.5 mg, the physician may consider prescribing moexipril 3.75 mg/hydrochlorothiazide 6.25 mg.

Replacement Therapy: The combination may be substituted for the titrated individual active ingredients.

Use in Renal Impairment: The usual dosage regimen of uniretic® does not need to be adjusted as long as the patient's creatinine clearance is $>$ 40 mL/min/1.73 m^2 (serum creatinine approximately $\leq$ 3 mg/dL or 265 µmol/L). In patients with more severe renal impairment, loop diuretics are preferred to thiazides, so uniretic® is not recommended (see PRECAUTIONS, General).

HOW SUPPLIED

uniretic® (moexipril hydrochloride/hydrochlorothiazide) 7.5 mg / 12.5 mg tablets are yellow, oval, film-coated and scored with engraved code 712 on the unscored side and S and P on either side of the score. They are supplied as follows:

Bottles of 100 NDC 0091-3712-01

uniretic® (moexipril hydrochloride/hydrochlorothiazide) 15 mg / 12.5 mg tablets are white, oval, film-coated and scored with engraved code 720 on the unscored side and S and P on either side of the score. They are supplied as follows:

Bottles of 100 NDC 0091-3720-01

uniretic® (moexipril hydrochloride/hydrochlorothiazide) 15 mg / 25 mg tablets are yellow, oval, film-coated and scored with engraved code 725 on the unscored side and S and P on either side of the score. They are supplied as follows:

Bottles of 100 NDC 0091-3725-01

Store, tightly closed, at controlled room temperature 20°–25°C (68°–77°F). Protect from excessive moisture.

If product package is subdivided, dispense in tight containers as described in USP-NF.

PC2459G Rev. 05/03

Shown in Product Identification Guide, page 333

UNIVASC® ℞
(moexipril hydrochloride)
tablets
℞ Only

USE IN PREGNANCY
When used in pregnancy during the second and third trimesters, ACE inhibitors can cause injury and even death to the developing fetus. When pregnancy is detected, univasc® should be discontinued as soon as possible. **See WARNINGS, Fetal/Neonatal Morbidity and Mortality.**

DESCRIPTION

univasc® (moexipril hydrochloride), the hydrochloride salt of moexipril, has the empirical formula $C_{27}H_{34}N_2O_7 \cdot HCl$ and a molecular weight of 535.04. It is chemically described as [3S-[2[R*(R*)],3R*]]-2-[2-[[1-(ethoxycarbonyl)-3-phenylpropyl]amino]-1-oxopropyl]-1,2,3,4-tetrahydro-6,7-dimethoxy-3-isoquinolinecarboxylic acid, monohydrochloride. It is a non-sulfhydryl containing precursor of the active angiotensin-converting enzyme (ACE) inhibitor moexiprilat and its structural formula is:

OCH_3 COOH CH_3 $COOC_2H_5$ N NH O OCH_3 • HCl

Moexipril hydrochloride is a fine white to off-white powder. It is soluble (about 10% weight-to-volume) in distilled water at room temperature.

univasc® is supplied as scored, coated tablets containing 7.5 mg and 15 mg of moexipril hydrochloride for oral administration. In addition to the active ingredient, moexipril hydrochloride, the tablet core contains the following inactive ingredients: lactose, magnesium oxide, crospovidone, magnesium stearate and gelatin. The film coating contains hypromellose, hydroxypropyl cellulose, polyethylene glycol 6000, magnesium stearate, titanium dioxide, and ferric oxide.

CLINICAL PHARMACOLOGY

Mechanism of Action

Moexipril hydrochloride is a prodrug for moexiprilat, which inhibits ACE in humans and animals. The mechanism through which moexiprilat lowers blood pressure is believed to be primarily inhibition of ACE activity. ACE is a peptidyl dipeptidase that catalyzes the conversion of the inactive decapeptide angiotensin I to the vasoconstrictor substance angiotensin II. Angiotensin II is a potent peripheral vasoconstrictor that also stimulates aldosterone secretion by the adrenal cortex and provides negative feedback on renin secretion. ACE is identical to kininase II, an enzyme that degrades bradykinin, an endothelium-dependent vasodilator. Moexiprilat is about 1000 times as potent as moexipril in inhibiting ACE and kininase II. Inhibition of ACE results in decreased angiotensin II formation, leading to decreased vasoconstriction, increased plasma renin activity, and decreased aldosterone secretion. The latter results in diuresis and natriuresis and a small increase in serum potassium concentration (mean increases of about 0.25 mEq/L were seen when moexipril was used alone, see PRECAUTIONS). Whether increased levels of bradykinin, a potent vasodepressor peptide, play a role in the therapeutic effects of moexipril remains to be elucidated. Although the principal mechanism of moexipril in blood pressure reduction is believed to be through the renin-angiotensin-aldosterone system, ACE inhibitors have some effect on blood pressure even in apparent low-renin hypertension. As is the case with other ACE inhibitors, however, the antihypertensive effect of moexipril is considerably smaller in black patients, a predominantly low-renin population, than in non-black hypertensive patients.

Pharmacokinetics and Metabolism

Pharmacokinetics: Moexipril's antihypertensive activity is almost entirely due to its deesterified metabolite, moexiprilat. Bioavailability of oral moexipril is about 13% compared to intravenous (I.V.) moexipril (both measuring the metabolite moexiprilat), and is markedly affected by food, which reduces the peak plasma level (C_{max}) and AUC (see Absorption). Moexipril should therefore be taken in a fasting state. The time of peak plasma concentration (T_{max}) of moexiprilat is about 1½ hours and elimination half-life (t½) is estimated at 2 to 9 hours in various studies, the variability reflecting a complex elimination pattern that is not simply exponential. Like all ACE inhibitors, moexiprilat has a prolonged terminal elimination phase, presumably reflecting slow release of drug bound to the ACE. Accumulation of moexiprilat with repeated dosing is minimal, about 30%, compatible with a functional elimination t½ of about 12 hours. Over the dose range of 7.5 to 30 mg, pharmacokinetics are approximately dose proportional.

Absorption: Moexipril is incompletely absorbed, with bioavailability as moexiprilat of about 13%. Bioavailability varies with formulation and food intake which reduces C_{max} and AUC by about 70% and 40% respectively after the ingestion of a low-fat breakfast or by 80% and 50% respectively after the ingestion of a high-fat breakfast.

Distribution: The clearance (CL) for moexipril is 441 mL/min and for moexiprilat 232 mL/min with a t½ of 1.3 and 9.8 hours, respectively. Moexipril is about 50% protein bound. The volume of distribution of moexiprilat is about 183 liters.

Metabolism and Excretion: Moexipril is relatively rapidly converted to its active metabolite moexiprilat, but persists longer than some other ACE inhibitor prodrugs, such that its t½ is over one hour and it has a significant AUC. Both moexipril and moexiprilat are converted to diketopiperazine derivatives and unidentified metabolites. After I.V. administration of moexipril, about 40% of the dose appears in urine as moexiprilat, about 26% as moexipril, with small amounts of the metabolites; about 20% of the I.V. dose appears in feces, principally as moexiprilat. After oral administration, only about 7% of the dose appears in urine as moexiprilat, about 1% as moexipril, with about 5% as other metabolites. Fifty-two percent of the dose is recovered in feces as moexiprilat and 1% as moexipril.

Special Populations:

Decreased Renal Function: The effective elimination t½ and AUC of both moexipril and moexiprilat are increased with decreasing renal function. There is insufficient information available to characterize this relationship fully, but at creatinine clearances in the range of 10 to 40 mL/min, the t½ of moexiprilat is increased by a factor of 3 to 4.

Decreased Hepatic Function: In patients with mild to moderate cirrhosis given single 15 mg doses of moexipril, the C_{max} of moexipril was increased by about 50% and the AUC increased by about 120%, while the C_{max} for moexiprilat was decreased by about 50% and the AUC increased by almost 300%.

Elderly Patients: In elderly male subjects (65–80 years old) with clinically normal renal and hepatic function, the AUC and C_{max} of moexiprilat is about 30% greater than those of younger subjects (19–42 years old).

Pharmacokinetic Interactions With Other Drugs:

No clinically important pharmacokinetic interactions occurred when univasc® was administered concomitantly with hydrochlorothiazide, digoxin, or cimetidine.

Pharmacodynamics and Clinical Effect

Single and multiple doses of 15 mg or more of univasc® gives sustained inhibition of plasma ACE activity of 80–90%, beginning within 2 hours and lasting 24 hours (80%).

In controlled trials, the peak effects of orally administered moexipril increased with the dose administered over a dose range of 7.5 to 60 mg, given once a day. Antihypertensive effects were first detectable about 1 hour after dosing, with a peak effect between 3 and 6 hours after dosing. Just before dosing (i.e., at trough), the antihypertensive effects were less prominently related to dose and the antihypertensive effect tended to diminish during the 24-hour dosing interval when the drug was administered once a day.

In multiple dose studies in the dose range of 7.5 to 30 mg once daily, univasc® lowered sitting diastolic and systolic blood pressure effects at trough by 3 to 6 mmHg and 4 to 11 mmHg more than placebo, respectively. There was a tendency toward increased response with higher doses over this range. These effects are typical of ACE inhibitors but, to date, there are no trials of adequate size comparing moexipril with other antihypertensive agents.

The trough diastolic blood pressure effects of moexipril were approximately 3 to 6 mmHg in various studies. Generally, higher doses of moexipril leave a greater fraction of the peak blood pressure effect still present at trough. During dose titration, any decision as to the adequacy of a dosing regimen should be based on trough blood pressure measurements. If diastolic blood pressure control is not adequate at the end of the dosing interval, the dose can be increased or given as a divided (BID) regimen.

During chronic therapy, the antihypertensive effect of any dose of univasc® is generally evident within 2 weeks of treatment, with maximal reduction after 4 weeks. The antihypertensive effects of univasc® have been proven to continue during therapy for up to 24 months.

univasc®, like other ACE inhibitors, is less effective in decreasing trough blood pressures in blacks than in non-blacks. Placebo-corrected trough group mean diastolic blood pressure effects in blacks in the proposed dose range varied between +1 to −3 mmHg compared with responses in non-blacks of −4 to −6 mmHg.

The effectiveness of univasc® was not significantly influenced by patient age, gender, or weight. univasc® has been shown to have antihypertensive activity in both pre- and postmenopausal women who have participated in placebo-controlled clinical trials.

Formal interaction studies with moexipril have not been carried out with antihypertensive agents other than thiazide diuretics. In these studies, the added effect of moexipril was similar to its effect as monotherapy. In general, ACE inhibitors have less than additive effects with beta-adrenergic blockers, presumably because both work by inhibiting the renin-angiotensin system.

INDICATIONS AND USAGE

univasc® is indicated for treatment of patients with hypertension. It may be used alone or in combination with thiazide diuretics.

In using univasc®, consideration should be given to the fact that another ACE inhibitor, captopril, has caused agranulocytosis, particularly in patients with renal impairment or collagen-vascular disease. Available data are insufficient to show that univasc® does not have a similar risk (see WARNINGS).

In considering use of univasc®, it should be noted that in controlled trials ACE inhibitors have an effect on blood pressure that is less in black patients than in non-blacks. In addition, ACE inhibitors (for which adequate data are available) cause a higher rate of angioedema in black than in non-black patients (see WARNINGS, Angioedema).

CONTRAINDICATIONS

univasc® is contraindicated in patients who are hypersensitive to this product and in patients with a history of angioedema related to previous treatment with an ACE inhibitor.

WARNINGS

Anaphylactoid and Possibly Related Reactions

Presumably because angiotensin-converting enzyme inhibitors affect the metabolism of eicosanoids and polypeptides, including endogenous bradykinin, patients receiving ACE inhibitors, including univasc®, may be subject to a variety of adverse reactions, some of them serious.

Head and Neck Angioedema: Angioedema involving the face, extremities, lips, tongue, glottis, and/or larynx has been reported in patients treated with ACE inhibitors, including univasc®. Symptoms suggestive of angioedema or facial edema occurred in <0.5% of moexipril-treated patients in placebo-controlled trials. None of the cases were considered life-threatening and all resolved either without treatment or with medication (antihistamines or glucocorticoids). One patient treated with hydrochlorothiazide alone experienced laryngeal edema. No instances of angioedema were reported in placebo-treated patients.

In cases of angioedema, treatment should be promptly discontinued and the patient carefully observed until the swelling disappears. In instances where swelling has been confined to the face and lips, the condition has generally resolved without treatment, although antihistamines have been useful in relieving symptoms.

Angioedema associated with involvement of the tongue, glottis, or larynx, may be fatal due to airway obstruction. Appropriate therapy, e.g., subcutaneous epinephrine solution 1:1000 (0.3 to 0.5 mL) and/or measures to ensure a patent airway, should be promptly provided (see ADVERSE REACTIONS).

Intestinal Angioedema: Intestinal angioedema has been reported in patients treated with ACE inhibitors. These patients presented with abdominal pain (with or without nausea or vomiting); in some cases there was no prior history of facial angioedema and C-1 esterase levels were normal. The angioedema was diagnosed by procedures including abdominal CT scan or ultrasound, or at surgery, and symptoms resolved after stopping the ACE inhibitor. Intestinal angioedema should be included in the differential diagnosis of patients on ACE inhibitors presenting with abdominal pain.

Anaphylactoid Reactions During Desensitization: Two patients undergoing desensitizing treatment with hymenoptera venom while receiving ACE inhibitors sustained life-threatening anaphylactoid reactions. In the same patients, these reactions did not occur when ACE inhibitors were temporarily withheld, but they reappeared when the ACE inhibitors were inadvertently readministered.

Anaphylactoid Reactions During Membrane Exposure: Anaphylactoid reactions have been reported in patients dialyzed with high-flux membranes and treated concomitantly with an ACE inhibitor. Anaphylactoid reactions have also been reported in patients undergoing low-density lipoprotein apheresis with dextran sulfate absorption.

Hypotension

univasc® can cause symptomatic hypotension, although, as with other ACE inhibitors, this is unusual in uncomplicated hypertensive patients treated with univasc® alone. Symptomatic hypotension was seen in 0.5% of patients given moexipril and led to discontinuation of therapy in about 0.25%. Symptomatic hypotension is most likely to occur in patients who have been salt- and volume-depleted as a result of prolonged diuretic therapy, dietary salt restriction, dialysis, diarrhea, or vomiting. Volume- and salt-depletion should be corrected and, in general, diuretics stopped, before initiating therapy with univasc® (see PRECAUTIONS, Drug Interactions, and ADVERSE REACTIONS).

In patients with congestive heart failure, with or without associated renal insufficiency, ACE inhibitor therapy may cause excessive hypotension, which may be associated with oliguria or progressive azotemia, and rarely, with acute renal failure and death. In these patients, univasc® therapy should be started under close medical supervision, and patients should be followed closely for the first two weeks of treatment and whenever the dose of moexipril or an accompanying diuretic is increased. Care in avoiding hypotension should also be taken in patients with ischemic heart disease, aortic stenosis, or cerebrovascular disease, in whom an excessive decrease in blood pressure could result in a myocardial infarction or a cerebrovascular accident.

If hypotension occurs, the patient should be placed in a supine position and, if necessary, treated with an intravenous infusion of normal saline. univasc® treatment usually can be continued following restoration of blood pressure and volume.

Neutropenia/Agranulocytosis

Another ACE inhibitor, captopril, has been shown to cause agranulocytosis and bone marrow depression, rarely in patients with uncomplicated hypertension, but more frequently in hypertensive patients with renal impairment, especially if they also have a collagen-vascular disease such as systemic lupus erythematosus or scleroderma. Although there were no instances of severe neutropenia (absolute neutrophil count <500/mm^3) among patients given univasc®, as with other ACE inhibitors, monitoring of white blood cell counts should be considered for patients who have collagen-vascular disease, especially if the disease is associated with impaired renal function. Available data from clinical trials of univasc® are insufficient to show that univasc® does not cause agranulocytosis at rates similar to captopril.

Fetal/Neonatal Morbidity and Mortality

ACE inhibitors can cause fetal and neonatal morbidity and death when administered to pregnant women. Several dozen cases have been reported in the world literature. When pregnancy is detected, ACE inhibitors should be discontinued as soon as possible.

The use of ACE inhibitors during the second and third trimesters of pregnancy has been associated with fetal and neonatal injury, including hypotension, neonatal skull hypoplasia, anuria, reversible or irreversible renal failure, and death. Oligohydramnios has also been reported, presumably resulting from decreased fetal renal function; oligohydramnios in this setting has been associated with fetal limb contractures, craniofacial deformation, and hypoplastic lung development. Prematurity, intrauterine growth retardation, and patent ductus arteriosus have also been reported, although it is not clear whether these were caused by the ACE inhibitor exposure.

Fetal and neonatal morbidity do not appear to have resulted from intrauterine ACE inhibitor exposure limited to the first trimester. Mothers who have used ACE inhibitors only during the first trimester should be informed of this. Nonetheless, when patients become pregnant, physicians should make every effort to discontinue the use of moexipril as soon as possible. Rarely (probably less often than once in every thousand pregnancies), no alternative to ACE inhibitors will be found. In these rare cases, the mothers should be apprised of the potential hazards to their fetuses, and serial ultrasound examinations should be performed to assess the intraamniotic environment.

If oligohydramnios is observed, moexipril should be discontinued unless it is considered life-saving for the mother. Contraction stress testing (CST), a non-stress test (NST), or biophysical profiling (BPP) may be appropriate, depending upon the week of pregnancy. Patients and physicians should be aware, however, that oligohydramnios may not be detected until after the fetus has sustained irreversible injury. Infants with histories of *in utero* exposure to ACE inhibitors should be closely observed for hypotension, oliguria, and hyperkalemia. If oliguria occurs, attention should be directed toward support of blood pressure and renal perfusion. Exchange transfusion or peritoneal dialysis may be required as means of reversing hypotension and/or substituting for disordered renal function.

Theoretically, the ACE inhibitor could be removed from the neonatal circulation by exchange transfusion, but no experience with this procedure has been reported.

No embryotoxic, fetotoxic, or teratogenic effects were seen in rats or in rabbits treated with up to 90.9 and 0.7 times, respectively, the Maximum Recommended Human Dose (MRHD) on a mg/m^2 basis.

Hepatic Failure

Rarely, ACE inhibitors have been associated with a syndrome that starts with cholestatic jaundice and progresses to fulminant hepatic necrosis and sometimes death. The mechanism of this syndrome is not understood. Patients receiving ACE inhibitors who develop jaundice or marked elevations of hepatic enzymes should discontinue the ACE inhibitor and receive appropriate medical follow-up.

PRECAUTIONS

General

Impaired Renal Function: As a consequence of inhibition of the renin-angiotensin-aldosterone system, changes in renal function may be anticipated in susceptible individuals. There is no clinical experience of univasc® in the treatment of hypertension in patients with renal failure.

Some hypertensive patients with no apparent preexisting renal vascular disease have developed increases in blood urea nitrogen and serum creatinine, usually minor and transient, especially when univasc® has been given conomitantly with a thiazide diuretic. This is more likely to occur in patients with preexisting renal impairment. There may be a need for dose adjustment of univasc® and/or the discontinuation of the thiazide diuretic.

Evaluation of hypertensive patients should always include assessment of renal function (see DOSAGE AND ADMINISTRATION).

Hypertensive Patients With Congestive Heart Failure: In hypertensive patients with severe congestive heart failure, whose renal function may depend on the activity of the renin-angiotensin-aldosterone system, treatment with ACE inhibitors, including univasc®, may be associated with oliguria and/or progressive azotemia and, rarely, acute renal failure and/or death.

Hypertensive Patients With Renal Artery Stenosis: In hypertensive patients with unilateral or bilateral renal artery stenosis, increases in blood urea nitrogen and serum creatinine have been observed in some patients following ACE inhibitor therapy. These increases were almost always reversible upon discontinuation of the ACE inhibitor and/or diuretic therapy. In such patients, renal function should be monitored during the first few weeks of therapy.

Hyperkalemia: In clinical trials, persistent hyperkalemia (serum potassium above 5.4 mEq/L) occurred in approximately 1.3% of hypertensive patients receiving univasc®. Risk factors for the development of hyperkalemia with ACE inhibitors include renal insufficiency, diabetes mellitus, and the concomitant use of potassium-sparing diuretics, potassium supplements, and/or potassium-containing salt substitutes, which should be used cautiously, if at all, with univasc® (see PRECAUTIONS, Drug Interactions).

Surgery/Anesthesia: In patients undergoing major surgery or during anesthesia with agents that produce hypotension, moexipril may block the effects of compensatory renin release. If hypotension occurs in this setting and is considered to be due to this mechanism, it can be corrected by volume expansion.

Cough: Presumably due to the inhibition of the degradation of endogenous bradykinin, persistent nonproductive cough has been reported with all ACE inhibitors, always resolving after discontinuation of therapy. ACE inhibitor-induced cough should be considered in the differential diagnosis of cough. In controlled trials with moexipril, cough was present in 6.1% of moexipril patients and 2.2% of patients given placebo.

Information for Patients

Food: Patients should be advised to take moexipril one hour before meals (see CLINICAL PHARMACOLOGY and DOSAGE AND ADMINISTRATION).

Angioedema: Angioedema, including laryngeal edema, may occur with treatment with ACE inhibitors, usually occurring early in therapy (within the first month). Patients should be so advised and told to report immediately any signs or symptoms suggesting angioedema (swelling of the face, extremities, eyes, lips, tongue, difficulty in breathing) and to take no more univasc® until they have consulted with the prescribing physician.

Symptomatic Hypotension: Patients should be cautioned that lightheadedness can occur with univasc®, especially during the first few days of therapy. If fainting occurs, the patient should stop taking univasc® and consult the prescribing physician.

All patients should be cautioned that excessive perspiration and dehydration may lead to an excessive fall in blood pressure because of reduction in fluid volume. Other causes of volume depletion such as vomiting or diarrhea may also lead to a fall in blood pressure; patients should be advised to consult their physician if they develop these conditions.

Hyperkalemia: Patients should be told not to use potassium supplements or salt substitutes containing potassium without consulting their physician.

Neutropenia: Patients should be told to report promptly any indication of infection (e.g., sore throat, fever) that could be a sign of neutropenia.

Pregnancy: Female patients of childbearing age should be told about the consequences of second- and third-trimester exposure to ACE inhibitors and should also be told that these consequences do not appear to have resulted from intrauterine ACE inhibitor exposure that has been limited to the first trimester. Patients should be asked to report pregnancies to their physicians as soon as possible.

Drug Interactions

Diuretics: Excessive reductions in blood pressure may occur in patients on diuretic therapy when ACE inhibitors are started. The possibility of hypotensive effects with univasc® can be minimized by discontinuing diuretic therapy for several days or cautiously increasing salt intake before initiation of treatment with univasc®. If this is not possible, the starting dose of moexipril should be reduced. (See WARNINGS and DOSAGE AND ADMINISTRATION).

Potassium Supplements and Potassium-Sparing Diuretics: univasc® can increase serum potassium because it decreases aldosterone secretion. Use of potassium-sparing diuretics (spironolactone, triamterene, amiloride) or potassium supplements concomitantly with ACE inhibitors can increase the risk of hyperkalemia. Therefore, if concomitant use of such agents is indicated, they should be given with caution and the patient's serum potassium should be monitored.

Oral Anticoagulants: Interaction studies with warfarin failed to identify any clinically important effect on the serum concentrations of the anticoagulant or on its anticoagulant effect.

Lithium: Increased serum lithium levels and symptoms of lithium toxicity have been reported in patients receiving ACE inhibitors during therapy with lithium. These drugs should be coadministered with caution, and frequent monitoring of serum lithium levels is recommended. If a diuretic is also used, the risk of lithium toxicity may be increased.

Other Agents: No clinically important pharmacokinetic interactions occurred when univasc® was administered concomitantly with hydrochlorothiazide, digoxin, or cimetidine. univasc® has been used in clinical trials concomitantly with calcium-channel-blocking agents, diuretics, H_2 blockers, digoxin, oral hypoglycemic agents, and cholesterol-lowering agents. There was no evidence of clinically important adverse interactions.

Carcinogenesis, Mutagenesis, Impairment of Fertility

No evidence of carcinogenicity was detected in long-term studies in mice and rats at doses up to 14 or 27.3 times the Maximum Recommended Human Dose (MRHD) on a mg/m^2 basis.

No mutagenicity was detected in the Ames test and microbial reverse mutation assay, with and without metabolic activation, or in an *in vivo* nucleus anomaly test. However, increased chromosomal aberration frequency in Chinese hamster ovary cells was detected under metabolic activation conditions at a 20-hour harvest time.

Reproduction studies have been performed in rabbits at oral doses up to 0.7 times the MRHD on a mg/m^2 basis, and in rats up to 90.9 times the MRHD on a mg/m^2 basis. No indication of impaired fertility, reproductive toxicity, or teratogenicity was observed.

Pregnancy

Pregnancy Categories C (first trimester) and D (second and third trimesters). See WARNINGS, Fetal/Neonatal Morbidity and Mortality.

Continued on next page

Univasc—Cont.

Nursing Mothers

It is not known whether univasc® is excreted in human milk. Because many drugs are excreted in human milk, caution should be exercised when univasc® is given to a nursing mother.

Pediatric Use

Safety and effectiveness of univasc® in pediatric patients have not been established.

Geriatric Use

Clinical studies of univasc® did not include sufficient numbers of subjects aged 65 and over to determine whether they respond differently from younger subjects. Other reported clinical experience has not identified differences in responses between the elderly and younger patients. In general, dose selection for an elderly patient should be cautious, usually starting at the low end of the dosing range, reflecting the greater frequency of decreased hepatic, renal, or cardiac function, and of concomitant disease or other drug therapy.

ADVERSE REACTIONS

univasc® has been evaluated for safety in more than 2500 patients with hypertension; more than 250 of these patients were treated for approximately one year. The overall incidence of reported adverse events was only slightly greater in patients treated with univasc® than patients treated with placebo.

Reported adverse experiences were usually mild and transient, and there were no differences in adverse reaction rates related to gender, race, age, duration of therapy, or total daily dosage within the range of 3.75 mg to 60 mg. Discontinuation of therapy because of adverse experiences was required in 3.4% of patients treated with univasc® and in 1.8% of patients treated with placebo. The most common reasons for discontinuation in patients treated with univasc® were cough (0.7%) and dizziness (0.4%).

All adverse experiences considered at least possibly related to treatment that occurred at any dose in placebo-controlled trials of once-daily dosing in more than 1% of patients treated with univasc® alone and that were at least as frequent in the univasc® group as in the placebo group are shown in the following table:

ADVERSE EVENTS IN PLACEBO-CONTROLLED STUDIES

ADVERSE EVENT	UNIVASC (N=674)	PLACEBO (N=226)
	N (%)	N (%)
Cough Increased	41 (6.1)	5 (2.2)
Dizziness	29 (4.3)	5 (2.2)
Diarrhea	21 (3.1)	5 (2.2)
Flu Syndrome	21 (3.1)	0 (0)
Fatigue	16 (2.4)	4 (1.8)
Pharyngitis	12 (1.8)	2 (0.9)
Flushing	11 (1.6)	0 (0)
Rash	11 (1.6)	2 (0.9)
Myalgia	9 (1.3)	0 (0)

Other adverse events occurring in more than 1% of patients on moexipril that were at least as frequent on placebo include: headache, upper respiratory infection, pain, rhinitis, dyspepsia, nausea, peripheral edema, sinusitis, chest pain, and urinary frequency. See WARNINGS and PRECAUTIONS for discussion of anaphylactoid reactions, angioedema, hypotension, neutropenia/agranulocytosis, second and third trimester fetal/neonatal morbidity and mortality, hyperkalemia, and cough.

Other potentially important adverse experiences reported in controlled or uncontrolled clinical trials in less than 1% of moexipril patients or that have been attributed to other ACE inhibitors include the following:

Cardiovascular: Symptomatic hypotension, postural hypotension, or syncope were seen in 9/1750 (0.51%) patients; these reactions led to discontinuation of therapy in controlled trials in 3/1254 (0.24%) patients who had received univasc® monotherapy and in 1/344 (0.3%) patients who had received univasc® with hydrochlorothiazide (see PRECAUTIONS and WARNINGS). Other adverse events included angina/myocardial infarction, palpitations, rhythm disturbances, and cerebrovascular accident.

Renal: Of hypertensive patients with no apparent preexisting renal disease, 1% of patients receiving univasc® alone and 2% of patients receiving univasc® with hydrochlorothiazide experienced increases in serum creatinine to at least 140% of their baseline values (see PRECAUTIONS and DOSAGE AND ADMINISTRATION).

Gastrointestinal: Abdominal pain, constipation, vomiting, appetite/weight change, dry mouth, pancreatitis, hepatitis.

Respiratory: Bronchospasm, dyspnea, eosinophilic pneumonitis.

Urogenital: Renal insufficiency, oliguria.

Dermatologic: Apparent hypersensitivity reactions manifested by urticaria, rash, pemphigus, pruritus, photosensitivity, alopecia.

Neurological and Psychiatric: Drowsiness, sleep disturbances, nervousness, mood changes, anxiety.

Other: Angioedema (see WARNINGS), taste disturbances, tinnitus, sweating, malaise, arthralgia, hemolytic anemia.

Clinical Laboratory Test Findings

Serum Electrolytes: Hyperkalemia (see PRECAUTIONS), hyponatremia.

Creatinine and Blood Urea Nitrogen: As with other ACE inhibitors, minor increases in blood urea nitrogen or serum creatinine, reversible upon discontinuation of therapy, were observed in approximately 1% of patients with essential hypertension who were treated with univasc®. Increases are more likely to occur in patients receiving concomitant diuretics and in patients with compromised renal function (see PRECAUTIONS, General).

Other (causal relationship unknown): Clinically important changes in standard laboratory tests were rarely associated with univasc® administration.

Elevations of liver enzymes and uric acid have been reported. In trials, less than 1% of moexipril-treated patients discontinued univasc® treatment because of laboratory abnormalities. The incidence of abnormal laboratory values with moexipril was similar to that in the placebo-treated group.

OVERDOSAGE

Human overdoses of moexipril have not been reported. In case reports of overdoses with other ACE inhibitors, hypotension has been the principal adverse effect noted. Single oral doses of 2 g/kg moexipril were associated with significant lethality in mice. Rats, however, tolerated single oral doses of up to 3 g/kg.

No data are available to suggest that physiological maneuvers (e.g., maneuvers to change the pH of the urine) would accelerate elimination of moexipril and its metabolites. The dialyzability of moexipril is not known.

Angiotensin II could presumably serve as a specific antagonist-antidote in the setting of moexipril overdose, but angiotensin II is essentially unavailable outside of research facilities. Because the hypotensive effect of moexipril is achieved through vasodilation and effective hypovolemia, it is reasonable to treat moexipril overdose by infusion of normal saline solution. In addition, renal function and serum potassium should be monitored.

DOSAGE AND ADMINISTRATION

Hypertension

The recommended initial dose of univasc® in patients not receiving diuretics is 7.5 mg, one hour prior to meals, once daily. Dosage should be adjusted according to blood pressure response. The antihypertensive effect of univasc® may diminish towards the end of the dosing interval. Blood pressure should, therefore, be measured just prior to dosing to determine whether satisfactory blood pressure control is obtained. If control is not adequate, increased dose or divided dosing can be tried. The recommended dose range is 7.5 to 30 mg daily, administered in one or two divided doses one hour before meals. Total daily doses above 60 mg a day have not been studied in hypertensive patients.

In patients who are currently being treated with a diuretic, symptomatic hypotension may occasionally occur following the initial dose of univasc®. The diuretic should, if possible, be discontinued for 2 to 3 days before therapy with univasc® is begun, to reduce the likelihood of hypotension (see WARNINGS). If the patient's blood pressure is not controlled with univasc® alone, diuretic therapy may then be reinstituted. If diuretic therapy cannot be discontinued, an initial dose of 3.75 mg of univasc® should be used with medical supervision until blood pressure has stabilized (see WARNINGS and PRECAUTIONS, Drug Interactions).

Dosage Adjustment in Renal Impairment

For patients with a creatinine clearance ≤40 mL/min/1.73 m^2, an initial dose of 3.75 mg once daily should be given cautiously. Doses may be titrated upward to a maximum daily dose of 15 mg.

HOW SUPPLIED

univasc® (moexipril hydrochloride) 7.5 mg tablets are pink colored, biconvex, film-coated and scored with engraved code **707** on the unscored side and **SP** above and 7.5 below the score. They are supplied as follows:

Bottles of 90 (Unit-of-Use) NDC 0091-3707-09
Bottles of 100 NDC 0091-3707-01

univasc® (moexipril hydrochloride) 15 mg tablets are salmon colored, biconvex, film-coated, and scored with engraved code **715** on the unscored side and **SP** above and **15** below the score. They are supplied as follows:

Bottles of 90 (Unit-of-Use) NDC 0091-3715-09
Bottles of 100 NDC 0091-3715-01

Store, tightly closed, at controlled room temperature. Protect from excessive moisture.

If product package is subdivided, dispense in tight containers as described in USP-NF.

SCHWARZ
PHARMA
Milwaukee, WI 53201, USA

PC1879L
Rev. 02/03

VERELAN® ℞

[vĕr'ă-lăn]
(Verapamil HCl)
Sustained-Release Pellet Filled Capsules
Rx Only

DESCRIPTION

VERELAN (verapamil hydrochloride capsules) is a calcium ion influx inhibitor (slow channel blocker or calcium ion antagonist). VERELAN is available for oral administration as a 360 mg hard gelatin capsule (lavender cap/yellow body), a 240 mg hard gelatin capsule (dark blue cap/yellow body), a 180 mg hard gelatin capsule (light grey cap/yellow body), and a 120 mg hard gelatin capsule (yellow cap/yellow body). These pellet filled capsules provide a sustained-release of the drug in the gastrointestinal tract.

The structural formula of verapamil HCl is given below:

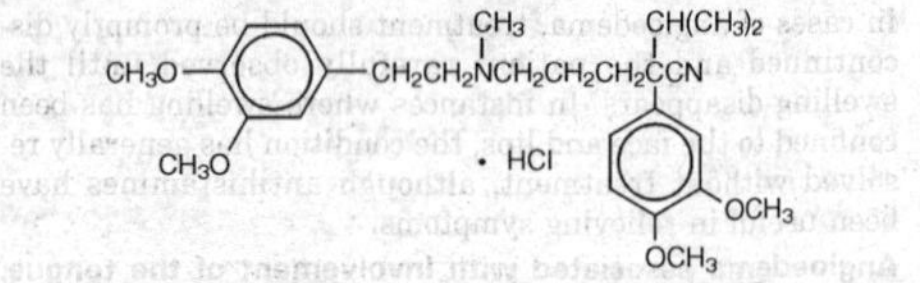

$C_{27}H_{38}N_2O_4 \cdot HCl$ M.W. 491.07

Chemical name: Benzeneacetonitrile, α-[3-[[2-(3,4-dimethoxyphenyl)-ethyl]methylamino]propyl]-3,4-dimethoxy-α-(1-methylethyl) monohydrochloride.

Verapamil HCl is an almost white, crystalline powder, practically free of odor, with a bitter taste. It is soluble in water, chloroform, and methanol. Verapamil HCl is not structurally related to other cardioactive drugs.

In addition to verapamil HCl the VERELAN capsule contains the following inactive ingredients: fumaric acid, talc, sugar spheres, povidone, shellac, gelatin, FD&C red #40, yellow iron oxide, titanium dioxide, methylparaben, propylparaben, silicon dioxide, and sodium lauryl sulfate. In addition, the VERELAN 240 mg and 360 mg capsules contain FD&C blue #1 and D&C red #28; and the VERELAN 180 mg capsule contains black iron oxide.

HOW SUPPLIED

VERELAN® verapamil HCl sustained-release pellet filled capsules are supplied in four dosage strengths:

120 mg—Two-piece, size 2 hard gelatin capsule (yellow cap/yellow body), printed with SCHWARZ above 2490 on left and VERELAN above 120 mg on right side of the capsule in black ink, supplied as follows:
NDC 0091-2490-23—Bottle of 100s

180 mg—Two-piece, size 1 elongated hard gelatin capsule (light grey cap/yellow body), printed with SCHWARZ above 2489 on left and VERELAN above 180 mg on right side of the capsule in black ink, supplied as follows:
NDC 0091-2489-23–Bottle of 100s

240 mg—Two-piece, size 0 hard gelatin capsule (dark blue cap/yellow body), printed with SCHWARZ above 2491 on left and VERELAN above 240 mg on right side of the capsule in black ink, supplied as follows:
NDC 0091-2491-23—Bottle of 100s

360 mg—Two-piece, size 00 hard gelatin capsule (lavender cap/yellow body), printed with SCHWARZ above 2495 on left and VERELAN above 360 mg on right side of the capsule in black ink, supplied as follows:
NDC 0091-2495-23—Bottle of 100s.

Store at controlled room temperature 20°–25°C (68°–77°F) [See USP]. Avoid excessive heat. Brief digressions above 25°C, while not detrimental, should be avoided. Protect from moisture.

Dispense in tight, light-resistant container as defined in USP.

Manufactured for:
SCHWARZ
PHARMA
Milwaukee, WI 53201
by
ELAN HOLDINGS, INC.
Gainesville, GA 30504

PC3799B Rev. 4/2000

VERELAN® PM Capsules ℞

[vĕr'ă-lăn]
(verapamil hydrochloride)
extended-release capsules controlled-onset
Rx Only

DESCRIPTION

Verelan® PM (verapamil hydrochloride) is a calcium ion influx inhibitor (slow channel blocker or calcium ion antagonist). Verelan® PM is available for oral administration as a 100 mg hard gelatin capsule (white opaque cap/amethyst body), a 200 mg hard gelatin capsule (amethyst opaque cap/amethyst body), and as a 300 mg hard gelatin capsule (lavender opaque cap/amethyst body). Verapamil is administered as a racemic mixture of the R and S enantiomers.

The structural formulae of the verapamil HCl enantiomers are:

[See chemical structure at top of next column]

Chemical name: Benzeneacetonitrile, α-[3-[[2-(3,4-dimethoxyphenyl)ethyl]methylamino]propyl]-3,4-dimethoxy-α-(1-methylethyl)-, monohydrochloride,(±)-.

S-verapamil

R-verapamil

$C_{27}H_{38}N_2O_4$•HCl M.W.=491.07

Verapamil HCl is an almost white, crystalline powder, practically free of odor, with a bitter taste. It is soluble in water, chloroform and methanol. Verapamil HCl is not structurally related to other cardioactive drugs.

In addition to verapamil HCl the Verelan® PM capsule contains the following inactive ingredients: D&C Red #28, FD & C Blue #1, FD&C red #40, fumaric acid, gelatin, povidone, shellac, silicon dioxide, sodium lauryl sulfate, starch, sugar spheres, talc, and titanium dioxide.

CLINICAL PHARMACOLOGY

Verapamil is a calcium ion influx inhibitor (L-type calcium channel blocker or calcium channel antagonist). Verapamil exerts its pharmacologic effects by selectively inhibiting the transmembrane influx of ionic calcium into arterial smooth muscle as well as in conductile and contractile myocardial cells without altering serum calcium concentrations.

System Components and Performance: Verelan® PM uses the proprietary CODAS™ (Chronotherapeutic Oral Drug Absorption System) technology, which is designed for bedtime dosing, incorporating a 4 to 5-hour delay in drug delivery. The controlled-onset delivery system results in a maximum plasma concentration (C_{max}) of verapamil in the morning hours. These pellet filled capsules provide for extended-release of the drug in the gastrointestinal tract. The Verelan® PM formulation has been designed to initiate the release of verapamil 4–5 hours after ingestion. This delay is introduced by the level of non-enteric release-controlling polymer applied to drug loaded beads. The release-controlling polymer is a combination of water soluble and water insoluble polymers. As water from the gastrointestinal tract comes into contact with the polymer coated beads, the water soluble polymer slowly dissolves and the drug diffuses through the resulting pores in the coating. The water insoluble polymer continues to act as a barrier, maintaining the controlled release of the drug. The rate of release is essentially independent of pH, posture and food. Multiparticulate systems such as Verelan® PM have been shown to be independent of gastrointestinal motility.

Mechanism of Action

In vitro: Verapamil binding is voltage-dependent with affinity increasing as the vascular smooth muscle membrane potential is reduced. In addition, verapamil binding is frequency dependent and apparent affinity increases with increased frequency of depolarizing stimulus.

The L-type calcium channel is an oligomeric structure consisting of five putative subunits designated alpha-1, alpha-2, beta, tau, and epsilon. Biochemical evidence points to separate binding sites for 1,4-dihydropyridines, phenylalkylamines, and the benzothiazepines (all located on the alpha-1 subunit). Although they share a similar mechanism of action, calcium channel blockers represent three heterogeneous categories of drugs with differing vascular-cardiac selectivity ratios.

Essential hypertension: Verapamil produces its antihypertensive effect by a combination of vascular and cardiac effects. It acts as a vasodilator with selectivity for the arterial portion of the peripheral vasculature. As a result the systemic vascular resistance is reduced and usually without orthostatic hypotension or reflex tachycardia. Bradycardia (rate less than 50 beats/min) is uncommon. During isometric or dynamic exercise verapamil does not alter systolic cardiac function in patients with normal ventricular function. Verapamil does not alter total serum calcium levels. However, one report has suggested that calcium levels above the normal range may alter the therapeutic effect of verapamil. Verapamil regularly reduces the total systemic resistance (afterload) against which the heart works both at rest and at a given level of exercise by dilating peripheral arterioles.

Effects in hypertension: Verelan® PM was evaluated in two placebo-controlled, parallel design, double-blind studies of patients with mild to moderate hypertension. In the clinical trials, 413 evaluable patients were randomized to either placebo, 100 mg, 200 mg, 300 mg, or 400 mg and treated for up to 8 weeks. Verelan® PM or placebo was given once daily between 9 pm and 11 pm (nighttime) and blood pressure changes were measured with 36-hour ambulatory blood pressure monitoring (ABPM). The results of these studies demonstrate that Verelan® PM, at 200, 300 and 400 mg, is a consistently and significantly more effective antihypertensive agent than placebo in reducing ambulatory blood pressures. Over this dose range, the placebo-subtracted net decreases in diastolic BP at trough (averaged over 6–10 pm) were dose-related, and ranged from 3.8 to 10.0 mm Hg after 8 weeks of therapy. Although Verelan® PM 100 mg was not effective in reducing diastolic BP at trough when measured by ABPM, efficacy was demonstrated in reducing diastolic BP when measured manually at trough and peak and, from 6 am to 12 noon and over 24 hours when measured by ABPM (See **DOSAGE AND ADMINISTRATION** for titration schedule).

There were no apparent treatment differences between patient subgroups of different age (older or younger than 65 years), sex and race. For severity of hypertension, "moderate" hypertensives (mean daytime diastolic BP ≥ 105 mm Hg and ≤ 114 mm Hg) appeared to respond better than "mild" hypertensives (mean daytime diastolic BP ≥ 90 mm Hg and ≤ 104 mm Hg). However, sample size for the subgroup comparisons were limited.

Electrophysiologic effects: Electrical activity through the AV node depends, to a significant degree, upon the transmembrane influx of extracellular calcium through the L-type (slow) channel. By decreasing the influx of calcium, verapamil prolongs the effective refractory period within the AV node and slows AV conduction in a rate-related manner.

Normal sinus rhythm is usually not affected, but in patients with sick sinus syndrome, verapamil may interfere with sinus-node impulse generation and may induce sinus arrest or sinoatrial block. Atrioventricular block can occur in patients without pre-existing conduction defects (See **WARNINGS**).

Verapamil does not alter the normal atrial action potential or intraventricular conduction time, but depresses amplitude, velocity of depolarization, and conduction in depressed atrial fibers. Verapamil may shorten the antegrade effective refractory period of the accessory bypass tract. Acceleration of ventricular rate and/or ventricular fibrillation has been reported in patients with atrial flutter or atrial fibrillation and a coexisting accessory AV pathway following administration of verapamil (See **WARNINGS**).

Verapamil has a local anesthetic action that is 1.6 times that of procaine on an equimolar basis. It is not known whether this action is important at the doses used in man.

Pharmacokinetics and metabolism: Verapamil is administered as a racemic mixture of the R and S enantiomers. The systemic concentrations of R and S enantiomers, as well as overall bioavailability, are dependent upon the route of administration and the rate and extent of release from the dosage forms. Upon oral administration, there is rapid stereoselective biotransformation during the first pass of verapamil through the portal circulation. In a study in 5 subjects with oral immediate-release verapamil, the systemic bioavailability was from 33% to 65% for the R enantiomer and from 13% to 34% for the S enantiomer. Following oral administration of an immediately releasing formulation every 8 hours in 24 subjects, the relative systemic availability of the S enantiomer compared to the R enantiomer was approximately 13% following a single day's administration and approximately 18% following administration to steady-state. The degree of stereoselectivity of metabolism for Verelan® PM was similar to that for the immediately releasing formulation. The R and S enantiomers have differing levels of pharmacologic activity. In studies in animals and humans, the S enantiomer has 8 to 20 times the activity of the R enantiomer in slowing AV conduction. In animal studies, the S enantiomer has 15 to 50 times the activity of the R enantiomer in reducing myocardial contractility in isolated blood-perfused dog papillary muscle, respectively, and twice the effect in reducing peripheral resistance. In isolated septal strip preparations from 5 patients, the S enantiomer was 8 times more potent than the R in reducing myocardial contractility. Dose escalation study data indicate that verapamil concentrations increase disproportionally to dose as measured by relative peak plasma concentrations (C_{max}) or areas under the plasma concentration vs time curves (AUC). Although some evidence of lack of dose linearity was observed for Verelan® PM, this non-linearity was enantiomer specific, with the R enantiomer showing the greatest degree of non-linearity.

[See table above]

Pharmacokinetic Characteristics of Verapamil Enantiomers After Administration of Escalating Doses of Verelan® PM

	ISOMER	200	300	400
Dose Ratio		1	1.5	2
Relative Cmax	R	1	1.89	2.34
	S	1	1.88	2.5
Relative AUC	R	1	1.67	2.34
	S	1	1.35	2.20

Racemic verapamil is released from Verelan® PM by diffusion following the gradual solubilization of the water soluble polymer. The rate of solubilization of the water soluble polymer produces a lag period in drug release for approximately 4–5 hours. The drug release phase is prolonged with the peak plasma concentration (C_{max}) occurring approximately 11 hours after administration. Trough concentrations occur approximately 4 hours after bedtime dosing while the patient is sleeping. Steady-state pharmacokinetics were determined in healthy volunteers. Steady-state concentration is achieved by day 5 of dosing.

In healthy volunteers, following administration of Verelan® PM (200 mg per day), steady-state pharmacokinetics of the R and S enantiomers of verapamil is as follows: Mean C_{max} of the R isomer was 77.8 ng/ml and 16.8 ng/ml for the S isomer; AUC (0–24h) of the R isomer was 1037 ng.h/ml and 195 ng.h/ml for the S isomer.

In general, bioavailability of verapamil is higher and half life longer in older (>65 yrs) subjects. Lean body weight also affects its pharmacokinetics inversely. It was not possible to observe a gender difference in the clinical trials of Verelan® PM due to the small sample size. However, there are conflicting data in the literature suggesting that verapamil clearance decreased with age in women to a greater degree than in men.

Consumption of a high fat meal just prior to dosing in the morning had no effect on the extent of absorption and a modest effect on the rate of absorption from Verelan® PM. The rate of absorption was not affected by whether the volunteers were supine two hours after night-time dosing or non-supine for four hours following morning dosing. Administering Verelan® PM in the morning increased the extent of absorption of verapamil and/or decreased the metabolism to norverapamil.

Orally administered verapamil undergoes extensive metabolism in the liver. Verapamil is metabolized by O-demethylation (25%) and N-dealkylation (40%), and is subject to presystemic hepatic metabolism with elimination of up to 80% of the dose. The metabolism is mediated by hepatic cytochrome P_{450}, and animal studies have implied that the mono-oxygenase is the specific isoenzyme of the P_{450} family. Thirteen metabolites have been identified in urine. Norverapamil enantiomers can reach steady-state plasma concentrations approximately equal to those of the enantiomers of the parent drug. For Verelan® PM, the norverapamil R enantiomer reached steady-state plasma concentrations similar to the verapamil R enantiomer, but the norverapamil S enantiomer concentrations were approximately twice that of the verapamil S enantiomer concentrations. The cardiovascular activity of norverapamil appears to be approximately 20% that of verapamil. Approximately 70% of an administered dose is excreted as metabolites in the urine and 16% or more in the feces within 5 days. About 3% to 4% is excreted in the urine as unchanged drug.

R verapamil is 94% bound to plasma albumin, while S verapamil is 88% bound. In addition, R verapamil is 92% and S verapamil 86% bound to alpha-1 acid glycoprotein. In patients with hepatic insufficiency, metabolism of immediate-release verapamil is delayed and elimination half-life prolonged up to 14 to 16 hours because of the extensive hepatic metabolism (See **PRECAUTIONS**). In addition, in these patients there is a reduced first pass effect, and verapamil is more bioavailable. Verapamil clearance values suggest that patients with liver dysfunction may attain therapeutic verapamil plasma concentrations with one third of the oral daily dose required for patients with normal liver function.

After four weeks of oral dosing of immediate-release verapamil (120 mg q.i.d.), verapamil and norverapamil levels were noted in the cerebrospinal fluid with estimated partition coefficient of 0.06 for verapamil and 0.04 for norverapamil.

Geriatric Use: The pharmacokinetics of verapamil GITS were studied after 5 consecutive nights of dosing 180 mg in 30 healthy young (19–43 years) versus 30 healthy elderly (65–80 years) male and female subjects. Older subjects had significantly higher mean verapamil C_{max}, C_{min} and $AUC_{(0-24h)}$ compared to younger subjects. Older subjects had mean AUCs that were approximately 1.7–2.0 times higher than those of younger subjects as well as a longer average verapamil $t_{1/2}$ (approximately 20 hr vs 13 hr).

Hemodynamics: Verapamil reduces afterload and myocardial contractility. In most patients, including those with organic cardiac disease, the negative inotropic action of verapamil is countered by reduction of afterload and cardiac index remains unchanged. During isometric or dynamic exercise, verapamil does not alter systolic cardiac function in patients with normal ventricular function. Improved left ventricular diastolic function in patients with IHSS and those with coronary heart disease has also been observed with verapamil. In patients with severe left ventricular dysfunction (e.g., pulmonary wedge pressure above 20 mm Hg or ejection fraction less than 30%), or in patients taking beta-adrenergic blocking agents or other cardiodepressant drugs, deterioration of ventricular function may occur (See **Drug Interactions**).

Pulmonary function: Verapamil does not induce bronchoconstriction and, hence, does not impair ventilatory function.

Verapamil has been shown to have either a neutral or relaxant effect on bronchial smooth muscle.

INDICATIONS AND USAGE

Verelan® PM is indicated for the management of essential hypertension.

Continued on next page

Verelan PM—Cont.

CONTRAINDICATIONS

Verapamil is contraindicated in:
1. Severe left ventricular dysfunction (See **WARNINGS**).
2. Hypotension (less than 90 mm Hg systolic pressure) or cardiogenic shock.
3. Sick sinus syndrome (except in patients with a functioning artifical ventricular pacemaker).
4. Second- or third-degree AV block (except in patients with a functioning artificial ventricular pacemaker).
5. Patients with atrial flutter or atrial fibrillation and an accessory bypass tract (e.g., Wolff-Parkinson-White, Lown-Ganong-Levine syndromes) (See **WARNINGS**).
6. Patients with known hypersensitivity to verapamil hydrochloride.

WARNINGS

Heart failure: Verapamil has a negative inotropic effect which, in most patients, is compensated by its afterload reduction (decreased systemic vascular resistance) properties without a net impairment of ventricular performance. In previous clinical experience with 4,954 patients primarily with immediate-release verapamil, 87 (1.8%) developed congestive heart failure or pulmonary edema. Verapamil should be avoided in patients with severe left ventricular dysfunction (e.g., ejection fraction less than 30% or moderate to severe symptoms of cardiac failure) and in patients with any degree of ventricular dysfunction if they are receiving a beta-adrenergic blocker (See **Drug Interactions**). Patients with milder ventricular dysfunction should, if possible, be controlled with optimum doses of digitalis and/or diuretics before verapamil treatment is started (See **PRECAUTIONS, Drug Interactions, Digitalis**).

Hypotension: Occasionally, the pharmacologic action of verapamil may produce a decrease in blood pressure below normal levels which may result in dizziness or symptomatic hypotension. The incidence of hypotension observed in 4,954 patients enrolled in clinical trials was 2.5%. In hypertensive patients, decreases in blood pressure below normal are unusual. Tilt table testing (60 degrees) was not able to induce orthostatic hypotension. In clinical studies of Verelan® PM, 1.7% of the patients developed significant hypotension.

Elevated liver enzymes: Elevations of transaminases with and without concomitant elevations in alkaline phosphatase and bilirubin have been reported. Such elevations have sometimes been transient and may disappear even in the face of continued verapamil treatment.

Several cases of hepatocellular injury related to verapamil have been proven by rechallenge; half of these had clinical symptoms (malaise, fever, and/or right upper quadrant pain) in addition to elevations of SGOT, SGPT and alkaline phosphatase. Periodic monitoring of liver function in patients receiving verapamil is therefore prudent.

Accessory bypass tract (Wolff-Parkinson-White or Lown-Ganong Levine): Some patients with paroxysmal and/or chronic atrial flutter or atrial fibrillation and a coexisting accessory AV pathway have developed increased antegrade conduction across the accessory pathway bypassing the AV node, producing a very rapid ventricular response or ventricular fibrillation after receiving intravenous verapamil (or digitalis). Although a risk of this occurring with oral verapamil has not been established, such patients receiving oral verapamil may be at risk and its use in these patients is contraindicated (See **CONTRAINDICATIONS**).

Treatment is usually DC-cardioversion. Cardioversion has been used safely and effectively after oral verapamil.

Atrioventricular block

The effect of verapamil on AV conduction and the SA node may lead to asymptomatic first-degree AV block and transient bradycardia, sometimes accompanied by nodal escape rhythms. PR interval prolongation is correlated with verapamil plasma concentrations, especially during the early titration phase of therapy. Higher degrees of AV block, however, were infrequently (0.8%) observed in previous verapamil clinical trials.

Marked first-degree block or progressive development to second- or third-degree AV block requires a reduction in dosage or, in rate instances, discontinuation of verapamil and institution of appropriate therapy depending upon the clinical situation.

Patients with hypertrophic cardiomyopathy (IHSS)

In 120 patients with hypertrophic cardiomyopathy (most of them refractory or intolerant to propranolol) who received therapy with verapamil at doses up to 720 mg/day, a variety of serious adverse effects were seen. Three patients died in pulmonary edema; all had severe left ventricular outflow obstruction and a past history of left ventricular dysfunction. Eight other patients had pulmonary edema and/or severe hypotension; abnormally high (over 20 mm Hg) pulmonary capillary wedge pressure and a marked left ventricular outflow obstruction were present in most of these patients. Concomitant administration of quinidine (See **Drug Interactions**) preceded the severe hypotension in 3 of the 8 patients (2 of whom developed pulmonary edema). Sinus bradycardia occurred in 11% of the patients, second-degree AV block in 4% and sinus arrest in 2%. It must be appreciated that this group of patients had a serious disease with a high mortality rate. Most adverse effects responded well to dose reduction and only rarely did verapamil have to be discontinued.

PRECAUTIONS

THE CONTENTS OF THE Verelan® PM CAPSULE SHOULD NOT BE CRUSHED OR CHEWED.

General

Use in patients with impaired hepatic function: Since verapamil is highly metabolized by the liver, it should be administered cautiously to patients with impaired hepatic function. Severe liver dysfunction prolongs the elimination half-life of immediate-release verapamil to about 14 to 16 hours; hence, approximately 30% of the dose given to patients with normal liver function should be administered to these patients. Careful monitoring for abnormal prolongation of the PR interval or other signs of excessive pharmacologic effects (See **OVERDOSAGE**) should be carried out.

Use in patients with attenuated (decreased) neuromuscular transmission: It has been reported that verapamil decreases neuromuscular transmission in patients with Duchenne's muscular dystrophy, and that verapamil prolongs recovery from the neuromuscular blocking agent vecuronium and causes a worsening of myasthenia gravis. It may be necessary to decrease the dosage of verapamil when it is administered to patients with attenuated neuromuscular transmission.

Use in patients with impaired renal function: About 70% of an administered dose of verapamil is excreted as metabolites in the urine. Until further data are available, verapamil should be administered cautiously to patients with impaired renal function. These patients should be carefully monitored for abnormal prolongation of the PR interval or other signs of overdosage (See **OVERDOSAGE**).

Drug-Drug Interactions

Drug Interactions: Effects of other drugs on verapamil pharmacokinetics: *In vitro* metabolic studies indicate that verapamil is metabolized by cytochrome P450 CYP3A4, CYP1A2, and CYP2C. Clinically significant interactions have been reported with inhibitors of CYP3A4 (eg, erythromycin, ritonavir) causing elevation of plasma levels of verapamil while inducers of CYP3A4 (eg, rifampin) have caused a lowering of plasma levels of verapamil.

Alcohol: Verapamil has been found to significantly inhibit ethanol elimination resulting in elevated blood ethanol concentrations that may prolong the intoxicating effects of alcohol.

Antineoplastic agents: Verapamil can increase the efficacy of doxorubicin both in tissue culture systems and in patients. It raises the serum doxorubicin levels. The absorption of verapamil can be reduced by the cyclophosphamide, oncovin, procarbazine, prednisone (COPP) and the vindesine, adriamycin, cisplatin (VAC) cytotoxic drug regimens. Concomitant administration of R verapamil can decrease the clearance of paclitaxel.

Aspirin: In a few reported cases, coadministration of verapamil with aspirin has led to increased bleeding times greater than observed with aspirin alone.

Beta blockers: Concomitant therapy with beta-adrenergic blockers and verapamil may result in additive negative effects on heart rate, atrioventricular conduction, and/or cardiac contractility. The combination of extended-release verapamil and beta-adrenergic blocking agents has not been studied. However, there have been reports of excess bradycardia and AV block, including complete heart block, when the combination has been used for the treatment of hypertension. For hypertensive patients, the risk of combined therapy may outweigh the potential benefits. The combination should be used only with caution and close monitoring. Asymptomatic bradycardia (36 beats/min) with a wandering atrial pacemaker has been observed in a patient receiving concomitant timolol (a beta-adrenergic blocker) eyedrops and oral verapamil.

A decrease in metoprolol and propranolol clearance has been observed when either drug is administered concomitantly with verapamil. A variable effect has been seen when verapamil and atenolol were given together.

Digitalis: Clinical use of verapamil in digitalized patients has shown the combination to be well tolerated if digoxin doses are properly adjusted. However, chronic verapamil treatment can increase serum digoxin levels by 50% to 75% during the first week of therapy, and this can result in digitalis toxicity. In patients with hepatic cirrhosis the influence of verapamil on digoxin kinetics is magnified. Verapamil may reduce total body clearance and extrarenal clearance of digitoxin by 27% and 29%, respectively. Maintenance and digitalization doses should be reduced when verapamil is administered, and the patient should be reassessed to avoid over- or underdigitalization. Whenever overdigitalization is suspected, the daily dose of digoxin should be reduced or temporarily discontinued. On discontinuation of verapamil use, the patient should be reassessed to avoid underdigitalization. In previous clinical trials with other verapamil formulations related to the control of ventricular response in digitalized patients who had atrial fibrillation or atrial flutter, ventricular rates below 50/min at rest occurred in 15% of patients, and asymptomatic hypotension occurred in 5% of patients.

Antihypertensive agents

Verapamil administered concomitantly with oral antihypertensive agents (e.g., vasodilators, angiotensin-converting enzyme inhibitors, diuretics, beta blockers) will usually have an additive effect on lowering blood pressure. Patients receiving these combinations should be appropriately monitored. Concomitant use of agents that attenuate alpha-adrenergic function with verapamil may result in reduction in blood pressure that is excessive in some patients. Such an effect was observed in one study following the concomitant administration of verapamil and prazosin.

Antiarrhythmic agents

Disopyramide: Until data on possible interactions between verapamil and disopyramide are obtained, disopyramide should not be administered within 48 hours before or 24 hours after verapamil administration.

Flecainide: A study in healthy volunteers showed that the concomitant administration of flecainide and verapamil may have additive effects on myocardial contractility, AV conduction, and repolarization. Concomitant therapy with flecainide and verapamil may result in additive negative inotropic effect and prolongation of atrioventricular conduction.

Quinidine: In a small number of patients with hypertrophic cardiomyopathy (IHSS), concomitant use of verapamil and quinidine resulted in significant hypotension. Until further data are obtained, combined therapy of verapamil and quinidine in patients with hypertrophic cardiomyopathy should probably be avoided.

The electrophysiological effects of quinidine and verapamil on AV conduction were studied in 8 patients. Verapamil significantly counteracted the effects of quinidine on AV conduction. There has been a report of increased quinidine levels during verapamil therapy.

Other

Nitrates: Verapamil has been given concomitantly with short- and long-acting nitrates without any undesirable drug interactions. The pharmacologic profile of both drugs and the clinical experience suggest beneficial interactions.

Cimetidine: The interaction between cimetidine and chronically administered verapamil has not been studied. Variable results on clearance have been obtained in acute studies of healthy volunteers; clearance of verapamil was either reduced or unchanged.

Grapefruit juice: Grapefruit juice may significantly increase concentrations of verapamil. Grapefruit juice given to nine healthy volunteers increased S- and R- verapamil AUC_{0-12} by 36% and 28%, respectively. Steady state C_{max} and C_{min} of S-verapamil increased by 57% and 16.7%, respectively with grapefruit juice compared to control. Similarly, C_{max} and C_{min} of R-verapamil increased by 40% and 13%, respectively. Grapefruit juice did not affect half-life, nor was there a significant change in AUC_{0-12} ratio R/S compared to control. Grapefruit juice did not cause a significant difference in the PK of norverapamil. This increase in verapamil plasma concentration is not expected to have any clinical consequences.

Lithium: Increased sensitivity to the effects of lithium (neurotoxicity) has been reported during concomitant verapamil-lithium therapy with either no change or an increase in serum lithium levels. However, the addition of verapamil has also resulted in the lowering of serum lithium levels in patients receiving chronic stable oral lithium. Patients receiving both drugs must be monitored carefully.

Carbamazepine: Verapamil therapy may increase carbamazepine concentrations during combined therapy. This may produce carbamazepine side effects such as diplopia, headache, ataxia, or dizziness.

Rifampin: Therapy with rifampin may markedly reduce oral verapamil bioavailability.

Phenobarbital: Phenobarbital therapy may increase verapamil clearance.

Cyclosporine: Verapamil therapy may increase serum levels of cyclosporine.

Theophylline: Verapamil may inhibit the clearance and increase the plasma levels of theophylline.

Inhalation anesthetics: Animal experiments have shown that inhalation anesthetics depress cardiovascular activity by decreasing the inward movement of calcium ions. When used concomitantly, inhalation anesthetics and calcium antagonists, such as verapamil, should each be titrated carefully to avoid excessive cardiovascular depression.

Neuromuscular blocking agents: Clinical data and animal studies suggest that verapamil may potentiate the activity of neuromuscular blocking agents (curare-like and depolarizing). It may be necessary to decrease the dose of verapamil and/or the dose of the neuromuscular blocking agent when the drugs are used concomitantly.

Carcinogenesis, Mutagenesis, Impairment of Fertility

An 18-month toxicity study in rats, at a low multiple (6-fold) of the maximum recommended human dose, and not the maximum tolerated dose, did not suggest a tumorigenic potential. There was no evidence of a carcinogenic potential of verapamil administered in the diet of rats for two years at doses of 10, 35 and 120 mg/kg/day or approximately 1.3, 4.4 and 15 times, respectively, the maximum recommended human daily dose (400 mg/day or 8 mg/kg/day).

Verapamil was not mutagenic in the Ames test in 5 test strains at 3 mg per plate, with or without metabolic activation.

Studies in female rats at daily dietary doses up to 6.9 times (55 mg/kg/day) the maximum recommended human dose did not show impaired fertility. Effects on male fertility have not been determined.

Pregnancy

Pregnancy Category C. Reproduction studies have been performed in rabbits and rats at oral doses up to 1.9 (15 mg/kg/day) and 7.5 (60 mg/kg/day) times the human oral daily dose, respectively, and have revealed no evidence of teratogenicity. In the rat, however, this multiple of the human dose was embryocidal and retarded fetal growth and development, probably because of adverse maternal effects reflected in reduced weight gains of the dams. This oral dose has also been shown to cause hypotension in rats. There are no adequate and well-controlled studies in pregnant women. Because animal reproduction studies are not always predictive of human response, this drug should be used during pregnancy only if clearly needed. Verapamil crosses the placental barrier and can be detected in umbilical vein blood at delivery.

Labor and Delivery

It is not known whether the use of verapamil during labor or delivery has immediate or delayed adverse effects on the fetus, or whether it prolongs the duration of labor or increases the need for forceps delivery or other obstetric intervention. Such adverse experiences have not been reported in the literature, despite a long history of use of verapamil in Europe in the treatment of cardiac side effects of beta-adrenergic agonist agents use to treat premature labor.

Nursing Mothers

Verapamil is excreted in human milk. Because of the potential for adverse reactions in nursing infants from verapamil, nursing should be discontinued while verapamil is administered.

Pediatric Use

Safety and effectiveness in pediatric patients have not been established.

Geriatric Use

Clinical studies of Verelan® PM were not adequate to determine if subjects aged 65 or over respond differently from younger patients. Other reported clinical experience has not identified differences in response between the elderly and younger patients; however, greater sensitivity to Verelan® PM by some older individuals cannot be ruled out.

Aging may affect the pharmacokinetics of verapamil. Elimination half-life may be prolonged in the elderly (See **CLINICAL PHARMACOLOGY, Pharmacokinetics and metabolism**).

Verapamil is highly metabolized by the liver, and about 70% of the administered dose is excreted as metabolites in the urine. Clinical circumstances, some of which may be more common in the elderly, such as hepatic or renal impairment, should be considered (See **PRECAUTIONS, General**). In general, lower initial doses of Verelan® PM may be warranted in the elderly (See **DOSAGE AND ADMINISTRATION, Essential Hypertension**).

Animal Pharmacology and/or Animal Toxicology

In chronic animal toxicology studies verapamil caused lenticular and/or suture line changes at 30 mg/kg/day or greater and frank cataracts at 62.5 mg/kg/day or greater in the beagle dog but not in the rat. Development of cataracts due to verapamil has not been reported in man.

ADVERSE REACTIONS

Serious adverse reactions are uncommon when verapamil therapy is initiated with upward dose titration within the recommended single and total daily dose.

The following reactions to orally administered Verelan® PM occurred at rates of 2.0% or greater or occurred at lower rates but appeared to be drug-related in clinical trials in hypertension.

[See first table above]

See **WARNINGS** for discussion of heart failure, hypotension, elevated liver enzymes, AV block, and rapid ventricular response. Reversible (upon discontinuation of verapamil) non-obstructive, paralytic ileus has been infrequently reported in association with the use of verapamil.

In previous experience with other formulations of verapamil (N=4,954) the following reactions have occurred at rates greater than 1.0% or occurred at lower rates but appeared clearly drug related in clinical trials in 4,954 patients.

[See second table above]

In clinical trials related to the control of ventricular response in digitalized patients who had atrial fibrillation or atrial flutter, ventricular rate below 50/min at rest occurred in 15% of patients and asymptomatic hypotension occurred in 5% of patients.

The following reactions, reported with orally administered verapamil in 2.0% or less of patients, occurred under conditions (open trials, marketing experience) where a causal relationship is uncertain; they are listed to alert the physician to a possible relationship:

Cardiovascular: angina pectoris, atrioventricular dissociation, chest pain, claudication, myocardial infarction, palpitations, purpura (vasculitis), syncope.

Digestive System: diarrhea, dry mouth, gastrointestinal distress, gingival hyperplasia.

Hemic and Lymphatic: ecchymosis or bruising.

Nervous System: cerebrovascular accident, confusion, equilibrium disorders, extrapyramidal symptoms, insomnia, muscle cramps, paresthesia, psychotic symptoms, shakiness, somnolence.

Respiratory: dyspnea.

Skin: arthralgia and rash, exanthema, hair loss, hyperkeratosis, macules, sweating, urticaria, Stevens-Johnson syndrome, erythema multiforme.

Special Senses: blurred vision, tinnitus.

Urogenital: gynecomastia, galactorrhea/hyperprolactinemia, impotence, increased urination, spotty menstruation.

Other: allergy aggravated.

Treatment of Acute Cardiovascular Adverse Reactions

The frequency of cardiovascular adverse reactions that require therapy is rare; hence, experience with their treatment is limited. Whenever severe hypotension or complete AV block occurs following oral administration of verapamil, the appropriate emergency measures should be applied immediately; e.g., intravenously administered norepinephrine bitartrate, atropine sulfate, isoproterenol HCl (all in the usual doses), or calcium gluconate (10% solution). In pa-

	Placebo N = 116 %	All Doses Studied N = 297 %
Headache	11.2	12.1
Infection	6.9	12.1*
Constipation	0.9	8.8*
Flu Syndrome	2.6	3.7
Peripheral edema	0.9	3.7
Dizziness	0.9	3.0
Pharyngitis	2.6	3.0
Sinusitis	2.6	3.0
Dyspepsia	1.7	2.7
Rhinitis	2.6	2.7
Diarrhea	1.7	2.4
Pain	1.7	2.4
Rash	2.6	2.4
Asthenia	3.4	2.0
ECG Abnormal	3.4	2.0
Hypertension	2.0	1.7
Edema	0.0	1.7
Nausea	0.0	1.7
Accidental Injury	0.0	1.5

*Infection, primarily upper respiratory infection (URI) and unrelated to study medication. Constipation was typically mild and easily manageable. At the usual once-daily dose of 200 mg, the observed incidence of constipation was 3.9%.

Constipation	7.3%
Dizziness	3.3%
Nausea	2.7%
Hypotension	2.5%
Headache	2.2%
Edema	1.9%
CHF/Pulmonary Edema	1.8%
Fatigue	1.7%
Bradycardia (HR<50/min)	1.4%
Rash	1.2%
AV block (total 1°, 2°, 3°)	1.2%
AV block (2° and 3°)	0.8%
Flushing	0.6%
Elevated Liver Enzymes (See **WARNINGS**)	

tients with hypertrophic cardiomyopathy (IHSS), alpha-adrenergic agents (phenylephrine HCl, metaraminol bitartrate, or methoxamine HCl) should be used to maintain blood pressure, and isoproterenol and norepinephrine should be avoided. If further support is necessary, inotropic agents (dopamine HCl or dobutamine HCl) may be administered. Actual treatment and dosage should depend on the severity of the clinical situation and the judgment and experience of the treating physician.

OVERDOSAGE

There is no specific antidote for verapamil overdosage; treatment should be supportive. Delayed pharmacodynamic consequences may occur with sustained-release formulations, and patients should be observed for at least 48 hours, preferably under continuous hospital care. Reported effects include hypotension, bradycardia, cardiac conduction defects, arrhythmias, hyperglycemia, and decreased mental status. In addition, there have been literature reports of noncardiogenic pulmonary edema in patients taking large overdoses of verapamil (up to approximately 9g).

In acute overdosage, gastrointestinal decontamination with cathartics and whole bowel irrigation should be considered. Calcium, inotropes (i.e., isoproterenol HCl, dopamine HCl, and glucagon), atropine sulfate, vasopressors (i.e., norepinephrine, and epinephrine), and cardiac pacing have been used with variable results to reverse hypotension and myocardial depression. In a few reported cases, overdose with calcium channel blockers that was initially refractory to atropine became more responsive to this treatment when the patients received large doses (close to 1 gram/hour for more than 24 hours) of calcium chloride.

Calcium chloride is preferred to calcium gluconate since it provides 3 times more calcium per volume. Asystole should be handled by the usual measures including cardiopulmonary resuscitation. Verapamil cannot be removed by hemodialysis.

DOSAGE AND ADMINISTRATION

Essential Hypertension

Verelan® PM should be administered once daily at bedtime. Clinical trials studied doses of 100 mg, 200 mg, 300 mg and 400 mg. The usual daily dose of extended-release Verelan® PM in clinical trials has been 200 mg given by mouth once daily at bedtime. In rare instances, initial doses of 100 mg a day may be warranted in patients who have an increased response to verapamil [e.g. patients with impaired renal function (See **PRECAUTIONS**), impaired hepatic function, elderly, small people, etc.]. Upward titration should be based on therapeutic efficacy and safety evaluated approximately 24 hours after dosing. The antihypertensive effects of Verelan® PM are evident within the first week of therapy.

If an adequate response is not obtained with 200 mg of Verelan® PM, the dose may be titrated upward in the following manner:

a) 300 mg each evening

b) 400 mg each evening (2 × 200 mg)

When Verelan® PM is administered at bedtime, office evaluation of blood pressure during morning and early afternoon hours is essentially a measure of peak effect. The usual evaluation of trough effect, which sometimes might be needed to evaluate the appropriateness of any given dose of Verelan® PM would be just prior to bedtime.

As with immediate-release and sustained-release verapamil, dosages of Verelan® PM capsules should be individualized and titration may be needed in some patients.

HOW SUPPLIED

Verelan® PM (verapamil hydrochloride) extended-release pellet filled capsules are supplied in three dosage strengths:

100 mg: Two piece size 2 hard gelatin capsule, white opaque cap imprinted SCHWARZ/4085 and amethyst body imprinted with 100 mg. Product identification printed in black ink, supplied as follows:
NDC 0091-4085-01 Bottle of 100s

200 mg: Two piece size 0 hard gelatin capsule, amethyst opaque cap imprinted SCHWARZ/4086 and amethyst body imprinted with 200 mg. Product identification printed in black ink, supplied as follows:
NDC 0091-4086-01 Bottle of 100s

300 mg: Two piece size 00 hard gelatin capsule, lavender opaque cap imprinted SCHWARZ/4087 and amethyst body imprinted with 300 mg. Product identification printed in black ink, supplied as follows:
NDC 0091-4087-01 Bottle of 100s

Store at 25°C (77°F); excursions permitted to 15–30°C (59–86°F). [See USP Controlled Room Temperature]. Protect from moisture. Dispense in tight, light-resistant container as defined in USP.

Rx only

Manufactured for:
SCHWARZ
PHARMA
Milwaukee, WI 53201, USA
by
élan
ELAN HOLDINGS, INC.
Gainesville, GA 30504, USA

U.S. Patent No.: 4,863,742

Printed in USA

Verelan® is a registered trademark of Elan Corporation, plc.

CODAS™ is a trademark of Elan Corporation, plc.

PC3810C Rev. 03/03

Shown in Product Identification Guide, page 333

G.D. Searle & Co.

A Division of Pfizer
235 EAST 42ND STREET
NEW YORK, NY 10017-5755

For updates to the product information listed below, please check the Pfizer Web site: http://www.pfizer.com, or call (800) 438-1985. For complete product listing, please see the Manufacturers' Index.

For Medical Information, Contact:
(800) 438-1985
24 hours a day, seven days a week

Distribution:
1855 Shelby Oaks Drive North
Memphis, TN 38134
(901) 387-5200
Customer Service:
(800) 533-4535

Alphabetic Product Listing
Product, ID# (NDC*), Form, Strength

Celebrex, 7767, (1520), Capsule, 100 mg
Celebrex, 7767, (1525), Capsule, 200 mg
Covera-HS 180, (2011), Tablets, 180 mg
Covera-HS 240, (2021), Tablets, 240 mg

*When the product ID # is not the same as the NDC #, the NDC # appears in parentheses.

CELEBREX® ℞

[*sĕ-lĕ-brĕks*]
celecoxib capsules

DESCRIPTION

CELEBREX (celecoxib) is chemically designated as 4-[5-(4-methylphenyl)-3-(trifluoromethyl)-1H-pyrazol-1-yl] benze-

Continued on next page

Celebrex—Cont.

nesulfonamide and is a diaryl-substituted pyrazole. It has the following chemical structure:

The empirical formula for celecoxib is $C_{17}H_{14}F_3N_3O_2S$, and the molecular weight is 381.38.

CELEBREX oral capsules contain either 100 mg, 200 mg or 400 mg of celecoxib.

The inactive ingredients in CELEBREX capsules include: croscarmellose sodium, edible inks, gelatin, lactose monohydrate, magnesium stearate, povidone, sodium lauryl sulfate and titanium dioxide.

CLINICAL PHARMACOLOGY

Mechanism of Action: CELEBREX is a nonsteroidal anti-inflammatory drug that exhibits anti-inflammatory, analgesic, and antipyretic activities in animal models. The mechanism of action of CELEBREX is believed to be due to inhibition of prostaglandin synthesis, primarily via inhibition of cyclooxygenase-2 (COX-2), and at therapeutic concentrations in humans, CELEBREX does not inhibit the cyclooxygenase-1 (COX-1) isoenzyme. In animal colon tumor models, celecoxib reduced the incidence and multiplicity of tumors.

Pharmacokinetics:

Absorption

Peak plasma levels of celecoxib occur approximately 3 hrs after an oral dose. Under fasting conditions, both peak plasma levels (C_{max}) and area under the curve (AUC) are roughly dose proportional up to 200 mg BID; at higher doses there are less than proportional increases in C_{max} and AUC (see Food Effects). Absolute bioavailability studies have not been conducted. With multiple dosing, steady state conditions are reached on or before day 5.

The pharmacokinetic parameters of celecoxib in a group of healthy subjects are shown in Table 1.

[See table 1 below]

Food Effects

When CELEBREX capsules were taken with a high fat meal, peak plasma levels were delayed for about 1 to 2 hours with an increase in total absorption (AUC) of 10% to 20%. Under fasting conditions, at doses above 200 mg, there is less than a proportional increase in C_{max} and AUC, which is thought to be due to the low solubility of the drug in aqueous media. Coadministration of CELEBREX with an aluminum- and magnesium-containing antacid resulted in a reduction in plasma celecoxib concentrations with a decrease of 37% in C_{max} and 10% in AUC. CELEBREX, at doses up to 200 mg BID can be administered without regard to timing of meals. Higher doses (400 mg BID) should be administered with food to improve absorption.

Distribution

In healthy subjects, celecoxib is highly protein bound (~97%) within the clinical dose range. *In vitro* studies indicate that celecoxib binds primarily to albumin and, to a lesser extent, α_1-acid glycoprotein. The apparent volume of distribution at steady state (V_{ss}/F) is approximately 400 L, suggesting extensive distribution into the tissues. Celecoxib is not preferentially bound to red blood cells.

Metabolism

Celecoxib metabolism is primarily mediated via cytochrome P450 2C9. Three metabolites, a primary alcohol, the corresponding carboxylic acid and its glucuronide conjugate, have been identified in human plasma. These metabolites are inactive as COX-1 or COX-2 inhibitors. Patients who are known or suspected to be P450 2C9 poor metabolizers based on a previous history should be administered celecoxib with caution as they may have abnormally high plasma levels due to reduced metabolic clearance.

Excretion

Celecoxib is eliminated predominantly by hepatic metabolism with little (<3%) unchanged drug recovered in the urine and feces. Following a single oral dose of radiolabeled drug, approximately 57% of the dose was excreted in the feces and 27% was excreted into the urine. The primary metabolite in both urine and feces was the carboxylic acid metabolite (73% of dose) with low amounts of the glucuronide also appearing in the urine. It appears that the low solubility of the drug prolongs the absorption process making terminal half-life ($t_{1/2}$) determinations more variable. The effective half-life is approximately 11 hours under fasted conditions. The apparent plasma clearance (CL/F) is about 500 mL/min.

Special Populations

Geriatric: At steady state, elderly subjects (over 65 years old) had a 40% higher C_{max} and a 50% higher AUC compared to the young subjects. In elderly females, celecoxib C_{max} and AUC are higher than those for elderly males, but these increases are predominantly due to lower body weight in elderly females. Dose adjustment in the elderly is not generally necessary. However, for patients of less than 50 kg in body weight, initiate therapy at the lowest recommended dose.

Pediatric: CELEBREX capsules have not been investigated in pediatric patients below 18 years of age.

Race: Meta-analysis of pharmacokinetic studies has suggested an approximately 40% higher AUC of celecoxib in Blacks compared to Caucasians. The cause and clinical significance of this finding is unknown.

Hepatic Insufficiency: A pharmacokinetic study in subjects with mild (Child-Pugh Class A) and moderate (Child-Pugh Class B) hepatic impairment has shown that steady-state celecoxib AUC is increased about 40% and 180%, respectively, above that seen in healthy control subjects. Therefore, the daily recommended dose of CELEBREX capsules should be reduced by approximately 50% in patients with moderate (Child-Pugh Class B) hepatic impairment. Patients with severe hepatic impairment (Child-Pugh Class C) have not been studied. The use of CELEBREX in patients with severe hepatic impairment is not recommended.

Renal Insufficiency: In a cross-study comparison, celecoxib AUC was approximately 40% lower in patients with chronic renal insufficiency (GFR 35-60 mL/min) than that seen in subjects with normal renal function. No significant relationship was found between GFR and celecoxib clearance. Patients with severe renal insufficiency have not been studied. Similar to other NSAIDs, CELEBREX is not recommended in patients with severe renal insufficiency (see WARNINGS – Advanced Renal Disease).

Drug Interactions

Also see **PRECAUTIONS – Drug Interactions.**

General: Significant interactions may occur when celecoxib is administered together with drugs that inhibit P450 2C9. *In vitro* studies indicate that celecoxib is not an inhibitor of cytochrome P450 2C9, 2C19 or 3A4.

Clinical studies with celecoxib have identified potentially significant interactions with fluconazole and lithium. Experience with nonsteroidal anti-inflammatory drugs (NSAIDs) suggests the potential for interactions with furosemide and ACE inhibitors. The effects of celecoxib on the pharmacokinetics and/or pharmacodynamics of glyburide, ketoconazole, methotrexate, phenytoin, and tolbutamide have been studied *in vivo* and clinically important interactions have not been found.

CLINICAL STUDIES

Osteoarthritis (OA): CELEBREX has demonstrated significant reduction in joint pain compared to placebo. CELEBREX was evaluated for treatment of the signs and the symptoms of OA of the knee and hip in approximately 4,200 patients in placebo- and active-controlled clinical trials of up to 12 weeks duration. In patients with OA, treatment with CELEBREX 100 mg BID or 200 mg QD resulted in improvement in WOMAC (Western Ontario and McMaster Universities) osteoarthritis index, a composite of pain, stiffness, and functional measures in OA. In three 12-week studies of pain accompanying OA flare, CELEBREX doses of 100 mg BID and 200 mg BID provided significant reduction of pain within 24-48 hours of initiation of dosing. At doses of 100 mg BID or 200 mg BID the effectiveness of CELEBREX was shown to be similar to that of naproxen 500 mg BID. Doses of 200 mg BID provided no additional benefit above that seen with 100 mg BID. A total daily dose of 200 mg has been shown to be equally effective whether administered as 100 mg BID or 200 mg QD.

Rheumatoid Arthritis (RA): CELEBREX has demonstrated significant reduction in joint tenderness/pain and joint swelling compared to placebo. CELEBREX was evaluated for treatment of the signs and symptoms of RA in approximately 2,100 patients in placebo- and active-controlled clinical trials of up to 24 weeks in duration. CELEBREX was shown to be superior to placebo in these studies, using the ACR20 Responder Index, a composite of clinical, laboratory, and functional measures in RA. CELEBREX doses of 100 mg BID and 200 mg BID were similar in effectiveness and both were comparable to naproxen 500 mg BID.

Although CELEBREX 100 mg BID and 200 mg BID provided similar overall effectiveness, some patients derived additional benefit from the 200 mg BID dose. Doses of 400 mg BID provided no additional benefit above that seen with 100-200 mg BID.

Analgesia, including primary dysmenorrhea: In acute analgesic models of post-oral surgery pain, post-orthopedic surgical pain, and primary dysmenorrhea, CELEBREX relieved pain that was rated by patients as moderate to severe. Single doses (see DOSAGE AND ADMINISTRATION) of CELEBREX provided pain relief within 60 minutes.

Familial Adenomatous Polyposis (FAP): CELEBREX was evaluated to reduce the number of adenomatous colorectal polyps. A randomized double-blind placebo-controlled study was conducted in 83 patients with FAP. The study population included 58 patients with a prior subtotal or total colectomy and 25 patients with an intact colon. Thirteen patients had the attenuated FAP phenotype.

One area in the rectum and up to four areas in the colon were identified at baseline for specific follow-up, and polyps were counted at baseline and following six months of treatment. The mean reduction in the number of colorectal polyps was 28% for CELEBREX 400 mg BID, 12% for CELEBREX 100 mg BID and 5% for placebo. The reduction in polyps observed with CELEBREX 400 mg BID was statistically superior to placebo at the six-month timepoint (p=0.003). (See Figure 1.)

Figure 1
Percent Change from Baseline in Number of Colorectal Polyps (FAP Patients)

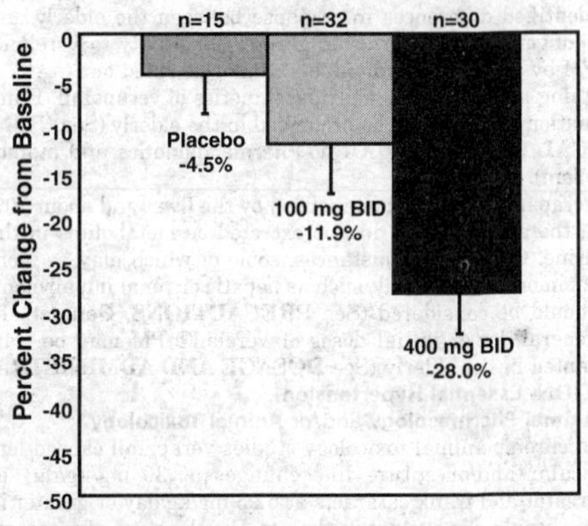

*p=0.003 versus placebo

Special Studies

Endoscopic Studies: Scheduled upper GI endoscopic evaluations were performed in over 4,500 arthritis patients who were enrolled in five controlled randomized 12-24 week trials using active comparators, two of which also included placebo controls. There was no consistent relationship between the incidence of gastroduodenal ulcers and the dose of CELEBREX over the range studied.

Table 2 summarizes the incidence of endoscopic ulcers in two 12-week studies that enrolled patients in whom baseline endoscopies revealed no ulcers.

Table 2
Incidence of Gastroduodenal Ulcers from Endoscopic Studies in OA and RA Patients

	3 Month Studies	
	Study 1 (n = 1108)	**Study 2 (n = 1049)**
Placebo	2.3% (5/217)	2.0% (4/200)
Celebrex 50 mg BID	3.4% (8/233)	—
Celebrex 100 mg BID	3.1% (7/227)	4.0% (9/223)
Celebrex 200 mg BID	5.9% (13/221)	2.7% (6/219)
Celebrex 400 mg BID	—	4.1% (8/197)
Naproxen 500 mg BID	16.2% (34/210)*	17.6% (37/210)*

*p≤0.05 vs all other treatments

Table 3 summarizes data from two 12-week studies that enrolled patients in whom baseline endoscopies revealed no ulcers. Patients underwent interval endoscopies every 4 weeks to give information on ulcer risk over time.

[See table 3 at top of next page]

One randomized and double-blind 6-month study in 430 RA patients was conducted in which an endoscopic examination was performed at 6 months. The incidence of endoscopic ulcers in patients taking CELEBREX 200 mg BID was 4% vs 15% for patients taking diclofenac SR 75 mg BID (p<0.001).

In 4 of the 5 endoscopic studies, approximately 11% of patients (440/4,000) were taking aspirin (≤325 mg/day). In the CELEBREX groups, the endoscopic ulcer rate appeared to be higher in aspirin users than in non-users. However, the increased rate of ulcers in these aspirin users was less than the endoscopic ulcer rates observed in the active comparator groups, with or without aspirin.

The correlation between findings of endoscopic studies, and the relative incidence of clinically significant serious upper GI events has not been established. Serious clinically significant upper GI bleeding has been observed in patients receiving CELEBREX in controlled and open-labeled trials, albeit infrequently (see *Use with Aspirin* and WARNINGS — Gastrointestinal (GI) Effects).

Use with Aspirin: The Celecoxib Long-Term Arthritis Safety Study (CLASS) was a prospective long-term safety outcome study conducted postmarketing in approximately

Table 1
Summary of Single Dose (200 mg) Disposition Kinetics of Celecoxib in Healthy Subjects[1]

Mean (%CV) PK Parameter Values				
C_{max}, ng/mL	**T_{max}, hr**	**Effective $t_{1/2}$, hr**	**V_{ss}/F, L**	**CL/F, L/hr**
705 (38)	2.8 (37)	11.2 (31)	429 (34)	27.7 (28)

[1]Subjects under fasting conditions (n=36, 19-52 yrs.)

5,800 OA patients and 2,200 RA patients. Patients received CELEBREX 400 mg BID (4-fold and 2-fold the recommended OA and RA doses, respectively, and the approved dose for FAP), ibuprofen 800 mg TID or diclofenac 75 mg BID (common therapeutic doses). Median exposures for CELEBREX (n = 3,987) and diclofenac (n = 1,996) were 9 months while ibuprofen (n = 1,985) was 6 months. The Kaplan-Meier cumulative rates at 9 months are provided for all analyses. The primary endpoint of this outcome study was the incidence of *complicated ulcers* (gastrointestinal bleeding, perforation or obstruction). Patients were allowed to take concomitant low-dose (≤ 325 mg/day) aspirin (ASA) for cardiovascular prophylaxis (ASA subgroups: CELEBREX, n = 882; diclofenac, n = 445; ibuprofen, n = 412). Differences in the incidence of *complicated ulcers* between CELEBREX and the combined group of ibuprofen and diclofenac were not statistically significant. Those patients on CELEBREX and concomitant low-dose ASA experienced 4-fold higher rates of *complicated ulcers* compared to those not on ASA (see WARNINGS — Gastrointestinal (GI) Effects). The results for CELEBREX are displayed in Table 4. For *complicated and symptomatic ulcer* rates, see WARNINGS — Gastrointestinal (GI) Effects – Risk of GI Ulceration, Bleeding, and Perforation.

Table 4
Effects of Co-Administration of Low-Dose Aspirin on *Complicated Ulcer* Rates with CELEBREX 400 mg BID (Kaplan-Meier Rates at 9 months [%])

	Non-Aspirin Users n=3105	Aspirin Users n=882
Complicated Ulcers	0.32	1.12

Platelets: In clinical trials, CELEBREX at single doses up to 800 mg and multiple doses of 600 mg BID for up to 7 days duration (higher than recommended therapeutic doses) had no effect on platelet aggregation and bleeding time. Comparators (naproxen 500 mg BID, ibuprofen 800 mg TID, diclofenac 75 mg BID) significantly reduced platelet aggregation and prolonged bleeding time.

Because of its lack of platelet effects, CELEBREX is not a substitute for aspirin for cardiovascular prophylaxis.

INDICATIONS AND USAGE

CELEBREX is indicated:

1) For relief of the signs and symptoms of osteoarthritis.
2) For relief of the signs and symptoms of rheumatoid arthritis in adults.
3) For the management of acute pain in adults (see CLINICAL STUDIES).
4) For the treatment of primary dysmenorrhea.
5) To reduce the number of adenomatous colorectal polyps in familial adenomatous polyposis (FAP), as an adjunct to usual care (e.g., endoscopic surveillance, surgery). It is not known whether there is a clinical benefit from a reduction in the number of colorectal polyps in FAP patients. It is also not known whether the effects of CELEBREX treatment will persist after CELEBREX is discontinued. The efficacy and safety of CELEBREX treatment in patients with FAP beyond six months have not been studied (see CLINICAL STUDIES, WARNINGS and PRECAUTIONS sections).

CONTRAINDICATIONS

CELEBREX is contraindicated in patients with known hypersensitivity to celecoxib.

CELEBREX should not be given to patients who have demonstrated allergic-type reactions to sulfonamides.

CELEBREX should not be given to patients who have experienced asthma, urticaria, or allergic-type reactions after taking aspirin or other NSAIDs. Severe, rarely fatal, anaphylactic-like reactions to NSAIDs have been reported in such patients (see WARNINGS — Anaphylactoid Reactions, and PRECAUTIONS — Preexisting Asthma).

WARNINGS

Gastrointestinal (GI) Effects—Risk of GI Ulceration, Bleeding, and Perforation

Serious gastrointestinal toxicity such as bleeding, ulceration, and perforation of the stomach, small intestine or large intestine, can occur at any time, with or without warning symptoms, in patients treated with nonsteroidal anti-inflammatory drugs (NSAIDs). Minor upper gastrointestinal problems, such as dyspepsia, are common and may also occur at any time during NSAID therapy. Therefore, physicians and patients should remain alert for ulceration and bleeding, even in the absence of previous GI tract symptoms (see PRECAUTIONS – Hematological Effects). Patients should be informed about the signs and/or symptoms of serious GI toxicity and the steps to take if they occur. The utility of periodic laboratory monitoring has not been demonstrated, nor has it been adequately assessed. Only one in five patients who develop a serious upper GI adverse event on NSAID therapy is symptomatic. It has been demonstrated that upper GI ulcers, gross bleeding or perforation, caused by NSAIDs, appear to occur in approximately 1% of patients treated for 3-6 months, and in about 2-4% of patients treated for one year. These trends continue thus, increasing the likelihood of developing a serious GI event at some time during the course of therapy. However, even short-term therapy is not without risk.

NSAIDs should be prescribed with extreme caution in patients with a prior history of ulcer disease or gastrointestinal bleeding. Most spontaneous reports of fatal GI events are in elderly or debilitated patients and therefore special care should be taken in treating this population. **To minimize the potential risk for an adverse GI event, the lowest effective dose should be used for the shortest possible duration.** For high risk patients, alternate therapies that do not involve NSAIDs should be considered.

Table 3
Incidence of Gastroduodenal Ulcers from 3-Month Serial Endoscopy Studies in OA and RA Patients

	Week 4	Week 8	Week 12	Final
Study 3 (n=523)				
Celebrex 200 mg BID	4.0% (10/252)*	2.2% (5/227)*	1.5% (3/196)*	7.5% (20/266)*
Naproxen 500 mg BID	19.0% (47/247)	14.2% (26/182)	9.9% (14/141)	34.6% (89/257)
Study 4 (n=1062)				
Celebrex 200 mg BID	3.9% (13/337)†	2.4% (7/296)†	1.8% (5/274)†	7.0% (25/356)†
Diclofenac 75 mg BID	5.1% (18/350)	3.3% (10/306)	2.9% (8/278)	9.7% (36/372)
Ibuprofen 800 mg TID	13.0% (42/323)	6.2% (15/241)	9.6% (21/219)	23.3% (78/334)

*p≤0.05 Celebrex vs. naproxen based on interval and cumulative analyses
†p≤0.05 Celebrex vs. ibuprofen based on interval and cumulative analyses

Studies have shown that patients with a *prior history of peptic ulcer disease and/or gastrointestinal bleeding* and who use NSAIDs, have a greater than 10-fold higher risk for developing a GI bleed than patients with neither of these risk factors. In addition to a past history of ulcer disease, pharmacoepidemiological studies have identified several other co-therapies or co-morbid conditions that may increase the risk for GI bleeding such as: treatment with oral corticosteroids, treatment with anticoagulants, longer duration of NSAID therapy, smoking, alcoholism, older age, and poor general health status.

CLASS Study: The estimated cumulative rates at 9 months of *complicated and symptomatic ulcers* (an adverse event similar but not identical to the "upper GI ulcers, gross bleeding or perforation" described in the preceding paragraphs) for patients treated with CELEBREX 400 mg BID (see Special Studies – *Use with Aspirin*) are described in Table 5. Table 5 also displays results for patients less than or greater than or equal to the age of 65 years. The differences in rates between CELEBREX alone and CELEBREX with ASA groups may be due to the higher risk for GI events in ASA users.

Table 5
***Complicated and Symptomatic Ulcer* Rates in Patients Taking CELEBREX 400 mg BID (Kaplan-Meier Rates at 9 months [%]) Based on Risk Factors**

	Complicated and Symptomatic Ulcer Rates
All Patients	
Celebrex alone (n=3105)	0.78
Celebrex with ASA (n=882)	2.19
Patients <65 Years	
Celebrex alone (n=2025)	0.47
Celebrex with ASA (n=403)	1.26
Patients ≥65 Years	
Celebrex alone (n=1080)	1.40
Celebrex with ASA (n=479)	3.06

In a small number of patients with a history of ulcer disease, the *complicated and symptomatic ulcer* rates in patients taking CELEBREX alone or CELEBREX with ASA were, respectively, 2.56% (n=243) and 6.85% (n=91) at 48 weeks. These results are to be expected in patients with a prior history of ulcer disease (see WARNINGS – Gastrointestinal (GI) Effects – Risk of GI Ulceration, Bleeding, and Perforation).

Anaphylactoid Reactions

As with NSAIDs in general, anaphylactoid reactions have occurred in patients without known prior exposure to CELEBREX. In post-marketing experience, rare cases of anaphylactic reactions and angioedema have been reported in patients receiving CELEBREX. CELEBREX should not be given to patients with the aspirin triad. This symptom complex typically occurs in asthmatic patients who experience rhinitis with or without nasal polyps, or who exhibit severe, potentially fatal bronchospasm after taking aspirin or other NSAIDs (see CONTRAINDICATIONS and PRECAUTIONS — Preexisting Asthma). Emergency help should be sought in cases where an anaphylactoid reaction occurs.

Advanced Renal Disease

No information is available from controlled clinical studies regarding the use of CELEBREX in patients with advanced kidney disease. Therefore, treatment with CELEBREX is not recommended in these patients with advanced kidney disease. If CELEBREX therapy must be initiated, close monitoring of the patient's kidney function is advisable (see PRECAUTIONS — Renal Effects).

Pregnancy

In late pregnancy CELEBREX should be avoided because it may cause premature closure of the ductus arteriosus (see PRECAUTIONS – Pregnancy).

Familial Adenomatous Polyposis (FAP): Treatment with CELEBREX in FAP has not been shown to reduce the risk of gastrointestinal cancer or the need for prophylactic colectomy or other FAP-related surgeries. Therefore, the usual care of FAP patients should not be altered because of the concurrent administration of CELEBREX. In particular, the frequency of routine endoscopic surveillance should not be decreased and prophylactic colectomy or other FAP-related surgeries should not be delayed.

PRECAUTIONS

General: CELEBREX cannot be expected to substitute for corticosteroids or to treat corticosteroid insufficiency. Abrupt discontinuation of corticosteroids may lead to exacerbation of corticosteroid-responsive illness. Patients on prolonged corticosteroid therapy should have their therapy tapered slowly if a decision is made to discontinue corticosteroids.

The pharmacological activity of CELEBREX in reducing inflammation, and possibly fever, may diminish the utility of these diagnostic signs in detecting infectious complications of presumed noninfectious, painful conditions.

Hepatic Effects: Borderline elevations of one or more liver associated enzymes may occur in up to 15% of patients taking NSAIDs, and notable elevations of ALT or AST (approximately 3 or more times the upper limit of normal) have been reported in approximately 1% of patients in clinical trials with NSAIDs. These laboratory abnormalities may progress, may remain unchanged, or may be transient with continuing therapy. Rare cases of severe hepatic reactions, including jaundice and fatal fulminant hepatitis, liver necrosis and hepatic failure (some with fatal outcome) have been reported with NSAIDs, including CELEBREX (see ADVERSE REACTIONS – post-marketing experience). In controlled clinical trials of CELEBREX, the incidence of borderline elevations (greater than or equal to 1.2 times and less than 3 times the upper limit of normal) of liver associated enzymes was 6% for CELEBREX and 5% for placebo, and approximately 0.2% of patients taking CELEBREX and 0.3% of patients taking placebo had notable elevations of ALT and AST.

A patient with symptoms and/or signs suggesting liver dysfunction, or in whom an abnormal liver test has occurred, should be monitored carefully for evidence of the development of a more severe hepatic reaction while on therapy with CELEBREX. If clinical signs and symptoms consistent with liver disease develop, or if systemic manifestations occur (e.g., eosinophilia, rash, etc.), CELEBREX should be discontinued.

Renal Effects: Long-term administration of NSAIDs has resulted in renal papillary necrosis and other renal injury. Renal toxicity has also been seen in patients in whom renal prostaglandins have a compensatory role in the maintenance of renal perfusion. In these patients, administration of a nonsteroidal anti-inflammatory drug may cause a dose-dependent reduction in prostaglandin formation and, secondarily, in renal blood flow, which may precipitate overt renal decompensation. Patients at greatest risk of this reaction are those with impaired renal function, heart failure, liver dysfunction, those taking diuretics and ACE inhibitors, and the elderly. Discontinuation of NSAID therapy is usually followed by recovery to the pretreatment state. Clinical trials with CELEBREX have shown renal effects similar to those observed with comparator NSAIDs.

Caution should be used when initiating treatment with CELEBREX in patients with considerable dehydration. It is advisable to rehydrate patients first and then start therapy with CELEBREX. Caution is also recommended in patients with preexisting kidney disease (see WARNINGS—Advanced Renal Disease).

Hematological Effects: Anemia is sometimes seen in patients receiving CELEBREX. In controlled clinical trials the incidence of anemia was 0.6% with CELEBREX and 0.4% with placebo. Patients on long-term treatment with CELEBREX should have their hemoglobin or hematocrit checked if they exhibit any signs or symptoms of anemia or blood loss. CELEBREX does not generally affect platelet counts, prothrombin time (PT), or partial thromboplastin time (PTT), and does not inhibit platelet aggregation at indicated dosages (see CLINICAL STUDIES—Special Studies—Platelets).

Fluid Retention, Edema, and Hypertension: Fluid retention and edema have been observed in some patients taking CELEBREX (see ADVERSE REACTIONS). In the CLASS

Continued on next page

Table 6
Adverse Events Occurring in ≥2% of CELEBREX Patients From CELEBREX Premarketing Controlled Arthritis Trials

	CELEBREX (100-200 mg BID or 200 mg QD) (n=4146)	Placebo (n=1864)	Naproxen 500 mg BID (n=1366)	Diclofenac 75 mg BID (n=387)	Ibuprofen 800 mg TID (n=345)
Gastrointestinal					
Abdominal Pain	4.1%	2.8%	7.7%	9.0%	9.0%
Diarrhea	5.6%	3.8%	5.3%	9.3%	5.8%
Dyspepsia	8.8%	6.2%	12.2%	10.9%	12.8%
Flatulence	2.2%	1.0%	3.6%	4.1%	3.5%
Nausea	3.5%	4.2%	6.0%	3.4%	6.7%
Body as a whole					
Back Pain	2.8%	3.6%	2.2%	2.6%	0.9%
Peripheral edema	2.1%	1.1%	2.1%	1.0%	3.5%
Injury-accidental	2.9%	2.3%	3.0%	2.6%	3.2%
Central and peripheral nervous system					
Dizziness	2.0%	1.7%	2.6%	1.3%	2.3%
Headache	15.8%	20.2%	14.5%	15.5%	15.4%
Psychiatric					
Insomnia	2.3%	2.3%	2.9%	1.3%	1.4%
Respiratory					
Pharyngitis	2.3%	1.1%	1.7%	1.6%	2.6%
Rhinitis	2.0%	1.3%	2.4%	2.3%	0.6%
Sinusitis	5.0%	4.3%	4.0%	5.4%	5.8%
Upper respiratory tract infection	8.1%	6.7%	9.9%	9.8%	9.9%
Skin					
Rash	2.2%	2.1%	2.1%	1.3%	1.2%

CELEBREX (100-200 mg BID or 200 mg QD)	
Gastrointestinal:	Constipation, diverticulitis, dysphagia, eructation, esophagitis, gastritis, gastroenteritis, gastroesophageal reflux, hemorrhoids, hiatal hernia, melena, dry mouth, stomatitis, tenesmus, tooth disorder, vomiting
Cardiovascular:	Aggravated hypertension, angina pectoris, coronary artery disorder, myocardial infarction
General:	Allergy aggravated, allergic reaction, asthenia, chest pain, cyst NOS, edema generalized, face edema, fatigue, fever, hot flushes, influenza-like symptoms, pain, peripheral pain
Resistance mechanism disorders:	Herpes simplex, herpes zoster, infection bacterial, infection fungal, infection soft tissue, infection viral, moniliasis, moniliasis genital, otitis media
Central, peripheral nervous system:	Leg cramps, hypertonia, hypoesthesia, migraine, neuralgia, neuropathy, paresthesia, vertigo
Female reproductive:	Breast fibroadenosis, breast neoplasm, breast pain, dysmenorrhea, menstrual disorder, vaginal hemorrhage, vaginitis
Male reproductive:	Prostatic disorder
Hearing and vestibular:	Deafness, ear abnormality, earache, tinnitus
Heart rate and rhythm:	Palpitation, tachycardia
Liver and biliary system:	Hepatic function abnormal, SGOT increased, SGPT increased
Metabolic and nutritional:	BUN increased, CPK increased, diabetes mellitus, hypercholesterolemia, hyperglycemia, hypokalemia, NPN increase, creatinine increased, alkaline phosphatase increased, weight increase
Musculoskeletal:	Arthralgia, arthrosis, bone disorder, fracture accidental, myalgia, neck stiffness, synovitis, tendinitis
Platelets (bleeding or clotting):	Ecchymosis, epistaxis, thrombocythemia
Psychiatric:	Anorexia, anxiety, appetite increased, depression, nervousness, somnolence
Hemic:	Anemia
Respiratory:	Bronchitis, bronchospasm, bronchospasm aggravated, coughing, dyspnea, laryngitis, pneumonia
Skin and appendages:	Alopecia, dermatitis, nail disorder, photosensitivity reaction, pruritus, rash erythematous, rash maculopapular, skin disorder, skin dry, sweating increased, urticaria
Application site disorders:	Cellulitis, dermatitis contact, injection site reaction, skin nodule
Special senses:	Taste perversion
Urinary system:	Albuminuria, cystitis, dysuria, hematuria, micturition frequency, renal calculus, urinary incontinence, urinary tract infection
Vision:	Blurred vision, cataract, conjunctivitis, eye pain, glaucoma

Celebrex—Cont.

study (see Special Studies – *Use with Aspirin*), the Kaplan-Meier cumulative rates at 9 months of peripheral edema in patients on CELEBREX 400 mg BID (4-fold and 2-fold the recommended OA and RA doses, respectively, and the approved dose for FAP), ibuprofen 800 mg TID and diclofenac 75 mg BID were 4.5%, 6.9% and 4.7%, respectively. The rates of hypertension in the CELEBREX, ibuprofen and diclofenac treated patients were 2.4%, 4.2% and 2.5%, respectively. As with other NSAIDs, CELEBREX should be used with caution in patients with fluid retention, hypertension, or heart failure.

Preexisting Asthma: Patients with asthma may have aspirin-sensitive asthma. The use of aspirin in patients with aspirin-sensitive asthma has been associated with severe bronchospasm which can be fatal. Since cross reactivity, including bronchospasm, between aspirin and other nonsteroidal anti-inflammatory drugs has been reported in such aspirin-sensitive patients, CELEBREX should not be administered to patients with this form of aspirin sensitivity and should be used with caution in patients with preexisting asthma.

Information for Patients: CELEBREX can cause discomfort and, rarely, more serious side effects, such as gastrointestinal bleeding, which may result in hospitalization and even fatal outcomes. Although serious GI tract ulcerations and bleeding can occur without warning symptoms, patients should be alert for the signs and symptoms of ulcerations and bleeding, and should ask for medical advice when observing any indicative signs or symptoms. Patients should be apprised of the importance of this follow-up (see WARNINGS — Gastrointestinal (GI) Effects – Risk of Gastrointestinal Ulceration, Bleeding, and Perforation).

Patients should promptly report signs or symptoms of gastrointestinal ulceration or bleeding, skin rash, unexplained weight gain, or edema to their physicians.

Patients should be informed of the warning signs and symptoms of hepatotoxicity (e.g., nausea, fatigue, lethargy, pruritus, jaundice, right upper quadrant tenderness, and "flu-like" symptoms). If these occur, patients should be instructed to stop therapy and seek immediate medical therapy.

Patients should also be instructed to seek immediate emergency help in the case of an anaphylactoid reaction (see WARNINGS).

In late pregnancy CELEBREX should be avoided because it may cause premature closure of the ductus arteriosus.

Patients with familial adenomatous polyposis (FAP) should be informed that CELEBREX has not been shown to reduce colorectal, duodenal or other FAP-related cancers, or the need for endoscopic surveillance, prophylactic or other FAP-related surgery. Therefore, all patients with FAP should be instructed to continue their usual care while receiving CELEBREX.

Laboratory Tests: Because serious GI tract ulcerations and bleeding can occur without warning symptoms, physicians should monitor for signs or symptoms of GI bleeding.

In controlled clinical trials, elevated BUN occurred more frequently in patients receiving CELEBREX compared with patients on placebo. This laboratory abnormality was also seen in patients who received comparator NSAIDs in these studies. The clinical significance of this abnormality has not been established.

Drug Interactions

General: Celecoxib metabolism is predominantly mediated via cytochrome P450 2C9 in the liver. Co-administration of celecoxib with drugs that are known to inhibit 2C9 should be done with caution.

In vitro studies indicate that celecoxib, although not a substrate, is an inhibitor of cytochrome P450 2D6. Therefore, there is a potential for an *in vivo* drug interaction with drugs that are metabolized by P450 2D6.

ACE-inhibitors: Reports suggest that NSAIDs may diminish the antihypertensive effect of Angiotensin Converting Enzyme (ACE) inhibitors. This interaction should be given consideration in patients taking CELEBREX concomitantly with ACE-inhibitors.

Furosemide: Clinical studies, as well as post marketing observations, have shown that NSAIDs can reduce the natriuretic effect of furosemide and thiazides in some patients. This response has been attributed to inhibition of renal prostaglandin synthesis.

Aspirin: CELEBREX can be used with low-dose aspirin. However, concomitant administration of aspirin with CELEBREX increases the rate of GI ulceration or other complications, compared to use of CELEBREX alone (see CLINICAL STUDIES — Special Studies — *Use with Aspirin* and WARNINGS – Gastrointestinal (GI) Effects – Risk of GI Ulceration, Bleeding, and Perforation – CLASS Study).

Because of its lack of platelet effects, CELEBREX is not a substitute for aspirin for cardiovascular prophylaxis.

Fluconazole: Concomitant administration of fluconazole at 200 mg QD resulted in a two-fold increase in celecoxib plasma concentration. This increase is due to the inhibition of celecoxib metabolism via P450 2C9 by fluconazole (see Pharmacokinetics — Metabolism). CELEBREX should be introduced at the lowest recommended dose in patients receiving fluconazole.

Lithium: In a study conducted in healthy subjects, mean steady-state lithium plasma levels increased approximately 17% in subjects receiving lithium 450 mg BID with CELEBREX 200 mg BID as compared to subjects receiving lithium alone. Patients on lithium treatment should be closely monitored when CELEBREX is introduced or withdrawn.

Methotrexate: In an interaction study of rheumatoid arthritis patients taking methotrexate, CELEBREX did not have a significant effect on the pharmacokinetics of methotrexate.

Warfarin: Anticoagulant activity should be monitored, particularly in the first few days, after initiating or changing CELEBREX therapy in patients receiving warfarin or similar agents, since these patients are at an increased risk of bleeding complications. The effect of celecoxib on the anticoagulant effect of warfarin was studied in a group of healthy subjects receiving daily doses of 2-5 mg of warfarin. In these subjects, celecoxib did not alter the anticoagulant effect of warfarin as determined by prothrombin time. However, in post-marketing experience, bleeding events have been reported, predominantly in the elderly, in association with increases in prothrombin time in patients receiving CELEBREX concurrently with warfarin.

Carcinogenesis, mutagenesis, impairment of fertility: Celecoxib was not carcinogenic in rats given oral doses up to 200 mg/kg for males and 10 mg/kg for females (approximately 2- to 4-fold the human exposure as measured by the AUC_{0-24} at 200 mg BID) or in mice given oral doses up to 25 mg/kg for males and 50 mg/kg for females (approximately equal to human exposure as measured by the AUC_{0-24} at 200 mg BID) for two years.

Celecoxib was not mutagenic in an Ames test and a mutation assay in Chinese hamster ovary (CHO) cells, nor clastogenic in a chromosome aberration assay in CHO cells and an *in vivo* micronucleus test in rat bone marrow.

Celecoxib did not impair male and female fertility in rats at oral doses up to 600 mg/kg/day (approximately 11-fold human exposure at 200 mg BID based on the AUC_{0-24}).

Pregnancy

Teratogenic effects: Pregnancy Category C. Celecoxib at oral doses ≥150 mg/kg/day (approximately 2-fold human exposure at 200 mg BID as measured by AUC_{0-24}), caused an increased incidence of ventricular septal defects, a rare event, and fetal alterations, such as ribs fused, sternebrae fused and sternebrae misshapen when rabbits were treated throughout organogenesis. A dose-dependent increase in diaphragmatic hernias was observed when rats were given celecoxib at oral doses ≥30 mg/kg/day (approximately 6-fold human exposure based on the AUC_{0-24} at 200 mg BID) throughout organogenesis. There are no studies in pregnant women. CELEBREX should be used during pregnancy only if the potential benefit justifies the potential risk to the fetus.

Nonteratogenic effects: Celecoxib produced pre-implantation and post-implantation losses and reduced embryo/fetal survival in rats at oral dosages ≥50 mg/kg/day (approximately 6-fold human exposure based on the AUC_{0-24} at 200 mg BID). These changes are expected with inhibition of prostaglandin synthesis and are not the result of permanent alteration of female reproductive function, nor are they expected at clinical exposures. No studies have been conducted to evaluate the effect of celecoxib on the closure of the ductus arteriosus in humans. Therefore, use of CELEBREX during the third trimester of pregnancy should be avoided.

Labor and delivery: Celecoxib produced no evidence of delayed labor or parturition at oral doses up to 100 mg/kg in rats (approximately 7-fold human exposure as measured by the AUC_{0-24} at 200 mg BID). The effects of CELEBREX on labor and delivery in pregnant women are unknown.

Nursing mothers: Celecoxib is excreted in the milk of lactating rats at concentrations similar to those in plasma. Limited data from one subject indicate that celecoxib is also excreted in human milk. Because many drugs are excreted in human milk and because of the potential for serious adverse reactions in nursing infants from CELEBREX, a decision should be made whether to discontinue nursing or to discontinue the drug, taking into account the importance of the drug to the mother.

Pediatric Use

Safety and effectiveness in pediatric patients below the age of 18 years have not been evaluated.

Geriatric Use

Of the total number of patients who received CELEBREX in clinical trials, more than 3,300 were 65-74 years of age, while approximately 1,300 additional patients were 75 years and over. No substantial differences in effectiveness were observed between these subjects and younger subjects. In clinical studies comparing renal function as measured by the GFR, BUN and creatinine, and platelet function as measured by bleeding time and platelet aggregation, the results were not different between elderly and young volunteers. However, as with other NSAIDs, including those that selectively inhibit COX-2, there have been more spontaneous post-marketing reports of fatal GI events and acute renal failure in the elderly than in younger patients (see WARNINGS – Gastrointestinal (GI) Effects – Risk of GI Ulceration, Bleeding, and Perforation).

ADVERSE REACTIONS

Of the CELEBREX treated patients in the premarketing controlled clinical trials, approximately 4,250 were patients with OA, approximately 2,100 were patients with RA, and approximately 1,050 were patients with post-surgical pain. More than 8,500 patients have received a total daily dose of CELEBREX of 200 mg (100 mg BID or 200 mg QD) or more, including more than 400 treated at 800 mg (400 mg BID). Approximately 3,900 patients have received CELEBREX at these doses for 6 months or more; approximately 2,300 of these have received it for 1 year or more and 124 of these have received it for 2 years or more.

Adverse events from CELEBREX premarketing controlled arthritis trials: Table 6 lists all adverse events, regardless of causality, occurring in ≥2% of patients receiving CELEBREX from 12 controlled studies conducted in patients with OA or RA that included a placebo and/or a positive control group.

[See table 6 at top of previous page]

In placebo- or active-controlled clinical trials, the discontinuation rate due to adverse events was 7.1% for patients receiving CELEBREX and 6.1% for patients receiving placebo. Among the most common reasons for discontinuation due to adverse events in the CELEBREX treatment groups were dyspepsia and abdominal pain (cited as reasons for discontinuation in 0.8% and 0.7% of CELEBREX patients, respectively). Among patients receiving placebo, 0.6% discontinued due to dyspepsia and 0.6% withdrew due to abdominal pain.

The following adverse events occurred in 0.1-1.9% of patients regardless of causality.

[See second table on previous page]

Other serious adverse reactions which occur rarely (estimated <0.1%), regardless of causality: The following serious adverse events have occurred rarely in patients taking CELEBREX. Cases reported only in the post-marketing experience are indicated in italics.

[See table above]

Safety Data from CLASS Study:

Hematological Events:

During this study (see Special Studies – *Use with Aspirin*), the incidence of clinically significant decreases in hemoglobin (>2 g/dL) confirmed by repeat testing was lower in patients on CELEBREX 400 mg BID (4-fold and 2-fold the recommended OA and RA doses, respectively, and the approved dose for FAP) compared to patients on either diclofenac 75 mg BID or ibuprofen 800 mg TID: 0.5%, 1.3% and 1.9%, respectively. The lower incidence of events with CELEBREX was maintained with or without ASA use (see CLINICAL STUDIES – Special Studies – Platelets).

Withdrawals/Serious Adverse Events:

Kaplan-Meier cumulative rates at 9 months for withdrawals due to adverse events for CELEBREX, diclofenac and ibuprofen were 24%, 29%, and 26%, respectively. Rates for serious adverse events (i.e. those causing hospitalization or felt to be life threatening or otherwise medically significant) regardless of causality were not different across treatment groups, respectively, 8%, 7%, and 8%.

Based on Kaplan-Meier cumulative rates for investigator-reported serious cardiovascular thromboembolic adverse events*, there were no differences between the CELEBREX, diclofenac, or ibuprofen treatment groups. The rates in all patients at 9 months for CELEBREX, diclofenac, and ibuprofen were 1.2%, 1.4%, and 1.1%, respectively. The rates for non-ASA users in each of the three treatment groups were less than 1%. The rates for myocardial infarction in each of the three non-ASA treatment groups were less than 0.2%.

*includes myocardial infarction, pulmonary embolism, deep venous thrombosis, unstable angina, transient ischemic attacks or ischemic cerebrovascular accidents.

Adverse events from analgesia and dysmenorrhea studies: Approximately 1,700 patients were treated with CELEBREX in analgesia and dysmenorrhea studies. All patients in post-

Cardiovascular:	Syncope, congestive heart failure, ventricular fibrillation, pulmonary embolism, cerebrovascular accident, peripheral gangrene, thrombophlebitis, *vasculitis*
Gastrointestinal:	Intestinal obstruction, intestinal perforation, gastrointestinal bleeding, colitis with bleeding, esophageal perforation, pancreatitis, ileus
Liver and biliary system:	Cholelithiasis, *hepatitis, jaundice, liver failure*
Hemic and lymphatic:	Thrombocytopenia, *agranulocytosis, aplastic anemia, pancytopenia, leukopenia*
Metabolic:	*Hypoglycemia, hyponatremia*
Nervous system:	*Aseptic meningitis,* ataxia, suicide
Renal:	Acute renal failure, *interstitial nephritis*
Skin:	*Erythema multiforme, exfoliative dermatitis, Stevens-Johnson syndrome, toxic epidermal necrolysis*
General:	Sepsis, sudden death, *anaphylactoid reaction, angioedema*

oral surgery pain studies received a single dose of study medication. Doses up to 600 mg/day of CELEBREX were studied in primary dysmenorrhea and post-orthopedic surgery pain studies. The types of adverse events in the analgesia and dysmenorrhea studies were similar to those reported in arthritis studies. The only additional adverse event reported was post-dental extraction alveolar osteitis (dry socket) in the post-oral surgery pain studies.

Adverse events from the controlled trial in familial adenomatous polyposis: The adverse event profile reported for the 83 patients with familial adenomatous polyposis enrolled in the randomized, controlled clinical trial was similar to that reported for patients in the arthritis controlled trials. Intestinal anastomotic ulceration was the only new adverse event reported in the FAP trial, regardless of causality, and was observed in 3 of 58 patients (one at 100 mg BID, and two at 400 mg BID) who had prior intestinal surgery.

OVERDOSAGE

No overdoses of CELEBREX were reported during clinical trials. Doses up to 2400 mg/day for up to 10 days in 12 patients did not result in serious toxicity. Symptoms following acute NSAID overdoses are usually limited to lethargy, drowsiness, nausea, vomiting, and epigastric pain, which are generally reversible with supportive care. Gastrointestinal bleeding can occur. Hypertension, acute renal failure, respiratory depression and coma may occur, but are rare. Anaphylactoid reactions have been reported with therapeutic ingestion of NSAIDs, and may occur following an overdose. Patients should be managed by symptomatic and supportive care following an NSAID overdose. There are no specific antidotes. No information is available regarding the removal of celecoxib by hemodialysis, but based on its high degree of plasma protein binding (>97%) dialysis is unlikely to be useful in overdose. Emesis and/or activated charcoal (60 to 100 g in adults, 1 to 2 g/kg in children) and/or osmotic cathartic may be indicated in patients seen within 4 hours of ingestion with symptoms or following a large overdose. Forced diuresis, alkalinization of urine, hemodialysis, or hemoperfusion may not be useful due to high protein binding.

DOSAGE AND ADMINISTRATION

For osteoarthritis and rheumatoid arthritis, the lowest dose of CELEBREX should be sought for each patient. These doses can be given without regard to timing of meals.

Osteoarthritis: For relief of the signs and symptoms of osteoarthritis the recommended oral dose is 200 mg per day administered as a single dose or as 100 mg twice per day.

Rheumatoid arthritis: For relief of the signs and symptoms of rheumatoid arthritis the recommended oral dose is 100 to 200 mg twice per day.

Management of Acute Pain and Treatment of Primary Dysmenorrhea: The recommended dose of CELEBREX is 400 mg initially, followed by an additional 200 mg dose if needed on the first day. On subsequent days, the recommended dose is 200 mg twice daily as needed.

Familial adenomatous polyposis (FAP): Usual medical care for FAP patients should be continued while on CELEBREX. To reduce the number of adenomatous colorectal polyps in patients with FAP, the recommended oral dose is 400 mg twice per day to be taken with food.

Special Populations

Hepatic insufficiency: The daily recommended dose of CELEBREX capsules in patients with moderate hepatic impairment (Child-Pugh Class B) should be reduced by approximately 50% (see CLINICAL PHARMACOLOGY – Special Populations).

HOW SUPPLIED

CELEBREX 100-mg capsules are white, reverse printed white on blue band of body and cap with markings of 7767 on the cap and 100 on the body, supplied as:

NDC Number	Size
0025-1520-31	bottle of 100
0025-1520-51	bottle of 500
0025-1520-34	carton of 100 unit dose

CELEBREX 200-mg capsules are white, with reverse printed white on gold band with markings of 7767 on the cap and 200 on the body, supplied as:

NDC Number	Size
0025-1525-31	bottle of 100
0025-1525-51	bottle of 500
0025-1525-34	carton of 100 unit dose

CELEBREX 400-mg capsules are white, with reverse printed white on green band with markings of 7767 on the cap and 400 on the body, supplied as:

NDC Number	Size
0025-1530-02	bottle of 60
0025-1530-01	carton of 100 unit dose

Store at 25°C (77°F); excursions permitted to 15-30°C (59-86°F) [see USP Controlled Room Temperature].

Rx only Revised: January 2004

Manufactured for: G.D. Searle LLC
A subsidiary of Pharmacia Corporation
Chicago, IL 60680, USA
Pfizer Inc
New York, NY 10017, USA
by: Searle Ltd.
Caguas, PR 00725

PHARMACIA Pfizer
CELEBREX®
celecoxib capsules
819 059 006 PS4025-7

Shown in Product Identification Guide, page 333

COVERA-HS® ℞

[*cō-vər' ə*]
(verapamil hydrochloride)
Extended-Release Tablets
Controlled-Onset

DESCRIPTION

Covera-HS (verapamil hydrochloride) is a calcium ion influx inhibitor (slow-channel blocker or calcium ion antagonist). Covera-HS is available for oral administration as pale yellow, round, film-coated tablets containing 240 mg of verapamil hydrochloride and as lavender, round, film-coated tablets containing 180 mg of verapamil hydrochloride. Verapamil is administered as a racemic mixture of the R and S enantiomers. The structural formulae of the verapamil HCl enantiomers are:

S-verapamil

R-verapamil

$C_{27}H_{38}N_2O_4 \cdot HCl$ M.W. = 491.07

Benzeneacetonitrile, (±)-α[3[[2-(3,4-dimethoxyphenyl) ethyl]methylamino]propyl]-3,4-dimethoxy-α-(1-methylethyl) hydrochloride

Verapamil HCl is an almost white, crystalline powder, practically free of odor, with a bitter taste. It is soluble in water, chloroform, and methanol. Verapamil HCl is not chemically related to other cardioactive drugs.

Inactive ingredients are black ferric oxide, BHT, cellulose acetate, hydroxyethyl cellulose, hydroxypropyl cellulose, hypromellose, magnesium stearate, polyethylene glycol, polyethylene oxide, polysorbate 80, povidone, sodium chloride, titanium dioxide, and coloring agents: 240-mg—FD&C Blue No. 2 Lake and D&C Yellow No. 10 Lake; 180-mg—FD&C Blue No. 2 Lake and D&C Red No. 30 Lake.

System components and performance: The Covera-HS formulation has been designed to initiate the release of verapamil 4–5 hours after ingestion. This delay is introduced by a layer between the active drug core and outer semipermeable membrane. As water from the gastrointestinal tract enters the tablet, this delay coating is solubilized and released. As tablet hydration continues, the osmotic layer expands and pushes against the drug layer, releasing drug through precision laser-drilled orifices in the outer membrane at a constant rate. This controlled rate of drug delivery in the gastrointestinal lumen is independent of posture, pH, gastrointestinal motility, and fed or fasting conditions.

The biologically inert components of the delivery system remain intact during GI transit and are eliminated in the feces as an insoluble shell.

CLINICAL PHARMACOLOGY

Covera-HS has a unique delivery system, designed for bedtime dosing, incorporating a 4 to 5-hour delay in drug delivery. The unique controlled-onset, extended-release (COER) delivery system, which is designed for bedtime dosing, results in a maximum plasma concentration (C_{max}) of verapamil in the morning hours.

Verapamil is a calcium ion influx inhibitor (L-type calcium channel blocker or calcium channel antagonist). Verapamil exerts its pharmacologic effects by selectively inhibiting the transmembrane influx of ionic calcium into arterial smooth

Continued on next page

Covera-HS—Cont.

muscle as well as in conductile and contractile myocardial cells without altering serum calcium concentrations.

Mechanism of action

In vitro: Verapamil binding is voltage-dependent with affinity increasing as the vascular smooth muscle membrane potential is reduced. In addition, verapamil binding is frequency dependent and apparent affinity increases with increased frequency of depolarizing stimulus.

The L-type calcium channel is an oligomeric structure consisting of five putative subunits designated alpha-1, alpha-2, beta, tau, and epsilon. Biochemical evidence points to separate binding sites for 1,4-dihydropyridines, phenylalkylamines, and the benzothiazepines (all located on the alpha-1 subunit). Although they share a similar mechanism of action, calcium channel blockers represent three heterogeneous categories of drugs with differing vascular-cardiac selectivity ratios.

Essential hypertension: Verapamil produces its antihypertensive effect by a combination of vascular and cardiac effects. It acts as a vasodilator with selectivity for the arterial portion of the peripheral vasculature. As a result the systemic vascular resistance is reduced and usually without orthostatic hypotension or reflex tachycardia. Bradycardia (rate less than 50 beats/min) is uncommon (<1% with Covera-HS as assessed by ECG). During isometric or dynamic exercise Covera-HS does not alter systolic cardiac function in patients with normal ventricular function.

Covera-HS does not alter total serum calcium levels. However, one report has suggested that calcium levels above the normal range may alter the therapeutic effect of verapamil. Covera-HS regularly reduces the total systemic resistance (afterload) against which the heart works both at rest and at a given level of exercise by dilating peripheral arterioles.

Effects in hypertension: Covera-HS was evaluated in two placebo-controlled, parallel design, double-blind studies of 382 patients with mild to moderate hypertension.

In a clinical trial, 287 patients were randomized to placebo, 120 mg, 180 mg, 360 mg, or 540 mg and treated for 8 weeks (the two higher doses were titrated from low doses and maintained for 6 and 4 weeks, respectively). Covera-HS or placebo was given once daily at 10 pm and blood pressure changes were measured with 36-hour ambulatory blood pressure monitoring (ABPM). The results of these studies demonstrate that Covera-HS, at 180–540 mg, is a consistently and significantly more effective antihypertensive agent than placebo in reducing ambulatory blood pressures. Over this dose range, the placebo-subtracted net decreases in diastolic BP at trough (averaged over 6–10 pm) were dose-related, ranged from 4.5 to 11.2 mm Hg after 4–8 weeks of therapy, and correlated well with sitting cuff blood pressures.

These studies demonstrate that clinically and statistically significant blood pressure reductions are achieved with Covera-HS throughout the 24-hour dosing period.

There were no significant treatment differences between patient subgroups of different age (older or younger than 65 years), sex, race (Caucasian and non-Caucasian) and severity of hypertension at baseline (cuff BP below and above 105 mm Hg).

Angina: Verapamil dilates the main coronary arteries and coronary arterioles, both in normal and ischemic regions, and is a potent inhibitor of coronary artery spasm, whether spontaneous or ergonovine-induced. This property increases myocardial oxygen delivery in patients with coronary artery spasm and is responsible for the effectiveness of verapamil in vasospastic (Prinzmetal's or variant) as well as unstable angina at rest. Whether this effect plays any role in classical effort angina is not clear, but studies of exercise tolerance have not shown an increase in the maximum exercise rate-pressure product, a widely accepted measure of oxygen utilization. This suggests that, in general, relief of spasm or dilation of coronary arteries is not an important factor in classical angina.

Verapamil regularly reduces the total systemic resistance (afterload) against which the heart works both at rest and at a given level of exercise by dilating peripheral arterioles.

Effect in chronic stable angina: Covera-HS was evaluated in two placebo-controlled, parallel design, double-blind studies of 453 patients with chronic stable angina.

In the first clinical trial 277 patients were randomized to placebo, 180 mg, 360 mg, or 540 mg and treated for 4 weeks (the two higher doses were titrated from low doses and maintained for 3 and 2 weeks, respectively). A single dose of 240 mg was compared to placebo in a separate study of 176 patients. In these studies Covera-HS was significantly more effective than placebo in improvement of exercise tolerance. Placebo-adjusted net increases in median exercise times at the end of the dosing interval were 0.1 to 1.0 minute for symptom limited duration, 0.3 to 1.4 minutes for time to angina, and 0.1 to 1.1 minutes for time to ST change. Increases in exercise tolerance were in general greater at higher doses, but dose-response relationship was not well defined due to shorter treatment duration for high doses.

In addition, in the first study, 24 to 34% of patients treated with Covera-HS did not experience exercise-limiting angina on exercise treadmill testing (ETT) versus 12% of patients on placebo.

Electrophysiologic effects: Electrical activity through the AV node depends, to a significant degree, upon the transmembrane influx of extracellular calcium through the L-type (slow) channel. By decreasing the influx of calcium, verapamil prolongs the effective refractory period within the AV node and slows AV conduction in a rate-related manner.

Normal sinus rhythm is usually not affected, but in patients with sick sinus syndrome, verapamil may interfere with sinus-node impulse generation and may induce sinus arrest or sinoatrial block. Atrioventricular block can occur in patients without preexisting conduction defects (see *Warnings*).

Covera-HS does not alter the normal atrial action potential or intraventricular conduction time, but depresses amplitude, velocity of depolarization, and conduction in depressed atrial fibers. Verapamil may shorten the antegrade effective refractory period of the accessory bypass tract. Acceleration of ventricular rate and/or ventricular fibrillation has been reported in patients with atrial flutter or atrial fibrillation and a coexisting accessory AV pathway following administration of verapamil (see *Warnings*).

Verapamil has a local anesthetic action that is 1.6 times that of procaine on an equimolar basis. It is not known whether this action is important at the doses used in man.

Pharmacokinetics and metabolism: Verapamil is administered as a racemic mixture of the R and S enantiomers. The systemic concentrations of R and S enantiomers, as well as overall bioavailability, are dependent upon the route of administration and the rate and extent of release from the dosage forms. Upon oral administration, there is rapid stereoselective biotransformation during the first pass of verapamil through the portal circulation. In a study in 5 subjects with oral immediate-release verapamil, the systemic bioavailability was from 33% to 65% for the R enantiomer and from 13% to 34% for the S enantiomer. The R and S enantiomers have differing levels of pharmacologic activity. In studies in animals and humans, the S enantiomer has 8 to 20 times the activity of the R enantiomer in slowing AV conduction. In animal studies, the S enantiomer has 15 and 50 times the activity of the R enantiomer in reducing myocardial contractility in isolated blood-perfused dog papillary muscle and isolated rabbit papillary muscle, respectively, and twice the effect in reducing peripheral resistance. In isolated septal strip preparations from 5 patients, the S enantiomer was 8 times more potent than the R in reducing myocardial contractility. Dose escalation study data indicate that verapamil concentrations increase disproportionally to dose as measured by relative peak plasma concentrations (C_{max}) or areas under the plasma concentration vs time curves (AUC).

Pharmacokinetic Characteristics of Verapamil Enantiomers After Administration of Escalating Doses

		Total Dose of Racemic Verapamil (mg)			
	Isomer	120	180	360	540
Dose Ratio	—	1	1.5	3	4.5
Relative C_{max}	R	1	1.55	4.47	7.06
	S	1	1.62	5.17	9.21
Relative AUC	R	1	1.59	6.14	11.1
	S	1	1.89	8.17	15.9

Pharmacokinetic Characteristics of Verapamil Enantiomers After Administration of a Single 180 mg Dose and at Steady State

	Isomer	First Dose (Verapamil-naive subject)	Steady State (Current verapamil exposure)
C_{max} (ng/ml)	R	59.4	90.5
	S	11.7	21.2
AUC (0-24h) (ng·hr/ml)	R	644	1,223
	S	111	266

Racemic verapamil is released from Covera-HS at a constant rate following solubilization and release of the delay coat through the tablet orifices. This delay coat produces a lag period in drug release for approximately 4–5 hours. The drug release phase is prolonged with the peak plasma concentration (C_{max}) occurring approximately 11 hours after administration. Trough concentrations occur approximately 4 hours after bedtime dosing while the patient is sleeping. Steady-state pharmacokinetics were determined in healthy volunteers. Steady-state concentration is reached by the third or fourth day of dosing.

Steady-State Pharmacokinetics of Verapamil Enantiomers in Healthy Humans

		Verapamil Dose (mg)	
	Isomer	180	240
Mean C_{max} (ng/ml)	R	90.5	120
	S	21.2	28.7
AUC (0-24h) (ng·hr/ml)	R	1,223	1,470
	S	266	322

Consumption of a high fat meal just prior to dosing at night had no effect on the pharmacokinetics of Covera-HS. The pharmacokinetics were also not affected by whether the volunteers were supine or ambulatory for the 8 hours following dosing. Administering Covera-HS in the morning led to a slower rate of absorption and/or elimination, but did not affect the extent of absorption or extent of metabolism to norverapamil.

Orally administered verapamil undergoes extensive metabolism in the liver. Thirteen metabolites have been identified in urine. Norverapamil enantiomers can reach steady-state plasma concentrations approximately equal to those of the enantiomers of the parent drug. The cardiovascular activity of norverapamil appears to be approximately 20% that of verapamil. Approximately 70% of an administered dose is excreted as metabolites in the urine and 16% or more in the feces within 5 days. About 3% to 4% is excreted in the urine as unchanged drug. R-verapamil is 94% bound to plasma albumin, while S-verapamil is 88% bound. In addition, R-verapamil is 92% and S-verapamil 86% bound to alpha-1 acid glycoprotein. In patients with hepatic insufficiency, metabolism of immediate-release verapamil is delayed and elimination half-life prolonged up to 14 to 16 hours because of the extensive hepatic metabolism (see *Precautions*). In addition, in these patients there is a reduced first pass effect, and verapamil is more bioavailable. Verapamil clearance values suggest that patients with liver dysfunction may attain therapeutic verapamil plasma concentrations with one third of the oral daily dose required for patients with normal liver function.

After four weeks of oral dosing of immediate release verapamil (120 mg q.i.d.), verapamil and norverapamil levels were noted in the cerebrospinal fluid with estimated partition coefficient of 0.06 for verapamil and 0.04 for norverapamil.

Geriatric use: The pharmacokinetics of Covera-HS were studied after 5 consecutive nights of dosing 180 mg in 30 healthy young (19-43 years) versus 30 healthy elderly (65-80 years) male and female subjects. Older subjects had significantly higher mean verapamil C_{max}, C_{min}, and $AUC_{(0-24h)}$ compared to younger subjects. Older subjects had mean AUCs that were approximately 1.7-2.0 times higher than those of younger subjects as well as a longer average verapamil $t_{1/2}$ (approximately 20 hr vs 13 hr). These results were typical of the age-related differences seen with many drug products in clinical medicine. Lean body mass was inversely related to AUC, but no gender difference was observed in the clinical trials of Covera-HS. However, there are conflicting data in the literature suggesting that verapamil clearance may decrease with age in women to a greater degree than in men. Mean T_{max} was similar in young and elderly subjects.

Hemodynamics: Verapamil reduces afterload and myocardial contractility. In most patients, including those with organic cardiac disease, the negative inotropic action of verapamil is countered by reduction of afterload and cardiac index remains unchanged. During isometric or dynamic exercise, verapamil does not alter systolic cardiac function in patients with normal ventricular function. Improved left ventricular diastolic function in patients with IHSS and those with coronary heart disease has also been observed with verapamil. In patients with severe left ventricular dysfunction (eg, pulmonary wedge pressure above 20 mm Hg or ejection fraction less than 30%), or in patients taking beta-adrenergic blocking agents or other cardiodepressant drugs, deterioration of ventricular function may occur (see *Drug Interactions*).

Pulmonary function: Verapamil does not induce bronchoconstriction and, hence, does not impair ventilatory function.

Verapamil has been shown to have either a neutral or relaxant effect on bronchial smooth muscle.

INDICATIONS AND USAGE

Covera-HS is indicated for the management of hypertension and angina.

CONTRAINDICATIONS

Covera-HS is contraindicated in:

1. Severe left ventricular dysfunction (see *Warnings*)
2. Hypotension (systolic pressure less than 90 mm Hg) or cardiogenic shock
3. Sick sinus syndrome (except in patients with a functioning artificial ventricular pacemaker)
4. Second- or third-degree AV block (except in patients with a functioning artificial ventricular pacemaker)
5. Patients with atrial flutter or atrial fibrillation and an accessory bypass tract (eg, Wolff-Parkinson-White, Lown-Ganong-Levine syndromes). (See *Warnings*.)
6. Patients with known hypersensitivity to verapamil hydrochloride.

WARNINGS

Heart failure: Verapamil has a negative inotropic effect, which in most patients is compensated by its afterload reduction (decreased systemic vascular resistance) properties without a net impairment of ventricular performance. In previous clinical experience with 4,954 patients primarily with immediate-release verapamil, 1.8% developed congestive heart failure or pulmonary edema. Verapamil should be avoided in patients with severe left ventricular dysfunction (eg, ejection fraction less than 30%) or moderate to severe symptoms of cardiac failure and in patients with any degree of ventricular dysfunction if they are receiving a beta-adrenergic blocker (see *Drug Interactions*). Patients with milder ventricular dysfunction should, if possible, be controlled with optimum doses of digitalis and/or diuretics before verapamil treatment is started. (**Note interactions with digoxin under *Precautions*.**)

Hypotension: Occasionally, the pharmacologic action of verapamil may produce a decrease in blood pressure below normal levels, which may result in dizziness or symptomatic hypotension. In previous verapamil clinical trials the incidence observed in 4,954 patients was 2.5%. In clinical studies of Covera-HS, 0.4% of hypertensive patients and 1.0% of angina patients developed significant hypotension. In hypertensive patients, decreases in blood pressure below normal are unusual. Tilt-table testing (60 degrees) was not able to induce orthostatic hypotension.

Elevated liver enzymes: Elevations of transaminases with and without concomitant elevations in alkaline phosphatase and bilirubin have been reported. Such elevations have sometimes been transient and may disappear even in the face of continued verapamil treatment. Several cases of hepatocellular injury related to verapamil have been proven by rechallenge; half of these had clinical symptoms (malaise, fever, and/or right upper quadrant pain) in addition to elevation of SGOT, SGPT, and alkaline phosphatase. Periodic monitoring of liver function in patients receiving verapamil is therefore prudent.

Accessory bypass tract (Wolff-Parkinson-White or Lown-Ganong-Levine): Some patients with paroxysmal and/or chronic atrial fibrillation or atrial flutter and a coexisting accessory AV pathway have developed increased antegrade conduction across the accessory pathway bypassing the AV node, producing a very rapid ventricular response or ventricular fibrillation after receiving intravenous verapamil (or digitalis). Although a risk of this occurring with oral verapamil has not been established, such patients receiving oral verapamil may be at risk and its use in these patients is contraindicated (see *Contraindications*). Treatment is usually DC-cardioversion. Cardioversion has been used safely and effectively after oral verapamil.

Atrioventricular block: The effect of verapamil on AV conduction and the SA node may cause asymptomatic first-degree AV block and transient bradycardia, sometimes accompanied by nodal escape rhythms. PR-interval prolongation is correlated with verapamil plasma concentrations, especially during the early titration phase of therapy. Higher degrees of AV block, however, were infrequently (0.8%) observed in previous verapamil clinical trials. Marked first-degree block or progressive development to second- or third-degree AV block requires a reduction in dosage or, in rare instances, discontinuation of verapamil HCl and institution of appropriate therapy, depending upon the clinical situation.

Patients with hypertrophic cardiomyopathy (IHSS): In 120 patients with hypertrophic cardiomyopathy (most of them refractory or intolerant to propranolol) who received therapy with verapamil at doses up to 720 mg/day, a variety of serious adverse effects were seen. Three patients died in pulmonary edema; all had severe left ventricular outflow obstruction and a past history of left ventricular dysfunction. Eight other patients had pulmonary edema and/or severe hypotension; abnormally high (greater than 20 mm Hg) pulmonary wedge pressure and a marked left ventricular outflow obstruction were present in most of these patients. Concomitant administration of quinidine (see *Drug Interactions*) preceded the severe hypotension in 3 of the 8 patients (2 of whom developed pulmonary edema). Sinus bradycardia occurred in 11% of the patients, second-degree AV block in 4%, and sinus arrest in 2%. It must be appreciated that this group of patients had a serious disease with a high mortality rate. Most adverse effects responded well to dose reduction, and only rarely did verapamil use have to be discontinued.

PRECAUTIONS

General

Formulation specific: As with any other non-deformable dosage form caution should be used when administering Covera-HS in patients with preexisting severe gastrointestinal narrowing (pathologic or iatrogenic). In patients with extremely short GI transit time (<7 hrs), pharmacokinetic data are not available and dosage adjustment may be required.

Use in patients with impaired hepatic function: Since verapamil is highly metabolized by the liver, it should be administered cautiously to patients with impaired hepatic function. Severe liver dysfunction prolongs the elimination half-life of immediate-release verapamil to about 14 to 16 hours; hence, approximately 30% of the dose given to patients with normal liver function should be administered to these patients. Careful monitoring for abnormal prolongation of the PR interval or other signs of excessive pharmacologic effects (see *Overdosage*) should be carried out.

Use in patients with attenuated (decreased) neuromuscular transmission: It has been reported that verapamil decreases neuromuscular transmission in patients with Duchenne's muscular dystrophy, prolongs recovery from the neuromuscular blocking agent vecuronium, and causes a worsening of myasthenia gravis. It may be necessary to decrease the dosage of verapamil when it is administered to patients with attenuated neuromuscular transmission.

Use in patients with impaired renal function: About 70% of an administered dose of verapamil is excreted as metabolites in the urine. Verapamil is not removed by hemodialysis. Until further data are available, verapamil should be administered cautiously to patients with impaired renal function. These patients should be carefully monitored for abnormal prolongation of the PR interval or other signs of overdosage (see *Overdosage*).

Information for patients: Covera-HS tablets should be swallowed whole; do not break, crush, or chew. The medication in the Covera-HS tablet is released slowly through an outer shell that does not dissolve. The patient should not be concerned they occasionally observe this outer shell in their stool as it passes from the body.

Drug-Drug Interactions

Drug interactions: Effects other drugs on verapamil pharmacokinetics: In vitro metabolic studies indicate verapamil is metabolized by cytochrome P450 CYP3A4, CYP1A2, and CYP2C. Clinically significant interactions have been reported with inhibitors of CYP3A4 (eg, erythromycin, ritonavir) causing elevation of plasma levels of verapamil while inducers of CYP3A4 (eg, rifampin) have caused a lowering plasma levels of verapamil.

Alcohol: Verapamil may increase blood alcohol concentrations and prolong its effects.

Aspirin: In a few reported cases, coadministration of verapamil with aspirin has led to increased bleeding times greater than observed with aspirin alone.

Grapefruit juice: Grapefruit juice may significantly increase concentrations of verapamil. Grapefruit juice given to nine healthy volunteers increased S- and R- verapamil AUC_{0-12} by 36% and 28%, respectively. Steady state C_{max} and C_{min} of S-verapamil increased by 57% and 16.7%, respectively, with grapefruit juice compared to control. Similarly, C_{max} and C_{min} of R-verapamil increased by 40% and 13%, respectively. Grapefruit juice did not affect half-life, nor was there a significant change in AUC_{0-12} ratio R/S compared to control. Grapefruit juice did not cause a significant difference in the PK of norverapamil. This increase in verapamil plasma concentration is not expected to have any clinical consequences.

Beta-blockers: Concomitant therapy with beta-adrenergic blockers and verapamil may result in additive negative effects on heart rate, atrioventricular conduction and/or cardiac contractility. The combination of sustained-release verapamil and beta-adrenergic blocking agents has not been studied. However, there have been reports of excessive bradycardia and AV block, including complete heart block, when the combination has been used for the treatment of hypertension. For hypertensive patients, the risks combined therapy may outweigh the potential benefits. The combination should used only with caution and close monitoring.

Asymptomatic bradycardia (36 beats/min) with a wandering atrial pacemaker has been observed in a patient receiving concomitant timolol (a beta-adrenergic blocker) eyedrops and oral verapamil.

A decrease in metoprolol and propranolol clearance has been observed when either drug is administered concomitantly with verapamil. A variable effect has been seen when verapamil and atenolol were given together.

Digitalis: Clinical use of verapamil in digitalized patients has shown the combination to be well tolerated if digoxin doses are properly adjusted. However, chronic verapamil treatment can increase serum digoxin levels by 50% to 75% during the first week of therapy, and this can result in digitalis toxicity. In patients with hepatic cirrhosis the influence of verapamil on digoxin kinetics is magnified. Verapamil may reduce total body clearance and extrarenal clearance digitoxin by 27% and 29%, respectively. Maintenance and digitalization doses should be reduced when verapamil is administered, and the patient should be reassessed to avoid over- to underdigitalization. Whenever overdigitalization is suspected, the daily dose of digitalis should be reduced or temporarily discontinued. On discontinuation of verapamil use, the patient should be reassessed to avoid underdigitalization. In previous clinical trials with other verapamil formulations related to the control of ventricular response in digitalized patients who had atrial or atrial flutter, ventricular rates below 50/min at rest occurred in 15% of patients, and asymptomatic hypotension occurred in 5% of patients.

Antihypertensive agents: Verapamil administered concomitantly with oral antihypertensive agents (eg, vasodilators, angiotensin-converting enzyme inhibitors, diuretics, beta-blockers) will usually have an additive effect on lowering blood pressure. Patients receiving these combinations should be appropriately monitored. Concomitant use of agents that attenuate alpha-adrenergic function with verapamil may result in a reduction in blood pressure that is excessive in some patients. Such an effect was observed in one study following the concomitant administration of verapamil and prazosin.

Antiarrhythmic agents:

Disopyramide: Until data on possible interactions between verapamil and disopyramide are obtained, disopyramide should not be administered within 48 hours before or 24 hours after verapamil administration.

Flecainide: A study in healthy volunteers showed that the concomitant administration of flecainide and verapamil may have additive effects on myocardial contractility, AV conduction, and repolarization. Concomitant therapy with flecainide and verapamil may result in additive negative inotropic effect and prolongation of atrioventricular conduction.

Quinidine: In a small number of patients with hypertrophic cardiomyopathy (IHSS), concomitant use of verapamil and quinidine resulted in significant hypotension. Until further data are obtained, combined therapy of verapamil and quinidine in patients with hypertrophic cardiomyopathy should probably be avoided.

The electrophysiologic effects of quinidine and verapamil on AV conduction were studied in 8 patients. Verapamil significantly counteracted the effects of quinidine on AV conduction. There has been a report of increased quinidine levels during verapamil therapy.

Other:

Nitrates: Verapamil has been given concomitantly with short- and long-acting nitrates without any undesirable drug interactions. The pharmacologic profile of both drugs and clinical experience suggest beneficial interactions.

Cimetidine: The interaction between cimetidine and chronically administered verapamil has not been studied. Variable results on clearance have been obtained in acute studies of healthy volunteers; clearance of verapamil was either reduced or unchanged.

Lithium: Increased sensitivity to the effects of lithium (neurotoxicity) has been reported during concomitant verapamil-lithium therapy; lithium levels have been observed sometimes to increase, sometimes to decrease, and sometimes to be unchanged. Patients receiving both drugs must be monitored carefully.

Carbamazepine: Verapamil therapy may increase carbamazepine concentrations during combined therapy. This may produce carbamazepine side effects such as diplopia, headache, ataxia, or dizziness.

Rifampin: Therapy with rifampin may markedly reduce oral verapamil bioavailability.

Phenobarbital: Phenobarbital therapy may increase verapamil clearance.

Cyclosporin: Verapamil therapy may increase serum levels of cyclosporin.

Theophylline: Verapamil may inhibit the clearance and increase the plasma levels of theophylline.

Inhalation anesthetics: Animal experiments have shown that inhalation anesthetics depress cardiovascular activity by decreasing the inward movement of calcium ions. When used concomitantly, inhalation anesthetics and calcium channel blocking agents, such as verapamil, should each be titrated carefully to avoid excessive cardiovascular depression.

Neuromuscular blocking agents: Clinical data and animal studies suggest that verapamil may potentiate the activity of neuromuscular blocking agents (curare-like and depolarizing). It may be necessary to decrease the dose of verapamil and/or the dose of the neuromuscular blocking agent when the drugs are used concomitantly.

Carcinogenesis, mutagenesis, impairment of fertility: An 18-month toxicity study in rats, at a low multiple (6-fold) of the maximum recommended human dose, not the maximum tolerated dose, did not suggest a tumorigenic potential. There was no evidence of a carcinogenic potential of verapamil administered in the diet of rats for two years at doses of 10, 35, and 120 mg/kg/day or approximately 1, 3.5, and 12 times, respectively, the maximum recommended human daily dose (480 mg/day or 9.6 mg/kg/day).

Verapamil was not mutagenic in the Ames test in 5 test strains at 3 mg per plate with or without metabolic activation.

Studies in female rats at daily dietary doses up to 5.5 times (55 mg/kg/day) the maximum recommended human dose did not show impaired fertility. Effects on male fertility have not been determined.

Pregnancy: Pregnancy Category C. Reproduction studies have been performed in rabbits and rats at oral doses up to 1.5 (15 mg/kg/day) and 6 (60 mg/kg/day) times the human oral daily dose, respectively, and have revealed no evidence of teratogenicity. In the rat, however, this multiple of the human dose was embryocidal and retarded fetal growth and development, probably because of adverse maternal effects reflected in reduced weight gains of the dams. This oral dose has also been shown to cause hypotension in rats. There are no adequate and well-controlled studies in pregnant women. Because animal reproduction studies are not always predictive of human response, this drug should be used during pregnancy only if clearly needed. Verapamil crosses the placental barrier and can be detected in umbilical vein blood at delivery.

Labor and delivery: It is not known whether the use of verapamil during labor or delivery has immediate or delayed adverse effects on the fetus, or whether it prolongs the duration of labor or increases the need for forceps delivery or other obstetric intervention. Such adverse experiences have not been reported in the literature, despite a long history of use of verapamil in Europe in the treatment of cardiac side effects of beta-adrenergic agonist agents used to treat premature labor.

Nursing mothers: Verapamil is excreted in human milk. Because of the potential for adverse reactions in nursing infants from verapamil, nursing should be discontinued while verapamil is administered.

Pediatric use: Safety and effectiveness in pediatric patients have not been established.

Geriatric use: Clinical studies of Covera-HS did not include sufficient numbers of subjects aged under 65 to determine whether they responded differently from older subjects. Other reported clinical experience has not identified differences in responses between the elderly and younger

Continued on next page

Covera-HS—Cont.

and quinidine resulted in significant hypotension. Until further data are obtained, combined therapy of verapamil and quinidine in patients with hypertrophic cardiomyopathy should probably be avoided.

patients. In general, dose selection for an elderly patient should be cautious, usually starting at the low end of the dosing range, reflecting the greater frequency of decreased hepatic, renal, or cardiac function, and of concomitant disease or other drug therapy.

Animal pharmacology and/or animal toxicology: In chronic animal toxicology studies verapamil caused lenticular and/or suture line changes at 30 mg/kg/day or greater, and frank cataracts at 62.5 mg/kg/day or greater in the beagle dog but not in the rat. Development of cataracts due to verapamil has not been reported in man.

ADVERSE REACTIONS

Serious adverse reactions are uncommon when verapamil therapy is initiated with upward dose titration within the recommended single and total daily dose. See *Warnings* for discussion of heart failure, hypotension, elevated liver enzymes, AV block, and rapid ventricular response. Reversible (upon discontinuation of verapamil) non-obstructive, paralytic ileus has been infrequently reported in association with the use of verapamil. The following reactions to orally administered Covera-HS occurred at rates greater than 2.0% or occurred at lower rates but appeared drug-related in clinical trials in hypertension and angina:

	Placebo n=261 %	All doses studied n=572 %
Constipation	2.7	11.7*
Headache	7.3	6.6
Upper respiratory infection	4.6	5.4
Dizziness	2.7	4.7
Fatigue	3.8	4.5
Edema	3.1	3.0
Nausea	1.9	2.1
AV block (1°)	0.0	1.7
Elevated liver enzymes (see *Warnings*)	0.8	1.4
Bradycardia	0.4	1.4
Paresthesia	0.0	1.0
Flushing	0.3	0.8
Hypotension	0.0	0.7
Postural hypotension	0.3	0.4

*Constipation was typically mild, easily manageable, and the incidence usually diminished within about one week. At a typical once-daily dose of 240 mg, the observed incidence was 7.2%.

In previous experience with other formulations of verapamil, the following reactions occurred at rates greater than 1.0% or occurred at lower rates but appeared clearly drug related in clinical trials in 4,954 patients.

Constipation	7.3%
Dizziness	3.3%
Nausea	2.7%
Hypotension	2.5%
Headache	2.2%
Edema	1.9%
CHF/Pulmonary Edema	1.8%
Fatigue	1.7%
Dyspnea	1.4%
Bradycardia (HR <50/min)	1.4%
AV Block (total 1°,2°,3°)	1.2%
AV Block 2° and 3°	0.8%
Rash	1.2%
Flushing	0.6%
Elevated liver enzymes (see *Warnings*)	

The following reactions, reported with orally administered verapamil in 2% or less of patients, occurred under conditions (open trials, marketing experience) where a causal relationship is uncertain; they are listed to alert the physician to a possible relationship:

Cardiovascular: angina pectoris, AV block (2° & 3°), atrioventricular dissociation, CHF, pulmonary edema, chest pain, claudication, myocardial infarction, palpitations, purpura (vasculitis), syncope.

Digestive system: diarrhea, dry mouth, gastrointestinal distress, gingival hyperplasia.

Hemic and lymphatic: ecchymosis or bruising.

Nervous system: cerebrovascular accident, confusion, equilibrium disorders, insomnia, muscle cramps, psychotic symptoms, shakiness, somnolence, extrapyramidal symptoms.

Skin: arthralgia and rash, exanthema, hair loss, hyperkeratosis, macules, sweating, urticaria, Stevens-Johnson syndrome, erythema multiforme.

Special senses: blurred vision, tinnitus.

Urogenital: gynecomastia, galactorrhea/hyperprolactinemia, increased urination, spotty menstruation, impotence.

Other: allergy aggravated, dyspnea.

Treatment of acute cardiovascular adverse reactions: The frequency of cardiovascular adverse reactions that require therapy is rare; hence, experience with their treatment is limited. Whenever severe hypotension or complete AV block occurs following oral administration of verapamil, the appropriate emergency measures should be applied immediately; eg, intravenously administered norepinephrine bitartrate, atropine sulfate, isoproterenol HCl (all in usual doses), or calcium gluconate (10% solution). In patients with hypertrophic cardiomyopathy (IHSS), alpha-adrenergic agents (phenylephrine HCl, metaraminol bitartrate, or methoxamine HCl) should be used to maintain blood pressure, and isoproterenol and norepinephrine should be avoided. If further support is necessary, dopamine HCl or dobutamine HCl may be administered. Actual treatment and dosage should depend on the severity of the clinical situation and the judgement and experience of the treating physician.

OVERDOSAGE

Treat all verapamil overdoses as serious and maintain observation for at least 48 hours (especially sustained-release verapamil products), preferably under continuous hospital care. Delayed pharmacodynamic consequences may occur with the sustained-release formulations. Verapamil is known to decrease gastrointestinal transit time.

Treatment of overdosage should be supportive. Beta-adrenergic stimulation or parenteral administration of calcium solutions may increase calcium ion flux across the slow channel and have been used effectively in treatment of deliberate overdosage with verapamil. In a few reported cases, overdose with calcium channel blockers has been associated with hypotension and bradycardia, initially refractory to atropine but becoming more responsive to this treatment when the patients received large doses (close to 1 gram/hour for more than 24 hours) calcium chloride. Verapamil cannot be removed by hemodialysis. Clinically significant hypotensive reactions or high degree AV block should be treated with vasopressor agents or cardiac pacing, respectively. Asystole should be handled by the usual measures including cardiopulmonary resuscitation.

DOSAGE AND ADMINISTRATION

Covera-HS should be administered once daily at bedtime. Clinical trials explored dose ranges between 180 mg and 540 mg given at bedtime and found effects to persist throughout the dosing interval.

Covera-HS tablets should be swallowed whole and not chewed, broken, or crushed.

For both hypertension and angina the dose of Covera-HS should be individualized by titration. Initiate therapy with 180 mg of Covera-HS.

If an adequate response is not obtained with 180 mg of Covera-HS, the dose may be titrated upward in the following manner:

a) 240 mg each evening
b) 360 mg each evening (2 × 180 mg)
c) 480 mg each evening (2 × 240 mg)

When Covera-HS is administered at bedtime, office evaluation of blood pressure during morning and early afternoon hours is essentially a measure of peak effect. The usual evaluation of trough effect, which sometimes might be needed to evaluate the appropriateness of any given dose of Covera-HS, would be just prior to bedtime.

HOW SUPPLIED

Covera-HS 240-mg tablets are pale yellow, round, film coated with COVERA–HS 2021 printed on one side, supplied as:

NDC Number	Size
0025-2021-31	bottle of 100
0025-2021-34	carton of 100 unit dose

Covera-HS 180-mg tablets are lavender, round, film coated, with COVERA-HS 2011 printed on one side, supplied as:

NDC Number	Size
0025-2011-31	bottle of 100
0025-2011-34	carton of 100 unit dose

Store at controlled room temperature 20°–25°C (68°–77°F) [see USP]. Dispense in tight, light-resistant containers.

℞ only Revised: July 2003

Manufactured for:
G.D. Searle LLC
A subsidiary of Pharmacia Corporation
Chicago, IL 60680, USA
by: Alza Corporation
Palo Alto, CA 94303, USA

PHARMACIA

Covera-HS®
(verapamil hydrochloride)
Extended-Release Tablets
Controlled-Onset

818 875 102 P04027-3

Shown in Product Identification Guide, page 333

NOTICE

Before prescribing or administering any product described in PHYSICIANS' DESK REFERENCE check the **PDR Supplements** for revised information.

Sepracor Inc.

84 WATERFORD DRIVE
MARLBOROUGH, MA 01752

For Medical Information for Healthcare Professionals Contact:
1-800-739-0565
For Direct Inquiries to the Customer Assistance Center (CAC) Contact:
1-888-394-7377
FAX 1-508-357-7589
E-mail CAC@sepracor.com
or write to Sepracor CAC at the address above.

XOPENEX® ℞
[*zō' pə-neks"*]
(levalbuterol HCl) Inhalation Solution,
0.31 mg*, 0.63 mg*, 1.25 mg*
***Potency expressed as levalbuterol**

PRESCRIBING INFORMATION

DESCRIPTION

Xopenex (levalbuterol HCl) Inhalation Solution is a sterile, clear, colorless, preservative-free solution of the hydrochloride salt of levalbuterol, the (R)-enantiomer of the drug substance racemic albuterol. Levalbuterol HCl is a relatively selective beta$_2$-adrenergic receptor agonist (see **CLINICAL PHARMACOLOGY**). The chemical name for levalbuterol HCl is (R)-α^1-[[(1,1-dimethylethyl)amino]methyl]-4-hydroxy-1,3-benzenedimethanol hydrochloride, and its established chemical structure is as follows:

The molecular weight of levalbuterol HCl is 275.8, and its empirical formula is $C_{13}H_{21}NO_3$•HCl. It is a white to off-white, crystalline solid, with a melting point of approximately 187°C and solubility of approximately 180 mg/mL in water.

Levalbuterol HCl is the USAN modified name for (R)-albuterol HCl in the United States.

Xopenex (levalbuterol HCl) Inhalation Solution is supplied in unit-dose vials and requires no dilution before administration by nebulization. Each 3 mL unit-dose vial contains either 0.31 mg of levalbuterol (as 0.36 mg of levalbuterol HCl) or 0.63 mg of levalbuterol (as 0.73 mg of levalbuterol HCl) or 1.25 mg of levalbuterol (as 1.44 mg of levalbuterol HCl), sodium chloride to adjust tonicity, and sulfuric acid to adjust the pH to 4.0 (3.3 to 4.5).

CLINICAL PHARMACOLOGY

Activation of beta$_2$-adrenergic receptors on airway smooth muscle leads to the activation of adenylcyclase and to an increase in the intracellular concentration of cyclic-3', 5'-adenosine monophosphate (cyclic AMP). This increase in cyclic AMP leads to the activation of protein kinase A, which inhibits the phosphorylation of myosin and lowers intracellular ionic calcium concentrations, resulting in relaxation. Levalbuterol relaxes the smooth muscles of all airways, from the trachea to the terminal bronchioles. Levalbuterol acts as a functional antagonist to relax the airway irrespective of the spasmogen involved, thus protecting against all bronchoconstrictor challenges. Increased cyclic AMP concentrations are also associated with the inhibition of release of mediators from mast cells in the airway.

While it is recognized that beta$_2$-adrenergic receptors are the predominant receptors on bronchial smooth muscle, data indicate that there is a population of beta$_2$-receptors in the human heart that comprise between 10% and 50% of cardiac beta-adrenergic receptors. The precise function of these receptors has not been established (see **WARNINGS**). However, all beta-adrenergic agonist drugs can produce a significant cardiovascular effect in some patients, as measured by pulse rate, blood pressure, symptoms, and/or electrocardiographic changes.

Preclinical Studies

Results from an *in vitro* study of binding to human beta-adrenergic receptors demonstrated that levalbuterol has approximately 2-fold greater binding affinity than racemic albuterol and approximately 100-fold greater binding affinity than (S)-albuterol. In guinea pig airways, levalbuterol HCl and racemic albuterol decreased the response to spasmogens (e.g., acetylcholine and histamine), whereas (S)-albuterol was ineffective. These results suggest that most of the bronchodilatory effect of racemic albuterol is due to the (R)-enantiomer.

Intravenous studies in rats with racemic albuterol sulfate have demonstrated that albuterol crosses the blood-brain barrier and reaches brain concentrations amounting to approximately 5.0% of the plasma concentrations. In structures outside the blood-brain barrier (pineal and pituitary glands), albuterol concentrations were found to be 100 times those in the whole brain.

Studies in laboratory animals (minipigs, rodents, and dogs) have demonstrated the occurrence of cardiac arrhythmias and sudden death (with histologic evidence of myocardial necrosis) when beta-agonists and methylxanthines are administered concurrently. The clinical significance of these findings is unknown.

Pharmacokinetics (Adults and Adolescents ≥12 years old)

The inhalation pharmacokinetics of Xopenex Inhalation Solution were investigated in a randomized cross-over study in 30 healthy adults following administration of a single dose of 1.25 mg and a cumulative dose of 5 mg of Xopenex Inhalation Solution and a single dose of 2.5 mg and a cumulative dose of 10 mg of racemic albuterol sulfate inhalation solution by nebulization using a PARI LC Jet™ nebulizer with a Dura-Neb® 2000 compressor.

Following administration of a single 1.25 mg dose of Xopenex Inhalation Solution, exposure to (R)-albuterol (AUC of 3.3 ng•hr/mL) was approximately 2-fold higher than following administration of a single 2.5 mg dose of racemic albuterol inhalation solution (AUC of 1.7 ng•hr/mL) (see **Table 1**). Following administration of a cumulative 5 mg dose of Xopenex Inhalation Solution (1.25 mg given every 30 minutes for a total of four doses) or a cumulative 10 mg dose of racemic albuterol inhalation solution (2.5 mg given every 30 minutes for a total of four doses), C_{max} and AUC of (R)-albuterol were comparable (see **Table 1**).

[See table 1 at right]

Pharmacokinetics (Children 6–11 years old)

The pharmacokinetic parameters of (R)- and (S)-albuterol in children with asthma were obtained using population pharmacokinetic analysis. These data are presented in Table 2. For comparison, adult data obtained by conventional pharmacokinetic analysis from a different study are also presented in Table 2.

In children, AUC and C_{max} of (R)-albuterol following administration of 0.63 mg Xopenex Inhalation Solution were comparable to that following administration of 1.25 mg racemic albuterol sulfate inhalation solution.

Given the same dose of 0.63 mg of Xopenex to children and adults, the predicted C_{max} of (R)-albuterol in children was similar to that in adults (0.52 vs. 0.56 ng/mL), while predicted AUC in children (2.55 ng•hr/mL) was about 1.5-fold higher than that in adults (1.65 ng•hr/mL). These data support lower doses for children 6–11 years old compared to the adult doses (see **Dosage and Administration**).

[See table 2 at right]

Pharmacodynamics

(Adults and Adolescents ≥12 years old)

In a randomized, double-blind, placebo-controlled, cross-over study, 20 adults with mild-to-moderate asthma received single doses of Xopenex Inhalation Solution (0.31, 0.63, and 1.25 mg) and racemic albuterol sulfate inhalation solution (2.5 mg). All doses of active treatment produced a significantly greater degree of bronchodilation (as measured by percent change from pre-dose in mean FEV_1) than placebo, and there were no significant differences between any of the active treatment arms. The bronchodilator responses to 1.25 mg of Xopenex Inhalation Solution and 2.5 mg of racemic albuterol sulfate inhalation solution were clinically comparable over the 6-hour evaluation period, except for a slightly longer duration of action (>15% increase in FEV_1 from baseline) after administration of 1.25 mg of Xopenex Inhalation Solution. Systemic beta-adrenergic adverse effects were observed with all active doses and were generally dose-related for (R)-albuterol. Xopenex Inhalation Solution at a dose of 1.25 mg produced a slightly higher rate of systemic beta-adrenergic adverse effects than the 2.5 mg dose of racemic albuterol sulfate inhalation solution.

In a randomized, double-blind, placebo-controlled, cross-over study, 12 adults with mild-to-moderate asthma were challenged with inhaled methacholine chloride 20 and 180 minutes following administration of a single dose of either 2.5 mg of racemic albuterol sulfate, 1.25 mg of Xopenex, 1.25 mg of (S)-albuterol, or placebo using a PARI LC Jet™ nebulizer. Racemic albuterol sulfate, Xopenex, and (S)-albuterol had a protective effect against methacholine-induced bronchoconstriction 20 minutes after administration, although the effect of (S)-albuterol was minimal. At 180 minutes after administration, the bronchoprotective effect of 1.25 mg of Xopenex was comparable to that of 2.5 mg of racemic albuterol sulfate. At 180 minutes after administration, 1.25 mg of (S)-albuterol had no bronchoprotective effect.

In a clinical study in adults with mild-to-moderate asthma, comparable efficacy (as measured by change from baseline in FEV_1) and safety (as measured by heart rate, blood pressure, ECG, serum potassium, and tremor) were demonstrated after a cumulative dose of 5 mg of Xopenex Inhalation Solution (four consecutive doses of 1.25 mg administered every 30 minutes) and 10 mg of racemic albuterol sulfate inhalation solution (four consecutive doses of 2.5 mg administered every 30 minutes).

Clinical Trials (Adults and Adolescents ≥12 years old)

The safety and efficacy of Xopenex Inhalation Solution were evaluated in a 4-week, multicenter, randomized, double-blind, placebo-controlled, parallel group study in 362 adult and adolescent patients 12 years of age and older, with mild-to-moderate asthma (mean baseline FEV_1 60% of predicted). Approximately half of the patients were also receiving inhaled corticosteroids. Patients were randomized to receive Xopenex 0.63 mg, Xopenex 1.25 mg, racemic albuterol sulfate 1.25 mg, racemic albuterol sulfate 2.5 mg, or placebo three times a day administered via a PARI LC Plus™ nebulizer and a Dura-Neb® portable compressor. Racemic albuterol delivered by a chlorofluorocarbon (CFC) metered dose inhaler (MDI) was used on an as-needed basis as the rescue medication.

Table 1: Mean (SD) Values for Pharmacokinetic Parameters in Healthy Adults

	Single Dose		Cumulative Dose	
	Xopenex 1.25 mg	Racemic albuterol sulfate 2.5 mg	Xopenex 5 mg	Racemic albuterol sulfate 10 mg
C_{max} (ng/mL) (R)-albuterol	1.1 (0.45)	0.8 (0.41)**	4.5 (2.20)	4.2 (1.51)**
T_{max} (h)$^{\gamma}$ (R)-albuterol	0.2 (0.17, 0.37)	0.2 (0.17, 1.50)	0.2 (−0.18*, 1.25)	0.2 (−0.28*, 1.00)
AUC (ng•h/mL) (R)-albuterol	3.3 (1.58)	1.7 (0.99)**	17.4 (8.56)	16.0 (7.12)**
$T_{½}$ (h) (R)-albuterol	3.3 (2.48)	1.5 (0.61)	4.0 (1.05)	4.1 (0.97)

γ Median (Min, Max) reported for T_{max}.
* A negative T_{max} indicates C_{max} occurred between first and last nebulizations.
**Values reflect only (R)-albuterol and do not include (S)-albuterol.

Table 2: (R)-Albuterol Exposure in Adults and Pediatric Subjects (6–11 years)

	Children 6–11 years				Adults ≥12 years	
Treatment	Xopenex 0.31 mg	Xopenex 0.63 mg	Racemic albuterol 1.25 mg	Racemic albuterol 2.5 mg	Xopenex 0.63 mg	Xopenex 1.25 mg
$AUC_{0-\infty}$ (ng•hr/mL) [c]	1.36	2.55	2.65	5.02	1.65 [a]	3.3 [b]
C_{max} (ng/mL) [d]	0.303	0.521	0.553	1.08	0.56 [a]	1.1 [b]

[a] The values are predicted by assuming linear pharmacokinetics
[b] The data obtained from Table 1
[c] Area under the plasma concentration curve from time 0 to infinity
[d] Maximum plasma concentration

Efficacy, as measured by the mean percent change from baseline in FEV_1, was demonstrated for all active treatment regimens compared with placebo on day 1 and day 29. On both day 1 (see **Figure 1**) and day 29 (see **Figure 2**), 1.25 mg of Xopenex demonstrated the largest mean percent change from baseline in FEV_1 compared to the other active treatments. A dose of 0.63 mg of Xopenex and 2.5 mg of racemic albuterol sulfate produced a clinically comparable mean percent change from baseline in FEV_1 on both day 1 and day 29.

Figure 1: Mean Percent Change from Baseline FEV_1 on Day 1, Adults and Adolescents ≥ 12 years old

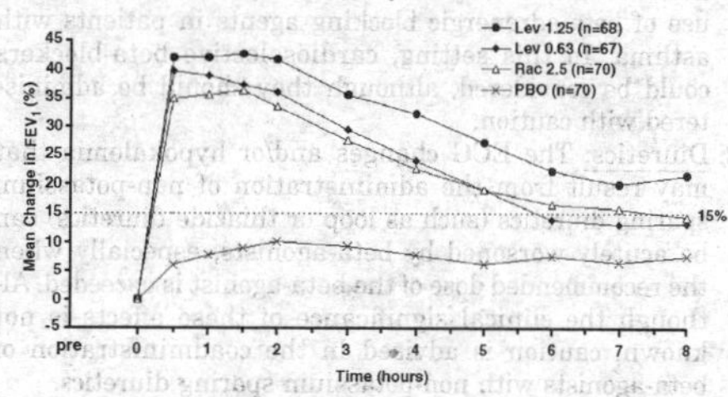

Figure 2: Mean Percent Change from Baseline FEV_1 on Day 29, Adults and Adolescents ≥ 12 years old

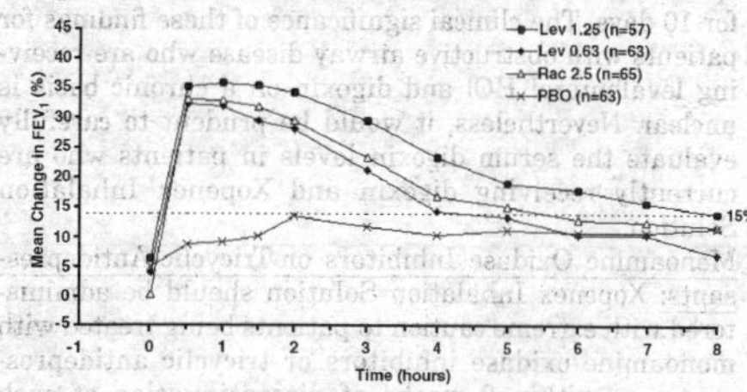

The mean time to onset of a 15% increase in FEV_1 over baseline for levalbuterol at doses of 0.63 mg and 1.25 mg was approximately 17 minutes and 10 minutes, respectively, and the mean time to peak effect for both doses was approximately 1.5 hours after 4 weeks of treatment. The mean duration of effect, as measured by a >15% increase from baseline in FEV_1, was approximately 5 hours after administration of 0.63 mg of levalbuterol and approximately 6 hours after administration of 1.25 mg of levalbuterol after 4 weeks of treatment. In some patients, the duration of effect was as long as 8 hours.

Clinical Trials (Children 6–11 years old)

A multi-center, randomized, double-blind, placebo- and active-controlled study was conducted in children with mild-to-moderate asthma (mean baseline FEV_1 73% of predicted) (n=316). Following a one week placebo run-in, subjects were randomized to Xopenex (0.31 or 0.63 mg), racemic albuterol (1.25 or 2.5 mg), or placebo, which were delivered three times a day for three weeks using a PARI LC Plus™ nebulizer and a Dura-Neb® 3000 compressor.

Efficacy, as measured by mean peak percent change from baseline in FEV_1, was demonstrated for all active treatment regimens compared with placebo on day 1 and day 21. Time profile FEV_1 curves for day 1 and day 21 are shown in Figure 3 and Figure 4, respectively. The onset of effect (time to a 15% increase in FEV_1 over test day baseline) and duration of effect (maintenance of a >15% increase in FEV_1 over test day baseline) of levalbuterol were clinically comparable to those of racemic albuterol.

Figure 3: Mean Percent Change from Baseline FEV_1 on Day 1, Children 6-11 Years of Age

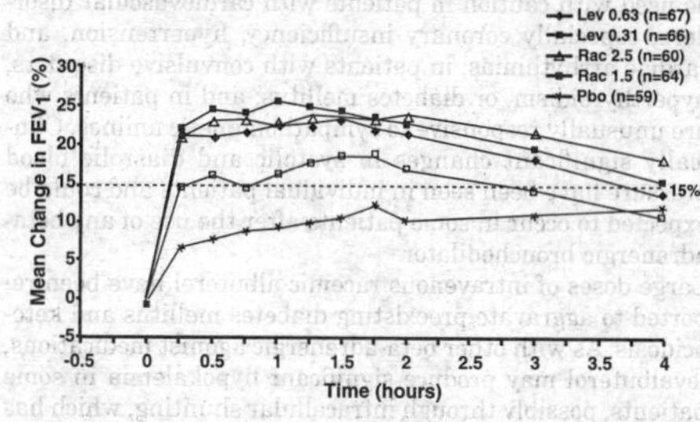

Figure 4: Mean Percent Change from Baseline FEV_1 on Day 21, Children 6-11 Years of Age

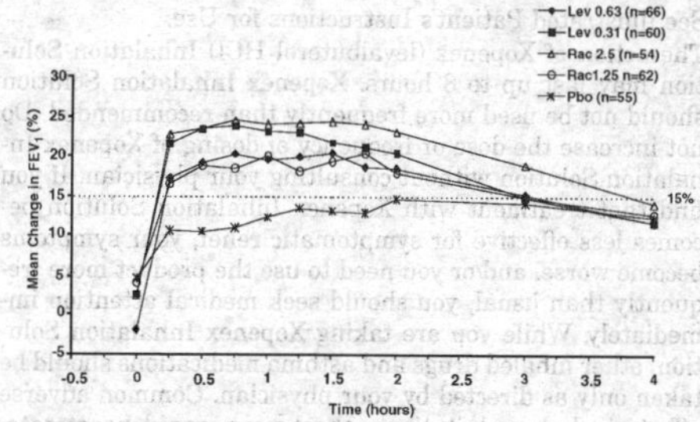

INDICATIONS AND USAGE

Xopenex (levalbuterol HCl) Inhalation Solution is indicated for the treatment or prevention of bronchospasm in adults, adolescents and children 6 years of age and older with reversible obstructive airway disease.

CONTRAINDICATIONS

Xopenex (levalbuterol HCl) Inhalation Solution is contraindicated in patients with a history of hypersensitivity to levalbuterol HCl or racemic albuterol.

WARNINGS

1. Paradoxical Bronchospasm: Like other inhaled beta-adrenergic agonists, Xopenex Inhalation Solution can produce paradoxical bronchospasm, which may be life threatening. If paradoxical bronchospasm occurs, Xopenex Inhalation Solution should be discontinued immediately and alternative therapy instituted. It should be recognized that paradoxical bronchospasm, when associated with inhaled formulations, frequently occurs with the first use of a new canister or vial.
2. Deterioration of Asthma: Asthma may deteriorate acutely over a period of hours or chronically over several days or longer. If the patient needs more doses of Xopenex Inhalation Solution than usual, this may be a marker of destabilization of asthma and requires reevaluation of the patient and treatment regimen, giving special consideration to the possible need for anti-inflammatory treatment, e.g., corticosteroids.

Continued on next page

Xopenex—Cont.

3. Use of Anti-Inflammatory Agents: The use of beta-adrenergic agonist bronchodilators alone may not be adequate to control asthma in many patients. Early consideration should be given to adding anti-inflammatory agents, e.g., corticosteroids, to the therapeutic regimen.
4. Cardiovascular Effects: Xopenex Inhalation Solution, like all other beta-adrenergic agonists, can produce a clinically significant cardiovascular effect in some patients, as measured by pulse rate, blood pressure, and/or symptoms. Although such effects are uncommon after administration of Xopenex Inhalation Solution at recommended doses, if they occur, the drug may need to be discontinued. In addition, beta-agonists have been reported to produce ECG changes, such as flattening of the T wave, prolongation of the QTc interval, and ST segment depression. The clinical significance of these findings is unknown. Therefore, Xopenex Inhalation Solution, like all sympathomimetic amines, should be used with caution in patients with cardiovascular disorders, especially coronary insufficiency, cardiac arrhythmias, and hypertension.
5. Do Not Exceed Recommended Dose: Fatalities have been reported in association with excessive use of inhaled sympathomimetic drugs in patients with asthma. The exact cause of death is unknown, but cardiac arrest following an unexpected development of a severe acute asthmatic crisis and subsequent hypoxia is suspected.
6. Immediate Hypersensitivity Reactions: Immediate hypersensitivity reactions may occur after administration of racemic albuterol, as demonstrated by rare cases of urticaria, angioedema, rash, bronchospasm, anaphylaxis, and oropharyngeal edema. The potential for hypersensitivity must be considered in the clinical evaluation of patients who experience immediate hypersensitivity reactions while receiving Xopenex Inhalation Solution.

PRECAUTIONS

General

Levalbuterol HCl, like all sympathomimetic amines, should be used with caution in patients with cardiovascular disorders, especially coronary insufficiency, hypertension, and cardiac arrhythmias; in patients with convulsive disorders, hyperthyroidism, or diabetes mellitus; and in patients who are unusually responsive to sympathomimetic amines. Clinically significant changes in systolic and diastolic blood pressure have been seen in individual patients and could be expected to occur in some patients after the use of any beta-adrenergic bronchodilator.

Large doses of intravenous racemic albuterol have been reported to aggravate preexisting diabetes mellitus and ketoacidosis. As with other beta-adrenergic agonist medications, levalbuterol may produce significant hypokalemia in some patients, possibly through intracellular shunting, which has the potential to produce adverse cardiovascular effects. The decrease is usually transient, not requiring supplementation.

Information for Patients

See illustrated Patient's Instructions for Use.

The action of Xopenex (levalbuterol HCl) Inhalation Solution may last up to 8 hours. Xopenex Inhalation Solution should not be used more frequently than recommended. Do not increase the dose or frequency of dosing of Xopenex Inhalation Solution without consulting your physician. If you find that treatment with Xopenex Inhalation Solution becomes less effective for symptomatic relief, your symptoms become worse, and/or you need to use the product more frequently than usual, you should seek medical attention immediately. While you are taking Xopenex Inhalation Solution, other inhaled drugs and asthma medications should be taken only as directed by your physician. Common adverse effects include palpitations, chest pain, rapid heart rate, headache, dizziness, and tremor or nervousness. If you are pregnant or nursing, contact your physician about the use of Xopenex Inhalation Solution.

Effective and safe use of Xopenex Inhalation Solution requires consideration of the following information in addition to that provided under Patient's Instructions for Use:

Xopenex Inhalation Solution single-use low-density polyethylene (LDPE) vials should be protected from light and excessive heat. Store in the protective foil pouch between 20°C and 25°C (68°F and 77°F) [see USP Controlled Room Temperature]. Do not use after the expiration date stamped on the container. Unused vials should be stored in the protective foil pouch. Once the foil pouch is opened, the vials should be used within two weeks. Vials removed from the pouch, if not used immediately, should be protected from light and used within one week. Discard any vial if the solution is not colorless.

The drug compatibility (physical and chemical), efficacy, and safety of Xopenex Inhalation Solution when mixed with other drugs in a nebulizer have not been established.

Drug Interactions

Other short-acting sympathomimetic aerosol bronchodilators or epinephrine should be used with caution with levalbuterol. If additional adrenergic drugs are to be administered by any route, they should be used with caution to avoid deleterious cardiovascular effects.

1. Beta-blockers: Beta-adrenergic receptor blocking agents not only block the pulmonary effect of beta-agonists such as Xopenex (levalbuterol HCl) Inhalation Solution, but may also produce severe bronchospasm in asthmatic patients. Therefore, patients with asthma should not normally be treated with beta-blockers. However, under certain circumstances, e.g., as prophylaxis after myocardial infarction, there may be no acceptable alternatives to the use of beta-adrenergic blocking agents in patients with asthma. In this setting, cardioselective beta-blockers could be considered, although they should be administered with caution.
2. Diuretics: The ECG changes and/or hypokalemia that may result from the administration of non-potassium sparing diuretics (such as loop or thiazide diuretics) can be acutely worsened by beta-agonists, especially when the recommended dose of the beta-agonist is exceeded. Although the clinical significance of these effects is not known, caution is advised in the coadministration of beta-agonists with non-potassium sparing diuretics.
3. Digoxin: Mean decreases of 16% and 22% in serum digoxin levels were demonstrated after single-dose intravenous and oral administration of racemic albuterol, respectively, to normal volunteers who had received digoxin for 10 days. The clinical significance of these findings for patients with obstructive airway disease who are receiving levalbuterol HCl and digoxin on a chronic basis is unclear. Nevertheless, it would be prudent to carefully evaluate the serum digoxin levels in patients who are currently receiving digoxin and Xopenex Inhalation Solution.
4. Monoamine Oxidase Inhibitors or Tricyclic Antidepressants: Xopenex Inhalation Solution should be administered with extreme caution to patients being treated with monoamine oxidase inhibitors or tricyclic antidepressants, or within 2 weeks of discontinuation of such agents, because the action of levalbuterol HCl on the vascular system may be potentiated.

Table 4: Adverse Events Reported in a 4-Week, Controlled Clinical Trial in Adults and Adolescents ≥12 years old

Body System Preferred Term	Percent of Patients Placebo (n=75)	 Xopenex 1.25 mg (n=73)	 Xopenex 0.63 mg (n=72)	 Racemic albuterol 2.5 mg (n=74)
Body as a Whole				
Allergic reaction	1.3	0	0	2.7
Flu syndrome	0	1.4	4.2	2.7
Accidental injury	0	2.7	0	0
Pain	1.3	1.4	2.8	2.7
Back pain	0	0	0	2.7
Cardiovascular System				
Tachycardia	0	2.7	2.8	2.7
Migraine	0	2.7	0	0
Digestive System				
Dyspepsia	1.3	2.7	1.4	1.4
Musculoskeletal System				
Leg cramps	1.3	2.7	0	1.4
Central Nervous System				
Dizziness	1.3	2.7	1.4	0
Hypertonia	0	0	0	2.7
Nervousness	0	9.6	2.8	8.1
Tremor	0	6.8	0	2.7
Anxiety	0	2.7	0	0
Respiratory System				
Cough increased	2.7	4.1	1.4	2.7
Infection viral	9.3	12.3	6.9	12.2
Rhinitis	2.7	2.7	11.1	6.8
Sinusitis	2.7	1.4	4.2	2.7
Turbinate edema	0	1.4	2.8	0

Table 5: Mean Changes from Baseline in Heart Rate at 15 Minutes and in Glucose and Potassium at 1 Hour after First Dose (Day 1) in Adults and Adolescents ≥12 years old

Treatment	Mean Changes (day 1) Heart Rate (bpm)	 Glucose (mg/dL)	 Potassium (mEq/L)
Xopenex 0.63 mg, n=72	2.4	4.6	−0.2
Xopenex 1.25 mg, n=73	6.9	10.3	−0.3
Racemic albuterol 2.5 mg, n=74	5.7	8.2	−0.3
Placebo, n=75	−2.8	−0.2	−0.2

Carcinogenesis, Mutagenesis, and Impairment of Fertility

No carcinogenesis or impairment of fertility studies have been carried out with levalbuterol HCl alone. However, racemic albuterol sulfate has been evaluated for its carcinogenic potential and ability to impair fertility.

In a 2-year study in Sprague-Dawley rats, racemic albuterol sulfate caused a significant dose-related increase in the incidence of benign leiomyomas of the mesovarium at and above dietary doses of 2 mg/kg (approximately 2 times the maximum recommended daily inhalation dose of levalbuterol HCl for adults and children on a mg/m^2 basis). In another study, this effect was blocked by the coadministration of propranolol, a nonselective beta-adrenergic antagonist. In an 18-month study in CD-1 mice, racemic albuterol sulfate showed no evidence of tumorigenicity at dietary doses up to 500 mg/kg (approximately 260 times the maximum recommended daily inhalation dose of levalbuterol HCl for adults and children on a mg/m^2 basis). In a 22-month study in the Golden hamster, racemic albuterol sulfate showed no evidence of tumorigenicity at dietary doses up to 50 mg/kg (approximately 35 times the maximum recommended daily inhalation dose of levalbuterol HCl for adults and children on a mg/m^2 basis).

Levalbuterol HCl was not mutagenic in the Ames test or the CHO/HPRT Mammalian Forward Gene Mutation Assay. Although levalbuterol HCl has not been tested for clastogenicity, racemic albuterol sulfate was not clastogenic in a human peripheral lymphocyte assay or in an AH1 strain mouse micronucleus assay. Reproduction studies in rats using racemic albuterol sulfate demonstrated no evidence of impaired fertility at oral doses up to 50 mg/kg (approximately 55 times the maximum recommended daily inhalation dose of levalbuterol HCl for adults on a mg/m^2 basis).

Teratogenic Effects—Pregnancy Category C

A reproduction study in New Zealand White rabbits demonstrated that levalbuterol HCl was not teratogenic when administered orally at doses up to 25 mg/kg (approximately 110 times the maximum recommended daily inhalation dose of levalbuterol HCl for adults on a mg/m^2 basis). However, racemic albuterol sulfate has been shown to be teratogenic in mice and rabbits. A study in CD-1 mice given racemic albuterol sulfate subcutaneously showed cleft palate formation in 5 of 111 (4.5%) fetuses at 0.25 mg/kg (less than the maximum recommended daily inhalation dose of levalbuterol HCl for adults on a mg/m^2 basis) and in 10 of 108 (9.3%) fetuses at 2.5 mg/kg (approximately equal to the maximum recommended daily inhalation dose of levalbuterol HCl for adults on a mg/m^2 basis). The drug did not induce cleft palate formation when administered subcutaneously at a dose of 0.025 mg/kg (less than the maximum recommended daily inhalation dose of levalbuterol HCl for adults on a mg/m^2 basis). Cleft palate also occurred in 22 of 72 (30.5%) fetuses from females treated subcutaneously with 2.5 mg/kg of isoproterenol (positive control).

A reproduction study in Stride Dutch rabbits revealed cranioschisis in 7 of 19 (37%) fetuses when racemic albuterol sulfate was administered orally at a dose of 50 mg/kg (approximately 110 times the maximum recommended daily inhalation dose of levalbuterol HCl for adults on a mg/m^2 basis).

A study in which pregnant rats were dosed with radiolabeled racemic albuterol sulfate demonstrated that drug-related material is transferred from the maternal circulation to the fetus.

There are no adequate and well-controlled studies of Xopenex Inhalation Solution in pregnant women. Because animal reproduction studies are not always predictive of human response, Xopenex Inhalation Solution should be used during pregnancy only if the potential benefit justifies the potential risk to the fetus.

During marketing experience of racemic albuterol, various congenital anomalies, including cleft palate and limb defects, have been rarely reported in the offspring of patients being treated with racemic albuterol. Some of the mothers were taking multiple medications during their pregnancies. No consistent pattern of defects can be discerned, and a relationship between racemic albuterol use and congenital anomalies has not been established.

Use in Labor and Delivery

Because of the potential for beta-adrenergic agonists to interfere with uterine contractility, the use of Xopenex Inhalation Solution for the treatment of bronchospasm during labor should be restricted to those patients in whom the benefits clearly outweigh the risk.

Tocolysis

Levalbuterol HCl has not been approved for the management of preterm labor. The benefit:risk ratio when levalbuterol HCl is administered for tocolysis has not been established. Serious adverse reactions, including maternal pulmonary edema, have been reported during or following treatment of premature labor with beta$_2$-agonists, including racemic albuterol.

Nursing Mothers

Plasma levels of levalbuterol after inhalation of therapeutic doses are very low in humans, but it is not known whether levalbuterol is excreted in human milk.

Because of the potential for tumorigenicity shown for racemic albuterol in animal studies and the lack of experience with the use of Xopenex Inhalation Solution by nursing mothers, a decision should be made whether to discontinue nursing or to discontinue the drug, taking into account the importance of the drug to the mother. Caution should be exercised when Xopenex Inhalation Solution is administered to a nursing woman.

Pediatrics

The safety and efficacy of Xopenex (levalbuterol HCl) Inhalation Solution have been established in pediatric patients 6 years of age and older in one adequate and well-controlled clinical trial (see **CLINICAL PHARMACOLOGY; Pharmacodynamics and Clinical Trials**). Use of Xopenex in children is also supported by evidence from adequate and well-controlled studies of Xopenex in adults, considering that the pathophysiology and the drug's exposure level and effects in pediatric and adult patients are substantially similar. Safety and effectiveness of Xopenex in pediatric patients below the age of 6 years have not been established.

Geriatrics

Data on the use of Xopenex in patients 65 years of age and older are very limited. A very small number of patients 65 years of age and older were treated with Xopenex Inhalation Solution in a 4-week clinical study (see **CLINICAL PHARMACOLOGY; Clinical Trials**) (n=2 for 0.63 mg and n=3 for 1.25 mg). In these patients, bronchodilation was observed after the first dose on day 1 and after 4 weeks of treatment. There are insufficient data to determine if the safety and efficacy of Xopenex Inhalation Solution are different in patients < 65 years of age and patients 65 years of age and older. In general, patients 65 years of age and older should be started at a dose of 0.63 mg of Xopenex Inhalation Solution. If clinically warranted due to insufficient bronchodilator response, the dose of Xopenex Inhalation Solution may be increased in elderly patients as tolerated, in conjunction with frequent clinical and laboratory monitoring, to the maximum recommended daily dose (see **DOSAGE AND ADMINISTRATION**).

ADVERSE REACTIONS

(Adults and Adolescents ≥12 years old)

Adverse events reported in ≥2% of patients receiving Xopenex Inhalation Solution or racemic albuterol and more frequently than in patients receiving placebo in a 4-week, controlled clinical trial are listed in **Table 4**.

[See table 4 at top of previous page]

The incidence of certain systemic beta-adrenergic adverse effects (e.g., tremor, nervousness) was slightly less in the Xopenex 0.63 mg group as compared to the other active treatment groups. The clinical significance of these small differences is unknown.

Changes in heart rate 15 minutes after drug administration and in plasma glucose and potassium one hour after drug administration on day 1 and day 29 were clinically comparable in the Xopenex 1.25 mg and the racemic albuterol 2.5 mg groups (see **Table 5**). Changes in heart rate and plasma glucose were slightly less in the Xopenex 0.63 mg group compared to the other active treatment groups (see **Table 5**). The clinical significance of these small differences is unknown. After 4 weeks, effects on heart rate, plasma glucose, and plasma potassium were generally diminished compared with day 1 in all active treatment groups.

[See table 5 at top of previous page]

No other clinically relevant laboratory abnormalities related to administration of Xopenex Inhalation Solution were observed in this study.

In the clinical trials, a slightly greater number of serious adverse events, discontinuations due to adverse events, and clinically significant ECG changes were reported in patients who received Xopenex 1.25 mg compared to the other active treatment groups.

The following adverse events, considered potentially related to Xopenex, occurred in less than 2% of the 292 subjects who received Xopenex and more frequently than in patients who received placebo in any clinical trial:

Body as a Whole:	chills, pain, chest pain
Cardiovascular System:	ECG abnormal, ECG change, hypertension, hypotension, syncope
Digestive System:	diarrhea, dry mouth, dry throat, dyspepsia, gastroenteritis, nausea
Hemic and Lymphatic System:	lymphadenopathy
Musculoskeletal System:	leg cramps, myalgia
Nervous System:	anxiety, hypesthesia of the hand, insomnia, paresthesia, tremor
Special Senses:	eye itch

Table 6: Most Frequently Reported Adverse Events (≥2% in Any Treatment Group) and More Frequently Than Placebo During the Double-Blind Period (ITT Population, 6–11 Years Old)

Body System Preferred Term	Percent of Patients Placebo (n=59)	 Xopenex 0.31 mg (n=66)	 Xopenex 0.63 mg (n=67)	 Racemic albuterol 1.25 mg (n=64)	 Racemic albuterol 2.5 mg (n=60)
Body as a Whole					
Abdominal pain	3.4	0	1.5	3.1	6.7
Accidental injury	3.4	6.1	4.5	3.1	5.0
Asthenia	0	3.0	3.0	1.6	1.7
Fever	5.1	9.1	3.0	1.6	6.7
Headache	8.5	7.6	11.9	9.4	3.3
Pain	3.4	3.0	1.5	4.7	6.7
Viral Infection	5.1	7.6	9.0	4.7	8.3
Digestive System					
Diarrhea	0	1.5	6.0	1.6	0
Hemic and Lymphatic					
Lymphadenopathy	0	3.0	0	1.6	0
Musculoskeletal System					
Myalgia	0	0	1.5	1.6	3.3
Respiratory System					
Asthma	5.1	9.1	9.0	6.3	10.0
Pharyngitis	6.8	3.0	10.4	0	6.7
Rhinitis	1.7	6.1	10.4	3.1	5.0
Skin and Appendages					
Eczema	0	0	0	0	3.3
Rash	0	0	7.5	1.6	0
Urticaria	0	0	3.0	0	0
Special Senses					
Otitis Media	1.7	0	0	0	3.3

Note: Subjects may have more than one adverse event per body system and preferred term.

Table 7: Mean Changes from Baseline in Heart Rate at 30 Minutes and in Glucose and Potassium at 1 Hour after First Dose (Day 1) and Last Dose (Day 21) in Children 6–11 years old

Treatment	Mean Changes (Day 1) Heart Rate (bpm)	 Glucose (mg/dL)	 Potassium (mEq/L)
Xopenex 0.31 mg, n=66	0.8	4.9	−0.31
Xopenex 0.63 mg, n=67	6.7	5.2	−0.36
Racemic albuterol 1.25 mg, n=64	6.4	8.0	−0.27
Racemic albuterol 2.5 mg, n=60	10.9	10.8	−0.56
Placebo, n=59	−1.8	0.6	−0.05
	Mean Changes (Day 21) Heart Rate (bpm)	 Glucose (mg/dL)	 Potassium (mEq/L)
Xopenex 0.31 mg, n=60	0	2.6	−0.32
Xopenex 0.63 mg, n=66	3.8	5.8	−0.34
Racemic albuterol 1.25 mg, n=62	5.8	1.7	−0.18
Racemic albuterol 2.5 mg, n=54	5.7	11.8	−0.26
Placebo, n=55	−1.7	1.1	−0.04

The following events, considered potentially related to Xopenex, occurred in less than 2% of the treated subjects but at a frequency less than in patients who received placebo: asthma exacerbation, cough increased, wheezing, sweating, and vomiting.

ADVERSE REACTIONS (Children 6-11 years old)

Adverse events reported in ≥2% of patients in any treatment group and more frequently than in patients receiving placebo in a 3-week, controlled clinical trial are listed in Table 6.

[See table 6 above]

Changes in heart rate, plasma glucose, and serum potassium are shown in Table 7. The clinical significance of these small differences is unknown.

[See table 7 above]

OVERDOSAGE

The expected symptoms with overdosage are those of excessive beta-adrenergic receptor stimulation and/or occurrence or exaggeration of any of the symptoms listed under **ADVERSE REACTIONS**, e.g., seizures, angina, hypertension or hypotension, tachycardia with rates up to 200 beats/min., arrhythmias, nervousness, headache, tremor, dry mouth, palpitation, nausea, dizziness, fatigue, malaise, and sleeplessness. Hypokalemia also may occur. As with all sympathomimetic medications, cardiac arrest and even death may be associated with the abuse of Xopenex Inhalation Solution. Treatment consists of discontinuation of Xopenex Inhalation Solution together with appropriate symptomatic therapy. The judicious use of a cardioselective beta-receptor blocker may be considered, bearing in mind that such medication can produce bronchospasm. There is insufficient evidence to determine if dialysis is beneficial for overdosage of Xopenex Inhalation Solution.

The intravenous median lethal dose of levalbuterol HCl in mice is approximately 66 mg/kg (approximately 70 times the maximum recommended daily inhalation dose of levalbuterol HCl for adults and children on a mg/m^2 basis). The inhalation median lethal dose has not been determined in animals.

DOSAGE AND ADMINISTRATION

Children 6–11 years old: The recommended dosage of Xopenex (levalbuterol HCl) Inhalation Solution for patients 6–11 years old is 0.31 mg administered three times a day, by nebulization. Routine dosing should not exceed 0.63 mg three times a day.

Adults and Adolescents ≥12 years old: The recommended starting dosage of Xopenex (levalbuterol HCl) Inhalation Solution for patients 12 years of age and older is 0.63 mg administered three times a day, every 6 to 8 hours, by nebulization.

Patients 12 years of age and older with more severe asthma or patients who do not respond adequately to a dose of 0.63 mg of Xopenex Inhalation Solution may benefit from a dosage of 1.25 mg three times a day.

Patients receiving the highest dose of Xopenex Inhalation Solution should be monitored closely for adverse systemic effects, and the risks of such effects should be balanced against the potential for improved efficacy.

The use of Xopenex Inhalation Solution can be continued as medically indicated to control recurring bouts of bronchospasm. During this time, most patients gain optimal benefit from regular use of the inhalation solution.

If a previously effective dosage regimen fails to provide the expected relief, medical advice should be sought immediately, since this is often a sign of seriously worsening asthma that would require reassessment of therapy.

The drug compatibility (physical and chemical), efficacy, and safety of Xopenex Inhalation Solution when mixed with other drugs in a nebulizer have not been established.

The safety and efficacy of Xopenex Inhalation Solution have been established in clinical trials when administered using the PARI LC Jet™ and the PARI LC Plus™ nebulizers, and the PARI Master® Dura-Neb® 2000 and Dura-Neb® 3000 compressors. The safety and efficacy of Xopenex Inhalation Solution when administered using other nebulizer systems have not been established.

HOW SUPPLIED

Xopenex (levalbuterol HCl) Inhalation Solution is supplied in 3 mL unit-dose, low-density polyethylene (LDPE) vials as

Continued on next page

Xopenex—Cont.

a clear, colorless, sterile, preservative-free, aqueous solution in three different strengths of levalbuterol (0.31 mg, 0.63 mg, 1.25 mg). Each strength of Xopenex Inhalation Solution is available in a shelf-carton containing one or more foil pouches, each containing 12 unit-dose LDPE vials.

Xopenex (levalbuterol HCl) Inhalation Solution, 0.31 mg *(foil pouch label color green)* contains 0.31 mg of levalbuterol (as 0.36 mg of levalbuterol HCl) and is available in cartons of 24 unit-dose LDPE vials (NDC 63402-511-24).

Xopenex (levalbuterol HCl) Inhalation Solution, 0.63 mg *(foil pouch label color yellow)* contains 0.63 mg of levalbuterol (as 0.73 mg of levalbuterol HCl) and is available in cartons of 24 unit-dose LDPE vials (NDC 63402-512-24).

Xopenex (levalbuterol HCl) Inhalation Solution, 1.25 mg *(foil pouch label color red)* contains 1.25 mg of levalbuterol (as 1.44 mg of levalbuterol HCl) and is available in cartons of 24 unit-dose LDPE vials (NDC 63402-513-24).

CAUTION

Federal law (U.S.) prohibits dispensing without prescription.

Store the Xopenex (levalbuterol HCl) Inhalation Solution in the protective foil pouch at 20–25°C (68–77°F) [see USP Controlled Room Temperature]. Protect from light and excessive heat. Keep unopened vials in the foil pouch. Once the foil pouch is opened, the vials should be used within two weeks. Vials removed from the pouch, if not used immediately, should be protected from light and used within one week. Discard any vial if the solution is not colorless.

Manufactured for:
Sepracor Inc.
Marlborough, MA 01752 USA
by Automatic Liquid Packaging, Woodstock, IL 60098 USA
1-877-SEPRACOR
To report adverse events, call 1-877-737-7226.
For medical information, call 1-800-739-0565.
January 2002
400437-R2

PHARMACIST—DETACH HERE AND GIVE INSTRUCTIONS TO PATIENT

Patient's Instructions for Use

Xopenex® (levalbuterol HCl) Inhalation Solution; 0.31 mg*, 0.63 mg*, 1.25 mg*; 3 mL Unit-Dose Vials

***Potency expressed as levalbuterol**

Read complete instructions carefully before using.

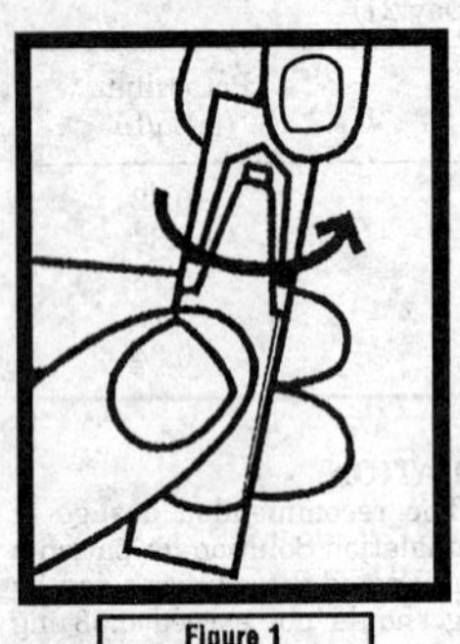

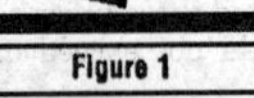

Figure 1

1. Open the foil pouch by tearing on the serrated edge along the seam of the pouch. Remove one unit-dose vial for immediate use. Keep the rest of the unused unit-dose vials in the foil pouch to protect them from light.
2. Carefully twist open the top of one unit-dose vial (**Figure 1**) and squeeze the entire contents into the nebulizer reservoir.

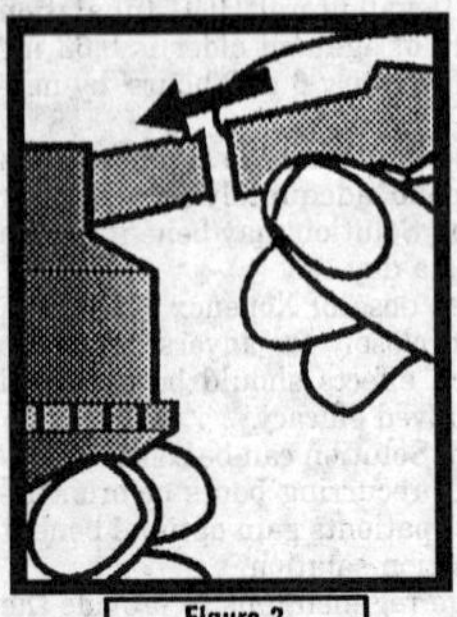

Figure 2

3. Connect the nebulizer reservoir to the mouthpiece or face mask (**Figure 2**).
4. Connect the nebulizer to the compressor.

Figure 3

5. Sit in a comfortable, upright position. Place the mouthpiece in your mouth (**Figure 3**) (or put on the face mask) and turn on the compressor.
6. Breathe as calmly, deeply, and evenly as possible until no more mist is formed in the nebulizer reservoir (about 5 to 15 minutes). At this point, the treatment is finished.
7. Clean the nebulizer (see manufacturer's instructions).

Note: Xopenex (levalbuterol HCl) Inhalation Solution should be used in a nebulizer only under the direction of a physician. More frequent administration or higher doses are not recommended without first discussing with your doctor. This solution should not be injected or administered orally. Protect from light and excessive heat. Store in the protective foil pouch at 20–25°C (68–77°F) [see USP Controlled Room Temperature]. Keep unopened vials in the foil pouch. Once the foil pouch is opened, the vials should be used within two weeks. Vials removed from the pouch, if not used immediately, should be protected from light and used within one week. Discard any vial if the solution is not colorless.

The safety and effectiveness of Xopenex Inhalation Solution have not been determined when one or more drugs are mixed with it in a nebulizer. Check with your doctor before mixing any medications in your nebulizer.

Manufactured for:
Sepracor Inc.
Marlborough, MA 01752 USA
by Automatic Liquid Packaging, Woodstock, IL 60098 USA
1-877-SEPRACOR
To report adverse events, call 1-877-737-7226.
For medical information, call 1-800-739-0565.
January 2002
400437-R2

Shown in Product Identification Guide, page 333

Serono, Inc.
**ONE TECHNOLOGY PLACE
ROCKLAND, MA 02370**

Direct Inquiries to:
Customer Service, Sales and Ordering
(888) 398-4567
(781) 982-9000

For Medical Information or to report Adverse Drug Experiences Contact the U.S. Medical Information or U.S. Product Surveillance Department at
(888) 275-7376
(781) 982-9000
www.howkidsgrow.com
www.novantrone.com
www.rebif.com
www.seronofertility.com
www.seronousa.com
www.serostim.com
www.zorbtive.com

Serono, Inc. will be pleased to answer inquiries about the following products:

CETROTIDE®
[cĕtrō-tīde]
(cetrorelix acetate for injection)
0.25 mg and 3 mg
FOR SUBCUTANEOUS USE ONLY

DESCRIPTION

Cetrotide® (cetrorelix acetate for injection) is a synthetic decapeptide with gonadotropin-releasing hormone (GnRH) antagonistic activity. Cetrorelix acetate is an analog of native GnRH with substitutions of amino acids at positions 1, 2, 3, 6, and 10. The molecular formula is Acetyl-*D*-3-(2′-naphtyl)-alanine-*D*-4-chlorophenylalanine-*D*-3-(3′-pyridyl)-alanine-*L*-serine-*L*-tyrosine-*D*-citruline-*L*-leucine-*L*-arginine-*L*-proline-*D*-alanine-amide, and the molecular weight is 1431.06, calculated as the anhydrous free base. The structural formula is as follows:

Cetrorelix acetate

[See chemical structure below]

Cetrotide® (cetrorelix acetate for injection) 0.25 mg or 3 mg is a sterile lyophilized powder intended for subcutaneous injection after reconstitution with Sterile Water for Injection, USP (pH 5–8), that comes supplied in either a 1.0 mL (for 0.25 mg vial) or 3.0 mL (for 3 mg vial) pre-filled syringe. Each vial of Cetrotide® 0.25 mg (multiple dose regimen) contains 0.26–0.27 mg cetrorelix acetate, equivalent to 0.25 mg cetrorelix, and 54.80 mg mannitol. Each vial of Cetrotide® 3 mg (single dose regimen) contains 3.12–3.24 mg cetrorelix acetate, equivalent to 3 mg cetrorelix, and 164.40 mg mannitol.

CLINICAL PHARMACOLOGY

GnRH induces the production and release of luteinizing hormone (LH) and follicle stimulating hormone (FSH) from the gonadotrophic cells of the anterior pituitary. Due to a positive estradiol (E_2) feedback at midcycle, GnRH liberation is enhanced resulting in an LH-surge. This LH-surge induces the ovulation of the dominant follicle, resumption of oocyte meiosis and subsequently luteinization as indicated by rising progesterone levels.

Cetrotide® competes with natural GnRH for binding to membrane receptors on pituitary cells and thus controls the release of LH and FSH in a dose-dependent manner. The onset of LH suppression is approximately one hour with the 3 mg dose and two hours with the 0.25 mg dose. This suppression is maintained by continuous treatment and there is a more pronounced effect on LH than on FSH. An initial release of endogenous gonadotropins has not been detected with Cetrotide®, which is consistent with an antagonist effect.

The effects of Cetrotide® on LH and FSH are reversible after discontinuation of treatment. In women, Cetrotide® delays the LH-surge, and consequently ovulation, in a dose-dependent fashion. FSH levels are not affected at the doses used during controlled ovarian stimulation. Following a single 3 mg dose of Cetrotide®, duration of action of at least 4 days has been established. A dose of Cetrotide® 0.25 mg every 24 hours has been shown to maintain the effect.

Pharmacokinetics

The pharmacokinetic parameters of single and multiple doses of Cetrotide® (cetrorelix acetate for injection) in adult healthy female subjects are summarized in Table 1.

[See table 1 at top of next page]

Absorption

Cetrotide® is rapidly absorbed following subcutaneous injection, maximal plasma concentrations being achieved approximately one to two hours after administration. The mean absolute bioavailability of Cetrotide® following subcutaneous administration to healthy female subjects is 85%.

Distribution

The volume of distribution of Cetrotide® following a single intravenous dose of 3 mg is about 1 l/kg. *In vitro* protein binding to human plasma is 86%.

Cetrotide® concentrations in follicular fluid and plasma were similar on the day of oocyte pick-up in patients undergoing controlled ovarian stimulation. Following subcutaneous administration of Cetrotide® 0.25 mg and 3 mg, plasma concentrations of cetrorelix were below or in the range of the lower limit of quantitation on the day of oocyte pick up and embryo transfer.

Metabolism

After subcutaneous administration of 10 mg Cetrotide® to females and males, Cetrotide® and small amounts of (1–9), (1–7), (1–6), and (1–4) peptides were found in bile samples over 24 hours.

In *in-vitro* studies, Cetrotide® was stable against phase I- and phase II-metabolism. Cetrotide® was transformed by peptidases, and the (1–4) peptide was the predominant metabolite.

Excretion

Following subcutaneous administration of 10 mg cetrorelix to males and females, only unchanged cetrorelix was detected in urine. In 24 hours, cetrorelix and small amounts of the (1–9), (1–7), (1–6), and (1–4) peptides were found in bile samples. 2–4% of the dose was eliminated in the urine as unchanged cetrorelix, while 5–10% was eliminated as cetrorelix and the four metabolites in bile. Therefore, only 7–14% of the total dose was recovered as unchanged cetrorelix and metabolites in urine and bile up to 24 hours. The remaining portion of the dose may not have been recovered since bile and urine were not collected for a longer period of time.

Special Populations

Pharmacokinetic investigations have not been performed either in subjects with impaired renal or liver function, or in the elderly, or in children (see PRECAUTIONS).

Pharmacokinetic differences in different races have not been determined.

There is no evidence of differences in pharmacokinetic parameters for Cetrotide® between healthy subjects and patients undergoing controlled ovarian stimulation.

Drug-Drug Interactions

No formal drug-drug interaction studies have been performed with Cetrotide® (see PRECAUTIONS).

Clinical Studies

Seven hundred thirty two (732) patients were treated with Cetrotide® (cetrorelix acetate for injection) in five (two Phase 2 dose-finding and three Phase 3) clinical trials. The clinical trial population consisted of Caucasians (95.5%) and Black, Asian, Arabian and Others (4.5%). Women were between 19 and 40 years of age (mean: 32). The studies excluded subjects with polycystic ovary syndrome (PCOS), subjects with low or no ovarian reserve, and subjects with stage III-IV endometriosis.

Two dose regimens were investigated in these clinical trials, either a single dose per treatment cycle or multiple dosing.

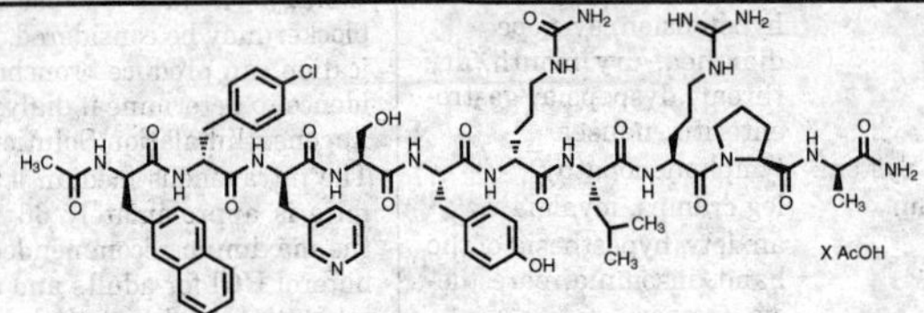

(Ac-*D*-Nal1-*D*-Cpa2-*D*-Pal3-Ser4-Tyr5-*D*-Cit6-Leu7-Arg8-Pro9-*D*-Ala10-NH_2)

In the Phase 2 studies, a single dose of 3 mg was established as the minimal effective dose for the inhibition of premature LH surges with a protection period of a least 4 days. When Cetrotide® is administered in a multidose regimen, 0.25 mg was established as the minimal effective dose. The extent and duration of LH-suppression is dose dependent.

In the Phase 3 program, efficacy of the single 3 mg dose regimen of Cetrotide® and the multiple 0.25 mg dose regimen of Cetrotide® was established separately in two adequate and well controlled clinical studies utilizing active comparators. A third non-comparative clinical study evaluated only the multiple 0.25 mg dose regimen of Cetrotide®. The ovarian stimulation treatment with recombinant FSH or human menopausal gonadotropin (hMG) was initiated on day 2 or 3 of a normal menstrual cycle. The dose of gonadotropins was administered according to the individual patient's disposition and response.

In the single dose regimen study, Cetrotide® 3 mg was administered on the day of controlled ovarian stimulation when adequate estradiol levels (400 pg/ml) were obtained, usually on day 7 (range day 5–12). If hCG was not given within 4 days of the 3 mg dose of Cetrotide®, then 0.25 mg of Cetrotide® was administered daily beginning 96 hours after the 3 mg injection until and including the day of hCG administration.

In the two multiple dose regimen studies, Cetrotide® 0.25 mg was started on day 5 or 6 of controlled ovarian stimulation (COS). Both gonadotropins and Cetrotide® were continued daily (multiple dose regimen) until the injection of human chorionic gonadotropin (hCG).

Oocyte pick-up (OPU) followed by *in vitro* fertilization (IVF) or intracytoplasmic sperm injection (ICSI) as well as embryo transfer (ET) were subsequently performed. The results for Cetrotide® are summarized below in Table 2.

[See table 2 at right]

In addition to IVF and ICSI, one pregnancy was obtained after intrauterine insemination. In the five Phase 2 and Phase 3 clinical trials, 184 pregnancies have been reported out of a total of 732 patients (including 21 pregnancies following the replacement of frozen-thawed embryos).

In the 3 mg regimen, 9 patients received an additional dose of 0.25 mg of Cetrotide® and two other patients received two additional doses of 0.25 mg Cetrotide®. The median number of days of Cetrotide® multiple dose treatment was 5 (range 1–15) in both studies.

No drug related allergic reactions were reported from these clinical studies.

INDICATIONS AND USAGE

Cetrotide® (cetrorelix acetate for injection) is indicated for the inhibition of premature LH surges in women undergoing controlled ovarian stimulation.

CONTRAINDICATIONS

Cetrotide® (cetrorelix acetate for injection) is contraindicated under the following conditions:

1. Hypersensitivity to cetrorelix acetate, extrinsic peptide hormones or mannitol.
2. Known hypersensitivity to GnRH or any other GnRH analogs.
3. Known or suspected pregnancy, and lactation (see PRECAUTIONS)
4. Severe renal impairment

WARNINGS

Cetrotide® (cetrorelix acetate for injection) should be prescribed by physicians who are experienced in fertility treatment. Before starting treatment with Cetrotide®, pregnancy must be excluded (see CONTRAINDICATIONS and PRECAUTIONS).

PRECAUTIONS

General

Caution is advised in patients with hypersensitivity to GnRH. These patients should be carefully monitored after the first injection. A severe anaphylactic reaction associated with cough, rash and hypotension, was observed in one patient after seven months of treatment with Cetrotide® (10 mg/day) in a study for an indication unrelated to infertility.

Special care should be taken in women with signs and symptoms of active allergic conditions or known history of allergic predisposition. Treatment with Cetrotide® is not advised in women were severe allergic conditions.

Information for Patients

Prior to therapy with Cetrotide® (cetrorelix acetate for injection), patients should be informed of the duration of treatment and monitoring procedures that will be required. The risk of possible adverse reactions should be discussed (see ADVERSE REACTIONS). Cetrotide® should not be prescribed if a patient is pregnant.

If Cetrotide® is prescribed to patients for self-administration, information for proper use is given in the Patient Leaflet (see below).

Laboratory Tests

After the exclusion of preexisting conditions, enzyme elevations (ALT, AST, GGT, alkaline phosphatase) were found in 1–2% of patients receiving Cetrotide® during controlled ovarian stimulation. The elevations ranged up to three times the upper limit of normal. The clinical significance of these findings was not determined.

During stimulation with human menopausal gonadotropin, Cetrotide® had no notable effects on hormone levels aside from inhibition of LH surges.

Table 1: Pharmacokinetic parameters of Cetrotide® following 3 mg single or 0.25 mg single and mulitple (daily for 14 days) subcutaneous (sc) administration.

	Single dose 3 mg	Single dose 0.25 mg	Multiple dose 0.25 mg
No. of subjects	12	12	12
t_{max}* [h]	1.5 (0.5–2)	1.0 (0.5–1.5)	1.0 (0.5–2)
$t_{1/2}$* [h]	62.8 (38.2–108)	5.0 (2.4–48.8)	20.6 (4.1–179.3)
C_{max} [ng/ml]	28.5 (22.5–36.2)	4.97 (4.17–5.92)	6.42 (5.18–7.96)
AUC [ng•h/ml]	536 (451–636)	31.4 (23.4–42.0)	44.5 (36.7–54.2)
CL† [ml/min•kg]	1.28[a]		
V_z† [l/kg]	1.16[a]		

Geometric mean (95%CI_{1n}), †arithmetic mean, or *mean (min-max)

t_{max} Time to reach observed maximum plasma concentration
$t_{1/2}$ Elimination half-life
C_{max} Maxinum plasma concentration; multiple dose $C_{ss,\ max}$
AUC Area under the curve; single dose $AUC_{0\text{-}inf}$, multiple dose AUC_{τ}
CL Total plasma clearance
V_z Volume of distribution
a Based on iv administration (n=, separate study 0013)

Table 2: Results of Phase 3 Clinical Studies with Cetrotide® (cetrorelix acetate for injection) 3 mg in a single dose (sd) regimen and 0.25 mg in a multiple dose (md) regimen.

Parameter	Cetrotide® 3mg (sd, active comparator study)	Cetrotide® 0.25 mg (md, active comparator study)	Cetrotide® 0.25 mg (md, non-comparative study)
No. of subjects	115	159	303
hCG administered [%]	98.3	96.2	96.0
Oocyte pick-up [%]	98.3	94.3	93.1
LH-surge [%] (LH ≥10 U/L and P[a] ≥ 1 ng/mL)[b]	0.0	1.9	1.0
Serum E_2 [pg/ml] at day hCG[c,d]	1125 (470–2952)	1064 (341–2531)	1185 (311–3676)
Serum LH [U/L] at day hCG[c,d]	1.0 (0.5–2.5)	1.5 (0.5–7.6)	1.1 (0.5–3.5)
No. of follicles ≥11 mm at day hCG[e]	11.2 ± 5.5	10.8 ± 5.2	10.4 ± 4.5
No. of oocytes: IVF[e] / ICSI[e]	9.2 ± 5.2 / 10.0 ± 4.2	7.6 ± 4.3 / 10.1 ± 5.6	8.5 ± 5.1 / 9.3 ± 5.9
Fertilization rate: IVF[e] / ICSI[e]	0.48 ± 0.33 / 0.66 ± 0.29	0.62 ± 0.26 / 0.63 ± 0.29	0.60 ± 0.26 / 0.61 ± 0.25
No. of embroys transferred[e]	2.6 ± 0.9	2.1 ± 0.6	2.7 ± 1.0
Clinical pregnancy rate [%]			
per attempt	22.6	20.8	19.8
per subject with ET	26.3	24.1	23.3

[a] Progesterone
[b] Following initiation of Cetrotide® therapy
[c] Morning values
[d] Median with 5th–95th percentiles
[e] Mean ± standard deviation

Drug Interactions

No formal drug interaction studies have been performed with Cetrotide®.

Carcinogenesis, Mutagenesis, Impairment of Fertility

Long-term carcinogenicity studies in animals have not been performed with cetrorelix acetate. Cetrorelix acetate was not genotoxic *in vitro* (Ames test, HPRT test, chromosome aberration test) or *in vivo* (chromosome aberration test, mouse micronucleus test). Cetrorelix acetate induced polyploidy in CHL-Chinese hamster lung fibroblasts, but not in V79-Chinese hamster lung fibroblasts, cultured peripheral human lymphocytes or in an *in-vitro* micronucleus test in the CHL-cell line. Treatment with 0.46 mg/kg cetrorelix acetate for 4 weeks resulted in complete infertility in female rats which was reversed 8 weeks after cessation of treatment.

Pregnancy Category X (see CONTRAINDICATIONS)

Cetrotide® is contraindicated in pregnant women.

When administered to rats for the first seven days of pregnancy, cetrorelix acetate did not affect the development of the implanted conceptus at doses up to 38 µg/kg (approximately 1 times the recommended human therapeutic dose based on body surface area). However, a dose of 139 µg/kg (approximately 4 times the human dose) resulted in a resorption rate and a postimplantation loss of 100%.

When administered from day 6 to near term to pregnant rats and rabbits, very early resorptions and total implantation losses were seen in rats at doses from 4.6 µg/kg (0.2 times the human dose) and in rabbits at doses from 6.8 µg/kg (0.4 times the human dose). In animals that maintained their pregnancy, there was no increase in the incidence of fetal abnormalities.

The fetal resorption observed in animals is a logical consequence of the alteration in hormonal levels effected by the antigonadotrophic properties of Cetrotide®, which could result in fetal loss in humans as well. Therefore, this drug should not be used in pregnant women.

Nursing Mothers

It is not known whether Cetrotide® is excreted in human milk. Because many drugs are excreted in human milk, and because the effects of Cetrotide® on lactation and/or the breast-fed child have not been determined, Cetrotide® should not be used by nursing mothers.

Geriatric Use

Cetrotide® is not intended to be used in subjects aged 65 and over.

ADVERSE REACTIONS

The safety of Cetrotide® (cetrorelix acetate for injection) in 949 patients undergoing controlled ovarian stimulation in clinical studies was evaluated. Women were between 19 and 40 years of age (mean: 32). 94.0% of them were Caucasian. Cetrotide® was given in doses ranging from 0.1 mg to 5 mg as either a single or multiple dose.

Table 3 shows systemic adverse events reported in clinical studies without regard to causality from the beginning of

Continued on next page

Cetrotide—Cont.

Cetrotide® treatment until confirmation of pregnancy by ultrasound at an incidence ≥1% in Cetrotide® treated subjects undergoing COS.

Table 3: Adverse Events in ≥1% (WHO preferred term)	**Cetrotide® N=949 % (n)**
Ovarian Hyperstimulation Syndrome#	3.5 (33)
Nausea	1.3 (12)
Headache	1.1 (10)

Intensity moderate or severe, or WHO Grade II or III, respectively

Local site reactions (e.g. redness, erythema, bruising, itching, swelling and pruritus) were reported. Usually, they were of a transient nature, mild intensity and short duration. During post-marketing surveillance, rare cases of hypersensitivity reactions including anaphylactoid reactions have been reported.

Two stillbirths were reported in Phase 3 studies of Cetrotide®.

Congenital Anomalies

Clinical follow-up studies of 316 newborns of women administered Cetrotide® were reviewed. One infant of a set of twin neonates was found to have anencephaly at birth and died after four days. The other twin was normal. Development findings from ongoing baby follow-up included a child with a ventricular septal defect and another child with bilateral congenital glaucoma.

Four pregnancies that resulted in therapeutic abortion in Phase 2 and Phase 3 controlled ovarian stimulation studies had major anomalies (diaphragmatic hernia, trisomy 21, Klinefelter syndrome, polymalformation, and trisomy 18). In three of these four cases, intracytoplasmic sperm injection (ICSI) was the fertilization method employed; in the fourth case, *in-vitro* fertilization (IVF) was the method employed.

The minor congenital anomalies reported include: supernumerary nipple, bilateral strabismus, imperforate hymen, congenital nevi, hemangiomata, and QT syndrome.

The causal relationship between the reported anomalies and Cetrotide® is unknown. Multiple factors, genetic and others (including, but not limited to ICSI, IVF, gonadotropins, and progesterone) make causal attribution difficult to study.

OVERDOSAGE

There have been no reports of overdosage with Cetrotide® 0.25 mg or 3 mg in humans. Single doses up to 120 mg Cetrotide® have been well tolerated in patients treated for other indications without signs of overdosage.

DOSAGE AND ADMINISTRATION

Ovarian stimulation therapy with gonadotropins (FSH, HMG) is started on cycle Day 2 or 3. The dose of gonadotropins should be adjusted according to individuals response. Cetrotide® (cetrorelix acetate for injection) may be administered subcutaneously either once daily (0.25 mg dose) or once (3 mg dose) during the early- to mid-follicular phase.

In the single dose regimen, 3 mg of Cetrotide® is administered when the serum estradiol level is indicative of an appropriate stimulation response, usually on stimulation day 7 (range day 5–9). If hCG has not been administered within four days after injection of Cetrotide® 3 mg, Cetrotide® 0.25 mg should be administered once daily until the day of hCG administration.

In the multiple dose regimen, 0.25 mg of Cetrotide® is administered on either stimulation day 5 (morning or evening) or day 6 (morning) and continued daily until the day of hCG administration.

When assessment by ultrasound shows a sufficient number of follicles of adequate size, hCG is administered to induce ovulation and final maturation of the oocytes. No hCG should be administered if the ovaries show an excessive response to the treatment with gonadotropins to reduce the chance of developing ovarian hyperstimulation syndrome (OHSS).

Administration

Cetrotide® 0.25 mg and 3 mg can be administered by the patient herself after appropriate instructions by her doctor.

Directions for using Cetrotide® 0.25 mg and 3 mg:

1. Wash hands thoroughly with soap and water.
2. Flip off the plastic cover of the vial and wipe the aluminum ring and the rubber stopper with an alcohol swab.
3. Twist the injection needle with the yellow mark (20 gauge) on the pre-filled syringe.
4. Push the needle through the center of the rubber stopper of the vial and slowly inject the solvent into the vial.
5. Leaving the syringe in the vial, gently swirl the vial until the solution is clear and without residues. Avoid forming bubbles.
6. Draw the total contents of the vial into the syringe. If necessary, invert the vial and pull back the needle as far as needed to withdraw the entire contents of the vial.
7. Replace the needle with the yellow mark by the injection needle with the grey mark (27 gauge).
8. Invert the syringe and push the plunger until all air bubbles have been expelled.
9. Choose an injection site at the lower abdominal area, preferably around, but staying at least one inch away from the navel. If you are on a multiple dose (0.25 mg) regimen, choose a different injection site each day to minimize local irritation. Use the second alcohol swab to clean the skin at the injection site and allow alcohol to dry. Gently pinch up the skin surrounding the site of injection.
10. Inject the prescribed dose as directed by your doctor, nurse or pharmacist.
11. Use the syringe and needles only once. Dispose of the syringe and needles properly after use. If available, use a medical waste container for disposal.

HOW SUPPLIED

Cetrotide® (cetrorelix acetate for injection) 0.25 mg is available in a carton of one packaged tray (NDC 44087-1225-1). Each packaged tray contains: one glass vial containing 0.26–0.27 mg cetrorelix acetate (corresponding to 0.25 mg cetrorelix), one pre-filled glass syringe with 1 mL of Sterile Water of Injection, USP (pH 5-8), one 20 gauge needle (yellow), one 27 gauge needle (grey), and two alcohol swabs.

Cetrotide® (cetrorelix acetate for injection) 3 mg is available in a carton of one packaged tray (NDC 44087-1203-1). Each packaged tray contains: one glass vial containing 3.12–3.24 mg cetrorelix acetate (corresponding to 3 mg cetrorelix), one pre-filled glass syringe with 3 mL of Sterile Water for Injection, USP (pH 5-8), one 20 gauge needle (yellow), one 27 gauge needle (grey), and two alcohol swabs.

Storage

Cetrotide® 3 mg:

Store at 25°C (77°F); excursions permitted to 15–30°C (59–86°F) [see USP Controlled Room Temperature]. Store the packaged tray in the outer carton.

Cetrotide® 0.25 mg:

Store refrigerated, 2–8°C (36–46°F). Store the packaged tray in the outer carton.

℞ only

June 2004

Manufactured for: Serono, Inc., Rockland, MA 02370, USA

CRINONE® 4% ℞
CRINONE® 8%

[*crĭ 'nōn*]

(progesterone gel)

DESCRIPTION

Crinone® (progesterone gel) is a bioadhesive vaginal gel containing micronized progesterone in an emulsion system, which is contained in single use, one piece polyethylene vaginal applicators. The carrier vehicle is an oil in water emulsion containing the water swellable, but insoluble polymer, polycarbophil. The progesterone is partially soluble in both the oil and water phase of the vehicle, with the majority of the progesterone existing as a suspension. Physically, Crinone® has the appearance of a soft, white to off-white gel.

The active ingredient, progesterone, is present in either a 4% or an 8% concentration (w/w). The chemical name for progesterone is pregn-4-ene-3,20-dione. It has an empirical formula of $C_{21}H_{30}O_2$ and a molecular weight of 314.5. The structural formula is:

Progesterone exists in two polymorphic forms. Form 1, which is the form used in Crinone®, exists as white orthorhombic prisms with a melting point of 127-131°C.

Each applicator delivers 1.125 grams of Crinone® gel containing either 45 mg (4% gel) or 90 mg (8% gel) of progesterone in a base containing glycerin, mineral oil, polycarbophil, carbomer 934P, hydrogenated palm oil glyceride, sorbic acid, purified water, and may contain sodium hydroxide.

CLINICAL PHARMACOLOGY

Progesterone is a naturally occurring steroid that is secreted by the ovary, placenta, and adrenal gland. In the presence of adequate estrogen, progesterone transforms a proliferative endometrium into a secretory endometrium. Progesterone is essential for the development of decidual tissue, and the effect of progesterone on the differentiation of glandular epithelia and stroma has been extensively studied. Progesterone is necessary to increase endometrial receptivity for implantation of an embryo. Once an embryo is implanted, progesterone acts to maintain the pregnancy. Normal or near-normal endometrial responses to oral estradiol and intramuscular progesterone have been noted in functionally agonadal women through the sixth decade of life. Progesterone administration decreases the circulatory levels of gonadotropins.

Pharmacokinetics

Absorption

Due to the sustained release properties of Crinone®, progesterone absorption is prolonged with an absorption half-life of approximately 25-50 hours, and an elimination half-life of 5-20 minutes. Therefore, the pharmacokinetics of Crinone® are rate-limited by absorption rather than by elimination.

The bioavailability of progesterone in Crinone® was determined relative to progesterone administered intramuscularly. In a single dose cross-over study, 20 healthy, estrogenized postmenopausal women received 45 mg or 90 mg progesterone vaginally in Crinone® 4% or Crinone® 8%, or 45 mg or 90 mg progesterone intramuscularly. The pharmacokinetic parameters (mean ± standard deviation) are shown in Table 1.

[See table 1 below]

The multiple dose pharmacokinetics of Crinone® 4% and Crinone® 8% administered every other day and Crinone® 8% administered daily or twice daily for 12 days were studied in 10 healthy, estrogenized postmenopausal women in two separate studies. Steady state was achieved within the first 24 hours after initiation of treatment. The pharmacokinetic parameters (mean ± standard deviation) after the last administration of Crinone® 4% or 8% derived from these studies are shown in Table 2.

[See table 2 at top of next page]

Distribution

Progesterone is extensively bound to serum proteins (~96-99%), primarily to serum albumin and corticosteroid binding globulin.

Metabolism

The major urinary metabolite of oral progesterone is 5β-pregnan-3α, 20α-diol glucuronide which is present in plasma in the conjugated form only. Plasma metabolites also include 5β-pregnan-3α-ol-20-one (5β-pregnanolone) and 5α-pregnan-3α-ol-20-one (5α-pregnanolone).

Excretion

Progesterone undergoes both biliary and renal elimination. Following an injection of labeled progesterone, 50-60% of the excretion of progesterone metabolites occurs via the kidney; approximately 10% occurs via the bile and feces, the second major excretory pathway. Overall recovery of labeled material accounts for 70% of an administered dose, with the remainder of the dose not characterized with respect to elimination. Only a small portion of unchanged progesterone is excreted in the bile.

CLINICAL STUDIES

Assisted Reproductive Technology

In a single-center, open-label study (COL1620-007US), 99 women (aged 28-47 years) with either partial (n=84) or pre-

TABLE 1
Single Dose Relative Bioavailability

	Crinone® 4%	45 mg Intramuscular Progesterone	Crinone® 8%	90 mg Intramuscular Progesterone
C_{max} (ng/mL)	13.15 ± 6.49	39.06 ± 13.68	14.87 ± 6.32	53.76 ± 14.9
$C_{avg\ 0\text{-}24}$ (ng/mL)	6.94 ± 4.24	22.41 ± 4.92	6.98 ± 3.21	28.98 ± 8.75
$AUC_{0\text{-}96}$ (ng•hr/mL)	288.63 ± 273.72	806.26 ± 102.75	296.78 ± 129.90	1378.91 ± 176.39
T_{max} (hr)	5.6 ± 1.84	8.2 ± 6.43	6.8 ± 3.3	9.2 ± 2.7
$t_{1/2}$ (hr)	55.13 ± 28.04	28.05 ± 16.87	34.8 ± 11.3	19.6 ± 6.0
F (%)	27.6		19.8	

C_{max} – maximum progesterone serum concentration
$C_{avg\ 0\text{-}24}$ – average progesterone serum concentration over 24 hours
$AUC_{0\text{-}96}$ – area under the drug concentration versus time curve from 0-96 hours post dose
T_{max} – time to maximum progesterone concentration
$t_{1/2}$ – elimination half-life
F – relative bioavailability

mature ovarian failure (n=15) who were candidates to receive a donor oocyte transfer as an Assisted Reproductive Technology ("ART") procedure were randomized to receive either Crinone® 8% twice daily (n=68) or intramuscular progesterone 100 mg daily (n=31). The study was divided into three phases (Pilot, Donor Egg and Treatment). The first phase of the study consisted of a test Pilot Cycle to ensure that the administration of transdermal estradiol and progesterone would adequately prime the endometrium to receive the donor egg. The second phase was the Donor Egg Cycle during which a fertilized oocyte was implanted. Crinone® 8% was administered beginning the evening of Day 14 of the Pilot and Donor Egg cycles. Subjects with partial ovarian function also underwent a Pre-Pilot Cycle and a Pre-Donor Egg Cycle during which time they were administered only leuprolide acetate to suppress remaining ovarian function. The Pre-Pilot Cycle, Pilot Cycle, Pre-Donor Egg Cycle, and Donor Egg Cycle each lasted approximately 34 days. The third phase of the study consisted of a 10-week treatment period to maintain a pregnancy until placental autonomy was achieved.

Sixty-one women received Crinone® 8% as part of the Pilot Cycle to determine their endometrial response. Of the 55 evaluable endometrial biopsies in the Crinone® 8% group performed on Day 25-27, all were histologically "in-phase", consistent with luteal phase biopsy specimens of menstruating women at comparable time intervals. Fifty-four women who received Crinone® 8% and had a histologically "in-phase" biopsy received a donor oocyte transfer. Among these 54 Crinone®-treated women, clinical pregnancies (assessed about week 10 after transfer by clinical examination, ultrasound and/or β-hCG levels) occurred in 26 women (48%). In these 54 women, 17 women (31%) delivered a total of 25 newborns, seven women (13%) had spontaneous abortions and two women (4%) had elective abortions.

In a second study (COL1620-F01), Crinone® 8% was used in luteal phase support of women with tubal or idiopathic infertility due to endometriosis and normal ovulatory cycles, undergoing *in vitro* fertilization ("IVF") procedures. All women received a GnRH analog to suppress endogenous progesterone, human menopausal gonadotropins, and human chorionic gonadotropin. In this multi-center, open-label study, 139 women (aged 22-38 years) received Crinone® 8% once daily beginning within 24 hours of embryo transfer and continuing through Day 30 post-transfer. Clinical pregnancies assessed at Day 90 post-transfer were seen in 36 (26%) of women. Thirty-two women (23%) delivered newborns and four women (3%) had spontaneous abortions. (See **PRECAUTIONS**, subsection **Pregnancy**)

Secondary Amenorrhea

In three parallel, open-label studies (COL1620-004US, COL1620-005US, COL1620-009US), 127 women (aged 18-44) with hypothalamic amenorrhea or premature ovarian failure were randomized to receive either Crinone® 4% (n=62) or Crinone® 8% (n=65). All women were treated with either conjugated estrogens 0.625 mg daily (n=100) or transdermal estradiol (delivering 50 mcg/day) twice weekly (n=27).

Estrogen therapy was continuous for the entire three 28-day cycle studies. At Day 15 of the second cycle (six weeks after initiating estrogen replacement), women who demonstrated adequate response to estrogen therapy (by ultrasound) and who continued to be amenorrheic received Crinone® every other day for six doses (Day 15 through Day 25 of the cycle).

In cycle 2, Crinone® 4% induced bleeding in 79% of women and Crinone® 8% induced bleeding in 77% of women. In the third cycle, estrogen was continued and Crinone® was administered every other day beginning on Day 15 for six doses. On Day 24 an endometrial biopsy was performed. In 53 women who received Crinone® 4%, biopsy results were as follows: 7% proliferative, 40% late secretory, 19% mid secretory, 13% early secretory, 7% atrophic, 6% menstrual endometrium, 6% inactive endometrium and 2% negative endometrium. In 54 women who received Crinone® 8%, biopsy results were as follows: 44% late secretory, 19% mid secretory, 11% early secretory, 19% atrophic, 5% menstrual endometrium and 2% "oral contraceptive like" endometrium.

INDICATIONS AND USAGE

Assisted Reproductive Technology

Crinone® 8% is indicated for progesterone supplementation or replacement as part of an Assisted Reproductive Technology ("ART") treatment for infertile women with progesterone deficiency.

Secondary Amenorrhea

Crinone® 4% is indicated for the treatment of secondary amenorrhea.

Crinone® 8% is indicated for use in women who have failed to respond to treatment with Crinone® 4%.

CONTRAINDICATIONS

Crinone® should not be used in individuals with any of the following conditions:

1. Known sensitivity to Crinone® (progesterone or any of the other ingredients)
2. Undiagnosed vaginal bleeding
3. Liver dysfunction or disease
4. Known or suspected malignancy of the breast or genital organs
5. Missed abortion
6. Active thrombophlebitis or thromboembolic disorders, or a history of hormone-associated thrombophlebitis or thromboembolic disorders.

TABLE 2
Multiple Dose Pharmacokinetics

	Assisted Reproductive Technology		Secondary Amenorrhea	
	Daily Dosing 8%	Twice Daily Dosing 8%	Every Other Day Dosing 4%	Every Other Day Dosing 8%
C_{max} (ng/mL)	15.97 ± 5.05	14.57 ± 4.49	13.21 ± 9.46	13.67 ± 3.58
C_{avg} (ng/mL)	8.99 ± 3.53	11.6 ± 3.47	4.05 ± 2.85	6.75 ± 2.83
T_{max} (hr)	5.40 ± 0.97	3.55 ± 2.48	6.67 ± 3.16	7.00 ± 2.88
$AUC_{0-\tau}$ (ng•hr/mL)	391.98 ± 153.28	138.72 ± 41.58	242.15 ± 167.88	438.36 ± 223.36
$t_{1/2}$ (hr)	45.00 ± 34.70	25.91 ± 6.15	49.87 ± 31.20	39.08 ± 12.88

WARNINGS

The physician should be alert to the earliest manifestations of thrombotic disorders (thrombophlebitis, cerebrovascular disorders, pulmonary embolism, and retinal thrombosis). Should any of these occur or be suspected, the drug should be discontinued immediately.

Progesterone and progestins have been used to prevent miscarriage in women with a history of recurrent spontaneous pregnancy losses. No adequate evidence is available to show that they are effective for this purpose.

PRECAUTIONS

General

1. The pretreatment physical examination should include special reference to breast and pelvic organs, as well as Papanicolaou smear.
2. In cases of breakthrough bleeding, as in all cases of irregular vaginal bleeding, nonfunctional causes should be considered. In cases of undiagnosed vaginal bleeding, adequate diagnostic measures should be undertaken.
3. Because progestogens may cause some degree of fluid retention, conditions which might be influenced by this factor (e.g., epilepsy, migraine, asthma, cardiac or renal dysfunction) require careful observation.
4. The pathologist should be advised of progesterone therapy when relevant specimens are submitted.
5. Patients who have a history of psychic depression should be carefully observed and the drug discontinued if the depression recurs to a serious degree.
6. A decrease in glucose tolerance has been observed in a small percentage of patients on estrogen-progestin combination drugs. The mechanism of this decrease is not known. For this reason, diabetic patients should be carefully observed while receiving progestin therapy.

Information for Patients

The product should not be used concurrently with other local intravaginal therapy. If other local intravaginal therapy is to be used concurrently, there should be at least a 6-hour period before or after Crinone® administration. Small, white globules may appear as a vaginal discharge possibly due to gel accumulation, even several days after usage.

Drug Interactions

No drug interactions have been assessed with Crinone®.

Carcinogenesis, Mutagenesis, Impairment of Fertility

Nonclinical toxicity studies to determine the potential of Crinone® to cause carcinogenicity or mutagenicity have not been performed. The effect of Crinone® on fertility has not been evaluated in animals.

Pregnancy (See **CLINICAL PHARMACOLOGY**, subsection **Clinical Studies**)

Crinone® 8% has been used to support embryo implantation and maintain pregnancies through its use as part of ART treatment regimens in two clinical studies (studies COL1620-007US and COL1620-F01). In the first study (COL1620-007US), 54 Crinone®-treated women had donor oocyte transfer procedures, and clinical pregnancies occurred in 26 women (48%). The outcomes of these 26 pregnancies were as follows: one woman had an elective termination of pregnancy at 19 weeks due to congenital malformations (omphalocele) associated with a chromosomal abnormality; one woman pregnant with triplets had an elective termination of her pregnancy; seven women had spontaneous abortions; and 17 women delivered 25 apparently normal newborns.

In the second study (COL1620-F01), Crinone® 8% was used in the luteal phase support of women undergoing *in vitro* fertilization ("IVF") procedures. In this multi-center, open-label study, 139 women received Crinone® 8% once daily beginning within 24 hours of embryo transfer and continuing through Day 30 post-transfer.

Clinical pregnancies assessed at Day 90 post-transfer were seen in 36 (26%) of women. Thirty-two women (23%) delivered newborns and four women (3%) had spontaneous abortions. Of the 47 newborns delivered, one had a teratoma associated with a cleft palate; one had respiratory distress syndrome; 44 were apparently normal and one was lost to follow-up.

Geriatric Use

The safety and effectiveness in geriatric patients (over age 65) have not been established.

Pediatric Use

Safety and effectiveness in pediatric patients have not been established.

Nursing Mothers

Detectable amounts of progestins have been identified in the milk of mothers receiving them. The effect of this on the nursing infant has not been determined.

ADVERSE REACTIONS

Assisted Reproductive Technology

In a study of 61 women with ovarian failure undergoing a donor oocyte transfer procedure receiving Crinone® 8% twice daily, treatment-emergent adverse events occurring in 5% or more of the women are shown in Table 3.

TABLE 3
Treatment-Emergent Adverse Events
in ≥5% of Women Receiving Crinone® 8%
Twice Daily
Study COL1620-007US (n=61)

Body as a Whole	
Bloating	7%
Cramps NOS	15%
Pain	8%
Central and Peripheral Nervous System	
Dizziness	5%
Headache	13%
Gastro-Intestinal System	
Nausea	7%
Reproductive, Female	
Breast Pain	13%
Moniliasis Genital	5%
Vaginal Discharge	7%
Skin and Appendages	
Pruritus Genital	5%

In a second clinical study of 139 women using Crinone® 8% once daily for luteal phase support while undergoing an *in vitro* fertilization procedure, treatment-emergent adverse events reported in ≥5% of the women are shown in Table 4.

TABLE 4
Treatment-Emergent Adverse Events
in ≥5% of Women Receiving Crinone® 8%
Once Daily
Study COL1620-F01 (n=139)

Body as a Whole	
Abdominal Pain	12%
Perineal Pain Female	17%
Central and Periphal Nervous System	
Headache	17%
Gastro-Intestinal System	
Constipation	27%
Diarrhea	8%
Nausea	22%

Continued on next page

Crinone—Cont.

Vomiting	5%
Musculo-Skeletal System	
Arthralgia	8%
Psychiatric	
Depression	11%
Libido Decreased	10%
Nervousness	16%
Somnolence	27%
Reproductive, Female	
Breast Enlargement	40%
Dyspareunia	6%
Urinary System	
Nocturia	13%

Secondary Amenorrhea

In three studies, 127 women with secondary amenorrhea received estrogen replacement therapy and Crinone® 4% or 8% every other day for six doses. Treatment emergent adverse events during estrogen and Crinone® treatment that occurred in 5% or more of women are shown in Table 5.

TABLE 5
Treatment Emergent Adverse Events in ≥5% of Women Receiving Estrogen Treatment and Crinone® Every Other Day
Studies COL1620-004US, COL1620-005US, COL1620-009US

	Estrogen +Crinone® 4% n=62	Estrogen +Crinone® 8% n=65
Body as a Whole		
Abdominal Pain	3 (5%)	6 (9%)
Appetite Increased	3 (5%)	5 (8%)
Bloating	8 (13%)	8 (12%)
Cramps NOS	12 (19%)	17 (26%)
Fatigue	13 (21%)	14 (22%)
Central and Peripheral Nervous System		
Headache	12 (19%)	10 (15%)
Gastro-Intestinal System		
Nausea	5 (8%)	4 (6%)
Musculo-Skeletal System		
Back Pain	5 (8%)	2 (3%)
Myalgia	5 (8%)	0 (0%)
Psychiatric		
Depression	12 (19%)	10 (15%)
Emotional Lability	14 (23%)	14 (22%)
Sleep Disorder	11 (18%)	12 (18%)
Reproductive, Female		
Vaginal Discharge	7 (11%)	2 (3%)
Resistance Mechanism		
Upper Respiratory Tract Infection	3 (5%)	5 (8%)
Skin and Appendages		
Pruritis genital	1 (2%)	4 (6%)

Additional adverse events reported in women at a frequency <5% in Crinone® ART and secondary amenorrhea studies and not listed in the tables above include:
Autonomic Nervous System–mouth dry, sweating increased
Body as a Whole–abnormal crying, allergic reaction, allergy, appetite decreased, asthenia, edema, face edema, fever, hot flushes, influenza-like symptoms, water retention, xerophthalmia
Cardiovascular, General–syncope
Central and Peripheral Nervous System–migraine, tremor
Gastro-Intestinal–dyspepsia, eructation, flatulence, gastritis, toothache
Metabolic and Nutritional–thirst
Musculo-Skeletal System–cramps legs, leg pain, skeletal pain
Neoplasm–benign cyst
Platelet, Bleeding & Clotting–purpura
Psychiatric–aggressive reactions, forgetfulness, insomnia
Red Blood Cell–anemia
Reproductive, Female–dysmenorrhea, premenstrual tension, vaginal dryness
Resistance Mechanism–infection, pharyngitis, sinusitis, urinary tract infection
Respiratory System–asthma, dyspnea, hyperventilation, rhinitis
Skin and Appendages–acne, pruritus, rash, seborrhea, skin discoloration, skin disorder, urticaria
Urinary System–cystitis, dysuria, micturition frequency
Vision Disorders–conjunctivitis

OVERDOSAGE

There have been no reports of overdosage with Crinone®. In the case of overdosage, however, discontinue Crinone®, treat the patient symptomatically, and institute supportive measures.

As with all prescription drugs, this medicine should be kept out of the reach of children.

DOSAGE AND ADMINISTRATION

Assisted Reproductive Technology—Crinone® 8% is administered vaginally at a dose of 90 mg once daily in women who require progesterone supplementation. Crinone® 8% is administered vaginally at a dose of 90 mg twice daily in women with partial or complete ovarian failure who require progesterone replacement. If pregnancy occurs, treatment may be continued until placental autonomy is achieved, up to 10-12 weeks.

Secondary Amenorrhea—Crinone® 4% is administered vaginally every other day up to a total of six doses. For women who fail to respond, a trial of Crinone® 8% every other day up to a total of six doses may be instituted.

It is important to note that a dosage increase from the 4% gel can only be accomplished by using the 8% gel. Increasing the volume of gel administered does not increase the amount of progesterone absorbed.

SEE Crinone® PATIENT INFORMATION SHEET—HOW TO USE Crinone®. Note: The PATIENT INFORMATION SHEET contains special instructions for using the applicator at altitudes above 2500 feet in order to avoid a partial release of Crinone® before vaginal insertion.

HOW SUPPLIED

Crinone® is available in the following strengths:
4% gel (45 mg) in a single use, one piece, disposable, white polyethylene vaginal applicator with a twist-off top. Each applicator contains 1.45 g of gel and delivers 1.125 g of gel.
NDC - 44087-0804-6 - 6 Single-use prefilled applicators.
8% gel (90 mg) in a single use, one piece, disposable, white polyethylene vaginal applicator with a twist-off top. Each applicator contains 1.45 g of gel and delivers 1.125 g of gel.
NDC - 44087-0808-6 - 6 Single-use prefilled applicators.
NDC - 44087-0818-8 - 18 Single-use prefilled applicators
Each applicator is wrapped and sealed in a foil overwrap.
Store at 25°C (77°F); excursions permitted to 15-30°C (59-86°F).
Rx only.
U.S. Patent Numbers 4,615,697 and 5,543,150.
Manufactured for:
Serono, Inc.
Rockland, MA 02370, U.S.A.
Code: 40405010002

Revised July 2004

PATIENT INFORMATION

Crinone® 8%
(progesterone gel)
For Vaginal Use Only

FOR PROGESTERONE SUPPLEMENTATION OR REPLACEMENT AS PART OF AN ASSISTED REPRODUCTIVE TECHNOLOGY ("ART") TREATMENT FOR INFERTILE WOMEN WITH PROGESTERONE DEFICIENCY

Please read this information carefully before you start to use Crinone® and each time your prescription is renewed, in case anything has changed. This leaflet does not take the place of discussions with your doctor. If you still have any questions, ask your doctor or health-care provider.

What Crinone® is

Crinone® is a specially formulated gel that you insert in your vagina. It contains the natural female hormone called progesterone. Crinone® 8% is used as part of a program for women who are undergoing fertility treatment.

Understanding the role of Crinone® in your infertility treatment

Progesterone is one of the hormones essential for maintaining a pregnancy. If you are undergoing ART treatment and your doctor has determined your body does not produce enough progesterone on its own, Crinone® may be prescribed to provide the progesterone you need.

The progesterone in Crinone® will help prepare the lining of your uterus so that it is ready to receive and nourish a fertilized egg. If pregnancy occurs, Crinone® may be supplemented for 10-12 weeks until production of progesterone by the placenta is adequate.

When you should not use Crinone®

- *If you are allergic to progesterone, progesterone-like drugs, or any of the inactive ingredients in the gel (ask a pharmacist if you are not sure about the inactive ingredients in Crinone®).*
- *If you have unusual vaginal bleeding which has not been evaluated by a doctor.*
- *If you have a liver disease.*
- *If you have known or suspected cancer of the breast or genital organs.*
- *If you have a miscarriage and your physician suspects some tissue is still in the uterus.*
- *If you have or have had blood clots in the legs, lungs, eyes, or elsewhere.*

Risks of Crinone®

- *Risk to the fetus.* Birth defects have been reported in the offspring of women who were using Crinone® during early pregnancy. These included an abdominal wall defect and a cleft palate. A causal association has been neither confirmed nor refuted. You should check with your doctor about the risks to your unborn child of any medication used during pregnancy.
- *Blood clots and related health problems.* Blood clots have been reported with the use of estrogens and progestational drugs (alone or in combination). If blood clots do form in your bloodstream, they can cut off the blood supply to vital organs, causing serious problems. These problems may include a stroke (by cutting off blood to part of the brain), a heart attack (by cutting off blood to part of the heart), a pulmonary embolus (by cutting off blood to part of the lungs), or other problems. Any of these conditions may cause death or serious long-term disability. Call your doctor immediately if you suspect you have any of these conditions. He or she may advise you to stop using this drug.

PRECAUTIONS

Be alert for unusual signs and symptoms. If any of these warning signals (or any other unusual symptoms) happen while you are using Crinone®, call your doctor immediately:

- Abnormal bleeding from the vagina.
- Pains in the calves or chest, a sudden shortness of breath or coughing blood indicating possible clots in the legs, heart, or lungs.
- Severe headache or vomiting, dizziness, faintness, or changes in vision or speech, weakness or numbness of an arm or leg indicating possible clots in the brain or eye.
- Breast lumps, which could be associated with fibrocystic disorders, fibroadenoma, or breast cancer. (Ask your doctor or health-care provider to show you how to examine your breasts monthly.)
- Yellowing of the skin and/or white of the eyes indicating possible liver problems.

You should also notify your doctor if you experience depression, worsening of your diabetic condition, or fluid retention.

Possible side effects of Crinone®

In addition to the risks listed above, the following side effects have been reported with Crinone® used either for progesterone supplementation or for replacement as part of an ART treatment for infertile women with progesterone deficiency. Consult your doctor if you experience any of the side effects mentioned below, or other side effects.

SIDE EFFECTS REPORTED AT A FREQUENCY OF 5% OR GREATER

- abdominal pain; perineal pain (the perineum is the area between the vagina and the rectum)
- headache
- constipation; diarrhea; nausea
- joint pain
- depression; decreased libido; nervousness; sleepiness*
- breast enlargement
- excessive urination at night

SIDE EFFECTS REPORTED AT A FREQUENCY RANGING FROM 1% TO 5%

- allergy; bloating; cramps; fatigue; pain
- dizziness*
- vomiting
- mood swings
- breast pain
- difficult or painful intercourse; genital itching; genital yeast infection; vaginal discharge
- urinary tract infection

SIDE EFFECTS REPORTED AT A FREQUENCY OF LESS THAN 1%

- fever; flu-like symptoms
- water retention+
- gastrointestinal discomfort; gas; abdominal swelling
- back pain; leg pain
- insomnia
- sinusitis; upper respiratory tract infection
- asthma
- acne; itching
- painful or difficult urination; frequent urination

*If you experience dizziness or sleepiness, do not drive or operate machinery.
+This may worsen some conditions such as asthma, epilepsy, migraine, heart disease, or kidney disease.

How Crinone® works

Crinone® has been formulated to be administered through the vagina. The moisturizing gel in Crinone® forms a coating on the walls of the vagina which allows for absorption of progesterone through the vaginal tissue.

Small, white globules may appear as a vaginal discharge possibly due to gel accumulation, even several days after usage. Crinone® contains no irritating perfumes or dyes.

Other information
1. Your doctor has prescribed this drug for you and you alone. Do not give this drug to anyone else.
2. This medication was prescribed for your particular medical condition. Do not use it for another condition.
3. Keep this and all drugs out of the reach of children.

How to use Crinone®
The dosage is one application of the 8% gel (90 mg of progesterone) vaginally, daily or twice daily as directed by your doctor. If you become pregnant, your doctor may decide to continue treatment for up to 10 to 12 weeks.
Crinone® is to be applied directly from the specially designed sealed applicator into the vagina. The applicator is designed to deliver a premeasured dose of Crinone®. A small amount of gel will be left in the tube after usage. Do not be concerned because you will still be receiving the appropriate dosage.

1. Remove the applicator from the sealed wrapper. DO NOT remove the twist-off tab at this time. *For use at altitudes above 2500 feet, see special instructions below.*

2. Hold the applicator between the thumb and forefinger along the seam on the sides of the bulb. Shake down vigorously 3 to 4 times (like a thermometer) to ensure that the contents are at the thin end of the applicator.

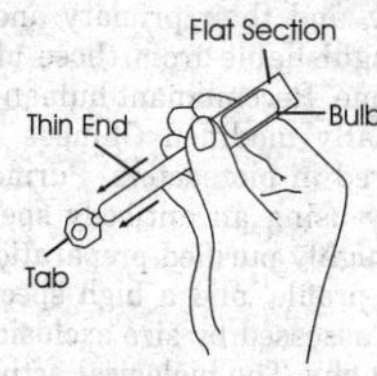

3. Hold the applicator by the flat section of the bulb. Twist off the tab at the thin end and throw away. DO NOT squeeze the bulb while twisting the tab. This could force some gel to be released before it is inserted.

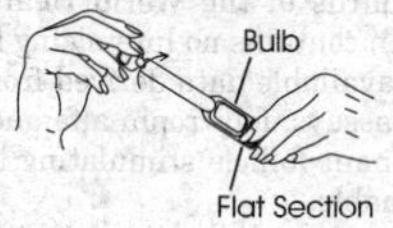

4. The applicator may be inserted into the vagina while you are in a sitting position or when lying on your back with your knees bent. Gently insert the thin end well into the vagina.

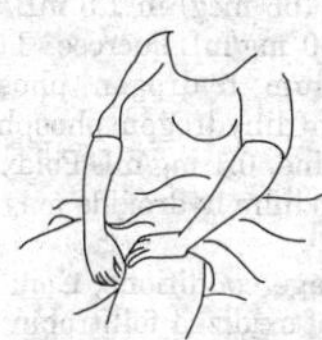

5. Squeeze the bulb of the applicator to deposit the gel into the vagina. Remove the applicator and throw it away in a waste container. Do not be concerned if a small amount of gel is left in the applicator. You will still be receiving the appropriate dosage.

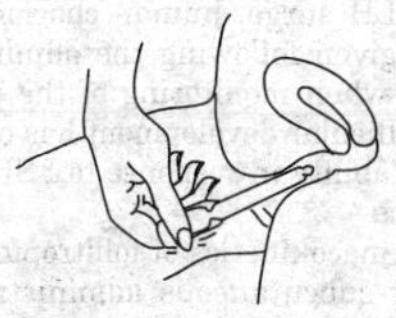

SPECIAL INSTRUCTIONS FOR USE AT ALTITUDES ABOVE 2500 FEET

1. Remove the applicator from the sealed wrapper. DO NOT remove the twist-off tab at this time. *Hold the applicator on both sides of the "bubble" in the bulb, as shown. Using a lancet, make a single puncture in the flat part of the "bubble." This will relieve the difference in air pressure between the inside and outside of the applicator caused by high altitudes. It will not affect the amount of gel administered.* You will still receive the prescribed dose.

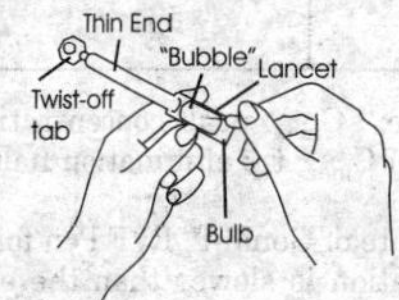

2. See Step 2 above.

3. See Step 3 above.

4. See Step 4 above.

5. *Place your thumb or finger over the puncture that you made in the "bubble" at the bulb of the applicator.* Squeeze the bulb of the applicator to deposit the gel into the vagina. Remove the applicator and throw it away in a waste container. Do not be concerned if a small amount of gel is left in the applicator. You will still be receiving the appropriate dosage.

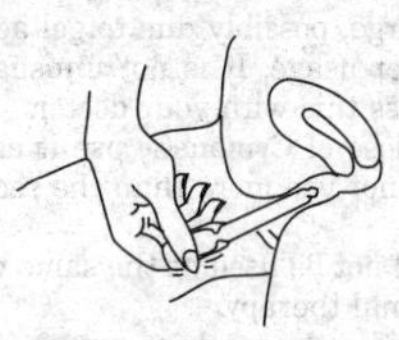

Crinone® coats the vaginal lining to provide long-lasting release of progesterone. Small, white globules may appear as a vagina discharge, possibly due to gel accumulation even several days after usage. It is not unusual, but if you are concerned, discuss this with your doctor.
If you forget a dose of Crinone®, use it as soon as you remember, but do not use more than the recommended daily dose.
Crinone® should not be used at the same time that you are using other vaginal therapy.
This leaflet provides the most important information about Crinone®. If you want to read more, ask your doctor or pharmacist to let you read the professional leaflet. You may need their help to understand some of the information.

How Supplied
Crinone® is available as 8% gel (90 mg of progesterone). Each box of the 8% gel contains either six or eighteen single use, disposable vaginal applicators with a twist-off tab. Each applicator is wrapped and sealed in a foil overwrap.
Crinone® should be stored at 25°C (77°F); excursions permitted to 15-30°C (59-86°F).
Do not use Crinone® after the expiration date which is printed on the box.
Manufactured for:
Serono, Inc.
Rockland, MA 02370, U.S.A.
Code 40405010002 Revised July 2004

PATIENT INFORMATION
Crinone® **4% and**
Crinone® **8%**
(progesterone gel)
For Vaginal Use Only
FOR THE TREATMENT OF SECONDARY AMENORRHEA (ABSENCE OF MENSES IN WOMEN WHO HAVE PREVIOUSLY HAD A MENSTRUAL PERIOD)
Please read this information carefully before you start to use Crinone® and each time your prescription is renewed, in case anything has changed. This leaflet does not take the place of discussions with your doctor. If you still have any questions, ask your doctor or health-care provider.

What Crinone® is
Crinone® is a specially formulated gel that you insert in your vagina. It contains the natural female hormone called progesterone. The 4% gel is used for women whose menstrual cycle has stopped. The 8% gel is to be used when the 4% gel has not worked.

Understanding the role of Crinone® in the treatment of your menstrual irregularities
Progesterone is one of the hormones essential for regular menstrual periods. If your doctor has determined your body does not produce enough progesterone on its own, Crinone® may be prescribed to provide the progesterone you need. When you do not produce enough progesterone, menstrual irregularities can occur. Crinone® can provide you with the progesterone needed during a normal menstrual cycle.

When you should not use Crinone®
- *If you are allergic to progesterone, progesterone-like drugs, or any of the inactive ingredients in the gel (ask a pharmacist if you are not sure about the inactive ingredients in Crinone®).*
- *If you have unusual vaginal bleeding which has not been evaluated by a doctor.*
- *If you have a liver disease.*
- *If you have known or suspected cancer of the breast or genital organs.*
- *If you have a miscarriage and your physician suspects some tissue is still in the uterus.*
- *If you have or have had blood clots in the legs, lungs, eyes, or elsewhere.*

Risks of Crinone®
- *Risk to the fetus.* Birth defects have been reported in the offspring of women who were using Crinone® during early pregnancy. These included an abdominal wall defect and a cleft palate. A causal association has been neither confirmed nor refuted. You should check with your doctor about the risks to your unborn child of any medication used during pregnancy.
- *Blood clots and related health problems.* Blood clots have been reported with the use of estrogens and progestational drugs (alone or in combination). If blood clots do form in your bloodstream, they can cut off the blood supply to vital organs, causing serious problems. These problems may include a stroke (by cutting off blood to part of the brain), a heart attack (by cutting off blood to part of the heart), a pulmonary embolus (by cutting off blood to part of the lungs), or other problems. Any of these conditions may cause death or serious long-term disability. Call your doctor immediately if you suspect you have any of these conditions. He or she may advise you to stop using this drug.

PRECAUTIONS
Be alert for unusual signs and symptoms. If any of these warning signals (or any other unusual symptoms) happen while you are using Crinone®, call your doctor immediately:
- Abnormal bleeding from the vagina.
- Pains in the calves or chest, a sudden shortness of breath or coughing blood indicating possible clots in the legs, heart, or lungs.
- Severe headache or vomiting, dizziness, faintness, or changes in vision or speech, weakness or numbness of an arm or leg indicating possible clots in the brain or eye.
- Breast lumps, which could be associated with fibrocystic disorders, fibroadenoma, or breast cancer. (Ask your doctor or health-care provider to show you how to examine your breasts monthly.)
- Yellowing of the skin and/or white of the eyes indicating possible liver problems.

You should also notify your doctor if you experience depression, worsening of your diabetic condition, or fluid retention.

Possible side effects of Crinone®
In addition to the risks listed above, the following side effects have been reported in studies with Crinone® used for the treatment of menstrual irregularities due to progesterone deficiency. In these studies, women were treated with estrogen prior to and during Crinone® therapy. All side effects reported at a frequency of 5% or greater after Crinone® was added to estrogen therapy also were reported with estrogen therapy alone. Consult your doctor if you experience any of the side effects mentioned below, or other side effects.

SIDE EFFECTS REPORTED AT A FREQUENCY OF 5% OR GREATER
- abdominal pain; increased appetite; bloating; cramps; fatigue
- headache
- nausea
- back pain
- depression; mood swings; sleep disorder
- vaginal discharge
- upper respiratory tract infection

SIDE EFFECTS REPORTED AT A FREQUENCY RANGING FROM 1% TO 5%
- increased sweating
- allergy; flu-like symptoms; hot flushes; pain
- dizziness*
- migraine; tremor
- gas; gastrointestinal discomfort
- thirst
- leg pain; muscle pain
- insomnia; nervousness; sleepiness*
- breast pain; painful menstruation
- infection; genital yeast infection
- acne; genital itching; rash; skin disorder
- frequent urination

SIDE EFFECTS REPORTED AT A FREQUENCY OF LESS THAN 1%
- dry mouth
- abnormal crying; allergic reaction; decreased appetite; dry eyes; swelling; face swelling; perineal pain (the perineum is the area between the vagina and the rectum); water retention+; weakness
- fainting
- abdominal swelling; gastritis; toothache
- joint pain; leg cramps; skeletal pain
- non-cancerous cyst
- bruising
- aggressive reaction; forgetfulness
- anemia
- premenstrual syndrome; vaginal dryness
- sore throat
- rapid, shallow breathing; shortness of breath; runny nose
- hives; itching; oily or dry scaly skin; skin discoloration
- bladder inflammation; painful or difficult urination
- "pink eye"

* If you experience dizziness or sleepiness, do not drive or operate machinery.
+ This may worsen some conditions such as asthma, epilepsy, migraine, heart disease, or kidney disease.

How Crinone® works
Crinone® has been formulated to be administered through the vagina. The moisturizing gel in Crinone® forms a coating on the walls of the vagina which allows for absorption of progesterone through the vaginal tissue.
Small, white globules may appear as a vaginal discharge possibly due to gel accumulation, even several days after usage. Crinone® contains no irritating perfumes or dyes.

Other information
1. Your doctor has prescribed this drug for you and you alone. Do not give this drug to anyone else.

Continued on next page

Crinone—Cont.

2. This medication was prescribed for your particular medical condition. Do not use it for another condition.
3. Keep this and all drugs out of the reach of children.

How to use Crinone®

The dosage is one application of the 4% gel (45 mg of progesterone), vaginally, every other day as directed by your doctor, for a total of six doses. In some cases, your doctor may prescribe the 8% gel (90 mg of progesterone) every other day, for a total of six doses.

It is important to note that a dosage increase from the 4% gel can only be accomplished by using the 8% gel. Increasing the volume of gel administered does not increase the amount of progesterone absorbed.

Crinone® is to be applied directly from the specially designed sealed applicator into the vagina. The applicator is designed to deliver a premeasured dose of Crinone®. A small amount of gel will be left in the tube after usage. Do not be concerned because you will still be receiving the appropriate dosage.

1. Remove the applicator from the sealed wrapper. DO NOT remove the twist-off tab at this time. *For use at altitudes above 2500 feet, see special instructions below.*

2. Hold the applicator between the thumb and forefinger along the seam on the sides of the bulb. Shake down vigorously 3 to 4 times (like a thermometer) to ensure that the contents are at the thin end of the applicator.

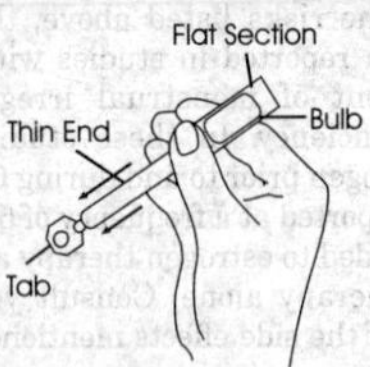

3. Hold the applicator by the flat section of the thick end. Twist off and throw away the tab at the other end. DO NOT squeeze the thick end while twisting the tab. This could force some gel to be released before it is inserted.

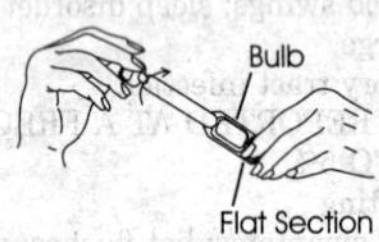

4. The applicator may be inserted into the vagina while you are in a sitting position or when lying on your back with your knees bent. Gently insert the thin end well into the vagina.

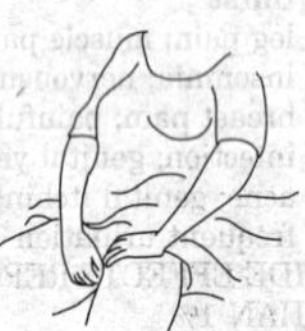

5. Squeeze the bulb of the applicator to deposit the gel into the vagina. Remove the applicator and throw it away in a waste container. Do not be concerned if a small amount of gel is left in the applicator. You will still be receiving the appropriate dosage.

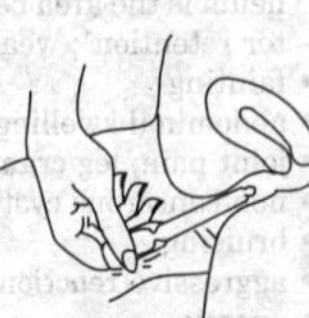

SPECIAL INSTRUCTIONS FOR USE AT ALTITUDES ABOVE 2500 FEET

1. Remove the applicator from the sealed wrapper. DO NOT remove the twist-off tab at this time. *Hold the applicator on both sides of the "bubble" in the bulb, as shown. Using a lancet, make a single puncture in the flat part of the "bubble." This will relieve the difference in air pressure between the inside and outside of the applicator caused by high altitudes. It will not affect the amount of gel administered.* You will still receive the prescribed dose.

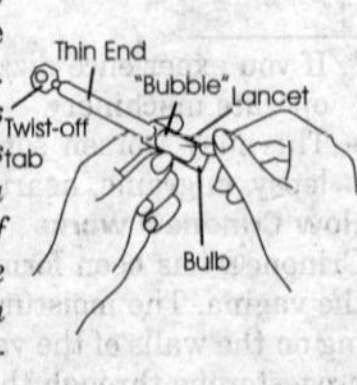

2. See Step 2 above.
3. See Step 3 above.
4. See Step 4 above.
5. *Place your thumb or finger over the puncture that you made in the "bubble" at the bulb of the applicator.* Squeeze the bulb of the applicator to deposit the gel into the vagina. Remove the applicator and throw it away in a waste container. Do not be concerned if a small amount of gel is left in the applicator. You will still be receiving the appropriate dosage.

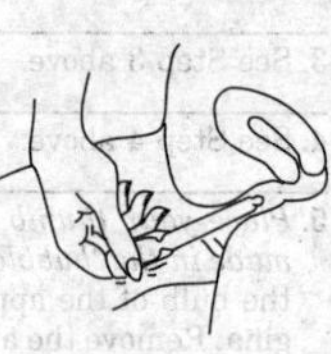

Crinone® coats the vaginal lining to provide long-lasting release of progesterone. Small, white globules may appear as a vaginal discharge, possibly due to gel accumulation even several days after usage. It is not unusual, but if you are concerned, discuss this with your doctor.

If you forget a dose of Crinone®, use it as soon as you remember, but do not use more than the recommended daily dose.

Crinone® should not be used at the same time that you are using other vaginal therapy.

This leaflet provides the most important information about Crinone®. If you want to read more, ask your doctor or pharmacist to let you read the professional leaflet. You may need their help to understand some of the information.

How Supplied

Crinone® is available in two strengths: 4% gel (45 mg of progesterone) and 8% gel (90 mg of progesterone).

Each box of the 4% gel contains six single use, disposable vaginal applicators with a twist-off tab. Each box of the 8% gel contains either six or eighteen single use, disposable vaginal applicators with a twist-off tab. Each applicator is wrapped and sealed in a foil overwrap.

Crinone® should be stored at 25°C (77°F); excursions permitted to 15-30°C (59-86°F).

Do not use Crinone® after the expiration date which is printed on the box.

Manufactured for:
Serono, Inc.
Rockland, MA 02370, U.S.A.
Code: 40405010002 Revised July 2004

GONAL-F® ℞

[gŏn al-ĕf]
(follitropin alfa for injection)
For subcutaneous injection

DESCRIPTION

Gonal-F® (follitropin alfa for injection) is a human follicle stimulating hormone (FSH) preparation of recombinant DNA origin, which consists of two non-covalently linked, non-identical glycoproteins designated as the α- and β-subunits. The α- and β-subunits have 92 and 111 amino acids, respectively, and their primary and tertiary structure are indistinguishable from those of human follicle stimulating hormone. Recombinant FSH production occurs in genetically modified Chinese Hamster Ovary (CHO) cells cultured in bioreactors. Purification by immunochromatography using an antibody specifically binding FSH results in a highly purified preparation with a consistent FSH isoform profile, and a high specific activity. The biological activity of follitropin alfa is determined by measuring the increase in ovary weight in female rats. The *in vivo* biological activity of follitropin alfa has been calibrated against the first International Standard for Recombinant Human Follicle Stimulating Hormone established in 1955 by the Expert Committee on Biological Standards of the World Health Organization. Gonal-F® contains no luteinizing hormone (LH) activity. Based on available data derived from physico-chemical tests and bioassays, follitropin alfa and follitropin beta, another recombinant follicle stimulating hormone product, are indistinguishable.

Gonal-F® is a sterile, lyophilized powder intended for subcutaneous injection after reconstitution.

Each Gonal-F® Multi-Dose vial is filled with 600 IU (44 µg) follitropin alfa to deliver 450 IU (33 µg) follitropin alfa, and contains 30 mg sucrose, 1.11 mg dibasic sodium phosphate dihydrate and 0.45 mg monobasic sodium phosphate monohydrate. O-phosphoric acid and/or sodium hydroxide may be used prior to lyophilization for pH adjustment. Multiple Dose vials are reconstituted with Bacteriostatic Water for Injection (0.9% benzyl alcohol), USP.

Under current storage conditions, Gonal-F® may contain up to 10% of oxidized follitropin alfa.

Therapeutic Class: Infertility

HOW SUPPLIED

Gonal-F® (follitropin alfa for injection) is supplied in a sterile, lyophilized form in multiple dose vials filled with 600 IU in order to deliver 450 IU FSH, after reconstitution with diluent (Bacteriostatic Water for Injection, USP, containing 0.9% benzyl alcohol as a preservative). Each carton contains syringes with mounted 27G × 0.5 inch needle, calibrated in FSH units (IU FSH) which should be used for administration.

Lyophilized Multi-Dose vials may be stored refrigerated or at room temperature (2°–25°C/36°–77°F). Following reconstitution, the Multi-Dose vial may be stored refrigerated or at room temperature (2°–25°C/36°–77°F). Protect from light. Discard unused reconstituted solution after 28 days.

The following package combinations are available:

— 1 vial Gonal-F® Multi-Dose 450 IU, 1 pre-filled syringe of Bacteriostatic Water for Injection, USP (0.9% benzyl alcohol), 1 mL and 6 syringes calibrated in FSH Units (IU FSH) for injection NDC 44087-9030-1

Rx only

Manufactured for: SERONO, INC., Rockland, MA 02370 U.S.A.
Revised: May 2004 v3

GONAL-F® RFF PEN ℞

[gŏn-əl F]
(follitropin alfa injection)
***revised formulation female**
For subcutaneous injection

DESCRIPTION

Gonal-f® RFF Pen (follitropin alfa injection) is a human follicle stimulating hormone (FSH) preparation of recombinant DNA origin, which consists of two non-covalently linked, non-identical glycoproteins designated as the α- and β-subunits. The α- and β-subunits have 92 and 111 amino acids, respectively, and their primary and tertiary structures are indistinguishable from those of human follicle stimulating hormone. Recombinant human FSH production occurs in genetically modified Chinese Hamster Ovary (CHO) cells cultured in bioreactors. Purification by immunochromatography using an antibody specifically binding FSH results in a highly purified preparation with a consistent FSH isoform profile, and a high specific activity. The protein content is assessed by size exclusion high pressure liquid chromatography. The biological activity of follitropin alfa is determined by measuring the increase in ovary weight in female rats. The *in vivo* biological activity of follitropin alfa has been calibrated against the first International Standard for recombinant human follicle stimulating hormone established in 1995 by the Expert Committee on Biological Standards of the World Health Organization.

Gonal-f® RFF Pen contains no luteinizing hormone (LH) activity. Based on available data derived from physico-chemical tests and bioassays, follitropin alfa and follitropin beta, another recombinant follicle stimulating hormone product, are indistinguishable.

Gonal-f® RFF Pen is a disposable, prefilled drug delivery system intended for the subcutaneous injection of multiple and variable doses of a liquid formulation of follitropin alfa. Each Gonal-f® RFF Pen is filled with 415 IU (30 mcg), 568 IU (41 mcg), or 1026 IU (75 mcg) follitropin alfa to deliver at least 300 IU (22 mcg) in 0.5 mL, 450 IU (33 mcg) in 0.75 mL, or 900 IU (66 mcg) in 1.5 mL, respectively. Each Pen also contains 60 mg/mL sucrose, 3.0 mg/mL m-cresol, 1.1 mg/mL di-sodium hydrogen phosphate dihydrate, 0.45 mg/mL sodium dihydrogen phosphate monohydrate, 0.1 mg/mL methionine, 0.1 mg/mL Poloxamer 188. O-phosphoric acid and/or sodium hydroxide may be used for pH adjustment.

Under current storage conditions, Gonal-f® RFF Pen may contain up to 10% of oxidized follitropin alfa.

Therapeutic Class: Infertility

CLINICAL PHARMACOLOGY

Gonal-f® RFF Pen (follitropin alfa injection) stimulates ovarian follicular growth in women who do not have primary ovarian failure. FSH, the active component of Gonal-f® RFF Pen is the primary hormone responsible for follicular recruitment and development. In order to effect final maturation of the follicle and ovulation in the absence of an endogenous LH surge, human chorionic gonadotropin (hCG) must be given following the administration of Gonal-f® RFF Pen when monitoring of the patient indicates that sufficient follicular development has occurred. There is interpatient variability in response to FSH administration.

Pharmacokinetics

Single-dose pharmacokinetics of follitropin alfa were determined following subcutaneous administration of 300 IU Gonal-f® RFF Pen to 21 pre-menopausal healthy female volunteers who were pituitary down-regulated with a GnRH agonist.

The descriptive statistics for the pharmacokinetic parameters are presented in Table 1.

Table 1: Pharmacokinetic parameters of FSH following administration of Gonal-f® RFF Pen

Population Dose (IU)	Healthy Volunteers (n=21) 300 IU SC in a single dose	
	Mean	**%CV**
AUC_{last} (IU·hr/L)	884	20%
C_{max} (IU/L)	9.83	23%
t_{max} (hr)	15.5	43%
$t_{1/2}$ (hr)	53	52%

Abbreviations are: C_{max}: peak concentration (above baseline); t_{max}: time of C_{max}; $t_{1/2}$: elimination half life

Absorption

The absorption rate of Gonal-f® RFF Pen following subcutaneous administration is slower than the elimination rate. Hence, the pharmacokinetics of Gonal-f® RFF Pen are absorption rate-limited.

Distribution
Human tissue or organ distribution of FSH has not been determined for Gonal-f® RFF Pen.
Metabolism/Excretion
FSH metabolism and excretion following administration of Gonal-f® RFF Pen have not been studied in humans.
Special populations: Safety, efficacy, and pharmacokinetics of Gonal-f® RFF Pen in patients with renal or hepatic insufficiency have not been established.
Drug-Drug Interactions: No drug-drug interaction studies have been conducted (see PRECAUTIONS).

CLINICAL STUDIES:

The safety and efficacy of Gonal-f® RFF have been examined in two clinical studies: one study (Study 22240) for ovulation induction and one study (Study 21884) for assisted reproductive technologies (ART).

1. Ovulation Induction (OI):
Study 22240 was a phase III, assessor-blind, randomized, comparative, multinational, multicenter study in oligo-anovulatory infertile women undergoing ovulation induction. Patients were randomized to either Gonal-f® RFF (n=83), administered subcutaneously, or a comparator recombinant human FSH. The use of insulin- sensitizing agents was allowed during the study. Efficacy was assessed using the mean ovulation rate in the first cycle of treatment. The cycle 1 ovulation rate (primary outcome) for Gonal-f® RFF is presented in Table 2. Additionally, this table includes cumulative secondary outcome results from cycle 1 through 3. Study 22240 was not powered to demonstrate differences in these secondary outcomes.

Table 2: Cumulative Ovulation and Clinical Pregnancy Rates in Ovulation Induction

Study 22240	n=83
Cumulative[a] Ovulation Rate	
Cycle 1	72%[b]
Cycle 2	89%[d]
Cycle 3	92%[d]
Cumulative[a] Clinical Pregnancy[c] Rate	
Cycle 1	28%[d]
Cycle 2	41%[d]
Cycle 3	45%[d]

a Cumulative rates were determined per patient over cycles 1, 2, and 3.
b Non-inferior to comparator recombinant human FSH based on a two-sided 95% confidence interval, intent-to-treat analysis.
c A clinical pregnancy was defined as a pregnancy during which a fetal sac (with or without heart activity) was visualized by ultrasound on day 34-36 after hCG administration.
d Secondary efficacy parameter. Study 22240 was not powered to demonstrate differences in this parameter.

2. Assisted Reproductive Technologies (ART):
Study 21884 was a phase III, assessor-blind, randomized, comparative, multinational, multicenter study in ovulatory, infertile women undergoing stimulation of multiple follicles for Assisted Reproductive Technologies (ART) after pituitary down-regulation with a GnRH agonist. Patients were randomized to either Gonal-f® RFF (n=237), administered subcutaneously, or a comparator recombinant human FSH. Randomization was stratified by insemination technique [conventional *in-vitro* fertilization (IVF) vs. intra-cytoplasmic sperm injection (ICSI)]. Efficacy was assessed using the mean number of fertilized oocytes the day after insemination. The initial doses of Gonal-f® RFF were 150 IU a day for patients < 35 years old and 225 IU for patients ≥ 35 years old. The maximal dose allowed for both age groups was 450 IU per day. Treatment outcomes for Gonal-f® RFF are summarized in Table 3.

Table 3: Treatment Outcomes in ART

Study 21884	value (n)
Mean number of 2PN oocytes per patient	6.3 (237)[a]
Mean number of 2PN oocytes per patient receiving IVF	6.1 (88)[b]
Mean number of 2PN oocytes per patient receiving ICSI	6.5 (132)[b]
Clinical pregnancy[c] rate per attempt	33.5% (218)[d]
Clinical pregnancy[c] rate per embryo transfer	35.8% (204)[d]
Mean treatment duration in days (range)	9.7 [3-21] (230)[d]

a Non-inferior to comparator recombinant human FSH based on a two-sided 95% confidence interval, intent-to-treat analysis.
b Study 21884 was not powered to demonstrate differences in subgroups.
c A clinical pregnancy was defined as a pregnancy during which a fetal sac (with or without heart activity) was visualized by ultrasound on day 35-42 after hCG administration.
d Secondary efficacy parameter. Study 21884 was not powered to demonstrate differences in this parameter.

INDICATIONS AND USAGE

Gonal-f® RFF Pen (follitropin alfa injection) is indicated for the induction of ovulation and pregnancy in the oligo-anovulatory infertile patient in whom the cause of infertility is functional and not due to primary ovarian failure. Gonal-f® RFF Pen is also indicated for the development of multiple follicles in the ovulatory patient participating in an Assisted Reproductive Technology (ART) program.

Selection of Patients:

1. Before treatment with Gonal-f® RFF Pen is instituted, a thorough gynecologic and endocrinologic evaluation must be performed. This should include an assessment of pelvic anatomy. Patients with tubal obstruction should receive Gonal-f® RFF Pen only if enrolled in an *in vitro* fertilization program.
2. Primary ovarian failure should be excluded by the determination of gonadotropin levels.
3. Appropriate evaluation should be performed to exclude pregnancy.
4. Patients in later reproductive life have a greater predisposition to endometrial carcinoma as well as a higher incidence of anovulatory disorders. A thorough diagnostic evaluation should always be performed in patients who demonstrate abnormal uterine bleeding or other signs of endometrial abnormalities before starting Gonal-f® RFF Pen therapy.
5. Evaluation of the partner's fertility potential should be included in the initial evaluation.

CONTRAINDICATIONS

Gonal-f® RFF Pen (follitropin alfa injection) is contraindicated in women who exhibit:

1. Prior hypersensitivity to recombinant FSH preparations or one of their excipients.
2. High levels of FSH indicating primary gonadal failure.
3. Uncontrolled thyroid or adrenal dysfunction.
4. Sex hormone dependent tumors of the reproductive tract and accessory organs.
5. An organic intracranial lesion such as a pituitary tumor.
6. Abnormal uterine bleeding of undetermined origin (see "Selection of Patients").
7. Ovarian cyst or enlargement of undetermined origin, not due to polycystic ovary syndrome (see "Selection of Patients").
8. Pregnancy.

WARNINGS

Gonal-f® RFF Pen (follitropin alfa injection) should only be used by physicians who are thoroughly familiar with infertility problems and their management.
Gonal-f® RFF Pen is a potent gonadotropic substance capable of causing Ovarian Hyperstimulation Syndrome (OHSS) in women with or without pulmonary or vascular complications. Gonadotropin therapy requires a certain time commitment by physicians and supportive health professionals, and requires the availability of appropriate monitoring facilities (see "Precautions/Laboratory Tests"). Safe and effective use of Gonal-f® RFF Pen in women requires monitoring of ovarian response with serum estradiol and vaginal ultrasound on a regular basis. The lowest effective dose should be used.

Overstimulation of the Ovary During FSH Therapy:
Ovarian Enlargement: Mild to moderate uncomplicated ovarian enlargement which may be accompanied by abdominal distention and/or abdominal pain occurs in approximately 20% of those treated with urofollitropin and hCG, and generally regresses without treatment within two or three weeks. Careful monitoring of ovarian response can further minimize the risk of overstimulation.
If the ovaries are abnormally enlarged on the last day of Gonal-f® RFF Pen therapy, hCG should not be administered in this course of therapy. This will reduce the chances of development of Ovarian Hyperstimulation Syndrome.
Ovarian Hyperstimulation Syndrome (OHSS): OHSS is a medical event distinct from uncomplicated ovarian enlargement. Severe OHSS may progress rapidly (within 24 hours to several days) to become a serious medical event. It is characterized by an apparent dramatic increase in vascular permeability which can result in a rapid accumulation of fluid in the peritoneal cavity, thorax, and potentially, the pericardium. The early warning signs of development of OHSS are severe pelvic pain, nausea, vomiting, and weight gain. The following symptomatology has been seen with cases of OHSS: abdominal pain, abdominal distension, gastrointestinal symptoms including nausea, vomiting and diarrhea, severe ovarian enlargement, weight gain, dyspnea, and oliguria. Clinical evaluation may reveal hypovolemia, hemoconcentration, electrolyte imbalances, ascites, hemoperitoneum, pleural effusions, hydrothorax, acute pulmonary distress, and thromboembolic events (see "Pulmonary and Vascular Complications"). Transient liver function test abnormalities suggestive of hepatic dysfunction, which may be accompanied by morphologic changes on liver biopsy, have been reported in association with Ovarian Hyperstimulation Syndrome (OHSS).
OHSS occurred in 6 of 83 (7.2%) Gonal-f® RFF treated women in Study 22240 (ovulation induction); none were classified as severe. In Study 21884 (ART), OHSS occurred in 11 of 237 (4.6%) Gonal-f® RFF treated women and 1 (0.42%) was classified as severe. OHSS may be more severe and more protracted if pregnancy occurs. OHSS develops rapidly; therefore, patients should be followed for at least two weeks after hCG administration. Most often, OHSS occurs after treatment has been discontinued and reaches its maximum at about seven to ten days following treatment. Usually, OHSS resolves spontaneously with the onset of menses. If there is evidence that OHSS may be developing prior to hCG administration (see "Precautions / Laboratory Tests"), the hCG must be withheld.
If severe OHSS occurs, treatment must be stopped and the patient should be hospitalized.
A physician experienced in the management of this syndrome, or who is experienced in the management of fluid and electrolyte imbalances should be consulted.

Pulmonary and Vascular Complications:
Serious pulmonary conditions (e.g., atelectasis, acute respiratory distress syndrome and exacerbation of asthma) have been reported. In addition, thromboembolic events both in association with, and separate from Ovarian Hyperstimulation Syndrome have been reported. Intravascular thrombosis and embolism can result in reduced blood flow to critical organs or the extremities. Sequelae of such events have included venous thrombophlebitis, pulmonary embolism, pulmonary infarction, cerebral vascular occlusion (stroke), and arterial occlusion resulting in loss of limb. In rare cases, pulmonary complications and/or thromboembolic events have resulted in death.
Multiple Births: Reports of multiple births have been associated with Gonal-f® RFF treatment. In Study 22240 for women receiving Gonal-f® RFF over three treatment cycles, 20% of live births were multiple births. In Study 21884, 35.1% of live births were multiple births in women receiving Gonal-f® RFF. The rate of multiple births is dependent on the number of embryos transferred. The patient should be advised of the potential risk of multiple births before starting treatment.

PRECAUTIONS

General: Careful attention should be given to the diagnosis of infertility in candidates for Gonal-f® RFF Pen (follitropin alfa injection) therapy (see "Indications and Usage/ Selection of Patients").
Information for Patients: Prior to therapy with Gonal-f® RFF Pen, patients should be informed of the duration of treatment and monitoring of their condition that will be required. The risks of Ovarian Hyperstimulation Syndrome and multiple births in women (see **WARNINGS**) and other possible adverse reactions (see "**Adverse Reactions**") should also be discussed.
A 'Patient's Information Leaflet' is provided for patients prescribed Gonal-f® RFF Pen.
Laboratory Tests: In most instances, treatment of women with Gonal-f® RFF Pen results only in follicular recruitment and development. In the absence of an endogenous LH surge, hCG is given when monitoring of the patient indicates that sufficient follicular development has occurred. This may be estimated by ultrasound alone or in combination with measurement of serum estradiol levels. The combination of both ultrasound and serum estradiol measurement are useful for monitoring the development of follicles, for timing of the ovulatory trigger, as well as for detecting ovarian enlargement and minimizing the risk of the Ovarian Hyperstimulation Syndrome and multiple gestation. It is recommended that the number of growing follicles be confirmed using ultrasonography because plasma estrogens do not give an indication of the size or number of follicles.
The clinical confirmation of ovulation, with the exception of pregnancy, is obtained by direct and indirect indices of progesterone production. The indices most generally used are as follows:

1. A rise in basal body temperature;
2. Increase in serum progesterone; and
3. Menstruation following a shift in basal body temperature.

When used in conjunction with the indices of progesterone production, sonographic visualization of the ovaries will assist in determining if ovulation has occurred. Sonographic evidence of ovulation may include the following:

1. Fluid in the cul-de-sac;
2. Ovarian stigmata;
3. Collapsed follicle; and
4. Secretory endometrium.

Accurate interpretation of the indices of follicle development and maturation require a physician who is experienced in the interpretation of these tests.
Drug Interactions: No drug/drug interaction studies have been performed.
Carcinogenesis, Mutagenesis, Impairment of Fertility: Long-term studies in animals have not been performed to evaluate the carcinogenic potential of Gonal-f® RFF Pen. However, follitropin alfa showed no mutagenic activity in a series of tests performed to evaluate its potential genetic toxicity including, bacterial and mammalian cell mutation tests, a chromosomal aberration test and a micronucleus test. Impaired fertility has been reported in rats, exposed to pharmacological doses of follitropin alfa (≥40 IU/kg/day) for extended periods, through reduced fecundity.

Continued on next page

Gonal-f RFF Pen—Cont.

Pregnancy: Pregnancy Category X. See CONTRAINDICATIONS.

Nursing Mothers: It is not known whether this drug is excreted in human milk. Because many drugs are excreted in human milk and because of the potential for serious adverse reactions in the nursing infant from Gonal-f® RFF Pen, a decision should be made whether to discontinue nursing or to discontinue the drug, taking into account the importance of the drug to the mother.

Pediatric Use: Safety and effectiveness in pediatric patients have not been established.

ADVERSE REACTIONS

The safety of Gonal-f® RFF was examined in two clinical studies [(one ovulation induction study (n=83) and one study in ART (n=237)].

Adverse events (without regard to causality assessment) occurring in at least 2.0% of patients in Study 22240 (ovulation induction) are listed in Table 4.

Table 4: Safety Profile in Ovulation Induction Study 22240

Body System Preferred Term	Patients (%) Experiencing Events Treatment cycles = 176* n=83†
Central and Peripheral Nervous System	
Headache	22 (26.5%)
Dizziness	2 (2.4%)
Migraine	3 (3.6%)
Gastro-intestinal System	
Abdominal Pain	10 (12.0%)
Nausea	3 (3.6%)
Flatulence	3 (3.6%)
Diarrhea	3 (3.6%)
Toothache	3 (3.6%)
Dyspepsia	2 (2.4%)
Constipation	2 (2.4%)
Stomatitis Ulcerative	2 (2.4%)
Neoplasm	
Ovarian Cyst	3 (3.6%)
Reproductive, Female	
Ovarian Hyperstimulation	6 (7.2%)
Breast Pain Female	5 (6.0%)
Vaginal Haemorrhage	5 (6.0%)
Gynecological-related pain	2 (2.4%)
Uterine haemorrhage	2 (2.4%)
Respiratory System	
Sinusitis	5 (6.0%)
Pharyngitis	6 (7.2%)
Rhinitis	6 (7.2%)
Coughing	2 (2.4%)
Application Site	
Injection Site Pain	4 (4.8%)
Injection Site Inflammation	2 (2.4%)
Body as a Whole- General	
Back Pain	3 (3.6%)
Pain	2 (2.4%)
Fever	2 (2.4%)
Hot Flushes	2 (2.4%)
Malaise	2 (2.4%)
Skin and Appendages	
Acne	3 (3.6%)
Urinary System	
Micturition Frequency	2 (2.4%)
Cystitis	2 (2.4%)
Resistance Mechanism	
Infection viral	2 (2.4%)

* up to 3 cycles of therapy
† total patients treated with Gonal-f® RFF

Headache occurred in greater than 20% of patients receiving Gonal-f® RFF in this study.

Adverse events (without regard to causality assessment) occurring in at least 2.0% of patients in Study 21884 (ART) are listed in Table 5.

Table 5: Safety Profile in Assisted Reproductive Technologies Study 21884

Body System Preferred Term	Patients (%) Experiencing Events n=237†
Gastro-intestinal System	
Abdominal Pain	55 (23.2%)
Nausea	19 (8.0%)
Body as a Whole- General	
Abdomen Enlarged	33 (13.9%)
Pain	7 (3.0%)
Central and Peripheral Nervous System	
Headache	44 (18.6%)
Dizziness	5 (2.1%)
Application Site Disorders	
Injection site bruising	23 (9.7%)
Injection site pain	13 (5.5%)
Injection site inflammation	10 (4.2%)
Injection site reaction	10 (4.2%)
Application site edema	6 (2.5%)
Reproductive, Female	
Ovarian Hyperstimulation	11 (4.6%)
Intermenstrual Bleeding	9 (3.8%)

† total patients treated with Gonal-f® RFF

Headache and abdomen enlargement occurred in more than 10% of patients and abdominal pain occurred in more than 20% of patients. The following medical events have been reported subsequent to pregnancies resulting from Gonal-f® RFF therapy in controlled clinical studies:

1. Spontaneous Abortion
2. Ectopic Pregnancy
3. Premature Labor
4. Postpartum Fever

There are no indications that use of gonadotropins during ART is associated with an increased risk of congenital malformations.

The following adverse reactions have been previously reported during Gonal-f® RFF therapy:

1. Pulmonary and vascular complications (see "WARNINGS"),
2. Adnexal torsion (as a complication of ovarian enlargement),
3. Mild to moderate ovarian enlargement,
4. Hemoperitoneum

There have been infrequent reports of ovarian neoplasms, both benign and malignant, in women who have undergone multiple drug regimens for ovulation induction; however, a causal relationship has not been established.

Post Marketing Reports

During post-market surveillance, reports of hypersensitivity reactions including anaphylactoid reactions have been reported with the use of Gonal-f® RFF.

OVERDOSAGE

Aside from possible ovarian hyperstimulation and multiple gestations (see "WARNINGS"), there is no information on the consequences of acute overdosage with Gonal-f® RFF Pen (follitropin alfa injection).

DOSAGE AND ADMINISTRATION

The Gonal-f® RFF Pen delivery system delivers at least 300 IU, 450 IU, or 900 IU, equivalent to a maximum of four 75 IU injections, six 75 IU injections or twelve 75 IU injections, respectively. The minimum dose that can be set is 37.5 IU; the maximum dose that can be set is 300 IU (for 300 IU delivery system) or 450 IU (for 450 IU and 900 IU delivery system).

Dosage:

Infertile Patients with Oligo-Anovulation: The dose of Gonal-f® RFF Pen (follitropin alfa injection) to stimulate development of the follicle must be individualized for each patient.

The lowest dose consistent with the expectation of good results should be used. Over the course of treatment, doses of Gonal-f® RFF Pen may range up to 300 IU per day depending on the individual patient response. Gonal-f® RFF Pen should be administered until adequate follicular development is indicated by serum estradiol and vaginal ultrasonography. A response is generally evident after 5 to 7 days. Subsequent monitoring intervals should be based on individual patient response.

It is recommended that the initial dose of the first cycle be 75 IU of Gonal-f® RFF Pen per day, administered subcutaneously. An incremental adjustment in dose of up to 37.5 IU may be considered after 14 days. Further dose increases of the same magnitude could be made, if necessary, every seven days. Treatment duration should not exceed 35 days unless an E2 rise indicates imminent follicular development. To complete follicular development and effect ovulation in the absence of an endogenous LH surge, chorionic gonadotropin, hCG, should be given after the last dose of Gonal-f® RFF Pen. Chorionic gonadotropin should be withheld if the serum estradiol is greater than 2,000 pg/mL. If the ovaries are abnormally enlarged or abdominal pain occurs, Gonal-f® RFF Pen treatment should be discontinued, hCG should not be administered, and the patient should be advised not to have intercourse; this may reduce the chance of development of the Ovarian Hyperstimulation Syndrome and, should spontaneous ovulation occur, reduce the chance of multiple gestation. A follow-up visit should be conducted in the luteal phase.

The initial dose administered in the subsequent cycles should be individualized for each patient based on her response in the preceding cycle. Doses larger than 300 IU of FSH per day are not routinely recommended. As in the initial cycle, hCG must be given after the last dose of Gonal-f® RFF Pen to complete follicular development and induce ovulation. The precautions described above should be followed to minimize the chance of development of the Ovarian Hyperstimulation Syndrome.

The couple should be encouraged to have intercourse daily, beginning on the day prior to the administration of hCG until ovulation becomes apparent from the indices employed for the determination of progestational activity. Care should be taken to ensure insemination. In light of the indices and parameters mentioned, it should become obvious that, unless a physician is willing to devote considerable time to these patients and be familiar with and conduct the necessary laboratory studies, he/she should not use Gonal-f® RFF Pen.

Assisted Reproductive Technologies: As in the treatment of patients with oligo-anovulatory infertility, the dose of Gonal-f® RFF Pen to stimulate development of the follicle must be individualized for each patient. For Assisted Reproductive Technologies, therapy with Gonal-f® RFF Pen should be initiated in the early follicular phase (cycle day 2 or 3) at a dose of 150 IU per day administered subcutaneously, until sufficient follicular development is attained. In most cases, therapy should not exceed ten days.

In patients undergoing ART under 35 years old, whose endogenous gonadotropin levels are suppressed, Gonal-f® RFF Pen should be initiated at a dose of 150 IU per day. In patients 35 years old and older whose endogenous gonadotropin levels are suppressed, Gonal-f® RFF Pen should be initiated at a dose of 225 IU per day. Treatment should be continued until adequate follicular development is indicated as determined by ultrasound in combination with measurement of serum estradiol levels. Adjustments to dose may be considered after five days based on the patient's response; subsequently dosage should be adjusted no more frequently than every 3-5 days and by no more than 75-150 IU additionally at each adjustment. Doses greater than 450 IU per day are not recommended. Once adequate follicular development is evident, hCG should be administered to induce final follicular maturation in preparation for oocyte retrieval. The administration of hCG must be withheld in cases where the ovaries are abnormally enlarged on the last day of therapy. This should reduce the chance of developing OHSS.

Administration:

Administer subcutaneously in the abdomen as described in the 'Patient's Information Leaflet' provided for patients prescribed Gonal-f® RFF Pen.

Patient Instructions for Use

Make sure you have all the supplies listed below before you begin.

1. Gonal-f® RFF Pen
   - Make sure the Gonal-f® RFF Pen is at room temperature before using.
   - Make sure the liquid in the Pen is clear. Do not use the Gonal-f® RFF Pen if it contains any particles. Get a replacement from your doctor, nurse or pharmacist.

[See figure above]

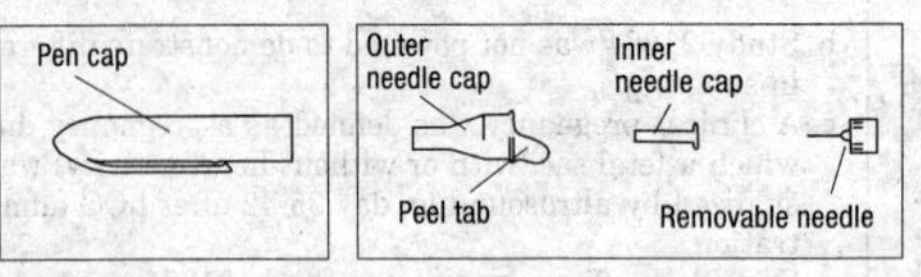

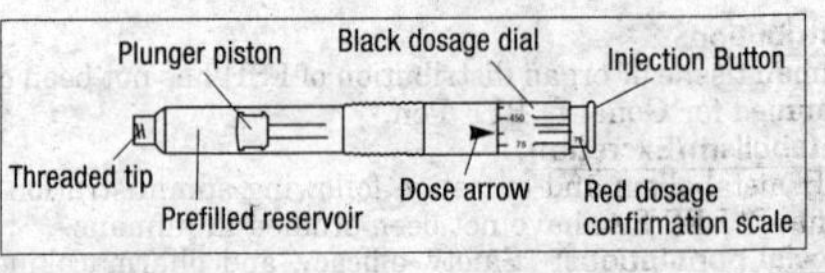

2. One new single-use, disposable administration needle supplied with the Gonal-f® RFF Pen.
3. Alcohol wipes.
4. Safety container (hard plastic or metal container) to use for safe disposal of used needles.

Before you start, wash your hands with soap and water. On a clean surface, layout everything you need.

Preparing the Pen

1. Remove the protective pen cap.
2. Take a single-use disposable needle provided in the Gonal-f® RFF Pen carton. If the peel tab of the needle is damaged or loose, do not use it. Discard the needle and take a new one. Remove the peel tab from the outer needle cap.
3. With the tab removed, hold the outer needle cap firmly in one hand and hold the Pen firmly in the other hand. Press the threaded tip of the Gonal-f® RFF Pen into the open end of the needle cap and twist it clockwise until it is securely fixed.
4. Once the needle is securely attached, remove the outer needle cap by gently pulling it straight off. Do NOT remove the inner needle cap—leave it where it is. Do NOT throw away the outer needle cap—you will need it when you are ready to remove the needle following your injection.

Note: Use only the single-use disposable needles provided within the Gonal-f® RFF Pen carton or compatible needles distributed separately by Serono.

Step 5 only needs to be performed before the first use of each new pen; Otherwise, proceed to Step 6.

5. You must prime the Pen before the first use. You only need to prime the first time you use a new pen. Do the following steps to get your pen ready for use:
   - Check to make sure the dose arrow is set at 37.5. If not, turn the dosage dial (black numbers) to align the dose arrow with 37.5.
   - Pull out the injection button as far as it will go.
   - Remove the inner needle cap and hold the Pen with the needle pointing upwards.
   - Tap the drug reservoir gently with your finger so that any air bubbles rise up towards the needle. (If a few small air bubbles remain, do not worry; this is normal).

- Keep the needle pointing upright and push in the injection button completely. Stop pushing after you hear the first click. A small amount of liquid should come out of the needle indicating that the Pen is ready for use. The amount of liquid seen at the needle tip is part of the extra medicine from the pen. If no liquid appears the first time, repeat these steps until liquid comes out of the needle tip.
- Replace the inner needle cap.

6. Select your prescribed dose by turning the dosage dial (black numbers) to the proper dose mark on the dial in front of the arrow mark. Carefully check the dosage dial before proceeding. Once you have set the dose correctly, load the Pen by pulling out the injection button as far as it will go.
7. Check the red dosage confirmation scale on the injection button to ensure the correct dose has been loaded and that the accurate dose will be injected. The loaded dose is shown by the last mark (flat arrow) on the red dosage confirmation scale that is fully visible.

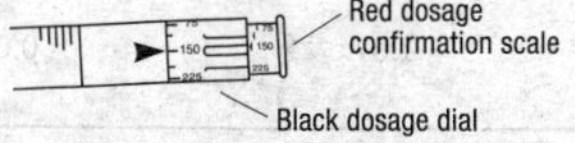

- If you accidentally pull out the injection button with an incorrect dose setting, do not inject. If the set dose is lower than the correct dose to be administered, you can turn the dosage dial to the correct dose and pull out the injection button again. If the set dose is higher than the dose to be administered, discard the dose by pushing all the liquid out into the safety container and repeat the previous steps for setting the dose.

Injecting the dose

Suitable injection sites on the stomach will be advised by your fertility specialist. Occasionally, your fertility specialist may suggest an alternative site.

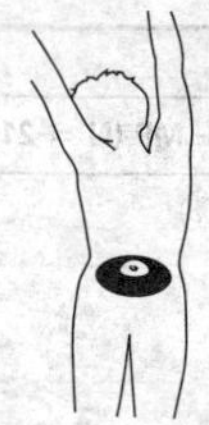

8. Clean the injection site with an alcohol swab and allow it to air dry.
9. Remove the inner needle cap from the needle on the pen. Do not touch the needle or allow the needle to touch any surface.
10. To inject, insert the needle into the skin at a 90° angle and push the injection button—you will hear the button clicking. After the last click, stop applying pressure on the injection button. Allow the needle to remain in the skin for at least 5 seconds. This will ensure that you inject the full dose.

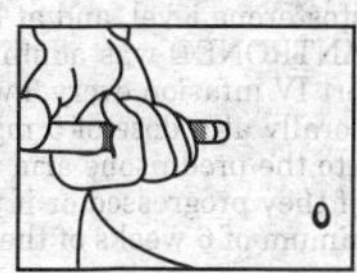

11. After the injection is complete, remove the needle out of your skin and apply pressure using a gauze pad.
12. Each time you finish an injection, remove and discard the used needle as follows. Hold the Gonal-f® RFF Pen firmly by the drug reservoir. Carefully replace the outer needle cap onto the needle. Gripping the outer needle cap firmly, remove the needle by unscrewing the pen counter-clockwise and dispose of the needle in your safety container.
13. Replace the pen cap and store properly. See "HOW SUPPLIED."

Parenteral drug products should be inspected visually for particulate matter and discoloration prior to administration, whenever solution and container permit.

HOW SUPPLIED

Gonal-f® RFF Pen (follitropin alfa injection) is a disposable, prefilled multiple-dose delivery system containing a sterile, ready-to-use liquid formulation of follitropin alfa. Each Gonal-f® RFF Pen is filled with 415 IU, 568 IU, or 1026 IU follitropin alfa to deliver a minimum total of 300 IU in 0.5 mL, 450 IU in 0.75 mL, or 900 IU in 1.5 mL, respectively. Each Pen is supplied in a carton containing 29G × 1/2 inch disposable needles to be used for administration.

The following package combinations are available:

NDC 44087-1113-1 One Gonal-f® RFF Pen contains 415 IU to deliver a minimum total of 300 IU/0.5 mL and 5 single-use disposable 29G × ½" needles

NDC 44087-1112-1 One Gonal-f® RFF Pen contains 568 IU to deliver a minimum total of 450 IU/0.75 mL and 7 single-use disposable 29G × ½" needles

NDC 44087-1114-1 One Gonal-f® RFF Pen contains 1026 IU to deliver a minimum total of 900 IU/1.5 mL and 14 single-use disposable 29G × ½" needles

Store the Gonal-f® RFF Pen refrigerated (2°-8°C/36°-46°F) until dispensed. Upon dispensing, the patient may store the pen refrigerated (2°-8°C/36°-46°F) until the expiration date, or at room temperature (20°-25°C/68°-77°F) for up to one month or until the expiration date, whichever occurs first. After the first injection, the pen may be stored refrigerated (2°-8°C/36°-46°F) or at room temperature (20°-25°C/68°-77°F) for up to 28 days. Protect from light. Do not freeze. Discard unused material after 28 days.

Rx only

Manufactured for: SERONO, INC., Rockland, MA 02370 U.S.A.

Revised: May 2004

Shown in Product Identification Guide, page 333

GONAL-F® RFF ℞

(follitropin alfa for injection)
***revised formulation female**
For subcutaneous injection

DESCRIPTION

Gonal-f® RFF (follitropin alfa for injection) is a human follicle stimulating hormone (FSH) preparation of recombinant DNA origin, which consists of two non-covalently linked, non-identical glycoproteins designated as the α- and β-subunits. The α- and β-subunits have 92 and 111 amino acids, respectively, and their primary and tertiary structure are indistinguishable from those of human follicle stimulating hormone. Recombinant FSH production occurs in genetically modified Chinese Hamster Ovary (CHO) cells cultured in bioreactors. Purification by immunochromatography using an antibody specifically binding FSH results in a highly purified preparation with a consistent FSH isoform profile, and a high specific activity. The biological activity of follitropin alfa is determined by measuring the increase in ovary weight in female rats. The *in vivo* biological activity of follitropin alfa has been calibrated against the first International Standard for recombinant human follicle stimulating hormone established in 1995 by the Expert Committee on Biological Standards of the World Health Organization. Gonal-f® RFF contains no luteinizing hormone (LH) activity. Based on available data derived from physico-chemical tests and bioassays, follitropin alfa and follitropin beta, another recombinant follicle stimulating hormone product, are indistinguishable.

Gonal-f® RFF is a sterile, lyophilized powder intended for subcutaneous injection after reconstitution.

Each Gonal-f® RFF single-dose vial is filled with 82 IU (6 µg) follitropin alfa to deliver 75 IU (5.5 µg) and contains 30 mg sucrose, 1.11 mg dibasic sodium phosphate dihydrate, 0.45 mg monobasic sodium phosphate monohydrate, 0.1 mg methionine, and 0.05 mg polysorbate 20. Phosphoric acid and/or sodium hydroxide may be used prior to lyophilization for pH adjustment. Vials are reconstituted with Sterile Water for Injection, USP.

Under current storage conditions, Gonal-f® RFF may contain up to 10% of oxidized follitropin alfa.

Therapeutic Class: Infertility

HOW SUPPLIED

Gonal-f® RFF (follitropin alfa for injection) is supplied in a sterile, lyophilized form in single-dose vials containing 82 IU with diluent (Sterile Water for Injection, USP) in a pre-filled syringe. Following reconstitution with the diluent as described, upon administration each vial will deliver a dose of 75 IU.

Lyophilized vials may be stored refrigerated or at room temperature (2°–25°C/36°–77°F). Protect from light. Use immediately after reconstitution. Discard unused material.

Sterile Water for Injection, USP is provided in a pre-filled syringe. Separate needles are provided for reconstitution (18 G) and administration (27 G).

Note: No antimicrobial or other substance has been added to the Sterile Water for Injection for the single-dose vials. Sterile Water for Injection is not suitable for intravascular injection without its first having been made approximately isotonic by the addition of a suitable solute.

The following package combinations are available:

1 vial Gonal-f® RFF 75 IU and 1 pre-filled syringe Sterile Water for Injection, USP, 1 mL, 1 reconstitution needle (18 gauge), 1 administration needle (27 gauge), NDC 44087-9005-1

10 vials Gonal-f® RFF 75 IU and 10 pre-filled syringes Sterile Water for Injection, USP, 1 mL, 10 reconstitution needles (18 gauge), 10 administration needles (27 gauge), NDC 44087-9005-6

Rx only

Manufactured for: SERONO, INC., Rockland, MA 02370 U.S.A.

Revised: May 2004

NOVANTRONE® ℞

[nō văn trōne]
(mitoxantrone)
for injection concentrate

WARNING

NOVANTRONE® (mitoxantrone for injection concentrate) should be administered under the supervision of a physician experienced in the use of cytotoxic chemotherapy agents.

NOVANTRONE® should be given slowly into a freely flowing intravenous infusion. It must never be given subcutaneously, intramuscularly, or intra-arterially. Severe local tissue damage may occur if there is extravasation during administration. (See **ADVERSE REACTIONS, General,** Cutaneous and **DOSAGE AND ADMINISTRATION, Preparation and Administration Precautions**).

NOT FOR INTRATHECAL USE. Severe injury with permanent sequelae can result from intrathecal administration. (See **WARNINGS, General**)

Except for the treatment of acute nonlymphocytic leukemia, NOVANTRONE® therapy generally should not be given to patients with baseline neutrophil counts of less than 1,500 cells/mm^3. In order to monitor the occurrence of bone marrow suppression, primarily neutropenia, which may be severe and result in infection, it is recommended that frequent peripheral blood cell counts be performed on all patients receiving NOVANTRONE®.

Myocardial toxicity, manifested in its most severe form by potentially fatal congestive heart failure (CHF), may occur either during therapy with NOVANTRONE® or months to years after termination of therapy. Use of NOVANTRONE® has been associated with cardiotoxicity; this risk increases with cumulative dose. In cancer patients, the risk of symptomatic congestive heart failure (CHF) was estimated to be 2.6% for patients receiving up to a cumulative dose of 140 mg/m^2. For this reason, patients should be monitored for evidence of cardiac toxicity and questioned about symptoms of heart failure prior to initiation of treatment. Patients with multiple sclerosis who reach a cumulative dose of 100 mg/m^2 should be monitored for evidence of cardiac toxicity prior to each subsequent dose. Ordinarily, patients with multiple sclerosis should not receive a cumulative dose greater than 140 mg/m^2. Active or dormant cardiovascular disease, prior or concomitant radiotherapy to the mediastinal/pericardial area, previous therapy with other anthracyclines or anthracenediones, or concomitant use of other cardiotoxic drugs may increase the risk of cardiac toxicity. Cardiac toxicity with NOVANTRONE® may occur at lower cumulative doses whether or not cardiac risk factors are present. For additional information, see **WARNINGS, Cardiac Effects,** and **DOSAGE AND ADMINISTRATION.**

Secondary acute myelogenous leukemia (AML) has been reported in cancer patients treated with anthracyclines. NOVANTRONE® is an anthracenedione, a related drug. Secondary AML has also been reported in cancer patients and multiple sclerosis patients who have been treated with NOVANTRONE®. The occurrence of refractory secondary leukemia is more common when anthracyclines are given in combination with DNA-damaging antineoplastic agents, when patients have been heavily pretreated with cytotoxic drugs, or when doses of anthracyclines have been escalated. The cumulative risk of developing treatment-related AML, in 1774 patients with breast cancer who received NOVANTRONE® concomitantly with other cytotoxic agents and radiotherapy, was estimated as 1.1% and 1.6% at 5 and 10 years, respectively (see **WARNINGS** section).

DESCRIPTION

NOVANTRONE® (mitoxantrone hydrochloride) is a synthetic antineoplastic anthracenedione for intravenous use. The molecular formula is $C_{22}H_{28}N_4O_6 \cdot 2HCl$ and the molecular weight is 517.41. It is supplied as a concentrate that MUST BE DILUTED PRIOR TO INJECTION. The concentrate is a sterile, nonpyrogenic, dark blue aqueous solution containing mitoxantrone hydrochloride equivalent to 2 mg/mL mitoxantrone free base, with sodium chloride (0.80% w/v), sodium acetate (0.005% w/v), and acetic acid (0.046% w/v) as inactive ingredients. The solution has a pH of 3.0 to 4.5 and contains 0.14 mEq of sodium per mL. The product does not contain preservatives. The chemical name is 1,4-dihydroxy-5,8-bis[[2-[(2-hydroxyethyl) amino] ethyl]amino]-9,10-anthracenedione dihydrochloride and the structural formula is:

OH O NHCH2CH2NHCH2CH2OH
2HCl
OH O NHCH2CH2NHCH2CH2OH

CLINICAL PHARMACOLOGY

Mechanism of Action: Mitoxantrone, a DNA-reactive agent that intercalates into deoxyribonucleic acid (DNA) through hydrogen bonding, causes crosslinks and strand breaks. Mitoxantrone also interferes with ribonucleic acid (RNA) and is a potent inhibitor of topoisomerase II, an enzyme responsible for uncoiling and repairing damaged DNA. It has a cytocidal effect on both proliferating and nonproliferating cultured human cells, suggesting lack of cell cycle phase specificity.

Continued on next page

Novantrone—Cont.

NOVANTRONE® has been shown in vitro to inhibit B cell, T cell, and macrophage proliferation and impair antigen presentation, as well as the secretion of interferon gamma, TNFα, and IL-2.

Pharmacokinetics: Pharmacokinetics of mitoxantrone in patients following a single intravenous administration of NOVANTRONE® can be characterized by a three-compartment model. The mean alpha half-life of mitoxantrone is 6 to 12 minutes, the mean beta half-life is 1.1 to 3.1 hours and the mean gamma (terminal or elimination) half-life is 23 to 215 hours (median approximately 75 hours). Pharmacokinetic studies have not been performed in humans receiving multiple daily dosing. Distribution to tissues is extensive: steady-state volume of distribution exceeds 1,000 L/m^2. Tissue concentrations of mitoxantrone appear to exceed those in the blood during the terminal elimination phase. In the healthy monkey, distribution to brain, spinal cord, eye, and spinal fluid is low.

In patients administered 15–90 mg/m^2 of NOVANTRONE® intravenously, there is a linear relationship between dose and the area under the concentration-time curve (AUC).

Mitoxantrone is 78% bound to plasma proteins in the observed concentration range of 26–455 ng/mL. This binding is independent of concentration and is not affected by the presence of phenytoin, doxorubicin, methotrexate, prednisone, prednisolone, heparin, or aspirin.

Metabolism and Elimination: Mitoxantrone is excreted in urine and feces as either unchanged drug or as inactive metabolites. In human studies, 11% and 25% of the dose were recovered in urine and feces, respectively, as either parent drug or metabolite during the 5-day period following drug administration. Of the material recovered in urine, 65% was unchanged drug. The remaining 35% was composed of monocarboxylic and dicarboxylic acid derivatives and their glucuronide conjugates. The pathways leading to the metabolism of NOVANTRONE® have not been elucidated.

Special Populations:

Gender—The effect of gender on mitoxantrone pharmacokinetics is unknown.

Geriatric—In elderly patients with breast cancer, the systemic mitoxantrone clearance was 21.3 L/hr/m^2, compared with 28.3 L/hr/m^2 and 16.2 L/hr/m^2 for non-elderly patients with nasopharyngeal carcinoma and malignant lymphoma, respectively.

Pediatric—Mitoxantrone pharmacokinetics in the pediatric population are unknown.

Race —The effect of race on mitoxantrone pharmacokinetics is unknown.

Renal Impairment—Mitoxantrone pharmacokinetics in patients with renal impairment are unknown.

Hepatic Impairment—Mitoxantrone clearance is reduced by hepatic impairment. Patients with severe hepatic dysfunction (bilirubin > 3.4 mg/dL) have an AUC more than three times greater than that of patients with normal hepatic function receiving the same dose. Patients with multiple sclerosis who have hepatic impairment should ordinarily not be treated with NOVANTRONE®. Other patients with hepatic impairment should be treated with caution and dosage adjustment may be required.

Drug Interactions: In vitro drug interaction studies have demonstrated that mitoxantrone did not inhibit CYP450 1A2, 2A6, 2C9, 2C19, 2D6, 2E1, and 3A4 across a broad concentration range. The results of in vitro induction studies are inconclusive, but suggest that mitoxantrone may be a weak inducer of CYP450 2E1 activity.

Pharmacokinetic studies of the interaction of NOVANTRONE with concomitantly administered medications in humans have not been performed. The pathways leading to the metabolism of NOVANTRONE have not been elucidated. To date, post-marketing experience has not revealed any significant drug interactions in patients who have received NOVANTRONE for treatment of cancer. Information on drug interactions in patients with multiple sclerosis is limited.

CLINICAL TRIALS

Multiple Sclerosis: The safety and efficacy of NOVANTRONE® in multiple sclerosis were assessed in two randomized, multicenter clinical studies.

One randomized, controlled study (Study 1) was conducted in patients with secondary progressive or progressive relapsing multiple sclerosis. Patients in this study demonstrated significant neurological disability based on the Kurtzke Expanded Disability Status Scale (EDSS). The EDSS is an ordinal scale with 0.5 point increments ranging from 0.0 to 10.0 (increasing score indicates worsening) and based largely on ambulatory impairment in its middle range (EDSS 4.5 to 7.5 points). Patients in this study had experienced a mean deterioration in EDSS of about 1.6 points over the 18 months prior to enrollment.

Patients were randomized to receive placebo, 5 mg/m^2 NOVANTRONE®, or 12 mg/m^2 NOVANTRONE® administered IV every 3 months for 2 years. High-dose methylprednisolone was administered to treat relapses. The intent-to-treat analysis cohort consisted of 188 patients; 149 completed the 2-year study. Patients were evaluated every 3 months, and clinical outcome was determined after 24 months. In addition, a subset of patients was assessed with magnetic resonance imaging (MRI) at baseline, Month 12, and Month 24. Neurologic assessments and MRI reviews were performed by evaluators blinded to study drug and clinical outcome, although the diagnosis of relapse and the decision to treat relapses with steroids were made by unblinded treating physicians. A multivariate analysis of five clinical variables (EDSS, Ambulation Index [AI], number of relapses requiring treatment with steroids, months to first relapse needing treatment with steroids, and Standard Neurological Status [SNS]) was used to determine primary efficacy. The AI is an ordinal scale ranging from 0 to 9 in one point increments to define progressive ambulatory impairment. The SNS provides an overall measure of neurologic impairment and disability, with scores ranging from 0 (normal neurologic examination) to 99 (worst possible score).

Results of Study 1 are summarized in Table 1.

[See table 1 above]

Table 1: Efficacy Results at Month 24: Study 1

Primary Endpoints	Placebo (N = 64)	NOVANTRONE® 5 mg/m^2 (N = 64)	NOVANTRONE® 12 mg/m^2 (N = 60)	p-value Placebo vs 12 mg/m^2 NOVANTRONE®
Primary efficacy multivariate analysis*	–	–	–	< 0.0001
Primary clinical variables analyzed:				
EDSS change** (mean)	0.23	−0.23	−0.13	0.0194
Ambulation index change** (mean)	0.77	0.41	0.30	0.0306
Mean number of relapses per patient requiring corticosteroid treatment (adjusted for discontinuation)	1.20	0.73	0.40	0.0002
Months to first relapse requiring corticosteroid treatment (median [1st quartile])	14.2 [6.7]	NR [6.9]	NR [20.4]	0.0004
Standard Neurological Status change** (mean)	0.77	−0.38	−1.07	0.0269
MRI‡				
No. of patients with new Gd-enhancing lesions	5/32 (16%)	4/37 (11%)	0/31	0.022
Change in number of T2-weighted lesions, mean (n)**	1.94 (32)	0.68 (34)	0.29 (28)	0.027

NR = not reached within 24 months; MRI = magnetic resonance imaging.
* Wei-Lachin test.
**Month 24 value minus baseline.
‡ A subset of 110 patients was selected for MRI analysis. MRI results were not available for all patients at all time points.

A second randomized, controlled study (Study 2) evaluated NOVANTRONE® in combination with methylprednisolone (MP) and was conducted in patients with secondary progressive or worsening relapsing-remitting multiple sclerosis who had residual neurological deficit between relapses. All patients had experienced at least two relapses with sequelae or neurological deterioration within the previous 12 months. The average deterioration in EDSS was 2.2 points during the previous 12 months. During the screening period, patients were treated with two monthly doses of 1 g of IV MP and underwent monthly MRI scans. Only patients who developed at least one new Gd-enhancing MRI lesion during the 2-month screening period were eligible for randomization. A total of 42 evaluable patients received monthly treatments of 1 g of IV MP alone (n = 21) or ~12 mg/m^2 of IV NOVANTRONE® plus 1 g of IV MP (n = 21) (NOV + MP) for 6 months. Patients were evaluated monthly, and study outcome was determined after 6 months. The primary measure of effectiveness in this study was a comparison of the proportion of patients in each treatment group who developed no new Gd-enhancing MRI lesions at 6 months; these MRIs were assessed by a blinded panel. Additional outcomes were measured, including EDSS and number of relapses, but all clinical measures in this trial were assessed by an unblinded treating physician. Five patients, all in the MP alone arm, failed to complete the study due to lack of efficacy.

The results of this trial are displayed in Table 2.

[See table 2 above]

Table 2: Efficacy Results. Study 2

Primary Endpoint	MP alone (N = 21)	NOV + MP (N = 21)	p-value
Patients (%) without new Gd-enhancing lesions on MRIs (primary endpoint)*	5 (31%)	19 (90%)	0.001
Secondary Endpoints			
EDSS change (Month 6 minus baseline)* (mean)	−0.1	−1.1	0.013
Annualized relapse rate (mean per patient)	3.0	0.7	0.003
Patients (%) without relapses	7 (33%)	14 (67%)	0.031

MP = methylprednisolone; NOV + MP = NOVANTRONE® plus methylprednisolone.
*Results at Month 6, not including data for 5 withdrawals in the MP alone group.

Advanced Hormone-Refractory Prostate Cancer: A multicenter Phase 2 trial of NOVANTRONE® and low-dose prednisone (N + P) was conducted in 27 symptomatic patients with hormone-refractory prostate cancer. Using NPCP (National Prostate Cancer Project) criteria for disease response, there was one partial responder and 12 patients with stable disease. However, nine patients or 33% achieved a palliative response defined on the basis of reduction in analgesic use or pain intensity.

These findings led to the initiation of a randomized multicenter trial (CCI-NOV22) comparing the effectiveness of (N + P) to low-dose prednisone alone (P). Eligible patients were required to have metastatic or locally advanced disease that had progressed on standard hormonal therapy, a castrate serum testosterone level, and at least mild pain at study entry. NOVANTRONE® was administered at a dose of 12 mg/m^2 by short IV infusion every 3 weeks. Prednisone was administered orally at a dose of 5 mg twice a day. Patients randomized to the prednisone arm were crossed over to the N + P arm if they progressed or if they were not improved after a minimum of 6 weeks of therapy with prednisone alone.

A total of 161 patients were randomized, 80 to the N + P arm and 81 to the P arm. The median NOVANTRONE® dose administered was 12 mg/m^2 per cycle. The median cumulative NOVANTRONE® dose administered was 73 mg/m^2 (range of 12 to 212 mg/m^2).

A primary palliative response (defined as a 2-point decrease in pain intensity in a 6-point pain scale, associated with stable analgesic use, and lasting a minimum of 6 weeks) was achieved in 29% of patients randomized to N + P compared to 12% of patients randomized to P alone (p = 0.011). Two responders left the study after meeting primary response criterion for two consecutive cycles. For the purposes of this analysis, these two patients were assigned a response duration of zero days. A secondary palliative response was defined as a 50% or greater decrease in analgesic use, associated with stable pain intensity, and lasting a minimum of 6 weeks. An overall palliative response (defined as primary plus secondary responses) was achieved in 38% of patients randomized to N + P compared to 21% of patients randomized to P (p = 0.025).

The median duration of primary palliative response for patients randomized to N + P was 7.6 months compared to 2.1 months for patients randomized to P alone (p = 0.0009). The median duration of overall palliative response for patients randomized to N + P was 5.6 months compared to 1.9 months for patients randomized to P alone (p = 0.0004).

Time to progression was defined as a 1-point increase in pain intensity, or a > 25% increase in analgesic use, or evidence of disease progression on radiographic studies, or requirement for radiotherapy. The median time to progression for all patients randomized to N + P was 4.4 months compared to 2.3 months for all patients randomized to P alone (p = 0.0001). Median time to death was 11.3 months for all patients on the N + P arm compared to 10.8 months for all patients on P alone (p = 0.2324).

Forty-eight patients on the P arm crossed over to receive N + P. Of these, thirty patients had progressed on P, while 18 had stable disease on P. The median cycle of crossover was 5 cycles (range of 2 to 16 cycles). Time trends for pain intensity prior to crossover were significantly worse for patients who crossed over than for those who remained on P alone (p = 0.012). Nine patients (19%) demonstrated a palliative response on N + P after crossover. The median time to death for patients who crossed over to N + P was 12.7 months.

The clinical significance of a fall in prostate-specific antigen (PSA) concentrations after chemotherapy is unclear. On the CCI-NOV22 trial, a PSA fall of 50% or greater for two consecutive follow-up assessments after baseline was reported in 33% of all patients randomized to the N + P arm and 9% of all patients randomized to the P arm. These findings should be interpreted with caution since PSA responses were not defined prospectively. A number of patients were inevaluable for response, and there was an imbalance between treatment arms in the numbers of evaluable patients. In addition, PSA reduction did not correlate precisely with palliative response, the primary efficacy endpoint of this study. For example, among the 26 evaluable patients randomized to the N + P arm who had ≥ 50% reduction in PSA, only 13 had a primary palliative response. Also, among 42 evaluable patients on this arm who did not have this reduction in PSA, 8 nonetheless had a primary palliative response.

Investigators at Cancer and Leukemia Group B (CALGB) conducted a Phase 3 comparative trial of NOVANTRONE® plus hydrocortisone (N + H) versus hydrocortisone alone (H) in patients with hormone-refractory prostate cancer (CALGB 9182). Eligible patients were required to have metastatic disease that had progressed despite at least one hormonal therapy. Progression at study entry was defined on the basis of progressive symptoms, increases in measurable or osseous disease, or rising PSA levels. NOVANTRONE® was administered intravenously at a dose of 14 mg/m^2 every 21 days and hydrocortisone was administered orally at a daily dose of 40 mg. A total of 242 subjects were randomized, 119 to the N + H arm and 123 to the H arm. There were no differences in survival between the two arms, with a median of 11.1 months in the N + H arm and 12 months in the H arm (p = 0.3298).

Using NPCP criteria for response, partial responses were achieved in 10 patients (8.4%) randomized to the N + H arm compared with 2 patients (1.6%) randomized to the H arm (p = 0.018). The median time to progression, defined by NPCP criteria, for patients randomized to the N + H arm was 7.3 months compared to 4.1 months for patients randomized to H alone (p = 0.0654).

Approximately 60% of patients on each arm required analgesics at baseline. Analgesic use was measured in this study using a 5-point scale. The best percent change from baseline in mean analgesic use was -17% for 61 patients with available data on the N + H arm, compared with +17% for 61 patients on H alone (p = 0.014). A time trend analysis for analgesic use in individual patients also showed a trend favoring the N + H arm over H alone but was not statistically significant.

Pain intensity was measured using the Symptom Distress Scale (SDS) Pain Item 2 (a 5-point scale). The best percent change from baseline in mean pain intensity was -14% for 37 patients with available data on the N + H arm, compared with +8% for 38 patients on H alone (p = 0.057). A time trend analysis for pain intensity in individual patients showed no difference between treatment arms.

Acute Nonlymphocytic Leukemia: In two large randomized multicenter trials, remission induction therapy for acute nonlymphocytic leukemia (ANLL) with NOVANTRONE® 12 mg/m^2 daily for 3 days as a 10-minute intravenous infusion and cytarabine 100 mg/m^2 for 7 days given as a continuous 24-hour infusion was compared with daunorubicin 45 mg/m^2 daily by intravenous infusion for 3 days plus the same dose and schedule of cytarabine used with NOVANTRONE®. Patients who had an incomplete antileukemic response received a second induction course in which NOVANTRONE® or daunorubicin was administered for 2 days and cytarabine for 5 days using the same daily dosage schedule. Response rates and median survival information for both the U.S. and international multicenter trials are given in Table 3:

[See table 3 above]

Table 3: Response Rates, Time to Response, and Survival in U.S. and International Trials

Trial	% Complete Response (CR)		Median Time to CR (days)		Survival (days)	
	NOV	DAUN	NOV	DAUN	NOV	DAUN
U.S.	63 (62/98)	53 (54/102)	35	42	312	237
International	50 (56/112)	51 (62/123)	36	42	192	230

NOV = NOVANTRONE® + cytarabine
DAUN = daunorubicin + cytarabine

In these studies, two consolidation courses were administered to complete responders on each arm. Consolidation therapy consisted of the same drug and daily dosage used for remission induction, but only 5 days of cytarabine and 2 days of NOVANTRONE® or daunorubicin were given. The first consolidation course was administered 6 weeks after the start of the final induction course if the patient achieved a complete remission. The second consolidation course was generally administered 4 weeks later. Full hematologic recovery was necessary for patients to receive consolidation therapy. For the U.S. trial, median granulocyte nadirs for patients receiving NOVANTRONE® + cytarabine for consolidation courses 1 and 2 were 10/mm^3 for both courses, and for those patients receiving daunorubicin + cytarabine nadirs were 170/mm^3 and 260/mm^3, respectively. Median platelet nadirs for patients who received NOVANTRONE® + cytarabine for consolidation courses 1 and 2 were 17,000/mm^3 and 14,000/mm^3, respectively, and were 33,000/mm^3 and 22,000/mm^3 in courses 1 and 2 for those patients who received daunorubicin + cytarabine. The benefit of consolidation therapy in ANLL patients who achieve a complete remission remains controversial. However, in the only well-controlled prospective, randomized multicenter trials with NOVANTRONE® in ANLL, consolidation therapy was given to all patients who achieved a complete remission. During consolidation in the U.S. study, two myelosuppression-related deaths occurred on the NOVANTRONE® arm and one on the daunorubicin arm. However, in the international study there were eight deaths on the NOVANTRONE® arm during consolidation which were related to the myelosuppression and none on the daunorubicin arm where less myelosuppression occurred.

INDICATIONS AND USAGE

NOVANTRONE® is indicated for reducing neurologic disability and/or the frequency of clinical relapses in patients with secondary (chronic) progressive, progressive relapsing, or worsening relapsing-remitting multiple sclerosis (i.e., patients whose neurologic status is significantly abnormal between relapses). NOVANTRONE® is not indicated in the treatment of patients with primary progressive multiple sclerosis.

The clinical patterns of multiple sclerosis in the studies were characterized as follows: secondary progressive and progressive relapsing disease were characterized by gradual increasing disability with or without superimposed clinical relapses, and worsening relapsing-remitting disease was characterized by clinical relapses resulting in a step-wise worsening of disability.

NOVANTRONE® in combination with corticosteroids is indicated as initial chemotherapy for the treatment of patients with pain related to advanced hormone-refractory prostate cancer.

NOVANTRONE® in combination with other approved drug(s) is indicated in the initial therapy of acute nonlymphocytic leukemia (ANLL) in adults. This category includes myelogenous, promyelocytic, monocytic, and erythroid acute leukemias.

CONTRAINDICATIONS

NOVANTRONE® is contraindicated in patients who have demonstrated prior hypersensitivity to it.

WARNINGS

WHEN NOVANTRONE® IS USED IN HIGH DOSES (> 14 mg/m^2/d x 3 days) SUCH AS INDICATED FOR THE TREATMENT OF LEUKEMIA, SEVERE MYELOSUPPRESSION WILL OCCUR. THEREFORE, IT IS RECOMMENDED THAT NOVANTRONE® BE ADMINISTERED ONLY BY PHYSICIANS EXPERIENCED IN THE CHEMOTHERAPY OF THIS DISEASE. LABORATORY AND SUPPORTIVE SERVICES MUST BE AVAILABLE FOR HEMATOLOGIC AND CHEMISTRY MONITORING AND ADJUNCTIVE THERAPIES, INCLUDING ANTIBIOTICS. BLOOD AND BLOOD PRODUCTS MUST BE AVAILABLE TO SUPPORT PATIENTS DURING THE EXPECTED PERIOD OF MEDULLARY HYPOPLASIA AND SEVERE MYELOSUPPRESSION. PARTICULAR CARE SHOULD BE GIVEN TO ASSURING FULL HEMATOLOGIC RECOVERY BEFORE UNDERTAKING CONSOLIDATION THERAPY (IF THIS TREATMENT IS USED) AND PATIENTS SHOULD BE MONITORED CLOSELY DURING THIS PHASE. NOVANTRONE® ADMINISTERED AT ANY DOSE CAN CAUSE MYELOSUPPRESSION.

General: Patients with preexisting myelosuppression as the result of prior drug therapy should not receive NOVANTRONE® unless it is felt that the possible benefit from such treatment warrants the risk of further medullary suppression.

The safety of NOVANTRONE® (mitoxantrone for injection concentrate) in patients with hepatic insufficiency is not established (see **CLINICAL PHARMACOLOGY**).

Safety for use by routes other than intravenous administration has not been established.

NOVANTRONE® is not indicated for subcutaneous, intramuscular, or intra-arterial injection. There have been reports of local/ regional neuropathy, some irreversible, following intra-arterial injection.

NOVANTRONE® must not be given by intrathecal injection. There have been reports of neuropathy and neurotoxicity, both central and peripheral, following intrathecal injection. These reports have included seizures leading to coma and severe neurologic sequelae, and paralysis with bowel and bladder dysfunction.

Topoisomerase II inhibitors, including NOVANTRONE®, have been associated with the development of acute leukemia and myelodysplasia.

Cardiac Effects: Because of the possible danger of cardiac effects in patients previously treated with daunorubicin or doxorubicin, the benefit-to-risk ratio of NOVANTRONE® therapy in such patients should be determined before starting therapy.

Functional cardiac changes including decreases in left ventricular ejection fraction (LVEF) and irreversible congestive heart failure can occur with NOVANTRONE®. Cardiac toxicity may be more common in patients with prior treatment with anthracyclines, prior mediastinal radiotherapy, or with preexisting cardiovascular disease. Such patients should have regular cardiac monitoring of LVEF from the initiation of therapy. Cancer patients who received cumulative doses of 140 mg/m^2 either alone or in combination with other chemotherapeutic agents had a cumulative 2.6% probability of clinical congestive heart failure. In comparative oncology trials, the overall cumulative probability rate of moderate or severe decreases in LVEF at this dose was 13%.

Multiple Sclerosis: Functional cardiac changes may occur in patients with multiple sclerosis treated with NOVANTRONE®. In one controlled trial (Study 1, see **CLINICAL TRIALS, Multiple Sclerosis**), two patients (2%) of 127 receiving NOVANTRONE®, one receiving a 5 mg/m^2 dose and the other receiving the 12 mg/m^2 dose, had LVEF values that decreased to below 50%. An additional patient receiving 12 mg/m^2, who did not have LVEF measured, had a decrease in another echocardiographic measurement of ventricular function (fractional shortening) that led to discontinuation from the trial (see **ADVERSE REACTIONS, Multiple Sclerosis**). There were no reports of congestive heart failure in either controlled trial.

Evaluation of LVEF (by echocardiogram or MUGA) is recommended prior to administration of the initial dose of NOVANTRONE®. Ordinarily, multiple sclerosis patients with a baseline LVEF of < 50% should not be treated with NOVANTRONE®. Subsequent LVEF evaluations are recommended if signs or symptoms of congestive heart failure develop, and prior to all doses administered to patients who have received a cumulative dose of ≥ 100 mg/m^2. NOVANTRONE® should not ordinarily be administered to multiple sclerosis patients who have received a cumulative lifetime dose of ≥ 140 mg/m^2, or those with either LVEF of < 50% or a clinically significant reduction in LVEF.

Leukemia: Acute congestive heart failure may occasionally occur in patients treated with NOVANTRONE® for ANLL. In first-line comparative trials of NOVANTRONE® + cytarabine vs daunorubicin + cytarabine in adult patients with previously untreated ANLL, therapy was associated with congestive heart failure in 6.5% of patients on each arm. A causal relationship between drug therapy and cardiac effects is difficult to establish in this setting since myocardial function is frequently depressed by the anemia, fever and infection, and hemorrhage that often accompany the underlying disease.

Hormone-Refractory Prostate Cancer: Functional cardiac changes such as decreases in LVEF and congestive heart failure may occur in patients with hormone-refractory prostate cancer treated with NOVANTRONE®. In a randomized comparative trial of NOVANTRONE® plus low-dose prednisone vs low-dose prednisone, 7 of 128 patients (5.5 %) treated with NOVANTRONE® had a cardiac event defined as any decrease in LVEF below the normal range, congestive heart failure (n = 3), or myocardial ischemia. Two patients had a prior history of cardiac disease. The total NOVANTRONE® dose administered to patients with cardiac effects ranged from > 48 to 212 mg/m^2.

Among 112 patients evaluable for safety on the NOVANTRONE® + hydrocortisone arm of the CALGB trial, 18 patients (19%) had a reduction in cardiac function, 5 patients (5%) had cardiac ischemia, and 2 patients (2%) experienced pulmonary edema. The range of total NOVANTRONE® doses administered to these patients is not available.

Pregnancy: NOVANTRONE® may cause fetal harm when administered to a pregnant woman. Women of childbearing potential should be advised to avoid becoming pregnant. Mitoxantrone is considered a potential human teratogen because of its mechanism of action and the developmental effects demonstrated by related agents. Treatment of pregnant rats during the organogenesis period of gestation was associated with fetal growth retardation at doses ≥ 0.1 mg/kg/day (0.01 times the recommended human dose on a mg/m^2 basis). When pregnant rabbits were treated during organogenesis, an increased incidence of premature delivery was observed at doses ≥ 0.1 mg/kg/day (0.01 times the recommended human dose on a mg/m^2 basis). No teratogenic effects were observed in these studies, but the maximum doses tested were well below the recommended human dose (0.02 and 0.05 times in rats and rabbits, respectively, on a mg/m^2 basis). There are no adequate and well-controlled studies in pregnant women. Women with multiple sclerosis who are biologically capable of becoming pregnant should have a pregnancy test prior to each dose, and the results should be known prior to administration of the drug. If this drug is used during pregnancy or if the patient becomes pregnant while taking this drug, the patient should be apprised of the potential risk to the fetus.

Secondary Leukemia: Secondary leukemia has been reported in cancer patients and multiple sclerosis patients

Continued on next page

Novantrone—Cont.

treated with NOVANTRONE®. The largest published report involved 1774 patients with breast cancer treated with NOVANTRONE® in combination with methotrexate with or without mitomycin. In this study, the cumulative probability of developing secondary leukemia was estimated to be 1.1% and 1.6% at 5 and 10 years, respectively. The second largest report involved 449 patients with breast cancer treated with NOVANTRONE®, usually in combination with radiotherapy and/or other cytotoxic agents. In this study, the cumulative probability of developing secondary leukemia was estimated to be 2.2% at 4 years.

There are insufficient long-term follow-up data to estimate the risk of leukemia or myelodysplasia in patients with multiple sclerosis treated with NOVANTRONE®.

PRECAUTIONS

General: Therapy with NOVANTRONE® should be accompanied by close and frequent monitoring of hematologic and chemical laboratory parameters, as well as frequent patient observation.

Systemic infections should be treated concomitantly with or just prior to commencing therapy with NOVANTRONE®.

Information for Patients: NOVANTRONE® may impart a blue-green color to the urine for 24 hours after administration, and patients should be advised to expect this during therapy. Bluish discoloration of the sclera may also occur. Patients should be advised of the signs and symptoms of myelosuppression.

Patients with multiple sclerosis should be provided with the Patient Package Insert at the time that the decision is made to treat with NOVANTRONE® and prior to and in close temporal proximity to each treatment. In addition, the physician should discuss the issues addressed in the Patient Package Insert with the patient.

Laboratory Tests: A complete blood count, including platelets, should be obtained prior to each course of NOVANTRONE® and in the event that signs and symptoms of infection develop. Liver function tests should also be performed prior to each course of therapy. NOVANTRONE® therapy in multiple sclerosis patients with abnormal liver function tests is not recommended because NOVANTRONE® clearance is reduced by hepatic impairment and no laboratory measurement can predict drug clearance and dose adjustments.

In leukemia treatment, hyperuricemia may occur as a result of rapid lysis of tumor cells by NOVANTRONE®. Serum uric acid levels should be monitored and hypouricemic therapy instituted prior to the initiation of antileukemic therapy.

Women with multiple sclerosis who are biologically capable of becoming pregnant, even if they are using birth control, should have a pregnancy test, and the results should be known, before receiving each dose of NOVANTRONE® (see **WARNINGS, Pregnancy**).

Carcinogenesis, Mutagenesis, Impairment of Fertility:

Carcinogenesis—Intravenous treatment of rats and mice, once every 21 days for 24 months, with NOVANTRONE® resulted in an increased incidence of fibroma and external auditory canal tumors in rats at a dose of 0.03 mg/kg (0.02 fold the recommended human dose, on a mg/m^2 basis), and hepatocellular adenoma in male mice at a dose of 0.1 mg/kg (0.03 fold the recommended human dose, on a mg/m^2 basis). Intravenous treatment of rats, once every 21 days for 12 months with NOVANTRONE® resulted in an increased incidence of external auditory canal tumors in rats at a dose of 0.3 mg/kg (0.15 fold the recommended human dose, on a mg/m^2 basis).

Mutagenesis—NOVANTRONE® was clastogenic in the in vivo rat bone marrow assay. NOVANTRONE® was also clastogenic in two in vitro assays; it induced DNA damage in primary rat hepatocytes and sister chromatid exchanges in Chinese hamster ovary cells. NOVANTRONE® was mutagenic in bacterial and mammalian test systems (Ames/ Salmonella and E. coli and L5178Y TK+/-mouse lymphoma).

Drug Interactions: Mitoxantrone and its metabolites are excreted in bile and urine, but it is not known whether the metabolic or excretory pathways are saturable, may be inhibited or induced, or if mitoxantrone and its metabolites undergo enterohepatic circulation. To date, post-marketing experience has not revealed any significant drug interactions in patients who have received NOVANTRONE® for treatment of cancer. Information on drug interactions in patients with multiple sclerosis is limited.

Following concurrent administration of NOVANTRONE® with corticosteroids, no evidence of drug interactions has been observed.

Special Populations:

Hepatic Impairment—Patients with multiple sclerosis who have hepatic impairment should ordinarily not be treated with NOVANTRONE®. NOVANTRONE® should be administered with caution to other patients with hepatic impairment. In patients with severe hepatic impairment, the AUC is more than three times greater than the value observed in patients with normal hepatic function.

Pregnancy: Pregnancy Category D (see **WARNINGS**).

Nursing Mothers: NOVANTRONE® is excreted in human milk and significant concentrations (18 ng/mL) have been reported for 28 days after the last administration. Because of the potential for serious adverse reactions in infants from

Table 4a: Adverse Events of Any Intensity Occurring in ≥ 5% of Patients on Any Dose of NOVANTRONE® and That Were Numerically Greater Than in the Placebo Group Study 1

Preferred Term	Placebo (N = 64)	Percent of Patients 5 mg/m^2 NOVANTRONE® (N = 65)	12 mg/m^2 NOVANTRONE® (N = 62)
Nausea	20	55	76
Alopecia	31	38	61
Menstrual disorder*	26	51	61
Amenorrhea*	3	28	43
Upper respiratory tract infection	52	51	53
Urinary tract infection	13	29	32
Stomatitis	8	15	19
Arrhythmia	8	6	18
Diarrhea	11	25	16
Urine abnormal	6	5	11
ECG abnormal	3	5	11
Constipation	6	14	10
Back pain	5	6	8
Sinusitis	2	3	6
Headache	5	6	6

*Percentage of female patients.

Table 4b: Laboratory Abnormalities Occurring in ≥ 5% of Patients* on Either Dose of NOVANTRONE® and That Were More Frequent Than in the Placebo Group Study 1

Event	Placebo (N = 64)	Percent of Patients 5 mg/m^2 NOVANTRONE® (N = 65)	12 mg/m^2 NOVANTRONE® (N = 62)
Leukopenia[a]	0	9	19
Gamma-GT increased	3	3	15
SGOT increased	8	9	8
Granulocytopenia[b]	2	6	6
Anemia	2	9	6
SGPT increased	3	6	5

*Assessed using World Health Organization (WHO) toxicity criteria.
a. < 4000 cells/mm^3
b. < 2000 cells/mm^3

NOVANTRONE®, breast feeding should be discontinued before starting treatment.

Pediatric Use: Safety and effectiveness in pediatric patients have not been established.

Geriatric Use: Multiple Sclerosis: Clinical studies of Novantrone did not include sufficient numbers of patients aged 65 and over to determine whether they respond differently from younger patients. Other reported clinical experience has not identified differences in responses between the elderly and younger patients.

Hormone-Refractory Prostate Cancer: One hundred forty-six patients aged 65 and over and 52 younger patients (<65 years) have been treated with Novantrone in controlled clinical studies. These studies did not include sufficient numbers of younger patients to determine whether they respond differently from older patients. However, greater sensitivity of some older individuals cannot be ruled out.

Acute Nonlymphocytic Leukemia: Although definitive studies with Novantrone have not been performed in geriatric patients with ANLL, toxicity may be more frequent in the elderly. Elderly patients are more likely to have age-related comorbidities due to disease or disease therapy.

ADVERSE REACTIONS

Multiple Sclerosis: NOVANTRONE® has been administered to 149 patients with multiple sclerosis in two randomized clinical trials, including 21 patients who received NOVANTRONE® in combination with corticosteroids.

In Study 1, the proportion of patients who discontinued treatment due to an adverse event was 9.7% (n = 6) in the 12 mg/m^2 NOVANTRONE® arm (leukopenia, depression, decreased LV function, bone pain and emesis, renal failure, and one discontinuation to prevent future complications from repeated urinary tract infections) compared to 3.1% (n = 2) in the placebo arm (hepatitis and myocardial infarction). The following clinical adverse experiences were significantly more frequent in the NOVANTRONE® groups: nausea, alopecia, urinary tract infection, and menstrual disorders, including amenorrhea.

Table 4a summarizes clinical adverse events of all intensities occurring in ≥ 5% of patients in either dose group of NOVANTRONE® and that were numerically greater on drug than on placebo in Study 1. The majority of these events were of mild to moderate intensity, and nausea was the only adverse event that occurred with severe intensity in more than one patient (three patients [5%] in the 12 mg/m^2 group). Of note, alopecia consisted of mild hair thinning.

Two of the 127 patients treated with NOVANTRONE® in Study 1 had decreased LVEF to below 50% at some point during the 2 years of treatment. An additional patient receiving 12 mg/m^2 did not have LVEF measured, but had another echocardiographic measure of ventricular function (fractional shortening) that led to discontinuation from the study.

[See table 4a above]

The proportion of patients experiencing any infection during Study 1 was 67% for the placebo group, 85% for the 5 mg/m^2 group, and 81% for the 12 mg/m^2 group. However, few of these infections required hospitalization: one placebo patient (tonsillitis), three 5 mg/m^2 patients (enteritis, urinary tract infection, viral infection), and four 12 mg/m^2 patients (tonsillitis, urinary tract infection [two], endometritis).

Table 4b summarizes laboratory abnormalities that occurred in ≥ 5% of patients in either NOVANTRONE® dose group, and that were numerically more frequent than in the placebo group.

[See table 4b above]

There was no difference among treatment groups in the incidence or severity of hemorrhagic events.

In Study 2, NOVANTRONE® was administered once a month. Clinical adverse events most frequently reported in the NOVANTRONE® group included amenorrhea (53% of female patients), alopecia (33% of patients), nausea (29% of patients), and asthenia (24% of patients). Tables 5a and 5b respectively summarize adverse events and laboratory abnormalities occurring in > 5% of patients in the NOVANTRONE® group and numerically more frequent than in the control group.

Table 5a: Adverse Events of Any Intensity Occurring in > 5% of Patient* in the NOVANTRONE® Group and Numerically More Frequent Than in the Control Group Study 2

Event	Percent of Patients MP (n = 21)	N + MP (n = 21)
Amenorrhea[a]	0	53
Alopecia	0	33
Nausea	0	29
Asthenia	0	24
Pharyngitis/throat infection	5	19
Gastraigia/stomach burn/epigastric pain	5	14
Aphthosis	0	10
Cutaneous mycosis	0	10
Rhinitis	0	10
Menorrhagia[a]	0	7

N = NOVANTRONE®, MP = methylprednisolone
*Assessed using National Cancer Institute (NCI) common toxicity criteria
a. Percentage of female patients.

Table 5b: Laboratory Abnormalities Occurring in > 5% of Patients* in the NOVANTRONE® Group and Numerically More Frequent Than in the Control Group Study 2

Event	Percent of Patients MP (n = 21)	N + MP (n = 21)
WBC low[a]	14	100
ANC low[b]	10	100
Lymphocyte low	43	95
Hemoglobin low	48	43
Platelets low[c]	0	33

SGOT high	5	15
SGPT high	10	15
Glucose high	5	10
Potassium low	0	10

N = NOVANTRONE®, MP = methylprednisolone

* Assessed using National Cancer Institute (NCI) common toxicity criteria.

a. < 4000 cells/mm^3

b. < 1500 cells/mm^3

c. < 100,000 cells/mm^3

Leukopenia and neutropenia were reported in the N +MP group (see Table 5b). Neutropenia occurred within 3 weeks after NOVANTRONE® administration and was always reversible. Only mild to moderate intensity infections were reported in 9 of 21 patients in the N +MP group and in 3 of 21 patients in the MP group; none of these required hospitalization. There was no difference among treatment groups in the incidence or severity of hemorrhagic events. There were no withdrawals from Study 2 for safety reasons.

Leukemia: NOVANTRONE® has been studied in approximately 600 patients with ANLL. Table 6 represents the adverse reaction experience in the large U.S. comparative study of mitoxantrone + cytarabine vs daunorubicin + cytarabine. Experience in the large international study was similar. A much wider experience in a variety of other tumor types revealed no additional important reactions other than cardiomyopathy (see **WARNINGS**). It should be appreciated that the listed adverse reaction categories include overlapping clinical symptoms related to the same condition, e.g., dyspnea, cough and pneumonia. In addition, the listed adverse reactions cannot all necessarily be attributed to chemotherapy as it is often impossible to distinguish effects of the drug and effects of the underlying disease. It is clear, however, that the combination of NOVANTRONE® + cytarabine was responsible for nausea and vomiting, alopecia, mucositis/stomatitis, and myelosuppression.

Table 6 summarizes adverse reactions occurring in patients treated with NOVANTRONE® + cytarabine in comparison with those who received daunorubicin + cytarabine for therapy of ANLL in a large multicenter randomized prospective U.S. trial.

Adverse reactions are presented as major categories and selected examples of clinically significant subcategories

[See table 6 at right]

Hormone-Refractory Prostate Cancer: Detailed safety information is available for a total of 353 patients with hormone-refractory prostate cancer treated with NOVANTRONE®, including 274 patients who received NOVANTRONE® in combination with corticosteroids.

Table 7 summarizes adverse reactions of all grades occurring in ≥ 5% of patients in Trial CCI-NOV22.

Table 7: Adverse Events of Any Intensity Occurring in ≥ 5% of Patients Trial CCI-NOV22

Event	N + P (n = 80) %	P (n = 81) %
Nausea	61	35
Fatigue	39	14
Alopecia	29	0
Anorexia	25	6
Constipation	16	14
Dyspnea	11	5
Nail bed changes	11	0
Edema	10	4
Systemic infection	10	7
Mucositis	10	0
UTI	9	4
Emesis	9	5
Pain	8	9
Fever	6	3
Hemorrhage/bruise	6	1
Anemia	5	3
Cough	5	0
Decreased LVEF	5	0
Anxiety/depression	5	3
Dyspepsia	5	6
Skin infection	5	3
Blurred vision	3	5

N = NOVANTRONE®, P = prednisone.

No nonhematologic adverse events of Grade 3/4 were seen in > 5% of patients.

Table 8 summarizes adverse events of all grades occurring in ≥ 5% of patients in Trial CALGB 9182.

[See table 8 at right]

General:

Allergic Reaction—Hypotension, urticaria, dyspnea, and rashes have been reported occasionally. Anaphylaxis/anaphylactoid reactions have been reported rarely.

Cutaneous—Extravasation at the infusion site has been reported, which may result in erythema, swelling, pain, burning, and/or blue discoloration of the skin. Extravasation can result in tissue necrosis with resultant need for debridement and skin grafting. Phlebitis has also been reported at the site of the infusion.

Hematologic—Topoisomerase II inhibitors, including NOVANTRONE®, in combination with other antineoplastic agents, have been associated with the development of acute leukemia (see **WARNINGS**).

Table 6: Adverse Events Occurring in ANLL Patients Receiving NAVANTRONE® or Daunorubicin

Event	Induction [% pts entering induction] NOV N = 102	Induction DAUN N = 102	Consolidation [% pts entering induction] NOV N = 55	Consolidation DAUN N = 49
Cardiovascular	26	28	11	24
CHF	5	6	0	0
Arrhythmias	3	3	4	4
Bleeding	37	41	20	6
GI	16	12	2	2
Petechiae/ecchymoses	7	9	11	2
Gastrointestinal	88	85	58	51
Nausea/vomiting	72	67	31	31
Diarrhea	47	47	18	8
Abdominal pain	15	9	9	4
Mucositis/stomatitis	29	33	18	8
Hepatic	10	11	14	2
Jaundice	3	8	7	0
Infections	66	73	60	43
UTI	7	2	7	2
Pneumonia	9	7	9	0
Sepsis	34	36	31	18
Fungal infections	15	13	9	6
Renal failure	8	6	0	2
Fever	78	71	24	18
Alopecia	37	40	22	16
Pulmonary	43	43	24	14
Cough	13	9	9	2
Dyspnea	18	20	6	0
CNS	30	30	34	35
Seizures	4	4	2	8
Headache	10	9	13	8
Eye	7	6	2	4
Conjunctivitis	5	1	0	0

NOV = NOVANTRONE®, DAUN = daunorubicin.

Table 8. Adverse Events of Any Intensity Occurring in ≥ 5% of Patients, Trial CALGB 9182

Event	N + H (n = 112) N	%	H (n = 113) n	%
Decreased WBC	96	87	4	4
Granulocytes/bands	88	79	3	8
Decreased hemoglobin	83	75	42	39
Lymphocytes	78	72	27	25
Pain	45	41	44	39
Platelets	43	39	8	7
Alkaline Phosphatase	41	37	42	38
Malaise/fatigue	37	34	16	14
Hyperglycemia	33	31	32	30
Edema	31	30	15	14
Nausea	28	26	9	8
Anorexia	24	22	16	14
BUN	24	22	22	20
Transaminase	22	20	16	14
Alopecia	20	20	1	1
Cardiac function	19	18	0	0
Infection	18	17	4	4
Weight loss	18	17	13	12
Dyspnea	16	15	9	8
Diarrhea	16	14	4	4
Fever in absence of infection	15	14	7	6
Weight gain	15	14	16	15
Creatinine	14	13	11	10
Other gastrointestinal	13	14	11	11
Vomiting	12	11	6	5
Other neurologic	11	11	5	5
Hypocalcemia	10	10	5	5
Hematuria	9	11	5	6
Hyponatremia	9	9	3	3
Sweats	9	9	2	2
Other liver	8	8	8	8
Stomatitis	8	8	1	1
Cardiac dysrhythmia	7	7	3	3
Hypokalemia	7	7	4	4
Neuro/constipation	7	7	2	2
Neuro/motor	7	7	3	3
Neuro/mood	6	6	2	2
Skin	6	6	4	4
Cardiac ischemia	5	5	1	1
Chills	5	5	0	0
Hemorrhage	5	5	3	3
Myalgias/arthralgias	5	5	3	3
Other kidney/bladder	5	5	3	3
Other endocrine	5	6	3	4
Other pulmonary	5	5	3	3
Hypertension	4	4	5	5
Impotence/libido	4	7	2	3
Proteinuria	4	6	2	3
Sterility	3	5	2	3

N= NOVANTRONE®, H= hydrocortisone

Leukemia—Myelosuppression is rapid in onset and is consistent with the requirement to produce significant marrow hypoplasia in order to achieve a response in acute leukemia. The incidences of infection and bleeding seen in the U.S. trial are consistent with those reported for other standard induction regimens.

Hormone-Refractory Prostate Cancer—In a randomized study where dose escalation was required for neutrophil counts greater than 1000/mm^3, Grade 4 neutropenia (ANC < 500 /mm^3) was observed in 54% of patients treated with

Continued on next page

Novantrone—Cont.

NOVANTRONE® + low-dose prednisone. In a separate randomized trial where patients were treated with 14 mg/m^2, Grade 4 neutropenia in 23% of patients treated with NOVANTRONE® + hydrocortisone was observed. Neutropenic fever/infection occurred in 11% and 10% of patients receiving NOVANTRONE® + corticosteroids, respectively, on the two trials. Platelets < 50,000/mm^3 were noted in 4% and 3% of patients receiving NOVANTRONE® + corticosteroids on these trials, and there was one patient death on NOVANTRONE® + hydrocortisone due to intracranial hemorrhage after a fall.

Gastrointestinal—Nausea and vomiting occurred acutely in most patients and may have contributed to reports of dehydration, but were generally mild to moderate and could be controlled through the use of antiemetics. Stomatitis/mucositis occurred within 1 week of therapy.

Cardiovascular—Congestive heart failure, tachycardia, EKG changes including arrhythmias, chest pain, and asymptomatic decreases in left ventricular ejection fraction have occurred. (See **WARNINGS**)

Pulmonary—Interstitial pneumonitis has been reported in cancer patients receiving combination chemotherapy that included NOVANTRONE®.

OVERDOSAGE

There is no known specific antidote for NOVANTRONE®. Accidental overdoses have been reported. Four patients receiving 140–180 mg/m^2 as a single bolus injection died as a result of severe leukopenia with infection. Hematologic support and antimicrobial therapy may be required during prolonged periods of severe myelosuppression.

Although patients with severe renal failure have not been studied, NOVANTRONE® is extensively tissue bound and it is unlikely that the therapeutic effect or toxicity would be mitigated by peritoneal or hemodialysis.

DOSAGE AND ADMINISTRATION

(SEE ALSO **WARNINGS**)

Multiple Sclerosis: The recommended dosage of NOVANTRONE® is 12 mg/m^2 given as a short (approximately 5 to 15 minutes) intravenous infusion every 3 months.

Evaluation of LVEF (by echocardiogram or MUGA) is recommended prior to administration of the initial dose of NOVANTRONE®. Subsequent LVEF evaluations are recommended if signs or symptoms of congestive heart failure develop, and prior to all doses administered to patients who have received a cumulative dose of ≥ 100 mg/m^2. NOVANTRONE® should not ordinarily be administered to multiple sclerosis patients who have received a cumulative lifetime dose of ≥ 140 mg/m^2, or those with either LVEF of < 50% or a clinically-significant reduction in LVEF.

Complete blood counts, including platelets, should be monitored prior to each course of NOVANTRONE® and in the event that signs or symptoms of infection develop. NOVANTRONE® generally should not be administered to multiple sclerosis patients with neutrophil counts less than 1500 cells/mm^3. Liver function tests should also be monitored prior to each course. NOVANTRONE® therapy in multiple sclerosis patients with abnormal liver function tests is not recommended because NOVANTRONE® clearance is reduced by hepatic impairment and no laboratory measurement can predict drug clearance and dose adjustments.

Women with multiple sclerosis who are biologically capable of becoming pregnant, even if they are using birth control, should have a pregnancy test, and the results should be known, before receiving each dose of NOVANTRONE® (see **WARNINGS, Pregnancy**).

Hormone-Refractory Prostate Cancer: Based on data from two Phase 3 comparative trials of NOVANTRONE® plus corticosteroids versus corticosteroids alone, the recommended dosage of NOVANTRONE® is 12 to 14 mg/m^2 given as a short intravenous infusion every 21 days.

Combination Initial Therapy for ANLL in Adults: For induction, the recommended dosage is 12 mg/m^2 of NOVANTRONE® daily on Days 1–3 given as an intravenous infusion, and 100 mg/m^2 of cytarabine for 7 days given as a continuous 24 hour infusion on Days 1–7.

Most complete remissions will occur following the initial course of induction therapy. In the event of an incomplete antileukemic response, a second induction course may be given. NOVANTRONE® should be given for 2 days and cytarabine for 5 days using the same daily dosage levels.

If severe or life-threatening nonhematologic toxicity is observed during the first induction course, the second induction course should be withheld until toxicity resolves.

Consolidation therapy which was used in two large randomized multicenter trials consisted of NOVANTRONE®, 12 mg/m^2 given by intravenous infusion daily on Days 1 and 2 and cytarabine, 100 mg/m^2 for 5 days given as a continuous 24-hour infusion on Days 1–5. The first course was given approximately 6 weeks after the final induction course, the second was generally administered 4 weeks after the first. Severe myelosuppression occurred. (See **CLINICAL PHARMACOLOGY**)

Hepatic Impairment: For patients with hepatic impairment, there is at present no laboratory measurement that allows for dose adjustment recommendations. (See **CLINICAL PHARMACOLOGY, Special Populations**, Hepatic Impairment)

Preparation and Administration Precautions

NOVANTRONE® CONCENTRATE MUST BE DILUTED PRIOR TO USE.

Parenteral drug products should be inspected visually for particulate matter and discoloration prior to administration whenever solution and container permit.

The dose of NOVANTRONE® should be diluted to at least 50 mL with either 0.9% Sodium Chloride Injection (USP) or 5% Dextrose Injection (USP). NOVANTRONE® may be further diluted into Dextrose 5% in Water, Normal Saline or Dextrose 5% with Normal Saline and used immediately. DO NOT FREEZE.

NOVANTRONE® should not be mixed in the same infusion as heparin since a precipitate may form. Because specific compatibility data are not available, it is recommended that NOVANTRONE® not be mixed in the same infusion with other drugs. The diluted solution should be introduced slowly into the tubing as a freely running intravenous infusion of 0.9% Sodium Chloride Injection (USP) or 5% Dextrose Injection (USP) over a period of not less than 3 minutes. Unused infusion solutions should be discarded immediately in an appropriate fashion. In the case of multidose use, after penetration of the stopper, the remaining portion of the undiluted NOVANTRONE® concentrate should be stored not longer than 7 days between 15°–25°C (59°–77°F) or 14 days under refrigeration. DO NOT FREEZE. CONTAINS NO PRESERVATIVE.

Care in the administration of NOVANTRONE® will reduce the chance of extravasation. NOVANTRONE® should be administered into the tubing of a freely running intravenous infusion of Sodium Chloride Injection, USP (0.9%) or 5% Dextrose Injection, USP. The tubing should be attached to a Butterfly needle or other suitable device and inserted preferably into a large vein. If possible, avoid veins over joints or in extremities with compromised venous or lymphatic drainage. Care should be taken to avoid extravasation at the infusion site and to avoid contact of NOVANTRONE® with the skin, mucous membranes, or eyes. NOVANTRONE® SHOULD NOT BE ADMINISTERED SUBCUTANEOUSLY. If any signs or symptoms of extravasation have occurred, including burning, pain, pruritis, erythema, swelling, blue discoloration, or ulceration, the injection or infusion should be immediately terminated and restarted in another vein. During intravenous administration of NOVANTRONE® extravasation may occur with or without an accompanying stinging or burning sensation even if blood returns well on aspiration of the infusion needle. If it is known or suspected that subcutaneous extravasation has occurred, it is recommended that intermittent ice packs be placed over the area of extravasation and that the affected extremity be elevated. Because of the progressive nature of extravasation reactions, the area of injection should be frequently examined and surgery consultation obtained early if there is any sign of a local reaction.

Skin accidentally exposed to NOVANTRONE® should be rinsed copiously with warm water and if the eyes are involved, standard irrigation techniques should be used immediately. The use of goggles, gloves, and protective gowns is recommended during preparation and administration of the drug.

Procedures for proper handling and disposal of anticancer drugs should be considered. Several guidelines on this subject have been published.[1–7] There is no general agreement that all of the procedures recommended in the guidelines are necessary or appropriate.

REFERENCES

1. Recommendations for the Safe Handling of Parenteral Antineoplastic Drugs. NIH Publication No. 83-2621. For sale by the Superintendent of Documents, US Government Printing Office, Washington, DC 20402.
2. AMA Council Report. Guidelines for Handling Parenteral Antineoplastics. JAMA 1985;253:1590.
3. National Study Commission on Cytotoxic Exposure - Recommendations for Handling Cytotoxic Agents. Available from Louis P. Jeffrey, Sc D, Chairman, National Study Commission on Cytotoxic Exposure, Massachusetts College of Pharmacy and Allied Health Sciences, 179 Longwood Avenue, Boston, Massachusetts 02115.
4. Clinical Oncological Society of Australia: Guidelines and recommendations for safe handling of antineoplastic agents. Med J Australia 1983;1:426.
5. Jones RB, et al. Safe handling of chemotherapeutic agents: A report from the Mount Sinai Medical Center. CA Cancer J Clin 1983;33:258.
6. American Society of Hospital Pharmacists technical assistance bulletin on handling cytotoxic and hazardous drugs. Am J Hosp Pharm 1990;47:1033.
7. Controlling occupational exposure to hazardous drugs. Am J Health-SystemPharm 1996;53:1669.

HOW SUPPLIED

NOVANTRONE® (mitoxantrone for injection concentrate) is a sterile aqueous solution containing mitoxantrone hydrochloride at a concentration equivalent to 2 mg mitoxantrone free base per mL supplied in vials for multidose use as follows:

NDC 44087-1520-1—10 mL/multidose vial (20 mg)
NDC 44087-1525-1—12.5 mL/multidose vial (25 mg)
NDC 44087-1530-1—15 mL/multidose vial (30 mg)

NOVANTRONE® (mitoxantrone for injection concentrate) should be stored between 15°–25°C (59°–77°F). DO NOT FREEZE.

Issue Date 4/2003

Manufactured for: Serono Inc. Rockland, MA 02370, USA

CI 7833-2

Marketed by:
Serono, Inc.
For Multiple Sclerosis*
Marketed by:
(osi)™ oncology
For Oncology*

*See Indications
(osi) oncology is a trademark of OSI Pharmaceuticals Inc., Melville, NY 11747, USA

OVIDREL® PreFilled Syringe ℞

[*ō-vĭ-drĕl*]

(choriogonadotropin alfa injection)
FOR SUBCUTANEOUS USE

DESCRIPTION

Ovidrel® PreFilled Syringe (choriogonadotropin alfa injection) is a sterile liquid preparation of choriogonadotropin alfa (recombinant human Chorionic Gonadotropin, r-hCG). Choriogonadotropin alfa is a water soluble glycoprotein consisting of two non-covalently linked subunits - designated α and β - consisting of 92 and 145 amino acid residues, respectively, with carbohydrate moieties linked to ASN-52 and ASN-78 (on alpha subunit) and ASN-13, ASN-30, SER-121, SER-127, SER-132 and SER-138 (on beta subunit). The primary structure of the α - chain of r-hCG is identical to that of the α - chain of hCG, FSH and LH. The glycoform pattern of the α - subunit of r-hCG is closely comparable to urinary derived hCG (u-hCG), the differences mainly being due to the branching and sialylation extent of the oligosaccharides. The β - chain has both O- and N-glycosylation sites and its structure and glycosylation pattern are also very similar to that of u-hCG.

The production process involves expansion of genetically modified Chinese Hamster Ovary (CHO) cells from an extensively characterized cell bank into large scale cell culture processing. Choriogonadotropin alfa is secreted by the CHO cells directly into the cell culture medium that is then purified using a series of chromatographic steps. This process yields a product with a high level of purity and consistent product characteristics including glycoforms and biological activity. The biological activity of choriogonadotropin alfa is determined using the seminal vesicle weight gain test in male rats described in the "Chorionic Gonadotrophins" monograph of the European Pharmacopoeia. The *in vivo* biological activity of choriogonadotropin alfa has been calibrated against the third international reference preparation IS75/587 for chorionic gonadotropin.

Ovidrel® PreFilled Syringe is a sterile, liquid intended for subcutaneous (SC) injection. Each Ovidrel® PreFilled Syringe is filled with 0.515 mL containing 257.5 µg of choriogonadotropin alfa, 28.1mg mannitol, 505 µg 85% O-phosphoric acid, 103 µg L-methionine, 51.5 µg Poloxamer 188, Sodium Hydroxide (for pH adjustment), and Water for Injection to deliver 250 µg of choriogonadotropin alfa in 0.5 mL. The pH of the solution is 6.5 to 7.5.

Therapeutic Class: Infertility

CLINICAL PHARMACOLOGY

The physicochemical, immunological, and biological activities of recombinant hCG are comparable to those of placental and human pregnancy urine-derived hCG. Choriogonadotropin alfa stimulates late follicular maturation and resumption of oocyte meiosis, and initiates rupture of the pre-ovulatory ovarian follicle. Choriogonadotropin alfa, the active component of Ovidrel® PreFilled Syringe, is an analogue of Luteinizing Hormone (LH) and binds to the LH/hCG receptor of the granulosa and theca cells of the ovary to effect these changes in the absence of an endogenous LH surge. In pregnancy, hCG, secreted by the placenta, maintains the viability of the corpus luteum to provide the continued secretion of estrogen and progesterone necessary to support the first trimester of pregnancy. Ovidrel® PreFilled Syringe is administered when monitoring of the patient indicates that sufficient follicular development has occurred in response to FSH treatment for ovulation induction.

Pharmacokinetics

When given by intravenous administration, the pharmacokinetic profile of Ovidrel® followed a biexponential model and was linear over a range of 25 µg to 1000 µg. Pharmacokinetic parameter estimates following SC administration of Ovidrel® 250 µg to females are presented in Table 1.

Table 1: Pharmacokinetic Parameters (mean ± SD) of r-hCG after Single-Dose Administration of Ovidrel® in Healthy Female Volunteers

	Ovidrel® 250 µg SC
C_{max} (IU/L)	121 ± 44
t_{max} (h)*	24 (12–24)
AUC (h•IU/L)	7701 ± 2101
t½ (h)	29 ± 6
F	0.4 ± 0.1

C_{max}: peak concentration (above baseline), t_{max}: time of C_{max}, AUC: total area under the curve, t½: elimination half-life, F: bioavailability
* median (range)

Table 2 Summary of Ovidrel® PreFilled Syringe Pharmacokinetics Parameters

Parameter	C_{max} (mIU/mL)	AUC_{last} (mIU·h/mL)	AUC (mIU·h/mL)	$AUC_{extrapolated}$ (%)	t_{max} (h)
Mean (Min - Max)	125 (68.0-294)	10050 (5646-14850)	10350 (5800-15100)	2.85 (1.08-6.27)	20.0 (9.00-48.0)

Abbreviations are: C_{max} peak concentration (about baseline); t_{max}: time of C_{max}

Absorption
Following subcutaneous administration of Ovidrel® 250 µg, maximum serum concentration (121 ± 44 IU/L) is reached after approximately 12 to 24 hours. The mean absolute bioavailability of Ovidrel® following a single subcutaneous injection to healthy female volunteers is about 40%.
Distribution
Following intravenous administration of Ovidrel® 250 µg to healthy down-regulated female volunteers, the serum profile of hCG is described by a two-compartment model with an initial half-life of 4.5 ± 0.5 hours. The volume of the central compartment is 3.0 ± 0.5 L and the steady state volume of distribution is 5.9 ± 1.0 L.
Metabolism/Excretion
Following subcutaneous administration of Ovidrel®, hCG is eliminated from the body with a mean terminal half-life of about 29 ± 6 hours. After intravenous administration of Ovidrel® 250 µg to healthy down-regulated females, the mean terminal half-life is 26.5 ± 2.5 hours and the total body clearance is 0.29 ± 0.04 L/h. One-tenth of the dose is excreted in the urine.
Pharmacodynamics
In female subjects on oral contraception after an initial latency period, Ovidrel® induced a clear increase in androstenedione serum levels by 24 hours after dosing. Pharmacodynamic studies in females determined that the relationship of Ovidrel® pharmacokinetics to pharmacologic effect of Ovidrel® are complex and vary with the pharmacodynamic marker examined. In general pharmacologic effects are not proportional to exposure and in some cases appear to be near maximal at a 250 µg dose.
Population pharmacokinetics and pharmacodynamics
In patients undergoing *in-vitro* fertilization/embryo transfer given Ovidrel® subcutaneously to trigger ovulation, the results of a population PK/PD analysis generally supported the data obtained in healthy subjects. Pharmacokinetic parameters for Ovidrel® include a median elimination half-life of 29.2 hours, median apparent clearance (Cl/F) of 0.51 L/hr and median apparent volume of distribution (V/F) of 21.4 L.
Bioequivalence of Formulations
Ovidrel® PreFilled Syringe (choriogonadotropin alfa injection) has been determined to be bioequivalent to Ovidrel® (choriogonadotropin alfa for injection) based on the statistical evaluation of AUC and C_{max}. A summary of the Ovidrel® PreFilled Syringe pharmacokinetic parameters is presented in Table 2.
[See table 2 above]
Special populations: Safety, efficacy, and pharmacokinetics of Ovidrel® PreFilled Syringe in patients with renal or hepatic insufficiency have not been established.
Drug-Drug Interactions: No drug-drug interaction studies have been conducted. Administration of Ovidrel® PreFilled Syringe may interfere with the interpretation of pregnancy tests. (see PRECAUTIONS.)
Clinical Studies:
The safety and efficacy of Ovidrel® have been examined in three well-controlled studies in women; two studies for assisted reproductive technologies (ART) and one study for ovulation induction (OI).
Assisted Reproductive Technologies (ART)
The safety and efficacy of Ovidrel® 250 µg and Ovidrel® 500 µg administered subcutaneously versus 10,000 USP Units of an approved urinary-derived hCG product administered intramuscularly were assessed in a randomized, open-label, multicenter study in infertile women undergoing *in vitro* fertilization and embryo transfer (Study 7927). The study was conducted in 20 U.S. centers.
The primary efficacy parameter in this single-cycle study was the number of oocytes retrieved. 297 patients entered the study, of whom 94 were randomized to receive Ovidrel® 250 µg. The number of oocytes retrieved was similar for the Ovidrel® and urinary-derived hCG (10,000 USP Units) treatment groups. The efficacy of Ovidrel® 250 µg and Ovidrel® 500 µg were both found to be clinically and statistically equivalent to that of the approved urinary-derived hCG product and to each other. The efficacy results for the patients who received Ovidrel® 250 µg are summarized in Table 3.

Table 3: Efficacy Outcomes of r-hCG in ART (Study 7927)

Parameter	Ovidrel® 250 µg (n = 94)
Mean number of oocytes retrieved per patient	13.60
Mean number of mature oocytes retrieved per patient	7.6
Mean number of 2 PN fertilized oocytes per patient	7.2
Mean number of 2 PN or cleaved embryos per patient	7.6
Implantation rate per embryo transferred (%)	18.7
Mean mid-luteal serum progesterone levels (nmol/L)*	423
Clinical pregnancy rate per initiated treatment cycle (%)†	35.1
Clinical pregnancy rate per transfer (%)†	36.3

†Clinical pregnancy was defined as a pregnancy during which a fetal sac (with or without heartbeat activity) was detected by ultrasound on day 35-42 after hCG administration)
*nmol/L ÷ 3.18 = ng/mL

For the 33 patients who achieved a clinical pregnancy with Ovidrel® 250 µg, the outcomes of the pregnancies are presented in Table 4.

Table 4: Pregnancy Outcomes of r-hCG in ART (Study 7927)

Parameter	Ovidrel® 250 µg (n = 33)
Clinical pregnancies not reaching term	4 (12.1%)
Live births	29 (87.9%)
Singleton	*20 (69.0%)*
Multiple birth	*9 (31.0%)*

The safety and efficacy of Ovidrel® 250 µg administered subcutaneously versus 5,000 IU of an approved urinary-derived hCG product administered subcutaneously were assessed in a second, randomized, multicenter study in infertile women undergoing *in vitro* fertilization and embryo transfer (Study 7648). This double-blinded study was conducted in nine centers in Europe and Israel.
The primary efficacy parameter in this single-cycle study was the number of oocytes retrieved per patient. 205 patients entered the study, of whom 97 received Ovidrel® 250 µg. The efficacy of Ovidrel® 250 µg was found to be clinically and statistically equivalent to that of the approved urinary-derived hCG product. The results for the 97 patients who received Ovidrel® 250 µg are summarized in Table 5.

Table 5: Efficacy Outcomes of r-hCG in ART (Study 7648)

Parameter	Ovidrel® 250 µg (n = 97)
Mean number of oocytes retrieved per patient	10.6
Mean number of mature oocytes retrieved per patient	10.1
Mean number of 2 PN fertilized oocytes per patient	5.7
Mean number of 2 PN or cleaved embryos per patient	5.1
Implantation rate per embryo transferred (%)	17.4
Mean mid-luteal serum progesterone levels (nmol/L)*	394
Clinical pregnancy rate per initiated treatment cycle (%)†	33
Clinical pregnancy rate per transfer (%)†	37.6

†Clinical pregnancy was defined as a pregnancy during which a fetal sac (with or without heartbeat activity) was detected by ultrasound on day 35-42 after hCG administration)
*nmol/L ÷ 3.18 = ng/mL

For the 32 patients who achieved a clinical pregnancy with Ovidrel® 250 µg, the outcomes of the pregnancies are presented in Table 6.

Table 6: Pregnancy Outcomes of r-hCG in ART (Study 7648)

Parameter	Ovidrel® 250 µg (n = 32)
Clinical Pregnancies not reaching term	6 (18.8%)
Live births	26 (81.2%)
Singleton	*18 (69.2%)*
Multiple birth	*8 (30.8%)*

Ovulation Induction (OI)
The safety and efficacy of Ovidrel® 250 µg administered subcutaneously versus 5,000 IU of an approved urinary-derived hCG product administered intramuscularly were assessed in a double-blind, randomized, multicenter study in anovulatory infertile women (Study 8209) which was conducted in 19 centers in Australia, Canada, Europe and Israel.
The primary efficacy parameter in this single-cycle study was the patient ovulation rate. 242 patients entered the study, of whom 99 received Ovidrel® 250 µg. The efficacy of Ovidrel® 250 µg was found to be clinically and statistically equivalent to that of the approved urinary-derived hCG product. The results of those patients who received Ovidrel® 250 µg are summarized in Table 7.

Table 7: Efficacy Outcomes of r-hCG in OI (Study 8209)

Parameter	Ovidrel® 250 µg (n = 99)
Ovulation Rate	91 (91.9%)
Clinical Pregnancy Rate†	22 (22%)

†Clinical pregnancy was defined as a pregnancy during which a fetal sac (with or without heartbeat activity) was detected by ultrasound on day 35-42 after hCG administration.

For the 22 patients who had a clinical pregnancy with Ovidrel® 250 µg, the outcome of the pregnancy is presented in Table 8.

Table 8: Pregnancy Outcomes of r-hCG in OI (Study 8209)

Parameter	Ovidrel® 250 µg (n = 22)
Clinical pregnancies not reaching term	7 (31.8%)
Live births	15 (68.2%)
Singleton	*13 (86.7%)*
Multiple birth	*2 (13.3%)*

INDICATIONS AND USAGE

Ovidrel® PreFilled Syringe (choriogonadotropin alfa injection) is indicated for the induction of final follicular maturation and early luteinization in infertile women who have undergone pituitary desensitization and who have been appropriately pretreated with follicle stimulating hormones as part of an Assisted Reproductive Technology (ART) program such as *in vitro* fertilization and embryo transfer. Ovidrel® PreFilled Syringe is also indicated for the induction of ovulation (OI) and pregnancy in anovulatory infertile patients in whom the cause of infertility is functional and not due to primary ovarian failure.
Selection of Patients:
1. Before treatment with gonadotropins is instituted, a thorough gynecologic and endocrinologic evaluation must be performed. This should include an assessment of pelvic anatomy. Patients with tubal obstruction should receive Ovidrel® PreFilled Syringe only if enrolled in an *in vitro* fertilization program.
2. Primary ovarian failure should be excluded by the determination of gonadotropin levels.
3. Appropriate evaluation should be performed to exclude pregnancy.
4. Patients in later reproductive life have a greater predisposition to endometrial carcinoma as well as a higher incidence of anovulatory disorders. A thorough diagnostic evaluation should always be performed in patients who demonstrate abnormal uterine bleeding or other signs of endometrial abnormalities before starting FSH and Ovidrel® PreFilled Syringe therapy.
5. Evaluation of the partner's fertility potential should be included in the initial evaluation.

Continued on next page

Ovidrel—Cont.

CONTRAINDICATIONS

Ovidrel® PreFilled Syringe (choriogonadotropin alfa injection) is contraindicated in women who exhibit:

1. Prior hypersensitivity to hCG preparations or one of their excipients.
2. Primary ovarian failure.
3. Uncontrolled thyroid or adrenal dysfunction.
4. An uncontrolled organic intracranial lesion such as a pituitary tumor.
5. Abnormal uterine bleeding of undetermined origin (see "Selection of Patients").
6. Ovarian cyst or enlargement of undetermined origin (see "Selection of Patients").
7. Sex hormone dependent tumors of the reproductive tract and accessory organs.
8. Pregnancy.

WARNINGS

Gonadotropins, including Ovidrel® PreFilled Syringe (choriogonadotropin alfa injection), should only be used by physicians who are thoroughly familiar with infertility problems and their management. Like other hCG products, Ovidrel® PreFilled Syringe is a potent gonadotropic substance capable of causing Ovarian Hyperstimulation Syndrome (OHSS) in women with or without pulmonary or vascular complications. Gonadotropin therapy requires a certain time commitment by physicians and supportive health professionals, and requires the availability of appropriate monitoring facilities (see "Precautions/Laboratory Tests"). Safe and effective induction of ovulation and use of Ovidrel® PreFilled Syringe in women requires monitoring of ovarian response with serum estradiol and transvaginal ultrasound on a regular basis.

Overstimulation of the Ovary Following hCG Therapy:

Ovarian Enlargement:

Mild to moderate uncomplicated ovarian enlargement which may be accompanied by abdominal distention and/or abdominal pain may occur in patients treated with FSH and hCG, and generally regresses without treatment within two or three weeks. Careful monitoring of ovarian response can further minimize the risk of overstimulation.

If the ovaries are abnormally enlarged on the last day of FSH therapy, choriogonadotropin alfa should not be administered in this course of therapy. This will reduce the risk of development of Ovarian Hyperstimulation Syndrome.

Ovarian Hyperstimulation Syndrome (OHSS):

OHSS is a medical event distinct from uncomplicated ovarian enlargement. Severe OHSS may progress rapidly (within 24 hours to several days) to become a serious medical event. It is characterized by an apparent dramatic increase in vascular permeability which can result in a rapid accumulation of fluid in the peritoneal cavity, thorax, and potentially, the pericardium. The early warning signs of development of OHSS are severe pelvic pain, nausea, vomiting, and weight gain. The following symptomatology has been seen with cases of OHSS: abdominal pain, abdominal distension, gastrointestinal symptoms including nausea, vomiting and diarrhea, severe ovarian enlargement, weight gain, dyspnea, and oliguria. Clinical evaluation may reveal hypovolemia, hemoconcentration, electrolyte imbalances, ascites, hemoperitoneum, pleural effusions, hydrothorax, acute pulmonary distress, and thromboembolic events (see "Pulmonary and Vascular Complications"). Transient liver function test abnormalities suggestive of hepatic dysfunction, which may be accompanied by morphologic changes on liver biopsy, have been reported in association with Ovarian Hyperstimulation Syndrome (OHSS).

OHSS occurred in 4 of 236 (1.7 %) patients treated with Ovidrel® 250 µg during clinical trials for ART and 3 of 99 (3.0%) patients treated in the OI trial. OHSS occurred in 8 of 89 (9.0%) patients who received Ovidrel® 500 µg. Two patients treated with Ovidrel® 500 µg developed severe OHSS.

OHSS may be more severe and more protracted if pregnancy occurs. OHSS develops rapidly; therefore, patients should be followed for at least two weeks after hCG administration. Most often, OHSS occurs after treatment has been discontinued and reaches its maximum at about seven to ten days following treatment. Usually, OHSS resolves spontaneously with the onset of menses. If there is evidence that OHSS may be developing prior to hCG administration (see "Precautions/Laboratory Tests"), the hCG must be withheld.

If severe OHSS occurs, treatment with gonadotropins must be stopped and the patient should be hospitalized.

A physician experienced in the management of this syndrome, or who is experienced in the management of fluid and electrolyte imbalances should be consulted.

Multiple Births: As with other hCG products, reports of multiple births have been associated with Ovidrel® treatment. In ART, the risk of multiple births correlates to the number of embryos transferred. Multiple births occurred in 17 of 55 live deliveries (30.9 %) experienced by women receiving Ovidrel® 250 µg in the ART studies. In the ovulation induction clinical trial, 2 of 15 live deliveries (13.3%) were associated with multiple births in women receiving Ovidrel®. The patient should be advised of the potential risk of multiple births before starting treatment.

Pulmonary and Vascular Complications: As with other hCG products, a potential for the occurrence of arterial thromboembolism exists.

PRECAUTIONS

General: Careful attention should be given to the diagnosis of infertility in candidates for hCG therapy. (see "Indications and Usage/Selection of Patients"). After the exclusion of pre-existing conditions, elevations in ALT were found in 10 (3%) of 335 patients receiving Ovidrel® 250 mg, 9 (10%) of 89 patients receiving Ovidrel® 500 mg and in 16 (4.8%) of 328 patients receiving urinary-derived hCG. The elevations ranged up to 1.2 times the upper limit of normal. The clinical significance of these findings is not known.

Information for Patients: Prior to therapy with hCG, patients should be informed of the duration of treatment and monitoring of their condition that will be required. The risks of ovarian hyperstimulation syndrome and multiple births in women (see **WARNINGS**) and other possible adverse reactions (see "**Adverse Reactions**") should also be discussed.

Laboratory Tests: In most instances, treatment of women with FSH results only in follicular recruitment and development. In the absence of an endogenous LH surge, hCG is given when monitoring of the patient indicates that sufficient follicular development has occurred. This may be estimated by ultrasound alone or in combination with measurement of serum estradiol levels. The combination of both ultrasound and serum estradiol measurement are useful for monitoring the development of follicles, for timing of the ovulatory trigger, as well as for detecting ovarian enlargement and minimizing the risk of the Ovarian Hyperstimulation Syndrome and multiple gestation. It is recommended that the number of growing follicles be confirmed using ultrasonography because serum estrogens do not give an indication of the size or number of follicles.

Human chorionic gonadotropins can crossreact in the radioimmunoassay of gonadotropins, especially luteinizing hormone. Each individual laboratory should establish the degree of crossreactivity with their gonadotropin assay. Physicians should make the laboratory aware of patients on hCG if gonadotropin levels are requested.

The clinical confirmation of ovulation, with the exception of pregnancy, is obtained by direct and indirect indices of progesterone production. The indices most generally used are as follows:

1. A rise in basal body temperature
2. Increase in serum progesterone and
3. Menstruation following a shift in basal body temperature

When used in conjunction with the indices of progesterone production, sonographic visualization of the ovaries will assist in determining if ovulation has occurred. Sonographic evidence of ovulation may include the following:

1. Fluid in the cul-de-sac
2. Ovarian stigmata
3. Collapsed follicle
4. Secretory endometrium

Accurate interpretation of the indices of ovulation require a physician who is experienced in the interpretation of these tests.

Carcinogenesis, Mutagenesis, Impairment of Fertility: Long-term studies to evaluate the carcinogenic potential of Ovidrel® in animals have not been performed. *In-vitro* genotoxicity testing of Ovidrel® in bacteria and mammalian cell lines, chromosome aberration assay in human lymphocytes and in-vivo mouse micronucleus have shown no indication of genetic defects.

Pregnancy: Pregnancy Category X. Intrauterine death and impaired parturition were observed in pregnant rats given a dose of urinary-hCG (500 IU) equivalent to three times the maximum human dose of 10,000 USP, based on body surface area.

Nursing Mothers: It is not known whether this drug is excreted in human milk. Because many drugs are excreted in human milk, caution should be exercised if hCG is administered to a nursing woman.

Pediatric Patients: Safety and effectiveness in pediatric patients has not been established.

Geriatric Patients: Safety and effectiveness in geriatric patients has not been established.

ADVERSE REACTIONS

(see **WARNINGS**)

The safety of Ovidrel® was examined in four clinical studies that treated 752 patients of whom 335 received Ovidrel® 250 µg following follicular recruitment with gonadotropins. When patients enrolled in four clinical studies (3 in ART and one in OI) were injected subcutaneously with either Ovidrel® or an approved urinary-derived hCG, 14.6 % (49 of 335 patients) in the Ovidrel® 250 µg group experienced application site disorders compared to 28% (92 of 328 patients) in the approved u-hCG group. Adverse events reported for Ovidrel® 250 µg occurring in at least 2% of patients (regardless of causality) are listed in Table 9 for the 3 ART studies and in Table 10 for the single OI study.

Table 9: Incidence of Adverse Events of r-hCG in ART (Studies 7648, 7927, 9073)

Body System Preferred Term	Ovidrel® 250 µg (n=236) Incidence Rate % (n)
At Least One Adverse Event	33.1% (78)
APPLICATION SITE DISORDERS	14.0% (33)
INJECTION SITE PAIN	7.6% (18)
INJECTION SITE BRUISING	4.7% (11)
GASTRO-INTESTINAL SYSTEM DISORDERS	8.5% (20)
ABDOMINAL PAIN	4.2% (10)
NAUSEA	3.4% (8)
VOMITING	2.5% (6)
SECONDARY TERMS (POST-OPERATIVE PAIN)	4.7% (11)
POST-OPERATIVE PAIN	4.7% (11)

Adverse events not listed in Table 9 that occurred in less than 2% of patients treated with Ovidrel® 250 µg whether or not considered causally related to Ovidrel®, included: injection site inflammation and reaction, flatulence, diarrhea, hiccup, ectopic pregnancy, breast pain, intermenstrual bleeding, vaginal hemorrhage, cervical lesion, leukorrhea, ovarian hyperstimulation, uterine disorders, vaginitis, vaginal discomfort, body pain, back pain, fever, dizziness, headache, hot flashes, malaise, paraesthesias, rash, emotional lability, insomnia, upper respiratory tract infection, cough, dysuria, urinary tract infection, urinary incontinence, albuminuria, cardiac arrhythmia, genital moniliasis, genital herpes, leukocytosis, heart murmur and cervical carcinoma.

Table 10: Incidence of Adverse Events of r-hCG in Ovulation Induction (Study 8209)

Body System Preferred Term	Ovidrel® 250 µg (n=236) Incidence Rate % (n)
At Least One Adverse Event	26.2% (26)
APPLICATION SITE DISORDERS	16.2% (16)
INJECTION SITE INFLAMMATION	2.0% (2)
INJECTION SITE BRUISING	3.0% (3)
INJECTION SITE REACTION	3.0% (3)
REPRODUCTIVE DISORDERS, FEMALE	7.1% (7)
OVARIAN CYST	3.0% (3)
OVARIAN HYPERSTIMULATION	3.0% (3)
GASTRO-INTESTINAL SYSTEM DISORDERS	4.0% (4)
ABDOMINAL PAIN	3.0% (3)

Additional adverse events not listed in Table 10 that occurred in less than 2% of patients treated with Ovidrel® 250 µg, whether or not considered causally related to Ovidrel®, included: breast pain, flatulence, abdominal enlargement, pharyngitis, upper respiratory tract infection, hyperglycemia and pruritis.

The following medical events have been reported subsequent to pregnancies resulting from hCG therapy in controlled clinical studies:

1. Spontaneous Abortion
2. Ectopic Pregnancy
3. Premature Labor
4. Postpartum Fever
5. Congenital abnormalities

Of 125 clinical pregnancies reported following treatment with FSH and Ovidrel® 250 µg or 500 µg, three were associated with a congenital anomaly of the fetus or newborn. Among patients receiving Ovidrel® 250 µg, cranial malformation was detected in the fetus of one woman and a chromosomal abnormality (47, XXX) in another. These events were judged by the investigators to be of unlikely or unknown relation to treatment. These three events represent an incidence of major congenital malformations of 2.4%, which is consistent with the reported rate for pregnancies resulting from natural or assisted conception. In a woman who received Ovidrel® 500 µg, one birth in a set of triplets was associated with Down's syndrome and atrial septal defect. This event was considered to be unrelated to the study drug.

The following adverse reactions have been previously reported during menotropin therapy:

1. Pulmonary and vascular complications (see "**Warnings**")
2. Adnexal torsion (as a complication of ovarian enlargement)
3. Mild to moderate ovarian enlargement
4. Hemoperitoneum

There have been infrequent reports of ovarian neoplasms, both benign and malignant, in women who have undergone multiple drug regimens for ovulation induction; however, a causal relationship has not been established.

DOSAGE AND ADMINISTRATION

For Subcutaneous Use Only

Infertile Women Undergoing Assisted Reproductive Technologies (ART)

Ovidrel® PreFilled Syringe 250 µg should be administered one day following the last dose of the follicle stimulating agent. Ovidrel® PreFilled Syringe should not be administered until adequate follicular development is indicated by serum estradiol and vaginal ultrasonography. Administration should be withheld in situations where there is an excessive ovarian response, as evidenced by clinically significant ovarian enlargement or excessive estradiol production.

Infertile Women Undergoing Ovulation Induction (OI)

Ovidrel® PreFilled Syringe should not be administered until adequate follicular development is indicated by serum estradiol and vaginal ultrasonography.

Ovidrel® PreFilled Syringe 250 µg should be administered one day following the last dose of the follicle stimulating agent.

Ovidrel® PreFilled Syringe administration should be withheld in situations where there is an excessive ovarian response, as evidenced by multiple follicular development, clinically significant ovarian enlargement or excessive estradiol production.

Directions for Administration of Ovidrel® Prefilled Syringe:

Ovidrel® PreFilled Syringe is intended for a single subcutaneous injection. Any unused material should be discarded.

Ovidrel® PreFilled Syringe may be self-administered by the patient. Follow the directions below for injecting Ovidrel® PreFilled Syringe.

Step 1: Wash your hands thoroughly with soap and water.

Step 2: Carefully clean the injection site.

Make yourself comfortable by sitting or lying down. Carefully clean the injection site on the stomach with an alcohol wipe and allow it to air-dry.

Step 3: Administer your injection.

Carefully remove the needle cap from the syringe. Do not touch the needle or allow the needle to touch any surface. Inject the prescribed dose as directed by your doctor, nurse or pharmacist.

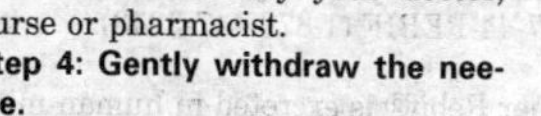

Step 4: Gently withdraw the needle.

Discard the needle and syringe into your safety container. Place gauze over the injection site. If any bleeding occurs, apply gentle pressure. If bleeding does not stop within a few minutes, place a clean piece of gauze over the injection site and cover it with an adhesive bandage.

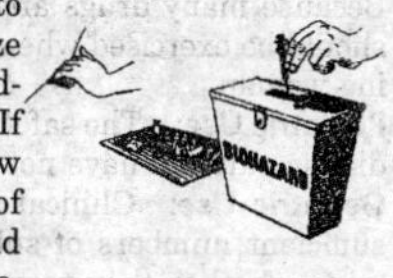

Step 5: Storage and clean up.

Remember that your injection materials must be kept sterile and cannot be reused.

HOW SUPPLIED

Ovidrel® PreFilled Syringe (choriogonadotropin alfa injection) is supplied in a sterile, liquid single dose pre-filled 1 mL syringe. Each Ovidrel® PreFilled Syringe is filled with 0.515 mL containing 257.5 µg of choriogonadotropin alfa, 28.1 mg mannitol, 505 µg 85% O-phosphoric acid, 103 µg L-methionine, 51.5 µg Poloxamer 188, Sodium Hydroxide (for pH adjustment), and Water for Injection to deliver 250 µg of choriogonadotropin alfa in 0.5 mL.

The following package combination is available:

- 1 prefilled syringe containing 250 µg Ovidrel® PreFilled Syringe NDC 44087-1150-1

Storage: The Ovidrel® PreFilled Syringe must be stored refrigerated between 2-8°C (36-46°F) before being dispensed to the patient. Patients should store the prefilled syringe refrigerated to allow the product to be used until the expiry date shown on the syringe or carton. The Ovidrel® PreFilled Syringe may be stored by the patient for no more than 30 days at room temperature [up to 25°C (77°F)] but must be used within those 30 days.

Protect from light.

Store in original package. Discard unused material.

Rx Only

Manufactured For:

Serono, Inc. Rockland, MA 02370

January, 2004

Shown in Product Identification Guide, page 333

REBIF® ℞

[rē'-bif]

(interferon beta-1a)

DESCRIPTION

Rebif® (interferon beta-1a) is a purified 166 amino acid glycoprotein with a molecular weight of approximately 22,500 daltons. It is produced by recombinant DNA technology using genetically engineered Chinese Hamster Ovary cells into which the human interferon beta gene has been introduced. The amino acid sequence of Rebif® is identical to that of natural fibroblast derived human interferon beta. Natural interferon beta and interferon beta-1a (Rebif®) are glycosylated with each containing a single N-linked complex carbohydrate moiety.

Using a reference standard calibrated against the World Health Organization natural interferon beta standard (Second International Standard for Interferon, Human Fibroblast GB 23 902 531), Rebif® has a specific activity of approximately 270 million international units (MIU) of antiviral activity per mg of interferon beta-1a determined specifically by an in vitro cytopathic effect bioassay using WISH cells and Vesicular Stomatitis virus. Rebif® 22 mcg and 44 mcg contains approximately 6 MIU or 12 MIU, respectively, of antiviral activity using this method.

Rebif® (interferon beta-1a) is formulated as a sterile solution in a prefilled syringe intended for subcutaneous (sc) injection. Each 0.5 ml (0.5 cc) of Rebif® contains either 22 mcg or 44 mcg of interferon beta-1a, 2 or 4 mg albumin (human) USP, 27.3 mg mannitol USP, 0.4 mg sodium acetate, Water for Injection USP.

CLINICAL PHARMACOLOGY

General

Interferons are a family of naturally occurring proteins that are produced by eukaryotic cells in response to viral infection and other biological inducers. Interferons possess immunomodulatory, antiviral and antiproliferative biological activities. They exert their biological effects by binding to specific receptors on the surface of cells. Three major groups of interferons have been distinguished: alpha, beta, and gamma. Interferons alpha and beta form the Type I interferons and interferon gamma is a Type II interferon. Type I interferons have considerably overlapping but also distinct biological activities. Interferon beta is produced naturally by various cell types including fibroblasts and macrophages. Binding of interferon beta to its receptors initiates a complex cascade of intracellular events that leads to the expression of numerous interferon-induced gene products and markers, including 2', 5'-oligoadenylate synthetase, beta 2-microglobulin and neopterin, which may mediate some of the biological activities. The specific interferon-induced proteins and mechanisms by which interferon beta-1a exerts its effects in multiple sclerosis have not been fully defined.

Pharmacokinetics

The pharmacokinetics of Rebif® (interferon beta-1a) in people with multiple sclerosis have not been evaluated. In healthy volunteer subjects, a single subcutaneous (sc) injection of 60 mcg of Rebif® (liquid formulation), resulted in a peak serum concentration (C_{max} of 5.1 ± 1.7 IU/mL (mean ± SD), with a median time of peak serum concentration (T_{max}) of 16 hours. The serum elimination half-life ($t_{1/2}$) was 69 ± 37 hours, and the area under the serum concentration versus time curve (AUC) from zero to 96 hours was 294 ± 81 IU·h/mL. Following every other day sc injections in healthy volunteer subjects, an increase in AUC of approximately 240% was observed, suggesting that accumulation of interferon beta-1a occurs after repeat administration. Total clearance is approximately 33–55 L/hours. There have been no observed gender-related effects on pharmacokinetic parameters. Pharmacokinetics of Rebif® in pediatric and geriatric patients or patients with renal or hepatic insufficiency have not been established.

Pharmacodynamics

Biological response markers (e.g., 2', 5'-OAS activity, neopterin and beta 2-microglobulin) are induced by interferon beta-1a following parenteral doses administered to healthy volunteer subjects and to patients with multiple sclerosis. Following a single sc administration of 60 mcg of Rebif® intracellular 2', 5'-OAS activity peaked between 12 to 24 hours and beta-2-microglobulin and neopterin serum concentrations showed a maximum at approximately 24 to 48 hours. All three markers remained elevated for up to four days. Administration of Rebif® 22 mcg three times per week (tiw) inhibited mitogen-induced release of pro-inflammatory cytokines (IFN-γ, IL-1, IL-6, TNF-α and TNF-β) by peripheral blood mononuclear cells that, on average, was near double that observed with Rebif® administered once per week (qw) at either 22 or 66 mcg.

The relationships between serum interferon beta-1a levels and measurable pharmacodynamic activities to the mechanism(s) by which Rebif® exerts its effects in multiple sclerosis are unknown. No gender-related effects on pharmacodynamic parameters have been observed.

CLINICAL STUDIES

Two multicenter studies evaluated the safety and efficacy of Rebif® in patients with relapsing-remitting multiple sclerosis.

Study 1 was a randomized, double-blind, placebo controlled study in patients with multiple sclerosis for at least one year, Kurtzke Expanded Disability Status Scale (EDSS) scores ranging from 0 to 5, and at least 2 acute exacerbations in the previous 2 years.[1] Patients with secondary progressive multiple sclerosis were excluded from the study. Patients received sc injections of either placebo (n = 187), Rebif® 22 mcg (n = 189), or Rebif® 44 mcg (n = 184) administered tiw for two years. Doses of study agents were progressively increased to their target doses during the first 4 to 8 weeks for each patient in the study (see DOSAGE AND ADMINISTRATION).

The primary efficacy endpoint was the number of clinical exacerbations. Numerous secondary efficacy endpoints were also evaluated and included exacerbation-related parameters, effects of treatment on progression of disability and magnetic resonance imaging (MRI)-related parameters. Progression of disability was defined as an increase in the EDSS score of at least 1 point sustained for at least 3 months. Neurological examinations were completed every 3 months, during suspected exacerbations, and coincident with MRI scans. All patients underwent proton density T2-weighted (PD/T2) MRI scans at baseline and every 6 months. A subset of 198 patients underwent PD/T2 and T1-weighted gadolinium-enhanced (Gd)-MRI scans monthly for the first 9 months. Of the 560 patients enrolled, 533 (95%) provided 2 years of data and 502 (90%) received 2 years of study agent.

Study results are shown in Table 1 and Figure 1. Rebif® at doses of 22 mcg and 44 mcg administered sc tiw significantly reduced the number of exacerbations per patient as compared to placebo. Differences between the 22 mcg and 44 mcg groups were not significant (p >0.05).

The exact relationship between MRI findings and the clinical status of patients is unknown. Changes in lesion area often do not correlate with changes in disability progression. The prognostic significance of the MRI findings in these studies has not been evaluated.

[See table 1 above]

Table 1: Clinical and MRI Endpoints from Study 1

	Placebo	22 mcg tiw	44 mcg tiw
	n = 187	n = 189	n = 184
Exacerbation-related			
Mean number of exacerbations per patient over 2 years[1,2]	2.56	1.82**	1.73***
(Percent reduction)		(29%)	(32%)
Percent (%) of patients exacerbation-free at 2 years[3]	15%	25%*	32%***
Median time to first exacerbation (months)[1,4]	4.5	7.6**	9.6***
MRI	n = 172	n = 171	n = 171
Median percent (%) change of MRI PD-T2 lesion area at 2 years[5]	11.0	-1.2***	-3.8***
Median number of active lesions per patient per scan (PD/T2; 6 monthly)[5]	2.25	0.75***	0.5***

* p<0.05 compared to placebo
** p<0.001 compared to placebo
*** p<0.0001 compared to placebo
(1) Intent-to-treat analysis.
(2) Poisson regression model adjusted for center and time on study
(3) Logistic regression adjusted for center. Patients lost to follow-up prior to an exacerbation were excluded from this analysis (n = 185, 183, and 184 for the placebo, 22 mcg tiw, and 44 mcg tiw groups, respectively).
(4) Cox proportional hazard model adjusted for center
(5) ANOVA on ranks adjusted for center. Patients with missing scans were excluded from this analysis

The time to onset of progression in disability sustained for three months was significantly longer in patients treated with Rebif® than in placebo-treated patients. The Kaplan-Meier estimates of the proportions of patients with sustained disability are depicted in Figure 1.

Figure 1: Proportions of Patients with Sustained Disability Progression

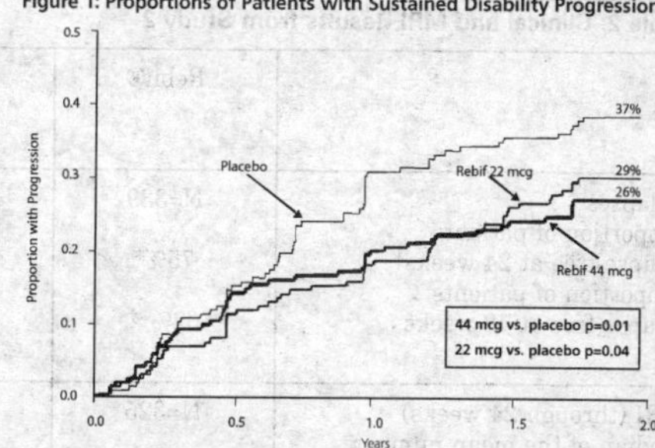

The safety and efficacy of treatment with Rebif® beyond 2 years have not been established.

Study 2 was a randomized, open-label, evaluator-blinded, active comparator study[2]. Patients with relapsing-remitting multiple sclerosis with EDSS scores ranging from 0 to 5.5, and at least 2 exacerbations in the previous 2 years

Continued on next page

Rebif—Cont.

were eligible for inclusion. Patients with secondary progressive multiple sclerosis were excluded from the study. Patients were randomized to treatment with Rebif® 44 mcg tiw by sc injection (n=339) or Avonex® 30 mcg qw by intramuscular (im) injection (n=338). Study duration was 48 weeks.

The primary efficacy endpoint was the proportion of patients who remained exacerbation-free at 24 weeks. The principal secondary endpoint was the mean number per patient per scan of combined unique active MRI lesions through 24 weeks, defined as any lesion that was T1 active or T2 active. Neurological examinations were performed every three months by a neurologist blinded to treatment assignment. Patient visits were conducted monthly, and mid-month telephone contacts were made to inquire about potential exacerbations. If an exacerbation was suspected, the patient was evaluated with a neurological examination. MRI scans were performed monthly and analyzed in a treatment–blinded manner.

Patients treated with Rebif® 44 mcg sc tiw were more likely to remain relapse-free at 24 and 48 weeks than were patients treated with Avonex® 30 mcg im qw (Table 2). This study does not support any conclusion regarding effects on the accumulation of physical disability.

[See table 2 below]

The adverse reactions over 48 weeks were generally similar between the two treatment groups. Exceptions included injection site disorders (83% of patients on Rebif® vs. 28% of patients on Avonex®), hepatic function disorders (18% on Rebif® vs. 10% on Avonex®), and leukopenia (6% on Rebif® vs. <1% on Avonex®), which were observed with greater frequency in the Rebif® group compared to the Avonex® group.

INDICATIONS AND USAGE

Rebif® (interferon-beta-1a) is indicated for the treatment of patients with relapsing forms of multiple sclerosis to decrease the frequency of clinical exacerbations and delay the accumulation of physical disability. Efficacy of Rebif® in chronic progressive multiple sclerosis has not been established.

CONTRAINDICATIONS

Rebif® (interferon beta-1a) is contraindicated in patients with a history of hypersensitivity to natural or recombinant interferon, human albumin, or any other component of the formulation.

WARNINGS

Depression

Rebif® (interferon beta-1a) should be used with caution in patients with depression, a condition that is common in people with multiple sclerosis. Depression, suicidal ideation, and suicide attempts have been reported to occur with increased frequency in patients receiving interferon compounds, including Rebif®. Patients should be advised to report immediately any symptoms of depression and/or suicidal ideation to the prescribing physician. If a patient develops depression, cessation of treatment with Rebif® should be considered.

Hepatic Injury

Severe liver dysfunction, leading to hepatic failure requiring liver transplantation, has been reported very rarely in patients taking Rebif®. Symptomatic hepatic dysfunction, including hepatitis, primarily presenting as jaundice, has been reported as a rare complication of Rebif® use. Asymptomatic elevation of hepatic transaminases (particularly SGPT) is common with interferon therapy (see ADVERSE REACTIONS). Rebif® should be initiated with caution in patients with active liver disease, alcohol abuse, increased serum SGPT (> 2.5 times ULN), or a history of significant liver disease. Dose reduction should be considered if SGPT rises above 5 times the upper limit of normal. The dose may be gradually re-escalated when enzyme levels have normalized. Treatment with Rebif® should be stopped if jaundice or other clinical symptoms of liver dysfunction appear.

Anaphylaxis

Anaphylaxis has been reported as a rare complication of Rebif® use. Other allergic reactions have included skin rash and urticaria, and have ranged from mild to severe without a clear relationship to dose or duration of exposure. Several allergic reactions, some severe, have occurred after prolonged use.

Albumin (Human)

This product contains albumin, a derivative of human blood. Based on effective donor screening and product manufacturing processes, it carries an extremely remote risk for transmission of viral diseases. A theoretical risk for transmission of Creutzfeldt-Jakob disease (CJD) also is considered extremely remote. No cases of transmission of viral diseases or CJD have ever been identified for albumin.

PRECAUTIONS

General

Caution should be exercised when administering Rebif® to patients with pre-existing seizure disorders. Seizures have been associated with the use of beta interferons. A relationship between occurrence of seizures and the use of Rebif® has not been established. Leukopenia and new or worsening thyroid abnormalities have developed in some patients treated with Rebif® (see ADVERSE REACTIONS). Regular monitoring for these conditions is recommended (see PRECAUTIONS: Laboratory Tests).

Information for Patients

All patients should be instructed to read the Rebif® Medication Guide supplied to them. Patients should be cautioned not to change the dosage or the schedule of administration without medical consultation.

Patients should be informed of the most common and the most severe adverse reactions associated with the use of Rebif® (see WARNINGS and ADVERSE REACTIONS). Patients should be advised of the symptoms associated with these conditions, and to report them to their physician.

Female patients should be cautioned about the abortifacient potential of Rebif® (see PRECAUTIONS: Pregnancy).

Patients should be instructed in the use of aseptic technique when administering Rebif®. Appropriate instruction for self-injection or injection by another person should be provided, including careful review of the Rebif® Medication Guide. If a patient is to self-administer Rebif®, the physical and cognitive ability of that patient to self-administer and properly dispose of syringes should be assessed. The initial injection should be performed under the supervision of an appropriately qualified health care professional. Patients should be advised of the importance of rotating sites of injection with each dose, to minimize the likelihood of severe injection site reactions or necrosis. A puncture-resistant container for disposal of used needles and syringes should be supplied to the patient along with instructions for safe disposal of full containers. Patients should be instructed in the technique and importance of proper syringe disposal and be cautioned against reuse of these items.

Laboratory Tests

In addition to those laboratory tests normally required for monitoring patients with multiple sclerosis, blood cell counts and liver function tests are recommended at regular intervals (1, 3, and 6 months) following introduction of Rebif® therapy and then periodically thereafter in the absence of clinical symptoms. Thyroid function tests are recommended every 6 months in patients with a history of thyroid dysfunction or as clinically indicated. Patients with myelosuppression may require more intensive monitoring of complete blood cell counts, with differential and platelet counts.

Drug Interactions

No formal drug interaction studies have been conducted with Rebif®. Due to its potential to cause neutropenia and lymphopenia, proper monitoring of patients is required if Rebif® is given in combination with myelosuppressive agents.

Carcinogenesis, Mutagenesis, Impairment of Fertility

Carcinogenesis: No carcinogenicity data for Rebif® are available in animals or humans.

Mutagenesis: Rebif® was not mutagenic when tested in the Ames bacterial test and in an *in vitro* cytogenetic assay in human lymphocytes in the presence and absence of metabolic activation.

Impairment of Fertility: No studies have been conducted to evaluate the effects of Rebif® on fertility in humans. In studies in normally cycling female cynomolgus monkeys given daily sc injections of Rebif® for six months at doses of up to 9 times the recommended weekly human dose (based on body surface area), no effects were observed on either menstrual cycling or serum estradiol levels. The validity of extrapolating doses used in animal studies to human doses is not established. In male monkeys, the same doses of Rebif® had no demonstrable adverse effects on sperm count, motility, morphology, or function.

Pregnancy Category C

Rebif® treatment has been associated with significant increases in embryolethal or abortifacient effects in cynomolgus monkeys administered doses approximately 2 times the cumulative weekly human dose (based on either body weight or surface area) either during the period of organogenesis (gestation day 21–89) or later in pregnancy. There were no fetal malformations or other evidence of teratogenesis noted in these studies. These effects are consistent with the abortifacient effects of other type I interferons. There are no adequate and well-controlled studies of Rebif® in pregnant women. However, in Studies 1 and 2, there were 2 spontaneous abortions observed and 5 fetuses carried to term among 7 women in the Rebif® groups. If a woman becomes pregnant or plans to become pregnant while taking Rebif®, she should be informed about the potential hazards to the fetus and discontinuation of Rebif® should be considered.

A pregnancy registry has been established to monitor pregnancy outcomes of women exposed to Rebif® while pregnant. Health care providers are encouraged to register patients on line at rebifpregnancyregistry.com or by calling MS LifeLines at 1-877-44-REBIF (1-877-447-3243).

Nursing Mothers

It is not known whether Rebif® is excreted in human milk. Because many drugs are excreted in human milk, caution should be exercised when Rebif® is administered to a nursing woman.

Pediatric Use: The safety and effectiveness of Rebif® in pediatric patients have not been studied.

Geriatric Use: Clinical studies of Rebif® did not include sufficient numbers of subjects aged 65 and over to determine whether they respond differently than younger subjects. In general, dose selection for an elderly patient should be cautious, usually starting at the low end of the dosing range, reflecting the greater frequency of decreased hepatic, renal or cardiac function, and of concomitant disease or other drug therapy.

ADVERSE REACTIONS

The most frequently reported serious adverse reactions with Rebif® were psychiatric disorders including depression and suicidal ideation or attempt (see WARNINGS). The incidence of depression of any severity in the Rebif®-treated groups and placebo-treated group was approximately 25%. The most commonly reported adverse reactions were injection site disorders, influenza-like symptoms (headache, fatigue, fever, rigors, chest pain, back pain, myalgia), abdominal pain, depression, elevation of liver enzymes and hematologic abnormalities. The most frequently reported adverse reactions resulting in clinical intervention (e.g., discontinuation of Rebif®, adjustment in dosage, or the need for concomitant medication to treat an adverse reaction symptom) were injection site disorders, influenza-like symptoms, depression and elevation of liver enzymes (see WARNINGS).

In Study 1, 6 patients randomized to Rebif® 44 mcg tiw (3%), and 2 patients who received Rebif® 22 mcg tiw (1%) developed injection site necrosis during two years of therapy. Rebif® was continued in 7 patients and interrupted briefly in one patient. There was one report of injection site necrosis in Study 2 during 48 weeks of Rebif® treatment. All events resolved with conservative management; none required skin debridement or grafting.

The rates of adverse reactions and association with Rebif® in patients with relapsing-remitting multiple sclerosis are drawn from the placebo-controlled study (n = 560) and the active comparator-controlled study (n = 339).

The population encompassed an age range from 18 to 55 years. Nearly three-fourths of the patients were female, and more than 90% were Caucasian, largely reflecting the general demographics of the population of patients with multiple sclerosis.

Because clinical trials are conducted under widely varying conditions, adverse reaction rates observed in the clinical trials of Rebif® cannot be directly compared to rates in the clinical trials of other drugs and may not reflect the rates observed in practice.

Table 3 enumerates adverse events and laboratory abnormalities that occurred at an incidence that was at least 2% more in either Rebif®-treated group than was observed in the placebo group.

[See table 3 at top of next page]

The adverse reactions were generally similar in Studies 1 and 2, taking into account the disparity in study durations.

Immunogenicity

As with all therapeutic proteins, there is a potential for immunogenicity. In study 1, the presence of neutralizing antibodies (NAb) to Rebif® was determined by collecting and analyzing serum pre-study and at 6 month time intervals during the 2 years of the clinical trial. Serum NAb were de-

Table 2: Clinical and MRI Results from Study 2

	Rebif®	Avonex®	Absolute Difference	Risk of relapse on Rebif® relative to Avonex®
Relapses	N=339	N=338	12%	0.68
Proportion of patients relapse-free at 24 weeks[1]	75%*	63%	(95% CI: 5%, 19%)	(95% CI: 0.54, 0.86)
Proportion of patients relapse-free at 48 weeks	62%**	52%	10% (95% CI: 2%, 17%)	0.81 (95% CI: 0.68, 0.96)
MRI (through 24 weeks)	N=325	N=325		
Median of the mean number of combined unique MRI lesions per patient per scan[2] (25th, 75th percentiles)	0.17* (0.00, 0.67)	0.33 (0.00, 1.25)		

* p <0.001, and ** p = 0.009, Rebif® compared to Avonex®

(1) Logistic regression model adjusted for treatment and center, intent to treat analysis

(2) Nonparametric ANCOVA model adjusted for treatment and center, with baseline combined unique lesions as the single covariate.

Table 3. Adverse Reactions and Laboratory Abnormalities in Study 1

Body System Preferred Term	Placebo tiw (n=187)	Rebif® 22 mcg tiw (n=189)	Rebif® 44 mcg tiw (n=184)
BODY AS A WHOLE			
Influenza-like symptoms	51%	56%	59%
Headache	63%	65%	70%
Fatigue	36%	33%	41%
Fever	16%	25%	28%
Rigors	5%	6%	13%
Chest Pain	5%	6%	8%
Malaise	1%	4%	5%
INJECTION SITE DISORDERS			
Injection Site Reaction	39%	89%	92%
Injection Site Necrosis	0%	1%	3%
CENTRAL & PERIPH NERVOUS SYSTEM DISORDERS			
Hypertonia	5%	7%	6%
Coordination Abnormal	2%	5%	4%
Convulsions	2%	5%	4%
ENDOCRINE DISORDERS			
Thyroid Disorder	3%	4%	6%
GASTROINTESTINAL SYSTEM DISORDERS			
Abdominal Pain	17%	22%	20%
Dry Mouth	1%	1%	5%
LIVER AND BILIARY SYSTEM DISORDERS			
SGPT Increased	4%	20%	27%
SGOT Increased	4%	10%	17%
Hepatic Function Abnormal	2%	4%	9%
Bilirubinaemia	1%	3%	2%
MUSCULO-SKELETAL SYSTEM DISORDERS			
Myalgia	20%	25%	25%
Back Pain	20%	23%	25%
Skeletal Pain	10%	15%	10%
HEMATOLOGIC DISORDERS			
Leukopenia	14%	28%	36%
Lymphadenopathy	8%	11%	12%
Thrombocytopenia	2%	2%	8%
Anemia	3%	3%	5%
PSYCHIATRIC DISORDERS			
Somnolence	1%	4%	5%
SKIN DISORDERS			
Rash Erythematous	3%	7%	5%
Rash Maculo-Papular	2%	5%	4%
URINARY SYSTEM DISORDERS			
Micturition Frequency	4%	2%	7%
Urinary Incontinence	2%	4%	2%
VISION DISORDERS			
Vision Abnormal	7%	7%	13%
Xerophthalmia	0%	3%	1%

Table 4: Schedule for Patient Titration

	Recommended Titration (% of final dose)	Titration dose for Rebif® 22 mcg	Titration dose for Rebif® 44 mcg	Injection Volume
Weeks 1–2	20 %	4.4 mcg	8.8 mcg	0.1 mL
Weeks 3–4	50 %	11 mcg	22 mcg	0.25 mL
Weeks 5+	100 %	22 mcg	44 mcg	0.5 mL

tected in 59/189 (31%) and 45/184 (24%) of Rebif®-treated patients at the 22 mcg and 44 mcg tiw doses, respectively, at one or more times during the study. The clinical significance of the presence of NAb to Rebif® is unknown.

The data reflect the percentage of patients whose test results were considered positive for antibodies to Rebif® using an antiviral cytopathic effect assay, and are highly dependent on the sensitivity and specificity of the assay. Additionally, the observed incidence of NAb positivity in an assay may be influenced by several factors including sample handling, timing of sample collection, concomitant medications and underlying disease. For these reasons, comparison of the incidence of antibodies to Rebif® with the incidence of antibodies to other products may be misleading.

Anaphylaxis and other allergic reactions have been observed with the use of Rebif® (see WARNINGS: Anaphylaxis).

DRUG ABUSE AND DEPENDENCE

There is no evidence that abuse or dependence occurs with Rebif® therapy. However, the risk of dependence has not been systematically evaluated.

OVERDOSAGE

Safety of doses higher than 44 mcg sc tiw have not been adequately evaluated. The maximum amount of Rebif® that can be safely administered has not been determined.

DOSAGE AND ADMINISTRATION

Dosages of Rebif® shown to be safe and effective are 22 mcg and 44 mcg injected subcutaneously three times per week. Rebif® should be administered, if possible, at the same time (preferably in the late afternoon or evening) on the same three days (e.g. Monday, Wednesday, and Friday) at least 48 hours apart each week (see CLINICAL STUDIES). Generally, patients should be started at 20% of the prescribed dose tiw and increased over a 4-week period to the targeted dose, either 22 mcg or 44 mcg tiw (see Table 4). Following the administration of each dose, any residual product remaining in the syringe should be discarded in a safe and proper manner.

[See table 4 above]

Leukopenia or elevated liver function tests may necessitate dose reductions of 20–50% until toxicity is resolved (see WARNINGS: Hepatic Injury and PRECAUTIONS: General).

Rebif® is intended for use under the guidance and supervision of a physician. It is recommended that physicians or qualified medical personnel train patients in the proper technique for self-administering subcutaneous injections using the prefilled syringe. Patients should be advised to rotate sites for sc injections (see PRECAUTIONS: Information for Patients). Concurrent use of analgesics and/or antipyretics may help ameliorate flu-like symptoms on treatment days. Rebif® should be inspected visually for particulate matter and discoloration prior to administration.

Stability and Storage

Rebif® should be stored refrigerated between 2-8°C (36-46°F). DO NOT FREEZE. If a refrigerator is not available, Rebif® may be stored at or below 25° C/77° F for up to 30 days and away from heat and light.

Do not use beyond the expiration date printed on packages. Rebif® contains no preservatives. Each syringe is intended for single use. Unused portions should be discarded.

HOW SUPPLIED

Rebif® is supplied as a sterile, preservative-free solution packaged in graduated, ready to use 0.5 mL prefilled syringes with 29-gauge, 0.5 inch needle for subcutaneous injection. The following package presentations are available.

Rebif® (interferon beta -1a) 22 mcg Prefilled syringe

- One Rebif® 22 mcg prefilled syringe, NDC 44087-0022-1
- Twelve Rebif® 22 mcg prefilled syringes, NDC 44087-0022-3

Rebif® (interferon beta -1a) 44 mcg Prefilled syringe

- One Rebif® 44 mcg prefilled syringe, NDC 44087-0044-1
- Twelve Rebif® 44 mcg prefilled syringes, NDC 44087-0044-3

RX only.

REFERENCES

1. PRISMS Study Group. Randomized double-blind placebo-controlled study of interferon β-1a in relapsing/remitting multiple sclerosis. Lancet 1998; 352: 1498–1504.
2. Panitch H. Goodin DS, Francis G, et al. Randomized, comparative study of interferon β-1a treatment regimens in MS. The EVIDENCE Trial. Neurology 2002 59:1496–1506

Manufacturer: Serono, Inc. Rockland, MA 02370
U.S. License # 1574
Co-Marketed by:
Serono, Inc.
Rockland, MA 02370
Pfizer Inc.
New York, NY 10017
Revised: March 2004

*Avonex® is a registered trademark of Biogen, Inc.

N6700101B

Medication Guide

Rebif (Re-bif)

Interferon beta-1a

(in-ter-feer-on beta-one-â)

Please read this leaflet carefully before you start to use Rebif® and each time your prescription is refilled since there may be new information. The information in this medication guide does not take the place of regularly talking with your doctor or healthcare professional.

What is the most important information I should know about Rebif®?

Rebif® will not cure multiple sclerosis (MS) but it has been shown to decrease the number of flare-ups and slow the occurrence of some of the physical disability that is common in people with MS. Rebif® can cause serious side effects, so before you start taking Rebif®, you should talk with your doctor about the possible benefits of Rebif® and its possible side effects to decide if Rebif® is right for you. Potential serious side effects include:

- **Depression.** Some patients treated with interferons, including Rebif®, have become seriously depressed (feeling sad). Some patients have thought about or have attempted to kill themselves. Depression (a sinking of spirits or sadness) is not uncommon in people with multiple sclerosis. However, if you are feeling noticeably sadder or helpless, or feel like hurting yourself or others, you should tell a family member or friend right away and call your doctor as soon as possible. Your doctor may ask that you stop using Rebif®. You should also tell your doctor if you have ever had any mental illness, including depression, and if you take any medications for depression.
- **Liver problems.** Your liver may be affected by taking Rebif® and a few patients have developed severe liver injury. Your healthcare provider may ask you to have regular blood tests to make sure that your liver is working properly. If your skin or the whites of your eyes become yellow or if you are bruising easily you should call your doctor right away.
- **Risk to pregnancy.** If you become pregnant while taking Rebif® you should stop using Rebif® immediately and call your doctor. Rebif® may cause you to lose your baby (miscarry) or may cause harm to your unborn child. You and your doctor will need to decide whether the potential benefit of taking Rebif® is greater than the risks are to your unborn child.

  A pregnancy registry has been established to monitor pregnancy outcomes of women exposed to Rebif® while pregnant. Patients are encouraged to have their health care provider register them at rebifpregnancyregistry.com or by calling MS LifeLines at 1-877-44-REBIF (1-877-447-3243).
- **Allergic reactions.** Some patients taking Rebif® have had severe allergic reactions leading to difficulty breathing, and loss of consciousness. Allergic reactions can happen after your first dose or may not happen until after you have taken Rebif® many times. Less severe allergic reactions such as itching, flushing or skin bumps can also happen at any time. If you think you are having an allergic reaction, stop using Rebif® immediately and call your doctor.
- **Injection site problems.** Rebif® may cause redness, pain or swelling at the place where an injection was given. A few patients have developed skin infections or areas of severe skin damage (necrosis). If one of your injection sites becomes swollen and painful or the area looks infected and it doesn't heal within a few days, you should call your doctor.

What is Rebif®?

Rebif® is a type of protein called beta interferon that occurs naturally in the body. It is used to treat relapsing forms of multiple sclerosis. It will not cure your MS but may decrease the number of flare-ups of the disease and slow the occurrence of some of the physical disability that is common in people with MS. MS is a life-long disease that affects your nervous system by destroying the protective covering (myelin) that surrounds your nerve fibers. The way Rebif® works in MS is not known.

Continued on next page

Rebif—Cont.

Who should not take Rebif®?

Do not take Rebif® if you:

- have had an allergic reaction such as difficulty breathing, flushing or hives to another interferon beta or to human albumin.

If you have any of the following conditions or serious medical problems, you should tell your doctor *before* taking Rebif®:

- Depression (a sinking feeling or sadness), anxiety (feeling uneasy or fearful for no reason), or trouble sleeping
- Liver diseases
- Problems with your thyroid gland
- Blood problems such as bleeding or bruising easily and anemia (low red blood cells) or low white blood cells
- Epilepsy
- Are planning to become pregnant

Tell your doctor about all medicines you take, including prescription and non-prescription medicines, vitamins and herbal supplements. Rebif® and other medicines may affect each other causing serious side effects. Talk to your doctor before you take any new medicines

How should I take Rebif®?

Rebif® is given by injection under the skin (subcutaneous injection) on the same three days a week (for example, Monday, Wednesday and Friday). Your injections should be at least 48 hours apart so it is best to take them the same time each day. Your doctor will tell you what dose of Rebif® to use, and may change the dose based on how your body responds. You should not change the dose without talking with your doctor.

If you miss a dose, you should take your next dose as soon as you remember or are able to take it, then skip the following day. **Do not take Rebif® on two consecutive days.** You should return to your regular schedule the following week. If you accidentally take more than your prescribed dose, or take it on two consecutive days, call your doctor right away. You should always follow your doctor's instructions and advice about how to take this medication. If your doctor feels that you, or a family member or friend may give you the injections then you and/or the other person should be trained by your doctor or healthcare provider in how to give an injection. Do not try to give yourself (or have another person give you) injections at home until you (or both of you) understand and are comfortable with how to prepare your dose and give the injections.

Always use a new, unopened, prefilled syringe of Rebif® for each injection. Never reuse syringes.

It is important that you change your injection site each time Rebif® is injected. This will lessen the chance of your having a serious skin reaction at the spot where you inject Rebif®. You should always avoid injecting Rebif into an area of skin that is sore, reddened, infected or otherwise damaged.

At the end of this leaflet there are detailed instructions on how to prepare and give an injection of Rebif®. You should become familiar with these instructions and follow your doctor's orders before injecting Rebif®.

What should I avoid while taking Rebif®?

- **Pregnancy.** You should avoid becoming pregnant while taking Rebif® until you have talked with your doctor. Rebif® can cause you to lose your baby (miscarry).
- **Breast feeding.** You should talk to your doctor if you are breast feeding an infant. It is not known if the interferon in Rebif® can be passed to an infant in mother's milk, and it is not known whether the drug could harm the infant if it is passed to an infant.
- Rebif® and other medicines may affect each other causing serious side effects. Talk to your doctor before you take any new medicines.

What are the possible side effects of Rebif®?

- **Flu-like symptoms.** Most patients have flu-like symptoms (fever, chills, sweating, muscle aches and tiredness). For many patients, these symptoms will lessen or go away over time. You should talk to your doctor about whether you should take an over the counter medication for pain or fever reduction before or after taking your dose of Rebif®.
- **Skin reactions.** Soreness, redness, pain, bruising or swelling may occur at the place of injection. (see: "*What is the most important information I should know about Rebif®?*")
- **Depression and anxiety.** Some patients taking interferons have become very depressed and or anxious. There have been patients taking interferons who have had thoughts about killing themselves. If you feel sad or hopeless you should tell a friend or family member right away and call your doctor immediately. (see: "*What is the most important information I should know about Rebif®?*")
- **Liver problems.** Your liver function may be affected. If you develop symptoms of changes in your liver, includeing yellowing of the skin and whites of the eyes and easy bruising, call your doctor immediately. (see: "*What is the most important information I should know about Rebif®?*")
- **Blood problems.** You may have a drop in the levels of infection-fighting blood cells, red blood cells or cells that help to form blood clots. If the drop in levels are severe, they can lessen your ability to fight infections, make you feel tired or sluggish or cause you to bruise or bleed easily.
- **Thyroid** problems: Your thyroid function may change. Symptoms of changes in the function of your thyroid include feeling cold or hot all the time, change in your weight (gain or loss) without a change in your diet or amount of exercise you are getting.
- **Allergic reactions:** Some patients have had hives, rash, skin bumps or itching while they were taking Rebif®. Other patients have had more serious allergic reactions such as difficulty breathing, or feeling light-headed. You should tell your doctor if you think you are having an allergic reaction. (see: "*What is the most important information I should know about Rebif®?*")

Whether you experience any of these side effects or not, you and your doctor should periodically talk about your general health. Your doctor may want to monitor you more closely and ask you to have blood tests done more frequently.

Storage Conditions

Rebif® is packaged in prefilled syringes with needles already attached to the syringe.

Rebif® should be stored refrigerated between 2–8°C (36–46°F). DO NOT FREEZE.

If a refrigerator is not available, Rebif® may be stored at or below 25° C/77° F for up to 30 days and away from heat and light.

General Information About Prescription Medicines

Medicines are sometimes prescribed for purposes other than those listed in a Medication Guide. This medication has been prescribed for your particular medical condition. Do not use it for another condition or give this drug to anyone else. If you have any questions you should speak with your doctor or health care professional. You may also ask your doctor or pharmacist for a copy of the information provided to them with the product.

Keep this and all drugs out of the reach of children.

Instructions for Preparing and Giving Yourself an Injection of Rebif®

Before you begin, gather all of the supplies listed below:

- Rebif® prefilled syringe with 27 gauge needle. You may wish to remove your syringe from the refrigerator at least 30 minutes prior to use and let it adjust to room temperature so the liquid is not cold. Do not heat or microwave a syringe.
- Alcohol swabs (wipes) or cotton balls and rubbing alcohol
- Small adhesive bandage strip (if desired)
- Puncture resistant safety container for disposal of used syringes
- Antibacterial soap
- An over-the-counter pain or fever reducing medication, if your doctor has recommended that you take this prior to, at the same time, or after you give yourself Rebif® to help minimize the fever, chills, sweating and muscle aches (flu-like symptoms) that may occur.

When first starting treatment with Rebif®, your doctor may prescribe either the 22 mcg or 44 mcg dose of Rebif®. It is advised to gradually increase the dose over 4 weeks, starting at 20% for 2 weeks, 50% for 2 weeks and then the targeted dose.

Preparing for an injection:

- Check the expiration date; **do not use if the medication is expired.** The expiration date is printed on the syringe, plastic syringe packaging and carton.
- Be sure that the dose, either 22 mcg or 44 mcg, described on the carton is the same as the dose prescribed by your doctor.
- Remove the Rebif® syringe from the plastic packaging. Keep the needle capped.
- Examine the contents of the syringe carefully. The liquid should be clear to slightly yellow. **Do not use if the liquid is cloudy, discolored or contains particles.**
- Choose the injection site. The best sites for giving yourself an injection are those areas with a layer of fat between the skin and muscle, like your thigh, the outer surface of your upper arm, your stomach or buttocks. Do not use the area near your navel or waistline. If you are very thin, use only the thigh or outer surface of the arm for injection. Use a different site each time you inject (thigh, hip, stomach or upper arm, see Figure below). Do not inject Rebif® into an area of your body where the skin is irritated, reddened, bruised, infected or abnormal in any way.
- Keep a record of the date and location of each injection.
- Wash your hands thoroughly with antibacterial soap before preparing to inject the medication.
- Clean the injection site with an alcohol swab (wipe) or cotton ball with rubbing alcohol using a circular motion. To avoid stinging, you should let your skin dry before you inject Rebif®.

[See first figure at top of next column]

Giving yourself an injection of Rebif®

- Remove the needle cap from the syringe needle.
- If your doctor has told you to use less than the full 0.5ml dose, slowly push the plunger in until the amount of medication left in the syringe is the amount your doctor told you to use.

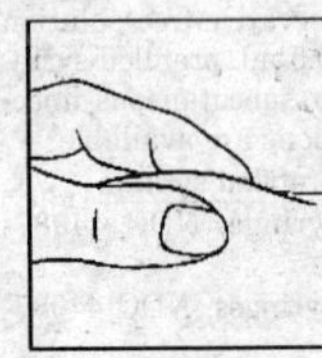

- Use your thumb and forefinger to pinch a pad of skin surrounding the cleaned injection site (see figure below). Hold the syringe like a pencil with your other hand.

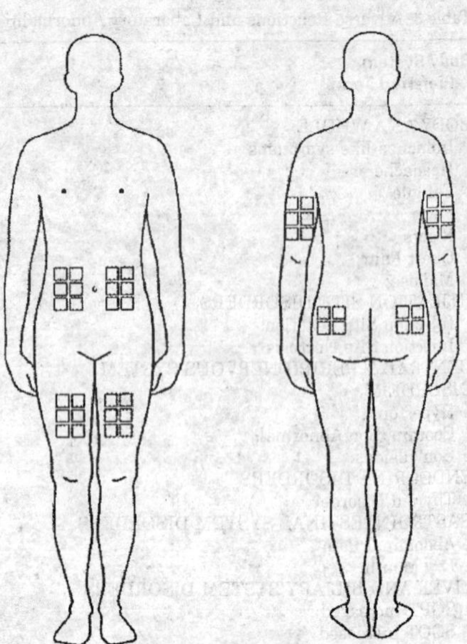

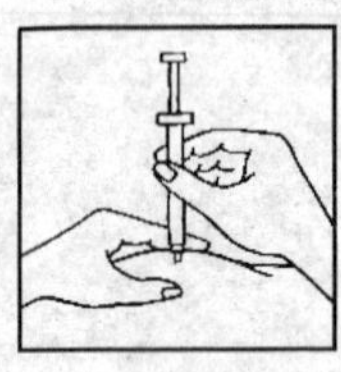

- While still pinching the skin, swiftly insert the needle like a dart at about a 90 degree angle (just under the skin) into the pad of tissue as shown.

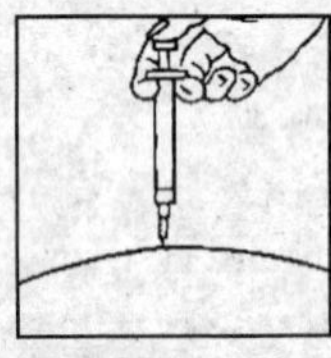

- After the needle is in, remove the hand that you used to pinch your skin and inject the drug using a slow, steady push on the plunger until all the medication is injected and the syringe is empty.

- Withdraw the needle and apply gentle pressure to the injection site with a dry cotton ball or sterile gauze. Applying a cold compress or ice pack to the injection site after injection may help reduce local skin reactions.
- Put a small adhesive bandage strip over the injection site, if desired.
- After 2 hours, check the injection site for redness, swelling, or tenderness. If you have a skin reaction and it doesn't clear up in a few days, contact your doctor or nurse.

Disposing of Needles and Syringes

There are special state or local laws for properly disposing used needles and syringes. Your doctor or health care professional will instruct you on how to discard your used syringe and needle and may provide you with a puncture resistant syringe disposal container called a Sharps container. Always keep your disposal container out of the reach of children.

DO NOT throw the needle and syringe in the household trash or recycle.

This Medication Guide has been approved by the U.S. Food and Drug Administration.

Manufactured by:
Serono, Inc.
Rockland, MA 02370
U.S. License 1574
Co-Marketed by:
Serono, Inc.
Rockland, MA 02370
Pfizer Inc
New York, NY 10017
Rev (3), March 2004

Shown in Product Identification Guide, page 333

SAIZEN® ℞

[sī- zen]

[somatropin (rDNA origin) for injection]
For subcutaneous or intramuscular injection

DESCRIPTION

Saizen® [somatropin (rDNA origin) for injection] is a human growth hormone produced by recombinant DNA technology. Saizen® has 191 amino acid residues and a molecular weight of 22,125 daltons. Its amino acid sequence and structure are identical to the dominant form of human pituitary growth hormone. Saizen® is produced by a mammalian cell line (mouse C127) that has been modified by the addition of the human growth hormone gene. Saizen®, with the correct three-dimensional configuration, is secreted directly through the cell membrane into the cell-culture medium for collection and purification.

Saizen® is a highly purified preparation. Biological potency is determined by measuring the increase in body weight induced in hypophysectomized rats.

Saizen® is a sterile, non-pyrogenic, white, lyophilized powder intended for subcutaneous or intramuscular injection after reconstitution with Bacteriostatic Water for Injection, USP (0.9% Benzyl Alcohol). The reconstituted solution has a pH of 6.5 to 8.5.

Saizen® is available in 5 mg and 8.8 mg vials. The quantitative composition per vial is:

5 mg (approximately 15 IU) vial:

Each vial contains 5.0 mg somatropin (approximately 15 IU), 34.2 mg sucrose and 1.165 mg O-phosphoric acid. The pH is adjusted with sodium hydroxide or O-phosphoric acid.

8.8 mg (approximately 26.4 IU) vial:

Each vial contains 8.8 mg somatropin (approximately 26.4 IU), 60.2 mg sucrose and 2.05 mg O-phosphoric acid. The pH is adjusted with sodium hydroxide or O-phosphoric acid.

The diluent is Bacteriostatic Water for Injection, USP containing 0.9% Benzyl Alcohol added as an antimicrobial preservative.

Saizen® is also available for use with the one.click auto injector pen and click.easy reconstitution device. The quantitative composition per vial contained in the click.easy reconstitution device is:

8.8 mg (approximately 26.4 IU) vial contained in the click.easy device:

Each vial contains 8.8 mg somatropin (approximately 26.4 IU), 60.2 mg sucrose and 2.05 mg O-phosphoric acid. The pH is adjusted with sodium hydroxide or O-phosphoric acid.

The diluent contained in the click.easy device is Bacteriostatic Water for Injection, USP containing 0.3% (w/v) metacresol added as an antimicrobial preservative.

HOW SUPPLIED

Saizen can be administered using (1) a standard, sterile, disposable syringe and needle, (2) the cool.click™ needle-free growth hormone delivery device or (3) the one.click autoinjector pen with the click.easy reconstitution device. For proper use, refer to the Instructions for Use provided with either the cool.click™ needle-free device or the one.click™ autoinjector pen / click.easy™ reconstitution device.

Saizen® [somatropin (rDNA origin) for injection] is a sterile, non-pyrogenic, white, lyophilized powder supplied in packages containing:

1 vial of 5 mg (approximately 15 IU) Saizen® and 1 vial of 10 mL Bacteriostatic Water for Injection, USP (0.9% Benzyl Alcohol) NDC 44087-1005-2

1 vial of 8.8 mg (approximately 26.4 IU) Saizen® and 1 vial of 10 mL Bacteriostatic Water for Injection, USP (0.9% Benzyl Alcohol) NDC 44087-1088-1

℞ Only

1 click.easy cartridge of 8.8 mg (approximately 26.4 IU) Saizen and 1.37 mL Bacteriostatic Water for Injection (0.3% (w/v) metacresol) NDC 44087-1080-1

5 click.easy cartridges of 8.8 mg (approximately 26.4 IU) Saizen and 1.37 mL Bacteriostatic Water for Injection (0.3% (w/v) metacresol) NDC 44087-1080-2

July, 2004

Manufactured for: Serono, Inc., Rockland, MA 02370

®-Registered trademark of Serono Inc., Rockland, MA 02370

SEROPHENE® ℞

[*se 'ro-fēn*]

(clomiPHENE citrate tablets, USP)

DESCRIPTION

ClomiPHENE citrate is an orally administered, nonsteroidal, ovulatory stimulant designated chemically as 2-[p-(2-chloro-1,2-diphenylvinyl)phenoxy] triethylamine citrate (1:1). It has a molecular formula of $C_{26}H_{28}ClNO \cdot C_6H_8O_7$ and a molecular weight of 598.09. It is represented structurally as:

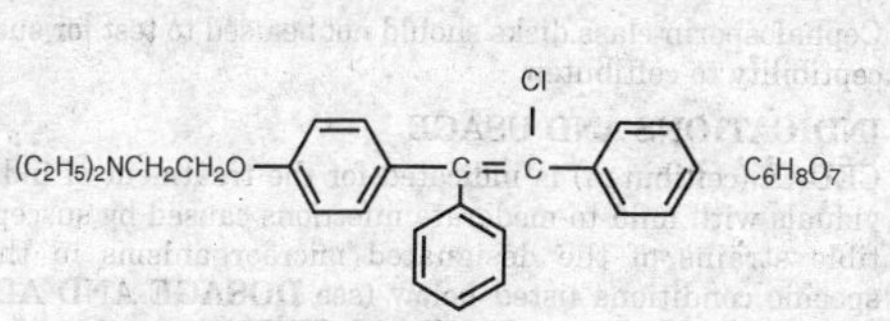

ClomiPHENE citrate is a white to pale yellow, essentially odorless, crystalline powder. It is freely soluble in methanol; soluble in ethanol; slightly soluble in acetone, water, and chloroform; and insoluble in ether.

ClomiPHENE citrate is a mixture of two geometric isomers [cis (zuclomiPHENE) and trans (enclomiPHENE)] containing between 30% and 50% of the cis-isomer.

Each white scored tablet contains 50 mg clomiPHENE citrate USP. The tablet also contains the following inactive ingredients: lactose, microcrystalline cellulose, starch, colloidal silicon dioxide, magnesium stearate and sodium starch glycolate.

HOW SUPPLIED

Serophene® (clomiPHENE citrate tablets USP) is available as 50 mg scored white tablets in the following package combinations:

- 1 carton 10 tablets, NDC 44087-8090-6
  Each carton contains 2 strips of 5 tablets each.
- 1 carton 30 tablets, NDC 44087-8090-1
  Each carton contains 3 strips of 10 tablets, each in a 2 × 5 arrangement.

Store tablets at controlled room temperature 59–86°F (15–30°C) [See USP]. Protect from heat, light, excessive humidity, and store in closed containers.

Rx Only

Manufactured for:
Serono, Inc.
Rockland, MA 02370
Revised: Dec. 2002

SEROSTIM® ℞

[*sē-rō-stĭm*]

[somatropin (rDNA origin) for injection]

DESCRIPTION

Serostim® [somatropin (rDNA origin) for injection] is a human growth hormone (hGH) produced by recombinant DNA technology. Serostim® has 191 amino acid residues and a molecular weight of 22,125 daltons. Its amino acid sequence and structure are identical to the dominant form of human pituitary GH. Serostim® is produced by a mammalian cell line (mouse C127) that has been modified by the addition of the hGH gene. Serostim® is secreted directly through the cell membrane into the cell-culture medium for collection and purification.

Serostim® is a highly purified preparation. Biological potency is determined by measuring the increase in the body weight induced in hypophysectomized rats.

Serostim® is available in 4 mg, 5 mg and 6 mg vials for single dose administration.

Each 4 mg vial contains 4.0 mg (approximately 12 IU) somatropin, 27.3 mg sucrose, 0.9 mg phosphoric acid. Each 5 mg vial contains 5.0 mg (approximately 15 IU) somatropin, 34.2 mg sucrose and 1.2 mg phosphoric acid. Each 6 mg vial contains 6.0 mg (approximately 18 IU) somatropin, 41.0 mg sucrose and 1.4 mg phosphoric acid. The pH is adjusted with sodium hydroxide or phosphoric acid to give a pH of 7.4 to 8.5 after reconstitution.

HOW SUPPLIED

Serostim® [somatropin (rDNA origin) for injection] is available in the following forms: Serostim® vials containing 4 mg (approximately 12 IU) somatropin (mammalian-cell) with Sterile Water for Injection, USP. Package of 7 vials. NDC 44087-0004-7

Serostim® vials containing 5 mg (approximately 15 IU) somatropin (mammalian-cell) with Sterile Water for Injection, USP. Package of 7 vials. NDC 44087-0005-7

Serostim® vials containing 6 mg (approximately 18 IU) somatropin (mammalian-cell) with Sterile Water for Injection, USP. Package of 7 vials. NDC 44087-0006-7

Manufactured for: Serono, Inc., Rockland, MA 02370

Rx Only **BX Rated**

August 2003

ZORBTIVE™ ℞

[*zorb-tiv*]

[somatropin (rDNA origin) for injection]

Rx Only BX Rated

DESCRIPTION

Zorbtive™ [somatropin (rDNA origin) for injection] is a human growth hormone (hGH) produced by recombinant DNA technology. Zorbtive™ has 191 amino acid residues and a molecular weight of 22,125 daltons. It's amino acid sequence and structure are identical to the dominant form of human pituitary GH. Zorbtive™ is produced by a mammalian cell line (mouse C127) that has been modified by the addition of the hGH gene. Zorbtive™ is secreted directly through the cell membrane into the cell-culture medium for collection and purification.

Zorbtive™ is a highly purified preparation. Biological potency is determined by measuring the increase in the body weight induced in hypophysectomized rats.

Zorbtive™ is available in 8.8 mg vials for multi-dose administration. Each 8.8 mg vial contains 8.8 mg (approximately 26.4 IU) somatropin, 60.19 mg sucrose and 2.05 mg phosphoric acid. The pH is adjusted with sodium hydroxide or phosphoric acid to give a pH of 7.4 to 8.5 after reconstitution.

HOW SUPPLIED

Zorbtive™ [somatropin (rDNA origin) for injection] is available in the following form:

Zorbtive™ vial containing 8.8 mg (approximately 26.4 IU) somatropin (mammalian-cell) with Bacteriostatic Water for Injection, USP (0.9% Benzyl Alcohol), 10 mL, Package of 7 vials.

NDC 44087-3388-7

Manufactured for: Serono, Inc., Rockland, MA 02370

January 2004

EDUCATIONAL MATERIAL

Access the Serono website www.seronousa.com for product, educational, and service information for practitioners and consumers.

To receive available educational and medical literature about Serono products, or the conditions they treat, phone inquiries can be made by calling the U.S. Medical Information Group at (888) 275-7376 or (781) 982-9000.

To obtain information about scientific, medical, nursing and consumer educational meetings and materials, please contact Serono Symposia USA, Inc., (800) 283-8088, X 2352.

Shionogi USA

100 CAMPUS DRIVE
FLORHAM PARK, NJ 07932

Direct Inquiries to:
Phone (973) 966-6900
Fax (973) 966-2820

CEDAX® ℞

[*sē-dăks*]

(ceftibuten capsules)
and
(ceftibuten for oral suspension)
FOR ORAL USE ONLY

DESCRIPTION

CEDAX (ceftibuten capsules) and (ceftibuten for oral suspension) contain the active ingredient ceftibuten as ceftibuten dihydrate. Ceftibuten dihydrate is a semisynthetic cephalosporin antibiotic for oral administration. Chemically, it is (+)-(6R,7R)-7-[(Z)-2-(2-Amino-4-thiazolyl)-4-carboxycroton-amido]-8-oxo-5-thia-1-azabicyclo[4.2.0]oct-2-ene-2-carboxylic acid, dihydrate. Its molecular formula is $C_{15}H_{14}N_4O_6S_2 \cdot 2H_2O$. Its molecular weight is 446.43 as the dihydrate.

Ceftibuten dihydrate has the following structural formula:

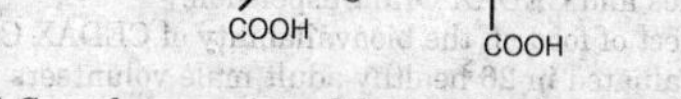

CEDAX Capsules contain ceftibuten dihydrate equivalent to 400 mg of ceftibuten. Inactive ingredients contained in the capsule formulation include: magnesium stearate, microcrystalline cellulose, and sodium starch glycolate. The capsule shell and/or band contains gelatin, sodium lauryl sulfate, titanium dioxide, and polysorbate 80. The capsule shell may also contain benzyl alcohol, sodium propionate, edetate calcium disodium, butylparaben, propylparaben, and methylparaben.

CEDAX Oral Suspension after reconstitution contains ceftibuten dihydrate equivalent to 90 mg of ceftibuten per 5 mL. CEDAX Oral Suspension is cherry flavored and contains the inactive ingredients: cherry flavoring, polysorbate 80, silicon dioxide, simethicone, sodium benzoate, sucrose (approximately 1 g/5 mL), titanium dioxide, and xanthan gum.

CLINICAL PHARMACOLOGY

PHARMACOKINETICS

Absorption:

CEDAX CAPSULES

Ceftibuten is rapidly absorbed after oral administration of CEDAX Capsules. The plasma concentrations and pharmacokinetic parameters of ceftibuten after a single 400-mg dose of CEDAX Capsules to 12 healthy adult male volunteers (20 to 39 years of age) are displayed in the table below. When CEDAX Capsules were administered once daily for 7 days, the average C_{max} was 17.9 µg/mL on day 7. Therefore, ceftibuten accumulation in plasma is about 20% at steady state.

CEDAX ORAL SUSPENSION

Ceftibuten is rapidly absorbed after oral administration of CEDAX Oral Suspension. The plasma concentrations and pharmacokinetic parameters of ceftibuten after a single 9-mg/kg dose of CEDAX Oral Suspension to 32 fasting pediatric patients (6 months to 12 years of age) are displayed in the following table:

[See table at top of next page]

The absolute bioavailability of CEDAX Oral Suspension has not been determined. The plasma concentrations of ceftibuten in pediatric patients are dose proportional following single doses of CEDAX Capsules of 200 mg and 400 mg and of CEDAX Oral Suspension between 4.5 mg/kg and 9 mg/kg.

Distribution:

CEDAX CAPSULES

The average apparent volume of distribution (V/F) of ceftibuten in 6 adult subjects is 0.21 L/kg (± 1 SD = 0.03 L/kg).

Continued on next page

Cedax—Cont.

CEDAX ORAL SUSPENSION
The average apparent volume of distribution (V/F) of ceftibuten in 32 fasting pediatric patients is 0.5 L/kg (± 1 SD = 0.2 L/kg).

Protein Binding:
Ceftibuten is 65% bound to plasma proteins. The protein binding is independent of plasma ceftibuten concentration.

Tissue Penetration:
Bronchial secretions: In a study of 15 adults administered a single 400-mg dose of ceftibuten and scheduled to undergo bronchoscopy, the mean concentrations in epithelial lining fluid and bronchial mucosa were 15% and 37%, respectively, of the plasma concentrations.
Sputum: Ceftibuten sputum levels average approximately 7% of the concomitant plasma ceftibuten level. In a study of 24 adults administered ceftibuten 200 mg bid or 400 mg qd, the average C_{max} in sputum (1.5 μg/mL) occurred at 2 hours postdose and the average C_{max} in plasma (17 μg/mL) occurred at 2 hours postdose.
Middle-ear fluid (MEF): In a study of 12 pediatric patients administered 9 mg/kg, ceftibuten MEF area under the curve (AUC) averaged approximately 70% of the plasma AUC. In the same study, C_{max} values were 14.3 ± 2.7 μg/mL in MEF at 4 hours postdose and 14.5 ± 3.7 μg/mL in plasma at 2 hours postdose.
Tonsillar tissue: Data on ceftibuten penetration into tonsillar tissue are not available.
Cerebrospinal fluid: Data on ceftibuten penetration into cerebrospinal fluid are not available.

Metabolism and Excretion:
A study with radiolabeled ceftibuten administered to 6 healthy adult male volunteers demonstrated that *cis*-ceftibuten is the predominant component in both plasma and urine. About 10% of ceftibuten is converted to the *trans*-isomer. The *trans*-isomer is approximately 1/8 as antimicrobially potent as the *cis*-isomer.
Ceftibuten is excreted in the urine; 95% of the administered radioactivity was recovered either in urine or feces. In 6 healthy adult male volunteers, approximately 56% of the administered dose of ceftibuten was recovered from urine and 39% from the feces within 24 hours. Because renal excretion is a significant pathway of elimination, patients with renal dysfunction and patients undergoing hemodialysis require dosage adjustment (see **DOSAGE AND ADMINISTRATION**).

Food Effect on Absorption:
Food affects the bioavailability of ceftibuten from CEDAX Capsules and CEDAX Oral Suspension.
The effect of food on the bioavailability of CEDAX Capsules was evaluated in 26 healthy adult male volunteers who ingested 400 mg of CEDAX Capsules after an overnight fast or immediately after a standardized breakfast. Results showed that food delays the time of C_{max} by 1.75 hours, decreases the C_{max} by 18%, and decreases the extent of absorption (AUC) by 8%.
The effect of food on the bioavailability of CEDAX Oral Suspension was evaluated in 18 healthy adult male volunteers who ingested 400 mg of CEDAX Oral Suspension after an overnight fast or immediately after a standardized breakfast. Results obtained demonstrated a decrease in C_{max} of 26% and an AUC of 17% when CEDAX Oral Suspension was administered with a high-fat breakfast, and a decrease in C_{max} of 17% and in AUC of 12% when CEDAX Oral Suspension was administered with a low-calorie nonfat breakfast (see **PRECAUTIONS**).

Bioequivalence of Dosage Formulations:
A study in 18 healthy adult male volunteers demonstrated that a 400-mg dose of CEDAX Capsules produced equivalent concentrations to a 400-mg dose of CEDAX Oral Suspension. Average C_{max} values were 15.6 (3.1) μg/mL for the capsule and 17.0 (3.2) μg/mL for the suspension. Average AUC values were 80.1 (14.4) μg•hr/mL for the capsule and 87.0 (12.2) μg•hr/mL for the suspension.

Special Populations:
Geriatric patients: Ceftibuten pharmacokinetics have been investigated in elderly (65 years of age and older) men (n = 8) and women (n = 4). Each volunteer received ceftibuten 200-mg capsules twice daily for 3½ days. The average C_{max} was 17.5 (3.7) μg/mL after 3½ days of dosing compared to 12.9 (2.1) μg/mL after the first dose; ceftibuten accumulation in plasma was 40% at steady state. Information regarding the renal function of these volunteers was not available; therefore, the significance of this finding for clinical use of CEDAX Capsules in elderly patients is not clear. Ceftibuten dosage adjustment in elderly patients may be necessary (see **DOSAGE AND ADMINISTRATION**).
Patients with renal insufficiency: Ceftibuten pharmacokinetics have been investigated in adult patients with renal dysfunction. The ceftibuten plasma half-life increased and apparent total clearance (CI/F) decreased proportionately with increasing degree of renal dysfunction. In 6 patients with moderate renal dysfunction (creatinine clearance 30 to 49 mL/min), the plasma half-life of ceftibuten increased to 7.1 hours and CI/F decreased to 30 mL/min. In 6 patients with severe renal dysfunction (creatinine clearance 5 to 29 mL/min), the half-life increased to 13.4 hours and CI/F decreased to 16 mL/min. In 6 functionally anephric patients (creatinine clearance <5 mL/min), the half-life increased to 22.3 hours and CI/F decreased to 11 mL/min (a 7- to 8-fold change compared to healthy volunteers). Hemodialysis removed 65% of the drug from the blood in 2 to 4 hours. These

Parameter	Average Plasma Concentration (in μg/mL of ceftibuten after a single 400-mg dose) and Derived Pharmacokinetic Parameters (± 1 SD) (n = 12 healthy adult males)	Average Plasma Concentration (in μg/mL of ceftibuten after a single 9-mg/kg dose) and Derived Pharmacokinetic Parameters (± 1 SD) (n = 32 pediatric patients)
1.0 h	6.1 (5.1)	9.3 (6.3)
1.5 h	9.9 (5.9)	8.6 (4.4)
2.0 h	11.3 (5.2)	11.2 (4.6)
3.0 h	13.3 (3.0)	9.0 (3.4)
4.0 h	11.2 (2.9)	6.6 (3.1)
6.0 h	5.8 (1.6)	3.8 (2.5)
8.0 h	3.2 (1.0)	1.6 (1.3)
12.0 h	1.1 (0.4)	0.5 (0.4)
C_{max}, μg/mL	15.0 (3.3)	13.4 (4.9)
T_{max}, h	2.6 (0.9)	2.0 (1.0)
AUC, μg•h/mL	73.7 (16.0)	56.0 (16.9)
T½, h	2.4 (0.2)	2.0 (0.6)
Total body clearance (CI/F) mL/min/kg	1.3 (0.3)	2.9 (0.7)

changes serve as the basis for dosage adjustment recommendations in adult patients with mild to severe renal dysfunction (see **DOSAGE AND ADMINISTRATION**).

Microbiology:
Ceftibuten exerts its bactericidal action by binding to essential target proteins of the bacterial cell wall. This binding leads to inhibition of cell-wall synthesis.
Ceftibuten is stable in the presence of most plasmid-mediated beta-lactamases, but it is not stable in the presence of chromosomally-mediated cephalosporinases produced in organisms such as *Bacteroides, Citrobacter, Enterobacter, Morganella,* and *Serratia.* Like other beta-lactam agents, ceftibuten should not be used against strains resistant to beta-lactams due to general mechanisms such as permeability or penicillin-binding protein changes like penicillin-resistant *S. pneumoniae.*
Ceftibuten has been shown to be active against most strains of the following organisms both *in vitro* and in clinical infections (see **INDICATIONS AND USAGE**):

Gram-positive aerobes:
Streptococcus pneumoniae (penicillin-susceptible strains only)
Streptococcus pyogenes

Gram-negative aerobes:
Haemophilus influenzae (including β-lactamase-producing strains)
Moraxella catarrhalis (including β-lactamase-producing strains)

There are no known organisms which are potential pathogens in the indications approved for ceftibuten for which ceftibuten exhibits *in vitro* activity but for which the safety and efficacy of ceftibuten in treating clinical infections due to these organisms, have not been established in adequate and well-controlled trials.
NOTE: Ceftibuten is INACTIVE *in vitro* against *Acinetobacter, Bordetella, Campylobacter, Enterobacter, Enterococcus, Flavobacterium, Hafnia, Listeria, Pseudomonas, Staphylococcus,* and *Streptococcus* (except *pneumoniae* and *pyogenes*) species. In addition, it shows little *in vitro* activity against most anaerobes, including most species of *Bacteroides.*

Susceptibility Testing:
Dilution Techniques: Quantitative methods are used to determine antimicrobial minimal inhibitory concentrations (MICs). These MICs provide estimates of the susceptibility of bacteria to antimicrobial compounds. The MICs should be determined using a standardized procedure. Standardized procedures are based on a dilution method (broth, agar, or microdilution) or equivalent with standardized inoculum concentrations and standardized concentrations of ceftibuten powder. The MIC values should be interpreted according to the following criteria when testing *Haemophilus* species using Haemophilus Test Media (HTM):

MIC (μg/mL)	Interpretation
≤ 2	(S) Susceptible

The current absence of resistant strains precludes defining any categories other than "Susceptible". Strains yielding results suggestive of a "Nonsusceptible" category should be submitted to a reference laboratory for further testing.
A report of "Susceptible" implies that an infection due to the strain may be appropriately treated with the dosage of antimicrobial agent recommended for that type of infection and infecting species, unless otherwise contraindicated.
Ceftibuten is indicated for penicillin-susceptible only strains of *Streptococcus pneumoniae.* A pneumococcal isolate that is susceptible to penicillin (MIC ≤ 0.06 μg/mL) can be considered susceptible to ceftibuten for approved indications. Testing of ceftibuten against penicillin-intermediate or penicillin-resistant isolates is not recommended. Reliable interpretive criteria for ceftibuten are not currently available. Physicians should be informed that clinical response rates with ceftibuten may be lower in strains that are not penicillin-susceptible.
Standardized susceptibility test procedures require the use of laboratory control microorganisms to control the technical aspect of laboratory procedures. Standard ceftibuten powder should provide the following MIC values:

Organism	MIC range (μg/mL)
Haemophilus influenzae ATCC 49247	0.25-1.0

Diffusion Techniques: Quantitative methods that require measurement of zone diameters also provide estimates of the susceptibility of bacteria to antimicrobial compounds. One such standardized procedure requires the use of standardized inoculum concentrations. This procedure uses paper disks impregnated with 30 μg of ceftibuten to test the susceptibility of microorganisms to ceftibuten.
Reports from the laboratory providing results of the standard single-disk susceptibility test with a 30-μg ceftibuten disk should be interpreted according to the following criteria when testing *Haemophilus* species using Haemophilus Test Media (HTM):

Zone diameter (mm)	Interpretation
≥ 28	(S) Susceptible

The current absence of resistant strains precludes defining any categories other than "Susceptible". Strains yielding results suggestive of a "Nonsusceptible" category should be submitted to a reference laboratory for further testing.
Interpretation should be as stated above for results using dilution techniques.
Ceftibuten is indicated for penicillin-susceptible only strains of *Streptococcus pneumoniae.* Pneumococcal isolates with oxacillin zone sizes of ≥ 20 mm are susceptible to penicillin and can be considered susceptible for approved indications. Reliable disk diffusion tests for ceftibuten do not yet exist.
As with standardized dilution techniques, diffusion methods require the use of laboratory control microorganisms that are used to control the technical aspects of the laboratory procedures. For the diffusion technique, the 30-μg ceftibuten disk should provide the following zone diameters in these laboratory test quality control strains:

Organism	Zone diameter (mm)
Haemophilus influenzae ATCC 49247	29-35

Cephalosporin-class disks should not be used to test for susceptibility to ceftibuten.

INDICATIONS AND USAGE

CEDAX (ceftibuten) is indicated for the treatment of individuals with mild-to-moderate infections caused by susceptible strains of the designated microorganisms in the specific conditions listed below (see **DOSAGE AND ADMINISTRATION** and **CLINICAL STUDIES** sections).
Acute Bacterial Exacerbations of Chronic Bronchitis due to *Haemophilus influenzae* (including β-lactamase-producing strains), *Moraxella catarrhalis* (including β-lactamase-producing strains), or *Streptococcus pneumoniae* (penicillin-susceptible strains only).
NOTE: In acute bacterial exacerbations of chronic bronchitis clinical trials where *Moraxella catarrhalis* was isolated from infected sputum at baseline, ceftibuten clinical efficacy was 22% less than control.
Acute Bacterial Otitis Media due to *Haemophilus influenzae* (including β-lactamase-producing strains), *Moraxella catarrhalis* (including β-lactamase-producing strains), or *Streptococcus pyogenes.*

NOTE: Although ceftibuten used empirically was equivalent to comparators in the treatment of clinically and/or microbiologically documented acute otitis media, the efficacy against *Streptococcus pneumoniae* was 23% less than control. Therefore, ceftibuten should be given empirically **only** when adequate antimicrobial coverage against *Streptococcus pneumoniae* has been previously administered.

Pharyngitis and Tonsillitis due to *Streptococcus pyogenes*.

NOTE: Only penicillin by the intramuscular route of administration has been shown to be effective in the prophylaxis of rheumatic fever. Ceftibuten is generally effective in the eradication of *Streptococcus pyogenes* from the oropharynx; however, data establishing the efficacy of the CEDAX product for the prophylaxis of subsequent rheumatic fever are not available.

CONTRAINDICATIONS

CEDAX (ceftibuten) is contraindicated in patients with known allergy to the cephalosporin group of antibiotics.

WARNINGS

BEFORE THERAPY WITH THE CEDAX PRODUCT IS INSTITUTED, CAREFUL INQUIRY SHOULD BE MADE TO DETERMINE WHETHER THE PATIENT HAS HAD PREVIOUS HYPERSENSITIVITY REACTIONS TO CEFTIBUTEN OR ANY COMPONENTS, OTHER CEPHALOSPORINS OR ANY COMPONENTS, PENICILLINS, OR OTHER DRUGS. IF THIS PRODUCT IS TO BE GIVEN TO PENICILLIN-SENSITIVE PATIENTS, CAUTION SHOULD BE EXERCISED BECAUSE CROSS HYPERSENSITIVITY AMONG BETALACTAM ANTIBIOTICS HAS BEEN CLEARLY DOCUMENTED AND MAY OCCUR IN UP TO 10% OF PATIENTS WITH A HISTORY OF PENICILLIN ALLERGY. IF AN ALLERGIC REACTION TO THE CEDAX PRODUCT OCCURS, DISCONTINUE THE DRUG. SERIOUS ACUTE HYPERSENSITIVITY REACTIONS MAY REQUIRE TREATMENT WITH EPINEPHRINE AND OTHER EMERGENCY MEASURES, INCLUDING OXYGEN, INTRAVENOUS FLUIDS, INTRAVENOUS ANTIHISTAMINES, CORTICOSTEROIDS, PRESSOR AMINES, AND AIRWAY MANAGEMENT, AS CLINICALLY INDICATED.

Pseudomembranous colitis has been reported with nearly all antibacterial agents, including ceftibuten, and may range in severity from mild to life threatening. Therefore, it is important to consider this diagnosis in patients who present with diarrhea subsequent to the administration of antibacterial agents.

Treatment with antibacterial agents alters normal flora of the colon and may permit overgrowth of clostridia. Studies indicate that a toxin produced by *Clostridium difficile* is one primary cause of "antibiotic-associated colitis".

After the diagnosis of pseudomembranous colitis has been established, appropriate therapeutic measures should be initiated. Mild cases of pseudomembranous colitis usually respond to drug discontinuation alone. In moderate to severe cases, consideration should be given to management with fluids and electrolytes, protein supplementation, and treatment with an antibacterial drug clinically effective against *Clostridium difficile*.

PRECAUTIONS

General:

As with other broad-spectrum antibiotics, prolonged treatment may result in the possible emergence and overgrowth of resistant organisms. Careful observation of the patient is essential. If superinfection occurs during therapy, appropriate measures should be taken.

The dose of ceftibuten may require adjustment in patients with varying degrees of renal insufficiency, particularly in patients with creatinine clearance less than 50 mL/min or undergoing hemodialysis (see **DOSAGE AND ADMINISTRATION**). Ceftibuten is readily dialyzable. Dialysis patients should be monitored carefully, and administration of ceftibuten should occur immediately following dialysis.

Ceftibuten should be prescribed with caution to individuals with a history of gastrointestinal disease, particularly colitis.

Information to Patients:

Patients should be informed that:

- If the patient is diabetic, he/she should be informed that CEDAX Oral Suspension contains 1 gram sucrose per teaspoon of suspension.
- CEDAX Oral Suspension should be taken at least 2 hours before a meal or at least 1 hour after a meal (see **CLINICAL PHARMACOLOGY, Food Effect on Absorption**).

Drug Interactions:

Theophylline: Twelve healthy male volunteers were administered one 200-mg ceftibuten capsule twice daily for 6 days. With the morning dose of ceftibuten on day 6, each volunteer received a single intravenous infusion of theophylline (4 mg/kg). The pharmacokinetics of theophylline were not altered. The effect of ceftibuten on the pharmacokinetics of theophylline administered orally has not been investigated.

Antacids or H2-receptor antagonists: The effect of increased gastric pH on the bioavailability of ceftibuten was evaluated in 18 healthy adult volunteers. Each volunteer was administered one 400-mg ceftibuten capsule. A single dose of liquid antacid did not affect the C_{max} or AUC of ceftibuten; however, 150 mg of ranitidine q12h for 3 days increased the ceftibuten C_{max} by 23% and ceftibuten AUC by 16%. The clinical relevance of these increases is not known.

Drug/Laboratory Test Interactions:

There have been no chemical or laboratory test interactions with ceftibuten noted to date. False-positive direct Coombs' tests have been reported during treatment with other cephalosporins. Therefore, it should be recognized that a positive Coombs' test could be due to the drug. The results of assays using red cells from healthy subjects to determine whether ceftibuten would cause direct Coombs' reactions *in vitro* showed no positive reaction at ceftibuten concentrations as high as 40 µg/mL.

Carcinogenesis, Mutagenesis, Impairment of Fertility:

Long-term animal studies have not been performed to evaluate the carcinogenic potential of ceftibuten. No mutagenic effects were seen in the following studies: *in vitro* chromosome assay in human lymphocytes, *in vivo* chromosome assay in mouse bone marrow cells, Chinese Hamster Ovary (CHO) cell point mutation assay at the hypoxanthine-guanine phosphoribosyl transferase (HGPRT) locus, and in a bacterial reversion point mutation test (Ames). No impairment of fertility occurred when rats were administered ceftibuten orally up to 2000 mg/kg/day (approximately 43 times the human dose based on $mg/m^2/day$).

Pregnancy: Teratogenic effects: Pregnancy Category B:

Ceftibuten was not teratogenic in the pregnant rat at oral doses up to 400 mg/kg/day (approximately 8.6 times the human dose based on $mg/m^2/day$). Ceftibuten was not teratogenic in the pregnant rabbit at oral doses up to 40 mg/kg/day (approximately 1.5 times the human dose based on $mg/m^2/day$) and has revealed no evidence of harm to the fetus. There are no adequate and well-controlled studies in pregnant women. Because animal reproduction studies are not always predictive of human response, this drug should be used during pregnancy only if clearly needed.

Labor and Delivery:

Ceftibuten has not been studied for use during labor and delivery. Its use during such clinical situations should be weighed in terms of potential risk and benefit to both mother and fetus.

Nursing Mothers:

It is not known whether ceftibuten (at recommended dosages) is excreted in human milk. Because many drugs are excreted in human milk, caution should be exercised when ceftibuten is administered to a nursing woman.

Pediatric Use:

The safety and efficacy of ceftibuten in infants less than 6 months of age has not been established.

Geriatric Patients:

The usual adult dosage recommendation may be followed for patients in this age group. However, these patients should be monitored closely, particularly their renal function, as dosage adjustment may be required.

ADVERSE EVENTS

Clinical Trials:

CEDAX CAPSULES (adult patients)

In clinical trials, 1728 adult patients (1092 US and 636 international) were treated with the recommended dose of ceftibuten capsules (400 mg per day). There were no deaths or permanent disabilities thought due to drug toxicity in any of the patients in these studies. Thirty-six of 1728 (2%) patients discontinued medication due to adverse events thought by the investigators to be possibly, probably, or almost certainly related to drug toxicity. The discontinuations were primarily for gastrointestinal disturbances, usually diarrhea, vomiting, or nausea. Six of 1728 (0.3%) patients were discontinued due to rash or pruritus thought related to ceftibuten administration.

In the US trials, the following adverse events were thought by the investigators to be possibly, probably, or almost certainly related to ceftibuten capsules in multiple-dose clinical trials (n = 1092 ceftibuten-treated patients).

[See first table above]

ADVERSE REACTIONS
CEFTIBUTEN CAPSULES
US CLINICAL TRIALS IN ADULT PATIENTS (n = 1092)

Incidence equal to or greater than 1%	Nausea	4%
	Headache	3%
	Diarrhea	3%
	Dyspepsia	2%
	Dizziness	1%
	Abdominal Pain	1%
	Vomiting	1%
Incidence less than 1% but greater than 0.1%	Anorexia	
	Constipation	
	Dry mouth	
	Dyspnea	
	Dysuria	
	Eructation	
	Fatigue	
	Flatulence	
	Loose stools	
	Moniliasis	
	Nasal congestion	
	Paresthesia	
	Pruritus	
	Rash	
	Somnolence	
	Taste perversion	
	Urticaria	
	Vaginitis	

LABORATORY VALUE CHANGES*
CEFTIBUTEN CAPSULES
US CLINICAL TRIALS IN ADULT PATIENTS

Incidence equal to or greater than 1%	↑ BUN	4%
	↑ Eosinophils	3%
	↓ Hemoglobin	2%
	↑ ALT (SGPT)	1%
	↑ Bilirubin	1%
Incidence less than 1% but greater than 0.1%	↑ Alk phosphatase	
	↑ Creatinine	
	↑ Platelets	
	↓ Platelets	
	↓ Leukocytes	
	↑ AST (SGOT)	

*Changes in laboratory values with possible clinical significance regardless of whether or not the investigator thought that the change was due to drug toxicity.

CEDAX ORAL SUSPENSION (pediatric patients)

In clinical trials, 1152 pediatric patients (772 US and 380 international), 97% of whom were younger than 12 years of age, were treated with the recommended dose of ceftibuten (9 mg/kg once daily up to a maximum dose of 400 mg per day) for 10 days. There were no deaths, life-threatening adverse events, or permanent disabilities in any of the patients in these studies. Eight of 1152 (<1%) patients discontinued medication due to adverse events thought by the investigators to be possibly, probably, or almost certainly related to drug toxicity. The discontinuations were primarily (7 out of 8) for gastrointestinal disturbances, usually diarrhea or vomiting. One patient was discontinued due to a cutaneous rash thought possibly related to ceftibuten administration.

In the US trials, the following adverse events were thought by the investigators to be possibly, probably, or almost certainly related to ceftibuten oral suspension in multiple-dose clinical trials (n = 772 ceftibuten-treated patients).

[See first table at top of next page]

In Post-marketing Experience:

The following adverse experiences have been reported during worldwide post-marketing surveillance: aphasia, jaundice, melena, psychosis, serum sickness-like reactions, stridor, toxic epidermal necrolysis, and very rarely were transient elevations in LDH.

Cephalosporin-class Adverse Reactions:

In addition to the adverse reactions listed above that have been observed in patients treated with ceftibuten capsules, the following adverse events and altered laboratory tests have been reported for cephalosporin-class antibiotics: allergic reactions, anaphylaxis, drug fever, Stevens-Johnson syndrome, erythema multiforme, renal dysfunction, toxic

Continued on next page

Cedax—Cont.

nephropathy, hepatic cholestasis, aplastic anemia, hemolytic anemia, hemorrhage, false-positive test for urinary glucose, neutropenia, pancytopenia, and agranulocytosis. Pseudomembranous colitis; onset of symptoms may occur during or after antibiotic treatment (see **WARNINGS**). Several cephalosporins have been implicated in triggering seizures, particularly in patients with renal impairment when the dosage was not reduced (see **DOSAGE AND ADMINISTRATION** and **OVERDOSAGE**). If seizures associated with drug therapy occur, the drug should be discontinued. Anticonvulsant therapy can be given if clinically indicated.

OVERDOSAGE

Overdosage of cephalosporins can cause cerebral irritation leading to convulsions. Ceftibuten is readily dialyzable and significant quantities (65% of plasma concentrations) can be removed from the circulation by a single hemodialysis session. Information does not exist with regard to removal of ceftibuten by peritoneal dialysis.

DOSAGE AND ADMINISTRATION

The recommended doses of CEDAX Oral Suspension are presented in the table below. **CEDAX Oral Suspension must be administered at least 2 hours before or 1 hour after a meal.**

[See second table at right]

CEFTIBUTEN ORAL SUSPENSION
PEDIATRIC DOSAGE CHART

CHILD'S WEIGHT		90 mg/5 mL
10 kg	22 lbs	1 tsp QD
20 kg	44 lbs	2 tsp QD
40 kg	88 lbs	4 tsp QD

Pediatric patients weighing more than 45 kg should receive the maximum daily dose of 400 mg.

Renal Impairment:

CEDAX Capsules and CEDAX Oral Suspension may be administered at normal doses in the presence of impaired renal function with creatinine clearance of 50 mL/min or greater. The recommendations for dosing in patients with varying degrees of renal insufficiency are presented in the following table.

Creatinine Clearance (mL/min)	Recommended Dosing Schedules
>50	9 mg/kg or 400 mg Q24h (normal dosing schedule)
30-49	4.5 mg/kg or 200 mg Q24h
5-29	2.25 mg/kg or 100 mg Q24h

Hemodialysis Patients:

In patients undergoing hemodialysis two or three times weekly, a single 400-mg dose of ceftibuten capsules or a single dose of 9 mg/kg (maximum of 400 mg of ceftibuten) oral suspension may be administered at the end of each hemodialysis session.

[See third table at right]

After mixing, the suspension may be kept for 14 days and must be stored in the refrigerator. Keep tightly closed. Shake well before each use. Discard any unused portion after 14 days.

HOW SUPPLIED

CEDAX Capsules, containing 400 mg of ceftibuten (as ceftibuten dihydrate) are white, opaque capsules imprinted with the product name and strength, are available as follows:

20 Capsules/Bottle (NDC 64455-691-01)
100 Capsules/Bottle (NDC 64455-691-02)

Store the capsules between 2° and 25°C (36° and 77°F). Replace cap securely after each opening.

CEDAX Oral Suspension is an off-white to cream-colored powder that, when reconstituted as directed, contains ceftibuten equivalent to 90 mg/5 mL, supplied as follows:

90 mg/5 mL	
18 mg/mL	30-mL Bottle (NDC 64455-777-03)
18 mg/mL	60-mL Bottle (NDC 64455-777-01)
18 mg/mL	90-mL Bottle (NDC 64455-777-04)
18 mg/mL	120-mL Bottle (NDC 64455-777-02)

Prior to reconstitution, the powder must be stored between 2° and 25°C (36° and 77°F). Once it is reconstituted, the oral suspension is stable for 14 days when stored in the refrigerator between 2° and 8°C (36° and 46°F).

CLINICAL STUDIES

Acute Bacterial Exacerbations of Chronic Bronchitis:

Three clinical trials (two domestic, the third abroad) have been conducted testing ceftibuten in the treatment of acute exacerbations of chronic bronchitis (AECB). Overall, the clinical outcome among patients who had signs and symptoms of AECB, who had a gram stain showing a predominance of PMNs and few epithelial cells, and who were evaluated at approximately 1 to 2 weeks after completing therapy were equivalent to comparators. The bacterial eradication rates of specific pathogens are presented below.

BACTERIOLOGICAL OUTCOME
ACUTE BACTERIAL EXACERBATIONS
OF CHRONIC BRONCHITIS

	Ceftibuten 400 mg QD	Control
Bacteriological Eradication Rates		
Haemophilus influenzae	45/62 (73%)	23/36 (72%)
H. parainfluenzae	10/10	4/6
Moraxella catarrhalis	33/46 (72%)	32/34 (94%)
Streptococcus pneumoniae	23/35 (66%)	14/20 (70%)

Acute Bacterial Otitis Media:

Four clinical trials (three domestic, the fourth abroad) have been conducted testing ceftibuten in the treatment of acute bacterial otitis media. Overall, the clinical outcome among patients who had signs and symptoms of acute bacterial otitis media and who were evaluated at approximately 1 to 2 weeks after completing therapy were equivalent to comparators. Tympanocentesis was performed on patients in three of the above-mentioned studies; the bacterial eradication rates of specific pathogens are presented below.

BACTERIOLOGICAL OUTCOME
ACUTE BACTERIAL OTITIS MEDIA

	Ceftibuten 9 mg/kg QD	Control
Bacteriological Eradication Rates		
Haemophilus influenzae	56/67 (81%)	29/38 (76%)
Moraxella catarrhalis	20/26 (77%)	13/17 (77%)
Streptococcus pneumoniae	68/105 (65%)	35/40 (88%)
Streptococcus pyogenes	13/15 (87%)	5/5

REFERENCES

1. National Committee for Clinical Laboratory Standards. Methods for Dilution Antimicrobial Susceptibility Tests for Bacteria that Grow Aerobically – Third Edition. Approved Standard NCCLS Document M7-A3, Vol. 13, No. 25, NCCLS, Villanova, PA. December 1993.

ADVERSE REACTIONS
CEFTIBUTEN ORAL SUSPENSION
US CLINICAL TRIALS IN PEDIATRIC PATIENTS (n = 772)

Incidence equal to or greater than 1%	Diarrhea*	4%
	Vomiting	2%
	Abdominal pain	2%
	Loose stools	2%
Incidence less than 1% but greater than 0.1%	Agitation Anorexia Dehydration Diaper dermatitis Dizziness Dyspepsia Fever Headache Hematuria Hyperkinesia Insomnia Irritability Nausea Pruritus Rash Rigors Urticaria	

*NOTE: The incidence of diarrhea in pediatric patients ≤2 years old was 8% (23/301) compared with 2% (9/471) in pediatric patients >2 years old.

LABORATORY VALUE CHANGES*
CEFTIBUTEN ORAL SUSPENSION
US CLINICAL TRIALS IN PEDIATRIC PATIENTS

Incidence equal to or greater than 1%	↑ Eosinophils	3%
	↑ BUN	2%
	↓ Hemoglobin	1%
	↑ Platelets	1%
Incidence less than 1% but greater than 0.1%	↑ ALT (SGPT) ↑ AST (SGOT) ↑ Alk phosphatase ↑ Bilirubin ↑ Creatinine	

*Changes in laboratory values with possible clinical significance regardless of whether or not the investigator thought that the change was due to drug toxicity.

Type of infection (as qualified in the **INDICATIONS AND USAGE** section of this labeling)	Daily Maximum Dose	Dose and Frequency	Duration
ADULTS (12 years of age and older): Acute Bacterial Exacerbations of Chronic Bronchitis due to *H. influenzae* (including β-lactamase-producing strains), *M. catarrhalis* (including β-lactamase-producing strains), or *Streptococcus pneumoniae* (penicillin-susceptible strains only). (See **INDICATIONS AND USAGE—NOTE.**) Pharyngitis and tonsillitis due to *S. pyogenes*. Acute Bacterial Otitis Media due to *H. influenzae* (including β-lactamase-producing strains), *M. catarrhalis* (including β-lactamase-producing strains), or *S. pyogenes*. (See **INDICATIONS AND USAGE—NOTE.**)	400 mg	400 mg QD	10 days
PEDIATRIC PATIENTS: Pharyngitis and tonsillitis due to *S. pyogenes*. Acute Bacterial Otitis Media due to *H. influenzae* (including β-lactamase-producing strains), and *M. catarrhalis* (including β-lactamase-producing strains), or *S. pyogenes*. (See **INDICATIONS AND USAGE—NOTE.**)	400 mg	9 mg/kg QD	10 days

Directions for Mixing CEDAX Oral Suspension:

DIRECTIONS FOR MIXING CEDAX ORAL SUSPENSION

Final Concentration	Bottle Size	Amount of Water	Directions
90 mg per 5 mL	30 mL	Suspend in 28 mL of water	First tap the bottle to loosen powder. Then add water in two portions, shaking well after each aliquot.
	60 mL	Suspend in 53 mL of water	
	90 mL	Suspend in 78 mL of water	
	120 mL	Suspend in 103 mL of water	

2. National Committee for Clinical Laboratory Standards. Performance Standards for Antimicrobial Disk Susceptibility Tests – Fifth Edition. Approved Standard NCCLS Document M2-A5, Vol. 13, No. 24, NCCLS, Villanova, PA. December, 1993.

SHIONOGI USA, INC.
For Medical Information Monday Through Friday 9 a.m. –7 p.m. (Eastern Standard Time)
Tel: (800) 454-6149
Fax: (800) 881-6092
Shionogi USA, Inc., Florham Park, NJ 07932
Manufactured by Schering Corporation CED01PIB02
Distributed by Shionogi USA, Inc.

Shire US Inc.

ONE RIVERFRONT PLACE
NEWPORT, KY 41071-4570

Direct Inquiries to:
Customer Service
(800) 828-2088
(859) 669-8000
FAX: (859) 669-8420

For Medical Information Contact:
(800) 828-2088

ADDERALL® TABLETS Ⓒ℞

5 mg, 7.5 mg, 10 mg, 12.5 mg, 15 mg, 20 mg & 30 mg TABLETS
℞ Only

AMPHETAMINES HAVE A HIGH POTENTIAL FOR ABUSE. ADMINISTRATION OF AMPHETAMINES FOR PROLONGED PERIODS OF TIME MAY LEAD TO DRUG DEPENDENCE AND MUST BE AVOIDED. PARTICULAR ATTENTION SHOULD BE PAID TO THE POSSIBILITY OF SUBJECTS OBTAINING AMPHETAMINES FOR NON-THERAPEUTIC USE OR DISTRIBUTION TO OTHERS, AND THE DRUGS SHOULD BE PRESCRIBED OR DISPENSED SPARINGLY.

DESCRIPTION

A single entity amphetamine product combining the neutral sulfate salts of dextroamphetamine and amphetamine, with the dextro isomer of amphetamine saccharate and d, l-amphetamine aspartate.

EACH TABLET CONTAINS:	5 mg	7.5 mg	10 mg	12.5 mg	15 mg	20 mg	30 mg
Dextroamphetamine Saccharate	1.25 mg	1.875 mg	2.5 mg	3.125 mg	3.75 mg	5 mg	7.5 mg
Amphetamine Aspartate	1.25 mg	1.875 mg	2.5 mg	3.125 mg	3.75 mg	5 mg	7.5 mg
Dextroamphetamine Sulfate USP	1.25 mg	1.875 mg	2.5 mg	3.125 mg	3.75 mg	5 mg	7.5 mg
Amphetamine Sulfate USP	1.25 mg	1.875 mg	2.5 mg	3.125 mg	3.75 mg	5 mg	7.5 mg
Total amphetamine base equivalence	3.13 mg	4.7 mg	6.3 mg	7.8 mg	9.4 mg	12.6 mg	18.8 mg

[See table above]

Inactive Ingredients: acacia, corn starch, lactose, magnesium stearate, and sucrose.

Colors: ADDERALL 5 mg, 7.5 mg and 10 mg contain FD & C Blue #1.
ADDERALL 12.5 mg, 15 mg, 20 mg and 30 mg contain FD & C Yellow #6 as a color additive.

CLINICAL PHARMACOLOGY

Amphetamines are non-catecholamine sympathomimetic amines with CNS stimulant activity. Peripheral actions include elevation of systolic and diastolic blood pressures and weak bronchodilator and respiratory stimulant action.

There is neither specific evidence which clearly establishes the mechanism whereby amphetamine produces mental and behavioral effects in children, nor conclusive evidence regarding how these effects relate to the condition of the central nervous system.

INDICATIONS

Attention Deficit Disorder with Hyperactivity: Adderall is indicated as an integral part of a total treatment program which typically includes other remedial measures (psychological, educational, social) for a stabilizing effect in children with behavioral syndrome characterized by the following group of developmentally inappropriate symptoms: moderate to severe distractibility, short attention span, hyperactivity, emotional lability, and impulsivity. The diagnosis of this syndrome should not be made with finality when these symptoms are only of comparatively recent origin. Nonlocalizing (soft) neurological signs, learning disability and abnormal EEG may or may not be present, and a diagnosis of central nervous system dysfunction may or may not be warranted.

In Narcolepsy

CONTRAINDICATIONS

Advanced arteriosclerosis, symptomatic cardiovascular disease, moderate to severe hypertension, hyperthyroidism, known hypersensitivity or idiosyncrasy to the sympathomimetic amines, glaucoma.

Agitated states.

Patients with a history of drug abuse.

During or within 14 days following the administration of monoamine oxidase inhibitors (hypertensive crises may result).

WARNINGS

Clinical experience suggests that in psychotic children, administration of amphetamine may exacerbate symptoms of behavior disturbance and thought disorder. Data are inadequate to determine whether chronic administration of amphetamine may be associated with growth inhibition; therefore, growth should be monitored during treatment.

Usage in Nursing Mothers: Amphetamines are excreted in human milk. Mothers taking amphetamines should be advised to refrain from nursing.

PRECAUTIONS

General: Caution is to be exercised in prescribing amphetamines for patients with even mild hypertension. The least amount feasible should be prescribed or dispensed at one time in order to minimize the possibility of overdosage.

Information for Patients: Amphetamines may impair the ability of the patient to engage in potentially hazardous activities such as operating machinery or vehicles; the patient should therefore be cautioned accordingly.

Drug Interactions: *Acidifying agents*—Gastrointestinal acidifying agents (guanethidine, reserpine, glutamic acid HCl, ascorbic acid, fruit juices, etc.) lower absorption of amphetamines.

Urinary acidifying agents—
(ammonium chloride, sodium acid phosphate, etc.) Increase the concentration of the ionized species of the amphetamine molecule, thereby increasing urinary excretion. Both groups of agents lower blood levels and efficacy of amphetamines.

Adrenergic blockers—
Adrenergic blockers are inhibited by amphetamines.

Alkalinizing agents—
Gastrointestinal alkalinizing agents (sodium bicarbonate, etc.) increase absorption of amphetamines. Urinary alkalinizing agents (acetazolamide, some thiazides) increase the concentration of the non-ionized species of the amphetamine molecule, thereby decreasing urinary excretion. Both groups of agents increase blood levels and therefore potentiate the actions of amphetamines.

Antidepressants, tricyclic—
Amphetamines may enhance the activity of tricyclic or sympathomimetic agents; d-amphetamine with desipramine or protriptyline and possibly other tricyclics cause striking and sustained increases in the concentration of d-amphetamine in the brain; cardiovascular effects can be potentiated.

MAO inhibitors—
MAOI antidepressants, as well as a metabolite of furazolidone, slow amphetamine metabolism. This slowing potentiates amphetamines, increasing their effect on the release of norepinephrine and other monoamines from adrenergic nerve endings; this can cause headaches and other signs of hypertensive crisis. A variety of neurological toxic effects and malignant hyperpyrexia can occur, sometimes with fatal results.

Antihistamines—
Amphetamines may counteract the sedative effect of antihistamines.

Antihypertensives—
Amphetamines may antagonize the hypotensive effects of antihypertensives.

Chlorpromazine—
Chlorpromazine blocks dopamine and norepinephrine receptors, thus inhibiting the central stimulant effects of amphetamines, and can be used to treat amphetamine poisoning.

Ethosuximide—
Amphetamines may delay intestinal absorption of ethosuximide.

Haloperidol—
Haloperidol blocks dopamine receptors, thus inhibiting the central stimulant effects of amphetamines.

Lithium carbonate—
The anorectic and stimulatory effects of amphetamines may be inhibited by lithium carbonate.

Meperidine—
Amphetamines potentiate the analgesic effect of meperidine.

Methenamine therapy—
Urinary excretion of amphetamines is increased, and efficacy is reduced, by acidifying agents used in methenamine therapy.

Norepinephrine—
Amphetamines enhance the adrenergic effect of norepinephrine.

Phenobarbital—
Amphetamines may delay intestinal absorption of phenobarbital; co-administration of phenobarbital may produce a synergistic anticonvulsant action.

Phenytoin—
Amphetamines may delay intestinal absorption of phenytoin; co-administration of phenytoin may produce a synergistic anticonvulsant action.

Propoxyphene—
In cases of propoxyphene overdosage, amphetamine CNS stimulation is potentiated and fatal convulsions can occur.

Veratrum alkaloids—
Amphetamines inhibit the hypotensive effect of veratrum alkaloids.

Drug/Laboratory Test Interactions:

- Amphetamines can cause a significant elevation in plasma corticosteroid levels. This increase is greatest in the evening.
- Amphetamines may interfere with urinary steroid determinations.

Carcinogenesis/Mutagenesis: Mutagenicity studies and long-term studies in animals to determine the carcinogenic potential of amphetamine, have not been performed.

Pregnancy—Teratogenic Effects: Pregnancy Category C. Amphetamine has been shown to have embryotoxic and teratogenic effects when administered to A/Jax mice and C57BL mice in doses approximately 41 times the maximum human dose. Embryotoxic effects were not seen in New Zealand white rabbits given the drug in doses 7 times the human dose nor in rats given 12.5 times the maximum human dose. While there are no adequate and well-controlled studies in pregnant women, there has been one report of severe congenital bony deformity, tracheoesophageal fistula, and anal atresia (vater association) in a baby born to a woman who took dextroamphetamine sulfate with lovastatin during the first trimester of pregnancy. Amphetamines should be used during pregnancy only if the potential benefit justifies the potential risk to the fetus.

Nonteratogenic Effects: Infants born to mothers dependent on amphetamines have an increased risk of premature delivery and low birth weight. Also, these infants may experience symptoms of withdrawal as demonstrated by dysphoria, including agitation, and significant lassitude.

Pediatric Use: Long-term effects of amphetamines in children have not been well established. Amphetamines are not recommended for use in children under 3 years of age with Attention Deficit Disorder with Hyperactivity described under INDICATIONS AND USAGE.

Amphetamines have been reported to exacerbate motor and phonic tics and Tourette's syndrome. Therefore, clinical evaluation for tics and Tourette's syndrome in children and their families should precede use of stimulant medications.

Drug treatment is not indicated in all cases of Attention Deficit Disorder with Hyperactivity and should be considered only in light of the complete history and evaluation of the child. The decision to prescribe amphetamines should depend on the physician's assessment of the chronicity and severity of the child's symptoms and their appropriateness for his/her age. Prescription should not depend solely on the presence of one or more of the behavioral characteristics. When these symptoms are associated with acute stress reactions, treatment with amphetamines is usually not indicated.

ADVERSE REACTIONS

Cardiovascular: Palpitations, tachycardia, elevation of blood pressure. There have been isolated reports of cardiomyopathy associated with chronic amphetamine use.

Central Nervous System: Psychotic episodes at recommended doses (rare), overstimulation, restlessness, dizziness, insomnia, euphoria, dyskinesia, dysphoria, tremor, headache, exacerbation of motor and phonic tics and Tourette's syndrome.

Gastrointestinal: Dryness of the mouth, unpleasant taste, diarrhea, constipation, other gastrointestinal disturbances. Anorexia and weight loss may occur as undesirable effects when amphetamines are used for other than the anorectic effect.

Allergic: Urticaria.

Endocrine: Impotence, changes in libido.

DRUG ABUSE AND DEPENDENCE

Dextroamphetamine sulfate is a Schedule II controlled substance.

Amphetamines have been extensively abused. Tolerance, extreme psychological dependence, and severe social disability have occurred. There are reports of patients who have increased the dosage to many times that recommended. Abrupt cessation following prolonged high dosage administration results in extreme fatigue and mental depression; changes are also noted on the sleep EEG. Manifestations of chronic intoxication with amphetamines include severe dermatoses, marked insomnia, irritability, hyperactivity, and personality changes. The most severe manifestation of chronic intoxication is psychosis, often clinically indistinguishable from schizophrenia. This is rare with oral amphetamines.

OVERDOSAGE

Individual patient response to amphetamines varies widely. While toxic symptoms occasionally occur as an idiosyncrasy at doses as low as 2 mg, they are rare with doses of less than 15 mg; 30 mg can produce severe reactions, yet doses of 400 to 500 mg are not necessarily fatal.

In rats, the oral LD_{50} of dextroamphetamine sulfate is 96.8 mg/kg.

Continued on next page

Adderall Tablets—Cont.

Symptoms: Manifestations of acute overdosage with amphetamines include restlessness, tremor, hyperreflexia, rapid respiration, confusion, assaultiveness, hallucinations, panic states, hyperpyrexia and rhabdomyolysis.
Fatigue and depression usually follow the central stimulation.
Cardiovascular effects include arrhythmias, hypertension or hypotension and circulatory collapse.
Gastrointestinal symptoms include nausea, vomiting, diarrhea, and abdominal cramps. Fatal poisoning is usually preceded by convulsions and coma.
Treatment: Consult with a Certified Poison Control Center for up to date guidance and advice. Management of acute amphetamine intoxication is largely symptomatic and includes gastric lavage, administration of activated charcoal, administration of a cathartic and sedation. Experience with hemodialysis or peritoneal dialysis is inadequate to permit recommendation in this regard. Acidification of the urine increases amphetamine excretion, but is believed to increase risk of acute renal failure if myoglobinuria is present. If acute, severe hypertension complicates amphetamine overdosage, administration of intravenous phentolamine has been suggested. However, a gradual drop in blood pressure will usually result when sufficient sedation has been achieved. Chlorpromazine antagonizes the central stimulant effects of amphetamines and can be used to treat amphetamine intoxication.

DOSAGE AND ADMINISTRATION

Regardless of indication, amphetamines should be administered at the lowest effective dosage and dosage should be individually adjusted. Late evening doses should be avoided because of the resulting insomnia.
Attention Deficit Disorder with Hyperactivity: Not recommended for children under 3 years of age. In children from 3 to 5 years of age, start with 2.5 mg daily; daily dosage may be raised in increments of 2.5 mg at weekly intervals until optimal response is obtained.
In children 6 years of age and older, start with 5 mg once or twice daily; daily dosage may be raised in increments of 5 mg at weekly intervals until optimal response is obtained. Only in rare cases will it be necessary to exceed a total of 40 mg per day. Give first dose on awakening; additional doses (1 or 2) at intervals of 4 to 6 hours.
Where possible, drug administration should be interrupted occasionally to determine if there is a recurrence of behavioral symptoms sufficient to require continued therapy.
Narcolepsy: Usual dose 5 mg to 60 mg per day in divided doses, depending on the individual patient response.
Narcolepsy seldom occurs in children under 12 years of age; however, when it does, dextroamphetamine sulfate may be used. The suggested initial dose for patients aged 6–12 is 5 mg daily; daily dose may be raised in increments of 5 mg at weekly intervals until optimal response is obtained. In patients 12 years of age and older, start with 10 mg daily; daily dosage may be raised in increments of 10 mg at weekly intervals until optimal response is obtained. If bothersome adverse reactions appear (e.g., insomnia or anorexia), dosage should be reduced. Give first dose on awakening; additional doses (1 or 2) at intervals of 4 to 6 hours.

HOW SUPPLIED

ADDERALL® 5 mg: Blue double-scored tablet, debossed "AD" on one side and "5" on the other side
(NDC 54092-031-01)
ADDERALL® 7.5 mg: Blue double-scored tablet, debossed "AD" on one side and "7.5" on the other side
(NDC 54092-076-01)
ADDERALL® 10 mg: Blue double-scored tablet, debossed "AD" on one side and "10" on the other side
(NDC 54092-032-01)
ADDERALL® 12.5 mg: Orange double-scored tablet, debossed "AD" on one side and "12.5" on the other side
(NDC 54092-125-01)
ADDERALL® 15 mg: Orange double-scored tablet, debossed "AD" on one side and "15" on the other side
(NDC 54092-150-01)
ADDERALL® 20 mg: Orange double-scored tablet, debossed "AD" on one side and "20" on the other side
(NDC 54092-033-01)
ADDERALL® 30 mg: Orange double-scored tablet, debossed "AD" on one side and "30" on the other side
(NDC 54092-034-01)
In bottles of 100 tablets.
Dispense in a tight, light-resistant container as defined in the USP.
Store at 25°C (77°F) excursions 15–30°C (59–86°F).
Rx only.
MG #10185
Mfg. for:
Shire
Shire US Inc.
One Riverfront Place
Newport, KY 41071
Made in U.S.A.
1-800-828-2088

Rev 12/02
Shown in Product Identification Guide, page 333

ADDERALL XR® Ⓒ℞

5 mg, 10 mg, 15 mg, 20 mg, 25 mg, 30 mg CAPSULES
(Mixed Salts of a Single-Entity Amphetamine Product)
Dextroamphetamine Sulfate Dextroamphetamine Saccharate Amphetamine Aspartate Monohydrate Amphetamine Sulfate

ADDERALL XR® CAPSULES

AMPHETAMINES HAVE A HIGH POTENTIAL FOR ABUSE. ADMINISTRATION OF AMPHETAMINES FOR PROLONGED PERIODS OF TIME MAY LEAD TO DRUG DEPENDENCE. PARTICULAR ATTENTION SHOULD BE PAID TO THE POSSIBILITY OF SUBJECTS OBTAINING AMPHETAMINES FOR NON-THERAPEUTIC USE OR DISTRIBUTION TO OTHERS AND THE DRUGS SHOULD BE PRESCRIBED OR DISPENSED SPARINGLY.

℞ only

DESCRIPTION

ADDERALL XR® is a once daily extended-release, single-entity amphetamine product. ADDERALL XR® combines the neutral sulfate salts of dextroamphetamine and amphetamine, with the dextro isomer of amphetamine saccharate and d,l-amphetamine aspartate monohydrate. The ADDERALL XR® capsule contains two types of drug-containing beads designed to give a double-pulsed delivery of amphetamines, which prolongs the release of amphetamine from ADDERALL XR® compared to the conventional ADDERALL® (immediate-release) tablet formulation.
[See table below]
Inactive Ingredients and Colors: The inactive ingredients in ADDERALL XR® capsules include: gelatin capsules, hydroxypropyl methylcellulose, methacrylic acid copolymer, opadry beige, sugar spheres, talc, and triethyl citrate. Gelatin capsules contain edible inks, kosher gelatin, and titanium dioxide. The 5 mg, 10 mg, and 15 mg capsules also contain FD&C Blue #2. The 20 mg, 25 mg, and 30 mg capsules also contain red iron oxide and yellow iron oxide.

CLINICAL PHARMACOLOGY

Pharmacodynamics
Amphetamines are non-catecholamine sympathomimetic amines with CNS stimulant activity. The mode of therapeutic action in Attention Deficit Hyperactivity Disorder (ADHD) is not known. Amphetamines are thought to block the reuptake of norepinephrine and dopamine into the presynaptic neuron and increase the release of these monoamines into the extraneuronal space.
Pharmacokinetics
Pharmacokinetic studies of ADDERALL XR® have been conducted in healthy adult and pediatric (6–12 yrs) subjects, and pediatric patients with ADHD. Both ADDERALL® (immediate-release) tablets and ADDERALL XR® capsules contain d-amphetamine and l-amphetamine salts in the ratio of 3:1. Following administration of ADDERALL® (immediate-release), the peak plasma concentrations occurred in about 3 hours for both d-amphetamine and l-amphetamine.
The time to reach maximum plasma concentration (T_{max}) for ADDERALL XR® is about 7 hours, which is about 4 hours longer compared to ADDERALL® (immediate-release). This is consistent with the extended-release nature of the product.

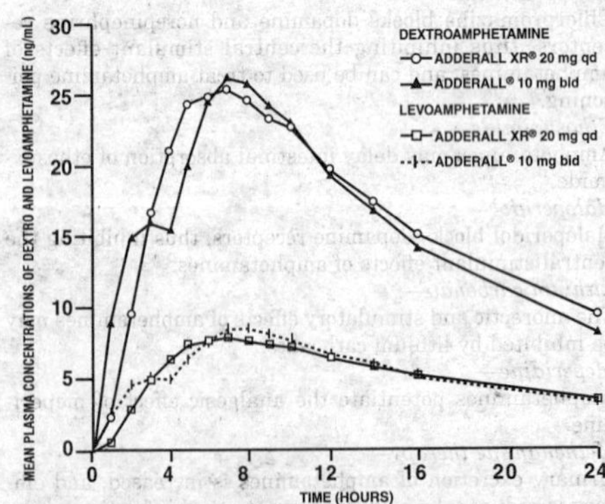

Figure 1 Mean d-amphetamine and l-amphetamine plasma concentrations following administration of ADDERALL XR® 20 mg (8 am) and ADDERALL® (immediate-release) 10 mg bid (8 am 12 noon) in the fed state.

A single dose of ADDERALL XR® 20 mg capsules provided comparable plasma concentration profiles of both d-amphetamine and l-amphetamine to ADDERALL® (immediate-release) 10 mg bid administered 4 hours apart. The mean elimination half-life is 1 hour shorter for d-amphetamine and 2 hours shorter for l-amphetamine in children aged 6 to 12 years compared to that in adults ($t_{1/2}$ is 10 hours for d-amphetamine and 13 hours for l-amphetamine in adults, and 9 hours and 11 hours, respectively, for children). ADDERALL XR® demonstrates linear pharmacokinetics over the dose range of 10 to 30 mg. There is no unexpected accumulation at steady state.
Food does not affect the extent of absorption of ADDERALL XR® capsules, but prolongs T_{max} by 2.5 hours (from 5.2 hrs at fasted state to 7.7 hrs after a high-fat meal). Opening the capsule and sprinkling the contents on applesauce results in comparable absorption to the intact capsule taken in the fasted state.
Special Populations
Pediatric Patients
Children eliminated amphetamine faster than adults. The elimination half-life ($t_{1/2}$) is approximately 1 hour shorter for d-amphetamine and 2 hours shorter for l-amphetamine in children than in adults. However, children had higher systemic exposure to amphetamine (C_{max} and AUC) than adults for a given dose of ADDERALL XR®, which was attributed to the higher dose administered to children on a mg/kg body weight basis compared to adults. Upon dose normalization on a mg/kg basis, children showed 30% less systemic exposure compared to adults.
Gender
Systemic exposure to amphetamine was 20–30% higher in women (N=20) than in men (N=20) due to the higher dose administered to women on a mg/kg body weight basis. When the exposure parameters (C_{max} and AUC) were normalized by dose (mg/kg), these differences diminished.
Race
Formal pharmacokinetic studies for race have not been conducted. However, amphetamine pharmacokinetics appeared to be comparable among Caucasians (N=33), Blacks (N=8) and Hispanics (N=10).
Clinical Trials
A double-blind, randomized, placebo-controlled, parallel-group study was conducted in children aged 6–12 (N=584) who met DSM-IV criteria for ADHD (either the combined type or the hyperactive-impulsive type). Patients were randomized to fixed dose treatment groups receiving final doses of 10, 20, or 30 mg of ADDERALL XR® or placebo once daily in the morning for three weeks. Significant improvements in patient behavior, based upon teacher ratings of attention and hyperactivity, were observed for all ADDERALL XR® doses compared to patients who received placebo, for all three weeks, including the first week of treatment, when all ADDERALL XR® subjects were receiving a dose of 10 mg/day. Patients who received ADDERALL XR® showed behavioral improvements in both morning and afternoon assessments compared to patients on placebo.
In a classroom analogue study, patients (N=51) receiving fixed doses of 10 mg, 20 mg or 30 mg ADDERALL XR® demonstrated statistically significant improvements in teacher-rated behavior and performance measures, compared to patients treated with placebo.

INDICATIONS

ADDERALL XR® is indicated for the treatment of Attention Deficit Hyperactivity Disorder (ADHD).
The efficacy of ADDERALL XR® in the treatment of ADHD was established on the basis of two controlled trials of children aged 6 to 12 who met DSM-IV criteria for ADHD (see CLINICAL PHARMACOLOGY), along with extrapolation from the known efficacy of ADDERALL®, the immediate-release formulation of this substance.
A diagnosis of Attention Deficit Hyperactivity Disorder (ADHD; DSM-IV) implies the presence of hyperactive-impulsive or inattentive symptoms that caused impairment and were present before age 7 years. The symptoms must cause clinically significant impairment, e.g., in social, academic, or occupational functioning, and be present in two or more settings, e.g., school (or work) and at home. The symptoms must not be better accounted for by another mental disorder. For the Inattentive Type, at least six of the following symptoms must have persisted for at least 6 months: lack of attention to details/careless mistakes; lack of sustained attention; poor listener; failure to follow through on tasks; poor organization; avoids tasks requiring sustained mental effort; loses things; easily distracted; forgetful. For the Hyperactive-Impulsive Type, at least six of the following symptoms must have persisted for at least 6 months: fidgeting/squirming; leaving seat; inappropriate running/climbing; difficulty with quiet activities; "on the go"; excessive talking; blurting answers; can't wait turn; intrusive. The Combined Type requires both inattentive and hyperactive-impulsive criteria to be met.
Special Diagnostic Considerations: Specific etiology of this syndrome is unknown, and there is no single diagnostic test. Adequate diagnosis requires the use not only of medical but of special psychological, educational, and social resources. Learning may or may not be impaired. The diagnosis must be based upon a complete history and evaluation of the child and not solely on the presence of the required number of DSM-IV characteristics.
Need for Comprehensive Treatment Program: ADDERALL XR® is indicated as an integral part of a total treatment program for ADHD that may include other measures (psycho-

EACH CAPSULE CONTAINS:	5 mg	10 mg	15 mg	20 mg	25 mg	30 mg
Dextroamphetamine Saccharate	1.25 mg	2.5 mg	3.75 mg	5.0 mg	6.25 mg	7.5 mg
Amphetamine Aspartate Monohydrate	1.25 mg	2.5 mg	3.75 mg	5.0 mg	6.25 mg	7.5 mg
Dextroamphetamine Sulfate USP	1.25 mg	2.5 mg	3.75 mg	5.0 mg	6.25 mg	7.5 mg
Amphetamine Sulfate USP	1.25 mg	2.5 mg	3.75 mg	5.0 mg	6.25 mg	7.5 mg
Total amphetamine base equivalent	3.1 mg	6.3 mg	9.4 mg	12.5 mg	15.6 mg	18.8 mg

logical, educational, social) for patients with this syndrome. Drug treatment may not be indicated for all children with this syndrome. Stimulants are not intended for use in the child who exhibits symptoms secondary to environmental factors and/or other primary psychiatric disorders, including psychosis. Appropriate educational placement is essential and psychosocial intervention is often helpful. When remedial measures alone are insufficient, the decision to prescribe stimulant medication will depend upon the physician's assessment of the chronicity and severity of the child's symptoms.

Long-Term Use: The effectiveness of ADDERALL XR® for long-term use, i.e., for more than 3 weeks, has not been systematically evaluated in controlled trials. Therefore, the physician who elects to use ADDERALL XR® for extended periods should periodically re-evaluate the long-term usefulness of the drug for the individual patient.

CONTRAINDICATIONS

Advanced arteriosclerosis, symptomatic cardiovascular disease, moderate to severe hypertension, hyperthyroidism, known hypersensitivity or idiosyncrasy to the sympathomimetic amines, glaucoma.

Agitated states.

Patients with a history of drug abuse.

During or within 14 days following the administration of monoamine oxidase inhibitors (hypertensive crises may result).

WARNINGS

Psychosis: Clinical experience suggests that, in psychotic patients, administration of amphetamine may exacerbate symptoms of behavior disturbance and thought disorder.

Long-Term Suppression of Growth: Data are inadequate to determine whether chronic use of stimulants in children, including amphetamine, may be causally associated with suppression of growth. Therefore, growth should be monitored during treatment, and patients who are not growing or gaining weight as expected should have their treatment interrupted.

PRECAUTIONS

General: The least amount of amphetamine feasible should be prescribed or dispensed at one time in order to minimize the possibility of overdosage.

Hypertension and other Cardiovascular Conditions: Caution is to be exercised in prescribing amphetamines for patients with even mild hypertension (see CONTRAINDICATIONS). Blood pressure and pulse should be monitored at appropriate intervals in patients taking ADDERALL XR®, especially patients with hypertension.

Tics: Amphetamines have been reported to exacerbate motor and phonic tics and Tourette's syndrome. Therefore, clinical evaluation for tics and Tourette's syndrome in children and their families should precede use of stimulant medications.

Information for Patients: Amphetamines may impair the ability of the patient to engage in potentially hazardous activities such as operating machinery or vehicles; the patient should therefore be cautioned accordingly.

Drug Interactions: *Acidifying agents*—Gastrointestinal acidifying agents (guanethidine, reserpine, glutamic acid HCl, ascorbic acid, etc.) lower absorption of amphetamines.

Urinary acidifying agents—These agents (ammonium chloride, sodium acid phosphate, etc.) increase the concentration of the ionized species of the amphetamine molecule, thereby increasing urinary excretion. Both groups of agents lower blood levels and efficacy of amphetamines.

Adrenergic blockers—Adrenergic blockers are inhibited by amphetamines.

Alkalinizing agents—Gastrointestinal alkalinizing agents (sodium bicarbonate, etc.) increase absorption of amphetamines. Co-administration of ADDERALL XR® and gastrointestinal alkalinizing agents, such as antacids, should be avoided. Urinary alkalinizing agents (acetazolamide, some thiazides) increase the concentration of the non-ionized species of the amphetamine molecule, thereby decreasing urinary excretion. Both groups of agents increase blood levels and therefore potentiate the actions of amphetamines.

Antidepressants, tricyclic—Amphetamines may enhance the activity of tricyclic antidepressants or sympathomimetic agents; d-amphetamine with desipramine or protriptyline and possibly other tricyclics cause striking and sustained increases in the concentration of d-amphetamine in the brain; cardiovascular effects can be potentiated.

MAO inhibitors—MAOI antidepressants, as well as a metabolite of furazolidone, slow amphetamine metabolism. This slowing potentiates amphetamines, increasing their effect on the release of norepinephrine and other monoamines from adrenergic nerve endings; this can cause headaches and other signs of hypertensive crisis. A variety of toxic neurological effects and malignant hyperpyrexia can occur, sometimes with fatal results.

Antihistamines—Amphetamines may counteract the sedative effect of antihistamines.

Antihypertensives—Amphetamines may antagonize the hypotensive effects of antihypertensives.

Chlorpromazine—Chlorpromazine blocks dopamine and norepinephrine receptors, thus inhibiting the central stimulant effects of amphetamines, and can be used to treat amphetamine poisoning.

Ethosuximide—Amphetamines may delay intestinal absorption of ethosuximide.

Table 1 Adverse Events Reported by More Than 1% of Patients Receiving ADDERALL XR® with Higher Incidence Than on Placebo in a 584 Patient Clinical Study

Body System	Preferred Term	ADDERALL XR™ (N=374)	Placebo (N=210)
General	Abdominal Pain (stomachache)	14%	10%
	Accidental injury	3%	2%
	Asthenia (fatigue)	2%	0%
	Fever	5%	2%
	Infection	4%	2%
	Viral Infection	2%	0%
Digestive System	Loss of Appetite	22%	2%
	Diarrhea	2%	1%
	Dyspepsia	2%	1%
	Nausea	5%	3%
	Vomiting	7%	4%
Nervous System	Dizziness	2%	0%
	Emotional Lability	9%	2%
	Insomnia	17%	2%
	Nervousness	6%	2%
Metabolic/Nutritional	Weight Loss	4%	0%

Haloperidol—Haloperidol blocks dopamine receptors, thus inhibiting the central stimulant effects of amphetamines.

Lithium carbonate—The anorectic and stimulatory effects of amphetamines may be inhibited by lithium carbonate.

Meperidine—Amphetamines potentiate the analgesic effect of meperidine.

Methenamine therapy—Urinary excretion of amphetamines is increased, and efficacy is reduced, by acidifying agents used in methenamine therapy.

Norepinephrine—Amphetamines enhance the adrenergic effect of norepinephrine.

Phenobarbital—Amphetamines may delay intestinal absorption of phenobarbital; co-administration of phenobarbital may produce a synergistic anticonvulsant action.

Phenytoin—Amphetamines may delay intestinal absorption of phenytoin; co-administration of phenytoin may produce a synergistic anticonvulsant action.

Propoxyphene—In cases of propoxyphene overdosage, amphetamine CNS stimulation is potentiated and fatal convulsions can occur.

Veratrum alkaloids—Amphetamines inhibit the hypotensive effect of veratrum alkaloids.

Drug/Laboratory Test Interactions:

Amphetamines can cause a significant elevation in plasma corticosteroid levels. This increase is greatest in the evening.

Amphetamines may interfere with urinary steroid determinations.

Carcinogenesis/Mutagenesis and Impairment of Fertility: No evidence of carcinogenicity was found in studies in which d,l-amphetamine (enantiomer ratio of 1:1) was administered to mice and rats in the diet for 2 years at doses of up to 30 mg/kg/day in male mice, 19 mg/kg/day in female mice, and 5 mg/kg/day in male and female rats. These doses are approximately 2.4, 1.5, and 0.8 times, respectively, the maximum recommended human dose of 30 mg/day on a mg/m^2 body surface area basis.

Amphetamine, in the enantiomer ratio present in ADDERALL® (immediate-release)(d- to l- ratio of 3:1), was not clastogenic in the mouse bone marrow micronucleus test *in vivo* and was negative when tested in the *E. coli* component of the Ames test *in vitro*. d,l-Amphetamine (1:1 enantiomer ratio) has been reported to produce a positive response in the mouse bone marrow micronucleus test, an equivocal response in the Ames test, and negative responses in the *in vitro* sister chromatid exchange and chromosomal aberration assays.

Amphetamine, in the enantiomer ratio present in ADDERALL® (immediate-release)(d- to l- ratio of 3:1), did not adversely affect fertility or early embryonic development in the rat at doses of up to 20 mg/kg/day (approximately 5 times the maximum recommended human dose of 30 mg/day on a mg/m^2 body surface area basis).

Pregnancy: Pregnancy Category C. Amphetamine, in the enantiomer ratio present in ADDERALL® (d- to l- ratio of 3:1), had no apparent effects on embryofetal morphological development or survival when orally administered to pregnant rats and rabbits throughout the period of organogenesis at doses of up to 6 and 16 mg/kg/day, respectively. These doses are approximately 1.5 and 8 times, respectively, the maximum recommended human dose of 30 mg/day on a mg/m^2 body surface area basis. Fetal malformations and death have been reported in mice following parenteral administration of d-amphetamine doses of 50 mg/kg/day (approximately 6 times the maximum recommended human dose of 30 mg/day on a mg/m^2 basis) or greater to pregnant animals. Administration of these doses was also associated with severe maternal toxicity.

A number of studies in rodents indicate that prenatal or early postnatal exposure to amphetamine (d- or d,l-), at doses similar to those used clinically, can result in long-term neurochemical and behavioral alterations. Reported behavioral effects include learning and memory deficits, altered locomotor activity, and changes in sexual function.

There are no adequate and well-controlled studies in pregnant women. There has been one report of severe congenital bony deformity, tracheo-esophageal fistula, and anal atresia (vater association) in a baby born to a woman who took dextroamphetamine sulfate with lovastatin during the first trimester of pregnancy. Amphetamines should be used during pregnancy only if the potential benefit justifies the potential risk to the fetus.

Nonteratogenic Effects: Infants born to mothers dependent on amphetamines have an increased risk of premature delivery and low birth weight. Also, these infants may experience symptoms of withdrawal as demonstrated by dysphoria, including agitation, and significant lassitude.

Usage in Nursing Mothers: Amphetamines are excreted in human milk. Mothers taking amphetamines should be advised to refrain from nursing.

Pediatric Use: ADDERALL XR® is indicated for use in children 6 years of age and older.

Use in Children Under Six Years of Age: Effects of ADDERALL XR® in 3–5 year olds have not been studied. Long-term effects of amphetamines in children have not been well established. Amphetamines are not recommended for use in children under 3 years of age.

Geriatric Use: ADDERALL XR® has not been studied in the geriatric population.

ADVERSE EVENTS

The premarketing development program for ADDERALL XR® included exposures in a total of 685 participants in clinical trials (615 patients, 70 healthy adult subjects). These participants received ADDERALL XR® at daily doses up to 30 mg. The 615 patients (ages 6 to 12) were evaluated in two controlled clinical studies, one open-label clinical study, and one single-dose clinical pharmacology study (N=20). Safety data on all patients are included in the discussion that follows. Adverse reactions were assessed by collecting adverse events, results of physical examinations, vital signs, weights, laboratory analyses, and ECGs.

Adverse events during exposure were obtained primarily by general inquiry and recorded by clinical investigators using terminology of their own choosing. Consequently, it is not possible to provide a meaningful estimate of the proportion of individuals experiencing adverse events without first grouping similar types of events into a smaller number of standardized event categories. In the tables and listings that follow, COSTART terminology has been used to classify reported adverse events.

The stated frequencies of adverse events represent the proportion of individuals who experienced, at least once, a treatment-emergent adverse event of the type listed.

Adverse events associated with discontinuation of treatment: In two placebo-controlled studies of up to 5 weeks duration, 2.4% (10/425) of ADDERALL XR® treated patients discontinued due to adverse events (including 3 patients with loss of appetite, one of whom also reported insomnia) compared to 2.7% (7/259) receiving placebo. The most frequent adverse events associated with discontinuation of ADDERALL XR® in controlled and uncontrolled, multiple-dose clinical trials (N=595) are presented below. Over half of these patients were exposed to ADDERALL XR® for 12 months or more.

Adverse event	% of patients discontinuing (N=595)
Anorexia (loss of appetite)	2.9
Insomnia	1.5
Weight loss	1.2
Emotional lability	1.0
Depression	0.7

Adverse events occurring in a controlled trial: Adverse events reported in a 3-week clinical trial of pediatric patients treated with ADDERALL XR® or placebo are presented in the table below.

The prescriber should be aware that these figures cannot be used to predict the incidence of adverse events in the course

Continued on next page

Adderall XR—Cont.

of usual medical practice where patient characteristics and other factors differ from those which prevailed in the clinical trials. Similarly, the cited frequencies cannot be compared with figures obtained from other clinical investigations involving different treatments, uses, and investigators. The cited figures, however, do provide the prescribing physician with some basis for estimating the relative contribution of drug and non-drug factors to the adverse event incidence rate in the population studied.

[See table 1 at top of previous page]

The following adverse reactions have been associated with amphetamine use:

Cardiovascular: Palpitations, tachycardia, elevation of blood pressure. There have been isolated reports of cardiomyopathy associated with chronic amphetamine use.

Central Nervous System: Psychotic episodes at recommended doses, overstimulation, restlessness, dizziness, insomnia, euphoria, dyskinesia, dysphoria, tremor, headache, exacerbation of motor and phonic tics and Tourette's syndrome.

Gastrointestinal: Dryness of the mouth, unpleasant taste, diarrhea, constipation, other gastrointestinal disturbances. Anorexia and weight loss may occur as undesirable effects.

Allergic: Urticaria.

Endocrine: Impotence, changes in libido.

DRUG ABUSE AND DEPENDENCE

ADDERALL XR® is a Schedule II controlled substance.

Amphetamines have been extensively abused. Tolerance, extreme psychological dependence, and severe social disability have occurred. There are reports of patients who have increased the dosage to many times that recommended. Abrupt cessation following prolonged high dosage administration results in extreme fatigue and mental depression; changes are also noted on the sleep EEG. Manifestations of chronic intoxication with amphetamines may include severe dermatoses, marked insomnia, irritability, hyperactivity, and personality changes. The most severe manifestation of chronic intoxication is psychosis, often clinically indistinguishable from schizophrenia.

OVERDOSAGE

Individual patient response to amphetamines varies widely. Toxic symptoms may occur idiosyncratically at low doses.

Symptoms: Manifestations of acute overdosage with amphetamines include restlessness, tremor, hyperreflexia, rapid respiration, confusion, assaultiveness, hallucinations, panic states, hyperpyrexia and rhabdomyolysis. Fatigue and depression usually follow the central nervous system stimulation. Cardiovascular effects include arrhythmias, hypertension or hypotension and circulatory collapse. Gastrointestinal symptoms include nausea, vomiting, diarrhea, and abdominal cramps. Fatal poisoning is usually preceded by convulsions and coma.

Treatment: Consult with a Certified Poison Control Center for up-to-date guidance and advice. Management of acute amphetamine intoxication is largely symptomatic and includes gastric lavage, administration of activated charcoal, administration of a cathartic and sedation. Experience with hemodialysis or peritoneal dialysis is inadequate to permit recommendation in this regard. Acidification of the urine increases amphetamine excretion, but is believed to increase risk of acute renal failure if myoglobinuria is present. If acute severe hypertension complicates amphetamine overdosage, administration of intravenous phentolamine has been suggested. However, a gradual drop in blood pressure will usually result when sufficient sedation has been achieved. Chlorpromazine antagonizes the central stimulant effects of amphetamines and can be used to treat amphetamine intoxication.

The prolonged release of mixed amphetamine salts from ADDERALL XR® should be considered when treating patients with overdose.

DOSAGE AND ADMINISTRATION

In children with ADHD who are 6 years of age and older and are either starting treatment for the first time or switching from another medication, start with 10 mg once daily in the morning; daily dosage may be raised in increments of 5 mg or 10 mg at weekly intervals. When in the judgement of the clinician a lower initial dose is appropriate, patients may begin treatment with 5 mg once daily in the morning. Dosage should be individualized according to the needs and response of the patient. Amphetamines should be administered at the lowest effective dosage. The maximum recommended dose is 30 mg/day; doses greater than 30 mg/day of ADDERALL XR® have not been studied. Amphetamines are not recommended for children under 3 years of age. ADDERALL XR® has not been studied in children under 6 years of age.

Patients Currently Using ADDERALL®—Based on bioequivalence data, patients taking divided doses of immediate-release ADDERALL®, for example twice a day, may be switched to ADDERALL XR® at the same total daily dose taken once daily. Titrate at weekly intervals to appropriate efficacy and tolerability as indicated.

ADDERALL XR® capsules may be taken whole, or the capsule may be opened and the entire contents sprinkled on applesauce. If the patient is using the sprinkle administration method, the sprinkled applesauce should be consumed immediately; it should not be stored. Patients should take the applesauce with sprinkled beads in its entirety without chewing. The dose of a single capsule should not be divided. The contents of the entire capsule should be taken, and patients should not take anything less than one capsule per day.

ADDERALL XR® should be given upon awakening. Afternoon doses should be avoided because of the potential for insomnia.

Where possible, drug administration should be interrupted occasionally to determine if there is a recurrence of behavioral symptoms sufficient to require continued therapy.

HOW SUPPLIED

ADDERALL XR® 5 mg Capsules: Clear/blue (imprinted ADDERALL XR 5 mg), bottles of 100, NDC 54092-381-01

ADDERALL XR® 10 mg Capsules: Blue/blue (imprinted Adderall XR 10 mg), bottles of 100, NDC 54092-383-01

ADDERALL XR® 15 mg Capsules: Blue/white (imprinted ADDERALL XR 15 mg), bottles of 100, NDC 54092-385-01

ADDERALL XR® 20 mg Capsules: Orange/orange (imprinted Adderall XR 20 mg), bottles of 100, NDC 54092-387-01

ADDERALL XR® 25 mg Capsules: Orange/white (imprinted ADDERALL XR 25 mg), bottles of 100, NDC 54092-389-01

ADDERALL XR® 30 mg Capsules: Natural/orange (imprinted Adderall XR 30 mg), bottles of 100, NDC 54092-391-01

Dispense in a tight, light-resistant container as defined in the USP.

Store at 25° C (77° F). Excursions permitted to 15–30°C (59–86° F) [see USP Controlled Room Temperature]

ANIMAL TOXICOLOGY

Acute administration of high doses of amphetamine (d- or d,l-) has been shown to produce long-lasting neurotoxic effects, including irreversible nerve fiber damage, in rodents. The significance of these findings to humans is unknown.

Manufactured by DSM Pharmaceuticals Inc., Greenville, North Carolina 27834. Distributed and marketed by Shire US Inc., Newport, KY 41071

For more information call 800-828-2088 or visit www.adderallxr.com

ADDERALL® is registered in the US Patent and Trademark Office

403958 (rev. 10/2002)

Shown in Product Identification Guide, page 333

AGRYLIN® ℞

[*ă-grĭ-lĭn*]

(anagrelide hydrochloride)

Capsules

Rx only

DESCRIPTION

Name: AGRYLIN® (anagrelide hydrochloride)

Dosage Form: 0.5 mg and 1 mg capsules for oral administration

Active Ingredient: AGRYLIN® Capsules contain either 0.5 mg or 1 mg of anagrelide base (as anagrelide hydrochloride).

Inactive Ingredients: Anhydrous Lactose NF, Crospovidone NF, Lactose Monohydrate NF, Magnesium Stearate NF, Microcrystalline Cellulose NF, Povidone USP.

Pharmacological Classification: Platelet-reducing agent.

Chemical Name: 6,7-dichloro-1,5-dihydroimidazo[2,1-b]quinazolin-2(3H)-one monohydrochloride monohydrate.

Molecular formula: $C_{10}H_7Cl_2N_3O \cdot HCl \cdot H_2O$

Molecular weight: 310.55

Structural formula:

Appearance: Off-white powder.

Solubility: Water .... Very slightly soluble
Dimethyl Sulfoxide .... Sparingly soluble
Dimethylformamide .... Sparingly soluble

CLINICAL PHARMACOLOGY

The mechanism by which anagrelide reduces blood platelet count is still under investigation. Studies in patients support a hypothesis of dose-related reduction in platelet production resulting from a decrease in megakaryocyte hypermaturation. In blood withdrawn from normal volunteers treated with anagrelide, a disruption was found in the postmitotic phase of megakaryocyte development and a reduction in megakaryocyte size and ploidy. At therapeutic doses, anagrelide does not produce significant changes in white cell counts or coagulation parameters, and may have a small, but clinically insignificant effect on red cell parameters. Platelet aggregation is inhibited in people at doses higher than those required to reduce platelet count. Anagrelide inhibits cyclic AMP phosphodiesterase, as well as ADP- and collagen-induced platelet aggregation.

Following oral administration of ^{14}C-anagrelide in people, more than 70% of radioactivity was recovered in urine. Based on limited data, there appears to be a trend toward dose linearity between doses of 0.5 mg and 2.0 mg. At fasting and at a dose of 0.5 mg of anagrelide, the plasma half-life is 1.3 hours. The available plasma concentration time data at steady state in patients showed that anagrelide does not accumulate in plasma after repeated administration. The drug is extensively metabolized; less than 1% is recovered in the urine as anagrelide.

When a 0.5 mg dose of anagrelide was taken after food, its bioavailability (based on AUC values) was modestly reduced by an average of 13.8% and its plasma half-life slightly increased (to 1.8 hours), when compared with drug administered to the same subjects in the fasted state. The peak plasma level was lowered by an average of 45% and delayed by 2 hours.

CLINICAL STUDIES

A total of 942 patients with myeloproliferative disorders including 551 patients with Essential Thrombocythemia (ET), 117 patients with Polycythemia Vera (PV), 178 patients with Chronic Myelogenous Leukemia (CML), and 96 patients with other myeloproliferative disorders (OMPD), were treated with anagrelide in three clinical trials. Patients with OMPD included 87 patients who had Myeloid Metaplasia with Myelofibrosis (MMM), and 9 patients who had unknown myeloproliferative disorders.

Clinical Studies

Patients with ET, PV, CML, or MMM were diagnosed based on the following criteria:

[See table below]

Patients were enrolled in clinical trials if their platelet count was ≥ 900,000/μL on two occasions or ≥ 650,000/μL on two occasions with documentation of symptoms associated with thrombocythemia. The mean duration of anagrelide therapy for ET, PV, CML, and OMPD patients was 65, 67, 40, and 44 weeks, respectively; 23% of patients received treatment for 2 years. Patients were treated with anagrelide starting at doses of 0.5-2.0 mg every 6 hours. The dose was increased if the platelet count was still high, but to no more than 12 mg each day. Efficacy was defined as reduction of platelet count to or near physiologic levels (150,000-400,000/μL). The criteria for defining subjects as "responders" were reduction in platelets for at least 4 weeks to ≤600,000/μL, or by at least 50% from baseline value. Subjects treated for less than 4 weeks were not considered evaluable. The results are depicted graphically below:

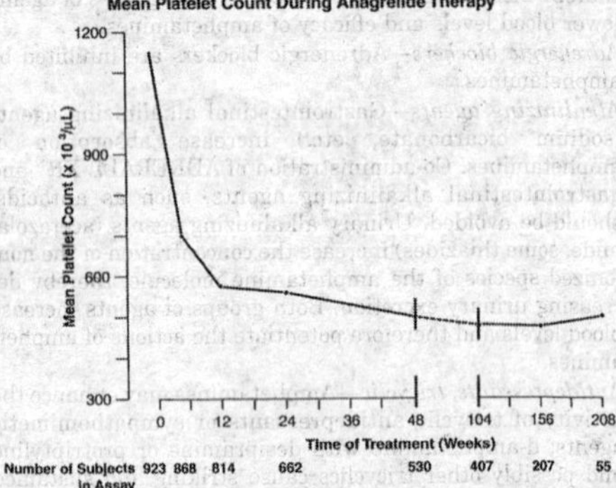

ET

- Platelet count ≥900,000/μL on two determinations
- Profound megakaryocytic hyperplasia in bone marrow
- Absence of Philadelphia chromosome
- Normal red cell mass
- Normal serum iron and ferritin and normal marrow iron stores

CML

- Persistent granulocyte count ≥50,000/μL without evidence of infection
- Absolute basophil count ≥ 100/μL
- Evidence for hyperplasia of the granulocytic line in the bone marrow
- Philadelphia chromosome present
- Leucocyte alkaline phophatase ≤ lower limit of the laboratory normal range

PV†

- A1 Increased red cell mass
- A2 Normal arterial oxygen saturation
- A3 Splenomegaly
- B1 Platelet count ≥ 400,000/μL, in absence of iron deficiency or bleeding
- B2 Leucocytosis (≥ 12,000/μL, in the absence of infection)
- B3 Elevated leucocyte alkaline phosphatase
- B4 Elevated Serum B_{12}

† Diagnosis positive if A1, A2, and A3 present; or, if no splenomegaly, diagnosis is positive if A1 and A2 are present with any two of B1, B2, or B3.

MMM

- Myelofibrotic (hypocellular, fibrotic) bone marrow
- Prominent megakaryocytic metaplasia in bone marrow
- Splenomegaly
- Moderate to severe normochromic normocytic anemia
- White cell count may be variable; (80,000–100,000/μL)
- Increased platelet count
- Variable red cell mass; teardrop poikilocytes
- Normal to high leucocyte alkaline phosphatase
- Absence of Philadelphia chromosome

	Time on Treatment							
		Weeks				Years		
	Baseline	4	12	24	48	2	3	4
Mean*	1131	683	575	526	484	460	437	457
N	923†	868	814	662	530	407	207	55

*x 10^3/μL

†Nine hundred and forty-two subjects with myeloproliferative disorders were enrolled in three research studies. Of these, 923 had platelet counts over the duration of the studies.

AGRYLIN® was effective in phlebotomized patients as well as in patients treated with other concomitant therapies including hydroxyurea, aspirin, interferon, radioactive phosphorus, and alkylating agents.

INDICATIONS AND USAGE

AGRYLIN® Capsules are indicated for the treatment of patients with thrombocythemia, secondary to myeloproliferative disorders, to reduce the elevated platelet count and the risk of thrombosis and to ameliorate associated symptoms including thrombo-hemorrhagic events (see CLINICAL STUDIES, DOSAGE and ADMINISTRATION).

WARNINGS

Cardiovascular

Anagrelide should be used with caution in patients with known or suspected heart disease, and only if the potential benefits of therapy outweigh the potential risks. Because of the positive inotropic effects and side-effects of anagrelide, a pre-treatment cardiovascular examination is recommended along with careful monitoring during treatment. In humans, therapeutic doses of anagrelide may cause cardiovascular effects, including vasodilation, tachycardia, palpitations, and congestive heart failure.

Renal

It is recommended that patients with renal insufficiency (creatinine $\geq$ 2mg/dL) receive anagrelide when, in the physician's judgment, the potential benefits of therapy outweigh the potential risks. These patients should be monitored closely for signs of renal toxicity while receiving anagrelide (see ADVERSE REACTIONS, Urogenital System).

Hepatic

It is recommended that patients with evidence of hepatic dysfunction (bilirubin, SGOT, or measures of liver function >1.5 times the upper limit of normal) receive anagrelide when, in the physician's judgment, the potential benefits of therapy outweigh the potential risks. These patients should be monitored closely for signs of hepatic toxicity while receiving anagrelide (see ADVERSE REACTIONS, Hepatic System).

PRECAUTIONS

Laboratory Tests: Anagrelide therapy requires close clinical supervision of the patient. While the platelet count is being lowered (usually during the first two weeks of treatment), blood counts (hemoglobin, white blood cells), liver function (SGOT, SGPT) and renal function (serum creatinine, BUN) should be monitored.

In 9 subjects receiving a single 5 mg dose of anagrelide, standing blood pressure fell an average of 22/15 mm Hg, usually accompanied by dizziness. Only minimal changes in blood pressure were observed following a dose of 2 mg.

Cessation of AGRYLIN® Treatment: In general, interruption of anagrelide treatment is followed by an increase in platelet count. After sudden stoppage of anagrelide therapy, the increase in platelet count can be observed within four days.

Drug Interactions: Bioavailability studies evaluating possible interactions between anagrelide and other drugs have not been conducted. The most common medications used concomitantly with anagrelide have been aspirin, acetaminophen, furosemide, iron, ranitidine, hydroxyurea, and allopurinol. The most frequently used concomitant cardiac medication has been digoxin. Although drug-to-drug interaction studies have not been conducted, there is no clinical evidence to suggest that anagrelide interacts with any of these compounds.

There is a single case report which suggests that sucralfate may interfere with anagrelide absorption.

Food has no clinically significant effect on the bioavailability of anagrelide.

Carcinogenesis, Mutagenesis, Impairment of Fertility: No long-term studies in animals have been performed to evaluate carcinogenic potential of anagrelide hydrochloride. Anagrelide hydrochloride was not genotoxic in the Ames test, the mouse lymphoma cell (L5178Y, $TK^{+/-}$) forward mutation test, the human lymphocyte chromosome aberration test, or the mouse micronucleus test. Anagrelide hydrochloride at oral doses up to 240 mg/kg/day (1,440 mg/m^2/day, 195 times the recommended maximum human dose based on body surface area) was found to have no effect on fertility and reproductive performance of male rats. However, in female rats, at oral doses of 60 mg/kg/day (360 mg/m^2/day, 49 times the recommended maximum human dose based on body surface area) or higher, it disrupted implantation when administered in early pregnancy and retarded or blocked parturition when administered in late pregnancy.

Pregnancy: Pregnancy Category C.

(i) Teratogenic Effects

Teratology studies have been performed in pregnant rats at oral doses up to 900 mg/kg/day (5,400 mg/m^2/day, 730 times the recommended maximum human dose based on body surface area) and in pregnant rabbits at oral doses up to 20 mg/kg/day (240 mg/m^2/day, 32 times the recommended maximum human dose based on body surface area) and have revealed no evidence of impaired fertility or harm to the fetus due to anagrelide hydrochloride.

(ii) Nonteratogenic Effects

A fertility and reproductive performance study performed in female rats revealed that anagrelide hydrochloride at oral doses of 60 mg/kg/day (360 mg/m^2/day, 49 times the recommended maximum human dose based on body surface area) or higher disrupted implantation and exerted adverse effect on embryo/fetal survival.

A perinatal and postnatal study performed in female rats revealed that anagrelide hydrochloride at oral doses of 60 mg/kg/day (360 mg/m^2/day, 49 times the recommended maximum human dose based on body surface area) or higher produced delay or blockage of parturition, deaths of nondelivering pregnant dams and their fully developed fetuses, and increased mortality in the pups born.

Five women became pregnant while on anagrelide treatment at doses of 1 to 4 mg/day. Treatment was stopped as soon as it was realized that they were pregnant. All delivered normal, healthy babies. There are no adequate and well-controlled studies in pregnant women. Anagrelide hydrochloride should be used during pregnancy only if the potential benefit justifies the potential risk to the fetus.

Anagrelide is not recommended in women who are or may become pregnant. If this drug is used during pregnancy, or if the patient becomes pregnant while taking this drug, the patient should be apprised of the potential harm to the fetus. Women of child-bearing potential should be instructed that they must not be pregnant and that they should use contraception while taking anagrelide. Anagrelide may cause fetal harm when administered to a pregnant woman.

Nursing Mothers: It is not known whether this drug is excreted in human milk. Because many drugs are excreted in human milk and because of the potential for serious adverse reaction in nursing infants from anagrelide hydrochloride, a decision should be made whether to discontinue nursing or to discontinue the drug, taking into account the importance of the drug to the mother.

Pediatric Use: The safety and efficacy of anagrelide in patients under the age of 16 years have not been established. Myeloproliferative disorders are uncommon in pediatric patients. Anagrelide has been used successfully in 12 pediatric patients (age range 6.8 to 17.4 years; 6 male and 6 female), including 8 patients with ET, 2 patients with CML, 1 patient with PV, and 1 patient with OMPD. Patients were started on therapy with 0.5 mg qid to a maximum daily dose of 10 mg. The median duration of treatment was 18.1 months with a range of 3.1 to 92 months. Three patients received treatment for greater than three years.

Geriatric Use: Of the total number of subjects in clinical studies of Agrylin, 42.1% were 65 years and over, while 14.9% were 75 years and over. No overall differences in safety or effectiveness were observed between these subjects and younger subjects, and other reported clinical experience has not identified differences in response between the elderly and younger patients, but greater sensitivity of some older individuals cannot be ruled out.

ADVERSE REACTIONS

Analysis of the adverse events in a population consisting of 942 patients diagnosed with myeloproliferative diseases of varying etiology (ET: 551; PV: 117; OMPD: 274) has shown that all disease groups have the same adverse event profile. While most reported adverse events during anagrelide therapy have been mild in intensity and have decreased in frequency with continued therapy, serious adverse events were reported in these patients. These include the following: congestive heart failure, myocardial infarction, cardiomyopathy, cardiomegaly, complete heart block, atrial fibrillation, cerebrovascular accident, pericarditis, pericardial effusion, pleural effusion, pulmonary infiltrates, pulmonary fibrosis, pulmonary hypertension, pancreatitis, gastric/duodenal ulceration, and seizure.

Of the 942 patients treated with anagrelide for a mean duration of approximately 65 weeks, 161 (17%) were discontinued from the study because of adverse events or abnormal laboratory test results. The most common adverse events for treatment discontinuation were headache, diarrhea, edema, palpitation, and abdominal pain. Overall, the occurrence rate of all adverse events was 17.9 per 1,000 treatment days. The occurrence rate of adverse events increased at higher dosages of anagrelide.

The most frequently reported adverse reactions to anagrelide (in 5% or greater of 942 patients with myeloproliferative disease) in clinical trials were:

Headache 43.5%
Palpitations 26.1%
Diarrhea 25.7%
Asthenia 23.1%
Edema, other 20.6%
Nausea 17.1%
Abdominal Pain 16.4%
Dizziness 15.4%
Pain, other 15.0%
Dyspnea 11.9%
Flatulence 10.2%
Vomiting 9.7%
Fever 8.9%
Peripheral Edema 8.5%
Rash, including urticaria 8.3%
Chest Pain 7.8%
Anorexia 7.7%
Tachycardia 7.5%
Pharyngitis 6.8%
Malaise 6.4%
Cough 6.3%
Paresthesia 5.9%
Back Pain 5.9%
Pruritus 5.5%
Dyspepsia 5.2%

Adverse events with an incidence of 1% to <5% included:

Body as a Whole System: Flu symptoms, chills, photosensitivity.

Cardiovascular System: Arrhythmia, hemorrhage, hypertension, cardiovascular disease, angina pectoris, heart failure, postural hypotension, thrombosis, vasodilatation, migraine, syncope.

Digestive System: Constipation, GI distress, GI hemorrhage, gastritis, melena, aphthous stomatitis, eructation.

Hemic & Lymphatic System: Anemia, thrombocytopenia, ecchymosis, lymphadenopathy.

Platelet counts below 100,000/μL occurred in 84 patients (ET: 35; PV: 9; OMPD: 40), reduction below 50,000/μL occurred in 44 patients (ET: 7; PV: 6; OMPD: 31) while on anagrelide therapy. Thrombocytopenia promptly recovered upon discontinuation of anagrelide.

Hepatic System: Elevated liver enzymes were observed in 3 patients (ET: 2; OMPD: 1) during anagrelide therapy.

Musculoskeletal System: Arthralgia, myalgia, leg cramps.

Nervous System: Depression, somnolence, confusion, insomnia, nervousness, amnesia.

Nutritional Disorders: Dehydration.

Respiratory System: Rhinitis, epistaxis, respiratory disease, sinusitis, pneumonia, bronchitis, asthma.

Skin and Appendages System: Skin disease, alopecia.

Special Senses: Amblyopia, abnormal vision, tinnitus, visual field abnormality, diplopia.

Urogenital System: Dysuria, hematuria.

Renal abnormalities occurred in 15 patients (ET: 10; PV: 4; OMPD: 1). Six ET, 4 PV and 1 with OMPD experienced renal failure (approximately 1%) while on anagrelide treatment; in 4 cases, the renal failure was considered to be possibly related to anagrelide treatment. The remaining 11 were found to have pre-existing renal impairment. Doses ranged from 1.5-6.0 mg/day, with exposure periods of 2 to 12 months. No dose adjustment was required because of renal insufficiency.

The adverse event profile for patients in clinical trials on anagrelide therapy (in 5% or greater of 942 patients with myeloproliferative diseases) is shown in the following bar graph:

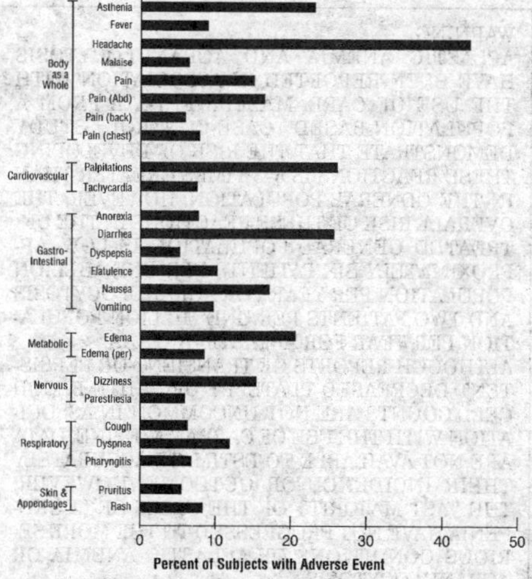

OVERDOSAGE

Acute Toxicity and Symptoms

Single oral doses of anagrelide hydrochloride at 2,500, 1,500 and 200 mg/kg in mice, rats and monkeys, respectively, were not lethal. Symptoms of acute toxicity were: decreased motor activity in mice and rats and softened stools and decreased appetite in monkeys.

There are no reports of overdosage with anagrelide hydrochloride. Platelet reduction from anagrelide therapy is dose-related; therefore, thrombocytopenia, which can potentially cause bleeding, is expected from overdosage. Should overdosage occur, cardiac and central nervous system toxicity can also be expected.

Management and Treatment

In case of overdosage, close clinical supervision of the patient is required; this especially includes monitoring of the platelet count for thrombocytopenia. Dosage should be decreased or stopped, as appropriate, until the platelet count returns to within the normal range.

Continued on next page

Agrylin—Cont.

DOSAGE AND ADMINISTRATION

Treatment with **AGRYLIN®** Capsules should be initiated under close medical supervision. The recommended starting dosage of **AGRYLIN®** is 0.5 mg qid or 1 mg bid, which should be maintained for at least one week. Dosage should then be adjusted to the lowest effective dosage required to reduce and maintain platelet count below 600,000/µL, and ideally to the normal range. The dosage should be increased by not more than 0.5 mg/day in any one week. Dosage should not exceed 10 mg/day or 2.5 mg in a single dose (see PRECAUTIONS). The decision to treat asymptomatic young adults with essential thrombocythemia should be individualized.

There are no special requirements for dosing the geriatric population.

To monitor the effect of anagrelide and prevent the occurrence of thrombocytopenia, platelet counts should be performed every two days during the first week of treatment and at least weekly thereafter until the maintenance dosage is reached.

Typically, platelet count begins to respond within 7 to 14 days at the proper dosage. The time to complete response, defined as platelet count ≤ 600,000/µL, ranged from 4 to 12 weeks. Most patients will experience an adequate response at a dose of 1.5 to 3.0 mg/day. Patients with known or suspected heart disease, renal insufficiency, or hepatic dysfunction should be monitored closely.

HOW SUPPLIED

AGRYLIN® is available as:

0.5 mg, opaque, white capsules imprinted "S 063" in black ink:

NDC 54092-063-01 = bottle of 100

1 mg, opaque, gray capsules imprinted "S 064" in black ink:

NDC 54092-064-01 = bottle of 100

Store at 25°C (77°F) excursions permitted to 15°-30°C (59-86°F), in a light-resistant container.

[See USP Controlled Room Temperature]

Manufactured for

Shire US Inc.

One Riverfront Place

Newport, KY 41071

By MALLINCKRODT INC.

Hobart, NY 13788

Rev. 4/03 063 0117 012

Printed in USA

Shown in Product Identification Guide, page 333

CARBATROL® ℞

[*căr-bō'trōl*]

(carbamazepine extended-release capsules)

100 mg • 200 mg • 300 mg

Prescribing information

WARNING

APLASTIC ANEMIA AND AGRANULOCYTOSIS HAVE BEEN REPORTED IN ASSOCIATION WITH THE USE OF CARBAMAZEPINE. DATA FROM A POPULATION-BASED CASE-CONTROL STUDY DEMONSTRATE THAT THE RISK OF DEVELOPING THESE REACTIONS IS 5–8 TIMES GREATER THAN IN THE GENERAL POPULATION. HOWEVER, THE OVERALL RISK OF THESE REACTIONS IN THE UNTREATED GENERAL POPULATION IS LOW. APPROXIMATELY SIX PATIENTS PER ONE MILLION POPULATION PER YEAR FOR AGRANULOCYTOSIS AND TWO PATIENTS PER ONE MILLION POPULATION PER YEAR FOR APLASTIC ANEMIA.

ALTHOUGH REPORTS OF TRANSIENT OR PERSISTENT DECREASED PLATELET OR WHITE BLOOD CELL COUNTS ARE NOT UNCOMMON IN ASSOCIATION WITH THE USE OF CARBAMAZEPINE, DATA ARE NOT AVAILABLE TO ESTIMATE ACCURATELY THEIR INCIDENCE OR OUTCOME. HOWEVER, THE VAST MAJORITY OF THE CASES OF LEUKOPENIA HAVE NOT PROGRESSED TO THE MORE SERIOUS CONDITIONS OF APLASTIC ANEMIA OR AGRANULOCYTOSIS.

BECAUSE OF THE VERY LOW INCIDENCE OF AGRANULOCYTOSIS AND APLASTIC ANEMIA, THE VAST MAJORITY OF MINOR HEMATOLOGIC CHANGES OBSERVED IN MONITORING OF PATIENTS ON CARBAMAZEPINE ARE UNLIKELY TO SIGNAL THE OCCURRENCE OF EITHER ABNORMALITY. NONETHELESS, COMPLETE PRETREATMENT HEMATOLOGICAL TESTING SHOULD BE OBTAINED AS A BASELINE. IF A PATIENT IN THE COURSE OF TREATMENT EXHIBITS LOW OR DECREASED WHITE BLOOD CELL OR PLATELET COUNTS, THE PATIENT SHOULD BE MONITORED CLOSELY. DISCONTINUATION OF THE DRUG SHOULD BE CONSIDERED IF ANY EVIDENCE OF SIGNIFICANT BONE MARROW DEPRESSION DEVELOPS.

Before prescribing Carbatrol, the physician should be thoroughly familiar with the details of this prescribing information, particularly regarding use with other drugs, especially those which accentuate toxicity potential.

DESCRIPTION

CARBATROL® is an anticonvulsant and specific analgesic for trigeminal neuralgia, available for oral administration as 100 mg, 200 mg and 300 mg extended-release capsules of Carbamazepine, USP. Carbamazepine is a white to off-white powder, practically insoluble in water and soluble in alcohol and in acetone. Its molecular weight is 236.27. Its chemical name is 5H-dibenz[b,f]azepine-5-carboxamide, and its structural formula is:

CARBAMAZEPINE

Carbatrol is a multi-component capsule formulation consisting of three different types of beads: immediate-release beads, extended-release beads, and enteric-release beads. The three bead types are combined in a specific ratio to provide twice daily dosing of Carbatrol.

Inactive ingredients: citric acid, colloidal silicon dioxide, lactose monohydrate, microcrystalline cellulose, polyethylene glycol, povidone, sodium lauryl sulfate, talc, triethyl citrate and other ingredients.

The 100 mg capsule shells contain gelatin-NF, FD&C Blue #2, Yellow Iron Oxide, and titanium dioxide and are imprinted with white ink; the 200 mg capsule shells contain gelatin-NF, FD&C Red #3, FD&C Yellow #6, Yellow Iron Oxide, FD&C Blue #2, and titanium dioxide, and are imprinted with white ink; and the 300 mg capsule shells contain gelatin-NF, FD&C Blue #2, FD&C Yellow #6, Red Iron Oxide, Yellow Iron Oxide, and titanium dioxide, and are imprinted with white ink.

CLINICAL PHARMACOLOGY

In controlled clinical trials, carbamazepine has been shown to be effective in the treatment of psychomotor and grand mal seizures, as well as trigeminal neuralgia.

Mechanism of Action

Carbamazepine has demonstrated anticonvulsant properties in rats and mice with electrically and chemically induced seizures. It appears to act by reducing polysynaptic responses and blocking the post-tetanic potentiation. Carbamazepine greatly reduces or abolishes pain induced by stimulation of the infraorbital nerve in cats and rats. It depresses thalamic potential and bulbar and polysynaptic reflexes, including the linguomandibular reflex in cats. Carbamazepine is chemically unrelated to other anticonvulsants or other drugs used to control the pain of trigeminal neuralgia. The mechanism of action remains unknown.

The principal metabolite of carbamazepine, carbamazepine-10,11-epoxide, has anticonvulsant activity as demonstrated in several *in vivo* animal models of seizures. Though clinical activity for the epoxide has been postulated, the significance of its activity with respect to the safety and efficacy of carbamazepine has not been established.

Pharmacokinetics

Carbamazepine (CBZ): Taken every 12 hours, carbamazepine extended-release capsules provide steady state plasma levels comparable to immediate-release carbamazepine tablets given every 6 hours, when administered at the same total mg daily dose. Following a single 200 mg oral extended-release dose of carbamazepine, peak plasma concentration was 1.9 ± 0.3 µg/mL and the time to reach the peak was 19 ± 7 hours. Following chronic administration (800 mg every 12 hours), the peak levels were 11.0 ± 2.5 µg/mL and the time to reach the peak was 5.9 ± 1.8 hours. The pharmacokinetics of extended-release carbamazepine is linear over the single dose range of 200–800 mg.

Carbamazepine is 76% bound to plasma proteins. Carbamazepine is primarily metabolized in the liver. Cytochrome P450 3A4 was identified as the major isoform responsible for the formation of carbamazepine-10,11-epoxide. Since carbamazepine induces its own metabolism, the half-life is also variable. Following a single extended-release dose of carbamazepine, the average half-life range from 35-40 hours and 12-17 hours on repeated dosing. The apparent oral clearance following a single dose was 25 ± 5 mL/min and following multiple dosing was 80 ± 30 mL/min.

After oral administration of ^{14}C-carbamazepine, 72% of the administered radioactivity was found in the urine and 28% in the feces. This urinary radioactivity was composed largely of hydroxylated and conjugated metabolites, with only 3% of unchanged carbamazepine.

Carbamazepine-10,11-epoxide (CBZ-E): Carbamazepine-10,11-epoxide is considered to be an active metabolite of carbamazepine. Following a single 200 mg oral extended-release dose of carbamazepine, the peak plasma concentration of carbamazepine-10,11-epoxide was 0.11 ± 0.012 µg/mL and the time to reach the peak was 36 ± 6 hours. Following chronic administration of a extended-release dose of carbamazepine (800 mg every 12 hours), the peak levels of carbamazepine-10,11-epoxide were 2.2 ± 0.9 µg/mL and the time to reach the peak was 14 ± 8 hours. The plasma half-life of carbamazepine-10,11-epoxide following administration of carbamazepine is 34 ± 9 hours. Following a single oral dose of extended-release carbamazepine (200-800 mg) the AUC and Cmax of carbamazepine-10,11-epoxide were less than 10% of carbamazepine. Following multiple dosing of extended-release carbamazepine (800-1600 mg daily for 14 days), the AUC and Cmax of carbamazepine-10,11-epoxide were dose related, ranging from 15.7 µg.hr/mL and 1.5 µg/mL at 800 mg/day to 32.6 µg.hr/mL and 3.2 µg/mL at 1600 mg/day, respectively, and were less than 30% of carbamazepine. Carbamazepine-10,11-epoxide is 50% bound to plasma proteins.

Food Effect: A high fat meal diet increased the rate of absorption of a single 400 mg dose (mean T_{max} was reduced from 24 hours, in the fasting state, to 14 hours and C_{max} increased from 3.2 to 4.3 µg/mL) but not the extent (AUC) of absorption. The elimination half-life remains unchanged between fed and fasting state. The multiple dose study conducted in the fed state showed that the steady-state C_{max} values were within the therapeutic concentration range. The pharmacokinetic profile of extended-release carbamazepine was similar when given by sprinkling the beads over applesauce compared to the intact capsule administered in the fasted state.

Special Populations

Hepatic Dysfunction: The effect of hepatic impairment on the pharmacokinetics of carbamazepine is not known. However, given that carbamazepine is primarily metabolized in the liver, it is prudent to proceed with caution in patients with hepatic dysfunction.

Renal Dysfunction: The effect of renal impairment on the pharmacokinetics of carbamazepine is not known.

Gender: No difference in the mean AUC and C_{max} of carbamazepine and carbamazepine-10,11-epoxide was found between males and females.

Age: Carbamazepine is more rapidly metabolized to carbamazepine-10,11-epoxide in young children than adults. In children below the age of 15, there is an inverse relationship between CBZ-E/CBZ ratio and increasing age.

Race: No information is available on the effect of race on the pharmacokinetics of carbamazepine.

INDICATIONS AND USAGE

Epilepsy

Carbatrol is indicated for use as an anticonvulsant drug. Evidence supporting efficacy of carbamazepine as an anticonvulsant was derived from active drug-controlled studies that enrolled patients with the following seizure types:

1. Partial seizures with complex symptomatology (psychomotor, temporal lobe). Patients with these seizures appear to show greater improvements than those with other types.
2. Generalized tonic-clonic seizures (grand mal).
3. Mixed seizure patterns which include the above, or other partial or generalized seizures. Absence seizures (petit mal) do not appear to be controlled by carbamazepine (see PRECAUTIONS, General).

Trigeminal Neuralgia

Carbatrol is indicated in the treatment of the pain associated with true trigeminal neuralgia. Beneficial results have also been reported in glossopharyngeal neuralgia. This drug is not a simple analgesic and should not be used for the relief of trivial aches or pains.

CONTRAINDICATIONS

Carbamazepine should not be used in patients with a history of previous bone marrow depression, hypersensitivity to the drug, or known sensitivity to any of the tricyclic compounds, such as amitriptyline, desipramine, imipramine, protriptyline and nortriptyline. Likewise, on theoretical grounds its use with monoamine oxidase inhibitors is not recommended. Before administration of carbamazepine, MAO inhibitors should be discontinued for a minimum of 14 days, or longer if the clinical situation permits.

WARNINGS

Usage in Pregnancy

Carbamazepine can cause fetal harm when administered to a pregnant woman.

Epidemiological data suggest that there may be an association between the use of carbamazepine during pregnancy and congenital malformations, including spina bifida. The prescribing physician will wish to weigh the benefits of therapy against the risks in treating or counseling women of childbearing potential. If this drug is used during pregnancy, or if the patient becomes pregnant while taking this drug, the patient should be apprised of the potential hazard to the fetus.

Retrospective case reviews suggest that, compared with monotherapy, there may be a higher prevalence of teratogenic effects associated with the use of anticonvulsants in combination therapy.

In humans, transplacental passage of carbamazepine is rapid (30–60 minutes), and the drug is accumulated in the fetal tissues, with higher levels found in liver and kidney than in brain and lung.

Carbamazepine has been shown to have adverse effects in reproduction studies in rats when given orally in dosages 10-25 times the maximum human daily dosage (MHDD) of 1200 mg on a mg/kg basis or 1.5-4 times the MHDD on a mg/m2 basis. In rat teratology studies, 2 of 135 offspring showed kinked ribs at 250 mg/kg and 4 of 119 offspring at 650 mg/kg showed other anomalies (cleft palate, 1; talipes, 1; anophthalmos, 2). In reproduction studies in rats, nursing offspring demonstrated a lack of weight gain and an unkempt appearance at a maternal dosage level of 200 mg/kg.

Antiepileptic drugs should not be discontinued abruptly in patients in whom the drug is administered to prevent major seizures because of the strong possibility of precipitating status epilepticus with attendant hypoxia and threat to life.

In individual cases where the severity and frequency of the seizure disorder are such that removal of medication does not pose a serious threat to the patient, discontinuation of the drug may be considered prior to and during pregnancy, although it cannot be said with any confidence that even minor seizures do not pose some hazard to the developing embryo or fetus.

Tests to detect defects using current accepted procedures should be considered a part of routine prenatal care in child-bearing women receiving carbamazepine.

General

Patients with a history of adverse hematologic reaction to any drug may be particularly at risk.

Severe dermatologic reactions, including toxic epidermal necrolysis (Lyell's syndrome) and Stevens-Johnson syndrome have been reported with carbamazepine. These reactions have been extremely rare. However, a few fatalities have been reported.

Carbamazepine has shown mild anticholinergic activity; therefore, patients with increased intraocular pressure should be closely observed during therapy.

Because of the relationship of the drug to other tricyclic compounds, the possibility of activation of a latent psychosis and, in elderly patients, of confusion or agitation should be considered.

PRECAUTIONS

General

Before initiating therapy, a detailed history and physical examination should be made.

Carbamazepine should be used with caution in patients with a mixed seizure disorder that includes atypical absence seizures, since in these patients carbamazepine has been associated with increased frequency of generalized convulsions (see INDICATIONS AND USAGE).

Therapy should be prescribed only after critical benefit-to-risk appraisal in patients with a history of cardiac, hepatic, or renal damage; adverse hematologic reaction to other drugs; or interrupted courses of therapy with carbamazepine.

Information for Patients

Patients should be made aware of the early toxic signs and symptoms of a potential hematologic problem, such as fever, sore throat, rash, ulcers in the mouth, easy bruising, petechial or purpuric hemorrhage, and should be advised to report to the physician immediately if any such signs or symptoms appear.

Since dizziness and drowsiness may occur, patients should be cautioned about the hazards of operating machinery or automobiles or engaging in other potentially dangerous tasks.

If necessary, the Carbatrol capsules can be opened and the contents sprinkled over food, such as a teaspoon of applesauce or other similar food products. Carbatrol capsules or their contents should not be crushed or chewed.

Laboratory Tests

Complete pretreatment blood counts, including platelets and possibly reticulocytes and serum iron, should be obtained as a baseline. If a patient in the course of treatment exhibits low or decreased white blood cell or platelet counts, the patient should be monitored closely. Discontinuation of the drug should be considered if any evidence of significant bone marrow depression develops.

Baseline and periodic evaluations of liver function, particularly in patients with a history of liver disease, must be performed during treatment with this drug since liver damage may occur. The drug should be discontinued immediately in cases of aggravated liver dysfunction or active liver disease.

Baseline and periodic eye examinations, including slit-lamp, funduscopy, and tonometry, are recommended since many phenothiazines and related drugs have been shown to cause eye changes.

Baseline and periodic complete urinalysis and BUN determinations are recommended for patients treated with this agent because of observed renal dysfunction.

Monitoring of blood levels (see CLINICAL PHARMACOLOGY) has increased the efficacy and safety of anticonvulsants. This monitoring may be particularly useful in cases of dramatic increase in seizure frequency and for verification of compliance. In addition, measurement of drug serum levels may aid in determining the cause of toxicity when more than one medication is being used.

Thyroid function tests have been reported to show decreased values with carbamazepine administered alone.

Hyponatremia has been reported in association with carbamazepine use, either alone or in combination with other drugs.

Interference with some pregnancy tests has been reported.

Drug Interactions

Clinically meaningful drug interactions have occurred with concomitant medications and include, but are not limited to the following:

Agents that may affect carbamazepine plasma levels:

CYP 3A4 inhibitors inhibit carbamazepine metabolism and can thus increase plasma carbamazepine levels.

Drugs that have been shown, or would be expected, to increase plasma carbamazepine levels include:

cimetidine, danazol, diltiazem, macrolides, erythromycin, troleandomycin, clarithromycin, fluoxetine, loratadine, terfenadine, isoniazid, niacinamide, nicotinamide, propoxyphene, ketoconazole, itraconazole, verapamil, valproate.*

CYP 3A4 inducers can increase the rate of carbamazepine metabolism and can thus decrease plasma carbamazepine levels. Drugs that have been shown, or would be expected, to decrease plasma carbamazepine levels include:

cisplatin, doxorubicin HCL, felbamate, rifampin*, phenobarbital, phenytoin, primidone, theophylline.

*increased levels of the active 10, 11-epoxide

Effect of carbamazepine on plasma levels of concomitant agents:

Carbatrol increases levels of clomipramine HCL, phenytoin and primidone.

Carbatrol induces hepatic CYP activity. Carbatrol causes, or would be expected to cause decreased levels of the following:

acetaminophen, alprazolam, clonazepam, clozapine, dicumarol, doxycycline, ethosuximide, haloperidol, methsuximide, oral contraceptives, phensuximide, phenytoin, theophylline, valproate, warfarin.

The doses of these drugs may therefore have to be increased when carbamazepine is added to the therapeutic regimen.

Concomitant administration of carbamazepine and lithium may increase the risk of neurotoxic side effects. Alterations of thyroid function have been reported in combination therapy with other anticonvulsant medications.

Breakthrough bleeding has been reported among patients receiving concomitant oral contraceptives and their reliability may be adversely affected.

Carcinogenesis, Mutagenesis, Impairment of Fertility

Administration of carbamazepine to Sprague-Dawley rats for two years in the diet at doses of 25, 75, and 250 mg/kg/day (low dose approximately 0.2 times the maximum human daily dose of 1200 mg on a mg/m^2 basis), resulted in a dose-related increase in the incidence of hepatocellular tumors in females and of benign interstitial cell adenomas in the testes of males.

Carbamazepine must, therefore, be considered to be carcinogenic in Sprague-Dawley rats. Bacterial and mammalian mutagenicity studies using carbamazepine produced negative results. The significance of these findings relative to the use of carbamazepine in humans is, at present, unknown.

Usage in Pregnancy

Pregnancy Category D (See WARNINGS)

Labor and Delivery

The effect of carbamazepine on human labor and delivery is unknown.

Nursing Mothers

Carbamazepine and its epoxide metabolite are transferred to breast milk and during lactation. The concentrations of carbamazepine and its epoxide metabolite are approximately 50% of the maternal plasma concentration. Because of the potential for serious adverse reactions in nursing infants from carbamazepine, a decision should be made whether to discontinue nursing or to discontinue the drug, taking into account the importance of the drug to the mother.

Pediatric Use

Substantial evidence of carbamazepine effectiveness for use in the management of children with epilepsy (see INDICATIONS for specific seizure types) is derived from clinical investigations performed in adults and from studies in several *in vitro* systems which support the conclusion that (1) the pathogenic mechanisms underlying seizure propagation are essentially identical in adults and children, and (2) the mechanism of action of carbamazepine in treating seizures is essentially identical in adults and children.

Taken as a whole, this information supports a conclusion that the generally acceptable therapeutic range of total carbamazepine in plasma (i.e., 4–12 μg/mL) is the same in children and adults.

The evidence assembled was primarily obtained from short-term use of carbamazepine. The safety of carbamazepine in children has been systematically studied up to 6 months. No longer term data from clinical trials is available.

Geriatric Use

No systematic studies in geriatric patients have been conducted.

ADVERSE REACTIONS

General: If adverse reactions are of such severity that the drug must be discontinued, the physician must be aware that abrupt discontinuation of any anticonvulsant drug in a responsive patient with epilepsy may lead to seizures or even status epilepticus with its life-threatening hazards.

The most severe adverse reactions previously observed with carbamazepine were reported in the hemopoietic system (see BOX WARNING), the skin, and the cardiovascular system.

The most frequently observed adverse reactions, particularly during the initial phases of therapy, are dizziness, drowsiness, unsteadiness, nausea, and vomiting. To minimize the possibility of such reactions, therapy should be initiated at the lowest dosage recommended.

The following additional adverse reactions were previously reported with carbamazepine:

Hemopoietic System: Aplastic anemia, agranulocytosis, pancytopenia, bone marrow depression, thrombocytopenia, leukopenia, leukocytosis, eosinophilia, acute intermittent porphyria.

Skin: Pruritic and erythematous rashes, urticaria, toxic epidermal necrolysis (Lyell's syndrome) (see WARNINGS), Stevens-Johnson syndrome (see WARNINGS), photosensitivity reactions, alterations in skin pigmentation, exfoliative dermatitis, erythema multiforme and nodosum, purpura, aggravation of disseminated lupus erythematosus, alopecia, and diaphoresis. In certain cases, discontinuation of therapy may be necessary. Isolated cases of hirsutism have been reported, but a causal relationship is not clear.

Cardiovascular System: Congestive heart failure, edema, aggravation of hypertension, hypotension, syncope and collapse, aggravation of coronary artery disease, arrhythmias and AV block, thrombophlebitis, thromboembolism, and adenopathy or lymphadenopathy. Some of these cardiovascular complications have resulted in fatalities. Myocardial infarction has been associated with other tricyclic compounds.

Liver: Abnormalities in liver function tests, cholestatic and hepatocellular jaundice, hepatitis.

Respiratory System: Pulmonary hypersensitivity characterized by fever, dyspnea, pneumonitis, or pneumonia.

Genitourinary System: Urinary frequency, acute urinary retention, oliguria with elevated blood pressure, azotemia, renal failure, and impotence. Albuminuria, glycosuria, elevated BUN, and microscopic deposits in the urine have also been reported.

Testicular atrophy occurred in rats receiving carbamazepine orally from 4-52 weeks at dosage levels of 50-400 mg/kg/day. Additionally, rats receiving carbamazepine in the diet for 2 years at dosage levels of 25, 75, and 250 mg/kg/day had a dose-related incidence of testicular atrophy and aspermatogenesis. In dogs, it produced a brownish discoloration, presumably a metabolite, in the urinary bladder at dosage levels of 50 mg/kg/day and higher. Relevance of these findings to humans is unknown.

Nervous System: Dizziness, drowsiness, disturbances of coordination, confusion, headache, fatigue, blurred vision, visual hallucinations, transient diplopia, oculomotor disturbances, nystagmus, speech disturbances, abnormal involuntary movements, peripheral neuritis and paresthesias, depression with agitation, talkativeness, tinnitus, and hyperacusis.

There have been reports of associated paralysis and other symptoms of cerebral arterial insufficiency, but the exact relationship of these reactions to the drug has not been established.

Isolated cases of neuroleptic malignant syndrome have been reported with concomitant use of psychotropic drugs.

Digestive System: Nausea, vomiting, gastric distress and abdominal pain, diarrhea, constipation, anorexia, and dryness of the mouth and pharynx, including glossitis and stomatitis.

Eyes: Scattered punctate cortical lens opacities, as well as conjunctivitis, have been reported. Although a direct causal relationship has not been established, many phenothiazines and related drugs have been shown to cause eye changes.

Musculoskeletal System: Aching joints and muscles, and leg cramps.

Metabolism: Fever and chills, inappropriate antidiuretic hormone (ADH) secretion syndrome has been reported. Cases of frank water intoxication, with decreased serum sodium (hyponatremia) and confusion have been reported in association with carbamazepine use (see PRECAUTIONS, Laboratory Tests). Decreased levels of plasma calcium have been reported.

Other: Isolated cases of a lupus erythematosus-like syndrome have been reported. There have been occasional reports of elevated levels of cholesterol, HDL cholesterol, and triglycerides in patients taking anticonvulsants.

A case of aseptic meningitis, accompanied by myoclonus and peripheral eosinophilia, has been reported in a patient taking carbamazepine in combination with other medications. The patient was successfully dechallenged, and the meningitis reappeared upon rechallenge with carbamazepine.

DRUG ABUSE AND DEPENDENCE

No evidence of abuse potential has been associated with carbamazepine, nor is there evidence of psychological or physical dependence in humans.

OVERDOSAGE

Acute Toxicity

Lowest known lethal dose: adults, >60 g (39-year-old man). Highest known doses survived: adults, 30 g (31-year-old woman); children, 10 g (6-year-old boy); small children, 5 g (3-year-old girl).

Oral LD_{50} in animals (mg/kg): mice, 1100-3750; rats, 3850-4025; rabbits, 1500–2680; guinea pigs, 920.

Signs and Symptoms

The first signs and symptoms appear after 1–3 hours. Neuromuscular disturbances are the most prominent. Cardiovascular disorders are generally milder, and severe cardiac complications occur only when very high doses (>60 g) have been ingested.

Respiration: Irregular breathing, respiratory depression.

Cardiovascular System: Tachycardia, hypotension or hypertension, shock, conduction disorders.

Nervous System and Muscles: Impairment of consciousness ranging in severity to deep coma. Convulsions, especially in small children. Motor restlessness, muscular twitching, tremor, athetoid movements, opisthotonos, ataxia, drowsiness, dizziness, mydriasis, nystagmus, adiadochokinesia, ballism, psychomotor disturbances, dysmetria. Initial hyperreflexia, followed by hyporeflexia.

Gastrointestinal Tract: Nausea, vomiting.

Kidneys and Bladder: Anuria or oliguria, urinary retention.

Continued on next page

Carbatrol—Cont.

Laboratory Findings: Isolated instances of overdosage have included leukocytosis, reduced leukocyte count, glycosuria, and acetonuria. EEG may show dysrhythmias.

Combined Poisoning: When alcohol, tricyclic antidepressants, barbiturates, or hydantoins are taken at the same time, the signs and symptoms of acute poisoning with carbamazepine may be aggravated or modified.

Treatment

The prognosis in cases of severe poisoning is critically dependent upon prompt elimination of the drug, which may be achieved by inducing vomiting, irrigating the stomach, and by taking appropriate steps to diminish absorption. If these measures cannot be implemented without risk on the spot, the patient should be transferred at once to a hospital, while ensuring that vital functions are safeguarded. There is no specific antidote.

Elimination of the Drug: Induction of vomiting.

Gastric lavage. Even when more than 4 hours have elapsed following ingestion of the drug, the stomach should be repeatedly irrigated, especially if the patient has also consumed alcohol.

Measures to Reduce Absorption: Activated charcoal, laxatives.

Measures to Accelerate Elimination: Forced diuresis.

Dialysis is indicated only in severe poisoning associated with renal failure. Replacement transfusion is indicated in severe poisoning in small children.

Respiratory Depression: Keep the airways free; resort, if necessary, to endotracheal intubation, artificial respiration, and administration of oxygen.

Hypotension, Shock: Keep the patient's legs raised and administer a plasma expander. If blood pressure fails to rise despite measures taken to increase plasma volume, use of vasoactive substances should be considered.

Convulsions: Diazepam or barbiturates.

Warning: Diazepam or barbiturates may aggravate respiratory depression (especially in children), hypotension, and coma. However, barbiturates should not be used if drugs that inhibit monoamine oxidase have also been taken by the patient either in overdosage or in recent therapy (within 1 week).

Surveillance: Respiration, cardiac function (ECG monitoring), blood pressure, body temperature, pupillary reflexes, and kidney and bladder function should be monitored for several days.

Treatment of Blood Count Abnormalities: If evidence of significant bone marrow depression develops, the following recommendations are suggested: (1) stop the drug, (2) perform daily CBC, platelet, and reticulocyte counts, (3) do a bone marrow aspiration and trephine biopsy immediately and repeat with sufficient frequency to monitor recovery.

Special periodic studies might be helpful as follows: (1) white cell and platelet antibodies, (2) ^{59}Fe-ferrokinetic studies, (3) peripheral blood cell typing, (4) cytogenetic studies on marrow and peripheral blood, (5) bone marrow culture studies for colony-forming units, (6) hemoglobin electrophoresis for A_2 and F hemoglobin, and (7) serum folic acid and B_{12} levels.

A fully developed aplastic anemia will require appropriate, intensive monitoring and therapy, for which specialized consultation should be sought.

DOSAGE AND ADMINISTRATION

Monitoring of blood levels has increased the efficacy and safety of anticonvulsants (see PRECAUTIONS, Laboratory Tests). Dosage should be adjusted to the needs of the individual patients. A low initial daily dosage with gradual increase is advised. As soon as adequate control is achieved, the dosage may be reduced very gradually to the minimum effective level. The Carbatrol capsules may be opened and the beads sprinkled over food, such as a teaspoon of applesauce or other similar food products if this method of administration is preferred. Carbatrol capsules or their contents should not be crushed or chewed. Carbatrol can be taken with or without meals.

Carbatrol is an extended-release formulation for twice a day administration. When converting patients from immediate release carbamazepine to Carbatrol extended-release capsules, the same total daily mg dose of carbamazepine should be administered.

Epilepsy (see INDICATIONS AND USAGE)

Adults and children over 12 years of age. Initial: 200 mg twice daily. Increase at weekly intervals by adding up to 200 mg/day until the optimal response is obtained. Dosage generally should not exceed 1000 mg per day in children 12-15 years of age, and 1200 mg daily in patients above 15 years of age. Doses up to 1600 mg daily have been used in adults. **Maintenance:** Adjust dosage to the minimum effective level, usually 800-1200 mg daily.

Children under 12 years of age: Children taking total daily dosages of immediate-release carbamazepine of 400 mg or greater may be converted to the same total daily dosage of Carbatrol extended-release capsules, using a twice daily regimen. Ordinarily, optimal clinical response is achieved at daily doses below 35 mg/kg. If satisfactory clinical response has not been achieved, plasma levels should be measured to determine whether or not they are in the therapeutic range. No recommendation regarding the safety of Carbatrol for use at doses above 35 mg/kg/24 hours can be made.

Combination Therapy: Carbatrol may be used alone or with other anticonvulsants. When added to existing anticonvulsant therapy, the drug should be added gradually while the other anticonvulsants are maintained or gradually decreased, except phenytoin, which may have to be increased (see PRECAUTIONS, Drug Interactions, and Pregnancy Category D).

Trigeminal Neuralgia (see INDICATIONS AND USAGE)

Initial: On the first day, start with one 200 mg capsule. This daily dose may be increased by up to 200 mg/day every 12 hours only as needed to achieve freedom from pain. Do not exceed 1200 mg daily. **Maintenance:** Control of pain can be maintained in most patients with 400-800 mg daily. However, some patients may be maintained on as little as 200 mg daily, while others may require as much as 1200 mg daily. At least once every 3 months throughout the treatment period, attempts should be made to reduce the dose to the minimum effective level or even to discontinue the drug.

HOW SUPPLIED

Carbatrol (carbamazepine extended-release capsules) is supplied in three dosage strengths.

100 mg-Two-piece hard gelatin capsule (bluish green opaque body and cap) printed with the Shire logo in white ink.

Supplied in bottles of 120 .... NDC 54092-171-12
Supplied in bottles of 14 .... NDC 54092-171-14

200 mg-Two-piece hard gelatin capsule (light gray opaque body with bluish green opaque cap) printed with the Shire logo in white ink.

Supplied in bottles of 120 .... NDC 54092-172-12
Supplied in bottles of 30 .... NDC 54092-172-30

300 mg-Two-piece hard gelatin capsule (black opaque body with bluish green opaque cap) printed with the Shire logo in white ink.

Supplied in bottles of 120 .... NDC 54092-173-12
Supplied in bottles of 30 .... NDC 54092-173-30

Store at 25°C (77°F). excursions 15-30°C (59-86°F).

Manufactured for:
Shire US Inc.
One River Front Place, Newport, KY 41071
1-800-828-2088, Made in U.S.A.
©2003 Shire US Inc.
172 1207 002 (Rev 8/2003)

Shown in Product Identification Guide, page 333

DEXTROSTAT® Ⓒ℞

[dĕks'trō-stăt]

Dextroamphetamine Sulfate Tablets, USP
Rx only

> WARNING
> AMPHETAMINES HAVE A HIGH POTENTIAL FOR ABUSE. ADMINISTRATION OF AMPHETAMINES FOR PROLONGED PERIODS OF TIME MAY LEAD TO DRUG DEPENDENCE AND MUST BE AVOIDED. PARTICULAR ATTENTION SHOULD BE PAID TO THE POSSIBILITY OF SUBJECTS OBTAINING AMPHETAMINES FOR NON-THERAPEUTIC USE OR DISTRIBUTION TO OTHERS, AND THE DRUGS SHOULD BE PRESCRIBED OR DISPENSED SPARINGLY.

DESCRIPTION

DextroStat® (dextroamphetamine sulfate) is the dextro isomer of the compound *d,l*-amphetamine sulfate, a sympathomimetic amine of the amphetamine group. Chemically, dextroamphetamine is *d*-alpha-methyl-phenethylamine, and is present in all forms of DextroStat® as the neutral sulfate. It has a chemical formula of $(C_9H_{13}N)_2 \bullet H_2SO_4$ and a molecular weight of 368.50.

Structural Formula:

$$\left[C_6H_5\text{–}CH_2\underset{\displaystyle CH_3}{\underset{|}{C}}HNH_2 \right]_2 \cdot H_2SO_4$$

Each tablet, for oral administration, contains dextroamphetamine sulfate USP, 5 mg or 10 mg. Each tablet also contains the following inactive ingredients: acacia, corn starch, lactose monohydrate, magnesium stearate, sucrose. 10 mg tablet contains sodium starch glycolate. 5 mg and 10 mg tablets contain FD&C Yellow #5 (tartrazine).

CLINICAL PHARMACOLOGY

Amphetamines are non-catecholamine, sympathomimetic amines with CNS stimulant activity. Peripheral actions include elevations of systolic and diastolic blood pressures and weak bronchodilator and respiratory stimulant action.

There is neither specific evidence which clearly establishes the mechanism whereby amphetamines produce mental and behavioral effects in children, nor conclusive evidence regarding how these effects relate to the condition of the central nervous system.

Pharmacokinetics

The single ingestion of two 5 mg tablets by healthy volunteers produced an average peak dextroamphetamine blood level of 29.2 ng/mL at 2 hours post-administration. The average half-life was 10.25 hours. The average urinary recovery was 45% in 48 hours.

INDICATIONS AND USAGE

Dextroamphetamine sulfate tablets are indicated:

1. **In Narcolepsy.**
2. **In Attention Deficit Disorder with Hyperactivity,** as an integral part of a total treatment program which typically includes other remedial measures (psychological, educational, social) for a stabilizing effect in pediatric patients (ages 3 to 16 years) with a behavioral syndrome characterized by the following group of developmentally inappropriate symptoms: moderate to severe distractibility, short attention span, hyperactivity, emotional lability, and impulsivity. The diagnosis of this syndrome should not be made with finality when these symptoms are only of comparatively recent origin. Nonlocalizing (soft) neurological signs, learning disability, and abnormal EEG may or may not be present, and a diagnosis of central nervous system dysfunction may or may not be warranted.

CONTRAINDICATIONS

Advanced arteriosclerosis, symptomatic cardiovascular disease, moderate to severe hypertension, hyperthyroidism, known hypersensitivity or idiosyncrasy to the sympathomimetic amines, glaucoma.

Agitated states.

Patients with a history of drug abuse.

During or within 14 days following the administration of monoamine oxidase inhibitors (hypertensive crises may result).

PRECAUTIONS

General: Caution is to be exercised in prescribing amphetamines for patients with even mild hypertension.

The least amount feasible should be prescribed or dispensed at one time in order to minimize the possibility of overdosage.

These products contain FD&C Yellow No. 5 (tartrazine), which may cause allergic-type reactions (including bronchial asthma) in certain susceptible individuals. Although the overall incidence of hypersensitivity in the general population is low, it is frequently seen in patients who also have aspirin hypersensitivity.

Information for Patients: Amphetamines may impair the ability of the patient to engage in potentially hazardous activities such as operating machinery or vehicles; the patient should therefore be cautioned accordingly.

Drug Interactions

Acidifying agents—Gastro-intestinal acidifying agents (guanethidine, reserpine, glutamic acid HCl, ascorbic acid, fruit juices, etc.) lower absorption of amphetamines. Urinary acidifying agents (ammonium chloride, sodium acid phosphate, etc.) increase the concentration of the ionized species of the amphetamine molecule, thereby increasing urinary excretion. Both groups of agents lower blood levels and efficacy of amphetamines.

Adrenergic blockers—Adrenergic blockers are inhibited by amphetamines.

Alkalinizing agents—Gastro-intestinal alkalinizing agents (sodium bicarbonate, etc.) increase absorption of amphetamines. Urinary alkalinizing agents (acetazolamide, some thiazides) increase the concentration of the non-ionized species of the amphetamine molecule, thereby decreasing urinary excretion. Both groups of agents increase blood levels and therefore potentiate the actions of amphetamines.

Antidepressants, tricyclic—Amphetamines may enhance the activity of tricyclic or sympathomimetic agents; *d*-amphetamine with desipramine or protriptyline and possibly other tricyclics cause striking and sustained increases in the concentration of *d*-amphetamine in the brain; cardiovascular effects can be potentiated.

MAO inhibitors—MAOI antidepressants, as well as a metabolite of furazolidone, slow amphetamine metabolism. This slowing potentiates amphetamines, increasing their effect on the release of norepinephrine and other monoamines from adrenergic nerve endings; this can cause headaches and other signs of hypertensive crisis. A variety of neurological toxic effects and malignant hyperpyrexia can occur, sometimes with fatal results.

Antihistamines—Amphetamines may counteract the sedative effect of antihistamines.

Antihypertensives—Amphetamines may antagonize the hypotensive effects of antihypertensives.

Chlorpromazine—Chlorpromazine blocks dopamine and norepinephrine reuptake, thus inhibiting the central stimulant effects of amphetamines, and can be used to treat amphetamine poisoning.

Ethosuximide—Amphetamines may delay intestinal absorption of ethosuximide.

Haloperidol—Haloperidol blocks dopamine and norepinephrine reuptake, thus inhibiting the central stimulant effects of amphetamines.

Lithium carbonate—The stimulatory effects of amphetamines may be inhibited by lithium carbonate.

Meperidine—Amphetamines potentiate the analgesic effect of meperidine.

Methenamine therapy—Urinary excretion of amphetamines is increased, and efficacy is reduced, by acidifying agents used in methenamine therapy.

Norepinephrine—Amphetamines enhance the adrenergic effect of norepinephrine.

Phenobarbital—Amphetamines may delay intestinal absorption of phenobarbital; co-administration of phenobarbital may produce a synergistic anticonvulsant action.
Phenytoin—Amphetamines may delay intestinal absorption of phenytoin; co-administration of phenytoin may produce a synergistic anticonvulsant action.
Propoxyphene—In cases of propoxyphene overdosage, amphetamine CNS stimulation is potentiated and fatal convulsions can occur.
Veratrum alkaloids—Amphetamines inhibit the hypotensive effect of veratrum alkaloids.

Drug/Laboratory Test Interactions

- Amphetamines can cause a significant elevation in plasma corticosteroid levels. This increase is greatest in the evening.
- Amphetamines may interfere with urinary steroid determinations.

Carcinogenesis/Mutagenesis: Mutagenicity studies and long-term studies in animals to determine the carcinogenic potential of DextroStat® (dextroamphetamine sulfate) have not been performed.

Pregnancy–Teratogenic Effects: Pregnancy Category C. Dextroamphetamine has been shown to have embryotoxic and teratogenic effects when administered to A/Jax mice and C57BL mice in doses approximately 41 times the maximum human dose. Embryotoxic effects were not seen in New Zealand white rabbits given the drug in doses 7 times the human dose nor in rats given 12.5 times the maximum human dose. While there are no adequate and well-controlled studies in pregnant women, there has been one report of severe congenital bony deformity, tracheoesophageal fistula, and anal atresia (Vater association) in a baby born to a woman who took dextroamphetamine sulfate with lovastatin during the first trimester of pregnancy. Dextroamphetamine should be used during pregnancy only if the potential benefit justifies the potential risk to the fetus.

Nonteratogenic Effects: Infants born to mothers dependent on amphetamines have an increased risk of premature delivery and low birth weight. Also, these infants may experience symptoms of withdrawal as demonstrated by dysphoria, including agitation, and significant lassitude.

Nursing Mothers: Amphetamines are excreted in human milk. Mothers taking amphetamines should be advised to refrain from nursing.

Pediatric Use: Long-term effects of amphetamines in pediatric patients have not been well established.
Amphetamines are not recommended for use in pediatric patients under 3 years of age with Attention Deficit Disorder with Hyperactivity described under INDICATIONS AND USAGE.
Clinical experience suggests that in psychotic pediatric patients, administration of amphetamines may exacerbate symptoms of behavior disturbance and thought disorder.
Amphetamines have been reported to exacerbate motor and phonic tics and Tourette's syndrome. Therefore, clinical evaluation for tics and Tourette's syndrome in pediatric patients and their families should precede use of stimulant medications.
Data are inadequate to determine whether chronic administration of amphetamines may be associated with growth inhibition; therefore, growth should be monitored during treatment.
Drug treatment is not indicated in all cases of Attention Deficit Disorder with Hyperactivity and should be considered only in light of the complete history and evaluation of the pediatric patient. The decision to prescribe amphetamines should depend on the physician's assessment of the chronicity and severity of the pediatric patient's symptoms and their appropriateness for his/her age. Prescription should not depend solely on the presence of one or more of the behavioral characteristics.
When these symptoms are associated with acute stress reactions, treatment with amphetamines is usually not indicated.

ADVERSE REACTIONS

Cardiovascular: Palpitations, tachycardia, elevation of blood pressure. There have been isolated reports of cardiomyopathy associated with chronic amphetamine use.

Central Nervous System:
Psychotic episodes at recommended doses (rare), overstimulation, restlessness, dizziness, insomnia, euphoria, dyskinesia, dysphoria, tremor, headache, exacerbation of motor and phonic tics and Tourette's syndrome.

Gastrointestinal: Dryness of the mouth, unpleasant taste, diarrhea, constipation, other gastrointestinal disturbances. Anorexia and weight loss may occur as undesirable effects.

Allergic: Urticaria.

Endocrine: Impotence, changes in libido.

DRUG ABUSE AND DEPENDENCE

Dextroamphetamine sulfate tablets are a Schedule II controlled substance.
Amphetamines have been extensively abused. Tolerance, extreme psychological dependence and severe social disability have occurred. There are reports of patients who have increased the dosage to many times that recommended. Abrupt cessation following prolonged high dosage administration results in extreme fatigue and mental depression; changes are also noted on the sleep EEG.
Manifestations of chronic intoxication with amphetamines include severe dermatoses, marked insomnia, irritability, hyperactivity and personality changes. The most severe manifestation of chronic intoxication is psychosis, often clinically indistinguishable from schizophrenia. This is rare with oral amphetamines.

OVERDOSAGE

Individual patient response to amphetamines varies widely. While toxic symptoms occasionally occur as an idiosyncrasy at doses as low as 2 mg, they are rare with doses of less than 15 mg; 30 mg can produce severe reactions, yet doses of 400 to 500 mg are not necessarily fatal.
In rats, the oral LD_{50} of dextroamphetamine sulfate is 96.8 mg/kg.
Manifestations of acute overdosage with amphetamines include restlessness, tremor, hyperreflexia, rhabdomyolysis, rapid respiration, hyperpyrexia, confusion, assaultiveness, hallucinations, panic states.
Fatigue and depression usually follow the central stimulation.
Cardiovascular effects include arrhythmias, hypertension or hypotension and circulatory collapse. Gastrointestinal symptoms include nausea, vomiting, diarrhea and abdominal cramps. Fatal poisoning is usually preceded by convulsions and coma.
TREATMENT—Consult with a Certified Poison Control Center for up-to-date guidance and advice. Management of acute amphetamine intoxication is largely symptomatic and includes gastric lavage, administration of activated charcoal, administration of a cathartic, and sedation. Experience with hemodialysis or peritoneal dialysis is inadequate to permit recommendation in this regard. Acidification of the urine increases amphetamine excretion, but is believed to increase risk of acute renal failure if myoglobinuria is present. If acute, severe hypertension complicates amphetamine overdosage, administration of intravenous phentolamine has been suggested. However, a gradual drop in blood pressure will usually result when sufficient sedation has been achieved.

DOSAGE AND ADMINISTRATION

Amphetamines should be administered at the lowest effective dosage and dosage should be individually adjusted. Late evening doses should be avoided because of the resulting insomnia.

Narcolepsy: Usual dose 5 to 60 mg per day in divided doses, depending on the individual patient response.
Narcolepsy seldom occurs in pediatric patients under 12 years of age; however, when it does, DextroStat® (dextroamphetamine sulfate) may be used. The suggested initial dose for patients aged 6 to 12 is 5 mg daily; daily dose may be raised in increments of 5 mg at weekly intervals until optimal response is obtained. In patients 12 years of age and older, start with 10 mg daily; daily dosage may be raised in increments of 10 mg at weekly intervals until optimal response is obtained. If bothersome adverse reactions appear (e.g., insomnia or anorexia), dosage should be reduced. Give first dose on awakening; additional doses (1 or 2) at intervals of 4 to 6 hours.

Attention Deficit Disorder with Hyperactivity: Not recommended for pediatric patients under 3 years of age.

In pediatric patients from 3 to 5 years of age, start with 2.5 mg daily; daily dosage may be raised in increments of 2.5 mg at weekly intervals until optimal response is obtained.

In pediatric patients 6 years of age and older, start with 5 mg once or twice daily; daily dosage may be raised in increments of 5 mg at weekly intervals until optimal response is obtained. Only in rare cases will it be necessary to exceed a total of 40 mg per day.
Give first dose on awakening; additional doses (1 or 2) at intervals of 4 to 6 hours.
Where possible, drug administration should be interrupted occasionally to determine if there is a recurrence of behavioral symptoms sufficient to require continued therapy.

HOW SUPPLIED

DextroStat®, (dextroamphetamine sulfate) Tablets are available as follows:
5 mg Yellow, Round, Scored Tablet debossed "RP" on one side and "51" on the other side.
NDC #: 54092-448-01 for 100s
10 mg Yellow, Round, Double-Scored Tablet debossed "RP" on one side and "52" on the other side.
NDC #: 54092-452-01 for 100s
Dispense in a tight container as defined in the USP. Store at 25°C (77°F) excursions 15-30°C (59-86°F).
DEA Order Form Required.
Manufactured by:
Shire US Inc.
One Riverfront Place
Newport, KY 41071
1-800-828-2088
Made in USA

448 0107 001
Rev 5/03

518164

Shown in Product Identification Guide, page 333

FARESTON® ℞

[*fă-rə-stŏn*]
(toremifene citrate)
Tablets
PRODUCT INFORMATION

DESCRIPTION

FARESTON (toremifene citrate) Tablets for oral administration each contain 88.5 mg of toremifene citrate, which is equivalent to 60 mg toremifene.
FARESTON is a nonsteroidal antiestrogen. The chemical name of toremifene is: 2-{p-[(Z)-4-chloro-1,2-diphenyl-1-butenyl]phenoxy}-N,N-dimethylethylamine citrate (1:1). The structural formula is:

and the molecular formula is $C_{26}H_{28}ClNO \cdot C_6H_8O_7$. The molecular weight of toremifene citrate is 598.10. The pK_a is 8.0. Water solubility at 37°C is 0.63 mg/mL and in 0.02N HCl at 37°C is 0.38 mg/mL.
FARESTON is available only as tablets for oral administration. Inactive ingredients: colloidal silicon dioxide, lactose, magnesium stearate, microcrystalline cellulose, povidone, sodium starch glycolate, and starch.

CLINICAL PHARMACOLOGY

Mechanism of Action: Toremifene is a nonsteroidal triphenylethylene derivative. Toremifene binds to estrogen receptors and may exert estrogenic, antiestrogenic, or both activities, depending upon the duration of treatment, animal species, gender, target organ, or endpoint selected. In general, however, nonsteroidal triphenylethylene derivatives are predominantly antiestrogenic in rats and humans and estrogenic in mice. In rats, toremifene causes regression of established dimethylbenzanthracene (DMBA)-induced mammary tumors. The antitumor effect of toremifene in breast cancer is believed to be mainly due to its antiestrogenic effects, ie, its ability to compete with estrogen for binding sites in the cancer, blocking the growth-stimulating effects of estrogen in the tumor.
Toremifene causes a decrease in the estradiol-induced vaginal cornification index in some postmenopausal women, indicative of its antiestrogenic activity. Toremifene also has estrogenic activity as shown by decreases in serum gonadotropin concentrations (FSH and LH).

Pharmacokinetics: The plasma concentration time profile of toremifene declines biexponentially after absorption with a mean distribution half-life of about 4 hours and an elimination half-life of about 5 days. Elimination half-lives of major metabolites, N-demethyltoremifene and (deaminohydroxy) toremifene were 6 and 4 days, respectively. Mean total clearance of toremifene was approximately 5L/h.

Absorption and Distribution: Toremifene is well absorbed after oral administration and absorption is not influenced by food. Peak plasma concentrations are obtained within 3 hours. Toremifene displays linear pharmacokinetics after single oral doses of 10 to 680 mg. After multiple dosing, dose proportionality was observed for doses of 10 to 400 mg. Steady-state concentrations were reached in about 4-6 weeks. Toremifene has an apparent volume of distribution of 580 L and binds extensively (>99.5%) to serum proteins, mainly to albumin.

Metabolism and Excretion: Toremifene is extensively metabolized, principally by CYP3A4 to N-demethyltoremifene, which is also antiestrogenic but with weak *in vivo* antitumor potency. Serum concentrations of N-demethyltoremifene are 2 to 4 times higher than toremifene at steady state. Toremifene is eliminated as metabolites predominantly in the feces, with about 10% excreted in the urine during a 1-week period. Elimination of toremifene is slow, in part because of enterohepatic circulation.

Special Populations: *Renal insufficiency:* The pharmacokinetics of toremifene and N-demethyltoremifene were similar in normals and in patients with impaired kidney function.
Hepatic insufficiency: The mean elimination half-life of toremifene was increased by less than twofold in 10 patients with hepatic impairment (cirrhosis or fibrosis) compared to subjects with normal hepatic function. The pharmacokinetics of N-demethyltoremifene were unchanged in these patients. Ten patients on anticonvulsants (phenobarbital, clonazepam, phenytoin, and carbamazepine) showed a twofold increase in clearance and a decrease in the elimination half-life of toremifene.
Geriatric patients: The pharmacokinetics of toremifene were studied in 10 healthy young males and 10 elderly females following a single 120 mg dose under fasting conditions. Increases in the elimination half-life (4.2 versus 7.2 days) and the volume of distribution (457 versus 627 L) of toremifene were seen in the elderly females without any change in clearance or AUC.
Race: The pharmacokinetics of toremifene in patients of different races has not been studied.
Drug-drug interactions: No formal drug-drug interaction studies with toremifene have been performed.

CLINICAL STUDIES

Three prospective, randomized, controlled clinical studies (North American, Eastern European, and Nordic) were conducted to evaluate the efficacy of FARESTON for the treatment of breast cancer in postmenopausal women. The patients were randomized to parallel groups receiving FARESTON 60 mg (FAR60) or tamoxifen 20 mg (TAM20) in the North American Study or tamoxifen 40 mg (TAM40) in

Continued on next page

Fareston—Cont.

the Eastern European and Nordic studies. The North American and Eastern European studies also included high-dose toremifene arms of 200 and 240 mg daily, respectively. The studies included postmenopausal patients with estrogen-receptor (ER) positive or estrogen-receptor (ER) unknown metastatic breast cancer. The patients had at least one measurable or evaluable lesion. The primary efficacy variables were response rate (RR) and time to progression (TTP). Survival (S) was also determined. Ninety-five percent confidence intervals (95% CI) were calculated for the difference in RR between FAR60 and TAM groups and the hazard ratio (relative risk for an unfavorable event, such as disease progression or death) between TAM and FAR60 for TTP and S. Two of the 3 studies showed similar results for all effectiveness endpoints. However, the Nordic Study showed a longer time to progression for tamoxifen (see table).

[See first table at right]

The high-dose groups, toremifene 200 mg daily in the North American Study and 240 mg daily in the Eastern European Study, were not superior to the lower toremifene dose groups, with response rates of 22.6% AND 28.7%, median times to progression of 5.6 and 6.1 months, and median survivals of 30.1 and 23.8 months, respectively. The median treatment duration in the three pivotal studies was 5 months (range 4.2-6.3 months).

CLINICAL STUDIES

Study	North American		Eastern European		Nordic	
Treatment Group	FAR60	TAM20	FAR60	TAM40	FAR60	TAM40
No. Patients	221	215	157	149	214	201
Responses						
CR[1] + PR[2]	14+33	11+30	7+25	3+28	19+48	19+56
RR[3] (CR + PR)%	21.3	19.1	20.4	20.8	31.3	37.3
Difference in RR	2.2		-0.4		-6.0	
95% CI[4] for Difference in RR	-5.8 to 10.2		-9.5 to 8.6		-15.1 to 3.1	
Time to Progression (TTP)						
Median TTP (mo.)	5.6	5.8	4.9	5.0	7.3	10.2
Hazard Ratio (TAM/FAR)	1.01		1.02		0.80	
95% CI[4] for Hazard Ratio (%)	0.81 to 1.26		0.79 to 1.31		0.64 to 1.00	
Survival (S)						
Median S (mo.)	33.6	34.0	25.4	23.4	33.0	38.7
Hazard Ratio (TAM/FAR)	0.94		0.96		0.94	
95% CI[4] for Hazard Ratio (%)	0.74 to 1.24		0.72 to 1.28		0.73 to 1.22	

[1]CR = complete response; [2]PR = partial response; [3]RR = response rate; [4]CI = confidence interval

Adverse Events	North American		Eastern European		Nordic	
	FAR60 n=221(%)	TAM20 n=215(%)	FAR60 n=157(%)	TAM40 n=149(%)	FAR60 n=214(%)	TAM40 n=201(%)
Cardiac						
Cardiac Failure	2 (1)	1 (<1)	–	1 (<1)	2 (1)	3 (1.5)
Myocardial Infarction	2 (1)	3 (1.5)	1 (<1)	2 (1)	–	1 (<1)
Arrhythmia	–	–	–	–	3 (1.5)	1 (<1)
Angina Pectoris	–	–	1 (<1)	–	1 (<1)	2 (1)
Ocular*						
Cataracts	22 (10)	16 (7.5)	–	–	–	5 (3)
Dry Eyes	20 (9)	16 (7.5)	–	–	–	–
Abnormal Visual Fields	8 (4)	10 (5)	–	–	–	1 (<1)
Corneal Keratopathy	4 (2)	2 (1)	–	–	–	–
Glaucoma	3 (1.5)	2 (1)	1 (<1)	–	–	1 (<1)
Abnormal Vision/ Diplopia	–	–	–	–	3 (1.5)	–
Thromboembolic						
Pulmonary Embolism	4 (2)	2 (1)	1 (<1)	–	–	1 (<1)
Thrombophlebitis	–	2 (1)	1 (<1)	1 (<1)	4 (2)	3 (1.5)
Thrombosis	–	1 (<1)	1 (<1)	–	3 (1.5)	4 (2)
CVA/TIA	1 (<1)	–	–	1 (<1)	4 (2)	4 (2)
Elevated Liver Tests**						
SGOT	11 (5)	4 (2)	30 (19)	22 (15)	32 (15)	35 (17)
Alkaline Phosphatase	41 (19)	24 (11)	16 (10)	13 (9)	18 (8)	31 (15)
Bilirubin	3 (1.5)	4 (2)	2 (1)	1 (<1)	2 (1)	3 (1.5)
Hypercalcemia	6 (3)	6 (3)	1 (<1)	–	–	–

* Most of the ocular abnormalities were observed in the North American Study in which on-study and biannual ophthalmic examinations were performed. No cases of retinopathy were observed in any arm.

** Elevated defined as follows: North American Study: SGOT >100 IU/L; alkaline phosphatase >200 IU/L; bilirubin >2 mg/dL. Eastern European and Nordic studies: SGOT, alkaline phosphatase, and bilirubin – WHO Grade 1 (1.25 times the upper limit of normal).

INDICATION AND USAGE

FARESTON is indicated for the treatment of metastatic breast cancer in postmenopausal women with estrogen-receptor positive or unknown tumors.

CONTRAINDICATIONS

FARESTON is contraindicated in patients with known hypersensitivity to the drug.

WARNINGS

Hypercalcemia and Tumor Flare: As with other antiestrogens, hypercalcemia and tumor flare have been reported in some breast cancer patients with bone metastases during the first weeks of treatment with FARESTON. Tumor flare is a syndrome of diffuse musculoskeletal pain and erythema with increased size of tumor lesions that later regress. It is often accompanied by hypercalcemia. Tumor flare does not imply failure of treatment or represent tumor progression. If hypercalcemia occurs, appropriate measures should be instituted and if hypercalcemia is severe, FARESTON treatment should be discontinued.

Tumorigenicity: Since most toremifene trials have been conducted in patients with metastatic disease, adequate data on the potential endometrial tumorigenicity of long-term treatment with FARESTON are not available. Endometrial hyperplasia has been reported. Some patients treated with FARESTON have developed endometrial cancer, but circumstances (short duration of treatment or prior antiestrogen treatment or premalignant conditions) make it difficult to establish the role of FARESTON.

Endometrial hyperplasia of the uterus was observed in monkeys following 52 weeks of treatment at ≥1 mg/kg and in dogs following 16 weeks of treatment at ≥3 mg/kg with toremifene (about 1/4 and 1.4 times, respectively, the daily maximum recommended human dose on a mg/m^2 basis).

Pregnancy: FARESTON may cause fetal harm when administered to pregnant women. Studies in rats at doses ≥1.0 mg/kg/day (about 1/4 the daily maximum recommended human dose on a mg/m^2 basis) administered during the period of organogenesis, have shown that toremifene is embryotoxic and fetotoxic, as indicated by intrauterine mortality, increased resorption, reduced fetal weight, and fetal anomalies; including malformation of limbs, incomplete ossification, misshapen bones, ribs/spine anomalies, hydroureter, hydronephrosis, testicular displacement, and subcutaneous edema. Fetal anomalies may have been a consequence of maternal toxicity. Toremifene has been shown to cross the placenta and accumulate in the rodent fetus.

In rodent models of fetal reproductive tract development, toremifene produced inhibition of uterine development in female pups similar to diethylstilbestrol (DES) and tamoxifen. The clinical relevance of these changes is not known.

Embryotoxicity and fetotoxicity were observed in rabbits at doses ≥1.25 mg/kg/day and 2.5 mg/kg/day, respectively (about 1/3 and 2/3 the daily maximum recommended human dose on a mg/m^2 basis); fetal anomalies included incomplete ossification and anencephaly.

There are no studies in pregnant women. If FARESTON is used during pregnancy, or if the patient becomes pregnant while receiving this drug, the patient should be apprised of the potential hazard to the fetus or potential risk for loss of the pregnancy.

PRECAUTIONS

General: Patients with a history of thromboembolic diseases should generally not be treated with FARESTON. In general, patients with preexisting endometrial hyperplasia should not be given long-term FARESTON treatment. Patients with bone metastases should be monitored closely for hypercalcemia during the first weeks of treatment (see **WARNINGS**). Leukopenia and thrombocytopenia have been reported rarely; leukocyte and platelet counts should be monitored when using FARESTON in patients with leukopenia and thrombocytopenia.

Information for Patients: Vaginal bleeding has been reported in patients using FARESTON. Patients should be informed about this and instructed to contact their physician if such bleeding occurs.

Patients with bone metastases should be informed about the typical signs and symptoms of hypercalcemia and instructed to contact their physician for further assessment if such signs or symptoms occur.

Laboratory Tests: Periodic complete blood counts, calcium levels, and liver function tests should be obtained.

Drug-drug Interactions: Drugs that decrease renal calcium excretion, eg, thiazide diuretics, may increase the risk of hypercalcemia in patients receiving FARESTON. There is a known interaction between antiestrogenic compounds of the triphenylethylene derivative class and coumarin-type anticoagulants (eg, warfarin), leading to an increased prothrombin time. When concomitant use of anticoagulants with FARESTON is necessary, careful monitoring of the prothrombin time is recommended.

Cytochrome P450 3A4 enzyme inducers, such as phenobarbital, phenytoin, and carbamazepine increase the rate of toremifene metabolism, lowering the steady-state concentration in serum. Metabolism of toremifene may be inhibited by drugs known to inhibit the CYP3A4-6 enzymes. Examples of such drugs are ketoconazole and similar antimycotics as well as erythromycin and similar macrolides. This interaction has not been studied and its clinical relevance is uncertain.

Carcinogenesis, Mutagenesis, and Impairment of Fertility: Conventional carcinogenesis studies in rats at doses of 0.12 to 12 mg/kg/day (about 1/100 to 1.5 times the daily maximum recommended human dose on a mg/m^2 basis) for up to 2 years did not show evidence of carcinogenicity. Studies in mice at doses of 1.0 to 30.0 mg/kg/day (about 1/15 to 2 times the daily maximum recommended human dose on a mg/m^2 basis) for up to 2 years revealed increased incidence of ovarian and testicular tumors, and increased incidence of osteoma and osteosarcoma. The significance of the mouse findings is uncertain because of the different role of estrogens in mice and the estrogenic effect of toremifene in mice. An increased incidence of ovarian and testicular tumors in mice has also been observed with other human antiestrogenic agents that have primarily estrogenic activity in mice.

Toremifene has not been shown to be mutagenic in *in vitro* tests (Ames and *E. coli* bacterial tests). Toremifene is clastogenic *in vitro* (chromosomal aberrations and micronuclei formation in human lymphoblastoid MCL-5 cells) and *in vivo* (chromosomal aberrations in rat hepatocytes). No significant adduct formation could be detected using ^{32}P post-labeling in liver DNA from rats administered toremifene when compared to tamoxifen at similar doses. A study in cultured human lymphocytes indicated that adducting activity of toremifene, detected by ^{32}P post-labeling, was about 1/6 that of tamoxifen at approximately equipotent concentrations. In addition, the DNA adducting activity of toremifene in salmon sperm, using ^{32}P post-labeling, was 1/6 and 1/4 that observed with tamoxifen at equivalent concentrations following activation by rat and human microsomal systems, respectively. However, toremifene exposure is fourfold the exposure of tamoxifen based on human AUC in serum at recommended clinical doses.

Toremifene produced impairment of fertility and conception in male and female rats at doses ≥25.0 and 0.14 mg/kg/day, respectively (about 3.5 times and 1/50 the daily maximum recommended human dose on a mg/m^2 basis). At these doses, sperm counts, fertility index, and conception rate were reduced in males with atrophy of seminal vesicles and prostate. In females, fertility and reproductive indices were markedly reduced with increased pre- and post-implantation loss. In addition, offspring of treated rats exhibited depressed reproductive indices. Toremifene produced ovarian atrophy in dogs administered doses ≥3 mg/kg/day (about 1.5 times the daily maximum recommended human dose on a mg/m^2 basis) for 16 weeks. Cystic ovaries and reduction in endometrial stromal cellularity were observed in monkeys at doses ≥1 mg/kg/day (about 1/4 the daily maximum recommended human dose on a mg/m^2 basis) for 52 weeks.

Pregnancy: *Pregnancy Category D:* (see **WARNINGS**).

Nursing mothers: Toremifene has been shown to be excreted in the milk of lactating rats. It is not known if this drug is excreted in human milk. (See **WARNINGS** and **PRECAUTIONS**).

Pediatric use: There is no indication for use of FARESTON in pediatric patients.

Geriatric use: The median ages in the three controlled studies ranged from 60 to 66 years. No significant age-related differences in FARESTON effectiveness or safety were noted.

Race: Fourteen percent of patients in the North American Study were non-Caucasian. No significant race-related differences in FARESTON effectiveness or safety were noted.

ADVERSE REACTIONS

Adverse drug reactions are principally due to the antiestrogenic hormonal actions of FARESTON and typically occur at the beginning of treatment.

The incidences of the following eight clinical toxicities were prospectively assessed in the North American Study. The incidence reflects the toxicities that were considered by the investigator to be drug related or possibly drug related.

	North American Study	
	FAR60 n = 221	TAM20 n = 215
Hot Flashes	35%	30%
Sweating	20%	17%
Nausea	14%	15%
Vaginal Discharge	13%	16%
Dizziness	9%	7%
Edema	5%	5%
Vomiting	4%	2%
Vaginal Bleeding	2%	4%

Approximately 1% of patients receiving FARESTON (n = 592) in the three controlled studies discontinued treatment as a result of adverse events (nausea and vomiting, fatigue, thrombophlebitis, depression, lethargy, anorexia, ischemic attack, arthritis, pulmonary embolism, and myocardial infarction).

Serious adverse events occurring in patients receiving FARESTON in the three major trials are listed in the table below.

[See second table on previous page]

Other adverse events of unclear causal relationship to FARESTON included leukopenia and thrombocytopenia, skin discoloration or dermatitis, constipation, dyspnea, paresis, tremor, vertigo, pruritis, anorexia, reversible corneal opacity (corneal verticulata), asthenia, alopecia, depression, jaundice, and rigors.

In the 200 and 240 mg FARESTON dose arms, the incidence of SGOT elevation and nausea was higher. Approximately 4% of patients were withdrawn for toxicity from the high-dose FARESTON treatment arms. Reasons for withdrawal included hypercalcemia, abnormal liver function tests, and one case each of toxic hepatitis, depression, dizziness, incoordination, ataxia, blurry vision, diffuse dermatitis, and a constellation of symptoms consisting of nausea, sweating, and tremor.

OVERDOSAGE

Lethality was observed in rats following single oral doses that were ≥1000 mg/kg (about 150 times the recommended human dose on a mg/m^2 basis) and was associated with gastric atony/dilatation leading to interference with digestion and adrenal enlargement.

Vertigo, headache, and dizziness were observed in healthy volunteer studies at a daily dose of 680 mg for 5 days. The symptoms occurred in two of the five subjects during the third day of the treatment and disappeared within 2 days of discontinuation of the drug. No immediate concomitant changes in any measured clinical chemistry parameters were found. In a study in postmenopausal breast cancer patients, toremifene 400 mg/m^2/day caused dose-limiting nausea, vomiting, and dizziness, as well as reversible hallucinations and ataxia in one patient.

Theoretically, overdose may be manifested as an increase of antiestrogenic effects, such as hot flashes; estrogenic effects, such as vaginal bleeding; or nervous system disorders, such as vertigo, dizziness, ataxia, and nausea. There is no specific antidote and the treatment is symptomatic.

DOSAGE AND ADMINISTRATION

The dosage of FARESTON is 60 mg, once daily, orally. Treatment is generally continued until disease progression is observed.

HOW SUPPLIED

FARESTON Tablets, containing toremifene citrate in an amount equivalent to 60 mg of toremifene, are round, convex, unscored, uncoated, and white, or almost white. FARESTON Tablets are identified with TO 60 embossed on one side.

FARESTON Tablets are available as:
NDC 54092-170-30 bottles of 30
NDC 54092-170-01 bottles of 100

Store at 25°C (77°F)
excursions permitted to 15-30°C (59-86°F)
[see USP Controlled Room Temperature].
Protect from heat and light.

Developed and Manufactured by
Orion Corporation, Espoo, Finland

Distributed by **Shire US Inc.**
Newport, KY 41071, USA
under license from Orion Corporation.
Product covered by Orion Product Patents and related patent numbers.

E702229US-2 170 0117 003 Rev. 5/03

Shown in Product Identification Guide, page 333

PENTASA®

(mesalamine)
Controlled-Release Capsules 250 mg ℞

Prescribing information as of June 1999
℞ only

DESCRIPTION

PENTASA (mesalamine) for oral administration is a controlled-release formulation of mesalamine, an aminosalicylate anti-inflammatory agent for gastrointestinal use.

Chemically, mesalamine is 5-amino-2-hydroxybenzoic acid. It has a molecular weight of 153.14.

The structural formula is:

COOH, OH, H_2N

Each capsule contains 250 mg of mesalamine. It also contains the following inactive ingredients: acetylated monoglyceride, castor oil, colloidal silicon dioxide, ethylcellulose, hydroxypropyl methylcellulose, starch, stearic acid, sugar, talc, and white wax. The capsule shell contains D&C Yellow #10, FD&C Blue #1, FD&C Green #3, gelatin, titanium dioxide, and other ingredients.

CLINICAL PHARMACOLOGY

Sulfasalazine is split by bacterial action in the colon into sulfapyridine (SP) and mesalamine (5-ASA). It is thought that the mesalamine component is therapeutically active in ulcerative colitis. The usual oral dose of sulfasalazine for active ulcerative colitis in adults is 2 to 4 g per day in divided doses. Four grams of sulfasalazine provide 1.6 g of free mesalamine to the colon.

The mechanism of action of mesalamine (and sulfasalazine) is unknown, but appears to be topical rather than systemic. Mucosal production of arachidonic acid (AA) metabolites, both through the cyclooxygenase pathways, ie, prostanoids, and through the lipoxygenase pathways, ie, leukotrienes (LTs) and hydroxyeicosatetraenoic acids (HETEs), is increased in patients with chronic inflammatory bowel disease, and it is possible that mesalamine diminishes inflammation by blocking cyclooxygenase and inhibiting prostaglandin (PG) production in the colon.

Human Pharmacokinetics and Metabolism

Absorption. PENTASA is an ethylcellulose-coated controlled-release formulation of mesalamine designed to release therapeutic quantities of mesalamine throughout the gastrointestinal tract. Based on urinary excretion data, 20% to 30% of the mesalamine in PENTASA is absorbed. In contrast, when mesalamine is administered orally as an unformulated 1-g aqueous suspension, mesalamine is approximately 80% absorbed.

Plasma mesalamine concentration peaked at approximately 1 μg/mL 3 hours following a 1-g PENTASA dose and declined in a biphasic manner. The literature describes a mean terminal half-life of 42 minutes for mesalamine following intravenous administration. Because of the continuous release and absorption of mesalamine from PENTASA throughout the gastrointestinal tract, the true elimination half-life cannot be determined after oral administration. N-acetylmesalamine, the major metabolite of mesalamine, peaked at approximately 3 hours at 1.8 μg/mL, and its concentration followed a biphasic decline. Pharmacological activities of N-acetylmesalamine are unknown, and other metabolites have not been identified.

Oral mesalamine pharmacokinetics were nonlinear when PENTASA capsules were dosed from 250 mg to 1 g four times daily, with steady-state mesalamine plasma concentrations increasing about nine times, from 0.14 μg/mL to 1.21 μg/mL, suggesting saturable first-pass metabolism. N-acetylmesalamine pharmacokinetics were linear.

Elimination. About 130 mg free mesalamine was recovered in the feces following a single 1-g PENTASA dose, which was comparable to the 140 mg of mesalamine recovered from the molar equivalent sulfasalazine tablet dose of 2.5 g. Elimination of free mesalamine and salicylates in feces increased proportionately with PENTASA dose. N-acetylmesalamine was the primary compound excreted in the urine (19% to 30%) following PENTASA dosing.

CLINICAL TRIALS

In two randomized, double-blind, placebo-controlled, dose-response trials (UC-1 and UC-2) of 625 patients with active mild to moderate ulcerative colitis, PENTASA, at an oral dose of 4 g/day given 1 g four times daily, produced consistent improvement in prospectively identified primary efficacy parameters, PGA, Tx F, and SI as shown in the table below.

The 4-g dose of PENTASA also gave consistent improvement in secondary efficacy parameters, namely the frequency of trips to the toilet, stool consistency, rectal bleeding, abdominal/rectal pain, and urgency. The 4-g dose of PENTASA induced remission as assessed by endoscopic and symptomatic endpoints.

In some patients, the 2-g dose of PENTASA was observed to improve efficacy parameters measured. However, the 2-g dose gave inconsistent results in primary efficacy parameters across the two adequate and well-controlled trials. [See table below]

INDICATIONS AND USAGE

PENTASA is indicated for the induction of remission and for the treatment of patients with mildly to moderately active ulcerative colitis.

CONTRAINDICATIONS

PENTASA is contraindicated in patients who have demonstrated hypersensitivity to mesalamine, any other components of this medication, or salicylates.

PRECAUTIONS

General

Caution should be exercised if PENTASA is administered to patients with impaired hepatic function.

Mesalamine has been associated with an acute intolerance syndrome that may be difficult to distinguish from a flare of inflammatory bowel disease. Although the exact frequency of occurrence cannot be ascertained, it has occurred in 3% of patients in controlled clinical trials of mesalamine or sulfasalazine. Symptoms include cramping, acute abdominal pain and bloody diarrhea, sometimes fever, headache, and rash. If acute intolerance syndrome is suspected, prompt withdrawal is required. If a rechallenge is performed later in order to validate the hypersensitivity, it should be carried out under close medical supervision at reduced dose and only if clearly needed.

Renal

Caution should be exercised if PENTASA is administered to patients with impaired renal function. Single reports of nephrotic syndrome and interstitial nephritis associated with mesalamine therapy have been described in the foreign literature. There have been rare reports of interstitial nephritis in patients receiving PENTASA. In animal studies, a 13-week oral toxicity study in mice and 13-week and 52-week oral toxicity studies in rats and cynomolgus monkeys have shown the kidney to be the major target organ of mesalamine toxicity. Oral daily doses of 2400 mg/kg in mice and 1150 mg/kg in rats produced renal lesions including granular and hyaline casts, tubular degeneration, tubular dilation, renal infarct, papillary necrosis, tubular necrosis, and interstitial nephritis. In cynomolgus monkeys, oral daily doses of 250 mg/kg or higher produced nephrosis, pap-

Continued on next page

	Clinical Trial UC-1			Clinical Trial UC-2		
		PENTASA			PENTASA	
Parameter Evaluated	PL (n=90)	4 g/day (n=95)	2 g/day (n=97)	PL (n=83)	4 g/day (n=85)	2 g/day (n=83)
PGA	36%	59%*	57%*	31%	55%*	41%
Tx F	22%	9%*	18%	31%	9%*	17%*
SI	−2.5	−5.0*	−4.3*	−1.6	−3.8*	−2.6
Remission†	12%	26%*	24%*	12%	27%*	12%

* $p < 0.05$ vs placebo.

PGA: Physician Global Assessment: proportion of patients with complete or marked improvement.

Tx F: Treatment Failure: proportion of patients developing severe or fulminant UC requiring steroid therapy or hospitalization or worsening of the disease at 7 days of therapy, or lack of significant improvement by 14 days of therapy.

SI: Sigmoidoscopic Index: an objective measure of disease activity rated by a standard (15-point) scale that includes mucosal vascular pattern, erythema, friability, granularity/ulcerations, and mucopus: improvement over baseline.

† Defined as complete resolution of symptoms plus improvement of endoscopic endpoints. To be considered in remission, patients had a "1" score for one of the endoscopic components (mucosal vascular pattern, erythema, granularity, or friability) and "0" for the others.

Pentasa—Cont.

illary edema, and interstitial fibrosis. Patients with pre-existing renal disease, increased BUN or serum creatinine, or proteinuria should be carefully monitored.

Carcinogenesis, Mutagenesis, Impairment of Fertility

In a 104-week dietary carcinogenicity study of mesalamine, CD-1 mice were treated with doses up to 2500 mg/kg/day and it was not tumorigenic. For a 50 kg person of average height (1.46 m^2 body surface area), this represents 2.5 times the recommended human dose on a body surface area basis (2960 mg/m^2/day). In a 104-week dietary carcinogenicity study in Wistar rats, mesalamine up to a dose of 800 mg/kg/day was not tumorigenic. This dose represents 1.5 times the recommended human dose on a body surface area basis.

No evidence of mutagenicity was observed in an in vitro Ames test and an in vivo mouse micronucleus test.

No effects on fertility or reproductive performance were observed in male or female rats at oral doses of mesalamine up to 400 mg/kg/day (0.8 times the recommended human dose based on body surface area).

Semen abnormalities and infertility in men, which have been reported in association with sulfasalazine, have not been seen with PENTASA capsules during controlled clinical trials.

Pregnancy

Category B. Reproduction studies have been performed in rats at doses up to 1000 mg/kg/day (5900 mg/M^2) and rabbits at doses of 800 mg/kg/day (6856 mg/M^2) and have revealed no evidence of teratogenic effects or harm to the fetus due to mesalamine. There are, however, no adequate and well-controlled studies in pregnant women. Because animal reproduction studies are not always predictive of human response, PENTASA should be used during pregnancy only if clearly needed.

Mesalamine is known to cross the placental barrier.

Nursing Mothers

Minute quantities of mesalamine were distributed to breast milk and amniotic fluid of pregnant women following sulfasalazine therapy. When treated with sulfasalazine at a dose equivalent to 1.25 g/day of mesalamine, 0.02 μg/mL to 0.08 μg/mL and trace amounts of mesalamine were measured in amniotic fluid and breast milk, respectively. N-acetylmesalamine, in quantities of 0.07 μg/mL to 0.77 μg/mL and 1.13 μg/mL to 3.44 μg/mL, was identified in the same fluids, respectively.

Caution should be exercised when PENTASA is administered to a nursing woman.

Pediatric Use

Safety and efficacy of PENTASA in pediatric patients have not been established.

ADVERSE REACTIONS

In combined domestic and foreign clinical trials, more than 2100 patients with ulcerative colitis or Crohn's disease received PENTASA therapy. Generally, PENTASA therapy was well tolerated. The most common events (ie, greater than or equal to 1%) were diarrhea (3.4%), headache (2.0%), nausea (1.8%), abdominal pain (1.7%), dyspepsia (1.6%), vomiting (1.5%), and rash (1.0%).

In two domestic placebo-controlled trials involving over 600 ulcerative colitis patients, adverse events were fewer in PENTASA-treated patients than in the placebo group (PENTASA 14% vs placebo 18%) and were not dose-related. Events occurring at 1% or more are shown in the table below. Of these, only nausea and vomiting were more frequent in the PENTASA group. Withdrawal from therapy due to adverse events was more common on placebo than PENTASA (7% vs 4%).

[See table 1 below]

Clinical laboratory measurements showed no significant abnormal trends for any test, including measurement of hematologic, liver, and kidney function.

The following adverse events, presented by body system, were reported infrequently (ie, less than 1%) during domestic ulcerative colitis and Crohn's disease trials. In many cases, the relationship to PENTASA has not been established.

Gastrointestinal: abdominal distention, anorexia, constipation, duodenal ulcer, dysphagia, eructation, esophageal ulcer, fecal incontinence, GGTP increase, GI bleeding, increased alkaline phosphatase, LDH increase, mouth ulcer, oral moniliases, pancreatitis, rectal bleeding, SGOT increase, SGPT increase, stool abnormalities (color or texture change), thirst

Dermatological: acne, alopecia, dry skin, eczema, erythema nodosum, nail disorder, photosensitivity, pruritus, sweating, urticaria

Nervous System: depression, dizziness, insomnia, somnolence, paresthesia

Cardiovascular: palpitations, pericarditis, vasodilation

Other: albuminuria, amenorrhea, amylase increase, arthraligia, asthenia, breast pain, conjunctivitis, ecchymosis, edema, fever, hematuria, hypomenorrhea, Kawasaki-like syndrome, leg cramps, lichen planus, lipase increase, malaise, menorrhagia, metrorrhagia, myalgia, pulmonary infiltrates, thrombocythemia, thrombocytopenia, urinary frequency

One week after completion of an 8-week ulcerative colitis study, a 72-year-old male, with no previous history of pulmonary problems, developed dyspnea. The patient was subsequently diagnosed with interstitial pulmonary fibrosis without eosinophilia by one physician and bronchiolitis obliterans with organizing pneumonitis by a second physician. A causal relationship between this event and mesalamine therapy has not been established.

Published case reports and/or spontaneous postmarketing surveillance have described infrequent instances of pericarditis, fatal myocarditis, chest pain and T-wave abnormalities, hypersensitivity pneumonitis, pancreatitis, nephrotic syndrome, interstitial nephritis, hepatitis, aplastic anemia, pancytopenia, leukopenia, agranulocytosis, or anemia while receiving mesalamine therapy. Anemia can be a part of the clinical presentation of inflammatory bowel disease. Allergic reactions, which could involve eosinophilia, can be seen in connection with PENTASA therapy.

Postmarketing Reports

The following events have been identified during post-approval use of products which contain (or are metabolized to) mesalamine in clinical practice. Because they are reported voluntarily from a population of unknown size, estimates of frequency cannot be made. These events have been chosen for inclusion due to a combination of seriousness, frequency of reporting, or potential causal connection to mesalamine:

Gastrointestinal: Reports of hepatotoxicity, including elevated liver function tests (SGOT/AST, SGPT/ALT, GGT, LDH, alkaline phosphatase, bilirubin), jaundice, cholestatic jaundice, cirrhosis, and possible hepatocellular damage including liver necrosis and liver failure. Some of these cases were fatal. One case of Kawasaki-like syndrome which included hepatic function changes was also reported.

OVERDOSAGE

Single oral doses of mesalamine up to 5 g/kg in pigs or a single intravenous dose of mesalamine at 920 mg/kg in rats were not lethal.

There is no clinical experience with PENTASA overdosage. PENTASA is an aminosalicylate, and symptoms of salicylate toxicity may be possible, such as: tinnitus, vertigo, headache, confusion, drowsiness, sweating, hyperventilation, vomiting, and diarrhea. Severe intoxication with salicylates can lead to disruption of electrolyte balance and blood pH, hyperthermia, and dehydration.

Treatment of Overdosage. Since PENTASA is an aminosalicylate, conventional therapy for salicylate toxicity may be beneficial in the event of acute overdosage. This includes prevention of further gastrointestinal tract absorption by emesis and, if necessary, by gastric lavage. Fluid and electrolyte imbalance should be corrected by the administration of appropriate intravenous therapy. Adequate renal function should be maintained.

DOSAGE AND ADMINISTRATION

The recommended dosage for the induction of remission and the symptomatic treatment of mildly to moderately active ulcerative colitis is 1 g (4 PENTASA capsules) four times a day for a total daily dose of 4 g. Treatment duration in controlled trials was up to 8 weeks.

HOW SUPPLIED

PENTASA controlled-release capsules are supplied in bottles of 240 capsules (NDC 54092-189-81); and blister packs of 80 capsules (NDC 54092-189-80). Each green and blue capsule contains 250 mg of mesalamine in controlled-release beads. PENTASA controlled-release capsules are identified with a pentagonal starburst logo and the number 2010 on the green portion and PENTASA 250 mg on the blue portion of the capsules.

Store at 25°C (77°F) excursions permitted to 15–30°C (59–86°F)

[see USP Controlled Room Temperature]

Manufactured for

Shire US Inc.

Newport, KY 41071, USA

Prescribing information as of June 1999

Licensed from Ferring A/S, Denmark

U.S. Patent Nos. B1 4,496,553 and 4,980,173

 Rev. 2/03

189 0107 005A 50019194

Shown in Product Identification Guide, page 333

Table 1. Adverse Events Occurring in More Than 1% of Either Placebo or PENTASA Patients in Domestic Placebo-controlled Ulcerative Colitis Trials. (PENTASA Comparison to Placebo)

Event	PENTASA n=451	Placebo n=173
Diarrhea	16 (3.5%)	13 (7.5%)
Headache	10 (2.2%)	6 (3.5%)
Nausea	14 (3.1%)	—
Abdominal Pain	5 (1.1%)	7 (4.0%)
Melena (Bloody Diarrhea)	4 (0.9%)	6 (3.5%)
Rash	6 (1.3%)	2 (1.2%)
Anorexia	5 (1.1%)	2 (1.2%)
Fever	4 (0.9%)	2 (1.2%)
Rectal Urgency	1 (0.2%)	4 (2.3%)
Nausea and Vomiting	5 (1.1%)	—
Worsening of Ulcerative Colitis	2 (0.4%)	2 (1.2%)
Acne	1 (0.2%)	2 (1.2%)

PROAMATINE® ℞

[prō-ă-mă-tin]

(midodrine hydrochloride)

2.5-mg tablet • 5-mg tablet • 10-mg tablet

> WARNING
>
> **Because ProAmatine® can cause marked elevation of supine blood pressure, it should be used in patients whose lives are considerably impaired despite standard clinical care. The indication for use of ProAmatine® in the treatment of symptomatic orthostatic hypotension is based primarily on a change in a surrogate marker of effectiveness, an increase in systolic blood pressure measured one minute after standing, a surrogate marker considered likely to correspond to a clinical benefit. At present, however, clinical benefits of ProAmatine®, principally improved ability to carry out activities of daily living, have not been verified.**

DESCRIPTION

Name: ProAmatine® (midodrine hydrochloride) Tablets

Dosage Form: 2.5-mg, 5-mg and 10-mg tablets for oral administration

Active Ingredient: Midodrine hydrochloride, 2.5 mg, 5 mg and 10 mg

Inactive Ingredients: Colloidal Silicone Dioxide NF, Corn Starch NF, FD&C Blue No. 2 Lake (10-mg tablets), FD&C Yellow No. 6 Lake (5-mg tablet), Magnesium Stearate NF, Microcrystalline Cellulose NF, Talc USP

Pharmacological Classification: Vasopressor/Antihypotensive

Chemical Names (USAN: Midodrine Hydrochloride): (1) Acetamide, 2-amino-*N*-[2-(2,5-dimethoxyphenyl)-2-hydroxyethyl]-monohydrochloride, (±)-; (2) (±) -2-amino-*N*-(β-hydroxy-2,5-dimethoxyphenethyl)acetamide monohydrochloride BAN, INN, JAN: Midodrine

Structural formula:

Molecular formula: $C_{12}H_{18}N_2O_4HCl$;

Molecular Weight: 290.7

Organoleptic Properties: Odorless, white, crystalline powder

Solubility:	Water:	Soluble
	Methanol:	Sparingly soluble

pKa: 7.8 (0.3% aqueous solution)

pH: 3.5 to 5.5 (5% aqueous solution)

Melting Range: 200 to 203°C

CLINICAL PHARMACOLOGY

Mechanism of Action: **ProAmatine®** forms an active metabolite, desglymidodrine, that is an $alpha_1$-agonist, and exerts its actions via activation of the alpha-adrenergic receptors of the arteriolar and venous vasculature, producing an increase in vascular tone and elevation of blood pressure. Desglymidodrine does not stimulate cardiac beta-adrenergic receptors. Desglymidodrine diffuses poorly across the blood-brain barrier, and is therefore not associated with effects on the central nervous system.

Administration of **ProAmatine®** results in a rise in standing, sitting, and supine systolic and diastolic blood pressure in patients with orthostatic hypotension of various etiologies. Standing systolic blood pressure is elevated by approximately 15 to 30 mmHg at 1 hour after a 10-mg dose of midodrine, with some effect persisting for 2 to 3 hours. **ProAmatine®** has no clinically significant effect on standing or supine pulse rates in patients with autonomic failure.

Pharmacokinetics: **ProAmatine®** is a prodrug, i.e., the therapeutic effect of orally administered midodrine is due to the major metabolite desglymidodrine, formed by deglycination of midodrine. After oral administration, **ProAmatine®** is rapidly absorbed. The plasma levels of the prodrug peak after about half an hour, and decline with a half-life of approximately 25 minutes, while the metabolite reaches peak blood concentrations about 1 to 2 hours after a dose of midodrine and has a half-life of about 3 to 4 hours. The absolute bioavailability of midodrine (measured as desglymidodrine) is 93%. The bioavailability of desglymidodrine is not affected by food. Approximately the same amount of desglymidodrine is formed after intravenous and oral administration of midodrine. Neither midodrine nor desglymidodrine is bound to plasma proteins to any significant extent.

Metabolism and Excretion: Thorough metabolic studies have not been conducted, but it appears that deglycination of midodrine to desglymidodrine takes place in many tissues, and both compounds are metabolized in part by the liver. Neither midodrine nor desglymidodrine is a substrate for monoamine oxidase.

Renal elimination of midodrine is insignificant. The renal clearance of desglymidodrine is of the order of 385 mL/minute, most, about 80%, by active renal secretion. The actual mechanism of active secretion has not been studied, but it is possible that it occurs by the base-secreting pathway responsible for the secretion of several other drugs that are bases (see also **Potential for Drug Interactions**).

Clinical Studies

Midodrine has been studied in 3 principal controlled trials, one of 3-weeks duration and 2 of 1 to 2 days duration. All studies were randomized, double-blind and parallel-design trials in patients with orthostatic hypotension of any etiology and supine-to-standing fall of systolic blood pressure of at least 15 mmHg accompanied by at least moderate dizziness/lightheadedness. Patients with pre-existing sustained supine hypertension above 180/110 mmHg were routinely excluded. In a 3-week study in 170 patients, most previously untreated with midodrine, the midodrine-treated patients (10 mg t.i.d., with the last dose not later than 6 P.M.) had significantly higher (by about 20 mmHg) 1-minute standing systolic pressure 1 hour after dosing (blood pressures were not measured at other times) for all 3 weeks. After week 1, midodrine-treated patients had small improvements in dizziness/lightheadedness/unsteadiness scores and global evaluations, but these effects were made difficult to interpret by a high early drop-out rate (about 25% vs 5% on placebo). Supine and sitting blood pressure rose 16/8 and 20/10 mmHg, respectively, on average. In a 2-day study, after open-label midodrine, known midodrine responders received midodrine 10 mg or placebo at 0, 3, and 6 hours. One-minute standing systolic blood pressures were increased 1 hour after each dose by about 15 mmHg and 3 hours after each dose by about 12 mmHg; 3-minute standing pressures were increased also at 1, but not 3, hours after dosing. There were increases in standing time seen intermittently 1 hour after dosing, but not at 3 hours.

In a 1-day, dose-response trial, single doses of 0, 2.5, 10, and 20 mg of midodrine were given to 25 patients. The 10- and 20-mg doses produced increases in standing 1-minute systolic pressure of about 30 mmHg at 1 hour; the increase was sustained in part for 2 hours after 10 mg and 4 hours after 20 mg. Supine systolic pressure was ≥200 mmHg in 22% of patients on 10 mg and 45% of patients on 20 mg; elevated pressures often lasted 6 hours or more.

Special Populations

A study with 16 patients undergoing hemodialysis demonstrated that **ProAmatine®** is removed by dialysis.

INDICATIONS AND USAGE

ProAmatine® is indicated for the treatment of symptomatic orthostatic hypotension (OH). Because **ProAmatine®** can cause marked elevation of supine blood pressure (BP>200 mmHg systolic), it should be used in patients whose lives are considerably impaired despite standard clinical care, including non-pharmacologic treatment (such as support stockings), fluid expansion, and lifestyle alterations. The indication is based on **ProAmatine®**'s effect on increases in 1-minute standing systolic blood pressure, a surrogate marker considered likely to correspond to a clinical benefit. At present, however, clinical benefits of **ProAmatine®**, principally improved abitlity to perform life activities, have not been established. Further clinical trials are underway to verify and describe the clinical benefits of **ProAmatine®**. After initiation of treatment, **ProAmatine®** should be continued only for patients who report significant symptomatic improvement.

CONTRAINDICATIONS

ProAmatine® is contraindicated in patients with severe organic heart disease, acute renal disease, urinary retention, pheochromocytoma or thyrotoxicosis. **ProAmatine®** should not be used in patients with persistent and excessive supine hypertension.

WARNINGS

Supine Hypertension: The most potentially serious adverse reaction associated with ProAmatine® therapy is marked elevation of supine arterial blood pressure (supine hypertension). Systolic pressure of about 200 mmHg were seen overall in about 13.4% of patients given 10 mg of ProAmatine®. Systolic elevations of this degree were most likely to be observed in patients with relatively elevated pre-treatment systolic blood pressures (mean 170 mmHg). There is no experience in patients with initial supine systolic pressure above 180 mmHg, as those patients were excluded from the clinical trials. Use of ProAmatine® in such patients is not recommended. Sitting blood pressures were also elevated by ProAmatine® therapy. It is essential to monitor supine and sitting blood pressures in patients maintained on ProAmatine®.

PRECAUTIONS

General: The potential for supine and sitting hypertension should be evaluated at the beginning of **ProAmatine®** therapy. Supine hypertension can often be controlled by preventing the patient from becoming fully supine, i.e., sleeping with the head of the bed elevated. The patient should be cautioned to report symptoms of supine hypertension immediately. Symptoms may include cardiac awareness, pounding in the ears, headache, blurred vision, etc. The patient should be advised to discontinue the medication immediately if supine hypertension persists.

Blood pressure should be monitored carefully when **ProAmatine®** is used concomitantly with other agents that cause vasoconstriction, such as phenylephrine, ephedrine, dihydroergotamine, phenylpropanolamine, or pseudoephedrine.

A slight slowing of the heart rate may occur after administration of **ProAmatine®**, primarily due to vagal reflex. Caution should be exercised when **ProAmatine®** is used concomitantly with cardiac glycosides (such as digitalis), psychopharmacologic agents, beta blockers or other agents that directly or indirectly reduce heart rate. Patients who experience any signs or symptoms suggesting bradycardia (pulse slowing, increased dizziness, syncope, cardiac awareness) should be advised to discontinue **ProAmatine®** and should be re-evaluated.

ProAmatine® should be used cautiously in patients with urinary retention problems, as desglymidodrine acts on the alpha-adrenergic receptors of the bladder neck. **ProAmatine®** should be used with caution in orthostatic hypotensive patients who are also diabetic, as well as those with a history of visual problems who are also taking fludrocortisone acetate, which is known to cause an increase in intraocular pressure and glaucoma. **ProAmatine®** use has not been studied in patients with renal impairment. Because desglymidodrine is eliminated via the kidneys, and higher blood levels would be expected in such patients, **ProAmatine®** should be used with caution in patients with renal impairment, with a starting dose of 2.5 mg (see **DOSAGE AND ADMINISTRATION**). Renal function should be assessed prior to initial use of **ProAmatine®**.

ProAmatine® use has not been studied in patients with hepatic impairment. **ProAmatine®** should be used with caution in patients with hepatic impairment, as the liver has a role in the metabolism of midodrine.

Information for Patients: Patients should be told that certain agents in over-the-counter products, such as cold remedies and diet aids, can elevate blood pressure, and therefore, should be used cautiously with **ProAmatine®**, as they may enhance or potentiate the pressor effects of **ProAmatine®** (see **Drug Interactions**). Patients should also be made aware of the possibility of supine hypertension. They should be told to avoid taking their dose if they are to be supine for any length of time, i.e., they should take their last daily dose of **ProAmatine®** 3 to 4 hours before bedtime to minimize nighttime supine hypertension.

Laboratory Tests: Since desglymidodrine is eliminated by the kidneys and the liver has a role in its metabolism, evaluation of the patient should include assessment of renal and hepatic function prior to initiating therapy and subsequently, as appropriate.

Drug Interactions: When administered concomitantly with **ProAmatine®**, cardiac glycosides may enhance or precipitate bradycardia, A.V. block or arrhythmia. The use of drugs that stimulate alpha-adrenergic receptors (e.g., phenylephrine, pseudoephedrine, ephedrine, phenylpropanolamine or dihydroergotamine) may enhance or potentiate the pressor effects of **ProAmatine®**. Therefore, caution should be used when **ProAmatine®** is administered concomitantly with agents that cause vasoconstriction.

ProAmatine® has been used in patients concomitantly treated with salt-retaining steroid therapy (i.e., fludrocortisone acetate), with or without salt supplementation. The potential for supine hypertension should be carefully monitored in these patients and may be minimized by either reducing the dose of fludrocortisone acetate or decreasing the salt intake prior to initiation of treatment with **ProAmatine®**. Alpha-adrenergic blocking agents, such as prazosin, terazosin, and doxazosin, can antagonize the effects of **ProAmatine®**.

Potential for Drug Interaction: It appears possible, although there is no supporting experimental evidence, that the high renal clearance of desyglymidodrine (a base) is due to active tubular secretion by the base-secreting system also responsible for the secretion of such drugs as metformin, cimetidine, ranitidine, procainamide, triamterene, flecainide, and quinidine. Thus there may be a potential for drug-drug interactions with these drugs.

Carcinogenesis, Mutagenesis, Impairment of Fertility: Long-term studies have been conducted in rats and mice at dosages 3 to 4 times the maximum recommended daily human dose on a mg/m^2 basis, with no indication of carcinogenic effects related to **ProAmatine®**. Studies investigating the mutagenic potential of **ProAmatine®** revealed no evidence of mutagenicity. Other than the dominant lethal assay in male mice, where no impairment of fertility was observed, there have been no studies on the effects of **ProAmatine®** on fertility.

Pregnancy: *Pregnancy Category C.* **ProAmatine®** increased the rate of embryo resorption, reduced fetal body weight in rats and rabbits, and decreased fetal survival in rabbits when given in doses 13 (rat) and 7 (rabbit) times the maximum human dose based on body surface area (mg/m^2). There are no adequate and well-controlled studies in pregnant women. **ProAmatine®** should be used during pregnancy only if the potential benefit justifies the potential risk to the fetus. No teratogenic effects have been observed in studies in rats and rabbits.

Nursing Mothers: It is not known whether this drug is excreted in human milk. Because many drugs are excreted in human milk, caution should be exercised when **ProAmatine®** is administered to nursing women.

Pediatric Use: Safety and effectiveness in pediatric patients have not been established.

ADVERSE REACTIONS

The most frequent adverse reactions seen in controlled trials were supine and sitting hypertension; paresthesia and pruritus, mainly of the scalp; goosebumps; chills; urinary urge; urinary retention and urinary frequency.

The frequency of these events in a 3-week placebo-controlled trial is shown in the following table:

Adverse Events

	Placebo n=88		Midodrine n=82	
Event	# of reports	% of patients	# of reports	% of patients
Total # of reports	22		77	
Paresthesia[1]	4	4.5	15	18.3
Piloerection	0	0	11	13.4
Dysuria[2]	0	0	11	13.4
Pruritus[3]	2	2.3	10	12.2
Supine hypertension[4]	0	0	6	7.3
Chills	0	0	4	4.9
Pain[5]	0	0	4	4.9
Rash	1	1.1	2	2.4

1 Includes hyperesthesia and scalp paresthesia

2 Includes dysuria (1), increased urinary frequency (2), impaired urination (1), urinary retention (5), urinary urgency (2)

3 Includes scalp pruritus

4 Includes patients who experienced an increase in supine hypertension

5 Includes abdominal pain and pain increase

Less frequent adverse reactions were headache; feeling of pressure/fullness in the head; vasodilation/flushing face; confusion/thinking abnormality; dry mouth; nervousness/anxiety and rash. Other adverse reactions that occurred rarely were visual field defect; dizziness; skin hyperesthesia; insomnia; somnolence; erythema multiforme; canker sore; dry skin; dysuria; impaired urination; asthenia; backache; pyrosis; nausea; gastrointestinal distress; flatulence and leg cramps. The most potentially serious adverse reaction associated with **ProAmatine®** therapy is supine hypertension. The feelings of paresthesia, pruritus, piloerection and chills are pilomotor reactions associated with the action of midodrine on the alpha-adrenergic receptors of the hair follicles. Feelings of urinary urgency, retention and frequency are associated with the action of midodrine on the alpha-receptors of the bladder neck.

OVERDOSAGE

Symptoms of overdose could include hypertension, piloerection (goosebumps), a sensation of coldness and urinary retention. There are 2 reported cases of overdosage with **ProAmatine®**, both in young males. One patient ingested **ProAmatine®** drops, 250 mg, experienced systolic blood pressure greater than 200 mmHg, was treated with an IV injection of 20 mg of phentolamine, and was discharged the same night without any complaints. The other patient ingested 205 mg of **ProAmatine®** (41 5-mg tablets), and was found lethargic and unable to talk, unresponsive to voice but responsive to painful stimuli, hypertensive and bradycardic. Gastric lavage was performed, and the patient recovered fully by the next day without sequelae.

The single doses that would be associated with symptoms of overdosage or would be potentially life-threatening are unknown. The oral LD_{50} is approximately 30 to 50 mg/kg in rats, 675 mg/kg in mice, and 125 to 160 mg/kg in dogs. Desglymidodrine is dialyzable. Recommended general treatment, based on the pharmacology of the drug, includes induced emesis and administration of alpha-sympatholytic drugs (e.g., phentolamine).

DOSAGE AND ADMINISTRATION

The recommended dose of **ProAmatine®** is 10 mg, 3 times daily. Dosing should take place during the daytime hours when the patient needs to be upright, pursuing the activities of daily living. A suggested dosing schedule of approximately 4-hour intervals is as follows: shortly before, or upon arising in the morning, midday and late afternoon (not later than 6 P.M.). Doses may be given in 3-hour intervals, if re-

Continued on next page

Proamatine—Cont.

quired, to control symptoms, but not more frequently. Single doses as high as 20 mg have been given to patients, but severe and persistent systolic supine hypertension occurs at a high rate (about 45%) at this dose. In order to reduce the potential for supine hypertension during sleep, **ProAmatine®** should not be given after the evening meal or less than 4 hours before bedtime. Total daily doses greater than 30 mg have been tolerated by some patients, but their safety and usefulness have not been studied systematically or established. Because of the risk of supine hypertension, **ProAmatine®** should be continued only in patients who appear to attain symptomatic improvement during initial treatment.
The supine and standing blood pressure should be monitored regulary, and the administration of **ProAmatine®** should be stopped if supine blood pressure increases excessively.
Because desglymidodrine is excreted renally, dosing in patients with abnormal renal function should be cautious; although this has not been systematically studied, it is recommended that treatment of these patients be initiated using 2.5-mg doses.
Dosing in children has not been adequately studied.
Blood levels of midodrine and desglymidodrine were similar when comparing levels in patients 65 or older vs. younger than 65 and when comparing males vs. females, suggesting dose modifications for these groups are not necessary.

HOW SUPPLIED

ProAmatine® is supplied as 2.5-mg, 5-mg and 10-mg tablets for oral administration. The 2.5-mg tablet is white, round, and biplanar, with a bevelled edge, and is scored on one side with "RPC" above and "2.5" below the score, and "003" on the other side. The 5-mg tablet is orange, round, and biplanar, with a bevelled edge, and is scored on one side with "RPC" above and "5" below the score, and "004" on the other side. The 10-mg is blue, round, and biplanar, with a bevelled edge, and is scored on one side with "RPC" above and "10" below the score, and "007" on the other side.

2.5-milligram Tablets:	NDC 54092-003-01	Bottle of 100
5.0-milligram Tablets:	NDC 54092-004-01	Bottle of 100
10-milligram Tablets:	NDC 54092-007-01	Bottle of 100

Store at 25°C (77°F)
Excursions permitted to 15–30°C (59–86°F)
[see USP Controlled Room Temperature]
Manufactured for
Shire US Inc., One Riverfront Place, Newport, KY, 41071, USA
By NYCOMED Austria GmbH

Rev. 10/03 **Rx only**
003 0107 006
Shown in Product Identification Guide, page 333

Sigma-Tau Pharmaceuticals, Inc.
800 SOUTH FREDERICK AVENUE, SUITE 300
GAITHERSBURG, MARYLAND 20877

Direct Inquiries to:
TEL: (301) 948-1041
800-447-0169
Fax: (301) 948-3194

CARNITOR® ℞

[*căr-nĭ-tor*]
(levocarnitine) Injection
1 g per 5 mL vial
FOR INTRAVENOUS USE ONLY.

DESCRIPTION

CARNITOR® (levocarnitine) is a carrier molecule in the transport of long-chain fatty acids across the inner mitochondrial membrane.
The chemical name of levocarnitine is 3-carboxy-2(*R*)-hydroxy-N,N,N-trimethyl-1-propanaminium, inner salt. Levocarnitine is a white crystalline, hygroscopic powder. It is readily soluble in water, hot alcohol, and insoluble in acetone. The specific rotation of levocarnitine is between -29° and -32°. Its chemical structure is:

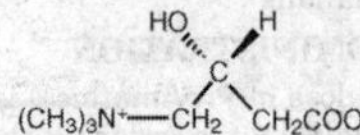

Empirical Formula: $C_7H_{15}NO_3$
Molecular Weight: 161.20

CARNITOR® (levocarnitine) Injection is a sterile aqueous solution containing 1 g of levocarnitine per 5 mL vial. The pH is adjusted to 6.0–6.5 with hydrochloric acid or sodium hydroxide.

Adverse Events with a Frequency ≥5% Regardless of Causality by Body System

	Placebo (n=63)	Levocarnitine 10 mg (n=34)	Levocarnitine 20 mg (n=62)	Levocarnitine 40 mg (n=34)	Levocarnitine 10, 20 & 40 mg (n=130)
Body as Whole					
Abdominal pain	17	21	5	6	9
Accidental injury	10	12	8	12	10
Allergic reaction	5	6			2
Asthenia	8	9	8	12	9
Back pain	10	9	8	6	8
Chest pain	14	6	15	12	12
Fever	5	6	5	12	7
Flu syndrome	40	15	27	29	25
Headache	16	12	37	3	22
Infection	17	15	10	24	15
Injection site reaction	59	38	27	38	33
Pain	49	21	32	35	30
Cardiovascular					
Arrhythmia	5	3		3	2
Atrial fibrillation			2	6	2
Cardiovascular disorder	6	3	5	6	5
Electrocardiogram abnormal		3		6	2
Hemorrhage	6	9	2	3	4
Hypertension	14	18	21	21	20
Hypotension	19	15	19	3	14
Palpitations		3	8		5
Tachycardia	5	6	5	9	6
Vascular disorder	2		2	6	2
Digestive					
Anorexia	3	3	5	6	5
Constipation	6	3	3	3	3
Diarrhea	19	9	10	35	16
Dyspepsia	10	9	6		5
Gastrointestinal disorder	2	3		6	2
Melena	3	6			2
Nausea	10	9	5	12	8
Stomach atony	5				
Vomiting	16	9	16	21	15
Endocrine System					
Parathyroid disorder	2	6	2	6	4
Hemic/Lymphatic					
Anemia	3	3	5	12	6
Metabolic/Nutritional					
Hypercalcemia	3	15	8	6	9
Hyperkalemia	6	6	6	6	6
Hypervolemia	17	3	3	12	5
Peripheral edema	3	6	5	3	5
Weight decrease	3	3	8	3	5
Weight increase	2	3		6	2

(Table continued on next page)

CLINICAL PHARMACOLOGY

CARNITOR® (levocarnitine) is a naturally occurring substance required in mammalian energy metabolism. It has been shown to facilitate long-chain fatty acid entry into cellular mitochondria, thereby delivering substrate for oxidation and subsequent energy production. Fatty acids are utilized as an energy substrate in all tissues except the brain. In skeletal and cardiac muscle, fatty acids are the main substrate for energy production.
Primary systemic carnitine deficiency is characterized by low concentrations of levocarnitine in plasma, RBC, and/or tissues. It has not been possible to determine which symptoms are due to carnitine deficiency and which are due to an

underlying organic acidemia, as symptoms of both abnormalities may be expected to improve with CARNITOR®. The literature reports that carnitine can promote the excretion of excess organic or fatty acids in patients with defects in fatty acid metabolism and/or specific organic acidopathies that bioaccumulate acylCoA esters.[1–6]

Secondary carnitine deficiency can be a consequence of inborn errors of metabolism or iatrogenic factors such as hemodialysis. CARNITOR® may alleviate the metabolic abnormalities of patients with inborn errors that result in accumulation of toxic organic acids. Conditions for which this effect has been demonstrated are: glutaric aciduria II, methyl malonic aciduria, propionic acidemia, and medium chain fatty acylCoA dehydrogenase deficiency.[7,8] Autointoxication occurs in these patients due to the accumulation of acylCoA compounds that disrupt intermediary metabolism. The subsequent hydrolysis of the acylCoA compound to its free acid results in acidosis which can be life-threatening. Levocarnitine clears the acylCoA compound by formation of acylcarnitine, which is quickly excreted. Carnitine deficiency is defined biochemically as abnormally low plasma concentrations of free carnitine, less than 20 µmol/L at one week post term and may be associated with low tissue and/or urine concentrations. Further, this condition may be associated with a plasma concentration ratio of acylcarnitine/levocarnitine greater than 0.4 or abnormally elevated concentrations of acylcarnitine in the urine. In premature infants and newborns, secondary deficiency is defined as plasma levocarnitine concentrations below age-related normal concentrations.

End Stage Renal Disease (ESRD) patients on maintenance hemodialysis may have low plasma carnitine concentrations and an increased ratio of acylcarnitine/carnitine because of reduced intake of meat and dairy products, reduced renal synthesis and dialytic losses. Certain clinical conditions common in hemodialysis patients such as malaise, muscle weakness, cardiomyopathy and cardiac arrhythmias may be related to abnormal carnitine metabolism.

Pharmacokinetic and clinical studies with CARNITOR® have shown that administration of levocarnitine to ESRD patients on hemodialysis results in increased plasma levocarnitine concentrations.

PHARMACOKINETICS

In a relative bioavailability study in 15 healthy adult male volunteers, CARNITOR® Tablets were found to be bio-equivalent to CARNITOR® Oral Solution. Following 4 days of dosing with 6 tablets of CARNITOR® 330 mg b.i.d. or 2 g of CARNITOR® oral solution b.i.d., the maximum plasma concentration (C_{max}) was about 80 µmol/L and the time to maximum plasma concentration (T_{max}) occurred at 3.3 hours.

The plasma concentration profiles of levocarnitine after a slow 3 minute intravenous bolus dose of 20 mg/kg of CARNITOR® were described by a two-compartment model. Following a single i.v. administration, approximately 76% of the levocarnitine dose was excreted in the urine during the 0–24h interval. Using plasma concentrations uncorrected for endogenous levocarnitine, the mean distribution half life was 0.585 hours and the mean apparent terminal elimination half life was 17.4 hours.

The absolute bioavailability of levocarnitine from the two oral formulations of CARNITOR®, calculated after correction for circulating endogenous plasma concentrations of levocarnitine, was 15.1 ± 5.3% for CARNITOR® Tablets and 15.9 ± 4.9% for CARNITOR® Oral Solution.

Total body clearance of levocarnitine (Dose/AUC including endogenous baseline concentrations) was a mean of 4.00 L/h.

Levocarnitine was not bound to plasma protein or albumin when tested at any concentration or with any species including the human.[9]

In a 9-week study, 12 ESRD patients undergoing hemodialysis for at least 6 months received CARNITOR® 20 mg/kg three times per week after dialysis. Prior to initiation of CARNITOR® therapy, mean plasma levocarnitine concentrations were approximately 20 µmol/L pre-dialysis and 6 µmol/L post-dialysis. The table summarizes the pharmacokinetic data (mean ± SD µmol/L) after the first dose of CARNITOR® and after 8 weeks of CARNITOR® therapy.

N=12	Baseline	Single dose	8 weeks
C_{max}	–	1139 ± 240	1190 ± 270
Trough (pre-dialysis, pre-dose)	21.3 ± 7.7	68.4 ± 26.1	190 ± 55

After one week of CARNITOR® therapy (3 doses), all patients had trough concentrations between 54 and 180 µmol/L (normal 40–50 µmol/L) and concentrations remained relatively stable or increased over the course of the study.

In a similar study in ESRD patients also receiving 20 mg/kg CARNITOR® 3 times per week after hemodialysis, 12- and 24-week mean pre-dialysis (trough) levocarnitine concentrations were 189 (N=25) and 243 (N=23) µmol/L, respectively.

In a dose-ranging study in ESRD patients undergoing hemodialysis, patients received 10, 20, or 40 mg/kg CARNITOR® 3 times per week following dialysis (N~30 for each dose group). Mean ± SD trough levocarnitine concentrations (µmol/L) by dose after 12 and 24 weeks of therapy are summarized in the table.

Adverse Events with a Frequency ≥5% Regardless of Causality by Body System *(cont.)*

	Placebo (n=63)	*Levocarnitine 10 mg (n=34)*	*Levocarnitine 20 mg (n=62)*	*Levocarnitine 40 mg (n=34)*	*Levocarnitine 10, 20 & 40 mg (n=130)*
Musculo-Skeletal					
Leg cramps	13		8		4
Myalgia	6				
Nervous					
Anxiety	5		2		1
Depression	3	6	5	6	5
Dizziness	11	18	10	15	13
Drug dependence	2	6			2
Hypertonia	5	3			1
Insomnia	6	3	6		4
Paresthesia	3	3	3	12	5
Vertigo		6			2
Respiratory					
Brochitis			5	3	3
Cough increase	16		10	18	9
Dyspnea	19	3	11	3	7
Pharyngitis	33	24	27	15	23
Respiratory disorder	5				
Rhinitis	10	6	11	6	9
Sinusitis	5		2	3	2
Skin And Appendages					
Pruritus	13		8	3	5
Rash	3		5	3	3
Special Senses					
Amblyopia	2		6		3
Eye disorder	3	6	3		3
Taste perversion			2	9	3
Urogenital					
Urinary tract infect	6	3	3		2
Kidney failure	5	6	6	6	6

	12 weeks	24 weeks
10 mg/kg	116 ± 69	148 ± 50
20 mg/kg	210 ± 58	240 ± 60
40 mg/kg	371 ± 111	456 ± 162

While the efficacy of CARNITOR® to increase carnitine concentrations in patients with ESRD undergoing dialysis has been demonstrated, the effects of supplemental carnitine on the signs and symptoms of carnitine deficiency and on clinical outcomes in this population have not been determined.

METABOLISM AND EXCRETION

In a pharmacokinetic study where five normal adult male volunteers received an oral dose of [^{3}H-methyl]-L-carnitine following 15 days of a high carnitine diet and additional carnitine supplement, 58 to 65% of the administered radioactive dose was recovered in the urine and feces in 5 to 11 days. Maximum concentration of [^{3}H-methyl]-L-carnitine in serum occurred from 2.0 to 4.5 hr after drug administration. Major metabolites found were trimethylamine N-oxide, primarily in urine (8% to 49% of the administered dose) and [^{3}H]-γ-butyrobetaine, primarily in feces (0.44% to 45% of the administered dose). Urinary excretion of levocarnitine was about 4 to 8% of the dose. Fecal excretion of total carnitine was less than 1% of the administered dose.[10]

After attainment of steady state following 4 days of oral administration of CARNITOR® Tablets (1980 mg q12h) or Oral Solution (2000 mg q12h) to 15 healthy male volunteers, the mean urinary excretion of levocarnitine during a single dosing interval (12h) was about 9% of the orally administered dose (uncorrected for endogenous urinary excretion).

INDICATIONS AND USAGE

For the acute and chronic treatment of patients with an inborn error of metabolism which results in secondary carnitine deficiency.

For the prevention and treatment of carnitine deficiency in patients with end stage renal disease who are undergoing dialysis. (US Patent Nos. 6,335,369; 6,429,230; 6,696,493)

CONTRAINDICATIONS

None known.

WARNINGS

None.

PRECAUTIONS

The safety and efficacy of oral levocarnitine has not been evaluated in patients with renal insufficiency. Chronic administration of high doses of oral levocarnitine in patients with severely compromised renal function or in ESRD patients on dialysis may result in accumulation of the potentially toxic metabolites, trimethylamine (TMA) and trimethylamine-N-oxide (TMAO), since these metabolites are normally excreted in the urine.

Carcinogenesis, mutagenesis, impairment of fertility

Mutagenicity tests performed in *Salmonella typhimurium*, *Saccharomyces cerevisiae*, and *Schizosaccharomyces pombe* indicate that levocarnitine is not mutagenic. No long-term animal studies have been performed to evaluate the carcinogenic potential of levocarnitine.

Pregnancy

Pregnancy Category B.

Reproductive studies have been performed in rats and rabbits at doses up to 3.8 times the human dose on the basis of surface area and have revealed no evidence of impaired fertility or harm to the fetus due to CARNITOR®. There are, however, no adequate and well controlled studies in pregnant women.

Because animal reproduction studies are not always predictive of human response, this drug should be used during pregnancy only if clearly needed.

Nursing Mothers

Levocarnitine supplementation in nursing mothers has not been specifically studied.

Continued on next page

Carnitor Injection—Cont.

Studies in dairy cows indicate that the concentration of levocarnitine in milk is increased following exogenous administration of levocarnitine. In nursing mothers receiving levocarnitine, any risks to the child of excess carnitine intake need to be weighed against the benefits of levocarnitine supplementation to the mother. Consideration may be given to discontinuation of nursing or of levocarnitine treatment.

Pediatric Use

See Dosage and Administration.

ADVERSE REACTIONS

Transient nausea and vomiting have been observed. Less frequent adverse reactions are body odor, nausea, and gastritis. An incidence for these reactions is difficult to estimate due to the confounding effects of the underlying pathology.

Seizures have been reported to occur in patients, with or without pre-existing seizure activity, receiving either oral or intravenous levocarnitine. In patients with pre-existing seizure activity, an increase in seizure frequency and/or severity has been reported.

The table below lists the adverse events that have been reported in two double-blind, placebo-controlled trials in patients on chronic hemodialysis. Events occurring at ≥5% are reported without regard to causality.

[See table on pages 3144 and 3145]

OVERDOSAGE

There have been no reports of toxicity from levocarnitine overdosage. Levocarnitine is easily removed from plasma by dialysis. The intravenous LD_{50} of levocarnitine in rats is 5.4 g/kg and the oral LD_{50} of levocarnitine in mice is 19.2 g/kg. Large doses of levocarnitine may cause diarrhea.

DOSAGE AND ADMINISTRATION

CARNITOR® Injection is administered intravenously.

Metabolic Disorders

The recommended dose is 50 mg/kg given as a slow 2–3 minute bolus injection or by infusion. Often a loading dose is given in patients with severe metabolic crisis, followed by an equivalent dose over the following 24 hours. It should be administered q3h or q4h, and never less than q6h either by infusion or by intravenous injection. All subsequent daily doses are recommended to be in the range of 50 mg/kg or as therapy may require. The highest dose administered has been 300 mg/kg.

It is recommended that a plasma carnitine concentration be obtained prior to beginning this parenteral therapy. Weekly and monthly monitoring is recommended as well. This monitoring should include blood chemistries, vital signs, plasma carnitine concentrations (the plasma free carnitine concentration should be between 35 and 60 µmol/L) and overall clinical condition.

ESRD Patients on Hemodialysis

The recommended starting dose is 10–20 mg/kg dry body weight as a slow 2–3 minute bolus injection into the venous return line after each dialysis session. Initiation of therapy may be prompted by trough (pre-dialysis) plasma levocarnitine concentrations that are below normal (40–50 µmol/L). Dose adjustments should be guided by trough (pre-dialysis) levocarnitine concentrations, and downward dose adjustments (e.g. to 5 mg/kg after dialysis) may be made as early as the third or fourth week of therapy.

Parenteral drug products should be inspected visually for particulate matter and discoloration prior to administration, whenever solution and container permit.

COMPATIBILITY AND STABILITY

CARNITOR® Injection is compatible and stable when mixed in parenteral solutions of Sodium Chloride 0.9% or Lactated Ringer's in concentrations ranging from 250 mg/500 mL (0.5 mg/mL) to 4200 mg/500 mL (8.0 mg/mL) and stored at room temperature (25°C) for up to 24 hours in PVC plastic bags.

HOW SUPPLIED

CARNITOR® (levocarnitine) Injection is available in 1 g per 5 mL single dose vials packaged 5 vials per carton (NDC 54482-147-01). CARNITOR® (levocarnitine) Injection 5 mL vial is manufactured for Sigma-Tau Pharmaceuticals, Inc. by Sigma-Tau S.p.A., 00040 Pomezia (Rome), Italy or Chesapeake Biological Laboratories, Inc. Baltimore, MD 21230-2591.

Store vials at controlled room temperature (25°C). See USP. Discard unused portion of an opened vial, as the formulation does not contain a preservative.

CARNITOR® (levocarnitine) is also available in the following dosage forms:

CARNITOR® (levocarnitine) Tablets are supplied as 330 mg tablets embossed with "CARNITOR ST" in blister packages, in boxes of 90 tablets (NDC 54482-144-07). Made in Italy.

CARNITOR® (levocarnitine) Oral Solution is supplied in 118 mL (4 FL. OZ.) multiple-unit plastic containers. The multiple-unit containers are packaged 24 per case (NDC 54482-145-08). CARNITOR® (levocarnitine) Oral Solution is manufactured for Sigma-Tau Pharmaceuticals, Inc. by Hi-Tech Pharmacal Co., Inc., Amityville, NY 11701.

Rx only.

REFERENCES

1. Bohmer, T., Rydning, A. and Solberg, H.E. 1974. Carnitine levels in human serum in health and disease. *Clin. Chim. Acta* 57:55–61.
2. Brooks, H., Goldberg, L., Holland, R. *et al.* 1977. Carnitine-induced effects on cardiac and peripheral hemodynamics. *J. Clin. Pharmacol.* 17:561–568.
3. Christiansen, R., Bremer, J. 1976. Active transport of butyrobetaine and carnitine into isolated liver cells. *Biochim. Biophys. Acta* 448:562–577.
4. Lindstedt, S. and Lindstedt, G. 1961. Distribution and excretion of carnitine in the rat. *Acta Chem. Scand.* 15: 701–702.
5. Rebouche, C.J. and Engel, A.G. 1983. Carnitine metabolism and deficiency syndromes. *Mayo Clin. Proc.* 58: 533–540.
6. Rebouche, C.J. and Paulson, D.J. 1986. Carnitine metabolism and function in humans. *Ann. Rev. Nutr.* 6:41–66.
7. Scriver, C.R., Beaudet, A.L., Sly, W.S. and Valle, D. 1989. *The Metabolic Basis of Inherited Disease.* New York: McGraw-Hill.
8. Schaub, J., Van Hoof, F. and Vis, H.L. 1991. *Inborn Errors of Metabolism.* New York: Raven Press.
9. Marzo, A., Arrigoni Martelli, E., Mancinelli, A., Cardace, G., Corbelletta, C., Bassani, E. and Solbiati, M.1991. Protein binding of L-carnitine family components. *Eur. J. Drug Met. Pharmacokin.*, Special Issue III: 364–368.
10. Rebouche, C.J. 1991. Quantitative estimation of absorption and degradation of a carnitine supplement by human adults. *Metabolism* 40:1305–1310.

sigma-tau
Pharmaceuticals, Inc.
Gaithersburg, MD 20877
PREVIOUS EDITION IS OBSOLETE
Date of Issue: 03/04 VPI(I)-10

CARNITOR® (levocarnitine) ℞

CARNITOR® (levocarnitine) Tablets (330 mg)
CARNITOR® (levocarnitine) Oral Solution (1 g per 10 mL multidose)

For oral use only. Not for parenteral use.

DESCRIPTION

CARNITOR® (levocarnitine) is a carrier molecule in the transport of long-chain fatty acids across the inner mitochondrial membrane.

The chemical name of levocarnitine is 3-carboxy-2(*R*)-hydroxy-N,N,N-trimethyl-1-propanaminium, inner salt. Levocarnitine is a white crystalline, hygroscopic powder. It is readily soluble in water, hot alcohol, and insoluble in acetone. The specific rotation of levocarnitine is between -29° and -32°. Its chemical structure is:

HO H
C
$(CH_3)_3N^+$—CH_2 CH_2COO^-

Empirical Formula: $C_7H_{15}NO_3$
Molecular Weight: 161.20

Each CARNITOR® (levocarnitine) Tablet contains 330 mg of levocarnitine and the inactive ingredients magnesium stearate, microcrystalline cellulose and povidone.

Each 118 mL container of CARNITOR® (levocarnitine) Oral Solution contains 1 g of levocarnitine/10 mL. Also contains: Artificial Cherry Flavor, D,L-Malic Acid, Purified Water, Sucrose Syrup. Methylparaben NF and Propylparaben NF are added as preservatives. The pH is approximately 5.

CLINICAL PHARMACOLOGY

CARNITOR® (levocarnitine) is a naturally occurring substance required in mammalian energy metabolism. It has been shown to facilitate long-chain fatty acid entry into cellular mitochondria, thereby delivering substrate for oxidation and subsequent energy production. Fatty acids are utilized as an energy substrate in all tissues except the brain. In skeletal and cardiac muscle, fatty acids are the main substrate for energy production.

Primary systemic carnitine deficiency is characterized by low concentrations of levocarnitine in plasma, RBC, and/or tissues. It has not been possible to determine which symptoms are due to carnitine deficiency and which are due to an underlying organic acidemia, as symptoms of both abnormalities may be expected to improve with CARNITOR®. The literature reports that carnitine can promote the excretion of excess organic or fatty acids in patients with defects in fatty acid metabolism and/or specific organic acidopathies that bioaccumulate acylCoA esters.[1–6]

Secondary carnitine deficiency can be a consequence of inborn errors of metabolism. CARNITOR® may alleviate the metabolic abnormalities of patients with inborn errors that result in accumulation of toxic organic acids. Conditions for which this effect has been demonstrated are: glutaric aciduria II, methyl malonic aciduria, propionic acidemia, and medium chain fatty acylCoA dehydrogenase deficiency.[7,8] Autointoxication occurs in these patients due to the accumulation of acylCoA compounds that disrupt intermediary metabolism. The subsequent hydrolysis of the acylCoA compound to its free acid results in acidosis which can be life-threatening. Levocarnitine clears the acylCoA compound by formation of acylcarnitine, which is quickly excreted. Carnitine deficiency is defined biochemically as abnormally low plasma concentrations of free carnitine, less than 20 µmol/L at one week post term and may be associated with low tissue and/or urine concentrations. Further, this condition may be associated with a plasma concentration ratio of acylcarnitine/levocarnitine greater than 0.4 or abnormally elevated concentrations of acylcarnitine in the urine. In premature infants and newborns, secondary deficiency is defined as plasma levocarnitine concentrations below age-related normal concentrations.

PHARMACOKINETICS

In a relative bioavailability study in 15 healthy adult male volunteers, CARNITOR® Tablets were found to be bio-equivalent to CARNITOR® Oral Solution. Following 4 days of dosing with 6 tablets of CARNITOR® 330 mg b.i.d. or 2 g of CARNITOR® oral solution b.i.d., the maximum plasma concentration (C_{max}) was about 80 µmol/L and the time to maximum plasma concentration (T_{max}) occurred at 3.3 hours.

The plasma concentration profiles of levocarnitine after a slow 3 minute intravenous bolus dose of 20 mg/kg of CARNITOR® were described by a two-compartment model. Following a single i.v. administration, approximately 76% of the levocarnitine dose was excreted in the urine during the 0–24h interval. Using plasma concentrations uncorrected for endogenous levocarnitine, the mean distribution half life was 0.585 hours and the mean apparent terminal elimination half life was 17.4 hours.

The absolute bioavailability of levocarnitine from the two oral formulations of CARNITOR®, calculated after correction for circulating endogenous plasma concentrations of levocarnitine, was 15.1 ± 5.3% for CARNITOR® Tablets and 15.9 ± 4.9% for CARNITOR® Oral Solution.

Total body clearance of levocarnitine (Dose/AUC including endogenous baseline concentrations) was a mean of 4.00 L/h.

Levocarnitine was not bound to plasma protein or albumin when tested at any concentration or with any species including the human.[9]

METABOLISM AND EXCRETION

In a pharmacokinetic study where five normal adult male volunteers received an oral dose of [^{3}H-methyl]-L-carnitine following 15 days of a high carnitine diet and additional carnitine supplement, 58 to 65% of the administered radioactive dose was recovered in the urine and feces in 5 to 11 days. Maximum concentration of [^{3}H-methyl]-L-carnitine in serum occurred from 2.0 to 4.5 hr after drug administration. Major metabolites found were trimethylamine N-oxide, primarily in urine (8% to 49% of the administered dose) and [^{3}H]-γ-butyrobetaine, primarily in feces (0.44% to 45% of the administered dose). Urinary excretion of levocarnitine was about 4 to 8% of the dose. Fecal excretion of total carnitine was less than 1% of the administered dose.[10]

After attainment of steady state following 4 days of oral administration of CARNITOR® Tablets (1980 mg q12h) or Oral Solution (2000 mg q12h) to 15 healthy male volunteers, the mean urinary excretion of levocarnitine during a single dosing interval (12h) was about 9% of the orally administered dose (uncorrected for endogenous urinary excretion).

INDICATIONS AND USAGE

CARNITOR® (levocarnitine) is indicated in the treatment of primary systemic carnitine deficiency. In the reported cases, the clinical presentation consisted of recurrent episodes of Reye-like encephalopathy, hypoketotic hypoglycemia, and/or cardiomyopathy. Associated symptoms included hypotonia, muscle weakness and failure to thrive. A diagnosis of primary carnitine deficiency requires that serum, red cell and/or tissue carnitine levels be low and that the patient does not have a primary defect in fatty acid or organic acid oxidation (see Clinical Pharmacology). In some patients, particularly those presenting with cardiomyopathy, carnitine supplementation rapidly alleviated signs and symptoms. Treatment should include, in addition to carnitine, supportive and other therapy as indicated by the condition of the patient.

CARNITOR® (levocarnitine) is also indicated for acute and chronic treatment of patients with an inborn error of metabolism which results in a secondary carnitine deficiency.

CONTRAINDICATIONS

None known.

WARNINGS

None.

PRECAUTIONS

General

CARNITOR® (levocarnitine) Oral Solution is for oral/internal use only.

Not for parenteral use.

Gastrointestinal reactions may result from a too rapid consumption of carnitine. CARNITOR® (levocarnitine) Oral Solution may be consumed alone, or dissolved in drinks or other liquid foods to reduce taste fatigue. It should be consumed slowly and doses should be spaced evenly throughout the day to maximize tolerance.

The safety and efficacy of oral levocarnitine has not been evaluated in patients with renal insufficiency. Chronic administration of high doses of oral levocarnitine in patients with severely compromised renal function or in ESRD patients on dialysis may result in accumulation of the potentially toxic metabolites, trimethylamine (TMA) and trimethylamine-N-oxide (TMAO), since these metabolites are normally excreted in the urine.

Carcinogenesis, mutagenesis, impairment of fertility

Mutagenicity tests performed in *Salmonella typhimurium*, *Saccharomyces cerevisiae*, and *Schizosaccharomyces pombe* indicate that levocarnitine is not mutagenic. No long-term animal studies have been performed to evaluate the carcinogenic potential of levocarnitine.

Pregnancy

Pregnancy Category B.

Reproductive studies have been performed in rats and rabbits at doses up to 3.8 times the human dose on the basis of surface area and have revealed no evidence of impaired fertility or harm to the fetus due to CARNITOR®. There are, however, no adequate and well controlled studies in pregnant women.

Because animal reproduction studies are not always predictive of human response, this drug should be used during pregnancy only if clearly needed.

Nursing Mothers

Levocarnitine supplementation in nursing mothers has not been specifically studied.

Studies in dairy cows indicate that the concentration of levocarnitine in milk is increased following exogenous administration of levocarnitine. In nursing mothers receiving levocarnitine, any risks to the child of excess carnitine intake need to be weighed against the benefits of levocarnitine supplementation to the mother. Consideration may be given to discontinuation of nursing or of levocarnitine treatment.

Pediatric Use

See Dosage and Administration.

ADVERSE REACTIONS

Various mild gastrointestinal complaints have been reported during the long-term administration of oral L- or D,L-carnitine; these include transient nausea and vomiting, abdominal cramps, and diarrhea. Mild myasthenia has been described only in uremic patients receiving D,L-carnitine. Gastrointestinal adverse reactions with CARNITOR® (levocarnitine) Oral Solution dissolved in liquids might be avoided by a slow consumption of the solution or by a greater dilution. Decreasing the dosage often diminishes or eliminates drug-related patient body odor or gastrointestinal symptoms when present. Tolerance should be monitored very closely during the first week of administration, and after any dosage increases.

Seizures have been reported to occur in patients with or without pre-existing seizure activity receiving either oral or intravenous levocarnitine. In patients with pre-existing seizure activity, an increase in seizure frequency and/or severity has been reported.

OVERDOSAGE

There have been no reports of toxicity from levocarnitine overdosage. Levocarnitine is easily removed from plasma by dialysis. The intravenous LD_{50} of levocarnitine in rats is 5.4 g/kg and the oral LD_{50} of levocarnitine in mice is 19.2 g/kg. Large doses of levocarnitine may cause diarrhea.

DOSAGE AND ADMINISTRATION

CARNITOR® (levocarnitine) Tablets.

Adults: The recommended oral dosage for adults is 990 mg two or three times a day using the 330 mg tablets, depending on clinical response.

Infants and children: The recommended oral dosage for infants and children is between 50 and 100 mg/kg/day in divided doses, with a maximum of 3 g/day. Dosage should begin at 50 mg/kg/day. The exact dosage will depend on clinical response.

Monitoring should include periodic blood chemistries, vital signs, plasma carnitine concentrations and overall clinical condition.

CARNITOR® (levocarnitine) Oral Solution.

For oral use only. **Not for parenteral use.**

Adults: The recommended dosage of levocarnitine is 1 to 3 g/day for a 50 kg subject, which is equivalent to 10 to 30 mL/day of CARNITOR® (levocarnitine) Oral Solution. Higher doses should be administered only with caution and only where clinical and biochemical considerations make it seem likely that higher doses will be of benefit. Dosage should start at 1 g/day, (10 mL/day), and be increased slowly while assessing tolerance and therapeutic response. Monitoring should include periodic blood chemistries, vital signs, plasma carnitine concentrations, and overall clinical condition.

Infants and children: The recommended dosage of levocarnitine is 50 to 100 mg/kg/day which is equivalent to 0.5 mL/kg/day CARNITOR® (levocarnitine) Oral Solution. Higher doses should be administered only with caution and only where clinical and biochemical considerations make it seem likely that higher doses will be of benefit. Dosage should start at 50 mg/kg/day, and be increased slowly to a maximum of 3 g/day (30 mL/day) while assessing tolerance and therapeutic response. Monitoring should include periodic blood chemistries, vital signs, plasma carnitine concentrations, and overall clinical condition.

CARNITOR® (levocarnitine) Oral Solution may be consumed alone or dissolved in drink or other liquid food. Doses should be spaced evenly throughout the day (every three or four hours) preferably during or following meals and should be consumed slowly in order to maximize tolerance.

HOW SUPPLIED

CARNITOR® (levocarnitine) Tablets are supplied as 330 mg tablets embossed with "CARNITOR ST" in individual blisters, packaged in boxes of 90 (NDC 54482-144-07). Store at controlled room temperature (25°C). See USP.

CARNITOR® (levocarnitine) Tablets are manufactured for Sigma-Tau Pharmaceuticals, Inc. by Sigma-Tau S.p.A., 00040 Pomezia (Rome), Italy.

CARNITOR® (levocarnitine) Oral Solution is supplied in 118 mL (4 FL. OZ.) multiple-unit plastic containers. The multiple-unit containers are packaged 24 per case (NDC 54482-145-08). Store at controlled room temperature (25°C). See USP. CARNITOR® (levocarnitine) Oral Solution is manufactured for Sigma-Tau Pharmaceuticals, Inc. by: Hi-Tech Pharmacal Co., Inc. Amityville, NY 11701.

CARNITOR® (levocarnitine) is also available in the following dosage forms for intravenous injection:

CARNITOR® (levocarnitine) Injection is available in 1 g per 5 mL single dose vials packaged 5 vials per carton (NDC 54482-147-01). CARNITOR® (levocarnitine) Injection 5 mL vial is manufactured for Sigma-Tau Pharmaceuticals, Inc. by Sigma-Tau S.p.A., 00040 Pomezia (Rome), Italy or Chesapeake Biological Laboratories, Inc. Baltimore, MD 21230-2591.

Rx only.

REFERENCES

1. Bohmer, T., Rydning, A. and Solberg, H.E. 1974. Carnitine levels in human serum in health and disease. *Clin. Chim. Acta* 57:55–61.
2. Brooks, H., Goldberg, L., Holland, R. *et al.* 1977. Carnitine-induced effects on cardiac and peripheral hemodynamics. *J. Clin. Pharmacol.* 17:561–568.
3. Christiansen, R., Bremer, J. 1976. Active transport of butyrobetaine and carnitine into isolated liver cells. *Biochim. Biophys. Acta* 448:562–577.
4. Lindstedt, S. and Lindstedt, G. 1961. Distribution and excretion of carnitine in the rat. *Acta Chem. Scand.* 15:701–702.
5. Rebouche, C.J. and Engel, A.G. 1983. Carnitine metabolism and deficiency syndromes. *Mayo Clin. Proc.* 58:533–540.
6. Rebouche, C.J. and Paulson, D.J. 1986. Carnitine metabolism and function in humans. *Ann. Rev. Nutr.* 6:41–66.
7. Scriver, C.R., Beaudet, A.L., Sly, W.S. and Valle, D. 1989. *The Metabolic Basis of Inherited Disease.* New York: McGraw-Hill.
8. Schaub, J., Van Hoof, F. and Vis, H.L. 1991. *Inborn Errors of Metabolism.* New York: Raven Press.
9. Marzo, A., Arrigoni Martelli, E., Mancinelli, A., Cardace, G., Corbelletta, C., Bassani, E. and Solbiati, M.1991. Protein binding of L-carnitine family components. *Eur. J. Drug Met. Pharmacokin.,* Special Issue III: 364–368.
10. Rebouche, C.J. 1991. Quantitative estimation of absorption and degradation of a carnitine supplement by human adults. *Metabolism* 40:1305–1310.

sigma-tau
Pharmaceuticals, Inc.
Gaithersburg, MD 20877
PREVIOUS EDITION IS OBSOLETE
Date of Issue: 03/04 OPI-6

MATULANE® ℞

[*măt' ū-lāne*]
brand of procarbazine hydrochloride Capsules

WARNING

It is recommended that MATULANE be given only by or under the supervision of a physician experienced in the use of potent antineoplastic drugs. Adequate clinical and laboratory facilities should be available to patients for proper monitoring of treatment.

DESCRIPTION

Matulane (procarbazine hydrochloride), a hydrazine derivative antineoplastic agent, is available as capsules containing the equivalent of 50 mg procarbazine as the hydrochloride. Each capsule also contains cornstarch, mannitol and talc. Gelatin capsule shells contain parabens (methyl and propyl), potassium sorbate, titanium dioxide, FD&C Yellow No. 6 and D&C Yellow No. 10.

Chemically, procarbazine hydrochloride is *N*-isopropyl-α-(2-methylhydrazino)-*p*-toluamide monohydrochloride. It is a white to pale yellow crystalline powder which is soluble but unstable in water or aqueous solutions. The molecular weight of procarbazine hydrochloride is 257.76 and the structural formula is:

$$(CH_3)_2CHNHC(=O)-C_6H_4-CH_2NHNHCH_3 \cdot HCl$$

CLINICAL PHARMACOLOGY

The precise mode of cytotoxic action of procarbazine has not been clearly defined. There is evidence that the drug may act by inhibition of protein, RNA and DNA synthesis. Studies have suggested that procarbazine may inhibit transmethylation of methyl groups of methionine into t-RNA. The absence of functional t-RNA could cause the cessation of protein synthesis and consequently DNA and RNA synthesis. In addition, procarbazine may directly damage DNA. Hydrogen peroxide, formed during the auto-oxidation of the drug, may attack protein sulfhydryl groups contained in residual protein which is tightly bound to DNA.

Procarbazine is metabolized primarily in the liver and kidneys. The drug appears to be auto-oxidized to the azo derivative with the release of hydrogen peroxide. The azo derivative isomerizes to the hydrazone, and following hydrolysis splits into a benzyl-aldehyde derivative and methylhydrazine. The methylhydrazine is further degraded to CO_2 and CH_4 and possibly hydrazine, whereas the aldehyde is oxidized to *N*-isopropylterephthalamic acid, which is excreted in the urine.

Procarbazine is rapidly and completely absorbed. Following oral administration of 30 mg of ^{14}C-labeled procarbazine, maximum peak plasma radioactive concentrations were reached within 60 minutes.

After intravenous injection, the plasma half-life of procarbazine is approximately 10 minutes. Approximately 70% of the radioactivity is excreted in the urine as *N*-isopropylterephthalamic acid within 24 hours following both oral and intravenous administration of ^{14}C-labeled procarbazine.

Procarbazine crosses the blood-brain barrier and rapidly equilibrates between plasma and cerebrospinal fluid after oral administration.

INDICATIONS AND USAGE

Matulane is indicated for use in combination with other anticancer drugs for the treatment of Stage III and IV Hodgkin's disease. Matulane is used as part of the MOPP (nitrogen mustard, vincristine, procarbazine, prednisone) regimen.

CONTRAINDICATIONS

Matulane is contraindicated in patients with known hypersensitivity to the drug or inadequate marrow reserve as demonstrated by bone marrow aspiration. Due consideration of this possible state should be given to each patient who has leukopenia, thrombocytopenia or anemia.

WARNINGS

To minimize CNS depression and possible potentiation, barbiturates, antihistamines, narcotics, hypotensive agents or phenothiazines should be used with caution. Ethyl alcohol should not be used since there may be an Antabuse (disulfiram)-like reaction. Because Matulane exhibits some monoamine oxidase inhibitory activity, sympathomimetic drugs, tricyclic antidepressant drugs (eg, amitriptyline HCl, imipramine HCl) and other drugs and foods with known high tyramine content, such as wine, yogurt, ripe cheese and bananas, should be avoided. A further phenomenon of toxicity common to many hydrazine derivatives is hemolysis and the appearance of Heinz-Ehrlich inclusion bodies in erythrocytes.

Pregnancy: *Teratogenic Effects:* Pregnancy Category D. Procarbazine hydrochloride can cause fetal harm when administered to a pregnant woman. While there are no adequate and well-controlled studies with procarbazine hydrochloride in pregnant women, there are case reports of malformations in the offspring of women who were exposed to procarbazine hydrochloride in combination with other antineoplastic agents during pregnancy. Matulane should be used during pregnancy only if the potential benefit justifies the potential risk to the fetus. If this drug is used during pregnancy, or if the patient becomes pregnant while taking this drug, the patient should be apprised of the potential hazard to the fetus. Women of childbearing potential should be advised to avoid becoming pregnant. Procarbazine hydrochloride is teratogenic in the rat when given at doses approximately 4 to 13 times the maximum recommended human therapeutic dose of 6 mg/kg/day.

Nonteratogenic Effects: Procarbazine hydrochloride has not been adequately studied in animals for its effects on peri- and postnatal development. However, neurogenic tumors were noted in the offspring of rats given intravenous injections of 125 mg/kg of procarbazine hydrochloride on day 22 of gestation. Compounds which inhibit DNA, RNA and protein synthesis might be expected to have adverse effects on peri- and postnatal development.

Carcinogenesis, Mutagenesis and Impairment of Fertility:

Carcinogenesis: The carcinogenicity of procarbazine hydrochloride in mice, rats and monkeys has been reported in a considerable number of studies. Instances of a second nonlymphoid malignancy, including lung cancer and acute myelocytic leukemia, have been reported in patients with Hodgkin's disease treated with procarbazine in combination with other chemotherapy and/or radiation. The risks of secondary lung cancer from treatment appear to be multiplied by tobacco use. The International Agency for Research on Cancer (IARC) considers that there is "sufficient evidence" for the human carcinogenicity of procarbazine hydrochloride when it is given in intensive regimens which include other antineoplastic agents but that there is inadequate evidence of carcinogenicity in humans given procarbazine hydrochloride alone.

Mutagenesis: Procarbazine hydrochloride has been shown to be mutagenic in a variety of bacterial and mammalian test systems.

Impairment of Fertility: Azoospermia and antifertility effects associated with procarbazine hydrochloride administration in combination with other chemotherapeutic agents for treating Hodgkin's disease have been reported in human clinical studies. Since these patients received multicombination therapy, it is difficult to determine to what extent procarbazine hydrochloride alone was involved in the male germ-cell damage. The usual Segment I fertility/reproduction studies in laboratory animals have not been carried out

Continued on next page

Matulane—Cont.

with procarbazine hydrochloride. However, compounds which inhibit DNA, RNA and/or protein synthesis might be expected to have adverse effects on gametogenesis. Unscheduled DNA synthesis in the testis of rabbits and decreased fertility in male mice treated with procarbazine hydrochloride have been reported.

PRECAUTIONS

General: Undue toxicity may occur if Matulane is used in patients with impairment of renal and/or hepatic function. When appropriate, hospitalization for the initial course of treatment should be considered.

If radiation or a chemotherapeutic agent known to have marrow-depressant activity has been used, an interval of one month or longer without such therapy is recommended before starting treatment with Matulane. The length of this interval may also be determined by evidence of bone marrow recovery based on successive bone marrow studies.

Prompt cessation of therapy is recommended if any one of the following occurs:

- Central nervous system signs or symptoms such as paresthesias, neuropathies or confusion.
- Leukopenia (white blood count under 4000).
- Thrombocytopenia (platelets under 100,000).
- Hypersensitivity reaction.
- Stomatitis–The first small ulceration or persistent spot soreness around the oral cavity is a signal for cessation of therapy.
- Diarrhea–Frequent bowel movements or watery stools.
- Hemorrhage or bleeding tendencies.

Bone marrow depression often occurs 2 to 8 weeks after the start of treatment. If leukopenia occurs, hospitalization of the patient may be needed for appropriate treatment to prevent systemic infection.

Information for Patients: Patients should be warned not to drink alcoholic beverages while on Matulane therapy since there may be an Antabuse (disulfiram)-like reaction. They should also be cautioned to avoid foods with known high tyramine content such as wine, yogurt, ripe cheese and bananas. Over-the-counter drug preparations which contain antihistamines or sympathomimetic drugs should also be avoided. Patients taking Matulane should also be warned against the use of prescription drugs without the knowledge and consent of their physician. Patients should be advised to discontinue tobacco use.

Laboratory Tests: Baseline laboratory data should be obtained prior to initiation of therapy. The hematologic status as indicated by hemoglobin, hematocrit, white blood count (WBC), differential, reticulocytes and platelets should be monitored closely–at least every 3 or 4 days.

Hepatic and renal evaluation are indicated prior to beginning therapy. Urinalysis, transaminase, alkaline phosphatase and blood urea nitrogen tests should be repeated at least weekly.

Drug Interactions: See WARNINGS section.

No cross-resistance with other chemotherapeutic agents, radio-therapy or steroids has been demonstrated.

Carcinogenesis, Mutagenesis and Impairment of Fertility: See WARNINGS section.

Pregnancy: Pregnancy Category D. See WARNINGS section.

Nursing Mothers: It is not known whether Matulane is excreted in human milk. Because of the potential for tumorigenicity shown for procarbazine hydrochloride in animal studies, mothers should not nurse while receiving this drug.

Pediatric Use: Undue toxicity, evidenced by tremors, coma and convulsions, has occurred in a few cases. Dosage, therefore, should be individualized (see DOSAGE AND ADMINISTRATION). Very close clinical monitoring is mandatory.

ADVERSE REACTIONS

Leukopenia, anemia and thrombopenia occur frequently. Nausea and vomiting are the most commonly reported side effects.

Other adverse reactions are:

Hematologic: Pancytopenia; eosinophilia; hemolytic anemia; bleeding tendencies such as petechiae, purpura, epistaxis and hemoptysis.

Gastrointestinal: Hepatic dysfunction, jaundice, stomatitis, hematemesis, melena, diarrhea, dysphagia, anorexia, abdominal pain, constipation, dry mouth.

Neurologic: Coma, convulsions, neuropathy, ataxia, paresthesia, nystagmus, diminished reflexes, falling, foot drop, headache, dizziness, unsteadiness.

Cardiovascular: Hypotension, tachycardia, syncope.

Ophthalmic: Retinal hemorrhage, papilledema, photophobia, diplopia, inability to focus.

Respiratory: Pneumonitis, pleural effusion, cough.

Dermatologic: Herpes, dermatitis, pruritus, alopecia, hyperpigmentation, rash, urticaria, flushing.

Allergic: Generalized allergic reactions.

Genitourinary: Hematuria, urinary frequency, nocturia.

Musculoskeletal: Pain, including myalgia and arthralgia; tremors.

Psychiatric: Hallucinations, depression, apprehension, nervousness, confusion, nightmares.

Endocrine: Gynecomastia in prepubertal and early pubertal boys.

Miscellaneous: Intercurrent infections, hearing loss, pyrexia, diaphoresis, lethargy, weakness, fatigue, edema, chills, insomnia, slurred speech, hoarseness, drowsiness.

Second nonlymphoid malignancies (including lung cancer, acute myelocytic leukemia and malignant myelosclerosis), and azoospermia have been reported in patients with Hodgkin's disease treated with procarbazine in combination with other chemotherapy and/or radiation. The risks of secondary lung cancer from treatment appear to be multiplied by tobacco use.

OVERDOSAGE

The major manifestations of overdosage with Matulane would be anticipated to be nausea, vomiting, enteritis, diarrhea, hypotension, tremors, convulsions and coma. Treatment should consist of either the administration of an emetic or gastric lavage. General supportive measures such as intravenous fluids are advised. Since the major toxicity of procarbazine hydrochloride is hematologic and hepatic, patients should have frequent complete blood counts and liver function tests throughout their period of recovery and for a minimum of two weeks thereafter. Should abnormalities appear in any of these determinations, appropriate measures for correction and stabilization should be immediately undertaken.

The estimated mean lethal dose of procarbazine hydrochloride in laboratory animals varied from approximately 150 mg/kg in rabbits to 1300 mg/kg in mice.

DOSAGE AND ADMINISTRATION

The following doses are for administration of the drug as a single agent. When used in combination with other anticancer drugs, the Matulane dose should be appropriately reduced, eg, in the MOPP regimen, the Matulane dose is 100 mg/m^2 daily for 14 days. All dosages are based on the patient's actual weight. However, the estimated lean body mass (dry weight) is used if the patient is obese or if there has been a spurious weight gain due to edema, ascites or other forms of abnormal fluid retention.

Adults: To minimize the nausea and vomiting experienced by a high percentage of patients beginning Matulane therapy, single or divided doses of 2 to 4 mg/kg/day for the first week are recommended. Daily dosage should then be maintained at 4 to 6 mg/kg/day until maximum response is obtained or until the white blood count falls below 4000/cmm or the platelets fall below 100,000/cmm. When maximum response is obtained, the dose may be maintained at 1 to 2 mg/kg/day. Upon evidence of hematologic or other toxicity (see PRECAUTIONS section), the drug should be discontinued until there has been satisfactory recovery. After toxic side effects have subsided, therapy may then be resumed at the discretion of the physician, based on clinical evaluation and appropriate laboratory studies, at a dosage of 1 to 2 mg/kg/day.

Pediatric Patients: Very close clinical monitoring is mandatory. Undue toxicity, evidenced by tremors, coma and convulsions, has occurred in a few cases. Dosage, therefore, should be individualized. The following dosage schedule is provided as a guideline only.

Fifty (50) mg per square meter of body surface per day is recommended for the first week. Dosage should then be maintained at 100 mg per square meter of body surface per day until maximum response is obtained or until leukopenia or thrombocytopenia occurs. When maximum response is attained, the dose may be maintained at 50 mg per square meter of body surface per day. Upon evidence of hematologic or other toxicity (see PRECAUTIONS section), the drug should be discontinued until there has been satisfactory recovery, based on clinical evaluation and appropriate laboratory tests. After toxic side effects have subsided, therapy may then be resumed.

Procedures for proper handling and disposal of anticancer drugs should be considered. Several guidelines on this subject have been published.[1–6] There is no general agreement that all of the procedures recommended in the guidelines are necessary or appropriate.

HOW SUPPLIED

Capsules, ivory, containing the equivalent of 50 mg procarbazine as the hydrochloride; bottles of 100 (NDC 54482-053-01). Imprint on capsules: Matulane σ sigma-tau.

REFERENCES

1. Recommendations for the safe handling of parenteral antineoplastic drugs. Washington, DC: U.S. Government Printing Office NIH Publication No. 83-2621.
2. AMA Council Report. Guidelines for handling parenteral antineoplastics. *JAMA*. Mar 15, 1985; 253:1590-1592.
3. National Study Commission on Cytotoxic Exposure: Recommendations for handling cytotoxic agents. Available from Louis P. Jeffrey, ScD, Director of Pharmacy Services, Rhode Island Hospital, 593 Eddy Street, Providence, Rhode Island 02902.
4. Clinical Oncological Society of Australia: Guidelines and recommendations for safe handling of antineoplastic agents. *Med J Aust*. Apr 30, 1983; 1;426-428.
5. Jones RB, Frank R, Mass T: Safe handling of chemotherapeutic agents: a report from the Mount Sinai Medical Center. *CA*. Sept-Oct 1983; 33:258-263.
6. ASHP technical assistance bulletin on handling cytotoxic drugs in hospitals. *Am J Hosp Pharm*. Jan 1985; 42:131-137.

Manufactured by
AAI Development Services
An *aaiPharma* Company
1726 North 23rd St.
Wilmington, NC 28405
for:
sigma-tau Pharmaceuticals, Inc.
800 S. Frederick Avenue
Gaithersburg, MD 20877

Revised: February 2004

16785-0204

Sirius Laboratories, Inc.

100 FAIRWAY DRIVE, SUITE 130
VERNON HILLS, IL 60061

Direct Inquiries to:
Customer Service:
866-292-2108
For Medical Emergencies Contact:
847-968-2424

AVAR™ GREEN ℞
AVAR™ GEL
AVAR™ CLEANSER
AVAR™-e
AVAR™-e GREEN

[a'var]
(sodium sulfacetamide 10% and sulfur 5%)
Rx Only

FOR DERMATOLOGICAL USE ONLY
NOT FOR OPHTHALMIC USE

DESCRIPTION

Each gram of AVAR™ Gel (sodium sulfacetamide 10% and sulfur 5%) contains 100 mg of sodium sulfacetamide and 50 mg of colloidal sulfur in an aqueous based emollient gel vehicle containing purified water USP, sodium magnesium silicate, emulsifying lipids, nicotinamide, disodium EDTA, sodium thiosulfate, zinc oxide, benzyl alcohol, phenoxyethanol, glycerin, xanthan gum, sodium lactate, polyacrylamide, C13-C14 isoparaffin, laureth-7, fragrance.

Each gram of AVAR™ Green (sodium sulfacetamide 10% and sulfur 5%) Color Corrective Gel contains 100 mg of sodium sulfacetamide and 50 mg of colloidal sulfur in an aqueous based emollient gel vehicle containing purified water USP, sodium magnesium silicate, emulsifying lipids, nicotinamide, disodium EDTA, sodium thiosulfate, zinc oxide, benzyl alcohol, phenoxyethanol, glycerin, xanthan gum, sodium lactate, polyacrylamide, C13-C14 isoparaffin, laureth-7, fragrance, chromium oxide green.

Each gram of AVAR™ Cleanser (sodium sulfacetamide 10% and sulfur 5%) contains 100 mg of sodium sulfacetamide and 50 mg of colloidal sulfur in a mild aqueous based cleansing vehicle containing purified water USP, sodium magnesium silicate, sodium thiosulfate, propylene glycol, sodium lauryl sulfate, cetyl alcohol, stearyl alcohol, phenoxyethanol, fragrance.

Each gram of AVAR™-*e* Emollient Cream (sodium sulfacetamide 10% and sulfur 5%) contains 100 mg of sodium sulfacetamide and 50 mg of colloidal sulfur in an emollient cream vehicle containing purified water, isostearyl palmitate, glyceryl stearate and PEG-100 stearate, sodium lactate USP, glycerin USP, self-emulsifying wax NF, zinc oxide USP, benzyl alcohol NF, nicotinamide, cetyl alcohol NF, dimethicone, sodium thiosulfate, phenoxyethanol, disodium EDTA, fragrance.

Each gram of AVAR™-*e* Green Cream (sodium sulfacetamide 10% and sulfur 5%) color corrective emollient cream contains 100 mg of sodium sulfacetamide and 50 mg of colloidal sulfur in an emollient cream vehicle containing purified water, isostearyl palmitate, glyceryl stearate and PEG-100 stearate, sodium lactate USP, glycerin USP, self-emulsifying wax NF, zinc oxide USP, benzyl alcohol NF, chromium oxide green, nicotinamide, cetyl alcohol NF, dimethicone, sodium thiosulfate, phenoxyethanol, disodium EDTA, fragrance.

Sodium sulfacetamide is a sulfonamide with antibacterial activity while sulfur acts as a keratolytic agent. Chemically sodium sulfacetamide is N-[(4-aminophenyl) sulfonyl]-acetamide, monosodium salt, monohydrate. The structural formula is:

$$H_2N-C_6H_4-SO_2N(Na)COCH_3 \cdot H_2O$$

CLINICAL PHARMACOLOGY

The most widely accepted mechanism of action of sulfonamides is the Woods-Fildes theory which is based on the fact that sulfonamides act as competitive antagonists to para-aminobenzoic acid (PABA), an essential component for bacterial growth. While absorption through intact skin has not been determined, sodium sulfacetamide is readily absorbed from the gastrointestinal tract when taken orally and excreted in the urine, largely unchanged. The biological half-life has variously been reported as 7 to 12.8 hours.

The exact mode of action of sulfur in the treatment of acne is unknown, but it has been reported that it inhibits the growth of Propionibacterium acnes and the formation of free fatty acids.

INDICATIONS

AVAR Gel, AVAR Green, AVAR Cleanser, AVAR-*e* Emollient Cream and AVAR-*e* Green Cream are indicated in the topical control of acne vulgaris, acne rosacea and seborrheic dermatitis.

CONTRAINDICATIONS

AVAR Gel, AVAR Green, AVAR Cleanser, AVAR-*e* Emollient Cream and AVAR-*e* Green Cream are contraindicated for use by patients having known hypersensitivity to sulfonamides, sulfur or any other component of these preparations. AVAR Gel, AVAR Green, AVAR Cleanser, AVAR-*e* Emollient Cream, and AVAR-*e* Green Cream are not to be used by patients with kidney disease.

WARNINGS

Although rare, sensitivity to sodium sulfacetamide may occur. Therefore, caution and careful supervision should be observed when prescribing this drug for patients who may be prone to hypersensitivity to topical sulfonamides. Systemic toxic reactions such as agranulocytosis, acute hemolytic anemia, purpura hemorrhagica, drug fever, jaundice, and contact dermatitis indicate hypersensitivity to sulfonamides. Particular caution should be employed if areas of denuded or abraded skin are involved.

FOR EXTERNAL USE ONLY. Keep away from eyes. Keep out of the reach of children. Keep containers tightly closed.

PRECAUTIONS

General: If irritation develops, use of the product should be discontinued and appropriate therapy instituted. Patients should be carefully observed for possible local irritation or sensitization during long-term therapy. The object of this therapy is to achieve desquamation without irritation, but sodium sulfacetamide and sulfur can cause reddening and scaling of epidermis. These side effects are not unusual in the treatment of acne vulgaris, but patients should be cautioned about the possibility.

Carcinogenesis, Mutagenesis and Impairment of Fertility: Long-term studies in animals have not been performed to evaluate carcinogenic potential.

Pregnancy: Category C. Animal reproduction studies have not been conducted with AVAR Gel, AVAR Green, AVAR Cleanser, AVAR-*e* Emollient Cream, or AVAR-*e* Green Cream. It is also not known whether AVAR Gel, AVAR Green, AVAR Cleanser, AVAR-*e* Emollient Cream, or AVAR-*e* Green Cream can cause fetal harm when administered to a pregnant woman or can affect reproduction capacity. AVAR Gel, AVAR Green, AVAR Cleanser, AVAR-*e* Emollient Cream, and AVAR-*e* Green Cream should be given to a pregnant woman only if clearly needed.

Nursing Mothers: It is not known whether sodium sulfacetamide is excreted in the human milk following topical use of AVAR Gel, AVAR Green, AVAR Cleanser, AVAR-*e* Emollient Cream, or AVAR-*e* Green Cream. However, small amounts of orally administered sulfonamides have been reported to be eliminated in human milk. In view of this and because many drugs are excreted in human milk, caution should be exercised when AVAR Gel, AVAR Green, AVAR Cleanser, AVAR-*e* Emollient Cream, or AVAR-*e* Green Cream are administered to a nursing woman.

Pediatric Use: Safety and effectiveness in children under the age of 12 have not been established.

ADVERSE REACTIONS

Although rare, sodium sulfacetamide may cause local irritation.

DOSAGE AND ADMINISTRATION

AVAR Gel: Apply a thin film of AVAR Gel to affected areas 1 to 3 times daily, or as directed by a physician.

AVAR Green Color Corrective Gel: Apply a thin layer of AVAR Green to affected areas 1 to 3 times daily, or as directed by a physician. Apply only a small amount of AVAR Green to affected area and massage the green gel completely and uniformly into the skin.

AVAR Cleanser: Wash affected areas with AVAR Cleanser 1 to 2 times daily, or as directed by a physician. Avoid contact with eyes or mucous membranes. Wet skin and liberally apply to areas to be cleansed, massage gently into skin for 10-20 seconds working into a full lather, rinse thoroughly and pat dry. If drying occurs, it may be controlled by rinsing cleanser off sooner or using cleanser less often.

AVAR-*e* Emollient Cream: Apply a thin film of AVAR-*e* Emollient Cream to affected areas 1 to 3 times daily, or as directed by a physician.

AVAR-*e* Green Cream: Apply a thin layer of AVAR-*e* Green Cream to affected areas 1 to 3 times daily, or as directed by a physician. Apply only a small amount of AVAR-*e* Green Cream to affected area and massage the green cream completely and uniformly into the skin.

HOW SUPPLIED

AVAR Gel - 45 g tubes (NDC 65880-001-45).
AVAR Green Color Corrective Gel - 45 g tubes (NDC 65880-002-45).
AVAR Cleanser - 8 oz. (226.8 g) bottles with a pump dispenser (NDC 65880-200-08)
AVAR-*e* Emollient Cream - 45 g tubes (NDC 65880-400-45)
AVAR-*e* Green Cream - 45 g tubes (NDC 65880-402-45)
Store between 15° and 25°C (59° and 77°F). Do not freeze.
Manufactured for:
Sirius Laboratories, Inc.
Vernon Hills, IL 60061
By: Harmony Laboratories Inc.
Landis, NC 28088

Patent Pending AVAR™ Gel, AVAR™ Green, AVAR™ Cleanser and AVAR™-*e* Green Cream
45011 0103 75151 1203

NICOMIDE® Tablets ℞

[*nī' kō-mīd*]
(nicotinamide, zinc, copper, and folic acid)
℞ only

DESCRIPTION

Nicomide® Tablets for oral administration are peach-colored; oval-shaped tablets imprinted "Sirius" 792 in blue ink on one side.

Each oral tablet provides:

Nicotinamide, USP	750 mg
Zinc Oxide, USP	25 mg
Cupric Oxide, USP	1.5 mg
Folic Acid, USP	500 mcg

Nicomide® has been designed to provide biphasic delivery of each of the active ingredients in order to minimize the potential for competitive antagonism in absorption of its ingredients. The biphasic delivery system facilitates the immediate release of 750 mg Nicotinamide, 1.5 mg Cupric Oxide, and 500 mcg Folic Acid, as well as, the sustained release of 25 mg Zinc Oxide. The biphasic delivery system also minimizes the potential for drug interaction induced deficiency states and impaired absorptions of other therapeutic agents.

Inactive Ingredients:

Carnauba wax powder, ethyl cellulose, FD&C Blue # 1, FD&C Yellow # 6 Aluminum Lake, hypromellose, magnesium stearate, microcrystalline cellulose, polyethylene glycol, polysorbate 80, propylene glycol, shellac, stearic acid, and titanium dioxide.

CLINICAL PHARMACOLOGY

Nicotinamide is a water-soluble component of the vitamin B complex group. In vivo, Nicotinamide is incorporated into nicotinamide adenine dinucleotide (NAD) and nicotinamide adenine dinucleotide phosphate (NADP). NAD and NADP function as coenzymes in a wide variety of enzymatic oxidation-reduction reactions essential for tissue respiration, lipid metabolism, and glycogenolysis.

Nicotinamide has demonstrated anti-inflammatory actions which may be of benefit in patients with inflammatory acne vulgaris, including but not limited to, suppression of antigen induced-lymphocytic transformation and inhibition of 3′–5′ cyclic AMP phosphodiesterase. Nicotinamide has demonstrated the ability to block the inflammatory actions of iodides known to precipitate or exacerbate inflammatory acne.

Nicotinamide lacks the vasodilator, gastrointestinal, hepatic, and hypolipemic actions of nicotinic acid or niacin. As such nicotinamide has not been shown to produce the flushing, itching and burning sensations of the skin as is commonly seen when large doses of nicotinic acid or niacin are administered orally.

(See **ADVERSE REACTIONS** section)

Zinc has been shown to inhibit the inflammatory polymorphonuclear leukocyte chemotaxis in acne patients. Zinc has also demonstrated an inhibitory effect on the lipase of the three Propionibacterium species found in human pilosebaceous follicles.

Patients with inflammatory acne have been shown to have significantly lower serum zinc levels than matched healthy controls.

Copper is an essential trace mineral in human nutrition. Although rare, copper deficiency has been induced by supplemental zinc therapy. Chronic zinc supplementation has been shown to reduce the intestinal absorption and utilization of copper, which can induce signs of copper deficiency in some patients. Symptoms of copper deficiency include anemia and decreased activity of cytochrome c oxidase. Heartbeat irregularities have also been reported in some studies. The biphasic delivery system is designed to address this issue by delivering supplemental copper with zinc in a manner that minimizes the potential for competitive antagonism in absorption.

Folic acid serves as an essential cofactor for the biosynthesis of thymidine and purine nucleotides required for normal cellular DNA synthesis. Deficiencies of folic acid have been demonstrated to occur in some cutaneous inflammatory disorders.

INDICATIONS AND USAGE

Indicated for non-pregnant patients with acne vulgaris or other inflammatory skin disorders who are deficient in, or at risk of deficiency in, one or more of the components of Nicomide®.

CONTRAINDICATIONS

Nicomide® is contraindicated in patients with hypersensitivity to any of its components.

Supplemental copper is contraindicated in those with Wilson's disease (hepatolenticular degeneration) a disease of abnormal copper accumulation.

WARNINGS

Folic Acid alone is improper treatment of pernicious anemia and other megaloblastic anemias where Vitamin B12 is deficient.

PRECAUTIONS

General: Large doses of nicotinamide should be administered with caution in patients with a history of jaundice, liver disease, or diabetes mellitus.

Folic Acid above 0.1 mg daily may obscure pernicious anemia (hematologic remission may occur while neurological manifestations remain progressive).

Those with chronic liver failure and chronic renal failure should exercise extreme caution in the use of supplements containing copper.

Drug Interactions: Nicotinamide: The clearance of primidone and carbamazepine may be reduced with the concomitant use of nicotinamide.

Zinc Oxide: The absorption of quinolones or tetracycline may be decreased with the concomitant use of zinc.

Cupric Oxide: Concomitant use of penicillamine and copper can cause decreased absorption of both substances.

Pregnancy: Large doses of nicotinamide, zinc, or copper should be avoided in pregnancy.

Nursing Mothers: Caution should be exercised when using Nicomide® in nursing mothers.

Pediatrics: Safety and effectiveness of Nicomide® in pediatric patients have not been established.

Geriatrics:

Clinical studies of Nicomide® have not been performed to determine whether elderly subjects respond differently than younger subjects. In general dose selection for an elderly patient should be cautious, usually starting at the low end of the dosing range, reflecting the greater frequency of decreased hepatic, renal, or cardiac function, and of concomitant disease or other drug therapy.

ADVERSE REACTIONS

Allergic sensitization has been reported rarely following oral and parenteral administration of Folic Acid.

At recommended doses, Nicomide® is expected to be well tolerated. Gastrointestinal distress such as nausea or vomiting have been associated with the administration of nicotinamide or zinc at doses greater than the recommended dose of Nicomide®.

Nicotinamide: Dizziness, headache, hyperglycemia, nausea, vomiting, diarrhea, elevations in liver function tests, hepatotoxicity, blurred vision, flushing, rash.

DOSAGE and ADMINISTRATION

Usual adult dose is one tablet taken once or twice a day or as prescribed by a physician.

HOW SUPPLIED

Is supplied in bottles of 60's—NDC 65880-792-60. Store between 15°-30°C (59°-86°F).
Manufactured for:
Sirius Laboratories, Inc.
Vernon Hills, IL 60061
New formula adopted February 2003. 0203 8357-00
Patent Pending

PSORIATEC™ ℞

[*sōr ī-ă-tek*]
(anthralin cream 1%, USP)
FOR DERMATOLOGICAL USE ONLY
NOT FOR OPHTHALMIC USE

DESCRIPTION

Psoriatec (anthralin cream 1.0%, USP) is a smooth, yellow cream containing 1% anthralin USP in an aqueous cream base of glyceryl monolaurate, glyceryl monomyristate, citric acid, sodium hydroxide and purified water. For topical dermatological use only.

The chemical name of anthralin is 1,8-dihydroxy-9-anthrone. The structure is:

OH O OH

CLINICAL PHARMACOLOGY

Psoriatec contains anthralin, a synthetic compound whose precise mechanism of anti-psoriatic action is not yet fully understood. Numerous studies, however, have demonstrated anti-proliferative and anti-inflammatory effects of anthralin on psoriatic and normal skin. The anti-proliferative effects of anthralin appear to result from both an inhibition of DNA synthesis as well as from its strong reducing properties. Recently, anthralin's effectiveness as an anti-psoriatic agent has also been in part attributed to its abilities to inactivate epidermal 12-lipoxygenase and reduce levels of endothelial adhesion molecules which are markedly elevated in psoriatic patients. Inactivation of 12-lipoxygenase by anthralin substantially reduces levels of 12-hydroperoxyeicosatetraenoic acid and its inflammatory metabolites, which are present in high concentrations in psoriatic plaques. Anthralin does not appear to affect liver microsomal enzyme activity. Systemic absorption of anthralin after topical application of Psoriatec has not been determined in humans.

Continued on next page

Psoriatec—Cont.

INDICATIONS AND USES

For the topical treatment of psoriasis.

CONTRAINDICATIONS

Psoriatec is contraindicated for patients with acute or actively inflamed psoriatic eruptions, or a history of hypersensitivity to any of the ingredients.

WARNINGS

For external use only. Avoid contact with the eyes or mucous membranes. Exercise care when applying Psoriatec cream to the face or intertriginous skin areas. Discontinue use if a sensitivity reaction occurs or if excessive irritation develops. Keep out of the reach of children.

PRECAUTIONS

General: To prevent the possibility of staining clothing or bed linen, it may be advisable to use protective dressings. To prevent discoloration of tub/shower, always rinse the tub/shower with cool to lukewarm water immediately after washing/showering and then use a suitable cleanser to remove any deposit on the surface of the tub or shower. Contact with fabrics, plastics and other materials may cause staining and should be avoided. Always wash hands thoroughly after use.

Carcinogenesis, Mutagenesis, Impairment of Fertility: Long-term studies in animals have not been performed to evaluate the carcinogenic potential of the drug. Although anthralin has been found to have tumor-promoting properties on mouse skin, there have been no reports to suggest carcinogenic effects in humans after many years of clinical use.

Pregnancy: Pregnancy Category C. Animal reproduction studies have not been conducted with Psoriatec cream. It is also not known whether Psoriatec cream can cause fetal harm when administered to a pregnant woman or can affect reproduction capacity. Psoriatec cream should be given to a pregnant woman only if clearly needed.

Nursing Mothers: It is not known whether this drug is excreted in human milk. Because many drugs are excreted in milk and because of the potential for tumorigenicity shown for anthralin in animal studies, a decision should be made whether to discontinue nursing or to discontinue the drug, taking into account the importance of the drug to the mother.

Pediatric Use: Safety and effectiveness in children have not been established.

ADVERSE REACTIONS

Very few instances of contact allergic reactions to anthralin have been reported. However, transient primary irritation of the normal skin or uninvolved skin surrounding the treated lesions is more frequently seen. If the initial treatment produces excessive soreness or if the lesions spread, reduce frequency of application and, in extreme cases, discontinue use and consult a physician.

Psoriatec cream may stain skin, hair or fabrics. Some temporary discoloration of hair and fingernails may arise during the period of treatment but should be minimized by careful application. Staining of fabrics may be permanent, so contact should be avoided.

DOSAGE AND ADMINISTRATION

Generally, it is recommended that Psoriatec cream be applied once a day. Anthralin is known to be a potential skin irritant. The irritant potential of anthralin is directly related to the strength being used, the time of contact, and each patient's individual tolerance.

Where the response to Psoriatec treatment has not previously been established, commence treatment using a short contact time for at least one week. When a short contact time is used initially, it can be increased stepwise to twenty to thirty minutes before removing the cream by washing or showering. The optimal period of contact will vary according to the patient's response to treatment. To open the tube, unscrew the cap and invert to puncture seal in tube. After use, replace cap in original position.

For the Skin: Apply sparingly only to the psoriatic lesions and rub gently and carefully into the skin. Avoid applying an excessive quantity which may cause unnecessary soiling and staining of the clothing and/or bed linen. At the end of each period of treatment, rinse the skin thoroughly with cool to lukewarm water before washing with soap. The margins of the lesions may gradually become stained purple/brown as treatment progresses, but this will disappear after cessation of treatment.

For the Scalp: Wash the hair with shampoo, rinse with water and apply Psoriatec cream while the hair is still damp. Rub the cream well into the psoriatic lesions. Keep Psoriatec cream away from the eyes. Care should be taken to avoid application of the cream to uninvolved scalp margins. Remove any unintended residue which may be deposited behind the ears. At the end of each period of contact, rinse hair and scalp thoroughly with cool to lukewarm water and then shampoo the hair and scalp to remove any surplus cream (which may have become red/brown in color). This treatment may be repeated on alternate days if necessary.

HOW SUPPLIED

Psoriatec (anthralin cream 1.0%, USP) is supplied in tubes. 50g NDC 65880-415-50

Keep container tightly capped when not in use. Avoid excessive heat.

Store at controlled room temperature: 59°F to 86°F (15°C to 30°C).

Rx only.

Date of preparation or last review: July 2001

Manufactured for:
Sirius Laboratories
100 Fairway Drive, Ste. 130
Vernon Hills, IL 60061
by Bioglan AB
Sweden

SkinMedica, Inc

5909 SEA LION PLACE
SUITE H
CARLSBAD, CA 92008

PH# 760-448-3600
FAX# 760-448-3601
website www.SkinMedica.com

EPIQUIN™ MICRO
EPIQUIN™ MICRO XD ℞

[*ĕ-pĭ-kwĭn*]
(hydroquinone USP 4%)
Skin Bleaching Moisturizing Topical Cream
Rx ONLY.
FOR EXTERNAL USE ONLY.

DESCRIPTION

EpiQuin™ Micro and EpiQuin™ Micro XD contain hydroquinone USP 4% and retinol (vitamin A) incorporated into patented porous microspheres (Microsponge®* System) composed of methyl methacrylate/glycol dimethacrylate crosspolymer. This polymeric system has been shown to provide gradual release of active ingredient into the skin.[1] Hydroquinone is 1,4-benzenediol. Hydroquinone is structurally related to monobenzone. Hydroquinone occurs as fine, white needles. The drug is freely soluble in water and in alcohol and has a pK_a of 9.96. Chemically, hydroquinone is designated as p-dihydroxybenzene; the empirical formula is $C_6H_6O_2$; molecular weight 110.1. The structural formula is:

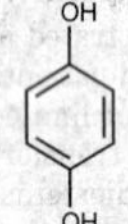

ACTIVE INGREDIENT:
Hydroquinone USP, 4%
OTHER INGREDIENTS:
Water, Caprylic/Capric Triglyceride, Emulsifying Wax, Dimethicone, Glycerin, C10-30 Cholesterol/Lanosterol Esters, Cetyl Alcohol, Cetyl Ricinoleate, Methyl Methacrylate/Glycol Dimethacrylate Crosspolymer, Retinol (Vitamin A), Tocopheryl Acetate (Vitamin E), Ascorbic Acid (Vitamin C), Ascorbyl Palmitate, Bisabolol, Cyclomethicone, PEG-10 Soy Sterol, Polyacrylamide, C13-14 Isoparaffin, Laureth-7, Magnesium Aluminum Silicate, TEA-Stearate, Cetyl Phosphate, Butylated Hydroxy Toluene, Propyl Gallate, Disodium EDTA, Benzyl Alcohol, Methylparaben, Phenoxyethanol, Polysorbate 20, Triethanolamine, Sodium Metabisulfite.

CLINICAL PHARMACOLOGY

Topical application of hydroquinone produces a reversible depigmentation of the skin by inhibition of the enzymatic oxidation of tyrosine to 3-(3,4-dihydroxyphenyl)alanine (dopa)[2] and suppression of other melanocyte metabolic processes.[3] Exposure to sunlight or ultraviolet light will cause repigmentation of the bleached areas.[4]

INDICATIONS AND USAGE

EpiQuin Micro and EpiQuin Micro XD are indicated for the gradual treatment of ultraviolet induced dyschromia and discoloration resulting from the use of oral contraceptives, pregnancy, hormone replacement therapy, or skin trauma.

CONTRAINDICATIONS

EpiQuin Micro and EpiQuin Micro XD are contraindicated in any patient with a prior history of hypersensitivity or allergic reaction to hydroquinone or any of the other ingredients. The safety of topical hydroquinone use during pregnancy or on children (12 years and under) has not been established.

WARNINGS

A. CAUTION: Hydroquinone is a depigmenting agent which may produce unwanted cosmetic effects if not used as directed. The physician should be familiar with the contents of this insert before prescribing or dispensing this medication.

B. Test for skin sensitivity before using EpiQuin Micro or EpiQuin Micro XD by applying a small amount to an unbroken patch of skin and check within 24 hours. Minor redness is not a contraindication, but where there is itching, vesicle formation, or excessive inflammatory response, further treatment is not advised. Close patient supervision is recommended. Contact with the eyes should be avoided. If no lightening effect is noted after 2 months of treatment, use of EpiQuin Micro or EpiQuin Micro XD should be discontinued.

C. Sunscreen use is an essential aspect of hydroquinone therapy, because even minimal sunlight sustains melanocytic activity. To prevent repigmentation during treatment and maintenance therapy, sun exposure on treated skin should be avoided by application of a broad spectrum sunscreen (SPF 15 or greater) or by use of protective clothing.

D. Keep this and all medications out of reach of children. In case of accidental ingestion, contact a physician or a poison control center immediately.

E. WARNING: Contains sodium metabisulfite, a sulfite which may cause serious allergic reactions (e.g., hives, itching, wheezing, anaphylaxis, severe asthma attack) in certain susceptible persons.

F. On rare occasions, a gradual blue-black darkening of the skin may occur, in which case, use of EpiQuin Micro and EpiQuin Micro XD should be discontinued and a physician contacted immediately.

PRECAUTIONS (SEE WARNINGS):

A. Pregnancy Category C: Animal reproduction studies have not been conducted with topical hydroquinone. It is also not known whether hydroquinone can cause fetal harm when used topically on a pregnant woman, or can affect reproductive capacity. It is not known to what degree, if any, topical hydroquinone is absorbed systemically. Topical hydroquinone should be used in pregnant women only when clearly indicated.

B. Nursing mothers: It is not known whether topical hydroquinone is absorbed or excreted in human milk. Caution is advised when hydroquinone is used by a nursing mother.

C. Pediatric usage: Safety and effectiveness in pediatric patients below the age of 12 years have not been established.

ADVERSE REACTIONS

No systemic reactions have been reported. Occasional cutaneous hypersensitivity (localized contact dermatitis) may occur, in which case the medication should be discontinued and the physician notified immediately.

OVERDOSAGE

There have been no systemic reactions reported from the use of topical hydroquinone. However, treatment should be limited to relatively small areas of the body at one time, since some patients experience a transient skin reddening and a mild burning sensation which does not preclude treatment.

DOSAGE AND ADMINISTRATION

EpiQuin Micro and EpiQuin Micro XD should be applied to the affected areas twice daily, morning and before bedtime, or as directed by a physician. To prevent repigmentation during and after the use of EpiQuin Micro and EpiQuin Micro XD, sun exposure should be limited and a sunscreen agent or sun-protective clothing should be used to cover the treated areas. There is no recommended dosage for pediatric patients under 12 years of age except under the advice and supervision of a physician.

If using EpiQuin Micro XD, hold the package (pouch) at the bottom with the sponge applicator facing upwards. Press or squeeze the pouch in the center where it says "Press Here" until the seal between the pouch and the sponge has been broken. Next, squeeze the pouch until the cream has emptied into the sponge. Immediately apply the cream by holding the pouch and rubbing the sponge applicator on the affected area. Single use only.

HOW SUPPLIED

EpiQuin Micro is supplied as follows:
SIZE: 1 oz tube (30g)
NDC NUMBER: 67402-010-30
EpiQuin Micro XD is supplied as follows:
SIZE: 1 box of 60 pouches (30g)
NDC NUMBER: 67402-010-06
Store at 25°C (77°F); excursions permitted to 15°-30°C (59°-86°F) (see USP Controlled Room Temperature)

REFERENCES

1. Data on file. Flash Topical Technologies, Cardinal Health. Somerset, NJ.
2. Denton C, Lerner AB, Fitzpatrick TB. Inhibition of melanin formation by chemical agents. *J Invest Dermatol.* 1952;18:119-135.
3. Jimbow K, Obata M, Pathak M, Fitzpatrick TB. Mechanism of depigmentation by hydroquinone. *J Invest Dermatol.* 1974;62:436-449.
4. Parrish JA, Anderson RR, Urbach F, Pitts D. UVA, *Biological Effects of Ultraviolet Radiation with Emphasis on Human Responses to Longwave Ultraviolet.* New York and London: Plenum Press; 1978:151.

Distributed by SkinMedica, Inc. Carlsbad, CA 92008
Covered by US Patent Numbers:
4,690,825; 5,145,675; 5,851,538 and 6,007,264

*Microsponge is a registered trademark of Cardinal Health, Inc. or one of its subsidiaries.
70172A

NEOBENZ™ MICRO ℞

[*nē-ō-bĕnz*]
(benzoyl peroxide cream)
Rx ONLY.
FOR EXTERNAL USE ONLY.

DESCRIPTION

NeoBenz Micro 3.5%, 5.5% and 8.5% creams are topical preparations containing benzoyl peroxide as the active in-

gredient incorporated into patented porous microspheres (Microsponge®* System) composed of methyl methacrylate/glycol dimethacrylate crosspolymer. This polymeric system has been shown to provide gradual release of active ingredient into the skin.[1] Other ingredients for all strengths include: water, glycerin, ethylhexyl palmitate, sorbitol, cetyl alcohol, glyceryl dilaurate, stearyl alcohol, magnesium aluminum silicate, silica, citric acid, xanthan gum, methylparaben, sodium citrate, propylparaben, polyacrylamide, C13-14 isoparaffin, laureth-7, sodium lauryl sulfate. The 8.5% cream also contains dimethicone.
Benzoyl peroxide is an oxidizing agent that possesses antibacterial properties and is classified as a keratolytic. Benzoyl peroxide ($C_{14}H_{10}O_4$) is represented by the following structure:

CLINICAL PHARMACOLOGY

The exact method of action of benzoyl peroxide in acne vulgaris is not known. Benzoyl peroxide is an antibacterial agent with demonstrated activity against Propionibacterium acnes. This action, combined with the mild keratolytic effect of benzoyl peroxide is believed to be responsible for its usefulness in acne. Benzoyl peroxide is absorbed by the skin where it is metabolized to benzoic acid and excreted as benzoate in the urine.

INDICATIONS AND USAGE

NeoBenz Micro is indicated for use in the topical treatment of mild to moderate acne vulgaris.

CONTRAINDICATIONS

NeoBenz Micro should not be used in patients who have shown hypersensitivity to benzoyl peroxide or to any of the other ingredients in the products.

WARNINGS

When using this product, avoid unnecessary sun exposure and use a sunscreen.

PRECAUTIONS

General—For external use only. Avoid contact with eyes and mucous membranes. If severe irritation develops, discontinue use and institute appropriate therapy.
Information for Patients: Avoid contact with eyes, eyelids, lips and mucous membranes. If accidental contact occurs, rinse with water. AVOID CONTACT WITH HAIR, FABRICS OR CARPETING AS BENZOYL PEROXIDE WILL CAUSE BLEACHING OR DISCOLORATION. If excessive irritation develops, discontinue use and consult your physician.
Carcinogenesis, Mutagenesis, Impairment of Fertility: Based upon all available evidence, benzoyl peroxide is not considered to be a carcinogen. However, data from a study using mice known to be highly susceptible to cancer suggest that benzoyl peroxide acts as a tumor promoter. The clinical significance of the findings is not known.
Pregnancy: Category C—Animal reproduction studies have not been conducted with benzoyl peroxide. It is also not known whether benzoyl peroxide can cause fetal harm when administered to a pregnant woman or can affect reproduction capacity. Benzoyl peroxide should be used by a pregnant woman only if clearly needed.
Nursing Mothers: It is not known whether this drug is excreted in human milk. Because many drugs are excreted in human milk, caution should be exercised when benzoyl peroxide is administered to a nursing woman.
Pediatric Use: Safety and effectiveness in children below the age of 12 have not been established.

ADVERSE REACTIONS

Allergic contact dermatitis and dryness have been reported with topical benzoyl peroxide therapy.

OVERDOSAGE

If excessive scaling, erythema or edema occurs, the use of these preparations should be discontinued. To hasten resolution of the adverse effects, cool compresses may be used. After symptoms and signs subside, a reduced dosage schedule may be cautiously tried if the reaction is judged to be due to excessive use and not allergenicity.

DOSAGE AND ADMINISTRATION

NeoBenz Micro should be applied once or twice daily to the affected area. Frequency of use should be adjusted to obtain the desired clinical response. Gentle cleansing of the affected areas prior to application may be beneficial. Clinically visible improvement will normally occur by the third week of therapy. Maximum lesion reduction may be expected after approximately eight to twelve weeks of drug use. Continuing use of the drug is normally required to maintain a satisfactory clinical response.

HOW SUPPLIED

NeoBenz Micro 3.5% Cream 45 gram tube
NDC 67402-020-45
NeoBenz Micro 5.5% Cream 45 gram tube
NDC 67402-021-45
NeoBenz Micro 8.5% Cream 45 gram tube
NDC 67402-022-45
Store at 15°-25°C (59°-77° F)

REFERENCE

1. Data on file. Flash Topical Technologies, Cardinal Health. Somerset, NJ

Distributed by SkinMedica, Inc., Carlsbad, CA 92008
Covered by US Patents: 4,690,825; 5,145,675; 5,879,716.

* Microsponge® is a registered trademark of Cardinal Health, Inc. or one of its subsidiaries.

70122B February 2004

VANIQA® ℞

(eflornithine hydrochloride) Cream, 13.9%
For topical dermatological use only.
Not for ophthalmic, oral or intravaginal use.
℞ only

DESCRIPTION

VANIQA® is a cream containing 13.9% (139 mg/g) of anhydrous eflornithine hydrochloride as eflornithine hydrochloride monohydrate (150 mg/g).
Chemically, eflornithine hydrochloride is (±) -2-(difluoromethyl) ornithine monohydrochloride monohydrate, with the empirical formula $C_6H_{12}F_2N_2O_2 \bullet HCl \bullet H_2O$, a molecular weight of 236.65 and the following structural formula:

Anhydrous eflornithine hydrochloride has an empirical formula $C_6H_{12}F_2N_2O_2 \bullet HCl$ and a molecular weight of 218.65. Other ingredients include: ceteareth-20, cetearyl alcohol, dimethicone, glyceryl stearate, methylparaben, mineral oil, PEG-100 stearate, phenoxyethanol, propylparaben, stearyl alcohol and water.

CLINICAL PHARMACOLOGY

Pharmacodynamics

There are no studies examining the inhibition of the enzyme ornithine decarboxylase (ODC) in human skin following the application of topical eflornithine. However, there are studies in the literature that report the inhibition of ODC activity in skin following oral eflornithine. It is postulated that topical eflornithine hydrochloride irreversibly inhibits skin ODC activity. This enzyme is necessary in the synthesis of polyamines. Animal data indicate that inhibition of ornithine decarboxylase inhibits cell division and synthetic functions, which affect the rate of hair growth. VANIQA (eflorithine hydrochloride) Cream, 13.9% has been shown to retard the rate of hair growth in non-clinical and clinical studies.

Pharmacokinetics

The mean percutaneous absorption of eflornithine in women with unwanted facial hair, from a 13.9% w/w cream formulation, is < 1% of the radioactive dose, following either single or multiple doses under conditions of clinical use, that included shaving within 2 hrs before radiolabeled dose application in addition to other forms of cutting or plucking and tweezing to remove facial hair. Steady state was reached within four days of twice-daily application. The apparent steady-state plasma $t_{1/2}$ of eflornithine was approximately 8 hours. Following twice-daily application of 0.5 g of the cream (total dose 1.0 g/day; 139 mg as anhydrous eflornithine hydrochloride), under conditions of clinical use in women with unwanted facial hair (n=10), the steady-state C_{max}, C_{trough} and AUC_{12hr} were approximately 10 ng/mL, 5 ng/mL, and 92 ng•hr/mL, respectively, expressed in terms of the anhydrous free base of eflornithine hydrochloride. At steady state, the dose-normalized peak concentrations (C_{max}) and the extent of daily systemic exposure (AUC) of eflornithine following twice-daily application of 0.5 g of the cream (total dose 1.0 g/day) is estimated to be approximately 100- and 60-fold lower, when compared to 370 mg/day once-daily oral doses. This compound is not known to be metabolized and is primarily excreted unchanged in the urine.

INDICATIONS AND USAGE

VANIQA (eflornithine hydrochloride) Cream, 13.9% is indicated for the reduction of unwanted facial hair in women. VANIQA has only been studied on the face and adjacent involved areas under the chin of affected individuals. Usage should be limited to these areas of involvement.

CLINICAL TRIALS

Results of topical dermal studies for contact sensitization, photocontact sensitization, and photocontact irritation reveal that under conditions of clinical use, VANIQA is not expected to cause contact sensitization, phototoxic, or photosensitization reactions. Results of the topical dermal study for contact irritation did reveal that VANIQA could cause irritation reactions in clinical use in susceptible individuals or under conditions of exaggerated use.
Two randomized double-blind studies involving 594 female patients (393 treated with VANIQA, 201 with vehicle) treated twice daily for up to 24 weeks evaluated the efficacy of VANIQA in the reduction of unwanted facial hair in women. Women in the trial had a customary frequency of removal of facial hair two or more times per week. Women with facial conditions such as severe inflammatory acne, women who were pregnant, and nursing mothers were excluded from the studies. Physicians assessed the improvement or worsening from the baseline condition (Physician's Global Assessment [PGA]), 48 hours after shaving, of all treated areas. Statistically significant improvement for VANIQA (eflornithine hydrochloride) Cream, 13.9% versus vehicle was seen in each of these studies for "marked improvement" or greater response (24-week time point; $p \leq 0.001$). Marked improvement was seen consistently at 8 weeks after initiation of treatment and continued throughout the 24 weeks of treatment. Hair growth approached pretreatment levels within 8 weeks of treatment withdrawal. The success rate over time is graphically presented below for each pivotal trial.

Physician's Global Assessment
Success Defined as Marked or Better Improvement

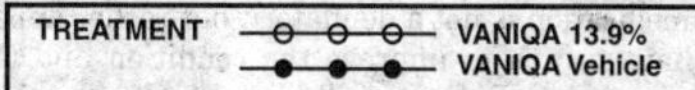

Study 1

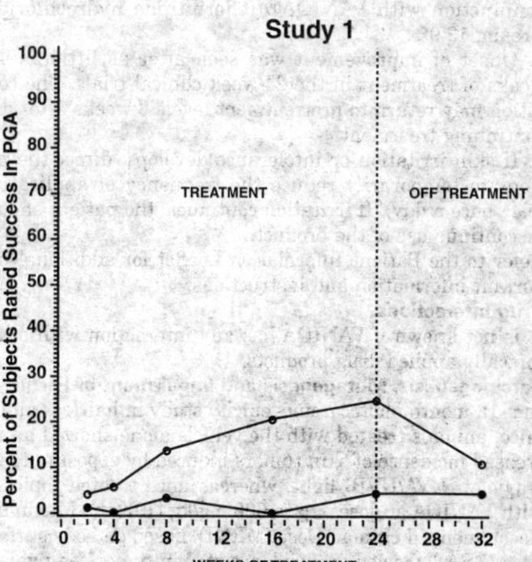

Study 2

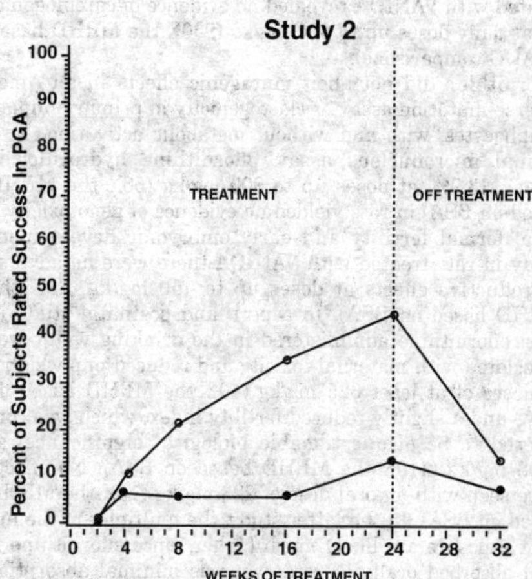

Approximately 32% of patients showed marked improvement or greater (protocol definition of clinical success) after 24 weeks of treatment with VANIQA (eflornithine hydrochloride) Cream, 13.9%, compared to 8% with the vehicle. Combined results of these two trials through 24 weeks are presented below.

PGA Outcome	VANIQA	Vehicle
Clear/almost clear	5%	0%
Marked improvement	27%	8%
Improved	26%	26%
No improvement/worse/missing	42%	66%

Subgroup analyses appeared to suggest greater benefit for Whites than non-Whites (37% vs. 22% success, respectively; p=0.017). However, non-Whites, mostly Black subjects, did have significant treatment benefit with 22% graded as success on VANIQA compared to 5% on vehicle.
About 12% of women in the clinical trials were postmenopausal. Significant improvement in PGA outcome versus vehicle was seen in postmenopausal women (38% compared to 0%, $p \leq 0.001$).
VANIQA statistically significantly reduced how bothered patients felt by their facial hair and by the time spent removing, treating, or concealing facial hair. These patient-observable differences were seen as early as 8 weeks after initiating treatment. Hair growth approached pretreatment levels within 8 weeks of treatment withdrawal.
Clinical trials with VANIQA involved over 1370 women with unwanted facial hair of skin types I-VI, of whom 68% were White, 17% Black, 11% Hispanic-Latino, 2% Asian-Pacific Islander, 0.6% American Native, and 1.3% other.

CONTRAINDICATIONS

VANIQA is contraindicated in patients with a history of sensitivity to any components of the preparation.

Continued on next page

Vaniqa—Cont.

WARNINGS

Discontinue use if hypersensitivity occurs.

PRECAUTIONS

General

For external use only.

Transient stinging or burning may occur when applied to abraded or broken skin.

Information For Patients

Patients using VANIQA should receive the following information and instructions:

1. This medication is not a depilatory, but rather appears to retard hair growth to improve the condition and the patient's appearance. Patients will likely need to continue using a hair removal method (e.g., shaving, plucking, etc.) in conjunction with VANIQA® (eflornithine hydrochloride) Cream, 13.9%.
2. Onset of improvement was seen after as little as 4-8 weeks of treatment in the 24-week clinical trials. The condition may return to pretreatment levels 8 weeks after discontinuing treatment.
3. If skin irritation or intolerance develops, direct the patient to temporarily reduce the frequency of application (e.g., once a day). If irritation continues, the patient should discontinue use of the product.

Refer to the Patient Information Leaflet for additional important information and instructions.

Drug Interactions

It is not known if VANIQA has any interaction with other topically applied drug products.

Carcinogenesis, Mutagenesis and Impairment of Fertility

In a 12-month photocarcinogenicity study in hairless albino mice, animals treated with the vehicle alone showed an increased incidence of skin tumors induced by exposure to ultraviolet (UVA/UVB) light, whereas mice treated topically with VANIQA at doses up to 600 mg/kg [19X the Maximum Recommended Human Dose (MRHD) based on body surface area (BSA)] showed an incidence of skin tumors equivalent to untreated-control animals.

A two-year dermal carcinogenicity study in CD-1 mice treated with VANIQA revealed no evidence of carcinogenicity at daily doses up to 600 mg/kg (950X the MRHD based on AUC comparisons).

Eflornithine did not elicit mutagenic effects in an Ames reverse-mutation assay or clastogenicity in primary human lymphocytes, with and without metabolic activation. In a dermal micronucleus assay, eflornithine hydrochloride cream, 13.9%, at doses up to 900 mg/kg (58X the MRHD based on BSA) in rats yielded no evidence of genotoxicity.

In a dermal fertility and early embryonic development study in rats treated with VANIQA there were no adverse reproductive effects at doses up to 450 mg/kg (29X the MRHD based on BSA). In a peri- and postnatal study in rats, eflornithine administered in the drinking water was associated with maternal toxicity and reduced pup weights at doses of at least 625 mg/kg (40X the MRHD based on BSA) and a slightly reduced fertility index, which was considered to be of questionable biological significance, at 1698 mg/kg (110X the MRHD based on BSA). No effects were seen with an oral dose of 223 mg/kg (14X the MRHD based on BSA). In the latter study, the multiples of the human exposure are likely much higher, since eflornithine is well absorbed orally in rats, whereas minimal absorption occurs in humans treated topically.

Pregnancy

Teratogenic Effects: Pregnancy Category C

In the first dermal embryo-fetal development study in rats treated with eflornithine hydrochloride cream, 13.9% (in which no precautions were taken to prevent ingestion of drug from application sites), maternal toxicity and fetal effects including reduced numbers of live fetuses, decreased fetal weights, and delayed ossification and development of the viscera were observed at doses of 225 and 450 mg/kg (15X and 29X the MRHD based on BSA, respectively). When the study was repeated under conditions that avoided ingestion from application sites, no maternal, fetal or teratogenic effects were observed at doses up to 450 mg/kg (29X the MRHD based on BSA). In the first study in which no precautions were taken to prevent ingestion, circulating plasma levels were 11- to 14-fold higher than in the second study in which ingestion was prevented. In a dermal embryo-fetal development study in rabbits treated with VANIQA (eflornithine hydrochloride) Cream, 13.9% no adverse maternal or fetal effects occurred at doses up to 90 mg/kg (11X the MRHD based on BSA). Significant dermal irritation, as well as possible ingestion of VANIQA occurred at 300 mg/kg/day (36X the MRHD based on BSA) and was associated with maternal deaths, abortions, increased fetal resorptions, and reduced fetal weights. Fetotoxicity in the absence of maternal toxicity has been reported in oral studies with eflornithine with fetal no-effect doses of 80 mg/kg in rats and 45 mg/kg in rabbits. In these studies, no evidence of teratogenicity was observed in rats given up to 200 mg/kg or in rabbits given up to 135 mg/kg. Although VANIQA was not formally studied in pregnant patients, 22 pregnancies occurred during the trials. Nineteen of these pregnancies occurred while patients were using VANIQA. Of the 19 pregnancies, there were 9 healthy infants, 4 spontaneous abortions, 5 induced/elective abortions, and 1 birth defect (Down's Syndrome to a 35-year-old). Because there are no adequate and well-controlled studies in pregnant women, the risk/benefit ratio of using VANIQA in women with unwanted facial hair who are pregnant should be weighed carefully with serious consideration for either not implementing or discontinuing use of VANIQA.

Nursing Mothers

It is not known whether or not eflornithine hydrochloride is excreted in human milk. Caution should be exercised when VANIQA is administered to a nursing woman.

Pediatric Use

The safety and effectiveness of this product have not been established in pediatric patients less than 12 years of age.

Geriatric Use

Of the 1373 patients on active treatment in clinical studies of VANIQA, approximately 7% were 65 years or older and approximately 1% were 75 or older. No apparent differences in safety were observed between older patients and younger patients.

ADVERSE REACTIONS

Adverse events reported for most body systems occurred at similar frequencies in VANIQA (eflornithine hydrochloride) Cream, 13.9% and vehicle control groups. The most frequent adverse events related to treatment with VANIQA were skin-related. The following table notes the percentage of adverse events associated with the use of VANIQA or its vehicle that occurred at greater than 1% in both the vehicle-controlled studies and the open-label safety studies up to 1 year of continuous use.

	Vehicle-Controlled Studies		Vehicle-Controlled and Open-Label Studies
Adverse Event Term	*VANIQA (n=393)*	*Vehicle (n=201)*	*VANIQA (n=1373)*
Acne	21.3	21.4	10.8
Pseudofolliculitis Barbae	16.3	15.4	4.9
Stinging Skin	7.9	2.5	4.1
Headache	3.8	5.0	4.0
Burning Skin	4.3	2.0	3.5
Dry Skin	1.8	3.0	3.3
Pruritus (itching)	3.8	4.0	3.1
Erythema (redness)	1.3	0.0	2.5
Tingling Skin	3.6	1.5	2.2
Dyspepsia	2.5	2.0	1.9
Skin Irritation	1.0	1.0	1.8
Rash	2.8	0.0	1.5
Alopecia	1.5	2.5	1.3
Dizziness	1.5	1.5	1.3
Folliculitis	0.5	0.0	1.0
Hair Ingrown	0.3	2.0	0.9
Facial edema	0.3	3.0	0.7
Anorexia	1.0	2.0	0.7
Nausea	0.5	1.0	0.7
Asthenia	0.0	1.0	0.3
Vertigo	0.3	1.0	0.1

Treatment related skin adverse events that occurred in less than 1% of the subjects treated with VANIQA are: bleeding skin, cheilitis, contact dermatitis, swelling of lips, herpes simplex, numbness and rosacea.

Adverse events were primarily mild in intensity and generally resolved without medical treatment or discontinuation of VANIQA. Only 2% of subjects discontinued studies due to an adverse event related to use of VANIQA.

Laboratory Test Abnormalities

No laboratory test abnormalities have been consistently found to be associated with VANIQA. In an open labeled study, some patients showed an increase in their transaminases; however, the clinical significance of these findings is not known.

OVERDOSAGE

Overdosage information with VANIQA is unavailable. Given the low percutaneous penetration of this drug, overdosage via the topical route is not expected (see **CLINICAL PHARMACOLOGY**). However, should very high topical doses (e.g., multiple tubes per day) or oral ingestion be encountered (a 30 g tube contains 4.2 g of eflornithine hydrochloride), the patient should be monitored, and appropriate supportive measures administered as necessary.

(Note: Use of an intravenous formulation of eflornithine hydrochloride at high doses (400 mg/kg/day or approximately 24 g/day) for the treatment of *Trypanosoma brucei gambiense* infection (African sleeping sickness) has been associated with adverse events and laboratory abnormalities. Adverse events in this setting have included hair loss, facial swelling, seizures, hearing impairment, stomach upset, loss of appetite, headache, weakness and dizziness. A variety of hematological toxicities, including anemia, thrombocytopenia and leukopenia have also been observed, but these were usually reversible upon discontinuation of treatment.)

DOSAGE AND ADMINISTRATION

Apply a thin layer of VANIQA (eflornithine hydrochloride) Cream, 13.9% to affected areas of the face and adjacent involved areas under the chin and rub in thoroughly. Do not wash treated area for at least 4 hours. Use twice daily at least 8 hours apart or as directed by a physician. The patient should continue to use hair removal techniques as needed in conjunction with VANIQA. (VANIQA should be applied at least 5 minutes after hair removal.) Cosmetics or sunscreens may be applied over treated areas after cream has dried.

HOW SUPPLIED

VANIQA® (eflornithine hydrochloride) Cream, 13.9% is available as:

30 gram tube

NDC 67402-040-30

STORAGE

Store at 25° C (77° F); excursions permitted to 15° C-30° C (59° F-86° F) [See USP Controlled Room Temperature] Do not freeze. See tube crimp and carton end for expiration date and lot number.

skin
MEDICA

Distributed By:
SkinMedica, Inc.
Carlsbad, CA 92008
www.skinmedica.com
U.S. Patent Numbers:
5,648,394 and 4,720,489
Revised 07/2004 03-6075

Patient Information Leaflet for

VANIQA®

(eflornithine hydrochloride) Cream, 13.9%

INFORMATION FOR PATIENTS

This section contains important information about VANIQA that you should read before you begin treatment. This section does not list all the benefits and risks of VANIQA and does not take the place of discussions with your doctor or healthcare professional about your condition or your treatment. If you have questions, talk with your healthcare professional. The medicine described here can only be prescribed by a licensed healthcare professional. Only your healthcare professional can determine if VANIQA is right for you.

What is VANIQA?

VANIQA (pronounced "VAN-i-ka") is a prescription medication applied to the skin for the reduction of unwanted facial hair in women.

The active ingredient in VANIQA is eflornithine hydrochloride. VANIQA also contains ceteareth-20, cetearyl alcohol, dimethicone, glyceryl stearate, methylparaben, mineral oil, PEG-100 stearate, phenoxyethanol, propylparaben, stearyl alcohol and water.

How does VANIQA work?

VANIQA interferes with an enzyme found in the hair follicle of the skin needed for hair growth. This results in slower hair growth and improved appearance where VANIQA is applied.

VANIQA does not permanently remove hair or "cure" unwanted facial hair. It is not a depilatory. Your treatment program should include continuation of any hair removal technique you are currently using. VANIQA will help you manage your condition and improve your appearance.

Improvement in the condition occurs gradually. Don't be discouraged if you see no immediate improvement. Be patient. Improvement may be seen as early as 4 to 8 weeks of treatment. Improvement may take longer in some individuals. If no improvement is seen after 6 months of use, discontinue use. Clinical studies show that in about 8 weeks after stopping treatment with VANIQA, the hair will return to the same condition as before beginning treatment.

Who should not use VANIQA?

You should not use VANIQA if you are allergic to any of the ingredients in the cream. All ingredients are listed on the tube and at the beginning of this leaflet.

You should not use VANIQA if you are less than 12 years of age.

What should you tell your doctor before using VANIQA?

If you are allergic to any of the ingredients, tell your doctor.

If you are pregnant or plan to become pregnant, discuss with your doctor whether you should use VANIQA during pregnancy. No clinical studies have been performed in pregnant women.

If you are breast feeding, consult your doctor before using VANIQA. It is not known if VANIQA is passed to infants through breast milk.

If you are taking any prescription medicines, non-prescription medicines or using any facial or skin creams, check with your physician before use of VANIQA.

How should I use VANIQA?
Use VANIQA only for the condition for which it was prescribed by your doctor. Do not give it to other people or allow other people to use it.
You will need to continue your normal procedures for hair removal until desired results have been achieved. You may then be less bothered by the time spent in removing hair or the frequency of hair removal. VANIQA is to be used twice daily, at least eight hours apart, or as directed by your doctor. VANIQA is for external use only.
Follow the instructions for application of VANIQA carefully. Apply a thin layer of VANIQA to the affected areas of the face and adjacent involved areas under the chin and rub in thoroughly. You should not wash the treatment areas for at least 4 hours after application of VANIQA.
VANIQA® may cause temporary redness, rash, burning, stinging or tingling, especially when the skin is damaged. If irritation continues, stop use of VANIQA and contact your doctor. Avoid getting the medication in your eyes or inside your nose or mouth. If the product gets in your eyes, rinse thoroughly with water and contact your doctor.
If you forget or miss a dose of VANIQA do not try to "make it up". Return to your normal application schedule as soon as you can.
You may use your normal cosmetics or sunscreen after applying VANIQA, but you should wait a few minutes to allow the treatment to be absorbed before applying them.
If your condition gets worse with treatment, stop use of VANIQA and contact your doctor.

What are the possible side effects of VANIQA?
VANIQA may cause temporary redness, stinging, burning, tingling or rash on areas of the skin where it is applied. Folliculitis (hair bumps) may also occur. If these persist, consult your doctor.

How should VANIQA be stored?
VANIQA should be stored at 15° C–30° C (59° F–86° F). Do not freeze.
Keep this and all medicines out of the reach of children.
This medicine was prescribed for your particular condition. Do not use it for another condition or give it to anyone else. This summary does not include everything there is to know about VANIQA. If you have questions or concerns, or want more information about VANIQA, your doctor or pharmacist has the comlete prescribing information upon which this leaflet is based. You may want to read it and discuss it with your doctor or healthcare professional. Remember, no written summary can replace careful discussion with your doctor.

℞ only
skin MEDICA

Distributed By:
SkinMedica, Inc.
Carlsbad, CA 92008
www.skinmedica.com
U.S. Patent Numbers:
5,648,394 and 4,720,489
Revised 07/2004 03-6075

Solvay Pharmaceuticals, Inc.

901 SAWYER ROAD
MARIETTA, GA 30062

www.solvaypharmaceuticals-us.com
For Medical Information Contact:
Generally:
Medical Information Department
800-241-1643
Sales and Ordering:
Orders may be placed by calling this toll free number:
(800) 241-1643
Fax # 770 578-5901
Mail orders should be sent to:
Solvay Pharmaceuticals
Order Entry Department
901 Sawyer Road
Marietta, GA 30062

ACEON® ℞
[ā-sē-ŏn]
(perindopril erbumine) Tablets
℞ only

> **USE IN PREGNANCY**
> When used in pregnancy during the second and third trimesters, ACE inhibitors can cause injury and even death to the developing fetus. When pregnancy is detected, ACEON® Tablets should be discontinued as soon as possible. See **WARNINGS: Fetal/Neonatal Morbidity and Mortality.**

DESCRIPTION
ACEON® (perindopril erbumine) Tablets is the tert-butylamine salt of perindopril, the ethyl ester of a non-sulfhydryl angiotensin-converting enzyme (ACE) inhibitor. Perindopril erbumine is chemically described as (2S,3∝S,7∝S)-1-[(S)-N-[(S)-1-Carboxybutyl]alanyl]hexahydro-2-indolinecarboxylic acid, 1-ethyl ester, compound with tert-butylamine (1:1). Its molecular formula is $C_{19}H_{32}N_2O_5C_4H_{11}N$. Its structural formula is:

CO_2H • $H_2N{-}C(CH_3)_3$
$C{-}CH{-}NH{-}CH{-}CH_2CH_2CH_3$
CH_3 $CO_2CH_2CH_3$

Perindopril erbumine is a white, crystalline powder with a molecular weight of 368.47 (free acid) or 441.61 (salt form). It is freely soluble in water (60% w/w), alcohol and chloroform.
Perindopril is the free acid form of perindopril erbumine, is a pro-drug and metabolized *in vivo* by hydrolysis of the ester group to form perindoprilat, the biologically active metabolite.
ACEON® Tablets is available in 2 mg, 4 mg and 8 mg strengths for oral administration. In addition to perindopril erbumine, each tablet contains the following inactive ingredients: colloidal silica (hydrophobic), lactose, magnesium stearate and microcrystalline cellulose. The 4 and 8 mg tablets also contain iron oxide.

CLINICAL PHARMACOLOGY
Mechanism of Action: ACEON® (perindopril erbumine) Tablets is a pro-drug for perindoprilat, which inhibits ACE in human subjects and animals. The mechanism through which perindoprilat lowers blood pressure is believed to be primarily inhibition of ACE activity. ACE is a peptidyl dipeptidase that catalyzes conversion of the inactive decapeptide, angiotensin I, to the vasoconstrictor, angiotensin II. Angiotensin II is a potent peripheral vasoconstrictor, which stimulates aldosterone secretion by the adrenal cortex, and provides negative feedback on renin secretion. Inhibition of ACE results in decreased plasma angiotensin II, leading to decreased vasoconstriction, increased plasma renin activity and decreased aldosterone secretion. The latter results in diuresis and natriuresis and may be associated with a small increase of serum potassium.
ACE is identical to kininase II, an enzyme that degrades bradykinin. Whether increased levels of bradykinin, a potent vasodepressor peptide, play a role in the therapeutic effects of ACEON® Tablets remains to be elucidated.
While the principal mechanism of perindopril in blood pressure reduction is believed to be through the renin-angiotensin-aldosterone system, ACE inhibitors have some effect even in apparent low-renin hypertension. Perindopril has been studied in relatively few black patients, usually a low-renin population, and the average response of diastolic blood pressure to perindopril was about half the response seen in nonblacks, a finding consistent with previous experience of other ACE inhibitors.
After administration of perindopril, ACE is inhibited in a dose and blood concentration-related fashion, with the maximal inhibition of 80 to 90% attained by 8 mg persisting for 10 to 12 hours. Twenty-four hour ACE inhibition is about 60% after these doses. The degree of ACE inhibition achieved by a given dose appears to diminish over time (the ID_{50} increases). The pressor response to an angiotensin I infusion is reduced by perindopril, but this effect is not as persistent as the effect on ACE; there is about 35% inhibition at 24 hours after a 12 mg dose.
Pharmacokinetics: Oral administration of ACEON® (perindopril erbumine) Tablets results in its rapid absorption with peak plasma concentrations occurring at approximately 1 hour. The absolute oral bioavailability of perindopril is about 75%. Following absorption, approximately 30 to 50% of systemically available perindopril is hydrolyzed to its active metabolite, perindoprilat, which has a mean bioavailability of about 25%. Peak plasma concentrations of perindoprilat are attained 3 to 7 hours after perindopril administration. The presence of food in the gastrointestinal tract does not affect the rate or extent of absorption of perindopril but reduces bioavailability of perindoprilat by about 35%. (See **PRECAUTIONS: *Food Interaction.***)
With 4, 8 and 16 mg doses of ACEON® Tablets, Cmax and AUC of perindopril and perindoprilat increase in a linear and dose-proportional manner following both single oral dosing and at steady state during a once-a-day multiple dosing regimen.
Perindopril exhibits multiexponential pharmacokinetics following oral administration. The mean half-life of perindopril associated with most of its elimination is approximately 0.8 to 1.0 hours. At very low plasma concentrations of perindopril (<3 ng/mL), there is a prolonged terminal elimination half-life, similar to that seen with other ACE inhibitors, that results from slow dissociation of perindopril from plasma/tissue ACE binding sites. Perindopril does not accumulate with a once-a-day multiple dosing regimen. Mean total body clearance of perindopril is 219 to 362 mL/min and its mean renal clearance is 23.3 to 28.6 mL/min.
Perindopril is extensively metabolized following oral administration, with only 4 to 12% of the dose recovered unchanged in the urine. Six metabolites resulting from hydrolysis, glucuronidation and cyclization via dehydration have been identified. These include the active ACE inhibitor, perindoprilat (hydrolyzed perindopril), perindopril and perindoprilat glucuronides, dehydrated perindopril and the diastereoisomers of dehydrated perindoprilat. In humans, hepatic esterase appears to be responsible for the hydrolysis of perindopril.
The active metabolite, perindoprilat, also exhibits multiexponential pharmacokinetics following the oral administration of ACEON® Tablets. Formation of perindoprilat is gradual with peak plasma concentrations occurring between 3 and 7 hours. The subsequent decline in plasma concentration shows an apparent mean half-life of 3 to 10 hours for the majority of the elimination, with a prolonged terminal elimination half-life of 30 to 120 hours resulting from slow dissociation of perindoprilat from plasma/tissue ACE binding sites. During repeated oral once-daily dosing with perindopril, perindoprilat accumulates about 1.5 to 2.0 fold and attains steady state plasma levels in 3 to 6 days. The clearance of perindoprilat and its metabolites is almost exclusively renal.
Approximately 60% of circulating perindopril is bound to plasma proteins, and only 10 to 20% of perindoprilat is bound. Therefore, drug interactions mediated through effects on protein binding are not anticipated.
At usual antihypertensive dosages, little radioactivity (<5% of the dose) was distributed to the brain after administration of ^{14}C-perindopril to rats.
Radioactivity was detectable in fetuses and in milk after administration of ^{14}C-perindopril to pregnant and lactating rats.
Elderly Patients: Plasma concentrations of both perindopril and perindoprilat in elderly patients (>70 yrs) are approximately twice those observed in younger patients, reflecting both increased conversion of perindopril to perindoprilat and decreased renal excretion of perindoprilat. (See **PRECAUTIONS: Geriatric Use.**)
Heart Failure Patients: Perindoprilat clearance is reduced in congestive heart failure patients, resulting in a 40% higher dose interval AUC. (See **DOSAGE AND ADMINISTRATION.**)
Patients with Renal Insufficiency: With perindopril erbumine doses of 2 to 4 mg, perindoprilat AUC increases with decreasing renal function. At creatinine clearances of 30 to 80 mL/min, AUC is about double that of 100 mL/min. When creatinine clearance drops below 30 mL/min, AUC increases more markedly.
In a limited number of patients studied, perindopril dialysis clearance ranged from 41.7 to 76.7 mL/min (mean 52.0 mL/min). Perindoprilat dialysis clearance ranged from 37.4 to 91.0 mL/min (mean 67.2 mL/min). (See **DOSAGE AND ADMINISTRATION.**)
Patients with Hepatic Insufficiency: The bioavailability of perindoprilat is increased in patients with impaired hepatic function. Plasma concentrations of perindoprilat in patients with impaired liver function were about 50% higher than those observed in healthy subjects or hypertensive patients with normal liver function.
Pharmacodynamics: In placebo-controlled studies of perindopril monotherapy (2 to 16 mg q.d.) in patients with a mean blood pressure of about 150/100 mm Hg, 2 mg had little effect, but doses of 4 to 16 mg lowered blood pressure. The 8 and 16 mg doses were indistinguishable, and both had a greater effect than the 4 mg dose. The magnitude of the blood pressure effect was similar in the standing and supine positions, generally about 1 mm Hg greater on standing. In these studies, doses of 8 and 16 mg per day gave supine, trough blood pressure reductions of 9 to 15/5 to 6 mm Hg. When once-daily and twice-daily dosing were compared, the B.I.D. regimen was generally slightly superior, but by not more than about 0.5 to 1 mm Hg. After 2 to 16 mg doses of perindopril, the trough mean systolic and diastolic blood pressure effects were approximately equal to the peak effects (measured 3 to 7 hours after dosing.). Trough effects were about 75 to 100% of peak effects. When perindopril was given to patients receiving 25 mg HCTZ, it had an added effect similar in magnitude to its effect as monotherapy, but 2 to 8 mg doses were approximately equal in effectiveness. In general, the effect of perindopril occurred promptly, with effects increasing slightly over several weeks.
In hemodynamic studies carried out in animal models of hypertension, blood pressure reduction after perindopril administration was accompanied by a reduction in peripheral arterial resistance and improved arterial wall compliance. In studies carried out in patients with essential hypertension, the reduction in blood pressure was accompanied by a reduction in peripheral resistance with no significant changes in heart rate or glomerular filtration rate. An increase in the compliance of large arteries was also observed, suggesting a direct effect on arterial smooth muscle, consistent with the results of animal studies.
Formal interaction studies of ACEON® Tablets have not been carried out with antihypertensive agents other than thiazides. Limited experience in controlled and uncontrolled trials coadministering ACEON® Tablets with a calcium channel blocker, a loop diuretic or triple therapy (beta-blocker, vasodilator and a diuretic), does not suggest any unexpected interactions. In general, ACE inhibitors have less than additive effects when given with beta-adrenergic blockers, presumably because both work in part through the renin angiotensin system. A controlled pharmacokinetic study has shown no effect on plasma digoxin concentrations when coadministered with ACEON® Tablets. (See **PRECAUTIONS: Drug Interactions.**)
In uncontrolled studies in patients with insulin-dependent diabetes, perindopril did not appear to affect glycemic control. In long-term use, no effect on urinary protein excretion was seen in these patients.

Continued on next page

Aceon—Cont.

The effectiveness of ACEON® Tablets was not influenced by sex and it was less effective in blacks than in nonblacks. In elderly patients (≥60 years), the mean blood pressure effect was somewhat smaller than in younger patients, although the difference was not significant.

INDICATIONS AND USAGE

ACEON® (perindopril erbumine) Tablets is indicated for the treatment of patients with essential hypertension. ACEON® Tablets may be used alone or given with other classes of antihypertensives, especially thiazide diuretics.

When using ACEON® Tablets, consideration should be given to the fact that another angiotensin converting enzyme inhibitor (captopril) has caused agranulocytosis, particularly in patients with renal impairment or collagen vascular disease. Available data are insufficient to determine whether ACEON® Tablets has a similar potential. (See **WARNINGS**.)

In considering use of ACEON® Tablets, it should be noted that in controlled trials ACE inhibitors have an effect on blood pressure that is less in black patients than in nonblacks. In addition, it should be noted that black patients receiving ACE inhibitor monotherapy have been reported to have a higher incidence of angioedema compared to nonblacks. (See **WARNINGS:** ***Head and Neck Angioedema.***)

CONTRAINDICATIONS

ACEON® (perindopril erbumine) Tablets is contraindicated in patients known to be hypersensitive to this product or to any other ACE inhibitor. ACEON® Tablets is also contraindicated in patients with a history of angioedema related to previous treatment with an ACE inhibitor.

WARNINGS

Anaphylactoid and Possibly Related Reactions: Presumably because angiotensin-converting enzyme inhibitors affect the metabolism of eicosanoids and polypeptides, including endogenous bradykinin, patients receiving ACE inhibitors (including ACEON® Tablets) may be subject to a variety of adverse reactions, some of them serious.

Head and Neck Angioedema: Angioedema involving the face, extremities, lips, tongue, glottis and/or larynx has been reported in patients treated with ACE inhibitors, including ACEON® (perindopril erbumine) Tablets (0.1% of patients treated with ACEON® Tablets in U.S. clinical trials). In such cases, ACEON® Tablets should be promptly discontinued and the patient carefully observed until the swelling disappears. In instances where swelling has been confined to the face and lips, the condition has generally resolved without treatment, although antihistamines have been useful in relieving symptoms. Angioedema associated with involvement of the tongue, glottis or larynx may be fatal due to airway obstruction. Appropriate therapy, such as subcutaneous epinephrine solution 1:1000 (0.3 to 0.5 mL), should be promptly administered. Patients with a history of angioedema unrelated to ACE inhibitor therapy may be at increased risk of angioedema while receiving an ACE inhibitor.

Intestinal Angioedema: Intestinal angioedema has been reported in patients treated with ACE inhibitors. These patients presented with abdominal pain (with or without nausea or vomiting); in some cases there was no prior history of facial angioedema and C-1 esterase levels were normal. The angioedema was diagnosed by procedures including abdominal CT scan or ultrasound, or at surgery, and symptoms resolved after stopping the ACE inhibitor. Intestinal angioedema should be included in the differential diagnosis of patients on ACE inhibitors presenting with abdominal pain.

Anaphylactoid Reactions During Desensitization: Two patients undergoing desensitizing treatment with hymenoptera venom while receiving ACE inhibitors sustained life-threatening anaphylactoid reactions. In the same patients, these reactions were avoided when ACE inhibitors were temporarily withheld, but they reappeared upon inadvertent rechallenge.

Anaphylactoid Reactions During Membrane Exposure: Anaphylactoid reactions have been reported in patients dialyzed with high-flux membranes and treated concomitantly with an ACE inhibitor. Anaphylactoid reactions have also been reported in patients undergoing low-density lipoprotein apheresis with dextran sulfate absorption.

Hypotension: Like other ACE inhibitors, ACEON® Tablets can cause symptomatic hypotension. ACEON® Tablets has been associated with hypotension in 0.3% of uncomplicated hypertensive patients in U.S. placebo-controlled trials. Symptoms related to orthostatic hypotension were reported in another 0.8% of patients.

Symptomatic hypotension associated with the use of ACE inhibitors is more likely to occur in patients who have been volume and/or salt-depleted, as a result of prolonged diuretic therapy, dietary salt restriction, dialysis, diarrhea or vomiting. Volume and/or salt depletion should be corrected before initiating therapy with ACEON® Tablets. (See **DOSAGE AND ADMINISTRATION**.)

In patients with congestive heart failure, with or without associated renal insufficiency, ACE inhibitors may cause excessive hypotension, and may be associated with oliguria or azotemia, and rarely with acute renal failure and death. In patients with ischemic heart disease or cerebrovascular disease such an excessive fall in blood pressure could result in a myocardial infarction or a cerebrovascular accident.

In patients at risk of excessive hypotension, ACEON® Tablets therapy should be started under very close medical supervision. Patients should be followed closely for the first two weeks of treatment and whenever the dose of ACEON® Tablets and/or diuretic is increased.

If excessive hypotension occurs, the patient should be placed immediately in a supine position and, if necessary, treated with an intravenous infusion of physiological saline. ACEON® Tablets treatment can usually be continued following restoration of volume and blood pressure.

Neutropenia/Agranulocytosis: Another ACE inhibitor, captopril, has been shown to cause agranulocytosis and bone marrow depression, rarely in uncomplicated patients but more frequently in patients with renal impairment, especially patients with a collagen vascular disease such as systemic lupus erythematosus or scleroderma. Available data from clinical trials of ACEON® Tablets are insufficient to show whether ACEON® Tablets causes agranulocytosis at similar rates.

Fetal/Neonatal Morbidity and Mortality: ACE inhibitors can cause fetal and neonatal morbidity and death when administered to pregnant women. Several dozen cases have been reported in the world literature. When pregnancy is detected, ACE inhibitors should be discontinued as soon as possible.

The use of ACE inhibitors during the second and third trimesters of pregnancy has been associated with fetal and neonatal injury, including hypotension, neonatal skull hypoplasia, anuria, reversible or irreversible renal failure and death. Oligohydramnios has also been reported, presumably resulting from decreased fetal renal function; oligohydramnios in this setting has been associated with fetal limb contractures, craniofacial deformation and hypoplastic lung development. Prematurity, intrauterine growth retardation and patent ductus arteriosus have also been reported, although it is not clear whether these occurrences were due to the ACE-inhibitor exposure.

These adverse effects do not appear to have resulted from intrauterine ACE-inhibitor exposure that has been limited to the first trimester. Mothers whose embryos and fetuses are exposed to ACE inhibitors only during the first trimester should be so informed. Nonetheless, when patients become pregnant, physicians should make every effort to discontinue the use of ACEON® Tablets as soon as possible.

Rarely (probably less often than once in every thousand pregnancies), no alternative to ACE inhibitors will be found. In these rare cases, the mothers should be apprised of the potential hazards to their fetuses, and serial ultrasound examinations should be performed to assess the intraamniotic environment.

If oligohydramnios is observed, Tablets should be discontinued unless it is considered life-saving for the mother. Contraction stress testing (CST), a non-stress test (NST) or biophysical profiling (BPP) may be appropriate, depending upon the week of pregnancy. Patients and physicians should be aware, however, that oligohydramnios may not appear until after the fetus has sustained irreversible injury.

Infants with histories of *in utero* exposure to ACE inhibitors should be closely observed for hypotension, oliguria and hyperkalemia. If oliguria occurs, attention should be directed toward support of blood pressure and renal perfusion. Exchange transfusion or dialysis may be required as means of reversing hypotension and/or substituting for disordered renal function. Perindopril, which crosses the placenta, can theoretically be removed from the neonatal circulation by these means, but limited experience has not shown that such removal is central to the treatment of these infants.

No teratogenic effects of perindopril were seen in studies of pregnant rats, mice, rabbits and cynomolgus monkeys. On a mg/m^2 basis, the doses used in these studies were 6 times (in mice), 670 times (in rats), 50 times (in rabbits) and 17 times (in monkeys) the maximum recommended human dose (assuming a 50 kg adult). On a mg/kg basis, these multiples are 60 times (in mice), 3,750 times (in rats), 150 times (in rabbits) and 50 times (in monkeys) the maximum recommended human dose.

Hepatic Failure: Rarely, ACE inhibitors have been associated with a syndrome that starts with cholestatic jaundice and progresses to fulminant hepatic necrosis and (sometimes) death. The mechanism of this syndrome is not understood. Patients receiving ACE inhibitors who develop jaundice or marked elevations of hepatic enzymes should discontinue the ACE inhibitor and receive appropriate medical follow-up.

PRECAUTIONS

General: ***Impaired Renal Function:*** As a consequence of inhibiting the renin-angiotensin-aldosterone system, changes in renal function may be anticipated in susceptible individuals.

Hypertensive Patients with Congestive Heart Failure: In patients with severe congestive heart failure, where renal function may depend on the activity of the renin-angiotensin-aldosterone system, treatment with ACE inhibitors, including ACEON® Tablets, may be associated with oliguria and/or progressive azotemia, and rarely with acute renal failure and/or death.

Hypertensive Patients with Renal Artery Stenosis: In hypertensive patients with unilateral or bilateral renal artery stenosis, increases in blood urea nitrogen and serum creatinine may occur. Experience with ACE inhibitors suggests that these increases are usually reversible upon discontinuation of the drug. In such patients, renal function should be monitored during the first few weeks of therapy.

Some hypertensive patients without apparent pre-existing renal vascular disease have developed increases in blood urea nitrogen and serum creatinine, usually minor and transient. These increases are more likely to occur in patients treated concomitantly with a diuretic and in patients with pre-existing renal impairment. Reduction of dosages of ACEON® Tablets, the diuretic or both may be required. In some cases, discontinuation of either or both drugs may be necessary.

Evaluation of hypertensive patients should always include an assessment of renal function. (See **DOSAGE AND ADMINISTRATION**.)

Hyperkalemia: Elevations of serum potassium have been observed in some patients treated with ACE inhibitors, including ACEON® Tablets. In U.S. controlled clinical trials, 1.4% of the patients receiving ACEON® Tablets and 2.3% of patients receiving placebo showed increased serum potassium levels to greater than 5.7 mEq/L. Most cases were isolated single values that did not appear clinically relevant and were rarely a cause for withdrawal. Risk factors for the development of hyperkalemia include renal insufficiency, diabetes mellitus and the concomitant use of agents such as potassium-sparing diuretics, potassium supplements and/or potassium-containing salt substitutes. Drugs associated with increases in serum potassium should be used cautiously, if at all, with ACEON® Tablets. (See **PRECAUTIONS: Drug Interactions.**)

Cough: Presumably due to the inhibition of the degradation of endogenous bradykinin, persistent nonproductive cough has been reported with all ACE inhibitors, always resolving after discontinuation of therapy. ACE inhibitor-induced cough should be considered in the differential diagnosis of cough. In controlled trials with perindopril, cough was present in 12% of perindopril patients and 4.5% of patients given placebo.

Surgery/Anesthesia: In patients undergoing surgery or during anesthesia with agents that produce hypotension, ACEON® Tablets may block angiotensin II formation that would otherwise occur secondary to compensatory renin release. Hypotension attributable to this mechanism can be corrected by volume expansion.

Information for Patients: ***Angioedema:*** Angioedema, including laryngeal edema, can occur with ACE inhibitor therapy, especially following the first dose. Patients should be told to report immediately signs or symptoms suggesting angioedema (swelling of face, extremities, eyes, lips, tongue, hoarseness or difficulty in swallowing or breathing) and to take no more drug before consulting a physician.

Symptomatic Hypotension: As with any antihypertensive therapy, patients should be cautioned that lightheadedness can occur, especially during the first few days of therapy and that it should be reported promptly. Patients should be told that if fainting occurs, ACEON® Tablets should be discontinued and a physician consulted.

All patients should be cautioned that inadequate fluid intake or excessive perspiration, diarrhea or vomiting can lead to an excessive fall in blood pressure in association with ACE inhibitor therapy.

Hyperkalemia: Patients should be advised not to use potassium supplements or salt substitutes containing potassium without a physician's advice.

Neutropenia: Patients should be told to report promptly any indication of infection (*e.g.,* sore throat, fever) which could be a sign of neutropenia.

Pregnancy: Female patients of childbearing age should be told about the consequences of second and third trimester exposure to ACE inhibitors, and they should also be told that these consequences do not appear to have resulted from intrauterine ACE-inhibitor exposure that has been limited to the first trimester. These patients should be asked to report pregnancies to their physicians as soon as possible.

Drug Interactions: ***Diuretics:*** Patients on diuretics, and especially those started recently, may occasionally experience an excessive reduction of blood pressure after initiation of ACEON® Tablets therapy. The possibility of hypotensive effects can be minimized by either discontinuing the diuretic or increasing the salt intake prior to initiation of treatment with perindopril. If diuretics cannot be interrupted, close medical supervision should be provided with the first dose of ACEON® Tablets, for at least two hours and until blood pressure has stabilized for another hour. (See **WARNINGS** and **DOSAGE AND ADMINISTRATION**.)

The rate and extent of perindopril absorption and elimination are not affected by concomitant diuretics. The bioavailability of perindoprilat was reduced by diuretics, however, and this was associated with a decrease in plasma ACE inhibition.

Potassium Supplements and Potassium-Sparing Diuretics: ACEON® Tablets may increase serum potassium because of its potential to decrease aldosterone production. Use of potassium-sparing diuretics (spironolactone, amiloride, triamterene and others), potassium supplements or other drugs capable of increasing serum potassium (indomethacin, heparin, cyclosporine and others) can increase the risk of hyperkalemia. Therefore, if concomitant use of such agents is indicated, they should be given with caution and the patient's serum potassium should be monitored frequently.

Lithium: Increased serum lithium and symptoms of lithium toxicity have been reported in patients receiving concomitant lithium and ACE inhibitor therapy. These drugs should be coadministered with caution and frequent monitoring of serum lithium concentration is recommended. Use of a diuretic may further increase the risk of lithium toxicity.

Digoxin: A controlled pharmacokinetic study has shown no effect on plasma digoxin concentrations when coadministered with ACEON® Tablets, but an effect of digoxin on the plasma concentration of perindopril/perindoprilat has not been excluded.

Gentamicin: Animal data have suggested the possibility of interaction between perindopril and gentamicin. However, this has not been investigated in human studies. Coadministration of both drugs should proceed with caution.

Food Interaction: Oral administration of ACEON® Tablets with food does not significantly lower the rate or extent of perindopril absorption relative to the fasted state. However, the extent of biotransformation of perindopril to the active metabolite, perindoprilat, is reduced approximately 43%, resulting in a reduction in the plasma ACE inhibition curve of approximately 20%, probably clinically insignificant. In clinical trials, perindopril was generally administered in a non-fasting state.

Carcinogenesis, Mutagenesis, Impairment of Fertility: ***Carcinogenesis:*** No evidence of carcinogenic effect was observed in studies in rats and mice when perindopril was administered at dosages up to 20 times (mg/kg) or 2 to 4 times (mg/m^2 the maximum proposed clinical doses (16 mg/day) for 104 weeks.

Mutagenesis: No genotoxic potential was detected for ACEON® Tablets, perindoprilat and other metabolites in various *in vitro* and *in vivo* investigations, including the Ames test, the *Saccharomyces cerevisiae* D4 test, cultured human lymphocytes, TK ± mouse lymphoma assay, mouse and rat micronucleus tests and Chinese hamster bone marrow assay.

Impairment of Fertility: There was no meaningful effect on reproductive performance or fertility in the rat given up to 30 times (mg/kg) or 6 times (mg/m^2) the proposed maximum clinical dosage of ACEON® Tablets during the period of spermatogenesis in males or oogenesis and gestation in females.

Pregnancy: Pregnancy Categories C (first trimester) and D (second and third trimesters). (See **WARNINGS: Fetal/Neonatal Morbidity and Mortality.**)

Nursing Mothers: Milk of lactating rats contained radioactivity following administration ^{14}C-perindopril. It is not known whether perindopril is secreted in human milk. Because many drugs are secreted in human milk, caution should be exercised when ACEON® Tablets is given to nursing mothers.

Pediatric Use: Safety and effectiveness of ACEON® Tablets in pediatric patients have not been established.

Geriatric Use: The mean blood pressure effect of perindopril was somewhat smaller in patients over 60 than in younger patients, although the difference was not significant. Plasma concentrations of both perindopril and perindoprilat were increased in elderly patients compared to concentrations in younger patients. No adverse effects were clearly increased in older patients with the exception of dizziness and possibly rash. Experience with ACEON® Tablets in elderly patients at daily doses exceeding 8 mg is limited.

ADVERSE REACTIONS

ACEON® (perindopril erbumine) Tablets has been evaluated for safety in approximately 3,400 patients with hypertension in U.S. and foreign clinical trials. ACEON® Tablets was in general well-tolerated in the patient populations studied, the side effects were usually mild and transient. Although dizziness was reported more frequently in placebo patients (8.5%) than in perindopril patients (8.2%), the incidence appeared to increase with an increase in perindopril dose.

The data presented here are based on results from the 1,417 ACEON® Tablets-treated patients who participated in the U.S. clinical trials. Over 220 of these patients were treated with ACEON® Tablets for at least one year.

In placebo-controlled U.S. clinical trials, the incidence of premature discontinuation of therapy due to adverse events was 6.5% in patients treated with ACEON® Tablets and 6.7% in patients treated with placebo. The most common causes were cough, headache, asthenia and dizziness.

Among 1,012 patients in placebo-controlled U.S. trials, the overall frequency of reported adverse events was similar in patients treated with ACEON® Tablets and in those treated with placebo (approximately 75% in each group). Adverse events that occurred in 1% or greater of the patients and that were more common for perindopril than placebo by at least 1% (regardless of whether they were felt to be related to study drug) are shown in the first two columns below. Of these adverse events, those considered possibly or probably related to study drug are shown in the last two columns.

[See table above]

FREQUENCY OF ADVERSE EVENTS (%)

	All Adverse Events		Possibly – or Probably – Related Adverse Events	
	Perindopril n=789	Placebo n=223	Perindopril n=789	Placebo n=223
Cough	12.0	4.5	6.0	1.8
Back Pain	5.8	3.1	0.0	0.0
Sinusitis	5.2	3.6	0.6	0.0
Viral Infection	3.4	1.6	0.3	0.0
Upper Extremity Pain	2.8	1.4	0.2	0.0
Hypertonia	2.7	1.4	0.2	0.0
Dyspepsia	1.9	0.9	0.3	0.0
Fever	1.5	0.5	0.3	0.0
Proteinuria	1.5	0.5	1.0	0.5
Ear Infection	1.3	0.0	0.0	0.0
Palpitation	1.1	0.0	0.9	0.0

Of these, cough was the reason for withdrawal in 1.3% of perindopril and 0.4% of placebo patients. While dizziness was not reported more frequently in the perindopril group (8.2%) than in the placebo group (8.5%), it was clearly increased with dose, suggesting a causal relationship with perindopril. Other commonly reported complaints (1% or greater), regardless of causality, include: headache (23.8%), upper respiratory infection (8.6%), asthenia (7.9%), rhinitis (4.8%), low extremity pain (4.7%), diarrhea (4.3%), edema (3.9%), pharyngitis (3.3%), urinary tract infection (2.8%), abdominal pain (2.7%), sleep disorder (2.5%), chest pain (2.4%), injury, paresthesia, nausea, rash (each 2.3%), seasonal allergy, depression (each 2.0%), abnormal ECG (1.8%), ALT increase (1.7%), tinnitus, vomiting (each 1.5%), neck pain, male sexual dysfunction (each 1.4%), triglyceride increase, somnolence (each 1.3%), joint pain, nervousness, myalgia, menstrual disorder (each 1.1%), flatulence and arthritis (each 1.0%), but none of those was more frequent by at least 1% on perindopril than on placebo. Depending on the specific adverse event, approximately 30 to 70% of the common complaints were considered possibly or probably related to treatment.

Below is a list (by body system) of adverse experiences reported in 0.3 to 1% of patients in U.S. placebo-controlled studies without regard to attribution to therapy. Less frequent but medically important adverse events are also included; the incidence of these events is given in parentheses.

Body as a Whole: malaise, pain, cold/hot sensation, chills, fluid retention, orthostatic symptoms, anaphylactic reaction, facial edema, angioedema (0.1%).

Gastrointestinal: constipation, dry mouth, dry mucous membrane, appetite increased, gastroenteritis.

Respiratory: posterior nasal drip, bronchitis, rhinorrhea, throat disorder, dyspnea, sneezing, epistaxis, hoarseness, pulmonary fibrosis (<0.1%).

Urogenital: vaginitis, kidney stone, flank pain, urinary frequency, urinary retention.

Cardiovascular: hypotension, ventricular extrasystole, myocardial infarction, vasodilation, syncope, abnormal conduction, heart murmur, orthostatic hypotension.

Endocrine: gout.

Hematology: hematoma, ecchymosis.

Musculoskeletal: arthralgia, myalgia.

CNS: migraine, amnesia, vertigo, cerebral vascular accident (0.2%).

Psychiatric: anxiety, psychosexual disorder.

Dermatology: sweating, skin infection, tinea, pruritus, dry skin, erythema, fever blisters, purpura (0.1%).

Special Senses: conjunctivitis, earache.

Laboratory: potassium decrease, uric acid increase, alkaline phosphatase increase, cholesterol increase, AST increase, creatinine increase, hematuria, glucose increase.

When ACEON® Tablets was given concomitantly with thiazide diuretics, adverse events were generally reported at the same rate as those for ACEON® Tablets alone, except for a higher incidence of abnormal laboratory findings known to be related to treatment with thiazide diuretics alone (*e.g.*, increases in serum uric acid, triglycerides and cholesterol and decreases in serum potassium).

Potential Adverse Effects Reported with ACE Inhibitors: Other medically important adverse effects reported with other available ACE inhibitors include: cardiac arrest, eosinophilic pneumonitis, neutropenia/agranulocytosis, pancytopenia, anemia (including hemolytic and aplastic), thrombocytopenia, acute renal failure, nephritis, hepatic failure, jaundice (hepatocellular or cholestatic), symptomatic hyponatremia, bullous pemphigus, acute pancreatitis, exfoliative dermatitis and a syndrome which may include: arthralgia/arthritis, vasculitis, serositis, myalgia, fever, rash or other dermatologic manifestations, a positive ANA, leukocytosis, eosinophilia or an elevated ESR. Many of these adverse effects have also been reported for perindopril.

Fetal/Neonatal Morbidity and Mortality: See **WARNINGS: Fetal/Neonatal Morbidity and Mortality.**

Clinical Laboratory Test Findings: Hematology, clinical chemistry and urinalysis parameters have been evaluated in U.S. placebo-controlled trials. In general, there were no clinically significant trends in laboratory test findings.

Hyperkalemia: In clinical trials, 1.4% of the patients receiving ACEON® Tablets and 2.3% of the patients receiving placebo showed serum potassium levels greater than 5.7 mEq/L. (See **PRECAUTIONS.**)

BUN/Serum Creatinine Elevations: Elevations, usually transient and minor, of BUN and serum creatinine have been observed. In placebo-controlled clinical trials, the proportion of patients experiencing increases in serum creatinine were similar in the ACEON® Tablets and placebo treatment groups. Rapid reduction of long-standing or markedly elevated blood pressure by any antihypertensive therapy can result in decreases in the glomerular filtration rate and, in turn, lead to increases in BUN or serum creatinine. (See **PRECAUTIONS.**)

Hematology: Small decreases in hemoglobin and hematocrit occur frequently in hypertensive patients treated with ACEON® Tablets, but are rarely of clinical importance. In controlled clinical trials, no patient was discontinued from therapy due to the development of anemia. Leukopenia (including neutropenia) was observed in 0.1% of patients in U.S. clinical trials (See **WARNINGS.**)

Liver Function Tests: Elevations in ALT (1.6% ACEON® Tablets vs 0.9% placebo) and AST (0.5% ACEON® Tablets vs 0.4% placebo) have been observed in U.S. placebo-controlled clinical trials. The elevations were generally mild and transient and resolved after discontinuation of therapy.

OVERDOSAGE

In animals, doses of perindopril up to 2500 mg/kg in mice, 3000 mg/kg in rats and 1600 mg/kg in dogs were non-lethal. Past experiences were scant but suggested that overdosage with other ACE inhibitors was also fairly well tolerated by humans. The most likely manifestation is hypotension, and treatment should be symptomatic and supportive. Therapy with the ACE inhibitor should be discontinued, and the patient should be observed. Dehydration, electrolyte imbalance and hypotension should be treated by established procedures.

However, of the reported cases of perindopril overdosage, one (dosage unknown) required assisted ventilation and the other developed hypothermia, circulatory arrest and died following ingestion of up to 180 mg of perindopril. The intervention for perindopril overdose may require vigorous support (see below).

Laboratory determinations of serum levels of perindopril and its metabolites are not widely available, and such determinations have, in any event, no established role in the management of perindopril overdose.

No data are available to suggest physiological maneuvers (*e.g.*, maneuvers to change the pH of the urine) that might accelerate elimination of perindopril and its metabolites. Perindopril can be removed by hemodialysis, with clearance of 52 mL/min for perindopril and 67 mL/min for perindoprilat.

Angiotensin II could presumably serve as a specific antagonist-antidote in the settling of perindopril overdose, but angiotensin II is essentially unavailable outside of scattered research facilities. Because the hypotensive effect of perindopril is achieved through vasodilation and effective hypovolemia, it is reasonable to treat perindopril overdose by infusion of normal saline solution.

DOSAGE AND ADMINISTRATION

Use in Uncomplicated Hypertensive Patients: In patients with essential hypertension, the recommended initial dose is 4 mg once a day. The dosage may be titrated upward until blood pressure, when measured just before the next dose, is controlled or to a maximum of 16 mg per day. The usual maintenance dose range is 4 to 8 mg administered as a single daily dose. ACEON® Tablets may also be administered in two divided doses. When once-daily dosing was compared to twice-daily dosing in clinical studies, the B.I.D. regimen was generally slightly superior, but not by more than about 0.5 to 1.0 mm Hg.

Use in the Elderly Patients: As in younger patients, the recommended initial daily dosage of ACEON® Tablets for the elderly (>65 years) is 4 mg daily, given in one or two divided doses. The daily dosage may be titrated upward until blood pressure, when measured just before the next dose, is controlled, but experience with ACEON® Tablets is limited in the elderly at doses exceeding 8 mg. Dosages above 8 mg should be administered with caution and under close medical supervision. (See **PRECAUTIONS: Geriatric Use.**)

Use in Concomitant Diuretics: If blood pressure is not adequately controlled with perindopril alone, a diuretic may be added. In patients currently being treated with a diuretic, symptomatic hypotension occasionally can occur following the initial dose of perindopril. To reduce likelihood of such reaction, the diuretic should, if possible, be discontinued 2 to 3 days prior to the beginning of ACEON® Tablets therapy. (See **WARNINGS.**) Then, if blood pressure is not controlled with ACEON® Tablets alone, the diuretic should be resumed.

If the diuretic cannot be discontinued, an initial dose of 2 to 4 mg daily in one or in two divided doses should be used with careful medical supervision for several hours and until blood pressure has stabilized. The dosage should then be titrated as described above. (See **WARNINGS** and **PRECAUTIONS: Drug Interactions.**)

Use in Patients with Impaired Renal Function: Kinetic data indicate that perindoprilat elimination is decreased in

Continued on next page

Aceon—Cont.

renally impaired patients, with a marked increase in accumulation when creatinine clearance drops below 30 mL/min. In such patients (creatinine clearance <30 mL/min), safety and efficacy of ACEON® Tablets have not been established. For patients with lesser degrees of impairment (creatinine clearance above 30 mL/min), the initial dosage should be 2 mg/day and dosage should not exceed 8 mg/day due to limited clinical experience. During dialysis, perindopril is removed with the same clearance as in patients with normal renal function.

HOW SUPPLIED

Tablets 2 mg: Scored one side, white, oblong (debossed "ACN 2" on one side and debossed with "SLV" on both sides of score on the other side)
Bottles of 100 .... NDC 0032-1101-01
Tablets 4 mg: Scored one side, pink, oblong (debossed "ACN 4" on one side and debossed with "SLV" on both sides of score on the other side)
Bottles of 100 .... NDC 0032-1102-01
Tablets 8 mg: Scored one side, salmon-colored, oblong (debossed "ACN 8" on one side and debossed with "SLV" on both sides of score on the other side)
Bottles of 100 .... NDC 0032-1103-01
Storage Conditions: Store at controlled room temperature 20° to 25°C (68° to 77°F) [see USP]. Protect from moisture. Keep out of the reach of children.
Manufactured by:
Patheon Pharmaceuticals, Inc.
Cincinnati, OH 45215 USA
Marketed by:
Solvay Pharmaceuticals, Inc.
Marietta, GA 30062

500063/500064 10E Rev 3/2003
Shown in Product Identification Guide, page 333

CREON® 5 ℞
[*krē-ōn*]
MINIMICROSPHERES®
(Pancrelipase Delayed-release Capsules, USP)
PRESCRIBING INFORMATION

DESCRIPTION

CREON® 5 Capsules are orally administered and contain delayed-release MINIMI-CROSPHERES® of pancrelipase, which is of porcine pancreatic origin. Each CREON® 5 Capsule contains lipase 5,000 USP Units, protease 18,750 USP Units and amylase 16,600 USP Units.
Inactive ingredients include dibutyl phthalate, dimethicone, hydroxypropylmethylcellulose phthalate, light mineral oil and polyethylene glycol. The capsule shells contain gelatin, red iron oxide, titanium dioxide, yellow iron oxide and FD & C blue No. 2. The capsule imprinting ink contains dimethicone, 2-ethoxyethanol, shellac, soya lecithin, and titanium dioxide.

CLINICAL PHARMACOLOGY

The pancreatic enzymes in CREON® 5 Capsules are enteric-coated to resist gastric destruction or inactivation. The pancreatic enzymes catalyze the hydrolysis of fats to glycerol and fatty acids, protein into proteoses and derived substances and starch into dextrins and short chain sugars.

INDICATIONS

CREON® 5 Capsules are indicated for patients with pancreatic exocrine insufficiency as is often associated with:
- cystic fibrosis
- chronic pancreatitis
- post-pancreatectomy
- post-gastrointestinal bypass surgery (e.g., Billroth II gastroenterostomy)
- ductal obstruction from neoplasm (e.g.,of the pancreas or common bile duct)

CONTRAINDICATIONS

CREON® 5 Capsules are contraindicated in the early stages of acute pancreatitis or in patients who are known to be hypersensitive to pork protein.

WARNINGS

Should symptoms of hypersensitivity appear, discontinue medication and initiate symptomatic and supportive therapy if necessary.
Strictures in the ileo-cecal region and/or ascending colon have been reported in cystic fibrosis patients treated with high doses of high-potency pancreatic enzyme supplements containing 20,000 or greater USP units of lipase per capsule. The underlying mechanism is unknown, but caution should be exercised when doses in excess of 6,000 USP units lipase per kg per meal fail to resolve symptoms, especially in patients with a history of intestinal complications such as meconium ileus equivalent, short bowel syndrome, surgery or Crohn's disease. If symptoms suggestive of gastrointestinal obstruction occur, the possibility of bowel stricture should be investigated including evaluation of pancreatic enzyme therapy.

PRECAUTIONS

CREON® 5 Capsules MINIMICROSPHERES® SHOULD NOT BE CRUSHED OR CHEWED or placed on foods having a pH greater than 5.5. These can dissolve the protective enteric coating resulting in early release of enzymes, irritation of oral mucosa, and/or loss of enzyme activity.

Information for Patients

CREON® 5 Capsules are a pancreatic enzyme product prescribed to promote improved digestion of foods, especially fat. The prescribed dosage should be taken with each meal and snack or as directed by the physician. The capsules can be swallowed whole, or the contents poured on soft, bland food. Care should be taken to avoid chewing or crushing of the capsule contents, which can result in early release of enzymes, irritation of oral mucosa, and/or loss of enzyme activity. Patients should maintain adequate fluid intake. The prescribed dose range should not be exceeded without calling your doctor.
The most common adverse reactions involve the stomach and intestine including diarrhea, nausea, vomiting, bloating, constipation, stomach cramps or pain. If these symptoms are persistent, contact your doctor.

Carcinogenesis, Mutagenesis, Impairment of Fertility

Long-term studies in animals have not been performed to evaluate carcinogenic potential.

Pregnancy, Category C

Animal reproduction studies have not been conducted with pancrelipase. It is also not known whether pancrelipase can cause fetal harm when administered to a pregnant woman or can affect reproduction capacity. CREON® 5 Capsules should be given to a pregnant woman only if clearly needed.

Nursing Mothers

It is not known whether this drug is excreted in human milk. Because many drugs are excreted in human milk, caution should be exercised when CREON® 5 Capsules are administered to a nursing mother.

ADVERSE REACTIONS

The most frequently reported adverse reactions to pancreatic enzyme-containing products are gastrointestinal in nature which may include nausea, vomiting, bloating, cramping, constipation or diarrhea. Less frequently, allergic-type reactions have also been observed. Very high doses of pancreatin have been associated with hyperuricosuria and hyperuricemia.

DOSAGE AND ADMINISTRATION

Clinical experience should dictate initial starting dose. Doses should be taken during meals or snacks, not before or after. Do not take without food.

Adults and Children Over 6 Years Old

Usual initial starting dosage is two to four CREON® 5 Capsules per meal or snack.

Children Under 6 Years Old

The exact dosage of CREON® 5 Capsules should be selected based on clinical experience for this age group. Patients can be started on one to two capsules per meal or snack.
For cystic fibrosis patients, typical doses are 1,500-3,000 USP lipase units/kg/meal. Dosage should be adjusted according to the severity of the disease, control of steatorrhea and maintenance of good nutritional status. Doses in excess of 6,000 USP lipase units/kg/meal are not recommended.
Dose increases, if required, should occur with careful monitoring of body weight and stool fat content. When changing strengths of pancreatic enzyme products, care should be taken to maintain equivalent lipase units for each divided dosage.
It is important to ensure adequate hydration of patients at all times while taking pancreatic enzymes.
Where swallowing of capsules is difficult, the capsules may be carefully opened and the MINIMICROSPHERES® added to a small amount of soft food, with a pH less than 5.5. The soft food should be swallowed immediately without chewing and followed with a glass of water or juice to insure swallowing.

HOW SUPPLIED

CREON® 5 MINIMICROSPHERES® (Pancrelipase Delayed-release Capsules, USP) are available in a two-piece gelatin capsule (orange opaque top half, blue opaque bottom half) imprinted in white with "SOLVAY" and "1205". Each capsule contains tan-colored delayed-release MINIMICROSPHERES® of pancrelipase supplied in bottles of:
100 .... NDC 0032-1205-01
250 .... NDC 0032-1205-07
CREON® 5 Capsules must be stored at 25°C (77°F); excursions permitted to 15°-30°C (59°-86°F). [See USP Controlled Room Temperature.] PROTECT FROM MOISTURE. DO NOT REFRIGERATE. Dispense in tight, light-resistant containers. For human consumption only.
Manufactured By:
Solvay Pharmaceuticals GmbH,
Hannover, Germany
Marketed by:
Solvay
Pharmaceuticals, Inc.
Marietta, GA 30062
0814
4E Rev 6/98

CREON® 10
MINIMICROSPHERES®
(Pancrelipase Delayed-release Capsules, USP)
PRESCRIBING INFORMATION

DESCRIPTION

CREON® 10 Capsules are orally administered and contain delayed-release MINIMICROSPHERES® of pancrelipase, which is of porcine pancreatic origin. Each CREON® 10 Capsule contains lipase 10,000 USP Units, protease 37,500 USP Units and amylase 33,200 USP Units.
Inactive ingredients include dibutyl phthalate, dimethicone, hydroxypropylmethylcellulose phthalate, light mineral oil and polyethylene glycol. The capsule shells contain black iron oxide, gelatin, red iron oxide, titanium dioxide, and yellow iron oxide. The capsule imprinting ink contains dimethicone, 2-ethoxyethanol, shellac, soya lecithin, and titanium dioxide.

CLINICAL PHARMACOLOGY

The pancreatic enzymes in CREON® 10 Capsules are enteric-coated to resist gastric destruction or inactivation. The pancreatic enzymes catalyze the hydrolysis of fats to glycerol and fatty acids, protein into proteoses and derived substances and starch into dextrins and short chain sugars.

INDICATIONS

CREON® 10 Capsules are indicated for patients with pancreatic exocrine insufficiency as is often associated with:
- cystic fibrosis
- chronic pancreatitis
- post-pancreatectomy
- post-gastrointestinal bypass surgery (e.g., Billroth II gastroenterostomy)
- ductal obstruction from neoplasm (e.g., of the pancreas or common bile duct)

CONTRAINDICATIONS

CREON® 10 Capsules are contraindicated in the early stages of acute pancreatitis or in patients who are known to be hypersensitive to pork protein.

WARNINGS

Should symptoms of hypersensitivity appear, discontinue medication and initiate symptomatic and supportive therapy if necessary.
Strictures in the ileo-cecal region and/or ascending colon have been reported in cystic fibrosis patients treated with high doses of high-potency pancreatic enzyme supplements containing 20,000 or greater USP units of lipase per capsule. The underlying mechanism is unknown, but caution should be exercised when doses in excess of 6,000 USP units lipase per kg per meal fail to resolve symptoms, especially in patients with a history of intestinal complications such as meconium ileus equivalent, short bowel syndrome, surgery or Crohn's disease. If symptoms suggestive of gastrointestinal obstruction occur, the possibility of bowel stricture should be investigated including evaluation of pancreatic enzyme therapy.

PRECAUTIONS

CREON® 10 Capsules MINIMICROSPHERES® SHOULD NOT BE CRUSHED OR CHEWED or placed on foods having a pH greater than 5.5. These can dissolve the protective enteric coating resulting in early release of enzymes, irritation of oral mucosa, and/or loss of enzyme activity.

Information for Patients

CREON® 10 Capsules are a pancreatic enzyme product prescribed to promote improved digestion of foods, especially fat. The prescribed dosage should be taken with each meal and snack or as directed by the physician. The capsules can be swallowed whole, or the contents poured on soft, bland food. Care should be taken to avoid chewing or crushing of the capsule contents, which can result in early release of enzymes, irritation of oral mucosa, and/or loss of enzyme activity. Patients should maintain adequate fluid intake. The prescribed dose range should not be exceeded without calling your doctor.
The most common adverse reactions involve the stomach and intestine including diarrhea, nausea, vomiting, bloating, constipation, stomach cramps or pain. If these symptoms are persistent, contact your doctor.

Carcinogenesis, Mutagenesis, Impairment of Fertility

Long-term studies in animals have not been performed to evaluate carcinogenic potential.

Pregnancy, Category C

Animal reproduction studies have not been conducted with pancrelipase. It is also not known whether pancrelipase can cause fetal harm when administered to a pregnant woman or can affect reproduction capacity. CREON® 10 Capsules should be given to a pregnant woman only if clearly needed.

Nursing Mothers

It is not known whether this drug is excreted in human milk. Because many drugs are excreted in human milk, caution should be exercised when CREON® 10 Capsules are administered to a nursing mother.

ADVERSE REACTIONS

The most frequently reported adverse reactions to pancreatic enzyme-containing products are gastrointestinal in nature which may include nausea, vomiting, bloating, cramping, constipation or diarrhea. Less frequently, allergic-type reactions have also been observed. Very high doses of pancreatin have been associated with hyperuricosuria and hyperuricemia.

DOSAGE AND ADMINISTRATION

Clinical experience should dictate initial starting dose. Doses should be taken during meals or snacks, not before or after. Do not take without food.

Adults and Children Over 6 Years Old

Usual initial starting dosage is one to two CREON® 10 Capsules per meal or snack.

Children Under 6 Years Old

Usual initial starting dosage is up to one CREON® 10 Capsule per meal or snack.

For cystic fibrosis patients, typical doses are 1,500-3,000 USP lipase units/kg/meal. Dosage should be adjusted according to the severity of the disease, control of steatorrhea and maintenance of good nutritional status. Doses in excess of 6,000 USP lipase units/kg/meal are not recommended.

Dose increases, if required, should occur with careful monitoring of body weight and stool fat content. When changing strengths of pancreatic enzyme products, care should be taken to maintain equivalent lipase units for each divided dosage.

It is important to ensure adequate hydration of patients at all times while taking pancreatic enzymes.

Where swallowing of capsules is difficult, the capsules may be carefully opened and the MINIMICROSPHERES® added to a small amount of soft food, with a pH less than 5.5. The soft food should be swallowed immediately without chewing and followed with a glass of water or juice to insure swallowing.

HOW SUPPLIED

CREON® 10 MINIMICROSPHERES® (Pancrelipase Delayed-release Capsules, USP) are available in a two-piece gelatin capsule (brown opaque top half, natural transparent bottom half) imprinted in white with "SOLVAY" and "1210". Each capsule contains tan-colored delayed-release MINIMICROSPHERES® of pancrelipase supplied in bottles of:

100 .... NDC 0032-1210-01
250 .... NDC 0032-1210-07

CREON® 10 Capsules must be stored at 25°C (77°F); excursions permitted to 15°-30°C (59°-86°F). [See USP Controlled Room Temperature.] PROTECT FROM MOISTURE. DO NOT REFRIGERATE. Dispense in tight, light-resistant containers. For human consumption only.

Manufactured By:
Solvay Pharmaceuticals GmbH
Hannover, Germany
Marketed by:
Solvay
Pharmaceuticals, Inc.
Marietta, GA 30062
0850
8E Rev 6/98

CREON® 20
MINIMICROSPHERES®
(Pancrelipase Delayed-release Capsules, USP)
PRESCRIBING INFORMATION

DESCRIPTION

CREON® 20 Capsules are orally administered and contain delayed-release MINIMICROSPHERES® of pancrelipase, which is of porcine pancreatic origin. Each CREON® 20 Capsule contains lipase 20,000 USP Units, protease 75,000 USP Units and amylase 66,400 USP Units.

Inactive ingredients include dibutyl phthalate, dimethicone, hydroxypropylmethylcellulose phthalate, light mineral oil and polyethylene glycol. The capsule shells contain gelatin, red iron oxide, titanium dioxide and yellow iron oxide. The capsule imprinting ink contains dimethicone, 2-ethoxyethanol, shellac, soya lecithin, and titanium dioxide.

CLINICAL PHARMACOLOGY

The pancreatic enzymes in CREON® 20 Capsules are enteric-coated to resist gastric destruction or inactivation. The pancreatic enzymes catalyze the hydrolysis of fats to glycerol and fatty acids, protein into proteoses and derived substances and starch into dextrins and short chain sugars.

INDICATIONS

CREON® 20 Capsules are indicated for patients with pancreatic exocrine insufficiency as is often associated with:

- cystic fibrosis
- chronic pancreatitis
- post-pancreatectomy
- post-gastrointestinal bypass surgery (e.g., Billroth II gastroenterostomy)
- ductal obstruction from neoplasm (e.g.,of the pancreas or common bile duct)

CONTRAINDICATIONS

CREON® 20 Capsules are contraindicated in the early stages of acute pancreatitis or in patients who are known to be hypersensitive to pork protein.

WARNINGS

Should symptoms of hypersensitivity appear, discontinue medication and initiate symptomatic and supportive therapy if necessary.

Strictures in the ileo-cecal region and/or ascending colon have been reported in cystic fibrosis patients treated with high doses of high-potency pancreatic enzyme supplements containing 20,000 or greater USP units of lipase per capsule. The underlying mechanism is unknown, but caution should be exercised when doses in excess of 6,000 USP units lipase per kg per meal fail to resolve symptoms, especially in patients with a history of intestinal complications such as meconium ileus equivalent, short bowel syndrome, surgery or Crohn's disease. If symptoms suggestive of gastrointestinal obstruction occur, the possibility of bowel stricture should be investigated including evaluation of pancreatic enzyme therapy.

PRECAUTIONS

CREON® 20 Capsules MINIMICROSPHERES® SHOULD NOT BE CRUSHED OR CHEWED or placed on foods having a pH greater than 5.5. These can dissolve the protective enteric coating resulting in early release of enzymes, irritation of oral mucosa, and/or loss of enzyme activity.

Information for Patients

CREON® 20 Capsules are a pancreatic enzyme product prescribed to promote improved digestion of foods, especially fat. The prescribed dosage should be taken with each meal and snack or as directed by the physician. The capsules can be swallowed whole, or the contents poured on soft, bland food. Care should be taken to avoid chewing or crushing of the capsule contents, which can result in early release of enzymes, irritation of oral mucosa, and/or loss of enzyme activity. Patients should maintain adequate fluid intake. The prescribed dose range should not be exceeded without calling your doctor.

The most common adverse reactions involve the stomach and intestine including diarrhea, nausea, vomiting, bloating, constipation, stomach cramps or pain. If these symptoms are persistent, contact your doctor.

Carcinogenesis, Mutagenesis, Impairment of Fertility

Long-term studies in animals have not been performed to evaluate carcinogenic potential.

Pregnancy, Category C

Animal reproduction studies have not been conducted with pancrelipase. It is also not known whether pancrelipase can cause fetal harm when administered to a pregnant woman or can affect reproduction capacity. CREON® 20 Capsules should be given to a pregnant woman only if clearly needed.

Nursing Mothers

It is not known whether this drug is excreted in human milk. Because many drugs are excreted in human milk, caution should be exercised when CREON® 20 Capsules are administered to a nursing mother.

ADVERSE REACTIONS

The most frequently reported adverse reactions to pancreatic enzyme-containing products are gastrointestinal in nature which may include nausea, vomiting, bloating, cramping, constipation or diarrhea. Less frequently, allergic-type reactions have also been observed. Very high doses of pancreatin have been associated with hyperuricosuria and hyperuricemia.

DOSAGE AND ADMINISTRATION

Clinical experience should dictate initial starting dose. Doses should be taken during meals or snacks, not before or after. Do not take without food.

Adults and Children Over 6 Years Old

Usual initial starting dosage is one CREON® 20 Capsule per meal or snack.

Children Under 6 Years Old

The exact dosage of CREON® 20 Capsules should be selected based on clinical experience for this age group.

For cystic fibrosis patients, typical doses are 1,500-3,000 USP lipase units/kg/meal. Dosage should be adjusted according to the severity of the disease, control of steatorrhea and maintenance of good nutritional status. Doses in excess of 6,000 USP lipase units/kg/meal are not recommended.

Dose increases, if required, should occur with careful monitoring of body weight and stool fat content. When changing strengths of pancreatic enzyme products, care should be taken to maintain equivalent lipase units for each divided dosage.

It is important to ensure adequate hydration of patients at all times while taking pancreatic enzymes.

Where swallowing of capsules is difficult, the capsules may be carefully opened and the MINIMICROSPHERES® added to a small amount of soft food, with a pH less than 5.5. The soft food should be swallowed immediately without chewing and followed with a glass of water or juice to insure swallowing.

HOW SUPPLIED

CREON® 20 MINIMICROSPHERES® (Pancrelipase Delayed-release Capsules, USP) are available in a two-piece gelatin capsule (orange opaque top half, natural transparent bottom half) imprinted in white with "SOLVAY" and "1220". Each capsule contains tan-colored delayed-release MINIMICROSPHERES® of pancrelipase supplied in bottles of:

100 .... NDC 0032-1220-01
250 .... NDC 0032-1220-07

CREON® 20 Capsules must be stored at 25°C (77°F); excursions permitted to 15°-30°C (59°-86°F). [See USP Controlled Room Temperature.] PROTECT FROM MOISTURE. DO NOT REFRIGERATE. Dispense in tight, light-resistant containers. For human consumption only.

Manufactured By:
Solvay Pharmaceuticals GmbH,
Hannover, Germany
Marketed by:
Solvay
Pharmaceuticals, Inc.
Marietta, GA 30062
0810
5E Rev 6/98

Shown in Product Identification Guide, page 333

ESTRATEST®‡ ℞
and
ESTRATEST® H.S.‡ ℞
[*ĕ′strā-tĕst*]
(Esterified Estrogens and Methyltestosterone) Tablets
℞ only

WARNINGS

1. **ESTROGENS HAVE BEEN REPORTED TO INCREASE THE RISK OF ENDOMETRIAL CARCINOMA.**
   Three independent case control studies have reported an increased risk of endometrial cancer in postmenopausal women exposed to exogenous estrogens for prolonged periods.[1-3] This risk was independent of the other known risk factors for endometrial cancer. These studies are further supported by the finding that incidence rates of endometrial cancer have increased sharply since 1969 in eight different areas of the United States with population-based cancer reporting systems, an increase which may be related to the rapidly expanding use of estrogens during the last decade.[4]
   The three case control studies reported that the risk of endometrial cancer in estrogen users was about 4.5 to 13.9 times greater than in nonusers. The risk appears to depend on both duration of treatment[1] and on estrogen dose.[3] In view of these findings, when estrogens are used for the treatment of menopausal symptoms, the lowest dose that will control symptoms should be utilized and medication should be discontinued as soon as possible. When prolonged treatment is medically indicated, the patient should be reassessed on at least a semiannual basis to determine the need for continued therapy. Although the evidence must be considered preliminary, one study suggests that cyclic administration of low doses of estrogen may carry less risk than continuous administration,[3] it therefore appears prudent to utilize such a regimen.
   Close clinical surveillance of all women taking estrogens is important. In all cases of undiagnosed persistent or recurring abnormal vaginal bleeding, adequate diagnostic measures should be undertaken to rule out malignancy.
   There is no evidence at present that "natural" estrogens are more or less hazardous than "synthetic" estrogens at equiestrogenic doses.
2. **ESTROGENS SHOULD NOT BE USED DURING PREGNANCY.**
   The use of female sex hormones, both estrogens and progestogens, during early pregnancy may seriously damage the offspring. It has been shown that females exposed in utero to diethylstilbestrol, a non-steroidal estrogen, have an increased risk of developing in later life a form of vaginal or cervical cancer that is ordinarily extremely rare.[5,6] This risk has been estimated as not greater than 4 per 1000 exposures.[7] Furthermore, a high percentage of such exposed women (from 30 to 90 percent) have been found to have vaginal adenosis,[8-12] epithelial changes of the vagina and cervix. Although these changes are histologically benign, it is not known whether they are precursors of malignancy. Although similar data are not available with the use of other estrogens, it cannot be presumed they would not induce similar changes.
   Several reports suggest an association between intrauterine exposure to female sex hormones and congenital anomalies, including congenital heart defects and limb reduction defects.[13-16] One case control study[16] estimated a 4.7-fold increased risk of limb reduction defects in infants exposed in utero to sex hormones (oral contraceptives, hormone withdrawal tests for pregnancy, or attempted treatment for threatened abortion). Some of these exposures were very short and involved only a few days of treatment. The data suggest that the risk of limb reduction defects in exposed fetuses is somewhat less than 1 per 1000.
   In the past, female sex hormones have been used during pregnancy in an attempt to treat threatened or habitual abortion. There is considerable evidence that estrogens are ineffective for these indications, and there is no evidence from well controlled studies that progestogens are effective for these uses.
   If ESTRATEST® or ESTRATEST® H.S. is used during pregnancy, or if the patient becomes pregnant while taking this drug, she should be apprised of the potential risks to the fetus, and the advisability of pregnancy continuation.
3. **CARDIOVASCULAR AND OTHER RISKS**
   ESTRATEST® and ESTRATEST® H.S. Tablets do not contain a progestin. ESTRATEST® and ESTRATEST® H.S. Tablets are an Estrogen/Androgen product.
   Estrogens with or without progestins should not be used for the prevention of cardiovascular disease.
   The Women's Health Initiative (WHI) study reported increased risks of myocardial infarction, stroke, invasive breast cancer, pulmonary emboli, and deep vein thrombosis in postmenopausal women during 5 years of treatment with conjugated equine estrogens (CE

Continued on next page

Estratest/Estratest H.S.—Cont.

0.625 mg) combined with medroxyprogesterone acetate (MPA 2.5 mg) relative to placebo (see **CLINICAL PHARMACOLOGY, Clinical Studies**). Other doses of conjugated estrogens with medroxyprogesterone and other combinations of estrogens and progestins were not studied in the WHI and, in the absence of comparable data, these risks should be assumed to be similar. Because of these risks, estrogens with or without progestins should be prescribed at the lowest effective doses and for the shortest duration consistent with treatment goals and risks for the individual woman.

DESCRIPTION

ESTRATEST® Each dark green, capsule shaped, sugar-coated oral tablet contains: 1.25 mg of Esterified Estrogens, USP and 2.5 mg of Methyltestosterone.

ESTRATEST® H.S. (Half-Strength): Each light green, capsule shaped, sugar-coated oral tablet contains: 0.625 mg of Esterified Estrogens, USP and 1.25 mg of Methyltestosterone.

Esterified Estrogens

Esterified Estrogens, USP is a mixture of the sodium salts of the sulfate esters of the estrogenic substances, principally estrone, that are of the type excreted by pregnant mares. Esterified Estrogens contain not less than 75.0 percent and not more than 85.0 percent of sodium estrone sulfate, and not less than 6.0 percent and not more than 15.0 percent of sodium equilin sulfate, in such proportion that the total of these two components is not less than 90.0 percent.

Category: Estrogens

Methyltestosterone

Methyltestosterone, USP is an androgen. Androgens are derivatives of cyclopentano-perhydrophenanthrene. Endogenous androgens are C-19 steroids with a side chain at C-17, and with two angular methyl groups. Testosterone is the primary endogenous androgen. Fluoxymesterone and methyltestosterone are synthetic derivatives of testosterone.

Methyltestosterone is a white to light yellow crystalline substance that is virtually insoluble in water but soluble in organic solvents. It is stable in air but decomposes in light.

Methyltestosterone structural formula:

$C_{20}H_{30}O_2$ 302.46

Androst-4-en-3-one, 17-hydroxy-17-methyl-, (17β)- Category: Androgen.

ESTRATEST® and ESTRATEST® H.S. Tablets contain the following inactive ingredients: acacia, calcium carbonate, citric acid, colloidal silicon dioxide, gelatin, lactose, magnesium stearate, methylparaben, propylparaben, microcrystalline cellulose, pharmaceutical glaze, povidone, sodium benzoate, sodium bicarbonate, carboxymethylcellulose sodium, sorbic acid, sucrose, starch, talc, titanium dioxide, tribasic calcium phosphate, alcohol denatured 3A and purified water.

ESTRATEST® Tablets also contain: FD&C Blue No. 1 Lake, FD&C Yellow No. 6 Lake, and D&C Yellow No. 10 Lake.

ESTRATEST® H.S. Tablets also contain: D&C Yellow No. 10 Lake, FD&C Blue No. 1 Lake, FD&C Blue No. 2 Lake, FD&C Yellow No. 6 Lake, and FD&C Red No. 40 Lake.

CLINICAL PHARMACOLOGY

Estrogens: Estrogens are important in the development and maintenance of the female reproductive system and secondary sex characteristics. They promote growth and development of the vagina, uterus, and fallopian tubes, and enlargement of the breasts. Indirectly, they contribute to the shaping of the skeleton, maintenance of tone and elasticity of urogenital structures, changes in the epiphyses of the long bones that allow for the pubertal growth spurt and its termination, growth of axillary and pubic hair, and pigmentation of the nipples and genitals. Decline of estrogenic activity at the end of the menstrual cycle can bring on menstruation, although the cessation of progesterone secretion is the most important factor in the mature ovulatory cycle. However, in the preovulatory or nonovulatory cycle, estrogen is the primary determinant in the onset of menstruation. Estrogens also affect the release of pituitary gonadotropins.

The pharmacologic effects of esterified estrogens are similar to those of endogenous estrogens. They are soluble in water and are well absorbed from the gastrointestinal tract.

In responsive tissues (female genital organs, breasts, hypothalamus, pituitary) estrogens enter the cell and are transported into the nucleus. As a result of estrogen action, specific RNA and protein synthesis occurs.

Estrogen Pharmacokinetics

Metabolism and inactivation occur primarily in the liver. Some estrogens are excreted into the bile; however they are reabsorbed from the intestine and returned to the liver through the portal venous system. Water soluble esterified estrogens are strongly acidic and are ionized in body fluids, which favor excretion through the kidneys since tubular reabsorption is minimal.

Androgens: Endogenous androgens are responsible for the normal growth and development of the male sex organs and for maintenance of secondary sex characteristics. These effects include the growth and maturation of prostate, seminal vesicles, penis, and scrotum; the development of male hair distribution, such as beard, pubic, chest, and axillary hair, laryngeal enlargement, vocal cord thickening, alterations in body musculature, and fat distribution. Drugs in this class also cause retention of nitrogen, sodium, potassium, phosphorus, and decreased urinary excretion of calcium. Androgens have been reported to increase protein anabolism and decrease protein catabolism. Nitrogen balance is improved only when there is sufficient intake of calories and protein. Androgens are responsible for the growth spurt of adolescence and for the eventual termination of linear growth which is brought about by fusion of the epiphyseal growth centers. In children, exogenous androgens accelerate linear growth rates, but may cause a disproportionate advancement in bone maturation. Use over long periods may result in fusion of the epiphyseal growth centers and termination of growth process. Androgens have been reported to stimulate the production of red blood cells by enhancing the production of erythropoietic stimulating factor.

Androgen Pharmacokinetics

Testosterone given orally is metabolized by the gut and 44 percent is cleared by the liver in the first pass. Oral doses as high as 400 mg per day are needed to achieve clinically effective blood levels for full replacement therapy. The synthetic androgens (methyltestosterone and fluoxymesterone) are less extensively metabolized by the liver and have longer half-lives. They are more suitable than testosterone for oral administration.

Testosterone in plasma is 98 percent bound to a specific testosterone-estradiol binding globulin, and about 2 percent is free. Generally, the amount of this sex-hormone binding globulin in the plasma will determine the distribution of testosterone between free and bound forms, and the free testosterone concentration will determine its half-life.

About 90 percent of a dose of testosterone is excreted in the urine as glucuronic and sulfuric acid conjugates of testosterone and its metabolites; about 6 percent of a dose is excreted in the feces, mostly in the unconjugated form. Inactivation of testosterone occurs primarily in the liver. Testosterone is metabolized to various 17-keto steroids through two different pathways. There are considerable variations of the half-life of testosterone as reported in the literature, ranging from 10 to 100 minutes.

In many tissues the activity of testosterone appears to depend on reduction to dihydrotestosterone, which binds to cytosol receptor proteins. The steroid-receptor complex is transported to the nucleus where it initiates transcription events and cellular changes related to androgen action.

INDICATIONS AND USAGE

ESTRATEST® and ESTRATEST® H.S. are indicated in the treatment of:

Moderate to severe vasomotor symptoms associated with the menopause in those patients not improved by estrogens alone. (There is no evidence that estrogens are effective for nervous symptoms or depression without associated vasomotor symptoms, and they should not be used to treat such conditions.)

ESTRATEST® and ESTRATEST® H.S. HAVE NOT BEEN SHOWN TO BE EFFECTIVE FOR ANY PURPOSE DURING PREGNANCY AND ITS USE MAY CAUSE SEVERE HARM TO THE FETUS (See **BOXED WARNINGS**).

CONTRAINDICATIONS

Estrogens should not be used in women with any of the following conditions:

1. Known or suspected cancer of the breast except in appropriately selected patients being treated for metastatic disease.
2. Known or suspected estrogen-dependent neoplasia.
3. Known or suspected pregnancy (See **BOXED WARNINGS**).
4. Undiagnosed abnormal genital bleeding.
5. Active thrombophlebitis or thromboembolic disorders.
6. A past history of thrombophlebitis, thrombosis, or thromboembolic disorders associated with previous estrogen use (except when in treatment of breast malignancy).

Methyltestosterone should not be used in:

1. The presence of severe liver damage.
2. Pregnancy and in breast-feeding mothers because of the possibility of masculinization of the female fetus or breast-fed infant.

WARNINGS

See BOXED WARNINGS.

Associated with Estrogens

1. **Breast Cancer** (See **BOXED WARNINGS**).
2. **Induction of Malignant Neoplasms:** Long-term continuous administration of natural and synthetic estrogens in certain animal species increases the frequency of carcinomas of the breast, cervix, vagina, and liver. There is now evidence that estrogens increase the risk of carcinoma of the endometrium in humans (See **BOXED WARNINGS**). At the present time there is no satisfactory evidence that estrogens given to postmenopausal women increase the risk of cancer of the breast,[17] although a recent long-term follow-up of a single physician's practice has raised this possibility.[18] Because of the animal data, there is a need for caution in prescribing estrogens for women with a strong family history of breast cancer or who have breast nodules, fibrocystic disease, or abnormal mammograms.
3. **Cardiovascular Disorders:** Estrogen with progestogen therapy has been associated with an increased risk of cardiovascular events such as myocardial infarction and stroke, as well as venous thrombosis and pulmonary embolism) venous thromboembolism or VTE). Should any of these occur or be suspected, estrogen with progestogens should be discontinued immediately.
   Risk factors for cardiovascular disease (e.g., hypertension, diabetes mellitus, tobacco use, hypercholesterolemia, and obesity) should be managed appropriately.
   If feasible, estrogens with progestins should be discontinued at least 4 to 6 weeks before surgery of the type associated with an increased risk of thromboembolism, or during periods of prolonged immobilization.
4. **Gallbladder Disease:** A recent study has reported a 2- to 3-fold increase in the risk of surgically confirmed gallbladder disease in women receiving postmenopausal estrogens,[17] similar to the 2-fold increase previously noted in users of oral contraceptives.[19-24] In the case of oral contraceptives the increased risk appeared after two years of use.[24]
5. **Effects similar to those caused by estrogen-progestogen oral contraceptives:** There are several serious adverse effects of oral contraceptives, most of which have not, up to now, been documented as consequences of postmenopausal estrogen therapy. This may reflect the comparatively low doses of estrogen used in postmenopausal women. It would be expected that the larger doses of estrogen used to treat prostatic or breast cancer or postpartum breast engorgement are more likely to result in these adverse effects, and, in fact, it has been shown that there is an increased risk of thrombosis in men receiving estrogens for prostatic cancer and women for postpartum breast engorgement.[20-23]
   Thromboembolic Disease: It is now well established that users of oral contraceptives have an increased risk of various thromboembolic and thrombotic vascular diseases, such as thrombophlebitis, pulmonary embolism, stroke, and myocardial infarction.[24-31] Cases of retinal thrombosis, mesenteric thrombosis, and optic neuritis have been reported in oral contraceptive users. There is evidence that the risk of several of these adverse reactions is related to the dose of the drug.[32,33] An increased risk of postsurgery thromboembolic complications has also been reported in users of oral contraceptives.[34,35] If feasible, estrogen should be discontinued at least 4 weeks before surgery of the type associated with an increased risk of thromboembolism, or during periods of prolonged immobilization.
   While an increased rate of thromboembolic and thrombotic disease in postmenopausal users of estrogens has not been found,[18-36] this does not rule out the possibility that such an increase may be present or that subgroups of women who have underlying risk factors or who are receiving relatively large doses of estrogens may have increased risk. Therefore estrogens should not be used in persons with active thrombophlebitis or thromboembolic disorders, and they should not be used (except in treatment of malignancy) in persons with a history of such disorders in association with estrogen use. They should be used with caution in patients with cerebral vascular or coronary artery disease and only for those in whom estrogens are clearly needed.
   Large doses of estrogen (5 mg esterified estrogens per day), comparable to those used to treat cancer of the prostate and breast, have been shown in a large prospective clinical trial in men[37] to increase the risk of nonfatal myocardial infarction, pulmonary embolism and thrombophlebitis. When estrogen doses of this size are used, any of the thromboembolic and thrombotic adverse effects associated with oral contraceptive use should be considered a clear risk.
   Hepatic Adenoma: Benign hepatic adenomas appear to be associated with the use of oral contraceptives.[38-40] Although benign and rare, these may rupture and may cause death through intra-abdominal hemorrhage. Such lesions have not yet been reported in association with other estrogen or progestogen preparations but should be considered in estrogen users having abdominal pain and tenderness, abdominal mass, or hypovolemic shock. Hepatocellular carcinoma has also been reported in women taking estrogen-containing oral contraceptives.[39] The relationship of this malignancy to these drugs is not known at this time.
   Elevated Blood Pressure: Increased blood pressure is not uncommon in women using oral contraceptives. There is now a report that this may occur with use of estrogens in the menopause[41] and blood pressure should be monitored with estrogen use, especially if high doses are used.
   Glucose Tolerance: A worsening of glucose tolerance has been observed in a significant percentage of patients of estrogen-containing oral contraceptives. For this reason, diabetic patients should be carefully observed while receiving estrogens.
6. **Hypercalcemia:** Administration of estrogens may lead to severe hypercalcemia in patients with breast cancer and bone metastases. If this occurs, the drug should be stopped and appropriate measures taken to reduce the serum calcium level.

Associated with Methyltestosterone

In patients with breast cancer, androgen therapy may cause hypercalcemia by stimulating osteolysis. In this case the drug should be discontinued.

Prolonged use of high doses of androgens has been associated with the development of peliosis hepatis and hepatic neoplasms including hepatocellular carcinoma. (See **PRECAUTIONS – *Carcinogenesis*)**. Peliosis hepatis can be a life-threatening or fatal complication.

Cholestatic hepatitis and jaundice occur with 17-alpha-alkylandrogens at a relatively low dose. If cholestatic hepatitis with jaundice appears or if liver function tests become abnormal, the androgen should be discontinued and the etiology should be determined. Drug-induced jaundice is reversible when the medication is discontinued.

Edema with or without heart failure may be a serious complication in patients with preexisting cardiac, renal, or hepatic disease. In addition to discontinuation of the drug, diuretic therapy may be required.

PRECAUTIONS

Associated with Estrogens

General Precautions

1. A complete medical and family history should be taken prior to the initiation of any estrogen therapy. The pretreatment and periodic physical examinations should include special reference to blood pressure, breasts, abdomen, and pelvic organs, and should include a Papanicolaou smear. As a general rule, estrogens should not be prescribed for longer than one year without another physical examination being performed.
2. Fluid retention–Because estrogens may cause some degree of fluid retention, conditions which might be influenced by this factor such as asthma, epilepsy, migraine, and cardiac or renal dysfunction, require careful observation.
3. Certain patients may develop undesirable manifestations of excessive estrogenic stimulation, such as abnormal or excessive uterine bleeding, mastodynia, etc.
4. Oral contraceptives appear to be associated with an increased incidence of mental depression.[24] Although it is not clear whether this is due to the estrogenic or progestogenic component of the contraceptive, patients with a history of depression should be carefully observed.
5. Preexisting uterine leiomyomata may increase in size during estrogen use.
6. The pathologist should be advised of estrogen therapy when relevant specimens are submitted.
7. Patients with a past history of jaundice during pregnancy have an increased risk of recurrence of jaundice while receiving estrogen-containing oral contraceptive therapy. If jaundice develops in any patient receiving estrogen, the medication should be discontinued while the cause is investigated.
8. Estrogens may be poorly metabolized in patients with impaired liver function and they should be administered with caution in such patients.
9. Because estrogens influence the metabolism of calcium and phosphorus, they should be used with caution in patients with metabolic bone diseases that are associated with hypercalcemia or in patients with renal insufficiency.
10. Because of the effects of estrogens on epiphyseal closure, they should be used judiciously in young patients in whom bone growth is not complete.
11. Certain endocrine and liver function tests may be affected by estrogen-containing oral contraceptives. The following similar changes may be expected with larger doses of estrogen:
    a. Increased sulfobromophthalein retention.
    b. Increased prothrombin and factors VII, VIII, IX and X; decreased antithrombin 3: increased norepinephrine-induced platelet aggregability.
    c. Increased thyroxine-binding globulin (TBG) leading to increased circulating total thyroid hormone, as measured by PBI, T4 by column, or T4 by radioimmunoassay. Free T3 resin uptake is decreased, reflecting the elevated TBG; free T4 concentration is unaltered.
    d. Impaired glucose tolerance.
    e. Decreased pregnanediol excretion.
    f. Reduced response to metyrapone test.
    g. Reduced serum folate concentration.
    h. Increased serum triglyceride and phospholipid concentration.

Information for the Patient

See text of Patient Package Insert which appears after the **REFERENCES**.

Pregnancy Category X

(See **CONTRAINDICATIONS** and **BOXED WARNINGS**).

Nursing Mothers

As a general principle, the administration of any drug to nursing mothers should be done only when clearly necessary since many drugs are excreted in human milk.

Associated with Methyltestosterone

General Precautions

1. Women should be observed for signs of virilization (deepening of the voice, hirsutism, acne, clitoromegaly, and menstrual irregularities). Discontinuation of drug therapy at the time of evidence of mild virilism is necessary to prevent irreversible virilization. Such virilization is usual following androgen use at high doses.
2. Prolonged dosage of androgen may result in sodium and fluid retention. This may present a problem, especially in patients with compromised cardiac reserve or renal disease.
3. Hypersensitivity may occur rarely.
4. PBI may be decreased in patients taking androgens.
5. Hypercalcemia may occur. If this does occur, the drug should be discontinued.

Information for the Patient

The physician should instruct patients to report any of the following side effects of androgens:

Women: Hoarseness, acne, changes in menstrual periods, or more hair on the face.

All Patients: Any nausea, vomiting, changes in skin color or ankle swelling.

Laboratory Tests

1. Women with disseminated breast carcinoma should have frequent determination of urine and serum calcium levels during the course of androgen therapy (see **WARNINGS**).
2. Because of the hepatotoxicity associated with the use of 17-alpha-alkylated androgens, liver function tests should be obtained periodically.
3. Hemoglobin and hematocrit should be checked periodically for polycythemia in patients who are receiving high doses of androgens.

Drug Interactions

1. ***Anticoagulants:*** C-17 substituted derivatives of testosterone, such as methandrostenolone, have been reported to decrease the anticoagulant requirements of patients receiving oral anticoagulants. Patients receiving oral anticoagulant therapy require close monitoring, especially when androgens are started or stopped.
2. ***Oxyphenbutazone:*** Concurrent administration of oxyphenbutazone and androgens may result in elevated serum levels of oxyphenbutazone.
3. ***Insulin:*** In diabetic patients, the metabolic effects of androgens may decrease blood glucose and insulin requirements.

Drug/Laboratory Test Interferences

Androgens may decrease levels of thyroxine-binding globulin, resulting in decreased T4 serum levels and increased resin uptake of T3 and T4. Free thyroid hormone levels remain unchanged, however, and there is no clinical evidence of thyroid dysfunction.

Carcinogenesis

Animal Data: Testosterone has been tested by subcutaneous injection and implantation in mice and rats. The implant induced cervical-uterine tumors in mice, which metastasized in some cases. There is suggestive evidence that injection of testosterone into some strains of female mice increases their susceptibility to hepatoma. Testosterone is also known to increase the number of tumors and decrease the degree of differentiation of chemically induced carcinomas of the liver in rats.

Human Data: There are rare reports of hepatocellular carcinoma in patients receiving long-term therapy with androgens in high doses. Withdrawal of the drugs did not lead to regression of the tumors in all cases.

Geriatric patients treated with androgens may be at increased risk for the development of prostatic hypertrophy and prostatic carcinoma.

Pregnancy

Teratogenic Effects: Pregnancy Category X (see **CONTRAINDICATIONS**).

Nursing Mothers

It is not known whether androgens are excreted in human milk. Because many drugs are excreted in human milk and because of the potential for serious adverse reactions in nursing infants from androgens, a decision should be made whether to discontinue nursing or to discontinue the drug, taking into account the importance of the drug to the mother.

ADVERSE REACTIONS

Associated with Estrogens

(See **WARNINGS** regarding induction of neoplasia, adverse effects on the fetus, increased incidence of gallbladder disease, and adverse effects similar to those of oral contraceptives, including thromboembolism). The following additional adverse reactions have been reported with estrogenic therapy, including oral contraceptives:

1. **Genitourinary system:** Breakthrough bleeding; spotting; change in menstrual flow; dysmenorrhea; premenstrual-like syndrome; amenorrhea during and after treatment; increase in size of uterine fibromyomata; vaginal candidiasis; change in cervical erosion and in degree of cervical secretion; cystitis-like syndrome.
2. **Breasts:** Tenderness; enlargement; secretion.
3. **Gastrointestinal:** Nausea; vomiting; abdominal cramps; bloating; cholestatic jaundice.
4. **Skin:** Chloasma or melasma which may persist when drug is discontinued; erythema multiforme; erythema nodosum; hemorrhagic eruption; loss of scalp hair; hirsutism.
5. **Eyes:** Steepening of corneal curvature; intolerance to contact lenses.
6. **Central Nervous System:** Headache, migraine, dizziness; mental depression; chorea.
7. **Miscellaneous:** Increase or decrease in weight; reduced carbohydrate tolerance; aggravation of porphyria; edema; changes in libido.

Associated with Methyltestosterone

Endocrine and Urogenital.

1. **Female:** The most common side effects of androgen therapy are amenorrhea and other menstrual irregularities, inhibition of gonadotropin secretion, and virilization, including deepening of the voice and clitoral enlargement. The latter usually is not reversible after androgens are discontinued. When administered to a pregnant woman androgens cause virilization of external genitalia of the female fetus.
2. **Skin and Appendages:** Hirsutism, male pattern of baldness, and acne.
3. **Fluid and Electrolyte Disturbances:** Retention of sodium, chloride, water, potassium, calcium, and inorganic phosphates.
4. **Gastrointestinal:** Nausea, cholestatic jaundice, alterations in liver function test, rarely hepatocellular neoplasms, and peliosis hepatis (see **WARNINGS**).
5. **Hematologic:** Suppression of clotting factors II, V, VII, and X, bleeding in patients on concomitant anticoagulant therapy, and polycythemia.
6. **Nervous System.** Increased or decreased libido, headache, anxiety, depression, and generalized paresthesia.
7. **Metabolic:** Increased serum cholesterol.
8. **Miscellaneous:** Inflammation and pain at the site of intramuscular injection or subcutaneous implantation of testosterone containing pellets, stomatitis with buccal preparations, and rarely anaphylactoid reactions.

OVERDOSAGE

Numerous reports of ingestion of large doses of estrogen-containing oral contraceptives by young children indicate that serious ill effects do not occur. Overdosage of estrogen may cause nausea, and withdrawal bleeding may occur in females.

There have been no reports of acute overdosage with the androgens.

DOSAGE AND ADMINISTRATION

Given cyclically for short-term use only:

For treatment of moderate to severe vasomotor symptoms associated with the menopause in patients not improved by estrogen alone.

The lowest dose that will control symptoms should be chosen and medication should be discontinued as promptly as possible.

Administration should be cyclic (e.g., three weeks on and one week off). Attempts to discontinue or taper medication should be made at three to six month intervals.

Usual Dosage Range:

1 tablet of ESTRATEST® or 1 to 2 tablets of ESTRATEST® H.S. daily as recommended by the physician.

Treated patients with an intact uterus should be monitored closely for signs of endometrial cancer and appropriate diagnostic measures should be taken to rule out malignancy in the event of persistent or recurring abnormal vaginal bleeding.

HOW SUPPLIED

ESTRATEST® (Imprinted "SOLVAY 1026")

Bottles of 100 .... NDC 0032-1026-01

Bottles of 1000 .... NDC 0032-1026-10

ESTRATEST® (dark green, capsule shaped, sugar-coated oral tablets) contains: 1.25 mg of Esterified Estrogens, USP and 2.5 mg of Methyltestosterone, USP.

ESTRATEST® H.S. (Imprinted "SOLVAY 1023")

Bottles of 100 .... NDC 0032-1023-01

ESTRATEST® H.S. "Half-Strength" (light green, capsule shaped, sugar-coated oral tablets) contains: 0.625 mg of Esterified Estrogens, USP and 1.25 mg of Methyltestosterone, USP.

Store at controlled room temperature 15° to 30°C (59° to 86°F).

REFERENCES

1. Ziel HK, et al. *N Engl J Med.* 1975;293:1167-1170.
2. Smith DC, et al. *N Engl J Med.* 1975;293:1164-1167.
3. Mack TM, et al. *N Engl J Med.* 1976;294:1262-1267.
4. Weiss NS, et al. *N Engl J Med.* 1976;294:1259-1262.
5. Herbst AL, et al. *N Engl J Med.* 1971;284:878-881.
6. Greenwald P, et al. *N Engl J Med.* 1971;285:390-392.
7. Lanier A, et al. *Mayo Clin Proc.* 1973;48:793-799.
8. Herbst A, et al. *Obstet Gynecol.* 1972;40:287-298.
9. Herbst A, et al. *Am J Obstet Gynecol.* 1974;118:607-615.
10. Herbst A, et al. *N Engl J Med.* 1975;292:334-339.
11. Stafl A, et al. *Obstet Gynecol.* 1974;43:118-128.
12. Sherman AI, et al. *Obstet Gynecol.* 1974;44:531-545.
13. Gal I, et al. *Nature.* 1967;216:83.
14. Levy EP, et al. *Lancet.* 1973;1:611.
15. Nora J, et al. *Lancet.* 1973;1:941-942.
16. Janerich DT, et al. *N Engl J Med.* 1974;291:697-700.
17. Boston Collaborative Drug Surveillance Program. *N Engl J Med.* 1974;290:15-19.
18. Hoover R, et al. *N Engl J Med.* 1976;295:401-405.
19. Boston Collaborative Drug Surveillance Program. *Lancet.* 1973;1:1399-1404.
20. Daniel DG, et al. *Lancet.* 1967;2:287-289.
21. The Veterans Administration Cooperative Urological Research Group. *J Urol.* 1967;98:516-522.
22. Bailar JC. *Lancet.* 1967;2:560.
23. Blackard C, et al. *Cancer.* 1970;26:249-256.
24. Royal College of General Practitioners: *J Coll Gen Practit.* 1967;13:267-279.
25. Inman WHW, et al. *Br Med J.* 1968;2:193-199.
26. Vessey MP, et al. *Br Med J.* 1969;2:651-657.
27. Sartwell PE, et al. *Am J Epidemiol.* 1969;90:365-380.
28. Collaborative Group for the Study of Stroke in Young Women. *N Engl J Med.* 1973;288:871-878.
29. Collaborative Group for the Study of Stroke in Young Women. *JAMA.* 1975;231:718-722.
30. Mann JI, et al. *Br Med J.* 1975;2:245-248.

Continued on next page

Estratest/Estratest H.S.—Cont.

31. Mann JI, et al. *Br Med J.* 1975;2:241-245.
32. Inman WHW, et al. *Br Med J.* 1970;2:203-209.
33. Stolley PD, et al. *Am J Epidemiol.* 1975;102:197-208.
34. Vessey MP, et al. *Br Med J.* 1970;3:123-126.
35. Greene GR, et al. *Am J Public Health.* 1972;62:680-685.
36. Rosenberg L, et al. *N Engl J Med.* 1976;294:1256-1259.
37. Coronary Drug Project Research Group. *JAMA.* 1970;214:1303-1313.
38. Baum J, et al. *Lancet.* 1973;2:926-928.
39. Mays ET, et al. *JAMA.* 1976;235:730-732.
40. Edmondson HA, et al. *N Engl J Med.* 1976;294:470-472.
41. Pfeffer RI, et al. *Am J Epidemiol.* 1976;103:445-456.

‡This product has not obtained FDA pre-market approval applicable for new drugs.

INFORMATION FOR THE PATIENT‡

WHAT YOU SHOULD KNOW ABOUT ESTROGENS

Estrogens are female hormones produced by the ovaries. The ovaries make several different kinds of estrogens. In addition, scientists have been able to make a variety of synthetic estrogens. As far as we know, all these estrogens have similar properties and therefore much the same usefulness, side effects, and risks. This leaflet is intended to help you understand what estrogens are used for, the risks involved in their use, and how to use them as safely as possible.

This leaflet includes the most important information about estrogens, but not all the information. If you want to know more, you can ask your doctor or pharmacist to let you read the package insert prepared for the doctor.

USES OF ESTROGEN

Estrogens are prescribed by doctors for a number of purposes, including:

1. To provide estrogen during a period of adjustment when a woman's ovaries no longer produce it, in order to prevent certain uncomfortable symptoms of estrogen deficiency. (All women normally stop producing estrogens, generally between the ages of 45 and 55; this is called the menopause).
2. To prevent symptoms of estrogen deficiency when a woman's ovaries have been removed surgically before the natural menopause.
3. To prevent pregnancy. (Estrogens are given along with a progestogen, another female hormone; these combinations are called oral contraceptives or birth control pills. Patient labeling is available to women taking oral contraceptives and they will not be discussed in this leaflet.)
4. To treat certain cancers in women and men.

THERE IS NO PROPER USE OF ESTROGENS IN A PREGNANT WOMAN.

ESTROGENS IN THE MENOPAUSE

In the natural course of their lives, all women eventually experience a decrease in estrogen production. This usually occurs between ages 45 and 55 but may occur earlier or later. Sometimes the ovaries may need to be removed before natural menopause by an operation, producing a "surgical menopause."

When the amount of estrogen in the blood begins to decrease, many women may develop typical symptoms: Feelings of warmth in the face, neck, and chest or sudden intense episodes of heat and sweating throughout the body (called "hot flashes" or "hot flushes"). These symptoms are sometimes very uncomfortable. A few women eventually develop changes in the vagina (called "atrophic vaginitis") which cause discomfort, especially during and after intercourse.

Estrogens can be prescribed to treat these symptoms of the menopause. It is estimated that considerably more than half of all women undergoing the menopause have only mild symptoms or no symptoms at all and therefore do not need estrogens. Other women may need estrogens for a few months, while their bodies adjust to lower estrogen levels. Sometimes the need will be for periods longer than six months. In an attempt to avoid overstimulation of the uterus (womb), estrogens are usually given cyclically during each month of use, that is three weeks of pills followed by one week without pills.

Sometimes women experience nervous symptoms or depression during menopause. There is no evidence that estrogens are effective for such symptoms and they should not be used to treat them, although other treatment may be needed.

You may have heard that taking estrogens for long periods (years) after the menopause will keep your skin soft and supple and keep you feeling young. There is no evidence that this is so, however, and such long-term treatment carries important risks.

THE DANGERS OF ESTROGENS

1. **Cancer of the Uterus:** If estrogens are used in the post-menopausal period for more than a year, there is an increased risk of **endometrial cancer** (cancer of the uterus). Women taking estrogens have roughly 5 to 10 times as great a chance of getting this cancer as women who take no estrogens. To put this another way, while a postmenopausal woman not taking estrogens has 1 chance in 1,000 each year of getting cancer of the uterus, a woman taking estrogens has 5 to 10 chances in 1,000 each year. For this reason **it is important to take estrogens only when you really need them.**
   The risk of this cancer is greater the longer estrogens are used and also seems to be greater when larger doses are taken. For this reason, **it is important to take the lowest dose of estrogen that will control symptoms and to take it only as long as it is needed.** If estrogens are needed for longer periods of time, your doctor will want to reevaluate your need for estrogens at least every six months.
   Women using estrogens should report any irregular vaginal bleeding to their doctors; such bleeding may be of no importance, but it can be an early warning of cancer of the uterus. If you have undiagnosed vaginal bleeding, you should not use estrogens until a diagnosis is made and you are certain there is no cancer of the uterus.
2. **Other Possible Cancers:** Estrogens can cause development of other tumors in animals, such as tumors of the breast, cervix, vagina, or liver, when given for a long time. This is a further reason to use estrogens only when clearly needed. While you are taking estrogens, it is important that you go to your doctor at least once a year for a physical examination. Also, if members of your family have had breast cancer or if you have breast nodules or abnormal mammograms (breast x-rays), your doctor may wish to carry out more frequent examinations of your breasts.
3. **Gallbladder Disease:** Women who use estrogens after menopause are more likely to develop gallbladder disease needing surgery as women who do not use estrogens. Birth control pills have a similar effect.
4. **Abnormal Blood Clotting:** Oral contraceptives increase the risk of blood clotting in various parts of the body. This can result in a stroke (if the clot is in the brain), a heart attack (clot in a blood vessel of the heart), or pulmonary embolus (a clot which forms in the legs or pelvis, then breaks off and travels to the lungs). Any of these can be fatal. At this time use of estrogens in the menopause is not known to cause such blood clotting, but this has not been fully studied and there could still prove to be such a risk. It is recommended that if you have had clotting in the legs or lungs or a heart attack or stroke while you were using estrogens or birth control pills, you should not use estrogens (unless they are being used to treat cancer of the breast or prostate). If you have had a stroke or heart attack or if you have angina pectoris, estrogens should be used with great caution and only if clearly needed (for example, if you have severe symptoms of the menopause).
   The larger doses of estrogen used to prevent swelling of the breasts after pregnancy have been reported to cause clotting in the legs and lungs.
5. **Other Potential Risks:** Using estrogens and progestins may increase your chances of getting heart attacks, strokes, breast cancer, or blood clots.

SPECIAL WARNING ABOUT PREGNANCY

You should not receive estrogen if you are pregnant. If this should occur, there is a greater than usual chance that the developing child will be born with a birth defect, although the possibility remains fairly small. A female child may have an increased risk of developing cancer of the vagina or cervix later in life (in the teens or twenties). Every possible effort should be made to avoid exposure to estrogens during pregnancy. If exposure occurs, see your doctor.

OTHER EFFECTS OF ESTROGENS

In addition to the serious known risks of estrogens described above, estrogens have the following side effects and potential risks:

1. **Nausea and vomiting:** The most common side effect of estrogen therapy is nausea. Vomiting is less common.
2. **Effects on breasts:** Estrogens may cause breast tenderness or enlargement and may cause the breasts to secrete a liquid. These effects are not dangerous.
3. **Effects on the uterus:** Estrogens may cause benign fibroid tumors of the uterus to get larger.
   Some women will have menstrual bleeding when estrogens are stopped. But if the bleeding occurs on days you are still taking estrogens you should report this to your doctor.
4. **Effects on liver:** Women taking oral contraceptives develop on rare occasions a benign tumor of the liver which can rupture and bleed into the abdomen. So far, these tumors have not been reported in women using estrogens in the menopause, but you should report any swelling or unusual pain or tenderness in the abdomen to your doctor immediately.
   Women with a past history of jaundice (yellowing of the skin and white parts of the eyes) may get jaundice again during estrogen use. If this occurs, stop taking estrogens and see your doctor.
5. **Other effects:** Estrogens may cause excess fluid to be retained in the body. This may make some conditions worse, such as epilepsy, migraine, heart disease, or kidney disease.

SUMMARY

Estrogens have important uses, but they have serious risks as well. You must decide, with your doctor, whether the risks are acceptable to you in view of the benefits of the treatment. Except where your doctor has prescribed estrogens for use in special cases of cancer of the breast or prostate, you should not use estrogens if you have cancer of the breast or uterus, are pregnant, have undiagnosed abnormal vaginal bleeding, or have had a stroke, heart attack or angina, or clotting in the legs or lungs in the past while you were taking estrogens.

You can use estrogens as safely as possible by understanding that your doctor will require regular physical examinations while you are taking them and will try to discontinue the drug as soon as possible and use the smallest dose possible. Be alert for signs of trouble including:

1. Abnormal bleeding from the vagina.
2. Pains in the calves or chest or sudden shortness of breath, or coughing blood (indicating possible clots in the legs, heart, or lungs).
3. Severe headache, dizziness, faintness, or changes in vision (indicating possible developing clots in the brain or eye).
4. Breast lumps (you should ask your doctor how to examine your own breasts).
5. Jaundice (yellowing of the skin).
6. Mental depression.

Based on his or her assessment of your medical needs, your doctor has prescribed this drug for you. Do not give the drug to anyone else.

HOW SUPPLIED

ESTRATEST® H.S. is a combination of Esterified Estrogens and Methyltestosterone. Each capsule-shaped light green sugar-coated tablet contains: 0.625 mg of Esterified Estrogens, USP and 1.25 mg of Methyltestosterone, USP.

ESTRATEST® is a combination of Esterified Estrogens and Methyltestosterone. Each capsule-shaped dark green sugar-coated tablet contains: 1.25 mg of Esterified Estrogens, USP and 2.5 mg of Methyltestosterone, USP.

‡ This product has not obtained FDA pre-market approval applicable for new drugs.

0978
11E Rev 2/2004
Solvay
Pharmaceuticals, Inc.
Marietta, GA 30062

Shown in Product Identification Guide, page 333

ESTROGEL® 0.06% ℞

[s-tro-gel]
(estradiol gel)
℞ only

ESTROGENS INCREASE THE RISK OF ENDOMETRIAL CANCER

Close clinical surveillance of all women taking estrogens is important. Adequate diagnostic measures, including endometrial sampling when indicated, should be undertaken to rule out malignancy in all cases of undiagnosed persistent or recurring abnormal vaginal bleeding. There is no evidence that the use of "natural" estrogens results in a different endometrial risk profile than synthetic estrogens at equivalent estrogen doses.

CARDIOVASCULAR AND OTHER RISKS

Estrogens with or without progestins should not be used for the prevention of cardiovascular disease.

The Women's Health Initiative (WHI) study reported increased risks of myocardial infarction, stroke, invasive breast cancer, pulmonary emboli, and deep vein thrombosis in postmenopausal women (50 to 79 years of age) during 5 years of treatment with oral conjugated estrogens (CE 0.625 mg) combined with medroxyprogesterone acetate (MPA 2.5 mg) relative to placebo. (See **CLINICAL PHARMACOLOGY, Clinical Studies.**)

Other doses of conjugated estrogens with medroxyprogesterone and other combinations and dosage forms of estrogens and progestins were not studied in the WHI clinical trials, and in the absence of comparable data, these risks should be assumed to be similar. Because of these risks, estrogens with or without progestins should be prescribed at the lowest effective doses and for the shortest duration consistent with treatment goals and risks for the individual woman.

DESCRIPTION

EstroGel® (estradiol gel) contains 0.06% estradiol in an absorptive hydroalcoholic gel base formulated to provide a controlled release of the active ingredient. The gel is applied over a large area (750 cm^2) of the skin in a thin layer. The recommended area of application is the arm, from wrist to shoulder. An EstroGel unit dose of 1.25 g contains 0.75 mg of estradiol.

Estradiol is a white crystalline powder, chemically described as estra-1,3,5(10)-triene-3,17 β-diol. It has an empirical formula of $C_{18}H_{24}O_2$ and molecular weight of 272.39. The structural formula is:

The active component of the transdermal gel is estradiol. The remaining components of the gel (purified water, alcohol, triethanolamine and carbomer 934P) are pharmacologically inactive.

CLINICAL PHARMACOLOGY

EstroGel provides systemic estrogen replacement therapy by releasing estradiol, the major estrogenic hormone secreted by the human ovary.

Endogenous estrogens are largely responsible for the development and maintenance of the female reproductive system and secondary sexual characteristics. Although circulating estrogens exist in a dynamic equilibrium of metabolic interconversions, estradiol is the principal intracellular human estrogen and is substantially more potent than its metabolites, estrone and estriol, at the receptor level. The primary source of estrogen in normally cycling adult women is the ovarian follicle, which secretes 70 to 500 mcg of estradiol daily, depending on the phase of the menstrual cycle. After menopause, most endogenous estrogen is produced by conversion of androstenedione, secreted by the adrenal cortex, to estrone by peripheral tissues. Thus, estrone and the sulfate-conjugated form, estrone sulfate, are the most abundant circulating estrogens in postmenopausal women.

Estrogens act through binding to nuclear receptors in estrogen-responsive tissues. To date, two estrogen receptors have been identified. These vary in proportion from tissue to tissue.

Circulating estrogens modulate the pituitary secretion of the gonadotropins, luteinizing hormone (LH) and follicle stimulating hormone (FSH) through a negative feedback mechanism. Estrogens act to reduce the elevated levels of these hormones seen in postmenopausal women.

Pharmacokinetics

Percutaneous administration of EstroGel produces plasma concentrations of estradiol and estrone that are similar to those observed in the follicular phase of the ovulatory cycle. Typical therapeutic levels of estradiol range from 40 to 80 pg/mL for relief of vasomotor symptoms.

Absorption

Estradiol is transported across intact skin and into the systemic circulation by a passive diffusion process. The rate of diffusion across the stratum corneum is the rate limiting factor. When EstroGel is applied on skin, it dries in 2 to 5 minutes.

EstroGel 1.25 g was administered to 24 postmenopausal women once daily on the posterior surface of one arm from wrist to shoulder for 14 consecutive days. Mean maximal serum concentrations of estradiol and estrone on day 14 were 46.4 pg/mL and 64.2 pg/mL, respectively. The time-averaged serum estradiol and estrone concentration over the 24-hour dose interval after administration of 1.25 g EstroGel on Day 14 are 28.3 pg/mL and 48.6 pg/mL, respectively. Mean concentrations-time profiles for unadjusted estradiol and estrone on Day 14 are shown in Figure 1.

FIGURE 1

Mean serum concentration-time profiles for unadjusted estradiol and estrone after multiple dose applications of 1.25 g EstroGel for 14 days

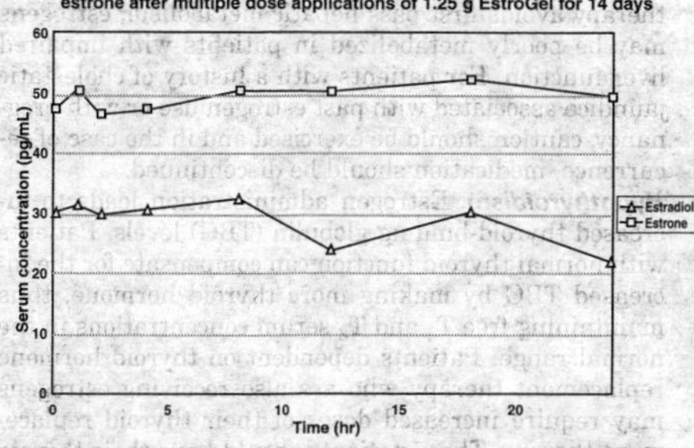

The serum concentrations of estradiol following 2.5 g EstroGel applications (1.25 g on each arm from wrist to shoulder) appeared to reach steady state after the third daily application.

Distribution

The distribution of exogenous estrogens is similar to that of endogenous estrogens. Estrogens are widely distributed in the body and are generally found in higher concentrations in the sex hormone target organs. Estrogens circulate in blood largely bound to sex hormone binding globulin (SHBG) and albumin.

Metabolism

Exogenous estrogens are metabolized in the same manner as endogenous estrogens. Circulating estrogens exist in a dynamic equilibrium of metabolic interconversions. These transformations take place mainly in the liver. Estradiol is converted reversibly to estrone, and both can be converted to estriol, which is the major urinary metabolite. Estrogens also undergo enterohepatic recirculation via sulfate and glucuronide conjugation in the liver, biliary secretion of conjugates into the intestine, and hydrolysis in the gut followed by reabsorption. In postmenopausal women, a significant proportion of the circulating estrogens exist as sulfate conjugates, especially estrone sulfate, which serves as a circulating reservoir for the formation of more active estrogens. Although the clinical significance has not been determined, estradiol from EstroGel does not go through the first pass liver metabolism.

Excretion

Estradiol, estrone and estriol are excreted in the urine along with glucuronide and sulfate conjugates.

The apparent terminal exponential half-life for estradiol was about 36 hours following administration of 1.25 g EstroGel.

Special Populations

EstroGel has been studied only in postmenopausal women. No pharmacokinetic studies were conducted in special populations, including patients with renal or hepatic impairment.

TABLE 1
Mean Change from Baseline in the Number and Severity of Hot Flushes Per Day, ITT Population, LOCF

	Number of Hot Flushes/Day (Moderate to Severe)		Severity Score/Day (Mild, Moderate, Severe)	
	Placebo n=73	EstroGel 1.25 g n=72	Placebo n=73	EstroGel 1.25 g n=72
Baseline				
Mean (SD)	11.01 (5.66)	10.33 (3.07)	2.30 (0.24)	2.36 (0.29)
Week 4◊				
Mean (SD)	5.95 (5.17)	4.43 (4.13)	2.00 (0.63)	1.73 (0.73)
Mean Change from Baseline (SD)	-5.06 (4.91)	-5.91 (3.68)	-0.31 (0.62)	-0.63 (0.71)
Diff. vs Placebo		0.85		0.32
p-value*		0.019**		0.005**
Week 8				
Mean (SD)	5.36 (5.78)	3.44 (4.40)	1.89 (0.77)	1.44 (0.90)
Mean Change from Baseline (SD)	-5.65 (4.11)	-6.89 (3.80)	-0.41 (0.78)	-0.92 (0.89)
Diff. vs Placebo		1.24		0.51
Week 12◊				
Mean (SD)	5.17 (6.52)	2.79 (3.70)	1.76 (0.84)	1.33 (0.97)
Mean Change from Baseline (SD)	-5.84 (4.52)	-7.55 (3.52)	-0.54 (0.84)	-1.03 (0.94)
Diff. vs Placebo		1.71		0.49
p-value*		0.043**		<0.001**

* p-values from Van Elteren's non-parametric test
** Statistically significantly different from placebo.
◊ Primary Timepoint

TABLE 2
Relative and Absolute Risk Seen in the CE/MPA Substudy of WHI[a]

Event[c]	Relative Risk CE/MPA vs. Placebo at 5.2 Years (95% CI*)	Placebo n = 8102	CE/MPA n = 8506
		Absolute Risk per 10,000 Person-years	
CHD events	1.29 (1.02-1.63)	30	37
Non-fatal MI	*1.32 (1.02-1.72)*	*23*	*30*
CHD death	*1.18 (0.70-1.97)*	*6*	*7*
Invasive breast cancer[b]	1.26 (1.00-1.59)	30	38
Stroke	1.41 (1.07-1.85)	21	29
Pulmonary embolism	2.13 (1.39-3.25)	8	16
Colorectal cancer	0.63 (0.43-0.92)	16	10
Endometrial cancer	0.83 (0.47-1.47)	6	5
Hip fracture	0.66 (0.45-0.98)	15	10
Death due to causes other than the events above	0.92 (0.74-1.14)	40	37
Global Index[c]	1.15 (1.03-1.28)	151	170
Deep vein thrombosis[d]	2.07 (1.49-2.87)	13	26
Vertebral fractures[d]	0.66 (0.44-0.98)	15	9
Other osteoporotic fractures[d]	0.77 (0.69-0.86)	170	131

[a] adapted from *JAMA*, 2002; 288:321-333
[b] includes metastatic and non-metastatic breast cancer with the exception of *in situ* breast cancer
[c] a subset of the events was combined in a "global index," defined as the earliest occurrence of CHD events, invasive breast cancer, stroke, pulmonary embolism, endometrial cancer, colorectal cancer, hip fracture, or death due to other causes
[d] not included in Global Index
* nominal confidence intervals unadjusted for multiple looks and multiple comparisons

Drug Interactions

Drug interactions have not been assessed for EstroGel.

In vitro and *in vivo* studies have shown that estrogens are metabolized partially by cytochrome P450 3A4 (CYP3A4). Therefore, inducers or inhibitors of CYP3A4 may affect estrogen drug metabolism. Inducers of CYP3A4 such as St. John's Wort preparations (Hypericum perforatum), phenobarbital, carbamazepine, and rifampin may reduce plasma concentrations of estrogens, possibly resulting in a decrease in therapeutic effects and/or changes in the uterine bleeding profile. Inhibitors of CYP3A4 such as erythromycin, clarithromycin, ketoconazole, itraconazole, ritonavir and grapefruit juice may increase plasma concentrations of estrogens and may result in side effects.

Clinical Studies

Effects on vasomotor symptoms

In a placebo-controlled study, 145 postmenopausal women between 29 and 67 years of age (81.4% were Caucasian) were randomly assigned to receive 1.25 g of EstroGel (containing 0.75 mg of estradiol) or placebo gel for 12 weeks. Efficacy was assessed at 4 and 12 weeks of treatment. A statistically significant reduction in the frequency and severity of moderate to severe hot flushes was shown at weeks 4 and 12. (See Table 1.)

[See table 1 above]

Effects on vasomotor symptoms

Effects on vulvar and vaginal atrophy Results of the vaginal wall cytology showed a significant ($p \leq 0.001$) increase from baseline in the percent of superficial epithelial cells at week 12 for 1.25 g EstroGel. In contrast, no significant change from baseline was observed in the placebo group.

Transdermal Effects

In two controlled clinical trials, application site reactions were reported by 0.6% of patients who received 1.25 g of EstroGel. Other skin reactions, such as pruritus and rash, were also noted. (See Table 3.)

Estradiol Transfer

The effect of estradiol transfer was evaluated in 24 healthy postmenopausal women who topically applied 1.25 g of EstroGel once daily on the posterior surface of one arm from wrist to shoulder for a period of 14 consecutive days. On each day, one hour after gel application, a cohort of 24 non-dosed healthy postmenopausal females directly contacted the dosed cohort at the site of gel application for 15 minutes. No change in endogenous mean serum concentrations of estradiol was observed in the non-dosed cohort after direct skin-to-skin contact with subjects administered EstroGel.

Effect of Application Site Washing

The effect of application site washing on the serum concentrations of estradiol was determined in 24 healthy postmenopausal females who applied 1.25 g of EstroGel once daily for 14 consecutive days. Site washing one hour after the application resulted in a 22% mean decrease in average 24-hour serum concentrations of estradiol.

Continued on next page

Estrogel—Cont.

Women's Health Initiative Studies

The Women's Health Initiative (WHI) enrolled a total of 27,000 predominantly healthy postmenopausal women to assess the risks and benefits of either the use of 0.625 mg conjugated estrogens (CE) per day alone or the use of 0.625 mg conjugated equine estrogens plus 2.5 mg medroxyprogesterone acetate (MPA) per day compared to placebo in the prevention of certain chronic diseases. The primary endpoint was the incidence of coronary heart disease (CHD) (nonfatal myocardial infarction and CHD death), with invasive breast cancer as the primary adverse outcome studied. A "global index" included the earliest occurrence of CHD events, invasive breast cancer, stroke, pulmonary embolism (PE), endometrial cancer, colorectal cancer, hip fracture, or death due to other causes. The study did not evaluate the effects of CE or CE/MPA on menopausal symptoms.

The CE-only substudy is continuing and results have not been reported. The CE/MPA substudy was stopped early because, according to predefined stopping rule, the increased risk of breast cancer and cardiovascular events exceeded the specified benefits included in the "global index." Results of the CE/MPA substudy, which included 16,608 women (average age of 63 years, range 50 to 79; 83.9% White, 6.5% Black, 5.5% Hispanic), after an average follow-up of 5.2 years are presented in Table 2.

[See table 2 on previous page]

For those outcomes included in the "global index," absolute excess risks per 10,000 person-years in the group treated with CE/MPA were 7 more CHD events, 8 more strokes, 8 more PEs, and 8 more invasive breast cancers, while absolute risk reductions per 10,000 women-years were 6 fewer colorectal cancers and 5 fewer hip fractures. The absolute excess risk of events included in the "global index" was 19 per 10,000 women-years. There was no difference between the groups in terms of all-cause mortality. (See **BOXED WARNINGS, WARNINGS**, and **PRECAUTIONS**.)

INDICATIONS AND USAGE

EstroGel is indicated in the:

1. Treatment of moderate to severe vasomotor symptoms associated with the menopause.
2. Treatment of moderate to severe symptoms of vulvar and vaginal atrophy associated with the menopause. When prescribing solely for the treatment of symptoms of vulvar and vaginal atrophy, topical vaginal products should be considered.

CONTRAINDICATIONS

Estrogens should not be used in individuals with any of the following conditions:

1. Undiagnosed abnormal genital bleeding.
2. Known, suspected, or history of cancer of the breast.
3. Known or suspected estrogen-dependent neoplasia
4. Active deep vein thrombosis, pulmonary embolism, or history of these conditions.
5. Active or recent (e.g., within the past year) arterial thromboembolic disease (e.g., stroke, myocardial infarction).
6. Liver dysfunction or disease.
7. EstroGel therapy should not be used in patients with known hypersensitivity to its ingredients.
8. Known or suspected pregnancy. There is no indication for EstroGel in pregnancy. There appears to be little or no increased risk of birth defects in children born to women who have used estrogens and progestins from oral contraceptives inadvertently during early pregnancy. (See **PRECAUTIONS**.)

WARNINGS

See BOXED WARNINGS.

1. Cardiovascular Disorders

Estrogen and estrogen/progestin therapy has been associated with an increased risk of cardiovascular events such as myocardial infarction and stroke, as well as venous thrombosis and pulmonary embolism (venous thromboembolism or VTE). Should any of these occur or be suspected, estrogens should be discontinued immediately.

Risk factors for arterial vascular disease (e.g., hypertension, diabetes mellitus, tobacco use, hypercholesterolemia, and obesity) and/or thromboembolism (e.g., personal history or family history of VTE, obesity, and systemic lupus erythematosus) should be managed appropriately.

a. *Coronary Heart Disease and Stroke:* In the Women's Health Initiative (WHI) study, an increase in the number of myocardial infarctions and strokes has been observed in women receiving CE compared to placebo. These observations are preliminary and the study is continuing. (See **CLINICAL PHARMACOLOGY, Clinical Studies.**)

In the CE/MPA substudy of WHI, an increased risk of coronary heart disease (CHD) events (defined as non-fatal myocardial infarction and CHD death) was observed in women receiving CE/MPA compared to women receiving placebo (37 vs. 30 per 10,000 women-years). The increase in risk was observed in year one and persisted.

In the same substudy of WHI, an increased risk of stroke was observed in women receiving CE/MPA compared to women receiving placebo (29 vs. 21 per 10,000 women-years). The increase in risk was observed after the first year and persisted.

In postmenopausal women with documented heart disease (n = 2,763, average age 66.7 years), a controlled clinical trial of secondary prevention of cardiovascular disease (Heart and Estrogen/Progestin Replacement Study; HERS) treatment with CE/MPA-0.625 mg/2.5 mg per day demonstrated no cardiovascular benefit. During an average follow-up of 4.1 years, treatment with CE/MPA did not reduce the overall rate of CHD events in postmenopausal women with established coronary heart disease. There were more CHD events in the CE/MPA-treated group than in the placebo group in year 1, but not during the subsequent years. Two thousand three hundred and twenty-one women from the original HERS trial agreed to participate in an open label extension of HERS, HERS II. Average follow-up in HERS II was an additional 2.7 years, for a total of 6.8 years overall. Rates of CHD events were comparable among women in the CE/MPA group and the placebo group in HERS, HERS II, and overall.

Large doses of estrogen (5 mg conjugated estrogens per day), comparable to those used to treat cancer of the prostate and breast, have been shown in a large prospective clinical trial in men to increase the risks of nonfatal myocardial infarction, pulmonary embolism, and thrombophlebitis.

b. *Venous Thromboembolism (VTE):* In the Women's Health Initiative (WHI) study, an increase in VTE has been observed in women receiving CE compared to placebo. These observations are preliminary, and the study is continuing. (See **CLINICAL PHARMACOLOGY, Clinical Studies.**)

In the CE/MPA substudy of WHI, a 2-fold greater rate of VTE, including deep venous thrombosis and pulmonary embolism, was observed in women receiving CE/MPA compared to women receiving placebo. The rate of VTE was 34 per 10,000 women-years in the CE/MPA group compared to 16 per 10,000 women-years in the placebo group. The increase in VTE risk was observed during the first year and persisted.

If feasible, estrogens should be discontinued at least 4 to 6 weeks before surgery of the type associated with an increased risk of thromboembolism, or during periods of prolonged immobilization.

2. Malignant Neoplasms

a. *Endometrial Cancer:* The use of unopposed estrogens in women with intact uteri has been associated with endometrial cancer. The reported endometrial cancer risk among unopposed estrogen users is about 2- to 12-fold greater than in non-users, and appears dependent on duration of treatment and on estrogen dose. Most studies show no significant increased risk associated with use of estrogens for less than one year. The greatest risk appears associated with prolonged use, with increased risks of 15- to 24-fold for 5 to 10 years or more, and this risk has been shown to persist for at least 8 to 15 years after estrogen therapy is discontinued.

Clinical surveillance of all women taking estrogen/progestin combinations is important. Adequate diagnostic measures, including endometrial sampling when indicated, should be undertaken to rule out malignancy in all cases of undiagnosed persistent or recurring abnormal vaginal bleeding. There is no evidence that the use of natural estrogens results in a different endometrial risk profile than synthetic estrogens of equivalent estrogen dose. Adding a progestin to estrogen therapy has been shown to reduce the risk of endometrial hyperplasia, which may be a precursor to endometrial cancer.

b. *Breast Cancer:* Estrogen and estrogen/progestin therapy in postmenopausal women has been associated with an increased risk of breast cancer. In the CE/MPA substudy of the Women's Health Initiative (WHI) study, a 26% increase of invasive breast cancer (38 vs. 30 per 10,000 women-years) after an average of 5.2 years of treatment was observed in women receiving CE/MPA compared to women receiving placebo. The increased risk of breast cancer became apparent after 4 years on CE/MPA. The women reporting prior postmenopausal use of estrogens and/or estrogen with progestin had a higher relative risk for breast cancer associated with CE/MPA than those who had never used these hormones. (See **CLINICAL PHARMACOLOGY, Clinical Studies.**)

In the WHI, no increased risk of breast cancer in CE-treated women compared to placebo was reported after an average of 5.2 years of therapy. These data are preliminary and that substudy of WHI is continuing.

Epidemiologic studies have reported an increased risk of breast cancer in association with increasing duration of postmenopausal treatment with estrogens with or without a progestin. This association was reanalyzed in original data from 51 studies that involved various doses and types of estrogens, with and without progestins. In the reanalysis, an increased risk of having breast cancer diagnosed became apparent after about 5 years of continued treatment, and subsided after treatment had been discontinued for 5 years or longer. Some later studies have suggested that postmenopausal treatment with estrogens and progestins increase the risk of breast cancer more than treatment with estrogen alone.

A postmenopausal woman without a uterus who requires estrogen should receive estrogen-alone therapy, and should not be exposed unnecessarily to progestins. All postmenopausal women should receive yearly breast exams by a healthcare provider and perform monthly self-examinations. In addition, mammography examinations should be scheduled based on patient age and risk factors.

3. Gallbladder Disease

A 2- to 4-fold increase in the risk of gallbladder disease requiring surgery in postmenopausal women receiving estrogens has been reported.

4. Hypercalcemia

Estrogen administration may lead to severe hypercalcemia in patients with breast cancer and bone metastases. If hypercalcemia occurs, use of the drug should be stopped and appropriate measures taken to reduce the serum calcium level.

5. Visual Abnormalities

Retinal vascular thrombosis has been reported in patients receiving estrogens. Discontinue medication pending examination if there is sudden partial or complete loss of vision, or a sudden onset of proptosis, diplopia, or migraine. If examination reveals papilledema or retinal vascular lesions, estrogens should be permanently discontinued.

6. Alcohol based gels are flammable. Avoid fire, flame, or smoking until the gel has dried.

PRECAUTIONS

A. General

1. ***Addition of a progestin when a woman has not had a hysterectomy.*** Studies of the addition of a progestin for 10 or more days of a cycle of estrogen administration, or daily with estrogen in a continuous regimen, have reported a lowered incidence of endometrial hyperplasia than would be induced by estrogen treatment alone. Endometrial hyperplasia may be a precursor to endometrial cancer.
   There are, however, possible risks that may be associated with the use of progestins with estrogens compared to estrogen-alone regimens. These include a possible increased risk of breast cancer, adverse effects on lipoprotein metabolism (e.g., lowering HDL, raising LDL), and impairment of glucose tolerance.
2. ***Elevated blood pressure.*** In a small number of case reports, substantial increases in blood pressure have been attributed to idiosyncratic reactions to estrogens. In a large, randomized, placebo-controlled clinical trial, a generalized effect of estrogens on blood pressure was not seen. Blood pressure should be monitored at regular intervals with estrogen use.
3. ***Hypertriglyceridemia.*** In patients with pre-existing hypertriglyceridemia, estrogen therapy may be associated with elevations of plasma triglycerides leading to pancreatitis and other complications.
4. ***Impaired liver function and past history of cholestatic jaundice.*** Although topically administered estrogen therapy avoids first pass hepatic metabolism, estrogens may be poorly metabolized in patients with impaired liver function. For patients with a history of cholestatic jaundice associated with past estrogen use or with pregnancy, caution should be exercised and in the case of recurrence, medication should be discontinued.
5. ***Hypothyroidism.*** Estrogen administration leads to increased thyroid-binding globulin (TBG) levels. Patients with normal thyroid function can compensate for the increased TBG by making more thyroid hormone, thus maintaining free T_4 and T_3 serum concentrations in the normal range. Patients dependent on thyroid hormone replacement therapy who are also receiving estrogens may require increased doses of their thyroid replacement therapy. These patients should have their thyroid function monitored in order to maintain their free thyroid hormone levels in an acceptable range.
6. ***Fluid retention.*** Because estrogens may cause some degree of fluid retention, patients with conditions that might be influenced by this factor, such as a cardiac or renal dysfunction, warrant careful observation when estrogens are prescribed.
7. ***Hypocalcemia.*** Estrogens should be used with caution in individuals with severe hypocalcemia.
8. ***Ovarian cancer.*** Use of estrogen-only products, in particular for 10 or more years, has been associated with an increased risk of ovarian cancer in some epidemiological studies. Other studies did not show a significant association. Data are insufficient to determine whether there is an increased risk with combined estrogen/progestin therapy in postmenopausal women.
9. ***Exacerbation of endometriosis.*** Endometriosis may be exacerbated with administration of estrogen-therapy.
   A few cases of malignant transformation of residual endometrial implants have been reported in women treated post-hysterectomy with estrogen-alone therapy. For patients known to have residual endometriosis post-hysterectomy, the addition of progestin should be considered.
10. ***Exacerbation of other conditions.*** Estrogens may cause an exacerbation of asthma, diabetes mellitus, epilepsy, migraine, porphyria, systemic lupus erythematosus, and hepatic hemangiomas and should be used with caution in women with these conditions.
11. ***Photosensitivity/Photoallergy.*** Increased sensitivity to direct exposure to the sun on areas of EstroGel application has not been evaluated.
12. ***Effect of sunscreen application.*** The effects of concomitant application of EstroGel and a sunscreen lotion have not been evaluated.

B. Patient Information

Physicians are advised to discuss the PATIENT INFORMATION leaflet with patients for whom they prescribe EstroGel.

C. Laboratory Tests

Estrogen administration should be initiated at the lowest dose approved for the indication and then guided by clinical response rather than by serum hormone levels (e.g., estradiol, FSH).

D. Drug and Laboratory Test Interactions

1. Accelerated prothrombin time, partial thromboplastin time, and platelet aggregation time; increased platelet count; increased factors II, VII antigen, VIII antigen, VIII coagulant activity, IX, X, XII, VII-X complex, II-VII-X complex, and beta-thromboglobulin; decreased levels of anti-factor Xa and antithrombin III, decreased antithrombin III activity; increased levels of fibrinogen and fibrinogen activity; increased plasminogen antigen and activity.
2. Increased thyroid-binding globulin (TBG) leading to increased circulating total thyroid hormone levels, as measured by protein-bound iodine (PBI), T_4 levels (by column or by radioimmunoassay) or T_3 levels by radioimmunoassay. T_3 resin uptake is decreased, reflecting the elevated TBG. Free T_4 and T_3 concentrations are unaltered. Patients on thyroid replacement therapy may require higher doses of thyroid hormone.
3. Other binding proteins may be elevated in serum, i.e., corticosteroid binding globulin (CBG), sex hormone-binding globulin (SHBG), leading to increased total circulating corticosteroids and sex steroids, respectively. Free hormone concentrations may be decreased. Other plasma proteins may be increased (angiotensinogen/renin substrate, alpha-1-antitrypsin, ceruloplasmin).
4. Increased plasma HDL and HDL_2 cholesterol subfraction concentrations, reduced LDL cholesterol concentration, increased triglyceride levels.
5. Impaired glucose tolerance.
6. Reduced response to metyrapone test.

E. Carcinogenesis, Mutagenesis, Impairment of Fertility

Long-term continuous administration of estrogen, with and without progestin, in women, with and without a uterus, has shown an increased risk of endometrial cancer, breast cancer, and ovarian cancer. (See **BOXED WARNINGS, WARNINGS** and **PRECAUTIONS**.)

Long-term, continuous administration of natural and synthetic estrogens in certain animal species increases the frequency of carcinomas of the breast, uterus, cervix, vagina, testis and liver.

F. Pregnancy

EstroGel should not be used in pregnancy. (See **CONTRAINDICATIONS**.)

G. Nursing Mothers

Estrogen administration to nursing mothers has been shown to decrease the quantity and quality of the milk. Detectable amounts of estrogens have been identified in the milk of mothers receiving this drug. Caution should be exercised when EstroGel is administered to a nursing woman.

H. Pediatric Use

EstroGel is not indicated for use in children.

I. Geriatric Use

There have not been sufficient numbers of geriatric patients involved in studies utilizing EstroGel to determine whether those over 65 years of age differ from younger subjects in their response to EstroGel.

ADVERSE REACTIONS

See **BOXED WARNINGS, WARNINGS** and **PRECAUTIONS**.

Because clinical trials are conducted under widely varying conditions, adverse reaction rates observed in the clinical trials of a drug cannot be directly compared to rates in the clinical trials of another drug and may not reflect the rates observed in practice. The adverse reaction information from clinical trials does, however, provide a basis for identifying the adverse events that appear to be related to drug use and for approximating rates.

EstroGel 1.25 g was studied in two well-controlled 12-week clinical trials. Incidence of adverse experiences ≥5% for 1.25 g EstroGel and placebo is given below in Table 3.

[See table 3 at right]

TABLE 3
Incidence of Treatment-Emergent Signs and Symptoms ≥5% By COSTART Body System and by Descending Frequency of Occurrence in the EstroGel Treatment Group for the Intent-to-Treat Safety Population in Two Well-Controlled Clinical Studies (Expressed as % of Treatment Group)

BODY SYSTEM/Treatment-Emergent Signs and Symptoms	EstroGel 1.25 g day (n=168)	Placebo (n=73)
BODY AS A WHOLE		
Headache	20.2	17.8
Infection[a]	17.3	6.8
Pain[b]	7.1	11.0
Abdominal Pain	7.7	1.4
Back Pain	4.8	4.1
Flu Syndrome	5.4	1.4
Asthenia	4.8	4.1
CARDIOVASCULAR SYSTEM		
Palpitations	0.6	1.4
DIGESTIVE SYSTEM		
Nausea	6.0	4.1
Flatulence	6.5	5.5
Diarrhea	4.2	0.0
METABOLIC and NUTRITIONAL SYSTEMS		
Weight Gain	2.4	0.0
NERVOUS SYSTEM		
Nervousness	2.4	1.4
Depression	3.0	2.7
Anxiety	1.8	0.0
RESPIRATORY SYSTEM		
Sinusitis	3.6	1.4
Rhinitis	2.4	6.8
SKIN AND APPENDAGES		
Rash[c]	7.1	5.5
Pruritus[c]	4.8	2.7
Application Site Reaction	0.6	0.0
UROGENITAL		
Breast Pain	12.5	9.6
Metrorrhagia	3.0	0.0
Endometrial Disorder[d]	1.8	1.4
Vaginitis	8.9	4.1
Pap Smear Suspicious[e]	5.4	2.7
Vaginal Hemorrhage	1.2	0.0

[a] Infection: upper respiratory infection, common cold, eye infection.
[b] Pain: generalized and extremity aches/pains, cramps.
[c] Rash and Pruritus: More than half of the EstroGel treated patients who had pruritus reported itching at a body site other than the arms or reported generalized itching or itching skin. Similarly, most of the EstroGel treated patients with rash had rash on one or more areas of the body in addition to the arms.
[d] Endometrial Disorder: proliferative endometrium, benign endometrial disorders.
[e] Pap Smear Suspicious: atypical squamous cells of undetermined significance, inflammatory changes, epithelial cell abnormality.

The following additional adverse reactions have been reported with estrogen and/or progestin therapy.

1. **Genitourinary system:** Changes in vaginal bleeding pattern and abnormal withdrawal bleeding or flow; breakthrough bleeding; spotting; dysmenorrhea; increase in size of uterine leiomyomata; vaginitis, including vaginal candidiasis; change in amount of cervical secretion; changes in cervical ectropion; ovarian cancer; endometrial hyperplasia; endometrial cancer.
2. **Breasts:** Tenderness; enlargement, pain, nipple discharge, galactorrhea; fibrocystic breast changes; breast cancer.
3. **Cardiovascular:** Deep and superficial venous thrombosis; pulmonary embolism; thrombophlebitis; myocardial infarction; stroke; increase in blood pressure.
4. **Gastrointestinal:** Nausea; bloating; diarrhea; dyspepsia; constipation; vomiting; abdominal cramps; cholestatic jaundice; increased incidence of gallbladder disease; pancreatitis, enlargement of hepatic hemangiomas.
5. **Skin:** Chloasma or melasma, which may persist when drug is discontinued; erythema multiforme; erythema nodosum; hemorrhagic eruption; loss of scalp hair; hirsutism; pruritus, rash.
6. **Eyes:** Retinal vascular thrombosis, intolerance to contact lenses.
7. **Central Nervous System:** Headache; migraine; dizziness; mental depression; chorea; nervousness; mood disturbances; irritability; exacerbation of epilepsy.
8. **Miscellaneous:** Increase or decrease in weight; reduced carbohydrate tolerance; aggravation of porphyria; edema; arthralgias; leg cramps; changes in libido; anaphylactoid/anaphylactic reactions; hypocalcemia; exacerbation of asthma; increased triglycerides.

OVERDOSAGE

Serious ill effects have not been reported following acute ingestion of large doses of estrogen-containing products by young children. Overdosage of estrogen may cause nausea and vomiting, and withdrawal bleeding may occur in females.

DOSAGE AND ADMINISTRATION

EstroGel 1.25 g is the single approved dose for the treatment of moderate to severe vasomotor symptoms and/or moderate to severe symptoms of vulvar and vaginal atrophy associated with the menopause. The lowest effective dose of EstroGel for these indications has not been determined. When prescribing solely for the treatment of moderate to severe symptoms of vulvar and vaginal atrophy, topical vaginal products should be considered.

When estrogen is prescribed for a postmenopausal woman with a uterus, a progestin should also be initiated to reduce the risk of endometrial cancer. A woman without a uterus does not need progestin. Use of estrogen, alone or in combination with a progestin, should be limited to the shortest duration consistent with treatment goals and risks for the individual woman. Patients should be reevaluated periodically as clinically appropriate (e.g., 3-month to 6-month intervals) to determine if treatment is still necessary (see **BOXED WARNINGS** and **WARNINGS**). For women who have a uterus, adequate diagnostic measures, such as endometrial sampling, when indicated, should be undertaken to rule out malignancy in cases of undiagnosed persistent or recurring abnormal vaginal bleeding.

Continued on next page

Estrogel—Cont.

HOW SUPPLIED

EstroGel is a clear, colorless, hydroalcoholic 0.06% estradiol gel supplied in a non-aerosol, metered-dose pump. The pump consists of a LDPE inner liner encased in rigid plastic with a resealable polypropylene cap. Each individually packaged pump contains 93 grams of gel and is capable of delivering 64 metered 1.25 g doses.

NDC 0051-1028-58 .... (93 grams Pump)

Keep out of reach of children.

Store at 20° to 25°C (68° to 77°F); excursions permitted to 15° to 30°C (59° to 86°F) [See USP Controlled Room Temperature].

Manufactured for:

Unimed Pharmaceuticals, Inc.
A Solvay Pharmaceuticals, Inc. company
Marietta, GA 30062
By Laboratoires Besins International
Montrouge, France
500123
3E Rev 3/2004

PATIENT INFORMATION

(Updated March 2004)

EstroGel ®

(estradiol gel)

℞ **only**

Read this PATIENT INFORMATION before you start taking EstroGel and read the patient information each time you refill your EstroGel prescription. There may be new information. This information does not take the place of talking to your healthcare provider about your medical condition or your treatment.

WHAT IS THE MOST IMPORTANT INFORMATION I SHOULD KNOW ABOUT EstroGel (AN ESTROGEN HORMONE)?

- Estrogens increase the chances of getting cancer of the uterus.

Report any unusual vaginal bleeding right away while you are taking estrogens. Vaginal bleeding after menopause may be a warning sign of cancer of the uterus (womb). Your healthcare provider should check any unusual vaginal bleeding to find out the cause.

- Do not use estrogens with or without progestins to prevent heart disease, heart attacks, or strokes.

Using estrogens with or without progestins may increase your chances of getting heart attack, strokes, breast cancer, and blood clots. You and your healthcare provider should talk regularly about whether you still need treatment with EstroGel.

What is EstroGel?

EstroGel is a clear, colorless gel medicine that contains an estrogen hormone (estradiol) which is absorbed through the skin into the bloodstream. The estrogen hormone in EstroGel is a synthetic estrogen made from a plant source.

What is EstroGel used for?

EstroGel is used after menopause to:

- **reduce moderate to severe hot flashes**

Estrogens are hormones made by a woman's ovaries. The ovaries normally stop making estrogens when a woman is between 45 and 55 years old. This drop in body estrogen levels causes the "change of life" or menopause (the end of monthly menstrual periods). Sometimes, both ovaries are removed during an operation before natural menopause takes place. The sudden drop in estrogen levels causes "surgical menopause."

When the estrogen levels begin dropping, some women get very uncomfortable symptoms, such as feelings of warmth in the face, neck, and chest, or sudden intense episodes of heat and sweating ("hot flashes" or "hot flushes"). In some women, the symptoms are mild, and they will not need estrogens. In other women, symptoms can be more severe. You and your healthcare provider should talk regularly about whether you still need treatment with EstroGel.

- **treat moderate to severe dryness, itching, and burning in and around your vagina**

You and your healthcare provider should talk regularly about whether you still need treatment with EstroGel to control these problems. If you use EstroGel only to treat your dryness, itching, and burning in and around your vagina, talk with your healthcare provider about whether a topical vaginal product would be better for you.

Who should not use EstroGel?

Do not start using EstroGel if you:

- **have unusual vaginal bleeding**
- **currently have or have had certain cancers**

Estrogens may increase the chances of getting certain types of cancer, including cancer of the breast or uterus. If you have or have had cancer, talk with your healthcare provider about whether you should use EstroGel.

- **had a stroke or heart attack in the past year**
- **currently have or have had blood clots**
- **currently have or have had liver problems**
- **are allergic to EstroGel or any of its ingredients**

See the end of this leaflet for a list of ingredients in EstroGel.

- **think you may be pregnant**

Tell your healthcare provider:

- **if you are breastfeeding**

The hormone in EstroGel can pass into your breast milk.

- **about all your medical problems**

Your healthcare provider may need to check you more carefully if you have certain conditions, such as asthma (wheezing), epilepsy (seizures), migraine, endometriosis, lupus, or problems with your heart, liver, thyroid, kidneys, or have high calcium levels in your blood.

- **about all the medicines you take**

This includes prescription and nonprescription medicines, vitamins, and herbal supplements. Some medicines may affect how EstroGel works. EstroGel may also affect how your other medicines work.

- **if you are going to have surgery or will be on bed rest**

You may need to stop taking estrogens.

How is EstroGel supplied?

EstroGel is available in a metered dose pump that delivers 1.25 grams (g) of a gel containing 0.75 milligrams (mg) of estradiol each time the pump is depressed.

Please refer to the chart below to determine the number of full pump depressions required for the daily dose prescribed by your healthcare provider:

Prescribed Daily Dose of EstroGel	Number of Pump Depressions	Amount of estradiol Applied	Application Area
1.25 g	1	0.75 mg	One Arm

How should I use the EstroGel pump?

It is important that you read and follow these directions on how to use the EstroGel pump properly.

1. **Before using the pump for the first time, it must be primed.** Remove the large pump cover and fully depress the pump twice. Discard the unused gel by thoroughly rinsing down the sink or placing it in the household trash in a manner that avoids accidental exposure or ingestion by household members or pets. **After priming, the pump is ready to use,** and one complete pump depression will dispense the same amount of EstroGel each time.
2. **Apply EstroGel at the same time each day.** You should apply your daily dose of gel to clean, dry, unbroken skin. If you take a bath or shower or use a sauna, apply your EstroGel dose after your bath, shower, or sauna. If you go swimming, try to leave as much time as possible between applying your EstroGel dose and going swimming.
3. **Be sure your skin is completely dry before applying EstroGel.**
4. To apply the dose, collect the gel into the palm of your hand by pressing the pump firmly and fully with one fluid motion without hesitation, as illustrated.

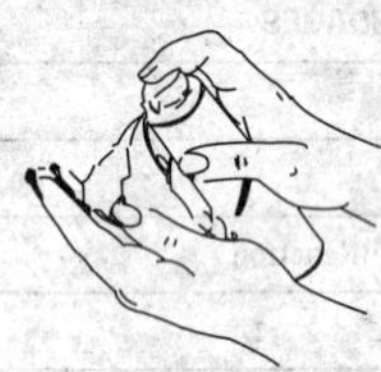

5. Apply the gel to one arm using your hand. Spread the gel as thinly as possible over the entire area on the inside and outside of your arm from wrist to shoulder, as illustrated.

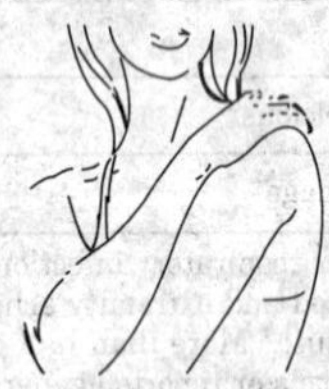

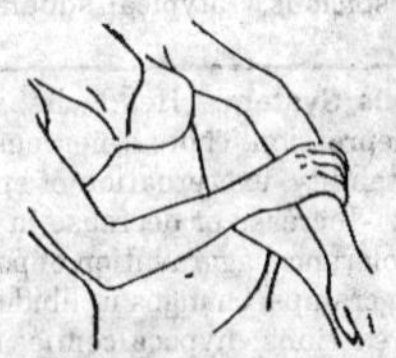

6. Always place the small protective cap back on the tip of the pump, and the large pump cover over the top of the pump after each use.
7. **Wash your hands with soap and water after applying the gel to reduce the chance that the medicine will spread from your hands to other people.**
8. It is not necessary to massage or rub in EstroGel. Simply allow the gel to dry for up to five minutes before dressing.
9. **Alcohol based gels are flammable. Avoid fire, flame or smoking until the gel has dried.**
10. Once dry, EstroGel is odorless.
11. **Never apply EstroGel directly to the breast.** Do not allow others to apply the gel for you.
12. The EstroGel pump contains enough product to allow for initial priming of the pump twice and to deliver 64 daily doses. After you have initially primed the pump twice and dispensed 64 doses, you will need to discard the pump.

What should I do if someone else is exposed to EstroGel?

If someone else is exposed to EstroGel by direct contact with the gel, that person should wash the area of contact with soap and water as soon as possible. The longer the gel is in contact with the skin before washing, the greater is the chance that the other person will absorb some of the estrogen hormone. This is especially important for men and children.

What should I do if I get EstroGel in my eyes?

If you get EstroGel in your eyes, rinse your eyes right away with warm clean water to flush out any EstroGel. Seek medical attention if needed.

What should I do if I miss a dose?

If you miss a dose, do not double the dose on the next day to catch up. If your next dose is less than 12 hours away, it is best just to wait and apply your normal dose the next day. If it is more than 12 hours until the next dose, apply the dose you missed and resume your normal dosing the next day.

What should I avoid while using EstroGel?

It is important that you do not spread the medicine to others, especially men and children. Be sure to wash your hands after applying EstroGel. Do not allow others to make contact with the area of skin where you applied the gel for at least one hour after application. **Alcohol based gels are flammable. Avoid fire, flame or smoking until the gel has dried.**

What are the possible side effects of estrogens?

Less common but serious side effects include:

- Breast cancer
- Cancer of the uterus
- Stroke
- Heart attack
- Blood clots
- Gallbladder disease
- Ovarian cancer

These are some of the warning signs of serious side effects:

- Breast lumps
- Unusual vaginal bleeding
- Dizziness and faintness
- Changes in speech
- Severe headaches
- Chest pain
- Shortness of breath
- Pains in your legs
- Changes in vision
- Vomiting

Call your healthcare provider right away if you get any of these warning signs, or any other unusual symptoms that concerns you.

Common side effects include:

- Headache
- Breast pain
- Irregular vaginal bleeding or spotting
- Stomach/abdominal cramps, bloating
- Nausea and vomiting
- Hair loss

Other side effects include:

- High blood pressure
- Liver problems
- High blood sugar
- Fluid retention
- Enlargement of benign tumors of the uterus ("fibroids")
- Vaginal yeast infection

These are not all the possible side effects of EstroGel. For more information, ask your healthcare provider or pharmacist.

What can I do to lower my chances of getting a serious side effect with EstroGel?

Talk with your healthcare provider regularly about whether you should continue using EstroGel. If you have a uterus, talk with your healthcare provider about whether the addition of a progestin is right for you. See your healthcare provider right away if you get vaginal bleeding while using EstroGel. Have a breast exam and mammogram (breast X-ray) every year unless your healthcare provider tells you something else. If members of your family have had breast cancer or if you have ever had breast lumps or an abnormal mammogram, you may need to have breast exams more often. If you have high blood pressure, high cholesterol (fat in the blood), diabetes, are overweight, or if you use tobacco, you may have higher chances of getting heart disease. Ask your healthcare provider for ways to lower your chances of getting heart disease.

General information about the safe and effective use of EstroGel

Medicines are sometimes prescribed for conditions that are not mentioned in patient information leaflets. Do not use EstroGel for conditions for which it was not prescribed. Do not give EstroGel to other people, even if they have the same symptoms you have. It may harm them. **Keep EstroGel out of the reach of children.**

This leaflet provides a summary of the most important information about EstroGel. If you would like more information, talk with your healthcare provider or pharmacist. You can ask for information about EstroGel that is written for health professionals. You can get more information by calling the toll free number 800-241-1643.

What are the ingredients of EstroGel?

EstroGel contains estradiol, purified water, alcohol, triethanolamine, and carbomer 934P.

EstroGel should be stored with the cap on securely. Store at 20° to 25°C (68° to 77°F); excursions permitted to 15° to 30°C (59° to 86°F) [See USP Controlled Room Temperature]. Do not freeze. The gel should not be used after the date printed on the end of the metered-dose pump after the term "Exp." (expiry date).

Manufactured for:

Unimed Pharmaceuticals, Inc.
A Solvay Pharmaceuticals, Inc. company
Marietta, GA 30062
By Laboratoires Besins International
Montrouge, France
500123 3E Rev 3/2004

Shown in Product Identification Guide, page 333

PROMETRIUM® ℞

[*pro-mē-trē-um*]
(progesterone, USP)
Capsules 100 mg
Capsules 200 mg

DESCRIPTION

PROMETRIUM® (progesterone, USP) Capsules contain micronized progesterone for oral administration. Progesterone has a molecular weight of 314.47 and an empirical formula of $C_{21}H_{30}O_2$. Progesterone (pregn-4-ene-3, 20-dione) is a white or creamy white, odorless, crystalline powder practically insoluble in water, soluble in alcohol, acetone and dioxane and sparingly soluble in vegetable oils, stable in air, melting between 126° and 131°C. The structural formula is:

Progesterone is synthesized from a starting material from a plant source and is chemically identical to progesterone of human ovarian origin. PROMETRIUM Capsules are available in multiple strengths to afford dosage flexibility for optimum management. PROMETRIUM Capsules contain 100 mg or 200 mg micronized progesterone.

The inactive ingredients for PROMETRIUM Capsules 100 mg include: peanut oil NF, gelatin NF, glycerin USP, lecithin NF, titanium dioxide USP, D&C Yellow No. 10, and FD&C Red No. 40.

The inactive ingredients for PROMETRIUM Capsules 200 mg include: peanut oil NF, gelatin NF, glycerin USP, lecithin NF, titanium dioxide USP, D&C Yellow No. 10, and FD&C Yellow No. 6.

CLINICAL PHARMACOLOGY

PROMETRIUM Capsules are an oral dosage form of micronized progesterone which is chemically identical to progesterone of ovarian origin. The oral bioavailability of progesterone is increased through micronization.

Pharmacokinetics

Absorption

After oral administration of progesterone as a micronized soft gelatin capsule formulation, maximum serum concentrations were attained within 3 hours. The absolute bioavailability of micronized progesterone is not known. Table 1 summarizes the mean pharmacokinetic parameters in postmenopausal women after five oral daily doses of PROMETRIUM Capsules 100 mg as a micronized soft-gelatin capsule formulation.

[See table 1 above]

Serum progesterone concentrations appeared linear and dose proportional following multiple dose administration of PROMETRIUM Capsules 100 mg over the dose range 100 mg/day to 300 mg/day in postmenopausal women. Although doses greater than 300 mg/day were not studied in females, serum concentrations from a study in male volunteers appeared linear and dose proportional between 100 mg/day and 400 mg/day. The pharmacokinetic parameters in male volunteers were generally consistent with those seen in postmenopausal women.

Distribution

Progesterone is approximately 96%-99% bound to serum proteins, primarily to serum albumin (50%-54%) and transcortin (43%-48%).

Metabolism

Progesterone is metabolized primarily by the liver largely to pregnanediols and pregnanolones. Pregnanediols and pregnanolones are conjugated in the liver to glucuronide and sulfate metabolites. Progesterone metabolites which are excreted in the bile may be deconjugated and may be further metabolized in the gut via reduction, dehydroxylation, and epimerization.

Excretion

The glucuronide and sulfate conjugates of pregnanediol and pregnanolone are excreted in the bile and urine.

Table 1

Parameter	PROMETRIUM Capsules Dose QD		
	100 mg	200 mg	300 mg
Cmax (ng/ml)	17.3±21.9[a]	38.1±37.8	60.6±72.5
Tmax (hr)	1.5±0.8	2.3±1.4	1.7±0.6
AUC (0-10) (ng•hr/ml)	43.3±30.8	101.2±66.0	175.7±170.3

[a] Mean ± S.D.

Table 2

Mean (±S.D.) Pharmacokinetic Parameters for Estradiol, Estrone and Equilin Following Coadministration of Conjugated Estrogens 0.625 mg and PROMETRIUM Capsules 200mg for 12 Days to Postmenopausal Women

	Conjugated Estrogens			Conjugated Estrogens plus PROMETRIUM Capsules		
Drug	Cmax (ng/mL)	Tmax (hr)	AUC(0-24h) (ng•h/mL)	Cmax (ng/mL)	Tmax (hr)	AUC(0-24h) (ng•h/mL)
Estradiol	0.037 ±0.048	12.7 ±9.1	0.676 ±0.737	0.030 ±0.032	17.32 ±1.21	0.561 ±0.572
Estrone Total[a]	3.68 ±1.55	10.6 ±6.8	61.3 ±26.36	4.93 ±2.07	7.5 ±3.8	85.9 ±41.2
Equilin Total[a]	2.27 ±0.95	6.0 ±4.0	28.8 ±13.0	3.22 ±1.13	5.3 ±2.6	38.1 ±20.2

[a] Total estrogens is the sum of conjugated and unconjugated estrogen.

Table 3

Incidence of Endometrial Hyperplasia in Women Receiving 3 Years of Treatment

Endometrial Diagnosis	Treatment Group					
	Conjugated Estrogens 0.625 mg + PROMETRIUM Capsules 200 mg (cyclical)		Conjugated Estrogens 0.625 mg (only)		Placebo	
	Number of patients	% of patients	number of patients	% of patients	number of patients	% of patients
	N=117		N=115		N=116	
Hyperplasia[a]	7	6	74	64	3	3
Adenocarcinoma	0	0	0	0	1	1
Atypical hyperplasia	1	1	14	12	0	0
Complex hyperplasia	0	0	27	23	1	1
Simple hyperplasia	6	5	33	29	1	1

a: Most advanced result to least advanced result:
Adenocarcinoma > atypical hyperplasia > complex hyperplasia > simple hyperplasia

Progesterone metabolites which are excreted in the bile may undergo enterohepatic recycling or may be excreted in the feces.

Special Populations

The pharmacokinetics of PROMETRIUM Capsules have not been assessed in low body weight or obese patients.

Race:

There is insufficient information available from trials conducted with PROMETRIUM Capsules to compare progesterone pharmacokinetics in different racial groups.

Hepatic Insufficiency:

No formal studies have evaluated the effect of hepatic disease on the disposition of progesterone. However, since progesterone is metabolized by the liver, use in patients with severe liver dysfunction or disease is contraindicated (see **CONTRAINDICATIONS**). If treatment with progesterone is indicated in patients with mild to moderate hepatic dysfunction, these patients should be monitored carefully.

Renal Insufficiency:

No formal studies have evaluated the effect of renal disease on the disposition of progesterone. Since progesterone metabolites are eliminated mainly by the kidneys, PROMETRIUM Capsules should be used with caution and only with careful monitoring in patients with renal dysfunction. (see **PRECAUTIONS**)

Food-Drug Interaction:

Concomitant food ingestion increased the bioavailability of PROMETRIUM Capsules relative to a fasting state when administered to postmenopausal women at a dose of 200 mg.

Drug-Drug Interaction:

The metabolism of progesterone by human liver microsomes was inhibited by ketoconazole (IC_{50}<0.1 μM). Ketoconazole is a known inhibitor of cytochrome P450 3A4, hence these data suggest that ketoconazole or other known inhibitors of this enzyme may increase the bioavailability of progesterone. The clinical relevance of the *in vitro* findings is unknown.

Coadministration of conjugated estrogens and PROMETRIUM Capsules to 29 postmenopausal women over a 12 day period resulted in an increase in total estrone concentrations (Cmax 3.68 ng/ml to 4.93 ng/ml) and total equilin concentrations (Cmax 2.27 ng/ml to 3.22 ng/ml) and a decrease in circulating 17β estradiol concentrations (Cmax 0.037 ng/ml to 0.030 ng/ml). The half-life of the conjugated estrogens was similar with coadministration of PROMETRIUM Capsules. Table 2 summarizes the pharmacokinetic parameters.

[See table 2 above]

Clinical Studies

Endometrial Protection

In a randomized double-blind clinical trial, 358 postmenopausal women, each with an intact uterus, received treatment for up to 36 months. The treatment groups were: PROMETRIUM Capsules at the dose of 200 mg/day for 12 days per 28 day cycle in combination with conjugated estrogens 0.625 mg/day (n=120); conjugated estrogens 0.625 mg/day only (n=119); or placebo (n=119). The subjects in all three treatment groups were primarily Caucasian women (87% or more of each group). The results for the incidence of endometrial hyperplasia in women receiving up to 3 years of treatment are shown in Table 3. A comparison of the PROMETRIUM Capsules plus conjugated estrogens treatment group to the conjugated estrogens only group showed a significantly lower rate of hyperplasia (6% combination

Continued on next page

Prometrium—Cont.

product vs. 64% estrogen alone) in the PROMETRIUM Capsules plus conjugated estrogens treatment group throughout 36 months of treatment.

[See table 3 on previous page]

The times to diagnosis of endometrial hyperplasia over 36 months of treatment are shown in Figure 1. This figure illustrates graphically that the proportion of patients with hyperplasia was significantly greater for the conjugated estrogens group (64%) compared to the conjugated estrogens plus PROMETRIUM Capsules group (6%).

Figure 1

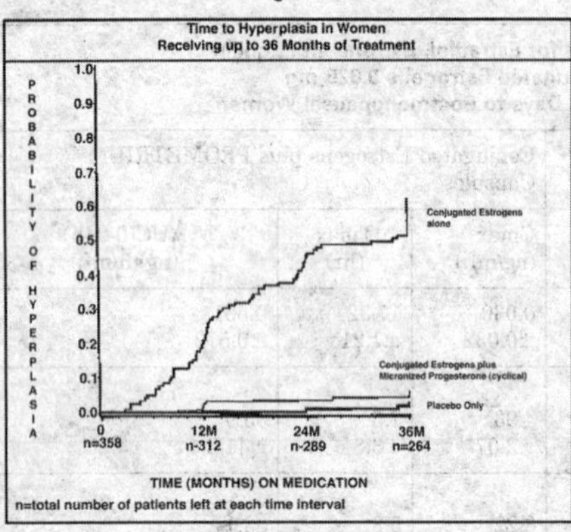

The discontinuation rates due to hyperplasia over the 36 months of treatment are as shown in Table 4. For any degree of hyperplasia, the discontinuation rate for patients who received conjugated estrogens plus PROMETRIUM Capsules was similar to that of the placebo only group, while the discontinuation rate for patients who received conjugated estrogens alone was significantly higher. Women who permanently discontinued treatment due to hyperplasia were similar in demographics to the overall study population.

[See table 4 above]

In the same three year clinical trial, postmenopausal women were treated with PROMETRIUM Capsules in combination with conjugated estrogens, conjugated estrogens only, or placebo. There was no statistically significant difference between the PROMETRIUM Capsules plus conjugated estrogens group and the conjugated estrogens only group in increases of HDL-C and triglycerides, or in decreases of LDL-C. The changes observed in lipid profiles are shown in Table 5.

[See table 5 at right]

Secondary Amenorrhea

In a single-center, randomized, double-blind clinical study that included premenopausal women with secondary amenorrhea for at least 90 days, administration of 10 days of PROMETRIUM Capsules therapy resulted in 80% of women experiencing withdrawal bleeding within 7 days of the last dose of PROMETRIUM Capsules, 300 mg/day (n=20), compared to 10% of women experiencing withdrawal bleeding in the placebo group (n=21).

The rate of secretory transformation was evaluated in a multicenter, randomized, double-blind clinical study in estrogen-primed postmenopausal women. PROMETRIUM Capsules administered orally for 10 days at 400 mg/day (n=22) induced complete secretory changes in the endometrium in 45% of women compared to 0% in the placebo group (n=23).

Table 4

Discontinuation Rate Due to Hyperplasia Over 36 Months of Treatment

Most Advanced Biopsy Result Through 36 Months of Treatment	Treatment Group					
	Conjugated Estrogens + PROMETRIUM Capsules (cyclical)		Conjugated Estrogens (only)		Placebo	
	N=120		N=119		N=119	
	Number of patients	% of patients	number of patients	% of patients	number of patients	% of patients
Adenocarcinoma	0	0	0	0	1	1
Atypical hyperplasia	1	1	10	8	0	0
Complex hyperplasia	0	0	21	18	1	1
Simple hyperplasia	1	1	13	11	0	0

Table 5

Mean Changes from Baseline in Lipid Profiles After 36 Months of Treatment

Parameter	Treatment Group Mean (Mean % Change)					
	Conjugated Estrogens 0.625 mg + PROMETRIUM Capsules 200 mg (cyclical)[a]		Conjugated Estrogens 0.625 mg (only)		Placebo	
	N= 176 to 177[b]		N=171 to 173[b]		N=171	
	Mean change	Mean % change	Mean change	mean % change	Mean change	mean % change
LIPID PROFILE						
HDL-C (mmol/L)	0.07	5.1	0.10	7.2	-0.05	-2
LDL-C (mmol/L)	-0.43	-11.8	-0.36	-9.5	-0.14	-2.9
Cholesterol (mmol/L)	-0.26	-4.0	-0.22	-3.6	-0.15	-1.8
Triglyceride (mmol/L)[c]	0.20	17.8	0.15	13.7	0.01	0.6

a: There are no significant changes ($p<0.05$) from conjugated estrogens values
b: Number of subjects (N) varies by parameter
c: Computed from log transformed data

Table 6

Mean Changes from Baseline in Insulin and Glucose Levels After 36 Months of Treatment

Parameter		Treatment Group Mean (Mean % Change)					
		Conjugated Estrogens 0.625 mg + PROMETRIUM Capsules 200 mg (cyclical)[a] N= 173 to 176[b]		Conjugated Estrogens 0.625 mg (only) N=170 to 172[b]		Placebo N=171	
		mean	mean % change	mean	mean % change	mean	mean % change
OGTT							
Insulin(pmol/L)	fasting	-2.2	-6.2	-1.1	-3.2	5.1	14.2
	2 hour	-45.2	-14.5	-23.9	-7.9	-29.7	-9.1
Glucose(mg/dL)	fasting	-3.0	-2.9	-2.7	-2.7	-1.0	-0.9
	2 hour	3.6	5.2	5.0	7.8	2.1	3.9

a: There are no significant changes ($p<0.05$) from conjugated estrogens values
b: Number of subjects (N) varies by parameter

INDICATIONS AND USAGE

PROMETRIUM Capsules are indicated for use in the prevention of endometrial hyperplasia in non-hysterectomized postmenopausal women who are receiving conjugated estrogens tablets. They are also indicated for use in secondary amenorrhea.

CONTRAINDICATIONS

1. **Known sensitivity to PROMETRIUM Capsules or its ingredients. PROMETRIUM Capsules contain peanut oil and should never be used by patients allergic to peanuts.**
2. Known or suspected pregnancy.
3. Thrombophlebitis, thromboembolic disorders, cerebral apoplexy, or patients with a past history of these conditions.
4. Severe liver dysfunction or disease.
5. Known or suspected malignancy of breast or genital organs.
6. Undiagnosed vaginal bleeding.
7. Missed abortion.
8. As a diagnostic test for pregnancy.

WARNINGS

1. The physician should be alert to the earliest manifestations of thrombotic disorders (thrombophlebitis, cerebrovascular disorders, pulmonary embolism, and retinal thrombosis). Should any of these occur or be suspected, the drug should be discontinued immediately.
2. Discontinue medication pending examination if there is sudden partial or complete loss of vision, or if there is a sudden onset of proptosis, diplopia or migraine. If examination reveals papilledema or retinal vascular lesions, medication should be withdrawn.
3. The administration of any drug to nursing mothers should be done only when clearly necessary since many drugs are excreted in human milk. Detectable amounts of progestin have been identified in the milk of mothers receiving progestins. The effect of this on the nursing infant has not been determined.
4. Retrospective studies of morbidity and mortality in Great Britain and studies of morbidity in the United States have shown a statistically significant association between thrombophlebitis, pulmonary embolism, cerebral thrombosis and embolism, and the use of oral contraceptives. The estimate of the relative risk of thromboembolism in the study by Vessey and Doll was about seven fold, while Sartwell and associates in the United States found a relative risk of 4.4, meaning that the users are several times as likely to undergo thromboembolic disease without evident cause as nonusers. The American study also indicated that the risk did not persist after discontinuation of administration, and that it was not enhanced by long-continued administration. The American study was not designed to evaluate a difference between products.

PRECAUTIONS

General

1. The pretreatment physical examination should include special reference to breast and pelvic organs, as well as Papanicolaou smear.
2. Because progesterone may cause some degree of fluid retention, conditions which might be influenced by this factor, such as epilepsy, migraine, asthma, cardiac or renal dysfunction, require careful observation.
3. In cases of breakthrough bleeding, as in any cases of irregular bleeding per vaginum, nonfunctional causes should be borne in mind. In cases of undiagnosed vaginal bleeding, adequate diagnostic measures are indicated.

4. Patients who have a history of psychic depression should be carefully observed and the drug discontinued if the depression recurs to a serious degree.
5. Any possible influence of prolonged progestin therapy on pituitary, ovarian, adrenal, hepatic or uterine functions awaits further study.
6. Although concomitant use of conjugated estrogens and PROMETRIUM Capsules did not result in a decrease in glucose tolerance, diabetic patients should be carefully observed while receiving estrogen-progestin therapy.
7. The pathologist should be advised of progestin therapy when relevant specimens are submitted.
8. Because of the occurrence of thrombotic disorders (thrombophlebitis, pulmonary embolism, retinal thrombosis, and cerebrovascular disorders) in patients taking estrogen-progestin combinations, the physician should be alert to the earliest manifestation of these disorders.
9. Transient dizziness may occur in some patients. Use caution when driving a motor vehicle or operating machinery. A small percentage of women may experience extreme dizziness and/or drowsiness during initial therapy. For these women, bedtime dosing is advised.
10. Rare instances of syncope and hypotension of possible orthostatic origin have been observed in patients taking PROMETRIUM Capsules.

Information for the Patient

See accompanying Patient Insert.

General: This product contains peanut oil and should not be used if you are allergic to peanuts.

Drug Lab Test Interactions

The following laboratory results may be altered by the use of estrogen-progestin combination drugs:

Increased sulfobromophthalein retention and other hepatic function tests.

Coagulation tests: increase in prothrombin factors VII, VIII, IX and X.

Metyrapone test.

Pregnanediol determination.

Thyroid function: increase in PBI, and butanol extractable protein bound iodine and decrease in T3 uptake values.

Fasting and 2-hour plasma insulin and glucose levels following an oral glucose tolerance test (OGTT) and fibrinogen levels were measured in patients receiving PROMETRIUM Capsules at a dose of 200 mg/day for 12 days per 28 day cycle in combination with conjugated estrogens 0.625 mg/day (n=120). Table 6 summarizes this data. Plasma insulin levels 2 hours post-OGTT were decreased from baseline. The fasting plasma glucose and fasting plasma insulin levels were also decreased from baseline. Glucose levels 2 hours post-OGTT were increased slightly. There was no effect on fibrinogen levels.

For information on changes in lipid profile, see the Clinical Studies subsection, Table 5.

[See table 6 on previous page]

Carcinogenesis, Mutagenesis, Impairment of Fertility

Progesterone has not been tested for carcinogenicity in animals by the oral route of administration. When implanted into female mice, progesterone produced mammary carcinomas, ovarian granulosa cell tumors and endometrial stromal sarcomas (1). In dogs, long-term intramuscular injections produced nodular hyperplasia and benign and malignant mammary tumors (2). Subcutaneous or intramuscular injections of progesterone decreased the latency period and increased the incidence of mammary tumors in rats previously treated with a chemical carcinogen (3).

Progesterone did not show evidence of genotoxicity in *in vitro* studies for point mutations or for chromosomal damage. *In vivo* studies for chromosome damage have yielded positive results in mice at oral doses of 1000 mg/kg and 2000 mg/kg (4). Exogenously administered progesterone has been shown to inhibit ovulation in a number of species and it is expected that high doses given for an extended duration would impair fertility until the cessation of treatment.

Pregnancy Category B

Reproductive studies have been performed in mice at doses up to 9 times the human oral dose (5, 6), in rats at doses up to 44 times the human oral dose (7, 8), in rabbits at a dose of 10 µg/day delivered locally within the uterus by an implanted device (9), in guinea pigs at doses of approximately one-half the human oral dose (10) and in rhesus monkeys (11) at doses approximately the human dose, all based on body surface area, and have revealed little or no evidence of impaired fertility or harm to the fetus due to progesterone. Several studies in women exposed to progesterone have not demonstrated any significant increase in fetal malformations (12). A single case of cleft palate was observed in the child of a woman using PROMETRIUM Capsules in early pregnancy, although definitive causality has not been established. Rare instances of fetal death have been reported in pregnant women prescribed PROMETRIUM Capsules for unapproved indications. Because the studies in humans cannot rule out the possibility of harm, PROMETRIUM Capsules should be used during pregnancy only if indicated (see **CONTRAINDICATIONS**).

Nursing Mothers

The administration of any drug to nursing mothers should be done only when clearly necessary since many drugs are excreted in human milk. Detectable amounts of progestin have been identified in the milk of nursing mothers receiving progestins. The effect of this on the nursing infant has not been determined.

Pediatric Use

The safety and effectiveness of PROMETRIUM Capsules in pediatric patients have not been established.

Table 7

Adverse Experiences (≥2%) Reported in an 875 Patient Placebo-Controlled Trial in Postmenopausal Women over a 3-Year Period (Percentage(%) of Patients Reporting)

	PROMETRIUM Capsules 200 mg with Conjugated Estrogens 0.625 mg (N=178)	Conjugated Estrogens 0.625 mg (only) (N=175)	Placebo (N=174)
Headache	31	30	27
Breast Tenderness	27	16	6
Joint Pain	20	22	29
Depression	19	18	12
Dizziness	15	5	9
Abdominal Bloating	12	10	5
Hot Flashes	11	14	35
Urinary Problems	11	10	9
Abdominal Pain	10	13	10
Vaginal Discharge	10	10	3
Nausea / Vomiting	8	6	7
Worry	8	5	4
Chest Pain	7	4	5
Diarrhea	7	7	4
Night Sweats	7	5	17
Breast Pain	6	6	2
Swelling of Hands and Feet	6	9	9
Vaginal Dryness	6	8	10
Constipation	3	3	2
Breast Carcinoma	2	<1	<1
Breast Excisional Biopsy	2	1	<1
Cholecystectomy	2	<1	<1

Table 8

Adverse Experiences (≥5%) Reported in Patients Using 400 mg/day in a Placebo-Controlled Trial in Estrogen-Primed Postmenopausal Women

Adverse Experience	PROMETRIUM Capsules 400 mg N=25	Placebo N=24
	Percentage (%) of Patients	
Fatigue	8	4
Headache	16	8
Dizziness	24	4
Abdominal Distention (Bloating)	8	8
Abdominal Pain (Cramping)	20	13
Diarrhea	8	4
Nausea	8	0
Back Pain	8	8
Musculoskeletal Pain	12	4
Irritability	8	4
Breast Pain	16	8
Infection Viral	12	0
Coughing	8	0

ADVERSE REACTIONS

Endometrial Protection

Table 7 lists adverse experiences which were reported in ≥2% of patients (regardless of relationship to treatment) who received cyclic PROMETRIUM Capsules, 200 mg daily (12 days per calendar month cycle) with daily 0.625 mg conjugated estrogen, in a multicenter, randomized, double-blind, placebo-controlled clinical trial in 875 postmenopausal women.

[See table 7 above]

Secondary Amenorrhea

Table 8 lists adverse experiences which were reported in ≥5% of patients receiving PROMETRIUM Capsules, 400 mg/day, in a multicenter, randomized, double-blind, placebo-controlled clinical trial in estrogen-primed (6 weeks) postmenopausal women receiving conjugated estrogens 0.625 mg/day and cyclic (10 days per calendar month cycle) PROMETRIUM Capsules at a dose of 400 mg/day, for three cycles.

[See table 8 above]

The most common adverse experiences reported in ≥5% of patients in all PROMETRIUM Capsules dosage groups studied in this trial (100 mg/day to 400 mg/day) were: dizziness (16%), breast pain (11%), headache (10%), abdominal pain (10%), fatigue (9%), viral infection (7%), abdominal dis-

Continued on next page

Prometrium—Cont.

tention (6%), musculoskeletal pain (6%), emotional lability (6%), irritability (5%), and upper respiratory tract infection (5%).

Other adverse events reported in <5% of patients taking PROMETRIUM Capsules include:

Autonomic Nervous System Disorders: dry mouth
Body As A Whole: accidental injury, chest pain, fever
Cardiovascular System Disorders: hypertension
Central and Peripheral Nervous System Disorders: confusion, somnolence, speech disorder
Gastrointestinal System Disorders: constipation, dyspepsia, gastroenteritis, hemorrhagic rectum, hiatus hernia, vomiting
Hearing and Vestibular Disorders: earache
Heart Rate and Rhythm Disorders: palpitation
Metabolic and Nutritional Disorders: edema, edema peripheral
Musculoskeletal System Disorders: arthritis, leg cramps, hypertonia, muscle disorder, myalgia
Myo/Endo/Pericardial and Valve Disorders: angina pectoris
Psychiatric Disorders: anxiety, impaired concentration, insomnia, personality disorder
Reproductive System Disorders: leukorrhea, uterine fibroid, vaginal dryness, fungal vaginitis, vaginitis
Resistance Mechanism Disorders: abscess, herpes simplex
Respiratory System Disorders: bronchitis, nasal congestion, pharyngitis, pneumonitis, sinusitis
Skin and Appendages Disorders: acne, verruca, wound debridement
Urinary System Disorders: urinary tract infection
Vision Disorders: abnormal vision
White Cell and Resistance Disorders: lymphadenopathy

The following adverse experiences have been reported with PROMETRIUM Capsules in other U.S. clinical trials: increased sweating, asthenia, tooth disorder, anorexia, increased appetite, nervousness, and breast enlargement.

The following spontaneous adverse events have been reported during the marketing of PROMETRIUM Capsules: reversible cases of hepatitis and elevated transaminases. These events occurred mainly in patients receiving high doses of up to 1200 mg. Additionally, rare instances of syncope with and without hypotension have been reported.

The following additional adverse experiences have been observed in women taking progestins in general: breakthrough bleeding, spotting, change in menstrual flow, amenorrhea, changes in weight (increase or decrease), changes in the cervical squamo-columnar junction and cervical secretions, cholestatic jaundice, anaphylactoid reactions and anaphylaxis, rash (allergic) with and without pruritus, melasma or chloasma, pyrexia, and insomnia.

OVERDOSAGE

No studies on overdosage have been conducted in humans. In the case of overdosage, PROMETRIUM Capsules should be discontinued, and the patient should be treated symptomatically.

DOSAGE AND ADMINISTRATION

Prevention of endometrial hyperplasia—PROMETRIUM Capsules should be given as a single daily dose in the evening, 200 mg orally for 12 days sequentially per 28 day cycle, to postmenopausal women with a uterus who are receiving daily conjugated estrogens tablets.

Secondary Amenorrhea—PROMETRIUM Capsules may be given as a single daily dose of 400 mg in the evening for 10 days.

HOW SUPPLIED

PROMETRIUM® (progesterone, USP) Capsules 100 mg are round, peach-colored capsules branded with black imprint "SV", available in bottles of 100 capsules (NDC0032-1708-01).

PROMETRIUM® (progesterone, USP) Capsules 200 mg are oval, pale yellow-colored capsules branded with black imprint "SV2", available in bottles of 100 capsules (NDC0032-1711-01).

Store at 25°C Excursions permitted to 15-30°C (59-86°F).
Dispense in tight, light-resistant container as defined in USP/NF, accompanied by a Patient Insert.
Protect from excessive moisture.

References:

1. International Agency for Research on Cancer (IARC) V.6, 1974; IARC V.21, 1979.
2. K.S. Larrson and D. Machin, Safety requirements for contraceptive steroids. F. Michal (ed.) Cambridge University Press, Cambridge. pp. 30-269, 1989.
3. Sixth Annual Report on Carcinogens V.2, pp 693-696, 1991.
4. Med. Sci. Res. 1987; 15:703-704.
5. Johnstone, E.E. and Franklin, R.R. (1964). Assay of progestins for fetal virilizing properties using the mouse. *Obstet Gynecol*. 23:359-62.
6. Seegmiller, R.E., Nelson, G.W. and Johnson, C.K. (1983) Evaluation of the teratogenic potential of Delalutin (17-hydroxyprogesterone caproate) in mice. *Teratology* 28: 201-8.
7. Suchowsky, G.K. and Junkmann, K. (1961). A study of the virilizing effects of progesterone on the female rat fetus. *Endocrinolgy* 68:341-9.
8. Scholer, H.F.L. and de Wachter, A.M. (1961). Evaluation of androgenic properties of progestational compounds in the rat by the female foetal masculinization test. *Acta. Endocrinol* 38:128-36.
9. Hudson, R., Pharriss, B.B., Tillson, S.A. and Reno, F. (1978). Preclinical evaluation of intrauterine progesterone as a contraceptive agent. III. Embryology and toxicology. Contraception 17:489-97.
10. Foote, W.D., Foote, W.C., and Foote, L.H. (1968). Influence of certain natural and synthetic steroids on genital development in guinea pigs. Fertil. Steril. 19:606-15.
11. Wharton, L.R. Jr. and Scott, R.B. (1964). Experimental production of genital lessions with norethindrone. Am J. Obstet. Gynecol. 89:701-15
12. Scialli, A.R. (1988). Developmental effects of progesterone and its derivatives. Reproductive Toxicol. 2:3-11.

Manufactured by: R. P. Scherer North America, St. Petersburg, FL 33716
Marketed by: Solvay Pharmaceuticals, Inc., Marietta, GA 30062.

9563 4E Rev 7/2000
Shown in Product Identification Guide, page 333

ROWASA® ℞

[*rō-wă-să*]
(Mesalamine)
Rectal Suspension Enema
4.0 grams/unit (60 mL)
℞ only

DESCRIPTION

The active ingredient in ROWASA® (Mesalamine) Rectal Suspension Enema, a disposable (60 mL) unit, is mesalamine, also known as 5-aminosalicylic acid (5-ASA). Chemically, mesalamine is 5-amino-2-hydroxybenzoic acid. The empirical formula is $C_7H_7NO_3$, representing a molecular weight of 153.14. The structural formula is:

Each rectal suspension enema unit contains 4 grams of mesalamine. In addition to mesalamine the preparation contains the inactive ingredients carbomer 934P, edetate disodium, potassium acetate, potassium metabisulfite, purified water and xanthan gum. Sodium benzoate is added as a preservative. The disposable unit consists of an applicator tip protected by a polyethylene cover and lubricated with USP white petrolatum. The unit has a one-way valve to prevent back flow of the dispensed product.

CLINICAL PHARMACOLOGY

Sulfasalazine is split by bacterial action in the colon into sulfapyridine (SP) and mesalamine (5-ASA). It is thought that the mesalamine component is therapeutically active in ulcerative colitis [A.K. Azad Khan *et al*, **Lancet** 2:892-895 (1977)]. The usual oral dose of sulfasalazine for active ulcerative colitis in adults is two to four grams per day in divided doses. Four grams of sulfasalazine provide 1.6 g of free mesalamine to the colon. Each ROWASA® (Mesalamine) Rectal Suspension Enema delivers up to 4 g of mesalamine to the left side of the colon.

The mechanism of action of mesalamine (and sulfasalazine) is unknown, but appears to be topical rather than systemic. Mucosal production of arachidonic acid (AA) metabolites, both through the cyclooxygenase pathways, i.e., prostanoids, and through the lipoxygenase pathways, i.e., leukotrienes (LTs) and hydroxyeicosatetraenoic acids (HETEs) is increased in patients with chronic inflammatory bowel disease, and it is possible that mesalamine diminishes inflammation by blocking cyclooxygenase and inhibiting prostaglandin (PG) production in the colon.

Preclinical Toxicology

Preclinical studies have shown the kidney to be the major target organ for mesalamine toxicity. Adverse renal function changes were observed in rats after a single 600 mg/kg oral dose, but not after a 200 mg/kg dose. Gross kidney lesions, including papillary necrosis, were observed after a single oral >900 mg/kg dose, and after i.v. doses of >214 mg/kg. Mice responded similarly. In a 13-week oral (gavage) dose study in rats, the high dose of 640 mg/kg/day mesalamine caused deaths, probably due to renal failure, and dose-related renal lesions (papillary necrosis and/or multifocal tubular injury) were seen in most rats given the high dose (males and females) as well as in males receiving lower doses 160 mg/kg/day. Renal lesions were not observed in the 160 mg/kg/day female rats. Minimal tubular epithelial damage was seen in the 40 mg/kg/day males and was reversible. In a six-month oral study in dogs, the no-observable dose level of mesalamine was 40 mg/kg/day and doses of 80 mg/kg/day and higher caused renal pathology similar to that described for the rat. In a combined 52-week toxicity and 127-week carcinogenicity study in rats, degeneration in kidneys was observed at doses of 100 mg/kg/day and above admixed with diet for 52 weeks, and at 127 weeks increased incidence of kidney degeneration and hyalinization of basement membranes and Bowman's capsule were seen at 100 mg/kg/day and above. In the 12 month eye toxicity study in dogs, Keratoconjunctivitis Sicca (KCS) occurred at oral doses of 40 mg/kg/day and above. The oral preclinical studies were done with a highly bioavailable suspension where absorption throughout the gastrointestinal tract occurred. The human dose of 4 grams represents approximately 80 mg/kg but when mesalamine is given rectally as a suspension, absorption is poor and limited to the distal colon (see **Pharmacokinetics**). Overt renal toxicity has not been observed (see **ADVERSE REACTIONS** and **PRECAUTIONS**), but the potential must be considered.

Pharmacokinetics

Mesalamine administered rectally as ROWASA® (Mesalamine) Rectal Suspension Enema is poorly absorbed from the colon and is excreted principally in the feces during subsequent bowel movements. The extent of absorption is dependent upon the retention time of the drug product, and there is considerable individual variation. At steady state, approximately 10 to 30% of the daily 4-gram dose can be recovered in cumulative 24-hour urine collections. Other than the kidney, the organ distribution and other bioavailability characteristics of absorbed mesalamine in man are not known. It is known that the compound undergoes acetylation but whether this process takes place at colonic or systemic sites has not been elucidated.

Whatever the metabolic site, most of the absorbed mesalamine is excreted in the urine as the N-acetyl-5-ASA metabolite. The poor colonic absorption of rectally administered mesalamine is substantiated by the low serum concentration of 5-ASA and N-acetyl-5-ASA seen in ulcerative colitis patients after dosage with mesalamine. Under clinical conditions patients demonstrated plasma levels 10 to 12 hours post mesalamine administration of 2 μg/mL, about two-thirds of which was the N-acetyl metabolite. While the elimination half-life of mesalamine is short (0.5 to 1.5 h), the acetylated metabolite exhibits a half-life of 5 to 10 hours [U. Klotz, **Clin. Pharmacokin.** 10:285-302 (1985)]. In addition, steady state plasma levels demonstrated a lack of accumulation of either free or metabolized drug during repeated daily administrations.

Efficacy

In a placebo-controlled, international, multicenter trial of 153 patients with active distal ulcerative colitis, proctosigmoiditis or proctitis, ROWASA® (Mesalamine) Rectal Suspension Enema reduced the overall disease activity index (DAI) and individual components as follows:

[See first table at top of next page]

Differences between ROWASA® and placebo were also statistically different in subgroups of patients on concurrent sulfasalazine and in those having an upper disease boundary between 5 and 20 or 20 and 40 cm. Significant differences between ROWASA® and placebo were not achieved in those subgroups of patients on concurrent prednisone or with an upper disease boundary between 40 and 50 cm.

INDICATIONS AND USAGE

ROWASA® (Mesalamine) Rectal Suspension Enema is indicated for the treatment of active mild to moderate distal ulcerative colitis, proctosigmoiditis or proctitis.

CONTRAINDICATIONS

ROWASA® (Mesalamine) Rectal Suspension Enema is contraindicated for patients known to have hypersensitivity to the drug or any component of this medication.

WARNINGS

ROWASA® (Mesalamine) Rectal Suspension Enema contains potassium metabisulfite, a sulfite that may cause allergic-type reactions including anaphylactic symptoms and life-threatening or less severe asthmatic episodes in certain susceptible people. The overall prevalence of sulfite sensitivity in the general population is unknown but probably low. Sulfite sensitivity is seen more frequently in asthmatic or in atopic nonasthmatic persons. Epinephrine is the preferred treatment for serious allergic or emergency situations even though epinephrine injection contains sodium or potassium metabisulfite with the above-mentioned potential liabilities. The alternatives to using epinephrine in a life-threatening situation may not be satisfactory. The presence of a sulfite(s) in epinephrine injection should not deter the administration of the drug for treatment of serious allergic or other emergency situations.

PRECAUTIONS

Mesalamine has been implicated in the production of an acute intolerance syndrome characterized by cramping, acute abdominal pain and bloody diarrhea, sometimes fever, headache and a rash; in such cases prompt withdrawal is required. The patient's history of sulfasalazine intolerance, if any, should be re-evaluated. If a rechallenge is performed later in order to validate the hypersensitivity it should be carried out under close supervision and only if clearly needed, giving consideration to reduced dosage. In the literature one patient previously sensitive to sulfasalazine was rechallenged with 400 mg oral mesalamine; within eight hours she experienced headache, fever, intensive abdominal colic, profuse diarrhea and was readmitted as an emergency. She responded poorly to steroid therapy and two weeks later a pancolectomy was required.

Although renal abnormalities were not noted in the clinical trials with ROWASA® (Mesalamine) Rectal Suspension Enema, the possibility of increased absorption of mesalamine and concomitant renal tubular damage as noted in the preclinical studies must be kept in mind. Patients on ROWASA® (Mesalamine) Rectal Suspension Enema, especially those on concurrent oral products which liberate mesalamine and those with preexisting renal disease, should be carefully monitored with urinalysis, BUN and creatinine studies.

In a clinical trial most patients who were hypersensitive to sulfasalazine were able to take mesalamine enemas without evidence of any allergic reaction. Nevertheless, caution should be exercised when mesalamine is initially used in patients known to be allergic to sulfasalazine. These patients should be instructed to discontinue therapy if signs of rash or fever become apparent.

While using ROWASA® (Mesalamine) Rectal Suspension Enema some patients have developed pancolitis. However, extension of upper disease boundary and/or flare-ups occurred less often in the ROWASA® (Mesalamine) Rectal Suspension Enema treated group than in the placebo-treated group.

Rare instances of pericarditis have been reported with mesalamine containing products including sulfasalazine. Cases of pericarditis have also been reported as manifestations of inflammatory bowel disease. In the cases reported with ROWASA® (Mesalamine) Rectal Suspension Enema there have been positive rechallenges with mesalamine or mesalamine containing products. In one of these cases, however, a second rechallenge with sulfasalazine was negative throughout a 2 month follow-up. Chest pain or dyspnea in patients treated with ROWASA® (Mesalamine) Rectal Suspension Enema should be investigated with this information in mind. Discontinuation of ROWASA® (Mesalamine) Rectal Suspension Enema may be warranted in some cases, but rechallenge with mesalamine can be performed under careful clinical observation should the continued therapeutic need for mesalamine be present.

Carcinogenesis, Mutagenesis, Impairment of Fertility

Mesalamine caused no increase in the incidence of neoplastic lesions over controls in a two-year study of Wistar rats fed up to 320 mg/kg/day of mesalamine admixed with diet. Mesalamine is not mutagenic to Salmonella typhimurium tester strains TA98, TA100, TA1535, TA1537, TA1538. There were no reverse mutations in an assay using E. coli strain WP2UVRA. There were no effects in an *in vivo* mouse micronucleus assay at 600 mg/kg and in an *in vivo* sister chromatid exchange at doses up to 610 mg/kg. No effects on fertility were observed in rats receiving up to 320 mg/kg/day. The oligospermia and infertility in men associated with sulfasalazine have not been reported with mesalamine.

Pregnancy (Category B)

Teratologic studies have been performed in rats and rabbits at oral doses up to five and eight times respectively, the maximum recommended human dose, and have revealed no evidence of harm to the embryo or the fetus. There are, however, no adequate and well controlled studies in pregnant women for either sulfasalazine or 5-ASA. Because animal reproduction studies are not always predictive of human response, 5-ASA should be used during pregnancy only if clearly needed.

Nursing Mothers

It is not known whether mesalamine or its metabolite(s) are excreted in human milk. As a general rule, nursing should not be undertaken while a patient is on a drug since many drugs are excreted in human milk.

Pediatric Use

Safety and effectiveness in pediatric patients have not been established.

ADVERSE REACTIONS

Clinical Adverse Experience

ROWASA® (Mesalamine) Rectal Suspension Enema is usually well tolerated. Most adverse effects have been mild and transient.

[See second table at right]

In addition, the following adverse events have been identified during post-approval use of products which contain (or are metabolized to) mesalamine in clinical practice: nephrotoxicity, pancreatitis, fibrosing alveolitis and elevated liver enzymes. Cases of pancreatitis and fibrosing alveolitis have been reported as manifestations of inflammatory bowel disease as well. Published case reports and/or spontaneous post marketing surveillance have described rare instances of aplastic anemia, agranulocytosis, thrombocytopenia, or eosinophilia. Anemia, leukocytosis, and thrombocytosis can be part of the clinical presentation of inflammatory bowel disease.

Hair Loss

Mild hair loss characterized by "more hair in the comb" but no withdrawal from clinical trials has been observed in seven of 815 mesalamine patients but none of the placebo-treated patients. In the literature there are at least six additional patients with mild hair loss who received either mesalamine or sulfasalazine. Retreatment is not always associated with repeated hair loss.

OVERDOSAGE

There have been no documented reports of serious toxicity in man resulting from massive overdosing with mesalamine. Under ordinary circumstances, mesalamine absorption from the colon is limited.

DOSAGE AND ADMINISTRATION

The usual dosage of ROWASA® (Mesalamine) Rectal Suspension Enema in 60 mL units is one rectal instillation (4 grams) once a day, preferably at bedtime, and retained for approximately eight hours. While the effect of ROWASA® (Mesalamine) Rectal Suspension Enema may be seen within three to twenty-one days, the usual course of therapy would be from three to six weeks depending on symptoms and sigmoidoscopic findings. Studies available to date have not assessed if ROWASA® (Mesalamine) Rectal Suspension Enema will modify relapse rates after the 6-week short-term treatment. ROWASA® (Mesalamine) Rectal Suspension Enema is for rectal use only.

Patients should be instructed to shake the bottle well to make sure the suspension is homogeneous. The patient should remove the protective sheath from the applicator tip. Holding the bottle at the neck will not cause any of the medication to be discharged. The position most often used is obtained by lying on the left side (to facilitate migration into the sigmoid colon); with the lower leg extended and the upper right leg flexed forward for balance. An alternative is the knee-chest position. The applicator tip should be gently inserted in the rectum pointing toward the umbilicus. A steady squeezing of the bottle will discharge most of the preparation. The preparation should be taken at bedtime with the objective of retaining it all night. Patient instructions are included with every seven units.

HOW SUPPLIED

ROWASA® (Mesalamine) Rectal Suspension Enema for rectal administration is an off-white to tan colored suspension. Each disposable enema bottle contains 4.0 grams of mesalamine in 60 mL aqueous suspension. Enema bottles are supplied in boxed, foil-wrapped trays as follows:.

NDC 0032-1924-82 (Carton of 7 Bottles)
NDC 0032-1924-28 (Carton of 28 Bottles)

ROWASA® (Mesalamine) Rectal Suspension Enemas are for rectal use only.

Patient instructions are included.

STORAGE

Store at controlled room temperature 20 to 25°C (68 to 77°F). Once the foil-wrapped unit of seven bottles is opened, all enemas should be used promptly as directed by your physician. **Contents of enemas removed from the foil pouch may darken with time. Slight darkening will not affect potency, however, enemas with dark brown contents should be discarded.**

NOTE: ROWASA® (Mesalamine) Rectal Suspension Enema will cause staining of direct contact surfaces, including but not limited to fabrics, flooring, painted surfaces, marble, granite, vinyl, and enamel. Take care in choosing a suitable location for administration of this product.

EFFECT OF TREATMENT ON SEVERITY OF DISEASE
DATA FROM U.S.-CANADA TRIAL
COMBINED RESULTS OF EIGHT CENTERS
Activity Indices, mean

		N	Baseline	Day 22	EndPoint	Change Baseline to Endpoint†
Overall DAI	ROWASA®	76	7.42	4.05**	3.37***	-55.07%***
	Placebo	77	7.40	6.03	5.83	-21.58%
Stool Frequency	ROWASA®		1.58	1.11*	1.01**	-0.57*
	Placebo		1.92	1.47	1.50	-0.41
Rectal Bleeding	ROWASA®		1.82	0.59***	0.51***	-1.30***
	Placebo		1.73	1.21	1.11	-0.61
Mucosal Inflammation	ROWASA®		2.17	1.22**	0.96***	-1.21**
	Placebo		2.18	1.74	1.61	-0.56
Physician's Assessment of Disease Severity	ROWASA®		1.86	1.13***	0.88***	-0.97***
	Placebo		1.87	1.62	1.55	-0.30

Each parameter has a 4-point scale with a numerical rating:
0=normal, 1=mild, 2=moderate, 3=severe. The four parameters are added together to produce a maximum overall DAI of 12.
† Percent change for overall DAI only (calculated by taking the average of the change for each individual patient).
* Significant ROWASA®/placebo difference. $p<0.05$
** Significant ROWASA®/placebo difference. $p<0.01$
*** Significant ROWASA®/placebo difference. $p<0.001$

ADVERSE REACTIONS OCCURRING IN MORE THAN 0.1%
OF ROWASA® (MESALAMINE) RECTAL SUSPENSION ENEMA
TREATED PATIENTS (COMPARISON TO PLACEBO)

SYMPTOM	ROWASA® N=815 N	%	PLACEBO N=128 N	%
Abdominal Pain/Cramps/Discomfort	66	8.10	10	7.81
Headache	53	6.50	16	12.50
Gas/Flatulence	50	6.13	5	3.91
Nausea	47	5.77	12	9.38
Flu	43	5.28	1	0.78
Tired/Weak/Malaise/Fatigue	28	3.44	8	6.25
Fever	26	3.19	0	0.00
Rash/Spots	23	2.82	4	3.12
Cold/Sore Throat	19	2.33	9	7.03
Diarrhea	17	2.09	5	3.91
Leg/Joint Pain	17	2.09	1	0.78
Dizziness	15	1.84	3	2.34
Bloating	12	1.47	2	1.56
Back Pain	11	1.35	1	0.78
Pain on Insertion of Enema Tip	11	1.35	1	0.78
Hemorrhoids	11	1.35	0	0.00
Itching	10	1.23	1	0.78
Rectal Pain	10	1.23	0	0.00
Constipation	8	0.98	4	3.12
Hair Loss	7	0.86	0	0.00
Peripheral Edema	5	0.61	11	8.59
UTI/Urinary Burning	5	0.61	4	3.12
Rectal Pain/Soreness/Burning	5	0.61	3	2.34
Asthenia	1	0.12	4	3.12
Insomnia	1	0.12	3	2.34

0645
15E Rev 5/2003

U.S. Pat. Nos. 4657900 and RE33239

Solvay
Pharmaceuticals, Inc.
Marietta, GA 30062

PATIENT INSTRUCTIONS

How to Use this Medication.

Best results are achieved if the bowel is emptied immediately before the medication is given.

NOTE: ROWASA® (Mesalamine) Rectal Suspension Enema will cause staining of direct contact surfaces, including but not limited to fabrics, flooring, painted surfaces, marble, granite, vinyl, and enamel. Take care in choosing a suitable location for administration of this product.

1. Remove the Bottles

a. Remove the bottles from the protective foil pouch by tearing or by using scissors as shown, being careful not to squeeze or puncture bottles. ROWASA® (Mesalamine) Rectal Suspension Enema is an off-white to tan colored suspension. Once the foil-wrapped unit of seven bottles is opened, all enemas should be used promptly as directed by your physician. **Contents of enemas removed from the foil pouch may darken with time. Slight darkening will not affect potency, however, enemas with dark brown contents should be discarded.**

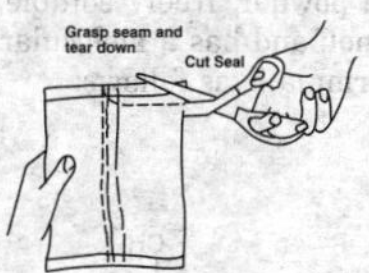

2. Prepare the Medication for Administration

a. Shake the bottle well to make sure that the medication is thoroughly mixed.

Continued on next page

Rowasa—Cont.

b. Remove the protective sheath from the applicator tip. Hold the bottle at the neck so as not to cause any of the medication to be discharged.

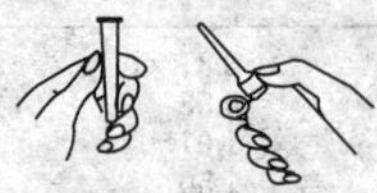

3. Assume the Correct Body Position

a. Best results are obtained by lying on the left side with the left leg extended and the right leg flexed forward for balance.

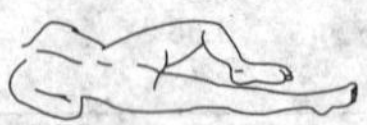

b. An alternative to lying on the left side is the "knee-chest" position as shown here.

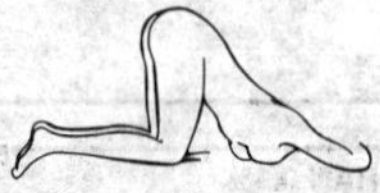

4. Administer the Medication

a. Gently insert the lubricated applicator tip into the rectum to prevent damage to the rectal wall, pointed slightly toward the navel.

b. Grasp the bottle firmly, then tilt slightly so that the nozzle is aimed toward the back, squeeze slowly to instill the medication. Steady hand pressure will discharge most of the medication. After administering, withdraw and discard the bottle.

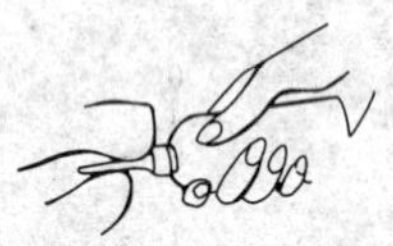

c. Remain in position for at least 30 minutes to allow thorough distribution of the medication internally. Retain the medication all night, if possible.

0645
15E Rev 5/2003

Solvay
Pharmaceuticals, Inc.
Marietta, GA 30062
Shown in Product Identification Guide, page 333

Somerset Pharmaceuticals, Inc.

2202 NORTH WESTSHORE BOULEVARD
SUITE 450
TAMPA, FLORIDA 33607

For Medical Information Contact:
Generally:
Professional Services Department
(813) 288-0040
FAX: (813) 282-3804
In Emergencies:
(800) 892-8889
FAX: (813) 282-0287

ELDEPRYL® ℞
(SELEGILINE HYDROCHLORIDE)
CAPSULES
℞ Only

DESCRIPTION

ELDEPRYL (selegiline hydrochloride) is a levorotatory acetylenic derivative of phenethylamine. It is commonly referred to in the clinical and pharmacological literature as l-deprenyl.

The chemical name is: (R)-(-)-*N*,2-dimethyl-*N*-2-propynylphenethylamine hydrochloride. It is a white to near white crystalline powder, freely soluble in water, chloroform, and methanol, and has a molecular weight of 223.75. The structural formula is as follows:

CH_3; H; $NCH_2C{\equiv}CH$ · HCl; C; CH_2; CH_3

Each aqua blue capsule is band imprinted with the Somerset logo on the cap and "Eldepryl 5 mg" on the body. Each capsule contains 5 mg selegiline hydrochloride. Inactive ingredients are citric acid, lactose, magnesium stearate, and microcrystalline cellulose.

CLINICAL PHARMACOLOGY

The mechanisms accounting for selegiline's beneficial adjunctive action in the treatment of Parkinson's disease are not fully understood. Inhibition of monoamine oxidase, type B, activity is generally considered to be of primary importance; in addition, there is evidence that selegiline may act through other mechanisms to increase dopaminergic activity.

Selegiline is best known as an irreversible inhibitor of monoamine oxidase (MAO), an intracellular enzyme associated with the outer membrane of mitochondria. Selegiline inhibits MAO by acting as a 'suicide' substrate for the enzyme; that is, it is converted by MAO to an active moiety which combines irreversibly with the active site and/or the enzyme's essential FAD cofactor. Because selegiline has greater affinity for type B rather than for type A active sites, it can serve as a selective inhibitor of MAO type B if it is administered at the recommended dose.

MAOs are widely distributed throughout the body; their concentration is especially high in liver, kidney, stomach, intestinal wall, and brain. MAOs are currently subclassified into two types, A and B, which differ in their substrate specificity and tissue distribution. In humans, intestinal MAO is predominantly type A, while most of that in brain is type B. In CNS neurons, MAO plays an important role in the catabolism of catecholamines (dopamine, norepinephrine and epinephrine) and serotonin. MAOs are also important in the catabolism of various exogenous amines found in a variety of foods and drugs. MAO in the GI tract and liver (primarily type A), for example, is thought to provide vital protection from exogenous amines (e.g., tyramine) that have the capacity, if absorbed intact, to cause a 'hypertensive crisis,' the so-called 'cheese reaction.' (If large amounts of certain exogenous amines gain access to the systemic circulation - e.g., from fermented cheese, red wine, herring, over-the-counter cough/cold medications, etc. - they are taken up by adrenergic neurons and displace norepinephrine from storage sites within membrane bound vesicles. Subsequent release of the displaced norepinephrine causes the rise in systemic blood pressure, etc.)

In theory, since MAO A of the gut is not inhibited, patients treated with selegiline at a dose of 10 mg a day should be able to take medications containing pharmacologically active amines and consume tyramine-containing foods without risk of uncontrolled hypertension. Although rare, a few reports of hypertensive reactions have occurred in patients receiving Eldepryl at the recommended dose, with tyramine-containing foods. In addition, one case of hypertensive crisis has been reported in a patient taking the recommended dose of selegiline and a sympathomimetic medication, ephedrine. The pathophysiology of the 'cheese reaction' is complicated and, in addition to its ability to inhibit MAO B selectively, selegiline's relative freedom from this reaction has been attributed to an ability to prevent tyramine and other indirect acting sympathomimetics from displacing norepinephrine from adrenergic neurons. However, until the pathophysiology of the cheese reaction is more completely understood, it seems prudent to assume that selegiline can ordinarily only be used safely without dietary restrictions at doses where it presumably selectively inhibits its MAO B (e.g., 10 mg/day).

In short, attention to the dose dependent nature of selegiline's selectivity is critical if it is to be used without elaborate restrictions being placed on diet and concomitant drug use although, as noted above, a few cases of hypertensive reactions have been reported at the recommended dose. (See WARNINGS and PRECAUTIONS.)

It is important to be aware that selegiline may have pharmacological effects unrelated to MAO B inhibition. As noted above, there is some evidence that it may increase dopaminergic activity by other mechanisms, including interfering with dopamine re-uptake at the synapse. Effects resulting from selegiline administration may also be mediated through its metabolites. Two of its three principal metabolites, amphetamine and methamphetamine, have pharmacological actions of their own; they interfere with neuronal uptake and enhance release of several neurotransmitters (e.g., norepinephrine, dopamine, serotonin). However, the extent to which these metabolites contribute to the effects of selegiline are unknown.

Rationale for the Use of a Selective Monoamine Oxidase Type B Inhibitor in Parkinson's Disease: Many of the prominent symptoms of Parkinson's disease are due to a deficiency of striatal dopamine that is the consequence of a progressive degeneration and loss of a population of dopaminergic neurons which originate in the substantia nigra of the midbrain and project to the basal ganglia or striatum. Early in the course of Parkinson's Disease, the deficit in the capacity of these neurons to synthesize dopamine can be overcome by administration of exogenous levodopa, usually given in combination with a peripheral decarboxylase inhibitor (carbidopa).

With the passage of time, due to the progression of the disease and/or the effect of sustained treatment, the efficacy and quality of the therapeutic response to levodopa diminishes. Thus, after several years of levodopa treatment, the response, for a given dose of levodopa, is shorter, has less predictable onset and offset (i.e., there is 'wearing off'), and is often accompanied by side effects (e.g., dyskinesia, akinesias, on-off phenomena, freezing, etc.).

This deteriorating response is currently interpreted as a manifestation of the inability of the ever decreasing population of intact nigrostriatal neurons to synthesize and release adequate amounts of dopamine.

MAO B inhibition may be useful in this setting because, by blocking the catabolism of dopamine, it would increase the net amount of dopamine available (i.e., it would increase the pool of dopamine). Whether or not this mechanism or an alternative one actually accounts for the observed beneficial effects of adjunctive selegiline is unknown.

Selegiline's benefit in Parkinson's disease has only been documented as an adjunct to levodopa/carbidopa. Whether or not it might be effective as a sole treatment is unknown, but past attempts to treat Parkinson's disease with non-selective MAOI monotherapy are reported to have been unsuccessful. It is important to note that attempts to treat Parkinsonian patients with combinations of levodopa and currently marketed non-selective MAO inhibitors were abandoned because of multiple side effects including hypertension, increase in involuntary movement, and toxic delirium.

Pharmacokinetic Information (Absorption, Distribution, Metabolism and Elimination—ADME):

The absolute bioavailability of selegiline following oral dosing is not known; however, selegiline undergoes extensive metabolism (presumably attributable to presystemic clearance in gut and liver). The major plasma metabolites are N-desmethylselegiline, L-amphetamine and L-methamphetamine. Only N-desmethylselegiline has MAO-B inhibiting activity. The peak plasma levels of these metabolites following a single oral dose of 10 mg are from 4 to almost 20 times greater than that of the maximum plasma concentration of selegiline [1 ng/mL]. The maximum concentrations of amphetamine and methamphetamine, however, are far below those ordinarily expected to produce clinically important effects.

Single oral dose studies do not predict multiple dose kinetics, however. At steady state the peak plasma level of selegiline is 4 fold that obtained following a single dose. Metabolite concentrations increase to a lesser extent, averaging 2 fold that seen after a single dose.

The bioavailability of selegiline is increased 3 to 4 fold when it is taken with food.

The extent of systemic exposure to selegiline at a given dose varies considerably among individuals. Estimates of systemic clearance of selegiline are not available. Following a single oral dose, the mean elimination half-life of selegiline is two hours. Under steady state conditions the elimination half-life increases to ten hours.

Because selegiline's inhibition of MAO-B is irreversible, it is impossible to predict the extent of MAO-B inhibition from steady state plasma levels. For the same reason, it is not possible to predict the rate of recovery of MAO-B activity as a function of plasma levels. The recovery of MAO-B activity is a function of de novo protein synthesis; however, information about the rate of de novo protein synthesis is not yet available. Although platelet MAO-B activity returns to the normal range within 5 to 7 days of selegiline discontinuation, the linkage between platelet and brain MAO-B inhibition is not fully understood nor is the relationship of MAO-B inhibition to the clinical effect established (see Clinical Pharmacology).

Special Populations:

Renal Impairment:

No pharmacokinetic information is available on selegiline or its metabolites in renally impaired subjects.

Hepatic Impairment:

No pharmacokinetic information is available on selegiline or its metabolites in hepatically impaired subjects.

Age:

Although a general conclusion about the effects of age on the pharmacokinetics of selegiline is not warranted because of the size of the sample evaluated (12 subjects greater than 60 years of age, 12 subjects between the ages of 18 to 30), systemic exposure was about twice as great in older as compared to a younger population given a single oral dose of 10 mg.

Gender:

No information is available on the effects of gender on the pharmacokinetics of selegiline.

INDICATIONS AND USAGE

ELDEPRYL is indicated as an adjunct in the management of Parkinsonian patients being treated with levodopa/carbidopa who exhibit deterioration in the quality of their response to this therapy. There is no evidence from controlled studies that selegiline has any beneficial effect in the absence of concurrent levodopa therapy.

Evidence supporting this claim was obtained in randomized controlled clinical investigations that compared the effects of added selegiline or placebo in patients receiving levodopa/carbidopa. Selegiline was significantly superior to placebo on all three principal outcome measures employed: change from baseline in daily levodopa/carbidopa dose, the amount of 'off' time, and patient self-rating of treatment success. Beneficial effects were also observed on other measures of treatment success (e.g., measures of reduced end of dose akinesia, decreased tremor and sialorrhea, improved speech and dressing ability and improved overall disability as assessed by walking and comparison to previous state).

CONTRAINDICATIONS

ELDEPRYL is contraindicated in patients with a known hypersensitivity to this drug.

ELDEPRYL is contraindicated for use with meperidine (DEMEROL & other trade names). This contraindication is often extended to other opioids. (See Drug Interactions.)

WARNINGS

Selegiline should not be used at daily doses exceeding those recommended (10 mg/day) because of the risks associated with nonselective inhibition of MAO. (See CLINICAL PHARMACOLOGY.)

The selectivity of selegiline for MAO B may not be absolute even at the recommended daily dose of 10 mg a day. Rare cases of hypertensive reactions associated with ingestion of tyramine-containing foods have been reported in patients taking the recommended daily dose of selegiline. The selectivity is further diminished with increasing daily doses. The precise dose at which selegiline becomes a non-selective inhibitor of all MAO is unknown, but may be in the range of 30 to 40 mg a day.

Severe CNS toxicity associated with hyperpyrexia and death have been reported with the combination of tricyclic antidepressants and non-selective MAOIs (NARDIL, PARNATE). A similar reaction has been reported for a patient on amitriptyline and ELDEPRYL. Another patient receiving protriptyline and ELDEPRYL developed tremors, agitation, and restlessness followed by unresponsiveness and death two weeks after ELDEPRYL was added. Related adverse events including hypertension, syncope, asystole, diaphoresis, seizures, changes in behavioral and mental status, and muscular rigidity have also been reported in some patients receiving ELDEPRYL and various tricyclic antidepressants.

Serious, sometimes fatal, reactions with signs and symptoms that may include hyperthermia, rigidity, myoclonus, autonomic instability with rapid fluctuations of the vital signs, and mental status changes that include extreme agitation progressing to delirium and coma have been reported with patients receiving a combination of fluoxetine hydrochloride (PROZAC) and non-selective MAOIs. Similar signs have been reported in some patients on the combination of ELDEPRYL (10 mg a day) and selective serotonin reuptake inhibitors including fluoxetine, sertraline and paroxetine.

Since the mechanisms of these reactions are not fully understood, it seems prudent, in general, to avoid this combination of ELDEPRYL and tricyclic antidepressants as well as ELDEPRYL and selective serotonin reuptake inhibitors. At least 14 days should elapse between discontinuation of ELDEPRYL and initiation of treatment with a tricyclic antidepressant or selective serotonin reuptake inhibitors. Because of the long half-lives of fluoxetine and its active metabolite, at least five weeks (perhaps longer, especially if fluoxetine has been prescribed chronically and/or at higher doses) should elapse between discontinuation of fluoxetine and initiation of treatment with ELDEPRYL.

PRECAUTIONS

General:

Some patients given selegiline may experience an exacerbation of levodopa associated side effects, presumably due to the increased amounts of dopamine reaction with super sensitive, post-synaptic receptors. These effects may often be mitigated by reducing the dose of levodopa/carbidopa by approximately 10 to 30%.

The decision to prescribe selegiline should take into consideration that the MAO system of enzymes is complex and incompletely understood and there is only a limited amount of carefully documented clinical experience with selegiline. Consequently, the full spectrum of possible responses to selegiline may not have been observed in pre-marketing evaluation of the drug. It is advisable, therefore, to observe patients closely for atypical responses.

Information for Patients:

Patients should be advised of the possible need to reduce levodopa dosage after the initiation of ELDEPRYL therapy.

Patients (or their families if the patient is incompetent) should be advised not to exceed the daily recommended dose of 10 mg. The risk of using higher daily doses of selegiline should be explained, and a brief description of the 'cheese reaction' provided. Rare hypertensive reactions with selegiline at recommended doses associated with dietary influences have been reported.

Consequently, it may be useful to inform patients (or their families) about the signs and symptoms associated with MAOI induced hypertensive reactions. In particular, patients should be urged to report, immediately, any severe headache or other atypical or unusual symptoms not previously experienced.

Laboratory Tests:

No specific laboratory tests are deemed essential for the management of patients on ELDEPRYL. Periodic routine evaluation of all patients, however, is appropriate.

Drug Interactions:

The occurrence of stupor, muscular rigidity, severe agitation, and elevated temperature has been reported in some patients receiving the combination of selegiline and meperidine. Symptoms usually resolve over days when the combination is discontinued. This is typical of the interaction of meperidine and MAOIs. Other serious reactions (including severe agitation, hallucinations, and death) have been reported in patients receiving this combination (see **CONTRAINDICATIONS**). Severe toxicity has also been reported in patients receiving the combination of tricyclic antidepressants and ELDEPRYL and selective serotonin reuptake inhibitors and ELDEPRYL. (See **WARNINGS** for details). One case of hypertensive crisis has been reported in a patient taking the recommended doses of selegiline and a sympathomimetic medication (ephedrine).

Carcinogenesis, Mutagenesis, and Impairment of Fertility:

Assessment of the carcinogenic potential of selegiline in mice and rats is ongoing.

Selegiline did not induce mutations or chromosomal damage when tested in the bacterial mutation assay in Salmonella typhimurium and in an *in vivo* chromosomal aberration assay. While these studies provide some reassurance that selegiline is not mutagenic or clastogenic, they are not definitive because of methodological limitations. No definitive *in vitro* chromosomal aberration or *in vitro* mammalian gene mutation assays have been performed.

The effect of selegiline on fertility has not been adequately assessed.

Pregnancy:

Pregnancy Category C: No teratogenic effects were observed in a study of embryo-fetal development in Sprague-Dawley rats at oral doses of 4, 12, and 36 mg/kg or 4, 12 and 35 times the human therapeutic dose on a mg/m^2 basis. No teratogenic effects were observed in a study of embryo-fetal development in New Zealand White rabbits at oral doses of 5, 25, and 50 mg/kg or 10, 48, and 95 times the human therapeutic dose on a mg/m^2 basis; however, in this study, the number of litters produced at the two higher doses was less than recommended for assessing teratogenic potential. In the rat study, there was a decrease in fetal body weight at the highest dose tested. In the rabbit study, increases in total resorptions and % post-implantation loss, and a decrease in the number of live fetuses per dam occurred at the highest dose tested. In a peri- and postnatal development study in Sprague-Dawley rats (oral doses of 4, 16, and 64 mg/kg or 4, 15, and 62 times the human therapeutic dose on a mg/m^2 basis), an increase in the number of stillbirths and decreases in the number of pups per dam, pup survival, and pup body weight (at birth and throughout the lactation period) were observed at the two highest doses. At the highest dose tested, no pups born alive survived to Day 4 postpartum. Postnatal development at the highest dose tested in dams could not be evaluated because of the lack of surviving pups. The reproductive performance of the untreated offspring was not assessed.

There are no adequate and well-controlled studies in pregnant women. Selegiline should be used during pregnancy only if the potential benefit justifies the potential risk to the fetus.

Nursing Mothers:

It is not known whether selegiline hydrochloride is excreted in human milk. Because many drugs are excreted in human milk, consideration should be given to discontinuing the use of all but absolutely essential drug treatments in nursing women.

Pediatric Use:

The effects of selegiline hydrochloride in children have not been evaluated.

ADVERSE REACTIONS

Introduction:

The number of patients who received selegiline in prospectively monitored pre-marketing studies is limited. While other sources of information about the use of selegiline are available (e.g., literature reports, foreign post-marketing reports, etc.) they do not provide the kind of information necessary to estimate the incidence of adverse events. Thus, overall incidence figures for adverse reactions associated with the use of selegiline cannot be provided. Many of the adverse reactions seen have also been reported as symptoms of dopamine excess.

Moreover, the importance and severity of various reactions reported often cannot be ascertained. One index of relative importance, however, is whether or not a reaction caused treatment discontinuation. In prospective pre-marketing studies, the following events led, in decreasing order of frequency, to discontinuation of treatment with selegiline: nausea, hallucinations, confusion, depression, loss of balance, insomnia, orthostatic hypotension, increased akinetic involuntary movements, agitation, arrhythmia, bradykinesia, chorea, delusions, hypertension, new or increased angina pectoris, and syncope. Events reported only once as a cause of discontinuation are ankle edema, anxiety, burning lips/mouth, constipation, drowsiness/lethargy, dystonia, excess perspiration, increased freezing, gastrointestinal bleeding, hair loss, increased tremor, nervousness, weakness, and weight loss.

Experience with ELDEPRYL obtained in parallel, placebo controlled, randomized studies provides only a limited basis for estimates of adverse reaction rates. The following reactions that occurred with greater frequency among the 49 patients assigned to selegiline as compared to the 50 patients assigned to placebo in the only parallel, placebo controlled trial performed in patients with Parkinson's disease are shown in the following Table. None of these adverse reactions led to a discontinuation of treatment.

INCIDENCE OF TREATMENT-EMERGENT ADVERSE EXPERIENCES IN THE PLACEBO-CONTROLLED CLINICAL TRIAL

Adverse Event	Number of Patients Reporting Events	
	selegiline hydrochloride N=49	placebo N=50
Nausea	10	3
Dizziness/Lightheaded/Fainting	7	1
Abdominal Pain	4	2
Confusion	3	0
Hallucinations	3	1
Dry mouth	3	1
Vivid Dreams	2	0
Dyskinesias	2	5
Headache	2	1
The following events were reported once in either or both groups:		
Ache, generalized	1	0
Anxiety/Tension	1	1
Anemia	0	1
Diarrhea	1	0
Hair Loss	0	1
Insomnia	1	1
Lethargy	1	0
Leg pain	1	0
Low back pain	1	0
Malaise	0	1
Palpitations	1	0
Urinary Retention	1	0
Weight Loss	1	0

In all prospectively monitored clinical investigations, enrolling approximately 920 patients, the following adverse events, classified by body system, were reported.

Central Nervous System:

Motor/Coordination/Extrapyramidal:

increased tremor, chorea, loss of balance, restlessness, blepharospasm, increased bradykinesia, facial grimace, falling down, heavy leg, muscle twitch*, myoclonic jerks*, stiff neck, tardive dyskinesia, dystonic symptoms, dyskinesia, involuntary movements, freezing, festination, increased apraxia, muscle cramps.

Mental Status/Behavioral/Psychiatric:

hallucinations, dizziness, confusion, anxiety, depression, drowsiness, behavior/mood change, dreams/nightmares, tiredness, delusions, disorientation, lightheadedness, impaired memory*, increased energy*, transient high*, hollow feeling, lethargy/malaise, apathy, overstimulation, vertigo, personality change, sleep disturbance, restlessness, weakness, transient irritability.

Pain/Altered Sensation:

headache, back pain, leg pain, tinnitus, migraine, supraorbital pain, throat burning, generalized ache, chills, numbness of toes/fingers, taste disturbance.

Autonomic Nervous System:

dry mouth, blurred vision, sexual dysfunction.

Cardiovascular:

orthostatic hypotension, hypertension, arrhythmia, palpitations, new or increased angina pectoris, hypotension, tachycardia, peripheral edema, sinus bradycardia, syncope.

Gastrointestinal:

nausea/vomiting, constipation, weight loss, anorexia, poor appetite, dysphagia, diarrhea, heartburn, rectal bleeding, bruxism*, gastrointestinal bleeding (exacerbation of preexisting ulcer disease).

Genitourinary/Gynecologic/Endocrine:

slow urination, transient anorgasmia*, nocturia, prostatic hypertrophy, urinary hesitancy, urinary retention, decreased penile sensation*, urinary frequency.

Skin and Appendages:

increased sweating, diaphoresis, facial hair, hair loss, hematoma, rash, photosensitivity.

Miscellaneous:

asthma, diplopia, shortness of breath, speech affected.

Postmarketing Reports:

The following experiences were described in spontaneous post-marketing reports. These reports do not provide sufficient information to establish a clear causal relationship with the use of ELDEPRYL.

CNS:

Seizure in dialyzed chronic renal failure patient on concomitant medications.

*indicates events reported only at doses greater than 10 mg/day.

OVERDOSAGE

Selegiline:

No specific information is available about clinically significant overdoses with ELDEPRYL. However, experience gained during selegiline's development reveals that some individuals exposed to doses of 600 mg of d,l-selegiline suffered severe hypotension and psychomotor agitation.

Continued on next page

Eldepryl—Cont.

Since the selective inhibition of MAO B by selegiline hydrochloride is achieved only at doses in the range recommended for the treatment of Parkinson's disease (e.g., 10 mg/day), overdoses are likely to cause significant inhibition of both MAO A and MAO B. Consequently, the signs and symptoms of overdose may resemble those observed with marketed non-selective MAO inhibitors [e.g., tranylcypromine (PARNATE), isocarboxazide (MARPLAN), and phenelzine (NARDIL)].

Overdose with Non-Selective MAO Inhibition:
NOTE:
This section is provided for reference; it does not describe events that have actually been observed with selegiline in overdose.
Characteristically, signs and symptoms of non-selective MAOI overdose may not appear immediately. Delays of up to 12 hours between ingestion of drug and the appearance of signs may occur. Importantly, the peak intensity of the syndrome may not be reached for upwards of a day following the overdose. Death has been reported following overdosage. Therefore, immediate hospitalization, with continuous patient observation and monitoring for a period of at least two days following the ingestion of such drugs in overdose, is strongly recommended.
The clinical picture of MAOI overdose varies considerably; its severity may be a function of the amount of drug consumed. The central nervous and cardiovascular systems are prominently involved.
Signs and symptoms of overdosage may include, alone or in combination, any of the following: drowsiness, dizziness, faintness, irritability, hyperactivity, agitation, severe headache, hallucinations, trismus, opisthotonos, convulsions, and coma; rapid and irregular pulse, hypertension, hypotension and vascular collapse; precordial pain, respiratory depression and failure, hyperpyrexia, diaphoresis, and cool, clammy skin.

Treatment Suggestions For Overdose:
NOTE:
Because there is no recorded experience with selegiline overdose, the following suggestions are offered based upon the assumption that selegiline overdose may be modeled by non-selective MAOI poisoning. In any case, up-to-date information about the treatment of overdose can often be obtained from a certified Regional Poison Control Center. Telephone numbers of certified Poison Control Centers are listed in the Physicians' Desk Reference (PDR).

Treatment of overdose with non-selective MAOIs is symptomatic and supportive. Induction of emesis or gastric lavage with instillation of charcoal slurry may be helpful in early poisoning, provided the airway has been protected against aspiration. Signs and symptoms of central nervous system stimulation, including convulsions, should be treated with diazepam, given slowly intravenously. Phenothiazine derivatives and central nervous system stimulants should be avoided. Hypotension and vascular collapse should be treated with intravenous fluids and, if necessary, blood pressure titration with an intravenous infusion of a dilute pressor agent. It should be noted that adrenergic agents may produce a markedly increased pressor response.

Respiration should be supported by appropriate measures, including management of the airway, use of supplemental oxygen, and mechanical ventilatory assistance, as required.

Body temperature should be monitored closely. Intensive management of hyperpyrexia may be required. Maintenance of fluid and electrolyte balance is essential.

DOSAGE AND ADMINISTRATION

ELDEPRYL is intended for administration to Parkinsonian patients receiving levodopa/carbidopa therapy who demonstrate a deteriorating response to this treatment. The recommended regimen for the administration of ELDEPRYL is 10 mg per day administered as divided doses of 5 mg each taken at breakfast and lunch. There is no evidence that additional benefit will be obtained from the administration of higher doses. Moreover, higher doses should ordinarily be avoided because of the increased risk of side effects.
After two to three days of selegiline treatment, an attempt may be made to reduce the dose of levodopa/carbidopa. A reduction of 10 to 30% was achieved with the typical participant in the domestic placebo controlled trials who was assigned to selegiline treatment. Further reductions of levodopa/carbidopa may be possible during continued selegiline therapy.

HOW SUPPLIED

ELDEPRYL capsules are available containing 5 mg of selegiline hydrochloride. Each aqua blue capsule is band imprinted with the Somerset logo on the cap and "Eldepryl 5 mg" on the body.
They are available as:
NDC 39506-022-60 bottles of 60 capsules.
NDC 39506-022-30 bottles of 300 capsules.
Store at controlled room temperature, 59° to 86°F (15° to 30°C).

SOMERSET
PHARMACEUTICALS, INC.
Tampa, FL 33607
Literature issued February 2003
ELD:R17C

Shown in Product Identification Guide, page 333

Star Pharmaceuticals, Inc.

1881 W. STATE ROAD 84, SUITE 101
FORT LAUDERDALE, FLORIDA 33315

Direct Inquiries to:
Roseanne Branciforte R. PH., MBA, President
(954) 971-9704
For Medical Information Contact:
Roseanne Branciforte
(800) 845-7827
Sales and Ordering:
(800) 845-7827
FAX: (954) 971-7718
http://www.starpharm.com
email info@starpharm.com

APHRODYNE® ℞
[*af"ro-din'*]
brand of yohimbine hydrochloride

DESCRIPTION

Yohimbine is a 3a-15a-20β-17a- hydroxy Yohimbine-16a-carboxylic acid methyl ester. The alkaloid is found in Rubaceae and related trees and is also found in Rauwolfia Serpentina (L) Benth.
Yohimbine is an indolalkylamine alkaloid with chemical similarity to reserpine. It is a crystalline powder, odorless. Each compressed caplet contains 5.4 mg (1/12 gr.) of Yohimbine Hydrochloride.

HOW SUPPLIED

APHRODYNE® scored caplets are aqua, debossed with APHRO DYNE. They are available in bottles of 100 NDC 0076-0401-03) and 1000 (NDC 0076-0401-04).

PROSED®/DS ℞
[*prō-sĕd DS*]

DESCRIPTION

PROSED®/DS is a dark blue, round, sugar-coated compressed tablet for oral administration imprinted with **PROSED®/DS.**

Methenamine	81.6 mg
Phenyl Salicylate	36.2 mg
Methylene Blue	10.8 mg
Benzoic Acid	9.0 mg
Atropine Sulfate	0.06 mg
Hyoscyamine Sulfate	0.06 mg

METHENAMINE (Hexamethylenetetramine) exists as colorless, lustrous crystals or white crystalline powder. Its solutions are alkaline to litmus. Freely soluble in water; soluble in alcohol and in chloroform.
PHENYL SALICYLATE (2-hydroxybenzoic acid phenyl ester) exists as white crystals with a melting point of 40–43°C. It is very slightly soluble in water and freely soluble in alcohol.
METHYLENE BLUE (methylthionine chloride) exists as dark green crystals. It is soluble in water and in chloroform; sparingly soluble in alcohol.
BENZOIC ACID (benzenecarboxylic acid) exists as white crystals, scales or needles. It has a slight odor and is slightly soluble in water; freely soluble in alcohol, in chloroform and in ether.
ATROPINE SULFATE (d/tropyl tropate) is an alkaloid of belladonna. It exists as a odorless, white crystalline powder that is slowly affected by light. It is very soluble in water and freely soluble in alcohol.
HYOSCYAMINE SULFATE (*l*-tropyl tropate) is an alkaloid of belladonna. It exists as a white crystalline powder. Its solutions are alkaline to litmus and affected by light. It is slightly soluble in water; freely soluble in alcohol; sparingly soluble in ether.
PROSED®/DS tablets contain the inactive ingredients calcium sulfate, dicalcium phosphate anhydrous, talc, kaolin, polyvinylpyrollidone, magnesium stearate, methylparaben, propylparaben, FD&C Blue #1 Aluminum Lake, FD&C Blue #2 Aluminum Lake, titanium dioxide, sodium benzoate, acacia, gelatin, sugar, white beeswax, carnauba, polyvinyl acetate phthalate, triethyl citrate, stearic acid.

CLINICAL PHARMACOLOGY

METHENAMINE degrades in an acidic urine environment releasing formaldehyde which provides bactericidal or bacteriostatic action. It is well absorbed from the gastrointestinal tract. 70 to 90% reaches the urine unchanged at which point it is hydrolyzed if the urine is acidic. Within 24 hours it is almost completely (90%) excreted; of this amount at pH 5, approximately 20% is formaldehyde. Protein binding—some formaldehyde is bound to substances in the urine and surrounding tissues. Methenamine is freely distributed to body tissue and fluids but is not clinically significant as it does not hydrolyze at a pH greater than 6.8.
PHENYL SALICYLATE releases salicylate, a mild analgesic for pain.
METHYLENE BLUE possesses weak antiseptic properties. It is well absorbed by the gastrointestinal tract and is rapidly reduced to leukomethylene blue which is stabilized in some combination form in the urine. 75% is excreted unchanged.
BENZOIC ACID has mild antibacterial and antifungal action. It also helps maintain an acid pH in the urine necessary for the degradation of methenamine.
ATROPINE SULFATE AND HYOSCYAMINE SULFATE are parasympatholytic drugs which relax smooth muscles. Protein binding for both atropine sulfate and hyoscyamine sulfate is moderate. Biotransformation for both atropine sulfate and hyoscyamine sulfate is hepatic. They are well absorbed from the gastrointestinal tract. Atropine sulfate is excreted 30 to 50% unchanged and the majority of hyoscyamine sulfate is excreted unchanged.

INDICATIONS AND USAGE

PROSED®/DS is indicated for the relief of discomfort of the lower urinary tract caused by hypermotility resulting from inflammation or diagnostic procedures and in the treatment of cystitis, urethritis and trigonitis when caused by organisms which maintain or produce an acid urine and are susceptible to formaldehyde.

CONTRAINDICATIONS

Risk-benefit should be considered when the following medical problems exist: glaucoma, urinary bladder neck obstruction, pyloric or duodenal obstruction or cardiospasm. Hypersensitivity to any of the ingredients.

WARNINGS

Do not exceed recommended dosage. If rapid pulse, dizziness, or blurring of vision occurs, discontinue use immediately.

PRECAUTIONS

Cross sensitivity and/or related problems: patients intolerant of other belladonna alkaloids or other salicylates may be intolerant of this medication also. Delay in gastric emptying could complicate the management of gastric ulcers.
Pregnancy/Reproduction (FDA Pregnancy Category C): Atropine, hyoscyamine and methenamine cross the placenta. Studies have not been done in either animals or humans. It is not known whether **PROSED®/DS** tablets can cause fetal harm when administered to a pregnant woman or can affect reproduction capacity. **PROSED®/DS** tablets should be given to a pregnant woman only if clearly needed.
Nursing mothers: Methenamine and traces of atropine and hyoscyamine are excreted in breast milk. Caution should be exercised when **PROSED®/DS** tablets are administered to a nursing mother.
Prolonged use: There have been no studies to establish the safety of prolonged use in humans. No known long-term animal studies have been performed to evaluate carcinogenic potential.
Pediatric: Infants and young children are especially susceptible to the toxic effect of the belladonna alkaloids.
Geriatric: Use with caution in elderly patients as they may respond to the usual doses of the belladonna alkaloids with excitement, agitation, drowsiness, or confusion.
Drug Interactions: As a result of atropine's and hyoscamine's effects on gastrointestinal motility and gastric emptying, absorption of other oral medications may be decreased during concurrent use with this combination medication.
Urinary alkalizers and thiazide diuretics: May cause the urine to become alkaline reducing the effectiveness of methenamine by inhibiting its conversion to formaldehyde.
Antimuscarinics: Concurrent use may intensify antimuscarinic effects of atropine and hyoscyamine because of secondary antimuscarinic activities of these medications.
Antacids/antidiarrheals: Concurrent use may reduce absorption of atropine and hyoscyamine resulting in decreased therapeutic effectiveness. Concurrent use with antacids may cause urine to become alkaline reducing the effectiveness of methenamine by inhibiting its conversion to formaldehyde. Doses of these medications should be spaced 1 hour apart from doses of atropine and hyoscyamine.
Antimyasthenics: Concurrent use with atropine and hyoscyamine may further reduce intestinal motility, therefore, caution is recommended.
Ketoconazole-atropine and hyoscyamine may cause increased gastrointestinal pH. Concurrent administration with atropine and hyoscyamine may result in marked reduction in the absorption of ketoconazole. Patients should be advised to take this combination at least 2 hours after ketoconazole.
Monoamine oxidase (MAO) inhibitors: Concurrent use with atropine and hyoscyamine may intensify antimuscarinic side effects.
Opioid (narcotic) analgesics may result in increased risk of severe constipation.
Sulfonamides: These drugs may precipitate with formaldehyde in the urine increasing the danger of crystalluria.
Patients should be advised that the urine and/or stools may become blue to blue-green as a result of the excretion of methylene blue.

ADVERSE REACTIONS

Cardiovascular—rapid pulse, flushing
Central Nervous System—blurred vision, dizziness
Respiratory—shortness of breath or troubled breathing
Genitourinary—difficult micturition, acute urinary retention
Gastrointestinal—dry mouth, nausea/vomiting.

DRUG ABUSE AND DEPENDENCE

A dependence on the use of **PROSED®/DS** has not been reported and due to the nature of its ingredients, abuse of **PROSED®/DS** is not expected.

OVERDOSAGE

Emesis or gastric lavage. Slow intravenous administration of physostigmine in doses of 1 to 4 mg (0.5 to 1 mg in children) repeated as needed in one to two hours to reverse severe antimuscarinic symptoms. Administration of small doses of diazepam to control excitement and seizures. Artificial respiration with oxygen if needed for respiratory depression. Adequate hydration. Symptomatic treatment as necessary.

DOSAGE AND ADMINISTRATION

Adults: One tablet orally 4 times per day followed by liberal fluid intake.
Older children: Dosage must be individualized by physician. Not recommended for use in children up to 12 years of age.

HOW SUPPLIED

Round, deep blue, sugar-coated tablets imprinted with **"PROSED®/DS"**. Bottles of 100 (NDC 0076-0108-03), and 1000 (NDC 0076-0108-04) tablets.
NDC 0076-0108-03
STORAGE
Store in a dry place between 15° and 30°C (59° to 86°F). Keep container tightly closed.
Code#STA108-031

PROSED® EC ℞

[*prō-sĕd*]
(www.Prosed.com)

DESCRIPTION

PROSED® EC (Enteric Coated) is a delayed release, dark blue tablet for oral administration. Each tablet contains: Methenamine 81.6 mg, Phenyl Salicylate 36.2 mg, Methylene Blue 10.8 mg, Benzoic Acid 9.0 mg, Atropine Sulfate 0.06 mg, and Hyoscyamine Sulfate 0.06 mg.
METHENAMINE (Hexamethylenetetramine) exists as colorless, lustrous crystals or white crystalline powder. Its solutions are alkaline to litmus. Freely soluble in water; soluble in alcohol and in chloroform.
PHENYL SALICYLATE (2-hydroxybenzoic acid phenyl ester) exists as white crystals with a melting point of 40-43°C. It is very slightly soluble in water and freely soluble in alcohol.
METHYLENE BLUE (methylthionine chloride) exists as dark green crystals. It is soluble in water and in chloroform; sparingly soluble in alcohol.
BENZOIC ACID (benzenecarboxylic acid) exists as white crystals, scales or needles. It has a slight odor and is slightly soluble in water; freely soluble in alcohol, in chloroform and in ether.
ATROPINE SULFATE (d/tropyl tropate) is an alkaloid of belladonna. It exists as an odorless, white crystalline powder that is slowly affected by light. It is very soluble in water and freely soluble in alcohol.
HYOSCYAMINE SULFATE (l-tropyl tropate) is an alkaloid of belladonna. It exists as a white crystalline powder. Its solutions are alkaline to litmus and affected by light. It is slightly soluble in water; freely soluble in alcohol; sparingly soluble in ether.

INDICATIONS AND USAGE

PROSED® EC is indicated for the relief of discomfort of the lower urinary tract caused by hypermotility resulting from inflammation or diagnostic procedures and in the treatment of cystitis, urethritis and trigonitis when caused by organisms which maintain or produce an acid urine and are susceptible to formaldehyde.

CONTRAINDICATIONS

Risk-benefit should be considered when the following medical problems exist: glaucoma, urinary bladder neck obstruction, pyloric or duodenal obstruction or cardiospasm. Hypersensitivity to any of the ingredients.

WARNINGS

Do not exceed recommended dosage. If rapid pulse, dizziness, or blurring of vision occurs, discontinue use immediately.

PRECAUTIONS

Cross sensitivity and/or related problems: Patients intolerant of other belladonna alkaloids or other salicylates may be intolerant of this medication also. Delay in gastric emptying could complicate the management of gastric ulcers.
Pregnancy/Reproduction (FDA Pregnancy Category C): Atropine, hyoscyamine and methenamine cross the placenta. Studies have not been done in either animals or humans. It is not known whether **PROSED® EC** tablets can cause fetal harm when administered to a pregnant woman or can affect reproduction capacity. **PROSED® EC** tablets should be given to a pregnant woman only if clearly needed.
Nursing mothers: Methenamine and traces of atropine and hyoscyamine are excreted in breast milk. Caution should be exercised when **PROSED® EC** tablets are administered to a nursing mother.
Prolonged use: There have been no studies to establish the safety of prolonged use in humans. No known long-term animal studies have been performed to evaluate carcinogenic potential.
Pediatric: Infants and young children are especially susceptible to the toxic effect of the belladonna alkaloids.
Geriatric: Use with caution in elderly patients as they may respond to the usual doses of the belladonna alkaloids with excitement, agitation, drowsiness, or confusion.
Drug Interactions: As a result of atropine's and hyoscyamine's effects on gastrointestinal motility and gastric emptying, absorption of other oral medications may be decreased during concurrent use with this combination medication.
Urinary alkalizers and thiazide diuretics: May cause the urine to become alkaline reducing the effectiveness of methenamine by inhibiting its conversion to formaldehyde.
Antimuscarinics: Concurrent use may intensify antimuscarinic effects of atropine and hyoscyamine because of secondary antimuscarinic activities of these medications.
Antacids/antidiarrheals: Concurrent use may reduce absorption of atropine and hyoscyamine resulting in decreased therapeutic effectiveness. Concurrent use with antacids may cause urine to become alkaline reducing the effectiveness of methenamine by inhibiting its conversion to formaldehyde. Doses of these medications should be spaced 1 hour apart from doses of atropine and hyoscyamine.
Antimyasthenics: Concurrent use with atropine and hyoscyaminemay further reduce intestinal motility, therefore, caution is recommended.
Ketoconazole-atropine and hyoscyamine may cause increased gastrointestinal pH.
Concurrent administration with atropine and hyoscyamine may result in marked reduction in the absorption of ketoconazole. Patients should be advised to take this combination at least 2 hours after ketoconazole.
Monoamine oxidase (MAO) inhibitors: Concurrent use with atropine and hyoscyamine may intensify antimuscarinic side effects.
Opioid (narcotic) analgesics may result in increased risk of severe constipation.
Sulfonamides: These drugs may precipitate with formaldehyde in the urine increasing the danger of crystalluria.
Patients should be advised that the urine and/or stools may become blue to blue-green as a result of the excretion of methylene blue.

ADVERSE REACTIONS

Cardiovascular—rapid pulse, flushing
Central Nervous System—blurred vision, dizziness
Respiratory—shortness of breath or troubled breathing
Genitourinary—difficult micturition, acute urinary retention
Gastrointestinal—dry mouth, nausea/vomiting

DRUG ABUSE AND DEPENDENCE

A dependence on the use of **PROSED® EC** has not been reported and due to the nature of its ingredients, abuse of **PROSED® EC** is not expected.

OVERDOSAGE

Emesis or gastric lavage. Slow intravenous administration of physostigmine in doses of 1 to 4 mg (0.5 to 1 mg in children) repeated as needed in one to two hours to reverse severe antimuscarinic symptoms. Administration of small doses of diazepam to control excitement and seizures. Artificial respiration with oxygen if needed for respiratory depression. Adequate hydration. Symptomatic treatment as necessary.

DOSAGE AND ADMINISTRATION

Adults: One tablet orally 4 times per day followed by liberal fluid intake.
Older children: Dosage must be individualized by physician. Not recommended for use in children up to 12 years of age.

HOW SUPPLIED

Round, deep blue, sugar-coated tablets imprinted with **"PROSED® EC"**. Bottles of 90
STORAGE
Store in a dry place between 15° and 30°C (59° to 86°F). Keep container tightly closed. Code#STA108-031 Rev. 4/04
FREE STARTER SAMPLES
1 (800) 845-7827
FAX (954) 971-7718
e-mail: info@Prosed.com
Manufactured For:
STAR PHARMACEUTICALS, INC.
Fort Lauderdale, FL 33315
www.StarPharm.com
Manufactured By:
CONTRACT PHARMACAL CORP.
Hauppage, NY 11788
www.cpchealth.com
STAR
PHARMACEUTICALS, INC.

URO-KP-NEUTRAL® Caplet ℞

[*ū 'ro-kp-nū 'tral*]

DESCRIPTION

Each light peach caplet contains 258 mg phosphorous, 49.4 mg potassium and 262.4 mg sodium derived from sodium phosphate monobasic anhydrous, dipotassium phosphate anhydrous, and disodium phosphate anhydrous.

HOW SUPPLIED

Light peach, film coated caplet with the Star logo and number 109 debossed on each caplet. Bottles of 100 caplets (NDC 0076-0109-03).

UROLENE BLUE® ℞

[*ū 'ro-lene blue*]
Methylene Blue Tablets

Each blue coated tablet contains Methylene blue USP 65 mg.

HOW SUPPLIED

Bottles of 100 and 1000.
NDC 0076-0501-03 & 04

VIRILON® Ⓒ℞

[*vir 'i-lon*]
Methyltestosterone Capsules
Oral Androgen

Each capsule contains Methyltestosterone ..... USP 10 mg. In a special base. Each black and white capsule contains Methyltestosterone .... USP 10 mg., available only from Star Pharmaceuticals.

HOW SUPPLIED

Bottles of 100 and 1000.
NDC 0076-0301-03 & 04

Stiefel Laboratories, Inc.

255 ALHAMBRA CIRCLE
CORAL GABLES, FL 33134

Direct Inquiries to:
Professional Services Department
1-888-STIEFEL

BREVOXYL®-4 Gel ℞

[*brĕv-ăhx-il*]
(benzoyl peroxide 4%)

BREVOXYL®-8 Gel ℞

(benzoyl peroxide 8%)

DESCRIPTION

Brevoxyl-4 Gel and Brevoxyl-8 Gel are topical preparations containing benzoyl peroxide 4% and 8%, respectively, as the active ingredient in a gel vehicle containing purified water, cetyl alcohol, dimethyl isosorbide, fragrance, simethicone, stearyl alcohol and ceteareth-20. The structural formula of benzoyl peroxide is:

$$C_6H_5-\overset{O}{\overset{\|}{C}}-O-O-\overset{O}{\overset{\|}{C}}-C_6H_5$$

CLINICAL PHARMACOLOGY

The exact method of action of benzoyl peroxide in acne vulgaris is not known. Benzoyl peroxide is an antibacterial agent with demonstrated activity against *Propionibacterium acnes.* This action, combined with the mild keratolytic effect of benzoyl peroxide is believed to be responsible for its usefulness in acne.
Benzoyl peroxide is absorbed by the skin where it is metabolized to benzoic acid and excreted as benzoate in the urine.

INDICATIONS AND USAGE

Brevoxyl-4 Gel and Brevoxyl-8 Gel are indicated for use in the topical treatment of mild to moderate acne vulgaris. Brevoxyl-4 Gel or Brevoxyl-8 Gel may be used as an adjunct in acne treatment regimens including antibiotics, retinoic acid products, and sulfur/salicylic acid containing preparations.

CONTRAINDICATIONS

Brevoxyl-4 Gel and Brevoxyl-8 Gel should not be used in patients who have shown hypersensitivity to benzoyl peroxide or to any of the other ingredients in the product.

PRECAUTIONS

General—For external use only. Avoid contact with eyes and mucous membranes. **AVOID CONTACT WITH HAIR, FABRICS OR CARPETING AS BENZOYL PEROXIDE WILL CAUSE BLEACHING.**
Carcinogenesis, Mutagenesis, Impairment of Fertility—Based upon all available evidence, benzoyl peroxide is not considered to be a carcinogen. However, data from a study using mice known to be highly susceptible to cancer suggest that benzoyl peroxide acts as a tumor promoter. The clinical significance of the findings is not known.
Pregnancy: Category C—Animal reproduction studies have not been conducted with benzoyl peroxide. It is also not

Continued on next page

Brevoxyl Gel—Cont.

known whether benzoyl peroxide can cause fetal harm when administered to a pregnant woman or can affect reproduction capacity. Benzoyl peroxide should be used by a pregnant woman only if clearly needed.

Nursing Mothers—It is not known whether this drug is excreted in human milk. Because many drugs are excreted in human milk, caution should be exercised when benzoyl peroxide is administered to a nursing woman.

Pediatric Use—Safety and effectiveness in children below the age of 12 have not been established.

ADVERSE REACTIONS

Contact sensitization reactions are associated with the use of topical benzoyl peroxide products and may be expected to occur in 10 to 25 of 1000 patients. The most frequent adverse reactions associated with benzoyl peroxide use are excessive erythema and peeling which may be expected to occur in 5 of 100 patients. Excessive erythema and peeling most frequently appear during the initial phase of drug use and may normally be controlled by reducing frequency of use.

DOSAGE AND ADMINISTRATION

Therapy may be initiated with either Brevoxyl-4 Gel or Brevoxyl-8 Gel. The medication should be applied once or twice daily to affected areas. Frequency of use should be adjusted to obtain the desired clinical response. Gentle cleansing of the affected areas prior to application of Brevoxyl-4 or Brevoxyl-8 may be beneficial. Clinically visible improvement will normally occur by the third week of therapy. Maximum lesion reduction may be expected after approximately eight to twelve weeks of drug use. Continuing use of the drug is normally required to maintain a satisfactory clinical response.

HOW SUPPLIED

Brevoxyl-4 Gel and Brevoxyl-8 Gel are supplied in 42.5 g (1.5 oz) and 90 g (3.1 oz) tubes.
Brevoxyl-4 Gel
42.5 g tube NDC 0145-2374-06
90 g tube NDC 0145-2374-08
Brevoxyl-8 Gel
42.5 g tube NDC 0145-2384-06
90 g tube NDC 0145-2384-08
Store at controlled room temperature 15°–30°C (59°–86°F).
U.S. Patent Nos. 4,923,900, 5,086,075

BREVOXYL®-4 Cleansing Lotion ℞

[brev-ăhx-il]
(benzoyl peroxide 4%)

BREVOXYL®-8 Cleansing Lotion ℞

(benzoyl peroxide 8%)

DESCRIPTION

Brevoxyl-4 and Brevoxyl-8 Cleansing Lotions are topical preparations containing benzoyl peroxide as the active ingredient.

Brevoxyl-4 and Brevoxyl-8 Cleansing Lotions contain benzoyl peroxide 4% and 8%, respectively, in a lathering vehicle containing purified water, cetyl alcohol, citric acid, dimethyl isosorbide, docusate sodium, hydroxypropyl methylcellulose, laureth-12, magnesium aluminum silicate, propylene glycol, sodium hydroxide, sodium lauryl sulfoacetate, and sodium octoxynol-2 ethane sulfonate.

The structural formula of benzoyl peroxide is:

CLINICAL PHARMACOLOGY

The exact method of action of benzoyl peroxide in acne vulgaris is not known. Benzoyl peroxide is an antibacterial agent with demonstrated activity against *Propionibacterium acnes*. This action, combined with the mild keratolytic effect of benzoyl peroxide is believed to be responsible for its usefulness in acne.

Benzoyl peroxide is absorbed by the skin where it is metabolized to benzoic acid and excreted as benzoate in the urine.

INDICATIONS AND USAGE

Brevoxyl-4 and Brevoxyl-8 Cleansing Lotions are indicated for use in the topical treatment of mild to moderate acne vulgaris. Brevoxyl-4 or Brevoxyl-8 Cleansing Lotion may be used as an adjunct in acne treatment regimens including antibiotics, retinoic acid products, and sulfur/salicylic acid containing preparations.

CONTRAINDICATIONS

Brevoxyl-4 and Brevoxyl-8 Cleansing Lotions should not be used in patients who have shown hypersensitivity to benzoyl peroxide or to any of the other ingredients in the product.

PRECAUTIONS

General—For external use only. Avoid contact with eyes and mucous membranes. **AVOID CONTACT WITH HAIR, FABRICS OR CARPETING AS BENZOYL PEROXIDE WILL CAUSE BLEACHING.**

Carcinogenesis, Mutagenesis, Impairment of Fertility—Based upon all available evidence, benzoyl peroxide is not considered to be a carcinogen. However, data from a study using mice known to be highly susceptible to cancer suggest that benzoyl peroxide acts as a tumor promoter. The clinical significance of the findings is not known.

Pregnancy: Category C—Animal reproduction studies have not been conducted with benzoyl peroxide. It is also not known whether benzoyl peroxide can cause fetal harm when administered to a pregnant woman or can affect reproduction capacity. Benzoyl peroxide should be used by a pregnant woman only if clearly needed.

Nursing Mothers—It is not known whether this drug is excreted in human milk. Because many drugs are excreted in human milk, caution should be exercised when benzoyl peroxide is administered to a nursing woman.

Pediatric Use—Safety and effectiveness in children below the age of 12 have not been established.

ADVERSE REACTIONS

Contact sensitization reactions are associated with the use of topical benzoyl peroxide products and may be expected to occur in 10 to 25 of 1000 patients. The most frequent adverse reactions associated with benzoyl peroxide use are excessive erythema and peeling which may be expected to occur in 5 of 100 patients. Excessive erythema and peeling most frequently appear during the initial phase of drug use and may normally be controlled by reducing frequency of use.

DOSAGE AND ADMINISTRATION

Shake well before using. Wash the affected areas once a day during the first week, and twice a day thereafter as tolerated. Wet skin areas to be treated; apply Brevoxyl-4 or Brevoxyl-8 Cleansing Lotion, work to a full lather, rinse thoroughly and pat dry. Frequency of use should be adjusted to obtain the desired clinical response. Clinically visible improvement will normally occur by the third week of therapy. Maximum lesion reduction may be expected after approximately eight to twelve weeks of drug use. Continuing use of the drug is normally required to maintain a satisfactory clinical response.

HOW SUPPLIED

Brevoxyl-4 Cleansing Lotion is supplied in 297 g (10.5 oz) plastic bottles NDC 0145-2310-05.
Brevoxyl-8 Cleansing Lotion is supplied in 297 g (10.5 oz) plastic bottles NDC 0145-2410-05.
Store at controlled room temperature 15°–30°C (59°–86°F).

BREVOXYL®-4 ℞

[brev 'ăhx-il]

Creamy Wash

(benzoyl peroxide 4%)

BREVOXYL®-8 ℞

Creamy Wash

(benzoyl peroxide 8%)
ACNE WASH FOR TOPICAL USE

DESCRIPTION

Brevoxyl-4 Creamy Wash and Brevoxyl-8 Creamy Wash are topical preparations containing benzoyl peroxide as the active ingredient. Brevoxyl-4 Creamy Wash and Brevoxyl-8 Creamy Wash contain: 4% and 8% Benzoyl Peroxide, respectively, in a lathering cream vehicle containing Cetostearyl Alcohol, Cocamidopropyl Betaine, Corn Starch, Dimethyl Isosorbide, Glycerin, Glycolic Acid, Hydrogenated Castor Oil, Imidurea, Methylparaben, Mineral Oil, PEG-14M, Purified Water, Sodium Hydroxide, Sodium PCA, Sodium Potassium Lauryl Sulfate, Titanium Dioxide.

The structural formula of benzoyl peroxide is:

CLINICAL PHARMACOLOGY

The exact method of action of benzoyl peroxide in acne vulgaris is not known. Benzoyl peroxide is an antibacterial agent with demonstrated activity against *Propionibacterium acnes*. This action, combined with the mild keratolytic effect of benzoyl peroxide is believed to be responsible for its usefulness in acne.

Benzoyl peroxide is absorbed by the skin where it is metabolized to benzoic acid and excreted as benzoate in the urine.

INDICATIONS AND USAGE

Brevoxyl-4 Creamy Wash and Brevoxyl-8 Creamy Wash are indicated for use in the topical treatment of mild to moderate acne vulgaris. Brevoxyl-4 Creamy Wash and Brevoxyl-8 Creamy Wash may be used as an adjunct in acne treatment regimens including antibiotics, retinoic acid products, and sulfur/salicylic acid containing preparations.

CONTRAINDICATIONS

Brevoxyl-4 Creamy Wash and Brevoxyl-8 Creamy Wash should not be used in patients who have shown hypersensitivity to benzoyl peroxide or to any of the other ingredients in the product.

PRECAUTIONS

General—For external use only. Avoid contact with eyes and mucous membranes. **AVOID CONTACT WITH HAIR, FABRICS OR CARPETING AS BENZOYL PEROXIDE WILL CAUSE BLEACHING.**

Carcinogenesis, Mutagenesis, Impairment of Fertility—Based upon all available evidence, benzoyl peroxide is not considered to be a carcinogen. However, data from a study using mice known to be highly susceptible to cancer suggest that benzoyl peroxide acts as a tumor promoter. The clinical significance of the findings is not known.

Pregnancy: Category C—Animal reproduction studies have not been conducted with benzoyl peroxide. It is also not known whether benzoyl peroxide can cause fetal harm when administered to a pregnant woman or can affect reproduction capacity. Benzoyl peroxide should be used by a pregnant woman only if clearly needed.

Nursing Mothers—It is not known whether this drug is excreted in human milk. Because many drugs are excreted in human milk, caution should be exercised when benzoyl peroxide is administered to a nursing woman.

Pediatric Use—Safety and effectiveness in children below the age of 12 have not been established.

ADVERSE REACTIONS

Contact sensitization reactions are associated with the use of topical benzoyl peroxide products and may be expected to occur in 10 to 25 of 1000 patients. The most frequent adverse reactions associated with benzoyl peroxide use are excessive erythema and peeling which may be expected to occur in 5 of 100 patients. Excessive erythema and peeling most frequently appear during the initial phase of drug use and may normally be controlled by reducing frequency of use.

DOSAGE AND ADMINISTRATION

Shake well before using. Wash the affected areas once a day during the first week, and twice a day thereafter as tolerated. Wet skin areas to be treated; apply Brevoxyl-4 Creamy Wash or Brevoxyl-8 Creamy Wash, work to a full lather, rinse thoroughly and pat dry. Frequency of use should be adjusted to obtain the desired clinical response. Clinically visible improvement will normally occur by the third week of therapy. Maximum lesion reduction may be expected after approximately eight to twelve weeks of drug use. Continuing use of the drug is normally required to maintain a satisfactory clinical response.

HOW SUPPLIED

Brevoxyl-4 Creamy Wash is supplied in 170.1 g (6.0 oz) tubes NDC 0145-2474-06.
Brevoxyl-8 Creamy Wash is supplied in 170.1 g (6.0 oz) tubes NDC 0145-2484-06.
Store at controlled room temperature, 15°–30°C (59°–86°F).
U.S. Patent No. 6,433,024

CLARIPEL™ CREAM ℞

With Sunscreens
[klăr'i-pĕl]
(Hydroquinone USP, 4%)
FOR EXTERNAL USE ONLY

I. DESCRIPTION

Hydroquinone is 1,4-benzenediol. Hydroquinone is structurally related to monobenzone. Hydroquinone occurs as fine, white needles. The drug is freely soluble in water and in alcohol and has a pKa of 9.96. Chemically, hydroquinone is designated as p-dihydroxybenzene; the empirical formula is $C_6H_6O_2$; molecular weight 110.1. The structural formula is:

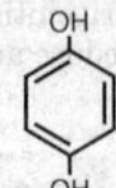

CONTENTS:

ACTIVE INGREDIENT: Hydroquinone USP 4%

OTHER INGREDIENTS: Avobenzone, Ceteareth-20, Cetostearyl Alcohol, Citric Acid, Diethylaminoethyl Stearate, Dimethicone, Edetate Disodium, Glyceryl Dilaurate, Glyceryl Monostearate, Glyceryl Stearate, PEG-100 Stearate, Hydroxyethyl Cellulose, Methylparaben, Octyldodecyl Stearoyl Stearate, Octinoxate, Oxybenzone, Polysorbate 80, Propylene Glycol, Propyl Gallate, Propylparaben, Purified Water, Quaternium-26, Sodium Metabisulfite, Sodium PCA, Squalane, Ubiquinone, Stearyl Alcohol, Water, Glycerin, *Rumex occidentalis* extract.

II. CLINICAL PHARMACOLOGY

Topical application of hydroquinone produces a reversible depigmentation of the skin by inhibition of the enzymatic oxidation of tyrosine to 3-(3,4-dihydroxyphenyl) alanine (dopa)[1] and suppression of other melanocyte metabolic processes.[2] Exposure to sunlight or ultraviolet light will cause repigmentation which may be prevented by the broad spectrum sunscreen agents contained in Claripel Cream.[3]

III. INDICATIONS AND USAGE

Claripel Cream is indicated for the gradual treatment of ultraviolet induced dyschromia and discoloration resulting from the use of oral contraceptives, pregnancy, hormone replacement therapy, or skin trauma.

IV. DOSAGE AND ADMINISTRATION

Claripel Cream should be applied to the affected areas twice daily or as directed by a physician. There is no recommended dosage for pediatric patients under 12 years of age except under the advice and supervision of a physician.

V. CONTRAINDICATIONS

Claripel Cream is contraindicated in any patient that has a prior history of hypersensitivity or allergic reaction to hydroquinone or any of the other ingredients. The safety of topical hydroquinone use during pregnancy or on children (12 years and under) has not been established.

VI. WARNINGS

A. CAUTION: Hydroquinone is a depigmenting agent which may produce unwanted cosmetic effects if not used as directed. The physician should be familiar with the contents of this insert before prescribing or dispensing this medication.

B. Test for skin sensitivity before using Claripel Cream by applying a small amount to an unbroken patch of skin and check within 24 hours. Minor redness is not a contraindication, but where there is itching, vesicle formation, or excessive inflammatory response further treatment is not advised. Close patient supervision is recommended. Contact with the eyes should be avoided. If no lightening effect is noted after two months of treatment, use of Claripel Cream should be discontinued. Claripel Cream is formulated for use as a treatment for dyschromia and should not be used for the prevention of sunburn.

C. Sunscreen use is an essential aspect of hydroquinone therapy, because even minimal sunlight sustains melanocytic activity. The sunscreens in Claripel Cream provide the necessary sun protection during therapy. During and after the use of Claripel Cream, sun exposure should be limited or sun-protective clothing should be used to cover the treated areas to prevent repigmentation.

D. Keep this and all medications out of the reach of children. In case of accidental ingestion, contact a physician or a poison control center immediately.

E. WARNING: Contains sodium metabisulfite, a sulfite that may cause allergic-type reactions including anaphylactic symptoms and life-threatening or less severe asthmatic episodes in certain susceptible people. The overall prevalence of sulfite sensitivity in the general population is unknown and probably low. Sulfite sensitivity is seen more frequently in asthmatic than in non-asthmatic people.

F. On rare occasions, a gradual blue-black darkening of the skin may occur. In which case, use of Claripel Cream should be discontinued and a physician contacted immediately.

VII. PRECAUTIONS

SEE WARNINGS

A. Pregnancy Category C: Animal reproduction studies have not been conducted with topical hydroquinone. It is also not known whether hydroquinone can cause fetal harm when used topically on a pregnant woman or can affect reproductive capacity. It is not known to what degree, if any, topical hydroquinone is absorbed systemically. Topical hydroquinone should be used in pregnant women only where clearly indicated.

B. Nursing mothers: It is not known whether topical hydroquinone is absorbed or excreted in human milk. Caution is advised when hydroquinone is used by a nursing mother.

C. Pediatric usage: Safety and effectiveness in pediatric patients below the age of 12 years have not been established.

VIII. ADVERSE REACTIONS

No systemic reactions have been reported. Occasional cutaneous hypersensitivity (localized contact dermatitis) may occur, in which case the medication should be discontinued and the physician notified immediately.

IX. OVERDOSAGE

There have been no systemic reactions reported from the use of topical hydroquinone. However, treatment should be limited to relatively small areas of the body at one time, since some patients experience a transient skin reddening and a mild burning sensation which does not preclude treatment.

X. HOW SUPPLIED

Claripel Cream is available as follows:

Tube Size	NDC Number
28 gram	0145-2516-03
45 gram	0145-2516-05

REFERENCES

1. Denton, C., A.B. Lerner, and T.B. Fitzpatrick. "Inhibition of Melanin Formation by Chemical Agents." *Journal of Investigative Dermatology.* 1952; 18:119–135.

2. Jimbow, K., H. Obata, M. Pathak, and T.B. Fitzpatrick. "Mechanism of Depigmentation by Hydroquinone." *Journal of Investigative Dermatology.* 1974; 62:436–449.

3. Parrish, J.A., R.R. Anderson, F. Urbach, and D. Pitts. *UVA, Biological Effects of Ultraviolet Radiation with Emphasis on Human Responses to Longwave Ultraviolet.* Plenum Press, New York and London, 1978, p. 151.

Claripel Cream should be stored at controlled room temperature: 15°–30° C (59°–86° F).

Patent Pending

CLINDETS® ℞

[*klĭn-dĕtz'*]

(Clindamycin Phosphate Pledgets)
1%*
***equivalent to 1% clindamycin**
(10 mg/mL)
FOR EXTERNAL USE ONLY

DESCRIPTION

Clindets® (Clindamycin Phosphate Pledgets) contain clindamycin phosphate, USP at a concentration equivalent to 10 mg clindamycin per milliliter in a vehicle of isopropyl alcohol 52% v/v, propylene glycol and water. Each Clindets® pledget applicator contains approximately 1 mL of Clindamycin Phosphate Topical Solution. Clindamycin Phosphate Topical Solution has a pH range between 4.0 and 7.0.

Clindamycin phosphate is a water soluble ester of the semi-synthetic antibiotic produced by a 7(S)-chloro-substitution of the 7(R)-hydroxyl group of the parent antibiotic lincomycin. It occurs as a white to off-white, hygroscopic, crystalline powder. It is freely soluble in water, slightly soluble in dehydrated alcohol, very slightly soluble in acetone and practically insoluble in chloroform, benzene, and ether. Clindamycin phosphate is odorless or practically odorless, and has a bitter taste.

Chemically, clindamycin phosphate is $C_{18}H_{34}ClN_2O_8PS$. It has the following structural formula:

The chemical name for clindamycin phosphate is Methyl 7-chloro-6,7,8-trideoxy-6-(1-methyl-*trans*-4-propyl-L-2-pyrrolidinecarboxamido)-1-thio-L-*threo*-α-D-*galacto*-octopyranoside 2-(dihydrogen phosphate). (MW=504.97)

CLINICAL PHARMACOLOGY

Although clindamycin phosphate is inactive *in vitro*, rapid *in vivo* hydrolysis converts this compound to the antibacterially active clindamycin.

Cross resistance has been demonstrated between clindamycin and lincomycin.

Antagonism has been demonstrated between clindamycin and erythromycin.

Following multiple topical applications of clindamycin phosphate at a concentration equivalent to 10 mg clindamycin per mL in an isopropyl alcohol and water solution, very low levels of clindamycin are present in the serum (0-3 ng/mL) and less than 0.2% of the dose is recovered in urine as clindamycin.

Clindamycin activity has been demonstrated in comedones from acne patients. The mean concentration of antibiotic activity in extracted comedones after application of a Clindamycin Phosphate Pledget for 4 weeks was 597 mcg/g of comedonal material (range 0-1490). Clindamycin *in vitro* inhibits all *Propionibacterium acnes* cultures tested (MICs 0.4 mcg/mL). Free fatty acids on the skin surface have been decreased from approximately 14% to 2% following application of clindamycin.

INDICATIONS AND USAGE

Clindets are indicated in the treatment of acne vulgaris. In view of the potential for diarrhea, bloody diarrhea and pseudomembranous colitis, the physician should consider whether other agents are more appropriate. (See CONTRAINDICATIONS, WARNINGS, and ADVERSE REACTIONS.)

CONTRAINDICATIONS

Clindets are contraindicated in individuals with a history of hypersensitivity to preparations containing clindamycin or lincomycin, a history of regional enteritis or ulcerative colitis, or a history of antibiotic-associated colitis.

WARNINGS

Orally and parenterally administered clindamycin has been associated with severe colitis which may result in patient death. Use of the topical formulation of clindamycin results in absorption of the antibiotic from the skin surface. Diarrhea, bloody diarrhea, and colitis (including pseudomembranous colitis) have been reported with the use of topical and systemic clindamycin.

Studies indicate a toxin(s) produced by *clostridia* is one primary cause of antibiotic-associated colitis. The colitis is usually characterized by severe persistent diarrhea and severe abdominal cramps and may be associated with the passage of blood and mucus. Endoscopic examination may reveal pseudomembranous colitis. Stool culture for *Clostridium difficile* and stool assay for *C. difficile* toxin may be helpful diagnostically.

When significant diarrhea occurs, the drug should be discontinued. Large bowel endoscopy should be considered to establish a definitive diagnosis in cases of severe diarrhea.

Antiperistaltic agents such as opiates and diphenoxylate with atropine may prolong and/or worsen the condition. Vancomycin has been found to be effective in the treatment of antibiotic-associated pseudomembranous colitis produced by *Clostridium difficile*. The usual adult dosage is 500 milligrams to 2 grams of vancomycin orally per day in three to four divided doses administered for 7 to 10 days. Cholestyramine or colestipol resins bind to vancomycin *in vitro*. If both a resin and vancomycin are to be administered concurrently, it may be advisable to separate the time of administration of each drug.

Diarrhea, colitis, and pseudomembranous colitis have been observed to begin up to several weeks following cessation of oral and parenteral therapy with clindamycin.

PRECAUTIONS

General

Clindets contain an alcohol base which will cause burning and irritation of the eyes. In the event of accidental contact with sensitive surfaces (eye, abraded skin, mucous membranes), bathe with copious amounts of cool tap water. The solution has an unpleasant taste and caution should be exercised when applying medication around the mouth.

Clindets should be prescribed with caution in atopic individuals.

Drug Interactions

Clindamycin has been shown to have neuromuscular blocking properties that may enhance the action of other neuromuscular blocking agents. Therefore, it should be used with caution in patients receiving such agents.

Pregnancy: Teratogenic effects-Pregnancy Category B

Reproduction studies have been performed in rats and mice using subcutaneous and oral doses of clindamycin ranging from 100 to 600 mg/kg/day and have revealed no evidence of impaired fertility or harm to the fetus due to clindamycin. There are, however, no adequate and well-controlled studies in pregnant women. Because animal reproduction studies are not always predictive of human response, this drug should be used during pregnancy only if clearly needed.

Nursing Mothers

It is not known whether clindamycin is excreted in human milk following use of Clindets. However, orally and parenterally administered clindamycin has been reported to appear in breast milk. Because of the potential for serious adverse reactions in nursing infants, a decision should be made whether to discontinue nursing or to discontinue the drug, taking into account the importance of the drug to the mother.

Pediatric Use

Safety and effectiveness in the pediatric population under the age of 12 has not been established.

ADVERSE REACTIONS

In 18 clinical studies of various topical formulations of clindamycin phosphate using placebo vehicle and/or active comparator drugs as controls, patients experienced a number of treatment emergent adverse dermatological events (see table below).

[See table below]

OVERDOSAGE

Topically applied Clindamycin Phosphate formulations can be absorbed in sufficient amounts to produce systemic effects. (See WARNINGS.)

DOSAGE AND ADMINISTRATION

Apply a thin film using a Clindets applicator for the application of Clindamycin Phosphate Topical Solution twice daily to affected area. More than one pledget may be used. Each pledget should be used only once and then discarded. Remove pledget from foil just before use. Do not use if the seal is broken.

Discard after single use.

Continued on next page

Treatment Emergent Adverse Event	Number of patients reporting events Solution n=553 (%)	Gel n=148 (%)	Lotion n=160 (%)
Burning	62 (11)	15 (10)	17 (11)
Itching	36 (7)	15 (10)	17 (11)
Burning/Itching	60 (11)	# (-)	# (-)
Dryness	105 (19)	34 (23)	29 (18)
Erythema	86 (16)	10 (7)	22 (14)
Oiliness/Oily Skin	8 (1)	26 (18)	12* (10)
Peeling	61 (11)	# (-)	11 (7)

\# not recorded * of 126 subjects

Clindets—Cont.

HOW SUPPLIED

Clindets® (Clindamycin Phosphate Pledgets) 1%* * equivalent to 1% clindamycin (10 mg/mL) is available in the following size:
69 pledget container — NDC 0145-2472-80
Store at controlled room temperature, 15°–30°C (59°–86°F).

CLOBEVATE® ℞

[klō' bə-vāt]
(Clobetasol Propionate Gel)
0.05%*
***potency expressed as clobetasol propionate**
FOR TOPICAL DERMATOLOGIC USE ONLY—
NOT FOR OPHTHALMIC, ORAL, OR
INTRAVAGINAL USE

DESCRIPTION

Clobevate® (Clobetasol Propionate Gel) contains the active compound clobetasol propionate, a synthetic corticosteroid, for topical dermatologic use. Clobetasol, an analog of prednisolone, has a high degree of glucocorticoid activity and a slight degree of mineralocorticoid activity.
Chemically, clobetasol propionate is 21-Chloro-9-fluoro-11β,17-dihydroxy-16β-methylpregna-1,4-diene-3,20-dione 17-propionate, and it has the following structural formula:

[Structural formula: CH_2Cl, C=O, $OCOCH_2CH_3$, CH_3, HO, F, H]

Clobetasol propionate has the molecular formula $C_{25}H_{32}ClFO_5$ and a molecular weight of 466.98. It is a white to cream-colored crystalline powder insoluble in water.
Each gram, for topical administration, contains clobetasol propionate 0.5 mg in a base of propylene glycol, carbomer 934P, sodium hydroxide, and purified water.

CLINICAL PHARMACOLOGY

Like other topical corticosteroids, clobetasol propionate has anti-inflammatory, antipruritic, and vasoconstrictive properties. The mechanism of the anti-inflammatory activity of the topical steroids, in general, is unclear. However, corticosteroids are thought to act by the induction of phospholipase A_2 inhibitory proteins, collectively called lipocortins. It is postulated that these proteins control the biosynthesis of potent mediators of inflammation such as prostaglandins and leukotrienes by inhibiting the release of their common precursor, arachidonic acid. Arachidonic acid is released from membrane phospholipids by phospholipase A_2.
Pharmacokinetics: The extent of percutaneous absorption of topical corticosteroids is determined by many factors, including the vehicle and the integrity of the epidermal barrier. Occlusive dressing with hydrocortisone for up to 24 hours has not been demonstrated to increase penetration; however, occlusion of hydrocortisone for 96 hours markedly enhances penetration. Topical corticosteroids can be absorbed from normal intact skin, while inflammation and/or other disease processes in the skin may increase percutaneous absorption. Greater absorption was observed for the clobetasol propionate gel formulation as compared to the cream formulation in *in vitro* human skin penetration studies.
Studies performed with Clobevate indicate that it is in the super-high range of potency as compared with other topical corticosteroids.

INDICATIONS AND USAGE

Clobevate is a super-high potency corticosteroid formulation indicated for the relief of the inflammatory and pruritic manifestations of corticosteroid-responsive dermatoses.
Treatment beyond 2 consecutive weeks is not recommended, and the total dosage should not exceed 50 g per week because of the potential for the drug to suppress the hypothalamic-pituitary-adrenal (HPA) axis. Use in children under 12 years of age is not recommended.

CONTRAINDICATIONS

Clobevate is contraindicated in those patients with a history of hypersensitivity to any of the components of the preparation.

PRECAUTIONS

General: Clobetasol propionate is a highly potent topical corticosteroid that has been shown to suppress the HPA axis at doses as low as 2 g per day.
Systemic absorption of topical corticosteroids can produce reversible HPA axis suppression with the potential for glucocorticosteroid insufficiency after withdrawal from treatment. Manifestations of Cushing's syndrome, hyperglycemia, and glucosuria can also be produced in some patients by systemic absorption of topical corticosteroids while on therapy.
Patients receiving a large dose applied to a large surface area should be evaluated periodically for evidence of HPA axis suppression. This may be done by using the ACTH stimulation, a.m. plasma cortisol, and urinary free cortisol tests. Patients receiving super-potent corticosteroids should not be treated for more than 2 weeks at a time, and only small areas should be treated at any one time due to the increased risk of HPA suppression.
If HPA axis suppression is noted, an attempt should be made to withdraw the drug, to reduce the frequency of application, or to substitute a less potent corticosteroid. Recovery of HPA axis function is generally prompt and complete upon discontinuation of topical corticosteroids. Infrequently, signs and symptoms of glucocorticosteroid insufficiency may occur that require supplemental systemic corticosteroids. For information on systemic supplementation, see prescribing information for those products.
Children may be more susceptible to systemic toxicity from equivalent doses due to their larger skin surface to body mass ratios (see PRECAUTIONS: Pediatric Use).
If irritation develops, Clobevate should be discontinued and appropriate therapy instituted. Allergic contact dermatitis with corticosteroids is usually diagnosed by observing *failure to heal* rather than noting a clinical exacerbation as with most topical products not containing corticosteroids. Such an observation should be corroborated with appropriate diagnostic patch testing.
If concomitant skin infections are present or develop, an appropriate antifungal or antibacterial agent should be used. If a favorable response does not occur promptly, use of Clobevate should be discontinued until the infection has been adequately controlled.
Clobevate should not be used in the treatment of rosacea or perioral dermatitis, and should not be used on the face, groin, or axillae.
Information for Patients: Patients using topical corticosteroids should receive the following information and instructions:

1. This medication is to be used as directed by the physician. It is for external use only. Avoid contact with the eyes.
2. This medication should not be used for any disorder other than that for which it was prescribed.
3. The treated skin area should not be bandaged or otherwise covered or wrapped so as to be occlusive unless directed by the physician.
4. Patients should report any signs of local adverse reactions to the physician.
5. Patients should inform their physicians that they are using Clobevate if surgery is contemplated.

Laboratory Tests: The following tests may be helpful in evaluating patients for HPA axis suppression:
ACTH stimulation test
A.M. plasma cortisol test
Urinary free cortisol test
Carcinogenesis, Mutagenesis, Impairment of Fertility: Long-term animal studies have not been performed to evaluate the carcinogenic potential of clobetasol propionate.
Studies in the rat following oral administration at dosage levels up to 50 mg/kg per day revealed no significant effect on the males. The females exhibited an increase in the number of resorbed embryos and a decrease in the number of living fetuses at the highest dose.
Clobetasol propionate was nonmutagenic in three different test systems: the Ames test, the *Saccharomyces cerevisiae* gene conversion assay, and the *E. coli* B WP2 fluctuation test.
Pregnancy: ***Teratogenic Effects: Pregnancy Category C:*** Corticosteroids have been shown to be teratogenic in laboratory animals when administered systemically at relatively low dosage levels. Some corticosteroids have been shown to be teratogenic after dermal application to laboratory animals.
Clobetasol propionate has not been tested for teratogenicity by this route; however, it is absorbed percutaneously, and when administered subcutaneously it was a significant teratogen in both the rabbit and mouse. Clobetasol propionate has greater teratogenic potential than steroids that are less potent.
Teratogenicity studies in mice using the subcutaneous routes resulted in fetotoxicity at the highest dose tested (1 mg/kg) and teratogenicity at all dose levels tested down to 0.03 mg/kg. These doses are approximately 0.33 and 0.01 times, respectively, the human topical dose of Clobevate. Abnormalities seen included cleft palate and skeletal abnormalities.
In rabbits, clobetasol propionate given by the same route was teratogenic at doses of 3 and 10 mcg/kg. These doses are approximately 0.001 and 0.003 times, respectively, the human topical dose of Clobevate. Abnormalities seen included cleft palate, cranioschisis, and other skeletal abnormalities.
There are no adequate and well-controlled studies of the teratogenic potential of clobetasol propionate in pregnant women. Clobevate should be used during pregnancy only if the potential benefit justifies the potential risk to the fetus.
Nursing Mothers: Systemically administered corticosteroids appear in human milk and could suppress growth, interfere with endogenous corticosteroid production, or cause other untoward effects. It is not known whether topical administration of corticosteroids could result in sufficient systemic absorption to produce detectable quantities in human milk. Because many drugs are excreted in human milk, caution should be exercised when Clobevate is administered to a nursing woman.
Pediatric Use: Safety and effectiveness of Clobevate in children and infants have not been established; therefore, use in children under 12 years of age is not recommended. Because of a higher ratio of skin surface area to body mass, children are at a greater risk than adults of HPA axis suppression when they are treated with topical corticosteroids. They are therefore also at greater risk of glucocorticosteroid insufficiency after withdrawal of treatment and of Cushing's syndrome while on treatment. Adverse effects including striae have been reported with inappropriate use of topical corticosteroids in infants and children (see PRECAUTIONS).
HPA axis suppression, Cushing's syndrome, and intracranial hypertension have been reported in children receiving topical corticosteroids. Manifestations of adrenal suppression in children include linear growth retardation, delayed weight gain, low plasma cortisol levels, and absence of response to ACTH stimulation. Manifestations of intracranial hypertension include bulging fontanelles, headaches, and bilateral papilledema.

ADVERSE REACTIONS

In a controlled trial with Clobevate, the only reported adverse reaction that was considered to be drug related was a report of burning sensation (1.8% of treated patients).
In larger controlled clinical trials with other clobetasol propionate formulations, the most frequently reported adverse reactions have included burning, stinging, irritation, pruritus, erythema, folliculitis, cracking and fissuring of the skin, numbness of the fingers, skin atrophy, and telangiectasia (all less than 2%).
Cushing's syndrome has been reported in infants and adults as a result of prolonged use of topical clobetasol propionate formulations.
The following additional local adverse reactions are reported infrequently with topical corticosteroids, but may occur more frequently with super-high potency corticosteroids such as Clobevate. These reactions are listed in approximate decreasing order of occurrence: dryness, hypertrichosis, acneiform eruptions, hypopigmentation, perioral dermatitis, allergic contact dermatitis, secondary infection, irritation, striae, and miliaria.

OVERDOSAGE

Topically applied Clobevate can be absorbed in sufficient amounts to produce systemic effects (see PRECAUTIONS).

DOSAGE AND ADMINISTRATION

Apply a thin layer of Clobevate to the affected areas twice daily and rub in gently and completely (see INDICATIONS AND USAGE).
Clobevate is a super-high potency topical corticosteroid; therefore, **treatment should be limited to 2 consecutive weeks, and amounts greater than 50 g per week should not be used.**
As with other highly active corticosteroids, therapy should be discontinued when control has been achieved. If no improvement is seen within 2 weeks, reassessment of diagnosis may be necessary.
Clobevate should not be used with occlusive dressings.

HOW SUPPLIED

Clobevate (Clobetasol Propionate Gel) 0.05% is supplied in 45-g (NDC 0145-2790-04) tubes.
Store between 15° and 30°C (59° and 86°F). Clobevate should not be refrigerated.

DUAC® TOPICAL GEL ℞

[dū'ăk]
(clindamycin, 1% - benzoyl peroxide, 5%)
For Dermatological Use Only.
Not for Ophthalmic Use.

DESCRIPTION

Duac® Topical Gel contains clindamycin phosphate, (7(S)-chloro-7-deoxylincomycin-2-phosphate), equivalent to 1% clindamycin, and 5% benzoyl peroxide.
Clindamycin phosphate is a water soluble ester of the semi-synthetic antibiotic produced by a 7(S)-chloro-substitution of the 7(R)-hydroxyl group of the parent antibiotic lincomycin.
Clindamycin phosphate is $C_{18}H_{34}ClN_2O_8PS$. The structural formula for clindamycin phosphate is represented below:

[Structural formula: CH_3, N, C_3H_7, C(=O)–NH–C–H, H–C–Cl, CH_3, HO, O, OH, SCH_3, O–P(=O)–OH, OH]

Clindamycin phosphate has a molecular weight of 504.97 and its chemical name is methyl 7-chloro-6,7,8-trideoxy-6-(1-methyl-*trans*-4-propyl-L-2-pyrrolidinecarboxamido)-1-thio-L-*threo*-α-D-*galacto*-octopyranoside 2-(dihydrogen phosphate).
Benzoyl peroxide is $C_{14}H_{10}O_4$. It has the following structural formula:
[See chemical structure at top of next column]
Benzoyl peroxide has a molecular weight of 242.23.
Each gram of Duac Topical Gel contains 10 mg (1%) clindamycin, as phosphate, and 50 mg (5%) benzoyl

peroxide in a base consisting of carbomer 940, dimethicone, disodium lauryl sulfosuccinate, edetate disodium, glycerin, silicon dioxide, methylparaben, poloxamer, purified water, and sodium hydroxide.

CLINICAL PHARMACOLOGY

A comparative study of the pharmacokinetics of Duac Topical Gel and 1% clindamycin solution alone in 78 patients indicated that mean plasma clindamycin levels during the four week dosing period were < 0.5 ng/ml for both treatment groups.

Benzoyl peroxide has been shown to be absorbed by the skin where it is converted to benzoic acid. Less than 2% of the dose enters systemic circulation as benzoic acid.

Microbiology:

Mechanism of Action

Clindamycin binds to the 50S ribosomal subunits of susceptible bacteria and prevents elongation of peptide chains by interfering with peptidyl transfer, thereby suppressing protein synthesis.

Benzoyl peroxide is a potent oxidizing agent.

***In Vivo* Activity**

No microbiology studies were conducted in the clinical trials with this product.

***In Vitro* Activity**

The clindamycin and benzoyl peroxide components individually have been shown to have *in vitro* activity against *Propionibacterium acnes*, an organism which has been associated with acne vulgaris; however, the clinical significance of this is not known.

Drug Resistance

There are reports of an increase of *P. acnes* resistance to clindamycin in the treatment of acne. In patients with *P. acnes* resistant to clindamycin, the clindamycin component may provide no additional benefit beyond benzoyl peroxide alone.

CLINICAL STUDIES

In five randomized, double-blind clinical studies of 1,319 patients, 397 used Duac, 396 used benzoyl peroxide, 349 used clindamycin and 177 used vehicle. Duac applied once daily for 11 weeks was significantly more effective than vehicle, benzoyl peroxide, and clindamycin in the treatment of inflammatory lesions of moderate to moderately severe facial acne vulgaris in three of the five studies (Studies 1, 2, and 5).

Patients were evaluated and acne lesions counted at each clinical visit: weeks 2, 5, 8, 11. The primary efficacy measures were the lesion counts and the investigator's global assessment evaluated at week 11. Patients were instructed to wash the face, wait 10 to 20 minutes, and then apply medication to the entire face, once daily, in the evening before retiring. Percent reductions in inflammatory lesion counts after treatment for 11 weeks in these five studies are shown in the following table:

[See first table above]

The Duac group showed greater overall improvement in the investigator's global assessment than the benzoyl peroxide, clindamycin and vehicle groups in three of the five studies (Studies 1, 2, and 5).

Clinical studies have not adequately demonstrated the effectiveness of Duac versus benzoyl peroxide alone in the treatment of non-inflammatory lesions of acne.

INDICATIONS AND USAGE

Duac Topical Gel is indicated for the topical treatment of inflammatory acne vulgaris.

Duac Topical Gel has not been demonstrated to have any additional benefit when compared to benzoyl peroxide alone in the same vehicle when used for the treatment of non-inflammatory acne.

CONTRAINDICATIONS

Duac Topical Gel is contraindicated in those individuals who have shown hypersensitivity to any of its components or to lincomycin. It is also contraindicated in those having a history of regional enteritis, ulcerative colitis, pseudomembranous colitis, or antibiotic-associated colitis.

WARNINGS

ORALLY AND PARENTERALLY ADMINISTERED CLINDAMYCIN HAS BEEN ASSOCIATED WITH SEVERE COLITIS WHICH MAY RESULT IN PATIENT DEATH. USE OF THE TOPICAL FORMULATION OF CLINDAMYCIN RESULTS IN ABSORPTION OF THE ANTIBIOTIC FROM THE SKIN SURFACE. DIARRHEA, BLOODY DIARRHEA, AND COLITIS (INCLUDING PSEUDOMEMBRANOUS COLITIS) HAVE BEEN REPORTED WITH THE USE OF TOPICAL AND SYSTEMIC CLINDAMYCIN. STUDIES INDICATE A TOXIN(S) PRODUCED BY CLOSTRIDIA IS ONE PRIMARY CAUSE OF ANTIBIOTIC-ASSOCIATED COLITIS. THE COLITIS IS USUALLY CHARACTERIZED BY SEVERE PERSISTENT DIARRHEA AND SEVERE ABDOMINAL CRAMPS AND MAY BE ASSOCIATED WITH THE PASSAGE OF BLOOD AND MUCUS. ENDOSCOPIC EXAMINATION MAY REVEAL PSEUDOMEMBRANOUS COLITIS. STOOL CULTURE FOR *Clostridium difficile* AND STOOL ASSAY FOR *Clostridium difficile* TOXIN MAY BE HELPFUL DIAGNOSTICALLY. WHEN SIGNIFICANT DIARRHEA OCCURS, THE DRUG SHOULD BE DISCONTINUED. LARGE BOWEL ENDOSCOPY SHOULD BE CONSIDERED TO ESTABLISH A DEFINITIVE DIAGNOSIS IN CASES OF SEVERE DIARRHEA. ANTIPERISTALTIC AGENTS SUCH AS OPIATES AND DIPHENOXYLATE WITH ATROPINE MAY PROLONG AND/OR WORSEN THE CONDITION. DIARRHEA, COLITIS AND PSEUDOMEMBRANOUS COLITIS HAVE BEEN OBSERVED TO BEGIN UP TO SEVERAL WEEKS FOLLOWING CESSATION OF ORAL AND PARENTERAL THERAPY WITH CLINDAMYCIN.

Mean percent reduction in inflammatory lesion counts

	Study 1 (n=120)	Study 2 (n=273)	Study 3 (n=280)	Study 4 (n=288)	Study 5 (n=358)
Duac	65%	56%	42%	57%	52%
Benzoyl Peroxide	36%	37%	32%	57%	41%
Clindamycin	34%	30%	38%	49%	33%
Vehicle	19%	–0.4%	29%	29%	29%

Local reactions with use of Duac Topical Gel
% of patients using Duac Topical Gel with symptom present
Combined results from 5 studies (n = 397)

	Before Treatment (Baseline)			During Treatment		
	Mild	Moderate	Severe	Mild	Moderate	Severe
Erythema	28%	3%	0	26%	5%	0
Peeling	6%	<1%	0	17%	2%	0
Burning	3%	<1%	0	5%	<1%	0
Dryness	6%	<1%	0	15%	1%	0

(Percentages derived by # subjects with symptom score/# enrolled Duac subjects, n = 397).

Mild cases of pseudomembranous colitis usually respond to drug discontinuation alone. In moderate to severe cases, consideration should be given to management with fluids and electrolytes, protein supplementation and treatment with an antibacterial drug clinically effective against *Clostridium difficile* colitis.

PRECAUTIONS

General: For dermatological use only; not for ophthalmic use. Concomitant topical acne therapy should be used with caution because a possible cumulative irritancy effect may occur, especially with the use of peeling, desquamating, or abrasive agents.

The use of antibiotic agents may be associated with the overgrowth of nonsusceptible organisms, including fungi. If this occurs, discontinue use of this medication and take appropriate measures.

Avoid contact with eyes and mucous membranes.

Clindamycin and erythromycin containing products should not be used in combination. *In vitro* studies have shown antagonism between these two antimicrobials. The clinical significance of this *in vitro* antagonism is not known.

Information for Patients: Patients using Duac Topical Gel should receive the following information and instructions:

1. Duac Topical Gel is to be used as directed by the physician. It is for external use only. Avoid contact with eyes, and inside the nose, mouth, and all mucous membranes, as this product may be irritating.
2. This medication should not be used for any disorder other than that for which it was prescribed.
3. Patients should not use any other topical acne preparation unless otherwise directed by their physician.
4. Patients should report any signs of local adverse reactions to their physician.
5. Duac Topical Gel may bleach hair or colored fabric.
6. Duac Topical Gel can be stored at room temperature up to 25°C (77°F) for up to 2 months. Do not freeze. Keep tube tightly closed. Keep out of the reach of small children. Discard any unused product after 2 months.
7. Before applying Duac Topical Gel to affected areas, wash the skin gently, rinse with warm water, and pat dry.
8. Excessive or prolonged exposure to sunlight should be limited. To minimize exposure to sunlight, a hat or other clothing should be worn.

Carcinogenesis, Mutagenesis, Impairment of Fertility: Benzoyl peroxide has been shown to be a tumor promoter and progression agent in a number of animal studies. The clinical significance of this is unknown.

Benzoyl peroxide in acetone at doses of 5 and 10 mg administered twice per week induced squamous cell skin tumors in transgenic TgAC mice in a study using 20 weeks of topical treatment.

Genotoxicity studies were not conducted with Duac Topical Gel. Clindamycin phosphate was not genotoxic in *Salmonella typhimurium* or in a rat micronucleus test. Benzoyl peroxide has been found to cause DNA strand breaks in a variety of mammalian cell types, to be mutagenic in *Salmonella typhimurium* tests by some but not all investigators, and to cause sister chromatid exchanges in Chinese hamster ovary cells. Studies have not been performed with Duac Topical Gel or benzoyl peroxide to evaluate the effect on fertility. Fertility studies in rats treated orally with up to 300 mg/kg/day of clindamycin (approximately 120 times the amount of clindamycin in the highest recommended adult human dose of 2.5 g Duac Topical Gel, based on mg/m^2) revealed no effects on fertility or mating ability.

Pregnancy: Teratogenic Effects: Pregnancy Category C: Animal reproduction studies have not been conducted with Duac Topical Gel or benzoyl peroxide. It is also not known whether Duac Topical Gel can cause fetal harm when administered to a pregnant woman or can affect reproduction capacity. Duac Topical Gel should be given to a pregnant woman only if clearly needed.

Developmental toxicity studies performed in rats and mice using oral doses of clindamycin up to 600 mg/kg/day (240 and 120 times the amount of clindamycin in the highest recommended adult human dose based on mg/m^2, respectively) or subcutaneous doses of clindamycin up to 250 mg/kg/day (100 and 50 times the amount of clindamycin in the highest recommended adult human dose based on mg/m^2, respectively) revealed no evidence of teratogenicity.

Nursing Women: It is not known whether Duac Topical Gel is secreted into human milk after topical application. However, orally and parenterally administered clindamycin has been reported to appear in breast milk. Because of the potential for serious adverse reactions in nursing infants, a decision should be made whether to discontinue nursing or to discontinue the drug, taking into account the importance of the drug to the mother.

Pediatric Use: Safety and effectiveness of this product in pediatric patients below the age of 12 have not been established.

ADVERSE REACTIONS

During clinical trials, all patients were graded for facial erythema, peeling, burning, and dryness on the following scale: 0 = absent, 1 = mild, 2 = moderate, and 3 = severe. The percentage of patients that had symptoms present before treatment (at baseline) and during treatment were as follows:

[See second table above]

DOSAGE AND ADMINISTRATION

Duac Topical Gel should be applied once daily, in the evening or as directed by the physician, to affected areas after the skin is gently washed, rinsed with warm water and patted dry.

HOW SUPPLIED

Duac® (clindamycin, 1% - benzoyl peroxide, 5%) Topical Gel is available in a 45 gram tube - NDC 0145-2371-05.

Prior to Dispensing: Store in a cold place, preferably in a refrigerator, between 2°C and 8°C (36°F and 46°F). Do not freeze.

Dispensing Instructions for the Pharmacist: Dispense Duac Topical Gel with a 60 day expiration date and specify "Store at room temperature up to 25°C (77°F). Do not freeze."

Keep tube tightly closed. Keep out of the reach of small children.

U.S. Patent Nos. 5,466,446, 5,446,028, 5,767,098, and 6,013,637

Patent Pending

LACTICARE®–HC Lotion 2$^1/_2$% ℞

[*läk 'tĭ-kār"*]

(hydrocortisone lotion, USP)

CONTAINS

Each mL of LactiCare-HC Lotion 2$^1/_2$% (hydrocortisone lotion, USP) contains 25 mg of hydrocortisone in a vehicle consisting of carbomer 940, sodium PCA, lactic acid, sodium hydroxide, stearyl alcohol (and) ceteareth-20, glyceryl stea-

Continued on next page

Lacticare-HC—Cont.

rate (and) PEG-100 stearate, cetyl alcohol, isopropyl palmitate, light mineral oil, myristyl lactate, DMDM hydantoin, dehydroacetic acid, fragrance and purified water.

HOW SUPPLIED

LactiCare®-HC Lotion 2$^1/_2$% (hydrocortisone lotion, USP) is available in the following sizes:

59 mL (2 fl oz) bottle NDC 0145-2538-02
118 mL (4 fl oz) bottle NDC 0145-2538-04

ROSAC® CREAM WITH SUNSCREENS ℞

[*rō' zăk*]

(sodium sulfacetamide 10% and sulfur 5%)

DESCRIPTION

Each gram of Rosac® Cream With Sunscreens contains 100 mg of sodium sulfacetamide and 50 mg of sulfur in a cream containing avobenzone, benzyl alcohol, C12-15 alkyl benzoate, cetostearyl alcohol, dimethicone, edetate disodium, emulsifying wax, monobasic sodium phosphate, octinoxate, propylene glycol, purified water, sodium thiosulfate, steareth-2, steareth-21.

Sodium sulfacetamide is a sulfonamide with antibacterial activity while sulfur acts as a keratolytic agent. Chemically, sodium sulfacetamide is N-[(4-aminophenyl) sulfonyl]-acetamide, monosodium salt, monohydrate. The structural formula is:

Na
NH_2–⟨benzene ring⟩–$SO_2NCOCH_3 \cdot H_2O$

CLINICAL PHARMACOLOGY

The most widely accepted mechanism of action of sulfonamides is the Woods-Fildes theory which is based on the fact that sulfonamides act as competitive antagonists to para-aminobenzoic acid (PABA), an essential component for bacterial growth. While absorption through intact skin has not been determined, sodium sulfacetamide is readily absorbed from the gastrointestinal tract when taken orally and excreted in the urine, largely unchanged. The biological half-life has variously been reported as 7 to 12.8 hours.

The exact mode of action of sulfur in the treatment of acne is unknown, but it has been reported that it inhibits the growth of *Propionibacterium acnes* and the formation of free fatty acids.

INDICATIONS AND USAGE

Rosac Cream With Sunscreens is indicated in the topical control of acne vulgaris, acne rosacea and seborrheic dermatitis.

CONTRAINDICATIONS

Rosac Cream With Sunscreens is contraindicated for use by patients having known hypersensitivity to sulfonamides, sulfur or any other component of this preparation. This drug is not to be used by patients with kidney disease.

WARNINGS

Although rare, sensitivity to sodium sulfacetamide may occur. Therefore, caution and careful supervision should be observed when prescribing this drug for patients who may be prone to hypersensitivity to topical sulfonamides. Systemic toxic reactions such as agranulocytosis, acute hemolytic anemia, purpura hemorrhagica, drug fever, jaundice, and contact dermatitis indicate hypersensitivity to sulfonamides. Particular caution should be employed if areas of denuded or abraded skin are involved.

PRECAUTIONS

General—If irritation develops, use of the product should be discontinued and appropriate therapy instituted. For external use only. Keep away from eyes. Patients should be carefully observed for possible local irritation or sensitization during long-term therapy. The object of this therapy is to achieve desquamation without irritation, but sodium sulfacetamide and sulfur can cause reddening and scaling of epidermis. These side effects are not unusual in the treatment of acne vulgaris, but patients should be cautioned about the possibility. Keep out of reach of children.

Carcinogenesis, Mutagenesis and Impairment of Fertility—Long-term studies in animals have not been performed to evaluate carcinogenic potential.

Pregnancy—Category C. Animal reproduction studies have not been conducted with Rosac Cream with Sunscreens. It is also not known whether this drug can cause fetal harm when administered to a pregnant woman or can affect reproduction capacity. It should be given to a pregnant woman only if clearly needed.

Nursing Mothers—It is not known whether sodium sulfacetamide is excreted in human milk following topical use of Rosac Cream With Sunscreens. However, small amounts of orally administered sulfonamides have been reported to be eliminated in human milk. In view of this and because many drugs are excreted in human milk, caution should be exercised when this drug is administered to a nursing woman.

Pediatric Use—Safety and effectiveness in children under the age of 12 have not been established.

ADVERSE REACTIONS

Although rare, sodium sulfacetamide may cause local irritation.

DOSAGE AND ADMINISTRATION

Apply a thin film of Rosac® Cream With Sunscreens to affected areas 1 to 3 times daily.

HOW SUPPLIED

45 g tubes (NDC 0145-2617-05)
Store at controlled room temperature 15°–30°C (59°–86°F).
Patent Pending

SULFOXYL® Lotion Regular ℞
SULFOXYL® Lotion Strong ℞

[*sul 'fox-ul*]

HOW SUPPLIED

Sulfoxyl Lotion Regular and Sulfoxyl Lotion Strong are supplied in 59 milliliter (2 fluid ounce) plastic bottles.

Sulfoxyl Lotion Regular	Sulfoxyl Lotion Strong
NDC 0145-3518-07	NDC 0145-3519-07

SuperGen, Inc.

4140 DUBLIN BLVD, SUITE 200
DUBLIN, CA 94568

For Placing Orders Contact:
Nipent: 800-222-6883
Mitomycin: 800-905-5474
For Customer Service:
Nipent
Mitomycin
800-353-1075 ext 184
For Medical or Drug Information Contact:
Medical Affairs:
888-437-8737
For Corporate Headquarters:
800-353-1075

MITOMYCIN ℞
FOR INJECTION, USP

DESCRIPTION

Mitomycin (also known as mitomycin-C) is an antibiotic isolated from the broth of *Streptomyces caespitosus* which has been shown to have antitumor activity. The compound is heat stable, has a high melting point, and is freely soluble in organic solvents.

Mitomycin for Injection is a sterile dry mixture of mitomycin and mannitol, which when reconstituted with Sterile Water for Injection provides a solution for intravenous administration. Mitomycin for Injection is supplied in vials containing 5 mg and 20 mg of mitomycin. Each 5 mg vial of Mitomycin for Injection contains mitomycin 5 mg and mannitol 10 mg. Each 20 mg vial of Mitomycin for Injection contains mitomycin 20 mg and mannitol 40 mg.

Mitomycin is a blue-violet crystalline powder with the molecular formula of $C_{15}H_{18}N_4O_5$ and a molecular weight of 334.33. Its chemical name is 7-amino-9α-methoxymitosane.

HOW SUPPLIED

Mitomycin for Injection, USP

NDC **62701-010-01**–5 mg mitomycin in an amber vial, individually packaged in single cartons.

NDC **62701-011-01**–20 mg mitomycin in an amber vial, individually packaged in single cartons.

Storage: Store dry powder at controlled room temperatures 15° to 30°C (59° to 86°F), protected from light. Protect reconstituted solution from light. Store solution under refrigeration 2° to 8°C (36° to 46°F), discard after 14 days. If unrefrigerated, discard after 7 days.

Rx Only

NIPENT® ℞
(pentostatin for injection)

WARNING

NIPENT should be administered under the supervision of a physician qualified and experienced in the use of cancer chemotherapeutic agents. The use of higher doses than those specified (see **DOSAGE AND ADMINISTRATION**) is not recommended. Dose-limiting severe renal, liver, pulmonary, and CNS toxicities occurred in Phase 1 studies that used NIPENT at higher doses (20–50 mg/m^2 in divided doses over 5 days) than recommended.

In a clinical investigation in patients with refractory chronic lymphocytic leukemia using NIPENT at the recommended dose in combination with fludarabine phosphate, 4 of 6 patients entered in the study had severe or fatal pulmonary toxicity. The use of NIPENT in combination with fludarabine phosphate is not recommended.

DESCRIPTION

NIPENT® (pentostatin for injection) is supplied as a sterile, apyrogenic, lyophilized powder in single-dose vials for intravenous administration. Each vial contains 10 mg of pentostain and 50 mg of Mannitol, USP. The pH of the final product is maintained between 7.0 and 8.5 by addition of sodium hydroxide or hydrochloric acid.

Pentostatin, also known as 2′-deoxycoformycin (DCF), is a potent inhibitor of the enzyme adenosine deaminase and is isolated from fermentation cultures of *Streptomyces antibioticus.* Pentostatin is known chemically as (R)-3-(2-deoxy-β-D-*erythro* -pentofuranosyl)-3,6,7,8-tetrahydroimidazo[4,5-*d*] [1,3]diazepin-8-ol with a molecular formula of $C_{11}H_{16}N_4O_4$ and a molecular weight of 268.27.

Pentostain is a white to off-white solid, freely soluble in distilled water.

The molecular structure of pentostatin is:

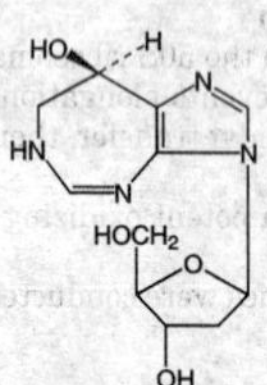

CLINICAL PHARMACOLOGY

Mechanism of Action

Pentostatin is a potent transition state inhibitor of the enzyme adenosine deaminase (ADA). The greatest activity of ADA is found in cells of the lymphoid system with T-cells having higher activity than B-cells and T-cell malignancies higher ADA activity than B-cell malignancies. Pentostatin inhibition of ADA, particularly in the presence of adenosine or deoxyadenosine, leads to cytotoxicity, and this is believed to be due to elevated intracellular levels of dATP which can block DNA synthesis through inhibition of ribonucleotide reductase. Pentostatin can also inhibit RNA synthesis as well as cause increased DNA damage. In addition to elevated dATP, these mechanisms may also contribute to the overall cytotoxic effect of pentostatin. The precise mechanism of pentostain's antitumor effect, however, in hairy cell leukemia is not known.

Pharmacokinetics/Drug Metabolism

A tissue distribution and whole-body autoradiography study in the rat revealed that radioactivity concentrations were highest in the kidneys with very little central nervous system penetration.

In man, following a single dose of 4 mg/m^2 of pentostain infused over 5 minutes, the distribution half-life was 11 minutes, the mean terminal half-life was 5.7 hours, the mean plasma clearance was 68 mL/min/m^2, and approximately 90% of the dose was excreted in the urine as unchanged pentostatin and/or metabolites as measured by adenosine deaminase inhibitory activity. The plasma protein binding of pentostain is low, approximately 4%.

A positive correlation was observed between pentostatin clearance and creatinine clearance (CrCl) in patients with creatinine clearance values ranging from 60 mL/min to 130 mL/min.[1] Pentostatin half-life in patients with renal impairment (CrCl <50 mL/min, n=2) was 18 hours, which was much longer than that observed in patients with normal renal function (CrCl >60 mL/min, n=14), about 6 hours.

CLINICAL STUDIES

The following table provides efficacy results for 4 groups (columns) of patients with hairy cell leukemia: patients who initially received NIPENT, patients who initially received alpha-interferon (IFN), and 2 different groups of patients who received NIPENT after proving to be refractory to, or intolerant of IFN therapy. The first 2 groups represent treatment results from the SWOG 8691 study, a large multicenter study comparing NIPENT and IFN in untreated (frontline) patients with confirmed hairy cell leukemia. The third group represents evaluable patients from the SWOG study who crossed over to NIPENT after initially receiving IFN. The fourth group, labeled NCI Phase 2 studies, displays pooled results of 2 noncomparative studies (MD Anderson and CALGB), in which NIPENT was used to treat patients with confirmed IFN-refractory disease.

In the SWOG 8691 study, NIPENT was administered at a dose of 4 mg/m^2 every 2 weeks. After 6 months of treatment, patients were evaluated for response. If a complete response was achieved, 2 additional doses of NIPENT were administered and then discontinued. If a partial response was achieved. NIPENT was continued for up to an additional 6 months. NIPENT was discontinued for stable disease after 6 months or progressive disease after 2 months of therapy. IFN was administered 3 million units subcutaneously 3 times per week. Patients who achieved a complete or partial response after 6 months of treatment continued on IFN for another 6 months. IFN was discontinued if patients did not achieve a complete or partial response after 6 months of initial treatment or progressed after 2 months. This study allowed crossover of patients intolerant of, or refractory to, initial treatment.

Interferon-refractory patients enrolled into the MD Anderson study received NIPENT at a dose of 4 mg/m^2 every other week for 3 months and responding patients received 3 additional months. CALGB patients received 4 mg/m^2 of NIPENT every other week for 3 months and responding patients were treated monthly for up to 9 additional months. Almost all patients had a PS of 0 to 2 in the Phase 2 and 3 studies.

For each study, a complete response (CR) required clearing of the peripheral blood and bone marrow of all hairy cells, normalization of organomegaly and lymphadenopathy by physical examination, and recovery of hemoglobin to at least 12 g/dL, platelet count to at least 100,000/mm^3, and granulocyte count to at least 1500/mm^3. A partial response (PR) required that the percentage of hairy cells in the blood and bone marrow decrease by more than 50%, enlarged organs and lymph nodes decrease by more than 50% by physical examination, and hematologic parameters had to meet the same criteria as for complete response. The table below reports the response rate for 2 groups of patients: (1) Evaluable, ie, patients who could be evaluated for response and (2) Intent-to-Treat, ie, patients diagnosed with hairy cell leukemia.

[See table above]

Parameter		FRONTLINE Evaluable NIPENT N=138	FRONTLINE Evaluable IFN N=130	IFN-REFRACTORY[a] SWOG 8691[b] Crossover N=79	IFN-REFRACTORY[a] NCI Phase 2 Studies N=44
Response Rates (%)					
Evaluable	CR	84	18	85	58
	PR	6	24	4	28
Intent-to-Treat		*N=170*	*N=170*		
	CR	*68*	*14*		
	PR	*5*	*18*		
Median Time to Response (months)					
	CR	6.6	11.5	6.0	4.2
	PR	4.0	6.2	5.8	—
Median Duration of Response (months)					
	CR	NR	8.3	NR	>7.7[c] (CALGB) >15.2[c] (MDA)
	PR	NR	15.2	NR	—
% Estimated to be in Response After 24 Months					
	CR	76	16	85	—
	PR	50	21	—	—
Median Time to Recovery (days)					
ANC (1500/mm^3)		70	106	—	—
Platelets (100,000/mm^3)		22	36	—	—

NR = Not reached by Kaplan-Meier method; ANC = Absolute neutrophil count.
[a]Evaluable patients
[b]Patients either refractory to, or intolerant of, IFN
[c]Kaplan-Meier estimate

The results show that frontline patients treated with NIPENT achieved a significantly higher rate of response than those treated with IFN. The time to recovery of neutrophil and platelet counts was shorter with NIPENT treatment and the estimated duration of response was longer. The response rate in IFN-refractory patients treated with NIPENT was similar to that in NIPENT-treated frontline patients. At a median follow-up duration of 46 months, there was no statistically significant difference in survival between hairy cell leukemia patients initially treated with NIPENT and those initially treated with IFN. However, no definite conclusions regarding survival can be made from these results because they are complicated by the fact that the majority of IFN patients crossed over to NIPENT treatment.

In the Phase 3 SWOG study, 25 patients with hairy cell leukemia died during treatment or follow-up: 18 patients had last received NIPENT (3 of whom had crossed over from IFN), and 7 patients had last received IFN (1 of whom crossed over from NIPENT). Eleven of the 25 deaths occurred within 60 days of the last dose of treatment. Of these, hairy cell leukemia was cited by the investigators as a contributory cause for 1 death in the NIPENT group and 3 deaths in the IFN group. Additionally, infection contributed to the deaths of 3 patients in the NIPENT group and 2 patients in the IFN group. Approximately 4% of hairy cell leukemia patients, in each arm, died more than 60 days after the last dose of either treatment and there was no outstanding cause of death among these patients.

INDICATIONS AND USAGE

NIPENT is indicated as single-agent treatment for both untreated and alpha-interferon-refractory hairy cell leukemia patients with active disease as defined by clinically significant anemia, neutropenia, thrombocytopenia, or disease-related symptoms.

CONTRAINDICATIONS

NIPENT is contraindicated in patients who have demonstrated hypersensitivity to NIPENT.

WARNINGS

See **Boxed Warning**.

Patients with hairy cell leukemia may experience myelosuppression primarily during the first few courses of treatment. Patients with infections prior to NIPENT treatment have in some cases developed worsening of their condition leading to death, whereas others have achieved complete response. Patients with infection should be treated only when the potential benefit of treatment justifies the potential risk to the patient. Efforts should be made to control the infection before treatment is initiated or resumed.

In patients with progressive hairy cell leukemia, the initial courses of NIPENT treatment were associated with worsening of neutropenia. Therefore, frequent monitoring of complete blood counts during this time is necessary. If severe neutropenia continues beyond the initial cycles, patients should be evaluated for disease status, including a bone marrow examination.

Elevations in liver function tests occurred during treatment with NIPENT and were generally reversible.

Renal toxicity was observed at higher doses in early studies; however, in patients treated at the recommended dose, elevations in serum creatinine were usually minor and reversible. There were some patients who began treatment with normal renal function who had evidence of mild to moderate toxicity at a final assessment. (See **DOSAGE AND ADMINISTRATION**.)

Rashes, occasionally severe, were commonly reported and may worsen with continued treatment. Withholding of treatment may be required (See **DOSAGE AND ADMINISTRATION**.)

Acute pulmonary edema and hypotension, leading to death, have been reported in the literature in patients treated with pentostatin in combination with carmustine, etoposide and high dose cyclophosphamide as part of the ablative regimen for bone marrow transplant.

Pregnancy Category D

Pentostatin can cause fetal harm when administered to a pregnant woman. Pentostatin was administered intravenously at doses of 0, 0.01, 0.1, or 0.75 mg/kg/day (0, 0.06, 0.6, and 4.5 mg/m^2) to pregnant rats on days 6 through 15 of gestation. Drug-related maternal toxicity occurred at doses of 0.1 and 0.75 mg/kg/day (0.6 and 4.5 mg/m^2). Teratogenic effects were observed at 0.75 mg/kg/day (4.5 mg/m^2) manifested by increased incidence of various skeletal malformations. In a dose range-finding study, pentostatin was administered intravenously to rats at doses of 0, 0.05, 0.1, 0.5, 0.75, or 1 mg/kg/day (0, 0.3, 0.6, 3, 4.5, 6 mg/m^2) on days 6 through 15 of gestation. Fetal malformations that were observed were an omphalocele at 0.05 mg/kg (0.3 mg/m^2), gastroschisis at 0.75 mg/kg and 1 mg/kg (4.5 and 6 mg/m^2), and a flexure defect of the hindlimbs at 0.75 mg/kg (4.5 mg/m^2). Pentostatin was also shown to be teratogenic in mice when administered as a single 2 mg/kg (6 mg/m^2) intraperitoneal injection on day 7 of gestation. Pentostatin was not teratogenic in rabbits when administered intravenously on days 6 through 18 of gestation at doses of 0, 0.005, 0.01, or 0.02 mg/kg/day (0, 0.015, 0.03, or 0.06 mg/m^2); however, maternal toxicity, abortions, early deliveries, and deaths occurred in all drug-treated groups. There are no adequate and well-controlled studies in pregnant women. If NIPENT is used during pregnancy, or if the patient becomes pregnant while taking (receiving) this drug, the patient should be apprised of the potential hazard to the fetus. Women of childbearing potential receiving NIPENT should be advised to avoid becoming pregnant.

PRECAUTIONS

General

Therapy with NIPENT requires regular patient observation and monitoring of hematologic parameters and blood chemistry values. If severe adverse reactions occur, the drug should be withheld (see **DOSAGE AND ADMINISTRATION**), and appropriate corrective measures should be taken according to the clinical judgment of the physician. NIPENT treatment should be withheld or discontinued in patients showing evidence of nervous system toxicity.

Information for Patients

Patients should be advised of the signs and symptoms of adverse events associated with NIPENT therapy. (See **ADVERSE REACTIONS**.)

Laboratory Tests

Prior to initiating therapy witn NIPENT, renal function should be assessed with a serum creatinine and/or a creatinine clearance assay. (See **CLINICAL PHARMACOLOGY** and **DOSAGE AND ADMINISTRATION**.) Complete blood counts and serum creatinine should be performed before each dose of NIPENT and at other appropriate periods during therapy (see **DOSAGE AND ADMINISTRATION**). Severe neutropenia has been observed following the early courses of treatment with NIPENT and therefore frequent monitoring of complete blood counts is recommended during this time. If hematologic parameters do not improve with subsequent courses, patients should be evaluated for disease status, including a bone marrow examination. Periodic monitoring of the peripheral blood for hairy cells should be performed to assess the response to treatment.

In addition, bone marrow aspirates and biopsies may be required at 2 to 3 month intervals to assess the response to treatment.

Drug Interactions

Allopurinol and NIPENT are both associated with skin rashes. Based on clinical studies in 25 refractory patients who received both NIPENT and allopurinol, the combined use of NIPENT and allopurinol did not appear to produce a higher incidence of skin rashes than observed with NIPENT alone. There has been a report of one patient who received both drugs and experienced a hypersensitivity vasculitis that resulted in death. It was unclear whether this adverse event and subsequent death resulted from the drug combination.

Biochemical studies have demonstrated that pentostatin enhances the effects of vidarabine, a purine nucleoside with antiviral activity. The combined use of vidarabine and NIPENT may result in an increase in adverse reactions associated with each drug. The therapeutic benefit of the drug combination has not been established.

The combined use of NIPENT and fludarabine phosphate is not recommended because it may be associated with an increased risk of fatal pulmonary toxicity (see **WARNINGS**).

Acute pulmonary edema and hypotension, leading to death, have been reported in the literature in patients treated with pentostatin in combination with carmustine, etoposide and high dose cyclophosphamide as part of the ablative regimen for bone marrow transplant.

Carcinogenesis, Mutagenesis, Impairment of Fertility

Carcinogenesis: No animal carcinogenicity studies have been conducted with pentostatin.

Mutagenesis: Pentostatin was nonmutagenic when tested in *Salmonella typhimurium* strains TA-98, TA-1535, TA-1537, and TA-1538. When tested with strain TA-100, a repeatable statistically significant response trend was observed with and without metabolic activation. The response was 2.1 to 2.2 fold higher than the background at 10 mg/plate, the maximum possible drug concentration. Formulated pentostatin was clastogenic in the *in vivo* mouse bone marrow micronucleus assay at 20, 120, and 240 mg/kg. Pentostatin was not mutagenic to V79 Chinese hamster lung cells at the HGPRT locus exposed 3 hours to concentrations of 1 to 3 mg/mL, with or without metabolic activation. Pentostatin did not significantly increase chromosomal aberrations in V79 Chinese hamster lung cells exposed 3 hours to 1 to 3 mg/mL in the presence or absence of metabolic activation.

Impairment of Fertility: No fertility studies have been conducted in animals; however, in a 5-day intravenous toxicity study in dogs, mild seminiferous tubular degeneration was observed with doses of 1 and 4 mg/kg. The possible adverse effects on fertility in humans have not been determined.

Pregnancy

Pregnancy Category D: (See **WARNINGS**)

Nursing Mothers

It is not known whether NIPENT is excreted in human milk. Because many drugs are excreted in human milk, and because of the potential for serious adverse reactions in nursing infants from pentostatin, a decision should be made whether to discontinue nursing or discontinue the drug, taking into account the importance of NIPENT to the mother.

Pediatric Use

Safety and effectiveness in children or adolescents have not been established.

ADVERSE REACTIONS

Most patients treated for hairy cell leukemia in the five NCI-sponsored Phase 2 and the Phase 3 SWOG study experienced an adverse event. The following table lists the most frequently occurring adverse events in patients treated with NIPENT (both frontline and IFN-refractory patients) compared with IFN (frontline only), regardless of drug association. The drug association of some adverse events is uncertain as they may be associated with the disease itself (eg, infection, hematologic suppression), but other events, such as the gastrointestinal symptoms, rashes, and abnormal liver function tests, can in many cases be attributed to the drug. Most adverse events that were asssessed for severity were either mild or moderate, and diminished in frequency with continued therapy.

Continued on next page

Nipent—Cont.

All Adverse Events[a]	Percent of Patients Frontline, Treated With NIPENT N=180	Frontline, Treated With IFN N=176	IFN-Refractory Treated With NIPENT N=197
Nausea and/or Vomiting	63	22	53[b]
Fever	46	59	42
Rash	43	30	26
Fatigue	42	55	29
Leukopenia	22	15	60
Pruritus	21	6	10
Coughing/Increased Cough	20	15	17
Myalgia	19	36	11
Chills	19	34	11
Headache	17	29	13
Diarrhea	17	17	15
Abdominal Pain	16	15	4
Anorexia	13	10	16
Upper Respiratory Infection	13	8	16
Asthenia	12	13	10
Stomatitis	12	7	5
Rhinitis	11	15	10
Dyspnea	11	13	8
Anemia	8	5	35
Pain	8	19	20
Pharyngitis	8	11	10
Sweating Increased/ Sweating	8	21	10
Viral Infection	8	17	NR
Infection	7[c]	2[c]	36
Arthralgia	6	14	3
Thrombocytopenia	6	6	32
Skin Disorder	4	5	17
Allergic Reaction	2	1	11
Hepatic Disorder/ Elevated Liver Function Tests[d]	2	2	19
Neurologic Disorder, CNS/CNS Toxicity	1	NR	11
Lung Disorder/ Disease	NR	1	12
Nausea	NR	NR	22
Genitourinary Disorder	NR	NR	15
Moniliasis, Oral	2	<1	
Mycotic Infection, Skin	<1	3	
Osteomyelitis	1	0	

NR = Not Reported

[a] Occurring in more than 10% of patients, in any group, regardless of drug association

[b] Includes only nausea with vomiting

[c] These figures represent only unspecified infections. Refer to infection table.

[d] Elevated liver enzymes and liver disorder for SWOG

The total incidence for all types of infections is considerably higher for both treatment groups in the SWOG 8691 study than is listed in the table above. An intent-to-treat analysis of infections found that 38% of patients treated with NIPENT and 34% of patients treated with IFN averaged 2.4 and 1.9 documented infections during treatment, respectively. The following table lists the different types of infections that were reported as adverse events during the initial phase of the SWOG study. There were no apparent differences in the types of infection between the 2 treatment groups, with the possible exception of herpes zoster which was reported more frequently for NIPENT (8%) than for IFN (1%).

Type of Infection	Percent of Patients Frontline, Treated With NIPENT N=180	Frontline, Treated With IFN N=176
Upper Respiratory Infection	13	8
Rhinitis	11	15
Herpes Zoster	8	1
Pharyngitis	8	11
Viral Infection	8	17
Infection (Unspecified)	7	2
Sinusitis	6	4
Cellulitis	6	3
Bacterial Infection	5	4
Pneumonia	5	7
Conjunctivitis	4	2
Furunculosis	4	<1
Herpes Simplex	4	1
Bronchitis	3	2
Sepsis	3	2
Urinary Tract Infection	3	3
Abscess, Skin	2	4

The drug relatedness of the adverse events listed below cannot be excluded. The following adverse events occurred in 3% to 10% of NIPENT-treated patients in the initial phase of the SWOG study:

Body as a Whole—Chest Pain, Death, Face Edema, Peripheral Edema

Cardiovascular System—Hemorrhage, Hypotension

Digestive System—Dental Abnormalities, Dyspepsia, Flatulence, Gingivitis

Hemic and Lymphatic System—Agranulocytosis

Laboratory Deviations—Elevated Creatinine

Musculoskeletal System—Arthralgia

Nervous System—Confusion, Dizziness, Insomnia, Paresthesia, Somnolence

Psychobiologic Function—Anxiety, Depression, Nervousness

Respiratory System—Asthma

Skin & Appendages—Skin Dry, Urticaria

The remaining adverse events which occurred in less than 3% of NIPENT-treated patients during the initial phase of the SWOG study:

Body as a Whole—Flu-like Symptoms, Hangover Effect, Neoplasm

Cardiovascular System—Angina Pectoris, Arrhythmia, A-V Block, Bradycardia, Extrasystoles Ventricular, Heart Arrest, Heart Failure, Hypertension, Pericardial Effusion, Phlebitis, Pulmonary Embolus, Sinus Arrest, Tachycardia, Thrombophlebitis Deep, Vasculitis

Digestive System—Constipation, Dysphagia, Glossitis, Ileus

Hemic and Lymphatic System—Acute Leukemia, Anemia-Hemolytic, Aplastic Anemia

Laboratory Deviations—Hypercalcemia, Hyponatremia

Musculoskeletal System—Arthritis, Gout

Nervous System—Amnesia, Ataxia, Convulsions, Dreaming Abnormal, Dysarthria, Encephalitis, Hyperkinesia, Meningism, Neuralgia, Neuritis, Neuropathy, Paralysis, Syncope, Twitching, Vertigo

Psychobiologic Function—Decrease/Loss Libido, Emotional Liability, Hallucination, Hostility, Neurosis, Thinking Abnormal

Respiratory System—Bronchospasm, Larynx Edema

Skin and Appendages—Acne, Alopecia, Eczema, Petechial Rash, Photosensitivity Reaction

Special Senses—Amblyopia, Deafness, Earache, Eyes Dry, Labyrinthitis, Lacrimation Disorder, Nonreactive Eye, Photophobia, Retinopathy, Tinnitus, Unusual Taste, Vision Abnormal, Watery Eyes

Urogenital System—Amenorrhea, Breast Lump, Impotence, Kidney Function Abnormal, Nephropathy, Renal Failure, Renal Insufficiency, Renal Stone

One patient with hairy cell leukemia treated with NIPENT during another clinical study developed unilateral uveitis with vision loss.

Nineteen (5%) patients withdrew from the Phase 3 SWOG 8691 study because of adverse events; 9 during initial NIPENT treatment, 4 during NIPENT crossover, 5 during initial IFN treatment, and 1 during both initial IFN treatment and NIPENT crossover. In the Phase 2 studies in IFN-refractory hairy cell leukemia, 11% of patients withdrew from treatment with NIPENT due to an adverse event.

OVERDOSAGE

No specific antidote for NIPENT overdose is known. NIPENT administered at higher doses (20 to 50 mg/m^2 in divided doses over 5 days) than recommended was associated with deaths due to severe renal, hepatic, pulmonary, and CNS toxicity. In case of overdose, management would include general supportive measures through any period of toxicity that occurs.

DOSAGE AND ADMINISTRATION

It is recommended that patients receive hydration with 500 to 1,000 mL of 5% Dextrose in 0.5 Normal Saline or equivalent before NIPENT administration. An additional 500 mL of 5% Dextrose or equivalent should be administered after NIPENT is given.

The recommended dosage of NIPENT for the treatment of hairy cell leukemia is 4 mg/m^2 every other week. NIPENT may be administered intravenously by bolus injection or diluted in a larger volume and given over 20 to 30 minutes. (See **Preparation of Intravenous Solution.**)

Higher doses are not recommended.

No extravasation injuries were reported in clinical studies.

The optimal duration of treatment has not been determined. In the absence of major toxicity and with observed continuing improvement, the patient should be treated until a complete response has been achieved. Although not established as required, the administration of two additional doses has been recommended following the achievement of a complete response.

All patients receiving NIPENT at 6 months should be assessed for response to treatment. If the patient has not achieved a complete or partial response, treatment with NIPENT should be discontinued.

If the patient has achieved a partial response, NIPENT treatment should be continued in an effort to achieve a complete response. At any time thereafter that a complete response is achieved, two additional doses of NIPENT are recommended. NIPENT treatment should then be stopped. If the best response to treatment at the end of 12 months is a partial response, it is recommended that treatment with NIPENT be stopped.

Withholding or discontinuation of individual doses may be needed when severe adverse reactions occur. Drug treatment should be withheld in patients with severe rash, and withheld or discontinued in patients showing evidence of nervous system toxicity.

NIPENT treatment should be withheld in patients with active infection occurring during the treatment but may be resumed when the infection is controlled.

Patients who have elevated serum creatinine should have their dose withheld and a creatinine clearance determined. There are insufficient data to recommend a starting or a subsequent dose for patients with impaired renal function (creatinine clearance <60 mL/min).

Patients with impaired renal function should be treated only when the potential benefit justifies the potential risk. Two patients with impaired renal function (creatinine clearances 50 to 60 mL/min) achieved complete response without unusual adverse events when treated with 2 mg/m^2.

No dosage reduction is recommended at the start of therapy with NIPENT in patients with anemia, neutropenia, or thrombocytopenia. In addition, dosage reductions are not recommended during treatment in patients with anemia and thrombocytopenia if patients can be otherwise supported hematologically. NIPENT should be temporarily withheld if the absolute neutrophil count falls during treatment below 200 cells/mm^3 in a patient who had an initial neutrophil count greater than 500 cells/mm^3 and may be resumed when the count returns to predose levels.

Preparation of Intravenous Solution

1. Procedures for proper handling and disposal of anticancer drugs should be followed. Several guidelines on this subject have been published.[2–7] There is no general agreement that all of the procedures recommended in the guidelines are necessary or appropriate. Spills and wastes should be treated with a 5% sodium hypochlorite solution prior to disposal.

2. Protective clothing including polyethylene gloves must be worn.

3. Transfer 5 mL of Sterile Water for Injection, USP to the vial containing NIPENT and mix thoroughly to obtain complete dissolution of a solution yielding 2 mg/mL. Parenteral drug products should be inspected visually for particulate matter and discoloration prior to administration.

4. NIPENT may be given intravenously by bolus injection or diluted in a larger volume (25 to 50 mL) with 5% Dextrose Injection, USP or 0.9% Sodium Chloride Injection, USP. Dilution of the entire contents of a reconstituted vial with 25 mL or 50 mL provides a pentostatin concentration of 0.33 mg/mL or 0.18 mg/mL, respectively, for the diluted solutions.

5. NIPENT solution when diluted for infusion with 5% Dextrose Injection, USP or 0.9% Sodium Chloride Injection, USP does not interact with PVC infusion containers or administration sets at concentrations of 0.18 mg/mL to 0.33 mg/mL.

Stability

NIPENT vials are stable at refrigerated storage temperature 2° to 8°C (36° to 46°F) for the period stated on the package. Vials reconstituted or reconstituted and further diluted as directed may be stored at room temperature and ambient light but should be used within 8 hours because NIPENT contains no preservatives.

HOW SUPPLIED

NIPENT (pentostatin for injection) is supplied as a sterile lyophilized white to off-white powder in single-dose vials containing 10 mg of pentostatin. The vials are packed in individual cartons. **NDC 62701-800-01**

Storage: Store NIPENT vials under refrigerated storage conditions 2° to 8°C (36° to 46°F).

Rx Only

REFERENCES

1. Malspeis L, et al. Clinical Pharmacokinetics of 2'-Deoxycoformycin. Cancer Treatment Symposia 2:7–15, 1984.

2. Recommendations for the safe handling of parenteral antineoplastic drugs. NIH publication 83-2621. For sale by the Superintendent of Documents, US Government Printing Office, Washington, NC 20402.

3. AMA council report. Guidelines for handling parenteral antineoplastics. JAMA 253:1590–2, 1985.

4. National Study Commission on Cytotoxic Exposure–Recommendations for handling cytotoxic agents. Available from Louis P. Jeffery, Sc.D., Chairman, National Study Commission on Cytotoxic Exposure, Massachusetts College of Pharmacy and Allied Health Sciences, 179 Longwood Ave, Boston, Massachusetts 02115.

5. Clinical Oncology Society of Australia: Guidelines and recommendations for safe handling of antineoplastic agents. Med J Australia 1:426–8, 1983.

6. Jones RB, et al. Safe handling of chemotherapeutic agents: A report from the Mount Sinai Medical Center. CA: A Cancer Journal for Clinicians 33:258–63, 1983.

7. American Society of Hospital Pharmacists technical assistance bulletin on handling cytotoxic and hazardous drugs. Am J Hosp Pharm 47:1033–49, 1990.

800P1 Rev. April, 1998

Swiss Bioceutical International, Ltd.

**2533 NORTH CARSON STREET
SUITE 3573
CARSON CITY, NV 89706**

Direct Inquiries to:
Executive Director
(775) 841-7020
FAX: (775) 883-2384
www.imuplus.net

IMUPLUS™ OTC

INTRACELLULAR GLUTATHIONE PRECURSOR
(A 99% non-denatured whey protein isolate)
Powder packets

DESCRIPTION

IMU*Plus*™ is a pharmaceutical grade (>99%) non-denatured whey protein isolate formula: a functional food that provides bioactive precursors for the intracellular production of glutathione, a critical constituent for the immune system and a vital antioxidant and detoxifying agent.

CLINICAL PHARMACOLOGY

Separation of whey components from the other constituents can result in significant denaturing of the bioactive whey proteins. IMU*Plus*™ utilizes a proprietary process to attain a product containing over 99% non-denatured whey protein, including bioactive lactoferrin, lysozyme, lactoperoxidase, glycomacropeptides, alpha lactalbumin and bovine serum albumin.

Non-denatured, bioactive whey proteins enhance intracellular glutathione by supplying to cells the dipeptides cysteine and glutamyl-cysteine. Glutathione has been found to enhance immune function, eliminate toxins and carcinogens, increases antioxidant and ionizing radiation protection and supports DNA synthesis and repair, protein prostaglandin and leukotriene synthesis, amino acid transport, and enzyme activity and regulation. Baruchel et al., have demonstrated that non-denatured whey protein isolate increased lymphocyte intracellular glutathione by greater than 120% in mice compared to mice fed standard, commercially available whey protein concentrates, or casein proteins. Similarly, Kennedy et al., demonstrated that non-denatured whey protein isolate increased glutathione in normal cells, but decreased glutathione in cancer cells. It has been proposed that cancer cells produce more intracellular glutathione than normal cells to protect themselves from various reactive oxygen species. Thus, it is possible that the ingestion of non-denatured whey protein isolates may oxidatively stress cancer cells, while protecting normal cells. This may be why carcinogen-treated mice fed non-denatured whey protein isolates had significantly smaller tumor burdens than controls. Wasting (cachexia) can also be a significant problem for the cancer patient. Although the mechanisms of cachexia are not fully understood, there are major metabolic alterations in the cancer patient and tumor cells usually resort to anaerobic rather than aerobic metabolism for the production of energy. This type of metabolism is grossly inefficient and generates large amounts of lactic acid that must, in turn, be regenerated back into glucose in the liver. Cachexia is also characterized by decreased appetite. IMU*Plus*™ supplies the patient with a perfectly balanced protein source without the need for large volumes of food and without the added burden of saturated fat solids or lactose associated with other milk protein sources.

CONTRAINDICATIONS and WARNINGS

IMU*Plus*™ is contraindicated in individuals who develop or have known hypersensitivity to specific milk proteins. IMU*Plus*™ contains <0.05% lactose and is generally well tolerated by lactose-intolerant individuals. Patients undergoing immunosuppressive therapy should discuss the use of this product with their health professional.

ADVERSE REACTIONS

Gastrointestinal bloating and cramps can occur if the product is not sufficiently rehydrated. Transient urticarial-like rash has been seen in rare individuals undergoing severe detoxification reaction. Such rashes were found to abate when product intake is stopped or reduced.

OVERDOSE

Overdosing on IMU*Plus*™ has not been reported. Unless hypersensitive to milk constituents, no toxicity of milk proteins has been described.

DOSAGES & ADMINISTRATION

Maintenance dose is 2 packets (20 grams) per day. For mild to moderate health challenges, higher doses are recommended. Clinical trials in patients with cancer, chronic fatigue syndrome, hepatitis and AIDS have used 30–50 grams per day.

DIRECTIONS

Take packet #1 at least 30 minutes before eating in the morning. Take packet #2 between 3-4 p.m. or, as directed by a health professional.

Fill a large glass with 6 ounces of distilled water -or- combine a compatible protein (milk, soy milk, almond milk and yogurt) with the distilled water. Empty a packet of IMU*Plus*™ into the liquid. Using a fork stir until mixture thickens. Let stand 5–10 minutes to rehydrate the formula, stir again and drink. (instructions are on packaging).

For easy mixing use our Portable Mixer designed to preserve the non-denatured quality of IMU*Plus*™.

CAUTION

Do not mix with fruit juice or heated liquids. Never mix in a conventional electric mixer/blender, as this will denature the IMU*Plus*™ bioactive proteins.

NOTE:- IMU*Plus*™ is a natural food supplement, and as such is limited from stating medical claims per se. Statements have not been evaluated by the FDA. As such, this product is not intended to diagnose, cure, prevent or treat any disease.

HOW SUPPLIED

One 600 gram carton contains 60, 10 gram packets.

- Gutman , J. Schettini, S., **The ultimate GSH 3. Handbook. Montreal**: Gutman and Schettini Enr. 1998
- Baruchel, S, Viav, G., Oliver. R., Bounous, G., Wainberg, MA. **Nutraceutical modulation of GSH with a humanized native milk serum protein isolate.** Marcel Deker Inc. New York, 1996
- Meister A. **New aspects of glutathione biochemistry and transport, selective alteration of glutathione metabolism.** *Nutr Rev* 42:397–410, 1984.
- Kaplowitz N, Aw T, Opkhtens M. **The regulation of hepatic glutathione.** *Ann Rev Pharmacol Toxicoil* 25:715-44, 1985.
- Kennedy R, Knok G, Bounous G, Baruchel S, Lee T. **The use of a whey protein in the treatment of patients with matastatic carcinoma: A phase i-ii clinical study.** *Anticancer Research* 15:2643–50.1995.
- Watanabe A, Higuichi K, Yasumura S, Shimizu Y, Kondo Y, Kohri H. **Nutritional modulation of glutathione level and cellular immunity in chronic hepatitis B and C.** *Hepatology.* 24:597A, 1996
- Lomaestro B. Malone M. **Glutathione in health and diseases: Pharmacotherapeutic Issues.** *Ann Pharmacother* 29:1267–73, 1995
- Lothian B, Grey V, Kimoff RJ, Lands LC. **Treatment of obstructive airway disease with a cysteine donor protein supplement:** a case report. *Chest* 117:914–916. 2000.

Distributed by:
SWISS BIOCEUTICAL INTERNATIONAL, LTD.
2533 N. Carson Street, Suite 3573
Carson City, Nevada 89706
Telephone: (775) 841-7020
Fax: (775) 883-2384
Web: www.imuplus.net

Product of USA — K-kosher seal
Packaged in USA — RedBook
Patent Pending — ADAP approved

Takeda Pharmaceuticals America, Inc.

**475 HALF DAY ROAD
LINCOLNSHIRE, IL 60069**

Direct Inquiries to:
Sales and Ordering:
Customer Service
(877) 5 TAKEDA
(877) 582-5332

For Medical Information Contact:
General:
(877) TAKEDA 7
(877) 825-3327

Adverse Drug Experiences:
(877) TAKEDA 7
(877) 825-3327

ACTOS® ℞

[*ăk'tōs*]
(pioglitazone hydrochloride) Tablets

DESCRIPTION

ACTOS (pioglitazone hydrochloride) is an oral antidiabetic agent that acts primarily by decreasing insulin resistance. ACTOS is used in the management of type 2 diabetes mellitus (also known as non-insulin-dependent diabetes mellitus [NIDDM] or adult-onset diabetes). Pharmacological studies indicate that ACTOS improves sensitivity to insulin in muscle and adipose tissue and inhibits hepatic gluconeogenesis. ACTOS improves glycemic control while reducing circulating insulin levels.

Pioglitazone [(±)-5-[[4-[2-(5-ethyl-2-pyridinyl)ethoxy]phenyl]methyl]-2,4-] thiazolidinedione monohydrochloride belongs to a different chemical class and has a different pharmacological action than the sulfonylureas, metformin, or the α-glucosidase inhibitors. The molecule contains one asymmetric carbon, and the compound is synthesized and used as the racemic mixture. The two enantiomers of pioglitazone interconvert in vivo. No differences were found in the pharmacologic activity between the two enantiomers. The structural formula is as shown:

[structural formula: CH_3 … N … O … S, O, NH, O • HCl]

Pioglitazone hydrochloride is an odorless white crystalline powder that has a molecular formula of $C_{19}H_{20}N_2O_3S \bullet HCl$ and a molecular weight of 392.90 daltons. It is soluble in N,N-dimethylformamide, slightly soluble in anhydrous ethanol, very slightly soluble in acetone and acetonitrile, practically insoluble in water, and insoluble in ether.

ACTOS is available as a tablet for oral administration containing 15 mg, 30 mg, or 45 mg of pioglitazone (as the base) formulated with the following excipients: lactose monohydrate NF, hydroxypropylcellulose NF, carboxymethylcellulose calcium NF, and magnesium stearate NF.

CLINICAL PHARMACOLOGY

Mechanism of Action

ACTOS is a thiazolidinedione antidiabetic agent that depends on the presence of insulin for its mechanism of action. ACTOS decreases insulin resistance in the periphery and in the liver resulting in increased insulin-dependent glucose disposal and decreased hepatic glucose output. Unlike sulfonylureas, pioglitazone is not an insulin secretagogue. Pioglitazone is a potent and highly selective agonist for peroxisome proliferator-activated receptor-gamma (PPARγ). PPAR receptors are found in tissues important for insulin action such as adipose tissue, skeletal muscle, and liver. Activation of PPARγ nuclear receptors modulates the transcription of a number of insulin responsive genes involved in the control of glucose and lipid metabolism.

In animal models of diabetes, pioglitazone reduces the hyperglycemia, hyperinsulinemia, and hypertriglyceridemia characteristic of insulin-resistant states such as type 2 diabetes. The metabolic changes produced by pioglitazone result in increased responsiveness of insulin-dependent tissues and are observed in numerous animal models of insulin resistance.

Since pioglitazone enhances the effects of circulating insulin (by decreasing insulin resistance), it does not lower blood glucose in animal models that lack endogenous insulin.

Pharmacokinetics and Drug Metabolism

Serum concentrations of total pioglitazone (pioglitazone plus active metabolites) remain elevated 24 hours after once daily dosing. Steady-state serum concentrations of both pioglitazone and total pioglitazone are achieved within 7 days. At steady-state, two of the pharmacologically active metabolites of pioglitazone, Metabolites III (M-III) and IV (M-IV), reach serum concentrations equal to or greater than pioglitazone. In both healthy volunteers and in patients with type 2 diabetes, pioglitazone comprises approximately 30% to 50% of the peak total pioglitazone serum concentrations and 20% to 25% of the total area under the serum concentration-time curve (AUC).

Maximum serum concentration (C_{max}), AUC, and trough serum concentrations (C_{min}) for both pioglitazone and total pioglitazone increase proportionally at doses of 15 mg and 30 mg per day. There is a slightly less than proportional increase for pioglitazone and total pioglitazone at a dose of 60 mg per day.

Absorption: Following oral administration, in the fasting state, pioglitazone is first measurable in serum within 30 minutes, with peak concentrations observed within 2 hours. Food slightly delays the time to peak serum concentration to 3 to 4 hours, but does not alter the extent of absorption.

Distribution: The mean apparent volume of distribution (Vd/F) of pioglitazone following single-dose administration is 0.63 ± 0.41 (mean ± SD) L/kg of body weight. Pioglitazone is extensively protein bound (> 99%) in human serum, principally to serum albumin. Pioglitazone also binds to other serum proteins, but with lower affinity. Metabolites M-III and M-IV also are extensively bound (> 98%) to serum albumin.

Metabolism: Pioglitazone is extensively metabolized by hydroxylation and oxidation; the metabolites also partly convert to glucuronide or sulfate conjugates. Metabolites M-II and M-IV (hydroxy derivatives of pioglitazone) and M-III (keto derivative of pioglitazone) are pharmacologically active in animal models of type 2 diabetes. In addition to pioglitazone, M-III and M-IV are the principal drug-related species found in human serum following multiple dosing. At steady-state, in both healthy volunteers and in patients with type 2 diabetes, pioglitazone comprises approximately 30% to 50% of the total peak serum concentrations and 20% to 25% of the total AUC.

In vitro data demonstrate that multiple CYP isoforms are involved in the metabolism of pioglitazone. The cytochrome P450 isoforms involved are CYP2C8 and, to a lesser degree, CYP3A4 with additional contributions from a variety of other isoforms including the mainly extrahepatic CYP1A1. In vivo studies of pioglitazone in combination with P450 inhibitors and substrates have been performed (see Drug Interactions). Urinary 6β-hydroxycortisol/cortisol ratios measured in patients treated with ACTOS showed that pioglitazone is not a strong CYP3A4 enzyme inducer.

Excretion and Elimination: Following oral administration, approximately 15% to 30% of the pioglitazone dose is recovered in the urine. Renal elimination of pioglitazone is negligible, and the drug is excreted primarily as metabolites

Continued on next page

Actos—Cont.

and their conjugates. It is presumed that most of the oral dose is excreted into the bile either unchanged or as metabolites and eliminated in the feces.

The mean serum half-life of pioglitazone and total pioglitazone ranges from 3 to 7 hours and 16 to 24 hours, respectively. Pioglitazone has an apparent clearance, CL/F, calculated to be 5 to 7 L/hr.

Special Populations

Renal Insufficiency: The serum elimination half-life of pioglitazone, M-III, and M-IV remains unchanged in patients with moderate (creatinine clearance 30 to 60 mL/min) to severe (creatinine clearance < 30 mL/min) renal impairment when compared to normal subjects. No dose adjustment in patients with renal dysfunction is recommended (see DOSAGE AND ADMINISTRATION).

Hepatic Insufficiency: Compared with normal controls, subjects with impaired hepatic function (Child-Pugh Grade B/C) have an approximate 45% reduction in pioglitazone and total pioglitazone mean peak concentrations but no change in the mean AUC values.

ACTOS therapy should not be initiated if the patient exhibits clinical evidence of active liver disease or serum transaminase levels (ALT) exceed 2.5 times the upper limit of normal (see PRECAUTIONS, Hepatic Effects).

Elderly: In healthy elderly subjects, peak serum concentrations of pioglitazone and total pioglitazone are not significantly different, but AUC values are slightly higher and the terminal half-life values slightly longer than for younger subjects. These changes were not of a magnitude that would be considered clinically relevant.

Pediatrics: Pharmacokinetic data in the pediatric population are not available.

Gender: The mean C_{max} and AUC values were increased 20% to 60% in females. As monotherapy and in combination with sulfonylurea, metformin, or insulin, ACTOS improved glycemic control in both males and females. In controlled clinical trials, hemoglobin A_{1c} (HbA_{1c}) decreases from baseline were generally greater for females than for males (average mean difference in HbA_{1c} 0.5%). Since therapy should be individualized for each patient to achieve glycemic control, no dose adjustment is recommended based on gender alone.

Ethnicity: Pharmacokinetic data among various ethnic groups are not available.

Drug-Drug Interactions

The following drugs were studied in healthy volunteers with a co-administration of ACTOS 45 mg once daily. Listed below are the results:

Oral Contraceptives: Co-administration of ACTOS (45 mg once daily) and an oral contraceptive (1 mg norethindrone plus 0.035 mg ethinyl estradiol once daily) for 21 days, resulted in 11% and 11-14% decrease in ethinyl estradiol AUC (0–24h) and C_{max} respectively. There were no significant changes in norethindrone AUC (0–24h) and C_{max}. In view of the high variability of ethinyl estradiol pharmacokinetics, the clinical significance of this finding is unknown.

Fexofenadine HCl: Co-administration of ACTOS for 7 days with 60 mg fexofenadine administered orally twice daily resulted in no significant effect on pioglitazone pharmacokinetics. ACTOS had no significant effect on fexofenadine pharmacokinetics.

Glipizide: Co-administration of ACTOS and 5 mg glipizide administered orally once daily for 7 days did not alter the steady-state pharmacokinetics of glipizide.

Digoxin: Co-administration of ACTOS with 0.25 mg digoxin administered orally once daily for 7 days did not alter the steady-state pharmacokinetics of digoxin.

Warfarin: Co-administration of ACTOS for 7 days with warfarin did not alter the steady-state pharmacokinetics of warfarin. ACTOS has no clinically significant effect on prothrombin time when administered to patients receiving chronic warfarin therapy.

Metformin: Co-administration of a single dose of metformin (1000 mg) and ACTOS after 7 days of ACTOS did not alter the pharmacokinetics of the single dose of metformin.

Midazolam: Administration of ACTOS for 15 days followed by a single 7.5 mg dose of midazolam syrup resulted in a 26% reduction in midazolam C_{max} and AUC.

Ranitidine HCl: Co-administration of ACTOS for 7 days with ranitidine administered orally twice daily for either 4 or 7 days resulted in no significant effect on pioglitazone pharmacokinetics. ACTOS showed no significant effect on ranitidine pharmacokinetics.

Nifedipine ER: Co-administration of ACTOS for 7 days with 30 mg nifedipine ER administered orally once daily for 4 days to male and female volunteers resulted in least square mean (90% CI) values for unchanged nifedipine of 0.83 (0.73-0.95) for C_{max} and 0.88 (0.80-0.96) for AUC. In view of the high variability of nifedipine pharmacokinetics, the clinical significance of this finding is unknown.

Ketoconazole: Co-administration of ACTOS for 7 days with ketoconazole 200 mg administered twice daily resulted in least square mean (90% CI) values for unchanged pioglitazone of 1.14 (1.06–1.23) for C_{max}, 1.34 (1.26–1.41) for AUC and 1.87 (1.71–2.04) for C_{min}.

Atorvastatin Calcium: Co-administration of ACTOS for 7 days with atorvastatin calcium (LIPITOR®) 80 mg once daily resulted in least square mean (90% CI) values for unchanged pioglitazone of 0.69 (0.57–0.85) for C_{max}, 0.76 (0.65–0.88) for AUC and 0.96 (0.87–1.05) for C_{min}. For unchanged atorvastatin the least square mean (90% CI) values were 0.77 (0.66–0.90) for C_{max}, 0.86 (0.78–0.94) for AUC and 0.92 (0.82–1.02) for C_{min}.

Theophylline: Co-administration of ACTOS for 7 days with theophylline 400 mg administered twice daily resulted in no change in the pharmacokinetics of either drug.

Cytochrome P450: See **PRECAUTIONS**

Pharmacodynamics and Clinical Effects

Clinical studies demonstrate that ACTOS improves insulin sensitivity in insulin-resistant patients. ACTOS enhances cellular responsiveness to insulin, increases insulin-dependent glucose disposal, improves hepatic sensitivity to insulin, and improves dysfunctional glucose homeostasis. In patients with type 2 diabetes, the decreased insulin resistance produced by ACTOS results in lower plasma glucose concentrations, lower plasma insulin levels, and lower HbA_{1c} values. Based on results from an open-label extension study, the glucose lowering effects of ACTOS appear to persist for at least one year. In controlled clinical trials, ACTOS in combination with sulfonylurea, metformin, or insulin had an additive effect on glycemic control.

Patients with lipid abnormalities were included in clinical trials with ACTOS. Overall, patients treated with ACTOS had mean decreases in triglycerides, mean increases in HDL cholesterol, and no consistent mean changes in LDL and total cholesterol.

In a 26-week, placebo-controlled, dose-ranging study, mean triglyceride levels decreased in the 15 mg, 30 mg, and 45 mg ACTOS dose groups compared to a mean increase in the placebo group. Mean HDL levels increased to a greater extent in patients treated with ACTOS than in the placebo-treated patients. There were no consistent differences for LDL and total cholesterol in patients treated with ACTOS compared to placebo (Table 1).

[See table 1 above]

Table 1 Lipids in a 26-Week Placebo-Controlled Monotherapy Dose-Ranging Study

	Placebo	ACTOS 15 mg Once Daily	ACTOS 30 mg Once Daily	ACTOS 45 mg Once Daily
Triglycerides (mg/dL)	N=79	N=79	N=84	N=77
Baseline (mean)	262.8	283.8	261.1	259.7
Percent change from baseline (mean)	4.8%	-9.0%	-9.6%	-9.3%
HDL Cholesterol (mg/dL)	N=79	N=79	N=83	N=77
Baseline (mean)	41.7	40.4	40.8	40.7
Percent change from baseline (mean)	8.1%	14.1%	12.2%	19.1%
LDL Cholesterol (mg/dL)	N=65	N=63	N=74	N=62
Baseline (mean)	138.8	131.9	135.6	126.8
Percent change from baseline (mean)	4.8%	7.2%	5.2%	6.0%
Total Cholesterol (mg/dL)	N=79	N=79	N=84	N=77
Baseline (mean)	224.6	220.0	222.7	213.7
Percent change from baseline (mean)	4.4%	4.6%	3.3%	6.4%

In the two other monotherapy studies (24 weeks and 16 weeks) and in combination therapy studies with sulfonylurea (24 weeks and 16 weeks) and metformin (24 weeks and 16 weeks), the results were generally consistent with the data above. In placebo-controlled trials, the placebo-corrected mean changes from baseline decreased 5% to 26% for triglycerides and increased 6% to 13% for HDL in patients treated with ACTOS. A similar pattern of results was seen in 24-week combination therapy studies of ACTOS with sulfonylurea or metformin.

In a combination therapy study with insulin (16 weeks), the placebo-corrected mean percent change from baseline in triglyceride values for patients treated with ACTOS was also decreased. A placebo-corrected mean change from baseline in LDL cholesterol of 7% was observed for the 15 mg dose group. Similar results to those noted above for HDL and total cholesterol were observed. A similar pattern of results was seen in a 24-week combination therapy study with ACTOS with insulin.

Clinical Studies

Monotherapy

In the U.S., three randomized, double-blind, placebo-controlled trials with durations from 16 to 26 weeks were conducted to evaluate the use of ACTOS as monotherapy in patients with type 2 diabetes. These studies examined ACTOS at doses up to 45 mg or placebo once daily in 865 patients.

In a 26-week dose-ranging study, 408 patients with type 2 diabetes were randomized to receive 7.5 mg, 15 mg, 30 mg, or 45 mg of ACTOS, or placebo once daily. Therapy with any previous antidiabetic agent was discontinued 8 weeks prior to the double-blind period. Treatment with 15 mg, 30 mg, and 45 mg of ACTOS produced statistically significant improvements in HbA_{1c} and fasting plasma glucose (FPG) at endpoint compared to placebo (see Figure 1, Table 2).

Figure 1 shows the time course for changes in FPG and HbA_{1c} for the entire study population in this 26-week study.

[See figure 1 above]

Figure 1 Mean Change from Baseline for FPG and HbA_{1c} in a 26-Week Placebo-Controlled Dose-Ranging Study

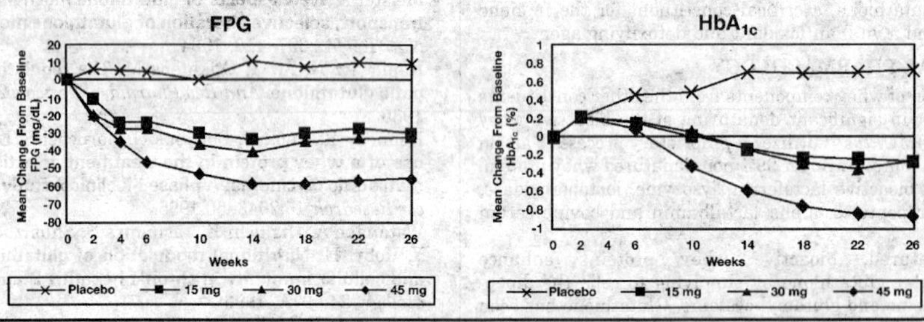

Table 2 shows HbA_{1c} and FPG values for the entire study population.

[See table 2 above]

Table 2 Glycemic Parameters in a 26-Week Placebo-Controlled Dose-Ranging Study

	Placebo	ACTOS 15 mg Once Daily	ACTOS 30 mg Once Daily	ACTOS 45 mg Once Daily
Total Population				
HbA_{1c} (%)	N=79	N=79	N=85	N=76
Baseline (mean)	10.4	10.2	10.2	10.3
Change from baseline (adjusted mean⁺)	0.7	-0.3	-0.3	-0.9
Difference from placebo (adjusted mean⁺)		-1.0*	-1.0*	-1.6*
FPG (mg/dL)	N=79	N=79	N=84	N=77
Baseline (mean)	268	267	269	276
Change from baseline (adjusted mean⁺)	9	-30	-32	-56
Difference from placebo (adjusted mean⁺)		-39*	-41*	-65*

⁺ Adjusted for baseline, pooled center, and pooled center by treatment interaction
* $p \leq 0.050$ vs. placebo

The study population included patients not previously treated with antidiabetic medication (naïve; 31%) and patients who were receiving antidiabetic medication at the time of study enrollment (previously treated; 69%). The data for the naïve and previously-treated patient subsets are shown in Table 3. All patients entered an 8 week wash-out/run-in period prior to double-blind treatment. This run-in period was associated with little change in HbA_{1c} and FPG values from screening to baseline for the naïve patients; however, for the previously-treated group, washout from previous antidiabetic medication resulted in deterioration of glycemic control and increases in HbA_{1c} and FPG. Although most patients in the previously-treated group had a decrease from baseline in HbA_{1c} and FPG with ACTOS, in many cases the values did not return to screening levels by the end of the study. The study design did not permit the evaluation of patients who switched directly to ACTOS from another antidiabetic agent.

[See table 3 at right]

In a 24-week placebo-controlled study, 260 patients with type 2 diabetes were randomized to one of two forced-titration ACTOS treatment groups or a mock titration placebo group. Therapy with any previous antidiabetic agent was discontinued 6 weeks prior to the double-blind period. In one ACTOS treatment group, patients received an initial dose of 7.5 mg once daily. After four weeks, the dose was increased to 15 mg once daily and after another four weeks, the dose was increased to 30 mg once daily for the remainder of the study (16 weeks). In the second ACTOS treatment group, patients received an initial dose of 15 mg once daily and were titrated to 30 mg once daily and 45 mg once daily in a similar manner. Treatment with ACTOS, as described, produced statistically significant improvements in HbA_{1c} and FPG at endpoint compared to placebo (see Table 4).

[See table 4 at right]

For patients who had not been previously treated with antidiabetic medication (24%), mean values at screening were 10.1% for HbA_{1c} and 238 mg/dL for FPG. At baseline, mean HbA_{1c} was 10.2% and mean FPG was 243 mg/dL. Compared with placebo, treatment with ACTOS titrated to a final dose of 30 mg and 45 mg resulted in reductions from baseline in mean HbA_{1c} of 2.3% and 2.6% and mean FPG of 63 mg/dL and 95 mg/dL, respectively. For patients who had been previously treated with antidiabetic medication (76%), this medication was discontinued at screening. Mean values at screening were 9.4% for HbA_{1c} and 216 mg/dL for FPG. At baseline, mean HbA_{1c} was 10.7% and mean FPG was 290 mg/dL. Compared with placebo, treatment with ACTOS titrated to a final dose of 30 mg and 45 mg resulted in reductions from baseline in mean HbA_{1c} of 1.3% and 1.4% and mean FPG of 55 mg/dL and 60 mg/dL, respectively. For many previously-treated patients, HbA_{1c} and FPG had not returned to screening levels by the end of the study.

In a 16-week study, 197 patients with type 2 diabetes were randomized to treatment with 30 mg of ACTOS or placebo once daily. Therapy with any previous antidiabetic agent was discontinued 6 weeks prior to the double-blind period. Treatment with 30 mg of ACTOS produced statistically significant improvements in HbA_{1c} and FPG at endpoint compared to placebo (see Table 5).

[See table 5 at right]

For patients who had not been previously treated with antidiabetic medication (40%), mean values at screening were 10.3% for HbA_{1c} and 240 mg/dL for FPG. At baseline, mean HbA_{1c} was 10.4% and mean FPG was 254 mg/dL. Compared with placebo, treatment with ACTOS 30 mg resulted in reductions from baseline in mean HbA_{1c} of 1.0% and mean FPG of 62 mg/dL. For patients who had been previously treated with antidiabetic medication (60%), this medication was discontinued at screening. Mean values at screening were 9.4% for HbA_{1c} and 216 mg/dL for FPG. At baseline, mean HbA_{1c} was 10.6% and mean FPG was 287 mg/dL. Compared with placebo, treatment with ACTOS 30 mg resulted in reductions from baseline in mean HbA_{1c} of 1.3% and mean FPG of 46 mg/dL. For many previously-treated patients, HbA_{1c} and FPG had not returned to screening levels by the end of the study.

Combination Therapy

Three 16-week, randomized, double-blind, placebo-controlled clinical studies and three 24-week randomized, double-blind, dose-controlled clinical studies were conducted to evaluate the effects of ACTOS on glycemic control in patients with type 2 diabetes who were inadequately controlled ($HbA_{1c} \geq 8\%$) despite current therapy with a sulfonylurea, metformin, or insulin. Previous diabetes treatment may have been monotherapy or combination therapy.

ACTOS Plus Sulfonylurea Studies

Two clinical studies were conducted with ACTOS in combination with a sulfonylurea. Both studies included patients with type 2 diabetes on a sulfonylurea, either alone or in combination with another antidiabetic agent. All other antidiabetic agents were withdrawn prior to starting study treatment. In the first study, 560 patients were randomized to receive 15 mg or 30 mg of ACTOS or placebo once daily for 16 weeks in addition to their current sulfonylurea regimen. When compared to placebo at Week 16, the addition of ACTOS to the sulfonylurea significantly reduced the mean HbA_{1c} by 0.9% and 1.3% and mean FPG by 39 mg/dL and 58 mg/dL for the 15 mg and 30 mg doses, respectively.

In the second study, 702 patients were randomized to receive 30 mg or 45 mg of ACTOS once daily for 24 weeks in addition to their current sulfonylurea regimen. The mean reductions from baseline at Week 24 in HbA_{1c} were 1.55% and 1.67% for the 30 mg and 45 mg doses, respectively. Mean reductions from baseline in FPG were 51.5 mg/dL and 56.1 mg/dL.

The therapeutic effect of ACTOS in combination with sulfonylurea was observed in patients regardless of whether the patients were receiving low, medium, or high doses of sulfonylurea.

Table 3 Glycemic Parameters in a 26-Week Placebo-Controlled Dose-Ranging Study

	Placebo	ACTOS 15 mg Once Daily	ACTOS 30 mg Once Daily	ACTOS 45 mg Once Daily
Naïve to Therapy				
HbA_{1c} (%)	N=25	N=26	N=26	N=21
Screening (mean)	9.3	10.0	9.5	9.8
Baseline (mean)	9.0	9.9	9.3	10.0
Change from baseline (adjusted mean*)	0.6	-0.8	-0.6	-1.9
Difference from placebo (adjusted mean*)		-1.4	-1.3	-2.6
FPG (mg/dL)	N=25	N=26	N=26	N=21
Screening (mean)	223	245	239	239
Baseline (mean)	229	251	225	235
Change from baseline (adjusted mean*)	16	-37	-41	-64
Difference from placebo (adjusted mean*)		-52	-56	-80
Previously Treated				
HbA_{1c} (%)	N=54	N=53	N=59	N=55
Screening (mean)	9.3	9.0	9.1	9.0
Baseline (mean)	10.9	10.4	10.4	10.6
Change from baseline (adjusted mean*)	0.8	-0.1	-0.0	-0.6
Difference from placebo (adjusted mean*)		-1.0	-0.9	-1.4
FPG (mg/dL)	N=54	N=53	N=58	N=56
Screening (mean)	222	209	230	215
Baseline (mean)	285	275	286	292
Change from baseline (adjusted mean*)	4	-32	-27	-55
Difference from placebo (adjusted mean*)		-36	-31	-59

* Adjusted for baseline and pooled center

Table 4 Glycemic Parameters in a 24-Week Placebo-Controlled Forced-Titration Study

	Placebo	ACTOS 30 mg+ Once Daily	ACTOS 45 mg+ Once Daily
Total Population			
HbA_{1c} (%)	N=83	N=85	N=85
Baseline (mean)	10.8	10.3	10.8
Change from baseline (adjusted mean++)	0.9	-0.6	-0.6
Difference from placebo (adjusted mean++)		-1.5*	-1.5*
FPG (mg/dL)	N=78	N=82	N=85
Baseline (mean)	279	268	281
Change from baseline (adjusted mean++)	18	-44	-50
Difference from placebo (adjusted mean++)		-62*	-68*

+ Final dose in forced titration

++ Adjusted for baseline, pooled center, and pooled center by treatment interaction

* $p \leq 0.050$ vs. placebo

Table 5 Glycemic Parameters in a 16-Week Placebo-Controlled Study

	Placebo	ACTOS 30 mg Once Daily
Total Population		
HbA_{1c} (%)	N=93	N=100
Baseline (mean)	10.3	10.5
Change from baseline (adjusted mean+)	0.8	-0.6
Difference from placebo (adjusted mean+)		-1.4*
FPG (mg/dL)	N=91	N=99
Baseline (mean)	270	273
Change from baseline (adjusted mean+)	8	-50
Difference from placebo (adjusted mean+)		-58*

+ Adjusted for baseline, pooled center, and pooled center by treatment interaction

* $p \leq 0.050$ vs. placebo

ACTOS Plus Metformin Studies

Two clinical studies were conducted with ACTOS in combination with metformin. Both studies included patients with type 2 diabetes on metformin, either alone or in combination with another antidiabetic agent. All other antidiabetic agents were withdrawn prior to starting study treatment. In the first study, 328 patients were randomized to receive either 30 mg of ACTOS or placebo once daily for 16 weeks in addition to their current metformin regimen. When compared to placebo at Week 16, the addition of ACTOS to metformin significantly reduced the mean HbA_{1c} by 0.8% and decreased the mean FPG by 38 mg/dL. In the second study, 827 patients were randomized to receive either 30 mg or 45 mg of ACTOS once daily for 24 weeks in addition to their current metformin regimen. The mean reductions from baseline at Week 24 in HbA_{1c} were 0.80% and 1.01% for the 30 mg and 45 mg doses, respectively. Mean reductions from baseline in FPG were 38.2 mg/dL and 50.7 mg/dL.

The therapeutic effect of ACTOS in combination with metformin was observed in patients regardless of whether the patients were receiving lower or higher doses of metformin.

ACTOS Plus Insulin Studies

Two clinical studies were conducted with ACTOS in combination with insulin. Both studies included patients with type 2 diabetes on insulin, either alone or in combination with another antidiabetic agent. All other antidiabetic agents were withdrawn prior to starting study treatment. In the first study, 566 patients receiving a median of 60.5 units per day of insulin were randomized to receive either 15 mg or 30 mg of ACTOS or placebo once daily for 16 weeks in addition to their insulin regimen. When compared to placebo at Week 16, the addition of ACTOS to insulin significantly reduced both HbA_{1c} by 0.7% and 1.0% and FPG by 35 mg/dL and 49 mg/dL for the 15 mg and 30 mg dose, respectively.

In the second study, 690 patients receiving a median of 60.0 units per day of insulin received either 30 mg or 45 mg of ACTOS once daily for 24 weeks in addition to their current insulin regimen. The mean reductions from baseline at Week 24 in HbA_{1c} were 1.17% and 1.46% for the 30 mg and 45 mg doses, respectively. Mean reductions from baseline in FPG were 31.9 mg/dL and 45.8 mg/dL. Improved glycemic control was accompanied by mean decreases from baseline in insulin dose requirements of 6.0% and 9.4% per day for the 30 mg and 45 mg dose, respectively.

The therapeutic effect of ACTOS in combination with insulin was observed in patients regardless of whether the patients were receiving lower or higher doses of insulin.

INDICATIONS AND USAGE

ACTOS is indicated as an adjunct to diet and exercise to improve glycemic control in patients with type 2 diabetes (non-insulin-dependent diabetes mellitus, NIDDM). ACTOS is indicated for monotherapy. ACTOS is also indicated for

Continued on next page

Actos—Cont.

use in combination with a sulfonylurea, metformin, or insulin when diet and exercise plus the single agent does not result in adequate glycemic control.

Management of type 2 diabetes should also include nutritional counseling, weight reduction as needed, and exercise. These efforts are important not only in the primary treatment of type 2 diabetes, but also to maintain the efficacy of drug therapy.

CONTRAINDICATIONS

ACTOS is contraindicated in patients with known hypersensitivity to this product or any of its components.

WARNINGS

Cardiac Failure and Other Cardiac Effects

ACTOS, like other thiazolidinediones, can cause fluid retention when used alone or in combination with other antidiabetic agents, including insulin. Fluid retention may lead to or exacerbate heart failure. Patients should be observed for signs and symptoms of heart failure (see Information for Patients). ACTOS should be discontinued if any deterioration in cardiac status occurs. Patients with New York Heart Association (NYHA) Class III and IV cardiac status were not studied during pre-approval clinical trials; ACTOS is not recommended in these patients (see PRECAUTIONS, Cardiovascular).

In one 16-week U.S. double-blind, placebo-controlled clinical trial involving 566 patients with type 2 diabetes, ACTOS at doses of 15 mg and 30 mg in combination with insulin was compared to insulin therapy alone. This trial included patients with long-standing diabetes and a high prevalence of pre-existing medical conditions as follows: arterial hypertension (57.2%), peripheral neuropathy (22.6%), coronary heart disease (19.6%), retinopathy (13.1%), myocardial infarction (8.8%), vascular disease (6.4%), angina pectoris (4.4%), stroke and/or transient ischemic attack (4.1%), and congestive heart failure (2.3%).

In this study two of the 191 patients receiving 15 mg ACTOS plus insulin (1.1%) and two of the 188 patients receiving 30 mg ACTOS plus insulin (1.1%) developed congestive heart failure compared with none of the 187 patients on insulin therapy alone. All four of these patients had previous histories of cardiovascular conditions including coronary artery disease, previous CABG procedures, and myocardial infarction. In a 24-week dose-controlled study in which ACTOS was coadministered with insulin, 0.3% of patients (1/345) on 30 mg and 0.9% (3/345) of patients on 45 mg reported CHF as a serious adverse event.

Analysis of data from these studies did not identify specific factors that predict increased risk of congestive heart failure on combination therapy with insulin.

In type 2 diabetes and congestive heart failure (systolic dysfunction)

A 24-week post-marketing safety study was performed to compare ACTOS (n=262) to glyburide (n=256) in uncontrolled diabetic patients (mean HbA_{1c} 8.8% at baseline) with NYHA Class II and III heart failure and ejection fraction less than 40% (mean EF 30% at baseline). Over the course of the study, overnight hospitalization for congestive heart failure was reported in 9.9% of patients on ACTOS compared to 4.7% of patients on glyburide with a treatment difference observed from 6 weeks. This adverse event associated with ACTOS was more marked in patients using insulin at baseline and in patients over 64 years of age. No difference in cardiovascular mortality between the treatment groups was observed.

ACTOS should be initiated at the lowest approved dose if it is prescribed for patients with type 2 diabetes and systolic heart failure (NYHA Class II). If subsequent dose escalation is necessary, the dose should be increased gradually only after several months of treatment with careful monitoring for weight gain, edema, or signs and symptoms of CHF exacerbation.

PRECAUTIONS

General

ACTOS exerts its antihyperglycemic effect only in the presence of insulin. Therefore, ACTOS should not be used in patients with type 1 diabetes or for the treatment of diabetic ketoacidosis.

Hypoglycemia: Patients receiving ACTOS in combination with insulin or oral hypoglycemic agents may be at risk for hypoglycemia, and a reduction in the dose of the concomitant agent may be necessary.

Cardiovascular: In U.S. placebo-controlled clinical trials that excluded patients with New York Heart Association (NYHA) Class III and IV cardiac status, the incidence of serious cardiac adverse events related to volume expansion was not increased in patients treated with ACTOS as monotherapy or in combination with sulfonylureas or metformin vs. placebo-treated patients. In insulin combination studies, a small number of patients with a history of previously existing cardiac disease developed congestive heart failure when treated with ACTOS in combination with insulin (see WARNINGS). Patients with NYHA Class III and IV cardiac status were not studied in these ACTOS clinical trials. ACTOS is not indicated in patients with NYHA Class III or IV cardiac status.

In postmarketing experience with ACTOS, cases of congestive heart failure have been reported in patients both with and without previously known heart disease.

Edema: ACTOS should be used with caution in patients with edema. In all U.S. clinical trials, edema was reported more frequently in patients treated with ACTOS than in placebo-treated patients and appears to be dose related (see ADVERSE REACTIONS). In postmarketing experience, reports of initiation or worsening of edema have been received.

Weight Gain: Dose related weight gain was seen with ACTOS alone and in combination with other hypoglycemic agents (Table 6). The mechanism of weight gain is unclear but probably involves a combination of fluid retention and fat accumulation.

[See table 6 below]

Ovulation: Therapy with ACTOS, like other thiazolidinediones, may result in ovulation in some premenopausal anovulatory women. As a result, these patients may be at an increased risk for pregnancy while taking ACTOS. Thus, adequate contraception in premenopausal women should be recommended. This possible effect has not been investigated in clinical studies so the frequency of this occurrence is not known.

Hematologic: ACTOS may cause decreases in hemoglobin and hematocrit. Across all clinical studies, mean hemoglobin values declined by 2% to 4% in patients treated with ACTOS. These changes primarily occurred within the first 4 to 12 weeks of therapy and remained relatively constant thereafter. These changes may be related to increased plasma volume and have rarely been associated with any significant hematologic clinical effects (see ADVERSE REACTIONS, Laboratory Abnormalities).

Hepatic Effects: In pre-approval clinical studies worldwide, over 4500 subjects were treated with ACTOS. In U.S. clinical studies, over 4700 patients with type 2 diabetes received ACTOS. There was no evidence of drug-induced hepatotoxicity or elevation of ALT levels in the clinical studies. During pre-approval placebo-controlled clinical trials in the U.S., a total of 4 of 1526 (0.26%) patients treated with ACTOS and 2 of 793 (0.25%) placebo-treated patients had ALT values ≥ 3 times the upper limit of normal. The ALT elevations in patients treated with ACTOS were reversible and were not clearly related to therapy with ACTOS.

In postmarketing experience with ACTOS, reports of hepatitis and of hepatic enzyme elevations to 3 or more times the upper limit of normal have been received. Very rarely, these reports have involved hepatic failure with and without fatal outcome, although causality has not been established.

Pioglitazone is structurally related to troglitazone, a thiazolidinedione no longer marketed in the United States, which was associated with idiosyncratic hepatotoxicity and cases of liver failure, liver transplants and death during postmarketing clinical use. In pre-approval controlled clinical trials in patients with type 2 diabetes, troglitazone was more frequently associated with clinically significant elevations of hepatic enzymes (ALT > 3 times the upper limit of normal) compared to placebo, and cases of reversible jaundice were reported.

Pending the availability of the results of additional large, long-term controlled clinical trials and additional postmarketing safety data, it is recommended that patients treated with ACTOS undergo periodic monitoring of liver enzymes.

Serum ALT (alanine aminotransferase) levels should be evaluated prior to the initiation of therapy with ACTOS in all patients and periodically thereafter per the clinical judgment of the health care professional. Liver function tests should also be obtained for patients if symptoms suggestive of hepatic dysfunction occur, e.g., nausea, vomiting, abdominal pain, fatigue, anorexia, or dark urine. The decision whether to continue the patient on therapy with ACTOS should be guided by clinical judgment pending laboratory evaluations. If jaundice is observed, drug therapy should be discontinued.

Therapy with ACTOS should not be initiated if the patient exhibits clinical evidence of active liver disease or the ALT levels exceed 2.5 times the upper limit of normal. Patients with mildly elevated liver enzymes (ALT levels at 1 to 2.5 times the upper limit of normal) at baseline or any time during therapy with ACTOS should be evaluated to determine the cause of the liver enzyme elevation. Initiation or continuation of therapy with ACTOS in patients with mildly elevated liver enzymes should proceed with caution and include appropriate clinical follow-up which may include more frequent liver enzyme monitoring. If serum transaminase levels are increased (ALT > 2.5 times the upper limit of normal), liver function tests should be evaluated more frequently until the levels return to normal or pretreatment values. If ALT levels exceed 3 times the upper limit of normal, the test should be repeated as soon as possible. If ALT levels remain > 3 times the upper limit of normal or if the patient is jaundiced, ACTOS therapy should be discontinued.

There are no data available to evaluate the safety of ACTOS in patients who experienced liver abnormalities, hepatic dysfunction, or jaundice while on troglitazone. ACTOS should not be used in patients who experienced jaundice while taking troglitazone.

Laboratory Tests

FPG and HbA_{1c} measurements should be performed periodically to monitor glycemic control and the therapeutic response to ACTOS.

Liver enzyme monitoring is recommended prior to initiation of therapy with ACTOS in all patients and periodically thereafter per the clinical judgment of the health care professional (see PRECAUTIONS, General, Hepatic Effects and ADVERSE REACTIONS, Serum Transaminase Levels).

Information for Patients

It is important to instruct patients to adhere to dietary instructions and to have blood glucose and glycosylated hemoglobin tested regularly. During periods of stress such as fever, trauma, infection, or surgery, medication requirements may change and patients should be reminded to seek medical advice promptly.

Patients who experience an unusually rapid increase in weight or edema or who develop shortness of breath or other symptoms of heart failure while on ACTOS should immediately report these symptoms to their physician.

Patients should be told that blood tests for liver function will be performed prior to the start of therapy and periodically thereafter per the clinical judgment of the health care professional. Patients should be told to seek immediate medical advice for unexplained nausea, vomiting, abdominal pain, fatigue, anorexia, or dark urine.

Patients should be told to take ACTOS once daily. ACTOS can be taken with or without meals. If a dose is missed on one day, the dose should not be doubled the following day.

When using combination therapy with insulin or oral hypoglycemic agents, the risks of hypoglycemia, its symptoms and treatment, and conditions that predispose to its development should be explained to patients and their family members.

Therapy with ACTOS, like other thiazolidinediones, may result in ovulation in some premenopausal anovulatory women. As a result, these patients may be at an increased risk for pregnancy while taking ACTOS. Thus, adequate contraception in premenopausal women should be recommended. This possible effect has not been investigated in clinical studies so the frequency of this occurrence is not known.

Drug Interactions

In vivo drug-drug interaction studies have suggested that pioglitazone may be a weak inducer of CYP 450 isoform 3A4 substrate (see CLINICAL PHARMACOLOGY, Metabolism and Drug-Drug Interactions).

Carcinogenesis, Mutagenesis, Impairment of Fertility

A two-year carcinogenicity study was conducted in male and female rats at oral doses up to 63 mg/kg (approximately 14 times the maximum recommended human oral dose of 45 mg based on mg/m^2). Drug-induced tumors were not observed in any organ except for the urinary bladder. Benign and/or malignant transitional cell neoplasms were observed in male rats at 4 mg/kg/day and above (approximately equal to the maximum recommended human oral dose based on mg/m^2). A two-year carcinogenicity study was conducted in male and female mice at oral doses up to 100 mg/kg/day (approximately 11 times the maximum recommended human oral dose based on mg/m^2). No drug-induced tumors were observed in any organ. Urinary tract tumors have been reported in rodents taking experimental drugs with dual PPAR α/γ activity; however, ACTOS is a selective agonist for PPARγ.

During prospective evaluation of urinary cytology involving more than 1800 patients receiving ACTOS in clinical trials up to one year in duration, no new cases of bladder tumors were identified. Occasionally, abnormal urinary cytology re-

Table 6 Weight Changes (kg) from Baseline during Double-Blind Clinical Trials with ACTOS

		Control Group (Placebo)	ACTOS 15 mg	ACTOS 30 mg	ACTOS 45 mg
		Median (25th / 75th percentile)	Median (25th / 75th percentile)	Median (25th / 75th percentile)	Median (25th / 75th percentile)
Monotherapy		-1.4 (-2.7/0.0) n=256	0.9 (-0.5/3.4) n=79	1.0 (-0.9/3.4) n=188	2.6 (0.2/5.4) n=79
Combination Therapy	Sulfonylurea	-0.5 (-1.8/0.7) n=187	2.0 (0.2/3.2) n=183	3.1 (1.1/5.4) n=528	4.1 (1.8/7.3) n=333
	Metformin	-1.4 (-3.2/0.3) n=160	N/A	0.9 (-0.3/3.2) n=567	1.8 (-0.9/5.0) n=407
	Insulin	0.2 (-1.4/1.4) n=182	2.3 (0.5/4.3) n=190	3.3 (0.9/6.3) n=522	4.1 (1.4/6.8) n=338

Note: Trial durations of 16 to 26 weeks

sults indicating possible malignancy were observed in both patients treated with ACTOS (0.72%) and patients treated with placebo (0.88%).
Pioglitazone HCl was not mutagenic in a battery of genetic toxicology studies, including the Ames bacterial assay, a mammalian cell forward gene mutation assay (CHO/HPRT and AS52/XPRT), an in vitro cytogenetics assay using CHL cells, an unscheduled DNA synthesis assay, and an in vivo micronucleus assay.
No adverse effects upon fertility were observed in male and female rats at oral doses up to 40 mg/kg pioglitazone HCl daily prior to and throughout mating and gestation (approximately 9 times the maximum recommended human oral dose based on mg/m^2).

Animal Toxicology

Heart enlargement has been observed in mice (100 mg/kg), rats (4 mg/kg and above) and dogs (3 mg/kg) treated orally with pioglitazone HCl (approximately 11, 1, and 2 times the maximum recommended human oral dose for mice, rats, and dogs, respectively, based on mg/m^2). In a one-year rat study, drug-related early death due to apparent heart dysfunction occurred at an oral dose of 160 mg/kg/day (approximately 35 times the maximum recommended human oral dose based on mg/m^2). Heart enlargement was seen in a 13-week study in monkeys at oral doses of 8.9 mg/kg and above (approximately 4 times the maximum recommended human oral dose based on mg/m^2), but not in a 52-week study at oral doses up to 32 mg/kg (approximately 13 times the maximum recommended human oral dose based on mg/m^2).

Pregnancy

Pregnancy Category C. Pioglitazone was not teratogenic in rats at oral doses up to 80 mg/kg or in rabbits given up to 160 mg/kg during organogenesis (approximately 17 and 40 times the maximum recommended human oral dose based on mg/m^2, respectively). Delayed parturition and embryotoxicity (as evidenced by increased postimplantation losses, delayed development and reduced fetal weights) were observed in rats at oral doses of 40 mg/kg/day and above (approximately 10 times the maximum recommended human oral dose based on mg/m^2). No functional or behavioral toxicity was observed in offspring of rats. In rabbits, embryotoxicity was observed at an oral dose of 160 mg/kg (approximately 40 times the maximum recommended human oral dose based on mg/m^2). Delayed postnatal development, attributed to decreased body weight, was observed in offspring of rats at oral doses of 10 mg/kg and above during late gestation and lactation periods (approximately 2 times the maximum recommended human oral dose based on mg/m^2).
There are no adequate and well-controlled studies in pregnant women. ACTOS should be used during pregnancy only if the potential benefit justifies the potential risk to the fetus.
Because current information strongly suggests that abnormal blood glucose levels during pregnancy are associated with a higher incidence of congenital anomalies, as well as increased neonatal morbidity and mortality, most experts recommend that insulin be used during pregnancy to maintain blood glucose levels as close to normal as possible.

Nursing Mothers

Pioglitazone is secreted in the milk of lactating rats. It is not known whether ACTOS is secreted in human milk. Because many drugs are excreted in human milk, ACTOS should not be administered to a breast-feeding woman.

Pediatric Use

Safety and effectiveness of ACTOS in pediatric patients have not been established.

Elderly Use

Approximately 500 patients in placebo-controlled clinical trials of ACTOS were 65 and over. No significant differences in effectiveness and safety were observed between these patients and younger patients.

ADVERSE REACTIONS

In worldwide clinical trials, over 5900 patients with type 2 diabetes have been treated with ACTOS. In U.S. clinical trials, over 4700 patients have received ACTOS, over 3300 patients have been treated for 6 months or longer, and over 450 patients for one year or longer.
The overall incidence and types of adverse events reported in placebo-controlled clinical trials of ACTOS monotherapy at doses of 7.5 mg, 15 mg, 30 mg, or 45 mg once daily are shown in Table 7.

Table 7 Placebo-Controlled Clinical Studies of ACTOS Monotherapy: Adverse Events Reported at a Frequency ≥ 5% of Patients Treated with ACTOS

(% of Patients)

	Placebo N=259	ACTOS N=606
Upper Respiratory Tract Infection	8.5	13.2
Headache	6.9	9.1
Sinusitis	4.6	6.3
Myalgia	2.7	5.4
Tooth Disorder	2.3	5.3
Diabetes Mellitus Aggravated	8.1	5.1
Pharyngitis	0.8	5.1

For most clinical adverse events the incidence was similar for groups treated with ACTOS monotherapy and those treated in combination with sulfonylureas, metformin, and insulin. There was an increase in the occurrence of edema in the patients treated with ACTOS and insulin compared to insulin alone.
In a 16-week, placebo-controlled ACTOS plus insulin trial (n=379), 10 patients treated with ACTOS plus insulin developed dyspnea and also, at some point during their therapy, developed either weight change or edema. Seven of these 10 patients received diuretics to treat these symptoms. This was not reported in the insulin plus placebo group.
The incidence of withdrawals from placebo-controlled clinical trials due to an adverse event other than hyperglycemia was similar for patients treated with placebo (2.8%) or ACTOS (3.3%).
In controlled combination therapy studies with either a sulfonylurea or insulin, mild to moderate hypoglycemia, which appears to be dose related, was reported (see PRECAUTIONS, General, Hypoglycemia and DOSAGE and ADMINISTRATION, Combination Therapy).
In U.S. double-blind studies, anemia was reported in ≥ 2% of patients treated with ACTOS plus sulfonylurea, metformin or insulin (see PRECAUTIONS, General, Hematologic).
In monotherapy studies, edema was reported for 4.8% of patients treated with ACTOS versus 1.2% of placebo-treated patients. In combination therapy studies, edema was reported for 7.2% of patients treated with ACTOS and sulfonylureas compared to 2.1% of patients on sulfonylureas alone. In combination therapy studies with metformin, edema was reported in 6.0% of patients on combination therapy compared to 2.5% of patients on metformin alone. In combination therapy studies with insulin, edema was reported in 15.3% of patients on combination therapy compared to 7.0% of patients on insulin alone. Most of these events were considered mild or moderate in intensity (see PRECAUTIONS, General, Edema).
In one 16-week clinical trial of insulin plus ACTOS combination therapy, more patients developed congestive heart failure on combination therapy (1.1%) compared to none on insulin alone (see WARNINGS, Cardiac Failure and Other Cardiac Effects).

Laboratory Abnormalities

Hematologic: ACTOS may cause decreases in hemoglobin and hematocrit. The fall in hemoglobin and hematocrit with ACTOS appears to be dose related. Across all clinical studies, mean hemoglobin values declined by 2% to 4% in patients treated with ACTOS. These changes generally occurred within the first 4 to 12 weeks of therapy and remained relatively stable thereafter. These changes may be related to increased plasma volume associated with ACTOS therapy and have rarely been associated with any significant hematologic clinical effects.
Serum Transaminase Levels: During all clinical studies in the U.S., 14 of 4780 (0.30%) patients treated with ACTOS had ALT values ≥ 3 times the upper limit of normal during treatment. All patients with follow-up values had reversible elevations in ALT. In the population of patients treated with ACTOS, mean values for bilirubin, AST, ALT, alkaline phosphatase, and GGT were decreased at the final visit compared with baseline. Fewer than 0.9% of patients treated with ACTOS were withdrawn from clinical trials in the U.S. due to abnormal liver function tests.
In pre-approval clinical trials, there were no cases of idiosyncratic drug reactions leading to hepatic failure (see PRECAUTIONS, Hepatic Effects).
CPK Levels: During required laboratory testing in clinical trials, sporadic, transient elevations in creatine phosphokinase levels (CPK) were observed. An isolated elevation to greater than 10 times the upper limit of normal was noted in 9 patients (values of 2150 to 11400 IU/L). Six of these patients continued to receive ACTOS, two patients had completed receiving study medication at the time of the elevated value and one patient discontinued study medication due to the elevation. These elevations resolved without any apparent clinical sequelae. The relationship of these events to ACTOS therapy is unknown.

OVERDOSAGE

During controlled clinical trials, one case of overdose with ACTOS was reported. A male patient took 120 mg per day for four days, then 180 mg per day for seven days. The patient denied any clinical symptoms during this period.
In the event of overdosage, appropriate supportive treatment should be initiated according to patient's clinical signs and symptoms.

DOSAGE AND ADMINISTRATION

ACTOS should be taken once daily without regard to meals. The management of antidiabetic therapy should be individualized. Ideally, the response to therapy should be evaluated using HbA_{1c} which is a better indicator of long-term glycemic control than FPG alone. HbA_{1c} reflects glycemia over the past two to three months. In clinical use, it is recommended that patients be treated with ACTOS for a period of time adequate to evaluate change in HbA_{1c} (three months) unless glycemic control deteriorates.

Monotherapy

ACTOS monotherapy in patients not adequately controlled with diet and exercise may be initiated at 15 mg or 30 mg once daily. For patients who respond inadequately to the initial dose of ACTOS, the dose can be increased in increments up to 45 mg once daily. For patients not responding adequately to monotherapy, combination therapy should be considered.

Combination Therapy

Sulfonylureas: ACTOS in combination with a sulfonylurea may be initiated at 15 mg or 30 mg once daily. The current sulfonylurea dose can be continued upon initiation of ACTOS therapy. If patients report hypoglycemia, the dose of the sulfonylurea should be decreased.
Metformin: ACTOS in combination with metformin may be initiated at 15 mg or 30 mg once daily. The current metformin dose can be continued upon initiation of ACTOS therapy. It is unlikely that the dose of metformin will require adjustment due to hypoglycemia during combination therapy with ACTOS.
Insulin: ACTOS in combination with insulin may be initiated at 15 mg or 30 mg once daily. The current insulin dose can be continued upon initiation of ACTOS therapy. In patients receiving ACTOS and insulin, the insulin dose can be decreased by 10% to 25% if the patient reports hypoglycemia or if plasma glucose concentrations decrease to less than 100 mg/dL. Further adjustments should be individualized based on glucose-lowering response.

Maximum Recommended Dose

The dose of ACTOS should not exceed 45 mg once daily in monotherapy or in combination with sulfonylurea, metformin, or insulin.
Dose adjustment in patients with renal insufficiency is not recommended (see CLINICAL PHARMACOLOGY, Pharmacokinetics and Drug Metabolism).
Therapy with ACTOS should not be initiated if the patient exhibits clinical evidence of active liver disease or increased serum transaminase levels (ALT greater than 2.5 times the upper limit of normal) at start of therapy (see PRECAUTIONS, General, Hepatic Effects and CLINICAL PHARMACOLOGY, Special Populations, Hepatic Insufficiency). Liver enzyme monitoring is recommended in all patients prior to initiation of therapy with ACTOS and periodically thereafter (see PRECAUTIONS, General, Hepatic Effects).
There are no data on the use of ACTOS in patients under 18 years of age; therefore, use of ACTOS in pediatric patients is not recommended.
No data are available on the use of ACTOS in combination with another thiazolidinedione.

HOW SUPPLIED

ACTOS is available in 15 mg, 30 mg, and 45 mg tablets as follows:
15 mg Tablet: white to off-white, round, convex, non-scored tablet with "ACTOS" on one side, and "15" on the other, available in:
NDC 64764-151-04 Bottles of 30
NDC 64764-151-05 Bottles of 90
NDC 64764-151-06 Bottles of 500
30 mg Tablet: white to off-white, round, flat, non-scored tablet with "ACTOS" on one side, and "30" on the other, available in:
NDC 64764-301-14 Bottles of 30
NDC 64764-301-15 Bottles of 90
NDC 64764-301-16 Bottles of 500
45 mg Tablet: white to off-white, round, flat, non-scored tablet with "ACTOS" on one side, and "45" on the other, available in:
NDC 64764-451-24 Bottles of 30
NDC 64764-451-25 Bottles of 90
NDC 64764-451-26 Bottles of 500

STORAGE

Store at 25°C (77°F); excursions permitted to 15–30°C (59–86°F) [see USP Controlled Room Temperature]. Keep container tightly closed, and protect from moisture and humidity.

Rx only

Manufactured by:
Takeda Pharmaceutical Company Limited
Osaka, Japan
Marketed by:
Takeda Pharmaceuticals America, Inc.
475 Half Day Road
Lincolnshire, IL 60069
and
Eli Lilly and Company
Lilly Corporate Center
Indianapolis, IN 46285

05-1113 Revised: August, 2004

Shown in Product Identification Guide, page 334

TAP Pharmaceuticals Inc.
LAKE FOREST, IL 60045

For Medical Information Contact:
(800) 622-2011 (LUPRON)

LUPRON® ℞
[*lew-prŏn*]
(leuprolide acetate) Injection

DESCRIPTION
LUPRON (leuprolide acetate) Injection is a synthetic nonapeptide analog of naturally occurring gonadotropin releasing hormone (GnRH or LH-RH). The analog possesses greater potency than the natural hormone. The chemical name is 5-Oxo-L-prolyl-L-histidyl-L-tryptophyl-L-seryl-L-tyrosyl-D-leucyl-L-leucyl-L-arginyl-N-ethyl-L-prolinamide acetate (salt) with the following structural formula:
[See chemical structure below]
LUPRON is a sterile, aqueous solution intended for subcutaneous injection. It is available in a 2.8 mL multiple-dose vial containing 5 mg/mL of leuprolide acetate, sodium chloride for tonicity adjustment, 9 mg/mL of benzyl alcohol as a preservative and water for injection. The pH may have been adjusted with sodium hydroxide and/or acetic acid.

CLINICAL PHARMACOLOGY
Leuprolide acetate, an LH-RH agonist, acts as a potent inhibitor of gonadotropin secretion when given continuously and in therapeutic doses. Animal and human studies indicate that following an initial stimulation, chronic administration of leuprolide acetate results in suppression of ovarian and testicular steroidogenesis. This effect is reversible upon discontinuation of drug therapy. Administration of leuprolide acetate has resulted in inhibition of the growth of certain hormone dependent tumors (prostatic tumors in Noble and Dunning male rats and DMBA-induced mammary tumors in female rats) as well as atrophy of the reproductive organs.
In humans, subcutaneous administration of single daily doses of leuprolide acetate results in an initial increase in circulation levels of luteinizing hormone (LH) and follicle stimulating hormone (FSH), leading to a transient increase in levels of the gonadal steroids (testosterone and dihydrotestosterone in males, and estrone and estradiol in premenopausal females). However, continuous daily administration of leuprolide acetate results in decreased levels of LH and FSH in all patients. In males, testosterone is reduced to castrate levels. In pre-menopausal females, estrogens are reduced to post-menopausal levels. These decreases occur within two to four weeks after initiation of treatment, and castrate levels of testosterone in prostatic cancer patients have been demonstrated for periods of up to five years.
Leuprolide acetate is not active when given orally. Bioavailability by subcutaneous administration is comparable to that by intravenous administration. Leuprolide acetate has a plasma half-life of approximately three hours. The metabolism, distribution and excretion of leuprolide acetate in man have not been determined.

INDICATIONS AND USAGE
LUPRON (leuprolide acetate) Injection is indicated in the palliative treatment of advanced prostatic cancer. It offers an alternative treatment of prostatic cancer when orchiectomy or estrogen administration are either not indicated or unacceptable to the patient. In a controlled study comparing LUPRON 1 mg/day given subcutaneously to DES (diethylstilbestrol), 3 mg/day, the survival rate for the two groups was comparable after two years treatment. The objective response to treatment was also similar for the two groups.

CONTRAINDICATIONS
A report of an anaphylactic reaction to synthetic GnRH (Factrel) has been reported in the medical literature.[1]
LUPRON is contraindicated in women who are or may become pregnant while receiving the drug. When administered on day 6 of pregnancy at test dosages of 0.00024, 0.0024, and 0.024 mg/kg (1/600 to 1/6 the human dose) to rabbits, LUPRON produced a dose-related increase in major fetal abnormalities. Similar studies in rats failed to demonstrate an increase in fetal malformations. There was increased fetal mortality and decreased fetal weights with the two higher doses of LUPRON in rabbits and with the highest dose in rats. The effects on fetal mortality are logical consequences of the alterations in hormonal levels brought about by this drug. Therefore, the possibility exists that spontaneous abortion may occur if the drug is administered during pregnancy.

WARNINGS
Isolated cases of worsening of signs and symptoms during the first weeks of treatment have been reported. Worsening of symptoms may contribute to paralysis with or without fatal complications.

PRECAUTIONS
Patients with metastatic vertebral lesions and/or with urinary tract obstruction should be closely observed during the first few weeks of therapy (see "ADVERSE REACTIONS" section).
Patients with known allergies to benzyl alcohol, an ingredient of the drug's vehicle, may present symptoms of hypersensitivity, usually local, in the form of erythema and induration at the injection site.
Information for Patients: See Information for Patients which appears after the "HOW SUPPLIED" section.
Laboratory Tests: Response to leuprolide acetate should be monitored by measuring serum levels of testosterone and acid phosphatase. In the majority of patients, testosterone levels increased above baseline during the first week, declining thereafter to baseline levels or below by the end of the second week of treatment. Castrate levels were reached within two to four weeks and once attained were maintained for as long as drug administration continued. Transient increases in acid phosphatase levels occurred sometimes early in treatment. However, by the fourth week, the elevated levels usually decreased to values at or near baseline.
Drug Interactions: None have been reported.
Carcinogenesis, Mutagenesis, Impairment of Fertility: Two-year carcinogenicity studies were conducted in rats and mice. In rats, a dose-related increase of benign pituitary hyperplasia and benign pituitary adenomas was noted at 24 months when the drug was administered subcutaneously at high daily doses (0.6 to 4 mg/kg). In mice no pituitary abnormalities were observed at a dose as high as 60 mg/kg for two years. Patients have been treated with leuprolide acetate for up to three years with doses as high as 10 mg/day and for two years with doses as high as 20 mg/day without demonstrable pituitary abnormalities.
Mutagenicity studies have been performed with leuprolide acetate using bacterial and mammalian systems. These studies provided no evidence of a mutagenic potential.
Clinical and pharmacologic studies with leuprolide acetate and similar analogs have shown full reversibility of fertility suppression when the drug is discontinued after continuous administration for periods of up to 24 weeks. However, no clinical studies have been conducted with leuprolide acetate to assess the reversibility of fertility suppression.
Pregnancy Category X. See "CONTRAINDICATIONS" section.
Pediatric Use: See labeling for LUPRON Injection for Pediatric Use for the safety and effectiveness in children with central precocious puberty.
Geriatric Use: In the clinical trials for LUPRON Injection, the majority (69%) of subjects studied were at least 65 years of age. Therefore, the labeling reflects the pharmacokinetics, efficacy and safety of LUPRON in this population.

ADVERSE REACTIONS
In the majority of patients testosterone levels increased above baseline during the first week, declining thereafter to baseline levels or below by the end of the second week of treatment. This transient increase was occasionally associated with a temporary worsening of signs and symptoms, usually manifested by an increase in bone pain (See "WARNINGS" section). In a few cases a temporary worsening of existing hematuria and urinary tract obstruction occurred during the first week. Temporary weakness and paresthesia of the lower limbs have been reported in a few cases.
Potential exacerbations of signs and symptoms during the first few weeks of treatment is a concern in patients with vertebral metastases and/or urinary obstruction which, if aggravated, may lead to neurological problems or increase the obstruction.
In a comparative trial of LUPRON (leuprolide acetate) Injection versus DES, in 5% or more of the patients receiving either drug, the following adverse reactions were reported to have a possible or probable relationship to drug as ascribed by the treating physician. Often, causality is difficult to assess in patients with metastatic prostate cancer. Reactions considered not drug related are excluded.

	LUPRON (N=98)	DES (N=101)
	Number of Reports	
Cardiovascular System		
Congestive heart failure	1	5
ECG changes/ischemia	19	22
High blood pressure	8	5
Murmur	3	8
Peripheral edema	12	30
Phlebitis/thrombosis	2	10
Gastrointestinal System		
Anorexia	6	5
Constipation	7	9
Nausea/vomiting	5	17
Endocrine System		
*Decreased testicular size	7	11
*Gynecomastia/breast tenderness or pain	7	63
*Hot flashes	55	12
*Impotence	4	12
Hemic and Lymphatic System		
Anemia	5	5
Musculoskeletal System		
Bone pain	5	2
Myalgia	3	9
Central/Peripheral Nervous System		
Dizziness/lightheadedness	5	7
General pain	13	13
Headache	7	4
Insomnia/sleep disorders	7	5
Respiratory System		
Dyspnea	2	8
Sinus congestion	5	6
Integumentary System		
Dermatitis	5	8
Urogenital System		
Frequency/urgency	6	8
Hematuria	6	4
Urinary tract infection	3	7
Miscellaneous		
Asthenia	10	10

*Physiologic effect of decreased testosterone.

In this same study, the following adverse reactions were reported in less than 5% of the patients on LUPRON.
Cardiovascular System—Angina, Cardiac arrhythmias, Myocardial infarction, Pulmonary emboli; *Gastrointestinal System*—Diarrhea, Dysphagia, Gastrointestinal bleeding, Gastrointestinal disturbance, Peptic ulcer, Rectal polyps; *Endocrine System*—Libido decrease, Thyroid enlargement; *Musculoskeletal System*—Joint pain; *Central/Peripheral Nervous System*—Anxiety, Blurred vision, Lethargy, Memory disorder, Mood swings, Nervousness, Numbness, Paresthesia, Peripheral neuropathy, Syncope/blackouts, Taste disorders; *Respiratory System*—Cough, Pleural rub, Pneumonia, Pulmonary fibrosis; *Integumentary System*—Carcinoma of skin/ear, Dry skin, Ecchymosis, Hair loss, Itching, Local skin reactions, Pigmentation, Skin lesions; *Urogenital System*—Bladder spasms, Dysuria, Incontinence, Testicular pain, Urinary obstruction; *Miscellaneous*—Depression, Diabetes, Fatigue, Fever/chills, Hypoglycemia, Increased BUN, Increased calcium, Increased creatinine, Infection/inflammation, Ophthalmologic disorders, Swelling (temporal bone).
The following additional adverse reactions have been reported with LUPRON or LUPRON DEPOT (leuprolide acetate for depot suspension) during other clinical trials and/or during postmarketing surveillance. Reactions considered as nondrug related by the treating physician are excluded.
Cardiovascular System—Hypotension, Transient ischemic attack/stroke; *Gastrointestinal System*—Hepatic dysfunction; *Endocrine System*—Libido increase; *Hemic and Lymphatic System*—Decreased WBC, Hemoptysis; *Musculoskeletal System*—Ankylosing spondylosis, Pelvic fibrosis; *Central/Peripheral Nervous System*—Hearing disorder, Peripheral neuropathy, Spinal fracture/paralysis; *Respiratory System*—Pulmonary infiltrate, Respiratory disorders; *Integumentary System*—Hair growth; *Urogenital System*—Penile swelling, Prostate pain; *Miscellaneous*—Hypoproteinemia, Hard nodule in throat, Weight gain, Increased uric acid.

OVERDOSAGE
In rats subcutaneous administration of 250 to 500 times the recommended human dose, expressed on a per body weight basis, resulted in dyspnea, decreased activity, and local irritation at the injection site. There is no evidence at present that there is a clinical counterpart of this phenomenon. In early clinical trials with leuprolide acetate doses as high as 20 mg/day for up to two years caused no adverse effects differing from those observed with the 1 mg/day dose.

DOSAGE AND ADMINISTRATION
The recommended dose is 1 mg (0.2 mL or 20 unit mark) administered as a single daily subcutaneous injection. As with other drugs administered chronically by subcutaneous injection, the injection site should be varied periodically.
NOTE: As with all parenteral products, inspect container's solution for discoloration and particulate matter before each use.

HOW SUPPLIED
LUPRON (leuprolide acetate) Injection is a sterile solution supplied in a 2.8 mL multiple-dose vial, NDC 0300-3612-28. Store below 77°F (25°C). Do not freeze. Protect from light—store vial in carton until use.

Each 0.2 mL contains 1 mg of leuprolide acetate, sodium chloride for tonicity adjustment, 1.8 mg of benzyl alcohol as preservative and water for injection. The pH may have been adjusted with sodium hydroxide and/or acetic acid.

℞ ONLY

U.S. Patent Nos. 4,005,063 and 4,005,194.

REFERENCE

1. MacLeod TL, Eisen A, Sussman GL, et al: Anaphylactic reaction to synthetic luteinizing hormone-releasing hormone. *Fertil Steril* 1987 Sept;48(3):500–502.

INFORMATION FOR PATIENTS

NOTE: Be sure to consult your physician with any questions you may have or for information about LUPRON (leuprolide acetate) Injection and its use.

WHAT IS LUPRON?

LUPRON (leuprolide acetate) Injection is chemically similar to gonadotropin releasing hormone (GnRH or LH-RH) a hormone which occurs naturally in your body.

Normally, your body releases small amounts of LH-RH and this leads to events which stimulate the production of sex hormones.

However, when you inject LUPRON (leuprolide acetate) Injection, the normal events that lead to sex hormone production are interrupted and testosterone is no longer produced by the testes.

LUPRON must be injected because, like insulin which is injected by diabetics, LUPRON is inactive when taken by mouth.

If you were to discontinue the drug for any reason, your body would begin making testosterone again.

DIRECTIONS FOR USING LUPRON

1. Wash hands thoroughly with soap and water.
2. If using a new bottle for the first time, flip off the plastic cover to expose the gray rubber stopper. Wipe metal ring and rubber stopper with an alcohol wipe each time you use LUPRON. Check the liquid in the container. If it is not clear or has particles in it, DO NOT USE IT. Exchange it at your pharmacy for another container.
3. Remove outer wrapping from one syringe. Pull plunger back until the tip of the plunger is at the 0.2 mL or 20 unit mark.
4. Take cover off needle. Push the needle through the center of the rubber stopper on the LUPRON bottle.
5. Push the plunger all the way in to inject air into the bottle.
6. Keep the needle in the bottle and turn the bottle upside down. Check to make sure the tip of the needle is in the liquid. Slowly pull back on the plunger, until the syringe fills to the 0.2 mL or 20 unit mark.
7. Toward the end of a two-week period, the amount of LUPRON left in the bottle will be small. Take special care to hold the bottle straight and to keep the needle tip in liquid while pulling back on the plunger.
8. Keeping the needle in the bottle and the bottle upside down, check for air bubbles in the syringe. If you see any, push the plunger *slowly* in to push the air bubble back into the bottle. Keep the tip of the needle in the liquid and pull the plunger back again to fill to the 0.2 mL or 20 unit mark.
9. Do this again if necessary to eliminate air bubbles. Remove needle from bottle and lay syringe down. DO NOT TOUCH THE NEEDLE OR ALLOW THE NEEDLE TO TOUCH ANY SURFACE.
10. To protect your skin, inject each daily dose at a different body spot.
11. Choose an injection spot. Cleanse the injection spot with another alcohol wipe.
12. Hold the syringe in one hand. Hold the skin taut, or pull up a little flesh with the other hand, as you were instructed.
13. Holding the syringe as you would a pencil, thrust the needle all the way into the skin at a 90° angle.
14. Hold an alcohol wipe down on your skin where the needle is inserted and withdraw the needle at the same angle it was inserted.
15. Use the disposable syringe only once and dispose of it properly as you were instructed. Needles thrown into a garbage bag could accidentally stick someone. NEVER LEAVE SYRINGES, NEEDLES OR DRUGS WHERE CHILDREN CAN REACH THEM.

SOME SPECIAL ADVICE

- You may experience hot flashes when using LUPRON (leuprolide acetate) Injection. During the first few weeks of treatment you may experience increased bone pain, increased difficulty in urinating, and less commonly but most importantly, you may experience the onset or aggravation of nerve symptoms. In any of these events, discuss the symptoms with your doctor.
- You may experience some irritation at the injection site, such as burning, itching or swelling. These reactions are usually mild and go away. If they do not, tell your doctor.
- Do not stop taking your injections because you feel better. You need an injection every day to make sure LUPRON keeps working for you.
- If you need to use an alternate to the syringe supplied with LUPRON, insulin syringes should be utilized.
- When the drug level gets low, take special care to hold the bottle straight up and down and to keep the needle tip in liquid while pulling back on the plunger.
- Do not try to get every last drop out of the bottle. This will increase the possibility of drawing air into the syringe and getting an incomplete dose. Some extra drug has been provided so that you can withdraw the recommended number of doses.
- Tell your pharmacist when you will need LUPRON so it will be at the pharmacy when you need it.
- Store below 77°F (25°C). Do not store near a radiator or other very warm place. Do not freeze. Protect from light - store vial in carton until use.
- Do not leave your drug or hypodermic syringes where anyone can pick them up.
- Keep this and all other medications out of reach of children.

Manufactured for
TAP Pharmaceuticals Inc.
Lake Forest, IL 60045
® – Registered
(No. 3612)
03-5273-R3, Rev. June, 2003

Shown in Product Identification Guide, page 334

For Pediatric Use

LUPRON® ℞

[lew-prŏn]

(leuprolide acetate) Injection

DESCRIPTION

Leuprolide acetate is a synthetic nonapeptide analog of naturally occurring gonadotropin releasing hormone (GnRH or LH-RH). The analog possesses greater potency than the natural hormone. The chemical name is 5-Oxo-L-prolyl-L-histidyl-L-tryptophyl-L-seryl-L-tyrosyl-D-leucyl-L-leucyl-L-arginyl-N-ethyl-L-prolinamide acetate (salt) with the following structural formula:

[See chemical structure below]

LUPRON Injection is a sterile, aqueous solution intended for daily subcutaneous injection.

- A 2.8 mL multiple dose vial contains leuprolide acetate (5 mg/mL), sodium chloride (6.3 mg/mL) for tonicity adjustment, benzyl alcohol as a preservative (9 mg/mL), and water for injection. The pH may have been adjusted with sodium hydroxide and/or acetic acid.

CLINICAL PHARMACOLOGY

Leuprolide acetate, a GnRH agonist, acts as a potent inhibitor of gonadotropin secretion when given continuously and in therapeutic doses. Human studies indicate that following an initial stimulation of gonadotropins, chronic stimulation with leuprolide acetate results in suppression or "downregulation" of these hormones and consequent suppression of ovarian and testicular steroidogenesis. These effects are reversible on discontinuation of drug therapy.

Leuprolide acetate is not active when given orally. In adults, bioavailability by subcutaneous administration is comparable to that by intravenous administration; and leuprolide acetate has a plasma half-life of approximately three hours. The metabolism, distribution and excretion of leuprolide acetate in humans have not been determined. A pharmacokinetic study of leuprolide acetate in children has not been performed.

In children with central precocious puberty (CPP), stimulated and basal gonadotropins are reduced to prepubertal levels. Testosterone and estradiol are reduced to prepubertal levels in males and females respectively. Reduction of gonadotropins will allow for normal physical and psychological growth and development. Natural maturation occurs when gonadotropins return to pubertal levels following discontinuation of leuprolide acetate.

The following physiologic effects have been noted with the chronic administration of leuprolide acetate in this patient population.

1. **Skeletal Growth.** A measurable increase in body length can be noted since the epiphyseal plates will not close prematurely.
2. **Organ growth.** Reproductive organs will return to a prepubertal state.
3. **Menses.** Menses, if present, will cease.

INDICATIONS AND USAGE

LUPRON Injection is indicated in the treatment of children with central precocious puberty. Children should be selected using the following criteria:

1. Clinical diagnosis of CPP (idiopathic or neurogenic) with onset of secondary sexual characteristics earlier than 8 years in females and 9 years in males.
2. Clinical diagnosis should be confirmed prior to initiation of therapy:
   - Confirmation of diagnosis by a pubertal response to a GnRH stimulation test. The sensitivity and methodology of this assay must be understood.
   - Bone age advanced one year beyond the chronological age.
3. Baseline evaluation should also include:
   - Height and weight measurements.
   - Sex steroid levels.
   - Adrenal steroid level to exclude congenital adrenal hyperplasia.
   - Beta human chorionic gonadotropin level to rule out a chorionic gonadotropin secreting tumor.
   - Pelvic/adrenal/testicular ultrasound to rule out a steroid secreting tumor.
   - Computerized tomography of the head to rule out intracranial tumor.

CONTRAINDICATIONS

LUPRON Injection is contraindicated in women who are or may become pregnant while receiving the drug. When administered on day 6 of pregnancy at test dosages of 0.00024, 0.0024, and 0.024 mg/kg (1/1200 to 1/12 the human pediatric dose) to rabbits, LUPRON produced a dose-related increase in major fetal abnormalities. Similar studies in rats failed to demonstrate an increase in fetal malformations. There was increased fetal mortality and decreased fetal weights with the two higher doses of LUPRON in rabbits and with the highest dose in rats. The effects on fetal mortality are logical consequences of the alterations in hormonal levels brought about by this drug. Therefore, the possibility exists that spontaneous abortion may occur if the drug is administered during pregnancy.

Leuprolide acetate is contraindicated in children demonstrating hypersensitivity to GnRH, GnRH agonist analogs, or any of the excipients.

A report of an anaphylactic reaction to synthetic GnRH (Factrel) has been reported in the medical literature.[1]

WARNINGS

During the early phase of therapy, gonadotropins and sex steroids rise above baseline because of the natural stimulatory effect of the drug. Therefore, an increase in clinical signs and symptoms may be observed (see "Clinical Pharmacology" section).

Noncompliance with drug regimen or inadequate dosing may result in inadequate control of the pubertal process. The consequences of poor control include the return of pubertal signs such as menses, breast development, and testicular growth. The long-term consequences of inadequate control of gonadal steroid secretion are unknown, but may include a further compromise of adult stature.

PRECAUTIONS

Patients with known allergies to benzyl alcohol, an ingredient of the vehicle of Lupron Injection, may present symptoms of hypersensitivity, usually local, in the form of erythema and induration at the injection site.

Laboratory Tests: Response to leuprolide acetate should be monitored 1–2 months after the start of therapy with a GnRH stimulation test and sex steroid levels. Measurement of bone age for advancement should be done every 6–12 months.

Sex steroids may increase or rise above prepubertal levels if the dose is inadequate (see "WARNINGS" section). Once a therapeutic dose has been established, gonadotropin and sex steroid levels will decline to prepubertal levels.

Drug Interactions: No pharmacokinetic-based drug-drug interaction studies have been conducted. However, because leuprolide acetate is a peptide that is primarily degraded by peptidase and not by cytochrome P-450 enzymes as noted in specific studies, and the drug is only about 46% bound to plasma proteins, drug interactions would not be expected to occur.

Drug/Laboratory Test Interactions: Administration of leuprolide acetate in therapeutic doses results in suppression of the pituitary-gonadal system. Normal function is usually restored within 4 to 12 weeks after treatment is discontinued.

Information for Parents: Prior to starting therapy with LUPRON Injection, the parent or guardian must be aware of the importance of continuous therapy. Adherence to daily drug administration schedules must be accepted if therapy is to be successful.

- During the first 2 months of therapy, a female may experience menses or spotting. If bleeding continues beyond the second month, notify the physician.
- Any irritation at the injection site should be reported to the physician immediately.

Continued on next page

Lupron IV—Cont.

• Report any unusual signs or symptoms to the physician.

Carcinogenesis, Mutagenesis, Impairment of Fertility: A two-year carcinogenicity study was conducted in rats and mice. In rats, a dose-related increase of benign pituitary hyperplasia and benign pituitary adenomas was noted at 24 months when the drug was administered subcutaneously at high daily doses (0.6 to 4 mg/kg). There was a significant but not dose-related increase of pancreatic islet-cell adenomas in females and of testes interstitial cell adenomas in males (highest incidence in the low dose group). In mice, no leuprolide acetate-induced tumors or pituitary abnormalities were observed at a dose as high as 60 mg/kg for two years. Adult patients have been treated with leuprolide acetate for up to three years with doses as high as 10 mg/day and for two years with doses as high as 20 mg/day without demonstrable pituitary abnormalities.

Although no clinical studies have been completed in children to assess the full reversibility of fertility suppression, animal studies (prepubertal and adult rats and monkeys) with leuprolide acetate and other GnRH analogs have shown functional recovery. However, following a study with leuprolide acetate, immature male rats demonstrated tubular degeneration in the testes even after a recovery period. In spite of the failure to recover histologically, the treated males proved to be as fertile as the controls. Also, no histologic changes were observed in the female rats following the same protocol. In both sexes, the offspring of the treated animals appeared normal. The effect of the treatment of the parents on the reproductive performance of the F1 generation was not tested. The clinical significance of these findings is unknown.

Pregnancy Category X. See **"CONTRAINDICATIONS"** section.

Nursing Mothers: It is not known whether leuprolide acetate is excreted in human milk. LUPRON should not be used by nursing mothers.

Geriatric Use: See labeling for LUPRON Injection for the pharmacokinetics, efficacy and safety of LUPRON in this population.

ADVERSE REACTIONS

Potential exacerbation of signs and symptoms during the first few weeks of treatment (See "PRECAUTIONS" section) is a concern in patients with rapidly advancing central precocious puberty.

In two studies of children with central precocious puberty, in 2% or more of the patients receiving the drug, the following adverse reactions were reported to have a possible or probable relationship to drug as ascribed by the treating physician. Reactions considered not drug related are excluded.

	Number of Patients N = 395	(Percent)
Body as a Whole		
General Pain	7	(2)
Integumentary System		
Acne/Seborrhea	7	(2)
Injection Site Reactions Including Abscess	21	(5)
Rash Including Erythema Multiforme	8	(2)
Urogenital System		
Vaginitis/Bleeding/ Discharge	7	(2)

In those same studies, the following adverse reactions were reported in less than 2% of the patients.

Body as a Whole - Body Odor, Fever, Headache, Infection; *Cardiovascular System* - Syncope, Vasodilation; *Digestive System* - Dysphagia, Gingivitis, Nausea/Vomiting; *Endocrine System* - Accelerated Sexual Maturity; *Metabolic and Nutritional Disorders* - Peripheral Edema, Weight Gain; *Nervous System* - Nervousness, Personality Disorder, Somnolence, Emotional Lability; *Respiratory System* - Epistaxis; *Integumentary System* - Alopecia, Skin Striae; *Urogenital System* - Cervix Disorder, Gynecomastia/Breast Disorders, Urinary Incontinence.

See other package inserts for adverse events reported in other patient populations.

OVERDOSAGE

In rats, subcutaneous administration of 125 to 250 times the recommended human pediatric dose, expressed on a per body weight basis, resulted in dyspnea, decreased activity, and local irritation at the injection site. There is no evidence at present that there is a clinical counterpart of this phenomenon. In early clinical trials using leuprolide acetate in adult patients, doses as high as 20 mg/day for up to two years caused no adverse effects differing from those observed with the 1 mg/day dose.

DOSAGE AND ADMINISTRATION

LUPRON INJECTION can be administered by a patient/parent or health care professional.

The dose of LUPRON Injection must be individualized for each child. The dose is based on a mg/kg ratio of drug to body weight. Younger children require higher doses on a mg/kg ratio.

For either dosage form, after 1-2 months of initiating therapy or changing doses, the child must be monitored with a GnRH stimulation test, sex steroids, and Tanner staging to confirm downregulation. Measurements of bone age for advancement should be monitored every 6-12 months. The dose should be titrated upward until no progression of the condition is noted either clinically and/or by laboratory parameters.

The first dose found to result in adequate downregulation can probably be maintained for the duration of therapy in most children. However, there are insufficient data to guide dosage adjustment as patients move into higher weight categories after beginning therapy at very young ages and low dosages. It is recommended that adequate downregulation be verified in such patients whose weight has increased significantly while on therapy.

As with other drugs administered by injection, the injection site should be varied periodically.

Discontinuation of LUPRON Injection should be considered before age 11 for females and age 12 for males.

The recommended starting dose is 50 mcg/kg/day administered as a single subcutaneous injection. If total downregulation is not achieved, the dose should be titrated upward by 10 mcg/kg/day. This dose will be considered the maintenance dose.

NOTE: As with other parenteral products, inspect container's solution for discoloration and particulate matter before each use.

HOW SUPPLIED

LUPRON (leuprolide acetate) Injection is a sterile solution.

- A 2.8 mL multiple dose vial (NDC 0300-3612-28) contains leuprolide acetate (5 mg/mL), sodium chloride (6.3 mg/mL) for tonicity adjustment, benzyl alcohol as a preservative (9 mg/mL), and water for injection. The pH may have been adjusted with sodium hydroxide and/or acetic acid.
- Store below 77°F (25°C). Do not freeze. Protect from light - store vial in carton until use.
- Use the syringes supplied with LUPRON Injection. Insulin syringes may be substituted for use with Lupron Injection. The volume of drug for the dose will vary depending on the syringe used and the concentration of drug.

Rx ONLY

U.S. Patent Nos. 4,005,063; 4,005,194.

REFERENCE

1. MacLeod TL, et al. Anaphylactic reaction to synthetic luteinizing hormone-releasing hormone. *Fertil Steril* 1987 Sept;48(3):500–502.

Manufactured for
TAP Pharmaceuticals Inc.
Lake Forest, IL 60045
® – Registered
(No. 3612)

This is combined labeling. Examples of different fonts appear below.
- General information
- Information on endometriosis
- **Information on uterine fibroids**

LUPRON DEPOT® 3.75 mg ℞

[lew-prŏn]

(leuprolide acetate for depot suspension)

This is combined labeling. Examples of different fonts appear below.
- General information
- Information on endometriosis
- Information on uterine fibroids

DESCRIPTION

Leuprolide acetate is a synthetic nonapeptide analog of naturally occurring gonadotropin-releasing hormone (GnRH or LH-RH). The analog possesses greater potency than the natural hormone. The chemical name is 5-oxo-L-prolyl-L-histidyl-L-tryptophyl-L-seryl-L-tyrosyl-D-leucyl-L-leucyl-L-arginyl-N-ethyl-L-prolinamide acetate (salt) with the following structural formula:

[See chemical structure below]

LUPRON DEPOT is available in a prefilled dual-chamber syringe containing sterile lyophilized microspheres which, when mixed with diluent, become a suspension intended as a monthly intramuscular injection.

The front chamber of LUPRON DEPOT 3.75 mg prefilled dual-chamber syringe contains leuprolide acetate (3.75 mg), purified gelatin (0.65 mg), DL-lactic and glycolic acids copolymer (33.1 mg), and D-mannitol (6.6 mg). The second chamber of diluent contains carboxymethylcellulose sodium (5 mg), D-mannitol (50 mg), polysorbate 80 (1 mg), water for injection, USP, and glacial acetic acid, USP to control pH. During the manufacture of LUPRON DEPOT 3.75 mg, acetic acid is lost, leaving the peptide.

CLINICAL PHARMACOLOGY

Leuprolide acetate is a long-acting GnRH analog. A single monthly injection of LUPRON DEPOT 3.75 mg results in an initial stimulation followed by a prolonged suppression of pituitary gonadotropins. Repeated dosing at monthly intervals results in decreased secretion of gonadal steroids; consequently, tissues and functions that depend on gonadal steroids for their maintenance become quiescent. This effect is reversible on discontinuation of drug therapy.

Leuprolide acetate is not active when given orally. Intramuscular injection of the depot formulation provides plasma concentrations of leuprolide over a period of one month.

Pharmacokinetics

Absorption A single dose of LUPRON DEPOT 3.75 mg was administered by intramuscular injection to healthy female volunteers. The absorption of leuprolide was characterized by an initial increase in plasma concentration, with peak concentration ranging from 4.6 to 10.2 ng/mL at four hours postdosing. However, intact leuprolide and an inactive metabolite could not be distinguished by the assay used in the study. Following the initial rise, leuprolide concentrations started to plateau within two days after dosing and remained relatively stable for about four to five weeks with plasma concentrations of about 0.30 ng/mL.

Distribution The mean steady-state volume of distribution of leuprolide following intravenous bolus administration to healthy male volunteers was 27 L. *In vitro* binding to human plasma proteins ranged from 43% to 49%.

Metabolism In healthy male volunteers, a 1 mg bolus of leuprolide administered intravenously revealed that the mean systemic clearance was 7.6 L/h, with a terminal elimination half-life of approximately 3 hours based on a two compartment model.

In rats and dogs, administration of ^{14}C-labeled leuprolide was shown to be metabolized to smaller inactive peptides, a pentapeptide (Metabolite I), tripeptides (Metabolites II and III) and a dipeptide (Metabolite IV). These fragments may be further catabolized.

The major metabolite (M-I) plasma concentrations measured in 5 prostate cancer patients reached maximum concentration 2 to 6 hours after dosing and were approximately 6% of the peak parent drug concentration. One week after dosing, mean plasma M-I concentrations were approximately 20% of mean leuprolide concentrations.

Excretion Following administration of LUPRON DEPOT 3.75 mg to 3 patients, less than 5% of the dose was recovered as parent and M-I metabolite in the urine.

Special Populations The pharmacokinetics of the drug in hepatically and renally impaired patients have not been determined.

Drug Interactions No pharmacokinetic-based drug-drug interaction studies have been conducted with LUPRON DEPOT. However, because leuprolide acetate is a peptide that is primarily degraded by peptidase and not by cytochrome P-450 enzymes as noted in specific studies, and the drug is only about 46% bound to plasma proteins, drug interactions would not be expected to occur.

CLINICAL STUDIES

Endometriosis: In controlled clinical studies, LUPRON DEPOT 3.75 mg monthly for six months was shown to be comparable to danazol 800 mg/day in relieving the clinical sign/symptoms of endometriosis (pelvic pain, dysmenorrhea, dyspareunia, pelvic tenderness, and induration) and in reducing the size of endometrial implants as evidenced by laparoscopy. The clinical significance of a decrease in endometriotic lesions is not known at this time, and in addition laparoscopic staging of endometriosis does not necessarily correlate with the severity of symptoms.

LUPRON DEPOT 3.75 mg monthly induced amenorrhea in 74% and 98% of the patients after the first and second treatment months respectively. Most of the remaining patients reported episodes of only light bleeding or spotting. In the first, second and third post-treatment months, normal menstrual cycles resumed in 7%, 71% and 95% of patients, respectively, excluding those who became pregnant.

Figure 1 illustrates the percent of patients with symptoms at baseline, final treatment visit and sustained relief at 6 and 12 months following discontinuation of treatment for the various symptoms evaluated during two controlled clinical studies. This included all patients at end of treatment and those who elected to participate in the follow-up period. This might provide a slight bias in the results at follow-up as 75% of the original patients entered the follow-up study, and 36% were evaluated at 6 months and 26% at 12 months.

[See figure 1 at top of next column]

Hormonal replacement therapy: Two clinical studies with a treatment duration of 12 months indicate that concurrent hormonal therapy (norethindrone acetate 5 mg daily) is effective in significantly re-

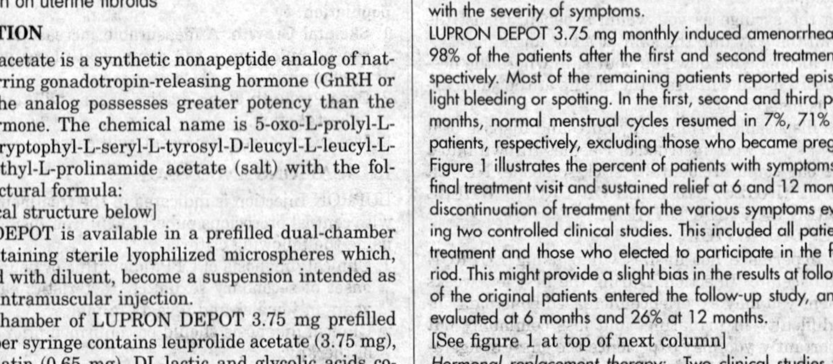

FIGURE 1–PERCENT OF PATIENTS WITH SIGN/SYMPTOMS AT BASELINE, FINAL TREATMENT VISIT, AND AFTER 6 AND 12 MONTHS OF FOLLOW-UP

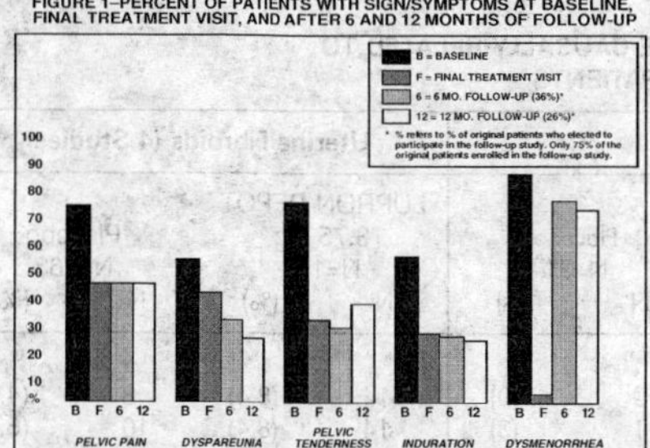

ducing the loss of bone mineral density associated with LUPRON, without compromising the efficacy of LUPRON in relieving symptoms of endometriosis. (All patients in these studies received calcium supplementation with 1000 mg elemental calcium). One controlled, randomized and double-blind study included 51 women treated with LUPRON DEPOT alone and 55 women treated with LUPRON plus norethindrone acetate 5 mg daily. The second study was an open label study in which 136 women were treated with LUPRON plus norethindrone acetate 5 mg daily. This study confirmed the reduction in loss of bone mineral density that was observed in the controlled study. Suppression of menses was maintained throughout treatment in 84% and 73% of patients receiving LD/N in the controlled study and open label study, respectively. The median time for menses resumption after treatment with LD/N was 8 weeks.

Figure 2 illustrates the mean pain scores for the LD/N group from the controlled study.

Figure 2
Treatment Period Mean Pain Scores for LD/N* Patients

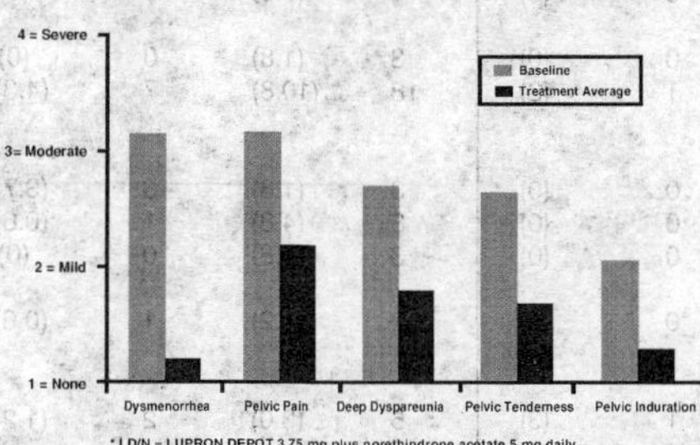

*LD/N = LUPRON DEPOT 3.75 mg plus norethindrone acetate 5 mg daily

Uterine Leiomyomata (Fibroids): In controlled clinical trials, administration of LUPRON DEPOT 3.75 mg for a period of three or six months was shown to decrease uterine and fibroid volume, thus allowing for relief of clinical symptoms (abdominal bloating, pelvic pain, and pressure). Excessive vaginal bleeding (menorrhagia and menometrorrhagia) decreased, resulting in improvement in hematologic parameters.

In three clinical trials, enrollment was not based on hematologic status. Mean uterine volume decreased by 41% and myoma volume decreased by 37% at final visit as evidenced by ultrasound or MRI. These patients also experienced a decrease in symptoms including excessive vaginal bleeding and pelvic discomfort. Benefit occurred by three months of therapy, but additional gain was observed with an additional three months of LUPRON DEPOT 3.75 mg. Ninety-five percent of these patients became amenorrheic with 61%, 25%, and 4% experiencing amenorrhea during the first, second, and third treatment months respectively.

Post-treatment follow-up was carried out for a small percentage of LUPRON DEPOT 3.75 mg patients among the 77% who demonstrated a ≥ 25% decrease in uterine volume while on therapy. Menses usually returned within two months of cessation of therapy. Mean time to return to pretreatment uterine size was 8.3 months. Regrowth did not appear to be related to pretreatment uterine volume.

In another controlled clinical study, enrollment was based on hematocrit ≤ 30% and/or hemoglobin ≤ 10.2 g/dL. Administration of LUPRON DEPOT 3.75 mg, concomitantly with iron, produced an increase of ≥ 6% hematocrit and ≥ 2 g/dL hemoglobin in 77% of patients at three months of therapy. The mean change in hematocrit was 10.1% and the mean change in hemoglobin was 4.2 g/dL. Clinical response was judged to be a hematocrit of ≥ 36% and hemoglobin of ≥ 12 g/dL, thus allowing for autologous blood donation prior to surgery. At three months, 75% of patients met this criterion.

At three months, 80% of patients experienced relief from either menorrhagia or menometrorrhagia. As with the previous studies, episodes of spotting and menstrual-like bleeding were noted in some patients.

In this same study, a decrease of ≥ 25% was seen in uterine and myoma volumes in 60% and 54% of patients respectively. LUPRON DEPOT 3.75 mg was found to relieve symptoms of bloating, pelvic pain, and pressure.

There is no evidence that pregnancy rates are enhanced or adversely affected by the use of LUPRON DEPOT 3.75 mg.

INDICATIONS AND USAGE

Endometriosis:

LUPRON DEPOT 3.75 mg is indicated for management of endometriosis, including pain relief and reduction of endometriotic lesions. LUPRON DEPOT monthly with norethindrone acetate 5 mg daily is also indicated for initial management of endometriosis and for management of recurrence of symptoms. (Refer also to norethindrone acetate prescribing information for WARNINGS, PRECAUTIONS, CONTRAINDICATIONS and ADVERSE REACTIONS associated with norethindrone acetate). Duration of initial treatment or retreatment should be limited to 6 months.

Uterine Leiomyomata (Fibroids):

LUPRON DEPOT 3.75 mg concomitantly with iron therapy is indicated for the preoperative hematologic improvement of patients with anemia caused by uterine leiomyomata. The clinician may wish to consider a one-month trial period on iron alone inasmuch as some of the patients will respond to iron alone. (See Table 1.) LUPRON may be added if the response to iron alone is considered inadequate. Recommended duration of therapy with LUPRON DEPOT 3.75 mg is **up to** three months.

Experience with LUPRON DEPOT in females has been limited to women 18 years of age and older.

Table 1
PERCENT OF PATIENTS ACHIEVING HEMOGLOBIN ≥ 12 GM/DL

Treatment Group	Week 4	Week 8	Week 12
LUPRON DEPOT 3.75 mg with Iron	41*	71**	79*
Iron Alone	17	40	56

* P-Value < 0.01
** P-Value < 0.001

CONTRAINDICATIONS

1. Hypersensitivity to GnRH, GnRH agonist analogs or any of the excipients in LUPRON DEPOT.
2. Undiagnosed abnormal vaginal bleeding.
3. LUPRON DEPOT is contraindicated in women who are or may become pregnant while receiving the drug. LUPRON DEPOT may cause fetal harm when administered to a pregnant woman. Major fetal abnormalities were observed in rabbits but not in rats after administration of LUPRON DEPOT throughout gestation. There was increased fetal mortality and decreased fetal weights in rats and rabbits. (See **Pregnancy** section.) The effects on fetal mortality are expected consequences of the alterations in hormonal levels brought about by the drug. If this drug is used during pregnancy, or if the patient becomes pregnant while taking this drug, the patient should be apprised of the potential hazard to the fetus.
4. Use in women who are breast-feeding. (See **Nursing Mothers** section.)
5. Norethindrone acetate is contraindicated in women with the following conditions:
   — Thrombophlebitis, thromboembolic disorders, cerebral apoplexy, or a past history of these conditions
   — Markedly impaired liver function or liver disease
   — Known or suspected carcinoma of the breast

WARNINGS

Safe use of leuprolide acetate or norethindrone acetate in pregnancy has not been established clinically. Before starting treatment with LUPRON DEPOT, pregnancy must be excluded.

When used monthly at the recommended dose, LUPRON DEPOT usually inhibits ovulation and stops menstruation. Contraception is not insured, however, by taking LUPRON DEPOT. Therefore, patients should use non-hormonal methods of contraception. Patients should be advised to see their physician if they believe they may be pregnant. If a patient becomes pregnant during treatment, the drug must be discontinued and the patient must be apprised of the potential risk to the fetus.

During the early phase of therapy, sex steroids temporarily rise above baseline because of the physiologic effect of the drug. Therefore, an increase in clinical signs and symptoms may be observed during the initial days of therapy, but these will dissipate with continued therapy.

Symptoms consistent with an anaphylactoid or asthmatic process have been rarely reported post-marketing.

The following applies to co-treatment with LUPRON and norethindrone acetate:

Norethindrone acetate treatment should be discontinued if there is a sudden partial or complete loss of vision or if there is sudden onset of proptosis, diplopia, or migraine. If examination reveals papilledema or retinal vascular lesions, medication should be withdrawn.

Because of the occasional occurrence of thrombophlebitis and pulmonary embolism in patients taking progestogens, the physician should be alert to the earliest manifestations of the disease in women taking norethindrone acetate.

Assessment and management of risk factors for cardiovascular disease is recommended prior to initiation of add-back therapy with norethindrone acetate. Norethindrone acetate should be used with caution in women with risk factors, including lipid abnormalities or cigarette smoking.

PRECAUTIONS

Information for Patients An information pamphlet for patients is included with the product. Patients should be aware of the following information:

1. Since menstruation usually stops with effective doses of LUPRON DEPOT, the patient should notify her physician if regular menstruation persists. Patients missing successive doses of LUPRON DEPOT may experience breakthrough bleeding.
2. Patients should not use LUPRON DEPOT if they are pregnant, breast feeding, have undiagnosed abnormal vaginal bleeding, or are allergic to any of the ingredients in LUPRON DEPOT.
3. Safe use of the drug in pregnancy has not been established clinically. Therefore, a non-hormonal method of contraception should be used during treatment. Patients should be advised that if they miss successive doses of LUPRON DEPOT, breakthrough bleeding or ovulation may occur with the potential for conception. If a patient becomes pregnant during treatment, she should discontinue treatment and consult her physician.
4. Adverse events occurring in clinical studies with LUPRON DEPOT that are associated with hypoestrogenism include: hot flashes, headaches, emotional lability, decreased libido, acne, myalgia, reduction in breast size, and vaginal dryness. Estrogen levels returned to normal after treatment was discontinued.
5. Patients should be counseled on the possibility of the development or worsening of depression and the occurrence of memory disorders.
6. The induced hypoestrogenic state **also** results in a loss in bone density over the course of treatment, some of which may not be reversible. For a period up to six months, this bone loss should not be clinically significant. Clinical studies show that concurrent hormonal therapy with norethindrone acetate 5 mg daily is effective in reducing loss of bone mineral density that occurs with LUPRON. (All patients received calcium supplementation with 1000 mg elemental calcium.) (See ***Changes in Bone Density*** section).
7. If the symptoms of endometriosis recur after a course of therapy, retreatment with a six-month course of LUPRON DEPOT and norethindrone acetate 5 mg daily may be considered. Retreatment beyond this one six month course cannot be recommended. It is recommended that bone density be assessed before retreatment begins to ensure that values are within normal limits. Retreatment with LUPRON DEPOT alone is not recommended.
8. In patients with major risk factors for decreased bone mineral content such as chronic alcohol and/or tobacco use, strong family history of osteoporosis, or chronic use of drugs that can reduce bone mass such as anticonvulsants or corticosteroids, LUPRON DEPOT therapy may pose an additional risk. In these patients, the risks and benefits must be weighed carefully before therapy with LUPRON DEPOT alone is instituted, and concomitant treatment with norethindrone acetate 5 mg daily should be considered. Retreatment with gonadotropin-releasing hormone analogs, including LUPRON is not advisable in patients with major risk factors for loss of bone mineral content.
9. Because norethindrone acetate may cause some degree of fluid retention, conditions which might be influenced by this factor, such as epilepsy, migraine, asthma, cardiac or renal dysfunctions require careful observation during norethindrone acetate add-back therapy.
10. Patients who have a history of depression should be carefully observed during treatment with norethindrone acetate and norethindrone acetate should be discontinued if severe depression occurs.

Laboratory Tests See **ADVERSE REACTIONS** section.

Drug Interactions See **CLINICAL PHARMACOLOGY, Pharmacokinetics.**

Drug/Laboratory Test Interactions Administration of LUPRON DEPOT in therapeutic doses results in suppression of the pituitary-gonadal system. Normal function is usually restored within three months after treatment is discontinued. Therefore, diagnostic tests of pituitary gonadotropic and gonadal functions conducted during treatment and for up to three months after discontinuation of LUPRON DEPOT may be misleading.

Carcinogenesis, Mutagenesis, Impairment of Fertility A two-year carcinogenicity study was conducted in rats and mice. In rats, a dose-related increase of benign pituitary hyperplasia and benign pituitary adenomas was noted at 24 months when the drug was administered subcutaneously at high daily doses (0.6 to 4 mg/kg). There was a significant but not dose-related increase of pancreatic islet-cell adenomas in females and of testicular interstitial cell adenomas in males (highest incidence in the low dose group). In mice, no leuprolide acetate-induced tumors or pituitary abnormalities were observed at a dose as high as 60 mg/kg for two years. Patients have been treated with leuprolide acetate for up to three years with doses as high as 10 mg/day and for two years with doses as high as 20 mg/day without demonstrable pituitary abnormalities.

Mutagenicity studies have been performed with leuprolide acetate using bacterial and mammalian systems. These studies provided no evidence of a mutagenic potential.

Clinical and pharmacologic studies in adults (>18 years) with leuprolide acetate and similar analogs have shown reversibility of fertility suppression when the drug is discontinued after continuous administration for periods of up to 24 weeks. Although no clinical studies have been completed in children to assess the full reversibility of fertility suppression, animal studies (prepubertal and adult rats and monkeys) with leuprolide acetate and other GnRH analogs have shown functional recovery.

Pregnancy, Teratogenic Effects Pregnancy Category X. (See **CONTRAINDICATIONS** section.) When administered on day 6 of pregnancy at test dosages of 0.00024, 0.0024, and 0.024 mg/kg (1/300 to 1/3 of the human dose) to rabbits, LUPRON DEPOT produced a dose-related increase

Continued on next page

Lupron Depot 3.75 mg—Cont.

in major fetal abnormalities. Similar studies in rats failed to demonstrate an increase in fetal malformations. There was increased fetal mortality and decreased fetal weights with the two higher doses of LUPRON DEPOT in rabbits and with the highest dose (0.024 mg/kg) in rats.

Nursing Mothers It is not known whether LUPRON DEPOT is excreted in human milk. Because many drugs are excreted in human milk, and because the effects of LUPRON DEPOT on lactation and/or the breast-fed child have not been determined, LUPRON DEPOT should not be used by nursing mothers.

Pediatric Use Experience with LUPRON DEPOT 3.75 mg for treatment of endometriosis has been limited to women 18 years of age and older. See LUPRON DEPOT-PED® (leuprolide acetate for depot suspension) labeling for the safety and effectiveness in children with central precocious puberty.

Geriatric Use This product has not been studied in women over 65 years of age and is not indicated in this population.

ADVERSE REACTIONS

Clinical Trials

Estradiol levels may increase during the first weeks following the initial injection of LUPRON, but then decline to menopausal levels. This transient increase in estradiol can be associated with a temporary worsening of signs and symptoms. (See **WARNINGS** section.)

As would be expected with a drug that lowers serum estradiol levels, the most frequently reported adverse reactions were those related to hypoestrogenism.

The **monthly formulation of LUPRON DEPOT 3.75 mg** was utilized in controlled clinical trials that studied the drug in 166 endometriosis and 166 uterine fibroids patients. Adverse events reported in ≥5% of patients in either of these populations and thought to be potentially related to drug are noted in the following table.

[See table 2 at right]

Table 2
ADVERSE EVENTS REPORTED TO BE CAUSALLY RELATED TO DRUG IN ≥ 5% OF PATIENTS

	Endometriosis (2 Studies)						Uterine Fibroids (4 Studies)			
	LUPRON DEPOT 3.75 mg N=166		Danazol N=136		Placebo N=31		LUPRON DEPOT 3.75 mg N=166		Placebo N=163	
	N	(%)	N	(%)	N	(%)	N	(%)	N	(%)
Body as a Whole										
Asthenia	5	(3)	9	(7)	0	(0)	14	(8.4)	8	(4.9)
General pain	31	(19)	22	(16)	1	(3)	14	(8.4)	10	(6.1)
Headache*	53	(32)	30	(22)	2	(6)	43	(25.9)	29	(17.8)
Cardiovascular System										
Hot flashes/ sweats*	139	(84)	77	(57)	9	(29)	121	(72.9)	29	(17.8)
Gastrointestinal System										
Nausea/vomiting	21	(13)	17	(13)	1	(3)	8	(4.8)	6	(3.7)
GI disturbances*	11	(7)	8	(6)	1	(3)	5	(3.0)	2	(1.2)
Metabolic and Nutritional Disorders										
Edema	12	(7)	17	(13)	1	(3)	9	(5.4)	2	(1.2)
Weight gain/loss	22	(13)	36	(26)	0	(0)	5	(3.0)	2	(1.2)
Endocrine System										
Acne	17	(10)	27	(20)	0	(0)	0	(0)	0	(0)
Hirsutism	2	(1)	9	(7)	1	(3)	1	(0.6)	0	(0)
Musculoskeletal System										
Joint disorder*	14	(8)	11	(8)	0	(0)	13	(7.8)	5	(3.1)
Myalgia*	1	(1)	7	(5)	0	(0)	1	(0.6)	0	(0)
Nervous System										
Decreased libido*	19	(11)	6	(4)	0	(0)	3	(1.8)	0	(0)
Depression/ emotional lability*	36	(22)	27	(20)	1	(3)	18	(10.8)	7	(4.3)
Dizziness	19	(11)	4	(3)	0	(0)	3	(1.8)	6	(3.7)
Nervousness*	8	(5)	11	(8)	0	(0)	8	(4.8)	1	(0.6)
Neuromuscular disorders*	11	(7)	17	(13)	0	(0)	3	(1.8)	0	(0)
Paresthesias	12	(7)	11	(8)	0	(0)	2	(1.2)	1	(0.6)
Skin and Appendages										
Skin reactions	17	(10)	20	(15)	1	(3)	5	(3.0)	2	(1.2)
Urogenital System										
Breast changes/ tenderness/pain*	10	(6)	12	(9)	0	(0)	3	(1.8)	7	(4.3)
Vaginitis*	46	(28)	23	(17)	0	(0)	19	(11.4)	3	(1.8)

In these same studies, symptoms reported in <5% of patients included: *Body as a Whole* - Body odor, Flu syndrome, Injection site reactions; *Cardiovascular System* - Palpitations, Syncope, Tachycardia; *Digestive System* - Appetite changes, Dry mouth, Thirst; *Endocrine System* - Androgen-like effects; *Hemic and Lymphatic System* - Ecchymosis, Lymphadenopathy; *Nervous System* - Anxiety*, Insomnia/Sleep disorders*, Delusions, Memory disorder, Personality disorder; *Respiratory System* - Rhinitis; *Skin and Appendages* - Alopecia, Hair disorder, Nail disorder; *Special Senses* - Conjunctivitis, Ophthalmologic disorders*, Taste perversion; *Urogenital System* - Dysuria*, Lactation, Menstrual disorders.

* = Possible effect of decreased estrogen.

In one controlled clinical trial utilizing the monthly formulation of LUPRON DEPOT, patients diagnosed with uterine fibroids received a higher dose (7.5 mg) of LUPRON DEPOT. Events seen with this dose that were thought to be potentially related to drug and were not seen at the lower dose included glossitis, hypesthesia, lactation, pyelonephritis, and urinary disorders. Generally, a higher incidence of hypoestrogenic effects was observed at the higher dose.

Table 3 lists the potentially drug-related adverse events observed in at least 5% of patients in any treatment group during the first 6 months of treatment in the add-back clinical studies.

[See table 3 at right]

Table 3
TREATMENT-RELATED ADVERSE EVENTS OCCURRING IN ≥ 5% OF PATIENTS

	Controlled Study				Open Label Study	
	LD-Only[1] N=51		LD/N[2] N=55		LD/N[2] N=136	
Adverse Events	N	(%)	N	(%)	N	(%)
Any Adverse Event	50	(98)	53	(96)	126	(93)
Body as a Whole						
Asthenia	9	(18)	10	(18)	15	(11)
Headache/Migraine	33	(65)	28	(51)	63	(46)
Injection Site Reaction	1	(2)	5	(9)	4	(3)
Pain	12	(24)	16	(29)	29	(21)
Cardiovascular System						
Hot flashes/sweats	50	(98)	48	(87)	78	(57)
Digestive System						
Altered Bowel Function	7	(14)	8	(15)	14	(10)
Changes in Appetite	2	(4)	0	(0)	8	(6)
GI Disturbance	2	(4)	4	(7)	6	(4)
Nausea/Vomiting	13	(25)	16	(29)	17	(13)
Metabolic and Nutritional Disorders						
Edema	0	(0)	5	(9)	9	(7)
Weight Changes	6	(12)	7	(13)	6	(4)
Nervous System						
Anxiety	3	(6)	0	(0)	11	(8)
Depression/Emotional Lability	16	(31)	15	(27)	46	(34)
Dizziness/Vertigo	8	(16)	6	(11)	10	(7)
Insomnia/Sleep Disorder	16	(31)	7	(13)	20	(15)
Libido Changes	5	(10)	2	(4)	10	(7)
Memory Disorder	3	(6)	1	(2)	6	(4)
Nervousness	4	(8)	2	(4)	15	(11)
Neuromuscular Disorder	1	(2)	5	(9)	4	(3)
Skin and Appendages						
Alopecia	0	(0)	5	(9)	4	(3)
Androgen-Like Effects	2	(4)	3	(5)	24	(18)
Skin/Mucous Membrane Reaction	2	(4)	5	(9)	15	(11)
Urogential System						
Breast Changes/Pain/Tenderness	3	(6)	7	(13)	11	(8)
Menstrual Disorders	1	(2)	0	(0)	7	(5)
Vaginitis	10	(20)	8	(15)	11	(8)

[1] LD-Only = LUPRON DEPOT 3.75 mg
[2] LD/N = LUPRON DEPOT 3.75 mg plus norethindrone acetate 5 mg

In the controlled clinical trial, 50 of 51 (98%) patients in the LD group and 48 of 55 (87%) patients in the LD/N group reported experiencing hot flashes on one or more occasions during treatment. During Month 6 of treatment, 32 of 37 (86%) patients in the LD group and 22 of 38 (58%) patients in the LD/N group reported having experienced hot flashes. The mean number of days on which hot flashes were reported during this month of treatment was 19 and 7 in the LD and LD/N treatment groups, respectively. The mean maximum number of hot flashes in a day during this month of treatment was 5.8 and 1.9 in the LD and LD/N treatment groups, respectively.

Changes in Bone Density

In controlled clinical studies, patients with endometriosis (six months of therapy) or uterine fibroids (three months of therapy) were treated with LUPRON DEPOT 3.75 mg. In endometriosis patients, vertebral bone density as measured by dual energy x-ray absorptiometry (DEXA) decreased by an average of 3.2% at six months compared with the pretreatment value. Clinical studies demonstrate that concurrent hormonal therapy (norethindrone acetate 5 mg daily) and calcium supplementation is effective in significantly reducing the loss of bone mineral density that occurs with LUPRON treatment, without compromising the efficacy of LUPRON in relieving symptoms of endometriosis.

LUPRON DEPOT 3.75 mg plus norethindrone acetate 5 mg daily was evaluated in two clinical trials. The results from this regimen were similar in both studies.

LUPRON DEPOT 3.75 mg was used as a control group in one study. The bone mineral density data of the lumbar spine from these two studies are presented in Table 4.

[See table 4 at top of next page]

When LUPRON DEPOT 3.75 mg was administered for three months in uterine fibroid patients, vertebral trabecular bone mineral density as assessed by quantitative digital radiography (QDR) revealed a mean decrease of 2.7% compared with baseline. Six months after discontinuation of therapy, a trend toward recovery was observed. Use of LUPRON DEPOT for longer than three months (uterine fibroids) or six months (endometriosis) or in the presence of other known risk factors for decreased bone mineral content may cause additional bone loss **and is not recommended.**

Changes in Laboratory Values During Treatment

Plasma Enzymes

Endometriosis: During early clinical trials with LUPRON DEPOT 3.75 mg, regular laboratory monitoring revealed that AST levels were more than twice the upper limit of normal in only one patient. There was no clinical or other laboratory evidence of abnormal liver function.

In two other clinical trials, 6 of 191 patients receiving LUPRON DEPOT 3.75 mg plus norethindrone acetate 5 mg daily for up to 12 months developed an elevated (at least twice the upper limit of normal) SGPT or GGT. Five of the 6 increases were observed beyond 6 months of treatment. None were associated with elevated bilirubin concentration.

Uterine Leiomyomata (Fibroids): In clinical trials with LUPRON DEPOT 3.75 mg, five (3%) patients had a post-treatment transaminase value that was at least twice the baseline value and above the upper limit of the normal range. None of the laboratory increases were associated with clinical symptoms.

Lipids

Endometriosis: In earlier clinical studies, 4% of the LUPRON DEPOT 3.75 mg patients and 1% of the danazol patients had total cholesterol values above the normal range at enrollment. These patients also had cholesterol values above the normal range at the end of treatment. Of those patients whose pretreatment cholesterol values were in the normal range, 7% of the LUPRON DEPOT 3.75 mg patients and 9% of the danazol patients had post-treatment values above the normal range.

The mean (±SEM) pretreatment values for total cholesterol from all patients were 178.8 (2.9) mg/dL in the LUPRON DEPOT 3.75 mg groups and 175.3 (3.0) mg/dL in the danazol group. At the end of treatment, the mean values for total cholesterol from all patients were 193.3 mg/dL in the LUPRON DEPOT 3.75 mg group and 194.4 mg/dL in the danazol group. These increases from the pretreatment values were statistically significant ($p<0.03$) in both groups.

Triglycerides were increased above the upper limit of normal in 12% of the patients who received LUPRON DEPOT 3.75 mg and in 6% of the patients who received danazol.

At the end of treatment, HDL cholesterol fractions decreased below the lower limit of the normal range in 2% of the LUPRON DEPOT 3.75 mg patients compared with 54% of those receiving danazol. LDL cholesterol fractions increased above the upper limit of the normal range in 6% of the patients receiving LUPRON DEPOT 3.75 mg compared with 23% of those receiving danazol. There was no increase in the LDL/HDL ratio in patients receiving LUPRON DEPOT 3.75 mg but there was approximately a two-fold increase in the LDL/HDL ratio in patients receiving danazol.

In two other clinical trials, LUPRON DEPOT 3.75 mg plus norethindrone acetate 5 mg daily was evaluated for 12 months of treatment. LUPRON DEPOT 3.75 mg was used as a control group in one study. Percent changes from baseline for serum lipids and percentages of patients with serum lipid values outside of the normal range in the two studies are summarized in the tables below.

[See table 5 at right]

Changes from baseline tended to be greater at Week 52. After treatment, mean serum lipid levels from patients with follow up data returned to pretreatment values.

[See table 6 at right]

Low HDL-cholesterol (<40 mg/dL) and elevated LDL-cholesterol (>160 mg/dL) are recognized risk factors for cardiovascular disease. The long-term significance of the observed treatment-related changes in serum lipids in women with endometriosis is unknown. Therefore assessment of cardiovascular risk factors should be considered prior to initiation of concurrent treatment with LUPRON and norethindrone acetate.

Uterine Leiomyomata (Fibroids): In patients receiving LUPRON DEPOT 3.75 mg, mean changes in cholesterol (+11 mg/dL to +29 mg/dL), LDL cholesterol (+8 mg/dL to +22 mg/dL), HDL cholesterol (0 to +6 mg/dL), and the LDL/HDL ratio (−0.1 to +0.5) were observed across studies. In the one study in which triglycerides were determined, the mean increase from baseline was 32 mg/dL.

Other Changes

Endometriosis: The following changes were seen in approximately 5% to 8% of patients. In the earlier comparative studies, LUPRON DEPOT 3.75 mg was associated with elevations of LDH and phosphorus, and decreases in WBC counts. Danazol therapy was associated with increases in hematocrit, platelet count, and LDH. In the hormonal add-back studies LUPRON DEPOT in combination with norethindrone acetate was associated with elevations of GGT and SGPT.

Uterine Leiomyomata (Fibroids):

Hematology: (See **CLINICAL STUDIES** section.) In LUPRON DEPOT 3.75 mg treated patients, although there were statistically significant mean decreases in platelet counts from baseline to final visit, the last mean platelet counts were within the normal range. Decreases in total WBC count and neutrophils were observed, but were not clinically significant.

Chemistry: Slight to moderate mean increases were noted for glucose, uric acid, BUN, creatinine, total protein, albumin, bilirubin, alkaline phosphatase, LDH, calcium, and phosphorus. None of these increases were clinically significant.

Postmarketing

During postmarketing surveillance, the following adverse events were reported. Like other drugs in this class, mood swings, including depression, have been reported. There have been rare reports of suicidal ideation and attempt. Many, but not all, of these patients had a history of depression or other psychiatric illness. Patients should be counseled on the possibility of development or worsening of depression during treatment with LUPRON.

Symptoms consistent with an anaphylactoid or asthmatic process have been rarely reported. Rash, urticaria, and photosensitivity reactions have also been reported.

Localized reactions including induration and abscess have been reported at the site of injection. Symptoms consistent with fibromyalgia (eg: joint and muscle pain, headaches, sleep disorder, gastrointestinal distress, and shortness of breath) have been reported individually and collectively.

Other events reported are:

Cardiovascular System - Hypotension, Pulmonary embolism; *Hemic and Lymphatic System* - Decreased WBC; *Central/Peripheral Nervous System* - Peripheral neuropathy, Spinal fracture/paralysis; *Musculoskeletal System* - Tenosynovitis-like symptoms; *Urogenital System* - Prostate pain. See other LUPRON DEPOT and LUPRON Injection package inserts for other events reported in different patient populations.

Table 4
MEAN PERCENT CHANGE FROM BASELINE IN BONE MINERAL DENSITY OF LUMBAR SPINE

	LUPRON DEPOT 3.75 mg		LUPRON DEPOT 3.75 mg plus norethindrone acetate 5 mg daily			
	Controlled Study		Controlled Study		Open Label Study	
	N	Change	N	Change	N	Change
Week 24[1]	41	-3.2%	42	-0.3%	115	-0.2%
Week 52[2]	29	-6.3%	32	-1.0%	84	-1.1%

[1] Includes on-treatment measurements that fell within 2–252 days after the first day of treatment.
[2] Includes on-treatment measurements >252 days after the first day of treatment.

Table 5
SERUM LIPIDS: MEAN PERCENT CHANGES FROM BASELINE VALUES AT TREATMENT WEEK 24

	LUPRON		LUPRON plus norethindrone acetate 5 mg daily			
	Controlled Study (n=39)		Controlled Study (n=41)		Open Label Study (n=117)	
	Baseline Value*	Wk 24 % Change	Baseline Value*	Wk 24 % Change	Baseline Value*	Wk 24 % Change
Total Cholesterol	170.5	9.2%	179.3	0.2%	181.2	2.8%
HDL Cholesterol	52.4	7.4%	51.8	-18.8%	51.0	-14.6%
LDL Cholesterol	96.6	10.9%	101.5	14.1%	109.1	13.1%
LDL/HDL Ratio	2.0**	5.0%	2.1**	43.4%	2.3**	39.4%
Triglycerides	107.8	17.5%	130.2	9.5%	105.4	13.8%

* mg/dL
** ratio

Table 6
PERCENTAGE OF PATIENTS WITH SERUM LIPID VALUES OUTSIDE OF THE NORMAL RANGE

	LUPRON		LUPRON plus norethindrone acetate 5 mg daily			
	Controlled Study (n=39)		Controlled Study (n=41)		Open Label Study (n=117)	
	Wk 0	Wk 24*	Wk 0	Wk 24*	Wk 0	Wk 24*
Total Cholesterol (>240 mg/dL)	15%	23%	15%	20%	6%	7%
HDL Cholesterol (<40 mg/dL)	15%	10%	15%	44%	15%	41%
LDL Cholesterol (>160 mg/dL)	0%	8%	5%	7%	9%	11%
LDL/HDL Ratio (>4.0)	0%	3%	2%	15%	7%	21%
Triglycerides (>200 mg/dL)	13%	13%	12%	10%	5%	9%

* Includes all patients regardless of baseline value.

OVERDOSAGE

In rats subcutaneous administration of 250 to 500 times the recommended human dose, expressed on a per body weight basis, resulted in dyspnea, decreased activity, and local irritation at the injection site. There is no evidence that there is a clinical counterpart of this phenomenon. In early clinical trials using daily subcutaneous leuprolide acetate in patients with prostate cancer, doses as high as 20 mg/day for up to two years caused no adverse effects differing from those observed with the 1 mg/day dose.

DOSAGE AND ADMINISTRATION

LUPRON DEPOT Must Be Administered Under The Supervision Of A Physician.

Endometriosis: The recommended duration of treatment with LUPRON DEPOT 3.75 mg alone or in combination with norethindrone acetate is six months. The choice of LUPRON DEPOT alone or LUPRON DEPOT plus norethindrone acetate therapy for initial management of the symptoms and signs of endometriosis should be made by the health care professional in consultation with the patient and should take into consideration the risks and benefits of the addition of norethindrone to LUPRON DEPOT alone.

If the symptoms of endometriosis recur after a course of therapy, retreatment with a six-month course of LUPRON DEPOT monthly and norethindrone acetate 5 mg daily may be considered. Retreatment beyond this one six-month course cannot be recommended. It is recommended that bone density be assessed before retreatment begins to ensure that values are within normal limits. LUPRON DEPOT alone is not recommended for retreatment. If norethindrone acetate is contraindicated for the individual patient, then retreatment is not recommended.

An assessment of cardiovascular risk and management of risk factors such as cigarette smoking is recommended before beginning treatment with LUPRON DEPOT and norethindrone acetate.

*Uterine Leiomyomata (Fibroids): Recommended duration of therapy with LUPRON DEPOT 3.75 mg is **up to** 3 months. The symptoms associated with uterine leiomyomata will recur following discontinuation of therapy. If additional treatment with LUPRON DEPOT 3.75 mg is contemplated, bone density should be assessed prior to initiation of therapy to ensure that values are within normal limits.*

The recommended dose of LUPRON DEPOT is 3.75 mg, incorporated in a depot formulation. The lyophilized microspheres are to be reconstituted and administered monthly as a single intramuscular injection. *For optimal performance of the prefilled dual chamber syringe (PDS), read and follow the following instructions:*

1. To prepare for injection, screw the white plunger into the end stopper until the stopper begins to turn.
2. Hold the syringe UPRIGHT. Release the diluent by SLOWLY PUSHING (6 to 8 seconds) the plunger until the first stopper is at the blue line in the middle of the barrel.
3. Keep the syringe UPRIGHT. Gently mix the microspheres (particles) thoroughly to form a uniform suspension. The suspension will appear milky.
4. Hold the syringe UPRIGHT. With the opposite hand pull the needle cap upward without twisting.
5. Keep the syringe UPRIGHT. Advance the plunger to expel the air from the syringe.
6. Inject the entire contents of the syringe intramuscularly at the time of reconstitution. The suspension settles very quickly following reconstitution; therefore, LUPRON DEPOT should be mixed and used immediately.

NOTE: Aspirated blood would be visible just below the luer lock connection if a blood vessel is accidentally penetrated. If present, blood can be seen through the transparent LuproLoc™ safety device.

AFTER INJECTION

7. Withdraw the needle. Immediately activate the LuproLoc™ safety device by pushing the arrow forward with the thumb or finger until the device is fully extended and a CLICK is heard or felt.

Since the product does not contain a preservative, the suspension should be discarded if not used immediately.

As with other drugs administered by injection, the injection site should be varied periodically.

HOW SUPPLIED

LUPRON DEPOT 3.75 mg is packaged as follows:

Kit with prefilled dual-chamber syringe NDC 0300-3641-01

Each syringe contains sterile lyophilized microspheres, which is leuprolide incorporated in a biodegradable copolymer of lactic and glycolic acids. When mixed with diluent, LUPRON DEPOT 3.75 mg is administered as a single monthly IM injection.

Store at 25°C (77°F); excursions permitted to 15-30°C (59-86°F) [See USP Controlled Room Temperature]

Rx only

Continued on next page

Lupron Depot 3.75 mg—Cont.

U.S. Patent Nos. 4,652,441; 4,677,191; 4,728,721; 4,849,228; 4,917,893; 5,330,767; 5,476,663; 5,575,987; 5,631,020; 5,631,021; 5,716,640; 5,823,997; 5,980,488; and 6,036,976.
Other patents pending.
Manufactured for
TAP Pharmaceuticals Inc.
Lake Forest, IL 60045, U.S.A.
by Takeda Chemical Industries, Ltd.
Osaka, JAPAN 541
™ - Trademark
® - Registered Trademark
(No. 3641)
03-5335-R17; Revised: February, 2004

Shown in Product Identification Guide, page 334

LUPRON DEPOT® 7.5 mg ℞

[lew-prŏn]
(leuprolide acetate for depot suspension)
Rx only

DESCRIPTION

Leuprolide acetate is a synthetic nonapeptide analog of naturally occurring gonadotropin-releasing hormone (GnRH or LH-RH). The analog possesses greater potency than the natural hormone. The chemical name is 5-oxo-L-prolyl-L-histidyl-L-tryptophyl-L-seryl-L-tyrosyl-D-leucyl-L-leucyl-L-arginyl-N-ethyl-L-prolinamide acetate (salt) with the following structural formula:
[See chemical structure below]
LUPRON DEPOT is available in a prefilled dual-chamber syringe containing sterile lyophilized microspheres which, when mixed with diluent, becomes a suspension intended as a monthly intramuscular injection.
The front chamber of LUPRON DEPOT 7.5 mg prefilled dual-chamber syringe contains leuprolide acetate (7.5 mg), purified gelatin (1.3 mg), DL-lactic and glycolic acids copolymer (66.2 mg), and D-mannitol (13.2 mg). The second chamber of diluent contains carboxymethylcellulose sodium (5 mg), D-mannitol (50 mg), polysorbate 80 (1 mg), water for injection, USP, and glacial acetic acid, USP to control pH.
During the manufacture of LUPRON DEPOT 7.5 mg, acetic acid is lost, leaving the peptide.

CLINICAL PHARMACOLOGY

Leuprolide acetate, an LH-RH agonist, acts as a potent inhibitor of gonadotropin secretion when given continuously and in therapeutic doses. Animal and human studies indicate that following an initial stimulation, chronic administration of leuprolide acetate results in suppression of ovarian and testicular steroidogenesis. This effect is reversible upon discontinuation of drug therapy. Administration of leuprolide acetate has resulted in inhibition of the growth of certain hormone dependent tumors (prostatic tumors in Noble and Dunning male rats and DMBA-induced mammary tumors in female rats) as well as atrophy of the reproductive organs.
In humans, administration of leuprolide acetate results in an initial increase in circulating levels of luteinizing hormone (LH) and follicle stimulating hormone (FSH), leading to a transient increase in levels of the gonadal steroids (testosterone and dihydrotestosterone in males, and estrone and estradiol in premenopausal females). However, continuous administration of leuprolide acetate results in decreased levels of LH and FSH. In males, testosterone is reduced to castrate levels. In premenopausal females, estrogens are reduced to postmenopausal levels. These decreases occur within two to four weeks after initiation of treatment. Castrate levels of testosterone in prostatic cancer patients have been demonstrated for up to 10 years.
Leuprolide acetate is not active when given orally.

Pharmacokinetics

Absorption Following a single injection of LUPRON DEPOT 7.5 mg to patients, mean plasma leuprolide concentration was almost 20 ng/mL at 4 hours and 0.36 ng/mL at 4 weeks. However, intact leuprolide and an inactive major metabolite could not be distinguished by the assay which was employed in the study. Nondetectable leuprolide plasma concentrations have been observed during chronic LUPRON DEPOT 7.5 mg administration, but testosterone levels appear to be maintained at castrate levels.

Distribution The mean steady-state volume of distribution of leuprolide following intravenous bolus administration to healthy male volunteers was 27 L. *In vitro* binding to human plasma proteins ranged from 43% to 49%.

Metabolism In healthy male volunteers, a 1 mg bolus of leuprolide administered intravenously revealed that the mean systemic clearance was 7.6 L/h, with a terminal elimination half-life of approximately 3 hours based on a two compartment model.
In rats and dogs, administration of ^{14}C-labeled leuprolide was shown to be metabolized to smaller inactive peptides, a pentapeptide (Metabolite I), tripeptides (Metabolites II and III) and a dipeptide (Metabolite IV). These fragments may be further catabolized.
The major metabolite (M-I) plasma concentrations measured in 5 prostate cancer patients reached maximum concentration 2 to 6 hours after dosing and were approximately 6% of the peak parent drug concentration. One week after dosing, mean plasma M-I concentrations were approximately 20% of mean leuprolide concentrations.

Excretion Following administration of LUPRON DEPOT 3.75 mg to 3 patients, less than 5% of the dose was recovered as parent and M-I metabolite in the urine.

Special Populations The pharmacokinetics of the drug in hepatically and renally impaired patients have not been determined.

Drug Interactions No pharmacokinetic-based drug-drug interaction studies have been conducted with LUPRON DEPOT. However, because leuprolide acetate is a peptide that is primarily degraded by peptidase and the drug is only about 46% bound to plasma proteins, drug interactions would not be expected to occur.

CLINICAL STUDIES

In an open-label, non-comparative, multicenter clinical study of LUPRON DEPOT 7.5 mg, 56 patients with stage D$_2$ prostatic adenocarcinoma and no prior systemic treatment were enrolled. The objectives were to determine if a 7.5 mg depot formulation of leuprolide injected once every 4 weeks would reduce and maintain serum testosterone to castrate range ($\leq$50 ng/dL), to evaluate objective clinical response, and to assess the safety of the formulation. During the initial 24 weeks, serum testosterone was measured weekly, biweekly, or every four weeks and objective tumor response assessments were performed at Weeks 12 and 24. Once the patient completed the initial 24-week treatment phase, treatment continued at the investigator's discretion. Data from the initial 24-week treatment phase are summarized in this section.
In the majority of patients, serum testosterone increased by 50% or more above baseline during the first week of treatment. Serum testosterone suppressed to the castrate range within 30 days of the initial depot injection in 94% (51/54) of patients for whom testosterone suppression was achieved (2 patients withdrew prior to onset of suppression) and within 66 days in all 54 patients. Mean serum testosterone suppressed to castrate level by Week 3. The median dosing interval between injections was 28 days. One escape from suppression (2 consecutive testosterone values >50 ng/dL after achieving castrate level) was noted at Week 18, associated with a substantial dosing delay. In this patient, serum testosterone returned to the castrate range at the next monthly measurement. Serum testosterone was minimally above the castrate range on a single occasion for 4 other patients. No clinical significance was attributed to these rises in testosterone.

Lupron Depot 7.5 mg
Mean Serum Testosterone Concentrations

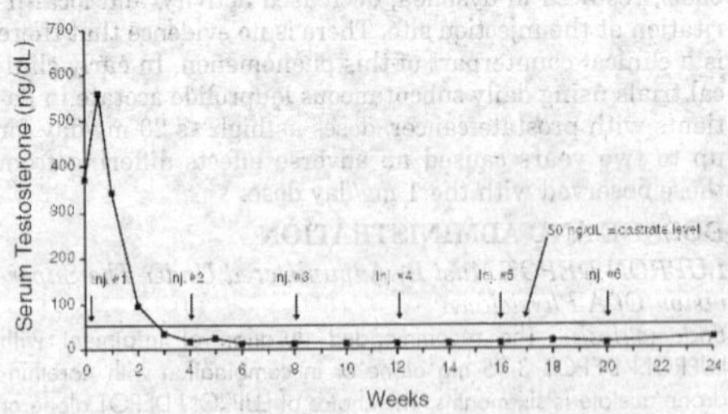

Secondary efficacy endpoints evaluated included objective tumor response, assessed by clinical evaluations of tumor burden (complete response, partial response, objectively stable, and progression), as well as changes in local disease status, assessed by digital rectal examination, and changes in prostatic acid phosphatase (PAP). These evaluations were performed at Weeks 12 and 24. The objective tumor response analysis showed a "no progression" (ie. complete or partial response, or stable disease) in 77% (40/52) of patients at Week 12, and in 84% (42/50) of patients at Week 24. Local disease improved or remained stable in all (42) patients evaluated at Week 12 and in 98% (41/42) of patients elevated at Week 24. PAP normalized or decreased at Week 12 and/or 24 in the majority of patients with elevated baseline PAP.
Periodic monitoring of serum testosterone and PSA levels is recommended, especially if the anticipated clinical or biochemical response to treatment has not been achieved. It should be noted that results of testosterone determinations are dependent on assay methodology. It is advisable to be aware of the type and precision of the assay methodology to make appropriate clinical and therapeutic decisions.

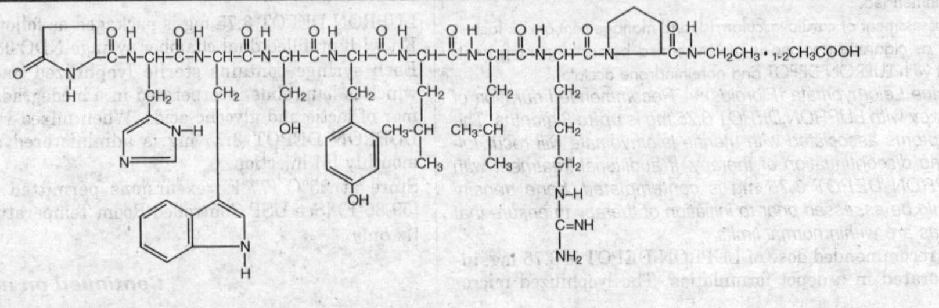

INDICATIONS AND USAGE

LUPRON DEPOT 7.5 mg is indicated in the palliative treatment of advanced prostatic cancer.

CONTRAINDICATIONS

1. Hypersensitivity to GnRH, GnRH agonist analogs or any of the excipients in LUPRON DEPOT. Reports of anaphylactic reactions to synthetic GnRH (Factrel) or GnRH agonist analogs have been reported in the medical literature.[1]
2. All formulations of LUPRON DEPOT are contraindicated in women who are or may become pregnant while receiving the drug. LUPRON DEPOT may cause fetal harm when administered to a pregnant woman. Major fetal abnormalities were observed in rabbits but not in rats after administration of LUPRON DEPOT throughout gestation. There was increased fetal mortality and decreased fetal weights in rats and rabbits. The effects on fetal mortality are expected consequences of the alterations in hormonal levels brought about by this drug. Therefore, the possibility exists that spontaneous abortion may occur. If this drug is administered during pregnancy or if the patient becomes pregnant while taking any formulation of LUPRON DEPOT, the patient should be apprised of the potential hazard to the fetus.

WARNINGS

Initially, LUPRON DEPOT, like other LH-RH agonists, causes increases in serum levels of testosterone to approximately 50% above baseline during the first week of treatment. Transient worsening of symptoms, or the occurrence of additional signs and symptoms of prostate cancer, may occasionally develop during the first few weeks of LUPRON DEPOT treatment. A small number of patients may experience a temporary increase in bone pain, which can be managed symptomatically. As with other LH-RH agonists, isolated cases of ureteral obstruction and spinal cord compression have been observed, which may contribute to paralysis with or without fatal complications.
For patients at risk, initiation of therapy with daily LUPRON® (leuprolide acetate) Injection (See **DOSAGE AND ADMINISTRATION** section in the LUPRON Injection labeling.) for the first two weeks to facilitate withdrawal of treatment may be considered. If spinal cord compression or renal impairment develops, standard treatment of these complications should be instituted.

PRECAUTIONS

Information for Patients An information pamphlet for patients is included with the product.

General Patients with metastatic vertebral lesions and/or with urinary tract obstruction should be closely observed during the first few weeks of therapy. (See **WARNINGS** section.)

Laboratory Tests Response to LUPRON DEPOT 7.5 mg should be monitored by measuring serum levels of testosterone as well as prostate-specific antigen. In the majority of patients, testosterone levels increased above baseline during the first week, declining thereafter to baseline levels or below by the end of the second week. Castrate levels were reached within two to four weeks and once achieved were maintained for the duration of treatment in all 54 patients. Minimal and transient increases to above the castrate level occurred in eight patients. (See **CLINICAL STUDIES** section.)

Drug Interactions (See **Pharmacokinetics.**)

Drug/Laboratory Test Interactions Administration of LUPRON DEPOT in therapeutic doses results in suppression of the pituitary-gonadal system. Normal function is usually restored within three months after treatment is discontinued. Due to the suppression of the pituitary-gonadal system by LUPRON DEPOT, diagnostic tests of pituitary gonadotropic and gonadal functions conducted during treatment and for up to three months after discontinuation of LUPRON DEPOT may be affected.

Carcinogenesis, Mutagenesis, Impairment of Fertility Two-year carcinogenicity studies were conducted in rats and mice. In rats, a dose-related increase of benign pituitary hyperplasia and benign pituitary adenomas was noted at 24 months when the drug was administered subcutaneously at high daily doses (0.6 to 4 mg/kg). There was a significant but not dose-related increase of pancreatic islet-cell adenomas in females and of testicular interstitial cell adenomas in males (highest incidence in the low dose group). In mice, no leuprolide acetate-induced tumors or pituitary abnormalities were observed at a dose as high as 60 mg/kg for two years. Patients have been treated with leuprolide acetate for up to three years with doses as high as 10 mg/day and for two years with doses as high as 20 mg/day without demonstrable pituitary abnormalities.
Mutagenicity studies have been performed with leuprolide acetate using bacterial and mammalian systems. These studies provided no evidence of a mutagenic potential.
Clinical and pharmacologic studies in adults ($\geq$ 18 years) with leuprolide acetate and similar analogs have shown re-

versibility of fertility suppression when the drug is discontinued after continuous administration for periods of up to 24 weeks.

Pregnancy Category X. See **CONTRAINDICATIONS** section.

Pediatric Use See LUPRON DEPOT-PED® (leuprolide acetate for depot suspension) labeling for the safety and effectiveness of the monthly formulation in children with central precocious puberty.

Geriatric Use In the clinical trials for LUPRON DEPOT, the majority (68%) of the subjects studied were at least 65 years of age. Therefore, the labeling reflects the pharmacokinetics, efficacy and safety of LUPRON DEPOT in this population.

ADVERSE REACTIONS

Clinical Trials

In the majority of patients testosterone levels increased above baseline during the first week, declining thereafter to baseline levels or below by the end of the second week of treatment.

Potential exacerbations of signs and symptoms during the first few weeks of treatment is a concern in patients with vertebral metastases and/or urinary obstruction or hematuria which, if aggravated, may lead to neurological problems such as temporary weakness and/or paresthesia of the lower limbs or worsening of urinary symptoms (See **WARNINGS** section.)

In a clinical trial of LUPRON DEPOT 7.5 mg, the following adverse reactions were reported in 5% or more of the patients during the initial 24-week treatment period regardless of causality.

LUPRON DEPOT 7.5 mg (N=56)		
	N	(%)
Body as a Whole		
General pain	13	(23.2)
Infection	3	(5.4)
Cardiovascular System		
Hot flashes/sweats*	32	(57.1)
Digestive System		
GI disorders	8	(14.3)
Metabolic and Nutritional Disorders		
Edema	8	(14.3)
Nervous System		
Libido decreased*	3	(5.4)
Respiratory System		
Respiratory disorder	6	(10.7)
Urogenital System		
Urinary disorder	7	(12.5)
Impotence*	3	(5.4)
Testicular atrophy*	3	(5.4)

*Due to the expected physiologic effect of decreased testosterone levels.

In this same study, the following adverse reactions were reported in less than 5% of the patients on LUPRON DEPOT 7.5 mg.

Body as a Whole—Asthenia, Cellulitis, Fever, Headache, Injection site reaction, Neoplasm; *Cardiovascular System*—Angina, Congestive heart failure; *Digestive System*—Anorexia, Dysphagia, Eructation, Peptic ulcer; *Hemic and Lymphatic System*—Ecchymosis; *Musculoskeletal System*—Myalgia; *Nervous System*—Agitation, Insomnia/sleep disorders, Neuromuscular disorders; *Respiratory System*—Emphysema, Hemoptysis, Lung edema, Sputum increased; *Skin and Appendages*—Hair disorder, Skin reaction; *Urogenital System*—Balanitis, Breast enlargement, Urinary tract infection.

Laboratory: Abnormalities of certain parameters were observed, but their relationship to drug treatment are difficult to assess in this population. The following were recorded in ≥5% of patients at final visit: Decreased albumin, decreased hemoglobin/hematocrit, decreased prostatic acid phosphatase, decreased total protein, decreased urine specific gravity, hyperglycemia, hyperuricemia, increased BUN, increased creatinine, increased liver function tests (AST, LDH), increased phosphorus, increased platelets, increased prostatic acid phosphatase, increased total cholesterol, increased urine specific gravity, leukopenia.

Postmarketing

During postmarketing surveillance, which includes other dosage forms and other patient populations, the following adverse events were reported.

Symptoms consistent with an anaphylactoid or asthmatic process have been rarely (incidence rate of about 0.002%) reported. Rash, urticaria, and photosensitivity reactions have also been reported.

Localized reactions including induration and abscess have been reported at the site of injection.

Symptoms consistent with fibromyalgia (eg, joint and muscle pain, headaches, sleep disorders, gastrointestinal distress, and shortness of breath) have been reported individually and collectively.

Cardiovascular System—Hypotension, Pulmonary embolism; *Hemic and Lymphatic System*—Decreased WBC; *Central/Peripheral Nervous System*—Peripheral neuropathy, Spinal fracture/paralysis; *Musculoskeletal System*—Tenosynovitis-like symptoms; *Urogenital System*—Prostate pain.

Changes in Bone Density: Decreased bone density has been reported in the medical literature in men who have had orchiectomy or who have been treated with an LH-RH agonist analog. In a clinical trial, 25 men with prostate cancer, 12 of whom had been treated previously with leuprolide acetate for at least six months, underwent bone density studies as a result of pain. The leuprolide-treated group had lower bone density scores than the nontreated control group. It can be anticipated that long periods of medical castration in men will have effects on bone density.

See other LUPRON DEPOT and LUPRON Injection package inserts for other events reported in women and pediatric populations.

OVERDOSAGE

In clinical trials using daily subcutaneous leuprolide acetate in patients with prostate cancer, doses as high as 20 mg/day for up to two years caused no adverse effects differing from those observed with the 1 mg/day dose.

DOSAGE AND ADMINISTRATION

LUPRON DEPOT Must Be Administered Under The Supervision Of A Physician.

The recommended dose of LUPRON DEPOT is 7.5 mg, incorporated in a depot formulation. The lyophilized microspheres are to be reconstituted and administered monthly as a single intramuscular injection. *For optimal performance of the prefilled dual chamber syringe (PDS), read and follow the following instructions:*

1. To prepare for injection, screw the white plunger into the end stopper until the stopper begins to turn.
2. Hold the syringe UPRIGHT. Release the diluent by SLOWLY PUSHING (6 to 8 seconds) the plunger until the first stopper is at the blue line in the middle of the barrel.
3. Keep the syringe UPRIGHT. Gently mix the microspheres (particles) thoroughly to form a uniform suspension. The suspension will appear milky.
4. Hold the syringe UPRIGHT. With the opposite hand pull the needle cap upward without twisting.
5. Keep the syringe UPRIGHT. Advance the plunger to expel the air from the syringe.
6. Inject the entire contents of the syringe intramuscularly at the time of reconstitution. The suspension settles very quickly following reconstitution; therefore, LUPRON DEPOT should be mixed and used immediately.

   NOTE: Aspirated blood would be visible just below the luer lock connection if a blood vessel is accidentally penetrated. If present, blood can be seen through the transparent LuproLoc™ safety device.

AFTER INJECTION

7. Withdraw the needle. Immediately activate the LuproLoc™ safety device by pushing the arrow forward with the thumb or finger until the device is fully extended and a CLICK is heard or felt.

Since the product does not contain a preservative, the suspension should be discarded if not used immediately.

As with other drugs administered by injection, the injection site should be varied periodically.

HOW SUPPLIED

LUPRON DEPOT 7.5 mg is packaged as follows:

Kit with prefilled dual-chamber syringe	NDC 0300-3642-01

Each syringe contains sterile lyophilized microspheres which is leuprolide incorporated in a biodegradable copolymer of lactic and glycolic acids. When mixed with diluent, LUPRON DEPOT 7.5 mg is administered as a single monthly IM injection.

An information pamphlet for patients is included with the kit.

Store at 25°C (77°F); excursions permitted to 15-30°C (59-86°F) [See USP Controlled Room Temperature]

REFERENCE

1. MacLeod TL, *et al.* Anaphylactic reaction to synthetic luteinizing hormone-releasing hormone. *Fertil Steril* 1987 Sept; 48(3):500–502.

U.S. Patent Nos. 4,652,441; 4,677,191; 4,728,721; 4,849,228; 4,917,893; 5,330,767; 5,476,663; 5,575,987; 5,631,020; 5,631,021; 5,716,640; 5,823,997; 5,980,488; and 6,036,976. Other patents pending.

Manufactured for
TAP Pharmaceuticals Inc.
Lake Forest, IL 60045, U.S.A.
by Takeda Chemical Industries, Ltd.
Osaka, JAPAN 541

™—Trademark
®—Registered Trademark
(No. 3642)
03-5308-R14; Revised September, 2003

Shown in Product Identification Guide, page 334

This is combined labeling. Examples of different fonts appear below.

- General information
- Information on endometriosis
- **Information on uterine fibroids**

LUPRON DEPOT®-3 Month 11.25 mg ℞

[*lew-prŏn*]

(leuprolide acetate for depot suspension)

3-MONTH FORMULATION

This is combined labeling. Examples of different fonts appear below.

- General information
- Information on endometriosis
- Information on uterine fibroids

DESCRIPTION

Leuprolide acetate is a synthetic nonapeptide analog of naturally occurring gonadotropin-releasing hormone (GnRH or LH-RH). The analog possesses greater potency than the natural hormone. The chemical name is 5-oxo-L-prolyl-L-histidyl-L-tryptophyl-L-seryl-L-tyrosyl-D-leucyl-L-leucyl-L-arginyl-N-ethyl-L-prolinamide acetate (salt) with the following structural formula:

[See chemical structure at top of next page]

LUPRON DEPOT–3 Month 11.25 mg is available in a prefilled dual-chamber syringe containing sterile lyophilized microspheres which, when mixed with diluent, become a suspension intended as an intramuscular injection to be given **ONCE EVERY THREE MONTHS.**

The front chamber of LUPRON DEPOT–3 Month 11.25 mg prefilled dual-chamber syringe contains leuprolide acetate (11.25 mg), polylactic acid (99.3 mg) and D-mannitol (19.45 mg). The second chamber of diluent contains carboxymethylcellulose sodium (7.5 mg), D-mannitol (75.0 mg), polysorbate 80 (1.5 mg), water for injection, USP, and glacial acetic acid, USP to control pH.

During the manufacture of LUPRON DEPOT–3 Month 11.25 mg, acetic acid is lost, leaving the peptide.

CLINICAL PHARMACOLOGY

Leuprolide acetate is a long-acting GnRH analog. A single injection of LUPRON DEPOT–3 Month 11.25 mg will result in an initial stimulation followed by a prolonged suppression of pituitary gonadotropins. Repeated dosing at quarterly (LUPRON DEPOT–3 Month 11.25 mg) intervals results in decreased secretion of gonadal steroids; consequently, tissues and functions that depend on gonadal steroids for their maintenance become quiescent. This effect is reversible on discontinuation of drug therapy.

Leuprolide acetate is not active when given orally.

Pharmacokinetics

Absorption Following a single injection of the three month formulation of LUPRON DEPOT–3 Month 11.25 mg in female subjects, a mean plasma leuprolide concentration of 36.3 ng/mL was observed at 4 hours. Leuprolide appeared to be released at a constant rate following the onset of steady-state levels during the third week after dosing and mean levels then declined gradually to near the lower limit of detection by 12 weeks. The mean (± standard deviation) leuprolide concentration from 3 to 12 weeks was 0.23 ± 0.09 ng/mL. However, intact leuprolide and an inactive major metabolite could not be distinguished by the assay which was employed in the study. The initial burst, followed by the rapid decline to a steady-state level, was similar to the release pattern seen with the monthly formulation.

Distribution The mean steady-state volume of distribution of leuprolide following intravenous bolus administration to healthy male volunteers was 27 L. *In vitro* binding to human plasma proteins ranged from 43% to 49%.

Metabolism In healthy male volunteers, a 1 mg bolus of leuprolide administered intravenously revealed that the mean systemic clearance was 7.6 L/h, with a terminal elimination half-life of approximately 3 hours based on a two compartment model.

In rats and dogs, administration of ^{14}C-labeled leuprolide was shown to be metabolized to smaller inactive peptides, a pentapeptide (Metabolite I), tripeptides (Metabolites II and III) and a dipeptide (Metabolite IV). These fragments may be further catabolized.

In a pharmacokinetic/pharmacodynamic study of endometriosis patients, intramuscular 11.25 mg LUPRON DEPOT (n=19) every 12 weeks or intramuscular 3.75 mg LUPRON DEPOT (n=15) every 4 weeks was administered for 24 weeks. There was no statistically significant difference in changes of serum estradiol concentration from baseline between the 2 treatment groups.

M-I plasma concentrations measured in 5 prostate cancer patients reached maximum concentration 2 to 6 hours after dosing and were approximately 6% of the peak parent drug concentration. One week after dosing, mean plasma M-I concentrations were approximately 20% of mean leuprolide concentrations.

Excretion Following administration of LUPRON DEPOT 3.75 mg to 3 patients, less than 5% of the dose was recovered as parent and M-I metabolite in the urine.

Special Populations The pharmacokinetics of the drug in hepatically and renally impaired patients have not been determined.

Drug Interactions No pharmacokinetic-based drug-drug interaction studies have been conducted with LUPRON DEPOT. However, because leuprolide acetate is a peptide that is primarily degraded by peptidase and not by cytochrome P-450 enzymes as noted in specific studies, and the drug is only about 46% bound to plasma proteins, drug interactions would not be expected to occur.

Continued on next page

Lupron Depot-3 Mo. 11.25 mg—Cont.

CLINICAL STUDIES

In a pharmacokinetic/pharmacodynamic study of healthy female subjects (N=20), the onset of estradiol suppression was observed for individual subjects between day 4 and week 4 after dosing. By the third week following the injection, the mean estradiol concentration (8 pg/mL) was in the menopausal range. Throughout the remainder of the dosing period, mean serum estradiol levels ranged from the menopausal to the early follicular range.

Serum estradiol was suppressed to ≤20 pg/mL in all subjects within four weeks and remained suppressed (≤40 pg/mL) in 80% of subjects until the end of the 12-week dosing interval, at which time two of these subjects had a value between 40 and 50 pg/mL. Four additional subjects had at least two consecutive elevations of estradiol (range 43–240 pg/mL) levels during the 12-week dosing interval, but there was no indication of luteal function for any of the subjects during this period.

LUPRON DEPOT–3 Month 11.25 mg induced amenorrhea in 85% (N=17) of subjects during the initial month and 100% during the second month following the injection. All subjects remained amenorrheic through the remainder of the 12-week dosing interval. Episodes of light bleeding and spotting were reported by a majority of subjects during the first month after the injection and in a few subjects at later time-points. Menses resumed on average 12 weeks (range 2.9 to 20.4 weeks) following the end of the 12-week dosing interval.

LUPRON DEPOT–3 Month 11.25 mg produced similar pharmacodynamic effects in terms of hormonal and menstrual suppression to those achieved with monthly injections of LUPRON DEPOT 3.75 mg during the controlled clinical trials for the management of endometriosis and the anemia caused by uterine fibroids.

Endometriosis: In a Phase IV pharmacokinetic/pharmacodynamic study of patients, LUPRON DEPOT–3 Month 11.25 mg (N=21) was shown to be comparable to monthly LUPRON DEPOT 3.75 mg (N=20) in relieving the clinical signs/symptoms of endometriosis (dysmenorrhea, non-menstrual pelvic pain, pelvic tenderness and pelvic induration). In both treatment groups, suppression of menses was achieved in 100% of the patients who remained in the study for at least 60 days. Suppression is defined as no new menses for at least 60 consecutive days.

In controlled clinical studies, LUPRON DEPOT 3.75 mg monthly for six months was shown to be comparable to danazol 800 mg/day in relieving the clinical sign/symptoms of endometriosis (pelvic pain, dysmenorrhea, dyspareunia, pelvic tenderness, and induration) and in reducing the size of endometrial implants as evidenced by laparoscopy.

The clinical significance of a decrease in endometriotic lesions is not known at this time, and in addition laparoscopic staging of endometriosis does not necessarily correlate with the severity of symptoms.

LUPRON DEPOT 3.75 mg monthly induced amenorrhea in 74% and 98% of the patients after the first and second treatment months respectively. Most of the remaining patients reported episodes of only light bleeding or spotting. In the first, second and third post-treatment months, normal menstrual cycles resumed in 7%, 71% and 95% of patients, respectively, excluding those who became pregnant.

Figure 1 illustrates the percent of patients with symptoms at baseline, final treatment visit and sustained relief at 6 and 12 months following discontinuation of treatment for the various symptoms evaluated during the two controlled clinical studies. A total of 166 patients received LUPRON DEPOT 3.75 mg. Seventy-five percent (N=125) of these elected to participate in the follow-up period. Of these patients, 36% and 24% are included in the 6 month and 12 month follow-up analysis, respectively. All the patients who had a pain evaluation at baseline and at a minimum of one treatment visit, are included in the Baseline (B) and final treatment visit (F) analysis.

FIGURE 1 – PERCENT OF PATIENTS WITH SIGN/SYMPTOMS OF ENDOMETRIOSIS AT BASELINE, FINAL TREATMENT VISIT, AND AFTER 6 AND 12 MONTHS OF FOLLOW-UP

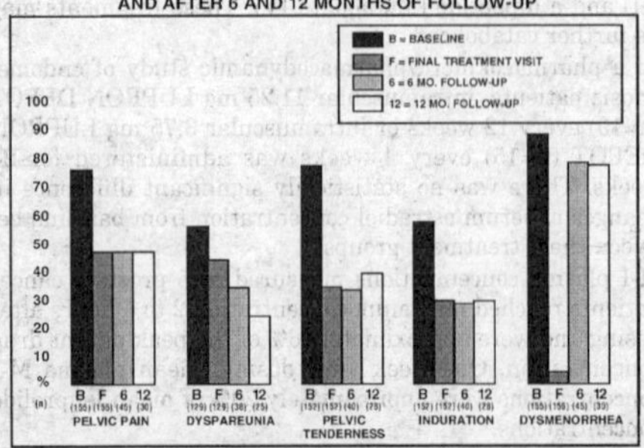

Hormonal add-back therapy: Two clinical studies with a treatment duration of 12 months indicate that concurrent hormonal therapy (norethindrone acetate 5 mg daily) is effective in significantly reducing the loss of bone mineral density associated with LUPRON, without compromising the efficacy of LUPRON in relieving symptoms of endometriosis. (All patients in these studies received calcium supplementation with 1000 mg elemental calcium). One controlled, randomized and double-blind study included 51 women treated with LUPRON DEPOT 3.75 mg alone and 55 women treated with LUPRON DEPOT 3.75 mg plus norethindrone acetate 5 mg (LD/N) daily. The second study was an open label study in which 136 women were treated with monthly LUPRON DEPOT 3.75 mg plus norethindrone acetate 5 mg daily. This study confirmed the reduction in loss of bone mineral density that was observed in the controlled study. Suppression of menses

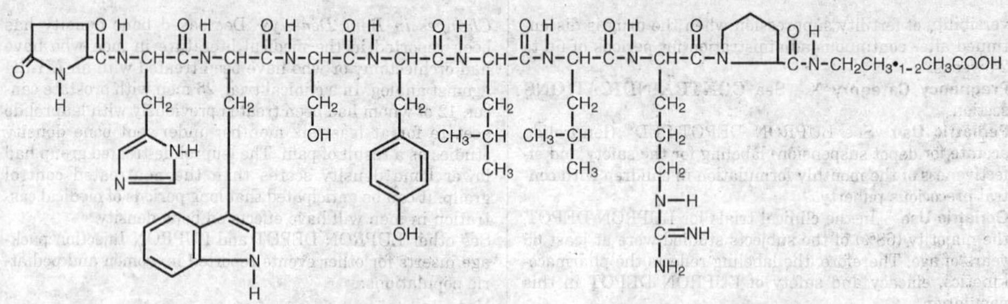

was maintained throughout treatment in 84% and 73% of patients receiving LD/N, in the controlled study and open label study, respectively. The median time for menses resumption after treatment with LD/N was 8 weeks.

Figure 2 illustrates the mean pain scores for the LD/N group from the controlled study.

Figure 2
Treatment Period Mean Pain Scores for LD/N* Patients

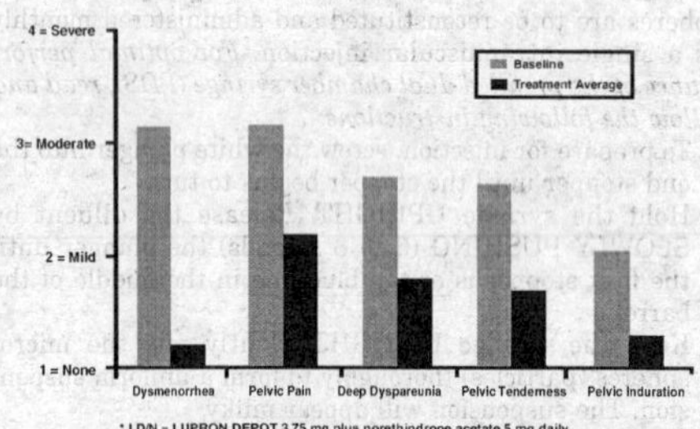

* LD/N = LUPRON DEPOT 3.75 mg plus norethindrone acetate 5 mg daily

Uterine Leiomyomata (Fibroids): LUPRON DEPOT 3.75 mg for a period of three to six months was studied in four controlled clinical trials.

In one of these clinical studies, enrollment was based on hematocrit ≤ 30% and/or hemoglobin ≤ 10.2 g/dL. Administration of LUPRON DEPOT 3.75 mg, concomitantly with iron, produced an increase of ≥ 6% hematocrit and ≥ 2 g/dL hemoglobin in 77% of patients at three months of therapy. The mean change in hematocrit was 10.1% and the mean change in hemoglobin was 4.2 g/dL. Clinical response was judged to be a hematocrit of ≥ 36% and hemoglobin of ≥ 12 g/dL, thus allowing for autologous blood donation prior to surgery. At two and three months respectively, 71% and 75% of patients met this criterion (Table 1). These data suggest however, that some patients may benefit from iron alone or 1 to 2 months of LUPRON DEPOT 3.75 mg.

Table 1
PERCENT OF PATIENTS ACHIEVING HEMATOCRIT ≥ 36% AND HEMOGLOBIN ≥ 12 GM/DL

Treatment Group	Week 4	Week 8	Week 12
LUPRON DEPOT 3.75 mg with Iron (N=104)	40*	71**	75*
Iron Alone (N=98)	17	39	49

* P-Value < 0.01
** P-Value < 0.001

Excessive vaginal bleeding (menorrhagia or menometrorrhagia) decreased in 80% of patients at three months. Episodes of spotting and menstrual-like bleeding were noted in 16% of patients at final visit.

In this same study, a decrease of ≥25% was seen in uterine and myoma volumes in 60% and 54% of patients respectively. The mean fibroid diameter was 6.3 cm at pretreatment and decreased to 5.6 cm at the end of treatment. LUPRON DEPOT 3.75 mg was found to relieve symptoms of bloating, pelvic pain, and pressure.

In three other controlled clinical trials, enrollment was not based on hematologic status. Mean uterine volume decreased by 41% and myoma volume decreased by 37% at final visit as evidenced by ultrasound or MRI. The mean fibroid diameter was 5.6 cm at pretreatment and decreased to 4.7 cm at the end of treatment. These patients also experienced a decrease in symptoms including excessive vaginal bleeding and pelvic discomfort. Ninety-five percent of these patients became amenorrheic with 61%, 25%, and 4% experiencing amenorrhea during the first, second, and third treatment months respectively.

In addition, posttreatment follow-up was carried out in one clinical trial for a small percentage of LUPRON DEPOT 3.75 mg patients (N=46) among the 77% who demonstrated a ≥25% decrease in uterine volume while on therapy. Menses usually returned within two months of cessation of therapy. Mean time to return to pretreatment uterine size was 8.3 months. Regrowth did not appear to be related to pretreatment uterine volume.

There is no evidence that pregnancy rates are enhanced or adversely affected by the use of LUPRON DEPOT.

INDICATIONS AND USAGE

Endometriosis: LUPRON DEPOT–3 Month 11.25 mg is indicated for management of endometriosis, including pain relief and reduction of endometriotic lesions. LUPRON DEPOT with norethindrone acetate 5 mg daily is also indicated for initial management of endometriosis and for management of recurrence of symptoms. (Refer also to norethindrone acetate prescribing information for WARNINGS, PRECAUTIONS, CONTRAINDICATIONS and ADVERSE REACTIONS associated with norethindrone acetate). Duration of initial treatment or retreatment should be limited to 6 months.

Uterine Leiomyomata (Fibroids): LUPRON DEPOT–3 Month 11.25 mg concomitantly with iron therapy is indicated for the preoperative hematologic improvement of patients with anemia caused by uterine leiomyomata. The clinician may wish to consider a one-month trial period on iron alone inasmuch as some of the patients will respond to iron alone. (See Table 1, **CLINICAL STUDIES** section.) LUPRON may be added if the response to iron alone is considered inadequate. Recommended therapy is a single injection of LUPRON DEPOT–3 Month 11.25 mg. This dosage form is indicated only for women for whom three months of hormonal suppression is deemed necessary.

Experience with LUPRON DEPOT–3 Month 11.25 mg in females has been limited to women 18 years of age and older treated for no more than 6 months.

CONTRAINDICATIONS

1. Hypersensitivity to GnRH, GnRH agonist analogs or any of the excipients in LUPRON DEPOT.
2. Undiagnosed abnormal vaginal bleeding.
3. LUPRON DEPOT is contraindicated in women who are or may become pregnant while receiving the drug. LUPRON DEPOT may cause fetal harm when administered to a pregnant woman. Major fetal abnormalities were observed in rabbits but not in rats after administration of LUPRON DEPOT throughout gestation. There was increased fetal mortality and decreased fetal weights in rats and rabbits. (See **Pregnancy** section.) The effects on fetal mortality are expected consequences of the alterations in hormonal levels brought about by the drug. If this drug is used during pregnancy or if the patient becomes pregnant while taking this drug, the patient should be apprised of the potential hazard to the fetus.
4. Use in women who are breast-feeding. (See **Nursing Mothers** section.)
5. Norethindrone acetate is contraindicated in women with the following conditions:
   — Thrombophlebitis, thromboembolic disorders, cerebral apoplexy, or a past history of these conditions
   — Markedly impaired liver function or liver disease
   — Known or suspected carcinoma of the breast

WARNINGS

1. As the effects of LUPRON DEPOT–3 Month 11.25 mg are present throughout the course of therapy, the drug should only be used in patients who require hormonal suppression for at least three months.
2. Experience with LUPRON DEPOT–3 Month 11.25 mg in females has been limited to six months; therefore, exposure should be limited to six months of therapy.
3. Safe use of leuprolide acetate or norethindrone acetate in pregnancy has not been established clinically. Before starting treatment with LUPRON DEPOT pregnancy must be excluded.
4. When used at the recommended dose and dosing interval, LUPRON DEPOT usually inhibits ovulation and stops menstruation. Contraception is not insured, however, by taking LUPRON DEPOT. Therefore, patients should use non-hormonal methods of contraception. Patients should be advised to see their physician if they believe they may be pregnant. If a patient becomes pregnant during treatment, the drug must be discontinued and the patient must be apprised of the potential risk to the fetus. (See **CONTRAINDICATIONS** section.)
5. During the early phase of therapy, sex steroids temporarily rise above baseline because of the physiologic effect of the drug. Therefore, an increase in clinical signs and symptoms may be observed during the initial days of therapy, but these will dissipate with continued therapy.
6. Symptoms consistent with an anaphylactoid or asthmatic process have been rarely reported post-marketing.
7. The following applies to co-treatment with LUPRON and norethindrone acetate:
   Norethindrone acetate treatment should be discontinued if there is a sudden partial or complete loss of vision or if there is sudden onset of proptosis, diplopia, or migraine. If examination reveals papilledema or retinal vascular lesions, medication should be withdrawn.
   Because of the occasional occurrence of thrombophlebitis and pulmonary embolism in patients taking progestogens, the physician should be alert to the earliest manifestations of the disease in women taking norethindrone acetate.
   Assessment and management of risk factors for cardiovascular disease is recommended prior to initiation of

add-back therapy with norethindrone acetate. Norethindrone acetate should be used with caution in women with risk factors, including lipid abnormalities or cigarette smoking.

PRECAUTIONS

Information for Patients An information pamphlet for patients is included with the product. Patients should be aware of the following information:

1. Since menstruation usually stops with effective doses of LUPRON DEPOT, the patient should notify her physician if regular menstruation persists. Patients missing successive doses of LUPRON DEPOT may experience breakthrough bleeding.
2. Patients should not use LUPRON DEPOT if they are pregnant, breast feeding, have undiagnosed abnormal vaginal bleeding, or are allergic to any of the ingredients in LUPRON DEPOT.
3. LUPRON DEPOT is contraindicated for use during pregnancy. Therefore, a non-hormonal method of contraception should be used during treatment. Patients should be advised that if they miss successive doses of LUPRON DEPOT, breakthrough bleeding or ovulation may occur with the potential for conception. If a patient becomes pregnant during treatment, she should discontinue treatment and consult her physician.
4. Adverse events occurring in clinical studies with LUPRON DEPOT that are associated with hypoestrogenism include: hot flashes, headaches, emotional lability, decreased libido, acne, myalgia, reduction in breast size, and vaginal dryness. Estrogen levels returned to normal after treatment was discontinued.
5. Patients should be counseled on the possibility of the development or worsening of depression and the occurrence of memory disorders.
6. The induced hypoestrogenic state **also** results in a loss in bone density over the course of treatment, some of which may not be reversible. For a period up to six months, this bone loss should not be clinically significant. Clinical studies show that concurrent hormonal therapy with norethindrone acetate 5 mg daily is effective in reducing loss of bone mineral density that occurs with LUPRON. (All patients received calcium supplementation with 1000 mg elemental calcium.) (See ***Changes in Bone Density*** section).
7. If the symptoms of endometriosis recur after a course of therapy, retreatment with a six-month course of LUPRON DEPOT and norethindrone acetate 5 mg daily may be considered. Retreatment beyond this one six-month course cannot be recommended. It is recommended that bone density be assessed before retreatment begins to ensure that values are within normal limits. Retreatment with LUPRON DEPOT alone is not recommended.
8. In patients with major risk factors for decreased bone mineral content such as chronic alcohol and/or tobacco use, strong family history of osteoporosis, or chronic use of drugs that can reduce bone mass such as anticonvulsants or corticosteroids, LUPRON DEPOT therapy may pose an additional risk. In these patients, the risks and benefits must be weighed carefully before therapy with LUPRON DEPOT alone is instituted, and concomitant treatment with norethindrone acetate 5 mg daily should be considered. Retreatment with gonadotropin-releasing hormone analogs, including LUPRON is not advisable in patients with major risk factors for loss of bone mineral content.
9. Because norethindrone acetate may cause some degree of fluid retention, conditions which might be influenced by this factor, such as epilepsy, migraine, asthma, cardiac or renal dysfunctions require careful observation during norethindrone acetate add-back therapy.
10. Patients who have a history of depression should be carefully observed during treatment with norethindrone acetate and norethindrone acetate should be discontinued if severe depression occurs.

Laboratory Tests See **ADVERSE REACTIONS** section.

Drug Interactions See **CLINICAL PHARMACOLOGY, Pharmacokinetics.**

Drug/Laboratory Test Interactions Administration of LUPRON DEPOT in therapeutic doses results in suppression of the pituitary-gonadal system. Normal function is usually restored within three months after treatment is discontinued. Therefore, diagnostic tests of pituitary gonadotropic and gonadal functions conducted during treatment and for up to three months after discontinuation of LUPRON DEPOT may be misleading.

Carcinogenesis, Mutagenesis, Impairment of Fertility A two-year carcinogenicity study was conducted in rats and mice. In rats, a dose-related increase of benign pituitary hyperplasia and benign pituitary adenomas was noted at 24 months when the drug was administered subcutaneously at high daily doses (0.6 to 4 mg/kg). There was a significant but not dose-related increase of pancreatic islet-cell adenomas in females and of testicular interstitial cell adenomas in males (highest incidence in the low dose group). In mice, no leuprolide acetate-induced tumors or pituitary abnormalities were observed at a dose as high as 60 mg/kg for two years. Patients have been treated with leuprolide acetate for up to three years with doses as high as 10 mg/day and for two years with doses as high as 20 mg/day without demonstrable pituitary abnormalities.

Mutagenicity studies have been performed with leuprolide acetate using bacterial and mammalian systems. These studies provided no evidence of a mutagenic potential.

Table 2
ADVERSE EVENTS REPORTED TO BE CAUSALLY RELATED TO DRUG IN ≥ 5% OF PATIENTS

	Endometriosis (2 Studies)						Uterine Fibroids (4 Studies)			
	LUPRON DEPOT 3.75 mg N=166		Danazol N=136		Placebo N=31		LUPRON DEPOT 3.75 mg N=166		Placebo N=163	
	N	(%)	N	(%)	N	(%)	N	(%)	N	(%)
Body as a Whole										
Asthenia	5	(3)	9	(7)	0	(0)	14	(8.4)	8	(4.9)
General pain	31	(19)	22	(16)	1	(3)	14	(8.4)	10	(6.1)
Headache*	53	(32)	30	(22)	2	(6)	43	(25.9)	29	(17.8)
Cardiovascular System										
Hot flashes/sweats*	139	(84)	77	(57)	9	(29)	121	(72.9)	29	(17.8)
Gastrointestinal System										
Nausea/vomiting	21	(13)	17	(13)	1	(3)	8	(4.8)	6	(3.7)
GI disturbances*	11	(7)	8	(6)	1	(3)	5	(3.0)	2	(1.2)
Metabolic and Nutritional Disorders										
Edema	12	(7)	17	(13)	1	(3)	9	(5.4)	2	(1.2)
Weight gain/loss	22	(13)	36	(26)	0	(0)	5	(3.0)	2	(1.2)
Endocrine System										
Acne	17	(10)	27	(20)	0	(0)	0	(0)	0	(0)
Hirsutism	2	(1)	9	(7)	1	(3)	1	(0.6)	0	(0)
Musculoskeletal System										
Joint disorder*	14	(8)	11	(8)	0	(0)	13	(7.8)	5	(3.1)
Myalgia*	1	(1)	7	(5)	0	(0)	1	(0.6)	0	(0)
Nervous System										
Decreased libido*	19	(11)	6	(4)	0	(0)	3	(1.8)	0	(0)
Depression/emotional lability*	36	(22)	27	(20)	1	(3)	18	(10.8)	7	(4.3)
Dizziness	19	(11)	4	(3)	0	(0)	3	(1.8)	6	(3.7)
Nervousness*	8	(5)	11	(8)	0	(0)	8	(4.8)	1	(0.6)
Neuromuscular disorders*	11	(7)	17	(13)	0	(0)	3	(1.8)	0	(0)
Paresthesias	12	(7)	11	(8)	0	(0)	2	(1.2)	1	(0.6)
Skin and Appendages										
Skin reactions	17	(10)	20	(15)	1	(3)	5	(3.0)	2	(1.2)
Urogenital System										
Breast changes/tenderness/pain*	10	(6)	12	(9)	0	(0)	3	(1.8)	7	(4.3)
Vaginitis*	46	(28)	23	(17)	0	(0)	19	(11.4)	3	(1.8)

Table 3
TREATMENT-RELATED ADVERSE EVENTS OCCURRING IN ≥ 5% OF PATIENTS

	Controlled Study				Open Label Study	
	LD - Only[1] N=51		LD/N[2] N=55		LD/N[2] N=136	
Adverse Events	N	(%)	N	(%)	N	(%)
Any Adverse Event	50	(98)	53	(96)	126	(93)
Body as a Whole						
Asthenia	9	(18)	10	(18)	15	(11)
Headache/Migraine	33	(65)	28	(51)	63	(46)
Injection Site Reaction	1	(2)	5	(9)	4	(3)
Pain	12	(24)	16	(29)	29	(21)
Cardiovascular System						
Hot flashes/Sweats	50	(98)	48	(87)	78	(57)
Digestive System						
Altered Bowel Function	7	(14)	8	(15)	14	(10)
Changes in Appetite	2	(4)	0	(0)	8	(6)
GI Disturbance	2	(4)	4	(7)	6	(4)
Nausea/Vomiting	13	(25)	16	(29)	17	(13)
Metabolic and Nutritional Disorders						
Edema	0	(0)	5	(9)	9	(7)
Weight Changes	6	(12)	7	(13)	6	(4)
Nervous System						
Anxiety	3	(6)	0	(0)	11	(8)
Depression/Emotional Lability	16	(31)	15	(27)	46	(34)
Dizziness/Vertigo	8	(16)	6	(11)	10	(7)
Insomnia/Sleep Disorder	16	(31)	7	(13)	20	(15)
Libido Changes	5	(10)	2	(4)	10	(7)
Memory Disorder	3	(6)	1	(2)	6	(4)
Nervousness	4	(8)	2	(4)	15	(11)
Neuromuscular Disorder	1	(2)	5	(9)	4	(3)
Skin and Appendages						
Alopecia	0	(0)	5	(9)	4	(3)
Androgen-Like Effects	2	(4)	3	(5)	24	(18)
Skin/Mucous Membrane Reaction	2	(4)	5	(9)	15	(11)
Urogenital System						
Breast Changes/Pain/Tenderness	3	(6)	7	(13)	11	(8)
Menstrual Disorders	1	(2)	0	(0)	7	(5)
Vaginitis	10	(20)	8	(15)	11	(8)

[1] LD-Only = LUPRON DEPOT 3.75 mg
[2] LD/N = LUPRON DEPOT 3.75 mg plus norethindrone acetate 5 mg

Clinical and pharmacologic studies in adults (> 18 years) with leuprolide acetate and similar analogs have shown reversibility of fertility suppression when the drug is discontinued after continuous administration for periods of up to 24 weeks. Although no clinical studies have been completed in children to assess the full reversibility of fertility suppression, animal studies (prepubertal and adult rats and monkeys) with leuprolide acetate and other GnRH analogs have shown functional recovery.

Pregnancy, Teratogenic Effects Pregnancy Category X. (See **CONTRAINDICATIONS** section.) When administered on day 6 of pregnancy at test dosages of 0.00024, 0.0024, and 0.024 mg/kg (1/300 to 1/3 of the human dose) to rabbits, LUPRON DEPOT produced a dose-related increase in major fetal abnormalities. Similar studies in rats failed to demonstrate an increase in fetal malformations. There was increased fetal mortality and decreased fetal weights with the two higher doses of LUPRON DEPOT in rabbits and with the highest dose (0.024 mg/kg) in rats.

Nursing Mothers It is not known whether LUPRON DEPOT is excreted in human milk. Because many drugs are excreted in human milk, and because the effects of LUPRON DEPOT on lactation and/or the breast-fed child have not been determined, LUPRON DEPOT should not be used by nursing mothers.

Pediatric Use Safety and effectiveness of LUPRON DEPOT–3 Month 11.25 mg have not been established in pediatric patients. Experience with LUPRON DEPOT for treatment of endometriosis has been limited to women 18 years of age and older. See LUPRON DEPOT-PED® (leupro-

Continued on next page

Lupron Depot-3 Mo. 11.25 mg—Cont.

lide acetate for depot suspension) labeling for the safety and effectiveness in children with central precocious puberty.

Geriatric Use This product has not been studied in women over 65 years of age and is not indicated in this population.

ADVERSE REACTIONS

Clinical Trials

The **monthly formulation of LUPRON DEPOT 3.75 mg** was utilized in controlled clinical trials that studied the drug in 166 endometriosis and 166 uterine fibroids patients. Adverse events reported in ≥5% of patients in either of these populations and thought to be potentially related to drug are noted in the following table.

[See table 2 at top of previous page]

In these same studies, symptoms reported in < 5% of patients included: *Body as a Whole* - Body odor, Flu syndrome, Injection site reactions; *Cardiovascular System* - Palpitations, Syncope, Tachycardia; *Digestive System* - Appetite changes, Dry mouth, Thirst; *Endocrine System* - Androgen-like effects; *Hemic and Lymphatic System* - Ecchymosis, Lymphadenopathy; *Nervous System* - Anxiety*, Insomnia/Sleep disorders*, Delusions, Memory disorder, Personality disorder; *Respiratory System* - Rhinitis; *Skin and Appendages* - Alopecia, Hair disorder, Nail disorder; *Special Senses* - Conjunctivitis, Ophthalmologic disorders*, Taste perversion; *Urogenital System* - Dysuria*, Lactation, Menstrual disorders.

* = Possible effect of decreased estrogen.

In one controlled clinical trial utilizing the monthly formulation of LUPRON DEPOT, patients diagnosed with uterine fibroids received a higher dose (7.5 mg) of LUPRON DEPOT. Events seen with this dose that were thought to be potentially related to drug and were not seen at the lower dose included glossitis, hypesthesia, lactation, pyelonephritis, and urinary disorders. Generally, a higher incidence of hypoestrogenic effects was observed at the higher dose.

In a pharmacokinetic trial involving 20 healthy female subjects receiving LUPRON DEPOT–3 Month 11.25 mg, a few adverse events were reported with this formulation that were not reported previously. These included face edema, agitation, laryngitis, and ear pain.

In a Phase IV study involving endometriosis patients receiving LUPRON DEPOT 3.75 mg (N=20) or LUPRON DEPOT–3 Month 11.25 mg (N=21), similar adverse events were reported by the two groups of patients. In general the safety profiles of the two formulations were comparable in this study.

Table 3 lists the potentially drug-related adverse events observed in at least 5% of patients in any treatment group, during the first 6 months of treatment in the add-back clinical studies, in which patients were treated with monthly LUPRON DEPOT 3.75 mg with or without norethindrone acetate co-treatment.

[See table 3 on previous page]

In the controlled clinical trial, 50 of 51 (98%) patients in the LD group (LUPRON DEPOT 3.75 mg) and 48 of 55 (87%) patients in the LD/N group (LUPRON DEPOT 3.75 mg plus norethindrone acetate 5 mg daily) reported experiencing hot flashes on one or more occasions during treatment. During Month 6 of treatment, 32 of 37 (86%) patients in the LD group and 22 of 38 (58%) patients in the LD/N group reported having experienced hot flashes. The mean number of days on which hot flashes were reported during this month of treatment was 19 and 7 in the LD and LD/N treatment groups, respectively. The mean maximum number of hot flashes in a day during this month of treatment was 5.8 and 1.9 in the LD and LD/N treatment groups, respectively.

Changes in Bone Density

In controlled clinical studies, patients with endometriosis (six months of therapy) or uterine fibroids (three months of therapy) were treated with LUPRON DEPOT 3.75 mg. In endometriosis patients, vertebral bone density as measured by dual energy x-ray absorptiometry (DEXA) decreased by an average of 3.2% at six months compared with the pretreatment value. Clinical studies demonstrate that concurrent hormonal therapy (norethindrone acetate 5 mg daily) and calcium supplementation is effective in significantly reducing the loss of bone mineral density that occurs with LUPRON treatment, without compromising the efficacy of LUPRON in relieving symptoms of endometriosis. LUPRON DEPOT 3.75 mg plus norethindrone acetate 5 mg daily was evaluated in two clinical trials. The results from this regimen were similar in both studies. LUPRON DEPOT 3.75 mg was used as a control group in one study. The bone mineral density data of the lumbar spine from these two studies are presented in Table 4.

[See table 4 above]

Table 4
MEAN PERCENT CHANGE FROM BASELINE IN BONE MINERAL DENSITY OF LUMBAR SPINE

	LUPRON DEPOT 3.75 mg		LUPRON DEPOT 3.75 mg plus norethindrone acetate 5 mg daily			
	Controlled Study		Controlled Study		Open Label Study	
	N	Change	N	Change	N	Change
Week 24[1]	41	−3.2%	42	−0.3%	115	−0.2%
Week 52[2]	29	−6.3%	32	−1.0%	84	−1.1%

[1] Includes on-treatment measurements that fell within 2-252 days after the first day of treatment.
[2] Includes on-treatment measurements >252 days after the first day of treatment.

In the Phase IV, six-month pharmacokinetic/pharmacodynamic study in endometriosis patients who were treated with LUPRON DEPOT 3.75 mg or LUPRON DEPOT–3 Month 11.25 mg, vertebral bone density measured by DEXA decreased compared with baseline by an average of 3.0% and 2.8% at six months for the two groups, respectively.

When LUPRON DEPOT 3.75 mg was administered for three months in uterine fibroid patients, vertebral trabecular bone mineral density as assessed by quantitative digital radiography (QDR) revealed a mean decrease of 2.7% compared with baseline. Six months after discontinuation of therapy, a trend toward recovery was observed. Use of LUPRON DEPOT for longer than three months (uterine fibroids) or six months (endometriosis) or in the presence of other known risk factors for decreased bone mineral content may cause additional bone loss **and is not recommended.**

Table 5
SERUM LIPIDS: MEAN PERCENT CHANGES FROM BASELINE VALUES AT TREATMENT WEEK 24

	LUPRON DEPOT 3.75 mg		LUPRON DEPOT 3.75 mg plus norethindrone acetate 5 mg daily			
	Controlled Study (n=39)		Controlled Study (n=41)		Open Label Study (n=117)	
	Baseline Value*	Wk 24 % Change	Baseline Value*	Wk 24 % Change	Baseline Value*	Wk 24 % Change
Total Cholesterol	170.5	9.2%	179.3	0.2%	181.2	2.8%
HDL Cholesterol	52.4	7.4%	51.8	−18.8%	51.0	−14.6%
LDL Cholesterol	96.6	10.9%	101.5	14.1%	109.1	13.1%
LDL/HDL Ratio	2.0**	5.0%	2.1**	43.4%	2.3**	39.4%
Triglycerides	107.8	17.5%	130.2	9.5%	105.4	13.8%

* mg/dL
** ratio

Table 6
PERCENTAGE OF PATIENTS WITH SERUM LIPID VALUES OUTSIDE OF THE NORMAL RANGE

	LUPRON DEPOT 3.75 mg		LUPRON DEPOT 3.75 mg plus norethindrone acetate 5 mg daily			
	Controlled Study (n=39)		Controlled Study (n=41)		Open Label Study (n=117)	
	Wk 0	Wk 24*	Wk 0	Wk 24*	Wk 0	Wk 24*
Total Cholesterol (>240 mg/dL)	15%	23%	15%	20%	6%	7%
HDL Cholesterol (<40 mg/dL)	15%	10%	15%	44%	15%	41%
LDL Cholesterol (>160 mg/dL)	0%	8%	5%	7%	9%	11%
LDL/HDL Ratio (>4.0)	0%	3%	2%	15%	7%	21%
Triglycerides (>200 mg/dL)	13%	13%	12%	10%	5%	9%

* Includes all patients regardless of baseline value.

Changes in Laboratory Values During Treatment

Liver Enzymes

Three percent of uterine fibroid patients treated with LUPRON DEPOT 3.75 mg, manifested posttreatment transaminase values that were at least twice the baseline value and above the upper limit of the normal range. None of the laboratory increases were associated with clinical symptoms.

In two other clinical trials, 6 of 191 patients receiving LUPRON DEPOT 3.75 mg plus norethindrone acetate 5 mg daily for up to 12 months developed an elevated (at least twice the upper limit of normal) SGPT or GGT. Five of the 6 increases were observed beyond 6 months of treatment. None were associated with an elevated bilirubin concentration.

Lipids

Triglycerides were increased above the upper limit of normal in 12% of the endometriosis patients who received LUPRON DEPOT 3.75 mg and in 32% of the subjects receiving LUPRON DEPOT–3 Month 11.25 mg.

Of those endometriosis and uterine fibroid patients whose pretreatment cholesterol values were in the normal range, mean change following therapy was +16 mg/dL to +17 mg/dL in endometriosis patients and +11 mg/dL to +29 mg/dL in uterine fibroid patients. In the endometriosis treated patients, increases from the pretreatment values were statistically significant ($p<0.03$). There was essentially no increase in the LDL/HDL ratio in patients from either population receiving LUPRON DEPOT 3.75 mg.

In two other clinical trials, LUPRON DEPOT 3.75 mg plus norethindrone acetate 5 mg daily were evaluated for 12 months of treatment. LUPRON DEPOT 3.75 mg was used as a control group in one study. Percent changes from baseline for serum lipids and percentages of patients with serum lipid values outside of the normal range in the two studies are summarized in the tables below.

[See table 5 above]

Changes from baseline tended to be greater at Week 52. After treatment, mean serum lipid levels from patients with follow up data returned to pretreatment values.

[See table 6 above]

Low HDL-cholesterol (<40 mg/dL) and elevated LDL-cholesterol (> 160 mg/dL) are recognized risk factors for cardiovascular disease. The long-term significance of the observed treatment-related changes in serum lipids in women with endometriosis is unknown. Therefore assessment of cardiovascular risk factors should be considered prior to initiation of concurrent treatment with LUPRON and norethindrone acetate.

Chemistry

Slight to moderate mean increases were noted for glucose, uric acid, BUN, creatinine, total protein, albumin, bilirubin, alkaline phosphatase, LDH, calcium, and phosphorus. None of these increases were clinically significant. In the hormonal add-back studies LUPRON DEPOT in combination with norethindrone acetate was associated with elevations of GGT and SGPT in 6% to 7% of patients.

Postmarketing

During postmarketing surveillance with other dosage forms and in the same and/or different populations, the following adverse events were reported. Like other drugs in this class, mood swings, including depression, have been reported. There have been rare reports of suicidal ideation and attempt. Many, but not all, of these patients had a history of depression or other psychiatric illness. Patients should be counseled on the possibility of development or worsening of depression during treatment with LUPRON.

Symptoms consistent with an anaphylactoid or asthmatic process have been rarely reported. Rash, urticaria, and photosensitivity reactions have also been reported.

Localized reactions including induration and abscess have been reported at the site of injection.

Symptoms consistent with fibromyalgia (eg: joint and muscle pain, headaches, sleep disorders, gastrointestinal distress, and shortness of breath) have been reported individually and collectively.

Other events reported are:

Cardiovascular System—Hypotension, Pulmonary embolism; *Hemic and Lymphatic System*—Decreased WBC; *Central/Peripheral Nervous System*—Peripheral neuropathy, Spinal fracture/paralysis; *Musculoskeletal System*—Tenosynovitis-like symptoms; *Urogenital System*—Prostate pain.

See other LUPRON DEPOT and LUPRON Injection package inserts for other events reported in the same and different patient populations.

OVERDOSAGE

In clinical trials using daily subcutaneous leuprolide acetate in patients with prostate cancer, doses as high as 20 mg/day for up to two years caused no adverse effects differing from those observed with the 1 mg/day dose.

DOSAGE AND ADMINISTRATION

LUPRON DEPOT Must Be Administered Under the Supervision of a Physician.

Endometriosis: The recommended duration of treatment with LUPRON DEPOT–3 Month 11.25 mg alone or in combination with norethindrone acetate is six months. The choice of LUPRON DEPOT alone or LUPRON DEPOT plus norethindrone acetate therapy for initial management of the symptoms and signs of endometriosis should be made by the health care professional in consultation with the patient and should take into consideration the risks and benefits of the addition of norethindrone to LUPRON DEPOT alone.

If the symptoms of endometriosis recur after a course of therapy, retreatment with a six-month course of LUPRON DEPOT and norethindrone acetate 5 mg daily may be considered. Retreatment beyond this one six-month course cannot be recommended. It is recommended that bone density be assessed before retreatment begins to ensure that values are within normal limits. LUPRON DEPOT alone is not recommended for retreatment. If norethindrone acetate is contraindicated for the individual patient, then retreatment is not recommended.

An assessment of cardiovascular risk and management of risk factors such as cigarette smoking is recommended before beginning treatment with LUPRON DEPOT and norethindrone acetate.

Uterine Leiomyomata (Fibroids): The recommended dose of LUPRON DEPOT–3 Month 11.25 mg is one injection. The symptoms associated with uterine leiomyomata will recur following discontinuation of therapy. If additional treatment with LUPRON DEPOT–3 Month 11.25 mg is contemplated, bone density should be assessed prior to initiation of therapy to ensure that values are within normal limits.

Due to different release characteristics, a fractional dose of the 3-month depot formulation is not equivalent to the same dose of the monthly formulation and should not be given.

Incorporated in a depot formulation, the lyophilized microspheres are to be reconstituted and administered as a single intramuscular injection. *For optimal performance of the prefilled dual chamber syringe (PDS), read and follow the following instructions:*

1. To prepare for injection, screw the white plunger into the end stopper until the stopper begins to turn.
2. Hold the syringe UPRIGHT. Release the diluent by SLOWLY PUSHING (6 to 8 seconds) the plunger until the first stopper is at the blue line in the middle of the barrel.
3. Keep the syringe UPRIGHT. Gently mix the microspheres (particles) thoroughly to form a uniform suspension. The suspension will appear milky.
4. Hold the syringe UPRIGHT. With the opposite hand pull the needle cap upward without twisting.
5. Keep the syringe UPRIGHT. Advance the plunger to expel the air from the syringe.
6. Inject the entire contents of the syringe intramuscularly at the time of reconstitution. The suspension settles very quickly following reconstitution; therefore, LUPRON DEPOT should be mixed and used immediately.

NOTE: Aspirated blood would be visible just below the luer lock connection if a blood vessel is accidentally penetrated. If present, blood can be seen through the transparent LuproLoc™ safety device.

AFTER INJECTION

7. Withdraw the needle. Immediately activate the LuproLoc™ safety device by pushing the arrow forward with the thumb or finger until the device is fully extended and a CLICK is heard or felt.

Since the product does not contain a preservative, the suspension should be discarded if not used immediately.

As with other drugs administered by injection, the injection site should be varied periodically.

HOW SUPPLIED

LUPRON DEPOT–3 Month 11.25 mg is packaged as follows:

Kit with prefilled dual-chamber syringe NDC 0300-3663-01

Each syringe contains sterile lyophilized microspheres which are leuprolide acetate incorporated in a biodegradable polymer of polylactic acid. When mixed with 1.5 mL of the diluent, LUPRON DEPOT–3 Month 11.25 mg is administered as a single IM injection **EVERY THREE MONTHS.**

Store at 25°C (77°F); excursions permitted to 15-30°C (59-86°F) [See USP Controlled Room Temperature]

Rx only

U.S. Patent Nos. 4,728,721; 4,849,228; 5,330,767; 5,476,663; 5,480,656; 5,575,987; 5,631,020; 5,631,021; 5,643,607; 5,716,640; 5,814,342; 5,823,997; 5,980,488; and 6,036,976.

Other patents pending.

Manufactured for
TAP Pharmaceuticals Inc.
Lake Forest, IL 60045, U.S.A.
by Takeda Chemical Industries, Ltd.
Osaka, JAPAN 541

™ - Trademark
® - Registered Trademark

(No. 3663)

03-5336-R12; Revised: February, 2004

Shown in Product Identification Guide, page 334

LUPRON DEPOT®–3 MONTH 22.5 MG ℞

[lew-prŏn]

(leuprolide acetate for depot suspension)
3-MONTH FORMULATION
Rx only

DESCRIPTION

Leuprolide acetate is a synthetic nonapeptide analog of naturally occurring gonadotropin-releasing hormone (GnRH or LH-RH). The analog possesses greater potency than the natural hormone. The chemical name is 5-oxo-L-prolyl-L-histidyl-L-tryptophyl-L-seryl-L-tyrosyl-D-leucyl-L-leucyl-L-arginyl-N-ethyl-L-prolinamide acetate (salt) with the following structural formula:

[See chemical structure below]

LUPRON DEPOT–3 Month 22.5 mg is available in a prefilled dual-chamber syringe containing sterile lyophilized microspheres which, when mixed with diluent, become a suspension intended as an intramuscular injection to be given **ONCE EVERY THREE MONTHS (84 days).**

The front chamber of LUPRON DEPOT–3 Month 22.5 mg prefilled dual-chamber syringe contains leuprolide acetate (22.5 mg), polylactic acid (198.6 mg) and D-mannitol (38.9 mg). The second chamber of diluent contains carboxymethylcellulose sodium (7.5 mg), D-mannitol (75.0 mg), polysorbate 80 (1.5 mg), water for injection, USP, and glacial acetic acid, USP to control pH.

During the manufacture of LUPRON DEPOT–3 Month 22.5 mg, acetic acid is lost, leaving the peptide.

CLINICAL PHARMACOLOGY

Leuprolide acetate, an LH-RH agonist, acts as a potent inhibitor of gonadotropin secretion when given continuously and in therapeutic doses. Animal and human studies indicate that following an initial stimulation, chronic administration of leuprolide acetate results in suppression of ovarian and testicular steroidogenesis. This effect is reversible upon discontinuation of drug therapy. Administration of leuprolide acetate has resulted in inhibition of the growth of certain hormone dependent tumors (prostatic tumors in Noble and Dunning male rats and DMBA-induced mammary tumors in female rats) as well as atrophy of the reproductive organs.

In humans, administration of leuprolide acetate results in an initial increase in circulating levels of luteinizing hormone (LH) and follicle stimulating hormone (FSH), leading to a transient increase in levels of the gonadal steroids (testosterone and dihydrotestosterone in males, and estrone and estradiol in premenopausal females). However, continuous administration of leuprolide acetate results in decreased levels of LH and FSH. In males, testosterone is reduced to castrate levels. In premenopausal females, estrogens are reduced to postmenopausal levels. These decreases occur within two to four weeks after initiation of treatment, and castrate levels of testosterone in prostatic cancer patients have been demonstrated for more than five years.

Leuprolide acetate is not active when given orally.

Pharmacokinetics

Absorption Following a single injection of the three month formulation of LUPRON DEPOT–3 Month 22.5 mg in patients, mean peak plasma leuprolide concentration of 48.9 ng/mL was observed at 4 hours and then declined to 0.67 ng/mL at 12 weeks. Leuprolide appeared to be released at a constant rate following the onset of steady-state levels during the third week after dosing, providing steady plasma concentrations through the 12-week dosing interval. However, intact leuprolide and an inactive major metabolite could not be distinguished by the assay which was employed in the study. Detectable levels of leuprolide were present at all measurement points in all patients. The initial burst, followed by the rapid decline to a steady-state level, was similar to the release pattern seen with the monthly formulation.

Distribution The mean steady-state volume of distribution of leuprolide following intravenous bolus administration to healthy male volunteers was 27 L. *In vitro* binding to human plasma proteins ranged from 43% to 49%.

Metabolism In healthy male volunteers, a 1 mg bolus of leuprolide administered intravenously revealed that the mean systemic clearance was 7.6 L/h, with a terminal elimination half-life of approximately 3 hours based on a two compartment model.

In rats and dogs, administration of ^{14}C-labeled leuprolide was shown to be metabolized to smaller inactive peptides, a pentapeptide (Metabolite I), tripeptides (Metabolites II and III) and a dipeptide (Metabolite IV). These fragments may be further catabolized.

The major metabolite (M-I) plasma concentrations measured in 5 prostate cancer patients reached maximum concentration 2 to 6 hours after dosing and were approximately 6% of the peak parent drug concentration. One week after dosing, mean plasma M-I concentrations were approximately 20% of mean leuprolide concentrations.

Excretion Following administration of LUPRON DEPOT® 3.75 mg to 3 patients, less than 5% of the dose was recovered as parent and M-I metabolite in the urine.

Special Populations The pharmacokinetics of the drug in hepatically and renally impaired patients have not been determined.

CLINICAL STUDIES

In clinical studies, serum testosterone was suppressed to castrate within 30 days in 87 of 92 (95%) patients and within an additional two weeks in three patients. Two patients did not suppress for 15 and 28 weeks, respectively. Suppression was maintained in all of these patients with the exception of transient minimal testosterone elevations in one of them, and in another an increase in serum testosterone to above the castrate range was recorded during the 12 hour observation period after a subsequent injection. This represents stimulation of gonadotropin secretion.

Lupron Depot – 3 Month 22.5 mg
Mean Serum Testosterone Concentrations

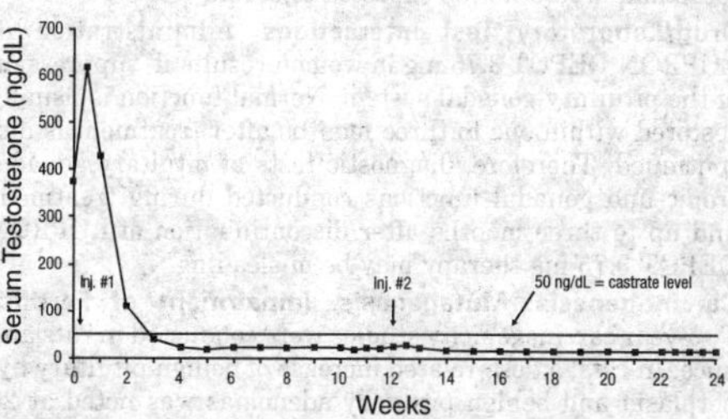

Note: Measurements were taken in a subset of patients from one study at Weeks 10.5, 11.5, 12.5, 22.5 and 23.5.

An 85% rate of "no progression" was achieved during the initial 24 weeks of treatment. A decrease from baseline in serum PSA of ≥90% was reported in 71% of the patients and a change to within the normal range (≤3.99 ng/mL) in 63% of the patients.

Periodic monitoring of serum testosterone and PSA levels is recommended, especially if the anticipated clinical or biochemical response to treatment has not been achieved. It should be noted that results of testosterone determinations are dependent on assay methodology. It is advisable to be aware of the type and precision of the assay methodology to make appropriate clinical and therapeutic decisions.

INDICATIONS AND USAGE

LUPRON DEPOT–3 Month 22.5 mg is indicated in the palliative treatment of advanced prostatic cancer. It offers an alternative treatment of prostatic cancer when orchiectomy or estrogen administration are either not indicated or unacceptable to the patient. In clinical trials, the safety and efficacy of LUPRON DEPOT–3 Month 22.5 mg were similar to that of the original daily subcutaneous injection and the monthly depot formulation.

CONTRAINDICATIONS

A report of an anaphylactic reaction to synthetic GnRH (Factrel) has been reported in the medical literature.[1]

LUPRON DEPOT is contraindicated in women who are or may become pregnant while receiving the drug. When administered on day 6 of pregnancy at test dosages of 0.00024, 0.0024, and 0.024 mg/kg (1/600 to 1/6 of the human dose) to rabbits, the monthly formulation of LUPRON DEPOT produced a dose-related increase in major fetal abnormalities. Similar studies in rats failed to demonstrate an increase in fetal malformations. There was increased fetal mortality and decreased fetal weights with the two higher doses of the monthly formulation of LUPRON DEPOT in rabbits and with the highest dose in rats. The effects on fetal mortality are logical consequences of the alterations in hormonal levels brought about by this drug. Therefore, the possibility exists that spontaneous abortion may occur if the drug is administered during pregnancy.

WARNINGS

Isolated cases of worsening of signs and symptoms during the first weeks of treatment have been reported with LH-RH analogs. Worsening of symptoms may contribute to paralysis with or without fatal complications. For patients at risk, the physician may consider initiating therapy with daily LUPRON® (leuprolide acetate) Injection for the first two weeks to facilitate withdrawal of treatment if that is considered necessary.

Continued on next page

Lupron Depot-3 Mo. 22.5 mg—Cont.

PRECAUTIONS

General Patients with metastatic vertebral lesions and/or with urinary tract obstruction should be closely observed during the first few weeks of therapy. (See **WARNINGS** section.)

Laboratory Tests Response to LUPRON DEPOT–3 Month 22.5 mg should be monitored by measuring serum levels of testosterone, as well as prostate-specific antigen and prostatic acid phosphatase. In the majority of patients, testosterone levels increased above baseline during the first week, declining thereafter to baseline levels or below by the end of the second week. Castrate levels were reached within two to four weeks and once achieved were maintained for as long as the patients received their injections.

Drug Interactions No pharmacokinetic-based drug-drug interaction studies have been conducted with LUPRON DEPOT. However, because leuprolide acetate is a peptide that is primarily degraded by peptidase and not by cytochrome P-450 enzymes as noted in specific studies, and the drug is only about 46% bound to plasma proteins, drug interactions would not be expected to occur.

Drug/Laboratory Test Interactions Administration of LUPRON DEPOT 3.75 mg in women results in suppression of the pituitary-gonadal system. Normal function is usually restored within one to three months after treatment is discontinued. Therefore, diagnostic tests of pituitary gonadotropic and gonadal functions conducted during treatment and up to three months after discontinuation of LUPRON DEPOT 3.75 mg therapy may be misleading.

Carcinogenesis, Mutagenesis, Impairment of Fertility Two-year carcinogenicity studies were conducted in rats and mice. In rats, a dose-related increase of benign pituitary hyperplasia and benign pituitary adenomas was noted at 24 months when the drug was administered subcutaneously at high daily doses (0.6 to 4 mg/kg). There was a significant but not dose-related increase of pancreatic islet-cell adenomas in females and of testicular interstitial cell adenomas in males (highest incidence in the low dose group). In mice no pituitary abnormalities were observed at a dose as high as 60 mg/kg for two years. Patients have been treated with leuprolide acetate for up to three years with doses as high as 10 mg/day and for two years with doses as high as 20 mg/day without demonstrable pituitary abnormalities.

Mutagenicity studies have been performed with leuprolide acetate using bacterial and mammalian systems. These studies provided no evidence of a mutagenic potential.

Clinical and pharmacologic studies in adults (≥ 18 years) with leuprolide acetate and similar analogs have shown reversibility of fertility suppression when the drug is discontinued after continuous administration for periods of up to 24 weeks.

Pregnancy, Teratogenic Effects Pregnancy Category X. (See **CONTRAINDICATIONS** section.)

Pediatric Use See LUPRON DEPOT-PED® (leuprolide acetate for depot suspension) labeling for the safety and effectiveness of the monthly formulation in children with central precocious puberty.

Geriatric Use In the clinical trials for LUPRON DEPOT–3 Month 22.5 mg, the majority (80%) of the subjects studied were at least 65 years of age. Therefore, the labeling reflects the pharmacokinetics, efficacy and safety of LUPRON DEPOT in this population.

ADVERSE REACTIONS

Clinical Trials

In the majority of patients testosterone levels increased above baseline during the first week, declining thereafter to baseline levels or below by the end of the second week of treatment.

Potential exacerbations of signs and symptoms during the first few weeks of treatment is a concern in patients with vertebral metastases and/or urinary obstruction or hematuria which, if aggravated, may lead to neurological problems such as temporary weakness and/or paresthesia of the lower limbs or worsening of urinary symptoms. (See **WARNINGS** section.)

In two clinical trials of LUPRON DEPOT–3 Month 22.5 mg, the following adverse reactions were reported to have a possible or probable relationship to drug as ascribed by the treating physician in 5% or more of the patients receiving the drug. **Often, causality is difficult to assess in patients with metastatic prostate cancer.** Reactions considered not drug-related are excluded.

	LUPRON DEPOT-3 Month 22.5 mg N=94	(%)
Body As A Whole		
Asthenia	7	(7.4)
General Pain	25	(26.6)
Headache	6	(6.4)
Injection Site Reaction	13	(13.8)
Cardiovascular System		
Hot flashes/Sweats*	55	(58.5)
Digestive System		
GI Disorders	15	(16.0)
Musculoskeletal System		
Joint Disorders	11	(11.7)
Central/Peripheral Nervous System		
Dizziness/Vertigo	6	(6.4)
Insomnia/Sleep Disorders	8	(8.5)
Neuromuscular Disorders	9	(9.6)
Respiratory System		
Respiratory Disorders	6	(6.4)
Skin and Appendages		
Skin Reaction	8	(8.5)
Urogenital System		
Testicular Atrophy*	19	(20.2)
Urinary Disorders	14	(14.9)

In these same studies, the following adverse reactions were reported in less than 5% of the patients on LUPRON DEPOT–3 Month 22.5 mg.

Body As A Whole – Enlarged abdomen, Fever; *Cardiovascular System* – Arrhythmia, Bradycardia, Heart failure, Hypertension, Hypotension, Varicose vein; *Digestive System* – Anorexia, Duodenal ulcer, Increased appetite, Thirst/dry mouth; *Hemic and Lymphatic System* – Anemia, Lymphedema; *Metabolic and Nutritional Disorders* – Dehydration, Edema; *Central/Peripheral Nervous System* – Anxiety, Delusions, Depression, Hypesthesia, Libido decreased*, Nervousness, Paresthesia; *Respiratory System* – Epistaxis, Pharyngitis, Pleural effusion, Pneumonia; *Special Senses* – Abnormal vision, Amblyopia, Dry eyes, Tinnitus; *Urogenital System* – Gynecomastia, Impotence*, Penis disorders, Testis disorders.

Laboratory: Abnormalities of certain parameters were observed, but are difficult to assess in this population. The following were recorded in ≥ 5% of patients: Increased BUN, Hyperglycemia, Hyperlipidemia (total cholesterol, LDL-cholesterol, triglycerides), Hyperphosphatemia, Abnormal liver function tests, Increased PT, Increased PTT. Additional laboratory abnormalities reported were: Decreased platelets, Decreased potassium and Increased WBC.

*Physiologic effect of decreased testosterone.

Postmarketing

During postmarketing surveillance, which includes other dosage forms and other patient populations, the following adverse events were reported.

Symptoms consistent with an anaphylactoid or asthmatic process have been rarely (incidence rate of about 0.002%) reported. Rash, urticaria, and photosensitivity reactions have also been reported.

Localized reactions including induration and abscess have been reported at the site of injection.

Symptoms consistent with fibromyalgia (eg, joint and muscle pain, headaches, sleep disorders, gastrointestinal distress, and shortness of breath) have been reported individually and collectively.

Cardiovascular System – Hypotension, Pulmonary embolism; *Hemic and Lymphatic System* – Decreased WBC; *Central/Peripheral Nervous System* – Peripheral neuropathy, Spinal fracture/paralysis; *Musculoskeletal System* – Tenosynovitis-like symptoms; *Urogenital System* – Prostate pain.

Changes in Bone Density: Decreased bone density has been reported in the medical literature in men who have had orchiectomy or who have been treated with an LH-RH agonist analog. In a clinical trial, 25 men with prostate cancer, 12 of whom had been treated previously with leuprolide acetate for at least six months, underwent bone density studies as a result of pain. The leuprolide-treated group had lower bone density scores than the nontreated control group. It can be anticipated that long periods of medical castration in men will have effects on bone density.

See other LUPRON DEPOT and LUPRON Injection package inserts for other events reported in women and pediatric populations.

OVERDOSAGE

In rats subcutaneous administration of 250 to 500 times the recommended human dose, expressed on a per body weight basis, resulted in dyspnea, decreased activity, and local irritation at the injection site. There is no evidence at present that there is a clinical counterpart of this phenomenon. In early clinical trials with daily subcutaneous leuprolide acetate, doses as high as 20 mg/day for up to two years caused no adverse effects differing from those observed with the 1 mg/day dose.

DOSAGE AND ADMINISTRATION

LUPRON DEPOT Must Be Administered Under The Supervision Of A Physician.

The recommended dose of LUPRON DEPOT–3 Month 22.5 mg to be administered is one injection every three months **(84 days)**. Due to different release characteristics, a fractional dose of this 3-month depot formulation is not equivalent to the same dose of the monthly formulation and should not be given.

Incorporated in a depot formulation, the lyophilized microspheres are to be reconstituted and administered every three months as a single intramuscular injection. *For optimal performance of the prefilled dual chamber syringe (PDS), read and follow the following instructions:*

1. To prepare for injection, screw the white plunger into the end stopper until the stopper begins to turn.
2. Hold the syringe UPRIGHT. Release the diluent by SLOWLY PUSHING (6 to 8 seconds) the plunger until the first stopper is at the blue line in the middle of the barrel.
3. Keep the syringe UPRIGHT. Gently mix the microspheres (particles) thoroughly to form a uniform suspension. The suspension will appear milky.
4. Hold the syringe UPRIGHT. With the opposite hand pull the needle cap upward without twisting.
5. Keep the syringe UPRIGHT. Advance the plunger to expel the air from the syringe.
6. Inject the entire contents of the syringe intramuscularly at the time of reconstitution. The suspension settles very quickly following reconstitution; therefore, LUPRON DEPOT should be mixed and used immediately.

NOTE: Aspirated blood would be visible just below the luer lock connection if a blood vessel is accidentally penetrated. If present, blood can be seen through the transparent LuproLoc™ safety device.

AFTER INJECTION

7. Withdraw the needle. Immediately activate the LuproLoc™ safety device by pushing the arrow forward with the thumb or finger until the device is fully extended and a CLICK is heard or felt.

Since the product does not contain a preservative, the suspension should be discarded if not used immediately.

As with other drugs administered by injection, the injection site should be varied periodically.

HOW SUPPLIED

LUPRON DEPOT–3 Month 22.5 mg is packaged as follows:

Kit with prefilled dual-chamber syringe NDC 0300-3346-01

Each syringe contains sterile lyophilized microspheres which is leuprolide acetate incorporated in a biodegradable polymer of polylactic acid. When mixed with 1.5 mL of accompanying diluent, LUPRON DEPOT–3 Month 22.5 mg is administered as a single IM injection **EVERY THREE MONTHS (84 days).**

An information pamphlet for patients is included with the kit.

Store at 25°C (77°F); excursions permitted to 15-30°C (59-86°F) [See USP Controlled Room Temperature]

REFERENCE

1. MacLeod TL, *et al.* Anaphylactic reaction to synthetic luteinizing hormone-releasing hormone. *Fertil Steril* 1987 Sept; 48(3):500-502.

U.S. Patent Nos. 4,728,721; 4,849,228; 5,330,767; 5,476,663; 5,480,656; 5,575,987; 5,631,020; 5,631,021; 5,643,607; 5,716,640; 5,814,342; 5,823,997; 5,980,488 and 6,036,976.
Other patents pending.
Manufactured for
TAP Pharmaceuticals Inc.
Lake Forest, IL 60045, U.S.A.
by Takeda Chemical Industries, Ltd.
Osaka, JAPAN 541
™-Trademark
® – Registered trademark
(No. 3346)
03-5307-R9; Revised September 2003

Shown in Product Identification Guide, page 334

LUPRON DEPOT®–4 MONTH 30 MG ℞

[*lew-prŏn*]

(leuprolide acetate for depot suspension)
4-MONTH FORMULATION
Rx only

DESCRIPTION

Leuprolide acetate is a synthetic nonapeptide analog of naturally occurring gonadotropin-releasing hormone (GnRH or LH-RH). The analog possesses greater potency than the natural hormone. The chemical name is 5-oxo-L-prolyl-L-histidyl-L-tryptophyl-L-seryl-L-tyrosyl-D-leucyl-L-leucyl-L-arginyl-N-ethyl-L-prolinamide acetate (salt) with the following structural formula:

[See chemical structure at top of next page]

LUPRON DEPOT-4 Month 30 mg is available in a prefilled dual-chamber syringe containing sterile lyophilized microspheres which, when mixed with diluent, become a suspension intended as an intramuscular injection to be given **ONCE EVERY FOUR MONTHS (16 weeks).**

The front chamber of LUPRON DEPOT-4 Month 30 mg prefilled dual-chamber syringe contains leuprolide acetate (30 mg), polylactic acid (264.8 mg) and D-mannitol (51.9 mg). The second chamber of diluent contains carboxymethylcellulose sodium (7.5 mg), D-mannitol (75.0 mg), polysorbate 80 (1.5 mg), water for injection, USP, and glacial acetic acid, USP to control pH.

During the manufacture of LUPRON DEPOT-4 Month 30 mg, acetic acid is lost, leaving the peptide.

CLINICAL PHARMACOLOGY

Leuprolide acetate, an LH-RH agonist, acts as a potent inhibitor of gonadotropin secretion when given continuously and in therapeutic doses. Animal and human studies indicate that following an initial stimulation, chronic administration of leuprolide acetate results in suppression of ovarian and testicular steroidogenesis. This effect is reversible upon discontinuation of drug therapy. Administration of leuprolide acetate has resulted in inhibition of the growth of certain hormone dependent tumors (prostatic tumors in Noble and Dunning male rats and DMBA-induced mammary tumors in female rats) as well as atrophy of the reproductive organs.

In humans, administration of leuprolide acetate results in an initial increase in circulating levels of luteinizing hormone (LH) and follicle stimulating hormone (FSH), leading to a transient increase in levels of the gonadal steroids (testosterone and dihydrotestosterone in males, and estrone and estradiol in premenopausal females). However, continuous administration of leuprolide acetate results in decreased levels of LH and FSH. In males, testosterone is reduced to castrate levels. In premenopausal females, estrogens are reduced to postmenopausal levels. These decreases occur within two to four weeks after initiation of treatment. Castrate levels of testosterone in prostatic cancer patients have been demonstrated for more than five years.

Leuprolide acetate is not active when given orally.

Pharmacokinetics

Absorption Following a single injection of LUPRON DEPOT-4 Month 30 mg in sixteen orchiectomized prostate cancer patients, mean plasma leuprolide concentration of 59.3 ng/mL was observed at 4 hours and the mean concentration then declined to 0.30 ng/mL at 16 weeks. The mean plasma concentration of leuprolide from weeks 3.5 to 16 was 0.44 ± 0.20 ng/mL (range: 0.20–1.06). Leuprolide appeared to be released at a constant rate following the onset of steady-state levels during the fourth week after dosing, providing steady plasma concentrations throughout the 16-week dosing interval. However, intact leuprolide and an inactive major metabolite could not be distinguished by the assay which was employed in the study. The initial burst, followed by the rapid decline to a steady-state level, was similar to the release pattern seen with the other depot formulations.

Distribution The mean steady-state volume of distribution of leuprolide following intravenous bolus administration to healthy male volunteers was 27 L. *In vitro* binding to human plasma proteins ranged from 43% to 49%.

Metabolism In healthy male volunteers, a 1 mg bolus of leuprolide administered intravenously revealed that the mean systemic clearance was 7.6 L/h, with a terminal elimination half-life of approximately 3 hours based on a two compartment model.

In rats and dogs, administration of ^{14}C-labeled leuprolide was shown to be metabolized to smaller inactive peptides, a pentapeptide (Metabolite I), tripeptides (Metabolites II and III) and a dipeptide (Metabolite IV). These fragments may be further catabolized.

The major metabolite (M-I) plasma concentrations measured in 5 prostate cancer patients reached maximum concentration 2 to 6 hours after dosing and were approximately 6% of the peak parent drug concentration. One week after dosing, mean plasma M-I concentrations were approximately 20% of mean leuprolide concentrations.

Excretion Following administration of LUPRON DEPOT® 3.75 mg to 3 patients, less than 5% of the dose was recovered as parent and M-I metabolite in the urine.

Special Populations The pharmacokinetics of the drug in hepatically and renally impaired patients have not been determined.

Drug Interactions No pharmacokinetic-based drug-drug interaction studies have been conducted with LUPRON DEPOT. However, because leuprolide acetate is a peptide that is primarily degraded by peptidase and the drug is only about 46% bound to plasma proteins, drug interactions would not be expected to occur.

CLINICAL STUDIES

In an open-label, noncomparative, multicenter clinical study of LUPRON DEPOT-4 Month 30 mg, 49 patients with stage D2 prostatic adenocarcinoma (with no prior treatment) were enrolled. The objectives were to determine whether a 30 mg depot formulation of leuprolide injected once every 16 weeks would reduce and maintain serum testosterone levels at castrate levels (≤ 50 ng/dL), and to assess the safety of the formulation. The study was divided into an initial 32-week treatment phase and a long-term treatment phase. Serum testosterone levels were determined biweekly or weekly during the first 32 weeks of treatment. Once the patient completed the initial 32-week treatment period, treatment continued at the investigator's discretion with serum testosterone levels being done every 4 months prior to the injection.

In the majority of patients, testosterone levels increased 50% or more above the baseline during the first week of treatment. Mean serum testosterone subsequently suppressed to castrate levels within 30 days of the first injection in 94% of patients and within 43 days in all 49 patients during the initial 32-week treatment period. The median dosing interval between injections was 112 days. One escape from suppression (two consecutive testosterone values > 50 ng/dL after castrate levels achieved) was noted at Week 16. In this patient, serum testosterone increased to above the castrate range following the second depot injection (Week 16) but returned to the castrate level by Week 18. No adverse events were associated with this rise in serum testosterone. A second patient had a rise in testosterone at Week 17, then returned to the castrate level by Week 18 and remained there through Week 32. In the long-term treatment phase two patients experienced testosterone elevations, both at Week 48. Testosterone for one patient returned to the castrate range at Week 52, and one patient discontinued the study at Week 48 due to disease progression.

Secondary efficacy endpoints evaluated in the study were the objective tumor response as assessed by clinical evaluations of tumor burden (complete response, partial response, objectively stable and progression) and evaluations of changes in prostatic involvement and prostate-specific antigen (PSA). These evaluations were performed at Weeks 16 and 32 of the treatment phase. The long-term treatment phase monitored PSA at each visit (every 16 weeks). The objective tumor response analysis showed "no progression" (i.e. complete or partial response, or stable disease) in 86% (37/43) of patients at Week 16, and in 77% (37/48) of patients at Week 32. Local disease improved or remained stable in all patients evaluated at Week 16 and/or 32. For patients with elevated baseline PSA, 50% (23/46) had a normal PSA (< 4.0 ng/mL) at Week 16, and 51% (19/37) had a normal PSA at Week 32.

Periodic monitoring of serum testosterone and PSA levels is recommended, especially if the anticipated clinical or biochemical response to treatment has not been achieved. It should be noted that results of testosterone determinations are dependent on assay methodology. It is advisable to be aware of the type and precision of the assay methodology to make appropriate clinical and therapeutic decisions.

Using historical comparisons, the safety and efficacy of LUPRON DEPOT-4 Month 30 mg appear similar to the other LUPRON DEPOT formulations.

Lupron Depot – 4 Month 30 mg
Mean Serum Testosterone Concentrations

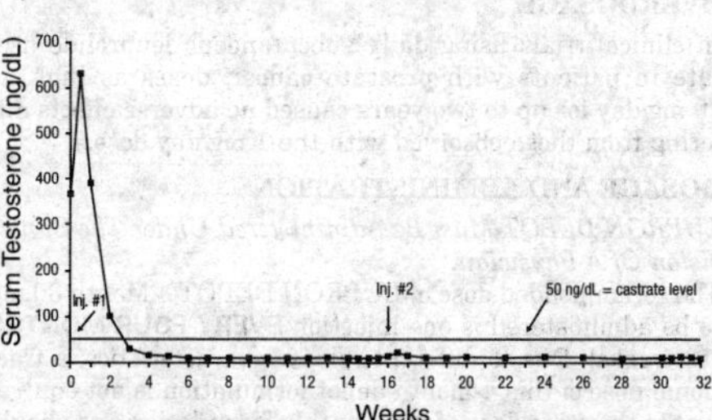

Note: Measurements were taken in a subset of patients at Weeks 14.5, 15.5, 16.5, 30.5, 31 and 31.5.

INDICATIONS AND USAGE

LUPRON DEPOT-4 Month 30 mg is indicated in the palliative treatment of advanced prostatic cancer.

CONTRAINDICATIONS

1. Hypersensitivity to GnRH, GnRH agonist analogs or any of the excipients in LUPRON DEPOT. Reports of anaphylactic reactions to synthetic GnRH (Factrel) or GnRH agonist analogs have been reported in the medical literature.
2. This formulation is not indicated for use in women. (See LUPRON DEPOT 3.75 mg and LUPRON DEPOT®–3 Month 11.25 mg package inserts.)
3. All formulations of LUPRON DEPOT are contraindicated in women who are or may become pregnant while receiving the drug. LUPRON DEPOT may cause fetal harm when administered to a pregnant woman. Major fetal abnormalities were observed in rabbits but not in rats after administration of LUPRON DEPOT throughout gestation. There was increased fetal mortality and decreased fetal weights in rats and rabbits. The effects on fetal mortality are expected consequences of the alterations in hormonal levels brought about by this drug. Therefore, the possibility exists that spontaneous abortion may occur. If this drug is used during pregnancy, or if the patient becomes pregnant while taking any formulation of LUPRON DEPOT, the patient should be apprised of the potential hazard to the fetus.

WARNINGS

Initially, LUPRON DEPOT, like other LH-RH agonists, causes increases in serum levels of testosterone to approximately 50% above baseline during the first week of treatment. Transient worsening of symptoms, or the occurrence of additional signs and symptoms of prostate cancer, may occasionally develop during the first few weeks of LUPRON DEPOT treatment. A small number of patients may experience a temporary increase in bone pain, which can be managed symptomatically. As with other LH-RH agonists, isolated cases of ureteral obstruction and spinal cord compression have been observed, which may contribute to paralysis with or without fatal complications.

For patients at risk, initiation of therapy with daily LUPRON® (leuprolide acetate) Injection (See **DOSAGE AND ADMINISTRATION** section in the LUPRON Injection labeling.) for the first two weeks to facilitate withdrawal of treatment may be considered. If spinal cord compression or renal impairment develops, standard treatment of these complications should be instituted.

PRECAUTIONS

Information for Patients An information pamphlet for patients is included with the product.

General Patients with metastatic vertebral lesions and/or with urinary tract obstruction should be closely observed during the first few weeks of therapy. (See **WARNINGS** section.)

Laboratory Tests Response to LUPRON DEPOT-4 Month 30 mg should be monitored by measuring serum levels of testosterone, as well as prostate-specific antigen. In the majority of patients, testosterone levels increased above baseline during the first week, declining thereafter to baseline levels or below by the end of the second week. Castrate levels were reached within two to four weeks and once achieved were maintained in most (45/49) patients for as long as the patients received their injections. (See **CLINICAL STUDIES** and **ADVERSE REACTIONS**.)

Drug Interactions See **CLINICAL PHARMACOLOGY, Pharmacokinetics.**

Drug/Laboratory Test Interactions Administration of LUPRON DEPOT in therapeutic doses results in suppression of the pituitary-gonadal system. Normal function is usually restored within three months after treatment is discontinued. Due to the suppression of the pituitary-gonadal system by LUPRON DEPOT, diagnostic tests of pituitary gonadotropic and gonadal functions conducted during treatment and for up to three months after discontinuation of LUPRON DEPOT may be affected.

Carcinogenesis, Mutagenesis, Impairment of Fertility Two-year carcinogenicity studies were conducted in rats and mice. In rats, a dose-related increase of benign pituitary hyperplasia and benign pituitary adenomas was noted at 24 months when the drug was administered subcutaneously at high daily doses (0.6 to 4 mg/kg). There was a significant but not dose-related increase of pancreatic islet-cell adenomas in females and of testicular interstitial cell adenomas in males (highest incidence in the low dose group). In mice no pituitary abnormalities were observed at a dose as high as 60 mg/kg for two years. Patients have been treated with leuprolide acetate for up to three years with doses as high as 10 mg/day and for two years with doses as high as 20 mg/day without demonstrable pituitary abnormalities.

Mutagenicity studies have been performed with leuprolide acetate using bacterial and mammalian systems. These studies provided no evidence of a mutagenic potential.

Clinical and pharmacologic studies in adults (≥ 18 years) with leuprolide acetate and similar analogs have shown reversibility of fertility suppression when the drug is discontinued after continuous administration for periods of up to 24 weeks.

Pregnancy, Teratogenic Effects. Pregnancy Category X. (See **CONTRAINDICATIONS** section.)

Pediatric Use Safety and effectiveness of LUPRON DEPOT-4 Month 30 mg have not been established in pediatric patients. See LUPRON DEPOT-PED® (leuprolide acetate for depot suspension) labeling for the safety and effectiveness of the monthly formulation in children with central precocious puberty.

Geriatric Use In the clinical trials for LUPRON DEPOT – 4 Month 30 mg, the majority (79%) of the subjects studied were at least 65 years of age. Therefore, the labeling reflects the pharmacokinetics, efficacy and safety of LUPRON DEPOT in this population.

ADVERSE REACTIONS

Clinical Trials

The 4-month formulation of LUPRON DEPOT 30 mg was utilized in clinical trials that studied the drug in 49 nonorchiectomized prostate cancer patients for 32 weeks or longer and in 24 orchiectomized prostate cancer patients for 20 weeks.

In the majority of nonorchiectomized patients, testosterone levels increased 50% or more above baseline during the first week of treatment with LUPRON DEPOT, declining thereafter to baseline levels or below by the end of the second week of treatment. Therefore, potential exacerbations of signs and symptoms during the first few weeks of treatment are of concern in patients with vertebral metastases and/or urinary obstruction or hematuria which, if aggravated, may lead to neurological problems such as temporary weakness and/or paresthesia of the lower limbs or worsening of urinary symptoms. (See **WARNINGS** section.)

In the above described clinical trials, the following adverse reactions were reported in ≥ 5% of the patients during the treatment period regardless of causality.

[See table at top of next page]

Continued on next page

Adverse Events Reported in ≥ 5% of Patients Regardless of Causality
LUPRON DEPOT-4 Month 30 mg

	Nonorchiectomized, N=49 Study 013		Orchiectomized, N=24 Study 012	
	N	(%)	N	(%)
Body As a Whole				
Asthenia	6	(12.2)	1	(4.2)
Flu Syndrome	6	(12.2)	0	(0.0)
General Pain	16	(32.7)	1	(4.2)
Headache	5	(10.2)	1	(4.2)
Injection Site Reaction	4	(8.2)	9	(37.5)
Cardiovascular System				
Hot flashes/Sweats*	23	(46.9)	2	(8.3)
Digestive System				
GI Disorders	5	(10.2)	3	(12.5)
Metabolic and Nutritional Disorders				
Dehydration	4	(8.2)	0	(0.0)
Edema	4	(8.2)	5	(20.8)
Musculoskeletal System				
Joint Disorder	8	(16.3)	1	(4.2)
Myalgia	4	(8.2)	0	(0.0)
Nervous System				
Dizziness/Vertigo	3	(6.1)	2	(8.3)
Neuromuscular Disorders	3	(6.1)	1	(4.2)
Paresthesia	4	(8.2)	1	(4.2)
Respiratory System				
Respiratory Disorder	4	(8.2)	1	(4.2)
Skin and Appendages				
Skin Reaction	6	(12.2)	0	(0.0)
Urogenital System				
Urinary Disorders	5	(10.2)	4	(16.7)

Lupron Depot-4 Mo. 30 mg—Cont.

In these same studies, the following adverse reactions were reported in less than 5% of the patients on LUPRON DEPOT-4 Month 30 mg.

Body As a Whole - Abscess, Accidental injury, Allergic reaction, Cyst, Fever, Generalized edema, Hernia, Neck pain, Neoplasm; *Cardiovascular System* - Atrial fibrillation, Deep thrombophlebitis, Hypertension; *Digestive System* - Anorexia, Eructation, Gastrointestinal hemorrhage, Gingivitis, Gum hemorrhage, Hepatomegaly, Increased appetite, Intestinal obstruction, Peridontal abscess; *Hemic and Lymphatic System* - Lymphadenopathy; *Metabolic and Nutritional Disorders* - Healing abnormal, Hypoxia, Weight loss; *Musculoskeletal System* - Leg cramps, Pathological fracture, Ptosis; *Nervous System* - Abnormal thinking, Amnesia, Confusion, Convulsion, Dementia, Depression, Insomnia/sleep disorders, Libido decreased*, Neuropathy, Paralysis; *Respiratory System* - Asthma, Bronchitis, Hiccup, Lung disorder, Sinusitis, Voice alteration; *Skin and Appendages* - Herpes zoster, Melanosis; *Urogenital System* - Bladder carcinoma, Epididymitis, Impotence*, Prostate disorder, Testicular atrophy*, Urinary incontinence, Urinary tract infection.

* Due to the expected physiologic effects of decreased testosterone levels.

Laboratory: Abnormalities of certain parameters were observed, but their relationship to drug treatment is difficult to assess in this population. The following were recorded in ≥ 5% of patients: Decreased bicarbonate, Decreased hemoglobin/hematocrit/RBC, Hyperlipidemia (total cholesterol, LDL-cholesterol, triglycerides), Decreased HDL-cholesterol, Eosinophilia, Increased glucose, Increased liver function tests (ALT, AST, GGTP, LDH), Increased phosphorus. Additional laboratory abnormalities were reported: Increased BUN and PT, Leukopenia, Thrombocytopenia, Uricaciduria.

Postmarketing

During postmarketing surveillance, which includes other dosage forms and other patient populations, the following adverse events were reported.

Symptoms consistent with an anaphylactoid or asthmatic process have been rarely (incidence rate of about 0.002%) reported. Rash, urticaria, and photosensitivity reactions have also been reported.

Localized reactions including induration and abscess have been reported at the site of injection.

Symptoms consistent with fibromyalgia (eg, joint and muscle pain, headaches, sleep disorders, gastrointestinal distress, and shortness of breath) have been reported individually and collectively.

Cardiovascular System - Hypotension, Pulmonary embolism; *Hemic and Lymphatic System* - Decreased WBC; *Central/Peripheral Nervous System* - Peripheral neuropathy, Spinal fracture/paralysis; *Musculoskeletal System* - Tenosynovitis-like symptoms; *Urogenital System* - Prostate pain.

Changes in Bone Density: Decreased bone density has been reported in the medical literature in men who have had orchiectomy or who have been treated with an LH-RH agonist analog. In a clinical trial, 25 men with prostate cancer, 12 of whom had been treated previously with leuprolide acetate for at least six months, underwent bone density studies as a result of pain. The leuprolide-treated group had lower bone density scores than the nontreated control group. It can be anticipated that long periods of medical castration in men will have effects on bone density.

See other LUPRON DEPOT and LUPRON Injection package inserts for other events reported in women and pediatric populations.

OVERDOSAGE

In clinical trials using daily subcutaneous leuprolide acetate in patients with prostate cancer, doses as high as 20 mg/day for up to two years caused no adverse effects differing from those observed with the 1 mg/day dose.

DOSAGE AND ADMINISTRATION

LUPRON DEPOT Must Be Administered Under The Supervision Of A Physician.

The recommended dose of LUPRON DEPOT-4 Month 30 mg to be administered is one injection **EVERY FOUR MONTHS (16 weeks)**. Due to different release characteristics, a fractional dose of this 4-month depot formulation is not equivalent to the same dose of the monthly formulation and should not be given.

Incorporated in a depot formulation, the lyophilized microspheres are to be reconstituted and administered **EVERY FOUR MONTHS (16 weeks)** as a single intramuscular injection.

For optimal performance of the prefilled dual chamber syringe (PDS), read and follow the following instructions:

1. To prepare for injection, screw the white plunger into the end stopper until the stopper begins to turn.
2. Hold the syringe UPRIGHT. Release the diluent by SLOWLY PUSHING (6 to 8 seconds) the plunger until the first stopper is at the blue line in the middle of the barrel.
3. Keep the syringe UPRIGHT. Gently mix the microspheres (particles) thoroughly to form a uniform suspension. The suspension will appear milky.
4. Hold the syringe UPRIGHT. With the opposite hand pull the needle cap upward without twisting.
5. Keep the syringe UPRIGHT. Advance the plunger to expel the air from the syringe.
6. Inject the entire contents of the syringe intramuscularly at the time of reconstitution. The suspension settles very quickly following reconstitution; therefore, LUPRON DEPOT should be mixed and used immediately.

NOTE: Aspirated blood would be visible just below the luer lock connection if a blood vessel is accidentally penetrated. If present, blood can be seen through the transparent LuproLoc™ safety device.

AFTER INJECTION

7. Withdraw the needle. Immediately activate the LuproLoc™ safety device by pushing the arrow forward with the thumb or finger until the device is fully extended and a CLICK is heard or felt.

Since the product does not contain a preservative, the suspension should be discarded if not used immediately.

As with other drugs administered by injection, the injection site should be varied periodically.

HOW SUPPLIED

LUPRON DEPOT-4 Month 30 mg is packaged as follows:
Kit with prefilled dual-chamber syringe NDC 0300-3683-01

Each syringe contains sterile lyophilized microspheres which is leuprolide acetate incorporated in a biodegradable polymer of polylactic acid. When mixed with 1.5 mL of accompanying diluent, LUPRON DEPOT-4 Month 30 mg is administered as a single IM injection **EVERY FOUR MONTHS (16 weeks).**

Store at 25°C (77°F); excursions permitted to 15-30°C (59-86°F) [See USP Controlled Room Temperature]

U.S. Patent Nos. 4,728,721; 4,849,228; 5,330,767; 5,476,663; 5,480,656; 5,575,987; 5,631,020; 5,631,021; 5,643,607; 5,716,640; 5,814,342; 5,823,997; 5,980,488; and 6,036,976. Other patents pending.

Manufactured for
TAP Pharmaceuticals Inc.
Lake Forest, IL 60045, U.S.A.
by Takeda Chemical Industries, Ltd.
Osaka, JAPAN 541
™ – Trademark
® – Registered Trademark
(No. 3683)
03-5306-R7; Revised September 2003

Shown in Product Identification Guide, page 334

LUPRON DEPOT-PED® ℞

[lew-prŏn]
(leuprolide acetate for depot suspension)
7.5 mg, 11.25 mg and 15 mg
Rx only

DESCRIPTION

Leuprolide acetate is a synthetic nonapeptide analog of naturally occurring gonadotropin-releasing hormone (GnRH or LH-RH). The analog possesses greater potency than the natural hormone. The chemical name is 5-oxo-L-prolyl-L-histidyl-L-tryptophyl-L-seryl-L-tyrosyl-D-leucyl-L-leucyl-L-arginyl-N-ethyl-L-prolinamide acetate (salt) with the following structural formula:

[See chemical structure at top of next page]

LUPRON DEPOT-PED is available in a prefilled dual-chamber syringe containing sterile lyophilized microspheres which, when mixed with diluent, become a suspension intended as a single intramuscular injection.

The front chamber of LUPRON DEPOT-PED 7.5 mg, 11.25 mg, and 15 mg prefilled dual-chamber syringe contains leuprolide acetate (7.5/11.25/15 mg), purified gelatin (1.3/1.95/2.6 mg), DL-lactic and glycolic acids copolymer (66.2/99.3/132.4 mg), and D-mannitol (13.2/19.8/26.4 mg). The second chamber of diluent contains carboxymethylcellulose sodium (5 mg), D-mannitol (50 mg), polysorbate 80 (1 mg), water for injection, USP, and glacial acetic acid, USP to control pH.

During the manufacture of LUPRON DEPOT-PED, acetic acid is lost, leaving the peptide.

CLINICAL PHARMACOLOGY

Leuprolide acetate, a GnRH agonist, acts as a potent inhibitor of gonadotropin secretion when given continuously and in therapeutic doses. Human studies indicate that following an initial stimulation of gonadotropins, chronic stimulation with leuprolide acetate results in suppression or "downregulation" of these hormones and consequent suppression of ovarian and testicular steroidogenesis. These effects are reversible on discontinuation of drug therapy.

Leuprolide acetate is not active when given orally.

Pharmacokinetics

Absorption Following a single LUPRON DEPOT 7.5 mg injection to adult patients, mean peak leuprolide plasma concentration was almost 20 ng/mL at 4 hours and then declined to 0.36 ng/mL at 4 weeks. However, intact leuprolide and an inactive major metabolite could not be distinguished by the assay which was employed in the study. Nondetectable leuprolide plasma concentrations have been observed during chronic LUPRON DEPOT 7.5 mg administration, but testosterone levels appear to be maintained at castrate levels.

Distribution The mean steady-state volume of distribution of leuprolide following intravenous bolus administration to healthy male volunteers was 27 L. *In vitro* binding to human plasma proteins ranged from 43% to 49%.

Metabolism In healthy male volunteers, a 1 mg bolus of leuprolide administered intravenously revealed that the mean systemic clearance was 7.6 L/h, with a terminal elimination half-life of approximately 3 hours based on a two compartment model.

In rats and dogs, administration of ^{14}C-labeled leuprolide was shown to be metabolized to smaller inactive peptides, a pentapeptide (Metabolite I), tripeptides (Metabolites II and III) and a dipeptide (Metabolite IV). These fragments may be further catabolized.

The major metabolite (M-I) plasma concentrations measured in 5 prostate cancer patients reached maximum concentration 2 to 6 hours after dosing and were approximately 6% of the peak parent drug concentration. One week after dosing, mean plasma M-I concentrations were approximately 20% of mean leuprolide concentrations.

Excretion Following administration of LUPRON DEPOT 3.75 mg to 3 patients, less than 5% of the dose was recovered as parent and M-I metabolite in the urine.

Special Populations The pharmacokinetics of the drug in hepatically and renally impaired patients have not been determined.

CLINICAL STUDIES

In children with central precocious puberty (CPP), stimulated and basal gonadotropins are reduced to prepubertal

levels. Testosterone and estradiol are reduced to prepubertal levels in males and females respectively. Reduction of gonadotropins will allow for normal physical and psychological growth and development. Natural maturation occurs when gonadotropins return to pubertal levels following discontinuation of leuprolide acetate.
The following physiologic effects have been noted with the chronic administration of leuprolide acetate in this patient population.

1. **Skeletal Growth.** A measurable increase in body length can be noted since the epiphyseal plates will not close prematurely.
2. **Organ Growth.** Reproductive organs will return to a prepubertal state.
3. **Menses.** Menses, if present, will cease.

In a study of 22 children with central precocious puberty, doses of LUPRON DEPOT were given every 4 weeks and plasma levels were determined according to weight categories as summarized below:
[See table above]

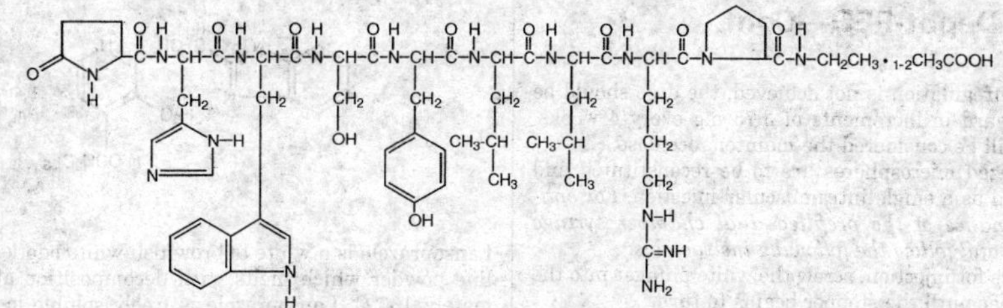

Patient Weight Range (kg)	Group Weight Average (kg)	Dose (mg)	Trough Plasma Leuprolide Level Mean ±SD (ng/mL)*
20.2–27.0	22.7	7.5	0.77±0.033
28.4–36.8	32.5	11.25	1.25±1.06
39.3–57.5	44.2	15.0	1.59±0.65

*Group average values determined at Week 4 immediately prior to leuprolide injection. Drug levels at 12 and 24 weeks were similar to respective 4 week levels.

INDICATIONS AND USAGE

LUPRON DEPOT-PED is indicated in the treatment of children with central precocious puberty. Children should be selected using the following criteria:

1. Clinical diagnosis of CPP (idiopathic or neurogenic) with onset of secondary sexual characteristics earlier than 8 years in females and 9 years in males.
2. Clinical diagnosis should be confirmed prior to initiation of therapy:
   - Confirmation of diagnosis by a pubertal response to a GnRH stimulation test. The sensitivity and methodology of this assay must be understood.
   - Bone age advanced one year beyond the chronological age.
3. Baseline evaluation should also include:
   - Height and weight measurements.
   - Sex steroid levels.
   - Adrenal steroid level to exclude congenital adrenal hyperplasia.
   - Beta human chorionic gonadotropin level to rule out a chorionic gonadotropin-secreting tumor.
   - Pelvic/adrenal/testicular ultrasound to rule out a steroid secreting tumor.
   - Computerized tomography of the head to rule out intracranial tumor.

CONTRAINDICATIONS

LUPRON DEPOT-PED is contraindicated in women who are or may become pregnant while receiving the drug. When administered on day 6 of pregnancy at test dosages of 0.00024, 0.0024, and 0.024 mg/kg (1/1200 to 1/12 of the human pediatric dose) to rabbits, LUPRON DEPOT produced a dose-related increase in major fetal abnormalities. Similar studies in rats failed to demonstrate an increase in fetal malformations. There was increased fetal mortality and decreased fetal weights with the two higher doses of LUPRON DEPOT in rabbits and with the highest dose in rats. The effects on fetal mortality are logical consequences of the alterations in hormonal levels brought about by this drug. Therefore, the possibility exists that spontaneous abortion may occur if the drug is administered during pregnancy.
Leuprolide acetate is contraindicated in children demonstrating hypersensitivity to GnRH, GnRH agonist analogs, or any of the excipients.
A report of an anaphylactic reaction to synthetic GnRH (Factrel) has been reported in the medical literature.[1]

WARNINGS

During the early phase of therapy, gonadotropins and sex steroids rise above baseline because of the natural stimulatory effect of the drug. Therefore, an increase in clinical signs and symptoms may be observed. (See **CLINICAL PHARMACOLOGY** section.)
Noncompliance with drug regimen or inadequate dosing may result in inadequate control of the pubertal process. The consequences of poor control include the return of pubertal signs such as menses, breast development, and testicular growth. The long-term consequences of inadequate control of gonadal steroid secretion are unknown, but may include a further compromise of adult stature.

PRECAUTIONS

Laboratory Tests Response to LUPRON DEPOT-PED should be monitored 1–2 months after the start of therapy with a GnRH stimulation test and sex steroid levels. Measurement of bone age for advancement should be done every 6–12 months.
Sex steroids may increase or rise above prepubertal levels if the dose is inadequate. (See **WARNINGS** section.) Once a therapeutic dose has been established, gonadotropin and sex steroid levels will decline to prepubertal levels.
Drug Interactions No pharmacokinetic-based drug-drug interaction studies have been conducted. However, because leuprolide acetate is a peptide that is primarily degraded by peptidase and not by cytochrome P-450 enzymes as noted in specific studies, and the drug is only about 46% bound to plasma proteins, drug interactions would not be expected to occur.
Drug/Laboratory Test Interactions Administration of LUPRON DEPOT 3.75 mg in women results in suppression of the pituitary-gonadal system. Normal function is usually restored within three months after treatment is discontinued. Therefore, diagnostic tests of pituitary gonadotropic and gonadal functions conducted during treatment and for up to three months after discontinuation of LUPRON DEPOT may be misleading.
Information for Parents Prior to starting therapy with LUPRON DEPOT-PED, the parent or guardian must be aware of the importance of continuous therapy. Adherence to 4 week drug administration schedules must be accepted if therapy is to be successful.

- During the first 2 months of therapy, a female may experience menses or spotting. If bleeding continues beyond the second month, notify the physician.
- Any irritation at the injection site should be reported to the physician immediately.
- Report any unusual signs or symptoms to the physician.

Carcinogenesis, Mutagenesis, Impairment of Fertility A two-year carcinogenicity study was conducted in rats and mice. In rats, a dose-related increase of benign pituitary hyperplasia and benign pituitary adenomas was noted at 24 months when the drug was administered subcutaneously at high daily doses (0.6 to 4 mg/kg). There was a significant but not dose-related increase of pancreatic islet-cell adenomas in females and of testicular interstitial cell adenomas in males (highest incidence in the low dose group). In mice, no leuprolide acetate-induced tumors or pituitary abnormalities were observed at a dose as high as 60 mg/kg for two years. Adult patients have been treated with leuprolide acetate for up to three years with doses as high as 10 mg/day and for two years with doses as high as 20 mg/day without demonstrable pituitary abnormalities.
Although no clinical studies have been completed in children to assess the full reversibility of fertility suppression, animal studies (prepubertal and adult rats and monkeys) with leuprolide acetate and other GnRH analogs have shown functional recovery. However, following a study with leuprolide acetate, immature male rats demonstrated tubular degeneration in the testes even after a recovery period. In spite of the failure to recover histologically, the treated males proved to be as fertile as the controls. Also, no histologic changes were observed in the female rats following the same protocol. In both sexes, the offspring of the treated animals appeared normal. The effect of the treatment of the parents on the reproductive performance of the F1 generation was not tested. The clinical significance of these findings is unknown.
Pregnancy, Teratogenic Effects Pregnancy Category X. (See **CONTRAINDICATIONS** section.)
Nursing Mothers It is not known whether leuprolide acetate is excreted in human milk. LUPRON should not be used by nursing mothers.
Geriatric Use See also the labeling for LUPRON DEPOT 7.5 mg which is indicated for the palliative treatment of advanced prostate cancer. For LUPRON DEPOT-PED 11.25 mg and LUPRON DEPOT-PED 15 mg, no clinical information has been established for persons aged 65 and over.

ADVERSE REACTIONS

Clinical Trials
Potential exacerbation of signs and symptoms during the first few weeks of treatment (See **PRECAUTIONS** section.) is a concern in patients with rapidly advancing central precocious puberty.
In two studies of children with central precocious puberty, in 2% or more of the patients receiving the drug, the following adverse reactions were reported to have a possible or probable relationship to drug as ascribed by the treating physician. Reactions which are not considered drug-related are excluded.

	Number of Patients N=395	(%)
Body as a Whole		
General Pain	7	(2)
Integumentary System		
Acne/Seborrhea	7	(2)
Injection Site Reactions Including Abscess	21	(5)
Rash Including Erythema Multiforme	8	(2)
Urogenital System		
Vaginitis/Bleeding/ Discharge	7	(2)

In those same studies, the following adverse reactions were reported in less than 2% of the patients.
Body as a Whole - Body Odor, Fever, Headache, Infection; *Cardiovascular System* - Syncope, Vasodilation; *Digestive System* - Dysphagia, Gingivitis, Nausea/Vomiting; *Endocrine System* - Accelerated Sexual Maturity; *Metabolic and Nutritional Disorders* - Peripheral Edema, Weight Gain; *Nervous System* - Emotional Lability, Nervousness, Personality Disorder, Somnolence; *Respiratory System* - Epistaxis; *Integumentary System* - Alopecia, Skin Striae; *Urogenital System* - Cervix Disorder, Gynecomastia/Breast Disorders, Urinary Incontinence.

Postmarketing
During postmarketing surveillance, which includes other dosage forms, the following adverse events were reported. Symptoms consistent with an anaphylactoid or asthmatic process have been rarely reported. Rash, urticaria, and photosensitivity reactions have also been reported.
Localized reactions including induration and abscess have been reported at the site of injection.
Cardiovascular System - Hypotension; *Hemic and Lymphatic System* - Decreased WBC; *Central/Peripheral Nervous System* - Peripheral neuropathy, Spinal fracture/paralysis; *Musculoskeletal System* - Tenosynovitis-like symptoms; *Urogenital System* - Prostate pain.
See other LUPRON DEPOT and LUPRON Injection package inserts for other events reported in different patient populations.

OVERDOSAGE

In rats, subcutaneous administration of 125 to 250 times the recommended human pediatric dose, expressed on a per body weight basis, resulted in dyspnea, decreased activity, and local irritation at the injection site. There is no evidence at present that there is a clinical counterpart of this phenomenon. In early clinical trials using leuprolide acetate in adult patients, doses as high as 20 mg/day for up to two years caused no adverse effects differing from those observed with the 1 mg/day dose.

DOSAGE AND ADMINISTRATION

LUPRON DEPOT-PED must be administered under the supervision of a physician.
The dose of LUPRON DEPOT-PED must be individualized for each child. The dose is based on a mg/kg ratio of drug to body weight. Younger children require higher doses on a mg/kg ratio.
For each dosage form, after 1–2 months of initiating therapy or changing doses, the child must be monitored with a GnRH stimulation test, sex steroids, and Tanner staging to confirm downregulation. Measurements of bone age for advancement should be monitored every 6–12 months. The dose should be titrated upward until no progression of the condition is noted either clinically and/or by laboratory parameters.
The first dose found to result in adequate downregulation can probably be maintained for the duration of therapy in most children. However, there are insufficient data to guide dosage adjustment as patients move into higher weight categories after beginning therapy at very young ages and low dosages. It is recommended that adequate downregulation be verified in such patients whose weight has increased significantly while on therapy.
Discontinuation of LUPRON DEPOT-PED should be considered before age 11 for females and age 12 for males.
The recommended starting dose is 0.3 mg/kg/4 weeks (minimum 7.5 mg) administered as a single intramuscular injection. The starting dose will be dictated by the child's weight.

≤ 25 kg	7.5 mg
> 25–37.5 kg	11.25 mg
> 37.5 kg	15 mg

Continued on next page

Lupron Depot-PED—Cont.

If total downregulation is not achieved, the dose should be titrated upward in increments of 3.75 mg every 4 weeks. This dose will be considered the maintenance dose.
The lyophilized microspheres are to be reconstituted and administered as a single intramuscular injection. *For optimal performance of the prefilled dual chamber syringe (PDS), read and follow the following instructions:*

1. To prepare for injection, screw the white plunger into the end stopper until the stopper begins to turn.
2. Hold the syringe UPRIGHT. Release the diluent by SLOWLY PUSHING (6 to 8 seconds) the plunger until the first stopper is at the blue line in the middle of the barrel.
3. Keep the syringe UPRIGHT. Gently mix the microspheres (particles) thoroughly to form a uniform suspension. The suspension will appear milky.
4. Hold the syringe UPRIGHT. With the opposite hand pull the needle cap upward without twisting.
5. Keep the syringe UPRIGHT. Advance the plunger to expel the air from the syringe.
6. Inject the entire contents of the syringe intramuscularly at the time of reconstitution. The suspension settles very quickly following reconstitution; therefore, LUPRON DEPOT should be mixed and used immediately.

NOTE: Aspirated blood would be visible just below the luer lock connection if a blood vessel is accidentally penetrated. If present, blood can be seen through the transparent LuproLoc™ safety device.
AFTER INJECTION

7. Withdraw the needle. Immediately activate the LuproLoc™ safety device by pushing the arrow forward with the thumb or finger until the device is fully extended and a CLICK is heard or felt.

Since the product does not contain a preservative, the suspension should be discarded if not used immediately.
As with other drugs administered by injection, the injection site should be varied periodically.

HOW SUPPLIED

LUPRON DEPOT-PED is packaged as follows:

Kit with prefilled dual-chamber syringe	7.5 mg	NDC 0300-2108-01
Kit with prefilled dual-chamber syringe	11.25 mg	NDC 0300-2282-01
Kit with prefilled dual-chamber syringe	15 mg	NDC 0300-2440-01

Each syringe contains sterile lyophilized microspheres which is leuprolide incorporated in a biodegradable copolymer of lactic and glycolic acids. When mixed with diluent, LUPRON DEPOT-PED is administered as a single IM injection.
An information pamphlet for parents is included with the kit.
Store at 25°C (77°F); excursions permitted to 15–30°C (59–86°F) [See USP Controlled Room Temperature]

REFERENCE

1. MacLeod TL, *et al.* Anaphylactic reaction to synthetic luteinizing hormone-releasing hormone. *Fertil Steril* 1987 Sept; 48(3):500–502.

U.S. Patent Nos. 4,652,441; 4,677,191; 4,728,721; 4,849,228; 4,917,893; 5,330,767; 5,476,663; 5,823,997; 5,980,488; and 6,036,976. Other patents pending.
Manufactured for
TAP Pharmaceuticals Inc.
Lake Forest, IL 60045, U.S.A.
by Takeda Chemical Industries, Ltd.
Osaka, JAPAN 541
™ -Trademark
®—Registered Trademark
(Nos. 2108, 2282, 2440)
03-5326-R11; Revised: November, 2003

Shown in Product Identification Guide, page 334

PREVACID® ℞
[*prē-va-sĭd*]
(lansoprazole)
Delayed-Release Capsules

PREVACID® ℞
(lansoprazole)
For Delayed-Release Oral Suspension

PREVACID® SOLUTAB™ ℞
(lansoprazole)
Delayed-Release Orally Disintegrating Tablets

DESCRIPTION

The active ingredient in PREVACID (lansoprazole) Delayed-Release Capsules, PREVACID (lansoprazole) for Delayed-Release Oral Suspension and PREVACID SoluTab (lansoprazole) Delayed-Release Orally Disintegrating Tablets is a substituted benzimidazole, 2-[[[3-methyl-4-(2,2,2-trifluoroethoxy)-2-pyridyl] methyl] sulfinyl] benzimidazole, a compound that inhibits gastric acid secretion. Its empirical formula is $C_{16}H_{14}F_3N_3O_2S$ with a molecular weight of 369.37. The structural formula is:

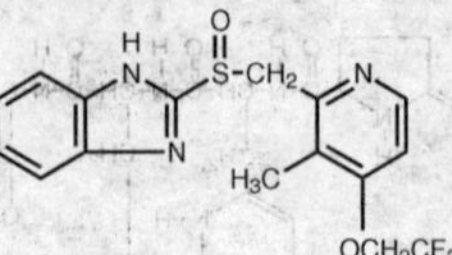

Lansoprazole is a white to brownish-white odorless crystalline powder which melts with decomposition at approximately 166°C. Lansoprazole is freely soluble in dimethylformamide; soluble in methanol; sparingly soluble in ethanol; slightly soluble in ethyl acetate, dichloromethane and acetonitrile; very slightly soluble in ether; and practically insoluble in hexane and water.
Lansoprazole is stable when exposed to light for up to two months. The rate of degradation of the compound in aqueous solution increases with decreasing pH. The degradation half-life of the drug substance in aqueous solution at 25°C is approximately 0.5 hour at pH 5.0 and approximately 18 hours at pH 7.0.
PREVACID is supplied in delayed-release capsules, in delayed-release orally disintegrating tablets for oral administration and in a packet for delayed-release oral suspension.
The delayed-release capsules contain the active ingredient, lansoprazole, in the form of enteric-coated granules and are available in two dosage strengths: 15 mg and 30 mg of lansoprazole per capsule. Each delayed-release capsule contains enteric-coated granules consisting of lansoprazole, hydroxypropyl cellulose, low substituted hydroxypropyl cellulose, colloidal silicon dioxide, magnesium carbonate, methacrylic acid copolymer, starch, talc, sugar sphere, sucrose, polyethylene glycol, polysorbate 80, and titanium dioxide. Components of the gelatin capsule include gelatin, titanium dioxide, D&C Red No. 28, FD&C Blue No. 1, FD&C Green No. 3*, and FD&C Red No. 40.
PREVACID for Delayed-Release Orally Disintegrating Tablets contain the active ingredient, lansoprazole in the form of enteric-coated microgranules. The tablets are available in 15 mg and 30 mg dosage strengths. Each tablet contains lansoprazole and the following inactive ingredients: lactose monohydrate, microcrystalline cellulose, magnesium carbonate, hydroxypropyl cellulose, hypromellose, titanium dioxide, talc, mannitol, methacrylic acid, polyacrylate, polyethylene glycol, glyceryl monostearate, polysorbate 80, triethyl citrate, ferric oxide, citric acid, crospovidone, aspartame**, artificial strawberry flavor and magnesium stearate.
PREVACID for Delayed-Release Oral Suspension is composed of the active ingredient, lansoprazole, in the form of enteric-coated granules and also contains inactive granules. The packets contain lansoprazole granules which are identical to those contained in PREVACID Delayed-Release Capsules and are available in 15 mg and 30 mg strengths. Inactive granules are composed of the following ingredients: confectioner's sugar, mannitol, docusate sodium, ferric oxide, colloidal silicon dioxide, xanthan gum, crospovidone, citric acid, sodium citrate, magnesium stearate, and artificial strawberry flavor. The lansoprazole granules and inactive granules, present in unit dose packets, are constituted with water to form a suspension and consumed orally.

* PREVACID 15-mg capsules only.
** **Phenylketonurics: Contains Phenylalanine 2.5 mg per 15 mg Tablet and 5.1 mg per 30 mg Tablet.**

CLINICAL PHARMACOLOGY

Pharmacokinetics and Metabolism
PREVACID Delayed-Release Capsules, PREVACID SoluTab Delayed-Release Orally Disintegrating Tablets and PREVACID for Delayed-Release Oral Suspension contain an enteric-coated granule formulation of lansoprazole. Absorption of lansoprazole begins only after the granules leave the stomach. Absorption is rapid, with mean peak plasma levels of lansoprazole occurring after approximately 1.7 hours. Peak plasma concentrations of lansoprazole (C_{max}) and the area under the plasma concentration curve (AUC) of lansoprazole are approximately proportional in doses from 15 mg to 60 mg after single-oral administration. Lansoprazole does not accumulate and its pharmacokinetics are unaltered by multiple dosing.
Absorption
The absorption of lansoprazole is rapid, with mean C_{max} occurring approximately 1.7 hours after oral dosing, and relatively complete with absolute bioavailability over 80%. In healthy subjects, the mean (±SD) plasma half-life was 1.5 (±1.0) hours. Both C_{max} and AUC are diminished by about 50% to 70% if the drug is given 30 minutes after food as opposed to the fasting condition. There is no significant food effect if the drug is given before meals.
Distribution
Lansoprazole is 97% bound to plasma proteins. Plasma protein binding is constant over the concentration range of 0.05 to 5.0 µg/mL.
Metabolism
Lansoprazole is extensively metabolized in the liver. Two metabolites have been identified in measurable quantities in plasma (the hydroxylated sulfinyl and sulfone derivatives of lansoprazole). These metabolites have very little or no antisecretory activity. Lansoprazole is thought to be transformed into two active species which inhibit acid secretion by (H^+,K^+)-ATPase within the parietal cell canaliculus, but are not present in the systemic circulation. The plasma elimination half-life of lansoprazole does not reflect its duration of suppression of gastric acid secretion. Thus, the plasma elimination half-life is less than two hours, while the acid inhibitory effect lasts more than 24 hours.
Elimination
Following single-dose oral administration of lansoprazole, virtually no unchanged lansoprazole was excreted in the urine. In one study, after a single oral dose of ^{14}C-lansoprazole, approximately one-third of the administered radiation was excreted in the urine and two-thirds was recovered in the feces. This implies a significant biliary excretion of the metabolites of lansoprazole.
Special Populations
Geriatric
The clearance of lansoprazole is decreased in the elderly, with elimination half-life increased approximately 50% to 100%. Because the mean half-life in the elderly remains between 1.9 to 2.9 hours, repeated once daily dosing does not result in accumulation of lansoprazole. Peak plasma levels were not increased in the elderly. No dosage adjustment is necessary in the elderly.
Pediatric
The pharmacokinetics of lansoprazole were studied in pediatric patients with GERD aged 1 to 11 years and 12 to 17 years in two separate clinical studies. In children aged 1 to 11 years, lansoprazole was dosed 15 mg q.d. for subjects weighing ≤ 30 kg and 30 mg q.d. for subjects weighing > 30 kg. Mean C_{max} and AUC values observed on Day 5 of dosing were similar between the two dose groups and were not affected by weight or age within each weight-adjusted dose group used in the study. In adolescent subjects aged 12 to 17 years, subjects were randomized to receive lansoprazole at 15 mg or 30 mg q.d. Mean C_{max} and AUC values of lansoprazole were not affected by body weight or age; and nearly dose-proportional increases in mean C_{max} and AUC values were observed between the two dose groups in the study. Overall, lansoprazole pharmacokinetics in pediatric patients aged 1 to 17 years were similar to those observed in healthy adult subjects.
Gender
In a study comparing 12 male and 6 female human subjects, no gender differences were found in pharmacokinetics and intragastric pH results. (Also see **Use in Women.**)
Renal Insufficiency
In patients with severe renal insufficiency, plasma protein binding decreased by 1.0%-1.5% after administration of 60 mg of lansoprazole. Patients with renal insufficiency had a shortened elimination half-life and decreased total AUC (free and bound). AUC for free lansoprazole in plasma, however, was not related to the degree of renal impairment, and C_{max} and T_{max} were not different from subjects with healthy kidneys. No dosage adjustment is necessary in patients with renal insufficiency.
Hepatic Insufficiency
In patients with various degrees of chronic hepatic disease, the mean plasma half-life of the drug was prolonged from 1.5 hours to 3.2-7.2 hours. An increase in mean AUC of up to 500% was observed at steady state in hepatically-impaired patients compared to healthy subjects. Dose reduction in patients with severe hepatic disease should be considered.
Race
The pooled mean pharmacokinetic parameters of lansoprazole from twelve U.S. Phase 1 studies (N=513) were compared to the mean pharmacokinetic parameters from two Asian studies (N=20). The mean AUCs of lansoprazole in Asian subjects were approximately twice those seen in pooled U.S. data; however, the inter-individual variability was high. The C_{max} values were comparable.
Pharmacodynamics
Mechanism of Action
Lansoprazole belongs to a class of antisecretory compounds, the substituted benzimidazoles, that do not exhibit anticholinergic or histamine H_2-receptor antagonist properties, but that suppress gastric acid secretion by specific inhibition of the (H^+,K^+)-ATPase enzyme system at the secretory surface of the gastric parietal cell. Because this enzyme system is regarded as the acid (proton) pump within the parietal cell, lansoprazole has been characterized as a gastric acid-pump inhibitor, in that it blocks the final step of acid production. This effect is dose-related and leads to inhibition of both basal and stimulated gastric acid secretion irrespective of the stimulus.
Antisecretory Activity
After oral administration, lansoprazole was shown to significantly decrease the basal acid output and significantly increase the mean gastric pH and percent of time the gastric pH was >3 and >4. Lansoprazole also significantly reduced meal-stimulated gastric acid output and secretion volume, as well as pentagastrin-stimulated acid output. In patients with hypersecretion of acid, lansoprazole significantly reduced basal and pentagastrin-stimulated gastric acid secretion. Lansoprazole inhibited the normal increases in secretion volume, acidity and acid output induced by insulin.
In a crossover study that included lansoprazole 15 and 30 mg for five days, the following effects on intragastric pH were noted:

Mean Antisecretory Effects After Single and Multiple Daily Dosing

Parameter	Baseline Value	PREVACID 15 mg Day 1	PREVACID 15 mg Day 5	PREVACID 30 mg Day 1	PREVACID 30 mg Day 5
Mean 24-Hour pH	2.1	2.7⁺	4.0⁺	3.6*	4.9*
Mean Nighttime pH	1.9	2.4	3.0⁺	2.6	3.8*
% Time Gastric pH>3	18	33⁺	59⁺	51*	72*
% Time Gastric pH>4	12	22⁺	49⁺	41*	66*

NOTE: An intragastric pH of >4 reflects a reduction in gastric acid by 99%.
*(p<0.05) versus baseline and lansoprazole 15 mg.
⁺(p<0.05) versus baseline only.

After the initial dose in this study, increased gastric pH was seen within 1-2 hours with lansoprazole 30 mg and 2-3 hours with lansoprazole 15 mg. After multiple daily dosing, increased gastric pH was seen within the first hour postdosing with lansoprazole 30 mg and within 1-2 hours postdosing with lansoprazole 15 mg.
Acid suppression may enhance the effect of antimicrobials in eradicating *Helicobacter pylori (H. pylori)*. The percentage of time gastric pH was elevated above 5 and 6 was evaluated in a crossover study of PREVACID given q.d., b.i.d. and t.i.d.

Mean Antisecretory Effects After 5 Days of b.i.d. and t.i.d. Dosing

Parameter	PREVACID 30 mg q.d.	PREVACID 15 mg b.i.d.	PREVACID 30 mg b.i.d.	PREVACID 30 mg t.i.d.
% Time Gastric pH>5	43	47	59⁺	77*
% Time Gastric pH>6	20	23	28	45*

⁺(p<0.05) versus PREVACID 30 mg q.d.
*(p<0.05) versus PREVACID 30 mg q.d., 15 mg b.i.d. and 30 mg b.i.d.

The inhibition of gastric acid secretion as measured by intragastric pH returns gradually to normal over two to four days after multiple doses. There is no indication of rebound gastric acidity.
Enterochromaffin-like (ECL) Cell Effects
During lifetime exposure of rats with up to 150 mg/kg/day of lansoprazole dosed seven days per week, marked hypergastrinemia was observed followed by ECL cell proliferation and formation of carcinoid tumors, especially in female rats. (See **PRECAUTIONS, Carcinogenesis, Mutagenesis, Impairment of Fertility.**)
Gastric biopsy specimens from the body of the stomach from approximately 150 patients treated continuously with lansoprazole for at least one year did not show evidence of ECL cell effects similar to those seen in rat studies. Longer term data are needed to rule out the possibility of an increased risk of the development of gastric tumors in patients receiving long-term therapy with lansoprazole.
Other Gastric Effects in Humans
Lansoprazole did not significantly affect mucosal blood flow in the fundus of the stomach. Due to the normal physiologic effect caused by the inhibition of gastric acid secretion, a decrease of about 17% in blood flow in the antrum, pylorus, and duodenal bulb was seen. Lansoprazole significantly slowed the gastric emptying of digestible solids. Lansoprazole increased serum pepsinogen levels and decreased pepsin activity under basal conditions and in response to meal stimulation or insulin injection. As with other agents that elevate intragastric pH, increases in gastric pH were associated with increases in nitrate-reducing bacteria and elevation of nitrite concentration in gastric juice in patients with gastric ulcer. No significant increase in nitrosamine concentrations was observed.
Serum Gastrin Effects
In over 2100 patients, median fasting serum gastrin levels increased 50% to 100% from baseline but remained within normal range after treatment with lansoprazole given orally in doses of 15 mg to 60 mg. These elevations reached a plateau within two months of therapy and returned to pretreatment levels within four weeks after discontinuation of therapy.
Endocrine Effects
Human studies for up to one year have not detected any clinically significant effects on the endocrine system. Hormones studied include testosterone, luteinizing hormone (LH), follicle stimulating hormone (FSH), sex hormone binding globulin (SHBG), dehydroepiandrosterone sulfate (DHEA-S), prolactin, cortisol, estradiol, insulin, aldosterone, parathormone, glucagon, thyroid stimulating hormone (TSH), triiodothyronine (T_3), thyroxine (T_4), and somatotropic hormone (STH). Lansoprazole in oral doses of 15 to 60 mg for up to one year had no clinically significant effect on sexual function. In addition, lansoprazole in oral doses of 15 to 60 mg for two to eight weeks had no clinically significant effect on thyroid function.
In 24-month carcinogenicity studies in Sprague-Dawley rats with daily dosages up to 150 mg/kg, proliferative changes in the Leydig cells of the testes, including benign neoplasm, were increased compared to control rates.

Other Effects
No systemic effects of lansoprazole on the central nervous system, lymphoid, hematopoietic, renal, hepatic, cardiovascular or respiratory systems have been found in humans. No visual toxicity was observed among 56 patients who had extensive baseline eye evaluations, were treated with up to 180 mg/day of lansoprazole and were observed for up to 58 months. Other rat-specific findings after lifetime exposure included focal pancreatic atrophy, diffuse lymphoid hyperplasia in the thymus, and spontaneous retinal atrophy.

MICROBIOLOGY

Lansoprazole, clarithromycin and/or amoxicillin have been shown to be active against most strains of *Helicobacter pylori in vitro* and in clinical infections as described in the **INDICATIONS AND USAGE** section.
Helicobacter
Helicobacter pylori
Pretreatment Resistance
Clarithromycin pretreatment resistance (≥2.0 μg/mL) was 9.5% (91/960) by E-test and 11.3% (12/106) by agar dilution in the dual and triple therapy clinical trials (M93-125, M93-130, M93-131, M95-392, and M95-399).
Amoxicillin pretreatment susceptible isolates (≤0.25 μg/mL) occurred in 97.8% (936/957) and 98.0% (98/100) of the patients in the dual and triple therapy clinical trials by E-test and agar dilution, respectively. Twenty-one of 957 patients (2.2%) by E-test and 2 of 100 patients (2.0%) by agar dilution had amoxicillin pretreatment MICs of >0.25 μg/mL. One patient on the 14-day triple therapy regimen had an unconfirmed pretreatment amoxicillin minimum inhibitory concentration (MIC) of >256 μg/mL by E-test and the patient was eradicated of *H. pylori.*

Clarithromycin Susceptibility Test Results and Clinical/Bacteriological Outcomes[a]

Clarithromycin Pretreatment Results	Clarithromycin Post-treatment Results: *H. pylori* negative – eradicated	*H. pylori* positive – not eradicated; Post-treatment susceptibility results: S[b]	I[b]	R[b]	No MIC
Triple Therapy 14-Day (lansoprazole 30 mg b.i.d./amoxicillin 1 gm b.i.d./clarithromycin 500 mg b.i.d.) (M95-399, M93-131, M95-392)					
Susceptible[b] 112	105				7
Intermediate[b] 3	3				
Resistant[b] 17	6			7	4
Triple Therapy 10-Day (lansoprazole 30 mg b.i.d./amoxicillin 1 gm b.i.d./clarithromycin 500 mg b.i.d.) (M95-399)					
Susceptible[b] 42	40	1		1	
Intermediate[b]					
Resistant[b] 4	1			3	

[a] Includes only patients with pretreatment clarithromycin susceptibility test results
[b] Susceptible (S) MIC ≤0.25 μg/mL, Intermediate (I) MIC 0.5-1.0 μg/mL, Resistant (R) MIC ≥2 μg/mL

Patients not eradicated of *H. pylori* following lansoprazole/amoxicillin/clarithromycin triple therapy will likely have clarithromycin resistant *H. pylori.* Therefore, for those patients who fail therapy, clarithromycin susceptibility testing should be done when possible. Patients with clarithromycin resistant *H. pylori* should not be treated with lansoprazole/amoxicillin/clarithromycin triple therapy or with regimens which include clarithromycin as the sole antimicrobial agent.
Amoxicillin Susceptibility Test Results and Clinical/Bacteriological Outcomes
In the dual and triple therapy clinical trials, 82.6% (195/236) of the patients that had pretreatment amoxicillin susceptible MICs (≤0.25 μg/mL) were eradicated of *H. pylori.* Of those with pretreatment amoxicillin MICs of >0.25 μg/mL, three of six had the *H. pylori* eradicated. A total of 30% (21/70) of the patients failed lansoprazole 30 mg t.i.d./amoxicillin 1 gm t.i.d. dual therapy and a total of 12.8% (22/172) of the patients failed the 10- and 14-day triple therapy regimens. Post-treatment susceptibility results were not obtained on 11 of the patients who failed therapy. Nine of the 11 patients with amoxicillin post-treatment MICs that failed the triple therapy regimen also had clarithromycin resistant *H. pylori* isolates.
Susceptibility Test for *Helicobacter pylori*
The reference methodology for susceptibility testing of *H. pylori* is agar dilution MICs.[1] One to three microliters of an inoculum equivalent to a No. 2 McFarland standard (1 × 10^7 – 1 × 10^8 CFU/mL for *H. pylori*) are inoculated directly onto freshly prepared antimicrobial-containing Mueller-Hinton agar plates with 5% aged defibrinated sheep blood (≥ 2 weeks old). The agar dilution plates are incubated at 35°C in a microaerobic environment produced by a gas generating system suitable for campylobacters. After 3 days of incubation, the MICs are recorded as the lowest concentration of antimicrobial agent required to inhibit growth of the organism. The clarithromycin and amoxicillin MIC values should be interpreted according to the following criteria:

Clarithromycin MIC (μg/mL)[a]	Interpretation
≤0.25	Susceptible (S)
0.5-1.0	Intermediate (I)
≥2.0	Resistant (R)
Amoxicillin MIC (μg/mL)[b]	**Interpretation**
≤0.25	Susceptible (S)

[a] These are tentative breakpoints for the agar dilution methodology and they should not be used to interpret results obtained using alternative methods.
[b] There were not enough organisms with MICs >0.25 μg/mL to determine a resistance breakpoint.

Standardized susceptibility test procedures require the use of laboratory control microorganisms to control the technical aspects of the laboratory procedures. Standard clarithromycin and amoxicillin powders should provide the following MIC values:

Microorganism	Antimicrobial Agent	MIC (μg/mL)[a]
H. pylori ATCC 43504	Clarithromycin	0.015-0.12 μg/mL
H. pylori ATCC 43504	Amoxicillin	0.015-0.12 μg/mL

[a] These are quality control ranges for the agar dilution methodology and they should not be used to control test results obtained using alternative methods.

REFERENCE

1. National Committee for Clinical Laboratory Standards. Summary Minutes, Subcommittee on Antimicrobial Susceptibility Testing, Tampa, FL, January 11-13, 1998.

CLINICAL STUDIES

Duodenal Ulcer

In a U.S. multicenter, double-blind, placebo-controlled, dose-response (15, 30, and 60 mg of PREVACID once daily) study of 284 patients with endoscopically documented duodenal ulcer, the percentage of patients healed after two and four weeks was significantly higher with all doses of PREVACID than with placebo. There was no evidence of a greater or earlier response with the two higher doses compared with PREVACID 15 mg. Based on this study and the second study described below, the recommended dose of PREVACID in duodenal ulcer is 15 mg per day.

Duodenal Ulcer Healing Rates

Week	PREVACID 15 mg q.d. (N=68)	PREVACID 30 mg q.d. (N=74)	PREVACID 60 mg q.d. (N=70)	Placebo (N=72)
2	42.4%*	35.6%*	39.1%*	11.3%
4	89.4%*	91.7%*	89.9%*	46.1%

*(p≤0.001) versus placebo.

PREVACID 15 mg was significantly more effective than placebo in relieving day and nighttime abdominal pain and in decreasing the amount of antacid taken per day.
In a second U.S. multicenter study, also double-blind, placebo-controlled, dose-comparison (15 and 30 mg of PREVACID once daily), and including a comparison with ranitidine, in 280 patients with endoscopically documented duodenal ulcer, the percentage of patients healed after four weeks was significantly higher with both doses of PREVACID than with placebo. There was no evidence of a greater or earlier response with the higher dose of PREVACID. Although the 15 mg dose of PREVACID was superior to ranitidine at 4 weeks, the lack of significant difference at 2 weeks and the absence of a difference between 30 mg of PREVACID and ranitidine leaves the comparative effectiveness of the two agents undetermined.

Duodenal Ulcer Healing Rates

Week	PREVACID 15 mg q.d. (N=80)	PREVACID 30 mg q.d. (N=77)	Ranitidine 300 mg h.s. (N=82)	Placebo (N=41)
2	35.0%	44.2%	30.5%	34.2%
4	92.3%**	80.3%*	70.5%*	47.5%

* (p≤0.05) versus placebo.
**(p≤0.05) versus placebo and ranitidine.

***H. pylori* Eradication to Reduce the Risk of Duodenal Ulcer Recurrence**

Randomized, double-blind clinical studies performed in the U.S. in patients with *H. pylori* and duodenal ulcer disease

Continued on next page

Prevacid—Cont.

(defined as an active ulcer or history of an ulcer within one year) evaluated the efficacy of PREVACID in combination with amoxicillin capsules and clarithromycin tablets as triple 14-day therapy or in combination with amoxicillin capsules as dual 14-day therapy for the eradication of *H. pylori*. Based on the results of these studies, the safety and efficacy of two different eradication regimens were established:

Triple therapy: PREVACID 30 mg b.i.d./
amoxicillin 1 gm b.i.d./
clarithromycin 500 mg b.i.d.

Dual therapy: PREVACID 30 mg t.i.d./
amoxicillin 1 gm t.i.d.

All treatments were for 14 days. *H. pylori* eradication was defined as two negative tests (culture and histology) at 4-6 weeks following the end of treatment.

Triple therapy was shown to be more effective than all possible dual therapy combinations. Dual therapy was shown to be more effective than both monotherapies. Eradication of *H. pylori* has been shown to reduce the risk of duodenal ulcer recurrence.

A randomized, double-blind clinical study performed in the U.S. in patients with *H. pylori* and duodenal ulcer disease (defined as an active ulcer or history of an ulcer within one year) compared the efficacy of PREVACID triple therapy for 10 and 14 days. This study established that the 10-day triple therapy was equivalent to the 14-day triple therapy in eradicating *H. pylori*.

H. pylori Eradication Rates – Triple Therapy
(PREVACID/amoxicillin/clarithromycin)
Percent of Patients Cured
[95% Confidence Interval]
(Number of patients)

Study	Duration	Triple Therapy Evaluable Analysis*	Triple Therapy Intent-to-Treat Analysis#
M93-131	14 days	92† [80.0-97.7] (N=48)	86† [73.3-93.5] (N=55)
M95-392	14 days	86‡ [75.7-93.6] (N=66)	83‡ [72.0-90.8] (N=70)
M95-399⁺	14 days	85 [77.0-91.0] (N=113)	82 [73.9-88.1] (N=126)
	10 days	84 [76.0-89.8] (N=123)	81 [73.9-87.6] (N=135)

*Based on evaluable patients with confirmed duodenal ulcer (active or within one year) and *H. pylori* infection at baseline defined as at least two of three positive endoscopic tests from CLOtest®, histology and/or culture. Patients were included in the analysis if they completed the study. Additionally, if patients dropped out of the study due to an adverse event related to the study drug, they were included in the evaluable analysis as failures of therapy.

Patients were included in the analysis if they had documented *H. pylori* infection at baseline as defined above and had a confirmed duodenal ulcer (active or within one year). All dropouts were included as failures of therapy.

† (p<0.05) versus PREVACID/amoxicillin and PREVACID/clarithromycin dual therapy

‡ (p<0.05) versus clarithromcyin/amoxicillin dual therapy

⁺ The 95% confidence interval for the difference in eradication rates, 10-day minus 14-day is (-10.5, 8.1) in the evaluable analysis and (-9.7, 9.1) in the intent-to-treat analysis.

H. pylori Eradication Rates – 14-Day Dual Therapy
(PREVACID/amoxicillin)
Percent of Patients Cured
[95% Confidence Interval]
(Number of patients)

Study	Dual Therapy Evaluable Analysis*	Dual Therapy Intent-to-Treat Analysis#
M93-131	77† [62.5-87.2] (N=51)	70† [56.8-81.2] (N=60)
M93-125	66‡ [51.9-77.5] (N=58)	61‡ [48.5-72.9] (N=67)

*Based on evaluable patients with confirmed duodenal ulcer (active or within one year) and *H. pylori* infection at baseline defined as at least two of three positive endoscopic tests from CLOtest®, histology and/or culture. Patients were included in the analysis if they completed the study. Additionally, if patients dropped out of the study due to an adverse event related to the study drug, they were included in the analysis as failures of therapy.

Patients were included in the analysis if they had documented *H. pylori* infection at baseline as defined above and had a confirmed duodenal ulcer (active or within one year). All dropouts were included as failures of therapy.

† (p<0.05) versus PREVACID alone.

‡ (p<0.05) versus PREVACID alone or amoxicillin alone.

Endoscopic Remission Rates

Trial	Drug	No. of Pts.	Percent in Endoscopic Remission 0-3 mo.	0-6 mo.	0-12 mo.
#1	PREVACID 15 mg q.d.	86	90%*	87%*	84%*
	Placebo	83	49%	41%	39%
#2	PREVACID 30 mg q.d.	18	94%*	94%*	85%*
	PREVACID 15 mg q.d.	15	87%*	79%*	70%*
	Placebo	15	33%	0%	0%

%=Life Table Estimate
* (p≤0.001) versus placebo.

Frequency of Heartburn

Variable	Placebo (n=43)	PREVACID 15 mg (n=80)	PREVACID 30 mg (n=86)
		—Median—	
% of Days without Hearburn			
Week 1	0%	71%*	46%*
Week 4	11%	81%*	76%*
Week 8	13%	84%*	82%*
% of Nights without Heartburn			
Week 1	17%	86%*	57%*
Week 4	25%	89%*	73%*
Week 8	36%	92%*	80%*

* (p<0.01) versus placebo.

Long-Term Maintenance Treatment of Duodenal Ulcers

PREVACID has been shown to prevent the recurrence of duodenal ulcers. Two independent, double-blind, multicenter, controlled trials were conducted in patients with endoscopically confirmed healed duodenal ulcers. Patients remained healed significantly longer and the number of recurrences of duodenal ulcers was significantly less in patients treated with PREVACID than in patients treated with placebo over a 12-month period.

[See first table above]

In trial #2, no significant difference was noted between PREVACID 15 mg and 30 mg in maintaining remission.

Gastric Ulcer

In a U.S. multicenter, double-blind, placebo-controlled study of 253 patients with endoscopically documented gastric ulcer, the percentage of patients healed at four and eight weeks was significantly higher with PREVACID 15 mg and 30 mg once a day than with placebo.

Gastric Ulcer Healing Rates

Week	PREVACID 15 mg q.d. (N=65)	30 mg q.d. (N=63)	60 mg q.d. (N=61)	Placebo (N=64)
4	64.6%*	58.1%*	53.3%*	37.5%
8	92.2%*	96.8%*	93.2%*	76.7%

* (p≤0.05) versus placebo.

Patients treated with any PREVACID dose reported significantly less day and night abdominal pain along with fewer days of antacid use and fewer antacid tablets used per day than the placebo group.

Independent substantiation of the effectiveness of PREVACID 30 mg was provided by a meta-analysis of published and unpublished data.

Healing of NSAID-Associated Gastric Ulcer

In two U.S. and Canadian multicenter, double-blind, active-controlled studies in patients with endoscopically confirmed NSAID-associated gastric ulcer who continued their NSAID use, the percentage of patients healed after 8 weeks was statistically significantly higher with 30 mg of PREVACID than with the active control. A total of 711 patients were enrolled in the study, and 701 patients were treated. Patients ranged in age from 18 to 88 years (median age 59 years), with 67% female patients and 33% male patients. Race was distributed as follows: 87% Caucasian, 8% Black, 5% other. There was no statistically significant difference between PREVACID 30 mg q.d. and the active control on symptom relief (i.e., abdominal pain).

NSAID-Associated Gastric Ulcer Healing Rates[1]

	PREVACID 30 mg q.d.	Active Control[2]
Study #1		
Week 4	60% (53/88)[3]	28% (23/83)
Week 8	79% (62/79)[3]	55% (41/74)
Study #2		
Week 4	53% (40/75)	38% (31/82)
Week 8	77% (47/61)[3]	50% (33/66)

[1] Actual observed ulcer(s) healed at time points ± 2 days
[2] Dose for healing of gastric ulcer
[3] (p≤0.05) versus the active control

Risk Reduction of NSAID-Associated Gastric Ulcer

In one large U.S., multicenter, double-blind, placebo- and misoprostol-controlled (misoprostol blinded only to the endoscopist) study in patients who required chronic use of an NSAID and who had a history of an endoscopically documented gastric ulcer, the proportion of patients remaining free from gastric ulcer at 4, 8, and 12 weeks was significantly higher with 15 or 30 mg of PREVACID than placebo. A total of 537 patients were enrolled in the study, and 535 patients were treated. Patients ranged in age from 23 to 89 years (median age 60 years), with 65% female patients and 35% male patients. Race was distributed as follows: 90% Caucasian, 6% Black, 4% other. The 30 mg dose of PREVACID demonstrated no additional benefit in risk reduction of the NSAID-associated gastric ulcer than the 15 mg dose.

NSAID-Associated Gastric Ulcer Risk Reduction Rates

% of Patients Remaining Gastric Ulcer-Free[1]

Week	PREVACID 15 mg q.d. (N=121)	PREVACID 30 mg q.d. (N=116)	Misoprostol 200 µg q.i.d. (N=106)	Placebo (N=112)
4	90%	92%	96%	66%
8	86%	88%	95%	60%
12	80%	82%	93%	51%

[1] % = Life Table Estimate
(p<0.001) PREVACID 15 mg q.d. versus placebo; PREVACID 30 mg q.d. versus placebo; and misoprostol 200 µg q.i.d. versus placebo.
(p<0.05) Misoprostol 200 µg q.i.d. versus PREVACID 15 mg q.d.; and misoprostol 200 µg q.i.d. versus PREVACID 30 mg q.d.

Gastroesophageal Reflux Disease (GERD)

Symptomatic GERD

In a U.S. multicenter, double-blind, placebo-controlled study of 214 patients with frequent GERD symptoms, but no esophageal erosions by endoscopy, significantly greater relief of heartburn associated with GERD was observed with the administration of lansoprazole 15 mg once daily up to 8 weeks than with placebo. No significant additional benefit from lansoprazole 30 mg once daily was observed.

The intent-to-treat analyses demonstrated significant reduction in frequency and severity of day and night heartburn. Data for frequency and severity for the 8-week treatment period were as follows:

[See second table above]
[See first figure at top of next column]
[See second figure at top of next column]

In two U.S., multicenter double-blind, ranitidine-controlled studies of 925 total patients with frequent GERD symptoms, but no esophageal erosions by endoscopy, lansoprazole 15 mg was superior to ranitidine 150 mg (b.i.d.) in decreasing the frequency and severity of day and night heartburn associated with GERD for the 8-week treatment period. No significant additional benefit from lansoprazole 30 mg once daily was observed.

Erosive Esophagitis

In a U.S. multicenter, double-blind, placebo-controlled study of 269 patients entering with an endoscopic diagnosis of

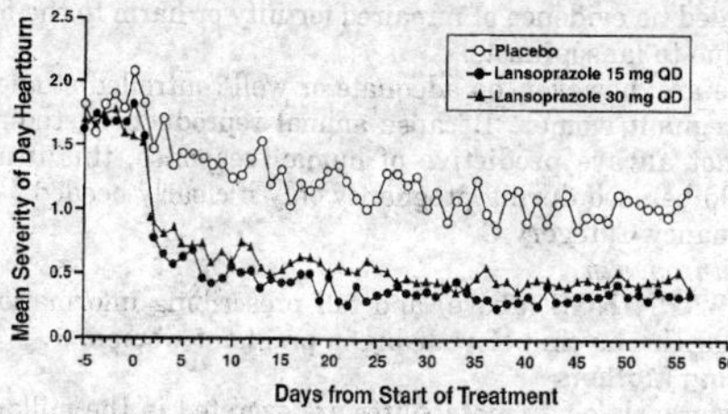

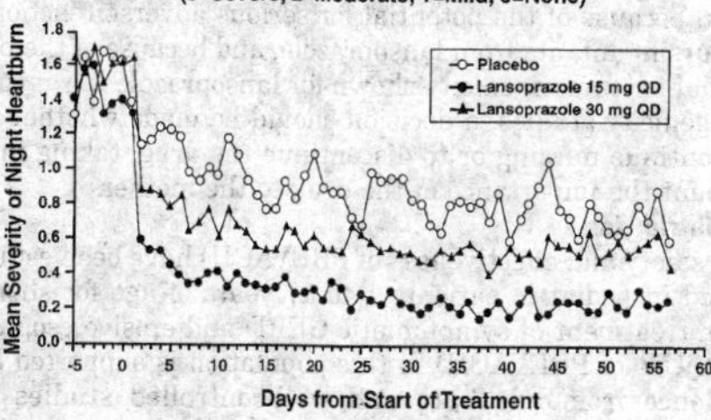

esophagitis with mucosal grading of 2 or more and grades 3 and 4 signifying erosive disease, the percentages of patients with healing were as follows:

Erosive Esophagitis Healing Rates

	PREVACID			Placebo
Week	15 mg q.d. (N=69)	30 mg q.d. (N=65)	60 mg q.d. (N=72)	(N=63)
4	67.6%*	81.3%*†	80.6%*†	32.8%
6	87.7%*	95.4%*	94.3%*	52.5%
8	90.9%*	95.4%*	94.4%*	52.5%

* ($p \leq 0.001$) versus placebo.
† ($p \leq 0.05$) versus PREVACID 15 mg.

In this study, all PREVACID groups reported significantly greater relief of heartburn and less day and night abdominal pain along with fewer days of antacid use and fewer antacid tablets taken per day than the placebo group.
Although all doses were effective, the earlier healing in the higher two doses suggests 30 mg q.d. as the recommended dose.
PREVACID was also compared in a U.S. multicenter, double-blind study to a low dose of ranitidine in 242 patients with erosive reflux esophagitis. PREVACID at a dose of 30 mg was significantly more effective than ranitidine 150 mg b.i.d. as shown below.

Erosive Esophagitis Healing Rates

Week	PREVACID 30 mg q.d. (N=115)	Ranitidine 150 mg b.i.d. (N=127)
2	66.7%*	38.7%
4	82.5%*	52.0%
6	93.0%*	67.8%
8	92.1%*	69.9%

* ($p \leq 0.001$) versus ranitidine.

In addition, patients treated with PREVACID reported less day and nighttime heartburn and took less antacid tablets for fewer days than patients taking ranitidine 150 mg b.i.d. Although this study demonstrates effectiveness of PREVACID in healing erosive esophagitis, it does not represent an adequate comparison with ranitidine because the recommended ranitidine dose for esophagitis is 150 mg q.i.d., twice the dose used in this study.
In the two trials described and in several smaller studies involving patients with moderate to severe erosive esophagitis, PREVACID produced healing rates similar to those shown above.
In a U.S. multicenter, double-blind, active-controlled study, 30 mg of PREVACID was compared with ranitidine 150 mg b.i.d. in 151 patients with erosive reflux esophagitis that was poorly responsive to a minimum of 12 weeks of treatment with at least one H_2-receptor antagonist given at the dose indicated for symptom relief or greater, namely, cimetidine 800 mg/day, ranitidine 300 mg/day, famotidine 40 mg/day or nizatidine 300 mg/day. PREVACID 30 mg was more effective than ranitidine 150 mg b.i.d. in healing reflux esophagitis, and the percentage of patients with healing were as follows. This study does not constitute a comparison of the effectiveness of histamine H_2-receptor antagonists with PREVACID, as all patients had demonstrated unresponsiveness to the histamine H_2-receptor antagonist mode of treatment. It does indicate, however, that PREVACID may be useful in patients failing on a histamine H_2-receptor antagonist.

Endoscopic Remission Rates

Trial	Drug	No. of Pts.	Percent in Endoscopic Remission 0-3 mo.	0-6 mo.	0-12 mo.
#1	PREVACID 15 mg q.d.	59	83%*	81%*	79%*
	PREVACID 30 mg q.d.	56	93%*	93%*	90%*
	Placebo	55	31%	27%	24%
#2	PREVACID 15 mg q.d.	50	74%*	72%*	67%*
	PREVACID 30 mg q.d.	49	75%*	72%*	55%*
	Placebo	47	16%	13%	13%

%=Life Table Estimate
* ($p \leq 0.001$) versus placebo.

Reflux Esophagitis Healing Rates in Patients Poorly Responsive to Histamine H_2-Receptor Antagonist Therapy

Week	PREVACID 30 mg q.d. (N=100)	Ranitidine 150 mg b.i.d. (N=51)
4	74.7%*	42.6%
8	83.7%*	32.0%

* ($p \leq 0.001$) versus ranitidine.

Long-Term Maintenance Treatment of Erosive Esophagitis
Two independent, double-blind, multicenter, controlled trials were conducted in patients with endoscopically confirmed healed esophagitis. Patients remained in remission significantly longer and the number of recurrences of erosive esophagitis was significantly less in patients treated with PREVACID than in patients treated with placebo over a 12-month period.
[See table above]
Regardless of initial grade of erosive esophagitis, PREVACID 15 mg and 30 mg were similar in maintaining remission.
In a U.S., randomized, double-blind, study, PREVACID 15 mg q.d. (n = 100) was compared with ranitidine 150 mg b.i.d. (n = 106), at the recommended dosage, in patients with endoscopically-proven healed erosive esophagitis over a 12-month period. Treatment with PREVACID resulted in patients remaining healed (Grade 0 lesions) of erosive esophagitis for significantly longer periods of time than those treated with ranitidine ($p<0.001$). In addition, PREVACID was significantly more effective than ranitidine in providing complete relief of both daytime and nighttime heartburn. Patients treated with PREVACID remained asymptomatic for a significantly longer period of time than patients treated with ranitidine.

Pathological Hypersecretory Conditions Including Zollinger-Ellison Syndrome
In open studies of 57 patients with pathological hypersecretory conditions, such as Zollinger-Ellison (ZE) syndrome with or without multiple endocrine adenomas, PREVACID significantly inhibited gastric acid secretion and controlled associated symptoms of diarrhea, anorexia and pain. Doses ranging from 15 mg every other day to 180 mg per day maintained basal acid secretion below 10 mEq/hr in patients without prior gastric surgery and below 5 mEq/hr in patients with prior gastric surgery.
Initial doses were titrated to the individual patient need, and adjustments were necessary with time in some patients. (See **DOSAGE AND ADMINISTRATION**.) PREVACID was well tolerated at these high dose levels for prolonged periods (greater than four years in some patients). In most ZE patients, serum gastrin levels were not modified by PREVACID. However, in some patients, serum gastrin increased to levels greater than those present prior to initiation of lansoprazole therapy.

INDICATIONS AND USAGE

PREVACID Delayed-Release Capsules, PREVACID SoluTab Delayed-Release Orally Disintegrating Tablets and PREVACID For Delayed-Release Oral Suspension are indicated for:

Short-Term Treatment of Active Duodenal Ulcer
PREVACID is indicated for short-term treatment (for 4 weeks) for healing and symptom relief of active duodenal ulcer.

***H. pylori* Eradication to Reduce the Risk of Duodenal Ulcer Recurrence**
Triple Therapy: PREVACID/amoxicillin/clarithromycin
PREVACID in combination with amoxicillin plus clarithromycin as triple therapy is indicated for the treatment of patients with *H. pylori* infection and duodenal ulcer disease (active or one-year history of a duodenal ulcer) to eradicate *H. pylori*. Eradication of *H. pylori* has been shown to reduce the risk of duodenal ulcer recurrence. (See **CLINICAL STUDIES** and **DOSAGE AND ADMINISTRATION**.)
Dual Therapy: PREVACID/amoxicillin
PREVACID in combination with amoxicillin as dual therapy is indicated for the treatment of patients with *H. pylori* infection and duodenal ulcer disease (active or one-year history of a duodenal ulcer) **who are either allergic or intolerant to clarithromycin or in whom resistance to clarithromycin is known or suspected.** (See the clarithromycin package insert, **MICROBIOLOGY** section.) Eradication of *H. pylori* has been shown to reduce the risk of duodenal ulcer recurrence. (See **CLINICAL STUDIES** and **DOSAGE AND ADMINISTRATION**.)

Maintenance of Healed Duodenal Ulcers
PREVACID is indicated to maintain healing of duodenal ulcers. Controlled studies do not extend beyond 12 months.

Short-Term Treatment of Active Benign Gastric Ulcer
PREVACID is indicated for short-term treatment (up to 8 weeks) for healing and symptom relief of active benign gastric ulcer.

Healing of NSAID-Associated Gastric Ulcer
PREVACID is indicated for the treatment of NSAID-associated gastric ulcer in patients who continue NSAID use. Controlled studies did not extend beyond 8 weeks.

Risk Reduction of NSAID-Associated Gastric Ulcer
PREVACID is indicated for reducing the risk of NSAID-associated gastric ulcers in patients with a history of a documented gastric ulcer who require the use of an NSAID. Controlled studies did not extend beyond 12 weeks.

Gastroesophageal Reflux Disease (GERD)
Short-Term Treatment of Symptomatic GERD
PREVACID is indicated for the treatment of heartburn and other symptoms associated with GERD.
Short-Term Treatment of Erosive Esophagitis
PREVACID is indicated for short-term treatment (up to 8 weeks) for healing and symptom relief of all grades of erosive esophagitis.
For patients who do not heal with PREVACID for 8 weeks (5-10%), it may be helpful to give an additional 8 weeks of treatment.
If there is a recurrence of erosive esophagitis an additional 8-week course of PREVACID may be considered.

Maintenance of Healing of Erosive Esophagitis
PREVACID is indicated to maintain healing of erosive esophagitis. Controlled studies did not extend beyond 12 months.

Pathological Hypersecretory Conditions Including Zollinger-Ellison Syndrome
PREVACID is indicated for the long-term treatment of pathological hypersecretory conditions, including Zollinger-Ellison syndrome.

CONTRAINDICATIONS

PREVACID is contraindicated in patients with known hypersensitivity to any component of the formulation of PREVACID.
Amoxicillin is contraindicated in patients with a known hypersensitivity to any penicillin.
Clarithromycin is contraindicated in patients with a known hypersensitivity to clarithromycin, erythromycin, and any of the macrolide antibiotics.
Concomitant administration of clarithromycin with cisapride, pimozide, astemizole, or terfenadine is contraindicated. There have been post-marketing reports of drug interactions when clarithromycin and/or erythromycin are co-administered with cisapride, pimozide, astemizole, or terfenadine resulting in cardiac arrhythmias (QT prolongation, ventricular tachycardia, ventricular fibrillation, and torsades de pointes) most likely due to inhibition of metabolism of these drugs by erythromycin and clarithromycin. Fatalities have been reported.
(Please refer to full prescribing information for amoxicillin and clarithromycin before prescribing.)

WARNINGS

CLARITHROMYCIN SHOULD NOT BE USED IN PREGNANT WOMEN EXCEPT IN CLINICAL CIRCUMSTANCES WHERE NO ALTERNATIVE THERAPY IS APPROPRIATE. IF PREGNANCY OCCURS WHILE TAKING CLARITHROMYCIN, THE PATIENT SHOULD BE APPRISED OF THE POTENTIAL HAZARD TO THE FETUS. (SEE **WARNINGS** IN PRESCRIBING INFORMATION FOR CLARITHROMYCIN.)
Pseudomembranous colitis has been reported with nearly all antibacterial agents, including clarithromycin and amoxicillin, and may range in severity from mild to life threatening. Therefore, it is important to consider this diagnosis in patients who present with diarrhea subsequent to the administration of antibacterial agents.
Treatment with antibacterial agents alters the normal flora of the colon and may permit overgrowth of clostridia. Studies indicate that a toxin produced by *Clostridium difficile* is a primary cause of "antibiotic-associated colitis."
After the diagnosis of pseudomembranous colitis has been established, therapeutic measures should be initiated. Mild cases of pseudomembranous colitis usually respond to discontinuation of the drug alone. In moderate to severe cases, consideration should be given to management with fluids and electrolytes, protein supplementation, and treatment with an antibacterial drug clinically effective against *Clostridium difficile* colitis.

Continued on next page

Prevacid—Cont.

Serious and occasionally fatal hypersensitivity (anaphylactic) reactions have been reported in patients on penicillin therapy. These reactions are more apt to occur in individuals with a history of penicillin hypersensitivity and/or a history of sensitivity to multiple allergens.

There have been well-documented reports of individuals with a history of penicillin hypersensitivity reactions who have experienced severe hypersensitivity reactions when treated with a cephalosporin. Before initiating therapy with any penicillin, careful inquiry should be made concerning previous hypersensitivity reactions to penicillins, cephalosporins, and other allergens. If an allergic reaction occurs, amoxicillin should be discontinued and the appropriate therapy instituted.

SERIOUS ANAPHYLACTIC REACTIONS REQUIRE IMMEDIATE EMERGENCY TREATMENT WITH EPINEPHRINE. OXYGEN, INTRAVENOUS STEROIDS, AND AIRWAY MANAGEMENT, INCLUDING INTUBATION, SHOULD ALSO BE ADMINISTERED AS INDICATED.

PRECAUTIONS

General

Symptomatic response to therapy with lansoprazole does not preclude the presence of gastric malignancy.

Information for Patients

PREVACID is available as a capsule, orally disintegrating tablet and oral suspension, and is available in 15 mg and 30 mg strengths. Directions for use specific to the route and available methods of administration for each of these dosage forms is presented below. PREVACID should be taken before eating. PREVACID products SHOULD NOT BE CRUSHED OR CHEWED.

Phenylketonurics: Contains Phenylalanine 2.5 mg per 15 mg Tablet and 5.1 mg per 30 mg Tablet.

Administration Options

1. PREVACID Delayed-Release Capsules

PREVACID Delayed-Release Capsules should be swallowed whole.

Alternatively, for patients who have difficulty swallowing capsules, PREVACID Delayed-Release Capsules can be opened and administered as follows:

- Open capsule.
- Sprinkle intact granules on one tablespoon of either applesauce, ENSURE® pudding, cottage cheese, yogurt or strained pears.
- Swallow immediately.

PREVACID Delayed-Release Capsules may also be emptied into a small volume of either apple juice, orange juice or tomato juice and administered as follows:

- Open capsule.
- Sprinkle intact granules into a small volume of either apple juice, orange juice or tomato juice (60 mL – approximately 2 ounces).
- Mix briefly.
- Swallow immediately.
- To ensure complete delivery of the dose, the glass should be rinsed with two or more volumes of juice and the contents swallowed immediately.

USE IN OTHER FOODS AND LIQUIDS HAS NOT BEEN STUDIED CLINICALLY AND IS THEREFORE NOT RECOMMENDED.

2. PREVACID SoluTab Delayed-Release Orally Disintegrating Tablets

PREVACID SoluTab should not be chewed. Place the tablet on the tongue and allow it to disintegrate, with or without water, until the particles can be swallowed. The tablet typically disintegrates in less than 1 minute.

Alternatively, for children or other patients who have difficulty swallowing tablets, PREVACID SoluTab can be delivered in two different ways.

PREVACID SoluTab – Oral Syringe

For administration via oral syringe, PREVACID SoluTab can be administered as follows:

- Place a 15 mg tablet in oral syringe and draw up approximately 4 mL of water, or place a 30 mg tablet in oral syringe and draw up approximately 10 mL of water.
- Shake gently to allow for a quick dispersal.
- After the tablet has dispersed, administer the contents within 15 minutes.
- Refill the syringe with approximately 2 mL (5 mL for the 30 mg tablet) of water, shake gently, and administer any remaining contents.

PREVACID SoluTab – Nasogastric Tube Administration (≥ 8 French)

For administration via a nasogastric tube, PREVACID SoluTab can be administered as follows:

- Place a 15 mg tablet in a syringe and draw up 4 mL of water, or place a 30 mg tablet in a syringe and draw up 10 mL of water.
- Shake gently to allow for a quick dispersal.
- After the tablet has dispersed, inject through the nasogastric tube into the stomach within 15 minutes.
- Refill the syringe with approximately 5 mL of water, shake gently, and flush the nasogastric tube.

3. PREVACID for Delayed-Release Oral Suspension

PREVACID for Delayed-Release Oral Suspension should be administered as follows:

- Open packet.
- To prepare a dose, empty the packet contents into a container containing 2 tablespoons of **WATER**. DO NOT USE OTHER LIQUIDS OR FOODS.
- Stir well, and drink immediately.
- If any material remains after drinking, add more water, stir, and drink immediately.
- **This product should not be given through enteral administration tubes.**

Drug Interactions

Lansoprazole is metabolized through the cytochrome P_{450} system, specifically through the CYP3A and CYP2C19 isozymes. Studies have shown that lansoprazole does not have clinically significant interactions with other drugs metabolized by the cytochrome P_{450} system, such as warfarin, antipyrine, indomethacin, ibuprofen, phenytoin, propranolol, prednisone, diazepam, or clarithromycin in healthy subjects. These compounds are metabolized through various cytochrome P_{450} isozymes including CYP1A2, CYP2C9, CYP2C19, CYP2D6, and CYP3A. When lansoprazole was administered concomitantly with theophylline (CYP1A2, CYP3A), a minor increase (10%) in the clearance of theophylline was seen. Because of the small magnitude and the direction of the effect on theophylline clearance, this interaction is unlikely to be of clinical concern. Nonetheless, individual patients may require additional titration of their theophylline dosage when lansoprazole is started or stopped to ensure clinically effective blood levels.

In a study of healthy subjects neither the pharmacokinetics of warfarin enantiomers nor prothrombin time were affected following single or multiple 60 mg doses of lansoprazole. However, there have been reports of increased International Normalized Ratio (INR) and prothrombin time in patients receiving proton pump inhibitors, including lansoprazole, and warfarin concomitantly. Increases in INR and prothrombin time may lead to abnormal bleeding and even death. Patients treated with proton pump inhibitors and warfarin concomitantly may need to be monitored for increases in INR and prothrombin time.

Lansoprazole has also been shown to have no clinically significant interaction with amoxicillin.

In a single-dose crossover study examining lansoprazole 30 mg and omeprazole 20 mg each administered alone and concomitantly with sucralfate 1 gram, absorption of the proton pump inhibitors was delayed and their bioavailability was reduced by 17% and 16%, respectively, when administered concomitantly with sucralfate. Therefore, proton pump inhibitors should be taken at least 30 minutes prior to sucralfate. In clinical trials, antacids were administered concomitantly with PREVACID Delayed-Release Capsules; this did not interfere with its effect.

Lansoprazole causes a profound and long-lasting inhibition of gastric acid secretion; therefore, it is theoretically possible that lansoprazole may interfere with the absorption of drugs where gastric pH is an important determinant of bioavailability (e.g., ketoconazole, ampicillin esters, iron salts, digoxin).

Carcinogenesis, Mutagenesis, Impairment of Fertility

In two 24-month carcinogenicity studies, Sprague-Dawley rats were treated orally with doses of 5 to 150 mg/kg/day, about 1 to 40 times the exposure on a body surface (mg/m^2) basis, of a 50-kg person of average height (1.46 m^2 body surface area) given the recommended human dose of 30 mg/day (22.2 mg/m^2). Lansoprazole produced dose-related gastric enterochromaffin-like (ECL) cell hyperplasia and ECL cell carcinoids in both male and female rats. It also increased the incidence of intestinal metaplasia of the gastric epithelium in both sexes. In male rats, lansoprazole produced a dose-related increase of testicular interstitial cell adenomas. The incidence of these adenomas in rats receiving doses of 15 to 150 mg/kg/day (4 to 40 times the recommended human dose based on body surface area) exceeded the low background incidence (range = 1.4 to 10%) for this strain of rat. Testicular interstitial cell adenoma also occurred in 1 of 30 rats treated with 50 mg/kg/day (13 times the recommended human dose based on body surface area) in a 1-year toxicity study.

In a 24-month carcinogenicity study, CD-1 mice were treated orally with doses of 15 to 600 mg/kg/day, 2 to 80 times the recommended human dose based on body surface area. Lansoprazole produced a dose-related increased incidence of gastric ECL cell hyperplasia. It also produced an increased incidence of liver tumors (hepatocellular adenoma plus carcinoma). The tumor incidences in male mice treated with 300 and 600 mg/kg/day (40 to 80 times the recommended human dose based on body surface area) and female mice treated with 150 to 600 mg/kg/day (20 to 80 times the recommended human dose based on body surface area) exceeded the ranges of background incidences in historical controls for this strain of mice. Lansoprazole treatment produced adenoma of rete testis in male mice receiving 75 to 600 mg/kg/day (10 to 80 times the recommended human dose based on body surface area).

Lansoprazole was not genotoxic in the Ames test, the *ex vivo* rat hepatocyte unscheduled DNA synthesis (UDS) test, the *in vivo* mouse micronucleus test or the rat bone marrow cell chromosomal aberration test. It was positive in *in vitro* human lymphocyte chromosomal aberration assays.

Lansoprazole at oral doses up to 150 mg/kg/day (40 times the recommended human dose based on body surface area) was found to have no effect on fertility and reproductive performance of male and female rats.

Pregnancy: Teratogenic Effects.

Pregnancy Category B

Lansoprazole

Teratology studies have been performed in pregnant rats at oral doses up to 150 mg/kg/day (40 times the recommended human dose based on body surface area) and pregnant rabbits at oral doses up to 30 mg/kg/day (16 times the recommended human dose based on body surface area) and have revealed no evidence of impaired fertility or harm to the fetus due to lansoprazole.

There are, however, no adequate or well-controlled studies in pregnant women. Because animal reproduction studies are not always predictive of human response, this drug should be used during pregnancy only if clearly needed.

Pregnancy Category C

Clarithromycin

See **WARNINGS** (above) and full prescribing information for clarithromycin before using in pregnant women.

Nursing Mothers

Lansoprazole or its metabolites are excreted in the milk of rats. It is not known whether lansoprazole is excreted in human milk. Because many drugs are excreted in human milk, because of the potential for serious adverse reactions in nursing infants from lansoprazole, and because of the potential for tumorigenicity shown for lansoprazole in rat carcinogenicity studies, a decision should be made whether to discontinue nursing or to discontinue the drug, taking into account the importance of the drug to the mother.

Pediatric Use

The safety and effectiveness of PREVACID have been established in pediatric patients 1 to 17 years of age for short-term treatment of symptomatic GERD and erosive esophagitis. Use of PREVACID in this population is supported by evidence from adequate and well-controlled studies of PREVACID in adults with additional clinical, pharmacokinetic, and pharmacodynamic studies performed in pediatric patients. The adverse events profile in pediatric patients is similar to that of adults. There were no adverse events reported in U.S. clinical studies that were not previously observed in adults. The safety and effectiveness of PREVACID in patients <1 year of age have not been established.

1 to 11 years of age

In an uncontrolled, open-label, U.S. multicenter study, 66 pediatric patients (1 to 11 years of age) with GERD were assigned, based on body weight, to receive an initial dose of either PREVACID 15 mg q.d. if ≤ 30 kg or PREVACID 30 mg q.d. if > 30 kg administered for 8 to 12 weeks. The PREVACID dose was increased (up to 30 mg b.i.d.) in 24 of 66 pediatric patients after 2 or more weeks of treatment if they remained symptomatic. At baseline 85% of patients had mild to moderate overall GERD symptoms (assessed by investigator interview), 58% had non-erosive GERD and 42% had erosive esophagitis (assessed by endoscopy).

After 8 to 12 weeks of PREVACID treatment, the intent-to-treat analysis demonstrated an approximate 50% reduction in frequency and severity of GERD symptoms.

Twenty-one of 27 erosive esophagitis patients were healed at 8 weeks and 100% of patients were healed at 12 weeks by endoscopy.

GERD symptom improvement and Erosive Esophagitis healing rates in pediatric patients age 1 to 11

GERD	Final Visit[a] % (n/N)
Symptomatic GERD	
Improvement in Overall GERD Symptoms[b]	76% (47/62[c])
Erosive Esophagitis	
Improvement in Overall GERD Symptoms[b]	81% (22/27)
Healing Rate	100% (27/27)

[a] At Week 8 or Week 12
[b] Symptoms assessed by patients diary kept by caregiver.
[c] No data were available for 4 pediatric patients.

In a study of 66 pediatric patients in the age group 1 year to 11 years old after treatment with PREVACID given orally in doses of 15 mg q.d. to 30 mg b.i.d., increases in serum gastrin levels were similar to those observed in adult studies. Median fasting serum gastrin levels increased 89% from 51 pg/mL at baseline to 97 pg/mL [interquartile range (25th-75th percentile) of 71-130 pg/mL] at the final visit.

The pediatric safety of PREVACID Delayed-Release Capsules has been assessed in 66 pediatric patients aged 1 to 11 years of age. Of the 66 patients with GERD 85% (56/66) took PREVACID for 8 weeks and 15% (10/66) took it for 12 weeks.

The most frequently reported (2 or more patients) treatment-related adverse events in patients 1 to 11 years of age (N=66) were constipation (5%) and headache (3%).

12 to 17 years of age

In an uncontrolled, open-label, U.S. multicenter study, 87 adolescent patients (12 to 17 years of age) with symptomatic GERD were treated with PREVACID for 8 to 12 weeks. Baseline upper endoscopies classified these patients into two groups: 64 (74%) nonerosive GERD and 23 (26%) erosive esophagitis (EE). The nonerosive GERD patients received PREVACID 15 mg q.d. for 8 weeks and the EE patients received PREVACID 30 mg q.d. for 8 to 12 weeks. At baseline, 89% of these patients had mild to moderate overall GERD symptoms (assessed by investigator interviews). During 8 weeks of PREVACID treatment, adolescent patients experienced a 63% reduction in frequency and a 69% reduction in severity of GERD symptoms based on diary results.

Twenty-one of 22 (95.5%) adolescent erosive esophagitis patients were healed after 8 weeks of PREVACID treatment. One patient remained unhealed after 12 weeks of treatment.

GERD symptom improvement and Erosive Esophagitis healing rates in pediatric patients age 12 to 17

GERD	Final Visit % (n/N)
Symptomatic GERD (All Patients) Improvement in Overall GERD Symptoms[a]	73.2% (60/82)[b]
Nonerosive GERD Improvement in Overall GERD Symptoms[a]	71.2% (42/59)[b]
Erosive Esophagitis Improvement in Overall GERD Symptoms[a]	78.3% (18/23)
Healing Rate[c]	95.5% (21/22)[c]

[a] Symptoms assessed by patient diary (parents/caregivers as necessary).
[b] No data available for 5 patients.
[c] Data from one healed patient was excluded from this analysis due to timing of final endoscopy.

In these 87 adolescent patients, increases in serum gastrin levels were similar to those observed in adult studies, median fasting serum gastrin levels increased 42% from 45 pg/mL at baseline to 64 pg/mL [interquartile range (25th–75th percentile) of 44–88 pg/mL] at the final visit. (Normal serum gastrin levels are 25 to 111 pg/mL.)

The safety of PREVACID Delayed-Release Capsules has been assessed in these 87 adolescent patients. Of the 87 adolescent patients with GERD, 6% (5/87) took PREVACID for <6 weeks, 93% (81/87) for 6–10 weeks, and 1% (1/87) for >10 weeks.

The most frequently reported (at least 3%) treatment-related adverse events in these patients were headache (7%), abdominal pain (5%), nausea (3%) and dizziness (3%). Treatment-related dizziness, reported in this package insert as occurring in <1% of adult patients, was reported in this study by 3 adolescent patients with nonerosive GERD, who had dizziness concurrently with other events (such as migraine, dyspnea, and vomiting).

Use in Women

Over 4,000 women were treated with lansoprazole. Ulcer healing rates in females were similar to those in males. The incidence rates of adverse events were also similar to those seen in males.

Use in Geriatric Patients

Ulcer healing rates in elderly patients are similar to those in a younger age group. The incidence rates of adverse events and laboratory test abnormalities are also similar to those seen in younger patients. For elderly patients, dosage and administration of lansoprazole need not be altered for a particular indication.

ADVERSE REACTIONS

Clinical

Worldwide, over 10,000 patients have been treated with lansoprazole in Phase 2-3 clinical trials involving various dosages and durations of treatment. The adverse reaction profiles for PREVACID Delayed-Release Capsules and PREVACID for Delayed-Release Oral Suspension are similar. In general, lansoprazole treatment has been well-tolerated in both short-term and long-term trials.

The following adverse events were reported by the treating physician to have a possible or probable relationship to drug in 1% or more of PREVACID-treated patients and occurred at a greater rate in PREVACID-treated patients than placebo-treated patients:

Incidence of Possibly or Probably Treatment-Related Adverse Events in Short-Term, Placebo-Controlled Studies

Body System/ Adverse Event	PREVACID (N=2768) %	Placebo (N=1023) %
Body as a Whole		
Abdominal Pain	2.1	1.2
Digestive System		
Constipation	1.0	0.4
Diarrhea	3.8	2.3
Nausea	1.3	1.2

Headache was also seen at greater than 1% incidence but was more common on placebo. The incidence of diarrhea was similar between patients who received placebo and patients who received lansoprazole 15 mg and 30 mg, but higher in the patients who received lansoprazole 60 mg (2.9%, 1.4%, 4.2%, and 7.4%, respectively).

The most commonly reported possibly or probably treatment-related adverse event during maintenance therapy was diarrhea.

In the risk reduction study of PREVACID for NSAID-associated gastric ulcers, the incidence of diarrhea for patients treated with PREVACID was 5%, misoprostol 22%, and placebo 3%.

Indication	Recommended Dose	Frequency	For Additional Information, See
Duodenal Ulcers			
Short-Term Treatment	15 mg	Once daily for 4 weeks	INDICATIONS AND USAGE CLINICAL STUDIES
Maintenance of Healed	15 mg	Once daily	
***H. pylori* Eradication to Reduce the Risk of Duodenal Ulcer Recurrence†**			
Triple Therapy:			INDICATIONS AND USAGE
PREVACID	30 mg	Twice daily (q12h) for 10 or 14 days	
Amoxicillin	1 gram	Twice daily (q12h) for 10 or 14 days	
Clarithromycin	500 mg	Twice daily (q12h) for 10 or 14 days	
Dual Therapy:			INDICATIONS AND USAGE
PREVACID	30 mg	Three times daily (q8h) for 14 days	
Amoxicillin	1 gram	Three times daily (q8h) for 14 days	
Benign Gastric Ulcer			
Short-Term Treatment	30 mg	Once daily for up to 8 weeks	CLINICAL STUDIES
NSAID-associated Gastric Ulcer			CLINICAL STUDIES
Healing	30 mg	Once daily for 8 weeks*	
Risk Reduction	15 mg	Once daily for up to 12 weeks*	
Gastroesophageal Reflux Disease (GERD)			
Short-Term Treatment of Symptomatic GERD	15 mg	Once daily for up to 8 weeks	CLINICAL STUDIES
Short-Term Treatment of Erosive Esophagitis	30 mg	Once daily for up to 8 weeks**	INDICATIONS AND USAGE
Pediatric (1 to 11 years of age) Short-Term Treatment of Symptomatic GERD and Short-Term Treatment of Erosive Esophagitis			PEDIATRIC USE
≤ 30 kg	15 mg	Once daily for up to 12 weeks+	
> 30 kg	30 mg	Once daily for up to 12 weeks+	
(12 to 17 years of age) Short-Term Treatment of Symptomatic GERD			
Nonerosive GERD	15 mg	Once daily for up to 8 weeks	
Erosive Esophagitis	30 mg	Once daily for up to 8 weeks	
Maintenance of Healing of Erosive Esophagitis	15 mg	Once daily	CLINICAL STUDIES
Pathological Hypersecretory Conditions Including Zollinger-Ellison Syndrome	60 mg	Once daily***	CLINICAL STUDIES

† Please refer to amoxicillin and clarithromycin full prescribing information for **CONTRAINDICATIONS** and **WARNINGS**, and for information regarding dosing in elderly and renally-impaired patients.
* Controlled studies did not extend beyond indicated duration.
** For patients who do not heal with PREVACID for 8 weeks (5–10%), it may be helpful to give an additional 8 weeks of treatment. If there is a recurrence of erosive esophagitis, an additional 8 week course of PREVACID may be considered.
*** Varies with individual patient. Recommended adult starting dose is 60 mg once daily. Doses should be adjusted to individual patient needs and should continue for as long as clinically indicated. Dosages up to 90 mg b.i.d. have been administered. Daily dose of greater than 120 mg should be administered in divided doses. Some patients with Zollinger-Ellison Syndrome have been treated continuously with PREVACID for more than 4 years.
+ The PREVACID dose was increased (up to 30 mg b.i.d.) in some pediatric patients after 2 or more weeks of treatment if they remained symptomatic. For pediatric patients unable to swallow an intact capsule please see **Administration Options**.

Additional adverse experiences occurring in <1% of patients or subjects in domestic trials are shown below. Refer to **Postmarketing** for adverse reactions occurring since the drug was marketed.

Body as a Whole – abdomen enlarged, allergic reaction, asthenia, back pain, candidiasis, carcinoma, chest pain (not otherwise specified), chills, edema, fever, flu syndrome, halitosis, infection (not otherwise specified), malaise, neck pain, neck rigidity, pain, pelvic pain; *Cardiovascular System* - angina, arrhythmia, bradycardia, cerebrovascular accident/cerebral infarction, hypertension/hypotension, migraine, myocardial infarction, palpitations, shock (circulatory failure), syncope, tachycardia, vasodilation; *Digestive System* – abnormal stools, anorexia, bezoar, cardiospasm, cholelithiasis, colitis, dry mouth, dyspepsia, dysphagia, enteritis, eructation, esophageal stenosis, esophageal ulcer, esophagitis, fecal discoloration, flatulence, gastric nodules/fundic gland polyps, gastritis, gastroenteritis, gastrointestinal anomaly, gastrointestinal disorder, gastrointestinal hemorrhage, glossitis, gum hemorrhage, hematemesis, increased appetite, increased salivation, melena, mouth ulceration, nausea and vomiting, nausea and vomiting and diarrhea, oral moniliasis, rectal disorder, rectal hemorrhage, stomatitis, tenesmus, thirst, tongue disorder, ulcerative colitis, ulcerative stomatitis; *Endocrine System* - diabetes mellitus, goiter, hypothyroidism; *Hemic and Lymphatic System* - anemia, hemolysis, lymphadenopathy; *Metabolic and Nutritional Disorders* - gout, dehydration, hyperglycemia/hypoglycemia, peripheral edema, weight gain/loss; *Musculoskeletal System* - arthralgia, arthritis, bone disorder, joint disorder, leg cramps, musculoskeletal pain, myalgia, myasthenia, synovitis; *Nervous System* – abnormal dreams, agitation, amnesia, anxiety, apathy, confusion, convulsion, depersonalization, depression, diplopia, dizziness, emotional lability, hallucinations, hemiplegia, hostility aggravated, hyperkinesia, hypertonia, hypesthesia, insomnia, libido decreased/increased, nervousness, neurosis, paresthesia, sleep disorder, somnolence, thinking abnormality, tremor, vertigo; *Respiratory System* - asthma, bronchitis, cough increased, dyspnea, epistaxis, hemoptysis, hiccup, laryngeal neoplasia, pharyngitis, pleural disorder, pneumonia, respiratory disorder, upper respiratory inflammation/infection, rhinitis, sinusitis, stridor; *Skin and Appendages* - acne, alopecia, contact dermatitis, dry skin, fixed eruption, hair disorder, maculopapular rash, nail disorder, pruritus, rash, skin carcinoma, skin disorder, sweating, urticaria; *Special Senses* – abnormal vision, blurred vision, conjunctivitis, deafness, dry eyes, ear disorder, eye pain, otitis media, parosmia, photophobia, retinal degeneration, taste loss, taste perversion, tinnitus, visual field defect; *Urogenital System* - abnormal menses, breast enlargement, breast pain, breast tenderness, dysmenorrhea, dysuria, gynecomastia, impotence, kidney calculus, kidney pain, leukorrhea, menorrhagia, menstrual disorder, penis disorder, polyuria, testis disorder, urethral pain, urinary frequency, urinary tract infection, urinary urgency, urination impaired, vaginitis.

Postmarketing

On-going Safety Surveillance: Additional adverse experiences have been reported since lansoprazole has been marketed. The majority of these cases are foreign-sourced and a relationship to lansoprazole has not been established. Because these events were reported voluntarily from a population of unknown size, estimates of frequency cannot be made. These events are listed below by COSTART body system.

Body as a Whole - anaphylactoid-like reaction; *Digestive System* - hepatotoxicity, pancreatitis, vomiting; *Hemic and Lymphatic System* - agranulocytosis, aplastic anemia, hemolytic anemia, leukopenia, neutropenia, pancytopenia, thrombocytopenia, and thrombotic thrombocytopenic purpura; *Skin and Appendages* – severe dermatologic reactions including erythema multiforme, Stevens-Johnson syn-

Continued on next page

Prevacid—Cont.

drome, toxic epidermal necrolysis (some fatal); *Special Senses* - speech disorder; *Urogenital System* - urinary retention.

Combination Therapy with Amoxicillin and Clarithromycin

In clinical trials using combination therapy with PREVACID plus amoxicillin and clarithromycin, and PREVACID plus amoxicillin, no adverse reactions peculiar to these drug combinations were observed. Adverse reactions that have occurred have been limited to those that had been previously reported with PREVACID, amoxicillin, or clarithromycin.

Triple Therapy: PREVACID/amoxicillin/clarithromycin

The most frequently reported adverse events for patients who received triple therapy for 14 days were diarrhea (7%), headache (6%), and taste perversion (5%). There were no statistically significant differences in the frequency of reported adverse events between the 10- and 14-day triple therapy regimens. No treatment-emergent adverse events were observed at significantly higher rates with triple therapy than with any dual therapy regimen.

Dual Therapy: PREVACID/amoxicillin

The most frequently reported adverse events for patients who received PREVACID t.i.d. plus amoxicillin t.i.d. dual therapy were diarrhea (8%) and headache (7%). No treatment-emergent adverse events were observed at significantly higher rates with PREVACID t.i.d. plus amoxicillin t.i.d. dual therapy than with PREVACID alone.

For more information on adverse reactions with amoxicillin or clarithromycin, refer to their package inserts, **ADVERSE REACTIONS** sections.

Laboratory Values

The following changes in laboratory parameters for lansoprazole were reported as adverse events:

Abnormal liver function tests, increased SGOT (AST), increased SGPT (ALT), increased creatinine, increased alkaline phosphatase, increased globulins, increased GGTP, increased/decreased/abnormal WBC, abnormal AG ratio, abnormal RBC, bilirubinemia, eosinophilia, hyperlipemia, increased/decreased electrolytes, increased/decreased cholesterol, increased glucocorticoids, increased LDH, increased/decreased/abnormal platelets, and increased gastrin levels. Urine abnormalities such as albuminuria, glycosuria, and hematuria were also reported. Additional isolated laboratory abnormalities were reported.

In the placebo controlled studies, when SGOT (AST) and SGPT (ALT) were evaluated, 0.4% (4/978) placebo patients and 0.4% (11/2677) lansoprazole patients had enzyme elevations greater than three times the upper limit of normal range at the final treatment visit. None of these lansoprazole patients reported jaundice at any time during the study.

In clinical trials using combination therapy with PREVACID plus amoxicillin and clarithromycin, and PREVACID plus amoxicillin, no increased laboratory abnormalities particular to these drug combinations were observed.

For more information on laboratory value changes with amoxicillin or clarithromycin, refer to their package inserts, **ADVERSE REACTIONS** section.

OVERDOSAGE

Oral doses up to 5000 mg/kg in rats (approximately 1300 times the recommended human dose based on body surface area) and mice (about 675.7 times the recommended human dose based on body surface area) did not produce deaths or any clinical signs.

Lansoprazole is not removed from the circulation by hemodialysis. In one reported case of overdose, the patient consumed 600 mg of lansoprazole with no adverse reaction.

DOSAGE AND ADMINISTRATION

PREVACID is available as a capsule, orally disintegrating tablet and oral suspension, and is available in 15 mg and 30 mg strengths. Directions for use specific to the route and available methods of administration for each of these dosage forms is presented below. PREVACID should be taken before eating. PREVACID products SHOULD NOT BE CRUSHED OR CHEWED. In the clinical trials, antacids were used concomitantly with PREVACID.

No dosage adjustment is necessary in patients with renal insufficiency or the elderly. For patients with severe liver disease, dosage adjustment should be considered.

[See table at top of previous page]

Administration Options

1. PREVACID Delayed-Release Capsules

PREVACID Capsules-Oral Administration

PREVACID Delayed-Release Capsules should be swallowed whole.

Alternatively, for patients who have difficulty swallowing capsules, PREVACID Delayed-Release Capsules can be opened and administered as follows:

- Open capsule.
- Sprinkle intact granules on one tablespoon of either applesauce, ENSURE® pudding, cottage cheese, yogurt or strained pears.
- Swallow immediately.

PREVACID Delayed-Release Capsules may also be emptied into a small volume of either apple juice, orange juice or tomato juice and administered as follows:

- Open capsule.
- Sprinkle intact granules into a small volume of either apple juice, orange juice or tomato juice (60 mL – approximately 2 ounces).
- Mix briefly.
- Swallow immediately.
- To ensure complete delivery of the dose, the glass should be rinsed with two or more volumes of juice and the contents swallowed immediately.

USE IN OTHER FOODS AND LIQUIDS HAS NOT BEEN STUDIED CLINICALLY AND IS THEREFORE NOT RECOMMENDED.

PREVACID Capsules - Nasogastric Tube Administration

For patients who have a nasogastric tube in place, PREVACID Delayed-Release Capsules can be administered as follows:

- Open capsule.
- Mix intact granules into 40 mL of apple juice. DO NOT USE OTHER LIQUIDS.
- Inject through the nasogastric tube into the stomach.
- Flush with additional apple juice to clear the tube.

2. PREVACID SoluTab Delayed-Release Orally Disintegrating Tablets

PREVACID SoluTab should not be chewed. Place the tablet on the tongue and allow it to disintegrate, with or without water, until the particles can be swallowed. The tablet typically disintegrates in less than 1 minute.

Alternatively, for children or other patients who have difficulty swallowing tablets, PREVACID SoluTab can be delivered in two different ways.

PREVACID SoluTab – Oral Syringe

For administration via oral syringe, PREVACID SoluTab can be administered as follows:

- Place a 15 mg tablet in oral syringe and draw up approximately 4 mL of water, or place a 30 mg tablet in oral syringe and draw up approximately 10 mL of water.
- Shake gently to allow for a quick dispersal.
- After the tablet has dispersed, administer the contents within 15 minutes.
- Refill the syringe with approximately 2 mL (5 mL for the 30 mg tablet) of water, shake gently, and administer any remaining contents.

PREVACID SoluTab – Nasogastric Tube Administration (≥ 8 French)

For administration via a nasogastric tube, PREVACID SoluTab can be administered as follows:

- Place a 15 mg tablet in a syringe and draw up 4 mL of water, or place a 30 mg tablet in a syringe and draw up 10 mL of water.
- Shake gently to allow for a quick dispersal.
- After the tablet has dispersed, inject through the nasogastric tube into the stomach within 15 minutes.
- Refill the syringe with approximately 5 mL of water, shake gently, and flush the nasogastric tube.

3. PREVACID for Delayed-Release Oral Suspension

PREVACID for Delayed-Release Oral Suspension should be administered as follows:

- Open packet.
- To prepare a dose, empty the packet contents into a container containing 2 tablespoons of **WATER**. DO NOT USE OTHER LIQUIDS OR FOODS.
- Stir well, and drink immediately.
- If any material remains after drinking, add more water, stir, and drink immediately.
- **This product should not be given through enteral administration tubes.**

HOW SUPPLIED

PREVACID Delayed-Release Capsules, 15 mg, are opaque, hard gelatin, colored pink and green with the TAP logo and "PREVACID 15" imprinted on the capsules. The 30 mg capsules are opaque, hard gelatin, colored pink and black with the TAP logo and "PREVACID 30" imprinted on the capsules. They are available as follows:

NDC 0300-1541-30 Unit of use bottles of 30: 15-mg capsules
NDC 0300-1541-19 Bottles of 1000: 15-mg capsules
NDC 0300-1541-11 Unit dose package of 100: 15-mg capsules
NDC 0300-3046-13 Bottles of 100: 30-mg capsules
NDC 0300-3046-19 Bottles of 1000: 30-mg capsules
NDC 0300-3046-11 Unit dose package of 100: 30-mg capsules

PREVACID for Delayed-Release Oral Suspension contains white to pale brownish lansoprazole granules and inactive pink granules in a unit dose packet. They are available as follows:

NDC 0300-7309-30 Unit dose carton of 30: 15-mg packets
NDC 0300-7311-30 Unit dose carton of 30: 30-mg packets

PREVACID SoluTab Delayed-Release Orally Disintegrating Tablets, 15 mg, are white to yellowish white uncoated tablets with orange to dark brown speckles, with "15" debossed on one side of the tablet. The 30 mg are white to yellowish white uncoated tablets with orange to dark brown speckles, with "30" debossed on one side of the tablet. The tablets are available as follows:

NDC 0300-1543-30 Unit dose packages of 30: 15-mg tablets
NDC 0300-1544-30 Unit dose packages of 30: 30-mg tablets

Store at 25°C (77°F); excursions permitted to 15-30°C (59-86°F). [See USP Controlled Room Temperature]

℞ only

U.S. Patent Nos. 4,628,098; 4,689,333; 5,013,743; 5,026,560; 5,045,321; 5,093,132; 5,433,959; 5,464,632; 6,123,962 and 6,328,994.

Distributed by
TAP Pharmaceuticals Inc.
Lake Forest, IL 60045, U.S.A.

ENSURE® is a registered trademark of Abbott Laboratories.
CLOtest® is a registered trademark of Delta West Ltd., Bentley, Australia.
03-5366-R24 Rev. July, 2004

IN-5216/S

Shown in Product Identification Guide, page 334

PREVACID® I.V. ℞

[pre-va-sid]
(lansoprazole)
for Injection
30 mg/vial
℞ only

DESCRIPTION

The active ingredient in PREVACID I.V. (lansoprazole) for Injection is a substituted benzimidazole, 2-[[[3-methyl-4-(2,2,2-trifluoroethoxy)-2-pyridyl] methyl] sulfinyl] benzimidazole, a compound that inhibits gastric acid secretion. Its empirical formula is $C_{16}H_{14}F_3N_3O_2S$ with a molecular weight of 369.37. The structural formula is:

[Structural formula: H, N, O, S-CH₂, N, N, H₃C, OCH₂CF₃]

Lansoprazole is a white to brownish-white odorless crystalline powder which melts with decomposition at approximately 166°C. Lansoprazole is freely soluble in dimethylformamide; soluble in methanol; sparingly soluble in ethanol; slightly soluble in ethyl acetate, dichloromethane and acetonitrile; very slightly soluble in ether; and practically insoluble in hexane and water.

Lansoprazole is stable when exposed to light for up to two months. The rate of degradation of the compound in aqueous solution increases with decreasing pH.

PREVACID I.V. for Injection contains 30 mg of the active ingredient lansoprazole, 60 mg mannitol, 10 mg meglumine, and 3.45 mg sodium hydroxide and is supplied as a sterile, lyophilized powder for I.V. (intravenous) use. The solution of PREVACID I.V. for Injection has a pH of approximately 11 following the first reconstitution with Sterile Water for Injection, USP, and approximately 10.2, 10.0, or 9.5 after further dilution with either 0.9% Sodium Chloride Injection, USP, Lactated Ringer's Injection, USP, or 5% Dextrose Injection, USP, respectively.

CLINICAL PHARMACOLOGY

Pharmacokinetics and Metabolism

Following the administration of 30 mg of lansoprazole by intravenous infusion over 30 minutes to healthy subjects, plasma concentrations of lansoprazole declined exponentially with a mean (± standard deviation) terminal elimination half-life of 1.3 (± 0.5) hours. The mean peak plasma concentration of lansoprazole (C_{max}) was 1705 (± 292) ng/mL and the mean area under the plasma concentration versus time curve (AUC) was 3192 (± 1745) ng·h/mL. The absolute bioavailability of lansoprazole following oral administration is over 80%, and C_{max} and AUC of lansoprazole are approximately proportional in doses from 15 mg to 60 mg after single oral administration. The pharmacokinetics of lansoprazole did not change with time after 7-day once daily repeated oral or intravenous administration of 30 mg lansoprazole.

Distribution

The apparent volume of distribution of lansoprazole is approximately 15.7 (± 1.9) L, distributing mainly in extracellular fluid. Lansoprazole is 97% bound to plasma proteins. Plasma protein binding is constant over the concentration range of 0.05 to 5.0 µg/mL.

Metabolism

Lansoprazole is extensively metabolized in the liver. Two metabolites have been identified in measurable quantities in plasma (the hydroxylated sulfinyl and sulfone derivatives of lansoprazole). These metabolites have very little or no antisecretory activity. Lansoprazole is thought to be transformed into two active species which inhibit acid secretion by (H^+,K^+)-ATPase within the parietal cell canaliculus, but are not present in the systemic circulation. The plasma elimination half-life of lansoprazole does not reflect its duration of suppression of gastric acid secretion. Thus, the plasma elimination half-life is less than two hours, while the acid inhibitory effect lasts more than 24 hours.

Elimination

Following an intravenous dose of lansoprazole, the mean clearance was 11.1 (± 3.8) L/h. Following single-dose oral administration of lansoprazole, virtually no unchanged lansoprazole was excreted in the urine. In one study, after a single oral dose of ^{14}C-lansoprazole, approximately one-third of the administered radiation was excreted in the urine and two-thirds was recovered in the feces. This implies a significant biliary excretion of the metabolites of lansoprazole.

Special Populations

Geriatric

Following oral administration, the clearance of lansoprazole is decreased in the elderly, with elimination half-life increased approximately 50% to 100%. Because the mean half-life in the elderly remains between 1.9 to 2.9 hours, repeated once daily dosing does not result in accumulation of lansoprazole. Peak plasma levels were not increased in the elderly. No intravenous dosage adjustment is needed.

Pediatric

The pharmacokinetics of intravenous lansoprazole have not been studied in pediatric patients. For further information, please see the PREVACID package insert for the oral formulations.

Gender

The pharmacokinetic data of intravenous lansoprazole in females is limited; however, in a study with oral lansoprazole comparing 12 male and 6 female human subjects, no gender differences were found in pharmacokinetics and intragastric pH results. No intravenous dosage adjustment is needed. (Also refer to **Use in Women.**)

Renal Insufficiency

In patients with severe renal insufficiency, plasma protein binding decreased by 1.0%-1.5% after oral administration of 60 mg of lansoprazole. Patients with renal insufficiency had a shortened elimination half-life and decreased total AUC (free and bound). AUC for free lansoprazole in plasma, however, was not related to the degree of renal impairment, and C_{max} and T_{max} were not different from subjects with healthy kidneys. No intravenous dosage adjustment is necessary in patients with renal insufficiency.

Hepatic Insufficiency

In patients with various degrees of chronic hepatic disease, the mean plasma half-life of the drug was prolonged from 1.5 hours to 3.2-7.2 hours after oral administration. An increase in mean AUC of up to 500% was observed at steady state in hepatically-impaired patients compared to healthy subjects. Intravenous dose reduction in patients with severe hepatic disease should be considered.

Race

The pooled mean pharmacokinetic parameters of orally administered lansoprazole from twelve U.S. Phase 1 studies (N=513) were compared to the mean pharmacokinetic parameters from two Asian studies (N=20). The mean AUCs of lansoprazole in Asian subjects were approximately twice those seen in pooled U.S. data; however, the inter-individual variability was high. The C_{max} values were comparable. Information for intravenous dosing is not available.

Pharmacodynamics

Mechanism of Action

Lansoprazole belongs to a class of antisecretory compounds, the substituted benzimidazoles, that do not exhibit anticholinergic or histamine H_2-receptor antagonist properties, but that suppress gastric acid secretion by specific inhibition of the (H^+,K^+)-ATPase enzyme system at the secretory surface of the gastric parietal cell. Because this enzyme system is regarded as the acid (proton) pump within the parietal cell, lansoprazole has been characterized as a gastric acid-pump inhibitor, in that it blocks the final step of acid production. This effect is dose-related and leads to inhibition of both basal and stimulated gastric acid secretion for at least 24 hours irrespective of the stimulus.

Antisecretory Activity

Acid Output

An open-label, single-center, two period study was conducted to evaluate the pharmacodynamics of 30 mg of intravenous lansoprazole and 30 mg of oral lansoprazole in 29 healthy subjects. The primary pharmacodynamic endpoints were pentagastrin stimulated maximum acid output (MAO) and basal acid output (BAO). Subjects received oral lansoprazole for 7 days in Period 1 and then were immediately switched to intravenous lansoprazole for 7 days in Period 2. MAO and BAO were measured at baseline and 21 hours following the last oral dose and the last intravenous dose of lansoprazole. This study demonstrated that 7 days of oral lansoprazole followed by 7 days of intravenous lansoprazole administration significantly suppressed gastric acid output as compared with baseline. Seven days of 30 mg of intravenous lansoprazole was equivalent to 30 mg of oral lansoprazole in the ability to maintain gastric acid output suppression.

Acid Output (mEq/hr)

		PREVACID 30 mg	
	Baseline	After 7 Days of Oral Dosing	After 7 Days of I.V. Dosing
Maximum Acid Output (Median)	11.26 n=27	4.76* n=28	5.13* n=28
Basal Acid Output (Median)	1.42 n=28	0.42* n=28	0.27* n=28

* Significantly ($p \leq 0.05$) less acid output as compared to baseline.

24-Hour Intragastric pH

A multiple-dose study was conducted in 36 healthy subjects comparing the pharmacokinetics and pharmacodynamics of lansoprazole after intravenous administration and oral administration. During the first-hour post-dosing interval, intravenous lansoprazole resulted in significantly higher mean intragastric pH than did oral lansoprazole. There were no statistically significant differences between oral and intravenous regimens in 24-hour mean intragastric pH for the percentage of time that the intragastric pH was above 3 and 4 after 1-day or 5-day once daily repeated administration of 30 mg lansoprazole. Gastric acid suppression was maintained throughout each treatment period. The pharmacodynamic results are summarized in the table below.

[See table above]

Mean Antisecretory Effects after Single and Multiple Daily Dosing

		PREVACID			
		30 mg q.d. Orally x 5 days		30 mg I.V. Infusion q.d. x 5 Days	
Parameter	Baseline Value	Day 1	Day 5	Day 1	Day 5
Mean 24-Hour pH	3.33	4.75	5.25	4.86	5.36
Mean first hour pH	4.44	2.74	4.79	4.64*	5.91*
% Time Gastric pH>3	45.27	74.08	83.92	78.36	85.54
% Time Gastric pH>4	31.07	67.18	77.61	70.51	79.68

*Significantly ($p \leq 0.05$) higher than the oral lansoprazole

Refer to **CLINICAL PHARMACOLOGY** for pharmacokinetic results.

Enterochromaffin-like (ECL) Cell Effects

During lifetime exposure of rats with up to 150 mg/kg/day of lansoprazole dosed orally seven days per week, marked hypergastrinemia was observed followed by ECL cell proliferation and formation of carcinoid tumors, especially in female rats. (Refer to **PRECAUTIONS, Carcinogenesis, Mutagenesis, Impairment of Fertility.**)

Gastric biopsy specimens from the body of the stomach from approximately 150 patients treated continuously with lansoprazole for at least one year did not show evidence of ECL cell effects similar to those seen in rat studies. Longer term data are needed to rule out the possibility of an increased risk of the development of gastric tumors in patients receiving long-term therapy with lansoprazole.

Other Gastric Effects In Humans

Lansoprazole did not significantly affect mucosal blood flow in the fundus of the stomach. Due to the normal physiologic effect caused by the inhibition of gastric acid secretion, a decrease of about 17% in blood flow in the antrum, pylorus, and duodenal bulb was seen. Lansoprazole significantly slowed the gastric emptying of digestible solids. Lansoprazole increased serum pepsinogen levels and decreased pepsin activity under basal conditions and in response to meal stimulation or insulin injection. As with other agents that elevate intragastric pH, increases in gastric pH were associated with increases in nitrate-reducing bacteria and elevation of nitrite concentration in gastric juice in patients with gastric ulcer. No significant increase in nitrosamine concentrations was observed.

Serum Gastrin Effects

In over 2,100 patients, median fasting serum gastrin levels increased 50% to 100% from baseline but remained within normal range after treatment with lansoprazole given orally in doses of 15 mg to 60 mg. These elevations reached a plateau within two months of therapy and returned to pretreatment levels within four weeks after discontinuation of therapy.

Endocrine Effects

Human studies for up to one year have not detected any clinically significant effects on the endocrine system. Hormones studied include testosterone, luteinizing hormone (LH), follicle stimulating hormone (FSH), sex hormone binding globulin (SHBG), dehydroepiandrosterone sulfate (DHEA-S), prolactin, cortisol, estradiol, insulin, aldosterone, parathormone, glucagon, thyroid stimulating hormone (TSH), triiodothyronine (T_3), thyroxine (T_4), and somatotropic hormone (STH). Lansoprazole in oral doses of 15 to 60 mg for up to one year had no clinically significant effect on sexual function. In addition, lansoprazole in oral doses of 15 to 60 mg for two to eight weeks had no clinically significant effect on thyroid function.

In 24-month carcinogenicity studies in Sprague-Dawley rats with daily dosages up to 150 mg/kg, proliferative changes in the Leydig cells of the testes, including benign neoplasm, were increased compared to control rates; these findings are rat specific.

Other Effects

No systemic effects of lansoprazole on the central nervous system, lymphoid, hematopoietic, renal, hepatic, cardiovascular or respiratory systems have been found in humans. No visual toxicity was observed among 56 patients who had extensive baseline eye evaluations, were treated with up to 180 mg/day of lansoprazole and were observed for up to 58 months.

Other rat-specific findings after lifetime exposure included focal pancreatic atrophy, diffuse lymphoid hyperplasia in the thymus and spontaneous retinal atrophy.

CLINICAL STUDIES

Erosive Esophagitis

A multicenter, double-blind, two-period placebo-controlled, pharmacodynamic study was conducted to assess the ability of PREVACID I.V. for Injection to maintain gastric acid suppression in patients switched from the oral dosage form of lansoprazole to the intravenous dosage form. Erosive esophagitis patients (n=87; 18 to 78 years of age; 28 female; 69 Caucasian/non-Hispanic, 14 Hispanic, 3 African-American, and 1 Native American) received 30 mg of oral lansoprazole for 7 days in Period 1. Patients were then immediately switched to receive either 30 mg of intravenous lansoprazole or intravenous placebo (normal saline) for 7 days in Period 2. MAO and BAO were determined 21 hours following the last dose of oral medication and the last dose of intravenous administration. MAO was calculated from two hours of continuous collection of gastric contents following a subcutaneous injection of 6.0 μg/kg of pentagastrin. BAO was calculated from one hour of continuous collection of gastric contents.

This study demonstrated that, after seven days of repeated oral administration followed by 7 days of intravenous administration, the oral and intravenous dosage forms of PREVACID were similar in their ability to suppress MAO and BAO in patients with erosive esophagitis (refer to the table below). Also, patients receiving oral PREVACID, who were switched to intravenous placebo, experienced a significant increase in acid output within 48 hours of their last oral dose.

Acid Output (mEq/h) in Erosive Esophagitis Patients

	PREVACID Oral (last oral dose)	PREVACID I.V. (last I.V. dose)	Placebo I.V. (last I.V. dose)
Maximum Acid Output (Median)	7.16 n=80	7.64 n=56	26.90** n=17
Basal Acid Output (Median)	0.77 n=81	0.51 n=55	3.19* n=16

*, ** Significantly different from PREVACID I.V. at p=0.005 and p<0.001 levels, respectively

INDICATIONS AND USAGE

When patients are unable to take the oral formulations, PREVACID I.V. for Injection is indicated as an alternative for the short-term treatment (up to 7 days) of all grades of erosive esophagitis. Once the patient is able to take medications orally, therapy can be switched to an oral formulation of PREVACID for a total of 6 to 8 weeks. The safety and efficacy of PREVACID I.V. for Injection as an initial treatment of erosive esophagitis have not been demonstrated. Refer to full prescribing information for the oral formulations of PREVACID.

CONTRAINDICATIONS

PREVACID I.V. for Injection is contraindicated in patients with known hypersensitivity to any component of the formulation.

PRECAUTIONS

GENERAL

Symptomatic response to therapy with lansoprazole does not preclude the presence of gastric malignancy.

Treatment with PREVACID I.V. for Injection should be discontinued as soon as the patient is able to resume treatment with PREVACID oral formulations.

Drug Interactions

Lansoprazole is metabolized through the cytochrome P_{450} system, specifically through the CYP3A and CYP2C19 isozymes. Studies have shown that lansoprazole does not have clinically significant interactions with other drugs metabolized by the cytochrome P_{450} system, such as warfarin, antipyrine, indomethacin, ibuprofen, phenytoin, propranolol, prednisone, diazepam, or clarithromycin in healthy subjects. These compounds are metabolized through various cytochrome P_{450} isozymes including CYP1A2, CYP2C9, CYP2C19, CYP2D6, and CYP3A. When lansoprazole was administered concomitantly with theophylline (CYP1A2, CYP3A), a minor increase (10%) in the clearance of theophylline was seen. Because of the small magnitude and the direction of the effect on theophylline clearance, this interaction is unlikely to be of clinical concern. Nonetheless, individual patients may require additional titration of their theophylline dosage when lansoprazole is started or stopped to ensure clinically effective blood levels.

In a study of healthy subjects neither the pharmacokinetics of warfarin enantiomers nor prothrombin time were affected following single or multiple 60 mg doses of lansoprazole. However, there have been reports of increased International Normalized Ratio (INR) and prothrombin time in patients receiving proton pump inhibitors, including lansoprazole, and warfarin concomitantly. Increases in INR and prothrombin time may lead to abnormal bleeding and even death. Patients treated with proton pump inhibitors and warfarin concomitantly may need to be monitored for increases in INR and prothrombin time.

Continued on next page

Prevacid I.V.—Cont.

Lansoprazole causes a profound and long-lasting inhibition of gastric acid secretion; therefore, it is theoretically possible that lansoprazole may interfere with the absorption of drugs where gastric pH is an important determinant of bioavailability (eg, ketoconazole, ampicillin esters, iron salts, digoxin).

Carcinogenesis, Mutagenesis, Impairment of Fertility

In two 24-month carcinogenicity studies, Sprague-Dawley rats were treated orally with doses of 5 to 150 mg/kg/day, about 1 to 40 times the exposure on a body surface (mg/m^2) basis, of a 50-kg person of average height (1.46 m^2 body surface area) given the recommended human dose of 30 mg/day (22.2 mg/m^2). Lansoprazole produced dose-related gastric enterochromaffin-like (ECL) cell hyperplasia and ECL cell carcinoids in both male and female rats. It also increased the incidence of intestinal metaplasia of the gastric epithelium in both sexes. In male rats, lansoprazole produced a dose-related increase of testicular interstitial cell adenomas. The incidence of these adenomas in rats receiving doses of 15 to 150 mg/kg/day (4 to 40 times the recommended human dose based on body surface area) exceeded the low background incidence (range = 1.4 to 10%) for this strain of rat. Testicular interstitial cell adenoma also occurred in 1 of 30 rats treated with 50 mg/kg/day (13 times the recommended human dose based on body surface area) in a 1-year toxicity study.

In a 24-month carcinogenicity study, CD-1 mice were treated orally with doses of 15 to 600 mg/kg/day, 2 to 80 times the recommended human dose based on body surface area. Lansoprazole produced a dose-related increased incidence of gastric ECL cell hyperplasia. It also produced an increased incidence of liver tumors (hepatocellular adenoma plus carcinoma). The tumor incidences in male mice treated with 300 and 600 mg/kg/day (40 to 80 times the recommended human dose based on body surface area) and female mice treated with 150 to 600 mg/kg/day (20 to 80 times the recommended human dose based on body surface area) exceeded the ranges of background incidences in historical controls for this strain of mice. Lansoprazole treatment produced adenoma of rete testis in male mice receiving 75 to 600 mg/kg/day (10 to 80 times the recommended human dose based on body surface area).

Lansoprazole was not genotoxic in the Ames test, the *ex vivo* rat hepatocyte unscheduled DNA synthesis (UDS) test, the *in vivo* mouse micronucleus test or the rat bone marrow cell chromosomal aberration test. It was positive in *in vitro* human lymphocyte chromosomal aberration assays.

Lansoprazole at intravenous doses of up to 30 mg/kg/day (approximately 8 times the recommended human dose based on body surface area) was found to have no effect on fertility and reproductive performance in male and female rats.

Pregnancy: Teratogenic Effects

Pregnancy Category B

Teratology studies have been conducted in rats and rabbits using intravenous doses of up to 30 mg/kg/day (approximately 8 times in rats and 16 times in rabbits of the recommended human dose based on body surface area). Treatment with lansoprazole did not result in any impairment of fertility or harm to the fetus.

However, there are no adequate and well-controlled studies in pregnant women using the intravenous route. Because animal reproduction studies are not always predicative of human response, this drug should be used during pregnancy only if clearly needed.

Nursing Mothers

Lansoprazole or its metabolites are excreted in the milk of rats. It is not known whether lansoprazole is excreted in human milk. Because many drugs are excreted in human milk, because of the potential for serious adverse reactions in nursing infants from lansoprazole, and because of the potential for tumorigenicity shown for lansoprazole in rodent carcinogenicity studies, a decision should be made whether to discontinue nursing or to discontinue the drug, taking into account the importance of the drug to the mother.

Pediatric Use

The safety and effectiveness of PREVACID I.V. for Injection have not been established for pediatric patients. For further information, please see the PREVACID package insert for the oral formulations.

Use in Women

Among intravenous lansoprazole treated subjects, similar percentages of adverse events were reported in males and females.

Over 4,000 women were treated with oral lansoprazole. Ulcer healing rates in females were similar to those in males. The incidence rates of adverse events were also similar to those seen in males.

Use in Geriatric Patients

Data in elderly patients administered intravenous lansoprazole is limited; however, with oral lansoprazole, ulcer healing rates in elderly patients are similar to those in a younger age group. The incidence rates of adverse events and laboratory test abnormalities are also similar to those seen in younger patients. For elderly patients, dosage and administration of lansoprazole need not be altered for a particular indication.

ADVERSE REACTIONS

Clinical Safety Experience with PREVACID I.V. for Injection

More than 1,000 patients and subjects have participated in domestic and foreign clinical trials. Treatment with PREVACID I.V. for Injection was well tolerated.

In four U.S. trials involving 161 subjects exposed to PREVACID I.V. for Injection, the following treatment-related adverse events were reported in ≥1% of subjects: headache (1.0%), injection site pain (1.0%), injection site reaction (1.0%) and nausea (1.3%). Treatment-related adverse events occurring in <1% of subjects included abdominal pain, vasodilatation, diarrhea, dyspepsia, vomiting, dizziness, paresthesia, rash, and taste perversion. No additional adverse drug reactions were reported with the intravenous formulation that had not been reported previously with the oral formulations.

Clinical Safety Experience with Oral Formulations of PREVACID

Worldwide, over 10,000 patients have been treated with oral lansoprazole in Phase 2-3 clinical trials involving various dosages and durations of treatment. In general, lansoprazole treatment has been well-tolerated in both short-term and long-term trials.

The following adverse events were reported by the treating physician to have a possible or probable relationship to drug in 1% or more of PREVACID-treated patients and occurred at a greater rate in PREVACID-treated patients than placebo-treated patients:

Incidence of Possibly or Probably Treatment-Related Adverse Events in Short-Term, Placebo-Controlled Studies

Body System/ Adverse Event	PREVACID Oral (N= 2768) %	Placebo (N= 1023) %
Body as a Whole		
Abdominal Pain	2.1	1.2
Digestive System		
Constipation	1.0	0.4
Diarrhea	3.8	2.3
Nausea	1.3	1.2

Headache was also seen at greater than 1% incidence but was more common on placebo. The incidence of diarrhea was similar between patients who received placebo and patients who received lansoprazole 15 mg and 30 mg, but higher in the patients who received lansoprazole 60 mg (2.9%, 1.4%, 4.2%, and 7.4%, respectively).

Additional adverse experiences occurring in <1% of patients or subjects in domestic trials are shown below. Refer to **Postmarketing** for adverse reactions occurring since the drug was marketed.

Body as a Whole - abdomen enlarged, allergic reaction, asthenia, back pain, candidiasis, carcinoma, chest pain (not otherwise specified), chills, edema, fever, flu syndrome, halitosis, infection (not otherwise specified), malaise, neck pain, neck rigidity, pain, pelvic pain; *Cardiovascular System* - angina, arrhythmia, bradycardia, cerebrovascular accident/cerebral infarction, hypertension/ hypotension, migraine, myocardial infarction, palpitations, shock (circulatory failure), syncope, tachycardia, vasodilation; *Digestive System* - abnormal stools, anorexia, bezoar, cardiospasm, cholelithiasis, colitis, dry mouth, dyspepsia, dysphagia, enteritis, eructation, esophageal stenosis, esophageal ulcer, esophagitis, fecal discoloration, flatulence, gastric nodules/ fundic gland polyps, gastritis, gastroenteritis, gastrointestinal anomaly, gastrointestinal disorder, gastrointestinal hemorrhage, glossitis, gum hemorrhage, hematemesis, increased appetite, increased salivation, melena, mouth ulceration, nausea and vomiting, nausea and vomiting and diarrhea, oral moniliasis, rectal disorder, rectal hemorrhage, stomatitis, tenesmus, thirst, tongue disorder, ulcerative colitis, ulcerative stomatitis; *Endocrine System* - diabetes mellitus, goiter, hypothyroidism; *Hemic and Lymphatic System* - anemia, hemolysis, lymphadenopathy; *Metabolic and Nutritional Disorders* - gout, dehydration, hyperglycemia/hypoglycemia, peripheral edema, weight gain/loss; *Musculoskeletal System* - arthralgia, arthritis, bone disorder, joint disorder, leg cramps, musculoskeletal pain, myalgia, myasthenia, synovitis; *Nervous System* - abnormal dreams, agitation, amnesia, anxiety, apathy, confusion, convulsion, depersonalization, depression, diplopia, dizziness, emotional lability, hallucinations, hemiplegia, hostility aggravated, hyperkinesia, hypertonia, hypesthesia, insomnia, libido decreased/increased, nervousness, neurosis, paresthesia, sleep disorder, somnolence, thinking abnormality, tremor, vertigo; *Respiratory System* - asthma, bronchitis, cough increased, dyspnea, epistaxis, hemoptysis, hiccup, laryngeal neoplasia, pharyngitis, pleural disorder, pneumonia, respiratory disorder, upper respiratory inflammation/ infection, rhinitis, sinusitis, stridor; *Skin and Appendages* - acne, alopecia, contact dermatitis, dry skin, fixed eruption, hair disorder, maculopapular rash, nail disorder, pruritus, rash, skin carcinoma, skin disorder, sweating, urticaria; *Special Senses* - abnormal vision, blurred vision, conjunctivitis, deafness, dry eyes, ear disorder, eye pain, otitis media, parosmia, photophobia, retinal degeneration, taste loss, taste perversion, tinnitus, visual field defect; *Urogenital System* - abnormal menses, breast enlargement, breast pain, breast tenderness, dysmenorrhea, dysuria, gynecomastia, impotence, kidney calculus, kidney pain, leukorrhea, menorrhagia, menstrual disorder, penis disorder, polyuria, testis disorder, urethral pain, urinary frequency, urinary tract infection, urinary urgency, urination impaired, vaginitis.

Postmarketing

On-going Safety Surveillance: Additional adverse experiences have been reported since oral lansoprazole has been marketed. The majority of these cases are foreign-sourced and a relationship to lansoprazole has not been established. Because these events were reported voluntarily from a population of unknown size, estimates of frequency cannot be made. These events are listed below by COSTART body system.

Body as a Whole - anaphylactoid-like reaction; *Digestive System* - hepatotoxicity, pancreatitis, vomiting; *Hemic and Lymphatic System* - agranulocytosis, aplastic anemia, hemolytic anemia, leukopenia, neutropenia, pancytopenia, thrombocytopenia, and thrombotic thrombocytopenic purpura; *Skin and Appendages* – severe dermatologic reactions including erythema multiforme, Stevens-Johnson syndrome, toxic epidermal necrolysis (some fatal); *Special Senses* - speech disorder; *Urogenital System* - urinary retention.

Laboratory Values

There were no clinically important changes identified in any laboratory parameter with PREVACID I.V. for Injection.

The following changes in laboratory parameters for oral lansoprazole were reported as adverse events:

Abnormal liver function tests, increased SGOT (AST), increased SGPT (ALT), increased creatinine, increased alkaline phosphatase, increased globulins, increased GGTP, increased/decreased/abnormal WBC, abnormal AG ratio, abnormal RBC, bilirubinemia, eosinophilia, hyperlipemia, increased/decreased electrolytes, increased/decreased cholesterol, increased glucocorticoids, increased LDH, increased/decreased/abnormal platelets, and increased gastrin levels. Urine abnormalities such as albuminuria, glycosuria, and hematuria were also reported. Additional isolated laboratory abnormalities were reported.

In the placebo controlled studies, when SGOT (AST) and SGPT (ALT) were evaluated, 0.4% (4/978) placebo patients and 0.4% (11/2677) lansoprazole patients had enzyme elevations greater than three times the upper limit of normal range at the final treatment visit. None of these lansoprazole patients reported jaundice at any time during the study.

OVERDOSAGE

Single intravenous doses of lansoprazole at 218 mg/kg in mice (approximately 30 times the recommended human dose based on body surface area) and 167 mg/kg in rats (approximately 46 times the recommended human dose based on body surface area) were lethal. The symptoms of acute toxicity were decreased locomotor response, ataxia, ptosis and tonic convulsions.

Lansoprazole is not removed from the circulation by hemodialysis.

DOSAGE AND ADMINISTRATION

PREVACID I.V. for Injection MUST be reconstituted with 5 mL of Sterile Water for Injection, USP. Failure to reconstitute with Sterile Water may result in formation of precipitation/particulates. PREVACID I.V. for Injection admixtures should be administered intravenously using the in-line filter provided. The filter must be used to remove precipitate that may form when the reconstituted drug product is mixed with I.V. solutions. Studies have shown that filtration does not alter the amount of drug that is available for administration. (See instructions below).

1. Reconstitution in vial

— Inject 5 mL of **ONLY Sterile Water for Injection, USP** into a 30 mg vial of PREVACID I.V. for Injection. The resulting solution will contain lansoprazole 6 mg/mL (30 mg/5 mL).

— Mix gently until the powder is dissolved.

The pH of this reconstituted solution is approximately 11. The reconstituted solution can be held for 1 hour when stored at 25°C (77°F) prior to further dilution.

2. Preparation of admixture

— Dilute the reconstituted solution in either 50 mL of 0.9% Sodium Chloride Injection, USP, Lactated Ringer's Injection, USP, or 5% Dextrose Injection, USP.

— The admixture should be stored at 25°C (77°F) and should be administered within the designated time period as listed in the Table below. No refrigeration is required.

Diluent	pH	Administer within:
0.9% Sodium Chloride Injection, USP	Approximately 10.2	24 hours
Lactated Ringer's Injection, USP	Approximately 10.0	24 hours
5% Dextrose Injection, USP	Approximately 9.5	12 hours

3. Instructions for priming and use of filter

TO PRIME FILTER

— Prime administration set in usual manner and close administration set clamp.

— Connect luer adapter of administration set to filter inlet using a twisting motion. Over-tightening should be avoided.

— Hold filter below the level of solution container.

— Open administration set clamp and slowly prime filter.
— Close administration set clamp. Verify no air bubbles are present on patient side of filter.
— If air bubbles are observed, open set clamp slightly to re-establish flow then gently tap filter housing. Observe that no air bubbles are present and close clamp.
— Connect to patient and regulate flow. Filter may be primed using a syringe and saline.
— The administration set can then be connected to inlet of filter.

PRECAUTIONS WITH USE OF FILTER
Follow instructions carefully:
— Use Aseptic technique. For single use only. Do not resterilize or reuse. Do not use if package is damaged.
— If repositioning of filter is required, loosen luer locking collar, reposition, then retighten locking collar firmly.
— Maximum working pressure is 1500 mmHg (30 psi, 2 bar). When the working limits of the filter are exceeded, causes of the added resistance should be investigated and corrected.
— The internal volume of the filter is approx. 0.7 mL.
— The administration set clamp should be closed during solution container change.
— It is recommended that this filter is changed at 24 hours.
— Pumps should not be used downstream of filter.

4. Administration
— IN-LINE FILTER MUST BE USED.
— Administer intravenously over 30 minutes.
— A dedicated line is not required; however, the intravenous line should be flushed before and after administration of PREVACID I.V. for Injection with either 0.9% Sodium Chloride Injection, USP, Lactated Ringer's Injection, USP, or 5% Dextrose Injection, USP.
— Do not administer with other drugs or diluents as this may cause incompatibilities.

Treatment of Erosive Esophagitis
The recommended adult dose (***when patients are unable to take the oral therapy***) is 30 mg of lansoprazole (1 vial of PREVACID I.V. for Injection) per day administered by I.V. infusion over 30 minutes for up to 7 days. Once the patient is able to take medications orally, therapy can be switched to an oral PREVACID formulation for a total of 6 to 8 weeks. Refer to full prescribing information for the oral formulations of PREVACID.
No dosage adjustment is necessary in patients with renal insufficiency or the elderly. For patients with severe liver disease, dosage adjustment should be considered.

HOW SUPPLIED
PREVACID I.V. for Injection contains 30 mg of lansoprazole as white to pale yellow friable masses and powder in a vial and is available as follows:
NDC 0300-3954-25 Tray containing 10 single dose vial packs: Each pack containing one 30-mg single dose vial of PREVACID I.V. for Injection and 1 required in-line filter (1.2 µm pore size).
Store PREVACID I.V. for Injection at 25°C (77°F); excursions permitted to 15-30°C (59-86°F). Protect from light. Use carton to protect contents from light.
U.S. Patent No. 4,628,098.
Distributed by
TAP Pharmaceuticals Inc.
Lake Forest, IL 60045, U.S.A.
(List 3954)
750035289R1, Rev. May, 2004

Shown in Product Identification Guide, page 334

PREVACID® NapraPAC™ 375 ℞
[pre'-va-sid]
(lansoprazole delayed-release 15 mg capsules and naproxen 375 mg tablets kit)
PREVACID® NapraPAC™ 500 ℞
(lansoprazole delayed-release 15 mg capsules and naproxen 500 mg tablets kit)

PREVACID® NapraPAC™ (375 or 500) is a combination package containing NAPROSYN® (naproxen) Tablets, a nonsteroidal anti-inflammatory drug (NSAID) with analgesic and antipyretic properties, and PREVACID® (lansoprazole) Delayed-Release Capsules, a proton pump inhibitor (PPI). The information described in this labeling concerns only the use of these products as indicated in this combination package and does not include all individual use information. For information on use of the components when dispensed as individual medications outside this combination package, please see the package inserts for NAPROSYN Tablets and PREVACID Delayed-Release Capsules.

DESCRIPTION
PREVACID® NapraPAC™ 375 is a combination package containing NAPROSYN 375 mg tablets and PREVACID 15 mg capsules. PREVACID® NapraPAC™ 500 is a combination package containing NAPROSYN 500 mg tablets and PREVACID 15 mg capsules.

NAPROSYN
Naproxen is a member of the arylacetic acid group of nonsteroidal anti-inflammatory drugs (NSAID).
The chemical name for naproxen is (S)-6-methoxy-α-methyl-2-naphthaleneacetic acid. Its empirical formula is $C_{14}H_{14}O_3$ with a molecular weight of 230.26. Naproxen has the following structure:

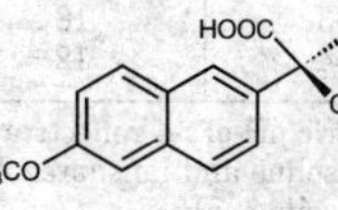

Naproxen is an odorless, white to off-white crystalline substance. It is lipid-soluble, practically insoluble in water at low pH and freely soluble in water at high pH. The octanol/water partition coefficient of naproxen at pH 7.4 is 1.6 to 1.8.
NAPROSYN tablets contain 250 mg, 375 mg or 500 mg of naproxen (active ingredient) and croscarmellose sodium, iron oxides, povidone and magnesium stearate (inactive ingredients).

PREVACID
The active ingredient in PREVACID capsules is a substituted benzimidazole, 2-[[[3-methyl-4-(2,2,2-trifluoroethoxy)-2-pyridyl]methyl] sulfinyl] benzimidazole, a compound that inhibits gastric acid secretion. Its empirical formula is $C_{16}H_{14}F_3N_3O_2S$ with a molecular weight of 369.37. The structural formula is:

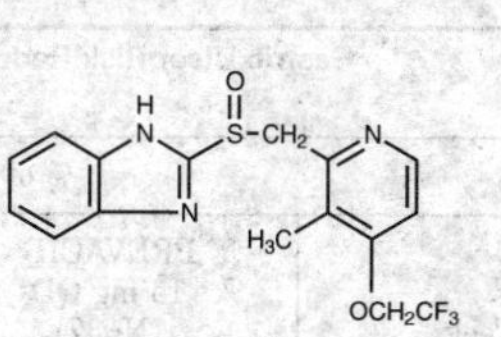

Lansoprazole is a white to brownish-white odorless crystalline powder which melts with decomposition at approximately 166°C. Lansoprazole is freely soluble in dimethylformamide; soluble in methanol; sparingly soluble in ethanol; slightly soluble in ethyl acetate, dichloromethane and acetonitrile; very slightly soluble in ether; and practically insoluble in hexane and water.
Lansoprazole is stable when exposed to light for up to two months. The rate of degradation of the compound in aqueous solution increases with decreasing pH. The degradation half-life of the drug substance in aqueous solution at 25°C is approximately 0.5 hour at pH 5.0 and approximately 18 hours at pH 7.0.
PREVACID capsules contain enteric-coated granules consisting of lansoprazole (15 mg) [active ingredient], hydroxypropyl cellulose, low substituted hydroxypropyl cellulose, colloidal silicon dioxide, magnesium carbonate, methacrylic acid copolymer, starch, talc, sugar sphere, sucrose, polyethylene glycol, polysorbate 80, and titanium dioxide [inactive ingredients]. Components of the gelatin capsule include gelatin, titanium dioxide, D&C Red No. 28, FD&C Blue No. 1, FD&C Green No. 3, and FD&C Red No. 40 [inactive ingredients].

CLINICAL PHARMACOLOGY
Pharmacokinetics
NAPROSYN
Absorption
Naproxen is rapidly and completely absorbed from the gastrointestinal tract, with an *in vivo* bioavailability of 95%. After administration of naproxen tablets, peak plasma levels are attained in 2 to 4 hours. The elimination half-life of naproxen ranges from 12 to 17 hours. Steady-state levels of naproxen are reached in 4 to 5 days, and the degree of naproxen accumulation is consistent with this half-life.
Distribution
Naproxen has a volume of distribution of 0.16 L/kg. At therapeutic levels, naproxen is greater than 99% albumin-bound. At doses of naproxen greater than 500 mg/day, there is a less than dose-proportional increase in plasma levels due to an increase in clearance caused by saturation of plasma protein binding at higher doses (average trough C_{ss} 36.5, 49.2 and 56.4 mg/L with 500, 1000 and 1500 mg daily doses of naproxen). However, the concentration of unbound naproxen continues to increase proportionally to dose.
Metabolism
Naproxen is extensively metabolized to 6-O-desmethyl naproxen, and both parent and metabolites do not induce metabolizing enzymes.
Elimination
The clearance of naproxen is 0.13 mL/min/kg. Approximately 95% of the naproxen from any dose is excreted in the urine, primarily as naproxen (less than 1%), 6-O-desmethyl naproxen (less than 1%) or their conjugates (66% to 92%). The plasma half-life of the naproxen anion in humans ranges from 12 to 17 hours. The corresponding half-lives of both naproxen's metabolites and conjugates are shorter than 12 hours, and their rates of excretion have been found to coincide closely with the rate of naproxen disappearance from the plasma. In patients with renal failure metabolites may accumulate.

Special Populations
Pediatric Use
The combination of naproxen and lansoprazole has not been studied in pediatric patients. (See **CLINICAL PHARMACOLOGY**, PREVACID Special Populations – *Pediatric Use.*)
Renal Insufficiency
Naproxen pharmacokinetics has not been determined in subjects with renal insufficiency. Given that naproxen, its metabolites and conjugates are primarily excreted by the kidney, the potential exists for naproxen to accumulate in the presence of renal insufficiency. (See **CLINICAL PHARMACOLOGY**, PREVACID Special Populations *-Renal Insufficiency.*)

PREVACID
PREVACID capsules contain an enteric-coated granule formulation of lansoprazole. Absorption of lansoprazole begins only after the granules leave the stomach. Absorption is rapid, with mean peak plasma levels of lansoprazole occurring after approximately 1.7 hours. Peak plasma concentrations of lansoprazole (C_{max}) and the area under the plasma concentration curve (AUC) of lansoprazole are approximately proportional in doses from 15 mg to 60 mg after single-dose oral administration. Lansoprazole does not accumulate and its pharmacokinetics are unaltered by multiple dosing.
Absorption
The absorption of lansoprazole is rapid, with mean C_{max} occurring approximately 1.7 hours after oral dosing, and relatively complete with absolute bioavailability over 80%. In healthy subjects, the mean (± SD) plasma half-life was 1.5 (± 1.0) hours. Both C_{max} and AUC are diminished by about 50–70% if the drug is given 30 minutes after food as opposed to the fasting condition. There is no significant food effect if the drug is given before meals.
Distribution
Lansoprazole is 97% bound to plasma proteins. Plasma protein binding is consistent over the concentration range of 0.05 to 5.0 µg/mL.
Metabolism
Lansoprazole is extensively metabolized in the liver. Two metabolites have been identified in measurable quantities in plasma (the hydroxylated sulfinyl and sulfone derivatives of lansoprazole). These metabolites have very little or no antisecretory activity. Lansoprazole is thought to be transformed into two active species which inhibit acid secretion by (H^+,K^+)-ATPase within the parietal cell canaliculus, but are not present in the systemic circulation. The plasma elimination half-life of lansoprazole does not reflect its duration of suppression of gastric acid secretion. Thus, the plasma elimination half-life is less than 2 hours while the acid inhibitory effect lasts more than 24 hours.
Elimination
Following single-dose oral administration of PREVACID, virtually no unchanged lansoprazole was excreted in the urine. In one study, after a single oral dose of ^{14}C-lansoprazole, approximately one-third of the administered radiation was excreted in the urine and two-thirds was recovered in the feces. This implies a significant biliary excretion of the metabolites of lansoprazole.
Special Populations
Pediatric Use
The combination of lansoprazole and naproxen has not been studied in pediatric patients. (See **CLINICAL PHARMACOLOGY**, NAPROSYN Special Populations – *Pediatric Use.*)
Geriatric Use
The clearance of lansoprazole is decreased in the elderly, with elimination half-life increased approximately 50% to 100%. Because the mean half-life in the elderly remains between 1.9 to 2.9 hours, repeated once daily dosing does not result in accumulation of lansoprazole. Peak plasma levels were not increased in the elderly.
Gender
In a study comparing 12 male and 6 female human subjects, no gender differences were found in pharmacokinetics and intragastric pH results. (See **PRECAUTIONS**, PREVACID **Use in Women.**)
Renal Insufficiency
In patients with severe renal insufficiency, plasma protein binding decreased by 1.0%-1.5% after administration of 60 mg of lansoprazole. Patients with renal insufficiency had a shortened elimination half-life and decreased total AUC (free and bound). AUC for free lansoprazole in plasma, however, was not related to the degree of renal impairment, and C_{max} and T_{max} were not different from subjects with healthy kidneys. (See **CLINICAL PHARMACOLOGY**, NAPROSYN Special Populations—*Renal Insufficiency.*)
Hepatic Insufficiency
In patients with various degrees of chronic hepatic disease, the mean plasma half-life of the drug was prolonged from 1.5 hours to 3.2–7.2 hours. An increase in mean AUC of up to 500% was observed at steady state in hepatically-impaired patients compared to healthy subjects. Dose reduction in patients with severe hepatic disease should be considered.
Race
The pooled pharmacokinetic parameters of PREVACID from twelve U.S. Phase I studies (N=513) were compared to the mean pharmacokinetic parameters from two Asian studies (N=20). The mean AUCs of PREVACID in Asian subjects are

Continued on next page

Prevacid NapraPAC—Cont.

approximately twice that seen in pooled U.S. data; however, the inter-individual variability is high. The C_{max} values are comparable.

Pharmacodynamics

NAPROSYN

Naproxen is an NSAID with analgesic and antipyretic properties. The naproxen anion inhibits prostaglandin synthesis but beyond this its mode of action is unknown.

PREVACID

Mechanism of Action

Lansoprazole belongs to a class of antisecretory compounds, the substituted benzimidazoles, that do not exhibit anticholinergic or histamine H2-receptor antagonist properties, but that suppress gastric acid secretion by specific inhibition of the (H^+,K^+)-ATPase enzyme system at the secretory surface of the gastric parietal cell. Because this enzyme system is regarded as the acid (proton) pump within the parietal cell, lansoprazole has been characterized as a gastric acid-pump inhibitor, in that it blocks the final step of acid production. This effect is dose-related and leads to inhibition of both basal and stimulated gastric acid secretion irrespective of the stimulus.

Antisecretory Activity

After oral administration, lansoprazole was shown to significantly decrease the basal acid output and significantly increase the mean gastric pH and percent of time the gastric pH was >3 and >4. Lansoprazole also significantly reduced meal-stimulated gastric acid output and secretion volume, as well as pentagastrin-stimulated acid output. In patients with hypersecretion of acid, lansoprazole significantly reduced basal and pentagastrin- stimulated gastric acid secretion. Lansoprazole inhibited the normal increases in secretion volume, acidity and acid output induced by insulin.

In a crossover study that included lansoprazole 15 and 30 mg for five days, the following effects on intragastric pH were noted:

[See table 1 above]

After the initial dose in this study, increased gastric pH was seen within 1-2 hours with lansoprazole 30 mg and 2-3 hours with lansoprazole 15 mg. After multiple daily dosing, increased gastric pH was seen within the first hour postdosing with lansoprazole 30 mg and within 1-2 hours postdosing with lansoprazole 15 mg.

The inhibition of gastric acid secretion as measured by intragastric pH returns gradually to normal over two to four days after multiple doses. There is no indication of rebound gastric acidity.

Enterochromaffin-like (ECL) Cell Effects

During lifetime exposure of rats with up to 150 mg/kg/day of lansoprazole dosed 7 days per week, marked hypergastrinemia was observed followed by ECL cell proliferation and formation of carcinoid tumors, especially in female rats. (See **PRECAUTIONS**, PREVACID **Carcinogenesis, Mutagenesis, Impairment of Fertility.**)

Gastric biopsy specimens from the body of the stomach from approximately 150 patients treated continuously with lansoprazole for at least one year did not show evidence of ECL cell effects similar to those seen in rat studies. Longer term data are needed to rule out the possibility of an increased risk of the development of gastric tumors in patients receiving long-term therapy with lansoprazole.

Other Gastric Effects in Humans

Lansoprazole did not significantly affect mucosal blood flow in the fundus of the stomach. Due to the normal physiologic effect caused by the inhibition of gastric acid secretion, a decrease of about 17% in blood flow in the antrum, pylorus, and duodenal bulb was seen. Lansoprazole significantly slowed the gastric emptying of digestible solids. Lansoprazole increased serum pepsinogen levels and decreased pepsin activity under basal conditions and in response to meal stimulation or insulin injection. As with other agents that elevate intragastric pH, increases in gastric pH were associated with increases in nitrate-reducing bacteria and elevation of nitrite concentration in gastric juice in patients with gastric ulcer. No significant increase in nitrosamine concentrations was observed.

Serum Gastrin Effects

In over 2100 patients, median fasting serum gastrin levels increased 50% to 100% from baseline but remained within normal range after treatment with lansoprazole given orally in doses of 15 mg to 60 mg. These elevations reached a plateau within two months of therapy and returned to pretreatment levels within four weeks after discontinuation of therapy.

Endocrine Effects

Human studies for up to one year have not detected any clinically significant effects on the endocrine system. Hormones studied include testosterone, luteinizing hormone (LH), follicle stimulating hormone (FSH), sex hormone binding globulin (SHBG), dehydroepiandrosterone sulfate (DHEA-S), prolactin, cortisol, estradiol, insulin, aldosterone, parathormone, glucagon, thyroid stimulating hormone (TSH), triiodothyronine (T_3), thyroxine (T_4), and somatotropic hormone (STH). Lansoprazole in oral doses of 15 to 60 mg for up to one year had no clinically significant effect on sexual function. In addition, lansoprazole in oral doses of 15 to 60 mg for two to eight weeks had no clinically significant effect on thyroid function.

In 24-month carcinogenicity studies in Sprague-Dawley rats with daily dosages up to 150 mg/kg, proliferative changes in the Leydig cells of the testes, including benign neoplasm, were increased compared to control rates.

Table 1 **Mean Antisecretory Effects After Single and Multiple Daily Dosing**

Parameter	Baseline Value	PREVACID 15 mg Day 1	PREVACID 15 mg Day 5	PREVACID 30 mg Day 1	PREVACID 30 mg Day 5
Mean 24-Hour pH	2.1	2.7⁺	4.0⁺	3.6*	4.9*
Mean Nighttime pH	1.9	2.4	3.0⁺	2.6	3.8*
% Time Gastric pH>3	18	33⁺	59⁺	51*	72*
% Time Gastric pH>4	12	22⁺	49⁺	41*	66*

NOTE: An intragastric pH of >4 reflects a reduction in gastric acid by 99%.
* (p<0.05) versus baseline and lansoprazole 15 mg.
⁺ (p<0.05) versus baseline only.

Table 2 **NSAID-Associated Gastric Ulcer Risk Reduction Rates**

Week	% of Patients Remaining Gastric Ulcer-Free[1] PREVACID 15 mg QD (N=121)	PREVACID 30 mg QD (N=116)	Misoprostol 200 µg QID (N=106)	Placebo (N=112)
4	90 %	92 %	96 %	66 %
8	86 %	88 %	95 %	60 %
12	80 %	82 %	93 %	51 %

[1] % = Life Table Estimate
(p<0.001) PREVACID 15 mg QD versus placebo; PREVACID 30 mg QD versus placebo; and misoprostol 200 µg QID versus placebo.
(p<0.05) Misoprostol 200 µg QID versus PREVACID 15 mg QD; and misoprostol 200 µg QID versus PREVACID 30 mg QD

Table 3 **Gastric Ulcer Risk Reduction Rates in Patients whose NSAID was Naproxen Only or Naproxen and Aspirin Only**

Week	% of Patients Remaining Gastric Ulcer-Free[1] PREVACID 15 mg QD (N=37)	PREVACID 30 mg QD (N=24)	Misoprostol 200 µg QID (N=28)	Placebo (N=30)
4	91%	83%	88%	52%
8	89%	83%	88%	52%
12	89%	83%	83%	33%

[1] % = Life Table Estimate
(p<0.001) PREVACID 15 mg QD versus placebo; PREVACID 30 mg QD versus placebo; and misoprostol 200 µg QID versus placebo.

Other Effects

No systemic effects of lansoprazole on the central nervous system, lymphoid, hematopoietic, renal, hepatic, cardiovascular or respiratory systems have been found in humans. No visual toxicity was observed among 56 patients who had extensive baseline eye evaluations, were treated with up to 180 mg/day of lansoprazole and were observed for up to 58 months. Other rat-specific findings after lifetime exposure included focal pancreatic atrophy, diffuse lymphoid hyperplasia in the thymus, and spontaneous retinal atrophy.

CLINICAL STUDIES

PREVACID® NapraPAC™ (375 or 500)

Risk Reduction of NSAID-Associated Gastric Ulcer

A large U.S., multicenter, double-blind, placebo- and misoprostol-controlled (misoprostol blinded only to the endoscopist) study was conducted in patients who required chronic use of an NSAID and had a history of an endoscopically documented gastric ulcer. Patients took one or more NSAIDs during the study. Concomitant aspirin use (≤ 325 mg) was allowed. The proportion of patients remaining free from gastric ulcer at 4, 8, and 12 weeks was significantly higher with 15 or 30 mg of PREVACID than placebo (see Table 2). A total of 537 patients were enrolled in the study, and 535 patients were treated. Patients ranged in age from 23 to 89 years (median age 60 years), with 65% female patients and 35% male patients. Race was distributed as follows: 90% Caucasian, 6% Black, 4% other. Concomitant aspirin was used in 20% of the patients. The 30 mg dose of PREVACID demonstrated no additional benefit in risk reduction of the NSAID-associated gastric ulcer than the 15 mg dose.

[See table 2 above]

A retrospective subset analysis of 119 patients whose NSAID was naproxen only or naproxen and aspirin only, was performed. Again, the proportion of patients remaining free from gastric ulcer at 4, 8, and 12 weeks was significantly higher with 15 or 30 mg of PREVACID than placebo (see Table 3). Patients ranged in age from 37 to 84 years (median age 58 years) with 61% female patients and 39% male patients. Race was distributed as follows: 88% Caucasian, 8% Black, 4% other. Concomitant aspirin was used in 15% of the patients. The 30 mg dose of PREVACID demonstrated no additional benefit in risk reduction of the NSAID-associated gastric ulcer than the 15 mg dose.

[See table 3 above]

For patients who received PREVACID the highest total daily dose of naproxen was as follows: 5 patients took < 750 mg/daily, 54 patients took 750 - 1000 mg daily. Only 2 patients who received PREVACID took greater than 1000 mg of naproxen.

NAPROSYN

General Information

Naproxen has been studied in patients with rheumatoid arthritis, osteoarthritis and ankylosing spondylitis. Improvement in patients treated for rheumatoid arthritis was demonstrated by a reduction in joint swelling, a reduction in duration of morning stiffness, a reduction in disease activity as assessed by both the investigator and patient, and by increased mobility as demonstrated by a reduction in walking time. Generally, response to naproxen has not been found to be dependent on age, sex, severity or duration of rheumatoid arthritis.

In patients with osteoarthritis, the therapeutic action of naproxen has been shown by a reduction in joint pain or tenderness, an increase in range of motion in knee joints, increased mobility as demonstrated by a reduction in walking time, and improvement in capacity to perform activities of daily living impaired by the disease.

In a clinical trial comparing standard formulations of naproxen 375 mg bid (750 mg a day) vs 750 mg bid (1500 mg/day), 9 patients in the 750 mg group terminated prematurely because of adverse events. Nineteen patients in the 1500 mg group terminated prematurely because of adverse events. Most of these adverse events were gastrointestinal events.

In clinical studies in patients with rheumatoid arthritis or osteoarthritis, naproxen has been shown to be comparable to aspirin and indomethacin in controlling the aforementioned measures of disease activity, but the frequency and severity of the milder gastrointestinal adverse effects (nausea, dyspepsia, heartburn) and nervous system adverse effects (tinnitus, dizziness, lightheadedness) were less in naproxen-treated patients than in those treated with aspirin or indomethacin.

In patients with ankylosing spondylitis, naproxen has been shown to decrease night pain, morning stiffness and pain at rest. In double-blind studies the drug was shown to be as effective as aspirin, but with fewer side effects.

Naproxen may be used safely in combination with gold salts and/or corticosteroids; however, in controlled clinical trials, when added to the regimen of patients receiving corticosteroids, it did not appear to cause greater improvement over that seen with corticosteroids alone. Whether naproxen has a "steroid-sparing" effect has not been adequately studied. When added to the regimen of patients receiving gold salts, naproxen did result in greater improvement. Its use in combination with salicylates is not recommended because there is evidence that aspirin increases the rate of excretion of naproxen and data are inadequate to demonstrate that naproxen and aspirin produce greater improvement over that achieved with aspirin alone. In addition, as with other NSAIDs, the combination may result in higher frequency of adverse events than demonstrated for either product alone.

In ^{51}Cr blood loss and gastroscopy studies with normal volunteers, daily administration of 1000 mg of naproxen has been demonstrated to cause statistically significantly less gastric bleeding and erosion than 3250 mg of aspirin.

INDICATIONS AND USAGE

PREVACID® NapraPAC™ (375 or 500) is indicated for reducing the risk of NSAID-associated gastric ulcers in patients with a history of documented gastric ulcer who require the use of an NSAID for treatment of the signs and symptoms of rheumatoid arthritis, osteoarthritis, and ankylosing spondylitis. (See **CLINICAL STUDIES** and **DOSAGE AND ADMINISTRATION**.) Controlled studies did not extend beyond 12 weeks.

CONTRAINDICATIONS

PREVACID® NapraPAC™ (375 or 500) is contraindicated in patients with known hypersensitivity or allergic reactions to any component of the formulations of PREVACID, NAPROSYN, or over-the-counter products containing naproxen.

Naproxen is also contraindicated in patients in whom aspirin or other nonsteroidal anti-inflammatory/analgesic drugs induce the syndrome of asthma, rhinitis, and nasal polyps. Both types of reactions have the potential of being fatal. Anaphylactoid reactions to naproxen, whether of the true allergic type or the pharmacologic idiosyncratic (eg, aspirin hypersensitivity syndrome) type, usually but not always occur in patients with a known history of such reactions. Therefore, careful questioning of patients for such things as asthma, nasal polyps, urticaria, and hypotension associated with nonsteroidal anti-inflammatory drugs before starting therapy is important. In addition, if such symptoms occur during therapy, treatment should be discontinued.

WARNINGS

NAPROSYN

Risk of GI Ulceration, Bleeding and Perforation With NSAID Therapy

Serious gastrointestinal toxicity such as bleeding, ulceration and perforation can occur at any time, with or without warning symptoms, in patients treated chronically with NSAID therapy. Although minor upper gastrointestinal problems, such as dyspepsia, are common, usually developing early in therapy, physicians should remain alert for ulceration and bleeding in patients treated chronically with NSAIDs even in the absence of previous GI tract symptoms. In patients observed in clinical trials of several months to 2 years' duration, symptomatic upper GI ulcers, gross bleeding or perforation appear to occur in approximately 1% of patients treated for 3 to 6 months and in about 2% to 4% of patients treated for 1 year.

Physicians should inform patients about the signs and/or symptoms of serious GI toxicity and what steps to take if they occur.

Studies to date with naproxen have not identified any subset of patients not at risk of developing peptic ulceration and bleeding. Except for a prior history of serious GI events and other risk factors known to be associated with peptic ulcer disease, such as alcoholism, smoking, etc., no risk factors (e.g., age, sex) have been associated with increased risk. Elderly or debilitated patients seem to tolerate ulceration or bleeding less well than other individuals and most spontaneous reports of fatal GI events are in this population. Studies to date are inconclusive concerning the relative risk of various NSAIDs in causing such reactions. High doses of any NSAID probably carry a greater risk of these reactions, although controlled clinical trials showing this do not exist in most cases. In considering the use of relatively large doses (within the recommended dosage range), sufficient benefit should be anticipated to offset the potential increased risk of GI toxicity.

Physicians should consider alternative treatment to NSAIDs in patients who have experienced a serious gastrointestinal toxicity associated with NSAID use. For patients who require the use of an NSAID, coadministration of PREVACID 15 mg Delayed-Release Capsules with NSAIDs has been proven effective to reduce the risk of gastric ulcers associated with NSAID use in patients with a previous history of documented gastric ulcers. (See **CLINICAL STUDIES**, PREVACID® NapraPAC™ (375 or 500), **Risk Reduction of NSAID-Associated Gastric Ulcer**.)

PRECAUTIONS

General

NAPROSYN

NAPROXEN-CONTAINING PRODUCTS SUCH AS NAPROSYN® (NAPROXEN) TABLETS, EC-NAPROSYN® (NAPROXEN) DELAYED-RELEASE TABLETS, ANAPROX®/ ANAPROX DS® (NAPROXEN SODIUM) TABLETS, NAPROSYN® (NAPROXEN) SUSPENSION, ALEVE® (NAPROXEN SODIUM), AND OTHER NAPROXEN PRODUCTS INCLUDING PREVACID® NapraPAC™ (375 or 500), SHOULD NOT BE USED CONCOMITANTLY SINCE THEY ALL CIRCULATE IN THE PLASMA AS THE NAPROXEN ANION.

NAPROSYN cannot be expected to substitute for corticosteroids or to treat corticosteroid insufficiency. If the steroid dose is reduced or eliminated during therapy, the steroid dosage should be reduced slowly and the patient should be observed closely for any evidence of adverse effects, including adrenal insufficiency and exacerbation of symptoms of arthritis.

Patients with initial hemoglobin values of 10 grams or less who are to receive long-term therapy should have hemoglobin values determined periodically.

The antipyretic and anti-inflammatory activities of the drug may reduce fever and inflammation, thus diminishing their utility as diagnostic signs in detecting complications of presumed noninfectious, noninflammatory painful conditions.

Because of adverse eye findings in animal studies with drugs of this class, it is recommended that ophthalmic studies be carried out if any change or disturbance in vision occurs.

PREVACID

Symptomatic response to therapy with lansoprazole does not preclude the presence of gastric malignancy.

Information for Patients

Each convenience package of PREVACID® NapraPAC™ (375 or 500) contains sufficient product for seven days of treatment. Each daily dose consists of one PREVACID 15 mg capsule and two NAPROSYN tablets, either 375 mg or 500 mg. Take the PREVACID capsule and one NAPROSYN tablet in the morning before eating with a glass of water. Take the second NAPROSYN tablet in the evening with a glass of water.

NAPROSYN, like other drugs of this class, is not free of side effects. The side effects of this formulation can cause discomfort and, rarely, there are more serious side effects, such as gastrointestinal bleeding, which may result in hospitalization and even fatal outcomes. PREVACID when taken with naproxen has been shown to reduce the risk of NSAID-associated gastric ulcers in patients with a history of ulcer. NSAIDs (Nonsteroidal Anti-Inflammatory Drugs) are often essential agents in the management of arthritis and have a major role in the treatment of pain. Naproxen as NAPROSYN is indicated for the treatment of rheumatoid arthritis, osteoarthritis, and ankylosing spondylitis.

Physicians may wish to discuss with their patients the potential risks (see **WARNINGS, PRECAUTIONS** and **ADVERSE REACTIONS**) and likely benefits of naproxen treatment, particularly when it is used for less serious conditions where treatment without NSAIDs may represent an acceptable alternative to both the patient and physician.

Caution should be exercised by patients whose activities require alertness if they experience drowsiness, dizziness, vertigo or depression during therapy with naproxen.

Renal Effects

NAPROSYN

As with other nonsteroidal anti-inflammatory drugs, long-term administration of naproxen to animals has resulted in renal papillary necrosis and other abnormal renal pathology. In humans, there have been reports of acute interstitial nephritis, hematuria, proteinuria and occasionally nephrotic syndrome associated with naproxen-containing products and other NSAIDs since they have been marketed.

A second form of renal toxicity has been seen in patients taking naproxen as well as other nonsteroidal anti-inflammatory drugs. In patients with prerenal conditions leading to a reduction in renal blood flow or blood volume, where the renal prostaglandins have a supportive role in the maintenance of renal perfusion, administration of a nonsteroidal anti-inflammatory drug may cause a dose-dependent reduction in prostaglandin formation and precipitate overt renal decompensation. Patients at greatest risk of this reaction are those with impaired renal function, heart failure, liver dysfunction, those taking diuretics and the elderly. Discontinuation of nonsteroidal anti- inflammatory therapy is typically followed by recovery to the pretreatment state.

Naproxen and its metabolites are eliminated primarily by the kidneys; therefore, the drug should be used with caution in patients with significantly impaired renal function, and the monitoring of serum creatinine and/or creatinine clearance is advised in these patients. Caution should be used if the drug is given to patients with creatinine clearance of less than 20 mL/minute because accumulation of naproxen metabolites has been seen in such patients.

Chronic alcoholic liver disease and probably other diseases with decreased or abnormal plasma proteins (albumin) reduce the total plasma concentration of naproxen, but the plasma concentration of unbound naproxen is increased. Caution is advised when high doses are required and some adjustment of dosage may be required in these patients. It is prudent to use the lowest effective dose.

Studies indicate that although total plasma concentration of naproxen is unchanged, the unbound plasma fraction of naproxen is increased in the elderly. Caution is advised when high doses are required and some adjustment of dosage may be required in elderly patients. As with other drugs used in the elderly, it is prudent to use the lowest effective dose.

Hepatic Function

NAPROSYN

As with other nonsteroidal anti-inflammatory drugs, borderline elevations of one or more liver tests may occur in up to 15% of patients. These abnormalities may progress, may remain essentially unchanged, or may be transient with continued therapy. The SGPT (ALT) test is probably the most sensitive indicator of liver dysfunction. Meaningful (3 times the upper limit of normal) elevations of SGPT or SGOT (AST) occurred in controlled clinical trials in less than 1% of patients. A patient with symptoms and/or signs suggesting liver dysfunction or in whom an abnormal liver test has occurred, should be evaluated for evidence of the development of more severe hepatic reaction while on therapy with naproxen. Severe hepatic reactions, including jaundice and cases of fatal hepatitis, have been reported with naproxen as with other nonsteroidal anti-inflammatory drugs. Although such reactions are rare, if abnormal liver tests persist or worsen, if clinical signs and symptoms consistent with liver disease develop, or if systemic manifestations occur (eg, eosinophilia, rash, etc.), naproxen should be discontinued.

Fluid Retention and Edema

NAPROSYN

Peripheral edema has been observed in some patients receiving naproxen.

Laboratory Tests

NAPROSYN

Because serious GI tract ulceration and bleeding can occur without warning symptoms, physicians should follow patients chronically treated with naproxen for signs and symptoms of ulceration and bleeding and should inform them of the importance of this follow-up and what they should do if certain signs and symptoms do appear (see **WARNINGS,** NAPROSYN **Risk of GI Ulcerations, Bleeding and Perforation With NSAID Therapy**).

Drug Interactions

NAPROSYN

The use of NSAIDs in patients who are receiving ACE inhibitors may potentiate renal disease states (see **PRECAUTIONS,** NAPROSYN **Renal Effects**).

In vitro studies have shown that naproxen anion, because of its affinity for protein, may displace from their binding sites other drugs that are also albumin-bound (see **CLINICAL PHARMACOLOGY,** NAPROSYN **Pharmacokinetics**).

Theoretically, the naproxen anion itself could likewise be displaced. Short-term controlled studies failed to show that taking the drug significantly affects prothrombin times when administered to individuals on coumarin-type anticoagulants. Caution is advised nonetheless, since interactions have been seen with other nonsteroidal agents of this class. Similarly, patients receiving the drug and a hydantoin, sulfonamide or sulfonylurea should be observed for signs of toxicity to these drugs (see **CLINICAL STUDIES,** NAPROSYN **General Information**).

Concomitant administration of naproxen and aspirin is not recommended because naproxen is displaced from its binding sites during the concomitant administration of aspirin, resulting in lower plasma concentrations and peak plasma levels.

The natriuretic effect of furosemide has been reported to be inhibited by some drugs of this class. Inhibition of renal lithium clearance leading to increases in plasma lithium concentrations has also been reported. Naproxen and other nonsteroidal anti-inflammatory drugs can reduce the antihypertensive effect of propranolol and other beta-blockers. Probenecid given concurrently increases naproxen anion plasma levels and extends its plasma half-life significantly. Caution should be used if naproxen is administered concomitantly with methotrexate. Naproxen, and other nonsteroidal anti-inflammatory drugs have been reported to reduce the tubular secretion of methotrexate in an animal model, possibly increasing the toxicity of methotrexate.

PREVACID

Lansoprazole is metabolized through the cytochrome P_{450} system, specifically through the CYP3A and CYP2C19 isozymes. Studies have shown that lansoprazole does not have clinically significant interactions with other drugs metabolized by the cytochrome P_{450} system, such as warfarin, antipyrine, indomethacin, ibuprofen, phenytoin, propranolol, prednisone, diazepam, or clarithromycin in healthy subjects. These compounds are metabolized through various cytochrome P_{450} isozymes including CYP1A2, CYP2C9, CYP2C19, CYP2D6, and CYP3A. When lansoprazole was administered concomitantly with theophylline (CYP1A2, CYP3A), a minor increase (10%) in the clearance of theophylline was seen. Because of the small magnitude and the direction of the effect on theophylline clearance, this interaction is unlikely to be of clinical concern. Nonetheless, individual patients may require additional titration of their theophylline dosage when lansoprazole is started or stopped to ensure clinically effective blood levels.

In a study of healthy subjects neither the pharmacokinetics of warfarin enantiomers nor prothrombin time were affected following single or multiple 60 mg doses of lansoprazole. However, there have been reports of increased International Normalized Ratio (INR) and prothrombin time in patients receiving proton pump inhibitors, including lansoprazole, and warfarin concomitantly. Increases in INR and prothrombin time may lead to abnormal bleeding and even death. Patients treated with proton pump inhibitors and warfarin concomitantly may need to be monitored for increases in INR and prothrombin time.

Lansoprazole has also been shown to have no clinically significant interaction with amoxicillin.

In a single-dose crossover study examining lansoprazole 30 mg and omeprazole 20 mg each administered alone and concomitantly with sucralfate 1 gram, absorption of the proton pump inhibitors was delayed and their bioavailability was reduced by 17% and 16%, respectively, when administered concomitantly with sucralfate. Therefore, proton pump inhibitors should be taken at least 30 minutes prior to sucralfate. In clinical trials, antacids were administered concomitantly with PREVACID Delayed-Release Capsules; this did not interfere with its effect.

Lansoprazole causes a profound and long-lasting inhibition of gastric acid secretion; therefore, it is theoretically possible that lansoprazole may interfere with the absorption of drugs where gastric pH is an important determinant of bioavailability (e.g., ketoconazole, ampicillin esters, iron salts, digoxin).

Drug/Laboratory Test Interactions

NAPROSYN

Naproxen may decrease platelet aggregation and prolong bleeding time. This effect should be kept in mind when bleeding times are determined.

Continued on next page

Prevacid NapraPAC—Cont.

The administration of naproxen may result in increased urinary values for 17-ketogenic steroids because of an interaction between the drug and/or its metabolites with m-dinitrobenzene used in this assay. Although 17-hydroxycorticosteroid measurements (Porter-Silber test) do not appear to be artifactually altered, it is suggested that therapy with naproxen be temporarily discontinued 72 hours before adrenal function tests are performed if the Porter-Silber test is to be used.

Naproxen may interfere with some urinary assays of 5-hydroxy indoleacetic acid (5HIAA).

Carcinogenesis, Mutagenesis, Impairment of Fertility

NAPROSYN

A 2-year study was performed in rats to evaluate the carcinogenic potential of naproxen at rat doses of 8, 16, and 24 mg/kg/day (50, 100, and 150 mg/m^2). The maximum dose used was 0.28 times the systemic exposure to humans at the recommended dose. No evidence of tumorigenicity was found.

PREVACID

In two 24-month carcinogenicity studies, Sprague-Dawley rats were treated orally with doses of 5 to 150 mg/kg/day, about 1 to 40 times the exposure on a body surface (mg/m^2) basis, of a 50-kg person of average height (1.46 m^2 body surface area) given the recommended human dose of 30 mg/day (22.2 mg/m^2). Lansoprazole produced dose-related gastric enterochromaffin-like (ECL) cell hyperplasia and ECL cell carcinoids in both male and female rats. It also increased the incidence of intestinal metaplasia of the gastric epithelium in both sexes. In male rats, lansoprazole produced a dose-related increase of testicular interstitial cell adenomas. The incidence of these adenomas in rats receiving doses of 15 to 150 mg/kg/day (4 to 40 times the recommended human dose based on body surface area) exceeded the low background incidence (range = 1.4 to 10%) for this strain of rat. Testicular interstitial cell adenoma also occurred in 1 of 30 rats treated with 50 mg/kg/day (13 times the recommended human dose based on body surface area) in a 1-year toxicity study.

In a 24-month carcinogenicity study, CD-1 mice were treated orally with doses of 15 to 600 mg/kg/day, 2 to 80 times the recommended human dose based on body surface area. Lansoprazole produced a dose-related increased incidence of gastric ECL cell hyperplasia. It also produced an increased incidence of liver tumors (hepatocellular adenoma plus carcinoma). The tumor incidences in male mice treated with 300 and 600 mg/kg/day (40 to 80 times the recommended human dose based on body surface area) and female mice treated with 150 to 600 mg/kg/day (20 to 80 times the recommended human dose based on body surface area) exceeded the ranges of background incidences in historical controls for this strain of mice. Lansoprazole treatment produced adenoma of rete testis in male mice receiving 75 to 600 mg/kg/day (10 to 80 times the recommended human dose based on body surface area).

Lansoprazole was not genotoxic in the Ames test, the *ex vivo* rat hepatocyte unscheduled DNA synthesis (UDS) test, the *in vivo* mouse micronucleus test or the rat bone marrow cell chromosomal aberration test. It was positive in *in vitro* human lymphocyte chromosomal aberration assays.

Lansoprazole at oral doses up to 150 mg/kg/day (40 times the recommended human dose based on body surface area) was found to have no effect on fertility and reproductive performance of male and female rats.

Pregnancy: Teratogenic Effects

Pregnancy Category B

PREVACID® NapraPAC™ (375 or 500)

There are no adequate and well-controlled studies in pregnant women. Because animal reproduction studies are not always predictive of human response, PREVACID® NapraPAC™ (375 or 500) should not be used during pregnancy unless clearly needed.

NAPROSYN

Reproduction studies have been performed in rats at 20 mg/kg/day (125 mg/m^2/day, 0.23 times the human systemic exposure), rabbits at 20 mg/kg/day (220 mg/m^2/day, 0.27 times the human systemic exposure), and mice at 170 mg/kg/day (510 mg/m^2/day, 0.28 times the human systemic exposure) with no evidence of impaired fertility or harm to the fetus due to the drug. There are no adequate and well-controlled studies in pregnant women. Because animal reproduction studies are not always predictive of human response, naproxen should not be used during pregnancy unless clearly needed.

PREVACID

Teratology studies have been performed in pregnant rats at oral doses up to 150 mg/kg/day (40 times the recommended human dose based on body surface area) and pregnant rabbits at oral doses up to 30 mg/kg/day (16 times the recommended human dose based on body surface area) and have revealed no evidence of impaired fertility or harm to the fetus due to lansoprazole.

Nonteratogenic Effects

NAPROSYN

There is some evidence to suggest that when inhibitors of prostaglandin synthesis are used to delay preterm labor there is an increased risk of neonatal complications such as necrotizing enterocolitis, patent ductus arteriosus and intracranial hemorrhage. Naproxen treatment given in late pregnancy to delay parturition has been associated with persistent pulmonary hypertension, renal dysfunction and abnormal prostaglandin E levels in preterm infants. Because of the known effect of drugs of this class on the human fetal cardiovascular system (closure of ductus arteriosus), use during third trimester should be avoided.

Nursing Mothers

PREVACID® NapraPAC™ (375 or 500)

No studies were conducted in this population with PREVACID® NapraPAC™, however, because of the possible adverse effects of prostaglandin-inhibiting drugs on neonates, use of PREVACID® NapraPAC™ (375 or 500) in nursing mothers should be avoided.

NAPROSYN

The naproxen anion has been found in the milk of lactating women at a concentration of approximately 1% of that found in plasma. Because of the possible adverse effects of prostaglandin-inhibiting drugs on neonates, use in nursing mothers should be avoided.

PREVACID

Lansoprazole or its metabolites are excreted in the milk of rats. It is not known whether lansoprazole is excreted in human milk. Because many drugs are excreted in human milk, because of the potential for serious adverse reactions in nursing infants from lansoprazole, and because of the potential for tumorigenicity shown for lansoprazole in rat carcinogenicity studies, a decision should be made whether to discontinue nursing or to discontinue the drug, taking into account the importance of the drug to the mother.

Pediatric Use

PREVACID® NapraPAC™ (375 or 500)

The safety and effectiveness of PREVACID® NapraPAC™ (375 or 500) in pediatric patients have not been established.

Geriatric Use

NAPROSYN

Studies indicate that although total plasma concentration of naproxen is unchanged, the unbound plasma fraction of naproxen is increased in the elderly. Caution is advised when high doses are required and some adjustment of dosage may be required in elderly patients. As with other drugs used in the elderly, it is prudent to use the lowest effective dose.

PREVACID

The incidence rates of adverse events and laboratory test abnormalities are also similar to those seen in younger patients. For elderly patients, dosage and administration of lansoprazole need not be altered.

Use in Women

PREVACID

Over 4,000 women were treated with lansoprazole. Ulcer healing rates in females were similar to those in males. The incidence rates of adverse events were also similar to those seen in males.

ADVERSE REACTIONS

NAPROSYN

The following adverse reactions are divided into three parts based on frequency and whether or not the possibility exists of a causal relationship between naproxen and these adverse events. In those reactions listed as "Probable Causal Relationship" there is at least 1 case for each adverse reaction where there is evidence to suggest that there is a causal relationship between drug usage and the reported event.

Adverse reactions reported in controlled clinical trials in 960 patients treated for rheumatoid arthritis or osteoarthritis are listed below. In general, reactions in patients treated chronically were reported 2 to 10 times more frequently than they were in short- term studies in the 962 patients treated for mild to moderate pain or for dysmenorrhea. The most frequent complaints reported related to the gastrointestinal tract.

A clinical study found gastrointestinal reactions to be more frequent and more severe in rheumatoid arthritis patients taking daily doses of 1500 mg naproxen compared to those taking 750 mg naproxen.

The following adverse reactions are divided into three parts based on frequency and causal relationship.

Incidence greater than 1% (Probable Causal Relationship): *Gastrointestinal* - constipation*, heartburn*, abdominal pain*, nausea*, dyspepsia, diarrhea, stomatitis; *Central Nervous System* - headache*, dizziness*, drowsiness*, lightheadedness, vertigo; *Dermatologic* - itching (pruritus)*, skin eruptions*, ecchymoses*, sweating, purpura; *Special Senses*- tinnitus*, hearing disturbances, visual disturbances; *Cardiovascular* - edema*, dyspnea*, palpitations; *General* - thirst

*Incidence of reported reaction between 3% and 9%. Those reactions occurring in less than 3% of the patients are unmarked.

Incidence less than 1% (Probable Causal Relationship): The following adverse reactions were reported less frequently than 1% during controlled clinical trials and through voluntary reports since marketing. Those reactions observed through voluntary reporting since marketing of NAPROSYN are underlined.

Gastrointestinal - abnormal liver function tests, colitis, gastrointestinal bleeding and/or perforation, hematemesis, jaundice, pancreatitis, melena, vomiting; *Renal* - glomerular nephritis, hematuria, hyperkalemia, interstitial nephritis, nephrotic syndrome, renal disease, renal failure, renal papillary necrosis; *Hematologic* - agranulocytosis, eosinophilia, granulocytopenia, leukopenia, thrombocytopenia; *Central Nervous System* - depression, dream abnormalities, inability to concentrate, insomnia, malaise, myalgia, muscle weakness; *Dermatologic* - alopecia, photosensitive dermatitis, urticaria, skin rashes, photosensitivity reactions resembling porphyria cutanea tarda, epidermolysis bullosa; *Special Senses* - hearing impairment; *Cardiovascular* - congestive heart failure; *Respiratory* - eosinophilic pneumonitis; *General* - anaphylactoid reactions, angioneurotic edema, menstrual disorders, pyrexia (chills and fever)

Incidence less than 1% (Causal Relationship Unknown): These observations are being listed to serve as alerting information to the physician. *Hematologic* - aplastic anemia, hemolytic anemia; *Central Nervous System* - aseptic meningitis, cognitive dysfunction; *Dermatologic* - epidermal necrolysis, erythema multiforme, Stevens-Johnson syndrome; *Gastrointestinal* - nonpeptic gastrointestinal ulceration, ulcerative stomatitis; *Cardiovascular* - vasculitis; *General* - hyperglycemia, hypoglycemia

PREVACID

Clinical

Worldwide, over 10,000 patients have been treated with lansoprazole in Phase 2-3 clinical trials involving various dosages and durations of treatment. The adverse reaction profiles for PREVACID Delayed-Release Capsules and PREVACID for Delayed-Release Oral Suspension are similar. In general, lansoprazole treatment has been well-tolerated in both short-term and long-term trials.

The following adverse events were reported by the treating physician to have a possible or probable relationship to drug in 1% or more of PREVACID-treated patients and occurred at a greater rate in PREVACID-treated patients than placebo-treated patients in Table 4.

Table 4 Incidence of Possibly or Probably Treatment-Related Adverse Events in Short-Term, Placebo-Controlled Studies

Body System/Adverse Event	PREVACID (N= 2768) %	Placebo (N= 1023) %
Body as a Whole		
Abdominal Pain	2.1	1.2
Digestive System		
Constipation	1.0	0.4
Diarrhea	3.8	2.3
Nausea	1.3	1.2

Headache was also seen at greater than 1% incidence but was more common on placebo. The incidence of diarrhea was similar between patients who received placebo and patients who received lansoprazole 15 mg and 30 mg, but higher in the patients who received lansoprazole 60 mg (2.9%, 1.4%, 4.2%, and 7.4%, respectively).

The most commonly reported possibly or probably treatment-related adverse event during maintenance therapy was diarrhea.

In the risk reduction study of PREVACID for NSAID-associated gastric ulcers, the incidence of diarrhea for patients treated with PREVACID was 5%, misoprostol 22%, and placebo 3%.

Additional adverse experiences occurring in <1% of patients or subjects in domestic trials are shown below. Refer to **Postmarketing** for adverse reactions occurring since the drug was marketed.

Body as a Whole—abdomen enlarged, allergic reaction, asthenia, back pain, candidiasis, carcinoma, chest pain (not otherwise specified), chills, edema, fever, flu syndrome, halitosis, infection (not otherwise specified), malaise, neck pain, neck rigidity, pain, pelvic pain; *Cardiovascular System* - angina, arrhythmia, bradycardia, cerebrovascular accident/cerebral infarction, hypertension/hypotension, migraine, myocardial infarction, palpitations, shock (circulatory failure), syncope, tachycardia, vasodilation; *Digestive System* – abnormal stools, anorexia, bezoar, cardiospasm, cholelithiasis, colitis, dry mouth, dyspepsia, dysphagia, enteritis, eructation, esophageal stenosis, esophageal ulcer, esophagitis, fecal discoloration, flatulence, gastric nodules/fundic gland polyps, gastritis, gastroenteritis, gastrointestinal anomaly, gastrointestinal disorder, gastrointestinal hemorrhage, glossitis, gum hemorrhage, hematemesis, increased appetite, increased salivation, melena, mouth ulceration, nausea and vomiting, nausea and vomiting and diarrhea, oral moniliasis, rectal disorder, rectal hemorrhage, stomatitis, tenesmus, thirst, tongue disorder, ulcerative colitis, ulcerative stomatitis; *Endocrine System* - diabetes mellitus, goiter, hypothyroidism; *Hemic and Lymphatic System* - anemia, hemolysis, lymphadenopathy; *Metabolic and Nutritional Disorders* - gout, dehydration, hyperglycemia/hypoglycemia, peripheral edema, weight gain/loss; *Musculoskeletal System* - arthralgia, arthritis, bone disorder, joint disorder, leg cramps, musculoskeletal pain, myalgia, myasthenia, synovitis; *Nervous System* - abnormal dreams, agitation, amnesia, anxiety, apathy, confusion, convulsion, depersonalization, depression, diplopia, dizziness, emotional lability, hallucinations, hemiplegia, hostility aggravated, hyperkinesia, hypertonia, hypesthesia, insomnia, libido decreased/increased, nervousness, neurosis, paresthesia, sleep disorder, somnolence, thinking abnormality, tremor, vertigo; *Respiratory System* - asthma, bronchitis, cough increased, dyspnea, epistaxis, hemoptysis, hiccup, laryngeal neoplasia, pharyngitis, pleural disorder, pneumonia, respiratory disorder, upper respiratory inflammation/infection, rhinitis, sinusitis, stridor; *Skin and Appendages* - acne, alopecia, contact dermatitis, dry skin, fixed eruption, hair disorder, maculopapular rash, nail disorder, pruritus, rash, skin carcinoma, skin disorder, sweating, urticaria; *Special Senses* -

abnormal vision, blurred vision, conjunctivitis, deafness, dry eyes, ear disorder, eye pain, otitis media, parosmia, photophobia, retinal degeneration, taste loss, taste perversion, tinnitus, visual field defect; *Urogenital System* - abnormal menses, breast enlargement, breast pain, breast tenderness, dysmenorrhea, dysuria, gynecomastia, impotence, kidney calculus, kidney pain, leukorrhea, menorrhagia, menstrual disorder, penis disorder, polyuria, testis disorder, urethral pain, urinary frequency, urinary tract infection, urinary urgency, urination impaired, vaginitis.

Postmarketing

On-going Safety Surveillance: Additional adverse experiences have been reported since lansoprazole has been marketed. The majority of these cases are foreign-sourced and a relationship to lansoprazole has not been established. Because these events were reported voluntarily from a population of unknown size, estimates of frequency cannot be made. These events are listed below by COSTART body system.

Body as a Whole—anaphylactoid-like reaction; *Digestive System* - hepatotoxicity, pancreatitis, vomiting; *Hemic and Lymphatic System* - agranulocytosis, aplastic anemia, hemolytic anemia, leukopenia, neutropenia, pancytopenia, thrombocytopenia, and thrombotic thrombocytopenic purpura; *Skin and Appendages* – severe dermatologic reactions including erythema multiforme, Stevens-Johnson syndrome, toxic epidermal necrolysis (some fatal); *Special Senses* - speech disorder; *Urogenital System* - urinary retention.

Laboratory Values

The following changes in laboratory parameters for lansoprazole were reported as adverse events:

Abnormal liver function tests, increased SGOT (AST), increased SGPT (ALT), increased creatinine, increased alkaline phosphatase, increased globulins, increased GGTP, increased/decreased/abnormal WBC, abnormal AG ratio, abnormal RBC, bilirubinemia, eosinophilia, hyperlipemia, increased/decreased electrolytes, increased/decreased cholesterol, increased glucocorticoids, increased LDH, increased/decreased/abnormal platelets, and increased gastrin levels. Urine abnormalities such as albuminuria, glycosuria, and hematuria were also reported. Additional isolated laboratory abnormalities were reported.

In the placebo controlled studies, when SGOT (AST) and SGPT (ALT) were evaluated, 0.4% (4/978) placebo patients and 0.4% (11/2677) lansoprazole patients had enzyme elevations greater than three times the upper limit of normal range at the final treatment visit. None of these lansoprazole patients reported jaundice at any time during the study.

OVERDOSAGE

PREVACID® NapraPAC™ (375 or 500)

In case of an overdose, patients should contact a physician, poison control center, or emergency room. There are no data suggesting increased toxicity of the combination of naproxen and lansoprazole compared with individual components.

NAPROSYN

Significant naproxen overdosage may be characterized by drowsiness, heartburn, indigestion, nausea or vomiting. In the event that ANAPROX/ANAPROX-DS, ALEVE, or naproxen sodium is taken with PREVACID® NapraPAC™ (375 or 500), earlier and higher blood levels may be anticipated due to the rapid absorption of naproxen sodium. A few patients have experienced seizures, but it is not clear whether or not these were drug-related. It is not known what dose of the drug would be life-threatening. The oral LD_{50} of the drug is 543 mg/kg in rats, 1234 mg/kg in mice, 4110 mg/kg in hamsters, and greater than 1000 mg/kg in dogs.

Should a patient ingest a large number of tablets, accidentally or purposefully, the stomach may be emptied and usual supportive measures employed. In animals 0.5 g/kg of activated charcoal was effective in reducing plasma levels of naproxen. Hemodialysis does not decrease the plasma concentration of naproxen because of the high degree of its protein binding.

PREVACID

Oral doses up to 5000 mg/kg in rats (approximately 1300 times the 30 mg human dose based on body surface area) and mice (about 675.7 times the 30 mg human dose based on body surface area) did not produce deaths or any clinical signs.

Lansoprazole is not removed from the circulation by hemodialysis. In one reported case of overdose, the patient consumed 600 mg of lansoprazole with no adverse reaction.

DOSAGE AND ADMINISTRATION

Risk Reduction of NSAID-Associated Gastric Ulcers in the Treatment of Osteoarthritis, Rheumatoid Arthritis, Ankylosing Spondylitis

Each convenience package of PREVACID® NapraPAC™ (375 or 500) contains sufficient product for seven days of treatment. Each daily dose consists of one PREVACID 15 mg capsule and two NAPROSYN tablets, either 375 mg or 500 mg. Take the PREVACID capsule and one NAPROSYN tablet in the morning before eating with a glass of water. Take the second NAPROSYN tablet in the evening with a glass of water.

The maximum daily naproxen dose of PREVACID® NapraPAC™ (375 or 500) is 1000 mg. Controlled studies for PREVACID® NapraPAC™ did not extend beyond 12 weeks.

For PREVACID® NapraPAC™ (375 or 500), no adjustment of the 15 mg PREVACID component is necessary in patients with renal insufficiency or for the elderly. Dosage adjustment for the NAPROSYN component should be considered for patients with renal insufficiency, liver disease or the elderly (see **PRECAUTIONS - Renal Effects** and **Hepatic Function**).

PREVACID Delayed-Release Capsules should be swallowed whole. The capsule should not be chewed or crushed.

HOW SUPPLIED

PREVACID® NapraPAC™ 375 is supplied as a weekly blister card packaged as a monthly (28 days) course of therapy. Each weekly blister card contains:

NAPROSYN
— fourteen pink, biconvex oval tablets, engraved with NPR LE 375 on one side.

PREVACID
— seven opaque, hard gelatin, pink and green PREVACID 15 mg capsules, with the TAP logo and "PREVACID 15" imprinted on the capsules.

PREVACID® NapraPAC™ 500 is supplied as a weekly blister card packaged as a monthly (28 days) course of therapy. Each weekly blister card contains:

NAPROSYN
— fourteen yellow, capsule-shaped tablets, engraved with NPR LE 500 on one side and scored on the other.

PREVACID
— seven opaque, hard gelatin, pink and green PREVACID 15 mg capsules, with the TAP logo and "PREVACID 15" imprinted on the capsules.

NDC 0300-1545-07 Weekly Blister Card, 375 mg
NDC 0300-1546-07 Weekly Blister Card, 500 mg
NDC 0300-1545-30 One Month Administration Pack, 375 mg
NDC 0300-1546-30 One Month Administration Pack, 500 mg

Storage: Protect from light and moisture.
Store at 25°C (77°F), excursions permitted to 15-30°C (59-86°F). [See USP Controlled Room Temperature]
Store and dispense in original container.

Rx only

U.S. Patent No. 6,047,829
Distributed by TAP Pharmaceuticals Inc.
Lake Forest, Illinois 60045, U.S.A.

ALEVE® is a registered trademark of Bayer-Roche L.L.C.
ANAPROX®/ANAPROX DS®, EC-NAPROSYN®, NAPROSYN®, and NAPROSYN® SUSPENSION are registered trademarks of and NapraPAC™ is a trademark of Syntex Pharmaceuticals International Ltd., A Bermuda Corporation
PREVACID® is a registered trademark of TAP Pharmaceuticals Inc.

3646-R3, Rev. November, 2003

Shown in Product Identification Guide, page 334

PREVPAC® ℞

[*prĕv'păk*]

(lansoprazole 30-mg capsules, amoxicillin 500-mg capsules, USP, and clarithromycin 500-mg tablets, USP)

To reduce the development of drug-resistant bacteria and maintain the effectiveness of PREVPAC and other antibacterial drugs, PREVPAC should be used only to treat or prevent infections that are proven or strongly suspected to be caused by bacteria.

THESE PRODUCTS ARE INTENDED ONLY FOR USE AS DESCRIBED. The individual products contained in this package should not be used alone or in combination for other purposes. The information described in this labeling concerns only the use of these products as indicated in this daily administration pack. For information on use of the individual components when dispensed as individual medications outside this combined use for treating *Helicobacter pylori (H. pylori)*, please see the package inserts for each individual product.

DESCRIPTION

PREVPAC consists of a daily administration pack containing two PREVACID 30-mg capsules, four amoxicillin 500-mg capsules, USP, and two clarithromycin 500-mg tablets, USP, for oral administration.

PREVACID® (lansoprazole) Delayed-Release Capsules

The active ingredient in PREVACID capsules is a substituted benzimidazole, 2-[[[3-methyl-4-(2,2,2-trifluoroethoxy)-2-pyridyl] methyl] sulfinyl] benzimidazole, a compound that inhibits gastric acid secretion. Its empirical formula is $C_{16}H_{14}F_3N_3O_2S$ with a molecular weight of 369.37. The structural formula is:

Lansoprazole is a white to brownish-white odorless crystalline powder which melts with decomposition at approximately 166°C. Lansoprazole is freely soluble in dimethylformamide; soluble in methanol; sparingly soluble in ethanol; slightly soluble in ethyl acetate, dichloromethane and acetonitrile; very slightly soluble in ether; and practically insoluble in hexane and water.

Each delayed-release capsule contains enteric-coated granules consisting of lansoprazole (30 mg), hydroxypropyl cellulose, low substituted hydroxypropyl cellulose, colloidal silicon dioxide, magnesium carbonate, methacrylic acid copolymer, starch, talc, sugar sphere, sucrose, polyethylene glycol, polysorbate 80, and titanium dioxide. Components of the gelatin capsule include gelatin, titanium dioxide, D&C Red No. 28, FD&C Blue No. 1, and FD&C Red No. 40.

TRIMOX® (amoxicillin, USP)

Amoxicillin, USP, (2*S*,5*R*,6*R*)-6-[(*R*)-(–)-2-Amino-2-(*p*-hydroxyphenyl) acetamido]-3,3-dimethyl-7-oxo-4-thia-1-azabicyclo[3.2.0] heptane-2-carboxylic acid trihydrate, is a semisynthetic penicillin, an analogue of ampicillin. It has the following chemical structure:

The empirical formula is $C_{16}H_{19}N_3O_5S \bullet 3H_2O$, and the molecular weight is 419.45.

The flesh body/maroon cap capsules contain amoxicillin trihydrate equivalent to 500 mg of amoxicillin. The inactive ingredient in the capsules is magnesium stearate.

BIAXIN® Filmtab® (clarithromycin tablets, USP)

Clarithromycin is a semi-synthetic macrolide antibiotic. Chemically, it is 6-*0*-methylerythromycin. The molecular formula is $C_{38}H_{69}NO_{13}$, and the molecular weight is 747.96. The structural formula is:

Clarithromycin is a white to off-white crystalline powder. It is soluble in acetone, slightly soluble in methanol, ethanol, and acetonitrile, and practically insoluble in water. Each yellow oval film-coated immediate-release tablet contains 500 mg of clarithromycin and the following inactive ingredients: hypromellose, hydroxypropyl cellulose, colloidal silicon dioxide, croscarmellose sodium, D&C Yellow No. 10, magnesium stearate, microcrystalline cellulose, povidone, propylene glycol, sorbic acid, sorbitan monooleate, titanium dioxide, and vanillin.

CLINICAL PHARMACOLOGY

Pharmacokinetics

Pharmacokinetics when all three of the PREVPAC components (PREVACID capsules, amoxicillin capsules, clarithromycin tablets) were coadministered has not been studied. Studies have shown no clinically significant interactions of PREVACID and amoxicillin or PREVACID and clarithromycin when administered together. There is no information about the gastric mucosal concentrations of PREVACID, amoxicillin and clarithromycin after administration of these agents concomitantly. The systemic pharmacokinetic information presented below is based on studies in which each product was administered alone.

PREVACID:

PREVACID capsules contain an enteric-coated granule formulation of lansoprazole. Absorption of lansoprazole begins only after the granules leave the stomach. Absorption is rapid, with mean peak plasma levels of lansoprazole occurring after approximately 1.7 hours. Peak plasma concentrations of lansoprazole (C_{max}) and the area under the plasma concentration curve (AUC) of lansoprazole are approximately proportional in doses from 15 mg to 60 mg after single-dose oral administration. Lansoprazole does not accumulate and its pharmacokinetics are unaltered by multiple dosing.

The absorption of lansoprazole is rapid, with mean C_{max} occurring approximately 1.7 hours after oral dosing, and relatively complete with absolute bioavailability over 80%. In healthy subjects, the mean (± SD) plasma half-life was 1.5 (± 1.0) hours. Both C_{max} and AUC are diminished by about 50% if the drug is given 30 minutes after food as opposed to the fasting condition. There is no significant food effect if the drug is given before meals.

Lansoprazole is 97% bound to plasma proteins. Plasma protein binding is consistent over the concentration range of 0.05 to 5.0 mcg/mL.

Lansoprazole is extensively metabolized in the liver. Two metabolites have been identified in measurable quantities in plasma (the hydroxylated sulfinyl and sulfone derivatives of lansoprazole). These metabolites have very little or no antisecretory activity. Lansoprazole is thought to be transformed into two active species which inhibit acid secretion by (H^+,K^+)-ATPase within the parietal cell canaliculus, but are not present in the systemic circulation. The plasma

Continued on next page

Prevpac—Cont.

elimination half-life of lansoprazole does not reflect its duration of suppression of gastric acid secretion. Thus, the plasma elimination half-life is less than two hours while the acid inhibitory effect lasts more than 24 hours.
Following single-dose oral administration of PREVACID, virtually no unchanged lansoprazole was excreted in the urine. In one study, after a single oral dose of ^{14}C-lansoprazole, approximately one-third of the administered radiation was excreted in the urine and two-thirds was recovered in the feces. This implies a significant biliary excretion of the metabolites of lansoprazole.

Special Populations

Geriatric

The clearance of lansoprazole is decreased in the elderly, with elimination half-life increased approximately 50% to 100%. Because the mean half-life in the elderly remains between 1.9 to 2.9 hours, repeated once daily dosing does not result in accumulation of lansoprazole. Peak plasma levels were not increased in the elderly.

Renal Insufficiency

In patients with severe renal insufficiency, plasma protein binding decreased by 1.0%–1.5% after administration of 60 mg of lansoprazole. Patients with renal insufficiency had a shortened elimination half-life and decreased total AUC (free and bound). AUC for free lansoprazole in plasma, however, was not related to the degree of renal impairment, and C_{max} and T_{max} were not different from subjects with healthy kidneys.

Hepatic Insufficiency

In patients with various degrees of chronic hepatic disease, the mean plasma half-life of the drug was prolonged from 1.5 hours to 3.2–7.2 hours. An increase in mean AUC of up to 500% was observed at steady state in hepatically-impaired patients compared to healthy subjects. Dose reduction in patients with severe hepatic disease should be considered.

Race

The pooled pharmacokinetic parameters of PREVACID from twelve U.S. Phase I studies (N=513) were compared to the mean pharmacokinetic parameters from two Asian studies (N=20). The mean AUCs of PREVACID in Asian subjects are approximately twice that seen in pooled U.S. data; however, the inter-individual variability is high. The C_{max} values are comparable.

Amoxicillin:

Amoxicillin is stable in the presence of gastric acid and may be given without regard to meals. It is rapidly absorbed after oral administration. It diffuses readily into most body tissues and fluids, with the exception of brain and spinal fluid, except when meninges are inflamed. The half-life of amoxicillin is 61.3 minutes. Most of the amoxicillin is excreted unchanged in the urine; its excretion can be delayed by concurrent administration of probenecid. Amoxicillin is not highly protein-bound. In blood serum, amoxicillin is approximately 20% protein-bound as compared to 60% for penicillin G.
Orally administered doses of 500-mg amoxicillin capsules result in average peak blood levels 1 to 2 hours after administration in the range of 5.5 mcg/mL to 7.5 mcg/mL.
Detectable serum levels are observed up to 8 hours after an orally administered dose of amoxicillin. Approximately 60% of an orally administered dose of amoxicillin is excreted in the urine within 6 to 8 hours.

Clarithromycin:

Clarithromycin is rapidly absorbed from the gastrointestinal tract after oral administration. The absolute bioavailability of 250 mg clarithromycin tablets was approximately 50%. For a single 500 mg dose of clarithromycin, food slightly delays the onset of clarithromycin absorption, increasing the peak time from approximately 2 to 2.5 hours. Food also increases the clarithromycin peak plasma concentration by about 24%, but does not affect the extent of clarithromycin bioavailability. Food does not affect the onset of formation of the antimicrobially active metabolite, 14-OH clarithromycin or its peak plasma concentration but does slightly increase the extent of metabolite formation, indicated by an 11% decrease in area under the plasma concentration-time curve (AUC). Therefore, BIAXIN tablets may be given without regard to food.
In nonfasting healthy human subjects (males and females), peak plasma concentrations were attained within 2 to 3 hours after oral dosing. Steady-state peak plasma clarithromycin concentrations were attained within 3 days and were approximately 3 to 4 µg/mL with a 500-mg dose administered every 8 to 12 hours. The elimination half-life of clarithromycin was 5 to 7 hours with 500 mg administered every 8 to 12 hours. The nonlinearity of clarithromycin pharmacokinetics is slight at the recommended dose of 500 mg administered every 8 to 12 hours. With a 500-mg every 8 to 12 hours dosing, the peak steady-state concentration of 14-OH clarithromycin is up to 1 µg/mL, and its elimination half-life is about 7 to 9 hours. The steady-state concentration of this metabolite is generally attained within 3 to 4 days.
After a 500-mg tablet every 12 hours, the urinary excretion of clarithromycin is approximately 30%. The renal clearance of clarithromycin approximates the normal glomerular filtration rate. The major metabolite found in urine is 14-OH clarithromycin, which accounts for an additional 10% to 15% of the dose with a 500-mg tablet administered every 12 hours.
The steady-state concentrations of clarithromycin in subjects with impaired hepatic function did not differ from those in normal subjects; however, the 14-OH clarithromycin concentrations were lower in the hepatically impaired subjects. The decreased formation of 14-OH clarithromycin was at least partially offset by an increase in renal clearance of clarithromycin in the subjects with impaired hepatic function when compared to healthy subjects.
The pharmacokinetics of clarithromycin was also altered in subjects with impaired renal function. (See **PRECAUTIONS** and **DOSAGE AND ADMINISTRATION**.)

Pharmacodynamics

MICROBIOLOGY

Lansoprazole, clarithromycin and/or amoxicillin have been shown to be active against most strains of *Helicobacter pylori in vitro* and in clinical infections as described in the **INDICATIONS AND USAGE** section.

Helicobacter

Helicobacter pylori

Pretreatment Resistance

Clarithromycin pretreatment resistance (≥2.0 µg/mL) was 9.5% (91/960) by E-test and 11.3% (12/106) by agar dilution in the dual and triple therapy clinical trials (M93-125, M93-130, M93-131, M95-392, and M95-399).
Amoxicillin pretreatment susceptible isolates (≤0.25 µg/mL) occurred in 97.8% (936/957) and 98.0% (98/100) of the patients in the dual and triple therapy clinical trials by E-test and agar dilution, respectively. Twenty-one of 957 patients (2.2%) by E-test and 2 of 100 patients (2.0%) by agar dilution had amoxicillin pretreatment MICs of >0.25 µg/mL. One patient on the 14-day triple therapy regimen had an unconfirmed pretreatment amoxicillin minimum inhibitory concentration (MIC) of >256 µg/mL by E-test and the patient was eradicated of *H. pylori*.

[See table below]

Patients not eradicated of *H. pylori* following lansoprazole/amoxicillin/clarithromycin triple therapy will likely have clarithromycin resistant *H. pylori*. Therefore, for those patients who fail therapy, clarithromycin susceptibility testing should be done when possible. Patients with clarithromycin resistant *H. pylori* should not be treated with lansoprazole/amoxicillin/clarithromycin triple therapy or with regimens which include clarithromycin as the sole antimicrobial agent.

Amoxicillin Susceptibility Test Results and Clinical/Bacteriological Outcomes

In the dual and triple therapy clinical trials, 82.6% (195/236) of the patients that had pretreatment amoxicillin susceptible MICs (≤0.25 µg/mL) were eradicated of *H. pylori*. Of those with pretreatment amoxicillin MICs of >0.25 µg/mL, three of six had the *H. pylori* eradicated. A total of 30% (21/70) of the patients failed lansoprazole 30 mg t.i.d./amoxicillin 1 gm t.i.d. dual therapy and a total of 12.8% (22/172) of the patients failed the 10- and 14-day triple therapy regimens. Post-treatment susceptibility results were not obtained on 11 of the patients who failed therapy. Nine of the 11 patients with amoxicillin post-treatment MICs that failed the triple therapy regimen also had clarithromycin resistant *H. pylori* isolates.

Susceptibility Test for *Helicobacter pylori*

The reference methodology for susceptibility testing of *H. pylori* is agar dilution MICs.[1] One to three microliters of an inoculum equivalent to a No. 2 McFarland standard ($1 \times 10^7 - 1 \times 10^8$ CFU/mL for *H. pylori*) are inoculated directly onto freshly prepared antimicrobial containing Mueller-Hinton agar plates with 5% aged defibrinated sheep blood (≥ 2 weeks old). The agar dilution plates are incubated at 35°C in a microaerobic environment produced by a gas generating system suitable for *Campylobacter* species. After 3 days of incubation, the MICs are recorded as the lowest concentration of antimicrobial agent required to inhibit growth of the organism. The clarithromycin and amoxicillin MIC values should be interpreted according to the following criteria:

Clarithromycin MIC (µg/mL)[a]	Interpretation
≤0.25	Susceptible (S)
0.5–1.0	Intermediate (I)
≥2.0	Resistant (R)

Amoxicillin MIC (µg/mL)[b]	Interpretation
≤0.25	Susceptible (S)

[a] These are tentative breakpoints for the agar dilution methodology and they should not be used to interpret results obtained using alternative methods.
[b] There were not enough organisms with MICs >0.25 µg/mL to determine a resistance breakpoint.

Standardized susceptibility test procedures require the use of laboratory control microorganisms to control the technical aspects of the laboratory procedures. Standard clarithromycin and amoxicillin powders should provide the following MIC values:

Microorganisms	Antimicrobial Agent	MIC (µg/mL)[a]
H. pylori ATCC 43504	Clarithromycin	0.015–0.12 µg/mL
H. pylori ATCC 43504	Amoxicillin	0.015–0.12 µg/mL

[a] These are quality control ranges for the agar dilution methodology and they should not be used to control test results obtained using alternative methods.

Reference

1. National Committee for Clinical Laboratory Standards. Summary Minutes, Subcommittee on Antimicrobial Susceptibility Testing, Tampa, FL, January 11–13, 1998.

Antisecretory activity

After oral administration, lansoprazole was shown to significantly decrease the basal acid output and significantly increase the mean gastric pH and percent of time the gastric pH was >3 and >4. Lansoprazole also significantly reduced meal-stimulated gastric acid output and secretion volume, as well as pentagastrin-stimulated acid output. In patients with hypersecretion of acid, lansoprazole significantly reduced basal and pentagastrin-stimulated gastric acid secretion. Lansoprazole inhibited the normal increases in secretion volume, acidity and acid output induced by insulin.
In a crossover study that included lansoprazole 15 and 30 mg for five days, the following effects on intragastric pH were noted:

[See first table at top of next page]

After the initial dose in this study, increased gastric pH was seen within 1–2 hours with lansoprazole 30 mg and 2–3 hours with lansoprazole 15 mg. After multiple daily dosing, increased gastric pH was seen within the first hour postdosing with lansoprazole 30 mg and within 1–2 hours postdosing with lansoprazole 15 mg.
Acid suppression may enhance the effect of antimicrobials in eradicating *Helicobacter pylori (H. pylori)*. The percentage of time gastric pH was elevated above 5 and 6 was evaluated in a crossover study of PREVACID given q.d., b.i.d. and t.i.d.

[See second table at top of next page]

The inhibition of gastric acid secretion as measured by intragastric pH returns gradually to normal over two to four days after multiple doses. There is no indication of rebound gastric acidity.

CLINICAL STUDIES

***H. pylori* Eradication to Reduce the Risk of Duodenal Ulcer Recurrence**

Randomized, double-blind clinical studies performed in the U.S. in patients with *H. pylori* and duodenal ulcer disease (defined as an active ulcer or history of an ulcer within one year) evaluated the efficacy of PREVPAC as triple 14-day therapy for the eradication of *H. pylori*. The triple therapy regimen (PREVACID 30 mg BID plus amoxicillin 1 gm BID plus clarithromycin 500 mg BID) produced statistically sig-

Clarithromycin Susceptibility Test Results and Clinical/Bacteriological Outcomes[a]

Clarithromycin Pretreatment Results	Clarithromycin Post-treatment Results				
	H. pylori negative –eradicated	*H. pylori* positive –not eradicated			
		Post-treatment susceptibility results			
		S[b]	I[b]	R[b]	No MIC
Triple Therapy 14-Day (lansoprazole 30 mg b.i.d./amoxicillin 1 gm b.i.d./clarithromycin 500 mg b.i.d.) (M95-399, M93-131, M95-392)					
Susceptible[b] 112	105				7
Intermediate[b] 3	3				
Resistant[b] 17	6			7	4
Triple Therapy 10-Day (lansoprazole 30 mg b.i.d./amoxicillin 1 gm b.i.d./clarithromycin 500 mg b.i.d.) (M95-399)					
Susceptible[b] 42	40	1		1	
Intermediate[b]					
Resistant[b] 4	1			3	

[a] Includes only patients with pretreatment clarithromycin susceptibility test results
[b] Susceptible (S) MIC ≤0.25 µg/mL, Intermediate (I) MIC 0.5–1.0 µg/mL, Resistant (R) MIC ≥2 µg/mL

nificantly higher eradication rates than PREVACID plus amoxicillin, PREVACID plus clarithromycin, and amoxicillin plus clarithromycin dual therapies.

H. pylori eradication was defined as two negative tests (culture and histology) at 4–6 weeks following the end of treatment.

Triple therapy was shown to be more effective than all possible dual therapy combinations. The combination of PREVACID plus amoxicillin and clarithromycin as triple therapy was effective in eradicating *H. pylori*. Eradication of *H. pylori* has been shown to reduce the risk of duodenal ulcer recurrence.

A randomized, double-blind clinical study performed in the U.S. in patients with *H. pylori* and duodenal ulcer disease (defined as an active ulcer or history of an ulcer within one year) compared the efficacy of PREVACID triple therapy for 10 and 14 days. This study established that the 10-day triple therapy was equivalent to the 14-day triple therapy in eradicating *H. pylori*.

H. pylori **Eradication Rates – Triple Therapy**
(PREVACID/amoxicillin/clarithromycin)
Percent of Patients Cured
[95% Confidence Interval]
(Number of patients)

Study	Duration	Triple Therapy Evaluable Analysis*	Triple Therapy Intent-to-Treat Analysis#
M93-131	14 days	92† [80.0–97.7] (N=48)	86† [73.3–93.5] (N=55)
M95-392	14 days	86‡ [75.7–93.6] (N=66)	83‡ [72.0–90.8] (N=70)
M95-399+	14 days	85 [77.0–91.0] (N=113)	82 [73.9–88.1] (N=126)
	10 days	84 [76.0–89.8] (N=123)	81 [73.9–87.6] (N=135)

*Based on evaluable patients with confirmed duodenal ulcer (active or within one year) and *H. pylori* infection at baseline defined as at least two of three positive endoscopic tests from CLOtest®, histology and/or culture. Patients were included in the analysis if they completed the study. Additionally, if patients dropped out of the study due to an adverse event related to the study drug, they were included in the evaluable analysis as failures of therapy.

#Patients were included in the analysis if they had documented *H. pylori* infection at baseline as defined above and had a confirmed duodenal ulcer (active or within one year). All dropouts were included as failures of therapy.

†($p<0.05$) versus PREVACID/amoxicillin and PREVACID/clarithromycin dual therapy

‡($p<0.05$) versus clarithromycin/amoxicillin dual therapy

+The 95% confidence interval for the difference in eradication rates, 10-day minus 14-day is (−10.5, 8.1) in the evaluable analysis and (−9.7, 9.1) in the intent-to-treat analysis.

Mean Antisecretory Effects after Single and Multiple Daily Dosing

Parameter	Baseline Value	PREVACID 15 mg Day 1	PREVACID 15 mg Day 5	PREVACID 30 mg Day 1	PREVACID 30 mg Day 5
Mean 24-Hour pH	2.1	2.7+	4.0+	3.6*	4.9*
Mean Nighttime pH	1.9	2.4	3.0+	2.6	3.8*
% Time Gastric pH>3	18	33+	59+	51*	72*
% Time Gastric pH>4	12	22+	49+	41*	66*

NOTE: An intragastric pH of >4 reflects a reduction in gastric acid by 99%.
* ($p<0.05$) versus baseline and lansoprazole 15 mg.
+ ($p<0.05$) versus baseline only.

Mean Antisecretory Effects After 5 Days of b.i.d. and t.i.d. Dosing

Parameter	PREVACID 30 mg q.d.	PREVACID 15 mg b.i.d.	PREVACID 30 mg b.i.d.	PREVACID 30 mg t.i.d.
% Time Gastric pH>5	43	47	59+	77*
% Time Gastric pH>6	20	23	28	45*

+ ($p<0.05$) versus PREVACID 30 mg q.d.
* ($p<0.05$) versus PREVACID 30 mg q.d., 15 mg b.i.d. and 30 mg b.i.d.

INDICATIONS AND USAGE

H. pylori Eradication to Reduce the Risk of Duodenal Ulcer Recurrence

The components in PREVPAC (PREVACID, amoxicillin, and clarithromycin) are indicated for the treatment of patients with *H. pylori* infection and duodenal ulcer disease (active or one-year history of a duodenal ulcer) to eradicate *H. pylori*. Eradication of *H. pylori* has been shown to reduce the risk of duodenal ulcer recurrence (See **CLINICAL STUDIES** and **DOSAGE AND ADMINISTRATION**).

To reduce the development of drug-resistant bacteria and maintain the effectiveness of PREVPAC and other antibacterial drugs, PREVPAC should be used only to treat or prevent infections that are proven or strongly suspected to be caused by susceptible bacteria. When culture and susceptibility information are available, they should be considered in selecting or modifying antibacterial therapy. In the absence of such data, local epidemiology and susceptibility patterns may contribute to the empiric selection of therapy.

CONTRAINDICATIONS

PREVPAC is contraindicated in patients with known hypersensitivity to any component of the formulation of PREVACID, any macrolide antibiotic, or any penicillin.

Concomitant administration of PREVPAC with cisapride, pimozide, astemizole, or terfenadine is contraindicated. There have been post-marketing reports of drug interactions when clarithromycin and/or erythromycin are co-administered with cisapride, pimozide, astemizole, or terfenadine resulting in cardiac arrhythmias (QT prolongation, ventricular tachycardia, ventricular fibrillation, and torsades de pointes) most likely due to inhibition of metabolism of these drugs by erythromycin and clarithromycin. Fatalities have been reported.

(Please refer to full prescribing information for amoxicillin and clarithromycin before prescribing.)

WARNINGS

Amoxicillin:

Serious and occasionally fatal hypersensitivity (anaphylactic) reactions have been reported in patients on penicillin therapy. Although anaphylaxis is more frequent following parenteral therapy, it has occurred in patients on oral penicillins. These reactions are more likely to occur in individuals with a history of penicillin hypersensitivity and/or a history of sensitivity to multiple allergens.

There have been reports of individuals with a history of penicillin hypersensitivity who have experienced severe reactions when treated with cephalosporins. Before initiating therapy with amoxicillin, careful inquiry should be made concerning previous hypersensitivity reactions to penicillins, cephalosporins, or other allergens. If an allergic reaction occurs, amoxicillin should be discontinued and appropriate therapy instituted.

SERIOUS ANAPHYLACTIC REACTIONS REQUIRE IMMEDIATE EMERGENCY TREATMENT WITH EPINEPHRINE. OXYGEN, INTRAVENOUS STEROIDS, AND AIRWAY MANAGEMENT, INCLUDING INTUBATION, SHOULD ALSO BE ADMINISTERED AS INDICATED.

Clarithromycin:

CLARITHROMYCIN SHOULD NOT BE USED IN PREGNANT WOMEN EXCEPT IN CLINICAL CIRCUMSTANCES WHERE NO ALTERNATIVE THERAPY IS APPROPRIATE. IF PREGNANCY OCCURS WHILE TAKING CLARITHROMYCIN, THE PATIENT SHOULD BE APPRISED OF THE POTENTIAL HAZARD TO THE FETUS. CLARITHROMYCIN HAS DEMONSTRATED ADVERSE EFFECTS OF PREGNANCY OUTCOME AND/OR EMBRYO-FETAL DEVELOPMENT IN MONKEYS, RATS, MICE, AND RABBITS AT DOSES THAT PRODUCED PLASMA LEVELS 2 TO 17 TIMES THE SERUM LEVELS ACHIEVED IN HUMANS TREATED AT THE MAXIMUM RECOMMENDED HUMAN DOSES. (See PRECAUTIONS - *Pregnancy*.)

Amoxicillin and/or Clarithromycin:

Pseudomembranous colitis has been reported with nearly all antibacterial agents, including clarithromycin and amoxicillin, and may range in severity from mild to life threatening. Therefore, it is important to consider this diagnosis in patients who present with diarrhea subsequent to the administration of antibacterial agents.

Treatment with antibacterial agents alters the normal flora of the colon and may permit overgrowth of clostridia. Studies indicate that a toxin produced by *Clostridium difficile* is a primary cause of "antibiotic-associated colitis."

After the diagnosis of pseudomembranous colitis has been established, therapeutic measures should be initiated. Mild cases of pseudomembranous colitis usually respond to discontinuation of the drug alone. In moderate to severe cases, consideration should be given to management with fluids and electrolytes, protein supplementation, and treatment with an antibacterial drug clinically effective against *Clostridium difficile* colitis.

PRECAUTIONS

Clarithromycin is principally excreted via the liver and kidney. Clarithromycin may be administered without dosage adjustment to patients with hepatic impairment and normal renal function. However, in the presence of severe renal impairment with or without coexisting hepatic impairment, decreased dosage or prolonged dosing intervals may be appropriate.

The possibility of superinfections with mycotic or bacterial pathogens should be kept in mind during therapy. If superinfections occur, PREVPAC should be discontinued and appropriate therapy instituted.

Symptomatic response to therapy with PREVACID does not preclude the presence of gastric malignancy.

Prescribing PREVPAC in the absence of a proven or strongly suspected bacterial infection or a prophylactic indication is unlikely to provide benefit to the patient and increases the risk of the development of drug-resistant bacteria.

Information for Patients: Each dose of PREVPAC contains four pills: one pink and black capsule (PREVACID), two flesh body/maroon cap capsules (amoxicillin) and one yellow tablet (clarithromycin). Each dose should be taken twice per day before eating. Patients should be instructed to swallow each pill whole.

Biaxin may interact with some drugs; therefore patients should be advised to report to their doctor the use of any other medications.

Patients should be counseled that antibacterial drugs including PREVPAC should only be used to treat bacterial infections. They do not treat viral infections (e.g., the common cold). When PREVPAC is prescribed to treat a bacterial infection, patients should be told that although it is common to feel better early in the course of therapy, the medication should be taken exactly as directed. Skipping doses or not completing the full course of therapy may (1) decrease the effectiveness of the immediate treatment and (2) increase the likelihood that bacteria will develop resistance and will not be treatable by PREVPAC or other antibacterial drugs in the future.

Drug Interactions

PREVACID:

PREVACID is metabolized through the cytochrome P_{450} system, specifically through the CYP3A and CYP2C19 isozymes. Studies have shown that PREVACID does not have clinically significant interactions with other drugs metabolized by the cytochrome P_{450} system, such as warfarin, antipyrine, indomethacin, ibuprofen, phenytoin, propranolol, prednisone, diazepam, or clarithromycin in healthy subjects. These compounds are metabolized through various cytochrome P_{450} isozymes including CYP1A2, CYP2C9, CYP2C19, CYP2D6, and CYP3A. When PREVACID was administered concomitantly with theophylline (CYP1A2, CYP3A), a minor increase (10%) in the clearance of theophylline was seen. Because of the small magnitude and the direction of the effect on theophylline clearance, this interaction is unlikely to be of clinical concern. Nonetheless, individual patients may require additional titration of their theophylline dosage when PREVACID is started or stopped to ensure clinically effective blood levels.

In a study of healthy subjects neither the pharmacokinetics of warfarin enantiomers nor prothrombin time were affected following single or multiple 60 mg doses of lansoprazole. However, there have been reports of increased International Normalized Ratio (INR) and prothrombin time in patients receiving proton pump inhibitors, including PREVACID, and warfarin concomitantly. Increases in INR and prothrombin time may lead to abnormal bleeding and even death. Patients treated with proton pump inhibitors and warfarin concomitantly may need to be monitored for increases in INR and prothrombin time.

PREVACID has also been shown to have no clinically significant interaction with amoxicillin.

In a single-dose crossover study examining PREVACID 30 mg and omeprazole 20 mg each administered alone and concomitantly with sucralfate 1 gram, absorption of the proton pump inhibitors was delayed and their bioavailability was reduced by 17% and 16%, respectively, when administered concomitantly with sucralfate. Therefore, proton pump inhibitors should be taken at least 30 minutes prior to sucralfate. In clinical trials, antacids were administered concomitantly with PREVACID Delayed-Release Capsules; this did not interfere with its effect.

PREVACID causes a profound and long-lasting inhibition of gastric acid secretion; therefore, it is theoretically possible that PREVACID may interfere with the absorption of drugs where gastric pH is an important determinant of bioavailability (e.g., ketoconazole, ampicillin esters, iron salts, digoxin).

Continued on next page

Prevpac—Cont.

Amoxicillin:
Probenecid decreases the renal tubular secretion of amoxicillin. Concurrent use with amoxicillin may result in increased and prolonged blood levels.
Chloramphenicol, erythromycins, sulfonamides, and tetracyclines may interfere with bactericidal effects of penicillin. This has been demonstrated *in vitro*; however, the clinical significance of this interaction is not well documented.
Clarithromycin:
Clarithromycin use in patients who are receiving theophylline may be associated with an increase of serum theophylline concentrations. Monitoring of serum theophylline concentrations should be considered for patients receiving high doses of theophylline or with baseline concentrations in the upper therapeutic range. In two studies in which theophylline was administered with clarithromycin (a theophylline sustained-release formulation was dosed at either 6.5 mg/kg or 12 mg/kg together with 250 or 500 mg q12h clarithromycin), the steady-state levels of C_{max}, C_{min}, and the area under the serum concentration time curve (AUC) of theophylline increased about 20%.
Concomitant administration of single doses of clarithromycin and carbamazepine has been shown to result in increased plasma concentrations of carbamazepine. Blood level monitoring of carbamazepine may be considered.
When clarithromycin and terfenadine were coadministered, plasma concentrations of the active acid metabolite of terfenadine were threefold higher, on average, than the values observed when terfenadine was administered alone. The pharmacokinetics of clarithromycin and the 14-hydroxy-clarithromycin were not significantly affected by coadministration of terfenadine once clarithromycin reached steady-state conditions. Concomitant administration of clarithromycin with terfenadine is contraindicated. (See **CONTRAINDICATIONS.**)
Spontaneous reports in the post-marketing period suggest that concomitant administration of clarithromycin and oral anticoagulants may potentiate the effects of the oral anticoagulants. Prothrombin times should be carefully monitored while patients are receiving clarithromycin and oral anticoagulants simultaneously.
Elevated digoxin serum concentrations in patients receiving clarithromycin and digoxin concomitantly have also been reported in post-marketing surveillance. Some patients have shown clinical signs consistent with digoxin toxicity, including potentially fatal arrhythmias. Serum digoxin levels should be carefully monitored while patients are receiving digoxin and clarithromycin simultaneously.
Erythromycin and clarithromycin are substrates and inhibitors of the 3A isoform subfamily of the cytochrome P450 enzyme system (CYP3A). Coadministration of erythromycin or clarithromycin and a drug primarily metabolized by CYP3A may be associated with elevations in drug concentrations that could increase or prolong both the therapeutic and adverse effects of the concomitant drug. Dosage adjustments may be considered, and when possible, serum concentrations of drugs primarily metabolized by CYP3A should be monitored closely in patients concurrently receiving clarithromycin or erythromycin.
The following are examples of some clinically significant CYP3A based drug interactions. Interactions with other drugs metabolized by the CYP3A isoform are also possible. Increased serum concentrations of carbamazepine and the active acid metabolite of terfenadine were observed in clinical trials with clarithromycin.
The following CYP3A based drug interactions have been observed with erythromycin products and/or with clarithromycin in post-marketing experience:

Antiarrhythmics: There have been post-marketing reports of torsades de pointes occurring with concurrent use of clarithromycin and quinidine or disopyramide. Electrocardiograms should be monitored for QTc prolongation during coadministration of clarithromycin with these drugs. Serum levels of these medications should also be monitored.

Ergotamine/dihydroergotamine: Concurrent use of erythromycin or clarithromycin and ergotamine or dihydroergotamine has been associated in some patients with acute ergot toxicity characterized by severe peripheral vasospasm and dysesthesia.

Triazolobenziodidiazepines (such as triazolam and alprazolam) and related benzodiazepines (such as midazolam): Erythromycin has been reported to decrease the clearance of triazolam and midazolam, and thus, may increase the pharmacologic effect of these benzodiazepines. There have been postmarketing reports of drug interactions and CNS effects (e.g., somnolence and confusion) with the concomitant use of clarithromycin and triazolam.

HMG-CoA Reductase Inhibitors: As with other macrolides, clarithromycin has been reported to increase concentrations of HMG-CoA reductase inhibitors (e.g., lovastatin and simvastatin). Rare reports of rhabdomyolysis have been reported in patients taking these drugs concomitantly.

Sildenafil (Viagra): Erythromycin has been reported to increase the systemic exposure (AUC) of sildenafil. A similar interaction may occur with clarithromycin; reduction of sildenafil dosage should be considered. (See Viagra package insert.) There have been spontaneous or published reports of CYP3A based interactions of erythromycin and/or clarithromycin with cyclosporine, carbamazepine, tacrolimus, alfentanil, disopyramide, rifabutin, quinidine, methylprednisolone, cilostazol, and bromocriptine.

Concomitant administration of clarithromycin with cisapride, pimozide, astemizole, or terfenadine is contraindicated (see **CONTRAINDICATIONS.**)

In addition, there have been reports of interactions of erythromycin or clarithromycin with drugs not thought to be metabolized by CYP3A, including hexobarbital, phenytoin, and valproate.
For information on interactions between clarithromycin in combination with other drugs which may be administered to HIV-infected patients, see the BIAXIN package insert, Drug Interactions, under the **PRECAUTIONS** section.

Carcinogenesis, Mutagenesis, Impairment of Fertility
PREVACID:
In two 24-month carcinogenicity studies, Sprague-Dawley rats were treated orally with doses of 5 to 150 mg/kg/day, about 1 to 40 times the exposure on a body surface (mg/m^2) basis, of a 50-kg person of average height (1.46 m^2 body surface area) given the recommended human dose of 30 mg/day (22.2 mg/m^2). Lansoprazole produced dose-related gastric enterochromaffin-like (ECL) cell hyperplasia and ECL cell carcinoids in both male and female rats. It also increased the incidence of intestinal metaplasia of the gastric epithelium in both sexes. In male rats, lansoprazole produced a dose-related increase of testicular interstitial cell adenomas. The incidence of these adenomas in rats receiving doses of 15 to 150 mg/kg/day (4 to 40 times the recommended human dose based on body surface area) exceeded the low background incidence (range = 1.4 to 10%) for this strain of rat. Testicular interstitial cell adenoma also occurred in 1 of 30 rats treated with 50 mg/kg/day (13 times the recommended human dose based on body surface area) in a 1-year toxicity study.
In a 24-month carcinogenicity study, CD-1 mice were treated orally with doses of 15 to 600 mg/kg/day, 2 to 80 times the recommended human dose based on body surface area. Lansoprazole produced a dose-related increased incidence of gastric ECL cell hyperplasia. It also produced an increased incidence of liver tumors (hepatocellular adenoma plus carcinoma). The tumor incidences in male mice treated with 300 and 600 mg/kg/day (40 to 80 times the recommended human dose based on body surface area) and female mice treated with 150 to 600 mg/kg/day (20 to 80 times the recommended human dose based on body surface area) exceeded the ranges of background incidences in historical controls for this strain of mice. Lansoprazole treatment produced adenoma of rete testis in male mice receiving 75 to 600 mg/kg/day (10 to 80 times the recommended human dose based on body surface area).
Lansoprazole was not genotoxic in the Ames test, the *ex vivo* rat hepatocyte unscheduled DNA synthesis (UDS) test, the *in vivo* mouse micronucleus test or the rat bone marrow cell chromosomal aberration test. It was positive in *in vitro* human lymphocyte chromosomal aberration assays.
Lansoprazole at oral doses up to 150 mg/kg/day (40 times the recommended human dose based on body surface area) was found to have no effect on fertility and reproductive performance of male and female rats.
Amoxicillin:
Long-term studies in animals have not been performed to evaluate carcinogenic potential. Studies to detect mutagenic potential of amoxicillin alone have not been conducted.
Clarithromycin:
The following *in vitro* mutagenicity tests have been conducted with clarithromycin:

- *Salmonella*/Mammalian Microsomes Test
- Bacterial Induced Mutation Frequency Test
- *In Vitro* Chromosome Aberration Test
- Rat Hepatocyte DNA Synthesis Assay
- Mouse Lymphoma Assay
- Mouse Dominant Lethal Study
- Mouse Micronucleus Test

All tests had negative results except the *In Vitro* Chromosome Aberration Test which was weakly positive in one test and negative in another.
In addition, a Bacterial Reverse-Mutation Test (Ames Test) has been performed on clarithromycin metabolites with negative results.
Fertility and reproduction studies have shown that daily doses of up to 160 mg/kg/day (1.3 times the recommended maximum human dose based on mg/m^2) to male and female rats caused no adverse effects on the estrous cycle, fertility, parturition, or number and viability of offspring. Plasma levels in rats after 150 mg/kg/day were 2 times the human serum levels.
In the 150 mg/kg/day monkey studies, plasma levels were 3 times the human serum levels. When given orally at 150 mg/kg/day (2.4 times the recommended maximum human dose based on mg/m^2), clarithromycin was shown to produce embryonic loss in monkeys. This effect has been attributed to marked maternal toxicity of the drug at this high dose.
In rabbits, *in utero* fetal loss occurred at an intravenous dose of 33 mg/m^2, which is 17 times less than the maximum proposed human oral daily dose of 618 mg/m^2.
Long-term studies in animals have not been performed to evaluate the carcinogenic potential of clarithromycin.

Pregnancy
Teratogenic Effects. Pregnancy Category C
Category C is based on the pregnancy category for clarithromycin.
Four teratogenicity studies in rats (three with oral doses and one with intravenous doses up to 160 mg/kg/day administered during the period of major organogenesis) and two in rabbits at oral doses up to 125 mg/kg/day (approximately 2 times the recommended maximum human dose based on mg/m^2) or intravenous doses of 30 mg/kg/day administered during gestation days 6 to 18 failed to demonstrate any teratogenicity from clarithromycin. Two additional oral studies in a different rat strain at similar doses and similar conditions demonstrated a low incidence of cardiovascular anomalies at doses of 150 mg/kg/day administered during gestation days 6 to 15. Plasma levels after 150 mg/kg/day were 2 times the human serum levels. Four studies in mice revealed a variable incidence of cleft palate following oral doses of 1000 mg/kg/day (2 and 4 times the recommended maximum human dose based on mg/m^2, respectively) during gestation days 6 to 15. Cleft palate was also seen at 500 mg/kg/day. The 1000 mg/kg/day exposure resulted in plasma levels 17 times the human serum levels. In monkeys, an oral dose of 70 mg/kg/day (an approximate equidose of the recommended maximum human dose based on mg/m^2) produced fetal growth retardation at plasma levels that were 2 times the human serum levels.
There were no adequate and well-controlled studies of PREVPAC in pregnant women. PREVPAC should be used during pregnancy only if the potential benefit justifies the potential risk to the fetus. (See **WARNINGS.**)

Labor and Delivery
Oral ampicillin-class antibiotics are poorly absorbed during labor. Studies in guinea pigs showed that intravenous administration of ampicillin slightly decreased the uterine tone and frequency of contractions, but moderately increased the height and duration of contractions. However, it is not known whether use of these drugs in humans during labor or delivery has immediate or delayed adverse effects on the fetus, prolongs the duration of labor, or increases the likelihood that forceps delivery or other obstetrical intervention or resuscitation of the newborn will be necessary.

Nursing Mothers
Lansoprazole or its metabolites are excreted in the milk of rats. It is not known whether lansoprazole is excreted in human milk. Penicillins have been shown to be excreted in human milk. Amoxicillin use by nursing mothers may lead to sensitization of infants. It is not known whether clarithromycin is excreted in human milk. It is known that clarithromycin is excreted in the milk of lactating animals and that other drugs of this class are excreted in human milk.
Due to the potential for serious adverse reactions in nursing infants from PREVPAC, and the potential for tumorigenicity shown for lansoprazole in rat carcinogenicity studies, a decision should be made whether to discontinue nursing or to discontinue PREVPAC, taking into account the importance of the therapy to the mother.

Pediatric Use
Safety and effectiveness of PREVPAC in pediatric patients infected with *H. pylori* have not been established. (See **CONTRAINDICATIONS** and **WARNINGS.**)

Use in Geriatric Patients
Elderly patients may suffer from asymptomatic renal and hepatic dysfunction. Care should be taken when administering PREVPAC to this patient population.

ADVERSE REACTIONS

The most common adverse reactions (≥3%) reported in clinical trials when all three components of this therapy were given concomitantly for 14 days are listed in the table below.

Adverse Reactions Most Frequently Reported in Clinical Trials (≥ 3%)

	Triple Therapy
Adverse Reaction	n=138 (%)
Diarrhea	7.0
Headache	6.0
Taste Perversion	5.0

The additional adverse reactions which were reported as possibly or probably related to treatment (<3%) in clinical trials when all three components of this therapy were given concomitantly are listed below and divided by body system: *Body as a Whole*—abdominal pain; *Digestive System*—dark stools, dry mouth/thirst, glossitis, rectal itching, nausea, oral moniliasis, stomatitis, tongue discoloration, tongue disorder, vomiting; *Musculoskeletal System*—myalgia; *Nervous System*—confusion, dizziness; *Respiratory System*—respiratory disorders; *Skin and Appendages*—skin reactions; *Urogenital System*—vaginitis, vaginal moniliasis. There were no statistically significant differences in the frequency of reported adverse events between the 10- and 14-day triple therapy regimens.
PREVACID:
The following adverse reactions from the labeling for lansoprazole are provided for information.
Worldwide, over 10,000 patients have been treated with lansoprazole in Phase 2–3 clinical trials involving various dos-

ages and durations of treatment. In general, lansoprazole treatment has been well-tolerated in both short-term and long-term trials.

Incidence in Clinical Trials

The following adverse events were reported by the treating physician to have a possible or probable relationship to drug in 1% or more of PREVACID-treated patients and occurred at a greater rate in PREVACID-treated patients than placebo-treated patients:

Incidence of Possibly or Probably Treatment-Related Adverse Events in Short-Term, Placebo-Controlled Studies

Body System/Adverse Event	PREVACID (N=2768) %	Placebo (N=1023) %
Body as a Whole		
Abdominal Pain	2.1	1.2
Digestive System		
Constipation	1.0	0.4
Diarrhea	3.8	2.3
Nausea	1.3	1.2

Headache was also seen at greater than 1% incidence but was more common on placebo. The incidence of diarrhea was similar between patients who received placebo and patients who received lansoprazole 15 mg and 30 mg, but higher in the patients who received lansoprazole 60 mg (2.9%, 1.4%, 4.2%, and 7.4%, respectively).

The most commonly reported possibly or probably treatment-related adverse event during maintenance therapy was diarrhea.

Additional adverse experiences occurring in <1% of patients or subjects in domestic trials are shown below. Refer to ***Postmarketing*** for adverse reactions occurring since the drug was marketed.

Body as a Whole—abdomen enlarged, allergic reaction, asthenia, back pain, candidiasis, carcinoma, chest pain (not otherwise specified), chills, edema, fever, flu syndrome, halitosis, infection (not otherwise specified), malaise, neck pain, neck rigidity, pain, pelvic pain; *Cardiovascular System*—angina, arrhythmia, bradycardia, cerebrovascular accident/cerebral infarction, hypertension/hypotension, migraine, myocardial infarction, palpitations, shock (circulatory failure), syncope, tachycardia, vasodilation; *Digestive System*—abnormal stools, anorexia, bezoar, cardiospasm, cholelithiasis, colitis, dry mouth, dyspepsia, dysphagia, enteritis, eructation, esophageal stenosis, esophageal ulcer, esophagitis, fecal discoloration, flatulence, gastric nodules/fundic gland polyps, gastritis, gastroenteritis, gastrointestinal anomaly, gastrointestinal disorder, gastrointestinal hemorrhage, glossitis, gum hemorrhage, hematemesis, increased appetite, increased salivation, melena, mouth ulceration, nausea and vomiting, nausea and vomiting and diarrhea, oral moniliasis, rectal disorder, rectal hemorrhage, stomatitis, tenesmus, thirst, tongue disorder, ulcerative colitis, ulcerative stomatitis; *Endocrine System*—diabetes mellitus, goiter, hypothyroidism; *Hemic and Lymphatic System*—anemia, hemolysis, lymphadenopathy; *Metabolic and Nutritional Disorders*—gout, dehydration, hyperglycemia/hypoglycemia, peripheral edema, weight gain/loss; *Musculoskeletal System*—arthralgia, arthritis, bone disorder, joint disorder, leg cramps, musculoskeletal pain, myalgia, myasthenia, synovitis; *Nervous System*—abnormal dreams, agitation, amnesia, anxiety, apathy, confusion, convulsion, depersonalization, depression, diplopia, dizziness, emotional lability, hallucinations, hemiplegia, hostility aggravated, hyperkinesia, hypertonia, hypesthesia, insomnia, libido decreased/increased, nervousness, neurosis, paresthesia, sleep disorder, somnolence, thinking abnormality, tremor, vertigo; *Respiratory System*—asthma, bronchitis, cough increased, dyspnea, epistaxis, hemoptysis, hiccup, laryngeal neoplasia, pharyngitis, pleural disorder, pneumonia, respiratory disorder, upper respiratory inflammation/infection, rhinitis, sinusitis, stridor; *Skin and Appendages*—acne, alopecia, contact dermatitis, dry skin, fixed eruption, hair disorder, maculopapular rash, nail disorder, pruritus, rash, skin carcinoma, skin disorder, sweating, urticaria; *Special Senses*—abnormal vision, blurred vision, conjunctivitis, deafness, dry eyes, ear disorder, eye pain, otitis media, parosmia, photophobia, retinal degeneration, taste loss, taste perversion, tinnitus, visual field defect; *Urogenital System*—abnormal menses, breast enlargement, breast pain, breast tenderness, dysmenorrhea, dysuria, gynecomastia, impotence, kidney calculus, kidney pain, leukorrhea, menorrhagia, menstrual disorder, penis disorder, polyuria, testis disorder, urethral pain, urinary frequency, urinary tract infection, urinary urgency, urination impaired, vaginitis.

Postmarketing

On-going Safety Surveillance: Additional adverse experiences have been reported since lansoprazole has been marketed. The majority of these cases are foreign-sourced and a relationship to lansoprazole has not been established. Because these events were reported voluntarily from a population of unknown size, estimates of frequency cannot be made. These events are listed below by COSTART body system.

Body as a Whole—anaphylactoid-like reaction; *Digestive System*—hepatotoxicity, pancreatitis, vomiting; *Hemic and Lymphatic System*—agranulocytosis, aplastic anemia, hemolytic anemia, leukopenia, neutropenia, pancytopenia, thrombocytopenia, and thrombotic thrombocytopenic purpura; *Skin and Appendages*—severe dermatologic reactions including erythema multiforme, Stevens-Johnson syndrome, toxic epidermal necrolysis, (some-fatal); *Special Senses*—speech disorder; *Urogenital System*—urinary retention.

Laboratory Values

The following changes in laboratory parameters for lansoprazole were reported as adverse events:

Abnormal liver function tests, increased SGOT (AST), increased SGPT (ALT), increased creatinine, increased alkaline phosphatase, increased globulins, increased GGTP, increased/decreased/abnormal WBC, abnormal AG ratio, abnormal RBC, bilirubinemia, eosinophilia, hyperlipemia, increased/decreased electrolytes, increased/decreased cholesterol, increased glucocorticoids, increased LDH, increased/decreased/abnormal platelets, and increased gastrin levels. Urine abnormalities such as albuminuria, glycosuria, and hematuria were also reported. Additional isolated laboratory abnormalities were reported.

In the placebo-controlled studies, when SGOT (AST) and SGPT (ALT) were evaluated, 0.4% (4/978) placebo patients and 0.4% (11/2677) lansoprazole patients had enzyme elevations greater than three times the upper limit of normal range at the final treatment visit. None of these lansoprazole patients reported jaundice at any time during the study.

Amoxicillin:

The following adverse reactions from the labeling for amoxicillin are provided for information.

As with other penicillins, it may be expected that untoward reactions will be essentially limited to sensitivity phenomena. They are more likely to occur in individuals who have previously demonstrated hypersensitivity to penicillins and in those with a history of allergy, asthma, hay fever, or urticaria.

The following adverse reactions have been reported as associated with the use of penicillins:

Gastrointestinal—Nausea, vomiting, diarrhea, and pseudomembranous colitis.

Onset of pseudomembranous colitis symptoms may occur during or after antibiotic treatment (See **WARNINGS.**)

Hypersensitivity Reactions—Erythematous maculopapular rashes, erythema multiforme, Stevens-Johnson Syndrome, toxic epidermal necrolysis, and urticaria have been reported. **Note:** These hypersensitivity reactions may be controlled with antihistamines and, if necessary, systemic corticosteroids. Whenever such reactions occur, amoxicillin should be discontinued unless, in the opinion of the physician, the condition being treated is life-threatening and amenable only to amoxicillin therapy.

Liver—A moderate rise in AST (SGOT) has been noted, but the significance of this finding is unknown.

Hemic and Lymphatic Systems—Anemia, thrombocytopenia, thrombocytopenic purpura, eosinophilia, leukopenia and agranulocytosis have been reported during therapy with penicillins. These reactions are usually reversible on discontinuation of therapy and are believed to be hypersensitivity phenomena.

Central Nervous System—Reversible hyperactivity, agitation, anxiety, insomnia, confusion, behavioral changes, and/or dizziness have been reported rarely.

Clarithromycin:

The following adverse reactions from the labeling for clarithromycin are provided for information.

The majority of side effects observed in clinical trials were of a mild and transient nature. Fewer than 3% of adult patients without mycobacterial infections discontinued therapy because of drug-related side effects.

The most frequently reported events in adults were diarrhea (3%), nausea (3%), abnormal taste (3%), dyspepsia (2%), abdominal pain/discomfort (2%), and headache (2%). Most of these events were described as mild or moderate in severity. Of the reported adverse events, only 1% was described as severe.

Postmarketing Experience:

Allergic reactions ranging from urticaria and mild skin eruptions to rare cases of anaphylaxis, Stevens-Johnson syndrome, and toxic epidermal necrolysis have occurred. Other spontaneously reported adverse events include glossitis, stomatitis, oral moniliasis, anorexia, vomiting, pancreatitis, tongue discoloration, thrombocytopenia, leukopenia, neutropenia, and dizziness. There have been reports of tooth discoloration in patients treated with clarithromycin. Tooth discoloration is usually reversible with professional dental cleaning. There have been isolated reports of hearing loss, which is usually reversible, occurring chiefly in elderly women. Reports of alterations of the sense of smell, usually in conjunction with taste perversion or taste loss have also been reported.

Transient CNS events including anxiety, behavioral changes, confusional states, convulsions, depersonalization, disorientation, hallucinations, insomnia, manic behavior, nightmares, psychosis, tinnitus, tremor, and vertigo have been reported during postmarketing surveillance. Events usually resolve with discontinuation of the drug.

Hepatic dysfunction, including increased liver enzymes, and hepatocellular and/or cholestatic hepatitis, with or without jaundice, has been infrequently reported with clarithromycin. This hepatic dysfunction may be severe and is usually reversible. In very rare instances, hepatic failure with fatal outcome has been reported and generally has been associated with serious underlying diseases and/or concomitant medications.

There have been rare reports of hypoglycemia, some of which have occurred in patients taking oral hypoglycemic agents or insulin.

As with other macrolides, clarithromycin has been associated with QT prolongation and ventricular arrhythmias, including ventricular tachycardia and torsades de pointes.

Changes in Laboratory Values: Changes in laboratory values with possible clinical significance were as follows: *Hepatic*—elevated SGPT (ALT) < 1%, SGOT (AST) < 1%, GGT < 1%, alkaline phosphatase < 1%, LDH < 1%, total bilirubin < 1%; *Hematologic*—decreased WBC < 1%, elevated prothrombin time 1%; *Renal*—elevated BUN 4%, elevated serum creatinine < 1%. GGT, alkaline phosphatase, and prothrombin time data are from adult studies only.

OVERDOSAGE

In case of an overdose, patients should contact a physician, poison control center, or emergency room. There is neither a pharmacologic basis nor data suggesting an increased toxicity of the combination compared to individual components.

Lansoprazole:

Oral doses up to 5000 mg/kg in rats (approximately 1300 times the 30 mg human dose based on body surface area) and mice (about 675.7 times the 30 mg human dose based on body surface area) did not produce deaths or any clinical signs.

Lansoprazole is not removed from the circulation by hemodialysis. In one reported case of overdose, the patient consumed 600 mg of lansoprazole with no adverse reaction.

Amoxicillin:

In case of overdosage, discontinue medication, treat symptomatically and institute supportive measures as required. If the overdosage is very recent and there is no contraindication, an attempt at emesis or other means of removal of drug from the stomach may be performed.

Interstitial nephritis resulting in oliguric renal failure has been reported in a small number of patients after overdosage with amoxicillin. Renal impairment appears to be reversible with cessation of drug administration. High blood levels may occur more readily in patients with impaired renal function because of decreased renal clearance of amoxicillin. Amoxicillin can be removed from circulation by hemodialysis.

Clarithromycin:

Overdosage of clarithromycin can cause gastrointestinal symptoms such as abdominal pain, vomiting, nausea, and diarrhea.

Adverse reactions accompanying overdosage should be treated by the prompt elimination of unabsorbed drug and supportive measures. As with other macrolides, clarithromycin serum levels are not expected to be appreciably affected by hemodialysis or peritoneal dialysis.

DOSAGE AND ADMINISTRATION

***H. pylori* Eradication to Reduce the Risk of Duodenal Ulcer Recurrence**

The recommended adult oral dose is 30 mg PREVACID, 1 g amoxicillin, and 500 mg clarithromycin administered together twice daily (morning and evening) for 10 or 14 days. (See **INDICATIONS AND USAGE.**)

PREVPAC is not recommended in patients with creatinine clearance less than 30 mL/min.

HOW SUPPLIED

PREVPAC is supplied as an individual daily administration pack, each containing:

PREVACID:

— two opaque, hard gelatin, black and pink PREVACID 30-mg capsules, with the TAP logo and "PREVACID 30" imprinted on the capsules.

TRIMOX:

— four flesh body/maroon cap amoxicillin 500-mg capsules, USP, printed with "BRISTOL 7279" in black ink on both body and cap.

BIAXIN Filmtab:

— two yellow oval film-coated clarithromycin 500-mg tablets, USP, debossed with the Abbott logo on one side and "KL" on the other side of the tablets.

NDC 0300-3702-01 Daily administration pack
NDC 0300-3702-11 Daily administration card

Storage: Protect from light and moisture.

Store at a controlled room temperature between 20°C and 25°C (68°F and 77°F).

Rx only

U.S. Patent No. 5,013,743

PREVPAC is distributed by TAP Pharmaceuticals Inc.
PREVACID® (lansoprazole) Delayed-Release Capsules
Distributed by TAP Pharmaceuticals Inc.
Lake Forest, IL 60045, U.S.A.

APOTHECON®
A BRISTOL-MYERS SQUIBB COMPANY
TRIMOX® (amoxicillin, USP)
Manufactured by APOTHECON®
A Bristol-Myers Squibb Company
Princeton, NJ 08540, U.S.A.
BIAXIN® Filmtab® (clarithromycin tablets, USP)
Manufactured by Abbott Laboratories
North Chicago, IL 60064, U.S.A.
03-5322-R6-Rev. October, 2003

Shown in Product Identification Guide, page 334

Targacept, Inc.

200 EAST FIRST STREET, SUITE 300
WINSTON SALEM, NC 27101

Direct Inquiries to:
phone: (336) 480-2233

INVERSINE® ℞
(MECAMYLAMINE HCl)
TABLETS

DESCRIPTION

INVERSINE® (Mecamylamine HCl) is a potent, oral antihypertension agent and ganglion blocker, and is a secondary amine. It is N,2,3,3-tetramethyl-bicyclo [2.2.1] heptan- 2 – amine hydrochloride. Its empirical formula is $C_{11}H_{21}N \cdot HCl$ and its structural formula is:

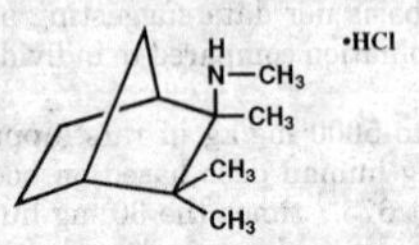

It is a white, odorless, or practically odorless, crystalline powder, is highly stable, soluble in water and has a molecular weight of 203.75.

INVERSINE is supplied as tablets for oral use, each containing 2.5 mg mecamylamine HCl. Inactive ingredients are acacia, calcium phosphate, D&C Yellow 10, FD&C Yellow 6, lactose, magnesium stearate, starch and talc.

CLINICAL PHARMACOLOGY

Mecamylamine reduces blood pressure in both normotensive and hypertensive individuals. It has a gradual onset of action (1/2 to 2 hours) and a longlasting effect (usually 6 to 12 hours or more). A small oral dosage often produces a smooth and predictable reduction of blood pressure. Although this antihypertensive effect is predominantly orthostatic, the supine blood pressure is also significantly reduced.

Pharmacokinetics and Metabolism

Mecamylamine is almost completely absorbed from the gastrointestinal tract, resulting in consistent lowering of blood pressure in most patients with hypertensive cardiovascular disease. Mecamylamine is excreted slowly in the urine in the unchanged form. The rate of its renal elimination is influenced markedly by urinary pH. Alkalinization of the urine reduces, and acidification promotes, renal excretion of mecamylamine.

Mecamylamine crosses the blood-brain and placental barriers.

INDICATIONS AND USAGE

For the management of moderately severe to severe essential hypertension and in uncomplicated cases of malignant hypertension.

CONTRAINDICATIONS

INVERSINE should not be used in mild, moderate, labile hypertension and may prove unsuitable in uncooperative patients. It is contraindicated in coronary insufficiency or recent myocardial infarction.

INVERSINE should be given with great discretion, if at all, when renal insufficiency is manifested by a rising or elevated BUN. The drug is contraindicated in uremia. Patients receiving antibiotics and sulfonamides should generally not be treated with ganglion blockers. Other contraindications are glaucoma, organic pyloric stenosis or hypersensitivity to the product.

WARNINGS

Mecamylamine, a secondary amine, readily penetrates into the brain and thus may produce central nervous system effects. Tremor, choreiform movements, mental aberrations, and convulsions may occur rarely. These have occurred most often when large doses of INVERSINE were used, especially in patients with cerebral or renal insufficiency.

When ganglion blockers or other potent antihypertensive drugs are discontinued suddenly, hypertensive levels return. In patients with malignant hypertension and others, this may occur abruptly and may cause fatal cerebral vascular accidents or acute congestive heart failure. When INVERSINE is withdrawn, this should be done gradually and other antihypertensive therapy usually must be substituted. On the other hand, the effects of INVERSINE sometimes may last from hours to days after therapy is discontinued.

PRECAUTIONS

General

The patient's condition should be evaluated carefully, particularly as to renal and cardiovascular function. When renal, cerebral, or coronary blood flow is deficient, any additional impairment, which might result from added hypotension, must be avoided. The use of INVERSINE in patients with marked cerebral and coronary arteriosclerosis or after a recent cerebral accident requires caution.

The action of INVERSINE may be potentiated by excessive heat, fever, infection, hemorrhage, pregnancy, anesthesia, surgery, vigorous exercise, other antihypertensive drugs, alcohol, and salt depletion as a result of diminished intake or increased excretion due to diarrhea, vomiting, excessive sweating, or diuretics.

During therapy with INVERSINE, sodium intake should not be restricted but, if necessary, the dosage of the ganglion blocker must be adjusted.

Since urinary retention may occur in patients on ganglion blockers, caution is required in patients with prostatic hypertrophy, bladder neck obstruction, and urethral stricture. Frequent loose bowel movements with abdominal distention and decreased borborygmi may be the first signs of paralytic ileus. If these are present, INVERSINE should be discontinued immediately and remedial steps taken.

Information for patients

INVERSINE may cause dizziness, lightheadedness, or fainting, especially when rising from a lying or sitting position. This effect may be increased by alcoholic beverages, exercise, or during hot weather. Getting up slowly may help alleviate such a reaction.

Drug Interactions

Patients receiving antibiotics and sulfonamides generally should not be treated with ganglion blockers.

The action of INVERSINE may be potentiated by anesthesia, other antihypertensive drugs and alcohol.

Carcinogenesis, Mutagenesis, Impairment of Fertility

Long-term studies in animals have not been performed to evaluate the effects upon fertility, mutagenic or carcinogenic potential of INVERSINE.

Pregnancy

Pregnancy Category C. Animal reproduction studies have not been conducted with INVERSINE. It is not known whether INVERSINE can cause fetal harm when given to a pregnant woman or can affect reproductive capacity. INVERSINE should be given to a pregnant woman only if clearly needed.

Nursing Mothers

Because of the potential for serious adverse reactions in nursing infants from INVERSINE, a decision should be made whether to discontinue nursing or to discontinue the drug, taking into account the importance of the drug to the mother.

Pediatric Use

Safety and effectiveness in pediatric patients have not been established.

ADVERSE REACTIONS

The following adverse reactions have been reported and within each category are listed in order of decreasing severity.

Gastrointestinal: Ileus, constipation (sometimes preceded by small, frequent liquid stools), vomiting, nausea, anorexia, glossitis and dryness of mouth.

Cardiovascular: Orthostatic dizziness and syncope, postural hypotension.

Nervous System/Psychiatric: Convulsions, choreiform movements, mental aberrations, tremor, and paresthesias (see WARNINGS).

Respiratory: Interstitial pulmonary edema and fibrosis.

Urogenital: Urinary retention, impotence, decreased libido.

Special Senses: Blurred vision, dilated pupils.

Miscellaneous: Weakness, fatigue, sedation.

OVERDOSAGE

Signs of overdosage include: hypotension (which may progress to peripheral vascular collapse), postural hypotension, nausea, vomiting, diarrhea, constipation, paralytic ileus, urinary retention, dizziness, anxiety, dry mouth, mydriasis, blurred vision, or palpitations. A rise in intraocular pressure may occur.

Pressor amines may be used to counteract excessive hypotension. Since patients being treated with ganglion blockers are more than normally reactive to pressor amines, small doses of the latter are recommended to avoid excessive response.

The oral LD_{50} of mecamylamine in the mouse is 92 mg/kg.

DOSAGE AND ADMINISTRATION

Therapy is usually started with one 2.5 mg tablet of INVERSINE twice a day. This initial dosage should be modified by increments of one 2.5 mg tablet at intervals of not less than 2 days until the desired blood pressure response occurs (the criterion being a dosage just under that which causes signs of mild postural hypotension).

The average total daily dosage of INVERSINE is 25 mg, usually in three divided doses. However, as little as 2.5 mg daily may be sufficient to control hypertension in some patients. A range of two to four or even more doses may be required in severe cases when smooth control is difficult to obtain. In severe or urgent cases, larger increments at smaller intervals may be needed. Partial tolerance may develop in certain patients, requiring an increase in the daily dosage of INVERSINE.

Administration of INVERSINE after meals may cause a more gradual absorption and smoother control of excessively high blood pressure. The timing of doses in relation to meals should be consistent. Since the blood pressure response to antihypertensive drugs is increased in the early morning, the larger dose should be given at noontime and perhaps in the evening. The morning dose, as a rule, should be relatively small and in some instances may even be omitted.

The *initial regulation of dosage* should be determined by blood pressure readings in the erect position at the time of maximal effect of the drug, as well as by other signs and symptoms of orthostatic hypotension.

The *effective maintenance dosage* should be regulated by blood pressure readings in the erect position and by limitation of dosage to that which causes slight faintness or dizziness in this position. If the patient or a relative can use a sphygmomanometer, instructions may be given to reduce or omit a dose if readings fall below a designated level or if faintness or lightheadedness occurs. *However, no change should be instituted without the knowledge of the physician.* Close supervision and education of the patient, as well as critical adjustment of dosage, are essential to successful therapy.

Other Antihypertensive Agents

When INVERSINE is given with other antihypertensive drugs, the dosage of these other agents, as well as that of INVERSINE, should be reduced to avoid excessive hypotension. However, thiazides should be continued in their usual dosage, while that of INVERSINE is decreased by at least 50 percent.

HOW SUPPLIED

Tablets INVERSINE, 2.5 mg, are slightly yellow, round, compressed tablets, coded LBS01. They are supplied as follows:

NDC 17205-0626-1 in bottles of 100.

STORAGE CONDITION

Store at 25°C (77°F); excursions permitted to 15–30°C (59–86°F)
[see USP Controlled Room [Temperature]
Manufactured by: Siegfried CMS Ltd., Zofingen, Switzerland for Targacept, Inc.
Winston-Salem, NC 27101
Inversine® is a registered trademark of Targacept, Inc.

Rev.7/02

Shown in Product Identification Guide, page 334

TaroPharma

5 SKYLINE DRIVE
HAWTHORNE, NY 10532

Direct Inquiries to:
1-800-544-1449

Product Name	Identification Code or Product Form*
Lustra 4% hydroquinone	C
Lustra-AF 4% hydroquinone	C
Ovide .5% ℞	L
Primsol 50 mg ℞	S
Topicort .25%	C.O
Topicort .05% ℞	G
Topicort LP .05% ℞	C
U-Cort 1% ℞	C

* C-Cream, O-Ointment, L-Lotion, G-Gel, S-Solution.

Taro Pharmaceuticals U.S.A., Inc.

5 SKYLINE DRIVE
HAWTHORNE, NY 10532

Direct Inquiries to:
1-888-TARO-USA

Product Name *Description* *Color, Shape*	Identification Code or Product Form† *(Front/Back)**
Acetazolamide Tablets USP, 125 mg Rx White, Round	T52/Scored
Acetazolamide Tablets USP, 250 mg Rx White, Round	T53/Scored in quarters
Acetic Acid 2% Otic Solution with Hydrocortisone 1% USP, Rx	OS

Alclometasone Dipropionate USP, 0.05%, Rx	O
Amcinonide 0.1% Rx	C, L
Amiodarone HCl Tablets, 200 mg Rx Light Orange, Round, Flat	TARO Scored/ 56/Blank
Ammonium Lactate 12%	C, L
Betamethasone Dipropionate USP, 0.05% Rx	C
Betamethasone Dipropionate (Augmented), 0.05%, Rx	C, G
Betamethasone Valerate USP, 0.1% Rx	C
Carbamazepine Tablets USP (Chewable), 100 mg Rx White, w/Pink Speckles, Cherry Odor Round	TARO/16/Blank
Carbamazepine Tablets USP, 200 mg Rx White, Round, Flat	TARO/11/Blank
Carbamazepine 100 mg/5mL Rx Orange Color & Flavor Oral Suspension	Susp
Clobetasol Propionate, USP 0.05% Rx	C,O,G,S
Clobetasol Propionate (Emollient) USP, 0.05% Rx	C,E
Clomipramine Hydrochloride Capsules, 25 mg Rx Dark Blue Cap, Light Blue Body	CLOM 25
Clomipramine Hydrochloride Capsules, 50 mg Rx Yellow Opaque	CLOM 50
Clomipramine Hydrochloride Capsules, 75 mg Rx White Opaque	CLOM 75
Clorazepate Dipotassium Tablets USP, 3.75 mg C-IV Rx Pale Violet, Slightly Mottled, Round, Flat	T Scored 45/Blank
Clorazepate Dipotassium Tablets USP, 7.5 mg C-IV Rx Orange, Slightly Mottled, Round, Flat	T Scored 46/Blank
Clorazepate Dipotassium Tablets USP, 15 mg C-IV Rx Pale Pink, Slightly Mottled, Round, Flat	T Scored 47/Blank
Clotrimazole 1% Rx	C,S
Clotrimazole and Betamethasone Dipropionate USP, Rx	C, L
Desonide 0.05% Rx	C,O
Desoximetasone USP, 0.05% Rx	C,G
Desoximetasone USP, 0.25% Rx	C,O
Diflorasone Diacetate 0.05% Rx	C,O
Econazole Nitrate Cream 1% Rx	C
Enalapril Maleate and Hydrochlorothiazide Tablets, USP 5/12.5 mg Rx Ivory, Caplet-Shaped Compressed Tablets	T4/Blank
Enalapril Maleate and Hydrochlorothiazide Tablets, USP 10/25 mg Rx Peach, Caplet-Shaped Compressed Tablets	T3/Blank
Enalapril Maleate Tablets, USP 2.5 mg Rx Yellow, Round, Biconvex	T Scored 2/Blank
Enalapril Maleate Tablets, USP 5 mg Rx Yellow, Round, Biconvex	T Scored 5/Blank
Enalapril Maleate Tablets, USP 10 mg Rx Pink, Round, Convex	T Scored 10/Blank
Enalapril Maleate Tablets, USP 20 mg Rx Orange, Round, Convex	T Scored 20/Blank
Etodolac Capsules USP, 200 mg Rx Dark Pink, Black Body	ETO 200
Etodolac Capsules USP, 300 mg Rx Pink, Black Body	ETO 300
Etodolac Tablets USP, 400 mg Rx Peach, Oval, Film Coated	T88/Blank
Etodolac Tablets USP, 500 mg Rx Blue, Oval, Film Coated	TARO/89
Etodolac Extended-Release Tablets, 400 mg Rx Pink, Round, Film Coated	T400/Blank
Etodolac Extended-Release Tablets, 500 mg Rx Green, Oblong, Convex	T500/Blank
Etodolac Extended-Release Tablets, 600 mg Rx Grey, Oval, Convex	T600/Blank
Fluconazole Tablets 50 mg Pink, Rectangular with rounded edge	FL50/TARO
Fluconazole Tablets 100 mg Pink, Rectangular with rounded edge	FL100/TARO
Fluconazole Tablets 150 mg Pink, Rectangular with rounded edge	FL150/TARO
Fluconazole Tablets 200 mg Pink, Rectangular with rounded edge	FL200/TARO
Fluocinonide USP, 0.05% Rx	C,O,G,S,
Fluocinonide USP, 0.05% (Emulsified Base) Rx	C,EB
Fluorouracil Topical 2% and 5% Rx	S
Fluticasone 0.05% Rx	C
Fluticasone 0.005% Rx	O
Gentamicin Sulfate USP, 0.1% Rx	C, O
Hydrocortisone USP, 1% Rx	C
Hydrocortisone USP, 2.5% Rx	C, L, O
Hydrocortisone Valerate USP, 0.2% Rx	C,O
Ketoconazole 2%	C
Ketoconazole Tablets USP, 200 mg Rx White to Off-White, Round, Flat	T Scored 57/Blank
Lidocaine USP, 5% Rx	O
Phenytoin USP, 125 mg/5mL Orange with orange-vanilla flavor	Susp
Nystatin USP, 100,000 units per gram Rx	C
Nystatin and Triamcinolone Acetonide USP, Rx	C,O
Terconazole Vaginal Cream 0.8% Rx	VC
Triamcinolone Acetonide USP, 0.1% Rx	DP
Warfarin Sodium Tablets, USP 1 mg Rx Pink, Capsule Shape, Flat	1/WARFARIN/TARO
Warfarin Sodium Tablets, USP 2 mg Rx Lavender, Capsule Shape, Flat	2/WARFARIN/TARO
Warfarin Sodium Tablets, USP 2.5 mg Rx Green, Capsule Shape, Flat	2½/WARFARIN/TARO
Warfarin Sodium Tablets, USP 3 mg Rx Tan, Capsule Shape, Flat	3/WARFARIN/TARO
Warfarin Sodium Tablets, USP 4 mg Rx Blue, Capsule Shape, Flat	4/WARFARIN/TARO
Warfarin Sodium Tablets, USP 5 mg Rx Peach, Capsule Shape, Flat	5/WARFARIN/TARO
Warfarin Sodium Tablets, USP 6 mg Rx Teal, Capsule Shape, Flat	6/WARFARIN/TARO
Warfarin Sodium Tablets, USP 7.5 mg Rx Yellow, Capsule Shape, Flat	7½/WARFARIN/TARO
Warfarin Sodium Tablets, USP 10 mg Rx White, Capsule Shape, Flat	10/WARFARIN/TARO

*Front/Back of Tablet & Body and Cap of Capsule
†C-Cream, O-Ointment, L-Lotion, G-Gel, OS-Otic Solution, S-Solution, Susp-Suspension, DP-Dental Paste, E-Emollient, EB-Emulsified Base, VC-Vaginal Cream

Teva Neuroscience, Inc.

901 E. 104TH STREET, SUITE 900
KANSAS CITY, MO 64131

For Company Inquiries Contact:
1-800-221-4026
For Medical Information Contact:
1-800-887-8100

COPAXONE®
(glatiramer acetate injection)

DESCRIPTION

COPAXONE® is the brand name for glatiramer acetate (formerly known as copolymer-1). Glatiramer acetate, the active ingredient of COPAXONE®, consists of the acetate salts of synthetic polypeptides, containing four naturally occurring amino acids: L-glutamic acid, L-alanine, L-tyrosine, and L-lysine with an average molar fraction of 0.141, 0.427, 0.095, and 0.338, respectively. The average molecular weight of glatiramer acetate is 5,000–9,000 daltons. Glatiramer acetate is identified by specific antibodies.
Chemically, glatiramer acetate is designated L-glutamic acid polymer with L-alanine, L-lysine and L-tyrosine, acetate (salt). Its structural formula is:

$$(Glu, Ala, Lys, Tyr)_x \bullet xCH_3COOH$$
$$(C_5H_9NO_4 \bullet C_3H_7NO_2 \bullet C_6H_{14}N_2O_2 \bullet C_9H_{11}NO_3)_x \bullet xC_2H_4O_2$$
CAS - 147245-92-9

COPAXONE® Injection is a clear, colorless to slightly yellow, sterile, non-pyrogenic solution for subcutaneous injection. Each 1.0 mL of solution contains 20 mg of glatiramer acetate and 40 mg of mannitol, USP. The pH range of the solution is approximately 5.5 to 7.0. The biological activity of COPAXONE® is determined by its ability to block the induction of EAE in mice.

CLINICAL PHARMACOLOGY

Mechanism of Action
The mechanism(s) by which glatiramer acetate exerts its effects in patients with Multiple Sclerosis (MS) is (are) not fully elucidated. However, it is thought to act by modifying immune processes that are currently believed to be responsible for the pathogenesis of MS. This hypothesis is supported by findings of studies that have been carried out to explore the pathogenesis of experimental allergic encephalomyelitis (EAE), a condition induced in several animal species through immunization against central nervous system derived material containing myelin and often used as an experimental animal model of MS. Studies in animals and *in vitro* systems suggest that upon its administration, glatiramer acetate-specific suppressor T-cells are induced and activated in the periphery.
Because glatiramer acetate can modify immune functions, concerns exist about its potential to alter naturally occurring immune responses. Results of a limited battery of tests designed to evaluate this risk produced no finding of concern; nevertheless, there is no logical way to absolutely exclude this possibility (see **PRECAUTIONS**).

Pharmacokinetics
Results obtained in pharmacokinetic studies performed in humans (healthy volunteers) and animals support the assumption that a substantial fraction of the therapeutic dose delivered to patients subcutaneously is hydrolyzed locally. Nevertheless, larger fragments of glatiramer acetate can be recognized by glatiramer acetate-reactive antibodies. Some fraction of the injected material, either intact or partially hydrolyzed, is presumed to enter the lymphatic circulation, enabling it to reach regional lymph nodes, and some may enter the systemic circulation intact.

Clinical Trials
Evidence supporting the effectiveness of glatiramer acetate in decreasing the frequency of relapses in patients with Relapsing-Remitting Multiple Sclerosis (RR MS) derives from two placebo-controlled trials, both of which used a glatiramer acetate dose of 20 mg/day. (No other dose or dosing regimen has been studied in placebo-controlled trials of RR MS.)
One trial was performed at a single center. It enrolled 50 patients who were randomized to receive daily doses of either glatiramer acetate, 20 mg subcutaneously, or placebo (glatiramer acetate, n=25; placebo, n=25). Patients were diagnosed with RR MS by standard criteria, and had had at least 2 exacerbations during the 2 years immediately preceding enrollment. Patients were ambulatory, as evidenced by a score of no more than 6 on the Kurtzke Disability Scale Score (DSS), a standard scale ranging from 0–Normal to 10–Death due to MS. A score of 6 is defined as one at which a patient is still ambulatory with assistance; a score of 7 means the patient must use a wheelchair.
Patients were examined every 3 months for 2 years, as well as within several days of a presumed exacerbation. To confirm an exacerbation, a blinded neurologist had to document objective neurologic signs, as well as document the existence of other criteria (e.g., the persistence of the neurological signs for at least 48 hours).

Continued on next page

Copaxone—Cont.

The protocol-specified primary outcome measure was the proportion of patients in each treatment group who remained exacerbation free for the 2 years of the trial, but two other important outcomes were also specified as endpoints: 1) the frequency of attacks during the trial, and 2) the change in the number of attacks compared with the number which occurred during the previous 2 years.

Table 1 presents the values of the three outcomes described above, as well as several protocol specified secondary measures. These values are based on the intent-to-treat population (i.e., all patients who received at least 1 dose of treatment and who had at least 1 on-treatment assessment):

[See table 1 at right]

The second trial was a multicenter trial of similar design which was performed in 11 US centers. A total of 251 patients (glatiramer acetate, 125; placebo, 126) were enrolled. The primary outcome measure was the Mean 2-Year Relapse Rate. The table below presents the values of this outcome for the intent-to-treat population, as well as several secondary measures:

[See table 2 at right]

In both studies glatiramer acetate exhibited a clear beneficial effect on relapse rate, and it is based on this evidence that glatiramer acetate is considered effective.

A third study was a multi-national study in which MRI parameters were used both as primary and secondary endpoints. A total of 239 patients with RR MS (119 on glatiramer acetate and 120 on placebo) were randomized. Inclusion criteria were similar to those in the second study with the additional criterion that patients had to have at least one Gd-enhancing lesion on the screening MRI. The patients were treated in a double-blind manner for nine months, during which they underwent monthly MRI scanning. The primary endpoint for the double-blind phase was the total cumulative number of T1 Gd-enhancing lesions over the nine months. Table 3 summarizes the results for the primary outcome measure monitored during the trial for the intent-to-treat cohort.

[See table 3 at right]

The following figure displays the results of the primary outcome on a monthly basis.

Figure 1: Median Cumulative Number of Gd-Enhancing Lesions

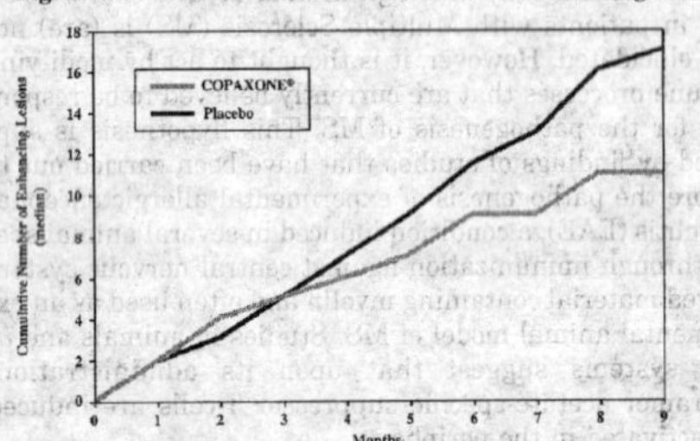

p= 0.0030 for the difference between the placebo-treated (n=120) and glatiramer acetate-treated (n=119) groups

INDICATIONS AND USAGE

COPAXONE® Injection is indicated for reduction of the frequency of relapses in patients with Relapsing-Remitting Multiple Sclerosis.

CONTRAINDICATIONS

COPAXONE® Injection is contraindicated in patients with known hypersensitivity to glatiramer acetate or mannitol.

WARNINGS

The only recommended route of administration of COPAXONE® Injection is the subcutaneous route. COPAXONE® Injection should not be administered by the intravenous route.

PRECAUTIONS

General

Patients should be instructed in self-injection techniques to assure the safe administration of COPAXONE® Injection (see **PRECAUTIONS: Information for Patients** and the **COPAXONE® INJECTION PATIENT INFORMATION** Leaflet). Current data indicate that no special caution is required for patients operating an automobile or using complex machinery.

Considerations Regarding the Use of a Product Capable of Modifying Immune Responses

Because glatiramer acetate can modify immune response, it could possibly interfere with useful immune functions. For example, treatment with glatiramer acetate might, in theory, interfere with the recognition of foreign antigens in a way that would undermine the body's tumor surveillance and its defenses against infection. There is no evidence that glatiramer acetate does this, but there has as yet been no systematic evaluation of this risk. Because glatiramer acetate is an antigenic material, it is possible that its use may lead to the induction of host responses that are untoward, but systematic surveillance for these effects has not been undertaken.

Although glatiramer acetate is intended to minimize the autoimmune response to myelin, there is the possibility that continued alteration of cellular immunity due to chronic treatment with glatiramer acetate might result in untoward effects.

Table 1: Study 1 Efficacy Results

Outcome	Glatiramer Acetate (N=25)	Placebo (N=25)	P-Value
% Relapse-Free Patients	14/25 (56%)	7/25 (28%)	0.085
Mean Relapse Frequency	0.6/2 years	2.4/2 years	0.005
Reduction in Relapse Rate Compared to Pre-Study	3.2	1.6	0.025
Median Time to First Relapse (days)	>700	150	0.03
% of Progression-Free* Patients	20/25 (80%)	13/25 (52%)	0.07

*Progression was defined as an increase of at least 1 point on the DSS, persisting for at least 3 consecutive months.

Table 2: Study 2 Efficacy Results

Outcome	Glatiramer Acetate (N=125)	Placebo (N=126)	P-Value
Mean No. of Relapses	1.19/2 years	1.68/2 years	0.055
% Relapse-Free Patients	42/125 (34%)	34/126 (27%)	0.25
Median Time to First Relapse (days)	287	198	0.23
% of Progression-Free Patients	98/125 (78%)	95/126 (75%)	0.48
Mean Change in DSS	-0.05	+0.21	0.023

Table 3: Study 3 MRI Results

Outcome	Glatiramer Acetate (N=119)	Placebo (N=120)	P-Value
Medians of the Cumulative Number of T1 Gd-Enhancing Lesions	11	17	0.0030

Glatiramer acetate-reactive antibodies are formed in practically all patients exposed to daily treatment with the recommended dose. Studies in both the rat and monkey have suggested that immune complexes are deposited in the renal glomeruli. Furthermore, in a controlled trial of 125 RR MS patients given glatiramer acetate, 20 mg, subcutaneously every day for 2 years, serum IgG levels reached at least 3 times baseline values in 80% of patients by 3 months of initiation of treatment. By 12 months of treatment, however, 30% of patients still had IgG levels at least 3 times baseline values, and 90% had levels above baseline by 12 months. The antibodies are exclusively of the IgG subtype-and predominantly of the IgG-1 subtype. No IgE type antibodies could be detected in any of the 94 sera tested; nevertheless, anaphylaxis can be associated with the administration of most any foreign substance, and therefore, this risk cannot be excluded.

Information for Patients

To assure safe and effective use of COPAXONE® Injection, the following information and instructions should be given to patients:

1. Inform your physician if you are pregnant, if you are planning to have a child, or if you become pregnant while taking this medication.
2. Inform your physician if you are nursing.
3. Do not change the dose or dosing schedule without consulting your physician.
4. Do not stop taking the drug without consulting your physician.

Patients should be instructed in the use of aseptic techniques when administering COPAXONE® Injection. Appropriate instructions for the self-injection of COPAXONE® Injection should be given, including a careful review of the **COPAXONE® INJECTION PATIENT INFORMATION** Leaflet. The first injection should be performed under the supervision of an appropriately qualified health care professional. Patient understanding and use of aseptic self-injection techniques and procedures should be periodically re-evaluated. Patients should be cautioned against the reuse of needles or syringes and instructed in safe disposal procedures. They should use a puncture-resistant container for disposal of used needles and syringes. Patients should be instructed on the safe disposal of full containers according to local laws.

Awareness of Adverse Reactions: Physicians are advised to counsel patients about adverse reactions associated with the use of COPAXONE® Injection (see **ADVERSE REACTIONS** section). In addition, patients should be advised to read the **COPAXONE® INJECTION PATIENT INFORMATION** Leaflet and resolve any questions regarding it prior to beginning COPAXONE® Injection therapy.

Laboratory Tests

Data collected during premarketing development do not suggest the need for routine laboratory monitoring.

Drug Interactions

Interactions between COPAXONE® Injection and other drugs have not been fully evaluated. Results from existing clinical trials do not suggest any significant interactions of COPAXONE® Injection with therapies commonly used in MS patients, including the concurrent use of corticosteroids for up to 28 days. COPAXONE® Injection has not been formally evaluated in combination with Interferon beta.

Drug/Laboratory Test Interactions

None are known.

Carcinogenesis, Mutagenesis, Impairment of Fertility

Carcinogenesis

In a two-year carcinogenicity study, mice were administered up to 60 mg/kg/day glatiramer acetate by subcutaneous injection (up to 15 times the human therapeutic dose on a mg/m^2 basis). No increase in systemic neoplasms was observed. In males of the high dose group (60 mg/kg/day), but not in females, there was an increased incidence of fibrosarcomas at the injection sites. These sarcomas were associated with skin damage precipitated by repetitive injections of an irritant over a limited skin area.

In a two-year carcinogenicity study, rats were administered up to 30 mg/kg/day glatiramer acetate by subcutaneous injection (up to 15 times the human therapeutic dose on a mg/m^2 basis). No increase in systemic neoplasms was observed.

Mutagenesis

Glatiramer acetate was not mutagenic in four strains of *Salmonella typhimurium* and two strains of *Escherichia coli* (Ames test) or in the *in vitro* mouse lymphoma assay in L5178Y cells. Glatiramer acetate was clastogenic in two separate *in vitro* chromosomal aberration assays in cultured human lymphocytes; it was not clastogenic in an *in vivo* mouse bone marrow micronucleus assay.

Impairment of Fertility

In a multigeneration reproduction and fertility study in rats, glatiramer acetate at subcutaneous doses of up to 36 mg/kg (18 times the human therapeutic dose on a mg/m^2 basis) had no adverse effects on reproductive parameters.

Pregnancy

Pregnancy Category B. No adverse effects on embryofetal development occurred in reproduction studies in rats and rabbits receiving subcutaneous doses of up to 37.5 mg/kg of glatiramer acetate during the period of organogenesis (18 and 36 times the therapeutic human dose on a mg/m^2 basis, respectively). In a prenatal and postnatal study in which rats received subcutaneous glatiramer acetate at doses of up to 36 mg/kg from day 15 of pregnancy throughout lactation, no significant effects on delivery or on offspring growth and development were observed.

There are no adequate and well-controlled studies in pregnant women. Because animal reproduction studies are not always predictive of human response, glatiramer acetate should be used during pregnancy only if clearly needed.

Labor and Delivery

In a prenatal and postnatal study, in which rats received subcutaneous glatiramer acetate at doses of up to 36 mg/kg from day 15 of pregnancy throughout lactation, no significant effects on delivery were observed. The relevance of these findings to humans is unknown.

Nursing Mothers

It is not known whether glatiramer acetate is excreted in human milk. Because many drugs are excreted in human milk, caution should be exercised when COPAXONE® is administered to a nursing woman.

Pediatric Use
The safety and efficacy of COPAXONE® Injection have not been established in individuals under 18 years of age.

Use in the Elderly
COPAXONE® Injection has not been studied specifically in elderly patients.

Use in Patients with Impaired Renal Function
The pharmacokinetics of glatiramer acetate in patients with impaired renal function have not been determined.

ADVERSE REACTIONS

During premarketing clinical trials approximately 900 individuals received at least one dose of glatiramer acetate.

In controlled clinical trials the most commonly observed adverse experiences associated with the use of glatiramer acetate and not seen at an equivalent frequency among placebo-treated patients were: injection site reactions, vasodilatation, chest pain, asthenia, infection, pain, nausea, arthralgia, anxiety, and hypertonia.

Approximately 8% of the 893 subjects receiving glatiramer acetate discontinued treatment because of an adverse reaction. The adverse reactions most commonly associated with discontinuation were: injection site reaction (6.5%), vasodilatation, unintended pregnancy, depression, dyspnea, urticaria, tachycardia, dizziness, and tremor.

Immediate Post-Injection Reaction
Approximately 10% of MS patients exposed to glatiramer acetate in premarketing studies experienced a constellation of symptoms immediately after injection that included flushing, chest pain, palpitations, anxiety, dyspnea, constriction of the throat, and urticaria. In clinical trials, the symptoms were generally transient and self-limited and did not require specific treatment. In general, these symptoms have their onset several months after the initiation of treatment, although they may occur earlier, and a given patient may experience one or several episodes of these symptoms. Whether or not any of these symptoms actually represent a specific syndrome is uncertain. During the postmarketing period, there have been reports of patients with similar symptoms who received emergency medical care.

Whether an immunologic or non-immunologic mechanism mediates these episodes, or whether several similar episodes seen in a given patient have identical mechanisms, is unknown.

Chest Pain
Approximately 21% of glatiramer acetate patients in the pre-marketing controlled studies (compared to 11% of placebo patients) experienced at least one episode of what was described as transient chest pain. While some of these episodes occurred in the context of the Immediate Post-Injection Reaction described above, many did not. The temporal relationship of this chest pain to an injection of glatiramer acetate was not always known. The pain was transient (usually lasting only a few minutes), often unassociated with other symptoms, and appeared to have no important clinical sequelae. There has been only one episode of chest pain during which a full EKG was performed; that EKG showed no evidence of ischemia. Some patients experienced more than one such episode, and episodes usually began at least 1 month after the initiation of treatment. The pathogenesis of this symptom is unknown.

Incidence in Controlled Clinical Studies: The following table lists treatment-emergent signs and symptoms that occurred in at least 2% of MS patients treated with glatiramer acetate in the pre-marketing placebo-controlled trials. These signs and symptoms were numerically more common in patients treated with glatiramer acetate than in patients treated with placebo. These trials include the first two controlled trials in RR MS patients and a controlled trial in patients with Chronic-Progressive MS. Adverse reactions were usually mild in intensity.

The prescriber should be aware that these figures cannot be used to predict the frequency of adverse experiences in the course of usual medical practice where patient characteristics and other factors may differ from those prevailing during clinical studies. Similarly, the cited frequencies cannot be directly compared with figures obtained from other clinical investigations involving different treatments, uses, or investigators. An inspection of these frequencies, however, does provide the prescriber with one basis on which to estimate the relative contribution of drug and nondrug factors to the adverse reaction incidences in the population studied. [See table above]

Other events which occurred in at least 2% of glatiramer acetate patients but were present at equal or greater rates in the placebo group included:

Body as a Whole: Headache, injection site ecchymosis, accidental injury, abdominal pain, allergic rhinitis, neck rigidity, and malaise.

Digestive System: Dyspepsia, constipation, dysphagia, fecal incontinence, flatulence, nausea and vomiting, gastritis, gingivitis, periodontal abscess, and dry mouth.

Musculoskeletal: Myasthenia and myalgia.

Nervous System: Dizziness, hypesthesia, paresthesia, insomnia, depression, dysesthesia, incoordination, somnolence, abnormal gait, amnesia, emotional lability, Lhermitte's sign, abnormal thinking, twitching, euphoria, and sleep disorder.

Respiratory System: Pharyngitis, sinusitis, increased cough, and laryngitis.

Skin and Appendages: Acne, alopecia, and nail disorder.

Special Senses: Abnormal vision, diplopia, amblyopia, eye pain, conjunctivitis, tinnitus, taste perversion, and deafness.

Controlled Trials in Patients with Multiple Sclerosis: Incidence of Glatiramer Acetate Adverse Reactions ≥2% and More Frequent than Placebo

Preferred Term	Glatiramer Acetate (N = 201)		Placebo (N = 206)	
	N	%	N	%
Body as a Whole				
Asthenia	83	41	78	38
Back Pain	33	16	30	15
Bacterial Infection	11	5	9	4
Chest Pain	43	21	22	11
Chills	8	4	2	1
Cyst	5	2	1	0
Face Edema	12	6	2	1
Fever	17	8	15	7
Flu Syndrome	38	19	35	17
Infection	101	50	99	48
Injection Site Erythema	132	66	40	19
Injection Site Hemorrhage	11	5	6	3
Injection Site Induration	26	13	1	0
Injection Site Inflammation	98	49	22	11
Injection Site Mass	54	27	21	10
Injection Site Pain	147	73	78	38
Injection Site Pruritus	80	40	12	6
Injection Site Urticaria	10	5	0	0
Injection Site Welt	22	11	5	2
Neck Pain	16	8	9	4
Pain	56	28	52	25
Cardiovascular System				
Migraine	10	5	5	2
Palpitations	35	17	16	8
Syncope	10	5	5	2
Tachycardia	11	5	8	4
Vasodilatation	55	27	21	10
Digestive System				
Anorexia	17	8	15	7
Diarrhea	25	12	23	11
Gastroenteritis	6	3	2	1
Gastrointestinal Disorder	10	5	8	4
Nausea	44	22	34	17
Vomiting	13	6	8	4
Hemic and Lymphatic System				
Ecchymosis	16	8	13	6
Lymphadenopathy	25	12	12	6
Metabolic and Nutritional				
Edema	5	3	1	0
Peripheral Edema	14	7	8	4
Weight Gain	7	3	0	0
Musculoskeletal System				
Arthralgia	49	24	39	19
Nervous System				
Agitation	8	4	4	2
Anxiety	46	23	40	19
Confusion	5	2	1	0
Foot Drop	6	3	4	2
Hypertonia	44	22	37	18
Nervousness	4	2	2	1
Nystagmus	5	2	2	1
Speech Disorder	5	2	3	1
Tremor	14	7	7	3
Vertigo	12	6	11	5
Respiratory System				
Bronchitis	18	9	12	6
Dyspnea	38	19	15	7
Laryngismus	10	5	7	3
Rhinitis	29	14	27	13
Skin and Appendages				
Erythema	8	4	4	2
Herpes Simplex	8	4	6	3
Pruritus	36	18	26	13
Rash	37	18	30	15
Skin Nodule	4	2	1	0
Sweating	31	15	21	10
Urticaria	9	4	5	2
Special Senses				
Ear Pain	15	7	12	6
Eye Disorder	8	4	1	0
Urogenital System				
Dysmenorrhea	12	6	10	5
Urinary Urgency	20	10	17	8
Vaginal Moniliasis	16	8	9	4

Urogenital System: Urinary tract infection, urinary frequency, urinary incontinence, urinary retention, dysuria, cystitis, metrorrhagia, breast pain, and vaginitis.

Data on adverse reactions occurring in the controlled clinical trials were analyzed to evaluate differences based on sex. No clinically significant differences were identified. Ninety-two percent of patients in these clinical trials were Caucasian. This percentage reflects the racial composition of the MS population. In addition, the vast majority of patients treated with COPAXONE® were between the ages of 18 and 45. Consequently, data are inadequate to perform an analysis of the adverse reaction incidence related to clinically relevant age subgroups.

Laboratory analyses were performed on all patients participating in the clinical program for glatiramer acetate. Clinically significant laboratory values for hematology, chemistry, and urinalysis were similar for both glatiramer acetate and placebo groups in blinded clinical trials. No patient receiving glatiramer acetate withdrew from any trial because of abnormal laboratory findings.

Other Adverse Events Observed During Clinical Trials
Glatiramer acetate was administered to 979 individuals during premarketing clinical trials, only some of which were placebo-controlled. During these trials, all adverse events were recorded by the clinical investigators, using terminology of their own choosing. To provide a meaningful estimate of the proportion of individuals having adverse events, similar types of events were grouped into standardized categories using COSTART dictionary terminology. All reported events occurring at least twice and potentially important events occurring once are listed below, except those already listed in the previous table, those too general to be informative, trivial events, and other reactions which occurred in at least 2% of treated patients and were present at equal or greater rates in the placebo group. Additional adverse reactions reported during the post-marketing period are included.

Events are further classified within body system categories and listed in order of decreasing frequency using the follow-

Continued on next page

Copaxone—Cont.

ing definitions: *Frequent* adverse events are defined as those occurring in at least 1/100 patients; *Infrequent* adverse events are those occurring in 1/100 to 1/1000 patients; *Rare* adverse events are those occurring in less than 1/1000 patients.

Body as a Whole:

◆ *Frequent:* Injection site edema, injection site atrophy, abscess, injection site hypersensitivity.

◆ *Infrequent:* Injection site hematoma, injection site fibrosis, moon face, cellulitis, generalized edema, hernia, injection site abscess, serum sickness, suicide attempt, injection site hypertrophy, injection site melanosis, lipoma, and photosensitivity reaction.

Cardiovascular:

◆ *Frequent:* Hypertension.

◆ *Infrequent:* Hypotension, midsystolic click, systolic murmur, atrial fibrillation, bradycardia, fourth heart sound, postural hypotension, and varicose veins.

Digestive:

◆ *Infrequent:* Dry mouth, stomatitis, burning sensation on tongue, cholecystitis, colitis, esophageal ulcer, esophagitis, gastrointestinal carcinoma, gum hemorrhage, hepatomegaly, increased appetite, melena, mouth ulceration, pancreas disorder, pancreatitis, rectal hemorrhage, tenesmus, tongue discoloration, and duodenal ulcer.

Endocrine:

◆ *Infrequent:* Goiter, hyperthyroidism, and hypothyroidism.

Gastrointestinal:

◆ *Frequent:* Bowel urgency, oral moniliasis, salivary gland enlargement, tooth caries, and ulcerative stomatitis.

Hemic and Lymphatic:

◆ *Infrequent:* Leukopenia, anemia, cyanosis, eosinophilia, hematemesis, lymphedema, pancytopenia, and splenomegaly.

Metabolic and Nutritional:

◆ *Infrequent:* Weight loss, alcohol intolerance, Cushing's syndrome, gout, abnormal healing, and xanthoma.

Musculoskeletal:

◆ *Infrequent:* Arthritis, muscle atrophy, bone pain, bursitis, kidney pain, muscle disorder, myopathy, osteomyelitis, tendon pain, and tenosynovitis.

Nervous:

◆ *Frequent:* Abnormal dreams, emotional lability, and stupor.

◆ *Infrequent:* Aphasia, ataxia, convulsion, circumoral paresthesia, depersonalization, hallucinations, hostility, hypokinesia, coma, concentration disorder, facial paralysis, decreased libido, manic reaction, memory impairment, myoclonus, neuralgia, paranoid reaction, paraplegia, psychotic depression, and transient stupor.

Respiratory:

◆ *Frequent:* Hyperventilation, hay-fever.

◆ *Infrequent:* Asthma, pneumonia, epistaxis, hypoventilation, and voice alteration.

Skin and Appendages:

◆ *Frequent:* Eczema, herpes zoster, pustular rash, skin atrophy, and warts.

◆ *Infrequent:* Dry skin, skin hypertrophy, dermatitis, furunculosis, psoriasis, angioedema, contact dermatitis, erythema nodosum, fungal dermatitis, maculopapular rash, pigmentation, benign skin neoplasm, skin carcinoma, skin striae, and vesiculobullous rash.

Special Senses:

◆ *Frequent:* Visual field defect.

◆ *Infrequent:* Dry eyes, otitis externa, ptosis, cataract, corneal ulcer, mydriasis, optic neuritis, photophobia, and taste loss.

Urogenital:

◆ *Frequent:* Amenorrhea, hematuria, impotence, menorrhagia, suspicious papanicolaou smear, urinary frequency and vaginal hemorrhage.

◆ *Infrequent:* Vaginitis, flank pain (kidney), abortion, breast engorgement, breast enlargement, carcinoma *in situ* cervix, fibrocystic breast, kidney calculus, nocturia, ovarian cyst, priapism, pyelonephritis, abnormal sexual function, and urethritis.

Postmarketing Clinical Experience

Postmarketing experience has shown an adverse event profile similar to that presented above. Reports of adverse reactions occurring under treatment with COPAXONE® (glatiramer acetate for injection) not mentioned above that have been received since market introduction and that may have or not have causal relationship to the drug include the following:

Body as a Whole: sepsis; LE syndrome; hydrocephalus; enlarged abdomen; injection site hypersensitivity; allergic reaction; anaphylactoid reaction

Cardiovascular System: thrombosis; peripheral vascular disease; pericardial effusion; myocardial infarct; deep thrombophlebitis; coronary occlusion; congestive heart failure; cardiomyopathy; cardiomegaly; arrhythmia; angina pectoris

Digestive System: tongue edema; stomach ulcer; hemorrhage; liver function abnormality; liver damage; hepatitis; eructation; cirrhosis of the liver; cholelithiasis

Hemic and Lymphatic System: thrombocytopenia; lymphoma-like reaction; acute leukemia

Metabolic and Nutritional Disorders: hypercholesterolemia

Musculoskeletal System: rheumatoid arthritis; generalized spasm

Nervous System: myelitis; meningitis; CNS neoplasm; cerebrovascular accident; brain edema; abnormal dreams; aphasia; convulsion; neuralgia

Respiratory System: pulmonary embolus; pleural effusion; carcinoma of lung; hay fever

Special Senses: glaucoma; blindness; visual field defect

Urogenital System: urogenital neoplasm; urine abnormality; ovarian carcinoma; nephrosis; kidney failure; breast carcinoma; bladder carcinoma; urinary frequency

DRUG ABUSE AND DEPENDENCE

No evidence or experience suggests that abuse or dependence occurs with COPAXONE® Injection therapy; however, the risk of dependence has not been systematically evaluated.

DOSAGE AND ADMINISTRATION

The recommended dose of COPAXONE® Injection for the treatment of RR MS is 20 mg/day injected subcutaneously.

Instructions for Use

Remove one blister with the syringe inside from the COPAXONE® Injection Pre-filled syringes package from the refrigerator. Let the pre-filled syringe package stand at room temperature for 20 minutes to allow the solution to warm up to room temperature. Store all unused syringes in the refrigerator. Inspect the product visually and discard or return the product to the pharmacist before use if it contains any particulate matter.

Sites for self-injection include arms, abdomen, hips, and thighs. The pre-filled syringe is suitable for single use only; unused portions should be discarded. (See the **COPAXONE® Injection PATIENT INFORMATION** Leaflet for **INSTRUCTIONS FOR INJECTING COPAXONE®**.)

HOW SUPPLIED

COPAXONE® Injection is supplied as a single-use pre-filled syringe containing 1.0 mL of a clear, colorless to slightly yellow, sterile, non-pyrogenic solution containing 20 mg of glatiramer acetate and 40 mg of mannitol, USP in cartons of 30 single-use pre-filled syringes, 33 alcohol preps (wipes) and instructions for use.

The recommended storage condition for the COPAXONE® Injection is refrigeration (2°C to 8°C / 36°F to 46°F). However, excursions from recommended storage conditions to room temperature conditions (15° to 30°C / 59° to 86°F) for up to one week have been shown to have no adverse impact on the product. Exposure to higher temperatures or intense light should be avoided.

COPAXONE® Injection contains no preservative. Do not use if the solution contains any particulate matter.

COPAXONE® Injection is available in packs of 30 single-use Pre-Filled Syringes (NDC 0088-1153-30).

Rx Only.

PATIENT INFORMATION

COPAXONE® (glatiramer acetate injection)

Read this information carefully before you use COPAXONE®. Read the information you get when you refill your COPAXONE® prescriptions because there may be new information. This information does not take the place of your doctor's advice. Ask your doctor or pharmacist if you do not understand some of this information or if you want to know more about this medicine.

What is COPAXONE®?

COPAXONE® (co-PAX-own) is a medicine you inject to treat Relapsing-Remitting Multiple Sclerosis. Although COPAXONE® is not a cure, patients treated with COPAXONE® have fewer relapses.

Who should not use COPAXONE®?

- COPAXONE® is not recommended for use in pregnancy. So, tell your doctor if you are pregnant or if you plan to become pregnant while taking this medicine.
- Tell your doctor if you are nursing. It is not known if COPAXONE® is passed through the breast milk to the baby.
- Do not use COPAXONE® if you are allergic to glatiramer acetate or mannitol.

What are the possible side effects of COPAXONE®?

- **Call your doctor right away if you develop any of the following symptoms: hives, skin rash with irritation, dizziness, sweating, chest pain, trouble breathing, or severe pain at the injection site.** Do not give yourself any more injections until your doctor tells you to begin again.
- The most common side effects of COPAXONE® are redness, pain, swelling, itching, or a lump at the injection site. These reactions are usually mild and seldom require medical care.
- Some patients report a short-term reaction right after injecting COPAXONE®. This reaction can involve flushing (feeling of warmth and/or redness), chest tightness or pain with heart palpitations, anxiety, and trouble breathing. These symptoms generally appear within minutes after an injection, last a few minutes, then go away by themselves without further problems.
- **If symptoms become severe, call the emergency phone number in your area.**

  Do not give yourself any more injections until your doctor tells you to begin again.

These are not all the possible side effects of COPAXONE®. For a complete list, ask your doctor or pharmacist. Tell your doctor about any side effects you have while taking COPAXONE®.

How should I use COPAXONE®?

- The recommended dose of COPAXONE® for the treatment of Relapsing-Remitting Multiple Sclerosis is 20 mg once a day injected subcutaneously (in the fatty layer under the skin).
- Look at the medicine in the pre-filled syringe. If the medicine is cloudy or has particles in it, do not use it. Instead, call Shared Solutions at 1-800-887-8100 for assistance.
- Have a friend or relative with you if you need help, especially when you first start giving yourself injections.
- Each pre-filled syringe should be used for only one injection. Do not reuse the pre-filled syringe. After use, throw it away properly.
- Do not change the dose or dosing schedule or stop taking the medicine without talking with your doctor.

How do I inject COPAXONE®?

There are 3 basic steps for injecting COPAXONE® pre-filled syringes:

1. Gather the materials.
2. Choose the injection site.
3. Give yourself the injection.

Step 1: Gather the materials

1. First, place each of the items you will need on a clean, flat surface in a well-lit area:
   - 1 blister pack with COPAXONE® Pre-Filled Syringe Remove only 1 blister pack from the COPAXONE® Pre-Filled Syringe carton. Keep all unused syringes in the Pre-Filled Syringe carton and store them in the refrigerator.
   - Alcohol prep (wipe)
   - Dry cotton ball (not supplied)
2. Let the blister pack with the syringe inside warm up to room temperature for 20 minutes.
3. To prevent infection, wash and dry your hands. Do not touch your hair or skin after washing.
4. There may be small air bubbles in the syringe. To avoid loss of medicine when using COPAXONE® pre-filled syringes, do not expel (or do not attempt to expel) the air bubble from the syringe before injecting the medicine.

Step 2: Choose the injection site

- There are 7 possible injection areas on your body: arms, thighs, hips and lower stomach area (abdomen) (See Figure 1).

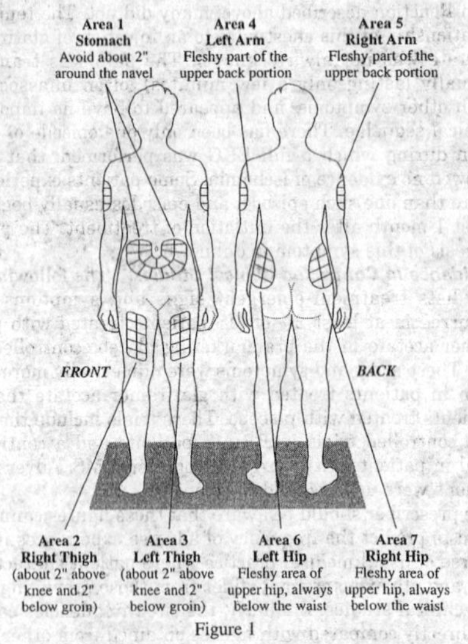

Figure 1

- Each day, pick a different injection area from one of the 7 areas. **Do not inject in the same area more than once a week.**
- Within each injection area there are multiple injection sites. Have a plan for rotating your injection sites. Keep a record of your injection sites, so you know where you have injected.
- There are some sites in your body that may be hard to reach for self-injection (like the back of your arm), and you may need help.

Step 3: Give yourself the injection

1. Remove the syringe from its protective blister pack by peeling back the paper label. Before use, look at the liquid in the syringe. If it is cloudy or contains any particles, do not use it and call Shared Solutions at 1-800-887-8100 for assistance. If the liquid is clear, place the syringe on the clean, flat surface.
2. Choose an injection site on your body. Clean the injection site with a new alcohol prep and let the site air dry to reduce stinging.
3. Pick up the syringe as you would a pencil. Remove the needle shield from the needle.

[See figure 2 at top of next column]

4. With your other hand, pinch about a 2-inch fold of skin between your thumb and index finger (See Figure 2).

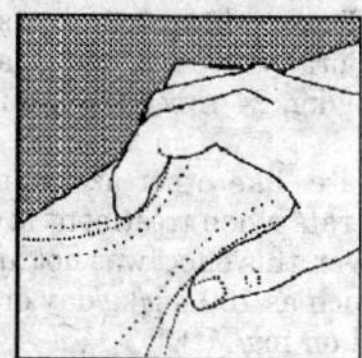

Figure 2

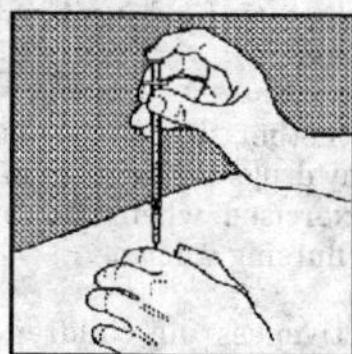

Figure 3

5. Insert the needle at a 90-degree angle (straight in), resting the heel of your hand against your body. When the needle is all the way in release the fold of skin (See Figure 3).
6. To inject the medicine, hold the syringe steady and push down the plunger.
7. When you have injected all of the medicine, pull the needle straight out.
8. Press a dry cotton ball on the injection site for a few seconds. **Do not rub the injection site.**
9. Throw away the syringe in a safe hard-walled plastic container.

What is the proper use and disposal of Pre-Filled Syringes?
Each Pre-Filled Syringe should be used for only 1 injection. Throw away all used Pre-Filled Syringes in a hard-walled plastic container, such as an empty liquid laundry detergent bottle. Keep the container closed tightly and out of the reach of children. When the container is full, check with your doctor, pharmacist, or nurse about proper disposal, as laws vary from state to state.

How should I store COPAXONE® Pre-Filled Syringes?
Keep the COPAXONE® Pre-Filled Syringe carton in the refrigerator, out of the reach of children.
The COPAXONE® package should be refrigerated as soon as you get it, at 36-46°F (2-8°C). If you cannot store COPAXONE® in a refrigerator, you can store it at room temperature, 59-86°F (15-30°C), for up to 7 days. Do not store COPAXONE® at room temperature for longer than 7 days. **Do not freeze COPAXONE®.** If a COPAXONE® pre-filled syringe freezes, throw it away in a proper container. COPAXONE® is light sensitive. Protect it from light when not injecting. Do not use the pre-filled syringe if the solution contains particles or is cloudy.

General advice about prescription medicines
Medicines are sometimes prescribed for conditions that are not mentioned in patient information leaflets. Do not use COPAXONE® for a condition for which it was not prescribed. Do not give COPAXONE® to other people, even if they have the same condition you have. It may harm them. This leaflet summarizes the most important information about COPAXONE®. If you would like more information, talk with your doctor. You can ask your pharmacist or doctor for information about COPAXONE® that is written for health professionals. Also, you can call Shared Solutions for any questions about COPAXONE® and its use. The phone number for Shared Solutions is 1-800-887-8100.
Manufactured in Israel by **TEVA Pharmaceutical Industries Ltd.**, Kfar-Saba 44102, Israel
Manufactured By: **Baxter Pharmaceutical Solutions LLC**, Bloomington, IN 47403
Manufactured For: **TEVA Neuroscience, Inc.**, Kansas City, MO 64131
Distributed by: **Aventis Pharmaceuticals Inc.**, Kansas City, MO 64137

Rev # 02/2004

Shown in Product Identification Guide, page 334

Ther-Rx Corporation

13622 LAKEFRONT DRIVE
ST. LOUIS, MISSOURI 63045

For Direct Inquiries Contact:
(314) 209-1517 phone
(314) 770-0371 fax

CHROMAGEN® ℞

[krō-mă-jĕn]
Soft Gelatin Capsules
Rx Only

DESCRIPTION

Each capsule contains:
Iron .... 70 mg Ferrochel® (elemental iron)*
Vitamin C .... 150 mg Ester-C®†
Vitamin B_{12} .... 10 mcg (cyanocobalamin)
Dessicated stomach substance .... 100 mg

Each capsule also contains soybean oil, gelatin, glycerine USP, yellow beeswax, lecithin – unbleached, titanium dioxide, methylparaben, ethyl vanillin, FD&C Red #40, FD&C Yellow #6, propylparaben, FD&C Blue #1.

INDICATIONS

For the treatment of all anemias responsive to oral iron therapy, such as hypochromic anemia associated with pregnancy, chronic or acute blood loss, dietary restriction, metabolic disease and post-surgical convalescence.

CONTRAINDICATIONS

Hemochromatosis and hemosiderosis are contraindications to iron therapy.

> WARNING
> **Accidental overdose of iron-containing products is a leading cause of fatal poisoning in children under 6. Keep this product out of reach of children. In case of accidental overdose, call a doctor or poison control center immediately.**

Allergy Alert: These gelcaps contain a soy product.

PRECAUTION

Pediatric Use: Safety and effectiveness in pediatric patients has not been established.

ADVERSE REACTIONS

Average capsule doses in sensitive individuals or excessive dosage may cause nausea, skin rash, vomiting, diarrhea, precordial pain, or flushing of the face or extremities.

DOSAGE AND ADMINISTRATION

Usual adult dose is 1 soft gelatin capsule daily.

HOW SUPPLIED

Chromagen® capsules for oral administration are supplied as red soft gelatin capsules, imprinted "THX 0129" in grey ink in child-resistant, unit-dose packages of 100 capsules (10 × 10 Unit Dose Packs) (NDC 64011-129-11).
Store at controlled room temperature 15°-30°C (59°-86°F). Avoid excessive heat 40°C (104°F). Avoid freezing.

* Ferrochel® (ferrous bis-glycinate chelate) is a registered trademark of Albion International, Inc., Clearfield, Utah, and is protected under US Patent Nos. 4,599,152 and 4,830,716.
† Ester-C® is a patented pharmaceutical grade material consisting of calcium ascorbate and calcium threonate. Ester-C® is a licensed trademark of Zila Nutraceuticals, Inc.
Manufactured by:
Accucaps Industries, Ltd.-Canada for
Ther-Rx Corporation
Saint Louis, MO 63044
P4223 Rev. 06/03

Shown in Product Identification Guide, page 334

CHROMAGEN® FA ℞

Soft Gelatin Capsules
℞ Only

DESCRIPTION

Each capsule contains:

Iron .... 70 mg Ferrochel® (elemental iron)*
Vitamin C .... 150 mg Ester-C®†
Folic Acid USP ..... 1 mg
Vitamin B_{12} .... 10 mcg (cyanocobalamin)

Each capsule also contains soybean oil, gelatin, glycerine USP, yellow beeswax, lecithin – unbleached, titanium dioxide, methylparaben, black ferric oxide, D&C Yellow #10, ethyl vanillin, propylparaben, FD&C Red #40, FD&C Blue #1.

INDICATIONS

For the treatment of all anemias responsive to oral iron therapy, such as hypochromic anemia associated with pregnancy, chronic or acute blood loss, dietary restriction, metabolic disease and post-surgical convalescence.

CONTRAINDICATIONS

Hemochromatosis and hemosiderosis are contraindications to iron therapy. Folic acid is contraindicated in patients with pernicious anemia (see PRECAUTIONS).

> WARNING
> **Accidental overdose of iron-containing products is a leading cause of fatal poisoning in children under 6. Keep this product out of reach of children. In case of accidental overdose, call a doctor or poison control center immediately.**

Allergy Alert: These gelcaps contain a soy product.

PRECAUTIONS

Folic acid alone is improper therapy in the treatment of pernicious anemia and other megaloblastic anemias where Vitamin B_{12} is deficient.
Folic acid in doses above 1.0 mg daily may obscure pernicious anemia in that hematologic remission can occur while neurological manifestations remain progressive.
Pediatric Use: Safety and effectiveness in pediatric patients has not been established.

ADVERSE REACTIONS

Average capsule doses in sensitive individuals or excessive dosage may cause nausea, skin rash, vomiting, diarrhea, precordial pain, or flushing of the face and extremities.

DOSAGE AND ADMINISTRATION

Usual adult dose is 1 soft gelatin capsule daily.

HOW SUPPLIED

Chromagen® FA capsules for oral administration are supplied as green and brown soft gelatin capsules, imprinted "THX 0130" in grey ink in child-resistant, unit-dose packages of 100 capsules (10 × 10 Unit Dose Packs) (NDC 64011-130-11).
Store at controlled room temperature 15°- 30°C (59°- 86°F). Avoid excessive heat 40°C (104°F). Avoid freezing.

* Ferrochel® (ferrous bis-glycinate chelate) is a registered trademark of Albion International, Inc., Clearfield, Utah, and is protected under US Patent Nos. 4,599,152 and 4,830,716.
† Ester-C® is a patented pharmaceutical grade material consisting of calcium ascorbate and calcium threonate. Ester-C® is a licensed trademark of Zila Nutraceuticals, Inc.
Manufactured by:
Accucaps Industries, Ltd.-Canada for
Ther-Rx Corporation
Saint Louis, MO 63044
P4224 Rev. 06/03

Shown in Product Identification Guide, page 334

CHROMAGEN® FORTE ℞

Soft Gelatin Capsules
℞ Only

DESCRIPTION

Each capsule contains:

Iron .... 70 mg Ferrochel® (elemental iron)*
.... 81 mg ferrous fumarate (elemental iron)
Vitamin C .... 60 mg Ester-C®†
Folic Acid USP .. 1 mg
Vitamin B_{12} ...... 10 mcg (cyanocobalamin)

Each capsule also contains soybean oil, gelatin, glycerine USP, yellow beeswax, lecithin – unbleached, titanium dioxide, methylparaben, ethyl vanillin, FD&C Red #40, FD&C Yellow #6, propylparaben, FD&C Blue #1.

INDICATIONS

For the treatment of all anemias responsive to oral iron therapy, such as hypochromic anemia associated with pregnancy, chronic or acute blood loss, dietary restriction, metabolic disease and post-surgical convalescence.

CONTRAINDICATIONS

Hemochromatosis and hemosiderosis are contraindications to iron therapy. Folic acid is contraindicated in patients with pernicious anemia (see PRECAUTIONS).

> WARNING
> **Accidental overdose of iron-containing products is a leading cause of fatal poisoning in children under 6. Keep this product out of reach of children. In case of accidental overdose, call a doctor or poison control center immediately.**

Allergy Alert: These gelcaps contain a soy product.

Continued on next page

Chromagen Forte—Cont.

PRECAUTIONS

Folic acid alone is improper therapy in the treatment of pernicious anemia and other megaloblastic anemias where Vitamin B_{12} is deficient.

Folic acid in doses above 1.0 mg daily may obscure pernicious anemia in that hematologic remission can occur while neurological manifestations remain progressive.

Pediatric Use: Safety and effectiveness in pediatric patients has not been established.

ADVERSE REACTIONS

Average capsule doses in sensitive individuals or excessive dosage may cause nausea, skin rash, vomiting, diarrhea, precordial pain, or flushing of the face and extremities.

DOSAGE AND ADMINISTRATION

Usual adult dose is 1 to 2 soft gelatin capsules daily, or as directed by a physician.

HOW SUPPLIED

Chromagen® Forte capsules for oral administration are supplied as brown soft gelatin capsules, imprinted "THX 0131" in grey ink in child-resistant, unit-dose packages of 100 capsules (10 × 10 Unit Dose Packs) (NDC 64011-131-11).

Store at controlled room temperature 15°-30°C (59°-86°F). Avoid excessive heat 40°C (104°F). Avoid freezing.

* Ferrochel® (ferrous bis-glycinate chelate) is a registered trademark of Albion International, Inc., Clearfield, Utah, and is protected under US Patent Nos. 4,599,152 and 4,830,716.

† Ester-C® is a patented pharmaceutical grade material consisting of calcium ascorbate and calcium threonate.

Ester-C® is a licensed trademark of Zila Nutraceuticals, Inc.

Manufactured by:
Accucaps Industries, Ltd.-Canada for
Ther-Rx Corporation
Saint Louis, MO 63044
P4225 Rev. 06/03

Shown in Product Identification Guide, page 334

GYNAZOLE•1® ℞

[gī-nă-zōl]

(butoconazole nitrate) Vaginal Cream, 2%
In one prefilled disposable applicator
Rx Only

DESCRIPTION

Gynazole•1® (butoconazole nitrate) vaginal cream, 2% contains butoconazole nitrate 2%, an imidazole derivative with antifungal activity. Its chemical name is (±)-1-[4-(p-chlorophenyl)-2-[(2,6-dichlorophenyl)thio]butyl] imidazole mononitrate, and it has the following chemical structure:

Cl · HNO_3 Cl S N N Cl

Butoconazole nitrate is a white to off-white crystalline powder with a molecular weight of 474.79. It is sparingly soluble in methanol; slightly soluble in chloroform, methylene chloride, acetone, and ethanol; very slightly soluble in ethyl acetate; and practically insoluble in water. It melts at about 159°C with decomposition.

Gynazole•1® contains 2% butoconazole nitrate in a cream of edetate disodium, glyceryl monoisostearate, methylparaben, mineral oil, polyglyceryl-3 oleate, propylene glycol, propylparaben, colloidal silicon dioxide, sorbitol solution, purified water, and microcrystalline wax.

CLINICAL PHARMACOLOGY

Following vaginal administration of butoconazole nitrate vaginal cream, 2% to 3 women, 1.7% (range 1.3–2.2%) of the dose was absorbed on average. Peak plasma levels (13.6–18.6 ng radioequivalents/mL of plasma) of the drug and its metabolites are attained between 12 and 24 hours after vaginal administration.

Microbiology

The exact mechanism of the antifungal action of butoconazole nitrate is unknown; however, it is presumed to function as other imidazole derivatives via inhibition of steroid synthesis. Imidazoles generally inhibit the conversion of lanosterol to ergosterol, resulting in a change in fungal cell membrane lipid composition. This structural change alters cell permeability and, ultimately, results in the osmotic disruption of growth inhibition of the fungal cell.

Butoconazole nitrate is an imidazole derivative that has fungicidal activity *in vitro* against *Candida* spp. and has been demonstrated to be clinically effective against vaginal infections due to *Candida albicans. Candida albicans* has been identified as the predominant species responsible for vulvovaginal candidiasis.

INDICATIONS AND USAGE

Gynazole•1® (butoconazole nitrate) vaginal cream, 2% is indicated for the local treatment of vulvovaginal candidiasis (infections caused by *Candida*). The diagnosis should be confirmed by KOH smears and/or cultures (see **CLINICAL STUDIES**).

Note: Gynazole•1® is safe and effective in non-pregnant women; however, the safety and effectiveness of this product in pregnant women has not been established. (See **PRECAUTIONS**: Pregnancy.)

CONTRAINDICATIONS

Gynazole•1® is contraindicated in patients with a history of hypersensitivity to any of the components of the product.

CLINICAL STUDIES

Vulvovaginal Candidiasis: Two studies were conducted that compared 2% butoconazole nitrate cream with clotrimazole tablets. There were 322 enrolled patients, 161 received 2.0% butoconazole vaginal cream and 161 patients inserted the 500-mg clotrimazole vaginal tablet. At the second follow-up visit (30 days post-therapy), 118 patients in the butoconazole group and 116 in the clotrimazole group were evaluable for efficacy analysis, respectively. All of these patients had infection caused by *Candida albicans*.

The efficacy of the study drugs was assessed by evaluating clinical, mycologic and therapeutic cure rates, which are summarized in Table 1.

The therapeutic cure is defined by a complete resolution of signs and symptoms of vaginal candidiasis (clinical cure) along with a negative KOH examination and negative culture for *Candida* spp. (microbiologic eradication) at the long term follow-up. The therapeutic cure rate was 67% in the butoconazole group and 61% in the clotrimazole group.

Table 1

	2% butoconazole nitrate cream	500-mg clotrimazole vaginal tablet
Enrolled	161	161
Evaluable at Late Follow-up	118	116
Clinical Cure	95/118 (81%)	93/116 (80%)
Mycologic Eradication*	87/118 (74%)	77/116 (66%)
Therapeutic Cure	79/118 (67%)	71/116 (61%)

*=*C. albicans* in the vaginal culture was proven at admission in all of the patients.

WARNINGS

This cream contains mineral oil. Mineral oil may weaken latex or rubber products such as condoms or vaginal contraceptive diaphragms; therefore, use of such products within 72 hours following treatment with Gynazole•1® is not recommended.

Recurrent vaginal yeast infections, especially those that are difficult to eradicate, can be an early sign of infection with the human immunodeficiency virus (HIV) in women who are considered at risk for HIV infection.

PRECAUTIONS

General:

If clinical symptoms persist, tests should be repeated to rule out other pathogens, to confirm the original diagnosis, and to rule out other conditions that may predispose a patient to recurrent vaginal fungal infections.

Carcinogenesis, Mutagenesis, Impairment of Fertility:

Carcinogenesis: Long term studies in animals have not been performed to evaluate the carcinogenic potential of this drug.

Mutagenicity: Butoconazole nitrate was not mutagenic when tested in the Ames bacterial test, yeast, chromosomal aberration assay in CHO cells, CHO/HGPRT point mutation assay, mouse micronucleus, and rat dominant lethal assays.

Impairment of Fertility: No impairment of fertility was seen in rabbits or rats administered butoconazole nitrate in oral doses up to 30 mg/kg/day (5 times the human dose based on mg/M^2) or 100 mg/kg/day (10 times the human dose based on mg/M^2), respectively.

Pregnancy:

Pregnancy Category C.

In pregnant rats administered 6 mg/kg/day of butoconazole nitrate intravaginally during the period of organogenesis, there was an increase in resorption rate and decrease in litter size; however, no teratogenicity was noted. This dose represents a 130- to 353-fold margin of safety based on serum levels achieved in rats following intravaginal administration compared to the serum levels achieved in humans following intravaginal administration of the recommended therapeutic dose of butoconazole nitrate.

Butoconazole nitrate has no apparent adverse effect when administered orally to pregnant rats throughout organogenesis at dose levels up to 50 mg/kg/day (5 times the human dose based on mg/M^2). Daily oral doses of 100, 300 or 750 mg/kg/day (10, 30 or 75 times the human dose based on mg/M^2 respectively) resulted in fetal malformations (abdominal wall defects, cleft palate), but maternal stress was also evident at these higher dose levels. There were, however, no adverse effects on litters of rabbits who received butoconazole nitrate orally, even at maternally stressful dose levels (e.g., 150 mg/kg, 24 times the human dose based on mg/M^2).

Butoconazole nitrate, like other azole anti-fungal agents, causes dystocia in rats when treatment is extended through parturition. However, this effect was not apparent in rabbits treated with as much as 100 mg/kg/day orally (16 times the human dose based on mg/M^2).

There are, however, no adequate and well-controlled studies in pregnant women. Gynazole•1® should be used during pregnancy only if the potential benefit justifies the potential risk to the fetus.

Nursing Mothers:

It is not known whether this drug is excreted in human milk. Because many drugs are excreted in human milk, caution should be exercised when butoconazole nitrate is administered to a nursing woman.

Pediatric Use:

Safety and effectiveness in children have not been established.

ADVERSE REACTIONS

Of the 314 patients treated with Gynazole•1® for 1 day in controlled clinical trials, 18 patients (5.7%) reported complaints such as vulvar/vaginal burning, itching, soreness and swelling, pelvic or abdominal pain or cramping, or a combination of two or more of these symptoms. In 3 patients (1%) these complaints were considered treatment-related. Five of the 18 patients reporting adverse events discontinued the study because of them.

DOSAGE AND ADMINISTRATION

The recommended dose of Gynazole•1® is one applicatorful of cream (approximately 5 grams of the cream) intravaginally. This amount of cream contains approximately 100 mg of butoconazole nitrate.

HOW SUPPLIED

Gynazole•1® (butoconazole nitrate) vaginal cream, 2% is available in cartons containing one single-dose prefilled disposable applicator (NDC 64011-001-08).

Store at 25°C (77°F); excursions permitted to 15°-30°C (59°-86°F). (See USP Controlled Room Temperature). Avoid heat above 30°C (86°F).

U.S. Patent Nos. 4,078,071, 4,551,148, 4,636,202 and 5,266,329

Manufactured for Ther-Rx Corporation
by KV Pharmaceutical Co.
St. Louis, MO 63044
P4249 08/03

Shown in Product Identification Guide, page 334

NIFEREX® Capsules OTC

Bisglycino iron amino acid chelate and polysaccharide iron complex

DOSAGE

Adults: 1 or 2 capsules twice daily
Pediatric patients age 6 and older: 1 capsule daily

SUPPLEMENT FACTS

Serving Size 1 or 2 capsules
Iron .... 40 mg Ferrochel® (elemental iron)*
.... 20 mg polysaccharide iron (elemental iron)

OTHER INGREDIENTS

FD&C blue #1, FD&C blue #1 aluminum lake, FD&C red #40, FD&C yellow #6, gelatin, lactose, magnesium stearate, pharmaceutical glaze, pharmaceutical shellac, silicon dioxide and titanium dioxide.

HOW SUPPLIED

Niferex® capsules for oral administration are supplied as brown (cap) and clear (body) capsules filled with grey powder, imprinted "THX" in white ink on the cap and "0134" in white ink on the body in child-resistant, unit-dose packages of 100 capsules (10 x 10 Unit Dose Packs) (NDC 64011-134-11).

Store at controlled room temperature 15°-30° C (59°-86° F).

If pregnant or breast-feeding, ask a health professional before use.

*Ferrochel® (ferrous bis-glycinate chelate) is a registered trademark of Albion International, Inc., Clearfield, Utah, and is protected under US Patent Nos. 4,599,152 and 4,830,716.

WARNING
Accidental overdose of iron-containing products is a leading cause of fatal poisoning in children under 6. Keep this product out of reach of children. In case of accidental overdose, call a doctor or poison control center immediately.

NOTICE: This product supplied in tamper-evident blisters. Do not use if outer foil is torn or missing.

Questions or comments? 1-877-567-7676

Manufactured by:
KV Pharmaceutical Co. for
Ther-Rx Corporation
Saint Louis, MO 63044
US Patent Nos.: 4,599,152; 4,830,716.
P4152-1 10/03

Shown in Product Identification Guide, page 334

NIFEREX®-150 CAPSULES **OTC**
Bisglycino iron amino acid chelate and polysaccharide iron complex

ADULT DOSAGE
1 or 2 capsules daily

SUPPLEMENT FACTS
Serving Size 1 or 2 capsules
Iron .... 80 mg Ferrochel® (elemental iron)*
.... 70 mg polysaccharide iron (elemental iron)
Vitamin C .... 50 mg Ester-C®†

OTHER INGREDIENTS
D&C red #28, D&C yellow #10, FD&C blue #1, FD&C red #40, gelatin, magnesium stearate, pharmaceutical glaze, silicon dioxide and titanium dioxide.

HOW SUPPLIED
Niferex®-150 capsules for oral administration are supplied as orange (cap) and clear (body) capsules filled with brown powder, imprinted "THX" in white ink on the cap and "0135" in white ink on the body in child-resistant, unit-dose packages of 100 capsules (10 × 10 Unit Dose Packs) (NDC 64011-135-11).
Store at controlled room temperature 15°–30° C (59°–86° F).

If pregnant or breast-feeding, ask a health professional before use.

*Ferrochel® (ferrous bis-glycinate chelate) is a registered trademark of Albion International, Inc., Clearfield, Utah, and is protected under US Patent Nos. 4,599,152 and 4,830,716.
†Ester-C® is a patented pharmaceutical grade material consisting of calcium ascorbate and calcium threonate. Ester-C® is a licensed trademark of Zila Nutraceuticals, Inc.

WARNING
Accidental overdose of iron-containing products is a leading cause of fatal poisoning in children under 6. Keep this product out of reach of children. In case of accidental overdose, call a doctor or poison control center immediately.

NOTICE: This product supplied in tamper-evident blisters. Do not use if outer foil is torn or missing.

Questions or comments? 1-877-567-7676
Manufactured by:
KV Pharmaceutical Co. for
Ther-Rx Corporation
Saint Louis, MO 63044
U.S. Patent Nos.: 4,599,152; 4,822,816; 4,830,716; 5,070,085.
P4155 05/03

Shown in Product Identification Guide, page 334

NIFEREX®-150 FORTE Capsules ℞
[ni 'fer "ex for 'ta]
℞ Only

DESCRIPTION
Each powder-filled capsule for oral administration contains:
Iron .... 80 mg Ferrochel® (elemental iron)*
.... 70 mg polysaccharide iron (elemental iron)
Vitamin C .... 60 mg Ester-C ®+
Folic Acid USP .... 1 mg
Vitamin B_{12} .... 25 mcg (cyanocobalamin)
Each capsule also contains the following inactive ingredients: D&C Red #28, FD&C Blue #1, FD&C Red # 40, gelatin, magnesium stearate, pharmaceutical glaze, silicon dioxide and titanium dioxide.

CLINICAL PHARMACOLOGY
Iron is an essential component in the formation of hemoglobin. Adequate amounts of iron are necessary for effective erythropoiesis. Iron also serves as a cofactor of several essential enzymes, including cytochromes that are involved in electron transport.
Folic acid is required for nucleoprotein synthesis and the maintenance of normal erythropoiesis. Folic acid is converted in the liver and plasma to its metabolically active form, tetrahydrofolic acid, by dihydrofolate reductase.
Vitamin B_{12} is required for the maintenance of normal erythropoiesis, nucleoprotein and myelin synthesis, cell reproduction and normal growth. Intrinsic factor, a glycoprotein secreted by the gastric mucosa, is required for active absorption of Vitamin B_{12} from the gastrointestinal tract.

INDICATIONS AND USAGE
niferex® -150 forte is indicated for the prevention and treatment of iron deficiency anemia and/or nutritional megaloblastic anemias.

CONTRAINDICATIONS
niferex® -150 forte is contraindicated in patients with a known hypersensitivity to any of the components of this product. Hemochromatosis and hemosiderosis are contraindications to iron therapy.

WARNINGS
Folic acid alone is improper therapy in the treatment of pernicious anemia and other megaloblastic anemias where Vitamin B_{12} is deficient.

WARNING: ACCIDENTAL OVERDOSE OF IRON-CONTAINING PRODUCTS IS A LEADING CAUSE OF FATAL POISONING IN CHILDREN UNDER 6. KEEP THIS PRODUCT OUT OF REACH OF CHILDREN. IN CASE OF ACCIDENTAL OVERDOSE, CALL A DOCTOR OR POISON CONTROL CENTER IMMEDIATELY.

PRECAUTIONS
General:
The type of anemia and the underlying cause or causes should be determined before starting therapy with niferex® -150 forte. Since the anemia may be a result of a systemic disturbance, such as recurrent blood loss, the underlying cause or causes should be corrected, if possible.
Folic acid in doses above 1.0 mg daily may obscure pernicious anemia in that hematologic remission can occur while neurological manifestations remain progressive.
Pediatric Use:
Safety and effectiveness in pediatric patients has not been established.
Information for Patients:
As with all oral iron preparations, niferex® -150 forte should be stored out of the reach of children to guard against accidental iron poisoning. Patients should not exceed the recommended dosage unless directed by the physician. Patients should be informed that iron therapy can cause black or dark stools.

ADVERSE REACTIONS
Adverse reactions with iron therapy may include constipation, diarrhea, nausea, vomiting, dark stools and abdominal pain. Adverse reactions with iron therapy are usually transient. Allergic sensitization has been reported following both oral and parenteral administration of folic acid.

OVERDOSAGE
ACCIDENTAL OVERDOSE OF IRON CONTAINING PRODUCTS IS A LEADING CAUSE OF FATAL POISONING IN CHILDREN UNDER 6. KEEP THIS PRODUCT OUT OF THE REACH OF CHILDREN. IN CASE OF ACCIDENTAL OVERDOSE, CALL A DOCTOR OR POISON CONTROL CENTER IMMEDIATELY.
The clinical course of acute iron overdosage can be variable. Initial symptoms may include abdominal pain, nausea, vomiting, diarrhea, tarry stools, melena, hematemesis, hypotension, tachycardia, metabolic acidosis, hyperglycemia, dehydration, drowsiness, pallor, cyanosis, lassitude, seizures, shock and coma.
The oral LD_{50} of polysaccharide-iron complex was estimated to be greater than 5000 mg iron/kg in the rat. Chronic toxicity studies in rats and dogs administered polysaccharide-iron complex showed that a daily dosage of 250 mg iron/kg for three months had no adverse effects.

DOSAGE AND ADMINISTRATION
Adults: 1 capsule daily or as directed by a physician.

HOW SUPPLIED
niferex® -150 forte capsules for oral administration are supplied as red (cap) and clear (body) capsules filled with brown powder imprinted "THX" in white ink on the cap and "0136" in white ink on the body in child-resistant, unit-dose packages of 100 capsules (10 × 10 Unit Dose Packs) (NDC 64011-136-11).
Store at controlled room temperature 15°–30°C (59°–86°F).

* Ferrochel® (ferrous bis-glycinate chelate) is a registered trademark of Albion International, Inc., Clearfield, Utah, and is protected under US Patent Nos. 4,599,152 and 4,830,716.
+ Ester-C® is a patented pharmaceutical grade material consisting of calcium ascorbate and calcium threonate. Ester-C® is a licensed trademark of Zila Nutraceuticals, Inc.
Manufactured by:
KV Pharmaceutical Co. for
Ther-Rx Corporation
St. Louis, MO 63044
P4206 Rev. 06/03

Shown in Product Identification Guide, page 334

PRECARE® Chewables ℞
Flavored Prenatal Multivitamin/ Mineral Tablet

Rx Only

DESCRIPTION
Each orange-colored tablet contains:
Vitamin C (as Ester-C®)* .... 50 mg
Calcium (as calcium carbonate) .... 250 mg
Iron (including MicroMask™ ferrous fumarate) ..... 40 mg
Vitamin D_3 (cholecalciferol) .... 6 mcg
Vitamin E (as dl-Alpha-Tocopheryl acetate) .... 3.5 mg
Vitamin B_6 (as pyridoxine HCl) .... 2 mg
Folic Acid, USP .... 1 mg
Magnesium (as magnesium oxide, USP) .... 50 mg
Zinc (as zinc oxide, USP) .... 15 mg
Copper (as cupric oxide) .... 2 mg
Inactive Ingredients: Citric acid, FD&C yellow No. 6 lake, flow agents, natural non-nutritive and nutritive sweetening agents, natural and artificial flavors.
KEEP THIS AND ALL DRUGS OUT OF THE REACH OF CHILDREN

*Ester-C® is a patented pharmaceutical grade material consisting of calcium ascorbate and calcium threonate. Ester-C® is a licensed trademark of Zila Nutraceuticals, Inc.

INDICATIONS
PreCare® Chewables are indicated to provide vitamin and mineral supplementation throughout pregnancy and during the postnatal period—for both lactating and non-lactating mothers. They are also useful for improving nutritional status prior to conception.

CONTRAINDICATIONS
This product is contraindicated in patients with a known hypersensitivity to any of the ingredients.

WARNINGS
Folic acid alone is improper therapy in the treatment of pernicious anemia and other megaloblastic anemias where Vitamin B_{12} is deficient.

Accidental overdose of iron-containing products is a leading cause of fatal poisoning in children under 6. Keep this product out of reach of children. In case of accidental overdose, call a doctor or poison control center immediately.

PRECAUTIONS
Folic acid in doses above 1.0 mg daily may obscure pernicious anemia, in that hematologic remission can occur while neurological manifestations remain progressive.

PEDIATRIC USE
Safety and effectiveness in pediatric patients has not been established.

GERIATRIC USE
Clinical studies on this product have not been performed to determine whether elderly subjects respond differently from younger subjects. In general, dose selection for an elderly patient should be cautious, usually starting at the low end of the dosing range, reflecting the greater frequency of decreased hepatic, renal, or cardiac function, and of concomitant disease or other drug therapy.

ADVERSE REACTIONS
Allergic sensitization has been reported following both oral and parenteral administration of folic acid.

DOSAGE AND ADMINISTRATION
Usual dosage is one tablet daily, or as prescribed by a physician.

HOW SUPPLIED
PreCare® Chewable tablets for oral administration are supplied as orange-colored, flavored tablets, debossed "Thx" on one side and "024" on the other side in child-resistant, unit dose packages of 100 tablets (10×10 Unit Dose Packs) (NDC 64011-024-11). Store at controlled room temperature, 15°–30°C (59°–86°F).
NOTICE: Contact with moisture may produce surface discoloration or erosion of the tablet.
P3881 01/02
Drug Delivery Technology Provided
and Product Manufactured by
KV Pharmaceutical Co.
for Ther-Rx Corporation
St. Louis, MO 63045
U.S. Patents No. 4,822,816, 5,070,085, 5,494,681, 6,228,388 and 6,261,600
Other U.S. Patent Pending

Shown in Product Identification Guide, page 334

PRECARE CONCEIVE® ℞
Prenatal/Preconception Multivitamin/Mineral Tablet
Rx only

DESCRIPTION
Each diamond shaped, film coated yellow tablet contains:
Vitamin C (as Ester-C®)* .... 60 mg

Continued on next page

PreCare Conceive—Cont.

Calcium (as Calcium Carbonate) .... 200 mg
Iron (as Ferrous Fumarate and Carbonyl Iron) ..... 30 mg
Vitamin E (as dl-Alpha-Tocopheryl Acetate) .... 30 IU
Thiamine (as Thiamine Mononitrate) .... 3 mg
Riboflavin (Riboflavin, USP) .... 3.4 mg
Niacin (as Niacinamide, USP) .... 20 mg
Pyridoxine (as Pyridoxine HCl, USP) .... 50 mg
Folic Acid, USP .... 1 mg
Magnesium (as Magnesium Oxide) .... 100 mg
Cyanocobalamin .... 12 mcg
Zinc (as Zinc Oxide) .... 15 mg
Copper (as Cupric Oxide) .... 2 mg

Inactive Ingredients: Cellulose polymers, flow agents, pigment, natural wax, D&C yellow #10 aluminum lake, FD&C yellow #6 aluminum lake, lactose and other ingredients.

*Ester-C® is a patented pharmaceutical grade material consisting of calcium ascorbate and calcium threonate. Ester-C® is a licensed trademark of Zila Nutraceuticals, Inc.

INDICATIONS

PreCare Conceive® tablets are indicated to provide vitamin and mineral supplementation which is useful to improve nutritional status prior to conception and throughout pregnancy.

CONTRAINDICATIONS

This product is contraindicated in patients with a known hypersensitivity to any of the ingredients.

WARNINGS

Folic acid alone is improper therapy in the treatment of pernicious anemia and other megaloblastic anemias where Vitamin B_{12} is deficient.

Accidental overdose of iron-containing products is a leading cause of fatal poisoning in children under 6. Keep this product out of reach of children. In case of accidental overdose, call a doctor or poison control center immediately.

PRECAUTIONS

Folic acid in doses above 1.0 mg daily may obscure pernicious anemia, in that hematologic remission can occur while neurological manifestations remain progressive.

PEDIATRIC USE

Safety and effectiveness in pediatric patients has not been established.

GERIATRIC USE

Clinical studies on this product have not been performed to determine whether elderly subjects respond differently from younger subjects. In general, dose selection for elderly patients should be cautious, usually starting at the low end of the dosing range, reflecting the greater frequency of decreased hepatic, renal, or cardiac function, and of concomitant disease or other drug therapy.

ADVERSE REACTIONS

Allergic sensitization has been reported following both oral and parenteral administration of folic acid.

DOSAGE AND ADMINISTRATION

Usual dosage is one tablet daily, or as prescribed by a physician.

HOW SUPPLIED

PreCare Conceive® tablets for oral administration are supplied as diamond shaped, film coated yellow tablets, debossed "Ther-Rx" on one side and "014" on the other side in child-resistant, unit dose packages of 100 tablets (10 × 10 Unit Dose Packs) (NDC 64011-014-11).
Store at controlled room temperature 15°–30°C (59°–86°F).
P3867 01/02

Drug Delivery Technology Provided
and Product Manufactured by
KV Pharmaceutical Co.
for Ther-Rx Corporation
St. Louis, MO 63045

U.S. Patents Nos. 4,822,816, 5,070,085 and 5,494,681
Other U.S. Patents Pending

Shown in Product Identification Guide, page 334

PRECARE® Prenatal ℞

Multivitamin/Mineral Film Coated Caplet

DESCRIPTION

Each peach film coated caplet contains:
Vitamin C (as Ester-C®)* .... 50 mg
Calcium (as CalciPure™ Calcium Carbonate) ...... 250 mg
Iron (as MicroMask™ Ferrous Fumarate) .... 40 mg
Vitamin E (as dl-Alpha-Tocopheryl Acetate) .... 3.5 mg
Vitamin D_3 (Cholecalciferol) .... 6 mcg
Thiamine (as Thiamine Mononitrate, USP) .... 3.0 mg
Riboflavin, USP .... 3.4 mg
Niacin (as Niacinamide, USP) .... 20 mg
Pyridoxine (as Pyridoxine HCl, USP) .... 50 mg
Folic Acid, USP .... 1 mg
Cyanocobalamin .... 12 mcg
Magnesium (as Magnesium Oxide, USP) .... 50 mg
Zinc (as Zinc Oxide, USP) .... 15 mg
Copper (as Cupric Oxide) .... 2 mg

Inactive Ingredients: Natural oils, natural wax, cellulose polymers, flow agents, and other ingredients. DYE FREE

*Ester-C® is a patented pharmaceutical grade material consisting of calcium ascorbate and calcium threonate. Ester-C® is a licensed trademark of Zila Nutraceuticals, Inc.

INDICATIONS

PreCare® Prenatal caplets are indicated to provide vitamin and mineral supplementation throughout pregnancy and during the postnatal period—for both lactating and nonlactating mothers. It is also useful for improving nutritional status prior to conception.

CONTRAINDICATIONS

This product is contraindicated in patients with a known hypersensitivity to any of the ingredients.

WARNINGS

Folic acid alone is improper therapy in the treatment of pernicious anemia and other megaloblastic anemias where Vitamin B_{12} is deficient.

Accidental overdose of iron-containing products is a leading cause of fatal poisoning in children under 6. Keep this product out of reach of children. In case of accidental overdose, call a doctor or poison control center immediately.

PRECAUTIONS

Folic acid in doses above 1.0 mg daily may obscure pernicious anemia, in that hematologic remission can occur while neurological manifestations remain progressive.

PEDIATRIC USE

Safety and effectiveness in pediatric patients has not been established.

GERIATRIC USE

Clinical studies on this product have not been performed to determine whether elderly subjects respond differently from younger subjects. In general, dose selection for elderly patients should be cautious, usually starting at the low end of the dosing range, reflecting the greater frequency of decreased hepatic, renal, or cardiac function, and of concomitant disease or other drug therapy.

ADVERSE REACTIONS

Allergic sensitization has been reported following both oral and parenteral administration of folic acid.

DOSAGE AND ADMINISTRATION

Usual dosage is one caplet daily, or as prescribed by a physician.

HOW SUPPLIED

PreCare® Prenatal Multivitamin/Mineral Caplets for oral administration are supplied as peach, film coated tablets, debossed "Ther-Rx" on one side and "118" with partial bisect on the other side in child-resistant, unit dose packages of 100 caplets (10×10 Unit Dose Packs) (NDC 64011-118-11). Store at controlled room temperature 15°–30°C (59°–86°F)
P3926 05/02

Manufactured by
KV Pharmaceutical Co.
for Ther-Rx Corporation
St. Louis, MO 63045

U.S. Patents Nos. 4,822,816 5,070,085 5,494,681 6,197,329 and 6,228,388

Shown in Product Identification Guide, page 334

PREMESISRX® ℞

Prenatal Multivitamin/Mineral Tablet with Controlled-Release Vitamin B_6

DESCRIPTION

Each blue tablet contains:
Vitamin B_6 (as pyridoxine HCl) .... 75 mg
Vitamin B_{12} (cyanocobalamin) .... 12 mcg
Folic Acid, USP .... 1 mg
Calcium (as calcium carbonate) .... 200 mg

Inactive Ingredients: Natural waxes, cellulose polymers, FD&C blue No. 1 aluminum lake, D&C yellow No. 10 aluminum lake, flow agents and other ingredients.

INDICATIONS

PremesisRx® tablets are indicated to provide vitamin and mineral supplementation during pregnancy and may be used in conjunction with a physician-prescribed regimen to minimize pregnancy related nausea.

CONTRAINDICATIONS

This product is contraindicated in patients with a known hypersensitivity to any of the ingredients.

WARNINGS

Folic acid alone is improper therapy in the treatment of pernicious anemia and other megaloblastic anemias where Vitamin B_{12} is deficient.

PRECAUTIONS

Folic acid in doses above 1.0 mg daily may obscure pernicious anemia, in that hematologic remission can occur while neurological manifestations remain progressive.

PEDIATRIC USE

Safety and effectiveness in pediatric patients has not been established.

GERIATRIC USE

Clinical studies on this product have not been performed to determine whether elderly subjects respond differently from younger subjects. In general, dose selection for elderly patients should be cautious, usually starting at the low end of the dosing range, reflecting the greater frequency of decreased hepatic, renal, or cardiac function, and of concomitant disease or other drug therapy.

ADVERSE REACTIONS

Allergic sensitization has been reported following both oral and parenteral administration of folic acid.

DOSAGE AND ADMINISTRATION

Usual dosage is one tablet daily, or as prescribed by a physician.

HOW SUPPLIED

PremesisRx® tablets for oral administration are supplied as blue, oval tablets, debossed "Ther-Rx" on one side and "019" on the other side in bottles of 100 tablets (NDC 64011-019-04). Store at controlled room temperature, 15°–30°C (59°–86°F).
P3264-3 02/02

Manufactured by
KV Pharmaceutical Co.
for Ther-Rx Corporation
St. Louis, MO 63045

U.S. Patent No. 6,197,329

Shown in Product Identification Guide, page 334

PRIMACARE® ℞

Prescription prenatal/postnatal multivitamin/mineral supplement with Essential Fatty Acids
℞ Only

DESCRIPTION

PrimaCare® is a prescription prenatal/ postnatal multivitamin/mineral capsule and tablet combination with essential fatty acids that consists of two dosage forms on each blister card designated as AM and PM, as follows:

AM dose is a white, dye-free, soft gelatin capsule containing the following ingredients:

Essential Fatty Acids (as OmegaNate™)
Omega-3 Fatty Acids .... 150 mg
Linoleic Acid .... 25 mg
Linolenic Acid .... 25 mg
Vitamins:
Vitamin D_3 (as cholecalciferol) .... 170 IU
Vitamin E (dl-alpha-tocopheryl acetate) .... 30 IU
Minerals:
Calcium (as calcium carbonate) .... 150 mg

PM dose is a pink, dye-free, oval shaped, film coated tablet containing the following ingredients:

Vitamins:
Biotin .... 35 mcg
Folic Acid, USP .... 1 mg
Vitamin B_1 / Thiamine (as thiamine mononitrate, USP) .... 3 mg
Vitamin B_2 / Riboflavin, USP .... 3.4 mg
Vitamin B_3 / Niacin (as niacinamide, USP) .... 20 mg
Vitamin B_6 / Pyridoxine (as pyridoxine HCl, USP) .... 10 mg
Vitamin B_{12} / Cyanocobalamin .... 12 mcg
Vitamin C (as *Ester-C®*)* .... 100 mg
Vitamin D_3 (as cholecalciferol) .... 230 IU
Vitamin K .... 90 mcg
Pantothenic Acid .... 7 mg
Minerals:
Calcium (as CalciPure™ calcium carbonate) ..... 250 mg
Chromium .... 45 mcg
Copper (as cupric oxide) .... 1.3 mg
Iron (as MicroMask™ ferrous fumarate) .... 30 mg
Molybdenum .... 50 mcg
Selenium .... 75 mcg
Zinc (as zinc oxide, USP) .... 11 mg

**Ester-C®* is a patented pharmaceutical grade material consisting of calcium ascorbate and calcium threonate. *Ester-C®* is a licensed trademark of Zila Nutraceuticals, Inc.

Inactive Ingredients: Capsule: Natural wax, natural oils, and other ingredients. **Tablet:** Cellulose polymers, flow agents, natural wax, natural oils, natural flavor and other ingredients.

INDICATIONS

PrimaCare® is indicated to provide vitamin/mineral and essential fatty acid supplementation throughout pregnancy, during the postnatal period for both lactating and nonlactating mothers, and throughout the childbearing years. It is also useful for improving nutritional status prior to conception.

CONTRAINDICATIONS

This product is contraindicated in patients with a known hypersensitivity to any of the ingredients.

WARNING

Folic acid alone is improper therapy in the treatment of pernicious anemia and other megaloblastic anemias where vitamin B_{12} is deficient.

> **WARNING: Accidental overdose of iron-containing products is a leading cause of fatal poisoning in children under 6. Keep this product out of reach of children. In case of accidental overdose, call a doctor or poison control center immediately.**

PRECAUTIONS

Folic acid in doses above 1.0 mg daily may obscure pernicious anemia, in that hematologic remission can occur while neurological manifestations remain progressive.

PEDIATRIC USE

Safety and effectiveness in pediatric patients has not been established.

GERIATRIC USE

Clinical studies on this product have not been performed to determine whether elderly subjects respond differently from younger subjects. In general, dose selection for elderly patients should be cautious, usually starting at the low end of the dosing range, reflecting the greater frequency of decreased hepatic, renal, or cardiac function, and of concomitant disease or other drug therapy.

ADVERSE REACTIONS

Allergic sensitization has been reported following both oral and parenteral administration of folic acid.

DOSAGE AND ADMINISTRATION

PrimaCare®'s patented Chronometric System™ dosing regimen, consisting of one "AM" dose taken in the morning and one "PM" dose taken at night, should be followed for improved nutrient absorption potential, or as prescribed by a physician.

HOW SUPPLIED

PrimaCare® is supplied as a morning and evening oral dosing regimen in child-resistant, unit-dose blister cards of 5 soft gelatin capsules and 5 tablets (6 unit-dose cards containing 2 × 5 tablets in a 30-day supply unit-of-use dispensing carton) as follows: PrimaCare® capsules are supplied as white, dye-free, soft gelatin capsules, imprinted "Ther-Rx" on one side in pink ink. PrimaCare® tablets are supplied as pink, dye-free, film coated tablets, debossed "Ther-Rx" on one side and "119" with partial bisect on the other side. (NDC 64011-015-31). Store at controlled room temperature 15°–30° C (59°–86° F).

P3846-3 12/02

Tablet Manufacturer: KV Pharmaceutical Co.

Capsule Manufacturer: Accucaps Industries, Ltd.-Canada for Ther-Rx Corporation

St. Louis, MO 63045

U.S. Patent Nos. 4,822,816. 5,070,085. 5,494,681. 5,945,123. 6,214,379. 6,258,846. 6,375,956. Other U.S. Patents Pending

Shown in Product Identification Guide, page 334

PRIMACARE® ONE ℞

[*prē-mă-kăr*]

Prescription prenatal/postnatal multivitamin/mineral supplement with Essential Fatty Acids

Rx Only

DESCRIPTION

PrimaCare® ONE is a prescription prenatal/postnatal multivitamin/mineral capsule with Essential Fatty Acids. Each purple soft gelatin capsule contains:

OmegaNate™ Essential Fatty Acids and Precursors:	
Omega-3 Fatty Acids	300 mg
Linoleic Acid	30 mg
Linolenic Acid	30 mg
Vitamins:	
Folic Acid, USP	1 mg
Vitamin B_6 (as pyridoxine HCl)	25 mg
Vitamin C (as *Ester-C*®)*	25 mg
Vitamin D_3 (from cholecalciferol)	170 IU
Vitamin E (from dl-alpha-tocopheryl acetate)	30 IU
Minerals:	
Calcium	150 mg
Iron (as carbonyl iron)	27 mg

**Ester-C*® is a patented pharmaceutical grade material consisting of calcium ascorbate and calcium threonate. *Ester-C*® is a licensed trademark of Zila Nutraceuticals, Inc.

Inactive Ingredients: Gelatin, vegetable shortening, glycerine, soybean oil, yellow beeswax, lecithin, titanium dioxide, methylparaben, ethylvanillin, D&C Red #33, propylparaben, FD&C Blue #1.

INDICATIONS

PrimaCare® ONE is indicated to provide vitamin/mineral and essential fatty acid supplementation throughout pregnancy, during the postnatal period for both lactating and non-lactating mothers, and throughout the childbearing years. It is also useful for improving nutritional status prior to conception.

CONTRAINDICATIONS

This product is contraindicated in patients with a known hypersensitivity to any of the ingredients.

WARNING

Folic acid alone is improper therapy in the treatment of pernicious anemia and other megaloblastic anemias where vitamin B_{12} is deficient.

> **WARNING: Accidental overdose of iron-containing products is a leading cause of fatal poisoning in children under 6. Keep this product out of reach of children. In case of accidental overdose, call a doctor or poison control center immediately.**

PRECAUTIONS

Folic acid in doses above 1.0 mg daily may obscure pernicious anemia, in that hematologic remission can occur while neurological manifestations remain progressive.

PEDIATRIC USE

Safety and effectiveness in pediatric patients has not been established.

GERIATRIC USE

Clinical studies on this product have not been performed to determine whether elderly subjects respond differently from younger subjects. In general, dose selection for elderly patients should be cautious, usually starting at the low end of the dosing range, reflecting the greater frequency of decreased hepatic, renal, or cardiac function, and of concomitant disease or other drug therapy.

ADVERSE REACTIONS

Allergic sensitization has been reported following both oral and parenteral administration of folic acid.

DOSAGE AND ADMINISTRATION

Usual dosage is one capsule daily, or as prescribed by a physician.

HOW SUPPLIED

PrimaCare® ONE prenatal/postnatal multivitamin/mineral capsules with essential fatty acids for oral administration are supplied as purple soft gelatin capsules imprinted "Ther-Rx 142" in white ink in bottles of 30 soft gelatin capsules (NDC 64011-142-19). Store at controlled room temperature 15°-30° C (59°-86° F).

KEEP THIS AND ALL DRUGS OUT OF THE REACH OF CHILDREN.

P4350 11/03

Mktd. by Ther-Rx Corp.

St. Louis, MO 63044

U.S. Patent Nos.: 4,822,816; 5,070,085; 6,197,329; 6,258,846; 6,569,857; 6,576,666.

Other U.S. Patents Pending

Shown in Product Identification Guide, page 334

STRONGSTART® CAPLETS ℞

℞ Only

USUAL ADULT DOSAGE

One caplet daily, or as directed by a physician. Each caplet contains:

Calcium (as CalciPure™ calcium carbonate)	225 mg
Vitamin C (as *Ester-C*®)*	50 mg
Iron (as MicroMask® ferrous fumarate)	40 mg
Vitamin E (dl-alpha-tocopheryl acetate)	30 IU
Vitamin B_6 (controlled-release, using pyridoxine HCl, USP)	75 mg
Zinc (zinc oxide, USP)	15 mg
Vitamin B_3 (as niacinamide)	20 mg
Pantothenic Acid	7 mg
Vitamin B_1 (as thiamine mononitrate, USP)	3.0 mg
Vitamin B_2 (riboflavin, USP)	3.4 mg
Folic Acid, USP	1 mg
Cyanocobalamin (vitamin B_{12})	12 mcg
Vitamin D_3 (cholecalciferol)	400 IU
Vitamin K	90 mcg
Biotin	35 mcg
Copper (cupric oxide)	2 mg
Selenium	75 mcg
Chromium	45 mcg
Molybdenum	50 mcg
Magnesium (magnesium oxide, USP)	30 mg
Docusate Sodium	25 mg

**Ester-C*® is a patented pharmaceutical grade material consisting of calcium ascorbate and calcium threonate. *Ester-C*® is a licensed trademark of Zila Nutraceuticals, Inc.

OTHER INGREDIENTS

Microcrystalline cellulose, croscarmellose sodium, silicon dioxide, hydrogenated vegetable oil, magnesium stearate, ethylcellulose, carnauba wax, hypromellose, titanium dioxide, polydextrose, triacetin, polyethylene glycol.

INDICATIONS

StrongStart® Caplets are indicated for vitamin and mineral dietary supplementation in women throughout their pregnancy and in the postnatal period for both lactating and non-lactating mothers. StrongStart® Caplets can also be administered to improve the nutritional status of women prior to conception.

PRECAUTIONS

Folic acid, in doses above 1.0 mg daily, may obscure pernicious anemia in that hematologic remission can occur while neurological manifestations remain progressive.

WARNING

The administration of folic acid alone is inadequate for the treatment of pernicious anemia and other megablastic anemias caused by vitamin B_{12} deficiency.

> **WARNING: Accidental overdose of iron-containing products is a leading cause of fatal poisoning in children under 6. Keep this product out of reach of children. In case of accidental overdose, call a doctor or Poison Control Center immediately.**

HOW SUPPLIED

StrongStart® Caplets for oral administration are supplied as modified oval, film coated white caplets debossed "Ther-Rx" on one side and "128" with a partial bisect on the other side in child-resistant, unit-dose packages of 30 caplets (3 × 10 Unit Dose Packs) (NDC 64011-128-22) or 100 caplets (10 × 10 Unit Dose Packs) (NDC 64011-128-11).

Store at controlled room temperature, 15°- 30°C (59°- 86°F).

Manufacturer:

KV Pharmaceutical

for Ther-Rx Corporation

St. Louis, MO 63044

U.S. Patent Nos. 4,822,816; 5,070,085; 5,494,681; 6,197,329; 6,228,388.

Shown in Product Identification Guide, page 334

STRONGSTART® CHEWABLE ℞

℞ Only

USUAL ADULT DOSAGE

One tablet daily, or as directed by a physician. Each tablet contains:

Calcium (calcium carbonate)	250 mg
Vitamin C (as *Ester-C*®)*	50 mg
Iron (as MicroMask® ferrous fumarate)	35 mg
Vitamin E (dl-alpha-tocopheryl acetate)	3.5 mg
Vitamin B_6 (as Descote® pyridoxine HCl)	50 mg
Zinc (zinc oxide, USP)	15 mg
Folic Acid, USP	1 mg
Vitamin D_3 (cholecalciferol)	6 mcg
Copper (cupric oxide)	2 mg
Magnesium (magnesium oxide, USP)	40 mg

**Ester-C*® is a patented pharmaceutical grade material consisting of calcium ascorbate and calcium threonate. *Ester-C*® is a licensed trademark of Zila Nutraceuticals, Inc.

OTHER INGREDIENTS

Magnesium stearate, FD&C Yellow #6 lake, citric acid, natural and artificial non-nutritive and artificial sweetening agents, natural and artificial flavors.

INDICATIONS

StrongStart® Chewable tablets are indicated for vitamin and mineral dietary supplementation in women throughout their pregnancy and in the postnatal period for both lactating and non-lactating mothers. StrongStart® Chewable tablets can also be administered to improve the nutritional status of women prior to conception.

PRECAUTIONS

Folic acid, in doses above 1.0 mg daily, may obscure pernicious anemia in that hematologic remission can occur while neurological manifestations remain progressive.

WARNING

Folic acid alone is improper therapy in the treatment of pernicious anemia and other megaloblastic anemias where vitamin B_{12} is deficient.

> **WARNING: Accidental overdose of iron-containing products is a leading cause of fatal poisoning in children under 6. Keep this product out of reach of children. In case of accidental overdose, call a doctor or Poison Control Center immediately.**

HOW SUPPLIED

StrongStart® Chewable tablets for oral administration are supplied as orange-colored, flavored tablets debossed "Ther-Rx" on one side and "137" on the other side in child-resistant, unit dose packages of 30 tablets (3 × 10 Unit Dose Packs) (NDC 64011-137-22) or 100 tablets (10 × 10 Unit Dose Packs) (NDC 64011-137-11).

Continued on next page

StrongStart Chewable—Cont.

Store at controlled room temperature, 15°- 30°C (59°- 86°F).
NOTICE: Contact with moisture may produce surface discoloration or erosion of the tablet.
Manufacturer:
KV Pharmaceutical
for Ther-Rx Corporation
St. Louis, MO 63044
U.S. Patent Nos.:
4,822,816; 5,070,085; 5,494,681; 6,197,329; 6,228,388; 6,261,600; 6,352,713.
Other U.S. Patent Pending
Shown in Product Identification Guide, page 334

Tibotec Therapeutics

Division of Ortho Biotech Products, L.P.
430 ROUTE 22 EAST
PO BOX 6914
BRIDGEWATER, NJ 08807

Direct Inquiries to:
(800) 325-7504
Prompt #1, Customer Service
Prompt #2, Medical Information
FAX: (908) 526-9230

DOXIL® ℞

[däk'sil]
(doxorubicin HCl liposome injection)
FOR INTRAVENOUS INFUSION ONLY

WARNINGS

1. Experience with Doxil® (doxorubicin HCl liposome injection) at high cumulative doses is too limited to have established its effects on the myocardium. It should therefore be assumed that Doxil® will have myocardial toxicity similar to conventional formulations of doxorubicin HCl. Irreversible myocardial toxicity leading to congestive heart failure often unresponsive to cardiac supportive therapy may be encountered as the total dosage of doxorubicin HCl approaches 550 mg/m^2. Prior use of other anthracyclines or anthracenediones will reduce the total dose of doxorubicin HCl that can be given without cardiac toxicity. Cardiac toxicity also may occur at lower cumulative doses in patients with prior mediastinal irradiation or who are receiving concurrent cyclophosphamide therapy.
   Doxil® should be administered to patients with a history of cardiovascular disease only when the benefit outweighs the risk to the patient.
2. Acute infusion-related reactions including, but not limited to, flushing, shortness of breath, facial swelling, headache, chills, back pain, tightness in the chest or throat, and/or hypotension have occurred in up to 10% of patients treated with Doxil®. In most patients, these reactions resolve over the course of several hours to a day once the infusion is terminated. In some patients, the reaction has resolved with slowing of the infusion rate. Serious and sometimes life-threatening or fatal allergic/anaphylactoid-like infusion reactions have been reported. Medications to treat such reactions, as well as emergency equipment, should be available for immediate use. Doxil® should be administered at an initial rate of 1 mg/min to minimize the risk of infusion reactions. (see **WARNINGS-Infusion Reactions**.)
3. Severe myelosuppression may occur. (see **WARNINGS-Myelosuppression**.)
4. Dosage should be reduced in patients with impaired hepatic function. (see **DOSAGE AND ADMINISTRATION**.)
5. Accidental substitution of Doxil® for doxorubicin HCl has resulted in severe side effects. Doxil® should not be substituted for doxorubicin HCl on a mg per mg basis. (see **DESCRIPTION** and **DOSAGE AND ADMINISTRATION**.)
6. Doxil® should be administered only under the supervision of a physician who is experienced in the use of cancer chemotherapeutic agents.

DESCRIPTION

Doxil® (doxorubicin HCl liposome injection) is doxorubicin hydrochloride (HCl) encapsulated in STEALTH® liposomes for intravenous administration.

Note: Liposomal encapsulation can substantially affect a drug's functional properties relative to those of the unencapsulated drug. In addition, different liposomal drug products may vary from one another in the chemical composition and physical form of the liposomes. Such differences can substantially affect the functional properties of liposomal drug products. DO NOT SUBSTITUTE.

Doxorubicin is a cytotoxic anthracycline antibiotic isolated from *Streptomyces peucetius* var. *caesius*.

Doxorubicin HCl, which is the established name for (8*S*,10*S*)-10-[(3-amino-2,3,6-trideoxy-α-L-*lyxo*-hexopyranosyl)oxy]-8-glycolyl-7,8,9,10-tetrahydro-6,8,11-trihydroxy-1-methoxy-5,12-naphthacenedione hydrochloride, has the following structure:

The molecular formula of the drug is $C_{27}H_{29}NO_{11}$•HCl; its molecular weight is 579.99.

Doxil® is provided as a sterile, translucent, red liposomal dispersion in 10-mL or 30-mL glass, single use vials. Each vial contains 20 mg or 50 mg doxorubicin HCl at a concentration of 2 mg/mL and a pH of 6.5. The STEALTH® liposome carriers are composed of N-(carbonyl-methoxypolyethylene glycol 2000)-1,2-distearoyl-*sn*-glycero-3-phosphoethanolamine sodium salt (MPEG-DSPE), 3.19 mg/mL; fully hydrogenated soy phosphatidylcholine (HSPC), 9.58 mg/mL; and cholesterol, 3.19 mg/mL. Each mL also contains ammonium sulfate, approximately 2 mg; histidine as a buffer; hydrochloric acid and/or sodium hydroxide for pH control; and sucrose to maintain isotonicity. Greater than 90% of the drug is encapsulated in the STEALTH® liposomes.

MPEG-DSPE has the following structural formula:

n = ca. 45

HSPC has the following structural formula:

m, n = 14 or 16

CLINICAL PHARMACOLOGY

Mechanism of Action

The active ingredient of Doxil® is doxorubicin HCl. The mechanism of action of doxorubicin HCl is thought to be related to its ability to bind DNA and inhibit nucleic acid synthesis. Cell structure studies have demonstrated rapid cell penetration and perinuclear chromatin binding, rapid inhibition of mitotic activity and nucleic acid synthesis, and induction of mutagenesis and chromosomal aberrations.

Doxil® is doxorubicin HCl encapsulated in long-circulating STEALTH® liposomes. Liposomes are microscopic vesicles composed of a phospholipid bilayer that are capable of encapsulating active drugs. The STEALTH® liposomes of Doxil® are formulated with surface-bound methoxypolyethylene glycol (MPEG), a process often referred to as pegylation, to protect liposomes from detection by the mononuclear phagocyte system (MPS) and to increase blood circulation time.

Representation of a STEALTH® liposome:

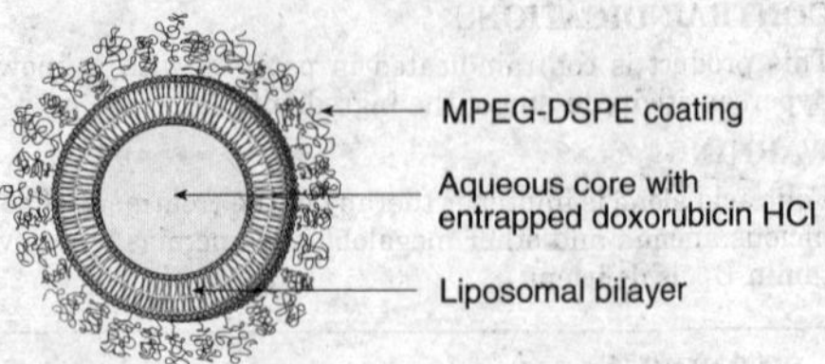

STEALTH® liposomes have a half-life of approximately 55 hours in humans. They are stable in blood, and direct measurement of liposomal doxorubicin shows that at least 90% of the drug (the assay used cannot quantify less than 5-10% free doxorubicin) remains liposome-encapsulated during circulation.

It is hypothesized that because of their small size (ca. 100 nm) and persistence in the circulation, the pegylated Doxil® liposomes are able to penetrate the altered and often compromised vasculature of tumors. This hypothesis is supported by studies using colloidal gold-containing STEALTH® liposomes, which can be visualized microscopically. Evidence of penetration of STEALTH® liposomes from blood vessels and their entry and accumulation in tumors has been seen in mice with C-26 colon carcinoma tumors and in transgenic mice with Kaposi's sarcoma-like lesions. Once the STEALTH® liposomes distribute to the tissue compartment, the encapsulated doxorubicin HCl becomes available. The exact mechanism of release is not understood.

Pharmacokinetics

The plasma pharmacokinetics of Doxil® were evaluated in 42 patients with AIDS-related Kaposi's sarcoma (KS) who received single doses of 10 or 20 mg/m^2 administered by a 30-minute infusion. Twenty-three of these patients received single doses of both 10 and 20 mg/m^2 with a 3-week washout period between doses. The pharmacokinetic parameter values of Doxil®, given for total doxorubicin (mostly liposomally bound), are presented in the following table.

[See table below]

Doxil® displayed linear pharmacokinetics over the range of 10 to 20 mg/m^2. Disposition occurred in two phases after Doxil® administration, with a relatively short first phase (≈ 5 hours) and a prolonged second phase (≈ 55 hours) that accounted for the majority of the area under the curve (AUC).

The pharmacokinetics of Doxil® at a 50 mg/m^2 dose is reported to be nonlinear. At this dose, the elimination half-life of Doxil® is expected to be longer and the clearance lower compared to a 20 mg/m^2 dose. The exposure (AUC) is thus expected to be more than proportional at a 50 mg/m^2 dose when compared with the lower doses.

Distribution: In contrast to the pharmacokinetics of doxorubicin, which displays a large volume of distribution, ranging from 700 to 1100 L/m^2, the small steady state volume of distribution of Doxil® shows that Doxil® is confined mostly to the vascular fluid volume. Plasma protein binding of Doxil® has not been determined; the plasma protein binding of doxorubicin is approximately 70%.

Metabolism: Doxorubicinol, the major metabolite of doxorubicin, was detected at very low levels (range: of 0.8 to 26.2 ng/mL) in the plasma of patients who received 10 or 20 mg/m^2 Doxil®.

Excretion: The plasma clearance of Doxil® was slow, with a mean clearance value of 0.041 L/h/m^2 at a dose of 20 mg/m^2. This is in contrast to doxorubicin, which displays a plasma clearance value ranging from 24 to 35 L/h/m^2. Because of its slower clearance, the AUC of Doxil®, primarily representing the circulation of liposome-encapsulated doxorubicin, is approximately two to three orders of magnitude larger than the AUC for a similar dose of conventional doxorubicin HCl as reported in the literature.

Special Populations: The pharmacokinetics of Doxil® have not been separately evaluated in women, in members of different ethnic groups, or in individuals with renal or hepatic insufficiency.

Drug-Drug Interactions: Although the patient populations for the current indications are on various medications, drug-drug interactions between Doxil® and other drugs, including antiviral agents, have not been evaluated.

Tissue Distribution

Kaposi's sarcoma lesions and normal skin biopsies were obtained at 48 and 96 hours postinfusion of 20 mg/m^2 Doxil® in 11 patients. The concentration of Doxil® in KS lesions was a median of 19 (range, 3-53) times higher than in normal skin at 48 hours posttreatment; however, this was not corrected for likely differences in blood content between KS lesions and normal skin. The corrected ratio may lie between 1 and 22 times. Thus, higher concentrations of Doxil® are delivered to KS lesions than to normal skin.

Clinical Studies

Ovarian Carcinoma

Doxil® (doxorubicin HCl liposome injection) was studied in three open-label, single-arm, clinical trials of 176 patients with metastatic ovarian carcinoma. One hundred forty-five

Pharmacokinetic Parameters of Doxil® in AIDS Patients with Kaposi's Sarcoma

Parameter (units)	Dose 10 mg/m^2	Dose 20 mg/m^2
Peak Plasma Concentration (μg/mL)	4.12 ± 0.215	8.34 ± 0.49
Plasma Clearance (L/h/m^2)	0.056 ± 0.01	0.041 ± 0.004
Steady State Volume of Distribution (L/m^2)	2.83 ± 0.145	2.72 ± 0.120
AUC (μg/mL•h)	277 ± 32.9	590 ± 58.7
First Phase (λ1) Half-Life (h)	4.7 ± 1.1	5.2 ± 1.4
Second Phase (λ2) Half-Life (h)	52.3 ± 5.6	55.0 ± 4.8

N = 23
Mean ± Standard Error

(145) of these patients were refractory to both paclitaxel- and platinum-based chemotherapy regimens. Refractory patients are defined as those having progressive disease while on treatment, or within 6 months of completing treatment. Patients in these studies received Doxil® at 50 mg/m^2 infused over one hour every 3 or 4 weeks for 3-6 cycles or longer in the absence of dose-limiting toxicity or progression of disease.

The baseline demographics and clinical characteristics of the refractory patients are shown in the following table.
[See first table above]

The primary efficacy parameter was response rate for the population of patients refractory to both paclitaxel and a platinum-containing regimen. Assessment of response was based on Southwest Oncology Group (SWOG) criteria, and required confirmation four weeks after the initial observation. Secondary efficacy parameters were time to response, duration of response, and time to progression.

The response rates for the individual phase 2 trials are given in the following table:
[See second table above]

When the data from the single arm trials are combined, the response rate for all patients refractory to paclitaxel and platinum agents was 13.8% (20/145) (95% CI 8.1% to 19.3%). The median time to progression was 15.9 weeks, the median time to response was 17.6 weeks, and the duration of response was 39.4 weeks.

Preliminary Results of Ovarian Cancer Randomized Trial

Data were also provided from an interim analysis of a randomized comparative study of Doxil®. Of the 44 patients in the Doxil® arm with tumors refractory to paclitaxel and platinum compounds, 6 had objective responses, a response rate of 13.6% (95% CI 5.2% to 27.4%).

AIDS-Related Kaposi's Sarcoma

Doxil® was studied in an open-label, single-arm, multicenter study utilizing Doxil® at 20 mg/m^2 by intravenous infusion every three weeks, generally until progression or intolerance occurred. In an interim analysis, the treatment history of 383 patients was reviewed, and a cohort of 77 patients was retrospectively identified as having disease progression on prior systemic combination chemotherapy (at least 2 cycles of a regimen containing at least two of three treatments: bleomycin, vincristine or vinblastine, or doxorubicin) or as being intolerant to such therapy. Forty-nine of the 77 (64%) patients had received prior doxorubicin HCl.

These 77 patients were predominantly white, homosexual males with a median CD4 count of 10 cells/mm^3. Their age ranged from 24 to 54 years, with a mean age of 38 years. Using the ACTG staging criteria,[1] 78% of the patients were at poor risk for tumor burden, 96% at poor risk for immune system, and 58% at poor risk for systemic illness at baseline. Their mean Karnofsky status score was 74%. All 77 patients had cutaneous or subcutaneous lesions, 40% also had oral lesions, 26% pulmonary lesions, and 14% of patients had lesions of the stomach/intestine. The majority of these patients had disease progression on prior systemic combination chemotherapy.

The median time on study for these 77 patients was 155 days and ranged from 1 to 456 days. The median cumulative dose was 154 mg/m^2 and ranged from 20 to 620 mg/m^2.

Two analyses of tumor response were used to evaluate the effectiveness of Doxil®: one analysis based on investigator assessment of changes in lesions over the entire body, and one analysis based on changes in indicator lesions.

Investigator Assessment

Investigator response was based on modified ACTG criteria.[1] Partial response was defined as no new lesions, sites of disease, or worsening edema; flattening of ≥ 50% of previously raised lesions or area of indicator lesions decreasing by ≥ 50%; and response lasting at least 21 days with no prior progression.

Indicator Lesion Assessment

A retrospectively defined analysis was conducted based on assessment of the response of up to five prospectively identified representative indicator lesions. A partial response was defined as flattening of ≥ 50% of previously raised indicator lesions, or > 50% decrease in the area of indicator lesions and lasting at least 21 days with no prior progression.

Only patients with adequate documentation of baseline status and follow-up assessments were considered evaluable for response. Patients who received concomitant KS treatment during study, who completed local radiotherapy to sites encompassing one or more of the indicator lesions within two months of study entry, who had less than four indicator lesions, or who had less than three raised indicator lesions at baseline (the latter applies solely to indicator lesion assessment) were considered nonevaluable for response. Of the 77 patients who had disease progression on prior systemic combination chemotherapy or who were intolerant to such therapy, 34 were evaluable for investigator assessment and 42 were evaluable for indicator lesion assessment.

Responses are summarized in the tables below.

Response in Refractory[a] AIDS-KS

Investigator Assessment	All Evaluable Patients (n = 34)	Evaluable Patients Who Received Prior Doxorubicin (n = 20)
Response[b]		
Partial (PR)	27%	30%
Stable	29%	40%
Progression	44%	30%
Duration of PR (days)		
Median	73	89
Range	42+–210 +	42+–210+
Time to PR (days)		
Median	43	53
Range	15–133	15–109

Indicator Lesion Assessment	All Evaluable Patients (n = 42)	Evaluable Patients Who Received Prior Doxorubicin (n = 23)
Response[b]		
Partial (PR)	48%	52%
Stable	26%	30%
Progression	26%	17%
Duration of PR (days)		
Median	71	79
Range	22+–210+	35–210+
Time to PR (days)		
Median	22	48
Range	15–109	15–109

[a] Patients with disease that progressed on prior combination chemotherapy or who were intolerant to such therapy.

[b] There were no complete responses in this population.

Patient Demographics for Refractory Patients from Phase 2 Ovarian Cancer Studies

	Study 1 (U.S.) (n = 27)	**Study 2 (U.S.) (n = 82)**	**Study 3 (non-U.S.) (n = 36)**
Age at diagnosis (years)			
Median	64	61.5	51.5
Range	46–75	34–85	22–80
Drug-Free Interval (months)			
Median	1.8	1.7	2.6
Range	0.5–15.6	0.6–7.0	0.7–15.2
Sum of Lesions at Baseline (cm^2)			
Median	25	18.3	32.4
Range	1.2–230.0	1.3–285.0	0.3–114.0
FIGO Staging			
I	1 (3.7%)	3 (3.7%)	4 (11.1%)
II	3 (11.1%)	3 (3.7%)	1 (2.8%)
III	15 (55.6%)	60 (73.2%)	24 (66.7%)
IV	8 (29.6%)	16 (19.5%)	6 (16.7%)
Not Specified	—	—	1 (2.8%)
CA-125 at Baseline			
Median	123.5	199.0	1004.5
Range	20–14,012	7–46,594	20–12,089
Number of Prior Chemotherapy Regimens			
1	7 (25.9%)	13 (15.9%)	9 (25.0%)
2	11 (40.7%)	44 (53.7%)	19 (52.8%)
3	6 (22.2%)	25 (30.5%)	8 (22.8%)
4	3 (11.1%)	—	—

Response Rates in Refractory Patients from Single Arm Ovarian Cancer Studies

	Study 1 (U.S.)	**Study 2 (U.S.)**	**Study 3 (non-U.S.)**
Response Rate	22.2% (6/27)	17.1% (14/82)	0% (0/36)
95% Confidence Interval	8.6%-42.3%	9.7%-27.0%	0.0%-9.7%

INDICATIONS AND USAGE

Doxil® (doxorubicin HCl liposome injection) is indicated for:

1. The treatment of metastatic carcinoma of the ovary in patients with disease that is refractory to both paclitaxel- and platinum-based chemotherapy regimens. Refractory disease is defined as disease that has progressed while on treatment, or within 6 months of completing treatment.
2. The treatment of AIDS-related Kaposi's sarcoma in patients with disease that has progressed on prior combination chemotherapy or in patients who are intolerant to such therapy.

These indications are based on objective tumor response rates. No results are available from controlled trials that demonstrate a clinical benefit resulting from this treatment, such as improvement in disease-related symptoms or increased survival.

CONTRAINDICATIONS

Doxil® (doxorubicin HCl liposome injection) is contraindicated in patients who have a history of hypersensitivity reactions to a conventional formulation of doxorubicin HCl or the components of Doxil®.

Doxil® is contraindicated in nursing mothers.

WARNINGS

Cardiac Toxicity

Experience with large cumulative doses of Doxil® (doxorubicin HCl liposome injection) is limited. Doxil's cardiac risk and its risk compared to conventional doxorubicin formulations have not been adequately evaluated. At present, therefore, warnings related to the use of conventional formulation doxorubicin HCl should be observed.

Special attention must be given to the cardiac toxicity exhibited by doxorubicin HCl. Acute left ventricular failure can occur with doxorubicin, particularly in patients who have received total doxorubicin dosage exceeding the currently recommended limit of 550 mg/m^2. Lower (400 mg/m^2) doses appear to cause heart failure in patients who have received radiotherapy to the mediastinal area or concomitant therapy with other potentially cardiotoxic agents such as cyclophosphamide.

Caution should be observed in patients who have received other anthracyclines, and the total dose of doxorubicin HCl given should take into account any previous or concomitant therapy with other anthracyclines or related compounds. Congestive heart failure and/or cardiomyopathy may be encountered after discontinuation of therapy. Patients with a history of cardiovascular disease should be administered Doxil® only when the potential benefit of treatment outweighs the risk.

Cardiac function should be carefully monitored in patients treated with Doxil®. The most definitive test for anthracycline myocardial injury is endomyocardial biopsy. Other methods, such as echocardiography or gated radionuclide scans, have been used to monitor cardiac function during anthracycline therapy. Any of these methods should be employed to monitor potential cardiac toxicity during Doxil® therapy. If these test results indicate possible cardiac injury associated with Doxil® therapy, the benefit of continued therapy must be carefully weighed against the risk of myocardial injury. (see **ADVERSE REACTIONS**; **cardiac events.**)

In the AIDS-KS studies, 68 (9.6%) patients experienced cardiac-related adverse events. In 30 patients (4.3%), the event was thought to be possibly or probably related to Doxil®. Nine cases of possibly or probably related cardiomyopathy and/or congestive heart failure were reported. Seven (1.0%) of the possibly or probably related cardiac events were severe. These severe events included arrhythmia (nonspecific), cardiomyopathy, heart failure, pericardial effusion, and tachycardia. Three patients discontinued study due to cardiac events.

Myelosuppression

In ovarian cancer patients, myelosuppression was generally moderate and reversible. Anemia was the most common hematologic adverse event (52.6%), followed by leukopenia (WBC < 4000 mm^3; 42.2%), thrombocytopenia (24.2%), and neutropenia [ANC < 1000] (19.0%) (see Hematology Data table in **ADVERSE REACTIONS Ovarian Cancer Patients.**)

In ovarian cancer patients, 3.3% received G-CSF (or GM-CSF) to support their blood counts. (See **DOSAGE AND ADMINISTRATION, Dose Modification Guidelines.**)

In AIDS-KS patients, who often present with baseline myelosuppression due to such factors as their HIV disease or concomitant medications, myelosuppression appears to be

Continued on next page

Doxil—Cont.

the dose-limiting adverse event, at the recommended dose of 20 mg/m^2 (see Hematology Data table in **ADVERSE REACTIONS, AIDS-KS Patients**). Leukopenia is the most common adverse event experienced in this population; anemia and thrombocytopenia can also be expected. Sepsis occurred in 5% of patients; for 0.7% of patients the event was considered possibly or probably related to Doxil®. Eleven patients (1.6%) discontinued study because of bone marrow suppression or neutropenia.

In all patients, because of the potential for bone marrow suppression, careful hematologic monitoring is required during use of Doxil®, including white blood cell, neutrophil, platelet counts, and Hgb/Hct. With the recommended dosage schedule, leukopenia is usually transient. Hematologic toxicity may require dose reduction or delay or suspension of Doxil® therapy. Persistent severe myelosuppression may result in superinfection, neutropenic fever, or hemorrhage. Development of sepsis in the setting of neutropenia has resulted in discontinuation of treatment and in rare cases, death.

Doxil® may potentiate the toxicity of other anticancer therapies. In particular, hematologic toxicity may be more severe when Doxil® is administered in combination with other agents that cause bone marrow suppression.

Infusion Reactions

Acute infusion-related reactions characterized by flushing, shortness of breath, facial swelling, headache, chills, chest pain, back pain, tightness in the chest and throat, fever, tachycardia, pruritus, rash, cyanosis, syncope, bronchospasm, asthma, apnea, and/or hypotension have occurred in up to 10% of patients treated with Doxil®. In most patients, these reactions resolve over the course of several hours to a day once the infusion is terminated. In some patients, the reaction resolves when the rate of infusion is slowed.

Six AIDS-KS patients (0.9%) and 13 (1.7%) solid tumor patients discontinued Doxil® therapy because of infusion-related reactions. Serious and sometimes life-threatening or fatal allergic/anaphylactoid-like infusion reactions have been reported. Medications to treat such reactions, as well as emergency equipment, should be available for immediate use.

The majority of infusion-related events occurred during the first infusion. Similar reactions have not been reported with conventional doxorubicin and they presumably represent a reaction to the Doxil® liposomes or one of its surface components.

The initial rate of infusion should be 1 mg/min to help minimize the risk of infusion reactions. (see **DOSAGE AND ADMINISTRATION.**)

Palmar-Plantar Erythrodysesthesia

In ovarian cancer patients, 37.4% of patients experienced PPE (developed palmar-plantar skin eruptions characterized by swelling, pain, erythema and, for some patients, desquamation of the skin on the hands and the feet), with 16.4% of the patients reporting Grade 3 or 4 events. Thirteen (3.5%) of the ovarian cancer patients discontinued treatment due to PPE or other skin toxicity. (see definitions of PPE grades in **DOSAGE AND ADMINISTRATION, Dose Modification Guidelines.**)

Among 705 patients with AIDS-related Kaposi's sarcoma treated with Doxil® at 20 mg/m^2, 24 (3.4%) developed PPE, with 3 (0.9%) discontinuing.

PPE was generally seen after 2 or 3 cycles of treatment but may occur earlier. In most patients the reaction is mild and resolves in one to two weeks so that prolonged delay of therapy need not occur. However, dose modification may be required to manage PPE. (see **DOSAGE AND ADMINISTRATION, Dose Modification Guidelines.**) The reaction can be severe and debilitating in some patients and may require discontinuation of treatment.

Pregnancy Category D

Doxil® can cause fetal harm when administered to a pregnant woman. Doxil® is embryotoxic at doses of 1 mg/kg/day in rats and is embryotoxic and abortifacient at 0.5 mg/kg/day in rabbits (both doses are about one-eighth the 50 mg/m^2 human dose on a mg/m^2 basis). Embryotoxicity was characterized by increased embryo-fetal deaths and reduced live litter sizes.

There are no adequate and well-controlled studies in pregnant women. If Doxil® is to be used during pregnancy, or if the patient becomes pregnant during therapy, the patient should be apprised of the potential hazard to the fetus. If pregnancy occurs in the first few months following treatment with Doxil, the prolonged half-life of the drug must be considered. Women of childbearing potential should be advised to avoid pregnancy.

Toxicity Potentiation

The doxorubicin in Doxil® may potentiate the toxicity of other anticancer therapies. Exacerbation of cyclophosphamide-induced hemorrhagic cystitis and enhancement of the hepatotoxicity of 6-mercaptopurine have been reported with the conventional formulation of doxorubicin HCl. Radiation-induced toxicity to the myocardium, mucosae, skin, and liver have been reported to be increased by the administration of doxorubicin HCl.

Injection Site Effects

Doxil® is not a vesicant, but should be considered an irritant and precautions should be taken to avoid extravasation. With intravenous administration of Doxil®, extravasation may occur with or without an accompanying stinging or burning sensation, even if blood returns well on aspiration of the infusion needle. (see **DOSAGE AND ADMINISTRATION.**) If any signs or symptoms of extravasation have occurred, the infusion should be immediately terminated and restarted in another vein. The application of ice over the site of extravasation for approximately 30 minutes may be helpful in alleviating the local reaction. **Doxil® must not be given by the intramuscular or subcutaneous route.**

In studies with rabbits, lesions that were induced by subcutaneous injection of Doxil® were minor and reversible compared to more severe and irreversible lesions and tissue necrosis that were induced after subcutaneous injection of conventional doxorubicin HCl.

Hepatic Impairment

The pharmacokinetics of Doxil® has not been adequately evaluated in patients with hepatic impairment. Doxorubicin is eliminated in large part by the liver. Thus, Doxil® dosage should be reduced in patients with impaired hepatic function. (see **DOSAGE AND ADMINISTRATION.**)

Prior to Doxil® administration, evaluation of hepatic function is recommended using conventional clinical laboratory tests such as SGOT, SGPT, alkaline phosphatase and bilirubin. (see **DOSAGE AND ADMINISTRATION.**)

Carcinogenesis, Mutagenesis, Impairment of Fertility

Secondary acute myelogenous leukemia has been reported in patients treated with topoisomerase II inhibitors, including anthracyclines.

Although no studies have been conducted with Doxil®, doxorubicin HCl and related compounds have been shown to have mutagenic and carcinogenic properties when tested in experimental models.

STEALTH® liposomes without drug were negative when tested in Ames, mouse lymphoma and chromosomal aberration assays in vitro, and mammalian micronucleus assay in vivo.

The possible adverse effects on fertility in males and females in humans or experimental animals have not been adequately evaluated. However, Doxil® resulted in mild to moderate ovarian and testicular atrophy in mice after a single dose of 36 mg/kg (about twice the 50 mg/m^2 human dose on a mg/m^2 basis). Decreased testicular weights and hypospermia were present in rats after repeat doses ≥ 0.25 mg/kg/day (about one thirtieth the 50 mg/m^2 human dose on a mg/m^2 basis), and diffuse degeneration of the seminiferous tubules and a marked decrease in spermatogenesis were observed in dogs after repeat doses of 1 mg/kg/day (about one half the 50 mg/m^2 human dose on a mg/m^2 basis).

PRECAUTIONS

General

Patients receiving therapy with Doxil® should be monitored by a physician experienced in the use of cancer chemotherapeutic agents. Most adverse events are manageable with dose reductions or delays. (see **DOSAGE AND ADMINISTRATION, Dose Modification Guidelines.**)

Laboratory Tests

Complete blood counts, including platelet counts, should be obtained frequently and at a minimum prior to each dose of Doxil®.

Drug Interactions

No formal drug interaction studies have been conducted with Doxil®. Until specific compatibility data are available, it is not recommended that Doxil® be mixed with other drugs. Doxil® may interact with drugs known to interact with the conventional formulation of doxorubicin HCl.

Pregnancy

Pregnancy Category D: (see **WARNINGS.**)

Nursing Mothers

It is not known whether this drug is excreted in human milk. Because many drugs, including anthracyclines, are excreted in human milk and because of the potential for serious adverse reactions in nursing infants from Doxil®, mothers should discontinue nursing prior to taking this drug.

Pediatric Use

The safety and effectiveness of Doxil® in pediatric patients have not been established.

Geriatric Use

Of the 373 ovarian cancer patients, 29% were 60 to 69 years old, while 22.8% were 70 years and over. No overall differences were observed between these subjects and younger subjects, but greater sensitivity of some older individuals cannot be ruled out. There are insufficient data for a comparative evaluation of efficacy according to age.

Radiation Therapy

Recall of skin reaction due to prior radiotherapy has occurred with Doxil® administration.

Information for the Patient

Patients and patients' caregivers should be informed of the expected adverse effects of Doxil®, particularly hand-foot syndrome, stomatitis, and neutropenia and its complications of neutropenic fever, infection, and sepsis.

Hand-Foot Syndrome (Palmar-Plantar Erythrodysesthesia): Patients who experience tingling or burning, redness, flaking, bothersome swelling, small blisters, or small sores on the palms of their hands or soles of their feet (symptoms of Hand-Foot Syndrome) should notify their physician.

Stomatitis: Patients who experience painful redness, swelling, or sores in the mouth (symptoms of stomatitis) should notify their physician.

Fever and Neutropenia: Patients who develop a fever of 100.5°F or higher should notify their physician.

Nausea, vomiting, tiredness, weakness, rash, or mild hair loss: Patients who develop any of these symptoms should notify their physician.

ADVERSE REACTIONS

Ovarian Cancer Patients

Safety data are available from 373 ovarian cancer patients treated with Doxil® in 4 clinical studies. The patient population was predominantly white (93.6%) with a median age of 60 years. Patients received a median cycle dose of 50 mg/m^2 administered with a median cycle length of 29.5 days. They remained on study drug for a median of 56 days and received a median cumulative dose of 137.5 mg/m^2. Patients received a median of 3 cycles of Doxil®, although some patients remained on study drug for a prolonged period, with 46 patients (12.3%) receiving more than 10 cycles of treatment.

Adverse events (AEs) were reported in all but 2 of the 361 patients who had at least one AE form collected. A total of 3,124 AEs were reported, an average of 8.6 AEs per patient. Most (91.7%) patients had AEs that were considered related to study drug.

Hematology Data Reported in Ovarian Cancer Patients

	% Ovarian Patients (n=373)
Neutropenia	
< 1000/mm^3	19.0
< 500/mm^3	8.3
Febrile neutropenia	0.3
Anemia	
< 10 g/dL	52.6
< 8 g/dL	25.0
RBC transfusions	12.9
Epoetin alpha support*	2.1
Thrombocytopenia	
< 150,000/mm^3	24.2
< 25,000/mm^3	1.1
Platelet transfusions*	1.4

*From concomitant medication or transfusion logs, not reported as AEs.

Drug-Related Non-Hematologic Adverse Events Reported in ≥ 5% of Ovarian Cancer Patients

Non-Hematologic Adverse Event	% Ovarian Patients (n=361)
Palmar-plantar erythrodysesthesia	
All Grades	37.4
Grade 3 & 4	16.4
Stomatitis	
All Grades	37.4
Grade 3 & 4	7.7
Nausea	
All Grades	37.7
Grade 3 & 4	4.2
Asthenia	33.0
Vomiting	22.4
Rash	21.6
Alopecia	15.2
Constipation	12.7
Anorexia	11.9
Mucous Membrane Disorder	11.6
Diarrhea	10.0
Abdominal Pain	8.0
Paresthesia	7.8
Pain	7.2
Fever	6.9
Pharyngitis	5.5
Dry Skin	5.5
Headache	5.3

The following additional (not in table) adverse events were observed in ovarian cancer patients with doses administered every four weeks; only events considered at least possibly drug-related by investigators are included.

Incidence 1% to 5%

Body as a Whole: allergic reaction, chills, infection, chest pain, back pain, abdomen enlarged, malaise.

Digestive System: dyspepsia, oral moniliasis, mouth ulceration, esophagitis, dysphagia.

Metabolic and Nutritional System: peripheral edema, dehydration.

Musculoskeletal System: myalgia.

Nervous System: somnolence, dizziness, depression, insomnia, anxiety.

Respiratory System: dyspnea, cough increased, rhinitis.

Cutaneous: pruritus, skin discoloration, skin disorder, vesiculobullous rash, maculopapular rash, exfoliative dermatitis, herpes zoster, sweating.

Special Senses: conjunctivitis, taste perversion.

Incidence Less Than 1%

Body As A Whole: cellulitis, anaphylactoid reaction, ascites, flu syndrome, neck pain, moniliasis, injection site pain, face edema, chills and fever, pelvic pain, chest pain substernal, injection site inflammation.

Cardiovascular System: hypertension, angina pectoris, pericardial effusion, postural hypotension, hypotension, palpitation, syncope, shock, bradycardia, arrhythmia, phlebitis, tachycardia, cardiomegaly, heart failure, hemorrhage.

Digestive System: gingivitis, eructation, increased salivation, melena, gastrointestinal hemorrhage, proctitis, jaundice, ileus, periodontal abscess, flatulence, aphthous stomatitis, gastritis, glossitis, gum hemorrhage.

Hemic and Lymphatic System: hypochromic anemia, lymphadenopathy, ecchymosis, petechia.
Metabolic/Nutritional Disorders: SGOT increase, creatinine increase, hypocalcemia, hyperglycemia, hypokalemia, hypermagnesemia, hyponatremia, weight gain, bilirubinemia, generalized edema, cachexia, hypochloremia.
Musculoskeletal System: arthralgia, bone pain, myasthenia.
Nervous System: peripheral neuritis, incoordination, thinking abnormal, confusion, hypertonia, nervousness, hyperesthesia, hypesthesia, neuropathy, ataxia.
Respiratory System: pleural effusion, asthma, hiccup, pneumothorax, laryngitis, sinusitis, voice alteration, epistaxis, pneumonia.
Skin and Appendages: skin ulcer, herpes simplex, contact dermatitis, fungal dermatitis, furunculosis, skin nodule, urticaria, acne.
Special Senses: amblyopia, blepharitis, parosmia, taste loss.
Urogenital System: urinary tract infection, leukorrhea, cystitis, nocturia, dysuria, breast pain, mastitis, oliguria, vaginitis, kidney function abnormal, vaginal hemorrhage, hydronephrosis, vaginal moniliasis.

AIDS-KS Patients

Information on adverse events is based on the experience reported in 753 patients with AIDS-related KS enrolled in four studies. The majority of patients were treated with 20 mg/m^2 of Doxil® (doxorubicin HCl liposome injection) every two to three weeks. The median time on study was 127 days and ranged from 1 to 811 days. The median cumulative dose was 120 mg/m^2 and ranged from 3.3 to 798.6 mg/m^2. Twenty-six patients (3.0%) received cumulative doses of greater than 450 mg/m^2.

Of these 753 patients, 61.2% were considered poor risk for KS tumor burden, 91.5% poor for immune system, and 46.9% for systemic illness; 36.2% were poor risk for all three categories. Patients' median CD4 count was 21.0 cells/mm^3, with 50.8% of patients having less than 50 cells/mm^3. The mean absolute neutrophil count at study entry was approximately 3000 cells/mm^3.

Patients received a variety of potentially myelotoxic drugs in combination with Doxil®. Of the 693 patients with concomitant medication information, 58.7% were on one or more antiretroviral medications; 34.9% patients were on zidovudine (AZT), 20.8% on didanosine (ddI), 16.5% on zalcitabine (ddC), and 9.5% on stavudine (D4T). A total of 85.1% patients were on PCP prophylaxis, most (54.4%) on sulfamethoxazole/trimethoprim. Eighty-five percent of patients were receiving antifungal medications, primarily fluconazole (75.8%). Seventy-two percent of patients were receiving antivirals, 56.3% acyclovir, 29% ganciclovir, and 16% foscarnet. In addition, 47.8% patients received colony-stimulating factors (sargramostim/filgrastim) sometime during their course of treatment.

Of the 753 patients enrolled in the Doxil® clinical trials, adverse event information was available for 705 patients. In many instances it was difficult to determine whether adverse events resulted from Doxil®, from concomitant therapy, or from the patients' underlying disease(s).

Eighty-three percent of the patients reported adverse events that were considered to be possibly or probably related to the treatment with Doxil®.

Adverse reactions only infrequently (5%) led to discontinuation of treatment. Those that did so included bone marrow suppression, cardiac adverse events, infusion-related reactions, toxoplasmosis, palmar-plantar erythrodysesthesia, pneumonia, cough/dyspnea, fatigue, optic neuritis, progression of a non-KS tumor, allergy to penicillin, and unspecified reasons.

Hematology Data Reported in AIDS-KS Patients

	Refractory or Intolerant AIDS-KS Patients (n=74)	Total AIDS-KS Patients (n=720)
Neutropenia		
< 1000/mm^3	34 (45.9%)	352 (48.9%)
< 500/mm^3	8 (10.8%)	96 (13.3%)
Anemia		
< 10 g/dL	43 (58.1%)	399 (55.4%)
< 8 g/dL	12 (16.2%)	131 (18.2%)
Thrombocytopenia		
< 150,000/mm^3	45 (60.8%)	439 (60.9%)
< 25,000/mm^3	1 (1.4%)	30 (4.2%)

Probably and Possibly Drug-Related Non-Hematologic *Adverse Events Reported in ≥ 5% of AIDS-KS Patients*

Adverse Event	Refractory or Intolerant AIDS-KS Patients (n=77)	Total AIDS-KS Patients (n=705)
Nausea	14 (18.2%)	119 (16.9%)
Asthenia	5 (6.5%)	70 (9.9%)
Fever	6 (7.8%)	64 (9.1%)
Alopecia	7 (9.1%)	63 (8.9%)
Alkaline Phosphatase Increase	1 (1.3%)	55 (7.8%)
Vomiting	6 (7.8%)	55 (7.8%)
Hypochromic Anemia	4 (5.2%)	69 (9.8%)
Diarrhea	4 (5.2%)	55 (7.8%)
Stomatitis	4 (5.2%)	48 (6.8%)
Oral Moniliasis	1 (1.3%)	39 (5.5%)

The following additional (not in table) adverse events were observed in AIDS-KS patients; only events considered at least possibly drug-related by investigators are included.

Incidence 1% to 5%

Body as a Whole: headache, back pain, infection, allergic reaction, chills.
Cardiovascular: chest pain, hypotension, tachycardia.
Cutaneous: Herpes simplex, rash, itching.
Digestive System: mouth ulceration, glossitis, constipation, aphthous stomatitis, anorexia, dysphagia, abdominal pain.
Hematologic: hemolysis, increased prothrombin time.
Metabolic/Nutritional: SGPT increase, weight loss, hypocalcemia, hyperbilirubinemia, hyperglycemia.
Other: dyspnea, albuminuria, pneumonia, retinitis, emotional lability, dizziness, somnolence.

Incidence Less Than 1%

Body As A Whole: face edema, cellulitis, sepsis, abscess, radiation injury, flu syndrome, moniliasis, hypothermia, injection site hemorrhage, injection site pain, cryptococcosis, ascites.
Cardiovascular System: thrombophlebitis, cardiomyopathy, pericardial effusion, hemorrhage, palpitation, syncope, bundle branch block, congestive heart failure, cardiomegaly, heart arrest, migraine, thrombosis, ventricular arrhythmia.
Digestive System: dyspepsia, cholestatic jaundice, gastritis, gingivitis, ulcerative proctitis, colitis, esophageal ulcer, esophagitis, gastrointestinal hemorrhage, hepatic failure, leukoplakia of mouth, pancreatitis, ulcerative stomatitis, hepatitis, hepatosplenomegaly, increased appetite, jaundice, sclerosing cholangitis, tenesmus, fecal impaction.
Endocrine System: diabetes mellitus.
Hemic and Lymphatic System: eosinophilia, lymphadenopathy, lymphangitis, lymphedema, petechia, thromboplastin decrease.
Metabolic/Nutritional Disorders: lactic dehydrogenase increase, hypernatremia, creatinine increase, BUN increase, dehydration, edema, hypercalcemia, hyperkalemia, hyperlipemia, hyperuricemia, hypoglycemia, hypokalemia, hypolipemia, hypomagnesemia, hyponatremia, hypophosphatemia, hypoproteinemia, ketosis, weight gain.
Musculoskeletal System: myalgia, arthralgia, bone pain, myositis.
Nervous System: paresthesia, insomnia, peripheral neuritis, depression, neuropathy, anxiety, convulsion, hypotonia, acute brain syndrome, confusion, hemiplegia, hypertonia, hypokinesia, vertigo.
Respiratory System: pleural effusion, asthma, bronchitis, cough increase, hyperventilation, pharyngitis, pneumothorax, rhinitis, sinusitis.
Skin and Appendages: maculopapular rash, skin ulcer, skin discoloration, herpes zoster, exfoliative dermatitis, cutaneous moniliasis, erythema multiforme, erythema nodosum, furunculosis, psoriasis, pustular rash, skin necrosis, urticaria, vesiculobullous rash.
Special Senses: otitis media, taste perversion, abnormal vision, blindness, conjunctivitis, eye pain, optic neuritis, tinnitus, visual field defect.
Urogenital System: hematuria, balanitis, cystitis, dysuria, genital edema, glycosuria, kidney failure.

OVERDOSAGE

Acute overdosage with doxorubicin HCl causes increases in mucositis, leukopenia and thrombocytopenia.

Treatment of acute overdosage consists of treatment of the severely myelosuppressed patient with hospitalization, antibiotics, platelet and granulocyte transfusions and symptomatic treatment of mucositis.

DOSAGE AND ADMINISTRATION

Ovarian Cancer Patients

Doxil® (doxorubicin HCl liposome injection) should be administered intravenously at a dose of 50 mg/m^2 (doxorubicin HCl equivalent) at an initial rate of 1 mg/min to minimize the risk of infusion reactions. If no infusion-related AEs are observed, the rate of infusion can be increased to complete administration of the drug over one hour. The patient should be dosed once every 4 weeks, for as long as the patient does not progress, shows no evidence of cardiotoxicity (see **WARNINGS**), and continues to tolerate treatment. A minimum of 4 courses is recommended because median time to response in clinical trials was 4 months. To manage adverse events such as PPE, stomatitis, or hematologic toxicity the doses may be delayed or reduced (see Dose Modification Guidelines below). Pretreatment with or concomitant use of antiemetics should be considered.

AIDS-KS Patients

Doxil® (doxorubicin HCl liposome injection) should be administered intravenously at a dose of 20 mg/m^2 (doxorubicin HCl equivalent) over 30 minutes, once every three weeks, for as long as patients respond satisfactorily and tolerate treatment.

General

Do not administer as a bolus injection or an undiluted solution. Rapid infusion may increase the risk of infusion-related reactions. (see **WARNINGS–Infusion Reactions.**)

Each 10-mL vial contains 20 mg doxorubicin HCl at a concentration of 2 mg/mL.

Each 30-mL vial contains 50 mg doxorubicin HCl at a concentration of 2 mg/mL.

Until specific compatibility data are available, it is not recommended that Doxil® be mixed with other drugs.

Doxil® should be considered an irritant and precautions should be taken to avoid extravasation. With intravenous administration of Doxil®, extravasation may occur with or without an accompanying stinging or burning sensation, even if blood returns well on aspiration of the infusion needle. If any signs or symptoms of extravasation have occurred, the infusion should be immediately terminated and restarted in another vein. The application of ice over the site of extravasation for approximately 30 minutes may be helpful in alleviating the local reaction. **Doxil® must not be given by the intramuscular or subcutaneous route.**

Dose Modification Guidelines

Doxil® exhibits nonlinear pharmacokinetics at 50 mg/m^2; therefore, dose adjustments may result in a non-proportional greater change in plasma concentration and exposure to the drug. (see **CLINICAL PHARMACOLOGY, Pharmacokinetics.**)

Patients should be carefully monitored for toxicity. Adverse events, such as PPE, hematologic toxicities, and stomatitis may be managed by dose delays and adjustments. Following the first appearance of a Grade 2 or higher adverse event, the dosing should be adjusted or delayed as described in the following tables. Once the dose has been reduced, it should not be increased at a later time.

Recommended Dose Modification Guidelines

PALMAR - PLANTAR ERYTHRODYSESTHESIA

Toxicity Grade	Dose Adjustment
1 (mild erythema, swelling, or desquamation not interfering with daily activities)	**Redose unless patient has experienced previous Grade 3 or 4 toxicity.** If so, delay up to 2 weeks and decrease dose by 25%. Return to original dose interval.
2 (erythema, desquamation, or swelling interfering with, but not precluding normal physical activities; small blisters or ulcerations less than 2 cm in diameter.)	**Delay dosing up to 2 weeks or until resolved to Grade 0–1.** If after 2 weeks there is no resolution, Doxil® should be discontinued.
3 (blistering, ulceration, or swelling interfering with walking or normal daily activities; cannot wear regular clothing)	**Delay dosing up to 2 weeks or until resolved to Grade 0-1.** Decrease dose by 25% and return to original dose interval. If after 2 weeks there is no resolution, Doxil® should be discontinued.
4 (diffuse or local process causing infectious complications, or a bed ridden state or hospitalization)	**Delay dosing up to 2 weeks or until resolved to Grade 0-1.** Decrease dose by 25% and return to original dose interval. If after 2 weeks there is no resolution, Doxil® should be discontinued.

HEMATOLOGICAL TOXICITY

GRADE	ANC	PLATELETS	MODIFICATION
1	1500 – 1900	75,000 – 150,000	Resume treatment with no dose reduction
2	1000 – <1500	50,000 – <75,000	Wait until ANC ≥ 1,500 and platelets ≥ 75,000; redose with no dose reduction
3	500 – 999	25,000 – <50,000	Wait until ANC ≥ 1,500 and platelets ≥ 75,000; redose with no dose reduction
4	<500	<25,000	Wait until ANC ≥ 1,500 and platelets ≥ 75,000; redose at 25% dose reduction or continue full dose with cytokine support.

[See table above]

Continued on next page

Doxil—Cont.

STOMATITIS

Toxicity Grade	Dose Adjustment
1 (painless ulcers, erythema, or mild soreness)	**Redose unless patient has experienced previous Grade 3 or 4 toxicity.** If so, delay up to 2 weeks and decrease dose by 25%. Return to original dose interval.
2 (painful erythema, edema, or ulcers, but can eat)	**Delay dosing up to 2 weeks or until resolved to Grade 0-1.** If after 2 weeks there is no resolution, Doxil® should be discontinued.
3 (painful erythema, edema, or ulcers, and cannot eat)	**Delay dosing up to 2 weeks or until resolved to Grade 0-1.** Decrease dose by 25% and return to original dose interval. If after 2 weeks there is no resolution, Doxil® should be discontinued.
4 (requires parenteral or enteral support)	**Delay dosing up to 2 weeks or until resolved to Grade 0-1.** Decrease dose by 25% and return to original dose interval. If after 2 weeks there is no resolution, Doxil® should be discontinued.

Patients with Impaired Hepatic Function
Limited clinical experience exists in treating hepatically impaired patients with Doxil®. Based on experience with doxorubicin HCl, it is recommended that Doxil® dosage be reduced if the bilirubin is elevated as follows: Serum bilirubin 1.2 to 3.0 mg/dL give ½ normal dose, >3 mg/dL give ¼ normal dose.
Preparation for Intravenous Administration
The appropriate dose of Doxil®, up to a maximum of 90 mg, must be diluted in 250 mL of 5% Dextrose Injection, USP prior to administration. Aseptic technique must be strictly observed since no preservative or bacteriostatic agent is present in Doxil®. Diluted Doxil® should be refrigerated at 2°C to 8°C (36°F to 46°F) and administered within 24 hours.
Do not use with in-line filters.
Do not mix with other drugs.
Do not use with any diluent other than 5% Dextrose Injection.
Do not use any bacteriostatic agent, such as benzyl alcohol.
Doxil® is not a clear solution but a translucent, red liposomal dispersion.
Parenteral drug products should be inspected visually for particulate matter and discoloration prior to administration, whenever solution and container permit. Do not use if a precipitate or foreign matter is present.
Storage and Stability
Refrigerate unopened vials of Doxil® at 2°C to 8°C (36°F to 46°F). Avoid freezing. Prolonged freezing may adversely affect liposomal drug products; however, short-term freezing (less than 1 month) does not appear to have a deleterious effect on Doxil®.
Procedure for Proper Handling and Disposal
Caution should be exercised in the handling and preparation of Doxil®.
The use of gloves is required.
If Doxil® comes into contact with skin or mucosa, immediately wash thoroughly with soap and water.
Doxil® should be considered an irritant and precautions should be taken to avoid extravasation. With intravenous administration of Doxil®, extravasation may occur with or without an accompanying stinging or burning sensation, even if blood returns well on aspiration of the infusion needle. If any signs or symptoms of extravasation have occurred, the infusion should be immediately terminated and restarted in another vein. Doxil® must not be given by the intramuscular or subcutaneous route.
Doxil® should be handled and disposed of in a manner consistent with other anticancer drugs. Several guidelines on this subject exist.[2-8]

HOW SUPPLIED

Doxil® (doxorubicin HCl liposome injection) is supplied as a sterile, translucent, red liposomal dispersion in 10-mL or 30-mL glass, single use vials.
Each 10-mL vial contains 20 mg doxorubicin HCl at a concentration of 2 mg/mL.
Each 30-mL vial contains 50 mg doxorubicin HCl at a concentration of 2 mg/mL.
Refrigerate at 2°-8°C. Avoid freezing. Prolonged freezing may adversely affect liposomal drug products; however, short-term freezing (less than 1 month) does not appear to have a deleterious effect on Doxil®.
The following packages of six individually cartoned vials are available:

mg in vial	fill volume	vial size	NDC#'s
20 mg vial	10-mL	10-mL	17314-9600-1
50 mg vial	25-mL	30-mL	17314-9600-2

REFERENCES

1. Krown et al. Kaposi's sarcoma in the acquired immune deficiency syndrome: A proposal for uniform evaluation, response, and staging criteria. J Clin Oncol. 1989; 7(9): 1201-1207.
2. Recommendations for the safe handling of cytotoxic drugs. NIH Publication No. 92-2621. US Government Printing Office, Washington, DC 20402.
3. OSHA Work-Practice guidelines for personnel dealing with cytotoxic (antineoplastic) drugs. Am J Hosp Pharm. 1986; 43:1193-1204.
4. American Society of Hospital Pharmacists Technical Assistance Bulletin on Handling Cytotoxic and Hazardous Drugs. Am J Hosp Pharm. 1985; 42:131-137.
5. National Study Commission on Cytotoxic Exposure—Recommendations for Handling Cytotoxic Agents. Available from Louis P. Jeffrey, Sc.D., Chairman, National Study Commission on Cytotoxic Exposure, Massachusetts College of Pharmacy and Allied Health Sciences, 179 Longwood Avenue, Boston, Massachusetts 02115.
6. AMA Council Report. Guidelines for handling parenteral antineoplastics. JAMA 1985; 253(11):1590-1592.
7. Clinical Oncologic Society of Australia: Guidelines and recommendation for safe handling of antineoplastic agents. Med. J. Australia 1983; 1:426-428.
8. Jones RB, et al. Safe handling of chemotherapeutic agents: a report from the Mount Sinai Medical Center. Ca–A Cancer Journal for Clinicians. 1983; Sept/Oct:258-263.

℞ only

Manufactured by:
Ben Venue Laboratories, Inc.
Bedford, OH 44146
Distributed by:
Ortho Biotech Products L.P.
Raritan, NJ 08869-0670
Last revised: February 2003
00122782
ORTHO BIOTECH
An ALZA STEALTH®
Technology Product
STEALTH® and Doxil® are registered trademarks of ALZA Corporation
Shown in Product Identification Guide, page 334

UCB Pharma, Inc.
1950 LAKE PARK DRIVE
SMYRNA, GA 30080

Direct Inquiries to:
UCB Pharma, Inc.
1950 Lake Park Drive
Smyrna, GA 30080
(800) 477-7877

For Medical Information Contact:
Medical Affairs Department
(800) 477-7877 Option 9
FAX: 770-970-8859

KEPPRA® ℞
[*kepp-ruh*]
(levetiracetam)
250 mg, 500 mg and 750 mg tablets
100 mg/mL oral solution
Rx only

DESCRIPTION

Keppra® (levetiracetam) is an antiepileptic drug available as 250 mg (blue), 500 mg (yellow) and 750 mg (orange) tablets and as a clear, colorless, grape-flavored liquid (100 mg/mL) for oral administration.
The chemical name of levetiracetam, a single enantiomer, is (-)-(S)-α-ethyl-2-oxo-1-pyrrolidine acetamide, its molecular formula is $C_8H_{14}N_2O_2$ and its molecular weight is 170.21. Levetiracetam is chemically unrelated to existing antiepileptic drugs (AEDs). It has the following structural formula:

CH_3CH_2 — N (pyrrolidinone, =O) — C — H, $CONH_2$

Levetiracetam is a white to off-white crystalline powder with a faint odor and a bitter taste. It is very soluble in water (104.0 g/100 mL). It is freely soluble in chloroform (65.3 g/100 mL) and in methanol (53.6 g/100 mL), soluble in ethanol (16.5 g/100 mL), sparingly soluble in acetonitrile (5.7 g/100 mL) and practically insoluble in n-hexane. (Solubility limits are expressed as g/100 mL solvent.)
Keppra® tablets contain the labeled amount of levetiracetam. Inactive ingredients: colloidal silicon dioxide, corn starch, hydroxypropyl methylcellulose, magnesium stearate, polyethylene glycol 4000, povidone, talc, titanium dioxide and coloring agents.
The individual tablets contain the following coloring agents:
250 mg tablets: FD&C Blue No. 2,
500 mg tablets: yellow iron oxide,
750 mg tablets: FD&C Blue No. 2, FD&C Yellow No. 6 and red iron oxide.
Keppra® oral solution contains 100 mg of levetiracetam per mL. Inactive ingredients: ammonium glycyrrhizinate, citric acid monohydrate, glycerin, maltitol solution, methylparaben, potassium acesulfame, propylparaben, purified water, sodium citrate dihydrate and natural and artificial flavor.

CLINICAL PHARMACOLOGY

Mechanism Of Action
The precise mechanism(s) by which levetiracetam exerts its antiepileptic effect is unknown. The antiepileptic activity of levetiracetam was assessed in a number of animal models of epileptic seizures. Levetiracetam did not inhibit single seizures induced by maximal stimulation with electrical current or different chemoconvulsants and showed only minimal activity in submaximal stimulation and in threshold tests. Protection was observed, however, against secondarily generalized activity from focal seizures induced by pilocarpine and kainic acid, two chemoconvulsants that induce seizures that mimic some features of human complex partial seizures with secondary generalization. Levetiracetam also displayed inhibitory properties in the kindling model in rats, another model of human complex partial seizures, both during kindling development and in the fully kindled state. The predictive value of these animal models for specific types of human epilepsy is uncertain.
In vitro and *in vivo* recordings of epileptiform activity from the hippocampus have shown that levetiracetam inhibits burst firing without affecting normal neuronal excitability, suggesting that levetiracetam may selectively prevent hypersynchronization of epileptiform burst firing and propagation of seizure activity.
Levetiracetam at concentrations of up to 10 μM did not demonstrate binding affinity for a variety of known receptors, such as those associated with benzodiazepines, GABA (gamma-aminobutyric acid), glycine, NMDA (N-methyl-D-aspartate), re-uptake sites, and second messenger systems. Furthermore, *in vitro* studies have failed to find an effect of levetiracetam on neuronal voltage-gated sodium or T-type calcium currents. Levetiracetam does not appear to directly facilitate GABAergic neurotransmission, but has been shown to oppose the activity of negative modulators of GABA- and glycine-gated currents in neuronal cell culture. A saturable and stereoselective neuronal binding site in rat brain tissue has been described for levetiracetam; however, the identification and function of this binding site is currently unknown.
Pharmacokinetics
The pharmacokinetics of levetiracetam have been studied in healthy adult subjects, adults and pediatric patients with epilepsy, elderly subjects and subjects with renal and hepatic impairment.
Overview
Levetiracetam is rapidly and almost completely absorbed after oral administration. Levetiracetam tablets and oral solution are bioequivalent. The pharmacokinetics are linear and time-invariant, with low intra- and inter-subject variability. The extent of bioavailability of levetiracetam is not affected by food. Levetiracetam is not protein-bound (<10% bound) and its volume of distribution is close to the volume of intracellular and extracellular water. Sixty-six percent (66%) of the dose is renally excreted unchanged. The major metabolic pathway of levetiracetam (24% of dose) is an enzymatic hydrolysis of the acetamide group. It is not liver cytochrome P450 dependent. The metabolites have no known pharmacological activity and are renally excreted. Plasma half-life of levetiracetam across studies is approximately 6-8 hours. It is increased in the elderly (primarily due to impaired renal clearance) and in subjects with renal impairment.
Absorption and Distribution
Absorption of levetiracetam is rapid, with peak plasma concentrations occurring in about an hour following oral administration in fasted subjects. The oral bioavailability of levetiracetam tablets is 100% and the tablets and oral solution are bioequivalent in rate and extent of absorption. Food does not affect the extent of absorption of levetiracetam but it decreases C_{max} by 20% and delays T_{max} by 1.5 hours. The pharmacokinetics of levetiracetam are linear over the dose range of 500-5000 mg. Steady state is achieved after 2 days of multiple twice-daily dosing. Levetiracetam and its major metabolite are less than 10% bound to plasma proteins; clinically significant interactions with other drugs through competition for protein binding sites are therefore unlikely.
Metabolism
Levetiracetam is not extensively metabolized in humans. The major metabolic pathway is the enzymatic hydrolysis of the acetamide group, which produces the carboxylic acid metabolite, ucb L057 (24% of dose) and is not dependent on any liver cytochrome P450 isoenzymes. The major metabolite is inactive in animal seizure models. Two minor metabolites were identified as the product of hydroxylation of the 2-oxo-pyrrolidine ring (2% of dose) and opening of the 2-oxo-pyrrolidine ring in position 5 (1% of dose). There is no enantiomeric interconversion of levetiracetam or its major metabolite.

Elimination
Levetiracetam plasma half-life in adults is 7 ± 1 hour and is unaffected by either dose or repeated administration. Levetiracetam is eliminated from the systemic circulation by renal excretion as unchanged drug which represents 66% of administered dose. The total body clearance is 0.96 mL/min/kg and the renal clearance is 0.6 mL/min/kg. The mechanism of excretion is glomerular filtration with subsequent partial tubular reabsorption. The metabolite ucb L057 is excreted by glomerular filtration and active tubular secretion with a renal clearance of 4 mL/min/kg. Levetiracetam elimination is correlated to creatinine clearance. Levetiracetam clearance is reduced in patients with impaired renal function (see Special Populations, Renal Impairment and DOSAGE AND ADMINISTRATION, Patients with Impaired Renal Function).

Pharmacokinetic Interactions
In vitro data on metabolic interactions indicate that levetiracetam is unlikely to produce, or be subject to, pharmacokinetic interactions. Levetiracetam and its major metabolite, at concentrations well above C_{max} levels achieved within the therapeutic dose range, are neither inhibitors of, nor high affinity substrates for, human liver cytochrome P450 isoforms, epoxide hydrolase or UDP-glucuronidation enzymes. In addition, levetiracetam does not affect the *in vitro* glucuronidation of valproic acid.
Potential pharmacokinetic interactions of or with levetiracetam were assessed in clinical pharmacokinetic studies (phenytoin, valproate, warfarin, digoxin, oral contraceptive, probenecid) and through pharmacokinetic screening in the placebo-controlled clinical studies in epilepsy patients (see PRECAUTIONS, Drug Interactions).

Special Populations
Elderly
Pharmacokinetics of levetiracetam were evaluated in 16 elderly subjects (age 61-88 years) with creatinine clearance ranging from 30 to 74 mL/min. Following oral administration of twice-daily dosing for 10 days, total body clearance decreased by 38% and the half-life was 2.5 hours longer in the elderly compared to healthy adults. This is most likely due to the decrease in renal function in these subjects.
Pediatric Patients
Pharmacokinetics of levetiracetam were evaluated in 24 pediatric patients (age 6-12 years) after single dose (20 mg/kg). The body weight adjusted apparent clearance of levetiracetam was approximately 40% higher than in adults.
Gender
Levetiracetam C_{max} and AUC were 20% higher in women (N=11) compared to men (N=12). However, clearances adjusted for body weight were comparable.
Race
Formal pharmacokinetic studies of the effects of race have not been conducted. Cross study comparisons involving Caucasians (N=12) and Asians (N=12), however, show that pharmacokinetics of levetiracetam were comparable between the two races. Because levetiracetam is primarily renally excreted and there are no important racial differences in creatinine clearance, pharmacokinetic differences due to race are not expected.
Renal Impairment
The disposition of levetiracetam was studied in subjects with varying degrees of renal function. Total body clearance of levetiracetam is reduced in patients with impaired renal function by 40% in the mild group (CLcr = 50-80 mL/min), 50% in the moderate group (CLcr = 30-50 mL/min) and 60% in the severe renal impairment group (CLcr <30 mL/min). Clearance of levetiracetam is correlated with creatinine clearance.
In anuric (end stage renal disease) patients, the total body clearance decreased 70% compared to normal subjects (CLcr >80mL/min). Approximately 50% of the pool of levetiracetam in the body is removed during a standard 4-hour hemodialysis procedure.
Dosage should be reduced in patients with impaired renal function receiving levetiracetam, and supplemental doses should be given to patients after dialysis (see PRECAUTIONS and DOSAGE AND ADMINISTRATION, Patients with Impaired Renal Function).
Hepatic Impairment
In subjects with mild (Child-Pugh A) to moderate (Child-Pugh B) hepatic impairment, the pharmacokinetics of levetiracetam were unchanged. In patients with severe hepatic impairment (Child-Pugh C), total body clearance was 50% that of normal subjects, but decreased renal clearance accounted for most of the decrease. No dose adjustment is needed for patients with hepatic impairment.

CLINICAL STUDIES

Effectiveness In Partial Onset Seizures
The effectiveness of Keppra® as adjunctive therapy (added to other antiepileptic drugs) in adults was established in three multicenter, randomized, double-blind, placebo-controlled clinical studies in patients who had refractory partial onset seizures with or without secondary generalization. The tablet formulation was used in all these studies. In these studies, 904 patients were randomized to placebo, 1000 mg, 2000 mg, or 3000 mg/day. Patients enrolled in Study 1 or Study 2 had refractory partial onset seizures for at least two years and had taken two or more classical AEDs. Patients enrolled in Study 3 had refractory partial onset seizures for at least 1 year and had taken one classical AED. At the time of the study, patients were taking a stable dose regimen of at least one and could take a maximum of two AEDs. During the baseline period, patients had to have experienced at least two partial onset seizures during each 4-week period.

Study 1
Study 1 was a double-blind, placebo-controlled, parallel-group study conducted at 41 sites in the United States comparing Keppra® 1000 mg/day (N=97), Keppra® 3000 mg/day (N=101), and placebo (N=95) given in equally divided doses twice daily. After a prospective baseline period of 12 weeks, patients were randomized to one of the three treatment groups described above. The 18-week treatment period consisted of a 6-week titration period, followed by a 12-week fixed dose evaluation period, during which concomitant AED regimens were held constant. The primary measure of effectiveness was a between group comparison of the percent reduction in weekly partial seizure frequency relative to placebo over the entire randomized treatment period (titration + evaluation period). Secondary outcome variables included the responder rate (incidence of patients with ≥ 50% reduction from baseline in partial onset seizure frequency). The results of the analysis of Study 1 are displayed in Table 1.

Table 1: Reduction In Weekly Frequency Of Partial Onset Seizures In Study 1

	Placebo (N=95)	Keppra® 1000 mg/day (N=97)	Keppra® 3000 mg/day (N=101)
Percent reduction in partial seizure frequency over placebo	–	26.1%*	30.1%*

*P<0.001

The percentage of patients (y-axis) who achieved ≥ 50% reduction in weekly seizure rates from baseline in partial onset seizure frequency over the entire randomized treatment period (titration + evaluation period) within the three treatment groups (x-axis) is presented in Figure 1.

Figure 1. Responder Rate (≥50% Reduction From Baseline) In Study 1

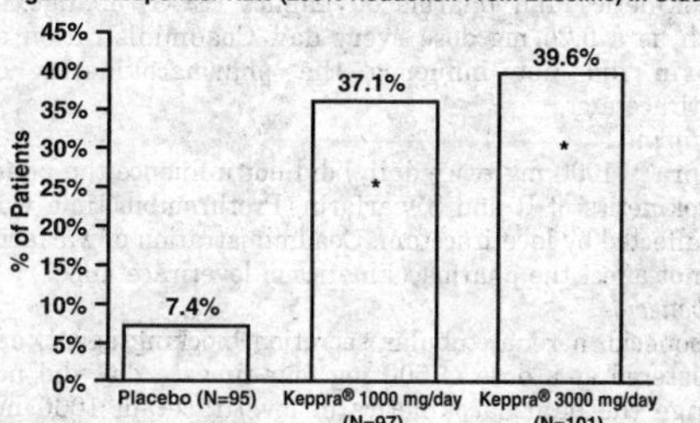

* P<0.001 versus placebo.

Study 2
Study 2 was a double-blind, placebo-controlled, crossover study conducted at 62 centers in Europe comparing Keppra® 1000 mg/day (N=106), Keppra® 2000 mg/day (N=105), and placebo (N=111) given in equally divided doses twice daily.
The first period of the study (Period A) was designed to be analyzed as a parallel-group study. After a prospective baseline period of up to 12 weeks, patients were randomized to one of the three treatment groups described above. The 16-week treatment period consisted of the 4-week titration period followed by a 12-week fixed dose evaluation period, during which concomitant AED regimens were held constant. The primary measure of effectiveness was a between group comparison of the percent reduction in weekly partial seizure frequency relative to placebo over the entire randomized treatment period (titration + evaluation period). Secondary outcome variables included the responder rate (incidence of patients with ≥50% reduction from baseline in partial onset seizure frequency). The results of the analysis of Period A are displayed in Table 2.

Table 2: Reduction In Weekly Frequency Of Partial Onset Seizures In Study 2: Period A

	Placebo (N=111)	Keppra® 1000 mg/day (N=106)	Keppra® 2000 mg/day (N=105)
Percent reduction in partial seizure frequency over placebo	–	17.1%*	21.4%*

*P≤0.001

The percentage of patients (y-axis) who achieved ≥ 50% reduction in weekly seizure rates from baseline in partial onset seizure frequency over the entire randomized treatment period (titration + evaluation period) within the three treatment groups (x-axis) is presented in Figure 2.
[See figure 2 at top of next column]
The comparison of Keppra® 2000 mg/day to Keppra® 1000 mg/day for responder rate was statistically significant (P=0.02). Analysis of the trial as a cross-over yielded similar results.

Figure 2. Responder Rate (≥50% Reduction From Baseline) In Study 2: Period A

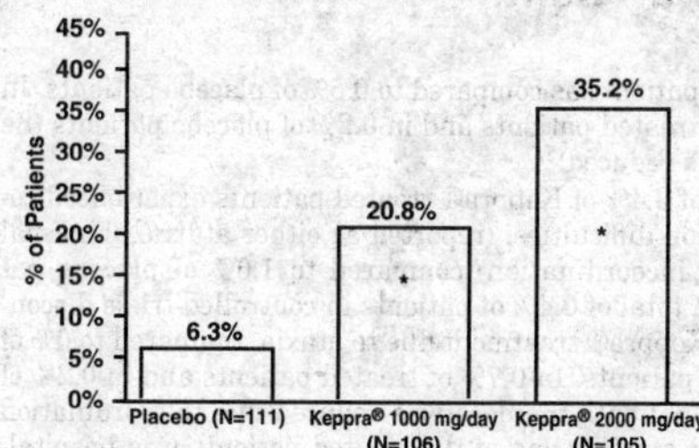

* P<0.001 versus placebo.

Study 3
Study 3 was a double-blind, placebo-controlled, parallel-group study conducted at 47 centers in Europe comparing Keppra® 3000 mg/day (N=180) and placebo (N=104) in patients with refractory partial onset seizures, with or without secondary generalization, receiving only one concomitant AED. Study drug was given in two divided doses. After a prospective baseline period of 12 weeks, patients were randomized to one of two treatment groups described above. The 16-week treatment period consisted of a 4-week titration period, followed by a 12-week fixed dose evaluation period, during which concomitant AED doses were held constant. The primary measure of effectiveness was a between group comparison of the percent reduction in weekly seizure frequency relative to placebo over the entire randomized treatment period (titration + evaluation period). Secondary outcome variables included the responder rate (incidence of patients with ≥50% reduction from baseline in partial onset seizure frequency). Table 3 displays the results of the analysis of Study 3.

Table 3: Reduction In Weekly Frequency Of Partial Onset Seizures In Study 3

	Placebo (N=104)	Keppra® 3000 mg/day (N=180)
Percent reduction in partial seizure frequency over placebo	–	23.0%*

*P<0.001

The percentage of patients (y-axis) who achieved ≥50% reduction in weekly seizure rates from baseline in partial onset seizure frequency over the entire randomized treatment period (titration + evaluation period) within the two treatment groups (x-axis) is presented in Figure 3.

Figure 3. Responder Rate (≥50% Reduction From Baseline) In Study 3

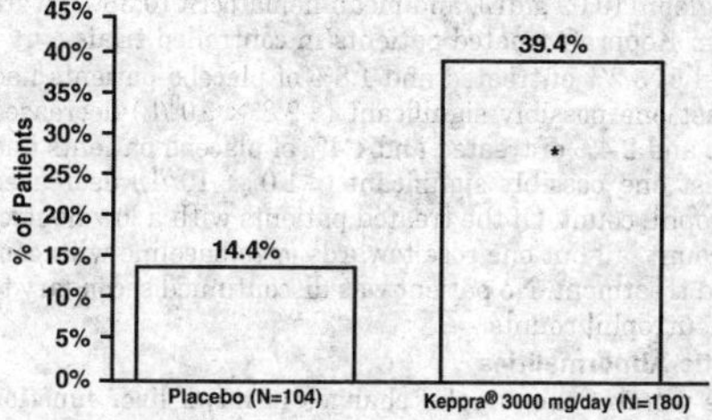

* P<0.001 versus placebo.

INDICATIONS AND USAGE

Keppra® (levetiracetam) is indicated as adjunctive therapy in the treatment of partial onset seizures in adults with epilepsy.

CONTRAINDICATIONS

This product should not be administered to patients who have previously exhibited hypersensitivity to levetiracetam or any of the inactive ingredients in Keppra® tablets or oral solution.

WARNINGS

Neuropsychiatric Adverse Events
Keppra® use is associated with the occurrence of central nervous system adverse events that can be classified into the following categories: 1) somnolence and fatigue, 2) coordination difficulties, and 3) behavioral abnormalities.
In controlled trials of patients with epilepsy, 14.8% of Keppra® treated patients reported somnolence, compared to 8.4% of placebo patients. There was no clear dose response up to 3000 mg/day. In a study where there was no titration, about 45% of patients receiving 4000 mg/day reported somnolence. The somnolence was considered serious in 0.3% of the treated patients, compared to 0% in the placebo group. About 3% of Keppra® treated patients discontinued treatment due to somnolence, compared to 0.7% of placebo patients. In 1.4% of treated patients and in 0.9% of placebo patients the dose was reduced, while 0.3% of the treated patients were hospitalized due to somnolence.
In controlled trials of patients with epilepsy, 14.7% of treated patients reported asthenia, compared to 9.1% of placebo patients. Treatment was discontinued in 0.8% of

Continued on next page

Keppra—Cont.

treated patients as compared to 0.5% of placebo patients. In 0.5% of treated patients and in 0.2% of placebo patients the dose was reduced.

A total of 3.4% of Keppra® treated patients experienced coordination difficulties, (reported as either ataxia, abnormal gait, or incoordination) compared to 1.6% of placebo patients. A total of 0.4% of patients in controlled trials discontinued Keppra® treatment due to ataxia, compared to 0% of placebo patients. In 0.7% of treated patients and in 0.2% of placebo patients the dose was reduced due to coordination difficulties, while one of the treated patients was hospitalized due to worsening of pre-existing ataxia.

Somnolence, asthenia and coordination difficulties occurred most frequently within the first 4 weeks of treatment.

In controlled trials of patients with epilepsy, 5 (0.7%) of Keppra® treated patients experienced psychotic symptoms compared to 1 (0.2%) placebo patient. Two (0.3%) Keppra® treated patients were hospitalized and their treatment was discontinued. Both events, reported as psychosis, developed within the first week of treatment and resolved within 1 to 2 weeks following treatment discontinuation. Two other events, reported as hallucinations, occurred after 1-5 months and resolved within 2-7 days while the patients remained on treatment. In one patient experiencing psychotic depression occurring within a month, symptoms resolved within 45 days while the patient continued treatment. A total of 13.3% of Keppra® patients experienced other behavioral symptoms (reported as aggression, agitation, anger, anxiety, apathy, depersonalization, depression, emotional lability, hostility, irritability etc.) compared to 6.2% of placebo patients. Approximately half of these patients reported these events within the first 4 weeks. A total of 1.7% of treated patients discontinued treatment due to these events, compared to 0.2% of placebo patients. The treatment dose was reduced in 0.8% of treated patients and in 0.5% of placebo patients. A total of 0.8% of treated patients had a serious behavioral event (compared to 0.2% of placebo patients) and were hospitalized.

In addition, 4 (0.5%) of treated patients attempted suicide compared to 0% of placebo patients. One of these patients successfully committed suicide. In the other 3 patients, the events did not lead to discontinuation or dose reduction. The events occurred after patients had been treated for between 4 weeks and 6 months.

Withdrawal Seizures

Antiepileptic drugs, including Keppra®, should be withdrawn gradually to minimize the potential of increased seizure frequency.

PRECAUTIONS

Hematologic Abnormalities

Minor, but statistically significant, decreases compared to placebo in total mean RBC count ($0.03 \times 10^6/mm^2$), mean hemoglobin (0.09 g/dL), and mean hematocrit (0.38%), were seen in Keppra® treated patients in controlled trials.

A total of 3.2% of treated and 1.8% of placebo patients had at least one possibly significant ($\leq 2.8 \times 10^9/L$) decreased WBC, and 2.4% of treated and 1.4% of placebo patients had at least one possibly significant ($\leq 1.0 \times 10^9/L$) decreased neutrophil count. Of the treated patients with a low neutrophil count, all but one rose towards or to baseline with continued treatment. No patient was discontinued secondary to low neutrophil counts.

Hepatic Abnormalities

There were no meaningful changes in mean liver function tests (LFT) in controlled trials; lesser LFT abnormalities were similar in drug and placebo treated patients in controlled trials (1.4%). No patients were discontinued from controlled trials for LFT abnormalities except for 1 (0.07%) epilepsy patient receiving open treatment.

Information For Patients

Patients should be instructed to take Keppra® only as prescribed.

Patients should be advised to notify their physician if they become pregnant or intend to become pregnant during therapy.

Patients should be advised that Keppra® may cause dizziness and somnolence. Accordingly, patients should be advised not to drive or operate machinery or engage in other hazardous activities until they have gained sufficient experience on Keppra® to gauge whether it adversely affects their performance of these activities.

Physicians should advise patients and caregivers to read the patient information leaflet which appears as the last section of the labeling.

Laboratory Tests

Although most laboratory tests are not systematically altered with Keppra® treatment, there have been relatively infrequent abnormalities seen in hematologic parameters and liver function tests.

Drug Interactions

In vitro data on metabolic interactions indicate that Keppra® is unlikely to produce, or be subject to, pharmacokinetic interactions. Levetiracetam and its major metabolite, at concentrations well above C_{max} levels achieved within the therapeutic dose range, are neither inhibitors of nor high affinity substrates for human liver cytochrome P450 isoforms, epoxide hydrolase or UDP-glucuronidation enzymes. In addition, levetiracetam does not affect the *in vitro* glucuronidation of valproic acid.

Levetiracetam circulates largely unbound (<10% bound) to plasma proteins; clinically significant interactions with other drugs through competition for protein binding sites are therefore unlikely.

Potential pharmacokinetic interactions were assessed in clinical pharmacokinetic studies (phenytoin, valproate, oral contraceptive, digoxin, warfarin, probenecid) and through pharmacokinetic screening in the placebo-controlled clinical studies in epilepsy patients.

Drug-Drug Interactions Between Keppra® And Other Antiepileptic Drugs (AEDs)

Phenytoin

Keppra® (3000 mg daily) had no effect on the pharmacokinetic disposition of phenytoin in patients with refractory epilepsy. Pharmacokinetics of levetiracetam were also not affected by phenytoin.

Valproate

Keppra® (1500 mg twice daily) did not alter the pharmacokinetics of valproate in healthy volunteers. Valproate 500 mg twice daily did not modify the rate or extent of levetiracetam absorption or its plasma clearance or urinary excretion. There also was no effect on exposure to and the excretion of the primary metabolite, ucb L057.

Potential drug interactions between Keppra® and other AEDs (carbamazepine, gabapentin, lamotrigine, phenobarbital, phenytoin, primidone and valproate) were also assessed by evaluating the serum concentrations of levetiracetam and these AEDs during placebo-controlled clinical studies. These data indicate that levetiracetam does not influence the plasma concentration of other AEDs and that these AEDs do not influence the pharmacokinetics of levetiracetam.

Other Drug Interactions

Oral Contraceptives

Keppra® (500 mg twice daily) did not influence the pharmacokinetics of an oral contraceptive containing 0.03 mg ethinyl estradiol and 0.15 mg levonorgestrel, or of the luteinizing hormone and progesterone levels, indicating that impairment of contraceptive efficacy is unlikely. Coadministration of this oral contraceptive did not influence the pharmacokinetics of levetiracetam.

Digoxin

Keppra® (1000 mg twice daily) did not influence the pharmacokinetics and pharmacodynamics (ECG) of digoxin given as a 0.25 mg dose every day. Coadministration of digoxin did not influence the pharmacokinetics of levetiracetam.

Warfarin

Keppra® (1000 mg twice daily) did not influence the pharmacokinetics of R and S warfarin. Prothrombin time was not affected by levetiracetam. Coadministration of warfarin did not affect the pharmacokinetics of levetiracetam.

Probenecid

Probenecid, a renal tubular secretion blocking agent, administered at a dose of 500 mg four times a day, did not change the pharmacokinetics of levetiracetam 1000 mg twice daily. C^{ss}_{max} of the metabolite, ucb L057, was approximately doubled in the presence of probenecid while the fraction of drug excreted unchanged in the urine remained the same. Renal clearance of ucb L057 in the presence of probenecid decreased 60%, probably related to competitive inhibition of tubular secretion of ucb L057. The effect of Keppra® on probenecid was not studied.

Carcinogenesis, Mutagenesis, Impairment Of Fertility

Carcinogenesis

Rats were dosed with levetiracetam in the diet for 104 weeks at doses of 50, 300 and 1800 mg/kg/day. The highest dose corresponds to 6 times the maximum recommended daily human dose (MRHD) of 3000 mg on a mg/m^2 basis and it also provided systemic exposure (AUC) approximately 6 times that achieved in humans receiving the MRHD. There was no evidence of carcinogenicity. A study was conducted in which mice received levetiracetam in the diet for 80 weeks at doses of 60, 240 and 960 mg/kg/day (high dose is equivalent to 2 times the MRHD on a mg/m^2 or exposure basis). Although no evidence for carcinogenicity was seen, the potential for a carcinogenic response has not been fully evaluated in that species because adequate doses have not been studied.

Mutagenesis

Levetiracetam was not mutagenic in the Ames test or in mammalian cells *in vitro* in the Chinese hamster ovary/HGPRT locus assay. It was not clastogenic in an *in vitro* analysis of metaphase chromosomes obtained from Chinese hamster ovary cells or in an *in vivo* mouse micronucleus assay. The hydrolysis product and major human metabolite of levetiracetam (ucb L057) was not mutagenic in the Ames test or the *in vitro* mouse lymphoma assay.

Impairment Of Fertility

No adverse effects on male or female fertility or reproductive performance were observed in rats at doses up to 1800 mg/kg/day (approximately 6 times the maximum recommended human dose on a mg/m^2 or exposure basis).

Pregnancy

Pregnancy Category C

In animal studies, levetiracetam produced evidence of developmental toxicity at doses similar to or greater than human therapeutic doses.

Administration to female rats throughout pregnancy and lactation was associated with increased incidences of minor fetal skeletal abnormalities and retarded offspring growth pre- and/or postnatally at doses ≥350 mg/kg/day (approximately equivalent to the maximum recommended human dose of 3000 mg [MRHD] on a mg/m^2 basis) and with increased pup mortality and offspring behavioral alterations at a dose of 1800 mg/kg/day (6 times the MRHD on a mg/m^2 basis). The developmental no effect dose was 70 mg/kg/day (0.2 times the MRHD on a mg/m^2 basis). There was no overt maternal toxicity at the doses used in this study.

Treatment of pregnant rabbits during the period of organogenesis resulted in increased embryofetal mortality and increased incidences of minor fetal skeletal abnormalities at doses ≥600 mg/kg/day (approximately 4 times MRHD on a mg/m^2 basis) and in decreased fetal weights and increased incidences of fetal malformations at a dose of 1800 mg/kg/day (12 times the MRHD on a mg/m^2 basis). The developmental no effect dose was 200 mg/kg/day (1.3 times the MRHD on a mg/m^2 basis). Maternal toxicity was also observed at 1800 mg/kg/day.

When pregnant rats were treated during the period of organogenesis, fetal weights were decreased and the incidence of fetal skeletal variations was increased at a dose of 3600 mg/kg/day (12 times the MRHD). 1200 mg/kg/day (4 times the MRHD) was a developmental no effect dose. There was no evidence of maternal toxicity in this study.

Treatment of rats during the last third of gestation and throughout lactation produced no adverse developmental or maternal effects at doses of up to 1800 mg/kg/day (6 times the MRHD on a mg/m^2 basis).

There are no adequate and well-controlled studies in pregnant women. Keppra® should be used during pregnancy only if the potential benefit justifies the potential risk to the fetus.

Pregnancy Exposure Registry

To facilitate monitoring fetal outcomes of pregnant women exposed to Keppra®, physicians should encourage patients to register, before fetal outcome is known (e.g., ultrasound, results of amniocentesis, etc.), in the Antiepileptic Drug Pregnancy Registry by calling (888) 233-2334 (toll free).

Labor And Delivery

The effect of Keppra® on labor and delivery in humans is unknown.

Nursing Mothers

Levetiracetam is excreted in breast milk. Because of the potential for serious adverse reactions in nursing infants from Keppra®, a decision should be made whether to discontinue nursing or discontinue the drug, taking into account the importance of the drug to the mother.

Pediatric Use

Safety and effectiveness in patients below the age of 16 have not been established.

Geriatric Use

Of the total number of subjects in clinical studies of levetiracetam, 347 were 65 and over. No overall differences in safety were observed between these subjects and younger subjects. There were insufficient numbers of elderly subjects in controlled trials of epilepsy to adequately assess the effectiveness of Keppra® in these patients.

A study in 16 elderly subjects (age 61-88 years) with oral administration of single dose and multiple twice-daily doses for 10 days showed no pharmacokinetic differences related to age alone.

Levetiracetam is known to be substantially excreted by the kidney, and the risk of adverse reactions to this drug may be greater in patients with impaired renal function. Because elderly patients are more likely to have decreased renal function, care should be taken in dose selection, and it may be useful to monitor renal function.

Use In Patients With Impaired Renal Function

Clearance of levetiracetam is decreased in patients with renal impairment and is correlated with creatinine clearance. Caution should be taken in dosing patients with moderate and severe renal impairment and in patients undergoing hemodialysis. The dosage should be reduced in patients with impaired renal function receiving Keppra® and supplemental doses should be given to patients after dialysis (see CLINICAL PHARMACOLOGY and DOSAGE AND ADMINISTRATION, Patients with Impaired Renal Function).

ADVERSE REACTIONS

In well-controlled clinical studies, the most frequently reported adverse events associated with the use of Keppra® in combination with other AEDs, not seen at an equivalent frequency among placebo-treated patients, were somnolence, asthenia, infection and dizziness.

Table 4 lists treatment-emergent adverse events that occurred in at least 1% of patients with epilepsy treated with Keppra® participating in placebo-controlled studies and were numerically more common in patients treated with Keppra® than placebo. In these studies, either Keppra® or placebo was added to concurrent AED therapy. Adverse events were usually mild to moderate in intensity. The prescriber should be aware that these figures, obtained when Keppra® was added to concurrent AED therapy, cannot be used to predict the frequency of adverse experiences in the course of usual medical practice where patient characteristics and other factors may differ from those prevailing during clinical studies. Similarly, the cited frequencies cannot be directly compared with figures obtained from other clinical investigations involving different treatments, uses, or investigators. An inspection of these frequencies, however, does provide the prescriber with one basis to estimate the relative contribution of drug and non-drug factors to the adverse event incidences in the population studied.

Table 4: Incidence (%) Of Treatment-Emergent Adverse Events In Placebo-Controlled, Add-On Studies By Body System (Adverse Events Occurred In At Least 1% Of Keppra®-Treated Patients And Occurred More Frequently Than Placebo-Treated Patients)

Body System/ Adverse Event	Keppra® (N=769) %	Placebo (N=439) %
Body as a Whole		
Asthenia	15	9
Headache	14	13
Infection	13	8
Pain	7	6
Digestive System		
Anorexia	3	2
Nervous System		
Amnesia	2	1
Anxiety	2	1
Ataxia	3	1
Depression	4	2
Dizziness	9	4
Emotional Lability	2	0
Hostility	2	1
Nervousness	4	2
Paresthesia	2	1
Somnolence	15	8
Vertigo	3	1
Respiratory System		
Cough Increased	2	1
Pharyngitis	6	4
Rhinitis	4	3
Sinusitis	2	1
Special Senses		
Diplopia	2	1

Other events reported by 1% or more of patients treated with Keppra® but as or more frequent in the placebo group were: abdominal pain, accidental injury, amblyopia, arthralgia, back pain, bronchitis, chest pain, confusion, constipation, convulsion, diarrhea, drug level increased, dyspepsia, ecchymosis, fever, flu syndrome, fungal infection, gastroenteritis, gingivitis, grand mal convulsion, insomnia, nausea, otitis media, rash, thinking abnormal, tremor, urinary tract infection, vomiting and weight gain.

Time Course Of Onset Of Adverse Events

Of the most frequently reported adverse events, asthenia, somnolence and dizziness appeared to occur predominantly during the first 4 weeks of treatment with Keppra®.

Discontinuation Or Dose Reduction In Well-Controlled Clinical Studies

In well-controlled clinical studies, 15.0% of patients receiving Keppra® and 11.6% receiving placebo either discontinued or had a dose reduction as a result of an adverse event. The adverse events most commonly associated (>1%) with discontinuation or dose reduction in either treatment group are presented in Table 5.

Table 5: Adverse Events Most Commonly Associated With Discontinuation Or Dose Reduction In Placebo-Controlled Studies In Patients With Epilepsy

	Number (%)	
	Keppra® (N=769)	Placebo (N=439)
Asthenia	10 (1.3%)	3 (0.7%)
Convulsion	23 (3.0%)	15 (3.4%)
Dizziness	11 (1.4%)	0
Somnolence	34 (4.4%)	7 (1.6%)
Rash	0	5 (1.1%)

$$CLcr = \frac{[140\text{-age (years)}] \times \text{weight (kg)}}{72 \times \text{serum creatinine (mg/dL)}} \quad (\times\ 0.85 \text{ for female patients})$$

Table 6: Dosing Adjustment Regimen for Patients with Impaired Renal Function

Group	Creatinine Clearance (mL/min)	Dosage (mg)	Frequency
Normal	>80	500 to 1,500	Every 12 h
Mild	50–80	500 to 1,000	Every 12 h
Moderate	30–50	250 to 750	Every 12 h
Severe	< 30	250 to 500	Every 12 h
ESRD patients using dialysis	—	500 to 1,000	[1]Every 24 h

[1]Following dialysis, a 250 to 500 mg supplemental dose is recommended.

Comparison Of Gender, Age And Race

The overall adverse experience profile of Keppra® was similar between females and males. There are insufficient data to support a statement regarding the distribution of adverse experience reports by age and race.

Postmarketing Experience

In addition to the adverse experiences listed above, the following have been reported in patients receiving marketed Keppra® worldwide. The listing is alphabetized: alopecia, leukopenia, neutropenia, pancreatitis, pancytopenia (with or without bone marrow depression) and thrombocytopenia. These adverse experiences have not been listed above, and data are insufficient to support an estimate of their incidence or to establish causation.

DRUG ABUSE AND DEPENDENCE

The abuse and dependence potential of Keppra® has not been evaluated in human studies.

OVERDOSAGE

Signs, Symptoms And Laboratory Findings Of Acute Overdosage In Humans

The highest known dose of Keppra® received in the clinical development program was 6000 mg/day. Other than drowsiness, there were no adverse events in the few known cases of overdose in clinical trials. Cases of somnolence, agitation, aggression, depressed level of consciousness, respiratory depression and coma were observed with Keppra® overdoses in postmarketing use.

Treatment Or Management Of Overdose

There is no specific antidote for overdose with Keppra®. If indicated, elimination of unabsorbed drug should be attempted by emesis or gastric lavage; usual precautions should be observed to maintain airway. General supportive care of the patient is indicated including monitoring of vital signs and observation of the patient's clinical status. A Certified Poison Control Center should be contacted for up to date information on the management of overdose with Keppra®.

Hemodialysis

Standard hemodialysis procedures result in significant clearance of levetiracetam (approximately 50% in 4 hours) and should be considered in cases of overdose. Although hemodialysis has not been performed in the few known cases of overdose, it may be indicated by the patient's clinical state or in patients with significant renal impairment.

DOSAGE AND ADMINISTRATION

Keppra® is indicated as adjunctive treatment of partial onset seizures in adults with epilepsy.

In clinical trials, daily doses of 1000 mg, 2000 mg, and 3000 mg, given as twice-daily dosing, were shown to be effective. Although in some studies there was a tendency toward greater response with higher dose (see CLINICAL STUDIES), a consistent increase in response with increased dose has not been shown.

Treatment should be initiated with a daily dose of 1000 mg/day, given as twice-daily dosing (500 mg BID). Additional dosing increments may be given (1000 mg/day additional every 2 weeks) to a maximum recommended daily dose of 3000 mg. Doses greater than 3000 mg/day have been used in open-label studies for periods of 6 months and longer. There is no evidence that doses greater than 3000 mg/day confer additional benefit.

Keppra® is given orally with or without food.

Patients With Impaired Renal Function

Keppra® dosing must be individualized according to the patient's renal function status. Recommended doses and adjustment for dose are shown in Table 6. To use this dosing table, an estimate of the patient's creatinine clearance (CLcr) in mL/min is needed. CLcr in mL/min may be estimated from serum creatinine (mg/dL) determination using the following formula:

[See first table above]

[See table 6 above]

HOW SUPPLIED

Keppra® (levetiracetam) tablets, 250 mg are blue, oblong-shaped, scored, film-coated tablets debossed with "ucb" and "250" on one side. They are supplied in containers of 120 tablets (NDC 50474-591-40).

Keppra® (levetiracetam) tablets, 500 mg are yellow, oblong-shaped, scored, film-coated tablets debossed with "ucb" and "500" on one side. They are supplied in containers of 120 tablets (NDC 50474-592-40).

Keppra® (levetiracetam) tablets, 750 mg are orange, oblong-shaped, scored, film-coated tablets debossed with "ucb" and "750" on one side. They are supplied in containers of 120 tablets (NDC 50474-593-40).

Keppra® (levetiracetam) oral solution 100 mg/mL is a clear, colorless, grape-flavored liquid. It is supplied in 16 fl oz white HDPE bottles (NDC 50474-001-48).

STORAGE

Store at 25°C (77°F); excursions permitted to 15-30°C (59-86°F).

[see USP Controlled Room Temperature]

FOR MEDICAL INFORMATION

Contact: Medical Affairs Department
Phone: (800) 477-7877
Fax: (770) 970-8859

Tablets Manufactured by
UCB S.A.
B-1420 Braine-l'Alleud (Belgium)
Oral Solution Manufactured by
Mallinckrodt Inc.
Hobart, NY 13788
For UCB Pharma, Inc.
Smyrna, GA 30080

PATIENT INFORMATION

KEPPRA® (pronounced *KEPP-ruh*) (levetiracetam) 250 mg, 500 mg and 750 mg tablets and 100 mg/mL oral solution

Read the Patient Information that comes with KEPPRA® before you start using it and each time you get a refill. There may be new information. This leaflet does not take the place of talking with your healthcare provider about your condition or your treatment.

Before taking your medicine, make sure you have received the correct medicine. Compare the name above with the name on your bottle and the appearance of your medicine with the description of KEPPRA® provided below. Contact your pharmacist immediately if you believe a dispensing error may have occurred.

What is KEPPRA®?

KEPPRA® is a medicine that is used to treat partial seizures in adults with epilepsy. It is used with other seizure medicines to help control your seizures. KEPPRA® comes in tablets and in liquid.

250 mg KEPPRA® tablets are blue, oblong-shaped, scored, film-coated tablets marked with "ucb" and "250" on one side.

500 mg KEPPRA® tablets are yellow, oblong-shaped, scored, film-coated tablets marked with "ucb" and "500" on one side.

750 mg KEPPRA® tablets are orange, oblong-shaped, scored, film-coated tablets marked with "ucb" and "750" on one side.

KEPPRA® oral solution is a clear, colorless, grape-flavored liquid.

Who should not take KEPPRA®?

Do not take KEPPRA® if you are allergic to any of its ingredients. The active ingredient is levetiracetam. See the end of this leaflet for a list of all the ingredients in KEPPRA®.

Tell your healthcare provider:

- **if you are pregnant or planning to become pregnant.** If you use KEPPRA® while you are pregnant, ask your healthcare provider about being in the Antiepileptic Drug Pregnancy Registry. You can join this registry by calling (888) 233-2334.
- **if you are breast feeding.** KEPPRA® can pass into your milk and may harm your baby. You should choose to either take KEPPRA® or breast feed, but not both.
- **if you have kidney disease.** You may need a lower dose of KEPPRA®.
- **about all the medicines you take,** including prescription, nonprescription, vitamins, and herbal supplements.

KEPPRA® has not been approved for children below the age of 16.

How should I take KEPPRA®?

- Take KEPPRA® exactly as prescribed. KEPPRA® is usually taken twice a day. Once in the morning and once at night. Take KEPPRA® at the same times each day.
- Your healthcare provider may start you on a lower dose of KEPPRA® and increase it as your body gets used to the medicine.

Continued on next page

Keppra—Cont.

- Take KEPPRA® with or without food. Swallow the tablets whole. Do not chew or crush tablets. Use the KEPPRA® oral solution if you cannot swallow tablets. Use a medicine dropper or medicine cup to measure KEPPRA® oral solution. **Do not use a teaspoon.** Ask your pharmacist for a medicine dropper or medicine cup to help you measure KEPPRA®.
- If you take too much KEPPRA® or overdose, call your local Poison Control Center or emergency room right away.
- Do not stop taking KEPPRA® or any other seizure medicine unless your healthcare provider told you to. Stopping a seizure medicine all at once can cause status epilepticus (seizures that will not stop), a very serious problem.
- Tell your healthcare provider if your seizures get worse or if you have any new types of seizures.
- Talk to your healthcare provider about what to do if you miss a dose.

What should I avoid while taking KEPPRA®?
Do not drive, operate complex machinery or participate in other hazardous activities until you know how KEPPRA® affects you. KEPPRA® may make you dizzy or sleepy.

What are the possible side effects of KEPPRA®?
KEPPRA® may cause the following serious problems. Call your healthcare provider right away if you get any of the following symptoms:

- **Extreme sleepiness, tiredness, and weakness.**
- **Problems with muscle coordination** (problems walking and moving).
- **Mood and behavior changes** such as aggression, agitation, anger, anxiety, apathy, depression, hostility, and irritability. Some people may get psychotic symptoms such as hallucinations (seeing or hearing things that are really not there). Some people may get thoughts of suicide (thoughts of killing yourself).

The most common side effects with KEPPRA® are:

- sleepiness
- weakness
- dizziness
- infection

These side effects could happen at any time but happen most often within the first four weeks of treatment except for infection.
These are not all the side effects of KEPPRA®. For more information, ask your healthcare provider or pharmacist. If you get any side effects that concern you, call your healthcare provider.

General information about KEPPRA®.
Medicines are sometimes prescribed for conditions other than those described in patient information leaflets. Do not use KEPPRA® for a condition for which it was not prescribed. Do not give your KEPPRA® to other people, even if they have the same symptoms that you have. It may harm them.
Store KEPPRA® at room temperature away from heat and light. **Keep KEPPRA® and all medicines out of the reach of children.**
This leaflet summarizes the most important information about KEPPRA®. If you would like more information, talk with your healthcare provider. You can ask your healthcare provider or pharmacist for information about KEPPRA® that is written for healthcare professionals. You can also get information about KEPPRA® at www.keppra.com.

What are the ingredients of KEPPRA®?
KEPPRA® tablets contain the labeled amount of levetiracetam. Inactive ingredients: colloidal silicon dioxide, corn starch, hydroxypropyl methylcellulose, magnesium stearate, polyethylene glycol 4000, povidone, talc, titanium dioxide and coloring agents.
The individual tablets contain the following coloring agents:
250 mg tablets: FD&C Blue No. 2,
500 mg tablets: yellow iron oxide,
750 mg tablets: FD&C Blue No. 2, FD&C Yellow No. 6 and red iron oxide.
KEPPRA® oral solution contains 100 mg of levetiracetam per mL. Inactive ingredients: ammonium glycyrrhizinate, citric acid monohydrate, glycerin, maltitol solution, methylparaben, potassium acesulfame, propylparaben, purified water, sodium citrate dihydrate and natural and artificial flavor.
KEPPRA® does not contain lactose or gluten. It does contain carbohydrates. The liquid is dye-free.

Rx Only
This patient leaflet has been approved by the US Food and Drug Administration.
Distributed by
UCB Pharma, Inc.
Smyrna, GA 30080

Printed in USA
Rev. 11E 10/2003

Shown in Product Identification Guide, page 334

LORTAB® ELIXIR Ⓒ℞

[lōr-tăb]
Hydrocodone Bitartrate and Acetaminophen Oral Solution
7.5 mg/500 mg per 15 mL
Rx only

DESCRIPTION

Hydrocodone bitartrate and acetaminophen is supplied in liquid form for oral administration.

WARNING: May be habit forming (see PRECAUTIONS, Information for Patients, and DRUG ABUSE AND DEPENDENCE).

Hydrocodone bitartrate is an opioid analgesic and antitussive and occurs as fine, white crystals or as a crystalline powder. It is affected by light. The chemical name is 4,5α-epoxy-3-methoxy-17-methylmorphinan-6-one tartrate (1:1) hydrate (2:5). It has the following structural formula:

$C_{18}H_{21}NO_3 \cdot C_4H_6O_6 \cdot 2\frac{1}{2}H_2O$ M.W. 494.490

Acetaminophen, 4'-hydroxyacetanilide, a slightly bitter, white, odorless, crystalline powder, is a non-opiate, non-salicylate analgesic and antipyretic. It has the following structural formula:

$C_8H_9NO_2$ MW = 151.16

Lortab Elixir contains:	Per 5 mL	Per 15 mL
Hydrocodone Bitartrate	2.5 mg	7.5 mg
Acetaminophen	167 mg	500 mg
Alcohol	7%	7%

In addition, the liquid contains the following inactive ingredients: citric acid anhydrous, ethyl maltol, glycerin, methylparaben, propylene glycol, propylparaben, purified water, saccharin sodium, sorbitol solution, sucrose, with D&C Yellow #10 and FD&C Yellow #6 as coloring and natural and artificial flavoring.

CLINICAL PHARMACOLOGY

Hydrocodone is a semisynthetic narcotic analgesic and antitussive with multiple actions qualitatively similar to those of codeine. Most of these involve the central nervous system and smooth muscle. The precise mechanism of action of hydrocodone and other opiates is not known, although it is believed to relate to the existence of opiate receptors in the central nervous system. In addition to analgesia, narcotics may produce drowsiness, changes in mood and mental clouding.
The analgesic action of acetaminophen involves peripheral influences, but the specific mechanism is as yet undetermined. Antipyretic activity is mediated through hypothalamic heat regulating centers. Acetaminophen inhibits prostaglandin synthetase. Therapeutic doses of acetaminophen have negligible effects on the cardiovascular or respiratory systems; however, toxic doses may cause circulatory failure and rapid, shallow breathing.

Pharmacokinetics
The behavior of the individual components is described below.

Hydrocodone
Following a 10 mg oral dose of hydrocodone administered to five adult male subjects, the mean peak concentration was 23.6 ± 5.2 ng/mL. Maximum serum levels were achieved at 1.3 ± 0.3 hours and the half-life was determined to be 3.8 ± 0.3 hours. Hydrocodone exhibits a complex pattern of metabolism including O-demethylation, N-demethylation and 6-keto reduction to the corresponding 6-α- and 6-β-hydroxymetabolites.
See OVERDOSAGE for toxicity information.

Acetaminophen
Acetaminophen is rapidly absorbed from the gastrointestinal tract and is distributed throughout most body tissues. The plasma half-life is 1.25 to 3 hours, but may be increased by liver damage and following overdosage. Elimination of acetaminophen is principally by liver metabolism (conjugation) and subsequent renal excretion of metabolites. Approximately 85% of an oral dose appears in the urine within 24 hours of administration, most as the glucuronide conjugate, with small amounts of other conjugates and unchanged drug.
See OVERDOSAGE for toxicity information.

INDICATIONS AND USAGE

Lortab Elixir (hydrocodone bitartrate and acetaminophen oral solution) is indicated for the relief of moderate to moderately severe pain.

CONTRAINDICATIONS

This product should not be administered to patients who have previously exhibited hypersensitivity to hydrocodone, acetaminophen, or any other component of this product.
Patients known to be hypersensitive to other opioids may exhibit cross sensitivity to hydrocodone.

WARNINGS

Respiratory Depression
At high doses or in sensitive patients, hydrocodone may produce dose-related respiratory depression by acting directly on the brain stem respiratory center. Hydrocodone also affects the center that controls respiratory rhythm, and may produce irregular and periodic breathing.
Infants may have increased sensitivity to the respiratory depressant effects of opioids (see PRECAUTIONS, Pediatric Use). If use of Lortab Elixir in such patients is contemplated, it should be administered cautiously, in substantially reduced initial doses, by personnel experienced in administering opioids to infants, and with intensive monitoring.

Head Injury and Increased Intracranial Pressure
The respiratory depressant effects of narcotics and their capacity to elevate cerebrospinal fluid pressure may be markedly exaggerated in the presence of head injury, other intracranial lesions or a preexisting increase in intracranial pressure. Furthermore, narcotics produce adverse reactions, which may obscure the clinical course of patients with head injuries.

Acute Abdominal Conditions
The administration of narcotics may obscure the diagnosis or clinical course of patients with acute abdominal conditions.

PRECAUTIONS

General
Special Risk Patients
As with any narcotic analgesic agent, Lortab Elixir should be used with caution in elderly or debilitated patients, and those with severe impairment of hepatic or renal function, hypothyroidism, Addison's disease, prostatic hypertrophy or urethral stricture. The usual precautions should be observed and the possibility of respiratory depression should be kept in mind.

Cough Reflex
Hydrocodone suppresses the cough reflex; as with all narcotics, caution should be exercised when Lortab Elixir are used postoperatively and in patients with pulmonary disease.

Information for Patients
Hydrocodone, like all narcotics, may impair mental and/or physical abilities required for the performance of potentially hazardous tasks such as driving a car or operating machinery. Such tasks should be avoided while taking this product.
Alcohol and other CNS depressants may produce an additive CNS depression, when taken with this combination product, and should be avoided.
Hydrocodone may be habit-forming. Patients should take the drug only for as long as it is prescribed, in the amounts prescribed, and no more frequently than prescribed.
Physicians should instruct patients and caregivers to read the patient information leaflet, which appears as the last section of the labeling.

Laboratory Tests
In patients with severe hepatic or renal disease, effects of therapy should be monitored with serial liver and/or renal function tests.

Drug Interactions
Patients receiving narcotics, antihistamines, antipsychotics, antianxiety agents, or other CNS depressants (including alcohol) concomitantly with hydrocodone bitartrate and acetaminophen oral solution may exhibit an additive CNS depression. When combined therapy is contemplated, the dose of one or both agents should be reduced.
The use of MAO inhibitors or tricyclic antidepressants with hydrocodone preparations may increase the effect of either the antidepressant or hydrocodone.

Drug/Laboratory Test Interactions
Acetaminophen may produce false-positive test results for urinary 5-hydroxyindoleacetic acid.

Carcinogenesis, Mutagenesis, Impairment of Fertility
No adequate studies have been conducted in animals to determine whether hydrocodone has a potential for carcinogenesis, mutagenesis, or impairment of fertility.
Hydrocodone has not demonstrated mutagenic potential using the Ames Salmonella-Microsomal Activation test, the Basc test on Drosophila germ cells, and the Micronucleus test on mouse bone marrow.
No adequate studies have been conducted in animals to determine whether acetaminophen has a potential for carcinogenesis, mutagenesis, or impairment of fertility.
Acetaminophen has not demonstrated mutagenic potential using the Ames Salmonella-Microsomal Activation test, the Basc test on Drosophila germ cells, and the Micronucleus test on mouse bone marrow.

Pregnancy
Teratogenic Effects
Pregnancy Category C
There are no adequate and well-controlled studies in pregnant women. Lortab Elixir should be used during pregnancy only if the potential benefit justifies the potential risk to the fetus.

Nonteratogenic Effects
Babies born to mothers who have been taking opioids regularly prior to delivery will be physically dependent. The withdrawal signs include irritability and excessive crying, tremors, hyperactive reflexes, increased respiratory rate, increased stools, sneezing yawning, vomiting and fever. These signs usually appear during the first few days of life. The intensity of the syndrome does not always correlate with the duration of maternal opioid use or dose. There is no consensus on the best method of managing withdrawal.

Labor and Delivery
Narcotic analgesics cross the placental barrier. The closer to delivery and the larger the dose used, the greater the pos-

sibility of respiratory depression in the newborn. Narcotic analgesics should be avoided during labor if delivery of a premature infant is anticipated. If the mother has received narcotic analgesics during labor, newborn infants should be observed closely for signs of respiratory depression. Resuscitation may be required (see OVERDOSAGE). The effect of hydrocodone, if any, on the later growth, development, and functional maturation of the child is unknown.

Nursing Mothers

Acetaminophen is excreted in breast milk in small amounts, but the significance of its effects on nursing infants is not known. It is not known whether hydrocodone is excreted in human milk. Because many drugs are excreted in human milk and because of the potential for serious adverse reactions in nursing infants from hydrocodone and acetaminophen, a decision should be made whether to discontinue nursing or to discontinue the drug, taking into account the importance of the drug to the mother.

Pediatric Use

Safety and effectiveness in the pediatric population below the age of two years have not been established. Use of Lortab Elixir in the pediatric population is supported by the evidence from adequate and well controlled studies of hydrocodone and acetaminophen combination products in adults with additional data which support the development of metabolic pathways in children two years of age and over (see DOSAGE AND ADMINISTRATION for pediatric dosage information).

Geriatric Use

Clinical studies of hydrocodone bitartrate and acetaminophen oral solution did not include sufficient numbers of subjects aged 65 and over to determine whether they respond differently from younger subjects. Other reported clinical experience has not identified differences in responses between the elderly and younger patients. In general, dose selection for an elderly patient should be cautious, usually starting at the low end of the dosing range, reflecting the greater frequency of decreased hepatic, renal, or cardiac function, and of concomitant disease or other drug therapy. Hydrocodone and the major metabolites of acetaminophen are known to be substantially excreted by the kidney. Thus the risk of toxic reactions may be greater in patients with impaired renal function due to the accumulation of the parent compound and/or metabolites in the plasma. Because elderly patients are more likely to have decreased renal function, care should be taken in dose selection, and it may be useful to monitor renal function.

Hydrocodone may cause confusion and over-sedation in the elderly; elderly patients generally should be started on low doses of hydrocodone bitartrate and acetaminophen oral solution and observed closely.

ADVERSE REACTIONS

Potential effects of high dosage are also listed in the OVERDOSAGE section.

Cardio-renal: Bradycardia, cardiac arrest, circulatory collapse, renal toxicity, renal tubular necrosis, hypotension.

Central Nervous System/Psychiatric: Anxiety, dizziness, drowsiness, dysphoria, euphoria, fear, general malaise, impairment of mental and physical performance, lethargy, light-headedness, mental clouding, mood changes, psychological dependence, sedation, somnolence progressing to stupor or coma.

Endocrine: Hypoglycemic coma.

Gastrointestinal System: Abdominal pain, constipation, gastric distress, heartburn, hepatic necrosis, hepatitis, occult blood loss, nausea, peptic ulcer, and vomiting.

Genitourinary System: Spasm of vesical sphincters, ureteral spasm, and urinary retention.

Hematologic: Agranulocytosis, hemolytic anemia, iron deficiency anemia, prolonged bleeding time, thrombocytopenia.

Hypersensitivity: Allergic reactions.

Musculoskeletal: Skeletal muscle flaccidity.

Respiratory Depression: Acute airway obstruction, apnea, dose-related respiratory depression (see OVERDOSAGE), shortness of breath.

Special Senses: Cases of hearing impairment or permanent loss have been reported predominantly in patients with chronic overdose.

Skin: Cold and clammy skin, diaphoresis, pruritus, rash.

DRUG ABUSE AND DEPENDENCE

Controlled Substance

Lortab Elixir (hydrocodone bitartrate and acetaminophen oral solution) is classified as a Schedule III controlled substance.

Abuse and Dependence

Hydrocodone can produce drug dependence of the morphine type and, therefore, has the potential for being abused. Psychological dependence, physical dependence, and tolerance may develop upon repeated administration of narcotics; therefore, this product should be prescribed and administered with caution appropriate to the use of other oral narcotic medications. However, psychological dependence is unlikely to develop when hydrocodone bitartrate and acetaminophen oral solution are used for a short time for the treatment of pain.

Physical dependence, the condition in which continued administration of the drug is required to prevent the appearance of a withdrawal syndrome, assumes clinically significant proportions only after several weeks of continued narcotic use, although some mild degree of physical dependence may develop after a few days of narcotic therapy. Tolerance, in which increasingly large doses are required in order to produce the same degree of analgesia, is manifested initially by a shortened duration of analgesic effect, and subsequently by decreases in the intensity of analgesia. The rate of development of tolerance varies among patients.

OVERDOSAGE

Following an acute overdosage, toxicity may result from hydrocodone or acetaminophen.

Signs and Symptoms

Toxicity from hydrocodone poisoning includes the opioid triad of loss of consciousness, pinpoint pupils, and respiratory depression (Cheyne-Stokes respiration, cyanosis, decrease in respiratory rate and/or tidal volume). Convulsions may occur.

The toxic dose of acetaminophen for adults is 10 grams. In adults, hepatic toxicity has rarely been reported with acute overdoses of less than 10 grams, or fatalities with less than 15 grams.

Early symptoms following a potentially hepatotoxic overdose of acetaminophen may include diaphoresis, general malaise, nausea, and vomiting. Clinical and laboratory evidence of hepatic toxicity may not be apparent until 48 to 72 hours post-ingestion.

Other signs and symptoms of overdose of this product include bradycardia, cold and clammy skin, extreme somnolence progressing to stupor or coma, hypoglycemic coma, hypotension, renal tubular necrosis, skeletal muscle flaccidity, thrombocytopenia.

In severe overdosage, apnea; circulatory collapse; cardiac arrest; dose-dependent, potentially fatal hepatic necrosis; and death may occur.

Treatment

A single or multiple overdose with hydrocodone and acetaminophen is a potentially lethal polydrug overdose, and consultation with a regional poison control center is recommended.

Immediate treatment includes support of cardiorespiratory function and measures to reduce drug absorption. Vomiting should be induced with syrup of ipecac, if the patient is alert (adequate pharyngeal and laryngeal reflexes). Oral activated charcoal (1 g/kg) should follow gastric emptying. The first dose should be accompanied by an appropriate cathartic. If repeated doses are used, the cathartic might be included with alternate doses as required. Hypotension is usually hypovolemic and should respond to fluids. Vasopressors and other supportive measures should be employed as indicated. A cuffed endo-tracheal tube should be inserted before gastric lavage of the unconscious patient and, when necessary, to provide assisted respiration.

Meticulous attention should be given to maintaining adequate pulmonary ventilation. In severe cases of intoxication, peritoneal dialysis, or preferably hemodialysis may be considered. If hypoprothrombinemia occurs due to acetaminophen overdose, vitamin K should be administered intravenously.

Naloxone, a narcotic antagonist, can reverse respiratory depression and coma associated with opioid overdose. Naloxone hydrochloride 0.4 mg to 2 mg is given parenterally. Since the duration of action of hydrocodone may exceed that of the naloxone, the patient should be kept under continuous surveillance and repeated doses of the antagonist should be administered as needed to maintain adequate respiration. A narcotic antagonist should not be administered in the absence of clinically significant respiratory or cardiovascular depression.

If the dose of acetaminophen may have exceeded 140 mg/kg, acetylcysteine should be administered as early as possible. Serum acetaminophen levels should be obtained, since levels four or more hours following ingestion help predict acetaminophen toxicity. Do not await acetaminophen assay results before initiating treatment. Hepatic enzymes should be obtained initially, and repeated at 24-hour intervals.

Methemoglobinemia over 30% should be treated with methylene blue by slow intravenous administration.

DOSAGE AND ADMINISTRATION

Dosage should be adjusted according to severity of pain and response of the patient. However, it should be kept in mind that tolerance to hydrocodone can develop with continued use and that the incidence of untoward effects is dose related.

The usual adult dosage is one tablespoonful every 4 to 6 hours as needed for pain. The total daily dosage for adults should not exceed 6 tablespoonfuls. The usual dosages for children are given by the table below, and are to be given every 4 to 6 hours as needed for pain. These dosages correspond to an average individual dose of 0.27 mL/kg of Lortab Elixir (providing 0.135 mg/kg of hydrocodone bitartrate and 9 mg/kg of acetaminophen). Dosing should be based on weight whenever possible.

BODY WEIGHT	APPROXIMATE AGE	DOSE Every 4 to 6 hours	MAXIMUM TOTAL DAILY DOSE (6 doses per day)
12 to 15 kg 27 to 34 lbs.	2 to 3 years	¾ teaspoonful = 3.75 mL	4½ teaspoonfuls = 22.5 mL
16 to 22 kg 35 to 50 lbs.	4 to 6 years	1 teaspoonful = 5 mL	6 teaspoonfuls = 30 mL
23 to 31 kg 51 to 69 lbs.	7 to 9 years	1½ teaspoonfuls = 7.5 mL	9 teaspoonfuls = 45 mL
32 to 45 kg 70 to 100 lbs.	10 to 13 years	2 teaspoonfuls = 10 mL	12 teaspoonfuls = 60 mL
46 kg and up 101 lbs. and up	14 years to adult	1 Tablespoonful = 15 mL	6 Tablespoonfuls = 90 mL

[See first table above]

BODY WEIGHT	APPROXIMATE AGE	DOSE Every 4 to 6 hours	MAXIMUM TOTAL DAILY DOSE (6 doses per day)
12 to 15 kg 27 to 34 lbs.	2 to 3 years	¾ teaspoonful = 3.75 mL	4½ teaspoonfuls = 22.5 mL
16 to 22 kg 35 to 50 lbs.	4 to 6 years	1 teaspoonful = 5 mL	6 teaspoonfuls = 30 mL
23 to 31 kg 51 to 69 lbs.	7 to 9 years	1½ teaspoonfuls = 7.5 mL	9 teaspoonfuls = 45 mL
32 to 45 kg 70 to 100 lbs.	10 to 13 years	2 teaspoonfuls = 10 mL	12 teaspoonfuls = 60 mL
46 kg and up 101 lbs. and up	14 years to adult	1 Tablespoonful = 15 mL	6 Tablespoonfuls = 90 mL

The total daily dosage for children should not exceed 6 doses per day. It is of utmost importance that the dose of Lortab Elixir be administered accurately. A household teaspoon or tablespoon is not an adequate measuring device, especially when one-half or three-fourths of a teaspoonful is to be measured. Given the inexactitude of the household spoon measure and the possibility of using a tablespoon instead of a teaspoon, which could lead to overdosage, it is strongly recommended that care givers obtain and use a calibrated measuring device. Health care providers should recommend a dropper that can measure and deliver the prescribed dose accurately, and instruct care givers to use extreme caution in measuring the dosage.

HOW SUPPLIED

Lortab ® Elixir (hydrocodone bitartrate and acetaminophen oral solution) is a yellow-colored tropical fruit punch flavored liquid containing hydrocodone bitartrate 7.5 mg and acetaminophen 500 mg per 15 mL, with 7% alcohol. It is supplied in containers of 1 pint (473 mL) NDC 50474-909-16

STORAGE

Store at 20 to 25° C (68 to 77° F). [see USP Controlled Room Temperature] Dispense in a tight, light-resistant container with a child-resistant closure.

A schedule CIII Narcotic.

Manufactured for
UCB Pharma, Inc.
Smyrna, GA 30080
Manufactured by
Mikart Inc.
Atlanta, GA 30318

Continued on next page

Lortab Elixir—Cont.

Patient Information Leaflet
LORTAB® ELIXIR ©III
(Hydrocodone Bitartrate and Acetaminophen Oral Solution)
7.5 mg/500 mg per 15 mL
Summary

Lortab (pronounced LOR-tab) is used to relieve moderate to moderately severe pain. You should not take Lortab Elixir if you are allergic to hydrocodone or acetaminophen. The most common side effects of Lortab Elixir are abdominal pain, dizziness, drowsiness, light-headedness, nausea, shortness of breath, unusual tiredness, and vomiting. Take this medicine as directed by your doctor. Do not take more of it, do not take it more often, and do not take it for a longer time than your doctor ordered.

Uses
Lortab Elixir is an analgesic used to relieve moderate to moderately severe pain. Lortab Elixir is a combination product containing hydrocodone (hye-droe-KO-done) bitartrate and acetaminophen (a-seat-a-MIN-oh-fen). Hydrocodone is a narcotic pain reliever and a cough suppressant. Acetaminophen is a non-narcotic pain reliever and fever reducer. A narcotic analgesic and acetaminophen used together may provide better pain relief than either product used alone. If you have any questions, please call your doctor or pharmacist.

General Cautions
- Do not take this drug if you have allergies or unusual reactions to narcotic pain relievers or acetaminophen because it is likely that you may also be allergic to Lortab Elixir.
- This product may inhibit your mental and physical abilities required for the performance of potentially hazardous tasks such as driving a car or operating machinery. Such tasks should be avoided while you are taking this product.
- This medicine may not be right for you. Check with your doctor or pharmacist, if you:
  - are pregnant.
  - are nursing.
  - are taking other medications; narcotic pain relievers; allergy medicines; antidepressant medicines; acetaminophen-containing medicines or other medicines that cause central nervous system depression, including alcohol.
  - have other medical problems: a history of drug or alcohol abuse; recent head injury; emphysema, asthma, or other chronic lung disease; liver disease, kidney disease; underactive thyroid, Addison's disease, enlarged prostate or difficulty urinating.

Proper Use
Take this medicine as directed by your doctor. Do not share it with anyone else. This medicine can cause drug dependence and has the potential for abuse. Do not take more of it, do not take it more often, and do not take it for a longer time than your doctor ordered. If you think that this medicine is not working properly after taking it for some time, do not increase the dose. Check with your doctor or pharmacist.

Dosing
The dose of this medication will be different for different patients. Follow the directions provided by your doctor. The following information includes only the average doses of this medication. *If your dose is different, do not change doses unless your doctor tells you to do so.*
[See second table at top of previous page]
It is very important that Lortab Elixir be dosed accurately. A household teaspoon or tablespoon is not an accurate measuring device, especially when one-half or three-fourths of a teaspoonful is to be measured.
Since a household teaspoon is not accurate and can be mixed-up with a tablespoon (which can cause overdosage), it is strongly recommended that you obtain and use a proper measuring device. Ask your doctor or pharmacist for help to find a dropper that can measure the needed dose properly and ask for help if you do not understand how to use the dropper.

Missed Dose
- To avoid a possible overdose, it is important that you do not take more than a single dosage at one time, or that you don't take doses at intervals less than 4 hours apart.
- If you miss taking a dose of Lortab Elixir, take it as soon as you remember. However, make sure to wait at least 4 hours before taking your next dose.
- If you missed taking a dose, and it is almost time for your next dose, skip the missed dose and take your medicine as scheduled.
- Do not double the prescribed dose.

Possible Side Effects
Side effects you may experience include abdominal pain, constipation, difficulty urinating, dizziness, drowsiness, fear, fuzzy thinking, general feeling of discomfort or illness, light-headedness, mood changes, nausea, nervousness, rash, shortness of breath, slower reactions, unusual tiredness, and vomiting.
Call your doctor if these effects continue or are bothersome.
Side effects not listed above may sometimes occur. If you notice any other effects, check with your doctor.

Storage
- Keep out of the reach of children.
- Store at room temperature (protect from heat, do not refrigerate).
- Keep in original labeled bottle.
- Discard medicines that are old or no longer needed.
- Even a single overdose of this medicine may be a life-threatening situation. If you suspect that you or someone else may have taken more than the prescribed dose of this medicine, contact your local poison control center or emergency room immediately. This medicine was prescribed for your particular condition. Do not use if for another condition or give the drug to others.
- This leaflet provides a summary of information about Lortab Elixir. If you have any questions or concerns, or want more information about Lortab Elixir, contact your doctor or pharmacist. Your pharmacist also has a longer leaflet about Lortab Elixir that is written for health professionals that you can ask to read.

Prepared by UCB Pharma, Inc. Rev. 6E 03/2004

LORTAB® TABLETS ©III ℞
Hydrocodone Bitartrate and Acetaminophen Tablets, USP
℞ only

DESCRIPTION
Hydrocodone bitartrate and acetaminophen is supplied in tablet form for oral administration.
WARNING: May be habit forming (see PRECAUTIONS, Information for Patients, and DRUG ABUSE AND DEPENDENCE).
Hydrocodone bitartrate is an opioid analgesic and antitussive and occurs as fine, white crystals or as a crystalline powder. It is affected by light. The chemical name is 4,5α-epoxy-3-methoxy-17-methylmorphinan-6-one tartrate (1:1) hydrate (2:5). It has the following structural formula:

$C_{18}H_{21}NO_3 \cdot C_4H_6O_6 \cdot 2^1/_2H_2O$ M.W. 494.490

Acetaminophen, 4′-hydroxyacetanilide, a slightly bitter, white, odorless, crystalline powder, is a non-opiate, non-salicylate analgesic and antipyretic. It has the following structural formula:

$C_8H_9NO_2$ M.W. 151.16

Each Lortab 2.5/500 tablet contains:
Hydrocodone Bitartrate .... 2.5 mg
Acetaminophen .... 500 mg
In addition, each tablet contains the following inactive ingredients: colloidal silicon dioxide, croscarmellose sodium, crospovidone, microcrystalline cellulose, povidone, pregelatinized starch, stearic acid and sugar spheres which are composed of starch derived from corn, sucrose, and FD&C Red #3. Meets USP dissolution test 1.

Each Lortab 5/500 tablet contains:
Hydrocodone Bitartrate .... 5 mg
Acetaminophen .... 500 mg
In addition, each tablet contains the following inactive ingredients: cornstarch, FD&C Blue # 1 Lake, gelatin, magnesium stearate, microcrystalline cellulose, povidone, pregelatinized starch, sodium starch glycolate, and sugar spheres. Meets USP dissolution test 1.

Each Lortab 7.5/500 tablet contains:
Hydrocodone Bitartrate .... 7.5 mg
Acetaminophen .... 500 mg
In addition, each tablet contains the following inactive ingredients: colloidal silicon dioxide, croscarmellose sodium, crospovidone, microcrystalline cellulose, povidone, pregelatinized starch, stearic acid, and sugar spheres which are composed of starch derived from corn, sucrose, FD&C Blue #1 and D&C Yellow #10. Meets USP dissolution test 1.

Each Lortab 10/500 tablet contains:
Hydrocodone Bitartrate .... 10 mg
Acetaminophen .... 500 mg
In addition, each tablet contains the following inactive ingredients: D&C Red No. 27 Aluminum Lake, D&C Red No. 30 Aluminum Lake, colloidal silicon dioxide, croscarmellose sodium, crospovidone, microcrystalline cellulose, povidone, pregelatinized starch, starch (corn), and stearic acid. Meets USP dissolution test 1.

CLINICAL PHARMACOLOGY
Hydrocodone is a semisynthetic narcotic analgesic and antitussive with multiple actions qualitatively similar to those of codeine. Most of these involve the central nervous system and smooth muscle. The precise mechanism of action of hydrocodone and other opiates is not known, although it is believed to relate to the existence of opiate receptors in the central nervous system. In addition to analgesia, narcotics may produce drowsiness, changes in mood and mental clouding.
The analgesic action of acetaminophen involves peripheral influences, but the specific mechanism is as yet undetermined. Antipyretic activity is mediated through hypothalamic heat regulating centers. Acetaminophen inhibits prostaglandin synthetase. Therapeutic doses of acetaminophen have negligible effects on the cardiovascular or respiratory systems; however, toxic doses may cause circulatory failure and rapid, shallow breathing.
Pharmacokinetics: The behavior of the individual components is described below.
Hydrocodone: Following a 10 mg oral dose of hydrocodone administered to five adult male subjects, the mean peak concentration was 23.6 ± 5.2 ng/mL. Maximum serum levels were achieved at 1.3 ± 0.3 hours and the half-life was determined to be 3.8 ± 0.3 hours. Hydrocodone exhibits a complex pattern of metabolism including O-demethylation, N-demethylation and 6-keto reduction to the corresponding 6-α- and 6-β-hydroxymetabolites.
See OVERDOSAGE for toxicity information.
Acetaminophen: Acetaminophen is rapidly absorbed from the gastrointestinal tract and is distributed throughout most body tissues. The plasma half-life is 1.25 to 3 hours, but may be increased by liver damage and following overdosage. Elimination of acetaminophen is principally by liver metabolism (conjugation) and subsequent renal excretion of metabolites. Approximately 85% of an oral dose appears in the urine within 24 hours of administration, most as the glucuronide conjugate, with small amounts of other conjugates and unchanged drug.
See OVERDOSAGE for toxicity information.

INDICATIONS AND USAGE
Lortab Tablets are indicated for the relief of moderate to moderately severe pain.

CONTRAINDICATIONS
This product should not be administered to patients who have previously exhibited hypersensitivity to hydrocodone or acetaminophen.
Patients known to be hypersensitive to other opioids may exhibit cross sensitivity to hydrocodone.

WARNINGS
Respiratory Depression: At high doses or in sensitive patients, hydrocodone may produce dose-related respiratory depression by acting directly on the brain stem respiratory center. Hydrocodone also affects the center that controls respiratory rhythm, and may produce irregular and periodic breathing.
Head Injury and Increased Intracranial Pressure: The respiratory depressant effects of narcotics and their capacity to elevate cerebrospinal fluid pressure may be markedly exaggerated in the presence of head injury, other intracranial lesions or a preexisting increase in intracranial pressure. Furthermore, narcotics produce adverse reactions which may obscure the clinical course of patients with head injuries.
Acute Abdominal Conditions: The administration of narcotics may obscure the diagnosis or clinical course of patients with acute abdominal conditions.

PRECAUTIONS
General: Special Risk Patients: As with any narcotic analgesic agent, Lortab Tablets should be used with caution in elderly or debilitated patients, and those with severe impairment of hepatic or renal function, hypothyroidism, Addison's disease, prostatic hypertrophy or urethral stricture. The usual precautions should be observed and the possibility of respiratory depression should be kept in mind.
Cough Reflex: Hydrocodone suppresses the cough reflex; as with all narcotics, caution should be exercised when Lortab Tablets are used postoperatively and in patients with pulmonary disease.
Information for Patients: Hydrocodone, like all narcotics, may impair mental and/or physical abilities required for the performance of potentially hazardous tasks such as driving a car or operating machinery; patients should be cautioned accordingly.
Alcohol and other CNS depressants may produce an additive CNS depression, when taken with this combination product, and should be avoided.
Hydrocodone may be habit-forming. Patients should take the drug only for as long as it is prescribed, in the amounts prescribed, and no more frequently than prescribed.
Laboratory Tests: In patients with severe hepatic or renal disease, effects of therapy should be monitored with serial liver and/or renal function tests.
Drug Interactions: Patients receiving narcotics, antihistamines, antipsychotics, antianxiety agents, or other CNS depressants (including alcohol) concomitantly with hydrocodone bitartrate and acetaminophen tablets may exhibit an additive CNS depression. When combined therapy is contemplated, the dose of one or both agents should be reduced.
The use of MAO inhibitors or tricyclic antidepressants with hydrocodone preparations may increase the effect of either the antidepressant or hydrocodone.
Drug/Laboratory Test Interactions: Acetaminophen may produce false-positive test results for urinary 5-hydroxyindoleacetic acid.
Carcinogenesis, Mutagenesis, Impairment of Fertility: No adequate studies have been conducted in animals to determine whether hydrocodone or acetaminophen have a poten-

tial for carcinogenesis, mutagenesis, or impairment of fertility.

Pregnancy:

Teratogenic Effects: Pregnancy Category C: There are no adequate and well-controlled studies in pregnant women. Lortab Tablets should be used during pregnancy only if the potential benefit justifies the potential risk to the fetus.

Nonteratogenic Effects: Babies born to mothers who have been taking opioids regularly prior to delivery will be physically dependent. The withdrawal signs include irritability and excessive crying, tremors, hyperactive reflexes, increased respiratory rate, increased stools, sneezing, yawning, vomiting, and fever. The intensity of the syndrome does not always correlate with the duration of maternal opioid use or dose. There is no consensus on the best method of managing withdrawal.

Labor and Delivery: As with all narcotics, administration of this product to the mother shortly before delivery may result in some degree of respiratory depression in the newborn, especially if higher doses are used.

Nursing Mothers: Acetaminophen is excreted in breast milk in small amounts, but the significance of its effects on nursing infants is not known. It is not known whether hydrocodone is excreted in human milk. Because many drugs are excreted in human milk and because of the potential for serious adverse reactions in nursing infants from hydrocodone and acetaminophen, a decision should be made whether to discontinue nursing or to discontinue the drug, taking into account the importance of the drug to the mother.

Pediatric Use: Safety and effectiveness in the pediatric population have not been established.

Geriatric Use: Clinical studies of hydrocodone bitartrate and acetaminophen tablets did not include sufficient numbers of subjects aged 65 and over to determine whether they respond differently from younger subjects. Other reported clinical experience has not identified differences in responses between the elderly and younger patients. In general, dose selection for an elderly patient should be cautious, usually starting at the low end of the dosage range, reflecting the greater frequency of decreased hepatic, renal or cardiac function, and of concomitant disease or other drug therapy.

Hydrocodone and the major metabolites of acetaminophen are known to be substantially excreted by the kidney. Thus the risk of toxic reactions may be greater in patients with impaired renal function due to the accumulation of the parent compound and/or metabolites in the plasma. Because elderly patients are more likely to have decreased renal function, care should be taken in dose selection, and it may be useful to monitor renal function.

Hydrocodone may cause confusion and over-sedation in the elderly; elderly patients generally should be started on low doses of hydrocodone bitartrate and acetaminophen tablets and observed closely.

ADVERSE REACTIONS

The most frequently reported adverse reactions are lightheadedness, dizziness, sedation, nausea and vomiting. These effects seem to be more prominent in ambulatory than in non-ambulatory patients, and some of these adverse reactions may be alleviated if the patient lies down.

Other adverse reactions include:

Central Nervous System: Drowsiness, mental clouding, lethargy, impairment of mental and physical performance, anxiety, fear, dysphoria, psychic dependence, mood changes.

Gastrointestinal System: Prolonged administration of Lortab Tablets may produce constipation.

Genitourinary System: Ureteral spasm, spasm of vesical sphincters and urinary retention have been reported with opiates.

Respiratory Depression: Hydrocodone bitartrate may produce dose-related respiratory depression by acting directly on brain stem respiratory centers (see OVERDOSAGE).

Special Senses: Cases of hearing impairment or permanent loss have been reported predominantly in patients with chronic overdose.

Dermatological: Skin rash, pruritus.

The following adverse drug events may be borne in mind as potential effects of acetaminophen: allergic reactions, rash, thrombocytopenia, agranulocytosis.

Potential effects of high dosage are listed in the OVERDOSAGE section.

DRUG ABUSE AND DEPENDENCE

Controlled Substance: Lortab Tablets are classified as Schedule III controlled substances.

Abuse and Dependence: Psychic dependence, physical dependence, and tolerance may develop upon repeated administration of narcotics; therefore, this product should be prescribed and administered with caution. However, psychic dependence is unlikely to develop when hydrocodone bitartrate and acetaminophen tablets are used for a short time for the treatment of pain.

Physical dependence, the condition in which continued administration of the drug is required to prevent the appearance of a withdrawal syndrome, assumes clinically significant proportions only after several weeks of continued narcotic use, although some mild degree of physical dependence may develop after a few days of narcotic therapy. Tolerance, in which increasingly large doses are required in order to produce the same degree of analgesia, is manifested initially by a shortened duration of analgesic effect, and subsequently by decreases in the intensity of analgesia. The rate of development of tolerance varies among patients.

OVERDOSAGE

Following an acute overdosage, toxicity may result from hydrocodone or acetaminophen.

Signs and Symptoms:

Hydrocodone: Serious overdose with hydrocodone is characterized by respiratory depression (a decrease in respiratory rate and/or tidal volume, Cheyne-Stokes respiration, cyanosis) extreme somnolence progressing to stupor or coma, skeletal muscle flaccidity, cold and clammy skin, and sometimes bradycardia and hypotension. In severe overdosage, apnea, circulatory collapse, cardiac arrest and death may occur.

Acetaminophen: In acetaminophen overdosage: dose-dependent, potentially fatal hepatic necrosis is the most serious adverse effect. Renal tubular necrosis, hypoglycemic coma and thrombocytopenia may also occur.

Early symptoms following a potentially hepatotoxic overdose may include: nausea, vomiting, diaphoresis and general malaise. Clinical and laboratory evidence of hepatic toxicity may not be apparent until 48 to 72 hours post-ingestion.

In adults, hepatic toxicity has rarely been reported with acute overdoses of less than 10 grams, or fatalities with less than 15 grams.

Treatment: A single or multiple overdose with hydrocodone and acetaminophen is a potentially lethal polydrug overdose, and consultation with a regional poison control center is recommended.

Immediate treatment includes support of cardiorespiratory function and measures to reduce drug absorption. Vomiting should be induced mechanically, or with syrup of ipecac, if the patient is alert (adequate pharyngeal and laryngeal reflexes). Oral activated charcoal (1 g/kg) should follow gastric emptying. The first dose should be accompanied by an appropriate cathartic. If repeated doses are used, the cathartic might be included with alternate doses as required. Hypotension is usually hypovolemic and should respond to fluids. Vasopressors and other supportive measures should be employed as indicated. A cuffed endo-tracheal tube should be inserted before gastric lavage of the unconscious patient and, when necessary, to provide assisted respiration.

Meticulous attention should be given to maintaining adequate pulmonary ventilation. In severe cases of intoxication, peritoneal dialysis, or preferably hemodialysis may be considered. If hypoprothrombinemia occurs due to acetaminophen overdose, vitamin K should be administered intravenously.

Naloxone, a narcotic antagonist, can reverse respiratory depression and coma associated with opioid overdose. Naloxone hydrochloride 0.4 mg to 2 mg is given parenterally. Since the duration of action of hydrocodone may exceed that of the naloxone, the patient should be kept under continuous surveillance and repeated doses of the antagonist should be administered as needed to maintain adequate respiration. A narcotic antagonist should not be administered in the absence of clinically significant respiratory or cardiovascular depression.

If the dose of acetaminophen may have exceeded 140 mg/kg, acetylcysteine should be administered as early as possible. Serum acetaminophen levels should be obtained, since levels four or more hours following ingestion help predict acetaminophen toxicity. Do not await acetaminophen assay results before initiating treatment. Hepatic enzymes should be obtained initially, and repeated at 24-hour intervals.

Methemoglobinemia over 30% should be treated with methylene blue by slow intravenous administration.

The toxic dose for adults for acetaminophen is 10 g.

DOSAGE AND ADMINISTRATION

Dosage should be adjusted according to severity of pain and response of the patient. However, it should be kept in mind that tolerance to hydrocodone can develop with continued use and that the incidence of untoward effects is dose related.

The usual adult dosage for **Lortab® 2.5/500** tablets is one or two tablets every four to six hours as needed for pain. The total daily dosage should not exceed 8 tablets.

The usual adult dosage for **Lortab® 5/500** tablets is one or two tablets every four to six hours as needed for pain. The total daily dosage should not exceed 8 tablets.

The usual adult dosage for **Lortab® 7.5/500** tablets is one tablet every four to six hours as needed for pain. The total daily dosage should not exceed 6 tablets.

The usual adult dosage for **Lortab® 10/500** tablets is one tablet every four to six hours as needed for pain. The total daily dosage should not exceed 6 tablets.

HOW SUPPLIED

Lortab® 2.5/500 tablets (Hydrocodone Bitartrate and Acetaminophen Tablets, USP, 2.5 mg/500 mg) contain hydrocodone bitartrate 2.5 mg and acetaminophen 500 mg. They are supplied as white with pink specks, capsule-shaped, bisected tablets debossed "ucb" on one side and "901" on the other side, in containers of 100 tablets NDC 50474-925-01 and 500 tablets NDC 50474-925-50.

Lortab® 5/500 tablets (Hydrocodone Bitartrate and Acetaminophen Tablets, USP, 5 mg/500 mg) contain hydrocodone bitartrate 5 mg and acetaminophen 500 mg. They are supplied as white with blue specks, capsule-shaped, bisected tablets debossed "ucb" on one side "902" on the other side, in containers of 100 tablets NDC 50474-902-01, 500 tablets NDC 50474-902-50, and in hospital unit-dose packages of 100 tablets [4×25] NDC 50474-902-60.

Lortab® 7.5/500 tablets (Hydrocodone Bitartrate and Acetaminophen Tablets, USP, 7.5 mg/500 mg) contain hydrocodone bitartrate 7.5 mg and acetaminophen 500 mg. They are supplied as white with green specks, capsule-shaped, bisected tablets debossed "ucb" on one side and "903" on the other side, in containers of 100 tablets NDC 50474-907-01, 500 tablets NDC 50474-907-50, and in hospital unit-dose packages of 100 tablets [4×25] NDC 50474-907-60.

Lortab® 10/500 tablets (Hydrocodone Bitartrate and Acetaminophen Tablets, USP, 10 mg/500 mg) contain hydrocodone bitartrate 10 mg and acetaminophen 500 mg. They are supplied as pink, capsule-shaped, bisected tablets, debossed "ucb" on one side "910" on the other side, in containers of 100 tablets NDC 50474-910-01, 500 tablets NDC 50474-910-50, and in hospital unit-dose packages of 100 tablets [4×25] NDC 50474-910-60.

Storage: Store at 20 to 25°C (68 to 77°F). [see USP Controlled Room Temperature]

Dispense in a tight, light-resistant container with a child-resistant closure.

A Schedule CIII Narcotic.

Manufactured for
UCB Pharma, Inc.
Smyrna, GA 30080

Lortab® 2.5/500, Lortab® 7.5/500
Manufactured by
Mikart, Inc.
Atlanta, GA 30318

Lortab® 5/500, Lortab® 10/500
Manufactured by
Mallinckrodt Inc.
Hobart, New York 13788

3E 03/2004

UCB Pharma, Inc.

THEO-24® ℞

(theophylline anhydrous)

Extended-release capsules 100, 200, 300, & 400 mg

℞ only

DESCRIPTION

Theophylline

Theophylline is structurally classified as a methylxanthine. It occurs as a white, odorless, crystalline powder with a bitter taste. Anhydrous theophylline has the chemical name 1H-Purine-2,6-dione,3,7-dihydro-1,3-dimethyl-, and is represented by the following structural formula:

The molecular formula of anhydrous theophylline is $C_7H_8N_4O_2$ with a molecular weight of 180.17.

Theo-24® is available as capsules intended for oral administration, containing 100 mg, 200 mg, 300 mg, or 400 mg of anhydrous theophylline per capsule, in an extended-release formulation which allows a 24-hour dosing interval for appropriate patients.

Inactive ingredients are edible ink (which contains synthetic black iron oxide, FD&C Blue No. 1, FD&C Blue No. 2, FD&C Yellow No. 6, D&C Yellow No. 10, FD&C Red No. 40), ethylcellulose, gelatin, pharmaceutical glaze, colloidal silicon dioxide, starch, sucrose, talc, titanium dioxide, and coloring agents: 100 mg—includes FD&C Yellow No. 6; 200 mg—FD&C Red No. 3 and D&C Yellow No. 10; 300 mg—FD&C Blue No.1 and FD&C Red No. 40; 400 mg—FD&C Red No. 40 and D&C Red No. 28.

Theo-24 Extended-release capsules meet Drug Release Test 6 as published in the current USP monograph for Theophylline Extended-release Capsules.

HOW SUPPLIED

Theo-24® (theophylline anhydrous) is supplied in extended-release capsules containing 100, 200, 300 or 400 mg of anhydrous theophylline.

Theo-24 100 mg capsules are yellow-orange and clear, with markings Theo-24, 100 mg, ucb, and 2832, supplied as:

NDC Number	Size
50474-100-01	bottle of 100

Theo-24 200 mg capsules are red-orange and clear, with markings Theo-24, 200 mg, ucb, and 2842, supplied as:

NDC Number	Size
50474-200-01	bottle of 100
50474-200-50	bottle of 500
50474-200-60	carton of 100 unit dose

Continued on next page

Theo-24—Cont.

Theo-24 300 mg capsules are red and clear, with markings Theo-24, 300 mg, ucb, and 2852, supplied as:

NDC Number	Size
50474-300-01	bottle of 100
50474-300-50	bottle of 500
50474-300-60	carton of 100 unit dose

Theo-24 400 mg capsules are pink and clear, with markings Theo-24, 400 mg, ucb, and 2902, supplied as:

NDC Number	Size
50474-400-01	bottle of 100
50474-400-50	bottle of 500

STORAGE

Store below 77 °F (25 °C).

FOR MEDICAL INFORMATION

Contact: Medical Affairs Department
Phone: (800) 477-7877
Fax: (770) 970-8859

Manufactured for:
UCB Pharma, Inc.
Smyrna, GA 30080
by:
Pfizer Co.
New York, NY 10017

Rev IE 10/2003

TRINSICON® Capsules ℞

[*tren 'sa-kon*]
Hematinic Concentrate With Intrinsic Factor
℞ only

DESCRIPTION

Each TRINSICON® capsule contains:

Special liver-stomach concentrate (containing intrinsic factor)	240 mg
Vitamin B_{12} (activity equivalent)	15 mcg
Iron, elemental (as ferrous fumarate)	110 mg
Ascorbic acid (vitamin C)	75 mg
Folic acid	0.5 mg

with other factors of vitamin B complex present in the liver-stomach concentrate.

Each capsule also contains FD&C Blue No. 1, D&C Red No. 28, FD&C Red No. 40, D&C Yellow No. 10, gelatin, silicon dioxide, corn starch, edible ink, silicone fluid, sodium lauryl sulfate and titanium dioxide.

HOW SUPPLIED

Dark pink and dark red capsules imprinted "ucb/364" in child-resistant, unit-dose packages of 60 capsules [6 × 10] (NDC 50474-364-23), and of 100 capsules [10 × 10] (NDC 50474-364-28).

Manufactured for
UCB Pharma, Inc.
Smyrna, GA 30080
By **Mallinckrodt Inc.**
Hobart, NY 13788

IE 12/2001

VICON FORTE® Capsules ℞

[*vī 'kon for 'tā*]
Therapeutic Vitamins-Minerals
℞ only

DESCRIPTION

Each black and orange VICON FORTE® capsule for oral administration contains:

Vitamin A	8,000 IU
Vitamin E	50 IU
Ascorbic acid	150 mg
Zinc sulfate, USP*	80 mg
Magnesium sulfate, USP†	70 mg
Niacinamide	25 mg
Thiamine mononitrate	10 mg
d-Calcium pantothenate	10 mg
Riboflavin	5 mg
Manganese chloride	4 mg
Pyridoxine hydrochloride	2 mg
Folic acid	1 mg
Vitamin B_{12} (Cyanocobalamin)	10 mcg

* As 50 mg dried zinc sulfate.
† As 50 mg dried magnesium sulfate.

Each capsule also contains edible ink, FD&C Blue No. 1, FD&C Red No. 40, FD&C Yellow No. 6, gelatin, lactose, magnesium stearate, silicon dioxide, sodium lauryl sulfate, and titanium dioxide.

HOW SUPPLIED

Orange and black capsules imprinted with "ucb" and "316" in bottles of 60 (NDC 50474-316-22) and 500 (NDC 50474-316-24) and unit-dose packs of 100 (NDC 50474-316-27).

Dispense in tight, light-resistant container with a child resistant closure.

Manufactured for
UCB Pharma, Inc.
Smyrna, GA 30080
by Mallinckrodt Inc.
Hobart, NY 13788

IE 10/2003

Unicity International

THE MAKE LIFE BETTER COMPANY
1201 NORTH 800 EAST
OREM, UT 84097

Direct Inquiries to:
(801) 226 2600
www.makelifebetter.com
science@unicity.net

Products of Unicity International, The Make Life Better Company are distributed through independent distributors.

CARDIOESSENTIALS® OTC

Caring for your heart

DESCRIPTION

CardioEssentials is Unicity's superior heart product.

Benefits and research

CardioEssentials provides nutrients for the heart muscle, and supports healthy heart function. The combination of L-carnithine, L-taurine, and Coenzyme Q10 has proven benefits to the heart. These ingredients are known to be important in providing adequate energy for the heart muscle. CardioEssentials provides adequate amounts of these ingredients, i.e. 100 mg of CoQ10. Hawthorn extract is traditionally used in supporting the heart function.*

SUGGESTED USE

Take three capsules twice daily with food.

Contents

CardioEssentials features a proprietary blend of L-carnitine, L-taurine, and Hawthorn, combined with 100 mg of Coenzyme Q10.

For detailed dietary information, please see www.unicity.net

SAFETY AND WARNINGS

CardioEssentials is well accepted. Some gastrointestinal discomfort may be experienced as with any dietary supplement.

REFERENCES

Jeejeebhoy, F *et al* (2002), "Nutritional supplementation with MyoVive repletes essential cardiac myocyte nutrients and reduces left ventricular size in patients with left ventricular dysfunction", *American Heart Journal* **143**, 1092-1100.

*THESE STATEMENTS HAVE NOT BEEN EVALUATED BY THE FOOD AND DRUG ADMINISTRATION. THIS PRODUCT IS NOT INTENDED TO DIAGNOSE, TREAT, CURE, OR PREVENT ANY DISEASE.

CM PLEX™ AND CM PLEX™ CREAM OTC

Proprietary fatty acid blend to help support joint health.*

DESCRIPTION

CM Plex and CM Plex Cream are an oral softgel, and topical cream product respectively, combining different fatty acids, in a proprietary blend of cetyl myristate, cetyl myristoleate, and other cetyl esters.

Benefits and research

Cetyl myristoleate and related fatty acids have been researched in relation to improving joint health. It is suggested that these fatty acids have anti-inflammatory effects. A clinical study with the proprietary fatty acid blend of CM Plex Softgels in 64 subjects indicated that subjects using the blend exhibited improvements in knee flexion and function compared to placebo. A second study in 40 subjects indicated a topical cream consisting of a blend of cetylated fatty acids is effective for improving knee range of motion, improving ability to climb stairs, rise from a chair, and walk, and improving balance, strength, and endurance.*

SUGGESTED USE

Softgels: Take one or two softgels three times daily with meals. Cream: Apply generously onto clean skin and gently massage until the cream disappears. Repeat 3 to 4 times daily as necessary. For maximum results combine both products.

Contents

CM Plex contains a proprietary blend of cetyl myristate, cetyl myristoleate, and other cetyl esters. For detailed dietary information, please see www.unicity.net

Safety and Warnings

CM Plex Softgels and Cream are well accepted. Some gastrointestinal discomfort may be experienced with CM Plex Softgels as with any dietary supplement.

REFERENCES

Hesslink, R *et al* (2002), "Cetylated fatty acids improve knee function in patients with osteoarthritis", *Journal of Rheumatology* **29**: 1708-1712.

Kraemer, WJ *et al* (2004), "Effect of a Cetylated Fatty Acid Topical Cream on Functional Mobility and Quality of Life of Patients with Osteoarthritis", *Journal of Rheumatology* **31**: 767-774.

*THESE STATEMENTS HAVE NOT BEEN EVALUATED BY THE FOOD AND DRUG ADMINISTRATION. THIS PRODUCT IS NOT INTENDED TO DIAGNOSE, TREAT, CURE, OR PREVENT ANY DISEASE.

LIFEHEALTH OTC

[*lif-hĕlth*]
Advanced Fiber and Nutrient Drink

DESCRIPTION

LifeHealth is Unicity's primary dietary supplement system that combines three advanced products that provide nutrients for the majority of health concerns in today's world. The individual products are described below.

CONTENTS

LifeHealth combines 60 packets of BiosLife 2®; 30 packets of Core Health™ (Male or Female); 60 capsules of Daily Produce 24™ Fruit Infusion and 60 capsules of Daily Produce 24™ Vegetable infusion.

BIOSLIFE 2®

Advanced Fiber and Nutrient Drink

DESCRIPTION

BiosLife 2 is a nutrient-rich fiber drink mix that contains a beneficial patented complex of soluble and insoluble fibers, vitamins and minerals.

BENEFITS AND RESEARCH

Studies show that people with relatively low blood cholesterol levels consume diets that are low in saturated fat and cholesterol and high in fiber sources such as fruits and vegetables. BiosLife 2—a good source of dietary fiber—when included as part of a healthy diet, may help lower your blood cholesterol levels and reduce your risk of heart disease. Eight weeks of BiosLife 2 showed a significant reduction in LDL-c compared to placebo. Moreover, levels of Apo protein B and homocysteine were also significantly reduced. The proposed mechanism of BiosLife 2 in cholesterol reduction is though bile-acid sequestration.

Research showed that a high intake of dietary fiber particularly of the soluble type, lowers plasma lipid concentrations. The gel forming characteristics of BiosLife 2 may lead to delayed gastric emptying that has beneficial effects on the body.

SUGGESTED USE

First users: dissolve the contents of one packet into 8 to 10 fl. oz. of liquid (water or juice), stir vigorously and drink immediately 5 to 10 minutes before the main meal. After fiber adjustment use as directed above up to three times daily before every meal.

CONTENTS

One packet of BiosLife 2 contains 4.5 gram fiber (guar gum, gum Arabic, locust bean gum, pectin, oat fiber) combining 4 gram soluble fiber and 0.5 gram insoluble fiber. Added to this fiber mix are optimal daily levels and bioavailable forms of vitamins A, C, E, B2, B6, B11, and B12, and the minerals chromium (as ChromeMate™), sodium, selenium, zinc, and calcium. Additional ingredients are beta-glucans, stevia (sweetener), maltodextrin, and biotin. BiosLife 2 is available in Natural, Original, and Tropical Fruit flavors. For detailed dietary information, please see www.unicity.net

SAFETY AND WARNINGS

BiosLife 2 is widely accepted. Some people report mild gastrointestinal discomfort after initial fiber intake. This is a normal effect of increased fiber intake and normally disappears within 30 days. Taking this product without adequate liquid can result in complications. If you are a diabetic, consult a physician for proper use of this product, which contains chromium. For maximum absorption, take medication at least one hour prior to using BiosLife 2.

REFERENCES

Sprecher, DL and Pearce GL (2002), "Fiber-multivitamin combination therapy: a beneficial influence on low-density lipoprotein and homocysteine", *Metabolism* **51**: 1166-70.

Freed, S and Joffe D (2004), "The Clinical Impact of Fiber Supplementation for the Reduction of Postprandial Blood Glucose and Risk Reduction of Complications from Diabetes II." *Manuscript in preparation*.

US Patent 4,883,788 and US Patent 4,824,672.

CORE HEALTH™

Daily multivitamin, mineral and phytonutrient supplement

DESCRIPTION

CoreHealth is Unicity's daily multivitamin, mineral and phytonutrient supplement that supplies all vitamins and minerals in optimal dosages, in highly bioavailable forms. Additionally, a wide selection of generally accepted phytonutrients is included. CoreHealth is available in a Male and a Female version.*

BENEFITS AND RESEARCH

CoreHealth provides nutrients that ensure adequate nourishment of the body and its metabolism, preventing deficiencies, and providing support for existing deficiencies. Unicity's commitment to efficacy of its products ensures the choice of ingredients with proven bioavailabilities, such as calcium citrate malate.

The phytonutrients in CoreHealth provide support for additional health concerns, such as prostate health with lycopene and ocular health with lutein, and extra natural antioxidant protection with ingredients such as green tea.*

SUGGESTED USE

One packet per day, preferably with breakfast.

CONTENTS

One packet of CoreHealth Male contains adequate levels and sources of vitamin A, B1, B2, B6, B11, B12, C, D2, E, K, choline, inositol, niacinamide, biotin, pantothenic acid, vanadium, iodine, chromium, manganese, copper, molybdenum, boron, selenium, zinc, calcium, magnesium, soy isoflavone extract, mixed carotenoids, lycopene, alpha tocopherols, green tea, potassium-D-glucarate, bioperine, cayenne pepper, ginger root, lutein, quercetin, and lemon bioflavonoids. CoreHealth Female contains the same ingredients as the Male version, and also iron. For detailed dietary information, please see www.unicity.net

SAFETY AND WARNINGS

CoreHealth is well accepted. Some gastrointestinal discomfort may be experienced as with any dietary supplement. Chromium has been known to affect blood sugar levels. If you are diabetic or taking a blood-thinning medication, consult a doctor before taking this product. Children, pregnant women, and women who may become pregnant should not take more than 10,000 IU per day of supplemental vitamin A (retinol) unless otherwise instructed by a physician.

DAILY PRODUCE 24™

Proprietary Fruit and Vegetable concentrate

DESCRIPTION

Daily Produce 24 comprises of two products: Fruit Infusion, and Vegetable Infusion. Both infusions combine 12 different kinds of fruits and vegetables that are concentrated using a proprietary cold-pressing technique, which prevents deterioration of the heat-sensitive phytonutrients.

BENEFITS AND RESEARCH

The American Dietetic Association advises that every adult consumes 5–9 servings of fruits and vegetables per day. Our lifestyles of today make it difficult to meet this recommendation. Even if adequate fruits and vegetables are consumed, the produce of today no longer provide comparable amounts of phytonutrients than that of decades ago, due to modernized and large-scale production techniques. Daily Produce 24 is designed to provide a daily boost of a very broad selection of plant and vegetable phytonutrients. Preliminary research has shown that Daily Produce 24 provides high ORAC values, indicating its antioxidant potential.*

SUGGESTED USE

Take two capsules Fruit Infusion with breakfast and two capsules Vegetable Infusion with dinner together with a large glass of water.

CONTENTS

Daily Produce 24 Fruit Infusion combines cold-pressed concentrates of plum, cranberry, blueberry, strawberry, blackberry, bilberry, cherry, apricot, papaya, orange, grape, and pineapple. Daily Produce 24 Vegetable Infusion combines cold-pressed concentrates of parsley, kale, spinach, wheat grass, Brussels sprouts, asparagus, broccoli, cauliflower, beet juice, carrot, cabbage, and garlic.

For detailed dietary information, please see www.unicity.net

SAFETY AND WARNINGS

Daily Produce 24 Fruit Infusion and Vegetable Infusion are well accepted. Some gastrointestinal discomfort may be experienced as with any dietary supplement.

*THESE STATEMENTS HAVE NOT BEEN EVALUATED BY THE FOOD AND DRUG ADMINISTRATION. THIS PRODUCT IS NOT INTENDED TO DIAGNOSE, TREAT, CURE, OR PREVENT ANY DISEASE.

VISUTEIN® OTC

[vī-su-tēn]

Clinically proven to support healthy eyes and vision.*

DESCRIPTION

VISUtein is Unicity's product providing key nutrients for the eye. The product is particularly high-dosed in lutein.

Benefits and research

The carotenoids lutein and zeaxanthin play an important role in eye health. Low concentrations of these phytonutrients in the retina have been associated with age-related macula degeneration (AMD). Studies have shown, that supplementation with high levels of lutein, as present in VISUtein, can restore the lutein concentration in the retina. The product further features important vitamins, and carotenoids that are detrimental in preserving overall eye health and supporting clear vision. N-acetyl cysteine is added to boost the glutathion levels. Low glutathion levels have been shown to reduce protection of the eye against oxidative stress. Bilberry is known to stimulate visual acuity, and provides anthocyanidins, strong eye-specific antioxidants. A recent clinical study with VISUtein has shown that AMD patients experience clear improvements in visual acuity, contrast sensitivity, and recovery from a flash.*

SUGGESTED USE

Take two capsules per day with a meal.

Contents

VISUtein provides 18 mg of lutein, along with 200 mg of N-acetyl cystein, and 60 mg anthocyanidins from bilberry. Other ingredients are mixed carotenoids, vitamins A, B2, and zinc. For detailed dietary information, please see www.unicity.net.

SAFETY AND WARNINGS

VISUtein is well accepted. Some gastrointestinal discomfort may be experienced as with any dietary supplement.

REFERENCES

Newsome, DA and Meyers, L (2004), "A Randomized Prospective Clinical Trial of Two Commercially Available Ocular Diet Supplements", *Submitted*.

*THESE STATEMENTS HAVE NOT BEEN EVALUATED BY THE FOOD AND DRUG ADMINISTRATION. THIS PRODUCT IS NOT INTENDED TO DIAGNOSE, TREAT, CURE, OR PREVENT ANY DISEASE.

Unimed Pharmaceuticals, Inc.

A Solvay Pharmaceuticals, Inc. Company
901 SAWYER ROAD
MARIETTA, GA 30062

Direct Inquiries to:
770 578-9000

ANADROL®-50 CIII ℞

[an-a-dral]

(oxymetholone)
50 mg Tablets
℞ only

DESCRIPTION

ANADROL® (oxymetholone) Tablets for oral administration each contain 50 mg of the steroid oxymetholone, a potent anabolic and androgenic drug.

The chemical name for oxymetholone is 17β-hydroxy-2-(hydroxymethylene)-17-methyl-5α-androstan-3-one. The structural formula is:

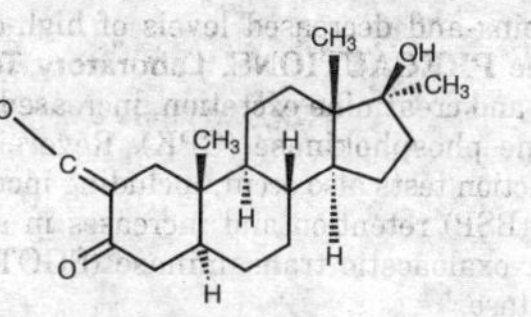

Inactive Ingredients: lactose
magnesium stearate
povidone
starch

CLINICAL PHARMACOLOGY

Anabolic steroids are synthetic derivatives of testosterone. Nitrogen balance is improved with anabolic agents but only when there is sufficient intake of calories and protein. Whether this positive nitrogen balance is of primary benefit in the utilization of protein-building dietary substances has not been established. Oxymetholone enhances the production and urinary excretion of erythropoietin in patients with anemias due to bone marrow failure and often stimulates erythropoiesis in anemias due to deficient red cell production.

Certain clinical effects and adverse reactions demonstrate the androgenic properties of this class of drugs. Complete dissociation of anabolic and androgenic effects has not been achieved. The actions of anabolic steroids are therefore similar to those of male sex hormones with the possibility of causing serious disturbances of growth and sexual development if given to young children. They suppress the gonadotropic functions of the pituitary and may exert a direct effect upon the testes.

INDICATIONS AND USAGE

ANADROL®-50 Tablets is indicated in the treatment of anemias caused by deficient red cell production. Acquired aplastic anemia, congenital aplastic anemia, myelofibrosis and the hypoplastic anemias due to the administration of myelotoxic drugs often respond. ANADROL®-50 Tablets should not replace other supportive measures such as transfusion, correction of iron, folic acid, vitamin B_{12} or pyridoxine deficiency, antibacterial therapy and the appropriate use of corticosteroids.

CONTRAINDICATIONS

1. Carcinoma of the prostate or breast in male patients.
2. Carcinoma of the breast in females with hypercalcemia; androgenic anabolic steroids may stimulate osteolytic resorption of bones.
3. Oxymetholone can cause fetal harm when administered to pregnant women. It is contraindicated in women who are or may become pregnant. If the patient becomes pregnant while taking the drug, she should be apprised of the potential hazard to the fetus.
4. Nephrosis or the nephrotic phase of nephritis.
5. Hypersensitivity to the drug.
6. Severe hepatic dysfunction.

WARNINGS

The following conditions have been reported in patients receiving androgenic anabolic steroids as a general class of drugs:

> Peliosis hepatis, a condition in which liver and sometimes splenic tissue is replaced with blood-filled cysts, has been reported in patients receiving androgenic anabolic steroid therapy. These cysts are sometimes present with minimal hepatic dysfunction, but at other times they have been associated with liver failure. They are often not recognized until life-threatening liver failure or intra-abdominal hemorrhage develops. Withdrawal of drug usually results in complete disappearance of lesions.
>
> Liver cell tumors are also reported. Most often these tumors are benign and androgen-dependent, but fatal malignant tumors have been reported. Withdrawal of drug often results in regression or cessation of progression of the tumor. However, hepatic tumors associated with androgens or anabolic steroids are much more vascular than other hepatic tumors and may be silent until life-threatening intra-abdominal hemorrhage develops.
>
> Blood lipid changes that are known to be associated with increased risk of atherosclerosis are seen in patients treated with androgens and anabolic steroids. These changes include decreased high density lipoprotein and sometimes increased low density lipoprotein. The changes may be very marked and could have a serious impact on the risk of atherosclerosis and coronary artery disease.

Cholestatic hepatitis and jaundice occur with 17-alpha-alkylated androgens at relatively low doses. Clinical jaundice may be painless, with or without pruritus. It may also be associated with acute hepatic enlargement and right upper-quadrant pain, which has been mistaken for acute (surgical) obstruction of the bile duct. Drug-induced jaundice is usually reversible when the medication is discontinued. Continued therapy has been associated with hepatic coma and death. Because of the hepatoxicity associated with oxymetholone administration, periodic liver function tests are recommended.

In patients with breast cancer, anabolic steroid therapy may cause hypercalcemia by stimulating osteolysis. In this case, the drug should be discontinued.

Edema with or without congestive heart failure may be a serious complication in patients with pre-existing cardiac, renal or hepatic disease. Concomitant administration with adrenal steroids or ACTH may add to the edema. This is generally controllable with appropriate diuretic and/or digitalis therapy.

Geriatric male patients treated with androgenic anabolic steroids may be at an increased risk for the development of prostate hypertrophy and prostatic carcinoma.

Anabolic steroids have not been shown to enhance athletic ability.

PRECAUTIONS

General:

Women should be observed for signs of virilization (deepening of the voice, hirsutism, acne and clitoromegaly). To prevent irreversible change, drug therapy must be discontinued when mild virilism is first detected. Such virilization is usual following androgenic anabolic steroid use at high doses. Some virilizing changes in women are irreversible even after prompt discontinuance of therapy and are not prevented by concomitant use of estrogens. Menstrual irregularities, including amenorrhea, may also occur.

The insulin or oral hypoglycemic dosage may need adjustment in diabetic patients who receive anabolic steroids.

Anabolic steroids may cause suppression of clotting factors II, V, VII and X, and an increase in prothrombin time.

Information for the Patient:

The physician should instruct patients to report any of the following side effects of androgens.

Adult or Adolescent Males: Too frequent or persistent erections of the penis, appearance or aggravation of acne.

Women: Hoarseness, acne, changes in menstrual periods or more hair on the face.

All Patients: Any nausea, vomiting, changes in skin color or ankle swelling.

Laboratory Tests:

Women with disseminated breast carcinoma should have frequent determination of urine and serum calcium levels during the course of androgenic anabolic steroid therapy (see **WARNINGS**).

Because of the hepatoxicity associated with the use of 17-alpha-alkylated androgens, liver function tests should be obtained periodically.

Periodic (every 6 months) x-ray examinations of bone age should be made during treatment of prepubertal patients to determine the rate of bone maturation and the effects of androgenic anabolic steroid therapy on the epiphyseal centers.

Anabolic steroids have been reported to lower the level of high-density lipoproteins and raise the level of low-density lipoproteins. These changes usually revert to normal on dis-

Continued on next page

Anadrol-50—Cont.

continuation of treatment. Increased low-density lipoproteins and decreased high-density lipoproteins are considered cardiovascular risk factors. Serum lipids and high-density lipoprotein cholesterol should be determined periodically.
Hemoglobin and hematocrit should be checked periodically for polycythemia in patients who are receiving high doses of anabolics.
Because iron deficiency anemia has been observed in some patients treated with oxymetholone, periodic determination of the serum iron and iron binding capacity is recommended. If iron deficiency is detected, it should be appropriately treated with supplementary iron.
Oxymetholone has been shown to decrease 17-ketosteroid excretion.

Drug Interactions:

Warfarin: Pharmacokinetic and pharmacodynamic interactions between anabolic steroids and warfarin have been reported in healthy volunteers. When anabolic steroid therapy is initiated in a patient already receiving treatment with warfarin, the INR (international normalized ratio) or prothrombin time (PT) should be monitored closely and the dose of warfarin adjusted as necessary until a stable target INR or PT has been achieved. In patients receiving both ANADROL® Tablets and warfarin, careful monitoring of the INR or PT and adjustment of the warfarin, if indicated, is recommended when the anabolic steroid dose is changed or discontinued. Patients should be closely monitored for signs and symptoms of occult bleeding.

Anticoagulants: Anabolic steroids may increase sensitivity to anticoagulants. Patients receiving oral anticoagulant therapy require close monitoring, especially when anabolic steroids are started or stopped.

Drug/Laboratory Test Interferences:

Therapy with androgenic anabolic steroids may decrease levels of thyroxine-binding globulin resulting in decreased total T_4 serum levels and increased resin uptake of T_3 and T_4. Free thyroid hormone levels remain unchanged and there is no clinical evidence of thyroid dysfunction. Altered tests usually persist for 2 to 3 weeks after stopping anabolic therapy.
Anabolic steroids may cause an increase in prothrombin time.
Anabolic steroids have been shown to alter fasting blood sugar and glucose tolerance tests.

Carcinogenesis, Mutagenesis, Impairment of Fertility:

A two-year carcinogenicity study in rats given oxymetholone orally was conducted under the auspices of the US National Toxicology Program (NTP). A wide spectrum of neoplastic and non-neoplastic effects was observed. In male rats, no effects were classified as neoplastic in response to doses up to 150 mg/kg/day (5 times therapeutic exposures with 5 mg/kg based on body surface area). Female rats given 30 mg/kg/day (1 fold the maximum recommended clinical dose of 5 mg/kg/day based on the body surface area) had increased incidences of lung alveolar/bronchiolar adenoma and adenoma or carcinoma combined. At 100 mg/kg/day (about 3 fold the maximum recommended clinical dose of 5 mg/kg/day based on BSA), female rats had increased incidences of hepatocellular adenoma and adenoma or carcinoma combined; the combined incidence of squamous cell carcinoma and carcinoma of the sweat glands also was increased.
Human data: There are rare reports of hepatocellular carcinoma in patients receiving long-term therapy with androgens in high doses. Withdrawal of the drugs did not lead to regression of the tumors in all cases.
Geriatric patients treated with androgens may be at an increased risk of developing prostatic hypertrophy and prostatic carcinoma although conclusive evidence to support this concept is lacking.
In studies conducted under the auspices of the US National Toxicology Program, no evidence of genotoxicity was found using standard assays for mutagenicity, chromosomal aberrations, or induction of micronuclei in erythrocytes.
Impairment of fertility was not tested directly in animal species. However, as noted below under **ADVERSE REACTIONS**, oligospermia in males and amenorrhea in females are potential adverse effects of treatment with ANADROL® Tablets. Therefore, impairment of fertility is a possible outcome of treatment with ANADROL® Tablets.

Pregnancy:

Pregnancy category X (see **CONTRAINDICATIONS**).

Nursing Mothers:

It is not known whether anabolics are excreted in human milk. Because of the potential for serious adverse reactions in nursed infants from anabolics, women who take oxymetholone should not nurse.

Pediatric Use:

Anabolic/androgenic steroids should be used very cautiously in children and only by specialists who are aware of their effects on bone maturation.
Anabolic agents may accelerate epiphyseal maturation more rapidly than linear growth in children, and the effect may continue for 6 months after the drug has been stopped. Therefore, therapy should be monitored by x-ray studies at 6-month intervals in order to avoid the risk of compromising the adult height.

Geriatric Use:

Clinical studies of ANADROL® Tablets did not include sufficient numbers of subjects aged 65 and over to determine whether they respond differently from younger subjects. Other reported clinical experience has not identified differences in responses between the elderly and younger patients. In general, dose selection for an elderly patient should be cautious, usually starting at the low end of the dosing range, reflecting the greater frequency of decreased hepatic, renal, or cardiac function, and of concomitant disease or other drug therapy.

ADVERSE REACTIONS

Hepatic: Cholestatic jaundice with, rarely, hepatic necrosis and death. Hepatocellular neoplasms and peliosis hepatis have been reported in association with long-term androgenic anabolic steroid therapy (see **WARNINGS**).

Genitourinary System:

In Men:

Prepubertal: Phallic enlargement and increased frequency of erections.
Postpubertal: Inhibition of testicular function, testicular atrophy and oligospermia, impotence, chronic priapism, epididymitis, bladder irritability and decrease in seminal volume.

In Women:

Clitoral enlargement, menstrual irregularities.

In Both Sexes:

Increased or decreased libido.

CNS: Excitation, insomnia.

Gastrointestinal: Nausea, vomiting, diarrhea.

Hematologic: Bleeding in patients on concomitant anticoagulant therapy, iron-deficiency anemia.

Leukemia has been observed in patients with aplastic anemia treated with oxymetholone. The role, if any, of oxymetholone is unclear because malignant transformation has been seen in blood dyscrasias and leukemia has been reported in patients with aplastic anemia who have not been treated with oxymetholone.

Breast: Gynecomastia.

Larynx: Deepening of the voice in women.

Hair: Hirsutism and male-pattern baldness in women, male-pattern of hair loss in postpubertal males.

Skin: Acne (especially in women and prepubertal boys).

Skeletal: Premature closure of epiphyses in children (see **PRECAUTIONS, Pediatric Use**), muscle cramps.

Body as a Whole: Chills.

Fluid and Electrolytes: Edema, retention of serum electrolytes (sodium, chloride, potassium, phosphate, calcium).

Metabolic/Endocrine: Decreased glucose tolerance (see **PRECAUTIONS**), increased serum levels of low-density lipoproteins and decreased levels of high-density lipoproteins (see **PRECAUTIONS, Laboratory Tests**), increased creatine and creatinine excretion, increased serum levels of creatinine phosphokinase (CPK). Reversible changes in liver function tests also occur, including increased Bromsulphalein (BSP) retention and increases in serum bilirubin, glutamic-oxaloacetic transaminase (SGOT), and alkaline phosphatase.

DRUG ABUSE AND DEPENDENCE

Controlled Substance:

ANADROL®-50 Tablets is considered to be a controlled substance and is listed in Schedule III.

OVERDOSAGE

There have been no reports of acute overdosage with anabolics.

DOSAGE AND ADMINISTRATION

The recommended daily dose in children and adults is 1-5 mg/kg body weight per day. The usual effective dose is 1-2 mg/kg/day but higher doses may be required, and the dose should be individualized. Response is not often immediate, and a minimum trial of three to six months should be given. Following remission, some patients may be maintained without the drug; others may be maintained on an established lower daily dosage. A continued maintenance dose is usually necessary in patients with congenital aplastic anemia.

HOW SUPPLIED

ANADROL®-50 (oxymetholone) Tablets is supplied in bottles of 100 white scored tablets imprinted with 8633 and UNIMED (NDC 0051-8633-33).
Store at controlled room temperature 20° to 25°C (68° to 77°F); excursions permitted to 15° to 30°C (59° to 86°F) [See USP].

Manufactured for
Unimed Pharmaceuticals, Inc.
by Solvay Pharmaceuticals, Inc
Marietta, GA 30062
Address medical inquiries to:
Unimed Pharmaceuticals, Inc.
901 Sawyer Road
Marietta, GA 30062
500031 5E Rev 2/2004

UNIMED
PHARMACEUTICALS, INC.
A Solvay Pharmaceuticals, Inc. Company
Marietta, GA 30062
Shown in Product Identification Guide, page 335

ANDROGEL® Ⓒ℞

[*ăn drō-jĕl*]
(testosterone gel) 1%

DESCRIPTION

AndroGel® (testosterone gel) is a clear, colorless hydroalcoholic gel containing 1% testosterone. AndroGel® provides continuous transdermal delivery of testosterone, the primary circulating endogenous androgen, for 24 hours following a single application to intact, clean, dry skin of the shoulders, upper arms and/or abdomen.
A daily application of AndroGel® 5 g, 7.5 g, or 10 g contains 50 mg, 75 mg, or 100 mg of testosterone, respectively, to be applied daily to the skin's surface. Approximately 10% of the applied testosterone dose is absorbed across skin of average permeability during a 24-hour period.
The active pharmacologic ingredient in AndroGel® is testosterone. Testosterone USP is a white to practically white crystalline powder chemically described as 17-beta hydroxyandrost-4-en-3-one.

Testosterone

$C_{19}H_{28}O_2$ MW 288.42

Inactive ingredients in AndroGel® are ethanol 67.0%, purified water, sodium hydroxide, carbomer 980 and isopropyl myristate; these ingredients are not pharmacologically active.

CLINICAL PHARMACOLOGY

AndroGel® (testosterone gel) delivers physiologic amounts of testosterone, producing circulating testosterone concentrations that approximate normal levels (298–1043 ng/dL) seen in healthy men.

Testosterone – General Androgen Effects:

Endogenous androgens, including testosterone and dihydrotestosterone (DHT), are responsible for the normal growth and development of the male sex organs and for maintenance of secondary sex characteristics. These effects include the growth and maturation of prostate, seminal vesicles, penis, and scrotum; the development of male hair distribution, such as facial, pubic, chest, and axillary hair; laryngeal enlargement, vocal chord thickening, alterations in body musculature, and fat distribution. Testosterone and DHT are necessary for the normal development of secondary sex characteristics. Male hypogonadism results from insufficient secretion of testosterone and is characterized by low serum testosterone concentrations. Symptoms associated with male hypogonadism include impotence and decreased sexual desire, fatigue and loss of energy, mood depression, regression of secondary sexual characteristics and osteoporosis. Hypogonadism is a risk factor for osteoporosis in men.
Drugs in the androgen class also promote retention of nitrogen, sodium, potassium, phosphorus, and decreased urinary excretion of calcium. Androgens have been reported to increase protein anabolism and decrease protein catabolism. Nitrogen balance is improved only when there is sufficient intake of calories and protein.
Androgens are responsible for the growth spurt of adolescence and for the eventual termination of linear growth brought about by fusion of the epiphyseal growth centers. In children, exogenous androgens accelerate linear growth rates but may cause a disproportionate advancement in bone maturation. Use over long periods may result in fusion of the epiphyseal growth centers and termination of the growth process. Androgens have been reported to stimulate the production of red blood cells by enhancing erythropoietin production.
During exogenous administration of androgens, endogenous testosterone release may be inhibited through feedback inhibition of pituitary luteinizing hormone (LH). At large doses of exogenous androgens, spermatogenesis may also be suppressed through feedback inhibition of pituitary follicle-stimulating hormone (FSH).
There is a lack of substantial evidence that androgens are effective in accelerating fracture healing or in shortening postsurgical convalescence.

Pharmacokinetics

Absorption: AndroGel® is a hydroalcoholic formulation that dries quickly when applied to the skin surface. The skin serves as a reservoir for the sustained release of testosterone into the systemic circulation. Approximately 10% of the testosterone dose applied on the skin surface from AndroGel® is absorbed into systemic circulation. Therefore, 5 g and 10 g of AndroGel® systemically delivers approximately 5 mg and 10 mg of testosterone, respectively. In a study with 10 g of AndroGel®, all patients showed an increase in serum testosterone within 30 minutes, and eight of nine patients had a serum testosterone concentration within normal range by 4 hours after the initial application. Absorption of testosterone into the blood continues for the entire 24-hour dosing interval. Serum concentrations approximate the steady-state level by the end of the first 24 hours and are at steady state by the second or third day of dosing.
With single daily applications of AndroGel®, follow-up measurements 30, 90 and 180 days after starting treatment

have confirmed that serum testosterone concentrations are generally maintained within the eugonadal range. Figure 1 summarizes the 24-hour pharmacokinetic profiles of testosterone for patients maintained on 5 g or 10 g of AndroGel® for 30 days. The average (± SD) daily testosterone concentration produced by AndroGel® 10 g on Day 30 was 792 (± 294) ng/dL and by AndroGel® 5 g 566 (± 262) ng/dL.

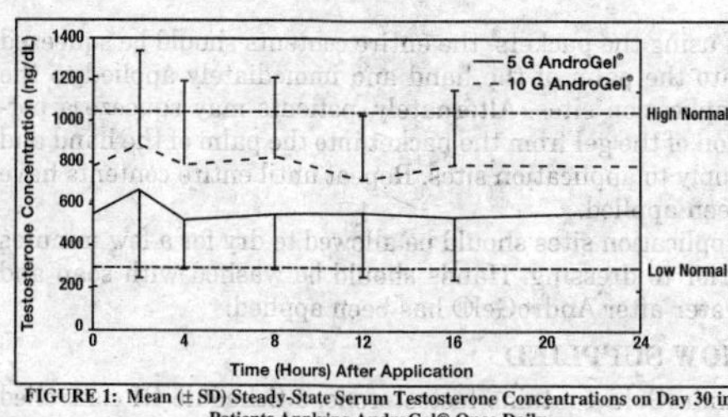

FIGURE 1: Mean (± SD) Steady-State Serum Testosterone Concentrations on Day 30 in Patients Applying AndroGel® Once Daily

When AndroGel® treatment is discontinued after achieving steady state, serum testosterone levels remain in the normal range for 24 to 48 hours but return to their pretreatment levels by the fifth day after the last application.

Distribution: Circulating testosterone is chiefly bound in the serum to sex hormone-binding globulin (SHBG) and albumin. The albumin-bound fraction of testosterone easily dissociates from albumin and is presumed to be bioactive. The portion of testosterone bound to SHBG is not considered biologically active. The amount of SHBG in the serum and the total testosterone level will determine the distribution of bioactive and nonbioactive androgen. SHBG-binding capacity is high in prepubertal children, declines during puberty and adulthood, and increases again during the later decades of life. Approximately 40% of testosterone in plasma is bound to SHBG, 2% remains unbound (free) and the rest is bound to albumin and other proteins.

Metabolism: There is considerable variation in the half-life of testosterone as reported in the literature, ranging from 10 to 100 minutes. Testosterone is metabolized to various 17-keto steroids through two different pathways. The major active metabolites of testosterone are estradiol and DHT. DHT binds with greater affinity to SHBG than does testosterone. In many tissues, the activity of testosterone depends on its reduction to DHT, which binds to cytosol receptor proteins. The steroid-receptor complex is transported to the nucleus where it initiates transcription and cellular changes related to androgen action. In reproductive tissues, DHT is further metabolized to 3-α and 3-β androstanediol. DHT concentrations increased in parallel with testosterone concentrations during AndroGel® treatment. After 180 days of treatment, mean DHT concentrations were within the normal range with 5 g AndroGel® and were about 7% above the normal range after a 10 g dose. The mean steady-state DHT/T ratio during 180 days of AndroGel® treatment remained within normal limits (as determined by the analytical laboratory involved with this clinical trial) and ranged from 0.23 to 0.29 (5 g/day) and from 0.27 to 0.33 (10 g/day).

Excretion: About 90% of a dose of testosterone given intramuscularly is excreted in the urine as glucuronic and sulfuric acid conjugates of testosterone and its metabolites; about 6% of a dose is excreted in the feces, mostly in the unconjugated form. Inactivation of testosterone occurs primarily in the liver.

Special Populations: In patients treated with AndroGel®, there are no observed differences in the average daily serum testosterone concentration at steady state based on age, cause of hypogonadism or body mass index. No formal studies were conducted involving patients with renal or hepatic insufficiencies.

Clinical Studies

AndroGel® 1% was evaluated in a multicenter, randomized, parallel-group, active-controlled, 180-day trial in 227 hypogonadal men. The study was conducted in 2 phases. During the Initial Treatment Period (Days 1-90), 73 patients were randomized to AndroGel® 5 g daily, 78 patients to AndroGel® 10 g daily, and 76 patients to a non-scrotal testosterone transdermal system. The study was double-blind for dose of AndroGel® but open-label for active control. Patients who were originally randomized to AndroGel® and who had single-sample serum testosterone levels above or below the normal range on Day 60 were titrated to 7.5 g daily on Day 91. During the Extended Treatment Period (Days 91-180), 51 patients continued on AndroGel® 5 g daily, 52 patients continued on AndroGel® 10 g daily, 41 patients continued on a non-scrotal testosterone transdermal system (5 mg daily), and 40 patients received AndroGel® 7.5 g daily.

Mean peak, trough and average serum testosterone concentrations within the normal range (298-1043 ng/dL) were achieved on the first day of treatment with doses of 5 g and 10 g. In patients continuing on AndroGel® 5 g and 10 g, these mean testosterone levels were maintained within the normal range for the 180-day duration of the study. Figure 2 summarizes the 24-hour pharmacokinetic profiles of testosterone administered as AndroGel® for 30, 90 and 180 days. Testosterone concentrations were maintained as long as the patient continued to properly apply the prescribed AndroGel® treatment.

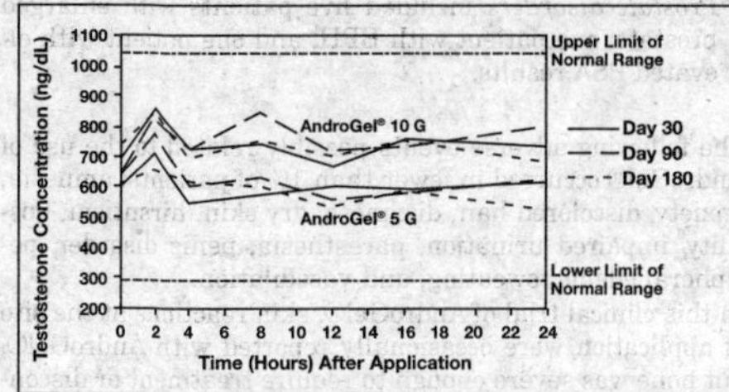

FIGURE 2: Mean Steady-State Testosterone Concentrations in Patients with Once-Daily AndroGel® Therapy

Table 1 summarizes the mean testosterone concentrations on Treatment Day 180 for patients receiving 5 g, 7.5 g, or 10 g of AndroGel®. The 7.5 g dose produced mean concentrations intermediate to those produced by 5 g and 10 g of AndroGel®.

TABLE 1: Mean (± SD) Steady-State Serum Testosterone Concentrations During Therapy (Day 180)

	5 g N = 44	7.5 g N = 37	10 g N = 48
Cavg	555 ± 225	601 ± 309	713 ± 209
Cmax	830 ± 347	901 ± 471	1083 ± 434
Cmin	371 ± 165	406 ± 220	485 ± 156

Of 129 hypogonadal men who were appropriately titrated with AndroGel® and who had sufficient data for analysis, 87% achieved an average serum testosterone level within the normal range on Treatment Day 180.

AndroGel® 5 g/day and 10 g/day resulted in significant increases over time in total body mass and total body lean mass, while total body fat mass and the percent body fat decreased significantly. These changes were maintained for 180 days of treatment. Changes in the 7.5 g dose group were similar. Bone mineral density in both hip and spine increased significantly from Baseline to Day 180 with 10 g AndroGel®.

AndroGel® treatment at 5 g/day and 10 g/day for 90 days produced significant improvement in libido (measured by sexual motivation, sexual activity and enjoyment of sexual activity as assessed by patient responses to a questionnaire). The degree of penile erection as subjectively estimated by the patients, increased with AndroGel® treatment, as did the subjective score for "satisfactory duration of erection." AndroGel® treatment at 5 g/day and 10 g/day produced positive effects on mood and fatigue. Similar changes were seen after 180 days of treatment and in the group treated with the 7.5 g dose. DHT concentrations increased in parallel with testosterone concentrations at AndroGel® doses of 5 g/day and 10 g/day, but the DHT/T ratio stayed within the normal range, indicating enhanced availability of the major physiologically active androgen. Serum estradiol (E2) concentrations increased significantly within 30 days of starting treatment with AndroGel® 5 or 10 g/day and remained elevated throughout the treatment period but remained within the normal range for eugonadal men. Serum levels of SHBG decreased very slightly (1 to 11%) during AndroGel® treatment. In men with hypergonadotropic hypogonadism, serum levels of LH and FSH fell in a dose- and time-dependent manner during treatment with AndroGel®.

Potential for Testosterone Transfer:

The potential for dermal testosterone transfer following AndroGel® use was evaluated in a clinical study between males dosed with AndroGel® and their untreated female partners. Two to 12 hours after AndroGel® (10 g) application by the male subjects, the couples (N=38 couples) engaged in daily, 15-minute sessions of vigorous skin-to-skin contact so that the female partners gained maximum exposure to the AndroGel® application sites. Under these study conditions, all unprotected female partners had a serum testosterone concentration > 2 times the baseline value at some time during the study. When a shirt covered the application site(s), the transfer of testosterone from the males to the female partners was completely prevented.

INDICATIONS AND USAGE

AndroGel® is indicated for replacement therapy in males for conditions associated with a deficiency or absence of endogenous testosterone:

1. Primary hypogonadism (congenital or acquired) – testicular failure due to cryptorchidism, bilateral torsion, orchitis, vanishing testis syndrome, orchiectomy, Klinefelter's syndrome, chemotherapy, or toxic damage from alcohol or heavy metals. These men usually have low serum testosterone levels and gonadotropins (FSH, LH) above the normal range.
2. Hypogonadotropic hypogonadism (congenital or acquired) – idiopathic gonadotropin or luteinizing hormone-releasing hormone (LHRH) deficiency or pituitary-hypothalamic injury from tumors, trauma, or radiation. These men have low testosterone serum levels but have gonadotropins in the normal or low range.

AndroGel® has not been clinically evaluated in males under 18 years of age.

CONTRAINDICATIONS

Androgens are contraindicated in men with carcinoma of the breast or known or suspected carcinoma of the prostate.

AndroGel® is not indicated for use in women, has not been evaluated in women, and must not be used in women.

Pregnant women should avoid skin contact with AndroGel® application sites in men. Testosterone may cause fetal harm. In the event that unwashed or unclothed skin to which AndroGel® has been applied does come in direct contact with the skin of a pregnant woman, the general area of contact on the woman should be washed with soap and water as soon as possible. *In vitro* studies show that residual testosterone is removed from the skin surface by washing with soap and water.

AndroGel® should not be used in patients with known hypersensitivity to any of its ingredients, including testosterone USP that is chemically synthesized from soy.

WARNINGS

1. Prolonged use of high doses of orally active 17-alpha-alkyl androgens (e.g., methyltestosterone) has been associated with serious hepatic adverse effects (peliosis hepatis, hepatic neoplasms, cholestatic hepatitis, and jaundice). Peliosis hepatis can be a life-threatening or fatal complication. Long-term therapy with testosterone enanthate, which elevates blood levels for prolonged periods, has produced multiple hepatic adenomas. Testosterone is not known to produce these adverse effects.
2. Geriatric patients treated with androgens may be at an increased risk for the development of prostatic hyperplasia and prostatic carcinoma.
3. Geriatric patients and other patients with clinical or demographic characteristics that are recognized to be associated with an increased risk of prostate cancer should be evaluated for the presence of prostate cancer prior to initiation of testosterone replacement therapy. In men receiving testosterone replacement therapy, surveillance for prostate cancer should be consistent with current practices for eugonadal men (see **PRECAUTIONS: Carcinogenesis, Mutagenesis, Impairment of Fertility** and **Laboratory Tests**).
4. Edema with or without congestive heart failure may be a serious complication in patients with preexisting cardiac, renal, or hepatic disease. In addition to discontinuation of the drug, diuretic therapy may be required.
5. Gynecomastia frequently develops and occasionally persists in patients being treated for hypogonadism.
6. The treatment of hypogonadal men with testosterone esters may potentiate sleep apnea in some patients, especially those with risk factors such as obesity or chronic lung diseases.
7. ALCOHOL BASED GELS ARE FLAMMABLE. AVOID FIRE, FLAME OR SMOKING UNTIL THE GEL HAS DRIED.

PRECAUTIONS

Transfer of testosterone to another person can occur when vigorous skin-to-skin contact is made with the application site (see **Clinical Studies**). The following precautions are recommended to minimize potential transfer of testosterone from AndroGel®-treated skin to another person:

- Patients should wash their hands immediately with soap and water after application of AndroGel®.
- Patients should cover the application site(s) with clothing after the gel has dried (e.g. a shirt).
- In the event that unwashed or unclothed skin to which AndroGel® has been applied does come in direct contact with the skin of another person, the general area of contact on the other person should be washed with soap and water as soon as possible. *In vitro* studies show that residual testosterone is removed from the skin surface by washing with soap and water.

Changes in body hair distribution, significant increase in acne, or other signs of virilization of the female partner should be brought to the attention of a physician.

General

The physician should instruct patients to report any of the following:

- Too frequent or persistent erections of the penis.
- Any nausea, vomiting, changes in skin color, or ankle swelling.
- Breathing disturbances, including those associated with sleep.

Information for Patients

Advise patients to carefully read the information brochure that accompanies each carton of 30 AndroGel® single-use packets or 88 g AndroGel® Pump.

Advise patients of the following:

- AndroGel® should not be applied to the scrotum.
- AndroGel® should be applied once daily to clean dry skin.
- After application of AndroGel®, it is currently unknown for how long showering or swimming should be delayed. For optimal absorption of testosterone, it appears reasonable to wait at least 5-6 hours after application prior to showering or swimming. Nevertheless, showering or swimming after just 1 hour should have a minimal effect on the amount of AndroGel® absorbed if done very infrequently.
- Since alcohol based gels are flammable, avoid fire, flame or smoking until the gel has dried.

Continued on next page

AndroGel—Cont.

Laboratory Tests

1. Hemoglobin and hematocrit levels should be checked periodically (to detect polycythemia) in patients on long-term androgen therapy.
2. Liver function, prostatic specific antigen, cholesterol, and high-density lipoprotein should be checked periodically.
3. To ensure proper dosing, serum testosterone concentrations should be measured (see **DOSAGE AND ADMINISTRATION**).

Drug Interactions

Oxyphenbutazone: Concurrent administration of oxyphenbutazone and androgens may result in elevated serum levels of oxyphenbutazone.

Insulin: In diabetic patients, the metabolic effects of androgens may decrease blood glucose and, therefore, insulin requirements.

Propranolol: In a published pharmacokinetic study of an injectable testosterone product, administration of testosterone cypionate led to an increased clearance of propranolol in the majority of men tested.

Corticosteroids: The concurrent administration of testosterone with ACTH or corticosteroids may enhance edema formation; thus, these drugs should be administered cautiously, particularly in patients with cardiac or hepatic disease.

Drug/Laboratory Test Interactions

Androgens may decrease levels of thyroxin-binding globulin, resulting in decreased total T4 serum levels and increased resin uptake of T3 and T4. Free thyroid hormone levels remain unchanged, however, and there is no clinical evidence of thyroid dysfunction.

Carcinogenesis, Mutagenesis, Impairment of Fertility

Animal Data: Testosterone has been tested by subcutaneous injection and implantation in mice and rats. In mice, the implant induced cervical-uterine tumors, which metastasized in some cases. There is suggestive evidence that injection of testosterone into some strains of female mice increases their susceptibility to hepatoma. Testosterone is also known to increase the number of tumors and decrease the degree of differentiation of chemically induced carcinomas of the liver in rats.

Human Data: There are rare reports of hepatocellular carcinoma in patients receiving long-term oral therapy with androgens in high doses. Withdrawal of the drugs did not lead to regression of the tumors in all cases.

Geriatric patients treated with androgens may be at an increased risk for the development of prostatic hyperplasia and prostatic carcinoma.

Geriatric patients and other patients with clinical or demographic characteristics that are recognized to be associated with an increased risk of prostate cancer should be evaluated for the presence of prostate cancer prior to initiation of testosterone replacement therapy.

In men receiving testosterone replacement therapy, surveillance for prostate cancer should be consistent with current practices for eugonadal men.

Pregnancy Category X (see **CONTRAINDICATIONS**) – Teratogenic Effects: AndroGel® is not indicated for women and must not be used in women.

Nursing Mothers: AndroGel® is not indicated for women and must not be used in women.

Pediatric Use: Safety and efficacy of AndroGel® in pediatric patients have not been established.

ADVERSE REACTIONS

In a controlled clinical study, 154 patients were treated with AndroGel® for up to 6 months (see **Clinical Studies**). Adverse Events possibly, probably or definitely related to the use of AndroGel® and reported by ≥1% of the patients are listed in Table 2.

TABLE 2: Adverse Events Possibly, Probably or Definitely Related to Use of AndroGel® in the Controlled Clinical Trial

Adverse Event	Dose of AndroGel®		
	5 g	7.5 g	10 g
Acne	1%	3%	8%
Alopecia	1%	0%	1%
Application Site Reaction	5%	3%	4%
Asthenia	0%	3%	1%
Depression	1%	0%	1%
Emotional Lability	0%	3%	3%
Gynecomastia	1%	0%	3%
Headache	4%	3%	0%
Hypertension	3%	0%	3%
Lab Test Abnormal*	6%	5%	3%
Libido Decreased	0%	3%	1%
Nervousness	0%	3%	1%
Pain Breast	1%	3%	1%
Prostate Disorder**	3%	3%	5%
Testis Disorder	3%	0%	0%

* *Lab test abnormal* occurred in nine patients with one or more of the following events: elevated hemoglobin or hematocrit, hyperlipidemia, elevated triglycerides, hypokalemia, decreased HDL, elevated glucose, elevated creatinine, or elevated total bilirubin.

** *Prostate disorders* included five patients with enlarged prostate, one patient with BPH, and one patient with elevated PSA results.

The following adverse events possibly related to the use of AndroGel® occurred in fewer than 1% of patients: amnesia, anxiety, discolored hair, dizziness, dry skin, hirsutism, hostility, impaired urination, paresthesia, penis disorder, peripheral edema, sweating, and vasodilation.

In this clinical trial of AndroGel®, skin reactions at the site of application were occasionally reported with AndroGel®, but none was severe enough to require treatment or discontinuation of drug.

Six (4%) patients in this trial had adverse events that led to discontinuation of AndroGel®. These events included the following: cerebral hemorrhage, convulsion (neither of which were considered related to AndroGel® administration), depression, sadness, memory loss, elevated prostate specific antigen and hypertension. No AndroGel® patients discontinued due to skin reactions.

In an uncontrolled pharmacokinetic study of 10 patients, two had adverse events associated with AndroGel®; these were asthenia and depression in one patient and increased libido and hyperkinesia in the other. Among 17 patients in foreign clinical studies there was 1 instance each of acne, erythema and benign prostate adenoma associated with a 2.5% testosterone gel formulation applied dermally.

One hundred six (106) patients have received AndroGel® for up to 12 months in a long-term follow-up study for patients who completed the controlled clinical trial. The preliminary safety results from this study are consistent with those reported for the controlled clinical trial. Table 3 summarizes those adverse events possibly, probably or definitely related to the use of AndroGel® and reported by at least 1% of the total number of patients during long-term exposure to AndroGel®.

TABLE 3: Incidence of Adverse Events Possibly, Probably or Definitely Related to the Use of AndroGel® in the Long-Term, Follow-up Study

Adverse Event	Dose of AndroGel®		
	5 g	7.5 g	10 g
Lab Test Abnormal*	4.2%	0.0%	6.3%
Peripheral Edema	1.4%	0.0%	3.1%
Acne	2.8%	0.0%	12.5%
Application Site Reaction	9.7%	10.0%	3.1%
Prostate Disorder**	2.8%	5.0%	18.8%
Urination Impaired	2.8%	0.0%	0.0%

* *Lab test abnormal* included one patient each with elevated GGTP, elevated hematocrit and hemoglobin, increased total bilirubin, worsened hyperlipidemia, decreased HDL, and hypokalemia.

** *Prostate disorders* included enlarged prostate, elevated PSA results, and in one patient, a new diagnosis of prostate cancer; three patients (one taking 7.5 g daily and two taking 10 g daily) discontinued AndroGel® treatment during the long-term study because of such disorders.

DRUG ABUSE AND DEPENDENCE

AndroGel® contains testosterone, a Schedule III controlled substance as defined by the Anabolic Steroids Control Act.

Oral ingestion of AndroGel® will not result in clinically significant serum testosterone concentrations due to extensive first-pass metabolism.

OVERDOSAGE

There is one report of acute overdosage by injection of testosterone enanthate: testosterone levels of up to 11,400 ng/dL were implicated in a cerebrovascular accident.

DOSAGE AND ADMINISTRATION

The recommended starting dose of AndroGel® 1% is 5 g delivering 5 mg of testosterone systemically, applied once daily (preferably in the morning) to clean, dry, intact skin of the shoulders and upper arms and/or abdomen. Serum testosterone levels should be measured approximately 14 days after initiation of therapy to ensure proper dosing. If the serum testosterone concentration is below the normal range, or if the desired clinical response is not achieved, the daily AndroGel® 1% dose may be increased from 5 g to 7.5 g and from 7.5 g to 10 g as instructed by the physician.

AndroGel® is available in either unit-dose packets or multiple-dose pumps. The metered-dose pump delivers 1.25 g of product when the pump mechanism is fully depressed once. AndroGel® must not be applied to the genitals.

If using the multi-dose AndroGel® Pump, patients should be instructed to prime the pump before using it for the first time by fully depressing the pump mechanism (actuation) 3 times and discard this portion of the product to assure precise dose delivery. After the priming procedure, patients should completely depress the pump one time (actuation) for every 1.25 g of product required to achieve the daily prescribed dosage. The product may be delivered directly into the palm of the hand and then applied to the desired application sites, either one pump actuation at a time or upon completion of all pump actuations required for the daily dose. Please refer to the chart below for specific dosing guidelines when the AndroGel® Pump is used.

Prescribed Daily Dose	Number of Pump Actuations
5 g	4 (once daily)
7.5 g	6 (once daily)
10 g	8 (once daily)

If using the packets, the entire contents should be squeezed into the palm of the hand and immediately applied to the application sites. Alternately, patients may squeeze a portion of the gel from the packet into the palm of the hand and apply to application sites. Repeat until entire contents have been applied.

Application sites should be allowed to dry for a few minutes prior to dressing. Hands should be washed with soap and water after AndroGel® has been applied.

HOW SUPPLIED

AndroGel® contains testosterone, a Schedule III controlled substance as defined by the Anabolic Steroids Control Act.

AndroGel® 1% is supplied in non-aerosol, metered-dose pumps. The pump is composed of plastic and stainless steel and an LDPE/aluminum foil inner liner encased in rigid plastic with a polypropylene cap. Each individual packaged 88 g AndroGel® Pump is capable of dispensing 75 g or 60 metered 1.25 g doses.

AndroGel® 1% is also supplied in unit-dose aluminum foil packets in cartons of 30. Each packet of 2.5 g or 5 g gel contains 25 mg or 50 mg testosterone, respectively.

NDC Number	Package Size
0051-8488-33	75 g pump (dispenses 60 metered 1.25 g doses)
0051-8488-88	2 × 75 g pumps (each pump dispenses 60 metered 1.25 g doses)
0051-8425-30	30 packets (2.5 g per packet)
0051-8450-30	30 packets (5 g per packet)

Keep AndroGel® out of the reach of children.

Storage

Store at 25°C (77°F); excursions permitted to 15° to 30°C (59° to 86°F) [see USP Controlled Room Temperature].

Disposal

Used AndroGel® pumps or used AndroGel® packets should be discarded in household trash in a manner that prevents accidental application or ingestion by children or pets. In addition, any discarded gel should be thoroughly rinsed down the sink or discarded in the household trash in a manner that prevents accidental application or ingestion by children or pets.

Manufactured by:
Laboratoires Besins International
Montrouge, France
For:
Unimed Pharmaceuticals, Inc.
A Solvay Pharmaceuticals, Inc. Company
Marietta, GA 30062-2224, USA
500122/500127
Rev Jun 2004
U.S. Patent No. 6,503,894

Patient Information and Instructions for Using

AndroGel® (CIII)
(testosterone gel) **1%**

Read this information carefully before using AndroGel® [AN drow jel]. The following information about AndroGel® should not take the place of your doctor's orders or recommendations. Your doctor will tell you exactly what dose to take, how to safely take it, and when to take it. Make sure you understand the benefits and risks of AndroGel® before you use it. If you have any other questions about your AndroGel® therapy, ask your doctor or pharmacist.

What is AndroGel®?

AndroGel® is a clear, colorless gel medicine that delivers testosterone into your body through your skin. Once AndroGel® is absorbed through your skin, it enters your bloodstream and helps your body reach normal testosterone levels. The type of testosterone delivered by AndroGel® is the same as the testosterone produced in your body.

Your doctor has prescribed this therapy because your body is not making enough testosterone. The medical term for this condition is hypogonadism. Testosterone helps the body produce sperm and the male sexual characteristics. Testosterone is also necessary for normal sexual function and sex drive.

Who should not take AndroGel®?

AndroGel® **must not be used by women** or by those individuals with known hypersensitivity to any of its components, including individuals who are hypersensitive to testosterone that is chemically synthesized from soy. Pregnant women should avoid skin contact with AndroGel® application sites in men. The active ingredient in AndroGel® is testosterone. (See "Inactive Ingredients" at the end of this leaflet for a list of the other ingredients.) Testosterone may cause fetal harm.

You should not use AndroGel® if you have any of the following conditions:

- prostate cancer (if your doctor knows for sure or suspects it)
- breast cancer (a rare condition for men)

How should I use the AndroGel® Pump?
It is important that you read and follow these directions on how to use the AndroGel® Pump properly.

1. **Apply AndroGel® at the same time each day (preferably every morning).** You should apply your daily dose of gel every morning to clean, dry, intact skin. If you take a bath or shower in the morning, use AndroGel® **after** your bath or shower. Your doctor will tell you how much AndroGel® to use each day.
2. **Be sure your skin is completely dry.**
3. Before using the pump for the first time, you must prime the AndroGel® pump by fully depressing the pump three times and discarding the gel. The unused gel should be discarded by thoroughly rinsing down the sink or discarding in the household trash in a manner to avoid accidental exposure or ingestion by household members or pets.
4. Each full pump depression delivers 1.25 g of AndroGel®. Please refer to the chart below to determine the number of full pump depressions required for the daily dose prescribed by your doctor:

Prescribed Daily Dose	Number of Pump Depressions
5 g	4 (once daily)
7.5 g	6 (once daily)
10 g	8 (once daily)

5. Fully depress the pump the appropriate number of times to deliver the daily dose prescribed by your doctor. The product may be delivered directly into the palm of your hand and then applied to the desired application sites, either one pump depression at a time or upon completion of all pump depressions required for the daily dose.

[See first figure above]

6. **Apply AndroGel® only to healthy, normal skin on your abdomen (stomach area), shoulders, or upper arms.** In this way your body will absorb the right amount of testosterone. **Never apply AndroGel® to your genitals (penis or scrotum) or to skin with open sores, wounds, or irritation.**
7. **Wash your hands with soap and water right away after application to reduce the chance that the medicine will spread from your hands to other people.**
8. **Let AndroGel® dry for a few minutes before you dress.** This prevents your clothing from wiping the gel off your skin. It ensures that your body will absorb the correct amount of testosterone.
9. **Allow gel to dry completely before smoking or going near an open flame.**
10. **Wait 5 to 6 hours before showering or swimming.** To ensure that the greatest amount of AndroGel® is absorbed into your system, you should wait 5 to 6 hours after application before showering or swimming. Once in a while, you may shower or swim as soon as 1 hour after applying AndroGel®. If done infrequently, this will have little effect on the amount of AndroGel® that is absorbed by your body.
11. **Maintain normal activities.** Once your hands are washed and the application site is covered with clothing, there is little risk of transferring testosterone to someone else's skin due to bodily contact. If, however, you expect direct skin contact with someone else, you should wash your application site(s) with soap and water before that encounter. This will reduce the chance that the medicine will transfer to the other person.
12. The AndroGel® pump contains enough product to allow for priming and a set number of precise doses. Please refer to the chart below to determine the number of days of treatment each pump will provide based on your individual dose. Discard pump afterwards.

	Prescribed Daily Dose	Number of Days of Treatment per Pump (after priming)
88 g Pump	5 g	15
	7.5 g	10
	10 g	7.5

How should I use AndroGel® packets?
It is important that you read and follow these directions on how to use AndroGel® properly.

1. **Apply AndroGel® at the same time each day (preferably every morning).** You should apply your daily dose of gel every morning to clean, dry, intact skin. If you take a bath or shower in the morning, use AndroGel® **after** your bath or shower. Your doctor will tell you how much AndroGel® to use each day.
2. **Be sure your skin is completely dry.**
3. **Open the packet.** Open one AndroGel® aluminum foil packet by folding the top edge at the perforation and tearing completely across the packet along the perforation.
4. **Remove the contents from the packet. Squeeze the contents into the palm of your hand.** Squeeze from the bottom of the packet toward the top. If you like, you may squeeze a portion of the gel from the packet into the palm of your hand and apply to application site(s). **Repeat until the entire contents of the packet have been applied.**

[See second figure above]

5. **Apply AndroGel® only to healthy, normal skin on your abdomen (stomach area), shoulders, or upper arms.** In this way your body will absorb the right amount of testosterone. **Never apply AndroGel® to your genitals (penis or scrotum) or to skin with open sores, wounds, or irritation.**
6. **Wash your hands with soap and water right away after application to reduce the chance that the medicine will spread from your hands to other people.**
7. **Let AndroGel® dry for a few minutes before you dress.** This prevents your clothing from wiping the gel off your skin. It ensures that your body will absorb the correct amount of testosterone.
8. **Allow gel to dry completely before smoking or going near an open flame.**
9. **Wait 5 to 6 hours before showering or swimming.** To ensure that the greatest amount of AndroGel® is absorbed into your system, you should wait 5 to 6 hours after application before showering or swimming. Once in a while, you may shower or swim as soon as 1 hour after applying AndroGel®. If done infrequently, this will have little effect on the amount of AndroGel® that is absorbed by your body.
10. **Maintain normal activities.** Once your hands are washed and the application site is covered with clothing, there is little risk of transferring testosterone to someone else's skin due to bodily contact. If, however, you expect direct skin contact with someone else, you should wash your application site(s) with soap and water before that encounter. This will reduce the chance that the medicine will transfer to the other person.

What to do if someone else is exposed to AndroGel®.
If someone else is exposed to AndroGel® either by direct contact with the gel itself or indirectly because of contact with your treated skin, that person should wash the area of contact with soap and water as soon as possible. The longer the gel is in contact with the skin before washing, the greater is the chance that some testosterone will be absorbed by the other person. This is especially important for women (especially pregnant women) and children. They have naturally low levels of testosterone and could be harmed by it.

Men should apply gel to starred (upper arm/shoulders) or shaded (abdomen) areas only.

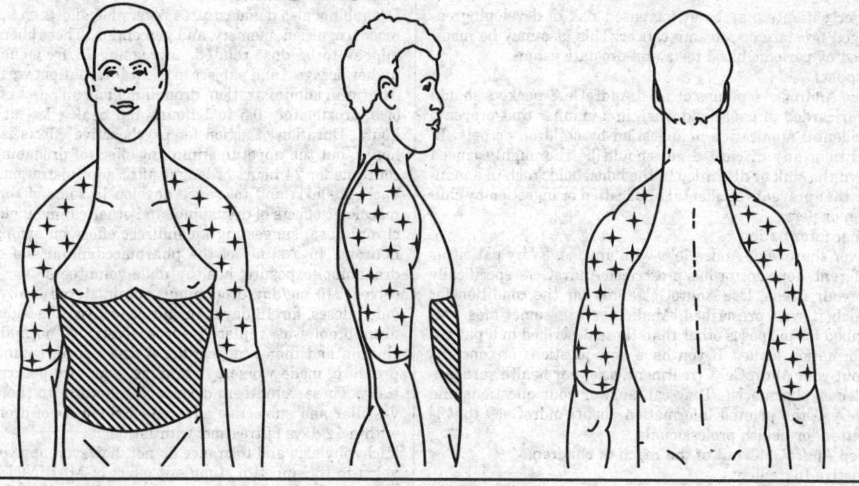

Men should apply gel to starred (upper arm/shoulders) or shaded (abdomen) areas only.

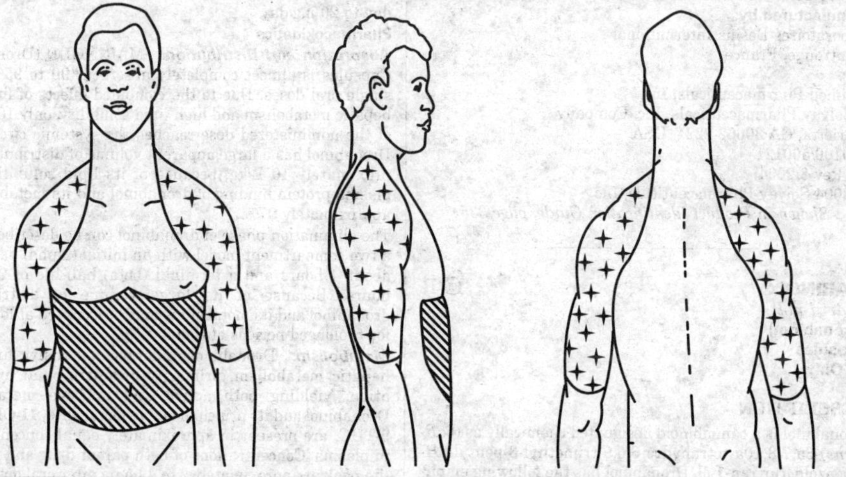

What to do if you get AndroGel® in your eyes.
If you get AndroGel® in your eyes, rinse your eyes right away with warm clean water to flush out any AndroGel®. Seek medical attention if needed.

What to do if you miss a dose.
If you miss a dose, do not double your next dose the next day to catch up. If your next dose is less than 12 hours away, it is best just to wait. Do not take the skipped dose. If it is more than 12 hours until your next dose, take the dose you missed. Resume your normal dosing the next day.

What should I avoid while using AndroGel®?
It is important that you do not spread the medicine to others, especially women and children. Be sure to wash your hands after applying AndroGel®. Do not allow other persons to contact your skin where you have applied AndroGel®, especially pregnant or nursing women. **Testosterone may harm the developing baby. ALCOHOL BASED GELS ARE FLAMMABLE. AVOID FIRE, FLAME OR SMOKING UNTIL THE GEL HAS DRIED.**

What are the possible side effects of AndroGel®?
AndroGel® may cause the following side effects:

- breast development and breast discomfort
- extra fluid in the body. This may cause serious problems for patients with heart, kidney, or liver damage.
- sleep disturbance called "sleep apnea." This is more likely in patients who are overweight or who have lung disease.
- prostate enlargement, sometimes accompanied by difficulty urinating
- emotional problems like depression
- changes in blood levels of cholesterol. This may be monitored and prevented by periodic blood tests.

Tell your doctor if you develop any of the following side effects:

- penis erections that are too frequent or continue too long
- nausea, vomiting, yellow or darker skin (jaundice), or ankle swelling
- breathing problems, including problems breathing while sleeping
- difficulty urinating
- any side effect that concerns you

Tell your doctor about other medicines you are taking. AndroGel® may affect how these medicines work, and you may need to have your doses adjusted.

Tell your doctor if your female partner develops changes in hair distribution, increases in acne, or other signs of masculinity.

Continued on next page

AndroGel—Cont.

Older patients may be at increased risk of developing enlarged prostate or prostate cancer. This also may be monitored by periodic blood tests and prostate exams.

Disposal

Used AndroGel® pumps or used AndroGel® packets should be discarded in household trash in a manner that prevents accidental application or ingestion by children or pets. In addition, any discarded gel should be thoroughly rinsed down the sink or discarded in the household trash in a manner that prevents accidental application or ingestion by children or pets.

Other Information

Never share your AndroGel® with anyone. Every patient is different. Your doctor has prescribed AndroGel® specifically for your needs. Use AndroGel® only for the condition for which it was prescribed. Medicines are sometimes prescribed for purposes other than those described in a patient information leaflet. If you have any questions or concerns about your AndroGel® treatment, ask your health care provider or pharmacist. They can answer your questions and give you the printed information about AndroGel® that is written for health professionals.

Keep AndroGel® out of the reach of children.

Inactive Ingredients

Ethanol, purified water, sodium hydroxide, carbomer 980 and isopropyl myristate.

Store at 25°C (77°F); excursions permitted to 15° to 30°C (59° to 86°F) [see USP Controlled Room Temperature].

Manufactured by:

Laboratoires Besins International
Montrouge, France
For:
Unimed Pharmaceuticals, Inc.
A Solvay Pharmaceuticals, Inc. Company
Marietta, GA 30062-2224, USA
500100/500121
3E Rev 3/2004

Shown in Product Identification Guide, page 335

MARINOL® Ⓒ℞

[măr' ĭ nol]
(Dronabinol)
Capsules
℞ Only

DESCRIPTION

Dronabinol is a cannabinoid designated chemically as (6a*R*-*trans*)-6a,7,8,10a-tetrahydro-6,6,9-trimethyl-3-pentyl-6*H*-dibenzo[*b,d*]pyran-1-ol. Dronabinol has the following empirical and structural formulas:

$C_{21}H_{30}O_2$ (molecular weight = 314.47)

Dronabinol, the active ingredient in MARINOL® Capsules, is synthetic delta-9-tetrahydrocannabinol (delta-9-THC). Delta-9-tetrahydrocannabinol is also a naturally occurring component of *Cannabis sativa L.* (Marijuana).

Dronabinol is a light yellow resinous oil that is sticky at room temperature and hardens upon refrigeration. Dronabinol is insoluble in water and is formulated in sesame oil. It has a pKa of 10.6 and an octanol-water partition coefficient: 6,000:1 at pH 7.

Capsules for oral administration: MARINOL® Capsules is supplied as round, soft gelatin capsules containing either 2.5 mg, 5 mg, or 10 mg dronabinol. Each MARINOL® Capsule is formulated with the following inactive ingredients: FD&C Blue No. 1 (5 mg), FD&C Red No. 40 (5 mg), FD&C Yellow No. 6 (5 mg and 10 mg), gelatin, glycerin, methylparaben, propylparaben, sesame oil, and titanium dioxide.

CLINICAL PHARMACOLOGY

Dronabinol is an orally active cannabinoid which, like other cannabinoids, has complex effects on the central nervous system (CNS), including central sympathomimetic activity. Cannabinoid receptors have been discovered in neural tissues. These receptors may play a role in mediating the effects of dronabinol and other cannabinoids.

Pharmacodynamics

Dronabinol-induced sympathomimetic activity may result in tachycardia and/or conjunctival injection. Its effects on blood pressure are inconsistent, but occasional subjects have experienced orthostatic hypotension and/or syncope upon abrupt standing.

Dronabinol also demonstrates reversible effects on appetite, mood, cognition, memory, and perception. These phenomena appear to be dose-related, increasing in frequency with higher dosages, and subject to great interpatient variability. After oral administration, dronabinol has an onset of action of approximately 0.5 to 1 hours and peak effect at 2 to 4 hours. Duration of action for psychoactive effects is 4 to 6 hours, but the appetite stimulant effect of dronabinol may continue for 24 hours or longer after administration.

Tachyphylaxis and tolerance develop to some of the pharmacologic effects of dronabinol and other cannabinoids with chronic use, suggesting an indirect effect on sympathetic neurons. In a study of the pharmacodynamics of chronic dronabinol exposure, healthy male volunteers (N = 12) received 210 mg/day dronabinol, administered orally in divided doses, for 16 days. An initial tachycardia induced by dronabinol was replaced successively by normal sinus rhythm and then bradycardia. A decrease in supine blood pressure, made worse by standing, was also observed initially. These volunteers developed tolerance to the cardiovascular and subjective adverse CNS effects of dronabinol within 12 days of treatment initiation.

Tachyphylaxis and tolerance do not, however, appear to develop to the appetite stimulant effect of MARINOL® Capsules. In studies involving patients with Acquired Immune Deficiency Syndrome (AIDS), the appetite stimulant effect of MARINOL® Capsules has been sustained for up to five months in clinical trials, at dosages ranging from 2.5 mg/day to 20 mg/day.

Pharmacokinetics

Absorption and Distribution: MARINOL® (Dronabinol) Capsules is almost completely absorbed (90 to 95%) after single oral doses. Due to the combined effects of first pass hepatic metabolism and high lipid solubility, only 10 to 20% of the administered dose reaches the systemic circulation. Dronabinol has a large apparent volume of distribution, approximately 10 L/kg, because of its lipid solubility. The plasma protein binding of dronabinol and its metabolites is approximately 97%.

The elimination phase of dronabinol can be described using a two compartment model with an initial (alpha) half-life of about 4 hours and a terminal (beta) half-life of 25 to 36 hours. Because of its large volume of distribution, dronabinol and its metabolites may be excreted at low levels for prolonged periods of time.

Metabolism: Dronabinol undergoes extensive first-pass hepatic metabolism, primarily by microsomal hydroxylation, yielding both active and inactive metabolites. Dronabinol and its principal active metabolite, 11-OH-delta-9-THC, are present in approximately equal concentrations in plasma. Concentrations of both parent drug and metabolite peak at approximately 2 to 4 hours after oral dosing and decline over several days. Values for clearance average about 0.2 L/kg-hr, but are highly variable due to the complexity of cannabinoid distribution.

Elimination: Dronabinol and its biotransformation products are excreted in both feces and urine. Biliary excretion is the major route of elimination with about half of a radio-labeled oral dose being recovered from the feces within 72 hours as contrasted with 10 to 15% recovered from urine. Less than 5% of an oral dose is recovered unchanged in the feces.

Following single dose administration, low levels of dronabinol metabolites have been detected for more than 5 weeks in the urine and feces.

In a study of MARINOL® Capsules involving AIDS patients, urinary cannabinoid/creatinine concentration ratios were studied bi-weekly over a six week period. The urinary cannabinoid/creatinine ratio was closely correlated with dose. No increase in the cannabinoid/creatinine ratio was observed after the first two weeks of treatment, indicating that steady-state cannabinoid levels had been reached. This conclusion is consistent with predictions based on the observed terminal half-life of dronabinol.

Special Populations: The pharmacokinetic profile of MARINOL® Capsules has not been investigated in either pediatric or geriatric patients.

CLINICAL TRIALS

Appetite Stimulation: The appetite stimulant effect of MARINOL® (Dronabinol) Capsules in the treatment of AIDS-related anorexia associated with weight loss was studied in a randomized, double-blind, placebo-controlled study involving 139 patients. The initial dosage of MARINOL® Capsules in all patients was 5 mg/day, administered in doses of 2.5 mg one hour before lunch and one hour before supper. In pilot studies, early morning administration of MARINOL® Capsules appeared to have been associated with an increased frequency of adverse experiences, as compared to dosing later in the day. The effect of MARINOL® Capsules on appetite, weight, mood, and nausea was measured at scheduled intervals during the six-week treatment period. Side effects (feeling high, dizziness, confusion, somnolence) occurred in 13 of 72 patients (18%) at this dosage level and the dosage was reduced to 2.5 mg/day, administered as a single dose at supper or bedtime.

As compared to placebo, MARINOL® Capsules treatment resulted in a statistically significant improvement in appetite as measured by visual analog scale (see figure). Trends toward improved body weight and mood, and decreases in nausea were also seen.

After completing the 6-week study, patients were allowed to continue treatment with MARINOL® Capsules in an open-label study, in which there was a sustained improvement in appetite.

Appetite Change from Baseline

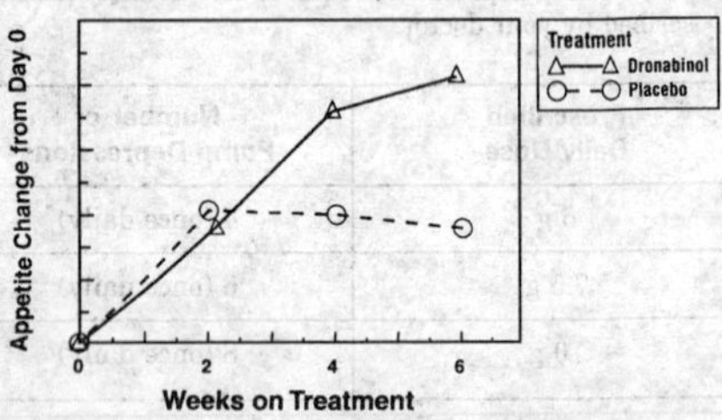

Antiemetic: MARINOL® (Dronabinol) Capsules treatment of chemotherapy-induced emesis was evaluated in 454 patients with cancer, who received a total of 750 courses of treatment of various malignancies. The antiemetic efficacy of MARINOL® Capsules was greatest in patients receiving cytotoxic therapy with MOPP for Hodgkin's and non-Hodgkin's lymphomas. MARINOL® Capsules dosages ranged from 2.5 mg/day to 40 mg/day, administered in equally divided doses every four to six hours (four times daily). As indicated in the following table, escalating the MARINOL® Capsules dose above 7 mg/m² increased the frequency of adverse experiences, with no additional antiemetic benefit.

[See table below]

Combination antiemetic therapy with MARINOL® Capsules and a phenothiazine (prochlorperazine) may result in synergistic or additive antiemetic effects and attenuate the toxicities associated with each of the agents.

INDIVIDUALIZATION OF DOSAGES

The pharmacologic effects of MARINOL® (Dronabinol) Capsules are dose-related and subject to considerable interpatient variability. Therefore, dosage individualization is critical in achieving the maximum benefit of MARINOL® Capsules treatment.

Appetite Stimulation: In the clinical trials, the majority of patients were treated with 5 mg/day MARINOL® Capsules, although the dosages ranged from 2.5 to 20 mg/day. For an adult:

1. Begin with 2.5 mg before lunch and 2.5 mg before supper. If CNS symptoms (feeling high, dizziness, confusion, somnolence) do occur, they usually resolve in 1 to 3 days with continued dosage.
2. If CNS symptoms are severe or persistent, reduce the dose to 2.5 mg before supper. If symptoms continue to be a problem, taking the single dose in the evening or at bedtime may reduce their severity.
3. When adverse effects are absent or minimal and further therapeutic effect is desired, increase the dose to 2.5 mg before lunch and 5 mg before supper or 5 and 5 mg. Although most patients respond to 2.5 mg twice daily, 10 mg twice daily has been tolerated in about half of the patients in appetite stimulation studies.

The pharmacologic effects of MARINOL® Capsules are reversible upon treatment cessation.

Antiemetic: Most patients respond to 5 mg three or four times daily. Dosage may be escalated during a chemotherapy cycle or at subsequent cycles, based upon initial results. Therapy should be initiated at the lowest recommended dosage and titrated to clinical response. Administration of MARINOL® Capsules with phenothiazines, such as prochlorperazine, has resulted in improved efficacy as compared to either drug alone, without additional toxicity.

Pediatrics: MARINOL® Capsules is not recommended for AIDS-related anorexia in pediatric patients because it has not been studied in this population. The pediatric dosage for the treatment of chemotherapy-induced emesis is the same as in adults. Caution is recommended in prescribing MARINOL® Capsules for children because of the psychoactive effects.

Geriatrics: Caution is advised in prescribing MARINOL® Capsules in elderly patients because they are generally more sensitive to the psychoactive effects of drugs. In antiemetic studies, no difference in tolerance or efficacy was apparent in patients >55 years old.

INDICATIONS AND USAGE

MARINOL® (Dronabinol) Capsules is indicated for the treatment of:

1. anorexia associated with weight loss in patients with AIDS; and

MARINOL® Capsules Dose: Response Frequency and Adverse Experiences*
(N = 750 treatment courses)

MARINOL® Capsules Dose	Response Frequency (%)			Adverse Events Frequency (%)		
	Complete	Partial	Poor	None	Nondysphoric	Dysphoric
<7 mg/m²	36	32	32	23	65	12
>7 mg/m²	33	31	36	13	58	28

*Nondysphoric events consisted of drowsiness, tachycardia, etc.

2. nausea and vomiting associated with cancer chemotherapy in patients who have failed to respond adequately to conventional antiemetic treatments.

CONTRAINDICATIONS

MARINOL® (Dronabinol) Capsules is contraindicated in any patient who has a history of hypersensitivity to any cannabinoid or sesame oil.

WARNINGS

Patients receiving treatment with MARINOL® Capsules should be specifically warned not to drive, operate machinery, or engage in any hazardous activity until it is established that they are able to tolerate the drug and to perform such tasks safely.

PRECAUTIONS

General: The risk/benefit ratio of MARINOL® (Dronabinol) Capsules use should be carefully evaluated in patients with the following medical conditions because of individual variation in response and tolerance to the effects of MARINOL® Capsules.

MARINOL® Capsules should be used with caution in patients with cardiac disorders because of occasional hypotension, possible hypertension, syncope, or tachycardia (see CLINICAL PHARMACOLOGY).

MARINOL® Capsules should be used with caution in patients with a history of substance abuse, including alcohol abuse or dependence, because they may be more prone to abuse MARINOL® Capsules as well. Multiple substance abuse is common and marijuana, which contains the same active compound, is a frequently abused substance.

MARINOL® Capsules should be used with caution and careful psychiatric monitoring in patients with mania, depression, or schizophrenia because MARINOL® Capsules may exacerbate these illnesses.

MARINOL® Capsules should be used with caution in patients receiving concomitant therapy with sedatives, hypnotics or other psychoactive drugs because of the potential for additive or synergistic CNS effects.

MARINOL® Capsules should be used with caution in pregnant patients, nursing mothers, or pediatric patients because it has not been studied in these patient populations.

Information for Patients: Patients receiving treatment with MARINOL® (Dronabinol) Capsules should be alerted to the potential for additive central nervous system depression if MARINOL® Capsules is used concomitantly with alcohol or other CNS depressants such as benzodiazepines and barbiturates.

Patients receiving treatment with MARINOL® Capsules should be specifically warned not to drive, operate machinery, or engage in any hazardous activity until it is established that they are able to tolerate the drug and to perform such tasks safely.

Patients using MARINOL® Capsules should be advised of possible changes in mood and other adverse behavioral effects of the drug so as to avoid panic in the event of such manifestations. Patients should remain under the supervision of a responsible adult during initial use of MARINOL® Capsules and following dosage adjustments.

Drug Interactions: In studies involving patients with AIDS and/or cancer, MARINOL® (Dronabinol) Capsules has been co-administered with a variety of medications (e.g., cytotoxic agents, anti-infective agents, sedatives, or opioid analgesics) without resulting in any clinically significant drug/drug interactions. Although no drug/drug interactions were discovered during the clinical trials of MARINOL® Capsules, cannabinoids may interact with other medications through both metabolic and pharmacodynamic mechanisms. Dronabinol is highly protein bound to plasma proteins, and therefore, might displace other protein-bound drugs. Although this displacement has not been confirmed *in vivo*, practitioners should monitor patients for a change in dosage requirements when administering dronabinol to patients receiving other highly protein-bound drugs. Published reports of drug/drug interactions involving cannabinoids are summarized in the following table.

CONCOMITANT DRUG	CLINICAL EFFECT(S)
Amphetamines, cocaine, other sympathomimetic agents	Additive hypertension, tachycardia, possibly cardiotoxicity
Atropine, scopolamine, antihistamines, other anticholinergic agents	Additive or super-additive tachycardia, drowsiness
Amitriptyline, amoxapine, desipramine, other tricyclic antidepressants	Additive tachycardia, hypertension, drowsiness
Barbiturates, benzodiazepines, ethanol, lithium, opioids, buspirone, antihistamines, muscle relaxants, other CNS depressants	Additive drowsiness and CNS depression
Disulfiram	A reversible hypomanic reaction was reported in a 28 y/o man who smoked marijuana; confirmed by dechallenge and rechallenge
Fluoxetine	A 21 y/o female with depression and bulimia receiving 20 mg/day fluoxetine X 4 wks became hypomanic after smoking marijuana; symptoms resolved after 4 days
Antipyrine, barbiturates	Decreased clearance of these agents, presumably via competitive inhibition of metabolism
Theophylline	Increased theophylline metabolism reported with smoking of marijuana; effect similar to that following smoking tobacco

Carcinogenesis, Mutagenesis, Impairment of Fertility: Carcinogenicity studies in mice and rats have been conducted under the US National Toxicology Program (NTP). In the 2-year carcinogenicity study in rats, there was no evidence of carcinogenicity at doses up to 50 mg/kg/day, about 20 times the maximum recommended human dose on a body surface area basis. In the 2-year carcinogenicity study in mice, treatment with dronabinol at 125 mg/kg/day, about 25 times the maximum recommended human dose on a body surface area basis, produced thyroid follicular cell adenoma in both male and female mice but not at 250 or 500 mg/kg/day.

Dronabinol was not genotoxic in the Ames tests, the *in vitro* chromosomal aberration test in Chinese hamster ovary cells, and the *in vivo* mouse micronucleus test. It, however, produced a weak positive response in a sister chromatid exchange test in Chinese hamster ovary cells.

In a long-term study (77 days) in rats, oral administration of dronabinol at doses of 30 to 150 mg/m^2, equivalent to 0.3 to 1.5 times maximum recommended human dose (MRHD) of 90 mg/m^2/day in cancer patients or 2 to 10 times MRHD of 15 mg/m^2/day in AIDS patients, reduced ventral prostate, seminal vesicle and epididymal weights and caused a decrease in seminal fluid volume. Decreases in spermatogenesis, number of developing germ cells, and number of Leydig cells in the testis were also observed. However, sperm count, mating success and testosterone levels were not affected. The significance of these animal findings in humans is not known.

Pregnancy: Pregnancy Category C. Reproduction studies with dronabinol have been performed in mice at 15 to 450 mg/m^2, equivalent to 0.2 to 5 times maximum recommended human dose (MRHD) of 90 mg/m^2/day in cancer patients or 1 to 30 times MRHD of 15 mg/m^2/day in AIDS patients, and in rats at 74 to 295 mg/m^2 (equivalent to 0.8 to 3 times MRHD of 90 mg/m^2 in cancer patients or 5 to 20 times MRHD of 15 mg/m^2/day in AIDS patients). These studies have revealed no evidence of teratogenicity due to dronabinol. At these dosages in mice and rats, dronabinol decreased maternal weight gain and number of viable pups and increased fetal mortality and early resorptions. Such effects were dose dependent and less apparent at lower doses which produced less maternal toxicity. There are no adequate and well-controlled studies in pregnant women. Dronabinol should be used only if the potential benefit justifies the potential risk to the fetus.

Nursing Mothers: Use of MARINOL® Capsules is not recommended in nursing mothers since, in addition to the secretion of HIV virus in breast milk, dronabinol is concentrated in and secreted in human breast milk and is absorbed by the nursing baby.

Geriatric Use: Clinical studies of MARINOL® (Dronabinol) Capsules in AIDS and cancer patients did not include the sufficient numbers of subjects aged 65 and over to determine whether they respond differently from younger subjects. Other reported clinical experience has not identified differences in responses between the elderly and younger patients. In general, dose selection for an elderly patient should be cautious usually starting at the low end of the dosing range, reflecting the greater frequency of decreased hepatic, renal, or cardiac function, increased sensitivity to psychoactive effects and of concomitant disease or other drug therapy.

ADVERSE REACTIONS

Adverse experiences information summarized in the tables below was derived from well-controlled clinical trials conducted in the US and US territories involving 474 patients exposed to MARINOL® (Dronabinol) Capsules. Studies of AIDS-related weight loss included 157 patients receiving dronabinol at a dose of 2.5 mg twice daily and 67 receiving placebo. Studies of different durations were combined by considering the first occurrence of events during the first 28 days. Studies of nausea and vomiting related to cancer chemotherapy included 317 patients receiving dronabinol and 68 receiving placebo.

A cannabinoid dose-related "high" (easy laughing, elation and heightened awareness) has been reported by patients receiving MARINOL® Capsules in both the antiemetic (24%) and the lower dose appetite stimulant clinical trials (8%) (see CLINICAL TRIALS).

The most frequently reported adverse experiences in patients with AIDS during placebo-controlled clinical trials involved the CNS and were reported by 33% of patients receiving MARINOL® Capsules. About 25% of patients reported a minor CNS adverse event during the first 2 weeks and about 4% reported such an event each week for the next 6 weeks thereafter.

PROBABLY CAUSALLY RELATED: Incidence greater than 1%.

Rates derived from clinical trials in AIDS-related anorexia (N=157) and chemotherapy-related nausea (N=317). Rates were generally higher in the anti-emetic use (given in parentheses).

Body as a whole: Asthenia.
Cardiovascular: Palpitations, tachycardia, vasodilation/facial flush.
Digestive: Abdominal pain*, nausea*, vomiting*.
Nervous system: (Amnesia), anxiety/nervousness, (ataxia), confusion, depersonalization, dizziness*, euphoria*, (hallucination), paranoid reaction*, somnolence*, thinking abnormal*.

*Incidence of events 3% to 10%

PROBABLY CAUSALLY RELATED: Incidence less than 1%.

Event rates derived from clinical trials in AIDS-related anorexia (N=157) and chemotherapy-related nausea (N=317).

Cardiovascular: Conjunctivitis*, hypotension*.
Digestive: Diarrhea*, fecal incontinence.
Musculoskeletal: Myalgias.
Nervous system: Depression, nightmares, speech difficulties, tinnitus.
Skin and Appendages: Flushing*.
Special senses: Vision difficulties.

*Incidence of events 0.3% to 1%

CAUSAL RELATIONSHIP UNKNOWN: Incidence less than 1%.

The clinical significance of the association of these events with MARINOL® Capsules treatment is unknown, but they are reported as alerting information for the clinician.

Body as a whole: Chills, headache, malaise.
Digestive: Anorexia, hepatic enzyme elevation.
Respiratory: Cough, rhinitis, sinusitis.
Skin and Appendages: Sweating.

DRUG ABUSE AND DEPENDENCE

MARINOL® (Dronabinol) Capsules is one of the psychoactive compounds present in cannabis, and is abusable and controlled [Schedule III (CIII)] under the Controlled Substances Act. Both psychological and physiological dependence have been noted in healthy individuals receiving dronabinol, but addiction is uncommon and has only been seen after prolonged high dose administration.

Chronic abuse of cannabis has been associated with decrements in motivation, cognition, judgement, and perception. The etiology of these impairments is unknown, but may be associated with the complex process of addiction rather than an isolated effect of the drug. No such decrements in psychological, social or neurological status have been associated with the administration of MARINOL® Capsules for therapeutic purposes.

In an open-label study in patients with AIDS who received MARINOL® Capsules for up to five months, no abuse, diversion or systematic change in personality or social functioning were observed despite the inclusion of a substantial number of patients with a past history of drug abuse.

An abstinence syndrome has been reported after the abrupt discontinuation of dronabinol in volunteers receiving dosages of 210 mg/day for 12 to 16 consecutive days. Within 12 hours after discontinuation, these volunteers manifested symptoms such as irritability, insomnia, and restlessness. By approximately 24 hours post-dronabinol discontinuation, withdrawal symptoms intensified to include "hot flashes", sweating, rhinorrhea, loose stools, hiccoughs and anorexia. These withdrawal symptoms gradually dissipated over the next 48 hours. Electroencephalographic changes consistent with the effects of drug withdrawal (hyperexcitation) were recorded in patients after abrupt dechallenge. Patients also complained of disturbed sleep for several weeks after discontinuing therapy with high dosages of dronabinol.

OVERDOSAGE

Signs and symptoms following MILD MARINOL® (Dronabinol) Capsules intoxication include drowsiness, euphoria, heightened sensory awareness, altered time perception, reddened conjunctiva, dry mouth and tachycardia; following MODERATE intoxication include memory impairment, depersonalization, mood alteration, urinary retention, and reduced bowel motility; and following SEVERE intoxication include decreased motor coordination, lethargy, slurred speech, and postural hypotension. Apprehensive patients may experience panic reactions and seizures may occur in patients with existing seizure disorders.

The estimated lethal human dose of intravenous dronabinol is 30 mg/kg (2100 mg/ 70 kg). Significant CNS symptoms in antiemetic studies followed oral doses of 0.4 mg/kg (28 mg/ 70 kg) of MARINOL® Capsules.

Management: A potentially serious oral ingestion, if recent, should be managed with gut decontamination. In unconscious patients with a secure airway, instill activated charcoal (30 to 100 g in adults, 1 to 2 g/kg in infants) via a nasogastric tube. A saline cathartic or sorbitol may be added

Continued on next page

Marinol—Cont.

to the first dose of activated charcoal. Patients experiencing depressive, hallucinatory or psychotic reactions should be placed in a quiet area and offered reassurance. Benzodiazepines (5 to 10 mg diazepam *po*) may be used for treatment of extreme agitation. Hypotension usually responds to Trendelenburg position and IV fluids. Pressors are rarely required.

DOSAGE AND ADMINISTRATION

Appetite Stimulation: Initially, 2.5 mg MARINOL® (Dronabinol) Capsules should be administered orally twice daily (b.i.d.), before lunch and supper. For patients unable to tolerate this 5 mg/day dosage of MARINOL® Capsules, the dosage can be reduced to 2.5 mg/day, administered as a single dose in the evening or at bedtime. If clinically indicated and in the absence of significant adverse effects, the dosage may be gradually increased to a maximum of 20 mg/day MARINOL® Capsules, administered in divided oral doses. Caution should be exercised in escalating the dosage of MARINOL® Capsules because of the increased frequency of dose-related adverse experiences at higher dosages (see **PRECAUTIONS**).

Antiemetic: MARINOL® Capsules is best administered at an initial dose of 5 mg/m^2, given 1 to 3 hours prior to the administration of chemotherapy, then every 2 to 4 hours after chemotherapy is given, for a total of 4 to 6 doses/day. Should the 5 mg/m^2 dose prove to be ineffective, and in the absence of significant side effects, the dose may be escalated by 2.5 mg/m^2 increments to a maximum of 15 mg/m^2 per dose. Caution should be exercised in dose escalation, however, as the incidence of disturbing psychiatric symptoms increases significantly at maximum dose (see **PRECAUTIONS**).

STORAGE CONDITIONS

MARINOL® (Dronabinol) Capsules should be packaged in a well-closed container and stored in a cool environment between 8° and 15°C (46° and 59°F) and alternatively could be stored in a refrigerator. Protect from freezing.

HOW SUPPLIED

MARINOL® Capsules (dronabinol solution in sesame oil in soft gelatin capsules)

2.5 mg white capsules (Identified UM or RL).
NDC 0051-0021-21 (Bottle of 60 capsules).

5 mg dark brown capsules (Identified UM or RL).
NDC 0051-0022-11 (Bottle of 25 capsules).

10 mg orange capsules (Identified UM or RL).
NDC 0051-0023-21 (Bottle of 60 capsules).

MARINOL® is a registered trademark of Unimed Pharmaceuticals, Inc. and is Manufactured by Banner Pharmacaps, Inc.
High Point, NC 27265
500012 4E Rev 5/2003
© UPI, 2003
UNIMED
PHARMACEUTICALS, INC.
A Solvay Pharmaceuticals, Inc. Company
Marietta, GA 30062

Shown in Product Identification Guide, page 335

Upsher-Smith Laboratories, Inc.

6701 EVENSTAD DRIVE
MINNEAPOLIS, MN 55369

For Medical Information Contact:
Write: Professional Services Department
or call: (800) 654-2299
(during business hours-8:00 am to 5:00 pm CST)

AMLACTIN AP® — OTC

[*ăm-lăk-tĭn*]
Anti-Itch Moisturizing Cream with 1% Pramoxine HCl

PRODUCT DESCRIPTION

AMLACTIN AP® Anti-Itch Moisturizing Cream is a special formulation containing 12% lactic acid neutralized with ammonium hydroxide to provide a cream pH of 4.5–5.5 with pramoxine HCl. Lactic acid, an alpha-hydroxy acid, is a naturally occurring humectant which moisturizes and softens rough, dry skin. Pramoxine HCl, USP, 1% is an effective antipruritic ingredient used to temporarily relieve itching associated with dry skin.

HOW SUPPLIED

AMLACTIN AP® is available in single 140g tubes packaged in an outer carton (NDC 0245-0025-14).

CLENIA™ — ℞

[*clĕn'ē-ə*]
(Sodium Sulfacetamide 10% and Sulfur 5%)
FOAMING WASH AND EMOLLIENT CREAM

PRODUCT DESCRIPTION

Clenia™ Foaming Wash and Emollient Cream contain 10% sodium sulfacetamide, which is a sulfonamide with antibacterial activity. They also contain 5% sulfur, which acts as a keratolytic agent.

HOW SUPPLIED

Clenia™ Foaming Wash is available in 6 oz (170 g) bottles (NDC 0245-0168-06) and 12 oz (340 g) bottles (NDC 0245-0168-12). Clenia™ Emollient Cream is available in 1 oz (28g) tubes (NDC 0245-0169-01).

Shown in Product Identification Guide, page 335

FOLGARD RX 2.2® Tablets — ℞

[*fōl-gärd*]
2.2mg Folic Acid, 25mg Vitamin B-6, 500mcg Vitamin B-12

DESCRIPTION

Folgard RX 2.2® Tablets are intended for oral administration. Folgard RX 2.2® is indicated for nutritional support and folic acid supplementation.

HOW SUPPLIED

Folgard RX 2.2® Tablets are oval, yellow and film-coated. Folgard RX 2.2® is available in bottles of 100 tablets (NDC 0245-0016-11).

Shown in Product Identification Guide, page 335

FOLGARD® Tablets — OTC

[*fōl'-gärd*]
Folic Acid, Vitamin B-6, Vitamin B-12 Combination Dietary Supplement

DESCRIPTION

Folgard® is a unique formulation of 800 mcg folic acid, 10 mg vitamin B-6 and 115 mcg vitamin B-12. Taking a folic acid supplement can mask a B-vitamin deficiency. Folgard® includes vitamin B-6 and B-12 to help ensure that this does not occur.

HOW SUPPLIED

Folgard® Tablets are available in bottles of 60 tablets: List 0245-0017-60

HEMRIL®-30 — ℞

[*hĕm' rĭl*]
(Hydrocortisone Acetate, 30 mg) Suppositories

DESCRIPTION

Each Hemril®-30 suppository contains 30 mg hydrocortisone acetate (a corticosteroid) in a hydrogenated vegetable oil base.

HOW SUPPLIED

Hemril®-30 suppositories are white, smooth surfaced, torpedo-shaped with one rounded end, supplied in cartons of 12 (NDC 0245-0112-12) and 24 (NDC 0245-0112-24).

JANTOVEN™ — ℞

[*jan'to-ven*]
(Warfarin Sodium Tablets, USP)

DESCRIPTION

Jantoven™ (crystalline warfarin sodium), is an anticoagulant which acts by inhibiting vitamin K-dependent coagulation factors. Chemically, it is 3-(α-acetonylbenzyl)-4-hydroxycoumarin and is a racemic mixture of the R- and S-enantiomers. Crystalline warfarin sodium is an isopropanol clathrate. The crystallization of warfarin sodium virtually eliminates trace impurities present in amorphous warfarin. Its empirical formula is $C_{19}H_{15}NaO_4$ and its structural formula may be represented by the following:

ONa CH₂COCH₃ M.W. 330.31

Crystalline warfarin sodium occurs as a white, odorless, crystalline powder, is discolored by light and is very soluble in water; freely soluble in alcohol; very slightly soluble in chloroform and in ether.

Jantoven™ (Warfarin Sodium Tablets, USP) for oral use contain: 1 mg, 2 mg, 2½ mg, 3 mg, 4 mg, 5 mg, 6 mg, 7½ mg or 10 mg of crystalline warfarin sodium, USP. They also contain:

All Strengths: Lactose monohydrate, magnesium stearate, povidone, and pregelatinized starch (corn).

1 mg:	FD&C Red #40 Aluminum Lake
2 mg:	FD&C Blue #2 Aluminum Lake and FD&C Red #40 Aluminum Lake
2½ mg:	D&C Yellow #10 Aluminum Lake and FD&C Blue #1 Aluminum Lake
3 mg:	Brown #75 Synthetic Brown Iron Oxide
4 mg:	FD&C Blue #1 Aluminum Lake
5 mg:	FD&C Yellow #6 Aluminum Lake
6 mg:	Yellow #10 Synthetic Yellow Iron Oxide, Black #85 Synthetic Black Iron Oxide and FD&C Blue #1 Aluminum Lake
7½ mg:	D&C Yellow #10 Aluminum Lake and FD&C Yellow #6 Aluminum Lake
10 mg:	Dye Free.

CLINICAL PHARMACOLOGY

Jantoven™ (Warfarin Sodium Tablets, USP) and other coumarin anticoagulants act by inhibiting the synthesis of vitamin K dependent clotting factors, which include Factors II, VII, IX and X, and the anticoagulant proteins C and S. Half-lives of these clotting factors are as follows: Factor II - 60 hours, VII - 4–6 hours, IX - 24 hours, and X - 48–72 hours. The half-lives of proteins C and S are approximately 8 hours and 30 hours, respectively. The resultant *in vivo* effect is a sequential depression of Factors VII, IX, X and II activities. Vitamin K is an essential cofactor for the post ribosomal synthesis of the vitamin K dependent clotting factors. The vitamin promotes the biosynthesis of γ-carboxyglutamic acid residues in the proteins which are essential for biological activity. Warfarin is thought to interfere with clotting factor synthesis by inhibition of the regeneration of vitamin K_1 epoxide. The degree of depression is dependent upon the dosage administered. Therapeutic doses of warfarin decrease the total amount of the active form of each vitamin K dependent clotting factor made by the liver by approximately 30% to 50%.

An anticoagulation effect generally occurs within 24 hours after drug administration. However, peak anticoagulant effect may be delayed 72 to 96 hours. The duration of action of a single dose of racemic warfarin is 2 to 5 days. The effects of **Jantoven™** may become more pronounced as effects of daily maintenance doses overlap. Anticoagulants have no direct effect on an established thrombus, nor do they reverse ischemic tissue damage. However, once a thrombus has occurred, the goal of anticoagulant treatment is to prevent further extension of the formed clot and prevent secondary thromboembolic complications which may result in serious and possibly fatal sequelae.

Pharmacokinetics: Jantoven™ is a racemic mixture of the R- and S-enantiomers. The S-enantiomer exhibits 2–5 times more anticoagulant activity than the R-enantiomer in humans, but generally has a more rapid clearance.

Absorption: Jantoven™ is essentially completely absorbed after oral administration with peak concentration generally attained within the first 4 hours.

Distribution: There are no differences in the apparent volumes of distribution after intravenous and oral administration of single doses of warfarin solution. Warfarin distributes into a relatively small apparent volume of distribution of about 0.14 liter/kg. A distribution phase lasting 6 to 12 hours is distinguishable after rapid intravenous or oral administration of an aqueous solution. Using a one compartment model, and assuming complete bioavailability, estimates of the volumes of distribution of R- and S- warfarin are similar to each other and to that of the racemate. Concentrations in fetal plasma approach the maternal values, but warfarin has not been found in human milk (see **WARNINGS-Lactation**). Approximately 99% of the drug is bound to plasma proteins.

Metabolism: The elimination of warfarin is almost entirely by metabolism. **Jantoven™** is stereoselectively metabolized by hepatic microsomal enzymes (cytochrome P-450) to inactive hydroxylated metabolites (predominant route) and by reductases to reduced metabolites (warfarin alcohols). The warfarin alcohols have minimal anticoagulant activity. The metabolites are principally excreted into the urine; and to a lesser extent into the bile. The metabolites of warfarin that have been identified include dehydrowarfarin, two diastereoisomer alcohols, 4'-, 6-, 7-, 8- and 10-hydroxywarfarin. The Cytochrome P-450 isozymes involved in the metabolism of warfarin include 2C9, 2C19, 2C8, 2C18,1A2, and 3A4. 2C9 is likely to be the principal form of human liver P-450 which modulates the *in vivo* anticoagulant activity of warfarin.

Excretion: The terminal half-life of warfarin after a single dose is approximately one week; however, the effective half-life ranges from 20 to 60 hours, with a mean of about 40 hours. The clearance of R-warfarin is generally half that of S-warfarin, thus as the volumes of distribution are similar, the half-life of R-warfarin is longer than that of S-warfarin. The half-life of R-warfarin ranges from 37 to 89 hours, while that of S-warfarin ranges from 21 to 43 hours. Studies with radiolabeled drug have demonstrated that up to 92% of the orally administered dose is recovered in urine. Very little warfarin is excreted unchanged in urine. Urinary excretion is in the form of metabolites.

Elderly: Patients 60 years or older appear to exhibit greater than expected PT/INR response to the anticoagulant effects of warfarin. The cause of the increased sensitivity to the anticoagulant effects of warfarin in this age group is unknown. This increased anticoagulant effect from warfarin may be due to a combination of pharmacokinetic and pharmacodynamic factors. Racemic warfarin clearance may be unchanged or reduced with increasing age. Limited information suggests there is no difference in the clearance of S-warfarin in the elderly versus young subjects. However, there may be a slight decrease in the clearance of R-warfarin in the elderly as compared to the young. Therefore, as patient age increases, a lower dose of warfarin is usually required to produce a therapeutic level of anticoagulation.

Asians: Asian patients may require lower initiation and maintenance doses of warfarin. One non-controlled study conducted in 151 Chinese outpatients reported a mean daily warfarin requirement of 3.3 ± 1.4 mg to achieve an INR of 2 to 2.5. These patients were stabilized on warfarin for various indications. Patient age was the most important determinant of warfarin requirement in Chinese patients with a progressively lower warfarin requirement with increasing age.

Renal Dysfunction: Renal clearance is considered to be a minor determinant of anticoagulant response to warfarin. No dosage adjustment is necessary for patients with renal failure.

Hepatic Dysfunction: Hepatic dysfunction can potentiate the response to warfarin through impaired synthesis of clotting factors and decreased metabolism of warfarin.

Clinical Trials

Atrial Fibrillation (AF): In five prospective randomized controlled clinical trials involving 3711 patients with non-rheumatic AF, warfarin significantly reduced the risk of systemic thromboembolism including stroke (See **Table 1**). The risk reduction ranged from 60% to 86% in all except one trial (CAFA: 45%) which stopped early due to published positive results from two of these trials. The incidence of major bleeding in these trials ranged from 0.6 to 2.7% (See **Table 1**). Meta-analysis findings of these studies revealed that the effects of warfarin in reducing thromboembolic events including stroke were similar at either moderately high INR (2.0–4.5) or low INR (1.4–3.0). There was a significant reduction in minor bleeds at the low INR. Similar data from clinical studies in valvular atrial fibrillation patients are not available.

[See table 1 above]

TABLE 1
CLINICAL STUDIES OF WARFARIN IN NON-RHEUMATIC AF PATIENTS*

Study	N Warfarin-Treated Patients	Control Patients	PT Ratio	INR	Thromboembolism % Risk Reduction	Thromboembolism p-value	% Major Bleeding Warfarin-Treated Patients	% Major Bleeding Control Patients
AFASAK	335	336	1.5–2.0	2.8–4.2	60	0.027	0.6	0.0
SPAF	210	211	1.3–1.8	2.0–4.5	67	0.01	1.9	1.9
BAATAF	212	208	1.2–1.5	1.5–2.7	86	<0.05	0.9	0.5
CAFA	187	191	1.3–1.6	2.0–3.0	45	0.25	2.7	0.5
SPINAF	260	265	1.2–1.5	1.4–2.8	79	0.001	2.3	1.5

*All study results of warfarin vs. control are based on intention-to-treat analysis and include ischemic stroke and systemic thromboembolism, excluding hemorrhage and transient ischemic attacks.

Myocardial Infarction: WARIS (The Warfarin Re-Infarction Study) was a double-blind, randomized study of 1214 patients 2 to 4 weeks post-infarction treated with warfarin to a target INR of 2.8 to 4.8. [But note that a lower INR was achieved and increased bleeding was associated with INR's above 4.0; (see **DOSAGE AND ADMINISTRATION**)]. The primary endpoint was a combination of total mortality and recurrent infarction. A secondary endpoint of cerebrovascular events was assessed. Mean follow-up of the patients was 37 months. The results for each endpoint separately, including an analysis of vascular death, are provided in the following table:

[See table 2 above]

TABLE 2

Event	Warfarin (N=607)	Placebo (N=607)	RR (95%CI)	% Risk Reduction (p-value)
Total Patient Years of Follow-up	2018	1944		
Total Mortality	94 (4.7/100 py)	123 (6.3/100 py)	0.76 (0.60, 0.97)	24 (p=0.030)
Vascular Death	82 (4.1/100 py)	105 (5.4/100 py)	0.78 (0.60, 1.02)	22 (p=0.068)
Recurrent MI	82 (4.1/100 py)	124 (6.4/100 py)	0.66 (0.51, 0.85)	34 (p=0.001)
Cerebrovascular Event	20 (1.0/100 py)	44 (2.3/100 py)	0.46 (0.28, 0.75)	54 (p=0.002)

RR = Relative risk; Risk reduction = (I-RR); CI = Confidence interval; MI = Myocardial infarction; py = patient years

Mechanical and Bioprosthetic Heart Valves: In a prospective, randomized, open label, positive-controlled study (Mok et al, 1985) in 254 patients, the thromboembolic-free interval was found to be significantly greater in patients with mechanical prosthetic heart valves treated with warfarin alone compared with dipyridamole-aspirin ($p<0.005$) and pentoxifylline-aspirin ($p<0.05$) treated patients. Rates of thromboembolic events in these groups were 2.2, 8.6, and 7.9/100 patient years, respectively. Major bleeding rates were 2.5, 0.0, and 0.9/100 patient years, respectively.

In a prospective, open label, clinical trial (Saour et al, 1990) comparing moderate (INR 2.65) vs. high intensity (INR 9.0) warfarin therapies in 258 patients with mechanical prosthetic heart valves, thromboembolism occurred with similar frequency in the two groups (4.0 and 3.7 events/100 patient years, respectively). Major bleeding was more common in the high intensity group (2.1 events/100 patient years) vs. 0.95 events/100 patient years in the moderate intensity group.

In a randomized trial (Turpie et al, 1988) in 210 patients comparing two intensities of warfarin therapy (INR 2.0–2.25 vs. INR 2.5–4.0) for a three-month period following tissue heart valve replacement, thromboembolism occurred with similar frequency in the two groups (major embolic events 2.0% vs. 1.9%, respectively and minor embolic events 10.8% vs.10.2%, respectively). Major bleeding complications were more frequent with the higher intensity (major hemorrhages 4.6%) vs. none in the lower intensity.

INDICATIONS AND USAGE

Jantoven™ (Warfarin Sodium Tablets, USP) is indicated for the prophylaxis and/or treatment of venous thrombosis and its extension, and pulmonary embolism.

Jantoven™ is indicated for the prophylaxis and/or treatment of the thromboembolic complications associated with atrial fibrillation and/or cardiac valve replacement.

Jantoven™ is indicated to reduce the risk of death, recurrent myocardial infarction, and thromboembolic events such as stroke or systemic embolization after myocardial infarction.

CONTRAINDICATIONS

Anticoagulation is contraindicated in any localized or general physical condition or personal circumstance in which the hazard of hemorrhage might be greater than the potential clinical benefits of anticoagulation, such as:

Pregnancy: Jantoven™ (Warfarin Sodium Tablets, USP) is contraindicated in women who are or may become pregnant because the drug passes through the placental barrier and may cause fatal hemorrhage to the fetus *in utero*. Furthermore, there have been reports of birth malformations in children born to mothers who have been treated with warfarin during pregnancy.

Embryopathy characterized by nasal hypoplasia with or without stippled epiphyses (chondrodysplasia punctata) has been reported in pregnant women exposed to warfarin during the first trimester. Central nervous system abnormalities also have been reported, including dorsal midline dysplasia characterized by agenesis of the corpus callosum, Dandy-Walker malformation, and midline cerebellar atrophy. Ventral midline dysplasia, characterized by optic atrophy, and eye abnormalities have been observed. Mental retardation, blindness, and other central nervous system abnormalities have been reported in association with second and third trimester exposure. Although rare, teratogenic reports following in utero exposure to warfarin include urinary tract anomalies such as single kidney, asplenia, anencephaly, spina bifida, cranial nerve palsy, hydrocephalus, cardiac defects and congenital heart disease, polydactyly, deformities of toes, diaphragmatic hernia, and corneal leukoma, cleft palate, cleft lip, schizencephaly, and microcephaly.

Spontaneous abortion and still birth are known to occur and a higher risk of fetal mortality is associated with the use of warfarin. Low birth weight and growth retardation have also been reported.

Women of childbearing potential who are candidates for anticoagulant therapy should be carefully evaluated and the indications critically reviewed with the patient. If the patient becomes pregnant while taking this drug, she should be apprised of the potential risks to the fetus, and the possibility of termination of the pregnancy should be discussed in light of those risks.

Hemorrhagic tendencies or blood dyscrasias.

Recent or contemplated surgery of: (1) central nervous system; (2) eye; (3) traumatic surgery resulting in large open surfaces.

Bleeding tendencies associated with active ulceration or overt bleeding of: (1) gastrointestinal, genitourinary or respiratory tracts; (2) cerebrovascular hemorrhage; (3) aneurysms-cerebral, dissecting aorta; (4) pericarditis and pericardial effusions; (5) bacterial endocarditis.

Threatened abortion, eclampsia and preeclampsia.

Inadequate laboratory facilities.

Unsupervised patients with senility, alcoholism, or psychosis or other lack of patient cooperation.

Spinal puncture and other diagnostic or therapeutic procedures with potential for uncontrollable bleeding.

Miscellaneous: major regional, lumbar block anesthesia, malignant hypertension and known hypersensitivity to warfarin or to any other component of this product.

WARNINGS

The most serious risks associated with anticoagulant therapy with warfarin sodium are hemorrhage in any tissue or organ and, less frequently (<0.1%), necrosis and/or gangrene of skin and other tissues. The risk of hemorrhage is related to the level of intensity and the duration of anticoagulant therapy. Hemorrhage and necrosis have in some cases been reported to result in death or permanent disability. Necrosis appears to be associated with local thrombosis and usually appears within a few days of the start of anticoagulant therapy. In severe cases of necrosis, treatment through debridement or amputation of the affected tissue, limb, breast or penis has been reported. Careful diagnosis is required to determine whether necrosis is caused by an underlying disease. Warfarin therapy should be discontinued when warfarin is suspected to be the cause of developing necrosis and heparin therapy may be considered for anticoagulation. Although various treatments have been attempted, no treatment for necrosis has been considered uniformly effective. See below for information on predisposing conditions. These and other risks associated with anticoagulant therapy must be weighed against the risk of thrombosis or embolization in untreated cases.

It cannot be emphasized too strongly that treatment of each patient is a highly individualized matter. **Jantoven™** (Warfarin Sodium Tablets, USP), a narrow therapeutic range (index) drug, may be affected by factors such as other drugs and dietary vitamin K. Dosage should be controlled by periodic determinations of prothrombin time (PT)/International Normalized Ratio (INR) or other suitable coagulation tests. Determinations of whole blood clotting and bleeding times are not effective measures for control of therapy. Heparin prolongs the one-stage PT. When heparin and **Jantoven™** are administered concomitantly, refer below to CONVERSION FROM HEPARIN THERAPY for recommendations.

Caution should be observed when **Jantoven™** is administered in any situation or in the presence of any predisposing condition where added risk of hemorrhage, necrosis and/or gangrene is present.

Anticoagulation therapy with **Jantoven™** may enhance the release of atheromatous plaque emboli, thereby increasing the risk of complications from systemic cholesterol microembolization, including the "purple toes syndrome." Discontinuation of **Jantoven™** therapy is recommended when such phenomena are observed.

Systemic atheroemboli and cholesterol microemboli can present with a variety of signs and symptoms including purple toes syndrome, livedo reticularis, rash, gangrene, abrupt and intense pain in the leg, foot, or toes, foot ulcers, myalgia, penile gangrene, abdominal pain, flank or back pain, hematuria, renal insufficiency, hypertension, cerebral ischemia, spinal cord infarction, pancreatitis, symptoms simulating polyarteritis, or any other sequelae of vascular compromise due to embolic occlusion. The most commonly involved visceral organs are the kidneys followed by the pancreas, spleen, and liver. Some cases have progressed to necrosis or death.

Purple toes syndrome is a complication of oral anticoagulation characterized by a dark, purplish or mottled color of the toes, usually occurring between 3–10 weeks, or later, after the initiation of therapy with warfarin or related compounds. Major features of this syndrome include purple color of plantar surfaces and sides of the toes that blanches on moderate pressure and fades with elevation of the legs; pain and tenderness of the toes; waxing and waning of the color over time. While the purple toes syndrome is reported to be reversible, some cases progress to gangrene or necrosis which may require debridement of the affected area, or may lead to amputation.

Heparin-induced thrombocytopenia: Jantoven™ should be used with caution in patients with heparin-induced thrombocytopenia and deep venous thrombosis. Cases of venous limb ischemia, necrosis and gangrene have occurred in patients with heparin-induced thrombocytopenia and deep venous thrombosis when heparin treatment was discontinued and warfarin therapy was started or continued. In some patients sequelae have included amputation of the involved area and/or death (Warkentin et al, 1997).

A severe elevation (>50 seconds) in activated partial thromboplastin time (aPTT) with a PT/INR in the desired range has been identified as an indication of increased risk of postoperative hemorrhage.

The decision to administer anticoagulants in the following conditions must be based upon clinical judgment in which the risks of anticoagulant therapy are weighed against the benefits:

Lactation: Based on very limited published data, warfarin has not been detected in the breast milk of mothers treated with warfarin. The same limited published data reports that breast-fed infants, whose mothers were treated with warfarin, had prolonged prothrombin times, although not as prolonged as those of the mothers. The decision to breast-feed should be undertaken only after careful consideration of the available alternatives. Women who are breastfeeding and anticoagulated with warfarin should be very carefully monitored so that recommended PT/INR values are not exceeded. It is prudent to perform coagulation tests and to

Continued on next page

Jantoven—Cont.

evaluate Vitamin K status in infants at risk for bleeding tendencies before advising women taking warfarin to breast-feed. Effects in premature infants have not been evaluated.

Severe to moderate hepatic or renal insufficiency.

Infectious diseases or disturbances of intestinal flora: sprue, antibiotic therapy.

Trauma which may result in internal bleeding.

Surgery or trauma resulting in large exposed raw surfaces.

Indwelling catheters.

Severe to moderate hypertension.

Known or suspected deficiency in protein C mediated anticoagulant response: Hereditary or acquired deficiencies of protein C or its cofactor, protein S, have been associated with tissue necrosis following warfarin administration. Not all patients with these conditions develop necrosis, and tissue necrosis occurs in patients without these deficiencies. Inherited resistance to activated protein C has been described in many patients with venous thromboembolic disorders but has not yet been evaluated as a risk factor for tissue necrosis. The risk associated with these conditions, both for recurrent thrombosis and for adverse reactions, is difficult to evaluate since it does not appear to be the same for everyone. Decisions about testing and therapy must be made on an individual basis. It has been reported that concomitant anticoagulation therapy with heparin for 5 to 7 days during initiation of therapy with **Jantoven™** may minimize the incidence of tissue necrosis. Warfarin therapy should be discontinued when warfarin is suspected to be the cause of developing necrosis and heparin therapy may be considered for anticoagulation.

Miscellaneous: polycythemia vera, vasculitis, and severe diabetes.

Minor and severe allergic/hypersensitivity reactions and anaphylactic reactions have been reported.

In patients with acquired or inherited warfarin resistance, decreased therapeutic responses to **Jantoven™** have been reported. Exaggerated therapeutic responses have been reported in other patients.

Patients with congestive heart failure may exhibit greater than expected PT/INR response to **Jantoven™**, thereby requiring more frequent laboratory monitoring, and reduced doses of **Jantoven™**.

Concomitant use of anticoagulants with streptokinase or urokinase is not recommended and may be hazardous. (Please note recommendations accompanying these preparations.)

PRECAUTIONS

Periodic determination of PT/INR or other suitable coagulation test is essential.

Numerous factors, alone or in combination, including travel, changes in diet, environment, physical state and medication, including botanicals, may influence response of the patient to anticoagulants. It is generally good practice to monitor the patient's response with additional PT/INR determinations in the period immediately after discharge from the hospital, and whenever other medications, including botanicals, are initiated, discontinued or taken irregularly. The following factors are listed for reference; however, other factors may also affect the anticoagulant response.

Drugs may interact with Jantoven™ (Warfarin Sodium Tablets, USP) through pharmacodynamic or pharmacokinetic mechanisms. Pharmacodynamic mechanisms for drug interactions with Jantoven™ are synergism (impaired hemostasis, reduced clotting factor synthesis), competitive antagonism (vitamin K), and altered physiologic control loop for vitamin K metabolism (hereditary resistance). Pharmacokinetic mechanisms for drug interactions with Jantoven™ are mainly enzyme induction, enzyme inhibition, and reduced plasma protein binding. It is important to note that some drugs may interact by more than one mechanism.

The following factors, alone or in combination, may be responsible for INCREASED PT/INR response:

ENDOGENOUS FACTORS:

[See first table above]

EXOGENOUS FACTORS:

Potential drug interactions with Jantoven™ are listed below by drug class and by specific drugs.

[See second table above]

[See third table above]

The following factors, alone or in combination, may be responsible for DECREASED PT/INR response:

ENDOGENOUS FACTORS:

edema	hypothyroidism
hereditary coumarin resistance	nephrotic syndrome
hyperlipemia	

EXOGENOUS FACTORS:

Potential drug interactions with Jantoven™ (Warfarin Sodium Tablets, USP) are listed below by drug class and by specific drugs.

[See fourth table at right]

[See first table at top of next page]

Because a patient may be exposed to a combination of the above factors, the net effect of **Jantoven™** on PT/INR response may be unpredictable. More frequent PT/INR moni-

blood dyscrasias - see **CONTRAINDICATIONS**	diarrhea	hyperthyroidism
cancer	elevated temperature	poor nutritional state
collagen vascular disease	hepatic disorders	steatorrhea
congestive heart failure	infectious hepatitis	vitamin K deficiency
	jaundice	

Classes of Drugs

5-lipoxygenase Inhibitor	Antineoplastics†	Fibric Acid Derivatives
Adrenergic Stimulants, Central	Antiparasitic/Antimicrobials	HMG-CoA Reductase Inhibitors†
Alcohol Abuse Reduction Preparations	Antiplatelet Drugs/Effects	Leukotriene Receptor Antagonist
Analgesics	Antithyroid Drugs†	Monoamine Oxidase Inhibitors
Anesthetics, Inhalation	Beta-Adrenergic Blockers	Narcotics, prolonged
Antiandrogen	Cholelitholytic Agents	Nonsteroidal Anti-Inflammatory Agents
Antiarrhythmics†	Diabetes Agents, Oral	Psychostimulants
Antibiotics†	Diuretics†	Pyrazolones
Aminoglycosides (oral)	Fungal Medications, Intravaginal,	Salicylates
Cephalosporins, parenteral	Systemic†	Selective Serotonin Reuptake Inhibitors
Macrolides	Gastric Acidity and Peptic Ulcer Agents†	Steroids, Adrenocortical†
Miscellaneous	Gastrointestinal Prokinetic Agents,	Steroids, Anabolic (17-Alkyl Testosterone Derivatives)
Penicillins, intravenous, high dose	Ulcerative Colitis Agents	Thrombolytics
Quinolones (fluoroquinolones)	Gout Treatment Agents	Thyroid Drugs
Sulfonamides, long acting	Hemorrheologic Agents	Tuberculosis Agents†
Tetracyclines	Hepatotoxic Drugs	Uricosuric Agents
Anticoagulants	Hyperglycemic Agents	Vaccines
Anticonvulsants†	Hypertensive Emergency Agents	Vitamins†
Antidepressants†	Hypnotics†	
Antimalarial Agents	Hypolipidemics†	
	Bile Acid-Binding Resins†	

Specific Drugs Reported

acetaminophen	dicumarol	mefenamic acid	propylthiouracil†
alcohol†	diflunisal	methimazole†	quinidine
allopurinol	disulfiram	methyldopa	quinine
aminosalicylic acid	doxycycline	methylphenidate	ranitidine†
amiodarone HCl	erythromycin	methylsalicylate ointment (topical)	rofecoxib
aspirin	ethacrynic acid	metronidazole	sertraline
atorvastatin†	fenofibrate	miconazole (intravaginal, systemic)	simvastatin
azithromycin	fenoprofen	moricizine hydrochloride†	stanozolol
capecitabine	fluconazole	nalidixic acid	streptokinase
cefamandole	fluorouracil	naproxen	sulfamethizole
cefazolin	fluoxetine	neomycin	sulfamethoxazole
cefoperazone	flutamide	norfloxacin	sulfinpyrazone
cefotetan	fluvastatin	ofloxacin	sulfisoxazole
cefoxitin	fluvoxamine	olsalazine	sulindac
ceftriaxone	gemfibrozil	omeprazole	tamoxifen
celecoxib	glucagon	oxaprozin	tetracycline
cerivastatin	halothane	oxymetholone	thyroid
chenodiol	heparin	paroxetine	ticarcillin
chloramphenicol	ibuprofen	penicillin G, intravenous	ticlopidine
chloral hydrate†	ifosfamide	pentoxifylline	tissue plasminogen activator (t-PA)
chlorpropamide	indomethacin	phenylbutazone	tolbutamide
cholestyramine†	influenza virus vaccine	phenytoin†	tramadol
cimetidine	itraconazole	piperacillin	trimethoprim/ sulfamethoxazole
ciprofloxacin	**Jantoven™** overdose	piroxicam	urokinase
cisapride	ketoprofen	pravastatin†	valproate
clarithromycin	ketorolac	prednisone†	vitamin E
clofibrate	levamisole	propafenone	zafirlukast
cyclophosphamide†	levofloxacin	propoxyphene	zileuton
danazol	levothyroxine	propranolol	
dextran	liothyronine		
dextrothyroxine	lovastatin		
diazoxide			
diclofenac			

also: other medications affecting blood elements which may modify hemostasis
dietary deficiencies
prolonged hot weather
unreliable PT/INR determinations

† Increased and decreased PT/INR responses have been reported.

Classes of Drugs

Adrenal Cortical Steroid Inhibitors	Antithyroid Drugs†	Bile Acid-Binding Resins†
Antacids	Barbiturates	HMG-CoA Reductase Inhibitors†
Antianxiety Agents	Diuretics†	Immunosuppressives
Antiarrhythmics†	Enteral Nutritional Supplements	Oral Contraceptives, Estrogen Containing
Antibiotics†	Fungal Medications, Systemic†	Selective Estrogen Receptor Modulators
Anticonvulsants†	Gastric Acidity and Peptic Ulcer Agents†	Steroids, Adrenocortical†
Antidepressants†	Hypnotics†	Tuberculosis Agents†
Antihistamines	Hypolipidemics†	Vitamins†
Antineoplastics†		
Antipsychotic Medications		

toring is therefore advisable. Medications of unknown interaction with coumarins are best regarded with caution. When these medications are started or stopped, more frequent PT/INR monitoring is advisable.

It has been reported that concomitant administration of warfarin and ticlopidine may be associated with cholestatic hepatitis. **Botanical (Herbal) Medicines:** Caution should be exercised when botanical medicines (botanicals) are taken concomitantly with **Jantoven™**. Few adequate, well-controlled studies exist evaluating the potential for metabolic and/or pharmacologic interactions between botanicals and **Jantoven™**. Due to a lack of manufacturing standardization with botanical medicinal preparations, the amount of active ingredients may vary. This could further confound the ability to assess potential interactions and effects on anticoagulation. It is good practice to monitor the patient's response with additional PT/INR determinations when initiating or discontinuing botanicals.

Specific botanicals reported to affect **Jantoven™** therapy include the following:

- Bromelains, danshen, dong quai (*Angelica sinensis*), garlic, Ginkgo biloba and ginseng are associated most often with an INCREASE in the effects of **Jantoven™**.

- Coenzyme Q_{10} (ubidecarenone) and St. John's wort are associated most often with a DECREASE in the effects of **Jantoven™**.

Some botanicals may cause bleeding events when taken alone (e.g., garlic and Ginkgo biloba) and may have anticoagulant, antiplatelet, and/or fibrinolytic properties. These effects would be expected to be additive to the anticoagulant effects of **Jantoven™**. Conversely, other botanicals may have coagulant properties when taken alone or may decrease the effects of **Jantoven™**.

Some botanicals that may affect coagulation are listed below for reference; however, this list should not be considered all-inclusive. Many botanicals have several common names and scientific names. The most widely recognized common botanical names are listed.

[See second table at right]
[See third table at right]
[See fourth table at right]
[See fifth table at right]
[See sixth table at right]

Effect on Other Drugs: Coumarins may also affect the action of other drugs. Hypoglycemic agents (chlorpropamide and tolbutamide) and anticonvulsants (phenytoin and phenobarbital) may accumulate in the body as a result of interference with either their metabolism or excretion.

Special Risk Patients: **Jantoven™** is a narrow therapeutic range (index) drug, and caution should be observed when warfarin sodium is administered to certain patients such as the elderly or debilitated or when administered in any situation or physical condition where added risk of hemorrhage is present.

Intramuscular (I.M.) injections of concomitant medications should be confined to the upper extremities which permits easy access for manual compression, inspections for bleeding and use of pressure bandages.

Caution should be observed when **Jantoven™** (or warfarin) is administered concomitantly with nonsteroidal anti-inflammatory drugs (NSAIDs), including aspirin, to be certain that no change in anticoagulation dosage is required. In addition to specific drug interactions that might affect PT/INR, NSAIDs, including aspirin, can inhibit platelet aggregation, and can cause gastrointestinal bleeding, peptic ulceration and/or perforation.

Acquired or inherited warfarin resistance should be suspected if large daily doses of **Jantoven™** are required to maintain a patient's PT/INR within a normal therapeutic range.

Information for Patients: The objective of anticoagulant therapy is to decrease the clotting ability of the blood so that thrombosis is prevented, while avoiding spontaneous bleeding. Effective therapeutic levels with minimal complications are in part dependent upon cooperative and well-instructed patients who communicate effectively with their physician. Patients should be advised: Strict adherence to prescribed dosage schedule is necessary. Do not take or discontinue any other medication, including salicylates (e.g., aspirin and topical analgesics), other over-the-counter medications, and botanical (herbal) products (e.g., bromelains, coenzyme Q_{10}, danshen, dong quai, garlic, Ginkgo biloba, ginseng and St. John's wort) except on advice of the physician. Avoid alcohol consumption. Do not take **Jantoven™** during pregnancy and do not become pregnant while taking it (see **CONTRAINDICATIONS**). Avoid any activity or sport that may result in traumatic injury. Prothrombin time tests and regular visits to physician or clinic are needed to monitor therapy. Carry identification stating that **Jantoven™** is being taken. If the prescribed dose of **Jantoven™** is forgotten, notify the physician immediately. Take the dose as soon as possible on the same day but do not take a double dose of **Jantoven™** the next day to make up for missed doses. The amount of vitamin K in food may affect therapy with **Jantoven™**. Eat a normal, balanced diet maintaining a consistent amount of vitamin K. Avoid drastic changes in dietary habits, such as eating large amounts of green leafy vegetables. Contact physician to report any illness, such as diarrhea, infection or fever. Notify physician immediately if any unusual bleeding or symptoms occur. Signs and symptoms of bleeding include: pain, swelling or discomfort, prolonged bleeding from cuts, increased menstrual flow or vaginal bleeding, nosebleeds, bleeding of gums from brushing, unusual bleeding or bruising, red or dark brown urine, red or tar black stools, headache, dizziness, or weakness. If therapy with **Jantoven™** is discontinued, patients should be cautioned that the anticoagulant effects of **Jantoven™** may persist for about 2 to 5 days. **Patients should be informed that all warfarin sodium, USP products represent the same medication, and should not be taken concomitantly, as overdosage may result.**

Carcinogenesis, Mutagenesis, Impairment of Fertility: Carcinogenicity and mutagenicity studies have not been performed with **Jantoven™**. The reproductive effects of **Jantoven™** have not been evaluated.

Use in Pregnancy: Pregnancy Category X - See **CONTRAINDICATIONS**.

Pediatric Use: Safety and effectiveness in pediatric patients below the age of 18 have not been established, in randomized, controlled clinical trials. However, the use of **Jantoven™** in pediatric patients is well-documented for the prevention and treatment of thromboembolic events. Difficulty achieving and maintaining therapeutic PT/INR ranges in the pediatric patient has been reported. More frequent PT/INR determinations are recommended because of possible changing warfarin requirements.

Specific Drugs Reported

alcohol†	cyclophosphamide†	phenytoin†
aminoglutethimide	dicloxacillin	pravastatin†
amobarbital	ethchlorvynol	prednisone†
atorvastatin†	glutethimide	primidone
azathioprine	griseofulvin	propylthiouracil†
butabarbital	haloperidol	raloxifene
butalbital	**Jantoven™** underdosage	ranitidine†
carbamazepine	meprobamate	rifampin
chloral hydrate†	6-mercaptopurine	secobarbital
chlordiazepoxide	methimazole†	spironolactone
chlorthalidone	moricizine hydrochloride†	sucralfate
cholestyramine†	nafcillin	trazodone
clozapine	paraldehyde	vitamin C (high dose)
corticotropin	pentobarbital	vitamin K
cortisone	phenobarbital	

also: diet high in vitamin K
unreliable PT/INR determinations

† Increased and decreased PT/INR responses have been reported.

Botanicals that contain coumarins with potential anticoagulant effects:

Alfalfa	Capsicum[2]	Horseradish	Red Clover
Angelica (Dong Quai)	Cassia[3]	Licorice[3]	Sweet Clover
Aniseed	Celery	Meadowsweet[1]	Sweet Woodruff
Arnica	Chamomile (German and Roman)	Nettle	Tonka Beans
Asa Foetida	Dandelion	Parsley	Wild Carrot
Bogbean[1]	Fenugreek	Passion Flower	Wild Lettuce
Boldo	Horse Chestnut	Prickly Ash (Northern)	
Buchu		Quassia	

Miscellaneous botanicals with anticoagulant properties:

Bladder Wrack (Fucus)	Pau d'arco

Botanicals that contain salicylate and/or have antiplatelet properties:

Agrimony[4]	Dandelion	Meadowsweet[1]
Aloe Gel	Feverfew	Onion[5]
Aspen	Garlic[5]	Policosanol
Black Cohosh	German Sarsaparilla	Poplar
Black Haw	Ginger	Senega
Bogbean[1]	Ginkgo Biloba	Tamarind
Cassia[3]	Ginseng (*Panax*)[5]	Willow
Clove	Licorice[3]	Wintergreen

Botanicals with fibrinolytic properties:

Bromelains	Garlic[5]	Inositol Nicotinate
Capsicum[2]	Ginseng (*Panax*)[5]	Onion[5]

Botanicals with coagulant properties:

Agrimony[4]	Mistletoe[5]
Goldenseal	Yarrow

[1] Contains coumarins and salicylate.
[2] Contains coumarins and has fibrinolytic properties.
[3] Contains coumarins and has antiplatelet properties.
[4] Contains salicylate and has coagulant properties.
[5] Has antiplatelet and fibrinolytic properties.

Geriatric Use: Patients 60 years or older appear to exhibit greater than expected PT/INR response to the anticoagulant effects of warfarin (see **CLINICAL PHARMACOLOGY**). **Jantoven™** is contraindicated in any unsupervised patient with senility. Caution should be observed with administration of warfarin sodium to elderly patients in any situation or physical condition where added risk of hemorrhage is present. Lower initiation and maintenance doses of **Jantoven™** are recommended for elderly patients (see **DOSAGE AND ADMINISTRATION**).

ADVERSE REACTIONS

Potential adverse reactions to **Jantoven™** (Warfarin Sodium Tablets, USP) may include:

- Fatal or nonfatal hemorrhage from any tissue or organ. This is a consequence of the anticoagulant effect. The signs, symptoms, and severity will vary according to the location and degree or extent of the bleeding. Hemorrhagic complications may present as paralysis; paresthesia; headache, chest, abdomen, joint, muscle or other pain; dizziness; shortness of breath, difficulty breathing or swallowing; unexplained swelling; weakness; hypotension; or unexplained shock. Therefore, the possibility of hemorrhage should be considered in evaluating the condition of any anticoagulated patient with complaints which do not indicate an obvious diagnosis. Bleeding during anticoagulant therapy does not always correlate with PT/INR. (See **OVERDOSAGE-Treatment**.)
- Bleeding which occurs when the PT/INR is within the therapeutic range warrants diagnostic investigation since it may unmask a previously unsuspected lesion, e.g., tumor, ulcer, etc.
- Necrosis of skin and other tissues. (See **WARNINGS**.)
- Adverse reactions reported infrequently include: hypersensitivity/allergic reactions, systemic cholesterol microembolization, purple toes syndrome, hepatitis, cholestatic hepatic injury, jaundice, elevated liver enzymes, vasculitis, edema, fever, rash, dermatitis, including bullous eruptions, urticaria, abdominal pain including cramping, flatulence/bloating, fatigue, lethargy, malaise, asthenia, nausea, vomiting, diarrhea, pain, headache, dizziness, taste perversion, pruritis, alopecia, cold intolerance, and paresthesia including feeling cold and chills.

Rare events of tracheal or tracheobronchial calcification have been reported in association with long-term warfarin therapy. The clinical significance of this event is unknown. Priapism has been associated with anticoagulant administration, however, a causal relationship has not been established.

OVERDOSAGE

Signs and Symptoms: Suspected or overt abnormal bleeding (e.g., appearance of blood in stools or urine, hematuria, excessive menstrual bleeding, melena, petechiae, excessive bruising or persistent oozing from superficial injuries) are early manifestations of anticoagulation beyond a safe and satisfactory level.

Treatment: Excessive anticoagulation, with or without bleeding, may be controlled by discontinuing **Jantoven™** (Warfarin Sodium Tablets, USP) therapy and if necessary, by administration of oral or parenteral vitamin K_1. (Please see recommendations accompanying vitamin K_1 preparations prior to use.)

Such use of vitamin K_1 reduces response to subsequent **Jantoven™** therapy. Patients may return to a pretreatment thrombotic status following the rapid reversal of a prolonged PT/INR. Resumption of **Jantoven™** administration reverses the effect of vitamin K, and a therapeutic PT/INR can again be obtained by careful dosage adjustment. If rapid anticoagulation is indicated, heparin may be preferable for initial therapy.

If minor bleeding progresses to major bleeding, give 5 to 25 mg (rarely up to 50 mg) parenteral vitamin K_1. In emer-

Continued on next page

Jantoven—Cont.

gency situations of severe hemorrhage, clotting factors can be returned to normal by administering 200 to 500 mL of fresh whole blood or fresh frozen plasma, or by giving commercial Factor IX complex.
A risk of hepatitis and other viral diseases is associated with the use of these blood products; Factor IX complex is also associated with an increased risk of thrombosis. Therefore, these preparations should be used only in exceptional or life-threatening bleeding episodes secondary to **Jantoven™** overdosage.
Purified Factor IX preparations should not be used because they cannot increase the levels of prothrombin. Factor VII and Factor X which are also depressed along with the levels of Factor IX as a result of **Jantoven™** treatment. Packed red blood cells may also be given if significant blood loss has occurred. Infusions of blood or plasma should be monitored carefully to avoid precipitating pulmonary edema in elderly patients or patients with heart disease.

DOSAGE AND ADMINISTRATION

The dosage and administration of **Jantoven™** (Warfarin Sodium Tablets, USP) must be individualized for each patient according to the particular patient's PT/INR response to the drug. The dosage should be adjusted based upon the patient's PT/INR. (See **LABORATORY CONTROL** below for full discussion on INR.)
Venous Thromboembolism (including pulmonary embolism): Available clinical evidence indicates that an INR of 2.0 to 3.0 is sufficient for prophylaxis and treatment of venous thromboembolism and minimizes the risk of hemorrhage associated with higher INRs. In patients with risk factors for recurrent venous thromboembolism including venous insufficiency, inherited thrombophilia, idiopathic venous thromboembolism, and a history of thrombotic events, consideration should be given to longer term therapy (Schulman et al, 1995 and Schulman et al, 1997).
Atrial Fibrillation: Five recent clinical trials evaluated the effects of warfarin in patients with non-valvular atrial fibrillation (AF). Meta-analysis findings of these studies revealed that the effects of warfarin in reducing thromboembolic events including stroke were similar at either moderately high INR (2.0–4.5) or low INR (1.4–3.0). There was a significant reduction in minor bleeds at the low INR. Similar data from clinical studies in valvular atrial fibrillation patients are not available. The trials in non-valvular atrial fibrillation support the American College of Chest Physicians' (ACCP) recommendation that an INR of 2.0–3.0 be used for long term warfarin therapy in appropriate AF patients.
Post-Myocardial Infarction: In post-myocardial infarction patients, **Jantoven™** therapy should be initiated early (2–4 weeks post-infarction) and dosage should be adjusted to maintain an INR of 2.5–3.5 long-term. The recommendation is based on the results of the WARIS study in which treatment was initiated 2 to 4 weeks after the infarction. In patients thought to be at an increased risk of bleeding complications or on aspirin therapy, maintenance of **Jantoven™** therapy at the lower end of this INR range is recommended.
Mechanical and Bioprosthetic Heart Valves: In patients with mechanical heart valve(s), long term prophylaxis with warfarin to an INR of 2.5–3.5 is recommended. In patients with bioprosthetic heart valve(s), based on limited data, the American College of Chest Physicians recommends warfarin therapy to an INR of 2.0–3.0 for 12 weeks after valve insertion. In patients with additional risk factors such as atrial fibrillation or prior thromboembolism, consideration should be given for longer term therapy.
Recurrent Systemic Embolism: In cases where the risk of thromboembolism is great, such as in patients with recurrent systemic embolism, a higher INR may be required.
An INR of greater than 4.0 appears to provide no additional therapeutic benefit in most patients and is associated with a higher risk of bleeding.
Initial Dosage: The dosing of **Jantoven™** must be individualized according to patient's sensitivity to the drug as indicated by the PT/INR. Use of a large loading dose may increase the incidence of hemorrhagic and other complications, does not offer more rapid protection against thrombi formation, and is not recommended. Lower initiation and maintenance doses are recommended for elderly and/or debilitated patients and patients with potential to exhibit greater than expected PT/INR response to **Jantoven™** (see **PRECAUTIONS**). Based on limited data, Asian patients may also require lower initiation and maintenance doses of **Jantoven™** (see **CLINICAL PHARMACOLOGY**). It is recommended that **Jantoven™** therapy be initiated with a dose of 2 to 5 mg per day with dosage adjustments based on the results of PT/INR determinations.
Maintenance: Most patients are satisfactorily maintained at a dose of 2 to 10 mg daily. Flexibility of dosage is provided by breaking scored tablets in half. The individual dose and interval should be gauged by the patient's prothrombin response.
Duration of Therapy: The duration of therapy in each patient should be individualized. In general, anticoagulant therapy should be continued until the danger of thrombosis and embolism has passed.
Missed Dose: The anticoagulant effect of **Jantoven™** persists beyond 24 hours. If the patient forgets to take the prescribed dose of **Jantoven™** at the scheduled time, the dose should be taken as soon as possible on the same day. The patient should not take the missed dose by doubling the daily dose to make up for the missed doses, but should refer back to his or her physician.
LABORATORY CONTROL: The PT reflects the depression of vitamin K dependent Factors VII, X and II. There are several modifications of the one-stage PT and the physician should become familiar with the specific method used in his laboratory. The degree of anticoagulation indicated by any range of PTs may be altered by the type of thromboplastin used; the appropriate therapeutic range must be based on the experience of each laboratory. The PT should be determined daily after the administration of the initial dose until PT/INR results stabilize in the therapeutic range. Intervals between subsequent PT/INR determinations should be based upon the physician's judgment of the patient's reliability and response to **Jantoven™** in order to maintain the individual within the therapeutic range. Acceptable intervals for PT/INR determinations are normally within the range of one to four weeks after a stable dosage has been determined. To ensure adequate control, it is recommended that additional PT tests are done when other warfarin products are interchanged with warfarin sodium tablets, USP, as well as whenever other medications are initiated, discontinued, or taken irregularly (see **PRECAUTIONS**). Different thromboplastin reagents vary substantially in their sensitivity to sodium warfarin-induced effects on PT. To define the appropriate therapeutic regimen it is important to be familiar with the sensitivity of the thromboplastin reagent used in the laboratory and its relationship to the International Reference Preparation (IRP), a sensitive thromboplastin reagent prepared from human brain.
A system of standardizing the PT in oral anticoagulant control was introduced by the World Health Organization in 1983. It is based upon the determination of an International Normalized Ratio (INR) which provides a common basis for communication of PT results and interpretations of therapeutic ranges. The INR system of reporting is based on a logarithmic relationship between the PT ratios of the test and reference preparation. The INR is the PT ratio that would be obtained if the International Reference Preparation (IRP), which has an ISI of 1.0, were used to perform the test. Early clinical studies of oral anticoagulants, which formed the basis for recommended therapeutic ranges of 1.5 to 2.5 times control mean normal PT, used sensitive human brain thromboplastin. When using the less sensitive rabbit brain thromboplastins commonly employed in PT assays today, adjustments must be made to the targeted PT range that reflect this decrease in sensitivity.
The INR can be calculated as: $INR = (\text{observed PT ratio})^{ISI}$ where the ISI (International Sensitivity Index) is the correction factor in the equation that relates the PT ratio of the local reagent to the reference preparation and is a measure of the sensitivity of a given thromboplastin to reduction of vitamin K-dependent coagulation factors; the lower the ISI, the more "sensitive" the reagent and the closer the derived INR will be to the observed PT ratio.[1]
The proceedings and recommendations of the 1992 National Conference on Antithrombotic Therapy[2–4] review and evaluate issues related to oral anticoagulant therapy and the sensitivity of thromboplastin reagents and provide additional guidelines for defining the appropriate therapeutic regimen.
The conversion of the INR to PT ratios for the less-intense (INR 2.0 to 3.0) and more intense (INR 2.5 to 3.5) therapeutic range recommended by the ACCP for thromboplastins over a range of ISI values is shown in TABLE 3.[5]
[See table 3 below]
TREATMENT DURING DENTISTRY AND SURGERY: The management of patients who undergo dental and surgical procedures requires close liaison between attending physicians, surgeons and dentists. PT/INR determination is recommended just prior to any dental or surgical procedure. In patients undergoing minimal invasive procedures who must be anticoagulated prior to, during, or immediately following these procedures, adjusting the dosage of **Jantoven™** to maintain the PT/INR at the low end of the therapeutic range may safely allow for continued anticoagulation. The operative site should be sufficiently limited and accessible to permit the effective use of local procedures for hemostasis. Under these conditions, dental and minor surgical procedures may be performed without undue risk of hemorrhage. Some dental or surgical procedures may necessitate the interruption of **Jantoven™** therapy. When discontinuing **Jantoven™** even for a short period of time, the benefits and risks should be strongly considered.
CONVERSION FROM HEPARIN THERAPY: Since the anticoagulant effect of **Jantoven™** is delayed, heparin is preferred initially for rapid anticoagulation. Conversion to **Jantoven™** may begin concomitantly with heparin therapy or may be delayed 3 to 6 days. To ensure continuous anticoagulation, it is advisable to continue full dose heparin therapy and that **Jantoven™** therapy be overlapped with heparin for 4 to 5 days, until **Jantoven™** has produced the desired therapeutic response as determined by PT/INR. When **Jantoven™** has produced the desired PT/INR or prothrombin activity, heparin may be discontinued.
Jantoven™ may increase the aPTT test, even in the absence of heparin. During initial therapy with **Jantoven™**, the interference with heparin anticoagulation is of minimal clinical significance.
As heparin may affect the PT/INR, patients receiving both heparin and **Jantoven™** should have blood for PT/INR determination drawn at least:

- 5 hours after the last IV bolus dose of heparin, or
- 4 hours after cessation of a continuous IV infusion of heparin, or
- 24 hours after the last subcutaneous heparin injection.

HOW SUPPLIED

Jantoven™ (Warfarin Sodium Tablets, USP) for oral use, are supplied in the following forms:

1 mg - Compressed tablet, pink, round; one side scored and debossed WRF & 1, one side debossed 832, in bottles of 100 and 1000 and in unit dose cartons of 100 tablets (10 cards containing 10 tablets each).
2 mg - Compressed tablet, lavender, round; one side scored and debossed WRF & 2, one side debossed 832, in bottles of 100 and 1000 and in unit dose cartons of 100 tablets (10 cards containing 10 tablets each).
2½ mg - Compressed tablet, green, round; one side scored and debossed WRF & 2½, one side debossed 832, in bottles of 100 and 1000 and in unit dose cartons of 100 tablets (10 cards containing 10 tablets each).
3 mg - Compressed tablet, tan, round; one side scored and debossed WRF & 3, one side debossed 832, in bottles of 100 and 1000 and in unit dose cartons of 100 tablets (10 cards containing 10 tablets each).
4 mg - Compressed tablet, blue, round; one side scored and debossed WRF & 4, one side debossed 832, in bottles of 100 and 1000 and in unit dose cartons of 100 tablets (10 cards containing 10 tablets each).
5 mg - Compressed tablet, peach, round; one side scored and debossed WRF & 5, one side debossed 832, in bottles of 100 and 1000 and in unit dose cartons of 100 tablets (10 cards containing 10 tablets each).
6 mg - Compressed tablet, teal, round; one side scored and debossed WRF & 6, one side debossed 832, in bottles of 100 and 1000 and in unit dose cartons of 100 tablets (10 cards containing 10 tablets each).
7½ mg - Compressed tablet, yellow, round; one side scored and debossed WRF & 7½, one side debossed 832, in bottles of 100 and 500 and in unit dose cartons of 100 tablets (10 cards containing 10 tablets each).
10 mg - Compressed tablet, white, round; one side scored and debossed WRF & 10, one side debossed 832, in bottles of 100 and 500 and in unit dose cartons of 100 tablets (10 cards containing 10 tablets each).

Store at 20–25°C (68–77°F) and excursions permitted to 15–30°C (59–86°F) [see USP Controlled Room Temperature]. Keep tightly closed. Protect from light and moisture. Dispense in a tight, light-resistant container with a child-resistant closure.
Keep out of reach of children.
Rx only

REFERENCES

1. Poller, L.: Laboratory Control of Anticoagulant Therapy. Seminars in Thrombosis and Hemostasis, Vol. 12, No. 1, pp. 13–19, 1986.
2. Hirsh, J.: Is the Dose of Warfarin Prescribed by American Physicians Unnecessarily High? *Arch Int Med*, Vol. 147, pp. 769–771, 1987.
3. Cook, D.J., Guyatt, H.G., Laupacis, A., Sackett, D.L.: Rules of Evidence and Clinical Recommendations on the Use of Antithrombotic Agents. Chest ACCP Consensus Conference on Antithrombotic Therapy. *Chest*, Vol. 102(Suppl), pp. 305S–311S, 1992.
4. Hirsh, J., Dalen, J., Deykin, D., Poller, L.: Oral Anticoagulants Mechanism of Action, Clinical Effectiveness, and Optimal Therapeutic Range. Chest ACCP Consensus Conference on Antithrombotic Therapy. *Chest*, Vol. 102(Suppl), pp. 312S–326S, 1992.
5. Hirsh, J., M.D., F.C.C.P.: Hamilton Civic Hospitals Research Center, Hamilton, Ontario, Personal Communication.

Manufactured by
UPSHER-SMITH LABORATORIES, INC.
Minneapolis, MN 55447
JAPI.1203-00 Revised 0703
Shown in Product Identification Guide, page 335

TABLE 3
Relationship Between INR and PT Ratios For Thromboplastins With Different ISI Values (Sensitivities)

	PT RATIOS				
	ISI 1.0	ISI 1.4	ISI 1.8	ISI 2.3	ISI 2.8
INR = 2.0–3.0	2.0–3.0	1.6–2.2	1.5–1.8	1.4–1.6	1.3–1.5
INR = 2.5–3.5	2.5–3.5	1.9–2.4	1.7–2.0	1.5–1.7	1.4–1.6

KLOR–CON® POWDER ℞
[*klōr 'kon*]
Potassium Chloride for Oral Solution, USP
20 mEq (1.5 g) per packet

DESCRIPTION
Each packet contains 1.5 g potassium chloride providing potassium 20 mEq and chloride 20 mEq. Fruit-flavored with artificial color and sweetener (saccharin) added.

HOW SUPPLIED
KLOR-CON® Powder 20 mEq: Cartons of 30 and 100 packets.
30's NDC 0245-0035-30, 100's NDC 0245-0035-01

KLOR-CON®/25 POWDER ℞
[*klōr 'kon*]
(Potassium Chloride for Oral Solution, USP)
25 mEq (1.875 g) per packet

DESCRIPTION
Each packet contains 1.875 g potassium chloride providing potassium 25 mEq and chloride 25 mEq. Fruit-flavored with artificial color and sweetener (saccharin) added.

HOW SUPPLIED
KLOR-CON®/25 Powder 25 mEq:
Cartons of 30 and 100.
30's NDC 0245-0037-30, 100's NDC 0245-0037-01

KLOR–CON® 8/KLOR–CON® 10 ℞
[*klōr 'kon*]
Potassium Chloride
Extended–release Tablets, USP
8 mEq and 10 mEq

DESCRIPTION
KLOR-CON® Extended-release Tablets, USP are a solid oral dosage form of potassium chloride. Each contains 600 mg or 750 mg of potassium chloride equivalent to 8 mEq or 10 mEq of potassium in a wax matrix tablet. This formulation is intended to slow the release of potassium so that the likelihood of a high localized concentration of potassium chloride within the gastrointestinal tract is reduced.

HOW SUPPLIED
Film coated, Klor-Con® 8 (blue), Klor-Con® 10 (yellow), imprinted round tablets containing:

600 mg potassium chloride (equivalent to 8 mEq) in bottles of 100 (NDC 0245-0040-11), bottles of 500 (NDC 0245-0040-15), unit-dose packages of 100 (NDC 0245-0040-01) and bulk packs of 5,000 for repack only (NDC 0245-0040-55).

750 mg potassium chloride (equivalent to 10 mEq) in bottles of 100 (NDC 0245-0041-11), bottles of 500 (NDC 0245-0041-15), unit-dose packages of 100 (NDC 0245-0041-01) and bulk packs of 5,000 for repack only (NDC 0245-0041-55).

Shown in Product Identification Guide, page 335

KLOR-CON®/EF 25mEq ℞
[*klōr 'kon*]
Potassium Bicarbonate Effervescent Tablets for Oral Solution, USP

DESCRIPTION
Each effervescent tablet in solution provides 25 mEq (978 mg) potassium as bicarbonate and citrate. Fruit-flavored with artificial color and sweetener (saccharin) added.

HOW SUPPLIED
KLOR-CON®/EF 25 mEq effervescent tablets in cartons of 30 and 100 individually wrapped tablets.
30's NDC 0245-0039-30, 100's NDC 0245-0039-01

KLOR-CON® M ℞
[*klōr'kŏn*]
(Potassium Chloride Extended-release Tablets, USP)
MICRO-DISPERSIBLE TECHNOLOGY®

DESCRIPTION
Klor-Con® M20 is an immediately dispersing extended-release oral dosage form of potassium chloride containing 1500 mg of microencapsulated potassium chloride, USP equivalent to 20 mEq of potassium in a tablet.
Klor-Con® M15 is an immediately dispersing extended-release oral dosage form of potassium chloride containing 1125 mg of microencapsulated potassium chloride, USP equivalent to 15 mEq of potassium in a tablet.
Klor-Con® M10 is an immediately dispersing extended-release oral dosage form of potassium chloride containing 750 mg of microencapsulated potassium chloride, USP equivalent to 10 mEq of potassium in a tablet.
These formulations are intended to slow the release of potassium so that the likelihood of a high localized concentration of potassium chloride within the gastrointestinal tract is reduced.
Klor-Con® M is an electrolyte replenisher. The chemical name of the active ingredient is potassium chloride, and the structural formula is KCl (molecular weight: 74.55). Potassium chloride, USP occurs as a white, granular powder or as colorless crystals. It is odorless and has a saline taste. Its solutions are neutral to litmus. It is freely soluble in water and insoluble in alcohol.
Klor-Con® M is a tablet formulation (not enteric coated or wax matrix) containing individually microencapsulated potassium chloride crystals which disperse upon tablet disintegration. In simulated gastric fluid at 37°C and in the absence of outside agitation, Klor-Con® M begins disintegrating into microencapsulated crystals within seconds and completely disintegrates within one minute. The microencapsulated crystals are formulated to provide an extended release of potassium chloride.
Inactive Ingredients: croscarmellose sodium, ethylcellulose and microcrystalline cellulose.

CLINICAL PHARMACOLOGY
The potassium ion is the principal intracellular cation of most body tissues. Potassium ions of participate in a number of essential physiological processes including the maintenance of intracellular tonicity, the transmission of nerve impulses, the contraction of cardiac, skeletal and smooth muscle and the maintenance of normal renal function.
The intracellular concentration of potassium is approximately 150 to 160 mEq per liter. The normal adult plasma concentration is 3.5 to 5 mEq per liter. An active ion transport system maintains this gradient across the plasma membrane.
Potassium is a normal dietary constituent and under steady state conditions the amount of potassium absorbed from the gastrointestinal tract is equal to the amount excreted in the urine. The usual dietary intake of potassium is 50 to 100 mEq per day.
Potassium depletion will occur whenever the rate of potassium loss through renal excretion and/or loss from the gastrointestinal tract exceeds the rate of potassium intake. Such depletion usually develops as a consequence therapy with diuretics, primary or secondary hyperaldosteronism, diabetic ketoacidosis or inadequate replacement of potassium in patients on prolonged parenteral nutrition. Depletion can develop rapidly with severe diarrhea, especially if associated with vomiting. Potassium depletion due to these causes is usually accompanied by a concomitant loss of chloride and is manifested by hypokalemia and metabolic alkalosis. Potassium depletion may produce weakness, fatigue, disturbances of cardiac rhythm (primarily ectopic beats), prominent U-waves in the electrocardiogram, and in advanced cases, flaccid paralysis and/or impaired ability to concentrate urine.
If potassium depletion associated with metabolic alkalosis cannot be managed by correcting the fundamental cause of the deficiency, e.g., where the patient requires long term diuretic therapy, supplemental potassium in the form of high potassium food or potassium chloride may be able to restore potassium levels.
In rare circumstances (e.g., patients with renal tubular acidosis) potassium depletion may be associated with metabolic acidosis and hyperchloremia. In such patients potassium replacement should be accomplished with potassium salts other than the chloride, such as potassium bicarbonate, potassium citrate, potassium acetate or potassium gluconate.

INDICATIONS AND USAGE
BECAUSE OF REPORTS OF INTESTINAL AND GASTRIC ULCERATION AND BLEEDING WITH EXTENDED-RELEASE POTASSIUM CHLORIDE PREPARATIONS, THESE DRUGS SHOULD BE RESERVED FOR THOSE PATIENTS WHO CANNOT TOLERATE OR REFUSE TO TAKE LIQUID OR EFFERVESCENT POTASSIUM PREPARATIONS OR FOR PATIENTS IN WHOM THERE IS A PROBLEM OF COMPLIANCE WITH THESE PREPARATIONS.

1. For the treatment of patients with hypokalemia with or without metabolic alkalosis, in digitalis intoxication and in patients with hypokalemic familial periodic paralysis. If hypokalemia is the result of diuretic therapy, consideration should be given to the use of a lower dose of diuretic, which may be sufficient without leading to hypokalemia.
2. For the prevention of hypokalemia in patients who would be at particular risk if hypokalemia were to develop, e.g., digitalized patients or patients with significant cardiac arrhythmias.

The use of potassium salts in patients receiving diuretics for uncomplicated essential hypertension is often unnecessary when such patients have a normal dietary pattern and when low doses of the diuretic are used. Serum potassium should be checked periodically, however, and if hypokalemia occurs, dietary supplementation with potassium-containing foods may be adequate to control milder cases. In more severe cases, and if dose adjustment of the diuretic is ineffective or unwarranted, supplementation with potassium salts may be indicated.

CONTRAINDICATIONS
Potassium supplements are contraindicated in patients with hyperkalemia since a further increase in serum potassium concentration in such patients can produce cardiac arrest. Hyperkalemia may complicate any of the following conditions: chronic renal failure, systemic acidosis, such as diabetic acidosis, acute dehydration, extensive tissue breakdown as in severe burns, adrenal insufficiency or the administration of a potassium-sparing diuretic (e.g., spironolactone, triamterene or amiloride) (see **OVERDOSAGE**).
Extended-release formulations of potassium chloride have produced esophageal ulceration in certain cardiac patients with esophageal compression due to enlarged left atrium. Potassium supplementation, when indicated in such patients, should be given as a liquid preparation or as an aqueous (water) suspension of Klor-Con® M (see **PRECAUTIONS;** *Information for Patients* and **DOSAGE AND ADMINISTRATION** sections).
All solid oral dosage forms of potassium chloride are contraindicated in any patient in whom there is structural, pathological (e.g., diabetic gastroparesis) or pharmacologic (use of anticholinergic agents or other agents with anticholinergic properties at sufficient doses to exert anticholinergic effects) cause for arrest or delay in tablet passage through the gastrointestinal tract.

WARNINGS
Hyperkalemia (see **OVERDOSAGE**)—In patients with impaired mechanisms for excreting potassium, the administration of potassium salts can produce hyperkalemia and cardiac arrest. This occurs most commonly in patients given potassium by the intravenous route but may also occur in patients given potassium orally. Potentially fatal hyperkalemia can develop rapidly and be asymptomatic. The use of potassium salts in patients with chronic renal disease or any other condition which impairs potassium excretion, requires particularly careful monitoring of the serum potassium concentration and appropriate dosage adjustment.
Interaction with Potassium-Sparing Diuretics—Hypokalemia should not be treated by the concomitant administration of potassium salts and a potassium-sparing diuretic (e.g., spironolactone, triamterene or amiloride) since the simultaneous administration of these agents can produce severe hyperkalemia.
Interaction with Angiotensin Converting Enzyme Inhibitors—Angiotensin converting enzyme (ACE) inhibitors (e.g., captopril, enalapril) will produce some potassium retention by inhibiting aldosterone production. Potassium supplements should be given to patients receiving ACE inhibitors only with close monitoring.
Gastrointestinal Lesions—Solid oral dosage forms of potassium chloride can produce ulcerative and/or stenotic lesions of the gastrointestinal tract. Based on spontaneous adverse reaction reports, enteric coated preparations of potassium chloride are associated with an increased frequency of small bowel lesions (40-50 per 100,000 patient years) compared to extended-release wax matrix formulations (less than one per 100,000 patient years). Because of the lack of extensive marketing experience with microencapsulated products, a comparison between such products and wax matrix or enteric coated products is not available. Klor-Con® M is a tablet formulated to provide an extended rate of release of microencapsulated potassium chloride and thus to minimize the possibility of a high local concentration of potassium near the gastrointestinal wall.
Prospective trials have been conducted in normal human volunteers in which the upper gastrointestinal tract was evaluated by endoscopic inspection before and after one week of solid oral potassium chloride therapy. The ability of this model to predict events occurring in usual clinical practice is unknown. Trials which approximated usual clinical practice did not reveal any clear differences between the wax matrix and microencapsulated dosage forms. In contrast, there was a higher incidence of gastric and duodenal lesions in subjects receiving a high dose of a wax matrix extended-release formulation under conditions which did not resemble usual or recommended clinical practice (i.e., 96 mEq per day in divided doses of potassium chloride administered to fasted patients, in the presence of an anticholinergic drug to delay gastric emptying). The upper gastrointestinal lesions observed by endoscopy were asymptomatic and were not accompanied by evidence of bleeding (Hemoccult testing). The relevance of these findings to the usual conditions (i.e., non-fasting, no anticholinergic agent, smaller doses) under which extended-release potassium chloride products are used is uncertain; epidemiologic studies have not identified an elevated risk, compared to microencapsulated products, for upper gastrointestinal lesions in patients receiving wax matrix formulations. Klor-Con® M should be discontinued immediately and the possibility of ulceration, obstruction or perforation considered if severe vomiting, abdominal pain, distention or gastrointestinal bleeding occurs.
Metabolic Acidosis—Hypokalemia in patients with metabolic acidosis should be treated with an alkalinizing potassium salt such as potassium bicarbonate, potassium citrate, potassium acetate or potassium gluconate.

PRECAUTIONS
General: The diagnosis of potassium depletion is ordinarily made by demonstrating hypokalemia in a patient with a clinical history suggesting some cause for potassium depletion. In interpreting the serum potassium level, the physician should be aware that acute alkalosis *per se* can produce hypokalemia in the absence of a deficit in total body potassium while acute acidosis *per se* can increase the

Continued on next page

Klor-Con M—Cont.

serum potassium concentration into the normal range even in the presence of a reduced total body potassium. The treatment of potassium depletion, particularly in the presence of cardiac disease, renal disease or acidosis requires careful attention to acid-base balance and appropriate monitoring of serum electrolytes, the electrocardiogram and the clinical status of the patient.

Information for Patients: Physicians should consider reminding the patient of the following:

To take each dose with meals and with a full glass of water or other liquid.

To take each dose without crushing, chewing or sucking the tablets. If those patients are having difficulty swallowing whole tablets, they may try one of the following alternate methods of administration:

a. Break the tablet in half and take each half separately with a glass of water.

b. Prepare an aqueous (water) suspension as follows:

1. Place the whole tablet(s) in approximately one-half glass of water (4 fluid ounces).
2. Allow approximately 2 minutes for the tablet(s) to disintegrate.
3. Stir for about half a minute after the tablet(s) has disintegrated.
4. Swirl the suspension and consume the entire contents of the glass immediately by drinking or by the use of a straw.
5. Add another one fluid ounce of water, swirl and consume immediately.
6. Then, add an additional one fluid ounce of water, swirl and consume immediately.

Aqueous suspension of Klor-Con® M extended-release tablet that is not taken immediately should be discarded. The use of other liquids for suspending Klor-Con® M tablets is not recommended.

To take this medicine follow the frequency and amount prescribed by the physician. This is especially important if the patient is also taking diuretics and/or digitalis preparations.

To check with the physician at once if tarry stools or other evidence of gastrointestinal bleeding is noticed.

Laboratory Tests: When blood is drawn for analysis of plasma potassium it is important to recognize that artifactual elevations can occur after improper venipuncture technique or as a result of *in-vitro* hemolysis of the sample.

Drug Interactions: Potassium-sparing diuretics, angiotensin converting enzyme inhibitors (see **WARNINGS**).

Carcinogenesis, Mutagenesis, Impairment of Fertility: Carcinogenicity, mutagenicity and fertility studies in animals have not been performed.

Potassium is a normal dietary constituent.

Pregnancy: Pregnancy Category C: Animal reproduction studies have not been conducted with Klor-Con® M. It is unlikely that potassium supplementation that does not lead to hyperkalemia would have an adverse effect on the fetus or would affect reproductive capacity.

Nursing Mothers: The normal potassium ion content of human milk is about 13 mEq per liter. Since oral potassium becomes part of the body potassium pool, so long as body potassium is not excessive, the contribution of potassium chloride supplementation should have little or no effect on the level in human milk.

Pediatric Use: Safety and effectiveness in pediatric patients have not been established.

ADVERSE REACTIONS

One of the most severe adverse effects is hyperkalemia (see **CONTRAINDICATIONS**, **WARNINGS** and **OVERDOSAGE**). There have also been reports of upper and lower gastrointestinal conditions including obstruction, bleeding, ulceration and perforation, (see **CONTRAINDICATIONS** and **WARNINGS**).

The most common adverse reactions to oral potassium salts are nausea, vomiting, flatulence, abdominal pain/discomfort and diarrhea. These symptoms are due to irritation of the gastrointestinal tract and are best managed by diluting the preparation further, taking the dose with meals or reducing the amount taken at one time.

OVERDOSAGE

The administration of oral potassium salts to persons with normal excretory mechanisms for potassium rarely causes serious hyperkalemia. However, if excretory mechanisms are impaired or if potassium is administered too rapidly intravenously, potentially fatal hyperkalemia can result (see **CONTRAINDICATIONS** and **WARNINGS**). It is important to recognize that hyperkalemia is usually asymptomatic and may be manifested only by an increased serum potassium concentration (6.5-8.0 mEq/L) and characteristic electrocardiographic changes (peaking of T-waves, loss of P-waves, depression of S-T segment and prolongation of the QT-interval). Late manifestations include muscle paralysis and cardiovascular collapse from cardiac arrest (9-12 mEq/L).

Treatment measures for hyperkalemia include the following:

1. Elimination of foods and medications containing potassium and of any agents with potassium-sparing properties.
2. Intravenous administration of 300 to 500 mL/hr of 10% dextrose injection containing 10-20 units of crystalline insulin per 1,000 mL.
3. Correction of acidosis, if present, with intravenous sodium bicarbonate.
4. Use of exchange resins, hemodialysis or peritoneal dialysis.

In treating hyperkalemia, it should be recalled that in patients who have been stabilized on digitalis, too rapid a lowering of the serum potassium concentration can produce digitalis toxicity.

DOSAGE AND ADMINISTRATION

The usual dietary intake of potassium by the average adult is 50 to 100 mEq per day. Potassium depletion sufficient to cause hypokalemia usually requires the loss of 200 or more mEq of potassium from the total body store.

Dosage must be adjusted to the individual needs of each patient. The dose for the prevention of hypokalemia is typically in the range of 20 mEq per day. Doses of 40-100 mEq per day or more are used for the treatment of potassium depletion. Dosage should be divided if more than 20 mEq per day is given such that no more than 20 mEq is given in a single dose.

Each Klor-Con® M20 tablet provides 1500 mg of potassium chloride equivalent to 20 mEq of potassium.

Each Klor-Con® M15 tablet provides 1125 mg of potassium chloride equivalent to 15 mEq of potassium.

Each Klor-Con® M10 tablet provides 750 mg of potassium chloride equivalent to 10 mEq of potassium.

Each Klor-Con® M tablets should be taken with meals and with a glass of water or other liquid. This product should not be taken on an empty stomach because of its potential for gastric irritation (see **WARNINGS**).

Patients having difficulty swallowing whole tablets may try one of the following alternate methods of administration:

a. Break the tablet in half and take each half separately with a glass of water.

b. Prepare an aqueous (water) suspension as follows:

1. Place the whole tablet(s) in approximately one-half glass of water (4 fluid ounces).
2. Allow approximately 2 minutes for the tablet(s) to disintegrate.
3. Stir for about half a minute after the tablet(s) has disintegrated.
4. Swirl the suspension and consume the entire contents of the glass immediately by drinking or by the use of a straw.
5. Add another one fluid ounce of water, swirl and consume immediately.
6. Then, add an additional one fluid ounce of water, swirl and consume immediately.

Aqueous suspension of Klor-Con® M extended-release tablet that is not taken immediately should be discarded. The use of other liquids for suspending Klor-Con® M tablets is not recommended.

HOW SUPPLIED

Klor-Con® M20 Extended-release Tablets, 1500 mg of potassium chloride (20 mEq of potassium) are available in bottles of 90 (NDC 0245-0058-90); bottles of 100 (NDC 0245-0058-11); bottles of 500 (NDC 0245-0058-15); bottles of 1000 (NDC 0245-0058-10) and cartons of 100 for unit dose dispensing (NDC 0245-0058-01). Klor-Con® M20 tablets are white, oblong, imprinted KC M20 and scored for flexibility of dosing.

Klor-Con® M15 Extended-release Tablets, 1125 mg of potassium chloride (15 mEq of potassium) are available in bottles of 100 (NDC 0245-0150-11); bottles of 1000 (NDC 0245-0150-10) and cartons of 100 for unit dose dispensing (NDC 0245-0150-01). Klor-Con® M15 tablets are white, oblong, imprinted M 15 and scored for flexibility of dosing.

Klor-Con® M10 Extended-release Tablets, 750 mg of potassium chloride (10 mEq of potassium) are available in bottles of 90 (NDC 0245-0057-90); bottles of 100 (NDC 0245-0057-11); bottles of 1000 (NDC 0245-0057-10) and cartons of 100 for unit dose dispensing (NDC 0245-0057-01). Klor-Con® M10 tablets are white, oblong, imprinted KC M10.

Storage Conditions: Keep tightly closed. Store at controlled room temperature, 15-30°C (59-86°F).

Manufactured by
UPSHER-SMITH LABORATORIES, INC.
Minneapolis, MN 55447

Certain manufacturing operations have been performed by other firms.

40-20150-00 Revised 0403

Shown in Product Identification Guide, page 335

PACERONE® ℞
(Amiodarone HCl)
Tablets

DESCRIPTION

Pacerone® (Amiodarone HCl) Tablets are a member of a new class of antiarrhythmic drugs with predominantly Class III (Vaughan Williams' classification) effects. Pacerone® Tablets are available in three strengths, containing 100 mg, 200 mg and 400 mg amiodarone hydrochloride, for oral administration. The 100 mg tablets are white tablets with the following inactive ingredients: anhydrous lactose, colloidal silicone dioxide, corn starch, magnesium stearate and povidone. The 200 mg tablets are pink, scored tablets with the following inactive ingredients: lactose monohydrate, magnesium stearate, povidone, pregelatinized corn starch, sodium starch glycolate, stearic acid, FD&C Red 40 and FD&C Yellow 6. The 400 mg tablets are light yellow, scored tablets with the following inactive ingredients: colloidal silicon dioxide, corn starch, lactose monohydrate, magnesium stearate, povidone and D&C Yellow 10 Aluminum Lake.

Amiodarone hydrochloride, the active ingredient in Pacerone®, is a benzofuran derivative: 2-butyl-3-benzofuranyl 4-[2-(diethylamino)-ethoxy]-3,5-diiodophenyl ketone hydrochloride. It is not chemically related to any other available antiarrhythmic drug.

The structural formula is as follows:

$(CH_2)_3CH_3$ $OCH_2CH_2N(C_2H_5)_2 \cdot HCl$

$C_{25}H_{29}I_2NO_3 \cdot HCl$ Molecular Weight: 681.8

Amiodarone HCl is a white to cream-colored crystalline powder. It is slightly soluble in water, soluble in alcohol and freely soluble in chloroform. It contains 37.3% iodine by weight.

CLINICAL PHARMACOLOGY

Electrophysiology/Mechanisms of Action

In animals, amiodarone HCl is effective in the prevention or suppression of experimentally-induced arrhythmias. The antiarrhythmic effect of amiodarone may be due to at least two major properties: 1) a prolongation of the myocardial cell-action potential duration and refractory period and 2) noncompetitive alpha- and beta-adrenergic inhibition.

Amiodarone prolongs the duration of the action potential of all cardiac fibers while causing minimal reduction of dV/dt (maximal upstroke velocity of the action potential). The refractory period is prolonged in all cardiac tissues. Amiodarone increases the cardiac refractory period without influencing resting membrane potential, except in automatic cells where the slope of the prepotential is reduced, generally reducing automaticity. These electrophysiologic effects are reflected in a decreased sinus rate of 15 to 20%, increased PR and QT intervals of about 10%, the development of U-waves and changes in T-wave contour. These changes should not require discontinuation of Pacerone® as they are evidence of its pharmacological action, although amiodarone can cause marked sinus bradycardia or sinus arrest and heart block. On rare occasions, QT prolongation has been associated with worsening of arrhythmia (see "**WARNINGS**").

Hemodynamics

In animal studies and after intravenous administration in man, amiodarone relaxes vascular smooth muscle, reduces peripheral vascular resistance (afterload) and slightly increases cardiac index. After oral dosing, however, amiodarone produces no significant change in left ventricular ejection fraction (LVEF), even in patients with depressed LVEF. After acute intravenous dosing in man, amiodarone may have a mild negative inotropic effect.

Pharmacokinetics

Following oral administration in man, amiodarone is slowly and variably absorbed. The bioavailability of amiodarone is approximately 50%, but has varied between 35 and 65% in various studies. Maximum plasma concentrations are attained 3 to 7 hours after a single dose. Despite this, the onset of action may occur in 2 to 3 days, but more commonly takes 1 to 3 weeks, even with loading doses. Plasma concentrations with chronic dosing at 100 to 600 mg/day are approximately dose proportional, with a mean 0.5 mg/L increase for each 100 mg/day. These means, however, include considerable individual variability. Food increases the rate and extent of absorption of amiodarone. The effects of food upon the bioavailability of amiodarone have been studied in 30 healthy subjects who received a single 600 mg dose immediately after consuming a high fat meal and following an overnight fast. The area under the plasma concentration-time curve (AUC) and the peak plasma concentration (C_{max}) of amiodarone increased by 2.3 (range 1.7 to 3.6) and 3.8 (range 2.7 to 4.4) times, respectively, in the presence of food. Food also increased the rate of absorption of amiodarone, decreasing the time to peak plasma concentration (T_{max}) by 37%. The mean AUC and mean C_{max} of desethylamiodarone increased by 55% (range 58 to 101%) and 32% (range 4 to 84%), respectively, but there was no change in the T_{max} in the presence of food.

Amiodarone has a very large but variable volume of distribution, averaging about 60 L/kg, because of extensive accumulation in various sites, especially adipose tissue and highly perfused organs, such as the liver, lung and spleen. One major metabolite of amiodarone, desethylamiodarone (DEA), has been identified in man; it accumulates to an even greater extent in almost all tissues. No data are available on the activity of DEA in humans, but in animals, it has significant electrophysiologic and antiarrhythmic effects generally similar to amiodarone itself. DEA's precise role and contribution to the antiarrhythmic activity of oral amiodarone are not certain. The development of maximal ventricular Class III effects after oral amiodarone adminis-

tration in humans correlates more closely with DEA accumulation over time than with amiodarone accumulation.
Amiodarone is eliminated primarily by hepatic metabolism and biliary excretion and there is negligible excretion of amiodarone or DEA in urine. Neither amiodarone nor DEA is dialyzable.
In clinical studies of 2 to 7 days, clearance of amiodarone after intravenous administration in patients with VT and VF ranged between 220 and 440 mL/hr/kg. Age, sex, renal disease and hepatic disease (cirrhosis) do not have marked effects on the disposition of amiodarone or DEA. Renal impairment does not influence the pharmacokinetics of amiodarone. After a single dose of intravenous amiodarone in cirrhotic patients, significantly lower C_{max} and average concentration values are seen for DEA, but mean amiodarone levels are unchanged. Normal subjects over 65 years of age show lower clearances (about 100 mL/hr/kg) than younger subjects (about 150 mL/hr/kg) and an increase in $t_{1/2}$ from about 20 to 47 days.
In patients with severe left ventricular dysfunction, the pharmacokinetics of amiodarone are not significantly altered but the terminal disposition $t_{1/2}$ of DEA is prolonged. Although no dosage adjustment for patients with renal, hepatic or cardiac abnormalities has been defined during chronic treatment with amiodarone, close clinical monitoring is prudent for elderly patients and those with severe left ventricular dysfunction.
Following single dose administration in 12 healthy subjects, amiodarone exhibited multi-compartmental pharmacokinetics with a mean apparent plasma terminal elimination half-life of 58 days (range 15 to 142 days) for amiodarone and 36 days (range 14 to 75 days) for the active metabolite (DEA). In patients, following discontinuation of chronic oral therapy, amiodarone has been shown to have a biphasic elimination with an initial one-half reduction of plasma levels after 2.5 to 10 days. A much slower terminal plasma-elimination phase shows a half-life of the parent compound ranging from 26 to 107 days, with a mean of approximately 53 days and most patients in the 40- to 55-day range. In the absence of a loading-dose period, steady-state plasma concentrations, at constant oral dosing, would therefore be reached between 130 and 535 days, with an average of 265 days. For the metabolite, the mean plasma-elimination half-life was approximately 61 days. These data probably reflect an initial elimination of drug from well-perfused tissue (the 2.5- to 10-day half-life phase), followed by a terminal phase representing extremely slow elimination from poorly perfused tissue compartments such as fat.
The considerable intersubject variation in both phases of elimination, as well as uncertainty as to what compartment is critical to drug effect, requires attention to individual responses once arrhythmia control is achieved with loading doses because the correct maintenance dose is determined, in part, by the elimination rates. Daily maintenance doses of Pacerone® should be based on individual patient requirements (see "**DOSAGE AND ADMINISTRATION**").
Amiodarone and its metabolite have a limited transplacental transfer of approximately 10 to 50%. The parent drug and its metabolite have been detected in breast milk.
Amiodarone is highly protein-bound (approximately 96%).
Although electrophysiologic effects, such as prolongation of QTc, can be seen within hours after a parenteral dose of amiodarone, effects on abnormal rhythms are not seen before 2 to 3 days and usually require 1 to 3 weeks, even when a loading dose is used. There may be a continued increase in effect for longer periods still. There is evidence that the time to effect is shorter when a loading-dose regimen is used.
Consistent with the slow rate of elimination, antiarrhythmic effects persist for weeks or months after Pacerone® is discontinued, but the time of recurrence is variable and unpredictable. In general, when the drug is resumed after recurrence of the arrhythmia, control is established relatively rapidly compared to the initial response, presumably because tissue stores were not wholly depleted at the time of recurrence.

Pharmacodynamics

There is no well-established relationship of plasma concentration to effectiveness, but it does appear that concentrations much below 1 mg/L are often ineffective and that levels above 2.5 mg/L are generally not needed. Within individuals, dose reductions and ensuing decreased plasma concentrations can result in loss of arrhythmia control. Plasma-concentration measurements can be used to identify patients whose levels are unusually low, and who might benefit from a dose increase, or unusually high, and who might have dosage reduction in the hope of minimizing side effects. Some observations have suggested a plasma concentration, dose or dose/duration relationship for side effects such as pulmonary fibrosis, liver-enzyme elevations, corneal deposits and facial pigmentation, peripheral neuropathy, gastrointestinal and central nervous system effects.

Monitoring Effectiveness

Predicting the effectiveness of any antiarrhythmic agent in long-term prevention of recurrent ventricular tachycardia and ventricular fibrillation is difficult and controversial, with highly qualified investigators recommending use of ambulatory monitoring, programmed electrical stimulation with various stimulation regimens, or a combination of these, to assess response. There is no present consensus on many aspects of how best to assess effectiveness, but there is a reasonable consensus on some aspects:
1. If a patient with a history of cardiac arrest does not manifest a hemodynamically unstable arrhythmia during electrocardiographic monitoring prior to treatment, assessment of the effectiveness of amiodarone requires some provocative approach, either exercise or programmed electrical stimulation (PES).
2. Whether provocation is also needed in patients who do manifest their life-threatening arrhythmia spontaneously is not settled, but there are reasons to consider PES or other provocation in such patients. In the fraction of patients whose PES-inducible arrhythmia can be made noninducible by amiodarone (a fraction that has varied widely in various series from less than 10 to almost 40%, perhaps due to different stimulation criteria), the prognosis has been almost uniformly excellent, with very low recurrence (ventricular tachycardia or sudden death) rates. More controversial is the meaning of continued inducibility. There has been an impression that continued inducibility in amiodarone patients may not foretell a poor prognosis but, in fact, many observers have found greater recurrence rates in patients who remain inducible than in those who do not. A number of criteria have been proposed, however, for identifying patients who remain inducible but who seem likely nonetheless to do well on Pacerone®. These criteria include increased difficulty of induction (more stimuli or more rapid stimuli), which has been reported to predict a lower rate of recurrence, and ability to tolerate the induced ventricular tachycardia without severe symptoms, a finding that has been reported to correlate with better survival but not with lower recurrence rates. While these criteria require confirmation and further study in general, *easier* inducibility or *poorer* tolerance of the induced arrhythmia should suggest consideration of a need to revise treatment.
Several predictors of success not based on PES have also been suggested, including complete elimination of all nonsustained ventricular tachycardia on ambulatory monitoring and very low premature ventricular-beat rates (less than 1 VPB/1,000 normal beats).
While these issues remain unsettled for amiodarone, as for other agents, the prescriber of Pacerone® should have access to (direct or through referral), and familiarity with, the full range of evaluatory procedures used in the care of patients with life-threatening arrhythmias.
It is difficult to describe the effectiveness rates of Pacerone®, as these depend on the specific arrhythmia treated, the success criteria used, the underlying cardiac disease of the patient, the number of drugs tried before resorting to Pacerone®, the duration of follow-up, the dose of amiodarone HCl, the use of additional antiarrhythmic agents and many other factors. As amiodarone has been studied principally in patients with refractory life-threatening ventricular arrhythmias, in whom drug therapy must be selected on the basis of response and cannot be assigned arbitrarily, randomized comparisons with other agents or placebo have not been possible. Reports of series of treated patients with a history of cardiac arrest and mean follow-up of one year or more have given mortality (due to arrhythmia) rates that were highly variable, ranging from less than 5 to over 30%, with most series in the range of 10 to 15%. Overall arrhythmia-recurrence rates (fatal and nonfatal) also were highly variable (and, as noted above, depended on response to PES and other measures), and depend on whether patients who do not seem to respond initially are included. In most cases, considering only patients who seemed to respond well enough to be placed on long-term treatment, recurrence rates have ranged from 20 to 40% in series with a mean follow-up of a year or more.

INDICATIONS AND USAGE

Because of its life-threatening side effects and the substantial management difficulties associated with amiodarone use (see "**WARNINGS**" below), Pacerone® (Amiodarone HCl) Tablets are indicated only for the treatment of the following documented, life-threatening recurrent ventricular arrhythmias when these have not responded to documented adequate doses of other available antiarrhythmics or when alternative agents could not be tolerated.
1. Recurrent ventricular fibrillation.
2. Recurrent hemodynamically unstable ventricular tachycardia.
As is the case for other antiarrhythmic agents, there is no evidence from controlled trials that the use of amiodarone HCl favorably affects survival.
Pacerone® (Amiodarone HCl) Tablets should be used only by physicians familiar with and with access to (directly or through referral) the use of all available modalities for treating recurrent life-threatening ventricular arrhythmias, and who have access to appropriate monitoring facilities, including in-hospital and ambulatory continuous electrocardiographic monitoring and electrophysiologic techniques. Because of the life-threatening nature of the arrhythmias treated, potential interactions with prior therapy and potential exacerbation of the arrhythmia, initiation of therapy with Pacerone® (Amiodarone HCl) Tablets should be carried out in the hospital.

CONTRAINDICATIONS

Pacerone® is contraindicated in severe sinus-node dysfunction, causing marked sinus bradycardia; second- and third-degree atrioventricular block; and when episodes of bradycardia have caused syncope (except when used in conjunction with a pacemaker).
Pacerone® is contraindicated in patients with a known hypersensitivity to the drug.

WARNINGS

Pacerone® is intended for use only in patients with the indicated life-threatening arrhythmias because amiodarone use is accompanied by substantial toxicity. Amiodarone has several potentially fatal toxicities, the most important of which is pulmonary toxicity (hypersensitivity pneumonitis or interstitial/alveolar pneumonitis) that has resulted in clinically manifest disease at rates as high as 10 to 17% in some series of patients with ventricular arrhythmias given doses around 400 mg/day, and as abnormal diffusion capacity without symptoms in a much higher percentage of patients. Pulmonary toxicity has been fatal about 10% of the time. Liver injury is common with amiodarone, but is usually mild and evidenced only by abnormal liver enzymes. Overt liver disease can occur, however, and has been fatal in a few cases. Like other antiarrhythmics, amiodarone can exacerbate the arrhythmia, e.g., by making the arrhythmia less well tolerated or more difficult to reverse. This has occurred in 2 to 5% of patients in various series, and significant heart block or sinus bradycardia has been seen in 2 to 5%. All of these events should be manageable in the proper clinical setting in most cases. Although the frequency of such proarrhythmic events does not appear greater with amiodarone than with many other agents used in this population, the effects are prolonged when they occur. Even in patients at high risk of arrhythmic death, in whom the toxicity of amiodarone is an acceptable risk, Pacerone® poses major management problems that could be life-threatening in a population at risk of sudden death, so that every effort should be made to utilize alternative agents first.
The difficulty of using Pacerone® effectively and safely itself poses a significant risk to patients. Patients with the indicated arrhythmias must be hospitalized while the loading dose of Pacerone® is given, and a response generally requires at least one week, usually two or more. Because absorption and elimination are variable, maintenance-dose selection is difficult, and it is not unusual to require dosage decrease or discontinuation of treatment. In a retrospective survey of 192 patients with ventricular tachyarrhythmias, 84 required dose reduction and 18 required at least temporary discontinuation because of adverse effects, and several series have reported 15 to 20% overall frequencies of discontinuation due to adverse reactions. The time at which a previously controlled life-threatening arrhythmia will recur after discontinuation or dose adjustment is unpredictable, ranging from weeks to months. The patient is obviously at great risk during this time and may need prolonged hospitalization. Attempts to substitute other antiarrhythmic agents when Pacerone® must be stopped will be made difficult by the gradually, but unpredictably, changing amiodarone body burden. A similar problem exists when amiodarone is not effective; it still poses the risk of an interaction with whatever subsequent treatment is tried.

Mortality

In the National Heart, Lung and Blood Institute's Cardiac Arrhythmia Suppression Trial (CAST), a long-term, multi-centered, randomized, double-blind study in patients with asymptomatic non-life-threatening ventricular arrhythmias who had had myocardial infarctions more than six days but less than two years previously, an excessive mortality or nonfatal cardiac arrest rate was seen in patients treated with encainide or flecainide (56/730) compared with that seen in patients assigned to matched placebo-treated groups (22/725). The average duration of treatment with encainide or flecainide in this study was ten months.
Amiodarone therapy was evaluated in two multi-centered, randomized, double-blind, placebo-controlled trials involving 1202 (Canadian Amiodarone Myocardial Infarction Arrhythmia Trial; CAMIAT) and 1486 (European Myocardial Infarction Amiodarone Trial; EMIAT) post-MI patients followed for up to 2 years. Patients in CAMIAT qualified with ventricular arrhythmias, and those randomized to amiodarone received weight- and response-adjusted doses of 200 to 400 mg/day. Patients in EMIAT qualified with ejection fraction <40%, and those randomized to amiodarone received fixed doses of 200 mg/day. Both studies had weeks-long loading dose schedules. Intent-to-treat all-cause mortality results were as follows:

	Placebo		Amiodarone		Relative Risk	
	N	Deaths	N	Deaths		95% CI
EMIAT	743	102	743	103	0.99	0.76–1.31
CAMIAT	596	68	606	57	0.88	0.58–1.16

These data are consistent with the results of a pooled analysis of smaller, controlled studies involving patients with structural heart disease (including myocardial infarction).

Pulmonary Toxicity

There have been postmarketing reports of acute-onset (days to weeks) pulmonary injury in patients treated with oral amiodarone with or without initial I.V. therapy. Findings have included pulmonary infiltrates on X-ray, bronchospasm, wheezing, fever, dyspnea, cough, hemoptysis, and hypoxia. Some cases have progressed to respiratory failure and/or death.

Continued on next page

Pacerone—Cont.

Amiodarone may cause a clinical syndrome of cough and progressive dyspnea accompanied by functional, radiographic, gallium scan and pathological data consistent with pulmonary toxicity, the frequency of which varies from 2 to 7% in most published reports, but is as high as 10 to 17% in some reports. Therefore, when Pacerone® therapy is initiated, a baseline chest X-ray and pulmonary-function tests, including diffusion capacity, should be performed. The patient should return for a history, physical exam and chest X-ray every 3 to 6 months.

Pulmonary toxicity secondary to amiodarone seems to result from either indirect or direct toxicity as represented by hypersensitivity pneumonitis or interstitial/alveolar pneumonitis, respectively.

Patients with preexisting pulmonary disease have a poorer prognosis if pulmonary toxicity develops.

Hypersensitivity pneumonitis usually appears earlier in the course of therapy and rechallenging these patients with Pacerone® results in a more rapid recurrence of greater severity. Bronchoalveolar lavage is the procedure of choice to confirm this diagnosis, which can be made when a T suppressor/cytotoxic (CD8-positive) lymphocytosis is noted. Steroid therapy should be instituted and Pacerone® therapy discontinued in these patients.

Interstitial/alveolar pneumonitis may result from the release of oxygen radicals and/or phospholipidosis and is characterized by findings of diffuse alveolar damage, interstitial pneumonitis or fibrosis in lung biopsy specimens. Phospholipidosis (foamy cells, foamy macrophages), due to inhibition of phospholipase, will be present in most cases of amiodarone-induced pulmonary toxicity; however, these changes also are present in approximately 50% of all patients on amiodarone therapy. These cells should be used as markers of therapy, but not as evidence of toxicity. A diagnosis of amiodarone-induced interstitial/alveolar pneumonitis should lead, at a minimum, to dose reduction or, preferably, to withdrawal of Pacerone® to establish reversibility, especially if other acceptable antiarrhythmic therapies are available. Where these measures have been instituted, a reduction in symptoms of amiodarone-induced pulmonary toxicity was usually noted within the first week, and a clinical improvement was greatest in the first two to three weeks. Chest X-ray changes usually resolve within two to four months. According to some experts, steroids may prove beneficial. Prednisone in doses of 40 to 60 mg/day or equivalent doses of other steroids have been given and tapered over the course of several weeks depending upon the condition of the patient. In some cases rechallenge with amiodarone at a lower dose has not resulted in return of toxicity. Reports suggest that the use of lower loading and maintenance doses of amiodarone are associated with a decreased incidence of amiodarone-induced pulmonary toxicity.

In a patient receiving Pacerone®, any new respiratory symptoms should suggest the possibility of pulmonary toxicity, and the history, physical exam, chest X-ray and pulmonary-function tests (with diffusion capacity) should be repeated and evaluated. A 15% decrease in diffusion capacity has a high sensitivity but only a moderate specificity for pulmonary toxicity; as the decrease in diffusion capacity approaches 30%, the sensitivity decreases but the specificity increases. A gallium scan also may be performed as part of the diagnostic workup.

Fatalities, secondary to pulmonary toxicity, have occurred in approximately 10% of cases. However, in patients with life-threatening arrhythmias, discontinuation of Pacerone® therapy due to suspected drug-induced pulmonary toxicity should be undertaken with caution, as the most common cause of death in these patients is sudden cardiac death. Therefore, every effort should be made to rule out other causes of respiratory impairment (i.e., congestive heart failure with Swan-Ganz catheterization if necessary, respiratory infection, pulmonary embolism, malignancy, etc.) before discontinuing Pacerone® in these patients. In addition, bronchoalveolar lavage, transbronchial lung biopsy and/or open lung biopsy may be necessary to confirm the diagnosis, especially in those cases where no acceptable alternative therapy is available.

If a diagnosis of amiodarone-induced hypersensitivity pneumonitis is made, Pacerone® should be discontinued, and treatment with steroids should be instituted. If a diagnosis of amiodarone-induced interstitial/alveolar pneumonitis is made, steroid therapy should be instituted and, preferably, Pacerone® discontinued or, at a minimum, reduced in dosage. Some cases of amiodarone-induced interstitial/alveolar pneumonitis may resolve following a reduction in Pacerone® dosage in conjunction with the administration of steroids. In some patients, rechallenge at a lower dose has not resulted in return of interstitial/alveolar pneumonitis; however, in some patients (perhaps because of severe alveolar damage) the pulmonary lesions have not been reversible.

Worsened Arrhythmia

Amiodarone, like other antiarrhythmics, can cause serious exacerbation of the presenting arrhythmia, a risk that may be enhanced by the presence of concomitant antiarrhythmics. Exacerbation has been reported in about 2 to 5% in most series, and has included new ventricular fibrillation, incessant ventricular tachycardia, increased resistance to cardioversion and polymorphic ventricular tachycardia associated with QTc prolongation (Torsade de Pointes). In addition, amiodarone has caused symptomatic bradycardia or sinus arrest with suppression of escape foci in 2 to 4% of patients.

The need to coadminister amiodarone with any other drug known to prolong the QTc interval must be based on a careful assessment of the potential risks and benefits of doing so for each patient. A careful assessment of the potential risks and benefits of administering Pacerone® must be made in patients with thyroid dysfunction due to the possibility of arrhythmia breakthrough or exacerbation of arrhythmia in these patients.

Liver Injury

Elevations of hepatic enzyme levels are seen frequently in patients exposed to amiodarone and in most cases are asymptomatic. If the increase exceeds three times normal, or doubles in a patient with an elevated baseline, discontinuation of Pacerone® or dosage reduction should be considered. In a few cases in which biopsy has been done, the histology has resembled that of alcoholic hepatitis or cirrhosis. Hepatic failure has been a rare cause of death in patients treated with amiodarone.

Loss of Vision

Cases of optic neuropathy and/or optic neuritis, usually resulting in visual impairment, have been reported in patients treated with amiodarone. In some cases, visual impairment has progressed to permanent blindness. Optic neuropathy and/or neuritis may occur at any time following initiation of therapy. A causal relationship to the drug has not been clearly established. If symptoms of visual impairment appear, such as changes in visual acuity and decreases in peripheral vision, prompt ophthalmic examination is recommended. Appearance of optic neuropathy and/or neuritis calls for re-evaluation of Pacerone® therapy. The risks and complications of antiarrhythmic therapy with Pacerone® must be weighed against its benefits in patients whose lives are threatened by cardiac arrhythmias. Regular ophthalmic examination, including fundoscopy and slit-lamp examination, is recommended during administration of Pacerone® (see "**ADVERSE REACTIONS**").

Neonatal Hypo- or Hyperthyroidism

Amiodarone can cause fetal harm when administered to a pregnant woman. Although amiodarone use during pregnancy is uncommon, there have been a small number of published reports of congenital goiter/hypothyroidism and hyperthyroidism. If Pacerone® (Amiodarone HCl) Tablets are used during pregnancy, or if the patient becomes pregnant while taking Pacerone®, the patient should be apprised of the potential hazard to the fetus.

In general, Pacerone® should be used during pregnancy only if the potential benefit to the mother justifies the unknown risk to the fetus.

In pregnant rats and rabbits, amiodarone HCl in doses of 25 mg/kg/day (approximately 0.4 and 0.9 times, respectively, the maximum recommended human maintenance dose*) had no adverse effects on the fetus. In the rabbit, 75 mg/kg/day (approximately 2.7 times the maximum recommended human maintenance dose*) caused abortions in greater than 90% of the animals. In the rat, doses of 50 mg/kg/day or more were associated with slight displacement of the testes and an increased incidence of incomplete ossification of some skull and digital bones; at 100 mg/kg/day or more, fetal body weights were reduced; at 200 mg/kg/day, there was an increased incidence of fetal resorption. (These doses in the rat are approximately 0.8, 1.6 and 3.2 times the maximum recommended human maintenance dose.*) Adverse effects on fetal growth and survival also were noted in one of two strains of mice at a dose of 5 mg/kg/day (approximately 0.04 times the maximum recommended human maintenance dose*).

*600 mg in a 50 kg patient (doses compared on a body surface area basis)

PRECAUTIONS

Impairment of Vision

Optic Neuropathy and/or Neuritis

Cases of optic neuropathy and optic neuritis have been reported (see "**WARNINGS**").

Corneal Microdeposits

Corneal microdeposits appear in the majority of adults treated with amiodarone. They are usually discernible only by slit-lamp examination, but give rise to symptoms such as visual halos or blurred vision in as many as 10% of patients. Corneal microdeposits are reversible upon reduction of dose or termination of treatment. Asymptomatic microdeposits alone are not a reason to reduce dose or discontinue treatment (see "**ADVERSE REACTIONS**").

Neurologic

Chronic administration of oral amiodarone in rare instances may lead to the development of peripheral neuropathy that may resolve when amiodarone is discontinued, but this resolution has been slow and incomplete.

Photosensitivity

Amiodarone has induced photosensitization in about 10% of patients; some protection may be afforded by the use of sun-barrier creams or protective clothing. During long-term treatment, a blue-gray discoloration of the exposed skin may occur. The risk may be increased in patients of fair complexion or those with excessive sun exposure, and may be related to cumulative dose and duration of therapy.

Thyroid Abnormalities

Amiodarone inhibits peripheral conversion of thyroxine (T_4) to triiodothyronine (T_3) and may cause increased thyroxine levels, decreased T_3 levels and increased levels of inactive reverse T_3 (rT_3) in clinically euthyroid patients. It is also a potential source of large amounts of inorganic iodine. Because of its release of inorganic iodine, or perhaps for other reasons, amiodarone can cause either hypothyroidism or hyperthyroidism. Thyroid function should be monitored prior to treatment and periodically thereafter, particularly in elderly patients, and in any patient with a history of thyroid nodules, goiter or other thyroid dysfunction. Because of the slow elimination of amiodarone and its metabolites, high plasma iodide levels, altered thyroid function and abnormal thyroid-function tests may persist for several weeks or even months following Pacerone® (Amiodarone HCl) Tablets withdrawal.

Hypothyroidism has been reported in 2 to 4% of patients in most series, but in 8 to 10% in some series. This condition may be identified by relevant clinical symptoms and particularly by elevated serum TSH levels. In some clinically hypothyroid amiodarone-treated patients, free thyroxine index values may be normal. Hypothyroidism is best managed by Pacerone® dose reduction and/or thyroid hormone supplement. However, therapy must be individualized, and it may be necessary to discontinue Pacerone® in some patients.

Hyperthyroidism occurs in about 2% of patients receiving amiodarone, but the incidence may be higher among patients with prior inadequate dietary iodine intake. Amiodarone-induced hyperthyroidism usually poses a greater hazard to the patient than hypothyroidism because of the possibility of arrhythmia breakthrough or aggravation which may result in death. In fact, IF ANY NEW SIGNS OF ARRHYTHMIA APPEAR, THE POSSIBILITY OF HYPERTHYROIDISM SHOULD BE CONSIDERED. Hyperthyroidism is best identified by relevant clinical symptoms and signs, accompanied usually by abnormally elevated levels of serum T_3 RIA, and further elevations of serum T_4, and a subnormal serum TSH level (using a sufficiently sensitive TSH assay). The finding of a flat TSH response to TRH is confirmatory of hyperthyroidism and may be sought in equivocal cases. Since arrhythmia breakthroughs may accompany amiodarone-induced hyperthyroidism, aggressive medical treatment is indicated, including, if possible, dose reduction or withdrawal of Pacerone®. The institution of antithyroid drugs, beta-adrenergic blockers and/or temporary corticosteroid therapy may be necessary. The action of antithyroid drugs may be especially delayed in amiodarone-induced thyrotoxicosis because of substantial quantities of preformed thyroid hormones stored in the gland. Radioactive iodine therapy is contraindicated because of the low radioiodine uptake associated with amiodarone-induced hyperthyroidism. Experience with thyroid surgery in this setting is extremely limited, and this form of therapy runs the theoretical risk of inducing thyroid storm. Amiodarone-induced hyperthyroidism may be followed by a transient period of hypothyroidism.

Surgery

Volatile Anesthetic Agents: Close perioperative monitoring is recommended in patients undergoing general anesthesia who are on amiodarone therapy as they may be more sensitive to the myocardial depressant and conduction effects of halogenated inhalational anesthetics.

Hypotension Postbypass: Rare occurrences of hypotension upon discontinuation of cardiopulmonary bypass during open-heart surgery in patients receiving amiodarone have been reported. The relationship of this event to Pacerone® therapy is unknown.

Adult Respiratory Distress Syndrome (ARDS): Postoperatively, occurrences of ARDS have been reported in patients receiving amiodarone therapy who have undergone either cardiac or noncardiac surgery. Although patients usually respond well to vigorous respiratory therapy, in rare instances the outcome has been fatal. Until further studies have been performed, it is recommended that FiO_2 and the determinants of oxygen delivery to the tissues (e.g., SaO_2, PaO_2) be closely monitored in patients on amiodarone.

Laboratory Tests

Elevations in liver enzymes (SGOT and SGPT) can occur. Liver enzymes in patients on relatively high maintenance doses should be monitored on a regular basis. Persistent significant elevations in the liver enzymes or hepatomegaly should alert the physician to consider reducing the maintenance dose of Pacerone® or discontinuing therapy.

Amiodarone alters the results of thyroid-function tests, causing an increase in serum T_4 and serum reverse T_3, and a decline in serum T_3 levels. Despite these biochemical changes, most patients remain clinically euthyroid.

Drug Interactions

Amiodarone is metabolized to desethylamiodarone by the cytochrome P450 (CYP450) enzyme group, specifically cytochrome P450 3A4 (CYP3A4). This isoenzyme is present in both the liver and intestines (see "**CLINICAL PHARMACOLOGY, Pharmacokinetics**"). Amiodarone is also known to be an inhibitor of CYP3A4. Therefore, amiodarone has the potential for interactions with drugs or substances that may be substrates, inhibitors or inducers of CYP3A4. While only a limited number of *in vivo* drug-drug interactions with amiodarone have been reported, the potential for other interactions should be anticipated. This is especially important for drugs associated with serious toxicity, such as other antiarrhythmics. If such drugs are needed, their dose should be reassessed and, where appropriate, plasma concentration measured.

In view of the long and variable half-life of amiodarone, potential for drug interactions exists not only with concomitant medication but also with drugs administered after discontinuation of amiodarone.

Since amiodarone is a substrate for CYP3A4, drugs/substances that inhibit CYP3A4 may decrease the metabolism and increase serum concentrations of amiodarone, with the potential for toxic effects. Reported examples of this interaction include the following:

Protease inhibitors:

Protease inhibitors are known to inhibit CYP3A4 to varying degrees. Inhibition of CYP3A4 by indinavir has been reported to result in increased serum concentrations of amiodarone. Monitoring for amiodarone toxicity and serial measurement of amiodarone serum concentration during concomitant protease inhibitor therapy should be considered.

Histamine H_2 antagonists:

Cimetidine inhibits CYP3A4 and can increase serum amiodarone levels.

Other substances:

Grapefruit juice inhibits CYP3A4-mediated metabolism of oral amiodarone in the intestinal mucosa, resulting in increased plasma levels of amiodarone; therefore, grapefruit juice should not be taken during treatment with oral amiodarone (see **"DOSAGE AND ADMINISTRATION"**).

Amiodarone may suppress certain CYP450 enzymes (enzyme inhibition). This can result in unexpectedly high plasma levels of other drugs which are metabolized by those CYP450 enzymes and may lead to toxic effects. Reported examples of this interaction include the following:

Immunosuppressives:

Cyclosporine (CYP3A4 substrate) administered in combination with oral amiodarone has been reported to produce persistently elevated plasma concentrations of cyclosporine resulting in elevated creatinine, despite reduction in dose of cyclosporine.

HMG-CoA Reductase Inhibitors:

Simvastatin (CYP3A4 substrate) in combination with amiodarone has been associated with reports of myopathy/rhabdomyolysis.

Cardiovasculars:

Cardiac glycosides: In patients receiving **digoxin** therapy, administration of oral amiodarone regularly results in an increase in the serum digoxin concentration that may reach toxic levels with resultant clinical toxicity. Amiodarone taken concomitantly with digoxin increases the serum digoxin concentration by 70% after one day. **On initiation of oral amiodarone, the need for digitalis therapy should be reviewed and the dose reduced by approximately 50% or discontinued.** If digitalis treatment is continued, serum levels should be closely monitored and patients observed for clinical evidence of toxicity. These precautions probably should apply to digitoxin administration as well.

Antiarrhythmics:

Other antiarrhythmic drugs, such as **quinidine, procainamide, disopyramide** and **phenytoin**, have been used concurrently with oral amiodarone.

There have been case reports of increased steady-state levels of quinidine, procainamide and phenytoin during concomitant therapy with amiodarone. Phenytoin decreases serum amiodarone levels. Amiodarone taken concomitantly with quinidine increases quinidine serum concentration by 33% after two days. Amiodarone taken concomitantly with procainamide for less than seven days increases plasma concentrations of procainamide and n-acetyl procainamide by 55% and 33%, respectively. Quinidine and procainamide doses should be reduced by one-third when either is administered with amiodarone. Plasma levels of **flecainide** have been reported to increase in the presence of oral amiodarone; because of this, the dosage of flecainide should be adjusted when these drugs are administered concomitantly. In general, any added antiarrhythmic drug should be initiated at a lower than usual dose with careful monitoring.

Combination of Pacerone® (Amiodarone HCl) Tablets with other antiarrhythmic therapy should be reserved for patients with life-threatening ventricular arrhythmias who are incompletely responsive to a single agent or incompletely responsive to amiodarone. During transfer to Pacerone®, the dose levels of previously administered agents should be reduced by 30 to 50% several days after the addition of Pacerone®, when arrhythmia suppression should be beginning. The continued need for the other antiarrhythmic agent should be reviewed after the effects of amiodarone have been established, and discontinuation ordinarily should be attempted. If the treatment is continued, these patients should be particularly carefully monitored for adverse effects, especially conduction disturbances and exacerbation of tachyarrhythmias, as Pacerone® is continued. In Pacerone® treated patients who require additional antiarrhythmic therapy, the initial dose of such agents should be approximately half of the usual recommended dose.

Antihypertensives:

Amiodarone should be used with caution in patients receiving **β-receptor blocking agents** (e.g., propranolol, a CYP3A4 inhibitor) or **calcium channel antagonists** (e.g., verapamil, a CYP3A4 substrate, and diltiazem, a CYP3A4 inhibitor) because of the possible potentiation of bradycardia, sinus arrest and AV block; if necessary, amiodarone can continue to be used after insertion of a pacemaker in patients with severe bradycardia or sinus arrest.

Anticoagulants:

Potentiation of **warfarin**-type (CYP2C9 and CYP3A4 substrate) anticoagulant response is almost always seen in patients receiving amiodarone and can result in serious or fatal bleeding. Since the concomitant administration of warfarin with amiodarone increases the prothrombin time by 100% after 3 to 4 days, **the dose of the anticoagulant should be reduced by one-third to one-half, and prothrombin times should be monitored closely.**

Some drugs/substances are known to accelerate the metabolism of amiodarone by stimulating the synthesis of CYP3A4 (enzyme induction). This may lead to low amiodarone serum levels and potential decrease in efficacy. Reported examples of this interaction include the following:

Antibiotics:

Rifampin is a potent inducer of CYP3A4. Administration of rifampin concomitantly with oral amiodarone has been shown to result in decreases in serum concentrations of amiodarone and desethylamiodarone.

Other substances, including herbal preparations:

St. John's Wort (Hypericum perforatum) induces CYP3A4. Since amiodarone is a substrate for CYP3A4, there is the potential that the use of St. John's Wort in patients receiving amiodarone could result in reduced amiodarone levels.

Other reported interactions with amiodarone:

Fentanyl (CYP3A4 substrate) in combination with amiodarone may cause hypotension, bradycardia, decreased cardiac output.

Sinus bradycardia has been reported with oral amiodarone in combination with **lidocaine** (CYP3A4 substrate) given for local anesthesia. Seizure, associated with increased lidocaine concentrations, has been reported with concomitant administration of intravenous amiodarone.

Dextromethorphan is a substrate for both CYP2D6 and CYP3A4. Amiodarone inhibits CYP2D6.

Cholestyramine increases enterohepatic elimination of amiodarone and may reduce serum levels and $t_{1/2}$.

Disopyramide increases QT prolongation which could cause arrhythmia.

Hemodynamic and electrophysiologic interactions have also been observed after concomitant administration with **propranolol, diltiazem** and **verapamil**.

Volatile Anesthetic Agents:

See **"PRECAUTIONS, Surgery,** *Volatile Anesthetic Agents*".

In addition to the interactions noted above, chronic (>2 weeks) ***oral*** amiodarone administration impairs metabolism of phenytoin, dextromethorphan and methotrexate.

Electrolyte Disturbances

Since antiarrhythmic drugs may be ineffective or may be arrhythmogenic in patients with hypokalemia, any potassium or magnesium deficiency should be corrected before instituting and during Pacerone® therapy. Use caution when coadministering Pacerone® with drugs which may induce hypokalemia and/or hypomagnesemia.

Carcinogenesis, Mutagenesis, Impairment of Fertility

Amiodarone HCl was associated with a statistically significant, dose-related increase in the incidence of thyroid tumors (follicular adenoma and/or carcinoma) in rats. The incidence of thyroid tumors was greater than control even at the lowest dose level tested, i.e., 5 mg/kg/day (approximately 0.08 times the maximum recommended human maintenance dose*).

Mutagenicity studies (Ames, micronucleus and lysogenic tests) with amiodarone were negative.

In a study in which amiodarone HCl was administered to male and female rats, beginning 9 weeks prior to mating, reduced fertility was observed at a dose level of 90 mg/kg/day (approximately 1.4 times the maximum recommended human maintenance dose*).

*600 mg in a 50 kg patient (dose compared on a body surface area basis)

Pregnancy: Pregnancy Category D

See **"WARNINGS, Neonatal Hypo- or Hyperthyroidism"**.

Labor and Delivery

It is not known whether the use of Pacerone® during labor or delivery has any immediate or delayed adverse effects. Preclinical studies in rodents have not shown any effect of amiodarone on the duration of gestation or on parturition.

Nursing Mothers

Amiodarone is excreted in human milk, suggesting that breast-feeding could expose the nursing infant to a significant dose of the drug. Nursing offspring of lactating rats administered amiodarone have been shown to be less viable and have reduced body-weight gains. Therefore, when Pacerone® therapy is indicated, the mother should be advised to discontinue nursing.

Pediatric Use

The safety and effectiveness of Pacerone® (Amiodarone HCl) Tablets in pediatric patients have not been established.

Geriatric Use

Clinical studies of amiodarone tablets did not include sufficient numbers of subjects aged 65 and over to determine whether they respond differently from younger subjects. Other reported clinical experience has not identified differences in responses between the elderly and younger patients. In general, dose selection for an elderly patient should be cautious, usually starting at the low end of the dosing range, reflecting the greater frequency of decreased hepatic, renal or cardiac function, and of concomitant disease or other drug therapy.

ADVERSE REACTIONS

Adverse reactions have been very common in virtually all series of patients treated with amiodarone HCl for ventricular arrhythmias with relatively large doses of drug (400 mg/day and above), occurring in about three-fourths of all patients and causing discontinuation in 7 to 18%. The most serious reactions are pulmonary toxicity, exacerbation of arrhythmia and rare serious liver injury (see **"WARNINGS"**), but other adverse effects constitute important problems. They are often reversible with dose reduction or cessation of amiodarone treatment. Most of the adverse effects appear to become more frequent with continued treatment beyond six months, although rates appear to remain relatively constant beyond one year. The time and dose relationships of adverse effects are under continued study.

Neurologic problems are extremely common, occurring in 20 to 40% of patients and including malaise and fatigue, tremor and involuntary movements, poor coordination and gait, and peripheral neuropathy; they are rarely a reason to stop therapy and may respond to dose reductions or discontinuation (see **"PRECAUTIONS"**).

Gastrointestinal complaints, most commonly nausea, vomiting, constipation and anorexia, occur in about 25% of patients but rarely require discontinuation of drug. These commonly occur during high-dose administration (i.e., loading dose) and usually respond to dose reduction or divided doses.

Ophthalmic abnormalities including optic neuropathy and/or optic neuritis, in some cases progressing to permanent blindness, papilledema, corneal degeneration, photosensitivity, eye discomfort, scotoma, lens opacities and macular degeneration have been reported (see **"WARNINGS"**).

Asymptomatic corneal microdeposits are present in virtually all adult patients who have been on drug for more than 6 months. Some patients develop eye symptoms of halos, photophobia and dry eyes. Vision is rarely affected and drug discontinuation is rarely needed.

Dermatological adverse reactions occur in about 15% of patients, with photosensitivity being most common (about 10%). Sunscreen and protection from sun exposure may be helpful, and drug discontinuation is not usually necessary. Prolonged exposure to amiodarone occasionally results in a blue-gray pigmentation. This is slowly and occasionally incompletely reversible on discontinuation of drug but is of cosmetic importance only.

Cardiovascular adverse reactions, other than exacerbation of the arrhythmias, include the uncommon occurrence of congestive heart failure (3%) and bradycardia. Bradycardia usually responds to dosage reduction but may require a pacemaker for control. CHF rarely requires drug discontinuation. Cardiac conduction abnormalities occur infrequently and are reversible on discontinuation of drug.

The following side-effect rates are based on a retrospective study of 241 patients treated for 2 to 1,515 days (mean 441.3 days).

The following side effects were each reported in 10 to 33% of patients:

Gastrointestinal: Nausea and vomiting.

The following side effects were each reported in 4 to 9% of patients:

Dermatologic: Solar dermatitis/photosensitivity.

Neurologic: Malaise and fatigue, tremor/abnormal involuntary movements, lack of coordination, abnormal gait/ataxia, dizziness, paresthesias.

Gastrointestinal: Constipation, anorexia.

Ophthalmologic: Visual disturbances.

Hepatic: Abnormal liver-function tests.

Respiratory: Pulmonary inflammation or fibrosis.

The following side effects were each reported in 1 to 3% of patients:

Thyroid: Hypothyroidism, hyperthyroidism.

Neurologic: Decreased libido, insomnia, headache, sleep disturbances.

Cardiovascular: Congestive heart failure, cardiac arrhythmias, SA node dysfunction.

Gastrointestinal: Abdominal pain.

Hepatic: Nonspecific hepatic disorders.

Other: Flushing, abnormal taste and smell, edema, abnormal salivation, coagulation abnormalities.

The following side effects were each reported in less than 1% of patients:

Blue skin discoloration, rash, spontaneous ecchymosis, alopecia, hypotension and cardiac conduction abnormalities.

In surveys of almost 5,000 patients treated in open U.S. studies and in published reports of treatment with amiodarone HCl, the adverse reactions most frequently requiring discontinuation of drug included pulmonary infiltrates or fibrosis, paroxysmal ventricular tachycardia, congestive heart failure and elevation of liver enzymes. Other symptoms causing discontinuations less often included visual disturbances, solar dermatitis, blue skin discoloration, hyperthyroidism and hypothyroidism.

Postmarketing Reports

In postmarketing surveillance, sinus arrest, hepatitis, cholestatic hepatitis, cirrhosis, epididymitis, impotence, vasculitis, pseudotumor cerebri, syndrome of inappropriate antidiuretic hormone secretion (SIADH), thrombocytopenia, angioedema, bronchiolitis obliterans organizing pneumonia (possibly fatal), bronchospasm, possibly fatal respiratory disorders (including distress, failure, arrest, and ARDS), fever, dyspnea, cough, hemoptysis, wheezing, hypoxia, pulmonary infiltrates, pleuritis, pancreatitis, toxic epidermal necrolysis, myopathy, rhabdomyolysis, hemolytic anemia, aplastic anemia, pancytopenia, neutropenia, erythema multiforme, Stevens-Johnson syndrome and exfoliative dermatitis also have been reported in patients receiving amiodarone.

Continued on next page

Pacerone—Cont.

OVERDOSAGE

There have been cases, some fatal, of amiodarone HCl overdose.

In addition to general supportive measures, the patient's cardiac rhythm and blood pressure should be monitored, and if bradycardia ensues, a β-adrenergic agonist or a pacemaker may be used. Hypotension with inadequate tissue perfusion should be treated with positive inotropic and/or vasopressor agents. Neither amiodarone nor its metabolite is dialyzable.

The acute oral LD_{50} of amiodarone HCI in mice and rats is greater than 3,000 mg/kg.

DOSAGE AND ADMINISTRATION

BECAUSE OF THE UNIQUE PHARMACOKINETIC PROPERTIES, DIFFICULT DOSING SCHEDULE AND SEVERITY OF THE SIDE EFFECTS IF PATIENTS ARE IMPROPERLY MONITORED, PACERONE® SHOULD BE ADMINISTERED ONLY BY PHYSICIANS WHO ARE EXPERIENCED IN THE TREATMENT OF LIFE-THREATENING ARRHYTHMIAS WHO ARE THOROUGHLY FAMILIAR WITH THE RISKS AND BENEFITS OF AMIODARONE THERAPY, AND WHO HAVE ACCESS TO LABORATORY FACILITIES CAPABLE OF ADEQUATELY MONITORING THE EFFECTIVENESS AND SIDE EFFECTS OF TREATMENT.

In order to insure that an antiarrhythmic effect will be observed without waiting several months, loading doses are required. A uniform, optimal dosage schedule for administration of Pacerone® has not been determined. Because of the food effect on absorption, Pacerone® should be administered consistently with regard to meals (see "**CLINICAL PHARMACOLOGY**"). Individual patient titration is suggested according to the following guidelines.

For life-threatening ventricular arrhythmias, such as ventricular fibrillation or hemodynamically unstable ventricular tachycardia: Close monitoring of the patients is indicated during the loading phase, particularly until risk of recurrent ventricular tachycardia or fibrillation has abated. Because of the serious nature of the arrhythmia and the lack of predictable time course of effect, loading should be performed in a hospital setting. Loading doses of 800 to 1,600 mg/day are required for 1 to 3 weeks (occasionally longer) until initial therapeutic response occurs. (Administration of Pacerone® in divided doses with meals is suggested for total daily doses of 1,000 mg or higher, or when gastrointestinal intolerance occurs.) If side effects become excessive, the dose should be reduced. Elimination of recurrence of ventricular fibrillation and tachycardia usually occurs within 1 to 3 weeks, along with reduction in complex and total ventricular ectopic beats.

Since grapefruit juice is known to inhibit CYP3A4-mediated metabolism of oral amiodarone in the intestinal mucosa, resulting in increased plasma levels of amiodarone, grapefruit juice should not be taken during treatment with oral amiodarone (see "**PRECAUTIONS, Drug Interactions**").

Upon starting Pacerone® therapy, an attempt should be made to gradually discontinue prior antiarrhythmic drugs (see "**PRECAUTIONS, Drug Interactions**"). When adequate arrhythmia control is achieved, or if side effects become prominent, Pacerone® dose should be reduced to 600 to 800 mg/day for one month and then to the maintenance dose, usually 400 mg/day (see "**CLINICAL PHARMACOLOGY, Monitoring Effectiveness**"). Some patients may require larger maintenance doses, up to 600 mg/day, and some can be controlled on lower doses. Pacerone® may be administered as a single daily dose, or in patients with severe gastrointestinal intolerance, as a b.i.d. dose. In each patient, the chronic maintenance dose should be determined according to antiarrhythmic effect as assessed by symptoms, Holter recordings and/or programmed electrical stimulation and by patient tolerance. Plasma concentrations may be helpful in evaluating nonresponsiveness or unexpectedly severe toxicity (see "**CLINICAL PHARMACOLOGY**").

The lowest effective dose should be used to prevent the occurrence of side effects. In all instances, the physician must be guided by the severity of the individual patient's arrhythmia and response to therapy.

When dosage adjustments are necessary, the patient should be closely monitored for an extended period of time because of the long and variable half-life of amiodarone and the difficulty in predicting the time required to attain a new steady-state level of drug. Dosage suggestions are summarized below:

	Loading Dose (Daily)	Adjustment and Maintenance Dose (Daily)	
Ventricular Arrhythmias	1 to 3 weeks	~1 month	usual maintenance
	800 to 1,600 mg	600 to 800 mg	400 mg

HOW SUPPLIED

Pacerone® (Amiodarone HCl) Tablets are available in three strengths, containing 100 mg, 200 mg and 400 mg amiodarone hydrochloride, for oral administration.

Pacerone® Tablets, 100 mg, are available in bottles of 30 tablets (NDC 0245-0144-30), and in unit dose cartons of 100 tablets (10 cards containing 10 tablets each) (NDC 0245-0144-01). The 100 mg tablets are white, round-shaped, flat-faced, uncoated tablets, debossed with "P" on one side, and "U-S" above "144" on the reverse side.

Pacerone® Tablets, 200 mg, are available in bottles of 60 tablets (NDC 0245-0147-60), bottles of 90 tablets (NDC 0245-0147-90), bottles of 500 tablets (NDC 0245-0147-15) and in unit dose cartons of 100 tablets (10 cards containing 10 tablets each) (NDC 0245-0147-01). The 200 mg tablets are pink, round-shaped, flat-faced, scored, uncoated tablets, debossed with "P_{200}" on the unscored side, and "U-S" above and "0147" below the score on the reverse side.

Pacerone® Tablets, 400 mg, are available in bottles of 30 tablets (NDC 0245-0145-30), bottles of 100 tablets (NDC 0245-0145-11), bottles of 500 tablets (NDC 0245-0145-15) and in unit dose cartons of 100 tablets (10 cards containing 10 tablets each) (NDC 0245-0145-01). The 400 mg tablets are light yellow, oval-shaped, scored, uncoated tablets, debossed with "P_{400}" on the unscored side, and "01" to the left and "45" to the right of the score on the reverse side.

Store at room temperature, approximately 25°C (77°F). Protect from light.

Dispense in a tight, light-resistant container with a child-resistant closure.

UPSHER-SMITH LABORATORIES, INC.
Minneapolis, MN 55447
US Patent 5,785,995
PCPI.0803-00 Revised 0803

Shown in Product Identification Guide, page 335

SLO-NIACIN® Tablets OTC

(polygel® controlled-release niacin)
Dietary Supplement

DESCRIPTION

Slo-Niacin® Tablets are manufactured utilizing a unique, patented polygel® controlled-release delivery system. This exclusive technology assures the gradual and measured release of niacin (nicotinic acid) and is designed to reduce the incidence of flushing and itching commonly associated with niacin use. Slo-Niacin® Tablets are available in 250 mg, 500 mg, and 750 mg strengths.

HOW SUPPLIED

250 mg tablets in bottles of 100: List 0245–0062–11
500 mg tablets in bottles of 100: List 0245–0063–11
750 mg tablets in bottles of 100: List 0245–0064–11
U.S. Patent No. 5,126,145 and 5,268,181

Shown in Product Identification Guide, page 335

U.S. Pharmaceutical Corporation

2401-C MELLON COURT
DECATUR, GA 30035

Direct Inquiries to:
Allison Krebs-Bensch
Vice President
(770) 987-4745
or
Clayton W. Bishop
National Sales Manager
(877) 775-2418
www.uspco.com

CENOGEN ULTRA® ℞

℞ ONLY
ADULTS ONLY

DESCRIPTION

Each capsule contains:

Ferrous Fumarate (anhydrous)	324 mg
(Equivalent to about 106 mg of Elemental Iron)	
Vitamin C (Sodium Ascorbate)	200 mg
Vitamin B_1 (Thiamine Mononitrate)	10 mg
Vitamin B_2 (Riboflavin)	6 mg
Vitamin B_6 (Pyridoxine HCl)	5 mg
Vitamin B_{12} (Cyanocobalamin Concentrate)	15 mcg
Folic Acid	1 mg
Niacinamide (Nicotinamide)	30 mg
Pantothenic Acid (Calcium Pantothenate)	10 mg
Manganese (Manganese Sulfate)	1.3 mg
Copper (Copper Sulfate)	0.8 mg

Inactive ingredients: Magnesium stearate, fumed silica dioxide, gelatin, titanium dioxide, FD&C Blue #2, FD&C Red #40.

HOW SUPPLIED

CenogenUltra® are blue and pink capsules imprinted with "US" logo and "CENOGEN ULTRA®/140". Available in child-resistant unit dose packs of 100 capsules, NDC 52747-40-60. Dispense in a tight, light resistant container as defined in the USP/NF with a child resistant closure.

Store at controlled room temperature 15°–30°C (59°–86°F). Keep in a cool, dry place.

CAUTION: ℞ only.

HEMOCYTE™ TABLETS OTC

[hē-mō-sīt]
(ferrous fumarate 324 mg.)

HOW SUPPLIED

Boxes of 100 child-proof tablets NDC 52747-307-70
Boxes of 30 child-proof tablets NDC 52747-307-30

HEMOCYTE PLUS® CAPSULES ℞

[hē-mō-cīte]
Iron-Vitamin-Mineral Complex Capsules
℞ ONLY
ADULTS ONLY

DESCRIPTION

Each capsule contains:

Iron (Ferrous Fumarate, anhydrous)	324 mg
(Equivalent to about 106 mg of Elemental Iron)	
Vitamin C (Sodium Ascorbate)	200 mg
Vitamin B_1 (Thiamine Mononitrate)	10 mg
Vitamin B_2 (Riboflavin)	6 mg
Vitamin B_6 (Pyridoxine HCl)	5 mg
Vitamin B_{12} (Cyanocobalamin Concentrate)	15 mcg
Folic Acid	1 mg
Niacinamide (Nicotinamide)	30 mg
Pantothenic Acid (Calcium Pantothenate)	10 mg
Zinc (Zinc Sulfate)	18.2 mg
Magnesium (Magnesium Sulfate)	6.9 mg
Manganese (Manganese Sulfate)	1.3 mg
Copper (Copper Sulfate)	0.8 mg

HOW SUPPLIED

Maroon cap and body printed "US" logo in black. Child resistant 10 × 10 blister packs in containers of 100 capsules (NDC 52747-800-60) and boxes of 10 × 3 blister packs in containers of 30 capsules (NDC 52747-800-30). Dispense in a tight, light-resistant container as defined in the USP/NF with a child resistant closure. Store at room temperature between 15°-30°C (59°-86°F). Keep in Cool Dry Place.

Rev. 02/2002
US Pharmaceutical Corporation
Decatur, GA 30035, USA

HEMOCYTE PLUS™ TABULES ℞

[hē-mō-cīt]
Iron-Vitamin-Mineral-Complex

DESCRIPTION

Each tabule contains:

Ferrous Fumarate (anhydrous)	324 mg.
[Equivalent to about 106 mg. of Elemental Iron]	
Sodium Ascorbate (Vit. C)	200 mg.
Vit. B-1—Thiamine Mononitrate	10 mg.
Vit. B-2—Riboflavin	6 mg.
Vit. B-6—Pyridoxine HCl	5 mg.
Vit. B-12—Cyanocobalamin Concentrate	5mcg.
Folic Acid	1 mg.
Niacinamide	30 mg.
Calcium Pantothenate	10 mg.
Zinc (as Zinc Sulfate)	18.2 mg.
Magnesium (as Magnesium Sulfate)	6.9 mg.
Manganese (as Manganese Sulfate)	1.3 mg.
Copper (as Copper Sulfate)	0.8 mg.

HOW SUPPLIED

Boxes of 100 child-proof tablets NDC 52747–308–70
Boxes of 30 child-proof tablets NDC 52747–308–30

HEMOCYTE-F ELIXIR ℞

[hē-mō-cīt]
Iron, Folic Acid, and Vitamin B12 Complex

DESCRIPTION

Each Teaspoon Contains:

Elemental Iron	100 mg
(As a polysaccharide-iron complex)	
Folic Acid	1 mg
Vitamin B12	25 mcg
Alcohol	10%
(Sugar Free)	

HOW SUPPLIED

Bottles of 16 oz. NDC 52747-404-90

HEMOCYTE-F TABLETS ℞
[*hē-mō-sīte*]

DESCRIPTION
Each tablet contains:

Ferrous Fumarate (anhydrous)	324 mg.
Folic Acid	1 mg.

HOW SUPPLIED
Boxes of 100 child proof tablets NDC 52747-306-70
Boxes of 30 child proof tablets NDC 52747-306-30

MEDIGESIC® Capsules ℞
[*mĕd-i-jē-sĭk*]

DESCRIPTION
Each capsule or tablet contains:

Butalbital*	50 mg
*WARNING: May be habit forming.	
Acetaminophen	325 mg
Caffeine	40 mg

HOW SUPPLIED
Capsules: Bottles of 100 NDC 52747-600-60

NOREL DM™ ℞
[*nō' rĕl*]
Antihistamine
Nasal Decongestant
Cough Suppressant
Alcohol Free • Sugar Free • Dye Free

DESCRIPTION
Each teaspoonful (5ml) contains:

Dextromethorphan hydrobromide	15 mg
Chloropheniramine maleate	4 mg
Phenylephrine hydrochloride	10 mg

HOW SUPPLIED
Bottles of 1 pint (16 fluid ounces)
NDC# 52747-410-90

NOVASAL™ ℞
[*nō-vă-săl*]
(Magnesium Salicylate Tetrahydrate)
℞ ONLY
ADULTS ONLY

DESCRIPTION
Each light-red, film coated, scored, oval-shaped tablet for oral administration contains:
Magnesium Salicylate Tetrahydrate .... 600 mg

HOW SUPPLIED
Each NOVASAL™ tablet contains magnesium salicylate 600 mg. NOVASAL™ tablets are light red film coated, oval shaped, debossed "0700/US" on one side, and are supplied in bottles of 100 tablets, NDC 52747-770-70.

USANA Health Sciences, Inc.
3838 WEST PARKWAY BOULEVARD
SALT LAKE CITY, UTAH 84120-6336

Direct Inquiries to:
Ph: (801) 954 7860
Fax: (801) 954 7658

ACTIVE CALCIUM™ OTC

COMPOSITION
Each Active Calcium tablet contains the following minerals:

Calcium (as citrate and carbonate)	200 mg
Magnesium (as citrate, aminoate* and oxide)	100 mg
Silicon (as aminoate*)	2.25 mg
Boron (as citrate)	330 mcg
Vitamin D_3 (cholecalciferol)	100 IU
Vitamin K (phylloquinone)	15 mcg

*Amino acid chelate from rice protein

ADVANTAGES
Each tablet contains a balanced blend of calcium, magnesium, vitamin D, vitamin K, boron and silicon; six nutrients required for bone development, bone remodeling and skeletal health. This non-prescription product meets USP guidelines for potency (as applicable), uniformity and disintegration, and is manufactured according to pharmaceutical cGMP standards.

RECOMMENDED USE
Take 4 tablets by mouth daily, preferably with meals.

SUPPLIED
Capsule-shaped tablet, mottled greenish-white color, with clear film coating, and with USANA imprint. In bottle of 112 tablets.

CHELATED MINERAL OTC
[*key'-lā-tĕd mineral*]

COMPOSITION
Each Chelated Mineral contains the following minerals:

Calcium (as citrate)	90 mg
Magnesium (as citrate, aminoate* and oxide)	100 mg
Zinc (as citrate)	6.7 mg
Manganese (as gluconate)	1.7 mg
Boron (as citrate)	1 mg
Copper (as gluconate)	1 mg
Chromium (as polynicotinate and picolinate)	100 mcg
Iodine (as potassium iodide)	75 mcg
Selenium (as L-selenomethionine and aminoate*)	66.7 mcg
Molybdenum (as citrate)	16.6 mcg
Vanadium (as vanadyl sulfate)	10 mcg
Silicon (as aminoate*)	1 mg
Trace minerals	1 mg

*amino acid chelate from rice protein.

ADVANTAGES
Each tablet contains a complete and balanced blend of essential minerals in bioavailable forms. The Chelated Mineral is designed to be taken with USANA's Mega Antioxidant to provide the full complement of essential nutrients required for health. This non-prescription product meets USP guidelines for potency (as applicable), uniformity and disintegration, and is manufactured according to pharmaceutical cGMP standards.

RECOMMENDED USE
Take 3 tablets by mouth daily, preferably with meals.

SUPPLIED
Oblong shaped tablet, off-white color, with clear film coating and with USANA imprint. In bottle of 84 tablets.
Shown in Product Identification Guide, page 335

COQUINONE® OTC
[*cō'-kwi-nōn*]

COMPOSITION
Each CoQuinone contains the following:

Coenzyme Q_{10}	30 mg
Alpha Lipoic Acid	12.5 mg

ADVANTAGES
CoQuinone contains a hydrosoluble form of Coenzyme Q_{10} (CoQ_{10}) that is 2.5 times more bioavailable than material supplied in dry tablet/capsule formulas. The higher blood levels of CoQ_{10} supplied enhance mitochondrial production of ATP. CoQ_{10} is a rate-limiting factor in the electron transport chain involved in mitochondrial production of ATP. It is also involved in neutralizing free radicals generated during ATP production. As such, CoQ_{10} helps the body maintain healthy skeletal and cardiac muscle. Alpha lipoic acid is included in the formula as a lipid-soluble antioxidant to recycle CoQ_{10} from the prooxidant form to the antioxidant form. This non-prescription product meets USP guidelines for uniformity and disintegration and is manufactured according to cGMP standards.

RECOMMENDED USE
Take 1 or 2 capsules by mouth daily.

SUPPLIED
Oval shaped, soft gelatin capsule, annatto-colored, opaque, imprinted with USANA in white edible ink. Capsules contain an orange colored liquid. In bottle of 56 soft-gel capsules.

MEGA ANTIOXIDANT OTC
[*mĕ-gă aenti-ŏk'-si-dĕnt*]

COMPOSITION
Each Mega Antioxidant contains the following vitamins and antioxidants:

Beta carotene	5000 IU
Vitamin C (as Poly C, a blend of calcium, zinc, potassium and magnesium ascorbates)	433 mg
Vitamin D_3 (Cholecalciferol)	150 IU
Vitamin E (d-alpha tocopheryl succinate)	150 IU
Vitamin K (phylloquinone)	20 mcg
Vitamin B1 (Thiamine HCl)	9 mg
Vitamin B2 (Riboflavin)	9 mg
Niacin and Niacinamide	13.3 mg
Vitamin B6 (Pyridoxine HCl)	9 mg
Folate (Folic Acid)	333 mcg
Vitamin B12 (Cyanocobalamin)	20 mcg
Biotin	100 mcg
Pantothenic Acid	30 mg
Olivol™ (Olive Extract)	10 mg
Bioflavonoid Complex (Rutin, Quercetin, Hesperidin, Green Tea Extract, Bilberry Extract)	64.5 mg
Inositol	50 mg
Choline Bitartrate	33.3 mg
N-Acetyl-L-Cysteine	21.7 mg
Bromelain	16.7 mg
Alpha-Lipoic Acid	5 mg
Coenzyme Q10	4 mg
Reduced Glutathione	3.3 mg
Turmeric Extract	5 mg
Lutein	200 mcg
Lycopene	0.33 mg
Broccoli Concentrate	5 mg

ADVANTAGES
A comprehensive and balanced formula containing the essential vitamins and antioxidants at levels substantially higher than RDA amounts. In addition to the traditionally recognized essential nutrients, the formula contains a unique blend of dietary antioxidants including carotenoids, a bioflavonoid complex, a glutathione complex, and USANA's patented Olivol™ to provide full-spectrum antioxidant protection. This formula is designed to be taken with USANA's Chelated Mineral to provide the full compliment of essential nutrients required for health. This non-prescription product meets USP guidelines for potency (as applicable), uniformity and disintegration, and is manufactured according to pharmaceutical cGMP standards.

RECOMMENDED USE
Three tablets by mouth daily, preferably with meals.

SUPPLIED
Oblong shaped tablets, mottled orange-brown color, with clear film coating and with USANA imprint. In bottle of 84 tablets.
Shown in Product Identification Guide, page 335

PROCOSA II OTC
[*prō-cō'-sə 2*]

COMPOSITION
Each Procosa II tablet contains the following:

Vitamin C (as calcium ascorbate)	75 mg
Manganese (as gluconate)	1.25 mg
Glucosamine Sulfate	500 mg
Silicon (as aminoate*)	0.75 mg
Turmeric Extract	125 mg

*Amino acid chelate from rice protein

ADVANTAGES
A comprehensive joint health formula combining a clinically proven dose of glucosamine sulfate with vitamin C, manganese, and silicon; three additional nutrients needed for cartilage synthesis. Procosa II also contains turmeric extract, a potent antioxidant that supports inflammation response. This non-prescription product meets USP guidelines for potency (as applicable), uniformity and disintegration, and is manufactured according to pharmaceutical cGMP standards.

RECOMMENDED USE
Take two tablets twice daily, preferably with meals

SUPPLIED
Oblong, orange-colored tablet, scored on one side. In bottle of 120 tablets.

PROFLAVANOL® 90 OTC
[*prō-flă' vi-nol*]

COMPOSITION
Each Proflavanol 90 contains the following:

Vitamin C (Poly C, a blend of calcium, zinc, potassium and magnesium ascorbates)	300 mg
Grape seed extract	90 mg
Ascorbyl palmitate	12 mg

ADVANTAGES
A potent antioxidant formula combining the proanthocyanidins (bioflavonoids) from standardized grape seed extract with vitamin C in the form of ascorbate salts and ascorbyl palmitate. Proflavanol 90 is designed to be taken as a stand-alone antioxidant, or preferably in combination with USANA's Mega Antioxidant and Chelated Mineral to provide additional antioxidant protection. This non-prescription product meets USP guidelines for uniformity and disintegration and is manufactured according to pharmaceutical cGMP standards.

Continued on next page

Proflavanol—Cont.

RECOMMENDED USE

Take 1–3 tablets by mouth daily.

SUPPLIED

Oblong, buff-colored tablet, with clear film coating, with USANA imprint. In bottles of 56 tablets.

Shown in Product Identification Guide, page 335

Valeant Pharmaceuticals International

3300 HYLAND AVENUE
COSTA MESA, CA 92626

For Medical Information, Contact:
(800) 548-5100, ext. 2286
FAX: (714) 641-7241

8-MOP® CAPSULES ℞

[*8-Mōp*]
(Methoxsalen Capsules, USP, 10 mg)

℞ only

CAUTION: METHOXSALEN IS A POTENT DRUG. READ ENTIRE BROCHURE PRIOR TO PRESCRIBING OR DISPENSING THIS MEDICATION.

Methoxsalen with UV radiation should be used only by physicians who have special competence in the diagnosis and treatment of psoriasis and vitiligo and who have special training and experience in photochemotherapy. Psoralen and ultraviolet radiation therapy should be under constant supervision of such a physician. For the treatment of patients with psoriasis, photochemotherapy should be restricted to patients with severe, recalcitrant, disabling psoriasis which is not adequately responsive to other forms of therapy, and only when the diagnosis is certain. Because of the possibilities of ocular damage, aging of the skin, and skin cancer (including melanoma), the patient should be fully informed by the physician of the risks inherent in this therapy. When methoxsalen is used in combination with photopheresis, refer to the UVAR* System Operator's Manual for specific warnings, cautions, indications, and instructions related to photopheresis.

CAUTION: 8-MOP® Capsules (Methoxsalen Hard Gelatin Capsules) may not be interchanged with Oxsoralen-Ultra® Capsules (Methoxsalen Soft Gelatin Capsules) without retitration of the patient.

I. DESCRIPTION

8-MOP (Methoxsalen, 8-Methoxypsoralen) Capsules, 10mg. Methoxsalen is a naturally occurring photoactive substance found in the seeds of the **Ammi majus** (Umbelliferae) plant and in the roots of **Heracleum Candicans**. It belongs to a group of compounds known as psoralens, or furocoumarins. The chemical name of methoxsalen is 9-methoxy-7 H-furo[3,2-g][1]-benzopyran-7-one; it has the following structure:

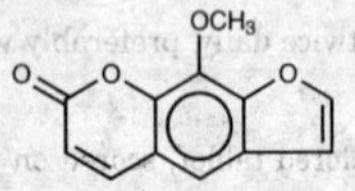

OCH_3

II. CLINICAL PHARMACOLOGY

The combination treatment regimen of psoralen (P) and ultraviolet radiation of 320-400 nm wavelength commonly referred to as UVA is known by the acronym, PUVA. Skin reactivity to UVA (320-400 nm) radiation is markedly enhanced by the ingestion of methoxsalen. The drug reaches its maximum bioavailability 1 1/2-3 hours after oral administration and may last for up to 8 hours (Pathak et al., 1974)[1]. Methoxsalen is reversibly bound to serum albumin and is also preferentially taken up by epidermal cells (Artuc et al. 1979)[2]. At a dose which is six times larger than that used in humans, it induces mixed function oxidases in the liver of mice (Mandula et al. 1978)[3]. In both mice and man, methoxsalen is rapidly metabolized. Approximately 95% of the drug is excreted as a series of metabolites in the urine within 24 hours (Pathak et al. 1977)[4].

The exact mechanism of action of methoxsalen with the epidermal melanocyctes and keratinocytes is not known. The best known biochemical reaction of methoxsalen is with DNA. Methoxsalen, upon photoactivation, conjugates and forms covalent bonds with DNA which leads to the formation of both monofunctional (addition to a single strand of DNA) and bifunctional adducts (crosslinking of psoralen to both strands of DNA) (Dall' Acqua et at., 1971[5]; Cole, 1970[6]; Musajo et al., 1974[7]; Dall' Acqua et al., 1979[8]). Reactions with proteins have also been described (Yoshikawa, et al., 1979[9]).

Methoxsalen acts as a photosensitizer. Administration of the drug and subsequent exposure to UVA can lead to cell injury. Orally administered methoxsalen reaches the skin via the blood and UVA penetrates well into the skin. If sufficient cell injury occurs in the skin, an inflammatory reaction occurs. The most obvious manifestation of this reaction is delayed erythema, which may not begin for several hours and peaks at 48–72 hours. The inflammation is followed, over several days to weeks, by repair which is manifested by increased melanization of the epidermis and thickening of the stratum corneum. The mechanisms of therapy are not known. In the treatment of vitiligo, it has been suggested that melanocytes in the hair follicle are stimulated to move up the follicle and to repopulate the epidermis (Ortonne et al, 1979[10]). In the treatment of psoriasis, the mechanism is most often assumed to be DNA photodamage and resulting decrease in cell proliferation but other vascular, leukocyte, or cell regulatory mechanisms may also be playing some role. Psoriasis is a hyperproliferative disorder and other agents known to be therapeutic for psoriasis are known to inhibit DNA synthesis.

III. INDICATIONS AND USAGE

A. Photochemotherapy (methoxsalen with long wave UVA radiation) is indicated for the symptomatic control of severe, recalcitrant, disabling psoriasis not adequately responsive to other forms of therapy and when the diagnosis has been supported by biopsy. Photochemotherapy is intended to be administered only in conjunction with a schedule of controlled doses of long wave ultraviolet radiation.

B. Photochemotherapy (methoxsalen with long wave ultraviolet radiation) is indicated for the repigmentation of idiopathic vitiligo.

C. Photopheresis (methoxsalen with long wave ultraviolet radiation of white blood cells) is indicated for use with the UVAR* System in the palliative treatment of the skin manifestations of cutaneous T-cell lymphoma (CTCL) in persons who have not been responsive to other forms of treatment. While this dosage form of methoxsalen has been approved for use in combination with photopheresis, Oxsoralen Ultra® Capsules have not been approved for that use.

IV. CONTRAINDICATIONS

A. Patients exhibiting idiosyncratic reactions to psoralen compounds.

B. Patients possessing a specific history of light sensitive disease states should not initiate methoxsalen therapy. Diseases associated with photosensitivity include lupus erythematosus, porphyria cutanea tarda, erythropoietic protoporphyria, variegate porphyria, xeroderma pigmentosum, and albinism.

C. Patients exhibiting melanoma or possessing a history of melanoma.

D. Patients exhibiting invasive squamous cell carcinomas.

E. Patients with aphakia, because of the significantly increased risk of retinal damage due to the absence of lenses.

V. WARNINGS—GENERAL

A. **SKIN BURNING:** Serious burns from either UVA or sunlight (even through window glass) can result if the recommended dosage of the drug and/or exposure schedules are not maintained.

B. **CARCINOGENICITY:**

1. ANIMAL STUDIES: Topical or intraperitoneal methoxsalen has been reported to be a potent photocarcinogen in albino mice and hairless mice. However, methoxsalen given by the oral route to albino mice or by any route in pigmented mice is considerably less phototoxic or carcinogenic (Hakim et at. 1960[11]; Pathak et al. 1959[12]).

2. HUMAN STUDIES: A prospective study of 1380 patients over 5 years revealed an approximately nine-fold increase in risks of squamous cell carcinoma among PUVA treated patients (Stern et al. 1979[13] and Stern et al. 1980[14]). This increase in risk appears greatest among patients who are fair skinned or had pre-PUVA exposure to 1) prolonged tar and UVB treatment, 2) ionizing radiation, or 3) arsenic.

In addition, an approximately two-fold increase in the risk of basal cell carcinoma was noted in this study. Roenigk et al. 1980[15] studied 690 patients for up to 4 years and found no increase in the risk of non-melanoma skin cancer. However, patients in this cohort had significantly less exposure to PUVA than in the Stern et al study. Recent analysis of new data in the Stern et al cohort (Stern et al., 1997[16]) has shown that these patients had an elevated relative risk of contracting melanoma. The relative risk for melanoma in these patients was 2.3 (95 percent confidence interval 1.1 to 4.1). The risk is particularly higher in those patients who have received more than 250 PUVA treatments and in those whose treatment has spanned greater than 15 years earlier. Some patients developing melanoma did so even after having ceased PUVA therapy over 5 years earlier. These observations indicate the need for monitoring of PUVA patients for skin tumors throughout their lives.

In a study in Indian patients treated for 4 years for vitiligo, 12 percent developed keratoses, but not cancer, in the depigmented, vitiliginous areas (Mosher, 1980[17]). Clinically, the keratoses were keratotic papules, actinic keratosis-like macules, nonscaling dome-shaped papules, and lichenoid porokeratotic-like papules.

C. **CATARACTOGENICITY:**

1. ANIMAL STUDIES: Exposure to large doses of UVA causes cataracts in animals, and this effect is enhanced by the administration of methoxsalen (Cloud et al. 1960[18]; Cloud et al. 1961[19]; Freeman et al. 1969[20]).

2. HUMAN STUDIES: It has been found that the concentration of methoxsalen in the lens is proportional to the serum level. If the lens is exposed to UVA during the time methoxsalen is present in the lens, photochemical action may lead to irreversible binding of methoxsalen to proteins and the DNA components of the lens (Lerman et al. 1980[21]). However, if the lens is shielded from UVA, the methoxsalen will diffuse out of the lens in a 24 hour period[21]. Patients should be told emphatically to wear UVA-absorbing, wraparound sunglasses for the twenty-four (24) hour period following ingestion of methoxsalen, whether exposed to direct or indirect sunlight in the open or through a window glass.

Among patients using proper eye protection, there is no evidence for a significantly increased risk of cataracts in association with PUVA therapy.[13] Thirty-five of 1380 patients have developed cataracts in the five years since their first PUVA treatment. This incidence is comparable to that expected in a population of this size and age distribution. No relationship between PUVA dose and cataract risk in this group has been noted.

D. **ACTINIC DEGENERATION:** Exposure to sunlight and/or ultraviolet radiation may result in "premature aging" of the skin.

E. **BASAL CELL CARCINOMAS:** Patients exhibiting multiple basal cell carcinomas or having a history of basal cell carcinomas should be diligently observed and treated.

F. **RADIATION THERAPY:** Patients having a history of previous x-ray therapy or grenz ray therapy should be diligently observed for signs of carcinoma.

G. **ARSENIC THERAPY:** Patients having a history of previous arsenic therapy should be diligently observed for signs of carcinoma.

H. **HEPATIC DISEASES:** Patients with hepatic insufficiency should be treated with caution since hepatic biotransformation is necessary for drug urinary excretion.

I. **CARDIAC DISEASES:** Patients with cardiac diseases or others who may be unable to tolerate prolonged standing or exposure to heat stress should not be treated in a vertical UVA chamber.

J. **TOTAL DOSAGE:** The total cumulative dose of UVA that can be given over long periods of time with safety has not as yet been established.

K. **CONCOMITANT THERAPY:** Special care should be exercised in treating patients who are receiving concomitant therapy (either topically or systemically) with known photosensitizing agents such as anthralin, coal tar or coal tar derivatives, griseofulvin, phenothiazines, nalidixic acid, fluoroquinolone antibiotics, halogenated salicylanilides (bacteriostatic soaps), sulfonamides, tetracyclines, thiazides, and certain organic staining dyes such as methylene blue, toluidine blue, rose bengal, and methyl orange.

VI. PRECAUTIONS

A. **GENERAL—APPLICABLE TO BOTH VITILIGO AND PSORIASIS TREATMENT:**

1. BEFORE METHOXSALEN INGESTION

Patients must not sunbathe during the 24 hours prior to methoxsalen ingestion and UV exposure. The presence of a sunburn may prevent an accurate evaluation of the patient's response to photochemotherapy.

2. AFTER METHOXSALEN INGESTION

a. UVA-absorbing wrap-around sunglasses should be worn during daylight for 24 hours after methoxsalen ingestion. The protective eyewear must be designed to prevent entry of stray radiation to the eyes, including that which may enter from the sides of the eyewear. The protective eyewear is used to prevent the irreversible binding of methoxsalen to the proteins and DNA components of the lens. Cataracts form when enough of the binding occurs. Visual discrimination should be permitted by the eyewear for patient well-being and comfort.

b. Patients must avoid sun exposure, even through window glass or cloud cover, for at least 8 hours after methoxsalen ingestion. If sun exposure cannot be avoided, the patient should wear protective devices such as a hat and gloves, and/or apply sunscreens which contain ingredients that filter out UVA radiation (e.g., sunscreens containing benzophenone and/or PABA esters which exhibit a sun protective factor equal to or greater than 15). These chemical sunscreens should be applied to all areas that might be exposed to the sun (including lips). Sunscreens should not be applied to areas affected by psoriasis until after the patient has been treated in the UVA chamber.

3. DURING PUVA THERAPY

a. Total UVA-absorbing/blocking goggles mechanically designed to give maximal ocular protection must be worn. Failure to do so may increase the risk of cataract formation. A reliable radiometer can be used to verify elimination of UVA transmission through the goggles.

b. Abdominal skin, breasts, genitalia, and other sensitive areas should be protected for approximately 1/3 of the initial exposure time until tanning occurs.

c. Unless affected by disease, male genitalia should be shielded.

4. AFTER COMBINED METHOXSALEN/UVA THERAPY

a. UVA-absorbing wrap-around sunglasses should be worn during the daylight for 24 hours after combined methoxsalen/UVA therapy.

b. Patients should not sunbathe for 48 hours after therapy. Erythema and/or burning due to photochemotherapy and sunburn due to sun exposure are additive.

5. VITILIGO THERAPY

a. The dosage of methoxsalen should not be increased above 0.6 mg/kg since overdosage may result in serious burning of the skin.

b. Eye and skin sun protection as described in the Precautions - General section should be observed.

B. INFORMATION FOR PATIENTS: See accompanying Patient Package Insert.

C. LABORATORY TESTS:

1. Patients should have an ophthalmologic examination prior to the start of therapy, and thence yearly.
2. Patients should have the following tests prior to the start of therapy and should be retested 6-12 months subsequently. Additional tests at more extended time periods should be conducted as clinically indicated.

a. Complete Blood Count (Hemoglobin or Hematocrit; White Blood Count - if abnormal, a differential count).

b. Anti-nuclear Antibodies.

c. Liver Function Tests.

d. Renal Function Tests (Creatinine or Blood Urea Nitrogen).

D. DRUG INTERACTIONS: See Warnings Section.

E. CARCINOGENESIS: See Warnings Section.

F. PREGNANCY:

Pregnancy Category C. Animal reproduction studies have not been conducted with methoxsalen. It is also not known whether methoxsalen can cause fetal harm when administered to a pregnant woman or can affect reproduction capacity. Methoxsalen should be given to a woman only if clearly needed.

G. NURSING MOTHERS:

It is not known whether this drug is excreted in human milk. Because many drugs are excreted in human milk, caution should be exercised when methoxsalen is administered to a nursing woman.

H. PEDIATRIC USE:

Safety in children has not been established. Potential hazards of long-term therapy include the possibilities of carcinogenicity and cataractogenicity as described in the Warnings Section as well as the probability of actinic degeneration which is also described in the Warnings Section.

VII. ADVERSE REACTIONS

A. METHOXSALEN:

The most commonly reported side effect of methoxsalen alone is nausea, which occurs with approximately 10% of all patients. This effect may be minimized or avoided by instructing the patient to take methoxsalen with milk or food, or to divide the dose into two portions, taken approximately one-half hour apart. Other effects include nervousness, insomnia, and psychological depression.

B. COMBINED METHOXSALEN/UVA THERAPY:

1. PRURITUS: This adverse reaction occurs with approximately 10% of all patients. In most cases, pruritus can be alleviated with frequent application of bland emollients or other topical agents; severe pruritus may require systemic treatment. If pruritus is unresponsive to these measures, shield pruritic areas from further UVA exposure until the condition resolves. If intractable pruritus is generalized, UVA treatment should be discontinued until the pruritus disappears.

2. ERYTHEMA: Mild, transient erythema at 24-48 hours after PUVA therapy is an expected reaction and indicates that a therapeutic interaction between methoxsalen and UVA occurred. Any area showing moderate erythema (greater than Grade 2 – See Table 1 for grades of erythema) should be shielded during subsequent UVA exposures until the erythema has resolved. Erythema greater than Grade 2 which appears within 24 hours after UVA treatment may signal a potentially severe burn. Erythema may become progressively worse over the next 24 hours, since the peak erythemal reaction characteristically occurs 48 hours or later after methoxsalen ingestion. The patient should be protected from further UVA exposures and sunlight, and should be monitored closely.

3. IMPORTANT DIFFERENCES BETWEEN PUVA ERYTHEMA AND SUNBURN: PUVA-induced inflammation differs from sunburn or UVB phototherapy in several ways. The **in situ** depth of photochemistry is deeper within the tissue because UVA is transmitted further into the skin. The DNA lesions induced by PUVA are very different from UV-induced thymine dimers and may lead to a DNA crosslink. This DNA lesion may be more problematic to the cell because crosslinks are more lethal and psoralen-DNA photoproducts may be "new" or unfamiliar substrates for DNA repair enzymes. DNA synthesis is also suppressed longer after PUVA. The time course of delayed erythema is different with PUVA and may not involve the usual mediators seen in sunburn. PUVA-induced redness may be just beginning at 24 hours, when UVB erythema has already passed its peak. The erythema dose-response curve is also steeper for PUVA. Compared to equally erythemogenic doses of UVB, the histologic alterations induced by PUVA show more dermal vessel damage and longer duration of epidermal and dermal abnormalities.

4. OTHER ADVERSE REACTIONS: Those reported include edema, dizziness, headache, malaise, depression, hypopigmentation, vesiculation and bullae formation, non-specific rash, herpes simplex, miliaria, urticaria, folliculitis, gastrointestinal disturbances, cutaneous tenderness, leg cramps, hypotension, and extension of psoriasis.

VIII. OVERDOSAGE

In the event of methoxsalen overdosage, induce emesis and keep the patient in a darkened room for at least 24 hours. Emesis is beneficial only within the first 2 to 3 hours after ingestion of methoxsalen, since maximum blood levels are reached by this time.

IX. DRUG DOSAGE & ADMINISTRATION

A: VITILIGO THERAPY

1. DRUG DOSAGE: Two capsules (10 mg each) in one dose taken with milk or in food two to four hours before ultraviolet light exposure.

2. LIGHT EXPOSURE: The exposure time to sunlight should comply with the following guide:

	Basic Skin Color		
	Light	**Medium**	**Dark**
Initial Exposure	15 min.	20 min.	25 min.
Second Exposure	20 min.	25 min.	30 min.
Third Exposure	25 min.	30 min.	35 min.
Fourth Exposure	30 min.	35 min.	40 min.

Subsequent Exposure: Gradually increase exposure based on erythema and tenderness of the amelanotic skin.

Therapy should be on alternate days and never two consecutive days.

B. PSORIASIS THERAPY

1. DRUG DOSAGE—INITIAL THERAPY: The methoxsalen capsules should be taken 2 hours before UVA exposure with some food or milk according to the following table:

Patient's Weight (kg)	(lbs)	Dose (mg)
<30	<66	10
30–50	66–110	20
51–65	112–143	30
66–80	146–176	40
81–90	179–198	50
91–115	201–254	60
>115	>254	70

Additional drug dosage directions are as follows:

a. Weight Change: In the event that the weight of a patient changes during treatment such that he/she falls into an adjacent weight range/dose category, no change in the dose of methoxsalen is usually required. If, in the physician's opinion, however, a weight change is sufficiently great to modify the drug dose, then an adjustment in the time of exposure to UVA should be made.

b. Dose/Week: The number of doses per week of methoxsalen capsules will be determined by the patient's schedule of UVA exposures. In no case should treatments be given more often than once every other day because the full extent of phototoxic reactions may not be evident until 48 hours after each exposure.

c. Dosage Increase: Dosage may be increased by 10 mg. after the fifteenth treatment under the conditions outlined in section XI.B.4.b.

X. UVA RADIATION SOURCE SPECIFICATIONS & INFORMATION

A. IRRADIANCE UNIFORMITY (For photopheresis, refer to the UVAR* System Operator's Manual.) The following specifications should be met with the window of the detector held in a vertical plane:

1. Vertical variation: For readings taken at any point along the vertical center axis of the chamber (to within 15 cm from the top and bottom), the lowest reading should not be less than 70 percent of the highest reading.

2. Horizontal variation: Throughout any specific horizontal plane, the lowest reading must be at least 80 percent of the highest reading, excluding the peripheral 3 cm of the patient treatment space.

B. PATIENT SAFETY FEATURES:

The following safety features should be present: (1) Protection from electrical hazard: All units should be grounded and conform to applicable electrical codes. The patient or operator should not be able to touch any live electrical parts. There should be ground fault protection. (2) Protective shielding of lamps: The patient should not be able to come in contact with the bare lamps. In the event of lamp breakage, the patient should not be exposed to broken lamp components. (3) Hand rails and hand holds: Appropriate supports should be available to the patient. (4) Patient viewing window: A window which blocks UV should be provided for viewing the patient during treatment. (5) Door and latches: Patients should be able to open the door from the inside with only slight pressure to the door. (6) Non-skid floor: The floor should be of a non-skid nature. (7) Thermoregulation: Sufficient air flow should be provided for patient safety and comfort, limiting temperature within the UVA radiator cabinet to approximately less than 100° F. (8) Timer: The irradiator should be equipped with an automatic timer which terminates the exposure at the conclusion of a pre-set time interval. (9) Patient alarm device: An alarm device within the UVA irradiator chamber should be accessible to the patient for emergency activation. (10) Danger label: The unit should have a label prominently displayed which reads as follows:

DANGER – Ultraviolet Radiation – Follow your physician's instructions – Failure to use protective eyewear may result in eye injury.

C. UVA EXPOSURE DOSIMETRY MEASUREMENTS:

The maximum radiant exposure or irradiance (within ±15 percent) of UVA (320–400 nm) delivered to the patient should be determined by using an appropriate radiometer calibrated to be read in Joules/cm^2 or mW/cm^2. In the absence of a standard measuring technique approved by the National Bureau of Standards, the system should use a detector corrected to a cosine spatial response. The use and recalibration frequency of such a radiometer for a specific UVA irradiator chamber should be specified by the manufacturer because the UVA dose (exposure) is determined by the design of the irradiator, the number of lamps, and the age of the lamps. If irradiance is measured, the radiometer reading in mW/cm^2 is used to calculate the exposure time in minutes to deliver the required UVA dose in Joules/cm^2 to a patient in the UVA irradiator cabinet. The equation is:

$$\text{Exposure Time in minutes} = \frac{\text{Desired UVA Dose (J/cm}^2)}{0.06 \times \text{Irradiance (mW/cm}^2)}$$

Overexposure due to human error should be minimized by using an accurate automatic timing device, which is set by the operator and controlled by energizing and de-energizing the UVA irradiator lamp. The timing device calibration interval should be specified by the manufacturer. Safety systems should be included to minimize the possibility of delivering a UVA exposure which exceeds the prescribed dose, in the event the timer or radiometer should malfunction.

D. UVA SPECTRAL OUTPUT DISTRIBUTION:

The spectral distributions of the lamps should meet the following specifications:

Wavelength Band (Nanometers)	Output[1]
<310	<1
310 to 320	1 to 3
320 to 330	4 to 8
330 to 340	11 to 17
340 to 350	18 to 25
350 to 360	19 to 28
360 to 370	15 to 23
370 to 380	8 to 12
380 to 390	3 to 7
390 to 400	1 to 3

[1]As a percentage of total irradiance between 320 and 400 nanometers.

XI. PUVA TREATMENT PROTOCOL

A. INITIAL EXPOSURE: The initial dosage and UVA exposure should be determined according to the guidelines presented previously under IX.B.1, and the information presented in this section.

Skin Type	History	Recommended Joules/cm^2
I	Always burn, never tan (Patients with Erythrodermic psoriasis are to be classed as Type I for determination of UVA dosage.)	0.5 J/cm^2
II	Always burn, but sometimes tan	1.0 J/cm^2
III	Sometimes burn, but always tan	1.5 J/cm^2
IV	Never burn, always tan	2.0 J/cm^2
	Physician Examination	
V*	Moderately pigmented	2.5 J/cm^2
VI*	Blacks	3.0 J/cm^2

[*Patients with natural pigmentation of these types should be classified into a lower skin type category if the sunburning history so indicates.]

B. CLEARING PHASE: Specific recommendations for patient treatment are as follows:

1. SKIN TYPES I, II & III: Patients with skin types I, II and III may be treated 2 or 3 times per week. UVA exposure may be held constant or increased by up to 1.0

Continued on next page

8-MOP—Cont.

Joule/cm² at each treatment, according to the patient's response. If erythema occurs, however, do not increase exposure time until erythema resolves. The severity and extent of the patient's erythema may be used to determine whether the next exposure should be shortened, omitted, or maintained at the previous dosage. See Adverse Reactions section for additional information.

2. SKIN TYPES IV, V & VI: Patients with skin types IV, V and VI may be treated 2 or 3 times per week. UVA exposure may be held constant or increased by up to 1.5 Joules/cm² at each treatment unless erythema occurs. If erythema occurs, follow instructions outlined above in the procedures for patients with skin types I, II and III.

3. ERYTHRODERMIC PSORIASIS: Patients with erythrodermic psoriasis should be treated with special attention because pre-existing erythema may obscure observations of possible treatment-related phototoxic erythema. These patients may be treated 2 or 3 times per week, as a Type I patient.

4. MISCELLANEOUS SITUATIONS:

a. If there is no response after a total of 10 treatments, the exposure of UVA energy may be increased by an additional 0.5–1.0 Joules/cm² above the prior incremental increases for each treatment. (Example: a patient whose exposure dosage is being increased by 1.0 Joule/cm² may now have all subsequent doses increased by 1.5–2.0 Joules/cm².)

b. If there is no response, or only minimal response, after 15 treatments, the dosage of methoxsalen may be increased by 10 mg. (a one-time increase in dosage). This increased dosage may be continued for the remainder of the course of treatment but should not be exceeded.

c. If a patient misses a treatment, the UVA exposure time of the next treatment should not be increased. If more than one treatment is missed, reduce the exposure by 0.5 Joule/cm² for each treatment missed.

d. If the lower extremities are not responding as well as the rest of the body and do not show erythema, cover all other body area and give 25 percent of the present exposure dose as an additional exposure to the lower extremities. This additional exposure to the lower extremities should be terminated if erythema develops on these areas.

e. Non-responsive psoriasis: If a patient's generalized psoriasis is not responding, or if the condition appears to be worsening during treatment, the possibility of a generalized phototoxic reaction should be considered. This may be confirmed by the improvement of the condition following temporary discontinuance of this therapy for two weeks. If no improvement occurs during the interruption of treatment, this patient may be considered a treatment failure.

C. ALTERNATIVE EXPOSURE SCHEDULE:

As an alternative to increasing the UVA exposure at each treatment, the following schedule may be followed; this schedule may reduce the total number of Joules/cm² received by the patient over the entire course of therapy.

1. Incremental increases in UVA exposure for all patients may range from 0.5 to 1.5 Joules/cm² according to the patient's response to therapy.

2. Once Grade 2 clearing (see Table 2) has been reached and the patient is progressing adequately, UVA dosage is held constant. This dosage is maintained until Grade 4 clearing is reached.

3. If the rate of clearing significantly decreases, exposure dosage may be increased at each treatment (0.1–1.5 Joules/cm²) until Grade 3 clearing and a satisfactory progress rate is attained. The UVA exposure will be held constant again until Grade 4 clearing is attained. These increases may be used also if the rate of clearing significantly decreases between Grade 3 and Grade 4 response. However, the possibility of a phototoxic reaction should be considered; see Non-responsive Psoriasis, above.

4. In summary, this schedule raises slightly the increments (Joules/cm²) of UVA dosage, but limits these increases to those periods when the patient is not responding adequately. Otherwise, the UVA exposure is held at the lowest effective dose.

D. MAINTENANCE PHASE:

The goal of maintenance treatment is to keep the patient as symptom-free as possible with the least amount of UVA exposure.

1. SCHEDULE OF EXPOSURES: When patients have achieved 95 percent clearing, or Grade 4 response (Table 2), they may be placed on the following maintenance schedules (M_1–M_4), in sequence. It is recommended that each maintenance schedule be adhered to for at least 2 treatments (unless erythema or psoriatic flare occurs, in which case see (2a) and (2b) below).

Maintenance Schedules

M_1 – once/week
M_2 – once/2 weeks
M_3 – once/3 weeks
M_4 – p.r.n. (i.e., for flares)

2. LENGTH OF EXPOSURE: The UVA exposure for the first maintenance treatment of any schedule (except M_4 as noted below) is the same as that of the patient's last treatment under the previous schedule. For skin types I–IV, however, it is recommended that the maximum UVA dosage during maintenance treatments not exceed the following:

Skin Types	Joules/cm²/treatment
I	12
II	14
III	18
IV	22

If the patient develops erythema or new lesions of psoriasis, proceed as follows:

a. Erythema: During maintenance therapy, the patient's tan and threshold dose for erythema may gradually decrease. If maintenance treatments produce significant erythema, the exposure to UVA should be decreased by 25 percent until further treatments no longer produce erythema.

b. Psoriasis: If the patient develops new areas of psoriasis during maintenance therapy (but still is classified as having a Grade 4 response), the exposure to UVA may be increased by 0.5–1.5 Joules/cm² at each treatment; this is appropriate for all types of patients. These increases are continued until the psoriasis is brought under control and the patient is again clear. The exposure being administered when this clearing is reached should be used for further maintenance treatment.

3. FLARES DURING MAINTENANCE: If the patient flares during maintenance treatment (i.e., develops psoriasis on more than 5 percent of the originally involved areas of the body) his maintenance treatment schedule may be changed to the preceding maintenance or clearing schedule. The patient may be kept on his schedule until again 95 percent clear. If the original maintenance treatment schedule is unable to control the psoriasis, the schedule may be changed to a more frequent regimen. If a flare occurs less than 6 weeks after the last treatment, 25 percent of the maximum exposure received during the clearing phase, may be used and then proceed with the clearing schedule previously followed for this patient. (At 95 percent clearing follow regular maintenance until the optimum maintenance schedule is determined for the patient.) If more than 6 weeks have elapsed since the last treatment was given, treat patients as if they were beginning therapy insofar as exposure dosages are concerned, since their threshold for erythema may have decreased.

Table 1. Grades of Erythema

Grade	Erythema Level
0	No erythema
1	Minimally perceptible erythema—faint pink
2	Marked erythema but with no edema
3	Fiery erythema with edema
4	Fiery erythema with edema and blistering

Table 2. Response to Therapy

Grade	Criteria	Percent Improvement (compared to original extent of (disease)
-1	Psoriasis worse	0
0	No change	0
1	Minimal improvement—slightly less scale and/or erythema	5–20
2	Definite improvement—partial flattening of all plaques—less scaling and less erythema	20–50
3	Considerable improvement—nearly complete flattening of all plaques but borders of plaques still palpable	50–95
4	Clearing; complete flattening of plaques including borders; plaques may be outlined by pigmentation	95

XII. HOW SUPPLIED

8-MOP Capsules, each containing 10 mg of methoxsalen (8-methoxypsoralen) are available in pink-colored hard gelatin capsules in amber glass bottles of 50 (NDC 0187-0651-42), with ICN imprinted on the cap of the capsule and 600 imprinted on the body of the capsule.

Store at 25°C (77°F); excursions permitted to 15°C–30°C (59°F–86°F).

BIBLIOGRAPHY

1. Pathak, M.A., Kramer, D.M., Fitzpatrick, T.B.: Photobiology and Photochemistry of Furocoumarins (Psoralens), SUNLIGHT AND MAN: Normal and Abnormal Photobiologic Responses. Edited by M.A. Pathak, L.C. Harbor, M. Seiji et al. University of Tokyo Press. 1974, pp. 335–368.
2. Artuc, M., Stuettgen, G., Schalla, W., Schaefer, H., and Gazith, J.: Reversible binding of 5- and 8-methoxypsoralen to human serum proteins (albumin) and to epidermis in vitro; Brit. J. Dermat. 101, pp. 669–677 (1979).
3. Mandula, B.B., Pathak, M.A., Nakayama, Y., and Davidson, S.J.: Induction of mixed-function oxidases in mouse liver by psoralens., Ibid, 99, pp. 687–692 (1978).
4. Pathak, M.A., Fitzpatrick, T.B., Parrish, J.A.: PSORIASIS, Proceedings of the Second International Symposium. Edited by E.M. Farber, A.J. Cox, Yorke Medical Books, pp. 262–265 (1977).
5. Dall'Acqua, F., Marciani, S., Ciavatta, L, Rodighiero, G.: Formation of interstrand cross-linkings in the photoreactions between furocoumarins and DNA; Z Naturforsch (B), 26, pp. 561–569 (1971).
6. Cole, R.S.: Light-induced cross-linkings of DNA in the presence of a furocoumarin (psoralen), Biochem. Biophys. Acta, 217, pp. 30–39 (1970).
7. Musajo, L., Rodighiero, G., Caporale, G., Dall'Acqua, F., Marciani, S., Bordin, F., Baccichetti, F., Bevilacqua, R.: Photoreactions between Skin-Photosensitizing Furocoumarins and Nucleic Acids, SUNLIGHT AND MAN; Normal and Abnormal Photobiologic Responses. Edited by M.A. Pathak, L.C. Harber, M. Seiji et al. University of Tokyo Press, pp. 369–387 (1974).
8. Dall'Acqua, F., Vedaldi, D., Bordin, F., and Rodighiero, G.: New studies in the interaction between 8-methoxypsoralen and DNA in vitro, J. Investigative Dermat., 73, pp. 191–197 (1979).
9. Yoshikawa, K., Mori, N., Sakakibara, S., Mizuno, N., Song, P.: Photo-Conjugation of 8-methoxypsoralen with Proteins; Photochem & Photobiol., 29, pp. 1127–1133 (1979).
10. Ortonne, J. P., MacDonald, D.M., Micoud, A., Thivolet, J.: PUVA-induced repigmentation of vitiligo: a histochemical (split-DOPA) and ultra-structural study: Brit. J. of Dermat., 101, pp. 1–12 (1979).
11. Hakim, R.E., Griffin, A.C., Knox, J.M.: Erythema and tumor formation in methoxsalen treated mice exposed to fluorescent light; Arch. Dermatol. 82, pp. 572–577 (1960).
12. Pathak, M.A., Daniels, F., Hopkins, C.E., Fitzpatrick, T.B.: Ultraviolet carcinogenesis in albino and pigmented mice receiving furocoumarins: psoralens and 8-methoxypsoralen, Nature 183, pp. 728–730 (1959).
13. Stern, R.S., Thibodeau, L.A., Kleinerman, R.A., Parrish, J.A., Fitzpatrick, T.B., and 22 Participating Investigators: Risk of Cutaneous Carcinoma in Patients Treated with Oral Methoxsalen Photochemotherapy for Psoriasis: NEJM 300. No. 15, pp. 809–813 (1979).
14. Stern, R.S., Parrish, J.A., Zierler, S.: Skin Carcinoma in Patients with Psoriasis Treated with Topical Tar and Artificial Ultraviolet Radiation. Lancet, 1, pp. 732–735 (1980).
15. Roenigk, Jr., H.H., and 12 Cooperating Investigators: Skin Cancer in the PUVA-48 Cooperative Study of Psoriasis. Program for Forty-First Annual Meeting for The Society of Investigative Dermatology, Inc., Sheraton Washington Hotel, Washington, D.C., May 12, 13, and 14, 1980. Abstracts JID, 74, No. 4, p. 250 (April, 1980).
16. Stern et al., Malignant melanoma in patients treated for psoriasis with methoxsalen (psoralen) and ultraviolet A radiation (PUVA). The PUVA Follow-up Study. New England Journal of Medicine, 336:1041–1045, (April 10, 1997).
17. Mosher, D.B., Pathak, M.A., Harris, T.J., Fitzpatrick, T.B.: Development of Cutaneous Lesions in Vitiligo During Long-Term PUVA Therapy. Program for Forty-First Annual Meeting for The Society for Investigative Dermatology, Inc., Sheraton Washington Hotel, Washington, D.C., May 12, 13, and 14, 1980. Abstracts JID, 74, No. 4, p. 259 (April, 1980).
18. Cloud, T.M., Hakim, R., Griffin, A.C.: Photosensitization of the eye with methoxsalen. I. Acute effects; Arch. Ophthalmol. 64, pp. 346–352 (1960).
19. Cloud, T.M., Hakim, R., Griffin, A.C.: Photosensitization of the eye with methoxsalen. II. Chronic effects, Ibid, 66, pp. 689–694 (1961).
20. Freeman, R.G., Troll, D.: Photosensitization of the eye by 8-methoxypsoralen, JID, 53, pp. 449–453 (1969).
21. Lerman, S., Megaw, J., Willis, I.: Potential ocular complications from PUVA therapy and their prevention; J. Invest. Dermtat., 74, pp. 197–199 (1980).

Valeant Pharmaceuticals International
3300 Hyland Ave.
Costa Mesa, CA 92626

2579-02 EL Rev. 4-03

ANCOBON® ℞

[an 'co-bon]
(flucytosine)
CAPSULES

WARNING

Use with extreme caution in patients with impaired renal function. Close monitoring of hematologic, renal and hepatic status of all patients is essential. These instructions should be thoroughly reviewed before administration of Ancobon.

DESCRIPTION

Ancobon (flucytosine), an antifungal agent, is available as 250-mg and 500-mg capsules for oral administration. Each capsule also contains corn starch, lactose and talc. Gelatin capsule shells contain parabens (butyl, methyl, propyl) and sodium propionate, with the following dye systems: 250-mg capsules — black iron oxide, FD&C Blue No. 1, FD&C Yellow No. 6, D&C Yellow No. 10 and titanium dioxide; 500-mg capsules — black iron oxide and titanium dioxide. Chemically, flucytosine is 5-fluorocytosine, a fluorinated pyrimidine which is related to fluorouracil and floxuridine. It is a white to off-white crystalline powder with a molecular weight of 129.09 and the following structural formula:

H
N O
F N
NH2

CLINICAL PHARMACOLOGY

Flucytosine is rapidly and virtually completely absorbed following oral administration. Bioavailability estimated by comparing the area under the curve of serum concentrations after oral and intravenous administration showed 78% to 89% absorption of the oral dose. Peak blood concentrations of 30 to 40 µg/mL were reached within 2 hours of administration of a 2-gm oral dose to normal subjects. The mean blood concentrations were approximately 70 to 80 µg/mL 1 to 2 hours after a dose in patients with normal renal function who received a 6-week regimen of flucytosine (150 mg/kg/day given in divided doses every 6 hours) in combination with amphotericin B. The half-life in the majority of normal subjects ranged between 2.4 and 4.8 hours. Flucytosine is excreted via the kidneys by means of glomerular filtration without significant tubular reabsorption. More than 90% of the total radioactivity after oral administration was recovered in the urine as intact drug. Flucytosine is deaminated (probably by gut bacteria) to 5-fluorouracil. The area under the curve (AUC) ratio of 5-fluorouracil to flucytosine is 4%. Approximately 1% of the dose is present in the urine as the α-fluoro-β-ureido-propionic acid metabolite. A small portion of the dose is excreted in the feces.

The half-life of flucytosine is prolonged in patients with renal insufficiency; the average half-life in nephrectomized or anuric patients was 85 hours (range: 29.9 to 250 hours). A linear correlation was found between the elimination rate constant of flucytosine and creatinine clearance.

In vitro studies have shown that 2.9% to 4% of flucytosine is protein-bound over the range of therapeutic concentrations found in the blood. Flucytosine readily penetrates the blood-brain barrier, achieving clinically significant concentrations in cerebrospinal fluid. Studies in pregnant rats have shown that flucytosine injected intraperitoneally crosses the placental barrier (see PRECAUTIONS).

Pharmacokinetics in Pediatric Patients: Limited data are available regarding the pharmacokinetics of Ancobon administered to neonatal patients being treated for systemic candidiasis. After five days of continuous therapy, median peak levels in infants were 19.6 µg/mL, 27.7 µg/mL, and 83.9 µg/mL at doses of 25 mg/kg (N=3), 50 mg/kg (N=4), and 100 mg/kg (N=3), respectively. Mean time to peak serum levels was of 2.5 ± 1.3 hours, similar to that observed in adult patients. A good deal of interindividual variability was noted, which did not correlate with gestational age. Some patients had serum levels > 100 µg/mL, suggesting a need for drug level monitoring during therapy. In another study, serum concentrations were determined during flucytosine therapy in two patients (total assays performed = 10). Median serum flucytosine concentrations at steady state were calculated to be 57 ± 10 µg/mL (doses of 50 to 125 mg/kg/day, normalized to 25 mg/kg per dose for comparison). In three infants receiving flucytosine 25 mg/kg/day (four divided doses), a median flucytosine half-life of 7.4 hours was observed, approximately double that seen in adult patients. The concentration of flucytosine in the cerebrospinal fluid of one infant was 43 µg/mL 3 hours after a 25 mg oral dose, and ranged from 20 to 67 mg/L in another neonate receiving oral doses of 120 to 150 mg/kg/day.

Microbiology: Flucytosine has *in vitro* and *in vivo* activity against Candida and Cryptococcus. Although the exact mode of action is unknown, it has been proposed that flucytosine acts directly on fungal organisms by competitive inhibition of purine and pyrimidine uptake and indirectly by intracellular metabolism to 5-fluorouracil. Flucytosine enters the fungal cell via cytosine permease; thus, flucytosine is metabolized to 5-fluorouracil within fungal organisms. The 5-fluorouracil is extensively incorporated into fungal RNA and inhibits synthesis of both DNA and RNA. The result is unbalanced growth and death of the fungal organism. Antifungal synergism between Ancobon and polyene antibiotics, particularly amphotericin B, has been reported.

Actions: Flucytosine has *in vitro* and *in vivo* activity against Candida and Cryptococcus. The exact mode of action against these fungi is not known. Ancobon is not metabolized significantly when given orally to man.

Susceptibility: *Cryptococcus:* Most strains initially isolated from clinical material have shown flucytosine minimal inhibitory concentrations (MIC's) ranging from .46 to 7.8 µg/mL. Any isolate with an MIC greater than 12.5 µg/mL is considered resistant. *In vitro* resistance has developed in originally susceptible strains during therapy. It is recommended that clinical cultures for susceptibility testing be taken initially and at weekly intervals during therapy. The initial culture should be reserved as a reference in susceptibility testing of subsequent isolates.

Candida: As high as 40% to 50% of the pretreatment clinical isolates of Candida have been reported to be resistant to flucytosine. It is recommended that susceptibility studies be performed as early as possible and be repeated during therapy. An MIC value greater than 100 µg/mL is considered resistant.

Interference with *in vitro* activity of flucytosine occurs in complex or semisynthetic media. In order to rely upon the recommended *in vitro* interpretations of susceptibility, it is essential that the broth medium and the testing procedure used be that described by Shadomy.[1]

INDICATIONS AND USAGE

Ancobon is indicated only in the treatment of serious infections caused by susceptible strains of Candida and/or Cryptococcus.

Candida: Septicemia, endocarditis and urinary system infections have been effectively treated with flucytosine. Limited trials in pulmonary infections justify the use of flucytosine.

Cryptococcus: Meningitis and pulmonary infections have been treated effectively. Studies in septicemias and urinary tract infections are limited, but good responses have been reported.

With the exception of urinary tract infection, Ancobon should be used in combination with amphotericin B for the treatment of systemic candidiasis and cryptococcosis because of rapid emergence of resistance to Ancobon in Candida and Cryptococcus isolates in patients receiving Ancobon alone.

CONTRAINDICATIONS

Ancobon should not be used in patients with a known hypersensitivity to the drug.

WARNINGS

Ancobon must be given with extreme caution to patients with impaired renal function. Since Ancobon is excreted primarily by the kidneys, renal impairment may lead to accumulation of the drug. Ancobon blood concentrations should be monitored to determine the adequacy of renal excretion in such patients.[1] Dosage adjustments should be made in patients with renal insufficiency to prevent progressive accumulation of active drug.

Ancobon must be given with extreme caution to patients with bone marrow depression. Patients may be more prone to depression of bone marrow function if they: 1) have a hematologic disease, 2) are being treated with radiation or drugs which depress bone marrow, or 3) have a history of treatment with such drugs or radiation. Bone marrow toxicity can be irreversible and may lead to death in immunosuppressed patients. Frequent monitoring of hepatic function and of the hematopoietic system is indicated during therapy.

PRECAUTIONS

General: Before therapy with Ancobon is instituted, electrolytes (because of hypokalemia) and the hematologic and renal status of the patient should be determined (see WARNINGS). Close monitoring of the patient during therapy is essential.

Laboratory Tests: Since renal impairment can cause progressive accumulation of the drug, blood concentrations and kidney function should be monitored during therapy. Hematologic status (leucocyte and thrombocyte count) and liver function (alkaline phosphatase, SGOT and SGPT) should be determined at frequent intervals during treatment as indicated.

Drug Interactions: Cytosine arabinoside, a cytostatic agent, has been reported to inactivate the antifungal activity of Ancobon by competitive inhibition. Drugs which impair glomerular filtration may prolong the biological half-life of flucytosine.

Drug/Laboratory Test Interactions: Measurement of serum creatinine levels should be determined by the Jaffé reaction, since Ancobon does not interfere with the determination of creatinine values by this method. Most automated equipment for measurement of creatinine makes use of the Jaffé reaction.

Carcinogenesis, Mutagenesis, Impairment of Fertility: Flucytosine has not undergone adequate animal testing to evaluate carcinogenic potential. The mutagenic potential of flucytosine was evaluated in Ames-type studies with five different mutants of *S. typhimurium* and no mutagenicity was detected in the presence or absence of activating enzymes. Flucytosine was nonmutagenic in three different repair assay systems (i.e., rec, uvr and pol).

There have been no adequate trials in animals on the effects of flucytosine on fertility or reproductive performance. The fertility and reproductive performance of the offspring (F_1 generation) of mice treated with 100 mg/kg/day (345 mg/M^2/day or 0.059 times the human dose), 200 mg/kg/day (690 mg/M^2/day or 0.118 times the human dose) or 400 mg/kg/day (1380 mg/M^2/day or 0.236 times the human dose) of flucytosine on days 7 to 13 of gestation was studied; the *in utero* treatment had no adverse effect on the fertility or reproductive performance of the offspring.

Pregnancy: Teratogenic Effects. Pregnancy Category C. Flucytosine was shown to be teratogenic (vertebral fusions) in the rat at doses of 40 mg/kg/day (298 mg/M^2/day or 0.051 times the human dose) administered on days 7 to 13 of gestation. At higher doses (700 mg/kg/day; 5208 mg/M^2/day or 0.89 times the human dose administered on days 9 to 12 of gestation), cleft lip and palate and micrognathia were reported. Flucytosine was not teratogenic in rabbits up to a dose of 100 mg/kg/day (1423 mg/M^2/day or 0.243 times the human dose) administered on days 6 to 18 of gestation. In mice, 400 mg/kg/day of flucytosine (1380 mg/M^2/day or 0.236 times the human dose) administered on days 7 to 13 of gestation was associated with a low incidence of cleft palate that was not statistically significant. There are no adequate and well-controlled studies in pregnant women. Ancobon should be used during pregnancy only if the potential benefit justifies the potential risk to the fetus.

Nursing Mothers: It is not known whether this drug is excreted in human milk. Because many drugs are excreted in human milk and because of the potential for serious adverse reactions in nursing infants from Ancobon, a decision should be made whether to discontinue nursing or to discontinue the drug, taking into account the importance of the drug to the mother.

Pediatric Use: The efficacy and safety of Ancobon have not been systematically studied in pediatric patients. A small number of neonates have been treated with 25 to 200 mg/kg/day of flucytosine, with and without the addition of amphotericin B, for systemic candidiasis. No unexpected adverse reactions were reported in these patients. It should be noted, however, that hypokalemia and acidemia were reported in one patient who received flucytosine in combination with amphotericin B, and anemia was observed in a second patient who received flucytosine alone. Transient thrombocytopenia was noted in two additional patients, one of whom also received amphotericin B.

ADVERSE REACTIONS

The adverse reactions which have occurred during treatment with Ancobon are grouped according to organ system affected.

Cardiovascular: Cardiac arrest, myocardial toxicity, ventricular dysfunction.

Respiratory: Respiratory arrest, chest pain, dyspnea.

Dermatologic: Rash, pruritus, urticaria, photosensitivity.

Gastrointestinal: Nausea, emesis, abdominal pain, diarrhea, anorexia, dry mouth, duodenal ulcer, gastrointestinal hemorrhage, acute hepatic injury with possible fatal outcome in debilitated patients, hepatic dysfunction, jaundice, ulcerative colitis, bilirubin elevation, increased hepatic enzymes.

Genitourinary: Azotemia, creatinine and BUN elevation, crystalluria, renal failure.

Hematologic: Anemia, agranulocytosis, aplastic anemia, eosinophilia, leukopenia, pancytopenia, thrombocytopenia.

Neurologic: Ataxia, hearing loss, headache, paresthesia, parkinsonism, peripheral neuropathy, pyrexia, vertigo, sedation, convulsions.

Psychiatric: Confusion, hallucinations, psychosis.

Miscellaneous: Fatigue, hypoglycemia, hypokalemia, weakness, allergic reactions, Lyell's syndrome.

OVERDOSAGE

There is no experience with intentional overdosage. It is reasonable to expect that overdosage may produce pronounced manifestations of the known clinical adverse reactions. Prolonged serum concentrations in excess of 100 µg/mL may be associated with an increased incidence of toxicity, especially gastrointestinal (diarrhea, nausea, vomiting), hematologic (leukopenia, thrombocytopenia) and hepatic (hepatitis).

In the management of overdosage, prompt gastric lavage or the use of an emetic is recommended. Adequate fluid intake should be maintained, by the intravenous route if necessary, since Ancobon is excreted unchanged via the renal tract. The hematologic parameters should be monitored frequently; liver and kidney function should be carefully monitored. Should any abnormalities appear in any of these parameters, appropriate therapeutic measures should be instituted.

Since hemodialysis has been shown to rapidly reduce serum concentrations in anuric patients, this method may be considered in the management of overdosage.

DOSAGE AND ADMINISTRATION

The usual dosage of Ancobon is 50 to 150 mg/kg/day administered in divided doses at 6-hour intervals. Nausea or vomiting may be reduced or avoided if the capsules are given a few at a time over a 15-minute period. If the BUN or the serum creatinine is elevated, or if there are other signs of renal impairment, the initial dose should be at the lower level (see WARNINGS).

HOW SUPPLIED

Capsules, 250 mg (gray and green), imprinted ANCOBON® 250 ICN, bottles of 100 (NDC 0187-3554-10). *Capsules,* 500 mg (gray and white), imprinted ANCOBON® 500 ICN, bottles of 100 (NDC 0187-3555-10).

Store at 25°C (77°F); excursions permitted to 15°C-30°C (59°F-86°F).

REFERENCE

1. Shadomy S. *Appl Microbiol.* June 1969, 17:871-877.

Valeant Pharmaceuticals International
Costa Mesa, CA 92626
3355497EX04 Rev. June 2003

BONTRIL® PDM Ⓒ℞

[*bōn 'tril*]
(phendimetrazine tartrate tablets, USP 35 mg)

HOW SUPPLIED

Three-layered green, white and yellow tablet with 48 on the scored side and the letter "A" on the other. Bontril® PDM tablets containing 35 mg of phendimetrazine tartrate are available in bottles of 100 (NDC 65234-048-10) and 1,000 (NDC 65234-048-90).

Continued on next page

Bontril PDM—Cont.

CAUTION
Rx only
See product insert for complete information.
Manufactured for Valeant Pharmaceuticals International
Shown in Product Identification Guide, page 335

BONTRIL® SLOW-RELEASE Ⓒ℞

[*bŏn 'tril*]
(brand of phendimetrazine tartrate slow–release capsules 105 mg)

HOW SUPPLIED
Bontril Slow Release Capsules (phendimetrazine tartrate 105 mg) is available as opaque green and clear yellow capsules, imprinted with the letter "A" and "047". Supplied in bottles of 100 capsules (NDC #65234-047-10) and 1000 capsules (NDC 65234-047-90).
Store at controlled room temperature, 15°–30°C (59°–86°F).
Rx only
Manufactured for Valeant Pharmaceuticals International
Shown in Product Identification Guide, page 335

CAPITAL® AND CODEINE ORAL SUSPENSION Ⓒ℞

(acetaminophen and codeine phosphate oral suspension USP)

HOW SUPPLIED
CAPITAL® AND CODEINE ORAL SUSPENSION contains 120 mg of acetaminophen and 12 mg of codeine phosphate/ 5 mL and is given orally. CAPITAL® AND CODEINE ORAL SUSPENSION is a fruit punch-flavored pink suspension available in 16 fluid oz. (473 mL) bottles, NDC 65234-046-16.
SHAKE WELL BEFORE USING
Store at controlled room temperature 15°–30°C (59°–86°F).
Dispense in tight, light-resistant glass container and label "Shake Well Before Using."
Rx only
See product insert for complete information.
Manufactured for Valeant Pharmaceuticals International
Shown in Product Identification Guide, page 335

DALMANE® Ⓒ℞

[*dăl'-măn*]
(flurazepam hydrochloride)
CAPSULES
For Relief of Insomnia

DESCRIPTION
Dalmane is available as capsules containing 15 mg or 30 mg flurazepam hydrochloride. Each 15-mg capsule also contains cornstarch, lactose, magnesium stearate and talc; gelatin capsule shells contain the following dye systems: D&C Red No. 28, FD&C Red No. 40, FD&C Yellow No. 6 and D&C Yellow No. 10. Each 30-mg capsule also contains cornstarch, lactose and magnesium stearate; gelatin capsule shells contain the following dye systems: FD&C Blue No. 1, FD&C Yellow No. 6, D&C Yellow No. 10 and either FD&C Red No. 3 or FD&C Red No. 40.
Flurazepam hydrochloride is chemically 7-chloro-1-[2-(diethylamino)ethyl]-5-(*o*-fluorophenyl)-1,3-dihydro-2*H*-1,4-benzodiazepin-2-one dihydrochloride. It is a pale yellow, crystalline compound, freely soluble in USP alcohol and very soluble in water. It has a molecular weight of 460.826 and the following structural formula:

$CH_2CH_2N(C_2H_5)_2$ · 2HCl

CLINICAL PHARMACOLOGY
Flurazepam hydrochloride is rapidly absorbed from the GI tract. Flurazepam is rapidly metabolized and is excreted primarily in the urine. Following a single oral dose, peak flurazepam plasma concentrations ranging from 0.5 to 4.0 ng/mL occur at 30 to 60 minutes post-dosing. The harmonic mean apparent half-life of flurazepam is 2.3 hours. The blood level profile of flurazepam and its major metabolites was determined in man following the oral administration of 30 mg daily for 2 weeks. The N_1-hydroxyethyl-flurazepam was measurable only during the early hours after a 30-mg dose and was not detectable after 24 hours. The major metabolite in blood was N_1-desalkyl-flurazepam, which reached steady-state (plateau) levels after 7 to 10 days of dosing, at levels approximately 5- to 6-fold greater than the 24-hour levels observed on Day 1. The half-life of elimination of N_1-desalkyl-flurazepam ranged from 47 to 100 hours. The major urinary metabolite is conjugated N_1-hydroxyethyl-flurazepam which accounts for 22% to 55% of the dose. Less than 1% of the dose is excreted in the urine as N_1-desalkyl-flurazepam.
This pharmacokinetic profile may be responsible for the clinical observation that flurazepam is increasingly effective on the second or third night of consecutive use and that for 1 or 2 nights after the drug is discontinued both sleep latency and total wake time may still be decreased.
Geriatric Pharmacokinetics: The single dose pharmacokinetics of flurazepam were studied in 12 healthy geriatric subjects (aged 61 to 85 years). The mean elimination half-life of desalkyl-flurazepam was longer in elderly male subjects (160 hours) compared with younger male subjects (74 hours), while mean elimination half-life was similar in geriatric female subjects (120 hours) and younger female subjects (90 hours). After multiple dosing, mean steady-state plasma levels of desalkyl-flurazepam were higher in elderly male subjects (81 ng/mL) compared with younger male subjects (53 ng/mL), while values were similar between elderly female subjects (85 ng/mL) and younger female subjects (86 ng/mL). The mean washout half-life of desalkyl-flurazepam was longer in elderly male and female subjects (126 and 158 hours, respectively) compared with younger male and female subjects (111 and 113 hours, respectively).[1]

INDICATIONS AND USAGE
Dalmane is a hypnotic agent useful for the treatment of insomnia characterized by difficulty in falling asleep, frequent nocturnal awakenings, and/or early morning awakening. Dalmane can be used effectively in patients with recurring insomnia or poor sleeping habits, and in acute or chronic medical situations requiring restful sleep. Sleep laboratory studies have objectively determined that Dalmane is effective for at least 28 consecutive nights of drug administration. Since insomnia is ofter transient and intermittent, short-term use is usually sufficient. Prolonged use of hypnotics is usually not indicated and should only be undertaken concomitantly with appropriate evaluation of the patient.

CONTRAINDICATIONS
Dalmane is contraindicated in patients with known hypersensitivity to the drug.
Usage in Pregnancy: Benzodiazepines may cause fetal damage when administered during pregnancy. An increased risk of congenital malformations associated with the use of diazepam and chlordiazepoxide during the first trimester of pregnancy has been suggested in several studies.
Dalmane is contraindicated in pregnant women. Symptoms of neonatal depression have been reported; a neonate whose mother received 30 mg of Dalmane nightly for insomnia during the 10 days prior to delivery appeared hypotonic and inactive during the first 4 days of life. Serum levels of N_1-desalkyl-flurazepam in the infant indicated transplacental circulation and implicate this long-acting metabolite in this case. If there is a likelihood of the patient becoming pregnant while receiving flurazepam, she should be warned of the potential risks to the fetus. Patients should be instructed to discontinue the drug prior to becoming pregnant. The possibility that a woman of childbearing potential may be pregnant at the time of institution of therapy should be considered.

WARNINGS
Patients receiving Dalmane should be cautioned about possible combined effects with alcohol and other CNS depressants. Also, caution patients that an additive effect may occur if alcoholic beverages are consumed during the day following the use of Dalmane for nighttime sedation. The potential for this interaction continues for several days following discontinuance of flurazepam, until serum levels of psychoactive metabolites have declined.
Patients should also be cautioned about engaging in hazardous occupations requiring complete mental alertness such as operating machinery or driving a motor vehicle after ingesting the drug, including potential impairment of the performance of such activities which may occur the day following ingestion of Dalmane.
Usage in Children: Clinical investigations of Dalmane have not been carried out in children. Therefore, the drug is not currently recommended for use in persons under 15 years of age.
Withdrawal symptoms of the barbiturate type have occurred after the discontinuation of benzodiazepines. (See DRUG ABUSE AND DEPENDENCE Section.)

PRECAUTIONS
Since the risk of the development of oversedation, dizziness, confusion and/or ataxia increases substantially with larger doses in elderly and debilitated patients, it is recommended that in such patients the dosage be limited to 15 mg. If Dalmane is to be combined with other drugs having known hypnotic properties or CNS-depressant effects, due consideration should be given to potential additive effects.
The usual precautions are indicated for severely depressed patients or those in whom there is any evidence of latent depression; particularly the recognition that suicidal tendencies may be present and protective measures may be necessary.
The usual precautions should be observed in patients with impaired renal or hepatic function and chronic pulmonary insufficiency.
Information for Patients: To assure the safe and effective use of benzodiazepines, patients should be informed that since benzodiazepines may produce psychological and physical dependence, it is advisable that they consult with their physician before either increasing the dose or abruptly discontinuing this drug.
Geriatric Use: Since the risk of the development of oversedation, dizziness, confusion and/or ataxia increases substantially with larger doses in elderly and debilitated patients, it is recommended that in such patients the dosage be limited to 15 mg. Staggering and falling have also been reported, particularly in geriatric patients.
Following single-dose administration of flurazepam, the elimination half-life for desalkyl-flurazepam was longer in elderly male subjects compared with younger male subjects, while values between elderly and young females were not significantly different. After multiple dosing, elimination half-life of desalkyl-flurazepam was longer in all elderly subjects compared with younger subjects, and mean steady-state serum concentrations were higher only in elderly male subjects relative to younger subjects (see CLINICAL PHARMACOLOGY: *Geriatric Pharmacokinetics*).

ADVERSE REACTIONS
Dizziness, drowsiness, light-headedness, staggering, ataxia and falling have occurred, particularly in elderly or debilitated persons. Severe sedation, lethargy, disorientation and coma, probably indicative of drug intolerance or overdosage, have been reported.
Also reported were headache, heartburn, upset stomach, nausea, vomiting, diarrhea, constipation, gastrointestinal pain, nervousness, talkativeness, apprehension, irritability, weakness, palpitations, chest pains, body and joint pains and genitourinary complaints. There have also been rare occurrences of leukopenia, granulocytopenia, sweating, flushes, difficulty in focusing, blurred vision, burning eyes, faintness, hypotension, shortness of breath, pruritus, skin rash, dry mouth, bitter taste, excessive salivation, anorexia, euphoria, depression, slurred speech, confusion, restlessness, hallucinations, and elevated SGOT, SGPT, total and direct bilirubins, and alkaline phosphatase. Paradoxical reactions, eg, excitement, stimulation and hyperactivity, have also been reported in rare instances.

DRUG ABUSE AND DEPENDENCE
Withdrawal symptoms, similar in character to those noted with barbiturates and alcohol (convulsions, tremor, abdominal and muscle cramps, vomiting and sweating), have occurred following abrupt discontinuance of benzodiazepines. The more severe withdrawal symptoms have usually been limited to those patients who had received excessive doses over an extended period of time. Generally milder withdrawal symptoms (eg, dysphoria and insomnia) have been reported following abrupt discontinuance of benzodiazepines taken continuously at therapeutic levels for several months. Consequently, after extended therapy, abrupt discontinuation should generally be avoided and a gradual dosage tapering schedule followed. Addiction-prone individuals (such as drug addicts or alcoholics) should be under careful surveillance when receiving flurazepam or other psychotropic agents because of the predisposition of such patients to habituation and dependence.

OVERDOSAGE
Manifestations of Dalmane overdosage include somnolence, confusion and coma. Respiration, pulse and blood pressure should be monitored as in all cases of drug overdosage. General supportive measures should be employed, along with immediate gastric lavage. Intravenous fluids should be administered and an adequate airway maintained. Hypotension and CNS depression may be combated by judicious use of appropriate therapeutic agents. The value of dialysis has not been determined. If excitation occurs in patients following Dalmane overdosage, barbiturates should not be used. As with the management of intentional overdosage with any drug, it should be borne in mind that multiple agents may have been ingested.
Flumazenil, a specific benzodiazepine-receptor antagonist, is indicated for the complete or partial reversal of the sedative effects of benzodiazepines and may be useful in situations when an overdose with a benzodiazepine is known or suspected. Prior to the administration of flumazenil, necessary measures should be instituted to secure airway, ventilation and intravenous access. Flumazenil is intended as an adjunct to, not as a substitute for, proper management of benzodiazepine overdose. Patients treated with flumazenil should be monitored for resedation, respiratory depression and other residual benzodiazepine effects for an appropriate period after treatement. **The prescriber should be aware of a risk of seizure in association with flumazenil treatment, particularly in long-term benzodiazepine users and in cyclic antidepressant overdose.** The complete flumazenil package insert, including CONTRAINDICATIONS, WARNINGS and PRECAUTIONS, should be consulted prior to use.

DOSAGE AND ADMINISTRATION
Dosage should be individualized for maximal beneficial effects. The usual adult dosage is 30 mg before retiring. In some patients, 15 mg may suffice. In elderly and/or debilitated patients, 15 mg is usually sufficient for a therapeutic response and it is therefore recommended that therapy be initiated with this dosage.

HOW SUPPLIED
Dalmane (flurazepam hydrochloride) Capsules are available in the following presentations:

15 mg hard gelatin capsules in bottles of 100 (NDC 0187-4051-10), with ICN logo imprinted on the opaque orange cap and Dalmane® 15 imprinted on the opaque ivory body.
30 mg hard gelatin capsules in bottles of 100 (NDC 0187-4052-10), with ICN logo imprinted on the opaque red cap and Dalmane® 30 imprinted on the opaque ivory body.
Store at 25°C (77°F); excursions permitted to 15°C–30°C (59°F–86°F).
[See USP Controlled Room Temperature]

REFERENCE

1. Greenblatt DJ, Divoll M, Harmatz JS, MacLauglin DS, Shader RI: Kinetics and clinical effects of flurazepam in young and elderly noninsomniacs. *Clin Pharmacol Ther* 30: 475–486, 1981.

Valeant Pharmaceuticals International
3300 Hyland Avenue
Costa Mesa, California 92626
714-545-0100
3405197EX04 Rev. March 2002

EFUDEX® ℞
[ef′u-dex]
(fluorouracil)
TOPICAL SOLUTIONS AND CREAM
For Topical Dermatological Use Only
Not for Ophthalmic Use or Application to Mucous Membranes, including Intravaginal Application

DESCRIPTION

Efudex Solutions and Cream are topical preparations containing the fluorinated pyrimidine 5-fluorouracil, an antineoplastic antimetabolite.
Efudex Solution consists of 2% or 5% fluorouracil on a weight/weight basis, compounded with propylene glycol, tris (hydroxymethyl) aminomethane, hydroxypropyl cellulose, parabens (methyl and propyl) and disodium edetate.
Efudex Cream contains 5% fluorouracil in a vanishing cream base consisting of white petrolatum, stearyl alcohol, propylene glycol, polysorbate 60 and parabens (methyl and propyl).
Chemically, fluorouracil is 5-fluoro-2,4(1*H*,3*H*)-pyrimidinedione. It is a white to practically white, crystalline powder which is sparingly soluble in water and slightly soluble in alcohol. One gram of fluorouracil is soluble in 100 mL of propylene glycol. The molecular weight of 5-fluorouracil is 130.08 and the structural formula is:

CLINICAL PHARMACOLOGY

There is evidence that the metabolism of fluorouracil in the anabolic pathway blocks the methylation reaction of deoxyuridylic acid to thymidylic acid. In this manner fluorouracil interferes with the synthesis of deoxyribonucleic acid (DNA) and to a lesser extent inhibits the formation of ribonucleic acid (RNA). Since DNA and RNA are essential for cell division and growth, the effect of fluorouracil may be to create a thymine deficiency which provokes unbalanced growth and death of the cell. The effects of DNA and RNA deprivation are most marked on those cells which grow more rapidly and take up fluorouracil at a more rapid rate. The catabolic metabolism of fluorouracil results in degradation products (eg, CO_2, urea, α-fluoro-β-alanine) which are inactive.
Systemic absorption studies of topically applied fluorouracil have been performed on patients with actinic keratoses using tracer amounts of ^{14}C-labeled fluorouracil added to a 5% preparation. All patients had been receiving nonlabeled fluorouracil until the peak of the inflammatory reaction occurred (2 to 3 weeks), ensuring that the time of maximum absorption was used for measurement. One gram of labeled preparation was applied to the entire face and neck and left in place for 12 hours. Urine samples were collected. At the end of 3 days, the total recovery ranged between 0.48% and 0.94% with an average of 0.76%, indicating that approximately 5.98% of the topical dose was absorbed systemically. If applied twice daily, this would indicate systemic absorption of topical fluorouracil to be in the range of 5 to 6 mg per daily dose of 100 mg. In an additional study, negligible amounts of labeled material were found in plasma, urine and expired CO_2 after 3 days of treatment with topically applied ^{14}C-labeled fluorouracil.

INDICATIONS AND USAGE

Efudex is recommended for the topical treatment of multiple actinic or solar keratoses. In the 5% strength it is also useful in the treatment of superficial basal cell carcinomas when conventional methods are impractical, such as with multiple lesions or difficult treatment sites. Safety and efficacy in other indications have not been established.
The diagnosis should be established prior to treatment, since this method has not been proven effective in other types of basal cell carcinomas. With isolated, easily accessible basal cell carcinomas, surgery is preferred since success with such lesions is almost 100%. The success rate with Efudex Cream and Solution is approximately 93%, based on 113 lesions in 54 patients. Twenty-five lesions treated with the solution produced 1 failure and 88 lesions treated with the cream produced 7 failures.

CONTRAINDICATIONS

Efudex may cause fetal harm when administered to a pregnant woman.
There are no adequate and well-controlled studies in pregnant women with either the topical or the parenteral forms of fluorouracil. One birth defect (cleft lip and palate) has been reported in the newborn of a patient using Efudex as recommended. One birth defect (ventricular septal defect) and cases of miscarriage have been reported when Efudex was applied to mucous membrane areas. Multiple birth defects have been reported in a fetus of a patient treated with intravenous fluorouracil.
Animal reproduction studies have not been conducted with Efudex. Fluorouracil administered parenterally has been shown to be teratogenic in mice, rats, and hamsters when given at doses equivalent to the usual human intravenous dose; however, the amount of fluorouracil absorbed systemically after topical administration to actinic keratoses is minimal (see CLINICAL PHARMACOLOGY). Fluorouracil exhibited maximum teratogenicity when given to mice as single intraperitoneal injections of 10 to 40 mg/kg on Day 10 or 12 of gestation. Similarly, intraperitoneal doses of 12 to 37 mg/kg given to rats between Days 9 and 12 of gestation and intramuscular doses of 3 to 9 mg/kg given to hamsters between Days 8 and 11 of gestation were teratogenic and/or embryotoxic (ie, resulted in increased resorptions or embryolethality). In monkeys, divided doses of 40 mg/kg given between Days 20 and 24 of gestation were not teratogenic. Doses higher than 40 mg/kg resulted in abortion.
Efudex is contraindicated in women who are or may become pregnant during therapy. If this drug is used during pregnancy, or if the patient becomes pregnant while using this drug, the patient should be apprised of the potential hazard to the fetus.
Efudex is also contraindicated in patients with known hypersensitivity to any of its components.
Efudex should not be used in patients with dihydropyrimidine dehydrogenase (DPD) enzyme deficiency. A large percentage of fluorouracil is catabolized by the DPD enzyme. DPD enzyme deficiency can result in shunting of fluorouracil to the anabolic pathway, leading to cytotoxic activity and potential toxicities. Rarely, life-threatening toxicities such as stomatitis, diarrhea, neutropenia, and neurotoxicity have been reported with intravenous administration of fluorouracil in patients with DPD enzyme deficiency.
One case of life-threatening systemic toxicity has been reported with the topical use of Efudex in a patient with DPD enzyme deficiency. Symptoms included severe abdominal pain, bloody diarrhea, vomiting, fever, and chills. Physical examination revealed stomatitis, erythematous skin rash, neutropenia, thrombocytopenia, inflammation of the esophagus, stomach, and small bowel. Although this case was observed with 5% fluorouracil cream, it is unknown whether patients with profound DPD enzyme deficiency would develop systemic toxicity with lower concentrations of topically applied fluorouracil.

WARNINGS

Application to mucous membranes should be avoided due to the possibility of local inflammation and ulceration. Additionally, cases of miscarriage and a birth defect (ventricular septal defect) have been reported when Efudex was applied to mucous membrane areas during pregnancy.
Occlusion of the skin with resultant hydration has been shown to increase precutaneous penetration of several topical preparations. If any occlusive dressing is used in treatment of basal cell carcinoma, there may be an increase in the severity of inflammatory reactions in the adjacent normal skin. A porous gauze dressing may be applied for cosmetic reasons without increase in reaction.
Exposure to ultraviolet rays should be minimized during and immediately following treatment with Efudex because the intensity of the reaction may be increased.
Patients should discontinue therapy with Efudex if symptoms of DPD enzyme deficiency develop (see CONTRAINDICATIONS section).

PRECAUTIONS

General: There is a possibility of increased absorption through ulcerated or inflamed skin.
Information for Patients: Patients should be forewarned that the reaction in the treated areas may be unsightly during therapy and, usually, for several weeks following cessation of therapy. Patients should be instructed to avoid exposure to ultraviolet rays during and immediately following treatment with Efudex because the intensity of the reaction may be increased. If Efudex is applied with the fingers, the hands should be washed immediately afterward. Efudex should not be applied on the eyelids or directly into the eyes, nose or mouth because irritation may occur.
Laboratory Tests: Solar keratoses which do not respond should be biopsied to confirm the diagnosis. Follow-up biopsies should be performed as indicated in the management of superficial basal cell carcinoma.
Carcinogenesis, Mutagenesis, Impairment of Fertility: Adequate long-term studies in animals to evaluate carcinogenic potential have not been conducted with fluorouracil. Studies with the active ingredient of Efudex, 5-fluorouracil, have shown positive effects in in vitro tests for mutagenicity and on impairment of fertility.
5-Fluorouracil was positive in three in vitro cell neoplastic transformation assays. In the C3H/10T½ clone 8 mouse embryo cell system, the resulting morphologically transformed cells formed tumors when inoculated into immunosuppressed syngeneic mice.
While no evidence for mutagenic activity was observed in the Ames test (3 studies), fluorouracil has been shown to be mutagenic in the survival count rec-assay with *Bacillus subtilis* and in the Drosophilia wing-hair spot test. Fluorouracil produced petite mutations in *Saccharomyces cerevisiae* and was positive in the micronucleus test (bone marrow cells of male mice).
Fluorouracil was clastogenic in vitro (ie, chromatid gaps, breaks and exchanges) in Chinese hamster fibroblasts at concentrations of 1.0 and 2.0 μg/mL and has been shown to increase sister chromatid exchange in vitro in human lymphocytes. In addition, 5-fluorouracil has been reported to produce an increase in numerical and structural chromosome aberrations in peripheral lymphocytes of patients treated with this product.
Doses of 125 to 250 mg/kg, administered intraperitoneally, have been shown to induce chromosomal aberrations and changes in chromosome organization of spermatogonia in rats. Spermatogonial differentiation was also inhibited by fluorouracil, resulting in transient infertility. However, in studies with a strain of mouse which is sensitive to the induction of sperm head abnormalities after exposure to a range of chemical mutagens and carcinogens, fluorouracil was inactive at oral doses of 5 to 80 mg/kg/day. In female rats, fluorouracil administered intraperitoneally at doses of 25 and 50 mg/kg during the preovulatory phase of oogenesis significantly reduced the incidence of fertile matings, delayed the development of preimplantation and postimplantation embryos, increased the incidence of preimplantation lethality and induced chromosomal anomalies in these embryos. Single dose intravenous and intraperitoneal injections of 5-fluorouracil have been reported to kill differentiated spermatogonia and spermatocytes (at 500 mg/kg) and to produce abnormalities in spermatids (at 50 mg/kg) in mice.
Pregnancy: **Teratogenic Effects: Pregnancy Category X:** See CONTRAINDICATIONS section.
Nursing Mothers: It is not known whether Efudex is excreted in human milk. Because there is some systemic absorption of fluorouracil after topical administration (see CLINICAL PHARMACOLOGY), because many drugs are excreted in human milk, and because of the potential for serious adverse reactions in nursing infants, a decision should be made whether to discontinue nursing or to discontinue use of the drug, taking into account the importance of the drug to the mother.
Pediatric Use: Safety and effectiveness in children have not been established.

ADVERSE REACTIONS

The most frequent adverse reactions to Efudex occur locally and are often related to an extension of the pharmacological activity of the drug. These include burning, crusting, allergic contact dermatitis, erosions, erythema, hyperpigmentation, irritation, pain, photosensitivity, pruritus, scarring, rash, soreness and ulceration. Ulcerations, other local reactions, cases of miscarriage and a birth defect (ventricular septal defect) have been reported when Efudex was applied to mucous membrane areas. Leukocytosis is the most frequent hematological side effect.
Although a causal relationship is remote, other adverse reactions which have been reported infrequently are:
Central Nervous System: Emotional upset, insomnia, irritability.
Gastrointestinal: Medicinal taste, stomatitis.
Hematological: Eosinophilia, thrombocytopenia, toxic granulation.
Integumentary: Alopecia, blistering, bullous pemphigoid, discomfort, ichthyosis, scaling, suppuration, swelling, telangiectasia, tenderness, urticaria, skin rash.
Special Senses: Conjunctival reaction, corneal reaction, lacrimation, nasal irritation.
Miscellaneous: Herpes simplex.

OVERDOSAGE

There have been no reports of overdosage with Efudex.
The oral LD_{50} for the 5% topical cream was 234 mg/kg in rats and 39 mg/kg in dogs. These doses represented 11.7 and 1.95 mg/kg of fluorouracil, respectively. Studies with a 5% topical solution yielded an oral LD_{50} of 214 mg/kg in rats and 28.5 mg/kg in dogs, corresponding to 10.7 and 1.43 mg/kg of fluorouracil, respectively. The topical application of the 5% cream to rats yielded an LD_{50} of greater than 500 mg/kg.

DOSAGE AND ADMINISTRATION

When Efudex is applied to a lesion, a response occurs with the following sequence: erythema, usually followed by vesiculation, desquamation, erosion and reepithelialization.
Efudex should be applied preferably with a nonmetal applicator or suitable glove. If Efudex is applied with the fingers, the hands should be washed immediately afterward.
Actinic or Solar Keratosis: Apply cream or solution twice daily in an amount sufficient to cover the lesions. Medication should be continued until the inflammatory response reaches the erosion stage, at which time use of the drug should be terminated. The usual duration of therapy is from

Continued on next page

Efudex—Cont.

2 to 4 weeks. Complete healing of the lesions may not be evident for 1 to 2 months following cessation of Efudex therapy.

Superficial Basal Cell Carcinomas: **Only the 5% strength is recommended.** Apply cream or solution twice daily in an amount sufficient to cover the lesions. Treatment should be continued for at least 3 to 6 weeks. Therapy may be required for as long as 10 to 12 weeks before the lesions are obliterated. As in any neoplastic condition, the patient should be followed for a reasonable period of time to determine if a cure has been obtained.

HOW SUPPLIED

Efudex Solution is available in 10-mL drop dispensers containing either 2% (NDC 0187-3202-10) or 5% (NDC 0187-3203-10) fluorouracil on a weight/weight basis compounded with propylene glycol, tris (hydroxymethyl) aminomethane, hydroxypropyl cellulose, parabens (methyl and propyl) and disodium edetate.

Efudex Cream is available in 25-gm tubes containing 5% fluorouracil (NDC 0187-3204-26) in a vanishing cream base consisting of white petrolatum, stearyl alcohol, propylene glycol, polysorbate 60 and parabens (methyl and propyl).

Store at 25°C (77°F); excursions permitted to 15°C – 30°C (59°F–86°F).

Valeant Pharmaceuticals International
3300 Hyland Avenue
Costa Mesa, CA 92626
3360097EX01 Rev. February 2003

GLYQUIN•XM™ ℞

[glȳ-quin XM]
(Hydroquinone USP, 4%)
Skin Bleaching Moisturizing Cream
with Sunscreens (SPF 15)
℞ only
FOR EXTERNAL USE ONLY

I. DESCRIPTION

Each gram of Glyquin•XM™ contains 40 mg Hydroquinone USP, 80 mg Octocrylene USP, 40 mg Oxybenzone USP and 30 mg Avobenzone USP in a vanishing cream base of purified water USP, glycolic acid, poloxamer 407 NF, propylene glycol USP, glycerol monostearate, triethanolamine NF, polyoxyl 4 lauryl ether, lemon extract, propyl gallate NF, ascorbyl palmitate NF, vitamin E USP, methylparaben NF, edetate disodium USP, benzalkonium chloride and hyaluronic acid.

II. CLINICAL PHARMACOLOGY

Topical application of hydroquinone produces a reversible depigmentation of the skin by inhibition of the enzymatic oxidation of tyrosine to 3,4-dihydroxyphenylalanine (dopa) (Denton, C. et al., 1952)[1] and suppression of other melanocyte metabolic processes (Jimbow, K. et al., 1974)[2].

III. INDICATIONS AND USAGE

Glyquin•XM™ is indicated for the gradual bleaching of hyperpigmented skin conditions such as chloasma, melasma, freckles, senile lentigines and other unwanted areas of melanin hyperpigmentation.

IV. CONTRAINDICATIONS

Prior history of sensitivity or allergic reaction to this product or any of its ingredients. The safety of topical hydroquinone use during pregnancy or in children (12 years and under) has not been established.

V. WARNINGS

A. CAUTION: Hydroquinone is a skin bleaching agent which may produce unwanted cosmetic effects if not used as directed. The physician should be familiar with the contents of this insert before prescribing or dispensing this medication.

B. Test for skin sensitivity before using Glyquin•XM™ by applying a small amount to an unbroken patch of skin and check in 24 hours. Minor redness is not a contraindication, but where there is itching or vesicle formation or excessive inflammatory response further treatment is not advised. Close patient supervision is recommended. Contact with the eyes should be avoided. If no bleaching or lightening effect is noted after 2 months of treatment use, Glyquin•XM™ should be discontinued. Glyquin•XM™ is formulated for use as a skin bleaching agent and should not be used for the prevention of sunburn.

C. Sunscreen use is an essential aspect of hydroquinone therapy because even minimal sunlight sustains melanocytic activity. The sunscreens in Glyquin•XM™ provide the necessary sun protection during skin bleaching therapy. After clearing and during maintenance therapy, sun exposure should be avoided on bleached skin by application of a sunscreen agent or protective clothing to prevent repigmentation.

D. Keep this and all medication out of the reach of children. In case of accidental ingestion, call a physician or a poison control center immediately.

VI. PRECAUTIONS

SEE WARNINGS

A. Pregnancy Category C. Animal reproduction studies have not been conducted with topical hydroquinone. It is also not known whether hydroquinone can cause fetal harm when used topically on a pregnant woman or affect reproductive capacity. It is not known to what degree, if any, topical hydroquinone is absorbed systemically. Topical hydroquinone should be used in pregnant women only when clearly indicated.

B. Nursing mothers. It is not known whether topical hydroquinone is absorbed or excreted in human milk. Caution is advised when topical hydroquinone is used by a nursing mother.

C. Pediatric usage. Safety and effectiveness in pediatric patients below the age of 12 years have not been established.

VII. ADVERSE REACTIONS

No systemic adverse reactions have been reported. Occasional hypersensitivity (localized contact dermatitis) may occur in which case the medication should be discontinued and the physician notified immediately.

VIII. OVERDOSAGE

There have been no systemic reactions from the use of topical hydroquinone in Glyquin•XM™. However, treatment should be limited to relatively small areas of the body at one time since some patients experience a transient skin reddening and a mild burning sensation which does not preclude treatment.

IX. DOSAGE AND ADMINISTRATION

Glyquin•XM™ should be applied to the affected area and rubbed in well twice daily or as directed by a physician. There is no recommended dosage for pediatric patients under 12 years of age except under the advice and supervision of a physician.

X. HOW SUPPLIED

GLYQUIN•XM™ (Hydroquinone USP, 4%) is available as follows:

SIZE	NDC
1 ounce jar (28 grams)	0187-0421-46

Store at 25°C (77°F); excursions permitted to 15°C–30°C (59°F–86°F).

REFERENCES

1. Denton, C., A.B. Lerner and T.B. Fitzpatrick, "Inhibition of Melanin Formation by Chemical Agents," **Journal of Investigative Dermatology**, 18:119–135, 1952.
2. Jimbow, K., H. Obata, M. Pathak, and T.B. Fitzpatrick, "Mechanism of Depigmentation by Hydroquinone," **Journal of Investigative Dermatology**, 62:436–449, 1974.

VALEANT
Manufactured by:
Valeant Pharmaceuticals International
3300 Hyland Avenue, Costa Mesa, CA 92626 U.S.A.
2669-00 EL
Orig. 6-02

LIBRIUM® Ⓒ ℞

[lĭb' –rē-um]
(chlordiazepoxide HCl)
CAPSULES

DESCRIPTION

Librium, the original chlordiazepoxide HCl and prototype for the benzodiazepine compounds, was synthesized and developed at Hoffmann-La Roche Inc. It is a versatile therapeutic agent of proven value for the relief of anxiety. Librium is among the safer of the effective psychopharmacologic compounds available, as demonstrated by extensive clinical evidence.

Librium is available as capsules containing 5 mg, 10 mg or 25 mg chlordiazepoxide HCl. Each capsule also contains corn starch, lactose and talc. Gelatin capsule shells may contain methyl and propyl parabens and potassium sorbate, with the following dye systems: 5-mg capsules – FD&C Yellow No. 6 plus D&C Yellow No. 10 and either FD&C Blue No. 1 or FD&C Green No. 3. 10-mg capsules – D&C Yellow No. 10 and either FD&C Blue No. 1 plus FD&C Red No. 3 or FD&C Green No.3 plus FD&C Red No. 40. 25-mg capsules–D&C Yellow No. 10 and either FD&C Green No. 3 or FD&C Blue No. 1.

Chlordiazepoxide hydrochloride is 7-chloro-2-(methylamino)-5-phenyl-3H-1,4-benzodiazepine 4-oxide hydrochloride. A white to practically white crystalline substance, it is soluble in water. It is unstable in solution and the powder must be protected from light. The molecular weight is 336.22. The structural formula of chlordiazepoxide hydrochloride is as follows:

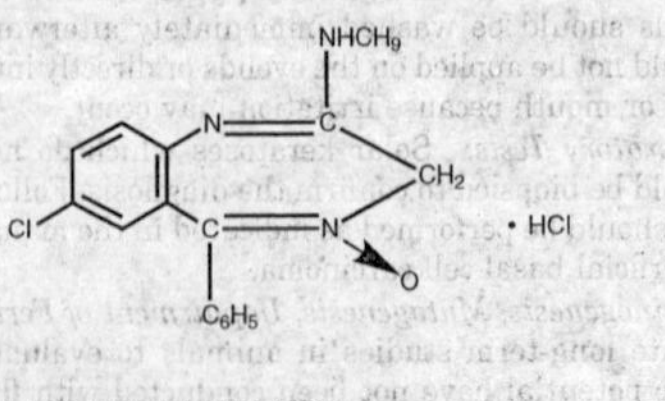

CLINICAL PHARMACOLOGY

Librium (chlordiazepoxide HCl) has antianxiety, sedative, appetite-stimulating and weak analgesic actions. The precise mechanism of action is not known. The drug blocks EEG arousal from stimulation of the brain stem reticular formation. It takes several hours for peak blood levels to be reached and the half-life of the drug is between 24 and 48 hours. After the drug is discontinued plasma levels decline slowly over a period of several days. Chlordiazepoxide is excreted in the urine, with 1% to 2% unchanged and 3% to 6% as conjugate.

Animal Pharmacology: The drug has been studied extensively in many species of animals and these studies are suggestive of action on the limbic system of the brain, which recent evidence indicates is involved in emotional responses.

Hostile monkeys were made tame by oral drug doses which did not cause sedation. Chlordiazepoxide HCl revealed a "taming" action with the elimination of fear and aggression. The taming effect of chlordiazepoxide HCl was further demonstrated in rats made vicious by lesions in the septal area of the brain. The drug dosage which effectively blocked the vicious reaction was well below the dose which caused sedation in these animals.

The LD_{50} of parenterally administered chlordiazepoxide HCl was determined in mice (72 hours) and rats (5 days), and calculated according to the method of Miller and Tainter, with the following results: mice, IV, 123±12mg/kg; mice, IM, 366±7mg/kg; rats, IV, 120±7 mg/kg; rats, IM, >160 mg/kg.

Effects on Reproduction: Reproduction studies in rats fed 10, 20 and 80 mg/kg daily and bred through one or two matings showed no congenital anomalies, nor were there adverse effects on lactation of the dams or growth of the newborn. However, in another study at 100 mg/kg daily there was noted a significant decrease in the fertilization rate and a marked decrease in the viability and body weight of offspring which may be attributable to sedative activity, thus resulting in lack of interest in mating and lessened maternal nursing and care of the young. One neonate in each of the first and second matings in the rat reproduction study at the 100 mg/kg dose exhibited major skeletal defects. Further studies are in progress to determine the significance of these findings.

INDICATIONS AND USAGE

Librium is indicated for the management of anxiety disorders or for the short term relief of symptoms of anxiety, withdrawal symptoms of acute alcoholism, and preoperative apprehension and anxiety. Anxiety or tension associated with the stress of everyday life usually does not require treatment with an anxiolytic.

The effectiveness of Librium in long-term use, that is, more than 4 months, has not been assessed by systematic clinical studies. The physician should periodically reassess the usefulness of the drug for the individual patient.

CONTRAINDICATIONS

Librium is contraindicated in patients with known hypersensitivity to the drug.

WARNINGS

Chlordiazepoxide HCl may impair the mental and/or physical abilities required for the performance of potentially hazardous tasks such as driving a vehicle or operating machinery. Similarly, it may impair mental alertness in children. The concomitant use of alcohol or other central nervous system depressants may have an additive effect. PATIENTS SHOULD BE WARNED ACCORDINGLY.

Usage in Pregnancy: An increased risk of congenital malformations associated with the use of minor tranquilizers (chlordiazepoxide, diazepam and meprobamate) during the first trimester of pregnancy has been suggested in several studies. Because use of these drugs is rarely a matter of urgency, their use during this period should almost always be avoided. The possibility that a woman of childbearing potential may be pregnant at the time of institution of therapy should be considered. Patients should be advised that if they become pregnant during therapy or intend to become pregnant they should communicate with their physicians about the desirability of discontinuing the drug.

Withdrawal symptoms of the barbiturate type have occurred after the discontinuation of benzodiazepines. (See DRUG ABUSE AND DEPENDENCE section.)

PRECAUTIONS

In elderly and debilitated patients, it is recommended that the dosage be limited to the smallest effective amount to preclude the development of ataxia or oversedation (10 mg or less per day initially, to be increased gradually as needed and tolerated). In general, the concomitant administration of Librium and other psychotropic agents is not recommended. If such combination therapy seems indicated, careful consideration should be given to the pharmacology of the agents to be employed – particularly when the known potentiating compounds such as MAO inhibitors and phenothiazines are to be used. The usual precautions in treating patients with impaired renal or hepatic function should be observed.

Paradoxical reactions, eg, excitement, stimulation and acute rage, have been reported in psychiatric patients and in hyperactive aggressive pediatric patients, and should be watched for during Librium therapy. The usual precautions are indicated when Librium is used in the treatment of anxiety states where there is any evidence of impending depression; it should be borne in mind that suicidal tendencies may be present and protective measures may be necessary.

Although clinical studies have not established a cause and effect relationship, physicians should be aware that variable effects on blood coagulation have been reported very rarely in patients receiving oral anticoagulants and Librium. In view of isolated reports associating chlordiazepoxide with exacerbation of porphyria, caution should be exercised in prescribing chlordiazepoxide to patients suffering from this disease.

Pediatric Use: Because of the varied response of pediatric patients to CNS-acting drugs, therapy should be initiated with the lowest dose and increased as required (see DOSAGE AND ADMINISTRATION). Since clinical experience with Librium in pediatric patients under 6 years of age is limited, use in this age group is not recommended. Hyperactive aggressive pediatric patients should be monitored for paradoxical reactions to Librium (see PRECAUTIONS).

Information for Patients: To assure the safe and effective use of benzodiazepines, patients should be informed that, since benzodiazepines may produce psychological and physical dependence, it is advisable that they consult with their physician before either increasing the dose or abruptly discontinuing this drug.

ADVERSE REACTIONS

The necessity of discontinuing therapy because of undesirable effects has been rare. Drowsiness, ataxia and confusion have been reported in some patients – particularly the elderly and debilitated. While these effects can be avoided in almost all instances by proper dosage adjustment, they have occasionally been observed at the lower dosage ranges. In a few instances syncope has been reported.

Other adverse reactions reported during therapy include isolated instances of skin eruptions, edema, minor menstrual irregularities, nausea and constipation, extrapyramidal symptoms, as well as increased and decreased libido. Such side effects have been infrequent, and are generally controlled with reduction of dosage. Changes in EEG patterns (low-voltage fast activity) have been observed in patients during and after Librium treatment.

Blood dyscrasias (including agranulocytosis), jaundice and hepatic dysfunction have occasionally been reported during therapy. When Librium treatment is protracted, periodic blood counts and liver function tests are advisable.

DRUG ABUSE AND DEPENDENCE

Chlordiazepoxide hydrochloride capsules are classified by the Drug Enforcement Administration as a Schedule IV controlled substance.

Withdrawal symptoms, similar in character to those noted with barbiturates and alcohol (convulsions, tremor, abdominal and muscle cramps, vomiting and sweating), have occurred following abrupt discontinuance of chlordiazepoxide. The more severe withdrawal symptoms have usually been limited to those patients who had received excessive doses over an extended period of time. Generally milder withdrawal symptoms (eg, dysphoria and insomnia) have been reported following abrupt discontinuance of benzodiazepines taken continuously at therapeutic levels for several months. Consequently, after extended therapy, abrupt discontinuation should generally be avoided and a gradual dosage tapering schedule followed. Addiction-prone individuals (such as drug addicts or alcoholics) should be under careful surveillance when receiving chlordiazepoxide or other psychotropic agents because of the predisposition of such patients to habituation and dependence.

OVERDOSAGE

Manifestations of Librium overdosage include somnolence, confusion, coma and diminished reflexes. Respiration, pulse and blood pressure should be monitored, as in all cases of drug overdosage, although, in general, these effects have been minimal following Librium overdosage. General supportive measures should be employed, along with immediate gastric lavage. Intravenous fluids should be administered and an adequate airway maintained. Hypotension may be combated by the use of Levophed® (norepinephrine) or Aramine (metaraminol). Dialysis is of limited value. There have been occasional reports of excitation in patients following chlordiazepoxide HCl overdosage; if this occurs barbiturates should not be used. As with the management of intentional overdosage with any drug, it should be borne in mind that multiple agents may have been ingested.

Flumazenil, a specific benzodiazepine-receptor antagonist, is indicated for the complete or partial reversal of the sedative effects of benzodiazepines and may be used in situations when an overdose with a benzodiazepine is known or suspected. Prior to the administration of flumazenil, necessary measures should be instituted to secure airway, ventilation and intravenous access. Flumazenil is intended as an adjunct to, not as a substitute for, proper management of benzodiazepine overdose. Patients treated with flumazenil should be monitored for resedation, respiratory depression and other residual benzodiazepine effects for an appropriate period after treatment. **The prescriber should be aware of a risk of seizure in association with flumazenil treatment, particularly in long-term benzodiazepine users and in cyclic antidepressant overdose.** The complete flumazenil package insert, including CONTRAINDICATIONS, WARNINGS and PRECAUTIONS, should be consulted prior to use.

DOSAGE AND ADMINISTRATION

Because of the wide range of clinical indications for Librium, the optimum dosage varies with the diagnosis and response of the individual patient. The dosage, therefore, should be individualized for maximum beneficial effects.

ADULTS	*USUAL DAILY DOSE*
Relief of Mild and Moderate Anxiety Disorders and Symptoms of Anxiety	5 mg or 10 mg, 3 or 4 times daily
Relief of Severe Anxiety Disorders and Symptoms of Anxiety	20 mg or 25 mg, 3 or 4 times daily
Geriatric Patients, or in the presence of debilitating disease.	5 mg, 2 to 4 times daily

Preoperative Apprehension and Anxiety: On days preceding surgery, 5 to 10 mg orally, 3 or 4 times daily. If used as preoperative medication, 50 to 100 mg IM* 1 hour prior to surgery.

PEDIATRIC PATIENTS	*USUAL DAILY DOSE*
Because of the varied response of pediatric patients to CNS-acting drugs, therapy should be initiated with the lowest dose and increased as required. Since clinical experience in pediatric patients under 6 years of age is limited, the use of the drug in this age group is not recommended.	*5 mg, 2 to 4 times daily (may be increased in some pediatric patients to 10 mg, 2 to 3 times daily)*

For the relief of withdrawal symptoms of acute alcoholism, the parenteral form* is usually used initially. If the drug is administered orally, the suggested initial dose is 50 to 100 mg, to be followed by repeated doses as needed until agitation is controlled – up to 300 mg per day. Dosage should then be reduced to maintenance levels.

* *See package insert for Injectable Librium (chlordiazepoxide HCl).*

HOW SUPPLIED

Librium (chlordiazepoxide HCl) Capsules are available in the following presentations:

5 mg hard gelatin capsules in bottles of 100 (NDC-0187-3750-10), with LIBRIUM 5 imprinted on the opaque green cap and ICN imprinted on the opaque yellow body.

10 mg hard gelatin capsules in bottles of 100 (NDC-0187-3751-10), with LIBRIUM 10 imprinted on the opaque black cap and ICN imprinted on the opaque green body.

25 mg hard gelatin capsules in bottles of 100 (NDC-0187-3758-10), with LIBRIUM 25 imprinted on the opaque green cap and ICN imprinted on the opaque white body.

Store at 25°C (77°F); excursions permitted to 15°C – 30°C (59°F – 86°F).

Valeant Pharmaceuticals International
Costa Mesa, CA 92626

Valeant
Valeant Pharmaceuticals International
3300 Hyland Avenue
Costa Mesa, CA 92626
714-545-0100
3375097EX03 Rev. September 2001

MESTINON® ℞

[mes 'tin-on]
(pyridostigmine bromide)
SYRUP, TABLETS, and TIMESPAN® TABLETS

DESCRIPTION

Mestinon (pyridostigmine bromide) is an orally active cholinesterase inhibitor. Chemically, pyridostigmine bromide is 3-hydroxy-1-methylpyridinium bromide dimethylcarbamate. Its structural formula is:

$[CH_3\text{–}N^+ \text{ pyridinium ring with } OCON(CH_3)_2]\ Br^-$

Mestinon is available in the following forms: *Syrup* containing 60 mg pyridostigmine bromide per teaspoonful in a vehicle containing 5% alcohol, glycerin, lactic acid, sodium benzoate, sorbitol, sucrose, FD&C Red No. 40, FD&C Blue No. 1, flavors and water. *Tablets* containing 60 mg pyridostigmine bromide; each tablet also contains lactose, silicon dioxide and stearic acid. *Timespan Tablets* containing 180 mg pyridostigmine bromide; each tablet also contains carnauba wax, corn-derived proteins, magnesium stearate, silica gel and tribasic calcium phosphate.

ACTIONS

Mestinon inhibits the destruction of acetylcholine by cholinesterase and thereby permits freer transmission of nerve impulses across the neuromuscular junction. Pyridostigmine is an analog of neostigmine (Prostigmin®), but differs from it in certain clinically significant respects; for example, pyridostigmine is characterized by a longer duration of action and fewer gastrointestinal side effects.

INDICATION

Mestinon is useful in the treatment of myasthenia gravis.

CONTRAINDICATIONS

Mestinon is contraindicated in mechanical intestinal or urinary obstruction, and particular caution should be used in its administration to patients with bronchial asthma. Care should be observed in the use of atropine for counteracting side effects, as discussed below.

WARNINGS

Although failure of patients to show clinical improvement may reflect underdosage, it can also be indicative of overdosage. As is true of all cholinergic drugs, overdosage of Mestinon may result in cholinergic crisis, a state characterized by increasing muscle weakness which, through involvement of the muscles of respiration, may lead to death. Myasthenic crisis due to an increase in the severity of the disease is also accompanied by extreme muscle weakness, and thus may be difficult to distinguish from cholinergic crisis on a symptomatic basis. Such differentiation is extremely important, since increases in doses of Mestinon or other drugs of this class in the presence of cholinergic crisis or of a refractory or "insensitive" state could have grave consequences. Osserman and Genkins[1] indicate that the differential diagnosis of the two types of crisis may require the use of Tensilon® (edrophonium chloride) as well as clinical judgment. The treatment of the two conditions obviously differs radically. Whereas the presence of myasthenic crisis suggests the need for more intensive anticholinesterase therapy, the diagnosis of cholinergic crisis, according to Osserman and Genkins,[1] calls for the prompt *withdrawal* of all drugs of this type. The immediate use of atropine in cholinergic crisis is also recommended.

Atropine may also be used to abolish or obtund gastrointestinal side effects or other muscarinic reactions; but such use, by masking signs of overdosage, can lead to inadvertent induction of cholinergic crisis.

For detailed information on the management of patients with myasthenia gravis, the physician is referred to one of the excellent reviews such as those by Osserman and Genkins,[2] Grob[3] or Schwab.[4,5]

Usage in Pregnancy: The safety of Mestinon during pregnancy or lactation in humans has not been established. Therefore, use of Mestinon in women who may become pregnant requires weighing the drug's potential benefits against its possible hazards to mother and child.

PRECAUTION

Pyridostigmine is mainly excreted unchanged by the kidney.[6,7,8] Therefore, lower doses may be required in patients with renal disease, and treatment should be based on titration of drug dosage to effect.[6,7]

Pediatric Use: Safety and effectiveness in pediatric patients have not been established.

ADVERSE REACTIONS

The side effects of Mestinon are most commonly related to overdosage and generally are of two varieties, muscarinic and nicotinic. Among those in the former group are nausea, vomiting, diarrhea, abdominal cramps, increased peristalsis, increased salivation, increased bronchial secretions, miosis and diaphoresis. Nicotinic side effects are comprised chiefly of muscle cramps, fasciculation and weakness. Muscarinic side effects can usually be counteracted by atropine, but for reasons shown in the preceding section the expedient is not without danger. As with any compound containing the bromide radical, a skin rash may be seen in an occasional patient. Such reactions usually subside promptly upon discontinuance of the medication.

DOSAGE AND ADMINISTRATION

Mestinon is available in three dosage forms:

Syrup —raspberry-flavored, containing 60 mg pyridostigmine bromide per teaspoonful (5 mL). This form permits accurate dosage adjustment for children and "brittle" myasthenic patients who require fractions of 60-mg doses. It is more easily swallowed, especially in the morning, by patients with bulbar involvement.

Conventional Tablets —each containing 60 mg pyridostigmine bromide.

Timespan Tablets —each containing 180 mg pyridostigmine bromide. This form provides uniformly slow release, hence prolonged duration of drug action; it facilitates control of myasthenic symptoms with fewer individual doses daily. The immediate effect of a 180-mg Timespan Tablet is about equal to that of a 60-mg Conventional Tablet; however, its duration of effectiveness, although varying in individual patients, averages $2^1/_2$ times that of a 60-mg dose.

Dosage: The size and frequency of the dosage must be adjusted to the needs of the individual patient.

Syrup and Conventional Tablets —The average dose is ten 60-mg tablets or ten 5-mL teaspoonfuls daily, spaced to provide maximum relief when maximum strength is needed. In severe cases as many as 25 tablets or teaspoonfuls a day may be required, while in mild cases one to six tablets or teaspoonfuls a day may suffice.

Timespan Tablets —One to three 180-mg tablets, once or twice daily, will usually be sufficient to control symptoms; however, the needs of certain individuals may vary mark-

Continued on next page

Mestinon—Cont.

edly from this average. The interval between doses should be at least 6 hours. For optimum control, it may be necessary to use the more rapidly acting regular tablets or syrup in conjunction with Timespan therapy.

Note: For information on a diagnostic test for myasthenia gravis, and for the evaluation and stabilization of therapy, please see product literature on Tensilon® (edrophonium chloride).

HOW SUPPLIED

Syrup, 60 mg pyridostigmine bromide per teaspoonful (5 mL) and 5% alcohol—bottles of 16 fluid ounces (1 pint) (NDC 0187-3012-20).

Tablets, scored, 60 mg pyridostigmine bromide each—bottles of 100 (NDC 0187-3010-30) and 500 (NDC 0187-3010-40).

Timespan Tablets, scored, 180 mg pyridostigmine bromide each—bottles of 30 (NDC 0187-3013-30).

Note: Because of the hygroscopic nature of the Timespan Tablets, mottling may occur. This does not affect their efficacy.

REFERENCES

1. Osserman KE, Genkins G. Studies in myasthenia gravis: Reduction in mortality rate after crisis. *JAMA.* Jan 1963; 183:97–101.
2. Osserman KE, Genkins G. Studies in myasthenia gravis. *NY State J. Med.* June 1961; 61:2076–2085.
3. Grob D. Myasthenia gravis. A review of pathogenesis and treatment. *Arch Intern Med.* Oct 1961; 108:615–638.
4. Schwab RS. Management of myasthenia gravis. *New Eng J Med.* Mar 1963; 268:596–597.
5. Schwab RS.Management of myasthenia gravis. *New Eng J Med.* Mar 1963; 268:717–719.
6. Cronnelly R, Stanski DR, Miller RD, Sheiner LB. Pyridostigmine kinetics with and without renal function. *Clin Pharmacol Ther.* 1980; 28:No. 1, 78–81.
7. Miller RD. Pharmacodynamics and pharmacokinetics of anticholinesterase. In: Ruegheimer E, Zindler M, ed. *Anaesthesiology.* (Hamburg, Germany: Congress; Sep 14–21, 1980; 222–223.) (Int Congr. No. 538), Amsterdam, Netherlands: Excerpta Medica; 1981.
8. Breyer-Pfaff U, Maier U, Brinkmann AM, Schumm F. Pyridostigmine kinetics in healthy subjects and patients with myasthenia gravis. *Clin Pharmacol Ther.* 1985;5: 495–501.

Valeant Pharmaceuticals International
3300 Hyland Avenue
Costa Mesa, CA 92626
(714) 545-0100

Rev. 8/00

Shown in Product Identification Guide, page 335

MOTOFEN® ©IV ℞

Tablets
(difenoxin hydrochloride with atropine sulfate)
antidiarrheal

HOW SUPPLIED

MOTOFEN® is available as a white, dye-free, five-sided, scored tablet with "74" on the scored side and "A" on the other. Each tablet contains 1.0 mg difenoxin (as the hydrochloride salt) and 0.025 mg atropine sulfate. Supplied in bottles of 100 tablets (NDC 65234-074-10) and in bottles of 50 tablets (NDC 65234-074-05).

Store at controlled room temperature, 15°–30°C (59°–86°F).

Rx only

Manufactured for: Valeant Pharmaceuticals International

Shown in Product Identification Guide, page 335

OXSORALEN® LOTION 1% ℞

[ox 'sore "a-len]
(methoxsalen USP, 1%)
Rx only

CAUTION: METHOXSALEN LOTION IS A POTENT TOPICAL DRUG. READ ENTIRE BROCHURE BEFORE PRESCRIBING OR USING THIS MEDICATION.

WARNING: METHOXSALEN LOTION IS A POTENT DRUG CAPABLE OF PRODUCING SEVERE BURNS IF IMPROPERLY USED. IT SHOULD BE APPLIED ONLY BY A PHYSICIAN UNDER CONTROLLED CONDITIONS FOR LIGHT EXPOSURE AND SUBSEQUENT LIGHT SHIELDING.

THIS PREPARATION SHOULD NEVER BE DISPENSED TO A PATIENT.

I. DESCRIPTION

Each ml. of Oxsoralen Lotion contains 10 mg methoxsalen in an inert vehicle containing alcohol (71% v/v), propylene glycol, acetone, and purified water.

Methoxsalen is a naturally occurring substance found in the seeds of the **Ammi majus** (Umbelliferae) plant and in the roots of **Heracleum Candicans.** It belongs to a group of compounds known as psoralens or furocoumarins. The chemical name of methoxsalen is 9-methoxy-7H-furo(3, 2g) (1)-benzopyran-7-one. It has the following structure:

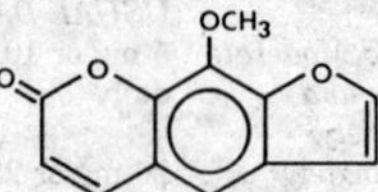

II. CLINICAL PHARMACOLOGY

The exact mechanism of action of methoxsalen with the epidermal melanocytes and keratinocytes is not known. Psoralens given orally are preferentially taken up by epidermal cells (Artuc et al, 1979).[1] The best known biochemical reaction of methoxsalen is with DNA. Methoxsalen, upon photoactivation, conjugates and forms covalent bonds with DNA which leads to the formation of both monofunctional (addition to a single strand of DNA) and bifunctional adducts (crosslinking of psoralen to both strands of DNA) (Dall'Acqua et al, 1971).[2] Reactions with proteins have also been described (Yoshikawa et al, 1979).[3]

Methoxsalen acts as a photosensitizer. Topical application of this drug and subsequent exposure to UVA, whether artificial or sunlight, can cause cell injury. If sufficient cell injury occurs in the skin an inflammatory reaction will result. The most obvious manifestation of this reaction is delayed erythema which may not begin for several hours and may not peak for 2 to 3 days or longer. It is crucial to realize that the length of time the skin remains sensitized or when the maximum erythema will occur is quite variable from person to person. The erythematous reaction is followed over several days or weeks by repair which is manifested by increased melanization of the epidermis and thickening of the stratum corneum. The exact mechanics are unknown but it has been suggested melanocytes in the hair follicles are stimulated to move up the follicle and to repopulate the epidermis. (Ortonne, et al, 1979).[4]

III. INDICATIONS AND USAGE

As a topical repigmenting agent in vitiligo in conjunction with controlled doses of ultraviolet A (320–400 nm) or sunlight.

IV. CONTRAINDICATIONS

A. Patients exhibiting idiosyncratic reactions to psoralen compounds or a history of sensitivity reactions to them.
B. Patients exhibiting melanoma or with a history of melanoma.
C. Patients exhibiting invasive skin carcinoma generally.
D. Patients with photosensitivity diseases such as porphyria, acute lupus erythematosus, xeroderma pigmentosum, etc.
E. Children under 12 since clinical studies to determine the efficacy and safety of treatment in this age group have not been done.

V. WARNINGS

A. **Skin Burns**

Serious skin burns from either UVA or sunlight (even through window glass) can result if recommended exposure schedule is exceeded and/or protective covering or sunscreens are not used. The blistering of the skin sometimes encountered after UVA exposure generally heals without complication or scarring. (Farrington Daniels, Jr, M.D., personal communication). Suitable covering of the area of application or a topical sunblock should follow the therapeutic UVA exposure.

B. **Carcinogenicity**

1. Animal Studies. Topical methoxsalen has been reported to be a potent photocarcinogen in certain strains of mice. (Pathak et al 1959).[5]

2. Human Studies. None of our clinical investigators reported skin cancer as a complication of topical treatment for vitiligo. However, it is recommended that caution be exercised when the patient is fair-skinned or has a history of prior coal tar UVA treatment, or has had ionizing radiation or taken arsenical compounds. Such patients who subsequently have **oral** psoralen—UVA treatment (PUVA) are at increased risk for developing skin cancer.

C. **Concomitant Therapy**

Special care should be exercised in treating patients who are receiving concomitant therapy (either topically or systemically) with known photosensitizing agents such as anthralin, coal tar or coal tar derivatives, griseofulvin, phenothiazines, nalidixic acid, halogenated salicylanilides (bacteriostatic soaps), sulfonamides, tetracyclines, thiazides, and certain organic staining dyes such as methylene blue, toluidine blue, rose bengal, and methyl orange.

VI. PRECAUTIONS

A. This product should be applied only in small well defined lesions and preferably on lesions which can be protected by clothing or a sunscreen from subsequent exposure to radiant UVA. If this product is used to treat vitiligo of face or hands, be very emphatic when instructing patient to keep the treated areas protected from light by use of protective clothing or sunscreening agents. The area of application may be highly photosensitive for several days and may result in severe burn injury if exposed to additional UV or sunlight.
B. CARCINOGENESIS: See Warning Section
C. Pregnancy Category C. Animal reproduction studies have not been conducted with topical methoxsalen. It is also not known whether methoxsalen can cause fetal harm when used topically on a pregnant woman or affect reproductive capacity. It is not known to what degree, if any, topical methoxsalen is absorbed systemically. Topical methoxsalen should be used in pregnant women only when clearly indicated.
D. Nursing Mothers. It is not known whether topical methoxsalen is absorbed or excreted in human milk. Caution is advised when topical methoxsalen is used in a nursing mother.
E. Pediatric Usage. Safety and effectiveness in children below the age of 12 years have not been established.

VII. ADVERSE REACTIONS

Systemic adverse reactions have not been reported. The most common adverse reaction is severe burns of the treated area from overexposure to UVA, including sunlight. TREATMENT MUST BE INDIVIDUALIZED. Minor blistering of the skin is not a contraindication to further treatment and generally heals without incident. Treatment would be the standard for burn therapy. Since 1953, many studies have demonstrated the safety and effectiveness of topical methoxsalen and UVA for the treatment of vitiligo when used as directed. (Lerner, A.B., et al, 1953)[6] (Fitzpatrick, T.B., et al, 1966)[7] (Fulton, James F. et al, 1969)[8].

VIII. OVERDOSAGE

This does not apply to topical usage. In the unlikely event that the lotion is ingested, standard procedures for poisoning should be followed, including gastric lavage. Protection from UVA or daylight for hours or days would also be necessary. The patient should be kept in a darkened room.

IX. ADMINISTRATION

OXSORALEN Lotion is applied to a well-defined area of vitiligo by the physician and the area is then exposed to a suitable source of UVA. Initial exposure time should be conservative and not exceed that which is predicted to be one-half the minimal erythema dose. Treatment intervals should be regulated by the erythema response; generally once a week is recommended or less often depending on the results. The hands and fingers of the person applying the medication should be protected by gloves or finger cots to avoid photosensitization and possible burns.

Pigmentation may begin after a few weeks but significant repigmentation may require up to 6 to 9 months of treatment. Periodic re-treatment may be necessary to retain all of the new pigment. Idiopathic vitiligo is reversible but not equally reversible in every patient. Treatment must be individualized. Repigmentation will vary in completeness, time of onset, and duration. Repigmentation occurs more rapidly in fleshy areas such as face, abdomen, and buttocks and less rapidly over less fleshy areas such as the dorsum of the hands or feet.

X. HOW SUPPLIED

Oxsoralen Lotion containing 1% methoxsalen (8-methoxypsoralen) packaged in 1 ounce (29.57 ml) amber glass bottles (NDC 0187-0402-31).

Store at 25°C (77°F); excursion permitted to 15°C–30°C (59°F–86°F).

REFERENCES

1. Artuc, M.; Stuettgen, G.; Schalla, W.; Schaefer, H.; Gazith, J.: Reversible binding of 5- and 8-methoxypsoralen to human serum proteins (albumin) and to epidermis **in vitro; Brit. J. Dermat., 101,** pp. 669–677 (1979).
2. Dall'Acqua, F.; Marciani, S.; Ciavatta, L.; Rodighiero, G.: formation of interstrand cross-linkings in the photoreactions between furocoumarins and DNA.; **Z Naturforsch** (B), **26,** pp. 561–569 (1971).
3. Yoshikawa, K; Mori, N.; Sakakibara, S.; Mizuno, N.; Song, P.: Photo-Conjugation of 8-methoxypsoralen with Proteins; **Photochem & Photobiol, 29,** pp. 1127–1133 (1979).
4. Ortonne, J.P.; MacDonald, D.M.; Micoud, A.; Thivolet, J.: PUVA-induced repigmentation of vitiligo: a histochemical (split-DOPA) and ultra-structural study; **Brit. J. Dermat., 101,** pp. 1–12 (1979).
5. Pathak, M.A.; Daniels, F.; Hopkins, C.E.; Fitzpatrick, T.B.: Ultraviolet carcinogenesis in albino and pigmented mice receiving furocoumarins: psoralens and 8-methoxypsoralen, **Nature, 183,** pp. 728–730 (1959).
6. Lerner, A.B.; Denton, C.R.; Fitzpatrick, T.B.: Clinical and experimental studies with 8-methoxypsoralen in vitiligo; **J. Invest. Derm., 20,** pp. 299–314 (April, 1953).
7. Fitzpatrick, T.B.; Arndt, K.A.; El Mofty, A.M.: Hydroquinone and psoralens in the therapy of hypermelanosis and vitiligo; **Arch Derm., 93,** pp. 589–599 (May, 1966).
8. Fulton, James F.; Leyden, James; Papa, Christopher: Treatment of vitiligo with topical methoxsalen and blacklite; **Arch. Derm., 101,** pp. 224–229 (1969).

2398-03 EL
Rev. 5-98

OXSORALEN-ULTRA® CAPSULES ℞

[ox '-sore "a-len]
(Methoxsalen Capsules, USP, 10 mg)
℞ only

CAUTION: METHOXSALEN IS A POTENT DRUG. READ ENTIRE BROCHURE PRIOR TO PRESCRIBING OR DISPENSING THIS MEDICATION.

Methoxsalen with UV radiation should be used only by physicians who have special competence in the diagnosis and treatment of psoriasis and who have special training and experience in photochemotherapy. The use of Psoralen and ultraviolet radiation therapy should be under constant supervision of such a physician. For the treatment of patients with psoriasis, photochemotherapy should be restricted to patients with severe, recalcitrant, disabling psoriasis which is not adequately responsive to other forms of therapy, and only when the diagnosis is certain. Because of the possibilities of ocular damage, aging of the skin, and skin cancer (including melanoma), the patient should be fully informed by the physician of the risks inherent in this therapy.

CAUTION: Oxsoralen-Ultra® (Methoxsalen Soft Gelatin Capsules) should not be used interchangeably with regular Oxsoralen® or 8-MOP® (Methoxsalen Hard Gelatin Capsules). This new dosage form of methoxsalen exhibits significantly greater bioavailability and earlier photosensitization onset time than previous methoxsalen dosage forms. Patients should be treated in accordance with the dosimetry specifically recommended for this product. The minimum phototoxic dose (MPD) and phototoxic peak time after drug administration prior to onset of photochemotherapy with this dosage form should be determined.

I. DESCRIPTION

Oxsoralen-Ultra (methoxsalen, 8-methoxypsoralen) Capsules, 10 mg. Methoxsalen is a naturally occurring photoactive substance found in the seeds of the **Ammi majus** (Umbelliferae) plant and in the roots of **Heracleum Candicans**. It belongs to a group of compounds known as psoralens, or furocoumarins. The chemical name of methoxsalen is 9-methoxy-7H-furo [3,2-g] [1]benzopyran-7-one; it has the following structure:

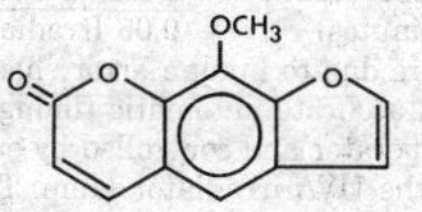

OCH_3

II. CLINICAL PHARMACOLOGY

The combination treatment regimen of psoralen (P) and ultraviolet radiation of 320-400 nm wavelength commonly referred to as UVA is known by the acronym, PUVA. Skin reactivity to UVA (320-400 nm) radiation is markedly enhanced by the ingestion of methoxsalen. In a well controlled bioavailability study, Oxsoralen-Ultra Capsules reached peak drug levels in the blood of test subjects between 0.5 and 4 hours (Mean = 1.8 hours) as compared to between 1.5 and 6 hours (Mean = 3.0 hours) for regular Oxsoralen when administered with 8 ounces of milk. Peak drug levels were 2 to 3 fold greater when the overall extent of drug absorption was approximately two fold greater for Oxsoralen-Ultra Capsules as compared to regular Oxsoralen Capsules. Detectable methoxsalen levels were observed up to 12 hours post dose. The drug half-life is approximately 2 hours. Photosensitivity studies demonstrate a shorter time of peak photosensitivity of 1.5 to 2.1 hours vs. 3.9 to 4.25 hours for regular Oxsoralen capsules. In addition, the mean minimal erythema dose (MED), J/cm^2, for the Oxsoralen-Ultra Capsules is substantially less than that required for regular Oxsoralen Capsules (Levins et al., 1984 and private communication[1]).

Methoxsalen is reversibly bound to serum albumin and is also preferentially taken up by epidermal cells (Artuc et al., 1979[2]). At a dose which is six times larger than that used in humans, it induces mixed function oxidases in the liver of mice (Mandula et al., 1978[3]). In both mice and man, methoxsalen is rapidly metabolized. Approximately 95% of the drug is excreted as a series of metabolites in the urine within 24 hours (Pathak et al., 1977[4]). The exact mechanism of action of methoxsalen with the epidermal melanocytes and keratinocytes is not known. The best known biochemical reaction of methoxsalen is with DNA. Methoxsalen, upon photoactivation, conjugates and forms covalent bonds with DNA which leads to the formation of both monofunctional (addition to a single strand of DNA) and bifunctional (crosslinking of psoralen to both strands of DNA) adducts (Dall'Acqua et al., 1971[5]; Cole, 1970[6]; Musajo et al., 1974[7]; Dall'Acqua et al., 1979[8]). Reactions with proteins have also been described (Yoshikawa, et al., 1979[9]).

Methoxsalen acts as a photosensitizer. Administration of the drug and subsequent exposure to UVA can lead to cell injury. Orally administered methoxsalen reaches the skin via the blood and UVA penetrates well into the skin. If sufficient cell injury occurs in the skin, an inflammatory reaction occurs. The most obvious manifestation of this reaction is delayed erythema, which may not begin for several hours and peaks at 48-72 hours. The inflammation is followed, over several days to weeks, by repair which is manifested by increased melanization of the epidermis and thickening of the stratum corneum. The mechanisms of therapy are not known. In the treatment of psoriasis, the mechanism is most often assumed to be DNA photodamage and resulting decrease in cell proliferation but other vascular, leukocyte, or cell regulatory mechanisms may also be playing some role. Psoriasis is a hyper-proliferative disorder and other agents known to be therapeutic for psoriasis are known to inhibit DNA synthesis.

III. INDICATIONS AND USAGE

Photochemotherapy (Methoxsalen with long wave UVA radiation) is indicated for the symptomatic control of severe, recalcitrant, disabling psoriasis not adequately responsive to other forms of therapy and when the diagnosis has been supported by biopsy. Methoxsalen is intended to be administered only in conjunction with a schedule of controlled doses of long wave ultraviolet radiation.

IV. CONTRAINDICATIONS

A. Patients exhibiting idiosyncratic reactions to psoralen compounds.
B. Patients possessing a specific history of light sensitive disease states should not initiate methoxsalen therapy except under special circumstances. Diseases associated with photosensitivity include lupus erythematosus, porphyria cutanea tarda, erythropoietic protoporphyria, variegate porphyria, xeroderma pigmentosum, and albinism.
C. Patients with melanoma or with a history of melanoma.
D. Patients with invasive squamous cell carcinomas.
E. Patients with aphakia, because of the significantly increased risk of retinal damage due to the absence of lenses.

V. WARNINGS—GENERAL

A. SKIN BURNING: Serious burns from either UVA or sunlight (even through window glass) can result if the recommended dosage of the drug and/or exposure schedules are exceeded.

B. CARCINOGENICITY:

1. ANIMAL STUDIES: Topical or intraperitoneal methoxsalen has been reported to be a potent photocarcinogen in albino mice and hairless mice (Hakim et al., 1960[10]). However, methoxsalen given by the oral route to Swiss albino mice suggests this agent exerts a protective effect against ultraviolet carcinogenesis; mice given 8-methoxypsoralen in their diet showed 38% ear tumors 180 days after the start of ultraviolet therapy compared to 62% for controls (O'Neal et al., 1957[11]).

2. HUMAN STUDIES: A 5.7 year prospective study of 1380 psoriasis patients treated with oral methoxsalen and ultraviolet A photochemotherapy (PUVA) demonstrated that the risk of cutaneous squamous-cell carcinoma developing at least 22 months following the first PUVA exposure was approximately 12.8 times higher in the high dose patients than in the low dose patients (Stern et al., 1979[12], Stern et al., 1980[13] and Stern et al., 1984[14]). The substantial dose-dependent increase was observed in patients with neither a prior history of skin cancer nor significant exposure to cutaneous carcinogens. Reduction in PUVA dosage significantly reduces the risk. No substantial dose related increase was noted for basal cell carcinoma according to Stern et al., 1984[14]. Increases appear greatest in patients who have pre-PUVA exposure to 1) prolonged tar and UVB treatment, 2) ionizing radiation, or 3) arsenic.

Roenigk et al., 1980[15], studied 690 patients for up to 4 years and found no increase in the risk of non-melanoma skin cancer, although patients in this cohort had significantly less exposure to PUVA than in the Stern et al. study. Recent analysis of new data in the Stern et al. cohort (Stern et al., 1997[16]) has shown that these patients had an elevated relative risk of contracting melanoma. The relative risk for melanoma in these patients was 2.3 (95 percent confidence interval 1.1 to 4.1). The risk is particularly higher in those patients who have received more than 250 PUVA treatments and in those whose treatment has spanned greater than 15 years earlier. Some patients developing melanoma did so even after having ceased PUVA therapy over 5 years earlier. These observations indicate the need for monitoring of PUVA patients for skin tumors throughout their lives.

In a study in Indian patients treated for 4 years for vitiligo, 12 percent developed keratoses, but not cancer, in the depigmented, vitiliginous areas (Mosher, 1980[17]). Clinically, the keratoses were keratotic papules, actinic keratosis-like macules, nonscaling dome-shaped papules, and lichenoid porokeratotic-like papules.

C. CATARACTOGENICITY:

1. ANIMAL STUDIES: Exposure to large doses of UVA causes cataracts in animals, and this effect is enhanced by the administration of methoxsalen (Cloud et al., 1960[18]; Cloud et al., 1961[19]; Freeman et al., 1969[20]).

2. HUMAN STUDIES: It has been found that the concentration of methoxsalen in the lens is proportional to the serum level. If the lens is exposed to UVA during the time methoxsalen is present in the lens, photochemical action may lead to irreversible binding of methoxsalen to proteins and the DNA components of the lens (Lerman et al., 1980[21]). However, if the lens is shielded from UVA, the methoxsalen will diffuse out of the lens in a 24 hour period (Lerman et al., 1980[21]). Patients should be told emphatically to wear UVA absorbing, wrap-around sunglasses for the twenty-four (24) hour period following ingestion of methoxsalen whether exposed to direct or indirect sunlight in the open or through a window glass.

Among patients using proper eye protection, there is no evidence for a significantly increased risk of cataracts in association with PUVA therapy (Stern et al., 1979[12]). Thirty-five of 1380 patients have developed cataracts in the five years since their first PUVA treatment. This incidence is comparable to that expected in a population of this size and age distribution. No relationship between PUVA dose and cataract risk in this group has been noted.

D. ACTINIC DEGENERATION: Exposure to sunlight and/or ultraviolet radiation may result in "premature aging" of the skin.

E. BASAL CELL CARCINOMAS: Patients exhibiting multiple basal cell carcinomas or having a history of basal cell carcinomas should be diligently observed and treated.

F. RADIATION THERAPY: Patients having a history of previous x-ray therapy or grenz ray therapy should be diligently observed for signs of carcinoma.

G. ARSENIC THERAPY: Patients having a history of previous arsenic therapy should be diligently observed for signs of carcinoma.

H. HEPATIC DISEASES: Patients with hepatic insufficiency should be treated with caution since hepatic biotransformation is necessary for drug urinary excretion.

I. CARDIAC DISEASES: Patients with cardiac diseases or others who may be unable to tolerate prolonged standing or exposure to heat stress should not be treated in a vertical UVA chamber.

J. ELDERLY PATIENTS: Caution should be used in elderly patients, especially those with a pre-existing history of cataracts, cardiovascular conditions, kidney and/or liver dysfunction, or skin cancer.

K. TOTAL DOSAGE: The total cumulative dose of UVA that can be given over long periods of time with safety has not as yet been established.

L. CONCOMITANT THERAPY: Special care should be exercised in treating patients who are receiving concomitant therapy (either topically or systemically) with known photosensitizing agents such as anthralin, coal tar or coal tar derivatives, griseofulvin, phenothiazines, nalidixic acid, fluoroquinolone antibiotics, halogenated salicylanilides (bacteriostatic soaps), sulfonamides, tetracyclines, thiazides, and certain organic staining dyes such as methylene blue, toluidine blue, rose bengal, and methyl orange.

VI. PRECAUTIONS

A. GENERAL—APPLICABLE TO PSORIASIS TREATMENT:

1. BEFORE METHOXSALEN INGESTION
Patients must not sunbathe during the 24 hours prior to methoxsalen ingestion and UV exposure. The presence of a sunburn may prevent an accurate evaluation of the patient's response to photochemotherapy.

2. AFTER METHOXSALEN INGESTION
a. UVA-absorbing wrap-around sunglasses should be worn during daylight for 24 hours after methoxsalen ingestion. The protective eyewear must be designed to prevent entry of stray radiation to the eyes, including that which may enter from the sides of the eyewear. The protective eyewear is used to prevent the irreversible binding of methoxsalen to the proteins and DNA components of the lens. Cataracts form when enough of the binding occurs. Visual discrimination should be permitted by the eyewear of patient well-being and comfort.
b. Patients must avoid sun exposure, even through window glass or cloud cover, for at least 8 hours after methoxsalen ingestion. If sun exposure cannot be avoided, the patient should wear protective devices such as a hat and gloves, and/or apply sunscreens which contain ingredients that filter out UVA radiation (e.g., sunscreens containing benzophenone and/or PABA esters which exhibit a sun protective factor equal to or greater than 15). These chemical sunscreens should be applied to all areas that might be exposed to the sun (including lips). Sunscreens should not be applied to areas affected by psoriasis until after the patient has been treated in the UVA chamber.

3. DURING PUVA THERAPY
a. Total UVA-absorbing/blocking goggles mechanically designed to give maximal ocular protection must be worn. Failure to do so may increase the risk of cataract formation. A reliable radiometer can be used to verify elimination of UVA transmission through the goggles.
b. Abdominal skin, breasts, genitalia, and other sensitive areas should be protected for approximately 1/3 of the initial exposure time until tanning occurs.
c. Unless affected by disease, male genitalia should be shielded.

4. AFTER COMBINED METHOXSALEN/UVA THERAPY
a. UVA-absorbing wrap-around sunglasses should be worn during daylight for 24 hours after combined methoxsalen/UVA therapy.
b. Patients should not sunbathe for 48 hours after therapy. Erythema and/or burning due to photochemotherapy and sunburn due to sun exposure are additive.

B. INFORMATION FOR PATIENTS: See accompanying Patient Package Insert.

C. LABORATORY TESTS:

1. Patients should have an ophthalmologic examination prior to start of therapy, and thence yearly.
2. Patients should have routine laboratory tests prior to the start of therapy and at regular periods thereafter if patients are on extended treatments.

D. DRUG INTERACTIONS: See Warnings Section.

E. CARCINOGENESIS: See Warnings Section.

Continued on next page

Oxsoralen-Ultra Caps—Cont.

F. PREGNANCY:
Pregnancy Category C. Animal reproduction studies have not been conducted with methoxsalen. It is also not known whether methoxsalen can cause fetal harm when administered to a pregnant woman or can affect reproduction capacity. Methoxsalen should be given to a woman with reproductive capacity only if clearly needed.

G. NURSING MOTHERS:
It is not known whether this drug is excreted in human milk. Because many drugs are excreted in human milk, either methoxsalen ingestion or nursing should be discontinued.

H. PEDIATRIC USE:
Safety in children has not been established. Potential hazards of long-term therapy include the possibilities of carcinogenicity and cataractogenicity as described in the Warnings Section as well as the probability of actinic degeneration which is also described in the Warnings Section.

I. GERIATRIC USE:
Clinical studies with Oxsoralen-Ultra capsules did not include sufficient numbers of subjects aged 65 and over to determine whether elderly subjects responded differently from younger subjects. Other reported clinical experience has not identified differences in response between the elderly and younger patients. In general, dose selection for an elderly patient should be cautious, usually starting at the low end of the dosing range, reflecting the greater frequency of decreased hepatic, renal, or cardiac function, and of concomitant disease or other drug therapy.

VII. ADVERSE REACTIONS

A. METHOXSALEN:
The most commonly reported side effect of methoxsalen alone is nausea, which occurs with approximately 10% of all patients. This effect may be minimized or avoided by instructing the patient to take methoxsalen in milk or food, or to divide the dose into two portions, taken approximately one-half hour apart. Other effects include nervousness, insomnia, and depression.

B. COMBINED METHOXSALEN/UVA THERAPY:
1. PRURITUS: This adverse reaction occurs with approximately 10% of all patients. In most cases, pruritus can be alleviated with frequent application of bland emollients or other topical agents; severe pruritus may require systemic treatment. If pruritus is unresponsive to these measures, shield pruritic areas from further UVA exposure until the condition resolves. If intractable pruritus is generalized, UVA treatment should be discontinued until the pruritus disappears.

2. ERYTHEMA: Mild, transient erythema at 24-48 hours after PUVA therapy is an expected reaction and indicates that a therapeutic interaction between methoxsalen and UVA occurred. Any area showing moderate erythema (greater than Grade 2—See Table 1 for grades of erythema) should be shielded during subsequent UVA exposures until the erythema has resolved. Erythema greater than Grade 2 which appears within 24 hours after UVA treatment may signal a potentially severe burn. Erythema may become progressively worse over the next 24 hours, since the peak erythemal reaction characteristically occurs 48 hours or later after methoxsalen ingestion. The patient should be protected from further UVA exposures and sunlight, and should be monitored closely.

3. IMPORTANT DIFFERENCES BETWEEN PUVA ERYTHEMA AND SUNBURN: PUVA-induced inflammation differs from sunburn or UVB phototherapy in several ways. The percent transmission of UVB varies between 0% to 34% through skin whereas UVA varies between 1% to 80% transmission; thus, UVA is transmitted to a larger percent through the skin. (Diffey, 1982[22]). The DNA lesions induced by PUVA are very different from UV-induced thymine dimers and may lead to a DNA crosslink. This DNA lesion may be more problematic to the cell because crosslinks are more lethal and psoralen-DNA photoproducts may be "new" or unfamiliar substrates for DNA repair enzymes. DNA synthesis is also suppressed longer after PUVA. The time course of delayed erythema is different with PUVA and may not involve the usual mediators seen in sunburn. PUVA-induced redness may be just beginning at 24 hours, when UVB erythema has already passed its peak. The erythema dose-response curve is also steeper for PUVA. Compared to equally erythemogenic doses of UVB, the histologic alterations induced by PUVA show more dermal vessel damage and longer duration of epidermal and dermal abnormalities.

4. OTHER ADVERSE REACTIONS: Those reported include edema, dizziness, headache, malaise, depression, hypopigmentation, vesiculation and bullae formation, non-specific rash, herpes simplex, miliaria, urticaria, folliculitis, gastrointestinal disturbances, cutaneous tenderness, leg cramps, hypotension, and extension of psoriasis.

VIII. OVERDOSAGE

In the event of methoxsalen overdosage, induce emesis and keep the patient in a darkened room for at least 24 hours. Emesis is most beneficial within the first 2 to 3 hours after ingestion of methoxsalen, since maximum blood levels are reached by this time.

IX. DRUG DOSAGE & ADMINISTRATION

CAUTION: Oxsoralen-Ultra represents a new dose form of methoxsalen. This new dosage form of methoxsalen exhibits significantly greater bioavailability and earlier photosensitization onset time than previous methoxsalen dosage forms. Each patient should be evaluated by determining the minimum phototoxic dose (MPD) and phototoxic peak time after drug administration prior to onset of photochemotherapy with this dosage form. Human bioavailability studies have indicated the following drug dosage and administration directions are to be used as a guideline only.

PSORIASIS THERAPY
1. DRUG DOSAGE - INITIAL THERAPY: The methoxsalen capsules should be taken 1 1/2 to 2 hours before UVA exposure with some low fat food or milk according to the following table:

Patient's Weight (kg)	(lbs)	Dose (mg)
<30	<66	10
30-50	66-110	20
51-65	112-143	30
66-80	146-176	40
81-90	179-198	50
91-115	201-254	60
>115	>254	70

Elderly patients should generally be started at the low end of the dose recommended according to body weight and closely monitored during PUVA therapy. Although clinical experience has not identified differences in response between elderly and younger patients, the use of methoxsalen in older individuals may be affected by the presence or preexisting medical conditions.

2. INITIAL EXPOSURE: The initial UVA exposure energy level and corresponding time of exposure is determined by the patient's skin characteristics for sunburning and tanning as follows:

Skin Type	History	Recommended Joules/cm²
I	Always burn, never tan (patients with erythrodermic psoriasis are to be classed as Type I for determination of UVA dosage.)	0.5 J/cm²
II	Always burn, but sometimes tan	1.0 J/cm²
III	Sometimes burn, but always tan	1.5 J/cm²
IV	Never burn, always tan	2.0 J/cm²
Skin Type	**Physician Examination**	**Joules/cm²**
V*	Moderately pigmented	2.5 J/cm²
VI*	Blacks	3.0 J/cm²

(*Patients with natural pigmentation of these types should be classified into a lower skin type category if the sunburning history so indicates.)

If the MPD is done, start at 1/2 MPD.

Additional drug dosage directions are as follows:

a. Weight Change: In the event that the weight of a patient changes during treatment such that he/she falls into an adjacent weight range/dose category, no change in the dose of methoxsalen is usually required. If, in the physician's opinion, however, a weight change is sufficiently great to modify the drug dose, then an adjustment in the time of exposure to UVA should be made.

b. Dose/Week: The number of doses per week of methoxsalen capsules will be determined by the patient's schedule of UVA exposures. In no case should treatments be given more often than once every other day because the full extent of phototoxic reactions may not be evident until 48 hours after each exposure.

c. Dosage Increase: Dosage may be increased by 10 mg. after the fifteenth treatment under the conditions outlined in section XI.B.4.b.

X. UVA RADIATION SOURCE SPECIFICATIONS & INFORMATION

A. IRRADIANCE UNIFORMITY:
The following specifications should be met with the window of the detector held in a vertical plane:

1. Vertical variation: For readings taken at any point along the vertical center axis of the chamber (to within 15 cm from the top and bottom), the lowest reading should not be less than 70 percent of the highest reading.

2. Horizontal variation: Throughout any specific horizontal plane, the lowest reading must be at least 80 percent of the highest reading, excluding the peripheral 3 cm of the patient treatment space.

B. PATIENT SAFETY FEATURES:
The following safety features should be present: (1) Protection from electrical hazard: All units should be grounded and conform to applicable electrical codes. The patient or operator should not be able to touch any live electrical parts. There should be ground fault protection. (2) Protective shielding of lamps: The patient should not be able to come in contact with the bare lamps. In the event of lamp breakage, the patient should not be exposed to broken lamp components. (3) Hand rails and hand holds: Appropriate supports should be available to the patient. (4) Patient viewing window: A window which blocks UV should be provided for viewing the patient during treatment. (5) Door and latches: Patients should be able to open the door from the inside with only slight pressure to the door. (6) Non-skid floor: The floor should be of a non-skid nature. (7) Thermoregulation: Sufficient air flow should be provided for patient safety and comfort, limiting temperature within the UVA radiator cabinet to approximately less than 100°F. (8) Timer: The irradiator should be equipped with an automatic timer which terminates the exposure at the conclusion of a preset time interval. (9) Patient alarm device: An alarm device within the UVA irradiator chamber should be accessible to the patient for emergency activation. (10) Danger label: The unit should have a label prominently displayed which reads as follows:

DANGER—Ultraviolet Radiation—Follow your physician's instructions

Failure to use protective eyewear may result in eye injury.

C. UVA EXPOSURE DOSIMETRY MEASUREMENTS:
The maximum radiant exposure or irradiance (within ± 15 percent) of UVA (320-400 nm) delivered to the patient should be determined by using an appropriate radiometer calibrated to be read in Joules/cm² or mW/cm². In the absence of a standard measuring technique approved by the National Bureau of Standards, the system should use a detector corrected to a cosine spatial response. The use and recalibration frequency of such a radiometer for a specific UVA irradiator chamber should be specified by the manufacturer because the UVA dose (exposure) is determined by the design of the irradiator, the number of lamps, and the age of the lamp. If irradiance is measured, the radiometer reading in mW/cm² is used to calculate the exposure time in minutes to deliver the required UVA in Joules/cm² to a patient in the UVA irradiator cabinet. The equation is:

$$\text{Exposure Time (minutes)} = \frac{\text{Desired UVA Dose (J/cm}^2\text{)}}{0.06 \text{ Irradiance (mW/cm}^2\text{)}}.$$

Overexposure due to human error should be minimized by using an accurate automatic timing device, which is set by the operator and controlled by energizing and de-energizing the UVA irradiator lamp. The timing device calibration interval should be specified by the manufacturer. Safety systems should be included to minimize the possibility of delivering a UVA exposure which exceeds the prescribed dose, in the event the timer or radiometer should malfunction.

D. UVA SPECTRAL OUTPUT DISTRIBUTION:
The spectral distributions of the lamps should meet the following specifications:

Wavelength band (nanometers)	Output[1]
<310	<1
310 to 320	1 to 3
320 to 330	4 to 8
330 to 340	11 to 17
340 to 350	18 to 25
350 to 360	19 to 28
360 to 370	15 to 23
370 to 380	8 to 12
380 to 390	3 to 7
390 to 400	1 to 3

[1] As a percentage of total irradiance between 320 and 400 nanometers.

XI. PUVA TREATMENT PROTOCOL

INTRODUCTION:
The Oxsoralen-Ultra® Capsules reach their maximum bioavailability in 1 1/2 to 2 hours after ingestion.

On average, the serum level achieved with Oxsoralen-Ultra is twice that obtained with 8-MOP (formerly Oxsoralen) and reach their peak concentration in less than 1/2 the time of the 8-MOP capsules.

As a result the mean MED J/cm² for the Oxsoralen-Ultra Capsules is substantially less than that required for 8-MOP (Levins et al., 1984 and private communication[1]).

Photosensitivity studies demonstrate a shorter time of peak photosensitivity of 1.5 to 2.1 hours vs. 3.9 to 4.25 hours for regular methoxsalen capsules.

A. INITIAL EXPOSURE: The initial UVA exposures should be conducted according to the guidelines presented previously under IX., Psoriasis Therapy, Drug Dosage-Initial Therapy and Initial Exposure.

B. CLEARING PHASE: Specific recommendations for patient treatment are as follows:

1. SKIN TYPES I, II, & III. Patients with skin types I, II, and III may be treated 2 or 3 times per week. UVA exposure may be held constant or increased by up to 1.0 Joule/cm² at each treatment, according to the patient's response. If erythema occurs, however, do not increase exposure time until erythema resolves. The severity and extent of the patient's erythema may be used to determine whether the next exposure should be shortened, omitted, or maintained at the previous dosage. See Adverse Reactions section for additional information.

2. SKIN TYPES IV, V, & VI. Patients with skin types IV, V, and VI may be treated 2 or 3 times per week. UVA exposure may be held constant or increased by up to 1.5 Joules/cm² at each treatment unless erythema occurs. If erythema occurs, follow instructions outlined above in the procedures for patients with skin types I, II, and III.

3. ERYTHRODERMIC PSORIASIS. Patients with erythrodermic psoriasis should be treated with special atten-

tion because pre-existing erythema may obscure observations of possible treatment-related phototoxic erythema. These patients may be treated 2 or 3 times per week, as a Type I patient.

4. MISCELLANEOUS SITUATIONS:

a. If there is no response after a total of 10 treatments, the exposure of UVA energy may be increased by an additional 0.5-1.0 Joules/cm^2 above the prior incremental increases for each treatment. (Example: a patient whose exposure dosage is being increased by 1.0 Joule/cm^2 may now have all subsequent doses increased by 1.5-2.0 Joules/cm^2.)

b. If there is no response, or only minimal response, after 15 treatments, the dosage of methoxsalen may be increased by 10 mg (a one-time increase in dosage). This increased dosage may be continued for the remainder of the course of treatment but should not be exceeded.

c. If a patient misses a treatment, the UVA exposure time of the next treatment should not be increased. If more than one treatment is missed, reduce the exposure by 0.5 Joules/cm^2 for each treatment missed.

d. If the lower extremities are not responding as well as the rest of the body and do not show erythema, cover all other body areas and give 25 percent of the present exposure dose as an additional exposure to the lower extremities. This additional exposure to the lower extremities should be terminated if erythema develops on these areas.

e. Non-responsive psoriasis: If a patient's generalized psoriasis is not responding, or if the condition appears to be worsening during treatment, the possibility of a generalized phototoxic reaction should be considered. This may be confirmed by the improvement of the condition following temporary discontinuance of this therapy for two weeks. If no improvement occurs during the interruption of treatment, this patient may be considered a treatment failure.

C. ALTERNATIVE EXPOSURE SCHEDULE:

As an alternative to increasing the UVA exposure at each treatment, the following schedule may be followed; this schedule may reduce the total number of Joules/cm^2 received by the patient over the entire course of therapy.

1. Incremental increases in UVA exposure for all patients may range from 0.5 to 1.5 Joules/cm^2 according to the patient's response to therapy.

2. Once Grade 2 clearing (see Table 2) has been reached and the patient is progressing adequately, UVA dosage is held constant. This dosage is maintained until Grade 4 clearing is reached.

3. If the rate of clearing significantly decreases, exposure dosage may be increased at each treatment (0.1-1.5 Joules/cm^2 until Grade 3 clearing and a satisfactory progress rate is attained. The UVA exposure will be held constant again until Grade 4 clearing is attained. These increases may be used also if the rate of clearing significantly decreases between Grade 3 and Grade 4 response. However, the possibility of a phototoxic reaction should be considered; see Non-responsive Psoriasis, above.

4. In summary, this schedule raises slightly the increments (Joules/cm^2) of UVA dosage, but limits these increases to those periods when the patient is not responding adequately. Otherwise, the UVA exposure is held at the lowest effective dose.

D. MAINTENANCE PHASE:

The goal of maintenance treatment is to keep the patient as symptom-free as possible with the least amount of UVA exposure.

1. SCHEDULE OF EXPOSURES: When patients have achieved 95 percent clearing, or Grade 4 response (Table 2), they may be placed on the following maintenance schedules (M_1-M_4), in sequence. It is recommended that each maintenance schedule be adhered to for at least 2 treatments (unless erythema or psoriatic flare occurs, in which case see (2a) and (2b) below).

Maintenance Schedules

M_1—once/week
M_2—once/2 weeks
M_3—once/3 weeks
M_4—p.r.n. (i.e., for flares)

2. LENGTH OF EXPOSURE: The UVA exposure for the first maintenance treatment of any schedule (except M_4 as noted below) is the same as that of the patient's last treatment under the previous schedule. For skin types I-IV, however, it is recommended that the maximum UVA dosage during maintenance treatments not exceed the following:

Skin Types	Joules/cm^2/treatment
I	12
II	14
III	18
IV	22

If the patient develops erythema or new lesions of psoriasis, proceed as follows:

a. Erythema: During maintenance therapy, the patient's tan and threshold dose for erythema may gradually decrease. If maintenance treatments produce significant erythema, the exposure to UVA should be decreased by 25 percent until further treatments no longer produce erythema.

b. Psoriasis: If the patient develops new areas of psoriasis during maintenance therapy (but still is classified as having a Grade 4 response), the exposure to UVA may be increased by 0.5-1.5 Joules/cm^2 at each treatment; this is appropriate for all types of patients. These increases are continued until the psoriasis is brought under control and the patient is again clear. The exposure being administered when this clearing is reached should be used for further maintenance treatment.

3. FLARES DURING MAINTENANCE: If the patient flares during maintenance treatment (i.e., develops psoriasis on more than 5 percent of the originally involved areas of the body), his maintenance treatment schedule may be changed to the preceding maintenance or clearing schedule. The patient may be kept on his schedule until again 95 percent clear. If the original maintenance treatment schedule is unable to control the psoriasis, the schedule may be changed to a more frequent regimen. If a flare occurs less than 6 weeks after the last treatment, 25 percent of the maximum exposure received during the clearing phase, with the clearing schedule received during the clearing phase, may be used and then proceed with the clearing schedule previously followed for this patient. (At 95 percent clearing, follow regular maintenance until the optimum maintenance schedule is determined for the patient.) If more than 6 weeks have elapsed since the last treatment was given, treat patients as if they were beginning therapy insofar as exposure dosages are concerned, since their threshold for erythema may have decreased.

Table 1. Grades of Erythema

Grades	Erythema
0	No erythema
1	Minimally perceptible erythema—faint pink
2	Marked erythema but with no edema
3	Fiery erythema with edema
4	Fiery erythema with edema and blistering

Table 2. Response to Therapy

Grade	Criteria	Percent Improvement (compared to original extent of disease)
-1	Psoriasis worse	0
0	No change	0
1	Minimal improvement—slightly less scale and/or erythema	5-20
2	Definite improvement—partial flattening of all plaques—less scaling and less erythema	20-50
3	Considerable improvement—nearly complete flattening of all plaques but borders of plaques still palpable	50-95
4	Clearing; complete flattening of plaques including borders; plaques may be outlined by pigmentation	95

XII. HOW SUPPLIED

Oxsoralen-Ultra Capsules, each containing 10 mg of methoxsalen (8-methoxypsoralen) are available in green soft gelatin capsules in amber glass bottles of 50 (NDC 0187-0650-42), with ICN imprinted on one side of the capsule and 650 imprinted on the other side.

Store at 25°C (77°F); excursions permitted to 15°C-30°C (59°F-86°F).

Valeant Pharmaceuticals International
3300 Hyland Ave.
Costa Mesa, CA 92626, U.S.A.

BIBLIOGRAPHY

1. Levins, P.C., Gange, R.W., Momtaz-T,K., Parrish, J.A., and Fitzpatrick, T.B.: A New Liquid Formulation of 8-Methoxypsoralen: Bioactivity and Effect of Diet: JID, *82,* No. 2, pp. 185-187 (1984) and private communication.
2. Artuc,M., Stuettgen, G., Schalla, W., Schaefer, H., and Gazith, J.: Reversible binding of 5-and 8-methoxypsoralen to human serum proteins (albumin) and to epidermis in vitro: Brit. J. Dermat. *101,* pp. 669-677 (1979).
3. Mandula, B.B., Pathak, M.A., Nakayama, T., and Davidson, S.J.: Induction of mixed-function oxidases in mouse liver by psoralens., Ibid, *99,* pp. 687-692 (1978).
4. Pathak, M.A., Fitzpatrick, T.B., Parrish, J.A.: PSORIASIS, Proceedings of the Second International Symposium. Edited by E.M. Farber, A.J. Cox, Yorke Medical Books, pp. 262-265 (1977).
5. Dall'Acqua, F., Marciani, S., Ciavatta, L., Rodighiero, G.: Formation of interstrand cross-linkings in the photoreactions between furocoumarins and DNA; Z Naturforsch (B), *26,* pp. 561-569 (1971).
6. Cole, R.S.: Light-induced cross-linkings of DNA in the presence of a furocoumarin (psoralen), Biochem. Biophys. Acta, *217,* pp. 30-39 (1970).
7. Musajo, L., Rodighiero, G., Caporale, G., Dall'Acqua, F., Marciani, S., Bordin, F., Baccichetti, F., Bevilacqua, R.: Photoreactions between Skin-Photosensitizing Furocoumarins and Nucleic Acids, *Sunlight and Man;* Normal and Abnormal Photobiologic Responses. Edited by M.A. Pathak, L.C. Harber, M. Seiji et al. University of Tokyo Press, pp. 369-387 (1974).
8. Dall'Acqua, F., Vedaldi, D., Bordin, F., and Rodighiero, G.: New studies in the interaction between 8-methoxypsoralen and DNA *in vitro:* JID, *73,* pp. 191-197 (1979).
9. Yoshikawa, K., Mori, N., Sakakibara, S., Mizuno, N., Song, P.: Photo Conjugation of 8-methoxypsoralen with Proteins; Photochem. & Photobiol. *29,* pp. 1127-1133 (1979).
10. Hakim, R.D., Griffin, A.C.: Knox, J.M.: Erythema and tumor formation in methoxsalen treated mice exposed to fluorescent light; Arch. Dermatol. *82,* pp. 572-577 (1960).
11. O'Neal, M.A., Griffin, A.C.: The Effect of Oxypsoralen upon Ultraviolet Carcinogenesis in Albino Mice, Cancer Res., *17,* pp. 911-916 (1957).
12. Stern, R.S., Unpublished personal communication.
13. Stern, R.S., Parrish, J.A., Zierler, S.: Skin Carcinoma in Patients with Psoriasis Treated with Topical Tar and Artificial Ultraviolet Radiation. Lancet, *1,* pp. 732-735 (1980).
14. Stern, R.S., Laird, N., Melski, J., Parrish, J.A., Fitzpatrick, T.B., Bleich, H.L.: Cutaneous Squamous-Cell Carcinoma in Patients Treated with PUVA: NEJM, *310,* No. 18, pp. 1156-1161 (1984).
15. Roenigk, Jr., H.H., and 12 Cooperating Investigators: Skin Cancer in the PUVA-48 Cooperative Study of Psoriasis. Program for Forty-First Annual Meeting for The Society of Investigative Dermatology, Inc., Sheraton Washington Hotel, Washington, D.C., May 12, 13, and 14, 1980. Abstracts JID, *74,* No. 4, p. 250 (April, 1980).
16. Stern et al., Malignant melanoma in patients treated for psoriasis with methoxsalen (psoralen) and ultraviolet A radiation (PUVA). The PUVA Follow-up Study. New England Journal of Medicine, 336:1041-1045, (April 10, 1997).
17. Mosher, D.B., Pathak, M.A., Harris, T.J., Fitzpatrick, T.B.: Development of Cutaneous Lesions in Vitiligo During Long-Term PUVA Therapy. Program for Forty-First Annual Meeting for The Society for Investigative Dermatology, Inc., Sheraton Washington Hotel, Washington, D.C., May 12, 13, and 14, 1980. Abstracts JID, *74,* No. 4, p. 259 (April, 1980).
18. Cloud, T.M., Hakim, R., Griffin, A.C.: Photosensitization of the eye with methoxsalen. I. Acute effects; Arch. Ophthalmol. *64,* pp. 346-352 (1960).
19. Cloud, T.M., Hakim, R., Griffin, A.C.: Photosensitization of the eye with methoxsalen. II. Chronic effects, Ibid, *66,* pp. 689-694 (1961).
20. Freeman, R.G., Troll, D.: Photosensitization of the eye by 8-methoxypsoralen, JID, *53,* pp. 449-453 (1969).
21. Lerman, S., Megaw, J., Willis, I.: Potential ocular complications from PUVA therapy and their prevention; JID *74,* pp. 197-199 (1980).
22. Diffey, B.L., Medical Physics Handbook 11, Ultraviolet Radiation In Medicine, Adam Hilger, Ltd., Bristol, p. 86 (1982).

Revised 4-03
2400-03 EL

Shown in Product Identification Guide, page 335

PERMAX® ℞
[*pĕr 'măks*]
(pergolide)
TABLETS

DESCRIPTION

Permax® (Pergolide Tablets, USP) is an ergot derivative dopamine receptor agonist at both D_1 and D_2 receptor sites. Pergolide mesylate is chemically designated as 8β-[(Methylthio)methyl]-6-propylergoline monomethanesulfonate; the structural formula is as follows:

H, CH_2SCH_3, H, $N-CH_2CH_2CH_3$, H, $\cdot\ CH_3SO_3H$, HN

The empirical formula is $C_{19}H_{26}N_2S \bullet CH_4O_3S$ representing a molecular weight of 410.60.

Permax is provided for oral administration in tablets containing 0.05 mg (0.159 μmol), 0.25 mg (0.795 μmol), or 1 mg (3.18 μmol) pergolide as the base. The tablets also contain croscarmellose sodium, iron oxide, lactose, magnesium stearate, and povidone. The 0.05 mg tablet also contains L-methionine, and the 0.25 mg tablet also contains FD&C Blue No. 2.

CLINICAL PHARMACOLOGY

Pharmacodynamic Information —Pergolide is a potent dopamine receptor agonist. Pergolide is 10 to 1000 times more potent than bromocriptine on a milligram per milligram basis in various in vitro and in vivo test systems. Pergolide

Continued on next page

Permax—Cont.

inhibits the secretion of prolactin in humans; it causes a transient rise in serum concentrations of growth hormone and a decrease in serum concentrations of luteinizing hormone. In Parkinson's disease, pergolide is believed to exert its therapeutic effect by directly stimulating postsynaptic dopamine receptors in the nigrostriatal system.

Pharmacokinetic Information (Absorption, Distribution, Metabolism, and Elimination) —Information on oral systemic bioavailability of pergolide is unavailable because of the lack of a sufficiently sensitive assay to detect the drug after the administration of a single dose. However, following oral administration of ^{14}C radiolabeled pergolide, approximately 55% of the administered radioactivity can be recovered from the urine and 5% from expired CO_2, suggesting that a significant fraction is absorbed. Nothing can be concluded about the extent of presystemic clearance, if any. Data on postabsorption distribution of pergolide are unavailable.

At least 10 metabolites have been detected, including N-despropylpergolide, pergolide sulfoxide, and pergolide sulfone. Pergolide sulfoxide and pergolide sulfone are dopamine agonists in animals. The other detected metabolites have not been identified, and it is not known whether any other metabolites are active pharmacologically.

The major route of excretion is the kidney.

Pergolide is approximately 90% bound to plasma proteins. This extent of protein binding may be important to consider when pergolide is coadministered with other drugs known to affect protein binding.

INDICATIONS AND USAGE

Permax is indicated as adjunctive treatment to levodopa/carbidopa in the management of the signs and symptoms of Parkinson's disease.

Evidence to support the efficacy of pergolide as an antiparkinsonian adjunct was obtained in a multicenter study enrolling 376 patients with mild to moderate Parkinson's disease who were intolerant to *l* -dopa/carbidopa as manifested by moderate to severe dyskinesia and/or on-off phenomena. On average, the patients evaluated had been on *l* -dopa/carbidopa for 3.9 years (range, 2 days to 16.8 years). The administration of pergolide permitted a 5% to 30% reduction in the daily dose of *l* -dopa. On average these patients treated with pergolide maintained an equivalent or better clinical status than they exhibited at baseline.

CONTRAINDICATIONS

Pergolide is contraindicated in patients who are hypersensitive to this drug or other ergot derivatives.

WARNINGS

Falling Asleep During Activities of Daily Living —Patients treated with Permax have reported falling asleep while engaged in activities of daily living, including the operation of motor vehicles which sometimes resulted in accidents. Although may of these patients reported somnolence while on Permax, some perceived that they had no warning signs such as excessive drowsiness, and believed that they were alert immediately prior to the event. Some of these events had been reported as late as 1 year after the initiation of treatment.

Somnolence is a common occurrence in patients receiving Permax. Many clinical experts believe that falling asleep while engaged in activities of daily living always occurs in a setting of preexisting somnolence, although patients may not give such a history. For this reason, prescribers should continually reassess patients for drowsiness or sleepiness, especially since some of the events occur well after the start of treatment. Prescribers should also be aware that patients may not acknowledge drowsiness or sleepiness until directly questioned about drowsiness or sleepiness during specific activities.

Before initiating treatment with Permax, patients should be advised of the potential to develop drowsiness and specifically asked about factors that may increase the risk with Permax such as concomitant sedating medications or the presence of sleep disorders. If a patient develops significant daytime sleepiness or episodes of falling asleep during activities that require participation (e.g., conversations, eating, etc.), Permax should ordinarily be discontinued. If a decision is made to continue Permax, patients should be advised to not drive and to avoid other potentially dangerous activities.

While dose reduction may reduce the degree of somnolence, there is insufficient information to establish that dose reduction will eliminate episodes of falling asleep while engaged in activities of daily living.

Symptomatic Hypotension —In clinical trials, approximately 10% of patients taking pergolide with *l* -dopa versus 7% taking placebo with *l* -dopa experienced symptomatic orthostatic and/or sustained hypotension, especially during initial treatment. With gradual dosage titration, tolerance to the hypotension usually develops. It is therefore important to warn patients of the risk, to begin therapy with low doses, and to increase the dosage in carefully adjusted increments over a period of 3 to 4 weeks (*see* Dosage and Administration).

Hallucinosis —In controlled trials, pergolide with *l* -dopa caused hallucinosis in about 14% of patients as opposed to 3% taking placebo with *l* -dopa. This was of sufficient severity to cause discontinuation of treatment in about 3% of those enrolled; tolerance to this untoward effect was not observed.

Fatalities —In the placebo-controlled trial, 2 of 187 patients treated with placebo died as compared with 1 of 189 patients treated with pergolide. Of the 2299 patients treated with pergolide in premarketing studies evaluated as of October 1988, 143 died while on the drug or shortly after discontinuing it. Because the patient population under evaluation was elderly, ill, and at high risk for death, it seems unlikely that pergolide played any role in these deaths, but the possibility that pergolide shortens survival of patients cannot be excluded with absolute certainty.

In particular, a case-by-case review of the clinical course of the patients who died failed to disclose any unique set of signs, symptoms, or laboratory results that would suggest that treatment with pergolide caused their deaths. Sixty-eight percent (68%) of the patients who died were 65 years of age or older. No death (other than a suicide) occurred within the first month of treatment; most of the patients who died had been on pergolide for years. A relative frequency of the causes of death by organ system are: Pulmonary failure/Pneumonia, 35%; Cardiovascular, 30%; Cancer, 11%; Unknown, 8.4%; Infection, 3.5%; Extrapyramidal syndrome, 3.5%; Stroke, 2.1%; Dysphagia, 2.1%; Injury, 1.4%; Suicide, 1.4%; Dehydration, 0.7%; Glomerulonephritis, 0.7%.

Serous Inflammation and Fibrosis —There have been rare reports of pulmonary fibrosis, pleuritis, pleural effusion, pleural fibrosis, pericarditis, pericardial effusion, cardiac valvulopathy, involving one or more valves, or retroperitoneal fibrosis in patients taking pergolide. In some cases, symptoms or manifestations of cardiac valvulopathy improved after discontinuation of pergolide.

Specific risk factors predisposing patients to developing fibrosis with ergot alkaloids have not been identified.

Before initiating treatment with pergolide, therapeutic benefits should be carefully weighed against potential risks taking into account the risk-benefit assessment of other ergot and non-ergot anti-Parkinsonian medication.

Pergolide should be used with caution in patients with a history of these conditions, particularly those patients who experienced the events while taking ergot derivatives. Patients with a history of such events should be carefully monitored clinically and with appropriate radiographic and laboratory studies while taking pergolide.

If a patient develops a fibrotic condition while on pergolide, the drug should be discontinued.

PRECAUTIONS

General —Caution should be exercised when administering pergolide to patients prone to cardiac dysrhythmias.

In a study comparing pergolide and placebo, patients taking pergolide were found to have significantly more episodes of atrial premature contractions (APCs) and sinus tachycardia.

The use of pergolide in patients on *l* -dopa may cause and/or exacerbate preexisting states of confusion and hallucinations (*see* Warnings) and preexisting dyskinesia. Also, the abrupt discontinuation of pergolide in patients receiving it chronically as an adjunct to *l*-dopa may precipitate the onset of hallucinations and confusion; these may occur within a span of several days. Discontinuation of pergolide should be undertaken gradually whenever possible, even if the patient is to remain on *l*-dopa.

A symptom complex resembling the neuroleptic malignant syndrome (NMS) (characterized by elevated temperature, muscular rigidity, altered consciousness, and autonomic instability), with no other obvious etiology, has been reported in association with rapid dose reduction, withdrawal of, or changes in antiparkinsonian therapy, including pergolide.

Information for Patients —Because pergolide may cause somnolence and the possibility of falling asleep during activities of daily living, patients should be cautioned about operating hazardous machinery, including automobiles, until they are reasonably certain that pergolide therapy does not affect them adversely. Patients should be advised that if increased somnolence or new episodes of falling asleep during activities of daily living (e.g., watching television, passenger in a car, etc.) are experienced at any time during treatment, they should not drive or participate in potentially dangerous activities until they have contacted their physician. Due to the possible additive sedative effects, caution should also be used when patients are taking other CNS depressants in combination with pergolide.

Patients and their families should be informed of the common adverse consequences of the use of pergolide (*see* Adverse Reactions) and the risk of hypotension (*see* Warnings).

Patients should be advised to notify their physician if they become pregnant or intend to become pregnant during therapy.

Patients should be advised to notify their physician if they are breast feeding an infant.

Laboratory Tests —No specific laboratory tests are deemed essential for the management of patients on Permax. Periodic routine evaluation of all patients, however, is appropriate.

Drug Interactions —Dopamine antagonists, such as the neuroleptics (phenothiazines, butyrophenones, thioxanthines) or metoclopramide, ordinarily should not be administered concurrently with Permax (a dopamine agonist); these agents may diminish the effectiveness of Permax.

Because pergolide is approximately 90% bound to plasma proteins, caution should be exercised if pergolide is coadministered with other drugs known to affect protein binding.

Carcinogenesis, Mutagenesis, and Impairment of Fertility —A 2-year carcinogenicity study was conducted in mice using dietary levels of pergolide equivalent to oral doses of 0.6, 3.7, and 36.4 mg/kg/day in males and 0.6, 4.4, and 40.8 mg/kg/day in females. A 2-year study in rats was conducted using dietary levels equivalent to oral doses of 0.04, 0.18, and 0.88 mg/kg/day in males and 0.05, 0.28, and 1.42 mg/kg/day in females. The highest doses tested in the mice and rats were approximately 340 and 12 times the maximum human oral dose administered in controlled clinical trials (6 mg/day equivalent to 0.12 mg/kg/day).

A low incidence of uterine neoplasms occurred in both rats and mice. Endometrial adenomas and carcinomas were observed in rats. Endometrial sarcomas were observed in mice. The occurrence of these neoplasms is probably attributable to the high estrogen/progesterone ratio that would occur in rodents as a result of the prolactin-inhibiting action of pergolide. The endocrine mechanisms believed to be involved in the rodents are not present in humans. However, even though there is no known correlation between uterine malignancies occurring in pergolide-treated rodents and human risk, there are no human data to substantiate this conclusion.

Pergolide was evaluated for mutagenic potential in a battery of tests that included an Ames bacterial mutation assay, a DNA repair assay in cultured rat hepatocytes, an in vitro mammalian cell gene mutation assay in cultured L5178Y cells, and a determination of chromosome alteration in bone marrow cells of Chinese hamsters. A weak mutagenic response was noted in the mammalian cell gene mutation assay only after metabolic activation with rat liver microsomes. No mutagenic effects were obtained in the 2 other in vitro assays and in the vivo assay. The relevance of these findings in humans is unknown.

A fertility study in male and female mice showed that fertility was maintained at 0.6 and 1.7 mg/kg/day but decreased at 5.6 mg/kg/day. Prolactin has been reported to be involved in stimulating and maintaining progesterone levels required for implantation in mice and, therefore, the impaired fertility at the high dose may have occurred because of depressed prolactin levels.

Usage in Pregnancy —Pregnancy Category B —Reproduction studies were conducted in mice at doses of 5, 16, and 45 mg/kg/day and in rabbits at doses of 2, 6, and 16 mg/kg/day. The highest doses tested in mice and rabbits were 375 and 133 times the 6 mg/day maximum human dose administered in controlled clinical trials. In these studies, there was no evidence of harm to the fetus due to pergolide.

There are, however, no adequate and well-controlled studies in pregnant women. Among women who received pergolide for endocrine disorders in premarketing studies, there were 33 pregnancies that resulted in healthy babies and 6 pregnancies that resulted in congenital abnormalities (3 major, 3 minor); a causal relationship has not been established. Because human data are limited and because animal reproduction studies are not always predictive of human response, this drug should be used during pregnancy only if clearly needed.

Nursing Mothers —It is not known whether this drug is excreted in human milk. The pharmacologic action of pergolide suggests that it may interfere with lactation. Because many drugs are excreted in human milk and because of the potential for serious adverse reactions to pergolide in nursing infants, a decision should be made whether to discontinue nursing or to discontinue the drug, taking into account the importance of the drug to the mother.

Pediatric Use —Safety and effectiveness in pediatric patients have not been established.

Geriatric Use —Of the total number of subjects in clinical studies of pergolide, 78 were 65 and over. There were no apparent differences in efficacy between these subjects and younger subjects. There was an increased incidence of confusion, somnolence, and peripheral edema in patients 65 and over. Other reported clinical experience has not identified differences in responses between the elderly and younger patients, but greater sensitivity of some older individuals cannot be ruled out. This drug is known to be substantially excreted by the kidney, and the risk of toxic reactions to this drug may be greater in patients with impaired renal function. Because elderly patients are more likely to have decreased renal function, care should be taken in dose selection, and it may be useful to monitor renal function.

ADVERSE REACTIONS

Commonly Observed —In premarketing clinical trials, the most commonly observed adverse events associated with use of pergolide which were not seen at an equivalent incidence among placebo-treated patients were: nervous system complaints, including dyskinesia, hallucinations, somnolence, insomnia; digestive complaints, including nausea, constipation, diarrhea, dyspepsia; and respiratory system complaints, including rhinitis.

Associated With Discontinuation of Treatment —Twenty-seven percent (27%) of approximately 1200 patients receiving pergolide for treatment of Parkinson's disease in premarketing clinical trials in the US and Canada discontinued treatment due to adverse events. The events most commonly causing discontinuation were related to the nervous system (15.5%), primarily hallucinations (7.8%) and confusion (1.8%).

Fatalities —*See* Warnings.

Incidence in Controlled Clinical Trials —The table that follows enumerates adverse events that occurred at a frequency of 1% or more among patients taking pergolide who participated in the premarketing controlled clinical trials comparing pergolide with placebo. In a double-blind, controlled study of 6 months' duration, patients with Parkinson's disease were continued on *l*-dopa/carbidopa and were randomly assigned to receive either pergolide or placebo as additional therapy.

The prescriber should be aware that these figures cannot be used to predict the incidence of side effects in the course of usual medical practice where patient characteristics and other factors differ from those which prevailed in the clinical trials. Similarly, the cited frequencies cannot be compared with figures obtained from other clinical investigations involving different treatments, uses, and investigators. The cited figures, however, do provide the prescribing physician with some basis for estimating the relative contribution of drug and nondrug factors to the side-effect incidence rate in the population studied.

[See table above]

Events Observed During the Premarketing Evaluation of Permax— This section reports event frequencies evaluated as of October 1988 for adverse events occurring in a group of approximately 1800 patients who took multiple doses of pergolide. The conditions and duration of exposure to pergolide varied greatly, involving well-controlled studies as well as experience in open and uncontrolled clinical settings. In the absence of appropriate controls in some of the studies, a causal relationship between these events and treatment with pergolide mesylate cannot be determined.

The following enumeration by organ system describes events in terms of their relative frequency of reporting in the data base. Events of major clinical importance are also described in the Warnings and Precautions sections.

The following definitions of frequency are used: frequent adverse events are defined as those occurring in at least 1/100 patients; infrequent adverse events are those occurring in 1/100 to 1/1000 patients; rare events are those occurring in fewer than 1/1000 patients.

Body as a Whole—*Frequent:* headache, asthenia, accidental injury, pain, abdominal pain, chest pain, back pain, flu syndrome, neck pain, fever; *Infrequent:* facial edema, chills, enlarged abdomen, malaise, neoplasm, hernia, pelvic pain, sepsis, cellulitis, moniliasis, abscess, jaw pain, hypothermia; *Rare:* acute abdominal syndrome, LE syndrome.

Cardiovascular System—*Frequent:* postural hypotension, syncope, hypertension, palpitations, vasodilatations, congestive heart failure; *Infrequent:* myocardial infarction, tachycardia, heart arrest, abnormal electrocardiogram, angina pectoris, thrombophlebitis, bradycardia, ventricular extrasystoles, cerebrovascular accident, ventricular tachycardia, cerebral ischemia, atrial fibrillation, varicose vein, pulmonary embolus, AV block, shock; *Rare:* vasculitis, pulmonary hypertension, pericarditis, migraine, heart block, cerebral hemorrhage.

Digestive System—*Frequent:* nausea, vomiting, dyspepsia, diarrhea, constipation, dry mouth, dysphagia; *Infrequent:* flatulence, abnormal liver function tests, increased appetite, salivary gland enlargement, thirst, gastroenteritis, gastritis, periodontal abscess, intestinal obstruction, nausea and vomiting, gingivitis, esophagitis, cholelithiasis, tooth caries, hepatitis, stomach ulcer, melena, hepatomegaly, hematemesis, eructation; *Rare:* sialadenitis, peptic ulcer, pancreatitis, jaundice, glossitis, fecal incontinence, duodenitis, colitis, cholecystitis, aphthous stomatitis, esophageal ulcer.

Endocrine System—*Infrequent:* hypothyroidism, adenoma, diabetes mellitus, ADH inappropriate; *Rare:* endocrine disorder, thyroid adenoma.

Hemic and Lymphatic System—*Frequent:* anemia; *Infrequent:* leukopenia, lymphadenopathy, leukocytosis, thrombocytopenia, petechia, megaloblastic anemia, cyanosis; *Rare:* purpura, lymphocytosis, eosinophilia, thrombocythemia, acute lymphoblastic leukemia, polycythemia, splenomegaly.

Metabolic and Nutritional System—*Frequent:* peripheral edema, weight loss, weight gain; *Infrequent:* dehydration, hypokalemia, hypoglycemia, iron deficiency anemia, hyperglycemia, gout, hypercholesteremia; *Rare:* electrolyte imbalance, cachexia, acidosis, hyperuricemia.

Musculoskeletal System—*Frequent:* twitching, myalgia, arthralgia; *Infrequent:* bone pain, tenosynovitis, myositis, bone sarcoma, arthritis; *Rare:* osteoporosis, muscle atrophy, osteomyelitis.

Nervous System—*Frequent:* dyskinesia, dizziness, hallucinations, confusion, somnolence, insomnia, dystonia, paresthesia, depression, anxiety, tremor, akinesia, extrapyramidal syndrome, abnormal gait, abnormal dreams, incoordination, psychosis, personality disorder, nervousness, choreoathetosis, amnesia, paranoid reaction, abnormal thinking; *Infrequent:* akathisia, neuropathy, neuralgia, hypertonia, delusions, convulsion, libido increased, euphoria, emotional lability, libido decreased, vertigo, myoclonus, coma, apathy, paralysis, neurosis, hyperkinesia, ataxia, acute brain syndrome, torticollis, meningitis, manic reaction, hypokinesia, hostility, agitation, hypotonia; *Rare:* stupor, neuritis, intracranial hypertension, hemiplegia, facial paralysis, brain edema, myelitis, hallucinations and confusion after abrupt discontinuation.

Respiratory System—*Frequent:* rhinitis, dyspnea, pneumonia, pharyngitis, cough increased; *Infrequent:* epistaxis, hiccup, sinusitis, bronchitis, voice alteration, hemoptysis, asthma, lung edema, pleural effusion, laryngitis, emphysema, apnea, hyperventilation; *Rare:* pneumothorax, lung fibrosis, larynx edema, hypoxia, hypoventilation, hemothorax, carcinoma of lung.

Skin and Appendages System—*Frequent:* sweating, rash; *Infrequent:* skin discoloration, pruritus, acne, skin ulcer, alopecia, dry skin, skin carcinoma, seborrhea, hirsutism, herpes simplex, eczema, fungal dermatitis, herpes zoster; *Rare:* vesiculobullous rash, subcutaneous nodule, skin nodule, skin benign neoplasm, lichenoid dermatitis.

Special Senses System—*Frequent:* abnormal vision, diplopia; *Infrequent:* otitis media, conjunctivitis, tinnitus, deafness, taste perversion, ear pain, eye pain, glaucoma, eye hemorrhage, photophobia, visual field defect; *Rare:* blindness, cataract, retinal detachment, retinal vascular disorder.

Urogenital System—*Frequent:* urinary tract infection, urinary frequency, urinary incontinence, hematuria, dysmenorrhea; *Infrequent:* dysuria, breast pain, menorrhagia, impotence, cystitis, urinary retention, abortion, vaginal hemorrhage, vaginitis, priapism, kidney calculus, fibrocystic breast, lactation, uterine hemorrhage, urolithiasis, salpingitis, pyuria, metrorrhagia, menopause, kidney failure, breast carcinoma, cervical carcinoma; *Rare:* amenorrhea, bladder carcinoma, breast engorgement, epididymitis, hypo-

Incidence of Treatment-Emergent Adverse Experiences in the Placebo-Controlled Clinical Trial

Body System/ Adverse Event*	Percentage of Patients Reporting Events Pergolide N = 189	Placebo N =187
Body as a Whole		
Pain	7.0	2.1
Abdominal pain	5.8	2.1
Injury, accident	5.8	7.0
Headache	5.3	6.4
Asthenia	4.2	4.8
Chest pain	3.7	2.1
Flu syndrome	3.2	2.1
Neck pain	2.7	1.6
Back pain	1.6	2.1
Surgical procedure	1.6	<1
Chills	1.1	0
Face edema	1.1	0
Infection	1.1	0
Cardiovascular		
Postural hypotension	9.0	7.0
Vasodilatation	3.2	<1
Palpitation	2.1	<1
Hypotension	2.1	<1
Syncope	2.1	1.1
Hypertension	1.6	1.1
Arrhythmia	1.1	<1
Myocardial infarction	1.1	<1
Digestive		
Nausea	24.3	12.8
Constipation	10.6	5.9
Diarrhea	6.4	2.7
Dyspepsia	6.4	2.1
Anorexia	4.8	2.7
Dry mouth	3.7	<1
Vomiting	2.7	1.6
Hemic and Lymphatic		
Anemia	1.1	<1
Metabolic and Nutritional		
Peripheral edema	7.4	4.3
Edema	1.6	0
Weight gain	1.6	0
Musculoskeletal		
Arthralgia	1.6	2.1
Bursitis	1.6	<1
Myalgia	1.1	<1
Twitching	1.1	0
Nervous System		
Dyskinesia	62.4	24.6
Dizziness	19.1	13.9
Hallucinations	13.8	3.2
Dystonia	11.6	8.0
Confusion	11.1	9.6
Somnolence	10.1	3.7
Insomnia	7.9	3.2
Anxiety	6.4	4.3
Tremor	4.2	7.5
Depression	3.2	5.4
Abnormal dreams	2.7	4.3
Personality disorder	2.1	<1
Psychosis	2.1	0
Abnormal gait	1.6	1.6
Akathisia	1.6	0
Extrapyramidal syndrome	1.6	1.1
Incoordination	1.6	<1
Paresthesia	1.6	3.2
Akinesia	1.1	1.1
Hypertonia	1.1	0
Neuralgia	1.1	<1
Speech disorder	1.1	1.6
Respiratory System		
Rhinitis	12.2	5.4
Dyspnea	4.8	1.1
Epistaxis	1.6	<1
Hiccup	1.1	0
Skin and Appendages		
Rash	3.2	2.1
Sweating	2.1	2.7
Special Senses		
Abnormal vision	5.8	5.4
Diplopia	2.1	0
Taste perversion	1.6	0
Eye disorder	1.1	0
Urogenital System		
Urinary frequency	2.7	6.4
Urinary tract infection	2.7	3.7
Hematuria	1.1	<1

* Events reported by at least 1% of patients receiving pergolide are included.

Continued on next page

Permax—Cont.

gonadism, leukorrhea, nephrosis, pyelonephritis, urethral pain, uricaciduria, withdrawal bleeding.

Postintroduction Reports—Voluntary reports of adverse events temporally associated with pergolide that have been received since market introduction and which may have no causal relationship with the drug, include the following: neuroleptic malignant syndrome.

OVERDOSAGE

There is no clinical experience with massive overdosage. The largest overdose involved a young hospitalized adult patient who was not being treated with pergolide but who intentionally took 60 mg of the drug. He experienced vomiting, hypotension, and agitation. Another patient receiving a daily dosage of 7 mg of pergolide unintentionally took 19 mg/day for 3 days, after which his vital signs were normal but he experienced severe hallucinations. Within 36 hours of resumption of the prescribed dosage level, the hallucinations stopped. One patient unintentionally took 14 mg/day for 23 days instead of her prescribed 1.4 mg/day dosage. She experienced severe involuntary movements and tingling in her arms and legs. Another patient who inadvertently received 7 mg instead of the prescribed 0.7 mg experienced palpitations, hypotension, and ventricular extrasystoles. The highest total daily dose (prescribed for several patients with refractory Parkinson's disease) has exceeded 30 mg.

Symptoms —Animal studies indicate that the manifestations of overdosage in man might include nausea, vomiting, convulsions, decreased blood pressure, and CNS stimulation. The oral median lethal doses in mice and rats were 54 and 15 mg/kg respectively.

Treatment —To obtain up-to-date information about the treatment of overdose, a good resource is your certified Regional Poison Control Center. Telephone numbers of certified poison control centers are listed in the *Physicians' Desk Reference (PDR)*. In managing overdosage, consider the possibility of multiple drug overdoses, interaction among drugs, and unusual drug kinetics in your patient.

Management of overdosage may require supportive measures to maintain arterial blood pressure. Cardiac function should be monitored; an antiarrhythmic agent may be necessary. If signs of CNS stimulation are present, a phenothiazine or other butyrophenone neuroleptic agent may be indicated; the efficacy of such drugs in reversing the effects of overdose has not been assessed.

Protect the patient's airway and support ventilation and perfusion. Meticulously monitor and maintain, within acceptable limits, the patient's vital signs, blood gases, serum electrolytes, etc. Absorption of drugs from the gastrointestinal tract may be decreased by giving activated charcoal, which, in many cases, is more effective than emesis or lavage; consider charcoal instead of or in addition to gastric emptying. Repeated doses of charcoal over time may hasten elimination of some drugs that have been absorbed. Safeguard the patient's airway when employing gastric emptying or charcoal.

There is no experience with dialysis or hemoperfusion, and these procedures are unlikely to be of benefit.

DOSAGE AND ADMINISTRATION

Administration of Permax should be initiated with a daily dosage of 0.05 mg for the first 2 days. The dosage should then be gradually increased by 0.1 or 0.15 mg/day every third day over the next 12 days of therapy. The dosage may then be increased by 0.25 mg/day every third day until an optimal therapeutic dosage is achieved.

Permax is usually administered in divided doses 3 times per day. During dosage titration, the dosage of concurrent *l*-dopa/carbidopa may be cautiously decreased.

In clinical studies, the mean therapeutic daily dosage of Permax was 3 mg/day. The average concurrent daily dosage of *l*-dopa/carbidopa (expressed as *l*-dopa) was approximately 650 mg/day. The efficacy of Permax at doses above 5 mg/day has not been systematically evaluated.

HOW SUPPLIED

Tablets (modified rectangle shape, scored):

0.05 mg, ivory, debossed with A 024, in bottles of 30 (UC5336)—NDC 65234-024-30

0.25 mg, green, debossed with A 025, in bottles of 100 (UC5337)—NDC 65234-025-10

1 mg, pink, debossed with A 026, in bottles of 100 (UC5338)—NDC 65234-026-10

Store at 25°C (77°F); excursions permitted to 15–30°C (59°–86°F) [See USP Controlled Room Temperature].

PERMAX is a registered trademark of Eli Lilly and Company, and licensed in the U.S. to Valeant Pharmaceuticals International.

Literature revised November 11, 2003.

Manufactured by:
Eli Lilly and Company
Indianapolis, IN 46285, USA

Distributed by:
Valeant Pharmaceuticals International
3300 Hyland Ave. Costa Mesa, CA 92626

Shown in Product Identification Guide, page 335

PHRENILIN® ℞
[fren 'ĭ-lin]
(Butalbital 50 mg and Acetaminophen 325 mg Tablet) and

PHRENILIN® FORTE ℞
(Butalbital 50 mg and Acetaminophen 650 mg Capsule)

HOW SUPPLIED

PHRENILIN®: Pale violet scored tablets with the letter A on one side and 50 on the other, in bottles of 100 (NDC 65234-050-10) in bottles of 500 (NDC 65234-050-50). Each tablet contains butalbital, USP 50 mg and acetaminophen USP 325 mg.

PHRENILIN® FORTE: Amethyst, opaque capsules imprinted with the letter A and 056, in bottles of 100 (NDC 65234-056-10) in bottles of 500 (NDC 65234-056-50). Each capsule contains butalbital, USP 50 mg and acetaminophen USP 650 mg.

Store PHRENILIN® and PHRENILIN® FORTE (Butalbital and Acetaminophen) at controlled room temperature, 15°–30°C (59°–86°F). Dispense in a tight container as defined in the USP.

Rx only

Manufactured for Valeant Pharmaceuticals International

Shown in Product Identification Guide, page 335

TASMAR® ℞
(tolcapone)
TABLETS

Before prescribing TASMAR, the physician should be thoroughly familiar with the details of this prescribing information.

TASMAR SHOULD NOT BE USED BY PATIENTS UNTIL THERE HAS BEEN A COMPLETE DISCUSSION OF THE RISKS AND THE PATIENT HAS PROVIDED WRITTEN INFORMED CONSENT (SEE PATIENT CONSENT SECTION).

WARNING:

Because of the risk of potentially fatal, acute fulminant liver failure, TASMAR (tolcapone) should ordinarily be used in patients with Parkinson's disease on l-dopa/carbidopa who are experiencing symptom fluctuations and are not responding satisfactorily to or are not appropriate candidates for other adjunctive therapies (see INDICATIONS and DOSAGE AND ADMINISTRATION sections).

Because of the risk of liver injury and because TASMAR, when it is effective, provides an observable symptomatic benefit, the patient who fails to show substantial clinical benefit within 3 weeks of initiation of treatment, should be withdrawn from TASMAR.

TASMAR therapy should not be initiated if the patient exhibits clinical evidence of liver disease or two SGPT/ALT or SGOT/AST values greater than the upper limit of normal. Patients with severe dyskinesia or dystonia should be treated with caution (see PRECAUTIONS: *Rhabdomyolysis*).

Patients who develop evidence of hepatocellular injury while on TASMAR and are withdrawn from the drug for any reason may be at increased risk for liver injury if TASMAR is reintroduced. Accordingly, such patients should not ordinarily be considered for retreatment.

Cases of severe hepatocellular injury, including fulminant liver failure resulting in death, have been reported in postmarketing use. As of October 1998, 3 cases of fatal fulminant hepatic failure have been reported from approximately 60,000 patients providing about 40,000 patient years of worldwide use. This incidence may be 10- to 100-fold higher than the background incidence in the general population. Underreporting of cases may lead to significant underestimation of the increased risk associated with the use of TASMAR.

A prescriber who elects to use TASMAR in face of the increased risk of liver injury is strongly advised to monitor patients for evidence of emergent liver injury. Patients should be advised of the need for self-monitoring for both the classical signs of liver disease (eg, clay colored stools, jaundice) and the nonspecific ones (eg, fatigue, loss of appetite, lethargy).

Although a program of frequent laboratory monitoring for evidence of hepatocellular injury is deemed essential, it is not clear that baseline and periodic monitoring of liver enzymes will prevent the occurrence of fulminant liver failure. However, it is generally believed that early detection of drug-induced hepatic injury along with immediate withdrawal of the suspect drug enhances the likelihood for recovery. It is also widely held, without a robust body of evidence, that patients with preexisting hepatic disease are more vulnerable to hepatotoxins. Accordingly, the following liver monitoring program is recommended.

Before starting treatment with TASMAR, the physician should conduct appropriate tests to exclude the presence of liver disease. In patients determined to be appropriate candidates for treatment with TASMAR, serum glutamic-pyruvic transaminase (SGPT/ALT) and serum glutamic-oxaloacetic transaminase (SGOT/AST) levels should be determined at baseline and then every 2 weeks for the first year of therapy, every 4 weeks for the next 6 months, and then every 8 weeks thereafter. If the dose is increased to 200 mg tid (see DOSAGE AND ADMINISTRATION section), liver enzyme monitoring should take place before increasing the dose and then be reinitiated at the frequency above.

TASMAR should be discontinued if SGPT/ALT or SGOT/AST exceeds the upper limit of normal or if clinical signs and symptoms suggest the onset of hepatic failure (persistent nausea, fatigue, lethargy, anorexia, jaundice, dark urine, pruritus, and right upper quadrant tenderness).

DESCRIPTION

TASMAR® is available as tablets containing 100 mg or 200 mg tolcapone.

Tolcapone, an inhibitor of catechol-*O*-methyltransferase (COMT), is used in the treatment of Parkinson's disease as an adjunct to levodopa/carbidopa therapy. It is a yellow, odorless, non-hygroscopic, crystalline compound with a relative molecular mass of 273.25. The chemical name of tolcapone is 3,4-dihydroxy-4'-methyl-5-nitrobenzophenone. Its empirical formula is $C_{14}H_{11}NO_5$.

Inactive ingredients: Core: lactose monohydrate, microcrystalline cellulose, dibasic calcium phosphate anhydrous, povidone K-30, sodium starch glycolate, talc and magnesium stearate. Film coating: hydroxypropyl methyl-cellulose, titanium dioxide, talc, ethylcellulose, triacetin and sodium lauryl sulfate, with the following dye systems: 100 mg—yellow and red iron oxide; 200 mg—red iron oxide.

CLINICAL PHARMACOLOGY

Mechanism of Action: Tolcapone is a selective and reversible inhibitor of catechol-*O*-methyltransferase (COMT).

In mammals, COMT is distributed throughout various organs. The highest activities are in the liver and kidney. COMT also occurs in the heart, lung, smooth and skeletal muscles, intestinal tract, reproductive organs, various glands, adipose tissue, skin, blood cells and neuronal tissues, especially in glial cells. COMT catalyzes the transfer of the methyl group of S-adenosyl-L-methionine to the phenolic group of substrates that contain a catechol structure. Physiological substrates of COMT include dopa, catecholamines (dopamine, norepinephrine, epinephrine) and their hydroxylated metabolites. The function of COMT is the elimination of biologically active catechols and some other hydroxylated metabolites. In the presence of a decarboxylase inhibitor, COMT becomes the major metabolizing enzyme for levodopa catalyzing the metabolism to 3-methoxy-4-hydroxy-L-phenylalanine (3-OMD) in the brain and periphery.

The precise mechanism of action of tolcapone is unknown, but it is believed to be related to its ability to inhibit COMT and alter the plasma pharmacokinetics of levodopa. When tolcapone is given in conjunction with levodopa and an aromatic amino acid decarboxylase inhibitor, such as carbidopa, plasma levels of levodopa are more sustained than after administration of levodopa and an aromatic amino acid decarboxylase inhibitor alone. It is believed that these sustained plasma levels of levodopa result in more constant dopaminergic stimulation in the brain, leading to greater effects on the signs and symptoms of Parkinson's disease in patients as well as increased levodopa adverse effects, sometimes requiring a decrease in the dose of levodopa. Tolcapone enters the CNS to a minimal extent, but has been shown to inhibit central COMT activity in animals.

Pharmacodynamics: *COMT Activity in Erythrocytes:* Studies in healthy volunteers have shown that tolcapone reversibly inhibits human erythrocyte catechol-*O*-methyltransferase (COMT) activity after oral administration. The inhibition is closely related to plasma tolcapone concentrations. With a 200-mg single dose of tolcapone, maximum inhibition of erythrocyte COMT activity is on average greater than 80%. During multiple dosing with tolcapone (200 mg tid), erythrocyte COMT inhibition at trough tolcapone blood concentrations is 30% to 45%.

Effect on the Pharmacokinetics of Levodopa and its Metabolites: When tolcapone is administered together with levodopa/carbidopa, it increases the relative bioavailability (AUC) of levodopa by approximately twofold. This is due to a decrease in levodopa clearance resulting in a prolongation of the terminal elimination half-life of levodopa (from approximately 2 hours to 3.5 hours). In general, the average peak levodopa plasma concentration (C_{max}) and the time of its occurrence (T_{max}) are unaffected. The onset of effect occurs after the first administration and is maintained during long-term treatment. Studies in healthy volunteers and Parkinson's disease patients have confirmed that the maximal effect occurs with 100 mg to 200 mg tolcapone. Plasma levels of 3-OMD are markedly and dose-dependently decreased by tolcapone when given with levodopa/carbidopa. Population pharmacokinetic analyses in patients with Parkinson's disease have shown the same effects of tolcapone on levodopa plasma concentrations that occur in healthy volunteers.

Pharmacokinetics of Tolcapone: Tolcapone pharmacokinetics are linear over the dose range of 50 mg to 400 mg, independent of levodopa/carbidopa coadministration. The elimination half-life of tolcapone is 2 to 3 hours and there is no significant accumulation. With tid dosing of 100 mg or 200 mg, C_{max} is approximately 3 μg/mL and 6 μg/mL, respectively.

Absorption: Tolcapone is rapidly absorbed, with a T_{max} of approximately 2 hours. The absolute bioavailability following oral administration is about 65%. Food given within 1 hour before and 2 hours after dosing of tolcapone decreases the relative bioavailability by 10% to 20% (see DOSAGE AND ADMINISTRATION).

Distribution: The steady-state volume of distribution of tolcapone is small (9 L). Tolcapone does not distribute widely into tissues due to its high plasma protein binding. The plasma protein binding of tolcapone is >99.9% over the concentration range of 0.32 to 210 µg/mL. In vitro experiments have shown that tolcapone binds mainly to serum albumin.

Metabolism and Elimination: Tolcapone is almost completely metabolized prior to excretion, with only a very small amount (0.5% of dose) found unchanged in urine. The main metabolic pathway of tolcapone is glucuronidation; the glucuronide conjugate is inactive. In addition, the compound is methylated by COMT to 3-*O*-methyl-tolcapone. Tolcapone is metabolized to a primary alcohol (hydroxylation of the methyl group), which is subsequently oxidized to the carboxylic acid. In vitro experiments suggest that the oxidation may be catalyzed by cytochrome P450 3A4 and P450 2A6. The reduction to an amine and subsequent *N*-acetylation occur to a minor extent. After oral administration of a ^{14}C-labeled dose of tolcapone, 60% of labeled material is excreted in urine and 40% in feces.

Tolcapone is a low-extraction-ratio drug (extraction ratio = 0.15) with a moderate systemic clearance of about 7 L/h.

Special Populations: Tolcapone pharmacokinetics are independent of sex, age, body weight, and race (Japanese, Black and Caucasian). Polymorphic metabolism is unlikely based on the metabolic pathways involved.

Hepatic Impairment: A study in patients with hepatic impairment has shown that moderate non-cirrhotic liver disease had no impact on the pharmacokinetics of tolcapone. In patients with moderate cirrhotic liver disease (Child-Pugh Class B), however, clearance and volume of distribution of unbound tolcapone was reduced by almost 50%. This reduction may increase the average concentration of unbound drug by twofold (see DOSAGE AND ADMINISTRATION). TASMAR therapy should not be initiated if the patient exhibits clinical evidence of active liver disease or two SGPT/ALT or SGOT/AST values greater than the upper limit of normal (see BOXED WARNING).

Renal Impairment: The pharmacokinetics of tolcapone have not been investigated in a specific renal impairment study. However, the relationship of renal function and tolcapone pharmacokinetics has been investigated using population pharmacokinetics during clinical trials. The data of more than 400 patients have confirmed that over a wide range of creatinine clearance values (30 mL/min to 130 mL/min) the pharmacokinetics of tolcapone are unaffected by renal function. This could be explained by the fact that only a negligible amount of unchanged tolcapone (0.5%) is excreted in the urine. The glucuronide conjugate of tolcapone is mainly excreted in the urine but is also excreted in the bile. Accumulation of this stable and inactive metabolite should not present a risk in renally impaired patients with creatinine clearance above 25 mL/min (see DOSAGE AND ADMINISTRATION). Given the very high protein binding of tolcapone, no significant removal of the drug by hemodialysis would be expected.

Drug Interactions: See PRECAUTIONS: *Drug Interactions.*

Clinical Studies: The effectiveness of TASMAR as an adjunct to levodopa in the treatment of Parkinson's disease was established in three multicenter randomized controlled trials of 13 to 26 weeks' duration, supported by four 6-week trials whose results were consistent with those of the longer trials. In two of the longer trials, tolcapone was evaluated in patients whose Parkinson's disease was characterized by deterioration in their response to levodopa at the end of a dosing interval (so-called fluctuating patients with wearing-off phenomena). In the remaining trial, tolcapone was evaluated in patients whose response to levodopa was relatively stable (so-called non-fluctuators).

Fluctuating Patients: In two 3-month trials, patients with documented episodes of wearing-off phenomena, despite optimum levodopa therapy, were randomized to receive placebo, tolcapone 100 mg tid or 200 mg tid. The formal double-blind portion of the trial was 3 months long, and the primary outcome was a comparison between treatments in the change from baseline in the amount of time spent "On" (a period of relatively good functioning) and "Off" (a period of relatively poor functioning). Patients recorded periodically, throughout the duration of the trial, the time spent in each of these states.

In addition to the primary outcome, patients were also assessed using sub-parts of the Unified Parkinson's Disease Rating Scale (UPDRS), a frequently used multi-item rating scale intended to evaluate mentation (Part I), activities of daily living (Part II), motor function (Part III), complications of therapy (Part IV), and disease staging (Parts V and VI); an Investigator's Global Assessment of Change (IGA), a subjective scale designed to assess global functioning in 5 areas of Parkinson's disease; the Sickness Impact Profile (SIP), a multi-item scale in 12 domains designed to assess the patient's functioning in multiple areas; and the change in daily levodopa/carbidopa dose.

In one of the studies, 202 patients were randomized in 11 centers in the United States and Canada. In this trial, all patients were receiving concomitant levodopa and carbidopa. In the second trial, 177 patients were randomized in 24 centers in Europe. In this trial, all patients were receiving concomitant levodopa and benserazide.

The following tables display the results of these 2 trials:

[See table 1 above]

[See table 2 at top of next page]

Table 1.
US/Canadian Fluctuator Study

Primary Measure

	Baseline (hrs)	**Change from Baseline at Month 3 (hrs)**	**p-value***
*Hours of Wake Time "Off"***			
Placebo	6.2	−1.2	—
100 mg tid	6.4	−2.0	0.169
200 mg tid	5.9	−3.0	<0.001
*Hours of Wake Time "On"***			
Placebo	8.7	1.4	—
100 mg tid	8.1	2.0	0.267
200 mg tid	9.1	2.9	0.008

Secondary Measures

	Baseline	**Change from Baseline at Month 3**	**p-value***
Levodopa Total Daily Dose (mg)			
Placebo	948	16	—
100 mg tid	788	−166	<0.001
200 mg tid	865	−207	<0.001
Global (overall) % Improved			
Placebo	—	42	—
100 mg tid	—	71	<0.001
200 mg tid	—	91	<0.001
UPDRS Motor			
Placebo	19.5	−0.4	—
100 mg tid	17.6	−1.9	0.217
200 mg tid	20.6	−2.0	0.210
UPDRS ADL			
Placebo	7.5	−0.3	—
100 mg tid	7.7	−0.8	0.487
200 mg tid	8.3	0.2	0.412
SIP (total)			
Placebo	14.7	−2.2	—
100 mg tid	14.9	−0.4	0.210
200 mg tid	17.6	−0.3	0.216

*Compared to placebo.
**Hours "Off" or "On" are based on the percent of waking day "Off" or "On", assuming a 16-hour waking day.

Effects on "Off" time and levodopa dose did not differ by age or sex.

Non-fluctuating Patients: In this study, 298 patients with idiopathic Parkinson's disease on stable doses of levodopa/carbidopa who were not experiencing wearing-off phenomena were randomized to placebo, tolcapone 100 mg tid, or tolcapone 200 mg tid for 6 months at 20 centers in the United States and Canada. The primary measure of effectiveness was the Activities of Daily Living portion (Subscale II) of the UPDRS. In addition, the change in daily levodopa dose, other subscales of the UPDRS, and the SIP were assessed as secondary measures. The results are displayed in the following table:

[See table 3 at top of next page]

Effects on Activities of Daily Living did not differ by age or sex.

INDICATIONS

TASMAR is indicated as an adjunct to levodopa and carbidopa for the treatment of the signs and symptoms of idiopathic Parkinson's disease. Because of the risk of potentially fatal, acute fulminant liver failure, TASMAR (tolcapone) should ordinarily be used in patients with Parkinson's disease on l-dopa/carbidopa who are experiencing symptom fluctuations and are not responding satisfactorily to or are not appropriate candidates for other adjunctive therapies. Because of the risk of liver injury and because TASMAR, when it is effective, provides an observable symptomatic benefit, the patient who fails to show substantial clinical benefit within 3 weeks of initiation of treatment, should be withdrawn from TASMAR.

The effectiveness of TASMAR was demonstrated in randomized controlled trials in patients receiving concomitant levodopa therapy with carbidopa or another aromatic amino acid decarboxylase inhibitor who experienced end of dose wearing-off phenomena as well as in patients who did not experience such phenomena (see CLINICAL PHARMACOLOGY: *Clinical Studies*).

CONTRAINDICATIONS

TASMAR tablets are contraindicated in patients with liver disease, in patients who were withdrawn from TASMAR because of evidence of TASMAR-induced hepatocellular injury or who have demonstrated hypersensitivity to the drug or its ingredients.

TASMAR is also contraindicated in patients with a history of non-traumatic rhabdomyolysis or hyperpyrexia and confusion possibly related to medication (see PRECAUTIONS: *Events Reported With Dopaminergic Therapy*).

WARNINGS

(SEE BOXED WARNING) Because of the risk of potentially fatal, acute fulminant liver failure, TASMAR (tolcapone) should ordinarily be used in patients with Parkinson's disease on l-dopa/carbidopa who are experiencing symptom fluctuations and are not responding satisfactorily to or are not appropriate candidates for other adjunctive therapies (see INDICATIONS and DOSAGE AND ADMINISTRATION sections).

Because of the risk of liver injury and because TASMAR, when it is effective, provides an observable symptomatic benefit, the patient who fails to show substantial clinical benefit within 3 weeks of initiation of treatment, should be withdrawn from TASMAR.

TASMAR therapy should not be initiated if the patient exhibits clinical evidence of liver disease or two SGPT/ALT or SGOT/AST values greater than the upper limit of normal. Patients with severe dyskinesia or dystonia should be treated with caution (see PRECAUTIONS: *Rhabdomyolysis*).

Patients who develop evidence of hepatocellular injury while on TASMAR and are withdrawn from the drug for any reason may be at increased risk for liver injury if TASMAR is reintroduced. Accordingly, such patients should not ordinarily be considered for retreatment.

In controlled Phase 3 trials, increases to more than 3 times the upper limit of normal in ALT or AST occurred in approximately 1% of patients at 100 mg tid and 3% of patients at 200 mg tid. Females were more likely than males to have an increase in liver enzymes (approximately 5% vs 2%). Approximately one third of patients with elevated enzymes had diarrhea. Increases to more than 8 times the upper limit of normal in liver enzymes occurred in 0.3% at 100 mg tid and 0.7% at 200 mg tid. Elevated enzymes led to discontinuation in 0.3% and 1.7% of patients treated with 100 mg tid and 200 mg tid, respectively. Elevations usually occurred within 6 weeks to 6 months of starting treatment. In about half the cases with elevated liver enzymes, enzyme levels returned to baseline values within 1 to 3 months while patients continued TASMAR treatment. When treatment was discontinued, enzymes generally declined within 2 to 3 weeks but in some cases took as long as 1 to 2 months to return to normal.

Monoamine oxidase (MAO) and COMT are the two major enzyme systems involved in the metabolism of catecholamines. It is theoretically possible, therefore, that the combination of TASMAR and a non-selective MAO inhibitor (eg, phenelzine and tranylcypromine) would result in inhibition of the majority of the pathways responsible for normal catecholamine metabolism. For this reason, patients should ordinarily not be treated concomitantly with TASMAR and a non-selective MAO inhibitor.

Tolcapone can be taken concomitantly with a selective MAO-B inhibitor (eg, selegiline).

PRECAUTIONS

Hypotension/Syncope: Dopaminergic therapy in Parkinson's disease patients has been associated with orthostatic hypotension. Tolcapone enhances levodopa bioavailability and, therefore, may increase the occurrence of orthostatic

Continued on next page

Tasmar—Cont.

hypotension. In TASMAR clinical trials, orthostatic hypotension was documented at least once in 8%, 14% and 13% of the patients treated with placebo, 100 mg and 200 mg TASMAR tid, respectively. A total of 2%, 5% and 4% of the patients treated with placebo, 100 mg and 200 mg TASMAR tid, respectively, reported orthostatic symptoms at some time during their treatment and also had at least one episode of orthostatic hypotension documented (however, the episode of orthostatic symptoms itself was invariably not accompanied by vital sign measurements). Patients with orthostasis at baseline were more likely than patients without symptoms to have orthostatic hypotension during the study, irrespective of treatment group. In addition, the effect was greater in tolcapone-treated patients than in placebo-treated patients. Baseline treatment with dopamine agonists or selegiline did not appear to increase the likelihood of experiencing orthostatic hypotension when treated with TASMAR. Approximately 0.7% of the patients treated with TASMAR (5% of patients who were documented to have had at least one episode of orthostatic hypotension) eventually withdrew from treatment due to adverse events presumably related to hypotension.

In controlled Phase 3 trials, approximately 5%, 4% and 3% of tolcapone 200 mg tid, 100 mg tid and placebo patients, respectively, reported at least one episode of syncope. Reports of syncope were generally more frequent in patients in all three treatment groups who had an episode of documented hypotension (although the episodes of syncope, obtained by history, were themselves not documented with vital sign measurement) compared to patients who did not have any episodes of documented hypotension.

Diarrhea: In clinical trials, diarrhea developed in approximately 8%, 16% and 18% of patients treated with placebo, 100 mg and 200 mg TASMAR tid, respectively. While diarrhea was generally regarded as mild to moderate in severity, approximately 3% to 4% of patients on tolcapone had diarrhea which was regarded as severe. Diarrhea was the adverse event which most commonly led to discontinuation, with approximately 1%, 5% and 6% of patients treated with placebo, 100 mg and 200 mg TASMAR tid, respectively, withdrawing from the trials prematurely. Discontinuing TASMAR for diarrhea was related to the severity of the symptom. Diarrhea resulted in withdrawal in approximately 8%, 40% and 70% of patients with mild, moderate and severe diarrhea, respectively. Although diarrhea generally resolved after discontinuation of TASMAR, it led to hospitalization in 0.3%, 0.7% and 1.7% of patients in the placebo, 100 mg and 200 mg TASMAR tid groups.

Typically, diarrhea presents 6 to 12 weeks after tolcapone is started, but it may appear as early as 2 weeks and as late as many months after the initiation of treatment. Clinical trial data suggested that diarrhea associated with tolcapone use may sometimes be associated with anorexia (decreased appetite).

No consistent description of tolcapone-induced diarrhea has been derived from clinical trial data, and the mechanism of action is currently unknown.

It is recommended that all cases of persistent diarrhea should be followed up with an appropriate work-up (including occult blood samples).

Hallucinations: In clinical trials, hallucinations developed in approximately 5%, 8% and 10% of patients treated with placebo, 100 mg and 200 mg TASMAR tid, respectively. Hallucinations led to drug discontinuation and premature withdrawal from clinical trials in 0.3%, 1.4% and 1.0% of patients treated with placebo, 100 mg and 200 mg TASMAR tid, respectively. Hallucinations led to hospitalization in 0.0%, 1.7% and 0.0% of patients in the placebo, 100 mg and 200 mg TASMAR tid groups, respectively.

In general, hallucinations present shortly after the initiation of therapy with tolcapone (typically within the first 2 weeks). Clinical trial data suggest that hallucinations associated with tolcapone use may be responsive to levodopa dose reduction. Patients whose hallucinations resolved had a mean levodopa dose reduction of 175 mg to 200 mg (20% to 25%) after the onset of the hallucinations. Hallucinations were commonly accompanied by confusion and to a lesser extent sleep disorder (insomnia) and excessive dreaming.

Dyskinesia: TASMAR may potentiate the dopaminergic side effects of levodopa and may cause and/or exacerbate preexisting dyskinesia. Although decreasing the dose of levodopa may ameliorate this side effect, many patients in controlled trials continued to experience frequent dyskinesias despite a reduction in their dose of levodopa. The rates of withdrawal for dyskinesia were 0.0%, 0.3% and 1.0% for placebo, 100 mg and 200 mg TASMAR tid, respectively.

Rhabdomyolysis: Cases of severe rhabdomyolysis, with one case of multiorgan system failure rapidly progressing to death, have been reported. The complicated nature of these cases makes it impossible to determine what role, if any, TASMAR played in their pathogenesis. Severe prolonged motor activity including dyskinesia may account for rhabdomyolysis. Some cases, however, included fever, alteration of consciousness and muscular rigidity. It is possible, therefore, that the rhabdomyolysis may be a result of the syndrome described in *Hyperpyrexia and Confusion* (see PRECAUTIONS: *Events Reported With Dopaminergic Therapy*).

Renal Impairment: No dosage adjustment is needed in patients with mild to moderate renal impairment, however, patients with severe renal impairment should be treated with caution (see CLINICAL PHARMACOLOGY: *Pharmacokinetics of Tolcapone* and DOSAGE AND ADMINISTRATION).

Table 2.
European Fluctuator Study

Primary Measure

	Baseline (hrs)	Change from Baseline at Month 3 (hrs)	p-value*
*Hours of Wake Time "Off"***			
Placebo	6.1	−0.7	—
100 mg tid	6.5	−2.0	0.008
200 mg tid	6.0	−1.6	0.081
*Hours of Wake Time "On"***			
Placebo	8.5	−0.1	—
100 mg tid	8.1	1.7	0.003
200 mg tid	8.4	1.7	0.003

Secondary Measures

	Baseline	Change from Baseline at Month 3	p-value*
Levodopa Total Daily Dose (mg)			
Placebo	660	−29	—
100 mg tid	667	−109	0.025
200 mg tid	675	−122	0.010
Global (overall) % Improved			
Placebo	—	37	—
100 mg tid	—	70	0.003
200 mg tid	—	78	<0.001
UPDRS Motor			
Placebo	24.0	−2.1	—
100 mg tid	22.4	−4.2	0.163
200 mg tid	22.4	−6.5	0.004
UPDRS ADL			
Placebo	7.9	−0.5	—
100 mg tid	7.5	−0.9	0.408
200 mg tid	7.7	−1.3	0.097
SIP (total)			
Placebo	21.6	−0.9	—
100 mg tid	16.6	−1.9	0.419
200 mg tid	18.4	−4.2	0.011

*Compared to placebo.
**Hours "Off" or "On" are based on the percent of waking day "Off" or "On", assuming a 16-hour waking day.

Table 3.
US/Canadian Non-fluctuator Study

Primary Measure

	Baseline	Change from Baseline at Month 6	p-value*
UPDRS ADL			
Placebo	8.5	0.1	—
100 mg tid	7.5	-1.4	<0.001
200 mg tid	7.9	-1.6	<0.001

Secondary Measures

	Baseline	Change from Baseline at Month 6	p-value*
Levodopa Total Daily Dose (mg)			
Placebo	364	47	—
100 mg tid	370	-21	<0.001
200 mg tid	381	-32	<0.001
UPDRS Motor			
Placebo	19.7	0.1	—
100 mg tid	17.3	-2.0	0.018
200 mg tid	16.0	-2.3	0.008
SIP (total)			
Placebo	6.9	0.4	—
100 mg tid	7.3	-0.9	0.044
200 mg tid	7.3	-0.7	0.078
Percent of Patients who Developed Fluctuations			
Placebo	—	26	—
100 mg tid	—	19	0.297
200 mg tid	—	14	0.047

* Compared to placebo.

Renal Toxicity: When rats were dosed daily for 1 or 2 years (exposures 6 times the human exposure or greater) there was a high incidence of proximal tubule cell damage consisting of degeneration, single cell necrosis, hyperplasia, karyocytomegaly and atypical nuclei. These effects were not associated with changes in clinical chemistry parameters, and there is no established method for monitoring for the possible occurrence of these lesions in humans. Although it has been speculated that these toxicities may occur as the result of a species-specific mechanism, experiments which would confirm that theory have not been conducted.

Hepatic Impairment: Because of the risk of liver injury, TASMAR therapy should not be initiated in any patient with liver disease. For similar reasons, treatment should not be initiated in patients who have two SGPT/ALT or SGOT/AST values greater than the upper limit of normal (see BOXED WARNING) or any other evidence of hepatocellular dysfunction.

Hematuria: The rates of hematuria in placebo-controlled trials were approximately 2%, 4% and 5% in placebo, 100 mg and 200 mg TASMAR tid, respectively. The etiology of the increase with TASMAR has not always been explained (for example, by urinary tract infection or coumadin therapy). In placebo-controlled trials in the United States (N=593) rates of microscopically confirmed hematuria were approximately 3%, 2% and 2% in placebo, 100 mg and 200 mg TASMAR tid, respectively.

Events Reported With Dopaminergic Therapy: The events listed below are known to be associated with the use of drugs that increase dopaminergic activity, although they are most often associated with the use of direct dopamine agonists. While cases of Hyperpyrexia and Confusion have been reported in association with tolcapone withdrawal (see paragraph below), the expected incidence of fibrotic complications is so low that even if tolcapone caused these complications at rates similar to those attributable to other dopaminergic therapies, it is unlikely that even a single example would have been detected in a cohort of the size exposed to tolcapone.

Hyperpyrexia and Confusion: In clinical trials, four cases of a symptom complex resembling the neuroleptic malignant syndrome (characterized by elevated temperature, muscular rigidity, and altered consciousness), similar to that reported in association with the rapid dose reduction or withdrawal of other dopaminergic drugs, have been reported in association with the abrupt withdrawal or lowering of the dose of tolcapone. In 3 of these cases, CPK was elevated as well. One patient died, and the other 3 patients recovered over periods of approximately 2, 4 and 6 weeks. Rare cases of this symptom complex have been reported during marketed use. These cases are of a complicated nature including the concomitant administration of several medications affecting brain monoaminergic (ie, MAO-I, tricyclic and selective serotonin reuptake inhibitors) and anticholinergic systems. It is difficult, therefore, to determine what role, if any, TASMAR played in the pathogenesis. It may, therefore, be prudent to be particularly cautious if several concomitant medications of these types are used.

Fibrotic Complications: Cases of retroperitoneal fibrosis, pulmonary infiltrates, pleural effusion, and pleural thickening have been reported in some patients treated with ergot derived dopaminergic agents. While these complications may resolve when the drug is discontinued, complete resolution does not always occur. Although these adverse events are believed to be related to the ergoline structure of these compounds, whether other, nonergot derived drugs (eg, tolcapone) that increase dopaminergic activity can cause them is unknown.

Three cases of pleural effusion, one with pulmonary fibrosis, occurred during clinical trials. These patients were also on concomitant dopamine agonists (pergolide or bromocriptine) and had a prior history of cardiac disease or pulmonary pathology (nonmalignant lung lesion).

Information for Patients: Patients should be instructed to take TASMAR only as prescribed.

TASMAR should not be used by patients until there has been a complete discussion of the risks and the patient has provided written informed consent (see PATIENT CONSENT section).

Patients should be informed of the clinical signs and symptoms that suggest the onset of hepatic injury (persistent nausea, fatigue, lethargy, anorexia, jaundice, dark urine, pruritus, and right upper quadrant tenderness) (**see WARNINGS**). If symptoms of hepatic failure occur, patients should be advised to contact their physician immediately.

Patients should be informed that hallucinations can occur.

Patients should be informed of the need to have regular blood tests to monitor liver enzymes.

Patients should be advised that they may develop postural (orthostatic) hypotension with or without symptoms such as dizziness, nausea, syncope, and sometimes sweating. Hypotension may occur more frequently during initial therapy. Accordingly, patients should be cautioned against rising rapidly after sitting or lying down, especially if they have been doing so for prolonged periods, and especially at the initiation of treatment with TASMAR.

Patients should be advised that they should neither drive a car nor operate other complex machinery until they have gained sufficient experience on TASMAR to gauge whether or not it affects their mental and/or motor performance adversely. Because of the possible additive sedative effects, caution should be used when patients are taking other CNS depressants in combination with TASMAR.

Patients should be informed that nausea may occur, especially at the initiation of treatment with TASMAR.

Patients should be advised of the possibility of an increase in dyskinesia and/or dystonia.

Although TASMAR has not been shown to be teratogenic in animals, it is always given in conjunction with levodopa/carbidopa, which is known to cause visceral and skeletal malformations in the rabbit. Accordingly, patients should be advised to notify their physicians if they become pregnant or intend to become pregnant during therapy (see PRECAUTIONS: *Pregnancy*).

Tolcapone is excreted into maternal milk in rats. Because of the possibility that tolcapone may be excreted into human maternal milk, patients should be advised to notify their physicians if they intend to breastfeed or are breastfeeding an infant.

Laboratory Tests: **Although a program of frequent laboratory monitoring for evidence of hepatocellular injury is deemed essential, it is not clear that baseline and periodic monitoring of liver enzymes will prevent the occurrence of fulminant liver failure. However, it is generally believed that early detection of drug-induced hepatic injury along with immediate withdrawal of the suspect drug enhances the likelihood for recovery. It is also widely held, without a robust body of evidence, that patients with preexisting hepatic disease are more vulnerable to hepatotoxins. Accordingly, the following liver monitoring program is recommended.**

Before starting treatment with TASMAR, the physician should conduct appropriate tests to exclude the presence of liver disease. In patients determined to be appropriate candidates for treatment with TASMAR, serum glutamic-pyruvic transaminase (SGPT/ALT) and serum glutamic-oxaloacetic transaminase (SGOT/AST) levels should be determined at baseline and then every 2 weeks for the first year of therapy, every 4 weeks for the next 6 months and then every 8 weeks thereafter.

If the dose is increased to 200 mg tid (see DOSAGE AND ADMINISTRATION section), liver enzyme monitoring should take place before increasing the dose and then be reinitiated at the frequency above.

TASMAR should be discontinued if SGPT/ALT or SGOT/AST exceeds the upper limit of normal or if clinical signs and symptoms suggest the onset of hepatic failure (persistent nausea, fatigue, lethargy, anorexia, jaundice, dark urine, pruritus, and right upper quadrant tenderness).

Special Populations: TASMAR therapy should not be initiated if the patient exhibits clinical evidence of active liver disease or two SGPT/ALT or SGOT/AST values greater than the upper limit of normal. Patients with severe dyskinesia or dystonia should be treated with caution (see PRECAUTIONS: *Rhabdomyolysis*). Patients with severe renal impairment should be treated with caution (see INDICATIONS, DOSAGE AND ADMINISTRATION, BOXED WARNING and WARNINGS).

Drug Interactions: *Protein Binding:* Although tolcapone is highly protein bound, in vitro studies have shown that tolcapone at a concentration of 50 µg/mL did not displace other highly protein-bound drugs from their binding sites at therapeutic concentrations. The experiments included warfarin (0.5 to 7.2 µg/mL), phenytoin (4.0 to 38.7 µg/mL), tolbutamide (24.5 to 96.1 µg/mL) and digitoxin (9.0 to 27.0 µg/mL).

Drugs Metabolized by Catechol-O-Methyltransferase (COMT): Tolcapone may influence the pharmacokinetics of drugs metabolized by COMT. However, no effects were seen on the pharmacokinetics of the COMT substrate carbidopa. The effect of tolcapone on the pharmacokinetics of other drugs of this class such as α-methyldopa, dobutamine, apomorphine, and isoproterenol has not been evaluated. A dose reduction of such compounds should be considered when they are coadministered with tolcapone.

Effect of Tolcapone on the Metabolism of Other Drugs: In vitro experiments have been performed to assess the potential of tolcapone to interact with isoenzymes of cytochrome P450 (CYP). No relevant interactions with substrates for CYP 2A6 (coumadin), CYP 1A2 (caffeine), CYP 3A4 (midazolam, terfenadine, cyclosporine), CYP 2C19 (S-mephenytoin) and CYP 2D6 (desipramine) were observed in vitro. The absence of an interaction with desipramine, a drug metabolized by cytochrome P450 2D6, was also confirmed in an in vivo study where tolcapone did not change the pharmacokinetics of desipramine.

Due to its affinity to cytochrome P450 2C9 in vitro, tolcapone may interfere with drugs, whose clearance is dependent on this metabolic pathway, such as tolbutamide and warfarin. However, in an in vivo interaction study, tolcapone did not change the pharmacokinetics of tolbutamide. Therefore, clinically relevant interactions involving cytochrome P450 2C9 appear unlikely. Similarly, tolcapone did not affect the pharmacokinetics of desipramine, a drug metabolized by cytochrome P450 2D6, indicating that interactions with drugs metabolized by that enzyme are unlikely. Since clinical information is limited regarding the combination of warfarin and tolcapone, coagulation parameters should be monitored when these two drugs are coadministered.

Drugs That Increase Catecholamines: Tolcapone did not influence the effect of ephedrine, an indirect sympathomimetic, on hemodynamic parameters or plasma catecholamine levels, either at rest or during exercise. Since tolcapone did not alter the tolerability of ephedrine, these drugs can be coadministered.

When TASMAR was given together with levodopa/carbidopa and desipramine, there was no significant change in blood pressure, pulse rate and plasma concentrations of desipramine. Overall, the frequency of adverse events increased slightly. These adverse events were predictable based on the known adverse reactions to each of the three drugs individually. Therefore, caution should be exercised when desipramine is administered to Parkinson's disease patients being treated with TASMAR and levodopa/carbidopa.

In clinical trials, patients receiving TASMAR/levodopa preparations reported a similar adverse event profile independent of whether or not they were also concomitantly administered selegiline (a selective MAO-B inhibitor).

Carcinogenesis, Mutagenesis and Impairment of Fertility: *Carcinogenesis:* Carcinogenicity studies in which tolcapone was administered in the diet were conducted in mice and rats. Mice were treated for 80 (female) or 95 (male) weeks with doses of 100, 300 and 800 mg/kg/day, equivalent to 0.8, 1.6 and 4 times human exposure (AUC = 80 µg·hr/mL) at the recommended daily clinical dose of 600 mg.

Rats were treated for 104 weeks with doses of 50, 250 and 450 mg/kg/day. Tolcapone exposures were 1, 6.3 and 13 times the human exposure in male rats and 1.7, 11.8 and 26.4 times the human exposure in female rats. There was an increased incidence of uterine adenocarcinomas in female rats at exposure equivalent to 26.4 times the human exposure. There was evidence of renal tubular injury and renal tubular tumor formation in rats. A low incidence of renal tubular cell adenomas occurred in middle- and high-dose female rats; tubular cell carcinomas occurred in middle- and high-dose male and high-dose female rats, with a statistically significant increase in high-dose males. Exposures were equivalent to 6.3 (males) or 11.8 (females) times the human exposure or greater; no renal tumors were observed at exposures of 1 (males) or 1.7 (females) times the human exposure. Minimal-to-marked damage to the renal tubules, consisting of proximal tubule cell degeneration, single cell necrosis, hyperplasia and karyocytomegaly, occurred at the doses associated with renal tumors. Renal tubule damage, characterized by proximal tubule cell degeneration and the presence of atypical nuclei, as well as one adenocarcinoma in a high-dose male, were observed in a 1-year study in rats receiving doses of tolcapone of 150 and 450 mg/kg/day. These histopathological changes suggest the possibility that renal tumor formation might be secondary to chronic cell damage and sustained repair, but this relationship has not been established, and the relevance of these findings to humans is not known. There was no evidence of carcinogenic effects in the long-term mouse study. The carcinogenic potential of tolcapone in combination with levodopa/carbidopa has not been examined.

Mutagenesis: Tolcapone was clastogenic in the in vitro mouse lymphoma/thymidine kinase assay in the presence of metabolic activation. Tolcapone was not mutagenic in the Ames test, the in vitro V79/HPRT gene mutation assay, or the unscheduled DNA synthesis assay. It was not clastogenic in an in vitro chromosomal aberration assay in cultured human lymphocytes, or in an in vivo micronucleus assay in mice.

Impairment of Fertility: Tolcapone did not affect fertility and general reproductive performance in rats at doses up to 300 mg/kg/day (5.7 times the human dose on a mg/m^2 basis).

Pregnancy: Pregnancy Category C. Tolcapone, when administered alone during organogenesis, was not teratogenic at doses of up to 300 mg/kg/day in rats or up to 400 mg/kg/day in rabbits (5.7 times and 15 times the recommended daily clinical dose of 600 mg, on a mg/m^2 basis, respectively). In rabbits, however, an increased rate of abortion occurred at a dose of 100 mg/kg/day (3.7 times the daily clinical dose on a mg/m^2 basis) or greater. Evidence of maternal toxicity (decreased weight gain, death) was observed at 300 mg/kg in rats and 400 mg/kg in rabbits. When tolcapone was administered to female rats during the last part of gestation and throughout lactation, decreased litter size and impaired growth and learning performance in female pups were observed at a dose of 250/150 mg/kg/day (dose reduced from 250 to 150 mg/kg/day during late gestation due to high rate of maternal mortality; equivalent to 4.8/2.9 times the clinical dose on a mg/m^2 basis).

Tolcapone is always given concomitantly with levodopa/carbidopa, which is known to cause visceral and skeletal malformations in rabbits. The combination of tolcapone (100 mg/kg/day) with levodopa/carbidopa (80/20 mg/kg/day) produced an increased incidence of fetal malformations (primarily external and skeletal digit defects) compared to levodopa/carbidopa alone when pregnant rabbits were treated throughout organogenesis. Plasma exposures to tolcapone (based on AUC) were 0.5 times the expected human exposure, and plasma exposures to levodopa were 6 times higher than those in humans under therapeutic conditions. In a combination embryo-fetal development study in rats, fetal body weights were reduced by the combination of tolcapone (10, 30 and 50 mg/kg/day) and levodopa/carbidopa (120/30 mg/kg/day) and by levodopa/carbidopa alone. Tolcapone exposures were 0.5 times expected human exposure or greater; levodopa exposures were 21 times the expected human exposure or greater. The high dose of 50 mg/kg/day of tolcapone given alone was not associated with reduced fetal body weight (plasma exposures of 1.4 times the expected human exposure).

There is no experience from clinical studies regarding the use of TASMAR in pregnant women. Therefore, TASMAR should be used during pregnancy only if the potential benefit justifies the potential risk to the fetus.

Nursing Women: In animal studies, tolcapone was excreted into maternal rat milk.

It is not known whether tolcapone is excreted in human milk. Because many drugs are excreted in human milk, caution should be exercised when tolcapone is administered to a nursing woman.

Pediatric Use: There is no identified potential use of tolcapone in pediatric patients.

ADVERSE REACTIONS

Cases of severe hepatocellular injury, including fulminant liver failure resulting in death, have been reported in postmarketing use. As of October 1998, 3 cases of fatal fulminant hepatic failure have been reported from approximately 60,000 patients providing about 40,000 patient years of worldwide use. This incidence may be 10- to 100-fold higher than the background incidence in the general population.

The imprecision of the estimated increase is due to uncertainties about the base rate and the actual number of cases occurring in association with TASMAR. The incidence of idiopathic potentially fatal fulminant hepatic failure (ie, not due to viral hepatitis or alcohol) is low. One estimate, based upon transplant registry data, is approximately 3/1,000,000 patients per year in the United States. Whether this estimate is an appropriate basis for estimating the increased risk of liver failure among TASMAR users is uncertain. TASMAR users, for example, differ in age and general health status from candidates for liver transplantation. Similarly, underreporting of cases may lead to significant underestimation of the increased risk associated with the use of TASMAR.

Continued on next page

Tasmar—Cont.

During the premarketing development of tolcapone, two distinct patient populations were studied, patients with end-of-dose wearing-off phenomena and patients with stable responses to levodopa therapy. All patients received concomitant treatment with levodopa preparations, however, and were similar in other clinical aspects. Adverse events are, therefore, shown for these two populations combined.
The most commonly observed adverse events (>5%) in the double-blind, placebo-controlled trials (N=892) associated with the use of TASMAR not seen at an equivalent frequency among the placebo-treated patients were dyskinesia, nausea, sleep disorder, dystonia, dreaming excessive, anorexia, cramps muscle, orthostatic complaints, somnolence, diarrhea, confusion, dizziness, headache, hallucination, vomiting, constipation, fatigue, upper respiratory tract infection, falling, sweating increased, urinary tract infection, xerostomia, abdominal pain, urine discoloration.
Approximately 16% of the 592 patients who participated in the double-blind, placebo-controlled trials discontinued treatment due to adverse events compared to 10% of the 298 patients who received placebo. Diarrhea was by far the most frequent cause of discontinuation (approximately 6% in tolcapone patients vs 1% on placebo).
Adverse Event Incidence in Controlled Clinical Studies: Table 4 lists treatment emergent adverse events that occurred in at least 1% of patients treated with tolcapone participating in the double-blind, placebo-controlled studies and were numerically more common in at least one of the tolcapone groups. In these studies, either tolcapone or placebo were added to levodopa/carbidopa (or benserazide).
The prescriber should be aware that these figures cannot be used to predict the incidence of adverse events in the course of usual medical practice where patient characteristics and other factors differ from those that prevailed in the clinical studies. Similarly, the cited frequencies cannot be compared with figures obtained from other clinical investigations involving different treatments, uses, and investigators. However, the cited figures do provide the prescriber with some basis for estimating the relative contribution of drug and nondrug factors to the adverse events incidence rate in the population studied.

Table 4.
Summary of Patients With Adverse Events After Start of Trial Drug Administration
(At Least 1% in TASMAR Group and at Least One TASMAR Dose Group > Placebo)

	Placebo	Tolcapone tid	
		100 mg	200 mg
	N = 298	N = 296	N = 298
Adverse Events	**(%)**	**(%)**	**(%)**
Dyskinesia	20	42	51
Nausea	18	30	35
Sleep Disorder	18	24	25
Dystonia	17	19	22
Dreaming Excessive	17	21	16
Anorexia	13	19	23
Cramps Muscle	17	17	18
Orthostatic Complaints	14	17	17
Somnolence	13	18	14
Diarrhea	8	16	18
Confusion	9	11	10
Dizziness	10	13	6
Headache	7	10	11
Hallucination	5	8	10
Vomiting	4	8	10
Constipation	5	6	8
Fatigue	6	7	3
Upper Respiratory Tract Infection	3	5	7
Falling	4	4	6
Sweating Increased	2	4	7
Urinary Tract Infection	4	5	5
Xerostomia	2	5	6
Abdominal Pain	3	5	6
Syncope	3	4	5
Urine Discoloration	1	2	7
Dyspepsia	2	4	3
Influenza	2	3	4
Dyspnea	2	3	3
Balance Loss	2	3	2
Flatulence	2	2	4
Hyperkinesia	1	3	2
Chest Pain	1	3	1
Hypotension	1	2	2
Paresthesia	2	3	1
Stiffness	1	2	2
Arthritis	1	2	1
Chest Discomfort	1	1	2
Hypokinesia	1	1	3
Micturition Disorder	1	2	1
Pain Neck	1	2	2
Burning	0	2	1
Sinus Congestion	0	2	1
Agitation	0	1	1
Bleeding Dermal	0	1	1
Irritability	0	1	1
Mental Deficiency	0	1	1
Hyperactivity	0	1	1
Malaise	0	1	0
Panic Reaction	0	1	0
Tumor Skin	0	1	0
Cataract	0	1	0
Euphoria	0	1	0
Fever	0	0	1
Alopecia	0	1	0
Eye Inflamed	0	1	0
Hypertonia	0	0	1
Tumor Uterus	0	1	0

Other events reported by 1% or more of patients treated with TASMAR but that were equally or more frequent in the placebo group were arthralgia, pain limbs, anxiety, micturition frequency, fractures, vision blurred, pneumonia, paresis, lethargy, asthenia, edema peripheral, gait abnormal, taste alteration, weight decrease and sinusitis.
Effects of Gender and Age on Adverse Reactions: Experience in clinical trials have suggested that patients greater than 75 years of age may be more likely to develop hallucinations than patients less than 75 years of age, while patients over 75 may be less likely to develop dystonia. Females may be more likely to develop somnolence than males.
Other Adverse Events Observed During All Trials in Patients With Parkinson's Disease: TASMAR has been administered in 1536 patients with Parkinson's disease in clinical trials. During these trials, all adverse events were recorded by the clinical investigators using terminology of their own choosing. To provide a meaningful estimate of the proportion of individuals having adverse events, similar types of adverse events were grouped into a smaller number of standardized categories using COSTART dictionary terminology. These categories are used in the listing below.
All reported events that occurred at least twice (or once for serious or potentially serious events), except those already listed above, trivial events and terms too vague to be meaningful are included, without regard to determination of a causal relationship to TASMAR.
Events are further classified within body system categories and enumerated in order of decreasing frequency using the following definitions: frequent adverse events are defined as those occurring in at least 1/100 patients; infrequent adverse events are defined as those occurring in between 1/100 and 1/1000 patients; and rare adverse events are defined as those occurring in fewer than 1/1000 patients.
Nervous System—frequent: depression, hypesthesia, tremor, speech disorder, vertigo, emotional lability; *infrequent:* neuralgia, amnesia, extrapyramidal syndrome, hostility, libido increased, manic reaction, nervousness, paranoid reaction, cerebral ischemia, cerebrovascular accident, delusions, libido decreased, neuropathy, apathy, choreoathetosis, myoclonus, psychosis, thinking abnormal, twitching; *rare:* antisocial reaction, delirium, encephalopathy, hemiplegia, meningitis.
Digestive System—frequent: tooth disorder; *infrequent:* dysphagia, gastrointestinal hemorrhage, gastroenteritis, mouth ulceration, increased salivation, abnormal stools, esophagitis, cholelithiasis, colitis, tongue disorder, rectal disorder; *rare:* cholecystitis, duodenal ulcer, gastrointestinal carcinoma, stomach atony.
Body as a Whole—frequent: flank pain, accidental injury, abdominal pain, infection; *infrequent:* hernia, pain, allergic reaction, cellulitis, infection fungal, viral infection, carcinoma, chills, infection bacterial, neoplasm, abscess, face edema; *rare:* death.
Cardiovascular System—frequent: palpitation; *infrequent:* hypertension, vasodilation, angina pectoris, heart failure, atrial fibrillation, tachycardia, migraine, aortic stenosis, arrhythmia, arteriospasm, bradycardia, cerebral hemorrhage, coronary artery disorder, heart arrest, myocardial infarct, myocardial ischemia, pulmonary embolus; *rare:* arteriosclerosis, cardiovascular disorder, pericardial effusion, thrombosis.
Musculoskeletal System—frequent: myalgia; *infrequent:* tenosynovitis, arthrosis, joint disorder.
Urogenital System—frequent: urinary incontinence, impotence; *infrequent:* prostatic disorder, dysuria, nocturia, polyuria, urinary retention, urinary tract disorder, hematuria, kidney calculus, prostatic carcinoma, breast neoplasm, oliguria, uterine atony, uterine disorder, vaginitis; *rare:* bladder calculus, ovarian carcinoma, uterine hemorrhage.
Respiratory System—frequent: bronchitis, pharyngitis; *infrequent:* cough increased, rhinitis, asthma, epistaxis, hyperventilation, laryngitis, hiccup; *rare:* apnea, hypoxia, lung edema.
Skin and Appendages—frequent: rash; *infrequent:* herpes zoster, pruritus, seborrhea, skin discoloration, eczema, erythema multiforme, skin disorder, furunculosis, herpes simplex, urticaria.
Special Senses—frequent: tinnitus; *infrequent:* diplopia, ear pain, eye hemorrhage, eye pain, lacrimation disorder, otitis media, parosmia; *rare:* glaucoma.
Metabolic and Nutritional—infrequent: edema, hypercholesteremia, thirst, dehydration.
Hemic and Lymphatic System—infrequent: anemia; *rare:* leukemia, thrombocytopenia.
Endocrine System—infrequent: diabetes mellitus.
Unclassified—infrequent: surgical procedure.

DRUG ABUSE AND DEPENDENCE

Tolcapone is not a controlled substance.
Studies conducted in rats and monkeys did not reveal any potential for physical or psychological dependence. Although clinical trials have not revealed any evidence of the potential for abuse, tolerance or physical dependence, systematic studies in humans designed to evaluate these effects have not been performed.

OVERDOSAGE

The highest dose of tolcapone administered to humans was 800 mg tid, with and without levodopa/carbidopa coadministration. This was in a 1-week study in elderly, healthy volunteers. The peak plasma concentrations of tolcapone at this dose were on average 30 μg/mL (compared to 3 μg/mL and 6 μg/mL with 100 mg and 200 mg tolcapone, respectively). Nausea, vomiting and dizziness were observed, particularly in combination with levodopa/carbidopa.
The threshold for the lethal plasma concentration for tolcapone based on animal data is >100 μg/mL. Respiratory difficulties were observed in rats at high oral (gavage) and intravenous doses and in dogs with rapidly injected intravenous doses.
Management of Overdose: Hospitalization is advised. General supportive care is indicated. Based on the physicochemical properties of the compound, hemodialysis is unlikely to be of benefit.

DOSAGE AND ADMINISTRATION

Because of the risk of potentially fatal, acute fulminant liver failure, TASMAR (tolcapone) should ordinarily be used in patients with Parkinson's disease on l-dopa/carbidopa who are experiencing symptom fluctuations and are not responding satisfactorily to or are not appropriate candidates for other adjunctive therapies (see INDICATIONS and DOSAGE AND ADMINISTRATION sections).
Because of the risk of liver injury and because TASMAR when it is effective provides an observable symptomatic benefit, the patient who fails to show substantial clinical benefit within 3 weeks of initiation of treatment, should be withdrawn from TASMAR.
TASMAR therapy should not be initiated if the patient exhibits clinical evidence of liver disease or two SGPT/ALT or SGOT/AST values greater than the upper limit of normal. Patients with severe dyskinesia or dystonia should be treated with caution (see PRECAUTIONS: *Rhabdomyolysis*).
Patients who develop evidence of hepatocellular injury while on TASMAR and are withdrawn from the drug for any reason may be at increased risk for liver injury if TASMAR is reintroduced. Accordingly, such patients should not ordinarily be considered for retreatment.
Treatment with TASMAR should always be initiated at a dose of 100 mg tid, always as an adjunct to levodopa/carbidopa therapy. The recommended daily dose of TASMAR is also 100 mg tid. In clinical trials, elevations in ALT occurred more frequently at the dose of 200 mg tid. While it is unknown whether the risk of acute fulminant liver failure is increased at the 200-mg dose, it would be prudent to use 200 mg only if the anticipated incremental clinical benefit is justified (see BOXED WARNING, WARNINGS, PRECAUTIONS: *Laboratory Tests*). If a patient fails to show the expected incremental benefit on the 200-mg dose after a total of 3 weeks of treatment (regardless of dose), TASMAR should be discontinued.
In clinical trials, the first dose of the day of TASMAR was always taken together with the first dose of the day of levodopa/carbidopa, and the subsequent doses of TASMAR were given approximately 6 and 12 hours later.
In clinical trials, the majority of patients required a decrease in their daily levodopa dose if their daily dose of levodopa was >600 mg or if patients had moderate or severe dyskinesias before beginning treatment.
To optimize an individual patient's response, reductions in daily levodopa dose may be necessary. In clinical trials, the average reduction in daily levodopa dose was about 30% in those patients requiring a levodopa dose reduction. (Greater than 70% of patients with levodopa doses above 600 mg daily required such a reduction.)
TASMAR can be combined with both the immediate and sustained release formulations of levodopa/carbidopa.
TASMAR may be taken with or without food (see CLINICAL PHARMACOLOGY).
Patients With Impaired Hepatic Function: TASMAR therapy should not be initiated if any patient with liver disease or two SGPT/ALT or SGOT/AST values greater than the upper limit of normal. (See BOXED WARNING, WARNINGS, and CLINICAL PHARMACOLOGY).
Patients With Impaired Renal Function: No dose adjustment of TASMAR is recommended for patients with mild to moderate renal impairment. However, patients with severe renal impairment should be treated with caution. The safety of tolcapone has not been examined in subjects who had creatinine clearance less than 25 mL/min (see CLINICAL PHARMACOLOGY).
Withdrawing Patients From TASMAR: As with any dopaminergic drug, withdrawal or abrupt reduction in the TASMAR dose may lead to emergence of signs and symptoms of Parkinson's disease or Hyperpyrexia and Confusion, a syndrome complex resembling the neuroleptic malignant syndrome (see PRECAUTIONS: *Events Reported With Dopaminergic Therapy*). If a decision is made to discontinue treatment with TASMAR, then it is recommended to closely monitor the patient and adjust other dopaminergic treat-

ments as needed. This syndrome should be considered in the differential diagnosis for any patient who develops a high fever or severe rigidity. Tapering TASMAR has not been systematically evaluated. As the duration of COMT inhibition with TASMAR is generally 5 to 6 hours on average, decreasing the frequency of dosage to twice or once a day may not in itself prevent withdrawal effects.

HOW SUPPLIED

TASMAR is supplied as film-coated tablets containing 100 mg or 200 mg tolcapone. The 100 mg beige tablet and the 200 mg reddish-brown tablet are hexagonal and biconvex. Imprinted with black ink on one side of the tablet is TASMAR and the tablet strength (100 or 200), on the other side is a V.

TASMAR 100 mg Tablets: bottles of 90 (NDC 0187-0938-01).
TASMAR 200 mg Tablets: bottles of 90 (NDC 0187-0939-01).

Storage: Store at controlled room temperature 20° to 25°C (68° to 77°F) in tight containers as defined in USP/NF.

PATIENT CONSENT

TASMAR SHOULD NOT BE USED BY PATIENTS UNTIL THERE HAS BEEN A COMPLETE DISCUSSION OF THE RISKS AND WRITTEN INFORMED CONSENT HAS BEEN OBTAINED.

IMPORTANT INFORMATION AND WARNING

Reports of potentially life threatening cases of severe hepatocellular injury, including fulminant liver failure resulting in death, have been reported in association with use of TASMAR.

PATIENT CONSENT

My, ________________, treatment with TASMAR has been personally described to me by Dr.______________.

The following points of information, among others, have been specifically discussed and made clear and I have had the opportunity to ask any questions concerning this information:

1. I. ________________ (patient's name) understand that TASMAR is used to treat certain types of patients with Parkinson's disease and my physician has told me that I am this type of patient.
   Initials: ____________
2. I understand that there is a serious risk that I could develop severe liver failure, which may be potentially fatal, by using TASMAR.
   Initials: ____________
3. I understand that there are no laboratory tests that will predict if I am at an increased risk for fatal liver failure.
   Initials: ____________
4. I understand that I should have the recommended blood work before my treatment with TASMAR is begun or continued and every 2 weeks for the first year, then every 4 weeks for the next 6 months, and then every 8 weeks thereafter while taking TASMAR. I understand that although this blood work may help detect if I develop liver failure it may do so only after significant, irreversible and potentially fatal damage has already occurred.
   Initials: ____________
5. I understand that I must immediately report any unusual symptoms to Dr. ____________ and be especially aware of persistent nausea, fatigue, lethargy, decreased appetite, jaundice (yellowing of skin or the whites of the eyes), dark urine, itchiness or right-sided abdominal pain.
   Initials: ____________

I now authorize Dr. ____________ to begin my treatment with TASMAR; OR, if my treatment has already begun with TASMAR, to continue such treatment.

Patient/Caretaker______________________

Address______________________

____

Telephone______________________

PHYSICIAN STATEMENT:

I have fully explained to the patient, ______________, the nature and purpose of the treatment with TASMAR (tolcapone) and the potential risks associated with that treatment. I have asked the patient if he/she has any questions regarding this treatment or the risks and have answered those questions to the best of my ability. I also acknowledge that I have read and understand the prescribing information listed above.

____

Physician Date

NOTE TO PHYSICIAN: It is strongly recommended that you retain a signed copy of the informed consent with the patient's medical records.

SUPPLY OF PATIENT CONSENT FORMS:

A supply of "Patient Consent" forms as printed above, is available, free of charge, from your local Valeant representative, or may be obtained by calling 1-800-321-4576. Permission to use the above Patient Consent by photocopy reproduction is also hereby granted by Valeant Pharmaceuticals International.

Manufactured for:
Valeant Pharmaceuticals International
3300 Hyland Ave., Costa Mesa CA 92626 USA
27898772 Revised: June 2004

Shown in Product Identification Guide, page 335

TESTRED® CIII ℞
MethylTESTOSTERone Capsules, USP 10 mg
Rx only

DESCRIPTION

The androgens are steroids that develop and maintain primary and secondary male sex characteristics.

Androgens are derivatives of cyclopentanoperhydrophenanthrene. Endogenous androgens are C-19 steroids with a side chain at C-17, and with two angular methyl groups. Testosterone is the primary endogenous androgen. In their active form, all drugs in the class have a 17-beta-hydroxy group. 17-alpha alkylation (methylTESTOSTERone) increases the pharmacologic activity per unit weight compared to testosterone when given orally.

MethylTESTOSTERone, a synthetic derivative of testosterone, is an androgenic preparation given by the oral route in a capsule form. Each capsule contains 10 mg of MethylTESTOSTERone USP. It has the following structural formula:

$C_{20}H_{30}O_2$ M.W. 302.46
17β-hydroxy-17-methylandrost-4-en-3-one

MethylTESTOSTERone occurs as white or creamy white crystals or powder, which is soluble in various organic solvents but is practically insoluble in water.

Each capsule, for oral administration, contains 10 mg of MethylTESTOSTERone. In addition, each capsule contains the following inactive ingredients: Corn starch NF, Gelatin NF, FD&C Blue #1, FD&C Red #40.

CLINICAL PHARMACOLOGY

Endogenous androgens are responsible for the normal growth and development of the male sex organs and for maintenance of secondary sex characteristics. These effects include the growth and maturation of prostate, seminal vesicles, penis, and scrotum. The development of male hair distribution, such as beard, pubic, chest, and axillary hair; laryngeal enlargement, vocal chord thickening, alterations in body musculature and fat distribution. Drugs in this class also cause retention of nitrogen, sodium, potassium, phosphorus, and decreased urinary excretion of calcium. Androgens have been reported to increase protein anabolism and decrease protein catabolism. Nitrogen balance is improved only when there is sufficient intake of calories and protein.

Androgens are responsible for the growth spurt of adolescence and for the eventual termination of linear growth which is brought about by fusion of the epiphyseal growth centers. In children, exogenous androgens accelerate linear growth rates, but may cause a disproportionate advancement in bone maturation. Use over long periods may result in fusion of the epiphyseal growth centers and termination of growth process. Androgens have been reported to stimulate the production of red blood cells by enhancing the production of erythropoietic stimulating factor.

During exogenous administration of androgens, endogenous testosterone release is inhibited through feedback inhibition of pituitary luteinizing hormone (LH). At large doses of exogenous androgens, spermatogenesis may also be suppressed through feedback inhibition of pituitary follicle stimulating hormone (FSH).

There is a lack of substantial evidence that androgens are effective in fractures, surgery, convalescence and functional uterine bleeding.

Pharmacokinetics

Testosterone given orally is metabolized by the gut and 44 percent is cleared by the liver of the first pass. Oral doses as high as 400 mg per day are needed to achieve clinically effective blood levels for full replacement therapy. The synthetic androgen, methylTESTOSTERone, is less extensively metabolized by the liver and has a longer half-life. It is more suitable than testosterone for oral administration.

Testosterone in plasma is 98 percent bound to a specific testosterone-estradiol binding globulin, and about 2 percent is free. Generally, the amount of this sex-hormone binding globulin in the plasma will determine the distribution of testosterone between free and bound forms, and the free testosterone concentration will determine its half-life.

About 90 percent of a dose of testosterone is excreted in the urine as glucuronic and sulfuric acid conjugates of testosterone and its metabolites; about 6 percent of a dose is excreted in the feces, mostly in the unconjugated form. Inactivation of testosterone occurs primarily in the liver. Testosterone is metabolized to various 17-keto steroids through two different pathways. There are considerable variations of the half-life of testosterone as reported in the literature, ranging from 10 to 100 minutes.

In many tissues the activity of testosterone appears to depend on reduction to dihydrotestosterone, which binds to cytosol receptor proteins. The steroid-receptor complex is transported to the nucleus where it initiates transcription events and cellular changes related to androgen action.

INDICATIONS AND USAGE

1. Males

Androgens are indicated for replacement therapy in conditions associated with a deficiency or absence of endogenous testosterone;

a. Primary hypogonadism (congenital or acquired)—testicular failure due to cryptorchidism, bilateral torsions, orchitis, vanishing testis syndrome; or orchidectomy.

b. Hypogonadotropic hypogonadism (congenital or acquired)—idiopathic gonadotropin or LHRH deficiency, or pituitary-hypothalamic injury from tumors, trauma or radiation.

If the above conditions occur prior to puberty, androgen replacement therapy will be needed during the adolescent years for development of secondary sexual characteristics. Prolonged androgen treatment will be required to maintain sexual characteristics in these and other males who develop testosterone deficiency after puberty.

c. Androgens may be used to stimulate puberty in carefully selected males with clearly delayed puberty. These patients usually have a familial pattern of delayed puberty that is not secondary to a pathological disorder; puberty is expected to occur spontaneously at a relatively late date. Brief treatment with conservative doses may occasionally be justified in these patients if they do not respond to psychological support. The potential adverse effect on bone maturation should be discussed with the patient and parents prior to androgen adminstration. An X-ray of the hand and wrist to determine bone age should be obtained every 6 months to assess the effect of treatment on the epiphyseal centers (see WARNINGS).

2. Females

Androgens may be used secondarily in women with advancing inoperable metastatic (skeletal) mammary cancer who are 1 to 5 years postmenopausal. Primary goals of therapy in these women include ablation of the ovaries. Other methods of counteracting estrogen activity are adrenalectomy, hypophysectomy, and/or antiestrogen therapy. This treatment has also been used in premenopausal women with breast cancer who have benefited from oophorectomy and are considered to have a hormone-responsive tumor. Judgment concerning androgen therapy should be made by an oncologist with expertise in this field.

CONTRAINDICATIONS

Androgens are contraindicated in men with carcinomas of the breast or with known or suspected carcinomas of the prostate, and in women who are or may become pregnant. When administered to pregnant women, androgens cause virilization of the external genitalia of the female fetus. This virilization includes clitoromegaly, abnormal vaginal development, and fusion of genital folds to form a scrotal-like structure. The degree of masculinization is related to the amount of drug given and the age of the fetus, and is most likely to occur in the female fetus when the drugs are given in the first trimester. If the patient becomes pregnant while taking these drugs, she should be apprised of the potential hazard to the fetus.

WARNINGS

In patients with breast cancer, androgen therapy may cause hypercalcemia by stimulating osteolysis. In this case, the drug should be discontinued.

Prolonged use of high doses of androgens has been associated with the development of peliosis hepatis and hepatic neoplasms including hepatocellular carcinoma. (See PRECAUTIONS-Carcinogenesis). Peliosis hepatis can be a life-threatening or fatal complication.

Cholestatic hepatitis and jaundice occur with 17-alpha-alkylandrogens at a relatively low dose. If cholestatic hepatitis with jaundice appears or if liver function tests become abnormal, the androgen should be discontinued and the etiology should be determined. Drug-induced jaundice is reversible when the medication is discontinued.

Geriatric patients treated with androgens may be at an increased risk for the development of prostatic hypertrophy and prostatic carcinoma.

Edema with or without congestive heart failure may be a serious complication in patients with preexisting cardiac, renal, or hepatic disease. In addition to discontinuation of the drug, diuretic therapy may be required.

Gynecomastia frequently develops and occasionally persists in patients being treated for hypogonadism.

Androgen therapy should be used cautiously in healthy males with delayed puberty. The effect on bone maturation should be monitored by assessing bone age of the wrist and hand every 6 months. In children, androgen treatment may accelerate bone maturation without producing compensatory gain in linear growth. This adverse effect may result in compromised adult stature. The younger the child the greater the risk of compromising final mature height.

This drug has not been shown to be safe and effective for the enhancement of athletic performance. Because of the potential risk of serious adverse health effects, this drug should not be used for such purpose.

PRECAUTIONS

General

Women should be observed for signs of virilization (deepening of the voice, hirsutism, acne, clitoromegaly and men-

Continued on next page

Testred—Cont.

strual irregularities). Discontinuation of drug therapy at the time of evidence of mild virilism is necessary to prevent irreversible virilization. Such virilization is usual following androgen use at high doses. A decision may be made by the patient and the physician that some virilization will be tolerated during treatment for breast carcinoma.

Information for the Patient

The physician should instruct patients to report any of the following side effects of androgens:

Adult or Adolescent Males:	Too frequent or persistent erections of the penis. Any male adolescent patient receiving androgens for delayed puberty should have bone development checked every six months.
Women:	Hoarseness, acne, changes in menstrual periods, or more hair on the face.
All Patients:	Any nausea, vomiting, changes in skin color or ankle swelling.

Laboratory Tests

1. Women with disseminated breast carcinoma should have frequent determination of urine and serum calcium levels during the course of androgen therapy. (See WARNINGS).
2. Because of the hepatotoxicity associated with the use of 17-alpha-alkylated androgens, liver function tests should be obtained periodically.
3. Periodic (every 6 months) x-ray examinations of bone age should be made during treatment of prepubertal males to determine the rate of bone maturation and the effects of androgen therapy on the epiphyseal centers.
4. Hemoglobin and hematocrit should be checked periodically for polycythemia in patients who are receiving high doses of androgens.

Drug Interactions

1. **Anticoagulants:** C-17 substituted derivatives of testosterone, such as methandrostenolone, have been reported to decrease the anticoagulant requirements of patients receiving oral anticoagulants. Patients receiving oral anticoagulant therapy require close monitoring, especially when androgens are started or stopped.
2. **Oxyphenbutazone:** Concurrent administration of oxyphenbutazone and androgens may result in elevated serum levels of oxyphenbutazone.
3. **Insulin:** In diabetic patients the metabolic effects of androgens may decrease blood glucose and insulin requirements.

Drug/Laboratory Test Interferences

Androgens may decrease levels of thyroxine-binding globulin, resulting in decreased total T4 serum levels and increased resin uptake of T3 and T4. Free thyroid hormone levels remain unchanged, however, and there is no clinical evidence of thyroid dysfunction.

Carcinogenesis

Animal Data

Testosterone has been tested by subcutaneous injection and implantation in mice and rats. The implant induced cervical-uterine tumors in mice, which metastasized in some cases. There is suggestive evidence that injection of testosterone into some strains of female mice increases their susceptibility to hepatoma. Testosterone is also known to increase the number of tumors and decrease the degree of differentiation of chemically induced carcinomas of the liver in rats.

Human Data

There are rare reports of hepatocellular carcinoma in patients receiving long-term therapy with androgens in high doses. Withdrawal of the drugs did not lead to regression of the tumors in all cases.

Geriatric patients treated with androgens may be at an increased risk for the development of prostatic hypertrophy and prostatic carcinoma.

Pregnancy

Teratogenic effects. Pregnancy Category X (See CONTRAINDICATIONS).

Nursing Mothers

It is not known whether androgens are excreted in human milk. Because many drugs are excreted in human milk and because of the potential for serious adverse reactions in nursing infants from androgens, a decision should be made whether to discontinue nursing or to discontinue the drug, taking into account the importance of the drug to the mother.

Pediatric Use

Androgen therapy should be used very cautiously in children and only by specialists who are aware of the adverse effects on bone maturation. Skeletal maturation must be monitored every six months by an x-ray of hand and wrist (See INDICATIONS AND USAGE and WARNINGS).

ADVERSE REACTIONS

Endocrine and Urogenital

Female: The most common side effects of androgen therapy are amenorrhea and other menstrual irregularities, inhibition of gonadotropin secretion, and virilization, including deepening of the voice and clitoral enlargement. The latter usually is not reversible after androgens are discontinued. When administered to a pregnant woman androgens cause virilization of external genitalia of the female fetus.

Male: Gynecomastia, and excessive frequency and duration of penile erections. Oligospermia may occur at high dosages (see CLINICAL PHARMACOLOGY).

Skin and appendages: Hirsutism, male pattern of baldness, and acne.

Fluid and Electrolyte Disturbances: Retention of sodium, chloride, water, potassium, calcium, and inorganic phosphates.

Gastrointestinal: Nausea, cholestatic jaundice, alterations in liver function tests, rarely hepatocellular neoplasms and peliosis hepatis (see WARNINGS).

Hematologic: Suppression of clotting factors II, V, VII, and X, bleeding in patients on concomitant anticoagulant therapy, and polycythemia.

Nervous System: Increased or decreased libido, headache, anxiety, depression, and generalized paresthesia.

Metabolic: Increased serum cholesterol.

Miscellaneous: Rarely anaphylactoid reactions.

DRUG ABUSE AND DEPENDENCE

MethylTESTOSTERone Capsules are classified as a schedule III Controlled Substance under the Anabolic Steroids Act of 1990.

OVERDOSAGE

There have been no reports of acute overdosage with the androgens.

DOSAGE AND ADMINISTRATION

MethylTESTOSTERone capsules are administered orally. The suggested dosage for androgens varies depending on the age, sex, and diagnosis of the individual patient. Dosage is adjusted according to the patient's response and the appearance of adverse reactions.

Replacement therapy in androgen-deficient males is 10 to 50 mg of methylTESTOSTERone daily. Various dosage regimens have been used to induce pubertal changes in hypogonadal males; some experts have advocated lower dosages initially, gradually increasing the dose as puberty progresses with or without a decrease to maintenance levels. Other experts emphasize that higher dosages are needed to induce pubertal changes and lower dosages can be used for maintenance after puberty. The chronological and skeletal ages must be taken into consideration, both in determining the initial dose and in adjusting the dose.

Doses used in delayed puberty generally are in the lower range of that given above, and for a limited duration, for example 4 to 6 months.

Women with metastatic breast carcinoma must be followed closely because androgen therapy occasionally appears to accelerate the disease. Thus, many experts prefer to use the shorter acting androgen preparations rather than those with prolonged activity for treating breast carcinoma, particularly during the early stages of androgen therapy. The dosage of methylTESTOSTERone for androgen therapy in breast carcinoma in females is from 50–200 mg daily.

HOW SUPPLIED

MethylTESTOSTERone capsules USP 10 mg are red capsules imprinted "ICN 0901" on both sections. They are available in bottles of 100 (NDC 0187-0901-01).

Store at 25°C (77°F); excursions permitted to 15°C–30°C (59°F–86°F).

7000092 Revision September 2001

Valeant Pharmaceuticals International
3300 Hyland Avenue
Costa Mesa, CA 92626
(714) 545-0100

Shown in Product Identification Guide, page 335

VIRAZOLE® ℞

[vira 'zahl ']

(Ribavirin for Inhalation Solution)

℞ only

PRESCRIBING INFORMATION

WARNINGS:

USE OF AEROSOLIZED VIRAZOLE IN PATIENTS REQUIRING MECHANICAL VENTILATOR ASSISTANCE SHOULD BE UNDERTAKEN ONLY BY PHYSICIANS AND SUPPORT STAFF FAMILIAR WITH THE SPECIFIC VENTILATOR BEING USED AND THIS MODE OF ADMINISTRATION OF THE DRUG. STRICT ATTENTION MUST BE PAID TO PROCEDURES THAT HAVE BEEN SHOWN TO MINIMIZE THE ACCUMULATION OF DRUG PRECIPITATE, WHICH CAN RESULT IN MECHANICAL VENTILATOR DYSFUNCTION AND ASSOCIATED INCREASED PULMONARY PRESSURES (SEE WARNINGS).

SUDDEN DETERIORATION OF RESPIRATORY FUNCTION HAS BEEN ASSOCIATED WITH INITIATION OF AEROSOLIZED VIRAZOLE USE IN INFANTS. RESPIRATORY FUNCTION SHOULD BE CAREFULLY MONITORED DURING TREATMENT. IF INITIATION OF AEROSOLIZED VIRAZOLE TREATMENT APPEARS TO PRODUCE SUDDEN DETERIORATION OF RESPIRATORY FUNCTION, TREATMENT SHOULD BE STOPPED AND REINSTITUTED ONLY WITH EXTREME CAUTION, CONTINUOUS MONITORING AND CONSIDERATION OF CONCOMITANT ADMINISTRATION OF BRONCHODILATORS (SEE WARNINGS).

VIRAZOLE IS NOT INDICATED FOR USE IN ADULTS. PHYSICIANS AND PATIENTS SHOULD BE AWARE THAT RIBAVIRIN HAS BEEN SHOWN TO PRODUCE TESTICULAR LESIONS IN RODENTS AND TO BE TERATOGENIC IN ALL ANIMAL SPECIES IN WHICH ADEQUATE STUDIES HAVE BEEN CONDUCTED (RODENTS AND RABBITS); (SEE CONTRAINDICATIONS).

DESCRIPTION

Virazole® is a brand name for ribavirin, a synthetic nucleoside with antiviral activity. VIRAZOLE for inhalation solution is a sterile, lyophilized powder to be reconstituted for aerosol administration. Each 100 mL glass vial contains 6 grams of ribavirin, and when reconstituted to the recommended volume of 300 mL with sterile water for injection or sterile water for inhalation (no preservatives added), will contain 20 mg of ribavirin per mL, pH approximately 5.5. Aerosolization is to be carried out in a Small Particle Aerosol Generator (SPAG-2) nebulizer only.

Ribavirin is 1-beta-D-ribofuranosyl-1H-1,2,4-triazole-3-carboxamide, with the following structural formula:

Ribavirin is a stable, white crystalline compound with a maximum solubility in water of 142 mg/mL at 25°C and with only a slight solubility in ethanol. The empirical formula is $C_8H_{12}N_4O_5$ and the molecular weight is 244.21.

CLINICAL PHARMACOLOGY

Mechanism of Action

In cell cultures the inhibitory activity of ribavirin for respiratory syncytial virus (RSV) is selective. The mechanism of action is unknown. Reversal of the *in vitro* antiviral activity by guanosine or xanthosine suggests ribavirin may act as an analogue of these cellular metabolites.

Microbiology

Ribavirin has demonstrated antiviral activity against RSV *in vitro*[1] and in experimentally infected cotton rats.[2] Several clinical isolates of RSV were evaluated for ribavirin susceptibility by plaque reduction in tissue culture. Plaques were reduced 85–98% by 16 µg/mL; however, results may vary with the test system. The development of resistance has not been evaluated *in vitro* or in clinical trials.

In addition to the above, ribavirin has been shown to have *in vitro* activity against influenza A and B viruses and herpes simplex virus, but the clinical significance of these data is unknown.

Immunologic Effects

Neutralizing antibody responses to RSV were decreased in aerosolized VIRAZOLE treated infants compared to placebo treated infants.[3] One study also showed that RSV-specific IgE antibody in bronchial secretions was decreased in patients treated with aerosolized VIRAZOLE. In rats, ribavirin administration resulted in lymphoid atrophy of the thymus, spleen, and lymph nodes. Humoral immunity was reduced in guinea pigs and ferrets. Cellular immunity was also mildly depressed in animal studies. The clinical significance of these observations is unknown.

Pharmacokinetics

Assay for VIRAZOLE in human materials is by a radioimmunoassay which detects ribavirin and at least one metabolite.

VIRAZOLE brand of ribavirin, when administered by aerosol, is absorbed systemically. Four pediatric patients inhaling VIRAZOLE aerosol administered by face mask for 2.5 hours each day for 3 days had plasma concentrations ranging from 0.44 to 1.55 µM, with a mean concentration of 0.76 µM. The plasma half-life was reported to be 9.5 hours. Three pediatric patients inhaling aerosolized VIRAZOLE administered by face mask or mist tent for 20 hours each day for 5 days had plasma concentrations ranging from 1.5 to 14.3 µM, with a mean concentration of 6.8 µM.

The bioavailability of aerosolized VIRAZOLE is unknown and may depend on the mode of aerosol delivery. After aerosol treatment, peak plasma concentrations of ribavirin are 85% to 98% less than the concentration that reduced RSV plaque formation in tissue culture. After aerosol treatment, respiratory tract secretions are likely to contain ribavirin in concentrations many fold higher than those required to reduce plaque formation. However, RSV is an intracellular virus and it is unknown whether plasma concentrations or respiratory secretion concentrations of the drug better reflect intracellular concentrations in the respiratory tract.

In man, rats, and rhesus monkeys, accumulation of ribavirin and/or metabolites in the red blood cells has been noted, plateauing in red cells in man in about 4 days and gradually declining with an apparent half-life of 40 days (the half-life of erythrocytes). The extent of accumulation of ribavirin following inhalation therapy is not well defined.

Animal Toxicology

Ribavirin, when administered orally or as an aerosol, produced cardiac lesions in mice, rats, and monkeys, when given at doses of 30, 36 and 120 mg/kg or greater for 4 weeks or more (estimated human equivalent doses of 4.8, 12.3 and 111.4 mg/kg for a 5 kg child, or 2.5, 5.1 and 40 mg/kg for a 60 kg adult, based on body surface area adjustment). Aerosolized ribavirin administered to developing ferrets at 60 mg/kg for 10 or 30 days resulted in inflammatory and possibly emphysematous changes in the lungs. Proliferative changes were seen in the lungs following exposure at 131 mg/kg for 30 days. The significance of these findings to human administration is unknown.

INDICATIONS AND USAGE

VIRAZOLE is indicated for the treatment of hospitalized infants and young children with severe lower respiratory tract infections due to respiratory syncytial virus. Treatment early in the course of severe lower respiratory tract infection may be necessary to achieve efficacy.

Only severe RSV lower respiratory tract infection should be treated with VIRAZOLE. The vast majority of infants and children with RSV infection have disease that is mild, self-limited, and does not require hospitalization or antiviral treatment. Many children with mild lower respiratory tract involvement will require shorter hospitalization than would be required for a full course of VIRAZOLE aerosol (3 to 7 days) and should not be treated with the drug. Thus the decision to treat with VIRAZOLE should be based on the severity of the RSV infection.

The presence of an underlying condition such as prematurity, immunosuppression or cardiopulmonary disease may increase the severity of clinical manifestations and complications of RSV infection.

Use of aerosolized VIRAZOLE in patients requiring mechanical ventilator assistance should be undertaken only by physicians and support staff familiar with this mode of administration and the specific ventilator being used (see WARNINGS, and DOSAGE AND ADMINISTRATION).

Diagnosis

RSV infection should be documented by a rapid diagnostic method such as demonstration of viral antigen in respiratory tract secretions by immunofluorescence[3,4] or ELISA[5] before or during the first 24 hours of treatment. Treatment may be initiated while awaiting rapid diagnostic test results. However, treatment should not be continued without documentation of RSV infection.

Non-culture antigen detection techniques may have false positive or false negative results. Assessment of the clinical situation, the time of year and other parameters may warrant reevaluation of the laboratory diagnosis.

Description of Studies

Non-Mechanically-Ventilated Infants: In two placebo controlled trials in infants hospitalized with RSV lower respiratory tract infection, aerosolized VIRAZOLE treatment had a therapeutic effect, as judged by the reduction in severity of clinical manifestations of disease by treatment day 3.[3,4] Treatment was most effective when instituted within the first 3 days of clinical illness. Virus titers in respiratory secretions were also significantly reduced with VIRAZOLE in one of these original studies.[4] Additional controlled studies conducted since these initial trials of aerosolized VIRAZOLE in the treatment of RSV infection have supported these data.

Mechanically-Ventilated Infants: A randomized, double-blind, placebo controlled evaluation of aerosolized VIRAZOLE at the recommended dose was conducted in 28 infants requiring mechanical ventilation for respiratory failure caused by documented RSV infection.[6] Mean age was 1.4 months (SD, 1.7 months). Seven patients had underlying diseases predisposing them to severe infection and 21 were previously normal. Aerosolized VIRAZOLE treatment significantly decreased the duration of mechanical ventilation required (4.9 vs. 9.9 days, p=0.01) and duration of required supplemental oxygen (8.7 vs 13.5 days, p=0.01). Intensive patient management and monitoring techniques were employed in this study. These included endotracheal tube suctioning every 1 to 2 hours; recording of proximal airway pressure, ventilatory rate, and F_1O_2 every hour; and arterial blood gas monitoring every 2 to 6 hours. To reduce the risk of VIRAZOLE precipitation and ventilator malfunction, heated wire tubing, two bacterial filters connected in series in the expiratory limb of the ventilator (with filter changes every 4 hours), and water column pressure release valves to monitor internal ventilator pressures were used in connecting ventilator circuits to the SPAG-2.

Employing these techniques, no technical difficulties with VIRAZOLE administration were encountered during the study. Adverse events consisted of bacterial pneumonia in one case, staphyloccus bacteremia in one case and two cases of post-extubation stridor. None were felt to be related to VIRAZOLE administration.

CONTRAINDICATIONS

VIRAZOLE is contraindicated in individuals who have shown hypersensitivity to the drug or its components, and in women who are or may become pregnant during exposure to the drug. Ribavirin has demonstrated significant teratogenic and/or embryocidal potential in all animal species in which adequate studies have been conducted (rodents and rabbits). Therefore, although clinical studies have not been performed, it should be assumed that VIRAZOLE may cause fetal harm in humans. Studies in which the drug has been administered systemically demonstrate that ribavirin is concentrated in the red blood cells and persists for the life of the erythrocyte.

WARNINGS

SUDDEN DETERIORATION OF RESPIRATORY FUNCTION HAS BEEN ASSOCIATED WITH INITIATION OF AEROSOLIZED VIRAZOLE USE IN INFANTS. Respiratory function should be carefully monitored during treatment. If initiation of aerosolized VIRAZOLE treatment appears to produce sudden deterioration of respiratory function, treatment should be stopped and reinstituted only with extreme caution, continuous monitoring, and consideration of concomitant administration of bronchodilators.

Use with Mechanical Ventilators

USE OF AEROSOLIZED VIRAZOLE IN PATIENTS REQUIRING MECHANICAL VENTILATOR ASSISTANCE SHOULD BE UNDERTAKEN ONLY BY PHYSICIANS AND SUPPORT STAFF FAMILIAR WITH THIS MODE OF ADMINISTRATION AND THE SPECIFIC VENTILATOR BEING USED. Strict attention must be paid to procedures that have been shown to minimize the accumulation of drug precipitate, which can result in mechanical ventilator dysfunction and associated increased pulmonary pressures. These procedures include the use of bacteria filters in series in the expiratory limb of the ventilator circuit with frequent changes (every 4 hours), water column pressure release valves to indicate elevated ventilator pressures, frequent monitoring of these devices and verification that ribavirin crystals have not accumulated within the ventilator circuitry, and frequent suctioning and monitoring of the patient (see Clinical Studies).

Those administering aerosolized VIRAZOLE in conjunction with mechanical ventilator use should be thoroughly familiar with detailed descriptions of these procedures as outlined in the SPAG-2 manual.

PRECAUTIONS

General: Patients with severe lower respiratory tract infection due to respiratory syncytial virus require optimum monitoring and attention to respiratory and fluid status (see SPAG-2 manual).

Drug Interactions

Clinical studies of interactions of VIRAZOLE with other drugs commonly used to treat infants with RSV infections, such as digoxin, bronchodilators, other antiviral agents, antibiotics, or anti-metabolites have not been conducted. Interference by VIRAZOLE with laboratory tests has not been evaluated.

Carcinogenesis and Mutagenesis

Ribavirin increased the incidence of cell transformations and mutations in mouse Balb/c 3T3 (fibroblasts) and L5178Y (lymphoma) cells at concentrations of 0.015 and 0.03–5.0 mg/mL, respectively (without metabolic activation.) Modest increases in mutation rates (3–4x) were observed at concentrations between 3.75–10.0 mg/mL in L5178Y cells *in vitro* with the addition of a metabolic activation fraction. In the mouse micronucleus assay, ribavirin was clastogenic at intravenous doses of 20–200 mg/kg, (estimated human equivalent of 1.67–16.7 mg/kg, based on body surface area adjustment for a 60 kg adult). Ribavirin was not mutagenic in a dominant lethal assay in rats at intraperitoneal doses between 50–200 mg/kg when administered for 5 days (estimated human equivalent of 7.14–28.6 mg/kg, based on body surface area adjustment; see Pharmacokinetics).

In vivo carcinogenicity studies with ribavirin are incomplete. However, results of a chronic feeding study with ribavirin in rats, at doses of 16–100 mg/kg/day (estimated human equivalent of 2.3–14.3 mg/kg/day, based on body surface area adjustment for the adult), suggest that ribavirin may induce benign mammary, pancreatic, pituitary and adrenal tumors. Preliminary results of 2 oral gavage oncogenicity studies in the mouse and rat (18–24 months; doses of 20–75 and 10–40 mg/kg/day, respectively [estimated human equivalent of 1.67–6.25 and 1.43–5.71 mg/kg/day, respectively, based on body surface area adjustment for the adult]) are inconclusive as to the carcinogenic potential of ribavirin (see Pharmacokinetics). However, these studies have demonstrated a relationship between chronic ribavirin exposure and increased incidences of vascular lesions (microscopic hemorrhages in mice) and retinal degeneration (in rats).

Impairment of Fertility

The fertility of ribavirin-treated animals (male or female) has not been fully investigated. However, in the mouse, administration of ribavirin at doses between 35–150 mg/kg/day (estimated human equivalent of 2.92–12.5 mg/kg/day, based on body surface area adjustment for the adult) resulted in significant seminiferous tubule atrophy, decreased sperm concentrations, and increased numbers of sperm with abnormal morphology. Partial recovery of sperm production was apparent 3–6 months following dose cessation. In several additional toxicology studies, ribavirin has been shown to cause testicular lesions (tubular atrophy), in adult rats at oral dose levels as low as 16 mg/kg/day (estimated human equivalent of 2.29 mg/kg/day, based on body surface area adjustment; see Pharmacokinetics). Lower doses were not tested. The reproductive capacity of treated male animals has not been studied.

Pregnancy: Category X

Ribavirin has demonstrated significant teratogenic and/or embryocidal potential in all animal species in which adequate studies have been conducted. Teratogenic effects were evident after single oral doses of 2.5 mg/kg or greater in the hamster, and after daily oral doses of 0.3 and 1.0 mg/kg in the rabbit and rat, respectively (estimated human equivalent doses of 0.12 and 0.14 mg/kg, based on body surface area adjustment for the adult). Malformations of the skull, palate, eye, jaw, limbs, skeleton, and gastrointestinal tract were noted. The incidence and severity of teratogenic effects increased with escalation of the drug dose. Survival of fetuses and offspring was reduced. Ribavirin caused embryolethality in the rabbit at daily oral dose levels as low as 1 mg/kg. No teratogenic effects were evident in the rabbit and rat administered daily oral doses of 0.1 and 0.3 mg/kg, respectively with estimated human equivalent doses of 0.01 and 0.04 mg/kg, based on body surface area adjustment (see Pharmacokinetics). These doses are considered to define the "No Observable Teratogenic Effects Level" (NOTEL) for ribavirin in the rabbit and rat.

Following oral administration of ribavirin in the pregnant rat (1.0 mg/kg) and rabbit (0.3 mg/kg), mean plasma levels of drug ranged from 0.10–0.20 μM [0.024–0.049 μg/mL] at 1 hour after dosing, to undetectable levels at 24 hours. At 1 hour following the administration of 0.3 or 0.1 mg/kg in the rat and rabbit (NOTEL), respectively, mean plasma levels of drug in both species were near or below the limit of detection (0.05 μM; see Pharmacokinetics),

Although clinical studies have not been performed, VIRAZOLE may cause fetal harm in humans. As noted previously, ribavirin is concentrated in red blood cells and persists for the life of the cell. Thus the terminal half-life for the systemic elimination of ribavirin is essentially that of the half-life of circulating erythrocytes. The minimum interval following exposure to VIRAZOLE before pregnancy may be safely initiated is unknown (see CONTRAINDICATIONS, WARNINGS, and Information for Health Care Personnel).

Nursing Mothers

VIRAZOLE has been shown to be toxic to lactating animals and their offspring. It is not known if VIRAZOLE is excreted in human milk.

Information for Health Care Personnel

Health care workers directly providing care to patients receiving aerosolized VIRAZOLE should be aware that ribavirin has been shown to be teratogenic in all animal species in which adequate studies have been conducted (rodents and rabbits). Although no reports of teratogenesis in offspring of mothers who were exposed to aerosolized VIRAZOLE during pregnancy have been confirmed, no controlled studies have been conducted in pregnant women. Studies of environmental exposure in treatment settings have shown that the drug can disperse into the immediate bedside area during routine patient care activities with highest ambient levels closest to the patient and extremely low levels outside of the immediate bedside area. Adverse reactions resulting from actual occupational exposure in adults are described below (see Adverse Events in Health Care Workers). Some studies have documented ambient drug concentrations at the bedside that could potentially lead to systemic exposures above those considered safe for exposure during pregnancy (1/1000 of the NOTEL dose in the most sensitive animal species).[7,8,9]

A 1992 study conducted by the National Institute of Occupational Safety and Health (NIOSH) demonstrated measurable urine levels of ribavirin in health care workers exposed to aerosol in the course of direct patient care.[7] Levels were lowest in workers caring for infants receiving aerosolized VIRAZOLE with mechanical ventilation and highest in those caring for patients being administered the drug via an oxygen tent or hood. This study employed a more sensitive assay to evaluate ribavirin levels in urine than was available for several previous studies of environmental exposure that failed to detect measurable ribavirin levels in exposed workers. Creatinine adjusted urine levels in the NIOSH study ranged from less than 0.001 to 0.140 μM of ribavirin per gram of creatinine in exposed workers. However, the relationship between urinary ribavirin levels in exposed workers, plasma levels in animal studies, and the specific risk of teratogenesis in exposed pregnant women is unknown.

It is good practice to avoid unnecessary occupational exposure to chemicals wherever possible. Hospitals are encouraged to conduct training programs to minimize potential occupational exposure to VIRAZOLE. Health care workers who are pregnant should consider avoiding direct care of patients receiving aerosolized VIRAZOLE. If close patient contact cannot be avoided, precautions to limit exposure should be taken. These include administration of VIRAZOLE in negative pressure rooms; adequate room ventilation (at least six air exchanges per hour); the use of VIRAZOLE aerosol scavenging devices; turning off the SPAG-2 device for 5 to 10 minutes prior to prolonged patient contact, and wearing appropriately fitted respirator masks. Surgical masks do not provide adequate filtration of VIRAZOLE particles. Further information is available from NIOSH's Hazard Evaluation and Technical Assistance Branch and additional recommendations have been published in an Aerosol Consensus Statement by the American Respiratory Care Foundation and the American Association for Respiratory Care.[10]

ADVERSE REACTIONS

The description of adverse reactions is based on events from clinical studies (approximately 200 patients) conducted prior to 1986, and the controlled trial of aerosolized VIRA-

Continued on next page

Virazole—Cont.

ZOLE conducted in 1989–1990. Additional data from spontaneous post-marketing reports of adverse events in individual patients have been available since 1986.

Deaths

Deaths during or shortly after treatment with aerosolized VIRAZOLE have been reported in 20 cases of patients treated with VIRAZOLE (12 of these patients were being treated for RSV infections). Several cases have been characterized as "possibly related" to VIRAZOLE by the treating physician; these were in infants who experienced worsening respiratory status related to bronchospasm while being treated with the drug. Several other cases have been attributed to mechanical ventilator malfunction in which VIRAZOLE precipitation within the ventilator apparatus led to excessively high pulmonary pressures and diminished oxygenation. In these cases the monitoring procedures described in the current package insert were not employed (see Description of Studies, WARNINGS, and DOSAGE AND ADMINISTRATION).

Pulmonary and Cardiovascular

Pulmonary function significantly deteriorated during aerosolized VIRAZOLE treatment in six of six adults with chronic obstructive lung disease and in four of six asthmatic adults. Dyspnea and chest soreness were also reported in the latter group. Minor abnormalities in pulmonary function were also seen in healthy adult volunteers.

In the original study population of approximately 200 infants who received aerosolized VIRAZOLE, several serious adverse events occurred in severely ill infants with life-threatening underlying diseases, many of whom required assisted ventilation. The role of VIRAZOLE in these events is indeterminate. Since the drug's approval in 1986, additional reports of similar serious, though non-fatal, events have been filed infrequently. Events associated with aerosolized VIRAZOLE use have included the following:

Pulmonary: Worsening of respiratory status, bronchospasm, pulmonary edema, hypoventilation, cyanosis, dyspnea, bacterial pneumonia, pneumothorax, apnea, atelectasis and ventilator dependence.

Cardiovascular: Cardiac arrest, hypotension, bradycardia and digitalis toxicity. Bigeminy, bradycardia and tachycardia have been described in patients with underlying congenital heart disease.

Some subjects requiring assisted ventilation experienced serious difficulties, due to inadequate ventilation and gas exchange. Precipitation of drug within the ventilatory apparatus, including the endotracheal tube, has resulted in increased positive end expiratory pressure and increased positive inspiratory pressure. Accumulation of fluid in tubing ("rain out") has also been noted. Measures to avoid these complications should be followed carefully (see DOSAGE AND ADMINISTRATION).

Hematologic

Although anemia was not reported with use of aerosolized VIRAZOLE in controlled clinical trials, most infants treated with the aerosol have not been evaluated 1 to 2 weeks post-treatment when anemia is likely to occur. Anemia has been shown to occur frequently with experimental oral and intravenous VIRAZOLE in humans. Also, cases of anemia (type unspecified), reticulocytosis and hemolytic anemia associated with aerosolized VIRAZOLE use have been reported through post-marketing reporting systems. All have been reversible with discontinuation of the drug.

Other

Rash and conjunctivitis have been associated with the use of aerosolized VIRAZOLE. These usually resolve within hours of discontinuing therapy. Seizures and asthenia associated with experimental intravenous VIRAZOLE therapy have also been reported.

Adverse Events in Health Care Workers

Studies of environmental exposure to aerosolized VIRAZOLE in health care workers administering care to patients receiving the drug have not detected adverse signs or symptoms related to exposure. However, 152 health care workers have reported experiencing adverse events through post-marketing surveillance. Nearly all were in individuals providing direct care to infants receiving aerosolized VIRAZOLE. Of 358 events from these 152 individual health care worker reports, the most common signs and symptoms were headache (51% of reports), conjunctivitis (32%), and rhinitis, nausea, rash, dizziness, pharyngitis, or lacrimation (10–20% each). Several cases of bronchospasm and/or chest pain were also reported, usually in individuals with known underlying reactive airway disease. Several case reports of damage to contact lenses after prolonged close exposure to aerosolized VIRAZOLE have also been reported. Most signs and symptoms reported as having occurred in exposed health care workers resolved within minutes to hours of discontinuing close exposure to aerosolized VIRAZOLE (also see Information for Health Care Personnel).

The symptoms of RSV in adults can include headache, conjunctivitis, sore throat and/or cough, fever, hoarseness, nasal congestion and wheezing, although RSV infections in adults are typically mild and transient. Such infections represent a potential hazard to uninfected hospital patients. It is unknown whether certain symptoms cited in reports from health care workers were due to exposure to the drug or infection with RSV. Hospitals should implement appropriate infection control procedures.

Overdosage

No overdosage with VIRAZOLE by aerosol administration has been reported in humans. The LD_{50} in mice is 2 g orally and is associated with hypoactivity and gastrointestinal symptoms (estimated human equivalent dose of 0.17 g/kg, based on body surface area conversion). The mean plasma half-life after administration of aerosolized VIRAZOLE for pediatric patients is 9.5 hours. VIRAZOLE is concentrated and persists in red blood cells for the life of the erythrocyte (see Pharmacokinetics).

DOSAGE AND ADMINISTRATION

BEFORE USE, READ THOROUGHLY THE ICN SMALL PARTICLE AEROSOL GENERATOR MODEL SPAG-2 OPERATOR'S MANUAL FOR SMALL PARTICLE AEROSOL GENERATOR OPERATING INSTRUCTIONS. AEROSOLIZED VIRAZOLE SHOULD NOT BE ADMINISTERED WITH ANY OTHER AEROSOL GENERATING DEVICE.

The recommended treatment regimen is 20 mg/mL VIRAZOLE as the starting solution in the drug reservoir of the SPAG-2 unit, with continuous aerosol administration for 12–18 hours per day for 3 to 7 days. Using the recommended drug concentration of 20 mg/mL the average aerosol concentration for a 12 hour delivery period would be 190 micrograms/liter of air. Aerosolized VIRAZOLE should not be administered in a mixture for combined aerosolization or simultaneously with other aerosolized medications.

Non-mechanically ventilated infants

VIRAZOLE should be delivered to an infant oxygen hood from the SPAG-2 aerosol generator. Administration by face mask or oxygen tent may be necessary if a hood cannot be employed (see SPAG-2 manual). However, the volume and condensation area are larger in a tent and this may alter delivery dynamics of the drug.

Mechanically ventilated infants

The recommended dose and administration schedule for infants who require mechanical ventilation is the same as for those who do not. Either a pressure or volume cycle ventilator may be used in conjunction with the SPAG-2. In either case, patients should have their endotracheal tubes suctioned every 1–2 hours, and their pulmonary pressures monitored frequently (every 2–4 hours). For both pressure and volume ventilators, heated wire connective tubing and bacteria filters in series in the expiratory limb of the system (which must be changed frequently, i.e., every 4 hours) must be used to minimize the risk of VIRAZOLE precipitation in the system and the subsequent risk of ventilator dysfunction. Water column pressure release valves should be used in the ventilator circuit for pressure cycled ventilators, and may be utilized with volume cycled ventilators (SEE SPAG-2 MANUAL FOR DETAILED INSTRUCTIONS).

Method of Preparation

VIRAZOLE brand of ribavirin is supplied as 6 grams of lyophilized powder per 100 mL vial for aerosol administration only. By sterile technique, reconstitute drug with a minimum of 75 mL of **sterile USP water for injection or inhalation** in the original 100 mL glass vial. Shake well. Transfer to the clean, sterilized 500 mL SPAG-2 reservoir and further dilute to a final volume of 300 mL with Sterile Water for Injection, USP, or Inhalation. The final concentration should be 20 mg/mL. **Important:** This water should NOT have had any antimicrobial agent or other substance added. The solution should be inspected visually for particulate matter and discoloration prior to administration. Solutions that have been placed in the SPAG-2 unit should be discarded at least every 24 hours and when the liquid level is low before adding newly reconstituted solution.

HOW SUPPLIED

VIRAZOLE (Ribavirin for Inhalation Solution, USP) is supplied in four packs containing 100 mL glass vials with 6 grams of Sterile, lyophilized drug (NDC 0187-0007-14) which is to be reconstituted with 300 mL Sterile Water for Injection or Sterile Water for Inhalation (no preservatives added) and administered only by a small particle aerosol generator (SPAG-2). Vials containing the lyophilized drug powder should be stored in a dry place at 25°C (77°F); excursions permitted to 15°C–30°C (59°F–86°F). Reconstituted solutions may be stored, under sterile conditions, at room temperature (20–30°C, 68–86°F) for 24 hours. Solutions which have been placed in the SPAG-2 unit should be discarded at least every 24 hours.

REFERENCES

1. Hruska JF, Bernstein JM, Douglas Jr., RG, and Hall CB. Effects of Virazole on respiratory syncytial virus in vitro. Antimicrob Agents Chemother 17:770–775, 1 1980.
2. Hruska JF, Morrow PE, Suffin SC, and Douglas Jr., RG. In vivo inhibition of respiratory syncytial virus by Virazole. Antimicrob Agents Chemother 21:125–130, 1982.
3. Taber LH, Knight V, Gilbert BE, McClung HW et al. Virazole aerosol treatment of bronchiolitis associated with respiratory tract infection in infants. Pediatrics 72:613–618, 1983.
4. Hall CB, McBride JT, Walsh EE, Bell DM et al. Aerosolized Virazole treatment of infants with respiratory syncytial viral infection. N Engl J Med 308:1443–7, 1983.
5. Hendry RM, McIntosh K, Fahnestock ML, and Pierik LT. Enzyme-linked immunosorbent assay for detection of respiratory syncytial virus infection. J Clin Microbiol 16:329–33, 1982.
6. Smith, David W., Frankel, Lorry R., Mather, Larry H., Tang, Allen T.S., Ariagno, Ronald L., Prober, Charles G. A Controlled Trial of Aerosolized Ribavirin in Infants Receiving Mechanical Ventilation for Severe Respiratory Syncytial Virus Infection. The New England Journal of Medicine 1991; 325:24–29.
7. Decker, John, Shultz, Ruth A., Health Hazard Evaluation Report: Florida Hospital, Orlando, Florida, Cincinnati OH: U.S. Department of Health and Human Services, Public Health Service, Centers for NIOSH Report No. HETA 91-104-2229.*
8. Barnes, D.J. and Doursew, M. Reference dose: Description and use in health risk assessments. Regul Tox. and Pharm. Vol. 8; p. 471–486, 1988.
9. Federal Register Vol. 53 No. 126 Thurs. June 30, 1988 p. 24834–24847.
10. American Association for Respirtory Care [1991]. Aerosol Consensus Statement-1991. Respiratory Care 36(9): 916–921.

*Copies of the Report may be purchased from National Technical Information Service, 5285 Port Royal Road, Springfield, VA 22161; Ask for Publication PB 93119-345.

1957-07 EL
Rev. 4-02
Manufactured for:
VALEANT PHARMACEUTICALS INTERNATIONAL
3300 Hyland Avenue
Costa Mesa, California 92626
714-545-0100

VISTAKON Pharmaceuticals LLC

7500 CENTURION PARKWAY
JACKSONVILLE, FL 32256

Direct Inquiries to:
Phone (866) 427-6815

ALAMAST® ℞

[ălă-măst]
(pemirolast potassium ophthalmic solution) 0.1%

DESCRIPTION

ALAMAST® (pemirolast potassium ophthalmic solution) is a sterile, aqueous ophthalmic solution with a pH of approximately 8.0 containing 0.1% of the mast cell stabilizer, pemirolast potassium, for topical administration to the eyes.

Pemirolast potassium is a slightly yellow, water-soluble powder with a molecular weight of 266.3.

The chemical structure is presented below:

K+
CH3
$C_{10}H_7KN_6O$

Chemical name:
9-methyl-3-(1H-tetrazol-5-yl)-4H-pyrido[1,2-α] pyrimidin-4-one potassium

Each mL contains: ACTIVE: pemirolast potassium 1 mg (0.1%); PRESERVATIVE: lauralkonium chloride 0.005%; INACTIVES: glycerin, dibasic sodium phosphate, monobasic sodium phosphate, phosphoric acid and/or sodium hydroxide to adjust pH, and purified water. The osmolality of ALAMAST® ophthalmic solution is approximately 240 mOsmol/kg.

CLINICAL PHARMACOLOGY

Mechanism of Action: Pemirolast potassium is a mast cell stabilizer that inhibits the *in vivo* Type I immediate hypersensitivity reaction.

In vitro and *in vivo* studies have demonstrated that pemirolast potassium inhibits the antigen-induced release of inflammatory mediators (e.g., histamine, leukotriene C_4, D_4, E_4) from human mast cells.

In addition, pemirolast potassium inhibits the chemotaxis of eosinophils into ocular tissue and blocks the release of mediators from human eosinophils.

Although the precise mechanism of action is unknown, the drug has been reported to prevent calcium influx into mast cells upon antigen stimulation.

Pharmacokinetics: Topical ocular administration of one to two drops of ALAMAST® ophthalmic solution in each eye four times daily in 16 healthy volunteers for two weeks resulted in detectable concentrations in the plasma. The mean (±SE) peak plasma level of 4.7 ± 0.8 ng/mL occurred at 0.42 ± 0.05 hours and the mean $t_{1/2}$ was 4.5 ± 0.2 hours. When a single 10 mg pemirolast potassium dose was taken orally, a peak plasma concentration of 0.723 μg/mL was reached. Following topical administration, about 10-15% of the dose was excreted unchanged in the urine.

CLINICAL STUDIES

In clinical environmental studies, ALAMAST® was significantly more effective than placebo after 28 days in preventing ocular itching associated with allergic conjunctivitis.

INDICATIONS AND USAGE

ALAMAST® ophthalmic solution is indicated for the prevention of itching of the eye due to allergic conjunctivitis. Symptomatic response to therapy (decreased itching) may be evident within a few days, but frequently requires longer treatment (up to four weeks).

CONTRAINDICATIONS

ALAMAST® ophthalmic solution is contraindicated in patients with previously demonstrated hypersensitivity to any of the ingredients of this product.

WARNINGS

For topical ophthalmic use only. Not for injection or oral use.

PRECAUTIONS

Information for patients: To prevent contaminating the dropper tip and solution, do not touch the eyelids or surrounding areas with the dropper tip. Keep the bottle tightly closed when not in use.

Patients should be advised not to wear contact lenses if their eyes are red. ALAMAST® should not be used to treat contact lens related irritation. The preservative in ALAMAST®, lauralkonium chloride, may be absorbed by soft contact lenses. Patients who wear soft contact lenses and whose eyes are not red should be instructed to wait at least ten minutes after instilling ALAMAST® before they insert their contact lenses.

Carcinogenesis, mutagenesis, impairment of fertility: Pemirolast potassium was not mutagenic or clastogenic when tested in a series of bacterial and mammalian tests for gene mutation and chromosomal injury *in vitro* nor was it clastogenic when tested *in vivo* in rats.

Pemirolast potassium had no effect on mating and fertility in rats at oral doses up to 250 mg/kg (approximately 20,000 fold the human dose at 2 drops/eye, 40 µL/drop, QID for a 50 kg adult). A reduced fertility and pregnancy index occurred in the F_1 generation when F_0 dams were treated with 400 mg/kg pemirolast potassium during late pregnancy and lactation period (approximately 30,000 fold the human dose).

Pregnancy:

***Teratogenic effects:* Pregnancy Category C.** Pemirolast potassium caused an increased incidence of thymic remnant in the neck, interventricular septal defect, fetuses with wavy rib, splitting of thoracic vertebral body, and reduced numbers of ossified sternebrae, sacral and caudal vertebrae, and metatarsi when rats were given oral doses ≥250 mg/kg (approximately 20,000 fold the human dose at 2 drops/eye, 40 µL/drop, QID for a 50 kg adult) during organogenesis. Increased incidence of dilation of renal pelvis/ureter in the fetuses and neonates was also noted when rats were given an oral dose of 400 mg/kg pemirolast potassium (approximately 30,000 fold the human dose). Pemirolast potassium was not teratogenic in rabbits given oral doses up to 150 mg/kg (approximately 12,000 fold the human dose) during the same time period. There are no adequate and well-controlled studies in pregnant women. Because animal reproductive studies are not always predictive of human response, ALAMAST® ophthalmic solution should be used during pregnancy only if the benefit outweighs the risk.

Non-teratogenic effects: Pemirolast potassium produced increased pre- and post-implantation losses, reduced embryo/fetal and neonatal survival, decreased neonatal body weight, and delayed neonatal development in rats receiving an oral dose at 400 mg/kg (approximately 30,000 fold the human dose). Pemirolast potassium also caused a reduction in the number of corpus lutea, the number of implantations, and number of live fetuses in the F_1 generation in rats when F_0 dams were given oral dosages ≥250 mg/kg (approximately 20,000 fold the human dose) during late gestation and the lactation period.

Nursing Mothers: Pemirolast potassium is excreted in the milk of lactating rats at concentrations higher than those in plasma. It is not known whether pemirolast potassium is excreted in human milk. Because many drugs are excreted in human milk, caution should be exercised when ALAMAST® ophthalmic solution is administered to a nursing woman.

Pediatric Use: Safety and effectiveness in pediatric patients below the age of 3 years have not been established.

ADVERSE REACTIONS

In clinical studies lasting up to 17 weeks with ALAMAST® ophthalmic solution, headache, rhinitis, and cold/flu symptoms were reported at an incidence of 10–25%. The occurrence of these side effects was generally mild. Some of these events were similar to the underlying ocular disease being studied.

The following ocular and non-ocular adverse reactions were reported at an incidence of less than 5%:

Ocular: burning, dry eye, foreign body sensation, and ocular discomfort.

Non-Ocular: allergy, back pain, bronchitis, cough, dysmenorrhea, fever, sinusitis, and sneezing/nasal congestion.

OVERDOSAGE

No accounts of ALAMAST® ophthalmic solution overdose were reported following topical ocular application.

Oral ingestion of the contents of a 10 mL bottle would be equivalent to 10 mg of pemirolast potassium.

DOSAGE AND ADMINISTRATION

The recommended dose is one to two drops in each affected eye four times daily.

Symptomatic response to therapy (decreased itching) may be evident within a few days, but frequently requires longer treatment (up to four weeks).

HOW SUPPLIED

ALAMAST® (pemirolast potassium ophthalmic solution) 0.1% is supplied as follows:

10 mL in a white, low density polyethylene bottle with a controlled dropper tip, and a white polyethylene screw cap.

NDC 68669-711-10 10 mL fill in 10 cc container

Storage: Store at 15°–25°C (59°–77°F).

Rx only

Manufactured by:
Parkedale Pharmaceuticals, Inc., Rochester, MI 48307, USA

2.5 mL Physician Sample Manufactured by:
Santen Oy, PO Box 33
FIN-33721 Tampere, Finland

Santen®

Marketed by:
VISTAKON® Pharmaceuticals, LLC
Jacksonville, FL 32256
Licensed from Mitsubishi Pharma Corporation
Tokyo, Japan
March 2004 Version
U.S. Patent No. 5,034,230
VISTAKON® Pharmaceuticals, LLC
III-03

Shown in Product Identification Guide, page 335

BETIMOL® ℞

[*bāt′-ī-mōl″*]

(timolol ophthalmic solution) 0.25%, 0.5%

DESCRIPTION

Betimol® (timolol ophthalmic solution), 0.25% and 0.5%, is a non-selective beta-adrenergic antagonist for ophthalmic use. The chemical name of the active ingredient is (S)-1-[(1,1-dimethylethyl)amino]-3-[[4-(4-morpholinyl)-1,2,5-thiadiazol-3-yl]oxy]-2-propanol. Timolol hemihydrate is the levo isomer. Specific rotation is $[\alpha]^{25}_{405nm} = -16°$ (C=10% as the hemihydrate form in 1N HCl).

The molecular formula of timolol is Formula $C_{13}H_{24}N_4O_3S$ and its structural formula is:

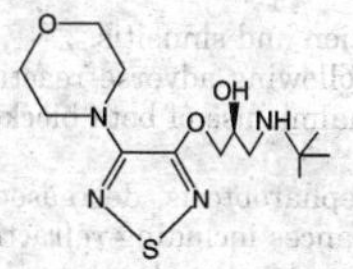

Timolol (as the hemihydrate) is a white, odorless, crystalline powder which is slightly soluble in water and freely soluble in ethanol. Timolol hemihydrate is stable at room temperature.

Betimol® is a clear, colorless, isotonic, sterile, microbiologically preserved phosphate buffered aqueous solution.

It is supplied in two dosage strengths, 0.25% and 0.5%.

Each mL of Betimol® 0.25% contains 2.56 mg of timolol hemihydrate equivalent to 2.5 mg timolol.

Each mL of Betimol® 05% contains 5.12 mg of timolol hemihydrate equivalent to 5.0 mg timolol.

Inactive ingredients: monosodium and disodium phosphate dihydrate to adjust pH (6.5 – 7.5) and water for injection, benzalkonium chloride 0.01% added as preservative.

The osmolality of Betimol® is 260 to 320 mOsmol/kg.

CLINICAL PHARMACOLOGY

Timolol is a non-selective beta-adrenergic antagonist.

It blocks both $beta_1$- and $beta_2$-adrenergic receptors. Timolol does not have significant intrinsic sympathomimetic activity, local anesthetic (membrane-stabilizing) or direct myocardial depressant activity.

Timolol, when applied topically in the eye, reduces normal and elevated intraocular pressure (IOP) whether or not accompanied by glaucoma. Elevated intraocular pressure is a major risk factor in the pathogenesis of glaucomatous visual field loss. The higher the level of IOP, the greater the likelihood of glaucomatous visual field loss and optic nerve damage. The predominant mechanism of ocular hypotensive action of topical beta-adrenergic blocking agents is likely due to a reduction in aqueous humor production.

In general, beta-adrenergic blocking agents reduce cardiac output both in healthy subjects and patients with heart diseases. In patients with severe impairment of myocardial function, beta-adrenergic receptor blocking agents may inhibit sympathetic stimulatory effect necessary to maintain adequate cardiac function. In the bronchi and bronchioles, beta-adrenergic receptor blockade may also increase airway resistance because of unopposed parasympathetic activity.

Pharmacokinetics

When given orally, timolol is well absorbed and undergoes considerable first pass metabolism. Timolol and its metabolites are primarily excreted in the urine. The half-life of timolol in plasma is approximately 4 hours.

Clinical Studies

In two controlled multicenter studies in the U.S., Betimol® 0.25% and 0.5% were compared with respective timolol maleate eyedrops. In these studies, the efficacy and safety profile of Betimol® was similar to that of timolol maleate.

INDICATIONS AND USAGE

Betimol® is indicated in the treatment of elevated intraocular pressure in patients with ocular hypertension or open-angle glaucoma.

CONTRAINDICATIONS

Betimol® is contraindicated in patients with overt heart failure, cardiogenic shock, sinus bradycardia, second- or third-degree atrioventricular block, bronchial asthma or history of bronchial asthma, or severe chronic obstructive pulmonary disease, or hypersensitivity to any component of this product.

WARNINGS

As with other topically applied ophthalmic drugs, Betimol® is absorbed systemically. The same adverse reactions found with systemic administration of beta-adrenergic blocking agents may occur with topical administration. For example, severe respiratory and cardiac reactions, including death due to bronchospasm in patients with asthma, and rarely, death in association with cardiac failure have been reported following systemic or topical administration of beta-adrenergic blocking agents.

Cardiac Failure: Sympathetic stimulation may be essential for support of the circulation in individuals with diminished myocardial contractility, and its inhibition by beta-adrenergic receptor blockade may precipitate more severe cardiac failure.

In patients without a history of cardiac failure, continued depression of the myocardium with beta-blocking agents over a period of time can, in some cases, lead to cardiac failure. Betimol® should be discontinued at the first sign or symptom of cardiac failure.

Obstructive Pulmonary Disease: Patients with chronic obstructive pulmonary disease (e.g. chronic bronchitis, emphysema) of mild or moderate severity, bronchospastic disease, or a history of bronchospastic disease (other than bronchial asthma or a history of bronchial asthma which are contraindications) should in general not receive beta-blocking agents.

Major Surgery: The necessity or desirability of withdrawal of beta-adrenergic blocking agents prior to a major surgery is controversial. Beta-adrenergic receptor blockade impairs the ability of the heart to respond to beta-adrenergically mediated reflex stimuli. This may augment the risk of general anesthesia in surgical procedures. Some patients receiving beta-adrenergic receptor blocking agents have been subject to protracted severe hypotension during anesthesia. Difficulty in restarting and maintaining the heartbeat has also been reported. For these reasons, in patients undergoing elective surgery, gradual withdrawal of beta-adrenergic receptor blocking agents is recommended. If necessary during surgery, the effects of beta-adrenergic blocking agents may be reversed by sufficient doses of beta-adrenergic agonists.

Diabetes Mellitus: Beta-adrenergic blocking agents should be administered with caution in patients subject to spontaneous hypoglycemia or to diabetic patients (especially those with labile diabetes) who are receiving insulin or oral hypoglycemic agents. Beta-adrenergic receptor blocking agents may mask the signs and symptoms of acute hypoglycemia.

Thyrotoxicosis: Beta-adrenergic blocking agents may mask certain clinical signs (e.g. tachycardia) of hyperthyroidism. Patients suspected of developing thyrotoxicosis should be managed carefully to avoid abrupt withdrawal of beta-adrenergic blocking agents which might precipitate a thyroid storm.

PRECAUTIONS

General

Because of the potential effects of beta-adrenergic blocking agents relative to blood pressure and pulse, these agents should be used with caution in patients with cerebrovascular insufficiency. If signs or symptoms suggesting reduced cerebral blood flow develop following initiation of therapy with Betimol®, alternative therapy should be considered.

There have been reports of bacterial keratitis associated with the use of multiple dose containers of topical ophthalmic products. These containers had been inadvertently contaminated by patients who, in most cases, had a concurrent corneal disease or a disruption of the ocular epithelial suface. (See PRECAUTIONS, Information for Patients.)

Muscle Weakness: Beta-adrenergic blockade has been reported to potentiate muscle weakness consistent with certain myasthenic symptoms (e.g. diplopia, ptosis, and generalized weakness). Beta-adrenergic blocking agents have been reported rarely to increase muscle weakness in some patients with myasthenia gravis or myasthenic symptoms.

In angle-closure glaucoma, the goal of the treatment is to reopen the angle. This requires constricting the pupil. Betimol® has no effect on the pupil. Therefore, if timolol is used in angle-closure glaucoma, it should always be combined with a miotic and not used alone.

Anaphylaxis: While taking beta-blockers, patients with a history of atopy or a history of severe anaphylactic reactions to a variety of allergens may be more reactive to repeated accidental, diagnostic, or therapeutic challenge with such allergens. Such patients may be unresponsive to the usual

Continued on next page

Betimol—Cont.

doses of epinephrine used to treat anaphylactic reactions.
The preservative benzalkonium chloride may be absorbed by soft contact lenses. Patients who wear soft contact lenses should wait 5 minutes after instilling Betimol® before they insert their lenses.

Information for Patients

Patients should be instructed to avoid allowing the tip of the dispensing container to contact the eye or surrounding structures.

Patients should also be instructed that ocular solutions can become contaminated by common bacteria known to cause ocular infections. Serious damage to the eye and subsequent loss of vision may result from using contaminated solutions. (See PRECAUTIONS, General.)

Patients requiring concomitant topical ophthalmic medications should be instructed to administer these at least 5 minutes apart.

Patients with bronchial asthma, a history of bronchial asthma, severe chronic obstructive pulmonary disease, sinus bradycardia, second- or third-degree atrioventricular block, or cardiac failure should be advised not to take this product (See CONTRAINDICATIONS.)

Drug Interactions

Beta-adrenergic blocking agents: Patients who are receiving a beta-adrenergic blocking agent orally and Betimol® should be observed for a potential additive effect either on the intraocular pressure or on the known systemic effects of beta-blockade.

Patients should not usually receive two topical ophthalmic beta-adrenergic blocking agents concurrently.

Catecholamine-depleting drugs: Close observation of the patient is recommended when a beta-blocker is administered to patients receiving catecholamine-depleting drugs such as reserpine, because of possible additive effects and the production of hypotension and/or marked bradycardia, which may produce vertigo, syncope, or postural hypotension.

Calcium antagonists: Caution should be used in the co-administration of beta-adrenergic blocking agents and oral or intravenous calcium antagonists, because of possible atrioventricular conduction disturbances, left ventricular failure, and hypotension. In patients with impaired cardiac function, co-administration should be avoided.

Digitalis and calcium antagonists The concomitant use of beta-adrenergic blocking agents with digitalis and calcium antagonists may have additive effects in prolonging atrioventricular conduction time.

Injectable Epinephrine: (See PRECAUTIONS, General, Anaphylaxis.)

Carcinogenesis, Mutagenesis, Impairment of Fertility

Carcinogenicity of timolol (as the maleate) has been studied in mice and rats. In a two-year study orally administrated timolol maleate (300mg/kg/day) (approximately 42,000 times the systemic exposure following the maximum recommended human ophthalmic dose) in male rats caused a significant increase in the incidence of adrenal pheochromocytomas; the lower doses, 25 mg or 100 mg/kg daily did not cause any changes.

In a life span study in mice the overall incidence of neoplasms was significantly increased in female mice at 500 mg/kg/day (approximately 71,000 times the systemic exposure following the maximum recommended human ophthalmic dose). Furthermore, significant increases were observed in the incidences of benign and malignant pulmonary tumors, benign uterine polyps, as well as mammary adenocarcinomas. These changes were not seen at the daily dose level of 5 or 50 mg/kg (approximately 700 or 7,000, respectively, times the systemic exposure following the maximum recommended human ophthalmic dose). For comparison, the maximum recommended human oral dose of timolol maleate is 1 mg/kg/day.

Mutagenic potential of timolol was evaluated *in vivo* in the micronucleus test and cytogenetic assay and *in vitro* in the neoplastic cell transformation assay and Ames test. In the bacterial mutagenicity test (Ames test) high concentrations of timolol maleate (5000 and 10,000 g/plate) statistically significantly increased the number of revertants in *Salmonella typhimurium* TA100, but not in the other three strains tested. However, no consistent dose-response was observed nor did the number of revertants reach the double of the control value, which is regarded as one of the criteria for a positive result in the Ames test. *In vivo* genotoxicity tests (the mouse micronucleus test and cytogenetic assay) and *in vitro* the neoplastic cell transformation assay were negative up to dose levels of 800 mg/kg and 100 g/mL, respectively.

No adverse effects on male and female fertility were reported in rats at timolol oral doses of up to 150 mg/kg/day (21,000 times the systemic exposure following the maximum recommended human ophthalmic dose).

Pregnancy Teratogenic effects:

Category C: Teratogenicity of timolol (as the maleate) after oral administration was studied in mice and rabbits. No fetal malformations were reported in mice or rabbits at a daily oral dose of 50 mg/kg (7,000 times the systemic exposure following the maximum recommended human ophthalmic dose). Although delayed fetal ossification was observed at this dose in rats, there were no adverse effects on postnatal development of offspring. Doses of 1000 mg/kg/day (142,000 times the systemic exposure following the maximum recommended human ophthalmic dose) were maternotoxic in mice and resulted in an increased number of fetal resorptions. Increased fetal resorptions were also seen in rabbits at doses of 14,000 times the systemic exposure following the maximum recommended human ophthalmic dose in this case without apparent maternotoxicity.

There are no adequate and well-controlled studies in pregnant women. Betimol® should be used during pregnancy only it the potential benefit justifies the potential risk to the fetus.

Nursing mothers:

Because of the potential for serious adverse reactions in nursing infants from timolol, a decision should be made whether to discontinue nursing or to discontinue the drug, taking into account the importance of the drug to the mother.

Pediatric use:

Safety and efficacy in pediatric patients have not been established.

ADVERSE REACTIONS

The most frequently reported ocular event in clinical trials was burning/stinging on instillation and was comparable between Betimol® and timolol maleate (approximately one in eight patients).

The following adverse events were associated with use of Betimol® in frequencies of more than 5% in two controlled, double-masked clinical studies in which 184 patients received 0.25% or 0.5% Betimol®:

OCULAR:

Dry eyes, itching, foreign body sensation, discomfort in the eye, eyelid erythema, conjunctival injection, and headache.

BODY AS A WHOLE:

Headache.

The following side effects were reported in frequencies of 1 to 5%:

OCULAR:

Eye pain, epiphora, photophobia, blurred or abnormal vision, corneal fluorescein staining, keratitis, blepharitis and cataract.

BODY AS A WHOLE:

Allergic reaction, asthenia, common cold and pain in extremities.

CARDIOVASCULAR:

Hypertension.

DIGESTIVE:

Nausea.

METABOLIC/NUTRITIONAL:

Peripheral edema.

NERVOUS SYSTEM/PSYCHIATRY:

Dizziness and dry mouth.

RESPIRATORY:

Respiratory infection and sinusitis.

In addition, the following adverse reactions have been reported with ophthalmic use of beta blockers:

OCULAR:

Conjunctivitis, blepharoptosis, decreased corneal sensitivity, visual disturbances including refractive changes, diplopia and retinal vascular disorder.

BODY AS A WHOLE:

Chest pain.

CARDIOVASCULAR:

Arrhythmia, palpitation, bradycardia, hypotension, syncope, heart block, cerebral vascular accident, cerebral ischemia, cardiac failure and cardiac arrest.

DIGESTIVE:

Diarrhea.

ENDOCRINE:

Masked symptoms of hypoglycemia in insulin dependent diabetics (See WARNINGS).

NERVOUS SYSTEM/PSYCHIATRY:

Depression, impotence, increase in signs and symptoms of myasthenia gravis and paresthesia.

RESPIRATORY:

Dyspnea, bronchospasm, respiratory failure and nasal congestion.

SKIN:

Alopecia, hypersensitivity including localized and generalized rash, urticaria.

OVERDOSAGE

No information is available on overdosage with Betimol®. Symptoms that might be expected with an overdose of a beta-adrenergic receptor blocking agent are bronchospasm, hypotension, bradycardia, and acute cardiac failure.

DOSAGE AND ADMINISTRATION

Betimol® Ophthalmic Solution is available in concentrations of 0.25 and 0.5 percent. The usual starting dose is one drop of 0.25 percent Betimol® in the affected eye(s) twice a day. If the clinical response is not adequate, the dosage may be changed to one drop of 0.5 percent solution in the affected eye(s) twice a day.

If the intraocular pressure is maintained at satisfactory levels, the dosage schedule may be changed to one drop once a day in the affected eye(s). Because of diurnal variations in intraocular pressure, satisfactory response to the once-a-day dose is best determined by measuring the intraocular pressure at different times during the day.

Since in some patients the pressure-lowering response to Betimol® may require a few weeks to stabilize, evaluation should include a determination of intraocular pressure after approximately 4 weeks of treatment with Betimol®.

Dosages above one drop of 0.5 percent Betimol® twice a day generally have not been shown to produce further reduction in intraocular pressure. If the patient's intraocular pressure is still not at a satisfactory level on this regimen, concomitant therapy with pilocarpine and other miotics, and/or epinephrine, and/or systemically administered carbonic anhydrase inhibitors, such as acetazolamide can be instituted.

HOW SUPPLIED

Betimol® (timolol ophthalmic solution) is a clear, colorless solution.

Betimol® 0.25% is supplied in a white, opaque, plastic, ophthalmic dispenser bottle with a controlled drop tip as follows:

NDC 68669-522-05 5.0mL fill in 5 cc container
NDC 68669-522-10 10mL fill in 11 cc container
NDC 68669-522-15 15mL fill in 15 cc container

Betimol® 0.5% is supplied in a white, opaque, plastic, ophthalmic dispenser bottle with a controlled drop tip as follows:

NDC 68669-525-05 5.0mL fill in 5 cc container
NDC 68669-525-10 10mL fill in 11 cc container
NDC 68669-525-15 15mL fill in 15 cc container

Rx Only

STORAGE

Store between 15-30°C (59-86°F). Do not freeze. Protect from light.

MARKETED BY:

VISTAKON® Pharmaceuticals, LLC
Jacksonville, FL 32256 USA

MANUFACTURED BY:

Santen Oy, P.O. Box 33
FIN-33721 Tampere, Finland

Santen®

March 2004 Version

VISTAKON® Pharmaceuticals, LLC

Shown in Product Identification Guide, page 335

QUIXIN® ℞

[*kwĭk-sĭn*]

(levofloxacin ophthalmic solution) 0.5%

DESCRIPTION

QUIXIN® (levofloxacin ophthalmic solution) 0.5% is a sterile topical ophthalmic solution. Levofloxacin is a fluoroquinolone antibacterial active against a broad spectrum of Gram-positive and Gram-negative ocular pathogens. Levofloxacin is the pure (-)-(*S*)-enantiomer of the racemic drug substance, ofloxacin. It is more soluble in water at neutral pH than ofloxacin.

Structural formula

levofloxacin hemihydrate

$C_{18}H_{20}FN_3O_4 \cdot 1/2\ H_2O$ Mol Wt 370.38

Chemical Name: (-)-(*S*)-9-fluoro-2,3-dihydro-3-methyl-10-(4-methyl-1-piperazinyl)-7-oxo-7*H*-pyrido[1,2,3-*de*]-1,4 benzoxazine-6-carboxylic acid hemihydrate.

Levofloxacin (hemihydrate) is a yellowish-white crystalline powder.

Each mL of QUIXIN® contains 5.12 mg of levofloxacin hemihydrate equivalent to 5 mg levofloxacin.

Contains: Active: Levofloxacin 0.5% (5 mg/mL); **Preservative:** benzalkonium chloride 0.005%; **Inactives:** sodium chloride and water. May also contain hydrochloric acid and/or sodium hydroxide to adjust pH.

QUIXIN® solution is isotonic and formulated at pH 6.5 with an osmolality of approximately 300 mOsm/kg. Levofloxacin is a fluorinated 4-quinolone containing a six-member (pyridobenzoxazine) ring from positions 1 to 8 of the basic ring structure.

CLINICAL PHARMACOLOGY

Pharmacokinetics: Levofloxacin concentration in plasma was measured in 15 healthy adult volunteers at various time points during a 15-day course of treatment with QUIXIN® solution. The mean levofloxacin concentration in plasma 1 hour postdose, ranged from 0.86 ng/mL on Day 1 to 2.05 ng/mL on Day 15. The highest maximum mean levofloxacin concentration of 2.25 ng/mL was measured on Day 4 following 2 days of dosing every 2 hours for a total of 8 doses per day. Maximum mean levofloxacin concentrations increased from 0.94 ng/mL on Day 1 to 2.15 ng/mL on Day 15, which is more than 1,000 times lower than those reported after standard oral doses of levofloxacin.

Levofloxacin concentration in tears was measured in 30 healthy adult volunteers at various time points following instillation of a single drop of QUIXIN® solution. Mean levofloxacin concentrations in tears ranged from 34.9 to 221.1 µg/mL during the 60-minute period following the single dose. The mean tear concentrations measured 4 and 6 hours postdose were 17.0 and 6.6 µg/mL. The clinical significance of these concentrations is unknown.

Microbiology: Levofloxacin is the *L*-isomer of the racemate, ofloxacin, a quinolone antimicrobial agent. The antibacterial activity of ofloxacin resides primarily in the *L*-isomer. The mechanism of action of levofloxacin and other fluoroquinolone antimicrobials involves the inhibition of bacterial topoisomerase IV and DNA gyrase (both of which are type II topoisomerases), enzymes required for DNA replication, transcription, repair, and recombination.

Levofloxacin has *in vitro* activity against a wide range of Gram-negative and Gram-positive microorganisms and is often bactericidal at concentrations equal to or slightly greater than inhibitory concentrations.

Fluoroquinolones, including levofloxacin, differ in chemical structure and mode of action from β-lactam antibiotics and aminoglycosides, and therefore may be active against bacteria resistant to β-lactam antibiotics and aminoglycosides. Additionally, β-lactam antibiotics and aminoglycosides may be active against bacteria resistant to levofloxacin.

Resistance to levofloxacin due to spontaneous mutation *in vitro* is a rare occurrence (range: 10^{-9} to 10^{-10}).

Levofloxacin has been shown to be active against most strains of the following microorganisms, both *in vitro* and in clinical infections as described in the INDICATIONS AND USAGE section:

AEROBIC GRAM-POSITIVE MICROORGANISMS

Corynebacterium species*
Staphylococcus aureus
Staphylococcus epidermidis
Streptococcus pneumoniae
Streptococcus (Groups C/F)
Streptococcus (Group G)
Viridans group streptococci

AEROBIC GRAM-NEGATIVE MICROORGANISMS

*Acinetobacter lwoffii**
Haemophilus influenzae
*Serratia marcescens**

*Efficacy for this organism was studied in fewer than 10 infections.

The following *in vitro* data are also available, but their clinical significance in ophthalmic infections is unknown. The safety and effectiveness of levofloxacin in treating ophthalmological infections due to these microorganisms have not been established in adequate and well-controlled trials.

These organisms are considered susceptible when evaluated using systemic breakpoints. However, a correlation between the *in vitro* systemic breakpoint and ophthalmological efficacy has not been established. The list of organisms is provided as guidance only in assessing the potential treatment of conjunctival infections. Levofloxacin exhibits *in vitro* minimal inhibitory concentrations (MICs) of 2 μg/mL or less (systemic susceptible breakpoint) against most (≥90%) strains of the following ocular pathogens.

AEROBIC GRAM-POSITIVE MICROORGANISMS

Enterococcus faecalis
Staphylococcus saprophyticus
Streptococcus agalactiae
Streptococcus pyogenes

AEROBIC GRAM-NEGATIVE MICROORGANISMS

Acinetobacter anitratus
Acinetobacter baumannii
Citrobacter diversus
Citrobacter freundii
Enterobacter aerogenes
Enterobacter agglomerans
Enterobacter cloacae
Escherichia coli
Haemophilus parainfluenzae
Klebsiella oxytoca
Klebsiella pneumoniae
Legionella pneumophila
Moraxella catarrhalis
Morganella morganii
Neisseria gonorrhoeae
Proteus mirabilis
Proteus vulgaris
Providencia rettgeri
Providencia stuartii
Pseudomonas aeruginosa
Pseudomonas fluorescens

Clinical Studies:

In randomized, double-masked, multicenter controlled clinical trials where patients were dosed for 5 days, QUIXIN® demonstrated clinical cures in 79% of patients treated for bacterial conjunctivitis on the final study visit day (day 6-10). Microbial outcomes for the same clinical trials demonstrated an eradication rate for presumed pathogens of 90%.

INDICATIONS AND USAGE

QUIXIN® solution is indicated for the treatment of bacterial conjunctivitis caused by susceptible strains of the following organisms:

AEROBIC GRAM-POSITIVE MICROORGANISMS

Corynebacterium species*
Staphylococcus aureus
Staphylococcus epidermidis
Streptococcus pneumoniae
Streptococcus (Groups C/F)
Streptococcus (Group G)
Viridans group streptococci

AEROBIC GRAM-NEGATIVE MICROORGANISMS

*Acinetobacter Iwoffii**
Haemophilus influenzae
*Serratia marcescens**

*Efficacy for this organism was studied in fewer than 10 infections.

CONTRAINDICATIONS

QUIXIN® solution is contraindicated in patients with a history of hypersensitivity to levofloxacin, to other quinolones, or to any of the components in this medication.

WARNINGS

NOT FOR INJECTION.

QUIXIN® solution should not be injected subconjunctivally, nor should it be introduced directly into the anterior chamber of the eye.

In patients receiving systemic quinolones, serious and occasionally fatal hypersensitivity (anaphylactic) reactions have been reported, some following the first dose. Some reactions were accompanied by cardiovascular collapse, loss of consciousness, angioedema (including laryngeal, pharyngeal or facial edema), airway obstruction, dyspnea, urticaria, and itching. If an allergic reaction to levofloxacin occurs, discontinue the drug. Serious acute hypersensitivity reactions may require immediate emergency treatment. Oxygen and airway management should be administered as clinically indicated.

PRECAUTIONS

General: As with other anti-infectives, prolonged use may result in overgrowth of non-susceptible organisms, including fungi. If superinfection occurs, discontinue use and institute alternative therapy. Whenever clinical judgment dictates, the patient should be examined with the aid of magnification, such as slit-lamp biomicroscopy, and, where appropriate, fluorescein staining.

Patients should be advised not to wear contact lenses if they have signs and symptoms of bacterial conjunctivitis.

Information for Patients: Avoid contaminating the applicator tip with material from the eye, fingers or other source. Systemic quinolones have been associated with hypersensitivity reactions, even following a single dose. Discontinue use immediately and contact your physician at the first sign of a rash or allergic reaction.

Drug Interactions: Specific drug interaction studies have not been conducted with QUIXIN®. However, the systemic administration of some quinolones has been shown to elevate plasma concentrations of theophylline, interfere with the metabolism of caffeine, and enhance the effects of the oral anticoagulant warfarin and its derivatives, and has been associated with transient elevations in serum creatinine in patients receiving systemic cyclosporine concomitantly.

Carcinogenesis, Mutagenesis, Impairment of Fertility: In a long term carcinogenicity study in rats, levofloxacin exhibited no carcinogenic or tumorigenic potential following daily dietary administration for 2 years; the highest dose (100 mg/kg/day) was 875 times the highest recommended human ophthalmic dose.

Levofloxacin was not mutagenic in the following assays: Ames bacterial mutation assay (*S. typhimurium* and *E. coli*), CHO/HGPRT forward mutation assay, mouse micronucleus test, mouse dominant lethal test, rat unscheduled DNA synthesis assay, and the *in vivo* mouse sister chromatid exchange assay. It was positive in the *in vitro* chromosomal aberration (CHL cell line) and *in vitro* sister chromatid exchange (CHL/IU cell line) assays.

Levofloxacin caused no impairment of fertility or reproduction in rats at oral doses as high as 360 mg/kg/day, corresponding to 3,150 times the highest recommended human ophthalmic dose.

Pregnancy: Teratogenic Effects. Pregnancy Category C: Levofloxacin at oral doses of 810 mg/kg/day in rats, which corresponds to approximately 7,000 times the highest recommended human ophthalmic dose, caused decreased fetal body weight and increased fetal mortality.

No teratogenic effect was observed when rabbits were dosed orally as high as 50 mg/kg/day, which corresponds to approximately 400 times the highest recommended maximum human ophthalmic dose, or when dosed intravenously as high as 25 mg/kg/day, corresponding to approximately 200 times the highest recommended human ophthalmic dose.

There are, however, no adequate and well-controlled studies in pregnant women. Levofloxacin should be used during pregnancy only if the potential benefit justifies the potential risk to the fetus.

Nursing Mothers: Levofloxacin has not been measured in human milk. Based upon data from ofloxacin, it can be presumed that levofloxacin is excreted in human milk. Caution should be exercised when QUIXIN® is administered to a nursing mother.

Pediatric Use: Safety and effectiveness in infants below the age of one year have not been established. Oral administration of quinolones has been shown to cause arthropathy in immature animals. There is no evidence that the ophthalmic administration of levofloxacin has any effect on weight bearing joints.

Geriatric Use: No overall differences in safety or effectiveness have been observed between elderly and other adult patients.

ADVERSE REACTIONS

The most frequently reported adverse events in the overall study population were transient decreased vision, fever, foreign body sensation, headache, transient ocular burning, ocular pain or discomfort, pharyngitis and photophobia. These events occurred in approximately 1-3% of patients. Other reported reactions occurring in less than 1% of patients included allergic reactions, lid edema, ocular dryness, and ocular itching.

DOSAGE AND ADMINISTRATION

Days 1 and 2: Instill one to two drops in the affected eye(s) every 2 hours while awake, up to 8 times per day.

Days 3 through 7: Instill one to two drops in the affected eye(s) every 4 hours while awake, up to 4 times per day.

HOW SUPPLIED

QUIXIN® (levofloxacin ophthalmic solution) 0.5% is supplied in a white, low density polyethylene bottle with a controlled dropper tip and a tan, high density polyethylene cap in the following size:

5 mL fill in 5cc container - NDC 68669-135-05

Storage: Store at 15° – 25°C (59° – 77°F).

Rx only

Manufactured by:
Santen Oy, P.O. Box 33, FIN-33721
Tampere, Finland
Licensed from:
Daiichi Pharmaceutical Co., Ltd.,
Tokyo, Japan
U.S. PAT. NO. 5,053,407

Marketed by:
VISTAKON® Pharmaceuticals, LLC
Jacksonville, FL 32256 USA
March 2004 Version

Shown in Product Identification Guide, page 335

VIVUS, Inc.

1172 CASTRO STREET
MOUNTAIN VIEW, CA 94040

Direct Inquiries to:
(888) 345-6873

For Medical Information or Emergencies Contact:
Medical Services Department @ VIVUS:
(650) 934-5200
FAX: (650) 934-5212

MUSE® ℞

(alprostadil)
urethral suppository

DESCRIPTION

MUSE® (alprostadil) is a single-use, medicated transurethral system for the delivery of alprostadil to the male urethra. Alprostadil is suspended in polyethylene glycol 1450 (as excipient) and is formed into a medicated pellet (microsuppository measuring 1.4 mm in diameter by 3 mm or 6 mm in length) that resides in the tip of a translucent hollow applicator. MUSE is administered by inserting the applicator stem into the urethra after urination. The pellet containing alprostadil is delivered by depressing the applicator button (**see Figure 1**). The components of the delivery system are constructed of medical grade polypropylene. Each MUSE system is packaged in an individual foil pouch.

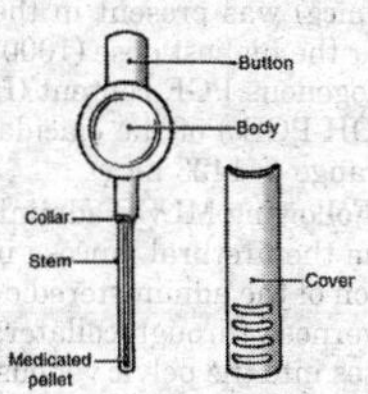

Figure 1: Diagram of the MUSE Transurethral System

The active ingredient in MUSE is alprostadil, which is chemically identical to the naturally occurring eicosanoid, prostaglandin E_1 (PGE_1). The chemical name for alprostadil is prost-13-en-1-oic acid, 11,15-dihydroxy-9-oxo-(11α,13E, 15S)-(1R,2R,3R)-3-hydroxy-2-[(E)-(3S)-3-hydroxy-1-octenyl]-5-oxo-cyclopentane heptanoic acid, and the molecular weight is 354.49. The empirical formula is $C_{20}H_{34}O_5$. The structural formula of alprostadil is represented below:

Alprostadil is a white to off-white crystalline powder with a melting point between 115° and 116°C. Its solubility at 35°C is 8000 mcg per 100 mL double-distilled water. The inactive ingredient in MUSE is polyethylene glycol 1450, USP. There are no other active agents or excipients in MUSE.

Continued on next page

MUSE—Cont.

MUSE is available in 4 dosage strengths: 125 mcg, 250 mcg, 500 mcg, and 1000 mcg.

CLINICAL PHARMACOLOGY

Mechanism of Action: Prostaglandin E_1 is a naturally occurring acidic lipid that is synthesized from fatty acid precursors by most mammalian tissues and has a variety of pharmacologic effects. Human seminal fluid is a rich source of prostaglandins, including PGE_1 and PGE_2, and the total concentration of prostaglandins in ejaculate has been estimated to be approximately 100–200 mcg/mL. In vitro, alprostadil (PGE_1) has been shown to cause dose-dependent smooth muscle relaxation in isolated corpus cavernosum and corpus spongiosum preparations. Additionally, vasodilation has been demonstrated in isolated cavernosal artery segments that were pre-contracted with either norepinephrine or prostaglandin $F_{2\alpha}$. When alprostadil was injected into the corpus cavernosum of pigtail monkeys in vivo, dose-dependent increases in cavernosal artery blood flow were observed.

In human studies using Doppler duplex ultrasonography, intraurethral administration of 500 mcg of MUSE resulted in an increase in cavernosal artery diameter and a 5- to 10-fold increase in peak systolic flow velocities. These results suggest that intraurethral alprostadil is absorbed from the urethra, transported throughout the erectile bodies by communicating vessels between the corpus spongiosum and corpora cavernosa, and able to induce vasodilation of the targeted vascular beds.

The vasodilatory effects of alprostadil on the cavernosal arteries and the trabecular smooth muscle of the corpora cavernosa result in rapid arterial inflow and expansion of the lacunar spaces within the corpora. As the expanded corporal sinusoids are compressed against the tunica albuginea, venous outflow through subtunical vessels is impeded and penile rigidity develops. This process is referred to as the corporal veno-occlusive mechanism.

The most notable systemic effects of alprostadil are vasodilation, inhibition of platelet aggregation, and stimulation of intestinal and uterine smooth muscle. Intravenous doses of 1 to 10 micrograms per kilogram of body weight lower blood pressure in mammals by decreasing peripheral resistance. Reflex increases in cardiac output and heart rate may accompany these effects.

Pharmacokinetics: About 80% of alprostadil administered by MUSE is absorbed within 10 minutes and is rapidly cleared from the systemic circulation by the lungs, leaving barely detectable systemic blood levels.

Absorption: MUSE is designed to deliver alprostadil directly to the urethral lining for transfer via the corpus spongiosum to the corpora cavernosa. Intraurethral administration of MUSE is preceded by urination, and the residual urine disperses the medicated pellet, permitting alprostadil to be absorbed by the urethral mucosa. The transurethral absorption of alprostadil after MUSE administration is biphasic. Initial absorption is rapid, with approximately 80% of an administered dose absorbed within 10 minutes. The mean time to the maximum plasma PGE_1 concentration after a 1000 mcg intraurethral dose of MUSE is approximately 16 minutes.

In 10 normal human volunteers, endogenous PGE_1 levels in the ejaculate averaged 31 mcg (range 0–161 mcg). In these same volunteers, an average of 123 mcg of additional PGE_1 (range 30–369 mcg) was present in the ejaculate obtained 10 minutes after the highest dose (1000 mcg) of MUSE. The mean total endogenous PGE content (PGE_1, PGE_2, 19-OH-PGE_1, and 19-OH-PGE_2) of the ejaculate in these subjects was 444 mcg (range 0–1423 mcg).

Distribution: Following MUSE administration, alprostadil is absorbed from the urethral mucosa into the corpus spongiosum. A portion of the administered dose is transported to the corpora cavernosa through collateral vessels, while the remainder passes into the pelvic venous circulation through veins draining the corpus spongiosum. The half-life of alprostadil in humans is short, varying between 30 seconds and 10 minutes, depending on the body compartment in which it is measured and the physiological status of the subject. Nearly all of the alprostadil entering the central venous circulation is removed in a single pass through the lungs; thus peripheral venous plasma levels of PGE_1 are low or undetectable (<2 picograms/mL) after MUSE administration. The mean maximum plasma PGE_1 concentration following intraurethral administration of the highest dose of MUSE (1000 mcg) was barely detectable (11.4 picograms/mL). In a study of 14 subjects, the plasma PGE_1 level was shown to be undetectable within 60 minutes of MUSE administration in most subjects.

Metabolism: Alprostadil is rapidly metabolized locally by enzymatic oxidation of the 15-hydroxyl group to 15-keto-PGE_1. The enzyme catalyzing this process has been isolated from many tissues in the lower genitourinary tract including the urethra, prostate, and corpus cavernosum. 15-keto-PGE_1 retains little (1–2%) of the biological activity of PGE_1. 15-keto-PGE_1 is rapidly reduced at the C_{13}–C_{14} position to form the most abundant metabolite in plasma, 13,14-dihydro,15-keto PGE_1 (DHK-PGE_1), which is biologically inactive. The majority of DHK-PGE_1 is further metabolized to smaller prostaglandin remnants that are cleared primarily by the kidney and liver. Between 60% and 90% of PGE_1 has been shown to be metabolized after 1 pass through the pulmonary capillary beds.

Excretion: After intravenous administration of tritium-labeled alprostadil in man, labeled drug disappears rapidly from the blood in the first 10 minutes, and by 1 hour radioactivity in the blood reaches a low level. The metabolites of alprostadil are excreted primarily by the kidney, with approximately 90% of an administered intravenous dose excreted in the urine within 24 hours of dosing. The remainder is excreted in the feces. There is no evidence of tissue retention of alprostadil or its metabolites following intravenous administration.

Pharmacokinetics in Special Populations:

Pulmonary Disease: The near-complete pulmonary first-pass metabolism of PGE_1 is the primary factor influencing the systemic pharmacokinetics of MUSE and is a reason that peripheral venous plasma levels of PGE_1 are low or undetectable (<2 picograms/mL) following MUSE administration. Patients with pulmonary disease therefore may have a reduced capacity to clear the drug. In patients with the adult respiratory distress syndrome (ARDS), pulmonary extraction of intravascularly administered alprostadil was reduced by approximately 15% compared to a control group of patients with normal respiratory function (66±3.2% vs. 78±2.4%).

Geriatrics: The effects of age on the pharmacokinetics of alprostadil have not been evaluated.

CLINICAL TRIALS

The MUSE system was evaluated in 7 placebo-controlled trials of various design in over 2500 patients with a history of erectile dysfunction of various etiologies. These trials assessed erectile function in the clinic and sexual intercourse in outpatient settings. In studies of sexual performance, patients were screened in the clinic, generally using doses of 125 mcg to 1000 mcg, for a satisfactory erectile response, then sent home with the selected dose or placebo for evaluation of sexual performance. Not all patients beginning titration had a successful dose and some patients could not tolerate MUSE, principally because of penile pain, so that the success rates in the studies described below must be understood to represent response rates only in patients who were successfully titrated.

In 2 identical multicenter, double-blind, placebo-controlled, parallel-group studies, 1511 monogamous and heterosexual patients with a mean 4-year history of erectile dysfunction and at least a 3-month history of no erections adequate for sexual intercourse without medical assistance, were enrolled and began dose titration in the clinic with doses between 125 mcg and 1000 mcg. 996 patients (66%) completed dose titration, achieved an erection sufficient for intercourse, and were randomized equally to placebo or active treatment and followed during at-home treatment for up to 3 months. 874 patients and partners completed 3 months of follow-up. About 10%, 20%, 30%, and 40% of patients were titrated to 125 mcg, 250 mcg, 500 mcg, and 1000 mcg, respectively. Couples on active therapy were more likely to have at least 1 successful sexual intercourse (65% vs. 19%) than were couples on placebo. Among patients who reported successful intercourse at least once with active treatment, approximately 7 of 10 MUSE systems resulted in successful sexual intercourse. Results were similar in patients with erectile dysfunction stemming from surgery or trauma, diabetes, vascular disease, or other etiologies, and were similar in Caucasians and non-Caucasians. In administrations resulting in sexual intercourse, the duration of erections sufficient for penetration was 6 minutes on placebo and 16 minutes on active drug. Successful therapy with MUSE was associated with improvement in the quality of life measures of "emotional well-being" for patients and "relationship with partner" for both patients and their female partners.

INDICATIONS AND USAGE

MUSE is indicated for the treatment of erectile dysfunction. Studies that established benefit demonstrated improvements in success rates for sexual intercourse compared with similarly administered placebo.

CONTRAINDICATIONS

MUSE is contraindicated in men with any of the following:

1. Known hypersensitivity to alprostadil.
2. Abnormal penile anatomy: MUSE is contraindicated in patients with urethral stricture, balanitis (inflammation/infection of the glans of the penis), severe hypospadias and curvature, and in patients with acute or chronic urethritis.
3. Sickle cell anemia or trait, thrombocythemia, polycythemia, multiple myeloma: MUSE is contraindicated in patients who are prone to venous thrombosis or who have a hyperviscosity syndrome and are therefore at increased risk of priapism (rigid erection lasting 6 or more hours).
4. MUSE should not be used in men for whom sexual activity is inadvisable (see General Precautions).
5. MUSE should not be used for sexual intercourse with a pregnant woman unless the couple uses a condom barrier.

WARNINGS

Because of the potential for symptomatic hypotension and syncope, which occurred in 3% and 0.4%, respectively, of patients during in-clinic dosing, MUSE titration should be carried out under medical supervision. During post-marketing surveillance syncope occurring within one hour of administration has been reported. Patients should be cautioned to avoid activities, such as driving or hazardous tasks, where injury could result if hypotension or syncope were to occur after MUSE administration.

PRECAUTIONS

General Precautions:

1. A complete medical history and physical examination should be undertaken to exclude reversible causes of erectile dysfunction prior to the initiation of MUSE therapy. In addition, underlying disorders that might preclude the use of MUSE (see CONTRAINDICATIONS) should be sought.
2. *Cardiovascular effects:* During in-clinic dosing, patients should be monitored for symptoms of hypotension, and the lowest effective dose of MUSE should be prescribed.
3. *Hematologic effects:* Patients administering MUSE improperly may be at risk of urethral abrasion resulting in minor bleeding or spotting. Patients on anticoagulant therapy or with bleeding disorders may be at higher risk of bleeding. Patients on anticoagulant therapy have been safely treated with MUSE; however, the risk/benefit ratio in these patients should be considered prior to prescribing MUSE.
4. *Resumption of sexual activity:* Sexual intercourse is considered a vigorous physical activity, and it increases heart rate as well as cardiac work. Physicians may want to examine the cardiac fitness of patients prior to treating erectile dysfunction.
5. *Priapism and prolonged erection:* In clinical trials of MUSE, priapism (rigid erection lasting ≥6 hours) and prolonged erection (rigid erection lasting 4 hours and <6 hours) were reported infrequently (<0.1% and 0.3% of patients, respectively). Nevertheless, these events are a potential risk of pharmacologic therapy and can cause penile injury. Physicians should lower the dose or consider discontinuing MUSE treatment in any patient who develops priapism or prolonged erection.
6. *Drug-Drug Interactions:* Because there are low or undetectable (<2 picograms/mL) amounts of alprostadil found in the peripheral venous circulation following MUSE administration, systemic drug-drug interactions with MUSE are unlikely. Although formal studies have not been conducted, the concomitant use of MUSE and antihypertensive medications may increase the risk of hypotension. It is therefore advised that caution be used in the administration of MUSE to individuals on anti-hypertensive medications. In addition, the presence of medications in the circulation that attenuate erectile function may influence the response to MUSE.
7. *Drug-Device Interactions:* Use of MUSE in patients with penile implants has not been studied.
8. *Sexual Preference:* There is no experience in homosexual men and no experience with other than vaginal intercourse.

Information for Patients: Patients should be informed that MUSE offers no protection from the transmission of sexually transmitted diseases. Patients and partners who use MUSE need to be counseled about the protective measures that are necessary to guard against the spread of sexually transmitted agents, including the human immunodeficiency virus (HIV).

Although unreported in clinical trials, there is the possibility that an overdosage of MUSE can cause priapism, a painful erection of the penis sustained for hours and unrelieved by sexual intercourse or masturbation. This condition is serious and, if untreated, it can lead to permanent inability to have an erection. Patients who experience a prolonged erection should seek prompt medical attention.

Patients should be instructed how to administer MUSE. A patient package insert must be given to each patient at the initiation of MUSE therapy.

Information for Partners: Partners of patients using MUSE should be informed that MUSE offers no protection from the transmission of sexually transmitted diseases. Patients and partners who use MUSE should be counseled about the protective measures that are necessary to guard against the spread of sexually transmitted agents, including the human immunodeficiency virus (HIV). Human semen contains PGE_1, but additional amounts may be present from MUSE administration (see CLINICAL PHARMACOLOGY). Partners who have experienced an extended period of sexual abstinence should be encouraged to seek advice from a health care professional prior to resuming sexual intercourse. The use of a water-based lubricant may facilitate vaginal penetration.

It is recommended that couples using MUSE employ adequate contraception if the female partner is of childbearing potential. There is no information on the effects on early pregnancy of PGE_1 at the levels received by female partners. MUSE has no contraceptive properties. MUSE should not be used if the female partner is pregnant, unless the couple uses a condom barrier.

Carcinogenesis, Mutagenesis, Impairment of Fertility: Long-term carcinogenicity studies of alprostadil have not been conducted. Alprostadil showed no evidence of mutagenicity in vitro in the Ames bacterial reverse mutation test, the unscheduled DNA synthesis assay in rat hepatocytes, or the Chinese hamster ovary forward gene mutation assay; nor was there evidence of mutagenicity in vivo in the mouse micronucleus assay. Alprostadil concentrations increased chromosomal aberrations above control incidence in the in vitro Chinese hamster ovary chromosomal aberration assay.

In dogs, sperm concentration, morphology, and motility were unaffected by daily intraurethral administration of up to 3000 mcg MUSE (alprostadil) for 13 weeks (200 mcg/kg/day or about 3.5 times the maximum recommended daily dose adjusted for body surface area). Alprostadil concentrations of 400 mcg/mL had no effect on human sperm motility or viability in vitro.

Pregnancy: Pregnancy Category C: Alprostadil has been shown to be embryotoxic (decreased fetal weight) when administered as a subcutaneous bolus to pregnant rats at doses as low as 500 mcg/kg/day. Doses of 2000 mcg/kg/day resulted in increased resorptions, reduced numbers of live fetuses, increased incidences of visceral and skeletal variations (primarily left umbilical artery and generalized reduction in ossification of the entire skeleton) and gross visceral and skeletal malformations (primarily edema, hydrocephaly, anophthalmia/microphthalmia, and skeletal anomalies). The latter dose produced maternal toxicity (ataxia, lethargy, diarrhea, and retarded body weight gain). When administered by continuous intravenous infusion, evidence of embryotoxicity (decreased fetal weight gain and increased incidence of hydroureter) was observed at 2000 mcg/kg/day, a dose that was also associated with a decrease in maternal weight gain. Intravaginal administration of up to 4000 mcg/day of MUSE (alprostadil) to pregnant rabbits (1100 mcg/kg/day or about 12.5 times the maximum recommended daily dose adjusted for body surface area) resulted in no evidence of harm to the fetus. MUSE should not be used for sexual intercourse with a pregnant woman unless the couple uses a condom barrier.

Nursing Mothers and Pediatric Use: MUSE is not indicated for use in newborns, children, or women.

ADVERSE REACTIONS

In-Clinic Titration: In the 2 largest double-blind, parallel, placebo-controlled trials, 1511 patients received MUSE at least 1 time in the clinic setting. The most frequently reported drug-related side effects during in-clinic titration included pain in the penis (36%), urethra (13%), or testes (5%). These discomforts were most commonly reported as mild and transient, but about 7% of patients withdrew at this stage because of adverse events. Urethral bleeding/spotting and other minor abrasions to the urethra were reported in approximately 3% of patients. Symptomatic lowering of blood pressure (hypotension) occurred in 3% of patients; in addition, some lowering of blood pressure may occur without symptoms. Dizziness was reported in 4% of patients. Syncope (fainting) was reported by 0.4% of patients. (See **WARNINGS**).

Home Treatment: 996 patients (66% of those who began titration) were studied during the home treatment portion of 2 Phase III placebo-controlled studies. Fewer than 2% of patients discontinued from these studies primarily because of adverse events. The following table summarizes the frequency of adverse events reported by patients using MUSE or placebo.

Adverse Events Reported by ≥2% of Patients Treated with MUSE and More Common than on Placebo At Home in Phase III Placebo-Controlled Clinical Studies for up to 3 Months

Event	MUSE n = 486	Placebo n = 511
UROGENITAL SYSTEM		
Penile Pain	32%	3%
Urethral Burning	12%	4%
Minor Urethral Bleeding/Spotting	5%	1%
Testicular Pain	5%	1%
NERVOUS SYSTEM		
Dizziness	2%	<1%
BODY AS A WHOLE		
Flu Symptoms	4%	2%
Headache	3%	2%
Pain	3%	1%
Accidental Injury	3%	2%
Back Pain	2%	1%
Pelvic Pain	2%	<1%
RESPIRATORY		
Rhinitis	2%	<1%
Infection	3%	2%

Other drug-related side effects observed during in-clinic titration and home treatment include swelling of leg veins, leg pain, perineal pain, and rapid pulse, each occurring in <2% of patients.

Female Partner Adverse Events: The most common drug-related adverse event reported by female partners during placebo-controlled clinical studies was vaginal burning/itching, reported by 5.8% of partners of patients on active vs. 0.8% of partners of patients on placebo. It is unknown whether this adverse event experienced by female partners was a result of the medication or a result of resuming sexual intercourse, which occurred much more frequently in partners of patients on active medication.

OVERDOSAGE

Overdosage has not been reported with MUSE. Overdosage with MUSE may result in hypotension, persistent penile pain, and possibly priapism (rigid erection lasting ≥6h). Priapism can result in permanent worsening of erectile function. Patients suspected of overdosage who develop these symptoms should be kept under medical supervision until systemic or local symptoms have resolved.

DOSAGE AND ADMINISTRATION

MUSE is a transurethral delivery system available in 4 dosage strengths: 125 mcg, 250 mcg, 500 mcg, and 1000 mcg. MUSE should be administered as needed to achieve an erection. The onset of effect is within 5–10 minutes after administration. The duration of effect is approximately 30–60 minutes. However, the actual duration will vary from patient to patient. Each patient should be instructed by a medical professional on proper technique for administering MUSE prior to self-administration. The maximum frequency of use is no more than 2 systems per 24-hour period.

Initiation of Therapy: Dose titration should be administered under the supervision of a physician to test a patient's responsiveness to MUSE, to demonstrate proper administration technique (see detailed instructions for MUSE administration in patient package insert), and to monitor for evidence of hypotension (see **WARNINGS**). Patients should be individually titrated to the lowest dose that is sufficient for sexual intercourse. The lower doses of MUSE (125 mcg or 250 mcg) are recommended for initial dosing. If necessary, the dose should be increased (or decreased) on separate occasions in a stepwise manner until the patient achieves an erection that is sufficient for sexual intercourse.

Home Treatment Regimen: MUSE should be used as needed to achieve an erection. The maximum frequency of use is 2 administrations per 24-hour period. Each MUSE is for single use only and should be properly discarded after use.

HOW SUPPLIED

MUSE is supplied in individual foil pouches containing one (1) system per pouch. MUSE is available in unit cartons containing six (6) systems. MUSE is available in the following 4 dosage strengths:

Dosage Strength	NDC Numbers Carton	Pouch	Identifying Package Color
125 mcg	62541-110-06	62541-110-01	Tan
250 mcg	62541-120-06	62541-120-01	Green
500 mcg	62541-130-06	62541-130-01	Blue
1000 mcg	62541-140-06	62541-140-01	Burgundy

STORAGE AND HANDLING

Store unopened foil pouches in a refrigerator at 2°–8°C (36°–46°F). Do not expose MUSE to temperatures above 30°C (86°F). MUSE may be kept by the patient at room temperature (below 30°C or 86°F) for up to 14 days prior to use.

Caution: Federal law prohibits dispensing without prescription.

Medical information line at VIVUS 1-888-345-MUSE (1-888-345-6873).

MUSE® IS A REGISTERED TRADEMARK OF VIVUS, INC. IN THE U.S. AND OTHER COUNTRIES.

Revised February 1998

PATIENT INFORMATION

Please read this pamphlet before using MUSE® (alprostadil). This pamphlet is a quick reference source on important information about MUSE for you and your partner. **Before administering MUSE, please review the patient video and education booklet. These materials provide visual instruction and more detailed information as well as practical tips on how to use MUSE.**

WHAT IS MUSE?

MUSE represents a unique approach for the treatment of erectile dysfunction, commonly called impotence. It is based on the discovery that the urethra (the normal pathway for urine) can absorb certain medications into the surrounding erectile tissues thereby creating an erection. There are 4 dose strengths available: 125, 250, 500, and 1000 micrograms. The MUSE applicator (Fig. 1) contained in each foil pouch is intended for 1 administration only. Your dose of MUSE will be determined by you and your physician. After administration, the erection process will begin within 5–10 minutes, and may last 30–60 minutes. However, the actual duration will vary from patient to patient.

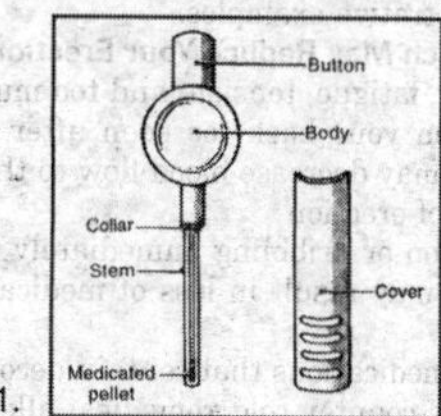

Figure 1.

WHAT IS MUSE USED FOR?

MUSE is indicated for the treatment of erectile dysfunction. Erectile dysfunction is the inability to attain or maintain an erection sufficient for sexual intercourse.

WHO SHOULD NOT USE MUSE?

You should not use MUSE if you have any of the following:

- Known hypersensitivity to alprostadil (the active medication in MUSE)
- An abnormally formed penis
- Have been advised not to undertake sexual activity
- Conditions that might result in long-lasting erections, such as sickle cell anemia or trait, leukemia, or tumor of the bone marrow (multiple myeloma)
- MUSE should not be used for sexual intercourse with a pregnant woman unless the couple uses a condom barrier.

WHAT ARE THE POSSIBLE SIDE EFFECTS OF MUSE?

The most common side effects that have been observed using MUSE follow:

- Aching in the penis, testicles, legs, and in the perineum (area between the penis and rectum)
- Warmth or burning sensation in the urethra
- Redness of the penis due to increased blood flow
- Minor urethral bleeding or spotting due to improper administration.

Side effects reported less frequently:

- Prolonged erection— PLEASE NOTE: IF YOUR ERECTION IS RIGID FOR MORE THAN 4 HOURS, CALL YOUR DOCTOR PROMPTLY.
- Swelling of leg veins
- Light-headedness/Dizziness
- Fainting— PLEASE NOTE: AFTER USING MUSE, YOU SHOULD AVOID ACTIVITIES, SUCH AS DRIVING OR HAZARDOUS TASKS, WHERE INJURY COULD RESULT IF DIZZINESS OR FAINTING WERE TO OCCUR. IN PATIENTS EXPERIENCING THESE SYMPTOMS, THE SYMPTOMS HAVE USUALLY OCCURRED DURING INITIATION OF THERAPY AND WITHIN ONE HOUR OF MUSE ADMINISTRATION.
- Rapid pulse.

If you have a history of fainting be sure to discuss this with your doctor prior to using MUSE. If you do experience dizziness or feel faint, this may be due to the lowering of your blood pressure. Lie down immediately and raise your legs. If symptoms persist, call your doctor promptly. Because of the potential for these side effects, MUSE titration should be carried out under medical supervision.

Changing Your Dosage

It is assumed that you and your doctor have determined the proper dose of MUSE. If you suspect that your dose needs to be increased or decreased to achieve the response that works best for you, please call your doctor to determine if your dose needs to be reevaluated. Do not use MUSE more than twice in a 24-hour period.

WHAT ARE THE POSSIBLE SIDE EFFECTS OF MUSE FOR YOUR PARTNER?

The most common reported side effects observed in women whose partners use MUSE are mild vaginal itching or burning. Using a water-based lubricant can help to make vaginal penetration easier. Your partner may want to consult her health care provider if she has not had sexual intercourse for an extended period of time.

IMPORTANT INFORMATION FOR YOU AND YOUR PARTNER

Pregnancy

MUSE has no contraceptive properties.

Because MUSE has not been tested during human pregnancy, it is recommended that couples use adequate contraception if the female partner is of childbearing potential. MUSE should not be used for sexual intercourse with a pregnant woman unless the couple uses a condom barrier.

Sexually Transmitted Diseases

MUSE will not protect you or your partner from sexually transmitted diseases like chlamydia, gonorrhea, herpes simplex virus, viral hepatitis, human immunodeficiency virus (HIV—the virus that causes AIDS), human papilloma virus (genital warts), and syphilis. Latex condoms can protect against these sexually transmitted diseases.

HOW SHOULD I STORE MUSE?

It is recommended that MUSE be stored in a refrigerator. MUSE may be kept at room temperature (less than 30°C/86°F) for up to 14 days prior to use. It is very important that MUSE not be exposed to temperatures above 30°C/86°F since this will make MUSE ineffective. MUSE should not be exposed to high temperatures or placed in direct sunlight.

Storage when traveling

When traveling, store MUSE in a portable ice pack or cooler. Do not store in the trunk of a car or in baggage storage areas where MUSE may be exposed to extremes in temperature.

HOW TO ADMINISTER MUSE:

1. Immediately prior to administration, urinate and gently shake the penis several times to remove excess urine. A moist urethra makes administration of MUSE easier. The medicated pellet has been specially developed to dissolve in the small quantity of urine that remains in the urethra after urination.
2. Open the foil pouch by tearing fully across the notched edge (Fig. 2). Let the MUSE slide out of the pouch. Save the pouch for discarding the MUSE applicator later.

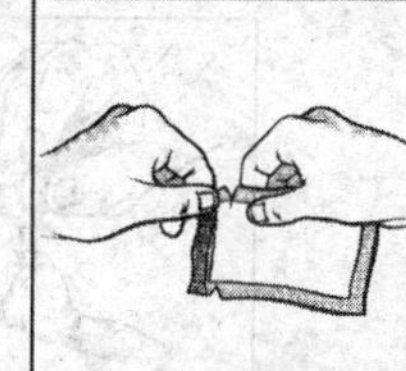

Figure 2.

3. To remove the protective cover from the applicator stem (Fig. 3), hold the body of the applicator with your thumb

Continued on next page

MUSE—Cont.

and forefinger. Twist the body and pull out the applicator from the cover, being careful not to push in or pull out the applicator button. Avoid touching the applicator stem and tip. Save the cover for discarding the MUSE applicator later.

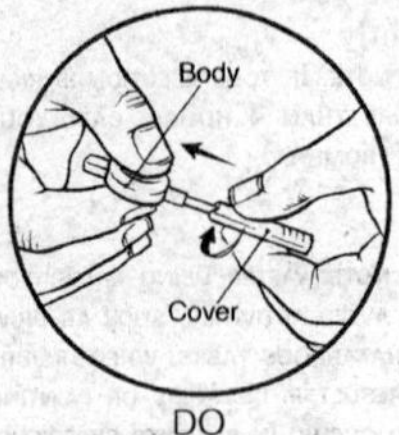

DO

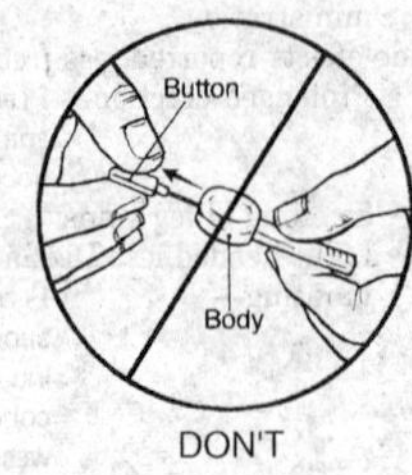

DON'T

Figure 3.

4. Visually inspect the MUSE. The MUSE system is see-through, and you will be able to see the medicated pellet at the end of the stem. Make sure that the pellet is present before insertion (Fig. 4).

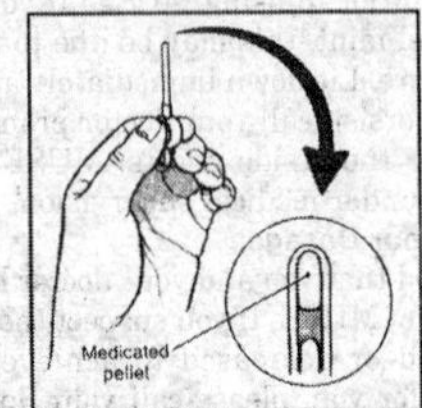

Figure 4.

5. Hold the applicator in a way which is the most comfortable for you (Fig. 5A and 5B).

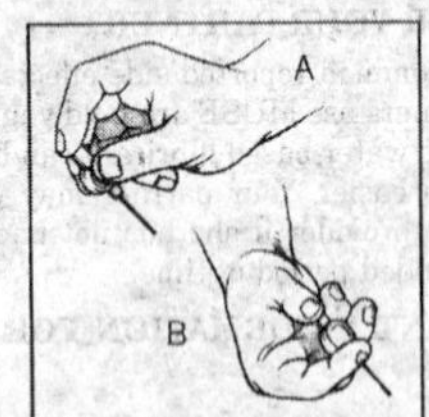

Figure 5.

6. Please review Figure 6A, the anatomy of the penis.

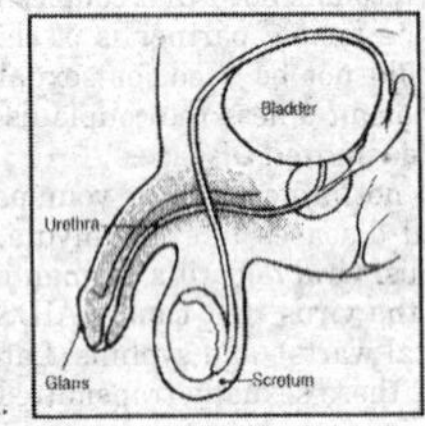

Figure 6A.

While sitting or standing, whichever is more comfortable for you, take several seconds to gently and slowly stretch the penis upward to its full length, with gentle compression from top to bottom of the glans (Fig. 6B). This straightens and opens the urethra. Slowly insert the MUSE stem into the urethra up to the collar (Fig. 6C). If you feel any discomfort or a pulling sensation, withdraw the applicator slightly and then gently reinsert.

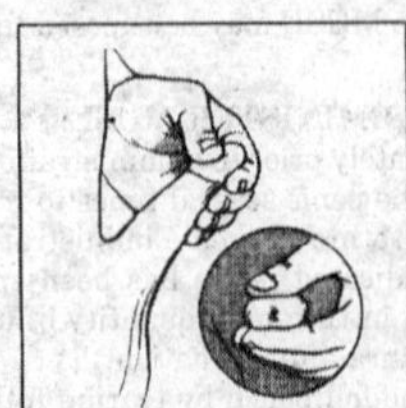
Figure 6B.

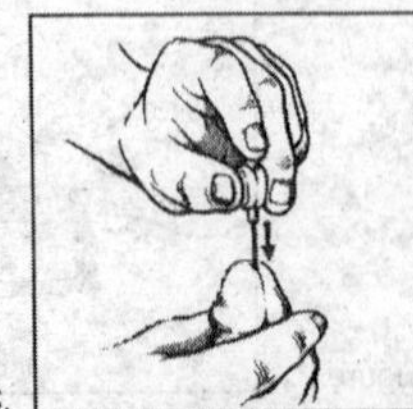
Figure 6C.

7. Gently and completely push down (Fig. 7) the button at the top of the applicator until it stops. It is important to do this to ensure that the medicated pellet is completely released. Hold the applicator in this position for 5 seconds.

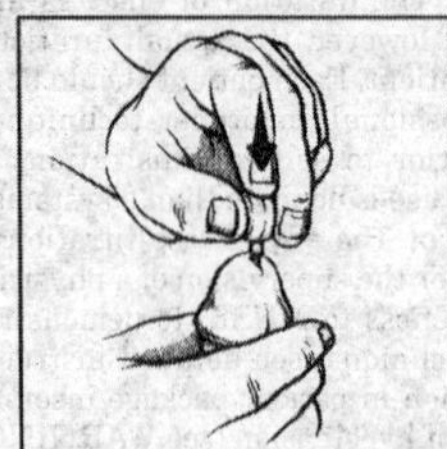
Figure 7.

8. Gently rock the applicator from side to side. This will separate the medicated pellet from the applicator tip (Fig. 8). If you apply too much pressure you may scratch the lining of the urethra causing it to bleed.

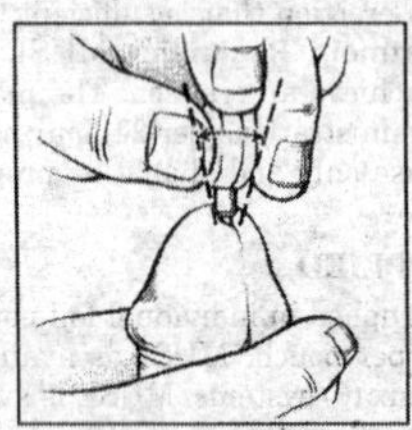
Figure 8.

9. Remove the applicator while keeping the penis upright.
10. Visually inspect the applicator tip to see that the medication is no longer in the applicator. Do not touch the stem. If you notice some residual medication in the end of the applicator, gently reinsert into the urethra and repeat steps 7, 8, and 9.
11. Holding the penis upright and stretched to its full length, roll the penis firmly between your hands for at least 10 seconds. This will ensure that the medication is adequately distributed along the walls of the urethra (Fig. 9). If you feel a burning sensation, it may help to continue to roll the penis for an additional 30–60 seconds or until the burning subsides.

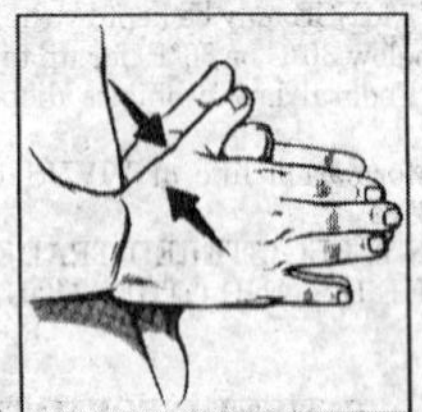
Figure 9.

12. Remember, each MUSE is good for a single administration only. Replace the cover on the MUSE applicator, place in the opened foil pouch, fold, and discard as normal household waste.

After you have administered MUSE, it is important to sit, or preferably stand or walk about for 10 minutes while the erection is developing. This increases blood flow to the penis and will enhance your erection.

ADDITIONAL INFORMATION AND PRACTICAL TIPS

Factors Which May Enhance Your Erection:

- Being well rested and relaxed
- Sexual foreplay with your partner or self-stimulation while sitting or standing
- Pelvic exercises (for example, Kegel exercises)—these consist of tightening and releasing your pelvic and buttock muscles. These are the muscles you use to stop urination
- Various positions that may favor blood flow into the penis. Please refer to the patient starter booklet and video for illustrative examples.

Factors Which May Reduce Your Erection:

- Anxiety, fatigue, tension, and too much alcohol
- Lying on your back too soon after administration of MUSE may decrease blood flow to the penis and result in loss of erection
- Urination or dribbling immediately following administration may result in loss of medication from the urethra
- Using medications that contain decongestants, such as over-the-counter cold remedies, allergy, sinus medications, and appetite suppressants, may block the effect of MUSE.

COMMONLY ASKED QUESTIONS ABOUT MUSE

Will insertion of MUSE hurt?
At first, you may feel some minor discomfort from insertion. Urinating prior to administration will reduce the chance of discomfort or abrasions and is important for dissolving the medicated pellet. Be sure to straighten your penis to its full length when inserting the MUSE applicator. With repeated use, administration will become much easier.

What are the side effects associated with MUSE?
Most of the side effects reported in men are relatively minor and include burning and aching in the penis and groin. Rarely noted are prolonged erection, light-headedness, dizziness, fainting, rapid pulse, and swelling of the leg veins. If you feel dizzy, light-headed, faint, or experience rapid pulse, lie down immediately and raise your legs. If symptoms persist, call your doctor promptly. Because of the potential for these side effects, MUSE titration should be carried out under medical supervision.
(See also: **"WHAT ARE THE POSSIBLE SIDE EFFECTS OF MUSE?"**)
In women, mild vaginal itching and burning have been observed.

After I administer MUSE, can we immediately lie down and begin sexual activity?
You can begin sexual activity, but having the man lie down, especially on his back shortly after administration, is not recommended. This will reduce blood flow to the penis and may reduce the erection. It is important to sit, stand or walk about for 10 minutes after administration. Many couples have used this time to incorporate various types of foreplay. After this initial period, you can assume different positions leading to sexual intercourse. Some couples have noticed that the erection is better maintained in positions that favor blood flow into the penis during intercourse.
Please review the video and patient starter booklet available from your doctor which illustrates various positions that will enhance your erection.

How long will the effect of MUSE last?
An erection should begin within 5–10 minutes after administering MUSE. The duration of effect is approximately 30–60 minutes. However, the actual duration will vary from patient to patient.

What will the erection be like? How will it compare to the erections I had when I was younger?
An effective dose of MUSE should produce an erection sufficient for sexual intercourse. MUSE may not create an erection such as those you experienced when you were younger. Some patients may experience some mild pain and aching in the penis or groin area. Also, your erection may continue after orgasm.

How do I know if I have the correct dose of MUSE?
You and your physician will determine the appropriate dose of MUSE. If your erection cannot be maintained for the time needed to have foreplay and sexual intercourse, you may need to have your dose increased. Similarly, an erection that lasts longer than desired may require a dose decrease. Call your doctor if you suspect you may require a dosing adjustment.

After my erection is over, will my penis feel sensitive?
Your penis may feel full, warm, and somewhat sensitive to the touch. These effects are normal and may last a few hours.

Can I reuse MUSE?
No. MUSE is intended for single-dose application only.

How do I dispose of the MUSE applicator?
After you have administered MUSE, replace the cap on the applicator, place in the opened foil pouch, fold, and discard as normal household waste.

If my erection lasts longer than desired, what should I do?
Note: Call your doctor promptly if you have a rigid erection that lasts more than 4 hours.
An application of ice packs to the inner thigh may shorten the duration of the erection, since the cold will restrict blood flow to the penis. If used, ice packs should be applied alternately to each inner thigh for a period not exceeding 10 minutes.

How often can I safely use MUSE?
MUSE should not be used more than twice per day.

If you have any additional questions about MUSE, please call the toll free patient information line at VIVUS 1-888-367-MUSE (1-888-367-6873).

MUSE® IS A REGISTERED TRADEMARK OF VIVUS, INC. IN THE U.S. AND OTHER COUNTRIES.
VIVUS, Inc.
Mountain View, CA 94040 February 1998
Shown in Product Identification Guide, page 335

Wallace Pharmaceuticals

for product information, please see MedPointe Pharmaceuticals

IDENTIFICATION PROBLEM?
Turn to the **Product Identification Guide,** where you'll find more than 1600 products pictured in actual size and full color.

Warner Chilcott, Inc.

100 ENTERPRISE DRIVE
ROCKAWAY, NJ 07866

Direct Inquiries to:
For Product Information:
(800) 521-8813
www.warnerchilcott.com
For Medical Information:
(800) 521-8813
For A Medical Emergency:
(800) 521-8813
After Hours and Weekends:
(303) 739-1110
For All Other Inquiries:
(800) 521-8813
www.warnerchilcott.com

Following is a list of Warner Chilcott products:

DORYX® Capsules, 75 mg and 100 mg ℞
(coated doxycycline hyclate pellets)

DOVONEX® Cream, 0.005% ℞
(calcipotriene cream)

DOVONEX® Ointment, 0.005% ℞
(calcipotriene ointment)

DOVONEX® Scalp Solution, 0.005% ℞
(calcipotriene solution)

DURICEF® Capsules, 500 mg ℞
(cefadroxil monohydrate, USP)

DURICEF® Tablets, 1 g ℞
(cefadroxil monohydrate, USP)

DURICEF® ℞
Oral Suspension, 250 mg/5 mL, 500 mg/5 mL
(cefadroxil monohydrate, USP)

ERYC® Capsules, 250 mg ℞
(Erythromycin Delayed-Release Capsules, USP)

ESTRACE® Vaginal Cream ℞
(estradiol vaginal cream, USP, 0.01%)

ESTRACE® Tablets 0.5 mg, 1 mg, 2 mg ℞
(estradiol tablets, USP)

ESTROSTEP® ℞
(norethindrone acetate and ethinyl estradiol tablets, USP and ferrous fumarate tablets)

FEMHRT® ℞
(norethindrone acetate/ethinyl estradiol tablets)

FEMRING®, 0.05 mg/day, 0.10 mg/day ℞
(estradiol acetate vaginal ring)

FEMTRACE®, 0.45 mg, 0.9 mg, 1.8 mg ℞
(estradiol acetate tablets)

LOESTRIN® 21 1/20 ℞
(norethindrone acetate and ethinyl estradiol tablets, USP)

LOESTRIN® 21 1.5/30 ℞
(norethindrone acetate and ethinyl estradiol tablets, USP)

LOESTRIN® Fe 1/20 ℞
(norethindrone acetate and ethinyl estradiol tablets, USP and ferrous fumarate tablets)

LOESTRIN® Fe 1.5/30 ℞
(norethindrone acetate and ethinyl estradiol tablets, USP and ferrous fumarate tablets)

MANDELAMINE® HAFGRAMS®, 0.5 g ℞
(Methenamine Mandelate, USP)

MANDELAMINE® Tablets, 1 g ℞
(Methenamine Mandelate, USP)

OVCON® 35 0.4 mg/35 mcg ℞
(norethindrone and ethinyl estradiol tablets, chewable)

OVCON® 35 0.4/35 ℞
(Norethindrone and Ethinyl Estradiol Tablets, USP)
21- and 28-DAY REGIMENS

OVCON® 50 ℞
(Norethindrone and Ethinyl Estradiol Tablets, USP)
28-DAY REGIMEN

PYRIDIUM® Tablets, 100 mg and 200 mg ℞
(Phenazopyridine Hydrochloride Tablets, USP)

PYRIDIUM® PLUS Tablets ℞
(phenazopyridine HCl, hyoscyamine HBr, butabarbital)

NATAFORT® ℞
Prenatal Multivitamin Tablet with Iron

NATACHEW® ℞
(Chewable Prenatal Multivitamin Tablet with Iron)

SARAFEM® ℞
(fluoxetine hydrochloride)

DOVONEX® ℞

[dōvă-nex]
(calcipotriene cream)
Cream, 0.005%
FOR TOPICAL DERMATOLOGIC USE ONLY.
Not for Ophthalmic, Oral or Intravaginal Use.
Rx only

DESCRIPTION

Dovonex® (calcipotriene cream) Cream, 0.005% contains calcipotriene monohydrate, a synthetic vitamin D_3 derivative, for topical dermatological use.

Chemically, calcipotriene monohydrate is (5Z,7E,22E,24S)-24-cyclopropyl-9,10-secochola-5,7,10(19), 22-tetraene-1α,3β,24-triol monohydrate, with the empirical formula $C_{27}H_{40}O_3 \bullet H_2O$, a molecular weight of 430.6, and the following structural formula:

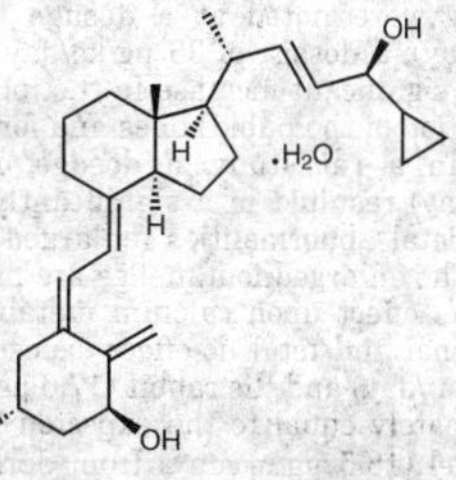

Calcipotriene monohydrate is a white or off-white crystalline substance. Dovonex Cream contains calcipotriene monohydrate equivalent to 50 µg/g anhydrous calcipotriene in a cream base of cetearyl alcohol, ceteth-20, diazolidinyl urea, dichlorobenzyl alcohol, dibasic sodium phosphate, edetate disodium, glycerin, mineral oil, petrolatum, and water.

CLINICAL PHARMACOLOGY

In humans, the natural supply of vitamin D depends mainly on exposure to the ultraviolet rays of the sun for conversion of 7-dehydrocholesterol to vitamin D_3 (cholecalciferol) in the skin. Calcipotriene is a synthetic analog of vitamin D_3.

Clinical studies with radiolabelled calcipotriene ointment indicate that approximately 6% (± 3%, SD) of the applied dose of calcipotriene is absorbed systemically when the ointment is applied topically to psoriasis plaques, or 5% (± 2.6%, SD) when applied to normal skin, and much of the absorbed active is converted to inactive metabolites within 24 hours of application. Systemic absorption of the cream has not been studied.

Vitamin D and its metabolites are transported in the blood, bound to specific plasma proteins. The active form of the vitamin, 1,25-dihydroxy vitamin D_3 (calcitriol), is known to be recycled via the liver and excreted in the bile. Calcipotriene metabolism following systemic uptake is rapid, and occurs via a similar pathway to the natural hormone.

CLINICAL STUDIES

Adequate and well-controlled trials of patients treated with Dovonex Cream have demonstrated improvement usually beginning after 2 weeks of therapy. This improvement continued with approximately 50% of patients showing at least marked improvement in the signs and symptoms of psoriasis after 8 weeks of therapy, but only approximately 4% showed complete clearing.

INDICATIONS AND USAGE

Dovonex Cream is indicated for the treatment of plaque psoriasis. The safety and effectiveness of topical calcipotriene in dermatoses other than psoriasis have not been established.

CONTRAINDICATIONS

Dovonex Cream is contraindicated in those patients with a history of hypersensitivity to any of the components of the preparation. It should not be used by patients with demonstrated hypercalcemia or evidence of vitamin D toxicity. Dovonex Cream should not be used on the face.

PRECAUTIONS

General: Use of Dovonex Cream may cause transient irritation of both lesions and surrounding uninvolved skin. If irritation develops, Dovonex Cream should be discontinued. Reversible elevation of serum calcium has occurred with use of topical calcipotriene. If elevation in serum calcium outside the normal range should occur, discontinue treatment until normal calcium levels are restored.

Information for Patients: Patients using Dovonex Cream should receive the following information and instructions:

1. This medication is to be used only as directed by the physician. It is for external use only. Avoid contact with the face or eyes. As with any topical medication, patients should wash their hands after application.
2. This medication should not be used for any disorder other than that for which it was prescribed.
3. Patients should report to their physician any signs of adverse reactions.

Carcinogenesis, Mutagenesis, Impairment of Fertility: Animal studies have not been conducted to evaluate the carcinogenic potential of calcipotriene. Studies in rats at doses up to 54 µg/kg/day (318 µg/m²/day) of calcipotriene indicated no impairment of fertility or general reproductive performance.

Calcipotriene did not elicit any mutagenic effects in the Ames mutagenicity assay, the mouse lymphoma TK locus assay, the human lymphocyte chromosome aberration test or the mouse micronucleus test.

Pregnancy: ***Teratogenic Effects: Pregnancy Category C:*** Studies of teratogenicity were done by the oral route where bioavailability is expected to be approximately 40–60% of the administered dose. Increased rabbit maternal and fetal toxicity was noted at 12 µg/kg/day (132 µg/m²/day). Rabbits administered 36 µg/kg/day (396 µg/m²/day) resulted in fetuses with a significant increase in the incidences of pubic bones, forelimb phalanges, and incomplete bone ossification. In a rat study, oral doses of 54 µg/kg/day (318 µg/m²/day) resulted in a significantly higher incidence of skeletal abnormalities consisting primarily of enlarged fontanelles and extra ribs. The enlarged fontanelles are most likely due to calcipotriene's effect upon calcium metabolism. The maternal and fetal calculated no-effect exposures in the rat (43.2 µg/m²/day) and rabbit (17.6 µg/m²/day) studies are approximately equal to the expected human systemic exposure level (18.5 µg/m²/day) from dermal application. There are no adequate and well-controlled studies in pregnant women. Therefore, Dovonex Cream should be used during pregnancy only if the potential benefit justifies the potential risk to the fetus.

Nursing Mothers: There is evidence that maternal 1,25-dihydroxy vitamin D_3 (calcitriol) may enter the fetal circulation, but it is not known whether it is excreted in human milk. The systemic disposition of calcipotriene is expected to be similar to that of the naturally occurring vitamin. Because many drugs are excreted in human milk, caution should be exercised when Dovonex Cream is administered to a nursing woman.

Pediatric Use: Safety and effectiveness of Dovonex Cream in pediatric patients have not been established. Because of a higher ratio of skin surface area to body mass, pediatric patients are at greater risk than adults of systemic adverse effects when they are treated with topical medication.

Geriatric Use: Of the total number of patients in clinical studies of calcipotriene cream, approximately 15% were 65 or older, while approximately 3% were 75 and over. There were no significant differences in adverse events for subjects over 65 years compared to those under 65 years of age. However, the greater sensitivity of older individuals cannot be ruled out.

ADVERSE REACTIONS

In controlled clinical trials, the most frequent adverse experiences reported for Dovonex Cream were cases of skin irritation, which occurred in approximately 10–15% of patients. Rash, pruritus, dermatitis and worsening of psoriasis were reported in 1 to 10% of patients.

OVERDOSAGE

Topically applied calcipotriene can be absorbed in sufficient amounts to produce systemic effects. Elevated serum calcium has been observed with excessive use of topical calcipotriene. If elevation in serum calcium should occur, discontinue treatment until normal calcium levels are restored. (See **PRECAUTIONS.**)

DOSAGE AND ADMINISTRATION

Apply a thin layer of Dovonex Cream to the affected skin twice daily and rub in gently and completely. The safety and efficacy of Dovonex Cream have been demonstrated in patients treated for eight weeks.

HOW SUPPLIED

Dovonex® (calcipotriene cream) Cream, 0.005% is available in:

60 gram aluminum tubes (NDC 0072-0260-06)
120 gram aluminum tubes (NDC 0072-0260-12).

STORAGE: Store at controlled room temperature 15°C–25°C (59°F–77°F).
Do not freeze.

Manufactured by
Leo Laboratories Ltd.,
Dublin, Ireland
Distributed by:
Bristol-Myers Squibb Company
Princeton, NJ 08543 U.S.A.
E6-B001A-04-01 J4687B
US Patent No. 4,866,048 Revised November 2000

DOVONEX® ℞

(calcipotriene ointment)
Ointment, 0.005%
Rx only
FOR TOPICAL DERMATOLOGIC USE ONLY.
Not for Ophthalmic, Oral or Intravaginal Use.

DESCRIPTION

Dovonex® (calcipotriene ointment) Ointment, 0.005% contains the compound calcipotriene, a synthetic vitamin D_3 derivative for topical dermatological use.

Chemically, calcipotriene is (5Z,7E,22E,24S)-24-cyclopropyl-9,10-secochola-5, 7, 10(19), 22-tetraene-1α, 3β, 24-triol-, with the empirical formula $C_{27}H_{40}O_3$, a molecular weight of 412.6, and the following structural formula:

Continued on next page

Dovonex Ointment—Cont.

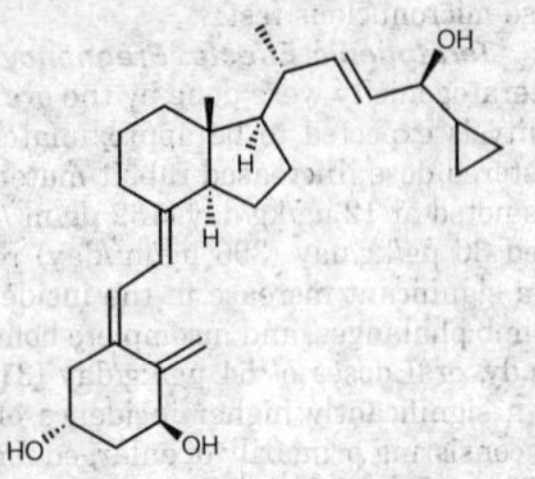

Calcipotriene is a white or off-white crystalline substance. Dovonex Ointment contains calcipotriene 50 µg/g in an ointment base of dibasic sodium phosphate, edetate disodium, mineral oil, petrolatum, propylene glycol, tocopherol, steareth-2 and water.

CLINICAL PHARMACOLOGY

In humans, the natural supply of vitamin D depends mainly on exposure to the ultraviolet rays of the sun for conversion of 7-dehydrocholesterol to vitamin D_3 (cholecalciferol) in the skin. Calcipotriene is a synthetic analog of vitamin D_3.
Clinical studies with radiolabelled ointment indicate that approximately 6% (±3%, SD) of the applied dose of calcipotriene is absorbed systemically when the ointment is applied topically to psoriasis plaques or 5% (±2.6%, SD) when applied to normal skin, and much of the absorbed active is converted to inactive metabolites within 24 hours of application.
Vitamin D and its metabolites are transported in the blood, bound to specific plasma proteins. The active form of the vitamin, 1,25-dihydroxy vitamin D_3 (calcitriol), is known to be recycled via the liver and excreted in the bile. Calcipotriene metabolism following systemic uptake is rapid, and occurs via a similar pathway to the natural hormone. The primary metabolites are much less potent than the parent compound.
There is evidence that maternal 1,25-dihydroxy vitamin D_3 (calcitriol) may enter the fetal circulation, but it is not known whether it is excreted in human milk. The systemic disposition of calcipotriene is expected to be similar to that of the naturally occurring vitamin.

CLINICAL STUDIES

Adequate and well-controlled trials of patients treated with Dovonex Ointment have demonstrated improvement usually beginning after two weeks of therapy. This improvement continued in patients using Dovonex Ointment once daily and twice daily. After 8 weeks of once daily Dovonex Ointment, 56.7% of patients showed at least marked improvement (6.4% showed complete clearing). After 8 weeks of twice daily Dovonex Ointment, 70.0% of patients showed at least marked improvement (11.3% showed complete clearing).
Subtracting percentages of patients using placebo (vehicle only) from percentages of patients using Dovonex Ointment who had at least marked improvement after 8 weeks yields 39.9% for once daily and 49.6% for twice daily. This adjustment for placebo effect indicates that what might appear to be differences between once and twice daily use may reflect differences in the studies independent from the frequency of dosing. Although there was a numerical difference in comparison across studies, twice daily dosing has not been shown to be superior in efficacy to once daily dosing.
Over 400 patients have been treated in open label clinical studies of Dovonex Ointment for periods of up to one year. In half of these studies, patients who previously had not responded well to Dovonex Ointment were excluded. The adverse events in these extended studies included skin irritation in approximately 25% of patients and worsening of psoriasis in approximately 10% of patients. In one of these open label studies, half of the patients no longer required Dovonex Ointment by 16 weeks of treatment, because of satisfactory therapeutic results.

INDICATIONS AND USAGE

Dovonex Ointment is indicated for the treatment of plaque psoriasis in adults. The safety and effectiveness of topical calcipotriene in dermatoses other than psoriasis have not been established.

CONTRAINDICATIONS

Dovonex Ointment is contraindicated in those patients with a history of hypersensitivity to any of the components of the preparation. It should not be used by patients with demonstrated hypercalcemia or evidence of vitamin D toxicity. Dovonex Ointment should not be used on the face.

PRECAUTIONS

General: Use of Dovonex Ointment may cause irritation of lesions and surrounding uninvolved skin. If irritation develops, Dovonex Ointment should be discontinued.
Transient, rapidly reversible elevation of serum calcium has occurred with use of Dovonex Ointment. If elevation in serum calcium outside the normal range should occur, discontinue treatment until normal calcium levels are restored.
Information for Patients: Patients using Dovonex Ointment should receive the following information and instructions:

1. This medication is to be used as directed by the physician. It is for external use only. Avoid contact with the face or eyes. As with any topical medication, patients should wash hands after application.
2. This medication should not be used for any disorder other than that for which it was prescribed.
3. Patients should report to their physician any signs of local adverse reactions.

Carcinogenesis, Mutagenesis, Impairment of Fertility: Long-term animal studies have not been conducted to evaluate the carcinogenic potential of calcipotriene. Studies in rats at doses up to 54 µg/kg/day (318 µg/m²/day) of calcipotriene indicated no impairment of fertility or general reproductive performance.
Calcipotriene did not elicit any mutagenic effects in the Ames mutagenicity assay, the mouse lymphoma TK locus assay, the human lymphocyte chromosome aberration test or the mouse micronucleus test.
Pregnancy: ***Teratogenic Effects: Pregnancy Category C:*** Studies of teratogenicity were done by the oral route where bioavailability is expected to be approximately 40–60% of the administered dose. In rabbits, increased maternal and fetal toxicity were noted at a dosage of 12 µg/kg/day (132 µg/m²/day); a dosage of 36 µg/kg/day (396 µg/m²/day) resulted in a significant increase in the incidence of incomplete ossification of the pubic bones and forelimb phalanges of fetuses. In a rat study, a dosage of 54 µg/kg/day (318 µg/m²/day) resulted in a significantly increased incidence of skeletal abnormalities (enlarged fontanelles and extra ribs). The enlarged fontanelles are most likely due to calcipotriene's effect upon calcium metabolism. The estimated maternal and fetal no-effect exposure levels in the rat (43.2 µg/m²/day) and the rabbit (17.6 µg/m²/day) studies are approximately equal to the expected human systemic exposure level (18.5 µg/m²/day) from dermal application. There are no adequate and well-controlled studies in pregnant women. Therefore, Dovonex Ointment should be used during pregnancy only if the potential benefit justifies the potential risk to the fetus.
Nursing Mothers: It is not known whether calcipotriene is excreted in human milk. Because many drugs are excreted in human milk, caution should be exercised when Dovonex Ointment is administered to a nursing woman.
Pediatric Use: Safety and effectiveness of Dovonex Ointment in children have not been established. Because of a higher ratio of skin surface area to body mass, children are at greater risk than adults of systemic adverse effects when they are treated with topical medication.
Geriatric Use: Of the total number of patients in clinical studies of calcipotriene ointment, approximately 12% were 65 or older, while approximately 4% were 75 and over. The results of an analysis of severity of skin-related adverse events showed a statistically significant difference for subjects over 65 years (more severe) compared to those under 65 years (less severe).

ADVERSE REACTIONS

In controlled clinical trials, the most frequent adverse reactions reported for Dovonex Ointment were burning, itching, and skin irritation, which occurred in approximately 10–15% of patients. Erythema, dry skin, peeling, rash, dermatitis, worsening of psoriasis including development of facial/scalp psoriasis were reported in 1 to 10% of patients. Other experiences reported in less than 1% of patients included skin atrophy, hyperpigmentation, hypercalcemia, and folliculitis. Once daily dosing has not been shown to be superior in safety to twice daily dosing.

OVERDOSAGE

Topically applied Dovonex Ointment can be absorbed in sufficient amounts to produce systemic effects. Elevated serum calcium has been observed with excessive use of Dovonex Ointment. (See **PRECAUTIONS.**)

DOSAGE AND ADMINISTRATION

Apply a thin layer of Dovonex Ointment to the affected skin once or twice daily and rub in gently and completely.

HOW SUPPLIED

Dovonex® (calcipotriene ointment) Ointment, 0.005% is available in:
60 gram aluminum tubes (NDC 0072-2540-06)
120 gram aluminum tubes (NDC 0072-2540-12).
STORAGE
Store at controlled room temperature 15°C – 25°C (59°F – 77°F).
Do not freeze.
Manufactured by
Leo Laboratories Ltd.,
Dublin, Ireland
Distributed by:
Bristol-Myers Squibb Company
Princeton, NJ 08543 U.S.A.
E6–B001B-04–01 J4688B
US Patent No. 4,866,048 Revised November 2000

DOVONEX® ℞

[*dōvănex*]
(calcipotriene solution)
Scalp Solution, 0.005%
FOR TOPICAL DERMATOLOGIC USE ONLY.
Not for Ophthalmic, Oral or Intravaginal Use.

DESCRIPTION

Dovonex® (calcipotriene solution) Scalp Solution 0.005%, is a colorless topical solution containing 0.005% calcipotriene in a vehicle of isopropanol (51% v/v) propylene glycol, hydroxypropyl cellulose, sodium citrate, menthol and water.
The chemical name of calcipotriene is (5Z, 7E, 22E, 24S)-24-cyclopropyl-9,10-secochola-5,7,10(19), 22-tetraene-1α,3β, 24-triol, with the empirical formula $C_{27}H_{40}O_3$, a molecular weight of 412.6, and the following structural formula:

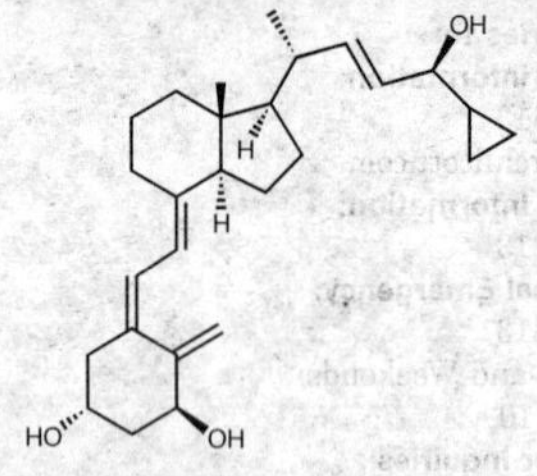

CLINICAL PHARMACOLOGY

In humans, the natural supply of vitamin D depends mainly on exposure to the ultraviolet rays of the sun for conversion of 7-dehydrocholesterol to vitamin D_3 (cholecalciferol) in the skin. Calcipotriene is a synthetic analog of vitamin D_3.
Although the precise mechanism of calcipotriene's antipsoriatic action is not fully understood, *in vitro* evidence suggests that calcipotriene is roughly equipotent to the natural vitamin in its effects on proliferation and differentiation of a variety of cell types. Calcipotriene has also been shown, in animal studies, to be 100–200 times less potent in its effects on calcium utilization than the natural hormone.
Clinical studies with radiolabelled calcipotriene solution indicate that less than 1% of the applied dose of calcipotriene is absorbed through the scalp when the solution (2.0 mL) is applied topically to normal skin or psoriasis plaques (160 cm²) for 12 hours, and that much of the absorbed calcipotriene is converted to inactive metabolites within 24 hours of application.
Vitamin D and its metabolites are transported in the blood, bound to specific plasma proteins. The active form of the vitamin, 1,25-dihydroxy vitamin D_3 (calcitriol), is known to be recycled via the liver and excreted in the bile. Calcipotriene metabolism following systemic uptake is rapid, and occurs via a similar pathway to the natural hormone. The primary metabolites are much less potent than the parent compound.
There is evidence that maternal 1,25-dihydroxy vitamin D_3 (calcitriol) may enter the fetal circulation, but it is not known whether it is excreted in human milk. The systemic disposition of calcipotriene is expected to be similar to that of the naturally occurring vitamin.

CLINICAL STUDIES

Adequate and well-controlled trials of patients treated with Dovonex Scalp Solution, 0.005%, have demonstrated improvement usually beginning after 2 weeks of therapy. This improvement continued with approximately 31% of patients appearing either cleared (14%) or almost cleared (17%) after 8 weeks of therapy.

INDICATIONS AND USAGE

Dovonex Scalp Solution, 0.005%, is indicated for the topical treatment of chronic, moderately severe psoriasis of the scalp. The safety and effectiveness of topical calcipotriene in dermatoses other than psoriasis have not been established.

CONTRAINDICATIONS

Dovonex Scalp Solution, 0.005%, is contraindicated in those patients with acute psoriatic eruptions or a history of hypersensitivity to any of the components of the preparation. It should not be used by patients with demonstrated hypercalcemia or evidence of vitamin D toxicity.

WARNINGS

Avoid contact with the eyes or mucous membranes. Discontinue use if a sensitivity reaction occurs or if excessive irritation develops on uninvolved skin areas.
Drug product is flammable. Keep away from open flame.

PRECAUTIONS

General: Use of Dovonex Scalp Solution, 0.005%, may cause transient irritation of both lesions and surrounding uninvolved skin. If irritation develops, Dovonex Scalp Solution, 0.005% should be discontinued.
For external use only. Keep out of the reach of children. Always wash hands thoroughly after use.
Reversible elevation of serum calcium has occurred with use of topical calcipotriene. If elevation in serum calcium outside the normal range should occur, discontinue treatment until normal calcium levels are restored.
Information for Patients: Patients using Dovonex Scalp Solution should receive the following information and instructions:

1. This medication is to be used only as directed by the physician. It is for external use only. Avoid contact with the face or eyes. As with any topical medication, patients should wash their hands after application.
2. This medication should not be used for any disorder other than that for which it was prescribed.
3. Patients should report to their physician any signs of adverse reactions.

Carcinogenesis, Mutagenesis, Impairment of Fertility: Animal studies have not been conducted to evaluate the carcinogenic potential of calcipotriene. Studies in rats at doses up to 54 µg/kg/day (318 µg/m²/day) of calcipotriene indicated no impairment of fertility or general reproductive performance.

Calcipotriene did not elicit any mutagenic effects in the Ames mutagenicity assay, the mouse lymphoma TK locus assay, the human lymphocyte chromosome aberration test or the mouse micronucleus test.

Pregnancy: Teratogenic Effects: Pregnancy Category C: Studies of teratogenicity were done by the oral route where bioavailability is expected to be approximately 40–60% of the administered dose. Increased rabbit maternal and fetal toxicity was noted at 12 µg/kg/day (132 µg/m²/day). Rabbits administered 36 µg/kg/day (396 µg/m²/day) resulted in fetuses with a significant increase in the incidences of pubic bones, forelimb phalanges, and incomplete bone ossification. In a rat study, oral doses of 54 µg/kg/day (318 µg/m²/day) resulted in a significantly higher incidence of skeletal abnormalities consisting primarily of enlarged fontanelles and extra ribs. The enlarged fontanelles are most likely due to calcipotriene's effect upon calcium metabolism. The maternal and fetal calculated no-effect exposures in the rat (43.2 µg/m²/day) and rabbit (17.6 µg/m²/day) studies are greater than the expected human systemic exposure level (0.13 µg/m²/day) from dermal application. There are no adequate and well-controlled studies in pregnant women. Therefore, Dovonex (calcipotriene solution) Scalp Solution, 0.005%, should be used during pregnancy only if the potential benefit justifies the potential risk to the fetus.

Nursing Mothers: There is evidence that maternal 1,25-dihydroxy vitamin D_3 (calcitriol) may enter the fetal circulation, but it is not known whether it is excreted in human milk. The systemic disposition of calcipotriene is expected to be similar to that of the naturally occurring vitamin. Because many drugs are excreted in human milk, caution should be exercised when Dovonex Scalp Solution, 0.005%, is administered to a nursing woman.

Pediatric Use: Safety and effectiveness of Dovonex Scalp Solution, 0.005%, in pediatric patients have not been specifically established. Because of a higher ratio of skin surface area to body mass, pediatric patients are at greater risk than adults of systemic adverse effects when they are treated with topical medication.

Geriatric Use: Of the total number of patients in clinical studies of calcipotriene solution, approximately 16% were 65 or older, while approximately 4% were 75 and over. The results of an analysis of severity of skin-related adverse events showed no differences for subjects over 65 years compared to those under 65 years, but greater sensitivity of some older individuals cannot be ruled out.

ADVERSE REACTIONS

In controlled clinical trials, the most frequent adverse reactions reported to be related to Dovonex Scalp Solution, 0.005%, use were transient burning, stinging and tingling, which occurred in approximately 23% of patients. Rash was reported in about 11% of patients. Dry skin, irritation and worsening of psoriasis was reported in 1–5% of patients. Skin atrophy, hyperpigmentation, hypercalcemia, and folliculitis were not observed in these studies, but cannot be excluded.

OVERDOSAGE

Topically applied calcipotriene can be absorbed in sufficient amounts to produce systemic effects. Elevated serum calcium has been observed with excessive use of topical calcipotriene. If elevation in serum calcium should occur, discontinue treatment until calcium levels are restored. (See PRECAUTIONS.)

DOSAGE AND ADMINISTRATION

Comb the hair to remove scaly debris and after suitably parting, apply Dovonex Scalp Solution, 0.005% twice daily, only to the lesions, and rub in gently and completely, taking care to prevent the solution spreading onto the forehead. The safety and efficacy of Dovonex Scalp Solution, 0.005%, have been demonstrated in patients treated for eight weeks. **Keep Dovonex Scalp Solution, 0.005%, well away from the eyes.** Avoid application of the solution to uninvolved scalp margins. **Always wash hands thoroughly after use.**

HOW SUPPLIED

Dovonex® (calcipotriene solution) Scalp Solution, 0.005%, is available in 60 mL plastic bottles (NDC 0072-1160-06).

STORAGE: Store at controlled room temperature 15°C – 25°C (59°F – 77°F). Avoid sunlight. Do not freeze

Manufactured by
Leo Pharmaceutical Products, Ltd.
Ballerup, Denmark
Distributed by
Bristol-Myers Squibb Company
Princeton, NJ 08543 U.S.A.
E6-B001C-04-01 J4686A
US Patent No. 4,866,048 Revised November 2000

FEMTRACE® ℞

[fĕm-trās]
(estradiol acetate tablets)
Rx Only

PRESCRIBING INFORMATION

ESTROGENS INCREASE THE RISK OF ENDOMETRIAL CANCER

Close clinical surveillance of all women taking estrogens is important. Adequate diagnostic measures, including endometrial sampling when indicated, should be undertaken to rule out malignancy in all cases of undiagnosed persistent or recurring abnormal vaginal bleeding. There is no evidence that the use of "natural" estrogens results in a different endometrial risk profile than synthetic estrogens at equivalent estrogen doses. (See **WARNINGS, Malignant neoplasms, *Endometrial cancer.***)

CARDIOVASCULAR AND OTHER RISKS

Estrogens with or without progestins should not be used for the prevention of cardiovascular disease. (See **WARNINGS, Cardiovascular disorders.**)

The Women's Health Initiative (WHI) study reported increased risks of myocardial infarction, stroke, invasive breast cancer, pulmonary emboli, and deep vein thrombosis in postmenopausal women (50 to 79 years of age) during 5 years of treatment with oral conjugated estrogens (CE 0.625 mg) combined with medroxyprogesterone acetate (MPA 2.5 mg) relative to placebo. (See **CLINICAL PHARMACOLOGY, Clinical Studies.**)

The Women's Health Initiative Memory Study (WHIMS), a substudy of WHI, reported increased risk of developing probable dementia in postmenopausal women 65 years of age or older during 4 years of treatment with oral conjugated estrogens plus medroxyprogesterone acetate relative to placebo. It is unknown whether this finding applies to younger postmenopausal women or to women taking estrogen alone therapy. (See **CLINICAL PHARMACOLOGY, Clinical Studies.**)

Other doses of oral conjugated estrogens with medroxyprogesterone acetate, and other combinations and dosage forms of estrogens and progestins were not studied in the WHI clinical trials and, in the absence of comparable data, these risks should be assumed to be similar. Because of these risks, estrogens with or without progestins should be prescribed at the lowest effective doses and for the shortest duration consistent with treatment goals and risks for the individual woman.

DESCRIPTION

Femtrace® (estradiol acetate tablets) for oral administration contains 0.45 mg, 0.9 mg or 1.8 mg estradiol acetate. Femtrace contains the following inactive ingredients: ferric oxide, povidone, lactose monohydrate, microcrystalline cellulose, croscarmellose sodium, silicon dioxide, magnesium stearate and acetic acid; ferric oxide, a coloring agent, is not an ingredient in the 0.9 mg tablets.

Estradiol acetate is chemically described as estra-1,3,5(10)-triene-3,17β-diol-3-acetate. The molecular formula of estradiol acetate is $C_{20}H_{26}O_3$ and the structural formula is:

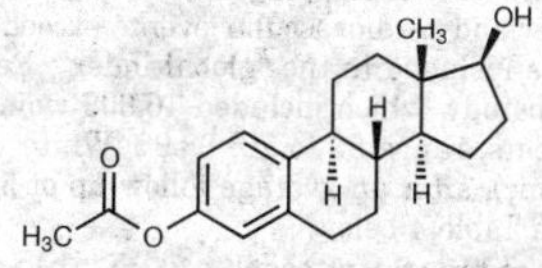

The molecular weight of estradiol acetate is 314.42.

CLINICAL PHARMACOLOGY

Endogenous estrogens are largely responsible for the development and maintenance of the female reproductive system and secondary sexual characteristics. Although circulating estrogens exist in a dynamic equilibrium of metabolic interconversions, estradiol is the principal intracellular human estrogen and is substantially more potent than its metabolites, estrone and estriol, at the receptor level.

The primary source of estrogen in normally cycling adult women is the ovarian follicle, which secretes 70 to 500 mcg of estradiol daily, depending on the phase of the menstrual cycle. After menopause, most endogenous estrogen is produced by conversion of androstenedione, secreted by the adrenal cortex, to estrone by peripheral tissues. Thus, estrone and the sulfate conjugated form, estrone sulfate, are the most abundant circulating estrogens in postmenopausal women.

Estrogens act through binding to nuclear receptors in estrogen-responsive tissues. To date, two estrogen receptors have been identified. These vary in proportion from tissue to tissue.

Circulating estrogens modulate the pituitary secretion of the gonadotropins, luteinizing hormone (LH) and follicle stimulating hormone (FSH) through a negative feedback mechanism. Estrogens act to reduce the elevated levels of these hormones seen in postmenopausal women.

Pharmacokinetics

In vitro studies suggest that within 5 minutes of administration, all estradiol acetate will be hydrolyzed to estradiol *in vivo*.

Absorption

Estradiol was rapidly absorbed following oral administration of estradiol acetate. Mean serum estradiol concentrations following multiple dosing are shown in Figure 1. Estradiol and estrone serum concentrations increased proportionally with increasing dose; the corresponding estradiol Cavg values were 23.5, 44.4 and 92.1 pg/mL for the 0.45, 0.9 and 1.8 mg doses, respectively (see Table 1).

Figure 1. Mean (± SD) Serum Estradiol Concentration Following Multiple-Dose Administration of Femtrace to Healthy Postmenopausal Women

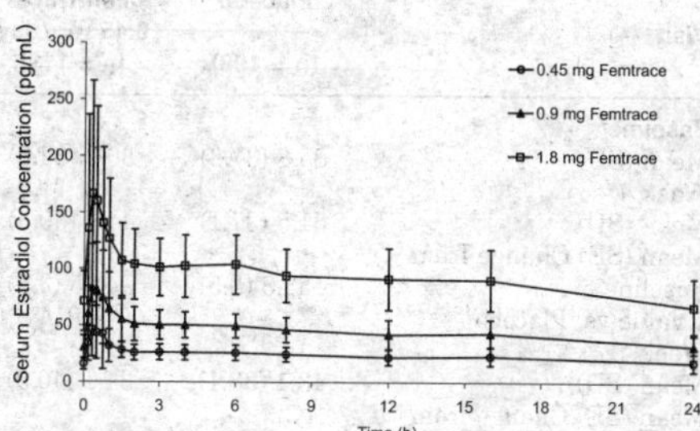

Table 1. Summary of Mean (%CV)* Pharmacokinetic Parameters Following Multiple-Dose Administration of Femtrace to Healthy Postmenopausal Women (n=18)

Estradiol Acetate Dose	Analyte	Cmax (pg/mL)	tmax** (hour)	AUC (0–τ) (pg·h/mL	t½**** (hour)
0.45 mg	Estradiol	56.7 (57)	0.50	565.0 (26)	25.9
	Estrone***	155.0 (40)	6.0	2363.8 (34)	15.9
0.9 mg	Estradiol	90.1 (51)	0.43	1066.5 (25)	22.2
	Estrone***	313.9 (25)	5.0	4980.9 (32)	16.1
1.8 mg	Estradiol	177.3 (55)	0.75	2211.3 (26)	21.4
	Estrone***	680.6 (25)	6.0	11510.8 (32)	17.6

* Coefficient of Variation
** Median value reported for Tmax
*** Baseline-adjusted values
**** Harmonic mean value reported for t½
Cmax: Maximum serum concentration
tmax: Time of Cmax
AUC(0–τ): Area under the serum concentration-time curve over the dosing interval
t½: Half-life

[See table 1 above]

Effect of Food

The maximum serum concentration (Cmax) of estradiol following administration of 1.8 mg estradiol acetate was 36% lower in the fed state compared to the fasted state. However, the area under the serum concentration versus time curve (AUC) was comparable among the fed and fasted states.

Distribution

The distribution of exogenous estrogens is similar to that of endogenous estrogens. Estrogens are widely distributed in the body and are generally found in higher concentrations in the sex hormone target organs. Estrogens circulate in the blood largely bound to sex hormone binding globulin (SHBG) and to albumin.

Metabolism

Estradiol acetate is hydrolyzed *in vivo* to estradiol. Exogenous estrogens are metabolized in the same manner as endogenous estrogens. Circulating estrogens exist in a dynamic equilibrium of metabolic interconversions. These transformations take place mainly in the liver. Estradiol is converted reversibly to estrone, and both can be converted to estriol, which is the major urinary metabolite. Estrogens also undergo enterohepatic recirculation via sulfate and glucuronide conjugation in the liver, biliary secretion of conjugates into the intestine, and hydrolysis in the gut followed by reabsorption. In postmenopausal women, a significant proportion of the circulating estrogens exist as sulfate conjugates, especially estrone sulfate, which serves as a circulating reservoir for the formation of more active estrogens.

Excretion

Estradiol, estrone, and estriol are excreted in the urine along with glucuronide and sulfate conjugates.

The estradiol apparent elimination half-life value is 21 to 26 hours.

Special Populations

No pharmacokinetic studies were conducted in special populations, including patients with renal or hepatic impairment.

Continued on next page

Femtrace—Cont.

Drug Interactions
No clinical drug-drug interaction studies with estradiol acetate have been performed. *In vitro* and *in vivo* studies have shown that estrogens are metabolized partially by cytochrome P450 3A4 (CYP3A4). Therefore, inducers or inhibitors of CYP3A4 may affect estrogen drug metabolism. Inducers of CYP3A4 such as St. John's Wort preparations (*Hypericum perforatum*), phenobarbital, carbamazepine and rifampin may reduce plasma concentrations of estrogens, possibly resulting in a decrease in therapeutic effects and/or changes in the uterine bleeding profile. Inhibitors of CYP3A4 such as erythromycin, clarithromycin, ketoconazole, itraconazole, ritonavir and grapefruit juice may increase plasma concentrations of estrogens and may result in side effects.

Clinical Studies
Effects on vasomotor symptoms.
Two 12-week double-blind, placebo-controlled clinical trials were conducted to evaluate the efficacy of Femtrace in the treatment of moderate to severe vasomotor symptoms in postmenopausal women who had at least 7 moderate to severe hot flushes daily or at least 60 moderate to severe hot flushes per week before randomization. In one study, 289 postmenopausal women (mean age 53.4 years [range 41 to 68 years], 78% Caucasian) were randomized to receive either placebo, Femtrace 0.9 mg/day or Femtrace 1.8 mg/day. In the second study, 221 postmenopausal women (mean age 52.2 years [range 36 to 80 years], 80% Caucasian) were randomized to receive either placebo or Femtrace 0.45 mg/day. The results in Tables 2a and 3a indicate that compared with placebo, Femtrace 0.9 mg/day and Femtrace 1.8 mg/day produced a reduction in both the frequency and severity of moderate to severe vasomotor symptoms at weeks 4 and 12. The results in Tables 2b and 3b indicate that compared with placebo, Femtrace 0.45 mg/day produced a reduction in the frequency of moderate to severe vasomotor symptoms at weeks 4 and 12, and a reduction in the severity of moderate to severe vasomotor symptoms at weeks 7 and 12.
[See table 2a above]

Table 2a. Mean Change from Baseline in the Number of Moderate to Severe Vasomotor Symptoms per Week – ITT Population, LOCF

Visit	Placebo (n = 94)	Femtrace 0.9 mg/day (n = 100)	Femtrace 1.8 mg/day (n = 95)
Baseline[1]			
Mean (SD)	86.1 (40.2)	78.5 (24.9)	82.4 (39.1)
Week 4*			
Mean (SD)	51.5 (47.2)	24.3 (28.4)	21.9 (25.9)
Mean (SE) Change from Baseline	–30.1 (3.3)	–56.5 (3.2)	–59.3 (3.4)
p value vs. Placebo[2]	–	<0.001	<0.001
Week 12*			
Mean (SD)	46.8 (54.6)	17.5 (28.9)	7.3 (15.2)
Mean (SE) Change from Baseline	–36.3 (3.5)	–63.9 (3.4)	–74.8 (3.6)
p value vs. Placebo[2]	–	<0.001	<0.001

*Primary endpoints
[1] The baseline number of moderate to severe vasomotor symptoms (MSVS) is the weekly average number of MSVS during the two weeks between screening and randomization
[2] p values were based on Wilcoxon rank sum test (van Elteren test)
ITT = intent to treat; LOCF = last observation carried forward; SD = standard deviation; SE = standard error

Table 3a. Mean Change from Baseline in the Severity of Moderate to Severe Vasomotor Symptoms per Week – ITT Population, LOCF

Visit	Placebo (n = 94)	Femtrace 0.9 mg/day (n = 100)	Femtrace 1.8 mg/day (n = 95)
Baseline[1]			
Mean (SD)	2.5 (0.2)	2.5 (0.2)	2.5 (0.2)
Week 4*			
Mean (SD)	2.3 (0.6)	1.8 (1.0)	1.9 (1.0)
Mean (SE) Change from Baseline	–0.2 (1.0)	–0.7 (0.1)	–0.7 (0.1)
p value vs. Placebo[2]	–	0.001	0.002
Week 12*			
Mean (SD)	2.2 (0.8)	1.4 (1.2)	1.0 (1.2)
Mean (SE) Change from Baseline	–0.3 (0.1)	–1.1 (0.1)	–1.5 (0.1)
p value vs. Placebo[2]	–	<0.001	<0.001

* Primary endpoints
[1] The baseline severity of moderate to severe vasomotor symptoms (MSVS) is the average severity of MSVS during the two weeks between screening and randomization
[2] p values were based on Wilcoxon rank sum test (van Elteren test)
Note: Hot flush severity was scored using the following scale: 1 = Mild, 2 = Moderate, 3 = Severe
ITT = intent to treat; LOCF = last observation carried forward; SD = standard deviation; SE = standard error

Table 2b. Mean Change from Baseline in the Number of Moderate to Severe Vasomotor Symptoms per Week – ITT (modified)[1] Population, LOCF

Visit	Placebo (n = 108)	Femtrace 0.45 mg/day (n = 113)
Baseline[2]		
Mean (SD)	85.8 (37.8)	86.2 (34.8)
Week 4*		
Mean (SD)	51.5 (37.1)	44.1 (39.5)
Mean (SE) Change from Baseline	–33.8 (3.5)	–41.5 (3.5)
p value vs. Placebo[3]	–	0.014
Week 12*		
Mean (SD)	43.1 (38.1)	34.1 (40.9)
Mean (SE) Change from Baseline	–41.5 (3.5)	–51.2 (3.5)
p value vs. Placebo[3]	–	0.005

*Primary endpoints
[1] ITT (modified): intent to treat modified by excluding 24 unblinded subjects
[2] The baseline number of moderate to severe vasomotor symptoms (MSVS) is the weekly average number of MSVS during the two weeks between screening and randomization
[3] p values were based on Wilcoxon rank sum test (van Elteren test)
ITT = intent to treat; LOCF = last observation carried forward; SD = standard deviation; SE = standard error

[See table 3a above]

Table 3b. Mean Change from Baseline in the Severity of Moderate to Severe Vasomotor Symptoms per Week – ITT (modified)[1] Population, LOCF

Visit	Placebo (n = 108)	Femtrace 0.45 mg/day (n = 113)
Baseline[2]		
Mean (SD)	2.6 (0.2)	2.5 (0.2)
Week 4*		
Mean (SD)	2.4 (0.5)	2.3 (0.7)
Mean (SE) Change from Baseline	–0.2 (0.1)	–0.3 (0.06)
p value vs. Placebo[3]	–	0.787
Week 12*		
Mean (SD)	2.3 (0.8)	1.9 (1.1)
Mean (SE) Change from Baseline	–0.3 (0.1)	–0.7 (0.1)
p value vs. Placebo[3]	–	0.016

*Primary endpoints
[1] ITT (modified): intent to treat modified by excluding 24 unblinded subjects
[2] The baseline severity of moderate to severe vasomotor symptoms (MSVS) is the average severity of MSVS during the two weeks between screening and randomization
[3] p values were based on Wilcoxon rank sum test (van Elteren test)
Note: Hot flush severity was scored using the following scale: 1 = Mild, 2 = Moderate, 3 = Severe
ITT = intent to treat; LOCF = last observation carried forward; SD = standard deviation; SE = standard error

Women's Health Initiative Studies
The Women's Health Initiative (WHI) study enrolled a total of 27,000 predominantly healthy postmenopausal women to assess the risks and benefits of either the use of oral 0.625 mg conjugated estrogens (CE) per day alone or the use of oral 0.625 mg conjugated estrogens plus 2.5 mg medroxyprogesterone acetate (MPA) per day compared to placebo in the prevention of certain chronic diseases. The primary endpoint was the incidence of coronary heart disease (CHD) (nonfatal myocardial infarction and CHD death), with invasive breast cancer as the primary adverse outcome studied. A "global index" included the earliest occurrence of CHD, invasive breast cancer, stroke, pulmonary embolism (PE), endometrial cancer, colorectal cancer, hip fracture or death due to other cause. The study did not evaluate the effects of CE or CE/MPA on menopausal symptoms.
The CE/MPA substudy was stopped early because, according to the predefined stopping rule, the increased risk of breast cancer and cardiovascular events exceeded the specified benefits included in the "global index". Results of the CE/MPA substudy, which included 16,608 women (average age of 63 years, range 50 to 79; 83.9% White, 6.5% Black, 5.5% Hispanic), after an average follow-up of 5.2 years are presented in Table 4 below.
[See table 4 at top of next page]
For those outcomes included in the "global index", the absolute excess risks per 10,000 women-years in the group treated with CE/MPA were 7 more CHD events, 8 more strokes, 8 more PEs, and 8 more invasive breast cancers, while the absolute risk reductions per 10,000 women-years were 6 fewer colorectal cancers and 5 fewer hip fractures. The absolute excess risk of events included in the "global index" was 19 per 10,000 women-years. There was no difference between the groups in terms of all-cause mortality. (See **BOXED WARNINGS**, **WARNINGS**, and **PRECAUTIONS**.)

Women's Health Initiative Memory Study
The Women's Health Initiative Memory Study (WHIMS), a substudy of WHI, enrolled 4,532 predominantly healthy postmenopausal women 65 years of age and older (47% were age 65 to 69 years, 35% were 70 to 74 years, and 18% were 75 years of age and older) to evaluate the effects of CE/MPA (0.625 mg conjugated estrogens plus 2.5 mg medroxyprogesterone acetate) on the incidence of probable dementia (primary outcome) compared with placebo.
After an average follow-up of 4 years, 40 women in the estrogen/progestin group (45 per 10,000 women-years) and 21 in the placebo group (22 per 10,000 women-years) were diagnosed with probable dementia. The relative risk of probable dementia in the hormone therapy group was 2.05 (95% CI, 1.21 to 3.48) compared to placebo. Differences between groups became apparent in the first year of treatment. It is unknown whether these findings apply to younger postmenopausal women. (See **BOXED WARNINGS** and **WARNINGS, Dementia**.)

INDICATIONS AND USAGE
Femtrace therapy is indicated in the treatment of moderate to severe vasomotor symptoms associated with the menopause.

CONTRAINDICATIONS
Femtrace should not be used in women with any of the following conditions:
1. Undiagnosed abnormal genital bleeding.
2. Known, suspected, or history of cancer of the breast.
3. Known or suspected estrogen-dependent neoplasia.
4. Active deep vein thrombosis, pulmonary embolism or history of these conditions.
5. Active or recent (e.g., within the past year) arterial thromboembolic disease (e.g., stroke, myocardial infarction).
6. Liver dysfunction or disease.
7. Femtrace should not be used in patients with known hypersensitivity to its ingredients.
8. Known or suspected pregnancy. There is no indication for Femtrace in pregnancy. There appears to be little or no increased risk of birth defects in children born to women who have used estrogens and progestins from oral contraceptives inadvertently during early pregnancy. (See **PRECAUTIONS**.)

WARNINGS
See **BOXED WARNINGS**.
1. Cardiovascular disorders
Estrogen and estrogen/progestin therapy has been associated with an increased risk of cardiovascular events such as myocardial infarction and stroke, as well as venous thrombosis and pulmonary embolism (venous thromboembolism or VTE). Should any of these occur or be suspected, estrogens should be discontinued immediately.
Risk factors for arterial vascular disease (e.g., hypertension, diabetes mellitus, tobacco use, hypercholesterolemia and obesity) and/or venous thromboembolism (e.g., personal history or family history of VTE, obesity and systemic lupus erythematosus) should be managed appropriately.
a. Coronary heart disease and stroke
In the Women's Health Initiative (WHI) study, an increase in the number of myocardial infarctions and strokes has been observed in women receiving CE compared to placebo. These observations are preliminary. (See **CLINICAL PHARMACOLOGY, Clinical Studies**.)

In the CE/MPA substudy of WHI, an increased risk of coronary heart disease (CHD) events (defined as non-fatal myocardial infarction and CHD death) was observed in women receiving CE/MPA compared to women receiving placebo (37 vs 30 per 10,000 women-years). The increase in risk was observed in year one and persisted.

In the same substudy of WHI, an increased risk of stroke was observed in women receiving CE/MPA compared to women receiving placebo (29 vs 21 per 10,000 women-years). The increase in risk was observed after the first year and persisted.

In postmenopausal women with documented heart disease (n = 2,763, average age 66.7 years) a controlled clinical trial of secondary prevention of cardiovascular disease (Heart and Estrogen/Progestin Replacement Study; HERS), treatment with CE/MPA (0.625 mg/2.5 mg per day) demonstrated no cardiovascular benefit. During an average follow-up of 4.1 years, treatment with CE/MPA did not reduce the overall rate of CHD events in postmenopausal women with established coronary heart disease. There were more CHD events in the CE/MPA-treated group than in the placebo group in year 1 but not during the subsequent years. Two thousand three hundred and twenty one women from the original HERS trial agreed to participate in an open label extension of HERS, HERS II. Average follow-up in HERS II was an additional 2.7 years, for a total of 6.8 years overall. Rates of CHD events were comparable among women in the CE/MPA group and the placebo group in HERS, HERS II and overall.

Large doses of estrogen (5 mg conjugated estrogens per day), comparable to those used to treat cancer of the prostate and breast, have been shown in a large prospective clinical trial in men to increase the risks of nonfatal myocardial infarction, pulmonary embolism and thrombophlebitis.

b. Venous thromboembolism (VTE)

In the Women's Health Initiative (WHI) study, an increase in VTE has been observed in women receiving CE compared to placebo. These observations are preliminary. (See **CLINICAL PHARMACOLOGY**, **Clinical Studies**.)

In the CE/MPA substudy of WHI, a 2-fold greater rate of VTE, including deep venous thrombosis and pulmonary embolism, was observed in women receiving CE/MPA compared to women receiving placebo. The rate of VTE was 34 per 10,000 women-years in the CE/MPA group compared to 16 per 10,000 women-years in the placebo group. The increase in VTE risk was observed during the first year and persisted.

If feasible, estrogens should be discontinued at least 4 to 6 weeks before surgery of the type associated with an increased risk of thromboembolism or during periods of prolonged immobilization.

2. Malignant neoplasms

a. Endometrial cancer

The use of unopposed estrogens in women with intact uteri has been associated with an increased risk of endometrial cancer. The reported endometrial cancer risk among unopposed estrogen users is about 2- to 12-fold greater than in non-users, and appears dependent on duration of treatment and on estrogen dose. Most studies show no significant increased risk associated with use of estrogens for less than one year. The greatest risk appears associated with prolonged use, with increased risks of 15- to 24-fold for five to ten years or more, and this risk has been shown to persist for at least 8 to 15 years after estrogen therapy is discontinued.

Clinical surveillance of all women taking estrogen/progestin combinations is important. Adequate diagnostic measures, including endometrial sampling when indicated, should be undertaken to rule out malignancy in all cases of undiagnosed persistent or recurring abnormal vaginal bleeding. There is no evidence that the use of natural estrogens results in a different endometrial risk profile than synthetic estrogens of equivalent estrogen dose. Adding a progestin to estrogen therapy has been shown to reduce the risk of endometrial hyperplasia which may be a precursor to endometrial cancer.

b. Breast cancer

The use of estrogens and progestins by postmenopausal women has been reported to increase the risk of breast cancer. The most important randomized clinical trial providing information about this issue is the Women's Health Initiative (WHI) substudy of CE/MPA (see **CLINICAL PHARMACOLOGY**, **Clinical Studies**). The results from observational studies are generally consistent with those of the WHI clinical trial and report no significant variation in the risk of breast cancer among different estrogens or progestins, doses, or routes of administration.

The CE/MPA substudy of WHI reported an increased risk of breast cancer in women who took CE/MPA for a mean follow-up of 5.6 years. Observational studies have also reported an increased risk for estrogen/progestin combination therapy and a smaller increased risk for estrogen alone therapy after several years of use. In the WHI trial and from observational studies, the excess risk increased with duration of use. From observational studies, the risk appeared to return to baseline in about five years after stopping treatment. In addition, observational studies suggest that the risk of breast cancer was greater, and became apparently earlier, with estrogen/progestin combination therapy as compared to estrogen alone therapy.

In the CE/MPA substudy, 26% of the women reported prior use of estrogen alone and/or estrogen/progestin combination hormone therapy. After a mean follow-up of 5.6 years during the clinical trial, the overall relative risk of invasive breast cancer was 1.24 (95% confidence interval 1.01–1.54) and the overall absolute risk was 41 vs 33 cases per 10,000 women-years, for CE/MPA compared with placebo. Among women who reported prior use of hormone therapy, the relative risk of invasive breast cancer was 1.86 and the absolute risk was 46 vs 25 cases per 10,000 women-years for CE/MPA compared with placebo. Among women who reported no prior use of hormone therapy, the relative risk of invasive breast cancer was 1.09 and the absolute risk was 40 vs 36 cases per 10,000 women-years for CE/MPA compared with placebo. In the same substudy, invasive breast cancers were larger and diagnosed at a more advanced stage in the CE/MPA group compared with the placebo group. Metastatic disease was rare with no apparent difference between the two groups. Other prognostic factors such as histologic subtype, grade and hormone receptor status did not differ between the groups.

Table 4. Relative and Absolute Risk Seen in the CE/MPA Substudy of WHI[a]

Event[c]	Relative Risk CE/MPA vs Placebo at 5.2 Years (95% CI*)	Placebo n = 8102	CE/MPA n = 8506
		Absolute Risk per 10,000 Women-years	
CHD events	1.29 (1.02–1.63)	30	37
Non-fatal MI	*1.32 (1.02–1.72)*	*23*	*30*
CHD death	*1.18 (0.70–1.97)*	*6*	*7*
Invasive breast cancer[b]	1.26 (1.00–1.59)	30	38
Stroke	1.41 (1.07–1.85)	21	29
Pulmonary embolism	2.13 (1.39–3.25)	8	16
Colorectal cancer	0.63 (0.43–0.92)	16	10
Endometrial cancer	0.83 (0.47–1.47)	6	5
Hip fracture	0.66 (0.45–0.98)	15	10
Death due to causes other than the events above	0.92 (0.74–1.14)	40	37
Global Index[c]	1.15 (1.03–1.28)	151	170
Deep vein thrombosis[d]	2.07 (1.49–2.87)	13	26
Vertebral fractures[d]	0.66 (0.44–0.98)	15	9
Other osteoporotic fractures[d]	0.77 (0.69–0.86)	170	131

[a] adapted from JAMA, 2002; 288:321–333
[b] includes metastatic and non-metastatic breast cancer with the exception of in situ breast cancer
[c] a subset of the events was combined in a "global index", defined as the earliest occurrence of CHD events, invasive breast cancer, stroke, pulmonary embolism, endometrial cancer, colorectal cancer, hip fracture, or death due to other causes
[d] not included in Global Index
*nominal confidence intervals unadjusted for multiple looks and multiple comparisons

The use of estrogen plus progestin has been reported to result in an increase in abnormal mammograms requiring further evaluation. All women should receive yearly breast examinations by a healthcare provider and perform monthly breast self-examinations. In addition, mammography examinations should be scheduled based on patient age, risk factors and prior mammogram results.

3. Dementia

In the Women's Health Initiative Memory Study (WHIMS), 4,532 generally healthy postmenopausal women 65 years of age and older were studied of whom 35% were 70 to 74 years of age and 18% were 75 or older. After an average follow-up of 4 years, 40 women being treated with CE/MPA (1.8%, n=2,229) and 21 women in the placebo group (0.9%, n=2,303) received diagnoses of probable dementia. The relative risk for CE/MPA versus placebo was 2.05 (95% confidence interval 1.21-3.48) and was similar for women with and without histories of menopausal hormone use before WHIMS. The absolute risk of probable dementia for CE/MPA versus placebo was 45 versus 22 cases per 10,000 women-years, and the absolute excess risk for CE/MPA was 23 cases per 10,000 women-years. It is unknown whether these findings apply to younger postmenopausal women. (See **CLINICAL PHARMACOLOGY**, **Clinical Studies** and **PRECAUTIONS**, **Geriatric Use**.)

It is unknown whether these findings apply to estrogen alone therapy.

4. Gallbladder disease

A 2- to 4-fold increase in the risk of gallbladder disease requiring surgery in postmenopausal women receiving estrogens has been reported.

5. Hypercalcemia

Estrogen administration may lead to severe hypercalcemia in patients with breast cancer and bone metastases. If hypercalcemia occurs, use of the drug should be stopped and appropriate measures taken to reduce the serum calcium level.

6. Visual abnormalities

Retinal vascular thrombosis has been reported in patients receiving estrogens. Discontinue medication pending examination if there is sudden partial or complete loss of vision, or a sudden onset of proptosis, diplopia or migraine. If examination reveals papilledema or retinal vascular lesions, estrogens should be permanently discontinued.

PRECAUTIONS

A. General

1. Addition of a progestin when a woman has not had a hysterectomy

Studies of the addition of a progestin for 10 or more days of a cycle of estrogen administration, or daily with estrogen in a continuous regimen, have reported a lowered incidence of endometrial hyperplasia than would be induced by estrogen treatment alone. Endometrial hyperplasia may be a precursor to endometrial cancer.

There are, however, possible risks that may be associated with the use of progestins with estrogens compared to estrogen-alone regimens. These include a possible increased risk of breast cancer.

2. Elevated blood pressure

In a small number of case reports, substantial increases in blood pressure have been attributed to idiosyncratic reactions to estrogens. In a large, randomized, placebo-controlled clinical trial, a generalized effect of estrogens on blood pressure was not seen. Blood pressure should be monitored at regular intervals with estrogen use.

3. Hypertriglyceridemia

In patients with pre-existing hypertriglyceridemia, estrogen therapy may be associated with elevations of plasma triglycerides leading to pancreatitis and other complications.

4. Impaired liver function and a past history of cholestatic jaundice

Estrogens may be poorly metabolized in patients with impaired liver function. For patients with a history of cholestatic jaundice associated with past estrogen use or with pregnancy, caution should be exercised and in the case of recurrence, medication should be discontinued.

5. Hypothyroidism

Estrogen administration leads to increased thyroid-binding globulin (TBG) levels. Patients with normal thyroid function can compensate for the increased TBG by making more thyroid hormone, thus maintaining free T_4 and T_3 serum concentrations in the normal range. Patients dependent on thyroid hormone replacement therapy who are also receiving estrogens may require increased doses of their thyroid replacement therapy. These patients should have their thyroid function monitored in order to maintain their free thyroid hormone levels in an acceptable range.

6. Fluid retention

Because estrogens may cause some degree of fluid retention, patients with conditions that might be influenced by this factor, such as cardiac or renal dysfunction, warrant careful observation when estrogens are prescribed.

7. Hypocalcemia

Estrogens should be used with caution in individuals with severe hypocalcemia.

8. Ovarian cancer

The CE/MPA substudy of WHI reported that estrogen plus progestin increased the risk of ovarian cancer. After an average follow-up of 5.6 years, the relative risk for ovarian cancer for CE/MPA versus placebo was 1.58 (95% confidence interval 0.77–3.24) but was not statistically significant. The absolute risk for CE/MPA versus placebo was 4.2 versus 2.7 cases per 10,000 women-years. In some epidemiologic stud-

Continued on next page

Femtrace—Cont.

ies, the use of estrogen alone, in particular for ten or more years, has been associated with an increased risk of ovarian cancer. Other epidemiologic studies have not found these associations.

9. Exacerbation of endometriosis

Endometriosis may be exacerbated with administration of estrogens. A few cases of malignant transformation of residual endometrial implants have been reported in women treated post-hysterectomy with estrogen alone therapy. For patients known to have residual endometriosis post-hysterectomy, the addition of progestin should be considered.

10. Exacerbation of other conditions

Estrogens may cause an exacerbation of asthma, diabetes mellitus, epilepsy, migraine or porphyria, systemic lupus erythematosus and hepatic hemangiomas, and should be used with caution in women with these conditions.

B. Patient Information

Physicians are advised to discuss the PATIENT INFORMATION leaflet with patients for whom they prescribe Femtrace.

C. Laboratory Tests

Estrogen administration should be initiated at the lowest dose approved for the indication and then guided by clinical response rather than by serum hormone levels (e.g., estradiol, FSH).

D. Drug/Laboratory Test Interactions

1. Accelerated prothrombin time, partial thromboplastin time, and platelet aggregation time; increased platelet count; increased factors II, VII antigen, VIII antigen, VIII coagulant activity, IX, X, XII, VII-X complex, II-VII-X complex, and beta-thromboglobulin; decreased levels of antifactor Xa and antithrombin III, decreased antithrombin III activity; increased levels of fibrinogen and fibrinogen activity; increased plasminogen antigen and activity.
2. Increased thyroid-binding globulin (TBG) levels leading to increased circulating total thyroid hormone levels as measured by protein-bound iodine (PBI), T_4 levels (by column or by radioimmunoassay) or T_3 levels by radioimmunoassay. T_3 resin uptake is decreased, reflecting the elevated TBG. Free T_4 and free T_3 concentrations are unaltered. Patients on thyroid replacement therapy may require higher doses of thyroid hormone.
3. Other binding proteins may be elevated in serum (i.e., corticosteroid binding globulin (CBG), sex hormone binding globulin (SHBG)) leading to increased total circulating corticosteroids and sex steroids, respectively. Free hormone concentrations may be decreased. Other plasma proteins may be increased (angiotensinogen/renin substrate, alpha-1-antitrypsin, ceruloplasmin).
4. Increased plasma HDL and HDL^2 cholesterol subfraction concentrations, reduced LDL cholesterol concentration, increased triglycerides levels.
5. Impaired glucose tolerance.
6. Reduced response to metyrapone test.

Carcinogenesis, Mutagenesis, Impairment of Fertility

Long-term continuous administration of estrogen, with or without progestin, in women with and without a uterus, has shown an increased risk of endometrial cancer, breast cancer and ovarian cancer. (See **BOXED WARNINGS, WARNINGS** and **PRECAUTIONS**.)

Long-term continuous administration of natural and synthetic estrogens in certain animal species increases the frequency of carcinomas of the breast, uterus, cervix, vagina, testis, and liver. Estradiol acetate was assayed for mutation in four histidine-requiring strains of *Salmonella typhimurium* and in one tryptophan-requiring strains of *Escherichia coli*. Estradiol acetate did not induce mutations in any of the bacterial strains tested under the conditions employed.

F. Pregnancy

Femtrace should not be used during pregnancy. (See **CONTRAINDICATIONS**.)

G. Nursing Mothers

Estrogen administration to nursing mothers has been shown to decrease the quantity and quality of the milk. Detectable amounts of estrogens have been identified in the milk of mothers receiving this drug. Caution should be exercised when Femtrace is administered to a nursing woman.

H. Pediatric Use

Safety and effectiveness in pediatric patients have not been established.

I. Geriatric Use

Clinical studies of Femtrace did not include sufficient numbers of subjects aged 65 and over to determine whether they respond differently from younger subjects. In general, dose selection for an elderly patient should be cautious, usually starting at the low end of the dosing range, reflecting the greatest frequency of decreased hepatic, renal or cardiac function, and of concomitant disease or other drug therapy.

In the Women's Health Initiative Memory Study, including 4,532 women 65 years of age and older, followed for an average of 4 years, 82% (n=3,729) were 65 to 74 while 18% (n=803) were 75 and over. Most women (80%) had no prior hormone therapy use. Women treated with conjugated estrogens plus medroxyprogesterone acetate were reported to have a two-fold increase in the risk of developing probable dementia. Alzheimer's disease was the most common classification of probable dementia in both the conjugated estrogens plus medroxyprogesterone acetate group and the placebo group. Ninety percent of the cases of probable dementia occurred in the 54% of women that were older than 70. (See **WARNINGS, Dementia.**)

It is unknown whether these findings apply to estrogen alone therapy.

ADVERSE REACTIONS

See **BOXED WARNINGS, WARNINGS** and **PRECAUTIONS**.

Because clinical trials are conducted under widely varying conditions, adverse reaction rates observed in the clinical trials of a drug cannot be directly compared to rates in the clinical trials of another drug and may not reflect the rates observed in practice. The adverse reaction information from clinical trials does, however, provide a basis for identifying the adverse events that appear to be related to drug use and for approximating rates.

In two 12-week clinical trials that included 327 postmenopausal women treated with Femtrace and 221 women treated with placebo tablets, adverse events that occurred in any treatment group at a rate of ≥ 2% regardless of drug relationship are summarized in Table 5.

[See table 5 below]

The following additional adverse reactions have been reported with estrogen and/or progestin therapy.

1. Genitourinary system

Changes in vaginal bleeding pattern and abnormal withdrawal bleeding or flow; breakthrough bleeding; spotting; dysmenorrhea; increase in size of uterine leiomyomata; vaginitis including vaginal candidiasis; change in amount of cervical secretion; changes in cervical ectropion; ovarian cancer; endometrial hyperplasia; endometrial cancer.

2. Breasts

Enlargement, pain, nipple discharge, galactorrhea; fibrocystic breast changes; breast cancer.

3. Cardiovascular

Deep and superficial venous thrombosis; pulmonary embolism; thrombophlebitis; myocardial infarction; stroke; increase in blood pressure.

4. Gastrointestinal

Vomiting, abdominal cramps, bloating; cholestatic jaundice; increased incidence of gallbladder disease; pancreatitis; enlargement of hepatic hemangiomas.

5. Skin

Chloasma or melasma that may persist when drug is discontinued; erythema multiforme; erythema nodosum; hemorrhagic eruption; loss of scalp hair; hirsutism; pruritis, rash.

6. Eyes

Retinal vascular thrombosis; intolerance to contact lenses.

7. Central nervous system

Migraine; dizziness; mental depression; chorea; nervousness; mood disturbances; irritability; exacerbation of epilepsy, dementia.

8. Miscellaneous

Increase or decrease in weight; reduced carbohydrate tolerance; aggravation of porphyria; edema; arthralgias; leg cramps; changes in libido; urticaria; angioedema; anaphylactoid/anaphylactic reactions; hypocalcemia; exacerbation of asthma; increased triglycerides.

OVERDOSAGE

Serious ill effects have not been reported following acute ingestion of large doses of estrogen-containing drug products by young children. Overdosage of estrogen may cause nausea and vomiting, and withdrawal bleeding may occur in females.

DOSAGE AND ADMINISTRATION

When estrogen is prescribed for a postmenopausal woman with a uterus, a progestin should also be initiated to reduce the risk of endometrial cancer. A woman without a uterus does not need progestin. Use of estrogen, alone or in combination with a progestin, should be with the lowest effective dose and for the shortest duration consistent with treatment goals and risks for the individual woman. Patients should be reevaluated periodically as clinically appropriate (e.g., 3-month to 6-month intervals) to determine if treatment is still necessary (see **BOXED WARNINGS** and **WARNINGS**). For women who have a uterus, adequate diagnostic measures, such as endometrial sampling, when indicated, should be undertaken to rule out malignancy in cases of undiagnosed persistent or recurring abnormal vaginal bleeding.

Femtrace therapy consists of a single tablet to be taken once daily.

Three doses of Femtrace are available, 0.45 mg/day, 0.9 mg/day and 1.8 mg/day, for the treatment of moderate to severe vasomotor symptoms associated with the menopause.

Patients should be started at the lowest dose.

HOW SUPPLIED

Femtrace (estradiol acetate tablets) is available in bottles of 100 tablets.

NDC 0430-0389-24 Femtrace 0.45 mg (estradiol acetate tablets) are cream, round tablets debossed with "WC 389" on one side and the tablet logo on the other side.

NDC 0430-0390-24 Femtrace 0.9 mg (estradiol acetate tablets) are white, round tablets debossed with "WC 390" on one side and the tablet logo on the other side.

NDC 0430-0391-24 Femtrace 1.8 mg (estradiol acetate tablets) are yellow, round tablets debossed with "WC 391" on one side and the tablet logo on the other side.

Keep out of reach of children.

STORAGE

Store at 25°C (77°F); excursions permitted to 15°–30°C (59°–86°F) [see USP Controlled Room Temperature]

Manufactured by: Pharmaceutics International, Inc., Hunt Valley, MD 21301

Marketed by: Warner Chilcott Inc., Rockaway, NJ 07866

WARNER CHILCOTT

0390G010

REVISED August 2004

Information on the preceding Warner Chilcott products is based on labeling in effect as of September 2004. Since the publication of this reference book, there may have been revisions to the labeling of these products.

For further product information and current package inserts please visit www.warnerchilcott.com or call 1-800-521-8813.

Table 5. Incidence of AEs Occurring in ≥ 2% of Subjects in Any Treatment Group Presented in Descending Frequency of Preferred Term

Adverse Event[a]	Placebo (n = 221)	Femtrace 0.45 mg/day (n = 132)	Femtrace 0.9 mg/day (n = 100)	Femtrace 1.8 mg/day (n = 95)
	n (%)	n (%)	n (%)	n (%)
Headache (NOS)	12 (5.4)	4 (3.0)	5 (5.0)	4 (4.2)
Vaginal Bleeding	3 (1.4)	1 (0.8)	4 (4.0)	7 (7.4)
Breast Tenderness	3 (1.4)	1 (0.8)	0 (0.0)	6 (6.3)
Influenza	3 (1.4)	3 (2.3)	0 (0.0)	4 (4.2)
Vaginal Discharge	0 (0.0)	3 (2.3)	4 (4.0)	3 (3.2)
Abdominal Pain (NOS)	4 (1.8)	1 (0.8)	0 (0.0)	3 (3.2)
Fungal Infection (NOS)	2 (0.9)	4 (3.0)	1 (1.0)	1 (1.1)
Nasopharyngitis	5 (2.3)	2 (1.5)	0 (0.0)	1 (1.1)
Nausea	3 (1.4)	3 (2.3)	0 (0.0)	2 (2.1)
Intermenstrual Bleeding	2 (0.9)	0 (0.0)	2 (2.0)	3 (3.2)
Sinusitis (NOS)	3 (1.4)	2 (1.5)	1 (1.0)	1 (1.1)
Upper Respiratory Tract Infection (NOS)	3 (1.4)	1 (0.8)	3 (3.0)	0 (0.0)
Back Pain	1 (0.5)	0 (0.0)	3 (3.0)	2 (2.1)
Bronchitis (NOS)	1 (0.5)	2 (1.5)	2 (2.0)	1 (1.1)

AE = adverse event; NOS = not otherwise specified
[a] Regardless of drug relationship

Watson Laboratories, Inc.

311 BONNIE CIRCLE
CORONA, CA 92880

Address Inquiries to:
Customer Support Department
Telephone: 800/272-5525
FAX: 909-493-5842

Product Listing (Generic Name) ℞

The following list of Watson Laboratories generic name products is provided to facilitate identification. It includes the color(s) and identification codes for all products.

Product/Color/Shape	Imprint
ACETAZOLAMIDE TABLETS 250MG White; Round; Scored	5430 DAN DAN
ACYCLOVIR CAPSULES 200MG OP light blue/op aqua	Watson / Acyclovir 200
ACYCLOVIR TABLETS 400MG White; Oval	Watson 335
ACYCLOVIR TABLETS 800MG White; Oval	Watson 336
AFEDITAB CR TABLETS 30MG Brick Red; Round, FC	ELN 30
AFEDITAB CR TABLETS 60MG Brick Red; Round, FC	ELN 60

ALLOPURINOL TABLETS 100MG — 5543 DAN DAN
White; Round; Scored

ALLOPURINOL TABLETS 300MG — 5544 DAN DAN
Orange; Round; Scored

AMOXAPINE TABLETS 100MG — DAN 100/5715
Blue; Round; Scored

AMOXAPINE TABLETS 150MG — DAN 150/5716
Orange; Round; Scored

AMOXAPINE TABLETS 25MG — DAN 25/5713
White; Round; Scored

AMOXAPINE TABLETS 50MG — DAN 50/5714
Orange; Round; Scored

ATENOLOL/CHLORTHALIDONE TABLETS 100MG-25MG — 5783 Dan
White; Round

ATENOLOL/CHLORTHALIDONE TABLETS 50MG-25MG — 5782 Dan
White; Round; Scored

ATENOLOL TABLETS 100MG — 5778 Dan 100
White; Round

ATENOLOL TABLETS 50MG — 5777 DAN 50
White; Round; Scored

BACLOFEN TABLETS 10MG — 5730 Dan 10
White; Round; Scored

BACLOFEN TABLETS 20MG — 5731 Dan 20
White; Round; Scored

BISOPROLOL/ HYDROCHLOROTHIAZIDE TABLETS 10/6.25MG — Watson / 843
White; Round;

BISOPROLOL/ HYDROCHLOROTHIAZIDE TABLETS 2.5/6.25MG — Watson / 841
Yellow; Round;

BISOPROLOL/ HYDROCHLOROTHIAZIDE TABLETS 5/6.25MG — Watson / 842
Pink; Round;

BUPROPION HCl SR TABLETS 100MG — WPI 858
White; Round, FC

BUPROPION HCl SR TABLETS 150MG — WPI 839
White; Round, FC

BUSPIRONE HCl TABLETS 10MG — WATSON 658
White; Oval; scored;

BUSPIRONE HCl TABLETS 15MG — Watson Logo - 718
White; Oval; bisected and trisected

BUSPIRONE HCl TABLETS 5MG — WATSON 657
White; Oval; scored;

BUTALBITAL/APAP/CAFFEINE TABLETS 50/325/40 MG — HD 567
White; Round

BUTALBITAL/APAP/CAFFEINE/ CODEINE CAPSULES 50/325/40/ 30MG C-III — Watson 3220
White / Dark Blue;

BUTALBITAL/ASA/CAFFEINE CAPSULES 50/325/40MG C-III — Watson 3219
Yellow / Green;

BUTALBITAL/ASA/CAFFEINE/ CODEINE CAPSULES 50/325/40/ 30MG C-III — Watson 425
Yellow/Blue;

CARISOPRODOL TABLETS 350MG — 5513 DAN
White; Round

CEFAZOLIN FOR INJECTION 10g — n/a

CEFAZOLIN FOR INJECTION 1g — n/a

CEFUROXIME AXETIL TABLETS 250MG — LUPIN 302
White/Off-White; capsule-shaped

CEFUROXIME AXETIL TABLETS 500MG — LUPIN 303
White/Off-White; capsule-shaped

CHLORDIAZEPOXIDE HCl/ CLIDINIUM Br CAPSULES, 5MG-2.5MG — A-018
Op Green;

CHLORDIAZEPOXIDE HCl CAPSULES 10MG C-IV — Watson 786/ 10mg
Black Op/Green Op;

CHLORDIAZEPOXIDE HCl CAPSULES 25MG C-IV — Watson 787/ 25mg
Green Op/White Op;

CHLORDIAZEPOXIDE HCl CAPSULES 5MG C-IV — Watson 785/5mg
Green Op/Yellow Op;

CLINDAMYCIN HCl CAPSULES 150MG — 5708 DAN
Op Grey/Op Pink;

CLINDAMYCIN HCl CAPSULES 300MG — DAN 3120
Pink;

CLOMIPHENE CITRATE TABLETS 50MG — Watson 781
Off White; Round, scored

CLONAZEPAM TABLETS 0.5MG C-IV — Watson 746
Yellow; Round; ; scored

CLONAZEPAM TABLETS 1MG C-IV — Watson 747
Aqua; Round; ; scored

CLONAZEPAM TABLETS 2MG C-IV — Watson 748
White; Round; ; scored

CLORAZEPATE DIPOTASSIUM TABLETS 15MG C-IV — Watson 365
Pink, round

CLORAZEPATE DIPOTASSIUM TABLETS 3.75MG C-IV — Watson 363
Light Blue; Round

CLORAZEPATE DIPOTASSIUM TABLETS 7.5MG C-IV — Watson 364
Lt Beige; Round; Bisected

COLCHICINE TABLETS 0.6MG (1/100 grain) — 944 DAN
White; Round

CYCLOBENZAPRINE HCl TABLETS 10MG — 5658 DAN
White; Round; Film Coated

DESIPRAMINE HCl TABLETS 100MG — Watston 545
Peach; Round, coated

DESIPRAMINE HCl TABLETS 25MG — Watson 808
Yellow; Round, coated

DESIPRAMINE HCl TABLETS 50MG — Watson 809
Green; Round, coated

DEXCHLORPHENIRAMINE MALEATE ER TABLETS 4MG — 014 Amide
Yellow; Oval

DEXCHLORPHENIRAMINE MALEATE ER TABLETS 6MG — 015 Amide
White; Oval

DIAZEPAM TABLETS 10MG C-IV
Lt Blue; Round; Scored

DIAZEPAM TABLETS 2MG C-IV — 5621 DAN 2
White; Round; Scored

DIAZEPAM TABLETS 5MG C-IV — 5619 DAN 5
Yellow; Round; Scored

DICLOFENAC SODIUM DR TABLETS 50MG — Watson 338
White; Round;

DICLOFENAC SODIUM DR TABLETS 75MG — Watson 339
White; Round;

DICLOFENAC SODIUM ER TABLETS 100MG — DX41
Pink; Round;

DICYCLOMINE HCl CAPSULES 10MG — Watson 794/ 10mg
Dk Blue/Dk Blue;

DICYCLOMINE HCl TABLETS 20MG — Watson/ 795
Blue; Round

DIETHYLPROPION ER TABLETS 75MG C-IV — Watson 782
White; capsule-shaped

DIETHYLPROPION TABLETS 25MG C-IV — Watson 783
White; Round

DILTIAZEM HCl TABLETS 120MG — Watson 778
White; Oblong; scored

DILTIAZEM HCl TABLETS 30MG — Watson 775
Blue; Round

DILTIAZEM HCl TABLETS 60MG — Watson 776
White; Round; Scored

DILTIAZEM HCl TABLETS 90MG — Watson 777
Blue; Oblong; scored

DISOPYRAMIDE PHOSPHATE CAPSULES, 100MG — 5560 DAN
Opaque Orange;

DISOPYRAMIDE PHOSPHATE CAPSULES, 150MG — 5561 DAN
Opaque Brown;

DOXEPIN HCl CAPSULES 100MG — 5633 DAN
Op White/Op Lt Grn;

DOXEPIN HCl CAPSULES 10MG — 5629 DAN
Buff;

DOXEPIN HCl CAPSULES 25MG — 5630 DAN
Op White/Op Ivory;

DOXEPIN HCl CAPSULES 50MG — 5631 DAN
Op Ivory;

DOXEPIN HCl CAPSULES 75MG — 5632 DAN
Op Lt Green;

DOXYCYCLINE HYCLATE CAPSULES, 100MG — 5440 DAN
Lt Blue;

DOXYCYCLINE HYCLATE CAPSULES, 50MG — 5535 DAN
Lt Blue/White;

DOXYCYCLINE HYCLATE TABLETS 100MG — 5553 DAN
Orange; Round; Film Coated

DOXYCYCLINE MONOHYDRATE CAPSULES 100MG — Watson 310/ 100mg
Green/Green;

DOXYCYCLINE MONOHYDRATE CAPSULES 50MG — Watson 309/ 50mg
Green/Yellow;

ENALAPRIL MALEATE TABLETS 10MG — Watson 670
White-Speckled Pink; Round;

ENALAPRIL MALEATE TABLETS 2.5MG — Watson 668
White/Off-White; Round; ; scored

ENALAPRIL MALEATE TABLETS 20MG — Watson 671
White-Speckled Peach; Round;

ENALAPRIL MALEATE TABLETS 5MG — Watson 669
White/Off-White; Round; ; scored

ESTAZOLAM TABLETS 1MG C-IV — Watson 744/1
White; Diamond Shape/scored

ESTAZOLAM TABLETS 2MG C-IV — Watson 745/2
Pink; Diamond Shape/scored

ESTRADIOL TABLETS 0.5MG — Watson 528
White; Round; Scored

ESTRADIOL TABLETS 1 MG — Watson 487
Gray; Round; Scored

ESTRADIOL TABLETS 2 MG — Watson 488
Lt Green; Round; Scored

ESTROPIPATE TABLETS 0.75MG — Watson 414
Yellow; Round; Scored

ESTROPIPATE TABLETS 1.5MG — Watson 415
Peach; Round; Scored

ESTROPIPATE TABLETS 3MG — Watson 416
Blue; Round; Scored

FOLIC ACID TABLETS 1MG — 5216 DAN DAN
Yellow; Round; Scored

GLIPIZIDE TABLETS 10MG — Watson 461
White; Round; Scored

GLIPIZIDE TABLETS 5MG — Watson 460
White; Round; Scored

GLIPIZIDE EXTENDED RELEASE TABLETS 5MG — WPI 844
Orange; Round; Film Coated

GLIPIZIDE EXTENDED RELEASE TABLETS 10MG — WPI 845
White/Off-White; Round; Film Coated

GUANFACINE TABLETS 1MG — Watson 444
Pink; Round

GUANFACINE TABLETS 2MG — Watson 453
Peach; Round

HALOTUSSIN-AC SYRUP SF C-V — N/A
Carmel; Syrup

HALOTUSSIN-DAC SYRUP SF C-V — N/A
Red/Cherry/Raspberry Flavored; Syrup

HYDROCHLOROTHIAZIDE CAPSULES 12.5MG — Watson 347/ 12.5mg
Teal Opaque/White Opaque

HYDROCODONE BITARTRATE/ ACETAMINOPHEN TABLETS 10/325MG C-III — Watson 853
Yellow; Capsule-Shaped; Bisected

HYDROCODONE BITARTRATE/ ACETAMINOPHEN TABLETS 10/500MG C-III — Watson 540
Blue; Capsule-Shaped; Bisected

HYDROCODONE BITARTRATE/ ACETAMINOPHEN TABLETS 10/650MG C-III — Watson 503
Lt Green; Capsule-Shaped; Bisected

HYDROCODONE BITARTRATE/ ACETAMINOPHEN TABLETS 2.5/500MG C-III — Watson 388
White; Oblong/Bisected

HYDROCODONE BITARTRATE/ ACETAMINOPHEN TABLETS 5/500MG C-III — Watson 349
White; Capsule-Shaped; Bisected

HYDROCODONE BITARTRATE/ ACETAMINOPHEN TABLETS 5/325MG C-III — Watson 3202
White w/orange specks; Capsule-Shaped; Bisected

HYDROCODONE BITARTRATE/ ACETAMINOPHEN TABLETS 7.5/500MG C-III — Watson 385
White; Capsule-Shaped; Bisected

HYDROCODONE BITARTRATE/ ACETAMINOPHEN TABLETS 7.5/650MG C-III — Watson 502
Pink; Capsule-Shaped; Bisected

HYDROCODONE BITARTRATE/ ACETAMINOPHEN TABLETS 7.5/750MG C-III — Watson 387
White; Oblong/Bisected

HYDROCODONE BITARTRATE/ ACETAMINOPHEN TABLETS 7.5/325MG C-III — Watson 3203
Light Orange; Capsule-Shaped; Bisected

HYDROXOCOBALAMIN Injection 1000MCG/ML — n/a

HYDROXYCHLORQUINE TABLETS 200MG — Watson 698/200
White; Oval, Bisected

HYDROXYZINE HCl TABLETS 10MG — 5522 DAN
Orange; Round; Film Coated

HYDROXYZINE HCl TABLETS 25MG — 5523 DAN
Green; Round; Film Coated

Continued on next page

Product List-Watson—Cont.

Product / Description	Imprint
HYDROXYZINE PAMOATE CAPSULES, 25MG Dk Green/Lt Green;	DAN 5726
HYDROXYZINE PAMOATE CAPSULES, 50MG Green Op/White Op;	Watson 801/ 50mg
IBUPROFEN TABLETS 400MG White; Oval ; Elongated, FC	WPI 4010
IBUPROFEN TABLETS 600MG White; Oval ; Elongated, FC	WPI 4011
IBUPROFEN TABLETS 800MG White; Oval ; Elongated, FC	WPI 2137
LABETALOL HCl TABLETS 100MG Beige; Round; scored; FC	Watson 605
LABETALOL HCl TABLETS 200MG White; Round; scored; FC	Watson 606
LABETALOL HCl TABLETS 300MG Blue; Round	Watson 607
LACTULOSE SOLUTION ORAL/ RECTAL, 10g/15ML Orange; Solution	n/a
LACTULOSE SOLUTION ORAL, 10g/15ML Orange; Solution	n/a
LISINOPRIL 10MG TABLETS Lt Blue; Round	WATSON 407
LISINOPRIL 2.5MG TABLETS White; Round	WATSON 405
LISINOPRIL 20MG TABLETS Yellow; Round	WATSON 408
LISINOPRIL 30MG TABLETS Yellow; Round	WATSON 885
LISINOPRIL 40MG TABLETS Yellow; Round	WATSON 409
LISINOPRIL 5MG TABLETS White; Capsule-Shaped	WATSON 406
LISINOPRIL/ HYDROCHLOROTHIAZIDE TABLETS 10MG/12.5MG Pink; Round	WATSON 860
LISINOPRIL/ HYDROCHLOROTHIAZIDE TABLETS 20MG/12.5MG Lt Blue; Round	WATSON 861
LISINOPRIL/ HYDROCHLOROTHIAZIDE TABLETS 20MG/25MG Pink; Round	WATSON 862
LORAZEPAM TABLETS 0.5MG C-IV White; Round; Scored	Watson 240/0.5
LORAZEPAM TABLETS 1MG C-IV White; Round; Scored	Watson 241/1
LORAZEPAM TABLETS 2MG C-IV White; Round; Scored	Watson 242/2
LOXAPINE CAPSULES 10MG Yellow/White;	Watson 370/ 10mg
LOXAPINE CAPSULES 25MG Green/White;	Watson 371/ 25mg
LOXAPINE CAPSULES 50MG Blue / White;	Watson 372/ 50mg
LOXAPINE CAPSULES 5MG White/White;	Watson 369/5mg
MECLIZINE HCl TABLETS 25MG Yellow/White layer tablet; Oval, partial score	Watson 803
MEPERIDINE HCl TABLETS 100MG C-II White; Round;	Watson 727/100
MEPERIDINE HCl TABLETS 50MG C-II White; Round;	Watson 726/50
MEPROBAMATE TABLETS C IV 200MG White; Round; Scored	591 - B
MEPROBAMATE TABLETS C IV 400MG White; Round; Scored	591 - A
METFORMIN HCl TABLETS 1000MG Light Peach; Capsule-Shaped, FC	WPI WPI; 24/55
METFORMIN HCl TABLETS 500MG Light Peach; Capsule-Shaped, FC	WP 2713
METFORMIN HCl TABLETS 850MG Light Peach; Capsule-Shaped, FC	WPI 2775
METHOCARBAMOL TABLETS 500MG White; Round; Scored	5381 DAN DAN
METHOCARBAMOL TABLETS 750MG White; Oval; Scored	5382 DAN DAN
METHYLPHENIDATE HCl TABLETS C II 10MG Lt Green; Round; Scored	5883 DAN 10
METHYLPHENIDATE HCl TABLETS C II 20MG Peach; Round; Scored	5884 DAN 20
METHYLPHENIDATE HCl TABLETS C II 5MG Lt Purple; Round	5882 DAN 5
METHYLPHENIDATE HCl TABLETS ER C-II 20MG White/Off-White; Oval	WPI 3111
METHYLPREDNISOLONE TABLETS 4MG White/Off-White; Oval Quadrisected	Watson 790
METOPROLOL TARTRATE TABLETS 100MG Blue; Round; Scored	Watson 463
METOPROLOL TARTRATE TABLETS 50MG Pink; Round; Scored	Watson 462
METOPROLOL TARTRATE INJECTION 1MG/ML	n/a
METRONIDAZOLE TABLETS 250MG White/Off-White; Round	5540 DAN
METRONIDAZOLE TABLETS 500MG White/Off-White; Round; Scored	5552 DAN DAN 50
MEXILETINE HCl CAPSULES 150MG Brown Opaque/Lt Brown;	Watson 491/ 150mg
MEXILETINE HCl CAPSULES 200MG Brown Opaque/Brown Opaque;	Watson 492/ 200mg
MEXILETINE HCl CAPSULES 250MG Brown Opaque/Lt Green;	Watson 493/ 250mg
MINOCYCLINE HCl CAPSULES, 100MG 50 Op Grey/Op Yellow;	5695 DAN MINOCYCLINE 100
MINOCYCLINE HCl CAPSULES, 50MG Op Yellow;	5694 DAN MINOCYCLINE 50
MINOCYCLINE HCl CAPSULES, 75MG White/Yellow;	WPI MINOCYCLINE 75
MINOXIDIL TABLETS 10MG White; Round; Scored	5643 DAN 10
MINOXIDIL TABLETS 2.5MG White; Round; Scored	5642 DAN 2.5
MIRTAZAPINE TABLETS 15MG White; Oval Coated	WPI 1117
MIRTAZAPINE TABLETS 30MG Yellow; Oval Coated	WPI 1118
MIRTAZAPINE TABLETS 45MG White; Oval Coated	WPI 1119
MORPHINE SULFATE ER 100MG TABLETS C-II Gray; Round	Watson 617
NANDROLONE DECANOATE INJECTION 100MG/ML C-III	n/a
NANDROLONE DECANOATE INJECTION 200MG/ML C-III	n/a
NAPROXEN SODIUM TABLETS 275MG White; Oval	Watson 792
NAPROXEN SODIUM TABLETS 550MG Green; Oval	Watson 793
NAPROXEN TABLETS 250MG White/Off-White; Round	Watson 821
NAPROXEN TABLETS 375MG Gray; Capsule-Shaped	Watson 822
NAPROXEN TABLETS 500MG White/Off-White; Capsule-Shaped	Watson 791
NEFAZODONE HCl TABLETS 100MG White; Capsule-Shaped	Watson logo 764
NEFAZODONE HCl TABLETS 150MG Orange; Capsule-Shaped	Watson logo 765
NEFAZODONE HCl TABLETS 200MG Yellow; Capsule-Shaped	Watson logo 766
NEFAZODONE HCl TABLETS 250MG White; Capsule-Shaped	Watson logo 767
NEPHRO-VITE RX TABLETS Yellow; Round	RD12
NICOTINE TRANSDERMAL SYSTEM, 14MG/24HR Tan, Opaque; Square, Round Edges	Nicotine 14 mg/ day (random over patch in brown print)
NICOTINE TRANSDERMAL SYSTEM, 21MG/24HR Tan, Opaque; Square, Round Edges	Nicotine 21 mg/ day (random over patch in brown print)
NICOTINE TRANSDERMAL SYSTEM, 7MG/24HR Tan, Opaque; Square, Round Edges	Nicotine 7 mg/ day (random over patch in brown print)
NITROFURANTOIN MONOHYDRATE/MACROCRYSTALS CAPSULES 100MG Opaque Yellow/Black;	Watson 3250
NITROFURANTOIN MACROCRYSTALS CAPSULES 50MG Opaque Yellow & White;	Watson 3253
NITROFURANTOIN MACROCRYSTALS CAPSULES 100MG Opaque Yellow;	Watson 3254
NIZATIDINE CAPSULES 150MG Cream;	WPI 3137
NIZATIDINE CAPSULES 300MG Lt. Brown;	WPI 3138
NORTRIPTYLINE HCl CAPSULES, 10MG Op Dk Grn/Op White;	Nortriptyline/ Dan 10mg
NORTRIPTYLINE HCl CAPSULES, 25MG Op Dk Grn/Op White;	Nortriptyline/ Dan 25mg
NORTRIPTYLINE HCl CAPSULES, 50MG Op White;	Nortriptyline/ Dan 50mg
NORTRIPTYLINE HCl CAPSULES, 75MG Dk Green;	Nortriptyline/ Dan 75mg
OXYBUTYNIN CHLORIDE TABLETS 5MG Pale Blue; Round, SCORED	Watson 779
OXYCODONE AND ACETAMINOPHEN TABLETS 10/650 C-II White; Capsule-Shaped; Scored	WATSON 825
OXYCODONE AND ACETAMINOPHEN TABLETS 7.5/500 C-II White; Capsule Shaped; Scored	WATSON 824
OXYCODONE AND ACETAMINOPHEN TABLETS 10/ 325MG C-II White; Round	WATSON 932
OXYCODONE AND ACETAMINOPHEN TABLETS 7.5/ 325MG C-II White; Round	WATSON 933
OXYCODONE AND ACETAMINOPHEN CAPSULES 5/500 C-II Opaque White, Opaque Red;	WATSON 737/5-500
OXYCODONE AND ACETAMINOPHEN TABLETS 5/325 C-II White; Round, SCORED	Watson 749
OXYCODONE AND ASPIRIN TABLETS 4.5/0.38/325MG C-II Yellow; Round, SCORED	Watson 820
PENTAZOCINE HCl/ ACETAMINOPHEN TABLETS 25/ 650MG C-IV Light Aqua; Capsule-Shaped; Scored	Watson 396 25/650
PENTAZOCINE HCl/NALOXONE HCl TABLETS 50/0.5MG C-IV Green; Capsule-Shaped; Scored	Watson 395/ 50-0.5mg
PODOFILOX 0.5% TOPICAL SOLUTION 3.5ML Clear Liquid in an Amber Glass Bottle; Solution	
POTASSIUM BICARBONATE EFFERVESCENT TABLETS 25MEQ Orange; Round	n/a
POTASSIUM CHLORIDE POWDER PACKET 20MEQ ; Powder	n/a
PREDNISOLONE SYRUP 15MG/5ML 8OZ ; Syrup	n/a
PREDNISOLONE TABLETS 5MG Peach; Round; Scored	5059 DAN DAN
PREDNISONE TABLETS 10MG White; Round; Scored	5442 DAN DAN
PREDNISONE TABLETS 20MG Peach; Round; Scored	5443 DAN DAN
PREDNISONE TABLETS 5MG White; Round; Scored	5052 DAN DAN
PRIMIDONE TABLETS 250MG White; Round; Scored	5321 DAN DAN
PROBENECID AND COLCHICINE TABLETS 500MG-0.5MG White; Capsule-Shaped; Scored	5325 DAN DAN
PROBENECID TABLETS 500MG Yellow; Capsule-Shaped; Scored; FC	5347 DAN DAN
PROGESTERONE INJECTION IN SESAME OIL 50 MG/ML	n/a
PROMETHAZINE HCl INJECTION 25MG/ML clear solution	n/a
PROMETHAZINE HCl INJECTION 50MG/ML clear solution	n/a
PROMETHAZINE HCl TABLETS 25MG White; Round; Scored	DAN 5307
PROMETHAZINE HCl TABLETS 50MG White; Round	DAN 5319
PROPAFENONE HCl TABLETS 150MG White; Round; Bisected	Watson 582
PROPAFENONE HCl TABLETS 225MG White; Round; Bisected	Watson 583
PROPOXYPHENE HCl/ ACETAMINOPHEN TABLETS 65/ 650MG C-IV Orange; Oblong	Watson 714/ 65-650
PROPRANOLOL HCl TABLETS 10MG Orange; Round; Scored	5554 DAN 10
PROPRANOLOL HCl TABLETS 20MG Lt Blue; Round; Scored	5555 DAN 20

Product/Color/Shape	Imprint
PROPRANOLOL HCl TABLETS 40MG Green; Round; Scored	5556 DAN 40
PROPRANOLOL HCl TABLETS 80MG Yellow; Round, scored	5557 DAN 80
PYRIDOSTIGMINE BROMIDE 60MG TABLETS White; Round, quadrisected	Watson 3191
QUINIDINE SULFATE TABLETS 200MG White; Round; Scored	5438 DAN DAN
QUINIDINE SULFATE TABLETS 300MG White; Round; Scored	5454 DAN DAN
QUININE SULFATE CAPSULES 325MG White Opaque;	Watson 716/ 325mg
QUININE SULFATE TABLETS 260MG White; Round	Watson / 715 260
RANITIDINE HCl TABLETS 150MG Beige; Round	WATSON 760
RANITIDINE HCl TABLETS 300MG Beige; Capsule-Shaped	WATSON 761
SILVER SULFADIAZINE 1% White; Cream	n/a
SUCRALFATE TABLETS 1g Lt Blue; Oblong; scored	Watson 780
SULFASALAZINE TABLETS 500MG Mustard; Round; partially bisected	Watson 796
SULINDAC TABLETS 150MG Yellow; Round	5661 DAN
SULINDAC TABLETS 200MG Yellow; Round; Scored	5660 DAN DAN
TERCONAZOLE CREAM 0.8% (3-day) White/Off-White; Cream	n/a
TESTOSTERONE CYPIONATE INJECTION 200MG/ML C-III Pale-Yellow OIL-Based Solution;	n/a
TESTOSTERONE ENANTHATE INJECTION 200MG/ML C-III Pale-Yellow Oil-Based Solution;	n/a
TRAMADOL HCl 50MG TABLETS White; Round	WATSON 466
TRAZODONE HCl TABLETS 150MG White; Round; Quadrisected	168 MP 25/25/ 50/50
TRAZODONE HCl TABLETS 100MG White; Round; scored	5599 DAN DAN
TRAZODONE HCl TABLETS 50MG White; Round; scored	5600 DAN DAN
TRIAMTERENE/ HYDROCHLOROTHIAZIDE TABLETS 37.5/25MG Lt. Green; Round; Scored	Watson 424
TRIAMTERENE/ HYDROCHLOROTHIAZIDE TABLETS 75/50MG Yellow; Round; Scored	Watson 348
TRIHEXYPHENIDYL HCl TABLETS 2MG White; Round; Scored	5335 DAN DAN
TRIHEXYPHENIDYL HCl TABLETS 5MG White; Round; Scored	5337 DAN DAN
TRIMETHOPRIM TABLETS 100MG White; Oval; Scored	5571 DAN DAN
URSODIOL CAPSULES 300MG Opaque White	Watson 3159
VALPROIC ACID CAPSULES, 250MG Off White;	Valproic 250-0364
VALPROIC ACID SYRUP 250 MG/5ML	n/a
VERAPAMIL HCl SR PELLET-FILLED CAPSULES 120MG Yellow Opaque;	60274/120mg
VERAPAMIL HCl SR PELLET-FILLED CAPSULES 180MG Lt Gray/Yellow Opaque;	60274/180mg
VERAPAMIL HCl SR PELLET-FILLED CAPSULES 240MG Dk Blue/Yellow Opaque;	60274/240mg
VERAPAMIL HCl SR PELLET-FILLED CAPSULES 360MG Lavender/Yellow Opaque;	60274/360mg
VERAPAMIL HCl TABLETS 120MG White; Round; Scored	Watson 345
VERAPAMIL HCl TABLETS 40MG Lt. Peach; Round	Watson 404
VERAPAMIL HCl TABLETS 80MG White; Round; Scored	Watson 343

Product Listing (Brand Name) ℞

The following list of Watson Laboratories generic name products is provided to facilitate identification. It includes the color(s) and identification codes for all products.

Product/Color/Shape	Imprint
ACTIGALL® CAPSULES 300MG (Ursodiol) Opaque/White/Pink;	Actigall 300 MG
ALORA® ETS PATCH 0.025MG/ DAY (Estradiol) Translucent; Rectangular	Alora 0.025mg/day estradiol
ALORA® ETS PATCH 0.05MG/ DAY (Estradiol) Translucent; Rectangular	Alora 0.05mg/day estradiol
ALORA® ETS PATCH 0.075MG/ DAY (Estradiol) Translucent; Rectangular	Alora 0.075mg/day estradiol
ALORA® ETS PATCH 0.1MG/ DAY (Estradiol) Translucent; Rectangular	Alora 0.1mg/day estradiol
ANDRODERM® PATCH 2.5MG C-III (Testosterone) Flesh Tone; Circular Reservoir 37cm^2	ANDRODERM 2.5MG/ DAY
ANDRODERM® PATCH 5MG C-III (Testosterone) Flesh Tone; Oblong Reservoir 44cm^2	ANDRODERM 5MG/ DAY
DILACOR® XR CAPSULES 120MG (Diltiazem HCl) Pink Opaque Cap/Flesh Opaque Body	"Watson logo"/Dilacor XR/120mg
DILACOR® XR CAPSULES 180MG (Diltiazem HCl) Lavender Opaque Cap/Flesh Opaque Body	"Watson logo"/Dilacor XR/180mg
DILACOR® XR CAPSULES 240MG (Diltiazem HCl) Lt. Blue Opaque Cap/Flesh Opaque Body	"Watson logo"/Dilacor XR/240mg
FERRLECIT® INJECTION 62.5MG/5ML (Sodium Ferric Gluconate Complex/Sucrose) NA	n/a Sodium Ferric Gluconate Complex/ Sucrose n/a
FIORICET® TABLETS (Butalbital/APAP/Caffeine) Light Blue Speckled; Round	FIORICET / Image = 3 head profile
FIORICET® WITH CODEINE CAPSULES C-III (Butalbital/ APAP/Caffeine/Codeine) Dark Blue & Grey	Fioricet/Codeine
FIORINAL® CAPSULES C-III (Butalbital/ASA/Caffeine) Kelly Green & Lime Green	Fiorinal 78-103
FIORINAL® WITH CODEINE CAPSULES C-III (Butalbital/ ASA/Caffeine/Codeine) Blue / Yellow	Sandoz logo FC/ Sandoz 78-107
INFED® VIAL 50MG/ML (Iron Dextran Complex) NA	n/a
LOXITANE® CAPSULES 5MG (Loxapine) Opaque Green	Watson logo/Watson/ Loxitane 5mg
LOXITANE® CAPSULES 10MG (Loxapine) Yellow/ Dk Green	Watson logo/Watson/ Loxitane/10mg
LOXITANE® CAPSULES 25MG (Loxapine) Light Green/ Dk Green	Watson logo/Watson/ Loxitane/25mg
LOXITANE® CAPSULES 50MG (Loxapine) Blue/Dark Green	Watson logo/Watson/ Loxitane 50mg
MAXIDONE® TABLETS 10MG/ 750MG C-III (Hydrocodone bitartrate/Acetaminophen) Yellow; Capsule-Shaped; Scored	Maxidone 634
MICROZIDE® CAPSULES 12.5MG (Hydrochlorothiazide) Teal opaque/Teal opaque	Microzide 12.5 mg
NORCO® TABLETS 5MG/325MG C-III (Hydrocodone/ Acetaminophen) White/Orange Specks; Capsule-Shaped; Bisected	Watson 913
NORCO® TABLETS 7.5MG/ 325MG C-III (Hydrocodone/ Acetaminophen) Light Orange, Capsule-Shaped; Bisected	Norco 729
NORCO® TABLETS 10MG/ 325MG C-III (Hydrocodone/ Acetaminophen) Yellow; Capsule-Shaped; Bisected	Norco 539
OXYTROL® (Oxybutynin Transdermal System) 3.9MG/DAY Transparent; Rectangular	OXYTROL 3.9mg/day OXYTROL

ORAL CONTRACEPTIVE PRODUCTS:

ETHYNODIOL DIACETATE AND ETHINYL ESTRADIOL TABLETS USP: ℞

ZOVIA® 1/35E (1 mg ethynodiol diacetate and 35 mcg ethinyl estradiol)	WATSON 383
ZOVIA® 1/50E (1 mg ethynodiol diacetate and 50 mcg ethinyl estradiol)	WATSON 384

LEVONORGESTREL AND ETHINYL ESTRADIOL TABLETS USP: ℞

LEVORA® 0.15/30–28 (levonorgestrel and ethinyl estradiol)	WATSON/15/30
TRIVORA®-28 (levonorgestrel and ethinyl estradiol)	WATSON/50/30 (6 tablets) WATSON/75/40 (5 tablets) WATSON/125/30 (10 tablets)

NORETHINDRONE ℞

JOLIVETTE® TABLETS: (norethindrone 0.35 mg)	WATSON/892
NOR-QD® Tablets (norethindrone 0.35 mg)	WATSON/235
Nora-BE® Tablets (norethindrone 0.35 mg)	WATSON 629

NORETHINDRONE AND ETHINYL ESTRADIOL TABLETS USP: ℞

BREVICON® (0.5 mg norethindrone and 35 mcg ethinyl estradiol)	WATSON/254
NORINYL® 1+35 (1 mg norethindrone and 35 mcg ethinyl estradiol)	WATSON/259
TRI-NORINYL® (norethindrone and ethinyl estradiol)	
NECON® 7/7/7 (7 tablets, each contains 0.5 mg norethindrone and 35 mcg ethinyl estradiol; 7 tablets, each contains 0.75 mg norethindrone and 35 mcg ethinyl estradiol; 7 tablets, each contains 1 mg norethindrone and 35 mcg ethinyl estradiol.)	WATSON/937 (7 tablets) WATSON/938 (7 tablets) WATSON/939 (7 tablets)
NECON® 0.5/35 (0.5 mg norethindrone and 35 mcg ethinyl estradiol)	WATSON/507
NECON® 1/35 (1 mg norethindrone and 35 mcg ethinyl estradiol)	WATSON/508
NECON® 10/11 (10 tablets—each contains 0.5 mg norethindrone and 35 mcg ethinyl estradiol; 11 tablets—each contains 1 mg norethindrone and 35 mcg ethinyl estradiol.)	WATSON/507 (10 tablets) and WATSON/508 (11 tablets)
MICROGESTIN® Fe 1/20 (1 mg norethindrone acetate and 20 mcg ethinyl estradiol)	WATSON/630 (21 tablets)
MICROGESTIN® 1/20	WATSON/630
MICROGESTIN® Fe 1.5/30 (1.5 mg norethindrone acetate and 30 mcg ethinyl estradiol)	WATSON/631 (21 tablets)
MICROGESTIN® 1.5/30	WATSON/631

NORETHINDRONE AND MESTRANOL TABLETS USP: ℞

NECON® 1/50 (1 mg norethindrone and 50 mcg mestranol)	WATSON/510
NORINYL® 1/50 (1 mg norethindrone and 50 mcg mestranol)	WATSON/265

NORGESTIMATE AND ETHINYL ESTRADIOL TABLETS, USP: ℞

MonoNessa® (norgestimate 0.25 mg and ethiny estradiol 35 mcg)	WATSON/526
TriNessa™ (7 tablets, each contains 0.18 mg norgestimate and 35 mcg ethinyl estradiol; 7 tablets, each contains 0.215 mg norgestimate and ethinyl estradiol 35 mcg; 7 tablets, each contains 0.25 mg norgestimate and 35 mcg ethinyl estradiol)	WATSON/524 (7 tablets) WATSON/525 (7 tablets) WATSON/526 (7 tablets)

NORGESTREL AND ETHINYL ESTRADIOL TABLETS USP: ℞

OGESTREL® (0.5 mg norgestrel and 0.05 mg ethinyl estradiol)	WATSON/848
LOW-OGESTREL® (0.3 mg norgestrel and 0.03 mg ethinyl estradiol)	WATSON/847

DERMATOLOGIC PRODUCTS: ℞

Condylox® Gel, 0.5%
Condylox® Topical Solution, 0.5%
Cordran® Lotion, 0.05%
Cordran® Ointment 0.05%
Cordran® SP Cream 0.05%
Cordran® Tape, 4 mcg per sq cm
Cormax® Cream, 0.05%
Cormax® Ointment, 0.05%
Cormax® Scalp Application, 0.05%
Monodox® Capsules 50 mg and 100 mg

PAIN PRODUCTS

The following list of Watson Laboratories pain products is provided to facilitate identification. It includes the color(s) and identification codes for all products.

Product/Color/Shape	Imprint
FIORICET® TABLETS (Butalbital/APAP/Caffeine) Light Blue Speckled; Round	FIORICET/Image-3 head profile
FIORICET® WITH CODEINE CAPSULES C-III (Butalbital/ APAP/Caffeine/Codeine) Dark Blue & Gray	Fioricet/Codeine
FIORINAL® CAPSULES C-III (Butalbital/ASA/Caffeine) Kelly Green/Lime Green	Fiorinal 78-103

Continued on next page

Watson-Pain Product Listing—Cont.

FIORINAL® WITH CODEINE CAPSULES C-III (Butalbital/ ASA/Caffeine/Codeine) Blue/Yellow	Sandoz logo FC/ Sandoz 78-107
MAXIDONE® TABLETS 10MG/ 750MG C-III (Hydrocodone bitartrate/Acetaminophen) Yellow, Capsule-Shaped; Scored	Maxidone 634
NORCO® TABLETS 10MG/ 325MG C-III (Hydrocodone/ Acetaminophen) Yellow; Capsule-Shaped; Bisected	Norco 539
NORCO® TABLETS 5MG/325MG C-III (Hydrocodone/ Acetaminophen) White/Orange Specks; Capsule-Shaped; Bisected	Watson 913
NORCO® TABLETS 7.5MG/ 325MG C-III (Hydrocodone/ Acetaminophen) Light Orange, Capsule-Shaped; Bisected	Norco 729
REPREXAIN (Hydrocodone Bitartrate & Ibuprofen 5 mg/200 mg) Oval, White, Bisected, Tablet	IP146

FERRLECIT® ℞

(sodium ferric gluconate complex in sucrose injection)

DESCRIPTION

Ferrlecit® (sodium ferric gluconate complex in sucrose injection) is a stable macromolecular complex with an apparent molecular weight on gel chromatography of 289,000–440,000 daltons. The macromolecular complex is negatively charged at alkaline pH and is present in solution with sodium cations. The product has a deep red color indicative of ferric oxide linkages.

The structural formula is considered to be $[NaFe_2O_3(C_6H_{11}O_7)(C_{12}H_{22}O_{11})_5]_{n\approx200}$.

Each ampule of 5 mL of Ferrlecit® for intravenous injection contains 62.5 mg (12.5 mg/mL) of elemental iron as the sodium salt of a ferric ion carbohydrate complex in an alkaline aqueous solution with approximately 20% sucrose w/v (195 mg/mL) in water for injection, pH 7.7–9.7.

Each mL contains 9 mg of benzyl alcohol as an inactive ingredient.

Therapeutic Class: Hematinic

CLINICAL PHARMACOLOGY

Ferrlecit® is used to replete the total body content of iron. Iron is critical for normal hemoglobin synthesis to maintain oxygen transport. Additionally, iron is necessary for metabolism and various enzymatic processes.

The total body iron content of an adult ranges from 2 to 4 grams. Approximately 2/3 is in hemoglobin and 1/3 is in reticuloendothelial (RE) storage (bone marrow, spleen, liver) bound to intracellular ferritin. The body highly conserves iron (daily loss of 0.03%) requiring supplementation of about 1 mg/day to replenish losses in healthy, non-menstruating adults. The etiology of iron deficiency in hemodialysis patients is varied and can include blood loss and/or increased iron utilization (e.g., from epoetin therapy). The administration of exogenous epoetin increases red blood cell production and iron utilization. The increased iron utilization and blood losses in the hemodialysis patient may lead to absolute or functional iron deficiency. Iron deficiency is absolute when hematological indicators of iron stores are low. Patients with functional iron deficiency do not meet laboratory criteria for absolute iron deficiency but demonstrate an increase in hemoglobin/hematocrit or a decrease in epoetin dosage with stable hemoglobin/hematocrit when parenteral iron is administered.

Pharmacokinetics

Multiple sequential single dose intravenous pharmacokinetic studies were performed on 14 healthy iron-deficient volunteers. Entry criteria included hemoglobin ≥10.5 gm/dL and transferrin saturation ≤15% (TSAT) or serum ferritin value ≤20 ng/mL. In the 1st stage, each subject was randomized 1:1 to undiluted Ferrlecit® injection of either 125 mg/hr or 62.5 mg/½ hr (2.1 mg/min). Five days after the 1st stage, each subject was re-randomized 1:1 to undiluted Ferrlecit® injection of either 125 mg/7 min or 62.5 mg/4 min (>15.5 mg/min).

Peak drug levels (C_{max}) varied significantly by dosage and by rate of administration with the highest C_{max} observed in the regimen in which 125 mg was administered in 7 minutes (19.0 mg/L). The initial volume of distribution (V_{Ferr}) of 6 L corresponds well to calculated blood volume. V_{Ferr} did not vary by dosage or rate of administration. The terminal elimination half-life (λ_z-HL) for drug bound iron was approximately 1 hour. λ_z-HL varied by dose but not by rate of administration. The shortest value (0.85 h) occurred in the 62.5 mg/4 min regimen; the longest value (1.45 h) occurred in the 125 mg/7 min regimen. Total clearance of Ferrlecit® was 3.02 to 5.35 L/h. There was no significant variation by rate of administration. The AUC for Ferrlecit® bound iron varied by dose from 17.5 mg-h/L (62.5 mg) to 35.6 mg-h/L (125 mg). There was no significant variation by rate of administration. Approximately 80% of drug bound iron was delivered to transferrin as a mononuclear ionic iron species within 24 hours of administration in each dosage regimen. Direct movement of iron from Ferrlecit® to transferrin was not observed. Mean peak transferrin saturation did not exceed 100% and returned to near baseline by 40 hours after administration of each dosage regimen.

In vitro experiments have shown that less than 1% of the iron species within Ferrlecit® can be dialyzed through membranes with pore sizes corresponding to 12,000 to 14,000 daltons over a period of up to 270 minutes. Human studies in renally competent subjects suggest the clinical insignificance of urinary excretion.

Drug-drug Interactions: Drug-drug interactions involving Ferrlecit® have not been studied. However, like other parenteral iron preparations, Ferrlecit® may be expected to reduce the absorption of concomitantly administered oral iron preparations.

CLINICAL STUDIES

Two clinical studies (Studies A and B) were conducted to assess the efficacy and safety of Ferrlecit®.

Study A

Study A was a three-center, randomized, open-label study of the safety and efficacy of two doses of Ferrlecit® administered intravenously to iron-deficient hemodialysis patients. The study included both a dose-response concurrent control and an historical control. Enrolled patients received a test dose of Ferrlecit® (25 mg of elemental iron) and were then randomly assigned to receive Ferrlecit® at cumulative doses of either 500 mg (low dose) or 1000 mg (high dose) of elemental iron. Ferrlecit® was given to both dose groups in eight divided doses during sequential dialysis sessions (a period of 16 to 17 days). At each dialysis session, patients in the low-dose group received Ferrlecit® 62.5 mg of elemental iron over 30 minutes, and those in the high-dose group received Ferrlecit® 125 mg of elemental iron over 60 minutes. The primary endpoint was the change in hemoglobin from baseline to the last available observation through Day 40. Eligibility for this study included chronic hemodialysis patients with a hemoglobin below 10 g/dL (or hematocrit at or below 32%) and either serum ferritin below 100 ng/mL or transferrin saturation below 18%. Exclusion criteria included significant underlying disease or inflammatory conditions or an epoetin requirement of greater than 10,000 units three times per week. Parenteral iron and red cell transfusion were not allowed for two months before the study. Oral iron and red cell transfusion were not allowed during the study for Ferrlecit®-treated patients.

The historical control population consisted of 25 chronic hemodialysis patients who received only oral iron supplementation for 14 months and did not receive red cell transfusion. All patients had stable epoetin doses and hematocrit values for at least two months before initiation of oral iron therapy.

The evaluated population consisted of 39 patients in the low-dose Ferrlecit® (sodium ferric gluconate complex in sucrose injection) group (50% female, 50% male; 74% white, 18% black, 5% Hispanic, 3% Asian; mean age 54 years, range 22–83 years), 44 patients in the high-dose Ferrlecit® group (50% female, 48% male, 2% unknown; 75% white, 11% black, 5% Hispanic, 7% other, 2% unknown; mean age 56 years, range 20–87 years), and 25 historical control patients (68% female, 32% male; 40% white, 32% black, 20% Hispanic, 4% Asian, 4% unknown; mean age 52 years, range 25–84 years).

The mean baseline hemoglobin and hematocrit were similar between treatment and historical control patients: 9.8 g/dL and 29% and 9.6 g/dL and 29% in low- and high-dose Ferrlecit®-treated patients, respectively, and 9.4 g/dL and 29% in historical control patients. Baseline serum transferrin saturation was 20% in the low-dose group, 16% in the high-dose group, and 14% in the historical control. Baseline serum ferritin was 106 ng/mL in the low-dose group, 88 ng/mL in the high-dose group, and 606 ng/mL in the historical control.

Patients in the high-dose Ferrlecit® group achieved significantly higher increases in hemoglobin and hematocrit than either patients in the low-dose Ferrlecit® group or patients in the historical control group (oral iron). Patients in the low-dose Ferrlecit® group did not achieve significantly higher increases in hemoglobin and hematocrit than patients receiving oral iron. See Table 1.

[See table 1 above]

TABLE 1
Hemoglobin, Hematocrit, and Iron Studies

Study A	Mean Change from Baseline to Two Weeks After Cessation of Therapy		
	Ferrlecit® 1000 mg IV (N=44)	Ferrlecit® 500 mg IV (N=39)	Historical Control-Oral Iron (N=25)
Hemoglobin (g/dL)	1.1*	0.3	0.4
Hematocrit (%)	3.6*	1.4	0.8
Transferrin Saturation (%)	8.5	2.8	6.1
Serum Ferritin (ng/mL)	199	132	NA

*p<0.01 versus both the 500 mg group and the historical control group

Cumulative Ferrlecit® Dose (mg of elemental iron)	62.5	250	375	562.5	625	750	1000	1125	1187.5
Patients (#)	1	1	2	1	10	4	12	6	1

Study B

Study B was a single-center, non-randomized, open-label, historically-controlled, study of the safety and efficacy of variable, cumulative doses of intravenous Ferrlecit® in iron-deficient hemodialysis patients. Ferrlecit® administration was identical to Study A. The primary efficacy variable was the change in hemoglobin from baseline to the last available observation through Day 50.

Inclusion and exclusion criteria were identical to those of Study A as was the historical control population. Sixty-three patients were evaluated in this study: 38 in the Ferrlecit®-treated group (37% female, 63% male; 95% white, 5% Asian; mean age 56 years, range 22–84 years) and 25 in the historical control group (68% female, 32% male; 40% white, 32% black, 20% Hispanic, 4% Asian, 4% unknown; mean age 52 years, range 25–84 years).

Ferrlecit®-treated patients were considered to have completed the study per protocol if they received at least eight Ferrlecit® doses of either 62.5 mg or 125 mg of elemental iron. A total of 14 patients (37%) completed the study per protocol. Twelve (32%) Ferrlecit®-treated patients received less than eight doses, and 12 (32%) patients had incomplete information on the sequence of dosing. Not all patients received Ferrlecit® at consecutive dialysis sessions and many received oral iron during the study.

[See second table above]

TABLE 2
Hemoglobin, Hematocrit, and Iron Studies

Study B	Mean Change from Baseline to One Month After Treatment	
	Ferrlecit® (N=38)	Oral Iron (N=25)
	change	change
Hemoglobin (g/dL)	1.3a,b	0.4
Hematocrit (%)	3.8a,b	0.2
Transferrin Saturation (%)	6.7b	1.7
Serum Ferritin (ng/mL)	73b	−145

a - p<0.05 on group comparison by the ANCOVA method
b - p<0.001 from baseline by the paired t-test method

Baseline hemoglobin and hematocrit values were similar between the treatment and control groups, and were 9.1 g/dL and 27.3%, respectively, for Ferrlecit®-treated patients. Serum iron studies were also similar between treatment and control groups, with the exception of serum ferritin, which was 606 ng/mL for historical control patients, compared to 77 ng/mL for Ferrlecit®-treated patients.

In this patient population, only the Ferrlecit®-treated group achieved significant increase in hemoglobin and hematocrit

from baseline. This increase was significantly greater than that seen in the historical oral iron treatment group. See Table 2.
[See table 2 at top of previous page]

INDICATIONS AND USAGE

Ferrlecit® (sodium ferric gluconate complex in sucrose injection) is indicated for treatment of iron deficiency anemia in patients undergoing chronic hemodialysis who are receiving supplemental epoetin therapy.

CONTRAINDICATIONS

- All anemias not associated with iron deficiency.
- Hypersensitivity to Ferrlecit® or any of its inactive components.
- Evidence of iron overload.

WARNINGS

Hypersensitivity reactions have been reported with injectable iron products. See PRECAUTIONS.

PRECAUTIONS

General: Iron is not easily eliminated from the body and accumulation can be toxic. Unnecessary therapy with parenteral iron will cause excess storage of iron with consequent possibility of iatrogenic hemosiderosis. Iron overload is particularly apt to occur in patients with hemoglobinopathies and other refractory anemias. Ferrlecit® should not be administered to patients with iron overload. See OVERDOSAGE.

Hypersensitivity Reactions: Serious hypersensitivity reactions have been reported rarely in patients receiving Ferrlecit®. One case of a life-threatening hypersensitivity reaction has been observed in 1,097 patients who received a single dose of Ferrlecit® in a post-marketing safety study. Three serious hypersensitivity reactions have been reported from the spontaneous reporting system in the United States. See ADVERSE REACTIONS.

Hypotension: Hypotension associated with light-headedness, malaise, fatigue, weakness or severe pain in the chest, back, flanks, or groin has been associated with administration of intravenous iron. These hypotensive reactions are not associated with signs of hypersensitivity and have usually resolved within one or two hours. Successful treatment may consist of observation or, if the hypotension causes symptoms, volume expansion. See ADVERSE REACTIONS.

Carcinogenesis, mutagenesis, impairment of fertility: Long term carcinogenicity studies in animals were not performed. Studies to assess the effects of Ferrlecit® on fertility were not conducted. Ferrlecit® was not mutagenic in the Ames test and the rat micronucleus test. It produced a clastogenic effect in an *in vitro* chromosomal aberration assay in Chinese hamster ovary cells.

Pregnancy Category B: Ferrlecit® was not teratogenic at doses of elemental iron up to 100 mg/kg/day (300 mg/m^2/day) in mice and 20 mg/kg/day (120 mg/m^2/day) in rats. On a body surface area basis, these doses were 1.3 and 3.24 times the recommended human dose (125 mg/day or 92.5 mg/m^2/day) for a person of 50 kg body weight, average height and body surface area of 1.46 m^2. There were no adequate and well-controlled studies in pregnant women. Ferrlecit® should be used during pregnancy only if the potential benefit justifies the potential risk to the fetus.

Nursing Mothers: It is not known whether this drug is excreted in human milk. Because many drugs are excreted in human milk, caution should be exercised when Ferrlecit® is administered to a nursing woman.

Pediatric Use: Safety and effectiveness of Ferrlecit® in pediatric patients have not been established. Ferrlecit® contains benzyl alcohol and therefore should not be used in neonates.

Geriatric Use: Clinical studies of Ferrlecit® did not include sufficient numbers of subjects aged 65 and over to determine whether they respond differently from younger subjects. Other reported clinical experience has not identified differences in responses between the elderly and younger patients. In particular, 51/159 hemodialysis patients in North American clinical studies were aged 65 years or older. Among these patients, no differences in safety or efficacy as a result of age were identified. In general, dose selection for an elderly patient should be cautious, usually starting at the low end of the dosing range, reflecting the greater frequency of decreased hepatic, renal, or cardiac function, and of concomitant disease or other drug therapy.

ADVERSE REACTIONS

Exposure to Ferrlecit® has been documented in over 1,400 patients on hemodialysis. This population included 1,097 Ferrlecit®-naïve patients who received a single-dose of Ferrlecit® in a placebo-controlled, cross-over, post-marketing safety study. Undiluted Ferrlecit® was administered over ten minutes (125 mg of Ferrlecit® at 12.5 mg/min). No test dose was used. From a total of 1,498 Ferrlecit®-treated patients in medical reports, North American trials, and post-marketing studies, twelve patients (0.8%) experienced serious reactions which precluded further therapy with Ferrlecit®.

Hypersensitivity Reactions: See PRECAUTIONS. In the single-dose, post-marketing, safety study one patient experienced a life-threatening hypersensitivity reaction (diaphoresis, nausea, vomiting, severe lower back pain, dyspnea, and wheezing for 20 minutes) following Ferrlecit® administration. Among 1,097 patients who received Ferrlecit® in this study, there were 9 patients (0.8%) who had an adverse reaction that, in the view of the investigator, precluded further Ferrlecit® administration (drug intolerance). These included one life-threatening reaction, six allergic reactions (pruritus x2, facial flushing, chills, dyspnea/chest pain, and rash), and two other reactions (hypotension and nausea). Another 2 patients experienced (0.2%) allergic reactions not deemed to represent drug intolerance (nausea/malaise and nausea/dizziness) following Ferrlecit® administration.

Seventy-two (7.0%) of the 1,034 patients who had prior iron dextran exposure had a sensitivity to at least one form of iron dextran (INFeD® or Dexferrum®). The patient who experienced a life-threatening adverse event following Ferrlecit® administration during the study had a previous severe anaphylactic reaction to dextran in both forms (INFeD® and Dexferrum®). The incidences of both drug intolerance and suspected allergic events following first dose Ferrlecit® administration were 2.8% in patients with prior iron dextran sensitivity compared to 0.8% in patients without prior iron dextran sensitivity.

In this study, 28% of the patients received concomitant angiotensin converting enzyme inhibitor (ACEi) therapy. The incidences of both drug intolerance or suspected allergic events following first dose Ferrlecit® administration were 1.6% in patients with concomitant ACEi use compared to 0.7% in patients without concomitant ACEi use. The patient with a life-threatening event was not on ACEi therapy. One patient had facial flushing immediately on Ferrlecit® exposure. No hypotension occurred and the event resolved rapidly and spontaneously without intervention other than drug withdrawal.

In multiple dose Studies A and B, no fatal hypersensitivity reactions occurred among the 126 patients who received Ferrlecit®. Ferrlecit®-associated hypersensitivity events in Study A resulting in premature study discontinuation occurred in three out of a total 88 (3.4%) Ferrlecit®-treated patients. The first patient withdrew after the development of pruritus and chest pain following the test dose of Ferrlecit®. The second patient, in the high-dose group, experienced nausea, abdominal and flank pain, fatigue and rash following the first dose of Ferrlecit®. The third patient, in the low-dose group, experienced a "red blotchy rash" following the first dose of Ferrlecit®. Of the 38 patients exposed to Ferrlecit® in Study B, none reported hypersensitivity reactions.

Many chronic renal failure patients experience cramps, pain, nausea, rash, flushing, and pruritus.

Three cases of serious hypersensitivity reactions have been reported from the spontaneous reporting system in the United States.

Hypotension: See PRECAUTIONS. In the single dose safety study post-administration hypotensive events were observed in 22/1,097 patients (2%) following Ferrlecit® administration. Hypotension has also been reported following administration of Ferrlecit® in European case reports. Of the 226 renal dialysis patients exposed to Ferrlecit® and reported in the literature, 3 (1.3%) patients experienced hypotensive events which were accompanied by flushing in two. All completely reversed after one hour without sequelae. Transient hypotension may occur during dialysis. Administration of Ferrlecit® may augment hypotension caused by dialysis.

Among the 126 patients who received Ferrlecit® in Studies A and B, one patient experienced a transient decreased level of consciousness without hypotension. Another patient discontinued treatment prematurely because of dizziness, lightheadedness, diplopia, malaise, and weakness without hypotension that resulted in a 3–4 hour hospitalization for observation following drug administration. The syndrome resolved spontaneously.

Adverse Laboratory Changes: No differences in laboratory findings associated with Ferrlecit® (sodium ferric gluconate complex in sucrose injection) were reported in North American clinical trials when normalized against a National Institute of Health database on laboratory findings in 1,100 hemodialysis patients.

Most Frequent Adverse Reactions: In the single-dose, post-marketing safety study, 11% of patients who received Ferrlecit® and 9.4% of patients who received placebo reported adverse reactions. The most frequent adverse reactions following Ferrlecit® were: hypotension (2%), nausea, vomiting and/or diarrhea (2%), pain (0.7%), hypertension (0.6%), allergic reaction (0.5%), chest pain (0.5%), pruritis (0.5%), and back pain (0.4%). Similar adverse reactions were seen following placebo administration. However, because of the high baseline incidence of adverse events in the hemodialysis patient population, insufficient number of exposed patients, and limitations inherent to the cross-over, single dose study design, no comparison of event rates between Ferrlecit® and placebo treatments can be made.

In multiple-dose Studies A and B, the most frequent adverse reactions following Ferrlecit® were:

Body as a Whole: injection site reaction (33%), chest pain (10%), pain (10%), asthenia (7%), headache (7%), abdominal pain (6%), fatigue (6%), fever (5%), malaise, infection, abscess, back pain, chills, rigors, arm pain, carcinoma, flu-like syndrome, sepsis.

Nervous System: cramps (25%), dizziness (13%), paresthesias (6%), agitation, somnolence.

Respiratory System: dyspnea (11%), coughing (6%), upper respiratory infections (6%), rhinitis, pneumonia.

Cardiovascular System: hypotension (29%), hypertension (13%), syncope (6%), tachycardia (5%), bradycardia, vasodilatation, angina pectoris, myocardial infarction, pulmonary edema.

Gastrointestinal System: nausea, vomiting and/or diarrhea (35%), anorexia, rectal disorder, dyspepsia, eructation, flatulence, gastrointestinal disorder, melena.

Musculoskeletal System: leg cramps (10%), myalgia, arthralgia.

Skin and Appendages: pruritus (6%), rash, increased sweating.

Genitourinary System: urinary tract infection.

Special Senses: conjunctivitis, abnormal vision, ear disorder.

Metabolic and Nutritional Disorders: hyperkalemia (6%), generalized edema (5%), leg edema, peripheral edema, hypoglycemia, edema, hypervolemia, hypokalemia.

Hematologic System: abnormal erythrocytes (11%), anemia, leukocytosis, lymphadenopathy.

Other Adverse Reactions Observed During Clinical Trials: In the single-dose post-marketing safety study in 1,097 patients receiving Ferrlecit®, the following additional events were reported in two or more patients: hypertonia, nervousness, dry mouth, and hemorrhage.

OVERDOSAGE

Dosages in excess of iron needs may lead to accumulation of iron in iron storage sites and hemosiderosis. Periodic monitoring of laboratory parameters of iron storage may assist in recognition of iron accumulation. Ferrlecit® should not be administered in patients with iron overload.

Serum iron levels greater than 300 µg/dL may indicate iron poisoning which is characterized by abdominal pain, diarrhea, or vomiting which progresses to pallor or cyanosis, lassitude, drowsiness, hyperventilation due to acidosis, and cardiovascular collapse. Caution should be exercised in interpreting serum iron levels in the 24 hours following the administration of Ferrlecit® since many laboratory assays will falsely overestimate serum or transferrin bound iron by measuring iron still bound to the Ferrlecit® complex. Additionally, in the assessment of iron overload, caution should be exercised in interpreting serum ferritin levels in the week following Ferrlecit® administration since, in clinical studies, serum ferritin exhibited a non-specific rise which persisted for five days.

The Ferrlecit® iron complex is not dialyzable.

Ferrlecit® at elemental iron doses of 125 mg/kg, 78.8 mg/kg, 62.5 mg/kg and 250 mg/kg caused deaths to mice, rats, rabbits, and dogs respectively. The major symptoms of acute toxicity were decreased activity, staggering, ataxia, increases in the respiratory rate, tremor, and convulsions.

DOSAGE AND ADMINISTRATION

The dosage of Ferrlecit® is expressed in terms of mg of elemental iron. Each 5 mL ampule contains 62.5 mg of elemental iron (12.5 mg/mL).

The recommended dosage of Ferrlecit® for the repletion treatment of iron deficiency in hemodialysis patients is 10 mL of Ferrlecit® (125 mg of elemental iron). Ferrlecit® may be diluted in 100 mL of 0.9% sodium chloride administered by intravenous infusion over 1 hour. Ferrlecit® may also be administered undiluted as a slow IV injection (at a rate of up to 12.5 mg/min). Most patients will require a minimum cumulative dose of 1.0 gram of elemental iron, administered over eight sessions at sequential dialysis treatments, to achieve a favorable hemoglobin or hematocrit response. Patients may continue to require therapy with intravenous iron at the lowest dose necessary to maintain target levels of hemoglobin, hematocrit, and laboratory parameters of iron storage within acceptable limits. Ferrlecit® has been administered at sequential dialysis sessions by infusion or by slow IV injection during the dialysis session itself.

Note: Do not mix Ferrlecit® with other medications, or add to parenteral nutrition solutions for intravenous infusion. The compatibility of Ferrlecit® with intravenous infusion vehicles other than 0.9% sodium chloride has not been evaluated. Parenteral drug products should be inspected visually for particulate matter and discoloration before administration, whenever the solution and container permit. If diluted in saline, use immediately after dilution.

HOW SUPPLIED

NDC# 52544-922-26

Ferrlecit® is supplied in colorless glass ampules. Each ampule contains 62.5 mg of elemental iron in 5 mL for intravenous use, packaged in cartons of 10 ampules.

Store at 20°C–25°C (68°F–77°F); excursions permitted to 15°C–30°C (59°F–86°F). Do not freeze. See USP Controlled Room Temperature.

Keep out of the reach of children.

Rx Only

© Watson Pharma Inc., a subsidiary of Watson Pharmaceuticals Inc., Corona, CA 92880. November 2001.

Shown in Product Identification Guide, page 335

INFED® ℞
(IRON DEXTRAN INJECTION, USP)

WARNING

THE PARENTERAL USE OF COMPLEXES OF IRON AND CARBOHYDRATES HAS RESULTED IN ANAPHYLACTIC-TYPE REACTIONS. DEATHS ASSOCIATED WITH SUCH ADMINISTRATION HAVE BEEN REPORTED. THEREFORE, INFeD SHOULD BE USED ONLY IN THOSE PATIENTS IN WHOM THE INDICATIONS HAVE BEEN CLEARLY ESTABLISHED AND LABORATORY INVESTI-

Continued on next page

INFeD—Cont.

GATIONS CONFIRM AN IRON DEFICIENT STATE NOT AMENABLE TO ORAL IRON THERAPY. BECAUSE FATAL ANAPHYLACTIC REACTIONS HAVE BEEN REPORTED AFTER ADMINISTRATION OF IRON DEXTRAN INJECTION, THE DRUG SHOULD BE GIVEN ONLY WHEN RESUSCITATION TECHNIQUES AND TREATMENT OF ANAPHYLACTIC AND ANAPHYLACTOID SHOCK ARE READILY AVAILABLE.

DESCRIPTION

INFeD (iron dextran injection, USP) is a dark brown, slightly viscous sterile liquid complex of ferric hydroxide and dextran for intravenous or intramuscular use.
Each mL contains the equivalent of 50 mg of elemental iron (as an iron dextran complex), approximately 0.9% sodium chloride, in water for injection. Sodium hydroxide and/or hydrochloric acid may have been used to adjust pH. The pH of the solution is between 5.2 and 6.5.
The iron dextran complex has an average apparent molecular weight of 165,000 g/mole with a range of approximately ±10%.
Therapeutic Class: Hematinic

CLINICAL PHARMACOLOGY

General: After intramuscular injection, iron dextran is absorbed from the injection site into the capillaries and the lymphatic system. Circulating iron dextran is removed from the plasma by cells of the reticuloendothelial system, which split the complex into its components of iron and dextran. The iron is immediately bound to the available protein moieties to form hemosiderin or ferritin, the physiological forms of iron, or to a lesser extent to transferrin. This iron which is subject to physiological control replenishes hemoglobin and depleted iron stores.
Dextran, a polyglucose, is either metabolized or excreted. Negligible amounts of iron are lost via the urinary or alimentary pathways after administration of iron dextran.
The major portion of intramuscular injections of iron dextran is absorbed within 72 hours; most of the remaining iron is absorbed over the ensuing 3 to 4 weeks.
Various studies involving intravenously administered ^{59}Fe iron dextran to iron deficient subjects, some of whom had coexisting diseases, have yielded half-life values ranging from 5 hours to more than 20 hours. The 5-hour value was determined for ^{59}Fe iron dextran from a study that used laboratory methods to separate the circulating ^{59}Fe iron dextran from the transferrin-bound ^{59}Fe. The 20-hour value reflects a half-life determined by measuring total ^{59}Fe, both circulating and bound. It should be understood that these half-life values do not represent clearance of iron from the body. Iron is not easily eliminated from the body and accumulation of iron can be toxic.
In vitro studies have shown that removal of iron dextran by dialysis is negligible.[1,2] Six different dialyzer membranes were investigated (polysulfone, cuprophane, cellulose acetate, cellulose triacetate, polymethylmethacrylate and polyacrylonitrile), including those considered high efficiency and high flux.

INDICATIONS AND USAGE

Intravenous or intramuscular injections of iron dextran are indicated for treatment of patients with documented iron deficiency in whom oral administration is unsatisfactory or impossible.

CONTRAINDICATIONS

Hypersensitivity to the product. All anemias not associated with iron deficiency.

WARNINGS

See BOXED WARNING.
A risk of carcinogenesis may attend the intramuscular injection of iron-carbohydrate complexes. Such complexes have been found under experimental conditions to produce sarcoma when large doses or small doses injected repeatedly at the same site were given to rats, mice, and rabbits, and possibly in hamsters.
The long latent period between the injection of a potential carcinogen and the appearance of a tumor makes it impossible to measure accurately the risk in man. There have, however, been several reports in the literature describing tumors at the injection site in humans who had previously received intramuscular injections of iron-carbohydrate complexes.
Large intravenous doses, such as used with total dose infusions (TDI), have been associated with an increased incidence of adverse effects. The adverse effects frequently are delayed (1–2 days) reactions typified by one or more of the following symptoms: arthralgia, backache, chills, dizziness, moderate to high fever, headache, malaise, myalgia, nausea, and vomiting. The onset is usually 24–48 hours after administration and symptoms generally subside within 3–4 days. These symptoms have also been reported following intramuscular injection and generally subside within 3–7 days. The etiology of these reactions is not known. The potential for a delayed reaction must be considered when estimating the risk/benefit of treatment.
The maximum daily dose should not exceed 2 mL undiluted iron dextran.
This preparation should be used with extreme care in patients with serious impairment of liver function.
It should not be used during the acute phase of infectious kidney disease.
Adverse reactions experienced following administration of INFeD may exacerbate cardiovascular complications in patients with pre-existing cardiovascular disease.

PRECAUTIONS

General: Unwarranted therapy with parenteral iron will cause excess storage of iron with the consequent possibility of exogenous hemosiderosis. Such iron overload is particularly apt to occur in patients with hemoglobinopathies and other refractory anemias that might be erroneously diagnosed as iron deficiency anemias.
INFeD should be used with caution in individuals with histories of significant allergies and/or asthma.
Anaphylaxis and other hypersensitivity reactions have been reported after uneventful test doses as well as therapeutic doses of iron dextran injection. Therefore, administration of subsequent test doses during therapy should be considered. (See DOSAGE AND ADMINISTRATION: Administration.)
Epinephrine should be immediately available in the event of acute hypersensitivity reactions. (Usual adult dose: 0.5 mL of a 1:1000 solution, by subcutaneous or intramuscular injection.) **Note:** Patients using beta-blocking agents may not respond adequately to epinephrine. Isoproterenol or similar beta-agonist agents may be required in these patients.
Patients with rheumatoid arthritis may have an acute exacerbation of joint pain and swelling following the administration of INFeD.
Reports in the literature from countries outside the United States (in particular, New Zealand) have suggested that the use of intramuscular iron dextran in neonates has been associated with an increased incidence of gram-negative sepsis, primarily due to *E. Coli.*
Information For Patients: Patients should be advised of the potential adverse reactions associated with the use of INFeD.
Drug/Laboratory Test Interactions: Large doses of iron dextran (5 mL or more) have been reported to give a brown color to serum from a blood sample drawn 4 hours after administration.
The drug may cause falsely elevated values of serum bilirubin and falsely decreased values of serum calcium.
Serum iron determinations (especially by colorimetric assays) may not be meaningful for 3 weeks following the administration of iron dextran.
Serum ferritin peaks approximately 7 to 9 days after an intravenous dose of INFeD and slowly returns to baseline after about 3 weeks.
Examination of the bone marrow for iron stores may not be meaningful for prolonged periods following iron dextran therapy because residual iron dextran may remain in the reticuloendothelial cells.
Bone scans involving 99m Tc-diphosphonate have been reported to show a dense, crescentic area of activity in the buttocks, following the contour of the iliac crest, 1 to 6 days after intramuscular injections of iron dextran.
Bone scans with 99m Tc-labeled bone seeking agents, in the presence of high serum ferritin levels or following iron dextran infusions, have been reported to show reduction of bony uptake, marked renal activity, and excessive blood pool and soft tissue accumulation.
Carcinogenesis, Mutagenesis, Impairment Of Fertility: See WARNINGS.
Pregnancy: *Pregnancy Category C:* Iron dextran has been shown to be teratogenic and embryocidal in mice, rats, rabbits, dogs, and monkeys when given in doses of about 3 times the maximum human dose.
No consistent adverse fetal effects were observed in mice, rats, rabbits, dogs and monkeys at doses of 50 mg iron/kg or less. Fetal and maternal toxicity has been reported in monkeys at a total intravenous dose of 90 mg iron/kg over a 14 day period. Similar effects were observed in mice and rats on administration of a single dose of 125 mg iron/kg. Fetal abnormalities in rats and dogs were observed at doses of 250 mg iron/kg and higher. The animals used in these tests were not iron deficient. There are no adequate and well-controlled studies in pregnant women. INFeD should be used during pregnancy only if the potential benefit justifies the potential risk to the fetus.
Placental Transfer: Various animal studies and studies in pregnant humans have demonstrated inconclusive results with respect to the placental transfer of iron dextran as iron dextran. It appears that some iron does reach the fetus, but the form in which it crosses the placenta is not clear.
Nursing Mothers: Caution should be exercised when INFeD is administered to a nursing woman. Traces of unmetabolized iron dextran are excreted in human milk.
Pediatric Use: Not recommended for use in infants under 4 months of age (See DOSAGE AND ADMINISTRATION).

ADVERSE REACTIONS

Severe/Fatal: Anaphylactic reactions have been reported with the use of iron dextran injection; on occasions these reactions have been fatal. Such reactions, which occur most often within the first several minutes of administration, have been generally characterized by sudden onset of respiratory difficulty and/or cardiovascular collapse. Because fatal anaphylactic reactions have been reported after administration of iron dextran injection, the drug should be given only when resuscitation techniques and treatment of anaphylactic and anaphylactoid shock are readily available. (See boxed WARNING and PRECAUTIONS: General, pertaining to immediate availability of epinephrine.)
Cardiovascular: Chest pain, chest tightness, shock, cardiac arrest, hypotension, hypertension, tachycardia, bradycardia, flushing, arrhythmias. (Flushing and hypotension may occur from too rapid injections by the intravenous route.)
Dermatologic: Urticaria, pruritus, purpura, rash, cyanosis.
Gastrointestinal: Abdominal pain, nausea, vomiting, diarrhea.
Hematologic/lymphatic: Leucocytosis, lymphadenopathy.
Musculoskeletal/soft tissue: Arthralgia, arthritis (may represent reactivation in patients with quiescent rheumatoid arthritis—See PRECAUTIONS: General), myalgia; backache; sterile abscess, atrophy/fibrosis (intramuscular injection site); brown skin and/or underlying tissue discoloration (staining), soreness or pain at or near intramuscular injection sites; cellulitis; swelling; inflammation; local phlebitis at or near intravenous injection site.
Neurologic: Convulsions, seizures, syncope, headache, weakness, unresponsiveness, paresthesia, febrile episodes, chills, dizziness, disorientation, numbness, unconsciousness.
Respiratory: Respiratory arrest, dyspnea, bronchospasm, wheezing.
Urologic: Hematuria.
Delayed reactions: Arthralgia, backache, chills, dizziness, fever, headache, malaise, myalgia, nausea, vomiting (See WARNINGS).
Miscellaneous: Febrile episodes, sweating, shivering, chills, malaise, altered taste.

OVERDOSAGE

Overdosage with iron dextran is unlikely to be associated with any acute manifestations. Dosages of iron dextran in excess of the requirements for restoration of hemoglobin and replenishment of iron stores may lead to hemosiderosis. Periodic monitoring of serum ferritin levels may be helpful in recognizing a deleterious progressive accumulation of iron resulting from impaired uptake of iron from the reticuloendothelial system in concurrent medical conditions such as chronic renal failure, Hodgkin's disease, and rheumatoid arthritis. The LD_{50} of iron dextran is not less than 500 mg/kg in the mouse.

DOSAGE AND ADMINISTRATION

Oral iron should be discontinued prior to administration of INFeD.
Dosage:
I. *Iron Deficiency Anemia:* Periodic hematologic determination (hemoglobin and hematocrit) is a simple and accurate technique for monitoring hematological response, and should be used as a guide in therapy. It should be recognized that iron storage may lag behind the appearance of normal blood morphology. Serum iron, total iron binding capacity (TIBC) and percent saturation of transferrin are other important tests for detecting and monitoring the iron deficient state.
After administration of iron dextran complex, evidence of a therapeutic response can be seen in a few days as an increase in the reticulocyte count.
Although serum ferritin is usually a good guide to body iron stores, the correlation of body iron stores and serum ferritin may not be valid in patients on chronic renal dialysis who are also receiving iron dextran complex.
Although there are significant variations in body build and weight distribution among males and females, the accompanying table and formula represent a convenient means for estimating the total iron required. This total iron requirement reflects the amount of iron needed to restore hemoglobin concentration to normal or near normal levels plus an additional allowance to provide adequate replenishment of iron stores in most individuals with moderately or severely reduced levels of hemoglobin. It should be remembered that iron deficiency anemia will not appear until essentially all iron stores have been depleted. Therapy, thus, should aim at not only replenishment of hemoglobin iron but iron stores as well.
Factors contributing to the formula are shown below.
[See first table at bottom of next page]
[See second table at bottom of next page]
The total amount of INFeD in mL required to treat the anemia and replenish iron stores may be approximated as follows:
Adults and Children over 15 kg (33 lbs): See Dosage Table.
Alternatively the total dose may be calculated:

Dose (mL) = 0.0442 (Desired Hb−Observed Hb) × LBW + (0.26 × LBW)

Based on: Desired Hb = the target Hb in g/dl.
Observed Hb = the patient's current hemoglobin in g/dl.
LBW = Lean body weight in kg. A patient's lean body weight (or actual body weight if less than lean body weight) should be utilized when determining dosage.
For males: LBW = 50 kg + 2.3 kg for each inch of patient's height over 5 feet
For females: LBW = 45.5 kg + 2.3 kg for each inch of patient's height over 5 feet
To calculate a patient's weight in kg when lbs are known:

$$\frac{\text{patient's weight in pounds}}{2.2} = \text{weight in kilograms}$$

Children 5–15 kg (11–33 lbs): See Dosage Table.
INFeD should not normally be given in the first four months of life. (See PRECAUTIONS: Pediatric Use.)
Alternatively the total dose may be calculated:
Dose (mL) = 0.0442 (Desired Hb−Observed Hb) × W + (0.26 × W)

Based on: Desired Hb = the target Hb in g/dl. (Normal Hb for Children 15 kg or less is 12 g/dl)
W = Weight in kg.

To calculate a patient's weight in kg when lbs are known:

$$\frac{\text{patient's weight in pounds}}{2.2} = \text{weight in kilograms}$$

II. *Iron Replacement for Blood Loss:* Some individuals sustain blood losses on an intermittent or repetitive basis. Such blood losses may occur periodically in patients with hemorrhagic diatheses (familial telangiectasia; hemophilia; gastrointestinal bleeding) and on a repetitive basis from procedures such as renal hemodialysis.

Iron therapy in these patients should be directed toward replacement of the equivalent amount of iron represented in the blood loss. The table and formula described under **I. *Iron Deficiency Anemia*** are ***not*** applicable for simple iron replacement values.

Quantitative estimates of the individual's periodic blood loss and hematocrit during the bleeding episode provide a convenient method for the calculation of the required iron dose.

The formula shown below is based on the approximation that 1 mL of normocytic, normochromic red cells contains 1 mg of elemental iron:

Replacement iron (in mg) = Blood loss (in mL) x hematocrit

Example: Blood loss of 500 mL with 20% hematocrit
Replacement Iron = 500 × 0.20 = 100 mg

$$\text{INFeD dose} = \frac{100 \text{ mg}}{50} = 2 \text{ mL}$$

Administration: The total amount of INFeD required for the treatment of iron deficiency anemia or iron replacement for blood loss is determined from the table or appropriate formula (See Dosage.)

1. *Intravenous Injection*—PRIOR TO RECEIVING THEIR FIRST INFeD THERAPEUTIC DOSE, ALL PATIENTS SHOULD BE GIVEN AN INTRAVENOUS TEST DOSE OF 0.5 mL. (See PRECAUTIONS: General.) THE TEST DOSE SHOULD BE ADMINISTERED AT A GRADUAL RATE OVER AT LEAST 30 SECONDS. Although anaphylactic reactions known to occur following INFeD administration are usually evident within a few minutes or sooner, it is recommended that a period of an hour or longer elapse before the remainder of the initial therapeutic dose is given.

Individual doses of 2 mL or less may be given on a daily basis until the calculated total amount required has been reached. INFeD is given undiluted at a **slow gradual rate** not to exceed 50 mg (1 mL) per minute.

2. *Intramuscular Injection*—PRIOR TO RECEIVING THEIR FIRST INFeD THERAPEUTIC DOSE, ALL PATIENTS SHOULD BE GIVEN AN INTRAMUSCULAR TEST DOSE OF 0.5 mL. (See PRECAUTIONS: General.) The test dose should be administered in the same recommended test site and by the same technique as described in the last paragraph of this section. Although anaphylactic reactions known to occur following INFeD administration are usually evident within a few minutes or sooner, it is recommended that at least an hour or longer elapse before the remainder of the initial therapeutic dose is given.

If no adverse reactions are observed, INFeD can be given according to the following schedule until the calculated total amount required has been reached. Each day's dose should ordinarily not exceed 0.5 mL (25 mg of iron) for infants under 5 kg (11 lbs); 1.0 mL (50 mg of iron) for children under 10 kg (22 lbs); and 2.0 mL (100 mg of iron) for other patients.

INFeD should be injected only into the muscle mass of the upper outer quadrant of the buttock—never into the arm or other exposed areas—and should be injected deeply, with a 2-inch or 3-inch 19 or 20 gauge needle. If the patient is standing, he/she should be bearing his/her weight on the leg opposite the injection site, or if in bed, he/she should be in the lateral position with injection site uppermost. To avoid injection or leakage into the subcutaneous tissue, a Z-track technique (displacement of the skin laterally prior to injection) is recommended.

NOTE: Do not mix INFeD with other medications or add to parenteral nutrition solutions for intravenous infusion.

Parenteral drug products should be inspected visually for particulate matter and discoloration prior to administration, whenever the solution and container permit.

HOW SUPPLIED

INFeD® (Iron Dextran Injection, USP) containing 50 mg of elemental iron per mL, is available in 2 mL single dose amber vials (for intramuscular or intravenous use) in cartons of 10 (NDC 52544-931-02).

Store at controlled room temperature 15°–30°C (59°–86°F).

Rx Only

REFERENCES

1. Hatton RC, Portales IT, Finlay A, Ross EA. Removal of Iron Dextran by Hemodialysis: An In Vitro Study. *Am J Kid Dis.* 1995; 26(2):327–330.
2. Manuel MA, Stewart WK, St. Clair Neill GD, Hutchinson F. Loss of Iron-Dextran through Cuprophane Membrane of a Disposable Coil Dialyser. *Nephron.* 1972;9:94–98.

Literature revised: February 2001
Product No.: 1001-02

$$\frac{\text{mg blood iron}}{\text{lb body weight}} = \frac{\text{mL blood}}{\text{lb body weight}} \times \frac{\text{g hemoglobin}}{\text{mL blood}} \times \frac{\text{mg iron}}{\text{g hemoglobin}}$$

a) Blood volume .... 65 mL/kg of body weight
b) Normal hemoglobin (males and females)
  over 15 kg (33 lbs) .... 14.8 g/dl
  15 kg (33 lbs) or less .... 12.0 g/dl
c) Iron content of hemoglobin 0.34%
d) Hemoglobin deficit
e) Weight

Based on the above factors, individuals with normal hemoglobin levels will have approximately 33 mg of blood iron per kilogram of body weight (15 mg/lb).

Note: The table and accompanying formula are applicable for dosage determinations only in patients with iron deficiency anemia; they are not to be used for dosage determinations in patients requiring iron replacement for blood loss.

TOTAL INFeD® REQUIREMENT FOR HEMOGLOBIN RESTORATION AND IRON STORES REPLACEMENT*

PATIENT LEAN BODY WEIGHT		Milliliter Requirement of INFeD Based On Observed Hemoglobin of							
kg	lb	3 (g/dl)	4 (g/dl)	5 (g/dl)	6 (g/dl)	7 (g/dl)	8 (g/dl)	9 (g/dl)	10 (g/dl)
5	11	3	3	3	3	2	2	2	2
10	22	7	6	6	5	5	4	4	3
15	33	10	9	9	8	7	7	6	5
20	44	16	15	14	13	12	11	10	9
25	55	20	18	17	16	15	14	13	12
30	66	23	22	21	19	18	17	15	14
35	77	27	26	24	23	21	20	18	17
40	88	31	29	28	26	24	22	21	19
45	99	35	33	31	29	27	25	23	21
50	110	39	37	35	32	30	28	26	24
55	121	43	41	38	36	33	31	28	26
60	132	47	44	42	39	36	34	31	28
65	143	51	48	45	42	39	36	34	31
70	154	55	52	49	45	42	39	36	33
75	165	59	55	52	49	45	42	39	35
80	176	63	59	55	52	48	45	41	38
85	187	66	63	59	55	51	48	44	40
90	198	70	66	62	58	54	50	46	42
95	209	74	70	66	62	57	53	49	45
100	220	78	74	69	65	60	56	52	47
105	231	82	77	73	68	63	59	54	50
110	242	86	81	76	71	67	62	57	52
115	253	90	85	80	75	70	64	59	54
120	264	94	88	83	78	73	67	62	57

* Table values were calculated based on a normal adult hemoglobin of 14.8 g/dl for weights greater than 15 kg (33 lbs) and a hemoglobin of 12.0 g/dl for weights less than or equal to 15 kg (33 lbs).

Watson Pharma, Inc.
a subsidiary of Watson Pharmaceuticals, Inc.
Morristown, NJ 07962 USA

OXYTROL® ℞

[*ŏks-ē-trōl*]
Oxybutynin Transdermal System
Rx only

DESCRIPTION

OXYTROL, oxybutynin transdermal system, is designed to deliver oxybutynin continuously and consistently over a 3- to 4-day interval after application to intact skin. **OXYTROL** is available as a 39 cm^2 system containing 36 mg of oxybutynin. **OXYTROL** has a nominal *in vivo* delivery rate of 3.9 mg oxybutynin per day through skin of average permeability (interindividual variation in skin permeability is approximately 20%).

Oxybutynin is an antispasmodic, anticholinergic agent. Oxybutynin is administered as a racemate of R- and S-isomers. Chemically, oxybutynin is d, l (racemic) 4-diethylamino-2-butynyl phenylcyclohexylglycolate. The empirical formula of oxybutynin is $C_{22}H_{31}NO_3$. Its structural formula is:

Oxybutynin is a white powder with a molecular weight of 357. It is soluble in alcohol, but relatively insoluble in water.

Transdermal System Components

OXYTROL is a matrix-type transdermal system composed of three layers as illustrated in Figure 1 below. Layer 1 (Backing Film) is a thin flexible polyester/ethylene-vinyl acetate film that provides the matrix system with occlusivity and physical integrity and protects the adhesive/drug layer. Layer 2 (Adhesive/Drug Layer) is a cast film of acrylic adhesive containing oxybutynin and triacetin, USP. Layer 3 (Release Liner) is two overlapped siliconized polyester strips that are peeled off and discarded by the patient prior to applying the matrix system.

Figure 1: Side and top views of the **OXYTROL** system. (Not to scale)

Side View

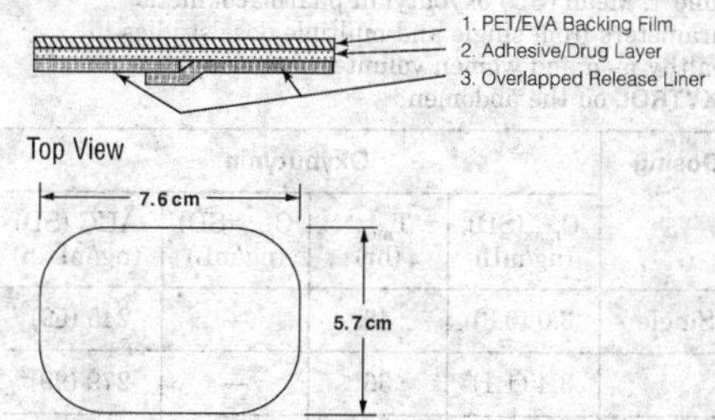

CLINICAL PHARMACOLOGY

The free base form of oxybutynin is pharmacologically equivalent to oxybutynin hydrochloride. Oxybutynin acts as a competitive antagonist of acetylcholine at postganglionic muscarinic receptors, resulting in relaxation of bladder smooth muscle. In patients with conditions characterized by involuntary detrusor contractions, cystometric studies have demonstrated that oxybutynin increases maximum urinary bladder capacity and increases the volume to first detrusor contraction. Oxybutynin thus decreases urinary urgency and the frequency of both incontinence episodes and voluntary urination.

Oxybutynin is a racemic (50:50) mixture of R- and S-isomers. Antimuscarinic activity resides predominantly in the R-isomer. The active metabolite, N-desethyloxybutynin, has pharmacological activity on the human detrusor muscle that is similar to that of oxybutynin in *in vitro* studies.

Pharmacokinetics

Absorption

Oxybutynin is transported across intact skin and into the systemic circulation by passive diffusion across the stratum corneum. The average daily dose of oxybutynin absorbed from the 39 cm^2 **OXYTROL** system is 3.9 mg. The average (SD) nominal dose, 0.10 (0.02) mg oxybutynin per cm^2 surface area, was obtained from analysis of residual oxybutynin content of systems worn over a continuous 4-day period during 303 separate occasions in 76 healthy volunteers. Following application of the first **OXYTROL** 3.9 mg/day system, oxybutynin plasma concentration increases for approximately 24 to 48 hours, reaching average maximum concentrations of 3 to 4 ng/mL. Thereafter, steady concentrations are maintained for up to 96 hours. Absorption of oxybutynin is bioequivalent when **OXYTROL** is applied to the abdomen, buttocks, or hip. Average plasma concentrations measured during a randomized, crossover study of the

Continued on next page

Oxytrol—Cont.

three recommended application sites in 24 healthy men and women are shown in Figure 2.

Figure 2: Average plasma oxybutynin concentrations (Cp) in 24 healthy male and female volunteers during single-dose application of **OXYTROL** 3.9 mg/day to the abdomen, buttock, and hip (System removal at 96 hours).

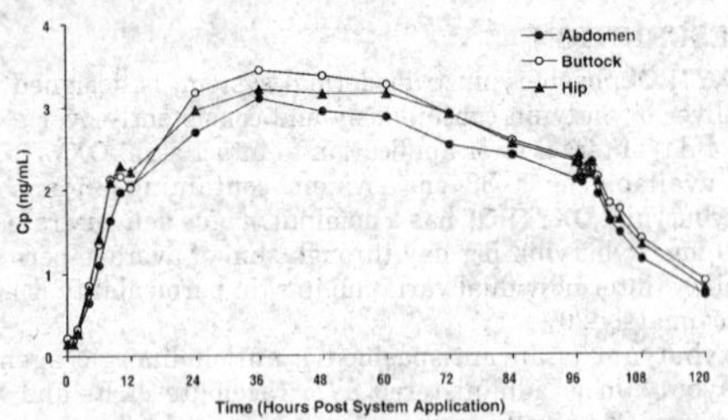

Steady-state conditions are reached during the second **OXYTROL** application. Average steady-state plasma concentrations were 3.1 ng/mL for oxybutynin and 3.8 ng/mL for N-desethyloxybutynin (Figure 3). Table 1 provides a summary of pharmacokinetic parameters of oxybutynin in healthy volunteers after single and multiple applications of **OXYTROL**.

Figure 3: Average (SEM) steady-state oxybutynin and N-desethyloxybutynin plasma concentrations (Cp) measured in 13 healthy volunteers following the second transdermal system application in a multiple-dose, randomized, crossover study.

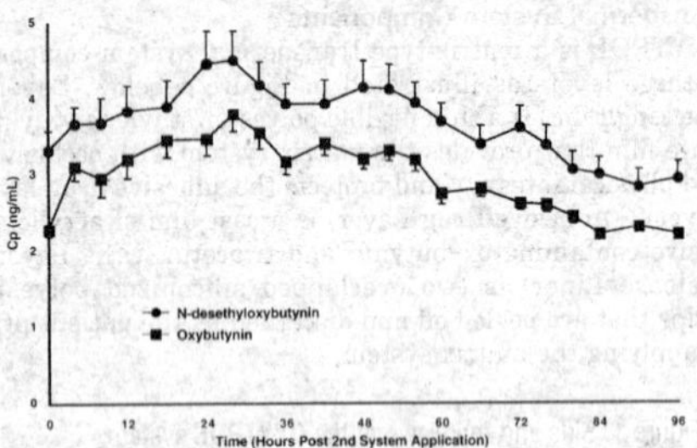

Table 1: Mean (SD) oxybutynin pharmacokinetic parameters from single and multiple dose studies in healthy men and women volunteers after application of **OXYTROL** on the abdomen.

Dosing	Oxybutynin			
	C_{max}(SD) (ng/mL)	T_{max}[1] (hr)	C_{avg} (SD) (ng/mL)	AUC (SD) (ng/mLxh)
Single	3.0 (0.8)	48	—	245 (59)[2]
	3.4 (1.1)	36	—	279 (99)[2]
Multiple	6.6 (2.4)	10	4.2 (1.1)	408 (108)[3]
	4.2 (1.0)	28	3.1 (0.7)	259 (57)[4]

[1] T_{max} given as median
[2] AUC_{inf}
[3] AUC_{0-96}
[4] AUC_{0-84}

Distribution

Oxybutynin is widely distributed in body tissues following systemic absorption. The volume of distribution was estimated to be 193 L after intravenous administration of 5 mg oxybutynin chloride.

Metabolism

Oxybutynin is metabolized primarily by the cytochrome P450 enzyme systems, particularly CYP3A4, found mostly in the liver and gut wall. Metabolites include phenylcyclohexylglycolic acid, which is pharmacologically inactive, and N-desethyloxybutynin, which is pharmacologically active.

After oral administration of oxybutynin, pre-systemic first-pass metabolism results in an oral bioavailability of approximately 6% and higher plasma concentration of the N-desethyl metabolite compared to oxybutynin (see Figure 4). The plasma concentration AUC ratio of N-desethyl metabolite to parent compound following a single 5 mg oral dose of oxybutynin chloride was 11.9:1.

Transdermal administration of oxybutynin bypasses the first-pass gastrointestinal and hepatic metabolism, reducing the formation of the N-desethyl metabolite (see Figure 4). Only small amounts of CYP3A4 are found in skin, limiting pre-systemic metabolism during transdermal absorption. The resulting plasma concentration AUC ratio of N-desethyl metabolite to parent compound following multiple **OXYTROL** applications was 1.3:1.

[See figure 4 at top of next column]

Following intravenous administration, the elimination half-life of oxybutynin is approximately 2 hours. Following re-

Figure 4: Average plasma concentrations (Cp) measured after a single, 96-hour application of the **OXYTROL** 3.9 mg/day system ($AUC_{inf}/96$) and a single, 5 mg, oral immediate-release dose of oxybutynin chloride ($AUC_{inf}/8$) in 16 healthy male and female volunteers.

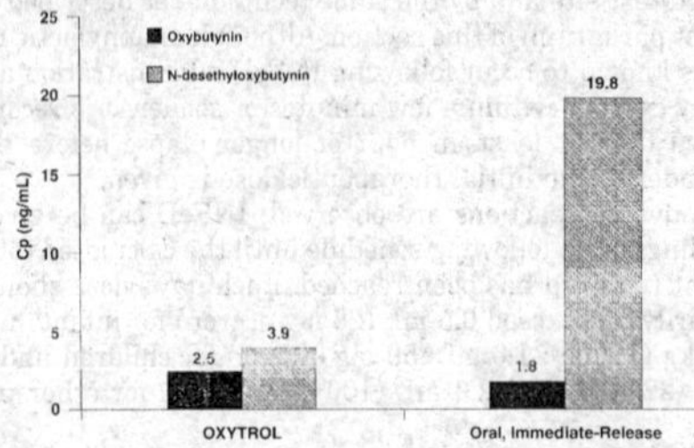

moval of **OXYTROL**, plasma concentrations of oxybutynin and N-desethyloxybutynin decline with an apparent half-life of approximately 7 to 8 hours.

Excretion

Oxybutynin is extensively metabolized by the liver, with less than 0.1% of the administered dose excreted unchanged in the urine. Also, less than 0.1% of the administered dose is excreted as the metabolite N-desethyloxybutynin.

Special Populations

Geriatric: The pharmacokinetics of oxybutynin and N-desethyloxybutynin were similar in all patients studied.

Pediatric: The pharmacokinetics of oxybutynin and N-desethyloxybutynin were not evaluated in individuals younger than 18 years of age. See **PRECAUTIONS: Pediatric Use.**

Gender: There were no significant differences in the pharmacokinetics of oxybutynin in healthy male and female volunteers following application of **OXYTROL**.

Race: Available data suggest that there are no significant differences in the pharmacokinetics of oxybutynin based on race in healthy volunteers following administration of **OXYTROL**. Japanese volunteers demonstrated a somewhat lower metabolism of oxybutynin to N-desethyloxybutynin compared to Caucasian volunteers.

Renal Insufficiency: There is no experience with the use of **OXYTROL** in patients with renal insufficiency.

Hepatic Insufficiency: There is no experience with the use of **OXYTROL** in patients with hepatic insufficiency.

Drug-Drug Interactions: See **PRECAUTIONS: Drug Interactions.**

Adhesion

Adhesion was periodically evaluated during the Phase 3 studies. Of the 4,746 **OXYTROL** evaluations in the Phase 3 trials, 20 (0.4%) were observed at clinic visits to have become completely detached and 35 (0.7%) became partially detached during routine clinic use. Similar to the pharmacokinetic studies, > 98% of the systems evaluated in the Phase 3 studies were assessed as being ≥ 75% attached and thus would be expected to perform as anticipated.

Clinical Studies

The efficacy and safety of **OXYTROL** were evaluated in patients with urge urinary incontinence in two Phase 3 controlled studies and one open-label extension. Study 1 was a Phase 3, placebo controlled study, comparing the safety and efficacy of **OXYTROL** at dose levels of 1.3, 2.6, and 3.9 mg/day to placebo in 520 patients. Open-label treatment was available for patients completing the study. Study 2 was a Phase 3 study, comparing the safety and efficacy of **OXYTROL** 3.9 mg/day versus active and placebo controls in 361 patients.

Study 1 was a randomized, double-blind, placebo-controlled, parallel group study of three dose levels of **OXYTROL** conducted in 520 patients. The 12-week double-blind treatment included **OXYTROL** doses of 1.3, 2.6, and 3.9 mg/day with matching placebo. An open-label, dose titration treatment extension allowed continued treatment for up to an additional 40 weeks for patients completing the double-blind period. The majority of patients were Caucasian (91%) and female (92%) with a mean age of 61 years (range, 20 to 88 years). Entry criteria required that patients have urge or mixed incontinence (with a predominance of urge), urge incontinence episodes of ≥ 10 per week, and ≥ 8 micturitions per day. The patient's medical history and a urinary diary during the treatment-free baseline period confirmed the diagnosis of urge incontinence. Approximately 80% of patients had no prior pharmacological treatment for incontinence. Reductions in weekly incontinence episodes, urinary frequency, and urinary void volume between placebo and active treatment groups are summarized in Table 2.

Table 2: Mean and median change from baseline to end of treatment (Week 12 or last observation carried forward) in incontinence episodes, urinary frequency, and urinary void volume in patients treated with **OXYTROL** 3.9 mg/day or placebo for 12 weeks (Study 1).

Parameter	Placebo (N=127)		OXYTROL 3.9 mg/day (N=120)	
	Mean (SD)	Median	Mean (SD)	Median
Weekly Incontinence Episodes				
Baseline	37.7 (24.0)	30	34.3 (18.2)	31
Reduction	19.2 (21.4)	15	21.0 (17.1)	19
p value vs. placebo		—	0.0265*	
Daily Urinary Frequency				
Baseline	12.3 (3.5)	11	11.8 (3.1)	11
Reduction	1.6 (3.0)	1	2.2 (2.5)	2
p value vs. placebo		—	0.0313*	
Urinary Void Volume (mL)				
Baseline	175.9 (69.5)	166.5	171.6 (65.1)	168
Increase	10.5 (56.9)	5.5	31.6 (65.6)	26
p value vs. placebo		—	0.0009**	

*Comparison significant if $p < 0.05$
**Comparison significant if $p \le 0.0167$

Study 2 was a randomized, double-blind, double-dummy, study of **OXYTROL** 3.9 mg/day versus active and placebo controls conducted in 361 patients. The 12-week double-blind treatment included an **OXYTROL** dose of 3.9 mg/day, an active comparator, and placebo. The majority of patients were Caucasian (95%) and female (93%) with a mean age of 64 years (range, 18 to 89 years). Entry criteria required that all patients have urge or mixed incontinence (with a predominance of urge) and had achieved a beneficial response from the anticholinergic treatment they were using at the time of study entry. The average duration of prior pharmacological treatment was greater than 2 years. The patient's medical history and a urinary diary during the treatment-free baseline period confirmed the diagnosis of urge incontinence. Reductions in daily incontinence episodes, urinary frequency, and urinary void volume between placebo and active treatment groups are summarized in Table 3.

Table 3: Mean and median change from baseline to end of treatment (Week 12 or last observation carried forward) in incontinence episodes, urinary frequency, and urinary void volume in patients treated with **OXYTROL** 3.9 mg/day or placebo for 12 weeks (Study 2).

Parameter	Placebo (N=117)		OXYTROL 3.9 mg/day (N=121)	
	Mean (SD)	Median	Mean (SD)	Median
Daily Incontinence Episodes				
Baseline	5.0 (3.2)	4	4.7 (2.9)	4
Reduction	2.1 (3.0)	2	2.9 (3.0)	3
p value vs. placebo		—	0.0137*	
Daily Urinary Frequency				
Baseline	12.3 (3.3)	12	12.4 (2.9)	12
Reduction	1.4 (2.7)	1	1.9 (2.7)	2
p value vs. placebo		—	0.1010*	
Urinary Void Volume (mL)				
Baseline	175.0 (68.0)	171.0	164.8 (62.3)	160
Increase	9.3 (63.1)	5.5	32.0 (55.2)	24
p value vs. placebo		—	0.0010*	

*Comparison significant if $p < 0.05$

INDICATIONS AND USAGE

OXYTROL is indicated for the treatment of overactive bladder with symptoms of urge urinary incontinence, urgency, and frequency.

CONTRAINDICATIONS

OXYTROL is contraindicated in patients with urinary retention, gastric retention, or uncontrolled narrow-angle glaucoma and in patients who are at risk for these conditions. **OXYTROL** is also contraindicated in patients who have demonstrated hypersensitivity to oxybutynin or other components of the product.

PRECAUTIONS

General

OXYTROL should be used with caution in patients with hepatic or renal impairment.

Urinary Retention: **OXYTROL** should be administered with caution to patients with clinically significant bladder outflow obstruction because of the risk of urinary retention (see **CONTRAINDICATIONS**).

Gastrointestinal Disorders: OXYTROL should be administered with caution to patients with gastrointestinal obstructive disorders because of the risk of gastric retention (see **CONTRAINDICATIONS**).

OXYTROL, like other anticholinergic drugs, may decrease gastrointestinal motility and should be used with caution in patients with conditions such as ulcerative colitis, intestinal atony, and myasthenia gravis. **OXYTROL** should be used with caution in patients who have gastroesophageal reflux and/or who are concurrently taking drugs (such as bisphosphonates) that can cause or exacerbate esophagitis.

Information for Patients

Patients should be informed that heat prostration (fever and heat stroke due to decreased sweating) can occur when anticholinergics such as oxybutynin are used in a hot environment. Because anticholinergic agents such as oxybutynin may produce drowsiness (somnolence) or blurred vision, patients should be advised to exercise caution. Patients should be informed that alcohol may enhance the drowsiness caused by anticholinergic agents such as oxybutynin.

OXYTROL should be applied to dry, intact skin on the abdomen, hip, or buttock. A new application site should be selected with each new system to avoid re-application to the same site within 7 days. Details on use of the system are explained in the patient information leaflet that should be dispensed with the product.

Drug Interactions

The concomitant use of oxybutynin with other anticholinergic drugs or with other agents that produce dry mouth, constipation, somnolence, and/or other anticholinergic-like effects may increase the frequency and/or severity of such effects. Anticholinergic agents may potentially alter the absorption of some concomitantly administered drugs due to anticholinergic effects on gastrointestinal motility. Pharmacokinetic studies have not been performed with patients concomitantly receiving cytochrome P450 enzyme inhibitors, such as antimycotic agents (e.g. ketoconazole, itraconazole, and miconazole) or macrolide antibiotics (e.g. erythromycin and clarithromycin). No specific drug-drug interaction studies have been performed with **OXYTROL**.

Carcinogenesis, Mutagenesis, Impairment of Fertility

A 24-month study in rats at dosages of oxybutynin chloride of 20, 80 and 160 mg/kg showed no evidence of carcinogenicity. These doses are approximately 6, 25 and 50 times the maximum exposure in humans taking an oral dose based on body surface area.

Oxybutynin chloride showed no increase of mutagenic activity when tested in *Schizosaccharomyces pompholiciformis, Saccharomyces cerevisiae*, and *Salmonella typhimurium* test systems. Reproduction studies with oxybutynin chloride in the mouse, rat, hamster, and rabbit showed no definite evidence of impaired fertility.

Pregnancy: Teratogenic Effects

Pregnancy Category B

Reproduction studies with oxybutynin chloride in the mouse, rat, hamster, and rabbit showed no definite evidence of impaired fertility or harm to the animal fetus. Subcutaneous administration to rats at doses up to 25 mg/kg (approximately 50 times the human exposure based on surface area) and to rabbits at doses up to 0.4 mg/kg (approximately 1 times the human exposure) revealed no evidence of harm to the fetus due to oxybutynin chloride. The safety of **OXYTROL** administration to women who are or who may become pregnant has not been established. Therefore, **OXYTROL** should not be given to pregnant women unless, in the judgment of the physician, the probable clinical benefits outweigh the possible hazards.

Nursing Mothers

It is not known whether oxybutynin is excreted in human milk. Because many drugs are excreted in human milk, caution should be exercised when **OXYTROL** is administered to a nursing woman.

Pediatric Use

The safety and efficacy of **OXYTROL** in pediatric patients have not been established.

Geriatric Use

Of the total number of patients in the clinical studies of **OXYTROL**, 49% were 65 and over. No overall differences in safety or effectiveness were observed between these subjects and younger subjects, and other reported clinical experience has not identified differences in response between elderly and younger patients, but greater sensitivity of some older individuals cannot be ruled out (see **CLINICAL PHARMACOLOGY, Pharmacokinetics, *Special Populations: Geriatric***).

ADVERSE REACTIONS

The safety of **OXYTROL** was evaluated in a total of 417 patients who participated in two Phase 3 clinical efficacy and safety studies and an open-label extension. Additional safety information was collected in Phase 1 and Phase 2 trials. In the two pivotal studies, a total of 246 patients received **OXYTROL** during the 12-week treatment periods. A total of 411 patients entered the open-label extension and of those, 65 patients and 52 patients received **OXYTROL** for at least 24 weeks and at least 36 weeks, respectively.

No deaths were reported during treatment. No serious adverse events related to treatment were reported.

Adverse events reported in the pivotal trials are summarized in Tables 4 and 5 below.

Table 4: Number (%) of adverse events occurring in ≥ 2% of **OXYTROL**-treated patients and greater in **OXYTROL** group than in placebo group (Study 1).

Adverse Event*	Placebo (N=132)		OXYTROL (3.9 mg/day) (N=125)	
	N	%	N	%
Application site pruritus	8	6.1%	21	16.8%
Dry mouth	11	8.3%	12	9.6%
Application site erythema	3	2.3%	7	5.6%
Application site vesicles	0	0.0%	4	3.2%
Diarrhea	3	2.3%	4	3.2%
Dysuria	0	0.0%	3	2.4%

*includes adverse events judged by the investigator as possibly, probably or definitely treatment-related.

Table 5: Number (%) of adverse events occurring in ≥ 2% of **OXYTROL**-treated patients and greater in **OXYTROL** group than in placebo group (Study 2).

Adverse Event*	Placebo (N=117)		OXYTROL (3.9 mg/day) (N=121)	
	N	%	N	%
Application site pruritus	5	4.3%	17	14.0%
Application site erythema	2	1.7%	10	8.3%
Dry mouth	2	1.7%	5	4.1%
Constipation	0	0.0%	4	3.3%
Application site rash	1	0.9%	4	3.3%
Application site macules	0	0.0%	3	2.5%
Abnormal vision	0	0.0%	3	2.5%

*includes adverse events judged by the investigator as possibly, probably or definitely treatment-related.

Other adverse events reported by > 1% of **OXYTROL**-treated patients, and judged by the investigator to be possibly, probably or definitely related to treatment include: abdominal pain, nausea, flatulence, fatigue, somnolence, headache, flushing, rash, application site burning and back pain.

Most treatment-related adverse events were described as mild or moderate in intensity. Severe application site reactions were reported by 6.4% of **OXYTROL**-treated patients in Study 1 and by 5.0% of **OXYTROL**-treated patients in Study 2.

Treatment-related adverse events that resulted in discontinuation were reported by 11.2% of **OXYTROL**-treated patients in Study 1 and 10.7% of **OXYTROL**-treated patients in Study 2. Most of these were secondary to application site reaction. In the two pivotal studies, no patient discontinued **OXYTROL** treatment due to dry mouth.

In the open-label extension, the most common treatment-related adverse events were: application site pruritus, application site erythema and dry mouth.

OVERDOSAGE

Plasma concentration of oxybutynin declines within 1 to 2 hours after removal of transdermal system(s). Patients should be monitored until symptoms resolve. Overdosage with oxybutynin has been associated with anticholinergic effects including CNS excitation, flushing, fever, dehydration, cardiac arrhythmia, vomiting, and urinary retention. Ingestion of 100 mg oral oxybutynin chloride in association with alcohol has been reported in a 13 year old boy who experienced memory loss, and in a 34 year old woman who developed stupor, followed by disorientation and agitation on awakening, dilated pupils, dry skin, cardiac arrhythmia, and retention of urine. Both patients recovered fully with symptomatic treatment.

DOSAGE AND ADMINISTRATION

OXYTROL should be applied to dry, intact skin on the abdomen, hip, or buttock. A new application site should be selected with each new system to avoid re-application to the same site within 7 days.

The dose of **OXYTROL** is one 3.9 mg/day system applied twice weekly (every 3 to 4 days).

HOW SUPPLIED

OXYTROL 3.9 mg/day (oxybutynin transdermal system). Each 39 cm^2 system imprinted with **OXYTROL** 3.9 mg/day contains 36 mg oxybutynin for nominal delivery of 3.9 mg oxybutynin per day when dosed in a twice weekly regimen.

NDC 52544-920-08 Patient Calendar Box of 8 Systems

Storage

Store at 25°C (77°F); excursions permitted to 15–30°C (59–86°F). Protect from moisture and humidity. Do not store outside the sealed pouch. Apply immediately after removal from the protective pouch. Discard used **OXYTROL** in household trash in a manner that prevents accidental application or ingestion by children, pets, or others.

WATSON Pharma, Inc.
A Subsidiary of Watson Pharmaceuticals, Inc.
Corona, CA 92880 USA
DATE OF ISSUANCE: FEBRUARY 2003
U.S. Patent Nos. 5,601,839 and 5,834,010

Shown in Product Identification Guide, page 336

WellSpring Pharmaceutical Corporation

1430 STATE ROUTE 34
NEPTUNE, NJ 07753-6807

Direct Inquiries to:
(732) 938-5885

DIBENZYLINE® ℞
brand of phenoxybenzamine hydrochloride Capsules
℞ only

DESCRIPTION

Each *Dibenzyline* capsule, with red cap and red body, is imprinted WPC 001 and 10 mg and contains phenoxybenzamine hydrochloride, 10 mg. Inactive ingredients consist of benzyl alcohol, cetylpyridinium chloride, D&C Red No. 33, FD&C Red No. 3, FD&C Yellow No. 6, gelatin, lactose, sodium lauryl sulfate and trace amounts of other inactive ingredients.

Dibenzyline is N-(2 Chloroethyl)-N-(1-methyl-2-phenoxyethyl)benzylamine hydrochloride:

$$C_6H_5\text{-}CH_2N(CH_2CH_2Cl)CH(CH_3)CH_2O\text{-}C_6H_5 \cdot HCl$$

Phenoxybenzamine hydrochloride is a colorless, crystalline powder with a molecular weight of 340.3 which melts between 136° and 141°C. It is soluble in water, alcohol and chloroform; insoluble in ether.

CLINICAL PHARMACOLOGY

Dibenzyline (phenoxybenzamine hydrochloride) is a long-acting, adrenergic, *alpha*-receptor blocking agent which can produce and maintain "chemical sympathectomy" by oral administration. It increases blood flow to the skin, mucosa and abdominal viscera, and lowers both supine and erect blood pressures. It has no effect on the parasympathetic system.

Twenty to 30 percent of orally administered phenoxybenzamine appears to be absorbed in the active form.[1]

The half-life of orally administered phenoxybenzamine hydrochloride is not known; however, the half-life of intravenously administered drug is approximately 24 hours. Demonstrable effects with intravenous administration persist for at least 3 to 4 days, and the effects of daily administration are cumulative for nearly a week.[1]

INDICATION AND USAGE

Pheochromocytoma, to control episodes of hypertension and sweating. If tachycardia is excessive, it may be necessary to use a beta-blocking agent concomitantly.

CONTRAINDICATIONS

Conditions where a fall in blood pressure may be undesirable.

WARNING

Dibenzyline-induced *alpha*-adrenergic blockade leaves *beta*-adrenergic receptors unopposed. Compounds that stimulate both types of receptors may therefore produce an exaggerated hypotensive response and tachycardia.

PRECAUTIONS

General—Administer with caution in patients with marked cerebral or coronary arteriosclerosis or renal damage. Adrenergic blocking effect may aggravate symptoms of respiratory infections.

Drug Interactions[2] Dibenzyline (phenoxybenzamine hydrochloride) may interact with compounds that stimulate

Continued on next page

Dibenzyline—Cont.

both *alpha*- and *beta*-adrenergic receptors (i.e., epinephrine) to produce an exaggerated hypotensive response and tachycardia (See WARNING.)

Dibenzyline blocks hyperthermia production by levarterenol, and blocks hypothermia production by reserpine.

Carcinogenesis and Mutagenesis—Phenoxybenzamine hydrochloride showed *in vitro* mutagenic activity in the Ames test and mouse lymphoma assay; it did not show mutagenic activity *in vivo* in the micronucleus test in mice. In rats and mice, repeated intraperitoneal administration of phenoxybenzamine hydrochloride (three times per week for up to 52 weeks) resulted in peritoneal sarcomas. Chronic oral dosing in rats (for up to 2 years) produced malignant tumors of the small intestine and non-glandular stomach, as well as ulcerative and/or erosive gastritis of the glandular stomach. Whereas squamous cell carcinomas of the non-glandular stomach were observed at all tested doses of phenoxybenzamine hydrochloride, there was a no observed effect level of 10 mg/kg for tumors (carcinomas and sarcomas) of the small intestine. This dose is, on a body surface area basis, about twice the maximum recommended human dosage of 20 mg b.i.d.

Pregnancy-Teratogenic Effects—Pregnancy Category C. Adequate reproductive studies in animals have not been performed with Dibenzyline (phenoxybenzamine hydrochloride). It is also not known whether *Dibenzyline* can cause fetal harm when administered to a pregnant woman. *Dibenzyline* should be given to a pregnant woman only if clearly needed.

Nursing Mothers—It is not known whether this drug is excreted in human milk. Because many drugs are excreted in human milk, and because of the potential for serious adverse reactions from phenoxybenzamine hydrochloride, a decision should be made whether to discontinue nursing or to discontinue the drug, taking into account the importance of the drug to the mother.

Pediatric Use—Safety and effectiveness in pediatric patients have not been established.

ADVERSE REACTIONS

The following adverse reactions have been observed, but there are insufficient data to support an estimate of their frequency.

Autonomic Nervous System*: Postural hypotension, tachycardia, inhibition of ejaculation, nasal congestion, miosis.

Miscellaneous: Gastrointestinal irritation, drowsiness, fatigue.

OVERDOSAGE

SYMPTOMS—These are largely the result of blocking of the sympathetic nervous system and of the circulating epinephrine. They may include postural hypotension resulting in dizziness or fainting; tachycardia, particularly postural; vomiting, lethargy; shock.

*These so-called "side effects" are actually evidence of adrenergic blockade and vary according to the degree of blockade.

TREATMENT—When symptoms and signs of overdosage exist, discontinue the drug. Treatment of circulatory failure, if present, is a prime consideration. In cases of mild overdosage, recumbent position with legs elevated usually restores cerebral circulation. In the more severe cases, the usual measures to combat shock should be instituted. Usual pressor agents are *not* effective. Epinephrine is contraindicated because it stimulates both *alpha* and *beta* receptors; since *alpha* receptors are blocked, the net effect of epinephrine administration is vasodilation and a further drop in blood pressure (epinephrine reversal).

The patient may have to be kept flat for 24 hours or more in the case of overdose, as the effect of the drug is prolonged. Leg bandages and an abdominal binder may shorten the period of disability.

I.V. infusion of levarterenol bitartrate** may be used to combat severe hypotensive reactions, because it stimulates *alpha* receptors primarily. Although Dibenzyline (phenoxybenzamine hydrochloride) is an *alpha*-adrenergic blocking agent, a sufficient dose of levarterenol bitartrate will overcome this effect.

The oral LD_{50} for phenoxybenzamine hydrochloride is approximately 2000 mg/kg in rats and approximately 500 mg/kg in guinea pigs.

DOSAGE AND ADMINISTRATION

The dosage should be adjusted to fit the needs of each patient. Small initial doses should be *slowly* increased until the desired effect is obtained or the side effects from blockade become troublesome. *After each increase, the patient should be observed on that level before instituting another increase.* The dosage should be carried to a point where symptomatic relief and/or objective improvement are obtained, but not so high that the side effects from blockade become troublesome.

Initially, 10 mg of Dibenzyline (phenoxybenzamine hydrochloride) twice a day. Dosage should be increased every other day, usually to 20 to 40 mg 2 or 3 times a day, until an optimal dosage is obtained, as judged by blood pressure control.

STORAGE

Store at 25°C (77°F); excursions permitted to 15°–30°C (59°–86°F) [See USP Controlled Room Temperature].

HOW SUPPLIED

Dibenzyline (phenoxybenzamine hydrochloride) capsules, 10 mg, in bottles of 100 (*NDC* 65197-001-01).

REFERENCES

1. Weiner, N.: Drugs That Inhibit Adrenergic Nerves and Block Adrenergic Receptors, in Goodman, L., and Gilman, A., *The Pharmacological Basis of Therapeutics,* ed. 6, New York, Macmillan Publishing Co., 1980, p. 179; p. 182.
2. Martin, E.W.: *Drug Interactions Index* 1978/1979, Philadelphia, J.B. Lippincott Co., 1978, pp. 209–210.

**Available as Levophed® Bitartrate (brand of norepinephrine bitartrate) from Abbott Laboratories.

DATE OF ISSUANCE JULY 2002

Manufactured for
WellSpring Pharmaceutical Corporation
Neptune, NJ 07753-6807
by **SmithKline Beecham Pharmaceuticals**
Cidra, Puerto Rico
DI:L4
731031

Shown in Product Identification Guide, page 336

DYRENIUM® ℞

brand of
triamterene
Capsules
50 mg and 100 mg
potassium-sparing diuretic
℞ only

DESCRIPTION

Dyrenium (triamterene) is a potassium-sparing diuretic.
Structural Formula

Triamterene

Triamterene is 2, 4, 7-triamino-6-phenyl-pteridine. Its molecular weight is 253.27. At 50°C, triamterene is slightly soluble in water. It is soluble in dilute ammonia, dilute aqueous sodium hydroxide and dimethylformamide. It is sparingly soluble in methanol.

Each capsule for oral use, with opaque red cap and body, contains triamterene, 50 or 100 mg, and is imprinted with the product name DYRENIUM, strength (50 or 100) and WPC 002 (for the 50 mg strength) and WPC 003 (for the 100 mg strength). Inactive ingredients consist of D&C Red No. 33, FD&C Yellow No. 6, gelatin, lactose, magnesium stearate, povidone, sodium lauryl sulfate, titanium dioxide and trace amounts of other inactive ingredients.

CLINICAL PHARMACOLOGY

Triamterene has a unique mode of action; it inhibits the reabsorption of sodium ions in exchange for potassium and hydrogen ions at that segment of the distal tubule under the control of adrenal mineralocorticoids (especially aldosterone). This activity is not directly related to aldosterone secretion or antagonism; it is a result of a direct effect on the renal tubule.

The fraction of filtered sodium reaching this distal tubular exchange site is relatively small, and the amount which is exchanged depends on the level of mineralocorticoid activity. Thus, the degree of natriuresis and diuresis produced by inhibition of the exchange mechanism is necessarily limited. Increasing the amount of available sodium and the level of mineralocorticoid activity by the use of more proximally acting diuretics will increase the degree of diuresis and potassium conservation.

Triamterene occasionally causes increases in serum potassium which can result in hyperkalemia. It does not produce alkalosis because it does not cause excessive excretion of titratable acid and ammonium.

Triamterene has been shown to cross the placental barrier and appear in the cord blood of animals.

Pharmacokinetics

Onset of action is 2 to 4 hours after ingestion. In normal volunteers the mean peak serum levels were 30 ng/mL at 3 hours. The average percent of drug recovered in the urine (0 to 48 hours) was 21%. Triamterene is primarily metabolized to the sulfate conjugate of hydroxytriamterene. Both the plasma and urine levels of this metabolite greatly exceed triamterene levels. Triamterene is rapidly absorbed, with somewhat less than 50% of the oral dose reaching the urine. Most patients will respond to Dyrenium (triamterene) during the first day of treatment. Maximum therapeutic effect, however, may not be seen for several days. Duration of diuresis depends on several factors, especially renal function, but it generally tapers off 7 to 9 hours after administration.

INDICATIONS AND USAGE

Dyrenium (triamterene) is indicated in the treatment of edema associated with congestive heart failure, cirrhosis of the liver and the nephrotic syndrome; also in steroid-induced edema, idiopathic edema and edema due to secondary hyperaldosteronism.

Dyrenium may be used alone or with other diuretics either for its added diuretic effect or its potassium-sparing potential. It also promotes increased diuresis when patients prove resistant or only partially responsive to thiazides or other diuretics because of secondary hyperaldosteronism.

Usage in Pregnancy. The routine use of diuretics in an otherwise healthy woman is inappropriate and exposes mother and fetus to unnecessary hazard. Diuretics do not prevent development of toxemia of pregnancy, and there is no satisfactory evidence that they are useful in the treatment of developed toxemia.

Edema during pregnancy may arise from pathological causes or from the physiologic and mechanical consequences of pregnancy. Diuretics are indicated in pregnancy when edema is due to pathologic causes, just as they are in the absence of pregnancy (however, see PRECAUTIONS below). Dependent edema in pregnancy, resulting from restriction of venous return by the expanded uterus, is properly treated through elevation of the lower extremities and use of support hose; use of diuretics to lower intravascular volume in this case is illogical and unnecessary. There is hypervolemia during normal pregnancy which is harmful to neither the fetus nor the mother (in the absence of cardiovascular disease), but which is associated with edema, including generalized edema, in the majority of pregnant women. If this edema produces discomfort, increased recumbency will often provide relief. In rare instances, this edema may cause extreme discomfort which is not relieved by rest. In these cases, a short course of diuretics may provide relief and may be appropriate.

CONTRAINDICATIONS

Anuria. Severe or progressive kidney disease or dysfunction with the possible exception of nephrosis.

Severe hepatic disease. Hypersensitivity to the drug.

Dyrenium (triamterene) should not be used in patients with pre-existing elevated serum potassium, as is sometimes seen in patients with impaired renal function or azotemia, or in patients who develop hyperkalemia while on the drug. Patients should not be placed on dietary potassium supplements, potassium salts or potassium-containing salt substitutes in conjunction with *Dyrenium.*

Dyrenium should not be given to patients receiving other potassium-sparing agents such as spironolactone, amiloride hydrochloride or other formulations containing triamterene. Two deaths have been reported in patients receiving concomitant spironolactone and *Dyrenium* or Dyazide®. Although dosage recommendations were exceeded in one case and in the other serum electrolytes were not properly monitored, these two drugs should not be given concomitantly.

WARNINGS

Abnormal elevation of serum potassium levels (greater than or equal to 5.5 mEq/liter) can occur with all potassium-sparing agents, including *Dyrenium.* Hyperkalemia is more likely to occur in patients with renal impairment and diabetes (even without evidence of renal impairment), and in the elderly or severely ill. Since uncorrected hyperkalemia may be fatal, serum potassium levels must be monitored at frequent intervals especially in patients receiving *Dyrenium,* when dosages are changed or with any illness that may influence renal function.

There have been isolated reports of hypersensitivity reactions; therefore, patients should be observed regularly for the possible occurrence of blood dyscrasias, liver damage or other idiosyncratic reactions.

Periodic BUN and serum potassium determinations should be made to check kidney function, especially in patients with suspected or confirmed renal insufficiency. It is particularly important to make serum potassium determinations in elderly or diabetic patients receiving the drug; these patients should be observed carefully for possible serum potassium increases.

If hyperkalemia is present or suspected, an electrocardiogram should be obtained. If the ECG shows no widening of the QRS or arrhythmia in the presence of hyperkalemia, it is usually sufficient to discontinue Dyrenium (triamterene) and any potassium supplementation and substitute a thiazide alone. Sodium polystyrene sulfonate (Kayexalate®, Winthrop) may be administered to enhance the excretion of excess potassium. **The presence of a widened QRS complex or arrhythmia in association with hyperkalemia requires prompt additional therapy.** For tachyarrhythmia, infuse 44 mEq of sodium bicarbonate or 10 mL of 10% calcium gluconate or calcium chloride over several minutes. For asystole, bradycardia or A-V block transvenous pacing is also recommended.

The effect of calcium and sodium bicarbonate is transient and repeated administration may be required. When indicated by the clinical situation, excess K^+ may be removed by dialysis or oral or rectal administration of Kayexalate®. Infusion of glucose and insulin has also been used to treat hyperkalemia.

PRECAUTIONS

General

Dyrenium (triamterene) tends to conserve potassium rather than to promote the excretion as do many diuretics and, occasionally, can cause increases in serum potassium which,

in some instances, can result in hyperkalemia. In rare instances, hyperkalemia has been associated with cardiac irregularities.
Electrolyte imbalance often encountered in such diseases as congestive heart failure, renal disease or cirrhosis may be aggravated or caused independently by any effective diuretic agent including *Dyrenium*. The use of full doses of a diuretic when salt intake is restricted can result in a low-salt syndrome.
Triamterene can cause mild nitrogen retention which is reversible upon withdrawal of the drug and is seldom observed with intermittent (every-other-day) therapy.
Triamterene may cause a decreasing alkali reserve with the possibility of metabolic acidosis.
By the very nature of their illness, cirrhotics with splenomegaly sometimes have marked variations in their blood pictures. Since triamterene is a weak folic acid antagonist, it may contribute to the appearance of megaloblastosis in cases where folic acid stores have been depleted. Therefore, periodic blood studies in these patients are recommended. They should also be observed for exacerbations of underlying liver disease.
Triamterene has elevated uric acid, especially in persons predisposed to gouty arthritis.
Triamterene has been reported in renal stones in association with other calculus components. *Dyrenium* should be used with caution in patients with histories of renal stones.

Information for Patients

To help avoid stomach upset, it is recommended that the drug be taken after meals.
If a single daily dose is prescribed, it may be preferable to take it in the morning to minimize the effect of increased frequency of urination on nighttime sleep.
If a dose is missed, the patient should not take more than the prescribed dose at the next dosing interval.

Laboratory Tests

Hyperkalemia will rarely occur in patients with adequate urinary output, but it is a possibility if large doses are used for considerable periods of time. If hyperkalemia is observed, Dyrenium (triamterene) should be withdrawn. The normal adult range of serum potassium is 3.5 to 5.0 mEq per liter with 4.5 mEq often being used for a reference point. Potassium levels persistently above 6 mEq per liter require careful observation and treatment. Normal potassium levels tend to be higher in neonates (7.7 mEq per liter) than in adults.
Serum potassium levels do not necessarily indicate true body potassium concentration. A rise in plasma pH may cause a decrease in plasma potassium concentration and an increase in the intracellular potassium concentration. Because *Dyrenium* conserves potassium, it has been theorized that in patients who have received intensive therapy or been given the drug for prolonged periods, a rebound kaliuresis could occur upon abrupt withdrawal. In such patients withdrawal of *Dyrenium* should be gradual.

Drug Interactions

Caution should be used when lithium and diuretics are used concomitantly because diuretic-induced sodium loss may reduce the renal clearance of lithium and increase serum lithium levels with risk of lithium toxicity. Patients receiving such combined therapy should have serum lithium levels monitored closely and the lithium dosage adjusted if necessary.
A possible interaction resulting in acute renal failure has been reported in a few subjects when indomethacin, a nonsteroidal anti-inflammatory agent, was given with triamterene. Caution is advised in administering nonsteroidal anti-inflammatory agents with triamterene.
The effects of the following drugs may be potentiated when given together with triamterene: antihypertensive medication, other diuretics, preanesthetic and anesthetic agents, skeletal muscle relaxants (nondepolarizing).
Potassium-sparing agents should be used with caution in conjunction with angiotensin-converting enzyme (ACE) inhibitors due to an increased risk of hyperkalemia.
The following agents, given together with triamterene, may promote serum potassium accumulation and possibly result in hyperkalemia because of the potassium-sparing nature of triamterene, especially in patients with renal insufficiency: blood from blood bank (may contain up to 30 mEq of potassium per liter of plasma or up to 65 mEq per liter of whole blood when stored for more than 10 days); low-salt milk (may contain up to 60 mEq of potassium per liter); potassium-containing medications (such as parenteral penicillin G potassium); salt substitutes (most contain substantial amounts of potassium).
Dyrenium (triamterene) may raise blood glucose levels; for adult onset diabetes, dosage adjustments of hypoglycemic agents may be necessary during and after therapy; concurrent use with chlorpropamide may increase the risk of severe hyponatremia.

Drug/Laboratory Test Interactions

Triamterene and quinidine have similar fluorescence spectra; thus, triamterene will interfere with the fluorescent measurement of quinidine.

Carcinogenesis, Mutagenesis, Impairment of Fertility

Carcinogenesis: In studies conducted under the auspices of the National Toxicology Program, groups of rats were fed diets containing 0, 150, 300 or 600 ppm triamterene, and groups of mice were fed diets containing 0, 100, 200 or 400 ppm triamterene. Male and female rats exposed to the highest tested concentration received triamterene at about 25 and 30 mg/kg/day, respectively. Male and female mice exposed to the highest tested concentration received triamterene at about 45 and 60 mg/kg/day, respectively.
There was an increased incidence of hepatocellular neoplasia (primarily adenomas) in male and female mice at the highest dosage level. These doses represent 7.5X and 10X the Maximum Recommended Human Dose (MRHD) of 300 mg/kg/day (or 6 mg/kg/day based on a 50 kg patient) for male and female mice, respectively, when based on body weight and 0.7X and 0.9X the MRHD when based on body-surface area.
Although hepatocellular neoplasia (exclusively adenomas) in the rat study was limited to triamterene-exposed males, incidence was not dose-dependent and there was no statistically significant difference from control incidence at any dose level.
Mutagenesis: Triamterene was not mutagenic in bacteria (*Salmonella typhimurium* strains TA98, TA100, TA1535 or TA1537) with or without metabolic activation. It did not induce chromosomal aberrations in Chinese hamster ovary (CHO) cells *in vitro* with or without metabolic activation, but it did induce sister chromatid exchanges in CHO cells *in vitro* with and without metabolic activation.
Impairment of Fertility: Studies of the effects of triamterene on animal reproductive function have not been conducted.
Pregnancy: Category C
Teratogenic Effects: Reproduction studies have been performed in rats at doses as high as 20 times the Maximum Recommended Human Dose (MRHD) on the basis of body weight, and 6 times the MRHD on the basis of body surface area without evidence of harm to the fetus due to triamterene. Because animal reproduction studies are not always predictive of human response, this drug should be used during pregnancy only if clearly needed.
Nonteratogenic Effects: Triamterene has been shown to cross the placental barrier and appear in the cord blood. The use of triamterene in pregnant women requires that the anticipated benefits be weighed against possible hazards to the fetus. These possible hazards include adverse reactions which have occurred in the adult.
Nursing Mothers: Triamterene has not been studied in nursing mothers. Triamterene appears in animal milk and is likely present in human milk. If use of the drug product is deemed essential, the patient should stop nursing.
Pediatric Use: Safety and effectiveness in pediatric patients have not been established.

ADVERSE REACTIONS

Adverse effects are listed in decreasing order of frequency, however, the most serious adverse effects are listed first regardless of frequency. All adverse effects occur rarely (that is, 1 in 1000, or less).
Hypersensitivity: anaphylaxis, rash, photosensitivity.
Metabolic: hyperkalemia, hypokalemia.
Renal: azotemia, elevated BUN and creatinine, renal stones, acute interstitial nephritis (rare), acute renal failure (one case of irreversible renal failure has been reported).
Gastrointestinal: jaundice and/or liver enzyme abnormalities, nausea and vomiting, diarrhea.
Hematologic: thrombocytopenia, megaloblastic anemia.
Central Nervous System: weakness, fatigue, dizziness, headache, dry mouth.

OVERDOSAGE

In the event of overdosage it can be theorized that electrolyte imbalance would be the major concern, with particular attention to possible hyperkalemia. Other symptoms that might be seen would be nausea and vomiting, other GI disturbances and weakness. It is conceivable that some hypotension could occur. As with an overdosage of any drug, immediate evacuation of the stomach should be induced through emesis and gastric lavage. Careful evaluation of the electrolyte pattern and fluid balance should be made. There is no specific antidote.
Reversible acute renal failure following ingestion of 50 tablets of a product containing a combination of 50 mg triamterene and 25 mg hydrochlorothiazide has been reported.
The oral LD_{50} in mice is 380 mg/kg. The amount of drug in a single dose ordinarily associated with symptoms of overdose or likely to be life-threatening is not known.
Although triamterene is 67% protein-bound, there may be some benefit to dialysis in cases of overdosage.

DOSAGE AND ADMINISTRATION

Adult Dosage

Dosage should be titrated to the needs of the individual patient. When used alone, the usual starting dose is 100 mg twice daily after meals. When combined with another diuretic or antihypertensive agent, the total daily dosage of each agent should usually be lowered initially and then adjusted to the patient's needs. The total daily dosage should not exceed 300 mg. Please refer to PRECAUTIONS—General.
When Dyrenium (triamterene) is added to other diuretic therapy or when patients are switched to *Dyrenium* from other diuretics, all potassium supplementation should be discontinued.

HOW SUPPLIED

Capsules: 50 mg in bottles of 100 and 100 mg in bottles of 100.
Store between 15° and 30°C (59° and 86°F). Protect from light.
50 mg 100's: NDC 65197-002-01
100 mg 100's: NDC 65197-003-01

DATE OF ISSUANCE June 2001

Manufactured for
WellSpring Pharmaceutical Corporation
Neptune, NJ 07753 USA
by **SmithKline Beecham Pharmaceuticals**
Cidra, Puerto Rico
DY:L3
731179

Shown in Product Identification Guide, page 336

Westlake Laboratories, Inc.

24700 CENTER RIDGE ROAD
CLEVELAND, OH 44145

Direct Inquiries to:
Customer Service
(888) WSTLAKE (978–5253)
Fax (440) 835–2177
Internet: www.westlake-labs.com

BEVITAMEL® — OTC

[*bē-vĭt 'ə-mĕl*]
Melatonin-B-Vitamin Supplement

DESCRIPTION

Each tablet contains:

	Amount	% U.S.RDA*
Melatonin	3 mg	***
Methylcobalamin (Vitamin B12)	1000 µg	16667
Folic Acid	400 µg	100

* U.S. Recommended Daily Amount (RDA) established by the U.S. Food and Drug Administration (FDA).
*** The U.S.RDA has not been established by the U.S. FDA.

INDICATIONS

Bevitamel can be used to enhance the natural sleep process. Vitamin B12 and Folic Acid can be used to assist the metabolism of blood homocysteine.

CONTRAINDICATIONS

Product NOT intended for the treatment of Pernicious anemia.

WARNINGS

Keep out of reach of children and store in a cool dry place. Tamper-resistant package, do not use if outer seal is missing or broken.

PRECAUTIONS

The dose size and timing may need to be adjusted by the physician to provide maximum effect for individual patients.
Individuals taking other medications, or with autoimmune, seizure or endocrine disorders and pregnant or lactating women, should consult a physician prior to use.

ADVERSE REACTIONS

None known.

DOSAGE AND ADMINISTRATION

One tablet sub-lingual approximately 30 minutes before bedtime as directed by a physician. Fractional tablets may be taken when indicated.

OVERDOSAGE

None known.

HOW SUPPLIED

BEVITAMEL is supplied as a pink bisected sub-lingual tablet (60 per bottle).

NOTICE
Before prescribing or administering
any product described in
PHYSICIANS' DESK REFERENCE
check the **PDR Supplements**
for revised information.

Winston Laboratories, Inc.

100 FAIRWAY DRIVE
VERNON HILLS, ILLINOIS 60061 USA

Direct Inquiries to:
Customer Service:
(877)-260-6534
Medical Information Contact:
(877)-260-6534

AXSAIN™ OTC

[*ăk-sān*]
Capsaicin Cream Ø.25% in Lidocare™ Vehicle
Topical Analgesic Cream

DESCRIPTION

Axsain contains capsaicin USP, in a patented emollient base containing benzyl alcohol, cetyl alcohol, glyceryl stearate, isopropyl myristate, lidocaine hydrochloride, PEG-100 stearate, purified water; sorbitol solution and white petrolatum. Capsaicin is designated chemically as trans-8-methyl-N-vanillyl-6-nonenamide with an empirical formula of $C_{18}H_{27}NO_3$ and molecular weight of 305.4. The structural formula is:

$CH_2NH{-}C(=O){-}(CH_2)_4CH{=}CH{-}CH(CH_3)_2$ (ring substituents: OCH_3, OH)

CLINICAL PHARMACOLOGY

Although the precise mechanism of action of Axsain (capsaicin) is not fully understood, current evidence suggests that capsaicin relieves neuralgia pain by depleting and preventing reaccumulation of substance P in peripheral sensory neurons. Substance P is thought to be the principal chemomediator of pain impulses from the periphery to the central nervous system. Initial release of substance P from sensory neurons is believed to be responsible for burning or stinging sensations experienced by some individuals. Such unpleasant sensations may be reduced or prevented by Axsain's patented Lidocare™ vehicle system which contains lidocaine.

CLINICAL STUDIES

A multi-center study was conducted to assess the clinical effectiveness and safety of Axsain for treatment of painful diabetic neuropathy (PDN) and postherpetic neuralgia (PHN). Eighty-three (83) patients with PDN (n=56) or PHN (n=27) who were taking oral antiepileptics or tricyclic antidepressants with incomplete pain relief were enrolled. Axsain was applied to painful areas three times daily for 6 weeks. Following 1, 3, and 6 weeks of treatment, pain was reduced by 21%, 40%, and 50%, respectively, in patients with PDN, and by 24%, 39%, and 51%, respectively, in patients with PHN. Following treatment, 90% of patients with PDN and 94% with PHN rated themselves as Improved. When evaluated by physicians, 89% of PDN and 88% of PHN patients were rated as Improved. Transient stinging/burning sensations at the application sites were the most commonly reported adverse events, while no serious adverse events related to study drug were observed.

INDICATIONS AND USAGES

Axsain is indicated for the temporary relief of neuralgia pain, *including painful diabetic neuropathy (PDN) and postherpetic neuralgia (PHN)*, when used under the supervision of a physician. Axsain is particularly useful as adjunctive therapy for PDN and PHN patients experiencing incomplete pain relief despite taking oral antiepileptics or tricyclic antidepressants.

WARNINGS

FOR EXTERNAL USE ONLY. Do not use if you have a known sensitivity to capsaicin, local anesthetics, or to any other ingredient in Axsain. Axsain should be used with caution in patients receiving Class I antiarrhythmic drugs (such as tocainide and mexiletine) since the toxic effects of these drugs are additive and potentially synergistic. Do not use on children under 10 years of age. When using this product, a burning sensation often occurs initially at the site of application, but generally diminishes or disappears with regular use as directed. Do not apply in large quantities or to wounds or damaged skin. Avoid contact with mucous membranes, eyes, or contact lenses. If this occurs, rinse the affected area thoroughly with cool water. Avoid inhaling airborne material from dried residue. This can result in coughing, sneezing, throat or respiratory irritation. Do not bandage tightly or apply heat to the Axsain-treated area immediately before or after use. Contact a physician immediately if difficulty breathing or swallowing occurs. If condition worsens, or does not improve with regular use, discontinue use of this product and consult your physician. If you are pregnant or breast feeding, check with your physician before using this product. **Keep out of reach of children.** If swallowed, get medical help or contact a Poison Control Center immediately.

DIRECTIONS

Apply a thin film of Axsain to the affected area 2 to 4 times daily or as directed by your doctor, and gently rub in until fully absorbed. Applications fewer than 2 times a day may cause the burning sensation to persist longer and may not provide optimum pain relief. It is recommended that disposable plastic gloves be worn when applying Axsain in order to reduce the chance of transferring residual cream to eyes, mucous membranes or other areas of the body. **Wash hands thoroughly with soap and water immediately after applying Axsain.**

HOW SUPPLIED

Axsain is available in 60g tubes (NDC 66358-100-60)
Store at controlled room temperature 15°–30°C (59°–86°F)
Manufactured for:
Rodlen Laboratories, Inc.
Subsidiary of Winston Laboratories, The Pain Company ®
Vernon Hills, Il 60061
Tel: (877) 260-6534
U.S. Patent No. 4,997,853 30100-60-00
0704

Axsain, Lidocare, and Winston Laboratories The Pain Company are all trademarks of Winston Laboratories, Inc.

Shown in Product Identification Guide, page 336

Wyeth Pharmaceuticals

Division of Wyeth
P.O. BOX 8299
PHILADELPHIA, PA 19101

For Product Information Contact:
(800) 934-5556
For Product Quality Contact:
(800) 999-9384
For Sales Representative Information Contact:
(800) 395-9938
For Customer Service and Ordering Information Contact:
Pharmaceuticals and Vaccines: (800) 666-7248
For Patient Assistance Program Contact:
(800) 568-9938
For All Other Inquiries:
(610) 688-4400
www.wyeth.com

Information on these Wyeth Pharmaceuticals products is based on labeling in effect as of July 2004. Since the publication of this reference book, there may have been revisions to the labeling of these products.
For further product information and current package inserts please visit www.wyeth.com or call our Global Medical Communications Department toll-free at 1-800-934-5556.

ALESSE® 28 TABLETS ℞

[*ă'lĕs*]
(levonorgestrel and ethinyl estradiol tablets)
℞ only

This product's label may have been revised after this insert was used in production. For further product information and current package insert, please visit www.wyeth.com or call our medical communications department toll-free at 1-800-934-5556.

Patients should be counseled that oral contraceptives do not protect against transmission of HIV (AIDS) and other sexually transmitted diseases (STDs) such as chlamydia, genital herpes, genital warts, gonorrhea, hepatitis B, and syphilis.

DESCRIPTION

21 pink active tablets each containing 0.10 mg of levonorgestrel, d(-)-13β-ethyl-17α-ethinyl-17β-hydroxygon-4-en-3-one, a totally synthetic progestogen, and 0.02 mg of ethinyl estradiol, 17α-ethinyl-1,3,5(10)-estratriene-3, 17β-diol. The inactive ingredients present are cellulose, hypromellose, iron oxide, lactose, magnesium stearate, polacrilin potassium, polyethylene glycol, titanium dioxide, and wax E.

7 light-green inert tablets, each containing cellulose, FD&C blue no. 1, hypromellose, iron oxide, lactose, magnesium stearate, polacrilin potassium, polyethylene glycol, titanium dioxide, and wax E.

Levonorgestrel
$C_{21}H_{28}O_2$ M.W. 312.45

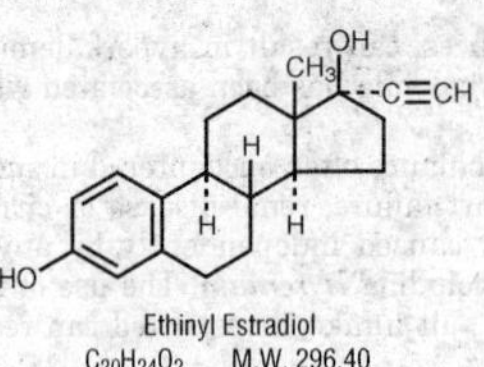

Ethinyl Estradiol
$C_{20}H_{24}O_2$ M.W. 296.40

CLINICAL PHARMACOLOGY

Mode of Action

Combination oral contraceptives act by suppression of gonadotropins. Although the primary mechanism of this action is inhibition of ovulation, other alterations include changes in the cervical mucus (which increase the difficulty of sperm entry into the uterus) and the endometrium (which reduce the likelihood of implantation).

Pharmacokinetics

Absorption

No specific investigation of the absolute bioavailability of Alesse in humans has been conducted. However, literature indicates that levonorgestrel is rapidly and completely absorbed after oral administration (bioavailability about 100%) and is not subject to first-pass metabolism. Ethinyl estradiol is rapidly and almost completely absorbed from the gastrointestinal tract but, due to first-pass metabolism in gut mucosa and liver, the bioavailability of ethinyl estradiol is between 38% and 48%.

After a single dose of Alesse to 22 women under fasting conditions, maximum serum concentrations of levonorgestrel are 2.8 ± 0.9 ng/mL (mean ± SD) at 1.6 ± 0.9 hours. At steady state, attained from day 19 onwards, maximum levonorgestrel concentrations of 6.0 ± 2.7 ng/mL are reached at 1.5 ± 0.5 hours after the daily dose. The minimum serum levels of levonorgestrel at steady state are 1.9 ± 1.0 ng/mL. Observed levonorgestrel concentrations increased from day 1 (single dose) to days 6 and 21 (multiple doses) by 34% and 96%, respectively (Figure 1). Unbound levonorgestrel concentrations increased from day 1 to days 6 and 21 by 25% and 83%, respectively. The kinetics of total levonorgestrel are non-linear due to an increase in binding of levonorgestrel to sex hormone binding globulin (SHBG), which is attributed to increased SHBG levels that are induced by the daily administration of ethinyl estradiol.

Following a single dose, maximum serum concentrations of ethinyl estradiol of 62 ± 21 pg/mL are reached at 1.5 ± 0.5 hours. At steady state, attained from at least day 6 onwards, maximum concentrations of ethinyl estradiol were 77 ± 30 pg/mL and were reached at 1.3 ± 0.7 hours after the daily dose. The minimum serum levels of ethinyl estradiol at steady state are 10.5 ± 5.1 pg/mL. Ethinyl estradiol concentrations did not increase from days 1 to 6, but did increase by 19% from days 1 to 21 (Figure 1).

[See figure 1 at top of next page]

Table I provides a summary of levonorgestrel and ethinyl estradiol pharmacokinetic parameters.

[See table I on next page]

Distribution

Levonorgestrel in serum is primarily bound to SHBG. Ethinyl estradiol is about 97% bound to plasma albumin. Ethinyl estradiol does not bind to SHBG, but induces SHBG synthesis.

Metabolism

Levonorgestrel: The most important metabolic pathway occurs in the reduction of the Δ4-3-oxo group and hydroxylation at positions 2α, 1β, and 16β, followed by conjugation. Most of the metabolites that circulate in the blood are sulfates of 3α,5β-tetrahydro-levonorgestrel, while excretion occurs predominantly in the form of glucuronides. Some of the parent levonorgestrel also circulates as 17β-sulfate. Metabolic clearance rates may differ among individuals by several-fold, and this may account in part for the wide variation observed in levonorgestrel concentrations among users.

Ethinyl estradiol: Cytochrome P450 enzymes (CYP3A4) in the liver are responsible for the 2-hydroxylation that is the major oxidative reaction. The 2-hydroxy metabolite is further transformed by methylation and glucuronidation prior to urinary and fecal excretion. Levels of Cytochrome P450 (CYP3A) vary widely among individuals and can explain the variation in rates of ethinyl estradiol 2-hydroxylation. Ethinyl estradiol is excreted in the urine and feces as glucuronide and sulfate conjugates, and undergoes enterohepatic circulation.

Excretion

The elimination half-life for levonorgestrel is approximately 36 ± 13 hours at steady state. Levonorgestrel and its metabolites are primarily excreted in the urine (40% to 68%) and about 16% to 48% are excreted in feces. The elimination half-life of ethinyl estradiol is 18 ± 4.7 hours at steady state.

Special Populations

Race

Based on the pharmacokinetic study with Alesse, there are no apparent differences in pharmacokinetic parameters among women of different races.

Hepatic insufficiency

No formal studies have evaluated the effect of hepatic disease on the disposition of Alesse. However, steroid hormones may be poorly metabolized in patients with impaired liver function.

Renal insufficiency

No formal studies have evaluated the effect of renal disease on the disposition of Alesse.

Drug-drug interactions
See **PRECAUTIONS** section - **Drug Interactions**

INDICATIONS AND USAGE

Oral contraceptives are indicated for the prevention of pregnancy in women who elect to use this product as a method of contraception.

Oral contraceptives are highly effective. Table II lists the typical accidental pregnancy rates for users of combination oral contraceptives and other methods of contraception. The efficacy of these contraceptive methods, except sterilization, the IUD, and Norplant® System, depends upon the reliability with which they are used. Correct and consistent use of methods can result in lower failure rates.

Table II: Percentage Of Women Experiencing An Unintended Pregnancy During The First Year Of Typical Use And The First Year Of Perfect Use Of Contraception And The Percentage Continuing Use At The End Of The First Year. United States.

Method (1)	% of Women Experiencing an Unintended Pregnancy within the First Year of Use: Typical Use[1] (2)	Perfect Use[2] (3)	% of Women Continuing Use at One Year[3] (4)
Chance[4]	85	85	
Spermicides[5]	26	6	40
Periodic abstinence	25		63
Calendar		9	
Ovulation Method		3	
Sympto-Thermal[6]		2	
Post-Ovulation		1	
Cap[7]			
Parous Women	40	26	42
Nulliparous Women	20	9	56
Sponge			
Parous Women	40	20	42
Nulliparous Women	20	9	56
Diaphragm[7]	20	6	56
Withdrawal	19	4	
Condom[8]			
Female (Reality)	21	5	56
Male	14	3	61
Pill	5		71
Progestin only		0.5	
Combined		0.1	
IUD			
Progesterone T	2.0	1.5	81
Copper T380A	0.8	0.6	78
LNg 20	0.1	0.1	81
Depo-Provera®	0.3	0.3	70
Levonorgestrel Implants (Norplant®)	0.05	0.05	88
Female Sterilization	0.5	0.5	100
Male Sterilization	0.15	0.10	100

Lactation Amenorrhea Method: LAM is a highly effective, temporary method of contraception.[9]

Source: Trussel J, Contraceptive efficacy. In: Hatcher RA, Trussel J, Stewart F, Cates W, Stewart GK, Kowel D, Guest F. Contraceptive Technology: Seventeenth Revised Edition. New York NY: Irvington Publishers; 1998.

1. Among *typical* couples who initiate use of a method (not necessarily for the first time), the percentage who experience an accidental pregnancy during the first year if they do not stop use for any other reason.
2. Among couples who initiate use of a method (not necessarily for the first time) and who use it perfectly (both consistently and correctly), the percentage who experience an accidental pregnancy during the first year if they do not stop use for any other reason.

FIGURE 1
Mean (SE) levonorgestrel and ethinyl estradiol serum concentrations in 22 subjects receiving Alesse (100 μg levonorgestrel and 20 μg ethinyl estradiol)

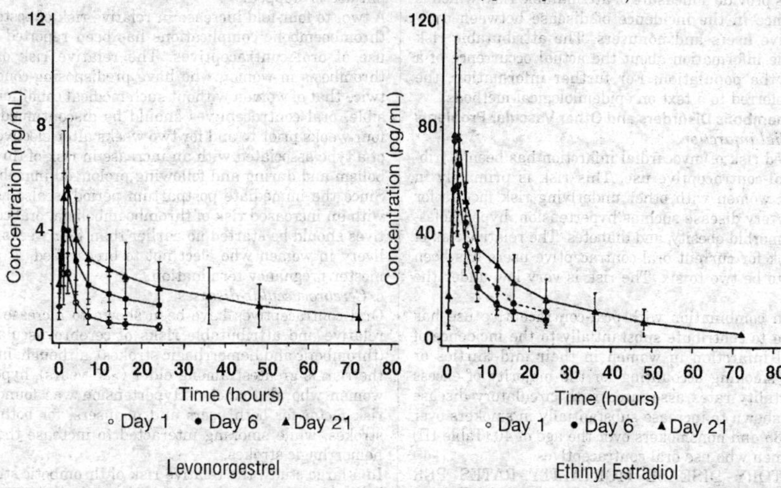

TABLE I: MEAN (SD) PHARMACOKINETIC PARAMETERS OF ALESSE OVER A 21-DAY DOSING PERIOD

Day	C_{max} ng/mL	T_{max} h	AUC ng•h/mL	CL/F mL/h/kg	Vλz/F L/kg	SHBG nmol/L
Levonorgestrel						
1	2.75 (0.88)	1.6 (0.9)	35.2 (12.8)	53.7 (20.8)	2.66 (1.09)	57 (18)
6	4.52 (1.79)	1.5 (0.7)	46.0 (18.8)	40.8 (14.5)	2.05 (0.86)	81 (25)
21	6.00 (2.65)	1.5 (0.5)	68.3 (32.5)	28.4 (10.3)	1.43 (0.62)	93 (40)
Unbound Levonorgestrel	pg/mL	h	pg•h/mL	L/h/kg	L/kg	fu %
1	51.2 (12.9)	1.6 (0.9)	654 (201)	2.79 (0.97)	135.9 (41.8)	1.92 (0.30)
6	77.9 (22.0)	1.5 (0.7)	794 (240)	2.24 (0.59)	112.4 (40.5)	1.80 (0.24)
21	103.6 (36.9)	1.5 (0.5)	1177 (452)	1.57 (0.49)	78.6 (29.7)	1.78 (0.19)
Ethinyl Estradiol	pg/mL	h	pg•h/mL	mL/h/kg	L/kg	
1	62.0 (20.5)	1.5 (0.5)	653 (227)	567 (204)	14.3 (3.7)	
6	76.7 (29.9)	1.3 (0.7)	604 (231)	610 (196)	15.5 (4.0)	
21	82.3 (33.2)	1.4 (0.6)	776 (308)	486 (179)	12.4 (4.1)	

3. Among couples attempting to avoid pregnancy, the percentage who continue to use a method for one year.
4. The percents becoming pregnant in columns (2) and (3) are based on data from populations where contraception is not used and from women who cease using contraception in order to become pregnant. Among such populations, about 89% become pregnant within one year. This estimate was lowered slightly (to 85%) to represent the percent who would become pregnant within one year among women now relying on reversible methods of contraception if they abandoned contraception altogether.
5. Foams, creams, gels, vaginal suppositories, and vaginal film.
6. Cervical mucus (ovulation) method supplemented by calendar in the pre-ovulatory and basal body temperature in the post-ovulatory phases.
7. With spermicidal cream or jelly.
8. Without spermicides.
9. However, to maintain effective protection against pregnancy, another method of contraception must be used as soon as menstruation resumes, the frequency or duration of breastfeeds is reduced, bottle feeds are introduced, or the baby reaches 6 months of age.

In a clinical trial with Alesse, (levonorgestrel and ethinyl estradiol tablets), 1,477 subjects had 7,720 cycles of use and a total of 5 pregnancies were reported. This represents an overall pregnancy rate of 0.84 per 100 woman-years. This rate includes patients who did not take the drug correctly. One or more pills were missed during 1,479 (18.8%) of the 7,870 cycles; thus all tablets were taken during 6,391 (81.2%) of the 7,870 cycles. Of the total 7,870 cycles, a total of 150 cycles were excluded from the calculation of the Pearl index due to the use of backup contraception and/or missing 3 or more consecutive pills.

CONTRAINDICATIONS

Combination oral contraceptives should not be used in women with any of the following conditions:

Thrombophlebitis or thromboembolic disorders
A past history of deep-vein thrombophlebitis or thromboembolic disorders
Cerebrovascular or coronary artery disease (current or past history)
Thrombogenic valvulopathies
Thrombogenic rhythm disorders
Major surgery with prolonged immobilization
Diabetes with vascular involvement
Headaches with focal neurological symptoms
Uncontrolled hypertension
Known or suspected carcinoma of the breast or personal history of breast cancer
Carcinoma of the endometrium or other known or suspected estrogen-dependent neoplasia
Undiagnosed abnormal genital bleeding
Cholestatic jaundice of pregnancy or jaundice with prior pill use
Hepatic adenomas or carcinomas, or active liver disease, as long as liver function has not returned to normal
Known or suspected pregnancy
Hypersensitivity to any of the components of Alesse

WARNINGS

Cigarette smoking increases the risk of serious cardiovascular side effects from oral-contraceptive use. This risk increases with age and with the extent of smoking (in epidemiologic studies, 15 or more cigarettes per day was associated with a significantly increased risk) and is quite marked in women over 35 years of age. Women who use oral contraceptives should be strongly advised not to smoke.

The use of oral contraceptives is associated with increased risks of several serious conditions including venous and arterial thrombotic and thromboembolic events (such as myocardial infarction, thromboembolism, and stroke), hepatic neoplasia, gallbladder disease, and hypertension, although the risk of serious morbidity or mortality is very small in healthy women without underlying risk factors. The risk of morbidity and mortality increases significantly in the presence of other underlying risk factors such as certain inherited or acquired thrombophilias, hypertension, hyperlipidemias, obesity, diabetes, and surgery or trauma with increased risk of thrombosis.

Practitioners prescribing oral contraceptives should be familiar with the following information relating to these risks.

The information contained in this package insert is principally based on studies carried out in patients who used oral contraceptives with higher formulations of estrogens and progestogens than those in common use today. The effect of long-term use of the oral contraceptives with lower doses of both estrogens and progestogens remains to be determined.

Throughout this labeling, epidemiological studies reported are of two types: retrospective or case control studies and prospective or cohort studies. Case control studies provide a measure of the relative risk of disease, namely, a ratio of the incidence of a disease among oral-contraceptive users to that among nonusers. The relative risk does not provide information on the actual clinical occurrence of a disease. Co-

Continued on next page

Alesse 28—Cont.

hort studies provide a measure of attributable risk, which is the difference in the incidence of disease between oral-contraceptive users and nonusers. The attributable risk does provide information about the actual occurrence of a disease in the population. For further information, the reader is referred to a text on epidemiological methods.

1. **Thromboembolic Disorders and Other Vascular Problems**

a. *Myocardial infarction*

An increased risk of myocardial infarction has been attributed to oral-contraceptive use. This risk is primarily in smokers or women with other underlying risk factors for coronary-artery disease such as hypertension, hypercholesterolemia, morbid obesity, and diabetes. The relative risk of heart attack for current oral-contraceptive users has been estimated to be two to six. The risk is very low under the age of 30.

Smoking in combination with oral-contraceptive use has been shown to contribute substantially to the incidence of myocardial infarction in women in their mid-thirties or older with smoking accounting for the majority of excess cases. Mortality rates associated with circulatory disease have been shown to increase substantially in smokers over the age of 35 and nonsmokers over the age of 40 (Table III) among women who use oral contraceptives.

CIRCULATORY DISEASE MORTALITY RATES PER 100,000 WOMAN YEARS BY AGE, SMOKING STATUS AND ORAL-CONTRACEPTIVE USE

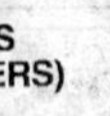
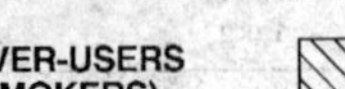
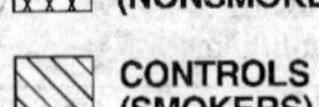

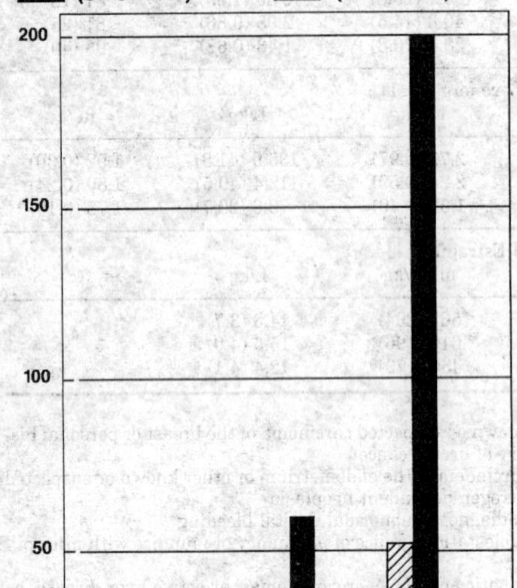

TABLE III. (Adapted from P.M. Layde and V. Beral, Lancet, *1*:541-546, 1981.)

Oral contraceptives may compound the effects of well-known risk factors, such as hypertension, diabetes, hyperlipidemias, age, and obesity. In particular, some progestogens are known to decrease HDL cholesterol and cause glucose intolerance, while estrogens may create a state of hyperinsulinism. Oral contraceptives have been shown to increase blood pressure among users (see section 9 in **WARNINGS**). Similar effects on risk factors have been associated with an increased risk of heart disease. Oral contraceptives must be used with caution in women with cardiovascular disease risk factors.

b. *Venous thrombosis and thromboembolism*

An increased risk of venous thromboembolic and thrombotic disease associated with the use of oral contraceptives is well established. Case control studies have found the relative risk of users compared to non-users to be 3 for the first episode of superficial venous thrombosis, 4 to 11 for deep-vein thrombosis or pulmonary embolism, and 1.5 to 6 for women with predisposing conditions for venous thromboembolic disease. Cohort studies have shown the relative risk to be somewhat lower, about 3 for new cases and about 4.5 for new cases requiring hospitalization. The approximate incidence of deep-vein thrombosis and pulmonary embolism in users of low dose (<50 mcg ethinyl estradiol) combination oral contraceptives is up to 4 per 10,000 woman-years compared to 0.5-3 per 10,000 woman-years for non-users. However, the incidence is substantially less than that associated with pregnancy (6 per 10,000 woman-years). The excess risk is highest during the first year a woman ever uses a combined oral contraceptive. Venous thromboembolism may be fatal. The risk of venous thrombotic and thromboembolic events is further increased in women with conditions predisposing for venous thrombosis and thromboembolism. The risk of thromboembolic disease due to oral contraceptives is not related to length of use and gradually disappears after pill use is stopped.

A two- to four-fold increase in relative risk of postoperative thromboembolic complications has been reported with the use of oral contraceptives. The relative risk of venous thrombosis in women who have predisposing conditions is twice that of women without such medical conditions. If feasible, oral contraceptives should be discontinued at least four weeks prior to and for two weeks after elective surgery of a type associated with an increase in risk of thromboembolism and during and following prolonged immobilization. Since the immediate postpartum period is also associated with an increased risk of thromboembolism, oral contraceptives should be started no earlier than four weeks after delivery in women who elect not to breast-feed, or a midtrimester pregnancy termination.

c. *Cerebrovascular diseases*

Oral contraceptives have been shown to increase both the relative and attributable risks of cerebrovascular events (thrombotic and hemorrhagic strokes), although, in general, the risk is greatest among older (>35 years), hypertensive women who also smoke. Hypertension was found to be a risk factor for both users and nonusers, for both types of strokes, while smoking interacted to increase the risk for hemorrhagic strokes.

In a large study, the relative risk of thrombotic strokes has been shown to range from 3 for normotensive users to 14 for users with severe hypertension. The relative risk of hemorrhagic stroke is reported to be 1.2 for nonsmokers who used oral contraceptives, 2.6 for smokers who did not use oral contraceptives, 7.6 for smokers who used oral contraceptives, 1.8 for normotensive users and 25.7 for users with severe hypertension. The attributable risk is also greater in older women. Oral contraceptives also increase the risk for stroke in women with other underlying risk factors such as certain inherited or acquired thrombophilias, hyperlipidemias, and obesity. Women with migraine (particularly migraine/headaches with focal neurological symptoms, see **CONTRAINDICATIONS**) who take combination oral contraceptives may be at an increased risk of stroke.

d. *Dose-related risk of vascular disease from oral contraceptives*

A positive association has been observed between the amount of estrogen and progestogen in oral contraceptives and the risk of vascular disease. A decline in serum high-density lipoproteins (HDL) has been reported with many progestational agents. A decline in serum high-density lipoproteins has been associated with an increased incidence of ischemic heart disease. Because estrogens increase HDL cholesterol, the net effect of an oral contraceptive depends on a balance achieved between doses of estrogen and progestogen and the nature and absolute amount of progestogen used in the contraceptive. The amount of both hormones should be considered in the choice of an oral contraceptive.

Minimizing exposure to estrogen and progestogen is in keeping with good principles of therapeutics. For any particular estrogen/progestogen combination, the dosage regimen prescribed should be one which contains the least amount of estrogen and progestogen that is compatible with a low failure rate and the needs of the individual patient. New acceptors of oral-contraceptive agents should be started on preparations containing the lowest estrogen content which is judged appropriate for the individual patient.

e. *Persistence of risk of vascular disease*

There are two studies which have shown persistence of risk of vascular disease for ever-users of oral contraceptives. In a study in the United States, the risk of developing myocardial infarction after discontinuing oral contraceptives persists for at least 9 years for women 40-49 years who had used oral contraceptives for five or more years, but this increased risk was not demonstrated in other age groups.

In another study in Great Britain, the risk of developing cerebrovascular disease persisted for at least 6 years after discontinuation of oral contraceptives, although excess risk was very small. However, both studies were performed with oral contraceptive formulations containing 50 mcg or higher of estrogens.

2. **Estimates of Mortality from Contraceptive Use**

One study gathered data from a variety of sources which have estimated the mortality rate associated with different methods of contraception at different ages (Table IV). These estimates include the combined risk of death associated with contraceptive methods plus the risk attributable to pregnancy in the event of method failure. Each method of contraception has its specific benefits and risks. The study concluded that with the exception of oral-contraceptive users 35 and older who smoke and 40 and older who do not smoke, mortality associated with all methods of birth control is less than that associated with childbirth. The observation of a possible increase in risk of mortality with age for oral-contraceptive users is based on data gathered in the 1970's — but not reported until 1983. However, current clinical practice involves the use of lower estrogen dose formulations combined with careful restriction of oral-contraceptive use to women who do not have the various risk factors listed in this labeling.

Because of these changes in practice and, also, because of some limited new data which suggest that the risk of cardiovascular disease with the use of oral contraceptives may now be less than previously observed, the Fertility and Maternal Health Drugs Advisory Committee was asked to review the topic in 1989. The Committee concluded that although cardiovascular disease risks may be increased with oral-contraceptive use after age 40 in healthy nonsmoking women (even with the newer low-dose formulations), there are greater potential health risks associated with pregnancy in older women and with the alternative surgical and medical procedures which may be necessary if such women do not have access to effective and acceptable means of contraception.

Therefore, the Committee recommended that the benefits of oral-contraceptive use by healthy nonsmoking women over 40 may outweigh the possible risks. Of course, older women, as all women who take oral contraceptives, should take the lowest possible dose formulation that is effective.

TABLE IV: ANNUAL NUMBER OF BIRTH-RELATED OR METHOD-RELATED DEATHS ASSOCIATED WITH CONTROL OF FERTILITY PER 100,000 NONSTERILE WOMEN, BY FERTILITY-CONTROL METHOD AND ACCORDING TO AGE

Method of control and outcome	15-19	20-24	25-29	30-34	35-39	40-44
No fertility-control methods*	7.0	7.4	9.1	14.8	25.7	28.2
Oral contraceptives nonsmoker**	0.3	0.5	0.9	1.9	13.8	31.6
Oral contraceptives smoker**	2.2	3.4	6.6	13.5	51.1	117.2
IUD**	0.8	0.8	1.0	1.0	1.4	1.4
Condom*	1.1	1.6	0.7	0.2	0.3	0.4
Diaphragm/ spermicide*	1.9	1.2	1.2	1.3	2.2	2.8
Periodic abstinence*	2.5	1.6	1.6	1.7	2.9	3.6

* Deaths are birth related
** Deaths are method related
Adapted from H.W. Ory, Family Planning Perspectives, *15*: 57-63, 1983.

3. **Carcinoma of the Reproductive Organs and Breasts**

Numerous epidemiological studies have been performed on the incidence of breast and cervical cancer in women using oral contraceptives.

The risk of having breast cancer diagnosed may be slightly increased among current and recent users of COCs. However, this excess risk appears to decrease over time after COC discontinuation and by 10 years after cessation the increased risk disappears. Some studies report an increased risk with duration of use while other studies do not and no consistent relationships have been found with dose or type of steroid. Some studies have reported a small increase in risk for women who first use COCs at a younger age. Most studies show a similar pattern of risk with COC use regardless of a woman's reproductive history or her family breast cancer history.

Breast cancers diagnosed in current or previous OC users tend to be less clinically advanced than in nonusers.

Women with known or suspected carcinoma of the breast or personal history of breast cancer should not use oral contraceptives because breast cancer is usually a hormonally-sensitive tumor.

Some studies suggest that oral contraceptive use has been associated with an increase in the risk of cervical intraepithelial neoplasia or invasive cervical cancer in some populations of women. However, there continues to be controversy about the extent to which such findings may be due to differences in sexual behavior and other factors.

In spite of many studies of the relationship between combination oral contraceptive use and breast and cervical cancers, a cause-and-effect relationship has not been established.

4. **Hepatic Neoplasia**

Benign hepatic adenomas are associated with oral-contraceptive use, although the incidence of these benign tumors is rare in the United States. Indirect calculations have estimated the attributable risk to be in the range of 3.3 cases/100,000 for users, a risk that increases after four or more years of use. Rupture of rare, benign, hepatic adenomas may cause death through intra-abdominal hemorrhage.

Studies from Britain have shown an increased risk of developing hepatocellular carcinoma in long-term (>8 years) oral-contraceptive users. However, these cancers are extremely rare in the U.S. and the attributable risk (the excess incidence) of liver cancers in oral-contraceptive users approaches less than one per million users.

5. **Ocular Lesions**

There have been clinical case reports of retinal thrombosis associated with the use of oral contraceptives that may lead to partial or complete loss of vision. Oral contraceptives should be discontinued if there is unexplained partial or complete loss of vision; onset of proptosis or diplopia; papilledema; or retinal vascular lesions. Appropriate diagnostic and therapeutic measures should be undertaken immediately.

6. **Oral-Contraceptive Use Before or During Early Pregnancy**

Extensive epidemiological studies have revealed no increased risk of birth defects in women who have used oral contraceptives prior to pregnancy. Studies also do not suggest a teratogenic effect, particularly insofar as cardiac anomalies and limb-reduction defects are concerned, when taken inadvertently during early pregnancy (see **CONTRAINDICATIONS** section).

The administration of oral contraceptives to induce withdrawal bleeding should not be used as a test for pregnancy. Oral contraceptives should not be used during pregnancy to treat threatened or habitual abortion.

It is recommended that for any patient who has missed two consecutive periods, pregnancy should be ruled out before continuing oral-contraceptive use. If the patient has not adhered to the prescribed schedule, the possibility of pregnancy should be considered at the time of the first missed period. Oral-contraceptive use should be discontinued if pregnancy is confirmed.

7. **Gallbladder Disease**

Combination oral contraceptives may worsen existing gallbladder disease and may accelerate the development of this disease in previously asymptomatic women. Earlier studies have reported an increased lifetime relative risk of gallbladder surgery in users of oral contraceptives and estrogens. More recent studies, however, have shown that the relative risk of developing gallbladder disease among oral-contraceptive users may be minimal. The recent findings of minimal risk may be related to the use of oral-contraceptive formulations containing lower hormonal doses of estrogens and progestogens.

8. **Carbohydrate and Lipid Metabolic Effects**

Oral contraceptives have been shown to cause glucose intolerance in a significant percentage of users. Oral contraceptives containing greater than 75 mcg of estrogens cause hyperinsulinism, while lower doses of estrogen cause less glucose intolerance. Progestogens increase insulin secretion and create insulin resistance, this effect varying with different progestational agents. However, in the nondiabetic woman, oral contraceptives appear to have no effect on fasting blood glucose. Because of these demonstrated effects, prediabetic and diabetic women should be carefully observed while taking oral contraceptives.

A small proportion of women will have persistent hypertriglyceridemia while on the pill. As discussed earlier (see **WARNINGS**, 1a. and 1d.; **PRECAUTIONS**, 3.), changes in serum triglycerides and lipoprotein levels have been reported in oral-contraceptive users.

9. **Elevated Blood Pressure**

An increase in blood pressure has been reported in women taking oral contraceptives and this increase is more likely in older oral-contraceptive users and with continued use. Data from the Royal College of General Practitioners and subsequent randomized trials have shown that the incidence of hypertension increases with increasing quantities of progestogens.

Women with a history of hypertension or hypertension-related diseases, or renal disease should be encouraged to use another method of contraception. If women with hypertension elect to use oral contraceptives, they should be monitored closely and if significant elevation of blood pressure occurs, oral contraceptives should be discontinued (see **CONTRAINDICATIONS** section). For most women, elevated blood pressure will return to normal after stopping oral contraceptives, and there is no difference in the occurrence of hypertension among ever- and never-users.

10. **Headache**

The onset or exacerbation of migraine or development of headache with a new pattern that is recurrent, persistent, or severe requires discontinuation of oral contraceptives and evaluation of the cause. (See **WARNINGS**, 1c. and **CONTRAINDICATIONS**.)

11. **Bleeding Irregularities**

Breakthrough bleeding and spotting are sometimes encountered in patients on oral contraceptives, especially during the first three months of use. The type and dose of progestogen may be important. If bleeding persists or recurs, nonhormonal causes should be considered and adequate diagnostic measures taken to rule out malignancy or pregnancy in the event of breakthrough bleeding, as in the case of any abnormal vaginal bleeding. If pathology has been excluded, time or a change to another formulation may solve the problem. In some women withdrawal bleeding may not occur during the "tablet free" or "inactive-tablet" interval. If the COC has not been taken according to directions prior to the first missed withdrawal bleed, or if two consecutive withdrawal bleeds are missed, tablet-taking should be discontinued and a nonhormonal method of contraception should be used until the possibility of pregnancy is excluded.

Some women may encounter post-pill amenorrhea or oligomenorrhea (possibly with anovulation), especially when such a condition was preexistent.

12. **Ectopic Pregnancy**

Ectopic as well as intrauterine pregnancy may occur in contraceptive failures.

PRECAUTIONS

1. **General**

Patients should be counseled that oral contraceptives do not protect against transmission of HIV (AIDS) and other sexually transmitted diseases (STDs) such as chlamydia, genital herpes, genital warts, gonorrhea, hepatitis B, and syphilis.

2. **Physical Examination and Follow-Up**

A periodic personal and family medical history and complete physical examination are appropriate for all women, including women using oral contraceptives. The physical examination, however, may be deferred until after initiation of oral contraceptives if requested by the woman and judged appropriate by the clinician. The physical examination should include special reference to blood pressure, breasts, abdomen, and pelvic organs, including cervical cytology, and relevant laboratory tests. In case of undiagnosed, persistent, or recurrent abnormal vaginal bleeding, appropriate diagnostic measures should be conducted to rule out malignancy. Women with a strong family history of breast cancer or who have breast nodules should be monitored with particular care.

3. **Lipid Disorders**

Women who are being treated for hyperlipidemias should be followed closely if they elect to use oral contraceptives. Some progestogens may elevate LDL levels and may render the control of hyperlipidemias more difficult. (See **WARNINGS**, 1a., 1d., and 8.)

In patients with elevated triglycerides, estrogen-containing preparations may be associated with rare but large elevations of plasma triglycerides which may lead to pancreatitis.

4. **Liver Function**

If jaundice develops in any woman receiving such drugs, the medication should be discontinued. Steroid hormones may be poorly metabolized in patients with impaired liver function.

5. **Fluid Retention**

Oral contraceptives may cause some degree of fluid retention. They should be prescribed with caution, and only with careful monitoring, in patients with conditions which might be aggravated by fluid retention.

6. **Emotional Disorders**

Patients becoming significantly depressed while taking oral contraceptives should stop the medication and use an alternate method of contraception in an attempt to determine whether the symptom is drug related. Women with a history of depression should be carefully observed and the drug discontinued if depression recurs to a serious degree.

7. **Contact Lenses**

Contact-lens wearers who develop visual changes or changes in lens tolerance should be assessed by an ophthalmologist.

8. **Gastrointestinal**

Diarrhea and/or vomiting may reduce hormone absorption resulting in decreased serum concentrations.

9. **Drug Interactions**

Changes in contraceptive effectiveness associated with coadministration of other products:

Contraceptive effectiveness may be reduced when hormonal contraceptives are coadministered with antibiotics, anticonvulsants, and other drugs that increase the metabolism of contraceptive steroids. This could result in unintended pregnancy or breakthrough bleeding. Examples include rifampin, rifabutin, barbiturates, primidone, phenylbutazone, phenytoin, dexamethasone, carbamazepine, felbamate, oxcarbazepine, topiramate, griseofulvin, and modafinil. Several cases of contraceptive failure and breakthrough bleeding have been reported in the literature with concomitant administration of antibiotics such as ampicillin and other penicillins, and tetracyclines, possibly due to a decrease of enterohepatic recirculation of estrogens. However, clinical pharmacology studies investigating drug interactions between combined oral contraceptives and these antibiotics have reported inconsistent results. Enterohepatic recirculation of estrogens may also be decreased by substances that reduce gut transit time.

Several of the anti-HIV protease inhibitors have been studied with co-administration of oral combination hormonal contraceptives; significant changes (increase and decrease) in the plasma levels of the estrogen and progestin have been noted in some cases. The safety and efficacy of oral contraceptive products may be affected with coadministration of anti-HIV protease inhibitors. Healthcare providers should refer to the label of the individual anti-HIV protease inhibitors for further drug-drug interaction information.

Herbal products containing St. John's Wort (Hypericum perforatum) may induce hepatic enzymes (cytochrome P 450) and p-glycoprotein transporter and may reduce the effectiveness of contraceptive steroids. This may also result in breakthrough bleeding.

During concomitant use of ethinyl estradiol containing products and substances that may lead to decreased plasma steroid hormone concentrations, it is recommended that a nonhormonal back-up method of birth control be used in addition to the regular intake of Alesse (levonorgestrel and ethinyl estradiol tablets). If the use of a substance which leads to decreased ethinyl estradiol plasma concentrations is required for a prolonged period of time, combination oral contraceptives should not be considered the primary contraceptive.

After discontinuation of substances that may lead to decreased ethinyl estradiol plasma concentrations, use of a nonhormonal back-up method of birth control is recommended for 7 days. Longer use of a back-up method is advisable after discontinuation of substances that have led to induction of hepatic microsomal enzymes, resulting in decreased ethinyl estradiol concentrations. It may take several weeks until enzyme induction has completely subsided, depending on dosage, duration of use, and rate of elimination of the inducing substance.

Increase in plasma levels associated with co-administered drugs:

Co-administration of atorvastatin and certain oral contraceptives containing ethinyl estradiol increases AUC values for ethinyl estradiol by approximately 20%. The mechanism of this interaction is unknown. Ascorbic acid and acetaminophen increase the bioavailability of ethinyl estradiol since these drugs act as competitive inhibitors for sulfation of ethinyl estradiol in the gastrointestinal wall, a known pathway of elimination for ethinyl estradiol. CYP 3A4 inhibitors such as indinavir, itraconazole, ketoconazole, fluconazole, and troleandomycin may increase plasma hormone levels. Troleandomycin may also increase the risk of intrahepatic cholestasis during coadministration with combination oral contraceptives.

Changes in plasma levels of co-administered drugs:

Combination hormonal contraceptives containing some synthetic estrogens (eg, ethinyl estradiol) may inhibit the metabolism of other compounds. Increased plasma concentrations of cyclosporin, prednisolone and other corticosteroids, and theophylline have been reported with concomitant administration of oral contraceptives. Decreased plasma concentrations of acetaminophen and increased clearance of temazepam, salicylic acid, morphine, and clofibric acid, due to induction of conjugation (particularly glucuronidation), have been noted when these drugs were administered with oral contraceptives.

The prescribing information of concomitant medications should be consulted to identify potential interactions.

10. **Interactions with Laboratory Tests**

Certain endocrine- and liver-function tests and blood components may be affected by oral contraceptives:

a. Increased prothrombin and factors VII, VIII, IX, and X; decreased antithrombin 3; increased norepinephrine-induced platelet aggregability.

b. Increased thyroid-binding globulin (TBG) leading to increased circulating total thyroid hormone, as measured by protein-bound iodine (PBI), T_4 by column or by radioimmunoassay. Free T_3 resin uptake is decreased, reflecting the elevated TBG; free T_4 concentration is unaltered.

c. Other binding proteins may be elevated in serum ie, corticosteroid binding globulin (CBG), sex hormone-binding globulins (SHBG) leading to increased levels of total circulating corticosteroids and sex steroids respectively. Free or biologically active hormone concentrations are unchanged.

d. Triglycerides may be increased and levels of various other lipids and lipoproteins may be affected.

e. Glucose tolerance may be decreased.

f. Serum folate levels may be depressed by oral-contraceptive therapy. This may be of clinical significance if a woman becomes pregnant shortly after discontinuing oral contraceptives.

11. **Carcinogenesis**

See **WARNINGS** section.

12. **Pregnancy**

Pregnancy Category X. See **CONTRAINDICATIONS** and **WARNINGS** sections.

13. **Nursing Mothers**

Small amounts of oral-contraceptive steroids and/or metabolites have been identified in the milk of nursing mothers, and a few adverse effects on the child have been reported, including jaundice and breast enlargement. In addition, combination oral contraceptives given in the postpartum period may interfere with lactation by decreasing the quantity and quality of breast milk. If possible, the nursing mother should be advised not to use combination oral contraceptives but to use other forms of contraception until she has completely weaned her child.

14. **Fertility Following Discontinuation**

Users of combination oral contraceptives may experience some delay in becoming pregnant after discontinuation of COCs, especially those women who had irregular menstrual cycles prior to use. Conception may be delayed an average of 1-2 months among women stopping COCs compared to women stopping nonhormonal contraceptive methods.

Women who do not wish to become pregnant after discontinuation of COCs should be advised to use another method of birth control.

15. **Pediatric Use**

Safety and efficacy of Alesse tablets have been established in women of reproductive age. Safety and efficacy are expected to be the same for postpubertal adolescents under the age of 16 and for users 16 years and older. Use of this product before menarche is not indicated.

16. **Geriatric use**

This product has not been studied in women over 65 years of age and is not indicated in this population.

17. **Information for the Patient**

See Patient Labeling Printed Below.

ADVERSE REACTIONS

An increased risk of the following serious adverse reactions (see **WARNINGS** section for additional information) has been associated with the use of oral contraceptives:

Thromboembolic and thrombotic disorders and other vascular problems (including thrombophlebitis and venous thrombosis with or without pulmonary embolism, arterial thromboembolism, myocardial infarction, cerebral hemorrhage, cerebral thrombosis), carcinoma of the reproductive organs and breasts, hepatic neoplasia (including hepatic adenomas or benign liver tumors), ocular lesions (including retinal vascular thrombosis), gallbladder disease, carbohydrate and lipid effects, elevated blood pressure, and headache.

The following adverse reactions have been reported in patients receiving oral contraceptives and are believed to be drug related (alphabetically listed):

Acne

Aggravation of varicose veins

Continued on next page

Alesse 28—Cont.

Amenorrhea
Anaphylactic/anaphylactoid reactions, including urticaria, angioedema, and severe reactions with respiratory and circulatory symptoms
Breakthrough bleeding
Breast changes: tenderness, pain, enlargement, secretion
Budd-Chiari syndrome
Change in cervical erosion and secretion
Change in corneal curvature (steepening)
Changes in libido
Change in menstrual flow
Change in weight or appetite (increase or decrease)
Cholestatic jaundice
Colitis
Decrease in serum folate levels
Diminution in lactation when given immediately postpartum
Dizziness
Edema/fluid retention
Erythema multiforme
Erythema nodosum
Exacerbation of chorea
Exacerbation of porphyria
Exacerbation of systemic lupus erythematosus
Gastrointestinal symptoms (such as abdominal pain, cramps, and bloating)
Hirsutism
Intolerance to contact lenses
Loss of scalp hair
Melasma/chloasma which may persist
Mesenteric thrombosis
Mood changes, including depression
Nausea
Nervousness
Pancreatitis
Rash (allergic)
Spotting
Temporary infertility after discontinuation of treatment
Vaginitis, including candidiasis
Vomiting

The following adverse reactions have been reported in users of oral contraceptives:

Cataracts
Cystitis-like syndrome
Dysmenorrhea
Hemolytic uremic syndrome
Hemorrhagic eruption
Impaired renal function
Optic neuritis, which may lead to partial or complete loss of vision
Premenstrual syndrome

OVERDOSAGE

Symptoms of oral contraceptive overdosage in adults and children may include nausea, vomiting, and drowsiness/fatigue; withdrawal bleeding may occur in females. There is no specific antidote and further treatment of overdose, if necessary, is directed to the symptoms.

NONCONTRACEPTIVE HEALTH BENEFITS

The following noncontraceptive health benefits related to the use of oral contraceptives are supported by epidemiological studies which largely utilized oral-contraceptive formulations containing doses exceeding 0.035 mg of ethinyl estradiol or 0.05 mg of mestranol.

Effects on menses:
Increased menstrual cycle regularity
Decreased blood loss and decreased incidence of iron-deficiency anemia
Decreased incidence of dysmenorrhea

Effects related to inhibition of ovulation:
Decreased incidence of functional ovarian cysts
Decreased incidence of ectopic pregnancies

Effects from long-term use:
Decreased incidence of fibroadenomas and fibrocystic disease of the breast
Decreased incidence of acute pelvic inflammatory disease
Decreased incidence of endometrial cancer
Decreased incidence of ovarian cancer

DOSAGE AND ADMINISTRATION

To achieve maximum contraceptive effectiveness, Alesse® (levonorgestrel and ethinyl estradiol tablets) must be taken exactly as directed and at intervals not exceeding 24 hours. The possibility of ovulation and conception prior to initiation of medication should be considered. The dispenser should be kept in the wallet supplied to avoid possible fading of the pills. If the pills fade, patients should continue to take them as directed.

The dosage of Alesse-28 is one pink tablet daily for 21 consecutive days, followed by one light-green inert tablet daily for 7 consecutive days, according to the prescribed schedule. It is recommended that Alesse-28 tablets be taken at the same time each day.

Sunday start:

During the first cycle of medication, the patient is instructed to begin taking Alesse-28 on the first Sunday after the onset of menstruation. If menstruation begins on a Sunday, the first tablet (pink) is taken that day. One pink tablet should be taken daily for 21 consecutive days, followed by one light-green inert tablet daily for seven consecutive days. Withdrawal bleeding should usually occur within three days following discontinuation of pink tablets and may not have finished before the next pack is started. During the first cycle, contraceptive reliance should not be placed on Alesse-28 until a pink tablet has been taken daily for 7 consecutive days, and a nonhormonal back-up method of birth control should be used during those 7 days. The possibility of ovulation and conception prior to initiation of medication should be considered.

The patient begins her next and all subsequent 28-day courses of tablets on the same day of the week (Sunday) on which she began her first course, following the same schedule: 21 days on pink tablets — 7 days on light-green inert tablets. If in any cycle the patient starts tablets later than the proper day, she should protect herself against pregnancy by using a nonhormonal back-up method of birth control until she has taken a pink tablet daily for 7 consecutive days.

Day 1 start:

During the first cycle of medication, the patient is instructed to begin taking Alesse-28 during the first 24 hours of her period (day one of her menstrual cycle). One pink tablet should be taken daily for 21 consecutive days, followed by one light-green inert tablet daily for seven consecutive days. Withdrawal bleeding should usually occur within three days following discontinuation of pink tablets and may not have finished before the next pack is started. If medication is begun on day one of the menstrual cycle, no back-up contraception is necessary. If Alesse-28 tablets are started later than day one of the first menstrual cycle or postpartum, contraceptive reliance should not be placed on Alesse-28 tablets until after the first 7 consecutive days of administration, and a nonhormonal back-up method of birth control should be used during those 7 days. The possibility of ovulation and conception prior to initiation of medication should be considered.

When the patient is switching from a 21-day regimen of tablets, she should wait 7 days after her last tablet before she starts Alesse. She will probably experience withdrawal bleeding during that week. She should be sure that no more than 7 days pass after her previous 21-day regimen. When the patient is switching from a 28-day regimen of tablets, she should start her first pack of Alesse on the day after her last tablet. She should not wait any days between packs. The patient may switch any day from a progestin-only pill and should begin Alesse the next day. If switching from an implant or injection, the patient should start Alesse on the day of implant removal or, if using an injection, the day the next injection would be due. In switching from a progestin-only pill, injection, or implant, the patient should be advised to use a nonhormonal back-up method of birth control for the first 7 days of tablet-taking.

If spotting or breakthrough bleeding occur, the patient is instructed to continue on the same regimen. This type of bleeding is usually transient and without significance; however, if the bleeding is persistent or prolonged, the patient is advised to consult her physician. While there is little likelihood of ovulation occurring if only one or two pink tablets are missed, the possibility of ovulation increases with each successive day that scheduled pink tablets are missed. Although the occurrence of pregnancy is unlikely if Alesse is taken according to directions, if withdrawal bleeding does not occur, the possibility of pregnancy must be considered. If the patient has not adhered to the prescribed schedule (missed one or more tablets or started taking them on a day later than she should have), the probability of pregnancy should be considered at the time of the first missed period and appropriate diagnostic measures taken before the medication is resumed. If the patient has adhered to the prescribed regimen and misses two consecutive periods, pregnancy should be ruled out before continuing the contraceptive regimen.

The risk of pregnancy increases with each active (pink) tablet missed. For additional patient instructions regarding missed tablets, see the **WHAT TO DO IF YOU MISS PILLS** section in the **DETAILED PATIENT LABELING** below.

Alesse may be initiated no earlier than day 28 postpartum in the nonlactating mother or after a second-trimester abortion due to the increased risk for thromboembolism (see **CONTRAINDICATIONS**, **WARNINGS**, and **PRECAUTIONS** concerning thromboembolic disease). The patient should be advised to use a nonhormonal back-up method for the first 7 days of tablet-taking. However, if intercourse has already occurred, pregnancy should be excluded before the start of combined oral contraceptive use or the patient must wait for her first menstrual period.

In the case of first-trimester abortion, if the patient starts Alesse immediately, additional contraceptive measures are not needed.

HOW SUPPLIED

Alesse®-28 tablets (0.10 mg levonorgestrel and 0.02 mg ethinyl estradiol) are available in packages of 3 MINI-PACK™ dispensers of 28 tablets each, NDC 0008-2576-02, as follows:

21 active tablets, NDC 0008-0912, pink, round tablet marked "W" and "912".

7 inert tablets, NDC 0008-0650, light-green, round tablet marked "W" and "650".

Store at controlled room temperature 20° to 25°C (68° to 77°F).

References available upon request.

Brief Summary Patient Package Insert

This product (like all oral contraceptives) is intended to prevent pregnancy. Oral contraceptives do not protect against transmission of HIV (AIDS) and other sexually transmitted diseases (STDs) such as chlamydia, genital herpes, genital warts, gonorrhea, hepatitis B, and syphilis.

Oral contraceptives, also known as "birth-control pills" or "the pill," are taken to prevent pregnancy, and when taken correctly, have a failure rate of approximately 1.0% per year when used without missing any pills. The average failure rate of large numbers of pill users is approximately 5% per year when women who miss pills are included. For most women oral contraceptives are also free of serious or unpleasant side effects. However, forgetting to take pills considerably increases the chances of pregnancy.

For the majority of women, oral contraceptives can be taken safely. But there are some women who are at high risk of developing certain serious diseases that can be life-threatening or may cause temporary or permanent disability or death. The risks associated with taking oral contraceptives increase significantly if you:

- smoke.
- have high blood pressure, diabetes, high cholesterol, or a tendency to form blood clots, or are obese.
- have or have had clotting disorders, heart attack, stroke, angina pectoris, cancer of the breast or sex organs, jaundice, malignant or benign liver tumors, or major surgery with prolonged immobilization.
- have headaches with neurological symptoms.

You should not take the pill if you suspect you are pregnant or have unexplained vaginal bleeding.

Cigarette smoking increases the risk of serious adverse effects on the heart and blood vessels from oral-contraceptive use. This risk increases with age and with the amount of smoking (15 or more cigarettes per day has been associated with a significantly increased risk) and is quite marked in women over 35 years of age. Women who use oral contraceptives should not smoke.

Most side effects of the pill are not serious. The most common such effects are nausea, vomiting, bleeding between menstrual periods, weight gain, breast tenderness, and difficulty wearing contact lenses. These side effects, especially nausea and vomiting, may subside within the first three months of use.

The serious side effects of the pill occur very infrequently, especially if you are in good health and do not smoke. However, you should know that the following medical conditions have been associated with or made worse by the pill:

1. Blood clots in the legs (thrombophlebitis), lungs (pulmonary embolism), stoppage or rupture of a blood vessel in the brain (stroke), blockage of blood vessels in the heart (heart attack and angina pectoris) or other organs of the body. As mentioned above, smoking increases the risk of heart attacks and strokes and subsequent serious medical consequences. Women with migraine also may be at increased risk of stroke with pill use.

2. Liver tumors, which may rupture and cause severe bleeding. A possible but not definite association has been found with the pill and liver cancer. However, liver cancers are extremely rare. The chance of developing liver cancer from using the pill is thus even rarer.

3. High blood pressure, although blood pressure usually returns to normal when the pill is stopped.

The symptoms associated with these serious side effects are discussed in the detailed leaflet given to you with your supply of pills. Notify your health-care provider if you notice any unusual physical disturbances while taking the pill. In addition, drugs such as rifampin, as well as some anticonvulsants and some antibiotics, herbal preparations containing St. John's Wort (Hypericum perforatum), and HIV/AIDS drugs may decrease oral-contraceptive effectiveness.

Various studies give conflicting reports on the relationship between breast cancer and oral contraceptive use.

Oral contraceptive use may slightly increase your chance of having breast cancer diagnosed, particularly if you started using hormonal contraceptives at a younger age.

After you stop using hormonal contraceptives, the chances of having breast cancer diagnosed begin to go down and disappear 10 years after stopping use of the pill. It is not known whether this slightly increased risk of having breast cancer diagnosed is caused by the pill. It may be that women taking the pill were examined more often, so that breast cancer was more likely to be detected.

You should have regular breast examinations by a health care professional and examine your own breasts monthly. Tell your health care professional if you have a family history of breast cancer or if you have had breast nodules or an abnormal mammogram. Women who currently have or have had breast cancer should not use oral contraceptives because breast cancer is usually a hormone-sensitive tumor.

Some studies have found an increase in the incidence of cancer of the cervix in women who use oral contraceptives. However, this finding may be related to factors other than the use of oral contraceptives. There is insufficient evidence to rule out the possibility that the pill may cause such cancers.

Taking the pill provides some important noncontraceptive benefits. These include less painful menstruation, less menstrual blood loss and anemia, fewer pelvic infections, and fewer cancers of the ovary and the lining of the uterus.

Be sure to discuss any medical condition you may have with your health-care provider. Your health-care provider will take a medical and family history before prescribing oral contraceptives and will examine you. The physical examination may be delayed to another time if you request it and the health-care provider believes that it is appropriate to postpone it. You should be reexamined at least once a year while taking oral contraceptives. The detailed patient information leaflet gives you further information which you should read and discuss with your health-care provider.

DETAILED PATIENT LABELING

This product (like all oral contraceptives) is intended to prevent pregnancy. Oral contraceptives do not protect against transmission of HIV (AIDS) and other sexually transmitted diseases (STDs) such as chlamydia, genital herpes, genital warts, gonorrhea, hepatitis B, and syphilis.

INTRODUCTION

Any woman who considers using oral contraceptives (the "birth-control pill" or "the pill") should understand the benefits and risks of using this form of birth control. This leaflet will give you much of the information you will need to make this decision and will also help you determine if you are at risk of developing any of the serious side effects of the pill. It will tell you how to use the pill properly so that it will be as effective as possible. However, this leaflet is not a replacement for a careful discussion between you and your health-care provider. You should discuss the information provided in this leaflet with him or her, both when you first start taking the pill and during your revisits. You should also follow your health-care provider's advice with regard to regular check-ups while you are on the pill.

EFFECTIVENESS OF ORAL CONTRACEPTIVES

Oral contraceptives or "birth-control pills" or "the pill" are used to prevent pregnancy and are more effective than other nonsurgical methods of birth control. When they are taken correctly, without missing any pills the chance of becoming pregnant is approximately 1.0% per year. Average failure rates are approximately 5% per year when women who miss pills are included. The chance of becoming pregnant increases with each missed pill during the menstrual cycle.

In comparison, average failure rates for other methods of birth control during the first year of use are as follows:

IUD: 0.1-2%	Female condom alone: 21%
Depo-Provera® (injectable progestogen): 0.3%	Cervical cap
Norplant® System (levonorgestrel implants): 0.05%	Never given birth: 20%
Diaphragm with spermicides: 20%	Given birth: 40%
Spermicides alone: 26%	Periodic abstinence: 25%
Male condom alone: 14%	No methods: 85%

WHO SHOULD NOT TAKE ORAL CONTRACEPTIVES

Cigarette smoking increases the risk of serious adverse effects on the heart and blood vessels from oral-contraceptive use. This risk increases with age and with the amount of smoking (15 or more cigarettes per day has been associated with a significantly increased risk) and is quite marked in women over 35 years of age. Women who use oral contraceptives should not smoke.

Some women should not use the pill. For example, you should not take the pill if you have any of the following conditions:

- Heart attack or stroke.
- Blood clots in the legs (thrombophlebitis), lungs (pulmonary embolism), or eyes.
- A history of blood clots in the deep veins of your legs.
- Chest pain (angina pectoris).
- Known or suspected breast cancer or cancer of the lining of the uterus, cervix or vagina, or certain hormonally-sensitive cancers.
- Unexplained vaginal bleeding (until a diagnosis is reached by your health-care provider).
- Liver tumor (benign or cancerous).
- Yellowing of the whites of the eyes or of the skin (jaundice) during pregnancy or during previous use of the pill.
- Known or suspected pregnancy.
- A need for surgery with prolonged bedrest.
- Heart valve or heart rhythm disorders that may be associated with formation of blood clots.
- Diabetes affecting your circulation.
- Headaches with neurological symptoms.
- Uncontrolled high blood pressure.
- Active liver disease with abnormal liver function tests.
- Allergy or hypersensitivity to any of the components of Alesse (levonorgestrel and ethinyl estradiol tablets).

Tell your health-care provider if you have had any of these conditions. Your health-care provider can recommend another method of birth control.

OTHER CONSIDERATIONS BEFORE TAKING ORAL CONTRACEPTIVES

Tell your health-care provider if you or any family member has ever had:

- Breast nodules, fibrocystic disease of the breast, an abnormal breast X-ray or mammogram.
- Diabetes.
- Elevated cholesterol or triglycerides.
- High blood pressure.
- A tendency to form blood clots.
- Migraine or other headaches or epilepsy.
- Mental depression.
- Gallbladder, liver, heart, or kidney disease.
- History of scanty or irregular menstrual periods.

Women with any of these conditions should be checked often by their health-care provider if they choose to use oral contraceptives. Also, be sure to inform your health-care provider if you smoke or are on any medications.

RISKS OF TAKING ORAL CONTRACEPTIVES

1. *Risk of developing blood clots*

Blood clots and blockage of blood vessels are the most serious side effects of taking oral contraceptives and can cause death or serious disability. In particular, a clot in the legs can cause thrombophlebitis and a clot that travels to the lungs can cause a sudden blocking of the vessel carrying blood to the lungs. Rarely, clots occur in the blood vessels of the eye and may cause blindness, double vision, or impaired vision.

Users of COCs have a higher risk of developing blood clots compared to non-users. This risk is highest during the first year of COC use.

If you take oral contraceptives and need elective surgery, need to stay in bed for a prolonged illness or injury, or have recently delivered a baby, you may be at risk of developing blood clots. You should consult your health-care provider about stopping oral contraceptives three to four weeks before surgery and not taking oral contraceptives for two weeks after surgery or during bed rest. You should also not take oral contraceptives soon after delivery of a baby or a midtrimester pregnancy termination. It is advisable to wait for at least four weeks after delivery if you are not breast-feeding. If you are breast-feeding, you should wait until you have weaned your child before using the pill. (See also the section on breast-feeding in GENERAL PRECAUTIONS.)

2. *Heart attacks and strokes*

Oral contraceptives may increase the tendency to develop strokes (stoppage or rupture of blood vessels in the brain) and angina pectoris and heart attacks (blockage of blood vessels in the heart). Any of these conditions can cause death or serious disability.

Smoking greatly increases the possibility of suffering heart attacks and strokes. Furthermore, smoking and the use of oral contraceptives greatly increase the chances of developing and dying of heart disease.

Women with migraine (especially migraine/headache with neurological symptoms) who take oral contraceptives also may be at higher risk of stroke.

3. *Gallbladder disease*

Oral-contraceptive users probably have a greater risk than nonusers of having gallbladder disease, although this risk may be related to pills containing high doses of estrogens. Oral-contraceptives may worsen existing gallbladder disease or accelerate the development of gallbladder disease in women previously without symptoms.

4. *Liver tumors*

In rare cases, oral contraceptives can cause benign but dangerous liver tumors. These benign liver tumors can rupture and cause fatal internal bleeding. In addition, a possible but not definite association has been found with the pill and liver cancers in two studies in which a few women who developed these very rare cancers were found to have used oral contraceptives for long periods. However, liver cancers are extremely rare. The chance of developing liver cancer from using the pill is thus even rarer.

5. *Cancer of the reproductive organs and breasts*

Various studies give conflicting reports on the relationship between breast cancer and oral contraceptive use.

Oral contraceptive use may slightly increase your chance of having breast cancer diagnosed, particularly if you started using hormonal contraceptives at a younger age.

After you stop using hormonal contraceptives, the chances of having breast cancer diagnosed begin to go down and disappear 10 years after stopping use of the pill. It is not known whether this slightly increased risk of having breast cancer diagnosed is caused by the pill. It may be that women taking the pill were examined more often, so that breast cancer was more likely to be detected.

You should have regular breast examinations by a health care professional and examine your own breasts monthly. Tell your health care professional if you have a family history of breast cancer or if you have had breast nodules or an abnormal mammogram. Women who currently have or have had breast cancer should not use oral contraceptives because breast cancer is usually a hormone-sensitive tumor.

Some studies have found an increase in the incidence of cancer of the cervix in women who use oral contraceptives. However, this finding may be related to factors other than the use of oral contraceptives. There is insufficient evidence to rule out the possibility that the pill may cause such cancers.

6. *Lipid metabolism and inflammation of the pancreas*

In patients with abnormal lipid levels, there have been reports of significant elevations of plasma triglycerides during estrogen therapy. This has led to pancreatitis in some cases.

ESTIMATED RISK OF DEATH FROM A BIRTH-CONTROL METHOD OR PREGNANCY

All methods of birth control and pregnancy are associated with a risk of developing certain diseases which may lead to disability or death. An estimate of the number of deaths associated with different methods of birth control and pregnancy has been calculated and is shown in the following table.

ANNUAL NUMBER OF BIRTH-RELATED OR METHOD-RELATED DEATHS ASSOCIATED WITH CONTROL OF FERTILITY PER 100,000 NONSTERILE WOMEN, BY FERTILITY-CONTROL METHOD AND ACCORDING TO AGE

Method of control and outcome	15-19	20-24	25-29	30-34	35-39	40-44
No fertility-control methods*	7.0	7.4	9.1	14.8	25.7	28.2
Oral contraceptives nonsmoker**	0.3	0.5	0.9	1.9	13.8	31.6
Oral contraceptives smoker**	2.2	3.4	6.6	13.5	51.1	117.2
IUD**	0.8	0.8	1.0	1.0	1.4	1.4
Condom*	1.1	1.6	0.7	0.2	0.3	0.4
Diaphragm/ spermicide*	1.9	1.2	1.2	1.3	2.2	2.8
Periodic abstinence*	2.5	1.6	1.6	1.7	2.9	3.6

* Deaths are birth related

** Deaths are method related

In the above table, the risk of death from any birth-control method is less than the risk of childbirth, except for oral-contraceptive users over the age of 35 who smoke and pill users over the age of 40 even if they do not smoke. It can be seen in the table that for women aged 15 to 39, the risk of death was highest with pregnancy (7 to 26 deaths per 100,000 women, depending on age). Among pill users who do not smoke, the risk of death was always lower than that associated with pregnancy for any age group, except for those women over the age of 40, when the risk increases to 32 deaths per 100,000 women, compared to 28 associated with pregnancy at that age. However, for pill users who smoke and are over the age of 35, the estimated number of deaths exceeds those for other methods of birth control. If a woman is over the age of 40 and smokes, her estimated risk of death is four times higher (117/100,000 women) than the estimated risk associated with pregnancy (28/100,000 women) in that age group.

The suggestion that women over 40 who do not smoke should not take oral contraceptives is based on information from older high-dose pills. An Advisory Committee of the FDA discussed this issue in 1989 and recommended that the benefits of oral-contraceptive use by healthy, nonsmoking women over 40 years of age may outweigh the possible risks. Older women, as all women, who take oral contraceptives, should take an oral contraceptive which contains the least amount of estrogen and progestogen that is compatible with the individual patient needs.

WARNING SIGNALS

If any of these adverse effects occur while you are taking oral contraceptives, call your health-care provider immediately:

- Sharp chest pain, coughing of blood, or sudden shortness of breath (indicating a possible clot in the lung).
- Pain in the calf (indicating a possible clot in the leg).
- Crushing chest pain or heaviness in the chest (indicating a possible heart attack).
- Sudden severe headache or vomiting, dizziness or fainting, disturbances of vision or speech, weakness, or numbness in an arm or leg (indicating a possible stroke).
- Sudden partial or complete loss of vision (indicating a possible clot in the eye).
- Breast lumps (indicating possible breast cancer or fibrocystic disease of the breast; ask your health-care provider to show you how to examine your breasts).
- Severe pain or tenderness in the stomach area (indicating a possibly ruptured liver tumor).
- Difficulty in sleeping, weakness, lack of energy, fatigue, or change in mood (possibly indicating severe depression).
- Jaundice or a yellowing of the skin or eyeballs, accompanied frequently by fever, fatigue, loss of appetite, dark-colored urine, or light-colored bowel movements (indicating possible liver problems).

SIDE EFFECTS OF ORAL CONTRACEPTIVES

1. *Vaginal bleeding*

Irregular vaginal bleeding or spotting may occur while you are taking the pills. Irregular bleeding may vary from slight staining between menstrual periods to breakthrough bleeding which is a flow much like a regular period. Irregular bleeding occurs most often during the first few months of oral-contraceptive use, but may also occur after you have been taking the pill for some time. Such bleeding may be temporary and usually does not indicate any serious problems. It is important to continue taking your pills on schedule. If the bleeding occurs in more than one cycle or lasts for more than a few days, talk to your health-care provider.

2. *Contact lenses*

If you wear contact lenses and notice a change in vision or an inability to wear your lenses, contact your health-care provider.

Continued on next page

Alesse 28—Cont.

3. *Fluid retention*
Oral contraceptives may cause edema (fluid retention) with swelling of the fingers or ankles and may raise your blood pressure. If you experience fluid retention, contact your health-care provider.
4. *Melasma*
A spotty darkening of the skin is possible, particularly of the face.
5. *Other side effects*
Other side effects may include nausea, breast tenderness, change in appetite, headache, nervousness, depression, dizziness, loss of scalp hair, rash, vaginal infections, inflammation of the pancreas, and allergic reactions.
If any of these side effects bother you, call your health-care provider.
GENERAL PRECAUTIONS
1. *Missed periods and use of oral contraceptives before or during early pregnancy*
There may be times when you may not menstruate regularly after you have completed taking a cycle of pills. If you have taken your pills regularly and miss one menstrual period, continue taking your pills for the next cycle but be sure to inform your health-care provider before doing so. If you have not taken the pills daily as instructed and missed a menstrual period, or if you missed two consecutive menstrual periods, you may be pregnant. Check with your health-care provider immediately to determine whether you are pregnant. Do not continue to take oral contraceptives until you are sure you are not pregnant, but continue to use another method of contraception.
There is no conclusive evidence that oral-contraceptive use is associated with an increase in birth defects, when taken inadvertently during early pregnancy. Previously, a few studies had reported that oral contraceptives might be associated with birth defects, but these studies have not been confirmed. Nevertheless, oral contraceptives should not be used during pregnancy. You should check with your health-care provider about risks to your unborn child of any medication taken during pregnancy.
2. *While breast-feeding*
If you are breast-feeding, consult your health-care provider before starting oral contraceptives. Some of the drug will be passed on to the child in the milk. A few adverse effects on the child have been reported, including yellowing of the skin (jaundice) and breast enlargement. In addition, oral contraceptives may decrease the amount and quality of your milk. If possible, do not use oral contraceptives while breast-feeding. You should use another method of contraception since breast-feeding provides only partial protection from becoming pregnant and this partial protection decreases significantly as you breast-feed for longer periods of time. You should consider starting oral contraceptives only after you have weaned your child completely.
3. *Laboratory tests*
If you are scheduled for any laboratory tests, tell your doctor you are taking birth-control pills. Certain blood tests may be affected by birth-control pills.
4. *Drug interactions*
Certain drugs may interact with birth-control pills to make them less effective in preventing pregnancy or cause an increase in breakthrough bleeding. Such drugs include rifampin, drugs used for epilepsy such as barbiturates (for example, phenobarbital) and phenytoin (Dilantin® is one brand of this drug), primidone (Mysoline®), topiramate (Topamax®), carbamazepine (Tegretol® is one brand of this drug), phenylbutazone (Butazolidin® is one brand), some drugs used for HIV or AIDS such as ritonavir (Norvir®), modafinil (Provigil®) and possibly certain antibiotics (such as ampicillin and other penicillins, and tetracyclines), and herbal products containing St. John's Wort (Hypericum perforatum). You may also need to use a nonhormonal method of contraception during any cycle in which you take drugs that can make oral contraceptives less effective.
You may be at higher risk of a specific type of liver dysfunction if you take troleandomycin and oral contraceptives at the same time.
You should inform your health-care provider about all medicines you are taking, including nonprescription products.
5. *Sexually transmitted diseases*
This product (like all oral contraceptives) is intended to prevent pregnancy. It does not protect against transmission of HIV (AIDS) and other sexually transmitted diseases such as chlamydia, genital herpes, genital warts, gonorrhea, hepatitis B, and syphilis.
HOW TO TAKE THE PILL
IMPORTANT POINTS TO REMEMBER
BEFORE YOU START TAKING YOUR PILLS:
1. BE SURE TO READ THESE DIRECTIONS:
Before you start taking your pills.
And
Anytime you are not sure what to do.
2. THE RIGHT WAY TO TAKE THE PILL IS TO TAKE ONE PILL EVERY DAY AT THE SAME TIME.
If you miss pills you could get pregnant. This includes starting the pack late. The more pills you miss, the more likely you are to get pregnant.
3. MANY WOMEN HAVE SPOTTING OR LIGHT BLEEDING, OR MAY FEEL SICK TO THEIR STOMACH DURING THE FIRST 1-3 PACKS OF PILLS.
If you feel sick to your stomach, do not stop taking the pill. The problem will usually go away. If it doesn't go away, check with your health-care provider.
4. MISSING PILLS CAN ALSO CAUSE SPOTTING OR LIGHT BLEEDING, even when you make up these missed pills.
On the days you take 2 pills to make up for missed pills, you could also feel a little sick to your stomach.
5. IF YOU HAVE VOMITING (within 4 hours after you take your pill), you should follow the instructions for WHAT TO DO IF YOU MISS PILLS. IF YOU HAVE DIARRHEA or IF YOU TAKE SOME MEDICINES, including some antibiotics, your pills may not work as well.
Use a back-up nonhormonal method (such as condoms and/or spermicide) until you check with your health-care provider.
6. IF YOU HAVE TROUBLE REMEMBERING TO TAKE THE PILL, talk to your health-care provider about how to make pill-taking easier or about using another method of birth control.
7. IF YOU HAVE ANY QUESTIONS OR ARE UNSURE ABOUT THE INFORMATION IN THIS LEAFLET, call your health-care provider.
***BEFORE* YOU START TAKING YOUR PILLS**
1. DECIDE WHAT TIME OF DAY YOU WANT TO TAKE YOUR PILL. It is important to take it at about the same time every day.
2. LOOK AT YOUR PILL PACK TO SEE IF IT HAS 21 OR 28 PILLS:
The *21-pill pack* has 21 "active" pink pills (with hormones) to take for 3 weeks, followed by 1 week without pills.
The *28-pill pack* has 21 "active" pink pills (with hormones) to take for 3 weeks, followed by 1 week of reminder light-green pills (without hormones).
3. ALSO FIND:
1) where on the pack to start taking pills, and
2) in what order to take the pills (follow the arrow).

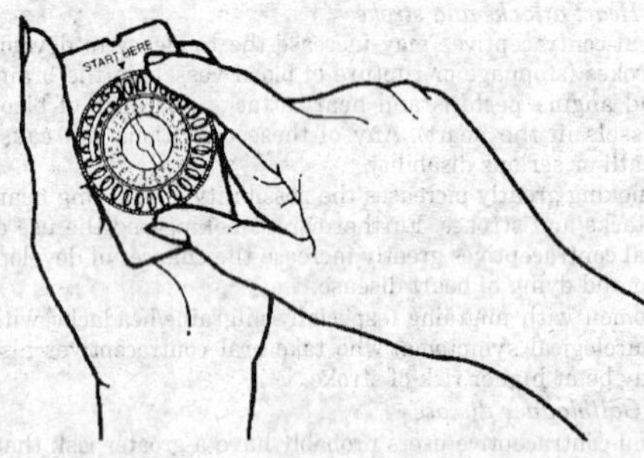

4. BE SURE YOU HAVE READY AT ALL TIMES:
ANOTHER KIND OF BIRTH CONTROL (such as condoms and/or spermicide) to use as a back-up in case you miss pills.
AN EXTRA, FULL PILL PACK.
WHEN TO START THE *FIRST* PACK OF PILLS
You have a choice of which day to start taking your first pack of pills.
Decide with your health-care provider which is the best day for you. Pick a time of day which will be easy to remember.
DAY 1 START:
1. Take the first "active" pink pill of the first pack during the *first 24 hours of your period.*
2. You will not need to use a back-up nonhormonal method of birth control, since you are starting the pill at the beginning of your period.
SUNDAY START:
1. Take the first "active" pink pill of the first pack on the *Sunday after your period starts,* even if you are still bleeding. If your period begins on Sunday, start the pack that same day.
2. Use a *nonhormonal method of birth control* (such as condoms and/or spermicide) as a back-up method if you have sex anytime from the Sunday you start your first pack until the next Sunday (7 days).
WHAT TO DO DURING THE MONTH
1. Take one pill at the same time every day until the pack is empty.
Do not skip pills even if you are spotting or bleeding between monthly periods or feel sick to your stomach (nausea).
Do not skip pills even if you do not have sex very often.
2. When you finish a pack or switch your brand of pills:
21 pills: Wait 7 days to start the next pack. You will probably have your period during that week. Be sure that no more than 7 days pass between 21-day packs.
28 pills: Start the next pack on the day after your last "reminder" pill. Do not wait any days between packs.
WHAT TO DO IF YOU MISS PILLS
The pill may not be as effective if you miss pink "active" pills, and particularly if you miss the first few or the last few pink "active" pills in a pack.
If you **MISS 1** pink "active" pill:
1. Take it as soon as you remember. Take the next pill at your regular time. This means you may take 2 pills in 1 day.
2. You COULD BECOME PREGNANT if you have sex in the *7 days* after you miss pills. You MUST use a nonhormonal birth-control method (such as condoms and/or spermicide) as a back-up for those 7 days.
If you **MISS 2** pink "active" pills in a row in **WEEK 1 OR WEEK 2** of your pack:
1. Take 2 pills on the day you remember and 2 pills the next day.
2. Then take 1 pill a day until you finish the pack.
3. You COULD BECOME PREGNANT if you have sex in the 7 days after you miss pills. You MUST use a nonhormonal birth-control method (such as condoms and/or spermicide) as a back-up for those 7 days.
If you **MISS 2** pink "active" pills in a row in **THE 3rd WEEK**:
1. ***If you are a Day 1 Starter:***
THROW OUT the rest of the pill pack and start a new pack that same day.
If you are a Sunday Starter:
Keep taking 1 pill every day until Sunday.
On Sunday, THROW OUT the rest of the pack and start a new pack of pills that same day.
2. You may not have your period this month but this is expected.
However, if you miss your period 2 months in a row, call your health-care provider because you might be pregnant.
3. You COULD BECOME PREGNANT if you have sex in the *7 days* after you miss pills. You MUST use a nonhormonal birth-control method (such as condoms and/or spermicide) as a back-up for those 7 days.
If you **MISS 3 OR MORE** pink "active" pills in a row (during the first 3 weeks):
1. ***If you are a Day 1 Starter:***
THROW OUT the rest of the pill pack and start a new pack that same day.
If you are a Sunday Starter:
Keep taking 1 pill every day until Sunday.
On Sunday, THROW OUT the rest of the pack and start a new pack of pills that same day.
2. You may not have your period this month but this is expected.
However, if you miss your period 2 months in a row, call your health-care provider because you might be pregnant.
3. You COULD BECOME PREGNANT if you have sex in the *7 days* after you miss pills. You MUST use a nonhormonal birth-control method (such as condoms and/or spermicide) as a back-up for those 7 days.
A REMINDER FOR THOSE ON 28-DAY PACKS
If you forget any of the 7 light-green "reminder" pills in Week 4:
THROW AWAY the pills you missed.
Keep taking 1 pill each day until the pack is empty.
You do not need a back-up nonhormonal birth-control method if you start your next pack on time.
FINALLY, IF YOU ARE STILL NOT SURE WHAT TO DO ABOUT THE PILLS YOU HAVE MISSED
Use a BACK-UP NONHORMONAL BIRTH-CONTROL METHOD anytime you have sex.
KEEP TAKING ONE PILL EACH DAY until you can reach your health-care provider.
PREGNANCY DUE TO PILL FAILURE
The incidence of pill failure resulting in pregnancy is approximately 1.0% if taken every day as directed, but the average failure rate is approximately 5% including women who do not always take the pill exactly as directed without missing any pills. If you do become pregnant, the risk to the fetus is minimal, but you should stop taking your pills and discuss the pregnancy with your health-care provider.
PREGNANCY AFTER STOPPING THE PILL
There may be some delay in becoming pregnant after you stop using oral contraceptives, especially if you had irregular menstrual cycles before you used oral contraceptives. It may be advisable to postpone conception until you begin menstruating regularly once you have stopped taking the pill and desire pregnancy.
There does not appear to be any increase in birth defects in newborn babies when pregnancy occurs soon after stopping the pill.
If you do not desire pregnancy, you should use another method of birth control immediately after stopping the oral contraceptive pill.
OVERDOSAGE
Overdosage may cause nausea, vomiting, and fatigue/drowsiness. Withdrawal bleeding may occur in females. In case of overdosage, contact your health-care provider or pharmacist.
OTHER INFORMATION
Your health-care provider will take a medical and family history before prescribing oral contraceptives and will examine you. The physical examination may be delayed to another time if you request it and the health-care provider believes that it is appropriate to postpone it. You should be reexamined at least once a year. Be sure to inform your health-care provider if there is a family history of any of the conditions listed previously in this leaflet. Be sure to keep all appointments with your health-care provider, because this is a time to determine if there are early signs of side effects of oral-contraceptive use.
Do not use the drug for any condition other than the one for which it was prescribed. This drug has been prescribed specifically for you; do not give it to others who may want birth-control pills.
HEALTH BENEFITS FROM ORAL CONTRACEPTIVES
In addition to preventing pregnancy, use of oral contraceptives may provide certain benefits. They are:
- Menstrual cycles may become more regular.
- Blood flow during menstruation may be lighter, and less iron may be lost. Therefore, anemia due to iron deficiency is less likely to occur.
- Pain or other symptoms during menstruation may be encountered less frequently.
- Ovarian cysts may occur less frequently.
- Ectopic (tubal) pregnancy may occur less frequently.

- Noncancerous cysts or lumps in the breast may occur less frequently.
- Acute pelvic inflammatory disease may occur less frequently.
- Oral-contraceptive use may provide some protection against developing two forms of cancer: cancer of the ovaries and cancer of the lining of the uterus.

If you want more information about birth-control pills, ask your health-care provider or pharmacist. They have a more technical leaflet called the Professional Labeling which you may wish to read.

Wyeth®
Wyeth Pharmaceuticals Inc.
Philadelphia, PA 19101

W10491C001
ET01
Rev 04/04

Shown in Product Identification Guide, page 336

ANTIVENIN (Crotalidae) ℞

[*ăn'-tī- vĕ"-nĭn*]

Polyvalent (equine origin)

IMPORTANT

Pit viper bites may cause severe tissue damage or fatal envenomation, or both. The physician responsible for treatment of an envenomated patient should be familiar with the contents of this brochure and the pertinent medical literature concerning current concepts of first-aid and general supportive therapy as presented in the references listed at the end of this pamphlet.

COMPOSITION

Antivenin (Crotalidae) Polyvalent, Wyeth, is a refined and concentrated preparation of serum globulins obtained by fractionating blood from healthy horses immunized with the following venoms: *Crotalus adamanteus* (Eastern diamond rattlesnake), *C. atrox* (Western diamond rattlesnake), *C. durissus terrificus* (tropical rattlesnake, Cascabel), and *Bothrops atrox* ("Fer-de-lance"). Phenol, 0.25%, and thimerosal, 0.005%, are added as preservatives. The product is standardized by its ability to neutralize the lethal action of standard venoms by intravenous injection in mice.[1] Dried from the frozen state, the lyophilized serum has a moisture content of less than 1% and is soluble on addition of the diluent contained in each package (Sterile Water for Injection, USP).

Antivenin (Crotalidae) Polyvalent, Wyeth (hereinafter referred to as Antivenin) contains protective substances capable of neutralizing the toxic effects of venoms of crotalids (pit vipers) native to North, Central, and South America, including rattlesnakes *(Crotalus, Sistrurus)*; copperhead and cottonmouth moccasins *(Agkistrodon)*, including *A. halys* of Korea and Japan; the Fer-de-lance and other species of *Bothrops*; the tropical rattler *(Crotalus durissus* and similar species); the Cantil *(A. bilineatus)*; and bushmaster *(Lachesis mutus)* of South and Central America.

INDICATION

Antivenin is indicated only for the treatment of envenomation caused by bites of those crotalids (pit vipers) specified in the immediately preceding paragraph.

Pit Viper Bites and Envenomation

The symptoms, signs, and severity of snake-venom poisoning resulting from pit viper bites depend on many factors, including, but not limited to, the following variables: species, age, and size of the biting snake; the number and location of bite(s); the depth of venom deposit by the snake's fangs; the condition of the snake's fangs and venom glands; the length of time the snake "hangs on"; the age, general health, and size of the victim; the type and efficacy of any first-aid treatment rendered in an attempt to remove venom and how soon such treatment was applied. In any venomous snake bite, the actual amount of venom introduced into the victim is always an unknown. Even the type of clothing or leg-footwear through which the snake's fangs pass may affect the amount of venom delivered by the bite. Although most North American pit vipers tend to bite and introduce venom superficially, their fangs may get hung-up in the subcutaneous tissues during the biting act and can penetrate deeper tissues during the attempt to release the bitten part. In some bites the fangs may penetrate into muscle. In such cases, the usual local superficial manifestations of envenomation may not appear early in the course of poisoning. In bites by some species, systemic evidence of envenomation may be present in the absence of significant local manifestations. It may be difficult to determine the severity of envenomation during the first several hours after a pit viper bite and estimates of severity may need to be revised as poisoning progresses. It must be remembered, too, that not all pit viper bites result in envenomation. In approximately 20% of rattlesnake bites, the snake may not inject any venom. The local and systemic symptoms and signs of envenomation include the following:

LOCAL:

Fang Puncture(s).

Swelling – edema is usually seen around the site of bite within five minutes. It may progress rapidly and involve the entire extremity within an hour. More than 95% of all snakebites are inflicted on extremities.[2] Generally, however, edema spreads more slowly, usually over a period of 8 or more hours. Swelling is usually most severe following envenomation by the Eastern diamondback; less severe after bites by the Western diamondback, prairie, timber, red, Pacific, Mojave, and blacktailed rattlers, the sidewinder and cottonmouth moccasins; least severe after bites by copperheads, massasaugas, and pygmy rattlers.

Ecchymosis and discoloration of the skin – often appear in the area of the bite within a few hours. Vesicules may form within a few hours and are usually present at 24 hours. Hemorrhagic blebs and petechiae are common. Necrosis may develop, necessitating amputation of an extremity or a portion thereof.

Pain – frequently a complaint of the victim beginning shortly after the bite by most pit vipers. Pain may be absent after bites by Mojave rattlers.

SYSTEMIC:

Weakness; faintness; nausea; sweating; numbness or tingling around the mouth, tongue, scalp, fingers, toes, site of bite; muscle fasciculations; hypotension; prolongation of bleeding and clotting times; hemoconcentration, early followed by a decrease in erythrocytes; thrombocytopenia; hematuria; proteinuria; vomiting, including hematemesis; melena; hemoptysis; epistaxis. In fatal poisoning, a frequent cause of death is associated with destruction of erythrocytes and changes in capillary permeability, especially of the pulmonary vascular system, leading to pulmonary edema; hemoconcentration usually occurs early, probably as a result of plasma loss secondary to vascular permeability; the hemoglobin may fall, and bleeding may occur throughout the body as early as 6 hours after the bite. Renal involvement is not uncommon. Mojave rattler venom may cause neuromuscular changes leading to respiratory failure.

An estimate of the severity of envenomation should be made as soon as possible and before any Antivenin is administered. The amount (volume) of the first dose of Antivenin is determined on this estimate of severity. Every symptom, sign, laboratory-test result, and any other pertinent information should be considered in estimating severity–local manifestations; systemic manifestations, including abnormal laboratory findings; species and size of the biting snake, if known; number and location of bite(s); size and health of the patient; type of first-aid treatment rendered; and interval between bite and arrival for treatment. Russell et al,[3,4] and Wingert and Wainschel[5] grade severity as follows:

No envenomation – no local or systemic manifestations.

Minimal envenomation – local swelling and other local changes; no systemic manifestations; normal laboratory findings.

Moderate envenomation – swelling progressing beyond the site of bite and one or more systemic manifestations; abnormal laboratory findings, for example, a fall in hematocrit or platelets.

Severe envenomation – marked local response, severe systemic manifestations and significant alteration in laboratory findings.

Parrish and Hayes,[6] McCollough and Gennaro,[7] and Watt and Gennaro[8] have used a Grade 0 (no envenomation) through Grade IV (very severe) classification of severity which was developed for the most part in treatment of envenomation by the Eastern diamondback and timber rattlers.

This classification is more dependent on local manifestations, or the absence thereof, as the venoms of these species seem to be more consistent in inducing local tissue damage.

Any suspected envenomation should be treated as a medical emergency, and until careful observation provides clear evidence that envenomation has not occurred or is minimal, the following procedures are recommended:

If practical, immobilize victim immediately and completely. Carry the victim to the nearest hospital as soon as possible. If complete immobilization is not practical, splint the bitten extremity to limit spread of venom. If the biting snake was killed, bring it to the hospital also.

Monitor vital signs at frequent intervals: Blood pressure, pulse, respiration.

Draw sufficient blood as soon as possible for baseline laboratory studies, including type and cross match, CBC, hematocrit, platelet count, prothrombin time, clot retraction, bleeding and coagulation times, BUN, electrolytes, bilirubin. Some of these studies may need to be repeated at daily intervals, or less, depending on the severity of envenomation and the response to treatment. During the first 4 or 5 days of severe envenomations, hemoglobin, hematocrit, and platelet counts should be carried out several times a day. Additional studies that may be useful include an electrocardiogram, chest radiograph, fibrinogen levels, fibrin split products and arterial blood gas analysis.[9]

Obtain urine samples at frequent intervals for analysis, with special attention to microscopic examination for presence of erythrocytes.

Chart fluid intake and urine output.

Measure and record the circumference of the bitten extremity just proximal to the bite and at one or more additional points each several inches closer to the trunk. Repeat measurements every 15 to 30 minutes to obtain information about progression of edema.

Have available and ready for immediate use: oxygen, resuscitation equipment including airway, tourniquet, epinephrine, injectable antihistaminic agents and corticosteroids.

Start an intravenous infusion in one or two extremities: one line to be used for supportive therapy, if needed, such as whole blood, plasma, packed red cells, specific clotting factors, platelet transfusion, plasma expanders; the other line to be used for administration of Antivenin (Crotalidae) Polyvalent (equine origin) and electrolytes.

Carry out and interpret a skin test for horse-serum sensitivity. (See **PRECAUTIONS** section below.)

CONTRAINDICATIONS

For persons with pit viper envenomations threatening life or limb, there are no contraindications to administration of Antivenin. However, administration to persons known to be allergic to horse serum, either by history or as a result of an appropriate sensitivity test, requires careful judgement and considerable experience in the use of antivenoms, as well as experience in the management of severe, immediate allergic reactions (anaphylaxis).[5,10,11,12]

Antivenin should never be administered prophylactically to asymptomatic patients.[13]

WARNINGS

There have been isolated reports of cardiac arrest and death associated with Antivenin use.

Patients sensitive to Antivenin or horse serum may develop anaphylaxis, therefore, it is essential that prior to intravenous (IV) or intramuscular (IM) Antivenin administration a proper skin test be performed, interpreted, and therapy modified if indicated.

PRECAUTIONS

General

Constant attendance and observation of the patient for untoward reactions are mandatory when Antivenin is administered.

Should any systemic reaction occur, administration should be discontinued immediately and appropriate treatment initiated. Those responsible for administration and/or monitoring administration of Antivenin should be familiar with current recommendations for treatment of severe, immediate, systemic reactions (anaphylaxis) associated with use of heterologous sera.

Therapy with beta-adrenergic blockers, including cardioselective agents, has been associated with an increased severity of acute anaphylaxis (See **Drug Interactions**).

Before administration of any product prepared from horse serum, appropriate measures must be taken in an effort to detect the presence of dangerous sensitivity: (1) A careful review of the patient's history, including any report of (a) asthma, hay fever, urticaria, or other allergic manifestations; (b) allergic reactions upon exposure to horses; and (c) prior injections of horse serum. (2) A suitable test for detection of sensitivity. A skin test should be performed in every patient prior to administration, regardless of clinical history.

Skin test – Inject intradermally 0.02 to 0.03 mL of a 1:10 dilution of Normal Horse Serum or Antivenin. A control test on the opposite extremity, using Sodium Chloride Injection, USP, facilitates interpretation. Use of larger amounts for the skin-test dose increases the likelihood of false-positive reactions, and in the exquisitely sensitive patient, increases the risk of a systemic reaction from the skin-test dose. A 10% rate of false negative skin test reactions has been reported.[14] A 1:100 or greater dilution should be used for preliminary skin testing if the history suggests sensitivity. A positive reaction to a skin test occurs within five to thirty minutes and is manifested by a wheal with or without pseudopodia and surrounding erythema. In general, the shorter the interval between injection and the beginning of the skin reaction, the greater the sensitivity.

If the history is negative for allergy and the result of a skin test is negative, proceed with administration of Antivenin as outlined below. If the history is positive and a skin test is strongly positive, administration may be dangerous, especially if the positive sensitivity test is accompanied by systemic allergic manifestations. In such instances, the risk of administering Antivenin must be weighed against the risk of withholding it, keeping in mind that severe envenomation can be fatal. (See last paragraph of this section.)

A negative allergic history and absence of reaction to a properly applied skin test do not rule out the possibility of an immediate reaction. Also, a negative skin test has no bearing on whether or not delayed serum reactions (serum sickness) will occur after administration of the full dose.

If the history is negative, and the skin test is mildly or questionably positive, administer as follows to reduce the risk of a severe immediate systemic reaction: (a) Prepare, in separate sterile vials or syringes, 1:100 and 1:10 dilutions of Antivenin. (b) Allow at least 15 minutes between injections and proceed with the next dose if no reaction follows the previous dose. (c) Inject subcutaneously, using a tuberculin-type syringe, 0.1, 0.2, and 0.5 mL of the 1:100 dilution at 15-minute intervals; repeat with the 1:10 dilution, and finally undiluted Antivenin. (d) If a systemic reaction occurs after any injection, place a tourniquet proximal to the site of injections and administer an appropriate dose of epinephrine, 1:1000, proximal to the tourniquet or into another extremity. Wait at least 30 minutes before injecting another dose. The amount of the next dose should be the same as the last that did not evoke a reaction. (e) If no reaction occurs after 0.5 mL of undiluted Antivenin has been administered, switch to the intramuscular route and continue doubling the dose at 15-minute intervals until the entire dose has been injected intramuscularly or proceed to the intravenous route as described below under **DOSAGE AND ADMINISTRATION**.

Obviously, if the just-described schedule is used, 3 to 5 or more hours would be required to administer the initial dose suggested for a moderate or severe envenomation, and time

Continued on next page

Antivenin (Crotalidae)—Cont.

is an important factor in neutralization of venom in a critically ill patient. Wingert and Wainschel[4] have described a procedure based on the experience of their group which they have used in some severely envenomated patients who have positive sensitivity tests: 50 to 100 mg of diphenhydramine hydrochloride is given intravenously, followed by slow intravenous infusion of diluted Antivenin for 15 to 20 minutes while carefully observing the patient for symptoms and signs of anaphylaxis; if anaphylaxis does not occur, Antivenin is continued, maintaining close observation of the patient. Patients who require Antivenin but develop signs of impending anaphylaxis in spite of this or the procedure described earlier present a difficult problem, and consultation should be sought.

Drug Interactions

Therapy with beta-adrenergic blockers, including cardioselective agents, has been associated with an increased severity of acute anaphylaxis.

Anaphylaxis may be prolonged and resistant to conventional treatment in patients receiving beta-adrenergic blockers. The pharmacotherapeutic actions of epinephrine and other adrenergic agents may be altered, and larger than usual doses may be required.[15]

DOSAGE AND ADMINISTRATION

Before administration, read **CONTRAINDICATIONS, PRECAUTIONS** and **ADVERSE REACTIONS** sections.

Since the possibility of a severe immediate reaction (anaphylaxis) exists whenever a horse-serum-containing product is administered, appropriate therapeutic agents, including a tourniquet, airway, oxygen, epinephrine, an injectable pressor amine, and corticosteroid, must be available and ready for immediate use. Constant attendance and observation of the patient for untoward reactions are mandatory when Antivenin (Crotalidae) Polyvalent (equine origin) is administered. Should any systemic reaction occur, administration should be discontinued immediately and appropriate treatment initiated.

The intravenous route of administration is preferred, and probably should always be used for moderate or severe envenomation. Intravenous administration is mandatory if venom-induced shock is present. To be most effective, Antivenin should be administered within 4 hours of the bite; it is less effective when given after 8 hours and may be of questionable value after 12 hours. However, it is recommended that Antivenin therapy be given in severe poisonings, even if 24 hours have elapsed since the time of the bite. It should be kept in mind that maximum blood levels of Antivenin may not be obtained for 8 or more hours after IM administration.

For intravenous-drip use, prepare a 1:1 to 1:10 dilution of reconstituted Antivenin in Sodium Chloride Injection, USP, or 5% Dextrose Injection, USP. To avoid foaming, mix by gently swirling rather than shaking. Allow the initial 5 to 10 mL to infuse over a 3- to 5-minute period, with careful observation of the patient for evidence of untoward reaction. If no symptoms or signs of an immediate systemic reaction appear, continue the infusion with delivery at the maximum safe rate for intravenous fluid administration. The dilution of Antivenin to be used, the type of electrolyte solution used for dilution, and the rate of intravenous delivery of the diluted Antivenin must take into consideration the age, weight, and cardiac status of the patient; the severity of envenomation; the total amount and type of parenteral fluids it is anticipated will be given or are needed; and the interval between bite and initiation of specific therapy.

It is important to begin administration of the entire initial dose of Antivenin as described above as soon as possible, based on the best estimate of the severity of envenomation at the time treatment is begun (see **PIT VIPER BITES AND ENVENOMATION**). The following initial doses are recommended:[3,4,5,16]

no envenomation–none.

minimal envenomation–20-40 mL (contents of 2 to 4 vials).

moderate envenomation–50-90 mL (contents of 5 to 9 vials).

severe envenomation–100-150 mL or more (contents of 10 to 15 or more vials).

These recommended initial-dosage volumes are in general accord with those of others.[10,17,18]

The need for additional Antivenin must be based on the clinical response to the initial dose and continuing assessment of the severity of poisoning. If swelling continues to progress or if systemic symptoms or signs of envenomation increase in severity or if new manifestations appear, for example, fall in hematocrit or hypotension, administer an additional 10 to 50 mL (contents of 1 to 5 vials) or more intravenously. For severe envenomation, a total of 200 to 400 mL (contents of 20 to 40 vials) may be necessary.[10,19,20,21,22] There is not a recommended maximum dose. The total required dose is the amount needed to neutralize the venom as determined by clinical response.[23]

Envenomation by large snakes in children or small adults requires larger doses of Antivenin. The amount administered to a child is not based on weight.

If Antivenin is given intramuscularly, it should be given into a large muscle mass, preferably the gluteal area, with care to avoid nerve trunks. Antivenin should never be injected into a finger or toe.

The effectiveness of corticosteroids in treatment of envenomation per se or venom shock is not resolved. Russell[3,4] and others[26,27] believe corticosteroids may mask the seriousness of hypovolemia in moderate or severe poisoning and have little, if any, effect on the local-tissue response to rattler venoms. Corticosteroids should not be given simultaneously with Antivenin on a routine basis or during the acute state of envenomation; however, their use may be necessary to treat immediate allergic reactions to Antivenin, and corticosteroids are the agents of choice for treating serious delayed reactions to Antivenin.

Intravascular envenomation characterized by extremely rapid (i.e., within several minutes) onset of severe signs and symptoms has occurred in rare instances. In such cases, neutralization with Antivenin must be instituted immediately.[24]

Snakes' mouths do not harbor *Clostridium tetani*. However, appropriate tetanus prophylaxis is indicated, since tetanus spores may be carried into the fang puncture wounds by dirt present on skin at time of bite or by nonsterile first-aid procedures.

A broad-spectrum antibiotic in adequate dosage is indicated if local tissue damage is evident.

Shock following envenomation is treated like shock resulting from hypovolemia from any cause, including administration of whole blood, plasma, albumin, or other plasma expanders, as indicated.

Aspirin or codeine is usually adequate for relieving pain. Sedation with phenobarbital or mild tranquilizers may be used if indicated, but not in the presence of respiratory failure.

The bitten extremity should not be packed in ice, and so-called "cryotherapy" is contraindicated.

Compartment syndromes may complicate pit viper envenomations, especially those caused by bites on the lower extremities. Prompt surgical consultation is indicated whenever a closed-compartment syndrome is suspected.[3,4,25]

Defibrination and disseminated intravascular coagulation (DIC) syndromes have been associated with envenomation caused by some pit vipers native to the United States, and appropriate therapy may be indicated.[3,4,26,27,28,29]

Technique for Reconstituting the Dried Antivenin

Pry off the small metal disc in the cap over the diaphragms of the vials of Antivenin and diluent. Swab the exposed surface of the rubber diaphragms of both vials with an appropriate germicide. With a sterile 10 mL syringe and needle, withdraw the diluent (Sterile Water for Injection, USP) from the vial of diluent and insert the needle through the stopper of the vacuum-containing vial of Antivenin. The vacuum in the Antivenin vial will pull the diluent out of the syringe into the vial. However, delivery of 10 mL of diluent may not always exhaust the vacuum in the Antivenin vial. If all vacuum is not exhausted, reconstitution may be more difficult. Therefore, either disconnect the needle from the syringe and allow room air to be pulled into the Antivenin vial until all vacuum is released from the container or withdraw the syringe with attached needle from the vial, pull 10 mL of room air into the syringe and reinsert needle with attached syringe containing room air through stopper and repeat, if necessary, to release any remaining vacuum. At the first introduction of diluent into the vaccine vial, it is important for the needle to be pointed at the center of the lyophilized pellet of Antivenin so that the diluent stream will wet the pellet. If the diluent stream is not directed at the pellet but allowed to run down the inside wall of the vial, the pellet will float up and adhere to the stopper thereby rendering complete reconstitution much more difficult. Agitate by swirling, NOT by shaking, for 1 minute, at 5-minute intervals. Shaking causes foaming and if the diluent stream is not properly directed as described earlier, pieces of the pellet may get caught in the foam and will be very difficult to wet. Complete reconstitution usually requires at least 30 minutes.

Parenteral drug products should be inspected visually for particulate matter and discoloration prior to administration, whenever solution and container permit. The color of reconstituted Antivenin may vary from clear to slight yellowish or greenish.

Before each administration, gently swirl the vial to dissolve the contents.

Before any Antivenin is administered, an appropriate horse-serum sensitivity test must be done so that, in case administration of Antivenin is subsequently required, a decision on how to proceed will have been made (see **PRECAUTIONS**).

ADVERSE REACTIONS

Immediate systemic reactions (allergic reactions or anaphylaxis) can occur whenever a horse-serum-containing product is administered. An immediate reaction (e.g. shock, anaphylaxis) usually occurs within 30 minutes. Symptoms and signs may develop before the needle is withdrawn and may include apprehension, flushing, itching, urticaria; edema of the face, tongue, and throat; cough, dyspnea, cyanosis, vomiting, and collapse. There have been isolated reports of cardiac arrest and death associated with Antivenin (Crotalidae) Polyvalent (equine origin) use. However, serious immediate reactions to Antivenin are rare. In skin-test-negative patients, Antivenin caused a true immediate sensitivity reaction in less than 1 percent of patients.[10]

Serum sickness usually occurs 5 to 24 days after administration and its frequency may be related to the number of Antivenin vials administered.[30] The incubation period may be less than 5 days, especially in those who have received horse-serum-containing preparations in the past. The usual symptoms and signs are malaise, fever, urticaria, lymphadenopathy, edema, arthralgia, nausea, and vomiting. Occasionally, neurological manifestations develop, such as meningismus or peripheral neuritis. Peripheral neuritis usually involves the shoulders and arms. Pain and muscle weakness are frequently present, and permanent atrophy may develop.

HOW SUPPLIED

Each combination package contains one vacuum vial to yield 10 mL of Antivenin (with preservatives: phenol 0.25% and thimerosal [mercury derivative] 0.005%) and one 1 mL vial of normal horse serum (diluted 1:10) as sensitivity testing material with preservatives: thimerosal (mercury derivative) 0.005% and phenol 0.35%.

Store original, unused *(not reconstituted)* vials at temperatures not exceeding 98°F (37°C) - Do not freeze.

Reconstituted Antivenin should be used as soon as possible but may be used up to 4 hours after reconstitution (but not yet diluted) if stored at 36°F to 46°F (2°C to 8°C).

Antivenin which has been *reconstituted and then diluted* should be used immediately. Any remaining after 12 hours or more after dilution should be discarded.

Gently swirl the vial of reconstituted Antivenin before each administration.

REFERENCES

1. GINGRICH, W. & HOHENADEL, J.: Standardization of polyvalent antivenin. "Venoms", edited by E. Buckley and N. Porges. Publication No. 44, Amer. Assoc. for the Advancement of Science, Washington, D.C., 1956, Pages 337-80.
2. PARRISH, H.: Incidence of treated snakebite in the United States. *Pub. Hlth. Rep. 81*:269, 1966.
3. RUSSELL, F. et al: Snake venom poisoning in the United States. Experiences with 550 cases. JAMA 233:341, 1975
4. RUSSELL, F.: Venomous bites and stings: Poisonous snakes. In The Merck Manual of Diagnosis and Therapy, pp. 2450-2456, 14th Ed., 1982.
5. WINGERT, W. and WAINSCHEL, J.: Diagnosis and management of envenomation by poisonous snakes. *South. Med. J. 68*:1015, 1975.
6. PARRISH, H. & HAYES, R.: Hospital management of pit viper venenations. Clinical Toxicol. 3:501, 1970.
7. McCOLLOUGH, N. & GENNARO, J.: Diagnosis, symptoms, treatment and sequelae of envenomation by Crotalus adamanteus and Genus Agkistrodon. *J. Florida Med. Assoc. 55*:327, 1968.
8. WATT, C. & GENNARO, J.: Pit viper bites in South Georgia and North Florida. *Tr. South. Surg. Assoc.* 77:378, 1966.
9. SEILER, J. et al: Venomous snake bite: Current concepts of treatment. *Orthopedics 17(8)*:707, 1994.
10. RUSSEL, F.: Snake venom poisoning. Scholium International, Inc., New York, 1983.
11. LOPRINZI, C. et al: Snake Antivenin administration in a patient allergic to horse serum. *South. Med. J. 76*:501, 1983.
12. OTTEN, E. & MCKIMM, D.: Venomous snakebite in a patient allergic to horse serum. *Ann. Emerg. Med. 12*:624, 1983.
13. BOWDEN, C. & KRENZELOK, E.: Clinical applications of commonly used contemporary antidotes, a US perspective. *Drug Safety 16(1)*:22-24, 1997.
14. JURKOVICH, G. et al: Complications of *Crotalidae* Antivenin therapy. *The J. of Trauma 28*:7, 1988.
15. TOOGOOD, J.: Beta-blocker therapy and the risk of anaphylaxis. *Can. Med. Assoc. J. 136*:929, 1987.
16. MINTON, S.: Venom Diseases: Snakebite. In Textbook of Medicine, P. Beeson and W. McDermott (Eds.), pp. 88-92: Saunders, Philadelphia, 1975.
17. WINGERT, W.: Rattlesnake bites. *West. J. Med. 140*:100, 1984.
18. PICCHIONI, A. et al: Management of poisonous snakebite. *Vet. Hum. Toxicol. 26*:139, 1984.
19. ARNOLD, R.: Rattlesnake venoms, their actions and treatment. Edited by Anthony Tu. Marcel Dekker Inc., New York, 1982. pp. 315-338.
20. ARNOLD, R.: Treatment of venomous snakebites in the Western Hemisphere. *Military Med. 149*:361, 1984.
21. WATT, C.: Treatment of poisonous snakebite with emphasis on digit dermotomy. *South. Med. J. 72*:694, 1985.
22. HENNESSEE, J.: Snakebite treatment. *South. Med. J. 77(2)*:280, 1984.
23. WINGERT, W. & CHAN, L.: Rattlesnake bites in Southern California and rationale for recommended treatment. *West. J. Med. 148(1)*:37, 1988.
24. DAVIDSON, T.: Intravenous rattlesnake envenomation. *West. J. Med. 148(1)*:45, 1988.
25. GARFIN, S. et al: Rattlesnake bites: Current concepts. Clin. Orthop. 140:50, 1979; Role of surgical decompression in treatment of rattlesnake bites. *Surg. Forum 30*:502, 1979.
26. VAN MIEROP, L.: Snakebite symposium. *J. Florida Med. Assoc. 63*:101, 1976.
27. ARNOLD, R.: Treatment of snakebite. JAMA 236:1843, 1976; Controversies and hazards in the treatment of pit viper bites. *South. Med. J. 72*:902, 1979.
28. VAN MIEROP, L. & KITCHENS, C.: Defibrination syndrome following bites by the Eastern diamondback rattlesnake. *J. Florida Med. Assoc. 67*:21, 1980.
29. SABBACK, M. et al: A study of the treatment of pit viper envenomization in 45 patients. *J. Trauma 17*:569, 1977.
30. LAWRENCE, W. et al: Pitviper bites: Rational management in which Copperheads and Cottonmouths predominate. *Annals of Plastic Surg. 36(3)*:276, 1996.

Wyeth Laboratories
A Wyeth-Ayerst Company
Marietta, PA 17547, USA
US Gov't License No. 3
CI 3285-4 Revised September 4, 2001

ANTIVENIN (Micrurus fulvius) ℞
[ăn'-tĭ-vĕ"-nĭn]
(Equine Origin)
North American
Coral Snake Antivenin

COMPOSITION

Antivenin (Micrurus fulvius), Wyeth, is a refined, concentrated, and lyophilized preparation of serum globulins obtained by fractionating blood from healthy horses that have been immunized with eastern coral snake (Micrurus fulvius fulvius) venom. Prior to lyophilization, the product contains 0.25% phenol and 0.005% thimerosal (mercury derivative).
Antivenin (Micrurus fulvius), Wyeth, is standardized for potency in mice in terms of its LD_{50} neutralizing capacity per milliliter as determined by intravenous injection of a graded series of Antivenin—M.f. fulvius venom mixtures. Based on this assay system, the reconstituted contents of each vial (10 ml) will neutralize approximately 250 mouse LD_{50} or approximately 2 mg of M.f. fulvius venom.
The results of cross-neutralization tests indicate that Antivenin (Micrurus fulvius), Wyeth, will neutralize the venom of M. fulvius tenere (Texas coral snake) but will NOT neutralize the venom of Micruroides euryxanthus (Arizona or Sonoran coral snake).

INDICATION

Antivenin (Micrurus fulvius) (equine origin) is indicated only for the treatment of envenomation caused by bites of those coral snakes specified in the following paragraph.

Coral Snakes and Bites

Two genera of coral snakes are found in the United States—Micrurus (including the eastern and Texas varieties) and Micruroides (the Sonoran or Arizona variety), found only in southeastern Arizona and southwestern New Mexico.
There are two subspecies of Micrurus fulvius native to the United States: 1) M.f. fulvius, found in the area from eastern North Carolina through the tip of Florida and in the Gulf coastal plain to the Mississippi River; 2) M.f. tenere, the Texas coral snake, found west of the Mississippi River in Louisiana, Arkansas, and Texas. These subspecies can be differentiated by experts but are very similar in appearance. The adult coral snake (M. fulvius) may vary between 20 to 44 inches in length, has a black snout, and yellow, black, and red bands encircling the body. The red and black rings are wider than the INTERPOSED yellow rings. However, melanistic (all black), albino (all white), and partially pigmented forms may be rarely seen. In contrast to the pit vipers (rattlesnakes, copperheads, cottonmouths), coral snakes have round pupils and lack facial pits. They are secretive and rarely bite unless disturbed or HANDLED. The fangs are short, erect, and fixed to the maxilla. Venom flows through the fang from a duct at its base. Pit vipers usually strike and then rapidly withdraw the head after insertion of the fangs. However, coral snakes, with their less efficient biting mechanism, may strike, hold on, and "chew", presumably so a sufficient amount of venom can be introduced to immobilize the prey. This "chewing" action may result in more than one "bite", and the victim MAY recall the colorful snake "hanging on" for a "minute" or so. Permitted to bite under laboratory conditions, M.f. fulvius have yielded 1 to 28 mg of venom.[1, 2] Fix and Minton,[2] after measuring the venom yields of 14 M.f. fulvius and the length of the individual snakes, found a positive linear relationship; six snakes measuring between 29 and 44 inches in length yielded 14 to 28 mg of dried venom, whereas eight measuring 21 to 28 inches in length yielded 2 to 10 mg. The adult human LD_{100} of M.f. fulvius venom has been estimated to be 4 to 5 mg of dried venom. Coral snake venom is chiefly paralytic (neurotoxic) in action, and usually only minimal-to-moderate tissue reaction and pain occur at the site of bite. Most coral snakebites are inflicted upon the upper extremities, especially the hands and fingers. The limited size of the biting apparatus makes it difficult for the coral snake to penetrate clothing or to successfully grasp any part of the body except the hands and feet. Hence, in areas where coral snakes are found, adherence to the simple practices of NEVER picking up colorful snakes, NEVER putting the hands where they cannot be seen (reaching behind rocks, logs, flowers, etc.), and always wearing leather shoes would substantially reduce the chances of a bite.
There are few published reports describing envenomation caused by coral snakebites.[1,3-7] It has been estimated that only 20±5 coral snakebites occur in the United States each year.[3] Although those persons who exhibit one or more fang punctures seem most likely to develop envenomation, there is NO way to predict which victim may be envenomated by a coral snakebite. Even a reliable observation that the biting snake did or did not "hang on" should NOT be used to predict the likelihood or possible severity of envenomation.
Coral snakebites, like bites by crotalids, are not always followed by envenomation. However, in contradistinction to crotalid bites, in which moderate-to-severe envenomation usually can be predicted by rapid onset of the local effects (e.g., pain, discoloration, edema), severe and even fatal envenomation from a coral snakebite can be present without any significant local tissue reaction.
Systemic signs and symptoms of envenomation usually begin from one to seven hours after the bite but may be delayed for as long as 18 hours. If envenomation occurs, the symptoms and signs may progress rapidly and precipitously. Paralysis has been observed within 2-1/2 hours post bite and appears to be of a bulbar type, involving cranial motor nerves. Death from respiratory paralysis has occurred within four hours of the accident.
SYSTEMIC signs and symptoms of envenomation may include euphoria, lethargy, weakness, nausea, vomiting, excessive salivation, ptosis of the eyelids, dyspnea, abnormal reflexes, convulsions, and motor weakness or paralysis, including complete respiratory paralysis. LOCAL signs and symptoms may include scratch marks or fang puncture wounds, no-to-moderate edema, erythema, pain at the bite site, and paresthesia in the bitten extremity.
TREATMENT OF CORAL SNAKEBITE: If practical, immobilize victim immediately and completely. Carry the victim to the nearest hospital as soon as possible. If complete immobilization is not practical, splint the bitten extremity to limit spread of venom. If the biting snake was killed, bring it to the hospital also.
ANY victim of a bite by a coral snake with ANY evidence of a break in the skin caused by the snake's teeth or fangs should be HOSPITALIZED for observation and/or treatment. Cleanse the bite area with germicidal soap and water to remove any venom remaining on the skin. If fang puncture wounds are present, application of a tourniquet and incision and suction over the fang punctures has been recommended,[1, 3] even though there is no evidence to indicate that incision and suction are or are not of value in removing coral snake venom. In addition to maintaining close observation of the patient for 24 hours, which should include checking the respiratory rate every 30 minutes, make sure the following will be available and ready for immediate use should need arise:
— a supply of Antivenin (Micrurus fulvius)
— an oxygen supply
— a mechanical respirator
— facilities and equipment for a tracheostomy
— the services of an anesthesiologist
Appropriate horse-serum sensitivity tests should be done so that, in case administration of Antivenin is subsequently required, a decision on how to proceed will have been made. Parrish and Khan[3] have recommended intravenous administration of coral snake antivenin to patients with one or more fang puncture wounds as soon as possible and before onset of symptoms and signs of envenomation.
If symptoms or signs of envenomation occur in a patient under observation or are already present at the time the patient is first seen, give Antivenin (Micrurus fulvius) promptly by the intravenous route. With vigorous treatment and careful observation, patients with complete respiratory paralysis have recovered, indicating that the respiratory paralysis is reversible.[4, 5] Hemoglobinuria has been observed in experimental animals envenomated by coral snakes. Hence, continuous bladder drainage is recommended with careful attention to urinary output and blood electrolyte balance.
Appropriate tetanus prophylaxis is indicated as for any other potentially contaminated puncture wound.

CONTRAINDICATIONS

For persons with coral snake envenomations threatening life or limb, there are no contraindications to administration of Antivenin. However, administration to persons known to be allergic to horse serum, either by history or as a result of an appropriate sensitivity test, requires careful judgement and considerable experience in the use of antivenoms of equine origin. Healthcare providers must be prepared to manage severe, immediate allergic reactions (anaphylaxis) seen with Antivenins of equine origin.[8,9,10,11]
Antivenin should never be administered prophylactically to asymptomatic patients.[12]

WARNINGS

Patients sensitive to Antivenin or horse serum may develop anaphylaxis. Therefore, it is essential that prior to intravenous (IV) or intramuscular (IM) Antivenin administration a proper skin test be performed, interpreted, and therapy modified if indicated.
There have been isolated reports of cardiac arrest and death associated with use of Antivenin (Crotalidae) Polyvalent (equine origin).[13] Although this experience has not been reported with Antivenin (coral snake), because of the similarity of these Antivenin products, this reaction cannot be ruled out for Antivenin (Micrurus fulvius) (equine origin).

PRECAUTIONS

General

Constant attendance and observation for untoward response is MANDATORY whenever horse serum is administered intravenously so that, should such occur, injection may be discontinued and appropriate treatment instituted immediately.
Those responsible for administration and/or monitoring administration of Antivenin should be familiar with current recommendations for treatment of severe, immediate, systemic reactions (anaphylaxis) associated with use of heterologous sera.
Therapy with beta-adrenergic blockers, including cardioselective agents, has been associated with an increased severity of acute anaphylaxis (see **Drug Interactions**).
Morphine or other narcotics that depress respiration are contraindicated. Sedatives should be used with extreme caution (see **Drug Interactions**).
The physician should be familiar with the package brochure and the pertinent published medical literature concerning envenomation resulting from coral snakebites, as well as the currently acceptable concepts of nonspecific treatment for venomous snakebites.

Precautions to be Taken in Administration of Horse Serum

Before administration of any product prepared from horse serum, appropriate measures must be taken in an effort to detect the presence of dangerous sensitivity: (1) A careful review of the patient's history, including any report of (a) asthma, hay fever, urticaria, or other allergic manifestations; (b) allergic reactions upon exposure to horses; and (c) prior injections of horse serum. (2) A suitable test for detection of sensitivity. A skin test should be performed in every patient prior to administration, regardless of clinical history.
Skin test–Inject intradermally 0.02 to 0.03 ml of a 1:10 dilution of Normal Horse Serum or Antivenin. A control test on the opposite extremity, using Sodium Chloride Injection, USP, facilitates interpretation. Use of larger amounts for the skin-test dose increases the likelihood of false-positive reactions, and in the exquisitely sensitive patient, increases the risk of a systemic reaction from the skin-test dose. A 10% rate of false negative skin test reactions has been reported with the use of Antivenin (Crotalidae) Polyvalent (equine origin).[14] Although this experience has not been reported with Antivenin (coral snake), because of the similarity of these Antivenin products, this reaction cannot be ruled out for Antivenin (Micrurus fulvius) (equine origin).
A 1:100 or greater dilution should be used for preliminary skin testing if the history suggests sensitivity. A positive reaction to a skin test occurs within five to thirty minutes and is manifested by a wheal with or without pseudopodia and surrounding erythema. In general, the shorter the interval between injection and the beginning of the skin reaction, the greater the sensitivity.
If the history is negative for allergy and the result of a skin test is negative, proceed with administration of Antivenin as outlined above. If the history is positive and a skin test is strongly positive, administration may be dangerous, especially if the positive sensitivity test is accompanied by systemic allergic manifestations. In such instances, the risk of administering Antivenin must be weighed against the risk of withholding it, keeping in mind that severe envenomation can be fatal. (See last paragraph of this section.)
A negative allergic history and absence of reaction to a properly applied skin test do not rule out the possibility of an immediate reaction. Also, a negative skin test has no bearing on whether or not delayed serum reactions (serum sickness) will occur after administration of the full dose.
If the history is negative, and the skin test is mildly or questionably positive, administer as follows to reduce the risk of a severe immediate systemic reaction: (a) Prepare, in separate sterile vials or syringes, 1:100 and 1:10 dilutions of Antivenin. (b) Allow at least 15 minutes between injections and proceed with the next dose if no reaction follows the previous dose. (c) Inject subcutaneously, using a tuberculin-type syringe, 0.1, 0.2, and 0.5 ml of the 1:100 dilution at 15-minute intervals; repeat with the 1:10 dilution, and finally undiluted Antivenin. (d) If a systemic reaction occurs after any injection, place a tourniquet proximal to the site of injections and administer an appropriate dose of epinephrine, 1:1000, proximal to the tourniquet or into another extremity. Wait at least 30 minutes before injecting another dose. The amount of the next dose should be the same as the last that did not evoke a reaction. (e) If no reaction occurs after 0.5 ml of undiluted Antivenin has been administered, switch to the intramuscular route and continue doubling the dose at 15-minute intervals until the entire dose has been injected intramuscularly or proceed to the intravenous route as described below under **Dosage and Administration**.

Drug Interactions

Morphine or other narcotics that depress respiration are contraindicated. Sedatives should be used with extreme caution.
Therapy with beta-adrenergic blockers, including cardioselective agents, has been associated with an increased severity of acute anaphylaxis.
Anaphylaxis may be prolonged and resistant to conventional treatment in patients receiving beta-adrenergic blockers. The pharmacotherapeutic actions of epinephrine and other adrenergic agents may be altered, and larger than usual doses may be required.[15]

DOSAGE AND ADMINISTRATION

IMPORTANT: Before administration, read sections on "**CONTRAINDICATIONS WARNINGS, PRECAUTIONS** and **Adverse Reactions**". Since the possibility of a severe immediate reaction (anaphylaxis) always exists whenever horse serum is administered, appropriate therapeutic agents, such as tourniquet, oxygen supply, epinephrine 1:1000, and another injectable pressor amine (NOT corticosteroids), must be ready for immediate use.
Start an intravenous drip of 250 to 500 ml of Sodium Chloride Injection, USP. If the results of appropriate tests have indicated the patient is not dangerously hypersensitive to horse serum, and depending on the nature and severity of the signs and symptoms of envenomation, administer the

Continued on next page

Antivenin (Micrurus fulvius)—Cont.

contents of 3 to 5 vials (30 to 50 ml) INTRAVENOUSLY by slow injection directly into the intravenous tubing or by adding to the reservoir bottle of the intravenous drip. (If added to reservoir bottle, mix by gentle swirling—DO NOT SHAKE.) In either case, the first 1 or 2 ml should be injected over a 3- to 5-minute period with careful observation of the patient for evidence of allergic reaction. If no signs or symptoms of anaphylaxis appear, continue the injection or intravenous infusion. The rate of delivery is regulated by the severity of signs and symptoms of envenomation and tolerance of Antivenin. However, until the equivalent of 30 to 50 ml of undiluted Antivenin has been given, administer at the maximum safe rate for intravenous fluids, based on body weight and general condition of the patient. For instance, if given by intravenous drip to a previously healthy adult, allow 250 or 500 ml to run in within 30 minutes; in small children, allow the first 100 ml to run in rapidly but then decrease to a rate not to exceed 4 ml per minute. Response to treatment may be rapid and dramatic. Observe the patient carefully and administer additional Antivenin intravenously as required.

According to the data reported by Fix and Minton[2] and cited above concerning venom yields obtained under artificial but probably physiological biting conditions, some envenomated patients may require administration of the contents of 10 or more vials to neutralize the venom dose injected by the biting snake if the entire venom load were delivered by the bite(s).

Snakes' mouths do not harbor *Clostridium tetani.* However, appropriate tetanus prophylaxis is indicated, since tetanus spores may be carried into the fang puncture wounds by dirt present on skin at time of bite or by nonsterile first-aid procedures.

A broad-spectrum antibiotic in adequate dosage is indicated if local tissue damage is evident.

Technique for Reconstituting the Dried Antivenin

Pry off the small metal disc in the cap over the diaphragms of the vials of Antivenin and diluent. Swab the exposed surface of the rubber diaphragms of both vials with an appropriate germicide. With a sterile 10 ml syringe and needle, withdraw the diluent (Sterile Water for Injection, USP) from the vial of diluent and insert the needle through the stopper of the vacuum-containing vial of Antivenin. The vacuum in the Antivenin vial will pull the diluent out of the syringe into the vial. However, delivery of 10 ml of diluent may not always exhaust the vacuum in the Antivenin vial. If all vacuum is not exhausted, reconstitution may be more difficult. Therefore, either disconnect the needle from the syringe and allow room air to be pulled into the Antivenin vial until all vacuum is released from the container or withdraw the syringe with attached needle from the vial, pull 10 ml of room air into the syringe and reinsert needle with attached syringe containing room air through stopper and repeat, if necessary, to release any remaining vacuum. At the first introduction of diluent into the vaccine vial, it is important for the needle to be pointed at the center of the lyophilized pellet of Antivenin so that the diluent stream will wet the pellet. If the diluent stream is not directed at the pellet but allowed to run down the inside wall of the vial, the pellet will float up and adhere to the stopper thereby rendering complete reconstitution much more difficult. Agitate by swirling, NOT by shaking, for 1 minute, at 5-minute intervals. Gentle agitation will hasten complete dissolution of the lyophilized Antivenin. Shaking causes foaming and if the diluent stream is not properly directed as described earlier, pieces of the pellet may get caught in the foam and will be very difficult to wet. Complete reconstitution usually requires at least 30 minutes.

Parenteral drug products should be inspected visually for particulate matter and discoloration prior to administration, whenever solution and container permit. The color of reconstituted Antivenin may vary from clear to slight yellowish or greenish.

Before each administration, gently swirl the vial to dissolve the contents.

Before any Antivenin is administered, an appropriate horse-serum sensitivity test must be done so that, in case administration of Antivenin is subsequently required, a decision on how to proceed will have been made (see **PRECAUTIONS**).

ADVERSE REACTIONS

Immediate systemic reactions (allergic reactions or anaphylaxis) can occur whenever a horse-serum-containing product is administered. An immediate reaction (shock, anaphylaxis) usually occurs within 30 minutes. Symptoms and signs may develop before the needle is withdrawn and may include apprehension, flushing, itching, urticaria; edema of the face, tongue, and throat; cough, dyspnea, cyanosis, vomiting, and collapse. There have been isolated reports of cardiac arrest and death associated with Antivenin (Crotalidae) Polyvalent (equine origin) use. However, serious immediate reactions to Antivenin are rare. In skin-test-negative patients, Antivenin caused a true immediate sensitivity reaction in less than 1 percent of patients.[9] Although this experience has not been reported with Antivenin (coral snake), because of the similarity of these Antivenin products, this reaction cannot be ruled out for Antivenin (Micrurus fulvius) (equine origin).

Serum sickness usually occurs 5 to 24 days after administration and its frequency may be related to the number of Antivenin vials administered.[16] The incubation period may be less than 5 days, especially in those who have received horse-serum-containing preparations in the past. The usual symptoms and signs are malaise, fever, urticaria, lymphadenopathy, edema, arthralgia, nausea, and vomiting. Occasionally, neurological manifestations develop, such as meningismus or peripheral neuritis. Peripheral neuritis usually involves the shoulders and arms. Pain and muscle weakness are frequently present, and permanent atrophy may develop.

HOW SUPPLIED

Each package contains one vacuum vial to yield 10 ml of Antivenin (with preservatives: phenol 0.25% and thimerosal [mercury derivative] 0.005%).

Store original, unused (not reconstituted) vials between 2 and 8 °C (36 and 46 °F). Do not freeze.

Gently swirl the vial of reconstituted Antivenin before each administration.

REFERENCES

1. MC COLLOUGH, N. and GENNARO, J.: Coral snakebites in the United States. J. Florida Med. Assn. *49*:968, 1963.
2. FIX, J. and MINTON, S.: Venom extraction and yields from the North American Coral Snake, Micrurus fulvius. Toxicon *14*:143, 1976.
3. PARRISH, H. and KAHN, M.: Bites by coral snakes: Report of 11 representative cases. Am. J. Med. Sci. *253*: 561, 1967.
4. MOSELY, T.: Coral snakebite: Recovery following symptoms of respiratory paralysis. Ann. Surg. *163*:943, 1966.
5. RAMSEY, G. and KLICKSTEIN, G.: Coral snakebite. Report of a case and suggested therapy. JAMA *182*:949, 1962.
6. NEILL, W.: Some misconceptions regarding the eastern coral snake, Micrurus fulvius. Herpetologica *13*:111, 1957.
7. RUSSELL, F.: Bites by the Sonoran coral snake, Micruroides euryxanthus. Toxicon *5*:39, 1967.
8. WINGERT, W. and WAINSCHEL, J.: Diagnosis and management of envenomation by poisonous snakes. South. Med. J. *68*:1015, 1975.
9. RUSSEL, F.: Snake venom poisoning. Scholium International, Inc., New York, 1983.
10. LOPRINZI, C. et al: Snake Antivenin administration in a patient allergic to horse serum. South. Med. J. *76*:501, 1983.
11. OTTEN, E. & MCKIMM, D.: Venomous snakebite in a patient allergic to horse serum. Ann. Emerg. Med. *12*: 624, 1983.
12. BOWDEN, C. & KRENZELOK, E.: Clinical applications of commonly used contemporary antidotes, a US perspective. Drug Safety *16(1)*:22-24, 1997.
13. Wyeth-Ayerst Data on File.
14. JURKOVICH, G. et al: Complications of Crotalidae Antivenin therapy. The J. of Trauma *28*:7, 1988.
15. TOOGOOD, J.: Beta-blocker therapy and the risk of anaphylaxis. Canc. Med. Assoc. J. *136*:929, 1987.
16. LAWRENCE, W. et al: Pitviper bites: Rational management in which Copperheads and Cottonmouths predominate. Annals of Plastic Surg. *36(3)*:276, 1996.

U.S. Govt. License No. 3
Wyeth Laboratories Inc., Marietta, PA 17547
CI3280-4 Revised August 31, 2001

BENEFIX® ℞

[*bĕnĕ-fĭks*]
COAGULATION FACTOR IX (RECOMBINANT)
USA: ℞ only

This product's label may have been revised after this insert was used in production. For further product information and current package insert, please visit www.wyeth.com or call our medical communications department toll-free at 1-800-934-5556.

DESCRIPTION

BeneFIX®, Coagulation Factor IX (Recombinant), is a purified protein produced by recombinant DNA technology for use in therapy of factor IX deficiency, known as hemophilia B or Christmas disease. Coagulation Factor IX (Recombinant) is a glycoprotein with an approximate molecular mass of 55,000 Da consisting of 415 amino acids in a single chain. It has a primary amino acid sequence that is identical to the Ala^{148} allelic form of plasma-derived factor IX, and has structural and functional characteristics similar to those of endogenous factor IX.

BeneFIX® is produced by a genetically engineered Chinese hamster ovary (CHO) cell line that is extensively characterized and shown to be free of known infectious agents. The stored cell banks are free of blood or plasma products. The CHO cell line secretes recombinant factor IX into a defined cell culture medium that does not contain any proteins derived from animal or human sources, and the recombinant factor IX is purified by a chromatography purification process that does not require a monoclonal antibody step and yields a high-purity, active product. A membrane filtration step that has the ability to retain molecules with apparent molecular weights >70,000 (such as large proteins and viral particles) is included for additional viral safety. BeneFIX® is predominantly a single component by SDS-polyacrylamide gel electrophoresis evaluation. The potency (in international units, IU) is determined using an *in vitro* one-stage clotting assay against the World Health Organization (WHO) International Standard for Factor IX concentrate. One international unit is the amount of factor IX activity present in 1 mL of pooled, normal human plasma. The specific activity of BeneFIX® is greater than or equal to 200 IU per milligram of protein. BeneFIX® is not derived from human blood and contains no preservatives or added animal or human components.

BeneFIX® is inherently free from the risk of transmission of human blood-borne pathogens such as HIV, hepatitis viruses, and parvovirus.

BeneFIX® is formulated as a sterile, nonpyrogenic, lyophilized powder preparation. BeneFIX® is intended for intravenous (IV) injection. It is available in single use vials containing the labeled amount of factor IX activity, expressed in international units (IU). Each vial contains nominally 250, 500, or 1000 IU of Coagulation Factor IX (Recombinant). After reconstitution of the lyophilized drug product, the concentrations of excipients in the 500 and 1000 IU dosage strengths are 10 mM L-histidine, 1% sucrose, 260 mM glycine, 0.005% polysorbate 80. The concentrations after reconstitution in the 250 IU dosage strength are half those of the other two dosage strengths. The 500 and 1000 IU dosage strengths are isotonic after reconstitution, and the 250 IU dosage strength has half the tonicity of the other two dosage strengths after reconstitution. All dosage strengths yield a clear, colorless solution upon reconstitution.

CLINICAL PHARMACOLOGY

Factor IX is activated by factor VII/tissue factor complex in the extrinsic coagulation pathway as well as by factor XIa in the intrinsic coagulation pathway. Activated factor IX, in combination with activated factor VIII, activates factor X. This results ultimately in the conversion of prothrombin to thrombin. Thrombin then converts fibrinogen to fibrin, and a clot can be formed.

Factor IX is the specific clotting factor deficient in patients with hemophilia B and in patients with acquired factor IX deficiencies. The administration of BeneFIX®, Coagulation Factor IX (Recombinant), increases plasma levels of factor IX and can temporarily correct the coagulation defect in these patients.

After single intravenous (IV) doses of 50 IU/kg of BeneFIX®, Coagulation Factor IX (Recombinant), in 37 previously treated adult patients (>15 years), each given as a 10-minute infusion, the mean increase from pre-infusion level in circulating factor IX activity was 0.8 ± 0.2 IU/dL per IU/kg infused (range 0.4 to 1.4 IU/dL per IU/kg) and the mean biologic half-life was 18.8 ± 5.4 hours (range 11 to 36 hours). In the randomized, cross-over pharmacokinetic study in previously treated patients (PTPs), the *in vivo* recovery using BeneFIX® was statistically significantly less (28% lower) than the recovery using a highly purified plasma-derived factor IX product. There was no significant difference in biological half-life. Structural differences of the BeneFIX® molecule compared with pdFIX were shown to contribute to the lower recovery. In subsequent evaluations for up to 24 months, the pharmacokinetic parameters were similar to the initial results.

For specific information regarding pediatric pharmacology, see **PRECAUTIONS, Pediatric Use.**

Clinical Studies

There are ongoing safety and efficacy studies of BeneFIX® in previously treated, previously untreated, and minimally treated patients.

In 4 clinical studies of BeneFIX®, a total of 128 subjects 56 previously treated patients [PTPs], 9 subjects participating only in the surgical study, and 63 previously untreated patients (PUPs) received more than 28 million IU administered over a period of up to 64 months. The studies included 121 HIV-negative and 7 HIV-positive subjects.

Fifty-six PTPs received approximately 20.9 million IU of BeneFIX® in two clinical studies. The median number of exposure days was 83.5. These PTPs who were treated for bleeding episodes on an on-demand basis or for the prevention of bleeds were followed over a median interval of 24 months (range 1 to 29 months; mean 23.4 ± 5.34 months). Fifty-five of these PTPs received a median of 42.8 IU/kg (range 6.5 to 224.6 IU/kg; mean 46.6 ± 23.5 IU/kg) per infusion for bleeding episodes. All subjects were evaluable for efficacy. One subject discontinued the study after one month of treatment due to bleeding episodes that were difficult to control; he did not have a detectable inhibitor. The subject's dose had not been adequately titrated. The remaining 55 subjects were treated successfully. Bleeding episodes that were managed successfully included hemarthroses and bleeding in soft tissue and muscle. Data concerning the severity of bleeding episodes were not reported. Eighty-eight percent of the total infusions administered for bleeding episodes were rated as providing an "excellent" or "good" response. Eighty-one percent of all bleeding episodes were managed with a single infusion of BeneFIX®. One subject developed a low titer, transient inhibitor (maximum titer 1.5 BU). This subject had previously received plasma-derived products without a history of inhibitor development. He was able to continue treatment with BeneFIX® with no anamnestic rise in inhibitor or anaphylaxis, however, increased frequency of BeneFIX® administration was required; subsequently the subject's factor IX inhibitor and its effect on the half-life of BeneFIX® resolved.

Forty-one of the subjects had measurements of fibrinopeptide A and prothrombin fragment 1 + 2 prior to infusion, 4 to 8 hours and then 24 hours following the infusion. Twenty-nine of the subjects had elevations in fibrinopeptide A with a maximum value of 35.3 nmol/L (22 of the 29 subjects had elevated baseline values). Ten of the subjects had elevated prothrombin fragment 1 + 2 with a maximum value of 1.82 nmol/L (3 of the 10 subjects had elevated baseline values).

A total of 20 PTPs were treated with BeneFIX® for secondary prophylaxis (the regular administration of FIX replacement therapy to prevent bleeding in patients who may have already demonstrated clinical evidence of hemophilic arthropathy or joint disease) at some regular interval during the study with a mean of 2.0 infusions per week. Nineteen subjects were administered BeneFIX® for routine secondary prophylaxis (at least twice weekly) for a total of 345 patient-months with a median follow-up period of 24 months per subject. The average dose used by these 19 subjects was 40.3 IU/kg, ranging from 13 to 78 IU/kg. One additional subject was treated weekly, using an average dose of 33.3 IU/kg, over a period of 21 months. Ninety-three percent of the responses were rated as "excellent" or "effective". These 20 PTPs received a total of 2985 infusions of BeneFIX® for routine prophylaxis. Seven of these PTPs experienced a total of 26 spontaneous bleeding episodes within 48 hours after an infusion.

Management of hemostasis was evaluated in the surgical setting. Thirty-six surgical procedures have been performed in 28 subjects. Thirteen (13) minor surgical procedures were performed in 12 subjects, including 7 dental procedures, 1 punch biopsy of the skin, 1 cyst removal, 1 male sterilization, 1 nevus ablation, and 2 ingrown toenail removals. Twenty-three (23) major surgical procedures were performed in 19 subjects including a liver transplant, splenectomy, 3 inguinal hernia repairs, 11 orthopedic procedures, a calf-debridement and 6 complicated dental extractions.

Twenty-three (23) subjects underwent 27 surgical procedures with a pulse-replacement regimen. The mean perioperative (preoperative and intraoperative) dose for these procedures was 85 ± 32.8 IU/kg (range 25-154.9 IU/kg). The mean total post-operative (inpatient and outpatient) dose was 63.1 ± 22.0 IU/kg (range 28.6-129.0).

Total BeneFIX® coverage during the surgical period for the major procedures ranged from 4230 to 385,800 IU. The preoperative dose for the major procedures ranged from 75 to 155 IU/kg. Nine of the major surgical procedures were performed in 8 subjects using a continuous infusion regimen. Following pre-operative bolus doses (94.1 -144.5 IU/kg), continuous infusion of BeneFIX® was administered at a median rate of 6.7 IU/kg/hr (range of average rates: 4.3-8.6 IU/kg/hr; mean 6.4 ± 1.5 IU/kg/hr for a median duration of 5 days (range 1-11 days; mean 4.9 ± 3.1). Six of the 8 subjects who had received continuous infusion of BeneFIX® in conjunction with major surgeries were switched over to intermittent pulse regimens at a median dose of 56.3 IU/kg (range 33.6-89.1 IU/kg; mean 57.8 ± 18.1 IU/kg SD) for a median of 3.5 exposure days (range 1-5 days, mean 3.3 ± 1.4 SD) during the post-operative period. Although circulating factor IX levels targeted to restore and maintain hemostasis were achieved with both pulse replacement and continuous infusion regimens, clinical trial experience with continuous infusion of BeneFIX® for surgical prophylaxis in hemophilia B has been too limited to establish the safety and clinical efficacy of administration of the product by continuous infusion. Subjects administered BeneFIX® by continuous infusion for surgical prophylaxis also received intermittent bolus infusions of the product.

Among the surgery subjects, the median increase in circulating factor IX activity was 0.7 IU/dL per IU/kg infused (range 0.3-1.2 IU/dL; mean 0.8 ± 0.2 IU/dL per IU/kg). The median elimination half-life for the surgery subjects was 19.4 hours (range 10-37 hours; mean 21.3 ± 8.1 hours).

Hemostasis was maintained throughout the surgical period, however, one subject required evacuation of a surgical wound site hematoma and another subject who received BeneFIX® after a tooth extraction required further surgical intervention due to oozing at the extraction site. There was no clinical evidence of thrombotic complications in any of the subjects. In seven subjects for whom fibrinopeptide A and prothrombin fragment 1 + 2 were measured pre-infusion, at 4 to 8 hours, and then daily up to 96 hours, there was no evidence of significant increase in coagulation activation. Data from two other subjects were judged to be not evaluable.

Sixty-three PUPs received approximately 6.2 million IU of BeneFIX® in an open-label safety and efficacy study over 89 median exposure days. These PUPs were followed over a median interval of 37 months (range 4 to 64 months; mean 38.1 ± 16.4 months). Fifty-four of these PUPs received a median dose of 62.7 IU/kg (range 8.2 to 292.0 IU/kg; mean 75.6 ± 42.5 IU/kg) per infusion for bleeding episodes. Data concerning the severity of bleeding episodes were not reported. Seventy-five percent of all bleeding episodes were managed with a single infusion of BeneFIX®. Three of these 54 subjects were not successfully treated; including one episode in a subject due to delayed time to infusion and insufficient dosing and in 2 subjects due to inhibitor formation. One subject developed a high titer inhibitor (maximum titer 42 BU) on exposure day 7. A second subject developed a high titer inhibitor (maximum titer 18 BU) after 15 exposure days. Both subjects experienced allergic manifestations in temporal association with their inhibitor development.

Thirty-two PUPs administered BeneFIX® for routine prophylaxis. Twenty-four PUPs administered BeneFIX® at least twice weekly for a total of 2587 infusions. The mean dose per infusion was 72.5 ± 37.1 IU/kg, and the mean duration of prophylaxis was 13.4 ± 8.2 months. Eight PUPs administered BeneFIX® once weekly for a total of 571 infusions. The mean dose per infusion was 75.9 ± 17.9 IU/kg, and the mean duration of prophylaxis was 17.6 ± 7.4 months. Five PUPs experienced a total of 6 spontaneous bleeding episodes within 48 hours after an infusion.

Twenty-three PUPs received BeneFIX® for surgical prophylaxis in 30 surgical procedures. All surgical procedures were minor except 2 hernia repairs. The preoperative bolus dose ranged from 32.3 IU/kg to 247.2 IU/kg. The perioperative total dose ranged from 385 to 23280 IU. Five of the surgical procedures were performed using a continuous infusion regimen over 3 to 5 days. Clinical trial experience with continuous infusion of BeneFIX® for surgical prophylaxis in hemophilia B has been too limited to establish the safety and clinical efficacy of administration of the product by continuous infusion.

INDICATIONS AND USAGE

BeneFIX®, Coagulation Factor IX (Recombinant), is indicated for the control and prevention of hemorrhagic episodes in patients with hemophilia B (congenital factor IX deficiency or Christmas disease), including control and prevention of bleeding in surgical settings.

BeneFIX®, Coagulation Factor IX (Recombinant), is not indicated for the treatment of other factor deficiencies (e.g., factors II, VII, VIII, and X), nor for the treatment of hemophilia A patients with inhibitors to factor VIII, nor for the reversal of coumarin-induced anticoagulation, nor for the treatment of bleeding due to low levels of liver-dependent coagulation factors.

CONTRAINDICATIONS

Because BeneFIX®, Coagulation Factor IX (Recombinant), is produced in a Chinese hamster ovary cell line, it may be contraindicated in patients with a known history of hypersensitivity to hamster protein.

WARNINGS

Allergic type hypersensitivity reactions, including anaphylaxis, have been reported for all factor IX products. Frequently, these events have occurred in close temporal association with the development of factor IX inhibitors. Patients should be informed of the early symptoms and signs of hypersensitivity reactions including hives, generalized urticaria, angioedema, chest tightness, dyspnea, wheezing, faintness, hypotension, tachycardia, and anaphylaxis. Patients should be advised to discontinue use of the product and contact their physician and/or seek immediate emergency care, depending on the type/severity of the reaction, if any of these symptoms occur (see **PRECAUTIONS**).

The diluent vial accompanying this product may contain dry natural rubber that may cause hypersensitivity reactions when handled by or administered to persons with known or possible latex sensitivity.

Nephrotic syndrome has been reported following immune tolerance induction with factor IX products in hemophilia B patients with factor IX inhibitors and a history of allergic reactions to factor IX. The safety and efficacy of using BeneFIX® for immune tolerance induction has not been established.

Since the use of factor IX complex concentrates has historically been associated with the development of thromboembolic complications, the use of factor IX-containing products may be potentially hazardous in patients with signs of fibrinolysis and in patients with disseminated intravascular coagulation (DIC).

PRECAUTIONS

General

Historically, the administration of factor IX complex concentrates derived from human plasma, containing factors II, VII, IX and X, has been associated with the development of thromboembolic complications.[1] Although BeneFIX® contains no coagulation factor other than factor IX, the potential risk of thrombosis and DIC observed with other products containing factor IX should be recognized. Because of the potential risk of thromboembolic complications, caution should be exercised when administering this product to patients with liver disease, to patients post-operatively, to neonates, or to patients at risk of thromboembolic phenomena or DIC. In each of these situations, the benefit of treatment with BeneFIX® should be weighed against the risk of these complications.

Twelve days after a dose of BeneFIX® for a bleeding episode, one hepatitis C antibody positive patient developed a renal infarct. The relationship of the infarct to prior administration of BeneFIX® is uncertain but was judged to be unlikely by the investigator. The patient continued to be treated with BeneFIX®.

Activity-neutralizing antibodies (inhibitors) have been detected in patients receiving factor IX-containing products. As with all factor IX products, patients using BeneFIX® should be monitored for the development of factor IX inhibitors (see **CLINICAL PHARMACOLOGY** and **WARNINGS**). Patients with factor IX inhibitors may be at an increased risk of anaphylaxis upon subsequent challenge with factor IX[2]. Patients experiencing allergic reactions should be evaluated for the presence of inhibitor. Preliminary information suggests a relationship may exist between the presence of major deletion mutations in a patient's factor IX gene and an increased risk of inhibitor formation and of acute hypersensitivity reactions. Patients known to have major deletion mutations of the factor IX gene should be observed closely for signs and symptoms of acute hypersensitivity reactions, particularly during the early phases of initial exposure to product. In view of the potential for allergic reactions with factor IX concentrates, the initial (approximately 10 - 20) administrations of factor IX should be performed under medical supervision where proper medical care for allergic reactions could be provided.

Dosing of BeneFIX® may differ from that of plasma-derived factor IX products (see **CLINICAL PHARMACOLOGY** and **DOSAGE AND ADMINISTRATION**).

Information for Patients

Patients should be informed of the early symptoms and signs of hypersensitivity reactions including hives, generalized urticaria, angioedema, chest tightness, dyspnea, wheezing, faintness, hypotension, tachycardia, and anaphylaxis. Patients should be advised to discontinue use of the product and contact their physician and/or seek immediate emergency care, depending on the type/severity of the reaction, if any of these symptoms occur. Patients experiencing allergic reactions should be evaluated for the presence of inhibitor.

Carcinogenesis, Mutagenesis, Impairment of Fertility

BeneFIX®, Coagulation Factor IX (Recombinant), has been shown to be nonmutagenic in the Ames assay and nonclastogenic in a chromosomal aberrations assay. No investigations on carcinogenesis or impairment of fertility have been conducted.

Pregnancy Category C

Animal reproduction and lactation studies have not been conducted with BeneFIX®, Coagulation Factor IX (Recombinant). It is not known whether BeneFIX® can affect reproductive capacity or cause fetal harm when given to pregnant women. BeneFIX® should be administered to pregnant and lactating women only if clearly indicated.

Pediatric Use

Additional safety and efficacy studies are ongoing in previously treated, minimally treated, and previously untreated pediatric patients (see **CLINICAL PHARMACOLOGY, WARNINGS** and **DOSAGE AND ADMINISTRATION**).

Data from BeneFIX® safety, efficacy, and pharmacokinetic studies have been evaluated in previously treated and previously untreated pediatric patients.

Nineteen (19) previously treated pediatric patients (range 4 to ≤15 years) underwent pharmacokinetic evaluations for up to 24 months. The mean increase in circulating factor IX activity was 0.7 ± 0.2 IU/dL per IU/kg infused (range 0.3 to 1.1 IU/dL per IU/kg; median of 0.6 IU/dL per IU/kg). The mean biological half-life was 20.2 ± 4.0 hours (range 14 to 28 hours).

Fifty-eight previously untreated patients [PUPs] less than 15 years of age at baseline [3 neonates (0-<1 month), 45 infants (≥1 month-<2 years), 9 children (≥2 years-<12 years) and 1 adolescent (>12 years)] underwent at least one recovery assessment within 30 minutes post-infusion in the presence or absence of hemorrhage during the study. The mean increase in circulating FIX activity was 0.7 ± 0.3 IU/dL per IU/kg infused (range 0.2 to 2.1 IU/dL per IU/kg; median of 0.6 IU/dL per IU/kg). In addition, there was no difference in the recoveries noted when data were evaluated by age group for infants (0.7 ± 0.4 IU/dL per IU/kg; range 0.2 to 2.1 IU/dL per IU/kg) and children (0.7 ± 0.2 IU/dL per IU/kg; range 0.2 to 1.5 IU/dL per IU/kg). The recoveries in these age groups were consistent with the recovery for the PUP study as a whole. There was insufficient sample size in the neonate and adolescent age groups to perform an analysis in these groups. Data from 57 subjects who underwent repeat recovery testing for up to 60 months demonstrated that the average incremental FIX recovery was consistent over time.

Geriatric Use

Clinical studies of BeneFIX® did not include sufficient numbers of subjects aged 65 and over to determine whether they respond differently from younger subjects. As with any patient receiving BeneFIX®, dose selection for an elderly patient should be individualized (see **DOSAGE AND ADMINISTRATION**).

ADVERSE REACTIONS

See also **CLINICAL PHARMACOLOGY: Clinical Studies.**

As with the intravenous administration of any protein product, the following reactions may be observed after administration: headache, fever, chills, flushing, nausea, vomiting, lethargy, or manifestations of allergic reactions. Should evidence of an acute hypersensitivity reaction be observed, the infusion should be stopped promptly and appropriate counter measures and supportive therapy should be administered.

During uncontrolled open-label clinical studies with BeneFIX®, Coagulation Factor IX (Recombinant), conducted in previously treated patients (PTPs), 131 adverse reactions with definite, probable, possible or unknown relation to BeneFIX® therapy were reported among 27 of 65 subjects (with some subjects reporting more than one event) who received a total of 7573 infusions. These adverse reactions are summarized in Table 1 below.

[See table 1 at top of next page]

One subject discontinued BeneFIX® due to pulmonary allergic-type symptoms.

In the 63 treated PUPS, who received a total of 5538 infusions, 22 adverse reactions were reported as having definite, probable, possible or unknown relationship to BeneFIX®. These events are summarized in Table 2 below.

[See table 2 on next page]

Continued on next page

BeneFix—Cont.

The following post-marketing adverse reactions have been reported for BeneFIX®, as well as for plasma-derived factor IX products: inadequate factor IX recovery, inadequate therapeutic response, inhibitor development (see **CLINICAL PHARMACOLOGY**), anaphylaxis (see **WARNINGS**), laryngeal edema, angioedema, cyanosis, dyspnea, hypotension, and thrombosis.

If any adverse reaction takes place that is thought to be related to the administration of BeneFIX®, the rate of infusion should be decreased or the infusion stopped.

DOSAGE AND ADMINISTRATION

Treatment with BeneFIX®, Coagulation Factor IX (Recombinant), should be initiated under the supervision of a physician experienced in the treatment of hemophilia B.

Dosage and duration of treatment for all factor IX products depend on the severity of the factor IX deficiency, the location and extent of bleeding, and the patient's clinical condition, age and recovery of factor IX.

To ensure that the desired factor IX activity level has been achieved, precise monitoring using the factor IX activity assay is advised. Doses should be titrated using the factor IX activity, pharmacokinetic parameters, such as half-life and recovery, as well as taking the clinical situation into consideration in order to adjust the dose as appropriate.

In an eleven subject, crossover, randomized PK evaluation of BeneFIX® and a single lot of high-purity plasma-derived factor IX, the recovery was lower for BeneFIX® (see **CLINICAL PHARMACOLOGY**). In the clinical efficacy studies, subjects were initially administered the same dose previously used for plasma-derived factor IX. Even in the absence of factor IX inhibitor, approximately half of the subjects increased their dose in these studies. Titrate the initial dose upward if necessary to achieve the desired clinical response. As with some plasma-derived factor IX products, subjects at the low end of the observed factor IX recovery may require upward dosage adjustment to as much as two times (2X) the initial empirically calculated dose in order to achieve the intended rise in circulating factor IX activity.

BeneFIX® is administered by IV infusion over several minutes after reconstitution of the lyophilized powder with Sterile Water for Injection (USP).

Method of Calculating Dose

The method of calculating the factor IX dose is shown in the following equation:

number of factor IX IU required (IU)	=	body weight (kg)	×	Desired factor IX increase (% or IU/dL)	×	reciprocal of observed recovery (IU/kg per IU/dL)

In the presence of an inhibitor, higher doses may be required.

Adult Patients

In adult PTPs, on average, one international unit of BeneFIX® per kilogram of body weight increased the circulating activity of factor IX by 0.8 ± 0.2 (range 0.4 to 1.4) IU/dL. The method of dose estimation is illustrated in the following example. If you use 0.8 IU/dL average increase of factor IX per IU/kg body weight administered, then:

number of factor IX IU required (IU)	=	body weight (kg)	×	desired factor IX increase (% or IU/dL)	×	1.2 (IU/kg per IU/dL)

Pediatric Patients (<15 years)

In pediatric patients, on average, one international unit of BeneFIX® per kilogram of body weight increased the circulating activity of factor IX by 0.7 ± 0.3 (range 0.2 to 2.1 IU/dL; median of 0.6 IU/dL per IU/kg). The method of dose estimation is illustrated in the following example. If you use 0.7 IU/dL average increase of factor IX per IU/kg body weight administered, then:

number of factor IX IU required (IU)	=	body weight (kg)	×	desired factor IX increase (% or IU/dL)	×	1.4 (IU/kg per IU/dL)

The following chart[3] may be used to guide dosing in bleeding episodes and surgery:

Type of Hemorrhage	Circulating Factor IX Activity Required [% or (IU/dL)]	Dosing Interval [hours]	Duration of Therapy [days]
Minor			
Uncomplicated hemarthroses, superficial muscle, or soft tissue	20-30	12-24	1-2
Moderate			
Intramuscle or soft tissue with dissection, mucous membranes, dental extractions, or hematuria	25-50	12-24	Treat until bleeding stops and healing begins; about 2 to 7 days
Major			
Pharynx, retropharynx, retroperitoneum, CNS, surgery	50-100	12-24	7-10

Adapted from: Roberts and Eberst[3]

Table 1: Adverse Events Reported for PTPs*

Reaction	Total number of events with definite, probable, possible or unknown relation to therapy (n=129)	Number and (%) of patients from which the reports originated (n=65)	Number and (%) of infusions temporally associated with the reaction[1] (n=7573)
Nausea	27	4 (6.2 %)	27 (0.36 %)
Taste perversion (Altered taste)	14	3 (4.6 %)	19 (0.25 %)
Hypoxia (Urge to cough with hypoxemia)	11	1 (1.5 %)	11 (0.15 %)
Injection site reaction	11	5 (7.7 %)	12 (0.16 %)
Injection site pain	10	4 (6.2 %)	16 (0.21 %)
Headache	10	7 (10.8 %)	13 (0.17 %)
Dizziness	7	5 (7.7 %)	8 (0.11 %)
Allergic rhinitis	7	3 (4.6 %)	9 (0.12 %)
Pain (Burning sensation in the jaw and skull)	6	1 (1.5 %)	7 (0.09 %)
Rash	6	5 (7.7 %)	7 (0.09 %)
Hives	3	2 (3.1 %)	3 (0.04 %)
Flushing	3	2 (3.1 %)	4 (0.05 %)
Fever	2	2 (3.1 %)	2 (0.03 %)
Shaking	2	2 (3.1 %)	1 (0.01 %)
Factor IX inhibitor[2]	1	1 (1.5 %)	2 (0.03 %)
Chest tightness	1	1 (1.5 %)	4 (0.05 %)
Drowsiness	1	1 (1.5 %)	1 (0.01 %)
Visual disturbance	1	1 (1.5 %)	1 (0.01 %)
Cellulitis at the IV site	1	1 (1.5 %)	7 (0.09 %)
Phlebitis at the IV site	1	1 (1.5 %)	7 (0.09 %)
Dry cough	1	1 (1.5 %)	0 (0.00 %)
Allergic reaction	1	1 (1.5 %)	1 (0.01 %)
Diarrhea	1	1 (1.5 %)	1 (0.01 %)
Lung disorder	1	1 (1.5 %)	1 (0.01 %)
Vomiting	1	1 (1.5 %)	1 (0.01 %)
Renal infarct[3]	1	1 (1.5 %)	1 (0.01 %)
Total	131	27/65 (41.5 %)	148/7573 (2.2 %)

*More than one event in the table could have been assoc. with an infusion; however, the total represents the actual number of infusions given.

1 Reaction occurring within 72 hours after infusion.

2 Low titer transient inhibitor formation.

3 The renal infarct developed in a hepatitis C antibody positive patient 12 days after a dose of BeneFIX® for a bleeding episode. The relationship of the infarct to the prior administration of BeneFIX® is uncertain. (See **PRECAUTIONS, General**).

Table 2: Adverse Events reported for PUPs*

Reaction	Total number of events with definite, probable, possible or unknown relation to therapy (n=22)	Number and (%) of patients from which the reports originated (n=63)	Number and (%) of infusions temporally associated with the reaction[1] (n=5538)
Diarrhea	5	1 (1.6 %)	11 (0.20 %)
Urticaria (hives)	3	3 (4.8 %)	3 (0.05 %)
Factor IX inhibitor[2]	2	2 (3.2 %)	4 (0.07 %)
Dyspnea (Respiratory distress)	2	2 (3.2 %)	2 (0.04 %)
Increased alkaline phosphatase	1	1 (1.6 %)	3 (0.05 %)
Elevated ALT	1	1 (1.6 %)	0 (0.00 %)
Rash (Body rash)	1	1 (1.6 %)	1 (0.02 %)
Elevated AST	1	1 (1.6 %)	0 (0.00 %)
Chills (Rigors)	1	1 (1.6 %)	3 (0.05 %)
Photosensitivity reaction	1	1 (1.6 %)	0 (0.00 %)
Injection site reaction	1	1 (1.6 %)	2 (0.04 %)
HAV seroconversion[3]	1	1 (1.6 %)	2 (0.04 %)
Parvovirus B19 seroconversion[4]	1	1 (1.6 %)	1 (0.02 %)
Asthma	1	1 (1.6 %)	1 (0.02 %)
Total	22	11/63 (17.5%)	27/5538 (0.60%)

*More than one event in the table could have been assoc. with an infusion; however, the total represents the actual number of infusions given.

1 Reaction occurring within 72 hours after infusion.

2 Two subjects developed high titer inhibitor formation during treatment with BeneFIX®.

3 Relationship of HAV seroconversion to BeneFIX® is unknown. HAV seroconversion was noted on 2 occasions in a single patient but was negative at final visit. The patient had no laboratory or clinical findings associated with active infection.

4 Relationship of Parvovirus B19 seroconversion to BeneFIX® is unknown. It was unlikely that seroconversion was related to BeneFIX® due to the frequency of community acquired infection and viral safeguards built into the manufacturing process (See **DESCRIPTION**).

INSTRUCTIONS FOR USE

The procedures below are provided as general guidelines for the reconstitution and administration of BeneFIX®. Patients should follow the specific reconstitution and administration procedures provided by their physicians.

Reconstitution

Always wash your hands before performing the following procedures. Aseptic technique should be used during the reconstitution procedure.

BeneFIX®, Coagulation Factor IX (Recombinant), will be administered by intravenous (IV) infusion after reconstitution with Sterile Water for Injection (diluent).

1. Allow the vials of lyophilized BeneFIX® and diluent to reach room temperature.
2. Remove the plastic flip-top caps from the BeneFIX® vial and the diluent vial to expose the central portions of the rubber stoppers.
3. Wipe the tops of both vials with the alcohol swab provided, or use another antiseptic solution, and allow to dry.
4. Remove the protective cover from the short end of the sterile double-ended needle and insert the short end into the diluent vial at the center of the stopper.
5. Remove the protective cover from the long end of the needle. Invert the solvent vial and, to minimize leakage, quickly insert the long end of the needle through the center of the stopper of the upright BeneFIX® vial.

Note: Point the double-ended needle toward the wall of the BeneFIX® vial to prevent excessive foaming.

6. The vacuum will draw the diluent into the BeneFIX® vial.
7. Once the transfer is complete, remove the long end of the needle from the BeneFIX® vial, and properly discard the needle with the diluent vial.
   Note: If the diluent does not transfer completely into the BeneFIX® vial, DO NOT USE the contents of the vial. Note that it is acceptable for a small amount of fluid to remain in the diluent vial after transfer.
8. Gently rotate the vial to dissolve the powder.
9. Parenteral drug products should be inspected visually for particulate matter and discoloration prior to administration, whenever solution and container permit. Reconstituted BeneFIX® should appear clear and colorless.

BeneFIX® should be administered within 3 hours after reconstitution. The reconstituted solution may be stored at room temperature prior to administration.

Administration (Intravenous Injection)

BeneFIX®, Coagulation Factor IX (Recombinant), should be administered using a single sterile disposable plastic syringe. In addition, the solution should be withdrawn from the vial using the sterile filter spike.

1. Using aseptic technique, attach the sterile filter spike to the sterile disposable syringe.
   Note: Do NOT inject air into the BeneFIX® vial. This may cause partial loss of product.
2. Insert the filter spike end into the stopper of the BeneFIX® vial.
3. Invert the vial and withdraw the reconstituted solution into the syringe.
4. Remove and discard the filter spike.
   Note: If you use more than one vial of BeneFIX®, the contents of multiple vials may be drawn into the same syringe through a separate, unused filter spike.
5. Attach the syringe to the Luer end of the infusion set tubing and perform venipuncture as instructed by your physician.
   Note: Agglutination of red blood cells in the tubing/syringe has been reported with the administration of BeneFIX®. No adverse events have been reported in association with this observation. To minimize the possibility of agglutination, it is important to limit the amount of blood entering the tubing. Blood should not enter the syringe. If red blood cell agglutination is observed in the tubing or syringe, discard all material (tubing, syringe and BeneFIX® solution) and resume administration with a new package.

After reconstitution, BeneFIX® should be injected intravenously over several minutes. The rate of administration should be determined by the patient's comfort level (see **ADVERSE REACTIONS**).

Dispose of all unused solution, empty vials, and used needles and syringes in an appropriate container for throwing away waste that might hurt others if not handled properly.

Storage

Product as packaged for sale: BeneFIX®, Coagulation Factor IX (Recombinant), should be stored under refrigeration at a temperature of 2 to 8°C (36 to 46°F). Prior to the expiration date, BeneFIX®, may also be stored at room temperature not to exceed 25°C (77°F) for up to 6 months. The patient should make note of the date the product was placed at room temperature in the space provided on the outer carton. Freezing should be avoided to prevent damage to the diluent vial. Do not use BeneFIX® after the expiry date on the label.

Product after reconstitution: The product does not contain a preservative and should be used within 3 hours.

HOW SUPPLIED

BeneFIX®, Coagulation Factor IX (Recombinant), is supplied in single use vials which contain nominally 250, 500, or 1000 IU per vial (NDC # 58394-003-01, 58394-002-01, and 58394-001-01, respectively) with sterile diluent, sterile double-ended needle for reconstitution, sterile filter spike for withdrawal, sterile infusion set, and two (2) alcohol swabs. Actual factor IX activity in IU is stated on the label of each vial.

REFERENCES

1. Lusher JM. Thrombogenicity associated with factor IX complex concentrates. *Semin Hematol.* 1991;28(3 Suppl. 6):3-5.
2. Shapiro AD, Ragni MV, Lusher JM, et al. Safety and efficacy of monoclonal antibody purified factor IX concentrate in previously untreated patients with hemophilia B. *Thromb Haemost.* 1996;75(1):30–35.
3. Roberts HR, Eberst ME. Current management of hemophilia B. *Hematol Oncol Clin North Am.* 1993;7(6):1269–1280.

Wyeth®

Manufactured by:
Wyeth Pharmaceuticals Inc.
Philadelphia, PA 19101
US Govt. License No. 3
Imported and Distributed in Canada by:
Wyeth Canada
Montreal, Canada

W10483C005
ET01
Rev 07/04

Shown in Product Identification Guide, page 336

EFFEXOR® ℞

[*ĕ-fĕks-ŏr*]
(venlafaxine hydrochloride)
Tablets
℞ only

This product's label may have been revised after this insert was used in production. For further product information and current package insert, please visit www.wyeth.com or call our medical communications department toll-free at 1-800-934-5556.

DESCRIPTION

Effexor (venlafaxine hydrochloride) is a structurally novel antidepressant for oral administration. It is designated (R/S)-1-[2-(dimethylamino)-1-(4-methoxyphenyl)ethyl] cyclohexanol hydrochloride or (±)-1-[α-[(dimethyl-amino) methyl]-p-methoxybenzyl] cyclohexanol hydrochloride and has the empirical formula of $C_{17}H_{27}NO_2$ HCl. Its molecular weight is 313.87. The structural formula is shown below.

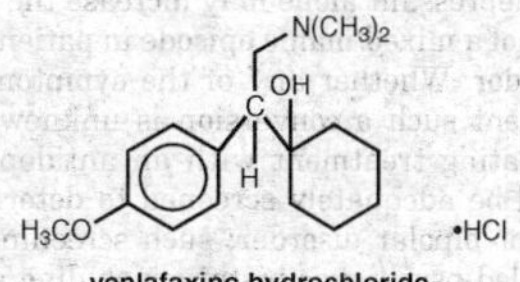

venlafaxine hydrochloride

Venlafaxine hydrochloride is a white to off-white crystalline solid with a solubility of 572 mg/mL in water (adjusted to ionic strength of 0.2 M with sodium chloride). Its octanol: water (0.2 M sodium chloride) partition coefficient is 0.43.

Compressed tablets contain venlafaxine hydrochloride equivalent to 25 mg, 37.5 mg, 50 mg, 75 mg, or 100 mg venlafaxine. Inactive ingredients consist of cellulose, iron oxides, lactose, magnesium stearate, and sodium starch glycolate.

CLINICAL PHARMACOLOGY

Pharmacodynamics

The mechanism of the antidepressant action of venlafaxine in humans is believed to be associated with its potentiation of neurotransmitter activity in the CNS. Preclinical studies have shown that venlafaxine and its active metabolite, O-desmethylvenlafaxine (ODV), are potent inhibitors of neuronal serotonin and norepinephrine reuptake and weak inhibitors of dopamine reuptake. Venlafaxine and ODV have no significant affinity for muscarinic, histaminergic, or α-1 adrenergic receptors in vitro. Pharmacologic activity at these receptors is hypothesized to be associated with the various anticholinergic, sedative, and cardiovascular effects seen with other psychotropic drugs. Venlafaxine and ODV do not possess monoamine oxidase (MAO) inhibitory activity.

Pharmacokinetics

Venlafaxine is well absorbed and extensively metabolized in the liver. O-desmethylvenlafaxine (ODV) is the only major active metabolite. On the basis of mass balance studies, at least 92% of a single dose of venlafaxine is absorbed. Approximately 87% of a venlafaxine dose is recovered in the urine within 48 hours as either unchanged venlafaxine (5%), unconjugated ODV (29%), conjugated ODV (26%), or other minor inactive metabolites (27%). Renal elimination of venlafaxine and its metabolites is the primary route of excretion. The relative bioavailability of venlafaxine from a tablet was 100% when compared to an oral solution. Food has no significant effect on the absorption of venlafaxine or on the formation of ODV.

The degree of binding of venlafaxine to human plasma is 27% ± 2% at concentrations ranging from 2.5 to 2215 ng/mL. The degree of ODV binding to human plasma is 30% ± 12% at concentrations ranging from 100 to 500 ng/mL. Protein-binding-induced drug interactions with venlafaxine are not expected.

Steady-state concentrations of both venlafaxine and ODV in plasma were attained within 3 days of multiple-dose therapy. Venlafaxine and ODV exhibited linear kinetics over the dose range of 75 to 450 mg total dose per day (administered on a q8h schedule). Plasma clearance, elimination half-life and steady-state volume of distribution were unaltered for both venlafaxine and ODV after multiple-dosing. Mean ± SD steady-state plasma clearance of venlafaxine and ODV is 1.3 ± 0.6 and 0.4 ± 0.2 L/h/kg, respectively; elimination half-life is 5 ± 2 and 11 ± 2 hours, respectively; and steady-state volume of distribution is 7.5 ± 3.7 L/kg and 5.7 ± 1.8 L/kg, respectively. When equal daily doses of venlafaxine were administered as either b.i.d. or t.i.d. regimens, the drug exposure (AUC) and fluctuation in plasma levels of venlafaxine and ODV were comparable following both regimens.

Age and Gender

A pharmacokinetic analysis of 404 venlafaxine-treated patients from two studies involving both b.i.d. and t.i.d. regimens showed that dose-normalized trough plasma levels of either venlafaxine or ODV were unaltered due to age or gender differences. Dosage adjustment based upon the age or gender of a patient is generally not necessary (see **DOSAGE AND ADMINISTRATION**).

Liver Disease

In 9 patients with hepatic cirrhosis, the pharmacokinetic disposition of both venlafaxine and ODV was significantly altered after oral administration of venlafaxine. Venlafaxine elimination half-life was prolonged by about 30%, and clearance decreased by about 50% in cirrhotic patients compared to normal subjects. ODV elimination half-life was prolonged by about 60% and clearance decreased by about 30% in cirrhotic patients compared to normal subjects. A large degree of intersubject variability was noted. Three patients with more severe cirrhosis had a more substantial decrease in venlafaxine clearance (about 90%) compared to normal subjects.

Dosage adjustment is necessary in these patients (see **DOSAGE AND ADMINISTRATION**).

Renal Disease

In a renal impairment study, venlafaxine elimination half-life after oral administration was prolonged by about 50% and clearance was reduced by about 24% in renally impaired patients (GFR = 10-70 mL/min), compared to normal subjects. In dialysis patients, venlafaxine elimination half-life was prolonged by about 180% and clearance was reduced by about 57% compared to normal subjects. Similarly, ODV elimination half-life was prolonged by about 40% although clearance was unchanged in patients with renal impairment (GFR = 10-70 mL/min) compared to normal subjects. In dialysis patients, ODV elimination half-life was prolonged by about 142% and clearance was reduced by about 56%, compared to normal subjects. A large degree of intersubject variability was noted.

Dosage adjustment is necessary in these patients (see **DOSAGE AND ADMINISTRATION**).

CLINICAL TRIALS

The efficacy of Effexor (venlafaxine hydrochloride) as a treatment for major depressive disorder was established in 5 placebo-controlled, short-term trials. Four of these were 6-week trials in adult outpatients meeting DSM-III or DSM-III-R criteria for major depression: two involving dose titration with Effexor in a range of 75 to 225 mg/day (t.i.d. schedule), the third involving fixed Effexor doses of 75, 225, and 375 mg/day (t.i.d. schedule), and the fourth involving doses of 25, 75, and 200 mg/day (b.i.d. schedule). The fifth was a 4-week study of adult inpatients meeting DSM-III-R criteria for major depression with melancholia whose Effexor doses were titrated in a range of 150 to 375 mg/day (t.i.d. schedule). In these 5 studies, Effexor was shown to be significantly superior to placebo on at least 2 of the following 3 measures: Hamilton Depression Rating Scale (total score), Hamilton depressed mood item, and Clinical Global Impression-Severity of Illness rating. Doses from 75 to 225 mg/day were superior to placebo in outpatient studies and a mean dose of about 350 mg/day was effective in inpatients. Data from the 2 fixed-dose outpatient studies were suggestive of a dose-response relationship in the range of 75 to 225 mg/day. There was no suggestion of increased response with doses greater than 225 mg/day.

While there were no efficacy studies focusing specifically on an elderly population, elderly patients were included among the patients studied. Overall, approximately 2/3 of all patients in these trials were women. Exploratory analyses for age and gender effects on outcome did not suggest any differential responsiveness on the basis of age or sex.

In one longer-term study, adult outpatients meeting DSM-IV criteria for major depressive disorder who had responded during an 8-week open trial on Effexor XR (75, 150, or 225 mg, qAM) were randomized to continuation of their same Effexor XR dose or to placebo, for up to 26 weeks of observation for relapse. Response during the open phase was defined as a CGI Severity of Illness item score of ≤3 and a HAM-D-21 total score of ≤10 at the day 56 evaluation. Relapse during the double-blind phase was defined as follows: (1) a reappearance of major depressive disorder as defined by DSM-IV criteria and a CGI Severity of Illness item score of ≥4 (moderately ill), (2) 2 consecutive CGI Severity of Illness item scores of ≥4, or (3) a final CGI Severity of Illness item score of ≥4 for any patient who withdrew from the study for any reason. Patients receiving continued Effexor XR treatment experienced significantly lower relapse rates over the subsequent 26 weeks compared with those receiving placebo.

In a second longer-term trial, adult outpatients meeting DSM-III-R criteria for major depression, recurrent type, who had responded (HAM-D-21 total score ≤12 at the day 56 evaluation) and continued to be improved [defined as the following criteria being met for days 56 through 180: (1) no HAM-D-21 total score ≥20; (2) no more than 2 HAM-D-21 total scores >10; and (3) no single CGI Severity of Illness item score ≥4 (moderately ill)] during an initial 26 weeks of treatment on Effexor (100 to 200 mg/day, on a b.i.d. schedule) were randomized to continuation of their same Effexor dose or to placebo. The follow-up period to observe patients for relapse, defined as a CGI Severity of Illness item score ≥4, was for up to 52 weeks. Patients receiving continued Effexor treatment experienced significantly lower relapse rates over the subsequent 52 weeks compared with those receiving placebo.

INDICATIONS AND USAGE

Effexor (venlafaxine hydrochloride) is indicated for the treatment of major depressive disorder.

The efficacy of Effexor in the treatment of major depressive disorder was established in 6-week controlled trials of adult outpatients whose diagnoses corresponded most closely to the DSM-III or DSM-III-R category of major depression and in a 4-week controlled trial of inpatients meeting diagnostic criteria for major depression with melancholia (see **CLINICAL TRIALS**).

Continued on next page

Effexor—Cont.

A major depressive episode implies a prominent and relatively persistent depressed or dysphoric mood that usually interferes with daily functioning (nearly every day for at least 2 weeks); it should include at least 4 of the following 8 symptoms: change in appetite, change in sleep, psychomotor agitation or retardation, loss of interest in usual activities or decrease in sexual drive, increased fatigue, feelings of guilt or worthlessness, slowed thinking or impaired concentration, and a suicide attempt or suicidal ideation.
The efficacy of Effexor XR in maintaining an antidepressant response for up to 26 weeks following 8 weeks of acute treatment was demonstrated in a placebo-controlled trial. The efficacy of Effexor in maintaining an antidepressant response in patients with recurrent depression who had responded and continued to be improved during an initial 26 weeks of treatment and were then followed for a period of up to 52 weeks was demonstrated in a second placebo-controlled trial (see **CLINICAL TRIALS**). Nevertheless, the physician who elects to use Effexor/Effexor XR for extended periods should periodically re-evaluate the long-term usefulness of the drug for the individual patient.

CONTRAINDICATIONS

Hypersensitivity to venlafaxine hydrochloride or to any excipients in the formulation.
Concomitant use in patients taking monoamine oxidase inhibitors (MAOIs) is contraindicated (see **WARNINGS**).

WARNINGS

Potential for Interaction with Monoamine Oxidase Inhibitors

Adverse reactions, some of which were serious, have been reported in patients who have recently been discontinued from a monoamine oxidase inhibitor (MAOI) and started on Effexor, or who have recently had Effexor therapy discontinued prior to initiation of an MAOI. These reactions have included tremor, myoclonus, diaphoresis, nausea, vomiting, flushing, dizziness, hyperthermia with features resembling neuroleptic malignant syndrome, seizures, and death. In patients receiving antidepressants with pharmacological properties similar to venlafaxine in combination with a monoamine oxidase inhibitor, there have also been reports of serious, sometimes fatal, reactions. For a selective serotonin reuptake inhibitor, these reactions have included hyperthermia, rigidity, myoclonus, autonomic instability with possible rapid fluctuations of vital signs, and mental status changes that include extreme agitation progressing to delirium and coma. Some cases presented with features resembling neuroleptic malignant syndrome. Severe hyperthermia and seizures, sometimes fatal, have been reported in association with the combined use of tricyclic antidepressants and MAOIs. These reactions have also been reported in patients who have recently discontinued these drugs and have been started on an MAOI. Therefore, it is recommended that Effexor not be used in combination with an MAOI, or within at least 14 days of discontinuing treatment with an MAOI. Based on the half-life of Effexor, at least 7 days should be allowed after stopping Effexor before starting an MAOI.

Clinical Worsening and Suicide Risk

Patients with major depressive disorder, both adult and pediatric, may experience worsening of their depression and/or the emergence of suicidal ideation and behavior (suicidality), whether or not they are taking antidepressant medications, and this risk may persist until significant remission occurs. Although there has been a long-standing concern that antidepressants may have a role in inducing worsening of depression and the emergence of suicidality in certain patients, a causal role for antidepressants in inducing such behaviors has not been established. **Nevertheless, patients being treated with antidepressants should be observed closely for clinical worsening and suicidality, especially at the beginning of a course of drug therapy, or at the time of dose changes, either increases or decreases.** Consideration should be given to changing the therapeutic regimen, including possibly discontinuing the medication, in patients whose depression is persistently worse or whose emergent suicidality is severe, abrupt in onset, or was not part of the patient's presenting symptoms.
Because of the possibility of co-morbidity between major depressive disorder and other psychiatric and nonpsychiatric disorders, the same precautions observed when treating patients with major depressive disorder should be observed when treating patients with other psychiatric and nonpsychiatric disorders.
The following symptoms, anxiety, agitation, panic attacks, insomnia, irritability, hostility (aggressiveness), impulsivity, akathisia (psychomotor restlessness), hypomania, and mania, have been reported in adult and pediatric patients being treated with antidepressants for major depressive disorder as well as for other indications, both psychiatric and nonpsychiatric. Although a causal link between the emergence of such symptoms and either the worsening of depression and/or the emergence of suicidal impulses has not been established, consideration should be given to changing the therapeutic regimen, including possibly discontinuing the medication, in patients for whom such symptoms are severe, abrupt in onset, or were not part of the patient's presenting symptoms.
Families and caregivers of patients being treated with antidepressants for major depressive disorder or other indications, both psychiatric and nonpsychiatric, should be alerted about the need to monitor patients for the emergence of agitation, irritability, and the other symptoms described above, as well as the emergence of suicidality, and to report such symptoms immediately to health care providers. Prescriptions for Effexor should be written for the smallest quantity of tablets consistent with good patient management, in order to reduce the risk of overdose.
If the decision has been made to discontinue treatment, medication should be tapered, as rapidly as is feasible, but with recognition that abrupt discontinuation can be associated with certain symptoms (see **PRECAUTIONS** and **DOSAGE AND ADMINISTRATION, Discontinuing Effexor**, for a description of the risks of discontinuation of Effexor).
It should be noted that Effexor is not approved for use in treating any indications in the pediatric population.
A major depressive episode may be the initial presentation of bipolar disorder. It is generally believed (though not established in controlled trials) that treating such an episode with an antidepressant alone may increase the likelihood of precipitation of a mixed/manic episode in patients at risk for bipolar disorder. Whether any of the symptoms described above represent such a conversion is unknown. However, prior to initiating treatment with an antidepressant, patients should be adequately screened to determine if they are at risk for bipolar disorder; such screening should include a detailed psychiatric history, including a family history of suicide, bipolar disorder, and depression. It should be noted that Effexor is not approved for use in treating bipolar depression.

Sustained Hypertension

Venlafaxine treatment is associated with sustained increases in blood pressure in some patients. (1) In a premarketing study comparing three fixed doses of venlafaxine (75, 225, and 375 mg/day) and placebo, a mean increase in supine diastolic blood pressure (SDBP) of 7.2 mm Hg was seen in the 375 mg/day group at week 6 compared to essentially no changes in the 75 and 225 mg/day groups and a mean decrease in SDBP of 2.2 mm Hg in the placebo group. (2) An analysis for patients meeting criteria for sustained hypertension (defined as treatment-emergent SDBP ≥ 90 mm Hg *and* ≥ 10 mm Hg above baseline for 3 consecutive visits) revealed a dose-dependent increase in the incidence of sustained hypertension for venlafaxine:

Probability of Sustained Elevation in SDBP
(Pool of Premarketing Venlafaxine Studies)

Treatment Group	Incidence of Sustained Elevation in SDBP
Venlafaxine	
< 100 mg/day	3%
101-200 mg/day	5%
201-300 mg/day	7%
> 300 mg/day	13%
Placebo	2%

An analysis of the patients with sustained hypertension and the 19 venlafaxine patients who were discontinued from treatment because of hypertension (<1% of total venlafaxine-treated group) revealed that most of the blood pressure increases were in a modest range (10 to 15 mm Hg, SDBP). Nevertheless, sustained increases of this magnitude could have adverse consequences. Therefore, it is recommended that patients receiving venlafaxine have regular monitoring of blood pressure. For patients who experience a sustained increase in blood pressure while receiving venlafaxine, either dose reduction or discontinuation should be considered.

PRECAUTIONS

General

Discontinuation of Treatment with Effexor

Discontinuation symptoms have been systematically evaluated in patients taking venlafaxine, to include prospective analyses of clinical trials in Generalized Anxiety Disorder and retrospective surveys of trials in major depressive disorder. Abrupt discontinuation or dose reduction of venlafaxine at various doses has been found to be associated with the appearance of new symptoms, the frequency of which increased with increased dose level and with longer duration of treatment. Reported symptoms include agitation, anorexia, anxiety, confusion, coordination impaired, diarrhea, dizziness, dry mouth, dysphoric mood, fasciculation, fatigue, headaches, hypomania, insomnia, nausea, nervousness, nightmares, sensory disturbances (including shock-like electrical sensations), somnolence, sweating, tremor, vertigo, and vomiting.
During marketing of Effexor, other SNRIs (Serotonin and Norepinephrine Reuptake Inhibitors), and SSRIs (Selective Serotonin Reuptake Inhibitors), there have been spontaneous reports of adverse events occurring upon discontinuation of these drugs, particularly when abrupt, including the following: dysphoric mood, irritability, agitation, dizziness, sensory disturbances (e.g. paresthesias such as electric shock sensations), anxiety, confusion, headache, lethargy, emotional lability, insomnia, hypomania, tinnitus, and seizures. While these events are generally self-limiting, there have been reports of serious discontinuation symptoms.
Patients should be monitored for these symptoms when discontinuing treatment with Effexor. A gradual reduction in the dose rather than abrupt cessation is recommended whenever possible. If intolerable symptoms occur following a decrease in the dose or upon discontinuation of treatment, then resuming the previously prescribed dose may be considered. Subsequently, the physician may continue decreasing the dose but at a more gradual rate (see **DOSAGE AND ADMINISTRATION**).

Anxiety and Insomnia

Treatment-emergent anxiety, nervousness, and insomnia were more commonly reported for venlafaxine-treated patients compared to placebo-treated patients in a pooled analysis of short-term, double-blind, placebo-controlled depression studies:

Symptom	Venlafaxine n = 1033	Placebo n = 609
Anxiety	6%	3%
Nervousness	13%	6%
Insomnia	18%	10%

Anxiety, nervousness, and insomnia led to drug discontinuation in 2%, 2%, and 3%, respectively, of the patients treated with venlafaxine in the Phase 2 and Phase 3 depression studies.

Changes in Weight

Adult Patients: A dose-dependent weight loss was noted in patients treated with venlafaxine for several weeks. A loss of 5% or more of body weight occurred in 6% of patients treated with venlafaxine compared with 1% of patients treated with placebo and 3% of patients treated with another antidepressant. However, discontinuation for weight loss associated with venlafaxine was uncommon (0.1% of venlafaxine-treated patients in the Phase 2 and Phase 3 depression trials).
The safety and efficacy of venlafaxine therapy in combination with weight loss agents, including phentermine, have not been established. Co-administration of Effexor and weight loss agents is not recommended. Effexor is not indicated for weight loss alone or in combination with other products.
Pediatric Patients: Weight loss has been observed in pediatric patients (ages 6-17) receiving Effexor XR. In a pooled analysis of four eight-week, double-blind, placebo-controlled, flexible dose outpatient trials for major depressive disorder (MDD) and generalized anxiety disorder (GAD), Effexor XR-treated patients lost an average of 0.45 kg (n = 333), while placebo-treated patients gained an average of 0.77 kg (n = 333). More patients treated with Effexor XR than with placebo experienced a weight loss of at least 3.5% in both the MDD and the GAD studies (18% of Effexor XR-treated patients vs. 3.6% of placebo-treated patients; $p<0.001$). Weight loss was not limited to patients with treatment-emergent anorexia (see **PRECAUTIONS, General**, *Changes in Appetite*).
The risks associated with longer-term Effexor XR use were assessed in an open-label study of children and adolescents who received Effexor XR for up to six months. The children and adolescents in the study had increases in weight that were less than expected based on data from age- and sex-matched peers. The difference between observed weight gain and expected weight gain was larger for children (<12 years old) than for adolescents (>12 years old).

Changes in Height

Pediatric Patients: During the eight-week placebo-controlled GAD studies, Effexor XR-treated patients (ages 6-17) grew an average of 0.3 cm (n = 122), while placebo-treated patients grew an average of 1.0 cm (n = 132); $p=0.041$. This difference in height increase was most notable in patients younger than twelve. During the eight-week placebo-controlled MDD studies, Effexor XR-treated patients grew an average of 0.8 cm (n = 146), while placebo-treated patients grew an average of 0.7 cm (n = 147). In the six-month open-label study, children and adolescents had height increases that were less than expected based on data from age- and sex-matched peers. The difference between observed growth rates and expected growth rates was larger for children (<12 years old) than for adolescents (>12 years old).

Changes in Appetite

Adult Patients: Treatment-emergent anorexia was more commonly reported for venlafaxine-treated (11%) than placebo-treated patients (2%) in the pool of short-term, double-blind, placebo-controlled depression studies.
Pediatric Patients: Decreased appetite has been observed in pediatric patients receiving Effexor XR. In the placebo-controlled trials for GAD and MDD, 10% of patients aged 6–17 treated with Effexor XR for up to eight weeks and 3% of patients treated with placebo reported treatment-emergent anorexia (decreased appetite). None of the patients receiving Effexor XR discontinued for anorexia or weight loss.

Activation of Mania/Hypomania

During Phase 2 and Phase 3 trials, hypomania or mania occurred in 0.5% of patients treated with venlafaxine. Activation of mania/hypomania has also been reported in a small proportion of patients with major affective disorder who were treated with other marketed antidepressants. As with all antidepressants, Effexor (venlafaxine hydrochloride) should be used cautiously in patients with a history of mania.

Hyponatremia
Hyponatremia and/or the syndrome of inappropriate antidiuretic hormone secretion (SIADH) may occur with venlafaxine. This should be taken into consideration in patients who are, for example, volume-depleted, elderly, or taking diuretics.
Mydriasis
Mydriasis has been reported in association with venlafaxine; therefore patients with raised intraocular pressure or at risk of acute narrow angle glaucoma should be monitored.
Seizures
During premarketing testing, seizures were reported in 0.26% (8/3082) of venlafaxine-treated patients. Most seizures (5 of 8) occurred in patients receiving doses of 150 mg/day or less. Effexor should be used cautiously in patients with a history of seizures. It should be discontinued in any patient who develops seizures.
Abnormal Bleeding
There have been reports of abnormal bleeding (most commonly ecchymosis) associated with venlafaxine treatment. While a causal relationship to venlafaxine is unclear, impaired platelet aggregation may result from platelet serotonin depletion and contribute to such occurrences.
Serum Cholesterol Elevation
Clinically relevant increases in serum cholesterol were recorded in 5.3% of venlafaxine-treated patients and 0.0% of placebo-treated patients treated for at least 3 months in placebo-controlled trials (see **ADVERSE REACTIONS–Laboratory Changes**). Measurement of serum cholesterol levels should be considered during long-term treatment.
Use in Patients with Concomitant Illness
Clinical experience with Effexor in patients with concomitant systemic illness is limited. Caution is advised in administering Effexor to patients with diseases or conditions that could affect hemodynamic responses or metabolism.
Effexor has not been evaluated or used to any appreciable extent in patients with a recent history of myocardial infarction or unstable heart disease. Patients with these diagnoses were systematically excluded from many clinical studies during the product's premarketing testing. Evaluation of the electrocardiograms for 769 patients who received Effexor in 4- to 6-week double-blind placebo-controlled trials, however, showed that the incidence of trial-emergent conduction abnormalities did not differ from that with placebo. The mean heart rate in Effexor-treated patients was increased relative to baseline by about 4 beats per minute.
The electrocardiograms for 357 patients who received Effexor XR (the extended-release form of venlafaxine) and 285 patients who received placebo in 8- to 12-week double-blind, placebo-controlled trials were analyzed. The mean change from baseline in corrected QT interval (QTc) for Effexor XR-treated patients was increased relative to that for placebo-treated patients (increase of 4.7 msec for Effexor XR and decrease of 1.9 msec for placebo). In these same trials, the mean change from baseline in heart rate for Effexor XR-treated patients was significantly higher than that for placebo (a mean increase of 4 beats per minute for Effexor XR and 1 beat per minute for placebo). In a flexible-dose study, with Effexor doses in the range of 200 to 375 mg/day and mean dose greater than 300 mg/day, Effexor-treated patients had a mean increase in heart rate of 8.5 beats per minute compared with 1.7 beats per minute in the placebo group.
As increases in heart rate were observed, caution should be exercised in patients whose underlying medical conditions might be compromised by increases in heart rate (eg, patients with hyperthyroidism, heart failure, or recent myocardial infarction), particularly when using doses of Effexor above 200 mg/day.
In patients with renal impairment (GFR=10 to 70 mL/min) or cirrhosis of the liver, the clearances of venlafaxine and its active metabolite were decreased, thus prolonging the elimination half-lives of these substances. A lower dose may be necessary (see **DOSAGE AND ADMINISTRATION**). Effexor (venlafaxine hydrochloride), like all antidepressants, should be used with caution in such patients.

Information for Patients
Physicians are advised to discuss the following issues with patients for whom they prescribe Effexor:
Patients and their families should be encouraged to be alert to the emergence of anxiety, agitation, panic attacks, insomnia, irritability, hostility, impulsivity, akathisia, hypomania, mania, worsening of depression, and suicidal ideation, especially early during antidepressant treatment. Such symptoms should be reported to the patient's physician, especially if they are severe, abrupt in onset, or were not part of the patient's presenting symptoms.
Interference with Cognitive and Motor Performance
Clinical studies were performed to examine the effects of venlafaxine on behavioral performance of healthy individuals. The results revealed no clinically significant impairment of psychomotor, cognitive, or complex behavior performance. However, since any psychoactive drug may impair judgment, thinking, or motor skills, patients should be cautioned about operating hazardous machinery, including automobiles, until they are reasonably certain that Effexor therapy does not adversely affect their ability to engage in such activities.
Pregnancy
Patients should be advised to notify their physician if they become pregnant or intend to become pregnant during therapy.
Nursing
Patients should be advised to notify their physician if they are breast-feeding an infant.
Concomitant Medication
Patients should be advised to inform their physicians if they are taking, or plan to take, any prescription or over-the-counter drugs, including herbal preparations, since there is a potential for interactions.
Alcohol
Although Effexor has not been shown to increase the impairment of mental and motor skills caused by alcohol, patients should be advised to avoid alcohol while taking Effexor.
Allergic Reactions
Patients should be advised to notify their physician if they develop a rash, hives, or a related allergic phenomenon.

Laboratory Tests
There are no specific laboratory tests recommended.

Drug Interactions
As with all drugs, the potential for interaction by a variety of mechanisms is a possibility.
Alcohol
A single dose of ethanol (0.5 g/kg) had no effect on the pharmacokinetics of venlafaxine or ODV when venlafaxine was administered at 150 mg/day in 15 healthy male subjects. Additionally, administration of venlafaxine in a stable regimen did not exaggerate the psychomotor and psychometric effects induced by ethanol in these same subjects when they were not receiving venlafaxine.
Cimetidine
Concomitant administration of cimetidine and venlafaxine in a steady-state study for both drugs resulted in inhibition of first-pass metabolism of venlafaxine in 18 healthy subjects. The oral clearance of venlafaxine was reduced by about 43%, and the exposure (AUC) and maximum concentration (C_{max}) of the drug were increased by about 60%. However, co-administration of cimetidine had no apparent effect on the pharmacokinetics of ODV, which is present in much greater quantity in the circulation than is venlafaxine. The overall pharmacological activity of venlafaxine plus ODV is expected to increase only slightly, and no dosage adjustment should be necessary for most normal adults. However, for patients with pre-existing hypertension, and for elderly patients or patients with hepatic dysfunction, the interaction associated with the concomitant use of venlafaxine and cimetidine is not known and potentially could be more pronounced. Therefore, caution is advised with such patients.
Diazepam
Under steady-state conditions for venlafaxine administered at 150 mg/day, a single 10 mg dose of diazepam did not appear to affect the pharmacokinetics of either venlafaxine or ODV in 18 healthy male subjects. Venlafaxine also did not have any effect on the pharmacokinetics of diazepam or its active metabolite, desmethyldiazepam, or affect the psychomotor and psychometric effects induced by diazepam.
Haloperidol
Venlafaxine administered under steady-state conditions at 150 mg/day in 24 healthy subjects decreased total oral-dose clearance (Cl/F) of a single 2 mg dose of haloperidol by 42%, which resulted in a 70% increase in haloperidol AUC. In addition, the haloperidol C_{max} increased 88% when coadministered with venlafaxine, but the haloperidol elimination half-life ($t_{1/2}$) was unchanged. The mechanism explaining this finding is unknown.
Lithium
The steady-state pharmacokinetics of venlafaxine administered at 150 mg/day were not affected when a single 600 mg oral dose of lithium was administered to 12 healthy male subjects. O-desmethylvenlafaxine (ODV) also was unaffected. Venlafaxine had no effect on the pharmacokinetics of lithium (see also *CNS-Active Drugs*, below).
Drugs Highly Bound to Plasma Protein
Venlafaxine is not highly bound to plasma proteins; therefore, administration of Effexor to a patient taking another drug that is highly protein bound should not cause increased free concentrations of the other drug.
Drugs that Inhibit Cytochrome P450 Isoenzymes
CYP2D6 Inhibitors: In vitro and in vivo studies indicate that venlafaxine is metabolized to its active metabolite, ODV, by CYP2D6, the isoenzyme that is responsible for the genetic polymorphism seen in the metabolism of many antidepressants. Therefore, the potential exists for a drug interaction between drugs that inhibit CYP2D6-mediated metabolism and venlafaxine. However, although imipramine partially inhibited the CYP2D6-mediated metabolism of venlafaxine, resulting in higher plasma concentrations of venlafaxine and lower plasma concentrations of ODV, the total concentration of active compounds (venlafaxine plus ODV) was not affected. Additionally, in a clinical study involving CYP2D6-poor and -extensive metabolizers, the total concentration of active compounds (venlafaxine plus ODV), was similar in the two metabolizer groups. Therefore, no dosage adjustment is required when venlafaxine is coadministered with a CYP2D6 inhibitor.
CYP3A4 Inhibitors: In vitro studies indicate that venlafaxine is likely metabolized to a minor, less active metabolite, N-desmethylvenlafaxine, by CYP3A4. Because CYP3A4 is typically a minor pathway relative to CYP2D6 in the metabolism of venlafaxine, the potential for a clinically significant drug interaction between drugs that inhibit CYP3A4-mediated metabolism and venlafaxine is small.
The concomitant use of venlafaxine with a drug treatment(s) that potently inhibits both CYP2D6 and CYP3A4, the primary metabolizing enzymes for venlafaxine, has not been studied. Therefore, caution is advised should a patient's therapy include venlafaxine and any agent(s) that produce potent simultaneous inhibition of these two enzyme systems.
Drugs Metabolized by Cytochrome P450 Isoenzymes
CYP2D6: In vitro studies indicate that venlafaxine is a relatively weak inhibitor of CYP2D6. These findings have been confirmed in a clinical drug interaction study comparing the effect of venlafaxine to that of fluoxetine on the CYP2D6-mediated metabolism of dextromethorphan to dextrorphan.
Imipramine—Venlafaxine did not affect the pharmacokinetics of imipramine and 2-OH-imipramine. However, desipramine AUC, C_{max}, and C_{min} increased by about 35% in the presence of venlafaxine. The 2-OH-desipramine AUCs increased by at least 2.5 fold (with venlafaxine 37.5 mg q12h) and by 4.5 fold (with venlafaxine 75 mg q12h). Imipramine did not affect the pharmacokinetics of venlafaxine and ODV. The clinical significance of elevated 2-OH-desipramine levels is unknown.
Risperidone—Venlafaxine administered under steady-state conditions at 150 mg/day slightly inhibited the CYP2D6-mediated metabolism of risperidone (administered as a single 1 mg oral dose) to its active metabolite, 9-hydroxyrisperidone, resulting in an approximate 32% increase in risperidone AUC. However, venlafaxine coadministration did not significantly alter the pharmacokinetic profile of the total active moiety (risperidone plus 9-hydroxyrisperidone).
CYP3A4: Venlafaxine did not inhibit CYP3A4 in vitro. This finding was confirmed in vivo by clinical drug interaction studies in which venlafaxine did not inhibit the metabolism of several CYP3A4 substrates, including alprazolam, diazepam, and terfenadine.
Indinavir—In a study of 9 healthy volunteers, venlafaxine administered under steady-state conditions at 150 mg/day resulted in a 28% decrease in the AUC of a single 800 mg oral dose of indinavir and a 36% decrease in indinavir C_{max}. Indinavir did not affect the pharmacokinetics of venlafaxine and ODV. The clinical significance of this finding is unknown.
CYP1A2: Venlafaxine did not inhibit CYP1A2 in vitro. This finding was confirmed in vivo by a clinical drug interaction study in which venlafaxine did not inhibit the metabolism of caffeine, a CYP1A2 substrate.
CYP2C9: Venlafaxine did not inhibit CYP2C9 in vitro. In vivo, venlafaxine 75 mg by mouth every 12 hours did not alter the pharmacokinetics of a single 500 mg dose of tolbutamide or the CYP2C9 mediated formation of 4-hydroxy-tolbutamide.
CYP2C19: Venlafaxine did not inhibit the metabolism of diazepam which is partially metabolized by CYP2C19 (see *Diazepam* above).
Monoamine Oxidase Inhibitors
See **CONTRAINDICATIONS** and **WARNINGS**.
CNS-Active Drugs
The risk of using venlafaxine in combination with other CNS-active drugs has not been systematically evaluated (except in the case of those CNS-active drugs noted above). Consequently, caution is advised if the concomitant administration of venlafaxine and such drugs is required. Based on the mechanism of action of venlafaxine and the potential for serotonin syndrome, caution is advised when venlafaxine is co-administered with other drugs that may affect the serotonergic neurotransmitter systems, such as triptans, serotonin reuptake inhibitors (SRIs), or lithium.
Electroconvulsive Therapy
There are no clinical data establishing the benefit of electroconvulsive therapy combined with Effexor treatment.
Postmarketing Spontaneous Drug Interaction Reports
See **ADVERSE REACTIONS, Postmarketing Reports.**

Carcinogenesis, Mutagenesis, Impairment of Fertility
Carcinogenesis
Venlafaxine was given by oral gavage to mice for 18 months at doses up to 120 mg/kg per day, which was 16 times, on a mg/kg basis, and 1.7 times on a mg/m^2 basis, the maximum recommended human dose. Venlafaxine was also given to rats by oral gavage for 24 months at doses up to 120 mg/kg per day. In rats receiving the 120 mg/kg dose, plasma levels of venlafaxine were 1 times (male rats) and 6 times (female rats) the plasma levels of patients receiving the maximum recommended human dose. Plasma levels of the O-desmethyl metabolite were lower in rats than in patients receiving the maximum recommended dose. Tumors were not increased by venlafaxine treatment in mice or rats.
Mutagenicity
Venlafaxine and the major human metabolite, O-desmethylvenlafaxine (ODV), were not mutagenic in the Ames reverse mutation assay in Salmonella bacteria or the CHO/HGPRT mammalian cell forward gene mutation assay. Venlafaxine was also not mutagenic in the in vitro BALB/c-3T3 mouse cell transformation assay, the sister chromatid exchange assay in cultured CHO cells, or the in vivo chromosomal aberration assay in rat bone marrow. ODV was not mutagenic in the in vitro CHO cell chromosomal aberration assay. There was a clastogenic response in the in vivo chromosomal aberration assay in rat bone marrow in male rats receiving 200 times, on a mg/kg basis, or 50 times, on a mg/m^2 basis, the maximum human daily dose. The no effect dose was 67 times (mg/kg) or 17 times (mg/m^2) the human dose.
Impairment of Fertility
Reproduction and fertility studies in rats showed no effects on male or female fertility at oral doses of up to 8 times the

Continued on next page

Effexor—Cont.

maximum recommended human daily dose on a mg/kg basis, or up to 2 times on a mg/m^2 basis.

Pregnancy

Teratogenic Effects—Pregnancy Category C

Venlafaxine did not cause malformations in offspring of rats or rabbits given doses up to 11 times (rat) or 12 times (rabbit) the maximum recommended human daily dose on a mg/kg basis, or 2.5 times (rat) and 4 times (rabbit) the human daily dose on a mg/m^2 basis. However, in rats, there was a decrease in pup weight, an increase in stillborn pups, and an increase in pup deaths during the first 5 days of lactation, when dosing began during pregnancy and continued until weaning. The cause of these deaths is not known. These effects occurred at 10 times (mg/kg) or 2.5 times (mg/m^2) the maximum human daily dose. The no effect dose for rat pup mortality was 1.4 times the human dose on a mg/kg basis or 0.25 times the human dose on a mg/m^2 basis. There are no adequate and well-controlled studies in pregnant women. Because animal reproduction studies are not always predictive of human response, this drug should be used during pregnancy only if clearly needed.

Non-teratogenic Effects

Neonates exposed to Effexor, other SNRIs (Serotonin and Norepinephrine Reuptake Inhibitors), or SSRIs (Selective Serotonin Reuptake Inhibitors), late in the third trimester have developed complications requiring prolonged hospitalization, respiratory support, and tube feeding. Such complications can arise immediately upon delivery. Reported clinical findings have included respiratory distress, cyanosis, apnea, seizures, temperature instability, feeding difficulty, vomiting, hypoglycemia, hypotonia, hypertonia, hyperreflexia, tremor, jitteriness, irritability, and constant crying. These features are consistent with either a direct toxic effect of SSRIs and SNRIs or, possibly, a drug discontinuation syndrome. It should be noted that, in some cases, the clinical picture is consistent with serotonin syndrome (see **PRECAUTIONS-Drug Interactions**-*CNS-Active Drugs*). When treating a pregnant woman with Effexor during the third trimester, the physician should carefully consider the potential risks and benefits of treatment (see **DOSAGE AND ADMINISTRATION**).

Labor and Delivery

The effect of Effexor® (venlafaxine hydrochloride) on labor and delivery in humans is unknown.

Nursing Mothers

Venlafaxine and ODV have been reported to be excreted in human milk. Because of the potential for serious adverse reactions in nursing infants from Effexor, a decision should be made whether to discontinue nursing or to discontinue the drug, taking into account the importance of the drug to the mother.

Pediatric Use

Effectiveness in pediatric patients has not been established. (See **WARNINGS-Clinical Worsening and Suicide Risk.**)

Although no studies have been designed to primarily assess Effexor XR's impact on the growth, development, and maturation of children and adolescents, the studies that have been done suggest that Effexor XR may adversely affect weight and height (see **PRECAUTIONS, General**, *Changes in Height* and *Changes in Weight*). Should the decision be made to treat a pediatric patient with Effexor, regular monitoring of weight and height is recommended during treatment, particularly if it is to be continued long term. The safety of Effexor XR treatment for pediatric patients has not been systematically assessed for chronic treatment longer than six months in duration.

In the studies conducted in pediatric patients (ages 6-17), the occurrence of blood pressure and cholesterol increases considered to be clinically relevant in pediatric patients was similar to that observed in adult patients. Consequently, the precautions for adults apply to pediatric patients (see **WARNINGS, Sustained Hypertension**, and **PRECAUTIONS, General**, *Serum Cholesterol Elevation*).

Geriatric Use

Of the 2,897 patients in Phase 2 and Phase 3 depression studies with Effexor, 12% (357) were 65 years of age or over. No overall differences in effectiveness or safety were observed between these patients and younger patients, and other reported clinical experience generally has not identified differences in response between the elderly and younger patients. However, greater sensitivity of some older individuals cannot be ruled out. As with other antidepressants, several cases of hyponatremia and syndrome of inappropriate antidiuretic hormone secretion (SIADH) have been reported, usually in the elderly.

The pharmacokinetics of venlafaxine and ODV are not substantially altered in the elderly (see **CLINICAL PHARMACOLOGY**). No dose adjustment is recommended for the elderly on the basis of age alone, although other clinical circumstances, some of which may be more common in the elderly, such as renal or hepatic impairment, may warrant a dose reduction (see **DOSAGE AND ADMINISTRATION**).

ADVERSE REACTIONS

Associated with Discontinuation of Treatment

Nineteen percent (537/2897) of venlafaxine patients in Phase 2 and Phase 3 depression studies discontinued treatment due to an adverse event. The more common events (≥ 1%) associated with discontinuation and considered to be drug-related (ie, those events associated with dropout at a rate approximately twice or greater for venlafaxine compared to placebo) included:

	Venlafaxine	Placebo
CNS		
Somnolence	3%	1%
Insomnia	3%	1%
Dizziness	3%	—
Nervousness	2%	—
Dry mouth	2%	—
Anxiety	2%	1%
Gastrointestinal		
Nausea	6%	1%
Urogenital		
Abnormal ejaculation*	3%	—
Other		
Headache	3%	1%
Asthenia	2%	—
Sweating	2%	—

* Percentages based on the number of males.
— Less than 1%

Incidence in Controlled Trials

Commonly Observed Adverse Events in Controlled Clinical Trials

The most commonly observed adverse events associated with the use of Effexor® (incidence of 5% or greater) and not seen at an equivalent incidence among placebo-treated patients (ie, incidence for Effexor at least twice that for placebo), derived from the 1% incidence table below, were asthenia, sweating, nausea, constipation, anorexia, vomiting, somnolence, dry mouth, dizziness, nervousness, anxiety, tremor, and blurred vision as well as abnormal ejaculation/orgasm and impotence in men.

Adverse Events Occurring at an Incidence of 1% or More Among Effexor-Treated Patients

The table that follows enumerates adverse events that occurred at an incidence of 1% or more, and were more frequent than in the placebo group, among Effexor-treated patients who participated in short-term (4- to 8-week) placebo-controlled trials in which patients were administered doses in a range of 75 to 375 mg/day. This table shows the percentage of patients in each group who had at least one episode of an event at some time during their treatment. Reported adverse events were classified using a standard COSTART-based Dictionary terminology.

The prescriber should be aware that these figures cannot be used to predict the incidence of side effects in the course of usual medical practice where patient characteristics and other factors differ from those which prevailed in the clinical trials. Similarly, the cited frequencies cannot be compared with figures obtained from other clinical investigations involving different treatments, uses and investigators. The cited figures, however, do provide the prescribing physician with some basis for estimating the relative contribution of drug and nondrug factors to the side effect incidence rate in the population studied.

[See table 1 at left]

TABLE 1
Treatment-Emergent Adverse Experience Incidence in 4- to 8-Week Placebo-Controlled Clinical Trials[1]

Body System	Preferred Term	Effexor (n=1033)	Placebo (n=609)
Body as a Whole	Headache	25%	24%
	Asthenia	12%	6%
	Infection	6%	5%
	Chills	3%	—
	Chest pain	2%	1%
	Trauma	2%	1%
Cardiovascular	Vasodilatation	4%	3%
	Increased blood pressure/hypertension	2%	—
	Tachycardia	2%	—
	Postural hypotension	1%	—
Dermatological	Sweating	12%	3%
	Rash	3%	2%
	Pruritus	1%	—
Gastrointestinal	Nausea	37%	11%
	Constipation	15%	7%
	Anorexia	11%	2%
	Diarrhea	8%	7%
	Vomiting	6%	2%
	Dyspepsia	5%	4%
	Flatulence	3%	2%
Metabolic	Weight loss	1%	—
Nervous System	Somnolence	23%	9%
	Dry mouth	22%	11%
	Dizziness	19%	7%
	Insomnia	18%	10%
	Nervousness	13%	6%
	Anxiety	6%	3%
	Tremor	5%	1%
	Abnormal dreams	4%	3%
	Hypertonia	3%	2%
	Paresthesia	3%	2%
	Libido decreased	2%	—
	Agitation	2%	—
	Confusion	2%	1%
	Thinking abnormal	2%	1%
	Depersonalization	1%	—
	Depression	1%	—
	Urinary retention	1%	—
	Twitching	1%	—
Respiration	Yawn	3%	—
Special Senses	Blurred vision	6%	2%
	Taste perversion	2%	—
	Tinnitus	2%	—
	Mydriasis	2%	—
Urogenital System	Abnormal ejaculation/orgasm	12%[2]	—[2]
	Impotence	6%[2]	—[2]
	Urinary frequency	3%	2%
	Urination impaired	2%	—
	Orgasm disturbance	2%[3]	—[3]

[1] Events reported by at least 1% of patients treated with Effexor (venlafaxine hydrochloride) are included, and are rounded to the nearest %. Events for which the Effexor incidence was equal to or less than placebo are not listed in the table, but included the following: abdominal pain, pain, back pain, flu syndrome, fever, palpitation, increased appetite, myalgia, arthralgia, amnesia, hypesthesia, rhinitis, pharyngitis, sinusitis, cough increased, and dysmenorrhea[3].

—Incidence less than 1%.

[2] Incidence based on number of male patients.

[3] Incidence based on number of female patients.

Dose Dependency of Adverse Events

A comparison of adverse event rates in a fixed-dose study comparing Effexor (venlafaxine hydrochloride) 75, 225, and 375 mg/day with placebo revealed a dose dependency for some of the more common adverse events associated with Effexor use, as shown in the table that follows. The rule for including events was to enumerate those that occurred at an incidence of 5% or more for at least one of the venlafaxine groups and for which the incidence was at least twice the placebo incidence for at least one Effexor group. Tests for potential dose relationships for these events (Cochran-Armitage Test, with a criterion of exact 2-sided p-value ≤ 0.05) suggested a dose-dependency for several adverse events in this list, including chills, hypertension, anorexia, nausea, agitation, dizziness, somnolence, tremor, yawning, sweating, and abnormal ejaculation.

[See table 2 at top of next page]

Adaptation to Certain Adverse Events

Over a 6-week period, there was evidence of adaptation to some adverse events with continued therapy (eg, dizziness and nausea), but less to other effects (eg, abnormal ejaculation and dry mouth).

Vital Sign Changes

Effexor (venlafaxine hydrochloride) treatment (averaged over all dose groups) in clinical trials was associated with a mean increase in pulse rate of approximately 3 beats per minute, compared to no change for placebo. In a flexible-dose study, with doses in the range of 200 to 375 mg/day and mean dose greater than 300 mg/day, the mean pulse was increased by about 2 beats per minute compared with a decrease of about 1 beat per minute for placebo.

In controlled clinical trials, Effexor was associated with mean increases in diastolic blood pressure ranging from 0.7 to 2.5 mm Hg averaged over all dose groups, compared to mean decreases ranging from 0.9 to 3.8 mm Hg for placebo. However, there is a dose dependency for blood pressure increase (see **WARNINGS**).

Laboratory Changes

Of the serum chemistry and hematology parameters monitored during clinical trials with Effexor, a statistically significant difference with placebo was seen only for serum cholesterol. In premarketing trials, treatment with Effexor tablets was associated with a mean final on-therapy increase in total cholesterol of 3 mg/dL.

Patients treated with Effexor tablets for at least 3 months in placebo-controlled 12-month extension trials had a mean final on-therapy increase in total cholesterol of 9.1 mg/dL compared with a decrease of 7.1 mg/dL among placebo-treated patients. This increase was duration dependent over the study period and tended to be greater with higher doses. Clinically relevant increases in serum cholesterol, defined as 1) a final on-therapy increase in serum cholesterol ≥50 mg/dL from baseline and to a value ≥261 mg/dL or 2) an average on-therapy increase in serum cholesterol ≥50 mg/dL from baseline and to a value ≥261 mg/dL, were recorded in 5.3% of venlafaxine-treated patients and 0.0% of placebo-treated patients (see **PRECAUTIONS-General-***Serum Cholesterol Elevation*).

ECG Changes

In an analysis of ECGs obtained in 769 patients treated with Effexor and 450 patients treated with placebo in controlled clinical trials, the only statistically significant difference observed was for heart rate, ie, a mean increase from baseline of 4 beats per minute for Effexor. In a flexible-dose study, with doses in the range of 200 to 375 mg/day and mean dose greater than 300 mg/day, the mean change in heart rate was 8.5 beats per minute compared with 1.7 beats per minute for placebo (see **PRECAUTIONS, General**, *Use in Patients with Concomitant Illness*).

Other Events Observed During the Premarketing Evaluation of Venlafaxine

During its premarketing assessment, multiple doses of Effexor were administered to 2897 patients in Phase 2 and Phase 3 studies. In addition, in premarketing assessment of Effexor XR (the extended release form of venlafaxine), multiple doses were administered to 705 patients in Phase 3 major depressive disorder studies and Effexor was administered to 96 patients. During its premarketing assessment, multiple doses of Effexor XR were also administered to 1381 patients in Phase 3 GAD studies and 277 patients in Phase 3 Social Anxiety Disorder studies. The conditions and duration of exposure to venlafaxine in both development programs varied greatly, and included (in overlapping categories) open and double-blind studies, uncontrolled and controlled studies, inpatient (Effexor only) and outpatient studies, fixed-dose and titration studies. Untoward events associated with this exposure were recorded by clinical investigators using terminology of their own choosing. Consequently, it is not possible to provide a meaningful estimate of the proportion of individuals experiencing adverse events without first grouping similar types of untoward events into a smaller number of standardized event categories.

In the tabulations that follow, reported adverse events were classified using a standard COSTART-based Dictionary terminology. The frequencies presented, therefore, represent the proportion of the 5356 patients exposed to multiple doses of either formulation of venlafaxine who experienced an event of the type cited on at least one occasion while receiving venlafaxine. All reported events are included except those already listed in Table 1 and those events for which a drug cause was remote. If the COSTART term for an event was so general as to be uninformative, it was replaced with a more informative term. It is important to emphasize that, although the events reported occurred during treatment with venlafaxine, they were not necessarily caused by it.

Events are further categorized by body system and listed in order of decreasing frequency using the following definitions: **frequent** adverse events are defined as those occurring on one or more occasions in at least 1/100 patients; **infrequent** adverse events are those occurring in 1/100 to 1/1000 patients; **rare** events are those occurring in fewer than 1/1000 patients.

Body as a whole—**Frequent**: accidental injury, chest pain substernal, neck pain; **Infrequent**: face edema, intentional injury, malaise, moniliasis, neck rigidity, pelvic pain, photosensitivity reaction, suicide attempt, withdrawal syndrome; **Rare**: appendicitis, bacteremia, carcinoma, cellulitis.

Cardiovascular system—**Frequent**: migraine; **Infrequent**: angina pectoris, arrhythmia, extrasystoles, hypotension, peripheral vascular disorder (mainly cold feet and/or cold hands), syncope, thrombophlebitis; **Rare**: aortic aneurysm, arteritis, first-degree atrioventricular block, bigeminy, bradycardia, bundle branch block, capillary fragility, cardiovascular disorder (mitral valve and circulatory disturbance), cerebral ischemia, coronary artery disease, congestive heart failure, heart arrest, mucocutaneous hemorrhage, myocardial infarct, pallor.

TABLE 2

Treatment-Emergent Adverse Experience Incidence in a Dose Comparison Trial

Body System/ Preferred Term	Placebo (n=92)	Effexor (mg/day) 75 (n=89)	225 (n=89)	375 (n=88)
Body as a Whole				
Abdominal pain	3.3%	3.4%	2.2%	8.0%
Asthenia	3.3%	16.9%	14.6%	14.8%
Chills	1.1%	2.2%	5.6%	6.8%
Infection	2.2%	2.2%	5.6%	2.3%
Cardiovascular System				
Hypertension	1.1%	1.1%	2.2%	4.5%
Vasodilatation	0.0%	4.5%	5.6%	2.3%
Digestive System				
Anorexia	2.2%	14.6%	13.5%	17.0%
Dyspepsia	2.2%	6.7%	6.7%	4.5%
Nausea	14.1%	32.6%	38.2%	58.0%
Vomiting	1.1%	7.9%	3.4%	6.8%
Nervous System				
Agitation	0.0%	1.1%	2.2%	4.5%
Anxiety	4.3%	11.2%	4.5%	2.3%
Dizziness	4.3%	19.1%	22.5%	23.9%
Insomnia	9.8%	22.5%	20.2%	13.6%
Libido decreased	1.1%	2.2%	1.1%	5.7%
Nervousness	4.3%	21.3%	13.5%	12.5%
Somnolence	4.3%	16.9%	18.0%	26.1%
Tremor	0.0%	1.1%	2.2%	10.2%
Respiratory System				
Yawn	0.0%	4.5%	5.6%	8.0%
Skin and Appendages				
Sweating	5.4%	6.7%	12.4%	19.3%
Special Senses				
Abnormality of accommodation	0.0%	9.1%	7.9%	5.6%
Urogenital System				
Abnormal ejaculation/orgasm	0.0%	4.5%	2.2%	12.5%
Impotence	0.0%	5.8%	2.1%	3.6%
(Number of men)	(n=63)	(n=52)	(n=48)	(n=56)

Digestive system—**Frequent**: eructation; **Infrequent**: bruxism, colitis, dysphagia, tongue edema, esophagitis, gastritis, gastroenteritis, gastrointestinal ulcer, gingivitis, glossitis, rectal hemorrhage, hemorrhoids, melena, oral moniliasis, stomatitis, mouth ulceration; **Rare**: cheilitis, cholecystitis, cholelithiasis, duodenitis, esophageal spasm, hematemesis, gastrointestinal hemorrhage, gum hemorrhage, hepatitis, ileitis, jaundice, intestinal obstruction, parotitis, periodontitis, proctitis, increased salivation, soft stools, tongue discoloration.

Endocrine system—**Rare**: goiter, hyperthyroidism, hypothyroidism, thyroid nodule, thyroiditis.

Hemic and lymphatic system—**Frequent**: ecchymosis; **Infrequent**: anemia, leukocytosis, leukopenia, lymphadenopathy, thrombocythemia, thrombocytopenia; **Rare**: basophilia, bleeding time increased, cyanosis, eosinophilia, lymphocytosis, multiple myeloma, purpura.

Metabolic and nutritional—**Frequent**: edema, weight gain; **Infrequent**: alkaline phosphatase increased, dehydration, hypercholesteremia, hyperglycemia, hyperlipemia, hypokalemia, SGOT (AST) increased, SGPT (ALT) increased, thirst; **Rare**: alcohol intolerance, bilirubinemia, BUN increased, creatinine increased, diabetes mellitus, glycosuria, gout, healing abnormal, hemochromatosis, hypercalcinuria, hyperkalemia, hyperphosphatemia, hyperuricemia, hypocholesteremia, hypoglycemia, hyponatremia, hypophosphatemia, hypoproteinemia, uremia.

Musculoskeletal system—**Infrequent**: arthritis, arthrosis, bone pain, bone spurs, bursitis, leg cramps, myasthenia, tenosynovitis; **Rare**: pathological fracture, myopathy, osteoporosis, osteosclerosis, plantar fasciitis, rheumatoid arthritis, tendon rupture.

Nervous system—**Frequent**: trismus, vertigo; **Infrequent**: akathisia, apathy, ataxia, circumoral paresthesia, CNS stimulation, emotional lability, euphoria, hallucinations, hostility, hyperesthesia, hyperkinesia, hypotonia, incoordination, libido increased, manic reaction, myoclonus, neuralgia, neuropathy, psychosis, seizure, abnormal speech, stupor; **Rare**: akinesia, alcohol abuse, aphasia, bradykinesia, buccoglossal syndrome, cerebrovascular accident, loss of consciousness, delusions, dementia, dystonia, facial paralysis, feeling drunk, abnormal gait, Guillain-Barre Syndrome, hyperchlorhydria, hypokinesia, impulse control difficulties, neuritis, nystagmus, paranoid reaction, paresis, psychotic depression, reflexes decreased, reflexes increased, suicidal ideation, torticollis.

Respiratory system—**Frequent**: bronchitis, dyspnea; **Infrequent**: asthma, chest congestion, epistaxis, hyperventilation, laryngismus, laryngitis, pneumonia, voice alteration; **Rare**: atelectasis, hemoptysis, hypoventilation, hypoxia, larynx edema, pleurisy, pulmonary embolus, sleep apnea.

Skin and appendages—**Infrequent**: acne, alopecia, brittle nails, contact dermatitis, dry skin, eczema, skin hypertrophy, maculopapular rash, psoriasis, urticaria; **Rare**: erythema nodosum, exfoliative dermatitis, lichenoid dermatitis, hair discoloration, skin discoloration, furunculosis, hirsutism, leukoderma, petechial rash, pustular rash, vesiculobullous rash, seborrhea, skin atrophy, skin striae.

Special senses—**Frequent**: abnormality of accommodation, abnormal vision; **Infrequent**: cataract, conjunctivitis, corneal lesion, diplopia, dry eyes, eye pain, hyperacusis, otitis media, parosmia, photophobia, taste loss, visual field defect; **Rare**: blepharitis, chromatopsia, conjunctival edema, deafness, exophthalmos, glaucoma, retinal hemorrhage, subconjunctival hemorrhage, keratitis, labyrinthitis, miosis, papilledema, decreased pupillary reflex, otitis externa, scleritis, uveitis.

Urogenital system—**Frequent**: metrorrhagia*, prostatic disorder (prostatitis and enlarged prostate)*, vaginitis*; **Infrequent**: albuminuria, amenorrhea*, cystitis, dysuria, hematuria, leukorrhea*, menorrhagia*, nocturia, bladder pain, breast pain, polyuria, pyuria, urinary incontinence, urinary urgency, vaginal hemorrhage*; **Rare**: abortion*, anuria, balanitis*, breast discharge, breast engorgement, breast enlargement, endometriosis*, fibrocystic breast, calcium crystalluria, cervicitis*, ovarian cyst*, prolonged erection*, gynecomastia (male)*, hypomenorrhea*, kidney calculus, kidney pain, kidney function abnormal, female lactation*, mastitis, menopause*, oliguria, orchitis*, pyelonephritis, salpingitis*, urolithiasis, uterine hemorrhage*, uterine spasm*, vaginal dryness*.

* Based on the number of men and women as appropriate.

Postmarketing Reports

Voluntary reports of other adverse events temporally associated with the use of venlafaxine that have been received since market introduction and that may have no causal relationship with the use of venlafaxine include the following: agranulocytosis, anaphylaxis, aplastic anemia, catatonia, congenital anomalies, CPK increased, deep vein thrombophlebitis, delirium, EKG abnormalities such as QT prolongation; cardiac arrhythmias including atrial fibrillation, supraventricular tachycardia, ventricular extrasystole, and rare reports of ventricular fibrillation and ventricular tachycardia, including torsade de pointes; epidermal necrosis/Stevens-Johnson Syndrome, erythema multiforme, extrapyramidal symptoms (including dyskinesia and tardive dyskinesia), hemorrhage (including eye and gastrointestinal bleeding), hepatic events (including GGT elevation; abnormalities of unspecified liver function tests; liver damage, necrosis, or failure; and fatty liver), involuntary movements, LDH increased, neuroleptic malignant syndrome-like events (including a case of a 10-year-old who may have been taking methylphenidate, was treated and recovered), neutropenia, night sweats, pancreatitis, pancytopenia, panic, prolactin increased, pulmonary eosinophilia, renal failure, rhabdomyolysis, serotonin syndrome, shock-like electrical sensations or tinnitus (in some cases, subsequent to the discontinuation of venlafaxine or tapering of dose), and syndrome of inappropriate antidiuretic hormone secretion (usually in the elderly).

There have been reports of elevated clozapine levels that were temporally associated with adverse events, including seizures, following the addition of venlafaxine. There have been reports of increases in prothrombin time, partial thromboplastin time, or INR when venlafaxine was given to patients receiving warfarin therapy.

DRUG ABUSE AND DEPENDENCE

Controlled Substance Class

Effexor (venlafaxine hydrochloride) is not a controlled substance.

Continued on next page

Effexor—Cont.

Physical and Psychological Dependence

In vitro studies revealed that venlafaxine has virtually no affinity for opiate, benzodiazepine, phencyclidine (PCP), or N-methyl-D-aspartic acid (NMDA) receptors.

Venlafaxine was not found to have any significant CNS stimulant activity in rodents. In primate drug discrimination studies, venlafaxine showed no significant stimulant or depressant abuse liability.

Discontinuation effects have been reported in patients receiving venlafaxine (see **DOSAGE AND ADMINISTRATION**).

While Effexor has not been systematically studied in clinical trials for its potential for abuse, there was no indication of drug-seeking behavior in the clinical trials. However, it is not possible to predict on the basis of premarketing experience the extent to which a CNS active drug will be misused, diverted, and/or abused once marketed. Consequently, physicians should carefully evaluate patients for history of drug abuse and follow such patients closely, observing them for signs of misuse or abuse of Effexor (eg, development of tolerance, incrementation of dose, drug-seeking behavior).

OVERDOSAGE

Human Experience

There were 14 reports of acute overdose with Effexor (venlafaxine hydrochloride), either alone or in combination with other drugs and/or alcohol, among the patients included in the premarketing evaluation. The majority of the reports involved ingestions in which the total dose of Effexor taken was estimated to be no more than several-fold higher than the usual therapeutic dose. The 3 patients who took the highest doses were estimated to have ingested approximately 6.75 g, 2.75 g, and 2.5 g. The resultant peak plasma levels of venlafaxine for the latter 2 patients were 6.24 and 2.35 µg/mL, respectively, and the peak plasma levels of O-desmethylvenlafaxine were 3.37 and 1.30 µg/mL, respectively. Plasma venlafaxine levels were not obtained for the patient who ingested 6.75 g of venlafaxine. All 14 patients recovered without sequelae. Most patients reported no symptoms. Among the remaining patients, somnolence was the most commonly reported symptom. The patient who ingested 2.75 g of venlafaxine was observed to have 2 generalized convulsions and a prolongation of QTc to 500 msec, compared with 405 msec at baseline. Mild sinus tachycardia was reported in 2 of the other patients.

In postmarketing experience, overdose with venlafaxine has occurred predominantly in combination with alcohol and/or other drugs. Electrocardiogram changes (eg, prolongation of QT interval, bundle branch block, QRS prolongation), sinus and ventricular tachycardia, bradycardia, hypotension, altered level of consciousness (ranging from somnolence to coma), rhabdomyolysis, seizures, vertigo, and death have been reported.

Management of Overdosage

Treatment should consist of those general measures employed in the management of overdosage with any antidepressant.

Ensure an adequate airway, oxygenation, and ventilation. Monitor cardiac rhythm and vital signs. General supportive and symptomatic measures are also recommended. Induction of emesis is not recommended. Gastric lavage with a large-bore orogastric tube with appropriate airway protection, if needed, may be indicated if performed soon after ingestion or in symptomatic patients. Activated charcoal should be administered. Due to the large volume of distribution of this drug, forced diuresis, dialysis, hemoperfusion and exchange transfusion are unlikely to be of benefit. No specific antidotes for venlafaxine are known.

In managing overdosage, consider the possibility of multiple drug involvement. The physician should consider contacting a poison control center for additional information on the treatment of any overdose. Telephone numbers for certified poison control centers are listed in the *Physicians' Desk Reference (PDR)*.

DOSAGE AND ADMINISTRATION

Initial Treatment

The recommended starting dose for Effexor is 75 mg/day, administered in two or three divided doses, taken with food. Depending on tolerability and the need for further clinical effect, the dose may be increased to 150 mg/day. If needed, the dose should be further increased up to 225 mg/day. When increasing the dose, increments of up to 75 mg/day should be made at intervals of no less than 4 days. In outpatient settings there was no evidence of usefulness of doses greater than 225 mg/day for moderately depressed patients, but more severely depressed inpatients responded to a mean dose of 350 mg/day. Certain patients, including more severely depressed patients, may therefore respond more to higher doses, up to a maximum of 375 mg/day, generally in three divided doses (see **PRECAUTIONS**, **General**, *Use in Patients with Concomitant Illness*).

Special Populations

Treatment of Pregnant Women During the Third Trimester

Neonates exposed to Effexor, other SNRIs, or SSRIs, late in the third trimester have developed complications requiring prolonged hospitalization, respiratory support, and tube feeding (see **PRECAUTIONS**). When treating pregnant women with Effexor during the third trimester, the physician should carefully consider the potential risks and benefits of treatment. The physician may consider tapering Effexor in the third trimester.

Dosage for Patients with Hepatic Impairment

Given the decrease in clearance and increase in elimination half-life for both venlafaxine and ODV that is observed in patients with hepatic cirrhosis compared to normal subjects (see **CLINICAL PHARMACOLOGY**), it is recommended that the total daily dose be reduced by 50% in patients with moderate hepatic impairment. Since there was much individual variability in clearance between patients with cirrhosis, it may be necessary to reduce the dose even more than 50%, and individualization of dosing may be desirable in some patients.

Dosage for Patients with Renal Impairment

Given the decrease in clearance for venlafaxine and the increase in elimination half-life for both venlafaxine and ODV that is observed in patients with renal impairment (GFR = 10 to 70 mL/min) compared to normals (see **CLINICAL PHARMACOLOGY**), it is recommended that the total daily dose be reduced by 25% in patients with mild to moderate renal impairment. It is recommended that the total daily dose be reduced by 50% and the dose be withheld until the dialysis treatment is completed (4 hrs) in patients undergoing hemodialysis. Since there was much individual variability in clearance between patients with renal impairment, individualization of dosing may be desirable in some patients.

Dosage for Elderly Patients

No dose adjustment is recommended for elderly patients on the basis of age. As with any antidepressant, however, caution should be exercised in treating the elderly. When individualizing the dosage, extra care should be taken when increasing the dose.

Maintenance Treatment

It is generally agreed that acute episodes of major depressive disorder require several months or longer of sustained pharmacological therapy beyond response to the acute episode. In one study, in which patients responding during 8 weeks of acute treatment with Effexor XR were assigned randomly to placebo or to the same dose of Effexor XR (75, 150, or 225 mg/day, qAM) during 26 weeks of maintenance treatment as they had received during the acute stabilization phase, longer-term efficacy was demonstrated. A second longer-term study has demonstrated the efficacy of Effexor in maintaining an antidepressant response in patients with recurrent depression who had responded and continued to be improved during an initial 26 weeks of treatment and were then randomly assigned to placebo or Effexor for periods of up to 52 weeks on the same dose (100 to 200 mg/day, on a b.i.d. schedule) (see **CLINICAL TRIALS**). Based on these limited data, it is not known whether or not the dose of Effexor/Effexor XR needed for maintenance treatment is identical to the dose needed to achieve an initial response. Patients should be periodically reassessed to determine the need for maintenance treatment and the appropriate dose for such treatment.

Discontinuing Effexor (venlafaxine hydrochloride)

Symptoms associated with discontinuation of Effexor, other SNRIs, and SSRIs, have been reported (see **PRECAUTIONS**). Patients should be monitored for these symptoms when discontinuing treatment. A gradual reduction in the dose rather than abrupt cessation is recommended whenever possible. If intolerable symptoms occur following a decrease in the dose or upon discontinuation of treatment, then resuming the previously prescribed dose may be considered. Subsequently, the physician may continue decreasing the dose but at a more gradual rate.

SWITCHING PATIENTS TO OR FROM A MONOAMINE OXIDASE INHIBITOR

At least 14 days should elapse between discontinuation of an MAOI and initiation of therapy with Effexor. In addition, at least 7 days should be allowed after stopping Effexor before starting an MAOI (see **CONTRAINDICATIONS** and **WARNINGS**).

HOW SUPPLIED

Effexor® (venlafaxine hydrochloride) Tablets are available as follows:

25 mg, peach, shield-shaped tablet with "25" and a "W" on one side and "701" on scored reverse side.

NDC 0008-0701-01, bottle of 100 tablets.

NDC 0008-0701-02, carton of 10 Redipak® blister strips of 10 tablets each.

37.5 mg, peach, shield-shaped tablet with "37.5" and a "W" on one side and "781" on scored reverse side.

NDC 0008-0781-01, bottle of 100 tablets.

NDC 0008-0781-02, carton of 10 Redipak® blister strips of 10 tablets each.

50 mg, peach, shield-shaped tablet with "50" and a "W" on one side and "703" on scored reverse side.

NDC 0008-0703-01, bottle of 100 tablets.

NDC 0008-0703-02, carton of 10 Redipak® blister strips of 10 tablets each.

75 mg, peach, shield-shaped tablet with "75" and a "W" on one side and "704" on scored reverse side.

NDC 0008-0704-01, bottle of 100 tablets.

NDC 0008-0704-02, carton of 10 Redipak® blister strips of 10 tablets each.

100 mg, peach, shield-shaped tablet with "100" and a "W" on one side and "705" on scored reverse side.

NDC 0008-0705-01, bottle of 100 tablets.

NDC 0008-0705-02, carton of 10 Redipak® blister strips of 10 tablets each.

The appearance of these tablets is a trademark of Wyeth Pharmaceuticals.

Store at controlled room temperature 20° to 25°C (68° to 77°F) in a dry place.

Dispense in a well-closed container as defined in the USP.

Wyeth®

Wyeth Pharmaceuticals Inc.
Philadelphia, PA 19101

W10402C008
ET01
Rev 05/04

Shown in Product Identification Guide, page 336

EFFEXOR® XR ℞

[*ĕ-fĕks-ōr*]
(venlafaxine hydrochloride)
Extended-Release Capsules
℞ only

This product's label may have been revised after this insert was used in production. For further product information and current package insert, please visit www.wyeth.com or call our medical communications department toll-free at 1-800-934-5556.

DESCRIPTION

Effexor XR is an extended-release capsule for oral administration that contains venlafaxine hydrochloride, a structurally novel antidepressant. It is designated (R/S)-1-[2-(dimethylamino)-1-(4-methoxyphenyl)ethyl] cyclohexanol hydrochloride or (±)-1-[α- [(dimethylamino)methyl]-p-methoxybenzyl] cyclohexanol hydrochloride and has the empirical formula of $C_{17}H_{27}NO_2$ HCl. Its molecular weight is 313.87. The structural formula is shown below.

$N(CH_3)_2$ OH C H H_3CO •HCl

venlafaxine hydrochloride

Venlafaxine hydrochloride is a white to off-white crystalline solid with a solubility of 572 mg/mL in water (adjusted to ionic strength of 0.2 M with sodium chloride). Its octanol: water (0.2 M sodium chloride) partition coefficient is 0.43.

Effexor XR is formulated as an extended-release capsule for once-a-day oral administration. Drug release is controlled by diffusion through the coating membrane on the spheroids and is not pH dependent. Capsules contain venlafaxine hydrochloride equivalent to 37.5 mg, 75 mg, or 150 mg venlafaxine. Inactive ingredients consist of cellulose, ethylcellulose, gelatin, hypromellose, iron oxide, and titanium dioxide.

CLINICAL PHARMACOLOGY

Pharmacodynamics

The mechanism of the antidepressant action of venlafaxine in humans is believed to be associated with its potentiation of neurotransmitter activity in the CNS. Preclinical studies have shown that venlafaxine and its active metabolite, O-desmethylvenlafaxine (ODV), are potent inhibitors of neuronal serotonin and norepinephrine reuptake and weak inhibitors of dopamine reuptake. Venlafaxine and ODV have no significant affinity for muscarinic cholinergic, H_1-histaminergic, or α_1-adrenergic receptors in vitro. Pharmacologic activity at these receptors is hypothesized to be associated with the various anticholinergic, sedative, and cardiovascular effects seen with other psychotropic drugs. Venlafaxine and ODV do not possess monoamine oxidase (MAO) inhibitory activity.

Pharmacokinetics

Steady-state concentrations of venlafaxine and ODV in plasma are attained within 3 days of oral multiple dose therapy. Venlafaxine and ODV exhibited linear kinetics over the dose range of 75 to 450 mg/day. Mean±SD steady-state plasma clearance of venlafaxine and ODV is 1.3±0.6 and 0.4±0.2 L/h/kg, respectively; apparent elimination half-life is 5±2 and 11±2 hours, respectively; and apparent (steady-state) volume of distribution is 7.5±3.7 and 5.7±1.8 L/kg, respectively. Venlafaxine and ODV are minimally bound at therapeutic concentrations to plasma proteins (27% and 30%, respectively).

Absorption

Venlafaxine is well absorbed and extensively metabolized in the liver. O-desmethylvenlafaxine (ODV) is the only major active metabolite. On the basis of mass balance studies, at least 92% of a single oral dose of venlafaxine is absorbed. The absolute bioavailability of venlafaxine is about 45%.

Administration of Effexor XR (150 mg q24 hours) generally resulted in lower C_{max} (150 ng/mL for venlafaxine and 260 ng/mL for ODV) and later T_{max} (5.5 hours for venlafaxine and 9 hours for ODV) than for immediate release venlafaxine tablets (C_{max}'s for immediate release 75 mg q12 hours were 225 ng/mL for venlafaxine and 290 ng/mL for ODV; T_{max}'s were 2 hours for venlafaxine and 3 hours for ODV). When equal daily doses of venlafaxine were administered as either an immediate release tablet or the extended-release capsule, the exposure to both venlafaxine and ODV was similar for the two treatments, and the fluctuation in plasma concentrations was slightly lower with the Effexor XR capsule. Effexor XR, therefore, provides a slower rate of absorption, but the same extent of absorption compared with the immediate release tablet.

Food did not affect the bioavailability of venlafaxine or its active metabolite, ODV. Time of administration (AM vs PM) did not affect the pharmacokinetics of venlafaxine and ODV from the 75 mg Effexor XR capsule.

Metabolism and Excretion

Following absorption, venlafaxine undergoes extensive presystemic metabolism in the liver, primarily to ODV, but also to N-desmethylvenlafaxine, N,O-didesmethylvenlafaxine, and other minor metabolites. In vitro studies indicate that the formation of ODV is catalyzed by CYP2D6; this has been confirmed in a clinical study showing that patients with low CYP2D6 levels ("poor metabolizers") had increased levels of venlafaxine and reduced levels of ODV compared to people with normal CYP2D6 ("extensive metabolizers"). The differences between the CYP2D6 poor and extensive metabolizers, however, are not expected to be clinically important because the sum of venlafaxine and ODV is similar in the two groups and venlafaxine and ODV are pharmacologically approximately equiactive and equipotent.

Approximately 87% of a venlafaxine dose is recovered in the urine within 48 hours as unchanged venlafaxine (5%), unconjugated ODV (29%), conjugated ODV (26%), or other minor inactive metabolites (27%). Renal elimination of venlafaxine and its metabolites is thus the primary route of excretion.

Special Populations

Age and Gender: A population pharmacokinetic analysis of 404 venlafaxine-treated patients from two studies involving both b.i.d. and t.i.d. regimens showed that dose-normalized trough plasma levels of either venlafaxine or ODV were unaltered by age or gender differences. Dosage adjustment based on the age or gender of a patient is generally not necessary (see **DOSAGE AND ADMINISTRATION**).

Extensive/Poor Metabolizers: Plasma concentrations of venlafaxine were higher in CYP2D6 poor metabolizers than extensive metabolizers. Because the total exposure (AUC) of venlafaxine and ODV was similar in poor and extensive metabolizer groups, however, there is no need for different venlafaxine dosing regimens for these two groups.

Liver Disease: In 9 patients with hepatic cirrhosis, the pharmacokinetic disposition of both venlafaxine and ODV was significantly altered after oral administration of venlafaxine. Venlafaxine elimination half-life was prolonged by about 30%, and clearance decreased by about 50% in cirrhotic patients compared to normal subjects. ODV elimination half-life was prolonged by about 60%, and clearance decreased by about 30% in cirrhotic patients compared to normal subjects. A large degree of intersubject variability was noted. Three patients with more severe cirrhosis had a more substantial decrease in venlafaxine clearance (about 90%) compared to normal subjects. Dosage adjustment is necessary in these patients (see **DOSAGE AND ADMINISTRATION**).

Renal Disease: In a renal impairment study, venlafaxine elimination half-life after oral administration was prolonged by about 50% and clearance was reduced by about 24% in renally impaired patients (GFR=10 to 70 mL/min), compared to normal subjects. In dialysis patients, venlafaxine elimination half-life was prolonged by about 180% and clearance was reduced by about 57% compared to normal subjects. Similarly, ODV elimination half-life was prolonged by about 40% although clearance was unchanged in patients with renal impairment (GFR=10 to 70 mL/min) compared to normal subjects. In dialysis patients, ODV elimination half-life was prolonged by about 142% and clearance was reduced by about 56% compared to normal subjects. A large degree of intersubject variability was noted. Dosage adjustment is necessary in these patients (see **DOSAGE AND ADMINISTRATION**).

Clinical Trials

Major Depressive Disorder

The efficacy of Effexor XR (venlafaxine hydrochloride) extended-release capsules as a treatment for major depressive disorder was established in two placebo-controlled, short-term, flexible-dose studies in adult outpatients meeting DSM-III-R or DSM-IV criteria for major depressive disorder.

A 12-week study utilizing Effexor XR doses in a range 75 to 150 mg/day (mean dose for completers was 136 mg/day) and an 8-week study utilizing Effexor XR doses in a range 75 to 225 mg/day (mean dose for completers was 177 mg/day) both demonstrated superiority of Effexor XR over placebo on the HAM-D total score, HAM-D Depressed Mood Item, the MADRS total score, the Clinical Global Impressions (CGI) Severity of Illness item, and the CGI Global Improvement item. In both studies, Effexor XR was also significantly better than placebo for certain factors of the HAM-D, including the anxiety/somatization factor, the cognitive disturbance factor, and the retardation factor, as well as for the psychic anxiety score.

A 4-week study of inpatients meeting DSM-III-R criteria for major depressive disorder with melancholia utilizing Effexor (the immediate release form of venlafaxine) in a range of 150 to 375 mg/day (t.i.d. schedule) demonstrated superiority of Effexor over placebo. The mean dose in completers was 350 mg/day.

Examination of gender subsets of the population studied did not reveal any differential responsiveness on the basis of gender.

In one longer-term study, adult outpatients meeting DSM-IV criteria for major depressive disorder who had responded during an 8-week open trial on Effexor XR (75, 150, or 225 mg, qAM) were randomized to continuation of their same Effexor XR dose or to placebo, for up to 26 weeks of observation for relapse. Response during the open phase was defined as a CGI Severity of Illness item score of ≤3 and a HAM-D-21 total score of ≤10 at the day 56 evaluation. Relapse during the double-blind phase was defined as follows: (1) a reappearance of major depressive disorder as defined by DSM-IV criteria and a CGI Severity of Illness item score of ≥4 (moderately ill), (2) 2 consecutive CGI Severity of Illness item scores of ≥4, or (3) a final CGI Severity of Illness item score of ≥4 for any patient who withdrew from the study for any reason. Patients receiving continued Effexor XR treatment experienced significantly lower relapse rates over the subsequent 26 weeks compared with those receiving placebo.

In a second longer-term trial, adult outpatients meeting DSM-III-R criteria for major depressive disorder, recurrent type, who had responded (HAM-D-21 total score ≤12 at the day 56 evaluation) and continued to be improved [defined as the following criteria being met for days 56 through 180: (1) no HAM-D-21 total score ≥20; (2) no more than 2 HAM-D-21 total scores >10, and (3) no single CGI Severity of Illness item score ≥4 (moderately ill)] during an initial 26 weeks of treatment on Effexor (100 to 200 mg/day, on a b.i.d. schedule) were randomized to continuation of their same Effexor dose or to placebo. The follow-up period to observe patients for relapse, defined as a CGI Severity of Illness item score ≥4, was for up to 52 weeks. Patients receiving continued Effexor treatment experienced significantly lower relapse rates over the subsequent 52 weeks compared with those receiving placebo.

Generalized Anxiety Disorder

The efficacy of Effexor XR capsules as a treatment for Generalized Anxiety Disorder (GAD) was established in two 8-week, placebo-controlled, fixed-dose studies, one 6-month, placebo-controlled, fixed-dose study, and one 6-month, placebo-controlled, flexible-dose study in adult outpatients meeting DSM-IV criteria for GAD.

One 8-week study evaluating Effexor XR doses of 75, 150, and 225 mg/day, and placebo showed that the 225 mg/day dose was more effective than placebo on the Hamilton Rating Scale for Anxiety (HAM-A) total score, both the HAM-A anxiety and tension items, and the Clinical Global Impressions (CGI) scale. While there was also evidence for superiority over placebo for the 75 and 150 mg/day doses, these doses were not as consistently effective as the highest dose.

A second 8-week study evaluating Effexor XR doses of 75 and 150 mg/day and placebo showed that both doses were more effective than placebo on some of these same outcomes; however, the 75 mg/day dose was more consistently effective than the 150 mg/day dose. A dose-response relationship for effectiveness in GAD was not clearly established in the 75 to 225 mg/day dose range utilized in these two studies.

Two 6-month studies, one evaluating Effexor XR doses of 37.5, 75, and 150 mg/day and the other evaluating Effexor XR doses of 75 to 225 mg/day, showed that daily doses of 75 mg or higher were more effective than placebo on the HAM-A total, both the HAM-A anxiety and tension items, and the CGI scale during 6 months of treatment. While there was also evidence for superiority over placebo for the 37.5 mg/day dose, this dose was not as consistently effective as the higher doses.

Examination of gender subsets of the population studied did not reveal any differential responsiveness on the basis of gender.

Social Anxiety Disorder (Social Phobia)

The efficacy of Effexor XR capsules as a treatment for Social Anxiety Disorder (also known as Social Phobia) was established in two double-blind, parallel group, 12-week, multicenter, placebo-controlled, flexible-dose studies in adult outpatients meeting DSM-IV criteria for Social Anxiety Disorder. Patients received doses in a range of 75 to 225 mg/day. Efficacy was assessed with the Liebowitz Social Anxiety Scale (LSAS). In these two trials, Effexor XR was significantly more effective than placebo on change from baseline to endpoint on the LSAS total score.

Examination of subsets of the population studied did not reveal any differential responsiveness on the basis of gender. There was insufficient information to determine the effect of age or race on outcome in these studies.

INDICATIONS AND USAGE

Major Depressive Disorder

Effexor XR (venlafaxine hydrochloride) extended-release capsules is indicated for the treatment of major depressive disorder.

The efficacy of Effexor XR in the treatment of major depressive disorder was established in 8- and 12-week controlled trials of adult outpatients whose diagnoses corresponded most closely to the DSM-III-R or DSM-IV category of major depressive disorder (see **Clinical Trials**).

A major depressive episode (DSM-IV) implies a prominent and relatively persistent (nearly every day for at least 2 weeks) depressed mood or the loss of interest or pleasure in nearly all activities, representing a change from previous functioning, and includes the presence of at least five of the following nine symptoms during the same two-week period: depressed mood, markedly diminished interest or pleasure in usual activities, significant change in weight and/or appetite, insomnia or hypersomnia, psychomotor agitation or retardation, increased fatigue, feelings of guilt or worthlessness, slowed thinking or impaired concentration, a suicide attempt or suicidal ideation.

The efficacy of Effexor (the immediate release form of venlafaxine) in the treatment of major depressive disorder in adult inpatients meeting diagnostic criteria for major depressive disorder with melancholia was established in a 4-week controlled trial (see **Clinical Trials**). The safety and efficacy of Effexor XR in hospitalized depressed patients have not been adequately studied.

The efficacy of Effexor XR in maintaining a response in major depressive disorder for up to 26 weeks following 8 weeks of acute treatment was demonstrated in a placebo-controlled trial. The efficacy of Effexor in maintaining a response in patients with recurrent major depressive disorder who had responded and continued to be improved during an initial 26 weeks of treatment and were then followed for a period of up to 52 weeks was demonstrated in a second placebo-controlled trial (see **Clinical Trials**). Nevertheless, the physician who elects to use Effexor/Effexor XR for extended periods should periodically re-evaluate the long-term usefulness of the drug for the individual patient (see **DOSAGE AND ADMINISTRATION**).

Generalized Anxiety Disorder

Effexor XR is indicated for the treatment of Generalized Anxiety Disorder (GAD) as defined in DSM-IV. Anxiety or tension associated with the stress of everyday life usually does not require treatment with an anxiolytic.

The efficacy of Effexor XR in the treatment of GAD was established in 8-week and 6-month placebo-controlled trials in adult outpatients diagnosed with GAD according to DSM-IV criteria (see **Clinical Trials**).

Generalized Anxiety Disorder (DSM-IV) is characterized by excessive anxiety and worry (apprehensive expectation) that is persistent for at least 6 months and which the person finds difficult to control. It must be associated with at least 3 of the following 6 symptoms: restlessness or feeling keyed up or on edge, being easily fatigued, difficulty concentrating or mind going blank, irritability, muscle tension, sleep disturbance.

Although the effectiveness of Effexor XR has been demonstrated in 6-month clinical trials in patients with GAD, the physician who elects to use Effexor XR for extended periods should periodically re-evaluate the long-term usefulness of the drug for the individual patient (see **DOSAGE AND ADMINISTRATION**).

Social Anxiety Disorder

Effexor XR is indicated for the treatment of Social Anxiety Disorder, also known as Social Phobia, as defined in DSM-IV (300.23).

Social Anxiety Disorder (DSM-IV) is characterized by a marked and persistent fear of 1 or more social or performance situations in which the person is exposed to unfamiliar people or to possible scrutiny by others. Exposure to the feared situation almost invariably provokes anxiety, which may approach the intensity of a panic attack. The feared situations are avoided or endured with intense anxiety or distress. The avoidance, anxious anticipation, or distress in the feared situation(s) interferes significantly with the person's normal routine, occupational or academic functioning, or social activities or relationships, or there is a marked distress about having the phobias. Lesser degrees of performance anxiety or shyness generally do not require psychopharmacological treatment.

The efficacy of Effexor XR in the treatment of Social Anxiety Disorder was established in two 12-week placebo-controlled trials in adult outpatients with Social Anxiety Disorder (DSM-IV). Effexor XR has not been studied in children or adolescents with Social Anxiety Disorder (see **Clinical Trials**).

The effectiveness of Effexor XR in the long-term treatment of Social Anxiety Disorder, ie, for more than 12 weeks, has not been systematically evaluated in adequate and well-controlled trials. Therefore, the physician who elects to use Effexor XR for extended periods should periodically re-evaluate the long-term usefulness of the drug for the individual patient (see **DOSAGE AND ADMINISTRATION**).

CONTRAINDICATIONS

Hypersensitivity to venlafaxine hydrochloride or to any excipients in the formulation.

Concomitant use in patients taking monoamine oxidase inhibitors (MAOIs) is contraindicated (see **WARNINGS**).

WARNINGS

Potential for Interaction with Monoamine Oxidase Inhibitors

Adverse reactions, some of which were serious, have been reported in patients who have recently been discontinued from a monoamine oxidase inhibitor (MAOI) and started on venlafaxine, or who have recently had venlafaxine therapy discontinued prior to initiation of an MAOI. These reactions have included tremor, myoclonus, diaphoresis, nausea, vomiting, flushing, dizziness, hyperthermia with features resembling neuroleptic malignant syndrome, seizures, and death. In patients receiving antidepressants with pharmacological properties similar to venlafaxine in combination with an MAOI, there have also been reports of serious, sometimes fatal, reactions. For a selective serotonin reuptake inhibitor, these reactions have included hyperthermia, rigidity, myoclonus, autonomic instability with possible rapid fluctuations of vital signs, and mental status changes that include extreme agitation progressing to delirium and coma. Some cases presented with features resembling neuroleptic malignant syndrome. Severe hyperthermia and seizures, sometimes fatal, have been reported

Continued on next page

Effexor XR—Cont.

in association with the combined use of tricyclic antidepressants and MAOIs. These reactions have also been reported in patients who have recently discontinued these drugs and have been started on an MAOI. The effects of combined use of venlafaxine and MAOIs have not been evaluated in humans or animals. Therefore, because venlafaxine is an inhibitor of both norepinephrine and serotonin reuptake, it is recommended that Effexor XR (venlafaxine hydrochloride) extended-release capsules not be used in combination with an MAOI, or within at least 14 days of discontinuing treatment with an MAOI. Based on the half-life of venlafaxine, at least 7 days should be allowed after stopping venlafaxine before starting an MAOI.

Clinical Worsening and Suicide Risk

Patients with major depressive disorder, both adult and pediatric, may experience worsening of their depression and/or the emergence of suicidal ideation and behavior (suicidality), whether or not they are taking antidepressant medications, and this risk may persist until significant remission occurs. Although there has been a long-standing concern that antidepressants may have a role in inducing worsening of depression and the emergence of suicidality in certain patients, a causal role for antidepressants in inducing such behaviors has not been established. **Nevertheless, patients being treated with antidepressants should be observed closely for clinical worsening and suicidality, especially at the beginning of a course of drug therapy, or at the time of dose changes, either increases or decreases.** Consideration should be given to changing the therapeutic regimen, including possibly discontinuing the medication, in patients whose depression is persistently worse or whose emergent suicidality is severe, abrupt in onset, or was not part of the patient's presenting symptoms.

Because of the possibility of co-morbidity between major depressive disorder and other psychiatric and nonpsychiatric disorders, the same precautions observed when treating patients with major depressive disorder should be observed when treating patients with other psychiatric and nonpsychiatric disorders.

The following symptoms, anxiety, agitation, panic attacks, insomnia, irritability, hostility (aggressiveness), impulsivity, akathisia (psychomotor restlessness), hypomania, and mania, have been reported in adult and pediatric patients being treated with antidepressants for major depressive disorder as well as for other indications, both psychiatric and nonpsychiatric. Although a causal link between the emergence of such symptoms and either the worsening of depression and/or the emergence of suicidal impulses has not been established, consideration should be given to changing the therapeutic regimen, including possibly discontinuing the medication, in patients for whom such symptoms are severe, abrupt in onset, or were not part of the patient's presenting symptoms.

Families and caregivers of patients being treated with antidepressants for major depressive disorder or other indications, both psychiatric and nonpsychiatric, should be alerted about the need to monitor patients for the emergence of agitation, irritability, and the other symptoms described above, as well as the emergence of suicidality, and to report such symptoms immediately to health care providers. Prescriptions for Effexor XR should be written for the smallest quantity of capsules consistent with good patient management, in order to reduce the risk of overdose.

If the decision has been made to discontinue treatment, medication should be tapered, as rapidly as is feasible, but with recognition that abrupt discontinuation can be associated with certain symptoms (see **PRECAUTIONS** and **DOSAGE AND ADMINISTRATION, Discontinuing Effexor XR**, for a description of the risks of discontinuation of Effexor XR).

It should be noted that Effexor XR is not approved for use in treating any indications in the pediatric population.

A major depressive episode may be the initial presentation of bipolar disorder. It is generally believed (though not established in controlled trials) that treating such an episode with an antidepressant alone may increase the likelihood of precipitation of a mixed/manic episode in patients at risk for bipolar disorder. Whether any of the symptoms described above represent such a conversion is unknown. However, prior to initiating treatment with an antidepressant, patients should be adequately screened to determine if they are at risk for bipolar disorder; such screening should include a detailed psychiatric history, including a family history of suicide, bipolar disorder, and depression. It should be noted that Effexor XR is not approved for use in treating bipolar depression.

Sustained Hypertension

Venlafaxine treatment is associated with sustained increases in blood pressure in some patients. Among patients treated with 75 to 375 mg/day of Effexor XR in premarketing studies in patients with major depressive disorder, 3% (19/705) experienced sustained hypertension [defined as treatment-emergent supine diastolic blood pressure (SDBP) $\geq$ 90 mm Hg and $\geq$ 10 mm Hg above baseline for 3 consecutive on-therapy visits]. Among patients treated with 37.5 to 225 mg/day of Effexor XR in premarketing GAD studies, 0.5% (5/1011) experienced sustained hypertension. Among patients treated with 75 to 225 mg/day of Effexor XR in premarketing Social Anxiety Disorder studies, 1.4% (4/277) experienced sustained hypertension. Experience with the immediate-release venlafaxine showed that sustained hypertension was dose-related, increasing from 3% to 7% at 100 to 300 mg/day to 13% at doses above 300 mg/day. An insufficient number of patients received mean doses of Effexor XR over 300 mg/day to fully evaluate the incidence of sustained increases in blood pressure at these higher doses.

In placebo-controlled premarketing studies in patients with major depressive disorder with Effexor XR 75 to 225 mg/day, a final on-drug mean increase in supine diastolic blood pressure (SDBP) of 1.2 mm Hg was observed for Effexor XR-treated patients compared with a mean decrease of 0.2 mm Hg for placebo-treated patients. In placebo-controlled premarketing GAD studies with Effexor XR 37.5 to 225 mg/day, up to 8 weeks or up to 6 months, a final on-drug mean increase in SDBP of 0.3 mm Hg was observed for Effexor XR-treated patients compared with a mean decrease of 0.9 and 0.8 mm Hg, respectively, for placebo-treated patients. In placebo-controlled premarketing Social Anxiety Disorder studies with Effexor XR 75 to 225 mg/day up to 12 weeks, a final on-drug mean increase in SDBP of 1.3 mm Hg was observed for Effexor XR-treated patients compared with a mean decrease of 1.3 mm Hg for placebo-treated patients.

In premarketing major depressive disorder studies, 0.7% (5/705) of the Effexor XR-treated patients discontinued treatment because of elevated blood pressure. Among these patients, most of the blood pressure increases were in a modest range (12 to 16 mm Hg, SDBP). In premarketing GAD studies up to 8 weeks and up to 6 months, 0.7% (10/1381) and 1.3% (7/535) of the Effexor XR-treated patients, respectively, discontinued treatment because of elevated blood pressure. Among these patients, most of the blood pressure increases were in a modest range (12 to 25 mm Hg, SDBP up to 8 weeks; 8 to 28 mm Hg up to 6 months). In premarketing Social Anxiety Disorder studies up to 12 weeks, 0.4% (1/277) of the Effexor XR-treated patients discontinued treatment because of elevated blood pressure. In this patient, the blood pressure increase was modest (13 mm Hg, SDBP).

Sustained increases of SDBP could have adverse consequences. Therefore, it is recommended that patients receiving Effexor XR have regular monitoring of blood pressure. For patients who experience a sustained increase in blood pressure while receiving venlafaxine, either dose reduction or discontinuation should be considered.

PRECAUTIONS

General

Discontinuation of Treatment with Effexor XR

Discontinuation symptoms have been systematically evaluated in patients taking venlafaxine, to include prospective analyses of clinical trials in Generalized Anxiety Disorder and retrospective surveys of trials in major depressive disorder. Abrupt discontinuation or dose reduction of venlafaxine at various doses has been found to be associated with the appearance of new symptoms, the frequency of which increased with increased dose level and with longer duration of treatment. Reported symptoms include agitation, anorexia, anxiety, confusion, coordination impaired, diarrhea, dizziness, dry mouth, dysphoric mood, fasciculation, fatigue, headaches, hypomania, insomnia, nausea, nervousness, nightmares, sensory disturbances (including shock-like electrical sensations), somnolence, sweating, tremor, vertigo, and vomiting.

During marketing of Effexor XR, other SNRIs (Serotonin and Norepinephrine Reuptake Inhibitors), and SSRIs (Selective Serotonin Reuptake Inhibitors), there have been spontaneous reports of adverse events occurring upon discontinuation of these drugs, particularly when abrupt, including the following: dysphoric mood, irritability, agitation, dizziness, sensory disturbances (e.g. paresthesias such as electric shock sensations), anxiety, confusion, headache, lethargy, emotional lability, insomnia, hypomania, tinnitus, and seizures. While these events are generally self-limiting, there have been reports of serious discontinuation symptoms.

Patients should be monitored for these symptoms when discontinuing treatment with Effexor XR. A gradual reduction in the dose rather than abrupt cessation is recommended whenever possible. If intolerable symptoms occur following a decrease in the dose or upon discontinuation of treatment, then resuming the previously prescribed dose may be considered. Subsequently, the physician may continue decreasing the dose but at a more gradual rate (see **DOSAGE AND ADMINISTRATION**).

Insomnia and Nervousness

Treatment-emergent insomnia and nervousness were more commonly reported for patients treated with Effexor XR (venlafaxine hydrochloride) extended-release capsules than with placebo in pooled analyses of short-term major depressive disorder, GAD, and Social Anxiety Disorder studies, as shown in Table 1.

[See table 1 below]

Table 1
Incidence of Insomnia and Nervousness in Placebo-Controlled Major Depressive Disorder, GAD, and Social Anxiety Disorder Trials

	Major Depressive Disorder		GAD		Social Anxiety Disorder	
Symptom	Effexor XR n = 357	Placebo n = 285	Effexor XR n = 1381	Placebo n = 555	Effexor XR n = 277	Placebo n = 274
Insomnia	17%	11%	15%	10%	23%	7%
Nervousness	10%	5%	6%	4%	11%	3%

Insomnia and nervousness each led to drug discontinuation in 0.9% of the patients treated with Effexor XR in major depressive disorder studies.

In GAD trials, insomnia and nervousness led to drug discontinuation in 3% and 2%, respectively, of the patients treated with Effexor XR up to 8 weeks and 2% and 0.7%, respectively, of the patients treated with Effexor XR up to 6 months.

In Social Anxiety Disorder trials, insomnia and nervousness led to drug discontinuation in 3% and 0%, respectively, of the patients treated with Effexor XR up to 12 weeks.

Changes in Weight

Adult Patients: A loss of 5% or more of body weight occurred in 7% of Effexor XR-treated and 2% of placebo-treated patients in the short-term placebo-controlled major depressive disorder trials. The discontinuation rate for weight loss associated with Effexor XR was 0.1% in major depressive disorder studies. In placebo-controlled GAD studies, a loss of 7% or more of body weight occurred in 3% of Effexor XR patients and 1% of placebo patients who received treatment for up to 6 months. The discontinuation rate for weight loss was 0.3% for patients receiving Effexor XR in GAD studies for up to eight weeks. In placebo-controlled Social Anxiety Disorder trials, 3% of the Effexor XR-treated and 0.4% of the placebo-treated patients sustained a loss of 7% or more of body weight during up to 12 weeks of treatment. None of the patients receiving Effexor XR in Social Anxiety Disorder studies discontinued for weight loss.

The safety and efficacy of venlafaxine therapy in combination with weight loss agents, including phentermine, have not been established. Co-administration of Effexor XR and weight loss agents is not recommended. Effexor XR is not indicated for weight loss alone or in combination with other products.

Pediatric Patients: Weight loss has been observed in pediatric patients (ages 6-17) receiving Effexor XR. In a pooled analysis of four eight-week, double-blind, placebo-controlled, flexible dose outpatient trials for major depressive disorder (MDD) and generalized anxiety disorder (GAD), Effexor XR-treated patients lost an average of 0.45 kg (n = 333), while placebo-treated patients gained an average of 0.77 kg (n = 333). More patients treated with Effexor XR than with placebo experienced a weight loss of at least 3.5% in both the MDD and the GAD studies (18% of Effexor XR-treated patients vs. 3.6% of placebo-treated patients; $p<0.001$). Weight loss was not limited to patients with treatment-emergent anorexia (see **PRECAUTIONS, General**, *Changes in Appetite*).

The risks associated with longer-term Effexor XR use were assessed in an open-label study of children and adolescents who received Effexor XR for up to six months. The children and adolescents in the study had increases in weight that were less than expected based on data from age- and sex-matched peers. The difference between observed weight gain and expected weight gain was larger for children (<12 years old) than for adolescents (>12 years old).

Changes in Height

Pediatric Patients: During the eight-week placebo-controlled GAD studies, Effexor XR-treated patients (ages 6-17) grew an average of 0.3 cm (n = 122), while placebo-treated patients grew an average of 1.0 cm (n = 132); p=0.041. This difference in height increase was most notable in patients younger than twelve. During the eight-week placebo-controlled MDD studies, Effexor XR-treated patients grew an average of 0.8 cm (n = 146), while placebo-treated patients grew an average of 0.7 cm (n = 147). In the six-month open-label study, children and adolescents had height increases that were less than expected based on data from age- and sex-matched peers. The difference between observed growth rates and expected growth rates was larger for children (<12 years old) than for adolescents (>12 years old).

Changes in Appetite

Adult Patients: Treatment-emergent anorexia was more commonly reported for Effexor XR-treated (8%) than placebo-treated patients (4%) in the pool of short-term, double-blind, placebo-controlled major depressive disorder studies. The discontinuation rate for anorexia associated with Effexor XR was 1.0% in major depressive disorder studies. Treatment-emergent anorexia was more commonly reported for Effexor XR-treated (8%) than placebo-treated patients (2%) in the pool of short-term, double-blind, placebo-controlled GAD studies. The discontinuation rate for anorexia was 0.9% for patients receiving Effexor XR for up to 8 weeks in GAD studies. Treatment-emergent anorexia was more commonly reported for Effexor XR-treated

(20%) than placebo-treated patients (2%) in the pool of short-term, double-blind, placebo-controlled Social Anxiety Disorder studies. The discontinuation rate for anorexia was 0.4% for patients receiving Effexor XR for up to 12 weeks in Social Anxiety Disorder studies.

Pediatric Patients: Decreased appetite has been observed in pediatric patients receiving Effexor XR. In the placebo-controlled trials for GAD and MDD, 10% of patients aged 6-17 treated with Effexor XR for up to eight weeks and 3% of patients treated with placebo reported treatment-emergent anorexia (decreased appetite). None of the patients receiving Effexor XR discontinued for anorexia or weight loss.

Activation of Mania/Hypomania

During premarketing major depressive disorder studies, mania or hypomania occurred in 0.3% of Effexor XR-treated patients and 0.0% placebo patients. In premarketing GAD studies, 0.0% of Effexor XR-treated patients and 0.2% of placebo-treated patients experienced mania or hypomania. In premarketing Social Anxiety Disorder studies, no Effexor XR-treated patients and no placebo-treated patients experienced mania or hypomania. In all premarketing major depressive disorder trials with Effexor, mania or hypomania occurred in 0.5% of venlafaxine-treated patients compared with 0% of placebo patients. Mania/hypomania has also been reported in a small proportion of patients with mood disorders who were treated with other marketed drugs to treat major depressive disorder. As with all drugs effective in the treatment of major depressive disorder, Effexor XR should be used cautiously in patients with a history of mania.

Hyponatremia

Hyponatremia and/or the syndrome of inappropriate antidiuretic hormone secretion (SIADH) may occur with venlafaxine. This should be taken into consideration in patients who are, for example, volume-depleted, elderly, or taking diuretics.

Mydriasis

Mydriasis has been reported in association with venlafaxine; therefore patients with raised intraocular pressure or those at risk of acute narrow-angle glaucoma should be monitored.

Seizures

During premarketing experience, no seizures occurred among 705 Effexor XR-treated patients in the major depressive disorder studies, among 1381 Effexor XR-treated patients in GAD studies, or among 277 Effexor XR-treated patients in Social Anxiety Disorder studies. In all premarketing major depressive disorder trials with Effexor, seizures were reported at various doses in 0.3% (8/3082) of venlafaxine-treated patients. Effexor XR, like many antidepressants, should be used cautiously in patients with a history of seizures and should be discontinued in any patient who develops seizures.

Abnormal Bleeding

There have been reports of abnormal bleeding (most commonly ecchymosis) associated with venlafaxine treatment. While a causal relationship to venlafaxine is unclear, impaired platelet aggregation may result from platelet serotonin depletion and contribute to such occurrences.

Serum Cholesterol Elevation

Clinically relevant increases in serum cholesterol were recorded in 5.3% of venlafaxine-treated patients and 0.0% of placebo-treated patients treated for at least 3 months in placebo-controlled trials (see **ADVERSE REACTIONS-Laboratory Changes**). Measurement of serum cholesterol levels should be considered during long-term treatment.

Use in Patients With Concomitant Illness

Premarketing experience with venlafaxine in patients with concomitant systemic illness is limited. Caution is advised in administering Effexor XR to patients with diseases or conditions that could affect hemodynamic responses or metabolism.

Venlafaxine has not been evaluated or used to any appreciable extent in patients with a recent history of myocardial infarction or unstable heart disease. Patients with these diagnoses were systematically excluded from many clinical studies during venlafaxine's premarketing testing. The electrocardiograms were analyzed for 275 patients who received Effexor XR and 220 patients who received placebo in 8- to 12-week double-blind, placebo-controlled trials in major depressive disorder, for 610 patients who received Effexor XR and 298 patients who received placebo in 8-week double-blind, placebo-controlled trials in GAD, and for 195 patients who received Effexor XR and 228 patients who received placebo in 12-week double-blind, placebo-controlled trials in Social Anxiety Disorder. The mean change from baseline in corrected QT interval (QTc) for Effexor XR-treated patients in major depressive disorder studies was increased relative to that for placebo-treated patients (increase of 4.7 msec for Effexor XR and decrease of 1.9 msec for placebo). The mean change from baseline in corrected QT interval (QTc) for Effexor XR-treated patients in the GAD studies did not differ significantly from that with placebo. The mean change from baseline in QTc for Effexor XR-treated patients in the Social Anxiety Disorder studies was increased relative to that for placebo-treated patients (increase of 2.8 msec for Effexor XR and decrease of 2.0 msec for placebo).

In these same trials, the mean change from baseline in heart rate for Effexor XR-treated patients in the major depressive disorder studies was significantly higher than that for placebo (a mean increase of 4 beats per minute for Effexor XR and 1 beat per minute for placebo). The mean change from baseline in heart rate for Effexor XR-treated patients in the GAD studies was significantly higher than that for placebo (a mean increase of 3 beats per minute for Effexor XR and no change for placebo). The mean change from baseline in heart rate for Effexor XR-treated patients in the Social Anxiety Disorder studies was significantly higher than that for placebo (a mean increase of 5 beats per minute for Effexor XR and no change for placebo).

In a flexible-dose study, with Effexor doses in the range of 200 to 375 mg/day and mean dose greater than 300 mg/day, Effexor-treated patients had a mean increase in heart rate of 8.5 beats per minute compared with 1.7 beats per minute in the placebo group.

As increases in heart rate were observed, caution should be exercised in patients whose underlying medical conditions might be compromised by increases in heart rate (eg, patients with hyperthyroidism, heart failure, or recent myocardial infarction), particularly when using doses of Effexor above 200 mg/day.

Evaluation of the electrocardiograms for 769 patients who received immediate release Effexor in 4- to 6-week double-blind, placebo-controlled trials showed that the incidence of trial-emergent conduction abnormalities did not differ from that with placebo.

In patients with renal impairment (GFR = 10 to 70 mL/min) or cirrhosis of the liver, the clearances of venlafaxine and its active metabolites were decreased, thus prolonging the elimination half-lives of these substances. A lower dose may be necessary (see **DOSAGE AND ADMINISTRATION**). Effexor XR, like all drugs effective in the treatment of major depressive disorder, should be used with caution in such patients.

Information for Patients

Physicians are advised to discuss the following issues with patients for whom they prescribe Effexor XR (venlafaxine hydrochloride) extended-release capsules:

Patients and their families should be encouraged to be alert to the emergence of anxiety, agitation, panic attacks, insomnia, irritability, hostility, impulsivity, akathisia, hypomania, mania, worsening of depression, and suicidal ideation, especially early during antidepressant treatment. Such symptoms should be reported to the patient's physician, especially if they are severe, abrupt in onset, or were not part of the patient's presenting symptoms.

Interference with Cognitive and Motor Performance

Clinical studies were performed to examine the effects of venlafaxine on behavioral performance of healthy individuals. The results revealed no clinically significant impairment of psychomotor, cognitive, or complex behavior performance. However, since any psychoactive drug may impair judgment, thinking, or motor skills, patients should be cautioned about operating hazardous machinery, including automobiles, until they are reasonably certain that venlafaxine therapy does not adversely affect their ability to engage in such activities.

Concomitant Medication

Patients should be advised to inform their physicians if they are taking, or plan to take, any prescription or over-the-counter drugs, including herbal preparations, since there is a potential for interactions.

Alcohol

Although venlafaxine has not been shown to increase the impairment of mental and motor skills caused by alcohol, patients should be advised to avoid alcohol while taking venlafaxine.

Allergic Reactions

Patients should be advised to notify their physician if they develop a rash, hives, or a related allergic phenomenon.

Pregnancy

Patients should be advised to notify their physician if they become pregnant or intend to become pregnant during therapy.

Nursing

Patients should be advised to notify their physician if they are breast-feeding an infant.

Laboratory Tests

There are no specific laboratory tests recommended.

Drug Interactions

As with all drugs, the potential for interaction by a variety of mechanisms is a possibility.

Alcohol

A single dose of ethanol (0.5 g/kg) had no effect on the pharmacokinetics of venlafaxine or O-desmethylvenlafaxine (ODV) when venlafaxine was administered at 150 mg/day in 15 healthy male subjects. Additionally, administration of venlafaxine in a stable regimen did not exaggerate the psychomotor and psychometric effects induced by ethanol in these same subjects when they were not receiving venlafaxine.

Cimetidine

Concomitant administration of cimetidine and venlafaxine in a steady-state study for both drugs resulted in inhibition of first-pass metabolism of venlafaxine in 18 healthy subjects. The oral clearance of venlafaxine was reduced by about 43%, and the exposure (AUC) and maximum concentration (C_{max}) of the drug were increased by about 60%. However, coadministration of cimetidine had no apparent effect on the pharmacokinetics of ODV, which is present in much greater quantity in the circulation than venlafaxine. The overall pharmacological activity of venlafaxine plus ODV is expected to increase only slightly, and no dosage adjustment should be necessary for most normal adults. However, for patients with pre-existing hypertension, and for elderly patients or patients with hepatic dysfunction, the interaction associated with the concomitant use of venlafaxine and cimetidine is not known and potentially could be more pronounced. Therefore, caution is advised with such patients.

Diazepam

Under steady-state conditions for venlafaxine administered at 150 mg/day, a single 10 mg dose of diazepam did not appear to affect the pharmacokinetics of either venlafaxine or ODV in 18 healthy male subjects. Venlafaxine also did not have any effect on the pharmacokinetics of diazepam or its active metabolite, desmethyldiazepam, or affect the psychomotor and psychometric effects induced by diazepam.

Haloperidol

Venlafaxine administered under steady-state conditions at 150 mg/day in 24 healthy subjects decreased total oral-dose clearance (Cl/F) of a single 2 mg dose of haloperidol by 42%, which resulted in a 70% increase in haloperidol AUC. In addition, the haloperidol C_{max} increased 88% when coadministered with venlafaxine, but the haloperidol elimination half-life ($t_{½}$) was unchanged. The mechanism explaining this finding is unknown.

Lithium

The steady-state pharmacokinetics of venlafaxine administered at 150 mg/day were not affected when a single 600 mg oral dose of lithium was administered to 12 healthy male subjects. ODV also was unaffected. Venlafaxine had no effect on the pharmacokinetics of lithium (see also *CNS-Active Drugs*, below).

Drugs Highly Bound to Plasma Proteins

Venlafaxine is not highly bound to plasma proteins; therefore, administration of Effexor XR to a patient taking another drug that is highly protein bound should not cause increased free concentrations of the other drug.

Drugs that Inhibit Cytochrome P450 Isoenzymes

CYP2D6 Inhibitors: In vitro and in vivo studies indicate that venlafaxine is metabolized to its active metabolite, ODV, by CYP2D6, the isoenzyme that is responsible for the genetic polymorphism seen in the metabolism of many antidepressants. Therefore, the potential exists for a drug interaction between drugs that inhibit CYP2D6-mediated metabolism of venlafaxine, reducing the metabolism of venlafaxine to ODV, resulting in increased plasma concentrations of venlafaxine and decreased concentrations of the active metabolite. CYP2D6 inhibitors such as quinidine would be expected to do this, but the effect would be similar to what is seen in patients who are genetically CYP2D6 poor metabolizers (see *Metabolism and Excretion* under **CLINICAL PHARMACOLOGY**). Therefore, no dosage adjustment is required when venlafaxine is coadministered with a CYP2D6 inhibitor.

The concomitant use of venlafaxine with drug treatment(s) that potentially inhibits both CYP2D6 and CYP3A4, the primary metabolizing enzymes for venlafaxine, has not been studied.

Therefore, caution is advised should a patient's therapy include venlafaxine and any agent(s) that produce simultaneous inhibition of these two enzyme systems.

Drugs Metabolized by Cytochrome P450 Isoenzymes

CYP2D6: In vitro studies indicate that venlafaxine is a relatively weak inhibitor of CYP2D6. These findings have been confirmed in a clinical drug interaction study comparing the effect of venlafaxine with that of fluoxetine on the CYP2D6-mediated metabolism of dextromethorphan to dextrorphan.

Imipramine—Venlafaxine did not affect the pharmacokinetics of imipramine and 2-OH-imipramine. However, desipramine AUC, C_{max}, and C_{min} increased by about 35% in the presence of venlafaxine. The 2-OH-desipramine AUC's increased by at least 2.5 fold (with venlafaxine 37.5 mg q12h) and by 4.5 fold (with venlafaxine 75 mg q12h). Imipramine did not affect the pharmacokinetics of venlafaxine and ODV. The clinical significance of elevated 2-OH-desipramine levels is unknown.

Risperidone—Venlafaxine administered under steady-state conditions at 150 mg/day slightly inhibited the CYP2D6-mediated metabolism of risperidone (administered as a single 1 mg oral dose) to its active metabolite, 9-hydroxyrisperidone, resulting in an approximate 32% increase in risperidone AUC. However, venlafaxine coadministration did not significantly alter the pharmacokinetic profile of the total active moiety (risperidone plus 9-hydroxyrisperidone).

CYP3A4: Venlafaxine did not inhibit CYP3A4 in vitro. This finding was confirmed in vivo by clinical drug interaction studies in which venlafaxine did not inhibit the metabolism of several CYP3A4 substrates, including alprazolam, diazepam, and terfenadine.

Indinavir—In a study of 9 healthy volunteers, venlafaxine administered under steady-state conditions at 150 mg/day resulted in a 28% decrease in the AUC of a single 800 mg oral dose of indinavir and a 36% decrease in indinavir C_{max}. Indinavir did not affect the pharmacokinetics of venlafaxine and ODV. The clinical significance of this finding is unknown.

CYP1A2: Venlafaxine did not inhibit CYP1A2 in vitro. This finding was confirmed in vivo by a clinical drug interaction study in which venlafaxine did not inhibit the metabolism of caffeine, a CYP1A2 substrate.

CYP2C9: Venlafaxine did not inhibit CYP2C9 in vitro. In vivo, venlafaxine 75 mg by mouth every 12 hours did not alter the pharmacokinetics of a single 500 mg dose of tolbutamide or the CYP2C9 mediated formation of 4-hydroxy-tolbutamide.

Continued on next page

Effexor XR—Cont.

CYP2C19: Venlafaxine did not inhibit the metabolism of diazepam, which is partially metabolized by CYP2C19 (see *Diazepam* above).

Monoamine Oxidase Inhibitors

See **CONTRAINDICATIONS** and **WARNINGS**.

CNS-Active Drugs

The risk of using venlafaxine in combination with other CNS-active drugs has not been systematically evaluated (except in the case of those CNS-active drugs noted above). Consequently, caution is advised if the concomitant administration of venlafaxine and such drugs is required. Based on the mechanism of action of venlafaxine and the potential for serotonin syndrome, caution is advised when venlafaxine is co-administered with other drugs that may affect the serotonergic neurotransmitter systems, such as triptans, serotonin reuptake inhibitors (SRIs), or lithium.

Electroconvulsive Therapy

There are no clinical data establishing the benefit of electroconvulsive therapy combined with Effexor XR (venlafaxine hydrochloride) extended-release capsules treatment.

Postmarketing Spontaneous Drug Interaction Reports

See **ADVERSE REACTIONS, Postmarketing Reports.**

Carcinogenesis, Mutagenesis, Impairment of Fertility

Carcinogenesis

Venlafaxine was given by oral gavage to mice for 18 months at doses up to 120 mg/kg per day, which was 1.7 times the maximum recommended human dose on a mg/m^2 basis. Venlafaxine was also given to rats by oral gavage for 24 months at doses up to 120 mg/kg per day. In rats receiving the 120 mg/kg dose, plasma concentrations of venlafaxine at necropsy were 1 times (male rats) and 6 times (female rats) the plasma concentrations of patients receiving the maximum recommended human dose. Plasma levels of the O-desmethyl metabolite were lower in rats than in patients receiving the maximum recommended dose. Tumors were not increased by venlafaxine treatment in mice or rats.

Mutagenesis

Venlafaxine and the major human metabolite, O-desmethylvenlafaxine (ODV), were not mutagenic in the Ames reverse mutation assay in Salmonella bacteria or the Chinese hamster ovary/HGPRT mammalian cell forward gene mutation assay. Venlafaxine was also not mutagenic or clastogenic in the in vitro BALB/c-3T3 mouse cell transformation assay, the sister chromatid exchange assay in cultured Chinese hamster ovary cells, or in the in vivo chromosomal aberration assay in rat bone marrow. ODV was not clastogenic in the in vitro Chinese hamster ovary cell chromosomal aberration assay, but elicited a clastogenic response in the in vivo chromosomal aberration assay in rat bone marrow.

Impairment of Fertility

Reproduction and fertility studies in rats showed no effects on male or female fertility at oral doses of up to 2 times the maximum recommended human dose on a mg/m^2 basis.

Pregnancy

Teratogenic Effects —Pregnancy Category C

Venlafaxine did not cause malformations in offspring of rats or rabbits given doses up to 2.5 times (rat) or 4 times (rabbit) the maximum recommended human daily dose on a mg/m^2 basis. However, in rats, there was a decrease in pup weight, an increase in stillborn pups, and an increase in pup deaths during the first 5 days of lactation, when dosing began during pregnancy and continued until weaning. The cause of these deaths is not known. These effects occurred at 2.5 times (mg/m^2) the maximum human daily dose. The no effect dose for rat pup mortality was 0.25 times the human dose on a mg/m^2 basis. There are no adequate and well-controlled studies in pregnant women. Because animal reproduction studies are not always predictive of human response, this drug should be used during pregnancy only if clearly needed.

Non-teratogenic Effects

Neonates exposed to Effexor XR, other SNRIs (Serotonin and Norepinephrine Reuptake Inhibitors), or SSRIs (Selective Serotonin Reuptake Inhibitors), late in the third trimester have developed complications requiring prolonged hospitalization, respiratory support, and tube feeding. Such complications can arise immediately upon delivery. Reported clinical findings have included respiratory distress, cyanosis, apnea, seizures, temperature instability, feeding difficulty, vomiting, hypoglycemia, hypotonia, hypertonia, hyperreflexia, tremor, jitteriness, irritability, and constant crying. These features are consistent with either a direct toxic effect of SSRIs and SNRIs or, possibly, a drug discontinuation syndrome. It should be noted that, in some cases, the clinical picture is consistent with serotonin syndrome (see **PRECAUTIONS-Drug Interactions**-*CNS-Active Drugs*). When treating a pregnant woman with Effexor XR during the third trimester, the physician should carefully consider the potential risks and benefits of treatment (see **DOSAGE AND ADMINISTRATION**).

Labor and Delivery

The effect of venlafaxine on labor and delivery in humans is unknown.

Nursing Mothers

Venlafaxine and ODV have been reported to be excreted in human milk. Because of the potential for serious adverse reactions in nursing infants from Effexor XR, a decision should be made whether to discontinue nursing or to discontinue the drug, taking into account the importance of the drug to the mother.

Pediatric Use

Effectiveness in pediatric patients has not been established. (See **WARNINGS-Clinical Worsening and Suicide Risk.**)

Although no studies have been designed to primarily assess Effexor XR's impact on the growth, development, and maturation of children and adolescents, the studies that have been done suggest that Effexor XR may adversely affect weight and height (see **PRECAUTIONS, General,** *Changes in Height and Changes in Weight*). Should the decision be made to treat a pediatric patient with Effexor XR, regular monitoring of weight and height is recommended during treatment, particularly if it is to be continued long term. The safety of Effexor XR treatment for pediatric patients has not been systematically assessed for chronic treatment longer than six months in duration.

In the studies conducted in pediatric patients (ages 6-17), the occurrence of blood pressure and cholesterol increases considered to be clinically relevant in pediatric patients was similar to that observed in adult patients. Consequently, the precautions for adults apply to pediatric patients (see **WARNINGS, Sustained Hypertension,** and **PRECAUTIONS, General,** *Serum Cholesterol Elevation*).

Geriatric Use

Approximately 4% (14/357), 6% (77/1381), and 2% (6/277) of Effexor XR-treated patients in placebo-controlled premarketing major depressive disorder, GAD, and Social Anxiety Disorder trials, respectively, were 65 years of age or over. Of 2,897 Effexor-treated patients in premarketing phase major depressive disorder studies, 12% (357) were 65 years of age or over. No overall differences in effectiveness or safety were observed between geriatric patients and younger patients, and other reported clinical experience generally has not identified differences in response between the elderly and younger patients. However, greater sensitivity of some older individuals cannot be ruled out. As with other antidepressants, several cases of hyponatremia and syndrome of inappropriate antidiuretic hormone secretion (SIADH) have been reported, usually in the elderly.

The pharmacokinetics of venlafaxine and ODV are not substantially altered in the elderly (see **CLINICAL PHARMACOLOGY**). No dose adjustment is recommended for the elderly on the basis of age alone, although other clinical circumstances, some of which may be more common in the elderly, such as renal or hepatic impairment, may warrant a dose reduction (see **DOSAGE AND ADMINISTRATION**).

ADVERSE REACTIONS

The information included in the **Adverse Findings Observed in Short-Term, Placebo-Controlled Studies with Effexor XR** subsection is based on data from a pool of three 8- and 12-week controlled clinical trials in major depressive disorder (includes two U.S. trials and one European trial), on data up to 8 weeks from a pool of five controlled clinical trials in GAD with Effexor XR®, and on data up to 12 weeks from a pool of two controlled clinical trials in Social Anxiety Disorder. Information on additional adverse events associated with Effexor XR in the entire development program for the formulation and with Effexor (the immediate release formulation of venlafaxine) is included in the **Other Adverse Events Observed During the Premarketing Evaluation of Effexor and Effexor XR** subsection (see also **WARNINGS** and **PRECAUTIONS**).

Adverse Findings Observed in Short-Term, Placebo-Controlled Studies with Effexor XR

Adverse Events Associated with Discontinuation of Treatment

Approximately 11% of the 357 patients who received Effexor® XR (venlafaxine hydrochloride) extended-release capsules in placebo-controlled clinical trials for major depressive disorder discontinued treatment due to an adverse experience, compared with 6% of the 285 placebo-treated patients in those studies. Approximately 18% of the 1381 patients who received Effexor XR capsules in placebo-controlled clinical trials for GAD discontinued treatment due to an adverse experience, compared with 12% of the 555 placebo-treated patients in those studies. Approximately 17% of the 277 patients who received Effexor XR capsules in placebo-controlled clinical trials for Social Anxiety Disorder discontinued treatment due to an adverse experience, compared with 5% of the 274 placebo-treated patients in those studies. The most common events leading to discontinuation and considered to be drug-related (ie, leading to discontinuation in at least 1% of the Effexor XR-treated patients at a rate at least twice that of placebo for either indication) are shown in Table 2.

[See table 2 at left]

Table 2
Common Adverse Events Leading to Discontinuation of Treatment in Placebo-Controlled Trials[1]

Adverse Event	Percentage of Patients Discontinuing Due to Adverse Event: Major Depressive Disorder Indication[2]		GAD Indication[3,4]		Social Anxiety Disorder Indication	
	Effexor XR n=357	Placebo n=285	Effexor XR n=1381	Placebo n=555	Effexor XR n=277	Placebo n=274
Body as a Whole						
Asthenia	—	—	3%	<1%	1%	<1%
Headache	—	—	—	—	2%	<1%
Digestive System						
Nausea	4%	<1%	8%	<1%	4%	0%
Anorexia	1%	<1%	—	—	—	—
Dry Mouth	1%	0%	2%	<1%	—	—
Vomiting	—	—	1%	<1%	—	—
Nervous System						
Dizziness	2%	1%	—	—	2%	0%
Insomnia	1%	<1%	3%	<1%	3%	<1%
Somnolence	2%	<1%	3%	<1%	2%	<1%
Nervousness	—	—	2%	<1%	—	—
Tremor	—	—	1%	0%	—	—
Anxiety	—	—	—	—	1%	<1%
Skin						
Sweating	—	—	2%	<1%	1%	0%
Urogenital System						
Impotence[5]	—	—	—	—	3%	0%

[1]Two of the major depressive disorder studies were flexible dose and one was fixed dose. Four of the GAD studies were fixed dose and one was flexible dose. Both of the Social Anxiety Disorder studies were flexible dose.

[2]In U.S. placebo-controlled trials for major depressive disorder, the following were also common events leading to discontinuation and were considered to be drug-related for Effexor XR-treated patients (% Effexor XR [n = 192], % Placebo [n = 202]): hypertension (1%, <1%); diarrhea (1%, 0%); paresthesia (1%, 0%); tremor (1%, 0%); abnormal vision, mostly blurred vision (1%, 0%); and abnormal, mostly delayed, ejaculation (1%, 0%).

[3]In two short-term U.S. placebo-controlled trials for GAD, the following were also common events leading to discontinuation and were considered to be drug-related for Effexor XR-treated patients (% Effexor XR [n = 476]), % Placebo [n = 201]): headache (4%, <1%); vasodilatation (1%, 0%); anorexia (2%, <1%); dizziness (4%, 1%); thinking abnormal (1%, 0%); and abnormal vision (1%, 0%).

[4]In long-term placebo-controlled trials for GAD, the following was also a common event leading to discontinuation and was considered to be drug-related for Effexor XR-treated patients (% Effexor XR [n = 535], % Placebo [n = 257]): decreased libido (1%, 0%).

[5]Incidence is based on the number of men (Effexor XR = 158, placebo = 153).

Adverse Events Occurring at an Incidence of 2% or More Among Effexor XR-Treated Patients

Tables 3, 4, and 5 enumerate the incidence, rounded to the nearest percent, of treatment-emergent adverse events that occurred during acute therapy of major depressive disorder (up to 12 weeks; dose range of 75 to 225 mg/day), of GAD (up to 8 weeks; dose range of 37.5 to 225 mg/day), and of Social Anxiety Disorder (up to 12 weeks; dose range of 75 to 225 mg/day), respectively, in 2% or more of patients treated with Effexor XR (venlafaxine hydrochloride) where the incidence in patients treated with Effexor XR was greater than the incidence for the respective placebo-treated patients. The table shows the percentage of patients in each group who had at least one episode of an event at some time during their treatment. Reported adverse events were classified using a standard COSTART-based Dictionary terminology. The prescriber should be aware that these figures cannot be used to predict the incidence of side effects in the course of usual medical practice where patient characteristics and other factors differ from those which prevailed in the clinical trials. Similarly, the cited frequencies cannot be compared with figures obtained from other clinical investigations involving different treatments, uses and investigators. The cited figures, however, do provide the prescribing physician with some basis for estimating the relative contribution of drug and nondrug factors to the side effect incidence rate in the population studied.

Commonly Observed Adverse Events from Tables 3, 4, and 5:

Major Depressive Disorder

Note in particular the following adverse events that occurred in at least 5% of the Effexor XR patients and at a rate at least twice that of the placebo group for all placebo-controlled trials for the major depressive disorder (Table 3): Abnormal ejaculation, gastrointestinal complaints (nausea, dry mouth, and anorexia), CNS complaints (dizziness, somnolence, and abnormal dreams), and sweating. In the two U.S. placebo-controlled trials, the following additional events occurred in at least 5% of Effexor XR-treated patients (n = 192) and at a rate at least twice that of the placebo group: Abnormalities of sexual function (impotence in men, anorgasmia in women, and libido decreased), gastrointestinal complaints (constipation and flatulence), CNS complaints (insomnia, nervousness, and tremor), problems of special senses (abnormal vision), cardiovascular effects (hypertension and vasodilatation), and yawning.

Generalized Anxiety Disorder

Note in particular the following adverse events that occurred in at least 5% of the Effexor XR patients and at a rate at least twice that of the placebo group for all placebo-controlled trials for the GAD indication (Table 4): Abnormalities of sexual function (abnormal ejaculation and impotence), gastrointestinal complaints (nausea, dry mouth, anorexia, and constipation), problems of special senses (abnormal vision), and sweating.

Social Anxiety Disorder

Note in particular the following adverse events that occurred in at least 5% of the Effexor XR patients and at a rate at least twice that of the placebo group for the 2 placebo-controlled trials for the Social Anxiety Disorder indication (Table 5): Asthenia, gastrointestinal complaints (anorexia, dry mouth, nausea), CNS complaints (anxiety, insomnia, libido decreased, nervousness, somnolence, dizziness), abnormalities of sexual function (abnormal ejaculation, orgasmic dysfunction, impotence), yawn, sweating, and abnormal vision.

Table 3
Treatment-Emergent Adverse Event Incidence in Short-Term Placebo-Controlled Effexor XR Clinical Trials in Patients with Major Depressive Disorder[1,2]

Body System Preferred Term	**% Reporting Event** **Effexor XR** (n=357)	**Placebo** (n=285)
Body as a Whole		
Asthenia	8%	7%
Cardiovascular System		
Vasodilatation[3]	4%	2%
Hypertension	4%	1%
Digestive System		
Nausea	31%	12%
Constipation	8%	5%
Anorexia	8%	4%
Vomiting	4%	2%
Flatulence	4%	3%
Metabolic/Nutritional		
Weight Loss	3%	0%
Nervous System		
Dizziness	20%	9%
Somnolence	17%	8%
Insomnia	17%	11%
Dry Mouth	12%	6%
Nervousness	10%	5%
Abnormal Dreams[4]	7%	2%
Tremor	5%	2%
Depression	3%	<1%
Paresthesia	3%	1%
Libido Decreased	3%	<1%
Agitation	3%	1%
Respiratory System		
Pharyngitis	7%	6%
Yawn	3%	0%
Skin		
Sweating	14%	3%
Special Senses		
Abnormal Vision[5]	4%	<1%
Urogenital System		
Abnormal Ejaculation (male)[6,7]	16%	<1%
Impotence[7]	4%	<1%
Anorgasmia (female)[8,9]	3%	<1%

[1]Incidence, rounded to the nearest %, for events reported by at least 2% of patients treated with Effexor XR, except the following events which had an incidence equal to or less than placebo: abdominal pain, accidental injury, anxiety, back pain, bronchitis, diarrhea, dysmenorrhea, dyspepsia, flu syndrome, headache, infection, pain, palpitation, rhinitis, and sinusitis.
[2]<1% indicates an incidence greater than zero but less than 1%.
[3]Mostly "hot flashes."
[4]Mostly "vivid dreams," "nightmares," and "increased dreaming."
[5]Mostly "blurred vision" and "difficulty focusing eyes."
[6]Mostly "delayed ejaculation."
[7]Incidence is based on the number of male patients.
[8]Mostly "delayed orgasm" or "anorgasmia."
[9]Incidence is based on the number of female patients.

Table 4
Treatment-Emergent Adverse Event Incidence in Short-Term Placebo-Controlled Effexor XR Clinical Trials in GAD Patients[1,2]

Body System Preferred Term	**% Reporting Event** **Effexor XR** (n=1381)	**Placebo** (n=555)
Body as a Whole		
Asthenia	12%	8%
Cardiovascular System		
Vasodilatation[3]	4%	2%
Digestive System		
Nausea	35%	12%
Constipation	10%	4%
Anorexia	8%	2%
Vomiting	5%	3%
Nervous System		
Dizziness	16%	11%
Dry Mouth	16%	6%
Insomnia	15%	10%
Somnolence	14%	8%
Nervousness	6%	4%
Libido Decreased	4%	2%
Tremor	4%	<1%
Abnormal Dreams[4]	3%	2%
Hypertonia	3%	2%
Paresthesia	2%	1%
Respiratory System		
Yawn	3%	<1%
Skin		
Sweating	10%	3%
Special Senses		
Abnormal Vision[5]	5%	<1%
Urogenital System		
Abnormal Ejaculation[6,7]	11%	<1%
Impotence[7]	5%	<1%
Orgasmic Dysfunction (female)[8,9]	2%	0%

[1]Adverse events for which the Effexor XR reporting rate was less than or equal to the placebo rate are not included. These events are: abdominal pain, accidental injury, anxiety, back pain, diarrhea, dysmenorrhea, dyspepsia, flu syndrome, headache, infection, myalgia, pain, palpitation, pharyngitis, rhinitis, tinnitus, and urinary frequency.
[2]<1% means greater than zero but less than 1%.
[3]Mostly "hot flashes."
[4]Mostly "vivid dreams," "nightmares," and "increased dreaming."
[5]Mostly "blurred vision" and "difficulty focusing eyes."
[6]Includes "delayed ejaculation" and "anorgasmia."
[7]Percentage based on the number of males (Effexor XR = 525, placebo = 220).
[8]Includes "delayed orgasm," "abnormal orgasm," and "anorgasmia."
[9]Percentage based on the number of females (Effexor XR = 856, placebo = 335).

Table 5
Treatment-Emergent Adverse Event Incidence in Short-Term Placebo-Controlled Effexor XR Clinical Trials in Social Anxiety Disorder Patients[1,2]

Body System Preferred Term	**% Reporting Event** **Effexor XR** (n=277)	**Placebo** (n=274)
Body as a Whole		
Headache	34%	33%
Asthenia	17%	8%
Flu Syndrome	6%	5%
Accidental Injury	5%	3%
Abdominal Pain	4%	3%
Cardiovascular System		
Hypertension	5%	4%
Vasodilatation[3]	3%	1%
Palpitation	3%	1%
Digestive System		
Nausea	29%	9%
Anorexia[4]	20%	1%
Constipation	8%	4%
Diarrhea	6%	5%
Vomiting	3%	2%
Eructation	2%	0%
Metabolic/Nutritional		
Weight Loss	4%	0%
Nervous System		
Insomnia	23%	7%
Dry Mouth	17%	4%
Dizziness	16%	8%
Somnolence	16%	8%
Nervousness	11%	3%
Libido Decreased	9%	<1%
Anxiety	5%	3%
Agitation	4%	1%
Tremor	4%	<1%
Abnormal Dreams[5]	4%	<1%
Paresthesia	3%	<1%
Twitching	2%	0%
Respiratory System		
Yawn	5%	<1%
Sinusitis	2%	1%
Skin		
Sweating	13%	2%
Special Senses		
Abnormal Vision[6]	6%	3%
Urogenital System		
Abnormal Ejaculation[7,8]	16%	1%
Impotence[8]	10%	1%
Orgasmic Dysfunction[9,10]	8%	0%

[1] Adverse events for which the Effexor XR reporting rate was less than or equal to the placebo rate are not included. These events are: back pain, depression, dysmenorrhea, dyspepsia, infection, myalgia, pain, pharyngitis, rash, rhinitis, and upper respiratory infection.
[2]<1% means greater than zero but less than 1%.
[3]Mostly "hot flashes."
[4]Mostly "decreased appetite" and "loss of appetite."
[5]Mostly "vivid dreams," "nightmares," and "increased dreaming."
[6]Mostly "blurred vision."
[7] Includes "delayed ejaculation" and "anorgasmia."
[8] Percentage based on the number of males (Effexor XR = 158, placebo = 153).
[9]Includes "abnormal orgasm" and "anorgasmia."
[10]Percentage based on the number of females (Effexor XR = 119, placebo = 121).

Vital Sign Changes

Effexor XR (venlafaxine hydrochloride) extended-release capsules treatment for up to 12 weeks in premarketing placebo-controlled major depressive disorder trials was associated with a mean final on-therapy increase in pulse rate of approximately 2 beats per minute, compared with 1 beat per minute for placebo. Effexor XR treatment for up to 8 weeks in premarketing placebo-controlled GAD trials was associated with a mean final on-therapy increase in pulse rate of approximately 2 beats per minute, compared with less than 1 beat per minute for placebo. Effexor XR treatment for up to 12 weeks in premarketing placebo-controlled Social Anxiety Disorder trials was associated with a mean final on-therapy increase in pulse rate of approximately 4 beats per minute, compared with an increase of 1 beat per minute for placebo. (See the **Sustained Hypertension** section of **WARNINGS** for effects on blood pressure.)

In a flexible-dose study, with Effexor doses in the range of 200 to 375 mg/day and mean dose greater than 300 mg/day, the mean pulse was increased by about 2 beats per minute compared with a decrease of about 1 beat per minute for placebo.

Laboratory Changes

Effexor XR (venlafaxine hydrochloride) extended-release capsules treatment for up to 12 weeks in premarketing placebo-controlled trials for major depressive disorder was associated with a mean final on-therapy increase in serum cholesterol concentration of approximately 1.5 mg/dL compared with a mean final decrease of 7.4 mg/dL for placebo. Effexor XR treatment for up to 8 weeks and up to 6 months in premarketing placebo-controlled GAD trials was associated with mean final on-therapy increases in serum cholesterol concentration of approximately 1.0 mg/dL and 2.3 mg/dL, respectively while placebo subjects experienced mean final decreases of 4.9 mg/dL and 7.7 mg/dL, respectively. Effexor XR treatment for up to 12 weeks in premarketing placebo-controlled Social Anxiety Disorder trials was associated with mean final on-therapy increases in serum cholesterol concentration of approximately 11.4 mg/dL compared with a mean final decrease of 2.2 mg/dL for placebo. Patients treated with Effexor tablets (the immediate-release form of venlafaxine) for at least 3 months in placebo-controlled 12-month extension trials had a mean final on-therapy increase in total cholesterol of 9.1 mg/dL compared with a decrease of 7.1 mg/dL among placebo-treated patients. This increase was duration dependent over the study period and tended to be greater with higher doses. Clinically relevant increases in serum cholesterol, defined as 1) a final on-therapy increase in serum cholesterol ≥50 mg/dL from baseline and to a value ≥261 mg/dL, or 2) an average on-therapy increase in serum cholesterol ≥50 mg/dL from baseline and to a value ≥261 mg/dL, were recorded in 5.3% of venlafaxine-treated patients and 0.0% of placebo-treated patients (see **PRECAUTIONS-General**-*Serum Cholesterol Elevation*).

ECG Changes

In a flexible-dose study, with Effexor doses in the range of 200 to 375 mg/day and mean dose greater than 300 mg/day, the mean change in heart rate was 8.5 beats per minute compared with 1.7 beats per minute for placebo.

(See the *Use in Patients with Concomitant Illness* section of **PRECAUTIONS**.)

Other Adverse Events Observed During the Premarketing Evaluation of Effexor and Effexor XR

During its premarketing assessment, multiple doses of Effexor XR were administered to 705 patients in Phase 3 major depressive disorder studies and Effexor was administered to 96 patients. During its premarketing assessment, multiple doses of Effexor XR were also administered to 1381 patients in Phase 3 GAD studies and 277 patients in Phase 3 Social Anxiety Disorder studies. In addition, in premarketing assessment of Effexor, multiple doses were administered to 2897 patients in Phase 2 to Phase 3 studies for ma-

Continued on next page

Effexor XR—Cont.

jor depressive disorder. The conditions and duration of exposure to venlafaxine in both development programs varied greatly, and included (in overlapping categories) open and double-blind studies, uncontrolled and controlled studies, inpatient (Effexor only) and outpatient studies, fixed-dose, and titration studies. Untoward events associated with this exposure were recorded by clinical investigators using terminology of their own choosing. Consequently, it is not possible to provide a meaningful estimate of the proportion of individuals experiencing adverse events without first grouping similar types of untoward events into a smaller number of standardized event categories.

In the tabulations that follow, reported adverse events were classified using a standard COSTART-based Dictionary terminology. The frequencies presented, therefore, represent the proportion of the 5356 patients exposed to multiple doses of either formulation of venlafaxine who experienced an event of the type cited on at least one occasion while receiving venlafaxine. All reported events are included except those already listed in Tables 3, 4, and 5 and those events for which a drug cause was remote. If the COSTART term for an event was so general as to be uninformative, it was replaced with a more informative term. It is important to emphasize that, although the events reported occurred during treatment with venlafaxine, they were not necessarily caused by it.

Events are further categorized by body system and listed in order of decreasing frequency using the following definitions: **frequent** adverse events are defined as those occurring on one or more occasions in at least 1/100 patients; **infrequent** adverse events are those occurring in 1/100 to 1/1000 patients; **rare** events are those occurring in fewer than 1/1000 patients.

Body as a whole—**Frequent:** chest pain substernal, chills, fever, neck pain; **Infrequent:** face edema, intentional injury, malaise, moniliasis, neck rigidity, pelvic pain, photosensitivity reaction, suicide attempt, withdrawal syndrome; **Rare:** appendicitis, bacteremia, carcinoma, cellulitis.

Cardiovascular system—**Frequent:** migraine, postural hypotension, tachycardia; **Infrequent:** angina pectoris, arrhythmia, extrasystoles, hypotension, peripheral vascular disorder (mainly cold feet and/or cold hands), syncope, thrombophlebitis; **Rare:** aortic aneurysm, arteritis, first-degree atrioventricular block, bigeminy, bradycardia, bundle branch block, capillary fragility, cerebral ischemia, coronary artery disease, congestive heart failure, heart arrest, cardiovascular disorder (mitral valve and circulatory disturbance), mucocutaneous hemorrhage, myocardial infarct, pallor.

Digestive system—**Frequent:** increased appetite; **Infrequent:** bruxism, colitis, dysphagia, tongue edema, esophagitis, gastritis, gastroenteritis, gastrointestinal ulcer, gingivitis, glossitis, rectal hemorrhage, hemorrhoids, melena, oral moniliasis, stomatitis, mouth ulceration; **Rare:** cheilitis, cholecystitis, cholelithiasis, esophageal spasms, duodenitis, hematemesis, gastrointestinal hemorrhage, gum hemorrhage, hepatitis, ileitis, jaundice, intestinal obstruction, parotitis, periodontitis, proctitis, increased salivation, soft stools, tongue discoloration.

Endocrine system—**Rare:** goiter, hyperthyroidism, hypothyroidism, thyroid nodule, thyroiditis.

Hemic and lymphatic system—**Frequent:** ecchymosis; **Infrequent:** anemia, leukocytosis, leukopenia, lymphadenopathy, thrombocythemia, thrombocytopenia; **Rare:** basophilia, bleeding time increased, cyanosis, eosinophilia, lymphocytosis, multiple myeloma, purpura.

Metabolic and nutritional—**Frequent:** edema, weight gain; **Infrequent:** alkaline phosphatase increased, dehydration, hypercholesteremia, hyperglycemia, hyperlipemia, hypokalemia, SGOT (AST) increased, SGPT (ALT) increased, thirst; **Rare:** alcohol intolerance, bilirubinemia, BUN increased, creatinine increased, diabetes mellitus, glycosuria, gout, healing abnormal, hemochromatosis, hypercalcinuria, hyperkalemia, hyperphosphatemia, hyperuricemia, hypocholesteremia, hypoglycemia, hyponatremia, hypophosphatemia, hypoproteinemia, uremia.

Musculoskeletal system—**Frequent:** arthralgia; **Infrequent:** arthritis, arthrosis, bone pain, bone spurs, bursitis, leg cramps, myasthenia, tenosynovitis; **Rare:** pathological fracture, myopathy, osteoporosis, osteosclerosis, plantar fasciitis, rheumatoid arthritis, tendon rupture.

Nervous system—**Frequent:** amnesia, confusion, depersonalization, hypesthesia, thinking abnormal, trismus, vertigo; **Infrequent:** akathisia, apathy, ataxia, circumoral paresthesia, CNS stimulation, emotional lability, euphoria, hallucinations, hostility, hyperesthesia, hyperkinesia, hypotonia, incoordination, libido increased, manic reaction, myoclonus, neuralgia, neuropathy, psychosis, seizure, abnormal speech, stupor; **Rare:** akinesia, alcohol abuse, aphasia, bradykinesia, buccoglossal syndrome, cerebrovascular accident, feeling drunk, loss of consciousness, delusions, dementia, dystonia, facial paralysis, abnormal gait, Guillain-Barre Syndrome, hyperchlorhydria, hypokinesia, impulse control difficulties, neuritis, nystagmus, paranoid reaction, paresis, psychotic depression, reflexes decreased, reflexes increased, suicidal ideation, torticollis.

Respiratory system—**Frequent:** cough increased, dyspnea; **Infrequent:** asthma, chest congestion, epistaxis, hyperventilation, laryngismus, laryngitis, pneumonia, voice alteration; **Rare:** atelectasis, hemoptysis, hypoventilation, hypoxia, larynx edema, pleurisy, pulmonary embolus, sleep apnea.

Skin and appendages—**Frequent:** pruritus; **Infrequent:** acne, alopecia, brittle nails, contact dermatitis, dry skin, eczema, skin hypertrophy, maculopapular rash, psoriasis, urticaria; **Rare:** erythema nodosum, exfoliative dermatitis, lichenoid dermatitis, hair discoloration, skin discoloration, furunculosis, hirsutism, leukoderma, petechial rash, pustular rash, vesiculobullous rash, seborrhea, skin atrophy, skin striae.

Special senses—**Frequent:** abnormality of accommodation, mydriasis, taste perversion; **Infrequent:** cataract, conjunctivitis, corneal lesion, diplopia, dry eyes, eye pain, hyperacusis, otitis media, parosmia, photophobia, taste loss, visual field defect; **Rare:** blepharitis, chromatopsia, conjunctival edema, deafness, exophthalmos, glaucoma, retinal hemorrhage, subconjunctival hemorrhage, keratitis, labyrinthitis, miosis, papilledema, decreased pupillary reflex, otitis externa, scleritis, uveitis.

Urogenital system—**Frequent:** metrorrhagia,* prostatic disorder (prostatitis and enlarged prostate),* urination impaired, vaginitis*; **Infrequent:** albuminuria, amenorrhea,* cystitis, dysuria, hematuria, leukorrhea,* menorrhagia,* nocturia, bladder pain, breast pain, polyuria, pyuria, urinary incontinence, urinary retention, urinary urgency, vaginal hemorrhage*; **Rare:** abortion,* anuria, breast discharge, breast engorgement, balanitis,* breast enlargement, endometriosis,* female lactation,* fibrocystic breast, calcium crystalluria, cervicitis,* orchitis,* ovarian cyst,* prolonged erection,* gynecomastia (male),* hypomenorrhea,* kidney calculus, kidney pain, kidney function abnormal, mastitis, menopause,* pyelonephritis, oliguria, salpingitis,* urolithiasis, uterine hemorrhage,* uterine spasm,* vaginal dryness.*

*Based on the number of men and women as appropriate.

Postmarketing Reports

Voluntary reports of other adverse events temporally associated with the use of venlafaxine that have been received since market introduction and that may have no causal relationship with the use of venlafaxine include the following: agranulocytosis, anaphylaxis, aplastic anemia, catatonia, congenital anomalies, CPK increased, deep vein thrombophlebitis, delirium, EKG abnormalities such as QT prolongation; cardiac arrhythmias including atrial fibrillation, supraventricular tachycardia, ventricular extrasystoles, and rare reports of ventricular fibrillation and ventricular tachycardia, including torsade de pointes; epidermal necrosis/Stevens-Johnson Syndrome, erythema multiforme, extrapyramidal symptoms (including dyskinesia and tardive dyskinesia), hemorrhage (including eye and gastrointestinal bleeding), hepatic events (including GGT elevation; abnormalities of unspecified liver function tests; liver damage, necrosis, or failure; and fatty liver), involuntary movements, LDH increased, neuroleptic malignant syndrome-like events (including a case of a 10-year-old who may have been taking methylphenidate, was treated and recovered), neutropenia, night sweats, pancreatitis, pancytopenia, panic, prolactin increased, pulmonary eosinophilia, renal failure, rhabdomyolysis, serotonin syndrome, shock-like electrical sensations or tinnitus (in some cases, subsequent to the discontinuation of venlafaxine or tapering of dose), and syndrome of inappropriate antidiuretic hormone secretion (usually in the elderly).

There have been reports of elevated clozapine levels that were temporally associated with adverse events, including seizures, following the addition of venlafaxine. There have been reports of increases in prothrombin time, partial thromboplastin time, or INR when venlafaxine was given to patients receiving warfarin therapy.

DRUG ABUSE AND DEPENDENCE

Controlled Substance Class

Effexor XR (venlafaxine hydrochloride) extended-release capsules is not a controlled substance.

Physical and Psychological Dependence

In vitro studies revealed that venlafaxine has virtually no affinity for opiate, benzodiazepine, phencyclidine (PCP), or N-methyl-D-aspartic acid (NMDA) receptors.

Venlafaxine was not found to have any significant CNS stimulant activity in rodents. In primate drug discrimination studies, venlafaxine showed no significant stimulant or depressant abuse liability.

Discontinuation effects have been reported in patients receiving venlafaxine (see **DOSAGE AND ADMINISTRATION**).

While venlafaxine has not been systematically studied in clinical trials for its potential for abuse, there was no indication of drug-seeking behavior in the clinical trials. However, it is not possible to predict on the basis of premarketing experience the extent to which a CNS active drug will be misused, diverted, and/or abused once marketed. Consequently, physicians should carefully evaluate patients for history of drug abuse and follow such patients closely, observing them for signs of misuse or abuse of venlafaxine (eg, development of tolerance, incrementation of dose, drug-seeking behavior).

OVERDOSAGE

Human Experience

Among the patients included in the premarketing evaluation of Effexor XR, there were 2 reports of acute overdosage with Effexor XR in major depressive disorder trials, either alone or in combination with other drugs. One patient took a combination of 6 g of Effexor XR and 2.5 mg of lorazepam. This patient was hospitalized, treated symptomatically, and recovered without any untoward effects. The other patient took 2.85 g of Effexor XR. This patient reported paresthesia of all four limbs but recovered without sequelae.

There were 2 reports of acute overdose with Effexor XR in GAD trials. One patient took a combination of 0.75 g of Effexor XR and 200 mg of paroxetine and 50 mg of zolpidem. This patient was described as being alert, able to communicate, and a little sleepy. This patient was hospitalized, treated with activated charcoal, and recovered without any untoward effects. The other patient took 1.2 g of Effexor XR. This patient recovered and no other specific problems were found. The patient had moderate dizziness, nausea, numb hands and feet, and hot-cold spells 5 days after the overdose. These symptoms resolved over the next week.

There were no reports of acute overdose with Effexor XR in Social Anxiety Disorder trials.

Among the patients included in the premarketing evaluation with Effexor, there were 14 reports of acute overdose with venlafaxine, either alone or in combination with other drugs and/or alcohol. The majority of the reports involved ingestion in which the total dose of venlafaxine taken was estimated to be no more than several-fold higher than the usual therapeutic dose. The 3 patients who took the highest doses were estimated to have ingested approximately 6.75 g, 2.75 g, and 2.5 g. The resultant peak plasma levels of venlafaxine for the latter 2 patients were 6.24 and 2.35 µg/mL, respectively, and the peak plasma levels of O-desmethylvenlafaxine were 3.37 and 1.30 µg/mL, respectively. Plasma venlafaxine levels were not obtained for the patient who ingested 6.75 g of venlafaxine. All 14 patients recovered without sequelae. Most patients reported no symptoms. Among the remaining patients, somnolence was the most commonly reported symptom. The patient who ingested 2.75 g of venlafaxine was observed to have 2 generalized convulsions and a prolongation of QTc to 500 msec, compared with 405 msec at baseline. Mild sinus tachycardia was reported in 2 of the other patients.

In postmarketing experience, overdose with venlafaxine has occurred predominantly in combination with alcohol and/or other drugs. Electrocardiogram changes (eg, prolongation of QT interval, bundle branch block, QRS prolongation), sinus and ventricular tachycardia, bradycardia, hypotension, altered level of consciousness (ranging from somnolence to coma), rhabdomyolysis, seizures, vertigo, and death have been reported.

Management of Overdosage

Treatment should consist of those general measures employed in the management of overdosage with any antidepressant.

Ensure an adequate airway, oxygenation, and ventilation. Monitor cardiac rhythm and vital signs. General supportive and symptomatic measures are also recommended. Induction of emesis is not recommended. Gastric lavage with a large bore orogastric tube with appropriate airway protection, if needed, may be indicated if performed soon after ingestion or in symptomatic patients.

Activated charcoal should be administered. Due to the large volume of distribution of this drug, forced diuresis, dialysis, hemoperfusion, and exchange transfusion are unlikely to be of benefit. No specific antidotes for venlafaxine are known. In managing overdosage, consider the possibility of multiple drug involvement. The physician should consider contacting a poison control center for additional information on the treatment of any overdose. Telephone numbers for certified poison control centers are listed in the *Physicians' Desk Reference® (PDR)*.

DOSAGE AND ADMINISTRATION

Effexor XR should be administered in a single dose with food either in the morning or in the evening at approximately the same time each day. Each capsule should be swallowed whole with fluid and not divided, crushed, chewed, or placed in water, or it may be administered by carefully opening the capsule and sprinkling the entire contents on a spoonful of applesauce. This drug/food mixture should be swallowed immediately without chewing and followed with a glass of water to ensure complete swallowing of the pellets.

Initial Treatment

Major Depressive Disorder

For most patients, the recommended starting dose for Effexor XR is 75 mg/day, administered in a single dose. In the clinical trials establishing the efficacy of Effexor XR in moderately depressed outpatients, the initial dose of venlafaxine was 75 mg/day. For some patients, it may be desirable to start at 37.5 mg/day for 4 to 7 days, to allow new patients to adjust to the medication before increasing to 75 mg/day. While the relationship between dose and antidepressant response for Effexor XR has not been adequately explored, patients not responding to the initial 75 mg/day dose may benefit from dose increases to a maximum of approximately 225 mg/day. Dose increases should be in increments of up to 75 mg/day, as needed, and should be made at intervals of not less than 4 days, since steady state plasma levels of venlafaxine and its major metabolites are achieved in most patients by day 4. In the clinical trials establishing efficacy, upward titration was permitted at intervals of 2 weeks or more; the average doses were about 140 to 180 mg/day (see **Clinical Trials** under **CLINICAL PHARMACOLOGY**).

It should be noted that, while the maximum recommended dose for moderately depressed outpatients is also 225 mg/day for Effexor (the immediate release form of venlafaxine), more severely depressed inpatients in one study of the development program for that product responded to a mean dose of 350 mg/day (range of 150 to 375 mg/day). Whether or not higher doses of Effexor XR are needed for more severely depressed patients is unknown; however, the experience with Effexor XR doses higher than 225 mg/day is very limited. (See **PRECAUTIONS-General**-*Use in Patients with Concomitant Illness*.)

Generalized Anxiety Disorder

For most patients, the recommended starting dose for Effexor XR is 75 mg/day, administered in a single dose. In clinical trials establishing the efficacy of Effexor XR in outpatients with Generalized Anxiety Disorder (GAD), the initial dose of venlafaxine was 75 mg/day. For some patients, it may be desirable to start at 37.5 mg/day for 4 to 7 days, to allow new patients to adjust to the medication before increasing to 75 mg/day. Although a dose-response relationship for effectiveness in GAD was not clearly established in fixed-dose studies, certain patients not responding to the initial 75 mg/day dose may benefit from dose increases to a maximum of approximately 225 mg/day. Dose increases should be in increments of up to 75 mg/day, as needed, and should be made at intervals of not less than 4 days. (See the *Use in Patients with Concomitant Illness* section of **PRECAUTIONS**.)

Social Anxiety Disorder (Social Phobia)

For most patients, the recommended starting dose for Effexor XR is 75 mg/day, administered in a single dose. In clinical trials establishing the efficacy of Effexor XR in outpatients with Social Anxiety Disorder, the initial dose of Effexor XR was 75 mg/day and the maximum dose was 225 mg/day. For some patients, it may be desirable to start at 37.5 mg/day for 4 to 7 days, to allow new patients to adjust to the medication before increasing to 75 mg/day. Although a dose-response relationship for effectiveness in patients with Social Anxiety Disorder was not clearly established in fixed-dose studies, certain patients not responding to the initial 75 mg/day dose may benefit from dose increases to a maximum of approximately 225 mg/day. Dose increases should be in increments of up to 75 mg/day, as needed, and should be made at intervals of not less than 4 days. (See the *Use in Patients with Concomitant Illness* section of **PRECAUTIONS**.)

Switching Patients from Effexor Tablets

Depressed patients who are currently being treated at a therapeutic dose with Effexor may be switched to Effexor XR at the nearest equivalent dose (mg/day), eg, 37.5 mg venlafaxine two-times-a-day to 75 mg Effexor XR once daily. However, individual dosage adjustments may be necessary.

Special Populations

Treatment of Pregnant Women During the Third Trimester

Neonates exposed to Effexor XR, other SNRIs, or SSRIs, late in the third trimester have developed complications requiring prolonged hospitalization, respiratory support, and tube feeding (see **PRECAUTIONS**). When treating pregnant women with Effexor XR during the third trimester, the physician should carefully consider the potential risks and benefits of treatment. The physician may consider tapering Effexor XR in the third trimester.

Patients with Hepatic Impairment

Given the decrease in clearance and increase in elimination half-life for both venlafaxine and ODV that is observed in patients with hepatic cirrhosis compared with normal subjects (see **CLINICAL PHARMACOLOGY**), it is recommended that the starting dose be reduced by 50% in patients with moderate hepatic impairment. Because there was much individual variability in clearance between patients with cirrhosis, individualization of dosage may be desirable in some patients.

Patients with Renal Impairment

Given the decrease in clearance for venlafaxine and the increase in elimination half-life for both venlafaxine and ODV that is observed in patients with renal impairment (GFR = 10 to 70 mL/min) compared with normal subjects (see **CLINICAL PHARMACOLOGY**), it is recommended that the total daily dose be reduced by 25% to 50%. In patients undergoing hemodialysis, it is recommended that the total daily dose be reduced by 50% and that the dose be withheld until the dialysis treatment is completed (4 hrs). Because there was much individual variability in clearance between patients with renal impairment, individualization of dosage may be desirable in some patients.

Elderly Patients

No dose adjustment is recommended for elderly patients solely on the basis of age. As with any drug for the treatment of major depressive disorder, Generalized Anxiety Disorder, or Social Anxiety Disorder, however, caution should be exercised in treating the elderly. When individualizing the dosage, extra care should be taken when increasing the dose.

Maintenance Treatment

There is no body of evidence available from controlled trials to indicate how long patients with major depressive disorder, Generalized Anxiety Disorder, or Social Anxiety Disorder should be treated with Effexor XR.

It is generally agreed that acute episodes of major depressive disorder require several months or longer of sustained pharmacological therapy beyond response to the acute episode. In one study, in which patients responding during 8 weeks of acute treatment with Effexor XR were assigned randomly to placebo or to the same dose of Effexor XR (75, 150, or 225 mg/day, qAM) during 26 weeks of maintenance treatment as they had received during the acute stabilization phase, longer-term efficacy was demonstrated. A second longer-term study has demonstrated the efficacy of Effexor in maintaining a response in patients with recurrent major depressive disorder who had responded and continued to be improved during an initial 26 weeks of treatment and were then randomly assigned to placebo or Effexor for periods of up to 52 weeks on the same dose (100 to 200 mg/day, on a b.i.d. schedule) (see **Clinical Trials** under **CLINICAL PHARMACOLOGY**). Based on these limited data, it is not known whether or not the dose of Effexor/Effexor XR needed for maintenance treatment is identical to the dose needed to achieve an initial response. Patients should be periodically reassessed to determine the need for maintenance treatment and the appropriate dose for such treatment.

In patients with Generalized Anxiety Disorder, Effexor XR has been shown to be effective in 6-month clinical trials. The need for continuing medication in patients with GAD who improve with Effexor XR treatment should be periodically reassessed.

In patients with Social Anxiety Disorder, there are no efficacy data beyond 12 weeks of treatment with Effexor XR. The need for continuing medication in patients with Social Anxiety Disorder who improve with Effexor XR treatment should be periodically reassessed.

Discontinuing Effexor XR

Symptoms associated with discontinuation of Effexor XR, other SNRIs, and SSRIs, have been reported (see **PRECAUTIONS**). Patients should be monitored for these symptoms when discontinuing treatment. A gradual reduction in the dose rather than abrupt cessation is recommended whenever possible. If intolerable symptoms occur following a decrease in the dose or upon discontinuation of treatment, then resuming the previously prescribed dose may be considered. Subsequently, the physician may continue decreasing the dose but at a more gradual rate. In clinical trials with Effexor XR, tapering was achieved by reducing the daily dose by 75 mg at 1 week intervals. Individualization of tapering may be necessary.

Switching Patients To or From a Monoamine Oxidase Inhibitor

At least 14 days should elapse between discontinuation of an MAOI and initiation of therapy with Effexor XR. In addition, at least 7 days should be allowed after stopping Effexor XR before starting an MAOI (see **CONTRAINDICATIONS** and **WARNINGS**).

HOW SUPPLIED

Effexor® XR (venlafaxine hydrochloride) extended-release capsules are available as follows:

37.5 mg, grey cap/peach body with **W** and "Effexor XR" on the cap and "37.5" on the body.

NDC 0008-0837-01, bottle of 100 capsules.

NDC 0008-0837-03, carton of 10 Redipak® blister strips of 10 capsules each.

Store at controlled room temperature, 20°C to 25°C (68°F to 77°F).

75 mg, peach cap and body with **W** and "Effexor XR" on the cap and "75" on the body.

NDC 0008-0833-01, bottle of 100 capsules.

NDC 0008-0833-03, carton of 10 Redipak® blister strips of 10 capsules each.

Store at controlled room temperature, 20°C to 25°C (68°F to 77°F).

150 mg, dark orange cap and body with **W** and "Effexor XR" on the cap and "150" on the body.

NDC 0008-0836-01, bottle of 100 capsules.

NDC 0008-0836-03, carton of 10 Redipak® blister strips of 10 capsules each.

Store at controlled room temperature, 20°C to 25°C (68°F to 77°F).

The appearance of these capsules is a trademark of Wyeth Pharmaceuticals.

Wyeth®

Wyeth Pharmaceuticals Inc. W10404C010
Philadelphia, PA 19101 ET01
Rev 05/04

Shown in Product Identification Guide, page 336

HibTITER® ℞

[hĭb-tī-tər]

HAEMOPHILUS b CONJUGATE VACCINE

(Diphtheria CRM_{197} Protein Conjugate)

℞ only

This product's label may have been revised after this insert was used in production. For further product information and current package insert, please visit www.wyeth.com or call our medical communications department toll-free at 1-800-934-5556.

DESCRIPTION

Haemophilus b Conjugate Vaccine (Diphtheria CRM_{197} Protein Conjugate) HibTITER is a sterile solution of a conjugate of oligosaccharides of the capsular antigen of *Haemophilus influenzae* type b (Haemophilus b) and diphtheria CRM_{197} protein (CRM_{197}) dissolved in 0.9% sodium chloride. The oligosaccharides are derived from highly purified capsular polysaccharide, polyribosylribitol phosphate, isolated from Haemophilus b strain Eagan grown in a chemically defined medium (a mixture of mineral salts, amino acids, and cofactors). The oligosaccharides are purified and sized by diafiltrations through a series of ultrafiltration membranes, and coupled by reductive amination directly to highly purified CRM_{197}.[1,2] CRM_{197} is a nontoxic variant of diphtheria toxin isolated from cultures of *Corynebacterium diphtheriae* C7 (β197) grown in a casamino acids and yeast extract-based medium that is ultrafiltered before use. CRM_{197} is purified through ultrafiltration, ammonium sulfate precipitation, and ion-exchange chromatography to high purity. The conjugate is purified to remove unreacted protein, oligosaccharides, and reagents; sterilized by filtration; and filled into vials. HibTITER is intended for intramuscular use.

The vaccine is a clear, colorless solution. Each single dose of 0.5 mL is formulated to contain 10 µg of purified Haemophilus b saccharide and approximately 25 µg of CRM_{197} protein. The potency of HibTITER is determined by chemical assay for polyribosylribitol.

CLINICAL PHARMACOLOGY

For several decades *Haemophilus influenzae* type b (Haemophilus b) was the most common cause of invasive bacterial disease, including meningitis, in young children in the United States. Although nonencapsulated *H. influenzae* are common and six capsular polysaccharide types are known, strains with the type b capsule caused most of the invasive Haemophilus diseases.[3]

Haemophilus b diseases occurred primarily in children under 5 years of age prior to immunization with *Haemophilus influenzae* type b vaccines. In the US, the cumulative risk of developing invasive Haemophilus b disease during the first 5 years of life was estimated to be about 1 in 200. Approximately 60% of cases were meningitis. Cellulitis, epiglottitis, pericarditis, pneumonia, sepsis, or septic arthritis made up the remaining 40%. An estimated 12,000 cases of Haemophilus b meningitis occurred annually prior to the routine use of conjugate vaccines in toddlers.[3,4] The mortality rate can be 5%, and neurologic sequelae have been observed in up to 38% of survivors.[5]

The incidence of invasive Haemophilus b disease peaks between 6 months and 1 year of age, and approximately 55% of disease occurs between 6 and 18 months of age.[3] Interpersonal transmission of Haemophilus b occurs and risk of invasive disease is increased in children younger than 4 years of age who are exposed in the household to a primary case of disease. Clusters of cases in children in day care have been reported and recent studies suggest that the rate of secondary cases may also be increased among children exposed to a primary case in the daycare setting.[3,6]

The incidence of invasive Haemophilus b disease is increased in certain children, such as those who are native Americans, black, or from lower socioeconomic status, and those with medical conditions such as asplenia, sickle cell disease, malignancies associated with immunosuppression, and antibody deficiency syndromes.[3,4,6]

The protective activity of antibody to Haemophilus b polysaccharide was demonstrated by passive antibody studies in animals and in children with agammaglobulinemia or with Haemophilus b disease[7] and confirmed with the efficacy study of Haemophilus b polysaccharide (HbPs) vaccine.[8] Data from passive antibody studies indicate that a preexisting titer of antibody to HbPs of 0.15 µg/mL correlates with protection.[9] Data from a Finnish field trial in children 18 to 71 months of age indicate that a titer of > 1.0 µg/mL 3 weeks after vaccination is associated with long-term protection.[10,11]

Linkage of Haemophilus b saccharides to a protein such as CRM_{197} converts the saccharide (HbO) to a T-dependent (HbOC) antigen, and results in an enhanced antibody response to the saccharide in young infants that primes for an anamnestic response and is predominantly of the IgG class.[12] Laboratory evidence indicates that the native state of the CRM_{197} protein and the use of oligosaccharides in the formulation of HibTITER enhances its immunogenicity.[13-15]

Prior to licensure, the immunogenicity of HibTITER was evaluated in US infants and children.[15] Infants 1 to 6 months of age at first immunization received three doses at approximately 2-month intervals.[16] Children 7 to 11 and 12 to 14 months of age received 2 doses at the same interval.[15] Children 15 to 23 months of age received a single dose.[17] HibTITER was highly immunogenic in all age groups studied, with 97% to 100% of 1,232 infants attaining titers of ≥ 1 µg/mL and 92% to 100% for bactericidal activity.[15-17]

Long-term persistence of the antibody response was observed. More than 80% of 235 infants who received three doses of vaccine had an anti-HbPs antibody level ≥ 1 µg/mL at 2 years of age.[18]

The vaccine generated an immune response characteristic of a protein antigen. IgG anti-HbPs antibodies of IgG_1 subclass predominated and the immune system was primed for a booster response to HibTITER. There is some evidence suggesting natural increases in antibody levels over time after vaccination, most probably the result of contact with Haemophilus type b organisms or cross-reactive antigens.[18] These studies were carried out at a time when significant levels of Haemophilus b disease were still present in the community.

Antibody generated by HibTITER has been found to have high avidity, a measure of the functional affinity of antibody to bind to antigen. High-avidity antibody is more potent than low-avidity antibody in serum bactericidal assays.[19] The contribution to clinical protection is unknown.

Immunogenicity of HibTITER was evaluated in 26 children 22 months to 5 years of age who had not responded to earlier vaccination with Haemophilus b polysaccharide vaccine. One dose of HibTITER was immunogenic in all 26 children and generated titers of ≥ 1 µg/mL in 25 of the 26 infants.[20] HibTITER has been found to be immunogenic in

Continued on next page

HibTITER—Cont.

children with sickle cell disease, a condition that may cause increased susceptibility to Haemophilus b disease.[21] HibTITER has also been shown to be immunogenic in native American infants, such as the group of 50 studied in Alaska who received three doses at 2, 4, and 6 months of age.[20] Antibody levels achieved were comparable to those seen in healthy US infants who received their first dose at 1 to 2 months of age and subsequent doses at 4 to 6 months of age.[15,16,20]

Postlicensure surveillance of immunogenicity was conducted during the distribution of the first 30 million doses of HibTITER and during the time period over which Haemophilus b disease in children has been decreasing significantly in areas of extensive vaccine usage.[20,22-29] After three doses, titers ranged from 2.37 to 8.45 μg/mL with 67% to 94% attaining ≥ 1 μg/mL.[20,24,25]

Persistence of antibody was examined in several cohorts of subjects that received either a selected commercial lot or that were part of the initial efficacy trial in northern California. Geometric mean titers for these cohorts were between 0.51 and 1.96 just prior to boosting at 15 to 18 months. These lots not only induced persistent antibody but also provided effective priming for a booster dose with commercial lots, with postboosting titers greater than 1.0 μg/mL in 80% to 97% of subjects.[20]

HibTITER (HbOC) was shown to be effective in a large-scale controlled clinical trial in a multiethnic population in northern California carried out between February 1988 and June 1990.[30,31] There were no (0) vaccine failures in infants who received three doses of HibTITER and 12 cases of Haemophilus b disease (6 cases of meningitis) in the control group. The estimate of efficacy is 100% ($P = .0002$) with 95% confidence intervals of 68% to 100%. Through the end of 1991, with an additional 49,000 person-years of follow-up, there were still no cases of Haemophilus b disease in fully vaccinated infants less than 2 years of age.[22,23] One case of disease has been reported in a 3 1/2-year-old child who did not receive a booster dose as recommended.

A comparative clinical trial was performed in Finland where approximately 53,000 infants received HibTITER at 4 and 6 months of age and a booster dose at 14 months in a trial conducted from January 1988 through December 1990. Only two children developed Haemophilus b disease after receiving the two-dose primary immunization schedule. One child became ill at 15 months of age and the other at 18 months of age; neither child received the scheduled booster at 14 months of age. No vaccine failure has been reported in children who received the two-dose primary series and the booster dose at 14 months of age. Based on more than 32,000 person-years of follow-up time, the estimate of efficacy is about 95% when compared to historical control groups followed between 1985 and 1988.[20] Historical controls were used since all infants received one of two Haemophilus b conjugate vaccines during the period of the trial.

Evidence of efficacy postlicensure includes significant reductions in Haemophilus b disease that are closely associated with increases in the net doses of Haemophilus b Conjugate Vaccine distributed in the US.[20,22-29] In the northern California Kaiser Permanente there has been a 94% decrease in Haemophilus disease incidence in 1991 for children younger than 18 months of age, compared to 1984-1988, when HibTITER was not available for this age group.[22,23] Furthermore, active surveillance by the Centers for Disease Control and Prevention (CDC) has shown a 71% decrease in Haemophilus b disease in children less than 15 months old, between 1989 and 1991, which corresponds temporally and geographically with increases in net doses of Haemophilus b conjugate vaccine distributed in the US.[26] As with all vaccines, this conjugate vaccine cannot be expected to be 100% effective. There have been rare reports to the Vaccine Adverse Event Reporting System (VAERS) of Haemophilus b disease following full primary immunization.

INDICATIONS AND USAGE

Haemophilus b Conjugate Vaccine (Diphtheria CRM_{197} Protein Conjugate) HibTITER is indicated for the immunization of children 2 months to 71 months of age against invasive diseases caused by *H. influenza* type b.

As with any vaccine, HibTITER may not protect 100% of individuals receiving the vaccine.

The American Academy of Pediatrics (AAP), the Advisory Committee on Immunization Practices (ACIP) and the American Academy of Family Physicians (AAFP) encourage the routine simultaneous administration of *Haemophilus influenzae* type b vaccines with other currently recommended vaccines, but at different sites (see **DRUG INTERACTIONS**).[32,33,34,35]

CONTRAINDICATIONS

Hypersensitivity to any component of the vaccine, including diphtheria toxoid, is a contraindication to the use of HibTITER.

The occurrence of an allergic or anaphylactic reaction following a prior dose of HibTITER is a contraindication to the use of HibTITER.

The decision to administer or delay vaccination because of a current or recent febrile illness depends largely on the severity of the symptoms and their etiology. Although a severe or even moderate febrile illness is sufficient reason to postpone vaccinations, minor illnesses, such as a mild respiratory infection with or without low-grade fever, are not generally contraindications.

WARNINGS

HibTITER WILL NOT PROTECT AGAINST *H. INFLUENZA* OTHER THAN TYPE b STRAINS, NOR WILL HibTITER PROTECT AGAINST OTHER MICROORGANISMS THAT CAUSE MENINGITIS OR SEPTIC DISEASE. AS WITH ANY INTRAMUSCULAR INJECTION, HibTITER SHOULD BE GIVEN WITH CAUTION TO INFANTS OR CHILDREN WITH THROMBOCYTOPENIA OR ANY COAGULATION DISORDER, OR TO THOSE RECEIVING ANTICOAGULANT THERAPY (SEE **DRUG INTERACTIONS**).

ANTIGENURIA HAS BEEN DETECTED FOLLOWING RECEIPT OF HAEMOPHILUS b CONJUGATE VACCINE[36] AND THEREFORE ANTIGEN DETECTION IN URINE MAY NOT HAVE DIAGNOSTIC VALUE IN SUSPECTED HAEMOPHILUS b DISEASE WITHIN 2 WEEKS OF IMMUNIZATION.

The vial stopper contains dry natural rubber that may cause hypersensitivity reactions when handled by or when the product is injected in persons with known or possible latex sensitivity.

PRECAUTIONS

GENERAL

1. CARE IS TO BE TAKEN BY THE HEALTH CARE PROVIDER FOR SAFE AND EFFECTIVE USE OF THIS PRODUCT.
2. PRIOR TO ADMINISTRATION OF ANY DOSE OF HibTITER, THE PARENT OR GUARDIAN SHOULD BE ASKED ABOUT THE PERSONAL HISTORY, FAMILY HISTORY, AND RECENT HEALTH STATUS OF THE VACCINE RECIPIENT. THE HEALTH CARE PROVIDER SHOULD ASCERTAIN PREVIOUS IMMUNIZATION HISTORY, CURRENT HEALTH STATUS, AND OCCURRENCE OF ANY SYMPTOMS AND/OR SIGNS OF AN ADVERSE EVENT AFTER PREVIOUS IMMUNIZATION IN THE CHILD TO BE IMMUNIZED, IN ORDER TO DETERMINE THE EXISTENCE OF ANY CONTRAINDICATION TO IMMUNIZATION WITH HibTITER AND TO ALLOW AN ASSESSMENT OF BENEFITS AND RISKS.
3. BEFORE THE INJECTION OF ANY BIOLOGICAL, THE HEALTH CARE PROVIDER SHOULD TAKE ALL PRECAUTIONS KNOWN FOR THE PREVENTION OF ALLERGIC OR ANY OTHER SIDE REACTIONS. This should include: a review of the patient's history regarding possible sensitivity; the ready availability of epinephrine 1:1,000 and other appropriate agents used for control of immediate allergic reactions; and a knowledge of the recent literature pertaining to use of the biological concerned, including the nature of side effects and adverse reactions that may follow its use.
4. Children with impaired immune responsiveness, whether due to the use of immunosuppressive therapy (including irradiation, corticosteroids, antimetabolites, alkylating agents, and cytotoxic agents), a genetic defect, human immunodeficiency virus (HIV) infection, or other causes, may have reduced antibody response to active immunization procedures.[37,38] Deferral of administration of vaccine may be considered in individuals receiving immunosuppressive therapy.[37] Other groups should receive this vaccine according to the usual recommended schedule.[37-39] (See **DRUG INTERACTIONS**.)
5. This product is not contraindicated based on the presence of human immunodeficiency virus infection.[40]
6. As reported with Haemophilus b polysaccharide vaccine, cases of Haemophilus b disease may occur prior to the onset of the protective effects of the vaccine.[3,41]
7. The vaccine should not be injected intradermally, subcutaneously, or intravenously since the safety and immunogenicity of these routes have not been evaluated. The vaccine should be given intramuscularly.
8. A separate sterile syringe and needle or a sterile disposable unit should be used for each individual patient to prevent transmission of infectious agents from one person to another. Needles should be disposed of properly and should not be recapped.
9. Special care should be taken to prevent injection into a blood vessel.
10. The vaccine is to be administered immediately after being drawn up into a syringe. Single dose 0.5 mL vial contains no preservative. Use one dose per vial; do not re-enter vial. Discard unused portions.

ALTHOUGH SOME ANTIBODY RESPONSE TO DIPHTHERIA TOXIN OCCURS, IMMUNIZATION WITH HibTITER DOES NOT SUBSTITUTE FOR ROUTINE DIPHTHERIA IMMUNIZATION.

The vial stopper contains dry natural rubber that may cause hypersensitivity reactions when handled by or when the product is injected in persons with known or possible latex sensitivity.

INFORMATION FOR PATIENT

PRIOR TO ADMINISTRATION OF HibTITER, HEALTH CARE PERSONNEL SHOULD INFORM THE PARENT, GUARDIAN OR OTHER RESPONSIBLE ADULT, OF THE RECOMMENDED IMMUNIZATION SCHEDULE FOR PROTECTION AGAINST HAEMOPHILUS b DISEASE AND THE BENEFITS AND RISKS TO THE CHILD RECEIVING THIS VACCINE. GUIDANCE SHOULD BE PROVIDED ON MEASURES TO BE TAKEN SHOULD ADVERSE EVENTS OCCUR, SUCH AS, ANTIPYRETIC MEASURES FOR ELEVATED TEMPERATURES AND THE NEED TO REPORT ADVERSE EVENTS TO THE HEALTH CARE PROVIDER. Parents should be provided with vaccine information pamphlets at the time of each vaccination, as stated in the National Childhood Vaccine Injury Act.[42]

PATIENTS, PARENTS, OR GUARDIANS SHOULD BE INSTRUCTED TO REPORT ANY SERIOUS ADVERSE REACTIONS TO THEIR HEALTH CARE PROVIDER.

DRUG INTERACTIONS

Children receiving therapy with immunosuppressive agents (large amounts of corticosteroids, antimetabolites, alkylating agents, cytotoxic agents) may not respond optimally to active immunization.[37,38,39] (See **PRECAUTIONS, GENERAL**.)

As with other intramuscular injections, HibTITER should be given with caution to children on anticoagulant therapy.

No impairment of the antibody response to the individual antigens was demonstrated when HibTITER was given at the same time but at separate sites as DTP plus OPV to children 2 to 20 months of age or MMR to children 15 ± 1 month of age.[20,43,44]

There are no clinical studies where a direct comparison of the immune responses to HibTITER was compared with the concurrent administration of diphtheria and tetanus toxoids and acellular pertussis vaccine (DTaP), hepatitis B vaccine (Hep B), inactivated poliovirus vaccine (IPV), 7-valent Conjugate Vaccine-Diphtheria CRM_{197} Protein (Prevnar), or Varicella vaccine. However, in clinical trials where HibTITER and DTaP or HibTITER, DTaP, IPV, and Hep B vaccines were administered concurrently with or without Prevnar in children at 2, 4, and 6 months of age, the percentage of children achieving Hib antibody levels of ≥0.15 or ≥1.0 μg/mL were similar.[45,46] In one study where children 12-15 months of age were administered a booster dose of HibTITER concurrently with DTaP and Prevnar, some suppression of the Hib antibody response was observed, but over 97% of children achieved titers of ≥1.0 μg/mL.[47,48] However, in another study where a booster dose of HibTITER was administered to children at 12-15 months of age concurrently with or without Prevnar the percentage of children achieving Hib antibody levels of ≥0.15 or ≥1.0 μg/mL was found to be similar.[49,50]

HibTITER and DTaP administered concurrently with and without Prevnar at 2, 4, and 6, and 12-15 months of age did not impair immune responses to the seven Pneumococcal vaccine serotypes in Prevnar.[47,48,51,52]

There are no clinical trials where the local and systemic reactogenicity of HibTITER was directly compared with the concurrent administration of DTaP, Hep B, IPV, Prevnar, or Varicella vaccines.

The American Academy of Pediatrics (AAP), the Advisory Committee on Immunization Practices (ACIP) and the American Academy of Family Physicians (AAFP) encourage routine simultaneous administration of DTaP, IPV, *Haemophilus influenzae* type b vaccine, pneumococcal conjugate vaccine, measles-mumps-rubella (MMR), varicella vaccine and hepatitis B vaccine for children who are the recommended age to receive these vaccines and for whom no specific contraindications exist at the time of the visit, unless, in the judgment of the provider, complete vaccination of the child will not be compromised by administering different vaccines at different visits. Simultaneous administration is particularly important if the child might not return for subsequent vaccinations.[32,33,34,35]

CARCINOGENESIS, MUTAGENESIS, IMPAIRMENT OF FERTILITY

HibTITER has not been evaluated for its carcinogenic, mutagenic potential, or impairment of fertility.

PREGNANCY

REPRODUCTIVE STUDIES— PREGNANCY CATEGORY C

Animal reproduction studies have not been conducted with HibTITER. It is also not known whether HibTITER can cause fetal harm when administered to a pregnant woman or can affect reproduction capability. HibTITER is NOT recommended for use in a pregnant woman.

GERIATRIC USE

This vaccine is NOT recommended for use in adult populations.

PEDIATRIC USE

The safety and effectiveness of HibTITER in children below the age of 6 weeks have not been established.

ADVERSE REACTIONS

Adverse reactions associated with HibTITER have been evaluated in 401 infants who were vaccinated initially at 1 to 6 months of age and were given 1,118 doses independent of DTP vaccine. Observations were made during the day of vaccination and days 1 and 2 postvaccination. A temperature > 38.3°C was recorded at least once during the observation period following 2% of the vaccinations. Local erythema, warmth, or swelling (≥ 2 cm) was observed following 3.3% of vaccinations. The incidence of temperature > 38.3°C was greater during the first postvaccination day than during the day of vaccination or the second postvaccination day. The incidence of local erythema, warmth, or swelling was similar during the day of vaccination and the first postvaccination day; it was lower during the second postvaccination day. All side effects have been infrequent, mild, and transient with no serious sequelae (Table 1). No difference in the rates of these complaints was reported after dose 1, 2, or 3.

[See table 1 at top of next page]

The following complaints were also observed after 1,118 vaccinations with HibTITER: irritability (133), sleepiness (91), prolonged crying [≥4 hours] (38), appetite loss (23), vomiting (9), diarrhea (2), and rash (1).

Additional safety data with HibTITER are available from the efficacy studies conducted in young infants.[30] There were 79,483 doses given to 30,844 infants at approximately 2, 4, and 6 months of age in California, usually at the same time as DTP (but at a separate injection site) and OPV; approximately 100,000 doses have been given to 53,000 infants at 4 and 6 months in Finland at the same time as a combined DTP and inactivated polio (IPV) vaccine (but at a separate injection site). The rate and type of reactions associated with the vaccinations were no different from those seen when DTP or DTP-IPV was administered alone. These included fever, local reactions, rash, and one hyporesponsive episode with a single seizure. The safety of HibTITER was also evaluated in the California study by direct phone questioning of the parents or guardians of 6,887 vaccine recipients. The incidence and type of side effects reported within 24 hours of vaccination were similar to those cited in Table 1. In addition, analysis of emergency room (ER) visits within 30 days and hospitalization within 60 days after receipt of 23,800 doses of HibTITER showed no increase in the rates of any type of ER visit or hospitalization.
Table 2 details the side effects associated with a single vaccination of HibTITER given (without DTP) to infants of 15 to 23 months of age.

TABLE 2
Selected Adverse Reactions* in Children of 15-23 Months of Age Following Vaccination with HibTITER

Adverse Reaction	No. of Subjects	Reaction Within 24 h	% Postvaccination At 48 h
Fever >38.3°C	354	1.4	0.6
Erythema	354	2.0	—
Swelling	354	1.7	—
Tenderness	354	3.7	0.3

*The following complaints were reported after vaccination of these 354 children in the indicated number of children: diarrhea (9), vomiting (5), prolonged crying [>4 hours] (4), and rashes (2).

Similar results have been observed in the analysis of 2,285 subjects of 18 to 60 months of age, vaccinated as part of a postmarketing safety study of HibTITER.[20] These data were collected by telephone survey 24 to 48 hours postvaccination. Additional observations included irritability, restless sleep, and Gl symptoms (diarrhea, vomiting, and loss of appetite) in the group that received HibTITER alone. A cause and effect relationship between these observations and the vaccinations has not been established.

Post Approval Experience

The following adverse reactions have been identified during post approval use of HibTITER. Because these reactions are reported voluntarily from a population of uncertain size, it is not always possible to reliably estimate their frequency or establish a causal relationship to drug exposure. Decisions to include these reactions in labeling are typically based on one or more of the following factors: (1) seriousness of the reaction, (2) frequency of reporting, or (3) strength of causal connection to the vaccine for post marketing surveillance information.

Injection Site Reactions

Injection site reactions including hypersensitivity (including urticaria), induration, inflammation, mass, and skin discoloration.

Systemic Events

Anaphylactoid/anaphylactic reactions (including shock), angioneurotic edema, convulsions,[53] erythema multiforme, facial edema, febrile seizures, Guillain-Barré syndrome,[54] headache, hives (urticaria), hypersensitivity reaction, lethargy, and malaise. Also reported, hypotonia or hyporesponsive-hypotonic-episodes (in many instances pertussis-containing vaccine was coadministered).

Reporting of Adverse Reactions

Any suspected adverse events following immunization should be reported by the healthcare professional to the US Department of Health and Human Services (DHHS). The National Vaccine Injury Compensation Program requires that the manufacturer and lot number of the vaccine administered be recorded by the healthcare professional in the vaccine recipient's permanent medical record (or in a permanent office log or file), along with the date of administration of the vaccine and the name, address, and title of the person administering the vaccine. The DHHS has established the Vaccine Adverse Event Reporting System (VAERS) to accept all reports of suspected adverse events after the administration of any vaccine, including but not limited to the reporting of events required by the National Childhood Vaccine Injury Act of 1986.[42] The VAERS FDA web site is:
http://www.fda.gov/cber/vaers/vaers.htm
The VAERS toll-free number for VAERS forms and information is 800-822-7967.
There have been spontaneous reports of apnea in temporal association with the administration of HibTITER. In most cases HibTITER was administered concomitantly with other vaccines including diphtheria tetanus pertussis vaccine (DTP), diphtheria tetanus acellular pertussis vaccine (DTaP), hepatitis B vaccine, inactivated polio vaccine (IPV), oral polio vaccine (OPV), pneumococcal 7-valent conjugate

TABLE 1
Number of Subjects (Percent) Manifesting Side Effects Associated with HibTITER Administered Independently from DTP* (Infants Vaccinated Initially at 1–6 Months of Age)

	Dose 1 n = 401			Dose 2 n = 383			Dose 3 n = 334		
Symptoms	Same Day As Vacc.	+1 Day	+2 Days	Same Day As Vacc.	+1 Day	+2 Days	Same Day As Vacc.	+1 Day	+2 Days
Temp > 38.3°C	0	2	2	2	3	2	2	6	5
	-	< 1%	< 1%	< 1%	< 1%	< 1%	< 1%	1.8%	1.5%
Redness ≥ 2 cm	1	0	0	1	6	0	5	4	0
	< 1%	-	-	< 1%	1.6%	-	1.5%	1.2%	-
Warmth ≥ 2 cm	1	1	0	2	1	0	1	6	0
	< 1%	< 1%	-	< 1%	< 1%	-	< 1%	1.8%	-
Swelling ≥ 2 cm	5	1	0	2	2	0	1	0	0
	1.2%	< 1%	-	< 1%	< 1%	-	< 1%	-	-

*DTP and HibTITER given 2 weeks apart with DTP having been given first.

vaccine, measles-mumps-rubella (MMR), and/or meningococcal group C conjugate vaccine (not licensed in the US). In addition, in some of the reports existing medical conditions such as prematurity and/or history of apnea were present.

OVERDOSAGE

There have been reports of overdose with HibTITER. Many cases were due to inadvertent coadministration with another Haemophilus b conjugate-containing vaccine. Most individuals were asymptomatic. In general, adverse events reported with overdosage have also been reported with recommended single doses of HibTITER.

DOSAGE AND ADMINISTRATION

HibTITER is for intramuscular use only.

Any parenteral drug product should be inspected visually for particulate matter and/or discoloration prior to administration whenever solution and container permit. If these conditions exist, or if cloudy, HibTITER should not be administered.
Before injection, the skin over the site to be injected should be cleansed with a suitable germicide. After insertion of the needle, aspirate to help avoid inadvertent injection into a blood vessel.
The vaccine should be injected intramuscularly, preferably into the midlateral muscles of the thigh or deltoid, with care to avoid major peripheral nerve trunks. Do not inject in the gluteal area.
The vaccine is to be administered immediately after being drawn up into a syringe. Single dose 0.5 mL vial contains no preservative. Use one dose per vial; do not re-enter vial. Discard unused portions.
HibTITER is indicated for children 2 months to 71 months of age for the prevention of invasive Haemophilus b disease.
For infants 2 to 6 months of age, the immunizing dose is three separate injections of 0.5 mL given at approximately 2-month intervals. Previously unvaccinated infants from 7 through 11 months of age should receive two separate injections approximately 2 months apart. Children from 12 through 14 months of age who have not been vaccinated previously receive one injection. All vaccinated children receive a single booster dose at 15 months of age or older, but not less than 2 months after the previous dose. Previously unvaccinated children 15 to 71 months of age receive a single injection of HibTITER.[32,33] Preterm infants should be vaccinated with HibTITER according to their chronological age, from birth.[32]

Recommended Immunization Schedule

Age at First Immunization (Mo)	No. of Doses	Booster
2–6	3	Yes
7–11	2	Yes
12–14	1	Yes
15 and over	1	No

Interruption of the recommended schedules with a delay between doses does not interfere with the final immunity achieved nor does it necessitate starting the series over again, regardless of the length of time elapsed between doses.[32,33]
Data support that HibTITER may be interchanged with other *Haemophilus influenzae* type b conjugate vaccines for the primary immunization series[55,56]
Each dose of 0.5 mL is formulated to contain 10 µg of purified Haemophilus b saccharide and approximately 25 µg of CRM_{197} protein.

STORAGE

DO NOT FREEZE. Store refrigerated away from freezer compartments at 2°C-8°C (36°F-46°F). Discard if the vaccine has been frozen.

HOW SUPPLIED

Vial, 1 Dose (5 per package) – Product No. 0005-0104-32

REFERENCES

1. United States Patent Number 4,902,506 by Anderson PW, Eby filed May 5, 1986 issued February 20, 1990.
2. Seid RC Jr, Boykins RA, Liu DF, et al. Chemical evidence for covalent linkage of a semi-synthetic glycoconjugate vaccine for *Haemophilus influenzae* type b disease. *Glycoconjugate J.* 1989;6:489–498.
3. Wenger JD, Ward JL, Broome CV. Prevention of *Haemophilus influenzae* type b disease: vaccines and passive prophylaxis. In: Remington JS, Swartz MS, eds. *Current Clinical Topics in Infectious Diseases*. New York, NY: McGraw-Hill Inc; 1989;10: 306–339.
4. Recommendation of the Immunization Practices Advisory Committee (ACIP) – polysaccharide vaccine for prevention of *Haemophilus influenzae* type b disease. *MMWR.* 1985;34:201–205.
5. Sell SH. Long term sequelae of bacterial meningitis in children. *Pediatr Infect Dis J.* 1983;2:90–93.
6. Broome CV. Epidemiology of *Haemophilus influenzae* type b infections in the United States. *Pediatr Infect Dis J.* 1987;6:779–782.
7. Alexander HE. The productive or curative element in type b *Haemophilus influenzae* rabbit serum. *Yale J Biol Med.* 1944;16:425–434.
8. Peltola H, Kayhty H, Sivonen A. *Haemophilus influenzae* type b capsular polysaccharide vaccine in children: a double-blind field study of 100,000 vaccinees 3 months to 5 years of age in Finland. *Pediatrics.* 1977;60:730–737.
9. Robbins JB, Parke JC Jr, Schneerson R. Quantitative measurement of "natural" and immunization-induced *Haemophilus influenzae* type b capsular polysaccharide antibodies. *Pediatr Res.* 1973;7:103–110.
10. Kayhty H, Peltola H, Karanko V, et al. The protective level of serum antibodies to the capsular polysaccharide of *Haemophilus influenzae* type b. *J Infect Dis.* 1983;147:1100.
11. Kayhty H, Karanko V, Peltola H, et al. Serum antibodies after vaccination with *Haemophilus influenzae* type b capsular polysaccharide and responses to reimmunization: no evidence immunologic tolerance or memory. *Pediatrics.* 1984;74:857–865.
12. Weinberg GA, Granoff DM. Polysaccharide-protein conjugate vaccines for the prevention of *Haemophilus influenzae* type b disease. *J Pediatr.* 1988;113:621–631.
13. Makela O, Péterfy F, Outshoorn IG, et al. Immunogenic properties of a (1-6) dextran, its protein conjugates, and conjugates of its breakdown products in mice. *Scand J Immunol.* 1984;19:541–550.
14. Anderson P, Pichichero ME, Insel RA. Immunogens consisting of oligosaccharides from *Haemophilus influenzae* type b coupled to diphtheria toxoid or the toxin protein CRM197. *J Clin Invest.* 1985;76:52–59.
15. Madore DV, Phipps DC, Eby R, et al. Immune response of young children vaccinated with *Haemophilus influenzae* type b conjugate vaccines. In: Cruse JM, Lewis RE, eds. *Contributions to Microbiology and Immunology: Conjugate Vaccines.* New York, NY: Karger Medical and Scientific Publishers; 1989;10:125–150.
16. Madore DV, Phipps DC, Eby R, et al. Safety and immunologic response to *Haemophilus influenzae* type b oligosaccharide-CRM197 conjugate vaccine in 1- to 6-month-old infants. *Pediatrics.* 1990;85:331–337.
17. Madore DV, Johnson CL, Phipps DC, et al. Safety and immunogenicity of *Haemophilus influenzae* type b oligosaccharide-CRM197 conjugate vaccine in infants aged 15–23 months. *Pediatrics.* 1990;86:527–534.
18. Rothstein EP, Madore DV, Long S. Antibody persistence four years after primary immunization of infants and toddlers with *Haemophilus influenzae* type b CRM197 conjugate vaccine. *J Pediatr.* 1991; 119:655–657.
19. Schlesinger Y, Granoff DM. Avidity and bactericidal activity of antibodies elicited by different *Haemophilus influenzae* type b conjugate vaccines. *JAMA.* 1992;267: 1489–1494.
20. Unpublished data available from Lederle Laboratories.
21. Gigliotti F, Feldman S, Wang WC, et al. Immunization of young infants with sickle cell disease with a *Haemophilus influenzae* type b saccharide-diphtheria CRM197 protein conjugate vaccine. *J Pediatr.* 1989;114:1006–1010.
22. Black SB, Shinefield HR, The Kaiser Permanente Pediatric Vaccine Study Group. Immunization with oligosaccharide conjugate *Haemophilus influenzae* type b (HbOC) vaccine on a large health maintenance organization population: extended follow-up and impact on *Haemophilus influenzae* disease epidemiology. *Pediatric Infect Dis J.* 1992;11:610–613.
23. Black SB, Shinefield HR, Fireman B, et al. Safety, immunogenicity, and efficacy in infancy of oligosaccharide

Continued on next page

HibTITER—Cont.

conjugate *Haemophilus influenzae* type b vaccine in a United States Population: possible implications for optimal use. *J Infect Dis.* 1992;165 (suppl 1):S139–S143.

24. Granoff DM, Anderson EL, Osterholm MT, et al. Differences in the immunogenicity of three *Haemophilus influenzae* type b conjugate vaccines in infants. *J Pediatr.* 1992;121:187–194.
25. Decker MD, Edwards KM, Bradley R, et al. Comparative trial in infants of four conjugate *Haemophilus influenzae* type b vaccines. *J Pediatr.* 1992;120:184–189.
26. Adams WG, Deaver KA, Cochi SL, et al. Decline of childhood *Haemophilus influenzae* type b (Hib) disease in the Hib vaccine era. *JAMA.* 1993;269:221–226.
27. Murphy TV, White KE, Pastor P, et al. Declining incidence of *Haemophilus influenzae* type b disease since introduction of vaccination. *JAMA.* 1993;269:246–248.
28. Broadhurst LE, Erickson RL, Kelley PW. Decreases in invasive *Haemophilus influenzae* diseases in US Army children, 1984 through 1991. *JAMA.* 1993;269:227–231.
29. Shapiro ED. Infections caused by *Haemophilus influenzae* type b: the beginning of the end? *JAMA.* 1993;269: 264–266.
30. Black SB, Shinefield HR, Lampert D, et al. Safety and immunogenicity of oligosaccharide conjugate *Haemophilus influenzae* type b (HbOC) vaccine in infancy. *Pediatr Infect Dis J.* 1991;10:92–96.
31. Black SB, Shinefield HR, Fireman B, et al. Efficacy in infancy of oligosaccharide conjugate *Haemophilus influenzae* type b (HbOC) vaccine in a United States Population of 61,080 children. *Pediatr Infect Dis J.* 1991;10:97–104.
32. Recommendations of the AAP: *Haemophilus influenzae* type b conjugate vaccines: recommendations for immunization of infants and children 2 months of age and older: update. *Pediatrics.* 1991;88:169–172.
33. Recommendation of the ACIP: Haemophilus b conjugate vaccines for prevention of *Haemophilus influenzae* type b disease among infants and children two months of age and older. *MMWR.* 1991;40:1–7.
34. Centers for Disease Control and Prevention. General recommendations on immunization: Recommendations of the Advisory Committee on Immunization Practices (ACIP) and the American Academy of Family Physicians (AAFP). *MMWR.* 2002;51(No. RR-2);1–36.
35. 2000 Red Book: Report of the Committee on Infectious Diseases. 25th ed. Elk Grove Village, IL: American Academy of Pediatrics; 2000: 26, 266–72.
36. Jones RG, Bass JW, Weisse ME, et al. Antigenuria after immunization with *Haemophilus influenzae* oligosaccharide CRM197 conjugate (HbOC) vaccine. *Pediatr Infect Dis J.* 1991;10:557–559.
37. American Academy of Pediatrics: Report of the Committee on Infectious Diseases. 22nd ed. Elk Grove Village, Ill: American Academy of Pediatrics; 1991.
38. Recommendation of the ACIP: Immunization of children infected with human T-lymphotrophic virus type III/lymphadenopathy-associated virus. *MMWR.* 1986; 35(38):595–606.
39. Immunization of children infected with human immunodeficiency virus – supplementary ACIP statement. *MMWR.* 1988;37(12):181–183.
40. General Recommendations on Immunization: Recommendations of the Immunization Practices Advisory Committee (ACIP). *MMWR.* 1989;38(13):221.
41. Spinola SM, Sheaffer CI, Philbrick KB, et al. Antigenuria after *Haemophilus influenzae* type b polysaccharide immunization: a prospective study. *J Pediatr.* 1986;109:835–837.
42. CDC. Vaccine Adverse Event Reporting System – United States. *MMWR.* 1990;39:730–733.
43. Paradiso PR. Combined childhood immunizations. *JAMA.* 1992;268:1685.
44. Paradiso PR, Hogerman DA, Madore DV, et al. Safety and immunogenicity of a combined diphtheria, tetanus, pertussis and *Haemophilus influenzae* type b vaccine in young infants. *Pediatrics.* 1993;92(6):827–32.
45. Wyeth Pharmaceuticals, Data on File: Prevnar Study D118-P12.
46. Wyeth Pharmaceuticals, Data on File: Prevnar Study D118-P16.
47. Wyeth Pharmaceuticals, Data on File: Prevnar Study D118-P7.
48. Shinefield H, Black S, Ray P, et al. Safety and immunogenicity of heptavalent pneumococcal CRM_{197} conjugate vaccine in infants and toddlers. *Pediatr Infect Dis J.* 1999;18:757–63.
49. Wyeth Pharmaceuticals, Data on File: Prevnar Study D118-P3.
50. Rennels MB, Edwards KM, Keyserling HL, et al. Safety and immunogenicity of heptavalent pneumococcal vaccine conjugated to CRM_{197} in United States infants. *Pediatrics.* 1998;101(4):604–11.
51. Wyeth Pharmaceuticals, Data on File: Prevnar Study D118-P8.
52. Black S, Shinefield H, Fireman B, et al. Efficacy, safety and immunogenicity of heptavalent pneumococcal conjugate vaccine in children. *Pediatr Infect Dis J.* 2000;19: 187–95.
53. Milstein JB, Gross TP, Kuritsky JN. Adverse reactions reported following receipt of *Haemophilus influenzae* type b vaccine: an analysis after one year of marketing. *Pediatrics.* 1987;80:270–274.
54. D'Cruz DF, Shapiro ED, Spiegelman KN, et al. Acute inflammatory demyelinating polyradiculoneuropathy (Guillain-Barré syndrome) after immunization with *Haemophilus influenzae* type b conjugate vaccine. *J Pediatr.* 1989;115:743–746.
55. Greenberg DP, Lieberman JM, Marcy SM, et al. Enhanced antibody responses in infants given different sequences of heterogenous *Haemophilus influenzae* type b conjugate vaccines. *J Pediatr.* 1995;126:206–11.
56. Anderson EL, Decker MD, Englund JA, et al. Interchangeability of conjugated *Haemophilus influenzae* type b vaccines in infants. *JAMA.* 1995;273:849–53.

Wyeth®
Manufactured by: W10461C003
Wyeth Pharmaceuticals Inc. ET02
Philadelphia, PA 19101 Rev 01/04
US Govt. License No. 3

INDERAL® LA ℞

[in 'der-ăl]
(propranolol hydrochloride)
Long-Acting Capsules
℞ only

This product's label may have been revised after this insert was used in production. For further product information and current package insert, please visit www.wyeth.com or call our medical communications department toll-free at 1-800-934-5556.

DESCRIPTION

Inderal (propranolol hydrochloride) is a synthetic beta-adrenergic receptor-blocking agent chemically described as 2-Propanol, 1-[(1-methylethyl)amino]-3-(1-naphthalenyloxy)-, hydrochloride. Its structural formula is:

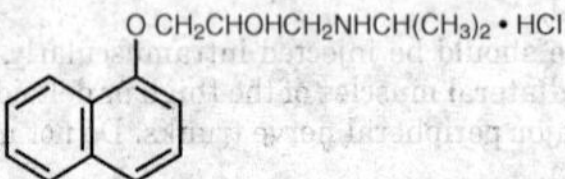

Propranolol hydrochloride is a stable, white, crystalline solid which is readily soluble in water and ethanol. Its molecular weight is 295.80.

Inderal LA is formulated to provide a sustained release of propranolol hydrochloride. Inderal LA is available as 60 mg, 80 mg, 120 mg, and 160 mg capsules.

Inderal LA capsules contain the following inactive ingredients: cellulose, ethylcellulose, gelatin capsules, hypromellose, and titanium dioxide. In addition, Inderal LA 60 mg, 80 mg, and 120 mg capsules contain D&C Red No. 28 and FD&C Blue No. 1; Inderal LA 160 mg capsules contain FD&C Blue No. 1.

These capsules comply with USP Drug Release Test 1.

CLINICAL PHARMACOLOGY

Inderal is a nonselective, beta-adrenergic receptor-blocking agent possessing no other autonomic nervous system activity. It specifically competes with beta-adrenergic receptor-stimulating agents for available receptor sites. When access to beta-receptor sites is blocked by Inderal, the chronotropic, inotropic, and vasodilator responses to beta-adrenergic stimulation are decreased proportionately.

Inderal LA Capsules (60, 80, 120, and 160 mg) release propranolol HCl at a controlled and predictable rate. Peak blood levels following dosing with Inderal LA occur at about 6 hours, and the apparent plasma half-life is about 10 hours. When measured at steady state over a 24-hour period the areas under the propranolol plasma concentration-time curve (AUCs) for the capsules are approximately 60% to 65% of the AUCs for a comparable divided daily dose of Inderal Tablets. The lower AUCs for the capsules are due to greater hepatic metabolism of propranolol, resulting from the slower rate of absorption of propranolol. Over a twenty-four (24) hour period, blood levels are fairly constant for about twelve (12) hours, then decline exponentially.

Inderal LA should not be considered a simple mg-for-mg substitute for conventional propranolol and the blood levels achieved do not match (are lower than) those of two to four times daily dosing with the same dose. When changing to Inderal LA from conventional propranolol, a possible need for retitration upwards should be considered, especially to maintain effectiveness at the end of the dosing interval. In most clinical settings, however, such as hypertension or angina where there is little correlation between plasma levels and clinical effect, Inderal LA has been therapeutically equivalent to the same mg dose of conventional Inderal as assessed by 24-hour effects on blood pressure and on 24-hour exercise responses of heart rate, systolic pressure, and rate pressure product. Inderal LA can provide effective beta blockade for a 24-hour period.

The mechanism of the antihypertensive effect of Inderal has not been established. Among the factors that may be involved in contributing to the antihypertensive action are: (1) decreased cardiac output, (2) inhibition of renin release by the kidneys, and (3) diminution of tonic sympathetic nerve outflow from vasomotor centers in the brain. Although total peripheral resistance may increase initially, it readjusts to or below the pretreatment level with chronic use. Effects on plasma volume appear to be minor and somewhat variable. Inderal has been shown to cause a small increase in serum potassium concentration when used in the treatment of hypertensive patients.

In angina pectoris, propranolol generally reduces the oxygen requirement of the heart at any given level of effort by blocking the catecholamine-induced increases in the heart rate, systolic blood pressure, and the velocity and extent of myocardial contraction. Propranolol may increase oxygen requirements by increasing left ventricular fiber length, end diastolic pressure, and systolic ejection period. The net physiologic effect of beta-adrenergic blockade is usually advantageous and is manifested during exercise by delayed onset of pain and increased work capacity.

In dosages greater than required for beta blockade, Inderal also exerts a quinidine-like or anesthetic-like membrane action which affects the cardiac action potential. The significance of the membrane action in the treatment of arrhythmias is uncertain.

The mechanism of the antimigraine effect of propranolol has not been established. Beta-adrenergic receptors have been demonstrated in the pial vessels of the brain.

Beta-receptor blockade can be useful in conditions in which, because of pathologic or functional changes, sympathetic activity is detrimental to the patient. But there are also situations in which sympathetic stimulation is vital. For example, in patients with severely damaged hearts, adequate ventricular function is maintained by virtue of sympathetic drive, which should be preserved. In the presence of AV block, greater than first degree, beta blockade may prevent the necessary facilitating effect of sympathetic activity on conduction. Beta blockade results in bronchial constriction by interfering with adrenergic bronchodilator activity, which should be preserved in patients subject to bronchospasm.

Propranolol is not significantly dialyzable.

INDICATIONS AND USAGE

Hypertension

Inderal LA is indicated in the management of hypertension; it may be used alone or used in combination with other antihypertensive agents, particularly a thiazide diuretic. Inderal LA is not indicated in the management of hypertensive emergencies.

Angina Pectoris Due to Coronary Atherosclerosis

Inderal LA is indicated for the long-term management of patients with angina pectoris.

Migraine

Inderal LA is indicated for the prophylaxis of common migraine headache. The efficacy of propranolol in the treatment of a migraine attack that has started has not been established, and propranolol is not indicated for such use.

Hypertrophic Subaortic Stenosis

Inderal LA is useful in the management of hypertrophic subaortic stenosis, especially for treatment of exertional or other stress-induced angina, palpitations, and syncope. Inderal LA also improves exercise performance. The effectiveness of propranolol hydrochloride in this disease appears to be due to a reduction of the elevated outflow pressure gradient, which is exacerbated by beta-receptor stimulation. Clinical improvement may be temporary.

CONTRAINDICATIONS

Inderal is contraindicated in 1) cardiogenic shock; 2) sinus bradycardia and greater than first-degree block; 3) bronchial asthma; 4) congestive heart failure (see "**WARNINGS**"), unless the failure is secondary to a tachyarrhythmia treatable with Inderal.

WARNINGS

Hypersensitivity reactions, including anaphylactic/anaphylactoid reactions, have been associated with the administration of propranolol (see "**ADVERSE REACTIONS**").

Cardiac Failure: Sympathetic stimulation may be a vital component supporting circulatory function in patients with congestive heart failure, and its inhibition by beta blockade may precipitate more severe failure. Although beta blockers should be avoided in overt congestive heart failure, if necessary, they can be used with close follow-up in patients with a history of failure who are well compensated and are receiving digitalis and diuretics. Beta-adrenergic blocking agents do not abolish the inotropic action of digitalis on heart muscle.

In Patients without a History of Heart Failure, continued use of beta blockers can, in some cases, lead to cardiac failure. Therefore, at the first sign or symptom of heart failure, the patient should be digitalized and/or treated with diuretics, and the response observed closely, or Inderal should be discontinued (gradually, if possible).

In Patients with Angina Pectoris, there have been reports of exacerbation of angina and, in some cases, myocardial infarction, following *abrupt* discontinuance of Inderal therapy. Therefore, when discontinuance of Inderal is planned, the dosage should be gradually reduced over at least a few weeks, and the patient should be cautioned against interruption or cessation of therapy without the physician's advice. If Inderal therapy is interrupted and exacerbation of angina occurs, it usually is advisable to reinstitute Inderal therapy and take other measures appropriate for the management of unstable angina pectoris. Since coronary artery disease may be unrecognized, it may be prudent to follow the above advice in patients considered at risk of having occult atherosclerotic heart disease who are given propranolol for other indications.

Nonallergic Bronchospasm (e.g., Chronic Bronchitis, Emphysema)—PATIENTS WITH BRONCHOSPASTIC DISEASES SHOULD IN GENERAL NOT RECEIVE BETA BLOCKERS. Inderal should be administered with caution since it may block bronchodilation produced by endogenous and exogenous catecholamine stimulation of beta receptors.

Major Surgery: The necessity or desirability of withdrawal of beta-blocking therapy prior to major surgery is controversial. It should be noted, however, that the impaired ability of the heart to respond to reflex adrenergic stimuli may augment the risks of general anesthesia and surgical procedures.

Inderal, like other beta blockers, is a competitive inhibitor of beta-receptor agonists and its effects can be reversed by administration of such agents, e.g., dobutamine or isoproterenol. However, such patients may be subject to protracted severe hypotension. Difficulty in starting and maintaining the heartbeat has also been reported with beta blockers.

Diabetes and Hypoglycemia: Beta-adrenergic blockade may prevent the appearance of certain premonitory signs and symptoms (pulse rate and pressure changes) of acute hypoglycemia in labile insulin-dependent diabetes. In these patients, it may be more difficult to adjust the dosage of insulin. Hypoglycemic attacks may be accompanied by a precipitous elevation of blood pressure in patients on propranolol.

Propranolol therapy, particularly in infants and children, diabetic or not, has been associated with hypoglycemia especially during fasting as in preparation for surgery. Hypoglycemia also has been found after this type of drug therapy and prolonged physical exertion and has occurred in renal insufficiency, both during dialysis and sporadically, in patients on propranolol.

Acute increases in blood pressure have occurred after insulin-induced hypoglycemia in patients on propranolol.

Thyrotoxicosis: Beta blockade may mask certain clinical signs of hyperthyroidism. Therefore, abrupt withdrawal of propranolol may be followed by an exacerbation of symptoms of hyperthyroidism, including thyroid storm. Propranolol may change thyroid-function tests, increasing T_4 and reverse T_3, and decreasing T_3.

In Patients with Wolff-Parkinson-White Syndrome, several cases have been reported in which, after propranolol, the tachycardia was replaced by a severe bradycardia requiring a demand pacemaker. In one case this resulted after an initial dose of 5 mg propranolol.

Skin Reactions: Cutaneous reactions, including Stevens-Johnson Syndrome, toxic epidermal necrolysis, exfoliative dermatitis, erythema multiforme, and urticaria, have been reported with use of propranolol (see **"ADVERSE REACTIONS"**).

PRECAUTIONS

General

Propranolol should be used with caution in patients with impaired hepatic or renal function. Inderal is not indicated for the treatment of hypertensive emergencies.

Beta-adrenoreceptor blockade can cause reduction of intraocular pressure. Patients should be told that Inderal may interfere with the glaucoma screening test. Withdrawal may lead to a return of increased intraocular pressure.

Risk of anaphylactic reaction. While taking beta blockers, patients with a history of severe anaphylactic reaction to a variety of allergens may be more reactive to repeated challenge, either accidental, diagnostic, or therapeutic. Such patients may be unresponsive to the usual doses of epinephrine used to treat allergic reaction.

Clinical Laboratory Tests

Elevated blood urea levels in patients with severe heart disease, elevated serum transaminase, alkaline phosphatase, lactate dehydrogenase.

Drug Interactions

Patients receiving catecholamine-depleting drugs such as reserpine should be closely observed if Inderal is administered. The added catecholamine-blocking action may produce an excessive reduction of resting sympathetic nervous activity which may result in hypotension, marked bradycardia, vertigo, syncopal attacks, or orthostatic hypotension.

Caution should be exercised when patients receiving a beta blocker are administered a calcium-channel-blocking drug, especially intravenous verapamil, for both agents may depress myocardial contractility or atrioventricular conduction. On rare occasions, the concomitant intravenous use of a beta blocker and verapamil has resulted in serious adverse reactions, especially in patients with severe cardiomyopathy, congestive heart failure or recent myocardial infarction.

Blunting of the antihypertensive effect of beta-adrenoceptor blocking agents by nonsteroidal anti-inflammatory drugs has been reported.

Hypotension and cardiac arrest have been reported with the concomitant use of propranolol and haloperidol.

Aluminum hydroxide gel greatly reduces intestinal absorption of propranolol.

Ethanol slows the rate of absorption of propranolol.

Phenytoin, phenobarbitone, and *rifampin* accelerate propranolol clearance.

Chlorpromazine, when used concomitantly with propranolol, results in increased plasma levels of both drugs.

Antipyrine and *lidocaine* have reduced clearance when used concomitantly with propranolol.

Thyroxine may result in a lower than expected T_3 concentration when used concomitantly with propranolol.

Cimetidine decreases the hepatic metabolism of propranolol, delaying elimination and increasing blood levels.

Theophylline clearance is reduced when used concomitantly with propranolol.

Carcinogenesis, Mutagenesis, Impairment of Fertility

In dietary administration studies in which mice and rats were treated with propranolol for up to 18 months at doses of up to 150 mg/kg/day, there was no evidence of drug-related tumorigenesis. In a study in which both male and female rats were exposed to propranolol in their diets at concentrations of up to 0.05%, from 60 days prior to mating and throughout pregnancy and lactation for two generations, there were no effects on fertility. Based on differing results from Ames Tests performed by different laboratories, there is equivocal evidence for a genotoxic effect of propranolol in bacteria (*S. typhimurium* strain TA 1538).

Pregnancy: Pregnancy Category C

In a series of reproductive and developmental toxicology studies, propranolol was given to rats by gavage or in the diet throughout pregnancy and lactation. At doses of 150 mg/kg/day (> 10 times the maximum recommended human daily dose of propranolol on a body weight basis), but not at doses of 80 mg/kg/day, treatment was associated with embryotoxicity (reduced litter size and increased resorption sites) as well as neonatal toxicity (deaths). Propranolol also was administered (in the feed) to rabbits (throughout pregnancy and lactation) at doses as high as 150 mg/kg/day (> 15 times the maximum recommended daily human dose). No evidence of embryo or neonatal toxicity was noted.

There are no adequate and well-controlled studies in pregnant women. Intrauterine growth retardation has been reported in neonates whose mothers received propranolol during pregnancy. Neonates whose mothers are receiving propranolol at parturition have exhibited bradycardia, hypoglycemia and respiratory depression. Adequate facilities for monitoring these infants at birth should be available. Inderal should be used during pregnancy only if the potential benefit justifies the potential risk to the fetus.

Nursing Mothers

Inderal is excreted in human milk. Caution should be exercised when Inderal is administered to a nursing woman.

Pediatric Use

Safety and effectiveness in pediatric patients have not been established.

Geriatric Use

Clinical studies of propranolol did not include sufficient numbers of subjects aged 65 and over to determine whether they respond differently from younger subjects. Other reported clinical experience has not identified differences in responses between the elderly and younger patients. In general, dose selection for an elderly patient should be cautious, usually starting at the low end of the dosing range, reflecting the greater frequency of the decreased hepatic, renal or cardiac function, and of concomitant disease or other drug therapy.

ADVERSE REACTIONS

Most adverse effects have been mild and transient and have rarely required the withdrawal of therapy.

Cardiovascular: Bradycardia; congestive heart failure; intensification of AV block; hypotension; paresthesia of hands; thrombocytopenic purpura; arterial insufficiency, usually of the Raynaud type.

Central Nervous System: Light-headedness; mental depression manifested by insomnia, lassitude, weakness, fatigue; reversible mental depression progressing to catatonia; visual disturbances; hallucinations; vivid dreams; an acute reversible syndrome characterized by disorientation for time and place, short-term memory loss, emotional lability, slightly clouded sensorium, and decreased performance on neuropsychometrics. For immediate formulations, fatigue, lethargy, and vivid dreams appear dose related.

Gastrointestinal: Nausea, vomiting, epigastric distress, abdominal cramping, diarrhea, constipation, mesenteric arterial thrombosis, and ischemic colitis.

Allergic: Hypersensitivity reactions, including anaphylactic/anaphylactoid reactions, pharyngitis and agranulocytosis, erythematous rash, fever combined with aching and sore throat, laryngospasm, and respiratory distress.

Respiratory: Bronchospasm.

Hematologic: Agranulocytosis, nonthrombocytopenic purpura, and thrombocytopenic purpura.

Autoimmune: In extremely rare instances, systemic lupus erythematosus has been reported.

Miscellaneous: Alopecia, LE-like reactions, psoriasiform rashes, dry eyes, male impotence, and Peyronie's disease have been reported rarely. Oculomucocutaneous reactions involving the skin, serous membranes, and conjunctivae reported for a beta blocker (practolol) have not been associated with propranolol.

Skin: Stevens-Johnson Syndrome, toxic epidermal necrolysis, exfoliative dermatitis, erythema multiforme, and urticaria.

DOSAGE AND ADMINISTRATION

Inderal® LA provides propranolol hydrochloride in a sustained-release capsule for administration once daily. If patients are switched from Inderal Tablets to Inderal LA Capsules, care should be taken to assure that the desired therapeutic effect is maintained. Inderal LA should not be considered a simple mg-for-mg substitute for Inderal. Inderal LA has different kinetics and produces lower blood levels. Retitration may be necessary, especially to maintain effectiveness at the end of the 24-hour dosing interval.

Hypertension

Dosage must be individualized. The usual initial dosage is 80 mg Inderal LA once daily, whether used alone or added to a diuretic. The dosage may be increased to 120 mg once daily or higher until adequate blood pressure control is achieved. The usual maintenance dosage is 120 to 160 mg once daily. In some instances a dosage of 640 mg may be required. The time needed for full hypertensive response to a given dosage is variable and may range from a few days to several weeks.

Angina Pectoris

Dosage must be individualized. Starting with 80 mg Inderal LA once daily, dosage should be gradually increased at three- to seven-day intervals until optimal response is obtained. Although individual patients may respond at any dosage level, the average optimal dosage appears to be 160 mg once daily. In angina pectoris, the value and safety of dosage exceeding 320 mg per day have not been established.

If treatment is to be discontinued, reduce dosage gradually over a period of a few weeks (see **"WARNINGS"**).

Migraine

Dosage must be individualized. The initial oral dose is 80 mg Inderal LA once daily. The usual effective dose range is 160 to 240 mg once daily. The dosage may be increased gradually to achieve optimal migraine prophylaxis. If a satisfactory response is not obtained within four to six weeks after reaching the maximal dose, Inderal LA therapy should be discontinued. It may be advisable to withdraw the drug gradually over a period of several weeks.

Hypertrophic Subaortic Stenosis

80 to 160 mg Inderal LA once daily.

Pediatric Dosage

At this time the data on the use of the drug in this age group are too limited to permit adequate directions for use.

OVERDOSAGE

Inderal is not significantly dialyzable. In the event of overdosage or exaggerated response, the following measures should be employed:

General

If ingestion is, or may have been, recent, evacuate gastric contents, taking care to prevent pulmonary aspiration.

Bradycardia

ADMINISTER ATROPINE (0.25 to 1.0 mg); IF THERE IS NO RESPONSE TO VAGAL BLOCKADE, ADMINISTER ISOPROTERENOL CAUTIOUSLY.

Cardiac Failure

DIGITALIZATION AND DIURETICS.

Hypotension

VASOPRESSORS, e.g., LEVARTERENOL OR EPINEPHRINE (THERE IS EVIDENCE THAT EPINEPHRINE IS THE DRUG OF CHOICE).

Bronchospasm

ADMINISTER ISOPROTERENOL AND AMINOPHYLLINE.

HOW SUPPLIED

Inderal® LA Capsules (propranolol hydrochloride)

Each white/light-blue capsule, identified by 3 narrow bands, 1 wide band, and "INDERAL LA 60," contains 60 mg of propranolol hydrochloride in bottles of 100 (NDC 0046-0470-81).

Each light-blue capsule, identified by 3 narrow bands, 1 wide band, and "INDERAL LA 80," contains 80 mg of propranolol hydrochloride in bottles of 100 (NDC 0046-0471-81).

Each light-blue/dark-blue capsule, identified by 3 narrow bands, 1 wide band, and "INDERAL LA 120," contains 120 mg of propranolol hydrochloride in bottles of 100 (NDC 0046-0473-81).

Each dark-blue capsule, identified by 3 narrow bands, 1 wide band, and "INDERAL LA 160," contains 160 mg of propranolol hydrochloride in bottles of 100 (NDC 0046-0479-81).

The appearance of these capsules is a registered trademark of Wyeth Pharmaceuticals.

Store at 20° to 25°C (68° to 77°F); excursions permitted to 15° to 30°C (59° to 86°F). [See USP Controlled Room Temperature]

Protect from light, moisture, freezing, and excessive heat. Dispense in a tight, light-resistant container as defined in the USP.

Wyeth®

Wyeth Pharmaceuticals Inc.
Philadelphia, PA 19101

W10478C003
ET01
Rev 07/04

Shown in Product Identification Guide, page 336

LO/OVRAL®-28 ℞

[lō'ōvrăl]

Tablets

(NORGESTREL AND ETHINYL ESTRADIOL TABLETS)

℞ only

This product's label may have been revised after this insert was used in production. For further product information

Continued on next page

Lo/Ovral-28—Cont.

and current package insert, please visit www.wyeth.com or call our medical communications department toll-free at 1-800-934-5556.

Patients should be counseled that oral contraceptives do not protect against transmission of HIV (AIDS) and other sexually transmitted diseases (STDs) such as chlamydia, genital herpes, genital warts, gonorrhea, hepatitis B, and syphilis.

DESCRIPTION

21 white LO/OVRAL tablets, each containing 0.3 mg of norgestrel (*dl*-13-beta-ethyl-17-alpha-ethinyl-17-beta-hydroxygon-4-en-3-one), a totally synthetic progestogen, and 0.03 mg of ethinyl estradiol (19-nor-17α-pregna-1,3,5 (10)-trien-20-yne-3,17-diol), and 7 pink inert tablets. The inactive ingredients present are cellulose, D&C Red 30, lactose, magnesium stearate, and polacrilin potassium.

Norgestrel $C_{21}H_{28}O_2$ M.W. 312.45

Ethinyl Estradiol $C_{20}H_{24}O_2$ M.W. 296.40

CLINICAL PHARMACOLOGY

Mode of Action

Combination oral contraceptives act by suppression of gonadotropins. Although the primary mechanism of this action is inhibition of ovulation, other alterations include changes in the cervical mucus (which increase the difficulty of sperm entry into the uterus) and the endometrium (which reduce the likelihood of implantation).

INDICATIONS AND USAGE

Oral contraceptives are indicated for the prevention of pregnancy in women who elect to use this product as a method of contraception.

Oral contraceptives are highly effective. Table I lists the typical accidental pregnancy rates for users of combination oral contraceptives and other methods of contraception. The efficacy of these contraceptive methods, except sterilization, the IUD, and implants depends upon the reliability with which they are used. Correct and consistent use of methods can result in lower failure rates.

[See table I at right]

CONTRAINDICATIONS

Combination oral contraceptives should not be used in women with any of the following conditions:

Thrombophlebitis or thromboembolic disorders
A past history of deep-vein thrombophlebitis or thromboembolic disorders
Cerebral-vascular or coronary-artery disease (current or history)
Thrombogenic valvulopathies
Thrombogenic rhythm disorders
Major surgery with prolonged immobilization
Diabetes with vascular involvement
Headaches with focal neurological symptoms
Uncontrolled hypertension
Known or suspected carcinoma of the breast or personal history of breast cancer
Carcinoma of the endometrium or other known or suspected estrogen-dependent neoplasia
Undiagnosed abnormal genital bleeding
Cholestatic jaundice of pregnancy or jaundice with prior pill use
Hepatic adenomas or carcinomas, or active liver disease, as long as liver function has not returned to normal
Known or suspected pregnancy
Hypersensitivity to any of the components of Lo/Ovral-28

WARNINGS

Cigarette smoking increases the risk of serious cardiovascular side effects from oral-contraceptive use. This risk increases with age and with the extent of smoking (in epidemiologic studies, 15 or more cigarettes per day was associated with a significantly increased risk) and is quite marked in women over 35 years of age. Women who use oral contraceptives should be strongly advised not to smoke.

The use of oral contraceptives is associated with increased risks of several serious conditions including venous and arterial thrombotic and thromboembolic events (such as myocardial infarction, thromboembolism, and stroke), hepatic neoplasia, gallbladder disease, and hypertension, although the risk of serious morbidity or mortality is very small in healthy women without underlying risk factors. The risk of morbidity and mortality increases significantly in the presence of other underlying risk factors such as certain inherited or acquired thrombophilias, hypertension, hyperlipidemias, obesity, diabetes, and surgery or trauma with increased risk of thrombosis.

Practitioners prescribing oral contraceptives should be familiar with the following information relating to these risks.

Table I: Percentage Of Women Experiencing An Unintended Pregnancy During The First Year Of Typical Use And The First Year Of Perfect Use Of Contraception And The Percentage Continuing Use At The End Of The First Year. United States.

Method (1)	% of Women Experiencing an Unintended Pregnancy within the First Year of Use: Typical Use[1] (2)	Perfect Use[2] (3)	% of Women Continuing Use at One Year[3] (4)
Chance[4]	85	85	
Spermicides[5]	26	6	40
Periodic abstinence	25		63
Calendar		9	
Ovulation Method		3	
Sympto-Thermal[6]		2	
Post-Ovulation		1	
Cap[7]			
Parous Women	40	26	42
Nulliparous Women	20	9	56
Sponge			
Parous Women	40	20	42
Nulliparous Women	20	9	56
Diaphragm[7]	20	6	56
Withdrawal	19	4	
Condom[8]			
Female (Reality)	21	5	56
Male	14	3	61
Pill	5		71
Progestin only		0.5	
Combined		0.1	
IUD			
Progesterone T	2.0	1.5	81
Copper T380A	0.8	0.6	78
LNg 20	0.1	0.1	81
Depo-Provera®	0.3	0.3	70
Levonorgestrel Implants (Norplant®)	0.05	0.05	88
Female Sterilization	0.5	0.5	100
Male Sterilization	0.15	0.10	100

Lactation Amenorrhea Method: LAM is a highly effective, temporary method of contraception.[9]

Source: Trussell J. Contraceptive efficacy. In: Hatcher RA, Trussell J, Stewart F, Cates W, Stewart GK, Kowel D, Guest F. Contraceptive Technology: Seventeenth Revised Edition. New York NY: Irvington Publishers; 1998.

1. Among *typical* couples who initiate use of a method (not necessarily for the first time), the percentage who experience an accidental pregnancy during the first year if they do not stop use for any other reason.
2. Among couples who initiate use of a method (not necessarily for the first time) and who use it *perfectly* (both consistently and correctly), the percentage who experience an accidental pregnancy during the first year if they do not stop use for any other reason.
3. Among couples attempting to avoid pregnancy, the percentage who continue to use a method for one year.
4. The percents becoming pregnant in columns (2) and (3) are based on data from populations where contraception is not used and from women who cease using contraception in order to become pregnant. Among such populations, about 89% become pregnant within one year. This estimate was lowered slightly (to 85%) to represent the percent who would become pregnant within one year among women now relying on reversible methods of contraception if they abandoned contraception altogether.
5. Foams, creams, gels, vaginal suppositories, and vaginal film.
6. Cervical mucus (ovulation) method supplemented by calendar in the pre-ovulatory and basal body temperature in the post-ovulatory phases.
7. With spermicidal cream or jelly.
8. Without spermicides.
9. However, to maintain effective protection against pregnancy, another method of contraception must be used as soon as menstruation resumes, the frequency or duration of breastfeeds is reduced, bottle feeds are introduced, or the baby reaches 6 months of age.

The information contained in this package insert is based principally on studies carried out in patients who used oral contraceptives with higher doses of estrogens and progestogens than those in common use today. The effect of long-term use of the oral contraceptives with lower doses of both estrogens and progestogens remains to be determined.

Throughout this labeling, epidemiological studies reported are of two types: retrospective or case control studies and prospective or cohort studies. Case control studies provide a measure of the relative risk of disease, namely, a ratio of the incidence of a disease among oral-contraceptive users to that among nonusers. The relative risk does not provide information on the actual clinical occurrence of a disease. Cohort studies provide a measure of attributable risk, which is the difference in the incidence of disease between oral-contraceptive users and nonusers. The attributable risk does provide information about the actual occurrence of a disease in the population. For further information, the reader is referred to a text on epidemiological methods.

1. **Thromboembolic Disorders And Other Vascular Problems**

a. *Myocardial infarction*

An increased risk of myocardial infarction has been attributed to oral-contraceptive use. This risk is primarily in smokers or women with other underlying risk factors for coronary-artery disease such as hypertension, hypercholesterolemia, morbid obesity, and diabetes. The relative risk of heart attack for current oral-contraceptive users has been estimated to be two to six. The risk is very low under the age of 30.

Smoking in combination with oral-contraceptive use has been shown to contribute substantially to the incidence of myocardial infarctions in women in their mid-thirties or older with smoking accounting for the majority of excess cases. Mortality rates associated with circulatory disease have been shown to increase substantially in smokers over the age of 35 and nonsmokers over the age of 40 (Table II) among women who use oral contraceptives.

CIRCULATORY DISEASE MORTALITY RATES PER 100,000 WOMAN YEARS BY AGE, SMOKING STATUS AND ORAL-CONTRACEPTIVE USE

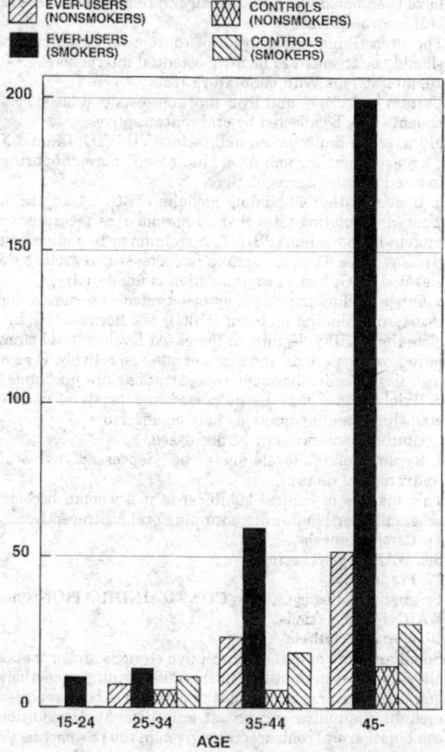

TABLE II. (Adapted from P.M. Layde and V. Beral, Lancet, *1*:541-546, 1981.)

Oral contraceptives may compound the effects of well-known risk factors, such as hypertension, diabetes, hyperlipidemias, age, and obesity. In particular, some progestogens are known to decrease HDL cholesterol and cause glucose intolerance, while estrogens may create a state of hyperinsulinism. Oral contraceptives have been shown to increase blood pressure among users (see section 9 in **WARNINGS**). Similar effects on risk factors have been associated with an increased risk of heart disease. Oral contraceptives must be used with caution in women with cardiovascular disease risk factors.

b. *Venous thrombosis and thromboembolism*

An increased risk of venous thromboembolic and thrombotic disease associated with the use of oral contraceptives is well established. Case control studies have found the relative risk of users compared to nonusers to be 3 for the first episode of superficial venous thrombosis, 4 to 11 for deep-vein thrombosis or pulmonary embolism, and 1.5 to 6 for women with predisposing conditions for venous thromboembolic disease. Cohort studies have shown the relative risk to be somewhat lower, about 3 for new cases and about 4.5 for new cases requiring hospitalization. The approximate incidence of deep-vein thrombosis and pulmonary embolism in users of low dose (<50 mcg ethinyl estradiol) combination oral contraceptives is up to 4 per 10,000 woman-years compared to 0.5-3 per 10,000 woman-years for non-users. However, the incidence is substantially less than that associated with pregnancy (6 per 10,000 woman-years). The excess risk is highest during the first year a woman ever uses a combined oral contraceptive. Venous thromboembolism may be fatal. The risk of venous thrombotic and thromboembolic events is further increased in women with conditions predisposing for venous thrombosis and thromboembolism. The risk of thromboembolic disease due to oral contraceptives is not related to length of use and gradually disappears after pill use is stopped.

A two- to four-fold increase in relative risk of postoperative thromboembolic complications has been reported with the use of oral contraceptives. The relative risk of venous thrombosis in women who have predisposing conditions is twice that of women without such medical conditions. If feasible, oral contraceptives should be discontinued at least four weeks prior to and for two weeks after elective surgery of a type associated with an increase in risk of thromboembolism and during and following prolonged immobilization. Since the immediate postpartum period is also associated with an increased risk of thromboembolism, oral contraceptives should be started no earlier than four weeks after delivery in women who elect not to breast-feed, or a midtrimester pregnancy termination.

c. *Cerebrovascular diseases*

Oral contraceptives have been shown to increase both the relative and attributable risks of cerebrovascular events (thrombotic and hemorrhagic strokes), although, in general, the risk is greatest among older (>35 years), hypertensive women who also smoke. Hypertension was found to be a risk factor for both users and nonusers, for both types of strokes, while smoking interacted to increase the risk for hemorrhagic strokes.

In a large study, the relative risk of thrombotic strokes has been shown to range from 3 for normotensive users to 14 for users with severe hypertension. The relative risk of hemorrhagic stroke is reported to be 1.2 for nonsmokers who used oral contraceptives, 2.6 for smokers who did not use oral contraceptives, 7.6 for smokers who used oral contraceptives, 1.8 for normotensive users, and 25.7 for users with severe hypertension. The attributable risk is also greater in older women. Oral contraceptives also increase the risk for stroke in women with other underlying risk factors such as certain inherited or acquired thrombophilias, hyperlipidemias, and obesity.

Women with migraine (particularly migraine/headaches with focal neurological symptoms, see **CONTRAINDICATIONS**) who take combination oral contraceptives may be at an increased risk of stroke.

d. *Dose-related risk of vascular disease from oral contraceptives*

A positive association has been observed between the amount of estrogen and progestogen in oral contraceptives and the risk of vascular disease. A decline in serum high-density lipoproteins (HDL) has been reported with many progestational agents. A decline in serum high-density lipoproteins has been associated with an increased incidence of ischemic heart disease. Because estrogens increase HDL cholesterol, the net effect of an oral contraceptive depends on a balance achieved between doses of estrogen and progestogen and the nature and absolute amount of progestogen used in the contraceptive. The amount of both hormones should be considered in the choice of an oral contraceptive.

Minimizing exposure to estrogen and progestogen is in keeping with good principles of therapeutics. For any particular estrogen/progestogen combination, the dosage regimen prescribed should be one which contains the least amount of estrogen and progestogen that is compatible with a low failure rate and the needs of the individual patient. New acceptors of oral-contraceptive agents should be started on preparations containing the lowest estrogen content which is judged appropriate for the individual patient.

e. *Persistence of risk of vascular disease*

There are two studies which have shown persistence of risk of vascular disease for ever-users of oral contraceptives. In a study in the United States, the risk of developing myocardial infarction after discontinuing oral contraceptives persists for at least 9 years for women 40 to 49 years who had used oral contraceptives for five or more years, but this increased risk was not demonstrated in other age groups. In another study in Great Britain, the risk of developing cerebrovascular disease persisted for at least 6 years after discontinuation of oral contraceptives, although excess risk was very small. However, both studies were performed with oral-contraceptive formulations containing 50 mcg or higher of estrogen.

2. Estimates of Mortality from Contraceptive Use

One study gathered data from a variety of sources which have estimated the mortality rate associated with different methods of contraception at different ages (Table III). These estimates include the combined risk of death associated with contraceptive methods plus the risk attributable to pregnancy in the event of method failure. Each method of contraception has its specific benefits and risks. The study concluded that with the exception of oral-contraceptive users 35 and older who smoke and 40 and older who do not smoke, mortality associated with all methods of birth control is less than that associated with childbirth. The observation of a possible increase in risk of mortality with age for oral-contraceptive users is based on data gathered in the 1970's—but not reported until 1983. However, current clinical practice involves the use of lower estrogen dose formulations combined with careful restriction of oral-contraceptive use to women who do not have the various risk factors listed in this labeling.

Because of these changes in practice and, also, because of some limited new data which suggest that the risk of cardiovascular disease with the use of oral contraceptives may now be less than previously observed, the Fertility and Maternal Health Drugs Advisory Committee was asked to review the topic in 1989. The Committee concluded that although cardiovascular-disease risks may be increased with oral-contraceptive use after age 40 in healthy nonsmoking women (even with the newer low-dose formulations), there are greater potential health risks associated with pregnancy in older women and with the alternative surgical and medical procedures which may be necessary if such women do not have access to effective and acceptable means of contraception.

Therefore, the Committee recommended that the benefits of oral-contraceptive use by healthy nonsmoking women over 40 may outweigh the possible risks. Of course, older women, as all women who take oral contraceptives, should take the lowest possible dose formulation that is effective.

TABLE III–ANNUAL NUMBER OF BIRTH-RELATED OR METHOD-RELATED DEATHS ASSOCIATED WITH CONTROL OF FERTILITY PER 100,000 NONSTERILE WOMEN, BY FERTILITY-CONTROL METHOD AND ACCORDING TO AGE

Method of control and outcome	15-19	20-24	25-29	30-34	35-39	40-44
No fertility-control methods*	7.0	7.4	9.1	14.8	25.7	28.2
Oral contraceptives nonsmoker**	0.3	0.5	0.9	1.9	13.8	31.6
Oral contraceptives smoker**	2.2	3.4	6.6	13.5	51.1	117.2
IUD**	0.8	0.8	1.0	1.0	1.4	1.4
Condom*	1.1	1.6	0.7	0.2	0.3	0.4
Diaphragm/ spermicide*	1.9	1.2	1.2	1.3	2.2	2.8
Periodic abstinence*	2.5	1.6	1.6	1.7	2.9	3.6

*Deaths are birth related
**Deaths are method related
Adapted from H.W. Ory, Family Planning Perspectives, *15*:57–63, 1983.

3. Carcinoma of the Reproductive Organs and Breasts

Numerous epidemiological studies have examined the association between the use of oral contraceptives and the incidence of breast and cervical cancer.

The risk of having breast cancer diagnosed may be slightly increased among current and recent users of COCs. However, this excess risk appears to decrease over time after COC discontinuation and by 10 years after cessation the increased risk disappears. Some studies report an increased risk with duration of use while other studies do not and no consistent relationships have been found with dose or type of steroid. Some studies have reported a small increase in risk for women who first use COCs at a younger age. Most studies show a similar pattern of risk with COC use regardless of a woman's reproductive history or her family breast cancer history.

Breast cancers diagnosed in current or previous OC users tend to be less clinically advanced than in nonusers.

Women with known or suspected carcinoma of the breast or personal history of breast cancer should not use oral contraceptives because breast cancer is usually a hormonally-sensitive tumor.

Some studies suggest that oral-contraceptive use has been associated with an increase in the risk of cervical intraepithelial neoplasia or invasive cervical cancer in some populations of women. However, there continues to be controversy about the extent to which such findings may be due to differences in sexual behavior and other factors.

In spite of many studies of the relationship between combination oral-contraceptive use and breast and cervical cancers, a cause-and-effect relationship has not been established.

4. Hepatic Neoplasia

Benign hepatic adenomas are associated with oral-contraceptive use, although the incidence of benign tumors is rare in the United States. Indirect calculations have estimated the attributable risk to be in the range of 3.3 cases/100,000 for users, a risk that increases after four or more years of use. Rupture of rare, benign, hepatic adenomas may cause death through intra-abdominal hemorrhage.

Studies from Britain have shown an increased risk of developing hepatocellular carcinoma in long-term (>8 years) oral-contraceptive users.

However, these cancers are extremely rare in the U.S., and the attributable risk (the excess incidence) of liver cancers in oral-contraceptive users approaches less than one per million users.

5. Ocular Lesions

There have been clinical case reports of retinal thrombosis associated with the use of oral contraceptives that may lead to partial or complete loss of vision. Oral contraceptives should be discontinued if there is unexplained partial or complete loss of vision; onset of proptosis or diplopia; papilledema; or retinal vascular lesions. Appropriate diagnostic and therapeutic measures should be undertaken immediately.

6. Oral-Contraceptive Use Before or During Early Pregnancy

Extensive epidemiological studies have revealed no increased risk of birth defects in infants born to women who have used oral contraceptives prior to pregnancy. Studies also do not suggest a teratogenic effect, particularly insofar as cardiac anomalies and limb-reduction defects are concerned, when taken inadvertently during early pregnancy (see **CONTRAINDICATIONS** section).

The administration of oral contraceptives to induce withdrawal bleeding should not be used as a test for pregnancy. Oral contraceptives should not be used during pregnancy to treat threatened or habitual abortion.

It is recommended that for any patient who has missed two consecutive periods, pregnancy should be ruled out before continuing oral-contraceptive use. If the patient has not adhered to the prescribed schedule, the possibility of pregnancy should be considered at the time of the first missed

Continued on next page

Lo/Ovral-28—Cont.

period. Oral-contraceptive use should be discontinued if pregnancy is confirmed.

7. **Gallbladder Disease**

Combination oral contraceptives may worsen existing gallbladder disease and may accelerate the development of this disease in previously asymptomatic women. Earlier studies have reported an increased lifetime relative risk of gallbladder surgery in users of oral contraceptives and estrogens. More recent studies, however, have shown that the relative risk of developing gallbladder disease among oral-contraceptive users may be minimal. The recent findings of minimal risk may be related to the use of oral-contraceptive formulations containing lower hormonal doses of estrogens and progestogens.

8. **Carbohydrate and Lipid Metabolic Effects**

Oral contraceptives have been shown to cause glucose intolerance in a significant percentage of users. Oral contraceptives containing greater than 75 mcg of estrogens cause hyperinsulinism, while lower doses of estrogen cause less glucose intolerance. Progestogens increase insulin secretion and create insulin resistance, this effect varying with different progestational agents. However, in the nondiabetic woman, oral contraceptives appear to have no effect on fasting blood glucose. Because of these demonstrated effects, prediabetic and diabetic women should be carefully observed while taking oral contraceptives.

A small proportion of women will have persistent hypertriglyceridemia while on the pill. As discussed earlier (see **WARNINGS**, 1a. and 1d.; **PRECAUTIONS**, 3.), changes in serum triglycerides and lipoprotein levels have been reported in oral-contraceptive users.

9. **Elevated Blood Pressure**

Women with uncontrolled hypertension should not be started on hormonal contraception. An increase in blood pressure has been reported in women taking oral contraceptives, and this increase is more likely in older oral-contraceptive users and with continued use. Data from the Royal College of General Practitioners and subsequent randomized trials have shown that the incidence of hypertension increases with increasing quantities of progestogens.

Women with a history of hypertension or hypertension-related diseases, or renal disease, should be encouraged to use another method of contraception. If women with hypertension elect to use oral contraceptives, they should be monitored closely, and if significant elevation of blood pressure occurs, oral contraceptives should be discontinued (see **CONTRAINDICATIONS** section). For most women, elevated blood pressure will return to normal after stopping oral contraceptives, and there is no difference in the occurrence of hypertension among ever- and never-users.

10. **Headache**

The onset or exacerbation of migraine or development of headache with a new pattern that is recurrent, persistent, or severe requires discontinuation of oral contraceptives and evaluation of the cause. (See **WARNINGS** 1c. and **CONTRAINDICATIONS**.)

11. **Bleeding Irregularities**

Breakthrough bleeding and spotting are sometimes encountered in patients on oral contraceptives, especially during the first three months of use. The type and dose of progestogen may be important. If bleeding persists or recurs, nonhormonal causes should be considered and adequate diagnostic measures taken to rule out malignancy or pregnancy in the event of breakthrough bleeding, as in the case of any abnormal vaginal bleeding. If pathology has been excluded, time or a change to another formulation may solve the problem. In some women withdrawal bleeding may not occur during the "tablet-free" or "inactive-tablet" interval. If the COC has not been taken according to directions prior to the first missed withdrawal bleed, or if two consecutive withdrawal bleeds are missed, tablet-taking should be discontinued and a nonhormonal method of contraception should be used until the possibility of pregnancy is excluded.

Some women may encounter post-pill amenorrhea or oligomenorrhea (possibly with anovulation), especially when such a condition was pre-existent.

12. **Ectopic Pregnancy**

Ectopic as well as intrauterine pregnancy may occur in contraceptive failures.

PRECAUTIONS

1. **General**

Patients should be counseled that oral contraceptives do not protect against transmission of HIV (AIDS) and other sexually transmitted diseases (STDs) such as chlamydia, genital herpes, genital warts, gonorrhea, hepatitis B, and syphilis.

2. **Physical Examination and Follow-Up**

A periodic personal and family medical history and complete physical examination are appropriate for all women, including women using oral contraceptives. The physical examination, however, may be deferred until after initiation of oral contraceptives if requested by the woman and judged appropriate by the clinician. The physical examination should include special reference to blood pressure, breasts, abdomen and pelvic organs, including cervical cytology, and relevant laboratory tests. In case of undiagnosed, persistent or recurrent abnormal vaginal bleeding, appropriate diagnostic measures should be conducted to rule out malignancy. Women with a strong family history of breast cancer or who have breast nodules should be monitored with particular care.

3. **Lipid Disorders**

Women who are being treated for hyperlipidemias should be followed closely if they elect to use oral contraceptives. Some progestogens may elevate LDL levels and may render the control of hyperlipidemias more difficult. (See **WARNINGS**, 1a., 1d., and 8.)

In patients with defects of lipoprotein metabolism, estrogen-containing preparations may be associated with rare but significant elevations of plasma triglycerides which may lead to pancreatitis.

4. **Liver Function**

If jaundice develops in any woman receiving hormonal contraceptives, the medication should be discontinued. Steroid hormones may be poorly metabolized in patients with impaired liver function.

5. **Fluid Retention**

Oral contraceptives may cause some degree of fluid retention. They should be prescribed with caution, and only with careful monitoring, in patients with conditions which might be aggravated by fluid retention.

6. **Emotional Disorders**

Patients becoming significantly depressed while taking oral contraceptives should stop the medication and use an alternate method of contraception in an attempt to determine whether the symptom is drug-related. Women with a history of depression should be carefully observed and the drug discontinued if significant depression occurs.

7. **Contact Lenses**

Contact-lens wearers who develop visual changes or changes in lens tolerance should be assessed by an ophthalmologist.

8. **Gastrointestinal**

Diarrhea and/or vomiting may reduce hormone absorption resulting in decreased serum concentrations.

9. **Drug Interactions**

Changes in contraceptive effectiveness associated with coadministration of other products:

Contraceptive effectiveness may be reduced when hormonal contraceptives are coadministered with antibiotics, anticonvulsants, and other drugs that increase the metabolism of contraceptive steroids. This could result in unintended pregnancy or breakthrough bleeding. Examples include rifampin, rifabutin, barbiturates, primidone, phenylbutazone, phenytoin, dexamethasone, carbamazepine, felbamate, oxcarbazepine, topiramate, griseofulvin, and modafinil.

Several cases of contraceptive failure and breakthrough bleeding have been reported in the literature with concomitant administration of antibiotics such as ampicillin and other penicillins, and tetracyclines, possibly due to a decrease of enterohepatic recirculation of estrogens. However, clinical pharmacology studies investigating drug interactions between combined oral contraceptives and these antibiotics have reported inconsistent results. Enterohepatic recirculation of estrogens may also be decreased by substances that reduce gut transit time.

Several of the anti-HIV protease inhibitors have been studied with coadministration of oral combination hormonal contraceptives; significant changes (increase and decrease) in the plasma levels of the estrogen and progestin have been noted in some cases. The safety and efficacy of oral contraceptive products may be affected with coadministration of anti-HIV protease inhibitors. Health-care professionals should refer to the label of the individual anti-HIV protease inhibitors for further drug-drug interaction information.

Herbal products containing St. John's Wort (Hypericum perforatum) may induce hepatic enzymes (cytochrome P 450) and p-glycoprotein transporter and may reduce the effectiveness of contraceptive steroids. This may also result in breakthrough bleeding.

During concomitant use of ethinyl estradiol containing products and substances that may lead to decreased plasma steroid hormone concentrations, it is recommended that a nonhormonal back-up method of birth control be used in addition to the regular intake of Lo/Ovral-28. If the use of a substance which leads to decreased ethinyl estradiol plasma concentrations is required for a prolonged period of time, combination oral contraceptives should not be considered the primary contraceptive.

After discontinuation of substances that may lead to decreased ethinyl estradiol plasma concentrations, use of a nonhormonal back-up method of birth control is recommended for 7 days. Longer use of a back-up method is advisable after discontinuation of substances that have led to induction of hepatic microsomal enzymes, resulting in decreased ethinyl estradiol concentrations. It may take several weeks until enzyme induction has completely subsided, depending on dosage, duration of use, and rate of elimination of the inducing substance.

Increase in plasma levels associated with coadministered drugs:

Coadministration of atorvastatin and certain oral contraceptives containing ethinyl estradiol increase AUC values for ethinyl estradiol by approximately 20%. The mechanism of this interaction is unknown. Ascorbic acid and acetaminophen increase the bioavailability of ethinyl estradiol since these drugs act as competitive inhibitors for sulfation of ethinyl estradiol in the gastrointestinal wall, a known pathway of elimination for ethinyl estradiol. CYP 3A4 inhibitors such as indinavir, itraconazole, ketoconazole, fluconazole, and troleandomycin may increase plasma hormone levels. Troleandomycin may also increase the risk of intrahepatic cholestasis during coadministration with combination oral contraceptives.

Changes in plasma levels of coadministered drugs:

Combination hormonal contraceptives containing some synthetic estrogens (eg, ethinyl estradiol) may inhibit the metabolism of other compounds. Increased plasma concentrations of cyclosporin, prednisolone and other corticosteroids, and theophylline have been reported with concomitant administration of oral contraceptives. Decreased plasma concentrations of acetaminophen and increased clearance of temazepam, salicylic acid, morphine, and clofibric acid, due to induction of conjugation (particularly glucuronidation), have been noted when these drugs were administered with oral contraceptives.

The prescribing information of concomitant medications should be consulted to identify potential interactions.

10. **Interactions With Laboratory Tests**

Certain endocrine- and liver-function tests and blood components may be affected by oral contraceptives:

a. Increased prothrombin and factors VII, VIII, IX, and X; decreased antithrombin 3; increased norepinephrine-induced platelet aggregability.

b. Increased thyroid-binding globulin (TBG) leading to increased circulating total thyroid hormone, as measured by protein-bound iodine (PBI), T_4 by column or by radioimmunoassay. Free T_3 resin uptake is decreased, reflecting the elevated TBG; free T_4 concentration is unaltered.

c. Other binding proteins may be elevated in serum ie, corticosteroid binding globulin (CBG), sex hormone-binding globulins (SHBG) leading to increased levels of total circulating corticosteroids and sex steroids respectively. Free or biologically active hormone concentrations are unchanged.

d. Triglycerides may be increased and levels of various other lipids and lipoproteins may be affected.

e. Glucose tolerance may be decreased.

f. Serum folate levels may be depressed by oral-contraceptive therapy.

This may be of clinical significance if a woman becomes pregnant shortly after discontinuing oral contraceptives.

11. **Carcinogenesis**

See **WARNINGS** section.

12. **Pregnancy**

Pregnancy Category X. See **CONTRAINDICATIONS** and **WARNINGS** sections.

13. **Nursing Mothers**

Small amounts of oral-contraceptive steroids and/or metabolites have been identified in the milk of nursing mothers, and a few adverse effects on the child have been reported, including jaundice and breast enlargement. In addition, combination oral contraceptives given in the postpartum period may interfere with lactation by decreasing the quantity and quality of breast milk. If possible, the nursing mother should be advised not to use combination oral contraceptives but to use other forms of contraception until she has completely weaned her child.

14. **Fertility Following Discontinuation**

Users of combination oral contraceptives may experience some delay in becoming pregnant after discontinuation of COCs, especially those women who had irregular menstrual cycles prior to use. Conception may be delayed an average of 1-2 months among women stopping COCs compared to women stopping nonhormonal contraceptive methods.

Women who do not wish to become pregnant after discontinuation of COCs should be advised to use another method of birth control.

15. **Pediatric Use**

Safety and efficacy of Lo/Ovral-28 tablets have been established in women of reproductive age. Safety and efficacy are expected to be the same for postpubertal adolescents under the age of 16 and for users 16 years and older. Use of this product before menarche is not indicated.

16. **Geriatric Use**

This product has not been studied in women over 65 years of age and is not indicated in this population.

Information for the Patient

See Patient Labeling Printed Below.

ADVERSE REACTIONS

An increased risk of the following serious adverse reactions (see **WARNINGS** section for additional information) has been associated with the use of oral contraceptives:

Thromboembolic and thrombotic disorders and other vascular problems (including thrombophlebitis and venous thrombosis with or without pulmonary embolism, mesenteric thrombosis, arterial thromboembolism, myocardial infarction, cerebral hemorrhage, cerebral thrombosis), carcinoma of the reproductive organs and breasts, hepatic neoplasia (including hepatic adenomas or benign liver tumors), ocular lesions (including retinal vascular thrombosis), gallbladder disease, carbohydrate and lipid effects, elevated blood pressure, and headache including migraine.

The following adverse reactions have been reported in patients receiving oral contraceptives and are believed to be drug-related (alphabetically listed):

Acne
Amenorrhea
Anaphylactic/anaphylactoid reactions, including urticaria, angioedema, and severe reactions with respiratory and circulatory symptoms
Breakthrough bleeding
Breast changes: tenderness, pain, enlargement, secretion
Budd-Chiari syndrome
Cervical erosion and secretion, change in

Cholestatic jaundice
Chorea, exacerbation of
Colitis
Corneal curvature (steepening), change in
Diminution in lactation when given immediately postpartum
Dizziness
Edema/fluid retention
Erythema multiforme
Erythema nodosum
Gastrointestinal symptoms (such as abdominal pain, cramps, and bloating)
Hirsutism
Intolerance to contact lenses
Libido, changes in
Loss of scalp hair
Melasma/chloasma which may persist
Menstrual flow, change in
Mood changes, including depression
Nausea
Nervousness
Pancreatitis
Porphyria, exacerbation of
Rash (allergic)
Serum folate levels, decrease in
Spotting
Systemic lupus erythematosus, exacerbation of
Temporary infertility after discontinuation of treatment
Vaginitis, including candidiasis
Varicose veins, aggravation of
Vomiting
Weight or appetite (increase or decrease), change in

The following adverse reactions have been reported in users of oral contraceptives:
Cataracts
Cystitis-like syndrome
Dysmenorrhea
Hemolytic uremic syndrome
Hemorrhagic eruption
Optic neuritis, which may lead to partial or complete loss of vision
Porphyria
Premenstrual syndrome
Renal function, impaired

OVERDOSAGE

Symptoms of oral contraceptive overdosage in adults and children may include nausea, vomiting, and drowsiness/fatigue; withdrawal bleeding may occur in females. There is no specific antidote and further treatment of overdose, if necessary, is directed to the symptoms.

NONCONTRACEPTIVE HEALTH BENEFITS

The following noncontraceptive health benefits related to the use of oral contraceptives are supported by epidemiological studies which largely utilized oral-contraceptive formulations containing doses exceeding 0.035 mg of ethinyl estradiol or 0.05 mg of mestranol.

Effects on menses:
Increased menstrual cycle regularity
Decreased blood loss and decreased incidence of iron-deficiency anemia
Decreased incidence of dysmenorrhea

Effects related to inhibition of ovulation:
Decreased incidence of functional ovarian cysts
Decreased incidence of ectopic pregnancies

Effects from long-term use:
Decreased incidence of fibroadenomas and fibrocystic disease of the breast
Decreased incidence of acute pelvic inflammatory disease
Decreased incidence of endometrial cancer
Decreased incidence of ovarian cancer

DOSAGE AND ADMINISTRATION

To achieve maximum contraceptive effectiveness, Lo/Ovral-28 must be taken exactly as directed and at intervals not exceeding 24 hours. The possibility of ovulation and conception prior to initiation of medication should be considered.

The dosage of Lo/Ovral-28 is one white tablet daily for 21 consecutive days, followed by one pink inert tablet daily for 7 consecutive days, according to prescribed schedule. It is recommended that tablets be taken at the same time each day.

During the first cycle of medication, the patient is instructed to begin taking Lo/Ovral-28 on the first Sunday after the onset of menstruation. If menstruation begins on a Sunday, the first tablet (white) is taken that day. One white tablet should be taken daily for 21 consecutive days followed by one pink inert tablet daily for 7 consecutive days. Withdrawal bleeding should usually occur within three days following discontinuation of white tablets and may not have finished before the next pack is started. During the first cycle, contraceptive reliance should not be placed on Lo/Ovral-28 until a white tablet has been taken daily for 7 consecutive days and a nonhormonal back-up method of birth control should be used during those 7 days. The possibility of ovulation and conception prior to initiation of medication should be considered.

The patient begins her next and all subsequent 28-day courses of tablets on the same day of the week (Sunday) on which she began her first course, following the same schedule: 21 days on white tablets—7 days on pink inert tablets. If in any cycle the patient starts tablets later than the proper day, she should protect herself against pregnancy by using a nonhormonal back-up method of birth control until she has taken a white tablet daily for 7 consecutive days.

When the patient is switching from a 21-day regimen of tablets, she should wait 7 days after her last tablet before she starts Lo/Ovral-28. She will probably experience withdrawal bleeding during that week. She should be sure that no more than 7 days pass after her previous 21-day regimen. When the patient is switching from a 28-day regimen of tablets, she should start her first pack of Lo/Ovral-28 on the day after her last tablet. She should not wait any days between packs. The patient may switch any day from a progestin-only pill and should begin Lo/Ovral-28 the next day. If switching from an implant or injection, the patient should start Lo/Ovral-28 on the day of implant removal or the day the next injection would be due. In switching from a progestin-only pill, injection, or implant, the patient should be advised to use a nonhormonal back-up method of birth control for the first 7 days of tablet-taking.

If spotting or breakthrough bleeding occurs, the patient is instructed to continue on the same regimen. This type of bleeding is usually transient and without significance; however, if the bleeding is persistent or prolonged, the patient is advised to consult her health-care professional. Although pregnancy is unlikely if Lo/Ovral-28 is taken according to directions, if withdrawal bleeding does not occur, the possibility of pregnancy must be considered. If the patient has not adhered to the prescribed schedule (missed one or more tablets or started taking them on a day later than she should have), the probability of pregnancy should be considered at the time of the first missed period and appropriate diagnostic measures taken. If the patient has adhered to the prescribed regimen and misses two consecutive periods, pregnancy should be ruled out. Hormone contraception should be discontinued if pregnancy is confirmed.

For additional patient instructions regarding missed tablets, see the **WHAT TO DO IF YOU MISS PILLS** section in the **DETAILED PATIENT LABELING** below.

Any time the patient misses two or more white tablets, she should also use another method of contraception until she has taken a white tablet daily for seven consecutive days. If the patient misses one or more pink tablets, she is still protected against pregnancy **provided** she begins taking white tablets again on the proper day.

If breakthrough bleeding occurs following missed white tablets, it will usually be transient and of no consequence. The possibility of ovulation increases with each successive day that scheduled white tablets are missed.

Lo/Ovral-28 may be initiated no earlier than day 28 postpartum in the nonlactating mother or after a second-trimester abortion due to the increased risk for thromboembolism (see **CONTRAINDICATIONS WARNINGS**, and **PRECAUTIONS** concerning thromboembolic disease). The patient should be advised to use a nonhormonal back-up method for the first 7 days of tablet-taking. However, if intercourse has already occurred, pregnancy should be excluded before the start of combined oral contraceptive use or the patient must wait for her first menstrual period. In the case of first-trimester abortion, if the patient starts Lo/Ovral-28 immediately, additional contraceptive measures are not needed.

HOW SUPPLIED

Lo/Ovral®-28 Tablets (0.3 mg norgestrel and 0.03 mg ethinyl estradiol) are available in packages of 6 PILPAK® dispensers, each containing 28 tablets as follows:

21 active tablets, NDC 0008-0078, white, round tablet marked "WYETH" and "78".

7 inert tablets, NDC 0008-0486, pink, round tablet marked "WYETH" and "486".

Store at controlled room temperature 20°C to to 25°C (68°F to 77°F).

References available upon request.

Brief Summary Patient Package Insert

This product (like all oral contraceptives) is intended to prevent pregnancy. Oral contraceptives do not protect against transmission of HIV (AIDS) and other sexually transmitted diseases (STDs) such as chlamydia, genital herpes, genital warts, gonorrhea, hepatitis B, and syphilis.

Oral contraceptives, also known as "birth-control pills" or "the pill," are taken to prevent pregnancy, and when taken correctly, have a failure rate of approximately 1% per year when taken without missing any pills. The average failure rate is approximately 5% per year when women who miss pills are included. For most women oral contraceptives are also free of serious or unpleasant side effects. However, forgetting to take pills considerably increases the chances of pregnancy.

For the majority of women, oral contraceptives can be taken safely. But there are some women who are at high risk of developing certain serious diseases that can be life-threatening or may cause temporary or permanent disability or death. The risks associated with taking oral contraceptives increase significantly if you:

- smoke
- have high blood pressure, diabetes, high cholesterol, or a tendency to form blood clots, or are obese
- have or have had clotting disorders, heart attack, stroke, angina pectoris, cancer of the breast or sex organs, jaundice, malignant or benign liver tumors, or major surgery with prolonged immobilization
- have headaches with neurological symptoms

You should not take the pill if you suspect you are pregnant or have unexplained vaginal bleeding.

Cigarette smoking increases the risk of serious adverse effects on the heart and blood vessels from oral-contraceptive use. This risk increases with age and with the amount of smoking (15 or more cigarettes per day has been associated with a significantly increased risk) and is quite marked in women over 35 years of age. Women who use oral contraceptives should not smoke.

Most side effects of the pill are not serious. The most common such effects are nausea, vomiting, bleeding between menstrual periods, weight gain, breast tenderness, and difficulty wearing contact lenses. These side effects, especially nausea and vomiting, may subside within the first three months of use.

The serious side effects of the pill occur very infrequently, especially if you are in good health and do not smoke. However, you should know that the following medical conditions have been associated with or made worse by the pill:

1. Blood clots in the legs (thrombophlebitis), lungs (pulmonary embolism), stoppage or rupture of a blood vessel in the brain (stroke), blockage of blood vessels in the heart (heart attack and angina pectoris) or other organs of the body. As mentioned above, smoking increases the risk of heart attacks and strokes and subsequent serious medical consequences. Women with migraine also may be at increased risk of stroke with pill use.

2. Liver tumors, which may rupture and cause severe bleeding. A possible but not definite association has been found with the pill and liver cancer. However, liver cancers are extremely rare. The chance of developing liver cancer from using the pill is thus even rarer.

3. High blood pressure, although blood pressure usually returns to normal when the pill is stopped.

The symptoms associated with these serious side effects are discussed in the detailed leaflet given to you with your supply of pills. Notify your health-care professional if you notice any unusual physical disturbances while taking the pill. In addition, drugs such as rifampin, as well as some anticonvulsants and some antibiotics, herbal preparations containing St. John's Wort (Hypericum perforatum), and HIV/AIDS drugs may decrease oral-contraceptive effectiveness.

Various studies give conflicting reports on the relationship between breast cancer and oral-contraceptive use.

Oral-contraceptive use may slightly increase your chance of having breast cancer diagnosed, particularly if you started using hormonal contraceptives at a younger age.

After you stop using hormonal contraceptives, the chances of having breast cancer diagnosed begin to go down and disappear 10 years after stopping use of the pill. It is not known whether this slightly increased risk of having breast cancer diagnosed is caused by the pill. It may be that women taking the pill were examined more often, so that breast cancer was more likely to be detected.

You should have regular breast examinations by a health-care professional and examine your own breasts monthly. Tell your health-care professional if you have a family history of breast cancer or if you have had breast nodules or an abnormal mammogram. Women who currently have or have had breast cancer should not use oral contraceptives because breast cancer is usually a hormone-sensitive tumor.

Some studies have found an increase in the incidence of cancer of the cervix in women who use oral contraceptives. However, this finding may be related to factors other than the use of oral contraceptives. There is insufficient evidence to rule out the possibility that the pill may cause such cancers.

Taking the combination pill provides some important noncontraceptive health benefits. These include less painful menstruation, less menstrual blood loss and anemia, fewer pelvic infections, and fewer cancers of the ovary and the lining of the uterus.

Be sure to discuss any medical condition you may have with your health-care professional. Your health-care professional will take a medical and family history before prescribing oral contraceptives and will examine you. The physical examination may be delayed to another time if you request it and the health-care professional believes that it is appropriate to postpone it. You should be reexamined at least once a year while taking oral contraceptives. The detailed patient information leaflet gives you further information which you should read and discuss with your health-care professional.

This product (like all oral contraceptives) is intended to prevent pregnancy. It does not protect against transmission of HIV (AIDS) and other sexually transmitted diseases such as chlamydia, genital herpes, genital warts, gonorrhea, hepatitis B, and syphilis.

DETAILED PATIENT LABELING

This product (like all oral contraceptives) is intended to prevent pregnancy. Oral contraceptives do not protect against transmission of HIV (AIDS) and other sexually transmitted diseases (STDs) such as chlamydia, genital herpes, genital warts, gonorrhea, hepatitis B, and syphilis.

INTRODUCTION

Any woman who considers using oral contraceptives (the "birth-control pill" or "the pill") should understand the benefits and risks of using this form of birth control. This leaflet will give you much of the information you will need to make

Continued on next page

Lo/Ovral-28—Cont.

this decision and will also help you determine if you are at risk of developing any of the serious side effects of the pill. It will tell you how to take the pill properly so that it will be as effective as possible. However, this leaflet is not a replacement for a careful discussion between you and your health-care professional. You should discuss the information provided in this leaflet with him or her, both when you first start taking the pill and during your revisits. You should also follow your health-care professional's advice with regard to regular check-ups while you are on the pill.

EFFECTIVENESS OF ORAL CONTRACEPTIVES

Oral contraceptives or "birth-control pills" or "the pill" are used to prevent pregnancy and are more effective than most other nonsurgical methods of birth control. When they are taken correctly without missing any pills, the chance of becoming pregnant is approximately 1% per year. Average failure rates are approximately 5% per year when women who miss pills are included. The chance of becoming pregnant increases with each missed pill during the menstrual cycle.

In comparison, average failure rates for other methods of birth control during the first year of use are as follows:

IUD: 0.1-2%	Female condom alone: 21%
Depo-Provera® (injectable progestogen): 0.3%	Cervical cap
Norplant® System (levonorgestrel implants): 0.05%	Never given birth: 20%
Diaphragm with spermicides: 20%	Given birth: 40%
Spermidices alone: 26%	Periodic abstinence: 25%
Male condom alone: 14%	No methods: 85%

WHO SHOULD NOT TAKE ORAL CONTRACEPTIVES

Cigarette smoking increases the risk of serious adverse effects on the heart and blood vessels from oral-contraceptive use. This risk increases with age and with the amount of smoking (15 or more cigarettes per day has been associated with a significantly increased risk) and is quite marked in women over 35 years of age. Women who use oral contraceptives should not smoke.

Some women should not take the pill. You should not take the pill if you have any of the following conditions:

- History of heart attack or stroke
- History of blood clots in the legs (thrombophlebitis), lungs (pulmonary embolism), or eyes
- History of blood clots in the deep veins of your legs
- Known or suspected breast cancer or cancer of the lining of the uterus, cervix, or vagina or certain hormonally-sensitive cancers
- Liver tumor (benign or cancerous)
- Chest pain (angina pectoris)
- Unexplained vaginal bleeding (until a diagnosis is reached by your health-care professional)
- Yellowing of the whites of the eyes or of the skin (jaundice) during pregnancy or during previous use of the pill
- Known or suspected pregnancy
- Heart valve or heart rhythm disorders that may be associated with formation of blood clots
- Diabetes affecting your circulation
- Headaches with neurological symptoms
- Uncontrolled high blood pressure
- Active liver disease with abnormal liver function tests
- Allergy or hypersensitivity to any of the components of Lo/Ovral-28
- A need for surgery with prolonged bedrest

Tell your health-care professional if you have any of these conditions. Your health-care professional can recommend another method of birth control.

OTHER CONSIDERATIONS BEFORE TAKING ORAL CONTRACEPTIVES

Tell your health-care professional if you or any family member has ever had:

- Breast nodules, fibrocystic disease of the breast, an abnormal breast X-ray or mammogram
- Diabetes
- Elevated cholesterol or triglycerides
- High blood pressure
- A tendency to form blood clots
- Migraine or other headaches or epilepsy
- Depression
- Gallbladder, liver, heart, or kidney disease
- History of scanty or irregular menstrual periods

Women with any of these conditions should be checked often by their health-care professional if they choose to use oral contraceptives. Also, be sure to inform your health-care professional if you smoke or are on any medications.

RISKS OF TAKING ORAL CONTRACEPTIVES

1. *Risk of developing blood clots*

Blood clots and blockage of blood vessels are the most serious side effects of taking oral contraceptives and can cause death or serious disability. In particular, a clot in the legs can cause thrombophlebitis and a clot that travels to the lungs can cause a sudden blocking of the vessel carrying blood to the lungs. Rarely, clots occur in the blood vessels of the eye and may cause blindness, double vision, or impaired vision.

Users of COCs have a higher risk of developing blood clots compared to nonusers. This risk is highest during the first year of COC use.

If you take oral contraceptives and need elective surgery, need to stay in bed for a prolonged illness or injury, or have recently delivered a baby, you may be at risk of developing blood clots. You should consult your health-care professional about stopping oral contraceptives three to four weeks before surgery and not taking oral contraceptives for two weeks after surgery or during bed rest. You should also not take oral contraceptives soon after delivery of a baby or a midtrimester pregnancy termination. It is advisable to wait for at least four weeks after delivery if you are not breast-feeding. If you are breast-feeding, you should wait until you have weaned your child before using the pill. (See also the section on breast-feeding in GENERAL PRECAUTIONS.)

2. *Heart attacks and strokes*

Oral contraceptives may increase the tendency to develop strokes (stoppage or rupture of blood vessels in the brain) and angina pectoris and heart attacks (blockage of blood vessels in the heart). Any of these conditions can cause death or serious disability.

Smoking greatly increases the possibility of suffering heart attacks and strokes. Furthermore, smoking and the use of oral contraceptives greatly increase the chances of developing and dying of heart disease.

Women with migraine (especially migraine/headache with neurological symptoms) who take oral contraceptives also may be at higher risk of stroke.

3. *Gallbladder disease*

Oral-contraceptive users probably have a greater risk than nonusers of having gallbladder disease. This risk may be related to pills containing high doses of estrogens. Oral contraceptives may worsen existing gallbladder disease or accelerate the development of gallbladder disease in women previously without symptoms.

4. *Liver tumors*

In rare cases, oral contraceptives can cause benign but dangerous liver tumors. These benign liver tumors can rupture and cause fatal internal bleeding. In addition, a possible but not definite association has been found with the pill and liver cancers in two studies in which a few women who developed these very rare cancers were found to have used oral contraceptives for long periods. However, liver cancers are extremely rare. The chance of developing liver cancer from using the pill is thus even rarer.

5. *Cancer of the reproductive organs and breasts*

Various studies give conflicting reports on the relationship between breast cancer and oral-contraceptive use.

Oral-contraceptive use may slightly increase your chance of having breast cancer diagnosed, particularly if you started using hormonal contraceptives at a younger age.

After you stop using hormonal contraceptives, the chances of having breast cancer diagnosed begin to go down and disappear 10 years after stopping use of the pill. It is not known whether this slightly increased risk of having breast cancer diagnosed is caused by the pill. It may be that women taking the pill were examined more often, so that breast cancer was more likely to be detected.

You should have regular breast examinations by a health-care professional and examine your own breasts monthly. Tell your health-care professional if you have a family history of breast cancer or if you have had breast nodules or an abnormal mammogram. Women who currently have or have had breast cancer should not use oral contraceptives because breast cancer is usually a hormone-sensitive tumor.

Some studies have found an increase in the incidence of cancer of the cervix in women who use oral contraceptives. However, this finding may be related to factors other than the use of oral contraceptives. There is insufficient evidence to rule out the possibility that the pill may cause such cancers.

6. *Lipid metabolism and inflammation of the pancreas*

In patients with abnormal lipid levels, there have been reports of significant increases in plasma triglycerides during estrogen therapy. This has led to inflammation of the pancreas in some cases.

ESTIMATED RISK OF DEATH FROM A BIRTH-CONTROL METHOD OR PREGNANCY

All methods of birth control and pregnancy are associated with a risk of developing certain diseases which may lead to disability or death. An estimate of the number of deaths associated with different methods of birth control and pregnancy has been calculated and is shown in the following table.

ANNUAL NUMBER OF BIRTH-RELATED OR METHOD-RELATED DEATHS ASSOCIATED WITH CONTROL OF FERTILITY PER 100,000 NONSTERILE WOMEN, BY FERTILITY-CONTROL METHOD AND ACCORDING TO AGE

Method of control and outcome	15-19	20-24	25-29	30-34	35-39	40-44
No fertility-control methods*	7.0	7.4	9.1	14.8	25.7	28.2
Oral contraceptives nonsmoker**	0.3	0.5	0.9	1.9	13.8	31.6
Oral contraceptives smoker**	2.2	3.4	6.6	13.5	51.1	117.2
IUD**	0.8	0.8	1.0	1.0	1.4	1.4
Condom*	1.1	1.6	0.7	0.2	0.3	0.4
Diaphragm/ spermicide*	1.9	1.2	1.2	1.3	2.2	2.8
Periodic abstinence*	2.5	1.6	1.6	1.7	2.9	3.6

*Deaths are birth related
**Deaths are method related

In the above table, the risk of death from any birth-control method is less than the risk of childbirth, except for oral-contraceptive users over the age of 35 who smoke and pill users over the age of 40 even if they do not smoke. It can be seen in the table that for women aged 15 to 39, the risk of death was highest with pregnancy (7 to 26 deaths per 100,000 women, depending on age). Among pill users who do not smoke, the risk of death was always lower than that associated with pregnancy for any age group, except for those women over the age of 40, when the risk increases to 32 deaths per 100,000 women, compared to 28 associated with pregnancy at that age. However, for pill users who smoke and are over the age of 35, the estimated number of deaths exceeds those for other methods of birth control. If a woman is over the age of 40 and smokes, her estimated risk of death is four times higher (117/100,000 women) than the estimated risk associated with pregnancy (28/100,000 women) in that age group.

The suggestion that women over 40 who do not smoke should not take oral contraceptives is based on information from older high-dose pills. An Advisory Committee of the FDA discussed this issue in 1989 and recommended that the benefits of oral-contraceptive use by healthy, nonsmoking women over 40 years of age may outweigh the possible risks. Older women, as all women who take oral contraceptives, should take an oral contraceptive which contains the least amount of estrogen and progestogen that is compatible with the individual patient needs.

WARNING SIGNALS

If any of these adverse effects occur while you are taking oral contraceptives, call your health-care professional immediately:

- Sharp chest pain, coughing of blood, or sudden shortness of breath (indicating a possible clot in the lung)
- Pain in the calf (indicating a possible clot in the leg)
- Crushing chest pain or heaviness in the chest (indicating a possible heart attack)
- Sudden severe headache or vomiting, dizziness or fainting, disturbances of vision or speech, weakness, or numbness in an arm or leg (indicating a possible stroke)
- Sudden partial or complete loss of vision (indicating a possible clot in the eye)
- Breast lumps (indicating possible breast cancer or fibrocystic disease of the breast; ask your health-care professional to show you how to examine your breasts)
- Severe pain or tenderness in the stomach area (indicating a possibly ruptured liver tumor)
- Difficulty in sleeping, weakness, lack of energy, fatigue, or change in mood (possibly indicating severe depression)
- Jaundice or a yellowing of the skin or eyeballs, accompanied frequently by fever, fatigue, loss of appetite, dark-colored urine, or light-colored bowel movements (indicating possible liver problems)

SIDE EFFECTS OF ORAL CONTRACEPTIVES

1. *Irregular vaginal bleeding*

Irregular vaginal bleeding or spotting may occur while you are taking the pills. Irregular bleeding may vary from slight staining between menstrual periods to breakthrough bleeding which is a flow much like a regular period. Irregular bleeding occurs most often during the first few months of oral-contraceptive use, but may also occur after you have been taking the pill for some time. Such bleeding may be temporary and usually does not indicate any serious problems. It is important to continue taking your pills on schedule. If the bleeding occurs in more than one cycle or lasts for more than a few days, talk to your health-care professional.

2. *Contact lenses*

If you wear contact lenses and notice a change in vision or an inability to wear your lenses, contact your health-care professional.

3. *Fluid retention*

Oral contraceptives may cause edema (fluid retention) with swelling of the fingers or ankles and may raise your blood pressure. If you experience fluid retention, contact your health-care professional.

4. *Melasma*

A spotty darkening of the skin is possible, particularly of the face.

5. *Other side effects*

Other side effects may include nausea, breast tenderness, change in appetite, headache, nervousness, depression, dizziness, loss of scalp hair, rash, vaginal infections, inflammation of the pancreas, and allergic reactions.

If any of these side effects bother you, call your health-care professional.

GENERAL PRECAUTIONS

1. *Missed periods and use of oral contraceptives before or during early pregnancy*

There may be times when you may not menstruate regularly after you have completed taking a cycle of pills. If you have taken your pills regularly and miss one menstrual period, continue taking your pills for the next cycle but be sure to inform your health-care professional. If you have not taken the pills daily as instructed and missed a menstrual period, or if you missed two consecutive menstrual periods, you may be pregnant. Check with your health-care professional immediately to determine whether you are pregnant. Stop taking oral contraceptives if pregnancy is confirmed.

There is no conclusive evidence that oral-contraceptive use is associated with an increase in birth defects when taken inadvertently during early pregnancy. Previously, a few studies had reported that oral contraceptives might be associated with birth defects, but these findings have not been confirmed in more recent studies. Nevertheless, oral contraceptives should not be used during pregnancy. You should check with your health-care professional about risks to your unborn child of any medication taken during pregnancy.

2. *While breast-feeding*

If you are breast-feeding, consult your health-care professional before starting oral contraceptives. Some of the drug will be passed on to the child in the milk. A few adverse effects on the child have been reported, including yellowing of the skin (jaundice) and breast enlargement. In addition, oral contraceptives may decrease the amount and quality of your milk. If possible, do not use oral contraceptives while breast-feeding. You should use another method of contraception since breast-feeding provides only partial protection from becoming pregnant, and this partial protection decreases significantly as you breast-feed for longer periods of time. You should consider starting oral contraceptives only after you have weaned your child completely.

3. *Laboratory tests*

If you are scheduled for any laboratory tests, tell your health-care professional you are taking birth-control pills. Certain blood tests may be affected by birth-control pills.

4. *Drug interactions*

Certain drugs may interact with birth-control pills to make them less effective in preventing pregnancy or cause an increase in breakthrough bleeding. Such drugs include rifampin, drugs used for epilepsy such as barbiturates (for example, phenobarbital) and phenytoin (Dilantin® is one brand of this drug), primidone (Mysoline®), topiramate (Topamax®), carbamazepine (Tegretol® is one brand of this drug), phenylbutazone (Butazolidin® is one brand of this drug), some drugs used for HIV or AIDS such as ritonavir (Norvir®), modafinil (Provigil®), possibly certain antibiotics (such as ampicillin and other penicillins, and tetracyclines), and herbal products containing St. John's Wort (Hypericum perforatum). You may also need to use a nonhormonal method of contraception (such as condoms and/or spermicide) during any cycle in which you take drugs that can make oral contraceptives less effective.

You may be at a higher risk of a specific type of liver dysfunction if you take troleandomycin and oral contraceptives at the same time.

Be sure to tell your health-care professional if you are taking or start taking any other medications, including nonprescription products or herbal products while taking birth control pills.

5. *Sexually transmitted diseases*

This product (like all oral contraceptives) is intended to prevent pregnancy. It does not protect against transmission of HIV (AIDS) and other sexually transmitted diseases such as chlamydia, genital herpes, genital warts, gonorrhea, hepatitis B, and syphilis.

HOW TO TAKE THE PILL

IMPORTANT POINTS TO REMEMBER

BEFORE YOU START TAKING YOUR PILLS:

1. BE SURE TO READ THESE DIRECTIONS:

Before you start taking your pills.

And

Anytime you are not sure what to do.

2. THE RIGHT WAY TO TAKE THE PILL IS TO TAKE ONE PILL EVERY DAY AT THE SAME TIME.

If you miss pills you could get pregnant. This includes starting the pack late. The more pills you miss, the more likely you are to get pregnant.

3. MANY WOMEN HAVE SPOTTING OR LIGHT BLEEDING, OR MAY FEEL SICK TO THEIR STOMACH DURING THE FIRST 1-3 PACKS OF PILLS.

If you feel sick to your stomach, do not stop taking the pill. The problem will usually go away. If it doesn't go away, check with your health-care professional.

4. MISSING PILLS CAN ALSO CAUSE SPOTTING OR LIGHT BLEEDING, even when you make up these missed pills.

On the days you take 2 pills to make up for missed pills, you could also feel a little sick to your stomach.

5. IF YOU HAVE VOMITING (within 4 hours after you take your pill), you should follow the instructions for WHAT TO DO IF YOU MISS PILLS. IF YOU HAVE DIARRHEA, or IF YOU TAKE SOME MEDICINES, including some antibiotics, your pills may not work as well. Use a back-up nonhormonal method (such as condoms and/or spermicide) until you check with your health-care professional.

6. IF YOU HAVE TROUBLE REMEMBERING TO TAKE THE PILL, talk to your health-care professional about how to make pill-taking easier or about using another method of birth control.

7. IF YOU HAVE ANY QUESTIONS OR ARE UNSURE ABOUT THE INFORMATION IN THIS LEAFLET, call your health-care professional.

LO/OVRAL® & LO/OVRAL®-28 TABLETS (norgestrel and ethinyl estradiol tablets).

BEFORE YOU START TAKING YOUR PILLS

1. DECIDE WHAT TIME OF DAY YOU WANT TO TAKE YOUR PILL.

It is important to take it at about the same time every day.

2. LOOK AT YOUR PILL PACK TO SEE IF IT HAS 21 OR 28 PILLS:

The *21-pill pack* has 21 "active" white pills (with hormones) to take for 3 weeks, followed by 1 week without pills.

The *28-pill pack* has 21 "active" white pills (with hormones) to take for 3 weeks, followed by 1 week of reminder pink pills (without hormones).

3. ALSO FIND:

1) where on the pack to start taking pills, and

2) in what order to take the pills (follow the arrows).

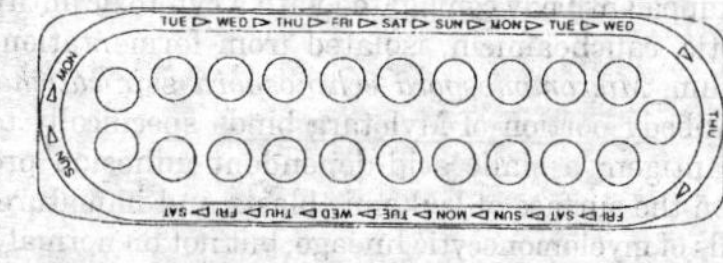

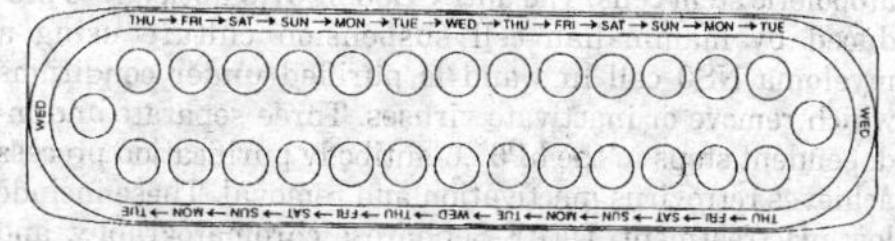

4. BE SURE YOU HAVE READY AT ALL TIMES:

ANOTHER KIND OF BIRTH CONTROL (such as condoms and/or spermicide) to use as a back-up in case you miss pills.

AN EXTRA, FULL PILL PACK.

WHEN TO START THE FIRST PACK OF PILLS

For the 21-day pill pack you have two choices of which day to start taking your first pack of pills. (See **DAY 1 START** or **SUNDAY START** directions below.) Decide with your health-care professional which is the best day for you. The 28-day pill pack accommodates a **SUNDAY START** only. For either pill pack pick a time of day which will be easy to remember.

DAY 1 START:

These instructions are for the 21-day pill pack only. The 28-day pill pack does not accommodate a **DAY 1 START** dosage regimen.

1. Take the first "active" white pill of the first pack during the *first 24 hours of your period.*

2. You will not need to use a back-up nonhormonal method of birth control, since you are starting the pill at the beginning of your period.

SUNDAY START:

These instructions are for either the 21-day or the 28-day pill pack.

1. Take the first "active" white pill of the first pack on the *Sunday after your period starts*, even if you are still bleeding. If your period begins on Sunday, start the pack that same day.

2. *Use a nonhormonal method of birth control* (such as condoms and/or spermicide) as a back-up method if you have sex anytime from the Sunday you start your first pack until the next Sunday (7 days).

WHAT TO DO DURING THE MONTH

1. TAKE ONE PILL AT THE SAME TIME EVERY DAY UNTIL THE PACK IS EMPTY.

Do not skip pills even if you are spotting or bleeding between monthly periods or feel sick to your stomach (nausea).

Do not skip pills even if you do not have sex very often.

2. WHEN YOU FINISH A PACK OR SWITCH YOUR BRAND OF PILLS:

21 pills: Wait 7 days to start the next pack. You will probably have your period during that week. Be sure that no more than 7 days pass between 21-day packs.

28 pills: Start the next pack on the day after your last "reminder" pill. Do not wait any days between packs.

WHAT TO DO IF YOU MISS PILLS

The pill may not be as effective if you miss white "active" pills, and particularly if you miss the first few or the last few white "active" pills in a pack.

If you **MISS 1** white "active" pill:

1. Take it as soon as you remember. Take the next pill at your regular time. This means you may take 2 pills in 1 day.

2. You COULD BECOME PREGNANT if you have sex in the *7 days* after you miss pills. You MUST use a nonhormonal birth-control method (such as condoms and/or spermicide) as a back-up for those 7 days.

If you **MISS 2** white "active" pills in a row in **WEEK 1 OR WEEK 2** of your pack:

1. Take 2 pills on the day you remember and 2 pills the next day.

2. Then take 1 pill a day until you finish the pack.

3. You COULD BECOME PREGNANT if you have sex in the *7 days* after you miss pills. You MUST use a nonhormonal birth-control method (such as condoms and/or spermicide) as a back-up for those 7 days.

If you **MISS 2** white "active" pills in a row in **THE 3rd WEEK:**

The ***Day 1 Starter*** instructions are for the 21-day pill pack only. The 28-day pill pack does not accommodate a **DAY 1 START** dosage regimen. The ***Sunday Starter*** instructions are for either the 21-day or 28-day pill pack.

1. ***If you are a Day 1 Starter:***

THROW OUT the rest of the pill pack and start a new pack that same day.

If you are a Sunday Starter:

Keep taking 1 pill every day until Sunday.

On Sunday, THROW OUT the rest of the pack and start a new pack of pills that same day.

2. You may not have your period this month but this is expected. However, if you miss your period 2 months in a row, call your health-care professional because you might be pregnant.

3. You COULD BECOME PREGNANT if you have sex in the *7 days* after you miss pills. You MUST use a nonhormonal birth-control method (such as condoms and/or spermicide) as a back-up for those 7 days.

If you **MISS 3 OR MORE** white "active" pills in a row (during the first 3 weeks):

The ***Day 1 Starter*** instructions are for the 21-day pill pack only. The 28-day pill pack does not accommodate a **DAY 1 START** dosage regimen. The ***Sunday Starter*** instructions are for either the 21-day or 28-day pill pack.

1. ***If you are a Day 1 Starter:***

THROW OUT the rest of the pill pack and start a new pack that same day.

If you are a Sunday Starter:

Keep taking 1 pill every day until Sunday.

On Sunday, THROW OUT the rest of the pack and start a new pack of pills that same day.

2. You may not have your period this month but this is expected. However, if you miss your period 2 months in a row, call your health-care professional because you might be pregnant.

3. You COULD BECOME PREGNANT if you have sex in the *7 days* after you miss pills. You MUST use a nonhormonal birth-control method (such as condoms and/or spermicide) as a back-up for those 7 days.

A REMINDER FOR THOSE ON 28-DAY PACKS

If you forget any of the 7 pink "reminder" pills in Week 4:

THROW AWAY the pills you missed.

Keep taking 1 pill each day until the pack is empty.

You do not need a back-up nonhormonal birth-control method if you start your next pack on time.

FINALLY, IF YOU ARE STILL NOT SURE WHAT TO DO ABOUT THE PILLS YOU HAVE MISSED

Use a BACK-UP NONHORMONAL BIRTH-CONTROL METHOD anytime you have sex.

KEEP TAKING ONE PILL EACH DAY until you can reach your health-care professional.

PREGNANCY DUE TO PILL FAILURE

The incidence of pill failure resulting in pregnancy is approximately 1% if taken every day as directed, but the average failure rate is approximately 5% including women who do not always take the pill exactly as directed without missing any pills. If you do become pregnant, the risk to the fetus is minimal, but you should stop taking your pills and discuss the pregnancy with your health-care professional.

PREGNANCY AFTER STOPPING THE PILL

There may be some delay in becoming pregnant after you stop using oral contraceptives, especially if you had irregular menstrual cycles before you used oral contraceptives. It may be advisable to postpone conception until you begin menstruating regularly once you have stopped taking the pill and desire pregnancy.

There does not appear to be any increase in birth defects in newborn babies when pregnancy occurs soon after stopping the pill.

If you do not desire pregnancy, you should use another method of birth control immediately after stopping the oral contraceptive pill.

OVERDOSAGE

Overdosage may cause nausea, vomiting, and fatigue/drowsiness. Withdrawal bleeding may occur in females. In case of overdosage, contact your health-care professional or pharmacist.

OTHER INFORMATION

Your health-care professional will take a medical and family history before prescribing oral contraceptives and will examine you. The physical examination may be delayed to another time if you request it and the health-care professional believes that it is appropriate to postpone it. You should be reexamined at least once a year. Be sure to inform your health-care professional if there is a family history of any of the conditions listed previously in this leaflet. Be sure to keep all appointments with your health-care professional, because this is a time to determine if there are early signs of side effects of oral-contraceptive use.

Continued on next page

Lo/Ovral-28—Cont.

Do not use the drug for any condition other than the one for which it was prescribed. This drug has been prescribed specifically for you; do not give it to others who may want birth-control pills.

HEALTH BENEFITS FROM ORAL CONTRACEPTIVES

In addition to preventing pregnancy, use of oral contraceptives may provide certain benefits. They are:

- Menstrual cycles may become more regular.
- Blood flow during menstruation may be lighter, and less iron may be lost. Therefore, anemia due to iron deficiency is less likely to occur.
- Pain or other symptoms during menstruation may be encountered less frequently.
- Ovarian cysts may occur less frequently.
- Ectopic (tubal) pregnancy may occur less frequently.
- Noncancerous cysts or lumps in the breast may occur less frequently.
- Acute pelvic inflammatory disease may occur less frequently.
- Oral-contraceptive use may provide some protection against developing two forms of cancer: cancer of the ovaries and cancer of the lining of the uterus.

If you want more information about birth-control pills, ask your health-care professional or pharmacist. They have a more technical leaflet called the Professional Labeling which you may wish to read.

Wyeth®
Wyeth Pharmaceuticals Inc.
Philadelphia, PA 19101

W10468C002
ET01
Rev 04/04

Shown in Product Identification Guide, page 336

MYLOTARG® ℞

[*mī'lō-tărg*]
(gemtuzumab ozogamicin for Injection)
FOR INTRAVENOUS USE ONLY
℞ only

This product's label may have been revised after this insert was used in production. For further product information and current package insert, please visit www.wyeth.com or call our medical communications department toll-free at 1-800-934-5556.

WARNINGS

Mylotarg should be administered under the supervision of physicians experienced in the treatment of acute leukemia and in facilities equipped to monitor and treat leukemia patients.

There are no controlled trials demonstrating efficacy and safety using Mylotarg in combination with other chemotherapeutic agents. Therefore, Mylotarg should only be used as single agent chemotherapy and not in combination chemotherapy regimens outside clinical trials.

Severe myelosuppression occurs when Mylotarg is used at recommended doses.

HYPERSENSITIVITY REACTIONS INCLUDING ANAPHYLAXIS, INFUSION REACTIONS, PULMONARY EVENTS

Mylotarg administration can result in severe hypersensitivity reactions (including anaphylaxis), and other infusion-related reactions which may include severe pulmonary events. Infrequently, hypersensitivity reactions and pulmonary events have been fatal. In most cases, infusion-related symptoms occurred during the infusion or within 24 hours of administration of Mylotarg and resolved. Mylotarg infusion should be interrupted for patients experiencing dyspnea or clinically significant hypotension. Patients should be monitored until signs and symptoms completely resolve. Discontinuation of Mylotarg treatment should be strongly considered for patients who develop anaphylaxis, pulmonary edema, or acute respiratory distress syndrome. Since patients with high peripheral blast counts may be at greater risk for pulmonary events and tumor lysis syndrome, physicians should consider leukoreduction with hydroxyurea or leukapheresis to reduce the peripheral white count to below 30,000/μL prior to administration of Mylotarg. (See **WARNINGS**.)

HEPATOTOXICITY:

Hepatotoxicity, including severe hepatic veno-occlusive disease (VOD), has been reported in association with the use of Mylotarg as a single agent, as part of a combination chemotherapy regimen, and in patients without a history of liver disease or hematopoietic stem-cell transplant (HSCT). Patients who receive Mylotarg either before or after HSCT, patients with underlying hepatic disease or abnormal liver function, and patients receiving Mylotarg in combinations with other chemotherapy are at increased risk for developing VOD, including severe VOD. Death from liver failure and from VOD has been reported in patients who received Mylotarg. Physicians should monitor their patients carefully for symptoms of hepatotoxicity, particularly VOD. These symptoms can include: rapid weight gain, right upper quadrant pain, hepatomegaly, ascites, elevations in bilirubin and/or liver enzymes. However, careful monitoring may not identify all patients at risk or prevent the complications of hepatotoxicity. (See **WARNINGS** and **ADVERSE REACTIONS** sections.)

TABLE 1: PERCENTAGE OF PATIENTS BY REMISSION CATEGORY AND PROGNOSTIC GROUP

	Age < 60 years	Age ≥ 60 years	First Remission < 6 months	First Remission 6 – 12 months	First Remission ≥ 12 months
Type of Remission	n = 120	n = 157	n = 37	n = 124	n = 116
CR (95% CI)	13 8, 21	12 7, 18	5 1, 18	10 5, 16	18 12, 26
CRp (95% CI)	14 8, 22	12 7, 18	5 1, 18	12 7, 19	16 10, 24
OR (CR + CRp) (95% CI)	28 20, 36	24 18, 32	11 3, 25	22 15, 30	35 26, 44

DESCRIPTION

Mylotarg® (gemtuzumab ozogamicin for Injection) is a chemotherapy agent composed of a recombinant humanized IgG4, kappa antibody conjugated with a cytotoxic antitumor antibiotic, calicheamicin, isolated from fermentation of a bacterium, *Micromonospora echinospora* ssp. *calichensis*. The antibody portion of Mylotarg binds specifically to the CD33 antigen, a sialic acid-dependent adhesion protein found on the surface of leukemic blasts and immature normal cells of myelomonocytic lineage, but not on normal hematopoietic stem cells. The anti-CD33 hP67.6 antibody is produced by mammalian cell suspension culture using a myeloma NS0 cell line and is purified under conditions which remove or inactivate viruses. Three separate and independent steps in the hP67.6 antibody purification process achieves retrovirus inactivation and removal. These include low pH treatment, DEAE-Sepharose chromatography, and viral filtration. Mylotarg contains amino acid sequences of which approximately 98.3% are of human origin. The constant region and framework regions contain human sequences while the complementarity-determining regions are derived from a murine antibody (p67.6) that binds CD33. This antibody is linked to N-acetyl-gamma calicheamicin via a bifunctional linker. Gemtuzumab ozogamicin has approximately 50% of the antibody loaded with 4-6 moles calicheamicin per mole of antibody. The remaining 50% of the antibody is not linked to the calicheamicin derivative. Gemtuzumab ozogamicin has a molecular weight of 151 to 153 kDa.

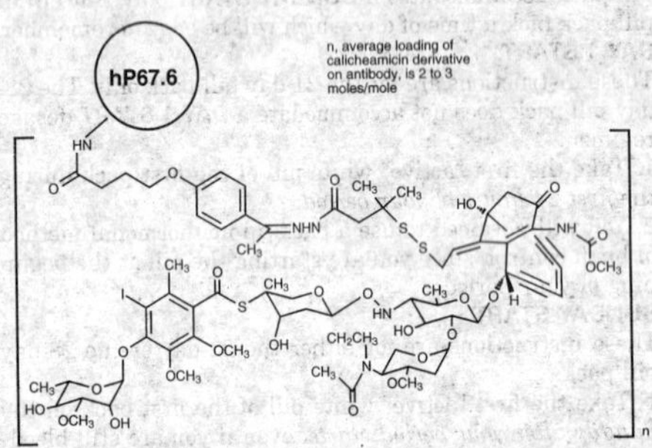

Mylotarg (gemtuzumab ozogamicin for Injection) is a sterile, white, preservative-free lyophilized powder containing 5 mg of drug conjugate (protein equivalent) in an amber vial. The drug product is light sensitive and must be protected from direct and indirect sunlight and unshielded fluorescent light during the preparation and administration of the infusion. The inactive ingredients are: dextran 40; sucrose; sodium chloride; monobasic and dibasic sodium phosphate.

CLINICAL PHARMACOLOGY

General

Gemtuzumab ozogamicin binds to the CD33 antigen. This antigen is expressed on the surface of leukemic blasts in more than 80% of patients with acute myeloid leukemia (AML). CD33 is also expressed on normal and leukemic myeloid colony-forming cells, including leukemic clonogenic precursors, but it is not expressed on pluripotent hematopoietic stem cells or on nonhematopoietic cells.

Mechanism of Action: Mylotarg is directed against the CD33 antigen expressed by hematopoietic cells. Binding of the anti-CD33 antibody portion of Mylotarg with the CD33 antigen results in the formation of a complex that is internalized. Upon internalization, the calicheamicin derivative is released inside the lysosomes of the myeloid cell. The released calicheamicin derivative binds to DNA in the minor groove resulting in DNA double strand breaks and cell death.

Gemtuzumab ozogamicin is cytotoxic to the CD33 positive HL-60 human leukemia cell line. Gemtuzumab ozogamicin produces significant inhibition of colony formation in cultures of adult leukemic bone marrow cells. The cytotoxic effect on normal myeloid precursors leads to substantial myelosuppression, but this is reversible because pluripotent hematopoietic stem cells are spared. In preclinical animal studies, gemtuzumab ozogamicin demonstrates antitumor effects in the HL-60 human promyelocytic leukemia xenograft tumor in athymic mice.

Human Pharmacokinetics

After administration of the first recommended 9 mg/m^2 dose of gemtuzumab ozogamicin, given as a 2 hour infusion, the elimination half lives of total and unconjugated calicheamicin were about 41 and 143 hours, respectively. After the second 9 mg/m^2 dose, the half life of total calicheamicin was increased to about 64 hours and the area under the concentration-time curve (AUC) was about twice that in the first dose period. The AUC for the unconjugated calicheamicin increased 30% after the second dose. Age, gender, body surface area (BSA), and weight did not affect the pharmacokinetics of Mylotarg.

Patients, especially patients previously treated with HSCT, have an underlying risk of VOD. The AUC of total calicheamicin was correlated with additional risk of hepatomegaly and the risk of veno-occlusive disease (VOD). There is no evidence that reducing Mylotarg dose will reduce the underlying risk of VOD. Metabolic studies indicate hydrolytic release of the calicheamicin derivative from gemtuzumab ozogamicin. Many metabolites of this derivative were found after *in vitro* incubation of gemtuzumab ozogamicin in human liver microsomes and cytosol, and in HL-60 promyelocytic leukemia cells. Metabolic studies characterizing the possible isozymes involved in the metabolic pathway of Mylotarg have not been performed.

CLINICAL STUDIES

The efficacy and safety of Mylotarg as a single agent have been evaluated in 277 patients in three single arm open-label studies in patients with CD33 positive AML in first relapse. The studies included 84, 95, and 98 patients. In studies 1 and 2 patients were ≥ 18 years of age with a first remission duration of at least 6 months. In study 3, only patients ≥ 60 were enrolled and their first remission had to have lasted for at least 3 months. Patients with secondary leukemia or white blood cell (WBC) counts ≥ 30,000/μL were excluded. Some patients were leukoreduced with hydroxyurea or leukapheresis to lower WBC counts below 30,000/μL in order to minimize the risk of tumor lysis syndrome. The treatment course included two 9 mg/m^2 doses separated by 14 days and a 28-day follow-up after the last dose. Although smaller doses had elicited responses in earlier studies, the 9 mg/m^2 was chosen because it would be expected to saturate all CD33 sites regardless of leukemic burden. A total of 157 patients were ≥ 60 years of age and older. The primary endpoint of the three clinical studies was the rate of complete remission (CR), which was defined as

a) leukemic blasts absent from the peripheral blood;
b) ≤ 5% blasts in the bone marrow, as measured by morphology studies;
c) hemoglobin (Hgb) ≥ 9 g/dL, platelets ≥ 100,000/μL, absolute neutrophil count (ANC) ≥ 1500/μL; and
d) red cell and platelet-transfusion independence (no red cell transfusions for 2 weeks; no platelet transfusions for 1 week).

In addition to CR, a second response category, CRp, was defined as patients satisfying the definition of CR, including platelet transfusion independence, with the exception of platelet recovery ≥100,000/μL. Remission status was determined at approximately 28 days after the last dose of Mylotarg. This category was added because Mylotarg appears to delay platelet recovery in some patients. Clinical equivalence between CR and CRp responses has not been established. Median time to recovery of platelet counts in patients who achieved a CR or a CRp is summarized in TABLE 4 (see **ADVERSE REACTIONS** section).

All patients were pre-medicated with acetaminophen 650-1000 mg and diphenhydramine 50 mg to decrease acute infusion-related symptoms. Growth factors and cytokines were not permitted. Use of prophylactic antibiotics was not specified.

Response Rate

The overall response (OR) rate for the three pooled monotherapy studies was 26% (71/277) consisting of 13% (35/277) of patients with CR and 13% (36/277) of patients with CRp. The median time to blast clearance in both CR and CRp patients was 28 days from the first dose of Mylotarg. The median time to remission was 60 days for both CR and CRp. Remission rates are shown in Table 1. Of the 157 patients who were ≥ 60 years old, the overall remission rate (OR = CR + CRp) was 24%. For the patients < 60 years old and all 277 patients the OR rates were 28% and 26%, respectively. Two of the most important determinants of response follow-

ing relapse are age and duration of first remission. Remission rates by prognostic category are outlined in Table 1.
[See table 1 at top of previous page]
The overall response rates were similar for females and males: 27% of females and 25% of males achieved remission. In the studies, 95% of the patients were white and 5% of the patients were non-white.

Survival

Overall survival was measured from date of first dose of gemtuzumab ozogamicin to date of death or data cut-off date (Table 2). Relapse-free survival (duration of remission) for patients in remission was defined as the time period from date of first documentation of maximum response (CR or CRp) to the first date of documentation of relapse (pathology report or complete blood count showing leukemic blast recurrence in peripheral blood or bone marrow), or death, or data cut-off date.

TABLE 2: SUMMARY OF RELAPSE FREE[a] and OVERALL SURVIVAL FOR PATIENTS WITH CR AND CRp

Remission Group	N	Relapse-Free Median months	Overall Survival Median months[c]
CR	35	6.4	12.0
CRp	36	4.5	12.7
OR[b]	71	5.2	12.4
Patients who responded to Mylotarg and received no further therapy			
CR	17	3.7	11.5
CRp	18	2.4	10.7
OR	35	2.4	11.1

a: Number of months after achieving CR or CRp.
b: Sixteen OR patients (6 CR and 10 CRp; 16/277; 5.7%) had a relapse-free survival at 12 months. 14/16 had stem cell transplants. 1/14 had a stem cell transplant prior to Mylotarg. The remaining 13 patients had stem cell transplants after Mylotarg. Six OR patients (3 CR and 3 CRp) had a relapse-free survival > 36 months. All 6 of these patients had subsequent stem cell transplants, representing 2.2% (6/277) of all patients.
c: The median overall survival was 3.3 months for NR patients; in all 277 patients it was 4.9 months.

Rates of Remission by Cytogenetic Risk

Patients in all three cytogenetic risk classification groups (poor, intermediate, favorable) responded to gemtuzumab ozogamicin.

Post-Remission Therapy

Twenty-five (25/71, 35%) OR patients (11 CR and 14 CRp patients) went on to hematopoietic stem cell transplantation (HSCT). Fourteen (14) received allogeneic HSCT and 11 received autologous HSCT.
Thirty-five (35/71, 49%) OR patients (17 CR and 18 CRp patients) who responded to treatment with Mylotarg received no additional therapy.

Repeat Courses

Twenty (20) patients have received more than 1 course of Mylotarg (gemtuzumab ozogamicin for Injection) in clinical trials. These patients were initially treated with Mylotarg, achieved remission, then subsequently relapsed and then received additional doses of Mylotarg.

Overview of Clinical Data

Available single arm trial data do not provide valid comparisons with various cytotoxic regimens that have been used in relapsed acute myeloid leukemia. Response rates are in the range of rates reported with such regimens only if the CRp responses are included. Nevertheless, treatment with Mylotarg can provide responses, including some of reasonable duration. The data support its use in patients for whom aggressive cytotoxic regimens would be considered unsuitable, such as many patients 60 years of age or older.

INDICATIONS AND USAGE

Mylotarg is indicated for the treatment of patients with CD33 positive acute myeloid leukemia in first relapse who are 60 years of age or older and who are not considered candidates for other cytotoxic chemotherapy. The safety and efficacy of Mylotarg in patients with poor performance status and organ dysfunction has not been established.
The effectiveness of Mylotarg is based on OR rates (see **CLINICAL STUDIES** section). There are no controlled trials demonstrating a clinical benefit, such as improvement in disease-related symptoms or increased survival, compared to any other treatment.

CONTRAINDICATIONS

Mylotarg is contraindicated in patients with a known hypersensitivity to gemtuzumab ozogamicin or any of its components: anti-CD33 antibody (hP67.6), calicheamicin derivatives, or inactive ingredients.

WARNINGS

Mylotarg should be administered under the supervision of physicians experienced in the treatment of acute leukemia and in facilities equipped to monitor and treat leukemia patients.

There are no controlled trials demonstrating efficacy and safety using Mylotarg in combination with other chemotherapeutic agents. Therefore, Mylotarg should only be used as single agent chemotherapy and not in combination chemotherapy regimens outside clinical trials.

Myelosuppression: Severe myelosuppression will occur in all patients given the recommended dose of this agent. Careful hematologic monitoring is required. Systemic infections should be treated.

Hypersensitivity Reactions Including Anaphylaxis, Infusion Reactions, Pulmonary Events: Mylotarg administration can result in severe hypersensitivity reactions (including anaphylaxis), and other infusion-related reactions which may include severe pulmonary events. Infrequently, hypersensitivity reactions and pulmonary events have been fatal. In most cases, infusion-related symptoms occurred during the infusion or within 24 hours of administration of Mylotarg and resolved.
Mylotarg (gemtuzumab ozogamicin for Injection) infusion should be interrupted for patients experiencing dyspnea or clinically significant hypotension. Patients should be monitored until signs and symptoms completely resolve. Discontinuation of further Mylotarg treatment should be strongly considered for patients who develop anaphylaxis, pulmonary edema, or acute respiratory distress syndrome. Since patients with high peripheral blast counts may be at greater risk for such reactions, physicians should consider leukoreduction with hydroxyurea or leukapheresis to reduce the peripheral white count to below 30,000/µL prior to administration of Mylotarg.

Infusion Reactions: Mylotarg can produce a post-infusion symptom complex of fever and chills, and less commonly hypotension and dyspnea that may occur during the first 24 hours after administration. Grade 3 or 4 non-hematologic infusion-related adverse events included chills, fever, hypotension, hypertension, hyperglycemia, hypoxia, and dyspnea. Most patients received the following prophylactic medications before administration: diphenhydramine 50 mg po and acetaminophen 650-1000 mg po; thereafter, two additional doses of acetaminophen 650-1000 mg po, one every 4 hours as needed. Vital signs should be monitored during infusion and for the four hours following infusion.
In clinical studies, these symptoms generally occurred after the end of the 2-hour intravenous infusion and resolved after 2 to 4 hours with a supportive therapy of acetaminophen, diphenhydramine, and IV fluids. Fewer infusion-related events were observed after the second dose.

Pulmonary Events: Severe pulmonary events leading to death have been reported infrequently with the use of Mylotarg in the postmarketing setting. Signs, symptoms and clinical findings include dyspnea, pulmonary infiltrates, pleural effusions, non-cardiogenic pulmonary edema, pulmonary insufficiency and hypoxia, and acute respiratory distress syndrome. These events occur as sequelae of infusion reactions; patients with WBC counts ≥ 30,000/µL may be at increased risk. (See **Infusion Reactions** section of **WARNINGS**.) Physicians should consider leukoreduction with hydroxyurea or leukapheresis to reduce the peripheral white count to below 30,000/µL prior to administration of Mylotarg. Patients with symptomatic intrinsic lung disease may also be at greater risk of severe pulmonary reactions.

Hepatotoxicity: Hepatotoxicity, including severe VOD, has been reported in association with the use of Mylotarg as a single agent, as part of a combination chemotherapy regimen, and in patients without a history of liver disease or HSCT. Patients who receive Mylotarg either before or after HSCT, patients with underlying hepatic disease or abnormal liver function, and patients receiving Mylotarg in combinations with other chemotherapy may be at increased risk for developing VOD, including severe VOD. Patients who had received HSCT before Mylotarg were at a higher risk of VOD (22%) than patients who had not been transplanted (1%). Patients who had received HSCT following Mylotarg were at a higher risk of VOD (15%) than patients who had not been transplanted (1%). Death from liver failure and from VOD has been reported in patients who received Mylotarg. Physicians should monitor their patients carefully for symptoms of hepatotoxicity, particularly VOD. These symptoms can include: rapid weight gain, right upper quadrant pain, hepatomegaly, ascites, elevations in bilirubin and/or liver enzymes. However, careful monitoring may not identify all patients at risk or prevent the complications of hepatotoxicity. (See **ADVERSE REACTIONS** section.)

Use in Patients with Hepatic Impairment: Mylotarg has not been studied in patients with bilirubin > 2 mg/dL. Extra caution should be exercised when administering Mylotarg in patients with hepatic impairment (see **ADVERSE REACTIONS** section).

Tumor Lysis Syndrome (TLS): TLS may be a consequence of leukemia treatment with any chemotherapeutic agent including Mylotarg. Renal failure secondary to TLS has been reported in association with the use of Mylotarg. Appropriate measures, (e.g. hydration and allopurinol), must be taken to prevent hyperuricemia. Physicians should consider leukoreduction with hydroxyurea or leukapheresis to reduce the peripheral white blood count to < 30,000/µL prior to administration of Mylotarg (see **CLINICAL STUDIES** section).

Pregnancy: Mylotarg may cause fetal harm when administered to a pregnant woman. Daily treatment of pregnant rats with gemtuzumab ozogamicin during organogenesis caused dose-related decreases in fetal weight in association with dose-related decreases in fetal skeletal ossification beginning at 0.025 mg/kg/day. Doses of 0.060 mg/kg/day (approximately 0.04 times the recommended human single dose on a mg/m^2 basis) produced increased embryo-fetal mortality (increased numbers of resorptions and decreased numbers of live fetuses per litter). Gross external, visceral, and skeletal alterations at the 0.060 mg/kg/day dose level included digital malformations (ectrodactyly, brachydactyly) in one or both hind feet, absence of the aortic arch, wavy ribs, anomalies of the long bones in the forelimb(s) (short/thick humerus, misshapen radius and ulna, and short/thick ulna), misshapen scapula, absence of vertebral centrum, and fused sternebrae. This dose was also associated with maternal toxicity (decreased weight gain, decreased food consumption). There are no adequate and well-controlled studies in pregnant women. If Mylotarg is used in pregnancy, or if the patient becomes pregnant while taking it, the patient should be apprised of the potential hazard to the fetus. Women of childbearing potential should be advised to avoid becoming pregnant while receiving treatment with Mylotarg.

PRECAUTIONS

DO NOT ADMINISTER AS AN INTRAVENOUS PUSH OR BOLUS

General

Treatment by Experienced Physicians: Mylotarg should be administered under the supervision of physicians experienced in the treatment of acute leukemia and in facilities equipped to monitor and treat leukemia patients.

Laboratory Monitoring: Electrolytes, tests of hepatic function, complete blood counts (CBCs) and platelet counts should be monitored during Mylotarg therapy.

Drug Interactions: There have been no formal drug-interaction studies performed with Mylotarg. The potential for drug-drug interaction with drugs affected by cytochrome P450 enzymes may not be ruled out.

Laboratory Test Interactions: Mylotarg is not known to interfere with any routine diagnostic tests.

Carcinogenesis, Mutagenesis, Impairment of Fertility: No long-term studies in animals have been performed to evaluate the carcinogenic potential of Mylotarg. Gemtuzumab ozogamicin was clastogenic in the mouse *in vivo* micronucleus test. This positive result is consistent with the known ability of calicheamicin to cause double-stranded breaks in DNA. Gemtuzumab ozogamicin adversely affected male, but not female, fertility in rats. Following daily administration of gemtuzumab ozogamicin to male rats for 28 days at doses of 0.02 to 0.16 mg/kg/day (approximately 0.01 to 0.11 times the human dose on a mg/m^2 basis) gemtuzumab ozogamicin caused: decreased fertility rates, epididymal sperm counts, and sperm motility; increased incidence of sperm abnormalities; and microscopic evidence of decreased spermatogonia and spermatocyte count. These findings did not resolve following a 9-week recovery period.

Pregnancy Category D: See **WARNINGS** section.

Nursing Mothers: It is not known if Mylotarg is excreted in human milk. Because many drugs, including immunoglobulins, are excreted in human milk, and because of the potential for serious adverse reactions in nursing infants from Mylotarg, a decision should be made whether to discontinue nursing or to discontinue the drug, taking into account the importance of the drug to the mother.

Pediatric Use: The safety and effectiveness of Mylotarg (gemtuzumab ozogamicin for Injection) in pediatric patients have not been established.

Use in Patients with Renal Impairment: Patients with renal impairment were not studied.

ADVERSE REACTIONS

Mylotarg has been administered to 277 patients with relapsed AML at 9 mg/m^2. Mylotarg was generally given as two intravenous infusions separated by 14 days.

Acute Infusion-Related Events (Table 3)

TABLE 3: NUMBER AND PERCENTAGE OF PATIENTS REPORTED TO HAVE ACUTE INFUSION-RELATED ADVERSE EVENTS (N = 277)

Adverse Event	Any Severity (%)	Grade 3 or 4 (%)
Fever	227 (82)	17 (6)
Nausea	188 (68)	8 (3)
Chills	183 (66)	21 (8)
Vomiting	162 (58)	3 (1)
Headache	102 (37)	2 (< 1)
Dyspnea	73 (26)	4 (1)
Hypotension	55 (20)	12 (4)
Hypertension	43 (16)	5 (2)
Hyperglycemia	29 (10)	3 (1)
Hypoxia	15 (5)	4 (1)

Fever and chills were commonly reported despite prophylactic treatment with acetaminophen and antihistamines (see **WARNINGS** section). Generally, these symptoms occurred at the end of the 2 hour infusion and resolved after 2 to 4

Continued on next page

Mylotarg—Cont.

hours with supportive therapy including acetaminophen, diphenhydramine, and intravenous fluids. These events all occurred on the same day as gemtuzumab ozogamicin infusion. Fewer infusion-related events were observed after the second dose. Methylprednisone given prior to Mylotarg infusion may ameliorate infusion-related symptoms.

Antibody Formation: Antibodies to gemtuzumab ozogamicin were not detected in any of the 277 patients, including the 20 patients who received more than 1 course of study drug, in the Phase 2 clinical studies. Two patients in a Phase 1 study developed antibody titers against the calicheamicin/calicheamicin-linker portion of gemtuzumab ozogamicin after three doses. One patient experienced transient fever, hypotension and dyspnea; the other patient had no clinical symptoms. No patient developed antibody responses to the hP67.6 antibody portion of Mylotarg.

Myelosuppression: Severe myelosuppression is the major toxicity associated with Mylotarg.

Neutropenia: During the treatment phase, 267/272 (98%) patients experienced Grade 3 or Grade 4 neutropenia. For all patients, the median times to ANC recovery at 500/µL for the CR and CRp patients were 40.0 and 43.0 days, respectively.

Anemia, Thrombocytopenia: During the treatment phase, 143/276 (52%) patients experienced Grade 3 or Grade 4 anemia and 272/276 (99%) patients experienced Grade 3 or Grade 4 thrombocytopenia. A summary of the platelet recovery for responding patients is provided in Table 4.

TABLE 4: MEDIAN TIME TO RECOVERY OF PLATELET COUNTS FOR ALL CR AND CRp PATIENTS (DAYS)

	CR		CRp	
Platelet levels	< 60 years of age	≥ 60 years of age	< 60 years of age	≥ 60 years of age
> 25,000/µL	35	38	39	75
50,000/µL	42	40	56	100
75,000/µL	48	42	122	NA
100,000/µL	56	50	NA	NA

Abbreviation: NA = Not Available

Infection: During the treatment phase, 84/277 (30%) patients experienced Grade 3 or Grade 4 infections, including opportunistic infections. The most frequent Grade 3 or Grade 4 infection-related treatment-emergent adverse events (TEAEs) were sepsis (17%), pneumonia (8%), shock (4%), infection (3%), stomatitis (2%), and herpes simplex (2%).

Bleeding: During the treatment phase, 36/277 (13%) patients experienced Grade 3 or Grade 4 bleeding. The most common bleeding events for all patients were epistaxis (3%), cerebral hemorrhage (2%), intracranial hemorrhage (1%), melena (1%), petechiae (1%), hematuria (1%), and disseminated intravascular coagulation (1%).

A greater proportion of NR patients (15%) experienced NCI grade 3 or 4 bleeding events compared with OR patients (7%). Among CR patients, 1 grade 3 bleeding event, epistaxis, was experienced. Bleeding events occurred in 1/35 CR patients and 4/36 CRp patients.

Transfusions: During the treatment phase, more transfusions were required in the NR and CRp patients compared with the CRs (Table 5):

[See table 5 above]

TABLE 5: NUMBER OF TRANSFUSIONS BY RESPONSE GROUP

Transfusions	All Patients	CR	CRp	NR
	N = 277	N = 35	N = 36	N = 206
Platelet transfusions				
Mean (SD)	NA	6.8 (7)	23.7 (67)	15.7 (20)
(95% CI)*	NA	(5.6, 8.0)	(12.5, 34.9)	(14.3, 17.1)
RBC transfusions				
Mean (SD)	NA	2.9 (3)	5.4 (4)	8.1 (22)
(95% CI)	NA	(2.4, 3.4)	(4.7, 10.1)	(8.0, 8.2)

* calculated - mean ± se where se = sd/sqr(n)

Mucositis: A total of 69/277 (25%) patients were reported to have a TEAE consistent with oral mucositis or stomatitis. During the treatment phase, 9/277 (3%) patients experienced Grade 3 or 4 stomatitis/mucositis after the first dose.

Hepatotoxicity: In clinical studies, 80/274 (29%) patients experienced Grade 3 or Grade 4 hyperbilirubinemia. 26/274 (9%) of patients experienced Grade 3 or Grade 4 abnormalities in levels of ALT, and 49/274 (18%) patients experienced Grade 3 or Grade 4 abnormalities in levels of AST. One patient died with liver failure in the setting of tumor lysis syndrome and multisystem organ failure 22 days after treatment. Another patient died after an episode of persistent jaundice and hepatosplenomegaly 156 days after treatment. Ascites, an event that can be associated with liver damage, was observed in 8 patients. Abnormalities of liver function were often transient and reversible.

VOD: A total of 299 courses of Mylotarg were administered in 277 relapsed patients and 16 episodes of VOD (in 15 patients) were identified (16/299, 5%). The incidence of VOD in patients treated with Mylotarg who had no prior or subsequent HSCT was 1.0%. The risk of developing VOD was 20% for patients with a history of HSCT prior to Mylotarg administration. In patients who received HSCT after Mylotarg administration, the risk of developing VOD was 15%. (See Table 6). In the 15 patients that developed VOD, 9 patients had fatal VOD or ongoing VOD at the time of death:

[See table 6 above]

TABLE 6: INCIDENCE OF VOD REPORTED BY TREATMENT GROUPS

	Number Courses of Mylotarg	Number Episodes of VOD	Incidence of VOD (episodes per courses)	Number Patients in Classification	Number Patients with VOD	Incidence of VOD (in patients)
Mylotarg Total	299	16	5%	277	15	5%
Mylotarg Only	215	2	1%	200	2	1%
HSCT with Mylotarg (total)[a]	84	14	17%	77	13	17%
HSCT prior to Mylotarg[b,c]	30	6	20%	27	6	22%
HSCT following Mylotarg[b,c]	54	8	15%	52	8	15%

a: 3 patients are included in more than one HSCT category.
b: 2 patients with a pre-trial history of HSCT each received HSCT after Mylotarg.
c: 1 patient received Mylotarg followed by HSCT and then received a second course of Mylotarg. This patient developed VOD after HSCT and again after the second course of Mylotarg.

Skin: Pruritus was reported in 18/277 (6%) patients, while rash occurred in 51/277 (18%) patients. Cutaneous herpes simplex was reported in 59/277 (21%) patients. No patient experienced alopecia.

TABLE 7: COMMONLY REPORTED (≥ 10%) TREATMENT-EMERGENT ADVERSE EVENTS BY AGE GROUP: NUMBER (%) OF PATIENTS

Body System Adverse Event	Patient Age in Years: Age ≥60 (n = 157)	Age <60 (n = 120)	Any Age (n = 277)
Any Adverse Event	157 (100)	119 (99)	276 (100)
Body as a whole			
Abdominal pain	41 (26)	47 (39)	88 (32)
Asthenia	56 (36)	44 (37)	100 (36)
Back pain	19 (12)	19 (16)	38 (14)
Chills	101 (64)	82 (68)	183 (66)
Fever	122 (78)	105 (88)	227 (82)
Headache	42 (27)	60 (50)	102 (37)
Infection	16 (10)	10 (8)	26 (9)
Neutropenic fever	30 (19)	18 (15)	48 (17)
Pain	28 (18)	21 (18)	49 (18)
Sepsis	40 (25)	33 (28)	73 (26)
Cardiovascular system			
Hemorrhage	14 (9)	16 (13)	30 (11)
Hypertension	27 (17)	16 (13)	43 (16)
Hypotension	28 (18)	27 (23)	55 (20)
Tachycardia	17 (11)	11 (9)	28 (10)
Digestive system			
Anorexia	43 (27)	26 (22)	69 (25)
Constipation	36 (23)	27 (23)	63 (23)
Diarrhea	47 (30)	43 (36)	90 (32)
Dyspepsia	13 (8)	15 (13)	28 (10)
Gum hemorrhage	8 (5)	17 (14)	25 (9)
Liver function tests abnormal	31 (20)	35 (29)	66 (24)
Nausea	99 (63)	89 (74)	188 (68)
Stomatitis	34 (22)	35 (29)	69 (25)
Vomiting	83 (53)	79 (66)	162 (58)
Hemic and lymphatic system			
Anemia	34 (22)	26 (22)	60 (22)
Ecchymosis	17 (11)	11 (9)	28 (10)
Leukopenia	67 (43)	62 (52)	129 (47)
Petechiae	30 (19)	24 (20)	54 (19)
Thrombocytopenia	77 (49)	62 (52)	139 (50)
Metabolic and nutritional			
Alkaline phosphatase increased	15 (10)	6 (5)	21 (8)
Bilirubinemia	18 (11)	15 (13)	33 (12)
Hyperglycemia	17 (11)	12 (10)	29 (10)
Hypocalcemia	15 (10)	14 (12)	29 (10)
Hypokalemia	38 (24)	35 (29)	73 (26)
Hypomagnesemia	4 (3)	12 (10)	16 (6)
Hypophosphatemia	9 (6)	12 (10)	21 (8)
Lactic dehydrogenase increased	28 (18)	17 (14)	45 (16)
Peripheral edema	30 (19)	10 (8)	40 (14)

(Table continued on next page)

Early Mortality in Clinical Studies

The overall mortality rate within 28 days of last dose was 16% (44/277). The mortality rate was 14% (17/120) for patients who were < 60 years old, and 17% (27/157) for patients who were ≥ 60 years old.

Retreatment Events: Twenty (20) patients received additional courses of Mylotarg in the studies. One (1) patient received a total of 4 courses of treatment.

Dose Relationship for Adverse Events: Dose-relationship data were generated from a small dose-escalation study. The most common clinical adverse event observed in this study was an infusion-related symptom complex of fever and chills. In general, the severity of fever, but not chills, increased as the dose level increased. Only one dose level of Mylotarg was studied in the Phase 2 clinical trials in relapsed AML.

Treatment-Emergent Adverse Events (TEAE): TEAEs (Grades 1-4) that occurred in ≥ 10% of the patients regardless of causality are listed in Table 7.

[See table 7 above and on next page]

TABLE 7 (cont.): COMMONLY REPORTED (≥ 10%) TREATMENT-EMERGENT ADVERSE EVENTS BY AGE GROUP: NUMBER (%) OF PATIENTS

Body System Adverse Event	Patient Age in Years Age ≥60 (n = 157)	Age <60 (n = 120)	Any Age (n = 277)
Musculoskeletal system			
Myalgia	5 (3)	13 (11)	18 (6)
Nervous system			
Anxiety	15 (10)	8 (7)	23 (8)
Depression	15 (10)	9 (8)	24 (9)
Dizziness	15 (10)	18 (15)	33 (12)
Insomnia	17 (11)	16 (13)	33 (12)
Respiratory system			
Cough increased	28 (18)	19 (16)	47 (17)
Dyspnea	41 (26)	32 (27)	73 (26)
Epistaxis	37 (24)	41 (34)	78 (28)
Pharyngitis	16 (10)	17 (14)	33 (12)
Pneumonia	20 (13)	15 (13)	35 (13)
Pulmonary physical finding	13 (8)	12 (10)	25 (9)
Rhinitis	11 (7)	12 (10)	23 (8)
Skin and apppendages			
Herpes simplex	29 (18)	30 (25)	59 (21)
Pruritus	6 (4)	12 (10)	18 (6)
Rash	29 (18)	22 (18)	51 (18)
Urogenital system			
Metrorrhagia	1 (2)	6 (10)	7 (3)
Vaginal hemorrhage	3 (5)	9 (15)	12 (4)
Adverse event associated with miscellaneous factors			
Local reaction to procedure	27 (17)	33 (28)	60 (22)

TABLE 8: NUMBER (%) OF PATIENTS REPORTING NCI GRADE 3 OR 4 TREATMENT-EMERGENT ADVERSE EVENTS DURING PART I BY AGE GROUP: EVENTS WITH INCIDENCE ≥ 10%

Body System Adverse Event	Patient Age in Years Age ≥ 60 (n = 157)	Age <60 (n = 120)	Any Age (n = 277)
Any adverse event	138 (88)	112 (93)	250 (90)
Body as a whole			
Chills	17 (11)	9 (8)	26 (9)
Fever	20 (13)	16 (13)	36 (13)
Sepsis	23 (15)	24 (20)	47 (17)
Digestive system			
Liver function tests abnormal	11 (7)	12 (10)	23 (8)
Hemic and lymphatic system			
Anemia	19 (12)	19 (16)	38 (14)
Leukopenia	67 (43)	60 (50)	127 (46)
Thrombocytopenia	75 (48)	61 (51)	136 (49)
Respiratory system			
Dyspnea	15 (10)	8 (7)	23 (8)

Abbreviation: NCI = National Cancer Institute.

TABLE 9: NUMBER (%[a]) OF PATIENTS WITH LABORATORY TEST RESULTS OF GRADE 3 OR 4 SEVERITY[b]

Test	Efficacy and Safety Studies Grades 3 – 4 Age ≥ 60 (n = 157)	Age < 60 (n = 120)	All Patients (n = 277)
Hematologic			
Hemoglobin	79/157 (50)	64/119 (54)	143/276 (52)
WBC	149/157 (95)	117/119 (98)	266/276 (96)
Total neutrophils, absolute	152/155 (98)	115/117 (98)	267/272 (98)
Lymphocytes	144/155 (93)	111/117 (95)	255/272 (94)
Platelet count	155/157 (99)	117/119 (98)	272/276 (99)
Prothrombin time	2/35 (6)	4/34 (12)	6/69 (9)
Partial thromboplastin time	1/66 (2)	1/61 (2)	2/127 (2)
Non-hematologic			
Glucose (hypo/hyper)	19/155 (12)	13/119 (11)	32/274 (12)
Creatinine	1/157 (<1)	4/119 (3)	5/276 (2)
Total bilirubin	45/156 (29)	35/118 (30)	80/274 (29)
AST	25/156 (16)	24/118 (20)	49/274 (18)
ALT	12/156 (8)	14/118 (12)	26/274 (9)
Alkaline phosphatase	4/156 (3)	7/118 (6)	11/274 (4)
Calcium (hypo/hyper)	14/157 (9)	21/119 (18)	35/276 (13)

a: Percentage is based on the number of patients receiving a particular laboratory test during the study as is indicated for each test.
b: Severity as defined by NCI common toxicity scale version 1.

TEAEs of NCI grade 3 or 4 severity that occurred in part I of studies with an incidence of ≥ 10% in at least 1 age subgroup, are presented in Table 8.
[See table 8 above]
Clinically important laboratory abnormalities with a Grade 3 or 4 severity are listed in Table 9.
[See table 9 above]
There were considered to be no clinically important differences in TEAEs between patients < 60 years of age and those patients ≥ 60.
There were considered to be no clinically important differences in TEAEs between female and male patients.

Other Clinical Experience:
In postmarketing experience and other clinical trials, additional cases of VOD have been reported, some in association with the use of other chemotherapeutic agents, underlying hepatic disease/abnormal liver function, or a history of prior or subsequent HSCT. Renal failure secondary to TLS, hypersensitivity reactions, anaphylaxis, pulmonary events, and gastrointestinal hemorrhage have also been reported in association with the use of Mylotarg (gemtuzumab ozogamicin for Injection). (See **WARNINGS** section).

OVERDOSAGE

No cases of overdose with Mylotarg were reported in clinical experience. Single doses higher than 9 mg/m² in adults were not tested. When a single dose of Mylotarg was administered to animals, mortality was observed in rats at the dose of 2 mg/kg (approximately 1.3-times the recommended human dose on a mg/m² basis), and in male monkeys at the dose of 4.5 mg/kg (approximately 6-times the recommended human dose on a mg/m² basis).

Signs and Symptoms: Signs of overdose with Mylotarg are unknown.

Recommended Treatment: General supportive measures should be followed in case of overdose. Blood pressure and blood counts should be carefully monitored. Gemtuzumab ozogamicin is not dialyzable.

DOSAGE AND ADMINISTRATION

The recommended dose of Mylotarg is 9 mg/m², administered as a 2-hour intravenous infusion. Physicians should consider leukoreduction with hydroxyurea or leukapheresis to reduce the peripheral white blood count to below 30,000/μL prior to administration of Mylotarg. Appropriate measures (e.g. hydration and allopurinol) must be taken to prevent hyperuricemia. Patients should receive the following prophylactic medications one hour before Mylotarg administration: diphenhydramine 50 mg po and acetaminophen 650-1000 mg po; thereafter, two additional doses of acetaminophen 650-1000 mg po, one every 4 hours as needed. Vital signs should be monitored during infusion and for four hours following infusion. The recommended treatment course with Mylotarg is a total of 2 doses with 14 days between the doses. Full recovery from hematologic toxicities is not a requirement for administration of the second dose. Methylprednisone given prior to Mylotarg infusion may ameliorate infusion-related symptoms.

Hepatic Insufficiency: Patients with hepatic impairment were not included in the clinical studies. (See **WARNINGS** section).

Renal Insufficiency: Patients with renal impairment were not included in the clinical studies.

Instructions for Reconstitution
The drug product is light sensitive and must be protected from direct and indirect sunlight and unshielded fluorescent light during the preparation and administration of the infusion. **All preparation should take place in a biologic safety hood with the fluorescent light off.** Prior to reconstitution, allow drug vials to come to room temperature. Reconstitute the contents of each vial with 5 mL Sterile Water for Injection, USP, using sterile syringes. Gently swirl each vial. Each vial should be inspected for complete solution and for particulate. The final concentration of drug in the vial is 1 mg/mL. While in the vial, the reconstituted drug may be stored refrigerated (2-8° C) and protected from light for up to 8 hours.

Instructions for Dilution
Withdraw the desired volume from each vial and inject into a 100 mL IV bag of 0.9% Sodium Chloride Injection. Place the 100-mL IV bag into an UV protectant bag. The resulting drug solution in the IV bag should be used immediately.

Administration
DO NOT ADMINISTER AS AN INTRAVENOUS PUSH OR BOLUS
Once the reconstituted Mylotarg is diluted into the IV bag containing normal saline, the resulting solution should be infused over a 2-hour period. A separate IV line equipped with a low protein-binding 1.2-micron terminal filter must be used for administration of the drug. Mylotarg may be given peripherally or through a central line. Premedication, consisting of acetaminophen and diphenhydramine, should be given before each infusion to reduce the incidence of a post-infusion symptom complex (see **ADVERSE REACTIONS, Acute Infusion-Related Events**).

Stability and Storage: Mylotarg should be stored refrigerated 2° to 8° C (36° to 46° F) and protected from light.

Instructions for Use, Handling and for Disposal: Mylotarg should be inspected visually for particulate matter and discoloration, following reconstitution and prior to administration. Protect from light and use an UV protective bag over the IV bag during infusion. Procedures for handling and disposal of anticancer drugs should be considered. Several guidelines on this subject have been published.[1,2,3]

HOW SUPPLIED

Mylotarg® (gemtuzumab ozogamicin for Injection) is supplied as a single-vial package with an amber glass vial containing 5 mg of Mylotarg lyophilized powder. Single-unit 5 mg package: each vial contains 5 mg of Mylotarg. NDC 0008-4510-01.

REFERENCES

[1] Recommendation for the Safe Handling of Parenteral Antineoplastic Drugs. NIH Publication No. 83-2621. For Sale by the Superintendent of Documents, US Government Printing Office, Washington, DC 20402.

[2] AMA Council Report. Guidelines for Handling Parenteral Antineoplastics. JAMA 1985; 253 (11): 1590-1592.

[3] National Study Commission on Cytotoxic Exposure–Recommendations for Handling Cytotoxic Agents. Available from Louis P. Jeffrey, ScD, Chairman, National Study Commission on Cytotoxic Exposure, Massachusetts College of Pharmacy and Allied Health Sciences, 179 Longwood Avenue, Boston, Massachusetts 02115.

Wyeth®
Wyeth Pharmaceuticals Inc.
Philadelphia, PA 19101

W10477C005
ET01
Rev 07/04

Shown in Product Identification Guide, page 336

NEUMEGA® ℞

[*nu-meg<a*]
(oprelvekin)
℞ only

This product's label may have been revised after this insert was used in production. For further product information and current package insert, please visit www.wyeth.com or call our medical communications department toll-free at 1-800-934-5556.

Continued on next page

Neumega—Cont.

BOXED WARNING

Allergic Reactions Including Anaphylaxis
Neumega has caused allergic or hypersensitivity reactions, including anaphylaxis. Administration of Neumega should be permanently discontinued in any patient who develops an allergic or hypersensitivity reaction (see **WARNINGS, CONTRAINDICATIONS, ADVERSE REACTIONS** and **ADVERSE REACTIONS, Immunogenicity**).

DESCRIPTION

Interleukin eleven (IL-11) is a thrombopoietic growth factor that directly stimulates the proliferation of hematopoietic stem cells and megakaryocyte progenitor cells and induces megakaryocyte maturation resulting in increased platelet production. IL-11 is a member of a family of human growth factors which includes human growth hormone, granulocyte colony-stimulating factor (G-CSF), and other growth factors.

Oprelvekin, the active ingredient in Neumega, is produced in *Escherichia coli (E. coli)* by recombinant DNA technology. The protein has a molecular mass of approximately 19,000 daltons, and is non-glycosylated. The polypeptide is 177 amino acids in length and differs from the 178 amino acid length of native IL-11 only in lacking the amino-terminal proline residue. This alteration has not resulted in measurable differences in bioactivity either *in vitro* or *in vivo*.

Neumega is formulated in single-use vials containing 5 mg of oprelvekin (specific activity approximately 8 x 10^6 Units/mg) as a sterile, lyophilized powder with 23 mg Glycine, USP, 1.6 mg Dibasic Sodium Phosphate Heptahydrate, USP, and 0.55 mg Monobasic Sodium Phosphate Monohydrate, USP. When reconstituted with 1 mL of Sterile Water for Injection, USP, the resulting solution has a pH of 7.0 and a concentration of 5 mg/mL.

CLINICAL PHARMACOLOGY

The primary hematopoietic activity of Neumega is stimulation of megakaryocytopoiesis and thrombopoiesis. Neumega has shown potent thrombopoietic activity in animal models of compromised hematopoiesis, including moderately to severely myelosuppressed mice and nonhuman primates. In these models, Neumega improved platelet nadirs and accelerated platelet recoveries compared to controls.

Preclinical trials have shown that mature megakaryocytes which develop during *in vivo* treatment with Neumega are ultrastructurally normal. Platelets produced in response to Neumega were morphologically and functionally normal and possessed a normal life span.

IL-11 has also been shown to have non-hematopoietic activities in animals including the regulation of intestinal epithelium growth (enhanced healing of gastrointestinal lesions), the inhibition of adipogenesis, the induction of acute phase protein synthesis, inhibition of pro-inflammatory cytokine production by macrophages, and the stimulation of osteoclastogenesis and neurogenesis. Non-hematopoietic pathologic changes observed in animals include fibrosis of tendons and joint capsules, periosteal thickening, papilledema, and embryotoxicity (see **PRECAUTIONS, Pediatric Use** and **PRECAUTIONS, Pregnancy Category C**).

IL-11 is produced by bone marrow stromal cells and is part of the cytokine family that shares the gp130 signal transducer. Primary osteoblasts and mature osteoclasts express mRNAs for both IL-11 receptor (IL-11R alpha) and gp130. Both bone-forming and bone-resorbing cells are potential targets of IL-11.(1)

Pharmacokinetics

The pharmacokinetics of Neumega have been evaluated in studies of healthy, adult subjects and cancer patients receiving chemotherapy. In a study in which a single 50 μg/kg subcutaneous dose was administered to eighteen healthy men, the peak serum concentration (C_{max}) of 17.4 ± 5.4 ng/mL (mean ± S.D.) was reached at 3.2 ± 2.4 hrs (T_{max}) following dosing. The terminal half-life was 6.9 ± 1.7 hrs. In a second study in which single 75 μg/kg subcutaneous and intravenous doses were administered to twenty-four healthy subjects, the pharmacokinetic profiles were similar between men and women. The absolute bioavailability of Neumega was >80%. In a study in which multiple, subcutaneous doses of both 25 and 50 μg/kg were administered to cancer patients receiving chemotherapy, Neumega did not accumulate and clearance of Neumega was not impaired following multiple doses.

In a dose escalation Phase 1 study, Neumega was also administered to 43 pediatric patients (ages 8 months to 18 years) and 1 adult patient receiving ICE (ifosfamide, carboplatin, etoposide) chemotherapy. Administered doses ranged from 25 to 125 μg/kg. Analysis of data from 40 pediatric patients showed that C_{max}, T_{max}, and terminal half-life were comparable to that in adults. The mean area under the concentration-time curve (AUC) for pediatric patients (8 months to 18 years), receiving 50 μg/kg was approximately half that achieved in healthy adults receiving 50 μg/kg. Available data suggest that clearance of oprelvekin decreases with increasing age.

In preclinical trials in rats, radiolabeled Neumega was rapidly cleared from the serum and distributed to highly perfused organs. The kidney was the primary route of elimination. The amount of intact Neumega in urine was low, indicating that the molecule was metabolized before excretion. In a clinical study, a single dose of Neumega was administered to subjects with severely impaired renal function (creatinine clearance <30 mL/min). The mean ± S.D. values for C_{max} and AUC were 30.8 ± 8.6 ng/mL and 373 ± 106 ng*hr/mL, respectively. When compared with control subjects in this study with normal renal function, the mean C_{max} was 2.2 fold higher and the mean AUC was 2.6 fold (95% confidence interval, 1.7%-3.8%) higher in the subjects with severe renal impairment. In the subjects with severe renal impairment, clearance was approximately 40% of the value seen in subjects with normal renal function. The average terminal half-life was similar in subjects with severe renal impairment and those with normal renal function.

A second clinical study of 24 subjects with varying degrees of renal function was also performed and confirmed the results observed in the first study. Single 50 μg/kg subcutaneous and intravenous doses were administered in a randomized fashion. As the degree of renal impairment increased, the Neumega AUC increased, although half-life remained unchanged. In the six patients with severe impairment, the mean ± S.D. C_{max} and AUC were 23.6 ± 6.7 ng/mL and 373 ± 55.2 ng*hr/mL, respectively, compared with 13.1 ± 3.8 ng/mL and 195 ± 49.3 ng*hr/mL, respectively, in the six subjects with normal renal function. A comparable increase in exposure was observed after intravenous administration of Neumega.

The pharmacokinetic studies suggest that overall exposure to oprelvekin increases as renal function decreases, indicating that a 50% dose reduction of Neumega is warranted for patients with severe renal impairment (see **PRECAUTIONS, Use in Patients with Renal Impairment** and **DOSAGE AND ADMINISTRATION**). No dosage reduction is required for smaller changes in renal function.

Pharmacodynamics

In a study in which Neumega was administered to non-myelosuppressed cancer patients, daily subcutaneous dosing for 14 days with Neumega increased the platelet count in a dose-dependent manner. Platelet counts began to increase relative to baseline between five and nine days after the start of dosing with Neumega. After cessation of treatment, platelet counts continued to increase for up to seven days then returned toward baseline within 14 days. No change in platelet reactivity as measured by platelet activation in response to ADP, and platelet aggregation in response to ADP, epinephrine, collagen, ristocetin and arachidonic acid has been observed in association with Neumega treatment.

In a randomized, double-blind, placebo-controlled study in normal volunteers, subjects receiving Neumega had a mean increase in plasma volume of >20%, and all subjects receiving Neumega had at least a 10% increase in plasma volume. Red blood cell volume decreased similarly (due to repeated phlebotomy) in the Neumega and placebo groups. As a result, whole blood volume increased approximately 10% and hemoglobin concentration decreased approximately 10% in subjects receiving Neumega compared with subjects receiving placebo. Mean 24 hour sodium excretion decreased, and potassium excretion did not increase, in subjects receiving Neumega compared with subjects receiving placebo.

CLINICAL STUDIES

Two randomized, double-blind, placebo-controlled trials in adults studied Neumega for the prevention of severe thrombocytopenia following single or repeated sequential cycles of various myelosuppressive chemotherapy regimens.

Study in Patients with Prior Chemotherapy-Induced Thrombocytopenia

One study evaluated the effectiveness of Neumega in eliminating the need for platelet transfusions in patients who had recovered from an episode of severe chemotherapy-induced thrombocytopenia (defined as a platelet count ≤20,000/μL), and were to receive one additional cycle of the same chemotherapy without dose reduction. Patients had various underlying non-myeloid malignancies, and were undergoing dose-intensive chemotherapy with a variety of regimens. Patients were randomized to receive Neumega at a dose of 25 μg/kg or 50 μg/kg, or placebo. The primary endpoint was whether the patient required one or more platelet transfusions in the subsequent chemotherapy cycle. Ninety-three patients were randomized. Five patients withdrew from the study prior to receiving the study drug. As a result, eighty-eight patients were included in a modified intent-to-treat analysis. The results for the Neumega 50 μg/kg and placebo groups are summarized in Table 1. The placebo group includes one patient who underwent chemotherapy dose reduction and who avoided platelet transfusions.

TABLE 1
STUDY RESULTS

	Placebo n=30	Neumega 50 μg/kg n=29
Number (%) of patients avoiding platelet transfusion	2 (7%)	8 (28%)
Number (%) of patients requiring platelet transfusion	28 (93%)	21 (72%)
Median (mean) number of platelet transfusion events	2.5 (3.3)	1 (2.2)

In the primary efficacy analysis, more patients avoided platelet transfusion in the Neumega 50 μg/kg arm than in the placebo arm (p = 0.04, Fisher's Exact test, 2-tailed). The difference in the proportion of patients avoiding platelet transfusions in the Neumega 50 μg/kg and placebo groups was 21% (95% confidence interval, 2%-40%). The results observed in patients receiving 25 μg/kg of Neumega were intermediate between those of the placebo and the 50 μg/kg groups.

Study in Patients Receiving Dose-Intensive Chemotherapy

A second study evaluated the effectiveness of Neumega in eliminating platelet transfusions over two dose-intensive chemotherapy cycles in breast cancer patients who had not previously experienced severe chemotherapy-induced thrombocytopenia. All patients received the same chemotherapy regimen (cyclophosphamide 3,200 mg/m^2 and doxorubicin 75 mg/m^2). All patients received concomitant filgrastim (G-CSF) in all cycles. The patients were stratified by whether or not they had received prior chemotherapy, and randomized to receive Neumega 50 μg/kg or placebo. The primary endpoint was whether or not a patient required one or more platelet transfusions in the two study cycles. Seventy-seven patients were randomized. Thirteen patients failed to complete both study cycles—eight of these had insufficient data to be evaluated for the primary endpoint. The results of this trial are summarized in Table 2. [See table 2 below]

TABLE 2
STUDY RESULTS

	Overall n=77		No Prior Chemotherapy n=54		Prior Chemotherapy n=23	
	Placebo n=37	Neumega n=40	Placebo n=27	Neumega n=27	Placebo n=10	Neumega n=13
Number (%) of patients avoiding platelet transfusion	15 (41%)	26 (65%)	14 (52%)	19 (70%)	1 (10%)	7 (54%)
Number (%) of patients requiring platelet transfusion	16 (43%)	12 (30%)	9 (33%)	7 (26%)	7 (70%)	5 (38%)
Number (%) of patients not evaluable	6 (16%)	2 (5%)	4 (15%)	1 (4%)	2 (20%)	1 (8%)

This study showed a trend in favor of Neumega, particularly in the subgroup of patients with prior chemotherapy. Open-label treatment with Neumega has been continued for up to four consecutive chemotherapy cycles without evidence of any adverse effect on the rate of neutrophil recovery or red blood cell transfusion requirements. Some patients continued to maintain platelet nadirs >20,000/μL for at least four sequential cycles of chemotherapy without the need for transfusions, chemotherapy dose reduction, or changes in treatment schedules.

Platelet activation studies done on a limited number of patients showed no evidence of abnormal spontaneous platelet activation, or an abnormal response to ADP. In an unblinded, retrospective analysis of the two placebo-controlled studies, 19 of 69 patients (28%) receiving Neumega 50 μg/kg and 34 of 67 patients (51%) receiving placebo reported at least one hemorrhagic adverse event which involved bleeding.

Study in Patients Following Myeloablative Chemotherapy

In a randomized, double-blind, placebo-controlled, Phase 2 study conducted in 80 women with high-risk breast cancer who received 0 (n=26), 25 μg/kg (n=28), or 50 μg/kg (n=26) Neumega following myeloablative chemotherapy and autologous bone marrow transplantation, the incidence of platelet transfusions and time to neutrophil and platelet engraftment were similar in the Neumega and placebo-treated arms. The study showed a statistically significant increased incidence in edema, conjunctival bleeding, hypotension, and tachycardia in patients receiving Neumega as compared to placebo.

In long term follow-up of patients, the distribution of survival and progression-free survival times was similar between patients randomized to Neumega therapy and those randomized to receive placebo.

INDICATIONS AND USAGE

Neumega is indicated for the prevention of severe thrombocytopenia and the reduction of the need for platelet transfusions following myelosuppressive chemotherapy in adult patients with nonmyeloid malignancies who are at high risk of severe thrombocytopenia. Efficacy was demonstrated in patients who had experienced severe thrombocytopenia following the previous chemotherapy cycle. Neumega is not indicated following myeloablative chemotherapy (see **WARNINGS, Increased Toxicity Following Myeloablative Therapy**. The safety and effectiveness of Neumega have not been established in pediatric patients.

CONTRAINDICATIONS

Neumega is contraindicated in patients with a history of hypersensitivity to Neumega or any component of the product (see **WARNINGS, Allergic Reactions Including Anaphylaxis**).

WARNINGS

Allergic Reactions Including Anaphylaxis

In the post-marketing setting, Neumega has caused allergic or hypersensitivity reactions, including anaphylaxis. The administration of Neumega should be attended by appropriate precautions in case allergic reactions occur. In addition, patients should be counseled about the symptoms for which they should seek medical attention (see **PRECAUTIONS, Information for Patients**). Signs and symptoms reported included edema of the face, tongue, or larynx; shortness of breath; wheezing; chest pain; hypotension (including shock); dysarthria; loss of consciousness; mental status changes; rash; urticaria; flushing and fever. Reactions occurred after the first dose or subsequent doses of Neumega. Administration of Neumega should be permanently discontinued in any patient who develops an allergic or hypersensitivity reaction (see **BOXED WARNING, CONTRAINDICATIONS, ADVERSE REACTIONS,** and **ADVERSE REACTIONS, Immunogenicity**).

Increased Toxicity Following Myeloablative Therapy

Neumega is not indicated following myeloablative chemotherapy. In a randomized, placebo-controlled Phase 2 study, the effectiveness Neumega was not demonstrated (see **CLINICAL STUDIES, Study in Patients Following Myeloablative Chemotherapy**). In this study, a statistically significant increased incidence in edema, conjunctival bleeding, hypotension, and tachycardia was observed in patients receiving Neumega as compared to placebo.

The following severe or fatal adverse reactions have been reported in post-marketing use in patients who received Neumega following bone marrow transplantation: fluid retention or overload (eg, facial edema, pulmonary edema), capillary leak syndrome, pleural and pericardial effusion, papilledema and renal failure.

Fluid Retention

Neumega is known to cause serious fluid retention that can result in peripheral edema, dyspnea on exertion, pulmonary edema, capillary leak syndrome, atrial arrhythmias, and exacerbation of pre-existing pleural effusions. Severe fluid retention, some cases resulting in death, was reported following recent bone marrow transplantation in patients who have received Neumega. Neumega is not indicated following myeloablative chemotherapy (see **CLINICAL PHARMACOLOGY, Pharmacodynamics; WARNINGS, Increased Toxicity Following Myeloablative Therapy; WARNINGS, Cardiovascular Events**; and **WARNINGS, Dilutional Anemia**). It should be used with caution in patients with clinically evident congestive heart failure, patients who may be susceptible to developing congestive heart failure, patients receiving aggressive hydration, patients with a history of heart failure who are well-compensated and receiving appropriate medical therapy, and patients who may develop fluid retention as a result of associated medical conditions or whose medical condition may be exacerbated by fluid retention.

Fluid retention is reversible within several days following discontinuation of Neumega. During dosing with Neumega, fluid balance should be monitored and appropriate medical management is advised.

Close monitoring of fluid and electrolyte status should be performed in patients receiving chronic diuretic therapy. Sudden deaths have occurred in oprelvekin-treated patients receiving chronic diuretic therapy and ifosfamide who developed severe hypokalemia (see **ADVERSE REACTIONS**).

Pre-existing fluid collections, including pericardial effusions or ascites, should be monitored. Drainage should be considered if medically indicated.

Dilutional Anemia

Moderate decreases in hemoglobin concentration, hematocrit, and red blood cell count (~10% to 15%) without a decrease in red blood cell mass have been observed. These changes are predominantly due to an increase in plasma volume (dilutional anemia) that is primarily related to renal sodium and water retention. The decrease in hemoglobin concentration typically begins within three to five days of the initiation of Neumega, and is reversible over approximately a week following discontinuation of Neumega (see **WARNINGS, Fluid Retention**).

Cardiovascular Events

Neumega use is associated with cardiovascular events including arrhythmias and pulmonary edema. Cardiac arrest has been reported, but the causal relationship to Neumega is uncertain. Use with caution in patients with a history of atrial arrhythmias, and only after consideration of the potential risks in relation to anticipated benefit. In clinical trials, cardiac events including atrial arrhythmias (atrial fibrillation or atrial flutter) occurred in 15% (23/157) of patients treated with Neumega at doses of 50 µg/kg. Arrhythmias were usually brief in duration; conversion to sinus rhythm typically occurred spontaneously or after rate-control drug therapy. Approximately one-half (11/24) of the patients who were rechallenged had recurrent atrial arrhythmias. Clinical sequelae, including stroke, have been reported in patients who experienced atrial arrhythmias while receiving Neumega.

The mechanism for induction of arrhythmias is not known. Neumega was not directly arrhythmogenic in animal models. In some patients, development of atrial arrhythmias may be due to increased plasma volume associated with fluid retention (see **WARNINGS, Fluid Retention**).

Nervous System Events

Stroke has been reported in the setting of patients who develop atrial fibrillation/flutter while receiving Neumega (see **WARNINGS, Cardiovascular Events**). Patients with a history of stroke or transient ischemic attack may also be at increased risk for these events.

Papilledema

Papilledema has been reported in 2% (10/405) of patients receiving Neumega in clinical trials following repeated cycles of exposure. The incidence was higher, 16% (7/43) in children than in adults, 1% (3/362). Nonhuman primates treated with Neumega at a dose of 1,000 µg/kg SC once daily for four to 13 weeks developed papilledema that was not associated with inflammation or any other histologic abnormality and was reversible after dosing was discontinued. Neumega should be used with caution in patients with pre-existing papilledema, or with tumors involving the central nervous system since it is possible that papilledema could worsen or develop during treatment (see **ADVERSE REACTIONS**).

PRECAUTIONS

General

Dosing with Neumega should begin 6 to 24 hours following the completion of chemotherapy dosing. The safety and efficacy of Neumega given immediately prior to or concurrently with cytotoxic chemotherapy or initiated at the time of expected nadir have not been established (see **DOSAGE AND ADMINISTRATION**).

The effectiveness of Neumega has not been evaluated in patients receiving chemotherapy regimens of greater than five days duration or regimens associated with delayed myelosuppression (eg, nitrosoureas, mitomycin-C).

Chronic Administration

Neumega has been administered safely using the recommended dosage schedule (see **DOSAGE AND ADMINISTRATION**) for up to six cycles following chemotherapy. The safety and efficacy of chronic administration of Neumega have not been established. Continuous dosage (two to 13 weeks) in nonhuman primates produced joint capsule and tendon fibrosis and periosteal hyperostosis (see **PRECAUTIONS, Pediatric Use**). The relevance of these findings to humans is unclear.

Information for Patients

Neumega should be used under the guidance and supervision of a health care professional. However, when the physician determines that Neumega may be used outside of the hospital or office setting, persons who will be administering Neumega should be instructed as to the proper dose, and the method for reconstituting and administering Neumega (see **DOSAGE AND ADMINISTRATION**). If home use is prescribed, patients should be instructed in the importance of proper disposal and cautioned against the reuse of needles, syringes, drug product, and diluent. A puncture resistant container should be used by the patient for the disposal of used needles.

Patients should be informed of the serious and most common adverse reactions associated with Neumega administration, including those symptoms related to allergic or hypersensitivity reactions (see **BOXED WARNING**). Patients should be advised to immediately seek medical attention if any of the following signs or symptoms develop: swelling of the face, tongue, or throat; difficulty breathing, swallowing or talking; shortness of breath; wheezing; chest pain; throat tightness; lightheadedness; loss of consciousness; confusion; drowsiness; rash; itching; hives; flushing and/or fever. Mild to moderate peripheral edema and shortness of breath on exertion can occur within the first week of treatment and may continue for the duration of administration of Neumega. Patients who have preexisting pleural or other effusions or a history of congestive heart failure should be advised to contact their physician for worsening of dyspnea (see **ADVERSE REACTIONS** and **WARNINGS, Fluid Retention**). Most patients who receive Neumega develop anemia. Patients should be advised to contact their physician if symptoms attributable to atrial arrhythmia develop. Female patients of childbearing potential should be advised of the possible risks to the fetus of Neumega (see **PRECAUTIONS, Pregnancy Category C**).

Laboratory Monitoring

A complete blood count should be obtained prior to chemotherapy and at regular intervals during Neumega therapy (see **DOSAGE AND ADMINISTRATION**). Platelet counts should be monitored during the time of the expected nadir and until adequate recovery has occurred (post-nadir counts ≥50,000/µL).

Drug Interactions

Most patients in trials evaluating Neumega were treated concomitantly with filgrastim (G-CSF) with no adverse effect of Neumega on the activity of G-CSF. No information is available on the clinical use of sargramostim (GM-CSF) with Neumega in human subjects. However, in a study in nonhuman primates in which Neumega and GM-CSF were coadministered, there were no adverse interactions between Neumega and GM-CSF and no apparent difference in the pharmacokinetic profile of Neumega.

Drug interactions between Neumega and other drugs have not been fully evaluated. Based on *in vitro* and nonclinical *in vivo* evaluations of Neumega, drug-drug interactions with known substrates of P450 enzymes would not be predicted.

Carcinogenesis, Mutagenesis, Impairment of Fertility

No studies have been performed to assess the carcinogenic potential of Neumega. *In vitro*, Neumega did not stimulate the growth of tumor colony-forming cells harvested from patients with a variety of human malignancies. Neumega has been shown to be non-genotoxic in *in vitro* studies. These data suggest that Neumega is not mutagenic. Although prolonged estrus cycles have been noted at two to 20 times the human dose, no effects on fertility have been observed in rats treated with Neumega at doses up to 1,000 µg/kg/day.

Pregnancy Category C

Neumega has been shown to have embryocidal effects in pregnant rats and rabbits when given in doses of 0.2 to 20 times the human dose. There are no adequate and well-controlled studies of Neumega in pregnant women. Neumega should be used during pregnancy only if the potential benefit justifies the potential risk to the fetus.

Neumega has been tested in studies of fertility, early embryonic development, and pre- and postnatal development in rats and in studies of organogenesis (teratogenicity) in rats and rabbits. Parental toxicity has been observed when Neumega is given at doses of two to 20 times the human dose (≥100 µg/kg/day) in the rat and at 0.02 to 2.0 times the human dose (≥1 µg/kg/day) in the rabbit. Findings in pregnant rats consisted of transient hypoactivity and dyspnea after administration (maternal toxicity), as well as prolonged estrus cycle, increased early embryonic deaths and decreased numbers of live fetuses. In addition, low fetal body weights and a reduced number of ossified sacral and caudal vertebrae (ie, retarded fetal development) occurred in rats at 20 times the human dose. Findings in pregnant rabbits consisted of decreased fecal/urine eliminations (the only toxicity noted at 1 µg/kg/day in dams) as well as decreased food consumption, body weight loss, abortion, increased embryonic and fetal deaths, and decreased numbers of live fetuses. No teratogenic effects of Neumega were observed in rabbits at doses up to 0.6 times the human dose (30 µg/kg/day).

Adverse effects in the first generation offspring of rats given Neumega at maternally toxic doses ≥2 times the human dose (≥100 µg/kg/day) during both gestation and lactation included increased newborn mortality, decreased viability index on day 4 of lactation, and decreased body weights during lactation. In rats given 20 times the human dose (1,000 µg/kg/day) during both gestation and lactation, maternal toxicity and growth retardation of the first generation offspring resulted in an increased rate of fetal death of the second generation offspring.

Nursing Mothers

It is not known if Neumega is excreted in human milk. Because many drugs are excreted in human milk and because of the potential for serious adverse reactions in nursing infants from Neumega, a decision should be made whether to discontinue nursing or to discontinue Neumega, taking into account the importance of the drug to the mother.

Pediatric Use

A safe and effective dose of Neumega has not been established in children. In a Phase 1, single arm, dose-escalation study, 43 pediatric patients were treated with Neumega at doses ranging from 25 to 125 µg/kg/day following ICE chemotherapy. All patients required platelet transfusions and the lack of a comparator arm made the study design inadequate to assess efficacy. The projected effective dose (based on comparable AUC observed for the effective dose in healthy adults) in children appears to exceed the maximum tolerated pediatric dose of 50 µg/kg/day (see **CLINICAL PHARMACOLOGY, Pharmacokinetics**). Papilledema was dose-limiting and occurred in 16% of children (see **WARNINGS, Papilledema**).

The most common adverse events seen in pediatric studies included tachycardia (84%), conjunctival injection (57%), radiographic and echocardiographic evidence of cardiomegaly (21%) and periosteal changes (11%). These events occurred at a higher frequency in children than adults. The incidence of other adverse events was generally similar to those observed using Neumega at a dose of 50 µg/kg in the randomized studies in adults receiving chemotherapy (see **ADVERSE REACTIONS**).

Studies in animals were predictive of the effect of Neumega on developing bone in children. In growing rodents treated with 100, 300, or 1,000 µg/kg/day for a minimum of 28 days, thickening of femoral and tibial growth plates was noted, which did not completely resolve after a 28-day non-treatment period. In a nonhuman primate toxicology study of Neumega, animals treated for two to 13 weeks at doses of 10 to 1000 µg/kg showed partially reversible joint capsule and tendon fibrosis and periosteal hyperostosis. An asymptomatic, laminated periosteal reaction in the diaphyses of the femur, tibia, and fibula has been observed in one patient during pediatric studies involving multiple courses of Neumega treatment. The relationship of these findings to treatment with Neumega is unclear. No studies have been performed to assess the long-term effects of Neumega on growth and development.

Use in Patients with Renal Impairment

Neumega is eliminated primarily by the kidneys. The pharmacokinetics of Neumega were studied in subjects with

Continued on next page

Neumega—Cont.

varying degrees of renal dysfunction. $AUC_{0-\infty}$ C_{max}, and absolute bioavailability were significantly increased in subjects with severe renal impairment (creatinine clearance < 30 mL/min) (see **DOSAGE AND ADMINISTRATION**). There were no significant changes in the pharmacokinetic parameters in subjects with mild or moderate impairment. A significant decrease in the hemoglobin concentration was noted on Day 2 after a single dose of Neumega in subjects with all degrees of renal impairment. By Day 14, the hemoglobin was decreased only in patients with severe renal impairment. Fluid retention associated with Neumega treatment has not been studied in patients with renal impairment, but fluid balance should be carefully monitored in these patients (see **WARNINGS, Fluid Retention**).

ADVERSE REACTIONS

Because clinical trials are conducted under widely varying conditions, adverse reaction rates observed in the clinical studies of a drug cannot be directly compared to rates in the clinical studies of another drug and may not reflect the rates observed in practice. The adverse reaction information from clinical trials does, however, provide a basis for identifying the adverse events that appear to be related to drug use and for approximating rates.

Three hundred twenty-four subjects, with ages ranging from eight months to 75 years, have been exposed to Neumega treatment in clinical studies. Subjects have received up to six (eight in pediatric patients) sequential courses of Neumega treatment, with each course lasting from one to 28 days. Apart from the sequelae of the underlying malignancy or cytotoxic chemotherapy, most adverse events were mild or moderate in severity and reversible after discontinuation of Neumega dosing.

In general, the incidence and type of adverse events were similar between Neumega 50 µg/kg and placebo groups. The most frequently reported serious adverse events were neutropenic fever, syncope, atrial fibrillation, fever and pneumonia. The most commonly reported adverse events were edema, dyspnea, tachycardia, conjunctival injection, palpitations, atrial arrhythmias, and pleural effusions. The most frequently reported adverse reactions resulting in clinical intervention (eg, discontinuation of Neumega, adjustment in dosage, or the need for concomitant medication to treat an adverse reaction symptom) were atrial arrhythmias, syncope, dyspnea, congestive heart failure, and pulmonary edema (see **WARNINGS, Fluid Retention** and **WARNINGS, Cardiovascular Events**). Selected adverse events that occurred in ≥10% of Neumega-treated patients are listed in Table 3.

TABLE 3
SELECTED ADVERSE EVENTS

Body System / Adverse Event	Placebo n=67 (%)	50 µg/kg n=69 (%)
Body as a Whole		
Edema*	10 (15)	41 (59)
Neutropenic fever	28 (42)	33 (48)
Headache	24 (36)	28 (41)
Fever	19 (28)	25 (36)
Cardiovascular System		
Tachycardia*	2 (3)	14 (20)
Vasodilatation	6 (9)	13 (19)
Palpitations*	2 (3)	10 (14)
Syncope	4 (6)	9 (13)
Atrial fibrillation/ flutter*	1 (1)	8 (12)
Digestive System		
Nausea/vomiting	47 (70)	53 (77)
Mucositis	25 (37)	30 (43)
Diarrhea	22 (33)	30 (43)
Oral moniliasis*	1 (1)	10 (14)
Nervous System		
Dizziness	19 (28)	26 (38)
Insomnia	18 (27)	23 (33)
Respiratory System		
Dyspnea*	15 (22)	33 (48)
Rhinitis	21 (31)	29 (42)
Cough increased	15 (22)	20 (29)
Pharyngitis	11 (16)	17 (25)
Pleural effusions*	0 (0)	7 (10)
Skin and Appendages		
Rash	11 (16)	17 (25)
Special Senses		
Conjunctival Injection*	2 (3)	13 (19)

*Occurred in significantly more Neumega-treated patients than in placebo-treated patients.

The following adverse events also occurred more frequently in cancer patients receiving Neumega than in those receiving placebo: amblyopia, paresthesia, dehydration, skin discoloration, exfoliative dermatitis, and eye hemorrhage; a statistically significant association of Neumega to these events has not been established. Other than a higher incidence of severe asthenia in Neumega treated patients (10 [14%] in Neumega patients versus two [3%] in placebo patients), the incidence of severe or life-threatening adverse events was comparable in the Neumega and placebo treatment groups.

$$CLcr \approx \frac{[140 - \text{age (years)}] \times \text{weight (kg)}}{72 \times \text{serum creatinine (mg/dL)}} \quad [\times 0.85 \text{ for female patients}]$$

Two patients with cancer treated with Neumega experienced sudden death that the investigator considered possibly or probably related to Neumega. Both deaths occurred in patients with severe hypokalemia (<3.0 mEq/L) who had received high doses of ifosfamide and were receiving daily doses of a diuretic (see **WARNINGS, Cardiovascular Events**).

Other serious events associated with Neumega were papilledema and cardiovascular events including atrial arrhythmias and stroke. In addition, cardiomegaly was reported in children.

The following adverse events, occurring in ≥10% of patients, were observed at equal or greater frequency in placebo-treated patients: asthenia, pain, chills, abdominal pain, infection, anorexia, constipation, dyspepsia, ecchymosis, myalgia, bone pain, nervousness, and alopecia. The incidence of fever, neutropenic fever, flu-like symptoms, thrombocytosis, thrombotic events, the average number of units of red blood cells transfused per patient, and the duration of neutropenia <500 cells/µL were similar in the Neumega 50 µg/kg and placebo groups.

Immunogenicity

In clinical studies that evaluated the immunogenicity of Neumega, two of 181 patients (1%) developed antibodies to Neumega. In one of these two patients, neutralizing antibodies to Neumega were detected in an unvalidated assay. The clinical relevance of the presence of these antibodies is unknown. In the post-marketing setting, cases of allergic reactions, including anaphylaxis have been reported (see **WARNINGS, Allergic Reactions Including Anaphylaxis**). The presence of antibodies to Neumega was not assessed in these patients.

The data reflect the percentage of patients whose test results were considered positive for antibodies to Neumega and are highly dependent on the sensitivity and specificity of the assay. Additionally the observed incidence of antibody positivity in an assay may be influenced by several factors including sample handling, concomitant medications, and underlying disease. For these reasons, comparisons of the incidence of antibodies to Neumega with incidence of antibodies to other products may be misleading.

Abnormal Laboratory Values

The most common laboratory abnormality reported in patients in clinical trials was a decrease in hemoglobin concentration predominantly as a result of expansion of the plasma volume (see **WARNINGS, Fluid Retention**). The increase in plasma volume is also associated with a decrease in the serum concentration of albumin and several other proteins (eg, transferrin and gamma globulins). A parallel decrease in calcium without clinical effects has been documented. After daily SC injections, treatment with Neumega resulted in a two-fold increase in plasma fibrinogen. Other acute-phase proteins also increased. These protein levels returned to normal after dosing with Neumega was discontinued. Von Willebrand factor (vWF) concentrations increased with a normal multimer pattern in healthy subjects receiving Neumega.

Post-marketing Reports

The following adverse reactions have been reported during the post-marketing use of Neumega: allergic reactions, anaphylaxis/anaphylactoid reactions, papilledema, capillary leak syndrome, renal failure, and injection site reactions described as dermatitis, pain, and discoloration (see **BOXED WARNING; WARNINGS, Allergic Reactions Including Anaphylaxis; WARNINGS, Increased Toxicity Following Myeloablative Therapy; WARNINGS, Papilledema,** and **CONTRAINDICATIONS**).

Because these reactions are reported voluntarily from a population of uncertain size, it is not always possible to reliably estimate their frequency or establish a causal relationship to drug exposure. Decisions to include these reactions in labeling are typically based on one or more of the following factors: (1) seriousness of the reactions, (2) frequency of reporting, or (3) strength of causal connection to Neumega.

OVERDOSAGE

Doses of Neumega above 125 µg/kg have not been administered to humans. While clinical experience is limited, doses of Neumega greater than 50 µg/kg may be associated with an increased incidence of cardiovascular events in adult patients (see **WARNINGS, Fluid Retention** and **Cardiovascular Events**). If an overdose of Neumega is administered, Neumega should be discontinued, and the patient should be closely observed for signs of toxicity (see **WARNINGS** and **ADVERSE REACTIONS**). Reinstitution of Neumega therapy should be based upon individual patient factors (eg, evidence of toxicity, continued need for therapy).

DOSAGE AND ADMINISTRATION

The recommended dose of Neumega in adults without severe renal impairment is 50 µg/kg given once daily. Neumega should be administered subcutaneously as a single injection in either the abdomen, thigh, or hip (or upper arm if not self-injecting). A safe and effective dose has not been established in children (see **PRECAUTIONS, Pediatric Use**).

The recommended dose of Neumega in adults with severe renal impairment (creatinine clearance <30 mL/min) is 25 µg/kg. An estimate of the patient's creatinine clearance (CLcr) in mL/min is required. CLcr in mL/min may be estimated from a spot serum creatinine (mg/dL) determination using the following formula:

[See table above]

Dosing should be initiated six to 24 hours after the completion of chemotherapy. Platelet counts should be monitored periodically to assess the optimal duration of therapy. Dosing should be continued until the post-nadir platelet count is ≥50,000/µL. In controlled clinical trials, doses were administered in courses of 10 to 21 days. Dosing beyond 21 days per treatment course is not recommended.

Treatment with Neumega should be discontinued at least two days before starting the next planned cycle of chemotherapy.

Preparation of Neumega

1. Neumega is a sterile, white, preservative-free, lyophilized powder for subcutaneous injection upon reconstitution. Neumega (5 mg vials) should be reconstituted aseptically with 1.0 mL of Sterile Water for Injection, USP (without preservative). The reconstituted Neumega solution is clear, colorless, isotonic, with a pH of 7.0, and contains 5 mg/mL of Neumega. The single-use vial should not be re-entered or reused. Any unused portion of either reconstituted Neumega solution or Sterile Water for Injection, USP should be discarded.
2. During reconstitution, the Sterile Water for Injection, USP should be directed at the side of the vial and the contents gently swirled. EXCESSIVE OR VIGOROUS AGITATION SHOULD BE AVOIDED.
3. Parenteral drug products should be inspected visually for particulate matter and discoloration prior to administration, whenever solution and container permit. If particulate matter is present or the solution is discolored, the vial should not be used.
4. Because neither Neumega powder for injection nor its accompanying diluent, Sterile Water for Injection, USP contains a preservative, Neumega should be used within 3 hours following reconstitution. Reconstituted Neumega may be refrigerated [2°C to 8°C (36°F to 46°F)] or at room temperature [up to 25°C (77°F)]. DO NOT FREEZE OR SHAKE THE RECONSTITUTED SOLUTION.

HOW SUPPLIED

Neumega is supplied as a sterile, white, preservative-free, lyophilized powder in vials containing 5 mg oprelvekin. Neumega is available in boxes containing one single-dose Neumega vial and one 1-mL vial of diluent for Neumega (Sterile Water for Injection, USP) - NDC 58394-004-01, and boxes containing seven single-dose Neumega vials and seven 1-mL vials of diluent for Neumega (Sterile Water for Injection, USP) - NDC 58394-004-02.

Storage

Lyophilized Neumega and diluent should be stored in a refrigerator at 2°C to 8°C (36°F to 46°F). Protect from light. DO NOT FREEZE. Reconstituted Neumega must be used within 3 hours of reconstitution and can be stored in the vial either at 2°C to 8°C (36°F to 46°F) or at room temperature up to 25°C (77°F).

REFERENCES

(1) Du, X. and Williams, D., Interleukin 11: review of molecular, cell biology and clinical use. *Blood*. 1997;89(11): 3897–3908.

Wyeth®

Wyeth Pharmaceuticals Inc.
Philadelphia, PA 19101
US Govt. License No. 3

W10439C007
ET01
Rev 06/04

Information for Patients
NEUMEGA®
[nu-meg<a]
(oprelvekin)
℞ only

This product's label may have been revised after this insert was used in production. For further product information and current package insert, please visit www.wyeth.com or call our medical communications department toll-free at 1-800-934-5556.

This patient package insert contains information and directions for patients and their caregivers who are getting or giving injections of Neumega at home. You should read this patient information each time you pick up your prescription in case new information has been added. This patient package insert does not take the place of talking with your doctor or other healthcare provider. If you have any questions about your treatment with Neumega you should talk to your doctor.

What is Neumega?

Neumega is a medicine that stimulates your body to make platelets, which are a type of blood cell. Neumega is for people who have received certain types of chemotherapy and is used to help prevent the number of platelets circulating in the blood from dropping dangerously low. Too few platelets can cause serious problems and even death. Platelets are needed to help clot your blood when you are cut or injured. People with very low platelet counts are more likely to bruise and may not be able to control their bleeding if they are cut or injured. Platelets that have been donated by other people (platelet transfusions) are often given to patients with very low platelet counts. Neumega may reduce the need for platelet transfusions after chemotherapy. If your platelet levels are still too low after taking Neumega, your doctor may recommend that you receive a platelet transfusion.

What is the most important information I should know about Neumega?

Neumega may have side effects; some of these side effects may be serious. The most serious possible side effects of treatment with Neumega include:

- **Allergic Reactions**

  Neumega can cause serious allergic reactions in some patients. Signs that you are having a serious allergic reaction include: swelling of your face, tongue or throat; difficulty breathing, swallowing or talking; shortness of breath; wheezing; chest pain; a tightness in your throat; feeling lightheaded; loss of consciousness; confusion; drowsiness; rash; itching; hives; flushing and/or fever. You or your caregiver should call your doctor immediately if you develop any of these signs or symptoms.

- **Heart Problems**

  Neumega can cause heart problems in some patients. If you feel like your heart is pounding, beating fast or skipping a beat, or you have chest pains or are short of breath, you should call your doctor immediately. If you have ever had heart problems, you should tell your doctor before you start treatment with Neumega.

  If you are taking a water pill (diuretic), you should tell your doctor, because the diuretic can cause your body to lose potassium. This is very important, because Neumega can cause heart problems and these heart problems could be more serious when the potassium in your blood is too low. Your doctor will be checking your blood for the amount of potassium in it. If your potassium level is low, your doctor may prescribe a potassium replacement medication to correct it.

- **Water Weight Gain**

  Neumega may cause you to retain water and gain weight from the extra fluid in your body. For some patients, water weight gain may cause serious problems that require medicine or hospitalization. A small amount of water weight gain will usually go away within several days after you stop taking Neumega. But, if you have a rapid weight gain over a few days, swelling of the legs and feet, dizziness, shortness of breath or chest pain, it could mean that you have a serious condition with fluid around the lungs and heart. If you have ever had heart failure or are taking medicine that may cause you to retain water, you should tell your doctor before you start treatment with Neumega.

- **Children Receiving Neumega**

  Because Neumega is approved only for use in adults, you should talk to your child's doctor about the reasons why Neumega has been prescribed for your child. You should talk to your child's doctor about the risks and side effects of using this medication in children. One of the side effects seen in children taking Neumega is a serious eye condition called papilledema which is a form of swelling in the back of the eye. Many children may not show any signs of papilledema. If your child complains that they have a headache or are having difficulty seeing, call your child's doctor right away. Other side effects that have been seen in children are fast heartbeat, redness of the eye, changes to the heart, and changes to bones that can be seen on x-ray.

- **Stop taking Neumega and call your doctor or healthcare provider immediately if you develop any of these symptoms:**
  - Shortness of breath or trouble breathing
  - Chest pains
  - Swelling in your face, hands, or feet
  - Rapid weight gain over a few days
  - You feel like your heart is pounding or beating out of your chest or skipping a beat, also referred to as palpitations

Before you start taking Neumega, you should tell your doctor the names of all of the medications you are taking including prescription and non-prescription drugs, vitamins, and nutritional supplements. If you have any of the following conditions or medical problems, tell your doctor or healthcare provider:

- You are pregnant or are planning to become pregnant
- Breast feeding
- You have heart problems
- You have kidney disease
- You have eye problems

Who should not take Neumega?

Do not take Neumega if you have ever had or think you have had an allergic reaction to Neumega. Talk to your doctor if you have any questions about this information.

What are the other possible side effects of Neumega?

The most common, but less serious side effects, are:

- Slight water weight gain
- Some swelling in the arms and/or legs
- Shortness of breath when walking or moving around
- Anemia (low red blood cell count)

These side effects may be caused by water retention. For most people, the water weight gain will go away a few days after the last injection of Neumega. Make sure you have read and understand the section called **"What is the most important information I should know about Neumega?"**, because many of these side effects could develop into a more serious condition.

Other side effects that you should tell your doctor about are:

- Blurred vision, headaches, or redness of the eyes
- Any swelling or bruising that doesn't go away in the location where you have injected Neumega

If you have any other problems, whether or not you think they are related to Neumega, you should call your doctor.

What important information do I need to know about taking Neumega at home?

To see if Neumega is working, your doctor will ask you to have blood tests done to measure the number of platelets in your body. After starting Neumega, it may take 10 to 21 days for your platelet numbers to increase. The amount of time it takes to increase the number of platelets varies from patient to patient. Neumega may not work for everyone and you may still need platelet transfusions or have bleeding even if you take Neumega as directed by your doctor. **You should always follow your doctor's instructions.**

If your doctor has recommended that you receive Neumega at home, then you and/or your caregiver should be instructed on how to prepare Neumega, how much Neumega to use, how to inject it, how often it should be injected, and how to dispose of the unused portions of each bottle. Do not inject Neumega until you are comfortable with the steps to prepare and inject Neumega at home.

It is important that you do not take any more or less of the amount of Neumega that your doctor prescribed. Too much Neumega might put you at risk for irregular heartbeats and water retention (including fluid around the heart and lungs). If you accidentally take too much Neumega, you should call your doctor immediately.

You should always change the site of your injections each day to avoid soreness at any one site. Your injections should be given about the same time each day. If you miss an injection on one day, you should not try to add it on the next day. Tell your doctor that you missed a dose and continue as usual with your next scheduled dose. The section **"How Do I Give Myself Neumega?"** gives you step-by-step instructions for preparing and injecting your dose of Neumega.

How Do I Give Myself Neumega?

Preparing the Neumega for Injection

1. First, make sure that you have all of the supplies that you will need:

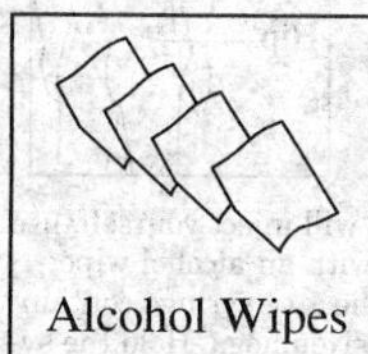

a) Four alcohol wipes.

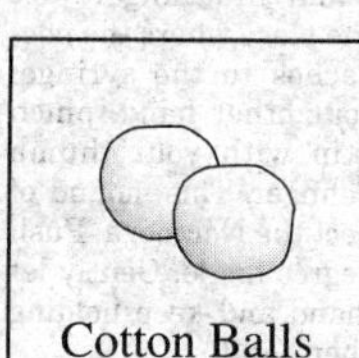
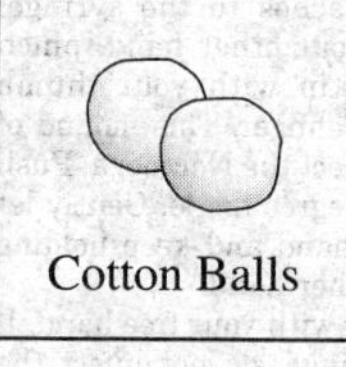

b) Two cotton balls.

3 cc
1 cc

c) Two syringes (plastic tube with lines on it).
A 3 cc (or 3 mL) syringe for adding the Sterile Water for Injection, USP to the Neumega powder
A 1 cc (or 1 mL) syringe for giving the injection

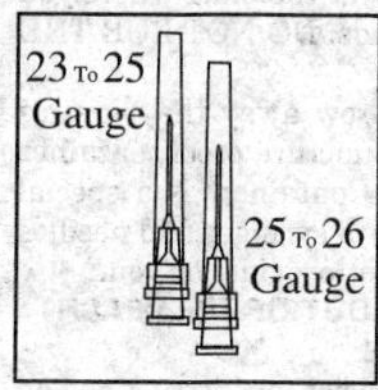

d) Two needles.
One needle to use with the 3 cc syringe: 23 to 25 gauge, ¾ to 1 inch needle
One needle to use with the 1 cc syringe: 25 to 26 gauge, ½ to 1 inch needle

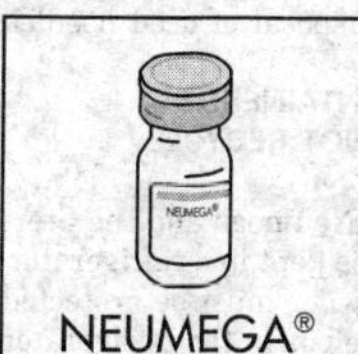

e) Bottle of Neumega powder.

STERILE WATER
FOR INJECTION, USP

f) Bottle of Sterile Water for Injection, USP.

g) A puncture proof container ("Sharps Container") for disposing needles and syringes.

2. You must use a new bottle of Neumega powder and a new bottle of Sterile Water for Injection, USP every time you give yourself a dose of Neumega.
   Look for the expiration date printed on each bottle. DO NOT USE the Neumega powder or the Sterile Water for Injection, USP if the current month and year is after the month and year on the bottles; this means that the Neumega or Sterile Water for Injection, USP have expired. Notify your doctor that the Neumega and/or the Sterile Water for Injection, USP have expired and that you need replacement bottles. If the Neumega powder and the Sterile Water for Injection, USP have not expired, then continue with the steps that follow.

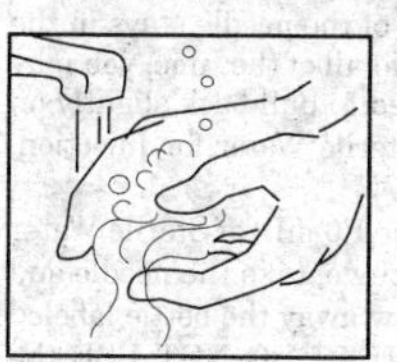

Wash your hands with soap and water.

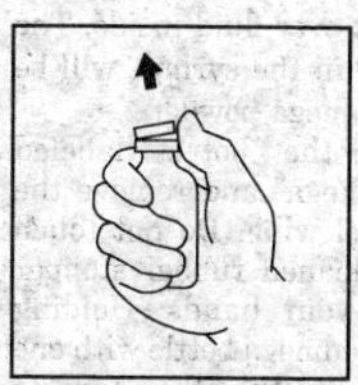

3. Pick up the bottle labeled "Sterile Water for Injection, USP" and flip off the white protective cap. Wipe the rubber stopper on the top of the bottle with a sterile alcohol wipe. Leave the wipe on top of the bottle.
4. Pick up the bottle labeled "Neumega" and flip off the orange protective cap. Wipe the rubber stopper on the top of the bottle with a sterile alcohol wipe. Leave the wipe on top of the bottle.
5. Remove the 3 cc syringe from its package.
   - The syringe has two parts:
     1) A clear plastic tube with lines on the outside and
     2) A plastic plunger that fits into the tube

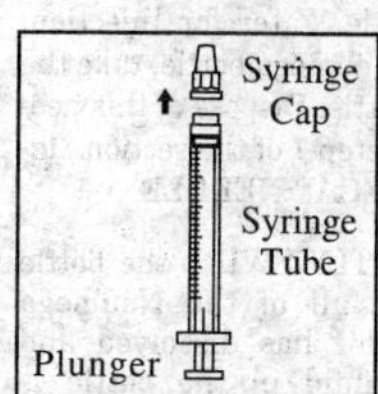

- Remove the protective cover (syringe cap) from the tip of this syringe. The needle attaches to this end of the syringe.

6. There are lines and numbers on the syringe, much like a measuring cup. The lines and numbers tell you how much fluid is in the syringe. If you hold the end of the plunger that sticks out, and move it in and out, you can adjust how much fluid you will pull into the syringe or inject out.

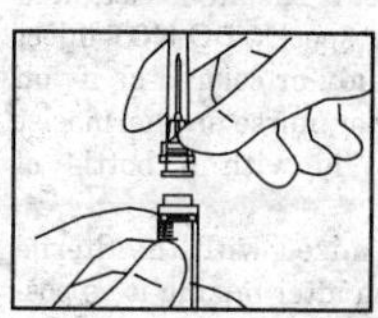

7. Remove the 23 to 25 gauge needle from its package. With the cap still on this needle, attach it to the 3 cc syringe. Remove the cap of this needle by gently pulling it off, but do not touch the needle with your hand or let it touch anything else. It is important to keep this needle sterile in order to prevent infection.

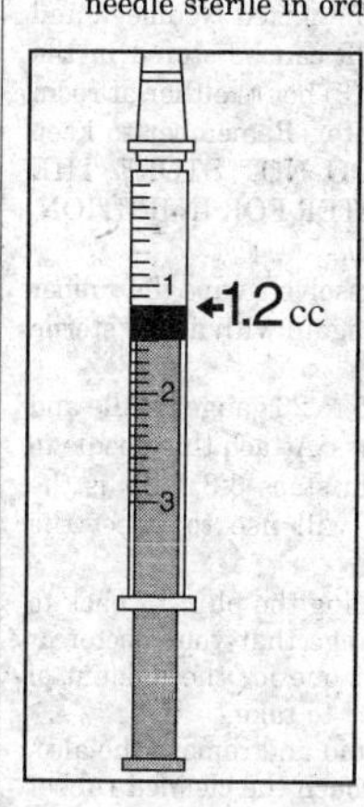

8. Holding the 3 cc syringe with the needle attached, carefully pull the plunger back until the end of the plunger that is inside the syringe is at the line that represents "1.2 cc" or 1.2 mL".

Continued on next page

Neumega—Cont.

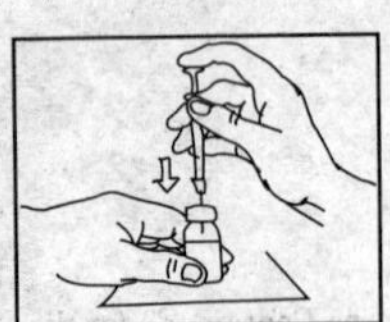

9. Take the bottle labeled "Sterile Water for Injection, USP" and remove the alcohol wipe. Do not touch the cleaned rubber stopper with your hands. Hold the bottle with one hand and push the needle through the center of the rubber stopper. Inject the air you pulled into the syringe (step 8) into the space at the top of the bottle. Do not inject the air into the water itself. Injecting the air directly into the sterile water will cause bubbles to form.

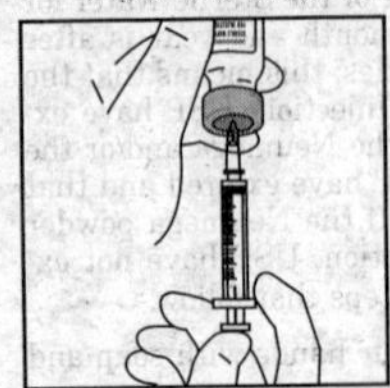

Keeping the needle inside the bottle, gently turn the bottle upside down. Slowly pull the plunger back to the black line marked "1.0 cc" or "1.0 mL" to remove 1.0 mL of Sterile Water for Injection, USP. To make sure that the tip of the needle stays in the fluid all of the time, you may need to pull back slightly on the syringe as you pull the Sterile Water for Injection, USP into the syringe.

10. After you have pulled 1.0 cc (or 1.0 mL) of Sterile Water for Injection, USP into the syringe, take the needle and syringe out of the bottle. Throw away the bottle labeled "Sterile Water for Injection, USP." DO NOT USE the bottle again, even if there is left over fluid inside. The Sterile Water for Injection, USP in the syringe will be added to the bottle with the Neumega powder.

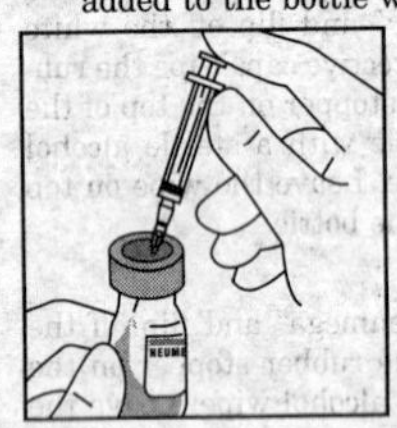

11. Take the bottle labeled "Neumega" and remove the alcohol wipe. Do not touch the cleaned rubber stopper with your hands. Holding the Neumega bottle with one hand, use the other hand to push the needle of the syringe that has the Sterile Water for Injection, USP through the middle of the rubber stopper. Press the plunger of the syringe SLOWLY. Gently aim the stream of Sterile Water for Injection, USP so that it runs down the inside wall of the bottle.

12. After injecting all of the Sterile Water for Injection, USP from the syringe into the Neumega bottle, take the needle and syringe out of the bottle. Dispose of this needle and syringe as described in step 7 of the section **"Injecting Neumega"**. DO NOT RECAP NEEDLE.

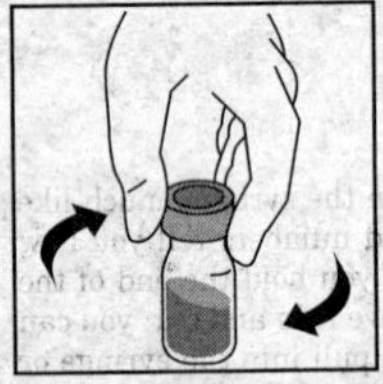

13. GENTLY SWIRL the bottle until all of the Neumega powder has dissolved and the fluid in the bottle is clear. **DO NOT SHAKE THE BOTTLE.** Shaking Neumega may damage the protein so it does not work properly.

Check the fluid inside the bottle. It should be clear and colorless without any powder or specks. **DO NOT** inject the Neumega if the fluid is cloudy or colored or if you see any particles. Call your doctor, nurse or pharmacist for instructions on what to do with a bottle of Neumega that you cannot use.

You should use the Neumega mixed with the Sterile Water for Injection, USP as soon after mixing it as possible. Do not let more than three (3) hours go by between the time you mix the Neumega and the water, and the time that you use it. The mixed Neumega and Sterile Water for Injection, USP can be stored in the Neumega bottle for up to three (3) hours either at room temperature or in the refrigerator. Remember to keep the bottle out of the light. DO NOT STORE THE NEUMEGA AND STERILE WATER FOR INJECTION, USP MIXTURE IN A SYRINGE.

14. After the Neumega powder is dissolved, wipe the rubber stopper on the top of the bottle again with a new sterile alcohol wipe.

15. Take the 1 cc syringe and the 25 to 26 gauge needle and remove them from their packages. Attach this needle to the 1 cc syringe as described in steps 6-8. This is the needle and syringe that you will use to inject the Neumega into your skin.

    Fill the syringe with air by pulling the plunger back to the line or number on the syringe that your doctor or nurse has told you is the right one for the amount of Neumega that you are supposed to take.

16. Take the bottle of Neumega liquid and remove the alcohol wipe from the top. Do not touch the cleaned rubber stopper with your hands. Hold the bottle with one hand and push the needle through the center of the rubber stopper. Inject the air from the syringe into the bottle.

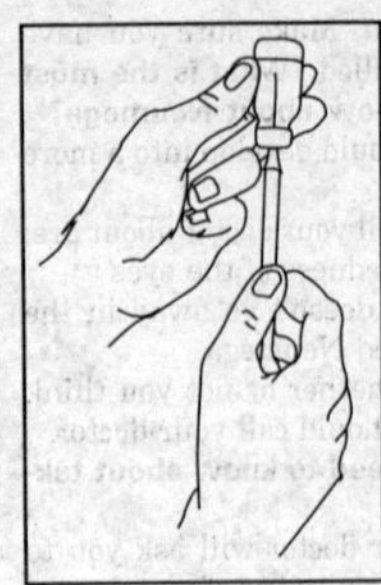

17. Turn the bottle and syringe upside down. Keep the tip of the needle in the fluid and slowly pull the plunger back. Stop when the fluid reaches the line or number that your doctor or nurse has told you is the right one for the amount of Neumega that you are supposed to take.

18. Check the syringe for bubbles. If you see bubbles in the syringe, push them back into the bottle by pushing in on the plunger. The fluid that is in the syringe should be clear and colorless, without any particles or bubbles.

    Check to be sure that the fluid is still at the line or number that your doctor or nurse has told you is the right one for the amount of Neumega that you are supposed to take. If it is too little, you will need to pull the plunger back to the mark. If it is too much, you will need to push the plunger in to the mark. Once you are sure you have the right amount, you can go on to step 19.

19. Take the needle out of the bottle. Hold the syringe with the needle pointing straight up and gently tap the side of the syringe with your fingers to bring remaining air bubbles to the top of the syringe.

20. Still holding the syringe and needle pointing up, press the plunger in a little to push any air out through the needle. If a small drop of fluid comes out, that's okay. DO NOT RECAP NEEDLE. Do not lay the syringe down or allow it to touch a surface.

Injecting Neumega

1. Neumega can be injected into the skin of your upper legs (thighs), your abdomen (stomach), your hip, or your upper arms if not self-injecting. You should inject the Neumega into one of these different places of your body every time you use it.

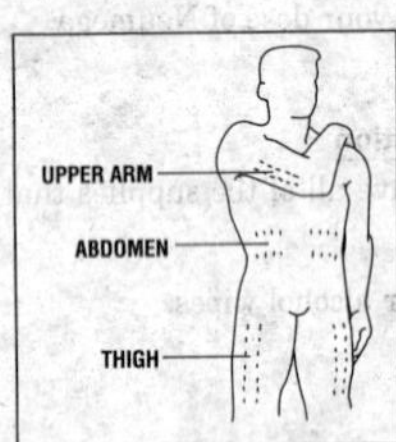

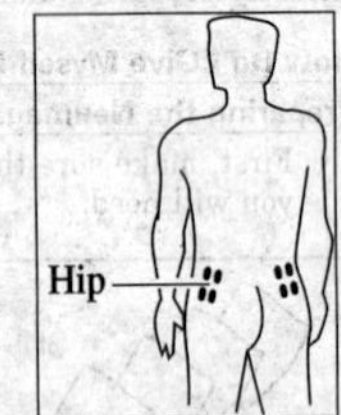

2. Once you have decided where you will inject yourself, use your free hand to clean the skin with an alcohol wipe.

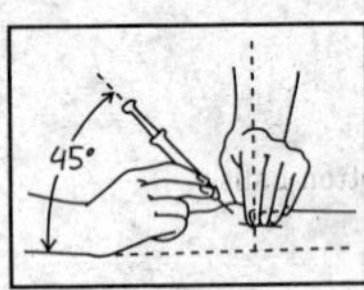

3. Take the 1 cc syringe containing the Neumega. Hold the syringe like a dart between the thumb and first finger just above the place where the needle attaches to the syringe. With your other hand, pinch your skin with your thumb and forefinger. This mound of skin is the place where you will inject the Neumega. Push the needle into the skin at a 45-degree angle. Gently let go of the pinched skin with one hand and keep holding the needle in the skin with the other hand.

4. GENTLY pull back on the plunger with your free hand. If you see blood come into the syringe, do not inject the Neumega. If this happens, take the syringe out of your skin, and discard this needle and syringe in a puncture proof container as outlined below in step 7 of this section. You will need to repeat all the above steps using new bottles of Sterile Water for Injection, USP and Neumega, with new syringes and needles and inject the Neumega at a new site.

5. If you do not see blood when you pull back the plunger, inject Neumega by slowly pushing the plunger all the way in.

6. Hold a cotton ball near the needle and pull the needle out of the skin. Press the cotton ball over the place where you made the injection for a few seconds. DO NOT RUB THE SITE.

7. DO NOT RECAP NEEDLES. Throw away the syringes with the needles on them into a puncture proof container ("Sharps Container"). A "Sharps Container" is a special box or other container for disposal of syringes and needles that your doctor or pharmacist can provide for you.

   ALWAYS KEEP THE CONTAINER OUT OF THE REACH OF CHILDREN.

   Ask your doctor, nurse, or pharmacist for instructions on how to properly dispose of a full container. There may be special state and local laws for disposal of used needles and syringes.

   DO NOT THROW THE CONTAINERS IN HOUSEHOLD TRASH. DO NOT RECYCLE.

How should I store Neumega?

Both the bottles with the powdered Neumega and the Sterile Water for Injection, USP should be kept in a refrigerator. **DO NOT FREEZE.** The Neumega powder must be protected from light. Keeping the bottles in the box in the refrigerator until you are ready to use them will help protect them.

Every time you give yourself a dose of Neumega, you must use a new bottle of Neumega powder and a new bottle of Sterile Water for Injection, USP. There is an expiration date printed on the bottles of the Neumega powder and on the Sterile Water for Injection, USP. Do not use the Neumega or the Sterile Water for Injection, USP if it is past the month and year on the bottles.

After you mix the Neumega with the Sterile Water for Injection, USP, you must use it as soon as possible. Do not let more than three (3) hours go by between the time you mix the Neumega and the water, and the time that you use it. The Neumega and Sterile Water for Injection, USP mixture can be stored in the Neumega bottle for up to three (3) hours either at room temperature or in the refrigerator. Remember to keep the bottle out of the light. DO NOT STORE THE NEUMEGA AND STERILE WATER MIXTURE IN A SYRINGE.

After you give yourself an injection of Neumega, if there is any left over in the bottle, or in the syringe, it should be thrown away. **DO NOT THROW THE CONTAINERS IN HOUSEHOLD TRASH. DO NOT RECYCLE.** Throw away these bottles into the same "Sharps Container" you put the needles and syringes in.

General Advice About Prescription Medicines

Medicines are sometimes prescribed for purposes other than those listed here. If you have any questions or concerns about Neumega talk to your doctor. Do not use Neumega for a condition or person other than for whom it is prescribed.

Wyeth®
Wyeth Pharmaceuticals Inc.
Philadelphia, PA 19101
US Govt. License No. 3

W10439C007
ET01
Rev 06/04

Shown in Product Identification Guide, page 336

OVRAL®-28 ℞

[*ō′vrăl*]
Tablets
(NORGESTREL AND ETHINYL ESTRADIOL TABLETS)
℞ only

Patients should be counseled that oral contraceptives do not protect against transmission of HIV (AIDS) and other sexually transmitted diseases (STDs) such as chlamydia, genital herpes, genital warts, gonorrhea, hepatitis B, and syphilis.

DESCRIPTION

21 white Ovral tablets, each containing 0.5 mg of norgestrel, (*dl*-13-beta-ethyl-17-alpha-ethinyl-17-beta-hydroxygon-4-en-3-one), a totally synthetic progestogen, and 0.05 mg of ethinyl estradiol, (19-nor-17α-pregna-1,3,5 (10)-trien-20-yne-3,17-diol), and 7 pink inert tablets. The inactive ingredients present are cellulose, D&C Red 30, lactose, magnesium stearate, and polacrilin potassium.

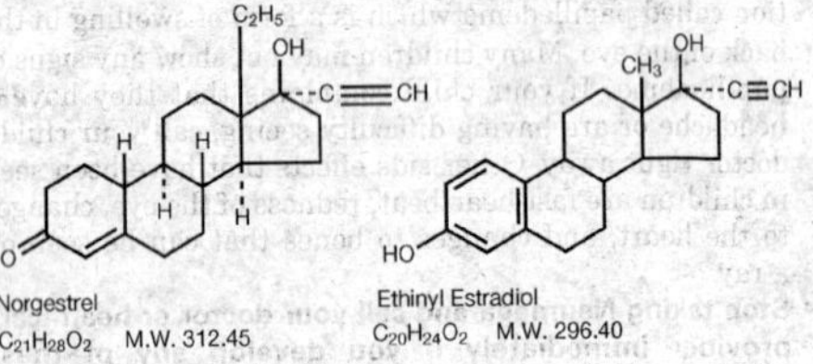

CLINICAL PHARMACOLOGY

Mode of Action

Combination oral contraceptives act by suppression of gonadotropins. Although the primary mechanism of this action is inhibition of ovulation, other alterations include changes in the cervical mucus (which increase the difficulty of sperm entry into the uterus) and the endometrium (which reduce the likelihood of implantation).

INDICATIONS AND USAGE

Oral contraceptives are indicated for the prevention of pregnancy in women who elect to use this product as a method of contraception. Oral contraceptive products such as Ovral® or Ovral®-28 (norgestrel and ethinyl estradiol tablets), which contain 50 mcg of estrogen, should not be used unless medically indicated.

Oral contraceptives are highly effective. Table I lists the typical accidental pregnancy rates for users of combination oral contraceptives and other methods of contraception. The efficacy of these contraceptive methods, except sterilization, the IUD, and implants depends upon the reliability with which they are used. Correct and consistent use of methods can result in lower failure rates.

[See table I at top of next page]

CONTRAINDICATIONS

Combination oral contraceptives should not be used in women with any of the following conditions:

Thrombophlebitis or thromboembolic disorders

Table I: Percentage Of Women Experiencing An Unintended Pregnancy During The First Year Of Typical Use And The First Year Of Perfect Use Of Contraception And The Percentage Continuing Use At The End Of The First Year. United States.

Method (1)	% of Women Experiencing an Unintended Pregnancy within the First Year of Use		% of Women Continuing Use at One Year[3]
	Typical Use[1] (2)	Perfect Use[2] (3)	(4)
Chance[4]	85	85	
Spermicides[5]	26	6	40
Periodic abstinence	25		63
Calendar		9	
Ovulation Method		3	
Sympto-Thermal[6]		2	
Post-Ovulation		1	
Cap[7]			
Parous Women	40	26	42
Nulliparous Women	20	9	56
Sponge			
Parous Women	40	20	42
Nulliparous Women	20	9	56
Diaphragm[7]	20	6	56
Withdrawal	19	4	
Condom[8]			
Female (Reality)	21	5	56
Male	14	3	61
Pill	5		71
Progestin only		0.5	
Combined		0.1	
IUD			
Progesterone T	2.0	1.5	81
Copper T380A	0.8	0.6	78
LNg 20	0.1	0.1	81
Depo-Provera®	0.3	0.3	70
Levonorgestrel Implants (Norplant®)	0.05	0.05	88
Female Sterilization	0.5	0.5	100
Male Sterilization	0.15	0.10	100

Lactation Amenorrhea Method: LAM is a highly effective, temporary method of contraception.[9]

Source: Trussell J. Contraceptive efficacy. In: Hatcher RA, Trussell J, Stewart F, Cates W, Stewart GK, Kowel D, Guest F. Contraceptive Technology: Seventeenth Revised Edition. New York NY: Irvington Publishers; 1998.

1. Among *typical* couples who initiate use of a method (not necessarily for the first time), the percentage who experience an accidental pregnancy during the first year if they do not stop use for any other reason.
2. Among couples who initiate use of a method (not necessarily for the first time) and who use it *perfectly* (both consistently and correctly), the percentage who experience an accidental pregnancy during the first year if they do not stop use for any other reason.
3. Among couples attempting to avoid pregnancy, the percentage who continue to use a method for one year.
4. The percents becoming pregnant in columns (2) and (3) are based on data from populations where contraception is not used and from women who cease using contraception in order to become pregnant. Among such populations, about 89% become pregnant within one year. This estimate was lowered slightly (to 85%) to represent the percent who would become pregnant within one year among women now relying on reversible methods of contraception if they abandoned contraception altogether.
5. Foams, creams, gels, vaginal suppositories, and vaginal film.
6. Cervical mucus (ovulation) method supplemented by calendar in the pre-ovulatory and basal body temperature in the post-ovulatory phases.
7. With spermicidal cream or jelly.
8. Without spermicides.
9. However, to maintain effective protection against pregnancy, another method of contraception must be used as soon as menstruation resumes, the frequency or duration of breastfeeds is reduced, bottle feeds are introduced, or the baby reaches 6 months of age.

A past history of deep-vein thrombophlebitis or thromboembolic disorders
Cerebral-vascular or coronary-artery disease (current or history)
Thrombogenic valvulopathies
Thrombogenic rhythm disorders
Major surgery with prolonged immobilization
Diabetes with vascular involvement
Headaches with focal neurological symptoms
Uncontrolled hypertension
Known or suspected carcinoma of the breast or personal history of breast cancer
Carcinoma of the endometrium or other known or suspected estrogen-dependent neoplasia
Undiagnosed abnormal genital bleeding
Cholestatic jaundice of pregnancy or jaundice with prior pill use
Hepatic adenomas or carcinomas, or active liver disease, as long as liver function has not returned to normal
Known or suspected pregnancy
Hypersensitivity to any of the components of Ovral-28

WARNINGS

Cigarette smoking increases the risk of serious cardiovascular side effects from oral-contraceptive use. This risk increases with age and with the extent of smoking (in epidemiologic studies, 15 or more cigarettes per day was associated with a significantly increased risk) and is quite marked in women over 35 years of age. Women who use oral contraceptives should be strongly advised not to smoke.

The use of oral contraceptives is associated with increased risks of several serious conditions including venous and arterial thrombotic and thromboembolic events (such as myocardial infarction, thromboembolism, and stroke), hepatic neoplasia, gallbladder disease, and hypertension, although the risk of serious morbidity or mortality is very small in healthy women without underlying risk factors. The risk of morbidity and mortality increases significantly in the presence of other underlying risk factors such as certain inherited or acquired thrombophilias, hypertension, hyperlipidemias, obesity, diabetes, and surgery or trauma with increased risk of thrombosis.

Practitioners prescribing oral contraceptives should be familiar with the following information relating to these risks. The information contained in this package insert is based principally on studies carried out in patients who used oral contraceptives with higher doses of estrogens and progestogens than those in common use today. The effect of long-term use of the oral contraceptives with lower doses of both estrogens and progestogens remains to be determined.

Throughout this labeling, epidemiological studies reported are of two types: retrospective or case control studies and prospective or cohort studies. Case control studies provide a measure of the relative risk of disease, namely, a ratio of the incidence of a disease among oral-contraceptive users to that among nonusers. The relative risk does not provide information on the actual clinical occurrence of a disease. Cohort studies provide a measure of attributable risk, which is the difference in the incidence of disease between oral-contraceptive users and nonusers. The attributable risk does provide information about the actual occurrence of a disease in the population. For further information, the reader is referred to a text on epidemiological methods.

1. Thromboembolic Disorders and Other Vascular Problems

a. Myocardial infarction

An increased risk of myocardial infarction has been attributed to oral-contraceptive use. This risk is primarily in smokers or women with other underlying risk factors for coronary-artery disease such as hypertension, hypercholesterolemia, morbid obesity, and diabetes. The relative risk of heart attack for current oral-contraceptive users has been estimated to be two to six. The risk is very low under the age of 30.

Smoking in combination with oral-contraceptive use has been shown to contribute substantially to the incidence of myocardial infarction in women in their mid-thirties or older with smoking accounting for the majority of excess cases. Mortality rates associated with circulatory disease have been shown to increase substantially in smokers over the age of 35 and nonsmokers over the age of 40 (Table II) among women who use oral contraceptives.

CIRCULATORY DISEASE MORTALITY RATES PER 100,000 WOMAN YEARS BY AGE, SMOKING STATUS AND ORAL-CONTRACEPTIVE USE

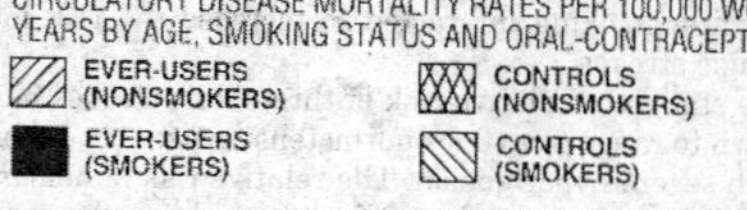

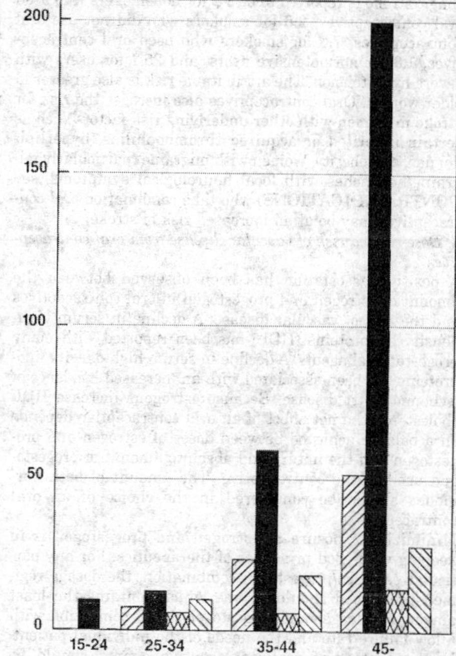

TABLE II. (Adapted From P.M. Layde And V. Beral, Lancet, *I*:541-546, 1981.)

Oral contraceptives may compound the effects of well-known risk factors, such as hypertension, diabetes, hyperlipidemias, age, and obesity. In particular, some progesto-

Continued on next page

Ovral-28—Cont.

gens are known to decrease HDL cholesterol and cause glucose intolerance, while estrogens may create a state of hyperinsulinism. Oral contraceptives have been shown to increase blood pressure among users (see section 9 in **WARNINGS**). Similar effects on risk factors have been associated with an increased risk of heart disease. Oral contraceptives must be used with caution in women with cardiovascular disease risk factors.

b. Venous thrombosis and thromboembolism

An increased risk of venous thromboembolic and thrombotic disease associated with the use of oral contraceptives is well established. Case control studies have found the relative risk of users compared to nonusers to be 3 for the first episode of superficial venous thrombosis, 4 to 11 for deep-vein thrombosis or pulmonary embolism, and 1.5 to 6 for women with predisposing conditions for venous thromboembolic disease. Cohort studies have shown the relative risk to be somewhat lower, about 3 for new cases and about 4.5 for new cases requiring hospitalization. Some epidemiological studies suggest that COCs with 50 mcg or more of ethinyl estradiol may be associated with a higher risk of such events than COCs with a lower dose of ethinyl estradiol. However, the incidence is substantially less than that associated with pregnancy (6 per 10,000 woman-years). The excess risk is highest during the first year a woman ever uses a combined oral contraceptive. Venous thromboembolism may be fatal. The risk of venous thrombotic and thromboembolic events is further increased in women with conditions predisposing for venous thrombosis and thromboembolism. The risk of thromboembolic disease due to oral contraceptives is not related to length of use and gradually disappears after pill use is stopped.

A two- to four-fold increase in relative risk of postoperative thromboembolic complications has been reported with the use of oral contraceptives. The relative risk of venous thrombosis in women who have predisposing conditions is twice that of women without such medical conditions. If feasible, oral contraceptives should be discontinued at least four weeks prior to and for two weeks after elective surgery of a type associated with an increase in risk of thromboembolism and during and following prolonged immobilization. Since the immediate postpartum period is also associated with an increased risk of thromboembolism, oral contraceptives should be started no earlier than four weeks after delivery in women who elect not to breast-feed, or a midtrimester pregnancy termination.

c. Cerebrovascular diseases

Oral contraceptives have been shown to increase both the relative and attributable risks of cerebrovascular events (thrombotic and hemorrhagic strokes), although, in general, the risk is greatest among older (>35 years), hypertensive women who also smoke. Hypertension was found to be a risk factor for both users and nonusers, for both types of strokes, while smoking interacted to increase the risk for hemorrhagic strokes.

In a large study, the relative risk of thrombotic strokes has been shown to range from 3 for normotensive users to 14 for users with severe hypertension. The relative risk of hemorrhagic stroke is reported to be 1.2 for nonsmokers who used oral contraceptives, 2.6 for smokers who did not use oral contraceptives, 7.6 for smokers who used oral contraceptives, 1.8 for normotensive users, and 25.7 for users with severe hypertension. The attributable risk is also greater in older women. Oral contraceptives also increase the risk for stroke in women with other underlying risk factors such as certain inherited or acquired thrombophilias, hyperlipidemias, and obesity. Women with migraine (particularly migraine/headaches with focal neurological symptoms, see **CONTRAINDICATIONS**) who take combination oral contraceptives may be at an increased risk of stroke.

d. Dose-related risk of vascular disease from oral contraceptives

A positive association has been observed between the amount of estrogen and progestogen in oral contraceptives and the risk of vascular disease. A decline in serum high-density lipoproteins (HDL) has been reported with many progestational agents. A decline in serum high-density lipoproteins has been associated with an increased incidence of ischemic heart disease. Because estrogens increase HDL cholesterol, the net effect of an oral contraceptive depends on a balance achieved between doses of estrogen and progestogen and the nature and absolute amount of progestogen used in the contraceptive. The amount of both hormones should be considered in the choice of an oral contraceptive.

Minimizing exposure to estrogen and progestogen is in keeping with good principles of therapeutics. For any particular estrogen/progestogen combination, the dosage regimen prescribed should be one which contains the least amount of estrogen and progestogen that is compatible with a low failure rate and the needs of the individual patient. New acceptors of oral-contraceptive agents should be started on preparations containing the lowest estrogen content which is judged appropriate for the individual patient. Products containing 50 mcg of estrogen should be used only when medically indicated.

e. Persistence of risk of vascular disease

There are two studies which have shown persistence of risk of vascular disease for ever-users of oral contraceptives. In a study in the United States, the risk of developing myocardial infarction after discontinuing oral contraceptives persists for at least 9 years for women 40 to 49 years who had used oral contraceptives for five or more years, but this increased risk was not demonstrated in other age groups. In another study in Great Britain, the risk of developing cerebrovascular disease persisted for at least 6 years after discontinuation of oral contraceptives, although excess risk was very small. Both studies were performed with oral-contraceptive formulations containing 50 mcg or higher of estrogen.

2. Estimates of Mortality from Contraceptive Use

One study gathered data from a variety of sources which have estimated the mortality rate associated with different methods of contraception at different ages (Table III). These estimates include the combined risk of death associated with contraceptive methods plus the risk attributable to pregnancy in the event of method failure. Each method of contraception has its specific benefits and risks. The study concluded that with the exception of oral-contraceptive users 35 and older who smoke and 40 and older who do not smoke, mortality associated with all methods of birth control is less than that associated with childbirth. The observation of a possible increase in risk of mortality with age for oral-contraceptive users is based on data gathered in the 1970's—but not reported until 1983. However, current clinical practice involves the use of lower estrogen dose formulations combined with careful restriction of oral-contraceptive use to women who do not have the various risk factors listed in this labeling.

Because of these changes in practice and, also, because of some limited new data which suggest that the risk of cardiovascular disease with the use of oral contraceptives may now be less than previously observed, the Fertility and Maternal Health Drugs Advisory Committee was asked to review the topic in 1989. The Committee concluded that although cardiovascular-disease risks may be increased with oral-contraceptive use after age 40 in healthy nonsmoking women (even with the newer low-dose formulations), there are greater potential health risks associated with pregnancy in older women and with the alternative surgical and medical procedures which may be necessary if such women do not have access to effective and acceptable means of contraception.

Therefore, the Committee recommended that the benefits of oral-contraceptive use by healthy nonsmoking women over 40 may outweigh the possible risks. Of course, older women, as all women who take oral contraceptives, should take the lowest possible dose formulation that is effective.

TABLE III–ANNUAL NUMBER OF BIRTH-RELATED OR METHOD-RELATED DEATHS ASSOCIATED WITH CONTROL OF FERTILITY PER 100,000 NONSTERILE WOMEN, BY FERTILITY-CONTROL METHOD AND ACCORDING TO AGE

Method of control and outcome	15-19	20-24	25-29	30-34	35-39	40-44
No fertility-control methods*	7.0	7.4	9.1	14.8	25.7	28.2
Oral contraceptives nonsmoker**	0.3	0.5	0.9	1.9	13.8	31.6
Oral contraceptives smoker**	2.2	3.4	6.6	13.5	51.1	117.2
IUD**	0.8	0.8	1.0	1.0	1.4	1.4
Condom*	1.1	1.6	0.7	0.2	0.3	0.4
Diaphragm/ spermicide*	1.9	1.2	1.2	1.3	2.2	2.8
Periodic abstinence*	2.5	1.6	1.6	1.7	2.9	3.6

*Deaths are birth related
**Deaths are method related
Adapted from H.W. Ory, Family Planning Perspectives, *15*:57-63, 1983.

3. Carcinoma of the Reproductive Organs and Breasts

Numerous epidemiological studies have examined the association between the use of oral contraceptives and the incidence of breast and cervical cancer.

The risk of having breast cancer diagnosed may be slightly increased among current and recent users of COCs. However, this excess risk appears to decrease over time after COC discontinuation and by 10 years after cessation the increased risk disappears. Some studies report an increased risk with duration of use while other studies do not and no consistent relationships have been found with dose or type of steroid. Some studies have reported a small increase in risk for women who first use COCs at a younger age. Most studies show a similar pattern of risk with COC use regardless of a woman's reproductive history or her family breast cancer history.

Breast cancers diagnosed in current or previous OC users tend to be less clinically advanced than in nonusers.

Women with known or suspected carcinoma of the breast or personal history of breast cancer should not use oral contraceptives because breast cancer is usually a hormonally-sensitive tumor.

Some studies suggest that oral-contraceptive use has been associated with an increase in the risk of cervical intraepithelial neoplasia or invasive cervical cancer in some populations of women. However, there continues to be controversy about the extent to which such findings may be due to differences in sexual behavior and other factors.

In spite of many studies of the relationship between combination oral-contraceptive use and breast and cervical cancers, a cause-and-effect relationship has not been established.

4. Hepatic Neoplasia

Benign hepatic adenomas are associated with oral-contraceptive use, although the incidence of benign tumors is rare in the United States. Indirect calculations have estimated the attributable risk to be in the range of 3.3 cases/100,000 for users, a risk that increases after four or more years of use. Rupture of rare, benign, hepatic adenomas may cause death through intra-abdominal hemorrhage.

Studies from Britain have shown an increased risk of developing hepatocellular carcinoma in long-term (>8 years) oral-contraceptive users.

However, these cancers are extremely rare in the U.S., and the attributable risk (the excess incidence) of liver cancers in oral-contraceptive users approaches less than one per million users.

5. Ocular Lesions

There have been clinical case reports of retinal thrombosis associated with the use of oral contraceptives that may lead to partial or complete loss of vision. Oral contraceptives should be discontinued if there is unexplained partial or complete loss of vision; onset of proptosis or diplopia; papilledema; or retinal vascular lesions. Appropriate diagnostic and therapeutic measures should be undertaken immediately.

6. Oral-Contraceptive Use Before or During Early Pregnancy

Extensive epidemiological studies have revealed no increased risk of birth defects in infants born to women who have used oral contraceptives prior to pregnancy. Studies also do not suggest a teratogenic effect, particularly insofar as cardiac anomalies and limb-reduction defects are concerned, when taken inadvertently during early pregnancy (see **CONTRAINDICATIONS** section).

The administration of oral contraceptives to induce withdrawal bleeding should not be used as a test for pregnancy. Oral contraceptives should not be used during pregnancy to treat threatened or habitual abortion.

It is recommended that for any patient who has missed two consecutive periods, pregnancy should be ruled out before continuing oral-contraceptive use. If the patient has not adhered to the prescribed schedule, the possibility of pregnancy should be considered at the time of the first missed period. Oral-contraceptive use should be discontinued if pregnancy is confirmed.

7. Gallbladder Disease

Combination oral contraceptives may worsen existing gallbladder disease and may accelerate the development of this disease in previously asymptomatic women. Earlier studies have reported an increased lifetime relative risk of gallbladder surgery in users of oral contraceptives and estrogens. More recent studies, however, have shown that the relative risk of developing gallbladder disease among oral-contraceptive users may be minimal. The recent findings of minimal risk may be related to the use of oral-contraceptive formulations containing lower hormonal doses of estrogens and progestogens.

8. Carbohydrate and Lipid Metabolic Effects

Oral contraceptives have been shown to cause glucose intolerance in a significant percentage of users. Oral contraceptives containing greater than 75 mcg of estrogens cause hyperinsulinism, while lower doses of estrogen cause less glucose intolerance. Progestogens increase insulin secretion and create insulin resistance, this effect varying with different progestational agents. However, in the nondiabetic woman, oral contraceptives appear to have no effect on fasting blood glucose. Because of these demonstrated effects, prediabetic and diabetic women should be carefully observed while taking oral contraceptives.

A small proportion of women will have persistent hypertriglyceridemia while on the pill. As discussed earlier (see **WARNINGS** 1a and 1d; **PRECAUTIONS** 3), changes in serum triglycerides and lipoprotein levels have been reported in oral-contraceptive users.

9. Elevated Blood Pressure

Women with uncontrolled hypertension should not be started on hormonal contraception. An increase in blood pressure has been reported in women taking oral contraceptives, and this increase is more likely in older oral-contraceptive users and with continued use. Data from the Royal College of General Practitioners and subsequent randomized trials have shown that the incidence of hypertension increases with increasing quantities of progestogens.

Women with a history of hypertension or hypertension-related diseases, or renal disease, should be encouraged to use another method of contraception. If women with hypertension elect to use oral contraceptives, they should be monitored closely, and if significant elevation of blood pressure occurs, oral contraceptives should be discontinued (see **CONTRAINDICATIONS** section). For most women, elevated blood pressure will return to normal after stopping oral contraceptives, and there is no difference in the occurrence of hypertension among ever- and never-users.

10. Headache

The onset or exacerbation of migraine or development of headache with a new pattern that is recurrent, persistent, or severe requires discontinuation of oral contraceptives and evaluation of the cause. (See **WARNINGS** 1c and **CONTRAINDICATIONS**.)

11. **Bleeding Irregularities**
Breakthrough bleeding and spotting are sometimes encountered in patients on oral contraceptives, especially during the first three months of use. The type and dose of progestogen may be important. If bleeding persists or recurs, nonhormonal causes should be considered and adequate diagnostic measures taken to rule out malignancy or pregnancy in the event of breakthrough bleeding, as in the case of any abnormal vaginal bleeding. If pathology has been excluded, time or a change to another formulation may solve the problem. In some women withdrawal bleeding may not occur during the "tablet-free" or "inactive-tablet" interval. If the COC has not been taken according to directions prior to the first missed withdrawal bleed, or if two consecutive withdrawal bleeds are missed, tablet-taking should be discontinued and a nonhormonal method of contraception should be used until the possibility of pregnancy is excluded.
Some women may encounter post-pill amenorrhea or oligomenorrhea (possibly with anovulation), especially when such a condition was preexistent.
12. **Ectopic Pregnancy**
Ectopic as well as intrauterine pregnancy may occur in contraceptive failures.

PRECAUTIONS

1. **General**
Patients should be counseled that oral contraceptives do not protect against transmission of HIV (AIDS) and other sexually transmitted diseases (STDs) such as chlamydia, genital herpes, genital warts, gonorrhea, hepatitis B, and syphilis.
2. **Physical Examination and Follow-Up**
A periodic personal and family medical history and complete physical examination are appropriate for all women, including women using oral contraceptives. The physical examination, however, may be deferred until after initiation of oral contraceptives if requested by the woman and judged appropriate by the clinician. The physical examination should include special reference to blood pressure, breasts, abdomen and pelvic organs, including cervical cytology, and relevant laboratory tests. In case of undiagnosed, persistent or recurrent abnormal vaginal bleeding, appropriate diagnostic measures should be conducted to rule out malignancy. Women with a strong family history of breast cancer or who have breast nodules should be monitored with particular care.
3. **Lipid Disorders**
Women who are being treated for hyperlipidemias should be followed closely if they elect to use oral contraceptives. Some progestogens may elevate LDL levels and may render the control of hyperlipidemias more difficult. (See **WARNINGS** 1a, 1d, and 8.)
In patients with defects of lipoprotein metabolism, estrogen-containing preparations may be associated with rare but significant elevations of plasma triglycerides which may lead to pancreatitis.
4. **Liver Function**
If jaundice develops in any woman receiving such drugs, the medication should be discontinued. Steroid hormones may be poorly metabolized in patients with impaired liver function.
5. **Fluid Retention**
Oral contraceptives may cause some degree of fluid retention. They should be prescribed with caution, and only with careful monitoring, in patients with conditions which might be aggravated by fluid retention.
6. **Emotional Disorders**
Patients becoming significantly depressed while taking oral contraceptives should stop the medication and use an alternate method of contraception in an attempt to determine whether the symptom is drug related. Women with a history of depression should be carefully observed and the drug discontinued if significant depression occurs.
7. **Contact Lenses**
Contact-lens wearers who develop visual changes or changes in lens tolerance should be assessed by an ophthalmologist.
8. **Gastrointestinal**
Diarrhea and/or vomiting may reduce hormone absorption resulting in decreased serum concentrations.
9. **Drug Interactions**
Changes in contraceptive effectiveness associated with coadministration of other products:
Contraceptive effectiveness may be reduced when hormonal contraceptives are coadministered with antibiotics, anticonvulsants, and other drugs that increase the metabolism of contraceptive steroids. This could result in unintended pregnancy or breakthrough bleeding. Examples include rifampin, rifabutin, barbiturates, primidone, phenylbutazone, phenytoin, dexamethasone, carbamazepine, felbamate, oxcarbazepine, topiramate, griseofulvin, and modafinil.
Several cases of contraceptive failure and breakthrough bleeding have been reported in the literature with concomitant administration of antibiotics such as ampicillin and other penicillins, and tetracyclines, possibly due to a decrease of enterohepatic recirculation of estrogens. However, clinical pharmacology studies investigating drug interactions between combined oral contraceptives and these antibiotics have reported inconsistent results. Enterohepatic recirculation of estrogens may also be decreased by substances that reduce gut transit time.
Several of the anti-HIV protease inhibitors have been studied with coadministration of oral combination hormonal contraceptives; significant changes (increase and decrease) in the plasma levels of the estrogen and progestin have been noted in some cases. The safety and efficacy of oral contraceptive products may be affected with coadministration of anti-HIV protease inhibitors. Health-care professionals should refer to the label of the individual anti-HIV protease inhibitors for further drug-drug interaction information.
Herbal products containing St. John's Wort (Hypericum perforatum) may induce hepatic enzymes (cytochrome P 450) and p-glycoprotein transporter and may reduce the effectiveness of contraceptive steroids. This may also result in breakthrough bleeding.
During concomitant use of ethinyl estradiol containing products and substances that may lead to decreased plasma steroid hormone concentrations, it is recommended that a nonhormonal back-up method of birth control be used in addition to the regular intake of Ovral. If the use of a substance which leads to decreased ethinyl estradiol plasma concentrations is required for a prolonged period of time, combination oral contraceptives should not be considered the primary contraceptive.
After discontinuation of substances that may lead to decreased ethinyl estradiol plasma concentrations, use of a nonhormonal back-up method of birth control is recommended for 7 days. Longer use of a back-up method is advisable after discontinuation of substances that have led to induction of hepatic microsomal enzymes, resulting in decreased ethinyl estradiol concentrations. It may take several weeks until enzyme induction has completely subsided, depending on dosage, duration of use, and rate of elimination of the inducing substance.
Increase in plasma levels associated with coadministered drugs:
Coadministration of atorvastatin and certain oral contraceptives containing ethinyl estradiol increase AUC values for ethinyl estradiol by approximately 20%. The mechanism of this interaction is unknown. Ascorbic acid and acetaminophen increase the bioavailability of ethinyl estradiol since these drugs act as competitive inhibitors for sulfation of ethinyl estradiol in the gastrointestinal wall, a known pathway of elimination for ethinyl estradiol. CYP 3A4 inhibitors such as indinavir, itraconazole, ketoconazole, fluconazole, and troleandomycin may increase plasma hormone levels. Troleandomycin may also increase the risk of intrahepatic cholestasis during coadministration with combination oral contraceptives.
Changes in plasma levels of coadministered drugs:
Combination hormonal contraceptives containing some synthetic estrogens (eg, ethinyl estradiol) may inhibit the metabolism of other compounds. Increased plasma concentrations of cyclosporin, prednisolone and other corticosteroids, and theophylline have been reported with concomitant administration of oral contraceptives. Decreased plasma concentrations of acetaminophen and increased clearance of temazepam, salicylic acid, morphine, and clofibric acid, due to induction of conjugation (particularly glucuronidation), have been noted when these drugs were administered with oral contraceptives.
The prescribing information of concomitant medications should be consulted to identify potential interactions.
10. **Interactions with Laboratory Tests**
Certain endocrine- and liver-function tests and blood components may be affected by oral contraceptives:
a. Increased prothrombin and factors VII, VIII, IX, and X; decreased antithrombin 3; increased norepinephrine-induced platelet aggregability.
b. Increased thyroid-binding globulin (TBG) leading to increased circulating total thyroid hormone, as measured by protein-bound iodine (PBI), T_4 by column or by radioimmunoassay. Free T_3 resin uptake is decreased, reflecting the elevated TBG; free T_4 concentration is unaltered.
c. Other binding proteins may be elevated in serum ie, corticosteroid binding globulin (CBG), sex hormone-binding globulins (SHBG) leading to increased levels of total circulating corticosteroids and sex steroids, respectively. Free or biologically active hormone concentrations are unchanged.
d. Triglycerides may be increased and levels of various other lipids and lipoproteins may be affected.
e. Glucose tolerance may be decreased.
f. Serum folate levels may be depressed by oral-contraceptive therapy. This may be of clinical significance if a woman becomes pregnant shortly after discontinuing oral contraceptives.
11. **Carcinogenesis**
See **WARNINGS** section.
12. **Pregnancy**
Pregnancy Category X. See **CONTRAINDICATIONS** and **WARNINGS** sections.
13. **Nursing Mothers**
Small amounts of oral-contraceptive steroids and/or metabolites have been identified in the milk of nursing mothers, and a few adverse effects on the child have been reported, including jaundice and breast enlargement. In addition, combination oral contraceptives given in the postpartum period may interfere with lactation by decreasing the quantity and quality of breast milk. If possible, the nursing mother should be advised not to use combination oral contraceptives but to use other forms of contraception until she has completely weaned her child.
14. **Fertility Following Discontinuation**
Users of combination oral contraceptives may experience some delay in becoming pregnant after discontinuation of COCs, especially those women who had irregular menstrual cycles prior to use. Conception may be delayed an average of 1–2 months among women stopping COCs compared to women stopping nonhormonal contraceptive methods.
Women who do not wish to become pregnant after discontinuation of COCs should be advised to use another method of birth control.
15. **Pediatric Use**
Safety and efficacy of Ovral-28 tablets have been established in women of reproductive age. Safety and efficacy are expected to be the same for postpubertal adolescents under the age of 16 and for users 16 years and older. Use of this product before menarche is not indicated.
16. **Geriatric Use**
This product has not been studied in women over 65 years of age and is not indicated in this population.
Information for the Patient
See Patient Labeling Printed Below.

ADVERSE REACTIONS

An increased risk of the following serious adverse reactions (see **WARNINGS** section for additional information) has been associated with the use of oral contraceptives:
Thromboembolic and thrombotic disorders and other vascular problems (including thrombophlebitis and venous thrombosis with or without pulmonary embolism, mesenteric thrombosis, arterial thromboembolism, myocardial infarction, cerebral hemorrhage, cerebral thrombosis), carcinoma of the reproductive organs and breasts, hepatic neoplasia (including hepatic adenomas or benign liver tumors), ocular lesions (including retinal vascular thrombosis), gallbladder disease, carbohydrate and lipid effects, elevated blood pressure, and headache including migraine.
The following adverse reactions have been reported in patients receiving oral contraceptives and are believed to be drug related (alphabetically listed):
Acne
Amenorrhea
Anaphylactic/anaphylactoid reactions, including urticaria, angioedema, and severe reactions with respiratory and circulatory symptoms
Breakthrough bleeding
Breast changes: tenderness, pain, enlargement, secretion
Budd-Chiari syndrome
Cervical erosion and secretion, change in
Cholestatic jaundice
Chorea, exacerbation of
Colitis
Corneal curvature (steepening), change in
Diminution in lactation when given immediately postpartum
Dizziness
Edema/fluid retention
Erythema multiforme
Erythema nodosum
Gastrointestinal symptoms (such as abdominal pain, cramps, and bloating)
Hirsutism
Intolerance to contact lenses
Libido, changes in
Loss of scalp hair
Melasma/chloasma which may persist
Menstrual flow, change in
Mood changes, including depression
Nausea
Nervousness
Pancreatitis
Porphyria, exacerbation of
Rash (allergic)
Serum folate levels, decrease in
Spotting
Systemic lupus erythematosus, exacerbation of
Temporary infertility after discontinuation of treatment
Vaginitis, including candidiasis
Varicose veins, aggravation of
Vomiting
Weight or appetite (increase or decrease), change in

The following adverse reactions have been reported in users of oral contraceptives:
Cataracts
Cystitis-like syndrome
Dysmenorrhea
Hemolytic uremic syndrome
Hemorrhagic eruption
Optic neuritis, which may lead to partial or complete loss of vision
Porphyria
Premenstrual syndrome
Renal function, impaired

OVERDOSAGE

Symptoms of oral contraceptive overdosage in adults and children may include nausea, vomiting, and drowsiness/fatigue; withdrawal bleeding may occur in females. There is no specific antidote and further treatment of overdose, if necessary, is directed to the symptoms.

NONCONTRACEPTIVE HEALTH BENEFITS

The following noncontraceptive health benefits related to the use of oral contraceptives are supported by epidemiological studies which largely utilized oral-contraceptive formulations containing doses exceeding 0.035 mg of ethinyl estradiol or 0.05 mg of mestranol.

Continued on next page

Ovral-28—Cont.

Effects on menses:
Increased menstrual cycle regularity
Decreased blood loss and decreased incidence of iron-deficiency anemia
Decreased incidence of dysmenorrhea

Effects related to inhibition of ovulation:
Decreased incidence of functional ovarian cysts
Decreased incidence of ectopic pregnancies

Effects from long-term use:
Decreased incidence of fibroadenomas and fibrocystic disease of the breast
Decreased incidence of acute pelvic inflammatory disease
Decreased incidence of endometrial cancer
Decreased incidence of ovarian cancer

DOSAGE AND ADMINISTRATION

To achieve maximum contraceptive effectiveness, Ovral-28 must be taken exactly as directed and at intervals not exceeding 24 hours. The possibility of ovulation and conception prior to initiation of medication should be considered.
The dosage of Ovral-28 is one white tablet daily for 21 consecutive days, followed by one pink inert tablet daily for 7 consecutive days, according to prescribed schedule.
It is recommended that Ovral-28 tablets be taken at the same time each day.
During the first cycle of medication, the patient is instructed to begin taking Ovral-28 on the first Sunday after the onset of menstruation. If menstruation begins on a Sunday, the first tablet (white) is taken that day. One white tablet should be taken daily for 21 consecutive days followed by one pink inert tablet daily for 7 consecutive days. Withdrawal bleeding should usually occur within three days following discontinuation of white tablets and may not have finished before the next pack is started. During the first cycle, contraceptive reliance should not be placed on Ovral-28 until a white tablet has been taken daily for 7 consecutive days and a nonhormonal back-up method of birth control should be used during those 7 days. The possibility of ovulation and conception prior to initiation of medication should be considered.
The patient begins her next and all subsequent 28-day courses of tablets on the same day of the week (Sunday) on which she began her first course, following the same schedule: 21 days on white tablets—7 days on pink inert tablets. If in any cycle the patient starts tablets later than the proper day, she should protect herself against pregnancy by using a nonhormonal back-up method of birth control until she has taken a white tablet daily for 7 consecutive days.
When the patient is switching from a 21-day regimen of tablets, she should wait 7 days after her last tablet before she starts Ovral-28. She will probably experience withdrawal bleeding during that week. She should be sure that no more than 7 days pass after her previous 21-day regimen. When the patient is switching from a 28-day regimen of tablets, she should start her first pack of Ovral-28 on the day after her last tablet. She should not wait any days between packs. The patient may switch any day from a progestin-only pill and should begin Ovral-28 the next day. If switching from an implant or injection, the patient should start Ovral-28 on the day of implant removal or the day the next injection would be due. In switching from a progestin-only pill, injection, or implant, the patient should be advised to use a nonhormonal back-up method of birth control for the first 7 days of tablet-taking.
If spotting or breakthrough bleeding occurs, the patient is instructed to continue on the same regimen. This type of bleeding is usually transient and without significance; however, if the bleeding is persistent or prolonged, the patient is advised to consult her health-care professional. Although pregnancy is unlikely if Ovral-28 is taken according to directions, if withdrawal bleeding does not occur, the possibility of pregnancy must be considered. If the patient has not adhered to the prescribed schedule (missed one or more tablets or started taking them on a day later than she should have), the probability of pregnancy should be considered at the time of the first missed period and appropriate diagnostic measures taken. If the patient has adhered to the prescribed regimen and misses two consecutive periods, pregnancy should be ruled out. Hormone contraception should be discontinued if pregnancy is confirmed.
For additional patient instructions regarding missed tablets, see the "**WHAT TO DO IF YOU MISS PILLS**" section in the **DETAILED PATIENT LABELING** below.
Any time the patient misses two or more white tablets, she should also use another method of contraception until she has taken a white tablet daily for seven consecutive days. If the patient misses one or more pink tablets, she is still protected against pregnancy **provided** she begins taking white tablets again on the proper day.
If breakthrough bleeding occurs following missed white tablets, it will usually be transient and of no consequence. The possibility of ovulation increases with each successive day that scheduled white tablets are missed.
Ovral-28 may be initiated no earlier than day 28 postpartum in the nonlactating mother or after a second-trimester abortion due to the increased risk for thromboembolism (see **CONTRAINDICATIONS**, **WARNINGS**, and **PRECAUTIONS** concerning thromboembolic disease). The patient should be advised to use a nonhormonal back-up method for the first 7 days of tablet-taking. However, if intercourse has already occurred, pregnancy should be excluded before the start of combined oral contraceptive use or the patient must wait for her first menstrual period.
In the case of first-trimester abortion, if the patient starts Ovral-28 immediately, additional contraceptive measures are not needed.

HOW SUPPLIED

Ovral®-28 Tablets (0.5 mg norgestrel and 0.05 mg ethinyl estradiol) are available in packages of 6 PILPAK® dispensers, each containing 28 tablets as follows:
21 active tablets, NDC 0008-0056, white, round tablet marked "WYETH" and "56".
7 inert tablets, NDC 0008-0445, pink, round tablet marked "WYETH" and "445".
Store at controlled room temperature 20°C to 25°C (68°F to 77°F).
References available upon request.

Brief Summary Patient Package Insert

This product (like all oral contraceptives) is intended to prevent pregnancy. Oral contraceptives do not protect against transmission of HIV (AIDS) and other sexually transmitted diseases (STDs) such as chlamydia, genital herpes, genital warts, gonorrhea, hepatitis B, and syphilis.
Oral contraceptives, also known as "birth-control pills" or "the pill," are taken to prevent pregnancy, and when taken correctly, have a failure rate of approximately 1% per year when taken without missing any pills. The average failure rate of large numbers of pill users is approximately 5% per year when women who miss pills are included. For most women oral contraceptives are also free of serious or unpleasant side effects. However, forgetting to take pills considerably increases the chances of pregnancy.
For the majority of women, oral contraceptives can be taken safely. But there are some women who are at high risk of developing certain serious diseases that can be life-threatening or may cause temporary or permanent disability or death. The risks associated with taking oral contraceptives increase significantly if you:

- smoke
- have high blood pressure, diabetes, high cholesterol, or a tendency to form blood clots, or are obese
- have or have had clotting disorders, heart attack, stroke, angina pectoris, cancer of the breast or sex organs, jaundice, malignant or benign liver tumors, or major surgery with prolonged immobilization
- have headaches with neurological symptoms

You should not take the pill if you suspect you are pregnant or have unexplained vaginal bleeding.

Cigarette smoking increases the risk of serious adverse effects on the heart and blood vessels from oral-contraceptive use. This risk increases with age and with the amount of smoking (15 or more cigarettes per day has been associated with a significantly increased risk) and is quite marked in women over 35 years of age. Women who use oral contraceptives should not smoke.

Most side effects of the pill are not serious. The most common such effects are nausea, vomiting, bleeding between menstrual periods, weight gain, breast tenderness, and difficulty wearing contact lenses. These side effects, especially nausea and vomiting, may subside within the first three months of use.
The serious side effects of the pill occur very infrequently, especially if you are in good health and do not smoke. However, you should know that the following medical conditions have been associated with or made worse by the pill:
1. Blood clots in the legs (thrombophlebitis), lungs (pulmonary embolism), stoppage or rupture of a blood vessel in the brain (stroke), blockage of blood vessels in the heart (heart attack and angina pectoris) or other organs of the body. As mentioned above, smoking increases the risk of heart attacks and strokes and subsequent serious medical consequences. Women with migraine also may be at increased risk of stroke with pill use.
2. Liver tumors, which may rupture and cause severe bleeding. A possible but not definite association has been found with the pill and liver cancer. However, liver cancers are extremely rare. The chance of developing liver cancer from using the pill is thus even rarer.
3. High blood pressure, although blood pressure usually returns to normal when the pill is stopped.
The symptoms associated with these serious side effects are discussed in the detailed leaflet given to you with your supply of pills. Notify your health-care professional if you notice any unusual physical disturbances while taking the pill. In addition, drugs such as rifampin, as well as some anticonvulsants and some antibiotics, herbal preparations containing St. John's Wort (Hypericum perforatum), and HIV/AIDS drugs may decrease oral-contraceptive effectiveness.
Various studies give conflicting reports on the relationship between breast cancer and oral-contraceptive use.
Oral-contraceptive use may slightly increase your chance of having breast cancer diagnosed, particularly if you started using hormonal contraceptives at a younger age.
After you stop using hormonal contraceptives, the chances of having breast cancer diagnosed begin to go down and disappear 10 years after stopping use of the pill. It is not known whether this slightly increased risk of having breast cancer diagnosed is caused by the pill. It may be that women taking the pill were examined more often, so that breast cancer was more likely to be detected.
You should have regular breast examinations by a health-care professional and examine your own breasts monthly. Tell your health-care professional if you have a family history of breast cancer or if you have had breast nodules or an abnormal mammogram. Women who currently have or have had breast cancer should not use oral contraceptives because breast cancer is usually a hormone-sensitive tumor.
Some studies have found an increase in the incidence of cancer of the cervix in women who use oral contraceptives. However, this finding may be related to factors other than the use of oral contraceptives. There is insufficient evidence to rule out the possibility that the pill may cause such cancers.
Taking the combination pill provides some important non-contraceptive health benefits. These include less painful menstruation, less menstrual blood loss and anemia, fewer pelvic infections, and fewer cancers of the ovary and the lining of the uterus.
Be sure to discuss any medical condition you may have with your health-care professional. Your health-care professional will take a medical and family history before prescribing oral contraceptives and will examine you. The physical examination may be delayed to another time if you request it and the health-care professional believes that it is appropriate to postpone it. You should be reexamined at least once a year while taking oral contraceptives. The detailed patient information leaflet gives you further information which you should read and discuss with your health-care professional.
This product (like all oral contraceptives) is intended to prevent pregnancy. It does not protect against transmission of HIV (AIDS) and other sexually transmitted diseases such as chlamydia, genital herpes, genital warts, gonorrhea, hepatitis B, and syphilis.

DETAILED PATIENT LABELING

This product (like all oral contraceptives) is intended to prevent pregnancy. Oral contraceptives do not protect against transmission of HIV (AIDS) and other sexually transmitted diseases (STDs) such as chlamydia, genital herpes, genital warts, gonorrhea, hepatitis B, and syphilis.

INTRODUCTION

You should not use Ovral or Ovral-28, which contain higher doses of estrogen than other oral contraceptives, unless specifically recommended by your health-care professional. Any woman who considers using oral contraceptives (the "birth-control pill" or "the pill") should understand the benefits and risks of using this form of birth control. This leaflet will give you much of the information you will need to make this decision and will also help you determine if you are at risk of developing any of the serious side effects of the pill. It will tell you how to take the pill properly so that it will be as effective as possible. However, this leaflet is not a replacement for a careful discussion between you and your health-care professional. You should discuss the information provided in this leaflet with him or her, both when you first start taking the pill and during your revisits. You should also follow your health-care professional's advice with regard to regular check-ups while you are on the pill.

EFFECTIVENESS OF ORAL CONTRACEPTIVES

Oral contraceptives or "birth-control pills" or "the pill" are used to prevent pregnancy and are more effective than most other nonsurgical methods of birth control. When they are taken correctly, without missing any pills the chance of becoming pregnant is approximately 1% per year. Average failure rates are approximately 5% per year when women who miss pills are included. The chance of becoming pregnant increases with each missed pill during the menstrual cycle. In comparison, average failure rates for other methods of birth control during the first year of use are as follows:

IUD: 0.1-2%	Female condom alone: 21%
Depo-Provera® (injectable progestogen): 0.3%	Cervical cap
Norplant® System (levonorgestrel implants): 0.05%	Never given birth: 20%
Diaphragm with spermicides: 20%	Given birth: 40%
Spermidices alone: 26%	Periodic abstinence: 25%
Male condom alone: 14%	No methods: 85%

WHO SHOULD NOT TAKE ORAL CONTRACEPTIVES

Cigarette smoking increases the risk of serious adverse effects on the heart and blood vessels from oral-contraceptive use. This risk increases with age and with the amount of smoking (15 or more cigarettes per day has been associated with a significantly increased risk) and is quite marked in women over 35 years of age. Women who use oral contraceptives should not smoke.

Some women should not take the pill. You should not take the pill if you have any of the following conditions:

- History of heart attack or stroke
- History of blood clots in the legs (thrombophlebitis), lungs (pulmonary embolism), or eyes
- History of blood clots in the deep veins of your legs

- Chest pain (angina pectoris)
- Known or suspected breast cancer or cancer of the lining of the uterus, cervix, or vagina or certain hormonally-sensitive cancers
- Unexplained vaginal bleeding (until a diagnosis is reached by your health-care professional)
- Liver tumor (benign or cancerous)
- Yellowing of the whites of the eyes or of the skin (jaundice) during pregnancy or during previous use of the pill
- Known or suspected pregnancy
- A need for surgery with prolonged bedrest
- Heart valve or heart rhythm disorders that may be associated with formation of blood clots
- Diabetes affecting your circulation
- Headaches with neurological symptoms
- Uncontrolled high blood pressure
- Active liver disease with abnormal liver function tests
- Allergy or hypersensitivity to any of the components of Ovral-28

Tell your health-care professional if you have any of these conditions. Your health-care professional can recommend another method of birth control.

OTHER CONSIDERATIONS BEFORE TAKING ORAL CONTRACEPTIVES

Tell your health-care professional if you or any family member has ever had:

- Breast nodules, fibrocystic disease of the breast, an abnormal breast X-ray or mammogram
- Diabetes
- Elevated cholesterol or triglycerides
- High blood pressure
- A tendency to form blood clots
- Migraine or other headaches or epilepsy
- Depression
- Gallbladder, liver, heart, or kidney disease
- History of scanty or irregular menstrual periods

Women with any of these conditions should be checked often by their health-care professional if they choose to use oral contraceptives. Also, be sure to inform your health-care professional if you smoke or are on any medications.

RISKS OF TAKING ORAL CONTRACEPTIVES

1. *Risk of developing blood clots*

Blood clots and blockage of blood vessels are the most serious side effects of taking oral contraceptives and can cause death or serious disability. In particular, a clot in the legs can cause thrombophlebitis and a clot that travels to the lungs can cause a sudden blocking of the vessel carrying blood to the lungs. Rarely, clots occur in the blood vessels of the eye and may cause blindness, double vision, or impaired vision.

Users of COCs have a higher risk of developing blood clots compared to nonusers. This risk is highest during the first year of COC use.

If you take oral contraceptives and need elective surgery, need to stay in bed for a prolonged illness or injury, or have recently delivered a baby, you may be at risk of developing blood clots. You should consult your health-care professional about stopping oral contraceptives three to four weeks before surgery and not taking oral contraceptives for two weeks after surgery or during bed rest. You should also not take oral contraceptives soon after delivery of a baby or a midtrimester pregnancy termination. It is advisable to wait for at least four weeks after delivery if you are not breast-feeding. If you are breast-feeding, you should wait until you have weaned your child before using the pill. (See also the section on breast-feeding in GENERAL PRECAUTIONS.)

2. *Heart attacks and strokes*

Oral contraceptives may increase the tendency to develop strokes (stoppage or rupture of blood vessels in the brain) and angina pectoris and heart attacks (blockage of blood vessels in the heart). Any of these conditions can cause death or serious disability.

Smoking greatly increases the possibility of suffering heart attacks and strokes. Furthermore, smoking and the use of oral contraceptives greatly increase the chances of developing and dying of heart disease.

Women with migraine (especially migraine/headache with neurological symptoms) who take oral contraceptives also may be at higher risk of stroke.

3. *Gallbladder disease*

Oral-contraceptive users probably have a greater risk than nonusers of having gallbladder disease. This risk may be related to pills containing high doses of estrogens. Oral contraceptives may worsen existing gallbladder disease or accelerate the development of gallbladder disease in women previously without symptoms.

4. *Liver tumors*

In rare cases, oral contraceptives can cause benign but dangerous liver tumors. These benign liver tumors can rupture and cause fatal internal bleeding. In addition, a possible but not definite association has been found with the pill and liver cancers in two studies in which a few women who developed these very rare cancers were found to have used oral contraceptives for long periods. However, liver cancers are extremely rare. The chance of developing liver cancer from using the pill is thus even rarer.

5. *Cancer of the reproductive organs and breasts*

Various studies give conflicting reports on the relationship between breast cancer and oral-contraceptive use.

Oral-contraceptive use may slightly increase your chance of having breast cancer diagnosed, particularly if you started using hormonal contraceptives at a younger age.

After you stop using hormonal contraceptives, the chances of having breast cancer diagnosed begin to go down and disappear 10 years after stopping use of the pill. It is not known whether this slightly increased risk of having breast cancer diagnosed is caused by the pill. It may be that women taking the pill were examined more often, so that breast cancer was more likely to be detected.

You should have regular breast examinations by a health-care professional and examine your own breasts monthly. Tell your health-care professional if you have a family history of breast cancer or if you have had breast nodules or an abnormal mammogram. Women who currently have or have had breast cancer should not use oral contraceptives because breast cancer is usually a hormone-sensitive tumor.

Some studies have found an increase in the incidence of cancer of the cervix in women who use oral contraceptives. However, this finding may be related to factors other than the use of oral contraceptives. There is insufficient evidence to rule out the possibility that the pill may cause such cancers.

6. *Lipid metabolism and inflammation of the pancreas*

In patients with abnormal lipid levels, there have been reports of significant increases in plasma triglycerides during estrogen therapy. This has led to inflammation of the pancreas in some cases.

ESTIMATED RISK OF DEATH FROM A BIRTH-CONTROL METHOD OR PREGNANCY

All methods of birth control and pregnancy are associated with a risk of developing certain diseases which may lead to disability or death. An estimate of the number of deaths associated with different methods of birth control and pregnancy has been calculated and is shown in the following table.

ANNUAL NUMBER OF BIRTH-RELATED OR METHOD-RELATED DEATHS ASSOCIATED WITH CONTROL OF FERTILITY PER 100,000 NONSTERILE WOMEN, BY FERTILITY-CONTROL METHOD AND ACCORDING TO AGE

Method of control and outcome	15-19	20-24	25-29	30-34	35-39	40-44
No fertility-control methods*	7.0	7.4	9.1	14.8	25.7	28.2
Oral contraceptives nonsmoker**	0.3	0.5	0.9	1.9	13.8	31.6
Oral contraceptives smoker**	2.2	3.4	6.6	13.5	51.1	117.2
IUD**	0.8	0.8	1.0	1.0	1.4	1.4
Condom*	1.1	1.6	0.7	0.2	0.3	0.4
Diaphragm/ spermicide*	1.9	1.2	1.2	1.3	2.2	2.8
Periodic abstinence*	2.5	1.6	1.6	1.7	2.9	3.6

*Deaths are birth related
**Deaths are method related

In the above table, the risk of death from any birth-control method is less than the risk of childbirth, except for oral-contraceptive users over the age of 35 who smoke and pill users over the age of 40 even if they do not smoke. It can be seen in the table that for women aged 15 to 39, the risk of death was highest with pregnancy (7 to 26 deaths per 100,000 women, depending on age). Among pill users who do not smoke, the risk of death was always lower than that associated with pregnancy for any age group, except for those women over the age of 40, when the risk increases to 32 deaths per 100,000 women, compared to 28 associated with pregnancy at that age. However, for pill users who smoke and are over the age of 35, the estimated number of deaths exceeds those for other methods of birth control. If a woman is over the age of 40 and smokes, her estimated risk of death is four times higher (117/100,000 women) than the estimated risk associated with pregnancy (28/100,000 women) in that age group.

The suggestion that women over 40 who do not smoke should not take oral contraceptives is based on information from older high-dose pills. An Advisory Committee of the FDA discussed this issue in 1989 and recommended that the benefits of oral-contraceptive use by healthy, nonsmoking women over 40 years of age may outweigh the possible risks. Older women, as all women who take oral contraceptives, should take an oral contraceptive which contains the least amount of estrogen and progestogen that is compatible with the individual patient needs.

WARNING SIGNALS

If any of these adverse effects occur while you are taking oral contraceptives, call your health-care professional immediately:

- Sharp chest pain, coughing of blood, or sudden shortness of breath (indicating a possible clot in the lung)
- Pain in the calf (indicating a possible clot in the leg)
- Crushing chest pain or heaviness in the chest (indicating a possible heart attack)
- Sudden severe headache or vomiting, dizziness or fainting, disturbances of vision or speech, weakness, or numbness in an arm or leg (indicating a possible stroke)
- Sudden partial or complete loss of vision (indicating a possible clot in the eye)
- Breast lumps (indicating possible breast cancer or fibrocystic disease of the breast; ask your health-care professional to show you how to examine your breasts)
- Severe pain or tenderness in the stomach area (indicating a possibly ruptured liver tumor)
- Difficulty in sleeping, weakness, lack of energy, fatigue, or change in mood (possibly indicating severe depression)
- Jaundice or a yellowing of the skin or eyeballs, accompanied frequently by fever, fatigue, loss of appetite, dark-colored urine, or light-colored bowel movements (indicating possible liver problems)

SIDE EFFECTS OF ORAL CONTRACEPTIVES

1. *Irregular vaginal bleeding*

Irregular vaginal bleeding or spotting may occur while you are taking the pills. Irregular bleeding may vary from slight staining between menstrual periods to breakthrough bleeding which is a flow much like a regular period. Irregular bleeding occurs most often during the first few months of oral-contraceptive use, but may also occur after you have been taking the pill for some time. Such bleeding may be temporary and usually does not indicate any serious problems. It is important to continue taking your pills on schedule. If the bleeding occurs in more than one cycle or lasts for more than a few days, talk to your health-care professional.

2. *Contact lenses*

If you wear contact lenses and notice a change in vision or an inability to wear your lenses, contact your health-care professional.

3. *Fluid retention*

Oral contraceptives may cause edema (fluid retention) with swelling of the fingers or ankles and may raise your blood pressure. If you experience fluid retention, contact your health-care professional.

4. *Melasma*

A spotty darkening of the skin is possible, particularly of the face.

5. *Other side effects*

Other side effects may include nausea, breast tenderness, change in appetite, headache, nervousness, depression, dizziness, loss of scalp hair, rash, vaginal infections, inflammation of the pancreas, and allergic reactions.

If any of these side effects bother you, call your health-care professional.

GENERAL PRECAUTIONS

1. *Missed periods and use of oral contraceptives before or during early pregnancy*

There may be times when you may not menstruate regularly after you have completed taking a cycle of pills. If you have taken your pills regularly and miss one menstrual period, continue taking your pills for the next cycle but be sure to inform your health-care professional. If you have not taken the pills daily as instructed and missed a menstrual period, or if you missed two consecutive menstrual periods, you may be pregnant. Check with your health-care professional immediately to determine whether you are pregnant. Stop taking oral contraceptives if pregnancy is confirmed.

There is no conclusive evidence that oral-contraceptive use is associated with an increase in birth defects when taken inadvertently during early pregnancy. Previously, a few studies had reported that oral contraceptives might be associated with birth defects, but these findings have not been confirmed in more recent studies. Nevertheless, oral contraceptives should not be used during pregnancy. You should check with your health-care professional about risks to your unborn child of any medication taken during pregnancy.

2. *While breast-feeding*

If you are breast-feeding, consult your health-care professional before starting oral contraceptives. Some of the drug will be passed on to the child in the milk. A few adverse effects on the child have been reported, including yellowing of the skin (jaundice) and breast enlargement. In addition, oral contraceptives may decrease the amount and quality of your milk. If possible, do not use oral contraceptives while breast-feeding. You should use another method of contraception since breast-feeding provides only partial protection from becoming pregnant, and this partial protection decreases significantly as you breast-feed for longer periods of time. You should consider starting oral contraceptives only after you have weaned your child completely.

3. *Laboratory tests*

If you are scheduled for any laboratory tests, tell your health-care professional you are taking birth-control pills. Certain blood tests may be affected by birth-control pills.

4. *Drug interactions*

Certain drugs may interact with birth-control pills to make them less effective in preventing pregnancy or cause an increase in breakthrough bleeding. Such drugs include rifampin, drugs used for epilepsy such as barbiturates (for example, phenobarbital) and phenytoin (Dilantin® is one brand of this drug), primidone (Mysoline®), topiramate (Topamax®), carbamazepine (Tegretol® is one brand of this drug), phenylbutazone (Butazolidin® is one brand of this drug), some drugs used for HIV or AIDS such as ritonavir (Norvir®), modafinil (Provigil®) and possibly certain antibiotics (such as ampicillin and other penicillins, and tetracyclines), and herbal products containing St. John's Wort (Hypericum perforatum). You may also need to use a nonhormonal method of contraception (such as condoms and/or spermicide) during any cycle in which you take drugs that can make oral contraceptives less effective.

Continued on next page

Ovral-28—Cont.

You may be at higher risk of a specific type of liver dysfunction if you take troleandomycin and oral contraceptives at the same time.

Be sure to tell your health-care professional if you are taking or start taking any other medications, including nonprescription products or herbal products while taking birth control pills.

5. *Sexually transmitted diseases*

This product (like all oral contraceptives) is intended to prevent pregnancy. It does not protect against transmission of HIV (AIDS) and other sexually transmitted diseases such as chlamydia, genital herpes, genital warts, gonorrhea, hepatitis B, and syphilis.

HOW TO TAKE THE PILL

IMPORTANT POINTS TO REMEMBER

BEFORE YOU START TAKING YOUR PILLS:

1. BE SURE TO READ THESE DIRECTIONS:
Before you start taking your pills.
And
Anytime you are not sure what to do.

2. THE RIGHT WAY TO TAKE THE PILL IS TO TAKE ONE PILL EVERY DAY AT THE SAME TIME.
If you miss pills you could get pregnant. This includes starting the pack late. The more pills you miss, the more likely you are to get pregnant.

3. MANY WOMEN HAVE SPOTTING OR LIGHT BLEEDING, OR MAY FEEL SICK TO THEIR STOMACH DURING THE FIRST 1–3 PACKS OF PILLS.
If you feel sick to your stomach, do not stop taking the pill. The problem will usually go away. If it doesn't go away, check with your health-care professional.

4. MISSING PILLS CAN ALSO CAUSE SPOTTING OR LIGHT BLEEDING, even when you make up these missed pills.
On the days you take 2 pills to make up for missed pills, you could also feel a little sick to your stomach.

5. IF YOU HAVE VOMITING (within 4 hours after you take your pill), you should follow the instructions for WHAT TO DO IF YOU MISS PILLS. IF YOU HAVE DIARRHEA or IF YOU TAKE SOME MEDICINES, including some antibiotics, your pills may not work as well. Use a back-up nonhormonal method (such as condoms and/or spermicide) until you check with your health-care professional.

6. IF YOU HAVE TROUBLE REMEMBERING TO TAKE THE PILL, talk to your health-care professional about how to make pill-taking easier or about using another method of birth control.

7. IF YOU HAVE ANY QUESTIONS OR ARE UNSURE ABOUT THE INFORMATION IN THIS LEAFLET, call your health-care professional.

OVRAL® AND OVRAL®-28 (norgestrel and ethinyl estradiol tablets)

***BEFORE* YOU START TAKING YOUR PILLS**

1. DECIDE WHAT TIME OF DAY YOU WANT TO TAKE YOUR PILL.
It is important to take it at about the same time every day.

2. LOOK AT YOUR PILL PACK TO SEE IF IT HAS 21 OR 28 PILLS:
The *21-pill* pack has 21 "active" white pills (with hormones) to take for 3 weeks, followed by 1 week without pills.
The *28-pill* pack has 21 "active" white pills (with hormones) to take for 3 weeks, followed by 1 week of reminder pink pills (without hormones).

3. ALSO FIND:
1) where on the pack to start taking pills, and
2) in what order to take the pills (follow the arrows).

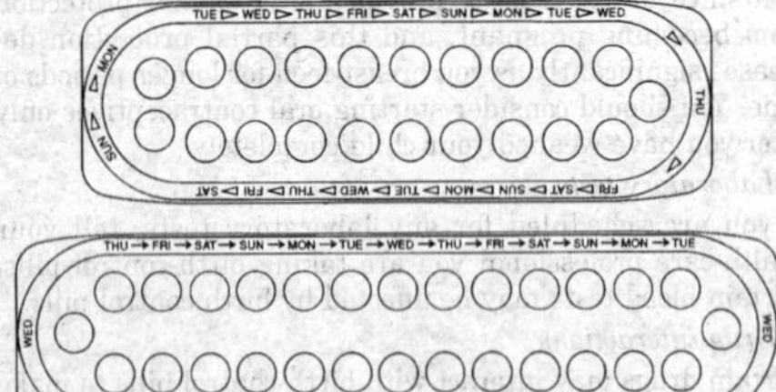

4. BE SURE YOU HAVE READY AT ALL TIMES:
ANOTHER KIND OF BIRTH CONTROL (such as condoms and/or spermicide) to use as a back-up in case you miss pills.
AN EXTRA, FULL PILL PACK.

WHEN TO START THE *FIRST* PACK OF PILLS

For the 21-day pill pack you have two choices of which day to start taking your first pack of pills. (See DAY 1 START or SUNDAY START directions below.) Decide with your health-care professional which is the best day for you. The 28-day pill pack accommodates a SUNDAY START only. For either pill pack pick a time of day which will be easy to remember.

DAY 1 START:
These instructions are for the 21-day pill pack only. The 28-day pill pack does not accommodate a **DAY 1 START** dosage regimen.
1. Take the first "active" white pill of the first pack during the *first 24 hours of your period.*
2. You will not need to use a back-up nonhormonal method of birth control, since you are starting the pill at the beginning of your period.

SUNDAY START:
These instructions are for either the 21-day or the 28-day pill pack.
1. Take the first "active" white pill of the first pack on the *Sunday after your period starts,* even if you are still bleeding. If your period begins on Sunday, start the pack that same day.
2. *Use a nonhormonal method of birth control* (such as condoms and/or spermicide) as a back-up method if you have sex anytime from the Sunday you start your first pack until the next Sunday (7 days).

WHAT TO DO DURING THE MONTH

1. TAKE ONE PILL AT THE SAME TIME EVERY DAY UNTIL THE PACK IS EMPTY.
Do not skip pills even if you are spotting or bleeding between monthly periods or feel sick to your stomach (nausea).
Do not skip pills even if you do not have sex very often.

2. WHEN YOU FINISH A PACK OR SWITCH YOUR BRAND OF PILLS:
21 pills: Wait 7 days to start the next pack. You will probably have your period during that week. Be sure that no more than 7 days pass between 21-day packs.
28 pills: Start the next pack on the day after your last "reminder" pill. Do not wait any days between packs.

WHAT TO DO IF YOU MISS PILLS

The pill may not be as effective if you miss white "active" pills, and particularly if you miss the first few or the last few white "active" pills in a pack.

If you **MISS 1** white "active" pill:
1. Take it as soon as you remember. Take the next pill at your regular time. This means you may take 2 pills in 1 day.
2. You COULD BECOME PREGNANT if you have sex in the *7 days* after you miss pills. You MUST use a nonhormonal birth-control method (such as condoms and/or spermicide) as a back-up for those 7 days.

If you **MISS 2** white "active" pills in a row in **WEEK 1 OR WEEK 2** of your pack:
1. Take 2 pills on the day you remember and 2 pills the next day.
2. Then take 1 pill a day until you finish the pack.
3. You COULD BECOME PREGNANT if you have sex in the *7 days* after you miss pills. You MUST use a nonhormonal birth-control method (such as condoms and/or spermicide) as a back-up for those 7 days.

If you **MISS 2** white "active" pills in a row in **THE 3rd WEEK:**
The ***Day 1 Starter*** instructions are for the 21-day pill pack only. The 28-day pill pack does not accommodate a **DAY 1 START** dosage regimen. The ***Sunday Starter*** instructions are for either the 21-day or 28-day pill pack.
1. ***If you are a Day 1 Starter:***
THROW OUT the rest of the pill pack and start a new pack that same day.
If you are a Sunday Starter:
Keep taking 1 pill every day until Sunday.
On Sunday, THROW OUT the rest of the pack and start a new pack of pills that same day.
2. You may not have your period this month but this is expected. However, if you miss your period 2 months in a row, call your health-care professional because you might be pregnant.
3. You COULD BECOME PREGNANT if you have sex in the *7 days* after you miss pills. You MUST use a nonhormonal birth-control method (such as condoms and/or spermicide) as a back-up for those 7 days.

If you **MISS 3 OR MORE** white "active" pills in a row (during the first 3 weeks):
The ***Day 1 Starter*** instructions are for the 21-day pill pack only. The 28-day pill pack does not accommodate a **DAY 1 START** dosage regimen. The ***Sunday Starter*** instructions are for either the 21-day or 28-day pill pack.
1. ***If you are a Day 1 Starter:***
THROW OUT the rest of the pill pack and start a new pack that same day.
If you are a Sunday Starter:
Keep taking 1 pill every day until Sunday.
On Sunday, THROW OUT the rest of the pack and start a new pack of pills that same day.
2. You may not have your period this month but this is expected. However, if you miss your period 2 months in a row, call your health-care professional because you might be pregnant.
3. You COULD BECOME PREGNANT if you have sex in the *7 days* after you miss pills. You MUST use a nonhormonal birth-control method (such as condoms and/or spermicide) as a back-up for those 7 days.

A REMINDER FOR THOSE ON 28-DAY PACKS
If you forget any of the 7 pink "reminder" pills in Week 4:
THROW AWAY the pills you missed.
Keep taking 1 pill each day until the pack is empty.
You do not need a back-up nonhormonal birth-control method if you start your next pack on time.

FINALLY, IF YOU ARE STILL NOT SURE WHAT TO DO ABOUT THE PILLS YOU HAVE MISSED
Use a BACK-UP NONHORMONAL BIRTH-CONTROL METHOD anytime you have sex.
KEEP TAKING ONE PILL EACH DAY until you can reach your health-care professional.

PREGNANCY DUE TO PILL FAILURE
The incidence of pill failure resulting in pregnancy is approximately 1% if taken every day as directed, but the average failure rate is approximately 5% including women who do not always take the pill exactly as directed without missing any pills. If you do become pregnant, the risk to the fetus is minimal, but you should stop taking your pills and discuss the pregnancy with your health-care professional.

PREGNANCY AFTER STOPPING THE PILL
There may be some delay in becoming pregnant after you stop using oral contraceptives, especially if you had irregular menstrual cycles before you used oral contraceptives. It may be advisable to postpone conception until you begin menstruating regularly once you have stopped taking the pill and desire pregnancy.
There does not appear to be any increase in birth defects in newborn babies when pregnancy occurs soon after stopping the pill.
If you do not desire pregnancy, you should use another method of birth control immediately after stopping the oral contraceptive pill.

OVERDOSAGE
Overdosage may cause nausea, vomiting, and fatigue/drowsiness. Withdrawal bleeding may occur in females. In case of overdosage, contact your health-care professional or pharmacist.

OTHER INFORMATION
Your health-care professional will take a medical and family history before prescribing oral contraceptives and will examine you. The physical examination may be delayed to another time if you request it and the health-care professional believes that it is appropriate to postpone it. You should be reexamined at least once a year. Be sure to inform your health-care professional if there is a family history of any of the conditions listed previously in this leaflet. Be sure to keep all appointments with your health-care professional, because this is a time to determine if there are early signs of side effects of oral-contraceptive use.
Do not use the drug for any condition other than the one for which it was prescribed. This drug has been prescribed specifically for you; do not give it to others who may want birth-control pills.

HEALTH BENEFITS FROM ORAL CONTRACEPTIVES
In addition to preventing pregnancy, use of oral contraceptives may provide certain benefits. They are:
- Menstrual cycles may become more regular.
- Blood flow during menstruation may be lighter, and less iron may be lost. Therefore, anemia due to iron deficiency is less likely to occur.
- Pain or other symptoms during menstruation may be encountered less frequently.
- Ovarian cysts may occur less frequently.
- Ectopic (tubal) pregnancy may occur less frequently.
- Noncancerous cysts or lumps in the breast may occur less frequently.
- Acute pelvic inflammatory disease may occur less frequently.
- Oral-contraceptive use may provide some protection against developing two forms of cancer: cancer of the ovaries and cancer of the lining of the uterus.

If you want more information about birth-control pills, ask your health-care professional or pharmacist. They have a more technical leaflet called the Professional Labeling which you may wish to read.

Wyeth®
Wyeth Pharmaceuticals Inc.
Philadelphia, PA 19101

W10442C003
ET02
Rev 08/03

Shown in Product Identification Guide, page 336

OVRETTE® Tablets ℞

[*ō'vrĕt*]
(norgestrel tablets)
℞ only

Patients should be counseled that oral contraceptives do not protect against transmission of HIV (AIDS) and other sexually transmitted diseases (STDs) such as chlamydia, genital herpes, genital warts, gonorrhea, hepatitis B, and syphilis.

DESCRIPTION
Each OVRETTE tablet contains 0.075 mg of norgestrel (*dl*-13-beta-ethyl-17-alpha-ethinyl-17-beta-hydroxygon-4-en-3-one). The inactive ingredients present are cellulose, FD&C Yellow 5, lactose, magnesium stearate, and polacrilin potassium.
Each OVRETTE tablet contains 0.075 mg of a single active steroid ingredient, norgestrel, a totally synthetic progestogen. The available data suggest that the d (-) enantiomeric

form of norgestrel is the biologically active portion. This form amounts to 0.0375 mg per OVRETTE tablet.

Norgestrel

$C_{21}H_{28}O_2$ M.W. 312.45

CLINICAL PHARMACOLOGY

1. Mode of Action

Progestin-only oral contraceptives such as OVRETTE prevent conception by suppressing ovulation in approximately half of users, thickening the midcycle mucus to inhibit sperm penetration, lowering the midcycle LH and FSH peaks, slowing the movement of the ovum through the fallopian tubes, and altering the endometrium.

2. Pharmacokinetics

Serum progestin levels peak about two hours after oral administration, followed by rapid distribution and elimination. By 24 hours after drug ingestion, serum levels are near baseline, making efficacy dependent upon rigid adherence to the dosing schedule. There are large variations in serum levels among individual users. Progestin-only administration results in lower steady-state progestin levels and a shorter elimination half-life than concomitant administration with estrogens.

INDICATIONS AND USAGE

1. Indications

Progestin-only oral contraceptives are indicated for the prevention of pregnancy.

2. Efficacy

Oral contraceptives are highly effective. Table 1 lists the typical accidental pregnancy rates for users of oral contraceptives and other methods of contraception. The efficacy of these contraceptive methods except sterilization, the IUD, and the NORPLANT System, depends upon the reliability with which they are used correctly. Consistent use of these methods can result in lower failure rates.

[See table 1 at right]

CONTRAINDICATIONS

Progestin-only oral contraceptives should not be used by women who currently have the following conditions:

- Known or suspected pregnancy
- Known or suspected carcinoma of the breast
- Undiagnosed abnormal genital bleeding
- Hypersensitivity to any component of this product
- Benign or malignant liver tumors
- Acute liver disease

WARNINGS

Cigarette smoking increases the risk of serious cardiovascular disease. Women who use oral contraceptives should be strongly advised not to smoke.

OVRETTE does not contain estrogen and, therefore, this insert does not discuss the serious health risks that have been associated with the estrogen component of combination oral contraceptives (COCs). The health-care professional is referred to the prescribing information of COCs for a discussion of those risks. The relationship between progestin-only oral contraceptives and these risks is not fully defined. The physician should remain alert to the earliest manifestation of symptoms of any serious disease and discontinue oral contraceptive therapy when appropriate.

1. Ectopic Pregnancy

The incidence of ectopic pregnancies for progestin-only oral contraceptive users is 5 per 1000 woman-years. Up to 10% of pregnancies reported in clinical studies of progestin-only oral contraceptive users are extrauterine. Although symptoms of ectopic pregnancy should be watched for, a history of ectopic pregnancy need not be considered a contraindication to use of this contraceptive method. Health-care professionals should be alert to the possibility of an ectopic pregnancy in women who become pregnant or complain of lower abdominal pain while on progestin-only oral contraceptives.

2. Delayed Follicular Atresia/Ovarian Cysts

If follicular development occurs, atresia of the follicle is sometimes delayed, and the follicle may continue to grow beyond the size it would attain in a normal cycle. Generally these enlarged follicles disappear spontaneously. Often they are asymptomatic; in some cases they are associated with mild abdominal pain. Rarely they may twist or rupture, requiring surgical intervention.

3. Irregular Genital Bleeding

Irregular menstrual patterns are common among women using progestin-only oral contraceptives. If genital bleeding is suggestive of infection, malignancy, pregnancy, or other conditions, such nonpharmacologic causes should be ruled out. If prolonged amenorrhea occurs, the possibility of pregnancy should be evaluated. If one menstrual period is missed and the progestin-only oral contraceptive has not been taken according to directions, or if two consecutive periods are missed, tablet-taking should be discontinued and a nonhormonal back-up method of contraception should be used until the possibility of pregnancy is excluded.

4. Carcinoma of the Breast and Reproductive Organs

Some epidemiological studies of oral contraceptive users have reported a slightly increased risk of having breast cancer diagnosed in women who were currently using combination oral contraceptives (COCs). The increased risk gradually disappeared within 10 years after stopping use of combination oral contraceptives. Breast cancers diagnosed in ever-users tend to be less clinically advanced than the cancers diagnosed in never-users. These studies have predominantly involved COCs and there are insufficient data to determine whether the use of progestin-only oral contraceptives similarly increases the risk. However, women with breast cancer should not use oral contraceptives because the role of female hormones in breast cancer has not been fully determined.

Some studies suggest that oral contraceptive use has been associated with an increase in the risk of cervical intraepithelial neoplasia or invasive cervical cancer in some populations of women. However, there continues to be controversy about the extent to which such findings may be due to differences in sexual behavior and other factors.

Table 1: Percentage Of Women Experiencing An Unintended Pregnancy During The First Year Of Typical Use And The First Year Of Perfect Use Of Contraception And The Percentage Continuing Use At The End Of The First Year United States

Method (1)	% of Women Experiencing an Unintended Pregnancy within the First Year of Use: Typical Use[1] (2)	Perfect Use[2] (3)	% of Women Continuing Use at One Year[3] (4)
Chance[4]	85	85	
Spermicides[5]	26	6	40
Periodic abstinence	25		63
Calendar		9	
Ovulation Method		3	
Sympto-Thermal[6]		2	
Post-Ovulation		1	
Cap[7]			
Parous Women	40	26	42
Nulliparous Women	20	9	56
Sponge			
Parous Women	40	20	42
Nulliparous Women	20	9	56
Diaphragm[7]	20	6	56
Withdrawal	19	4	
Condom[8]			
Female (Reality)	21	5	56
Male	14	3	61
Pill	5		71
Progestin only		0.5	
Combined		0.1	
IUD			
Progesterone T	2.0	1.5	81
Copper T380A	0.8	0.6	78
LNg 20	0.1	0.1	81
Depo-Provera®	0.3	0.3	70
Levonorgestrel Implants (Norplant®)	0.05	0.05	88
Female Sterilization	0.5	0.5	100
Male Sterilization	0.15	0.10	100

Lactation Amenorrhea Method: LAM is a highly effective, temporary method of contraception.[9]

Source: Trussell J, Contraceptive efficacy. In: Hatcher RA, Trussell J, Stewart F, Cates W, Stewart GK, Kowel D, Guest F. Contraceptive Technology: Seventeenth Revised Edition. New York NY: Irvington Publishers; 1998.

[1] Among *typical* couples who initiate use of a method (not necessarily for the first time), the percentage who experience an accidental pregnancy during the first year if they do not stop use for any other reason.

[2] Among couples who initiate use of a method (not necessarily for the first time) and who use it *perfectly* (both consistently and correctly), the percentage who experience an accidental pregnancy during the first year if they do not stop use for any other reason.

[3] Among couples attempting to avoid pregnancy, the percentage who continue to use a method for one year.

[4] The percents becoming pregnant in columns (2) and (3) are based on data from populations where contraception is not used and from women who cease using contraception in order to become pregnant. Among such populations, about 89% become pregnant within one year. This estimate was lowered slightly (to 85%) to represent the percent who would become pregnant within one year among women now relying on reversible methods of contraception if they abandoned contraception altogether.

[5] Foams, creams, gels, vaginal suppositories, and vaginal film.

[6] Cervical mucus (ovulation) method supplemented by calendar in the pre-ovulatory and basal body temperature in the post-ovulatory phases.

[7] With spermicidal cream or jelly.

[8] Without spermicides.

[9] However, to maintain effective protection against pregnancy, another method of contraception must be used as soon as menstruation resumes, the frequency or duration of breastfeeds is reduced, bottle feeds are introduced, or the baby reaches 6 months of age.

Ovrette—Cont.

There are insufficient data to determine whether the use of progestin-only oral contraceptives increases the risk of developing cervical intraepithelial neoplasia.

5. Hepatic Neoplasia/Liver Disease

Benign hepatic adenomas are associated with COC use, although the incidence of benign tumors is rare in the United States. Rupture of benign, hepatic adenomas may cause death through intra-abdominal hemorrhage.

Studies from Britain and the US have shown an increased risk of developing hepatocellular carcinoma in COC-users. However, these cancers are rare. There are insufficient data to determine whether progestin-only oral contraceptives increase the risk of developing hepatic neoplasia.

Women with a history of oral contraceptive related cholestasis or women with cholestasis during pregnancy are more likely to have this condition with oral contraceptive use. If these women receive a progestin-only oral contraceptive they should be carefully monitored and, if the condition recurs, progestin-only oral contraceptive use should be discontinued.

6. Thromboembolic Disorders and Other Vascular Problems

An increased risk of venous and arterial thrombotic and thromboembolic events have been found to be associated with the use of COCs. These events include superficial venous thrombosis, deep-vein thrombosis, pulmonary embolism, retinal vascular thrombosis, myocardial infarction, and cerebrovascular events (thrombotic and hemorrhagic strokes). There are insufficient data to determine whether the use of progestin-only contraceptives increases the risk of developing thrombotic disease and/or other vascular problems. However, there have been reports of some of these conditions coincident with the use of progestin-only oral contraceptives; therefore, the possibility of thrombosis should be considered.

Care should be used when prescribing progestin-only oral contraceptives to women predisposed to thromboembolic disorders (eg, a history of thromboembolic events, thrombophilia, cardiovascular disease; women who are obese or experience prolonged immobilization).

PRECAUTIONS

1. General

Patients should be counseled that oral contraceptives do not protect against transmission of HIV (AIDS) and other sexually transmitted diseases (STDs) such as chlamydia, genital herpes, genital warts, gonorrhea, hepatitis B, and syphilis.

2. Physical Examination and Follow Up

A complete personal and family medical history and physical examination is appropriate for all women, including women using oral contraceptives. The physical examination may be deferred until after initiation of oral contraceptives if requested by the woman and judged appropriate by the clinician. Such examinations should be repeated periodically during the use of progestin-only oral contraceptives.

3. Carbohydrate and Lipid Effects

Some progestin-only oral contraceptive users may experience slight deterioration in glucose tolerance with increases in plasma insulin, but women with diabetes mellitus who use progestin-only oral contraceptives do not generally experience changes in their insulin requirements. Nonetheless, diabetic women should be carefully observed while taking progestin-only oral contraceptives.

Lipid metabolism is occasionally affected in that HDL, HDL_2, and apolipoprotein A-I and A-II may be decreased; hepatic lipase may be increased. There is usually no effect on total cholesterol, HDL_3, LDL, or VLDL.

4. Drug Interactions

The effectiveness of progestin-only pills is reduced by hepatic enzyme-inducing drugs such as the anticonvulsants, phenytoin, carbamazepine; barbiturates; the antituberculosis drug rifampin; protease inhibitors; and herbal preparations containing St. John's Wort (hypericum perforatum). This could result in unintended pregnancy or breakthrough bleeding. There are anecdotal reports of reduced efficacy of combination oral contraceptives when used concomitantly with broad-spectrum antibiotics. No significant interaction has been found with progestin-only oral contraceptives and broad-spectrum antibiotics.

During concomitant use of OVRETTE and substances that may affect its efficacy, it is recommended that a nonhormonal back-up method of contraception be used in addition to the regular intake of OVRETTE. Use of a nonhormonal back-up method is advisable after discontinuation of substances that have led to induction of hepatic microsomal enzymes. It may take several weeks until enzyme induction has subsided, depending on dosage, duration of use, and rate of elimination of the inducing substance. For women receiving long-term therapy with hepatic enzyme inducers, another method of contraception should be considered.

Substances that reduce gastrointestinal transit time may affect contraceptive efficacy.

The product information of concomitant medications/substances should be consulted to identify potential interactions.

5. Interactions with Laboratory Tests

The following endocrine tests may be affected by progestin-only oral contraceptive use:

- Sex hormone-binding globulin (SHBG) concentrations may be decreased.
- Total thyroxine concentrations may be decreased, due to a decrease in thyroid binding globulin (TBG). However, free thyroxine level should remain unchanged.

6. Carcinogenesis

See **WARNINGS** section.

7. Pregnancy

Many epidemiological studies have found no effects on fetal development associated with long-term use of contraceptive doses of oral progestins. The few studies of infant growth and development that have been conducted have not demonstrated significant adverse effects. It is nonetheless prudent to rule out suspected pregnancy before initiating any hormonal contraceptive use. Epidemiological studies also do not suggest a teratogenic effect of oral contraceptives when taken inadvertently during early pregnancy. (See **CONTRAINDICATIONS**.)

8. Nursing Mothers

Small amounts of progestin pass into the breast milk, resulting in steroid levels in infant plasma. No adverse effects have been found on breastfeeding performance. Very rarely, adverse effects in the infant/child have been reported, including jaundice.

9. Fertility Following Discontinuation

The limited available data do not indicate a significant delay in the return of normal ovulation and fertility following discontinuation of progestin-only oral contraceptives.

10. Migraine/Headache

The onset or exacerbation of migraine, or development of headache with a new pattern that is recurrent, persistent, or severe requires discontinuation of oral contraceptives and evaluation of the cause.

Women with migraine (particularly migraine with aura) who take progestin-only oral contraceptives may be at increased risk of stroke.

11. Gastrointestinal

Diarrhea and/or vomiting may reduce hormone absorption.

12. Pediatric Use

Safety and efficacy of OVRETTE has been established in women of reproductive age. Safety and efficacy are expected to be the same for postpubertal adolescents under the age of 16 and users 16 and older. Use of this product before menarche is not indicated.

13. FD&C Yellow No. 5

This product contains FD&C Yellow No. 5 (tartrazine) which may cause allergic-type reactions (including bronchial asthma) in certain susceptible persons. Although the overall incidence of FD&C Yellow No. 5 (tartrazine) sensitivity in the general population is low, it is frequently seen in patients who also have aspirin hypersensitivity. (See **CONTRAINDICATIONS**.)

14. Geriatric Use

This product has not been studied in women over 65 years of age and is not indicated in this population.

INFORMATION FOR THE PATIENT

1. See **PATIENT LABELING** for detailed information.
2. Counseling issues

The following points should be discussed with prospective users before prescribing progestin-only oral contraceptives:

- The necessity of taking pills at the same time every day, including throughout all bleeding episodes.
- The need to use a nonhormonal back-up method of contraception (such as condoms and/or spermicides) for the next 48 hours whenever a progestin-only oral contraceptive is taken 3 or more hours late.
- The potential side effects of progestin-only oral contraceptives, particularly menstrual irregularities.
- The need to inform the clinician of prolonged episodes of bleeding, amenorrhea or severe abdominal pain.
- The importance of using a barrier method in addition to progestin-only oral contraceptives if a woman is at risk of contracting or transmitting STDs/HIV.

ADVERSE REACTIONS

An increased risk of the following adverse reactions has been reported with the use of progestin-only oral contraceptives (see **WARNINGS** section for additional information):

Ectopic pregnancy
Delayed follicular atresia/ovarian cysts
Menstrual irregularity, changes in menstrual flow; breakthrough bleeding/spotting; amenorrhea, prolonged bleeding

The following adverse reactions also have been reported with the use of progestin-only oral contraceptives:

Abdominal pain, cramps, distention
Acne
Alopecia
Anaphylactic/anaphylactoid reactions, including urticaria, throat tightness, and facial edema
Appetite increase or decrease
AST, ALT, bilirubin increase
Blood pressure increase
Breast pain, enlargement, secretion, and tenderness
Chloasma/melasma that may persist
Cholestasis
Dizziness
Edema
Fatigue
Galactorrhea
Glucose intolerance
HDL decrease
Hirsutism
Leg cramps/pain
Libido decrease
Migraine/headache
Mood disturbances, including depression
Myocardial infarction
Nausea
Nervousness
Rash
Stroke
Vaginal discharge
Vomiting
Weight change (increase or decrease)

See **WARNINGS** section for discussion of:
Carcinoma of the breast and reproductive organs
Hepatic neoplasia
Arterial and venous thromboembolic events

OVERDOSAGE

Symptoms of oral contraceptive overdosage may include nausea, vomiting, breast tenderness, dizziness, somnolence (drowsiness/fatigue), and withdrawal bleeding in females. There is no specific antidote and further treatment of overdose,.if necessary, is directed to the symptoms.

DOSAGE AND ADMINISTRATION

To achieve maximum contraceptive effectiveness, OVRETTE must be taken exactly as directed. One tablet is taken every day, at the same time. Administration is continuous, with no interruption between pill packs. See **PATIENT LABELING** for detailed instructions.

If one menstrual period is missed and the progestin-only oral contraceptive has not been taken according to directions, or if two consecutive periods are missed, tablet-taking should be discontinued and a nonhormonal back-up method of contraception should be used until the possibility of pregnancy is excluded.

HOW SUPPLIED

OVRETTE® tablets (0.075 mg norgestrel) are available in packages of 6 PILPAK® dispensers with 28 tablets each as follows: NDC 0008-0062-01, yellow, round tablet marked "WYETH" on one side and "62" on reverse side.

STORAGE

Store at controlled room temperature 20° to 25°C (68° to 77°F).

References available upon request.

DETAILED PATIENT LABELING

OVRETTE® (norgestrel) TABLETS

This product (like all oral contraceptives) is used to prevent pregnancy. It does not protect against HIV infection (AIDS) or other sexually transmitted diseases (STDs) such as chlamydia, genital herpes, genital warts, gonorrhea, hepatitis B, and syphilis.

DESCRIPTION

Each OVRETTE® tablet contains 0.075 mg of norgestrel. The inactive ingredients present are cellulose, FD&C Yellow 5, lactose, magnesium stearate, and polacrilin potassium.

INTRODUCTION

This leaflet is about birth control pills that contain one hormone, a progestin. Please read this leaflet before you begin to take your pills. It is meant to be used along with talking with your health-care professional.

Progestin-only pills are often called "POPs" or "the mini-pill." POPs have less progestin than the combined birth control pill (or "the pill") which contains both an estrogen and a progestin.

HOW EFFECTIVE ARE POPs?

POPs or "birth-control pills" or "the pill" are used to prevent pregnancy and are more effective than other nonsurgical methods of birth control. When they are taken correctly, without missing any pills the chance of becoming pregnant is approximately 1.0% per year. Average failure rates are approximately 5% per year when women who miss pills are included. The chance of becoming pregnant increases with each missed pill during the menstrual cycle.

In comparison, average failure rates for other methods of birth control during the first year of use are as follows:

IUD: 0.1-2%	Female condom alone: 21%
Depo-Provera® (injectable progestogen): 0.3%	Cervical cap
Norplant® System (levonorgestrel implants): 0.05%	Never given birth: 20%
Diaphragm with spermicides: 20%	Given birth: 40%
Spermicides alone: 26%	Periodic abstinence: 25%
Male condom alone: 14%	No methods: 85%

HOW DO POPs WORK?

POPs can prevent pregnancy in different ways including:

- They make the cervical mucus at the entrance to the womb (the uterus) too thick for the sperm to get through to the egg.
- They prevent ovulation (release of the egg from the ovary) in about half of the cycles.
- They also affect other hormones, the fallopian tubes, and the lining of the uterus.

YOU SHOULD NOT TAKE POPs

- If there is any chance you may be pregnant.
- If you have breast cancer.

- If you have bleeding between your periods which has not been diagnosed.
- If you are hypersensitive or allergic to any component of this product.
- If you have liver tumors, either non-cancerous or cancerous.
- If you have acute liver disease.

RISKS OF TAKING POPs

Cigarette smoking greatly increases the possibility of suffering heart attacks and strokes. Women who use oral contraceptives are strongly advised not to smoke.

Warning: If you have sudden or severe pain in your lower abdomen or stomach area, you may have an ectopic pregnancy or an ovarian cyst. If this happens, you should contact your health-care professional immediately.

Ectopic Pregnancy

An ectopic pregnancy is a pregnancy outside the womb. Because POPs protect against pregnancy, the chance of having a pregnancy outside the womb is very low. If you do get pregnant while taking POPs, you have a slightly higher chance that the pregnancy will be ectopic than do users of some other birth control methods.

Ovarian Cysts

These cysts are small sacs of fluid in the ovary. They are more common among POP-users than among users of most other birth control methods. They usually disappear without treatment and rarely cause problems.

Cancer of the Reproductive Organs and Breasts

Some studies reported a slightly increased risk of the diagnosis of breast cancer in women who were currently using oral contraceptives, which contained both estrogen and progestin. The risk gradually disappeared within 10 years after stopping use of the combination oral contraceptive. There is not enough information to determine whether the use of POPs increases this risk in a similar way.

Some studies have found an increase in the incidence of cancer or precancerous lesions of the cervix in women who use combination oral contraceptives (COCs). However, this finding may be related to factors other than the use of oral contraceptives and there is not enough information to determine whether the use of POPs increases the risk of developing cancer of the cervix.

Liver Tumors or Diseases

In rare cases, use of COCs has been associated with non-cancerous but dangerous liver tumors. These non-cancerous liver tumors can rupture and cause fatal internal bleeding. In addition, a possible association has been found with COCs and liver cancer in studies in which a few women who developed these very rare cancers were found to have used COCs for long periods of time. There is not enough information to determine if POPs increase the risk of liver tumors. Talk with your health-care professional if you have or have had liver problems.

Headache/Migraine

If you develop or have worsening of migraine or develop headache with a new pattern that is recurrent, persistent, or severe, you should discontinue taking oral contraceptives and see your health-care professional for an evaluation of the cause.

Women with migraine (particularly migraine with aura) who take POPs may be at increased risk of stroke.

Abnormal Blood Clotting

Changes in the blood clotting system have been reported in users of COCs. These changes allow the blood to clot more easily, possibly allowing clots to form in the bloodstream. If blood clots do form in the bloodstream, they can cause serious problems by cutting off the blood supply to vital organs. These problems may include a stroke (if the clot is in a blood vessel of the brain), a heart attack (if the clot is in a blood vessel of the heart), a pulmonary embolus (if the clot forms in the legs or pelvis, then breaks off and travels to the lungs), retinal thrombosis (if the clot is in a blood vessel of the eye) or other problems. Any of these conditions may cause death or serious long term disability.

There is not enough information to determine whether the use of POPs is associated with the development of blood clots, blockage of blood vessels, heart attack, and stroke. However, there have been reports of some of these conditions with the use of POPs. Therefore, the possibility of blood clots should be considered.

Diabetic Women

Diabetic women taking POPs do not generally require changes in the amount of insulin they are taking. However, your health-care professional may monitor you more closely under these conditions.

FD&C Yellow No. 5 (tartrazine)

Ovrette contains FD&C Yellow No. 5 (tartrazine) which may cause allergic-type reactions (including bronchial asthma) in certain susceptible persons. Although the overall incidence of FD&C Yellow No. 5 (tartrazine) sensitivity in the general population is low, it is frequently seen in patients who also have aspirin sensitivity.

SEXUALLY TRANSMITTED DISEASES (STDs)

Warning: POPs DO NOT PROTECT AGAINST GETTING OR GIVING SOMEONE HIV (AIDS) OR ANY OTHER STD SUCH AS CHLAMYDIA, GONORRHEA, GENITAL WARTS, HERPES, HEPATITIS B, AND SYPHILIS.

SIDE EFFECTS

An increased risk of the following side effects (see **RISKS OF TAKING POPs** for additional information) has been associated with the use of POPs:

Irregular bleeding - The most common side effect of POPs is a change in menstrual bleeding. Your periods may be either early or late, shorter or longer, heavier or lighter and/or you may have some spotting between periods. Taking pills late or missing pills can also result in some spotting or bleeding.

Ectopic pregnancy (pregnancy outside of the uterus)

Ovarian cysts

Other Side Effects:

Abdominal pain, cramps, bloating
Acne
Allergic/hypersensitivity reactions, including hives, rash, throat tightness, and facial swelling
Appetite increase or decrease
Blood pressure increase
Blood sugar increase
Breast pain, enlargement, secretion, and tenderness
Changes in liver function tests (AST, ALT, bilirubin increase)
Darkening areas of skin, especially on the face that may persist
Dizziness
Excessive hair growth on the face and body
Fatigue
Fluid retention
Hair loss
HDL decrease
Headache/migraine
Heart attack
Jaundice
Leg cramps/pain
Milky breast discharge
Mood disturbances, including depression
Nausea
Nervousness
Rash
Sex drive decrease
Stroke
Vaginal discharge
Vomiting
Weight changes (increase or decrease)

See also **RISKS OF TAKING POPs** for information on:
Abnormal blood clotting
Cancer of the reproductive organs and breast
Liver tumors

If you are concerned about any of these side effects, check with your health-care professional.

USING POPs WITH OTHER MEDICINES

Before taking a POP, inform your health-care professional if you are taking medicines for seizures (epilepsy), tuberculosis (TB), HIV/AIDS, or any other medication, including over-the-counter medicine and herbal products.

These medicines can make POPs less effective:

Medicines for seizures such as:
- Phenytoin (Dilantin®)
- Carbamazepine (Tegretol®)
- Phenobarbital

Medicine for TB:
- Rifampin (Rifadin®, Rimactane®)

Herbal Preparations such as:
- St. John's Wort (hypericum perforatum)

HIV/AIDS drugs such as:
- Zidovudine (Retrovir®)
- Indinavir (Crixivan®)

Before you begin taking any new medicines, be sure your health-care professional knows you are taking a progestin-only birth control pill.

HOW TO TAKE POPs

Important Points to Remember

- POPs must be taken at the same time every day, so choose a time and then take the pill at that same time every day. Every time you take a pill late, and especially if you miss a pill, you are more likely to get pregnant.
- Start the next pack the day after the last pack is finished. There is no break between packs. Always have your next pack of pills ready.
- You may have some bleeding between periods. Do not stop taking your pills if this happens. This is usually temporary and without significance; however, if bleeding is prolonged (more than 8 days) or unusually heavy, consult your health-care professional.
- If 1 menstrual period is missed and Ovrette has not been taken according to directions or if 2 consecutive periods are missed, tablet-taking should be discontinued and a nonhormonal back-up method of birth control (such as a condom and/or a spermicide) should be used until the possibility of pregnancy is excluded.
- If you vomit within 4 hours after taking a pill, or have diarrhea, absorption may not be complete; therefore, use a nonhormonal back-up method of birth control every time you have sex during the next 48 hours. (See **If You Are Late or Miss Taking Your POPs**.)
- If you want to stop taking POPs, you can do so at any time, but, if you remain sexually active and don't wish to become pregnant, be certain to use another birth control method.
- If you are not sure about how to take POPs, ask your health-care professional.

Starting POPs

- It's best to take your first POP on the first day of your menstrual period.
- If you decide to take your first POP on another day, use a nonhormonal back-up method of birth control (such as a condom and/or a spermicide) every time you have sex during the first 48 hours.
- If you have had a miscarriage, an abortion, or gave birth and are NOT breastfeeding, you can start POPs the next day. In addition, a nonhormonal back-up method of birth control should be used for the first 48 hours.

If You Are Late or Miss Taking Your POPs

- If one tablet is missed, but is less than three hours late, it should be taken as soon as it is remembered. Further tablets should be taken at the usual time.
- If one tablet is missed and is more than three hours late or if more than one consecutive tablet is missed, the last missed tablet should be taken as soon as it is remembered, even if this means taking two tablets in one day. Further tablets should be taken at the usual time, and a nonhormonal back-up method of birth control (such as a condom and/or a spermicide) should be used for the next 48 hours.
- In addition, if three or more tablets have been missed, the possibility of pregnancy should be considered before tablet-taking is resumed.
- If you are not sure what to do about the pills you have missed, keep taking POPs and use a nonhormonal back-up method of birth control until you can talk to your health-care professional.

If You Are Breastfeeding

- If you are breastfeeding (not giving your baby any food or formula), you may start your pills 6 weeks after delivery.
- When you begin taking your pills, a nonhormonal back-up method of birth control (such as a condom and/or a spermicide) should be used for the first 48 hours.

If You Are Switching Pills

- If you are switching from the combined pills to POPs, take the first POP the day after you finish the last active combined pill. Do not take any of the 7 inactive pills from the combined pill pack. You should know that many women have irregular periods after switching to POPs, but this is normal and to be expected.
- If you are switching from POPs to the combined pills, take the first active combined pill on the first day of your period, even if your POPs pack is not finished.
- If you switch to another brand of POPs, start the new brand anytime.
- If you are breastfeeding, you can switch to another method of birth control (such as a condom and/or a spermicide) at any time, except do not switch to the combined pills until you stop breastfeeding.

CHANGING FROM ANOTHER TYPE OF PROGESTIN-ONLY METHOD (IMPLANT, INJECTION)

Tablet-taking should start on the day of an implant removal or, if using an injection, the day the next injection would be due. In addition, a nonhormonal back-up method of birth control should be used for the first 48 hours.

PREGNANCY WHILE ON THE PILL

If you become pregnant or think you might be pregnant contact your health-care professional. You should stop taking POPs if pregnancy is confirmed. Even though POPs have not been shown to cause harm to the unborn baby, it is always best to avoid taking any drugs or medicines that you do not need when you are pregnant.

You should get a pregnancy test:
- If your period is late and you took one or more pills late or missed taking them and had sex without a nonhormonal back-up method of birth control.
- Anytime you miss 2 periods in a row.

WILL POPs AFFECT YOUR ABILITY TO GET PREGNANT LATER?

If you want to become pregnant, simply stop taking POPs. POPs will not delay your ability to get pregnant.

BREASTFEEDING

POPs have not been shown to affect breastfeeding performance. As with other medications taken while breastfeeding, small amounts of Ovrette can pass into the breast milk. Very rarely, adverse effects in the infant/child have been reported, including jaundice.

OVERDOSE

Overdosage may cause nausea, vomiting, breast tenderness, dizziness, somnolence (fatigue/drowsiness), and withdrawal bleeding in females. In case of overdosage, contact your health-care professional or pharmacist.

OTHER QUESTIONS OR CONCERNS

If you have any questions or concerns, check with your health-care professional. You can also ask for the more detailed "Professional Labeling" written for health-care professionals.

HOW TO STORE OVRETTE®

Store at controlled room temperature, 20° to 25°C (68° to 77°F).

Wyeth®
Wyeth Pharmaceuticals Inc.
Philadelphia, PA 19101

W10454C003
ET02
Rev 10/03

Shown in Product Identification Guide, page 336

Continued on next page

PHENERGAN® ℞

[fĕn-ər-jăn]

(promethazine HCl)

Tablets and Suppositories

℞ only

DESCRIPTION

Each tablet of Phenergan contains 12.5 mg, 25 mg, or 50 mg promethazine HCl. The inactive ingredients present are lactose, magnesium stearate, and methylcellulose. Each dosage strength also contains the following:

12.5 mg—FD&C Yellow 6 and saccharin sodium;

25 mg—saccharin sodium;

50 mg—FD&C Red 40.

Each rectal suppository of Phenergan contains 12.5 mg, 25 mg, or 50 mg promethazine HCl with ascorbyl palmitate, silicon dioxide, white wax, and cocoa butter. Phenergan Suppositories are for rectal administration only.

Promethazine HCl is a racemic compound; the empirical formula is $C_{17}H_{20}N_2S \cdot HCl$ and its molecular weight is 320.88.

Promethazine HCl, a phenothiazine derivative, is designated chemically as 10*H*-Phenothiazine-10-ethanamine, *N,N*,α-trimethyl-, monohydrochloride, (±)- with the following structural formula:

$CH_2CH(CH_3)N(CH_3)_2$

N S • HCl

Promethazine HCl occurs as a white to faint yellow, practically odorless, crystalline powder which slowly oxidizes and turns blue on prolonged exposure to air. It is freely soluble in water and soluble in alcohol.

CLINICAL PHARMACOLOGY

Promethazine is a phenothiazine derivative which differs structurally from the antipsychotic phenothiazines by the presence of a branched side chain and no ring substitution. It is thought that this configuration is responsible for its relative lack (1/10 that of chlorpromazine) of dopamine antagonist properties.

Promethazine is an H_1 receptor blocking agent. In addition to its antihistaminic action, it provides clinically useful sedative and antiemetic effects.

Promethazine is well absorbed from the gastrointestinal tract. Clinical effects are apparent within 20 minutes after oral administration and generally last four to six hours, although they may persist as long as 12 hours. Promethazine is metabolized by the liver to a variety of compounds; the sulfoxides of promethazine and N-demethylpromethazine are the predominant metabolites appearing in the urine.

INDICATIONS AND USAGE

Phenergan, either orally or by suppository, is useful for:

Perennial and seasonal allergic rhinitis.

Vasomotor rhinitis.

Allergic conjunctivitis due to inhalant allergens and foods.

Mild, uncomplicated allergic skin manifestations of urticaria and angioedema.

Amelioration of allergic reactions to blood or plasma.

Dermographism.

Anaphylactic reactions, as adjunctive therapy to epinephrine and other standard measures, after the acute manifestations have been controlled.

Preoperative, postoperative, or obstetric sedation.

Prevention and control of nausea and vomiting associated with certain types of anesthesia and surgery.

Therapy adjunctive to meperidine or other analgesics for control of post-operative pain.

Sedation in both children and adults, as well as relief of apprehension and production of light sleep from which the patient can be easily aroused.

Active and prophylactic treatment of motion sickness.

Antiemetic therapy in postoperative patients.

CONTRAINDICATIONS

Phenergan Tablets and Suppositories are contraindicated in comatose states, and in individuals known to be hypersensitive or to have had an idiosyncratic reaction to promethazine or to other phenothiazines.

Antihistamines are contraindicated for use in the treatment of lower respiratory tract symptoms including asthma.

WARNINGS

CNS Depression

Phenergan Tablets and Suppositories may impair the mental and/or physical abilities required for the performance of potentially hazardous tasks, such as driving a vehicle or operating machinery. The impairment may be amplified by concomitant use of other central-nervous-system depressants such as alcohol, sedatives/hypnotics (including barbiturates), narcotics, narcotic analgesics, general anesthetics, tricyclic antidepressants, and tranquilizers; therefore such agents should either be eliminated or given in reduced dosage in the presence of promethazine HCl (see **PRECAUTIONS—Information for Patients** and **Drug Interactions**).

Respiratory Depression

Phenergan Tablets and Suppositories may lead to potentially fatal respiratory depression.

Use of Phenergan Tablets and Suppositories in patients with compromised respiratory function (e.g., COPD, sleep apnea) should be avoided.

Lower Seizure Threshold

Phenergan Tablets and Suppositories may lower seizure threshold. It should be used with caution in persons with seizure disorders or in persons who are using concomitant medications, such as narcotics or local anesthetics, which may also affect seizure threshold.

Bone-Marrow Depression

Phenergan Tablets and Suppositories should be used with caution in patients with bone-marrow depression. Leukopenia and agranulocytosis have been reported, usually when Phenergan (promethazine HCl) has been used in association with other known marrow-toxic agents.

Neuroleptic Malignant Syndrome

A potentially fatal symptom complex sometimes referred to as Neuroleptic Malignant Syndrome (NMS) has been reported in association with promethazine HCl alone or in combination with antipsychotic drugs. Clinical manifestations of NMS are hyperpyrexia, muscle rigidity, altered mental status and evidence of autonomic instability (irregular pulse or blood pressure, tachycardia, diaphoresis and cardiac dysrhythmias).

The diagnostic evaluation of patients with this syndrome is complicated. In arriving at a diagnosis, it is important to identify cases where the clinical presentation includes both serious medical illness (e.g. pneumonia, systemic infection, etc.) and untreated or inadequately treated extrapyramidal signs and symptoms (EPS). Other important considerations in the differential diagnosis include central anticholinergic toxicity, heat stroke, drug fever and primary central nervous system (CNS) pathology.

The management of NMS should include 1) immediate discontinuation of promethazine HCl, antipsychotic drugs, if any, and other drugs not essential to concurrent therapy, 2) intensive symptomatic treatment and medical monitoring, and 3) treatment of any concomitant serious medical problems for which specific treatments are available. There is no general agreement about specific pharmacological treatment regimens for uncomplicated NMS.

Since recurrences of NMS have been reported with phenothiazines, the reintroduction of promethazine HCl should be carefully considered.

Use in Pediatric Patients

PHENERGAN TABLETS AND SUPPOSITORIES ARE NOT RECOMMENDED FOR USE IN PEDIATRIC PATIENTS LESS THAN TWO YEARS OF AGE.

CAUTION SHOULD BE EXERCISED WHEN ADMINISTERING PHENERGAN TABLETS AND SUPPOSITORIES TO PEDIATRIC PATIENTS 2 YEARS OF AGE AND OLDER BECAUSE OF THE POTENTIAL FOR FATAL RESPIRATORY DEPRESSION. ANTIEMETICS ARE NOT RECOMMENDED FOR TREATMENT OF UNCOMPLICATED VOMITING IN PEDIATRIC PATIENTS, AND THEIR USE SHOULD BE LIMITED TO PROLONGED VOMITING OF KNOWN ETIOLOGY. THE EXTRAPYRAMIDAL SYMPTOMS WHICH CAN OCCUR SECONDARY TO PHENERGAN TABLETS AND SUPPOSITORIES ADMINISTRATION MAY BE CONFUSED WITH THE CNS SIGNS OF UNDIAGNOSED PRIMARY DISEASE, e.g., ENCEPHALOPATHY OR REYE'S SYNDROME. THE USE OF PHENERGAN TABLETS AND SUPPOSITORIES SHOULD BE AVOIDED IN PEDIATRIC PATIENTS WHOSE SIGNS AND SYMPTOMS MAY SUGGEST REYE'S SYNDROME OR OTHER HEPATIC DISEASES.

Excessively large dosages of antihistamines, including Phenergan Tablets and Suppositories, in pediatric patients may cause sudden death (see **OVERDOSAGE**). Hallucinations and convulsions have occurred with therapeutic doses and overdoses of Phenergan in pediatric patients. In pediatric patients who are acutely ill associated with dehydration, there is an increased susceptibility to dystonias with the use of promethazine HCl.

Other Considerations

Administration of promethazine HCl has been associated with reported cholestatic jaundice.

PRECAUTIONS

General

Drugs having anticholinergic properties should be used with caution in patients with narrow-angle glaucoma, prostatic hypertrophy, stenosing peptic ulcer, pyloroduodenal obstruction, and bladder-neck obstruction.

Phenergan Tablets and Suppositories should be used cautiously in persons with cardiovascular disease or with impairment of liver function.

Information for Patients

Phenergan Tablets and Suppositories may cause marked drowsiness or impair the mental and/or physical abilities required for the performance of potentially hazardous tasks, such as driving a vehicle or operating machinery. The use of alcohol or other central-nervous-system depressants such as sedatives/hypnotics (including barbiturates), narcotics, narcotic analgesics, general anesthetics, tricyclic antidepressants, and tranquilizers, may enhance impairment (see **WARNINGS—CNS Depression** and **PRECAUTIONS—Drug Interactions**). Pediatric patients should be supervised to avoid potential harm in bike riding or in other hazardous activities.

Patients should be advised to report any involuntary muscle movements.

Avoid prolonged exposure to the sun.

Drug Interactions

CNS Depressants—Phenergan Tablets and Suppositories may increase, prolong, or intensify the sedative action of other central-nervous-system depressants, such as alcohol, sedatives/hypnotics (including barbiturates), narcotics, narcotic analgesics, general anesthetics, tricyclic antidepressants, and tranquilizers; therefore, such agents should be avoided or administered in reduced dosage to patients receiving promethazine HCl. When given concomitantly with Phenergan Tablets and Suppositories, the dose of barbiturates should be reduced by at least one-half, and the dose of narcotics should be reduced by one-quarter to one-half. Dosage must be individualized. Excessive amounts of promethazine HCl relative to a narcotic may lead to restlessness and motor hyperactivity in the patient with pain; these symptoms usually disappear with adequate control of the pain.

Epinephrine—Because of the potential for Phenergan to reverse epinephrine's vasopressor effect, epinephrine should NOT be used to treat hypotension associated with Phenergan Tablets and Suppositories overdose.

Anticholinergics—Concomitant use of other agents with anticholinergic properties should be undertaken with caution.

Monoamine Oxidase Inhibitors (MAOI)—Drug interactions, including an increased incidence of extrapyramidal effects, have been reported when some MAOI and phenothiazines are used concomitantly. This possibility should be considered with Phenergan Tablets and Suppositories.

Drug/Laboratory Test Interactions

The following laboratory tests may be affected in patients who are receiving therapy with promethazine HCl:

Pregnancy Tests

Diagnostic pregnancy tests based on immunological reactions between HCG and anti-HCG may result in false-negative or false-positive interpretations.

Glucose Tolerance Test

An increase in blood glucose has been reported in patients receiving promethazine HCl.

Carcinogenesis, Mutagenesis, Impairment of Fertility

Long-term animal studies have not been performed to assess the carcinogenic potential of promethazine, nor are there other animal or human data concerning carcinogenicity, mutagenicity, or impairment of fertility with this drug. Promethazine was nonmutagenic in the *Salmonella* test system of Ames.

Pregnancy

Teratogenic Effects—Pregnancy Category C

Teratogenic effects have not been demonstrated in rat-feeding studies at doses of 6.25 and 12.5 mg/kg of promethazine HCl. These doses are from approximately 2.1 to 4.2 times the maximum recommended total daily dose of promethazine for a 50-kg subject, depending upon the indication for which the drug is prescribed. Daily doses of 25 mg/kg intraperitoneally have been found to produce fetal mortality in rats.

Specific studies to test the action of the drug on parturition, lactation, and development of the animal neonate were not done, but a general preliminary study in rats indicated no effect on these parameters. Although antihistamines have been found to produce fetal mortality in rodents, the pharmacological effects of histamine in the rodent do not parallel those in man. There are no adequate and well-controlled studies of Phenergan® Tablets and Suppositories in pregnant women.

Phenergan (promethazine HCl) Tablets and Suppositories should be used during pregnancy only if the potential benefit justifies the potential risk to the fetus.

Nonteratogenic Effects

Phenergan Tablets and Suppositories administered to a pregnant woman within two weeks of delivery may inhibit platelet aggregation in the newborn.

Labor and Delivery

Promethazine HCl may be used alone or as an adjunct to narcotic analgesics during labor (see **DOSAGE AND ADMINISTRATION**). Limited data suggest that use of Phenergan during labor and delivery does not have an appreciable effect on the duration of labor or delivery and does not increase the risk of need for intervention in the newborn. The effect on later growth and development of the newborn is unknown. (See also *Nonteratogenic Effects*.)

Nursing Mothers

It is not known whether promethazine HCl is excreted in human milk. Because many drugs are excreted in human milk and because of the potential for serious adverse reactions in nursing infants from Phenergan Tablets and Suppositories, a decision should be made whether to discontinue nursing or to discontinue the drug, taking into account the importance of the drug to the mother.

Pediatric Use

Safety and effectiveness in children under 2 years of age have not been established.

Phenergan Tablets and Suppositories should be used with caution in pediatric patients 2 years of age and older (see **WARNINGS—Use in Pediatric Patients**).

Geriatric Use

Clinical studies of Phenergan formulations did not include sufficient numbers of subjects aged 65 and over to determine whether they respond differently from younger subjects. Other reported clinical experience has not identified differences in responses between the elderly and younger patients. In general, dose selection for an elderly patient should be cautious, usually starting at the low end of the dosing range, reflecting the greater frequency of decreased hepatic, renal or cardiac function, and of concomitant disease or other drug therapy.

Sedating drugs may cause confusion and over-sedation in the elderly; elderly patients generally should be started on low doses of Phenergan Tablets and Suppositories and observed closely.

ADVERSE REACTIONS

Central Nervous System

Drowsiness is the most prominent CNS effect of this drug. Sedation, somnolence, blurred vision, dizziness; confusion, disorientation, and extrapyramidal symptoms such as oculogyric crisis, torticollis, and tongue protrusion; lassitude, tinnitus, incoordination, fatigue, euphoria, nervousness, diplopia, insomnia, tremors, convulsive seizures, excitation, catatonic-like states, hysteria. Hallucinations have also been reported.

Cardiovascular—Increased or decreased blood pressure, tachycardia, bradycardia, faintness.

Dermatologic—Dermatitis, photosensitivity, urticaria.

Hematologic—Leukopenia, thrombocytopenia, thrombocytopenic purpura, agranulocytosis.

Gastrointestinal—Dry mouth, nausea, vomiting, jaundice.

Respiratory—Asthma, nasal stuffiness, respiratory depression (potentially fatal) and apnea (potentially fatal). (See **WARNINGS—Respiratory Depression.**)

Other—Angioneurotic edema. Neuroleptic malignant syndrome (potentially fatal) has also been reported. (See **WARNINGS—Neuroleptic Malignant Syndrome.**)

Paradoxical Reactions

Hyperexcitability and abnormal movements have been reported in patients following a single administration of promethazine HCl. Consideration should be given to the discontinuation of promethazine HCl and to the use of other drugs if these reactions occur. Respiratory depression, nightmares, delirium, and agitated behavior have also been reported in some of these patients.

OVERDOSAGE

Signs and symptoms of overdosage with promethazine HCl range from mild depression of the central nervous system and cardiovascular system to profound hypotension, respiratory depression, unconsciousness, and sudden death. Other reported reactions include hyperreflexia, hypertonia, ataxia, athetosis, and extensor-plantar reflexes (Babinski reflex).

Stimulation may be evident, especially in children and geriatric patients. Convulsions may rarely occur. A paradoxical-type reaction has been reported in children receiving single doses of 75 mg to 125 mg orally, characterized by hyperexcitability and nightmares.

Atropine-like signs and symptoms—dry mouth, fixed, dilated pupils, flushing, as well as gastrointestinal symptoms—may occur.

Treatment

Treatment of overdosage is essentially symptomatic and supportive. Only in cases of extreme overdosage or individual sensitivity do vital signs, including respiration, pulse, blood pressure, temperature, and EKG, need to be monitored. Activated charcoal orally or by lavage may be given, or sodium or magnesium sulfate orally as a cathartic. Attention should be given to the reestablishment of adequate respiratory exchange through provision of a patent airway and institution of assisted or controlled ventilation. Diazepam may be used to control convulsions. Acidosis and electrolyte losses should be corrected. Note that any depressant effects of promethazine HCl are not reversed by naloxone. Avoid analeptics which may cause convulsions.

The treatment of choice for resulting hypotension is administration of intravenous fluids, accompanied by repositioning if indicated. In the event that vasopressors are considered for the management of severe hypotension which does not respond to intravenous fluids and repositioning, the administration of norepinephrine or phenylephrine should be considered. EPINEPHRINE SHOULD NOT BE USED, since its use in patients with partial adrenergic blockade may further lower the blood pressure. Extrapyramidal reactions may be treated with anticholinergic antiparkinsonian agents, diphenhydramine, or barbiturates. Oxygen may also be administered.

Limited experience with dialysis indicates that it is not helpful.

DOSAGE AND ADMINISTRATION

Phenergan Tablets and Phenergan Rectal Suppositories are not recommended for children under 2 years of age (see **WARNINGS-Use in Pediatric Patients).**

Phenergan Suppositories are for rectal administration only.

Allergy

The average oral dose is 25 mg taken before retiring; however, 12.5 mg may be taken before meals and on retiring, if necessary. Single 25-mg doses at bedtime or 6.25 to 12.5 mg taken three times daily will usually suffice. After initiation of treatment in children or adults, dosage should be adjusted to the smallest amount adequate to relieve symptoms. The administration of promethazine HCl in 25-mg doses will control minor transfusion reactions of an allergic nature.

Motion Sickness

The average adult dose is 25 mg taken twice daily. The initial dose should be taken one-half to one hour before anticipated travel and be repeated 8 to 12 hours later, if necessary. On succeeding days of travel, it is recommended that 25 mg be given on arising and again before the evening meal. For children, Phenergan Tablets, Syrup, or Rectal Suppositories, 12.5 to 25 mg, twice daily, may be administered.

Nausea and Vomiting

Antiemetics should not be used in vomiting of unknown etiology in children and adolescents (see **WARNINGS-Use in Pediatric Patients**).

The average effective dose of Phenergan for the active therapy of nausea and vomiting in children or adults is 25 mg. When oral medication cannot be tolerated, the dose should be given parenterally (cf. Phenergan Injection) or by rectal suppository. 12.5- to 25-mg doses may be repeated, as necessary, at 4- to 6-hour intervals.

For nausea and vomiting in children, the usual dose is 0.5 mg per pound of body weight, and the dose should be adjusted to the age and weight of the patient and the severity of the condition being treated.

For prophylaxis of nausea and vomiting, as during surgery and the postoperative period, the average dose is 25 mg repeated at 4- to 6-hour intervals, as necessary.

Sedation

This product relieves apprehension and induces a quiet sleep from which the patient can be easily aroused. Administration of 12.5 to 25 mg Phenergan by the oral route or by rectal suppository at bedtime will provide sedation in children. Adults usually require 25 to 50 mg for nighttime, presurgical, or obstetrical sedation.

Pre- and Postoperative Use

Phenergan in 12.5- to 25-mg doses for children and 50-mg doses for adults the night before surgery relieves apprehension and produces a quiet sleep.

For preoperative medication, children require doses of 0.5 mg per pound of body weight in combination with an appropriately reduced dose of narcotic or barbiturate and the appropriate dose of an atropine-like drug. Usual adult dosage is 50 mg Phenergan with an appropriately reduced dose of narcotic or barbiturate and the required amount of a belladonna alkaloid.

Postoperative sedation and adjunctive use with analgesics may be obtained by the administration of 12.5 to 25 mg in children and 25- to 50-mg doses in adults.

Phenergan Tablets and Phenergan Rectal Suppositories are not recommended for children under 2 years of age.

HOW SUPPLIED

Phenergan® (promethazine HCl) Tablets are available as follows:

12.5 mg, orange tablet with "WYETH" on one side and "19" on the scored reverse side.

NDC 0008-0019-01, bottle of 100 tablets.

25 mg, white tablet with "WYETH" and "27" on one side and scored on the reverse side.

NDC 0008-0027-02, bottle of 100 tablets.

NDC 0008-0027-07, Redipak® carton of 100 tablets (10 blister strips of 10).

50 mg, pink tablet with "WYETH" on one side and "227" on the other side.

NDC 0008-0227-01, bottle of 100 tablets.

Keep tightly closed.

Store at controlled room temperature 20° to 25°C (68° to 77°F).

Protect from light.

Dispense in light-resistant, tight container.

Use carton to protect contents from light.

Phenergan® (promethazine HCl) Rectal Suppositories are available in boxes of 12 as follows:

12.5 mg, ivory, torpedo-shaped suppository wrapped in copper-colored foil, NDC 0008-0498-01.

25 mg, ivory, torpedo-shaped suppository wrapped in light-green foil, NDC 0008-0212-01.

50 mg, ivory, torpedo-shaped suppository wrapped in blue foil, NDC 0008-0229-01.

Store refrigerated between 2°-8°C (36°-46°F).

Dispense in well-closed container.

Wyeth Pharmaceuticals Inc.
Philadelphia, PA 19101

W10448C002
ET02
Rev 08/03

PREMARIN® ℞

[prĕ-mă-rĭn]

Intravenous

(conjugated estrogens, USP) for injection

Specially prepared for Intravenous & Intramuscular use

℞ only

ESTROGENS INCREASE THE RISK OF ENDOMETRIAL CANCER

Close clinical surveillance of all women taking estrogens is important. Adequate diagnostic measures, including endometrial sampling when indicated, should be undertaken to rule out malignancy in all cases of undiagnosed persistent or recurring abnormal vaginal bleeding. There is no evidence that the use of "natural" estrogens results in a different endometrial risk profile than synthetic estrogens of equivalent estrogen doses.

CARDIOVASCULAR AND OTHER RISKS

Estrogens with or without progestins should not be used for the prevention of cardiovascular disease.

The Women's Health Initiative (WHI) study reported increased risks of myocardial infarction, stroke, invasive breast cancer, pulmonary emboli, and deep vein thrombosis in postmenopausal women (50 to 79 years of age) during 5 years of treatment with oral conjugated estrogens (0.625 mg) combined with medroxyprogesterone acetate (2.5 mg) relative to placebo. (See **CLINICAL PHARMACOLOGY, Clinical Studies.**)

The Women's Health Initiative Memory Study (WHIMS), a substudy of WHI, reported increased risk of developing probable dementia in postmenopausal women 65 years of age or older during 4 years of treatment with conjugated estrogens plus medroxyprogesterone acetate relative to placebo. It is unknown whether this finding applies to younger postmenopausal women or to women taking estrogen alone therapy. (See **CLINICAL PHARMACOLOGY, Clinical Studies.**)

Other doses of conjugated estrogens and medroxyprogesterone acetate, and other combinations and dosage forms of estrogens and progestins were not studied in the WHI clinical trials and, in the absence of comparable data, these risks should be assumed to be similar. Because of these risks, estrogens with or without progestins should be prescribed at the lowest effective doses and for the shortest duration consistent with treatment goals and risks for the individual woman.

DESCRIPTION

Premarin® Intravenous (conjugated estrogens, USP) for injection contains a mixture of conjugated estrogens obtained exclusively from natural sources, occurring as the sodium salts of water-soluble estrogen sulfates blended to represent the average composition of materials derived from pregnant mares' urine. It is a mixture of sodium estrone sulfate and sodium equilin sulfate. It contains as concomitant components, as sodium sulfate conjugates, 17α-dihydroequilin, 17α-estradiol, and 17β-dihydroequilin.

Each Secule® vial contains 25 mg of conjugated estrogens, USP, in a sterile lyophilized cake which also contains lactose 200 mg, sodium citrate 12.2 mg, and simethicone 0.2 mg. The pH is adjusted with sodium hydroxide or hydrochloric acid. A sterile diluent (5 mL) containing 2% benzyl alcohol in sterile water is provided for reconstitution. The reconstituted solution is suitable for intravenous or intramuscular injection.

CLINICAL PHARMACOLOGY

Endogenous estrogens are largely responsible for the development and maintenance of the female reproductive system and secondary sexual characteristics. Although circulating estrogens exist in a dynamic equilibrium of metabolic interconversions, estradiol is the principal intracellular human estrogen and is substantially more potent than its metabolites, estrone and estriol, at the receptor level. The primary source of estrogen in normally cycling adult women is the ovarian follicle, which secretes 70 to 500 mcg of estradiol daily, depending on the phase of the menstrual cycle. After menopause, most endogenous estrogen is produced by conversion of androstenedione, secreted by the adrenal cortex, to estrone by peripheral tissues. Thus, estrone and the sulfate-conjugated form, estrone sulfate, are the most abundant circulating estrogen in postmenopausal women.

Estrogens act through binding to nuclear receptors in estrogen-responsive tissues. To date, two estrogen receptors have been identified. These vary in proportion from tissue to tissue.

Circulating estrogens modulate the pituitary secretion of the gonadotropins, luteinizing hormone (LH) and follicle stimulating hormone (FSH) through a negative feedback mechanism. Estrogens act to reduce the elevated levels of these gonadotropins seen in postmenopausal women.

Pharmacokinetics

Absorption

Conjugated estrogens are soluble in water and are well absorbed through the skin, mucous membranes, and gastrointestinal tract after release from the drug formulation.

Distribution

The distribution of exogenous estrogens is similar to that of endogenous estrogens. Estrogens are widely distributed in the body and are generally found in higher concentration in the sex hormone target organs. Estrogens circulate in the blood largely bound to sex hormone-binding globulin (SHBG) and albumin.

Metabolism

Exogenous estrogens are metabolized in the same manner as endogenous estrogens. Circulating estrogens exist in a dynamic equilibrium of metabolic interconversions. These transformations take place mainly in the liver. Estradiol is converted reversibly to estrone, and both can be converted to estriol, which is the major urinary metabolite. Estrogens also undergo enterohepatic recirculation via sulfate and glucuronide conjugation in the liver, biliary secretion of conjugates into the intestine, and hydrolysis in the gut followed by reabsorption. In postmenopausal women a significant proportion of the circulating estrogens exists as sulfate conjugates, especially estrone sulfate, which serves as a circulating reservoir for the formation of more active estrogens.

Excretion

Estradiol, estrone, and estriol are excreted in the urine along with glucuronide and sulfate conjugates.

Special Populations

No pharmacokinetic studies were conducted in special populations, including patients with renal or hepatic impairment.

Continued on next page

Premarin Intravenous—Cont.

Drug Interactions

Data from a single-dose drug-drug interaction study involving oral conjugated estrogens and medroxyprogesterone acetate indicate that the pharmacokinetic dispositions of both drugs are not altered when the drugs are coadministered. No other clinical drug-drug interaction studies have been conducted with conjugated estrogens.

In vitro and in vivo studies have shown that estrogens are metabolized partially by cytochrome P450 3A4 (CYP3A4). Therefore, inducers or inhibitors of CYP3A4 may affect estrogen drug metabolism. Inducers of CYP3A4 such as St. John's Wort preparations (Hypericum perforatum), phenobarbital, carbamazepine, and rifampin may reduce plasma concentrations of estrogens, possibly resulting in a decrease in therapeutic effects and/or changes in the uterine bleeding profile. Inhibitors of CYP3A4 such as erythromycin, clarithromycin, ketoconazole, itraconazole, ritonavir and grapefruit juice may increase plasma concentrations of estrogens and may result in side effects.

Clinical Studies

Women's Health Initiative Studies.

The Women's Health Initiative (WHI) enrolled a total of 27,000 predominantly healthy postmenopausal women to assess the risks and benefits of either the use of Premarin tablets (0.625 mg conjugated estrogens per day) alone or the use of PREMPRO™ tablets (0.625 mg conjugated estrogens plus 2.5 mg medroxyprogesterone acetate per day) compared to placebo in the prevention of certain chronic diseases. The primary endpoint was the incidence of coronary heart disease (CHD) (nonfatal myocardial infarction and CHD death), with invasive breast cancer as the primary adverse outcome studied. A "global index" included the earliest occurrence of CHD, invasive breast cancer, stroke, pulmonary embolism (PE), endometrial cancer, colorectal cancer, hip fracture, or death due to other cause. The study did not evaluate the effects of Premarin tablets or PREMPRO on menopausal symptoms.

The Premarin tablets-only substudy results have not been reported. The estrogen plus progestin substudy was stopped early because, according to the predefined stopping rule, the increased risk of breast cancer and cardiovascular events exceeded the specified benefits included in the "global index." Results of the estrogen plus progestin substudy, which included 16,608 women (average age of 63 years, range 50 to 79; 83.9% White, 6.5% Black, 5.5% Hispanic), after an average follow-up of 5.2 years, are presented in Table 1 below:

[See table 1 below]

For those outcomes included in the "global index", the absolute excess risks per 10,000 women-years in the group treated with PREMPRO were 7 more CHD events, 8 more strokes, 8 more PEs, and 8 more invasive breast cancers, while the absolute risk reductions per 10,000 women-years were 6 fewer colorectal cancers and 5 fewer hip fractures. The absolute excess risk of events included in the "global index" was 19 per 10,000 women-years. There was no difference between the groups in terms of all-cause mortality. (See **BOXED WARNINGS, WARNINGS,** and **PRECAUTIONS.**)

INDICATIONS AND USAGE

Premarin Intravenous (conjugated estrogens, USP) for injection is indicated in the treatment of abnormal uterine bleeding due to hormonal imbalance in the absence of organic pathology.

Premarin Intravenous is indicated for short-term use only, to provide a rapid and temporary increase in estrogen levels.

CONTRAINDICATIONS

Premarin Intravenous should not be used in individuals with any of the following conditions:

1. Undiagnosed abnormal genital bleeding.
2. Known, suspected, or history of cancer of the breast.
3. Known or suspected estrogen-dependent neoplasia.
4. Active deep vein thrombosis, pulmonary embolism or a history of these conditions.
5. Active or recent (e.g., within past year) arterial thromboembolic disease (e.g., stroke, myocardial infarction).
6. Liver dysfunction or disease.
7. Premarin Intravenous for injection should not be used in patients with known hypersensitivity to its ingredients.
8. Known or suspected pregnancy. There is no indication for Premarin Intravenous in pregnancy. There appears to be little or no increased risk of birth defects in children born to women who have used estrogen and progestins from oral contraceptives inadvertently during pregnancy. (See **PRECAUTIONS.**)

WARNINGS

See **BOXED WARNINGS.**

Premarin Intravenous is indicated for short-term use. However, warnings, precautions and adverse reactions associated with Premarin tablets should be taken into account.

1. **Cardiovascular disorders.**

Estrogen and estrogen/progestin therapy have been associated with an increased risk of cardiovascular events such as myocardial infarction and stroke, as well as venous thrombosis and pulmonary embolism (venous thromboembolism or VTE). Should any of these occur or be suspected, estrogens should be discontinued immediately.

Risk factors for arterial vascular disease (e.g., hypertension, diabetes mellitus, tobacco use, hypercholesterolemia, and obesity) and/or venous thromboembolism (e.g., personal history or family history of VTE, obesity, and systemic lupus erythematosus) should be managed appropriately.

a. Coronary heart disease and stroke. In the Premarin tablets substudy of the Women's Health Initiative (WHI) study, an increase in the number of myocardial infarctions and strokes has been observed in women receiving Premarin compared to placebo. These observations are preliminary. (See **CLINICAL PHARMACOLOGY, Clinical Studies.**)

In the estrogen plus progestin substudy of WHI, an increased risk of coronary heart disease (CHD) events (defined as nonfatal myocardial infarction and CHD death) was observed in women receiving PREMPRO compared to women receiving placebo (37 vs 30 per 10,000 women-years). The increase in risk was observed in year one and persisted.

In the same substudy of WHI, an increased risk of stroke was observed in women receiving PREMPRO compared to women receiving placebo (29 vs 21 per 10,000 women-years). The increase in risk was observed after the first year and persisted.

In postmenopausal women with documented heart disease (n = 2,763, average age 66.7 years) a controlled clinical trial of secondary prevention of cardiovascular disease (Heart and Estrogen/progestin Replacement Study; HERS) treatment with PREMPRO (0.625 mg conjugated estrogen plus 2.5 mg medroxyprogesterone acetate per day) demonstrated no cardiovascular benefit. During an average follow-up of 4.1 years, treatment with PREMPRO did not reduce the overall rate of CHD events in postmenopausal women with established coronary heart disease. There were more CHD events in the PREMPRO-treated group than in the placebo group in year 1, but not during the subsequent years. Two thousand three hundred and twenty one women from the original HERS trial agreed to participate in an open label extension of HERS, HERS II. Average follow-up in HERS II was an additional 2.7 years, for a total of 6.8 years overall. Rates of CHD events were comparable among women in the PREMPRO group and the placebo group in HERS, HERS II, and overall.

Large doses of estrogen (5 mg conjugated estrogens per day), comparable to those used to treat cancer of the prostate and breast, have been shown in a large prospective clinical trial in men to increase the risks of nonfatal myocardial infarction, pulmonary embolism, and thrombophlebitis.

b. Venous thromboembolism (VTE). In the Premarin tablets substudy of the Women's Health Initiative (WHI), an increase in VTE has been observed in women receiving Premarin compared to placebo. These observations are preliminary. (See **CLINICAL PHARMACOLOGY, Clinical Studies.**)

In the estrogen plus progestin substudy of WHI, a 2-fold greater rate of VTE, including deep venous thrombosis and pulmonary embolism, was observed in women receiving PREMPRO compared to women receiving placebo. The rate of VTE was 34 per 10,000 women-years in the PREMPRO group compared to 16 per 10,000 women-years in the placebo group. The increase in VTE risk was observed during the first year and persisted.

2. **Malignant neoplasms.**

a. Endometrial cancer. The use of unopposed estrogens in women with intact uteri has been associated with an increased risk of endometrial cancer. The reported endometrial cancer risk among unopposed estrogen users is about 2- to 12-fold greater than in non-users, and appears dependent on duration of treatment and on estrogen dose. Most studies show no significant increased risk associated with use of estrogens for less than one year. The greatest risk appears associated with prolonged use, with increased risks of 15- to 24-fold for five to ten years or more and this risk has been shown to persist for at least 8 to 15 years after estrogen therapy is discontinued.

b. Breast cancer. The use of estrogens and progestins by postmenopausal women has been reported to increase the risk of breast cancer. The most important randomized clinical trial providing information about this issue is the Women's Health Initiative (WHI) trial of estrogen plus progestin (see **CLINICAL PHARMACOLOGY, Clinical Studies**). The results from observational studies are generally consistent with those of the WHI clinical trial.

After a mean follow-up of 5.6 years, the WHI trial reported an increased risk of breast cancer in women who took estrogen plus progestin. Observational studies have also reported an increased risk for estrogen/progestin combination therapy, and a smaller increased risk for estrogen alone therapy, after several years of use. For both findings, the excess risk increased with duration of use, and appeared to return to baseline over about five years after stopping treatment (only the observational studies have substantial data on risk after stopping). In these studies, the risk of breast cancer was greater, and became apparent earlier, with estrogen/progestin combination therapy as compared to estrogen alone therapy. However, these studies have not found significant variation in the risk of breast cancer among different estrogens or among different estrogen/progestin combinations, doses, or routes of administration.

In the WHI trial of estrogen plus progestin, 26% of the women reported prior use of estrogen alone and/or estrogen/progestin combination hormone therapy. After a mean follow-up of 5.6 years during the clinical trial, the overall relative risk of invasive breast cancer was 1.24 (95% confidence interval 1.01-1.54), and the overall absolute risk was 41 vs. 33 cases per 10,000 women-years, for estrogen plus progestin compared with placebo. Among women who reported prior use of hormone therapy, the relative risk of invasive breast cancer was 1.86, and the absolute risk was 46 vs. 25 cases per 10,000 women-years, for estrogen plus progestin compared with placebo. Among women who reported no prior use of hormone therapy, the relative risk of invasive breast cancer was 1.09, and the absolute risk was 40 vs. 36 cases per 10,000 women-years for estrogen plus progestin compared with placebo. In the WHI trial, invasive breast cancers were larger and diagnosed at a more advanced stage in the estrogen plus progestin group compared with the placebo group. Metastatic disease was rare with no apparent difference between the two groups. Other prognostic factors such as histologic subtype, grade and hormone receptor status did not differ between the groups.

Table 1. RELATIVE AND ABSOLUTE RISK SEEN IN THE ESTROGEN PLUS PROGESTIN SUBSTUDY OF WHI[a]

Event[c]	Relative Risk Prempro vs Placebo at 5.2 Years (95% CI*)	Placebo n = 8102	Prempro n = 8506
		Absolute Risk per 10,000 Women-years	
CHD events	1.29 (1.02-1.63)	30	37
Non-fatal MI	*1.32 (1.02-1.72)*	*23*	*30*
CHD death	*1.18 (0.70-1.97)*	*6*	*7*
Invasive breast cancer[b]	1.26 (1.00-1.59)	30	38
Stroke	1.41 (1.07-185)	21	29
Pulmonary embolism	2.13 (1.39-3.25)	8	16
Colorectal cancer	0.63 (0.43-0.92)	16	10
Endometrial cancer	0.83 (0.47-1.47)	6	5
Hip fracture	0.66 (0.45-0.98)	15	10
Death due to causes other than the events above	0.92 (0.74-1.14)	40	37
Global Index[c]	1.15 (1.03-1.28)	151	170
Deep vein thrombosis[d]	2.07 (1.49-2.87)	13	26
Vertebral fractures[d]	0.66 (0.44-0.98)	15	9
Other osteoporotic fractures[d]	0.77 (0.69-0.86)	170	131

[a] adapted from JAMA, 2002; 288:321-333
[b] includes metastatic and non-metastatic breast cancer with the exception of in situ breast cancer
[c] a subset of the events was combined in a "global index", defined as the earliest occurrence of CHD events, invasive breast cancer, stroke, pulmonary embolism, endometrial cancer, colorectal cancer, hip fracture, or death due to other causes
[d] not included in Global Index
* nominal confidence intervals unadjusted for multiple looks and multiple comparisons

The observational Million Women Study in Europe reported an increased risk of mortality due to breast cancer among current users of estrogens alone or estrogens plus progestins compared to never users, while the estrogen plus progestin sub-study of WHI showed no effect on breast cancer mortality with a mean follow-up of 5.6 years.
The use of estrogen plus progestin has been reported to result in an increase in abnormal mammograms requiring further evaluation. All women should receive yearly breast examinations by a healthcare provider and perform monthly breast self-examinations. In addition, mammography examinations should be scheduled based on patient age, risk factors, and prior mammogram results.

3. **Gallbladder disease.**
A 2- to 4-fold increase in the risk of gallbladder disease requiring surgery in postmenopausal women receiving postmenopausal estrogens has been reported.

4. **Hypercalcemia.**
Estrogen administration may lead to severe hypercalcemia in patients with breast cancer and bone metastases. If hypercalcemia occurs, use of the drug should be stopped and appropriate measures taken to reduce the serum calcium level.

5. **Visual abnormalities.**
Retinal vascular thrombosis has been reported in patients receiving estrogens. Discontinue medication pending examination if there is sudden partial or complete loss of vision, or a sudden onset of proptosis, diplopia, or migraine. If examination reveals papilledema or retinal vascular lesions, estrogens should be discontinued.

PRECAUTIONS

A. General

Premarin Intravenous is indicated for short-term use. However, warnings, precautions and adverse reactions associated with Premarin tablets should be taken into account.

1. ***Addition of a progestin when a woman has not had a hysterectomy.***

Studies of the addition of a progestin for 10 or more days of a cycle of estrogen administration or daily with estrogen in a continuous regimen have reported a lowered incidence of endometrial hyperplasia than would be induced by estrogen treatment alone. Endometrial hyperplasia may be a precursor to endometrial cancer.
There are, however, possible risks which may be associated with the use of progestins with estrogens compared to estrogen-alone regimens. These include a possible increased risk of breast cancer, adverse effects on lipoprotein metabolism (e.g., lowering HDL, raising LDL) and impairment of glucose tolerance.

2. ***Elevated blood pressure.***

In a small number of case reports, substantial increases in blood pressure have been attributed to idiosyncratic reactions to estrogens. In a large, randomized, placebo-controlled clinical trial, a generalized effect of estrogen therapy on blood pressure was not seen. Blood pressure should be monitored at regular intervals with estrogen use.

3. ***Hypertriglyceridemia.***

In patients with pre-existing hypertriglyceridemia, estrogen therapy may be associated with elevations of plasma triglycerides leading to pancreatitis and other complications.

4. ***Impaired liver function and past history of cholestatic jaundice.***

Estrogens may be poorly metabolized in patients with impaired liver function. For patients with a history of cholestatic jaundice associated with past estrogen use or with pregnancy, caution should be exercised and in the case of recurrence, medication should be discontinued.

5. ***Hypothyroidism.***

Estrogen administration leads to increased thyroid-binding globulin (TBG) levels. Patients with normal thyroid function can compensate for the increased TBG by making more thyroid hormone, thus maintaining free T_4 and T_3 serum concentrations in the normal range. Patients dependent on thyroid hormone replacement therapy who are also receiving estrogens may require increased doses of their thyroid replacement therapy. These patients should have their thyroid function monitored in order to maintain their free thyroid hormone levels in an acceptable range.

6. ***Fluid retention.***

Because estrogens may cause some degree of fluid retention, patients with conditions that might be influenced by this factor, such as a cardiac or renal dysfunction, warrant careful observation when estrogens are prescribed.

7. ***Hypocalcemia.***

Estrogens should be used with caution in individuals with severe hypocalcemia.

8. ***Ovarian cancer.***

The estrogen plus progestin substudy of WHI reported that after an average follow-up of 5.6 years, the relative risk of ovarian cancer for estrogen plus progestin versus placebo was 1.58 (95% confidence interval 0.77 – 3.24) but was not statistically significant. The absolute risk for estrogen plus progestin versus placebo was 4.2 versus 2.7 cases per 10,000 women-years. In some epidemiologic studies, the use of estrogen-only products, in particular for ten or more years, has been associated with an increased risk of ovarian cancer. Other epidemiologic studies have not found these associations.

9. ***Exacerbation of endometriosis.***

Endometriosis may be exacerbated with administration of estrogen therapy.
A few cases of malignant transformation of residual endometrial implants have been reported in women treated post-hysterectomy with estrogen alone therapy. For patients known to have residual endometriosis post-hysterectomy, the addition of progestin should be considered.

10. ***Exacerbation of other conditions.***

Estrogen therapy may cause an exacerbation of asthma, diabetes mellitus, epilepsy, migraine, porphyria, systemic lupus erythematosus, and hepatic hemangiomas and should be used with caution in women with these conditions.

B. Patient Information

Physicians are advised to discuss the contents of the PATIENT INFORMATION leaflet with patients who are being treated with Premarin Intravenous.

C. Laboratory Tests

Estrogen administration should be guided by clinical response at the lowest dose, rather than laboratory monitoring.

D. Drug/Laboratory Test Interactions

1. Accelerated prothrombin time, partial thromboplastin time, and platelet aggregation time; increased platelet count; increased factors II, VII antigen, VIII antigen, VIII coagulant activity, IX, X, XII, VII-X complex, II-VII-X complex, and beta-thromboglobulin; decreased levels of anti-factor Xa and antithrombin III, decreased antithrombin III activity; increased levels of fibrinogen and fibrinogen activity; increased plasminogen antigen and activity.
2. Increased thyroid-binding globulin (TBG) leading to increased circulating total thyroid hormone, as measured by protein-bound iodine (PBI), T_4 levels (by column or by radioimmunoassay) or T_3 levels by radioimmunoassay. T_3 resin uptake is decreased, reflecting the elevated TBG. Free T_4 and free T_3 concentrations are unaltered. Patients on thyroid replacement therapy may require higher doses of thyroid hormone.
3. Other binding proteins may be elevated in serum, i.e., corticosteroid binding globulin (CBG), sex hormone-binding globulin (SHBG), leading to increased total circulating corticosteroids and sex steroids respectively. Free hormone concentrations may be decreased. Other plasma proteins may be increased (angiotensinogen/renin substrate, alpha-1-antitrypsin, ceruloplasmin).
4. Increased plasma HDL and HDL_2 subfraction concentrations, reduced LDL cholesterol concentration, increased triglyceride levels.
5. Impaired glucose tolerance.
6. Reduced response to metyrapone test.

E. Carcinogenesis, Mutagenesis, and Impairment of Fertility

(See **BOXED WARNINGS, WARNINGS,** and **PRECAUTIONS.**)
Long-term continuous administration of natural and synthetic estrogens in certain animal species increases the frequency of carcinomas of the breast, uterus, cervix, vagina, testis, and liver.

F. Pregnancy

Premarin Intravenous should not be used during pregnancy. (See **CONTRAINDICATIONS.**)

G. Nursing Mothers

Estrogen administration to nursing mothers has been shown to decrease the quantity and quality of breast milk. Detectable amounts of estrogens have been identified in the milk of mothers receiving the drug. Caution should be exercised when Premarin Intravenous is administered to a nursing woman.

H. Pediatric Use

Estrogen therapy has been used for the induction of puberty in adolescents with some forms of pubertal delay. Safety and effectiveness in pediatric patients have not otherwise been established.
Large and repeated doses of estrogen over an extended time period have been shown to accelerate epiphyseal closure, which could result in short adult stature if treatment is initiated before the completion of physiologic puberty in normally developing children. If estrogen is administered to patients whose bone growth is not complete, periodic monitoring of bone maturation and effects on epiphyseal centers is recommended during estrogen administration.
Estrogen treatment of prepubertal girls also induces premature breast development and vaginal cornification, and may induce vaginal bleeding. In boys, estrogen treatment may modify the normal pubertal process and induce gynecomastia.

I. Geriatric Use

Of the total number of subjects in the estrogen plus progestin substudy of the Women's Health Initiative study, 44% (n = 7,320) were 65 years and over, while 6.6% (n = 1,095) were 75 years and over (see **CLINICAL PHARMACOLOGY, Clinical Studies**). There was a higher incidence of stroke and invasive breast cancer in women 75 and over compared to women less than 75 years of age.
There have not been sufficient numbers of geriatric patients involved in studies utilizing Premarin to determine whether those over 65 years of age differ from younger subjects in their response to Premarin.

ADVERSE REACTIONS

See **BOXED WARNINGS, WARNINGS,** and **PRECAUTIONS.**
Premarin Intravenous is indicated for short-term use. However, the warnings, precautions and adverse reactions associated with Premarin tablets should be taken into account.

1. *Genitourinary system.*
   - Changes in vaginal bleeding pattern and abnormal withdrawal bleeding or flow; breakthrough bleeding, spotting.
   - Increase in size of uterine leiomyomata.
   - Vaginal candidiasis.
   - Change in amount of cervical secretion.
2. *Breasts.*
   - Pain, tenderness, enlargement.
3. *Cardiovascular.*
   - Venous thrombosis.
   - Pulmonary embolism.
   - Superficial thrombophlebitis.
   - Hypotension.
   - Myocardial infarction.
   - Stroke.
4. *Gastrointestinal.*
   - Nausea, vomiting.
   - Abdominal cramps, bloating.
   - Cholestatic jaundice.
   - Increased incidence of gallbladder disease.
   - Pancreatitis.
   - Enlargement of hepatic hemangiomas.
5. *Skin.*
   - Chloasma or melasma that may persist when drug is discontinued.
   - Erythema multiforme.
   - Erythema nodosum.
   - Hemorrhagic eruption.
   - Loss of scalp hair.
   - Hirsutism.
   - Pruritis.
   - Rash.
6. *Eyes.*
   - Retinal vascular thrombosis.
   - Intolerance to contact lenses.
7. *Central Nervous System.*
   - Headache.
   - Migraine.
   - Dizziness.
   - Mental depression.
   - Chorea.
   - Nervousness.
   - Exacerbation of epilepsy.
   - Dementia.
8. *Miscellaneous.*
   - Increase or decrease in weight.
   - Reduced carbohydrate tolerance.
   - Aggravation of porphyria.
   - Edema.
   - Changes in libido.
   - Anaphylactoid/anaphylactic reactions.
   - Urticaria.
   - Angioedema.
   - Injection site pain.
   - Injections site edema.
   - Phlebitis (injection site).
   - Exacerbation of asthma.

OVERDOSAGE

Serious ill effects have not been reported following acute ingestion of large doses of estrogen-containing drug products by young children. Overdosage of estrogen may cause nausea and vomiting, and withdrawal bleeding may occur in females.

DOSAGE AND ADMINISTRATION

For treatment of abnormal uterine bleeding due to hormonal imbalance in the absence of organic pathology:
One 25 mg injection, intravenously or intramuscularly. Intravenous use is preferred since more rapid response can be expected from this mode of administration. Repeat in 6 to 12 hours if necessary. The use of Premarin Intravenous for injection does not preclude the advisability of other appropriate measures.
One should adhere to the usual precautionary measures governing intravenous administration. Injection should be made SLOWLY to obviate the occurrence of flushes.
Infusion of Premarin Intravenous for injection with other agents is not generally recommended. In emergencies, however, when an infusion has already been started it may be expedient to make the injection into the tubing just distal to the infusion needle. If so used, compatibility of solutions must be considered.
COMPATIBILITY OF SOLUTIONS: Premarin Intravenous is compatible with normal saline, dextrose, and invert sugar solutions. **It is not compatible with protein hydrolysate, ascorbic acid, or any solution with an acid pH.**

DIRECTIONS FOR STORAGE AND RECONSTITUTION

STORAGE BEFORE RECONSTITUTION: Store package in refrigerator, 2° to 8°C (36° to 46°F).
TO RECONSTITUTE: First withdraw air from Secule® vial so as to facilitate introduction of sterile diluent. Then, flow the sterile diluent slowly against the side of Secule® vial and agitate gently. **Do not shake violently.**
STORAGE AFTER RECONSTITUTION: It is common practice to utilize the reconstituted solution within a few hours. If it is necessary to keep the reconstituted solution for more than a few hours, store the reconstituted solution under refrigeration (2° to 8°C). Under these conditions, the solution is stable for 60 days, and is suitable for use unless darkening or precipitation occurs.

Continued on next page

Premarin Intravenous—Cont.

HOW SUPPLIED

NDC 0046-0749-05–Each package provides: (1) One Secule® vial containing 25 mg of conjugated estrogens, USP, for injection (also lactose 200 mg, sodium citrate 12.2 mg, and simethicone 0.2 mg). The pH is adjusted with sodium hydroxide or hydrochloric acid. (2) One 5 mL ampul of sterile diluent with 2% benzyl alcohol in sterile water.

Premarin Intravenous (conjugated estrogens, USP) for injection is prepared by cryodesiccation.

SECULE®-Registered trademark to designate a vial containing an injectable preparation in dry form.

PATIENT INFORMATION

Updated July 6, 2004

Premarin® Intravenous (conjugated estrogens, USP) for injection

Read this PATIENT INFORMATION which describes the benefit and major risks of your treatment, as well as how and when treatment should be used. This information does not take the place of talking to your healthcare provider about your medical condition or your treatment.

What is the most important information I should know about Premarin Intravenous (an estrogen mixture)?

- Estrogens increase the chances of getting cancer of the uterus.
  Report any unusual vaginal bleeding right away while you are taking Premarin. Vaginal bleeding after menopause may be a warning sign of cancer of the uterus (womb). Your healthcare provider should check any unusual vaginal bleeding to find out the cause.
- Do not use estrogens with or without progestins to prevent heart disease, heart attacks, or strokes.
  Using estrogens with or without progestins may increase your chances of getting heart attacks, strokes, breast cancer, and blood clots. Using estrogens with progestins may increase your risk of dementia, based on a study of women age 65 years or older. You and your healthcare provider should talk regularly about whether you still need treatment with estrogens.

What is Premarin Intravenous?

Premarin Intravenous is a medicine that contains a mixture of estrogen hormones.

Premarin Intravenous is used to:

- treat certain types of abnormal uterine bleeding due to hormonal imbalance when your doctor has found no other cause of bleeding.

Who should not use Premarin Intravenous?

Premarin Intravenous should not be used if you:

- **have unusual vaginal bleeding that has not been evaluated by your healthcare provider.**
- **currently have or have had certain cancers.**
  Estrogens may increase the chances of getting certain types of cancers, including cancer of the breast or uterus. If you have or have had cancer, talk with your healthcare provider.
- **had a stroke or heart attack in the past year.**
- **currently have or have had blood clots.**
- **currently have liver problems.**
- **are allergic to Premarin Intravenous or any of its ingredients.**
- **think you may be pregnant.**

Tell your healthcare provider:

- **if you are breast feeding.** The hormones in Premarin Intravenous can pass into your milk.
- **about all of your medical problems.** Your healthcare provider may need to check you more carefully if you have certain conditions, such as asthma (wheezing), epilepsy (seizures), migraine, endometriosis, lupus, problems with your heart, liver, thyroid, kidneys, or have high calcium levels in your blood.
- **about all the medicines you take,** including prescription and nonprescription medicines, vitamins, and herbal supplements. Some medicines may affect how Premarin Intravenous works.

What are the possible side effects of Premarin Intravenous?

Premarin Intravenous is for short-term use only. However, the risks associated with Premarin tablets should be taken into account.

Less common but serious side effects include:

- Breast cancer
- Cancer of the uterus
- Stroke
- Heart attack
- Blood clots
- Dementia
- Gallbladder disease
- Ovarian cancer

These are some of the warning signs of serious side effects:

- Breast lumps
- Unusual vaginal bleeding
- Dizziness and faintness
- Changes in speech
- Severe headaches
- Chest pain
- Shortness of breath
- Pains in your legs
- Changes in vision
- Vomiting

Call your healthcare provider right away if you get any of these warning signs, or any other unusual symptom that concerns you.

Common side effects include:

- Headache
- Breast tenderness
- Irregular vaginal bleeding or spotting
- Stomach/abdominal cramps, bloating
- Nausea and vomiting
- Hair loss

Other side effects include:

- High blood pressure
- Liver problems
- High blood sugar
- Fluid retention
- Enlargement of benign tumors of the uterus ("fibroids")
- Vaginal yeast infections

These are not all the possible side effects of Premarin. For more information, ask your healthcare provider or pharmacist.

What can I do to lower my chances of getting a serious side effect with Premarin Intravenous?

- If you have high blood pressure, high cholesterol (fat in the blood), diabetes, are overweight, or if you use tobacco, you may have higher chances for getting heart disease. Ask your healthcare provider for ways to lower your chances for getting heart disease.

General information about the safe and effective use of Premarin Intravenous

Medicines are sometimes prescribed for conditions that are not mentioned in patient information leaflets. Do not use Premarin Intravenous for conditions for which it was not prescribed. Do not give Premarin Intravenous to other people, even if they have the same symptoms you have. It may harm them. **Keep Premarin Intravenous out of the reach of children.**

This leaflet provides a summary of the most important information about Premarin Intravenous. If you would like more information, talk with your healthcare provider or pharmacist. You can ask for information about Premarin Intravenous that is written for health professionals. You can get more information by calling the toll free number 1-800-934-5556.

What are the ingredients in Premarin IV?

Premarin Intravenous for injection contains a mixture of conjugated estrogens, which are a mixture of sodium estrone sulfate and sodium equilin sulfate including 17α-dihydroequilin, 17α-estradiol, and 17β-dihydroequilin salts. Premarin Intravenous for injection also contains lactose, sodium citrate, simethicone, and sodium hydroxide or hydrochloric acid in dry form. A sterile diluent containing benzyl alcohol in sterile water is provided for reconstitution. The reconstituted solution is suitable for intravenous or intramuscular injection.

Each Premarin Intravenous (conjugated estrogens, USP) for injection package provides 25 mg of conjugated estrogens, USP, in dry form and 5 mLs of sterile diluent for intravenous or intramuscular use.

This product's label may have been revised after this insert was used in production. For further product information and current package insert, please visit www.wyeth.com or call our medical communications department toll-free at 1-800-934-5556.

Wyeth®
Wyeth Pharmaceuticals Inc.
Philadelphia, PA 19101

W10411C003
ET01
Revised July 6, 2004

Shown in Product Identification Guide, page 336

PREMARIN® ℞

[prĕm'ă-rin]
(conjugated estrogens tablets, USP)
℞ **only**

ESTROGENS INCREASE THE RISK OF ENDOMETRIAL CANCER

Close clinical surveillance of all women taking estrogens is important. Adequate diagnostic measures, including endometrial sampling when indicated, should be undertaken to rule out malignancy in all cases of undiagnosed persistent or recurring abnormal vaginal bleeding. There is no evidence that the use of "natural" estrogens results in a different endometrial risk profile than synthetic estrogens of equivalent estrogen dose.

CARDIOVASCULAR AND OTHER RISKS

Estrogens with or without progestins should not be used for the prevention of cardiovascular disease or dementia.

The Women's Health Initiative (WHI) study reported increased risks of stroke and deep vein thrombosis in postmenopausal women (50 to 79 years of age) during 6.8 years of treatment with conjugated estrogens (0.625 mg) relative to placebo.

The WHI study reported increased risks of myocardial infarction, stroke, invasive breast cancer, pulmonary emboli, and deep vein thrombosis in postmenopausal women (50 to 79 years of age) during 5 years of treatment with conjugated estrogens (0.625 mg) combined with medroxyprogesterone acetate (2.5 mg) relative to placebo. (See **CLINICAL PHARMACOLOGY, Clinical Studies.**)

The Women's Health Initiative Memory Study (WHIMS), a substudy of WHI, reported increased risk of developing probable dementia in postmenopausal women 65 years of age or older during 4 to 5.2 years of treatment with conjugated estrogens, with or without medroxyprogesterone acetate, relative to placebo. It is unknown whether this finding applies to younger postmenopausal women.

Other doses of conjugated estrogens and medroxyprogesterone acetate, and other combinations and dosage forms of estrogens and progestins were not studied in the WHI clinical trials and, in the absence of comparable data, these risks should be assumed to be similar. Because of these risks, estrogens with or without progestins should be prescribed at the lowest effective doses and for the shortest duration consistent with treatment goals and risks for the individual woman.

DESCRIPTION

Premarin® (conjugated estrogens tablets, USP) for oral administration contains a mixture of conjugated estrogens obtained exclusively from natural sources, occurring as the sodium salts of water-soluble estrogen sulfates blended to represent the average composition of material derived from pregnant mares' urine. It is a mixture of sodium estrone sulfate and sodium equilin sulfate. It contains as concomitant components, as sodium sulfate conjugates, 17α-dihydroequilin, 17α-estradiol, and 17β-dihydroequilin. Tablets for oral administration are available in 0.3 mg, 0.45 mg, 0.625 mg, 0.9 mg, and 1.25 mg strengths of conjugated estrogens.

Premarin tablets contain the following inactive ingredients: calcium phosphate tribasic, calcium sulfate, carnauba wax, cellulose, glyceryl monooleate, lactose, magnesium stearate, methylcellulose, pharmaceutical glaze, polyethylene glycol, stearic acid (not present in 0.45 mg tablet), sucrose, and titanium dioxide.

— 0.3 mg tablets also contain: D&C Yellow No. 10, FD&C Blue No. 1, FD&C Blue No. 2, FD&C Yellow No. 6; these tablets comply with USP Drug Release Test 1.
— 0.45 mg tablets also contain: FD&C Blue No. 2; these tablets comply with USP Drug Release Test 1.
— 0.625 mg tablets also contain: FD&C Blue No. 2, D&C Red No. 27, FD&C Red No. 40; these tablets comply with USP Drug Release Test 1.
— 0.9 mg tablets also contain: D&C Red No. 6, D&C Red No. 7; these tablets comply with USP Drug Release Test 2.
— 1.25 mg tablets also contain: black iron oxide, D&C Yellow No. 10, FD&C Yellow No. 6; these tablets comply with USP Drug Release Test 3.

CLINICAL PHARMACOLOGY

Endogenous estrogens are largely responsible for the development and maintenance of the female reproductive system and secondary sexual characteristics. Although circulating estrogens exist in a dynamic equilibrium of metabolic interconversions, estradiol is the principal intracellular human estrogen and is substantially more potent than its metabolites, estrone and estriol, at the receptor level.

The primary source of estrogen in normally cycling adult women is the ovarian follicle, which secretes 70 to 500 mcg of estradiol daily, depending on the phase of the menstrual cycle. After menopause, most endogenous estrogen is produced by conversion of androstenedione, secreted by the adrenal cortex, to estrone by peripheral tissues. Thus, estrone and the sulfate-conjugated form, estrone sulfate, are the most abundant circulating estrogens in postmenopausal women.

Estrogens act through binding to nuclear receptors in estrogen-responsive tissues. To date, two estrogen receptors have been identified. These vary in proportion from tissue to tissue.

Circulating estrogens modulate the pituitary secretion of the gonadotropins, luteinizing hormone (LH) and follicle stimulating hormone (FSH) through a negative feedback mechanism. Estrogens act to reduce the elevated levels of these gonadotropins seen in postmenopausal women.

Pharmacokinetics

Absorption

Conjugated estrogens are soluble in water and are well absorbed from the gastrointestinal tract after release from the drug formulation. The Premarin tablet releases conjugated estrogens slowly over several hours. Table 1 summarizes the mean pharmacokinetic parameters for unconjugated and conjugated estrogens following administration of 2 × 0.3 mg, 2 × 0.45 mg, and 2 × 0.625 mg tablets to healthy postmenopausal women.

[See table 1 at top of next page]

Distribution

The distribution of exogenous estrogens is similar to that of endogenous estrogens. Estrogens are widely distributed in the body and are generally found in higher concentration in the sex hormone target organs. Estrogens circulate in the blood largely bound to sex hormone binding globulin (SHBG) and albumin.

Metabolism

Exogenous estrogens are metabolized in the same manner as endogenous estrogens. Circulating estrogens exist in a dynamic equilibrium of metabolic interconversions. These transformations take place mainly in the liver. Estradiol is converted reversibly to estrone, and both can be converted

TABLE 1. PHARMACOKINETIC PARAMETERS FOR PREMARIN

Pharmacokinetic Profile of Unconjugated Estrogens Following a Dose of 2 × 0.3 mg

PK Parameter Arithmetic Mean (%CV)	C_{max} (pg/mL)	t_{max} (h)	$t_{1/2}$ (h)	AUC (pg•h/mL)
Estrone	82 (33)	7.8 (27)	54.7 (42)	5390 (50)
Baseline-adjusted estrone	58 (42)	7.8 (27)	21.1 (45)	1467 (41)
Equilin	31 (47)	7.2 (28)	18.3 (110)	652 (68)

Pharmacokinetic Profile of Conjugated Estrogens Following a Dose of 2 × 0.3 mg

PK Parameter Arithmetic Mean (%CV)	C_{max} (ng/mL)	t_{max} (h)	$t_{1/2}$ (h)	AUC (ng•h/mL)
Estrone	2.5 (32)	6.5 (29)	25.4 (22)	61.0 (43)
Baseline-adjusted total estrone	2.4 (32)	6.5 (29)	16.2 (34)	40.8 (36)
Equilin	1.6 (40)	5.9 (27)	11.8 (21)	22.4 (42)

Pharmacokinetic Profile of Unconjugated Estrogens Following a Dose of 2 × 0.45 mg

PK Parameter Arithmetic Mean (%CV)	C_{max} (pg/mL)	t_{max} (h)	$t_{1/2}$ (h)	AUC (pg•h/mL)
Estrone	92 (32)	8.7 (28)	56.4 (68)	6344 (56)
Baseline-adjusted estrone	65 (40)	8.7 (28)	20.3 (38)	1940 (40)
Equilin	35 (49)	7.6 (33)	21.9 (113)	849 (60)

Pharmacokinetic Profile of Conjugated Estrogens Following a Dose of 2 × 0.45 mg

PK Parameter Arithmetic Mean (%CV)	C_{max} (ng/mL)	t_{max} (h)	$t_{1/2}$ (h)	AUC (ng•h/mL)
Total estrone	2.8 (46)	7.1 (27)	27.6 (35)	77 (34)
Baseline-adjusted total estrone	2.6 (46)	7.1 (27)	14.7 (42)	48 (38)
Total equilin	1.9 (53)	5.9 (32)	11.8 (32)	29 (55)

Pharmacokinetic Profile of Unconjugated Estrogens Following a Dose of 2 × 0.625 mg

PK Parameter Arithmetic Mean (%CV)	C_{max} (pg/mL)	t_{max} (h)	$t_{1/2}$ (h)	AUC (pg•h/mL)
Estrone	139 (37)	8.8 (20)	28.0 (30)	5016 (34)
Baseline-adjusted estrone	120 (41)	8.8 (20)	17.4 (37)	2956 (39)
Equilin	66 (42)	7.9 (19)	13.6 (52)	1210 (37)

Pharmacokinetic Profile of Conjugated Estrogens Following a Dose of 2 × 0.625 mg

PK Parameter Arithmetic Mean (%CV)	C_{max} (ng/mL)	t_{max} (h)	$t_{1/2}$ (h)	AUC (ng•h/mL)
Total estrone	7.3 (41)	7.3 (24)	15.0 (25)	134 (42)
Baseline-adjusted total estrone	7.1 (41)	7.3 (24)	13.6 (23)	122 (38)
Total equilin	5.0 (42)	6.2 (26)	10.1 (26)	65 (44)

TABLE 2. SUMMARY TABULATION OF THE NUMBER OF HOT FLUSHES PER DAY–MEAN VALUES AND COMPARISONS BETWEEN THE ACTIVE TREATMENT GROUPS AND THE PLACEBO GROUP: PATIENTS WITH AT LEAST 7 MODERATE TO SEVERE FLUSHES PER DAY OR AT LEAST 50 PER WEEK AT BASELINE, LOCF

Treatment (No. of Patients) Time Period (week)	No. of Hot Flushes/Day: Baseline Mean ± SD	Observed Mean ± SD	Mean Change± SD	p-Values vs. Placebo[a]
0.625 mg CE (n = 27)				
4	12.29 ± 3.89	1.95 ± 2.77	−10.34 ± 4.73	<0.001
12	12.29 ± 3.89	0.75 ± 1.82	−11.54 ± 4.62	<0.001
0.45 mg CE (n = 32)				
4	12.25 ± 5.04	5.04 ± 5.31	−7.21 ± 4.75	<0.001
12	12.25 ± 5.04	2.32 ± 3.32	−9.93 ± 4.64	<0.001
0.3 mg CE (n = 30)				
4	13.77 ± 4.78	4.65 ± 3.71	−9.12 ± 4.71	<0.001
12	13.77 ± 4.78	2.52 ± 3.23	−11.25 ± 4.60	<0.001
Placebo (n = 28)				
4	11.69 ± 3.87	7.89 ± 5.28	−3.80 ± 4.71	—
12	11.69 ± 3.87	5.71 ± 5.22	−5.98 ± 4.60	—

a: Based on analysis of covariance with treatment as factor and baseline as covariate.

to estriol, which is the major urinary metabolite. Estrogens also undergo enterohepatic recirculation via sulfate and glucuronide conjugation in the liver, biliary secretion of conjugates into the intestine, and hydrolysis in the gut followed by reabsorption. In postmenopausal women a significant proportion of the circulating estrogens exists as sulfate conjugates, especially estrone sulfate, which serves as a circulating reservoir for the formation of more active estrogens.

Excretion

Estradiol, estrone, and estriol are excreted in the urine along with glucuronide and sulfate conjugates.

Special Populations

No pharmacokinetic studies were conducted in special populations, including patients with renal or hepatic impairment.

Drug Interactions

Data from a single-dose drug-drug interaction study involving conjugated estrogens and medroxyprogesterone acetate indicate that the pharmacokinetic dispositions of both drugs are not altered when the drugs are coadministered. No other clinical drug-drug interaction studies have been conducted with conjugated estrogens.

In vitro and in vivo studies have shown that estrogens are metabolized partially by cytochrome P450 3A4 (CYP3A4). Therefore, inducers or inhibitors of CYP3A4 may affect estrogen drug metabolism. Inducers of CYP3A4 such as St. John's Wort preparations (Hypericum perforatum), phenobarbital, carbamazepine, and rifampin may reduce plasma concentrations of estrogens, possibly resulting in a decrease in therapeutic effects and/or changes in the uterine bleeding profile. Inhibitors of CYP3A4 such as erythromycin, clarithromycin, ketoconazole, itraconazole, ritonavir and grapefruit juice may increase plasma concentrations of estrogens and may result in side effects.

Clinical Studies

Effects on vasomotor symptoms.

In the first year of the Health and Osteoporosis, Progestin and Estrogen (HOPE) Study, a total of 2805 postmenopausal women (average age 53.3 ± 4.9 years) were randomly assigned to one of eight treatment groups, receiving either placebo or conjugated estrogens with or without medroxyprogesterone acetate. Efficacy for vasomotor symptoms was assessed during the first 12 weeks of treatment in a subset of symptomatic women (n = 241) who had at least 7 moderate to severe hot flushes daily or at least 50 moderate to severe hot flushes during the week before randomization. Premarin (0.3 mg, 0.45 mg, and 0.625 mg tablets) was shown to be statistically better than placebo at weeks 4 and 12 for relief of both the frequency and severity of moderate to severe vasomotor symptoms. Table 2 shows the adjusted mean number of hot flushes in the Premarin 0.3 mg, 0.45 mg, and 0.625 mg and placebo treatment groups over the initial 12-week period.

[See table 2 below]

Effects on vulvar and vaginal atrophy.

Results of vaginal maturation indexes at cycles 6 and 13 showed that the differences from placebo were statistically significant ($p<0.001$) for all treatment groups (conjugated estrogens alone and conjugated estrogens/medroxyprogesterone acetate treatment groups).

Effects on bone mineral density.

Health and Osteoporosis, Progestin and Estrogen (HOPE) Study

The HOPE study was a double-blind, randomized, placebo/active-drug-controlled, multicenter study of healthy postmenopausal women with an intact uterus. Subjects (mean age 53.3 ± 4.9 years) were 2.3 ± 0.9 years, on average, since menopause, and took one 600-mg tablet of elemental calcium (Caltrate) daily. Subjects were not given vitamin D supplements. They were treated with Premarin 0.625 mg, 0.45 mg, 0.3 mg, or placebo. Prevention of bone loss was assessed by measurement of bone mineral density (BMD), primarily at the anteroposterior lumbar spine (L_2 to L_4). Secondarily, BMD measurements of the total body, femoral neck, and trochanter were also analyzed. Serum osteocalcin, urinary calcium, and N-telopeptide were used as bone turnover markers (BTM) at cycles 6, 13, 19, and 26.

Intent-to-treat subjects

All active treatment groups showed significant differences from placebo in each of the 4 BMD endpoints at cycles 6, 13, 19, and 26. The mean percent increases in the primary efficacy measure (L_2 to L_4 BMD) at the final on-therapy evaluation (cycle 26 for those who completed and the last available evaluation for those who discontinued early) were 2.46% with 0.625 mg, 2.26% with 0.45 mg, and 1.13% with 0.3 mg. The placebo group showed a mean percent decrease from baseline at the final evaluation of 2.45%. These results show that the lower dosages of Premarin were effective in increasing L_2 to L_4 BMD compared with placebo and, therefore, support the efficacy of the lower doses.

The analysis for the other 3 BMD endpoints yielded mean percent changes from baseline in femoral trochanter that were generally larger than those seen for L_2 to L_4 and changes in femoral neck and total body that were generally smaller than those seen for L_2 to L_4. Significant differences between groups indicated that each of the Premarin treatments was more effective than placebo for all 3 of these additional BMD endpoints. With regard to femoral neck and total body, the active treatment groups all showed mean percent increases in BMD while placebo treatment was accompanied by mean percent decreases. For femoral trochanter, each of the Premarin dose groups showed a mean percent increase that was significantly greater than the small increase seen in the placebo group. The percent changes from baseline to final evaluation are shown in Table 3.

[See table 3 at top of next page]

Figure 1 shows the cumulative percentage of subjects with changes from baseline equal to or greater than the value shown on the x-axis.

Figure 1. CUMULATIVE PERCENT OF SUBJECTS WITH CHANGES FROM BASELINE IN SPINE BMD OF GIVEN MAGNITUDE OR GREATER IN PREMARIN AND PLACEBO GROUPS

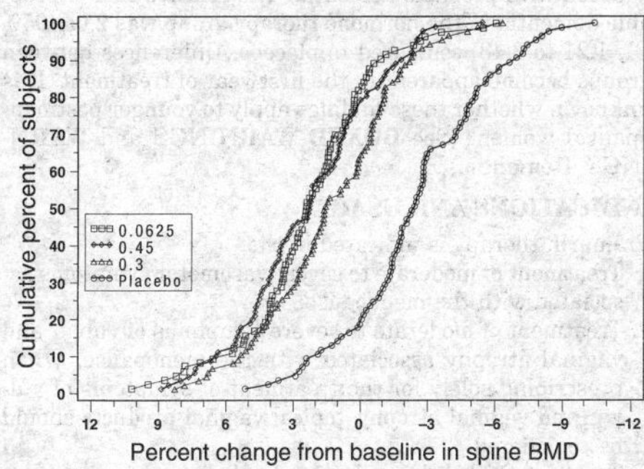

The mean percent changes from baseline in L_2 to L_4 BMD for women who completed the bone density study are shown with standard error bars by treatment group in Figure 2. Significant differences between each of the Premarin dosage groups and placebo were found at cycles 6, 13, 19, and 26.

[See figure 2 at top of next column]

The bone turnover markers serum osteocalcin and urinary N-telopeptide significantly decreased ($p<0.001$) in all active-treatment groups at cycles 6, 13, 19, and 26 compared with the placebo group. Larger mean decreases from baseline were seen with the active groups than with the placebo group. Significant differences from placebo were seen less frequently in urine calcium.

Continued on next page

Premarin Tablets—Cont.

Figure 2. ADJUSTED MEAN (SE) PERCENT CHANGE FROM BASELINE AT EACH CYCLE IN SPINE BMD: SUBJECTS COMPLETING IN PREMARIN GROUPS AND PLACEBO

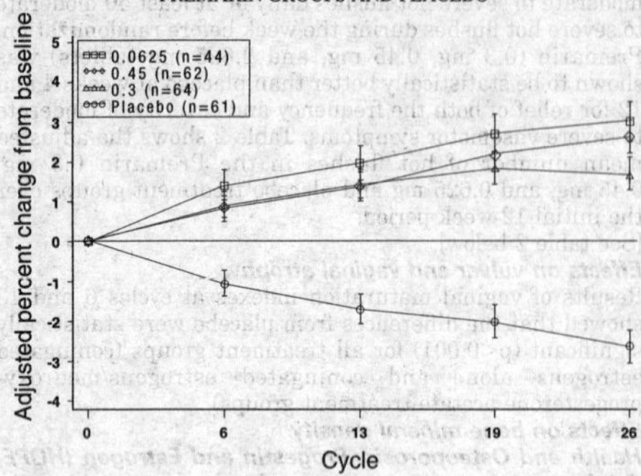

Women's Health Initiative Studies.

The Women's Health Initiative (WHI) enrolled a total of 27,000 predominantly healthy postmenopausal women to assess the risks and benefits of either the use of Premarin (0.625 mg conjugated estrogens per day) alone or the use of PREMPRO™ (0.625 mg conjugated estrogens plus 2.5 mg medroxyprogesterone acetate per day) compared to placebo in the prevention of certain chronic diseases. The primary endpoint was the incidence of coronary heart disease (CHD) (nonfatal myocardial infarction and CHD death), with invasive breast cancer as the primary adverse outcome studied. A "global index" included the earliest occurrence of CHD, invasive breast cancer, stroke, pulmonary embolism (PE), endometrial cancer, colorectal cancer, hip fracture, or death due to other cause. The study did not evaluate the effects of Premarin or PREMPRO on menopausal symptoms.

The estrogen plus progestin substudy was stopped early because, according to the predefined stopping rule, the increased risk of breast cancer and cardiovascular events exceeded the specified benefits included in the "global index." Results of the estrogen plus progestin substudy, which included 16,608 women (average age of 63 years, range 50 to 79; 83.9% White, 6.5% Black, 5.5% Hispanic), after an average follow-up of 5.2 years are presented in Table 4 below.

[See table 4 at right]

For those outcomes included in the "global index," the absolute excess risks per 10,000 women-years in the group treated with PREMPRO were 7 more CHD events, 8 more strokes, 8 more PEs, and 8 more invasive breast cancers, while the absolute risk reductions per 10,000 women-years were 6 fewer colorectal cancers and 5 fewer hip fractures. The absolute excess risk of events included in the "global index" was 19 per 10,000 women-years. There was no difference between the groups in terms of all-cause mortality. (See **BOXED WARNINGS**, **WARNINGS**, and **PRECAUTIONS**.)

Women's Health Initiative Memory Study.

The Women's Health Initiative Memory Study (WHIMS), a substudy of WHI, enrolled 4,532 predominantly healthy postmenopausal women 65 years of age and older (47% were age 65 to 69 years, 35% were 70 to 74 years, and 18% were 75 years of age and older) to evaluate the effects of PREMPRO (0.625 mg conjugated estrogens plus 2.5 mg medroxyprogesterone acetate) on the incidence of probable dementia (primary outcome) compared with placebo.

After an average follow-up of 4 years, 40 women in the estrogen/progestin group (45 per 10,000 women-years) and 21 in the placebo group (22 per 10,000 women-years) were diagnosed with probable dementia. The relative risk of probable dementia in the hormone therapy group was 2.05 (95% CI, 1.21 to 3.48) compared to placebo. Differences between groups became apparent in the first year of treatment. It is unknown whether these findings apply to younger postmenopausal women. (See **BOXED WARNINGS** and **WARNINGS, Dementia**.)

INDICATIONS AND USAGE

Premarin therapy is indicated in the:

1. Treatment of moderate to severe vasomotor symptoms associated with the menopause.
2. Treatment of moderate to severe symptoms of vulvar and vaginal atrophy associated with the menopause. When prescribing solely for the treatment of symptoms of vulvar and vaginal atrophy, topical vaginal products should be considered.
3. Treatment of hypoestrogenism due to hypogonadism, castration or primary ovarian failure.
4. Treatment of breast cancer (for palliation only) in appropriately selected women and men with metastatic disease.
5. Treatment of advanced androgen-dependent carcinoma of the prostate (for palliation only).
6. Prevention of postmenopausal osteoporosis. When prescribing solely for the prevention of postmenopausal osteoporosis, therapy should only be considered for women at significant risk of osteoporosis and for whom non-estrogen medications are not considered to be appropriate. (See **CLINICAL PHARMACOLOGY, Clinical Studies**.)

   The mainstays for decreasing the risk of postmenopausal osteoporosis are weight-bearing exercise, adequate calcium and vitamin D intake, and when indicated, pharmacologic therapy. Postmenopausal women require an average of 1500 mg/day of elemental calcium. Therefore, when not contraindicated, calcium supplementation may be helpful for women with suboptimal dietary intake. Vitamin D supplementation of 400–800 IU/day may also be required to ensure adequate daily intake in postmenopausal women.

TABLE 3. PERCENT CHANGE IN BONE MINERAL DENSITY: COMPARISON BETWEEN ACTIVE AND PLACEBO GROUPS IN THE INTENT-TO-TREAT POPULATION, LAST OBSERVATION CARRIED FORWARD

Region Evaluated Treatment Group[a]	No. of Subjects	Baseline (g/cm^2) Mean ± SD	Change from Baseline (%) Adjusted Mean ± SE	p-Value vs Placebo
L_2 to L_4 BMD				
0.625	83	1.17 ± 0.15	2.46 ± 0.37	<0.001
0.45	91	1.13 ± 0.15	2.26 ± 0.35	<0.001
0.3	87	1.14 ± 0.15	1.13 ± 0.36	<0.001
Placebo	85	1.14 ± 0.14	−2.45 ± 0.36	
Total Body BMD				
0.625	84	1.15 ± 0.08	0.68 ± 0.17	<0.001
0.45	91	1.14 ± 0.08	0.74 ± 0.16	<0.001
0.3	87	1.14 ± 0.07	0.40 ± 0.17	<0.001
Placebo	85	1.13 ± 0.08	−1.50 ± 0.17	
Femoral Neck BMD				
0.625	84	0.91 ± 0.14	1.82 ± 0.45	<0.001
0.45	91	0.89 ± 0.13	1.84 ± 0.44	<0.001
0.3	87	0.86 ± 0.11	0.62 ± 0.45	<0.001
Placebo	85	0.88 ± 0.14	−1.72 ± 0.45	
Femoral Trochanter BMD				
0.625	84	0.78 ± 0.13	3.82 ± 0.58	<0.001
0.45	91	0.76 ± 0.12	3.16 ± 0.56	0.003
0.3	87	0.75 ± 0.10	3.05 ± 0.57	0.005
Placebo	85	0.75 ± 0.12	0.81 ± 0.58	

a: Identified by dosage (mg) of Premarin or placebo.

TABLE 4. RELATIVE AND ABSOLUTE RISK SEEN IN THE ESTROGEN PLUS PROGESTIN SUBSTUDY OF WHI[a]

Event[c]	Relative Risk Prempro vs Placebo at 5.2 Years (95% CI*)	Placebo n = 8102	Prempro n = 8506
		Absolute Risk per 10,000 Women-years	
CHD events	1.29 (1.02–1.63)	30	37
Non-fatal MI	*1.32 (1.02–1.72)*	*23*	*30*
CHD death	*1.18 (0.70–1.97)*	*6*	*7*
Invasive breast cancer[b]	1.26 (1.00–1.59)	30	38
Stroke	1.41 (1.07–1.85)	21	29
Pulmonary embolism	2.13 (1.39–3.25)	8	16
Colorectal cancer	0.63 (0.43–0.92)	16	10
Endometrial cancer	0.83 (0.47–1.47)	6	5
Hip fracture	0.66 (0.45–0.98)	15	10
Death due to causes other than the events above	0.92 (0.74–1.14)	40	37
Global Index[c]	1.15 (1.03–1.28)	151	170
Deep vein thrombosis[d]	2.07 (1.49–2.87)	13	26
Vertebral fractures[d]	0.66 (0.44–0.98)	15	9
Other osteoporotic fractures[d]	0.77 (0.69–0.86)	170	131

a: adapted from JAMA, 2002; 288:321–333
b: includes metastatic and non-metastatic breast cancer with the exception of in situ breast cancer
c: a subset of the events was combined in a "global index," defined as the earliest occurrence of CHD events, invasive breast cancer, stroke, pulmonary embolism, endometrial cancer, colorectal cancer, hip fracture, or death due to other causes
d: not included in Global Index
* nominal confidence intervals unadjusted for multiple looks and multiple comparisons.

CONTRAINDICATIONS

Estrogens should not be used in individuals with any of the following conditions:

1. Undiagnosed abnormal genital bleeding.
2. Known, suspected, or history of cancer of the breast except in appropriately selected patients being treated for metastatic disease.
3. Known or suspected estrogen-dependent neoplasia.
4. Active deep vein thrombosis, pulmonary embolism or a history of these conditions.
5. Active or recent (e.g., within past year) arterial thromboembolic disease (e.g., stroke, myocardial infarction).
6. Liver dysfunction or disease.
7. Premarin tablets should not be used in patients with known hypersensitivity to their ingredients.
8. Known or suspected pregnancy. There is no indication for Premarin in pregnancy. There appears to be little or no increased risk of birth defects in children born to women who have used estrogen and progestins from oral contraceptives inadvertently during pregnancy. (See **PRECAUTIONS**.)

WARNINGS

See **BOXED WARNINGS**.

1. **Cardiovascular disorders.** Estrogen and estrogen/progestin therapy have been associated with an increased risk of cardiovascular events such as myocardial infarction and stroke, as well as venous thrombosis and pulmonary embolism (venous thromboembolism or VTE). Should any of these occur or be suspected, estrogens should be discontinued immediately.

   Risk factors for arterial vascular disease (e.g., hypertension, diabetes mellitus, tobacco use, hypercholesterolemia, and obesity) and/or venous thromboembolism (e.g., personal history or family history of VTE, obesity, and systemic lupus erythematosus) should be managed appropriately.

a. ***Coronary heart disease and stroke.*** In the Premarin substudy of the Women's Health Initiative (WHI) study, an increase in the number of myocardial infarctions and strokes has been observed in women receiving Premarin compared to placebo. (See **CLINICAL PHARMACOLOGY, Clinical Studies**.)

   In the estrogen plus progestin substudy of WHI, an increased risk of coronary heart disease (CHD) events (defined as nonfatal myocardial infarction and CHD death) was observed in women receiving PREMPRO (0.625 mg conjugated estrogens plus 2.5 mg medroxyprogesterone acetate) per day compared to women receiving placebo (37 vs 30 per 10,000 women-years). The increase in risk was observed in year one and persisted.

   In the same substudy of WHI, an increased risk of stroke was observed in women receiving PREMPRO compared to women receiving placebo (29 vs 21 per 10,000 women-years). The increase in risk was observed after the first year and persisted.

In postmenopausal women with documented heart disease (n = 2,763, average age 66.7 years) a controlled clinical trial of secondary prevention of cardiovascular disease (Heart and Estrogen/progestin Replacement Study; HERS) treatment with PREMPRO (0.625 mg conjugated estrogen plus 2.5 mg medroxyprogesterone acetate per day) demonstrated no cardiovascular benefit. During an average follow-up of 4.1 years, treatment with PREMPRO did not reduce the overall rate of CHD events in postmenopausal women with established coronary heart disease. There were more CHD events in the PREMPRO-treated group than in the placebo group in year 1, but not during the subsequent years. Two thousand three hundred and twenty one women from the original HERS trial agreed to participate in an open label extension of HERS, HERS II. Average follow-up in HERS II was an additional 2.7 years, for a total of 6.8 years overall. Rates of CHD events were comparable among women in the PREMPRO group and the placebo group in HERS, HERS II, and overall.

Large doses of estrogen (5 mg conjugated estrogens per day), comparable to those used to treat cancer of the prostate and breast, have been shown in a large prospective clinical trial in men to increase the risk of nonfatal myocardial infarction, pulmonary embolism, and thrombophlebitis.

b. ***Venous thromboembolism (VTE).*** In the Premarin substudy of the Women's Health Initiative (WHI), an increase in VTE has been observed in women receiving Premarin compared to placebo. (See **CLINICAL PHARMACOLOGY, Clinical Studies.**)

In the estrogen plus progestin substudy of WHI, a 2-fold greater rate of VTE, including deep venous thrombosis and pulmonary embolism, was observed in women receiving PREMPRO compared to women receiving placebo. The rate of VTE was 34 per 10,000 women-years in the PREMPRO group compared to 16 per 10,000 women-years in the placebo group. The increase in VTE risk was observed during the first year and persisted.

If feasible, estrogens should be discontinued at least 4 to 6 weeks before surgery of the type associated with an increased risk of thromboembolism, or during periods of prolonged immobilization.

2. **Malignant neoplasms.**

a. ***Endometrial cancer.*** The use of unopposed estrogens in women with intact uteri has been associated with an increased risk of endometrial cancer. The reported endometrial cancer risk among unopposed estrogen users with an intact uterus is about 2- to 12-fold greater than in non-users, and appears dependent on duration of treatment and on estrogen dose. Most studies show no significant increased risk associated with the use of estrogens for less than one year. The greatest risk appears associated with prolonged use, with increased risks of 15- to 24-fold for five to ten years or more, and this risk has been shown to persist for at least 8 to 15 years after estrogen therapy is discontinued.

Clinical surveillance of all women taking estrogen/progestin combinations is important. Adequate diagnostic measures, including endometrial sampling when indicated, should be undertaken to rule out malignancy in all cases of undiagnosed persistent or recurring abnormal vaginal bleeding. There is no evidence that the use of natural estrogens results in a different endometrial risk profile than synthetic estrogens of equivalent estrogen dose. Adding a progestin to postmenopausal estrogen therapy has been shown to reduce the risk of endometrial hyperplasia, which may be a precursor to endometrial cancer.

b. ***Breast cancer.*** In some studies, the use of estrogens and progestins by postmenopausal women has been reported to increase the risk of breast cancer. The most important randomized clinical trial providing information about this issue is the Women's Health Initiative (WHI) trial of estrogen plus progestin (see **CLINICAL PHARMACOLOGY, Clinical Studies**). The results from observational studies are generally consistent with those of the WHI clinical trial.

After a mean follow-up of 5.6 years, the WHI trial reported an increased risk of breast cancer in women who took estrogen plus progestin. Observational studies have also reported an increased risk for estrogen/progestin combination therapy, and a smaller increased risk for estrogen alone therapy, after several years of use. For both findings, the excess risk increased with duration of use, and appeared to return to baseline over about five years after stopping treatment (only the observational studies have substantial data on risk after stopping). In these studies, the risk of breast cancer was greater, and became apparent earlier, with estrogen/progestin combination therapy as compared to estrogen alone therapy. However, these studies have not found significant variation in the risk of breast cancer among different estrogens or among different estrogen/progestin combinations, doses, or routes of administration.

In the WHI trial of estrogen plus progestin, 26% of the women reported prior use of estrogen alone and/or estrogen/progestin combination hormone therapy. After a mean follow-up of 5.6 years during the clinical trial, the overall relative risk of invasive breast cancer was 1.24 (95% confidence interval 1.01–1.54), and the overall absolute risk was 41 vs. 33 cases per 10,000 women-years, for estrogen plus progestin compared with placebo. Among women who reported prior use of hormone therapy, the relative risk of invasive breast cancer was 1.86, and the absolute risk was 46 vs. 25 cases per 10,000 women-years, for estrogen plus progestin compared with placebo. Among women who reported no prior use of hormone therapy, the relative risk of invasive breast cancer was 1.09, and the absolute risk was 40 vs. 36 cases per 10,000 women-years for estrogen plus progestin compared with placebo. In the WHI trial, invasive breast cancers were larger and diagnosed at a more advanced stage in the estrogen plus progestin group compared with the placebo group. Metastatic disease was rare with no apparent difference between the two groups. Other prognostic factors such as histologic subtype, grade and hormone receptor status did not differ between the groups.

The observational Million Women Study in Europe reported an increased risk of mortality due to breast cancer among current users of estrogens alone or estrogens plus progestins compared to never users, while the estrogen plus progestin sub-study of WHI showed no effect on breast cancer mortality with a mean follow-up of 5.6 years.

The use of estrogen plus progestin has been reported to result in an increase in abnormal mammograms requiring further evaluation. All women should receive yearly breast examinations by a healthcare provider and perform monthly breast self-examinations. In addition, mammography examinations should be scheduled based on patient age, risk factors, and prior mammogram results.

3. **Dementia.** In the Women's Health Initiative Memory Study (WHIMS), an ancillary study of WHI, a population of 4,532 women aged 65 to 79 years was randomized to PREMPRO (0.625 mg/2.5 mg) or placebo. A population of 2,947 hysterectomized women, aged 65 to 79 years, was randomized to Premarin (0.625 mg) or placebo. In the planned analysis, pooling the events in women receiving Premarin or PREMPRO in comparison to those in women on placebo, the overall relative risk (RR) for probable dementia was 1.76 (95% CI 1.19–2.60). In the estrogen-alone group, after an average follow-up of 5.2 years a RR of 1.49 (95% CI 0.83–2.66) for probable dementia was observed compared to placebo. In the estrogen-plus-progestin group, after an average follow-up of 4 years, a RR of 2.05 (95% CI 1.21–3.48) for probable dementia was observed compared to placebo. Since this study was conducted in women aged 65 to 79 years, it is unknown whether these findings apply to younger postmenopausal women. (See **PRECAUTIONS, Geriatric Use.**)

4. **Gallbladder Disease.** A 2- to 4-fold increase in the risk of gallbladder disease requiring surgery in postmenopausal women receiving estrogens has been reported.

5. **Hypercalcemia.** Estrogen administration may lead to severe hypercalcemia in patients with breast cancer and bone metastases. If hypercalcemia occurs, use of the drug should be stopped and appropriate measures taken to reduce the serum calcium level.

6. **Visual abnormalities.** Retinal vascular thrombosis has been reported in patients receiving estrogens. Discontinue medication pending examination if there is sudden partial or complete loss of vision, or a sudden onset of proptosis, diplopia, or migraine. If examination reveals papilledema or retinal vascular lesions, estrogens should be discontinued.

PRECAUTIONS

A. General

1. ***Addition of a progestin when a woman has not had a hysterectomy.***

   Studies of the addition of a progestin for 10 or more days of a cycle of estrogen administration, or daily with estrogen in a continuous regimen, have reported a lowered incidence of endometrial hyperplasia than would be induced by estrogen treatment alone. Endometrial hyperplasia may be a precursor to endometrial cancer.

   There are, however, possible risks that may be associated with the use of progestins with estrogens compared to estrogen-alone regimens. These include: a possible increased risk of breast cancer, adverse effects on lipoprotein metabolism (e.g., lowering HDL, raising LDL) and impairment of glucose tolerance.

2. ***Elevated blood pressure.***

   In a small number of case reports, substantial increases in blood pressure have been attributed to idiosyncratic reactions to estrogens. In a large, randomized, placebo-controlled clinical trial, a generalized effect of estrogen therapy on blood pressure was not seen. Blood pressure should be monitored at regular intervals during estrogen use.

3. ***Hypertriglyceridemia.***

   In patients with pre-existing hypertriglyceridemia, estrogen therapy may be associated with elevations of plasma triglycerides leading to pancreatitis and other complications. In the HOPE study, the mean percent increase from baseline in serum triglycerides after one year of treatment with Premarin 0.625 mg, 0.45 mg, and 0.3 mg compared with placebo were 34.3, 30.2, 25.1, and 10.7, respectively. After two years of treatment, the mean percent changes were 47.6, 32.5, 19.0, and 5.5, respectively.

4. ***Impaired liver function and past history of cholestatic jaundice.***

   Estrogens may be poorly metabolized in patients with impaired liver function. For patients with a history of cholestatic jaundice associated with past estrogen use or with pregnancy, caution should be exercised and in the case of recurrence, medication should be discontinued.

5. ***Hypothyroidism.***

   Estrogen administration leads to increased thyroid-binding globulin (TBG) levels. Patients with normal thyroid function can compensate for the increased TBG by making more thyroid hormone, thus maintaining free T_4 and T_3 serum concentrations in the normal range. Patients dependent on thyroid hormone replacement therapy who are also receiving estrogens may require increased doses of their thyroid replacement therapy. These patients should have their thyroid function monitored in order to maintain their free thyroid hormone levels in an acceptable range.

6. ***Fluid retention.***

   Because estrogens may cause some degree of fluid retention, patients with conditions that might be influenced by this factor, such as cardiac or renal dysfunction, warrant careful observation when estrogens are prescribed.

7. ***Hypocalcemia.***

   Estrogens should be used with caution in individuals with severe hypocalcemia.

8. ***Ovarian cancer.***

   The estrogen plus progestin substudy of WHI reported that after an average follow-up of 5.6 years, the relative risk for ovarian cancer for estrogen plus progestin versus placebo was 1.58 (95% confidence interval 0.77–3.24) but was not statistically significant. The absolute risk of estrogen plus progestin versus placebo was 4.2 versus 2.7 cases per 10,000 women-years. In some epidemiologic studies, the use of estrogen-only products, in particular for ten or more years, has been associated with an increased risk of ovarian cancer. Other epidemiologic studies have not found these associations.

9. ***Exacerbation of endometriosis.***

   Endometriosis may be exacerbated with administration of estrogen therapy.

   A few cases of malignant transformation of residual endometrial implants have been reported in women treated post-hysterectomy with estrogen alone therapy. For patients known to have residual endometriosis post-hysterectomy, the addition of progestin should be considered.

10. ***Exacerbation of other conditions.***

    Estrogen therapy may cause an exacerbation of asthma, diabetes mellitus, epilepsy, migraine, porphyria, systemic lupus erythematosus, and hepatic hemangiomas and should be used with caution in patients with these conditions.

B. Patient Information

Physicians are advised to discuss the contents of the PATIENT INFORMATION leaflet with patients for whom they prescribe Premarin.

C. Laboratory Tests

Estrogen administration should be initiated at the lowest dose for the treatment of postmenopausal moderate to severe vasomotor symptoms and moderate to severe symptoms of postmenopausal vulvar and vaginal atrophy and then guided by clinical response rather than by serum hormone levels (e.g., estradiol, FSH). Laboratory parameters may be useful in guiding dosage for the treatment of hypoestrogenism due to hypogonadism, castration and primary ovarian failure.

D. Drug/Laboratory Test Interactions

1. Accelerated prothrombin time, partial thromboplastin time, and platelet aggregation time; increased platelet count; increased factors II, VII antigen, VIII antigen, VIII coagulant activity, IX, X, XII, VII-X complex, II-VII-X complex, and beta-thromboglobulin; decreased levels of anti-factor Xa and antithrombin III, decreased antithrombin III activity; increased levels of fibrinogen and fibrinogen activity; increased plasminogen antigen and activity.
2. Increased thyroid binding globulin (TBG) levels leading to increased circulating total thyroid hormone levels as measured by protein-bound iodine (PBI), T_4 levels (by column or by radioimmunoassay) or T_3 levels by radioimmunoassay. T_3 resin uptake is decreased, reflecting the elevated TBG. Free T_4 and free T_3 concentrations are unaltered. Patients on thyroid replacement therapy may require higher doses of thyroid hormone.
3. Other binding proteins may be elevated in serum, i.e., corticosteroid binding globulin (CBG), sex hormone binding globulin (SHBG), leading to increased total circulating corticosteroids and sex steroids, respectively. Free hormone concentrations may be decreased. Other plasma proteins may be increased (angiotensinogen/renin substrate, alpha-1-antitrypsin, ceruloplasmin).
4. Increased plasma HDL and HDL_2 cholesterol subfraction concentrations, reduced LDL cholesterol concentrations, increased triglyceride levels.
5. Impaired glucose tolerance.
6. Reduced response to metyrapone test.

E. Carcinogenesis, Mutagenesis, Impairment of Fertility

(See **BOXED WARNINGS, WARNINGS,** and **PRECAUTIONS.**)

Long term continuous administration of natural and synthetic estrogens in certain animal species increases the frequency of carcinomas of the breast, uterus, cervix, vagina, testis, and liver.

Continued on next page

Premarin Tablets—Cont.

F. Pregnancy

Premarin should not be used during pregnancy. (See **CONTRAINDICATIONS**).

G. Nursing Mothers

Estrogen administration to nursing mothers has been shown to decrease the quantity and quality of the milk. Detectable amounts of estrogens have been identified in the milk of mothers receiving this drug. Caution should be exercised when Premarin is administered to a nursing woman.

H. Pediatric Use

Estrogen therapy has been used for the induction of puberty in adolescents with some forms of pubertal delay. Safety and effectiveness in pediatric patients have not otherwise been established.

Large and repeated doses of estrogen over an extended time period have been shown to accelerate epiphyseal closure, which could result in short stature if treatment is initiated before the completion of physiologic puberty in normally developing children. If estrogen is administered to patients whose bone growth is not complete, periodic monitoring of bone maturation and effects on epiphyseal centers is recommended during estrogen administration.

Estrogen treatment of prepubertal girls also induces premature breast development and vaginal cornification, and may induce vaginal bleeding. In boys, estrogen treatment may modify the normal pubertal process and induce gynecomastia. See **INDICATIONS** and **DOSAGE AND ADMINISTRATION** sections.

I. Geriatric Use

Of the total number of subjects in the estrogen plus progestin substudy of the Women's Health Initiative study, 44% (n=7,320) were 65 years and over, while 6.6% (n=1,095) were 75 years and over (see **CLINICAL PHARMACOLOGY, Clinical Studies**). There was a higher relative risk (PREMPRO vs placebo) of stroke and invasive breast cancer in women 75 and over compared to women less than 75 years of age.

In the Women's Health Initiative Memory Study (WHIMS), an ancillary study of WHI, a population of 4,532 women aged 65 to 79 years was randomized to PREMPRO (0.625 mg/2.5 mg) or placebo. A population of 2,947 hysterectomized women, aged 65 to 79 years, was randomized to Premarin (0.625 mg) or placebo. In the planned analysis, pooling the events in women receiving Premarin or PREMPRO in comparison to those in women on placebo, the overall relative risk (RR) for probable dementia was 1.76 (95% CI 1.19–2.60). In the estrogen-alone group, after an average follow-up of 5.2 years a RR of 1.49 (95% CI 0.83–2.66) for probable dementia was observed compared to placebo. In the estrogen-plus-progestin group, after an average follow-up of 4 years, a RR of 2.05 (95% CI 1.21–3.48) for probable dementia was observed compared to placebo. Since this study was conducted in women aged 65 to 79 years, it is unknown whether these findings apply to younger postmenopausal women. (See **WARNINGS, Dementia.**)

With respect to efficacy in the approved indications, there have not been sufficient numbers of geriatric patients involved in studies utilizing Premarin to determine whether those over 65 years of age differ from younger subjects in their response to Premarin.

ADVERSE REACTIONS

See **BOXED WARNINGS, WARNINGS**, and **PRECAUTIONS.**

Because clinical trials are conducted under widely varying conditions, adverse reaction rates observed in the clinical trials of a drug cannot be directly compared to rates in the clinical trials of another drug and may not reflect the rates observed in practice. The adverse reaction information from clinical trials does, however, provide a basis for identifying the adverse events that appear to be related to drug use and for approximating rates.

During the first year of a 2-year clinical trial with 2333 postmenopausal women between 40 and 65 years of age (88% Caucasian), 1012 women were treated with conjugated estrogens and 332 were treated with placebo. Table 5 summarizes adverse events that occurred at a rate of ≥ 5%.

[See table below]

TABLE 5. NUMBER (%) OF PATIENTS REPORTING ≥ 5% TREATMENT EMERGENT ADVERSE EVENTS

Body System Adverse event	--Conjugated Estrogens Treatment Group-- 0.625 mg (n = 348)	0.45 mg (n = 338)	0.3 mg (n = 326)	Placebo (n = 332)
Any adverse event	323 (93%)	305 (90%)	292 (90%)	281 (85%)
Body as a Whole				
Abdominal pain	56 (16%)	50 (15%)	54 (17%)	37 (11%)
Accidental injury	21 (6%)	41 (12%)	20 (6%)	29 (9%)
Asthenia	25 (7%)	23 (7%)	25 (8%)	16 (5%)
Back pain	49 (14%)	43 (13%)	43 (13%)	39 (12%)
Flu syndrome	37 (11%)	38 (11%)	33 (10%)	35 (11%)
Headache	90 (26%)	109 (32%)	96 (29%)	93 (28%)
Infection	61 (18%)	75 (22%)	74 (23%)	74 (22%)
Pain	58 (17%)	61 (18%)	66 (20%)	61 (18%)
Digestive System				
Diarrhea	21 (6%)	25 (7%)	19 (6%)	21 (6%)
Dyspepsia	33 (9%)	32 (9%)	36 (11%)	46 (14%)
Flatulence	24 (7%)	23 (7%)	18 (6%)	9 (3%)
Nausea	32 (9%)	21 (6%)	21 (6%)	30 (9%)
Musculoskeletal System				
Arthralgia	47 (14%)	42 (12%)	22 (7%)	39 (12%)
Leg cramps	19 (5%)	23 (7%)	11 (3%)	7 (2%)
Myalgia	18 (5%)	18 (5%)	29 (9%)	25 (8%)
Nervous System				
Depression	25 (7%)	27 (8%)	17 (5%)	22 (7%)
Dizziness	19 (5%)	20 (6%)	12 (4%)	17 (5%)
Insomnia	21 (6%)	25 (7%)	24 (7%)	33 (10%)
Nervousness	12 (3%)	17 (5%)	6 (2%)	7 (2%)
Respiratory System				
Cough increased	13 (4%)	22 (7%)	14 (4%)	14 (4%)
Pharyngitis	35 (10%)	35 (10%)	40 (12%)	38 (11%)
Rhinitis	21 (6%)	30 (9%)	31 (10%)	42 (13%)
Sinusitis	22 (6%)	36 (11%)	24 (7%)	24 (7%)
Upper respiratory infection	42 (12%)	34 (10%)	28 (9%)	35 (11%)
Skin and Appendages				
Pruritus	14 (4%)	17 (5%)	16 (5%)	7 (2%)
Urogenital System				
Breast pain	38 (11%)	41 (12%)	24 (7%)	29 (9%)
Leukorrhea	18 (5%)	22 (7%)	13 (4%)	9 (3%)
Vaginal hemorrhage	47 (14%)	14 (4%)	7 (2%)	0
Vaginal moniliasis	20 (6%)	18 (5%)	17 (5%)	6 (2%)
Vaginitis	24 (7%)	20 (6%)	16 (5%)	4 (1%)

The following additional adverse reactions have been reported with estrogen and/or progestin therapy:

1. *Genitourinary system*
Changes in vaginal bleeding pattern and abnormal withdrawal bleeding or flow; breakthrough bleeding, spotting, dysmenorrhea
Increase in size of uterine leiomyomata
Vaginitis, including vaginal candidiasis
Change in amount of cervical secretion
Change in cervical ectropion
Ovarian cancer
Endometrial hyperplasia
Endometrial cancer

2. *Breasts*
Tenderness, enlargement, pain, discharge, galactorrhea
Fibrocystic breast changes
Breast cancer

3. *Cardiovascular*
Deep and superficial venous thrombosis
Pulmonary embolism
Thrombophlebitis
Myocardial infarction
Stroke
Increase in blood pressure

4. *Gastrointestinal*
Nausea, vomiting
Abdominal cramps, bloating
Cholestatic jaundice
Increased incidence of gallbladder disease
Pancreatitis
Enlargement of hepatic hemangiomas

5. *Skin*
Chloasma or melasma that may persist when drug is discontinued
Erythema multiforme
Erythema nodosum
Hemorrhagic eruption
Loss of scalp hair
Hirsutism
Pruritus, rash

6. *Eyes*
Retinal vascular thrombosis
Intolerance to contact lenses

7. *Central Nervous System*
Headache
Migraine
Dizziness
Mental depression
Chorea
Nervousness
Mood disturbances
Irritability
Exacerbation of epilepsy
Dementia

8. *Miscellaneous*
Increase or decrease in weight
Reduced carbohydrate tolerance
Aggravation of porphyria
Edema
Arthralgias
Leg cramps
Changes in libido
Urticaria, angioedema, anaphylactoid/anaphylactic reactions
Hypocalcemia
Exacerbation of asthma
Increased triglycerides

OVERDOSAGE

Serious ill effects have not been reported following acute ingestion of large doses of estrogen-containing drug products by young children. Overdosage of estrogen may cause nausea and vomiting, and withdrawal bleeding may occur in females.

DOSAGE AND ADMINISTRATION

When estrogen is prescribed for a postmenopausal woman with a uterus, progestin should also be initiated to reduce the risk of endometrial cancer. A woman without a uterus does not need progestin. Use of estrogen, alone or in combination with a progestin, should be with the lowest effective dose and for the shortest duration consistent with treatment goals and risks for the individual woman. Patients should be re-evaluated periodically as clinically appropriate (e.g., at 3-month to 6-month intervals) to determine if treatment is still necessary (see **BOXED WARNINGS** and **WARNINGS**). For women with a uterus, adequate diagnostic measures, such as endometrial sampling, when indicated, should be undertaken to rule out malignancy in cases of undiagnosed persistent or recurring abnormal vaginal bleeding.

1. For treatment of moderate to severe vasomotor symptoms and/or moderate to severe symptoms of vulvar and vaginal atrophy associated with the menopause. When prescribing solely for the treatment of moderate to severe symptoms of vulvar and vaginal atrophy, topical vaginal products should be considered.
   Patients should be treated with the lowest effective dose. Generally women should be started at 0.3 mg Premarin daily. Subsequent dosage adjustment may be made based upon the individual patient response. This dose should be periodically reassessed by the healthcare provider.
   Premarin therapy may be given continuously with no interruption in therapy, or in cyclical regimens (regimens such as 25 days on drug followed by five days off drug) as is medically appropriate on an individualized basis.
2. For prevention of postmenopausal osteoporosis:
   When prescribing solely for the prevention of postmenopausal osteoporosis, therapy should be considered only for women at significant risk of osteoporosis and for whom non-estrogen medications are not considered to be appropriate. Patients should be treated with the lowest effective dose. Generally women should be started at 0.3 mg Premarin daily. Subsequent dosage adjustment may be made based upon the individual clinical and bone mineral density responses. This dose should be periodically reassessed by the healthcare provider.
   Premarin therapy may be given continuously with no interruption in therapy, or in cyclical regimens (regimens such as 25 days on drug followed by five days off drug) as is medically appropriate on an individualized basis.
3. For treatment of female hypoestrogenism due to hypogonadism, castration, or primary ovarian failure:
   Female hypogonadism—0.3 mg or 0.625 mg daily, administered cyclically (e.g., three weeks on and one week off). Doses are adjusted depending on the severity of symptoms and responsiveness of the endometrium.
   In clinical studies of delayed puberty due to female hypogonadism, breast development was induced by doses as low as 0.15 mg. The dosage may be gradually titrated upward at 6 to 12 month intervals as needed to achieve appropriate bone age advancement and eventual epiphyseal closure. Clinical studies suggest that doses of 0.15 mg, 0.3 mg, and 0.6 mg are associated with mean ratios of bone age advancement to chronological age progression (ΔBA/ΔCA) of 1.1, 1.5, and 2.1, respectively. (Premarin in

the dose strength of 0.15 mg is not available commercially). Available data suggest that chronic dosing with 0.625 mg is sufficient to induce artificial cyclic menses with sequential progestin treatment and to maintain bone mineral density after skeletal maturity is achieved. Female castration or primary ovarian failure—1.25 mg daily, cyclically. Adjust dosage, upward or downward, according to severity of symptoms and response of the patient. For maintenance, adjust dosage to lowest level that will provide effective control.

4. For treatment of breast cancer, for palliation only, in appropriately selected women and men with metastatic disease:
   Suggested dosage is 10 mg three times daily for a period of at least three months.
5. For treatment of advanced androgen-dependent carcinoma of the prostate, for palliation only:
   1.25 mg to 2 × 1.25 mg three times daily. The effectiveness of therapy can be judged by phosphatase determinations as well as by symptomatic improvement of the patient.

HOW SUPPLIED

Premarin (conjugated estrogens tablets, USP)

— Each oval yellow tablet contains 1.25 mg, in bottles of 100 (NDC 0046-0866-81); and 1,000 (NDC 0046-0866-91).
— Each oval white tablet contains 0.9 mg, in bottles of 100 (NDC 0046-0864-81).
— Each oval maroon tablet contains 0.625 mg, in bottles of 100 (NDC 0046-0867-81); 1,000 (NDC 0046-0867-91); and Unit-Dose Packages of 100 (NDC 0046-0867-99).
— Each oval blue tablet contains 0.45 mg, in bottles of 100 (NDC 0046-0936-81).
— Each oval green tablet contains 0.3 mg, in bottles of 100 (NDC 0046-0868-81) and 1,000 (NDC 0046-0868-91).

The appearance of these tablets is a trademark of Wyeth Pharmaceuticals.

Store at 20–25° C (68–77° F); excursions permitted to 15–30° C (59–86° F) [see USP Controlled Room Temperature]. Dispense in a well-closed container as defined in the USP.

PATIENT INFORMATION

(Updated August 3, 2004)
Premarin®
(conjugated estrogens tablets, USP)

Read this PATIENT INFORMATION before you start taking Premarin and read what you get each time you refill Premarin. There may be new information. This information does not take the place of talking to your healthcare provider about your medical condition or your treatment.

What is the most important information I should know about Premarin (an estrogen mixture)?

- Estrogens increase the chances of getting cancer of the uterus.
  Report any unusual vaginal bleeding right away while you are taking Premarin. Vaginal bleeding after menopause may be a warning sign of cancer of the uterus (womb). Your healthcare provider should check any unusual vaginal bleeding to find out the cause.
- Do not use estrogens with or without progestins to prevent heart disease, heart attacks, strokes, or dementia.
  Using estrogens with or without progestins may increase your chances of getting heart attacks, strokes, breast cancer, and blood clots. Using estrogens, with or without progestins, may increase your risk of dementia, based on a study of women age 65 years or older. You and your healthcare provider should talk regularly about whether you still need treatment with Premarin.

What is Premarin?

Premarin is a medicine that contains a mixture of estrogen hormones.

Premarin is used after menopause to:

- **reduce moderate to severe hot flashes.** Estrogens are hormones made by a woman's ovaries. The ovaries normally stop making estrogens when a woman is between 45 and 55 years old. This drop in body estrogen levels causes the "change of life" or menopause (the end of monthly menstrual periods). Sometimes both ovaries are removed during an operation before natural menopause takes place. The sudden drop in estrogen levels causes "surgical menopause."
  When the estrogen levels begin dropping, some women get very uncomfortable symptoms, such as feelings of warmth in the face, neck, and chest, or sudden strong feelings of heat and sweating ("hot flashes" or "hot flushes"). In some women the symptoms are mild, and they will not need to take estrogens. In other women, symptoms can be more severe. You and your healthcare provider should talk regularly about whether you still need treatment with Premarin.
- **treat moderate to severe dryness, itching, and burning, in and around the vagina.** You and your healthcare provider should talk regularly about whether you still need treatment with Premarin to control these problems. If you use Premarin only to treat your dryness, itching, and burning in and around your vagina, talk with your healthcare provider about whether a topical vaginal product would be better for you.
- **help reduce your chances of getting osteoporosis (thin weak bones).** Osteoporosis from menopause is a thinning of the bones that makes them weaker and easier to break. If you use Premarin only to prevent osteoporosis from menopause, talk with your healthcare provider about whether a different treatment or medicine without estrogens might be better for you. You and your healthcare provider should talk regularly about whether you should continue with Premarin.
  Weight-bearing exercise, like walking or running, and taking calcium and vitamin D supplements may also lower your chances for getting postmenopausal osteoporosis. It is important to talk about exercise and supplements with your healthcare provider before starting them.

Premarin is also used to:

- **treat certain conditions in women before menopause if their ovaries do not make enough estrogen naturally.**
- **ease symptoms of certain cancers that have spread through the body, in men and women.**

Who should not take Premarin?

Do not start taking Premarin if you:

- **have unusual vaginal bleeding.**
- **currently have or have had certain cancers.** Estrogens may increase the chances of getting certain types of cancers, including cancer of the breast or uterus. If you have or have had cancer, talk with your healthcare provider about whether you should take Premarin.
- **had a stroke or heart attack in the past year.**
- **currently have or have had blood clots.**
- **currently have liver problems.**
- **are allergic to Premarin tablets or any of its ingredients.** See the end of this leaflet for a list of all the ingredients in Premarin.
- **think you may be pregnant.**

Tell your healthcare provider:

- **if you are breast feeding.** The hormones in Premarin can pass into your milk.
- **about all of your medical problems.** Your healthcare provider may need to check you more carefully if you have certain conditions, such as asthma (wheezing), epilepsy (seizures), migraine, endometriosis, lupus, problems with your heart, liver, thyroid, kidneys, or have high calcium levels in your blood.
- **about all the medicines you take,** including prescription and nonprescription medicines, vitamins, and herbal supplements. Some medicines may affect how Premarin works. Premarin may also affect how your other medicines work.
- **if you are going to have surgery or will be on bedrest.** You may need to stop taking estrogens.

How should I take Premarin?

- Take one Premarin tablet at the same time each day.
- If you miss a dose, take it as soon as possible. If it is almost time for your next dose, skip the missed dose and go back to your normal schedule. Do not take 2 doses at the same time.
- Estrogens should be used at the lowest dose possible for your treatment only as long as needed. You and your healthcare provider should talk regularly (for example, every 3 to 6 months) about the dose you are taking and whether you still need treatment with Premarin.

What are the possible side effects of Premarin?

Less common but serious side effects include:

- Breast cancer
- Cancer of the uterus
- Stroke
- Heart attack
- Blood clots
- Dementia
- Gallbladder disease
- Ovarian cancer

These are some of the warning signs of serious side effects:

- Breast lumps
- Unusual vaginal bleeding
- Dizziness and faintness
- Changes in speech
- Severe headaches
- Chest pain
- Shortness of breath
- Pains in your legs
- Changes in vision
- Vomiting

Call your healthcare provider right away if you get any of these warning signs, or any other unusual symptom that concerns you.

Common side effects include:

- Headache
- Breast pain
- Irregular vaginal bleeding or spotting
- Stomach/abdominal cramps, bloating
- Nausea and vomiting
- Hair loss

Other side effects include:

- High blood pressure
- Liver problems
- High blood sugar
- Fluid retention
- Enlargement of benign tumors of the uterus ("fibroids")
- Vaginal yeast infections

These are not all the possible side effects of Premarin. For more information, ask your healthcare provider or pharmacist.

What can I do to lower my chances of getting a serious side effect with Premarin?

- Talk with your healthcare provider regularly about whether you should continue taking Premarin.
- If you have a uterus, talk to your healthcare provider about whether the addition of a progestin is right for you. In general, the addition of a progestin is recommended for women with a uterus.
- See your healthcare provider right away if you get vaginal bleeding while taking Premarin.
- Have a breast exam and mammogram (breast X-ray) every year unless your healthcare provider tells you something else. If members of your family have had breast cancer or if you have ever had breast lumps or an abnormal mammogram, you may need to have breast exams more often.
- If you have high blood pressure, high cholesterol (fat in the blood), diabetes, are overweight, or if you use tobacco, you may have higher chances for getting heart disease. Ask your healthcare provider for ways to lower your chances for getting heart disease.

General information about the safe and effective use of Premarin

Medicines are sometimes prescribed for conditions that are not mentioned in patient information leaflets. Do not take Premarin for conditions for which it was not prescribed. Do not give Premarin to other people, even if they have the same symptoms you have. It may harm them.

Keep Premarin out of the reach of children.

This leaflet provides a summary of the most important information about Premarin. If you would like more information, talk with your healthcare provider or pharmacist. You can ask for information about Premarin that is written for health professionals. You can get more information by calling the toll free number 800-934-5556.

What are the ingredients in Premarin?

Premarin contains a mixture of conjugated estrogens, which are a mixture of sodium estrone sulfate and sodium equilin sulfate and other components including sodium sulfate conjugates, 17 α-dihydroequilin, 17 α-estradiol, and 17 β-dihydroequilin. Premarin also contains calcium phosphate tribasic, calcium sulfate, carnauba wax, cellulose, glyceryl monooleate, lactose, magnesium stearate, methylcellulose, pharmaceutical glaze, polyethylene glycol, stearic acid, sucrose, and titanium dioxide. The tablets come in different strengths and each strength tablet is a different color. The color ingredients are:

— 0.3 mg tablet (green color): D&C Yellow No. 10, FD&C Blue No. 1, FD&C Blue No. 2, and FD&C Yellow No. 6.
— 0.45 mg tablet (blue color): FD&C Blue No. 2.
— 0.625 mg tablet (maroon color): FD&C Blue No. 2, D&C Red No. 27, and FD&C Red No. 40.
— 0.9 mg tablet (white color): D&C Red No. 6 and D&C Red No. 7.
— 1.25 mg tablet (yellow color): black iron oxide, D&C Yellow No. 10, and FD&C Yellow No. 6.

The appearance of these tablets is a trademark of Wyeth Pharmaceuticals.

This product's label may have been revised after this insert was used in production. For further product information and current package insert, please visit www.wyeth.com or call our medical communications department toll-free at 1-800-934-5556.

Wyeth®
Wyeth Pharmaceuticals Inc.
Philadelphia, PA 19101

W10405C010
ET01
Revised August 3, 2004

Shown in Product Identification Guide, page 336

PREMARIN® ℞

[prĕ-măr-ĭn]
(conjugated estrogens)
Vaginal Cream in a nonliquefying base
℞ only

NOTE: PATIENT INFORMATION LEAFLET ATTACHED.

ESTROGENS INCREASE THE RISK OF ENDOMETRIAL CANCER

Close clinical surveillance of all women taking estrogens is important. Adequate diagnostic measures, including endometrial sampling when indicated, should be undertaken to rule out malignancy in all cases of undiagnosed persistent or recurring abnormal vaginal bleeding. There is no evidence that the use of "natural" estrogens results in a different endometrial risk profile than synthetic estrogens of equivalent estrogen dose.

CARDIOVASCULAR AND OTHER RISKS

Estrogens with or without progestins should not be used for the prevention of cardiovascular disease.

The Women's Health Initiative (WHI) reported increased risks of myocardial infarction, stroke, invasive breast cancer, pulmonary emboli, and deep vein thrombosis in postmenopausal women (50 to 79 years of age) during 5 years of treatment with oral conjugated estrogens (0.625 mg) combined with medroxyprogesterone acetate (2.5 mg) relative to placebo. (See **CLINICAL PHARMACOLOGY, Clinical Studies.**)

Continued on next page

Premarin Vaginal Cream—Cont.

The Women's Health Initiative Memory Study (WHIMS), a substudy of WHI, reported increased risk of developing probable dementia in postmenopausal women 65 years of age or older during 4 years of treatment with oral conjugated estrogens plus medroxyprogesterone acetate relative to placebo. It is unknown whether this finding applies to younger postmenopausal women or to women taking estrogen alone therapy. (See **CLINICAL PHARMACOLOGY, Clinical Studies.**)

Other doses of conjugated estrogens and medroxyprogesterone acetate, and other combinations and dosage forms of estrogens and progestins were not studied in the WHI clinical trials and, in the absence of comparable data, these risks should be assumed to be similar. Because of these risks, estrogens with or without progestins should be prescribed at the lowest effective doses and for the shortest duration consistent with treatment goals and risks for the individual woman.

DESCRIPTION

Each gram of Premarin® (conjugated estrogens) Vaginal Cream contains 0.625 mg conjugated estrogens, USP in a nonliquefying base containing cetyl esters wax, cetyl alcohol, white wax, glyceryl monostearate, propylene glycol monostearate, methyl stearate, benzyl alcohol, sodium lauryl sulfate, glycerin, and mineral oil. Premarin Vaginal Cream is applied intravaginally.

Premarin (conjugated estrogens) Vaginal Cream is a mixture of conjugated estrogens obtained exclusively from natural sources, occurring as the sodium salts of water-soluble estrogen sulfates blended to represent the average composition of material derived from pregnant mares' urine. It is a mixture of sodium estrone sulfate and sodium equilin sulfate. It contains estrone, equilin, and 17 α-dihydroequilin, together with smaller amounts of 17 α-estradiol, equilenin, and 17 α-dihydroequilenin as salts of their sulfate esters.

CLINICAL PHARMACOLOGY

Endogenous estrogens are largely responsible for the development and maintenance of the female reproductive system and secondary sexual characteristics. Although circulating estrogens exist in a dynamic equilibrium of metabolic interconversions, estradiol is the principal intracellular human estrogen and is substantially more potent than its metabolites, estrone and estriol, at the receptor level.

The primary source of estrogen in normally cycling adult women is the ovarian follicle, which secretes 70 to 500 mcg of estradiol daily, depending on the phase of the menstrual cycle. After menopause, most endogenous estrogen is produced by conversion of androstenedione, secreted by the adrenal cortex, to estrone by peripheral tissues. Thus, estrone and the sulfate-conjugated form, estrone sulfate, are the most abundant circulating estrogen in postmenopausal women.

Estrogens act through binding to nuclear receptors in estrogen-responsive tissues. To date, two estrogen receptors have been identified. These vary in proportion from tissue to tissue.

Circulating estrogens modulate the pituitary secretion of the gonadotropins, luteinizing hormone (LH) and follicle stimulating hormone (FSH) through a negative feedback mechanism. Estrogens act to reduce the elevated levels of these gonadotropins seen in postmenopausal women.

Pharmacokinetics

Absorption

Conjugated estrogens are soluble in water and are well absorbed through the skin, mucous membranes, and the gastrointestinal tract after release from the drug formulation.

Distribution

The distribution of exogenous estrogens is similar to that of endogenous estrogens. Estrogens are widely distributed in the body and are generally found in higher concentration in the sex hormone target organs. Estrogens circulate in the blood largely bound to sex hormone-binding globulin (SHBG) and albumin.

Metabolism

Exogenous estrogens are metabolized in the same manner as endogenous estrogens. Circulating estrogens exist in a dynamic equilibrium of metabolic interconversions. These transformations take place mainly in the liver. Estradiol is converted reversibly to estrone, and both can be converted to estriol, which is the major urinary metabolite. Estrogens also undergo enterohepatic recirculation via sulfate and glucuronide conjugation in the liver, biliary secretion of conjugates into the intestine, and hydrolysis in the gut followed by reabsorption. In postmenopausal women a significant proportion of the circulating estrogens exists as sulfate conjugates, especially estrone sulfate, which serves as a circulating reservoir for the formation of more active estrogens.

Excretion

Estradiol, estrone, and estriol are excreted in the urine along with glucuronide and sulfate conjugates.

Special Populations

No pharmacokinetic studies were conducted in special populations, including patients with renal or hepatic impairment.

Drug Interactions

Data from a single-dose drug-drug interaction study involving oral conjugated estrogens and medroxyprogesterone acetate indicate that the pharmacokinetic dispositions of both drugs are not altered when the drugs are coadministered. No other clinical drug-drug interaction studies have been conducted with conjugated estrogens.

In vitro and in vivo studies have shown that estrogens are metabolized partially by cytochrome P450 3A4 (CYP3A4). Therefore, inducers or inhibitors of CYP3A4 may affect estrogen drug metabolism. Inducers of CYP3A4 such as St. John's Wort preparations (Hypericum perforatum), phenobarbital, carbamazepine, and rifampin may reduce plasma concentrations of estrogens, possibly resulting in a decrease in therapeutic effects and/or changes in the uterine bleeding profile. Inhibitors of CYP3A4 such as erythromycin, clarithromycin, ketoconazole, itraconazole, ritonavir and grapefruit juice may increase plasma concentrations of estrogens and may result in side effects.

Clinical Studies

Women's Health Initiative Studies.

The Women's Health Initiative (WHI) enrolled a total of 27,000 predominantly healthy postmenopausal women to assess the risks and benefits of either the use of Premarin tablets (0.625 mg conjugated estrogens per day) alone or the use of PREMPRO™ tablets (0.625 mg conjugated estrogens plus 2.5 mg medroxyprogesterone acetate per day) compared to placebo in the prevention of certain chronic diseases. The primary endpoint was the incidence of coronary heart disease (CHD) (nonfatal myocardial infarction and CHD death), with invasive breast cancer as the primary adverse outcome studied. A "global index" included the earliest occurrence of CHD, invasive breast cancer, stroke, pulmonary embolism (PE), endometrial cancer, colorectal cancer, hip fracture, or death due to other cause. The study did not evaluate the effects of Premarin tablets or PREMPRO on menopausal symptoms.

The Premarin tablets-only substudy results have not been reported. The estrogen plus progestin substudy was stopped early because, according to the predefined stopping rule, the increased risk of breast cancer and cardiovascular events exceeded the specified benefits included in the "global index." Results of the estrogen plus progestin substudy, which included 16,608 women (average age of 63 years, range 50 to 79; 83.9% White, 6.5% Black, 5.5% Hispanic), after an average follow-up of 5.2 years, are presented in Table 1 below:

[See table below]

For those outcomes included in the "global index", the absolute excess risks per 10,000 women-years in the group treated with PREMPRO were 7 more CHD events, 8 more strokes, 8 more PEs, and 8 more invasive breast cancers, while the absolute risk reductions per 10,000 women-years were 6 fewer colorectal cancers and 5 fewer hip fractures. The absolute excess risk of events included in the "global index" was 19 per 10,000 women-years. There was no difference between the groups in terms of all-cause mortality. (See **BOXED WARNINGS, WARNINGS,** and **PRECAUTIONS.**)

Women's Health Initiative Memory Study.

The Women's Health Initiative Memory Study (WHIMS), a substudy of WHI, enrolled 4,532 predominantly healthy postmenopausal women 65 years of age and older (47% were age 65 to 69 years, 35% were 70 to 74 years, and 18% were 75 years of age and older) to evaluate the effects of PREMPRO (0.625 mg conjugated estrogens plus 2.5 mg medroxyprogesterone acetate) on the incidence of probable dementia (primary outcome) compared with placebo.

After an average follow-up of 4 years, 40 women in the estrogen/progestin group (45 per 10,000 women-years) and 21 in the placebo group (22 per 10,000 women-years) were diagnosed with probable dementia. The relative risk of probable dementia in the hormone therapy group was 2.05 (95% CI, 1.21 to 3.48) compared to placebo. Differences between groups became apparent in the first year of treatment. It is unknown whether these findings apply to younger postmenopausal women. (See **BOXED WARNING,** and **WARNINGS, Dementia.**)

INDICATIONS AND USAGE

Premarin (conjugated estrogens) Vaginal Cream is indicated in the treatment of atrophic vaginitis and kraurosis vulvae.

CONTRAINDICATIONS

Premarin Vaginal Cream should not be used in women with any of the following conditions:

1. Undiagnosed abnormal genital bleeding.
2. Known, suspected, or history of cancer of the breast.
3. Known or suspected estrogen-dependent neoplasia.
4. Active deep vein thrombosis, pulmonary embolism or a history of these conditions.
5. Active or recent (e.g., within past year) arterial thromboembolic disease (e.g., stroke, myocardial infarction).
6. Liver dysfunction or disease.
7. Premarin Vaginal Cream should not be used in patients with known hypersensitivity to its ingredients.
8. Known or suspected pregnancy. There is no indication for Premarin Vaginal Cream in pregnancy. There appears to be little or no increased risk of birth defects in children born to women who have used estrogen and progestins from oral contraceptives inadvertently during pregnancy. (See **PRECAUTIONS.**)

WARNINGS

See **BOXED WARNINGS.**

Systemic absorption may occur with the use of Premarin Vaginal Cream. The warnings, precautions, and adverse reactions associated with oral Premarin treatment should be taken into account.

1. **Cardiovascular disorders.**

Estrogen and estrogen/progestin therapy have been associated with an increased risk of cardiovascular events such as myocardial infarction and stroke, as well as venous thrombosis and pulmonary embolism (venous thromboembolism or VTE). Should any of these occur or be suspected, estrogens should be discontinued immediately.

Risk factors for arterial vascular disease (e.g., hypertension, diabetes mellitus, tobacco use, hypercholesterolemia, and obesity) and/or venous thromboembolism (e.g., personal history or family history of VTE, obesity, and systemic lupus erythematosus) should be managed appropriately.

a. Coronary heart disease and stroke. In the Premarin tablets substudy of the Women's Health Initiative (WHI) study, an increase in the number of myocardial infarctions and stroke has been observed in women receiving Premarin compared to placebo. These observations are preliminary. (See **CLINICAL PHARMACOLOGY, Clinical Studies.**)

Table 1. RELATIVE AND ABSOLUTE RISK SEEN IN THE ESTROGEN PLUS PROGESTIN SUBSTUDY OF WHI[a]

Event[c]	Relative Risk Prempro vs Placebo at 5.2 Years (95% CI*)	Placebo n = 8102	Prempro n = 8506
		Absolute Risk per 10,000 Women-years	
CHD events	1.29 (1.02–1.63)	30	37
Non-fatal MI	*1.32 (1.02–1.72)*	*23*	*30*
CHD death	*1.18 (0.70–1.97)*	*6*	*7*
Invasive breast cancer[b]	1.26 (1.00–1.59)	30	38
Stroke	1.41 (1.07–1.85)	21	29
Pulmonary embolism	2.13 (1.39–3.25)	8	16
Colorectal cancer	0.63 (0.43–0.92)	16	10
Endometrial cancer	0.83 (0.47–1.47)	6	5
Hip fracture	0.66 (0.45–0.98)	15	10
Death due to causes other than the events above	0.92 (0.74–1.14)	40	37
Global Index[c]	1.15 (1.03–1.28)	151	170
Deep vein thrombosis[d]	2.07 (1.49–2.87)	13	26
Vertebral fractures[d]	0.66 (0.44–0.98)	15	9
Other osteoporotic fractures[d]	0.77 (0.69–0.86)	170	131

[a] adapted from JAMA, 2002; 288:321–333

[b] includes metastatic and non-metastatic breast cancer with the exception of in situ breast cancer

[c] a subset of the events was combined in a "global index", defined as the earliest occurrence of CHD events, invasive breast cancer, stroke, pulmonary embolism, endometrial cancer, colorectal cancer, hip fracture, or death due to other causes

[d] not included in Global Index

*nominal confidence intervals unadjusted for multiple looks and multiple comparisons

In the estrogen plus progestin substudy of WHI, an increased risk of coronary heart disease (CHD) events (defined as nonfatal myocardial infarction and CHD death) was observed in women receiving PREMPRO compared to women receiving placebo (37 vs 30 per 10,000 women-years). The increase in risk was observed in year one and persisted.
In the same substudy of the WHI, an increased risk of stroke was observed in women receiving PREMPRO compared to women receiving placebo (29 vs 21 per 10,000 women-years). The increase in risk was observed after the first year and persisted.
In postmenopausal women with documented heart disease (n = 2,763, average age 66.7 years) a controlled clinical trial of secondary prevention of cardiovascular disease (Heart and Estrogen/progestin Replacement Study; HERS) treatment with PREMPRO (0.625 mg conjugated estrogen plus 2.5 mg medroxyprogesterone acetate per day) demonstrated no cardiovascular benefit. During an average follow-up of 4.1 years, treatment with PREMPRO did not reduce the overall rate of CHD events in postmenopausal women with established coronary heart disease. There were more CHD events in the PREMPRO-treated group than in the placebo group in year 1, but not during the subsequent years. Two thousand three hundred and twenty one women from the original HERS trial agreed to participate in an open label extension of HERS, HERS II. Average follow-up in HERS II was an additional 2.7 years, for a total of 6.8 years overall. Rates of CHD events were comparable among women in the PREMPRO group and the placebo group in HERS, HERS II, and overall.
Large doses of estrogen (5 mg conjugated estrogens per day), comparable to those used to treat cancer of the prostate and breast, have been shown in a large prospective clinical trial in men to increase the risks of nonfatal myocardial infarction, pulmonary embolism, and thrombophlebitis.

b. Venous thromboembolism (VTE). In the Premarin tablets substudy of the Women's Health Initiative (WHI), an increase in VTE has been observed in women receiving Premarin compared to placebo. These observations are preliminary. (See **CLINICAL PHARMACOLOGY, Clinical Studies.**)
In the estrogen plus progestin substudy of WHI, a 2-fold greater rate of VTE, including deep venous thrombosis and pulmonary embolism, was observed in women receiving PREMPRO compared to women receiving placebo. The rate of VTE was 34 per 10,000 women-years in the Prempro group compared to 16 per 10,000 women-years in the placebo group. The increase in VTE risk was observed during the first year and persisted.
If feasible, estrogens should be discontinued at least 4 to 6 weeks before surgery of the type associated with an increased risk of thromboembolism, or during periods of prolonged immobilization.

2. Malignant neoplasms.

a. Endometrial cancer. The use of unopposed estrogens in women with intact uteri has been associated with an increased risk of endometrial cancer. The reported endometrial cancer risk among unopposed estrogen users is about 2- to 12-fold greater than in non-users, and appears dependent on duration of treatment and on estrogen dose. Most studies show no significant increased risk associated with use of estrogens for less than one year. The greatest risk appears associated with prolonged use, with increased risks of 15- to 24-fold for five to ten years or more and this risk has been shown to persist for at least 8 to 15 years after estrogen therapy is discontinued.
Clinical surveillance of all women taking estrogen/progestin combinations is important. Adequate diagnostic measures, including endometrial sampling when indicated, should be undertaken to rule out malignancy in all cases of undiagnosed persistent or recurring abnormal vaginal bleeding. There is no evidence that the use of natural estrogens results in a different endometrial risk profile than synthetic estrogens of equivalent estrogen dose. Adding a progestin to postmenopausal estrogen therapy has been shown to reduce the risk of endometrial hyperplasia, which may be a precursor to endometrial cancer.

b. Breast cancer. The use of estrogens and progestins by postmenopausal women has been reported to increase the risk of breast cancer. The most important randomized clinical trial providing information about this issue is the Women's Health Initiative (WHI) trial of estrogen plus progestin (See **CLINICAL PHARMACOLOGY, Clinical Studies**). The results from observational studies are generally consistent with those of the WHI trial.
After a mean follow-up of 5.6 years, the WHI trial reported an increased risk of breast cancer in women who took estrogen plus progestin. Observational studies have also reported an increased risk for estrogen/progestin combination therapy, and a smaller increased risk for estrogen alone therapy, after several years of use. For both findings, the excess risk increased with duration of use, and appeared to return to baseline over about five years after stopping treatment (only the observational studies have substantial data on risk after stopping). In these studies, the risk of breast cancer was greater, and became apparent earlier, with estrogen/progestin combination therapy as compared to estrogen alone therapy. However, these studies have not found significant variation in the risk of breast cancer among different estrogens or among different estrogen/progestin combinations, doses, or routes of administration.
In the WHI trial of estrogen plus progestin, 26% of the women reported prior use of estrogen alone and/or estrogen/progestin combination hormone therapy. After a mean follow-up of 5.6 years during the clinical trial, the overall relative risk of invasive breast cancer was 1.24 (95% confidence interval 1.01-1.54), and the overall absolute risk was 41 vs. 33 cases per 10,000 women-years, for estrogen plus progestin compared with placebo. Among women who reported prior use of hormone therapy, the relative risk of invasive breast cancer was 1.86, and the absolute risk was 46 vs. 25 cases per 10,000 women-years, for estrogen plus progestin compared with placebo. Among women who reported no prior use of hormone therapy, the relative risk of invasive breast cancer was 1.09, and the absolute risk was 40 vs. 36 cases per 10,000 women-years for estrogen plus progestin compared with placebo. In the WHI trial, invasive breast cancers were larger and diagnosed at a more advanced stage in the estrogen plus progestin group compared with the placebo group. Metastatic disease was rare with no apparent difference between the two groups. Other prognostic factors such as histologic subtype, grade and hormone receptor status did not differ between the groups. The observational Million Women Study in Europe reported an increased risk of mortality due to breast cancer among current users of hormone therapy compared to never users, while the estrogen plus progestin sub-study of WHI showed no effect on breast cancer mortality with a mean follow-up of 5.6 years.
The observational Million Women Study in Europe reported an increased risk of mortality due to breast cancer among current users of estrogens alone or estrogens plus progestins compared to never users, while the estrogen plus progestin sub-study of WHI showed no effect on breast cancer mortality with a mean follow-up of 5.6 years.
The use of estrogen plus progestin has been reported to result in an increase in abnormal mammograms requiring further evaluation. All women should receive yearly breast examinations by a healthcare provider and perform monthly breast self-examinations. In addition, mammography examinations should be scheduled based on patient age, risk factors, and prior mammogram results.

3. Dementia.

In the Women's Health Initiative Memory Study (WHIMS), 4,532 generally healthy postmenopausal women 65 years of age and older were studied, of whom 35% were 70 to 74 years of age and 18% were 75 or older. After an average follow-up of 4 years, 40 women being treated with PREMPRO (1.8%, n = 2,229) and 21 women in the placebo group (0.9%, n = 2,303) received diagnoses of probable dementia. The relative risk for PREMPRO versus placebo was 2.05 (95% confidence interval 1.21 – 3.48), and was similar for women with and without histories of menopausal hormone use before WHIMS. The absolute risk of probable dementia for PREMPRO versus placebo was 45 versus 22 cases per 10,000 women-years, and the absolute excess risk for PREMPRO was 23 cases per 10,000 women-years. It is unknown whether these findings apply to younger postmenopausal women. (See **CLINICAL PHARMACOLOGY, Clinical Studies** and **PRECAUTIONS, Geriatric Use.**)
The results of the estrogen-alone sub-study of the Women's Health Initiative Memory Study have not been reported. It is unknown whether these findings apply to estrogen-alone therapy.

4. Gallbladder disease.

A 2- to 4-fold increase in the risk of gallbladder disease requiring surgery in postmenopausal women receiving postmenopausal estrogens has been reported.

5. Hypercalcemia.

Estrogen administration may lead to severe hypercalcemia in patients with breast cancer and bone metastases. If hypercalcemia occurs, use of the drug should be stopped and appropriate measures taken to reduce the serum calcium level.

6. Visual abnormalities.

Retinal vascular thrombosis has been reported in patients receiving estrogens. Discontinue medication pending examination if there is sudden partial or complete loss of vision, or a sudden onset of proptosis, diplopia, or migraine. If examination reveals papilledema or retinal vascular lesions, estrogens should be discontinued.

PRECAUTIONS

A. General

1. Addition of a progestin when a woman has not had a hysterectomy.
Studies of the addition of a progestin for 10 or more days of a cycle of estrogen administration or daily with estrogen in a continuous regimen have reported a lowered incidence of endometrial hyperplasia than would be induced by estrogen treatment alone. Endometrial hyperplasia may be a precursor to endometrial cancer.
There are, however, possible risks that may be associated with the use of progestins with estrogens compared to estrogen-alone regimens. These include a possible increased risk of breast cancer, adverse effects on lipoprotein metabolism (e.g., lowering HDL, raising LDL) and impairment of glucose tolerance.

2. Elevated blood pressure.
In a small number of case reports, substantial increases in blood pressure have been attributed to idiosyncratic reactions to estrogens. In a large, randomized, placebo-controlled clinical trial, a generalized effect of estrogen therapy on blood pressure was not seen. Blood pressure should be monitored at regular intervals with estrogen use.

3. Hypertriglyceridemia.
In patients with pre-existing hypertriglyceridemia, estrogen therapy may be associated with elevations of plasma triglycerides leading to pancreatitis and other complications.

4. Impaired liver function and past history of cholestatic jaundice.
Estrogens may be poorly metabolized in patients with impaired liver function. For patients with a history of cholestatic jaundice associated with past estrogen use or with pregnancy, caution should be exercised and in the case of recurrence, medication should be discontinued.

5. Hypothyroidism.
Estrogen administration leads to increased thyroid-binding globulin (TBG) levels. Patients with normal thyroid function can compensate for the increased TBG by making more thyroid hormone, thus maintaining free T_4 and T_3 serum concentrations in the normal range. Patients dependent on thyroid hormone replacement therapy who are also receiving estrogens may require increased doses of their thyroid replacement therapy. These patients should have their thyroid function monitored in order to maintain their free thyroid hormone levels in an acceptable range.

6. Fluid retention.
Because estrogens may cause some degree of fluid retention, patients with conditions that might be influenced by this factor, such as cardiac or renal dysfunction, warrant careful observation when estrogens are prescribed.

7. Hypocalcemia.
Estrogens should be used with caution in individuals with severe hypocalcemia.

8. Ovarian cancer.
The estrogen plus progestin substudy of WHI reported that after an average follow-up of 5.6 years, the relative risk for ovarian cancer for estrogen plus progestin versus placebo was 1.58 (95% confidence interval 0.77–3.24) but was not statistically significant. The absolute risk for estrogen plus progestin versus placebo was 4.2 versus 2.7 cases per 10,000 women-years. In some epidemiologic studies, the use of estrogen-only products, in particular for ten or more years, has been associated with an increased risk of ovarian cancer. Other epidemiologic studies have not found these associations.

9. Exacerbation of endometriosis.
Endometriosis may be exacerbated with administration of estrogen therapy.
A few cases of malignant transformation of residual endometrial implants have been reported in women treated post-hysterectomy with estrogen alone therapy. For patients known to have residual endometriosis post-hysterectomy, the addition of progestin should be considered.

10. Exacerbation of other conditions.
Estrogen therapy may cause an exacerbation of asthma, diabetes mellitus, epilepsy, migraine, porphyria, systemic lupus erythematosus, and hepatic hemangiomas and should be used with caution in women with these conditions.

11. Barrier contraceptives.
Premarin Vaginal Cream exposure has been reported to weaken latex condoms. The potential for Premarin Vaginal Cream to weaken and contribute to the failure of condoms, diaphragms, or cervical caps made of latex or rubber should be considered.

B. Patient Information

Physicians are advised to discuss the contents of the PATIENT INFORMATION leaflet with patients for whom they prescribe Premarin Vaginal Cream.

C. Laboratory Tests

Estrogen administration should be guided by clinical response at the lowest dose for the treatment of postmenopausal vulvar and vaginal atrophy.

D. Drug/Laboratory Test Interactions

1. Accelerated prothrombin time, partial thromboplastin time, and platelet aggregation time; increased platelet count; increased factors II, VII antigen, VIII antigen, VIII coagulant activity, IX, X, XII, VII-X complex, II-VII-X complex, and beta-thromboglobulin; decreased levels of antifactor Xa and antithrombin III, decreased antithrombin III activity; increased levels of fibrinogen and fibrinogen activity; increased plasminogen antigen and activity.
2. Increased thyroid-binding globulin (TBG) leading to increased circulating total thyroid hormone, as measured by protein-bound iodine (PBI), T_4 levels (by column or by radioimmunoassay) or T_3 levels by radioimmunoassay. T_3 resin uptake is decreased, reflecting the elevated TBG. Free T_4 and free T_3 concentrations are unaltered. Patients on thyroid replacement therapy may require higher doses of thyroid hormone.
3. Other binding proteins may be elevated in serum, i.e., corticosteroid binding globulin (CBG), sex hormone-binding globulin (SHBG), leading to increased total circulating corticosteroids and sex steroids, respectively. Free hormone concentrations may be decreased. Other plasma proteins may be increased (angiotensinogen/renin substrate, alpha-1-antitrypsin, ceruloplasmin).
4. Increased plasma HDL and HDL_2 cholesterol subfraction concentrations, reduced LDL cholesterol concentration, increased triglyceride levels.
5. Impaired glucose tolerance.
6. Reduced response to metyrapone test.

E. Carcinogenesis, Mutagenesis, Impairment of Fertility

(See **BOXED WARNINGS, WARNINGS,** and **PRECAUTIONS.**)
Long-term continuous administration of natural and synthetic estrogens in certain animal species increases the frequency of carcinomas of the breast, uterus, cervix, vagina, testis, and liver.

Continued on next page

Premarin Vaginal Cream—Cont.

F. Pregnancy
Premarin Vaginal Cream should not be used during pregnancy. (See **CONTRAINDICATIONS**.)
G. Nursing Mothers
Estrogen administration to nursing mothers has been shown to decrease the quantity and quality of breast milk. Detectable amounts of estrogens have been identified in the milk of mothers receiving the drug. Caution should be exercised when Premarin Vaginal Cream is administered to a nursing woman.
H. Pediatric Use
Estrogen therapy has been used for the induction of puberty in adolescents with some forms of pubertal delay. Safety and effectiveness in pediatric patients have not otherwise been established.
Large and repeated doses of estrogen over an extended time period have been shown to accelerate epiphyseal closure, which could result in short adult stature if treatment is initiated before the completion of physiologic puberty in normally developing children. If estrogen is administered to patients whose bone growth is not complete, periodic monitoring of bone maturation and effects on epiphyseal centers is recommended during estrogen administration.
Estrogen treatment of prepubertal girls also induces premature breast development and vaginal cornification, and may induce vaginal bleeding. In boys, estrogen treatment may modify the normal pubertal process and induce gynecomastia. See **INDICATIONS** and **DOSAGE AND ADMINISTRATION** sections.
I. Geriatric Use
Of the total number of subjects in the estrogen plus progestin substudy of the Women's Health Initiative study, 44% (n = 7,320) were 65 years and over, while 6.6% (n = 1,095) were 75 years and over (See **CLINICAL PHARMACOLOGY, Clinical Studies**). There was a higher incidence of stroke and invasive breast cancer in women 75 and over compared to women less than 75 years of age.
In the Women's Health Initiative Memory Study (WHIMS), including 4,532 women 65 years of age and older, followed for an average of 4 years, 82% (n = 3,729) were 65 to 74 while 18% (n = 803) were 75 and over. Most women (80%) had no prior hormone therapy use. Women treated with oral conjugated estrogens plus medroxyprogesterone acetate were reported to have a two-fold increase in the risk of developing probable dementia. Alzheimer's disease was the most common classification of probable dementia in both the conjugated estrogens plus medroxyprogesterone acetate group and the placebo group. Ninety percent of the cases of probable dementia occurred in the 54% of women that were older than 70. (See **WARNINGS, Dementia**).
There have not been sufficient numbers of geriatric patients involved in studies utilizing Premarin Vaginal Cream to determine whether those over 65 years of age differ from younger subjects in their response to Premarin Vaginal Cream.

ADVERSE REACTIONS

See **BOXED WARNINGS**, **WARNINGS**, and **PRECAUTIONS**.
Systemic absorption may occur with the use of Premarin Vaginal Cream. Warnings, precautions, and adverse reactions associated with oral Premarin treatment should be taken into account.
The following additional adverse reactions have been reported with estrogen and/or progestin therapy:

1. *Genitourinary system:* Breakthrough bleeding, spotting, change in menstrual flow; dysmenorrhea; premenstrual-like syndrome; amenorrhea during and after treatment; increase in size of uterine fibromyomata; vaginitis, including vaginal candidiasis; change in cervical erosion and in degree of cervical secretion; cystitis-like syndrome; application site reactions of vulvovaginal discomfort including burning and irritation; genital pruritus; ovarian cancer; endometrial hyperplasia; endometrial cancer; precocious puberty.
2. *Breasts:* Tenderness, pain, enlargement, secretion; breast cancer; fibrocystic breast changes.
3. *Cardiovascular:* Deep and superficial venous thrombosis, pulmonary embolism, myocardial infarction, stroke; increase in blood pressure.
4. *Gastrointestinal:* Nausea, vomiting, abdominal cramps, bloating; cholestatic jaundice; pancreatitis; increased incidence of gallbladder disease; enlargement of hepatic hemangiomas.
5. *Skin:* Chloasma or melasma which may persist when drug is discontinued; erythema multiforme; erythema nodosum; hemorrhagic eruption; loss of scalp hair; hirsutism; pruritis; rash; urticaria.
6. *Eyes:* Retinal vascular thrombosis; intolerance to contact lenses.
7. *Central Nervous System:* Headache; migraine; dizziness; nervousness; mood disturbances; irritability; mental depression; chorea; exacerbation of epilepsy; dementia.
8. *Miscellaneous:* Increase or decrease in weight; reduced carbohydrate tolerance; glucose intolerance; aggravation of porphyria; edema; changes in libido; anaphylactoid/anaphylactic reactions; hypocalcemia; exacerbation of asthma; angioedema; hypersensitivity; increased triglycerides; arthralgias; leg cramps.

OVERDOSAGE

Serious ill effects have not been reported following acute ingestion of large doses of estrogen/progestin containing drug products by young children. Overdosage of estrogens may cause nausea and vomiting, and withdrawal bleeding may occur in females.

DOSAGE AND ADMINISTRATION

Use of Premarin Vaginal Cream, alone or in combination with a progestin, should be limited to the shortest duration consistent with treatment goals and risks for the individual woman. Patients should be re-evaluated periodically as clinically appropriate (e.g., at 3-month to 6-month intervals) to determine if treatment is still necessary (See **BOXED WARNINGS** and **WARNINGS**). For women who have a uterus, adequate diagnostic measures, such as endometrial sampling, when indicated, should be undertaken to rule out malignancy in cases of undiagnosed persistent or recurring abnormal vaginal bleeding.
Given cyclically for short-term use only:
For treatment of atrophic vaginitis, or kraurosis vulvae. The lowest dose that will control symptoms should be chosen and medication should be discontinued as promptly as possible. Administration should be cyclic (e.g., three weeks on and one week off).
Usual Dosage Range:
½ to 2 g daily, intravaginally, depending on the severity of the condition.
Instructions For Use Of Gentle Measure™ Applicator
1. Remove cap from tube.
2. Screw nozzle end of applicator onto tube.
3. *Gently* squeeze tube from the *bottom* to force sufficient cream into the barrel to provide the prescribed dose. Use the marked stopping points on the applicator as a guideline to measure the correct dose.
4. Unscrew applicator from tube.
5. Lie on back with knees drawn up. To deliver medication, gently insert applicator deeply into vagina and press plunger downward to its original position.
To Cleanse: Pull plunger to remove it from barrel. Wash with mild soap and warm water.
DO NOT BOIL OR USE HOT WATER.

HOW SUPPLIED

Premarin® (conjugated estrogens) Vaginal Cream—Each gram contains 0.625 mg conjugated estrogens, USP.
Combination package: Each contains Net Wt. 1 ½ oz (42.5 g) tube with one plastic applicator calibrated in ½ g increments to a maximum of 2 g (NDC 0046-0872-93).
Also Available—Refill package: Each contains Net Wt. 1 ½ oz (42.5 g) tube (NDC 0046-0872-01).
Store at room temperature (approximately 25° C).

PATIENT INFORMATION

Updated July 6, 2004
Premarin® (conjugated estrogens) Vaginal Cream
Read this PATIENT INFORMATION before you start using Premarin Vaginal Cream and read what you get each time you refill Premarin Vaginal Cream. There may be new information. This information does not take the place of talking to your healthcare provider about your medical condition or your treatment.

What is the most important information I should know about Premarin (an estrogen mixture)?
- Estrogens increase the chances of getting cancer of the uterus.
  Report any unusual vaginal bleeding right away while you are taking Premarin. Vaginal bleeding after menopause may be a warning sign of cancer of the uterus (womb). Your healthcare provider should check any unusual vaginal bleeding to find out the cause.
- Do not use estrogens with or without progestins to prevent heart disease, heart attacks, or strokes.
  Using estrogens with or without progestins may increase your chances of getting heart attacks, strokes, breast cancer, and blood clots. Using estrogens with progestins may increase your risk of dementia based on a study of women age 65 years or older. You and your healthcare provider should talk regularly about whether you still need treatment with Premarin Vaginal Cream.

What is Premarin Vaginal Cream?
Premarin Vaginal Cream is a medicine that contains a mixture of estrogen hormones.
Premarin Vaginal Cream is used to:
- treat dryness, itching, and burning, in and around the vagina due to menopause. You and your healthcare provider should talk regularly about whether you still need treatment with Premarin Vaginal Cream to control these problems.

Who should not use Premarin Vaginal Cream?
Do not start using Premarin Vaginal Cream if you:
- **have unusual vaginal bleeding.**
- **currently have or have had certain cancers.**
  Estrogens may increase the chances of getting certain types of cancers, including cancer of the breast or uterus. If you have or have had cancer, talk with your healthcare provider about whether you should use Premarin Vaginal Cream.
- **had a stroke or heart attack in the past year.**
- **currently have or had blood clots.**
- **currently have liver problems.**
- **are allergic to Premarin Vaginal Cream or any of its ingredients.**
  See the end of this leaflet for a list of all the ingredients in Premarin Vaginal Cream.
- **think you may be pregnant.**

Tell your healthcare provider:
- **if you are breast feeding.** The hormones in Premarin Vaginal Cream can pass into your milk.
- **about all of your medical problems.** Your healthcare provider may need to check you more carefully if you have certain conditions, such as asthma (wheezing), epilepsy (seizures), migraine, endometriosis, lupus, or problems with your heart, liver, thyroid, kidneys, or have high calcium levels in your blood.
- **about all the medicines you take,** including prescription and nonprescription medicines, vitamins, and herbal supplements. Some medicines may affect how Premarin Vaginal Cream works. Premarin Vaginal Cream may also affect how your other medicines work.
- **if you are going to have surgery or will be on bedrest.** You may need to stop using Premarin Vaginal Cream.

How should I use Premarin Vaginal Cream?
The Gentle Measure™ Applicator has been specifically designed for comfortable, easy use.
1. Remove cap from tube.
2. Screw nozzle end of applicator onto tube.
3. *Gently* squeeze tube from the *bottom* to force sufficient cream into the barrel to provide the prescribed dose. Use the marked stopping points on the applicator as a guideline to measure the correct dose, as prescribed by your healthcare provider.
4. Unscrew applicator from tube.
5. Lie on back with knees drawn up. To deliver medication, gently insert applicator deeply into vagina and press plunger downward to its original position.

TO CLEANSE: Pull plunger to remove it from barrel. Wash with mild soap and warm water.
DO NOT BOIL OR USE HOT WATER.
Premarin Vaginal Cream should be used at the lowest possible dose for your treatment and only as long as needed. You and your healthcare provider should talk regularly (for example, every 3 to 6 months) about the dose you are taking and whether you still need treatment with Premarin Vaginal Cream.

What are the possible side effects of Premarin Vaginal Cream?
Although Premarin Vaginal Cream is only used in and around the vagina, the risks associated with Premarin tablets should be taken into account.
Less common but serious side effects of estrogens include:
- Breast cancer
- Cancer of the uterus
- Stroke
- Heart attack
- Blood clots
- Dementia
- Gallbladder disease
- Ovarian cancer

These are some of the warning signs of serious side effects:
- Breast lumps
- Unusual vaginal bleeding
- Dizziness and faintness
- Changes in speech
- Severe headaches
- Chest pain
- Shortness of breath
- Pains in your legs
- Changes in vision
- Vomiting

Call your healthcare provider right away if you get any of these warning signs, or any other unusual symptom that concerns you.
Common side effects of estrogens include:
- Headache
- Breast tenderness
- Irregular vaginal bleeding or spotting
- Stomach/abdominal cramps, bloating
- Nausea and vomiting
- Hair loss
- Reactions from inserting Premarin Vaginal Cream such as vaginal burning, irritation, and itching

Other side effects of estrogens include:
- High blood pressure
- Liver problems
- High blood sugar
- Fluid retention
- Enlargement of benign tumors of the uterus ("fibroids")
- Vaginal yeast infections
- Allergic Reactions

These are not all the possible side effects of Premarin Vaginal Cream. For more information, ask your healthcare provider or pharmacist.
What can I do to lower my chances of getting a serious side effect with Premarin Vaginal Cream?
- Talk with your healthcare provider regularly about whether you should continue using Premarin Vaginal Cream.
- See your healthcare provider right away if you get vaginal bleeding while using Premarin Vaginal Cream.
- Have a breast exam and mammogram (breast X-ray) every year unless your healthcare provider tells you something else. If members of your family have had breast can-

cer or if you have ever had breast lumps or an abnormal mammogram, you may need to have breast exams more often.

- If you have high blood pressure, high cholesterol (fat in the blood), diabetes, are overweight, or if you use tobacco, you may have higher chances for getting heart disease. Ask your health care provider for ways to lower your chances for getting heart disease.

General information about the safe and effective use of Premarin Vaginal Cream

Medicines are sometimes prescribed for conditions that are not mentioned in patient information leaflets. Do not use Premarin Vaginal Cream for conditions for which it was not prescribed. Do not give Premarin Vaginal Cream to other people, even if they have the same symptoms you have. It may harm them. **Keep Premarin Vaginal Cream out of the reach of children.**

This leaflet provides a summary of the most important information about Premarin Vaginal Cream. If you would like more information, talk with your healthcare provider or pharmacist. You can ask for information about Premarin Vaginal Cream that is written for health professionals. You can get more information by calling the toll free number 1-800-934-5556.

What are the ingredients in Premarin Vaginal Cream?

Premarin Vaginal Cream is a mixture of conjugated estrogens, which are a mixture of sodium estrone sulfate and sodium equilin sulfate and other components including estrone, equilin, and 17 α-dihydroequilin, together with smaller amounts of 17 α-estradiol, equile'nin, and 17 α-dihydroequilenin salts. Premarin Vaginal Cream also contains cetyl esters wax, cetyl alcohol, white wax, glyceryl monostearate, propylene glycol monostearate, methyl stearate, benzyl alcohol, sodium lauryl sulfate, glycerin, and mineral oil.

Premarin® (conjugated estrogens) Vaginal Cream—Each gram contains 0.625 mg conjugated estrogens, USP.

Combination package: Each contains Net Wt. 1 ½ oz (42.5 g) tube with one plastic applicator calibrated in ½ g increments to a maximum of 2 g (NDC 0046-0872-93).

Also Available—Refill package: Each contains Net Wt. 1 ½ oz (42.5 g) tube (NDC 0046-0872-01).

Store at room temperature (approximately 25° C).

Wyeth®

Wyeth Pharmaceuticals Inc.
Philadelphia, PA 19101

W10413C004
ET01
Revised July 6, 2004

Premarin® (conjugated estrogens)
Vaginal Cream in a nonliquefying base
℞ only

◄TEAR HERE

PATIENT INFORMATION

Read this PATIENT INFORMATION before you start using Premarin Vaginal Cream and read what you get each time you refill Premarin Vaginal Cream. There may be new information. This information does not take the place of talking to your healthcare provider about your medical condition or your treatment.

What is the most important information I should know about Premarin (an estrogen mixture)?

- Estrogens increase the chances of getting cancer of the uterus.
  Report any unusual vaginal bleeding right away while you are taking Premarin. Vaginal bleeding after menopause may be a warning sign of cancer of the uterus (womb). Your healthcare provider should check any unusual vaginal bleeding to find out the cause.
- Do not use estrogens with or without progestins to prevent heart disease, heart attacks, or strokes.
  Using estrogens with or without progestins may increase your chances of getting heart attacks, strokes, breast cancer, and blood clots. Using estrogens with progestins may increase your risk of dementia based on a study of women age 65 years or older. You and your healthcare provider should talk regularly about whether you still need treatment with Premarin Vaginal Cream.

What is Premarin Vaginal Cream?

Premarin Vaginal Cream is a medicine that contains a mixture of estrogen hormones.

Premarin Vaginal Cream is used to:

- treat dryness, itching, and burning, in and around the vagina due to menopause.

You and your healthcare provider should talk regularly about whether you still need treatment with Premarin Vaginal Cream to control these problems.

Who should not use Premarin Vaginal Cream?

Do not start using Premarin Vaginal Cream if you:

- **have unusual vaginal bleeding.**
- **currently have or have had certain cancers.**
  Estrogens may increase the chances of getting certain types of cancers, including cancer of the breast or uterus. If you have or have had cancer, talk with your healthcare provider about whether you should use Premarin Vaginal Cream.
- **had a stroke or heart attack in the past year.**
- **currently have or had blood clots.**
- **currently have liver problems.**
- **are allergic to Premarin Vaginal Cream or any of its ingredients.**
  See the end of this leaflet for a list of all the ingredients in Premarin Vaginal Cream.
- **think you may be pregnant.**

Tell your healthcare provider:

- **if you are breast feeding.** The hormones in Premarin Vaginal Cream can pass into your milk.
- **about all of your medical problems.** Your healthcare provider may need to check you more carefully if you have certain conditions, such as asthma (wheezing), epilepsy (seizures), migraine, endometriosis, lupus, problems with your heart, liver, thyroid, kidneys, or have high calcium levels in your blood.
- **about all the medicines you take,** including prescription and nonprescription medicines, vitamins, and herbal supplements. Some medicines may affect how Premarin Vaginal Cream works. Premarin Vaginal Cream may also affect how your other medicines work.
- **if you are going to have surgery or will be on bedrest.** You may need to stop using Premarin Vaginal Cream.

How should I use Premarin Vaginal Cream?

The Gentle Measure™ Applicator has been specifically designed for comfortable, easy use.

1. Remove cap from tube.
2. Screw nozzle end of applicator onto tube.
3. *Gently* squeeze tube from the *bottom* to force sufficient cream into the barrel to provide the prescribed dose. Use the marked stopping points on the applicator as a guideline to measure the correct dose.
4. Unscrew nozzle end of applicator onto tube.
5. Lie on back with knees drawn up. To deliver medication, gently insert applicator deeply into vagina and press plunger downward to its original position.

TO CLEANSE: Pull plunger to remove it from barrel. Wash with mild soap and warm water.

DO NOT BOIL OR USE HOT WATER.

Premarin Vaginal Cream should be used at the lowest dose possible for your treatment and only as long as needed. You and your healthcare provider should talk regularly (for example, every 3 to 6 months) about the dose you are taking and about whether you still need treatment with Premarin Vaginal Cream.

What are the possible side effects of Premarin Vaginal Cream?

Although Premarin Vaginal Cream is only used in and around vagina, the risks associated with Premarin tablets should be taken into account.

Less common but serious side effects of estrogens include:

- Breast cancer
- Cancer of the uterus
- Stroke
- Heart attack
- Dementia
- Blood clots
- Gallbladder disease
- Ovarian cancer

These are some of the warning signs of serious side effects:

- Breast lumps
- Unusual vaginal bleeding
- Dizziness and faintness
- Changes in speech
- Severe headaches
- Chest pain
- Shortness of breath
- Pains in your legs
- Changes in vision
- Vomiting

Call your healthcare provider right away if you get any of these warning signs, or any other unusual symptom that concerns you.

Common side effects of estrogens include:

- Headache
- Breast tenderness
- Irregular vaginal bleeding or spotting
- Stomach/abdominal cramps, bloating
- Nausea and vomiting
- Hair loss
- Reactions from inserting Premarin Vaginal Cream such as vaginal burning, irritation, and itching

Other side effects of estrogens include:

- High blood pressure
- Liver problems
- High blood sugar
- Fluid retention
- Enlargement of benign tumors of the uterus ("fibroids")
- Vaginal yeast infections
- Allergic reactions

These are not all the possible side effects of Premarin Vaginal Cream. For more information, ask your healthcare provider or pharmacist.

What can I do to lower my chances of getting a serious side effect with Premarin Vaginal Cream?

- Talk with your healthcare provider regularly about whether you should continue using Premarin Vaginal Cream.
- See your healthcare provider right away if you get vaginal bleeding while using Premarin Vaginal Cream.
- Have a breast exam and mammogram (breast X-ray) every year unless your healthcare provider tells you something else. If members of your family have had breast cancer or if you have ever had breast lumps or an abnormal mammogram, you may need to have breast exams more often.
- If you have high blood pressure, high cholesterol (fat in the blood), diabetes, are overweight, or if you use tobacco, you may have higher chances for getting heart disease. Ask your health care provider for ways to lower your chances for getting heart disease.

General information about the safe and effective use of Premarin Vaginal Cream

Medicines are sometimes prescribed for conditions that are not mentioned in patient information leaflets. Do not use Premarin Vaginal Cream for conditions for which it was not prescribed. Do not give Premarin Vaginal Cream to other people, even if they have the same symptoms you have. It may harm them. **Keep Premarin Vaginal Cream out of the reach of children.**

This leaflet provides a summary of the most important information about Premarin Vaginal Cream. If you would like more information, talk with your healthcare provider or pharmacist. You can ask for information about Premarin Vaginal Cream that is written for health professionals. You can get more information by calling the toll free number 800-934-5556.

What are the ingredients in Premarin Vaginal Cream?

Premarin Vaginal Cream is a mixture of conjugated estrogens, which are a mixture of sodium estrone sulfate and sodium equilin sulfate and other components including estrone, equilin, and 17 α-dihydroequilin, together with smaller amounts of 17 α-estradiol, equilenin, and 17 α-dihydroequilenin salts. Premarin Vaginal Cream also contains cetyl esters wax, cetyl alcohol, white wax, glyceryl monostearate, propylene glycol monostearate, methyl stearate, benzyl alcohol, sodium lauryl sulfate, glycerin, and mineral oil.

Premarin® (conjugated estrogens) Vaginal Cream—Each gram contains 0.625 mg conjugated estrogens, USP.

Combination package: Each contains Net Wt. 1 ½ oz (42.5 g) tube with one plastic applicator calibrated in ½ g increments to a maximum of 2 g (NDC 0046-0872-93).

Also Available—Refill package: Each contains Net Wt. 1 ½ oz (42.5 g) tube (NDC 0046-0872-01).

Store at room temperature (approximately 25° C).

This product's label may have been revised after this insert was used in production. For further product information and current package insert, please visit www.wyeth.com or call our medical communications department toll-free at 1-800-934-5556.

Wyeth®

Wyeth Pharmaceuticals Inc. W10413C004
Philadelphia, PA 19101 ET01
Revised July 6, 2004

Shown in Product Identification Guide, page 336

PREMPRO™ ℞

[prĕm-prō]

(conjugated estrogens/medroxyprogesterone acetate tablets)

PREMPHASE®

[prĕm-fāz]

(conjugated estrogens/medroxyprogesterone acetate tablets)

℞ only

WARNING

Estrogens and progestins should not be used for the prevention of cardiovascular disease.

The Women's Health Initiative (WHI) study reported increased risks of myocardial infarction, stroke, invasive breast cancer, pulmonary emboli, and deep vein thrombosis in postmenopausal women (50 to 79 years of age) during 5 years of treatment with conjugated estrogens (0.625 mg) combined with medroxyprogesterone acetate (2.5 mg) relative to placebo. (See **CLINICAL PHARMACOLOGY, Clinical Studies.**)

The Women's Health Initiative Memory Study (WHIMS), a substudy of WHI, reported increased risk of developing probable dementia in postmenopausal women 65 years of age or older during 4 years of treatment with conjugated estrogens plus medroxyprogesterone acetate relative to placebo. It is unknown whether this finding applies to younger postmenopausal women or to women taking estrogen alone therapy. (See **CLINICAL PHARMACOLOGY, Clinical Studies.**)

Other doses of conjugated estrogens and medroxyprogesterone acetate, and other combinations and dosage forms of estrogens and progestins were not studied in the WHI clinical trials and, in the absence of comparable data, these risks should be assumed to be similar.

Continued on next page

Prempro/Premphase—Cont.

Because of these risks, estrogens with or without progestins should be prescribed at the lowest effective doses and for the shortest duration consistent with treatment goals and risks for the individual woman.

DESCRIPTION

PREMPRO™ 0.3 mg/1.5 mg therapy consists of a single tablet containing 0.3 mg of the conjugated estrogens (CE) found in Premarin® tablets and 1.5 mg of medroxyprogesterone acetate (MPA) for oral administration.

PREMPRO 0.45 mg/1.5 mg therapy consists of a single tablet containing 0.45 mg of the conjugated estrogens found in Premarin tablets and 1.5 mg of medroxyprogesterone acetate for oral administration.

PREMPRO 0.625 mg/2.5 mg therapy consists of a single tablet containing 0.625 mg of the conjugated estrogens found in Premarin tablets and 2.5 mg of medroxyprogesterone acetate for oral administration.

PREMPRO 0.625 mg/5 mg therapy consists of a single tablet containing 0.625 mg of the conjugated estrogens found in Premarin tablets and 5 mg of medroxyprogesterone acetate for oral administration.

PREMPHASE® therapy consists of two separate tablets, a maroon Premarin tablet containing 0.625 mg of conjugated estrogens that is taken orally on days 1 through 14 and a light-blue tablet containing 0.625 mg of the conjugated estrogens found in Premarin tablets and 5 mg of medroxyprogesterone acetate that is taken orally on days 15 through 28.

The conjugated estrogens found in Premarin tablets are a mixture of sodium estrone sulfate and sodium equilin sulfate, obtained exclusively from natural sources and blended to represent the average composition of materials derived from pregnant mares' urine. They contain as concomitant components, as sodium sulfate conjugates, 17 α-dihydroequilin, 17 α-estradiol and 17 β-dihydroequilin.

Medroxyprogesterone acetate is a derivative of progesterone. It is a white to off-white, odorless, crystalline powder, stable in air, melting between 200°C and 210°C. It is freely soluble in chloroform, soluble in acetone and in dioxane, sparingly soluble in alcohol and in methanol, slightly soluble in ether, and insoluble in water. The chemical name for MPA is pregn-4-ene-3, 20-dione, 17-(acetyloxy)-6-methyl-, (6α)-. Its molecular formula is $C_{24}H_{34}O_4$, with a molecular weight of 386.53. Its structural formula is:

PREMPRO 0.3 mg/1.5 mg

Each cream tablet for oral administration contains 0.3 mg conjugated estrogens, 1.5 mg medroxyprogesterone acetate, and the following inactive ingredients: calcium phosphate tribasic, calcium sulfate, carnauba wax, cellulose, glyceryl monooleate, lactose, magnesium stearate, methylcellulose, pharmaceutical glaze, polyethylene glycol, sucrose, povidone, titanium dioxide, yellow ferric oxide.

PREMPRO 0.45 mg/1.5 mg

Each gold tablet for oral administration contains 0.45 mg conjugated estrogens, 1.5 mg medroxyprogesterone acetate and the following inactive ingredients: calcium phosphate tribasic, calcium sulfate, carnauba wax, cellulose, glyceryl monooleate, lactose, magnesium stearate, methylcellulose, pharmaceutical glaze, polyethylene glycol, sucrose, povidone, titanium dioxide, yellow ferric oxide.

PREMPRO 0.625 mg/2.5 mg

Each peach tablet for oral administration contains 0.625 mg conjugated estrogens, 2.5 mg of medroxyprogesterone acetate and the following inactive ingredients: calcium phosphate tribasic, calcium sulfate, carnauba wax, cellulose, glyceryl monooleate, lactose, magnesium stearate, methylcellulose, pharmaceutical glaze, polyethylene glycol, sucrose, povidone, titanium dioxide, red ferric oxide.

PREMPRO 0.625 mg/5 mg

Each light-blue tablet for oral administration contains 0.625 mg conjugated estrogens, 5 mg of medroxyprogesterone acetate and the following inactive ingredients: calcium phosphate tribasic, calcium sulfate, carnauba wax, cellulose, glyceryl monooleate, lactose, magnesium stearate, methylcellulose, pharmaceutical glaze, polyethylene glycol, sucrose, povidone, titanium dioxide, FD&C Blue No. 2.

PREMPHASE

Each maroon Premarin tablet for oral administration contains 0.625 mg of conjugated estrogens and the following inactive ingredients: calcium phosphate tribasic, calcium sulfate, carnauba wax, cellulose, glyceryl monooleate, lactose, magnesium stearate, methylcellulose, pharmaceutical glaze, polyethylene glycol, stearic acid, sucrose, titanium dioxide, FD&C Blue No. 2, D&C Red No. 27, FD&C Red No. 40. These tablets comply with USP Drug Release Test 1.

Each light-blue tablet for oral administration contains 0.625 mg of conjugated estrogens and 5 mg of medroxyprogesterone acetate and the following inactive ingredients:

TABLE 1. PHARMACOKINETIC PARAMETERS FOR UNCONJUGATED AND CONJUGATED ESTROGENS (CE) AND MEDROXYPROGESTERONE ACETATE (MPA)

DRUG	2 × 0.625 mg CE/2.5 mg MPA Combination Tablets (n=54)				2 × 0.625 mg CE/5 mg MPA Combination Tablets (n=51)			
PK Parameter Arithmetic Mean (%CV)	C_{max} (pg/mL)	t_{max} (h)	$t_{1/2}$ (h)	AUC (pg•h/mL)	C_{max} (pg/mL)	t_{max} (h)	$t_{1/2}$ (h)	AUC (pg•h/mL)
Unconjugated Estrogens								
Estrone	175 (23)	7.6 (24)	31.6 (23)	5358 (34)	124 (43)	10 (35)	62.2 (137)	6303 (40)
BA* -Estrone	159 (26)	7.6 (24)	16.9 (34)	3313 (40)	104 (49)	10 (35)	26.0 (100)	3136 (51)
Equilin	71 (31)	5.8 (34)	9.9 (35)	951 (43)	54 (43)	8.9 (34)	15.5 (53)	1179 (56)
PK Parameter Arithmetic Mean (%CV)	C_{max} (ng/mL)	t_{max} (h)	$t_{1/2}$ (h)	AUC (ng•h/mL)	C_{max} (ng/mL)	t_{max} (h)	$t_{1/2}$ (h)	AUC (ng•h/mL)
Conjugated Estrogens								
Total Estrone	6.6 (38)	6.1 (28)	20.7 (34)	116 (59)	6.3 (48)	9.1 (29)	23.6 (36)	151 (42)
BA* -Total Estrone	6.4 (39)	6.1 (28)	15.4 (34)	100 (57)	6.2 (48)	9.1 (29)	20.6 (35)	139 (40)
Total Equilin	5.1 (45)	4.6 (35)	11.4 (25)	50 (70)	4.2 (52)	7.0 (36)	17.2 (131)	72 (50)
PK Parameter Arithmetic Mean (%CV)	C_{max} (ng/mL)	t_{max} (h)	$t_{1/2}$ (h)	AUC (ng•h/mL)	C_{max} (ng/mL)	t_{max} (h)	$t_{1/2}$ (h)	AUC (ng•h/mL)
Medroxyprogesterone Acetate								
MPA	1.5 (40)	2.8 (54)	37.6 (30)	37 (30)	4.8 (31)	2.4 (50)	46.3 (39)	102 (28)

BA* = Baseline adjusted
C_{max} = peak plasma concentration
t_{max} = time peak concentration occurs
$t_{1/2}$ = apparent terminal-phase disposition half-life ($0.693/\lambda_z$)
AUC = total area under the concentration-time curve

TABLE 2. PHARMACOKINETIC PARAMETERS FOR UNCONJUGATED AND CONJUGATED ESTROGENS (CE) AND MEDROXYPROGESTERONE ACETATE (MPA)

DRUG	2 × 0.3 mg CE/1.5 mg MPA Combination (n = 30)				2 × 0.45 mg CE/1.5 mg MPA Combination (n = 61)			
PK Parameter Arithmetic Mean (%CV)	C_{max} (pg/mL)	t_{max} (h)	$t_{1/2}$ (h)	AUC (pg•h/mL)	C_{max} (pg/mL)	t_{max} (h)	$t_{1/2}$ (h)	AUC (pg•h/mL)
Unconjugated Estrogens								
Estrone	79 (35)	9.4 (86)	51.3 (30)	5029 (45)	91 (30)	9.8 (47)	48.9 (28)	5786 (42)
BA* -Estrone	56 (46)	9.4 (86)	19.8 (39)	1429 (49)	67 (37)	9.8 (47)	21.5 (49)	2042 (52)
Equilin	30 (43)	7.9 (42)	14.0 (75)	590 (42)	35 (40)	8.5 (34)	16.4 (49)	825 (44)
PK Parameter Arithmetic Mean (%CV)	C_{max} (ng/mL)	t_{max} (h)	$t_{1/2}$ (h)	AUC (ng•h/mL)	C_{max} (ng/mL)	t_{max} (h)	$t_{1/2}$ (h)	AUC (ng•h/mL)
Conjugated Estrogens								
Total Estrone	2.4 (38)	7.1 (27)	26.5 (33)	62 (48)	3.0 (37)	8.2 (39)	25.9 (23)	78 (40)
BA* -Total Estrone	2.2 (36)	7.1 (27)	16.3 (32)	41 (44)	2.8 (36)	8.2 (39)	16.9 (36)	56 (39)
Total Equilin	1.5 (47)	5.5 (29)	11.5 (24)	22 (41)	1.9 (42)	7.2 (33)	12.2 (25)	31 (52)
PK Parameter Arithmetic Mean (%CV)	C_{max} (ng/mL)	t_{max} (h)	$t_{1/2}$ (h)	AUC (ng•h/mL)	C_{max} (ng/mL)	t_{max} (h)	$t_{1/2}$ (h)	AUC (ng•h/mL)
Medroxyprogesterone Acetate								
MPA	1.2 (42)	2.8 (61)	42.3 (34)	29.4 (30)	1.2 (42)	2.7 (52)	47.2 (41)	32.0 (36)

BA* = Baseline adjusted
C_{max} = peak plasma concentration
t_{max} = time peak concentration occurs
$t_{1/2}$ = apparent terminal-phase disposition half-life ($0.693/\lambda_z$)
AUC = total area under the concentration-time curve

calcium phosphate tribasic, calcium sulfate, carnauba wax, cellulose, glyceryl monooleate, lactose, magnesium stearate, methylcellulose, pharmaceutical glaze, polyethylene glycol, sucrose, povidone, titanium dioxide, FD&C Blue No. 2.

CLINICAL PHARMACOLOGY

Endogenous estrogens are largely responsible for the development and maintenance of the female reproductive system and secondary sexual characteristics. Although circulating estrogens exist in a dynamic equilibrium of metabolic interconversions, estradiol is the principal intracellular human estrogen and is substantially more potent than its metabolites, estrone and estriol, at the receptor level.

The primary source of estrogen in normally cycling adult women is the ovarian follicle, which secretes 70 to 500 mcg of estradiol daily, depending on the phase of the menstrual cycle. After menopause, most endogenous estrogen is produced by conversion of androstenedione, secreted by the adrenal cortex, to estrone by peripheral tissues. Thus, estrone and the sulfate-conjugated form, estrone sulfate, are the most abundant circulating estrogens in postmenopausal women.

Estrogens act through binding to nuclear receptors in estrogen-responsive tissues. To date, two estrogen receptors have been identified. These vary in proportion from tissue to tissue.

Circulating estrogens modulate the pituitary secretion of the gonadotropins, luteinizing hormone (LH) and follicle stimulating hormone (FSH) through a negative feedback mechanism. Estrogens act to reduce the elevated levels of these gonadotropins seen in postmenopausal women.

Parenterally administered medroxyprogesterone acetate (MPA) inhibits gonadotropin production, which in turn prevents follicular maturation and ovulation, although available data indicate that this does not occur when the usually recommended oral dosage is given as single daily doses. MPA may achieve its beneficial effect on the endometrium in part by decreasing nuclear estrogen receptors and suppression of epithelial DNA synthesis in endometrial tissue. Androgenic and anabolic effects of MPA have been noted, but the drug is apparently devoid of significant estrogenic activity.

Pharmacokinetics

Absorption

Conjugated estrogens are soluble in water and are well absorbed from the gastrointestinal tract after release from the drug formulation. However, PREMPRO and PREMPHASE contain a formulation of medroxyprogesterone acetate (MPA) that is immediately released and conjugated estrogens that are slowly released over several hours. MPA is well absorbed from the gastrointestinal tract. Table 1 summarizes the mean pharmacokinetic parameters for unconjugated and conjugated estrogens, and medroxyprogesterone acetate following administration of 2 PREMPRO 0.625 mg/2.5 mg and 2 PREMPRO 0.625 mg/5 mg tablets to healthy postmenopausal women.

[See table 1 above]

Table 2 summarizes the mean pharmacokinetic parameters for unconjugated and conjugated estrogens and medroxyprogesterone acetate following administration of 2 PREMPRO 0.45 mg/1.5 mg and 2 PREMPRO 0.3 mg/1.5 mg tablets to healthy, postmenopausal women.

[See table 2 above]

Food-Effect: Single dose studies in healthy, postmenopausal women were conducted to investigate any potential drug interaction when PREMPRO or PREMPHASE is administered with a high fat breakfast. Administration with food decreased the C_{max} of total estrone by 18 to 34% and increased total equilin C_{max} by 38% compared to the fasting state, with no other effect on the rate or extent of absorption of other conjugated or unconjugated estrogens. Administration with food approximately doubles MPA C_{max} and increases MPA AUC by approximately 20 to 30%.

Dose Proportionality: The C_{max} and AUC values for MPA observed in two separate pharmacokinetic studies conducted with 2 PREMPRO 0.625 mg/2.5 mg or 2 PREMPRO or PREMPHASE 0.625 mg/5 mg tablets exhibited nonlinear dose proportionality; doubling the MPA dose from 2 × 2.5 to 2 × 5.0 mg increased the mean C_{max} and AUC by 3.2 and 2.8 folds, respectively.

The dose proportionality of estrogens and medroxyprogesterone acetate was assessed by combining pharmacokinetic data across another two studies totaling 61 healthy, postmenopausal women. Single conjugated estrogens doses of 2 × 0.3 mg, 2 × 0.45 mg, or 2 × 0.625 mg were administered either alone or in combination with medroxyprogesterone acetate doses of 2 × 1.5 mg or 2 × 2.5 mg. Most of the estrogen components demonstrated dose proportionality; however, several estrogen components did not. Medroxyprogesterone acetate pharmacokinetic parameters increased in a dose-proportional manner.

Distribution

The distribution of exogenous estrogens is similar to that of endogenous estrogens. Estrogens are widely distributed in the body and are generally found in higher concentrations in the sex hormone target organs. Estrogens circulate in the blood largely bound to sex hormone binding globulin (SHBG) and albumin. MPA is approximately 90% bound to plasma proteins but does not bind to SHBG.

Metabolism

Exogenous estrogens are metabolized in the same manner as endogenous estrogens. Circulating estrogens exist in a dynamic equilibrium of metabolic interconversions. These transformations take place mainly in the liver. Estradiol is converted reversibly to estrone, and both can be converted to estriol, which is the major urinary metabolite. Estrogens also undergo enterohepatic recirculation via sulfate and glucuronide conjugation in the liver, biliary secretion of conjugates into the intestine, and hydrolysis in the gut followed by reabsorption. In postmenopausal women a significant proportion of the circulating estrogens exists as sulfate conjugates, especially estrone sulfate, which serves as a circulating reservoir for the formation of more active estrogens. Metabolism and elimination of MPA occur primarily in the liver via hydroxylation, with subsequent conjugation and elimination in the urine.

Excretion

Estradiol, estrone, and estriol are excreted in the urine along with glucuronide and sulfate conjugates. Most metabolites of MPA are excreted as glucuronide conjugates with only minor amounts excreted as sulfates.

Special Populations

No pharmacokinetic studies were conducted in special populations, including patients with renal or hepatic impairment.

Drug Interactions

Data from a single-dose drug-drug interaction study involving conjugated estrogens and medroxyprogesterone acetate indicate that the pharmacokinetic disposition of both drugs is not altered when the drugs are coadministered. No other clinical drug-drug interaction studies have been conducted with conjugated estrogens.

In vitro and in vivo studies have shown that estrogens are metabolized partially by cytochrome P450 3A4 (CYP3A4). Therefore, inducers or inhibitors of CYP3A4 may affect estrogen drug metabolism. Inducers of CYP3A4 such as St. John's Wort preparations (Hypericum perforatum), phenobarbital, carbamazepine, and rifampin may reduce plasma concentrations of estrogens, possibly resulting in a decrease in therapeutic effects and/or changes in the uterine bleeding profile. Inhibitors of CYP3A4 such as erythromycin, clarithromycin, ketoconazole, itraconazole, ritonavir and grapefruit juice may increase plasma concentrations of estrogens and may result in side effects.

Clinical Studies

Effects on vasomotor symptoms.

In the first year of the Health and Osteoporosis, Progestin and Estrogen (HOPE) Study, a total of 2805 postmenopausal women (average age 53.3 ± 4.9 years) were randomly assigned to one of eight treatment groups of either placebo or conjugated estrogens with or without medroxyprogesterone acetate. Efficacy for vasomotor symptoms was assessed during the first 12 weeks of treatment in a subset of symptomatic women (n = 241) who had at least 7 moderate to severe hot flushes daily or at least 50 moderate to severe hot flushes during the week before randomization. PREMPRO 0.625 mg/2.5 mg, 0.45 mg/1.5 mg, and 0.3 mg/1.5 mg were shown to be statistically better than placebo at weeks 4 and 12 for relief of both the frequency and severity of moderate to severe vasomotor symptoms. Table 3 shows the adjusted mean number of hot flushes in the PREMPRO 0.625 mg/2.5 mg, 0.45 mg/1.5 mg, 0.3 mg/1.5 mg, and placebo groups during the initial 12-week period.

[See table 3 above]

Effects on vulvar and vaginal atrophy.

Results of vaginal maturation indexes at cycles 6 and 13 showed that the differences from placebo were statistically significant ($p < 0.001$) for all treatment groups (conjugated estrogens alone and conjugated estrogens/medroxyprogesterone acetate treatment groups).

Effects on the endometrium.

In a 1-year clinical trial of 1376 women (average age 54.0 ± 4.6 years) randomized to PREMPRO 0.625 mg/2.5 mg (n=340), PREMPRO 0.625 mg/5 mg (n=338), PREMPHASE 0.625 mg/5 mg (n=351), or Premarin 0.625 mg alone (n=347), results of evaluable biopsies at 12 months (n=279, 274, 277, and 283, respectively) showed a reduced risk of endometrial hyperplasia in the two PREMPRO treatment groups (less than 1%) and in the PREMPHASE treatment group (less than 1%; 1% when focal hyperplasia was included) compared to the Premarin group (8%; 20% when focal hyperplasia was included). See Table 4.

[See table 4 above]

In the first year of the Health and Osteoporosis, Progestin and Estrogen (HOPE) Study, 2001 women (average age 53.3 ± 4.9 years) of whom 88% were Caucasian were treated with either Premarin 0.625 mg alone (n = 348), Premarin 0.45 mg alone (n = 338), Premarin 0.3 mg alone (n = 326) or PREMPRO 0.625 mg/2.5 mg (n = 331), PREMPRO 0.45 mg/1.5 mg (n = 331) or PREMPRO 0.3 mg/1.5 mg (n = 327). Results of evaluable endometrial biopsies at 12 months showed a reduced risk of endometrial hyperplasia or cancer in the PREMPRO treatment groups compared with the corresponding Premarin alone treatment groups, except for the PREMPRO 0.3 mg/1.5 mg and Premarin 0.3 mg alone groups, in each of which there was only 1 case. See Table 5. No endometrial hyperplasia or cancer was noted in those patients treated with the continuous combined regimens who continued for a second year in the osteoporosis and metabolic substudy of the HOPE study. See Table 6.

[See table 5 above]

[See table 6 at top of next page]

Effects on uterine bleeding or spotting.

The effects of PREMPRO on uterine bleeding or spotting, as recorded on daily diary cards, were evaluated in 2 clinical trials. Results are shown in Figures 1 and 2.

TABLE 3. SUMMARY TABULATION OF THE NUMBER OF HOT FLUSHES PER DAY – MEAN VALUES AND COMPARISONS BETWEEN THE ACTIVE TREATMENT GROUPS AND THE PLACEBO GROUP – PATIENTS WITH AT LEAST 7 MODERATE TO SEVERE FLUSHES PER DAY OR AT LEAST 50 PER WEEK AT BASELINE, LOCF

Treatment[a] (No. of Patients) Time Period (week)	Baseline Mean ± SD	Observed Mean ± SD	Mean Change ± SD	p-Values vs. Placebo[b]
	No. of Hot Flushes/Day			
0.625 mg/2.5 mg (n=34)				
4	11.98 ± 3.54	3.19 ± 3.74	–8.78 ± 4.72	<0.001
12	11.98 ± 3.54	1.16 ± 2.22	–10.82 ± 4.61	<0.001
0.45 mg/1.5 mg (n=29)				
4	12.61 ± 4.29	3.64 ± 3.61	–8.98 ± 4.74	<0.001
12	12.61 ± 4.29	1.69 ± 3.36	–10.92 ± 4.63	<0.001
0.3 mg/1.5 mg (n=33)				
4	11.30 ± 3.13	3.70 ± 3.29	–7.60 ± 4.71	<0.001
12	11.30 ± 3.13	1.31 ± 2.82	–10.00 ± 4.60	<0.001
Placebo (n=28)				
4	11.69 ± 3.87	7.89 ± 5.28	–3.80 ± 4.71	–
12	11.69 ± 3.87	5.71 ± 5.22	–5.98 ± 4.60	–

a: Identified by dosage (mg) of Premarin/MPA or placebo.
b: There were no statistically significant differences between the 0.625 mg/2.5 mg, 0.45 mg/1.5 mg, and 0.3 mg/1.5 mg groups at any time period.

TABLE 4. INCIDENCE OF ENDOMETRIAL HYPERPLASIA AFTER ONE YEAR OF TREATMENT

	Groups			
	PREMPRO 0.625 mg/2.5 mg	PREMPRO 0.625 mg/5 mg	PREMPHASE 0.625 mg/5 mg	Premarin 0.625 mg
Total number of patients	340	338	351	347
Number of patients with evaluable biopsies	279	274	277	283
No. (%) of patients with biopsies				
• all focal and non-focal hyperplasia	2 (<1)*	0 (0)*	3 (1)*	57 (20)
• excluding focal cystic hyperplasia	2 (<1)*	0 (0)*	1 (<1)*	25 (8)

*Significant (p<0.001) in comparison with Premarin (0.625 mg) alone.

TABLE 5. INCIDENCE OF ENDOMETRIAL HYPERPLASIA/CANCER[a] AFTER ONE YEAR OF TREATMENT[b]

Patient	Groups					
	Prempro 0.625 mg/ 2.5 mg	Premarin 0.625 mg	Prempro 0.45 mg/ 1.5 mg	Premarin 0.45 mg	Prempro 0.3 mg/ 1.5 mg	Premarin 0.3 mg
Total number of patients	331	348	331	338	327	326
Number of patients with evaluable biopsies	278	249	272	279	271	269
No. (%) of patients with biopsies						
• hyperplasia/cancer[a] (consensus[c])	0 (0)[d]	20 (8)	1 (<1)[a,d]	9 (3)	(<1)[e]	1 (<1)[a]

a: All cases of hyperplasia/cancer were endometrial hyperplasia except for 1 patient in the Premarin 0.3 mg group diagnosed with endometrial cancer based on endometrial biopsy and 1 patient in the Premarin/MPA 0.45 mg/1.5 mg group diagnosed with endometrial cancer based on endometrial biopsy.
b: Two (2) primary pathologists evaluated each endometrial biopsy. Where there was lack of agreement on the presence or absence of hyperplasia/cancer between the two, a third pathologist adjudicated (consensus).
c: For an endometrial biopsy to be counted as consensus endometrial hyperplasia or cancer, at least 2 pathologists had to agree on the diagnosis.
d: Significant (p <0.05) in comparison with corresponding dose of Premarin alone.
e: Non-significant in comparison with corresponding dose of Premarin alone.

FIGURE 1. PATIENTS WITH CUMULATIVE AMENORRHEA OVER TIME PERCENTAGES OF WOMEN WITH NO BLEEDING OR SPOTTING AT A GIVEN CYCLE THROUGH CYCLE 13 INTENT-TO-TREAT POPULATION, LOCF

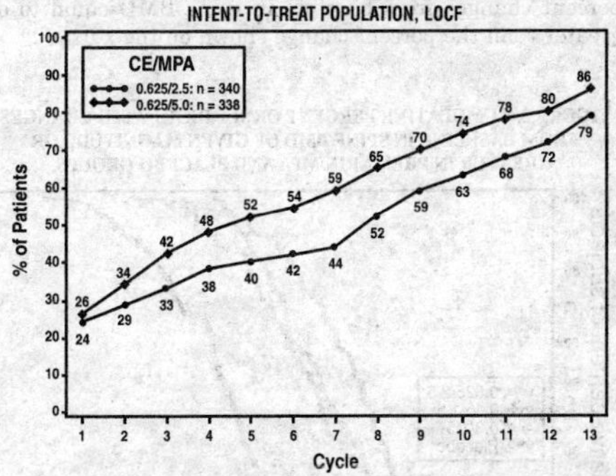

Note: The percentage of patients who were amenorrheic in a given cycle and through cycle 13 is shown. If data were

Continued on next page

Prempro/Premphase—Cont.

missing, the bleeding value from the last reported day was carried forward (LOCF).

FIGURE 2. PATIENTS WITH CUMULATIVE AMENORRHEA OVER TIME PERCENTAGES OF WOMEN WITH NO BLEEDING OR SPOTTING AT A GIVEN CYCLE THROUGH CYCLE 13 INTENT-TO-TREAT POPULATION, LOCF

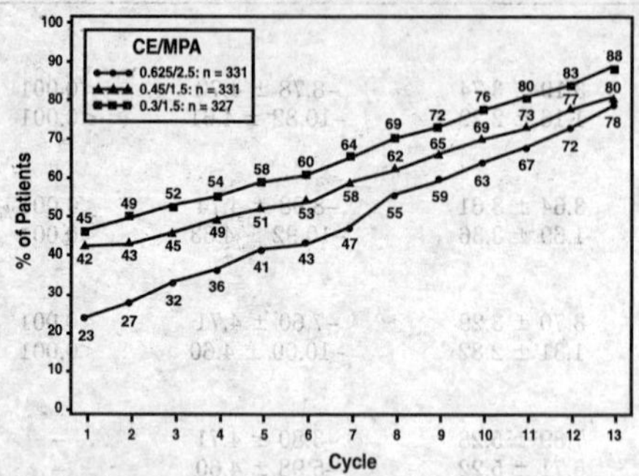

Note: The percentage of patients who were amenorrheic in a given cycle and through cycle 13 is shown. If data were missing, the bleeding value from the last reported day was carried forward (LOCF).

Effects on bone mineral density.

Health and Osteoporosis, Progestin and Estrogen (HOPE) Study

The HOPE study was a double-blind, randomized, placebo/active-drug-controlled, multicenter study of healthy postmenopausal women with an intact uterus. Subjects (mean age 53.3 ± 4.9 years) were 2.3 ± 0.9 years, on average, since menopause, and took one 600-mg tablet of elemental calcium (Caltrate) daily. Subjects were not given vitamin D supplements. They were treated with PREMPRO 0.625 mg/2.5 mg, 0.45 mg/1.5 mg or 0.3 mg/1.5 mg, comparable doses of Premarin alone, or placebo. Prevention of bone loss was assessed by measurement of bone mineral density (BMD), primarily at the anteroposterior lumbar spine (L_2 to L_4). Secondarily, BMD measurements of the total body, femoral neck, and trochanter were also analyzed. Serum osteocalcin, urinary calcium, and N-telopeptide were used as bone turnover markers (BTM) at cycles 6, 13, 19, and 26.

Intent-to-treat subjects

All active treatment groups showed significant differences from placebo in each of the 4 BMD endpoints. These significant differences were seen at cycles 6, 13, 19, and 26. With PREMPRO, the mean percent increases in the primary efficacy measure (L_2 to L_4 BMD) at the final on-therapy evaluation (cycle 26 for those who completed and the last available evaluation for those who discontinued early) were 3.28% with 0.625 mg/2.5 mg, 2.18% with 0.45 mg/1.5 mg, and 1.71% with 0.3 mg/1.5 mg. The placebo group showed a mean percent decrease from baseline at the final evaluation of 2.45%. These results show that the lower dose regimens of PREMPRO were effective in increasing L_2 to L_4 BMD compared with placebo and, therefore, support the efficacy of lower doses of PREMPRO.

The analysis for the other 3 BMD endpoints yielded mean percent changes from baseline in femoral trochanter that were generally larger than those seen for L_2 to L_4 and changes in femoral neck and total body that were generally smaller than those seen for L_2 to L_4. Significant differences between groups indicated that each of the PREMPRO treatment groups was more effective than placebo for all 3 of these additional BMD endpoints. With regard to femoral neck and total body, the continuous combined treatment groups all showed mean percent increases in BMD while the placebo group showed mean percent decreases. For femoral trochanter, each of the PREMPRO groups showed a mean percent increase that was significantly greater than the small increase seen in the placebo group. The percent changes from baseline to final evaluation are shown in Table 7.

[See table 7 above]

Figure 3 shows the cumulative percentage of subjects with percent changes from baseline in spine BMD equal to or greater than the percent change shown on the x-axis.

FIGURE 3. CUMULATIVE PERCENT OF SUBJECTS WITH CHANGES FROM BASELINE IN SPINE BMD OF GIVEN MAGNITUDE OR GREATER IN PREMARIN/MPA AND PLACEBO GROUPS

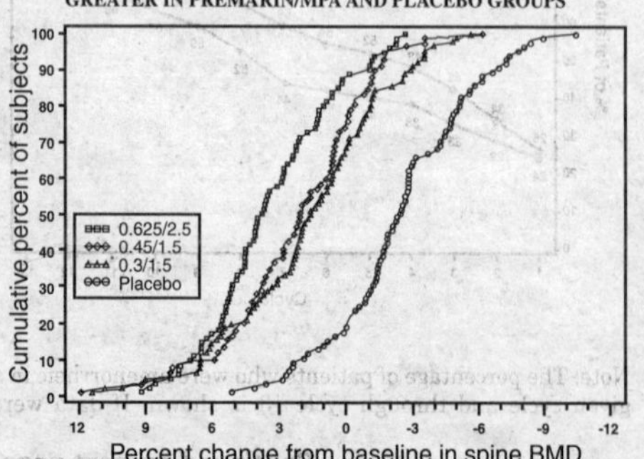

TABLE 6. OSTEOPOROSIS AND METABOLIC SUBSTUDY, INCIDENCE OF ENDOMETRIAL HYPERPLASIA/CANCER[a] AFTER TWO YEARS OF TREATMENT[b]

Patient	Groups: Prempro 0.625 mg/ 2.5 mg	Premarin 0.625 mg	Prempro 0.45 mg/ 1.5 mg	Premarin 0.45 mg	Prempro 0.3 mg/ 1.5 mg	Premarin 0.3 mg
Total number of patients	75	65	75	74	79	73
Number of patients with evaluable biopsies	62	55	69	67	75	63
No. (%) of patients with biopsies						
• hyperplasia/cancer[a] (consensus[c])	0 (0)[d]	15 (27)	0 (0)[d]	10 (15)	0 (0)[d]	2 (3)

a: All cases of hyperplasia/cancer were endometrial hyperplasia in patients who continued for a second year in the osteoporosis and metabolic substudy of the HOPE study.
b: Two (2) primary pathologists evaluated each endometrial biopsy. Where there was lack of agreement on the presence or absence of hyperplasia/cancer between the two, a third pathologist adjudicated (consensus).
c: For an endometrial biopsy to be counted as consensus endometrial hyperplasia or cancer, at least 2 pathologists had to agree on the diagnosis.
d: Significant ($p < 0.05$) in comparison with corresponding dose of Premarin alone.

TABLE 7. PERCENT CHANGE IN BONE MINERAL DENSITY: COMPARISON BETWEEN ACTIVE AND PLACEBO GROUPS IN THE INTENT-TO-TREAT POPULATION, LAST OBSERVATION CARRIED FORWARD

Region Evaluated Treatment Group[a]	No. of Subjects	Baseline (g/cm²) Mean ± SD	Change from Baseline (%) Adjusted Mean ± SE	p-Value vs Placebo
L_2 to L_4 BMD				
0.625/2.5	81	1.14 ± 0.16	3.28 ± 0.37	<0.001
0.45/1.5	89	1.16 ± 0.14	2.18 ± 0.35	<0.001
0.3/1.5	90	1.14 ± 0.15	1.71 ± 0.35	<0.001
Placebo	85	1.14 ± 0.14	−2.45 ± 0.36	
Total body BMD				
0.625/2.5	81	1.14 ± 0.08	0.87 ± 0.17	<0.001
0.45/1.5	89	1.14 ± 0.07	0.59 ± 0.17	<0.001
0.3/1.5	91	1.13 ± 0.08	0.60 ± 0.16	<0.001
Placebo	85	1.13 ± 0.08	−1.50 ± 0.17	
Femoral neck BMD				
0.625/2.5	81	0.89 ± 0.14	1.62 ± 0.46	<0.001
0.45/1.5	89	0.89 ± 0.12	1.48 ± 0.44	<0.001
0.3/1.5	91	0.86 ± 0.11	1.31 ± 0.43	<0.001
Placebo	85	0.88 ± 0.14	−1.72 ± 0.45	
Femoral trochanter BMD				
0.625/2.5	81	0.77 ± 0.14	3.35 ± 0.59	0.002
0.45/1.5	89	0.76 ± 0.12	2.84 ± 0.57	0.011
0.3/1.5	91	0.76 ± 0.12	3.93 ± 0.56	<0.001
Placebo	85	0.75 ± 0.12	0.81 ± 0.58	

a: Identified by dosage (mg/mg) of Premarin/MPA or placebo.

The mean percent changes from baseline in L_2 to L_4 BMD for women who completed the bone density study are shown with standard error bars by treatment group in Figure 4. Significant differences between each of the PREMPRO dosage groups and placebo were found at cycles 6, 13, 19, and 26.

FIGURE 4. ADJUSTED MEAN (SE) PERCENT CHANGE FROM BASELINE AT EACH CYCLE IN SPINE BMD: SUBJECTS COMPLETING IN PREMARIN/MPA GROUPS AND PLACEBO

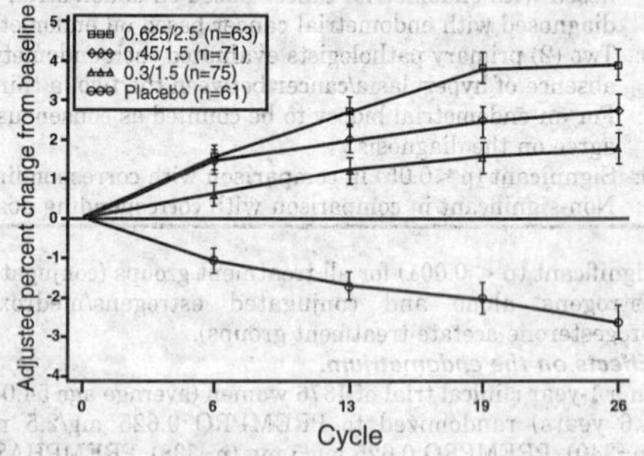

The bone turnover markers, serum osteocalcin and urinary N-telopeptide, significantly decreased ($p < 0.001$) in all active-treatment groups at cycles 6, 13, 19, and 26 compared with the placebo group. Larger mean decreases from baseline were seen with the active groups than with the placebo group. Significant differences from placebo were seen less frequently in urine calcium; only with PREMPRO 0.625 mg/2.5 mg and 0.45 mg/1.5 mg were there significantly larger mean decreases than with placebo at 3 or more of the 4 time points.

Women's Health Initiative Studies.

A substudy of the Women's Health Initiative (WHI) enrolled 16,608 predominantly healthy postmenopausal women (average age of 63 years, range 50 to 79; 83.9% White, 6.5% Black, 5.5% Hispanic) to assess the risks and benefits of the use of PREMPRO (0.625 mg conjugated estrogens plus 2.5 mg medroxyprogesterone acetate per day) compared to placebo in the prevention of certain chronic diseases. The primary endpoint was the incidence of coronary heart disease (CHD) (nonfatal myocardial infarction and CHD death), with invasive breast cancer as the primary adverse outcome studied. A "global index" included the earliest occurrence of CHD, invasive breast cancer, stroke, pulmonary embolism (PE), endometrial cancer, colorectal cancer, hip fracture, or death due to other cause. The study did not evaluate the effects of PREMPRO on menopausal symptoms. The estrogen plus progestin substudy was stopped early because, according to the predefined stopping rule, the increased risk of breast cancer and cardiovascular events exceeded the specified benefits included in the "global index." Results are presented in Table 8 below:

[See table 8 at bottom of next page]

For those outcomes included in the "global index", the absolute excess risks per 10,000 women-years in the group treated with PREMPRO were 7 more CHD events, 8 more strokes, 8 more PEs, and 8 more invasive breast cancers, while the absolute risk reductions per 10,000 women-years were 6 fewer colorectal cancers and 5 fewer hip fractures. The absolute excess risk of events included in the "global index" was 19 per 10,000 women-years. There was no difference between the groups in terms of all-cause mortality. (See **BOXED WARNING, WARNINGS,** and **PRECAUTIONS.**)

Women's Health Initiative Memory Study.

The Women's Health Initiative Memory Study (WHIMS), a substudy of WHI, enrolled 4,532 predominantly healthy postmenopausal women 65 years of age and older (47% were age 65 to 69 years, 35% were 70 to 74 years, and 18% were 75 years of age and older) to evaluate the effects of PREMPRO (0.625 mg conjugated estrogens plus 2.5 mg medroxyprogesterone acetate) on the incidence of probable dementia (primary outcome) compared with placebo.

After an average follow-up of 4 years, 40 women in the estrogen/progestin group (45 per 10,000 women-years) and 21 in the placebo group (22 per 10,000 women-years) were diagnosed with probable dementia. The relative risk of probable dementia in the hormone therapy group was 2.05 (95% CI, 1.21 to 3.48) compared to placebo. Differences between groups became apparent in the first year of treatment. It is unknown whether these findings apply to younger postmenopausal women or to women taking estrogen alone therapy. (See **BOXED WARNING** and **WARNINGS, Dementia.**)

INDICATIONS AND USAGE

PREMPRO or PREMPHASE therapy is indicated in women who have a uterus for the:

1. Treatment of moderate to severe vasomotor symptoms associated with the menopause.
2. Treatment of moderate to severe symptoms of vulvar and vaginal atrophy associated with the menopause. When prescribing solely for the treatment of symptoms of vulvar and vaginal atrophy, topical vaginal products should be considered.
3. Prevention of postmenopausal osteoporosis. When prescribing solely for the prevention of postmenopausal osteoporosis, therapy should only be considered for women at significant risk of osteoporosis and for whom non-

estrogen medications are not considered to be appropriate. (See **CLINICAL PHARMACOLOGY, Clinical Studies.**)

The mainstays for decreasing the risk of postmenopausal osteoporosis are weight-bearing exercise, adequate calcium and vitamin D intake, and when indicated, pharmacologic therapy. Postmenopausal women require an average of 1500 mg/day of elemental calcium. Therefore, when not contraindicated, calcium supplementation may be helpful for women with suboptimal dietary intake. Vitamin D supplementation of 400-800 IU/day may also be required to ensure adequate daily intake in postmenopausal women.

CONTRAINDICATIONS

Estrogens/progestins combined should not be used in women with any of the following conditions:

1. Undiagnosed abnormal genital bleeding.
2. Known, suspected, or history of cancer of the breast.
3. Known or suspected estrogen-dependent neoplasia.
4. Active deep vein thrombosis, pulmonary embolism or a history of these conditions.
5. Active or recent (e.g., within past year) arterial thromboembolic disease (e.g., stroke, myocardial infarction).
6. Liver dysfunction or disease.
7. PREMPRO or PREMPHASE therapy should not be used in patients with known hypersensitivity to their ingredients.
8. Known or suspected pregnancy. There is no indication for PREMPRO or PREMPHASE in pregnancy. There appears to be little or no increased risk of birth defects in children born to women who have used estrogen and progestins from oral contraceptives inadvertently during pregnancy. (See **PRECAUTIONS.**)

WARNINGS

See **BOXED WARNING.**

1. Cardiovascular disorders.

Estrogen/progestin therapy has been associated with an increased risk of cardiovascular events such as myocardial infarction and stroke, as well as venous thrombosis and pulmonary embolism (venous thromboembolism or VTE). Should any of these occur or be suspected, estrogen/progestin therapy should be discontinued immediately.

Risk factors for arterial vascular disease (e.g., hypertension, diabetes mellitus, tobacco use, hypercholesterolemia, and obesity) and/or venous thromboembolism (e.g., personal history or family history of VTE, obesity, and systemic lupus erythematosus) should be managed appropriately.

a. Coronary heart disease and stroke. In the estrogen plus progestin substudy of the Women's Health Initiative (WHI) study, an increased risk of coronary heart disease (CHD) events (defined as nonfatal myocardial infarction and CHD death) was observed in women receiving PREMPRO compared to women receiving placebo (37 vs 30 per 10,000 women-years). The increase in risk was observed in year one and persisted. (See **CLINICAL PHARMACOLOGY, Clinical Studies.**)

In the same substudy of WHI, an increased risk of stroke was observed in women receiving PREMPRO compared to women receiving placebo (29 vs 21 per 10,000 women-years). The increase in risk was observed after the first year and persisted.

In postmenopausal women with documented heart disease (n = 2,763, average age 66.7 years) a controlled clinical trial of secondary prevention of cardiovascular disease (Heart and Estrogen/progestin Replacement Study; HERS) treatment with PREMPRO (0.625 mg conjugated estrogens plus 2.5 mg medroxyprogesterone acetate per day) demonstrated no cardiovascular benefit. During an average follow-up of 4.1 years, treatment with PREMPRO did not reduce the overall rate of CHD events in postmenopausal women with established coronary heart disease. There were more CHD events in the PREMPRO-treated group than in the placebo group in year 1, but not during the subsequent years. Two thousand three hundred and twenty one women from the original HERS trial agreed to participate in an open label extension of HERS, HERS II. Average follow-up in HERS II was an additional 2.7 years, for a total of 6.8 years overall. Rates of CHD events were comparable among women in the PREMPRO group and the placebo group in HERS, HERS II, and overall.

Large doses of estrogen (5 mg conjugated estrogens per day), comparable to those used to treat cancer of the prostate and breast, have been shown in a large prospective clinical trial in men to increase the risk of nonfatal myocardial infarction, pulmonary embolism, and thrombophlebitis.

b. Venous thromboembolism (VTE). In the estrogen plus progestin substudy of WHI, a 2-fold greater rate of VTE, including deep venous thrombosis and pulmonary embolism, was observed in women receiving PREMPRO compared to women receiving placebo. The rate of VTE was 34 per 10,000 women-years in the PREMPRO group compared to 16 per 10,000 women-years in the placebo group. The increase in VTE risk was observed during the first year and persisted. (See **CLINICAL PHARMACOLOGY, Clinical Studies.**)

If feasible, estrogens should be discontinued at least 4 to 6 weeks before surgery of the type associated with an increased risk of thromboembolism, or during periods of prolonged immobilization.

2. Malignant neoplasms.

a. Breast cancer.

The use of estrogens and progestins by postmenopausal women has been reported to increase the risk of breast cancer. The most important randomized clinical trial providing information about this issue is the Women's Health Initiative (WHI) trial of estrogen plus progestin (see **CLINICAL PHARMACOLOGY, Clinical Studies.**) The results from observational studies are generally consistent with those of the WHI clinical trial.

After a mean follow-up of 5.6 years, the WHI trial reported an increased risk of breast cancer in women who took estrogen plus progestin. Observational studies have also reported an increased risk for estrogen/progestin combination therapy, and a smaller increased risk for estrogen alone therapy, after several years of use. For both findings, the excess risk increased with duration of use, and appeared to return to baseline over about five years after stopping treatment (only the observational studies have substantial data on risk after stopping). In these studies, the risk of breast cancer was greater, and became apparent earlier, with estrogen/progestin combination therapy as compared to estrogen alone therapy. However, these studies have not found significant variation in the risk of breast cancer among different estrogens or among different estrogen/progestin combinations, doses, or routes of administration.

TABLE 8. RELATIVE AND ABSOLUTE RISK SEEN IN THE ESTROGEN PLUS PROGESTIN SUBSTUDY OF WHI[a]

Event[c]	Relative Risk PREMPRO vs Placebo at 5.2 Years (95% CI*)	Placebo n=8102	PREMPRO n=8506
		Absolute Risk per 10,000 Women-years	
CHD events	1.29 (1.02–1.63)	30	37
Non-fatal MI	*1.32 (1.02–1.72)*	*23*	*30*
CHD death	*1.18 (0.70–1.97)*	*6*	*7*
Invasive breast cancer[b]	1.26 (1.00–1.59)	30	38
Stroke	1.41 (1.07–1.85)	21	29
Pulmonary embolism	2.13 (1.39–3.25)	8	16
Colorectal cancer	0.63 (0.43–0.92)	16	10
Endometrial cancer	0.83 (0.47–1.47)	6	5
Hip fracture	0.66 (0.45–0.98)	15	10
Death due to causes other than the events above	0.92 (0.74–1.14)	40	37
Global Index[c]	1.15 (1.03–1.28)	151	170
Deep vein thrombosis[d]	2.07 (1.49–2.87)	13	26
Vertebral fractures[d]	0.66 (0.44–0.98)	15	9
Other osteoporotic fractures[d]	0.77 (0.69–0.86)	170	131

a: adapted from JAMA, 2002; 288:321–333

b: includes metastatic and non-metastatic breast cancer with the exception of in situ breast cancer

c: a subset of the events was combined in a "global index," defined as the earliest occurrence of CHD events, invasive breast cancer, stroke, pulmonary embolism, endometrial cancer, colorectal cancer, hip fracture, or death due to other causes

d: not included in Global Index

*: nominal confidence intervals unadjusted for multiple looks and multiple comparisons.

In the WHI trial of estrogen plus progestin, 26% of the women reported prior use of estrogen alone and/or estrogen/progestin combination hormone therapy. After a mean follow-up of 5.6 years during the clinical trial, the overall relative risk of invasive breast cancer was 1.24 (95% confidence interval 1.01-1.54), and the overall absolute risk was 41 vs. 33 cases per 10,000 women-years, for estrogen plus progestin compared with placebo. Among women who reported prior use of hormone therapy, the relative risk of invasive breast cancer was 1.86, and the absolute risk was 46 vs. 25 cases per 10,000 women-years, for estrogen plus progestin compared with placebo. Among women who reported no prior use of hormone therapy, the relative risk of invasive breast cancer was 1.09, and the absolute risk was 40 vs. 36 cases per 10,000 women-years for estrogen plus progestin compared with placebo. In the WHI trial, invasive breast cancers were larger and diagnosed at a more advanced stage in the estrogen plus progestin group compared with the placebo group. Metastatic disease was rare with no apparent difference between the two groups. Other prognostic factors such as histologic subtype, grade and hormone receptor status did not differ between the groups.

The observational Million Women Study in Europe reported an increased risk of mortality due to breast cancer among current users of estrogens alone or estrogens plus progestins compared to never users, while the estrogen plus progestin sub-study of WHI showed no effect on breast cancer mortality with a mean follow-up of 5.6 years.

The use of estrogen plus progestin has been reported to result in an increase in abnormal mammograms requiring further evaluation. All women should receive yearly breast examinations by a healthcare provider and perform monthly breast self-examinations. In addition, mammography examinations should be scheduled based on patient age, risk factors, and prior mammogram results.

b. Endometrial cancer. The reported endometrial cancer risk among unopposed estrogen users is about 2- to 12-fold greater than in nonusers, and appears dependent on duration of treatment and on estrogen dose. Most studies show no significant increased risk associated with the use of estrogens for less than one year. The greatest risk appears associated with prolonged use, with increased risks of 15- to 24-fold for five to ten years or more, and this risk has been shown to persist for at least 8 to 15 years after estrogen therapy is discontinued.

Clinical surveillance of all women taking estrogen/progestin combinations is important. Adequate diagnostic measures, including endometrial sampling when indicated, should be undertaken to rule out malignancy in all cases of undiagnosed persistent or recurring abnormal vaginal bleeding. There is no evidence that the use of natural estrogens results in a different endometrial risk profile than synthetic estrogens of equivalent estrogen dose.

Endometrial hyperplasia (a possible precursor of endometrial cancer) has been reported to occur at a rate of approximately 1% or less with PREMPRO or PREMPHASE in two large clinical trials. In the two large clinical trials described above, two cases of endometrial cancer were reported to occur among women taking combination Premarin/medroxyprogesterone acetate therapy.

3. Dementia.

In the Women's Health Initiative Memory Study (WHIMS), 4,532 generally healthy postmenopausal women 65 years of age and older were studied, of whom 35% were 70 to 74 years of age and 18% were 75 or older. After an average follow-up of 4 years, 40 women being treated with PREMPRO (1.8%, n = 2,229) and 21 women in the placebo group (0.9%, n = 2,303) received diagnoses of probable dementia. The relative risk for PREMPRO versus placebo was 2.05 (95% confidence interval 1.21 – 3.48), and was similar for women with and without histories of menopausal hormone use before WHIMS. The absolute risk of probable dementia for PREMPRO versus placebo was 45 versus 22 cases per 10,000 women-years, and the absolute excess risk for PREMPRO was 23 cases per 10,000 women-years. It is unknown whether these findings apply to younger postmenopausal women. (See **CLINICAL PHARMACOLOGY, Clinical Studies** and **PRECAUTIONS, Geriatric Use.**)

The results of the estrogen alone sub-study of the Women's Health Initiative Memory Study have not been reported. It is unknown whether these findings apply to estrogen alone therapy.

4. Gallbladder Disease.

A 2- to 4-fold increase in the risk of gallbladder disease requiring surgery in postmenopausal women receiving estrogens has been reported.

5. Hypercalcemia.

Estrogen administration may lead to severe hypercalcemia in patients with breast cancer and bone metastases. If hypercalcemia occurs, use of the drug should be stopped and appropriate measures taken to reduce the serum calcium level.

6. Visual Abnormalities.

Retinal vascular thrombosis has been reported in patients receiving estrogens. Discontinue medication pending examination if there is sudden partial or complete loss of vision, or a sudden onset of proptosis, diplopia, or migraine. If examination reveals papilledema or retinal vascular lesions, estrogens should be discontinued.

Continued on next page

Prempro/Premphase—Cont.

PRECAUTIONS

A. General

1. Addition of a progestin when a woman has not had a hysterectomy.

Studies of the addition of a progestin for 10 or more days of a cycle of estrogen administration, or daily with estrogen in a continuous regimen, have reported a lowered incidence of endometrial hyperplasia than would be induced by estrogen treatment alone. Endometrial hyperplasia may be a precursor to endometrial cancer.

There are, however, possible risks that may be associated with the use of progestins with estrogens compared with estrogen-alone regimens. These include a possible increased risk of breast cancer, adverse effects on lipoprotein metabolism (e.g., lowering HDL, raising LDL) and impairment of glucose tolerance.

2. Elevated blood pressure.

In a small number of case reports, substantial increases in blood pressure have been attributed to idiosyncratic reactions to estrogens. In a large, randomized, placebo-controlled clinical trial, a generalized effect of estrogen therapy on blood pressure was not seen. Blood pressure should be monitored at regular intervals with estrogen use.

3. Hypertriglyceridemia.

In patients with pre-existing hypertriglyceridemia, estrogen therapy may be associated with elevations of plasma triglycerides leading to pancreatitis and other complications. In the HOPE study, the mean percent increase from baseline in serum triglycerides after one year of treatment with PREMPRO 0.625 mg/2.5 mg, 0.45 mg/1.5 mg, and 0.3 mg/1.5 mg compared with placebo were 32.8, 24.8, 23.3, and 10.7, respectively. After two years of treatment, the mean percent changes were 33.0, 17.1, 21.6, and 5.5, respectively.

4. Impaired liver function and past history of cholestatic jaundice.

Estrogens may be poorly metabolized in patients with impaired liver function. For patients with a history of cholestatic jaundice associated with past estrogen use or with pregnancy, caution should be exercised and in the case of recurrence, medication should be discontinued.

5. Hypothyroidism.

Estrogen administration leads to increased thyroid-binding globulin (TBG) levels. Patients with normal thyroid function can compensate for the increased TBG by making more thyroid hormone, thus maintaining free T_4 and T_3 serum concentrations in the normal range. Patients dependent on thyroid hormone replacement therapy who are also receiving estrogens may require increased doses of their thyroid replacement therapy. These patients should have their thyroid function monitored in order to maintain their free thyroid hormone levels in an acceptable range.

6. Fluid retention.

Because estrogens/progestins may cause some degree of fluid retention, patients with conditions that might be influenced by this factor, such as cardiac or renal dysfunction, warrant careful observation when estrogens are prescribed.

7. Hypocalcemia.

Estrogens should be used with caution in individuals with severe hypocalcemia.

8. Ovarian cancer.

The estrogen plus progestin substudy of WHI reported that after an average follow-up of 5.6 years, the relative risk of ovarian cancer for estrogen plus progestin versus placebo was 1.58 (95% confidence interval 0.77 – 3.24) but was not statistically significant. The absolute risk for estrogen plus progestin versus placebo was 4.2 versus 2.7 cases per 10,000 women-years. In some epidemiologic studies, the use of estrogen-only products, in particular for ten or more years, has been associated with an increased risk of ovarian cancer. Other epidemiologic studies have not found these associations.

9. Exacerbation of endometriosis.

Endometriosis may be exacerbated with administration of estrogen therapy.

10. Exacerbation of other conditions.

Estrogen therapy may cause an exacerbation of asthma, diabetes mellitus, epilepsy, migraine, porphyria, systemic lupus erythematosus, and hepatic hemangiomas and should be used with caution in women with these conditions.

B. Patient Information

Physicians are advised to discuss the contents of the PATIENT INFORMATION leaflet with patients for whom they prescribe PREMPRO or PREMPHASE.

C. Laboratory Tests

Estrogen administration should be initiated at the lowest dose approved for the indication and then guided by clinical response rather than by serum hormone levels (e.g., estradiol, FSH).

D. Drug/Laboratory Test Interactions

1. Accelerated prothrombin time, partial thromboplastin time, and platelet aggregation time; increased platelet count; increased factors II, VII antigen, VIII coagulant activity, IX, X, XII, VII-X complex, II-VII-X complex, and beta-thromboglobulin; decreased levels of anti-factor Xa and antithrombin III, decreased antithrombin III activity; increased levels of fibrinogen and fibrinogen activity; increased plasminogen antigen and activity.
2. Increased thyroid binding globulin (TBG) levels leading to increased circulating total thyroid hormone levels as measured by protein-bound iodine (PBI), T_4 levels (by column or by radioimmunoassay), or T_3 levels by radioimmunoassay. T_3 resin uptake is decreased, reflecting the elevated TBG. Free T_4 and free T_3 concentrations are unaltered. Patients on thyroid replacement therapy may require higher doses of thyroid hormone.

TABLE 9: ALL TREATMENT EMERGENT STUDY EVENTS REGARDLESS OF DRUG RELATIONSHIP REPORTED AT A FREQUENCY ≥ 5%

Body System Adverse event	PREMPRO 0.625 mg/2.5 mg continuous (n=340)	PREMPRO 0.625 mg/5.0 mg continuous (n=338)	PREMPHASE 0.625 mg/5.0 mg sequential (n=351)	PREMARIN 0.625 mg daily (n=347)
Body as a whole				
abdominal pain	16%	21%	23%	17%
accidental injury	5%	4%	5%	5%
asthenia	6%	8%	10%	8%
back pain	14%	13%	16%	14%
flu syndrome	10%	13%	12%	14%
headache	36%	28%	37%	38%
infection	16%	16%	18%	14%
pain	11%	13%	12%	13%
pelvic pain	4%	5%	5%	5%
Digestive system				
diarrhea	6%	6%	5%	10%
dyspepsia	6%	6%	5%	5%
flatulence	8%	9%	8%	5%
nausea	11%	9%	11%	11%
Metabolic and Nutritional				
peripheral edema	4%	4%	3%	5%
Musculoskeletal system				
arthralgia	9%	7%	9%	7%
leg cramps	3%	4%	5%	4%
Nervous system				
depression	6%	11%	11%	10%
dizziness	5%	3%	4%	6%
hypertonia	4%	3%	3%	7%
Respiratory system				
pharyngitis	11%	11%	13%	12%
rhinitis	8%	6%	8%	7%
sinusitis	8%	7%	7%	5%
Skin and appendages				
pruritus	10%	8%	5%	4%
rash	4%	6%	4%	3%
Urogenital system				
breast pain	33%	38%	32%	12%
cervix disorder	4%	4%	5%	5%
dysmenorrhea	8%	5%	13%	5%
leukorrhea	6%	5%	9%	8%
vaginal hemorrhage	2%	1%	3%	6%
vaginitis	7%	7%	5%	3%

3. Other binding proteins may be elevated in serum, i.e., corticosteroid binding globulin (CBG), sex hormone binding globulin (SHBG), leading to increased total circulating corticosteroids and sex steroids, respectively. Free hormone concentrations may be decreased. Other plasma proteins may be increased (angiotensinogen/renin substrate, alpha-1-antitrypsin, ceruloplasmin).
4. Increased plasma HDL and HDL_2 cholesterol subfraction concentrations, reduced LDL cholesterol concentration, increased triglyceride levels.
5. Impaired glucose tolerance.
6. Reduced response to metyrapone test.
7. Aminoglutethimide administered concomitantly with medroxyprogesterone acetate (MPA) may significantly depress the bioavailability of MPA.

E. Carcinogenesis, Mutagenesis, Impairment of Fertility

(See **BOXED WARNINGS**, **WARNINGS**, and **PRECAUTIONS**.)

Long-term continuous administration of natural and synthetic estrogens in certain animal species increases the frequency of carcinomas of the breasts, uterus, cervix, vagina, testis, and liver.

In a two-year oral study of medroxyprogesterone acetate (MPA) in which female rats were exposed to dosages of up to 5000 mcg/kg/day in their diets (50 times higher – based on AUC values – than the level observed experimentally in women taking 10 mg of MPA), a dose-related increase in pancreatic islet cell tumors (adenomas and carcinomas) occurred. Pancreatic tumor incidence was increased at 1000 and 5000 mcg/kg/day, but not at 200 mcg/kg/day.

A decreased incidence of spontaneous mammary gland tumors was observed in all three MPA-treated groups, compared with controls, in the two-year rat study. The mechanism for the decreased incidence of mammary gland tumors observed in the MPA-treated rats may be linked to the significant decrease in serum prolactin concentration observed in rats.

Beagle dogs treated with MPA developed mammary nodules, some of which were malignant. Although nodules occasionally appeared in control animals, they were intermittent in nature, whereas the nodules in the drug-treated animals were larger, more numerous, persistent, and there were some breast malignancies with metastases. It is known that progestogens stimulate synthesis and release of growth hormone in dogs. The growth hormone, along with the progestogen, stimulates mammary growth and tumors. In contrast, growth hormone in humans is not increased, nor does growth hormone have any significant mammotrophic role. No pancreatic tumors occurred in dogs.

F. Pregnancy

PREMPRO and PREMPHASE should not be used during pregnancy. (See **CONTRAINDICATIONS**.)

G. Nursing Mothers

Estrogen administration to nursing mothers has been shown to decrease the quantity and quality of the milk. Detectable amounts of estrogen and progestin have been identified in the milk of mothers receiving these drugs. Caution should be exercised when PREMPRO or PREMPHASE are administered to a nursing woman.

H. Pediatric Use

PREMPRO and PREMPHASE are not indicated in children.

I. Geriatric Use

Of the total number of subjects in the estrogen plus progestin substudy of the Women's Health Initiative study, 44% (n = 7320) were 65 years and over, while 6.6% (n = 1,095) were 75 years and over (see **CLINICAL PHARMACOLOGY, Clinical Studies**). There was a higher incidence of stroke and invasive breast cancer in women 75 and over compared to women less than 75 years of age.

In the Women's Health Initiative Memory Study (WHIMS), including 4,532 women 65 years of age and older, followed for an average of 4 years, 82% (n = 3,729) were 65 to 74 while 18% (n = 803) were 75 and over. Most women (80%) had no prior hormone therapy use. Women treated with conjugated estrogens plus medroxyprogesterone acetate were reported to have a two-fold increase in the risk of developing probable dementia. Alzheimer's disease was the most common classification of probable dementia in both the conjugated estrogens plus medroxyprogesterone acetate group and the placebo group. Ninety percent of the cases of probable dementia occurred in the 54% of women that were older than 70. (See **WARNINGS, Dementia**.)

With respect to efficacy in the approved indications, there have not been sufficient numbers of geriatric patients involved in studies utilizing Premarin and medroxyprogesterone acetate to determine whether those over 65 years of age differ from younger subjects in their response to PREMPRO or PREMPHASE.

ADVERSE REACTIONS

See **BOXED WARNING**, **WARNINGS**, and **PRECAUTIONS**.

Because clinical trials are conducted under widely varying conditions, adverse reaction rates observed in the clinical trials of a drug cannot be directly compared with rates in the clinical trials of another drug and may not reflect the rates observed in practice. The adverse reaction information from clinical trials does, however, provide a basis for identifying the adverse events that appear to be related to drug use and for approximating rates.

In a 1-year clinical trial that included 678 postmenopausal women treated with PREMPRO, 351 postmenopausal women treated with PREMPHASE, and 347 postmenopausal women treated with Premarin, the following adverse events occurred at a rate ≥ 5% (see Table 9):

[See table 9 at left]

During the first year of a 2-year clinical trial with 2333 postmenopausal women between 40 and 65 years of age (88% Caucasian), 2001 women received continuous regimens of either 0.625 mg of CE with or without 2.5 mg MPA, or 0.45 mg or 0.3 mg of CE with or without 1.5 mg MPA, and 332 received placebo tablets. Table 10 summarizes adverse events that occurred at a rate ≥ 5% in at least 1 treatment group.

[See table 10 at right]

TABLE 10. PERCENT OF PATIENTS WITH TREATMENT EMERGENT STUDY EVENTS REGARDLESS OF DRUG RELATIONSHIP REPORTED AT A FREQUENCY ≥ 5% DURING STUDY YEAR 1

Body System Adverse event	Premarin 0.625 mg daily (n=348)	Prempro 0.625 mg/ 2.5 mg continuous (n=331)	Premarin 0.45 mg daily (n=338)	Prempro 0.45 mg/ 1.5 mg continuous (n=331)	Premarin 0.3 mg daily (n=326)	Prempro 0.3 mg/ 1.5 mg continuous (n=327)	Placebo daily (n=332)
Any adverse event	93%	92%	90%	89%	90%	90%	85%
Body as a whole							
abdominal pain	16%	17%	15%	16%	17%	13%	11%
accidental injury	6%	10%	12%	9%	6%	9%	9%
asthenia	7%	8%	7%	8%	8%	6%	5%
back pain	14%	12%	13%	13%	13%	12%	12%
flu syndrome	11%	8%	11%	11%	10%	10%	11%
headache	26%	28%	32%	29%	29%	33%	28%
infection	18%	21%	22%	19%	23%	18%	22%
pain	17%	14%	18%	15%	20%	20%	18%
Digestive system							
diarrhea	6%	7%	7%	7%	6%	6%	6%
dyspepsia	9%	8%	9%	8%	11%	8%	14%
flatulence	7%	7%	7%	8%	6%	5%	3%
nausea	9%	7%	7%	10%	6%	8%	9%
Musculoskeletal system							
arthralgia	14%	9%	12%	13%	7%	10%	12%
leg cramps	5%	7%	7%	5%	3%	4%	2%
myalgia	5%	5%	5%	5%	9%	4%	8%
Nervous system							
anxiety	5%	4%	4%	5%	4%	2%	4%
depression	7%	11%	8%	5%	5%	8%	7%
dizziness	6%	3%	6%	5%	4%	5%	5%
insomnia	6%	6%	7%	7%	7%	6%	10%
nervousness	3%	3%	5%	2%	2%	2%	2%
Respiratory system							
cough increased	4%	8%	7%	5%	4%	6%	4%
pharyngitis	10%	11%	10%	8%	12%	9%	11%
rhinitis	6%	8%	9%	9%	10%	10%	13%
sinusitis	6%	8%	11%	8%	7%	10%	7%
upper respiratory infection	12%	10%	10%	9%	9%	11%	11%
Skin and appendages							
pruritus	4%	4%	5%	5%	5%	5%	2%
Urogenital system							
breast enlargement	<1%	5%	1%	3%	2%	2%	<1%
breast pain	11%	26%	12%	21%	7%	13%	9%
dysmenorrhea	4%	5%	3%	6%	1%	3%	<1%
leukorrhea	5%	4%	7%	5%	4%	3%	3%
vaginal hemorrhage	14%	6%	4%	4%	2%	2%	0%
vaginal moniliasis	6%	8%	5%	7%	5%	4%	2%
vaginitis	7%	5%	6%	6%	5%	4%	1%

The following additional adverse reactions have been reported with estrogen and/or progestin therapy:

1. *Genitourinary system*
Changes in vaginal bleeding pattern and abnormal withdrawal bleeding or flow, breakthrough bleeding, spotting, dysmenorrhea, change in amount of cervical secretion, premenstrual-like syndrome, cystitis-like syndrome, increase in size of uterine leiomyomata, vaginal candidiasis, amenorrhea, changes in cervical erosion, ovarian cancer, endometrial hyperplasia, endometrial cancer.

2. *Breasts*
Tenderness, enlargement, pain, nipple discharge, galactorrhea, fibrocystic breast changes, breast cancer.

3. *Cardiovascular*
Deep and superficial venous thrombosis, pulmonary embolism, thrombophlebitis, myocardial infarction, stroke, increase in blood pressure.

4. *Gastrointestinal*
Nausea, cholestatic jaundice, changes in appetite, vomiting, abdominal cramps, bloating, increased incidence of gallbladder disease, pancreatitis, enlargement of hepatic hemangiomas.

5. *Skin*
Chloasma or melasma that may persist when drug is discontinued, erythema multiforme, erythema nodosum, hemorrhagic eruption, loss of scalp hair, hirsutism, itching, urticaria, pruritus, generalized rash, rash (allergic) with and without pruritus, acne.

6. *Eyes*
Neuro-ocular lesions, e.g., retinal vascular thrombosis and optic neuritis, intolerance of contact lenses.

7. *Central Nervous System (CNS)*
Headache, dizziness, mental depression, mood disturbances, anxiety, irritability, nervousness, migraine, chorea, insomnia, somnolence, exacerbation of epilepsy, dementia.

8. *Miscellaneous*
Increase or decrease in weight, edema, changes in libido, fatigue, backache, reduced carbohydrate tolerance, aggravation of porphyria, pyrexia, urticaria, angioedema, anaphylactoid/anaphylactic reactions, hypocalcemia, exacerbation of asthma, increased triglycerides.

OVERDOSAGE

Serious ill effects have not been reported following acute ingestion of large doses of estrogen/progestin-containing drug products by young children. Overdosage of estrogen/progestin may cause nausea and vomiting, and withdrawal bleeding may occur in females.

DOSAGE AND ADMINISTRATION

Use of estrogens, alone or in combination with a progestin, should be with the lowest effective dose and for the shortest duration consistent with treatment goals and risks for the individual woman. Patients should be re-evaluated periodically as clinically appropriate (e.g., at 3-month to 6-month intervals) to determine if treatment is still necessary (see **BOXED WARNING** and **WARNINGS**.) For women who have a uterus, adequate diagnostic measures, such as endometrial sampling, when indicated, should be undertaken to rule out malignancy in cases of undiagnosed persistent or recurring abnormal vaginal bleeding.

PREMPRO therapy consists of a single tablet to be taken once daily.

1. For treatment of moderate to severe vasomotor symptoms and/or moderate to severe symptoms of vulvar and vaginal atrophy associated with the menopause. When prescribing solely for the treatment of symptoms of vulvar and vaginal atrophy, topical vaginal products should be considered.

- PREMPRO 0.3 mg/1.5 mg
- PREMPRO 0.45 mg/1.5 mg
- PREMPRO 0.625 mg/2.5 mg
- PREMPRO 0.625 mg/5 mg
- PREMPHASE

Patients should be treated with the lowest effective dose. Generally women should be started at 0.3 mg/1.5 mg PREMPRO daily. Subsequent dosage adjustment may be made based upon the individual patient response. In patients where bleeding or spotting remains a problem, after appropriate evaluation, consideration should be given to changing the dose level. This dose should be periodically reassessed by the healthcare provider.

2. For prevention of postmenopausal osteoporosis. When prescribing solely for the prevention of postmenopausal osteoporosis, therapy should be considered only for women at significant risk of osteoporosis and for whom non-estrogen medications are not considered to be appropriate.

- PREMPRO 0.3 mg/1.5 mg
- PREMPRO 0.45 mg/1.5 mg
- PREMPRO 0.625 mg/2.5 mg
- PREMPRO 0.625 mg/5 mg
- PREMPHASE

Patients should be treated with the lowest effective dose. Generally women should be started at 0.3 mg/1.5 mg PREMPRO daily. Dosage may be adjusted depending on individual clinical and bone mineral density responses. This dose should be periodically reassessed by the healthcare provider.

In patients where bleeding or spotting remains a problem, after appropriate evaluation, consideration should be given to changing the dose level. This dose should be periodically reassessed by the healthcare provider.

PREMPHASE therapy consists of two separate tablets; one maroon 0.625 mg Premarin tablet taken daily on days 1 through 14 and one light-blue tablet, containing 0.625 mg conjugated estrogens and 5 mg of medroxyprogesterone acetate, taken on days 15 through 28.

HOW SUPPLIED

PREMPRO therapy consists of a single tablet to be taken once daily.

PREMPRO 0.3 mg/1.5 mg
Each carton contains 3 EZ DIAL® dispensers containing 28 tablets. One EZ DIAL dispenser contains 28 oval, cream tablets containing 0.3 mg of the conjugated estrogens found in Premarin tablets and 1.5 mg medroxyprogesterone acetate for oral administration (NDC 0046-0938-09).

PREMPRO 0.45 mg/1.5 mg
Each carton includes 3 EZ DIAL dispensers containing 28 tablets. One EZ DIAL dispenser contains 28 oval, gold tablets containing 0.45 mg of the conjugated estrogens found in Premarin tablets and 1.5 mg medroxyprogesterone acetate for oral administration (NDC 0046-0937-09).

PREMPRO 0.625 mg/2.5 mg
Each carton includes 3 EZ DIAL dispensers containing 28 tablets. One EZ DIAL dispenser contains 28 oval, peach tablets containing 0.625 mg of the conjugated estrogens found in Premarin tablets and 2.5 mg of medroxyprogesterone acetate for oral administration (NDC 0046-0875-06).

PREMPRO 0.625 mg/5 mg
Each carton includes 3 EZ DIAL dispensers containing 28 tablets. One EZ DIAL dispenser contains 28 oval, light-blue tablets containing 0.625 mg of the conjugated estrogens found in Premarin tablets and 5 mg of medroxyprogesterone acetate for oral administration (NDC 0046-0975-06).

PREMPHASE therapy consists of two separate tablets; one maroon Premarin tablet taken daily on days 1 through 14 and one light-blue tablet taken on days 15 through 28.

Each carton includes 3 EZ DIAL dispensers containing 28 tablets. One EZ DIAL dispenser contains 14 oval, maroon Premarin tablets containing 0.625 mg of conjugated estrogens and 14 oval, light-blue tablets that contain 0.625 mg of the conjugated estrogens found in Premarin tablets and 5 mg of medroxyprogesterone acetate for oral administration (NDC 0046-2573-06).

The appearance of PREMPRO tablets is a trademark of Wyeth Pharmaceuticals.

The appearance of Premarin tablets is a trademark of Wyeth Pharmaceuticals. The appearance of the conjugated estrogens/medroxyprogesterone acetate combination tablets is a registered trademark.

Store at 20 - 25°C (68 - 77°F); excursions permitted to 15 - 30°C (59 - 86°F) [see USP Controlled Room Temperature].

PATIENT INFORMATION

PREMPRO™
(conjugated estrogens/medroxyprogesterone acetate tablets)
PREMPHASE®
(conjugated estrogens/medroxyprogesterone acetate tablets)

Read this PATIENT INFORMATION before you start taking PREMPRO or PREMPHASE and read what you get each time you refill PREMPRO or PREMPHASE. There may be new information. This information does not take the place of talking to your healthcare provider about your medical condition or your treatment.

What is the most important information I should know about PREMPRO and PREMPHASE (combinations of estrogens and a progestin)?

Do not use estrogens and progestins to prevent heart disease, heart attacks, or strokes.

Using estrogens and progestins may increase your chances of getting heart attacks, strokes, breast cancer, or blood clots. Using estrogens with progestins may increase your risk of dementia, based on a study of women age 65 years or older. You and your healthcare provider should talk regularly about whether you still need treatment with PREMPRO or PREMPHASE.

What is PREMPRO or PREMPHASE?

PREMPRO or PREMPHASE are medicines that contain two kinds of hormones, estrogens and a progestin.

PREMPRO or PREMPHASE is used after menopause to:

- **reduce moderate to severe hot flashes.** Estrogens are hormones made by a woman's ovaries. The ovaries normally stop making estrogens when a woman is between 45 and 55 years old. This drop in body estrogen levels causes the "change of life" or menopause (the end of monthly menstrual periods). Sometimes, both ovaries are removed during an operation before natural menopause takes place. The sudden drop in estrogen levels causes "surgical menopause."

When the estrogen levels begin dropping, some women get very uncomfortable symptoms, such as feelings of warmth in the face, neck, and chest, or sudden strong

Continued on next page

Prempro/Premphase—Cont.

feelings of heat and sweating ("hot flashes" or "hot flushes"). In some women the symptoms are mild, and they will not need to take estrogens. In other women, symptoms can be more severe. You and your healthcare provider should talk regularly about whether you still need treatment with PREMPRO or PREMPHASE.

- **treat moderate to severe dryness, itching, and burning, in and around the vagina.** You and your healthcare provider should talk regularly about whether you still need treatment with PREMPRO or PREMPHASE to control these problems. If you use Premarin only to treat your dryness, itching, and burning in and around your vagina, talk with your healthcare provider about whether a topical vaginal product would be better for you.
- **help reduce your chances of getting osteoporosis (thin weak bones).** Osteoporosis from menopause is a thinning of the bones that makes them weaker and easier to break. If you use PREMPRO or PREMPHASE only to prevent osteoporosis from menopause, talk with your healthcare provider about whether a different treatment or medicine without estrogens might be better for you. You and your healthcare provider should talk regularly about whether you should continue with PREMPRO or PREMPHASE. Weight-bearing exercise, like walking or running, and taking calcium and vitamin D supplements may also lower your chances of getting postmenopausal osteoporosis. It is important to talk about exercise and supplements with your healthcare provider before starting them.

Who should not take PREMPRO or PREMPHASE?

Do not take PREMPRO or PREMPHASE if you have had your uterus removed (hysterectomy).

PREMPRO and PREMPHASE contain a progestin to decrease the chances of getting cancer of the uterus. If you do not have a uterus, you do not need a progestin and you should not take PREMPRO or PREMPHASE.

Do not start taking PREMPRO or PREMPHASE if you:

- **have unusual vaginal bleeding.**
- **currently have or have had certain cancers.** Estrogens may increase the chances of getting certain types of cancers, including cancer of the breast or uterus. If you have or had cancer, talk with your healthcare provider about whether you should take PREMPRO or PREMPHASE.
- **had a stroke or heart attack in the past year.**
- **currently have or have had blood clots.**
- **currently have liver problems.**
- **are allergic to PREMPRO or PREMPHASE or any of their ingredients.** See the end of this leaflet for a list of all the ingredients in PREMPRO and PREMPHASE.
- **think you may be pregnant.**

Tell your healthcare provider:

- **if you are breastfeeding.** The hormones in PREMPRO and PREMPHASE can pass into your milk.
- **about all of your medical problems.** Your healthcare provider may need to check you more carefully if you have certain conditions, such as asthma (wheezing), epilepsy (seizures), migraine, endometriosis, lupus, problems with your heart, liver, thyroid, kidneys, or have high calcium levels in your blood.
- **about all the medicines you take,** including prescription and nonprescription medicines, vitamins, and herbal supplements. Some medicines may affect how PREMPRO or PREMPHASE works. PREMPRO or PREMPHASE may also affect how your other medicines work.
- **if you are going to have surgery or will be on bedrest.** You may need to stop taking estrogens and progestins.

How should I take PREMPRO or PREMPHASE?

- Take one PREMPRO or PREMPHASE tablet at the same time each day.
- If you miss a dose, take it as soon as possible. If it is almost time for your next dose, skip the missed dose and go back to your normal schedule. Do not take 2 doses at the same time.
- Estrogens should be used at the lowest dose possible for your treatment only as long as needed. You and your healthcare provider should talk regularly (for example, every 3 to 6 months) about the dose you are taking and whether you still need treatment with PREMPRO or PREMPHASE.

What are the possible side effects of PREMPRO or PREMPHASE?

Less common but serious side effects include:

- Breast cancer
- Cancer of the uterus
- Stroke
- Heart attack
- Blood clots
- Dementia
- Gallbladder disease
- Ovarian cancer

These are some of the warning signs of serious side effects:

- Breast lumps
- Unusual vaginal bleeding
- Dizziness and faintness
- Changes in speech
- Severe headaches
- Chest pain
- Shortness of breath
- Pains in your legs
- Changes in vision
- Vomiting

Call your healthcare provider right away if you get any of these warning signs, or any other unusual symptoms that concerns you.

Common side effects include:

- Headache
- Breast pain
- Irregular vaginal bleeding or spotting
- Stomach/abdominal cramps/bloating
- Nausea and vomiting
- Hair loss

Other side effects include:

- High blood pressure
- Liver problems
- High blood sugar
- Fluid retention
- Enlargement of benign tumors of the uterus ("fibroids")
- Vaginal yeast infections
- Mental depression

These are not all the possible side effects of PREMPRO or PREMPHASE. For more information, ask your healthcare provider or pharmacist.

What can I do to lower my chances of getting a serious side effect with PREMPRO or PREMPHASE?

- Talk with your healthcare provider regularly about whether you should continue taking PREMPRO or PREMPHASE.
- See your healthcare provider right away if you get vaginal bleeding while taking PREMPRO or PREMPHASE.
- Have a breast exam and mammogram (breast X-ray) every year unless your healthcare provider tells you something else. If members of your family have had breast cancer or if you have ever had breast lumps or an abnormal mammogram, you may need to have breast exams more often.
- If you have high blood pressure, high cholesterol (fat in the blood), diabetes, are overweight, or if you use tobacco, you may have higher chances for getting heart disease. Ask your healthcare provider for ways to lower your chances of getting heart attacks.

General Information about the safe and effective use of PREMPRO and PREMPHASE

Medicines are sometimes prescribed for conditions that are not mentioned in patient information leaflets. Do not take PREMPRO or PREMPHASE for conditions for which it was not prescribed. Do not give PREMPRO or PREMPHASE to other people, even if they have the same symptoms you have. It may harm them.

Keep PREMPRO and PREMPHASE out of the reach of children.

This leaflet provides a summary of the most important information about PREMPRO and PREMPHASE. If you would like more information, talk with your healthcare provider or pharmacist. You can ask for information about PREMPRO and PREMPHASE that is written for health professionals. You can get more information by calling the toll free number 800-934-5556.

What are the ingredients in PREMPRO and PREMPHASE?

PREMPRO contains the same conjugated estrogens found in Premarin which are a mixture of sodium estrone sulfate and sodium equilin sulfate and other components including sodium sulfate conjugates, 17α-dihydroequilin, 17α-estradiol and 17β-dihydroequilin. PREMPRO also contains either 1.5, 2.5, or 5 mg of medroxyprogesterone acetate. PREMPRO also contains calcium phosphate tribasic, calcium sulfate, carnauba wax, cellulose, glyceryl monooleate, lactose, magnesium stearate, methylcellulose, pharmaceutical glaze, polyethylene glycol, sucrose, povidone, titanium dioxide, and yellow ferric oxide or red ferric oxide or FD&C Blue No. 2.

PREMPHASE is two separate tablets. One tablet (maroon color) is 0.625 mg of Premarin which is a mixture of sodium estrone sulfate and sodium equilin sulfate and other components including sodium sulfate conjugates, 17 α-dihydroequilin, 17 α-estradiol and 17 β-dihydroequilin. The maroon tablet also contains calcium phosphate tribasic, calcium sulfate, carnauba wax, cellulose, glyceryl monooleate, lactose, magnesium stearate, methylcellulose, pharmaceutical glaze, polyethylene glycol, stearic acid, sucrose, titanium dioxide, FD&C Blue No. 2, D&C Red No. 27, FD&C Red No. 40. The second tablet (light blue color) contains 0.625 mg of the same ingredients as the maroon color tablet plus 5 mg of medroxyprogesterone acetate. The light blue tablet also contains calcium phosphate tribasic, calcium sulfate, carnauba wax, cellulose, glyceryl monooleate, lactose, magnesium stearate, methylcellulose, pharmaceutical glaze, polyethylene glycol, sucrose, povidone, titanium dioxide, FD&C Blue No. 2.

PREMPRO therapy consists of a single tablet to be taken once daily.

PREMPRO 0.3 mg/1.5 mg

Each carton includes 3 EZ DIAL® dispensers containing 28 tablets. One EZ DIAL dispenser contains 28 oval, cream tablets containing 0.3 mg of the conjugated estrogens found in Premarin tablets and 1.5 mg of medroxyprogesterone acetate for oral administration.

PREMPRO 0.45 mg/1.5 mg

Each carton includes 3 EZ DIAL dispensers containing 28 tablets. One EZ DIAL dispenser contains 28 oval, gold tablets containing 0.45 mg of the conjugated estrogens found in Premarin tablets and 1.5 mg of medroxyprogesterone acetate for oral administration.

PREMPRO 0.625 mg/2.5 mg

Each carton includes 3 EZ DIAL dispensers containing 28 tablets. One EZ DIAL dispenser contains 28 oval, peach tablets containing 0.625 mg of the conjugated estrogens found in Premarin tablets and 2.5 mg of medroxyprogesterone acetate for oral administration.

PREMPRO 0.625 mg/5 mg

Each carton includes 3 EZ DIAL dispensers containing 28 tablets. One EZ DIAL dispenser contains 28 oval, light-blue tablets containing 0.625 mg of the conjugated estrogens found in Premarin tablets and 5 mg of medroxyprogesterone acetate for oral administration.

PREMPHASE therapy consists of two separate tablets; one maroon Premarin tablet taken daily on days 1 through 14 and one light-blue tablet taken on days 15 through 28.

Each carton includes 3 EZ DIAL dispensers containing 28 tablets. One EZ DIAL dispenser contains 14 oval, maroon Premarin tablets containing 0.625 mg of conjugated estrogens and 14 oval, light-blue tablets that contain 0.625 mg of the conjugated estrogens found in Premarin tablets and 5 mg of medroxyprogesterone acetate for oral administration.

The appearance of PREMPRO tablets is a trademark of Wyeth Pharmaceuticals.

The appearance of Premarin tablets is a trademark of Wyeth Pharmaceuticals. The appearance of the conjugated estrogens/medroxyprogesterone acetate combination tablets is a registered trademark.

Store at 20 - 25°C (68 - 77°F); excursions permitted to 15 - 30°C (59 - 86°F) [see USP Controlled Room Temperature].

This product's label may have been revised after this insert was used in production. For further product information and current package insert, please visit www.wyeth.com or call our medical communications department toll-free at 1-800-934-5556.

Wyeth®

Wyeth Pharmaceuticals Inc.
Philadelphia, PA 19101

W10407C011
ET01
Revised April 28, 2004

Shown in Product Identification Guide, page 336

PREVNAR® ℞

[*prĕv' när*]

Pneumococcal 7-valent Conjugate Vaccine (Diphtheria CRM_{197} Protein)

FOR PEDIATRIC USE ONLY

℞ only

For Intramuscular Injection Only

This product's label may have been revised after this insert was used in production. For further product information and current package insert, please visit www.wyeth.com or call our medical communications department toll-free at 1-800-934-5556.

DESCRIPTION

Pneumococcal 7-valent Conjugate Vaccine (Diphtheria CRM_{197} Protein), Prevnar®, is a sterile solution of saccharides of the capsular antigens of *Streptococcus pneumoniae* serotypes 4, 6B, 9V, 14, 18C, 19F, and 23F individually conjugated to diphtheria CRM_{197} protein. Each serotype is grown in soy peptone broth. The individual polysaccharides are purified through centrifugation, precipitation, ultrafiltration, and column chromatography. The polysaccharides are chemically activated to make saccharides which are directly conjugated to the protein carrier CRM_{197} to form the glycoconjugate. This is effected by reductive amination. CRM_{197} is a nontoxic variant of diphtheria toxin isolated from cultures of *Corynebacterium diphtheriae* strain C7 (β197) grown in a casamino acids and yeast extract-based medium. CRM_{197} is purified through ultrafiltration, ammonium sulfate precipitation, and ion-exchange chromatography. The individual glycoconjugates are purified by ultrafiltration and column chromatography and are analyzed for saccharide to protein ratios, molecular size, free saccharide, and free protein.

The individual glycoconjugates are compounded to formulate the vaccine, Prevnar®. Potency of the formulated vaccine is determined by quantification of each of the saccharide antigens, and by the saccharide to protein ratios in the individual glycoconjugates.

Prevnar® is manufactured as a liquid preparation. Each 0.5 mL dose is formulated to contain: 2 µg of each saccharide for serotypes 4, 9V, 14, 18C, 19F, and 23F, and 4 µg of serotype 6B per dose (16 µg total saccharide); approximately 20 µg of CRM_{197} carrier protein; and 0.125 mg of aluminum per 0.5 mL dose as aluminum phosphate adjuvant.

After shaking, the vaccine is a homogeneous, white suspension.

CLINICAL PHARMACOLOGY

S. pneumoniae is an important cause of morbidity and mortality in persons of all ages worldwide. The organism causes invasive infections, such as bacteremia and meningitis, as well as pneumonia and upper respiratory tract infections including otitis media and sinusitis. In children older than 1 month, *S. pneumoniae* is the most common cause of invasive disease.[1] Data from community-based studies performed between 1986 and 1995, indicate that the overall annual incidence of invasive pneumococcal disease in the United States (US) is an estimated 10 to 30 cases per 100,000 persons, with the highest risk in children aged less than or equal to 2 years of age (140 to 160 cases per 100,000 persons).[2,3,4,5,6] Children in group child care have an increased risk for invasive pneumococcal disease.[7,8] Immunocompromised individuals with neutropenia, asplenia, sickle cell disease, disorders of complement and humoral immunity, human immunodeficiency virus (HIV) infections or chronic underlying disease are also at increased risk for invasive pneumococcal disease.[8] *S. pneumoniae* is the most common cause of bacterial meningitis in the US.[1] The annual incidence of pneumococcal meningitis in children between 1 to 23 months of age is approximately 7 cases per 100,000 persons.[1] Pneumococcal meningitis in childhood has been associated with 8% mortality and may result in neurological sequelae (25%) and hearing loss (32%) in survivors.[9]

Acute otitis media (AOM) is a common childhood disease, with more than 60% of children experiencing an episode by one year of age, and more than 90% of children experiencing an episode by age 5. Prior to the US introduction of Prevnar® in the year 2000, approximately 24.5 million ambulatory care visits and 490,000 procedures for myringotomy with tube placement were attributed to otitis media annually.[10,11] The peak incidence of AOM is 6 to 18 months of age.[12] Otitis media is less common, but occurs, in older children. In a 1990 surveillance by the Centers for Disease Control and Prevention (CDC), otitis media was the most common principal illness diagnosis in children 2-10 years of age.[13] Complications of AOM include persistent middle ear effusion, chronic otitis media, transient hearing loss, or speech delays and, if left untreated, may lead to more serious diseases such as mastoiditis and meningitis. *S. pneumoniae* is an important cause of AOM. It is the bacterial pathogen most commonly isolated from middle ear fluid, identified in 20% to 40% of middle ear fluid cultures in AOM.[14,15] Pneumococcal otitis media is associated with higher rates of fever, and is less likely to resolve spontaneously than AOM due to either nontypeable *H. influenzae* or *M. catarrhalis*.[16,17] Prior to the introduction of Prevnar®®, the seven serotypes contained in the vaccine accounted for approximately 60% of AOM due to *S. pneumoniae* (12%-24% of all AOM).[18]

The exact contribution of *S. pneumoniae* to childhood pneumonia is unknown, as it is often not possible to identify the causative organisms. In studies of children less than 5 years of age with community-acquired pneumonia, where diagnosis was attempted using serological methods, antigen testing, or culture data, 30% of cases were classified as bacterial pneumonia, and 70% of these (21% of total community-acquired pneumonia) were found to be due to *S. pneumoniae*.[19,20]

In the past decade the proportion of *S. pneumoniae* isolates resistant to antibiotics has been on the rise in the US and worldwide. In a multi-center US surveillance study, the prevalence of penicillin and cephalosporin-nonsusceptible (intermediate or high level resistance) invasive disease isolates from children was 21% (range <5% to 38% among centers), and 9.3% (range 0%-18%), respectively. Over the 3-year surveillance period (1993-1996), there was a 50% increase in penicillin-nonsusceptible *S. pneumoniae* (PNSP) strains and a three-fold rise in cephalosporin-nonsusceptible strains.[8] Although generally less common than PNSP, pneumococci resistant to macrolides and trimethoprim-sulfamethoxazole have also been observed.[4] Day care attendance, a history of ear infection, and a recent history of antibiotic exposure, have also been associated with invasive infections with PNSP in children 2 months to 59 months of age.[7,8] There has been no difference in mortality associated with PNSP strains.[8,9] However, the American Academy of Pediatrics (AAP) revised the antibiotic treatment guidelines in 1997 in response to the increased prevalence of antibiotic-resistant pneumococci.[21]

Approximately 90 serotypes of *S. pneumoniae* have been identified based on antigenic differences in their capsular polysaccharides. The distribution of serotypes responsible for disease differ with age and geographic location.[22]

Serotypes 4, 6B, 9V, 14, 18C, 19F, and 23F have been responsible for approximately 80% of invasive pneumococcal disease in children <6 years of age in the US.[18] These 7 serotypes also accounted for 74% of PNSP and 100% of pneumococci with high level penicillin resistance isolated from children <6 years with invasive disease during a 1993-1994 surveillance by the CDC.[23]

Results of Clinical Evaluations

Efficacy Against Invasive Disease

Efficacy was assessed in a randomized, double-blinded clinical trial in a multiethnic population at Northern California Kaiser Permanente (NCKP) from October 1995 through August 20, 1998, in which 37,816 infants were randomized to receive either Prevnar® or a control vaccine (an investigational meningococcal group C conjugate vaccine [MnCC]) at 2, 4, 6, and 12-15 months of age. Prevnar® was administered to 18,906 children and the control vaccine to 18,910 children. Routinely recommended vaccines were also administered which changed during the trial to reflect changing AAP and Advisory Committee on Immunization Practices (ACIP) recommendations. A planned interim analysis was performed upon accrual of 17 cases of invasive disease due to vaccine-type *S. pneumoniae* (August 1998). Ancillary endpoints for evaluation of efficacy against pneumococcal disease were also assessed in this trial.

Invasive disease was defined as isolation and identification of *S. pneumoniae* from normally sterile body sites in children presenting with an acute illness consistent with pneumococcal disease. Weekly surveillance of listings of cultures

TABLE 1
Efficacy of Prevnar® Against Invasive Disease Due to *S. pneumoniae* in Cases Accrued From October 15, 1995 Through August 20, 1998[24,25]

	Prevnar® Number of Cases	Control* Number of Cases	Efficacy	95% CI
Vaccine serotypes				
Per protocol	**0**	**17**	**100%**	**75.4, 100**
Intent-to-treat	**0**	**22**	**100%**	**81.7, 100**
All pneumococcal serotypes				
Per protocol	2	20	90.0%	58.3, 98.9
Intent-to-treat	3	27†	88.9%	63.8, 97.9

* Investigational meningococcal group C conjugate vaccine (MnCC).
† Includes one case in an immunocompromised subject.

TABLE 2
Efficacy of Prevnar® Against Otitis Media in the Finnish and NCKP Trials[24,25,26,27]

	Per Protocol		Intent-to-Treat	
	Vaccine Efficacy Estimate*	95% Confidence Interval	Vaccine Efficacy Estimate*	95% Confidence Interval
Finnish Trial	**N=1632**		**N=1662**	
AOM due to Vaccine Serotypes	**57%**	**44, 67**	**54%**	**41, 64**
All culture-confirmed pneumococcal AOM regardless of serotype	34%	21, 45	32%	19, 42
NCKP Trial	**N=23,746**		**N=34,146**	
All Otitis Media Episodes regardless of etiology†	**7%**	**4, 10**	**6%**	**4, 9**

* All vaccine efficacy estimates in the table are statistically significant.
† The vaccine efficacy against all AOM episodes in the Finnish trial, while not reaching statistical significance, was 6% (95% CI: -4, 16) in the per protocol population and 4% (95% CI: –7, 14) in the intent-to-treat population.

TABLE 3
Geometric Mean Concentrations (µg/mL) of Pneumococcal Antibodies Following the Third and Fourth Doses of Prevnar® or Control* When Administered Concurrently With DTP-HbOC in the Efficacy Study[24,25]

Serotype	Post dose 3 GMC† (95% CI for Prevnar®)		Post dose 4 GMC‡ (95% CI for Prevnar®)	
	Prevnar®§	Control*	Prevnar®§	Control*
	N=88	N=92	N=68	N=61
4	1.46 (1.19, 1.78)	0.03	2.38 (1.88, 3.03)	0.04
6B	4.70 (3.59, 6.14)	0.08	14.45 (11.17, 18.69)	0.17
9V	1.99 (1.64, 2.42)	0.05	3.51 (2.75, 4.48)	0.06
14	4.60 (3.70, 5.74)	0.05	6.52 (5.18, 8.21)	0.06
18C	2.16 (1.73, 2.69)	0.04	3.43 (2.70, 4.37)	0.07
19F	1.39 (1.16, 1.68)	0.09	2.07 (1.66, 2.57)	0.18
23F	1.85 (1.46, 2.34)	0.05	3.82 (2.85, 5.11)	0.09

* Control was investigational meningococcal group C conjugate vaccine (MnCC).
† Mean age of Prevnar® group was 7.8 months and of control group was 7.7 months. N is slightly less for some serotypes in each group.
‡ Mean age of Prevnar® group was 14.2 months and of control group was 14.4 months. N is slightly less for some serotypes in each group.
§ p<0.001 when Prevnar® compared to control for each serotype using a Wilcoxon's test.

from the NCKP Regional Microbiology database was conducted to assure ascertainment of all cases. The primary endpoint was efficacy against invasive pneumococcal disease due to vaccine serotypes. The per protocol analysis of the primary endpoint included cases which occurred ≥14 days after the third dose. The intent-to-treat (ITT) analysis included all cases of invasive pneumococcal disease due to vaccine serotypes in children who received at least one dose of vaccine. Secondary analyses of efficacy against all invasive pneumococcal disease, regardless of serotype, were also performed according to these same per protocol and ITT definitions. Results of these analyses are presented in Table 1.

[See table 1 above]

All 22 cases of invasive disease due to vaccine serotype strains in the ITT population were bacteremic. In addition, the following diagnoses were also reported: meningitis (2), pneumonia (2), and cellulitis (1).

Data accumulated through an extended follow-up period to April 20, 1999, resulted in a similar efficacy estimate (Per protocol: 1 case in Pneumococcal 7-valent Conjugate Vaccine (Diphtheria CRM_{197} Protein), Prevnar® group, 39 cases in control group; ITT: 3 cases in Prevnar® group, 49 cases in the control group).[25]

Efficacy Against Otitis Media

The efficacy of Prevnar® against otitis media was assessed in two clinical trials: a trial in Finnish infants at the National Public Health Institute and the invasive disease efficacy trial in US infants at Northern California Kaiser Permanente (NCKP).

The trial in Finland was a randomized, double-blind trial in which 1,662 infants were equally randomized to receive either Prevnar® or a control vaccine (Hepatitis B vaccine [Hep B]) at 2, 4, 6, and 12-15 months of age. All infants received

Continued on next page

Prevnar—Cont.

a DTP-Hib combination vaccine concurrently at 2, 4, and 6 months of age, and Inactivated Poliovirus Vaccine (IPV) concurrently at 12 months of age. Parents of study participants were asked to bring their children to the study clinics if the child had respiratory infections or symptoms suggesting acute otitis media (AOM). If AOM was diagnosed, tympanocentesis was performed, and the middle ear fluid was cultured. If *S. pneumoniae* was isolated, serotyping was performed.

AOM was defined as a visually abnormal tympanic membrane suggesting effusion in the middle ear cavity, concomitantly with at least one of the following symptoms of acute infection: fever, ear ache, irritability, diarrhea, vomiting, acute otorrhea not caused by external otitis, or other symptoms of respiratory infection. A new visit or "episode" was defined as a visit with a study physician at which time a diagnosis of AOM was made and at least 30 days had elapsed since any previous visit for otitis media. The primary endpoint was efficacy against AOM episodes caused by vaccine serotypes in the per protocol population.

In the NCKP invasive disease efficacy trial, the effectiveness of Prevnar® in reducing the incidence of otitis media was assessed from the beginning of the trial in October 1995 through April 1998. During this time, 34,146 infants were randomized to receive either Prevnar® (N=17,070), or the control, an investigational meningococcal group C conjugate vaccine (N=17,076), at 2, 4, 6, and 12-15 months of age. Physician visits for otitis media were identified by physician coding of outpatient encounter forms. Because visits may have included both acute and follow-up care, a new visit or "episode" was defined as a visit that was at least 21 days following a previous visit for otitis media (at least 42 days, if the visit appointment was made > 3 days in advance). Data on placement of ear tubes were collected from automated databases. No routine tympanocentesis was performed, and no standard definition of otitis media was used by study physicians. The primary otitis media endpoint was efficacy against all otitis media episodes in the per protocol population.

Table 2 presents the per protocol and intent-to-treat results of key otitis media analyses for both studies. The per protocol analyses include otitis media episodes that occurred ≥14 days after the third dose. The intent-to-treat analyses include all otitis media episodes in children who received at least one dose of vaccine.

[See table 2 at top of previous page]

The vaccine efficacy against AOM episodes due to vaccine-related serotypes (6A, 9N, 18B, 19A, 23A), also assessed in the Finnish trial, was 51% (95% CI: 27, 67) in the per protocol population and 44% (95% CI: 20, 62) in the intent-to-treat population. The vaccine efficacy against AOM episodes caused by serotypes unrelated to the vaccine was −33% (95% CI: -80, 1) in the per protocol population and −39% (95% CI: -86, -3) in the intent-to-treat population, indicating that children who received Prevnar® appear to be at increased risk of otitis media due to pneumococcal serotypes not represented in the vaccine, compared to children who received the control vaccine. However, vaccination with Prevnar® reduced pneumococcal otitis media episodes overall.

Several other otitis media endpoints were also assessed in the two trials. Recurrent AOM, defined as 3 episodes in 6 months or 4 episodes in 12 months, was reduced by 9% in both the per protocol and intent-to-treat populations (95% CI: 3, 15 in per protocol and 95% CI: 4, 14 in intent-to-treat) in the NCKP trial. This observation was supported by a similar trend, although not statistically significant, seen in the Finnish trial. The NCKP trial also demonstrated a 20% reduction (95% CI: 2, 35) in the placement of tympanostomy tubes in the per protocol population and a 21% reduction (95% CI: 4, 34) in the intent-to-treat population.

Data from the NCKP trial accumulated through an extended follow-up period to April 20, 1999, in which a total of 37,866 children were included (18,925 in Prevnar® group and 18,941 in MnCC control group), resulted in similar otitis media efficacy estimates for all endpoints.[28]

Immunogenicity

Routine Schedule

Subjects from a subset of selected study sites in the NCKP efficacy study were approached for participation in the immunogenicity portion of the study on a volunteer basis. Immune responses following three or four doses of Prevnar® or the control vaccine were evaluated in children who received either concurrent Diphtheria and Tetanus Toxoids and Pertussis Vaccine Adsorbed and Haemophilus b Conjugate Vaccine (Diphtheria CRM_{197} Protein Conjugate), (DTP-HbOC), or Diphtheria and Tetanus Toxoids and Acellular Pertussis Vaccine Adsorbed (DTaP), and Haemophilus b Conjugate Vaccine (Diphtheria CRM_{197} Protein Conjugate), (HbOC) vaccines at 2, 4, and 6 months of age. The use of Hepatitis B (Hep B), Oral Polio Vaccine (OPV), Inactivated Polio Vaccine (IPV), Measles-Mumps-Rubella (MMR), and Varicella vaccines were permitted according to the AAP and ACIP recommendations.

Table 3 presents the geometric mean concentrations (GMC) of pneumococcal antibodies following the third and fourth doses of Prevnar® or the control vaccine when administered concurrently with DTP-HbOC vaccine in the efficacy study.

[See table 3 on previous page]

In another randomized study (Manufacturing Bridging Study, 118-16), immune responses were evaluated following three doses of Pneumococcal 7-valent Conjugate Vaccine (Diphtheria CRM_{197} Protein), Prevnar® administered concomitantly with DTaP and HbOC vaccines at 2, 4, and 6 months of age, IPV at 2 and 4 months of age, and Hep B at 2 and 6 months of age. The control group received concomitant vaccines only. Table 4 presents the immune responses to pneumococcal polysaccharides observed in both this study and in the subset of subjects from the efficacy study that received concomitant DTaP and HbOC vaccines.

TABLE 4
Geometric Mean Concentrations (μg/mL) of Pneumococcal Antibodies Following the Third Dose of Prevnar® or Control* When Administered Concurrently With DTaP and HbOC in the Efficacy Study† and Manufacturing Bridging Study[24,25,29]

Serotype	Efficacy Study		Manufacturing Bridging Study	
	Post dose 3 GMC‡ (95% CI for Prevnar®)		Post dose 3 GMC§ (95% CI for Prevnar®)	
	Prevnar® ‖	Control*	Prevnar® ‖	Control*
	N=32	N=32	N=159	N=83
4	1.47 (1.08, 2.02)	0.02	2.03 (1.75, 2.37)	0.02
6B	2.18 (1.20, 3.96)	0.06	2.97 (2.43, 3.65)	0.07
9V	1.52 (1.04, 2.22)	0.04	1.18 (1.01, 1.39)	0.04
14	5.05 (3.32, 7.70)	0.04	4.64 (3.80, 5.66)	0.04
18C	2.24 (1.65, 3.02)	0.04	1.96 (1.66, 2.30)	0.04
19F	1.54 (1.09, 2.17)	0.10	1.91 (1.63, 2.25)	0.08
23F	1.48 (0.97, 2.25)	0.05	1.71 (1.44, 2.05)	0.05

*Control in efficacy study was investigational meningococcal group C conjugate vaccine (MnCC) and in Manufacturing Bridging Study was concomitant vaccines only.
† Sufficient data are not available to reliably assess GMCs following 4 doses of Prevnar® when administered with DTaP in the NCKP efficacy study.
‡ Mean age of the Prevnar® study group was 7.4 months and of the control group was 7.6 months. N is slightly less for some serotypes in each group.
§ Mean age of the Prevnar® study group and the control group was 7.2 months.
‖ p<0.001 when Prevnar® compared to control for each serotype using a Wilcoxon's test in the efficacy study and two-sample t-test in the Manufacturing Bridging Study.

[See table 4 above]

In all studies in which the immune responses to Prevnar® were contrasted to control, a significant antibody response was seen to all vaccine serotypes following three or four doses, although geometric mean concentrations of antibody varied among serotypes.[24,25,27,29,30,31,32,33,34] The minimum serum antibody concentration necessary for protection against invasive pneumococcal disease or against pneumococcal otitis media has not been determined for any serotype. Prevnar® induces functional antibodies to all vaccine serotypes, as measured by opsonophagocytosis following three doses.[34]

Previously Unvaccinated Older Infants and Children

To determine an appropriate schedule for children 7 months of age or older at the time of the first immunization with Prevnar®, 483 children in 4 ancillary studies received Prevnar® at various schedules and were evaluated for immunogenicity. GMCs attained using the various schedules among older infants and children were comparable to immune responses of children, who received concomitant DTaP, in the NCKP efficacy study (118-8) after 3 doses for most serotypes, as shown in Table 5. These data support the schedule for previously unvaccinated older infants and children who are beyond the age of the infant schedule. For usage in older infants and children, see **DOSAGE AND ADMINISTRATION.**

TABLE 5
Geometric Mean Concentrations (μg/mL) of Pneumococcal Antibodies Following Immunization of Children From 7 Months Through 9 Years of Age With Prevnar® [35]

Age group, Vaccinations	Study	Sample Size(s)	4	6B	9V	14	18C	19F	23F
7-11 mo. 3 doses	118-12	22	**2.34**	**3.66**	**2.11**	**9.33**	**2.31**	**1.60**	**2.50**
	118-16	39	**3.60**	**4.63**	**2.04**	**5.48**	**1.98**	**2.15**	**1.93**
12-17 mo. 2 doses	118-15*	82-84†	**3.91**	**4.67**	**1.94**	**6.92**	**2.25**	**3.78**	**3.29**
	118-18	33	**7.02**	**4.25**	**3.26**	**6.31**	**3.60**	**3.29**	**2.92**
18-23 mo. 2 doses	118-15*	52-54†	**3.36**	**4.92**	**1.80**	**6.69**	**2.65**	**3.17**	**2.71**
	118-18	45	**6.85**	**3.71**	**3.86**	**6.48**	**3.42**	**3.86**	**2.75**
24-35 mo. 1 dose	118-18	53	**5.34**	**2.90**	**3.43**	1.88	**3.03**	**4.07**	**1.56**
36-59 mo. 1 dose	118-18	52	**6.27**	**6.40**	**4.62**	**5.95**	**4.08**	**6.37**	**2.95**
5-9 yrs. 1 dose	118-18	101	**6.92**	**20.84**	**7.49**	**19.32**	**6.72**	**12.51**	**11.57**
118-8, DTaP	Post dose 3	31-32†	1.47	2.18	1.52	5.05	2.24	1.54	1.48

Bold = GMC not inferior to 118-8, DTaP post dose 3 (one-sided lower limit of the 95% CI of GMC ratio ≥0.50).
*Study in Navajo and Apache populations.
† Numbers vary with serotype.

[See table 5 above]

INDICATIONS AND USAGE

Prevnar® is indicated for active immunization of infants and toddlers against invasive disease caused by *S. pneumoniae* due to capsular serotypes included in the vaccine (4, 6B, 9V, 14, 18C, 19F, and 23F). The routine schedule is 2, 4, 6, and 12-15 months of age.

The decision to administer Pneumococcal 7-valent Conjugate Vaccine (Diphtheria CRM_{197} Protein), Prevnar® should be based primarily on its efficacy in preventing invasive pneumococcal disease. As with any vaccine, Prevnar® may not protect all individuals receiving the vaccine from invasive pneumococcal disease.

Prevnar® is also indicated for active immunization of infants and toddlers against otitis media caused by serotypes included in the vaccine. However, for vaccine serotypes, protection against otitis media is expected to be substantially lower than protection against invasive disease. Additionally, because otitis media is caused by many organisms other than serotypes of *S. pneumoniae* represented in the vaccine, protection against all causes of otitis media is expected to be low.

TABLE 6
Concurrent Administration of Prevnar® With Other Vaccines to Infants in Non-Efficacy Studies[29,32]

Antigen*	GMC*		% Responders†		Study	Vaccine Schedule‡	N	
	Prevnar®	Control§	Prevnar®	Control§		(mo.)	Prevnar®	Control§
Hib	6.2	4.4	99.5, 88.3	97.0, 88.1	118-12	2, 4, 6	214	67
Diphtheria	0.9	0.8	100	97.0				
Tetanus	3.5	4.1¶	100	100				
PT	19.1	17.8	74.0	69.7				
FHA	43.8	46.7	66.4	69.7				
Pertactin	40.1	50.9	65.6	77.3				
Fimbriae 2	3.3	4.2	44.7	62.5‖				
Hib	11.9	7.8‖	100, 96.9	98.8, 92.8	118-16	2, 4, 6	159	83
Hep B	—	—	99.4	96.2	118-16	0, 2, 6	156	80
IPV Type 1	—	—	89.0	93.6¶	118-16	2, 4	156	80
Type 2	—	—	94.2	93.6				
Type 3	—	—	83.8	80.8				

* Hib vaccine was HibTITER®, DTaP vaccine was Acel-Imune®. Hib (μg/mL) Dip, Tet (IU/mL); Pertussis Antigens (PT, FHA, Ptn, Fim) (units/mL).
† Responders = Hib (≥0.15 μg/mL, ≥1.0 μg/mL); Dip, Tet (≥0.1 IU/mL); Pertussis Antigens (PT, FHA, Ptn, Fim) [4-fold rise]; IPV (≥1:10); Hep B (≥10 mIU/mL).
‡ Schedule for concurrently administered vaccines; Pneumococcal 7-valent Conjugate Vaccine (Diphtheria CRM_{197} Protein), Prevnar® administered at 2, 4, 6 mos.; blood for antibody assessment attained 1 month after third dose, except for IPV (3 months post-immunization).
§ Concurrent vaccines only.
‖ $p<0.05$ when Prevnar® compared to control group using the following tests: ANCOVA for GMCs in 118-12; ANOVA for GMCs in 118-16; and Fisher's Exact test for % Responders in 118-12.
¶ Lower bound of 90% CI of difference >10%.

TABLE 7
Concurrent Administration of Prevnar® With Other Vaccines to Toddlers in a Non-Efficacy Study[31]

Antigen*	GMC*		% Responders†		Study‡	Vaccine Schedule§	N	
	Prevnar®	Control‖	Prevnar®	Control‖		(mo.)	Prevnar®	Control‖
Hib	22.7	47.9¶	100, 97.9	100, 100	118–7	12–15	47	26
Diphtheria	2.0	3.2¶	100	100				
Tetanus	14.4	18.8	100	100				
PT	68.6	121.2¶	68.1	73.1				
FHA	29.0	48.2¶	68.1	84.6				
Pertactin	84.4	83.0	83.0	96.2				
Fimbriae 2	5.2	3.8	63.8	50.0				

* Hib vaccine was HibTITER®, DTaP vaccine was Acel-Imune®. Hib (μg/mL); Dip, Tet (IU/mL); Pertussis Antigens (PT, FHA, Ptn, Fim) (units/mL).
† Responders = Hib (≥0.15 μg/mL, ≥1.0 μg/mL); Dip, Tet (≥0.1 IU/mL); Pertussis Antigens (PT, FHA, Ptn, Fim) [4-fold rise].
‡ Children received a primary series of DTP-HbOC (Tetramune®).
§ Blood for antibody assessment obtained 1 month after dose.
‖ Concurrent vaccines only.
¶ $p<0.05$ when Prevnar® compared to control group using a two-sample t-test.

TABLE 8
Percentage of Subjects Reporting Local Reactions Within 2 Days Following Immunization With Prevnar® and DTP-HbOC* Vaccines at 2, 4, 6, and 12-15 Months of Age[24,25]

Reaction	Dose 1		Dose 2		Dose 3		Dose 4	
	Prevnar® Site	DTP-HbOC Site	Prevnar® Site	DTP-HbOC Site†	Prevnar® Site	DTP-HbOC Site†	Prevnar® Site	DTP-HbOC Site†
	N=2890	N=2890	N=2725	N=2725	N=2538	N=2538	N=599	N=599
Erythema								
Any	12.4	21.9	14.3	25.1	15.2	26.5	12.7	23.4
>2.4 cm	1.2	4.6	1.0	2.9	2.0	4.4	1.7	6.4
Induration								
Any	10.9	22.4	12.3	23.0	12.8	23.3	11.4	20.5
>2.4 cm	2.6	7.2	2.4	5.6	2.9	6.7	2.8	7.2
Tenderness								
Any	28.0	36.4	25.2	30.5	25.6	32.8	36.5	45.1
Interfered with limb movement	7.9	10.7	7.4	8.4	7.8	10.0	18.5	22.2

* If Hep B vaccine was administered simultaneously, it was administered into the same limb as the DTP-HbOC vaccine. If reactions occurred at either or both sites on that limb, the more severe reaction was recorded.
† $p<0.05$ when Prevnar® site compared to the DTP-HbOC site using the sign test.

(See **CLINICAL PHARMACOLOGY** for estimates of efficacy against invasive disease and otitis media).
For additional information on usage, see **DOSAGE AND ADMINISTRATION**.
This vaccine is not intended to be used for treatment of active infection.

CONTRAINDICATIONS
Hypersensitivity to any component of the vaccine, including diphtheria toxoid, is a contraindication to use of this vaccine.
The decision to administer or delay vaccination because of a current or recent febrile illness depends largely on the severity of the symptoms and their etiology. Although a severe or even a moderate febrile illness is sufficient reason to postpone vaccinations, minor illnesses, such as a mild upper respiratory infection with or without low-grade fever, are not generally contraindications.[36,37]

WARNINGS
THIS VACCINE WILL NOT PROTECT AGAINST *S. PNEUMONIAE* DISEASE CAUSED BY SEROTYPES UNRELATED TO THOSE IN THE VACCINE, NOR WILL IT PROTECT AGAINST OTHER MICROORGANISMS THAT CAUSE INVASIVE INFECTIONS SUCH AS BACTEREMIA AND MENINGITIS OR NON-INVASIVE INFECTIONS SUCH AS OTITIS MEDIA.
This vaccine should not be given to infants or children with thrombocytopenia or any coagulation disorder that would contraindicate intramuscular injection unless the potential benefit clearly outweighs the risk of administration. If the decision is made to administer this vaccine to children with coagulation disorders, it should be given with caution. (See **DRUG INTERACTIONS**.)
Immunization with Prevnar® does not substitute for routine diphtheria immunization.
Healthcare professionals should prescribe and/or administer this product with caution to patients with a possible history of latex sensitivity since the packaging contains dry natural rubber.

PRECAUTIONS
Prevnar® is for intramuscular use only. Prevnar® SHOULD UNDER NO CIRCUMSTANCES BE ADMINISTERED INTRAVENOUSLY. The safety and immunogenicity for other routes of administration (eg, subcutaneous) have not been evaluated.
Fever, and rarely febrile seizure, have been reported in children receiving Prevnar®. For children at higher risk of seizures than the general population, acetaminophen or other appropriate antipyretics (dosed according to respective prescribing information) may be administered around the time of vaccination, to reduce the possibility of post-vaccination fever.

General
CARE IS TO BE TAKEN BY THE HEALTHCARE PROFESSIONAL FOR THE SAFE AND EFFECTIVE USE OF THIS PRODUCT.

1. PRIOR TO ADMINISTRATION OF ANY DOSE OF THIS VACCINE, THE PARENT OR GUARDIAN SHOULD BE ASKED ABOUT THE PERSONAL HISTORY, FAMILY HISTORY, AND RECENT HEALTH STATUS OF THE VACCINE RECIPIENT. THE HEALTHCARE PROFESSIONAL SHOULD ASCERTAIN PREVIOUS IMMUNIZATION HISTORY, CURRENT HEALTH STATUS, AND OCCURRENCE OF ANY SYMPTOMS AND/OR SIGNS OF AN ADVERSE EVENT AFTER PREVIOUS IMMUNIZATIONS IN THE CHILD TO BE IMMUNIZED, IN ORDER TO DETERMINE THE EXISTENCE OF ANY CONTRAINDICATION TO IMMUNIZATION WITH THIS VACCINE AND TO ALLOW AN ASSESSMENT OF RISKS AND BENEFITS.
2. BEFORE THE ADMINISTRATION OF ANY BIOLOGICAL, THE HEALTHCARE PROFESSIONAL SHOULD TAKE ALL PRECAUTIONS KNOWN FOR THE PREVENTION OF ALLERGIC OR ANY OTHER ADVERSE REACTIONS. This should include a review of the patient's history regarding possible sensitivity; the ready availability of epinephrine 1:1000 and other appropriate agents used for control of immediate allergic reactions; and a knowledge of the recent literature pertaining to use of the biological concerned, including the nature of side effects and adverse reactions that may follow its use.
3. Children with impaired immune responsiveness, whether due to the use of immunosuppressive therapy (including irradiation, corticosteroids, antimetabolites, alkylating agents, and cytotoxic agents), a genetic defect, HIV infection, or other causes, may have reduced antibody response to active immunization.[36,37,38] (See **DRUG INTERACTIONS**.)
4. The use of pneumococcal conjugate vaccine does not replace the use of 23-valent pneumococcal polysaccharide vaccine in children ≥ 24 months of age with sickle cell disease, asplenia, HIV infection, chronic illness or who are immunocompromised. Data on sequential vaccination with Prevnar® followed by 23-valent pneumococcal polysaccharide vaccine are limited. In a randomized study, 23 children ≥ 2 years of age with sickle cell disease were administered either 2 doses of Prevnar® followed by a dose of polysaccharide vaccine or a single dose of polysaccharide vaccine alone. In this small study, safety and immune responses with the combined schedule were similar to polysaccharide vaccine alone.[39]
5. Since this product is a suspension containing an aluminum adjuvant, shake vigorously immediately prior to use to obtain a uniform suspension prior to withdrawing the dose.
6. A separate sterile syringe and needle or a sterile disposable unit should be used for each individual to prevent transmission of hepatitis or other infectious agents from one person to another. Needles should be disposed of properly and should not be recapped.
7. The vaccine is to be administered immediately after being drawn up into a syringe.

Continued on next page

Prevnar—Cont.

8. Special care should be taken to prevent injection into or near a blood vessel or nerve.
9. Healthcare professionals should prescribe and/or administer this product with caution to patients with a possible history of latex sensitivity since the packaging contains dry natural rubber.

Information for Parents or Guardians

Prior to administration of this vaccine, the healthcare professional should inform the parent, guardian, or other responsible adult of the potential benefits and risks to the patient (see **ADVERSE REACTIONS** and **WARNINGS** sections), and the importance of completing the immunization series unless contraindicated. Parents or guardians should be instructed to report any suspected adverse reactions to their healthcare professional. The healthcare professional should provide vaccine information statements prior to each vaccination.

DRUG INTERACTIONS

Children receiving therapy with immunosuppressive agents (large amounts of corticosteroids, antimetabolites, alkylating agents, cytotoxic agents) may not respond optimally to active immunization.[37,38,40,41] (See **PRECAUTIONS, General.**)

As with other intramuscular injections, Prevnar® should be given with caution to children on anticoagulant therapy.

Simultaneous Administration with Other Vaccines

During clinical studies, Prevnar® was administered simultaneously with DTP-HbOC or DTaP and HbOC, OPV or IPV, Hep B vaccines, MMR, and Varicella vaccine. Thus, the safety experience with Prevnar® reflects the use of this product as part of the routine immunization schedule.[24,25,29,31,32,34]

The immune response to routine vaccines when administered with Prevnar® (at separate sites) was assessed in 3 clinical studies in which there was a control group for comparison. Results for the concurrent immunizations in infants are shown in Table 6 and for toddlers in Table 7. Enhancement of antibody response to HbOC in the infant series was observed. Some suppression of *Haemophilus influenzae* type b (Hib) response was seen at the 4th dose, but over 97% of children achieved titers ≥1 μg/mL. Although some inconsistent differences in response to pertussis antigens were observed, the clinical relevance is unknown. The response to 2 doses of IPV given concomitantly with Prevnar®, assessed 3 months after the second dose, was equivalent to controls for poliovirus Types 2 and 3, but lower for Type 1. MMR and Varicella immunogenicity data from controlled clinical trials with concurrent administration of Prevnar® are not available.

[See table 6 at top of previous page]
[See table 7 on previous page]

CARCINOGENESIS, MUTAGENESIS, IMPAIRMENT OF FERTILITY

Prevnar® has not been evaluated for any carcinogenic or mutagenic potential, or impairment of fertility.

PREGNANCY

Pregnancy Category C

Animal reproductive studies have not been conducted with this product. It is not known whether Prevnar® can cause fetal harm when administered to a pregnant woman or whether it can affect reproductive capacity. This vaccine is not recommended for use in pregnant women.

Nursing Mothers

It is not known whether vaccine antigens or antibodies are excreted in human milk. This vaccine is not recommended for use in a nursing mother.

PEDIATRIC USE

Prevnar® has been shown to be usually well-tolerated and immunogenic in infants. The safety and effectiveness of Prevnar® in children below the age of 6 weeks or on or after the 10th birthday have not been established. Immune responses elicited by Prevnar® among infants born prematurely have not been studied. See **DOSAGE AND ADMINISTRATION** for the recommended pediatric dosage.

GERIATRIC USE

This vaccine is NOT recommended for use in adult populations. It is not to be used as a substitute for the pneumococcal polysaccharide vaccine in geriatric populations.

ADVERSE REACTIONS

Pre-Licensure Clinical Trial Experience

The majority of the safety experience with Prevnar® comes from the NCKP Efficacy Trial in which 17,066 infants received 55,352 doses of Prevnar®, along with other routine childhood vaccines through April 1998 (see **CLINICAL PHARMACOLOGY** section). The number of Prevnar® recipients in the safety analysis differs from the number included in the efficacy analysis due to the different lengths of follow-up for these study endpoints. Safety was monitored in this study using several modalities. Local reactions and systemic events occurring within 48 hours of each dose of vaccine were ascertained by scripted telephone interview on a randomly selected subset of approximately 3,000 children in each vaccine group. The rate of relatively rare events requiring medical attention was evaluated across all doses in all study participants using automated databases. Specifically, rates of hospitalizations within 3, 14, 30, and 60 days of immunization, and of emergency room visits within 3, 14, and 30 days of immunization were assessed and compared between vaccine groups for each diagnosis. Seizures within 3 and 30 days of immunization were ascertained across multiple settings (hospitalizations, emergency room or clinic visits, telephone interviews). Deaths and SIDS were ascertained through April 1999. Hospitalizations due to diabetes, autoimmune disorders, and blood disorders were ascertained through August 1999.

In Tables 8 and 9 the rate of local reactions at the Prevnar® injection site is compared at each dose to the DTP or DTaP injection site in the same children.

[See table 8 on previous page]
[See table 9 above]

TABLE 9
Percentage of Subjects Reporting Local Reactions Within 2 Days Following Immunization With Prevnar®* and DTaP Vaccines† at 2, 4, 6, and 12-15 Months of Age[24,25]

Reaction	Dose 1		Dose 2		Dose 3		Dose 4	
	Prevnar® Site	DTaP Site	Prevnar® Site	DTaP Site	Prevnar® Site	DTaP Site	Prevnar® Site	DTPaP Site‡
	N=693	N=693	N=526	N=526	N=422	N=422	N=165	N=165
Erythema								
Any	10.0	6.7§	11.6	10.5	13.8	11.4	10.9	3.6§
>2.4 cm	1.3	0.4§	0.6	0.6	1.4	1.0	3.6	0.6
Induration								
Any	9.8	6.6§	12.0	10.5	10.4	10.4	12.1	5.5§
>2.4 cm	1.6	0.9	1.3	1.7	2.4	1.9	5.5	1.8
Tenderness								
Any	17.9	16.0	19.4	17.3	14.7	13.1	23.3	18.4
Interfered with limb movement	3.1	1.8§	4.1	3.3	2.9	1.9	9.2	8.0

*HbOC was administered in the same limb as Pneumococcal 7-valent Conjugate Vaccine (Diphtheria CRM_{197} Protein), Prevnar®. If reactions occurred at either or both sites on that limb, the more severe reaction was recorded.
† If Hep B vaccine was administered simultaneously, it was administered into the same limb as DTaP. If reactions occurred at either or both sites on that limb, the more severe reaction was recorded.
‡ Subjects may have received DTP or a mixed DTP/DTaP regimen for the primary series. Thus, this is the 4th dose of a pertussis vaccine, but not a 4th dose of DTaP.
§ $p<0.05$ when Prevnar® site compared to DTaP site using the sign test.

Table 10 presents the rates of local reactions in previously unvaccinated older infants and children.

[See table 10 above]

TABLE 10
Percentage of Subjects Reporting Local Reactions Within 3 Days of Immunization With Prevnar® in Infants and Children from 7 Months Through 9 Years of Age[35]

Age at 1st Vaccination	7-11 Mos.						12-23 Mos.			24-35 Mos.	36-59 Mos.	5-9 Yrs.
Study No.	118-12			118-16			118-9*	118-18		118-18	118-18	118-18
Dose Number	1	2	3†	1	2	3†	1	1	2	1	1	1
Number of Subjects	54	51	24	81	76	50	60	114	117	46	48	49
Reaction												
Erythema												
Any	16.7	11.8	20.8	7.4	7.9	14.0	48.3	10.5	9.4	6.5	29.2	24.2
>2.4 cm‡	1.9	0.0	0.0	0.0	0.0	0.0	6.7	1.8	1.7	0.0	8.3	7.1
Induration												
Any	16.7	11.8	8.3	7.4	3.9	10.0	48.3	8.8	6.0	10.9	22.9	25.5
>2.4 cm‡	3.7	0.0	0.0	0.0	0.0	0.0	3.3	0.9	0.9	2.2	6.3	9.3
Tenderness												
Any	13.0	11.8	12.5	8.6	10.5	12.0	46.7	25.7	26.5	41.3	58.3	82.8
Interfered with limb movement§	1.9	2.0	4.2	1.2	1.3	0.0	3.3	6.2	8.5	13.0	20.8	39.4

*For 118-9, 2 of 60 subjects were ≥24 months of age.
† For 118-12, dose 3 was administered at 15–18 mos. of age. For 118-16, dose 3 was administered at 12–15 mos. of age.
‡ For 118-16 and 118-18, ≥2 cm.
§ Tenderness interfering with limb movement.

Tables 11 and 12 present the rates of systemic events observed in the efficacy study when Prevnar® was administered concomitantly with DTP or DTaP.

[See table 11 on next page]
[See table 12 on next page]

Table 13 presents results from a second study (Manufacturing Bridging Study) conducted at Northern California and Denver Kaiser sites, in which children were randomized to receive one of three lots of Pneumococcal 7-valent Conjugate Vaccine (Diphtheria CRM_{197} Protein), Prevnar®, with concomitant vaccines including DTaP, or the same concomitant vaccines alone. Information was ascertained by scripted telephone interview, as described above.

[See table 13 at bottom of next page]

Fever (≥38.0°C) within 48 hours of a vaccine dose was reported by a greater proportion of subjects who received Prevnar®, compared to control (investigational meningococcal group C conjugate vaccine [MnCC]), after each dose when administered concurrently with DTP-HbOC or DTaP in the efficacy study. In the Manufacturing Bridging Study, fever within 48-72 hours was also reported more commonly after each dose compared to infants in the control group who received only recommended vaccines. When administered concurrently with DTaP in either study, fever rates among Prevnar® recipients ranged from 15% to 34%, and were greatest after the 2nd dose.

Table 14 presents the frequencies of systemic reactions in previously unvaccinated older infants and children.

[See table 14 at top of page 3388]

Of the 17,066 subjects who received at least one dose of Prevnar® in the efficacy trial, there were 24 hospitalizations (for 29 diagnoses) within 3 days of a dose from October 1995 through April 1998. Diagnoses were as follows: bronchiolitis (5); congenital anomaly (4); elective procedure, UTI (3 each); acute gastroenteritis, asthma, pneumonia (2 each); aspiration, breath holding, influenza, inguinal hernia repair, otitis media, febrile seizure, viral syndrome, well child/reassurance (1 each). There were 162 visits to the emergency room (for 182 diagnoses) within 3 days of a dose from October 1995 through April 1998. Diagnoses were as follows: febrile illness (20); acute gastroenteritis (19); trauma, URI (16 each); otitis media (15); well child (13); irritable child, viral syndrome (10 each); rash (8); croup, pneumonia (6 each); poisoning/ingestion (5); asthma, bronchiolitis (4 each); febrile seizure, UTI (3 each); thrush, wheezing, breath holding, choking, conjunctivitis, inguinal hernia repair, pharyngitis (2 each); colic, colitis, congestive heart failure, elective procedure, hives, influenza, ingrown toenail, local swelling, roseola, sepsis (1 each).[24,25]

In the large-scale efficacy study, urticaria-like rash was reported in 0.4%-1.4% of children within 48 hours following immunization with Prevnar® administered concurrently with other routine childhood vaccines. Urticaria-like rash was reported in 1.3%-6% of children in the period from 3 to 14 days following immunization, and was most often reported following the fourth dose when it was administered concurrently with MMR vaccine. Based on limited data, it appears that children with urticaria-like rash after a dose of Prevnar® may be more likely to report urticaria-like rash following a subsequent dose of Prevnar®.

One case of a hypotonic-hyporesponsive episode (HHE) was reported in the efficacy study following Prevnar® and concurrent DTP vaccines in the study period from October 1995 through April 1998. Two additional cases of HHE were reported in four other studies and these also occurred in children who received Prevnar® concurrently with DTP vaccine.[31,34]

In the Kaiser efficacy study in which 17,066 children received a total of 55,352 doses of Prevnar® and 17,080 children received a total of 55,387 doses of the control vaccine (investigational meningococcal group C conjugate vaccine [MnCC]), seizures were reported in 8 Prevnar® recipients and 4 control vaccine recipients within 3 days of immunization from October 1995 through April 1998. Of the 8 Prevnar® recipients, 7 received concomitant DTP-containing vaccines and one received DTaP. Of the 4 control vaccine recipients, 3 received concomitant DTP-containing vaccines and one received DTaP.[24,25] In the other 4 studies combined, in which 1,102 children were immunized with 3,347 doses of Prevnar® and 408 children were immunized with 1,310 doses of control vaccine (either investigational meningococcal group C conjugate vaccine [MnCC] or concurrent vaccines), there was one seizure event reported within 3 days of immunization.[32] This subject received Prevnar® concurrent with DTaP vaccine.

Twelve deaths (5 SIDS and 7 with clear alternative cause) occurred among subjects receiving Prevnar®, of which 11 (4 SIDS and 7 with clear alternative cause) occurred in the Kaiser efficacy study from October 1995 until April 20, 1999. In comparison, 21 deaths (8 SIDS, 12 with clear alternative cause and one SIDS-like death in an older child), occurred in the control vaccine group during the same time period in the efficacy study.[24,25,29] The number of SIDS deaths in the efficacy study from October 1995 until April 20, 1999 was similar to or lower than the age and season-adjusted expected rate from the California State data from 1995–1997 and are presented in Table 15.

[See table 15 on next page]

In a review of all hospitalizations that occurred between October 1995 and August 1999 in the efficacy study for the specific diagnoses of aplastic anemia, autoimmune disease, autoimmune hemolytic anemia, diabetes mellitus, neutropenia, and thrombocytopenia, the numbers of such cases were equal to or less than the expected numbers based on the 1995 Kaiser Vaccine Safety Data Link (VSD) data set.

Overall, the safety of Prevnar® was evaluated in a total of five clinical studies in the US in which 18,168 infants and children received a total of 58,699 doses of vaccine at 2, 4, 6, and 12-15 months of age. In addition, the safety of Prevnar® was evaluated in 831 Finnish infants using the same schedule, and the overall safety profile was similar to that in US infants. The safety of Prevnar® was also evaluated in 560 children from 4 ancillary studies in the US who started immunization at 7 months to 9 years of age. Tables 16 and 17 summarize systemic reactogenicity data within 2 or 3 days across 4,748 subjects in US studies (13,039 infant doses and 1,706 toddler doses) for whom these data were collected and according to the pertussis vaccine administered concurrently.

[See table 16 on next page]
[See table 17 at top of page 3389]

With vaccines in general, including Pneumococcal 7-valent Conjugate Vaccine (Diphtheria CRM_{197} Protein), Prevnar®, it is not uncommon for patients to note within 48 to 72 hours at or around the injection site the following minor reactions: edema; pain or tenderness; redness, inflammation or skin discoloration; mass; or local hypersensitivity reaction. Such local reactions are usually self-limited and require no therapy.

As with other aluminum-containing vaccines, a nodule may occasionally be palpable at the injection site for several weeks.[42]

Postmarketing Experience

Additional adverse reactions identified from postmarketing experience are listed below:

Administration site conditions: injection site dermatitis, injection site urticaria, injection site pruritus

Blood and lymphatic system disorders: lymphadenopathy localized to the region of the injection site

Immune system disorders: hypersensitivity reaction including face edema, dyspnea, bronchospasm; anaphylactic/anaphylactoid reaction including shock

Skin and subcutaneous tissue disorders: angioneurotic edema, erythema multiforme

There have been spontaneous reports of apnea in temporal association with the administration of Prevnar. In most cases Prevnar was administered concomitantly with other vaccines including diphtheria tetanus pertussis vaccine (DTP), diphtheria tetanus acellular pertussis vaccine (DTaP), hepatitis B vaccines, inactivated polio vaccine (IPV), *Haemophilus influenzae* type b vaccine (Hib), measles-mumps-rubella vaccine (MMR), and/or varicella

Continued on next page

TABLE 11
Percentage of Subjects* Reporting Systemic Events Within 2 Days Following Immunization With Prevnar® or Control† Vaccine Concurrently With DTP-HbOC Vaccine at 2, 4, 6, and 12-15 Months of Age[24,25]

Reaction	Dose 1		Dose 2		Dose 3		Dose 4	
	Prevnar®	Control†	Prevnar®	Control†	Prevnar®	Control†	Prevnar®	Control†
	N=2998	N=2982	N=2788	N=2761	N=2596	N=2591	N=709	N=733
Fever								
≥38.0°C	33.4	28.7‡	34.7	27.4‡	40.6	32.4‡	41.9	36.9
>39.0°C	1.3	1.3	3.0	1.6‡	5.3	3.4‡	4.5	4.5
Irritability	71.3	67.9‡	69.4	63.8‡	68.9	61.6‡	72.8	65.8‡
Drowsiness	49.2	50.6	32.5	33.6	25.9	23.4‡	21.3	22.7
Restless Sleep	18.1	17.9	27.3	24.3‡	33.3	30.1‡	29.9	28.0
Decreased Appetite	24.7	23.6	22.8	20.3‡	27.7	25.6	33.0	27.4‡
Vomiting	17.9	14.9‡	16.2	14.4	15.5	12.7‡	9.6	6.8
Diarrhea	12.0	10.7	10.9	9.9	11.5	10.4	12.1	11.2
Urticaria-like Rash	0.7	0.6	0.8	0.8	1.4	1.1	1.4	0.8

*Approximately 90% of subjects received prophylactic or therapeutic antipyretics within 48 hours of each dose.
† Investigational meningococcal group C conjugate vaccine (MnCC).
‡ $p<0.05$ when Prevnar® compared to control group using a Chi-Square test.

TABLE 12
Percentage of Subjects* Reporting Systemic Events Within 2 Days Following Immunization With Prevnar® or Control† Vaccine Concurrently With DTaP Vaccine at 2, 4, 6, and 12-15 Months of Age[24,25]

Reaction	Dose 1		Dose 2		Dose 3		Dose 4‡	
	Prevnar®	Control†	Prevnar®	Control†	Prevnar®	Control†	Prevnar®	Control†
	N=710	N=711	N=559	N=508	N=461	N=414	N=224	N=230
Fever								
≥38.0°C	15.1	9.4§	23.9	10.8§	19.1	11.8§	21.0	17.0
>39.0°C	0.9	0.3	2.5	0.8§	1.7	0.7	1.3	1.7
Irritability	48.0	48.2	58.7	45.3§	51.2	44.8	44.2	42.6
Drowsiness	40.7	42.0	25.6	22.8	19.5	21.9	17.0	16.5
Restless Sleep	15.3	15.1	20.2	19.3	25.2	19.0§	20.2	19.1
Decreased Appetite	17.0	13.5	17.4	13.4	20.7	13.8§	20.5	23.1
Vomiting	14.6	14.5	16.8	14.4	10.4	11.6	4.9	4.8
Diarrhea	11.9	8.4§	10.2	9.3	8.3	9.4	11.6	9.2
Urticaria-like Rash	1.4	0.3§	1.3	1.4	0.4	0.5	0.5	1.7

*Approximately 75% of subjects received prophylactic or therapeutic antipyretics within 48 hours of each dose.
† Investigational meningococcal group C conjugate vaccine (MnCC).
‡ Most of these children had received DTP for the primary series. Thus, this is a 4th dose of a pertussis vaccine, but not of DTaP.
§ $p<0.05$ when Prevnar® compared to control group using a Chi-Square test.

TABLE 13
Percentage of Subjects* Reporting Systemic Reactions Within 3 Days Following Immunization With Prevnar®, DTaP, HbOC, Hep B, and IPV vs. Control† in Manufacturing Bridging Study[29]

Reaction	Dose 1		Dose 2		Dose 3	
	Prevnar®	Control†	Prevnar®	Control†	Prevnar®	Control†
	N=498	N=108	N=452	N=99	N=445	N=89
Fever						
≥38.0°C	21.9	10.2‡	33.6	17.2‡	28.1	23.6
>39.0°C	0.8	0.9	3.8	0.0	2.2	0.0
Irritability	59.7	60.2	65.3	52.5‡	54.2	50.6
Drowsiness	50.8	38.9‡	30.3	31.3	21.2	20.2
Decreased Appetite	19.1	15.7	20.6	11.1‡	20.4	9.0‡

*Approximately 72% of subjects received prophylactic or therapeutic antipyretics within 48 hours of each dose.
† Control group received concomitant vaccines only in the same schedule as the Prevnar® group (DTaP, HbOC at dose 1, 2, 3; IPV at doses 1 and 2; Hep B at doses 1 and 3).
‡ $p<0.05$ when Prevnar® compared to control group using Fisher's Exact test.

Prevnar—Cont.

vaccine. In addition, in most of the reports existing medical conditions such as history of apnea, infection, prematurity, and/or seizure were present.

ADVERSE EVENT REPORTING

Any suspected adverse events following immunization should be reported by the healthcare professional to the US Department of Health and Human Services (DHHS). The National Vaccine Injury Compensation Program requires that the manufacturer and lot number of the vaccine administered be recorded by the healthcare professional in the vaccine recipient's permanent medical record (or in a permanent office log or file), along with the date of administration of the vaccine and the name, address, and title of the person administering the vaccine.

The US DHHS has established the Vaccine Adverse Event Reporting System (VAERS) to accept all reports of suspected adverse events after the administration of any vaccine including, but not limited to, the reporting of events required by the National Childhood Vaccine Injury Act of 1986. The FDA web site is: http://www.fda.gov/cber/vaers/vaers.htm.

The VAERS toll-free number for VAERS forms and information is 800-822-7967.[43]

OVERDOSAGE

There have been reports of overdose with Prevnar®, including cases of administration of a higher than recommended dose and cases of subsequent doses administered closer than recommended to the previous dose. Most individuals were asymptomatic. In general, adverse events reported with overdose have also been reported with recommended single doses of Prevnar®.

DOSAGE AND ADMINISTRATION

For intramuscular injection only. *Do not inject intravenously.*

The dose is 0.5 mL to be given intramuscularly.

Since this product is a suspension containing an adjuvant, shake vigorously immediately prior to use to obtain a uniform suspension in the vaccine container. The vaccine should not be used if it cannot be resuspended.

After shaking, the vaccine is a homogeneous, white suspension.

Parenteral drug products should be inspected visually for particulate matter and discoloration prior to administration (see **DESCRIPTION**). This product should not be used if particulate matter or discoloration is found.

The vaccine should be injected intramuscularly. The preferred sites are the anterolateral aspect of the thigh in infants or the deltoid muscle of the upper arm in toddlers and young children. The vaccine should not be injected in the gluteal area or areas where there may be a major nerve trunk and/or blood vessel. Before injection, the skin at the injection site should be cleansed and prepared with a suitable germicide. After insertion of the needle, aspirate and wait to see if any blood appears in the syringe, which will help avoid inadvertent injection into a blood vessel. If blood appears, withdraw the needle and prepare for a new injection at another site.

Vaccine Schedule

For infants, the immunization series of Prevnar® consists of three doses of 0.5 mL each, at approximately 2-month intervals, followed by a fourth dose of 0.5 mL at 12-15 months of age. The customary age for the first dose is 2 months of age, but it can be given as young as 6 weeks of age. The recommended dosing interval is 4 to 8 weeks. The fourth dose should be administered at least 2 months after the third dose.

Previously Unvaccinated Older Infants and Children

For previously unvaccinated older infants and children, who are beyond the age of the routine infant schedule, the following schedule applies:[35]

Age at First Dose	Total Number of 0.5 mL Doses
7-11 months of age	3*
12-23 months of age	2†
≥24 months through 9 years of age	1

*2 doses at least 4 weeks apart; third dose after the one-year birthday, separated from the second dose by at least 2 months.

† 2 doses at least 2 months apart.

(See **CLINICAL PHARMACOLOGY** section for the limited available immunogenicity data and **ADVERSE EVENTS** section for limited safety data corresponding to the previously noted vaccination schedule for older children).

Safety and immunogenicity data are either limited or not available for children in specific high risk groups for invasive pneumococcal disease (eg, persons with sickle cell disease, asplenia, HIV-infected).

HOW SUPPLIED

Vial, 1 Dose (5 per package) - NDC 0005-1970-67
CPT Code 90669

TABLE 14
Percentage of Subjects Reporting Systemic Reactions Within 3 Days of Immunization With Prevnar® in Infants and Children from 7 Months Through 9 Years of Age[35]

Age at 1st Vaccination	7-11 Mos.						12-23 Mos.			24-35 Mos.	36-59 Mos.	5-9 Yrs.
Study No.	118-12			118-16			118-9*	118-18		118-18	118-18	118-18
Dose Number	1	2	3†	1	2	3†	1	1	2	1	1	1
Number of Subjects	54	51	24	85	80	50	60	120	117	47	52	100
Reaction												
Fever ≥38.0°C	20.8	21.6	25.0	17.6	18.8	22.0	36.7	11.7	6.8	14.9	11.5	7.0
>39.0°C	1.9	5.9	0.0	1.6	3.9	2.6	0.0	4.4	0.0	4.2	2.3	1.2
Fussiness	29.6	39.2	16.7	54.1	41.3	38.0	40.0	37.5	36.8	46.8	34.6	29.3
Drowsiness	11.1	17.6	16.7	24.7	16.3	14.0	13.3	18.3	11.1	12.8	17.3	11.0
Decreased Appetite	9.3	15.7	0.0	15.3	15.0	30.0	25.0	20.8	16.2	23.4	11.5	9.0

*For 118-9, 2 of 60 subjects were ≥24 months of age.
† For 118-12, dose 3 was administered at 15-18 mos. of age. For 118-16, dose 3 was administered at 12-15 mos. of age.

TABLE 15
Age and Season-Adjusted Comparison of SIDS Rates in the NCKP Efficacy Trial With the Expected Rate from the California State Data for 1995-1997[24,25]

Vaccine	<One Week After Immunization		≤Two Weeks After Immunization		≤One Month After Immunization		≤One Year After Immunization	
	Exp	Obs	Exp	Obs	Exp	Obs	Exp	Obs
Prevnar®	1.06	1	2.09	2	4.28	2	8.08	4
Control*	1.06	2	2.09	3†	4.28	3†	8.08	8†

* Investigational meningococcal group C conjugate vaccine (MnCC).
† Does not include one additional case of SIDS-like death in a child older than the usual SIDS age (448 days).

TABLE 16
Overall Percentage of Doses Associated With Systemic Events Within 2 or 3 Days For The US Efficacy Study and All US Ancillary Studies When Prevnar® Administered To Infants As a Primary Series at 2, 4, and 6 Months of Age[24,25,29,31,32,33]

Systemic Event	Prevnar® Concurrently With DTP-HbOC (9,191 Doses)*	Prevnar® Concurrently With DTaP and HbOC (3,848 Doses)†	DTaP and HbOC Control (538 Doses)‡
Fever			
≥38.0°C	35.6	21.1	**14.2**
>39.0°C	3.1	1.8	**0.4**
Irritability	69.1	52.5	**45.2**
Drowsiness	36.9	32.9	**27.7**
Restless Sleep	25.8	20.6	**22.3**
Decreased Appetite	24.7	18.1	**13.6**
Vomiting	16.2	13.4	**9.8**
Diarrhea	11.4	9.8	**4.4**
Urticaria-like Rash	0.9	0.6	**0.3**

*Total from which reaction data are available varies between reactions from 8,874-9,191 doses. Data from studies 118-3, 118-7, 118-8.
† Total from which reaction data are available varies between reactions from 3,121-3,848 doses. Data from studies 118-8, 118-12, 118-16.
‡ Total from which reaction data are available varies between reactions from 295-538 doses. Data from studies 118-12 and 118-16.

STORAGE

DO NOT FREEZE. STORE REFRIGERATED, AWAY FROM FREEZER COMPARTMENT, AT 2°C TO 8°C (36°F TO 46°F).

REFERENCES

1. Schuchat A, Robinson K, Wenger JD, et al. Bacterial meningitis in the United States in 1995. N Engl J Med. 1997; 337:970–6.
2. Zangwill KM, Vadheim CM, Vannier AM, et al. Epidemiology of invasive pneumococcal disease in Southern California: implications for the design and conduct of a pneumococcal conjugate vaccine efficacy trial. J Infect Dis. 1996; 174:752–9.
3. Pastor P, Medley F, Murphy T. Invasive pneumococcal disease in Dallas County, Texas: results from population-based surveillance in 1995. Clin Infect Dis. 1998; 26:590–5.
4. Hofmann J, Cetron MS, Farley MM, et al. The prevalence of drug-resistant *Streptococcus pneumoniae* in Atlanta. N Engl J Med. 1995; 333:481–515.
5. Breiman R, Spika J, Navarro V, et al. Pneumococcal bacteremia in Charleston County, South Carolina. Arch Intern Med. 1990; 150:1401–5.
6. Plouffe J, Breiman R, Facklam R. Franklin County Study Group. Bacteremia with *Streptococcus pneumoniae* in adults-implications for therapy and prevention. JAMA. 1996; 275:194–8.
7. Levine O, Farley M, Harrison LH, et al. Risk factors for invasive pneumococcal disease in children: a population-based case-control study in North America. Pediatrics. 1999; 103:1–5.
8. Kaplan SL, Mason EO, Barson WJ, et al. Three-year multicenter surveillance of systemic pneumococcal infections in children. Pediatrics. 1998; 102:538–44.
9. Arditi M, Mason E, Bradley J, et al. Three-year multicenter surveillance of pneumococcal meningitis in children: clinical characteristics and outcome related to penicillin susceptibility and dexamethasone use. Pediatrics. 1998; 102:1087–97.
10. Shappert SM. Ambulatory care visits to physician offices, hospital outpatient departments, and emergency

TABLE 17
Overall Percentage of Doses Associated With Systemic Events Within 2 or 3 Days For The US Efficacy Study and All US Ancillary Studies When Prevnar® Administered To Toddlers as a Fourth Dose At 12 to 15 Months of Age[24,25,31]

Systemic Event	Prevnar® Concurrently With DTP-HbOC (709 Doses)*	Prevnar® Concurrently With DTaP and HbOC (270 Doses)†	Prevnar® Only No Concurrent Vaccines (727 Doses)‡
Fever			
≥38.0°C	41.9	19.6	13.4
>39.0°C	4.5	1.5	1.2
Irritability	72.8	45.9	45.8
Drowsiness	21.3	17.5	15.9
Restless Sleep	29.9	21.2	21.2
Decreased Appetite	33.0	21.1	18.3
Vomiting	9.6	5.6	6.3
Diarrhea	12.1	13.7	12.8
Urticaria-like Rash	1.4	0.7	1.2

*Total from which reaction data are available varies between reactions from 706-709 doses. Data from study 118-8.
†Total from which reaction data are available varies between reactions from 269-270 doses. Data from studies 118-7 and 118-8.
‡Total from which reaction data are available varies between reactions from 725-727 doses. Data from studies 118-7 and 118-8.

departments: United States, 1997. National Center for Health Statistics. Vital Health Sat. 1999; 13(143):1–41.
11. Hall MJ, Lawrence L. Ambulatory surgery in the United States, 1996. Adv Data Vital Health Stat. 1998; 300:1–16.
12. Teele DW, Klein JO, Rosner B, et al. Epidemiology of otitis media during the first seven years of life in children in greater Boston: a prospective, cohort study. J Infect Dis. 1989; 160:83–94.
13. Shappert, SM. Office visits for otitis media: United States, 1975-1990. Adv Data Vital Health Stat. 1992; 214:1–20.
14. Bluestone CD, Stephenson BS, Martin LM. Ten-year review of otitis media pathogens. Pediatr Infect Dis J. 1992; 11:S7–S11.
15. Giebink GS. The microbiology of otitis media. Pediatr Infect Dis J. 1989; 8:S18–S20.
16. Rodriguez WJ, Schwartz RH. Streptococcus pneumoniae causes otitis media with higher fever and more redness of tympanic membrane than Haemophilus influenzae or Moraxella catarrhalis. Pediatr Infect Dis J. 1999; 18: 942–4.
17. Barnett ED, Klein JO. The problem of resistant bacteria for the management of acute otitis media. Ped Clin North Am. 1995; 42:509–17.
18. Butler JC, Breiman RF, Lipman HB, et al. Serotype distribution of *Streptococcus pneumoniae* infections among preschool children in the United States, 1978-1994: implications for development of a conjugate vaccine. J Infect Dis. 1995; 171:885–9.
19. Paisley JW, Lauer BA, McIntosh K, et al. Pathogens associated with acute lower respiratory tract infection in young children. Pediatr Infect Dis J. 1984; 3:14–9.
20. Heiskanen-Kosma T, Korppi M, Jokinen C, et al. Etiology of childhood pneumonia: serologic results of a prospective, population-based study. Pediatr Infect Dis J. 1998; 17:986–91.
21. American Academy of Pediatrics Committee on Infectious Diseases. Therapy for children with invasive pneumococcal infections. Pediatrics. 1997; 99:289–300.
22. Hausdorff WP, Bryant J, Paradiso PR, Siber GR. Which pneumococcal serogroups cause the most invasive disease: implications for conjugate vaccine formulation and use, part I. Clin Infect Dis. 2000; 30:100–21.
23. Butler JC, Hoffman J, Cetron MS, et al. The continued emergence of drug-resistant *Streptococcus pneumoniae* in the United States. An Update from the Centers for Disease Control and Prevention's Pneumococcal Sentinel Surveillance System. J Infect Dis. 1996; 174:986–93.
24. Lederle Laboratories, Data on File: D118-P8.
25. Black S, Shinefield H, Ray P, et al. Efficacy, safety and immunogenicity of heptavalent pneumococcal conjugate vaccine in children. Pediatr Infect Dis J. 2000; 19:187–195.
26. Lederle Laboratories, Data on File: D118-P809.
27. Eskola J, Kilpi T, Palma A, et al. Efficacy of a pneumococcal conjugate vaccine against acute otitis media. N Engl J Med. 2001; 344:403–409.
28. Fireman B, Black S, Shinefield H, et al. The impact of the pneumococcal conjugate vaccine on otitis media. Pediatr Infect Dis J. In press.
29. Lederle Laboratories, Data on File: D118-P16.
30. Lederle Laboratories, Data on File: D118-P8 Addendum DTaP Immunogenicity.
31. Shinefield HR, Black S, Ray P. Safety and immunogenicity of heptavalent pneumococcal CRM_{197} conjugate vaccine in infants and toddlers. Pediatr Infect Dis J. 1999; 18:757–63.
32. Lederle Laboratories, Data on File: D118-P12.
33. Rennels MD, Edwards KM, Keyserling HL, et al. Safety and immunogenicity of heptavalent pneumococcal vaccine conjugated to CRM_{197} in United States infants. Pediatrics. 1998; 101(4):604–11.
34. Lederle Laboratories, Data on File: D118-P3.
35. Lederle Laboratories, Data on File: Integrated Summary on Catch-Up.
36. Report of the Committee on Infectious Diseases 24th Edition. Elk Grove Village, IL: American Academy of Pediatrics. 1997; 31–3.
37. Update: Vaccine Side Effects, Adverse Reactions, Contraindications, and Precautions. MMWR. 1996; 45 (RR-12):1–35.
38. Recommendations of the Advisory Committee on Immunization Practices (ACIP): use of vaccines and immunoglobulins in persons with altered immunocompetence. MMWR. 1993; 43(RR-4):1–18.
39. Vernacchio L, Neufeld EJ, MacDonald K, et al. Combined schedule of 7-valent pneumococcal conjugate vaccine followed by 23-valent pneumococcal vaccine in children and young adults with sickle cell disease. J Pediatr. 1998; 103:275–8.
40. Immunization of children infected with human immunodeficiency virus – supplementary ACIP statement. MMWR. 1988; 37(12):181–83.
41. Centers for Disease Control and Prevention. General recommendations on immunization. Recommendations of the Advisory Committee on Immunization Practices (ACIP) and the American Academy of Family Physicians (AAFP). MMWR. 2002; 51(RR-2):1–36.
42. Fawcett HA, Smith NP. Injection-site granuloma due to aluminum. Archives Dermatology. 1984; 120:1318–22.
43. Vaccines Adverse Event Reporting System – United States. MMWR. 1990; 39:730–3.

Wyeth®
Manufactured by:
Wyeth Pharmaceuticals Inc.
Philadelphia, PA 19101
US Govt. License No. 3

W10430C003
ET01
Rev 01/04

Shown in Product Identification Guide, page 337

PROTONIX® ℞

[*prō'tŏn-iks*]
(pantoprazole sodium)
Delayed-Release Tablets
℞ only

DESCRIPTION

The active ingredient in PROTONIX® (pantoprazole sodium) Delayed-Release Tablets is a substituted benzimidazole, sodium 5-(difluoromethoxy)-2-[[(3,4-dimethoxy-2-pyridinyl)methyl] sulfinyl]-1*H*-benzimidazole sesquihydrate, a compound that inhibits gastric acid secretion. Its empirical formula is $C_{16}H_{14}F_2N_3NaO_4S$ x 1.5 H_2O, with a molecular weight of 432.4. The structural formula is:
[See chemical structure at top of next column]
Pantoprazole sodium sesquihydrate is a white to off-white crystalline powder and is racemic. Pantoprazole has weakly basic and acidic properties. Pantoprazole sodium sesquihydrate is freely soluble in water, very slightly soluble in phosphate buffer at pH 7.4, and practically insoluble in n-hexane.

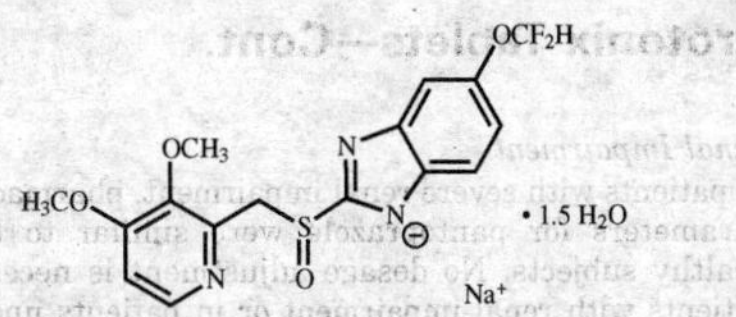

The stability of the compound in aqueous solution is pH-dependent. The rate of degradation increases with decreasing pH. At ambient temperature, the degradation half-life is approximately 2.8 hours at pH 5.0 and approximately 220 hours at pH 7.8.
PROTONIX is supplied as a delayed-release tablet for oral administration, available in 2 strengths. Each delayed-release tablet contains 45.1 mg or 22.6 mg of pantoprazole sodium sesquihydrate (equivalent to 40 mg or 20 mg pantoprazole, respectively) with the following inactive ingredients: calcium stearate, crospovidone, hypromellose, iron oxide, mannitol, methacrylic acid copolymer, polysorbate 80, povidone, propylene glycol, sodium carbonate, sodium lauryl sulfate, titanium dioxide, and triethyl citrate.

CLINICAL PHARMACOLOGY

Pharmacokinetics

PROTONIX is prepared as an enteric-coated tablet so that absorption of pantoprazole begins only after the tablet leaves the stomach. Peak serum concentration (C_{max}) and area under the serum concentration time curve (AUC) increase in a manner proportional to oral and intravenous doses from 10 mg to 80 mg. Pantoprazole does not accumulate and its pharmacokinetics are unaltered with multiple daily dosing. Following oral or intravenous administration, the serum concentration of pantoprazole declines biexponentially with a terminal elimination half-life of approximately one hour. In extensive metabolizers (see Metabolism section) with normal liver function receiving an oral dose of the enteric-coated 40 mg pantoprazole tablet, the peak concentration (C_{max}) is 2.5 μg/mL, the time to reach the peak concentration (t_{max}) is 2.5 h and the total area under the plasma concentration versus time curve (AUC) is 4.8 μg•hr/mL. When pantoprazole is given with food, its t_{max} is highly variable and may increase significantly. Following intravenous administration of pantoprazole to extensive metabolizers, its total clearance is 7.6-14.0 L/h and its apparent volume of distribution is 11.0-23.6L.

Absorption

The absorption of pantoprazole is rapid, with a C_{max} of 2.5 μg/mL that occurs approximately 2.5 hours after single or multiple oral 40-mg doses. Pantoprazole is well absorbed; it undergoes little first-pass metabolism resulting in an absolute bioavailability of approximately 77%. Pantoprazole absorption is not affected by concomitant administration of antacids. Administration of pantoprazole with food may delay its absorption up to 2 hours or longer; however, the C_{max} and the extent of pantoprazole absorption (AUC) are not altered. Thus, pantoprazole may be taken without regard to timing of meals.

Distribution

The apparent volume of distribution of pantoprazole is approximately 11.0-23.6L, distributing mainly in extracellular fluid. The serum protein binding of pantoprazole is about 98%, primarily to albumin.

Metabolism

Pantoprazole is extensively metabolized in the liver through the cytochrome P450 (CYP) system. Pantoprazole metabolism is independent of the route of administration (intravenous or oral). The main metabolic pathway is demethylation, by CYP2C19, with subsequent sulfation; other metabolic pathways include oxidation by CYP3A4. There is no evidence that any of the pantoprazole metabolites have significant pharmacologic activity. CYP2C19 displays a known genetic polymorphism due to its deficiency in some sub-populations (e.g. 3% of Caucasians and African-Americans and 17-23% of Asians). Although these sub-populations of slow pantoprazole metabolizers have elimination half-life values of 3.5 to 10.0 hours, they still have minimal accumulation (≤ 23%) with once daily dosing.

Elimination

After a single oral or intravenous dose of ^{14}C-labeled pantoprazole to healthy, normal metabolizer volunteers, approximately 71% of the dose was excreted in the urine with 18% excreted in the feces through biliary excretion. There was no renal excretion of unchanged pantoprazole.

Special Populations

Geriatric

Only slight to moderate increases in pantoprazole AUC (43%) and C_{max} (26%) were found in elderly volunteers (64 to 76 years of age) after repeated oral administration, compared with younger subjects. No dosage adjustment is recommended based on age.

Pediatric

The pharmacokinetics of pantoprazole have not been investigated in patients <18 years of age.

Gender

There is a modest increase in pantoprazole AUC and C_{max} in women compared to men. However, weight-normalized clearance values are similar in women and men. No dosage adjustment is needed based on gender (Also see **Use in Women**).

Continued on next page

Protonix Tablets—Cont.

Renal Impairment
In patients with severe renal impairment, pharmacokinetic parameters for pantoprazole were similar to those of healthy subjects. No dosage adjustment is necessary in patients with renal impairment or in patients undergoing hemodialysis.
Hepatic Impairment
In patients with mild to severe hepatic impairment, maximum pantoprazole concentrations increased only slightly (1.5-fold) relative to healthy subjects. Although serum half-life values increased to 7-9 hours and AUC values increased by 5- to 7-fold in hepatic-impaired patients, these increases were no greater than those observed in slow CYP2C19 metabolizers, where no dosage frequency adjustment is warranted. These pharmacokinetic changes in hepatic-impaired patients result in minimal drug accumulation following once daily multiple-dose administration. No dosage adjustment is needed in patients with mild to severe hepatic impairment. Doses higher than 40 mg/day have not been studied in hepatically-impaired patients.

Drug-Drug Interactions
Pantoprazole is metabolized mainly by CYP2C19 and to minor extents by CYPs 3A4, 2D6 and 2C9. In *in vivo* drug-drug interaction studies with CYP2C19 substrates (diazepam [also a CYP3A4 substrate] and phenytoin [also a CYP3A4 inducer]), nifedipine, midazolam, and clarithromycin (CYP3A4 substrates), metoprolol (a CYP2D6 substrate), diclofenac, naproxen and piroxicam (CYP2C9 substrates) and theophylline (a CYP1A2 substrate) in healthy subjects, the pharmacokinetics of pantoprazole were not significantly altered. It is, therefore, expected that other drugs metabolized by CYPs 2C19, 3A4, 2D6, 2C9 and 1A2 would not significantly affect the pharmacokinetics of pantoprazole. *In vivo* studies also suggest that pantoprazole does not significantly affect the kinetics of other drugs (cisapride, theophylline, diazepam [and its active metabolite, desmethyldiazepam], phenytoin, warfarin, metoprolol, nifedipine, carbamazepine, midazolam, clarithromycin, naproxen, piroxicam and oral contraceptives [levonorgestrel/ethinyl estradiol]) metabolized by CYPs 2C19, 3A4, 2C9, 2D6 and 1A2. Therefore, it is expected that pantoprazole would not significantly affect the pharmacokinetics of other drugs metabolized by these isozymes. Dosage adjustment of such drugs is not necessary when they are co-administered with pantoprazole. In other *in vivo* studies, digoxin, ethanol, glyburide, antipyrine, caffeine, metronidazole, and amoxicillin had no clinically relevant interactions with pantoprazole. Although no significant drug-drug interactions have been observed in clinical studies, the potential for significant drug-drug interactions with more than once daily dosing with high doses of pantoprazole has not been studied in poor metabolizers or individuals who are hepatically impaired.

Pharmacodynamics
Mechanism of Action
Pantoprazole is a proton pump inhibitor (PPI) that suppresses the final step in gastric acid production by covalently binding to the (H^+,K^+)-ATPase enzyme system at the secretory surface of the gastric parietal cell. This effect leads to inhibition of both basal and stimulated gastric acid secretion irrespective of the stimulus. The binding to the (H^+,K^+)-ATPase results in a duration of antisecretory effect that persists longer than 24 hours for all doses tested.
Antisecretory Activity
Under maximal acid stimulatory conditions using pentagastrin, a dose-dependent decrease in gastric acid output occurs after a single dose of oral (20-80 mg) or a single dose of intravenous (20-120 mg) pantoprazole in healthy volunteers. Pantoprazole given once daily results in increasing inhibition of gastric acid secretion. Following the initial oral dose of 40 mg pantoprazole, a 51% mean inhibition was achieved by 2.5 hours. With once a day dosing for 7 days the mean inhibition was increased to 85%. Pantoprazole suppressed acid secretion in excess of 95% in half of the subjects. Acid secretion had returned to normal within a week after the last dose of pantoprazole; there was no evidence of rebound hypersecretion.
In a series of dose-response studies pantoprazole, at oral doses ranging from 20 to 120 mg, caused dose-related increases in median basal gastric pH and in the percent of time gastric pH was > 3 and > 4. Treatment with 40 mg of pantoprazole produced optimal increases in gastric pH which were significantly greater than the 20-mg dose. Doses higher than 40 mg (60, 80, 120 mg) did not result in further significant increases in median gastric pH. The effects of pantoprazole on median pH from one double-blind crossover study are shown below.

Effect of Single Daily Doses of Oral Pantoprazole on Intragastric pH

Time	Median pH on day 7			
	Placebo	20 mg	40 mg	80 mg
8 a.m. - 8 a.m. (24 hours)	1.3	2.9*	3.8*#	3.9*#
8 a.m. - 10 p.m. (Daytime)	1.6	3.2*	4.4*#	4.8*#
10 p.m. - 8 a.m. (Nighttime)	1.2	2.1*	3.0*	2.6*

* Significantly different from placebo
\# Significantly different from 20 mg

Serum Gastrin Effects
Fasting serum gastrin levels were assessed in two double-blind studies of the acute healing of erosive esophagitis (EE) in which 682 patients with gastroesophageal reflux disease (GERD) received 10, 20, or 40 mg of PROTONIX for up to 8 weeks. At 4 weeks of treatment there was an increase in mean gastrin levels of 7%, 35%, and 72% over pretreatment values in the 10, 20, and 40 mg treatment groups, respectively. A similar increase in serum gastrin levels was noted at the 8 week visit with mean increases of 3%, 26%, and 84% for the three pantoprazole dose groups. Median serum gastrin levels remained within normal limits during maintenance therapy with PROTONIX (pantoprazole sodium) Delayed-Release Tablets.
In long-term international studies involving over 800 patients, a 2- to 3-fold mean increase from the pretreatment fasting serum gastrin level was observed in the initial months of treatment with pantoprazole at doses of 40 mg per day during GERD maintenance studies and 40 mg or higher per day in patients with refractory GERD. Fasting serum gastrin levels generally remained at approximately 2 to 3 times baseline for up to 4 years of periodic follow-up in clinical trials.
Following healing of gastric or duodenal ulcers with pantoprazole treatment, elevated gastrin levels return to normal by at least 3 months.
Enterochromaffin-Like (ECL) Cell Effects
In 39 patients treated with oral pantoprazole 40 mg to 240 mg daily (majority receiving 40 mg to 80 mg) for up to 5 years, there was a moderate increase in ECL-cell density starting after the first year of use which appeared to plateau after 4 years.
In a nonclinical study in Sprague-Dawley rats, lifetime exposure (24 months) to pantoprazole at doses of 0.5 to 200 mg/kg/day resulted in dose-related increases in gastric ECL-cell proliferation and gastric neuroendocrine (NE)-cell tumors. Gastric NE-cell tumors in rats may result from chronic elevation of serum gastrin concentrations. The high density of ECL cells in the rat stomach makes this species highly susceptible to the proliferative effects of elevated gastrin concentrations produced by proton pump inhibitors. However, there were no observed elevations in serum gastrin following the administration of pantoprazole at a dose of 0.5 mg/kg/day. In a separate study, a gastric NE-cell tumor without concomitant ECL-cell proliferative changes was observed in 1 female rat following 12 months of dosing with pantoprazole at 5 mg/kg/day and a 9 month off-dose recovery. (See **PRECAUTIONS, Carcinogenesis, Mutagenesis, Impairment of Fertility**).
Other Effects
No clinically relevant effects of pantoprazole on cardiovascular, respiratory, ophthalmic, or central nervous system function have been detected. In a clinical pharmacology study, pantoprazole 40 mg given once daily for 2 weeks had no effect on the levels of the following hormones: cortisol, testosterone, triiodothyronine (T3), thyroxine (T4), thyroid-stimulating hormone (TSH), thyronine-binding protein, parathyroid hormone, insulin, glucagon, renin, aldosterone, follicle-stimulating hormone, luteinizing hormone, prolactin and growth hormone.
In a 1-year study of GERD patients treated with pantoprazole 40 mg or 20 mg, there were no changes from baseline in overall levels of T3, T4, and TSH.

Clinical Studies
PROTONIX Delayed-Release Tablets were used in all clinical trials.
Erosive Esophagitis (EE) Associated with Gastroesophageal Reflux Disease (GERD)
A U.S. multicenter double-blind, placebo-controlled study of PROTONIX 10 mg, 20 mg, or 40 mg once daily was conducted in 603 patients with reflux symptoms and endoscopically diagnosed EE of grade 2 or above (Hetzel-Dent scale). In this study, approximately 25% of enrolled patients had severe EE of grade 3 and 10% had grade 4. The percentages of patients healed (per protocol, n=541) in this study were as follows:

Erosive Esophagitis Healing Rates (per protocol)

	PROTONIX			Placebo
Week	10 mg QD (n = 153)	20 mg QD (n = 158)	40 mg QD (n = 162)	(n = 68)
4	45.6%$^+$	58.4%$^+$#	75.0%$^+$*	14.3%
8	66.0%$^+$	83.5%$^+$#	92.6%$^+$*	39.7%

$^+$ ($p < 0.001$) PROTONIX versus placebo.
* ($p < 0.05$) versus 10 mg, or 20 mg PROTONIX
\# ($p < 0.05$) versus 10 mg PROTONIX

In this study, all PROTONIX treatment groups had significantly greater healing rates than the placebo group. This was true regardless of *H. pylori* status for the 40-mg and 20-mg PROTONIX treatment groups. The 40-mg dose of PROTONIX resulted in healing rates significantly greater than those found with either the 20- or 10-mg dose.
A significantly greater proportion of patients taking PROTONIX 40 mg experienced complete relief of daytime and nighttime heartburn and the absence of regurgitation starting from the first day of treatment compared with placebo. Patients taking PROTONIX consumed significantly fewer antacid tablets per day than those taking placebo.
PROTONIX 40 mg and 20 mg once daily were also compared with nizatidine 150 mg twice daily in a U.S. multicenter, double-blind study of 243 patients with reflux symptoms and endoscopically diagnosed EE of grade 2 or above. The percentages of patients healed (per protocol, n=212) were as follows:

Erosive Esophagitis Healing Rates (per protocol)

	PROTONIX		Nizatidine
Week	20 mg QD (n = 72)	40 mg QD (n = 70)	150 mg BID (n = 70)
4	61.4%$^+$	64.0%$^+$	22.2%
8	79.2%$^+$	82.9%$^+$	41.4%

$^+$ ($p < 0.001$) PROTONIX versus nizatidine.

Once daily treatment with PROTONIX 40 or 20 mg resulted in significantly superior rates of healing at both 4 and 8 weeks compared with twice daily treatment with 150 mg of nizatidine. For the 40 mg treatment group, significantly greater healing rates compared to nizatidine were achieved regardless of the *H. pylori* status.
A significantly greater proportion of the patients in the PROTONIX treatment groups experienced complete relief of nighttime heartburn and regurgitation starting on the first day and of daytime heartburn on the second day compared with those taking nizatidine 150 mg twice daily. Patients taking PROTONIX consumed significantly fewer antacid tablets per day than those taking nizatidine.

Long-Term Maintenance of Healing of Erosive Esophagitis
Two independent, multicenter, randomized, double-blind, comparator-controlled trials of identical design were conducted in GERD patients with endoscopically-confirmed healed erosive esophagitis to demonstrate efficacy of PROTONIX in long-term maintenance of healing. The two U.S. studies enrolled 386 and 404 patients, respectively, to receive either 10 mg, 20 mg, or 40 mg of PROTONIX (pantoprazole sodium) Delayed-Release Tablets once daily or 150 mg of ranitidine twice daily. As demonstrated in the table below, PROTONIX 40 mg and 20 mg were significantly superior to ranitidine at every time point with respect to the maintenance of healing. In addition, PROTONIX 40 mg was superior to all other treatments studied.

Long-Term Maintenance of Healing of Erosive Gastroesophageal Reflux Disease (GERD Maintenance): Percentage of Patients Who Remained Healed

	PROTONIX 20 mg QD	PROTONIX 40 mg QD	Ranitidine 150 mg BID
Study 1	n = 75	n = 74	n = 75
Month 1	91*	99*	68
Month 3	82*	93*#	54
Month 6	76*	90*#	44
Month 12	70*	86*#	35
Study 2	n = 74	n = 88	n = 84
Month 1	89*	92*#	62
Month 3	78*	91*#	47
Month 6	72*	88*#	39
Month 12	72*	83*	37

* ($p < 0.05$ vs ranitidine)
\# ($p < 0.05$ vs PROTONIX 20 mg)
Note: PROTONIX 10 mg was superior ($p < 0.05$) to ranitidine in study 2 but not study 1.

PROTONIX 40 mg was superior to ranitidine in reducing the number of daytime and nighttime heartburn episodes from the first through the twelfth month of treatment. PROTONIX 20 mg, administered once daily, was also effective in reducing episodes of daytime and nighttime heartburn in one trial.

Number of Episodes of Heartburn (mean ± SD)

		PROTONIX 40 mg QD	Ranitidine 150 mg BID
Month 1	Daytime	5.1 ± 1.6*	18.3 ± 1.6
	Nighttime	3.9 ± 1.1*	11.9 ± 1.1
Month 12	Daytime	2.9 ± 1.5*	17.5 ± 1.5
	Nighttime	2.5 ± 1.2*	13.8 ± 1.3

* ($p < 0.001$ vs ranitidine, combined data from the 2 U.S. studies)

Pathological Hypersecretory Conditions Including Zollinger-Ellison Syndrome
In a multicenter, open-label trial of 35 patients with pathological hypersecretory conditions, such as Zollinger-Ellison syndrome with or without multiple endocrine neoplasia-type I, PROTONIX successfully controlled gastric acid secretion. Doses ranging from 80 mg daily to 240 mg daily maintained gastric acid output below 10mEq/h in patients without prior acid-reducing surgery and below 5 mEq/h in patients with prior acid-reducing surgery.
Doses were initially titrated to the individual patient needs, and adjusted in some patients based on the clinical response

with time. (See DOSAGE AND ADMINISTRATION.) PROTONIX was well tolerated at these dose levels for prolonged periods (greater than 2 years in some patients).

INDICATIONS AND USAGE

Short-Term Treatment of Erosive Esophagitis Associated With Gastroesophageal Reflux Disease (GERD)

PROTONIX® (pantoprazole sodium) Delayed-Release Tablets are indicated for the short-term treatment (up to 8 weeks) in the healing and symptomatic relief of erosive esophagitis. For those patients who have not healed after 8 weeks of treatment, an additional 8 week course of PROTONIX may be considered.

Maintenance of Healing of Erosive Esophagitis

PROTONIX Delayed-Release Tablets are indicated for maintenance of healing of erosive esophagitis and reduction in relapse rates of daytime and nighttime heartburn symptoms in patients with gastroesophageal reflux disease (GERD). Controlled studies did not extend beyond 12 months.

Pathological Hypersecretory Conditions Including Zollinger-Ellison Syndrome

PROTONIX Delayed-Release Tablets are indicated for the long-term treatment of pathological hypersecretory conditions, including Zollinger-Ellison syndrome.

CONTRAINDICATIONS

PROTONIX Delayed-Release Tablets are contraindicated in patients with known hypersensitivity to any component of the formulation.

PRECAUTIONS

General

Symptomatic response to therapy with pantoprazole does not preclude the presence of gastric malignancy.

Owing to the chronic nature of erosive esophagitis, there may be a potential for prolonged administration of pantoprazole. In long-term rodent studies, pantoprazole was carcinogenic and caused rare types of gastrointestinal tumors. The relevance of these findings to tumor development in humans is unknown.

Generally, daily treatment with any acid-suppressing medications over a long period of time (e.g. longer than 3 years) may lead to malabsorption of cyanocobalamin (Vitamin B-12) caused by hypo- or achlorhydria. Rare reports of cyanocobalamin deficiency occurring with acid-suppressing therapy have been reported in the literature. This possibility should be considered if clinical symptoms consistent with cyanocobalamin deficiency are observed.

Information for Patients

Patients should be cautioned that PROTONIX Delayed-Release Tablets should not be split, crushed or chewed. The tablets should be swallowed whole, with or without food in the stomach. Concomitant administration of antacids does not affect the absorption of pantoprazole.

Drug Interactions

Pantoprazole is metabolized through the cytochrome P450 system, primarily the CYP2C19 and CYP3A4 isozymes, and subsequently undergoes Phase II conjugation. (See **CLINICAL PHARMACOLOGY, Drug-Drug Interactions.**)

Based on studies evaluating possible interactions of pantoprazole with other drugs, no dosage adjustment is needed with concomitant use of the following: theophylline, cisapride, antipyrine, caffeine, carbamazepine, diazepam (and its active metabolite, desmethyldiazepam), diclofenac, naproxen, piroxicam, digoxin, ethanol, glyburide, an oral contraceptive (levonorgestrel/ethinyl estradiol), metoprolol, nifedipine, phenytoin, warfarin (see below), midazolam, clarithromycin, metronidazole, or amoxicillin. Clinically relevant interactions of pantoprazole with other drugs with the same metabolic pathways are not expected. Therefore, when co-administered with pantoprazole, adjustment of the dosage of pantoprazole or of such drugs may not be necessary. There was also no interaction with concomitantly administered antacids. There have been postmarketing reports of increased INR and prothrombin time in patients receiving proton pump inhibitors, including pantoprazole, and warfarin concomitantly. Increases in INR and prothrombin time may lead to abnormal bleeding and even death. Patients treated with proton pump inhibitors and warfarin concomitantly should be monitored for increases in INR and prothrombin time.

Because of profound and long lasting inhibition of gastric acid secretion, pantoprazole may interfere with absorption of drugs where gastric pH is an important determinant of their bioavailability (e.g., ketoconazole, ampicillin esters, and iron salts).

Carcinogenesis, Mutagenesis, Impairment of Fertility

In a 24-month carcinogenicity study, Sprague-Dawley rats were treated orally with doses of 0.5 to 200 mg/kg/day, about 0.1 to 40 times the exposure on a body surface area basis, of a 50-kg person dosed at 40 mg/day. In the gastric fundus, treatment at 0.5 to 200 mg/kg/day produced enterochromaffin-like (ECL) cell hyperplasia and benign and malignant neuroendocrine cell tumors in a dose-related manner. In the forestomach, treatment at 50 and 200 mg/kg/day (about 10 and 40 times the recommended human dose on a body surface area basis) produced benign squamous cell papillomas and malignant squamous cell carcinomas. Rare gastrointestinal tumors associated with pantoprazole treatment included an adenocarcinoma of the duodenum at 50 mg/kg/day, and benign polyps and adenocarcinomas of the gastric fundus at 200 mg/kg/day. In the liver, treatment at 0.5 to 200 mg/kg/day produced dose-related increases in the incidences of hepatocellular adenomas and carcinomas. In the thyroid gland, treatment at 200 mg/kg/day produced increased incidences of follicular cell adenomas and carcinomas for both male and female rats.

Sporadic occurrences of hepatocellular adenomas and a hepatocellular carcinoma were observed in Sprague-Dawley rats exposed to pantoprazole in 6-month and 12-month toxicity studies.

In a 24-month carcinogenicity study, Fischer 344 rats were treated orally with doses of 5 to 50 mg/kg/day, approximately 1 to 10 times the recommended human dose based on body surface area. In the gastric fundus, treatment at 5 to 50 mg/kg/day produced enterochromaffin-like (ECL) cell hyperplasia and benign and malignant neuroendocrine cell tumors. Dose selection for this study may not have been adequate to comprehensively evaluate the carcinogenic potential of pantoprazole.

In a 24-month carcinogenicity study, B6C3F1 mice were treated orally with doses of 5 to 150 mg/kg/day, 0.5 to 15 times the recommended human dose based on body surface area. In the liver, treatment at 150 mg/kg/day produced increased incidences of hepatocellular adenomas and carcinomas in female mice. Treatment at 5 to 150 mg/kg/day also produced gastric fundic ECL cell hyperplasia.

A 26-week p53 +/- transgenic mouse carcinogenicity study was not positive.

Pantoprazole was positive in the *in vitro* human lymphocyte chromosomal aberration assays, in one of two mouse micronucleus tests for clastogenic effects, and in the *in vitro* Chinese hamster ovarian cell/HGPRT forward mutation assay for mutagenic effects. Equivocal results were observed in the *in vivo* rat liver DNA covalent binding assay. Pantoprazole was negative in the *in vitro* Ames mutation assay, the *in vitro* unscheduled DNA synthesis (UDS) assay with rat hepatocytes, the *in vitro* AS52/GPT mammalian cell-forward gene mutation assay, the *in vitro* thymidine kinase mutation test with mouse lymphoma L5178Y cells, and the *in vivo* rat bone marrow cell chromosomal aberration assay.

Pantoprazole at oral doses up to 500 mg/kg/day in male rats (98 times the recommended human dose based on body surface area) and 450 mg/kg/day in female rats (88 times the recommended human dose based on body surface area) was found to have no effect on fertility and reproductive performance.

Pregnancy

Teratogenic Effects

Pregnancy Category B

Teratology studies have been performed in rats at oral doses up to 450 mg/kg/day (88 times the recommended human dose based on body surface area) and rabbits at oral doses up to 40 mg/kg/day (16 times the recommended human dose based on body surface area) and have revealed no evidence of impaired fertility or harm to the fetus due to pantoprazole. There are, however, no adequate and well-controlled studies in pregnant women. Because animal reproduction studies are not always predictive of human response, this drug should be used during pregnancy only if clearly needed.

Nursing Mothers

Pantoprazole and its metabolites are excreted in the milk of rats. Pantoprazole excretion in human milk has been detected in a study of a single nursing mother after a single 40 mg oral dose. The clinical relevance of this finding is not known. Many drugs which are excreted in human milk have a potential for serious adverse reactions in nursing infants. Based on the potential for tumorigenicity shown for pantoprazole in rodent carcinogenicity studies, a decision should be made whether to discontinue nursing or to discontinue the drug, taking into account the benefit of the drug to the mother.

Pediatric Use

Safety and effectiveness in pediatric patients have not been established.

Use in Women

Erosive esophagitis healing rates in the 221 women treated with PROTONIX (pantoprazole sodium) Delayed-Release Tablets in U.S. clinical trials were similar to those found in men. In the 122 women treated long-term with PROTONIX 40 mg or 20 mg, healing was maintained at a rate similar to that in men. The incidence rates of adverse events were also similar for men and women.

Use in Elderly

In short-term U.S. clinical trials, erosive esophagitis healing rates in the 107 elderly patients (≥ 65 years old) treated with PROTONIX were similar to those found in patients under the age of 65. The incidence rates of adverse events and laboratory abnormalities in patients aged 65 years and older were similar to those associated with patients younger than 65 years of age.

Laboratory Tests

There have been reports of false-positive urine screening tests for tetrahydrocannabinol (THC) in patients receiving most proton pump inhibitors, including pantoprazole. An alternative confirmatory method should be considered to verify positive results.

ADVERSE REACTIONS

Worldwide, more than 11,100 patients have been treated with pantoprazole in clinical trials involving various dosages and duration of treatment. In general, pantoprazole has been well tolerated in both short-term and long-term trials.

In two U.S. controlled clinical trials involving PROTONIX 10-, 20-, or 40-mg doses for up to 8 weeks, there were no dose-related effects on the incidence of adverse events. The following adverse events considered by investigators to be possibly, probably or definitely related to drug occurred in 1% or more in the individual studies of GERD patients on therapy with PROTONIX.

Most Frequent Adverse Events Reported as Drug Related in Short-term Domestic Trials

	% Incidence			
	Study 300-US		Study 301-US	
Study Event	PROTONIX (n = 521)	Placebo (n = 82)	PROTONIX (n = 161)	Nizatidine (n = 82)
Headache	6	6	9	13
Diarrhea	4	1	6	6
Flatulence	2	2	4	0
Abdominal pain	1	2	4	4
Rash	<1	0	2	0
Eructation	1	1	0	0
Insomnia	<1	2	1	1
Hyperglycemia	1	0	<1	0

Note: Only adverse events with an incidence greater than or equal to the comparators are shown.

In international short-term double-blind or open-label, clinical trials involving 20 to 80 mg per day, the following adverse events were reported to occur in 1% or more of 2805 GERD patients receiving pantoprazole for up to 8 weeks.

Adverse Events in GERD Patients in Short-term International Trials

	% Incidence			
Study Event	Pantoprazole Total (N=2805)	Ranitidine 300 mg (N=594)	Omeprazole 20 mg (N=474)	Famotidine 40 mg (N=239)
Headache	2	3	2	1
Diarrhea	2	2	2	<1
Abdominal Pain	1	1	<1	<1

In two U.S. controlled clinical trials involving PROTONIX 10-, 20-, or 40-mg doses for up to 12 months, the following adverse events considered by investigators to be possibly, probably or definitely related to drug occurred in 1% or more of GERD patients on long-term therapy.

Most Frequent Adverse Events Reported as Drug Related in Long-term Domestic Trials

	% Incidence	
Study Event	PROTONIX (n = 536)	Ranitidine (n = 185)
Headache	5	2
Abdominal pain	3	1
Liver function tests abnormal	2	<1
Nausea	2	2
Vomiting	2	2

Note: Only adverse events with an incidence greater than or equal to the comparators are shown.

In addition, in these short- and long-term domestic and international trials, the following treatment-emergent events, regardless of causality, occurred at a rate of ≥ 1% in pantoprazole-treated patients: anxiety, arthralgia, asthenia, back pain, bronchitis, chest pain, constipation, cough increased, dizziness, dyspepsia, dyspnea, flu syndrome, gastroenteritis, gastrointestinal disorder, hyperlipemia, hypertonia, infection, liver function tests abnormal, migraine, nausea, neck pain, pain, pharyngitis, rectal disorder, rhinitis, SGPT increased, sinusitis, upper respiratory tract infection, urinary frequency, urinary tract infection, and vomiting.

Additional treatment-emergent adverse experiences occurring in <1% of pantoprazole-treated patients from these trials are listed below by body system. In most instances the relationship to pantoprazole was unclear.

BODY AS A WHOLE: abscess, allergic reaction, chills, cyst, face edema, fever, generalized edema, heat stroke, hernia, laboratory test abnormal, malaise, moniliasis, neoplasm, non-specified drug reaction, photosensitivity reaction.

CARDIOVASCULAR SYSTEM: abnormal electrocardiogram, angina pectoris, arrhythmia, atrial fibrillation/flutter, cardiovascular disorder, chest pain substernal, congestive heart failure, hemorrhage, hypertension, hypotension, myocardial infarction, myocardial ischemia, palpitation, retinal vascular disorder, syncope, tachycardia, thrombophlebitis, thrombosis, vasodilatation.

DIGESTIVE SYSTEM: anorexia, aphthous stomatitis, cardiospasm, colitis, dry mouth, duodenitis, dysphagia, enteritis, esophageal hemorrhage, esophagitis, gastrointestinal carcinoma, gastrointestinal hemorrhage, gastrointestinal moniliasis, gingivitis, glossitis, halitosis, hematemesis, increased appetite, melena, mouth ulceration, oral moniliasis, periodontal abscess, periodontitis, rectal hemorrhage, stomach ulcer, stomatitis, stools abnormal, tongue discoloration, ulcerative colitis.

Continued on next page

Protonix Tablets—Cont.

ENDOCRINE SYSTEM: diabetes mellitus, glycosuria, goiter.
HEPATO-BILIARY SYSTEM: biliary pain, hyperbilirubinemia, cholecystitis, cholelithiasis, cholestatic jaundice, hepatitis, alkaline phosphatase increased, gamma glutamyl transpeptidase increased, SGOT increased.
HEMIC AND LYMPHATIC SYSTEM: anemia, ecchymosis, eosinophilia, hypochromic anemia, iron deficiency anemia, leukocytosis, leukopenia, thrombocytopenia.
METABOLIC AND NUTRITIONAL: dehydration, edema, gout, peripheral edema, thirst, weight gain, weight loss.
MUSCULOSKELETAL SYSTEM: arthritis, arthrosis, bone disorder, bone pain, bursitis, joint disorder, leg cramps, neck rigidity, myalgia, tenosynovitis.
NERVOUS SYSTEM: abnormal dreams, confusion, convulsion, depression, dry mouth, dysarthria, emotional lability, hallucinations, hyperkinesia, hypesthesia, libido decreased, nervousness, neuralgia, neuritis, neuropathy, paresthesia, reflexes decreased, sleep disorder, somnolence, thinking abnormal, tremor, vertigo.
RESPIRATORY SYSTEM: asthma, epistaxis, hiccup, laryngitis, lung disorder, pneumonia, voice alteration.
SKIN AND APPENDAGES: acne, alopecia, contact dermatitis, dry skin, eczema, fungal dermatitis, hemorrhage, herpes simplex, herpes zoster, lichenoid dermatitis, maculopapular rash, pruritus, skin disorder, skin ulcer, sweating, urticaria.
SPECIAL SENSES: abnormal vision, amblyopia, cataract specified, deafness, diplopia, ear pain, extraocular palsy, glaucoma, otitis externa, taste perversion, tinnitus.
UROGENITAL SYSTEM: albuminuria, balanitis, breast pain, cystitis, dysmenorrhea, dysuria, epididymitis, hematuria, impotence, kidney calculus, kidney pain, nocturia, prostatic disorder, pyelonephritis, scrotal edema, urethral pain, urethritis, urinary tract disorder, urination impaired, vaginitis.

In an open-label US clinical trial conducted in 35 patients with pathological hypersecretory conditions treated with PROTONIX for up to 27 months, the adverse events reported were consistent with the safety profile of the drug in other populations.

Postmarketing Reports
There have been spontaneous reports of adverse events with the postmarketing use of pantoprazole. These reports include anaphylaxis (including anaphylactic shock); angioedema (Quincke's edema); anterior ischemic optic neuropathy; elevated CPK (creatine phosphokinase); severe dermatologic reactions, including erythema multiforme, Stevens-Johnson syndrome, and toxic epidermal necrolysis (TEN, some fatal); hepatocellular damage leading to jaundice and hepatic failure; interstitial nephritis; pancreatitis; pancytopenia; and rhabdomyolysis. In addition, also observed have been confusion, hypokinesia, speech disorder, increased salivation, vertigo, nausea, tinnitus, and blurred vision.

Laboratory Values
In two U.S. controlled, short-term trials in patients with erosive esophagitis associated with GERD, 0.4% of the patients on PROTONIX 40 mg experienced SGPT elevations of greater than three times the upper limit of normal at the final treatment visit. In two U.S. controlled, long-term trials in patients with erosive esophagitis associated with GERD, none of 178 patients (0%) on PROTONIX 40 mg and two of 181 patients (1.1%) on PROTONIX 20 mg, experienced significant transaminase elevations at 12 months (or earlier if a patient discontinued prematurely). Significant elevations of SGOT or SGPT were defined as values at least three times the upper limit of normal that were non-sporadic and had no clear alternative explanation. The following changes in laboratory parameters were reported as adverse events: creatinine increased, hypercholesterolemia, and hyperuricemia.

OVERDOSAGE

Experience in patients taking very high doses of pantoprazole is limited. There have been spontaneous reports of overdosage with pantoprazole, including a suicide in which pantoprazole 560 mg and undetermined amounts of chloroquine and zopiclone were also ingested. There have also been spontaneous reports of patients taking similar amounts of pantoprazole (400 and 600 mg) with no adverse effects.
Pantoprazole is not removed by hemodialysis. In case of overdosage, treatment should be symptomatic and supportive.
Single oral doses of pantoprazole at 709 mg/kg, 798 mg/kg and 887 mg/kg were lethal to mice, rats and dogs, respectively. The symptoms of acute toxicity were hypoactivity, ataxia, hunched sitting, limb-splay, lateral position, segregation, absence of ear reflex, and tremor.

DOSAGE AND ADMINISTRATION

Treatment of Erosive Esophagitis
The recommended adult oral dose is 40 mg given once daily for up to 8 weeks. For those patients who have not healed after 8 weeks of treatment, an additional 8-week course of PROTONIX may be considered. (See **INDICATIONS AND USAGE.**)

Maintenance of Healing of Erosive Esophagitis
The recommended adult oral dose is one PROTONIX 40 mg Delayed-Release Tablet, taken daily. (See **Clinical Studies.**)

Pathological Hypersecretory Conditions Including Zollinger-Ellison Syndrome
The dosage of PROTONIX in patients with pathological hypersecretory conditions varies with the individual patient. The recommended adult starting dose is 40 mg twice daily. Dosage regimens should be adjusted to individual patient needs and should continue for as long as clinically indicated. Doses up to 240 mg daily have been administered. Some patients have been treated continuously with PROTONIX for more than 2 years.
No dosage adjustment is necessary in patients with renal impairment, hepatic impairment, or for elderly patients. Doses higher than 40 mg/day have not been studied in hepatically-impaired patients. No dosage adjustment is necessary in patients undergoing hemodialysis.
PROTONIX delayed-release Tablets should be swallowed whole, with or without food in the stomach. If patients are unable to swallow a 40 mg tablet, two 20 mg tablets may be taken. Concomitant administration of antacids does not affect the absorption of PROTONIX.
Patients should be cautioned that PROTONIX delayed-release Tablets should not be split, chewed or crushed.

HOW SUPPLIED

PROTONIX® (pantoprazole sodium) Delayed-Release Tablets are supplied as 40 mg yellow oval biconvex delayed-release tablets imprinted with PROTONIX (brown ink) on one side.
They are available as follows:
NDC 0008-0841-10 bottles of 100
NDC 0008-0841-81 bottles of 90
NDC 0008-0841-91 bottles of 1000
NDC 0008-0841-99 carton of 10 Redipak® blister strips of 10 tablets each
PROTONIX is supplied as 20 mg yellow oval biconvex delayed-release tablets imprinted with P20 (brown ink) on one side.
They are available as follows:
NDC 0008-0843-81 bottles of 90

Storage
Store PROTONIX® delayed-release Tablets at 20°–25°C (68°–77°F); excursions permitted to 15°–30°C (59°–86°F). [See USP Controlled Room Temperature].
U.S. Patent No. 4,758,579
Packaged by Wyeth Laboratories
A Wyeth-Ayerst Company
Philadelphia, PA 19101
under license from
ALTANA Pharma
D78467 Konstanz, Germany

W10438C008
ET01
Rev 06/04

Shown in Product Identification Guide, page 337

PROTONIX® I.V. ℞

[*prō'tō-nĭks*]
(pantoprazole sodium)
for Injection
℞ only

DESCRIPTION

The active ingredient in PROTONIX® I.V. (pantoprazole sodium) for Injection is a substituted benzimidazole, sodium 5-(difluoromethoxy)-2-[[(3,4-dimethoxy-2-pyridinyl)methyl] sulfinyl]-1H-benzimidazole, a compound that inhibits gastric acid secretion. Its empirical formula is $C_{16}H_{14}F_2N_3NaO_4S$, with a molecular weight of 405.4. The structural formula is:

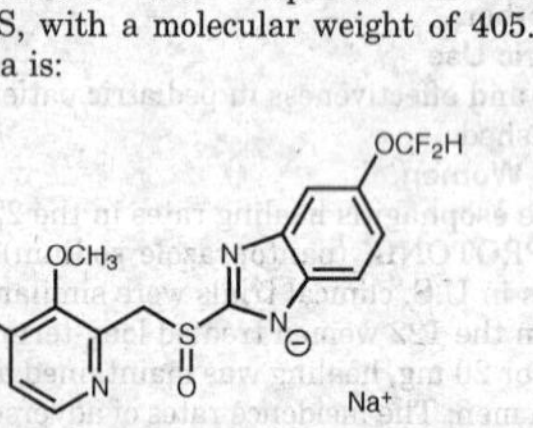

Pantoprazole sodium is a white to off-white crystalline powder and is racemic. Pantoprazole has weakly basic and acidic properties. Pantoprazole sodium is freely soluble in water, very slightly soluble in phosphate buffer at pH 7.4, and practically insoluble in n-hexane. The stability of the compound in aqueous solution is pH-dependent. The rate of degradation increases with decreasing pH. The reconstituted solution of PROTONIX I.V. for Injection is in the pH range 9.0 to 10.5.
PROTONIX I.V. for Injection is supplied as a freeze-dried powder in a clear glass vial fitted with a rubber stopper and crimp seal containing pantoprazole sodium, equivalent to 40 mg of pantoprazole, edetate disodium (1 mg), and sodium hydroxide to adjust pH.

CLINICAL PHARMACOLOGY

Pharmacokinetics
Pantoprazole peak serum concentration (C_{max}) and area under the serum concentration-time curve (AUC) increase in a manner proportional to intravenous doses from 10 mg to 80 mg. Pantoprazole does not accumulate and its pharmacokinetics are unaltered with multiple daily dosing. Following the administration of PROTONIX I.V. for Injection, the serum concentration of pantoprazole declines biexponentially with a terminal elimination half-life of approximately one hour. In extensive metabolizers (see **CLINICAL PHARMACOLOGY, Metabolism**) with normal liver function receiving a 40 mg dose of PROTONIX I.V. for Injection by constant rate over 15 minutes, the peak concentration (C_{max}) is 5.52 µg/mL and the total area under the plasma concentration versus time curve (AUC) is 5.4 µg · hr/mL. The total clearance is 7.6-14.0 L/h and the apparent volume of distribution is 11.0-23.6 L.

Distribution
The apparent volume of distribution of pantoprazole is approximately 11.0-23.6 L, distributing mainly in extracellular fluid. The serum protein binding of pantoprazole is about 98%, primarily to albumin.

Metabolism
Pantoprazole is extensively metabolized in the liver through the cytochrome P450 (CYP) system. Pantoprazole metabolism is independent of the route of administration (intravenous or oral). The main metabolic pathway is demethylation, by CYP2C19, with subsequent sulfation; other metabolic pathways include oxidation by CYP3A4. There is no evidence that any of the pantoprazole metabolites have significant pharmacologic activity. CYP2C19 displays a known genetic polymorphism due to its deficiency in some sub-populations (e.g., 3% of Caucasians and African-Americans and 17-23% of Asians). Although these sub-populations of slow pantoprazole metabolizers have elimination half-life values from 3.5 to 10.0 hours, they still have minimal accumulation (≤23%) with once daily dosing.

Elimination
After administration of a single intravenous dose of ^{14}C-labeled pantoprazole to healthy, normal metabolizer subjects, approximately 71% of the dose was excreted in the urine with 18% excreted in the feces through biliary excretion. There was no renal excretion of unchanged pantoprazole.

Special Populations
Geriatric
After repeated I.V. administration in elderly subjects (65 to 76 years of age), pantoprazole AUC and elimination half-life values were similar to those observed in younger subjects. No dosage adjustment is recommended based on age.
Pediatric
The pharmacokinetics of pantoprazole have not been investigated in patients <18 years of age.
Gender
After oral administration there is a modest increase in pantoprazole AUC and C_{max} in women compared to men. However, weight-normalized clearance values are similar in women and men. No dosage adjustment is warranted based on gender (also see **Use in Women**).
Renal Impairment
In patients with severe renal impairment, pharmacokinetic parameters for pantoprazole were similar to those of healthy subjects. No dosage adjustment is necessary in patients with renal impairment or in patients undergoing hemodialysis.
Hepatic Impairment
Oral administration studies (absolute bioavailability is approximately 70%) were performed in patients with mild to severe hepatic impairment. Maximum pantoprazole concentrations increased only slightly (1.5-fold) relative to healthy subjects. Although serum elimination half-life values increased to 7-9 hours and AUC values increased by 5- to 7-fold in hepatic-impaired patients, these increases were no greater than those observed in slow CYP2C19 metabolizers, where no dosage adjustment is warranted. These pharmacokinetic changes in hepatic-impaired patients result in minimal drug accumulation following once daily multiple-dose administration equal to or less than 21%. No dosage adjustment is needed in patients with mild to severe hepatic impairment. Doses higher than 40 mg/day have not been studied in hepatically-impaired patients.

Drug-Drug Interactions
Pantoprazole is metabolized mainly by CYP2C19 and to minor extents by CYPs 3A4, 2D6 and 2C9. In *in vivo* drug-drug interaction studies with CYP2C19 substrates (diazepam [also a CYP3A4 substrate] and phenytoin [also a CYP3A4 inducer]), nifedipine, midazolam, and clarithromycin (CYP3A4 substrates), metoprolol (a CYP2D6 substrate), diclofenac, naproxen and piroxicam (CYP2C9 substrates) and theophylline (a CYP1A2 substrate) in healthy subjects, the pharmacokinetics of pantoprazole were not significantly altered. It is, therefore, expected that other drugs metabolized by CYPs 2C19, 3A4, 2D6, 2C9 and 1A2 would not significantly affect the pharmacokinetics of pantoprazole. *In vivo* studies also suggest that pantoprazole does not significantly affect the kinetics of other drugs (cisapride, theophylline, diazepam [and its active metabolite, desmethyldiazepam], phenytoin, warfarin, metoprolol, nifedipine, carbamazepine, midazolam, clarithromycin, naproxen, piroxicam and oral contraceptives [levonorgestrel/ethinyl estradiol]) metabolized by CYPs 2C19, 3A4, 2D6, 2C9 and 1A2. Therefore, it is expected that pantoprazole would not significantly affect the pharmacokinetics of other drugs metabolized by these isozymes. Dosage adjustment of such drugs is not necessary when they are co-administered with pantoprazole. In other *in vivo* studies, digoxin, ethanol, glyburide, antipyrine, caffeine, metronidazole, and amoxicillin had no clinically relevant interactions with pantoprazole. Although no significant drug-drug interactions have been observed in clinical studies, the potential for significant drug-drug interactions

Gastric Acid Output (mEq/hr, Mean ± SD) and Percent Inhibition[a] (Mean ± SD) of Pentagastrin-Stimulated Acid Output Over 24 Hours Following a Single Dose of PROTONIX I.V. for Injection[b] in Healthy Subjects

Treatment Dose	—2 hours— Acid Output	% Inhibition	—4 hours— Acid Output	% Inhibition	—12 hours— Acid Output	% Inhibition	—24 hours— Acid Output	% Inhibition
0 mg (Placebo, n=4)	39 ± 21	NA	26 ± 14	NA	32 ± 20	NA	38 ± 24	NA
20 mg (n=4–6)	13 ± 18	47 ± 27	6 ± 8	83 ± 21	20 ± 20	54 ± 44	30 ± 23	45 ± 43
40 mg (n=8)	5 ± 5	82 ± 11	4 ± 4	90 ± 11	11 ± 10	81 ± 13	16 ± 12	52 ± 36
80 mg (n=8)	0.1 ± 0.2	96 ± 6	0.3 ± 0.4	99 ± 1	2 ± 2	90 ± 7	7 ± 4	63 ± 18

a: Compared to individual subject baseline prior to treatment with PROTONIX I.V. for Injection.
NA = not applicable.
b: Inhibition of gastric acid output and the percent inhibition of stimulated acid output in response to PROTONIX I.V. for Injection may be higher after repeated doses.

ANTISECRETORY EFFECTS (mEq/h) OF 40 mg PROTONIX I.V. for INJECTION AND 40 mg ORAL PROTONIX IN GERD PATIENTS WITH A HISTORY OF EROSIVE ESOPHAGITIS

Parameter	PROTONIX Delayed-Release Tablets DAY 10	PROTONIX I.V. for Injection DAY 7	Placebo I.V. DAY 7
Mean maximum acid output	6.49 n=30	6.62 n=23	29.19* n=7
Mean basal acid output	0.80 n=30	0.53 n=23	4.14* n=7

*P<0.0001 Significantly different from PROTONIX I.V. for Injection.

with more than once daily dosing with high doses of pantoprazole has not been studied in poor metabolizers or individuals who are hepatically impaired.

Pharmacodynamics

Mechanism of Action

Pantoprazole is a proton pump inhibitor (PPI) that suppresses the final step in gastric acid production by covalently binding to the (H^+, K^+)-ATPase enzyme system at the secretory surface of the gastric parietal cell. This effect leads to inhibition of both basal and stimulated gastric acid secretion irrespective of the stimulus. The binding to the (H^+, K^+)-ATPase results in a duration of antisecretory effect that persists longer than 24 hours for all doses tested.

Antisecretory Activity

The magnitude and time course for inhibition of pentagastrin-stimulated acid output (PSAO) by single doses (20 to 120 mg) of PROTONIX I.V. for Injection were assessed in a single-dose, open-label, placebo-controlled, dose-response study. The results of this study are shown in the table below. Healthy subjects received a continuous infusion for 25 hours of pentagastrin (PG) at 1 μg/kg/h, a dose known to produce submaximal gastric acid secretion. The placebo group showed a sustained, continuous acid output for 25 hours, validating the reliability of the testing model. PROTONIX I.V. for Injection had an onset of antisecretory activity within 15 to 30 minutes of administration. Doses of 20 to 80 mg of PROTONIX I.V. for Injection substantially reduced the 24-hour cumulative PSAO in a dose-dependent manner, despite a short plasma elimination half-life. Complete suppression of PSAO was achieved with 80 mg within approximately 2 hours and no further significant suppression was seen with 120 mg. The duration of action of PROTONIX I.V. for Injection was 24 hours.

[See first table above]

In one study of gastric pH in healthy subjects, pantoprazole was administered orally (40 mg enteric coated tablets) or intravenously (40 mg) once daily for 5 days and pH was measured for 24 hours following the fifth dose. The outcome measure was median percent of time that pH was ≥ 4 and the results were similar for intravenous and oral medications; however, the clinical significance of this parameter is unknown.

Serum Gastrin Effects

Serum gastrin concentrations were assessed in a placebo-controlled five-day study of oral pantoprazole with 40 and 60 mg doses in healthy subjects. Following the last dose on day 5, the median 24-hour serum gastrin concentrations were elevated by 3-4 fold compared to placebo in both 40 and 60 mg dose groups. However, by 24 hours following the last dose median serum gastrin concentrations for both groups returned to normal levels.

During 6 days of repeated administration of PROTONIX I.V. for Injection in patients with Zollinger-Ellison Syndrome, consistent changes of serum gastrin concentrations from baseline were not observed.

Enterochromaffin-Like (ECL) Cell Effects

There are no data available on the effects of intravenous pantoprazole on ECL cells.

In a nonclinical study in Sprague-Dawley rats, lifetime exposure (24 months) to pantoprazole at doses of 0.5 to 200 mg/kg/day resulted in dose-related increases in gastric ECL-cell proliferation and gastric neuroendocrine (NE)-cell tumors. Gastric NE-cell tumors in rats may result from chronic elevation of serum gastrin concentrations. The high density of ECL cells in the rat stomach makes this species highly susceptible to the proliferative effects of elevated gastrin concentrations produced by proton pump inhibitors. However, there were no observed elevations in serum gastrin following the administration of pantoprazole at a dose of 0.5 mg/kg/day. In a separate study, a gastric NE-cell tumor without concomitant ECL-cell proliferative changes was observed in 1 female rat following 12 months of dosing with pantoprazole at 5 mg/kg/day and a 9 month off-dose recovery (see **PRECAUTIONS, Carcinogenesis, Mutagenesis, Impairment of Fertility**).

Other Effects

No clinically relevant effects of pantoprazole on cardiovascular, respiratory, ophthalmic, or central nervous system function have been detected. In a clinical pharmacology study, pantoprazole 40 mg given orally once daily for 2 weeks had no effect on the levels of the following hormones: cortisol, testosterone, triiodothyronine (T3), thyroxine (T4), thyroid-stimulating hormone, thyronine-binding protein, parathyroid hormone, insulin, glucagon, renin, aldosterone, follicle-stimulating hormone, luteinizing hormone, prolactin and growth hormone.

Clinical Studies

Gastroesophageal Reflux Disease (GERD) Associated With a History of Erosive Esophagitis

A multicenter, double-blind, two-period placebo-controlled study was conducted to assess the ability of PROTONIX® I.V. (pantoprazole sodium) for Injection to maintain gastric acid suppression in patients switched from the oral dosage form of pantoprazole to the intravenous dosage form. Gastroesophageal reflux disease (GERD) patients (n=65, 26 to 64 years; 35 female; 9 black, 11 Hispanic, 44 white, 1 other) with a history of erosive esophagitis were randomized to receive either 20 or 40 mg of oral pantoprazole once per day for 10 days (period 1) and, then were switched in period 2 to either daily intravenous pantoprazole or placebo for 7 days, matching their respective dose level from period 1. Patients were administered all test medication with a light meal. Maximum acid output (MAO) and basal acid output (BAO) were determined 24 hours following the last day of oral medication (day 10), the first day (day 1) of intravenous administration and the last day of intravenous administration (day 7). MAO was estimated from a 1 hour continuous collection of gastric contents following subcutaneous injection of 6.0 μg/kg of pentagastrin.

This study demonstrated that, after 10 days of repeated oral administration followed by 7 days of intravenous administration, the oral and intravenous dosage forms of PROTONIX 40 mg are similar in their ability to suppress MAO and BAO in patients having GERD with a history of erosive esophagitis (see table below). Also, patients on oral PROTONIX who were switched to intravenous placebo experienced a significant increase in acid output within 48 hours of their last oral dose. However, at 48 hours after their last oral dose, patients treated with PROTONIX I.V. for Injection had a significantly lower mean basal acid output than those treated with placebo.

[See second table above]

Data comparing PROTONIX I.V. for Injection to other proton pump inhibitors (oral or I.V.) or H2 receptor antagonists (oral or I.V.) are limited, and therefore, are inadequate to support any conclusions regarding comparative efficacy.

Pathological Hypersecretion Associated with Zollinger-Ellison Syndrome

Two studies measured the pharmacodynamic effects of 6 day treatment with PROTONIX I.V. for Injection in patients with Zollinger-Ellison Syndrome (with and without multiple endocrine neoplasia type I). In one of these studies, an initial treatment with PROTONIX I.V. for Injection in 21 patients (29 to 75 years; 8 female; 4 black, 1 Hispanic, 16 white) reduced acid output to the target level (≤ 10 mEq/h) and significantly reduced H+ concentration and the volume of gastric secretions; target levels were achieved within 45 minutes of drug administration.

In the other study of 14 patients (38 to 67 years; 5 female; 2 black, 12 white) with Zollinger-Ellison Syndrome, treatment was switched from an oral proton pump inhibitor to PROTONIX I.V. for Injection. PROTONIX I.V. for Injection maintained or improved control of gastric acid secretion.

In both studies, PROTONIX I.V. for Injection 160 or 240 mg per day in divided doses maintained basal acid secretion below target levels in all patients. Target levels were 10 mEq/h in patients without prior gastric surgery, and 5 mEq/h in all patients with prior gastric acid-reducing surgery. Once gastric acid secretion was controlled, there was no evidence of tolerance during this 7 day study. Basal acid secretion was maintained below target levels for at least 24 hours in all patients and through the end of treatment in these studies (3 to 7 days) in all but 1 patient who required a dose adjustment guided by acid output measurements until acid control was achieved. In both studies, doses were adjusted to the individual patient need, but gastric acid secretion was controlled in greater than 80% of patients by a starting regimen of 80 mg q12h.

INDICATIONS AND USAGE

Treatment of Gastroesophageal Reflux Disease Associated With a History of Erosive Esophagitis

PROTONIX I.V. for Injection is indicated for short-term treatment (7 to 10 days) of patients having gastroesophageal reflux disease (GERD) with a history of erosive esophagitis, **as an alternative to oral therapy in patients who are unable to continue taking PROTONIX (pantoprazole sodium) Delayed-Release Tablets.** Safety and efficacy of PROTONIX I.V. for Injection as an initial treatment of patients having GERD with a history of erosive esophagitis have not been demonstrated.

Pathological Hypersecretion Associated with Zollinger-Ellison Syndrome

PROTONIX I.V. for Injection is indicated for the treatment of pathological hypersecretory conditions associated with Zollinger-Ellison Syndrome or other neoplastic conditions.

CONTRAINDICATIONS

PROTONIX I.V. for Injection is contraindicated in patients with known hypersensitivity to the formulation.

PRECAUTIONS

General

Immediate hypersensitivity reactions: Anaphylaxis has been reported with use of intravenous pantoprazole. This may require emergency medical treatment.

Injection site reactions: Thrombophlebitis was associated with the administration of intravenous pantoprazole.

Hepatic effects: Mild, transient transaminase elevations have been observed in clinical studies. The clinical significance of this finding in a large population of subjects administered intravenous pantoprazole is unknown. (See **ADVERSE REACTIONS** section).

Symptomatic response to therapy with pantoprazole does not preclude the presence of gastric malignancy.

As with any other intravenous product containing edetate disodium (the salt form of EDTA) which is a potent chelator of metal ions including zinc, zinc supplementation should be considered in patients treated with PROTONIX I.V. for Injection who are prone to zinc deficiency. Caution should be used when other EDTA containing products are also co-administered intravenously.

Treatment with PROTONIX® I.V. (pantoprazole sodium) for Injection should be discontinued as soon as the patient is able to resume treatment with PROTONIX Delayed-Release Tablets.

Drug Interactions

Pantoprazole is metabolized through the cytochrome P450 system, primarily the CYP2C19 and CYP3A4 isozymes, and subsequently undergoes Phase II conjugation. (See **CLINICAL PHARMACOLOGY, Drug-Drug Interactions.**)

Based on studies evaluating possible interactions of pantoprazole with other drugs, no dosage adjustment is needed with concomitant use of the following: theophylline, cisapride, antipyrine, caffeine, carbamazepine, diazepam (and its active metabolite, desmethyldiazepam), diclofenac, naproxen, piroxicam, digoxin, ethanol, glyburide, an oral contraceptive (levonorgestrel/ethinyl estradiol), metoprolol, nifedipine, phenytoin, warfarin (see below), midazolam, clarithromycin, metronidazole, or amoxicillin. Clinically relevant interactions of pantoprazole with other drugs with the same metabolic pathways are not expected. Therefore, when co-administered with pantoprazole, adjustment of the dosage of pantoprazole or of such drugs may not be necessary. There was also no interaction with concomitantly administered antacids. There have been postmarketing reports of increased INR and prothrombin time in patients receiving proton pump inhibitors, including pantoprazole, and warfarin concomitantly. Increases in INR and prothrombin time may lead to abnormal bleeding and even death. Patients treated with proton pump inhibitors and warfarin concomitantly should be monitored for increases in INR and prothrombin time.

Because of profound and long lasting inhibition of gastric acid secretion, pantoprazole may interfere with absorption of drugs where gastric pH is an important determinant of their bioavailability (e.g., ketoconazole, ampicillin esters, and iron salts).

Continued on next page

Protonix I.V.—Cont.

Carcinogenesis, Mutagenesis, Impairment of Fertility
In a 24-month carcinogenicity study, Sprague-Dawley rats were treated orally with doses of 0.5 to 200 mg/kg/day, about 0.1 to 40 times the exposure on a body surface area basis, of a 50-kg person dosed at 40 mg/day. In the gastric fundus, treatment at 0.5 to 200 mg/kg/day produced enterochromaffin-like (ECL) cell hyperplasia and benign and malignant neuroendocrine cell tumors in a dose-related manner. In the forestomach, treatment at 50 and 200 mg/kg/day (about 10 and 40 times the recommended human dose on a body surface area basis) produced benign squamous cell papillomas and malignant squamous cell carcinomas. Rare gastrointestinal tumors associated with pantoprazole treatment included an adenocarcinoma of the duodenum at 50 mg/kg/day, and benign polyps and adenocarcinomas of the gastric fundus at 200 mg/kg/day. In the liver, treatment at 0.5 to 200 mg/kg/day produced dose-related increases in the incidences of hepatocellular adenomas and carcinomas. In the thyroid gland, treatment at 200 mg/kg/day produced increased incidences of follicular cell adenomas and carcinomas for both male and female rats.
Sporadic occurrences of hepatocellular adenomas and a hepatocellular carcinoma were observed in Sprague-Dawley rats exposed to pantoprazole in 6-month and 12-month oral toxicity studies.
In a 24-month carcinogenicity study, Fischer 344 rats were treated orally with doses of 5 to 50 mg/kg/day, approximately 1 to 10 times the recommended human dose based on body surface area. In the gastric fundus, treatment at 5 to 50 mg/kg/day produced enterochromaffin-like (ECL) cell hyperplasia and benign and malignant neuroendocrine cell tumors. Dose selection for this study may not have been adequate to comprehensively evaluate the carcinogenic potential of pantoprazole.
In a 24-month carcinogenicity study, B6C3F1 mice were treated orally with doses of 5 to 150 mg/kg/day, 0.5 to 15 times the recommended human dose based on body surface area. In the liver, treatment at 150 mg/kg/day produced increased incidences of hepatocellular adenomas and carcinomas in female mice. Treatment at 5 to 150 mg/kg/day also produced gastric fundic ECL cell hyperplasia.
Pantoprazole was positive in the *in vitro* human lymphocyte chromosomal aberration assays, in one of two mouse micronucleus tests for clastogenic effects, and in the *in vitro* Chinese hamster ovarian cell/HGPRT forward mutation assay for mutagenic effects. Equivocal results were observed in the *in vivo* rat liver DNA covalent binding assay. Pantoprazole was negative in the *in vitro* Ames mutation assay, the *in vitro* unscheduled DNA synthesis (UDS) assay with rat hepatocytes, the *in vitro* AS52/GPT mammalian cell-forward gene mutation assay, the *in vitro* thymidine kinase mutation test with mouse lymphoma L5178Y cells, and the *in vivo* rat bone marrow cell chromosomal aberration assay. A 26-week p53 +/- transgenic mouse carcinogenicity study was not positive.
Pantoprazole at oral doses up to 500 mg/kg/day in male rats (98 times the recommended human dose based on body surface area) and 450 mg/kg/day in female rats (88 times the recommended human dose based on body surface area) was found to have no effect on fertility and reproductive performance.

Pregnancy
Teratogenic Effects
Pregnancy Category B
Teratology studies have been performed in rats at intravenous doses up to 20 mg/kg/day (4 times the recommended human dose based on body surface area) and rabbits at intravenous doses up to 15 mg/kg/day (6 times the recommended human dose based on body surface area) and have revealed no evidence of impaired fertility or harm to the fetus due to pantoprazole. There are, however, no adequate and well-controlled studies in pregnant women. Because animal reproduction studies are not always predictive of human response, this drug should be used during pregnancy only if clearly needed.

Nursing Mothers
Pantoprazole and its metabolites are excreted in the milk of rats. Pantoprazole excretion in human milk has been detected in a study of a single nursing mother after a single 40 mg oral dose. The clinical relevance of this finding is not known. Many drugs which are excreted in human milk have a potential for serious adverse reactions in nursing infants. Based on the potential for tumorigenicity shown for pantoprazole in rodent carcinogenicity studies, a decision should be made whether to discontinue nursing or to discontinue the drug, taking into account the benefit of the drug to the mother.

Pediatric Use
Safety and effectiveness in pediatric patients have not been established.

Use in Women
No gender-related differences in the safety profile of intravenous pantoprazole were seen in international trials involving 166 men and 120 women with erosive esophagitis associated with GERD. Erosive esophagitis healing rates in the 221 women treated with oral pantoprazole in U.S. clinical trials were similar to those found in men. The incidence rates of adverse events were also similar between men and women.

Use in Elderly
No age-related differences in the safety profile of intravenous pantoprazole were seen in international trials involving 86 elderly (≥ 65 years old) and 200 younger (< 65 years old) patients with erosive esophagitis associated with GERD. Erosive esophagitis healing rates in the 107 elderly patients (≥ 65 years old) treated with oral pantoprazole in U.S. clinical trials were similar to those found in patients under the age of 65. The incidence rates of adverse events and laboratory abnormalities in patients aged 65 years and older were similar to those associated with patients younger than 65 years of age.

Laboratory Tests
There have been reports of false-positive urine screening tests for tetrahydrocannabinol (THC) in patients receiving most proton pump inhibitors, including pantoprazole. An alternative confirmatory method should be considered to verify positive results.

ADVERSE REACTIONS

Safety Experience with Intravenous Pantoprazole
Intravenous pantoprazole has been studied in clinical trials in several populations including patients having GERD with a history of erosive esophagitis, patients with Zollinger-Ellison Syndrome and healthy subjects. Adverse experiences occurring in >1% of patients treated with intravenous pantoprazole (n=714) in domestic or international clinical trials are shown below by body system. In most instances, the relationship to pantoprazole was unclear.
BODY AS A WHOLE: abdominal pain, headache, injection site reaction (including thrombophlebitis and abscess).
DIGESTIVE SYSTEM: constipation, dyspepsia, nausea, diarrhea.
NERVOUS SYSTEM: insomnia.
RESPIRATORY SYSTEM: rhinitis.
Head-to-head comparative studies between PROTONIX I.V. for Injection and oral PROTONIX, other proton pump inhibitors (oral or I.V.), or H2 receptor antagonists (oral or I.V.) have been limited. The available information does not provide sufficient evidence to distinguish the safety profile of these regimens.

Safety Experience with Oral Pantoprazole
In short-term clinical trials in patients with erosive esophagitis associated with GERD treated with oral pantoprazole, the following adverse events, regardless of causality, occurred at a rate of ≥1%.
BODY AS A WHOLE: headache, asthenia, back pain, chest pain, neck pain, flu syndrome, infection, pain.
CARDIOVASCULAR SYSTEM: migraine.
DIGESTIVE SYSTEM: diarrhea, flatulence, abdominal pain, eructation, constipation, dyspepsia, gastroenteritis, gastrointestinal disorder, nausea, rectal disorder, vomiting.
HEPATO-BILIARY SYSTEM: liver function tests abnormal, SGPT increased.
METABOLIC AND NUTRITIONAL: hyperglycemia, hyperlipemia.
MUSCULOSKELETAL SYSTEM: arthralgia.
NERVOUS SYSTEM: insomnia, anxiety, dizziness, hypertonia.
RESPIRATORY SYSTEM: bronchitis, cough increased, dyspnea, pharyngitis, rhinitis, sinusitis, upper respiratory tract infection.
SKIN AND APPENDAGES: rash.
UROGENITAL SYSTEM: urinary frequency, and urinary tract infection.
Additional adverse experiences occurring in <1% of patients with erosive esophagitis associated with GERD receiving oral pantoprazole based on pooled results from either short-term domestic or international trials are shown below within each body system. In most instances, the relationship to pantoprazole was unclear.
BODY AS A WHOLE: abscess, allergic reaction, chills, cyst, face edema, fever, generalized edema, heat stroke, hernia, laboratory test abnormal, malaise, moniliasis, neoplasm, non-specified drug reaction.
CARDIOVASCULAR SYSTEM: abnormal electrocardiogram, angina pectoris, arrhythmia, cardiovascular disorder, chest pain substernal, congestive heart failure, hemorrhage, hypertension, hypotension, myocardial ischemia, palpitation, retinal vascular disorder, syncope, tachycardia, thrombophlebitis, thrombosis, vasodilatation.
DIGESTIVE SYSTEM: anorexia, aphthous stomatitis, cardiospasm, colitis, dry mouth, duodenitis, dysphagia, enteritis, esophageal hemorrhage, esophagitis, gastrointestinal carcinoma, gastrointestinal hemorrhage, gastrointestinal moniliasis, gingivitis, glossitis, halitosis, hematemesis, increased appetite, melena, mouth ulceration, oral moniliasis, periodontal abscess, periodontitis, rectal hemorrhage, stomach ulcer, stomatitis, stools abnormal, tongue discoloration, ulcerative colitis.
ENDOCRINE SYSTEM: diabetes mellitus, glycosuria, goiter.
HEPATO-BILIARY SYSTEM: biliary pain, hyperbilirubinemia, cholecystitis, cholelithiasis, cholestatic jaundice, hepatitis, alkaline phosphatase increased, gamma glutamyl transpeptidase increased, SGOT increased.
HEMIC AND LYMPHATIC SYSTEM: anemia, ecchymosis, eosinophilia, hypochromic anemia, iron deficiency anemia, leukocytosis, leukopenia, thrombocytopenia.
METABOLIC AND NUTRITIONAL: dehydration, edema, gout, peripheral edema, thirst, weight gain, weight loss.
MUSCULOSKELETAL SYSTEM: arthritis, arthrosis, bone disorder, bone pain, bursitis, joint disorder, leg cramps, neck rigidity, myalgia, tenosynovitis.
NERVOUS SYSTEM: abnormal dreams, confusion, convulsion, depression, dry mouth, dysarthria, emotional lability, hallucinations, hyperkinesia, hypesthesia, libido decreased, nervousness, neuralgia, neuritis, paresthesia, reflexes decreased, sleep disorder, somnolence, thinking abnormal, tremor, vertigo.
RESPIRATORY SYSTEM: asthma, epistaxis, hiccup, laryngitis, lung disorder, pneumonia, voice alteration.
SKIN AND APPENDAGES: acne, alopecia, contact dermatitis, dry skin, eczema, fungal dermatitis, hemorrhage, herpes simplex, herpes zoster, lichenoid dermatitis, maculopapular rash, pain, pruritus, skin disorder, skin ulcer, sweating, urticaria.
SPECIAL SENSES: abnormal vision, amblyopia, cataract specified, deafness, diplopia, ear pain, extraocular palsy, glaucoma, otitis externa, taste perversion, tinnitus.
UROGENITAL SYSTEM: albuminuria, balanitis, breast pain, cystitis, dysmenorrhea, dysuria, epididymitis, hematuria, impotence, kidney calculus, kidney pain, nocturia, prostatic disorder, pyelonephritis, scrotal edema, urethral pain, urethritis, urinary tract disorder, urination impaired, vaginitis.

Postmarketing Reports
The postmarketing safety profile of intravenous pantoprazole is not substantially different from that of oral pantoprazole (described below).
There have been spontaneous reports of adverse events with postmarketing use of intravenous or oral pantoprazole. These reports include anaphylaxis (including anaphylactic shock); angioedema (Quincke's edema); anterior ischemic optic neuropathy; elevated CPK (creatine phosphokinase); severe dermatologic reactions, including erythema multiforme, Stevens-Johnson syndrome, and toxic epidermal necrolysis (TEN, some fatal); hepatocellular damage leading to jaundice and hepatic failure; interstitial nephritis; pancreatitis; pancytopenia; and rhabdomyolysis. In addition, also observed have been confusion, hypokinesia, speech disorder, increased salivation, vertigo, nausea, tinnitus, and blurred vision.

Laboratory Values
In U.S. clinical trials of patients having GERD with a history of erosive esophagitis and international clinical trials of patients with erosive esophagitis associated with GERD, the overall percentages of transaminase elevations did not increase during treatment with intravenous pantoprazole. For other laboratory parameters, there were no clinically important changes identified.
In two U.S. controlled trials of oral pantoprazole in patients with erosive esophagitis associated with GERD, 0.4% of the patients on 40 mg oral pantoprazole experienced SGPT elevations of greater than three times the upper limit of normal at the final treatment visit. Except in those patients where there was a clear alternative explanation for a laboratory value change, such as intercurrent illness, the elevations tended to be mild and sporadic. The following changes in laboratory parameters were reported as adverse events: creatinine increased, hypercholesterolemia, and hyperuricemia.

OVERDOSAGE

Experience in patients taking very high doses of pantoprazole is limited. There have been spontaneous reports of overdosage with pantoprazole, including a suicide in which pantoprazole 560 mg and undetermined amounts of chloroquine and zopiclone were also ingested. There have also been spontaneous reports of patients taking similar amounts of pantoprazole (400 and 600 mg) with no adverse effects.
Pantoprazole is not removed by hemodialysis. In case of overdose, treatment should be symptomatic and supportive.
Single intravenous doses of pantoprazole at 378, 230, and 266 mg/kg (38, 46, and 177 times the recommended human dose based on body surface area) were lethal to mice, rats and dogs, respectively. The symptoms of acute toxicity were hypoactivity, ataxia, hunched sitting, limb-splay, lateral position, segregation, absence of ear reflex, and tremor.

DOSAGE AND ADMINISTRATION

PROTONIX I.V. for Injection may be administered intravenously through a dedicated line or through a Y-site. The intravenous line should be flushed before and after administration of PROTONIX I.V. for Injection with either 5% Dextrose Injection, USP, 0.9% Sodium Chloride Injection, USP, or Lactated Ringer's Injection, USP. When administered through a Y-site, PROTONIX I.V. for Injection is compatible with the following solutions: 5% Dextrose Injection, USP, 0.9% Sodium Chloride Injection, USP, or Lactated Ringer's Injection, USP.
Midazolam HCl has been shown to be incompatible with Y-site administration of PROTONIX I.V. for Injection. PROTONIX I.V. for Injection may not be compatible with products containing zinc. When PROTONIX I.V. for Injection is administered through a Y-site, immediately stop use if precipitation or discoloration occurs.
Parenteral drug products should be inspected visually for particulate matter and discoloration prior to and during administration whenever solution and container permit.
Treatment with PROTONIX I.V. for Injection should be discontinued as soon as the patient is able to resume treatment with PROTONIX Delayed-Release Tablets. Also, data on the safe and effective dosing for conditions other than those described in **INDICATIONS AND USAGE** such as life-threatening upper gastrointestinal bleeds, are not avail-

able. PROTONIX I.V. 40 mg once daily does not raise gastric pH to levels sufficient to contribute to the treatment of such life-threatening conditions.
Parenteral routes of administration other than intravenous are not recommended.
No dosage adjustment is necessary in patients with renal impairment, hepatic impairment, or for elderly patients. Doses higher than 40 mg/day have not been studied in hepatically-impaired patients. No dosage adjustment is necessary in patients undergoing hemodialysis.

Treatment of Gastroesophageal Reflux Disease Associated With a History of Erosive Esophagitis

The recommended adult dose, **as an alternative to continued oral therapy** is 40-mg pantoprazole given once daily by intravenous infusion for 7 to 10 days. Safety and efficacy of PROTONIX I.V. for Injection as a treatment of patients having GERD with a history of erosive esophagitis for more than 10 days have not been demonstrated (see **INDICATIONS AND USAGE**).

Fifteen Minute Infusion

PROTONIX I.V. for Injection should be reconstituted with 10 mL of 0.9% Sodium Chloride Injection, USP, and further diluted (admixed) with 100 mL of 5% Dextrose Injection, USP, 0.9% Sodium Chloride Injection, USP, or Lactated Ringer's Injection, USP, to a final concentration of approximately 0.4 mg/mL. The reconstituted solution may be stored for up to 2 hours at room temperature prior to further dilution; the admixed solution may be stored for up to 22 hours at room temperature prior to intravenous infusion. Both the reconstituted solution and the admixed solution do not need to be protected from light.
PROTONIX I.V. for Injection admixtures should be administered intravenously over a period of approximately 15 minutes at a rate of approximately 7 mL/min.

Two Minute Infusion

PROTONIX I.V. for Injection should be reconstituted with 10 mL of 0.9% Sodium Chloride Injection, USP, to a final concentration of approximately 4 mg/mL. The reconstituted solution may be stored for up to 2 hours at room temperature prior to intravenous infusion and does not need to be protected from light. PROTONIX I.V. for Injection should be administered intravenously over a period of at least 2 minutes.

Pathological Hypersecretion Associated with Zollinger-Ellison Syndrome

The dosage of PROTONIX I.V. for Injection in patients with pathological hypersecretory conditions associated with Zollinger-Ellison Syndrome or other neoplastic conditions varies with individual patients. The recommended adult dosage is 80 mg q12h. The frequency of dosing can be adjusted to individual patient needs based on acid output measurements. In those patients who need a higher dosage, 80 mg q8h is expected to maintain acid output below 10 mEq/h. Daily doses higher than 240 mg or administered for more than 6 days have not been studied. (See **Clinical Studies** section.) Transition from oral to I.V. and from I.V. to oral formulations of gastric acid inhibitors should be performed in such a manner to ensure continuity of effect of suppression of acid secretion. Patients with Zollinger-Ellison Syndrome may be vulnerable to serious clinical complications of increased acid production even after a short period of loss of effective inhibition.

Fifteen Minute Infusion

Each vial of PROTONIX I.V. for Injection should be reconstituted with 10 mL of 0.9% Sodium Chloride Injection, USP. The contents of the two vials should be combined and further diluted (admixed) with 80 mL of 5% Dextrose Injection, USP, 0.9% Sodium Chloride Injection, USP, or Lactated Ringer's Injection, USP, to a total volume of 100 mL with a final concentration of approximately 0.8 mg/mL. The reconstituted solution may be stored for up to 2 hours at room temperature prior to further dilution; the admixed solution may be stored for up to 22 hours at room temperature prior to intravenous infusion. Both the reconstituted solution and the admixed solution do not need to be protected from light.
PROTONIX I.V. for Injection should be administered intravenously over a period of approximately 15 minutes at a rate of approximately 7 mL/min.

Two Minute Infusion

PROTONIX I.V. for Injection should be reconstituted with 10 mL of 0.9% Sodium Chloride Injection, USP, per vial to a final concentration of approximately 4 mg/mL. The reconstituted solution may be stored for up to 2 hours at room temperature prior to intravenous infusion and does not need to be protected from light. The total volume from both vials should be administered intravenously over a period of at least 2 minutes.

HOW SUPPLIED

PROTONIX® I.V. (pantoprazole sodium) for Injection is supplied as a freeze-dried powder containing 40 mg of pantoprazole per vial.
PROTONIX I.V. for Injection is available as follows:
NDC 0008-0923-51 One carton containing 1 vial of PROTONIX I.V. for Injection (each vial containing 40-mg pantoprazole).

Storage

Store PROTONIX I.V. for Injection at 2°C-8°C (36°F-46°F) and protect from light.
Caution: the reconstituted product should not be frozen.
U.S. Patent No. 4,758,579
Marketed by Wyeth Pharmaceuticals Inc.
Philadelphia, PA 19101
under license from
ALTANA Pharma
D78467 Konstanz, Germany

W10447C009
ET01
Rev 06/04

Shown in Product Identification Guide, page 337

RAPAMUNE® ℞

[*răp-ă-mūn*]
(sirolimus)
Oral Solution and Tablets
℞ only

This product's label may have been revised after this insert was used in production. For further product information and current package insert, please visit www.wyeth.com or call our medical communications department toll-free at 1-800-934-5556.

WARNING:
Increased susceptibility to infection and the possible development of lymphoma may result from immunosuppression. Only physicians experienced in immunosuppressive therapy and management of renal transplant patients should use Rapamune®. Patients receiving the drug should be managed in facilities equipped and staffed with adequate laboratory and supportive medical resources. The physician responsible for maintenance therapy should have complete information requisite for the follow-up of the patient.

DESCRIPTION

Rapamune® (sirolimus) is an immunosuppressive agent. Sirolimus is a macrocyclic lactone produced by *Streptomyces hygroscopicus*. The chemical name of sirolimus (also known as rapamycin) is (3*S*,6*R*,7*E*,9*R*,10*R*,12*R*,14*S*,15*E*,17*E*,19*E*,21*S*,23*S*,26*R*,27*R*,34a*S*)-9,10,12,13,14,21,22,23,24,25,26,27,32,33,34,34a-hexadecahydro-9,27-dihydroxy-3-[(1*R*)-2-[(1*S*,3*R*,4*R*)-4-hydroxy-3-methoxycyclohexyl]-1-methylethyl]-10,21-dimethoxy-6,8,12,14,20,26-hexamethyl-23,27-epoxy-3*H*-pyrido[2,1-c][1,4] oxaazacyclohentriacontine-1,5,11,28,29 (4*H*,6*H*,31*H*)-pentone. Its molecular formula is $C_{51}H_{79}NO_{13}$ and its molecular weight is 914.2. The structural formula of sirolimus is shown below.

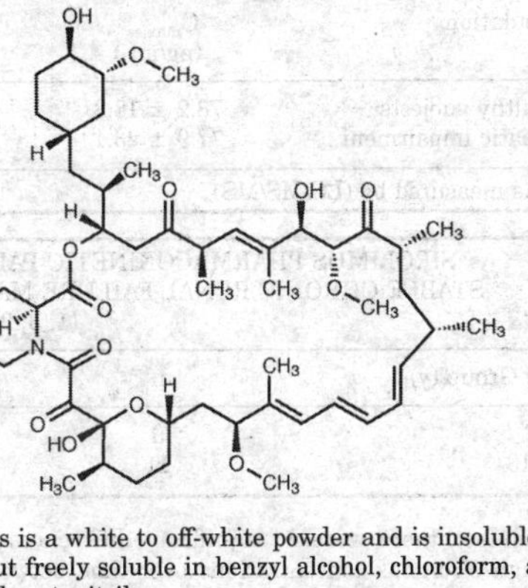

Sirolimus is a white to off-white powder and is insoluble in water, but freely soluble in benzyl alcohol, chloroform, acetone, and acetonitrile.
Rapamune® is available for administration as an oral solution containing 1 mg/mL sirolimus. Rapamune is also available as a white, triangular-shaped tablet containing 1-mg sirolimus, and as a yellow to beige triangular-shaped tablet containing 2-mg sirolimus.
The inactive ingredients in Rapamune® Oral Solution are Phosal 50 PG® (phosphatidylcholine, propylene glycol, mono- and di-glycerides, ethanol, soy fatty acids, and ascorbyl palmitate) and polysorbate 80. Rapamune Oral Solution contains 1.5%-2.5% ethanol.
The inactive ingredients in Rapamune® Tablets include sucrose, lactose, polyethylene glycol 8000, calcium sulfate, microcrystalline cellulose, pharmaceutical glaze, talc, titanium dioxide, magnesium stearate, povidone, poloxamer 188, polyethylene glycol 20,000, glyceryl monooleate, carnauba wax, and other ingredients. The 2 mg dosage strength also contains iron oxide yellow 10 and iron oxide brown 70.

CLINICAL PHARMACOLOGY

Mechanism of Action

Sirolimus inhibits T lymphocyte activation and proliferation that occurs in response to antigenic and cytokine (Interleukin [IL]-2, IL-4, and IL-15) stimulation by a mechanism that is distinct from that of other immunosuppressants. Sirolimus also inhibits antibody production. In cells, sirolimus binds to the immunophilin, FK Binding Protein-12 (FKBP-12), to generate an immunosuppressive complex. The sirolimus:FKBP-12 complex has no effect on calcineurin activity. This complex binds to and inhibits the activation of the mammalian Target Of Rapamycin (mTOR), a key regulatory kinase. This inhibition suppresses cytokine-driven T-cell proliferation, inhibiting the progression from the G_1 to the S phase of the cell cycle.
Studies in experimental models show that sirolimus prolongs allograft (kidney, heart, skin, islet, small bowel, pancreatico-duodenal, and bone marrow) survival in mice, rats, pigs, and/or primates. Sirolimus reverses acute rejection of heart and kidney allografts in rats and prolongs the graft survival in presensitized rats. In some studies, the immunosuppressive effect of sirolimus lasts up to 6 months after discontinuation of therapy. This tolerization effect is alloantigen specific.
In rodent models of autoimmune disease, sirolimus suppresses immune-mediated events associated with systemic lupus erythematosus, collagen-induced arthritis, autoimmune type I diabetes, autoimmune myocarditis, experimental allergic encephalomyelitis, graft-versus-host disease, and autoimmune uveoretinitis.

Pharmacokinetics

Sirolimus pharmacokinetic activity has been determined following oral administration in healthy subjects, pediatric dialysis patients, hepatically-impaired patients, and renal transplant patients.

Absorption

Following administration of Rapamune® Oral Solution, sirolimus is rapidly absorbed, with a mean time-to-peak concentration (t_{max}) of approximately 1 hour after a single dose in healthy subjects and approximately 2 hours after multiple oral doses in renal transplant recipients. The systemic availability of sirolimus was estimated to be approximately 14% after the administration of Rapamune Oral Solution. The mean bioavailability of sirolimus after administration of the tablet is about 27% higher relative to the oral solution. Sirolimus oral tablets are not bioequivalent to the oral solution; however, clinical equivalence has been demonstrated at the 2-mg dose level. (See **Clinical Studies** and **DOSAGE AND ADMINISTRATION**).
Sirolimus concentrations, following the administration of Rapamune Oral Solution to stable renal transplant patients, are dose proportional between 3 and 12 mg/m².
Food effects: In 22 healthy volunteers receiving Rapamune Oral Solution, a high-fat meal (861.8 kcal, 54.9% kcal from fat) altered the bioavailability characteristics of sirolimus. Compared with fasting, a 34% decrease in the peak blood sirolimus concentration (C_{max}), a 3.5-fold increase in the time-to-peak concentration (t_{max}), and a 35% increase in total exposure (AUC) was observed. After administration of Rapamune Tablets and a high-fat meal in 24 healthy volunteers, C_{max}, t_{max}, and AUC showed increases of 65%, 32%, and 23%, respectively. To minimize variability, both Rapamune Oral Solution and Tablets should be taken consistently with or without food (See **DOSAGE AND ADMINISTRATION**).

Distribution

The mean (± SD) blood-to-plasma ratio of sirolimus was 36 ± 18 in stable renal allograft recipients after administration of oral solution, indicating that sirolimus is extensively partitioned into formed blood elements. The mean volume of distribution (V_{ss}/F) of sirolimus is 12 ± 8 L/kg. Sirolimus is extensively bound (approximately 92%) to human plasma proteins. In man, the binding of sirolimus was shown mainly to be associated with serum albumin (97%), α_1-acid glycoprotein, and lipoproteins.

Metabolism

Sirolimus is a substrate for both cytochrome P450 IIIA4 (CYP3A4) and P-glycoprotein (P-gp). Sirolimus is extensively metabolized by the CYP3A4 isozyme in the intestinal wall and liver and undergoes counter-transport from enterocytes of the small intestine into the gut lumen by the P-gp drug efflux pump. Sirolimus is potentially recycled between enterocytes and the gut lumen to allow continued metabolism by CYP3A4. Therefore, absorption and subsequent elimination of systemically absorbed sirolimus may be influenced by drugs that affect these proteins. Inhibitors of CYP3A4 and P-gp increase sirolimus concentrations. Inducers of CYP3A4 and P-gp decrease sirolimus concentrations. (See **WARNINGS** and **PRECAUTIONS, Drug Interactions** and **Other Drug Interactions**). Sirolimus is extensively metabolized by O-demethylation and/or hydroxylation. Seven (7) major metabolites, including hydroxy, demethyl, and hydroxydemethyl, are identifiable in whole blood. Some of these metabolites are also detectable in plasma, fecal, and urine samples. Glucuronide and sulfate conjugates are not present in any of the biologic matrices. Sirolimus is the major component in human whole blood and contributes to more than 90% of the immunosuppressive activity.

Excretion

After a single dose of [^{14}C]sirolimus oral solution in healthy volunteers, the majority (91%) of radioactivity was recovered from the feces, and only a minor amount (2.2%) was excreted in urine.

Pharmacokinetics in renal transplant patients

Rapamune Oral Solution: Pharmacokinetic parameters for sirolimus oral solution given daily in combination with cyclosporine and corticosteroids in renal transplant patients are summarized below based on data collected at months 1, 3, and 6 after transplantation (Studies 1 and 2; see **CLINICAL STUDIES**). There were no significant differences in any of these parameters with respect to treatment group or month.
[See first table at top of next page]
Whole blood sirolimus trough concentrations (mean ± SD), as measured by immunoassay, for the 2 mg/day and 5 mg/day dose groups were 8.6 ± 4.0 ng/mL (n = 226) and

Continued on next page

Rapamune—Cont.

17.3 ± 7.4 ng/mL (n = 219), respectively. Whole blood trough sirolimus concentrations, as measured by LC/MS/MS, were significantly correlated (r^2 = 0.96) with $AUC_{\tau,ss}$. Upon repeated twice daily administration without an initial loading dose in a multiple-dose study, the average trough concentration of sirolimus increases approximately 2 to 3-fold over the initial 6 days of therapy at which time steady state is reached. A loading dose of 3 times the maintenance dose will provide near steady-state concentrations within 1 day in most patients. The mean ± SD terminal elimination half life ($t_{½}$) of sirolimus after multiple dosing in stable renal transplant patients was estimated to be about 62 ± 16 hours.

Rapamune Tablets: Pharmacokinetic parameters for sirolimus tablets administered daily in combination with cyclosporine and corticosteroids in renal transplant patients are summarized below based on data collected at months 1 and 3 after transplantation (Study 3; see **CLINICAL STUDIES**).

[See second table at right]

Whole blood sirolimus trough concentrations (mean ± SD), as measured by immunoassay, for 2 mg of oral solution and 2 mg of tablets over 6 months, were 8.9 ± 4.4 ng/mL (n = 172) and 9.5 ± 3.9 ng/mL (n = 179), respectively. Whole blood trough sirolimus concentrations, as measured by LC/MS/MS, were significantly correlated (r^2 = 0.85) with $AUC_{\tau,ss}$. Mean whole blood sirolimus trough concentrations in patients receiving either Rapamune Oral Solution or Rapamune Tablets with a loading dose of three times the maintenance dose achieved steady-state concentrations within 24 hours after the start of dose administration.

Average Rapamune doses and sirolimus whole blood trough concentrations for tablets administered daily in combination with cyclosporine and following cyclosporine withdrawal, in combination with corticosteroids in renal transplant patients (Study 4; see **CLINICAL STUDIES**) are summarized in the table below.

[See third table at right]

The withdrawal of cyclosporine and concurrent increases in sirolimus trough concentrations to steady-state required approximately 6 weeks. Larger Rapamune® doses were required due to the absence of the inhibition of sirolimus metabolism and transport by cyclosporine and to achieve higher target concentrations during concentration-controlled administration following cyclosporine withdrawal.

Special Populations

Hepatic impairment: Sirolimus oral solution (15 mg) was administered as a single oral dose to 18 subjects with normal hepatic function and to 18 patients with Child-Pugh classification A or B hepatic impairment, in which hepatic impairment was primary and not related to an underlying systemic disease. Shown below are the mean ± SD pharmacokinetic parameters following the administration of sirolimus oral solution.

[See fourth table at right]

Compared with the values in the normal hepatic group, the hepatic impairment group had higher mean values for sirolimus AUC (61%) and $t_{1/2}$ (43%) and had lower mean values for sirolimus CL/F/WT (33%). The mean $t_{1/2}$ increased from 79 ± 12 hours in subjects with normal hepatic function to 113 ± 41 hours in patients with impaired hepatic function. The rate of absorption of sirolimus was not altered by hepatic disease, as evidenced by C_{max} and t_{max} values. However, hepatic diseases with varying etiologies may show different effects and the pharmacokinetics of sirolimus in patients with severe hepatic dysfunction is unknown. Dosage adjustment is recommended for patients with mild to moderate hepatic impairment (see **DOSAGE AND ADMINISTRATION**).

Renal impairment: The effect of renal impairment on the pharmacokinetics of sirolimus is not known. However, there is minimal (2.2%) renal excretion of the drug or its metabolites.

Pediatric: Limited pharmacokinetic data are available in pediatric patients. The table below summarizes pharmacokinetic data obtained in pediatric dialysis patients with chronically impaired renal function.

[See fifth table above]

Geriatric: Clinical studies of Rapamune did not include a sufficient number of patients >65 years of age to determine whether they will respond differently than younger patients. After the administration of Rapamune Oral Solution, sirolimus trough concentration data in 35 renal transplant patients >65 years of age were similar to those in the adult population (n = 822) 18 to 65 years of age. Similar results were obtained after the administration of Rapamune Tablets to 12 renal transplant patients >65 years of age compared with adults (n = 167) 18 to 65 years of age.

Gender: After the administration of Rapamune Oral Solution, sirolimus oral dose clearance in males was 12% lower than that in females; male subjects had a significantly longer $t_{1/2}$ than did female subjects (72.3 hours versus 61.3 hours). A similar trend in the effect of gender on sirolimus oral dose clearance and $t_{1/2}$ was observed after the administration of Rapamune Tablets. Dose adjustments based on gender are not recommended.

Race: In large phase 3 trials (Studies 1 and 2) using Rapamune Oral Solution and cyclosporine oral solution (MODIFIED) (e.g., Neoral® Oral Solution) and/or cyclosporine capsules (MODIFIED) (e.g., Neoral® Soft Gelatin

SIROLIMUS PHARMACOKINETIC PARAMETERS (MEAN ± SD) IN RENAL TRANSPLANT PATIENTS (MULTIPLE DOSE ORAL SOLUTION)[a,b]

N	Dose	$C_{max,ss}$[c] (ng/mL)	$t_{max,ss}$ (h)	$AUC_{\tau,ss}$[c] (ng•h/mL)	CL/F/WT[d] (mL/h/kg)
19	2 mg	12.2 ± 6.2	3.01 ± 2.40	158 ± 70	182 ± 72
23	5 mg	37.4 ± 21	1.84 ± 1.30	396 ± 193	221 ± 143

a: Sirolimus administered four hours after cyclosporine oral solution (MODIFIED) (e.g., Neoral® Oral Solution) and/or cyclosporine capsules (MODIFIED) (e.g., Neoral® Soft Gelatin Capsules).
b: As measured by the Liquid Chromatographic/Tandem Mass Spectrometric Method (LC/MS/MS).
c: These parameters were dose normalized prior to the statistical comparison.
d: CL/F/WT = oral dose clearance.

SIROLIMUS PHARMACOKINETIC PARAMETERS (MEAN ± SD) IN RENAL TRANSPLANT PATIENTS (MULTIPLE DOSE TABLETS)[a,b]

n	Dose (2 mg/day)	$C_{max,ss}$[c] (ng/mL)	$t_{max,ss}$ (h)	$AUC_{\tau,ss}$[c] (ng•h/mL)	CL/F/WT[d] (mL/h/kg)
17	Oral solution	14.4 ± 5.3	2.12 ± 0.84	194 ± 78	173 ± 50
13	Tablets	15.0 ± 4.9	3.46 ± 2.40	230 ± 67	139 ± 63

a: Sirolimus administered four hours after cyclosporine oral solution (MODIFIED) (e.g., Neoral® Oral Solution) and/or cyclosporine capsules (MODIFIED) (e.g., Neoral® Soft Gelatin Capsules).
b: As measured by the Liquid Chromatographic/Tandem Mass Spectrometric Method (LC/MS/MS).
c: These parameters were dose normalized prior to the statistical comparison.
d: CL/F/WT = oral dose clearance.

AVERAGE RAPAMUNE DOSES AND SIROLIMUS TROUGH CONCENTRATIONS (MEAN ± SD) IN RENAL TRANSPLANT PATIENTS AFTER MULTIPLE DOSE TABLET ADMINISTRATION

	Rapamune with Cyclosporine Therapy[a]	Rapamune Following Cyclosporine Withdrawal[a]
Rapamune Dose (mg/day)		
Months 4 to 12	2.1 ± 0.7	8.2 ± 4.2
Months 12 to 24	2.0 ± 0.8	6.4 ± 3.0
Sirolimus C_{min} (ng/mL)[b]		
Months 4 to 12	10.7 ± 3.8	23.3 ± 5.0
Months 12 to 24	11.2 ± 4.1	22.5 ± 4.8

a: 215 patients were randomized to each group.
b: Expressed by immunoassay and equivalence.

SIROLIMUS PHARMACOKINETIC PARAMETERS (MEAN ± SD) IN 18 HEALTHY SUBJECTS AND 18 PATIENTS WITH HEPATIC IMPAIRMENT (15 MG SINGLE DOSE – ORAL SOLUTION)

Population	$C_{max,ss}$[a] (ng/mL)	t_{max} (h)	$AUC_{0-\infty}$ (ng•h/mL)	CL/F/WT (mL/h/kg)
Healthy subjects	78.2 ± 18.3	0.82 ± 0.17	970 ± 272	215 ± 76
Hepatic impairment	77.9 ± 23.1	0.84 ± 0.17	1567 ± 616	144 ± 62

[a]: As measured by (LC/MS/MS).

SIROLIMUS PHARMACOKINETIC PARAMETERS (MEAN ± SD) IN PEDIATRIC PATIENTS WITH STABLE CHRONIC RENAL FAILURE MAINTAINED ON HEMODIALYSIS OR PERITONEAL DIALYSIS (1, 3, 9, 15 MG/M^2 SINGLE DOSE)

Age Group (y)	n	t_{max} (h)	$t_{1/2}$ (h)	CL/F/WT (mL/h/kg)
5-11	9	1.1 ± 0.5	71 ± 40	580 ± 450
12-18	11	0.79 ± 0.17	55 ± 18	450 ± 232

Capsules), there were no significant differences in mean trough sirolimus concentrations over time between black (n = 139) and non-black (n = 724) patients during the first 6 months after transplantation at sirolimus doses of 2 mg/day and 5 mg/day. Similarly, after administration of Rapamune Tablets (2 mg/day) in a phase III trial, mean sirolimus trough concentrations over 6 months were not significantly different among black (n = 51) and non-black (n = 128) patients.

CLINICAL STUDIES

Rapamune® Oral Solution: The safety and efficacy of Rapamune® Oral Solution for the prevention of organ rejection following renal transplantation were assessed in two randomized, double-blind, multicenter, controlled trials. These studies compared two dose levels of Rapamune Oral Solution (2 mg and 5 mg, once daily) with azathioprine (Study 1) or placebo (Study 2) when administered in combination with cyclosporine and corticosteroids. Study 1 was conducted in the United States at 38 sites. Seven hundred nineteen (719) patients were enrolled in this trial and randomized following transplantation; 284 were randomized to receive Rapamune Oral Solution 2 mg/day, 274 were randomized to receive Rapamune Oral Solution 5 mg/day, and 161 to receive azathioprine 2-3 mg/kg/day. Study 2 was conducted in Australia, Canada, Europe, and the United States, at a total of 34 sites. Five hundred seventy-six (576) patients were enrolled in this trial and randomized before transplantation; 227 were randomized to receive Rapamune Oral Solution 2 mg/day, 219 were randomized to receive Rapamune Oral Solution 5 mg/day, and 130 to receive placebo. In both studies, the use of antilymphocyte antibody induction therapy was prohibited. In both studies, the primary efficacy endpoint was the rate of efficacy failure in the first 6 months after transplantation. Efficacy failure was defined as the first occurrence of an acute rejection episode (confirmed by biopsy), graft loss, or death. The tables below summarize the results of the primary efficacy analyses from these trials. Rapamune Oral Solution, at doses of 2 mg/day and 5 mg/day, significantly reduced the incidence of efficacy failure (statistically significant at the <0.025 level; nominal significance level adjusted for multiple [2] dose comparisons) at 6 months following transplantation compared with both azathioprine and placebo.

[See first table on next page]

[See second table on next page]

Patient and graft survival at 1 year were co-primary endpoints. The table below shows graft and patient survival at 1 and 2 years in Study 1 and 1 and 3 years in Study 2. The graft and patient survival rates were similar in patients treated with Rapamune and comparator-treated patients.

[See third table at bottom of next page]

The reduction in the incidence of first biopsy-confirmed acute rejection episodes in patients treated with Rapamune compared with the control groups included a reduction in all grades of rejection.

In Study 1, which was prospectively stratified by race within center, efficacy failure was similar for Rapamune Oral Solution 2 mg/day and lower for Rapamune Oral Solution 5 mg/day compared with azathioprine in black patients. In Study 2, which was not prospectively stratified by race, efficacy failure was similar for both Rapamune Oral Solution doses compared with placebo in black patients. The decision to use the higher dose of Rapamune Oral Solution in black patients must be weighed against the increased risk of dose-dependent adverse events that were observed with the Rapamune Oral Solution 5-mg dose (see **ADVERSE REACTIONS**).

[See fourth table at bottom of next page]

Mean glomerular filtration rates (GFR) post transplant were calculated by using the Nankivell equation at 12 and 24 months for Study 1, and 12 and 36 months for Study 2. Mean GFR was lower in patients treated with cyclosporine and Rapamune Oral Solution compared with those treated with cyclosporine and the respective azathioprine or placebo control.

[See first table at top of next page]

Within each treatment group in Studies 1 and 2, mean GFR at one year post transplant was lower in patients who experienced at least 1 episode of biopsy-proven acute rejection, compared with those who did not.

Renal function should be monitored and appropriate adjustment of the immunosuppression regimen should be considered in patients with elevated or increasing serum creatinine levels (see **PRECAUTIONS**).

Rapamune® Tablets: The safety and efficacy of Rapamune Oral Solution and Rapamune Tablets for the prevention of organ rejection following renal transplantation were compared in a randomized multicenter controlled trial (Study 3). This study compared a single dose level (2 mg, once daily) of Rapamune Oral Solution and Rapamune Tablets when administered in combination with cyclosporine and corticosteroids. The study was conducted at 30 centers in Australia, Canada, and the United States. Four hundred seventy-seven (477) patients were enrolled in this study and randomized before transplantation; 238 patients were randomized to receive Rapamune Oral Solution 2 mg/day and 239 patients were randomized to receive Rapamune Tablets 2 mg/day. In this study, the use of antilymphocyte antibody induction therapy was prohibited. The primary efficacy endpoint was the rate of efficacy failure in the first 3 months after transplantation. Efficacy failure was defined as the first occurrence of an acute rejection episode (confirmed by biopsy), graft loss, or death.

The table below summarizes the result of the efficacy failure analysis at 3 and 6 months from this trial. The overall rate of efficacy failure at 3 months, the primary endpoint, in the tablet treatment group was equivalent to the rate in the oral solution treatment group.

[See second table at top of next page]

Graft and patient survival at 12 months were co-primary endpoints. There was no significant difference between the oral solution and tablet formulations for both graft and patient survival. Graft survival was 92.0% and 88.7% for the oral solution and tablet treatment groups, respectively. The patient survival rates in the oral solution and tablet treatment groups were 95.8% and 96.2%, respectively.

The mean GFR at 12 months, calculated by the Nankivell equation, were not significantly different for the oral solution group and for the tablet group.

The table below summarizes the mean GFR at one-year post-transplantation for all patients in Study 3 who had serum creatinine measured at 12 months.

INCIDENCE (%) OF EFFICACY FAILURE AT 6 AND 24 MONTHS FOR STUDY 1[a,b]

Parameter	Rapamune® Oral Solution 2 mg/day (n = 284)	Rapamune® Oral Solution 5 mg/day (n = 274)	Azathioprine 2-3 mg/kg/day (n = 161)
Efficacy failure at 6 months[c]	18.7	16.8	32.3
Components of efficacy failure			
Biopsy-proven acute rejection	16.5	11.3	29.2
Graft loss	1.1	2.9	2.5
Death	0.7	1.8	0
Lost to follow-up	0.4	0.7	0.6
Efficacy failure at 24 months	32.8	25.9	36.0
Components of efficacy failure			
Biopsy-proven acute rejection	23.6	17.5	32.3
Graft loss	3.9	4.7	3.1
Death	4.2	3.3	0
Lost to follow-up	1.1	0.4	0.6

a: Patients received cyclosporine and corticosteroids.
b: Includes patients who prematurely discontinued treatment.
c: Primary endpoint.

INCIDENCE (%) OF EFFICACY FAILURE AT 6 AND 36 MONTHS FOR STUDY 2[a,b]

Parameter	Rapamune® Oral Solution 2 mg/day (n = 227)	Rapamune® Oral Solution 5 mg/day (n = 219)	Placebo (n = 130)
Efficacy failure at 6 months[c]	30.0	25.6	47.7
Components of efficacy failure			
Biopsy-proven acute rejection	24.7	19.2	41.5
Graft loss	3.1	3.7	3.9
Death	2.2	2.7	2.3
Lost to follow-up	0	0	0
Efficacy failure at 36 months	44.1	41.6	54.6
Components of efficacy failure			
Biopsy-proven acute rejection	32.2	27.4	43.9
Graft loss	6.2	7.3	4.6
Death	5.7	5.9	5.4
Lost to follow-up	0	0.9	0.8

a: Patients received cyclosporine and corticosteroids.
b: Includes patients who prematurely discontinued treatment.
c: Primary endpoint.

GRAFT AND PATIENT SURVIVAL (%) FOR STUDY 1 (12 AND 24 MONTHS) AND STUDY 2 (12 AND 36 MONTHS)[a,b]

Parameter	Rapamune® Oral Solution 2 mg/day	Rapamune® Oral Solution 5 mg/day	Azathioprine 2-3 mg/kg/day	Placebo
Study 1	(n = 284)	(n = 274)	(n = 161)	
Graft survival				
Month 12	94.7	92.7	93.8	
Month 24	85.2	89.1	90.1	
Patient survival				
Month 12	97.2	96.0	98.1	
Month 24	92.6	94.9	96.3	
Study 2	(n = 227)	(n = 219)		(n = 130)
Graft survival				
Month 12	89.9	90.9		87.7
Month 36	81.1	79.9		80.8
Patient survival				
Month 12	96.5	95.0		94.6
Month 36	90.3	89.5		90.8

a: Patients received cyclosporine and corticosteroids.
b: Includes patients who prematurely discontinued treatment.

PERCENTAGE OF EFFICACY FAILURE BY RACE AT 6 MONTHS[a,b]

Parameter	Rapamune® Oral Solution 2 mg/day	Rapamune® Oral Solution 5 mg/day	Azathioprine 2-3 mg/kg/day	Placebo
Study 1				
Black (n = 166)	34.9 (n = 63)	18.0 (n = 61)	33.3 (n = 42)	
Non-black (n = 553)	14.0 (n = 221)	16.4 (n = 213)	31.9 (n = 119)	
Study 2				
Black (n = 66)	30.8 (n = 26)	33.7 (n = 27)		38.5 (n = 13)
Non-black (n = 510)	29.9 (n = 201)	24.5 (n = 192)		48.7 (n = 117)

a: Patients received cyclosporine and corticosteroids.
b: Includes patients who prematurely discontinued treatment.

OVERALL CALCULATED GLOMERULAR FILTRATION RATES (CC/MIN) BY NANKIVELL EQUATION AT 12 MONTHS POST TRANSPLANT: STUDY 3[a,b]

	Rapamune® Oral Solution	Rapamune® Tablets
Mean ± SEM	53.1 ± 1.7 (n = 229)	51.7 ± 1.7 (n = 225)

a: Includes patients who prematurely discontinued treatment.
b: Patients who had a graft loss were included in the analysis with GFR set to 0.0.

In Study 4, the safety and efficacy of Rapamune as a maintenance regimen were assessed following cyclosporine withdrawal at 3 to 4 months post renal transplantation. Study 4 was a randomized, multicenter, controlled trial conducted at 57 centers in Australia, Canada, and Europe. Five hundred twenty-five (525) patients were enrolled. All patients in this study received the tablet formulation. This study compared patients who were administered Rapamune, cyclosporine, and corticosteroids continuously with patients who received the same standardized therapy for the first 3 months after transplantation (prerandomization period) followed by the withdrawal of cyclosporine. During cyclosporine withdrawal the Rapamune dosages were adjusted to achieve targeted sirolimus whole blood trough concentration ranges (20 to 30 ng/mL, experimental immunoassay). At 3 months, 430 patients were equally randomized to either Rapamune with cyclosporine therapy or Rapamune as a maintenance regimen following cyclosporine withdrawal. Eligibility for randomization included no Banff Grade 3 acute rejection episode or vascular rejection in the 4 weeks before random assignment; serum creatinine ≤ 4.5 mg/dL; and adequate renal function to support cyclosporine withdrawal (in the opinion of the investigator). The primary efficacy endpoint was graft survival at 12 months after transplantation. Secondary efficacy endpoints were the rate of biopsy-confirmed acute rejection, patient survival, incidence of efficacy failure (defined as the first occurrence of either biopsy-proven acute rejection, graft loss, or death), and treatment failure (defined as the first occurrence of either discontinuation, acute rejection, graft loss, or death).

The safety and efficacy of cyclosporine withdrawal in high-risk patients have not been adequately studied and it is therefore not recommended. This includes patients with Banff grade III acute rejection or vascular rejection prior to cyclosporine withdrawal, those who are dialysis-dependent, serum creatinine > 4.5 mg/dL, black patients, re-transplants, multi-organ transplants, or patients with high panel of reactive antibodies (See **INDICATIONS AND USAGE**).

The table below summarizes the resulting graft and patient survival at 12, 24, and 36 months for this trial. At 12, 24, and 36 months, graft and patient survival were similar for both groups.

GRAFT AND PATIENT SURVIVAL (%): STUDY 4[a]

Parameter	Rapamune with Cyclosporine Therapy (n = 215)	Rapamune Following Cyclosporine Withdrawal (n = 215)
Graft Survival		
Month 12[b]	95.8	97.2
Month 24	91.2	93.5
Month 36	85.1	91.2

Continued on next page

Rapamune—Cont.

Patient Survival		
Month 12	97.2	98.1
Month 24	94.0	95.3
Month 36	88.4	93.5

a: Includes patients who prematurely discontinued treatment.
b: Primary efficacy endpoint.

The table below summarizes the results of first biopsy-proven acute rejection at 12 and 36 months. There was a significant difference in first biopsy-proven rejection between the two groups during post-randomization through 12 months. Most of the post-randomization acute rejections occurred in the first 3 months following randomization.

INCIDENCE OF FIRST BIOPSY-PROVEN ACUTE REJECTION (%) BY TREATMENT GROUP AT 36 MONTHS: STUDY 4[a]

Period	Rapamune with Cyclosporine Therapy (n = 215)	Rapamune Following Cyclosporine withdrawal (n = 215)
Prerandomization[b]	9.3	10.2
Postrandomization through 12 months[b]	4.2	9.8
Postrandomization from 12 to 36 months	1.4	0.5
Postrandomization through 36 months	5.6	10.2
Total at 36 months	14.9	20.5

a: Includes patients who prematurely discontinued treatment.
b: Randomization occurred at 3 months ± 2 weeks.

Patients receiving renal allografts with ≥ 4 HLA mismatches experienced significantly higher rates of acute rejection following randomization to the cyclosporine withdrawal group compared with patients who continued cyclosporine (15.3% vs 3.0%). Patients receiving renal allografts with ≤ 3 HLA mismatches, demonstrated similar rates of acute rejection between treatment groups (6.8% vs 7.7%) following randomization.

The table below summarizes the mean calculated GFR in Study 4.

CALCULATED GLOMERULAR FILTRATION RATES (mL/min) BY NANKIVELL EQUATION AT 12, 24, AND 36 MONTHS POST TRANSPLANT: STUDY 4[a,b]

Parameter	Rapamune with Cyclosporine Therapy	Rapamune Following Cyclosporine Withdrawal
Month 12		
Mean ± SEM	53.2 ± 1.5 n = 208	59.3 ± 1.5 n = 203
Month 24		
Mean ± SEM	48.4 ± 1.7 n = 203	58.4 ± 1.6 n = 201
Month 36		
Mean ± SEM	47.3 ± 1.8 (n = 194)	59.4 ± 1.8 (n = 194)

a: Includes patients who prematurely discontinued treatment.
b: Patients who had a graft loss were included in the analysis and had their GFR set to 0.0.

The mean GFR at 12, 24, and 36 months, calculated by the Nankivell equation, was significantly higher for patients receiving Rapamune as a maintenance regimen following cyclosporine withdrawal than for those in the Rapamune with cyclosporine therapy group. Patients who had an acute rejection prior to randomization had a significantly higher GFR following cyclosporine withdrawal compared to those in the Rapamune with cyclosporine group. There was no significant difference in GFR between groups for patients who experienced acute rejection postrandomization.

INDICATIONS AND USAGE

Rapamune® (sirolimus) is indicated for the prophylaxis of organ rejection in patients receiving renal transplants. It is recommended that Rapamune be used initially in a regimen with cyclosporine and corticosteroids. In patients at low to moderate immunologic risk cyclosporine should be withdrawn 2 to 4 months after transplantation and Rapamune® dose should be increased to reach recommended blood concentrations (See **DOSAGE AND ADMINISTRATION**).

The safety and efficacy of cyclosporine withdrawal in high-risk patients have not been adequately studied and it is therefore not recommended. This includes patients with Banff grade III acute rejection or vascular rejection prior to cyclosporine withdrawal, those who are dialysis-dependent, or with serum creatinine > 4.5 mg/dL, black patients, retransplants, multi-organ transplants, patients with high panel of reactive antibodies (See **CLINICAL STUDIES**).

OVERALL CALCULATED GLOMERULAR FILTRATION RATES (Mean ± SEM, cc/min) BY NANKIVELL EQUATION POST TRANSPLANT[a,b]

Parameter	Rapamune® Oral Solution 2 mg/day	Rapamune® Oral Solution 5 mg/day	Azathioprine 2-3 mg/kg/day	Placebo
Study 1				
Month 12	57.4 ± 1.3 (n = 269)	54.6 ± 1.3 (n = 248)	64.1 ± 1.6 (n = 149)	
Month 24	58.4 ± 1.5 (n = 221)	52.6 ± 1.5 (n = 222)	62.4 ± 1.9 (n = 132)	
Study 2				
Month 12	52.4 ± 1.5 (n = 211)	51.5 ± 1.5 (n = 199)		58.0 ± 2.1 (n = 117)
Month 36	48.1 ± 1.8 (n = 183)	46.1 ± 2.0 (n = 177)		53.4 ± 2.7 (n = 102)

a: Includes patients who prematurely discontinued treatment.
b: Patients who had a graft loss were included in the analysis with GFR set to 0.0.

INCIDENCE (%) OF EFFICACY FAILURE AT 3 AND 6 MONTHS: STUDY 3[a,b]

	Rapamune® Oral Solution (n = 238)	Rapamune® Tablets (n = 239)
Efficacy Failure at 3 months[c]	23.5	24.7
Components of efficacy failure		
Biopsy-proven acute rejection	18.9	17.6
Graft loss	3.4	6.3
Death	1.3	0.8
Efficacy Failure at 6 months	26.1	27.2
Components of efficacy failure		
Biopsy-proven acute rejection	21.0	19.2
Graft loss	3.4	6.3
Death	1.7	1.7

a: Patients received cyclosporine and corticosteroids.
b: Includes patients who prematurely discontinued treatment.
c: Efficacy failure at 3 months was the primary endpoint.

CONTRAINDICATIONS

Rapamune is contraindicated in patients with a hypersensitivity to sirolimus or its derivatives or any component of the drug product.

WARNINGS

Increased susceptibility to infection and the possible development of lymphoma and other malignancies, particularly of the skin, may result from immunosuppression (see **ADVERSE REACTIONS**). Oversuppression of the immune system can also increase susceptibility to infection including opportunistic infections, fatal infections, and sepsis. Only physicians experienced in immunosuppressive therapy and management of organ transplant patients should use Rapamune. Patients receiving the drug should be managed in facilities equipped and staffed with adequate laboratory and supportive medical resources. The physician responsible for maintenance therapy should have complete information requisite for the follow-up of the patient.

Hypersensitivity reactions, including anaphylactic/anaphylactoid reactions, have been associated with the administration of sirolimus (see **ADVERSE REACTIONS**).

As usual for patients with increased risk for skin cancer, exposure to sunlight and UV light should be limited by wearing protective clothing and using a sunscreen with a high protection factor.

Increased serum cholesterol and triglycerides, that may require treatment, occurred more frequently in patients treated with Rapamune compared with azathioprine or placebo controls (see **PRECAUTIONS**).

In Studies 1 and 2, from month 6 through months 24 and 36, respectively, mean serum creatinine was increased and mean glomerular filtration rate was decreased in patients treated with Rapamune and cyclosporine compared with those treated with cyclosporine and placebo or azathioprine controls. The rate of decline in renal function was greater in patients receiving Rapamune and cyclosporine compared with control therapies (see **CLINICAL STUDIES**).

Renal function should be closely monitored during the administration of Rapamune® in combination with cyclosporine since long-term administration can be associated with deterioration of renal function. Appropriate adjustment of the immunosuppression regimen, including discontinuation of Rapamune and/or cyclosporine, should be considered in patients with elevated or increasing serum creatinine levels. Caution should be exercised when using other drugs which are known to impair renal function. In patients at low to moderate immunologic risk continuation of combination therapy with cyclosporine beyond 4 months following transplantation should only be considered when the benefits outweigh the risks of this combination for the individual patients (see **PRECAUTIONS**).

In clinical trials, Rapamune has been administered concurrently with corticosteroids and with the following formulations of cyclosporine:

Sandimmune® Injection (cyclosporine injection)
Sandimmune® Oral Solution (cyclosporine oral solution)
Sandimmune® Soft Gelatin Capsules (cyclosporine capsules)
Neoral® Soft Gelatin Capsules (cyclosporine capsules [MODIFIED])
Neoral® Oral Solution (cyclosporine oral solution [MODIFIED])

The efficacy and safety of the use of Rapamune in combination with other immunosuppressive agents has not been determined.

Liver Transplantation – Excess Mortality, Graft Loss, and Hepatic Artery Thrombosis (HAT):

The use of sirolimus in combination with tacrolimus was associated with excess mortality and graft loss in a study in de novo liver transplant recipients. Many of these patients had evidence of infection at or near the time of death.

In this and another study in de novo liver transplant recipients, the use of sirolimus in combination with cyclosporine or tacrolimus was associated with an increase in HAT; most cases of HAT occurred within 30 days post-transplantation and most led to graft loss or death.

Lung Transplantation – Bronchial Anastomotic Dehiscence:

Cases of bronchial anastomotic dehiscence, most fatal, have been reported in de novo lung transplant patients when sirolimus has been used as part of an immunosuppressive regimen.

The safety and efficacy of Rapamune® (sirolimus) as immunosuppressive therapy have not been established in liver or lung transplant patients, and therefore, such use is not recommended.

Co-administration of sirolimus with strong inhibitors of CYP3A4 and/or P-gp (such as ketoconazole, voriconazole, itraconazole, erythromycin, telithromycin, or clarithromycin) or strong inducers of CYP3A4 and/or P-gp (such as rifampin or rifabutin) is not recommended (see **CLINICAL PHARMACOLOGY, Metabolism,** and **PRECAUTIONS, Drug Interactions** and **Other drug interactions**).

PRECAUTIONS

General

Rapamune is intended for oral administration only.

Lymphocele, a known surgical complication of renal transplantation, occurred significantly more often in a dose-related fashion in patients treated with Rapamune. Appropriate operative measures should be considered to minimize this complication.

Lipids

The use of Rapamune® in renal transplant patients was associated with increased serum cholesterol and triglycerides that may require treatment.

In Studies 1 and 2, in *de novo* renal transplant recipients who began the study with normal, fasting, total serum cholesterol (<200 mg/dL) or normal, fasting, total serum triglycerides (<200 mg/dL), there was an increased incidence of hypercholesterolemia (fasting serum cholesterol >240 mg/dL) or hypertriglyceridemia (fasting serum triglycerides >500 mg/dL), respectively, in patients receiving both Rapamune® 2 mg and Rapamune® 5 mg compared with azathioprine and placebo controls.

Treatment of new-onset hypercholesterolemia with lipid-lowering agents was required in 42-52% of patients enrolled in the Rapamune arms of Studies 1 and 2 compared with 16% of patients in the placebo arm and 22% of patients in the azathioprine arm.

In Study 4 during the prerandomization period, mean fasting serum cholesterol and triglyceride values rapidly increased, and peaked at 2 months with mean cholesterol values > 240 mg/dL and triglycerides > 250 mg/dL. After randomization mean cholesterol and triglyceride values remained higher in the cyclosporine withdrawal arm compared to the Rapamune® and cyclosporine combination.

Renal transplant patients have a higher prevalence of clinically significant hyperlipidemia. Accordingly, the risk/benefit should be carefully considered in patients with established hyperlipidemia before initiating an immunosuppressive regimen including Rapamune.

Any patient who is administered Rapamune should be monitored for hyperlipidemia using laboratory tests and if hyperlipidemia is detected, subsequent interventions such as diet, exercise, and lipid-lowering agents, as outlined by the National Cholesterol Education Program guidelines, should be initiated.

In clinical trials, the concomitant administration of Rapamune and HMG-CoA reductase inhibitors and/or fibrates appeared to be well tolerated.

During Rapamune therapy with cyclosporine, patients administered an HMG-CoA reductase inhibitor and/or fibrate should be monitored for the possible development of rhabdomyolysis and other adverse effects as described in the respective labeling for these agents.

Renal Function

Patients treated with cyclosporine and Rapamune were noted to have higher serum creatinine levels and lower glomerular filtration rates compared with patients treated with cyclosporine and placebo or azathioprine controls (Studies 1 and 2). The rate of decline in renal function in these studies was greater in patients receiving Rapamune and cyclosporine compared with control therapies. In patients at low to moderate immunologic risk (See **CLINICAL STUDIES**) continuation of combination therapy with cyclosporine beyond 4 months following transplantation should only be considered when the benefits outweigh the risks of this combination for the individual patients. (see **WARNINGS**).

Renal function should be monitored during the administration of Rapamune® in combination with cyclosporine. Appropriate adjustment of the immunosuppression regimen, including discontinuation of Rapamune and/or cyclosporine, should be considered in patients with elevated or increasing serum creatinine levels. Caution should be exercised when using agents (e.g., aminoglycosides, and amphotericin B) that are known to have a deleterious effect on renal function.

Antimicrobial Prophylaxis

Cases of *Pneumocystis carinii* pneumonia have been reported in patients not receiving antimicrobial prophylaxis. Therefore, antimicrobial prophylaxis for *Pneumocystis carinii* pneumonia should be administered for 1 year following transplantation.

Cytomegalovirus (CMV) prophylaxis is recommended for 3 months after transplantation, particularly for patients at increased risk for CMV disease.

Interstitial Lung Disease

Cases of interstitial lung disease (including pneumonitis, and infrequently bronchiolitis obliterans organizing pneumonia [BOOP] and pulmonary fibrosis), some fatal, with no identified infectious etiology have occurred in patients receiving immunosuppressive regimens including Rapamune. In some cases, the interstitial lung disease has resolved upon discontinuation or dose reduction of Rapamune. The risk may be increased as the trough Rapamune concentration increases (see **ADVERSE REACTIONS, Other clinical experience**).

Information for Patients

Patients should be given complete dosage instructions (see **Patient Instructions**). Women of childbearing potential should be informed of the potential risks during pregnancy and that they should use effective contraception prior to initiation of Rapamune therapy, during Rapamune therapy and for 12 weeks after Rapamune therapy has been stopped (see **PRECAUTIONS: Pregnancy**).

Patients should be told that exposure to sunlight and UV light should be limited by wearing protective clothing and using a sunscreen with a high protection factor because of the increased risk for skin cancer (see **WARNINGS**).

Laboratory Tests

Whole blood sirolimus concentrations should be monitored in patients receiving concentration-controlled Rapamune. Monitoring is also necessary in patients likely to have altered drug metabolism, in patients ≥13 years who weigh less than 40 kg, in patients with hepatic impairment, and during concurrent administration of potent CYP3A4 inducers and inhibitors (see **PRECAUTIONS: Drug Interactions**).

Drug Interactions

Sirolimus is known to be a substrate for both cytochrome CYP3A4 and P-gp. The pharmacokinetic interaction between sirolimus and concomitantly administered drugs is discussed below. Drug interaction studies have not been conducted with drugs other than those described below.

Cyclosporine capsules MODIFIED:

Cyclosporine is a substrate and inhibitor of CYP3A4 and P-gp.

Because of the effect of cyclosporine capsules (MODIFIED), it is recommended that sirolimus should be taken 4 hours after administration of cyclosporine oral solution (MODIFIED) and/or cyclosporine capsules (MODIFIED) (see DOSAGE AND ADMINISTRATION).

Studies assessing the effect of concomitant administration of cyclosporine capsules (MODIFIED) with sirolimus oral solution and with sirolimus tablets are summarized below.

Rapamune Oral Solution: In a single dose drug-drug interaction study, 24 healthy volunteers were administered 10 mg sirolimus either simultaneously or 4 hours after a 300 mg dose of Neoral® Soft Gelatin Capsules (cyclosporine capsules [MODIFIED]). For simultaneous administration, the mean C_{max} and AUC of sirolimus were increased by 116% and 230%, respectively, relative to administration of sirolimus alone. However, when given 4 hours after Neoral® Soft Gelatin Capsules (cyclosporine capsules [MODIFIED]) administration, sirolimus C_{max} and AUC were increased by 37% and 80%, respectively, compared with administration of sirolimus alone.

In a single-dose cross-over drug-drug interaction study, 33 healthy volunteers received 5 mg sirolimus alone, 2 hours before, and 2 hours after a 300 mg dose of Neoral® Soft Gelatin Capsules (cyclosporine capsules [MODIFIED]). When given 2 hours before Neoral® Soft Gelatin Capsules (cyclosporine capsules [MODIFIED]) administration, sirolimus C_{max} and AUC were comparable to those with administration of sirolimus alone. However, when given 2 hours after, the mean C_{max} and AUC of sirolimus were increased by 126% and 141%, respectively, relative to administration of sirolimus alone.

Mean cyclosporine C_{max} and AUC were not significantly affected when sirolimus was given simultaneously or when administered 4 hours after Neoral® Soft Gelatin Capsules (cyclosporine capsules [MODIFIED]). However, after multiple-dose administration of sirolimus given 4 hours after Neoral® in renal post-transplant patients over 6 months, cyclosporine oral-dose clearance was reduced, and lower doses of Neoral® Soft Gelatin Capsules (cyclosporine capsules [MODIFIED]) were needed to maintain target cyclosporine concentration.

Rapamune Tablets: In a single-dose drug-drug interaction study, 24 healthy volunteers were administered 10 mg sirolimus (Rapamune Tablets) either simultaneously or 4 hours after a 300-mg dose of Neoral® Soft Gelatin Capsules (cyclosporine capsules [MODIFIED]). For simultaneous administration, mean C_{max} and AUC were increased by 512% and 148%, respectively, relative to administration of sirolimus alone. However, when given 4 hours after cyclosporine administration, sirolimus C_{max} and AUC were both increased by only 33% compared with administration of sirolimus alone.

Cyclosporine oral solution: In a multiple-dose study in 150 psoriasis patients, sirolimus 0.5, 1.5, and 3 mg/m^2/day was administered simultaneously with Sandimmune® Oral Solution (cyclosporine Oral Solution) 1.25 mg/kg/day. The increase in average sirolimus trough concentrations ranged between 67% to 86% relative to when sirolimus was administered without cyclosporine. The intersubject variability (%CV) for sirolimus trough concentrations ranged from 39.7% to 68.7%. There was no significant effect of multiple-dose sirolimus on cyclosporine trough concentrations following Sandimmune® Oral Solution (cyclosporine oral solution) administration. However, the %CV was higher (range 85.9%-165%) than those from previous studies.

Sandimmune® Oral Solution (cyclosporine oral solution) is not bioequivalent to Neoral® Oral Solution (cyclosporine oral solution MODIFIED), and should not be used interchangeably. Although there is no published data comparing Sandimmune® Oral Solution (cyclosporine oral solution) to SangCya® Oral Solution (cyclosporine oral solution [MODIFIED]), they should not be used interchangeably. Likewise, Sandimmune® Soft Gelatin Capsules (cyclosporine capsules) are not bioequivalent to Neoral® Soft Gelatin Capsules (cyclosporine capsules [MODIFIED]) and should not be used interchangeably.

Diltiazem: Diltiazem is a substrate and inhibitor of CYP3A4 and P-gp; sirolimus concentrations should be monitored and a dose adjustment may be necessary. The simultaneous oral administration of 10 mg of sirolimus oral solution and 120 mg of diltiazem to 18 healthy volunteers significantly affected the bioavailability of sirolimus. Sirolimus C_{max}, t_{max}, and AUC were increased 1.4-, 1.3-, and 1.6-fold, respectively. Sirolimus did not affect the pharmacokinetics of either diltiazem or its metabolites desacetyldiltiazem and desmethyldiltiazem.

Erythromycin: Erythromycin is a substrate and inhibitor of CYP3A4 and P-gp; co-administration of sirolimus oral solution or tablets and erythromycin is not recommended (see **WARNINGS**). The simultaneous oral administration of 2 mg daily of sirolimus oral solution and 800 mg q 8h of erythromycin as erythromycin ethylsuccinate tablets at steady state to 24 healthy volunteers significantly affected the bioavailability of sirolimus and erythromycin. Sirolimus C_{max} and AUC were increased 4.4- and 4.2-fold respectively and t_{max} was increased by 0.4 hr. Erythromycin C_{max} and AUC were increased 1.6- and 1.7-fold, respectively, and t_{max} was increased by 0.3 hr.

Ketoconazole: Ketoconazole is a strong inhibitor of CYP3A4 and P-gp; co-administration of sirolimus oral solution or tablets and ketoconazole is not recommended (see **WARNINGS**). Multiple-dose ketoconazole administration significantly affected the rate and extent of absorption and sirolimus exposure after administration of Rapamune® Oral Solution, as reflected by increases in sirolimus C_{max}, t_{max} and AUC of 4.3-fold, 38%, and 10.9-fold, respectively. However, the terminal $t_{1/2}$ of sirolimus was not changed. Single-dose sirolimus did not affect steady-state 12-hour plasma ketoconazole concentrations.

Rifampin: Rifampin is a strong inducer of CYP3A4 and P-gp; co-administration of sirolimus oral solution or tablets and rifampin is not recommended (see **WARNINGS**). Pretreatment of 14 healthy volunteers with multiple doses of rifampin, 600 mg daily for 14 days, followed by a single 20-mg dose of sirolimus oral solution, greatly increased sirolimus oral-dose clearance by 5.5-fold (range = 2.8 to 10), which represents mean decreases in AUC and C_{max} of about 82% and 71%, respectively. In patients where rifampin is indicated, alternative therapeutic agents with less enzyme induction potential should be considered.

Verapamil: Verapamil is a substrate and inhibitor of CYP3A4 and P-gp; sirolimus concentrations should be monitored and a dose adjustment may be necessary. The simultaneous oral administration of 2 mg daily of sirolimus oral solution and 180 mg q 12h of verapamil at steady state to 26 healthy volunteers significantly affected the bioavailability of sirolimus and verapamil. Sirolimus C_{max} and AUC were increased 2.3- and 2.2-fold, respectively, without substantial change in t_{max}. The C_{max} and AUC of the pharmacologically active S(-) enantiomer of verapamil were both increased 1.5-fold and t_{max} was decreased by 1.2 hr.

Drugs which may be coadministered without dose adjustment

Clinically significant pharmacokinetic drug-drug interactions were not observed in studies of drugs listed below. A synopsis of the type of study performed for each drug is provided. Sirolimus and these drugs may be coadministered without dose adjustments.

Acyclovir: Acyclovir, 200 mg, was administered once daily for 3 days followed by a single 10-mg dose of sirolimus oral solution on day 3 in 20 adult healthy volunteers.

Digoxin: Digoxin, 0.25 mg, was administered daily for 8 days and a single 10-mg dose of sirolimus oral solution was given on day 8 to 24 healthy volunteers.

Glyburide: single 5-mg dose of glyburide and a single 10-mg dose of sirolimus oral solution were administered to 24 healthy volunteers. Sirolimus did not affect the hypoglycemic action of glyburide.

Nifedipine: A single 60-mg dose of nifedipine and a single 10-mg dose of sirolimus oral solution were administered to 24 healthy volunteers.

Norgestrel/ethinyl estradiol (Lo/Ovral®): Sirolimus oral solution, 2 mg, was given daily for 7 days to 21 healthy female volunteers on norgestrel/ethinyl estradiol.

Prednisolone: Pharmacokinetic information was obtained from 42 stable renal transplant patients receiving daily doses of prednisone (5-20 mg/day) and either single or multiple doses of sirolimus oral solution (0.5-5 mg/m^2 q 12h).

Sulfamethoxazole/trimethoprim (Bactrim®): A single oral dose of sulfamethoxazole (400 mg)/trimethoprim (80 mg) was given to 15 renal transplant patients receiving daily oral doses of sirolimus (8 to 25 mg/m^2).

Other drug interactions

Co-administration of sirolimus with strong inhibitors of CYP3A4 and/or P-gp (such as ketoconazole, voriconazole, itraconazole, erythromycin, telithromycin, or clarithromycin) or strong inducers of CYP3A4 and/or P-gp (such as rifampin or rifabutin) is not recommended (see **WARNINGS**). Sirolimus is extensively metabolized by the CYP3A4 isoenzyme in the intestinal wall and liver and undergoes counter-transport from enterocytes of the small intestine into the gut lumen by the P-gp drug efflux pump. Sirolimus is potentially recycled between enterocytes and the gut lumen to allow continued metabolism by CYP3A4. Therefore, absorption and the subsequent elimination of systemically absorbed sirolimus may be influenced by drugs that affect these proteins. Strong inhibitors of CYP3A4 and P-gp significantly decrease the metabolism of sirolimus and increase sirolimus concentrations, while strong inducers of CYP3A4 and P-gp significantly increase the metabolism of sirolimus and decrease sirolimus concentrations.

In patients in whom strong inhibitors or inducers of CYP3A4 are indicated, alternative therapeutic agents with less potential for inhibition or induction of CYP3A4 should be considered.

Sirolimus is a substrate for the multidrug efflux pump, P-gp in the small intestine. Therefore, absorption of sirolimus may be influenced by drugs that affect P-gp.

Aside from those mentioned above, other drugs that increase sirolimus blood concentrations include (but are not limited to):

Calcium channel blockers: nicardipine.

Antifungal agents: clotrimazole, fluconazole.

Antibiotics: troleandomycin.

Gastrointestinal prokinetic agents: cisapride, metoclopramide.

Other drugs: bromocriptine, cimetidine, danazol, HIV-protease inhibitors (e.g., ritonavir, indinavir).

Aside from those mentioned above, other drugs that decrease sirolimus concentrations include (but are not limited to):

Anticonvulsants: carbamazepine, phenobarbital, phenytoin.

Antibiotics: rifapentine.

Continued on next page

Rapamune—Cont.

Care should be exercised when drugs or other substances that are metabolized by CYP3A4 are administered concomitantly with Rapamune. Grapefruit juice reduces CYP3A4-mediated metabolism of Rapamune and must not be used for dilution (see **DOSAGE AND ADMINISTRATION**).

Herbal Preparations

St. John's Wort (*hypericum perforatum*) induces CYP3A4 and P-gp. Since sirolimus is a substrate for both cytochrome CYP3A4 and P-gp, there is the potential that the use of St. John's Wort in patients receiving Rapamune could result in reduced sirolimus concentrations.

Vaccination

Immunosuppressants may affect response to vaccination. Therefore, during treatment with Rapamune, vaccination may be less effective. The use of live vaccines should be avoided; live vaccines may include, but are not limited to measles, mumps, rubella, oral polio, BCG, yellow fever, varicella, and TY21a typhoid.

Drug-Laboratory Test Interactions

There are no studies on the interactions of sirolimus in commonly employed clinical laboratory tests.

Carcinogenesis, Mutagenesis, and Impairment of Fertility

Sirolimus was not genotoxic in the in vitro bacterial reverse mutation assay, the Chinese hamster ovary cell chromosomal aberration assay, the mouse lymphoma cell forward mutation assay, or the in vivo mouse micronucleus assay.

Carcinogenicity studies were conducted in mice and rats. In an 86-week female mouse study at dosages of 0, 12.5, 25 and 50/6 (dosage lowered from 50 to 6 mg/kg/day at week 31 due to infection secondary to immunosuppression) there was a statistically significant increase in malignant lymphoma at all dose levels (approximately 16 to 135 times the clinical doses adjusted for body surface area) compared with controls. In a second mouse study at dosages of 0, 1, 3 and 6 mg/kg (approximately 3 to 16 times the clinical dose adjusted for body surface area), hepatocellular adenoma and carcinoma (males), were considered Rapamune related. In the 104-week rat study at dosages of 0, 0.05, 0.1, and 0.2 mg/kg/day (approximately 0.4 to 1 times the clinical dose adjusted for body surface area), there was a statistically significant increased incidence of testicular adenoma in the 0.2 mg/kg/day group.

There was no effect on fertility in female rats following the administration of sirolimus at dosages up to 0.5 mg/kg (approximately 1 to 3 times the clinical doses adjusted for body surface area). In male rats, there was no significant difference in fertility rate compared to controls at a dosage of 2 mg/kg (approximately 4 to 11 times the clinical doses adjusted for body surface area). Reductions in testicular weights and/or histological lesions (e.g., tubular atrophy and tubular giant cells) were observed in rats following dosages of 0.65 mg/kg (approximately 1 to 3 times the clinical doses adjusted for body surface area) and above and in a monkey study at 0.1 mg/kg (approximately 0.4 to 1 times the clinical doses adjusted for body surface area) and above. Sperm counts were reduced in male rats following the administration of sirolimus for 13 weeks at a dosage of 6 mg/kg (approximately 12 to 32 times the clinical doses adjusted for body surface area), but showed improvement by 3 months after dosing was stopped.

Pregnancy

Pregnancy Category C: Sirolimus was embryo/feto toxic in rats at dosages of 0.1 mg/kg and above (approximately 0.2 to 0.5 the clinical doses adjusted for body surface area). Embryo/feto toxicity was manifested as mortality and reduced fetal weights (with associated delays in skeletal ossification). However, no teratogenesis was evident. In combination with cyclosporine, rats had increased embryo/feto mortality compared with Rapamune alone. There were no effects on rabbit development at the maternally toxic dosage of 0.05 mg/kg (approximately 0.3 to 0.8 times the clinical doses adjusted for body surface area). There are no adequate and well controlled studies in pregnant women. Effective contraception must be initiated before Rapamune therapy, during Rapamune therapy, and for 12 weeks after Rapamune therapy has been stopped. Rapamune should be used during pregnancy only if the potential benefit outweighs the potential risk to the embryo/fetus.

Use during lactation

Sirolimus is excreted in trace amounts in milk of lactating rats. It is not known whether sirolimus is excreted in human milk. The pharmacokinetic and safety profiles of sirolimus in infants are not known. Because many drugs are excreted in human milk and because of the potential for adverse reactions in nursing infants from sirolimus, a decision should be made whether to discontinue nursing or to discontinue the drug, taking into account the importance of the drug to the mother.

Pediatric use

The safety and efficacy of Rapamune in pediatric patients below the age of 13 years have not been established.

Geriatric use

Clinical studies of Rapamune Oral Solution or Tablets did not include sufficient numbers of patients aged 65 years and over to determine whether safety and efficacy differ in this population from younger patients. Data pertaining to sirolimus trough concentrations suggest that dose adjustments based upon age in geriatric renal patients are not necessary.

ADVERSE EVENTS OCCURRING AT A FREQUENCY OF ≥ 20% IN ANY TREATMENT GROUP IN PREVENTION OF ACUTE RENAL REJECTION TRIALS (%) AT ≥ 12 MONTHS POST-TRANSPLANTATION FOR STUDIES 1 AND 2[a]

Body System	Rapamune® Oral Solution -------2 mg/day-------		Rapamune® Oral Solution -------5 mg/day-------		Azathioprine 2-3 mg/kg/day	Placebo
Adverse Event	Study 1 (n = 281)	Study 2 (n = 218)	Study 1 (n = 269)	Study 2 (n = 208)	Study 1 (n = 160)	Study 2 (n = 124)
Body As A Whole						
Abdominal pain	28	29	30	36	29	30
Asthenia	38	22	40	28	37	28
Back pain	16	23	26	22	23	20
Chest pain	16	18	19	24	16	19
Fever	27	23	33	34	33	35
Headache	23	34	27	34	21	31
Pain	24	33	29	29	30	25
Cardiovascular System						
Hypertension	43	45	39	49	29	48
Digestive System						
Constipation	28	36	34	38	37	31
Diarrhea	32	25	42	35	28	27
Dyspepsia	17	23	23	25	24	34
Nausea	31	25	36	31	39	29
Vomiting	21	19	25	25	31	21
Hemic And Lymphatic System						
Anemia	27	23	37	33	29	21
Leukopenia	9	9	15	13	20	8
Thrombocytopenia	13	14	20	30	9	9
Metabolic And Nutritional						
Creatinine increased	35	39	37	40	28	38
Edema	24	20	16	18	23	15
Hypercholesteremia (See **WARNINGS** and **PRECAUTIONS**)	38	43	42	46	33	23
Hyperkalemia	15	17	12	14	24	27
Hyperlipemia (See **WARNINGS** and **PRECAUTIONS**)	38	45	44	57	28	23
Hypokalemia	17	11	21	17	11	9
Hypophosphatemia	20	15	23	19	20	19
Peripheral edema	60	54	64	58	58	48
Weight gain	21	11	15	8	19	15
Musculoskeletal System						
Arthralgia	25	25	27	31	21	18
Nervous System						
Insomnia	14	13	22	14	18	8
Tremor	31	21	30	22	28	19
Respiratory System						
Dyspnea	22	24	28	30	23	30
Pharyngitis	17	16	16	21	17	22
Upper respiratory infection	20	26	24	23	13	23
Skin And Appendages						
Acne	31	22	20	22	17	19
Rash	12	10	13	20	6	6
Urogenital System						
Urinary tract infection	20	26	23	33	31	26

a: Patients received cyclosporine and corticosteroids.

ADVERSE REACTIONS

Rapamune® Oral Solution: The incidence of adverse reactions was determined in two randomized, double-blind, multicenter controlled trials in which 499 renal transplant patients received Rapamune Oral Solution 2 mg/day, 477 received Rapamune Oral Solution 5 mg/day, 160 received azathioprine, and 124 received placebo. All patients were treated with cyclosporine and corticosteroids. Data (≥ 12 months post-transplant) presented in the table below show the adverse reactions that occurred in any treatment group with an incidence of ≥ 20%.

Specific adverse reactions associated with the administration of Rapamune (sirolimus) Oral Solution occurred at a significantly higher frequency than in the respective control group. For both Rapamune Oral Solution 2 mg/day and 5 mg/day these include hypercholesterolemia, hyperlipemia, hypertension, and rash; for Rapamune Oral Solution 2 mg/day acne; and for Rapamune Oral Solution 5 mg/day anemia, arthralgia, diarrhea, hypokalemia, and thrombocytopenia. The elevations of triglycerides and cholesterol and decreases in platelets and hemoglobin occurred in a dose-related manner in patients receiving Rapamune.

Patients maintained on Rapamune Oral Solution 5 mg/day, when compared with patients on Rapamune Oral Solution 2 mg/day, demonstrated an increased incidence of the following adverse events: anemia, leukopenia, thrombocytopenia, hypokalemia, hyperlipemia, fever, and diarrhea.

In general, adverse events related to the administration of Rapamune were dependent on dose/concentration.

[See table below]

With longer term follow-up, the adverse event profile remained similar. Some new events became significantly different among the treatment groups. For events which occurred at a frequency of ≥ 20% by 24 months for Study 1 and 36 months for Study 2, only the incidence of edema became significantly higher in both Rapamune groups as compared with the control group. The incidence of headache became significantly more common in the Rapamune 5mg/day group as compared with control therapy.

At 24 months for Study 1, the following treatment-emergent infections were significantly different among the treatment groups: bronchitis, Herpes simplex, pneumonia, pyelonephritis, and upper respiratory infections. In each instance, the incidence was highest in the Rapamune 5 mg/day group, lower in the Rapamune 2 mg/day group and lowest in the azathioprine group. Except for upper respiratory infections in the Rapamune 5 mg/day cohort, the remainder of events occurred with a frequency of < 20%.

At 36 months in Study 2 only the incidence of treatment-emergent Herpes simplex was significantly different among the treatment groups, being higher in the Rapamune 5 mg/day group than either of the other groups.

The table below summarizes the incidence of malignancies in the two controlled trials for the prevention of acute rejection. At 24 (Study 1) and 36 months (Study 2) there were no significant differences among treatment groups.

[See first table at top of next page]

Among the adverse events that were reported at a rate of ≥3% and <20% at 12 months, the following were more prominent in patients maintained on Rapamune 5 mg/day, when compared with patients on Rapamune 2 mg/day: epistaxis, lymphocele, insomnia, thrombotic thrombocytopenic purpura (hemolytic-uremic syndrome), skin ulcer, increased LDH, hypotension, facial edema.

The following adverse events were reported with ≥3% and <20% incidence in patients in any Rapamune treatment group in the two controlled clinical trials for the prevention of acute rejection, BODY AS A WHOLE: abdomen enlarged, abscess, ascites, cellulitis, chills, face edema, flu syndrome, generalized edema, hernia, *Herpes zoster* infection, lymphocele, malaise, pelvic pain, peritonitis, sepsis; CARDIOVASCULAR SYSTEM: atrial fibrillation, congestive heart failure, hemorrhage, hypervolemia, hypotension, palpitation, peripheral vascular disorder, postural hypotension, syncope, tachycardia, thrombophlebitis, thrombosis, vasodilatation, venous thromboembolism; DIGESTIVE SYSTEM: anorexia, dysphagia, eructation, esophagitis, flatulence, gastritis, gastroenteritis, gingivitis, gum hyperplasia, ileus, liver function tests abnormal, mouth ulceration, oral moniliasis, stomatitis; ENDOCRINE SYSTEM: Cushing's syndrome, diabetes mellitus, glycosuria; HEMIC AND LYMPHATIC SYSTEM: ecchymosis, leukocytosis, lymphadenopathy, polycythemia, thrombotic thrombocytopenic purpura (hemolytic-uremic syndrome); METABOLIC AND NUTRITIONAL: acidosis, alkaline phosphatase increased,

BUN increased, creatine phosphokinase increased, dehydration, healing abnormal, hypercalcemia, hyperglycemia, hyperphosphatemia, hypocalcemia, hypoglycemia, hypomagnesemia, hyponatremia, lactic dehydrogenase increased, AST/SGOT increased, ALT/SGPT increased, weight loss; MUSCULOSKELETAL SYSTEM: arthrosis, bone necrosis, leg cramps, myalgia, osteoporosis, tetany; NERVOUS SYSTEM: anxiety, confusion, depression, dizziness, emotional lability, hypertonia, hypesthesia, hypotonia, insomnia, neuropathy, paresthesia, somnolence; RESPIRATORY SYSTEM: asthma, atelectasis, bronchitis, cough increased, epistaxis, hypoxia, lung edema, pleural effusion, pneumonia, rhinitis, sinusitis; SKIN AND APPENDAGES: fungal dermatitis, hirsutism, pruritus, skin hypertrophy, skin ulcer, sweating; SPECIAL SENSES: abnormal vision, cataract, conjunctivitis, deafness, ear pain, otitis media, tinnitus; UROGENITAL SYSTEM: albuminuria, bladder pain, dysuria, hematuria, hydronephrosis, impotence, kidney pain, kidney tubular necrosis, nocturia, oliguria, pyelonephritis, pyuria, scrotal edema, testis disorder, toxic nephropathy, urinary frequency, urinary incontinence, urinary retention.

Less frequently occurring adverse events included: mycobacterial infections, Epstein-Barr virus infections, and pancreatitis.

Among the events which were reported at an incidence of ≥ 3% and < 20% by 24 months for Study 1 and 36 months for Study 2, tachycardia and Cushing's syndrome were reported significantly more commonly in both Rapamune groups as compared with the control therapy. Events that were reported more commonly in the Rapamune 5 mg/day group than either the Rapamune 2 mg/day group and/or control group were: abnormal healing, bone necrosis, chills, congestive heart failure, dysuria, hernia, hirsutism, urinary frequency, and lymphadenopathy.

Rapamune® Tablets: The safety profile of the tablet did not differ from that of the oral solution formulation. The incidence of adverse reactions up to 12 months was determined in a randomized, multicenter controlled trial (Study 3) in which 229 renal transplant patients received Rapamune Oral Solution 2 mg once daily and 228 patients received Rapamune Tablets 2 mg once daily. All patients were treated with cyclosporine and corticosteroids. The adverse reactions that occurred in either treatment group with an incidence of ≥ 20% in Study 3 are similar to those reported for Studies 1 and 2. There was no notable difference in the incidence of these adverse events between treatment groups (oral solution versus tablets) in Study 3, with the exception of acne, which occurred more frequently in the oral solution group, and tremor which occurred more frequently in the tablet group, particularly in Black patients.

The adverse events that occurred in patients with an incidence of ≥3% and <20% in either treatment group in Study 3 were similar to those reported in Studies 1 and 2. There was no notable difference in the incidence of these adverse events between treatment groups (oral solution versus tablets) in Study 3, with the exception of hypertonia, which occurred more frequently in the oral solution group and diabetes mellitus which occurred more frequently in the tablet group. Hispanic patients in the tablet group experienced hyperglycemia more frequently than Hispanic patients in the oral solution group. In Study 3 alone, menorrhagia, metrorrhagia, and polyuria occurred with an incidence of ≥3% and <20%.

The clinically important opportunistic or common transplant-related infections were identical in all three studies and the incidences of these infections were similar in Study 3 compared with Studies 1 and 2. The incidence rates of these infections were not significantly different between the oral solution and tablet treatment groups in Study 3.

In Study 3 (at 12 months), there were two cases of lymphoma/lymphoproliferative disorder in the oral solution treatment group (0.8%) and two reported cases of lymphoma/lymphoproliferative disorder in the tablet treatment group (0.8%). These differences were not statistically significant and were similar to the incidences observed in Studies 1 and 2.

Rapamune following cyclosporine withdrawal: The incidence of adverse reactions was determined through 36 months in a randomized, multicenter controlled trial (Study 4) in which 215 renal transplant patients received Rapamune as a maintenance regimen following cyclosporine withdrawal and 215 patients received Rapamune with cyclosporine therapy. All patients were treated with corticosteroids. The safety profile prior to randomization (start of cyclosporine withdrawal) was similar to that of the 2-mg Rapamune groups in Studies 1, 2, and 3. Following randomization (at 3 months) patients who had cyclosporine eliminated from their therapy experienced significantly higher incidences of abnormal liver function tests (including increased AST/SGOT and increased ALT/SGPT), hypokalemia, thrombocytopenia, abnormal healing, ileus, and rectal disorder. Conversely, the incidence of hypertension, cyclosporine toxicity, increased creatinine, abnormal kidney function, toxic nephropathy, edema, hyperkalemia, hyperuricemia, and gum hyperplasia was significantly higher in patients who remained on cyclosporine than those who had cyclosporine withdrawn from therapy. Mean systolic and diastolic blood pressure improved significantly following cyclosporine withdrawal.

In Study 4, at 36 months, the incidence of Herpes zoster infection was significantly lower in patients receiving

INCIDENCE (%) OF MALIGNANCIES IN STUDIES 1 (24 MONTHS) AND STUDY 2 (36 MONTHS) POST-TRANSPLANT[a,b]

Malignancy	Rapamune® Oral Solution 2 mg/day Study 1 (n = 284)	Rapamune® Oral Solution 2 mg/day Study 2 (n = 227)	Rapamune® Oral Solution 5 mg/day Study 1 (n = 274)	Rapamune® Oral Solution 5 mg/day Study 2 (n = 219)	Azathioprine 2-3 mg/kg/day Study 1 (n = 161)	Placebo Study 2 (n = 130)
Lymphoma/ lymphoproliferative disease	**0.7**	**1.8**	**1.1**	**3.2**	**0.6**	**0.8**
Skin Carcinoma						
Any Squamous Cell[c]	0.4	2.7	2.2	0.9	3.8	3.0
Any Basal Cell[c]	0.7	2.2	1.5	1.8	2.5	5.3
Melanoma	0.0	0.4	0.0	1.4	0.0	0.0
Miscellaneous/Not Specified	0.0	0.0	0.0	0.0	0.0	0.8
Total	**1.1**	**4.4**	**3.3**	**4.1**	**4.3**	**7.7**
Other Malignancy	**1.1**	**2.2**	**1.5**	**1.4**	**0.6**	**2.3**

a: Patients received cyclosporine and corticosteroids.
b: Includes patients who prematurely discontinued treatment.
c: Patients may be counted in more than one category.

INCIDENCE (%) OF MALIGNANCIES IN STUDY 4 AT 36 MONTHS POST-TRANSPLANT[a,b]

Malignancy	Nonrandomized (n = 95)	Rapamune with Cyclosporine Therapy (n = 215)	Rapamune Following Cyclosporine Withdrawal (n = 215)
Lymphoma/lymphoproliferative disease	**1.1**	**1.4**	**0.5**
Skin Carcinoma			
Any Squamous Cell[c]	1.1	1.9	2.3
Any Basal Cell[c]	3.2	4.7	2.3
Melanoma	0.0	0.5	0.0
Miscellaneous/Not Specified	1.1	0.9	0.0
Total	**4.2**	**6.5**	**3.7**
Other Malignancy	**1.1**	**3.3**	**1.4**

a: Patients received cyclosporine and corticosteroids.
b: Includes patients who prematurely discontinued treatment.
c: Patients may be counted in more than one category.

Rapamune following cyclosporine withdrawal compared with patients who continued to receive Rapamune and cyclosporine.

The incidence of malignancies in Study 4 is presented in the table below. In Study 4, the incidence of lymphoma/lymphoproliferative disease was similar in all treatment groups. The overall incidence of malignancy was higher in patients receiving Rapamune plus cyclosporine compared with patients who had cyclosporine withdrawn.

[See second table above]

Other clinical experience: Cases of interstitial lung disease (including pneumonitis, and infrequently bronchiolitis obliterans organizing pneumonia [BOOP] and pulmonary fibrosis), some fatal, with no identified infectious etiology have occurred in patients receiving immunosuppressive regimens including Rapamune. In some cases, the interstitial lung disease has resolved upon discontinuation or dose reduction of Rapamune. The risk may be increased as the sirolimus trough concentration increases (see **PRECAUTIONS, General, *Interstitial Lung Disease***). There have been reports of neutropenia and rare reports of pancytopenia. Hypersensitivity reactions, including anaphylactic/anaphylactoid reactions, have been associated with the administration of sirolimus (see **WARNINGS**). Hepatotoxicity has been reported, including fatal hepatic necrosis with elevated sirolimus trough concentrations. Abnormal healing following transplant surgery has been reported, including fascial dehiscence and anastomotic disruption (e.g., wound, vascular, airway, ureteral, biliary).

The safety and efficacy of conversion from calcineurin inhibitors to sirolimus in maintenance renal transplant population has not been established. In an ongoing study evaluating the safety and efficacy of conversion from calcineurin inhibitors to sirolimus (target concentrations of 12-20 ng/mL) in maintenance renal transplant patients; enrollment was stopped in the subset of patients (n=90) with a baseline glomerular filtration rate of less than 40 mL/min. There was a higher rate of serious adverse events including pneumonia, acute rejection, graft loss and death in this sirolimus treatment arm.

OVERDOSAGE

Reports of overdose with Rapamune have been received; however, experience has been limited. In general, the adverse effects of overdose are consistent with those listed in the **ADVERSE REACTIONS** section (see **ADVERSE REACTIONS**).

General supportive measures should be followed in all cases of overdose. Based on the poor aqueous solubility and high erythrocyte and plasma protein binding of sirolimus, it is anticipated that sirolimus is not dialyzable to any significant extent. In mice and rats, the acute oral lethal dose was greater than 800 mg/kg.

DOSAGE AND ADMINISTRATION

It is recommended that Rapamune Oral Solution and Tablets be used initially in a regimen with cyclosporine and corticosteroids. Cyclosporine withdrawal is recommended 2 to 4 months after transplantation in patients at low to moderate immunologic risk.

The safety and efficacy of cyclosporine withdrawal in high-risk patients have not been adequately studied and it is therefore not recommended. This includes patients with Banff grade III acute rejection or vascular rejection prior to cyclosporine withdrawal, those who are dialysis-dependent, or with serum creatinine > 4.5 mg/dL, black patients, re-transplants, multi-organ transplants, patients with high panel of reactive antibodies (See **INDICATIONS AND USAGE** and **CLINICAL STUDIES**).

Two-mg of Rapamune oral solution has been demonstrated to be clinically equivalent to 2-mg Rapamune oral tablets and hence, are interchangeable on a mg to mg basis. However, it is not known if higher doses of Rapamune oral solution are clinically equivalent to higher doses of tablets on a mg to mg basis. (See **CLINICAL PHARMACOLOGY: Absorption**). Rapamune is to be administered orally once daily.

Rapamune and cyclosporine combination therapy: The initial dose of Rapamune should be administered as soon as possible after transplantation. For *de novo* transplant recipients, a loading dose of Rapamune of 3 times the maintenance dose should be given. A daily maintenance dose of 2-mg is recommended for use in renal transplant patients, with a loading dose of 6 mg. Although a daily maintenance dose of 5 mg, with a loading dose of 15 mg was used in clinical trials of the oral solution and was shown to be safe and effective, no efficacy advantage over the 2-mg dose could be established for renal transplant patients. Patients receiving 2 mg of Rapamune Oral Solution per day demonstrated an overall better safety profile than did patients receiving 5 mg of Rapamune Oral Solution per day.

Rapamune following cyclosporine withdrawal: Initially, patients considered for cyclosporine withdrawal should be receiving Rapamune and cyclosporine combination therapy. At 2 to 4 months following transplantation, cyclosporine should be progressively discontinued over 4 to 8 weeks and the Rapamune® dose should be adjusted to obtain whole blood trough concentrations within the range of 12 to 24 ng/mL (chromatographic method). Therapeutic drug monitoring should not be the sole basis for adjusting Rapamune therapy. Careful attention should be made to clinical signs/symptoms, tissue biopsy, and laboratory parameters. Cyclosporine inhibits the metabolism and transport of sirolimus, and consequently, sirolimus concentrations will decrease when cyclosporine is discontinued unless the Rapamune dose is increased. The Rapamune® dose will need to be approximately 4-fold higher to account for both the absence of the pharmacokinetic interaction (approximately 2-fold increase) and the augmented immunosuppressive requirement in the absence of cyclosporine (approximately 2-fold increase).

Frequent Rapamune® dose adjustments based on non-steady-state sirolimus concentrations can lead to overdosing or underdosing because sirolimus has a long half-life. Once Rapamune® maintenance dose is adjusted, patients should be retained on the new maintenance dose at least for 7 to 14 days before further dosage adjustment with concentration monitoring. In most patients dose adjustments can be based

Continued on next page

Rapamune—Cont.

on simple proportion: new Rapamune® dose = current dose x (target concentration/current concentration). A loading dose should be considered in addition to a new maintenance dose when it is necessary to considerably increase sirolimus trough concentrations: Rapamune® loading dose = 3 × (new maintenance dose - current maintenance dose). The maximum Rapamune® dose administered on any day should not exceed 40 mg. If an estimated daily dose exceeds 40 mg due to the addition of a loading dose, the loading dose should be administered over 2 days. Sirolimus trough concentrations should be monitored at least 3 to 4 days after a loading dose(s).

To minimize the variability of exposure to Rapamune, this drug should be taken consistently with or without food. Grapefruit juice reduces CYP3A4-mediated drug metabolism and potentially enhances P-gp mediated drug counter-transport from enterocytes of the small intestine. This juice must not be administered with Rapamune or used for dilution.

It is recommended that sirolimus be taken 4 hours after administration of cyclosporine oral solution (MODIFIED) and/or cyclosporine capsules (MODIFIED).

Dosage Adjustments

The initial dosage in patients ≥13 years who weigh less than 40 kg should be adjusted, based on body surface area, to 1 mg/m²/day. The loading dose should be 3 mg/m².

It is recommended that the maintenance dose of Rapamune be reduced by approximately one third in patients with hepatic impairment. It is not necessary to modify the Rapamune loading dose. Dosage need not be adjusted because of impaired renal function.

Blood Concentration Monitoring

Whole blood trough concentrations of sirolimus should be monitored in patients receiving concentration-controlled Rapamune®. Monitoring is also necessary in pediatric patients, in patients with hepatic impairment, during concurrent administration of CYP3A4 and/or P-gp inducers and inhibitors, and/or if cyclosporine dosage is markedly changed or discontinued (see **DOSAGE AND ADMINISTRATION**).

In controlled clinical trials with concomitant cyclosporine (Studies 1 and 2), mean sirolimus whole blood trough concentrations through month 12 following transplantation, as measured by immunoassay, were 9 ng/mL (range 4.5–14 ng/mL [10th to 90th percentile]) for the 2 mg/day treatment group, and 17 ng/mL (range 10-28 ng/mL [10th to 90th percentile]) for the 5 mg/day dose.

In a controlled clinical trial with cyclosporine withdrawal (Study 4), the mean sirolimus whole blood trough concentrations during months 4 through 12 following transplantation, as measured by immunoassay, were 10.7 ng/mL (range 6.3-16.0 ng/mL [10th to 90th percentile]) in the concomitant Rapamune and cyclosporine treatment group (n = 205) and were 23.3 ng/mL (range 17.0–29.0 ng/mL [10th to 90th percentile]) in the cyclosporine withdrawal treatment group (n = 200).

Results from other assays may differ from those with an immunoassay. On average, chromatographic methods (HPLC UV or LC/MS/MS) yield results that are approximately 20% lower than the immunoassay for whole blood concentration determinations. Adjustments to the targeted range should be made according to the assay utilized to determine sirolimus trough concentrations. Therefore, comparison between concentrations in the published literature and an individual patient concentration using current assays must be made with detailed knowledge of the assay methods employed. A discussion of the different assay methods is contained in *Clinical Therapeutics*, Volume 22, Supplement B, April 2000.

Instructions for Dilution and Administration of Rapamune® Oral Solution Bottles

The amber oral dose syringe should be used to withdraw the prescribed amount of Rapamune® Oral Solution from the bottle. Empty the correct amount of Rapamune from the syringe into only a glass or plastic container holding at least two (2) ounces (1/4 cup, 60 mL) of water or orange juice. No other liquids, including grapefruit juice, should be used for dilution. Stir vigorously and drink at once. Refill the container with an additional volume (minimum of four [4] ounces [1/2 cup, 120 mL]) of water or orange juice, stir vigorously, and drink at once.

Handling and Disposal

Since Rapamune is not absorbed through the skin, there are no special precautions. However, if direct contact with the skin or mucous membranes occurs, wash thoroughly with soap and water; rinse eyes with plain water.

HOW SUPPLIED

Rapamune® Oral Solution is supplied at a concentration of 1 mg/mL in:

Cartons:

NDC # 0008-1030-06, containing a 2 oz (60 mL fill) amber glass bottle.

In addition to the bottles, each carton is supplied with an oral syringe adapter for fitting into the neck of the bottle, sufficient disposable amber oral syringes and caps for daily dosing, and a carrying case.

Rapamune® Tablets are available as follows:

1 mg, white, triangular-shaped tablets marked "RAPAMUNE 1 mg" on one side.

NDC # 0008-1031-05 bottle of 100 tablets.

NDC # 0008-1031-10, Redipak® cartons of 100 tablets (10 blister cards of 10 tablets each).

2 mg, yellow to beige triangular-shaped tablets marked "RAPAMUNE 2 mg" on one side.

NDC # 0008-1032-05, bottle of 100 tablets.

NDC # 0008-1032-10, Redipak® cartons of 100 tablets (10 blister cards of 10 tablets each [2 x 5]).

Storage

Rapamune® Oral Solution bottles should be stored protected from light and refrigerated at 2°C to 8°C (36°F to 46°F). Once the bottle is opened, the contents should be used within one month. If necessary, the patient may store the bottles at room temperatures up to 25°C (77°F) for a short period of time (e.g., not more than 15 days for the bottles).

An amber syringe and cap are provided for dosing and the product may be kept in the syringe for a maximum of 24 hours at room temperatures up to 25°C (77°F) or refrigerated at 2°C to 8°C (36°F to 46°F). The syringe should be discarded after one use. After dilution, the preparation should be used immediately.

Rapamune Oral Solution provided in bottles may develop a slight haze when refrigerated. If such a haze occurs allow the product to stand at room temperature and shake gently until the haze disappears. The presence of this haze does not affect the quality of the product.

Rapamune® Tablets should be stored at 20° to 25°C (USP Controlled Room Temperature) (68° to 77°F). Use cartons to protect blister cards and strips from light. Dispense in a tight, light-resistant container as defined in the USP.

US Pat. Nos.: 5,100,899; 5,212,155; 5,308,847; 5,403,833; 5,536,729.

PATIENT INSTRUCTIONS FOR RAPAMUNE® (SIROLIMUS) ORAL SOLUTION

Bottles

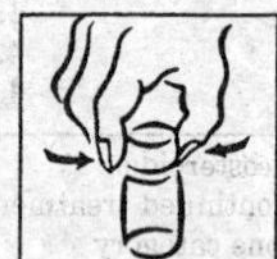

1. Open the solution bottle. Remove the safety cap by squeezing the tabs on the cap and twisting counter-clockwise.

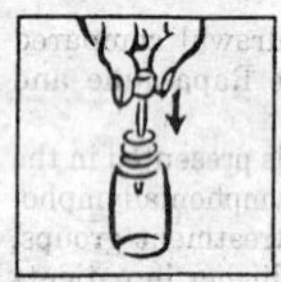

2. On first use, insert the adapter assembly (plastic tube with stopper) tightly into the bottle until it is even with the top of the bottle. Do not remove the adapter assembly from the bottle once inserted.

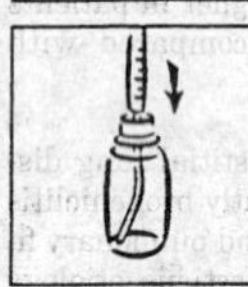

3. For each use, tightly insert one of the amber syringes with the plunger fully depressed into the opening in the adapter.

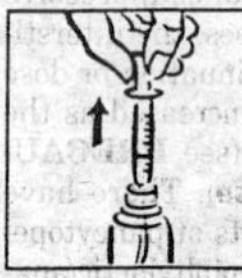

4. Withdraw the prescribed amount of Rapamune® Oral Solution by gently pulling out the plunger of the syringe until the bottom of the black line of the plunger is even with the appropriate mark on the syringe. Always keep the bottle in an upright position. If bubbles form in the syringe, empty the syringe into the bottle and repeat the procedure.

5. You may have been instructed to carry your medication with you. If it is necessary to carry the filled syringe, place a cap securely on the syringe – the cap should snap into place.

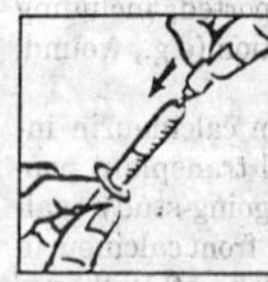

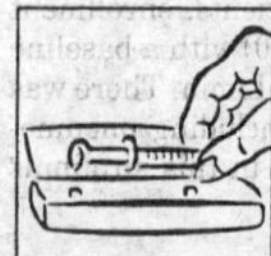

6. Then place the capped syringe in the enclosed carrying case. Once in the syringe, the medication may be kept at room temperature or refrigerated and should be used within 24 hours. Extreme temperatures (below 36°F and above 86°F) should be avoided. Remember to keep this medication out of the reach of children.

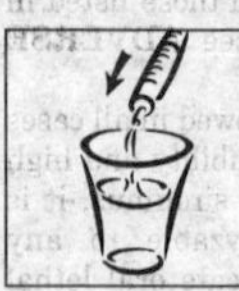

7. Empty the syringe into a glass or plastic cup containing at least 2 ounces (1/4 cup, 60 mL) of water or orange juice, stir vigorously for one (1) minute and drink immediately. Refill the container with at least 4 ounces (1/2 cup, 120 mL) of water or orange juice, stir vigorously again and drink the rinse solution. Apple juice, grapefruit juice, or other liquids are NOT to be used. Only glass or plastic cups should be used to dilute Rapamune® Oral Solution. The syringe and cap should be used once and then discarded.

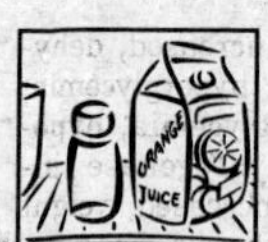

8. Always store the bottles of medication in the refrigerator. When refrigerated, a slight haze may develop in the solution. The presence of a haze does not affect the quality of the product. If this happens, bring the Rapamune® Oral Solution to room temperature and shake until the haze disappears. If it is necessary to wipe clean the mouth of the bottle before returning the product to the refrigerator, wipe with a dry cloth to avoid introducing water, or any other liquid, into the bottle.

Wyeth®

Wyeth Pharmaceuticals Inc. W10431C006
Philadelphia, PA 19101 ET01
Rev 08/04

Shown in Product Identification Guide, page 337

REFACTO® ℞

[*rē-făk'tō*]

Antihemophilic Factor, Recombinant

℞ only

This product's label may have been revised after this insert was used in production. For further product information and current package insert, please visit www.wyeth.com or call our medical communications department toll-free at 1-800-934-5556.

DESCRIPTION

ReFacto® Antihemophilic Factor (Recombinant) is a purified protein produced by recombinant DNA technology for use in therapy of factor VIII deficiency. ReFacto is a glycoprotein with an approximate molecular mass of 170 kDa consisting of 1438 amino acids. It has an amino acid sequence that is comparable to the 90 + 80 kDa form of factor VIII, and post-translational modifications that are similar to those of the plasma-derived molecule. ReFacto has *in vitro* functional characteristics comparable to those of endogenous factor VIII.

ReFacto is produced by a genetically engineered Chinese hamster ovary (CHO) cell line. The CHO cell line secretes B-domain deleted recombinant factor VIII into a defined cell culture medium that contains human serum albumin and recombinant insulin, but does not contain any proteins derived from animal sources. The protein is purified by a chromatography purification process that yields a high-purity, active product. The potency expressed in international units (IU) is determined using the European Pharmacopoeial chromogenic assay against the WHO standard. The specific activity of ReFacto is 9110-13700 IU per milligram of protein. ReFacto is not purified from human blood and contains no preservatives or added human components in the final formulation.

ReFacto is formulated as a sterile, nonpyrogenic, lyophilized powder preparation for intravenous (IV) injection. It is available in single-use vials containing the labeled amount of factor VIII activity (IU). Each vial contains nominally 250, 500, 1000 or 2000 IU of ReFacto per vial. The formulated product is a clear colorless solution upon reconstitution and contains sodium chloride, sucrose, L-histidine, calcium chloride, and polysorbate 80.

CLINICAL PHARMACOLOGY

Factor VIII is the specific clotting factor deficient in patients with hemophilia A (classical hemophilia). The administration of ReFacto® Antihemophilic Factor (Recombinant) increases plasma levels of factor VIII activity and can temporarily correct the *in vitro* coagulation defect in these patients.

Activated factor VIII acts as a cofactor for activated factor IX accelerating the conversion of factor X to activated factor X. Activated factor X converts prothrombin into thrombin. Thrombin then converts fibrinogen into fibrin and a clot is formed. Factor VIII activity is greatly reduced in patients with hemophilia A and therefore replacement therapy is necessary.

In a crossover pharmacokinetic study of eighteen (18) previously treated patients **using the chromogenic assay,** the circulating mean half-life for ReFacto was 14.5 ± 5.3 hours (ranged from 7.6-27.7 hours), which was not statistically significantly different from plasma-derived Antihemophilic Factor (Human) (pdAHF), which had a mean half-life of 13.7 ± 3.4 hours (ranged from 8.8-23.7 hours). Mean incremental recovery (K-value) of ReFacto in plasma was 2.4 ± 0.4 IU/dL per IU/kg (ranged from 1.9-3.3 IU/dL per IU/kg). This was comparable to the mean incremental recovery observed in plasma for pdAHF which was 2.3 ± 0.3 IU/dL per IU/kg (ranged from 1.7-2.9 IU/dL per IU/kg). **Results obtained from this controlled pharmacokinetic study, which used a central laboratory for the analysis of all plasma samples, showed that the one-stage factor VIII clotting assay gave results which were approximately 50% of the values obtained with the chromogenic assay** (see **DOSAGE AND ADMINISTRATION**).

In two additional clinical studies, pharmacokinetic parameters were evaluated for previously treated patients [PTPs] and previously untreated patients [PUPs]. In PTPs (n=87) ReFacto had a mean incremental recovery of 2.4 ± 0.4 IU/dL per IU/kg (ranged from 1.1-3.8 IU/dL per IU/kg) and an elimination half-life (n=67) of 10.7 ± 2.8 hours. In PUPs (n=45) ReFacto had a lower mean incremental recovery of 1.7 ± 0.4 IU/dL per IU/kg (ranged from 0.2-2.8 IU/dL per IU/kg) as compared to PTPs. Population pharmacokinetic modeling using data from 44 PUPs led to a mean estimated half-life of ReFacto in PUPs of 8.0 ± 2.2 hours. These parameters did not change over time (12 months) for PTPs or PUPs.

In clinical studies of ReFacto involving a total of 218 patients (117 PTPs including 4 who participated in the surgery study only, and 101 PUPs), more than 84 million IU were administered over a period of up to 54 months. The 117 PTPs were given a median of 230 injections (range of 4-1530 injections) over a median of 1200 days (range of 31-1640 days). The 101 PUPs were given a median of 26 injections (range of 1-490 injections) over a median of 830 days (range of 1-1298 days). One hundred thirteen PTPs and 99 PUPs were evaluated for efficacy in bleeding episodes. The 113 PTPs experienced a median of 54 bleeding episodes and the 99 PUPs experienced a median of 12 bleeding episodes. All were treated successfully on an on-demand basis or for the reduction of bleeding episodes except for one PTP and two PUPs who discontinued ReFacto treatment and switched to another product after the development of inhibitors. Bleeding episodes included hemarthroses, and bleeding in soft tissue, muscle, and other anatomical sites.

ReFacto has been studied in short-term routine prophylaxis. In uncontrolled clinical trials, an average dose of 27 ± 10 IU/kg in PTPs (n=77) and an average dose of 57 ± 20 IU/kg in PUPs (n=17) was given repeatedly at variable intervals longer than 2 weeks. In 64 patients who had both on-demand and prophylactic periods during their time on study, the mean rate of spontaneous musculoskeletal bleeding episodes was less during periods of routine prophylaxis. There were an average of 10 bleeding episodes per year during the prophylactic periods compared to an average of 37 bleeding episodes per year during the on-demand periods. The clinical trial experience with routine prophylaxis in PUPs is limited (n=17). These non-randomized trial results should be interpreted with caution, as the investigators exercised their own discretion in deciding when and in whom prophylaxis was to be initiated and terminated.

Management of hemostasis was evaluated in the surgical setting where 28 surgical procedures have been performed in 25 patients. The average preoperative dose in PTPs was 59 IU/kg. Procedures included orthopedic procedures, inguinal hernia repair, epidural hematoma evacuation, transposition ulnar nerve, and other minor procedures (e.g., venous access catheter placement and explantation, toenail removal). Circulatory factor VIII levels targeted to restore and maintain hemostasis were achieved. While the one-stage clotting assay was used most frequently in the surgical setting (24 versus 4 surgeries), hemostasis was maintained throughout the surgical period regardless of which assay was used. Hemostatic efficacy was rated as excellent or good in all procedures.

The occurrence of neutralizing antibody (inhibitors) is well known in the treatment of patients with hemophilia A[1,2,3]. Thirty out of 101 PUPs (30%) developed an inhibitor: 16 out of 101 (16%) with a high titer (≥ 5 BU) (11 of the 16 patients had peak values ≥ 10 BU) and 14 out of 101(14%) with a low titer (< 5 BU). In this study the incidence of inhibitor development to factor VIII using ReFacto is similar to that reported for other factor VIII products[1,2,3,5].

One of 113 (0.9%) previously treated patients (PTPs) developed a high titer inhibitor. Inhibitor development occurred in the same time frame as the development of monoclonal gammopathy of uncertain significance. The patient was noted initially to have low titer inhibitor at a local laboratory at 99 exposure days (1.2 BU) and became positive at the central laboratory at 113 exposure days, initially also with low titer inhibitor of 2 BU. After 14 months on continued treatment with ReFacto, the inhibitor level rose to nearly 13 BU and a bleeding episode failed to respond to ReFacto treatment. In this study the incidence of inhibitor development to factor VIII using ReFacto is similar to that reported for other factor VIII products[4]. Also there have been spontaneous post-marketing reports of high titer inhibitors involving previously treated patients (see also **PRECAUTIONS, General** and **ADVERSE REACTIONS**).

INDICATIONS AND USAGE

ReFacto® Antihemophilic Factor (Recombinant) is indicated for the control and prevention of hemorrhagic episodes and for surgical prophylaxis in patients with hemophilia A (congenital factor VIII deficiency or classic hemophilia).

ReFacto is indicated for short-term routine prophylaxis to reduce the frequency of spontaneous bleeding episodes. The effect of regular routine prophylaxis on long-term morbidity and mortality is unknown.

ReFacto can be of a significant therapeutic value for treatment of hemophilia A in certain patients with inhibitors to factor VIII[6]. In clinical studies of ReFacto, patients who developed inhibitors on study continued to manifest a clinical response when inhibitor titers were < 10 BU. When an inhibitor is present, the dosage requirement of factor VIII is variable. The dosage can be determined only by a clinical response and by monitoring of circulating factor VIII levels after treatment (see **DOSAGE AND ADMINISTRATION**).

ReFacto does not contain von Willebrand factor and therefore is not indicated in von Willebrand's disease.

Type of Hemorrhage	Factor VIII Level Required (IU/dL or % of normal)	Frequency of Doses (h)/ Duration of Therapy (d)
Minor		
Early hemarthrosis, minor muscle or oral bleeds.	20–40	Repeat every 12 to 24 hours as necessary until resolved. At least 1 day, depending upon the severity of the hemorrage.
Moderate		
Hemorrhages into muscles. Mild trauma capitis. Minor operations including tooth extraction. Hemorrhages into the oral cavity.	30–60	Repeat infusion every 12–24 hours for 3–4 days or until adequate local hemostasis is achieved. For tooth extraction a single infusion plus oral antifibrinolytic therapy within 1 hour may be sufficient.
Major		
Gastrointestinal bleeding. Intracranial, intra-abdominal or intrathoracic hemorrhages. Fractures. Major operations.	60–100	Repeat infusion every 8–24 hours until threat is resolved or in the case of surgery, until adequate local hemostasis is achieved.

CONTRAINDICATIONS

Known hypersensitivity to mouse, hamster, or bovine proteins may be a contraindication to the use of ReFacto® Antihemophilic Factor (Recombinant).

WARNINGS

As with any intravenous protein product, allergic type hypersensitivity reactions are possible. Patients should be informed of the early signs of hypersensitivity reactions including hives, generalized urticaria, tightness of the chest, wheezing, hypotension, and anaphylaxis. Patients should be advised to discontinue use of the product and contact their physicians if these symptoms occur.

PRECAUTIONS

General

Activity-neutralizing antibodies (inhibitors) have been detected in patients receiving factor VIII-containing products. Low titer inhibitors are common in previously untreated patients and in previously treated patients on factor VIII products, as are high titer inhibitors in previously untreated patients. High titer inhibitors, which are generally rare in previously treated patients, have been reported in previously treated patients on ReFacto. As with all coagulation factor VIII products, patients should be monitored for the development of inhibitors that should be titrated in Bethesda Units using appropriate biological testing.

Reports of lack of effect, mainly in prophylaxis patients, have been received in the clinical trials and in the post-marketing setting. The reported lack of effect has been described as bleeding into target joints, bleeding into new joints or a subjective feeling by the patient of new onset bleeding. When switching to ReFacto it is important to individually titrate and monitor each patient's dose in order to ensure an adequate therapeutic response (see **DOSAGE AND ADMINISTRATION**).

Formation of Antibodies to Mouse and Hamster Protein

As Antihemophilic Factor (Recombinant), ReFacto contains trace amounts of mouse protein (maximum of 5 ng/1000 IU) and hamster protein (maximum of 30 ng/1000 IU), the remote possibility exists that patients treated with this product may develop hypersensitivity to these non-human mammalian proteins.

Carcinogenicity, Mutagenicity, Impairment of Fertility

ReFacto® Antihemophilic Factor (Recombinant) has been shown to be nonmutagenic in the mouse micronucleus assay. No other mutagenicity studies and no investigations on carcinogenesis or impairment of fertility have been conducted.

Pregnancy Category C

Animal reproduction and lactation studies have not been conducted with ReFacto® Antihemophilic Factor (Recombinant). It is not known whether ReFacto can affect reproductive capacity or cause fetal harm when given to pregnant women. ReFacto should be administered to pregnant and lactating women only if clearly indicated.

Pediatric Use

ReFacto® Antihemophilic Factor (Recombinant) is appropriate for use in children of all ages, including newborns. Safety and efficacy studies have been performed both in previously treated children and adolescents (N=22, ages 8-15 years) and in previously untreated neonates, infants, and children (N=101, ages 0-52 months) (see **CLINICAL PHARMACOLOGY** and **PRECAUTIONS**).

Geriatric Use

Clinical studies of ReFacto did not include sufficient numbers of subjects aged 65 and over to determine whether they respond differently from younger subjects. Other reported clinical experience has not identified differences in responses between the elderly and younger patients. As with any patient receiving ReFacto, dose selection for an elderly patient should be individualized.

ADVERSE REACTIONS

As with the intravenous administration of any protein product, the following reactions may be observed after administration: headache, fever, chills, flushing, nausea, vomiting, lethargy, or manifestations of allergic reactions. During clinical studies with ReFacto® Antihemophilic Factor (Recombinant), 77 adverse reactions in 43 of 218 patients (20%) probably or possibly-related to therapy were reported for 64,363 infusions (0.12%). These were anaphylaxis (1), dyspnea (6), urticaria (1), nausea (11), headache (4), vasodilation (5), dizziness (4), permanent venous access catheter complications (3), asthenia (3), fever (3), taste perversion [altered taste] (3), bleeding/hematoma (3), infected hematoma (1), anorexia (2), diarrhea (2), injection site reaction (2), somnolence (2), rash (2), pruritus (2), angina pectoris (1), tachycardia (1), perspiration increased (1), chills (1), increased amino transferase (1), increased bilirubin (1), pain in finger (1), muscle weakness (1), CPK increase (1), cold sensation (1), eye disorder-vision abnormal (1), coughing (1), myalgia (1), gastroenteritis (1), abdominal pain (1), acne (1), and forehead bruises (1). If any adverse reaction takes place that is thought to be related to administration of ReFacto, the rate of infusion should be decreased or stopped.

Inhibitor development is a known adverse event associated with the treatment of patients with hemophilia A. In addition to the one report of high titer inhibitors in the clinical study of PTPs (see **CLINICAL PHARMACOLOGY**), there have been reports of high titer inhibitors in PTPs in the post-marketing setting. High and low titer inhibitors have been reported in PUPs in both clinical trials and the post-marketing setting (see **PRECAUTIONS, General**).

A total of 182 adverse reactions in 54 of 218 patients (25%) who received 32,013 infusions (0.6%) were reported by the investigator to have an "unlikely" or "not assessable" relationship to ReFacto administration. The study sponsor considered that the events may be of possible or of unknown relationship to therapy because of the temporal relationship to the infusion and/or the frequency of the event for a given patient and/or because insufficient information was available to assign another causality. In this category, 25 patients experienced the following 38 events which are different from the events described above: pain (10), rhinitis (10), vomiting (4), insomnia (3), constipation (2), pharyngitis (2), flushing (1), palpitation (1), sinusitis (1), gastritis (1), dyspepsia (1), hypotension (1), and URI (1).

Other adverse experiences that were reported during the clinical trials, but which were assessed by both the investigator and the sponsor as "unlikely" to be related to ReFacto administration included: dyspnea (3), rash (2), pruritus (1), neuropathy (1), arm weakness (1), and thrombophlebitis of upper arm (1).

DOSAGE AND ADMINISTRATION

Treatment with ReFacto® Antihemophilic Factor (Recombinant) should be initiated under the supervision of a physician experienced in the treatment of hemophilia A.

The labeled potency of ReFacto is based on the European Pharmacopoeial chromogenic substrate assay, whereas other factor VIII products are labeled based on the one-stage clotting assay. With recombinant factor VIII products, the chromogenic assay typically yields results which are higher than the results obtained with the one-stage clotting assay. When switching between products it is important to individually titrate each patient's dose in order to ensure an adequate therapeutic response (see **PRECAUTIONS, General**). Results obtained from a controlled pharmacokinetic study, which used one central laboratory for the analysis of all plasma samples, showed that the one-stage factor VIII clotting assay gave results that were approximately 50% of those obtained with the chromogenic substrate assay (see **CLINICAL PHARMACOLOGY**). In addition, in clinical trials of ReFacto use in the surgical setting in which multiple laboratories were used for plasma sample analysis, the ratio of factor VIII activity results obtained by the one-stage clotting and chromogenic substrate assays ranged between 20 and 80%.

When monitoring patients' factor VIII activity levels during treatment, the available clinical data suggest that either assay may be used. Most patients in clinical trials were monitored with the one-stage clotting assay (see **CLINICAL PHARMACOLOGY**). It is necessary to adhere to the incubation/activation times and other test conditions as specified by the assay manufacturers.

Dosage and duration of treatment depend on the severity of the factor VIII deficiency, the location and extent of bleeding, and the patient's clinical condition. Doses administered should be titrated to the patient's clinical response. In the presence of an inhibitor, higher doses may be required.

Precise monitoring of the replacement therapy by means of coagulation analysis (plasma factor VIII activity) is recommended, particularly for surgical intervention.

Continued on next page

ReFacto—Cont.

One international unit (IU) of factor VIII activity corresponds approximately to the quantity of factor VIII in one mL of normal human plasma. The calculation of the required dosage of factor VIII is based upon the empirical finding that, on average, 1 IU of factor VIII per kg body weight raises the plasma factor VIII activity by approximately 2 IU/dL per IU/kg administered. The required dosage is determined using the following formula:

Required units = body weight (kg)
× desired factor VIII rise (IU/dL or % of normal)
× 0.5 (IU/kg per IU/dL)

The following chart can be used to guide dosing in bleeding episodes and surgery:

[See table at top of previous page]

For short-term routine prophylaxis to prevent or reduce the frequency of spontaneous musculoskeletal hemorrhage in patients with hemophilia A, ReFacto should be given at least twice a week. In some cases, especially pediatric patients, shorter dosage intervals or higher doses may be necessary. Pharmacokinetic/pharmacodynamic modeling, based on pharmacokinetic data from 185 infusions in 102 PTPs, predicts that routine prophylactic dosing 3 times per week may be associated with a lower bleeding risk than with dosing twice weekly. No randomized comparison of different doses or frequency regimens of ReFacto for routine prophylaxis has been performed. In clinical studies in PTPs (ages 8-73 years) and PUPs (ages 9-52 months), the mean dose used for routine prophylaxis was 27 ± 10 IU/kg and 57 ± 20 IU/kg, respectively.

Patients using ReFacto should be monitored for the development of factor VIII inhibitors. If expected factor VIII activity plasma levels are not attained, or if bleeding is not controlled with an appropriate dose, an assay should be performed to determine if a factor VIII inhibitor is present. If the inhibitor is present at levels less than 5 Bethesda Units, administration of additional antihemophilic factor may neutralize the inhibitor.

ReFacto is administered by IV infusion after reconstitution of the lyophilized powder with Sodium Chloride Diluent (provided).

INSTRUCTIONS FOR USE

Patients should follow the specific reconstitution and administration procedures provided by their physicians. The procedures below are provided as general guidelines for the reconstitution and administration of ReFacto.

Reconstitution

Always wash your hands before performing the following procedures. Aseptic technique should be used during the reconstitution procedure.

ReFacto® Antihemophilic Factor (Recombinant) is administered by intravenous (IV) infusion after reconstitution with the supplied Sodium Chloride Diluent.

1. Allow the vials of lyophilized ReFacto and diluent to reach room temperature.
2. Remove the plastic flip-top caps from the ReFacto vial and the diluent vial to expose the central portions of the rubber stoppers.
3. Wipe the tops of both vials with the alcohol swab provided, or use another antiseptic solution, and allow to dry.
4. Remove the transparent protective cover from the short end of the sterile double-ended needle and insert that end into the diluent vial at the center of the stopper.
5. Remove the colored protective cover from the long end of the sterile double-ended needle. Invert the diluent vial and, to minimize leakage, quickly insert the long end of the needle through the center of the stopper of the upright ReFacto vial.
   Note: Point the double-ended needle toward the wall of the ReFacto vial to prevent excessive foaming.
6. The vacuum will draw the diluent into the ReFacto vial.
7. Once the transfer is complete, remove the double-ended needle from the ReFacto vial, and properly discard the needle with the diluent vial.
   Note: If the diluent does not transfer completely into the ReFacto vial, DO NOT USE the contents of the vial. Note that it is acceptable for a small amount of fluid to remain in the solvent vial after transfer.
8. Gently rotate the vial to dissolve the powder.
9. The final solution should be inspected visually for particulate matter before administration. The solution should appear clear and colorless.

ReFacto should be administered within 3 hours after reconstitution. The reconstituted solution may be stored at room temperature prior to administration.

Administration (Intravenous Injection)

ReFacto® Antihemophilic Factor (Recombinant) should be administered using a single sterile disposable plastic syringe. In addition, the solution should be withdrawn from the vial using the sterile filter needle.

1. Using aseptic technique, attach the sterile filter needle to the sterile disposable syringe. Pull back the syringe plunger to the 5 mL mark.
2. Insert the filter needle into the stopper of the ReFacto vial. Push plunger forward to inject air into the vial.
3. Invert the vial and withdraw the reconstituted solution into the syringe.
4. Remove and discard the filter needle.
   Note: If you use more than one vial of ReFacto, the contents of multiple vials may be drawn into the same syringe through a separate, unused filter needle.
5. Attach the syringe to the luer end of the infusion set tubing and perform venipuncture as instructed by your physician.

After reconstitution, ReFacto should be injected intravenously over several minutes. The rate of administration should be determined by the patient's comfort level.

Dispose of all unused solution, empty vials, and used needles and syringes in an appropriate container for throwing away waste that might hurt others if not handled properly.

Storage

Product as packaged for sale: ReFacto® Antihemophilic Factor (Recombinant) should be stored under refrigeration at a temperature of 2 to 8 °C (36 to 46 °F). ReFacto may also be stored at room temperature not to exceed 25 °C (77 °F) for up to 3 months. Freezing should be avoided to prevent damage to the diluent vial. During storage, avoid prolonged exposure of ReFacto® vial to light. Do not use ReFacto after the expiry date on the label.

Product after reconstitution: The product does not contain a preservative and should be used within 3 hours.

HOW SUPPLIED

ReFacto® Antihemophilic Factor (Recombinant) is supplied in single-use vials which contain nominally 250, 500, 1000 or 2000 IU per vial (NDC 58394-007-01, 58394-006-01, 58394-005-01, 58394-011-01, respectively) with sterile diluent, sterile double-ended needle for reconstitution, sterile filter needle for withdrawal, sterile infusion set, and two (2) alcohol swabs. Actual factor VIII activity in IU is stated on the label of each vial.

REFERENCES

1. Ehrenforth S, Kreuz W, Scharrer I, et al. Incidence of development of factor VIII and factor IX inhibitors in hemophiliacs. Lancet. 1992;339:594-598.
2. Bray GL, Gomperts ED, Courter S, et al. A multicenter study of recombinant factor VIII (Recombinate): safety, efficacy, and inhibitor risk in previously untreated patients with hemophilia A. Blood. 1994;83(9):2428-2435.
3. Lusher J, Arkin S, Abildgaard CF, Schwartz RS, Group TKPUPS. Recombinant factor VIII for the treatment of previously untreated patients with hemophilia A. N Engl J Med. 1993;328:453-459.
4. Kessler C, Sachse K. Factor VIII:C inhibitor associated with monoclonal-antibody purified FVIII concentrate. Lancet 1990; 335:1403.
5. Scharrer I, Bray G. Incidence of inhibitors in haemophilia A patients - a review of recent studies of recombinant and plasma-derived factor VIII concentrates. Hemophilia 1999; 5:145.
6. Kessler CM. An Introduction to Factor VIII Inhibitors: The Detection and Quantitation. American Journal of Medicine 91 1991, (Supplement 5A): 1S-5S.

Wyeth®
Wyeth Pharmaceuticals Inc.
Philadelphia, PA 19101
US Govt. License No. 3
Telephone: 1-800-934-5556

W10403C004
ET01
Rev 02/04

Shown in Product Identification Guide, page 337

SYNVISC® ℞

[sin'vĭsk]

HYLAN G-F 20

Caution: Federal law restricts this device to sale by or on the order of a physician (or properly licensed practitioner).

DESCRIPTION

Synvisc® (hylan G-F 20) is an elastoviscous fluid containing hylan polymers produced from chicken combs. Hylans are derivatives of hyaluronan (sodium hyaluronate), a natural complex sugar of the glycosaminoglycan family. Hyaluronan is a long-chain polymer containing repeating disaccharide units of Na-glucuronate-N-acetylglucosamine.

INDICATIONS

Synvisc is indicated for the treatment of pain in osteoarthritis (OA) of the knee in patients who have failed to respond adequately to conservative nonpharmacologic therapy and simple analgesics, e.g., acetaminophen.

CONTRAINDICATIONS

- Do not administer to patients with known hypersensitivity (allergy) to hyaluronan (sodium hyaluronate) preparations.
- Do not inject Synvisc in the knees of patients having knee joint infections or skin diseases or infections in the area of the injection site.

WARNINGS

- Do not concomitantly use disinfectants containing quaternary ammonium salts for skin preparation because hyaluronan can precipitate in their presence.
- Do not inject Synvisc extra-articularly or into the synovial tissues and capsule. Local and systemic adverse events, generally in the area of the injection, have occurred following extra-articular injection of Synvisc.
- Intravascular injections of Synvisc may cause systemic adverse events.

PRECAUTIONS

General

- The effectiveness of a single treatment cycle of less than three injections of Synvisc has not been established.
- The safety and effectiveness of Synvisc in locations other than the knee and for conditions other than osteoarthritis have not been established.
- Do not inject anesthetics or other medications into the knee joint during Synvisc therapy. Such medications may dilute Synvisc and affect its safety and effectiveness.
- Use caution when injecting Synvisc into patients who are allergic to avian proteins, feathers and egg products.
- The safety and effectiveness of Synvisc in severely inflamed knee joints have not been established.
- Strict aseptic administration technique must be followed.
- STERILE CONTENTS. The syringe is intended for single use. The contents of the syringe must be used immediately after its packaging is opened. Discard any unused Synvisc.
- Do not use Synvisc if package is opened or damaged. Store in original packaging (protected from light) at room temperature below 86°F (30°C). DO NOT FREEZE.
- Remove synovial fluid or effusion before each Synvisc injection.
- Synvisc should be used with caution when there is evidence of lymphatic or venous stasis in that leg.

Information for Patients

- Provide patients with a copy of the Patient Labeling prior to use.
- Transient pain, swelling and/or effusion of the injected joint may occur after intra-articular injection of Synvisc. In some cases the effusion may be considerable and can cause pronounced pain; cases where swelling is extensive should be discussed with the physician.
- As with any invasive joint procedure, it is recommended that the patient avoid any strenuous activities or prolonged weight-bearing activities such as jogging or tennis following the intra-articular injection.
- The packaging of this product contains dry natural rubber latex.

Use in Specific Populations

- **Pregnancy:** The safety and effectiveness of Synvisc have not been established in pregnant women.
- **Nursing mothers:** It is not known if Synvisc is excreted in human milk. The safety and effectiveness of Synvisc have not been established in lactating women.
- The safety and effectiveness of Synvisc have not been established in children.

ADVERSE EVENTS

Adverse Events Involving the Injected Joint

Clinical Trials: A total of 511 patients (559 knees) received 1771 injections in seven clinical trials of Synvisc. There were 39 reports in 37 patients (2.2% of injections, 7.2% of patients) of knee pain and/or swelling after these injections. Ten patients (10 knees) were treated with arthrocentesis and removal of joint effusion. Two additional patients (two knees) received treatment with intra-articular steroids. Two patients (two knees) received NSAIDs. One of these patients also received arthrocentesis. One patient was treated with arthroscopy. The remaining patients with adverse events localized to the knee received no treatment or only analgesics.

Postmarket Experience: The most common adverse events reported have been pain, swelling and/or effusion in the injected knee. In some cases the effusion was considerable and caused pronounced pain. In some instances, patients have presented with knees that were tender, warm and red. It is important to rule out infection or crystalline arthropathies in such cases. Synovial fluid aspirates of varying volumes have revealed a range of cell counts, from very few to over 50,000 cells/mm^3. Reported treatments included symptomatic therapy (e.g., rest, ice, heat, elevation, simple analgesics and NSAIDs) and/or arthrocentesis. Intra-articular corticosteroids have been used when infection was excluded. Rarely, arthroscopy has been performed. The occurrence of post-injection effusion may be associated with patient history of effusion, advanced stage of disease and/or the number of injections or treatment courses a patient receives. Reactions generally abate within a few days. Clinical benefit from the treatment may still occur after such reactions.

The clinical trials described above included 38 patients who received a second course of Synvisc injections (132 injections). There were twelve reports in nine patients (9.1% of injections, 23.7% of patients) of knee pain and/or swelling after these injections. Reports of two additional clinical trials in which patients received repeated courses of Synvisc treatment have appeared during the post-marketing period. One of these trials included 48 patients who received 210 injections during a second course of Synvisc treatment[1]; the other contained 71 patients who received 211 injections during a second course of Synvisc treatment.

A total of 157 patients have received 553 injections in the three clinical trials of repeated courses of Synvisc treatment. The reports in these trials describe a total of 48 reports of adverse events localized to the injected knee in 35 patients that occurred after injections that patients had received during their second course of treatment. These adverse events accounted for 6.3% of injections in 22.3% of patients as compared to 2.2% of injections in 7.2% of patients in a single course of Synvisc injections. In addition, reports of two retrospective studies during the post-marketing period have described adverse events localized to the injected knee that have occurred after 4.4% and 8.5% of injections that patients had received during one or more repeated courses of Synvisc treatment.[2,3]

Intra-articular infections did not occur in any of the clinical trials and have been reported only rarely during clinical use of Synvisc.

Other Adverse Events

Clinical Trials: In three concurrently controlled clinical trials with a total of 112 patients who received Synvisc and 110 patients who received either saline or arthrocentesis, there were no statistically significant differences in the numbers or types of adverse events between the group of patients that received Synvisc and the group that received control treatments.

Systemic adverse events each occurred in 10 (2.0%) of the Synvisc-treated patients. There was one case each of rash (thorax and back) and itching of the skin following Synvisc injections in these studies. These symptoms did not recur when these patients received additional Synvisc injections. The remaining generalized adverse events reported were calf cramps, hemorrhoid problems, ankle edema, muscle pain, tonsillitis with nausea, tachyarrythmia, phlebitis with varicosities and low back sprain.

Postmarket Experience: Other adverse events reported include: rash, *hives*, itching, *fever*, nausea, *headache*, *dizziness*, *chills*, muscle cramps, *paresthesia*, peripheral edema, *malaise*, *respiratory difficulties*, *flushing* and *facial swelling*. There have been rare reports of *thrombocytopenia* coincident with Synvisc injection. These medical events occurred under circumstances where causal relationship to Synvisc is uncertain. (Adverse events reported *only* in worldwide postmarketing experience, not seen in clinical trials, are considered more rare and are *italicized*.)

CLINICAL STUDIES

The safety and effectiveness of Synvisc were studied in patients ≥40 years old in the three concurrently controlled clinical trials. The three studies investigated a total of 136 women and 81 men. The demographics of trial participants were comparable across treatment groups with regard to age, gender and duration of osteoarthritis, except that there was a significantly greater (p = 0.04) number of men in the Synvisc group and women in the control group in one study (see Table 1).

One study was a multicenter study conducted at four sites in Germany. This was a randomized, double-blind prospective clinical trial with two treatment groups. The study compared the safety and effectiveness of three weekly intra-articular injections of Synvisc and of physiological saline in 103 subjects (109 knees) with osteoarthritis of the knee over a 26-week period.

A significantly greater number of saline-treated patients took concurrent osteoarthritis medications than did patients treated with Synvisc (see Table 2). While both the Synvisc and the saline-treated groups improved significantly as compared to baseline in all effectiveness measures, the Synvisc group showed a significantly greater improvement in all outcome measures than did the saline-treated patients over a 26-week period (see Tables 3A and 3B).

A second study conducted at a single center in Germany[4] was a concurrently controlled, randomized, double-blind prospective clinical trial with two treatment groups. This study compared the safety and effectiveness over a 26-week period of three weekly intra-articular injections of Synvisc and of physiological saline in 29 subjects (29 knees) with osteoarthritis of the knee. The results of the study were similar to those in the German multicenter study, except that the significance levels in most comparisons were smaller (see Tables 3A and 3B). In both of these studies the most pain relief and the greatest amount of treatment success occurred 8 to 12 weeks after Synvisc treatment began.

Investigators obtained data at 26 weeks by telephone interviews. A validation study suggested that the results obtained in telephone interviews are equivalent to those obtained in office visits. Since investigators did not follow patients beyond week 26, the duration of pain relief beyond 26 weeks is not known.

A third study was a prospective, concurrently controlled, randomized, double-blind multicenter study conducted in 90 subjects (103 knees) at five U.S. sites. The study compared the safety and effectiveness of three weekly intra-articular injections of Synvisc and of three weekly arthrocenteses in subjects with osteoarthritis of the knee over a four-week period after the first injection or arthrocentesis.

Both the Synvisc-treated and the arthrocentesis-treated groups improved significantly as compared to baseline in all effectiveness measures. However, there were no significant differences between the Synvisc-treated and arthrocentesis-treated patients at any time during the four-week evaluation period (see Tables 3A and 3B).

Covariate analyses with the covariates of center, presence or absence of previous treatments, baseline levels of outcome measures, age, gender, body mass, effusion, baseline X-ray score, duration of osteoarthritis, treatment of contralateral knee, and presence or absence of concurrent therapies, did not reveal any factors that significantly affected the results of any of the three studies.

The German studies and the U.S. study differed in several respects, including inclusion of patients with effusions, length of no treatment period prior to Synvisc injection, nature of control treatment, final evaluation time, mean duration of disease, mean weight, prior treatments for OA, pain and X-ray inclusion criteria. Thus, the German and the U.S. studies, which gave different results, investigated different patient populations and compared Synvisc with different control treatments.

Although success criteria for safety were not specified in any of the three studies, adverse events were enumerated in each study. These events are included in the "Adverse Events" section.

TABLE 2
CONCURRENT OSTEOARTHRITIS THERAPIES[1]

CONCURRENT MEDICATIONS[2]	TREATED KNEES: TOTAL	Synvisc	Control	P Synvisc/Control
German Multicenter	N[3]=109	N=52	N=57	
Medications [N (%)][4]	27 (25%)	5 (10%)	22 (39%)	0.001
NSAIDS	17 (16%)	4 (8%)	13 (23%)	0.03
Acetaminophen	7 (6%)	1 (2%)	6 (11%)	0.07
Other medications[5]	3 (3%)	3 (5%)	0 (0%)	0.09
German Single Center[6]	N=29	N=14	N=15	
Any concurrent medication [N (%)]	NA[7]	NA	NA	NA
U.S. Multicenter[8]	N=103	N=51	N=52	
Acetaminophen [N (%)]	100 (97%)	50 (98%)	50 (96%)	0.6

Footnotes:
[1] Patients ≥ 40 years old and received the complete treatment course
[2] Individual patients may be represented by more than one therapy
[3] N = number of knees
[4] Number and percentage of subjects
[5] Medications not approved in the U.S.
[6] No concurrent therapies were recorded
[7] Data not collected
[8] Only acetaminophen was allowed

TABLE 1
DEMOGRAPHIC DATA[1]

	Age	Gender [N[2] (%)] M	Gender [N[2] (%)] F	Duration of Osteoarthritis (years)
German Multicenter[3]				
Synvisc	62.3	21 (45%)	26 (55%)	5.4
Saline	64.7	13 (25%)	39 (75%)	5.6
P (Synvisc/Saline)	0.3	0.04		0.9
German Single Center				
Synvisc	59.8	10 (71%)	4 (29%)	2.4
Saline	59.5	8 (53%)	7 (47%)	2.5
P (Synvisc/Saline)	0.9	0.3		1.0
U.S. Multicenter[4]				
Synvisc	62.9	17 (39%)	27 (61%)	8.9
Arthrocenteses	67.1	12 (29%)	30 (71%)	7.9
P (Synvisc/Arthrocenteses)	0.06	0.3		0.5

Footnotes:
[1] Patients ≥ 40 years old and received the complete treatment course
[2] N = number of patients
[3] In addition, 1 male and 3 females were treated with Synvisc in one knee and saline in the other
[4] In addition, 4 females were treated with Synvisc in one knee and arthrocenteses in the other

[See table 2 above]
[See table 3A at top of next page]
[See table 3B on next page]

DETAILED DEVICE DESCRIPTION

Synvisc contains hylan A (average molecular weight 6,000,000) and hylan B hydrated gel in a buffered physiological sodium chloride solution, pH 7.2. Synvisc has an elasticity (storage modulus G′) at 2.5 Hz of 111 ± 13 Pascals (Pa) and a viscosity (loss modulus G″) of 25 ± 2 Pa (elasticity and viscosity of knee synovial fluid of 18 to 27-year-old humans measured with a comparable method at 2.5 Hz: G′ = 117 ± 13 Pa; G″ = 45 ± 8 Pa.)

Each syringe of Synvisc contains:

Hylan polymers (hylan A + hylan B)	16 mg
Sodium chloride	17 mg
Disodium hydrogen phosphate	0.32 mg
Sodium dihydrogen phosphate monohydrate	0.08 mg
Water for injection	q.s. to 2.0 mL

HOW SUPPLIED

Synvisc is supplied in a 2.25 mL glass syringe containing 2 mL Synvisc.

Product Number: 0008-9149-02 3 disposable syringes

The contents of the syringe are sterile and nonpyrogenic.

DIRECTIONS FOR USE

Synvisc is administered by intra-articular injection once a week (one week apart) for a total of three injections.

Precaution: Do not use Synvisc if the package has been opened or damaged. Store in original packaging (protected from light) at room temperature below 86°F (30°C). DO NOT FREEZE.

Precaution: Strict aseptic administration technique must be followed.

Precaution: Do not concomitantly use disinfectants containing quaternary ammonium salts for skin preparation because hyaluronan can precipitate in their presence.

Precaution: Remove synovial fluid or effusion before each Synvisc injection.

Do not use the same syringe for removing synovial fluid and for injecting Synvisc, but the same needle should be used.

Take particular care to remove the tip cap of the syringe and needle aseptically.

Twist the gray tip cap before pulling it off, as this will minimize product leakage.

Inject Synvisc into the knee joint through an 18 to 22 gauge needle.

To ensure a tight seal and prevent leakage during administration, secure the needle tightly while firmly holding the luer hub.

Precaution: Do not over tighten or apply excessive leverage when attaching the needle or removing the needle guard, as this may break the tip of the syringe.

Do not inject anesthetics or any other medications intra-articularly into the knee while administering Synvisc therapy. This may dilute Synvisc and affect its safety and effectiveness.

Precaution: The syringe containing Synvisc is intended for single use. The contents of the syringe must be used immediately after the syringe has been removed from its packaging. Inject the full 2 mL in one knee only. If treatment is bilateral, a separate syringe must be used for each knee. Discard any unused Synvisc.

DISTRIBUTED BY:
Wyeth-Ayerst Pharmaceuticals
Philadelphia, Pennsylvania 19101
Telephone: 1-800-99-WYETH

DEVELOPED AND MANUFACTURED BY:
Genzyme Biosurgery
a division of Genzyme Corporation
1125 Pleasant View Terrace
Ridgefield, New Jersey 07657

Covered by U.S. patents #4,636,524, #4,713,448, #5,099,013, #5,143,724.

SYNVISC and GENZYME are registered trademarks of Genzyme Corporation.

REFERENCES

1. Raynauld, J.P., Bellamy, N., Goldsmith, C.H., Tugwell, P., Torrance, G.W., Pericak, D., et al. (2002). An evaluation of the safety and effectiveness of repeat courses of hylan G-F 20 for treating patients with knee osteoarthritis. Os-

Continued on next page

TABLE 3A
EFFECTIVENESS OF WEIGHT-BEARING PAIN[1]
EVALUATED BY PATIENTS

	Baseline	Improvement (Change from Baseline)						
Week	0	1	2	3	4	8	12	26[6]
German Multicenter								
Synvisc-treated								
Mean[2]	69.7	12.0	26.5	37.9	NA[5]	45.9	46.5	34.0
P[3]		0.0001	0.0001	0.0001		0.0001	0.0001	0.0001
Saline-treated								
Mean	75.1	9.0	17.0	23.0	NA	16.8	16.4	19.1
P[3]		0.0001	0.0001	0.0001		0.0001	0.0002	0.0001
P[4]	0.1	0.3	0.01	0.0008	NA	<0.0001	<0.0001	0.005
German Single Center								
Synvisc-treated								
Mean	65.2	10.6	31.8	43.9	NA	51.7	53.5	44.5
P[3]		0.02	0.0001	0.0001		0.0001	0.0001	0.0001
Saline-treated								
Mean	69.8	5.4	19.3	25.4	NA	24.4	26.8	21.2
P[3]		0.01	0.0001	0.0001		0.0001	0.0001	0.002
P[4]	0.4	0.2	0.03	0.01	NA	0.0001	0.0001	0.001
U.S. Multicenter								
Synvisc-treated								
Mean	67.3	12.9	18.9	NA	21.3	NA	NA	NA
P[3]		0.0002	0.0001		0.0001			
Arthrocenteses								
Mean	69.4	9.4	21.2	NA	19.1	NA	NA	NA
P[3]		0.01	0.0001		0.0002			
P[4]	0.6	0.5	0.7	NA	0.7	NA	NA	NA

Footnotes:
[1] Patients ≥ 40 years old and received the complete treatment course
[2] Mean of assessments on VAS of 0 to 100 mm
[3] Significance from baseline
[4] Significance between Synvisc and control
[5] NA = no measurement taken
[6] Week 26 data based on patient telephone interviews rather than patient office visit

TABLE 3B
EFFECTIVENESS OF NIGHT PAIN[1]
EVALUATED BY PATIENTS

	Baseline	Improvement (Change from Baseline)						
Week	0	1	2	3	4	8	12	26[6]
German Multicenter								
Synvisc-treated								
Mean[2]	41.6	9.2	20.0	26.4	NA[5]	28.3	29.8	24.3
P[3]		0.0001	0.0001	0.0001		0.0001	0.0001	0.0001
Saline-treated								
Mean	45.7	9.5	15.2	21.2	NA	18.4	17.3	12.8
P[3]		0.0001	0.0001	0.0001		0.0001	0.0001	0.002
P[4]	0.5	0.9	0.2	0.3	NA	0.05	0.02	0.03
German Single Center								
Synvisc-treated								
Mean	31.8	8.4	17.7	24.8	NA	28.9	29.5	25.4
P[3]		0.04	0.005	0.004		0.005	0.005	0.004
Saline-treated								
Mean	33.3	4.5	13.1	16.1	NA	16.1	17.9	14.9
P[3]		0.1	0.001	0.0007		0.0001	0.0001	0.01
P[4]	0.9	0.4	0.4	0.3	NA	0.1	0.2	0.2
U.S. Multicenter								
Synvisc-treated								
Mean	61.0	19.0	17.9	NA	22.8	NA	NA	NA
P[3]		0.0001	0.0001		0.0001			
Arthrocenteses								
Mean	76.0	23.3	36.3	NA	29.8	NA	NA	NA
P[3]		0.0001	0.0001		0.0001			
P[4]	0.002	0.5	0.004	NA	0.3	NA	NA	NA

Footnotes:
[1] Patients ≥ 40 years old and received the complete treatment course
[2] Mean of assessments on VAS of 0 to 100 mm
[3] Significance from baseline
[4] Significance between Synvisc and control
[5] NA = no measurement taken
[6] Week 26 data based on patient telephone interviews rather than patient office visit

Synvisc—Cont.

teoarthritis Research Society International, 2002 OARSI World Congress on Osteoarthritis, Sydney, Australia [Paper reference # PS128]. Presentation on File.

2. Leopold, S.S., Warme, W.J., Pettis, P.D. and Shott, S. (2002). Increased frequency of acute local reaction to intra-articular Hylan GF-20 (Synvisc) in patients receiving more than one course of treatment. J. Bone Joint Surg. 84-A (9): 1619–1623.
3. Waddell, D.D., Estey, D.J. and Bricker, D. (2001). Retrospective tolerance of Hylan G-F 20 using fluoroscopically-confirmed injection and effectiveness of retreatment in knee osteoarthritis. Proceedings of the American College of Rheumatology Annual Meeting 2001. Presentation on File.
4. Scale, D., Wobig, and Wolpert, W. (1994). Viscosupplementation of osteoarthritic knees with hylan: a treatment schedule study. Curr. Ther. Res. 55: 220–232.

CI 6082-5 Revised October 7, 2003

Shown in Product Identification Guide, page 337

TRECATOR®-SC ℞

[trĕk"ă'tōr]

(ethionamide tablets, USP)
Sugar-Coated Tablets
℞ only

DESCRIPTION

Trecator® (ethionamide tablets, USP) is used in the treatment of tuberculosis. The chemical name for ethionamide is 2-ethylthioisonicotinamide with the following structural formula:

Ethionamide is a yellow crystalline, nonhygroscopic compound with a faint to moderate sulfide odor and a melting point of 162°C. It is practically insoluble in water and ether, but soluble in methanol and ethanol. It has a partition coefficient (octanol/water) Log P value of 0.3699. Trecator-SC tablets contain 250 mg of ethionamide. The inactive ingredients present are lactose, methylcellulose, magnesium stearate, polacrilin potassium, pharmaceutical glaze, talc, gelatin, acacia, sucrose, calcium carbonate, confectioners sugar, FD&C Yellow #6, povidone, sodium benzoate, titanium dioxide, white wax, and carnauba wax.

CLINICAL PHARMACOLOGY

Ethionamide is essentially completely absorbed following oral administration and is not subjected to any appreciable first pass metabolism.[1] Following a single 250 mg oral dose of ethionamide in healthy volunteers, peak plasma concentrations of about 2 µg/mL were attained at 2 hours in most cases. Normal serum concentrations of 1 to 5 µg/mL are usually seen 2 hours following doses of 250 mg to 500 mg.[2] These concentrations approximate the therapeutic range for this drug when the therapeutic range is defined by those serum concentrations associated with a high probability of success and a low probability of dose-related toxicity. The drug is approximately 30 percent bound to plasma proteins. Trecator-SC is rapidly and widely distributed into body tissues and fluids, with concentrations in plasma and various organs being approximately equal. Significant concentrations also are present in cerebrospinal fluid.

Ethionamide is extensively metabolized to active and inactive metabolites with less than 1% excreted as the free form in urine. Metabolism is presumed to occur in the liver and thus far 6 metabolites have been isolated: 2-ethylisonicotinamide, carbamoyl-dihydropyridine, thiocarbamoyl-dihydropyridine, S-oxocarbamoyl dihydropyridine, 2-ethylthioiso-nicotinamide, and ethionamide sulphoxide. The sulphoxide metabolite has been demonstrated to have antimicrobial activity against *Mycobacterium tuberculosis*. Trecator-SC has a plasma elimination half-life of approximately 2 hours after oral dosing.

Mechanism of Action

Ethionamide may be bacteriostatic or bactericidal in action, depending on the concentration of the drug attained at the site of infection and the susceptibility of the infecting organism. The exact mechanism of action of ethionamide has not been fully elucidated, but the drug appears to inhibit peptide synthesis in susceptible organisms.

Microbiology

In Vitro Activity

Ethionamide exhibits bacteriostatic activity against extracellular and intracellular *Mycobacterium tuberculosis* organisms. The development of ethionamide resistant *M. tuberculosis* isolates can be obtained by repeated subculturing in liquid or on solid media containing increasing concentrations of ethionamide. Multi-drug resistant strains of *M. tuberculosis* may have acquired resistance to both isoniazid and ethionamide. However, the majority of *M. tuberculosis* isolates that are resistant to one are usually susceptible to the other. There is no evidence of cross-resistance between ethionamide and para-aminosalicylic acid (PAS), streptomycin, or cycloserine. However, limited data suggest that cross-resistance may exist between ethionamide and thiosemicarbazones (i.e., thiacetazone) as well as isoniazid.

In Vivo Activity

Ethionamide administered orally initially decreased the number of culturable *Mycobacterium tuberculosis* organisms from the lungs of H37Rv infected mice. Drug resistance developed with continued ethionamide monotherapy, but did not occur when mice received ethionamide in combination with streptomycin or isoniazid.

SUSCEPTIBILITY TESTING

Ethionamide susceptibility testing should only be performed by qualified or reference laboratories.

Two standardized *in vitro* susceptibility methods are available for testing ethionamide against *M. tuberculosis* organisms. The modified proportion method (CDC or NCCLS M24-P) utilizes Middlebrook and Cohn 7H10 agar medium impregnated with ethionamide at a final concentration of 5.0 µg/mL. After 2 to 3 weeks of incubation, MIC_{99} values are calculated by comparing the quantity of organisms growing in the medium containing drug to the control cultures. Mycobacterial growth in the presence of drug, of at least 1% of the growth in the control culture, indicates resistance.

The radiometric broth method employs the BACTEC 460 machine to compare the growth index from untreated control cultures to cultures grown in the presence of 5.0 µg/mL of ethionamide. Strict adherence to the manufacturer's instructions for sample processing and data interpretation is required for this assay.

Susceptibility test results obtained by these two different methods cannot be compared unless equivalent drug concentrations are evaluated.

The clinical relevance of *in vitro* susceptibility test results for mycobacterial species other than *M. tuberculosis* using either the radiometric or the proportion method has not been determined.

INDICATIONS AND USAGE

Trecator-SC (ethionamide) is primarily indicated for the treatment of active tuberculosis in patients with *M. tuberculosis* resistant to isoniazid or rifampin, or when there is intolerance on the part of the patient to other drugs. Its use alone in the treatment of tuberculosis results in the rapid development of resistance. It is essential, therefore, to give a suitable companion drug or drugs, the choice being based on the results of susceptibility tests. If the susceptibility tests indicate that the patient's organism is resistant to one of the first-line antituberculosis drugs (i.e., isoniazid or rifampin) yet susceptible to ethionamide, ethionamide should be accompanied by at least one drug to which the *M. tuberculosis* isolate is known to be susceptible.[6] If the tuberculosis is resistant to both isoniazid and rifampin, yet susceptible to ethionamide, ethionamide should be accompanied by at least two other drugs to which the *M. tuberculosis* isolate is known to be susceptible.[6]

Patient nonadherence to prescribed treatment can result in treatment failure and in the development of drug-resistant tuberculosis, which can be life-threatening and lead to other serious health risks. It is, therefore, essential that patients adhere to the drug regimen for the full duration of treatment. Directly observed therapy is recommended for all patients receiving treatment for tuberculosis. Patients in whom drug-resistant *M. tuberculosis* organisms are isolated should be managed in consultation with an expert in the treatment of drug-resistant tuberculosis.

CONTRAINDICATIONS

Ethionamide is contraindicated in patients with severe hepatic impairment and in patients who are hypersensitive to the drug.

WARNINGS

The use of Trecator-SC (ethionamide) alone in the treatment of tuberculosis results in rapid development of resistance. It is essential, therefore, to give a suitable companion drug or drugs, the choice being based on the results of susceptibility testing. However, therapy may be initiated prior to receiving the results of susceptibility tests as deemed appropriate by the physician. Ethionamide should be administered with at least one, sometimes two, other drugs to which the organism is known to be susceptible (see **INDICATIONS AND USAGE**). Drugs which have been used as companion agents are rifampin, ethambutol, pyrazinamide, cycloserine, kanamycin, streptomycin, and isoniazid. The usual warnings, precautions, and dosage regimens for these companion drugs should be observed.

Patient compliance is essential to the success of the antituberculosis therapy and to prevent the emergence of drug-resistant organisms. Therefore, patients should adhere to the drug regimen for the full duration of treatment. It is recommended that directly observed therapy be practiced when patients are receiving antituberculous medication. Additional consultation from experts in the treatment of drug-resistant tuberculosis is recommended when patients develop drug-resistant organisms.

PRECAUTIONS

General

Ethionamide may potentiate the adverse effects of the other anti-tuberculous drugs administered concomitantly (see **Drug Interactions**). Ophthalmologic examinations (including ophthalmoscopy) should be performed before and periodically during therapy with Trecator-SC.

Information For Patients

Patients should be advised to consult their physician should blurred vision or any loss of vision, with or without eye pain, occur during treatment.

Excessive ethanol ingestion should be avoided because a psychotic reaction has been reported.[3]

Laboratory Tests

Determination of serum transaminases (SGOT, SGPT) should be made prior to initiation of therapy and should be monitored monthly. If serum transaminases become elevated during therapy, ethionamide and the companion antituberculosis drug or drugs may be discontinued temporarily until the laboratory abnormalities have resolved. Ethionamide and the companion antituberculosis medication(s) then should be reintroduced sequentially to determine which drug (or drugs) is (are) responsible for the hepatotoxicity.

Blood glucose determinations should be made prior to and periodically throughout therapy with Trecator®-SC. Diabetic patients should be particularly alert for episodes of hypoglycemia.

Periodic monitoring of thyroid function tests is recommended as hypothyroidism, with or without goiter, has been reported with ethionamide therapy.

Drug Interactions

Trecator-SC has been found to temporarily raise serum concentrations of isoniazid. Trecator-SC may potentiate the adverse effects of other antituberculous drugs administered concomitantly. In particular, convulsions have been reported when ethionamide is administered with cycloserine and special care should be taken when the treatment regimen includes both of these drugs. Excessive ethanol ingestion should be avoided because a psychotic reaction has been reported.

Carcinogenesis, Mutagenesis, Impairment of Fertility

Teratogenic Effects: Pregnancy Category C

Animal studies conducted with Trecator (ethionamide) indicate that the drug has teratogenic potential in rabbits and rats. The doses used in these studies on a mg/kg basis were considerably in excess of those recommended in humans. There are no adequate and well-controlled studies in pregnant women. Because of these animal studies, however, it must be recommended that Trecator-SC (ethionamide) be withheld from women who are pregnant, or who are likely to become pregnant while under therapy, unless the prescribing physician considers it to be an essential part of the treatment.

Labor and Delivery

The effect of Trecator-SC on labor and delivery in pregnant women is unknown.

Nursing Mothers

Because no information is available on the excretion of ethionamide in human milk, Trecator-SC should be administered to nursing mothers only if the benefits outweigh the risks. Newborns who are breast-fed by mothers who are taking Trecator-SC should be monitored for adverse effects.

Pediatric Use

Due to the fact that pulmonary tuberculosis resistant to primary therapy is rarely found in neonates, infants, and children, investigations have been limited in these age groups. At present, the drug should not be used in pediatric patients under 12 years of age except when the organisms are definitely resistant to primary therapy and systemic dissemination of the disease, or other life-threatening complications of tuberculosis, is judged to be imminent.

ADVERSE REACTIONS

Gastrointestinal: The most common side effects of ethionamide are gastrointestinal disturbances including nausea, vomiting, diarrhea, abdominal pain, excessive salivation, metallic taste, stomatitis, anorexia and weight loss. Adverse gastrointestinal effects appear to be dose related, with approximately 50% of patients unable to tolerate 1 gm as a single dose. Gastrointestinal effects may be minimized by decreasing dosage, by changing the time of drug administration, or by the concurrent administration of an antiemetic agent.

Nervous System: Psychotic disturbances (including mental depression), drowsiness, dizziness, restlessness, headache, and postural hypotension have been reported with ethionamide. Rare reports of peripheral neuritis, optic neuritis, diplopia, blurred vision, and a pellagra-like syndrome also have been reported. Concurrent administration of pyridoxine has been recommended to prevent or relieve neurotoxic effects.

Hepatic: Transient increases in serum bilirubin, SGOT, SGPT; Hepatitis (with or without jaundice).

Other: Hypersensitivity reactions including rash, photosensitivity, thrombocytopenia and purpura have been reported rarely. Hypoglycemia, gynecomastia, impotence, and acne also have occurred. The management of patients with diabetes mellitus may become more difficult in those receiving ethionamide.

OVERDOSAGE

No specific information is available on the treatment of overdosage with Trecator-SC. If it should occur, standard procedures to evacuate gastric contents and to support vital functions should be employed.

DOSAGE AND ADMINISTRATION

In the treatment of tuberculosis, a major cause of the emergence of drug-resistant organisms, and thus treatment failure, is patient nonadherence to prescribed treatment. Treatment failure and drug-resistant organisms can be life-threatening and may result in other serious health risks. It is, therefore, important that patients adhere to the drug regimen for the full duration of treatment. Directly observed therapy is recommended when patients are receiving treatment for tuberculosis. Consultation with an expert in the treatment of drug-resistant tuberculosis is advised for patients in whom drug-resistant tuberculosis is suspected or likely. Ethionamide should be administered with at least one, sometimes two, other drugs to which the organism is known to be susceptible (see **INDICATIONS AND USAGE**).

Trecator-SC (ethionamide) is administered orally. The usual adult dose is 15 to 20 mg/kg/day, administered once daily or, if patient exhibits poor gastrointestinal tolerance, in divided doses, with a maximum daily dosage of 1 gram. Thus far, there is insufficient evidence to indicate the lowest effective dosage levels. Therefore, in order to minimize the risk of resistance developing to the drug or to the companion drug, the principle of giving the highest tolerated dose (based on gastrointestinal intolerance) has been followed. In the adult this would seem to be between 0.5 and 1.0 gm daily, with an average of 0.75 gm daily.

The optimum dosage for pediatric patients has not been established. However, pediatric dosages of 10 to 20 mg/kg p.o. daily in 2 or 3 divided doses given after meals or 15 mg/kg/24 hrs as a single daily dose have been recommended.[4,5]

As with adults, ethionamide may be administered to pediatric patients once daily. It should be noted that in patients with concomitant tuberculosis and HIV infection, malabsorption syndrome may be present. Drug malabsorption should be suspected in patients who adhere to therapy, but who fail to respond appropriately. In such cases, consideration should be given to therapeutic drug monitoring (see **CLINICAL PHARMACOLOGY**).

The best times of administration are those which the individual patient finds most suitable in order to avoid or minimize gastrointestinal intolerance, which is usually at mealtimes. Every effort should be made to encourage patients to persevere with treatment when gastrointestinal side effects appear, since they may diminish in severity as treatment proceeds.

Initiation of therapy at a dose of 250 mg daily, with gradual titration to optimal doses as tolerated by the patient, also may be beneficial. A regimen of 250 mg daily for 1 or 2 days, followed by 250 mg twice daily for 1 or 2 days with a subsequent increase to 1 gm in 3 or 4 divided doses has been reported.[2]

Concomitant administration of pyridoxine is recommended.

Duration of treatment should be based on individual clinical response. In general, continue therapy until bacteriological conversion has become permanent and maximal clinical improvement has occurred.

HOW SUPPLIED

Trecator®-SC (ethionamide tablets, USP) are supplied in bottles of 100 tablets as follows:

250 mg, NDC 0008-4130, reddish orange, sugar-coated tablet marked WYETH and 4130.

Store at controlled room temperature 20° to 25°C (68° to 77°F). Dispense in a tight container.

REFERENCES

1) Jenner, P.J.: Plasma Levels of Ethionamide and Prothionamide in a Volunteer Following Intravenous and Oral Dosages, Lepr Rev 58:31-37, 1987.

2) Peloquin, C.A.: Pharmacology of the Antimycobacterial Drugs, Med Clin North Am 77(6):1253-1262, 1993.

3) Lansdown, F.S., Beran, M., Litwak, T.: Psychotoxic Reaction During Ethionamide Therapy, Am Rev Resp Dis 95(6): 1053-1055, 1967.

4) Feigin, R.D., and Cherry, J.D.: Textbook of Pediatric Infectious Diseases, 2nd Edition. Philadelphia, W.B. Saunders Co., 1987, pp. 1371-1372.

5) Nelson, W.E., Behrman, R.E., Vaughan, V.C. (eds.): Nelson Textbook of Pediatrics, 13th edition. Philadelphia, W.B. Saunders Co., 1987, p.636.

6) Treatment of Tuberculosis and Tuberculosis Infection in Adults and Children, Am J Respiratory and Critical Care Medicine, 149:1359-1374, 1994.

Wyeth Pharmaceuticals Inc.
Philadelphia, PA 19101
W10479C001
ET01
Rev 10/03

TRIPHASIL®–28 ℞

[*tri-'fā-sĭl*]

Tablets

(levonorgestrel and ethinyl estradiol tablets—triphasic regimen)

℞ only

This product's label may have been revised after this insert was used in production. For further product information and current package insert, please visit www.wyeth.com or call our medical communications department toll-free at 1-800-934-5556.

Patients should be counseled that this product does not protect against HIV infection (AIDS) and other sexually transmitted diseases.

DESCRIPTION

Each Triphasil cycle of 28 tablets consists of three different drug phases as follows: Phase 1 comprised of 6 brown tablets, each containing 0.050 mg of levonorgestrel (d(-)-13 beta-ethyl-17-alpha-ethinyl-17-beta-hydroxygon-4-en-3-one), a totally synthetic progestogen, and 0.030 mg of ethinyl estradiol (19-nor-17α-pregna-1,3,5(10)-trien-20-yne-3, 17-diol); phase 2 comprised of 5 white tablets, each containing 0.075 mg levonorgestrel and 0.040 mg ethinyl estradiol; and phase 3 comprised of 10 light-yellow tablets, each containing 0.125 mg levonorgestrel and 0.030 mg ethinyl estradiol; then followed by 7 light-green inert tablets. The inactive ingredients present are cellulose, FD&C Blue 1, iron oxides, lactose, magnesium stearate, polacrilin potassium, polyethylene glycol, titanium dioxide, and hydroxypropyl methylcellulose.

Continued on next page

Triphasil-28—Cont.

Levonorgestrel Ethinyl Estradiol

CLINICAL PHARMACOLOGY

Combination oral contraceptives primarily act by suppression of gonadotropins. Although the primary mechanism of this action is inhibition of ovulation, other alterations include changes in the cervical mucus (which increase the difficulty of sperm entry into the uterus) and the endometrium (which reduce the likelihood of implantation).

PHARMACOKINETICS

Absorption

Levonorgestrel is rapidly and completely absorbed after oral administration (bioavailability about 100%). Levonorgestrel is not subject to first-pass metabolism or enterohepatic circulation and therefore does not undergo variations in absorption after oral administration. Ethinyl estradiol is rapidly and almost completely absorbed from the gastrointestinal tract but, due to first-pass metabolism in gut mucosa and liver, the bioavailability of ethinyl estradiol is between 38% and 48%.

There have been no formal multiple-dose studies conducted using Triphasil. However, a multiple-dose study was done in 22 women using a monophasic, low dose combination of 0.10 mg levonorgestrel and 0.02 mg ethinyl estradiol. Maximum serum concentrations of levonorgestrel were found to be 2.8 ± 0.9 ng/mL (mean ± SD) at 1.6 ± 0.9 hours after a single dose, reaching a steady state at day 19. Observed levonorgestrel concentrations increased from day 1 to days 6 and 21 by 34% and 96%, respectively. Unbound levonorgestrel concentrations subsequently increased from day 1 to days 6 and 21 by 25% and 83%, respectively, however, the accumulation of unbound levonorgestrel was approximately 14% less than total levonorgestrel accumulation. The kinetics of total levonorgestrel were non-linear due to an increase in binding of levonorgestrel to SHBG, which is attributed to increased SHBG levels that are induced by the daily administration of ethinyl estradiol. Ethinyl estradiol reached maximum serum concentrations of 62 ± 21 pg/mL at 1.5 ± 0.5 hours after a single dose, reaching steady state at day 6. Ethinyl estradiol concentrations increased by 19% from days 1 to 21 consistent with an elimination half-life of 18 hours.

Single-dose studies with Triphasil have been conducted with the following data reported below in Table I. Plasma concentrations have been corrected below to reflect single tablet dosing/day.

[See table I above]

Distribution

Levonorgestrel is bound to SHBG and albumin. Levonorgestrel has high binding affinity for SHBG that is 60% of that of testosterone. Ethinyl estradiol is about 97% bound to plasma albumin. Ethinyl estradiol does not bind to SHBG, but will induce SHBG synthesis.

Metabolism

Levonorgestrel: The most important metabolic pathway occurs in the reduction of the Δ4-3-oxo group and hydroxylation at positions 2α, 1β, and 16β, followed by conjugation. Most of the metabolites that circulate in the blood are sulfates of 3α, 5β-tetrahydro-levonorgestrel, while excretion occurs predominately in the form of glucuronides. Some of the parent levonorgestrel also circulates as 17β-sulfate. Metabolic clearance rates may differ among individuals by several-fold, and this may account in part for the wide variation observed in levonorgestrel concentrations among users.

Ethinyl estradiol: Cytochrome P450 enzymes (CYP3A4) in the liver are responsible for the 2-hydroxylation that is the major oxidative reaction. The 2-hydroxy metabolite is further transformed by methylation and glucuronidation prior to urinary and fecal excretion. Levels of Cytochrome P450 (CYP3A) vary widely among individuals and can explain the variation in rates of ethinyl estradiol 2-hydroxylation. Ethinyl estradiol is excreted in the urine and feces as glucuronide and sulfate conjugates, and undergoes enterohepatic circulation.

Excretion

The elimination half-life for levonorgestrel is approximately 36 ± 13 hours at steady state. Levonorgestrel and its metabolites are primarily excreted in the urine (40% to 68%) and about 16% to 48% are excreted in the feces. The elimination half-life of ethinyl estradiol is 18 ± 4.7 hours at steady state.

SPECIAL POPULATIONS

Hepatic Insufficiency

No formal studies have evaluated the effect of hepatic disease on the disposition of Triphasil. However, steroid hormones may be poorly metabolized in patients with impaired liver function.

Renal Insufficiency

No formal studies have evaluated the effect of renal disease on the disposition of Triphasil.

TABLE I: MEAN (SE) PHARMACOKINETIC PARAMETERS OF TRIPHASIL IN SINGLE-DOSE STUDIES

Levonorgestrel (LNG)

Dose LNG/EE µg	C_{max} ng/mL	t_{max} h	$t_{1/2}$ h	AUC ng•h/mL
50/30	1.7 (0.1)	1.3 (0.1)	23 (2.2)	17 (1.5)
75/40	2.1 (0.2)	1.5 (0.2)	15 (1.2)	21 (2.0)
125/30	2.5 (0.2)	1.6 (0.1)	23 (1.4)	34 (3.0)

Ethinyl Estradiol (EE)

Dose LNG/EE µg	C_{max} pg/mL	t_{max} h	$t_{1/2}$ h	AUC pg•h/mL
50/30	141 (9)	1.4 (0.1)	8.1 (1.0)	1126 (113)
75/40	179 (13)	1.6 (0.2)	14 (1.7)	2177 (244)
125/30	115 (10)	1.5 (0.1)	8.8 (1.6)	1072 (170)

Drug-Drug Interactions

See **"Precautions"** section - DRUG INTERACTIONS

INDICATIONS AND USAGE

Oral contraceptives are indicated for the prevention of pregnancy in women who elect to use this product as a method of contraception.

Oral contraceptives are highly effective. Table II lists the typical accidental pregnancy rates for users of combination oral contraceptives and other methods of contraception. The efficacy of these contraceptive methods, except sterilization and the IUD, depends upon the reliability with which they are used. Correct and consistent use of methods can result in lower failure rates.

TABLE II: PERCENTAGE OF WOMEN EXPERIENCING AN UNINTENDED PREGNANCY DURING THE FIRST YEAR OF USE OF A CONTRACEPTIVE METHOD

Method	Perfect Use	Typical Use
Levonorgestrel implants	0.05	0.05
Male sterilization	0.1	0.15
Female sterilization	0.5	0.5
Depo-Provera® (injectable progestogen)	0.3	0.3
Oral contraceptives		5
Combined	0.1	NA
Progestin only	0.5	NA
IUD		
Progesterone	1.5	2.0
Copper T 380A	0.6	0.8
Condom (male) without spermicide	3	14
(Female) without spermicide	5	21
Cervical cap		
Nulliparous women	9	20
Parous women	26	40
Vaginal sponge		
Nulliparous women	9	20
Parous women	20	40
Diaphragm with spermicidal cream or jelly	6	20
Spermicides alone (foam, creams, jellies, and vaginal suppositories)	6	26
Periodic abstinence (all methods)	1-9*	25
Withdrawal	4	19
No contraception (planned pregnancy)	85	85

NA - not available

*Depending on method (calendar, ovulation, symptothermal, post-ovulation)

Adapted from Hatcher RA et al, *Contraceptive Technology: 17th Revised Edition.* NY, NY: Ardent Media, Inc., 1998.

CONTRAINDICATIONS

Combination oral contraceptives should not be used in women with any of the following conditions:

Thrombophlebitis or thromboembolic disorders.

A past history of deep-vein thrombophlebitis or thromboembolic disorders.

Cerebral-vascular or coronary-artery disease.

Thrombogenic valvulopathies.

Thrombogenic rhythm disorders.

Diabetes with vascular involvement.

Uncontrolled hypertension.

Known or suspected carcinoma of the breast.

Carcinoma of the endometrium or other known or suspected estrogen-dependent neoplasia.

Undiagnosed abnormal genital bleeding.

Cholestatic jaundice of pregnancy or jaundice with prior pill use.

Hepatic adenomas or carcinomas, or active liver disease, as long as liver function has not returned to normal.

Known or suspected pregnancy.

Hypersensitivity to any of the components of Triphasil (levonorgestrel and ethinyl estradiol tablets–triphasic regimen).

WARNINGS

Cigarette smoking increases the risk of serious cardiovascular side effects from oral-contraceptive use. This risk increases with age and with the extent of smoking (in epidemiologic studies, 15 or more cigarettes per day was associated with a significantly increased risk) and is quite marked in women over 35 years of age. Women who use oral contraceptives should be strongly advised not to smoke.

The use of oral contraceptives is associated with increased risks of several serious conditions including venous and arterial thrombotic and thromboembolic events (such as myocardial infarction, thromboembolism, and stroke), hepatic neoplasia, gallbladder disease, and hypertension, although the risk of serious morbidity or mortality is very small in healthy women without underlying risk factors. The risk of morbidity and mortality increases significantly in the presence of other underlying risk factors such as certain inherited or acquired thrombophilias, hypertension, hyperlipidemias, obesity, and diabetes.

Practitioners prescribing oral contraceptives should be familiar with the following information relating to these risks.

The information contained in this package insert is based principally on studies carried out in patients who used oral contraceptives with higher formulations of estrogens and progestogens than those in common use today. The effect of long-term use of the oral contraceptives with lower formulations of both estrogens and progestogens remains to be determined.

Throughout this labeling, epidemiological studies reported are of two types: retrospective or case control studies and prospective or cohort studies. Case control studies provide a measure of the relative risk of disease, namely, a ratio of the incidence of a disease among oral-contraceptive users to that among nonusers. The relative risk does not provide information on the actual clinical occurrence of a disease. Cohort studies provide a measure of attributable risk, which is the difference in the incidence of disease between oral-contraceptive users and nonusers. The attributable risk does provide information about the actual occurrence of a disease in the population. For further information, the reader is referred to a text on epidemiological methods.

1. THROMBOEMBOLIC DISORDERS AND OTHER VASCULAR PROBLEMS

a. Myocardial infarction

An increased risk of myocardial infarction has been attributed to oral-contraceptive use. This risk is primarily in smokers or women with other underlying risk factors for coronary-artery disease such as hypertension, hypercholesterolemia, morbid obesity, and diabetes. The relative risk of heart attack for current oral-contraceptive users has been estimated to be two to six. The risk is very low under the age of 30.

Smoking in combination with oral-contraceptive use has been shown to contribute substantially to the incidence of myocardial infarctions in women in their mid-thirties or older with smoking accounting for the majority of excess cases. Mortality rates associated with circulatory disease have been shown to increase substantially in smokers over the age of 35 and nonsmokers over the age of 40 (Table III) among women who use oral contraceptives.

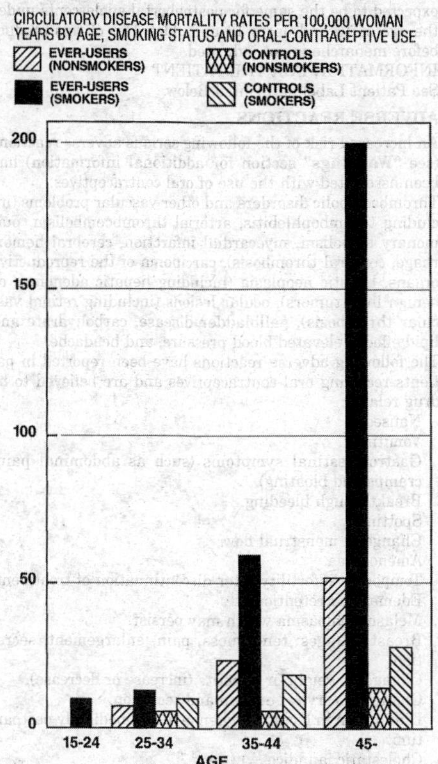

TABLE III. (Adapted from P.M. Layde and V. Beral, Lancet, *1*:541-546, 1981.)

Oral contraceptives may compound the effects of well-known risk factors, such as hypertension, diabetes, hyperlipidemias, age, and obesity. In particular, some progestogens are known to decrease HDL cholesterol and cause glucose intolerance, while estrogens may create a state of hyperinsulinism. Oral contraceptives have been shown to increase blood pressure among users (see section 9 in **"Warnings"**). Similar effects on risk factors have been associated with an increased risk of heart disease. Oral contraceptives must be used with caution in women with cardiovascular disease risk factors.

b. Thromboembolism

An increased risk of venous thromboembolic and thrombotic disease associated with the use of oral contraceptives is well established. Case control studies have found the relative risk of users compared to nonusers to be 3 for the first episode of superficial venous thrombosis, 4 to 11 for deep-vein thrombosis or pulmonary embolism, and 1.5 to 6 for women with predisposing conditions for venous thromboembolic disease. Cohort studies have shown the relative risk to be somewhat lower, about 3 for new cases and about 4.5 for new cases requiring hospitalization. The approximate incidence of deep-vein thrombosis and pulmonary embolism in users of low dose (<50µg ethinyl estradiol) combination oral contraceptives is up to 4 per 10,000 woman-years compared to 0.5-3 per 10,000 woman-years for non-users. However, the incidence is substantially less than that associated with pregnancy (6 per 10,000 woman-years). The risk of thromboembolic disease due to oral contraceptives is not related to length of use and disappears after pill use is stopped.

A two- to four-fold increase in relative risk of postoperative thromboembolic complications has been reported with the use of oral contraceptives. The relative risk of venous thrombosis in women who have predisposing conditions is twice that of women without such medical conditions. If feasible, oral contraceptives should be discontinued at least four weeks prior to and for two weeks after elective surgery of a type associated with an increase in risk of thromboembolism and during and following prolonged immobilization. Since the immediate postpartum period is also associated with an increased risk of thromboembolism, oral contraceptives should be started no earlier than four to six weeks after delivery in women who elect not to breast-feed, or a midtrimester pregnancy termination.

c. Cerebrovascular diseases

Oral contraceptives have been shown to increase both the relative and attributable risks of cerebrovascular events (thrombotic and hemorrhagic strokes), although, in general, the risk is greatest among older (>35 years), hypertensive women who also smoke. Hypertension was found to be a risk factor for both users and nonusers, for both types of strokes, while smoking interacted to increase the risk for hemorrhagic strokes.

In a large study, the relative risk of thrombotic strokes has been shown to range from 3 for normotensive users to 14 for users with severe hypertension. The relative risk of hemorrhagic stroke is reported to be 1.2 for nonsmokers who used oral contraceptives, 2.6 for smokers who did not use oral contraceptives, 7.6 for smokers who used oral contraceptives, 1.8 for normotensive users, and 25.7 for users with severe hypertension. The attributable risk is also greater in older women. Oral contraceptives also increase the risk for stroke in women with other underlying risk factors such as certain inherited or acquired thrombophilias, hyperlipidemias, and obesity.

Women with migraine (particularly migraine with aura) who take combination oral contraceptives may be at an increased risk of stroke.

d. Dose-related risk of vascular disease from oral contraceptives

A positive association has been observed between the amount of estrogen and progestogen in oral contraceptives and the risk of vascular disease. A decline in serum high-density lipoproteins (HDL) has been reported with many progestational agents. A decline in serum high-density lipoproteins has been associated with an increased incidence of ischemic heart disease. Because estrogens increase HDL cholesterol, the net effect of an oral contraceptive depends on a balance achieved between doses of estrogen and progestogen and the nature and absolute amount of progestogen used in the contraceptive. The amount of both hormones should be considered in the choice of an oral contraceptive.

Minimizing exposure to estrogen and progestogen is in keeping with good principles of therapeutics. For any particular estrogen/progestogen combination, the dosage regimen prescribed should be one which contains the least amount of estrogen and progestogen that is compatible with a low failure rate and the needs of the individual patient. New acceptors of oral-contraceptive agents should be started on preparations containing less than 50 mcg of estrogen.

e. Persistence of risk of vascular disease

There are two studies which have shown persistence of risk of vascular disease for ever-users of oral contraceptives. In a study in the United States, the risk of developing myocardial infarction after discontinuing oral contraceptives persists for at least 9 years for women 40 to 49 years who had used oral contraceptives for five or more years, but this increased risk was not demonstrated in other age groups. In another study in Great Britain, the risk of developing cerebrovascular disease persisted for at least 6 years after discontinuation of oral contraceptives, although excess risk was very small. However, both studies were performed with oral-contraceptive formulations containing 50 micrograms or higher of estrogens.

2. ESTIMATES OF MORTALITY FROM CONTRACEPTIVE USE

One study gathered data from a variety of sources which have estimated the mortality rate associated with different methods of contraception at different ages (Table IV). These estimates include the combined risk of death associated with contraceptive methods plus the risk attributable to pregnancy in the event of method failure. Each method of contraception has its specific benefits and risks. The study concluded that with the exception of oral-contraceptive users 35 and older who smoke and 40 and older who do not smoke, mortality associated with all methods of birth control is less than that associated with childbirth. The observation of a possible increase in risk of mortality with age for oral-contraceptive users is based on data gathered in the 1970's — but not reported until 1983. However, current clinical practice involves the use of lower estrogen dose formulations combined with careful restriction of oral-contraceptive use to women who do not have the various risk factors listed in this labeling.

Because of these changes in practice and, also, because of some limited new data which suggest that the risk of cardiovascular disease with the use of oral contraceptives may now be less than previously observed, the Fertility and Maternal Health Drugs Advisory Committee was asked to review the topic in 1989. The Committee concluded that although cardiovascular-disease risks may be increased with oral-contraceptive use after age 40 in healthy nonsmoking women (even with the newer low-dose formulations), there are greater potential health risks associated with pregnancy in older women and with the alternative surgical and medical procedures which may be necessary if such women do not have access to effective and acceptable means of contraception.

Therefore, the Committee recommended that the benefits of oral-contraceptive use by healthy nonsmoking women over 40 may outweigh the possible risks. Of course, older women, as all women who take oral contraceptives, should take the lowest possible dose formulation that is effective.

TABLE IV—ANNUAL NUMBER OF BIRTH-RELATED OR METHOD-RELATED DEATHS ASSOCIATED WITH CONTROL OF FERTILITY PER 100,000 NONSTERILE WOMEN, BY FERTILITY-CONTROL METHOD ACCORDING TO AGE

Method of control and outcome	15-19	20-24	25-29	30-34	35-39	40-44
No fertility-control methods*	7.0	7.4	9.1	14.8	25.7	28.2
Oral contraceptives nonsmoker**	0.3	0.5	0.9	1.9	13.8	31.6
Oral contraceptives smoker**	2.2	3.4	6.6	13.5	51.1	117.2
IUD**	0.8	0.8	1.0	1.0	1.4	1.4
Condom*	1.1	1.6	0.7	0.2	0.3	0.4
Diaphragm/ spermicide*	1.9	1.2	1.2	1.3	2.2	2.8
Periodic abstinence*	2.5	1.6	1.6	1.7	2.9	3.6

*Deaths are birth related
**Deaths are method related

Adapted from H.W. Ory, Family Planning Perspectives, *15*: 57-63, 1983.

3. CARCINOMA OF THE REPRODUCTIVE ORGANS

A meta-analysis from 54 epidemiological studies reported that there is a slightly increased relative risk (RR=1.24) of having breast cancer diagnosed in women who are currently using combination oral contraceptives compared to never-users. The increased risk gradually disappears during the course of the 10 years after cessation of combination oral-contraceptive use. These studies do not provide evidence for causation. The observed pattern of increased risk of breast cancer diagnosis may be due to earlier detection of breast cancer in combination oral contraceptive users, the biological effects of combination oral contraceptives, or a combination of both. Because breast cancer is rare in women under 40 years of age, the excess number of breast cancer diagnoses in current and recent combination oral contraceptive users is small in relation to the lifetime risk of breast cancer. Breast cancers diagnosed in ever-users tend to be less advanced clinically than the cancers diagnosed in never-users.

Some studies suggest that oral-contraceptive use has been associated with an increase in the risk of cervical intraepithelial neoplasia or invasive cervical cancer in some populations of women. However, there continues to be controversy about the extent to which such findings may be due to differences in sexual behavior and other factors.

In spite of many studies of the relationship between oral-contraceptive use and breast and cervical cancers, a cause-and-effect relationship has not been established.

4. HEPATIC NEOPLASIA

Benign hepatic adenomas are associated with oral-contraceptive use, although the incidence of benign tumors is rare in the United States. Indirect calculations have estimated the attributable risk to be in the range of 3.3 cases/100,000 for users, a risk that increases after four or more years of use. Rupture of rare, benign, hepatic adenomas may cause death through intra-abdominal hemorrhage.

Studies from Britain have shown an increased risk of developing hepatocellular carcinoma in long-term (>8 years) oral-contraceptive users. However, these cancers are extremely rare in the U.S., and the attributable risk (the excess incidence) of liver cancers in oral-contraceptive users approaches less than one per million users.

5. OCULAR LESIONS

There have been clinical case reports of retinal thrombosis associated with the use of oral contraceptives that may lead to partial or complete loss of vision. Oral contraceptives should be discontinued if there is unexplained partial or complete loss of vision; onset of proptosis or diplopia; papilledema; or retinal vascular lesions. Appropriate diagnostic and therapeutic measures should be undertaken immediately.

6. ORAL-CONTRACEPTIVE USE BEFORE OR DURING EARLY PREGNANCY

Extensive epidemiological studies have revealed no increased risk of birth defects in women who have used oral contraceptives prior to pregnancy. Studies also do not suggest a teratogenic effect, particularly insofar as cardiac anomalies and limb-reduction defects are concerned, when taken inadvertently during early pregnancy. (See **"Contraindications"** section).

The administration of oral contraceptives to induce withdrawal bleeding should not be used as a test for pregnancy. Oral contraceptives should not be used during pregnancy to treat threatened or habitual abortion.

It is recommended that for any patient who has missed two consecutive periods, pregnancy should be ruled out before continuing oral-contraceptive use. If the patient has not adhered to the prescribed schedule, the possibility of pregnancy should be considered at the time of the first missed period. Oral-contraceptive use should be discontinued if pregnancy is confirmed.

7. GALLBLADDER DISEASE

Earlier studies have reported an increased lifetime relative risk of gallbladder surgery in users of oral contraceptives and estrogens. More recent studies, however, have shown that the relative risk of developing gallbladder disease among oral-contraceptive users may be minimal. The recent findings of minimal risk may be related to the use of oral-contraceptive formulations containing lower hormonal doses of estrogens and progestogens.

8. CARBOHYDRATE AND LIPID METABOLIC EFFECTS

Oral contraceptives have been shown to cause glucose intolerance in a significant percentage of users. Oral contraceptives containing greater than 75 micrograms of estrogens cause hyperinsulinism, while lower doses of estrogen cause less glucose intolerance. Progestogens increase insulin secretion and create insulin resistance, this effect varying with different progestational agents. However, in the nondiabetic woman, oral contraceptives appear to have no effect

Continued on next page

Triphasil-28—Cont.

on fasting blood glucose. Because of these demonstrated effects, prediabetic and diabetic women should be carefully observed while taking oral contraceptives.
A small proportion of women will have persistent hypertriglyceridemia while on the pill. As discussed earlier (see **"Warnings,"** 1a. and 1d.), changes in serum triglycerides and lipoprotein levels have been reported in oral-contraceptive users.
9. ELEVATED BLOOD PRESSURE
An increase in blood pressure has been reported in women taking oral contraceptives, and this increase is more likely in older oral-contraceptive users and with continued use. Data from the Royal College of General Practitioners and subsequent randomized trials have shown that the incidence of hypertension increases with increasing quantities of progestogens.
Women with a history of hypertension or hypertension-related diseases, or renal disease, should be encouraged to use another method of contraception. If women with hypertension elect to use oral contraceptives, they should be monitored closely, and if significant elevation of blood pressure occurs, oral contraceptives should be discontinued (See **"Contraindications"** section). For most women, elevated blood pressure will return to normal after stopping oral contraceptives, and there is no difference in the occurrence of hypertension among ever- and never-users.
10. HEADACHE
The onset or exacerbation of migraine or development of headache with a new pattern that is recurrent, persistent, or severe requires discontinuation of oral contraceptives and evaluation of the cause. (See **"Warnings,"** 1c.)
11. BLEEDING IRREGULARITIES
Breakthrough bleeding and spotting are sometimes encountered in patients on oral contraceptives, especially during the first three months of use. The type and dose of progestogen may be important. If bleeding persists or recurs, nonhormonal causes should be considered and adequate diagnostic measures taken to rule out malignancy or pregnancy in the event of breakthrough bleeding, as in the case of any abnormal vaginal bleeding. If pathology has been excluded, time or a change to another formulation may solve the problem. In the event of amenorrhea, pregnancy should be ruled out if the oral contraceptive has not been taken according to directions prior to the first missed withdrawal bleed or if two consecutive withdrawal bleeds have been missed. Some women may encounter post-pill amenorrhea or oligomenorrhea (possibly with anovulation), especially when such a condition was preexistent.

PRECAUTIONS

1. GENERAL
Patients should be counseled that this product does not protect against HIV infection (AIDS) and other sexually transmitted diseases.
2. PHYSICAL EXAMINATION AND FOLLOW-UP
A periodic personal and family medical history and complete physical examination are appropriate for all women, including women using oral contraceptives. The physical examination, however, may be deferred until after initiation of oral contraceptives if requested by the woman and judged appropriate by the clinician. The physical examination should include special reference to blood pressure, breasts, abdomen and pelvic organs, including cervical cytology, and relevant laboratory tests. In case of undiagnosed, persistent, or recurrent abnormal vaginal bleeding, appropriate measures should be conducted to rule out malignancy. Women with a strong family history of breast cancer or who have breast nodules should be monitored with particular care.
3. LIPID DISORDERS
Women who are being treated for hyperlipidemias should be followed closely if they elect to use oral contraceptives. Some progestogens may elevate LDL levels and may render the control of hyperlipidemias more difficult. (See **"Warnings,"** 1d.)
In patients with familial defects of lipoprotein metabolism receiving estrogen-containing preparations, there have been case reports of significant elevations of plasma triglycerides leading to pancreatitis.
4. LIVER FUNCTION
If jaundice develops in any woman receiving such drugs, the medication should be discontinued. Steroid hormones may be poorly metabolized in patients with impaired liver function.
5. FLUID RETENTION
Oral contraceptives may cause some degree of fluid retention. They should be prescribed with caution, and only with careful monitoring, in patients with conditions which might be aggravated by fluid retention.
6. EMOTIONAL DISORDERS
Patients becoming significantly depressed while taking oral contraceptives should stop the medication and use an alternate method of contraception in an attempt to determine whether the symptom is drug related. Women with a history of depression should be carefully observed and the drug discontinued if depression recurs to a serious degree.
7. CONTACT LENSES
Contact-lens wearers who develop visual changes or changes in lens tolerance should be assessed by an ophthalmologist.
8. GASTROINTESTINAL MOTILITY
Diarrhea and/or vomiting may reduce hormone absorption.
9. DRUG INTERACTIONS
Interactions between ethinyl estradiol and other substances may lead to decreased or increased serum ethinyl estradiol concentrations.
Decreased ethinyl estradiol plasma concentrations may cause an increased incidence of breakthrough bleeding and menstrual irregularities and may possibly reduce efficacy of the combination oral contraceptive.
Reduced ethinyl estradiol concentrations have been associated with concomitant use of substances that induce hepatic microsomal enzymes, such as rifampin, rifabutin, barbiturates, phenylbutazone, phenytoin sodium, griseofulvin, topiramate, some protease inhibitors, modafinil, and possibly St. John's wort.
Substances that may decrease plasma ethinyl estradiol concentrations by other mechanisms include any substance that reduces gut transit time and certain antibiotics (e.g. ampicillin and other penicillins, tetracyclines) by a decrease of enterohepatic circulation of estrogens. During concomitant use of ethinyl estradiol containing products and substances that may lead to decreased plasma steroid hormone concentrations, it is recommended that a nonhormonal back-up method of birth control be used in addition to the regular intake of Triphasil (levonorgestrel and ethinyl estradiol tablets-triphasic regimen). If the use of a substance which leads to decreased ethinyl estradiol plasma concentrations is required for a prolonged period of time, combination oral contraceptives should not be considered the primary contraceptive.
After discontinuation of substances that may lead to deceased ethinyl estradiol plasma concentrations, use of a nonhormonal back-up method of birth control is recommended for 7 days. Longer use of a back-up method is advisable after discontinuation of substances that have led to induction of hepatic microsomal enzymes, resulting in decreased ethinyl estradiol concentrations. It may take several weeks until enzyme induction has completely subsided, depending on dosage, duration of use, and rate of elimination of the inducing substance.
Some substances may increase plasma ethinyl estradiol concentrations. These include:

- Competitive inhibitors for sulfation of ethinyl estradiol in the gastrointestinal wall, such as ascorbic acid (vitamin C) and acetaminophen.
- Substances that inhibit cytochrome P450 3A4 isoenzymes such as indinavir, fluconazole, and troleandomycin. Troleandomycin may increase the risk of intrahepatic cholestasis during coadministration with combination oral contraceptives.
- Atorvastatin (unknown mechanism).

Ethinyl estradiol may interfere with the mechanism of other drugs by inhibiting hepatic microsomal enzymes or by inducing hepatic drug conjugation, particularly glucuronidation. Accordingly, tissue concentrations may be either increased (e.g. cyclosporine, theophylline, corticosteroids) or decreased.
The prescribing information of concomitant medications should be consulted to identify potential interactions.
10. INTERACTIONS WITH LABORATORY TESTS
Certain endocrine- and liver-function tests and blood components may be affected by oral contraceptives:
a. Increased prothrombin and factors VII, VIII, IX, and X; decreased antithrombin 3; increased norepinephrine-induced platelet aggregability.
b. Increased thyroid-binding globulin (TBG) leading to increased circulating total thyroid hormone, as measured by protein-bound iodine (PBI), T_4 by column or by radioimmunoassay. Free T_3 resin uptake is decreased, reflecting the elevated TBG; free T_4 concentration is unaltered.
c. Other binding proteins may be elevated in serum.
d. Sex-binding globulins are increased and result in elevated levels of total circulating sex steroids and corticoids; however, free or biologically active levels remain unchanged.
e. Triglycerides may be increased.
f. Glucose tolerance may be decreased.
g. Serum folate levels may be depressed by oral-contraceptive therapy. This may be of clinical significance if a woman becomes pregnant shortly after discontinuing oral contraceptives.
11. CARCINOGENESIS
See **"Warnings"** section.
12. PREGNANCY
Pregnancy Category X. See **"Contraindications"** and **"Warnings"** sections.
13. NURSING MOTHERS
Small amounts of oral-contraceptive steroids and/or metabolites have been identified in the milk of nursing mothers, and a few adverse effects on the child have been reported, including jaundice and breast enlargement. In addition, combination oral contraceptives given in the postpartum period may interfere with lactation by decreasing the quantity and quality of breast milk. If possible, the nursing mother should be advised not to use combination oral contraceptives but to use other forms of contraception until she has completely weaned her child.
14. PEDIATRIC USE
Safety and efficacy of Triphasil-28 (levonorgestrel and ethinyl estradiol tablets—triphasic regimen) have been established in women of reproductive age. Safety and efficacy are expected to be the same for postpubertal adolescents under the age of 16 and users 16 and older. Use of this product before menarche is not indicated.
INFORMATION FOR THE PATIENT
See Patient Labeling Printed Below.

ADVERSE REACTIONS

An increased risk of the following serious adverse reactions (see **"Warnings"** section for additional information) has been associated with the use of oral contraceptives.
Thromboembolic disorders and other vascular problems (including thrombophlebitis, arterial thromboembolism, pulmonary embolism, myocardial infarction, cerebral hemorrhage, cerebral thrombosis), carcinoma of the reproductive organs, hepatic neoplasia (including hepatic adenomas or benign liver tumors), ocular lesions (including retinal vascular thrombosis), gallbladder disease, carbohydrate and lipid effects, elevated blood pressure, and headache.
The following adverse reactions have been reported in patients receiving oral contraceptives and are believed to be drug related:

Nausea.
Vomiting.
Gastrointestinal symptoms (such as abdominal pain, cramps and bloating).
Breakthrough bleeding.
Spotting.
Change in menstrual flow.
Amenorrhea.
Temporary infertility after discontinuation of treatment.
Edema/fluid retention.
Melasma/chloasma which may persist.
Breast changes: tenderness, pain, enlargement, secretion.
Change in weight or appetite (increase or decrease).
Change in cervical erosion and secretion.
Diminution in lactation when given immediately postpartum.
Cholestatic jaundice.
Rash (allergic).
Mood changes, including depression.
Vaginitis, including candidiasis.
Change in corneal curvature (steepening).
Intolerance to contact lenses.
Mesenteric thrombosis.
Decrease in serum folate levels.
Exacerbation of systemic lupus erythematosus.
Exacerbation of porphyria.
Exacerbation of chorea.
Aggravation of varicose veins.
Anaphylactic/anaphylactoid reactions, including urticaria, angioedema, and severe reactions with respiratory and circulatory symptoms.

The following adverse reactions have been reported in users of oral contraceptives, and the association has been neither confirmed nor refuted:

Congenital anomalies.
Premenstrual syndrome.
Cataracts.
Optic neuritis, which may lead to partial or complete loss of vision.
Cystitis-like syndrome.
Nervousness.
Dizziness.
Hirsutism.
Loss of scalp hair.
Erythema multiforme.
Erythema nodosum.
Hemorrhagic eruption.
Impaired renal function.
Hemolytic uremic syndrome.
Budd-Chiari syndrome.
Acne.
Changes in libido.
Colitis.
Sickle-cell disease.
Cerebral-vascular disease with mitral valve prolapse.
Lupus-like syndromes.
Pancreatitis.
Dysmenorrhea.

OVERDOSAGE

Serious ill effects have not been reported following acute ingestion of large doses of oral contraceptives by young children. Overdosage may cause nausea, and withdrawal bleeding may occur in females.
Noncontraceptive Health Benefits
The following noncontraceptive health benefits related to the use of oral contraceptives are supported by epidemiological studies which largely utilized oral-contraceptive formulations containing doses exceeding 0.035 mg of ethinyl estradiol or 0.05 mg of mestranol.
Effects on menses:
Increased menstrual cycle regularity.
Decreased blood loss and decreased incidence of iron-deficiency anemia.
Decreased incidence of dysmenorrhea.
Effects related to inhibition of ovulation:
Decreased incidence of functional ovarian cysts.
Decreased incidence of ectopic pregnancies.
Effects from long-term use:
Decreased incidence of fibroadenomas and fibrocystic disease of the breast.
Decreased incidence of acute pelvic inflammatory disease.
Decreased incidence of endometrial cancer.

Decreased incidence of ovarian cancer.

DOSAGE AND ADMINISTRATION

To achieve maximum contraceptive effectiveness, Triphasil®-28 Tablets (levonorgestrel and ethinyl estradiol tablets—triphasic regimen) must be taken exactly as directed and at intervals not exceeding 24 hours.

Triphasil-28 Tablets are a three-phase preparation plus 7 inert tablets. The dosage of Triphasil-28 Tablets is **one tablet daily** for 28 consecutive days per menstrual cycle in the following order: 6 brown tablets (phase 1), followed by 5 white tablets (phase 2), followed by 10 light-yellow tablets (phase 3), plus 7 light-green inert tablets, according to the prescribed schedule.

It is recommended that Triphasil-28 Tablets be taken at the same time each day, preferably after the evening meal or at bedtime. During the first cycle of medication, the patient should be instructed to take one Triphasil-28 Tablet daily in the order of 6 brown, 5 white, 10 light-yellow tablets, and then 7 light-green inert tablets for twenty-eight (28) consecutive days, beginning on day one (1) of her menstrual cycle. (The first day of menstruation is day one.) Withdrawal bleeding usually occurs within 3 days following the last light-yellow tablet and may not have finished before the next pack is started. (If Triphasil-28 Tablets are first taken later than the first day of the first menstrual cycle of medication or postpartum, contraceptive reliance should not be placed on Triphasil-28 Tablets until after the first 7 consecutive days of administration and a nonhormonal back-up method of birth control should be used during those 7 days. The possibility of ovulation and conception prior to initiation of medication should be considered.)

When switching from another oral contraceptive, Triphasil-28 Tablets should be started on the first day of bleeding following the last active tablet taken of the previous oral contraceptive.

The patient may switch any day from a progestin-only pill and should begin Triphasil-28 the next day. If switching from an implant or injection, the patient should start Triphasil-28 on the day of implant removal or, if using an injection, the day the next injection would be due. In switching from a progestin-only pill, injection, or implant, the patient should be advised to use a non-hormonal back-up method of birth control for the first 7 days of tablet-taking.

The patient begins her next and all subsequent 28-day courses of Triphasil-28 Tablets on the same day of the week that she began her first course, following the same schedule. She begins taking her brown tablets on the next day after ingestion of the last light-green tablet, regardless of whether or not a menstrual period has occurred or is still in progress. Any time a subsequent cycle of Triphasil-28 Tablets is started later than the next day, the patient should be protected by another means of contraception until she has taken a tablet daily for seven consecutive days.

If spotting or breakthrough bleeding occurs, the patient is instructed to continue on the same regimen. This type of bleeding is usually transient and without significance; however, if the bleeding is persistent or prolonged, the patient is advised to consult her physician. Although the occurrence of pregnancy is highly unlikely if Triphasil-28 Tablets are taken according to directions, if withdrawal bleeding does not occur, the possibility of pregnancy must be considered. If the patient has not adhered to the prescribed schedule (missed one or more tablets or started taking them on a day later than she should have), the probability of pregnancy should be considered at the time of the first missed period and appropriate diagnostic measures taken before the medication is resumed. If the patient has adhered to the prescribed regimen and misses two consecutive periods, pregnancy should be ruled out before continuing the contraceptive regimen.

The risk of pregnancy increases with each active (brown, white, or light-yellow) tablet missed. For additional patient instructions regarding missed pills, see the "WHAT TO DO IF YOU MISS PILLS" section in the DETAILED PATIENT LABELING below. If breakthrough bleeding occurs following missed active tablets, it will usually be transient and of no consequence. If the patient misses one or more light-green tablets, she is still protected against pregnancy **provided** she begins taking brown tablets again on the proper day.

Triphasil-28 may be initiated no earlier than day 28 postpartum in the non-lactating mother or after a second trimester abortion due to the increased risk for thromboembolism (see **"Contraindications," "Warnings,"** and **"Precautions"** concerning thromboembolic disease). The patient should be advised to use a nonhormonal back-up method for the first 7 days of tablet-taking. However, if intercourse has already occurred, pregnancy should be excluded before the start of combined oral contraceptive use or the patient must wait for her first menstrual period. In the case of first-trimester abortion, if the patient starts Triphasil-28 immediately, additional contraceptive measures are not needed. It is to be noted that early resumption of ovulation may occur if Parlodel® (bromocriptine mesylate) has been used for the prevention of lactation.

HOW SUPPLIED

Triphasil®-28 Tablets (levonorgestrel and ethinyl estradiol tablets—triphasic regimen), NDC 0008-2536, are available in packages of 3 dial dispensers. Each cycle contains 28 round, coated tablets as follows:

NDC 0008-0641, six brown tablets marked "W" and "641", each containing 0.050 mg levonorgestrel and 0.030 mg ethinyl estradiol;

NDC 0008-0642, five white to off-white tablets marked "W" and "642", each containing 0.075 mg levonorgestrel and 0.040 mg ethinyl estradiol;

NDC 0008-0643, ten light-yellow tablets marked "W" and "643", each containing 0.125 mg levonorgestrel and 0.030 mg ethinyl estradiol; and

NDC 0008-0650, seven light-green inert tablets marked "W" and "650".

Store at controlled room temperature 20° to 25°C (68° to 77°F).

References available upon request.

Brief Summary Patient Package Insert

This product (like all oral contraceptives) is intended to prevent pregnancy. It does not protect against HIV infection (AIDS) and other sexually transmitted diseases.

Oral contraceptives, also known as "birth-control pills" or "the pill," are taken to prevent pregnancy, and when taken correctly, have a failure rate of less than 1.0% per year when used without missing any pills. The average failure rate of large numbers of pill users is 5% per year when women who miss pills are included. For most women oral contraceptives are also free of serious or unpleasant side effects. However, forgetting to take pills considerably increases the chances of pregnancy.

For the majority of women, oral contraceptives can be taken safely. But there are some women who are at high risk of developing certain serious diseases that can be life-threatening or may cause temporary or permanent disability or death. The risks associated with taking oral contraceptives increase significantly if you:

- smoke.
- have high blood pressure, diabetes, high cholesterol, or a tendency to form blood clots, or are obese.
- have or have had clotting disorders, heart attack, stroke, angina pectoris, cancer of the breast or sex organs, jaundice, or malignant or benign liver tumors.

You should not take the pill if you suspect you are pregnant or have unexplained vaginal bleeding.

Cigarette smoking increases the risk of serious adverse effects on the heart and blood vessels from oral-contraceptive use. This risk increases with age and with the amount of smoking (15 or more cigarettes per day has been associated with a significantly increased risk) and is quite marked in women over 35 years of age. Women who use oral contraceptives should not smoke.

Most side effects of the pill are not serious. The most common such effects are nausea, vomiting, bleeding between menstrual periods, weight gain, breast tenderness, and difficulty wearing contact lenses. These side effects, especially nausea and vomiting, may subside within the first three months of use.

The serious side effects of the pill occur very infrequently, especially if you are in good health and do not smoke. However, you should know that the following medical conditions have been associated with or made worse by the pill:

1. Blood clots in the legs (thrombophlebitis), lungs (pulmonary embolism), stoppage or rupture of a blood vessel in the brain (stroke), blockage of blood vessels in the heart (heart attack and angina pectoris) or other organs of the body. As mentioned above, smoking increases the risk of heart attacks and strokes and subsequent serious medical consequences. Women with migraine also may be at increased risk of stroke.

2. Liver tumors, which may rupture and cause severe bleeding. A possible but not definite association has been found with the pill and liver cancer. However, liver cancers are extremely rare. The chance of developing liver cancer from using the pill is thus even rarer.

3. High blood pressure, although blood pressure usually returns to normal when the pill is stopped.

The symptoms associated with these serious side effects are discussed in the detailed leaflet given to you with your supply of pills. Notify your doctor or health-care provider if you notice any unusual physical disturbances while taking the pill. In addition, drugs such as rifampin, as well as some anticonvulsants and some antibiotics, and possibly St. John's wort, may decrease oral-contraceptive effectiveness.

Breast cancer has been diagnosed slightly more often in women who use the pill than in women of the same age who do not use the pill. This very small increase in the number of breast cancer diagnoses gradually disappears during the 10 years after stopping use of the pill. It is not known whether the difference is caused by the pill. It may be that women taking the pill were examined more often, so that breast cancer was more likely to be detected.

Some studies have found an increase in the incidence of cancer or precancerous lesions of the cervix in women who use the pill. However, this finding may be related to factors other than the use of the pill.

Taking the pill provides some important noncontraceptive benefits. These include less painful menstruation, less menstrual blood loss and anemia, fewer pelvic infections, and fewer cancers of the ovary and the lining of the uterus.

Be sure to discuss any medical condition you may have with your health-care provider. Your health-care provider will take a medical and family history before prescribing oral contraceptives and will examine you. The physical examination may be delayed to another time if you request it and the health-care provider believes that it is appropriate to postpone it. You should be reexamined at least once a year while taking oral contraceptives. The detailed patient information leaflet gives you further information which you should read and discuss with your health-care provider.

This product (like all oral contraceptives) is intended to prevent pregnancy. It does not protect against transmission of HIV (AIDS) and other sexually transmitted diseases such as chlamydia, genital herpes, genital warts, gonorrhea, hepatitis B, and syphilis.

DETAILED PATIENT LABELING

This product (like all oral contraceptives) is intended to prevent pregnancy. It does not protect against HIV infection (AIDS) and other sexually transmitted diseases.

INTRODUCTION

Any woman who considers using oral contraceptives (the birth-control pill or the pill) should understand the benefits and risks of using this form of birth control. This leaflet will give you much of the information you will need to make this decision and will also help you determine if you are at risk of developing any of the serious side effects of the pill. It will tell you how to use the pill properly so that it will be as effective as possible. However, this leaflet is not a replacement for a careful discussion between you and your health-care provider. You should discuss the information provided in this leaflet with him or her, both when you first start taking the pill and during your revisits. You should also follow your health-care provider's advice with regard to regular check-ups while you are on the pill.

EFFECTIVENESS OF ORAL CONTRACEPTIVES

Oral contraceptives or "birth-control pills" or "the pill" are used to prevent pregnancy and are more effective than other nonsurgical methods of birth control. When they are taken correctly, the chance of becoming pregnant is less than 1.0% when used perfectly, without missing any pills. Average failure rates are 5% per year. The chance of becoming pregnant increases with each missed pill during the menstrual cycle. In comparison, average failure rates for other nonsurgical methods of birth control during the first year of use are as follows:

TABLE: PERCENTAGE OF WOMEN EXPERIENCING AN UNINTENDED PREGNANCY DURING THE FIRST YEAR OF USE OF A CONTRACEPTIVE METHOD

Method	Perfect Use	Average Use
Levonorgestrel implants	0.05	0.05
Male sterilization	0.1	0.15
Female sterilization	0.5	0.5
Depo-Provera® (injectable progestogen)	0.3	0.3
Oral contraceptives		5
Combined	0.1	NA
Progestin only	0.5	NA
IUD		
Progesterone	1.5	2.0
Copper T 380A	0.6	0.8
Condom (male) without spermicide	3	14
(Female) without spermicide	5	21
Cervical cap		
Never given birth	9	20
Given birth	26	40
Vaginal sponge		
Never given birth	9	20
Given birth	20	40
Diaphragm with spermicidal cream or jelly	6	20
Spermicides alone (foam, creams, jellies, and vaginal suppositories)	6	26
Periodic abstinence (all methods)	1-9*	25
Withdrawal	4	19
No contraception (planned pregnancy)	85	85

NA - not available

*Depending on method (calendar, ovulation, symptothermal, post-ovulation)

Adapted from Hatcher RA et al, *Contraceptive Technology: 17th Revised Edition*. NY, NY: Ardent Media, Inc., 1998.

Continued on next page

Triphasil-28—Cont.

WHO SHOULD NOT TAKE ORAL CONTRACEPTIVES

Cigarette smoking increases the risk of serious adverse effects on the heart and blood vessels from oral-contraceptive use. This risk increases with age and with the amount of smoking (15 or more cigarettes per day has been associated with a significantly increased risk) and is quite marked in women over 35 years of age. Women who use oral contraceptives should not smoke.

Some women should not use the pill. For example, you should not take the pill if you are pregnant or think you may be pregnant. You should also not use the pill if you have had any of the following conditions:

- Heart attack or stroke.
- Blood clots in the legs (thrombophlebitis), lungs (pulmonary embolism), or eyes.
- Blood clots in the deep veins of your legs.
- Known or suspected breast cancer or cancer of the lining of the uterus, cervix, or vagina or certain hormonally-sensitive cancers.
- Liver tumor (benign or cancerous).

Or, if you have any of the following:

- Chest pain (angina pectoris).
- Unexplained vaginal bleeding (until a diagnosis is reached by your doctor).
- Yellowing of the whites of the eyes or of the skin (jaundice) during pregnancy or during previous use of the pill.
- Known or suspected pregnancy.
- Heart valve or heart rhythm disorders that may be associated with formation of blood clots.
- Diabetes affecting your circulation.
- Uncontrolled high blood pressure.
- Active liver disease with abnormal liver function tests.
- Allergy or hypersensitivity to any of the components of Triphasil (levonorgestrel and ethinyl estradiol tablets—triphasic regimen).

Tell your health-care provider if you have ever had any of these conditions. Your health-care provider can recommend another method of birth control.

OTHER CONSIDERATIONS BEFORE TAKING ORAL CONTRACEPTIVES

Tell your health-care provider if you or any family member has ever had:

- Breast nodules, fibrocystic disease of the breast, an abnormal breast X-ray or mammogram.
- Diabetes.
- Elevated cholesterol or triglycerides.
- High blood pressure.
- A tendency to form blood clots.
- Migraine or other headaches or epilepsy.
- Mental depression.
- Gallbladder, heart, or kidney disease.
- History of scanty or irregular menstrual periods.

Women with any of these conditions should be checked often by their health-care provider if they choose to use oral contraceptives. Also, be sure to inform your doctor or health-care provider if you smoke or are on any medications.

RISKS OF TAKING ORAL CONTRACEPTIVES

1. Risk of developing blood clots

Blood clots and blockage of blood vessels are the most serious side effects of taking oral contraceptives and can be fatal. In particular, a clot in the legs can cause thrombophlebitis and a clot that travels to the lungs can cause a sudden blocking of the vessel carrying blood to the lungs. Rarely, clots occur in the blood vessels of the eye and may cause blindness, double vision, or impaired vision.

If you take oral contraceptives and need elective surgery, need to stay in bed for a prolonged illness, or have recently delivered a baby, you may be at risk of developing blood clots. You should consult your doctor about stopping oral contraceptives three to four weeks before surgery and not taking oral contraceptives for two weeks after surgery or during bed rest. You should also not take oral contraceptives soon after delivery of a baby or a midtrimester pregnancy termination. It is advisable to wait for at least four weeks after delivery if you are not breast-feeding. If you are breast-feeding, you should wait until you have weaned your child before using the pill. (See also the section on breast-feeding in "GENERAL PRECAUTIONS.")

2. Heart attacks and strokes

Oral contraceptives may increase the tendency to develop strokes (stoppage or rupture of blood vessels in the brain) and angina pectoris and heart attacks (blockage of blood vessels in the heart). Any of these conditions can cause death or serious disability.

Smoking greatly increases the possibility of suffering heart attacks and strokes. Furthermore, smoking and the use of oral contraceptives greatly increase the chances of developing and dying of heart disease.

Women with migraine (especially migraine with aura) who take oral contraceptives also may be at higher risk of stroke.

3. Gallbladder disease

Oral-contraceptive users probably have a greater risk than nonusers of having gallbladder disease, although this risk may be related to pills containing high doses of estrogens.

4. Liver tumors

In rare cases, oral contraceptives can cause benign but dangerous liver tumors. These benign liver tumors can rupture and cause fatal internal bleeding. In addition, a possible but not definite association has been found with the pill and liver cancers in two studies in which a few women who developed these very rare cancers were found to have used oral contraceptives for long periods. However, liver cancers are extremely rare. The chance of developing liver cancer from using the pill is thus even rarer.

5. Cancer of the reproductive organs

Breast cancer has been diagnosed slightly more often in women who use the pill than in women of the same age who do not use the pill. This very small increase in the number of breast cancer diagnoses gradually disappears during the 10 years after stopping use of the pill. It is not known whether the difference is caused by the pill. It may be that women taking the pill were examined more often, so that breast cancer was more likely to be detected.

Some studies have found an increase in the incidence of cancer or precancerous lesions of the cervix in women who use oral contraceptives. However, this finding may be related to factors other than the use of oral contraceptives.

6. Lipid metabolism and inflammation of the pancreas

In patients with inherited defects of lipid metabolism, there have been reports of significant elevations of plasma triglycerides during estrogen therapy. This has led to pancreatitis in some cases.

ESTIMATED RISK OF DEATH FROM A BIRTH-CONTROL METHOD OR PREGNANCY

All methods of birth control and pregnancy are associated with a risk of developing certain diseases which may lead to disability or death. An estimate of the number of deaths associated with different methods of birth control and pregnancy has been calculated and is shown in the following table.

ANNUAL NUMBER OF BIRTH-RELATED OR METHOD-RELATED DEATHS ASSOCIATED WITH CONTROL OF FERTILITY PER 100,000 NONSTERILE WOMEN, BY FERTILITY-CONTROL METHOD ACCORDING TO AGE

Method of control and outcome	15-19	20-24	25-29	30-34	35-39	40-44
No fertility-control methods*	7.0	7.4	9.1	14.8	25.7	28.2
Oral contraceptives nonsmoker**	0.3	0.5	0.9	1.9	13.8	31.6
Oral contraceptives smoker**	2.2	3.4	6.6	13.5	51.1	117.2
IUD**	0.8	0.8	1.0	1.0	1.4	1.4
Condom*	1.1	1.6	0.7	0.2	0.3	0.4
Diaphragm/spermicide*	1.9	1.2	1.2	1.3	2.2	2.8
Periodic abstinence*	2.5	1.6	1.6	1.7	2.9	3.6

*Deaths are birth related
**Deaths are method related

In the above table, the risk of death from any birth-control method is less than the risk of childbirth, except for oral-contraceptive users over the age of 35 who smoke and pill users over the age of 40 even if they do not smoke. It can be seen in the table that for women aged 15 to 39, the risk of death was highest with pregnancy (7 to 26 deaths per 100,000 women, depending on age). Among pill users who do not smoke, the risk of death was always lower than that associated with pregnancy for any age group, except for those women over the age of 40, when the risk increases to 32 deaths per 100,000 women, compared to 28 associated with pregnancy at that age. However, for pill users who smoke and are over the age of 35, the estimated number of deaths exceeds those for other methods of birth control. If a woman is over the age of 40 and smokes, her estimated risk of death is four times higher (117/100,000 women) than the estimated risk associated with pregnancy (28/100,000 women) in that age group.

The suggestion that women over 40 who don't smoke should not take oral contraceptives is based on information from older high-dose pills and on less-selective use of pills than is practiced today. An Advisory Committee of the FDA discussed this issue in 1989 and recommended that the benefits of oral-contraceptive use by healthy, nonsmoking women over 40 years of age may outweigh the possible risks. However, all women, especially older women, are cautioned to use the lowest-dose pill that is effective.

WARNING SIGNALS

If any of these adverse effects occur while you are taking oral contraceptives, call your doctor immediately:

- Sharp chest pain, coughing of blood, or sudden shortness of breath (indicating a possible clot in the lung).
- Pain in the calf (indicating a possible clot in the leg).
- Crushing chest pain or heaviness in the chest (indicating a possible heart attack).
- Sudden severe headache or vomiting, dizziness or fainting, disturbances of vision or speech, weakness, or numbness in an arm or leg (indicating a possible stroke).
- Sudden partial or complete loss of vision (indicating a possible clot in the eye).
- Breast lumps (indicating possible breast cancer or fibrocystic disease of the breast; ask your doctor or health-care provider to show you how to examine your breasts).
- Severe pain or tenderness in the stomach area (indicating a possibly ruptured liver tumor).
- Difficulty in sleeping, weakness, lack of energy, fatigue, or change in mood (possibly indicating severe depression).
- Jaundice or a yellowing of the skin or eyeballs, accompanied frequently by fever, fatigue, loss of appetite, dark-colored urine, or light-colored bowel movements (indicating possible liver problems).

SIDE EFFECTS OF ORAL CONTRACEPTIVES

1. Vaginal bleeding

Irregular vaginal bleeding or spotting may occur while you are taking the pills. Irregular bleeding may vary from slight staining between menstrual periods to breakthrough bleeding which is a flow much like a regular period. Irregular bleeding occurs most often during the first few months of oral-contraceptive use, but may also occur after you have been taking the pill for some time. Such bleeding may be temporary and usually does not indicate any serious problems. It is important to continue taking your pills on schedule. If the bleeding occurs in more than one cycle or lasts for more than a few days, talk to your doctor or health-care provider.

2. Contact lenses

If you wear contact lenses and notice a change in vision or an inability to wear your lenses, contact your doctor or health-care provider.

3. Fluid retention

Oral contraceptives may cause edema (fluid retention) with swelling of the fingers or ankles and may raise your blood pressure. If you experience fluid retention, contact your doctor or health-care provider.

4. Melasma

A spotty darkening of the skin is possible, particularly of the face.

5. Other side effects

Other side effects may include nausea, breast tenderness, change in appetite, headache, nervousness, depression, dizziness, loss of scalp hair, rash, vaginal infections, inflammation of the pancreas, and allergic reactions.

If any of these side effects bother you, call your doctor or health-care provider.

GENERAL PRECAUTIONS

1. Missed periods and use of oral contraceptives before or during early pregnancy

There may be times when you may not menstruate regularly after you have completed taking a cycle of pills. If you have taken your pills regularly and miss one menstrual period, continue taking your pills for the next cycle but be sure to inform your health-care provider before doing so. If you have not taken the pills daily as instructed and missed a menstrual period, or if you missed two consecutive menstrual periods, you may be pregnant. Check with your health-care provider immediately to determine whether you are pregnant. Do not continue to take oral contraceptives until you are sure you are not pregnant, but continue to use another method of contraception.

There is no conclusive evidence that oral-contraceptive use is associated with an increase in birth defects when taken inadvertently during early pregnancy. Previously, a few studies had reported that oral contraceptives might be associated with birth defects, but these studies have not been confirmed. Nevertheless, oral contraceptives or any other drugs should not be used during pregnancy unless clearly necessary and prescribed by your doctor. You should check with your doctor about risks to your unborn child of any medication taken during pregnancy.

2. While breast-feeding

If you are breast-feeding, consult your doctor before starting oral contraceptives. Some of the drug will be passed on to the child in the milk. A few adverse effects on the child have been reported, including yellowing of the skin (jaundice) and breast enlargement. In addition, oral contraceptives may decrease the amount and quality of your milk. If possible, do not use oral contraceptives while breast-feeding. You should use another method of contraception since breast-feeding provides only partial protection from becoming pregnant, and this partial protection decreases significantly as you breast-feed for longer periods of time. You should consider starting oral contraceptives only after you have weaned your child completely.

3. Laboratory tests

If you are scheduled for any laboratory tests, tell your doctor you are taking birth-control pills. Certain blood tests may be affected by birth control pills.

4. Drug interactions

Certain drugs may interact with birth-control pills to make them less effective in preventing pregnancy or cause an increase in breakthrough bleeding. Such drugs include rifampin, drugs used for epilepsy such as barbiturates (for example, phenobarbital) and phenytoin (Dilantin® is one brand of this drug), primidone (Mysoline®), topiramate (Topamax®), phenylbutazone (Butazolidin® is one brand), some drugs used for HIV such as ritonavir (Norvir®), modafinil (Provigil®), and possibly certain antibiotics (such as ampicillin and other penicillins, and tetracyclines) and St. John's wort. You may need to use an additional method of contraception during any cycle in which you take drugs that can make oral contraceptives less effective.

You may be at higher risk of a specific type of liver dysfunction if you take troleandomycin and oral contraceptives at the same time.

You should inform your healthcare provider about all medicines you are taking, including nonprescription products.

5. Sexually transmitted diseases
This product (like all oral contraceptives) is intended to prevent pregnancy. It does not protect against transmission of HIV (AIDS) and other sexually transmitted diseases such as chlamydia, genital herpes, genital warts, gonorrhea, hepatitis B, and syphilis.
HOW TO TAKE THE PILL
IMPORTANT POINTS TO REMEMBER
BEFORE YOU START TAKING YOUR PILLS:
1. BE SURE TO READ THESE DIRECTIONS:
Before you start taking your pills.
Anytime you are not sure what to do.
2. THE RIGHT WAY TO TAKE THE PILL IS TO TAKE ONE PILL EVERY DAY AT THE SAME TIME.
If you miss pills you could get pregnant. This includes starting the pack late. The more pills you miss, the more likely you are to get pregnant.
3. MANY WOMEN HAVE SPOTTING OR LIGHT BLEEDING, OR MAY FEEL SICK TO THEIR STOMACH DURING THE FIRST 1-3 PACKS OF PILLS.
If you feel sick to your stomach, do not stop taking the pill. The problem will usually go away. If it doesn't go away, check with your doctor or clinic.
4. MISSING PILLS CAN ALSO CAUSE SPOTTING OR LIGHT BLEEDING, even when you make up these missed pills.
On the days you take 2 pills to make up for missed pills, you could also feel a little sick to your stomach.
5. IF YOU HAVE VOMITING (within 3 to 4 hours after you take your pill), you should follow the instructions for **WHAT TO DO IF YOU MISS PILLS**. IF YOU HAVE DIARRHEA, or IF YOU TAKE SOME MEDICINES, including some antibiotics, your pills may not work as well.
Use a back-up method (such as condoms, spermicide or sponge) until you check with your doctor or clinic.
6. IF YOU HAVE TROUBLE REMEMBERING TO TAKE THE PILL, talk to your doctor or clinic about how to make pill-taking easier or about using another method of birth control.
7. IF YOU HAVE ANY QUESTIONS OR ARE UNSURE ABOUT THE INFORMATION IN THIS LEAFLET, call your doctor or clinic.
BEFORE YOU START TAKING YOUR PILLS
1. DECIDE WHAT TIME OF DAY YOU WANT TO TAKE YOUR PILL.
It is important to take it at about the same time every day.
2. LOOK AT YOUR PILL PACK TO SEE IF IT HAS 21 OR 28 PILLS:
The *21-pill pack* has 21 "active" brown, white or light-yellow pills (with hormones) to take for 3 weeks, followed by 1 week without pills.
The *28-pill pack* has 21 "active" brown, white or light-yellow pills (with hormones) to take for 3 weeks, followed by 1 week of reminder light-green pills (without hormones).
3. ALSO FIND:
1) where on the pack to start taking pills, and
2) in what order to take the pills (follow the arrow).

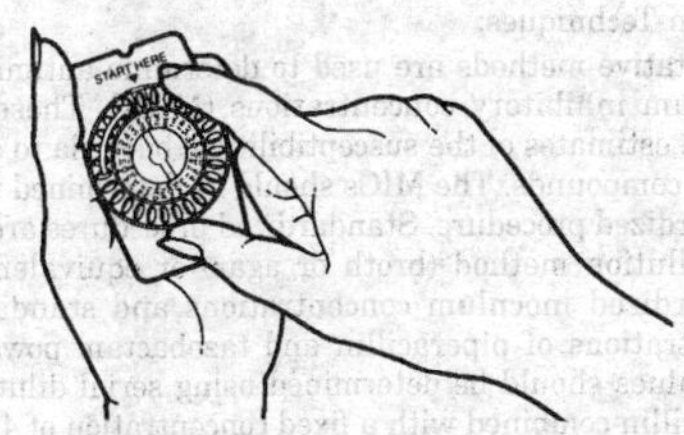

4. BE SURE YOU HAVE READY AT ALL TIMES:
ANOTHER KIND OF BIRTH CONTROL (such as condoms, spermicide, or sponge) to use as a back-up in case you miss pills.
AN EXTRA, FULL PILL PACK.
WHEN TO START THE *FIRST* PACK OF PILLS:
You have a choice of which day to start taking your first pack of pills. Decide with your doctor or clinic which is the best day for you. Pick a time of day which will be easy to remember.
DAY 1 START:
1. Take the first "active" brown pill of the first pack during the *first 24 hours of your period.*
2. You will not need to use a back-up method of birth control, since you are starting the pill at the beginning of your period.
SUNDAY START:
1. Take the first "active" brown pill of the first pack on the *Sunday after your period starts,* even if you are still bleeding. If your period begins on Sunday, start the pack that same day.
2. *Use another method of birth control* as a back-up method if you have sex anytime from the Sunday you start your first pack until the next Sunday (7 days). Condoms, spermicide, or the sponge are good back-up methods of birth control.
WHAT TO DO DURING THE MONTH:
1. TAKE ONE PILL AT THE SAME TIME EVERY DAY UNTIL THE PACK IS EMPTY.
Do not skip pills even if you are spotting or bleeding between monthly periods or feel sick to your stomach (nausea).
Do not skip pills even if you do not have sex very often.

2. WHEN YOU FINISH A PACK OR SWITCH YOUR BRAND OF PILLS:
21 pills: Wait 7 days to start the next pack. You will probably have your period during that week. Be sure that no more than 7 days pass between 21-day packs.
28 pills: Start the next pack on the day after your last "reminder" pill. Do not wait any days between packs.
WHAT TO DO IF YOU MISS PILLS
The pill may not be as effective if you miss brown, white or light-yellow "active" pills, and particularly if you miss the first few brown or the last few light-yellow "active" pills in a pack.
If you **MISS 1** brown, white or light-yellow "active" pill:
1. Take it as soon as you remember. Take the next pill at your regular time. This means you may take 2 pills in 1 day.
2. You do not need to use a back-up birth-control method if you have sex.
If you **MISS 2** brown, white or light-yellow "active" pills in a row in **WEEK 1 OR WEEK 2** of your pack:
1. Take 2 pills on the day you remember and 2 pills the next day.
2. Then take 1 pill a day until you finish the pack.
3. You MAY BECOME PREGNANT if you have sex in the 7 *days* after you miss pills. You MUST use another birth-control method (such as condoms, spermicide, or sponge) as a back-up for those 7 days.
If you **MISS 2** brown, white or light-yellow "active" pills in a row in **THE 3rd WEEK:**
1. ***If you are a Day 1 Starter:***
THROW OUT the rest of the pill pack and start a new pack that same day.
If you are a Sunday Starter:
Keep taking 1 pill every day until Sunday.
On Sunday, THROW OUT the rest of the pack and start a new pack of pills that same day.
2. You may not have your period this month but this is expected. However, if you miss your period 2 months in a row, call your doctor or clinic because you might be pregnant.
3. You MAY BECOME PREGNANT if you have sex in the 7 *days* after you miss pills. You MUST use another birth-control method (such as condoms, spermicide, or sponge) as a back-up for those 7 days.
If you **MISS 3 OR MORE** brown, white or light-yellow "active" pills in a row (during the first 3 weeks):
1. ***If you are a Day 1 Starter:***
THROW OUT the rest of the pill pack and start a new pack that same day.
If you are a Sunday Starter:
Keep taking 1 pill every day until Sunday.
On Sunday, THROW OUT the rest of the pack and start a new pack of pills that same day.
2. You may not have your period this month but this is expected. However, if you miss your period 2 months in a row, call your doctor or clinic because you might be pregnant.
3. You MAY BECOME PREGNANT if you have sex in the 7 *days* after you miss pills. You MUST use another birth-control method (such as condoms, spermicide, or sponge) as a back-up for those 7 days.
A REMINDER FOR THOSE ON 28-DAY PACKS:
If you forget any of the 7 light-green "reminder" pills in Week 4:
THROW AWAY the pills you missed.
Keep taking 1 pill each day until the pack is empty.
You do not need a back-up method if you start your next pack on time.
FINALLY, IF YOU ARE STILL NOT SURE WHAT TO DO ABOUT THE PILLS YOU HAVE MISSED:
Use a BACK-UP METHOD anytime you have sex.
KEEP TAKING ONE PILL EACH DAY until you can reach your doctor or clinic.
Pregnancy due to pill failure
The incidence of pill failure resulting in pregnancy is approximately less than 1.0% if taken every day as directed, but average failure rates are 5%. If you do become pregnant, the risk to the fetus is minimal, but you should stop taking your pills and discuss the pregnancy with your doctor.
Pregnancy after stopping the pill
There may be some delay in becoming pregnant after you stop using oral contraceptives, especially if you had irregular menstrual cycles before you used oral contraceptives. It may be advisable to postpone conception until you begin menstruating regularly once you have stopped taking the pill and desire pregnancy.
There does not appear to be any increase in birth defects in newborn babies when pregnancy occurs soon after stopping the pill.
Overdosage
Serious ill effects have not been reported following ingestion of large doses of oral contraceptives by young children. Overdosage may cause nausea and withdrawal bleeding in females. In case of overdosage, contact your health-care provider or pharmacist.
Other information
Your health-care provider will take a medical and family history before prescribing oral contraceptives and will examine you. The physical examination may be delayed to another time if you request it and the health-care provider believes that it is appropriate to postpone it. You should be reexamined at least once a year. Be sure to inform your health-care provider if there is a family history of any of the conditions listed previously in this leaflet. Be sure to keep all appointments with your health-care provider, because this is a time to determine if there are early signs of side effects of oral-contraceptive use.

Do not use the drug for any condition other than the one for which it was prescribed. This drug has been prescribed specifically for you; do not give it to others who may want birth-control pills.
HEALTH BENEFITS FROM ORAL CONTRACEPTIVES
In addition to preventing pregnancy, use of oral contraceptives may provide certain benefits. They are:
- Menstrual cycles may become more regular.
- Blood flow during menstruation may be lighter, and less iron may be lost. Therefore, anemia due to iron deficiency is less likely to occur.
- Pain or other symptoms during menstruation may be encountered less frequently.
- Ovarian cysts may occur less frequently.
- Ectopic (tubal) pregnancy may occur less frequently.
- Noncancerous cysts or lumps in the breast may occur less frequently.
- Acute pelvic inflammatory disease may occur less frequently.
- Oral-contraceptive use may provide some protection against developing two forms of cancer: cancer of the ovaries and cancer of the lining of the uterus.

If you want more information about birth-control pills, ask your doctor or pharmacist. They have a more technical leaflet called the Professional Labeling which you may wish to read.
Wyeth Pharmaceuticals Inc. W10508C001
Philadelphia, PA 19101 ET01
Rev 06/04
Shown in Product Identification Guide, page 337

ZOSYN® ℞
[zō'sĭn]
(Piperacillin and Tazobactam for Injection)
℞ only

To reduce the development of drug-resistant bacteria and maintain the effectiveness of Zosyn (piperacillin and tazobactam) injection and other antibacterial drugs, Zosyn (piperacillin and tazobactam) should be used only to treat or prevent infections that are proven or strongly suspected to be caused by bacteria.

DESCRIPTION
Zosyn (piperacillin and tazobactam for injection) is an injectable antibacterial combination product consisting of the semisynthetic antibiotic piperacillin sodium and the β-lactamase inhibitor tazobactam sodium for intravenous administration.
Piperacillin sodium is derived from D(-)-α-aminobenzyl-penicillin. The chemical name of piperacillin sodium is sodium (2*S*,5*R*,6*R*)-6-[(*R*)-2-(4-ethyl-2,3-dioxo-1-piperazine- carboxamido)-2-phenylacetamido]-3,3-dimethyl-7-oxo-4-thia-1-azabicyclo[3.2.0]heptane-2-carboxylate. The chemical formula is $C_{23}H_{26}N_5NaO_7S$ and the molecular weight is 539.5. The chemical structure of piperacillin sodium is:

Tazobactam sodium, a derivative of the penicillin nucleus, is a penicillanic acid sulfone. Its chemical name is sodium (2*S*,3*S*,5*R*)-3-methyl-7-oxo-3-(1*H*-1,2,3-triazol-1-ylmethyl)-4-thia-1-azabicyclo[3.2.0]heptane-2-carboxylate-4,4-dioxide. The chemical formula is $C_{10}H_{11}N_4NaO_5S$ and the molecular weight is 322.3. The chemical structure of tazobactam sodium is:

Zosyn, piperacillin/tazobactam parenteral combination, is a white to off-white sterile, cryodesiccated powder consisting of piperacillin and tazobactam as their sodium salts packaged in glass vials. The product does not contain excipients or preservatives.
Each Zosyn 2.25 g single dose vial or ADD-Vantage® vial contains an amount of drug sufficient for withdrawal of piperacillin sodium equivalent to 2 grams of piperacillin and tazobactam sodium equivalent to 0.25 g of tazobactam.
Each Zosyn 3.375 g single dose vial or ADD-Vantage® vial contains an amount of drug sufficient for withdrawal of piperacillin sodium equivalent to 3 grams of piperacillin and tazobactam sodium equivalent to 0.375 g of tazobactam.
Each Zosyn 4.5 g single dose vial or ADD-Vantage® vial contains an amount of drug sufficient for withdrawal of piperacillin sodium equivalent to 4 grams of piperacillin and tazobactam sodium equivalent to 0.5 g of tazobactam.
Zosyn (piperacillin and tazobactam for injection) is a monosodium salt of piperacillin and a monosodium salt of tazobactam containing a total of 2.35 mEq (54 mg) of Na^+ per gram of piperacillin in the combination product.

Continued on next page

Zosyn—Cont.

CLINICAL PHARMACOLOGY

Peak plasma concentrations of piperacillin and tazobactam are attained immediately after completion of an intravenous infusion of Zosyn. Piperacillin plasma concentrations, following a 30-minute infusion of Zosyn, were similar to those attained when equivalent doses of piperacillin were administered alone, with mean peak plasma concentrations of approximately 134, 242 and 298 μg/mL for the 2.25 g, 3.375 g and 4.5 g Zosyn (piperacillin/tazobactam) doses, respectively. The corresponding mean peak plasma concentrations of tazobactam were 15, 24 and 34 μg/mL, respectively. Following a 30-minute I.V. infusion of 3.375 g Zosyn every 6 hours, steady-state plasma concentrations of piperacillin and tazobactam were similar to those attained after the first dose. In like manner, steady-state plasma concentrations were not different from those attained after the first dose when 2.25 g or 4.5 g doses of Zosyn were administered via 30-minute infusions every 6 hours. Steady-state plasma concentrations after 30-minute infusions every 6 hours are provided in Table 1.

Following single or multiple Zosyn doses to healthy subjects, the plasma half-life of piperacillin and of tazobactam ranged from 0.7 to 1.2 hours and was unaffected by dose or duration of infusion.

Piperacillin is metabolized to a minor microbiologically active desethyl metabolite. Tazobactam is metabolized to a single metabolite that lacks pharmacological and antibacterial activities. Both piperacillin and tazobactam are eliminated via the kidney by glomerular filtration and tubular secretion. Piperacillin is excreted rapidly as unchanged drug with 68% of the administered dose excreted in the urine. Tazobactam and its metabolite are eliminated primarily by renal excretion with 80% of the administered dose excreted as unchanged drug and the remainder as the single metabolite. Piperacillin, tazobactam and desethyl piperacillin are also secreted into the bile.

Both piperacillin and tazobactam are approximately 30% bound to plasma proteins. The protein binding of either piperacillin or tazobactam is unaffected by the presence of the other compound. Protein binding of the tazobactam metabolite is negligible.

Piperacillin and tazobactam are widely distributed into tissues and body fluids including intestinal mucosa, gallbladder, lung, female reproductive tissues (uterus, ovary, and fallopian tube), interstitial fluid, and bile. Mean tissue concentrations are generally 50% to 100% of those in plasma. Distribution of piperacillin and tazobactam into cerebrospinal fluid is low in subjects with non-inflamed meninges, as with other penicillins.

After the administration of single doses of piperacillin/tazobactam to subjects with renal impairment, the half-life of piperacillin and of tazobactam increases with decreasing creatinine clearance. At creatinine clearance below 20 mL/min, the increase in half-life is twofold for piperacillin and fourfold for tazobactam compared to subjects with normal renal function. Dosage adjustments for Zosyn are recommended when creatinine clearance is below 40 mL/min in patients receiving the usual recommended daily dose of Zosyn (piperacillin and tazobactam for injection). (See **DOSAGE AND ADMINISTRATION** section for specific recommendations for the treatment of patients with renal insufficiency.)

Hemodialysis removes 30% to 40% of a piperacillin/tazobactam dose with an additional 5% of the tazobactam dose removed as the tazobactam metabolite. Peritoneal dialysis removes approximately 6% and 21% of the piperacillin and tazobactam doses, respectively, with up to 16% of the tazobactam dose removed as the tazobactam metabolite. For dosage recommendations for patients undergoing hemodialysis, see **DOSAGE AND ADMINISTRATION** section.

The half-life of piperacillin and of tazobactam increases by approximately 25% and 18%, respectively, in patients with hepatic cirrhosis compared to healthy subjects. However, this difference does not warrant dosage adjustment of Zosyn due to hepatic cirrhosis.

[See table 1 above]

Microbiology

Piperacillin sodium exerts bactericidal activity by inhibiting septum formation and cell wall synthesis of susceptible bacteria. In vitro, piperacillin is active against a variety of gram-positive and gram-negative aerobic and anaerobic bacteria. Tazobactam sodium has little clinically relevant in vitro activity against bacteria due to its reduced affinity to penicillin-binding proteins. It is, however, a β-lactamase inhibitor of the Richmond-Sykes class III (Bush class 2b & 2b') penicillinases and cephalosporinases. It varies in its ability to inhibit class II and IV (2a & 4) penicillinases. Tazobactam does not induce chromosomally-mediated β-lactamases at tazobactam concentrations achieved with the recommended dosage regimen.

Piperacillin/tazobactam has been shown to be active against most strains of the following microorganisms both in vitro and in clinical infections as described in the **INDICATIONS AND USAGE** section.

Aerobic and facultative Gram-positive microorganisms:

Staphylococcus aureus (excluding methicillin and oxacillin-resistant isolates)

Aerobic and facultative Gram-negative microorganisms:

Acinetobacter baumanii
Escherichia coli

TABLE 1
STEADY STATE MEAN PLASMA CONCENTRATIONS IN ADULTS AFTER 30-MINUTE INTRAVENOUS INFUSION OF PIPERACILLIN/TAZOBACTAM EVERY 6 HOURS

PIPERACILLIN

Piperacillin/ Tazobactam Dose[a]	No. of Evaluable Subjects	Plasma Concentrations** (μg/mL) 30 min	1 hr	2 hr	3 hr	4 hr	6 hr	AUC** (μg•hr/mL) AUC_{0-6}
2.25 g	8	134 (14)	57 (14)	17.1 (23)	5.2 (32)	2.5 (35)	0.9 (14)[b]	131 (14)
3.375 g	6	242 (12)	106 (8)	34.6 (20)	11.5 (19)	5.1 (22)	1.0 (10)	242 (10)
4.5 g	8	298 (14)	141 (19)	46.6 (28)	16.4 (29)	6.9 (29)	1.4 (30)	322 (16)

TAZOBACTAM

Piperacillin/ Tazobactam Dose[a]	No. of Evaluable Subjects	Plasma Concentrations** (μg/mL) 30 min	1 hr	2 hr	3 hr	4 hr	6 hr	AUC** (μg•hr/mL) AUC_{0-6}
2.25 g	8	14.8 (14)	7.2 (22)	2.6 (30)	1.1 (35)	0.7 (6)[c]	<0.5	16.0 (21)
3.375 g	6	24.2 (14)	10.7 (7)	4.0 (18)	1.4 (21)	0.7 (16)[b]	<0.5	25.0 (8)
4.5 g	8	33.8 (15)	17.3 (16)	6.8 (24)	2.8 (25)	1.3 (30)	<0.5	39.8 (15)

** Numbers in parentheses are coefficients of variation (CV%).
a: Piperacillin and tazobactam were given in combination.
b: N = 4
c: N = 3

TABLE 2
SUSCEPTIBILITY INTERPRETIVE CRITERIA FOR PIPERACILLIN/TAZOBACTAM

Pathogen	Susceptibility Test Result Interpretive Criteria: Minimal Inhibitory Concentration (MIC in μg/mL) S	I	R	Disk Diffusion (Zone Diameter in mm) S	I	R
Enterobacteriaceae and *Acinetobacter baumanii*	≤ 16	32 – 64	≥ 128	≥ 21	18 – 20	≤ 17
Haemophilus influenzae[a]	≤ 1	–	≥ 2	–	–	–
Pseudomonas aeruginosa	≤ 64	–	≥ 128	≥ 18	–	≤ 17
Staphylococcus aureus	≤ 8	–	≥ 16	≥ 20	–	≤ 19
Bacteroides fragilis group	≤ 32	64	≥ 128	–	–	–

a: These interpretive criteria for *Haemophilus influenzae* are applicable only to tests performed using Haemophilus Test Medium inoculated with a direct colony suspension and incubated at 35°C in ambient air for 20 to 24 hours.

Haemophilus influenzae (excluding β-lactamase negative, ampicillin-resistant isolates)
Klebsiella pneumoniae
Pseudomonas aeruginosa (given in combination with an aminoglycoside to which the isolate is susceptible)

Gram-negative anaerobes:

Bacteroides fragilis group (*B. fragilis, B. ovatus, B. thetaiotaomicron,* and *B. vulgatus*)

The following in vitro data are available, **but their clinical significance is unknown.**

At least 90% of the following microorganisms exhibit an in vitro minimum inhibitory concentration (MIC) less than or equal to the susceptible breakpoint for piperacillin/tazobactam. However, the safety and effectiveness of piperacillin/tazobactam in treating clinical infections due to these bacteria have not been established in adequate and well-controlled clinical trials.

Aerobic and facultative Gram-positive microorganisms:

Enterococcus faecalis (ampicillin or penicillin-susceptible isolates only)
Staphylococcus epidermidis (excluding methicillin and oxacillin resistant isolates)
Streptococcus agalactiae†
Streptococcus pneumoniae† (penicillin-susceptible isolates only)
Streptococcus pyogenes†
Viridans group streptococci†

Aerobic and facultative Gram-negative microorganisms:

Citrobacter koseri
Moraxella catarrhalis
Morganella morganii
Neisseria gonorrhoeae
Proteus mirabilis
Proteus vulgaris
Serratia marcescens
Providencia stuartii
Providencia rettgeri
Salmonella enterica

Gram-positive anaerobes:

Clostridium perfringens

Gram-negative anaerobes:

Bacteroides distasonis
Prevotella melaninogenica

†These are not β-lactamase producing bacteria and, therefore, are susceptible to piperacillin alone.

Susceptibility Testing Methods

As is recommended with all antimicrobials, the results of in vitro susceptibility tests, when available, should be provided to the physician as periodic reports, which describe the susceptibility profile of nosocomial and community-acquired pathogens. These reports should aid the physician in selecting the most effective antimicrobial.

Dilution Techniques:

Quantitative methods are used to determine antimicrobial minimum inhibitory concentrations (MICs). These MICs provide estimates of the susceptibility of bacteria to antimicrobial compounds. The MICs should be determined using a standardized procedure. Standardized procedures are based on a dilution method (broth or agar) or equivalent with standardized inoculum concentrations and standardized concentrations of piperacillin and tazobactam powders.[1,2] MIC values should be determined using serial dilutions of piperacillin combined with a fixed concentration of 4 μg/mL tazobactam. The MIC values obtained should be interpreted according to criteria provided in Table 2.

Diffusion Technique:

Quantitative methods that require measurement of zone diameters also provide reproducible estimates of the susceptibility of bacteria to antimicrobial compounds. One such standardized procedure[1,3] requires the use of standardized inoculum concentrations. This procedure uses paper disks impregnated with 100 μg of piperacillin and 10 μg of tazobactam to test the susceptibility of microorganisms to piperacillin/tazobactam. The disk diffusion interpreted criteria are provided in Table 2.

Anaerobic Techniques

For anaerobic bacteria, the susceptibility to piperacillin/tazobactam can be determined by the reference agar dilution method.[4]

[See table 2 above]

A report of S ("Susceptible") indicates that the pathogen is likely to be inhibited if the antimicrobial compound in the blood reaches the concentration usually achievable. A report of I ("Intermediate") indicates that the results should be considered equivocal, and if the microorganism is not fully susceptible to alternative, clinically feasible drugs, the test should be repeated. This category implies possible clinical applicability in body sites where the drug is physiologically concentrated or in situations where high dosage of drug can be used. This category also provides a buffer zone, which prevents small, uncontrolled technical factors from causing major discrepancies in interpretation. A report of R ("Resistant") indicates that the pathogen is not likely to be inhibited if the antimicrobial compound in the blood reaches the concentration usually achievable; other therapy should be considered.

Quality Control
Standardized susceptibility test procedures require the use of quality control microorganisms to control the technical aspects of the test procedures.[1,2,3,4] Standard piperacillin/tazobactam powder should provide the following ranges of values noted in Table 3. Quality control microorganisms are specific strains of microorganisms with intrinsic biological properties relating to resistance mechanisms and their genetic expression within the microorganism; the specific strains used for microbiological quality control are not clinically significant.
[See table 3 at right]

TABLE 3
ACCEPTABLE QUALITY CONTROL RANGES FOR PIPERACILLIN/TAZOBACTAM TO BE USED IN VALIDATION OF SUSCEPTIBILITY TEST RESULTS

	Acceptable Quality Control Ranges	
QC Strain	Minimum Inhibitory Concentration Range (MIC in μg/mL)	Disk Diffusion Zone Diameter Ranges in mm
Escherichia coli ATCC 25922	1 - 4	24 - 30
Escherichia coli ATCC 35218	0.5 - 2	24 - 30
Pseudomonas aeruginosa ATCC 27853	1 - 8	25 - 33
Haemophilus influenzae[a] ATCC 49247	0.06 - 0.5	-
Staphylococcus aureus ATCC 29213	0.25 - 2	-
Staphylococcus aureus ATCC 25923	-	27 - 36
Bacteroides fragilis ATCC 25285	0.12 - 0.5	-
Bacteroides thetaiotaomicron ATCC 29741	4 - 16	-

a: This quality control range for *Haemophilus influenzae* is applicable only to tests performed using Haemophilus Test Medium inoculated with a direct colony suspension and incubated at 35°C in ambient air for 20 to 24 hours.

INDICATIONS AND USAGE
Zosyn (piperacillin and tazobactam for injection) is indicated for the treatment of patients with moderate to severe infections caused by piperacillin-resistant, piperacillin/tazobactam-susceptible, β-lactamase producing strains of the designated microorganisms in the specified conditions listed below:
Appendicitis (complicated by rupture or abscess) and peritonitis caused by piperacillin-resistant, β-lactamase producing strains of *Escherichia coli* or the following members of the *Bacteroides fragilis* group: *B. fragilis, B. ovatus, B. thetaiotaomicron*, or *B. vulgatus*. The individual members of this group were studied in less than 10 cases.
Uncomplicated and complicated skin and skin structure infections, including cellulitis, cutaneous abscesses and ischemic/diabetic foot infections caused by piperacillin-resistant, β-lactamase producing strains of *Staphylococcus aureus*.
Postpartum endometritis or pelvic inflammatory disease caused by piperacillin-resistant, β-lactamase producing strains of *Escherichia coli*.
Community-acquired pneumonia (moderate severity only) caused by piperacillin-resistant, β-lactamase producing strains of *Haemophilus influenzae*.
Nosocomial pneumonia (moderate to severe) caused by piperacillin-resistant, β-lactamase producing strains of *Staphylococcus aureus* and by piperacillin/tazobactam-susceptible *Acinetobacter baumanii, Haemophilus influenzae, Klebsiella pneumoniae*, and *Pseudomonas aeruginosa* (Nosocomial pneumonia caused by *P. aeruginosa* should be treated in combination with an aminoglycoside). (See **DOSAGE AND ADMINISTRATION**.)
Zosyn (piperacillin and tazobactam for injection) is indicated only for the specified conditions listed above. Infections caused by piperacillin-susceptible organisms, for which piperacillin has been shown to be effective, are also amenable to Zosyn treatment due to its piperacillin content. The tazobactam component of this combination product does not decrease the activity of the piperacillin component against piperacillin-susceptible organisms. Therefore, the treatment of mixed infections caused by piperacillin-susceptible organisms and piperacillin-resistant, β-lactamase producing organisms susceptible to Zosyn should not require the addition of another antibiotic. (See **DOSAGE AND ADMINISTRATION**.)
Zosyn is useful as presumptive therapy in the indicated conditions prior to the identification of causative organisms because of its broad spectrum of bactericidal activity against gram-positive and gram-negative aerobic and anaerobic organisms.
Appropriate cultures should usually be performed before initiating antimicrobial treatment in order to isolate and identify the organisms causing infection and to determine their susceptibility to Zosyn. Antimicrobial therapy should be adjusted, if appropriate, once the results of culture(s) and antimicrobial susceptibility testing are known.
To reduce the development of drug-resistant bacteria and maintain the effectiveness of Zosyn (piperacillin and tazobactam) injection and other antibacterial drugs, Zosyn (piperacillin and tazobactam) should be used only to treat or prevent infections that are proven or strongly suspected to be caused by susceptible bacteria. When culture and susceptibility information are available, they should be considered in selecting or modifying antibacterial therapy. In the absence of such data, local epidemiology and susceptibility patterns may contribute to the empiric selection of therapy.

CONTRAINDICATIONS
Zosyn is contraindicated in patients with a history of allergic reactions to any of the penicillins, cephalosporins, or β-lactamase inhibitors.

WARNINGS
SERIOUS AND OCCASIONALLY FATAL HYPERSENSITIVITY (ANAPHYLACTIC/ANAPHYLACTOID) REACTIONS (INCLUDING SHOCK) HAVE BEEN REPORTED IN PATIENTS RECEIVING THERAPY WITH PENICILLINS INCLUDING ZOSYN. THESE REACTIONS ARE MORE LIKELY TO OCCUR IN INDIVIDUALS WITH A HISTORY OF PENICILLIN HYPERSENSITIVITY OR A HISTORY OF SENSITIVITY TO MULTIPLE ALLERGENS. THERE HAVE BEEN REPORTS OF INDIVIDUALS WITH A HISTORY OF PENICILLIN HYPERSENSITIVITY WHO HAVE EXPERIENCED SEVERE REACTIONS WHEN TREATED WITH CEPHALOSPORINS. BEFORE INITIATING THERAPY WITH ZOSYN, CAREFUL INQUIRY SHOULD BE MADE CONCERNING PREVIOUS HYPERSENSITIVITY REACTIONS TO PENICILLINS, CEPHALOSPORINS, OR OTHER ALLERGENS. IF AN ALLERGIC REACTION OCCURS, ZOSYN SHOULD BE DISCONTINUED AND APPROPRIATE THERAPY INSTITUTED. **SERIOUS ANAPHYLACTIC/ANAPHYLACTOID REACTIONS (INCLUDING SHOCK) REQUIRE IMMEDIATE EMERGENCY TREATMENT WITH EPINEPHRINE. OXYGEN, INTRAVENOUS STEROIDS, AND AIRWAY MANAGEMENT, INCLUDING INTUBATION, SHOULD ALSO BE ADMINISTERED AS INDICATED.**
Pseudomembranous colitis has been reported with nearly all antibacterial agents, including piperacillin/tazobactam, and may range in severity from mild to life-threatening. Therefore, it is important to consider this diagnosis in patients who present with diarrhea subsequent to the administration of antibacterial agents.
Treatment with antibacterial agents alters the normal flora of the colon and may permit overgrowth of clostridia. Studies indicate that a toxin produced by *Clostridium difficile* is one primary cause of "antibiotic-associated colitis."
After the diagnosis of pseudomembranous colitis has been established, therapeutic measures should be initiated. Mild cases of pseudomembranous colitis usually respond to drug discontinuation alone. In moderate to severe cases, consideration should be given to management with fluids and electrolytes, protein supplementation, and treatment with an antibacterial drug clinically effective against *Clostridium difficile* colitis.

PRECAUTIONS
General
Bleeding manifestations have occurred in some patients receiving β-lactam antibiotics, including piperacillin. These reactions have sometimes been associated with abnormalities of coagulation tests such as clotting time, platelet aggregation and prothrombin time, and are more likely to occur in patients with renal failure. If bleeding manifestations occur, Zosyn (piperacillin and tazobactam for injection) should be discontinued and appropriate therapy instituted.
The possibility of the emergence of resistant organisms that might cause superinfections should be kept in mind. If this occurs, appropriate measures should be taken.
As with other penicillins, patients may experience neuromuscular excitability or convulsions if higher than recommended doses are given intravenously (particularly in the presence of renal failure).
Zosyn is a monosodium salt of piperacillin and a monosodium salt of tazobactam and contains a total of 2.35 mEq (54 mg) of Na^+ per gram of piperacillin in the combination product. This should be considered when treating patients requiring restricted salt intake. Periodic electrolyte determinations should be performed in patients with low potassium reserves, and the possibility of hypokalemia should be kept in mind with patients who have potentially low potassium reserves and who are receiving cytotoxic therapy or diuretics.
As with other semisynthetic penicillins, piperacillin therapy has been associated with an increased incidence of fever and rash in cystic fibrosis patients.
In patients with creatinine clearance ≤ 40 mL/min and dialysis patients (hemodialysis and CAPD), the intravenous dose should be adjusted to the degree of renal function impairment. (See **DOSAGE AND ADMINISTRATION**.)
Prescribing Zosyn (piperacillin and tazobactam) in the absence of a proven or strongly suspected bacterial infection or a prophylactic indication is unlikely to provide benefit to the patient and increases the risk of development of drug-resistant bacteria.

Information for Patients
Patients should be counseled that antibacterial drugs including Zosyn should only be used to treat bacterial infections. They do not treat viral infections (e.g., the common cold). When Zosyn is prescribed to treat a bacterial infection, patients should be told that although it is common to feel better early in the course of therapy, the medication should be taken exactly as directed. Skipping doses or not completing the full course of therapy may (1) decrease the effectiveness of the immediate treatment and (2) increase the likelihood that bacteria will develop resistance and will not be treatable by Zosyn or other antibacterial drugs in the future.

Laboratory Tests
Periodic assessment of hematopoietic function should be performed, especially with prolonged therapy, ie, ≥ 21 days. (See **ADVERSE REACTIONS, Adverse Laboratory Events.**)

Drug Interactions
Aminoglycosides
The mixing of Zosyn with an aminoglycoside in vitro can result in substantial inactivation of the aminoglycoside. (See **DOSAGE AND ADMINISTRATION, Compatible Intravenous Diluent Solutions.**)
When Zosyn was co-administered with tobramycin, the area under the curve, renal clearance, and urinary recovery of tobramycin were decreased by 11%, 32%, and 38%, respectively. The alterations in the pharmacokinetics of tobramycin when administered in combination with piperacillin/tazobactam may be due to in vivo and in vitro inactivation of tobramycin in the presence of piperacillin/tazobactam. The inactivation of aminoglycosides in the presence of penicillin-class drugs has been recognized. It has been postulated that penicillin-aminoglycoside complexes form; these complexes are microbiologically inactive and of unknown toxicity. In patients with severe renal dysfunction (ie, chronic hemodialysis patients), the pharmacokinetics of tobramycin are significantly altered when tobramycin is administered in combination with piperacillin.[5] The alteration of tobramycin pharmacokinetics and the potential toxicity of the penicillin-aminoglycoside complexes in patients with mild to moderate renal dysfunction who are administered an aminoglycoside in combination with piperacillin/tazobactam are unknown.
Probenecid
Probenecid administered concomitantly with Zosyn prolongs the half-life of piperacillin by 21% and that of tazobactam by 71%.
Vancomycin
No pharmacokinetic interactions have been noted between Zosyn and vancomycin.
Heparin
Coagulation parameters should be tested more frequently and monitored regularly during simultaneous administration of high doses of heparin, oral anticoagulants, or other drugs that may affect the blood coagulation system or the thrombocyte function.
Vecuronium
Piperacillin when used concomitantly with vecuronium has been implicated in the prolongation of the neuromuscular blockade of vecuronium. Zosyn (piperacillin/tazobactam) could produce the same phenomenon if given along with vecuronium. Due to their similar mechanism of action, it is expected that the neuromuscular blockade produced by any of the non-depolarizing muscle relaxants could be prolonged in the presence of piperacillin. (See package insert for vecuronium bromide.)
Methotrexate
Limited data suggests that co-administration of methotrexate and piperacillin may reduce the clearance of methotrexate due to competition for renal secretion. The impact of tazobactam on the elimination of methotrexate has not been evaluated. If concurrent therapy is necessary, serum concentrations of methotrexate as well as the signs and symptoms of methotrexate toxicity should be frequently monitored.

Drug/Laboratory Test Interactions
As with other penicillins, the administration of Zosyn® (piperacillin and tazobactam for injection) may result in a false-positive reaction for glucose in the urine using a copper-

Continued on next page

Zosyn—Cont.

reduction method (CLINITEST®). It is recommended that glucose tests based on enzymatic glucose oxidase reactions (such as DIASTIX® or TES-TAPE®) be used.

There have been reports of positive test results using the Bio-Rad Laboratories Platelia *Aspergillus* EIA test in patients receiving piperacillin/tazobactam injection who were subsequently found to be free of *Aspergillus* infection. Cross-reactions with non-*Aspergillus* polysaccharides and polyfuranoses with the Bio-Rad Laboratories Platelia *Aspergillus* EIA test have been reported.

Therefore, positive test results in patients receiving piperacillin/tazobactam should be interpreted cautiously and confirmed by other diagnostic methods.

Carcinogenesis, Mutagenesis, Impairment of Fertility

Long-term carcinogenicity studies in animals have not been conducted with piperacillin/tazobactam, piperacillin, or tazobactam.

Piperacillin/Tazobactam

Piperacillin/tazobactam was negative in microbial mutagenicity assays at concentrations up to 14.84/1.86 μg/plate. Piperacillin/tazobactam was negative in the unscheduled DNA synthesis (UDS) test at concentrations up to 5689/711 μg/mL. Piperacillin/tazobactam was negative in a mammalian point mutation (Chinese hamster ovary cell HPRT) assay at concentrations up to 8000/1000 μg/mL. Piperacillin/tazobactam was negative in a mammalian cell (BALB/c-3T3) transformation assay at concentrations up to 8/1 μg/mL. In vivo, piperacillin/ tazobactam did not induce chromosomal aberrations in rats dosed I.V. with 1500/187.5 mg/kg; this dose is similar to the maximum recommended human daily dose on a body-surface-area basis (mg/m^2).

Piperacillin

Piperacillin was negative in microbial mutagenicity assays at concentrations up to 50 μg/plate. There was no DNA damage in bacteria (Rec assay) exposed to piperacillin at concentrations up to 200 μg/disk. Piperacillin was negative in the UDS test at concentrations up to 10,000 μg/mL. In a mammalian point mutation (mouse lymphoma cells) assay, piperacillin was positive at concentrations ≥2500 μg/mL. Piperacillin was negative in a cell (BALB/c-3T3) transformation assay at concentrations up to 3000 μg/mL. In vivo, piperacillin did not induce chromosomal aberrations in mice at I.V. doses up to 2000 mg/kg/day or rats at I.V. doses up to 1500 mg/kg/day. These doses are half (mice) or similar (rats) to the maximum recommended human daily dose based on body-surface area (mg/m^2). In another in vivo test, there was no dominant lethal effect when piperacillin was administered to rats at I.V. doses up to 2000 mg/kg/day, which is similar to the maximum recommended human daily dose based on body-surface area (mg/m^2). When mice were administered piperacillin at I.V. doses up to 2000 mg/kg/day, which is half the maximum recommended human daily dose based on body-surface area (mg/m^2), urine from these animals was not mutagenic when tested in a microbial mutagenicity assay. Bacteria injected into the peritoneal cavity of mice administered piperacillin at I.V. doses up to 2000 mg/kg/day did not show increased mutation frequencies.

Tazobactam

Tazobactam was negative in microbial mutagenicity assays at concentrations up to 333 μg/plate. Tazobactam was negative in the UDS test at concentrations up to 2000 μg/mL. Tazobactam was negative in a mammalian point mutation (Chinese hamster ovary cell HPRT) assay at concentrations up to 5000 μg/mL. In another mammalian point mutation (mouse lymphoma cells) assay, tazobactam was positive at concentrations ≥3000 μg/mL. Tazobactam was negative in a cell (BALB/c-3T3) transformation assay at concentrations up to 900 μg/mL. In an in vitro cytogenetics (Chinese hamster lung cells) assay, tazobactam was negative at concentrations up to 3000 μg/mL. In vivo, tazobactam did not induce chromosomal aberrations in rats at I.V. doses up to 5000 mg/kg, which is 23 times the maximum recommended human daily dose based on body-surface area (mg/m^2).

Pregnancy

Teratogenic effects—Pregnancy Category B

Piperacillin/tazobactam

Reproduction studies have been performed in rats and have revealed no evidence of impaired fertility due to piperacillin/tazobactam administered up to a dose which is similar to the maximum recommended human daily dose based on body-surface area (mg/m^2).

Teratology studies have been performed in mice and rats and have revealed no evidence of harm to the fetus due to piperacillin/tazobactam administered up to a dose which is 1 to 2 times and 2 to 3 times the human dose of piperacillin and tazobactam, respectively, based on body-surface area (mg/m^2).

Piperacillin and tazobactam cross the placenta in humans.

Piperacillin

Reproduction and teratology studies have been performed in mice and rats and have revealed no evidence of impaired fertility or harm to the fetus due to piperacillin administered up to a dose which is half (mice) or similar (rats) to the maximum recommended human daily dose based on body-surface area (mg/m^2).

Tazobactam

Reproduction studies have been performed in rats and have revealed no evidence of impaired fertility due to tazobactam administered at doses up to 3 times the maximum recommended human daily dose based on body-surface area (mg/m^2).

Teratology studies have been performed in mice and rats and have revealed no evidence of harm to the fetus due to tazobactam administered at doses up to 6 and 14 times, respectively, the human dose based on body-surface area (mg/m^2). In rats, tazobactam crosses the placenta. Concentrations in the fetus are less than or equal to 10% of those found in maternal plasma.

There are, however, no adequate and well-controlled studies with the piperacillin/tazobactam combination or with piperacillin or tazobactam alone in pregnant women. Because animal reproduction studies are not always predictive of the human response, this drug should be used during pregnancy only if clearly needed.

Nursing Mothers

Piperacillin is excreted in low concentrations in human milk; tazobactam concentrations in human milk have not been studied. Caution should be exercised when Zosyn (piperacillin and tazobactam for injection) is administered to a nursing woman.

Pediatric Use

Safety and efficacy in pediatric patients have not been established.

Geriatric Use

Patients over 65 years are <u>not</u> at an increased risk of developing adverse effects solely because of age. However, dosage should be adjusted in the presence of renal insufficiency. (See **DOSAGE AND ADMINISTRATION**.)

In general, dose selection for an elderly patient should be cautious, usually starting at the low end of the dosing range, reflecting the greater frequency of decreased hepatic, renal, or cardiac function, and of concomitant disease or other drug therapy.

Zosyn contains 54 mg (2.35 mEq) of sodium per gram of piperacillin in the combination product. At the usual recommended doses, patients would receive between 648 and 864 mg/day (28.2 and 37.6 mEq) of sodium. The geriatric population may respond with a blunted natriuresis to salt loading. This may be clinically important with regard to such diseases as congestive heart failure.

This drug is known to be substantially excreted by the kidney, and the risk of toxic reactions to this drug may be greater in patients with impaired renal function. Because elderly patients are more likely to have decreased renal function, care should be taken in dose selection, and it may be useful to monitor renal function.

ADVERSE REACTIONS

Adverse Events From Clinical Trials

During the initial clinical investigations, 2621 patients worldwide were treated with Zosyn (piperacillin and tazobactam for injection) in phase 3 trials. In the key North American clinical trials (n=830 patients), 90% of the adverse events reported were mild to moderate in severity and transient in nature. However, in 3.2% of the patients treated worldwide, Zosyn was discontinued because of adverse events primarily involving the skin (1.3%), including rash and pruritus; the gastrointestinal system (0.9%), including diarrhea, nausea, and vomiting; and allergic reactions (0.5%).

Adverse local reactions that were reported, irrespective of relationship to therapy with Zosyn, were phlebitis (1.3%), injection site reaction (0.5%), pain (0.2%), inflammation (0.2%), thrombophlebitis (0.2%), and edema (0.1%).

Based on patients from the North American trials (n=1063), the events with the highest incidence in patients, irrespective of relationship to Zosyn therapy, were diarrhea (11.3%); headache (7.7%); constipation (7.7%); nausea (6.9%); insomnia (6.6%); rash (4.2%), including maculopapular, bullous, urticarial, and eczematoid; vomiting (3.3%); dyspepsia (3.3%); pruritus (3.1%); stool changes (2.4%); fever (2.4%); agitation (2.1%); pain (1.7%); moniliasis (1.6%); hypertension (1.6%); dizziness (1.4%); abdominal pain (1.3%); chest pain (1.3%); edema (1.2%); anxiety (1.2%); rhinitis (1.2%); and dyspnea (1.1%).

Additional adverse systemic clinical events reported in 1.0% or less of the patients in the initial North American trials are listed below within each body system.

Autonomic nervous system—hypotension, ileus, syncope

Body as a whole—rigors, back pain, malaise

Cardiovascular—tachycardia, including supraventricular and ventricular; bradycardia; arrhythmia, including atrial fibrillation, ventricular fibrillation, cardiac arrest, cardiac failure, circulatory failure, myocardial infarction

Central nervous system—tremor, convulsions, vertigo

Gastrointestinal—melena, flatulence, hemorrhage, gastritis, hiccough, ulcerative stomatitis

Pseudomembranous colitis was reported in one patient during the clinical trials. The onset of pseudomembranous colitis symptoms may occur during or after antibacterial treatment. (See **WARNINGS**.)

Hearing and Vestibular System—tinnitus

Hypersensitivity—anaphylaxis

Metabolic and Nutritional—symptomatic hypoglycemia, thirst

Musculoskeletal—myalgia, arthralgia

Platelets, Bleeding, Clotting—mesenteric embolism, purpura, epistaxis, pulmonary embolism (See **PRECAUTIONS, General**).

Psychiatric—confusion, hallucination, depression

Reproductive, Female—leukorrhea, vaginitis

Respiratory—pharyngitis, pulmonary edema, bronchospasm, coughing

Skin and Appendages—genital pruritus, diaphoresis

Special senses—taste perversion

Urinary—retention, dysuria, oliguria, hematuria, incontinence

Vision—photophobia

Vascular (extracardiac)—flushing

Nosocomial Pneumonia Trials

In a completed study of nosocomial lower respiratory tract infections, 222 patients were treated with Zosyn in a dosing regimen of 4.5 g every 6 hours in combination with an aminoglycoside and 215 patients were treated with imipenem/cilastatin (500 mg/500 mg q6h) in combination with an aminoglycoside. In this trial, treatment-emergent adverse events were reported by 402 patients, 204 (91.9%) in the piperacillin/tazobactam group and 198 (92.1%) in the imipenem/cilastatin group. Twenty-five (11.0%) patients in the piperacillin/tazobactam group and 14 (6.5%) in the imipenem/cilastatin group ($p > 0.05$) discontinued treatment due to an adverse event.

In this study of Zosyn in combination with an aminoglycoside, adverse events that occurred in more than 1% patients and were considered by the investigator to be drug-related were: diarrhea (17.6%), fever (2.7%), vomiting (2.7%), urinary tract infection (2.7%), rash (2.3%), abdominal pain (1.8%), generalized edema (1.8%), moniliasis (1.8%), nausea (1.8%), oral moniliasis (1.8%), BUN increased (1.8%), creatinine increased (1.8%), peripheral edema (1.8%), abdomen enlarged (1.4%), headache (1.4%), constipation (1.4%), liver function tests abnormal (1.4%), thrombocythemia (1.4%), excoriations (1.4%), and sweating (1.4%).

Drug-related adverse events reported in 1% or less of patients in the nosocomial pneumonia study of Zosyn with an aminoglycoside were: acidosis, acute kidney failure, agitation, alkaline phosphatase increased, anemia, asthenia, atrial fibrillation, chest pain, CNS depression, colitis, confusion, convulsion, cough increased, thrombocytopenia, dehydration, depression, diplopia, drug level decreased, dry mouth, dyspepsia, dysphagia, dyspnea, dysuria, eosinophilia, fungal dermatitis, gastritis, glossitis, grand mal convulsion, hematuria, hyperglycemia, hypernatremia, hypertension, hypertonia, hyperventilation, hypochromic anemia, hypoglycemia, hypokalemia, hyponatremia, hypophosphatemia, hypoxia, ileus, injection site edema, injection site pain, injection site reaction, kidney function abnormal, leukocytosis, leukopenia, local reaction to procedure, melena, pain, prothrombin decreased, pruritus, respiratory disorder, SGOT increased, SGPT increased, sinus bradycardia, somnolence, stomatitis, stupor, tremor, tachycardia, ventricular extrasystoles, and ventricular tachycardia.

In a previous nosocomial pneumonia study conducted with a dosing regimen of 3.375 g given every 4 hours with an aminoglycoside, the following adverse events, irrespective of drug relationship, were observed: diarrhea (20%); constipation (8.4%); agitation (7.1%); nausea (5.8%); headache (4.5%); insomnia (4.5%); oral thrush (3.9%); erythematous rash (3.9%); anxiety (3.2%); fever (3.2%); pain (3.2%); pruritus (3.2%); hiccough (2.6%); vomiting (2.6%); dyspepsia (1.9%); edema (1.9%); fluid overload (1.9%); stool changes (1.9%); anorexia (1.3%); cardiac arrest (1.3%); confusion (1.3%); diaphoresis (1.3%); duodenal ulcer (1.3%); flatulence (1.3%); hypertension (1.3%); hypotension (1.3%); inflammation at injection site (1.3%); pleural effusion (1.3%); pneumothorax (1.3%); rash, not otherwise specified (1.3%); supraventricular tachycardia (1.3%); thrombophlebitis (1.3%); and urinary incontinence (1.3%).

Adverse events irrespective of drug relationship observed in 1% or less of patients in the above study with Zosyn and an aminoglycoside included: aggressive reaction (combative), angina, asthenia, atelectasis, balanoposthitis, cerebrovascular accident, chest pain, conjunctivitis, deafness, dyspnea, earache, ecchymosis, fecal incontinence, gastric ulcer, gout, hemoptysis, hypoxia, pancreatitis, perineal irritation/pain, urinary tract infection with trichomonas, vitamin B_{12} deficiency anemia, xerosis, and yeast in urine.

Post-Marketing Experience

Additional adverse events reported from worldwide marketing experience with Zosyn, occurring under circumstances where causal relationship to Zosyn is uncertain:

Gastrointestinal—hepatitis, cholestatic jaundice

Hematologic—hemolytic anemia, anemia, thrombocytosis, agranulocytosis, pancytopenia

Immune—hypersensitivity reactions, anaphylactic/anaphylactoid reactions (including shock)

Infections—candidal superinfections

Renal—interstitial nephritis, renal failure

Skin and Appendages—erythema multiforme, Stevens-Johnson syndrome, toxic epidermal necrolysis

Adverse Laboratory Events (Seen During Clinical Trials)

Of the studies reported, including that of nosocomial lower respiratory tract infections in which a higher dose of Zosyn (piperacillin and tazobactam for injection) was used in combination with an aminoglycoside, changes in laboratory parameters, without regard to drug relationship, include:

Hematologic—decreases in hemoglobin and hematocrit, thrombocytopenia, increases in platelet count, eosinophilia, leukopenia, neutropenia. The leukopenia/neutropenia associated with Zosyn administration appears to be reversible and most frequently associated with prolonged administration, ie, ≥21 days of therapy. These patients were withdrawn from therapy; some had accompanying systemic symptoms (eg, fever, rigors, chills).

Coagulation—positive direct Coombs' test, prolonged prothrombin time, prolonged partial thromboplastin time

Hepatic—transient elevations of AST (SGOT), ALT (SGPT), alkaline phosphatase, bilirubin

Renal—increases in serum creatinine, blood urea nitrogen

Urinalysis—proteinuria, hematuria, pyuria

Additional laboratory events include abnormalities in electrolytes (ie, increases and decreases in sodium, potassium, and calcium), hyperglycemia, decreases in total protein or albumin, blood glucose decreased, gamma-glutamyltransferase increased, hypokalemia, and bleeding time prolonged.

The following adverse reaction has also been reported for PIPRACIL® (piperacillin for injection):

Skeletal—prolonged muscle relaxation (See **PRECAUTIONS, Drug Interactions.**)

Piperacillin therapy has been associated with an increased incidence of fever and rash in cystic fibrosis patients.

OVERDOSAGE

There have been postmarketing reports of overdose with piperacillin/tazobactam. The majority of those events experienced, including nausea, vomiting, and diarrhea, have also been reported with the usual recommended dosages. Patients may experience neuromuscular excitability or convulsions if higher than recommended doses are given intravenously (particularly in the presence of renal failure).

Treatment should be supportive and symptomatic according the patient's clinical presentation. Excessive serum concentrations of either piperacillin or tazobactam may be reduced by hemodialysis. Following a single 3.375 g dose of piperacillin/tazobactam, the percentage of the piperacillin and tazobactam dose removed by hemodialysis was approximately 31% and 39%, respectively. (See **CLINICAL PHARMACOLOGY.**)

DOSAGE AND ADMINISTRATION

Zosyn should be administered by intravenous infusion over 30 minutes.

The usual total daily dose of Zosyn for adults is 3.375 g every six hours totaling 13.5 g (12.0 g piperacillin/1.5 g tazobactam).

Initial presumptive treatment of patients with nosocomial pneumonia should start with Zosyn at a dosage of 4.5 g every six hours plus an aminoglycoside, totaling 18.0 g (16.0 g piperacillin/2.0 g tazobactam). Treatment with the aminoglycoside should be continued in patients from whom *Pseudomonas aeruginosa* is isolated. If *Pseudomonas aeruginosa* is not isolated, the aminoglycoside may be discontinued at the discretion of the treating physician.

Renal Insufficiency

In patients with renal insufficiency (Creatinine Clearance ≤ 40 mL/min), the intravenous dose of Zosyn (piperacillin and tazobactam for injection) should be adjusted to the degree of actual renal function impairment. In patients with nosocomial pneumonia receiving concomitant aminoglycoside therapy, the aminoglycoside dosage should be adjusted according to the recommendations of the manufacturer. The recommended daily doses of Zosyn for patients with renal insufficiency are as follows:

[See table above]

For patients on hemodialysis, the maximum dose is 2.25 g every twelve hours for all indications other than nosocomial pneumonia and 2.25 g every eight hours for nosocomial pneumonia. Since hemodialysis removes 30% to 40% of the administered dose, an additional dose of 0.75 g Zosyn should be administered following each dialysis period on hemodialysis days. No additional dosage of Zosyn is necessary for CAPD patients.

Duration of Therapy

The usual duration of Zosyn treatment is from seven to ten days. However, the recommended duration of Zosyn treatment of nosocomial pneumonia is 7 to 14 days. In all conditions, the duration of therapy should be guided by the severity of the infection and the patient's clinical and bacteriological progress.

Directions for Reconstitution and Dilution for Use

Intravenous Administration

For conventional vials, reconstitute Zosyn per gram of piperacillin with 5 mL of a compatible reconstitution diluent from the list provided below.

2.25 g, 3.375 g, and 4.5 g Zosyn should be reconstituted with 10 mL, 15 mL, and 20 mL, respectively. Swirl until dissolved.

Pharmacy vials should be used immediately after reconstitution. Discard any unused portion after 24 hours if stored at room temperature (20°C to 25°C [68°F to 77°F]), or after 48 hours if stored at refrigerated temperature (2°C to 8°C [36°F to 46°F]).

Compatible Reconstitution Diluents

0.9% Sodium Chloride for Injection

Sterile Water for Injection‡

Dextrose 5%

Bacteriostatic Saline/Parabens

Bacteriostatic Water/Parabens

Bacteriostatic Saline/Benzyl Alcohol

Bacteriostatic Water/Benzyl Alcohol

Reconstituted Zosyn solution should be further diluted (recommended volume per dose of 50 mL to 150 mL) in a compatible intravenous diluent solution listed below. Administer by infusion over a period of at least 30 minutes. During the infusion it is desirable to discontinue the primary infusion solution.

Compatible Intravenous Diluent Solutions

0.9% Sodium Chloride for Injection

Sterile Water for Injection‡

Recommended Dosing of Zosyn in Patients with Normal Renal Function and Renal Insufficiency (As total grams piperacillin/tazobactam)

Renal Function (Creatinine Clearance, mL/min)	All Indications (except nosocomial pneumonia)	Nosocomial Pneumonia
>40 mL/min	3.375 q 6 h	4.5 q 6 h
20–40 mL/min*	2.25 q 6 h	3.375 q 6 h
<20 mL/min*	2.25 q 8 h	2.25 q 6 h
Hemodialysis**	2.25 q 12 h	2.25 q 8 h
CAPD	2.25 q 12 h	2.25 q 8 h

* Creatinine clearance for patients not receiving hemodialysis
** 0.75 g should be administered following each hemodialysis session on hemodialysis days

Dextrose 5%

Dextran 6% in Saline

‡Maximum recommended volume per dose of Sterile Water for Injection is 50 mL.

ADD-Vantage® System Admixtures

Dextrose 5% in Water (50 or 100 mL)

0.9% Sodium Chloride (50 or 100 mL)

For ADD-Vantage® vials reconstitution directions, see *INSTRUCTIONS FOR USE* sheet provided in the box.

Zosyn should not be mixed with other drugs in a syringe or infusion bottle since compatibility has not been established.

Zosyn is not chemically stable in solutions that contain only sodium bicarbonate and solutions that significantly alter the pH.

LACTATED RINGER'S SOLUTION IS NOT COMPATIBLE WITH ZOSYN.

Zosyn should not be added to blood products or albumin hydrolysates.

When concomitant therapy with aminoglycosides is indicated, Zosyn and the aminoglycoside should be reconstituted and administered separately, due to the in vitro inactivation of the aminoglycoside by the penicillin. (See PRECAUTIONS, Drug Interactions.)

Zosyn can be used in ambulatory intravenous infusion pumps.

Stability of Zosyn Following Reconstitution

Zosyn is stable in glass and plastic containers (plastic syringes, I.V. bags and tubing) when used with compatible diluents.

Pharmacy vials should be used immediately after reconstitution. Discard any unused portion after 24 hours if stored at room temperature (20°C to 25°C [68°F to 77°F]), or after 48 hours if stored at refrigerated temperature (2°C to 8°C [36°F to 46°F]). Vials should not be frozen after reconstitution.

Stability studies in the I.V. bags have demonstrated chemical stability (potency, pH of reconstituted solution and clarity of solution) for up to 24 hours at room temperature and up to one week at refrigerated temperature. Zosyn contains no preservatives. Appropriate consideration of aseptic technique should be used.

Stability of Zosyn in an ambulatory intravenous infusion pump has been demonstrated for a period of 12 hours at room temperature. Each dose was reconstituted and diluted to a volume of 37.5 mL or 25 mL. One-day supplies of dosing solution were aseptically transferred into the medication reservoir (I.V. bags or cartridge). The reservoir was fitted to a preprogrammed ambulatory intravenous infusion pump per the manufacturer's instructions. Stability of Zosyn is not affected when administered using an ambulatory intravenous infusion pump.

Stability studies with the admixed ADD-Vantage® system have demonstrated chemical stability (potency, pH and clarity) through 24 hours at room temperature. (Note: The admixed ADD-Vantage® should not be refrigerated or frozen after reconstitution.) Parenteral drug products should be inspected visually for particulate matter and discoloration prior to administration, whenever solution and container permit.

HOW SUPPLIED

Zosyn® (piperacillin and tazobactam for injection) is supplied in the following sizes:

Each Zosyn 2.25 g vial provides piperacillin sodium equivalent to 2 grams of piperacillin and tazobactam sodium equivalent to 0.25 g of tazobactam. Each vial contains 4.69 mEq (108 mg) of sodium.

Supplied 10 per box—NDC 0206-8452-16

Each Zosyn 3.375 g vial provides piperacillin sodium equivalent to 3 grams of piperacillin and tazobactam sodium equivalent to 0.375 g of tazobactam. Each vial contains 7.04 mEq (162 mg) of sodium.

Supplied 10 per box—NDC 0206-8454-55

Each Zosyn 4.5 g vial provides piperacillin sodium equivalent to 4 grams of piperacillin and tazobactam sodium equivalent to 0.5 g of tazobactam. Each vial contains 9.39 mEq (216 mg) of sodium.

Supplied 10 per box—NDC 0206-8455-25

Each Zosyn 2.25 g ADD-Vantage® vial provides piperacillin sodium equivalent to 2 grams of piperacillin and tazobactam sodium equivalent to 0.25 g of tazobactam. Each ADD-Vantage® vial contains 4.69 mEq (108 mg) of sodium.

Supplied 10 per box—NDC 0206-8452-17.

Each Zosyn 3.375 g ADD-Vantage® vial provides piperacillin sodium equivalent to 3 grams of piperacillin and tazobactam sodium equivalent to 0.375 g of tazobactam. Each ADD-Vantage® vial contains 7.04 mEq (162 mg) of sodium.

Supplied 10 per box—NDC 0206-8454-17.

Each Zosyn 4.5 g ADD-Vantage® vial provides piperacillin sodium equivalent to 4 grams of piperacillin and tazobactam sodium equivalent to 0.5 g of tazobactam. Each ADD-Vantage® vial contains 9.39 mEq (216 mg) of sodium.

Supplied 10 per box—NDC 0206-8455-17.

Zosyn conventional and ADD-Vantage® vials should be stored at controlled room temperature (20°C to 25°C [68°F to 77°F]) prior to reconstitution.

Also Available

Zosyn® (piperacillin and tazobactam injection) in Galaxy® Container (PL 2040 Plastic) is supplied as a frozen, iso-osmotic, sterile, nonpyrogenic solution in single dose plastic containers as follows:

2.25 g (piperacillin sodium equivalent to 2 g piperacillin/tazobactam sodium equivalent to 0.25 g tazobactam) in 50 mL. Each container has 5.7 mEq (131 mg) of sodium.

Supplied 24/box— NDC 0206-8820-02

3.375 g (piperacillin sodium equivalent to 3 g piperacillin/tazobactam sodium equivalent to 0.375 g tazobactam) in 50 mL. Each container has 8.6 mEq (197 mg) of sodium.

Supplied 24/box—NDC 0206-8821-02

4.5 g (piperacillin sodium equivalent to 4 g piperacillin/tazobactam sodium equivalent to 0.5 g tazobactam) in 100 mL. Each container has 11.4 mEq (263 mg) of sodium.

Supplied 12/box— NDC 0206-8822-02

Also Available

Zosyn (piperacillin and tazobactam for injection) is supplied as a powder in the pharmacy bulk vial as follows:

40.5 g pharmacy bulk vial containing piperacillin sodium equivalent to 36 grams of piperacillin and tazobactam sodium equivalent to 4.5 grams of tazobactam. Each pharmacy bulk vial contains 84.5 mEq (1,944 mg) of sodium.

NDC 0206-8620-11

REFERENCES

1. National Committee for Clinical Laboratory Standards, Performance Standards for Antimicrobial Susceptibility Testing; 13th Informational Supplement. NCCLS document M100-S13. NCCLS, Wayne, PA, 2003.
2. National Committee for Clinical Laboratory Standards, Methods for Dilution Antimicrobial Susceptibility Test for Bacteria that Grow Aerobically; Approved Standard—5th Edition. NCCLS document M7-A5. NCCLS, Wayne, PA, 2000.
3. National Committee for Clinical Laboratory Standards, Performance Standards for Antimicrobial Disk Susceptibility Test; Approved Standard—8th Edition. NCCLS document M2-A8. NCCLS, Wayne, PA, 2003.
4. National Committee for Clinical Laboratory Standards, Methods for Antimicrobial Susceptibility Testing of Anaerobic Bacteria; Approved Standard—5th ed. NCCLS document M11-A5. NCCLS, Wayne, PA, 2001.
5. Halstenson CE, Hirata CAI, Heim-Duthoy KL, Abraham PA, and Matzke GR. Effect of concomitant administration of piperacillin on the dispositions of netilmicin and tobramycin in patients with end-stage renal disease. Antimicrob Agents Chemother 34(1):128-133, 1990.

CLINITEST® and DIASTIX® are registered trademarks of Ames Division, Miles Laboratories, Inc.

TES-TAPE® is a registered trademark of Eli Lilly and Company.

Galaxy® is a registered trademark of Baxter International, Inc.

ADD-Vantage® is a registered trademark of Abbott Laboratories.

Wyeth®

Wyeth Pharmaceuticals Inc. W10414C005

Philadelphia, PA 19101 ET01

Rev 06/04

Shown in Product Identification Guide, page 337

Xanodyne Pharmaceuticals, Inc.
7300 TURFWAY ROAD, SUITE 300
FLORENCE, KY 41042

Direct Inquiries to:
1-877-XANODYNE (1-877-926-6396)
FAX: 1-859-371-6391
www.xanodyne.com

AMICAR® ℞
(aminocaproic acid)
Injection, Tablets, and Syrup
℞ only

DESCRIPTION

AMICAR (aminocaproic acid) is 6-aminohexanoic acid, which acts as an inhibitor of fibrinolysis.
Its chemical structure is:

$$H_2C(CH_2)_3CH_2COOH$$
$$NH_2$$

$C_6H_{13}NO_2$ M.W. 131.17

AMICAR is soluble in water, acid and alkaline solutions; it is sparingly soluble in methanol and practically insoluble in chloroform.

AMICAR (aminocaproic acid) Injection, for intravenous administration, is a sterile pyrogen-free solution containing 250 mg/mL of aminocaproic acid with benzyl alcohol 0.9% as preservative and Water for Injection. Hydrochloric acid may be added to adjust pH to approximately 6.8 during manufacture.

AMICAR (aminocaproic acid) Syrup, 25%, for oral administration, contains 250 mg/mL of aminocaproic acid with methylparaben 0.20%, propylparaben 0.05%, edetate disodium 0.30% as preservatives and the following inactive ingredients: sodium saccharin, sorbitol solution, citric acid anhydrous, natural and artificial raspberry flavor and an artificial bitterness modifier.

Each AMICAR (aminocaproic acid) Tablet, for oral administration contains 500 mg or 1000 mg of aminocaproic acid and the following inactive ingredients: povidone, crospovidone, stearic acid and magnesium stearate.

HOW SUPPLIED

AMICAR®
(aminocaproic acid)

AMICAR Injection
Each 20 mL vial contains 5 g of aminocaproic acid (250 mg/mL) as an aqueous solution with benzyl alcohol 0.9% as preservative.
20 mL vial – NDC 66479-025-39
Store Between 15°–30°C (59°–86°F); Do Not Freeze.

AMICAR Syrup, 25%
Each mL of raspberry-flavored syrup contains 250 mg of aminocaproic acid.
16 Fl. Oz. (473 mL) Bottle – NDC 66479-023-56
Store Between 15°–30°C (59°–86°F); Dispense in Tight Containers; Do Not Freeze.

AMICAR 500 mg Tablets
Each round, white tablet, engraved with XP on one side and scored on the other with A to the left of the score and 10 on the right, contains 500 mg of aminocaproic acid.
Bottle of 100 – NDC 66479-021-82
Store Between 15°–30°C (59°–86°F); Dispense in Tight Containers.

AMICAR 1000 mg Tablets
Each oblong, white tablet, engraved with XP on one side and scored on the other with A to the left of the score and 20 on the right, contains 1000 mg of aminocaproic acid
Bottle of 100 – NDC 66479-022-82
Store Between 15°–30°C (59°–86°F); Dispense in Tight Containers.

DUET® by StuartNatal® Tablet ℞
DUET® CHEWABLE by StuartNatal® ℞
DUET® DHA by StuartNatal® ℞

DESCRIPTION

Duet®:
Duet® is a yellow oval prenatal multi-vitamin and multi-mineral tablet imprinted with the StuartNatal® logo ("heart-in-a-heart") on one side and "828" on the other.

Duet® Chewable:
Duet® Chewable is a orange heart-shaped prenatal multi-vitamin and multi-mineral chewable tablet imprinted with the StuartNatal® logo ("heart-in-a-heart") on one side and "83" on the other.

Duet® DHA
Duet® DHA is a prescription regimen of prenatal multi-vitamin, multi-mineral, and omega-3 fatty acid supplements. Supplied as tablets and softgel capsules. Duet® is a yellow oval tablet imprinted with the StuartNatal® logo ("heart-in-a-heart") on one side and "828" on the other. The DHA softgel capsule is a translucent golden-colored oval softgel capsule imprinted with the StuartNatal® logo ("heart-in-a-heart").

HOW SUPPLIED

Duet® Tablet:
NDC 66479-828-01, bottle of 100 tablets.

Duet® Chewable:
NDC 66479-830-90, bottle of 90 chewable tablets.

Duet® DHA
NDC 66479-840-30. Duet DHA is supplied in child-resistant, unit-dose blister cards containing 6 Duet® tablets and 6 DHA softgel capsules per card. Each unit-of-use dispensing carton contains 5 unit-dose cards which is a 30-day supply.

HYCET ℂ ℞
[hi'-sĕt]
hydrocodone bitartrate and acetaminophen oral solution
7.5 mg/325 mg per 15 mL

DESCRIPTION

Hydrocodone bitartrate and acetaminophen is supplied in liquid form for oral administration.

HOW SUPPLIED

Hycet (hydrocodone bitartrate and acetaminophen oral solution), is a red-colored, tropical fruit punch flavored liquid containing hydrocodone bitartrate (WARNING: may be habit-forming) 7.5 mg and acetaminophen 325 mg per 15 mL, with 7% alcohol. It is supplied in containers of one pint (473 mL).
NDC 66479-574-16

URIMAX® ℞
[yur' i-măx]
URINARY ANTISEPTIC

DESCRIPTION

URIMAX® Enteric (delayed-release) film-coated tablets for oral administration.
Each tablet contains:

Methenamine	81.60 mg
Sodium Biphosphate	40.80 mg
Phenyl Salicylate	36.20 mg
Methylene Blue	10.80 mg
Hyoscyamine Sulfate	0.12 mg

HOW SUPPLIED

URIMAX® are round, magenta, enteric film-coated tablets, imprinted with logo **"URIMAX"** in black.
NDC 66479-860-01 Bottles of 100

ZLB Behring
1020 FIRST AVENUE
KING OF PRUSSIA, PA 19406-0901

Direct Inquiries to:
(610) 878-4000

For Medical Information Contact:
(800) 504-5434

Sales and Ordering:
Customer Support Center
(800) 683-1288
Fax: (610) 878-4888

CARIMUNE™ NF Nanofiltered ℞
[ka-ri-mewn]
Immune Globulin Intravenous (Human)
Lyophilized Preparation
Rx only

DESCRIPTION

Immune Globulin Intravenous (Human) (IGIV), Carimune™ NF Nanofiltered, is a sterile, highly purified polyvalent antibody product containing in concentrated form all the IgG antibodies which regularly occur in the donor population (1). This immunoglobulin preparation is produced by cold alcohol fractionation from the plasma of US donors. Part of the fractionation may be performed by another US-licensed manufacturer. Carimune™ NF is made suitable for intravenous use by treatment at acid pH in the presence of trace amounts of pepsin (2,3). The manufacturing process by which Carimune™ NF is prepared from plasma consists of fractionation and purification steps that comprise filtrations in the presence of filter aids. Four of these steps were validated for virus elimination of both enveloped and non-enveloped viruses. To complement the existing virus elimination / inactivation mechanism in the Carimune™ NF manufacturing process, nanofiltration (removing viruses via size-exclusion) was introduced as an additional virus removal step into the manufacturing process (4,5). Nanofiltration is performed prior to the viral inactivation step (pH 4 in presence of pepsin) in order to reduce the potential viral load before inactivation is performed. Treatment with pepsin at pH4 rapidly inactivates enveloped viruses (6).

The Carimune™ NF manufacturing process provides a significant viral reduction in in vivo studies. These studies results are summarized in Table 1, demonstrate virus clearance during Carimune™ NF manufacturing using model viruses for lipid enveloped and non-enveloped viruses. The LRFs (log10 reduction factors) from nanofiltration, and viral elimination and inactivation steps were:

[See table 1 at top of next page]

The preparation contains at least 96% of IgG and after reconstitution with a neutral unbuffered diluent has a pH of 6.6 ± 0.2. Most of the immunoglobulins are monomeric (7 S) IgG; the remainder consists of dimeric IgG and a small amount of polymeric IgG, traces of IgA and IgM and immunoglobulin fragments (7). The distribution of the IgG subclasses corresponds to that of normal serum (8,9,10,11). Final container lyophilized units are prepared so as to contain 1, 3, 6, or 12 g protein with 1.67 g sucrose and less than 20 mg NaCl per gram of protein. The lyophilized preparation contains no preservative and may be reconstituted with sterile water, 5% dextrose or 0.9% saline to a solution with protein concentrations ranging from 3% to 12% (see Table 3). The patient's fluid, electrolyte, caloric requirements and renal function should be considered in selecting an appropriate diluent and concentration.

Table 2
Calculated Carimune™ NF Osmolality (mOsm/kg)

	Concentration			
Diluent	3%	6%	9%	12%
0.9% NaCl	498	690	882	1074
5% Dextrose	444	636	828	1020
Sterile Water	192	384	576	768

CLINICAL PHARMACOLOGY

Carimune™ NF Nanofiltered contains a broad spectrum of antibody specificities against bacterial, viral, parasitic, and mycoplasma antigens, that are capable of both opsonization and neutralization of microbes and toxins. The 3 week half-life of Immune Globulin Intravenous (Human), Carimune™ NF, corresponds to that of Immune Globulin (Human) for intramuscular use, although individual variations in half-life have been observed (12,13). Appropriate doses of Carimune™ NF restore abnormally low immunoglobulin G levels to the normal range. One hundred percent of the infused dose of IGIV-products is available in the recipient's circulation immediately after infusion. After approximately 6 days, equilibrium is reached between the intra- and extravascular compartments, with immunoglobulin G being distributed approximately 50% intravascular and 50% extravascular. In comparison, after the intramuscular injection of immune globulin, the IgG requires 2-5 days to reach its maximum concentration in the intravascular compartment. This concentration corresponds to about 40% of the injected dose (13).

While Carimune™ NF has been shown to be effective in some cases of Immune Thrombocytopenic Purpura (ITP) (see INDICATIONS AND USAGE), the mechanism of action in ITP has not been fully elucidated. Toxicity from overdose has not been observed on regimens of 0.4 g/kg body weight each day for 5 days (14,15,16). Sucrose is added to Carimune™ NF for reasons of stability and solubility. Since sucrose is excreted unchanged in the urine when given intravenously, Carimune™ NF, may be given to diabetics without compensatory changes in insulin dosage regimen. Please see WARNINGS section.

INDICATIONS AND USAGE

Immunodeficiency
Immune Globulin Intravenous (Human), Carimune™ NF, is indicated for the maintenance treatment of patients with primary immunodeficiencies (PID), e.g., common variable immunodeficiency, X-linked agammaglobulinemia, severe combined immunodeficiency (15,17,18,19). Carimune™ NF is preferable to intramuscular Immune Globulin (Human) preparations in treating patients who require an immediate and large increase in the intravascular immunoglobulin level (13), in patients with limited muscle mass, and in patients with bleeding tendencies for whom intramuscular injections are contraindicated. The infusions must be repeated at regular intervals. Please see DOSAGE AND ADMINISTRATION section.

Immune Thrombocytopenic Purpura (ITP)
Acute
A controlled study was performed in children in which Immune Globulin Intravenous (Human), Carimune™, was compared with steroids for the treatment of acute (defined as less than 6 months duration) ITP. In this study sequential platelet levels of 30,000, 100,000, and 150,000/μL were all achieved faster with Carimune™ than with steroids and without any of the side effects associated with steroids (14,20). However, it should be noted that many cases of acute ITP in childhood resolve spontaneously within weeks to months. Carimune™ has been used with good results in the treatment of acute ITP in adult patients (21,22,23). In a study involving 10 adults with ITP of less than 16 weeks duration, Carimune™ therapy raised the platelet count to the normal range after a 5 day course. This effect lasted a mean of over 173 days, ranging from 30 to 372 days (24).

Chronic

Children and adults with chronic (defined as greater than 6 months duration) ITP have also shown an increase (sometimes temporary) in platelet counts upon administration of Immune Globulin Intravenous (Human), Carimune™, (20,24,25,26,27,28). Therefore, in situations that require a rapid rise in platelet count, for example prior to surgery or to control excessive bleeding, use of Carimune™ should be considered. In children with chronic ITP, Carimune™ therapy resulted in a mean rise in platelet count of 312,000/μL with a duration of increase ranging from 2 to 6 months (25,28). Carimune™ therapy may be considered as a means to defer or avoid splenectomy (27,28,29). In adults, Carimune™ therapy has been shown to be effective in maintaining the platelet count in an acceptable range with or without periodic booster therapy. The mean rise in platelet count was 93,000/μL and the average duration of the increase was 20–24 days (24,25). However, it should be noted that not all patients will respond. Even in those patients who do respond, this treatment should not be considered to be curative.

CONTRAINDICATIONS

As with all blood products containing IgA, Immune Globulin Intravenous (Human), Carimune™ NF, is contra-indicated in patients with selective IgA deficiency, who possess antibody to IgA. It may also be contraindicated in patients who have had severe systemic reactions to the intravenous or intramuscular administration of human immune globulin.

WARNINGS

Immune Globulin Intravenous (Human) (IGIV) products have been reported to be associated with renal dysfunction, acute renal failure, osmotic nephrosis, and death (30,31,32,33,34,35). Patients predisposed to acute renal failure include patients with:

1. any degree of pre-existing renal insufficiency
2. diabetes mellitus
3. age greater than 65
4. volume depletion
5. sepsis
6. paraproteinemia
7. patients receiving known nephrotoxic drugs

In such patients, IGIV products should be administered at the minimum concentration available and the minimum rate of infusion practicable. While these reports of renal dysfunction and acute renal failure have been associated with the use of many of the licensed IGIV products, those containing sucrose as a stabilizer accounted for a disproportionate share of the total number. See PRECAUTIONS and DOSAGE AND ADMINISTRATION sections for important information intended to reduce the risk of acute renal failure.

Immune Globulin Intravenous (Human), Carimune™ NF, is made from human plasma. Products made from human plasma may contain infectious agents, such as viruses, that can cause disease. The risk that such products will transmit an infectious agent has been reduced by screening plasma donors for prior exposure to certain viruses, by testing for the presence of certain current virus infections, and through the application of viral elimination/reduction steps such as alcohol fractionation in the presence of filter aids, nanofiltration and pH4/pepsin treatment (4,5,6; see Table 1). Despite these measures, such products may carry a risk of transmitting infectious agents, e.g., viruses, and theoretically, the Creutzfeldt-Jakob disease (CJD) agent. There is also the possibility that unknown infectious agents may be present in such products. ALL infections thought by a physician possibly to have been transmitted by this product should be reported by the physician or other healthcare provider to ZLB Bioplasma Inc., Tel. no: 866 244 29 52. The physician should discuss the risks and benefits of this product with the patient.

Patients with agamma- or extreme hypogammaglobulinemia who have never before received immunoglobulin substitution treatment or whose time from last treatment is greater than 8 weeks, may be at risk of developing inflammatory reactions on rapid infusion (greater than 1 mL per minute) of Immune Globulin Intravenous (Human), Carimune™ NF. These reactions are manifested by a rise in temperature, chills, nausea, and vomiting. The patient's vital signs should be monitored continuously. The patient should be carefully observed throughout the infusion, since these reactions on rare occasions may lead to shock. Epinephrine should be available for treatment of an acute anaphylactic reaction.

PRECAUTIONS

Please see DOSAGE AND ADMINISTRATION below, for important information on Immune Globulin Intravenous (Human), Carimune™ NF, compatibility with other medications or fluids. Patients should not be volume depleted prior to the initiation of the infusion of IGIV. Periodic monitoring of renal function tests and urine output is particularly important in patients judged to have a potential increased risk for developing acute renal failure. Renal function, including measurement of blood urea nitrogen (BUN) and serum creatinine, should be assessed prior to the initial infusion of Carimune™ NF and again at appropriate intervals thereafter. If renal function deteriorates, discontinuation of the product should be considered. For patients judged to be at risk for developing renal dysfunction, it may be prudent to reduce the amount of product infused per unit time by infusing Carimune™ NF at a rate less than 2 mg/kg/min.

Table 1
Viral Elimination and Inactivation

Virus	**HIV**	**BVDV**	**PRV**	**SFV**	**SV**	**BEV**
Genome	RNA	RNA	DNA	RNA	RNA	RNA
Envelope	Yes	Yes	Yes	Yes	Yes	No
Size (nm)	80-100	40-60	120-200	50-70	50-70	28-30
Fractionation&						
Depth filtration	15.5	nt	16.0	9.3	12.4	14.1
pH 4 / pepsin	> 6.1	> 4.4	> 5.3	> 6.8	nt	nt
Nanofiltration	> 4.9	> 4.5	> 4.4	nt	> 7.5	> 5.1
Overall reduction	> 26	> 9	> 25	> 16	> 19	> 19

HIV: Human immunodeficiency virus, model for HIV 1 and HIV 2
BVDV: Bovine viral diarrhea virus, model for HCV (Hepatitis C virus)
PRV: Pseudorabies virus, model for large, enveloped DNA viruses (e,g., herpes virus)
SFV: Semliki Forest virus, model for HCV
SV: Sindbis virus, model for HCV
BEV: Bovine enterovirus, model for HAV (Hepatitis A virus)
Nt: not tested
PRV and the two model viruses for HCV, BVDV and SFV, were inactivated within 1/10, and HIV within 1/2 of the incubation time (pH 4/pepsin treatment) used during production of Carimune™ NF.

Information for Patients

Patients should be instructed to immediately report symptoms of decreased urine output, sudden weight gain, fluid retention/edema, and/or shortness of breath (which may suggest kidney damage) to their physicians.

Pregnancy Category C

Animal reproduction studies have not been conducted with Immune Globulin Intravenous (Human), Carimune™ NF. It is also not known whether Carimune™ NF can cause fetal harm when administered to a pregnant woman or can affect reproduction capacity. Carimune™ NF should be given to a pregnant woman only if clearly needed (23). Intact immune globulins such as those contained in Carimune™ NF cross the placenta from maternal circulation increasingly after 30 weeks gestation (36,37). In cases of maternal ITP where Carimune™ NF was administered to the mother prior to delivery, the platelet response and clinical effect were similar in the mother and neonate (23,37-46).

Pediatric Use

High dose administration of Immune Globulin Intravenous (Human), Carimune™, in pediatric patients with acute or chronic Immune Thrombocytopenic Purpura did not reveal any pediatric-specific hazard (14). Antibodies in Immune Globulin Intravenous (Human) may impair the efficacy of live attenuated viral vaccines such as measles, rubella, and mumps (47,48,49). Immunizing physicians should be informed of recent therapy with Immune Globulin Intravenous (Human) so that appropriate precautions may be taken.

Aseptic Meningitis Syndrome

An aseptic meningitis syndrome (AMS) has been reported to occur infrequently in association with Immune Globulin Intravenous (Human) (IGIV) treatment. The syndrome usually begins within several hours to two days following IGIV treatment. It is characterized by symptoms and signs including severe headache, nuchal rigidity, drowsiness, fever, photophobia, painful eye movements, and nausea and vomiting. Cerebrospinal fluid (CSF) studies are frequently positive with pleocytosis. Patients exhibiting such symptoms and signs should receive a thorough neurological examination, including CSF studies, to rule out other causes of meningitis. AMS may occur more frequently in association with high dose (2 g/kg) IGIV treatment. Discontinuation of IGIV treatment has resulted in remission of AMS within several days without sequelae.

ADVERSE REACTIONS

Increases in creatinine and blood urea nitrogen (BUN) have been observed as soon as one to two days following infusion. Progression to oliguria or anuria, requiring dialysis has been observed. Types of severe renal adverse events that have been seen following IGIV therapy include: acute renal failure, acute tubular necrosis, proximal tubular nephropathy and osmotic nephrosis (30-35,50,60-62).Inflammatory adverse reactions have been described in agammaglobulinemic and hypogammaglobulinemic patients who have never received immunoglobulin substitution therapy before or in patients whose time from last treatment is greater than 8 weeks and whose initial infusion rate exceeds 1 mL per minute.

This occurs in approximately 10% of such cases. Such reactions may also be observed in some patients during chronic substitution therapy. These reactions, which generally become apparent only 30 minutes to 1 hour after the beginning of the infusion, are as follows: flushing of the face, feelings of tightness in the chest, chills, fever, dizziness, nausea, diaphoresis, and hypotension. In such cases the infusion should be temporarily stopped until the symptoms have subsided. Immediate anaphylactoid and hypersensitivity reactions due to previous sensitization of the recipient to certain antigens, most commonly IgA, may be observed in exceptional cases, described under CONTRAINDICATIONS (15,16,51). In patients with ITP, who receive higher doses (0.4 g/kg/day or greater), 2.9% of infusions may result in adverse reactions (20). Headache, generally mild, is the most common symptom noted, occurring during or following 2% of infusions. A few cases of usually mild hemolysis have been reported after infusion of intravenous immunoglobulin products (52,53). These were attributed to transferral of blood group (e.g., anti-D) antibodies (54,55).

DOSAGE AND ADMINISTRATION

It is generally advisable not to dilute plasma derivatives with other infusable drugs. Immune Globulin Intravenous (Human), Carimune™ NF, should be given by a separate infusion line. No other medications or fluids should be mixed with Carimune™ NF preparation.

Carimune™ NF should be used with caution in patients with pre-existing renal insufficiency and in patients judged to be at increased risk of developing renal insufficiency (including, but not limited to those with diabetes mellitus, age greater than 65, volume depletion, paraproteinemia, sepsis, and patients receiving known nephrotoxic drugs). In these cases especially it is important to assure that patients are not volume depleted prior to Carimune™ NF infusion. No prospective data are presently available to identify a maximum safe dose, concentration, and rate of infusion in patients determined to be at increased risk of acute renal failure. In the absence of prospective data, recommended doses should not be exceeded and the concentration and infusion rate selected should be the minimum practicable. The product should be infused at a rate less than 2 mg/kg/min.

Adult and Child Substitution Therapy

The usual dose of Immune Globulin Intravenous (Human), Carimune™ NF in immunodeficiency syndromes is 0.2 g/kg of body weight administered once a month by intravenous infusion. If the clinical response is inadequate, the dose may be increased to 0.3 g/kg of body weight or the infusion may be repeated more frequently than once a month (15,17,18,19).

The first infusion of Carimune™ NF in previously untreated agammaglobulinemic or hypogammaglobulinemic patients must be given as a 3% immunoglobulin solution (use the total volume of fluid provided, or see Table 3, to reconstitute the lyophilized product).

1. Start with a flow rate of 10-20 drops (0.5-1.0 mL) per minute.
2. After 15-30 minutes the rate of infusion may be further increased to 30-50 drops (1.5-2.5 mL) per minute.
3. After the first bottle of 3% solution is infused and the patient shows good tolerance, subsequent infusions may be administered at a higher rate or concentration. Such increases should be made gradually allowing 15-30 minutes before each increment.

The first infusion of Carimune™ NF in previously untreated agammaglobulinemic and hypogammaglobulinemic patients may lead to systemic side effects. The nature of these effects has not been fully elucidated. Some of them may be due to the release of proinflammatory cytokines by activated macrophages in immunodeficient recipients (56,57). Subsequent administration of Carimune™ NF to immunodeficient patients as well as to normal individuals usually does not cause further untoward side effects.

Therapy of Idiopathic Thrombocytopenic Purpura (ITP)

Induction

0.4 g/kg of body weight on 2–5 consecutive days.

Acute ITP-Childhood

In acute ITP of childhood, if an initial platelet count response to the first two doses is adequate (30–50,000/μL), therapy may be discontinued after the second day of the 5 day course (20).

Maintenance-Chronic ITP

In adults and children, if after induction therapy the platelet count falls to less than 30,000/μL and/or the patient manifests clinically significant bleeding, 0.4 g/kg of body weight may be given as a single infusion. If an adequate response does not result, the dose can be increased to 0.8-1.0 g/kg of body weight given as a single infusion (21,58,59).

Continued on next page

Carimune NF—Cont.

Reconstitution
(see also pictures next page)

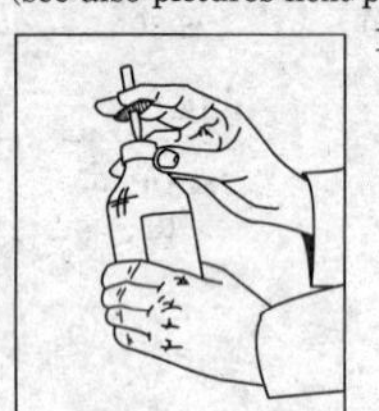

1. Remove the protective plastic caps from the lyophilisate and diluent bottles and disinfect both rubber stoppers with alcohol. Remove the protective cover from one end of the transfer set and insert the exposed needle through the rubber stopper into the bottle containing the diluent.

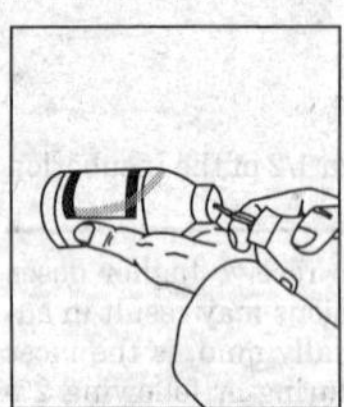

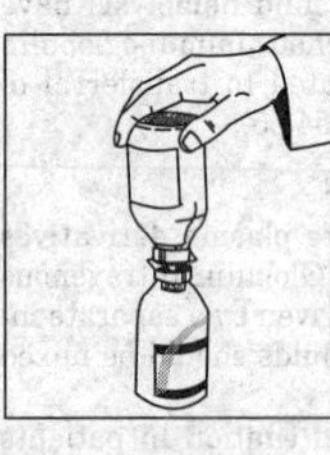

2. and 3. Remove the second protective cover from the other end of the transfer set. Grasp both bottles as shown in picture 2, quickly plunge the diluent bottle onto the lyophilisate bottle and bring the bottles into an upright position. Only if this is done quickly and the bottles are immediately brought into an upright position can the vacuum in the lyophilisate bottle be maintained, thus speeding up reconstitution and facilitating the transfer. Allow the diluent to flow into the lyophilisate bottle.

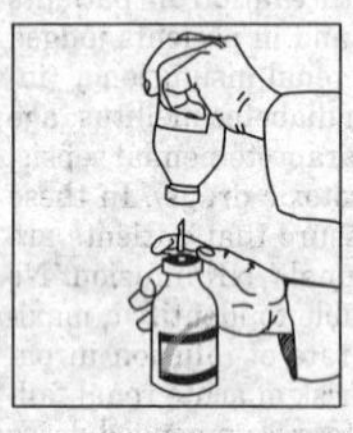

4. Once the appropriate amount of diluent is transferred (see Table 3), lift the diluent bottle off the spike to release the vacuum. This will reduce foaming and facilitate dissolution. Remove the spike.

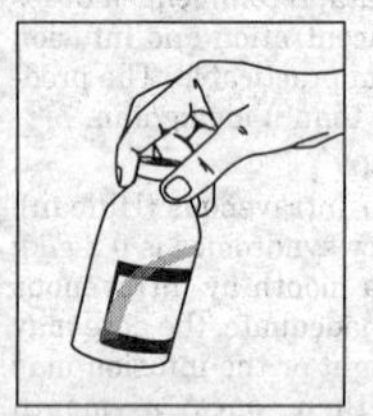

5. Swirl vigorously but do not shake, otherwise a foam will form which is very slow to subside. The lyophilisate dissolves within a few minutes.

To reconstitute Carimune™ NF from the individual vial package, or when using other diluents or higher concentrations, Table 3 indicates the volume of sterile diluent required. Observing aseptic technique, this volume should be drawn into a sterile hypodermic syringe and needle. The diluent is then injected into the corresponding Carimune™ NF vial size.

Table 3
Required Diluent Volume*

Concentration	1g Vial	3g Vial	6g Vial	12g Vial
3%	33.0cc	100cc	200cc	**
6%	16.5cc	50cc	100cc	200cc
9%	11.0cc	33cc	66cc	132cc
12%	8.3cc	25cc	50cc	100cc

* In patients judged to be at increased risk of developing renal insufficiency, the concentration and infusion rate of Carimune™ NF should be the minimum practicable.
**Container not large enough to permit this concentration.

If large doses of Carimune™ NF are to be administered, several reconstituted vials of identical concentration and diluent may be pooled in an empty sterile glass or plastic i.v. infusion container using aseptic technique. Carimune™ NF normally dissolves within a few minutes, though in exceptional cases it may take up to 20 minutes.

DO NOT SHAKE! Excessive shaking will cause foaming.

Any undissolved particles should respond to careful rotation of the bottle. Avoid foaming. Parenteral drug products should be inspected visually for particulate matter and discoloration prior to administration, whenever solution and container permit. Filtering of Carimune™ NF is acceptable but not required. Pore sizes of 15 microns or larger will be less likely to slow infusion, especially with higher Carimune™ NF concentrations. Antibacterial filters (0.2 microns) may be used. When reconstitution of Carimune™ NF occurs outside of sterile laminar air flow conditions, administration must begin promptly with partially used vials discarded. When reconstitution is carried out in a sterile laminar flow hood using aseptic technique, administration may begin within 24 hours provided the solution has been refrigerated during that time. Do not freeze Carimune™ NF solution.

PROCEED WITH INFUSION ONLY IF SOLUTION IS CLEAR AND AT APPROXIMATELY ROOM TEMPERATURE!

HOW SUPPLIED

Immune Globulin Intravenous (Human), Carimune™ NF Nanofiltered is available as a white lyophilized powder in 1, 3, 6 and 12 g size vials. The only diluents which may be used to reconstitute the product are sterile (0.9%) Sodium Chloride Injection USP, 5% Dextrose, or Sterile Water.

Carimune™ NF is available in individual vial packages.

1g Individual vial package (NDC 44206-415-01)
3g Individual vial package (NDC 44206-416-03)
6g Individual vial package (NDC 44206-417-06)
12g Individual vial package (NDC 44206-418-12)

Please see Table 2 for Calculated Carimune™ NF Osmolality (mOsmol/kg).

Store and Dispense

Immune Globulin Intravenous (Human), Carimune™ NF, should be stored at room temperature not exceeding 30 °C (86 °F). The preparation should not be used after the expiration date printed on the label.

REFERENCES

1. Gardi A: Quality control in the production of an immunoglobulin for intravenous use. Blut 1984; 48:337-344.
2. Römer J, Morgenthaler JJ, Scherz R, et al: Characterization of various immunoglobulin-preparations for intravenous application. I. Protein composition and antibody content. Vox Sang 1982; 42:62-73.
3. Römer J, Späth PJ, Skvaril F, et al: Characterization of various immunoglobulin preparations for intravenous application. II. Complement activation and binding to Staphylococcus protein A. Vox Sang 1982; 42:74-80.
4. Omar A, and Kempf C: Removal of neutralized model Parvoviruses and Enteroviruses in human IgG solutions by nanofiltration. Transfusion, in press (2002).
5. Späth P, Kempf C, and Gold R: Herstellung, Verträglichkeit und Virussicherheit von intravenösem Immunglobulin. In «Immunglobuline in der Neurobiologie» (P. Berlit, ed.), Steinkopff Verlag, Darmstadt, BRD, 2001, pp 1-42.
6. Kempf C, Morgenthaler JJ, Rentsch M, and Omar A: Viral safety and manufacturing of an intravenous immunoglobulin. In «Intravenous Immunoglobulin Research and Therapy» Kazatchkine and Morell, eds. Parthenon Publishing Group. 1996, pp. 11-18.
7. Römer J, Späth PJ: Molecular composition of immunoglobulin preparations and its relation to complement activation, in Nydegger UE (ed): Immunohemotherapy: A Guide to Immunoglobulin Prophylaxis and Therapy. London, Academic Press, 1981, pp 123-130.
8. Skvaril F, Roth-Wicky B, and Barandun S: IgG subclasses in human-g-globulin preparations for intravenous use and their reactivity with Staphylococcus protein A. Vox Sang 1980; 38:147.
9. Skvaril F: Qualitative and quantitative aspects of IgG subclasses in i.v. immunoglobulin preparations, in Nydegger UE (ed): Immunohemotherapy: A Guide to Immunoglobulin Prophylaxis and Therapy. London, Academic Press, 1981, pp 113-122.
10. Skvaril F, and Barandun S: In vitro characterization of immunoglobulins for intravenous use, in Alving BM, Finlayson JS (eds): Immunoglobulins: Characteristics and Uses of Intravenous Preparations, DHHS Publication No. (FDA)-80-9005. US Government Printing Office, 1980, pp 201-206.
11. Burckhardt JJ, Gardi A, Oxelius V, et al: Immunoglobulin G subclass distribution in three human intravenous immunoglobulin preparations. Vox Sang 1989; 57:10-14.
12. Morell A, and Skvaril F: Struktur und biologische Eigenschaften von Immunoglobulinen und g-Globulin-Präparaten. II. Eigenschaften von g-Globulin-Präparaten. Schweiz Med Wochenschr 1980; 110:80.
13. Morell A, Schürch B, Ryser D, et al: In vivo behaviour of gamma globulin preparations. Vox Sang 1980; 38:272.
14. Imbach P, Barandun S, d'Apuzzo V, et al: High-dose intravenous gamma globulin for idiopathic thrombocytopenic purpura in childhood. Lancet 1981; 1:1228.
15. Barandun S, Morell A, Skvaril F: Clinical experiences with immunoglobulin for intravenous use, in Alving BM, Finlayson JS (eds): Immunoglobulins: Characteristics and Uses of Intravenous Preparations. DHHS Publication No. (FDA)-80-9005. US Government Printing Office, 1980, pp 31-35.
16. Schiff R, Sedlak D, Buckley R: Rapid infusion of Sandoglobulin® in patients with primary humoral immunodeficiency. J Allergy Clin Immunol, 88:61, 1991.
17. Joller PW, Barandun S, Hitzig WH: Neue Möglichkeiten der Immunoglobulin-Ersatztherapie bei Antikörpermangel. Syndrom. Schweiz Med Wochenschr 1980; 110: 1451.
18. Barandun S, Imbach P, Morell A, et al: Clinical indications for immunoglobulin infusion, in Nydegger UE (ed): Immunohemotherapy: A Guide to Immunoglobulin Prophylaxis and Therapy. London, Academic Press, 1981, pp 275-282.
19. Cunningham-Rundles C, Smithwick EM, Siegal FP, et al: Treatment of primary humoral immunodeficiency disease with intravenous (pH 4.0 treated) gamma globulin, in Nydegger UE (ed): Guide to Immunoglobulin Prophylaxis and Therapy. London, Academic Press, 1981, pp 283-290.
20. Imbach P, Wagner HP, Berchtold W, et al: Intravenous immunoglobulin versus oral corticosteroids in acute immune thrombocytopenic purpura in childhood. Lancet 1985; 2:464.
21. Fehr J, Hofmann V, Kappeler U: Transient reversal of thrombocytopenia in idiopathic thrombocytopenic purpura by high-dose intravenous gamma globulin. N Engl J Med 1982; 306:1254.
22. Müller-Eckhardt C, Küenzlen E, Thilo-Körner D, et al: High-dose intravenous immunoglobulin for posttransfusion purpura. N Engl J Med 1983; 308:287.
23. Wenske G, Gaedicke G, Küenzlen E, et al: Treatment of idiopathic thrombocytopenic purpura in pregnancy by high-dose intravenous immunoglobulin. Blut 1983; 46: 347-353.
24. Newland AC, Treleaven JG, Minchinton B, et al: High-dose intravenous IgG in adults with autoimmune thrombocytopenia. Lancet 1983; 1:84-87.
25. Bussel JB, Kimberly RP, Inman RD, et al: Intravenous gammaglobulin for chronic idiopathic thrombocytopenic purpura. Blood 1983; 62:480-486.
26. Abe T, Matsuda J, Kawasugi K, et al: Clinical effect of intravenous immunoglobulin in chronic idiopathic thrombocytopenic purpura. Blut 1983; 47:69-75.
27. Bussel JB, Schulman I, Hilgartner MW, et al: Intravenous use of gamma globulin in the treatment of chronic immune thrombocytopenic purpura as a means to defer splenectomy. J Pediatr 1983; 103:651-654.
28. Imholz B, et al: Intravenous immunoglobulin (i.v. IgG) for previously treated acute or for chronic idiopathic thrombocytopenic purpura (ITP) in childhood: A prospective multicenter study. Blut 1988; 56:63-68.
29. Lusher JM, and Warrier I: Use of intravenous gamma globulin in children with idiopathic thrombocytopenic purpura and other immune thrombocytopenias. Am J Med 1987; 83 (suppl 4A):10-16.
30. Winward DB, Brophy MT: Acute renal failure after administration of intravenous immunoglobulin: Review of the literature and case report. Pharmacotherapy 1995; 15: 765-772.
31. Cantú TG, Hoehn-Saric EW, Burgess KM, Racusen L, Scheel P: Acute renal failure associated with immunoglobulin therapy. Am J. Kidney Dis. 1995; 25:228-234.
32. Cayco AV, Perazelly Ma, Hayslett JP: Renal insufficiency after intravenous immune globulin therapy: A Report of Two Cases and an Analysis of the Literature. J. Amer. Soc Nephrology. 1997; 8:1788-1793.
33. Rault R, Pirano B, Johston J, Oral A: Pulmonary and renal toxicity of intravenous immunoglobulin. Clin Nephrol: 1991, 36:83-86.
34. Michail S, Nakopoulou L, Stravrianopoulos I, Stamatiadis D, Avdikou K, Vaiopoulos G, Stathakis C: Acute renal failure associated with immunoglobulin administration. Nephrol Dial Transpalant. 1997; 12:1497-99.
35. Ashan N, Wiegand LA, Abendroth CS, Manning EC: Acute renal failure following immunoglobulin therapy. Am J Nephrol. 1996; 16:532-6.
36. Hammarstrom L, and Smith CI: Placental transfer of intravenous immunoglobulin. Lancet 1986; 1:681.
37. Sidiropoulos D, et al: Transplacental passage of intravenous immunoglobulin in the last trimester of pregnancy. J Pediatr 1986; 109:505-508.
38. Wenske G, et al: Idiopathic thrombocytopenic purpura in pregnancy and neonatal period. Blut 1984; 48:377-382.
39. Fabris P, et al: Successful treatment of a steroid-resistant form of idiopathic thrombocytopenic purpura in pregnancy with high doses of intravenous immunoglobulins. Acta Haemat 1987; 77:107-110.
40. Coller BS, et al: Management of severe ITP during pregnancy with intravenous immunoglobulin (IVIgG). Clin Res 1985; 33:545A.
41. Tchernia G, et al: Management of immune thrombocytopenia in pregnancy: Response to infusions of immunoglobulins. Am J Obstet Gynecol 1984; 148:225-226.
42. Newland AC, et al: Intravenous IgG for autoimmune thrombocytopenia in pregnancy. N Engl J Med 1984; 310:261-262.
43. Morgenstern GR, et al: Autoimmune thrombocytopenia in pregnancy: New approach to management. Br Med J 1983; 287:584.
44. Ciccimarra F, et al: Treatment of neonatal passive immune thrombocytopenia. J Pediat 1984; 105:677-678.
45. Rose VL, and Gordon LI: Idiopathic thrombocytopenic purpura in pregnancy. Successful management with immunoglobulin infusion. JAMA 1985; 254: 2626-2628.
46. Gounder MP, et al: Intravenous gammaglobulin therapy in the management of a patient with idiopathic thrombocytopenic purpura and a warm autoimmune erythrocyte panagglutinin during pregnancy. Obstet Gynecol 1986; 67:741-746.
47. Siber GR, Werner BG, Halsey NA, et al: Interference of immune globulin with measles and rubella immunisation. J. Pediatr. 1993; 122:204-211.
48. American Academy of Pediatrics, Committee on Infectious Diseases: Recommended timing of routine measles immunization for children who have recently received immune globulin preparations. Pediatrics 1994; 93:682-685.
49. Centers of Disease Control and Prevention Measles, mumps, and rubella-vaccine use and strategies for elimination of measles, rubella, and congenital rubella syndrome and control of mumps: recommendations of the

advisory commitee on immunization practices (ACIP). MMWR, Morbidity and Mortality Weekly Report. May 22, 1998; vol 47/No. RR-8, 1-57.
50. Phillips AO: Renal failure and intravenous immunoglobulin [letter; comment]. Clin Nephrol 1992; 36: 83-86.
51. Cunningham-Rundles C, Day NK, Wahn V, et al: Reactions to intravenous gamma globulin infusions and immune complex formation, in Nydegger UE (ed): Immunohemotherapy: A Guide to Immunoglobulin Prophylaxis and Therapy. London, Academic Press, 1981, pp 447-449.
52. Brox AG, Cournoyer D, et al: Hemolytic anemia following intravenous gamma globulin administration. Am J. Med. 1987; 82:633-635.
53. Kim HC, Park CL, Cowan JH, et al: Massive intravascular hemolysis associated with intravenous immunoglobulin in bone marrow transplant recipients. Am J. Ped. Hematol/Oncol 1988; 10:67-74.
54. Nicholls MD, Cummins JC, et al: Haemolysis induced by intravenously-administered immunoglobulin. Med J of Australia 1989; 150:404-406.
55. Copelan EA et al: Hemolysis following intravenous immune globulin therapy. Transfusion 1986; 26:410-412.
56. Aukrust P, Froland SS, N-B Liabakk, F. Müller, et al: Release of cytokines, soluble cytokine receptors, and interleukin-1 receptor antagonist after intravenous immunoglobulin administration in vivo. Blood 1994; 84: 2136-2143.
57. Bagdasarian A, Tonetta S, Harel W, Mamidi R. Uemura Y: IVIG adverse reactions: potential role of cytokines and vasoactive substances. Vox Sang 1998; 74:74-82.
58. Bussel JB, Pham LC, Hilgartner MW, et al: Long-term maintenance of adults with ITP using intravenous gamma globulin. Abstract, America Society of Hematology. New Orleans, December, 1985.
59. Imbach PA, Kühne T, Holländer G: Immunologic aspects in the pathogenesis and treatment of immune thrombocytopenic purpura in children. Current opinion in Pediatrics 1997; 9:35-40.
60. Anderson W, Bethea W: Renal lesions following administration of hypertonic solutions of sucrose. JAMA. 1940; 114:1983-1987.
61. Lindberg H, Wald A: Renal lesions following the administration of hypertonic solutions: Arch Intern Med. 1939; 63:907-918.
62. Rigdon RH, Cardwell ES: Renal lesions following the intravenous injection of hypertonic solution of sucrose: A clinical and experimental study. Arch Intern Med. 1942; 69:670-690.

Manufactured by:
ZLB Bioplasma AG
Wankdorfstrasse 10, 3000 Berne 22
Switzerland
US License No. 1598
Distributed by:
ZLB Bioplasma Inc.
Glendale, California 91203, USA
February 2003
R&W 02.03 20'000
04354/163

RHOPHYLAC® ℞

[rō-fī-lăk]

Rh_o(D) Immune Globulin Intravenous (Human)
1500 IU (300 µg)

Rx only

For Intravenous and Intramuscular Injection
Preservative free, ready to use pre-filled syringe

DESCRIPTION

Rhophylac® is a sterile Rh_o(D) Immune Globulin Intravenous (Human) solution in a prefilled, ready to use syringe for either intravenous or intramuscular injection. One syringe contains at least 1500 IU (300 µg) of IgG antibodies to Rh_o(D) in a 2 mL solution, sufficient to suppress the immune response to at least 15 mL of Rh-positive red blood cells[1]. The product potency is expressed in international units by comparison to the World Health Organization (WHO) standard, which is also the US and the European Pharmacopoeia standard[2].

Plasma donations are taken from Rh_o(D)-negative healthy donors who have been immunized with Rh_o(D)-positive red blood cells. The donors' histories have been carefully screened to reduce the risk of receipt of donations containing blood borne pathogens. Each plasma donation used for the manufacture of Rhophylac® is tested for the presence of hepatitis B virus (HBV) surface antigen (HBsAg), human immunodeficiency viruses (HIV) 1/2, and hepatitis C virus (HCV) antibodies as well as elevated alanine aminotransferase (ALT) activity. In addition, plasma used in the manufacture of this product was tested by FDA licensed Nucleic Acid Testing (NAT) for HIV and HCV and found to be negative. An investigational NAT for HBV was also performed on all Source Plasma used, and found to be negative; however, the significance of a negative result has not been established. The Source Plasma has been tested by NAT for hepatitis A virus (HAV) and parvovirus B19.

Rhophylac® is produced by an ion-exchange chromatography isolation procedure[3], using pooled plasma obtained by plasmapheresis of immunized Rh_o(D)-negative US donors. The manufacturing process includes a solvent detergent (S/D) treatment step (using tri-n-butyl phosphate and Triton® X-100) that is effective in inactivating enveloped viruses such as HBV, HCV, and HIV. Rhophylac® is nanofiltered using a Planova® 15 nm virus filter which has been validated to be effective in the removal of enveloped as well as non-enveloped viruses. Viral clearance and inactivation data from validation studies are presented below.

The donor selection criteria, testing of donations and manufacturing pools, together with purification steps and specific viral inactivation and removal steps are included to ensure the safety of this product with respect to potential contamination with blood borne pathogens.

[See table above]

Viral Inactivation and Removal

Virus	HIV	BVDV	PRV	MVM
Genome Envelope Size	RNA Yes 80-100nm	RNA YES 40-70nm	DNA YES 120-200nm	DNA No 18-24nm
S/D-treatment	≥ 6.0	≥ 5.4	≥ 5.6	Not tested
Chromatographic Process steps	4.5	1.6	≥ 3.9	≥ 2.6
Nanofiltration	≥ 6.3	≥ 5.5	≥ 5.6	3.4
Overall reduction (log_{10}units)	≥ 16.8	≥ 12.5	≥ 15.1	6.0

HIV: Model for HIV 1 and HIV 2.
BVDV: Bovine viral diarrhea virus, as a model for HCV.
PRV: Pseudorabies virus, as a model for large, enveloped DNA viruses (e.g., herpes virus).
MVM: Minute virus of mice, as a model for parvovirus B19 and other small, non-enveloped DNA viruses.

Rhophylac® contains a maximum of 30 mg/mL of human plasma proteins of which 10 mg/mL is human albumin, which is added as a stabilizer. Prior to the addition of the stabilizer, the product purity is greater than 95% IgG. The product contains less than 5 µg/mL IgA. Additional excipients are approximately 20 mg/mL of glycine and up to 0.25 M sodium chloride. Rhophylac® contains no preservative. Human albumin, added as a stabilizer, is manufactured from pooled plasma of US donors by cold ethanol fractionation, followed by pasteurization.

CLINICAL PHARMACOLOGY

Mechanism of Action

The mechanism by which Rh_o(D) Immune Globulin suppresses immunization to Rh_o(D)-positive red blood cells is not completely known. In a clinical study with Rh_o(D)-negative healthy male volunteers, both the intravenous and intramuscular administration of Rhophylac® 1500 IU (300 µg) at 24 hours after injection of 15 mL of Rh_o(D)-positive red blood cells resulted in an effective clearance of Rh_o(D)-positive red blood cells. While the intravenous administration of Rhophylac® caused an instant onset of red blood cell disappearance, the onset of elimination of red blood cells following intramuscular administration was delayed as anti-Rh_o(D) IgG had to be released from the injection site into the bloodstream. On average, 99% of injected red cells were cleared within 12 hours after intravenous administration. After intramuscular administration, a similar degree of red cell clearance was measured after 144 hours.[4]

Pharmacokinetics

In a clinical study of fourteen Rh_o(D)-negative women, a single injection of Rhophylac® 1500 IU (300 µg) was administered either intravenously or intramuscularly at week 28 of gestation and anti-Rh_o(D) IgG serum levels were measured until 11 weeks. Six women received Rhophylac® intravenously and eight women received Rhophylac® intramuscularly. Following intravenous injection in pregnant Rh_o(D)-negative women, peak serum levels ranged from 62 to 84 ng/mL after one day. The mean systemic clearance was 0.20 ± 0.03 mL/min and half-life was 16 ± 4 days.

Following intramuscular injection, peak serum concentrations of anti-Rh_o(D) IgG ranged from 7 to 46 ng/mL and were achieved between two and seven days. The mean apparent clearance was 0.29 ± 0.12 mL/min and half-life was 18 ± 5 days. The absolute bioavailability of intramuscular administration was 69%.

Regardless of the route of administration, anti-D IgG titers were measurable in all women up to at least nine weeks following administration of Rhophylac®.

INDICATION AND USAGE

Pregnancy and Obstetrical Conditions

Rhophylac® is recommended:

1. for the suppression of Rh isoimmunization in non-sensitized Rh_o(D)-negative (D-negative) women.
   The criteria for an Rh-incompatible pregnancy requiring administration of Rhophylac® at 28 to 30 weeks of gestation and within 72 hours after delivery are:
   — the mother must be Rh_o(D)-negative,
   — the mother is carrying a child whose father is either Rh_o(D)-positive or Rh_o(D) unknown,
   — the baby is either Rh_o(D)-positive or Rh_o(D) unknown, and the mother must not be previously sensitized to the Rh_o(D) factor.
2. for Rhesus prophylaxis in case of obstetric complications, e.g., miscarriage, abortion, threatened abortion, ectopic pregnancy or hydatidiform mole, transplacental hemorrhage resulting from antepartum hemorrhage.
3. for Rhesus prophylaxis in case of invasive procedures during pregnancy, e.g., amniocentesis, chorionic biopsy or obstetric manipulative procedures, e.g., external version, or abdominal trauma.

Incompatible Transfusions

Rhophylac® Rh_o(D) Immune Globulin Intravenous (Human), is recommended for the suppression of Rh isoimmunization in Rh_o(D)-negative individuals transfused with Rh_o(D)-positive RBCs or blood components containing Rh_o(D)-positive RBCs. Treatment should be initiated within 72 hours of exposure. Treatment should be given (without preceding exchange transfusion) only if the transfused Rh_o(D)-positive blood represents less than 20% of the total circulating red cells. A 1500 IU (300 µg) dose will suppress the immunizing potential of approximately 15 mL of Rh_o(D)-positive RBCs.

CLINICAL STUDIES

The efficacy, safety, tolerability and pharmacokinetics of Rhophylac® are supported by the results of two clinical studies in 446 Rh_o(D)-negative pregnant women[5,6]. In both studies, Rh_o(D)-negative women received Rhophylac® 1500 IU (300 µg) intravenously or intramuscularly in the 28th week of pregnancy. Mothers who gave birth to a Rh_o(D)-positive child received a further dose of Rhophylac® 1500 IU (300 µg) within 72 hours after the birth.

Eight out of 14 pregnant women from the above mentioned pharmacokinetic study gave birth to a Rh_o(D)-positive child and received Rhophylac® 1500 IU (300 µg) postpartum as well. The antibody tests performed 6 to 8 months later were negative for all mothers, which suggest that no Rh_o(D) immunization occurred.

In a second study at 22 centres in the United Kingdom and the USA, 432 pregnant women received Rhophylac® 1500 IU (300 µg) for antepartum rhesus prophylaxis. Two randomized groups of 216 women each received Rhophylac® 1500 IU (300 µg), either as an intravenous or intramuscular injection. Rhophylac® 1500 IU (300 µg) was also injected if there was a risk of fetomaternal hemorrhage between routine antepartum rhesus prophylaxis in the 28th week of pregnancy and birth, or if extensive fetomaternal hemorrhage was measured after birth. Of the 432 women who received Rhophylac® 1500 IU (300 µg) in the 28th week of pregnancy, 270 women delivered Rh_o(D)-positive children. 248 women were available for the investigation of Rh_o(D) immunization 6 to 11.5 months postpartum. None of those women developed antibodies against the Rh_o(D) antigen as assessed by the absence of anti-D antibodies.

CONTRAINDICATIONS

Rhophylac® is contraindicated in persons with hypersensitivity to human globulin. The concentration of IgA in Rhophylac® was found to be below the detection limit of 5 µg/mL. Nevertheless, the product may contain trace amounts of IgA. Although anti-D immunoglobulin has been used to treat selected IgA deficient individuals, the attending physician must weigh the benefit against the potential risk of hypersensitivity reactions. Individuals deficient in IgA have a potential for development of IgA antibodies and anaphylactic reactions after administration of blood components containing IgA.

WARNINGS

Rhophylac® is made from human plasma. Products made from human plasma may carry a risk of transmitting infectious agents, e.g., viruses, and theoretically, the CJD agent. The risk that such products will transmit an infectious agent has been reduced by screening plasma donors for prior exposure to certain viruses, by testing for the presence of certain current virus infections, and by inactivating and/or removing certain viruses during manufacturing. The Rhophylac® manufacturing process includes a solvent detergent treatment step (using tri-n-butyl phosphate and Triton® X-100) that is effective in inactivating enveloped viruses such as HBV, HCV, and HIV[7,8]. Rhophylac® is nanofiltered using a Planova® 15 nm virus filter that is effective in reducing the level of enveloped as well as non enveloped viruses[3]. These two processes are designed to increase product safety by reducing the risk of transmission of enveloped and non enveloped viruses, respectively. Despite these

Continued on next page

Indication	Dose (administer IM or IV)
Pregnancy	
Routine antepartum prevention (at 28 to 30 weeks of gestation)	1500 IU (300 μg)
Postpartum prevention (within 72 hrs)	1500 IU (300 μg)
Obstetric conditions	
Obstetric complications e.g. miscarriage, abortion, threatened abortion, ectopic pregnancy or hydatidiform mole, transplacental hemorrhage resulting from antepartum hemorrhage	1500 IU (300 μg)
Invasive procedures during pregnancy e.g., amniocentesis, chorionic biopsy or obstetric manipulative procedures, e.g., external version, or abdominal trauma	1500 IU (300 μg)
Incompatible transfusions	100 IU (20 μg) per 2 mL transfused blood or per 1 mL erythrocyte concentrate

Rhophylac—Cont.

measures, these products could still potentially transmit disease. There is also the possibility that unknown infectious agents may be present in such products. All infections thought by a physician possibly to have been transmitted by this product should be reported by the physician or other healthcare provider to ZLB Bioplasma Inc. at (866) 244 2952. The physician should discuss the risks and benefits of this product with the patient.

PRECAUTIONS

For postpartum use, Rhophylac® is intended for maternal administration. It should not be given to the newborn infant. The product is not intended for use in Rh_o(D)-positive individuals. Patients should be observed for at least 20 minutes after administration.

As with all pharmaceutical agents, allergic responses may occur. If symptoms of allergic or anaphylactic type reactions occur, immediately discontinue administration. Patients should be informed of the early signs of hypersensitivity reactions including hives, generalized urticaria, tightness of the chest, wheezing, hypotension and anaphylaxis. The treatment required depends on the nature and severity of the side effect. If necessary, the current medical standards for shock treatment should be observed.

The concentration of IgA in Rhophylac® was found to be below the detection limit of 5 μg/mL. Nevertheless, the product may contain trace amounts of IgA. Although anti-D immunoglobulin has been used to treat selected IgA deficient individuals, the attending physician must weigh the benefit against the potential risk of hypersensitivity reactions. Individuals deficient in IgA have a potential for development of IgA antibodies and anaphylactic reactions after administration of blood components containing IgA. Parenteral drug products should be inspected visually for particulate matter and discoloration prior to administration, whenever solution and container permit. The solution should be clear or slightly opalescent. Do not use solutions that are cloudy or have deposits.

Drug Interactions

Active immunization with live virus vaccines (e.g., measles, mumps, rubella or varicella) should be postponed until 3 months after the last administration of immunoglobulin products, as the efficacy of the live virus vaccine may be impaired. If immunoglobulin needs to be administered within 2–4 weeks of a live virus vaccination, then the efficacy of such a vaccination may be impaired.

The results of blood typing and antibody testing in neonates, including the Coombs or antiglobulin test, may be affected by the administration of anti-D immunoglobulin.

Rhophylac® can contain antibodies to other Rh antigens, e.g., anti-C antibodies, which might be detected by sensitive serological test methods following administration of the product.

Pregnancy Category C

This medicinal product is used in pregnancy. Animal reproduction studies have not been conducted with Rhophylac®. The available evidence suggests that Rhophylac® does not harm the fetus or affect future pregnancies or the reproduction capacity of the maternal recipient. Rh_o(D) Immune Globulin is not secreted in breast milk. No hazards are expected during breast-feeding.

ADVERSE REACTIONS

When anti-D immunoglobulins are administered by the intramuscular route, local pain and tenderness can be observed at the injection site; this can be prevented by dividing larger doses over several injection sites.

Mild and transient fever, malaise, headache, cutaneous reactions and chills occur occasionally. In rare cases, nausea, vomiting, hypotension, tachycardia, and allergic or anaphylactic type reactions, including dyspnea and shock are reported, even when the patient has shown no hypersensitivity to previous administration.

No data are available on overdosage. Patients with incompatible transfusion who receive an overdose of anti-D immunoglobulin should be monitored clinically and by biological parameters because of the risk of hemolytic reaction. In other Rh_o(D)-negative individuals overdosage should not lead to more frequent or more severe undesirable effects than the normal dose.

DOSAGE AND ADMINISTRATION

[See table above]

In case of known or suspected excessive feto-maternal hemorrhage, the number of fetal red blood cells in the maternal circulation should be determined. If excess transplacental bleeding is measured, extra anti-D immunoglobulin [100 IU (20 μg) for each 1 mL of fetal red blood cells] should be administered, preferably by the intravenous route. If testing is not feasible and an excessive feto-maternal hemorrhage cannot be excluded, a further 1500 IU (300 μg) should be administered. A 1500 IU (300 μg) dose will suppress the immunizing potential of at least 15 mL of Rh_o(D)-positive red blood cells[1].

Rhophylac® should be administered by intravenous or intramuscular injection as soon as possible within 72 hours of delivery, or of the at-risk event, in cases of obstetric complications or invasive procedures.

For incompatible transfusions, the recommended dose is 100 IU (20 μg) anti-D IgG per 2 mL of transfused Rh_o(D)-positive blood or per 1 mL of Rh_o(D)-positive erythrocyte concentrate. Rhophylac® should be brought to room or body temperature before use. Rhophylac® should be administered by slow intravenous or by intramuscular injection. If large doses (> 5 mL) are required and intramuscular injection is chosen, it is advisable to administer them in divided doses at different sites. Rhophylac® is for single use only. Any unused product or waste material should be disposed of in accordance with local requirements.

HOW SUPPLIED

Rhophylac®, Rh_o(D) Immune Globulin Intravenous (Human) 1500 IU (300 μg) is available in packages containing one or ten pre-filled 2 mL syringes.

STORAGE

Store at 2 °C to 8 °C (36 °F to 46 °F). If stored at this temperature, Rhophylac® has a shelf life of 36 months. Do not freeze. Protect from light. The preparation should not be used after the expiration date printed on the label.

REFERENCES

1. Pollack W, Ascari WQ, Kochesky RJ, O'Connor RR, Ho TY, Tripodi D. Studies on Rh prophylaxis. I. Relationship between doses of anti-Rh and size of antigenic stimulus. Transfusion 1971; 11: 333-39.
2. Thorpe SJ, Sands D, Fox B, Behr-Gross M-E, Schäffner G, and Yu MW. A Global standard for anti-D immunoglobulin: International collaborative study to evaluate a candidate preparation. Vox Sang 2003; 85: 313-21.
3. Stucki M, Moudry R, Kempf C, Omar A, Schlegel A, Lerch PG. Characterisation of a chromatographically produced anti-D immunoglobulin product. J Chromatogr B 1997; 700: 241-8.
4. Data on file at ZLB Bioplasma AG.
5. Bichler J, Schöndorfer G, Pabst G, Andresen I. Pharmacokinetics of anti-D IgG in pregnant RhD-negative women. BJOG 2003; 110: 39-45.
6. Data on file at ZLB Bioplasma AG.
7. Horowitz B, Chin S, Prince AM, Brotman B, Pascual D, Williams B. Preparation and characterization of S/D-FFP, a virus sterilized "fresh frozen plasma". Thromb Haemostas 1991; 65: 1163.
8. Horowitz B, Bonomo R, Prince AM, Chin SN, Brotman B, Shulman RW. Solvent detergent treated plasma: A virus-inactivated substitute for frozen plasma. Blood 1992; 79: 826-31.

Manufactured by:
ZLB Bioplasma AG
Wankdorfstrasse 10, 3000 Berne 22
Switzerland
US License No. 1598
Distributed by:
ZLB Bioplasma Inc.
Glendale, California 91203, USA
Last Revision: January 2004
Rhophylac®
Rh_o(D) Immune Globulin
Intravenous (Human)
Purity delivered

ZEMAIRA™ ℞

ALPHA$_1$-PROTEINASE INHIBITOR (HUMAN)

℞ **only**

DESCRIPTION

Alpha$_1$-Proteinase Inhibitor (Human), Zemaira™, is a sterile, stable, lyophilized preparation of highly purified human alpha$_1$-proteinase inhibitor (A_1-PI), also known as alpha$_1$-antitrypsin, derived from human plasma. Zemaira™ is manufactured from large pools of human plasma by cold ethanol fractionation according to a modified Cohn process followed by additional purification steps.

Zemaira™ is supplied as a sterile, white, lyophilized powder to be administered by the intravenous route. The specific activity of Zemaira™ is ≥0.7 mg of functional A_1-PI per milligram of total protein. The purity is ≥90% A_1-PI. Following reconstitution with 20 mL of Sterile Water for Injection, U.S.P., each vial contains approximately 1000 mg of functionally active A_1-PI, 81 mM sodium, 38 mM chloride, 17 mM phosphate, and 144 mM mannitol. Hydrochloric acid and/or sodium hydroxide may have been added to adjust the pH. Zemaira™ contains no preservatives.

Each vial of Zemaira™ contains the labeled amount of functionally active A_1-PI in milligrams as stated on the vial label as determined by its capacity to neutralize human neutrophil elastase.

The plasma used in the manufacture of this product has been tested and found to be nonreactive to HBsAg, nonreactive for antibody to Hepatitis C Virus (Anti-HCV), and negative for antibody to Human Immunodeficiency Virus (Anti-HIV-1/HIV-2).

Two viral reduction steps are employed in the manufacture of Zemaira™: pasteurization at 60°C for 10 hours in an aqueous solution with stabilizers and two sequential ultrafiltration steps. These viral reduction steps have been validated in a series of *in vitro* experiments for their capacity to inactivate/remove Human Immunodeficiency Virus (HIV), Hepatitis A Virus (HAV), and the following model viruses: Bovine Viral Diarrhea Virus (BVDV) as a model virus for HCV, Canine Parvovirus (CPV) as a model virus for Parvovirus B19, and Pseudorabies Virus (PRV) as a non-specific model virus to cover a wide range of physiochemical properties of the viruses studied. Total mean $\log_{10}$ reductions range from 6.8 to >12.2 $\log_{10}$ as shown in Table 1.

[See table 1 at top of next page]

CLINICAL PHARMACOLOGY

Alpha$_1$-proteinase inhibitor (A_1-PI) deficiency is a chronic, hereditary, autosomal, co-dominant disorder that is usually fatal in its severe form. Low blood levels of A_1-PI are most commonly associated with progressive, severe emphysema that becomes clinically apparent by the third to fourth decade of life. However, an unknown percentage of individuals with severe A_1-PI deficiency apparently never develop clinically evident emphysema during their lifetimes. A recent registry study showed 54% of A_1-PI deficient subjects had emphysema.[1] Another registry study showed 72% of A_1-PI deficient subjects had pulmonary symptoms.[2] Smoking is an important risk factor for the development of emphysema in patients with A_1-PI deficiency. Less commonly, low blood levels of A_1-PI are associated with liver disease and liver cirrhosis.[3,4,5]

Approximately 100 genetic variants of A_1-PI deficiency can be identified electrophoretically, only some of which are associated with the clinical disease.[6,7] Ninety-five percent of A_1-PI deficient individuals are of the severe PiZZ phenotype. Up to 39% of A_1-PI deficient patients may have an asthmatic component to their lung disease, as evidenced by symptoms and/or bronchial hyperreactivity.[1] Pulmonary infections, including pneumonia and acute bronchitis, are common in A_1-PI deficient patients and contribute significantly to the morbidity of the disease.

The most direct approach to therapy for A_1-PI deficiency in patients with emphysema has been to partially replace the missing protease inhibitor by intravenous infusion and, thus, attempt to ameliorate the imbalance in the anti-neutrophil elastase protection of the lower respiratory tract. Individuals with endogenous levels of A_1-PI below 11 μM, in general, manifest a significantly increased risk for development of emphysema above the general population background risk.[3,4,7,8] Therefore, the maintenance of blood serum levels of A_1-PI (antigenically measured) above 11 μM is historically thought to provide therapeutically relevant anti-neutrophil elastase protection.[9] However, the hypothesis that maintaining a serum level of antigenic A_1-PI will restore protease-antiprotease balance and prevent further lung damage has never been tested in an adequately-powered controlled clinical trial.

Mechanism of Action

Pulmonary disease, particularly emphysema, is the most frequent manifestation of A_1-PI deficiency.[7] The pathogenesis of emphysema is understood to evolve as described in the "protease-antiprotease imbalance" model. A_1-PI is now understood to be the primary antiprotease in the lower respiratory tract, where it inhibits neutrophil elastase (NE).[10] Normal healthy individuals produce sufficient A_1-PI to control the NE produced by activated neutrophils and are thus able to prevent inappropriate proteolysis of lung tissue by NE. Conditions that increase neutrophil accumulation and activation in the lung, such as respiratory infection and smoking, will in turn increase levels of NE. However, individuals who are severely deficient in endogenous A_1-PI are unable to maintain an appropriate antiprotease defense and are thereby subject to more rapid proteolysis of the alveolar walls leading to chronic lung disease. Zemaira™ serves as A_1-PI augmentation therapy in this patient population, acting to increase and maintain serum levels and lung epithelial lining fluid (ELF) levels of A_1-PI.

In 18 subjects treated with a single dose (60 mg/kg) of Zemaira™, the mean area under the curve (AUC) and standard deviation (SD) were 144 μM × day (SD 27), maximum serum concentration was 44.1 μM (SD 10.8), clearance was 603 mL per day (SD 129), and terminal half-life was 5.1 days (SD 2.4).

Weekly repeated infusions of A_1-PI at a dose of 60 mg/kg lead to serum A_1-PI levels above the historical target threshold of 11 μM.

CLINICAL STUDIES

Clinical studies were conducted with Zemaira™ in 89 subjects (59 males and 30 females). The subjects ranged in age from 29 to 68 years (median age 49 years). Ninety-seven percent of the treated subjects had the PiZZ phenotype of A_1-PI deficiency, and 3% had the M_{MALTON} phenotype. At screening, serum A_1-PI levels were between 3.2 and 10.1 μM (mean of 5.6 μM). The objectives of the clinical studies were to demonstrate that Zemaira™ augments and maintains serum levels of A_1-PI above 11 μM and increases A_1-PI levels in ELF of the lower lung.

In a double-blind, controlled clinical study to evaluate the safety and efficacy of Zemaira™, 44 subjects were randomized to receive 60 mg/kg of either Zemaira™ or Prolastin® (a commercially available Alpha$_1$-Proteinase Inhibitor [Human] product) once weekly for 10 weeks. After 10 weeks, all subjects received Zemaira™ for an additional 14 weeks. All subjects were followed for a total of 24 weeks to complete the safety evaluation. The mean trough serum A_1-PI levels at steady state (Weeks 7–11) in the Zemaira™-treated subjects were statistically equivalent to those in the Prolastin®-treated subjects. Both groups were maintained above 11 μM (80 mg/dL). The mean (range and standard deviation) of the steady state trough serum antigenic A_1-PI level for Zemaira™-treated subjects was 17.7 μM (range 13.9 to 23.2, SD 2.5) and for Prolastin®-treated subjects was 19.1 μM (range 14.7 to 23.1, SD 2.2). The difference between the Zemaira™ and the Prolastin® groups was not considered clinically significant and may be related to the higher specific activity of Zemaira™.

In a subgroup of subjects enrolled in the study (10 Zemaira™-treated subjects and 5 Prolastin®-treated subjects), bronchoalveolar lavage was performed at baseline and at Week 11. Four A_1-PI related analytes in ELF were measured: antigenic A_1-PI, A_1-PI:NE complexes, free NE, and functional A_1-PI (anti-neutrophil elastase capacity, ANEC). A blinded retrospective analysis, which revised the prospectively established acceptance criteria showed that within each treatment group, ELF levels of antigenic A_1-PI and A_1-PI:NE complexes increased from baseline to Week 11. Free elastase was immeasurably low in all samples. The post-treatment ANEC values in ELF were not significantly different between the Zemaira™-treated and Prolastin®-treated subjects (mean 1725 nM vs. 1418 nM). No conclusions can be drawn about changes of ANEC values in ELF during the study period as baseline values in the Zemaira™-treated subjects were unexpectedly high. No A_1-PI analytes showed any clinically significant differences between the Zemaira™ and Prolastin® treatment groups.

[See table 2 above]

Subjects were also monitored for the presence of antibodies to HIV and markers for viral hepatitis (HAV, HBV, and HCV). Subjects who were negative for Hepatitis B surface antigen (HBsAg) at screening were vaccinated against Hepatitis B. Zemaira™-treated subjects were tested six months after the end of treatment for HAV, HBV, HCV, HIV, and Parvovirus B19, and no evidence of viral transmission was observed. No subjects developed detectable antibodies to Zemaira™.

INDICATIONS AND USAGE

Zemaira™ is indicated for chronic augmentation and maintenance therapy in individuals with alpha$_1$-proteinase inhibitor (A_1-PI) deficiency and clinical evidence of emphysema.

Zemaira™ increases antigenic and functional (ANEC) serum levels and lung epithelial lining fluid levels of A_1-PI. Clinical data demonstrating the long-term effects of chronic augmentation therapy of individuals with Zemaira™ are not available.

Safety and effectiveness in pediatric patients have not been established.

Zemaira™ is not indicated as therapy for lung disease patients in whom severe congenital A_1-PI deficiency has not been established.

CONTRAINDICATIONS

Zemaira™ is contraindicated in individuals with a known hypersensitivity to any of its components. Zemaira™ is also contraindicated in individuals with a history of anaphylaxis or severe systemic response to A_1-PI products.

Individuals with selective IgA deficiencies who have known antibodies against IgA (anti-IgA antibodies) should not receive Zemaira™, since these patients may experience severe reactions, including anaphylaxis, to IgA that may be present in Zemaira™.

WARNINGS

Zemaira™ is made from human plasma. Products made from human plasma may contain infectious agents, such as viruses, that can cause disease. Because Zemaira™ is made from human blood, it may carry a risk of transmitting infectious agents, e.g., viruses, and theoretically the Creutzfeldt-Jakob disease (CJD) agent. The risk that such products will transmit an infectious agent has been reduced by screening plasma donors for prior exposure to certain viruses, by testing for the presence of certain current virus infections, and by inactivating and/or removing certain viruses during manufacture. (See **DESCRIPTION** section for viral reduction measures.) The manufacturing procedure for Zemaira™ includes processing steps designed to reduce further the risk of viral transmission. Stringent procedures utilized at plasma collection centers, plasma testing laboratories, and fractionation facilities are designed to reduce the risk of viral transmission. The primary viral reduction steps of the Zemaira™ manufacturing process are pasteurization (60°C for 10 hours) and two sequential ultrafiltration steps. Additional purification procedures used in the manufacture of Zemaira™ also potentially provide viral reduction. Despite these measures, such products may still potentially contain human pathogenic agents, including those not yet known or identified. Thus, the risk of transmission of infectious agents can not be totally eliminated. Any infections thought by a physician possibly to have been transmitted by this product should be reported by the physician or other healthcare provider to Aventis Behring at 800-504-5434. The physician should discuss the risks and benefits of this product with the patient.

Individuals who receive infusions of blood or plasma products may develop signs and/or symptoms of some viral infections (see **Information For Patients**).

During clinical studies, no cases of hepatitis A, B, C, or HIV viral infections were reported with the use of Zemaira™.

Table 1: Mean (cumulative) virus reduction factors

	Mean Reduction Factor Pasteurization [$\log_{10}$]	Mean Reduction Factor Two Ultrafiltration Steps [$\log_{10}$]	Cumulative Reduction Factor [$\log_{10}$]
HIV-1	≥ 6.7	≥ 5.5	≥ 12.2
BVDV	≥ 5.9	5.1	≥ 11.0
PRV	4.3	≥ 6.9	≥ 11.2
HAV	≥ 5.4	≥ 6.3	≥ 11.7
CPV	(0.9)	6.8	6.8

Table 2: ELF Analytes — change from baseline

Analyte	Treatment	Mean change from baseline	90% CI
A_1-PI (nM)	Zemaira™	1358.3	822.6 to 1894.0
	Prolastin®	949.9	460.0 to 1439.7
ANEC (nM)	Zemaira™	-588.1	-2032.3 to 856.1
	Prolastin®	497.5	-392.3 to 1387.2
A_1-PI:NE Complexes (nM)	Zemaira™	118.0	39.9 to 196.1
	Prolastin®	287.1	49.8 to 524.5

PRECAUTIONS

General — Infusion rates and the patient's clinical state should be monitored closely during infusion. The patient should be observed for signs of infusion-related reactions.

As with any colloid solution, there may be an increase in plasma volume following intravenous administration of Zemaira™. Caution should therefore be used in patients at risk for circulatory overload.

Information For Patients — Patients should be informed of the early signs of hypersensitivity reactions including hives, generalized urticaria, tightness of the chest, dyspnea, wheezing, faintness, hypotension, and anaphylaxis. Patients should be advised to discontinue use of the product and contact their physician and/or seek immediate emergency care, depending on the severity of the reaction, if these symptoms occur.

As with all plasma-derived products, some viruses, such as parvovirus B19, are particularly difficult to remove or inactivate at this time. Parvovirus B19 may most seriously affect pregnant women and immune-compromised individuals. Symptoms of parvovirus B19 include fever, drowsiness, chills, and runny nose followed two weeks later by a rash and joint pain. Patients should be encouraged to consult their physician if such symptoms occur.

Pregnancy Category C — Animal reproduction studies have not been conducted with Zemaira™. It is also not known whether Zemaira™ can cause fetal harm when administered to a pregnant woman or can affect reproduction capacity. Zemaira™ should be given to a pregnant woman only if clearly needed.

Nursing Mothers — It is not known whether Zemaira™ is excreted in human milk. Because many drugs are excreted in human milk, caution should be exercised when Zemaira™ is administered to a nursing woman.

Pediatric Use — Safety and effectiveness in the pediatric population have not been established.

Geriatric Use — Clinical studies of Zemaira™ did not include sufficient numbers of subjects aged 65 and over to determine whether they respond differently from younger subjects. As for all patients, dosing for geriatric patients should be appropriate to their overall situation.

ADVERSE REACTIONS

Intravenous administration of Zemaira™, 60 mg/kg weekly, has been shown to be generally well tolerated. In clinical studies, the following treatment-related adverse reactions were reported: asthenia, injection site pain, dizziness, headache, paresthesia, and pruritus. Each of these related adverse events was observed in 1 of 89 subjects (1%). The adverse reactions were mild.

Should evidence of an acute hypersensitivity reaction be observed, the infusion should be stopped promptly and appropriate countermeasures and supportive therapy should be administered.

Table 3 summarizes the adverse event data obtained with single and multiple doses during clinical trials with Zemaira™ and Prolastin®. No clinically significant differences were detected between the two treatment groups.

[See table 3 at top of next page]

The frequencies of adverse events per infusion that were ≥0.4% in Zemaira™-treated subjects, regardless of causality, were: headache (33 events per 1296 infusions, 2.5%), upper respiratory infection (1.6%), sinusitis (1.5%), injection site hemorrhage (0.9%), sore throat (0.9%), bronchitis (0.8%), asthenia (0.6%), fever (0.6%), pain (0.5%), rhinitis (0.5%), bronchospasm (0.5%), chest pain (0.5%), increased cough (0.4%), rash (0.4%), and infection (0.4%).

The following adverse events, regardless of causality, occurred at a rate of 0.2% to <0.4% per infusion: abdominal pain, diarrhea, dizziness, ecchymosis, myalgia, pruritus, vasodilation, accidental injury, back pain, dyspepsia, dyspnea, hemorrhage, injection site reaction, lung disorder, migraine, nausea, and paresthesia.

Diffuse interstitial lung disease was noted on a routine chest x-ray of one subject at Week 24. Causality could not be determined.

In a retrospective analysis, during the 10-week blinded portion of the 24-week clinical study, 6 subjects (20%) of the 30 treated with Zemaira™ had a total of 7 exacerbations of their chronic obstructive pulmonary disease (COPD). Nine subjects (64%) of the 14 treated with Prolastin® had a total of 11 exacerbations of their COPD. The observed difference between groups was 44% (95% confidence interval from 8% to 70%). Over the entire 24-week treatment period, of the 30 subjects in the Zemaira™ treatment group, 7 subjects (23%) had a total of 11 exacerbations of their COPD.

DOSAGE AND ADMINISTRATION

Each vial of Zemaira™ contains the labeled amount of functionally active A_1-PI in milligrams as stated on the vial label as determined by capacity to neutralize human neutrophil elastase. The recommended dose of Zemaira™ is 60 mg/kg body weight administered once weekly.

When reconstituted as directed, Zemaira™ may be administered intravenously at a rate of approximately 0.08 mL/kg/min as determined by the response and comfort of the patient. The recommended dosage of 60 mg/kg body weight will take approximately 15 minutes to infuse.

Preparation

Each product package contains one Zemaira™ single use vial, one 20 mL vial of Sterile Water for Injection, U.S.P. (diluent), one color-coded vented transfer device with air inlet filter, and one large volume 5 micron conical filter. Administer within three hours after reconstitution.

Reconstitution

1. Bring both product (green cap) vial and diluent (white cap) vial to room temperature prior to reconstitution.

Continued on next page

Table 3: Summary of Adverse Events

	Zemaira™	Prolastin®
No. of subjects treated	89	32
No. of subjects with adverse events regardless of causality (%)	69 (78%)	20 (63%)
No. of subjects with related adverse events (%)	5 (6%)	4 (13%)
No. of subjects with related serious adverse events	0	0
No. of infusions	1296	160
No. of adverse events regardless of causality (rates per infusion)	298 (0.230)	83 (0.519)
No. of related adverse events (rates per infusion)	6 (0.005)	5 (0.031)

Zemaira—Cont.

2. Remove the plastic flip-top caps from the vials. Aseptically cleanse the rubber stoppers with antiseptic solution and allow them to dry.

NOTE: The transfer device (Fig. 1) provided in the package is comprised of a white (diluent) end, which has a double orifice, and a green (product) end, which has a single orifice. Incorrect use of the transfer device will result in loss of vacuum and prevent transfer of the diluent, thereby preventing reconstitution of the product.

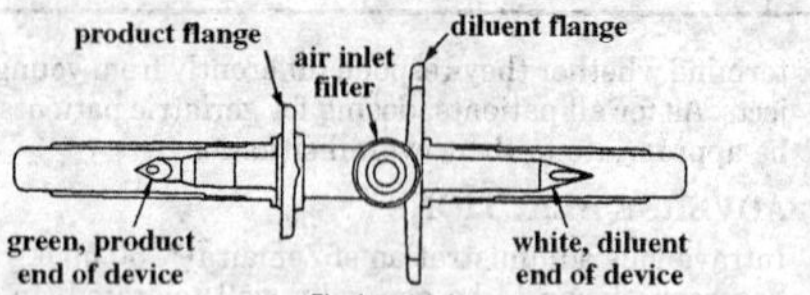

Fig.1

The transfer device is sterile. Do not touch the exposed ends of the spike after removing the protective covers.

3. Remove the protective cover from the white (diluent) end of the transfer device. Insert the white end of the transfer device into the center of the stopper of the upright diluent vial first. (Fig. 2)
4. Remove the protective cover from the green (product) end of the transfer device. Invert the diluent vial with the attached transfer device and, using minimum force, insert the green end of the transfer device into the center of the rubber stopper of the upright Zemaira™ vial (green top). (Fig. 3) The flange of the transfer device should rest on the surface of the stopper so that the diluent flows into the Zemaira™ vial.
5. Allow the vacuum in the Zemaira™ vial to pull the diluent into the Zemaira™ vial.
6. During diluent transfer, wet the lyophilized cake completely by gently tilting the Zemaira™ vial. (Fig. 4) Do not allow the air inlet filter to face downward. Care should be taken not to lose the vacuum, as this will prolong reconstitution of the product.
7. After diluent transfer is complete, the transfer device will allow filtered air into the Zemaira™ vial through the air filter. Additional venting of the product vial after diluent transfer is complete is not required. When diluent transfer is complete, withdraw the transfer device and diluent vial and properly discard in accordance with biohazard procedures.
8. Gently swirl the Zemaira™ vial until the powder is completely dissolved. (Fig. 5) **DO NOT SHAKE.**
9. Parenteral drug preparations should be inspected visually for particulate matter and discoloration prior to administration. Administer at room temperature within three hours after reconstitution.

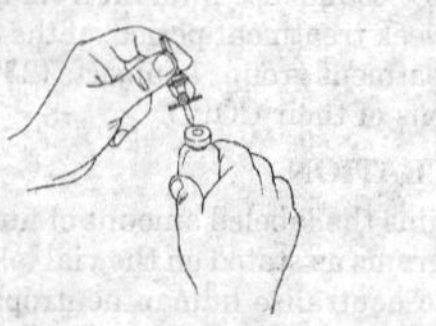
Fig. 2

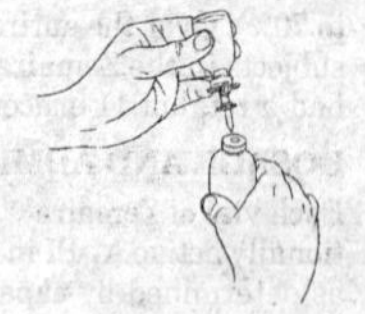
Fig. 3

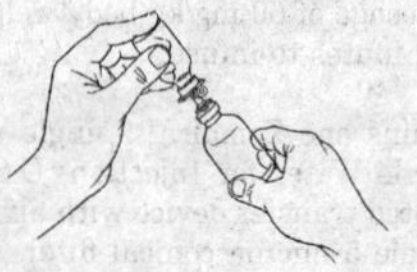
Fig. 4

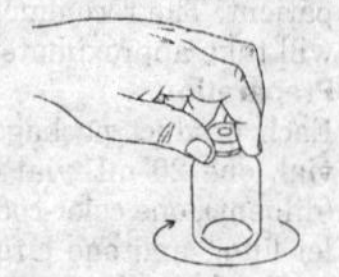
Fig. 5

Pooling Reconstituted Vials

If more than one vial of Zemaira™ is needed to achieve the required dose, use an aseptic technique to transfer the reconstituted solution from the vials into the administration container (e.g., empty I.V. bag or glass bottle).

Administration

Parenteral drug preparations should be inspected visually for particulate matter and discoloration prior to administration. Administer at room temperature within three hours after reconstitution.

The reconstituted solution should be filtered during administration. To ensure proper filtration of Zemaira™, place the large volume 5 micron conical filter (provided) between the distal end of the I.V. administration set and the infusion set. (Fig. 6) Follow the appropriate procedure for I.V. administration.

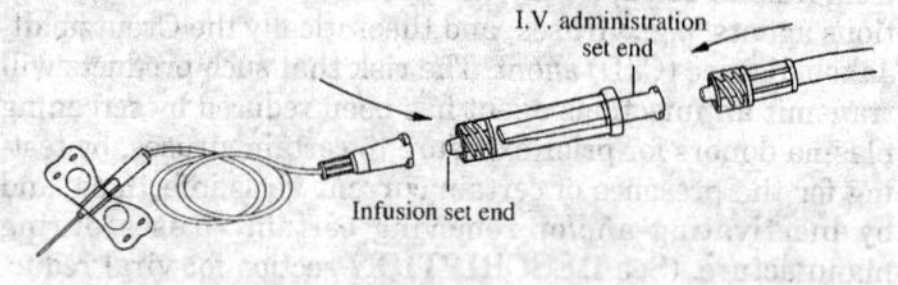

Fig. 6

After administration, any unused solution and administration equipment should be discarded in accordance with biohazard procedures.

HOW SUPPLIED

Zemaira™ is supplied in a single use vial containing the labeled amount of functionally active A_1-PI, as stated on the label. Each product package (NDC 0053-7201-02) contains one single use vial of Zemaira™, one 20 mL vial of Sterile Water for Injection, U.S.P. (diluent), one vented transfer device, and one large volume 5 micron conical filter.

STORAGE

When stored up to 25°C (77°F), Zemaira™ is stable for the period indicated by the expiration date on its label. Avoid freezing which may damage container for the diluent.

REFERENCES

1. Stoller JK, Brantly M, *et al.* Formation and current results of a patient-organized registry for α_1-antitrypsin deficiency. *Chest* 118(3):843–848, 2000.
2. McElvaney NG, Stoller JK, *et al.* Baseline Characteristics of Enrollees in the National Heart, Lung, and Blood Institute Registry of α_1-Antitrypsin Deficiency. *Chest* 111:394–403, 1997.
3. Eriksson S. Pulmonary Emphysema and Alpha$_1$-Antitrypsin Deficiency. *ACTA Med Scand* 175(2):197–205, 1964.
4. Eriksson S. Studies in α_1-antitrypsin deficiency. *ACTA Med Scan* Suppl. 432:1–85, 1965.
5. Morse JO. Alpha$_1$-Antitrypsin Deficiency. *N Engl J Med* 299:1045–1048; 1099–1105, 1978.
6. Crystal RG. α_1-Antitrypsin Deficiency, Emphysema, and Liver Disease; Genetic Basis and Strategies for Therapy. *J Clin Invest* 85:1343–1352, 1990.
7. World Health Organization. Alpha-1-Antitrypsin Deficiency; Report of a WHO Meeting. Geneva. 18–20 March 1996.
8. Gadek JE, Crystal RG. α_1-Antitrypsin Deficiency. In: The Metabolic Basis of Inherited Disease 5th ed. Stanbury JB, Wyngaarden JB, Frederickson DS, *et al.*, eds: New York, McGraw-Hill. 1983; pp. 1450–1467.
9. American Thoracic Society. Guidelines for the Approach to the Patient with Severe Hereditary Alpha-1-Antitrypsin Deficiency. *Am Rev Respir Dis* 140:1494–1497, 1989.
10. Gadek JE, Fells GA, Zimmerman RL, Rennard SI, Crystal RG. Antielastases of the Human Alveolar Structures; Implications for the Protease-Antiprotease Theory of Emphysema. *J Clin Invest* 68:889–898, 1981.

Prolastin® is a registered trademark of Bayer Corporation.

Manufactured by:
Aventis Behring L.L.C.
Kankakee, IL 60901 U.S.A.
U.S. License No. 1281
19131-02
Revised: December 2003

Bayer Pharmaceuticals Corporation

400 MORGAN LANE
WEST HAVEN, CT 06516

For Medical Information Contact:
Director, Medical Services
(800) 468-0894
(203) 812-2000

BILTRICIDE® TABLETS ℞

[*bĭl-trĭ-sīd*]
(praziquantel)

DESCRIPTION

BILTRICIDE® (praziquantel) is a trematodicide provided in tablet form for the oral treatment of schistosome infections and infections due to liver fluke.

BILTRICIDE® (praziquantel) is 2-(cyclohexylcarbonyl)-1,2,3,6,7,11b-hexahydro-4H-pyrazino [2, 1-a] isoquinolin-4-one with the molecular formula; $C_{19}H_{24}N_2O_2$. The structural formula is as follows:

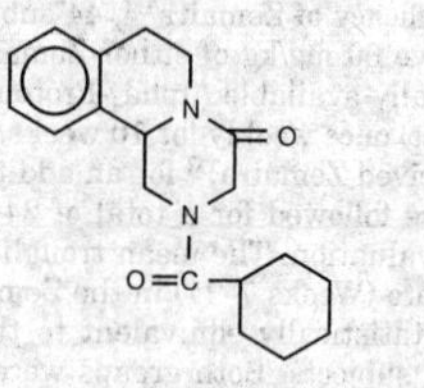

Praziquantel is a white to nearly white crystalline powder of bitter taste. The compound is stable under normal conditions and melts at 136-140°C with decomposition. The active substance is hygroscopic. Praziquantel is easily soluble in chloroform and dimethylsulfoxide, soluble in ethanol and very slightly soluble in water.

BILTRICIDE tablets contain 600 mg of praziquantel. Inactive ingredients: corn starch, magnesium stearate, microcrystalline cellulose, povidone, sodium lauryl sulfate, polyethylene glycol, titanium dioxide and hypromellose.

CLINICAL PHARMACOLOGY

Praziquantel induces a rapid contraction of schistosomes by a specific effect on the permeability of the cell membrane. The drug further causes vacuolization and disintegration of the schistosome tegument.

After oral administration BILTRICIDE® is rapidly absorbed (80%), subjected to a first pass effect, metabolized and eliminated by the kidneys. Maximal serum concentration is achieved 1-3 hours after dosing. The half-life of praziquantel in serum is 0.8-1.5 hours.

Special Populations: The pharmacokinetics of praziquantel were studied in 40 patients with *Schistosoma mansoni* infections with varying degrees of hepatic dysfunction (See table1). In patients with schistosomiasis, the pharmacokinetic parameters did not differ significantly between those with normal hepatic function (Group 1) and those with mild (Child-Pugh class A) hepatic impairment. However, in patients with moderate-to-severe hepatic dysfunction (Child-Pugh class B and C), praziquantel half-life, C_{max}, and AUC increased progressively with the degree of hepatic impairment. In Child-Pugh class B, the increases in mean half-life, C_{max}, and AUC relative to Group 1 were 1.58-fold, 1.76-fold, and 3.55-fold, respectively. The corresponding increases in Child-Pugh class C patients were 2.82-fold, 4.29-fold, and 15-fold for half-life, C_{max}, and AUC. [See table at top of next page]

INDICATIONS AND USAGE

BILTRICIDE® is indicated for the treatment of infections due to: all species of schistosoma (e.g. *Schistosoma mekongi*, *Schistosoma japonicum*, *Schistosoma mansoni* and *Schistosoma hematobium*), and infections due to the liver flukes, *Clonorchis sinensis/Opisthorchis viverrini* (approval of this indication was based on studies in which the two species were not differentiated).

CONTRAINDICATIONS

BILTRICIDE® must not be given to patients who previously have shown hypersensitivity to the drug. Since parasite destruction within the eye may cause irreparable lesions, ocular cysticercosis should not be treated with this compound.

WARNINGS

Therapeutically effective levels of praziquantel may not be achieved with concomitant administration of strong inducers of cytochrome P450 such as rifampin.

PRECAUTIONS

General:

Approximately 80% of a dose of praziquantel is excreted in the kidneys, almost exclusively (>99%) in the form of metabolites. Excretion might be delayed in patients with impaired renal function, but accumulation of unchanged drug would not be expected. Therefore, dose adjustment for renal impairment is not considered necessary. Nephrotoxic effects of praziquantel or its metabolites are not known.

Caution should be exercised in the administration of the usual recommended dose of praziquantel to hepatosplenic schistosomiasis patients with moderate to severe liver impairment (Child-Pugh class B and C). Reduced metabo-

Table 1: Pharmacokinetic parameters of praziquantel in four groups of patients with varying degrees of liver function following administration of 40 mg/kg under fasting conditions.

Patient Group	Half-life (hr)	T_{max} (hr)	C_{max} (μg/mL)	AUC (μg/mL* hr)
Normal hepatic function (Group 1)	2.99 ± 1.28	1.48 ± 0.74	0.83 ± 0.52	3.02 ± 0.59
Child-Pugh A (Group 2)	4.66 ± 2.77	1.37 ± 0.61	0.93 ± 0.58	3.87 ± 2.44
Child-Pugh B (Group 3)	4.74 ± 2.16[a]	2.21 ± 0.78[a,b]	1.47 ± 0.74[a,b]	10.72 ± 5.53[a,b]
Child-Pugh C (Group 4)	8.45 ± 2.62[a,b,c]	3.2 ± 1.05[a,b,c]	3.57 ± 1.30[a,b,c]	45.35 ± 17.50[a,b,c]

a) $p<0.05$ compared to Group 1
b) $p<0.05$ compared to Group 2
c) $p<0.05$ compared to Group 3

lism of praziquantel by the liver in these patients may lead to considerably higher and longer lasting plasma concentrations of unmetabolized praziquantel (See **CLINICAL PHARMACOLOGY/ Special Populations**).

Minimal increases in liver enzymes have been reported in some patients.

Patients suffering from cardiac irregularities should be monitored during treatment.

When schistosomiasis or fluke infection is found to be associated with cerebral cysticercosis it is advised to hospitalize the patient for the duration of treatment.

Information for Patients:

Patients should be warned not to drive a car and not to operate machinery on the day of BILTRICIDE® treatment and the following day.

Drug Interactions:

Concomitant administration of drugs that increase the activity of drug metabolizing liver enzymes (Cytochrome P450), e.g. antiepileptic drugs (phenytoin, phenobarbital and carbamazepine), dexamethasone, may reduce plasma levels of praziquantel.

Concomitant administration of rifampin should be avoided (see **WARNINGS**).

Concomitant administration of drugs that decrease the activity of drug metabolizing liver enzymes (Cytochrome P 450), e.g. cimetidine, ketoconazole, itraconazole, erythromycin may increase plasma levels of praziquantel.

Chloroquine, when taken simultaneously, may lead to lower concentrations of praziquantel in blood. The mechanism of this drug-drug interaction is unclear.

Grapefruit juice was reported to produce a 1.6-fold increase in the C_{max} and a 1.9-fold increase in the AUC of praziquantel. However, the effect of this exposure increase on the therapeutic effect and safety of praziquantel has not been systematically evaluated.

Mutagenesis, Carcinogenesis:

Mutagenic effects in Salmonella tests found by one laboratory have not been confirmed in the same tested strain by other laboratories. Long term carcinogenicity studies in rats and golden hamsters did not reveal any carcinogenic effect.

Pregnancy Category B:

Reproduction studies have been performed in rats and rabbits at doses up to 40 times the human dose and have revealed no evidence of impaired fertility or harm to the fetus due to praziquantel. There are, however, no adequate and well-controlled studies in pregnant women. An increase of the abortion rate was found in rats at three times the single human therapeutic dose. While animal reproduction studies are not always predictive of human response, this drug should be used during pregnancy only if clearly needed.

Nursing mothers:

Praziquantel appeared in the milk of nursing women at a concentration of about 1/4 that of maternal serum. Women should not nurse on the day of BILTRICIDE® treatment and during the subsequent 72 hours.

Pediatric use:

Safety in children under 4 years of age has not been established.

Geriatric use:

Clinical studies of praziquantel did not include a sufficient number of subjects ages 65 and over to determine whether they respond differently from younger subjects. Other reported clinical experience has not identified differences in responses between the elderly and younger patients, but greater sensitivity of some older patients cannot be ruled out.

This drug is known to be substantially excreted by the kidney. Because elderly patients are more likely to have decreased renal function, the risk of toxic reactions to this drug may be greater in these patients.

ADVERSE EVENTS

In general BILTRICIDE® is very well tolerated. Side effects are usually mild and transient and do not require treatment. The following side effects were observed generally in order of severity: malaise, headache, dizziness, abdominal discomfort with or without nausea, rise in temperature and, rarely, urticaria. Such symptoms can, however, also result from the infection itself. Such side effects may be more frequent and/or serious in patients with a heavy worm burden.

Post Marketing Adverse Event Reports:

Additional adverse events reported from worldwide post marketing experience and from publications with praziquantel include:

abdominal pain, allergic reaction (generalized hypersensitivity) including polyserositis, anorexia, arrhythmia (including bradycardia, ectopic rhythms, ventricular fibrillation, AV blocks), asthenia, bloody diarrhea, convulsion, myalgia, somnolence, vertigo, vomiting

OVERDOSAGE

In rats and mice the acute LD_{50} was about 2,500 mg/kg. No data are available in humans. In the event of overdose a fast-acting laxative should be given.

DOSAGE AND ADMINISTRATION

The dosage recommended for the treatment of schistosomiasis is: 20 mg/kg bodyweight three times a day as a one day treatment, at intervals of not less than 4 hours and not more than 6 hours. The recommended dose for clonorchiasis and opisthorchiasis is: 25 mg/kg bodyweight three times a day as a one day treatment, at intervals of not less than 4 hours and not more than 6 hours. The tablets should be washed down unchewed with water during meals. Keeping the tablets or segments thereof in the mouth can reveal a bitter taste which can promote gagging or vomiting.

HOW SUPPLIED

BILTRICIDE® is supplied as a 600 mg white to orange tinged, film-coated, oblong tablet with three scores. The tablet is coded with "BAYER" on one side and "LG" on the reverse side. When broken, each of the four segments contains 150 mg of active ingredient so that the dosage can be easily adjusted to the patient's bodyweight.

Segments are broken off by pressing the score (notch) with thumbnails. If 1/4 of a tablet is required, this is best achieved by breaking the segment from the outer end.

BILTRICIDE® is available in bottles of 6 tablets.

	Strength	NDC
Bottles of 6:	600 mg	0026-2521-06

Store below 86°F (30°C).

Bayer HealthCare
Bayer Pharmaceuticals Corporation
400 Morgan Lane
West Haven, CT 06516 USA
Made in Germany
℞ Only

08753760, R.1 8/04 EMBAY 8440 12400

Printed in U.S.A.

Dermik Laboratories
1050 WESTLAKES DRIVE
BERWYN, PA 19312

Direct Inquiries to:
Customer Service
Somerset Corporate Center, Blg 3
300 Somerset Corporate Blvd
Bridgewater, NJ 08807-2854
(800) 207-8049

For Medical Information Contact:
Medical Information Services
Somerset Corporate Center, Blg 3
300 Somerset Corporate Blvd
Bridgewater, NJ 08807-2854
(800) 633-1610
www.dermik.com

SCULPTRA™ ℞
injectable poly-L-lactic acid

Caution: Federal (USA) law restricts this device to sale by or on the order of a licensed physician, or properly licensed practitioner.

BEFORE USING PRODUCT, READ THE FOLLOWING INFORMATION THOROUGHLY.

DEVICE DESCRIPTION

SCULPTRA™ is an injectable implant that contains microparticles of poly-L-lactic acid, a biocompatible, biodegradable, synthetic polymer from the alpha-hydroxy-acid family. **SCULPTRA** is reconstituted prior to use by the addition of Sterile Water for Injection, USP (SWFI) to form a sterile non-pyrogenic suspension.

INTENDED USE / INDICATIONS

SCULPTRA is intended for restoration and/or correction of the signs of facial fat loss (lipoatrophy) in people with human immunodeficiency virus.

CONTRAINDICATIONS

- **SCULPTRA** should not be used in any person who has hypersensitivity to any of the components of the product.

WARNINGS

- Use of **SCULPTRA** in any person with active skin inflammation or infection in or near the treatment area should be deferred until the inflammatory or infectious process has been controlled.
- Do not overcorrect (overfill) a contour deficiency because the depression should gradually improve within several weeks as the treatment effect of **SCULPTRA** occurs (see **PATIENT TREATMENT**).
- Injection procedure reactions to **SCULPTRA** have been observed consisting mainly of hematoma, bruising, edema, discomfort, inflammation, and erythema. The most common device related adverse effect was the delayed occurrence of subcutaneous papules, which were confined to the injection site and were typically palpable, asymptomatic and non-visible. Refer to **ADVERSE EVENTS** for details.
- Special care should be taken to avoid injection into the blood vessels. An introduction into the vasculature may occlude the vessels and could cause infarction or embolism.

PRECAUTIONS

- **SCULPTRA** should only be used by health care providers with expertise in the correction of volume deficiencies in patients with human immunodeficiency virus after fully familiarizing themselves with the product, the product educational materials, and the entire package insert.
- **SCULPTRA** vials are for single patient use only. Do not reuse or resterilize the vial. Do not use if package or vial is opened or damaged.
- Long-term safety and effectiveness of **SCULPTRA** beyond two years have not been investigated. Dermik® is conducting a post approval study to evaluate the safety and effectiveness of **SCULPTRA** beyond two years.
- **SCULPTRA** should be used in the deep dermis or subcutaneous layer. Avoid superficial injections. Special care must be taken when using **SCULPTRA** in areas of thin skin. Refer to **PATIENT TREATMENT** for instructions regarding injection techniques.
- Safety and effectiveness of treatment in the periorbital area have not been established.
- As with all transcutaneous procedures, **SCULPTRA** injection carries a risk of infection. Standard precautions associated with injectable materials should be followed.
- As with all injections, patients treated with anti-coagulants may run the risk of a hematoma or localized bleeding at the injection site.
- Universal precautions must be observed when there is a potential for contact with patient body fluids. The injection session must be conducted with aseptic technique.
- After use, treatment syringes and needles may be potential biohazards. Handle accordingly and dispose of in accordance with accepted medical practice and applicable local, state and federal requirements.
- The safety of **SCULPTRA** for use during pregnancy, in breastfeeding females or in patients under 18 years has not been established.
- No studies of interactions of **SCULPTRA** with drugs or other substances or implants have been made.
- The safety and effectiveness data from clinical trials of **SCULPTRA** in non-Caucasians and women with human immunodeficiency virus are limited. Dermik® will conduct a post approval study in non-Caucasians and women with human immunodeficiency virus.
- The safety of using **SCULPTRA** in patients with increased susceptibility to keloid formation and hypertrophic scarring has not been studied. Dermik® will conduct a post approval study to determine the likelihood of keloid formation and hypertrophic scars in patients with human immunodeficiency virus receiving **SCULPTRA** injections.
- The patient should be informed that he or she should minimize exposure of the treatment area to excessive sun and UV lamp exposure until any initial swelling and redness has resolved.

ADVERSE EVENTS

Adverse event data from four clinical studies that included 277 patients are summarized in Tables 1 & 2 below.

Continued on next page

Sculptra—Cont.

TABLE 1:
NUMBER OF PATIENTS WITH TREATMENT-RELATED ADVERSE EVENTS OBSERVED IN CLINICAL STUDIES WITH TWO-YEAR FOLLOW-UP

	VEGA STUDY 50 Patients	C&W STUDY*** 29 Patients	AVERAGE DURATION (DAYS)
INJECTION PROCEDURE RELATED ADVERSE EVENTS			
Bruising	3(6%)	11(38%)	6
Edema	2(4%)	2(7%)	3
Discomfort	0	3(10%)	3
Hematoma	14(28%)	0	17
Inflammation	0	3(10%)	3
Erythema	0	3(10%)	3
DEVICE-RELATED ADVERSE EVENTS			**AVERAGE ONSET** (Months)**
Injection site subcutaneous papule*	26(52%)	9(31%)	7

*Subcutaneous papules refer to lesions of 5 mm or less, typically palpable, asymptomatic and non-visible.
**Onset data available from VEGA study only. Duration not noted for subcutaneous papules because most were ongoing at study completion.
*** Safety data were collected post hoc for 27 of the patients at approximately two years from study start.

TABLE 2:
NUMBER OF PATIENTS WITH TREATMENT-RELATED ADVERSE EVENTS OBSERVED IN CLINICAL STUDIES WITH ONE-YEAR FOLLOW-UP

	APEX 002 STUDY 99 Patients	BLUE PACIFIC STUDY 99 Patients
INJECTION PROCEDURE RELATED ADVERSE EVENTS		
Bruising	1(1%)	30(30%)
Edema	3(3%)	17(17%)
Discomfort	19(19%)	15(15%)
Erythema	0	3(3%)
DEVICE RELATED ADVERSE EVENTS		
Injection site subcutaneous papule	6(6%)	13(13%)

The duration of the adverse events in Table 2 was not collected. The most common device related adverse effect was the delayed occurrence of subcutaneous papules, which were confined to the injection site and were typically palpable, asymptomatic, and non-visible. The study protocols did not include evaluation of treatment for subcutaneous papules, therefore, no information is available on how the papules were treated. In the VEGA study, the average onset of subcutaneous papules was 7 months after initial injection (range 0.3–25 months). Subcutaneous papules resolved spontaneously in 6/26 patients (24%) during the study. No information of onset and duration of papules is available from the Chelsea & Westminster study.
Treatment related adverse events, not included in Table 1 & 2, observed in clinical studies with a frequency of less than 5% were: injection site tenderness, injection site lesion, injection site bleeding, injection site induration, injection site infection and fever.
The following adverse events, which were not observed in the clinical studies, were detected from post-marketing surveillance outside of the US and literature reports: visible nodules with or without inflammation or dyspigmentation, malaise, injection site abscess, allergic reaction, injection site atrophy, Quincke's edema, injection site fat atrophy, photosensitive reaction, fatigue, injection site granuloma, hypersensitivity reaction, skin rash, skin roughness, lack of effectiveness, injection site reaction, hypertrophy of skin, hair breakage, colitis not otherwise specified, brittle nails, application site discharge, angioedema, aching joints, ectropion, and telangiectasias.

CLINICAL STUDIES

Clinical data, including skin thickness measurements and serial photographs, were collected in four clinical studies.

Vega Study

This was a 96-week, open-label, uncontrolled, single-center study to determine the treatment effects of **SCULPTRA** on the signs of lipoatrophy of the face in 50 patients infected with human immunodeficiency virus. Patients had a mean age of 45 years (range 33-58), 84% were Caucasian and 98% were male. All patients had little or no adipose tissue in cheek area at baseline, indicating severe facial lipoatrophy (mean adipose thickness of 0.5±0.7 mm, ranging from 0.0 to 2.1 mm).

Treatment

Injection sessions were conducted at approximately two-week intervals, and the majority (86%) of the patients received four to five injection sessions. Generally, one vial of product was injected intradermally into multiple points of each cheek at each injection session. The quantity of injected product and number of injection sessions depended upon the severity of the facial depression.

Results

The mean increases from baseline in skin thickness are presented in Figure 1 below.

FIGURE 1
MEAN INCREASES ABOVE BASELINE IN SKIN THICKNESS (MM) OBSERVED IN THE VEGA STUDY

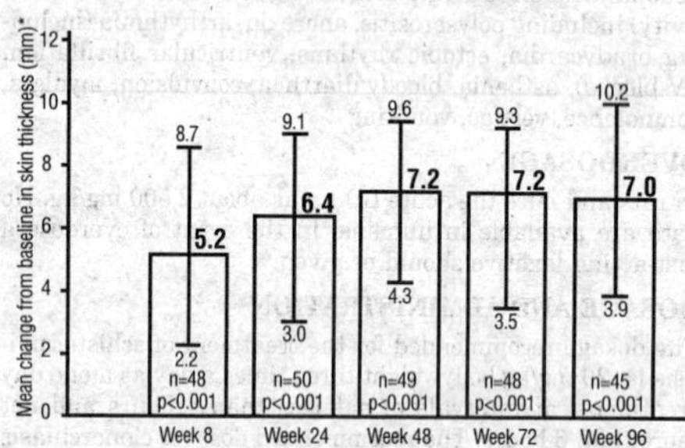

Bars represent maximum and minumum values; The p-value is based on the paired t-test.
* Baseline = 3.0 ± 0.6 mm

All patients experienced increases in skin thickness in the treatment area (minimum increase of 2.2 mm noted at Week 8 visit). Statistically significant increases above baseline values of mean skin thickness were noted at all time points (Weeks 8, 24, 48, 72 and 96) during the study. Increases in mean skin thickness changes above baseline persisted for up to 2 years.

Chelsea & Westminster (C&W) Study

This was a 24-week, open-label, single-center, uncontrolled study in 30 human immunodeficiency virus positive patients with facial lipoatrophy. Patients were placed into groups of 12 or 24 weeks of follow-up. Patients had a mean age of 41 (range 32–60), 72% were Caucasian and 93% were male.

Treatment

All patients received a fixed treatment regimen of three injection sessions conducted at two-week intervals. Each vial of **SCULPTRA** was reconstituted with 2 mLs of SWFI and 1 mL of 2% lidocaine to give a total volume of 3 mL. Up to 3 mL of the reconstituted product was injected bilaterally into multiple points into the cheek and nasolabial areas.

Results

Baseline skin thickness in the treatment areas ranged from 2.1 to 2.7 mm and are presented in the Table 3 below.

TABLE 3:
RANGE OF MEAN INCREASES IN SKIN THICKNESS FROM BASELINE

	12 WEEKS AFTER 1st TREATMENT N=27*	24 WEEKS AFTER 1st TREATMENT N=14*
Cheek Areas	3.9-5.7 mm	4.9mm
Nasolabial Areas	3.9-6.0 mm	4.9-5.3mm

Baselines ranged from 2.1 to 2.7 mm; all changes were significant ($p<0.001$).
*Number of patients varies dependent upon which group they were placed.

Significant changes from Baseline ($p<0.001$) in mean skin thickness were observed in the areas treated (left and right nasolabial and cheeks) with **SCULPTRA** in all patients. A mean increase in skin thickness of approximately 4-6 mm was observed twelve weeks after the initiation of treatment for all treated patients.

APEX 002 and Blue Pacific Studies

Data were obtained from two, single-center, open-label, 12-month investigator-initiated studies in human immunodeficiency virus positive patients with facial lipoatrophy. Ninety-nine patients between 31 and 65 years of age were enrolled in each study. The majority of patients were Caucasian males.

Treatment

Patients were treated with **SCULPTRA** injections at an interval of approximately 3 to 6 weeks and received up to 6 injection sessions.

Results

The results from these studies are shown in Table 2 and were provided for safety information only.

INDIVIDUALIZATION OF TREATMENT (see also Patient Treatment)

The quantity of **SCULPTRA** and the number of injection sessions will vary by patient. Treatment for severe facial fat loss typically requires the injection of one vial of **SCULPTRA** per cheek area per injection session. A typical treatment course for severe facial fat loss involves 3-6 injection sessions, with the sessions separated by two or more weeks. Full effects of the treatment course are evident within weeks to months. The patient should be reevaluated no sooner than two weeks after each injection session to determine if additional correction is needed. Patients should be advised that supplemental injection sessions may be required to maintain an optimal treatment effect.

HOW SUPPLIED

SCULPTRA is supplied as a sterile freeze-dried preparation for injection in a clear glass vial, which is sealed by a penetrable stopper, covered by an aluminum seal with a flip-off cap. Each carton of **SCULPTRA** contains two vials.

COMPOSITION OF SCULPTRA

The final composition of **SCULPTRA** consists of poly-L-lactic acid, sodium carboxymethylcellulose (USP), non-pyrogenic mannitol (USP), sterile water for injection (USP).

NHRIC 8313-1106-02

INSTRUCTIONS FOR USE

Reconstitution

The following supplies are used with **SCULPTRA** but are to be provided by the end-user:

- Sterile Water for Injection (SWFI), USP
- Single-use 5 mL sterile syringe
- Single-use 1-3 mL (depending on physician practitioner preference) sterile syringes (at least 2)
- 18 G sterile needles (at least 2)
- 26 G sterile needles (several should be available)
- Antiseptic

SCULPTRA is reconstituted in the following way:

1. Remove the flip-off cap from the vial and clean the penetrable stopper of the vial with an antiseptic. If the vial, seal, or flip-off cap are damaged, do not use, and call Aventis Pharmaceuticals Inc. at 1-800-633-1610.
2. Attach an 18 G sterile needle to a sterile single-use 5 mL syringe.
3. Draw 3-5 mLs of SWFI into the 5 mL syringe.
4. Introduce the 18 G sterile needle into the stopper of the vial and slowly add all SWFI into the vial.
5. **Let the vial stand for at least 2 hours to ensure complete hydration; do not shake during this period. SCULPTRA** can be stored at room temperature up to 30°C (86°F) during and after hydration. Refrigeration is not required.
6. After waiting at least 2 hours, agitate the vial until a uniform translucent suspension is obtained. A single vial swirling agitator may be used. Product should be agitated immediately prior to use. The reconstituted product is usable within 72 hours of reconstitution. Discard any material remaining after use or after 72 hours following reconstitution.
7. Clean the penetrable stopper of the vial with an antiseptic, and use a new 18 G sterile needle to withdraw an appropriate amount of the suspension (typically 1 mL) into a single–use 1-3 mL sterile syringe. Do not store the reconstituted product in the syringe.
8. Replace the 18 G needle with a 26 G sterile needle before injecting the product into the deep dermis or subcutaneous layer. Do not inject **SCULPTRA** using needles of an internal diameter smaller than 26 G.
9. To withdraw remaining contents of the vial, repeat steps 6 through 8.

Patient Treatment

1. <u>Patient Assessment.</u> Before treatment with **SCULPTRA**, the patient should be informed completely of the indications, contraindications, warnings, precautions for use, possible side effects and mode of administration of **SCULPTRA**. A complete medical history should be taken to determine if the treatment is appropriate. Patients should be informed that more than one injection session is typically necessary to achieve the desired results.
2. <u>Patient Preparation.</u> As with all injectable products, universal precautions must be observed when there is a potential for contact with patient body fluids. The injection session must be conducted with aseptic technique.
3. <u>The needle for injections.</u> **SCULPTRA** should be injected using a 26 G sterile needle. Do not inject with needles smaller than 26 G and do not bend the needle. Agitate the product in the syringe as needed to maintain a uniform suspension throughout the procedure. Before injecting, expel some drops of the product from the prepared syringe with 26 G needle attached to eliminate air and to check for needle blockage. If the 26 G needle becomes occluded or dull during an injection session replacement may be necessary. Draw a small amount of air into the syringe between needle changes to assist in removing clogged particles.
4. <u>The dermal plane.</u> **SCULPTRA** should be injected into the deep dermis or subcutaneous layer. In order to control the injection depth of **SCULPTRA**, stretch/pull the skin opposite to the direction of the injection to create a firm injection surface. The 26 G sterile needle, bevel up, should be introduced into the skin at an angle of approximately 30-40 degrees, until the desired skin depth is reached. A change in tissue resistance is evident when

the needle traverses the dermal-subcutaneous junction. If the needle is inserted at too shallow an angle [i.e., into the mid or superficial (papillary) dermis] the bevel of the needle may be visible through the skin. If product is injected too superficially it will be evident as immediate or slightly delayed blanching in the injected area. If this occurs, the needle should be removed and the treatment area gently massaged.

5. **Injecting: Threading or Tunneling**
   a. **Technique**. When the appropriate dermal plane is reached, the needle angle should be lowered to advance the needle in that dermal plane. Prior to depositing **SCULPTRA** in the skin, a reflux maneuver should be performed to assure that a blood vessel has not been entered. Using the threading or tunneling technique, a thin trail of **SCULPTRA** should then be deposited in the tissue plane as the needle is withdrawn. To avoid deposition in the superficial skin, deposition should be stopped before the needle bevel is visible in the skin.
   b. **Volume per injection**. The volume of **SCULPTRA** should be limited to approximately 0.1 mL-0.2 mL per each individual injection. Note that in areas such as the cheek, approximately 20 injections may be required to cover the targeted area.
   c. **Volume per treatment area**. The volume of product injected per treatment area will vary depending on the surface area to be treated. Treatment of an entire cheek typically requires injection of one vial of **SCULPTRA** per cheek per injection session. Multiple injections (typically administered in a grid or cross-hatched pattern) may be required to cover the targeted area. The total number of injections and thus total volume of **SCULPTRA** injected will vary based on the surface area to be corrected, not on the depth or severity of the deficiency to be corrected.
6. **Injecting: Depot**
   a. **Technique.** The depot technique is most appropriate for injections into areas of thin skin at the level of the upper zygoma or temples. When using this technique, **SCULPTRA** is injected as a small bolus. For the upper zygoma it is injected under the orbicularis oculi muscle. For the temples, it is injected in the temporal fascia.
   b. **Volume per injection.** The volume of **SCULPTRA** should be reduced to approximately 0.05 mL/injection. Following each injection, the area should be massaged.
7. **Massage during the injection session.** The treatment areas should be periodically massaged during the injection session to evenly distribute the product.
8. **Degree of correction.** The depressed area should never be overcorrected (overfilled) in an injection session. Limited correction of the treatment area allows for the gradual improvement of the depressed area over several weeks as the treatment effect occurs. Typically, patients will experience some degree of edema associated with the injection procedure itself, which will give the appearance of a full correction by the end of the injection session (within about 30 minutes). The patient should be informed that the injection-related edema typically resolves in several hours to a few days, resulting in the 'reappearance' of the original contour deficiency.
9. **Post-treatment care.** Immediately following an injection session with **SCULPTRA**, redness, swelling, and/or bruising may be noted in the treatment area. Refer to **ADVERSE EVENTS** for details. After the injection session, an ice pack (avoiding any direct contact of the ice with the skin) should be applied to the treatment area in order to reduce swelling. It is important to thoroughly massage the treatment area to evenly distribute the product. The patient should periodically massage the treatment area for several days after the injection session to promote a natural-looking correction.
10. **Treat, Wait, Assess.** During the first injection session with **SCULPTRA**, only a limited correction should be made. Do not overcorrect (overfill). The patient should be evaluated no sooner than two weeks after the injection session to determine if additional correction is needed. The original skin depression may initially reappear, but the depression should gradually improve within several weeks as the treatment effect of **SCULPTRA** occurs. The patient should be advised of the potential need for additional injection sessions at the first consultation.

PATIENT INSTRUCTIONS

It is recommended that the following information be shared with patients:

- To report any adverse reactions, call Aventis Pharmaceuticals Inc. at 1-800-633-1610.
- Within the first 24 hours, an ice pack (avoiding any direct contact of the ice with the skin) should be applied to the treatment area to reduce swelling. **SCULPTRA** may cause redness, swelling, or bruising when first injected into the skin, typically resolving in hours to one week. Hematoma may also occur, typically resolving in hours to about two weeks. Worsening or prolonged symptoms or signs should be reported to the health care provider. The original skin depression may initially reappear, but the depression should gradually improve within several weeks as the treatment effect of **SCULPTRA** occurs. The health care provider will assess the need for additional **SCULPTRA** injection sessions after two or more weeks.
- Massage the treatment area daily, for several days following any injection session.
- Treatment with **SCULPTRA** can result in small papules in the treatment area. These subcutaneous papules are typically not visible and asymptomatic and may be noticed only upon pressing on the treatment area. However, visible nodules, sometimes with redness or color change to the skin, have been reported. Patients should report any side effects to their health care provider.
- Make-up may be applied a few hours post-treatment if no complications are present (e.g. open wounds, bleeding, redness and swelling).
- Patients should minimize exposure of the treatment area to excessive sun and UV lamp exposure until any initial swelling and redness has resolved.

STORAGE

SCULPTRA can be stored at room temperature, up to 30°C (86°F).
DO NOT FREEZE.
Refrigeration is not required.

STERILITY

Each vial of **SCULPTRA** is packaged for single-use only. Do not resterilize.
IF THE VIAL, SEAL, OR THE FLIP-OFF CAP ARE DAMAGED, DO NOT USE AND CONTACT AVENTIS PHARMACEUTICALS INC. AT 1-800-633-1610.
Rx only.
ANY SIDE EFFECTS OR PRODUCT COMPLAINTS SHOULD BE REPORTED TO:
Aventis Pharmaceuticals Inc.
Bridgewater, NJ USA
1-800-633-1610
Pat. No. US 6,716,251
Prescribing Information as of August 2004.
Manufactured for:
Dermik Laboratories
A Division of Aventis Pharmaceuticals Inc.
1050 Westlakes Drive
Berwyn, PA 19312
USA
1-800-633-1610
Produced by:
Gruppo Lepetit S.p.A. 20020 Lainate, Italy

A PATIENT'S GUIDE TO TREATMENT WITH SCULPTRA™

SCULPTRA™
injectable poly-L-lactic acid

GLOSSARY

Anesthetic: A substance that causes loss of feeling or awareness. A topical or local anesthetic causes temporary loss of feeling in a part of the body.
Antiseptic: An agent that kills bacteria or prevents or slows growth of germs.
Biocompatible: A material that does not harm the body.
Biodegradable: Able to be broken down by the body.
Induration: Any hardening or thickening of tissue or skin.
Keloids: An overgrowth of scar tissue at the site of a skin injury. Keloids may occur around surgical cuts, traumatic wounds, vaccination sites, burns, or minor scratches.
Lipoatrophy: The loss of body fat.
Palpable: Able to be touched and felt.
Poly-L-lactic acid: A synthetic material that is biocompatible and bioabsorbable and has been used for over 25 years in dissolvable stitches, soft tissue implants and other implants.
Side effect: An undesirable event caused by use of the product.
Synthetic: "man-made."

BACKGROUND INFORMATION

WHAT IS SCULPTRA?

SCULPTRA is a synthetic injectable material known as "poly-L-lactic acid." Poly-L-lactic acid is a biocompatible, biodegradable material that has been widely used for many years in dissolvable stitches, soft tissue implants, and other types of implants.

WHO MIGHT BENEFIT FROM TREATMENT WITH SCULPTRA?

SCULPTRA is intended for restoration and/or correction of the signs of facial fat loss (lipoatrophy) in people with human immunodeficiency virus.

WHO SHOULD NOT USE SCULPTRA?

Talk to your health care provider about your medical history when deciding on treatment options.
You should not use **SCULPTRA** if:
- you are allergic to any ingredient of **SCULPTRA**.

ARE SKIN TESTS NEEDED BEFORE TREATMENT WITH SCULPTRA?

No skin testing is required prior to use.

HOW DOES SCULPTRA WORK?

SCULPTRA is injected below the surface of the skin in the area of fat loss.
SCULPTRA provides an increase in skin thickness. Visible results appear within the first few treatment sessions.
SCULPTRA will not correct the underlying cause of the facial fat loss, but will help improve the appearance by increasing skin thickness in the treated area.

ARE THE RESULTS FROM SCULPTRA IMMEDIATE?

No. At your first treatment visit it may appear that **SCULPTRA** worked immediately. That is because of swelling from the injections and the water used to dilute **SCULPTRA**. In a few days, when the swelling goes down and the water is absorbed by your body, you may look as you did before your treatment. **SCULPTRA** takes time to gradually correct the depression in your skin. Your health care provider will see you again in a few weeks to decide if you need more **SCULPTRA** injections.

HOW MANY TREATMENTS ARE REQUIRED?

Your health care provider will decide with you the number of treatment sessions and the amount of **SCULPTRA** you will need at each treatment session. Patients with **severe** facial fat loss may require three to six treatment sessions. Touch-up treatments may be needed to maintain the desired effect.

HOW OFTEN ARE TREATMENTS GIVEN?

Your health care provider will see you two or more weeks after each treatment to assess whether you need additional treatments.

HOW LONG DO TREATMENT EFFECTS LAST?

Treatment effects will differ for each person. In a clinical study the treatment results lasted for up to 2 years after the first treatment session, in most patients. Touch-up treatments may be needed to maintain the desired effect. Dermik® is studying the long-term effects beyond two years.

DO INJECTIONS OF SCULPTRA HURT?

As with any injection, injections with **SCULPTRA** may hurt. **SCULPTRA** is injected in small amounts using a very fine needle. Your health care provider may apply a topical or local anesthetic.

WHAT CAN I EXPECT TO HAPPEN AT A TREATMENT SESSION?

Your health care provider will answer all of your questions and prepare you for the treatment.
- Make-up should be removed.
- The area where the injections will be given will be cleaned with an antiseptic.
- You and your health care provider will determine if a topical or local anesthetic is needed.
- **SCULPTRA** will be injected in small amounts into the skin using a very fine needle. Multiple injections will be needed.
- An ice pack should be applied to the treatment area to help reduce swelling.
- After the treatment session, the area should be thoroughly massaged to disribute the product evenly.

WHAT ARE THE POSSIBLE SIDE EFFECTS OF TREATMENT WITH SCULPTRA?

Talk to your health care provider about the possible side effects of **SCULPTRA**.

TABLE 1:
NUMBER OF PATIENTS WITH TREATMENT-RELATED SIDE EFFECTS OBSERVED IN CLINICAL STUDIES WITH ONE TO TWO YEARS OF FOLLOW-UP

	277 Patients
INJECTION PROCEDURE RELATED SIDE EFFECTS	
Bruising	59 (21%)
Swelling*	27 (10%)
Pain	37 (13%)
Redness	6 (2%)
DEVICE-RELATED SIDE EFFECTS	
Small bumps under the skin	54 (19%)

*Occasionally accompanied with redness

The most common side effects with the use of **SCULPTRA** include injection-related side effects at the site of the injection, such as bleeding, tenderness or pain, redness, bruising, or swelling. These side effects generally last, on average, 3 to 17 days.
One possible delayed side effect with **SCULPTRA** can be small bumps under the skin in the treated area. These small bumps may not be visible, and you may notice them only when you press on the treated skin. These bumps tend to happen within the first six to twelve months after the first treatment. Occasionally, these bumps go away on their own. Visible bumps, sometimes with redness or color change to the treated area, have also been reported. As with all procedures that involve an injection through the skin, there is a risk of infection.
Report any side effects to your health care provider.

SHOULD I TELL MY HEALTHCARE PROVIDER WHAT MEDICATIONS I AM TAKING?

Yes. You should tell your healthcare provider about all the medicines you are taking, even over the counter medicines or treatments. If you are taking blood thinners or medications that may interfere with clotting of the blood, such as aspirin, you might be more likely to have bruising or bleeding at the injection site. There have been no studies of possible interactions between **SCULPTRA** and drugs or other substances or implants. Talk to your health care provider about your medical history when deciding on treatment options.

WHAT CAN I EXPECT AFTER TREATMENT?

Immediately following a treatment session with **SCULPTRA**, redness, swelling, pain, bruising or all of these

Continued on next page

Sculptra—Cont.

signs can happen in the treatment area. These signs usually go away in a few hours to a few days. Some have been known to last up to 17 days. Your health care provider will give you specific post-treatment care instructions. You should massage the treated area (a few times each day) for several days after the treatment session. Within the first 24 hours after treatment, an ice pack should be applied for a few minutes at a time to the treatment area to help reduce swelling. Wrap the ice in a cloth and avoid putting ice directly on your skin. Avoid excessive sun and UV lamp exposure until any initial swelling and redness has resolved. Report any worsening or longer-lasting symptoms or signs to your health care provider.

HOW QUICKLY CAN I GET BACK TO MY DAILY ACTIVITIES?
Most patients feel comfortable going back to their normal activities following treatment.

WHEN WILL I BE ABLE TO APPLY MAKE-UP AFTER TREATMENT?
Make-up may be applied a few hours after treatment if no complications are present (for example, open wounds or bleeding).

ADDITIONAL INFORMATION

What are my other options for treatment?
At present there are no other medical devices for restoration and/or correction of facial fat loss (lipoatrophy) in people with human immunodeficiency virus.

Prescribing Information as of August 2004.

Dermik Laboratories
A Division of Aventis Pharmaceuticals Inc.
1050 Westlakes Drive
Berwyn, PA 19312
Telephone: 1-800-633-1610

Forest Pharmaceuticals, Inc.

(Subsidiary of Forest Laboratories, Inc.)
13600 SHORELINE DRIVE
ST. LOUIS, MO 63045

Direct Inquiries to:
Professional Affairs Department
13600 Shoreline Drive
St. Louis, MO 63045
(800) 678-1605

CAMPRAL® ℞

[kăm-prəl]
(acamprosate calcium)
Delayed-Release Tablets
Rx Only

DESCRIPTION

CAMPRAL® (acamprosate calcium) is supplied in an enteric-coated tablet for oral administration. Acamprosate calcium is a synthetic compound with a chemical structure similar to that of the endogenous amino acid homotaurine, which is a structural analogue of the amino acid neurotransmitter γ-aminobutyric acid and the amino acid neuromodulator taurine. Its chemical name is calcium acetylaminopropane sulfonate. Its chemical formula is $C_{10}H_{20}N_2O_8S_2Ca$ and molecular weight is 400.48. Its structural formula is:

Acamprosate calcium is a white, odorless or nearly odorless powder. It is freely soluble in water, and practically insoluble in absolute ethanol and dichloromethane.

Each *CAMPRAL* tablet contains acamprosate calcium 333 mg, equivalent to 300 mg of acamprosate. Inactive ingredients in *CAMPRAL* tablets include: crospovidone, microcrystalline cellulose, magnesium silicate, sodium starch glycolate, colloidal anhydrous silica, magnesium stearate, talc, propylene glycol and Eudragit® L 30 D or equivalent. Sulfites were used in the synthesis of the drug substance and traces of residual sulfites may be present in the drug product.

CLINICAL PHARMACOLOGY

Pharmacodynamics
The mechanism of action of acamprosate in maintenance of alcohol abstinence is not completely understood. Chronic alcohol exposure is hypothesized to alter the normal balance between neuronal excitation and inhibition. *In vitro* and *in vivo* studies in animals have provided evidence to suggest acamprosate may interact with glutamate and GABA neurotransmitter systems centrally, and has led to the hypothesis that acamprosate restores this balance.

Pharmacodynamic studies have shown that acamprosate calcium reduces alcohol intake in alcohol-dependent animals in a dose-dependent manner and that this effect appears to be specific to alcohol and the mechanisms of alcohol dependence.

Acamprosate calcium has negligible observable central nervous system (CNS) activity in animals outside of its effects on alcohol dependence, exhibiting no anticonvulsant, antidepressant, or anxiolytic activity.

The administration of acamprosate calcium is not associated with the development of tolerance or dependence in animal studies.

CAMPRAL is not known to cause alcohol aversion and does not cause a disulfiram-like reaction as a result of ethanol ingestion.

Pharmacokinetics

Absorption
The absolute bioavailability of *CAMPRAL* after oral administration is about 11%. Steady-state plasma concentrations of acamprosate are reached within 5 days of dosing. Steady-state peak plasma concentrations after *CAMPRAL* doses of 2 × 333 mg tablets three times daily average 350 ng/mL and occur at 3-8 hours post-dose. Coadministration of *CAMPRAL* with food decreases bioavailability as measured by C_{max} and AUC, by approximately 42% and 23%, respectively. The food effect on absorption is not clinically significant and no adjustment of dose is necessary.

Distribution
The volume of distribution for acamprosate following intravenous administration is estimated to be 72-109 liters (approximately 1 L/kg). Plasma protein binding of acamprosate is negligible.

Metabolism
Acamprosate does not undergo metabolism.

Elimination
After oral dosing of 2 × 333 mg of *CAMPRAL*, the terminal half-life ranges from approximately 20-33 hours. Following oral administration of *CAMPRAL*, the major route of excretion is via the kidneys as acamprosate.

Special Populations

Gender: *CAMPRAL* does not exhibit any significant pharmacokinetic differences between male and female subjects.

Age: The pharmacokinetics of *CAMPRAL* have not been evaluated in a geriatric population. However, since renal function diminishes in elderly patients and acamprosate is excreted unchanged in urine, acamprosate plasma concentrations are likely to be higher in the elderly population compared to younger adults.

Pediatrics: The pharmacokinetics of *CAMPRAL* have not been evaluated in a pediatric population.

Renal Impairment: Peak plasma concentrations after administration of a single dose of 2 × 333 mg *CAMPRAL* tablets to patients with moderate or severe renal impairment were about 2-fold and 4-fold higher, respectively, compared to healthy subjects. Similarly, elimination half-life was about 1.8-fold and 2.6-fold longer, respectively, compared to healthy subjects. There is a linear relationship between creatinine clearance values and total apparent plasma clearance, renal clearance and plasma half-life of acamprosate. A dose of 1 × 333 mg *CAMPRAL*, three times daily, is recommended in patients with moderate renal impairment (creatinine clearance of 30-50 mL/min, see also **PRECAUTIONS**).

Patients with severe renal impairment (creatinine clearance ≤30 mL/min) should not be given *CAMPRAL* (see also **CONTRAINDICATIONS**).

Hepatic Impairment: Acamprosate is not metabolized by the liver and the pharmacokinetics of *CAMPRAL* are not altered in patients with mild to moderate hepatic impairment (groups A and B of the Child-Pugh classification). No adjustment of dosage is recommended in such patients.

Alcohol-dependent subjects: A cross-study comparison of *CAMPRAL* at doses of 2 × 333 mg three times daily indicated similar pharmacokinetics between alcohol-dependent subjects and healthy subjects.

Drug-Drug Interactions
Acamprosate had no inducing potential on the cytochrome CYP1A2 and 3A4 systems, and *in vitro* inhibition studies suggest that acamprosate does not inhibit *in vivo* metabolism mediated by cytochrome CYP1A2, 2C9, 2C19, 2D6, 2E1, or 3A4. The pharmacokinetics of *CAMPRAL* were unaffected when co-administered with alcohol, disulfiram or diazepam. Similarly, the pharmacokinetics of ethanol, diazepam and nordiazepam, imipramine and desipramine, naltrexone and 6-beta naltrexol were unaffected following co-administration with *CAMPRAL*. However, co-administration of *CAMPRAL* with naltrexone led to a 33% increase in the C_{max} and a 25% increase in the AUC of acamprosate. No adjustment of dosage is recommended in such patients.

CLINICAL STUDIES

The efficacy of *CAMPRAL* in the maintenance of abstinence was supported by three clinical studies involving a total of 998 patients who were administered at least one dose of *CAMPRAL* or placebo as an adjunct to psychosocial therapy. Each study was a double-blind, placebo-controlled trial in alcohol-dependent patients who had undergone inpatient detoxification and were abstinent from alcohol on the day of randomization. Study durations ranged from 90 days to 360 days. *CAMPRAL* proved superior to placebo in maintaining abstinence, as indicated by a greater percentage of subjects being assessed as continuously abstinent throughout treatment.

In a fourth study, the efficacy of *CAMPRAL* was evaluated in alcoholics, including patients with a history of polysubstance abuse and patients who had not undergone detoxification and were not required to be abstinent at baseline. This study failed to demonstrate superiority of *CAMPRAL* over placebo.

INDICATIONS AND USAGE

CAMPRAL is indicated for the maintenance of abstinence from alcohol in patients with alcohol dependence who are abstinent at treatment initiation. Treatment with *CAMPRAL* should be part of a comprehensive management program that includes psychosocial support.

The efficacy of *CAMPRAL* in promoting abstinence has not been demonstrated in subjects who have not undergone detoxification and not achieved alcohol abstinence prior to beginning *CAMPRAL* treatment. The efficacy of *CAMPRAL* in promoting abstinence from alcohol in polysubstance abusers has not been adequately assessed.

CONTRAINDICATIONS

CAMPRAL is contraindicated in patients who previously have exhibited hypersensitivity to acamprosate calcium or any of its components.

CAMPRAL is contraindicated in patients with severe renal impairment (creatinine clearance ≤30 mL/min).

PRECAUTIONS

Use of *CAMPRAL* does not eliminate or diminish withdrawal symptoms.

General

Renal Impairment: Treatment with *CAMPRAL* in patients with moderate renal impairment (creatinine clearance of 30-50 mL/min) requires a dose reduction. Patients with severe renal impairment (creatinine clearance of ≤30 mL/min) should not be given *CAMPRAL* (see also **CONTRAINDICATIONS**).

Suicidality: In controlled clinical trials of *CAMPRAL*, adverse events of a suicidal nature (suicidal ideation, suicide attempts, completed suicides) were infrequent overall, but were more common in *CAMPRAL*-treated patients than in patients treated with placebo (1.4% vs. 0.5% in studies of 6 months or less; 2.4% vs. 0.8% in year-long studies). Completed suicides occurred in 3 of 2272 (0.13%) patients in the pooled acamprosate group from all controlled studies and 2 of 1962 patients (0.10%) in the placebo group. Adverse events coded as "depression" were reported at similar rates in *CAMPRAL*-treated and placebo-treated patients. Although many of these events occurred in the context of alcohol relapse, no consistent pattern of relationship between the clinical course of recovery from alcoholism and the emergence of suicidality was identified. The interrelationship between alcohol dependence, depression and suicidality is well-recognized and complex. Alcohol-dependent patients, including those patients being treated with *CAMPRAL* should be monitored for the development of symptoms of depression or suicidal thinking. Families and caregivers of patients being treated with *CAMPRAL* should be alerted to the need to monitor patients for the emergence of symptoms of depression or suicidality, and to report such symptoms to the patient's health care provider.

Information for Patients
Physicians are advised to discuss the following issues with patients for whom they prescribe *CAMPRAL*.

Any psychoactive drug may impair judgment, thinking, or motor skills. Patients should be cautioned about operating hazardous machinery, including automobiles, until they are reasonably certain that *CAMPRAL* therapy does not affect their ability to engage in such activities.

Patients should be advised to notify their physician if they become pregnant or intend to become pregnant during therapy.

Patients should be advised to notify their physician if they are breast-feeding.

Patients should be advised to continue *CAMPRAL* therapy as directed, even in the event of relapse and should be reminded to discuss any renewed drinking with their physician.

Patients should be advised that *CAMPRAL* has been shown to help maintain abstinence only when used as a part of a treatment program that includes counseling and support.

Drug Interactions
The concomitant intake of alcohol and *CAMPRAL* does not affect the pharmacokinetics of either alcohol or acamprosate.

Pharmacokinetic studies indicate that administration of disulfiram or diazepam does not affect the pharmacokinetics of acamprosate. Co-administration of naltrexone with *CAMPRAL* produced a 25% increase in AUC and a 33% increase in the C_{max} of acamprosate. No adjustment of dosage is recommended in such patients.

The pharmacokinetics of naltrexone and its major metabolite 6-beta-naltrexol were unaffected following co-administration with *CAMPRAL*.

Other concomitant therapies: In clinical trials, the safety profile in subjects treated with *CAMPRAL* concomitantly with anxiolytics, hypnotics and sedatives (including benzodiazepines), or non-opioid analgesics was similar to that of subjects taking placebo with these concomitant medications. Patients taking *CAMPRAL* concomitantly with antidepressants more commonly reported both weight gain and weight loss, compared with patients taking either medication alone.

Carcinogenicity, Mutagenicity and Impairment of Fertility
A carcinogenicity study was conducted in which Sprague-Dawley rats received acamprosate calcium in their diet at doses of 25, 100 or 400 mg/kg/day (0.2, 0.7 or 2.5-fold the maximum recommended human dose based on an AUC

comparison). There was no evidence of an increased incidence of tumors in this carcinogenicity study in the rat. An adequate carcinogenicity study in the mouse has not been conducted.

Acamprosate calcium was negative in all genetic toxicology studies conducted. Acamprosate calcium demonstrated no evidence of genotoxicity in an *in vitro* bacterial reverse point mutation assay (Ames assay) or an *in vitro* mammalian cell gene mutation test using Chinese Hamster Lung V79 cells. No clastogenicity was observed in an *in vitro* chromosomal aberration assay in human lymphocytes and no chromosomal damage detected in an *in vivo* mouse micronucleus assay.

Acamprosate calcium had no effect on fertility after treatment for 70 days prior to mating in male rats and for 14 days prior to mating, throughout mating, gestation and lactation in female rats at doses up to 1000 mg/kg/day (approximately 4 times the maximum recommended human daily oral dose on a mg/m^2 basis). In mice, acamprosate calcium administered orally for 60 days prior to mating and throughout gestation in females at doses up to 2400 mg/kg/day (approximately 5 times the maximum recommended human daily oral dose on a mg/m^2 basis) had no effect on fertility.

Pregnancy Category C

Teratogenic effects: Acamprosate calcium has been shown to be teratogenic in rats when given in doses that are approximately equal to the human dose (on a mg/m^2 basis) and in rabbits when given in doses that are approximately 3 times the human dose (on a mg/m^2 basis). Acamprosate calcium produced a dose-related increase in the number of fetuses with malformations in rats at oral doses of 300 mg/kg/day or greater (approximately equal to the maximum recommended human daily oral dose on a mg/m^2 basis). The malformations included hydronephrosis, malformed iris, retinal dysplasia, and retroesophageal subclavian artery. No findings were observed at an oral dose of 50 mg/kg/day (approximately one-fifth the maximum recommended human daily oral dose on a mg/m^2 basis). An increased incidence of hydronephrosis was also noted in Burgundy Tawny rabbits at oral doses of 400 mg/kg/day or greater (approximately 3 times the maximum recommended human daily oral dose on a mg/m^2 basis). No developmental effects were observed in New Zealand white rabbits at oral doses up to 1000 mg/kg/day (approximately 8 times the maximum recommended human daily oral dose on a mg/m^2 basis). The findings in animals should be considered in relation to known adverse developmental effects of ethyl alcohol, which include the characteristics of fetal alcohol syndrome (craniofacial dysmorphism, intrauterine and postnatal growth retardation, retarded psychomotor and intellectual development) and milder forms of neurological and behavioral disorders in humans. There are no adequate and well controlled studies in pregnant women. *CAMPRAL* should be used during pregnancy only if the potential benefit justifies the potential risk to the fetus.

Nonteratogenic effects: A study conducted in pregnant mice that were administered acamprosate calcium by the oral route starting on Day 15 of gestation through the end of lactation on postnatal day 28 demonstrated an increased incidence of still-born fetuses at doses of 960 mg/kg/day or greater (approximately 2 times the maximum recommended human daily oral dose on a mg/m^2 basis). No effects were observed at a dose of 320 mg/kg/day (approximately one-half the maximum recommended human daily dose on a mg/m^2 basis).

Labor and Delivery

The potential for *CAMPRAL* to affect the duration of labor and delivery is unknown.

Nursing Mothers

In animal studies, acamprosate was excreted in the milk of lactating rats dosed orally with acamprosate calcium. The concentration of acamprosate in milk compared to blood was 1.3:1. It is not known whether acamprosate is excreted in human milk. Because many drugs are excreted in human milk, caution should be exercised when *CAMPRAL* is administered to a nursing woman.

Pediatric Use

The safety and efficacy of *CAMPRAL* have not been established in the pediatric population.

Geriatric Use

Forty-one of the 4234 patients in double-blind, placebo-controlled, clinical trials of *CAMPRAL* were 65 years of age or older, while none were 75 years of age or over. There were too few patients in the ≥65 age group to evaluate any differences in safety or effectiveness for geriatric patients compared to younger patients.

This drug is known to be substantially excreted by the kidney, and the risk of toxic reactions to this drug may be greater in patients with impaired renal function. Because elderly patients are more likely to have decreased renal function, care should be taken in dose selection, and it may be useful to monitor renal function (See **CLINICAL PHARMACOLOGY, ADVERSE REACTIONS,** and **DOSAGE AND ADMINISTRATION**).

ADVERSE REACTIONS

The adverse event data described below reflect the safety experience in over 7000 patients exposed to *CAMPRAL* for up to one year, including over 2000 *CAMPRAL*-exposed patients who participated in placebo-controlled trials.

Adverse Events Leading to Discontinuation

In placebo-controlled trials of 6 months or less, 8% of *CAMPRAL*-treated patients discontinued treatment due to an adverse event, as compared to 6% of patients treated with placebo. In studies longer than 6 months, the discontinuation rate due to adverse events was 7% in both the placebo-treated and the *CAMPRAL*-treated patients. Only diarrhea was associated with the discontinuation of more than 1% of patients (2% of *CAMPRAL*-treated vs. 0.7% of placebo-treated patients). Other events, including nausea, depression, and anxiety, while accounting for discontinuation in less than 1% of patients, were nevertheless more commonly cited in association with discontinuation in *CAMPRAL*-treated patients than in placebo-treated patients.

Table 1. Events Occurring at a Rate of at Least 3% and Greater than Placebo in any *CAMPRAL* Treatment Group in Controlled Clinical Trials with Spontaneously Reported Adverse Events

	Number of Patients (%) with Events			
Body System/ Preferred Term	***CAMPRAL* 1332 mg/day**	***CAMPRAL* 1998 mg/day[1]**	***CAMPRAL* Pooled[2]**	**Placebo**
Number of patients in Treatment Group	**397**	**1539**	**2019**	**1706**
Number (%) of patients with an AE	**248 (62%)**	**910 (59%)**	**1231 (61%)**	**955 (56%)**
Body as a Whole	**121 (30%)**	**513 (33%)**	**685 (34%)**	**517 (30%)**
Accidental Injury*	17 (4%)	44 (3%)	70 (3%)	52 (3%)
Asthenia	29 (7%)	79 (5%)	114 (6%)	93 (5%)
Pain	6 (2%)	56 (4%)	65 (3%)	55 (3%)
Digestive System	**85 (21%)**	**440 (29%)**	**574 (28%)**	**344 (20%)**
Anorexia	20 (5%)	35 (2%)	57 (3%)	44 (3%)
Diarrhea	39 (10%)	257 (17%)	329 (16%)	166 (10%)
Flatulence	4 (1%)	55 (4%)	63 (3%)	28 (2%)
Nausea	11 (3%)	69 (4%)	87 (4%)	58 (3%)
Nervous System	**150 (38%)**	**417 (27%)**	**598 (30%)**	**500 (29%)**
Anxiety**	32 (8%)	80 (5%)	118 (6%)	98 (6%)
Depression	33 (8%)	63 (4%)	102 (5%)	87 (5%)
Dizziness	15 (4%)	49 (3%)	67 (3%)	44 (3%)
Dry mouth	13 (3%)	23 (1%)	36 (2%)	28 (2%)
Insomnia	34 (9%)	94 (6%)	137 (7%)	121 (7%)
Paresthesia	11 (3%)	29 (2%)	40 (2%)	34 (2%)
Skin and Appendages	**26 (7%)**	**150 (10%)**	**187 (9%)**	**169 (10%)**
Pruritus	12 (3%)	68 (4%)	82 (4%)	58 (3%)
Sweating	11 (3%)	27 (2%)	40 (2%)	39 (2%)

*includes events coded as "fracture" by sponsor; **includes events coded as "nervousness" by sponsor

[1] includes 258 patients treated with acamprosate calcium 2000 mg/day, using a different dosage strength and regimen.

[2] includes all patients in the first two columns as well as 83 patients treated with acamprosate calcium 3000 mg/day, using a different dosage strength and regimen.

Common Adverse Events Reported in Controlled Trials

Common, non-serious adverse events were collected spontaneously in some controlled studies and using a checklist in other studies. The overall profile of adverse events was similar using either method. Table 1 shows those events that occurred in any *CAMPRAL* treatment group at a rate of 3% or greater and greater than the placebo group in controlled clinical trials with spontaneously reported adverse events. The reported frequencies of adverse events represent the proportion of individuals who experienced, at least once, a treatment-emergent adverse event of the type listed, without regard to the causal relationship of the events to the drug.

[See table 1 above]

Other Events Observed During the Premarketing Evaluation of *CAMPRAL*

Following is a list of terms that reflect treatment-emergent adverse events reported by patients treated with *CAMPRAL* in 20 clinical trials (4461 patients treated with *CAMPRAL*, 3526 of whom received the maximum recommended dose of 1998 mg/day for up to one year in duration). This listing does not include those events already listed above; events for which a drug cause was considered remote; event terms which were so general as to be uninformative; and events reported only once which were not likely to be acutely life- threatening.

Events are further categorized by body system and listed in order of decreasing frequency according to the following definitions: frequent adverse events are those occurring in at least 1/100 patients (only those not already listed in the summary of adverse events in controlled trials appear in this listing); infrequent adverse events are those occurring in 1/100 to 1/1000 patients; rare events are those occurring in fewer than 1/1000 patients.

Body as a Whole – *Frequent*: headache, abdominal pain, back pain, infection, flu syndrome, chest pain, chills, suicide attempt; *Infrequent*: fever, intentional overdose, malaise, allergic reaction, abscess, neck pain, hernia, intentional injury; *Rare*: ascites, face edema, photosensitivity reaction, abdomen enlarged, sudden death.

Cardiovascular System – *Frequent*: palpitation, syncope; *Infrequent*: hypotension, tachycardia, hemorrhage, angina pectoris, migraine, varicose vein, myocardial infarct, phlebitis, postural hypotension; *Rare*: heart failure, mesenteric arterial occlusion, cardiomyopathy, deep thrombophlebitis, shock.

Digestive System – *Frequent*: vomiting, dyspepsia, constipation, increased appetite; *Infrequent*: liver function tests abnormal, gastroenteritis, gastritis, dysphagia, eructation, gastrointestinal hemorrhage, pancreatitis, rectal hemorrhage, liver cirrhosis, esophagitis, hematemesis, nausea and vomiting, hepatitis; *Rare*: melena, stomach ulcer, cholecystitis, colitis, duodenal ulcer, mouth ulceration, carcinoma of liver.

Endocrine System – *Rare*: goiter, hypothyroidism.

Hemic and Lymphatic System – *Infrequent*: anemia, ecchymosis, eosinophilia, lymphocytosis, thrombocytopenia; *Rare*: leukopenia, lymphadenopathy, monocytosis.

Metabolic and Nutritional Disorders – *Frequent*: peripheral edema, weight gain; *Infrequent*: weight loss, hyperglycemia, SGOT increased, SGPT increased, gout, thirst, hyperuricemia, diabetes mellitus, avitaminosis, bilirubinemia; *Rare*: alkaline phosphatase increased, creatinine increased, hyponatremia, lactic dehydrogenase increased.

Musculoskeletal System – *Frequent*: myalgia, arthralgia; *Infrequent*: leg cramps; *Rare*: rheumatoid arthritis, myopathy.

Nervous System – *Frequent*: somnolence, libido decreased, amnesia, thinking abnormal, tremor, vasodilatation, hypertension; *Infrequent*: convulsion, confusion, libido increased, vertigo, withdrawal syndrome, apathy, suicidal ideation, neuralgia, hostility, agitation, neurosis, abnormal dreams, hallucinations, hypesthesia; *Rare*: alcohol craving, psychosis, hyperkinesia, twitching, depersonalization, increased salivation, paranoid reaction, torticollis, encephalopathy, manic reaction.

Respiratory System – *Frequent*: rhinitis, cough increased, dyspnea, pharyngitis, bronchitis; *Infrequent*: asthma, epistaxis, pneumonia; *Rare*: laryngismus, pulmonary embolus.

Skin and Appendages – *Frequent*: rash; *Infrequent*: acne, eczema, alopecia, maculopapular rash, dry skin, urticaria, exfoliative dermatitis, vesiculobullous rash; *Rare*: psoriasis.

Special Senses – *Frequent*: abnormal vision, taste perversion; *Infrequent*: tinnitus, amblyopia, deafness; *Rare*: ophthalmitis, diplopia, photophobia.

Continued on next page

Campral—Cont.

Urogenital System – *Frequent*: impotence; *Infrequent* – metrorrhagia, urinary frequency, urinary tract infection, sexual function abnormal, urinary incontinence, vaginitis; *Rare*: kidney calculus, abnormal ejaculation, hematuria, menorrhagia, nocturia, polyuria, urinary urgency.

Serious Adverse Events Observed During the Non-US Postmarketing Evaluation of *CAMPRAL* (acamprosate calcium)
Although no causal relationship to *CAMPRAL* has been found, the serious adverse event of acute kidney failure has been reported to be temporally associated with *CAMPRAL* treatment in at least 3 patients and is not described elsewhere in the labeling.

DRUG ABUSE AND DEPENDENCE

Controlled Substance Class
Acamprosate calcium is not a controlled substance.

Physical and Psychological Dependence
CAMPRAL did not produce any evidence of withdrawal symptoms in patients in clinical trials at therapeutic doses. Post marketing data, collected retrospectively outside the U.S., have provided no evidence of *CAMPRAL* abuse or dependence.

OVERDOSAGE

In all reported cases of acute overdosage with *CAMPRAL* (total reported doses of up to 56 grams of acamprosate calcium), the only symptom that could be reasonably associated with *CAMPRAL* was diarrhea. Hypercalcemia has not been reported in cases of acute overdose. A risk of hypercalcemia should be considered in chronic overdosage only. Treatment of overdose should be symptomatic and supportive.

DOSAGE AND ADMINISTRATION

The recommended dose of *CAMPRAL* is two 333 mg tablets (each dose should total 666 mg) taken three times daily. Although dosing may be done without regard to meals, dosing with meals was employed during clinical trials and is suggested as an aid to compliance in those patients who regularly eat three meals daily. A lower dose may be effective in some patients.
Treatment with *CAMPRAL* should be initiated as soon as possible after the period of alcohol withdrawal, when the patient has achieved abstinence, and should be maintained if the patient relapses. *CAMPRAL* should be used as part of a comprehensive psychosocial treatment program.

Dosage in Renal Impairment: For patients with moderate renal impairment (creatinine clearance of 30-50 mL/min), a starting dose of one 333 mg tablet taken three times daily is recommended. Patients with severe renal impairment (creatinine clearance of ≤30 mL/min) should not be given *CAMPRAL*.

HOW SUPPLIED

CAMPRAL 333 mg tablets are enteric-coated, white, round, biconvex tablets, identified with "333" debossed on one side.
Opaque HDPE bottles of 180-NDC #0456-3330-01
Dose Pak of 180-NDC #0456-3330-60
Storage:
Store at 25°C (77°F); excursions permitted to 15°-30°C (59°-86°F).
Manufactured by:
Merck Santé s.a.s.
Subsidiary of Merck KGaA, Darmstadt, Germany
37, rue Saint-Romain
69008 LYON FRANCE
Manufactured for FOREST PHARMACEUTICALS, Inc.
Subsidiary of Forest Laboratories, Inc.
St. Louis, MO 63045
07/04

Eli Lilly and Company

LILLY CORPORATE CENTER
INDIANAPOLIS, IN 46285

Direct Inquiries to:
Lilly Corporate Center
Indianapolis, IN 46285
(317) 276-2000
www.lilly.com

For Medical Information Contact:
Lilly Research Laboratories
Lilly Corporate Center
Indianapolis, IN 46285
(800) 545-5979

CYMBALTA® ℞

[*sĭm-băl-tă*]
(duloxetine hydrochloride) Delayed-release Capsules

DESCRIPTION

Cymbalta® (duloxetine hydrochloride) is a selective serotonin and norepinephrine reuptake inhibitor (SSNRI) for oral administration. Its chemical designation is (+)-(*S*)-*N*-methyl-γ-(1-naphthyloxy)-2-thiophenepropylamine hydrochloride. The empirical formula is $C_{18}H_{19}NOS \cdot HCl$, which corresponds to a molecular weight of 333.88. The structural formula is:

NH • HCl
CH3

Duloxetine hydrochloride is a white to slightly brownish white solid, which is slightly soluble in water.
Each capsule contains enteric-coated pellets of 22.4, 33.7, or 67.3 mg of duloxetine hydrochloride equivalent to 20, 30, or 60 mg of duloxetine, respectively. These enteric-coated pellets are designed to prevent degradation of the drug in the acidic environment of the stomach. Inactive ingredients include FD&C Blue No. 2, gelatin, hypromellose, hydroxypropyl methylcellulose acetate succinate, sodium lauryl sulfate, sucrose, sugar spheres, talc, titanium dioxide, and triethyl citrate. The 20 and 60 mg capsules also contain iron oxide yellow.

CLINICAL PHARMACOLOGY

Pharmacodynamics
Although the exact mechanisms of the antidepressant and central pain inhibitory action of duloxetine in humans are unknown, the antidepressant and pain inhibitory actions are believed to be related to its potentiation of serotonergic and noradrenergic activity in the CNS. Preclinical studies have shown that duloxetine is a potent inhibitor of neuronal serotonin and norepinephrine reuptake and a less potent inhibitor of dopamine reuptake. Duloxetine has no significant affinity for dopaminergic, adrenergic, cholinergic, histaminergic, opioid, glutamate, and GABA receptors *in vitro*. Duloxetine does not inhibit monoamine oxidase (MAO). Duloxetine undergoes extensive metabolism, but the major circulating metabolites have not been shown to contribute significantly to the pharmacologic activity of duloxetine.

Pharmacokinetics
Duloxetine has an elimination half-life of about 12 hours (range 8 to 17 hours) and its pharmacokinetics are dose proportional over the therapeutic range. Steady-state plasma concentrations are typically achieved after 3 days of dosing. Elimination of duloxetine is mainly through hepatic metabolism involving two P450 isozymes, CYP2D6 and CYP1A2.
Absorption and Distribution—Orally administered duloxetine hydrochloride is well absorbed. There is a median 2-hour lag until absorption begins (T_{lag}), with maximal plasma concentrations (C_{max}) of duloxetine occurring 6 hours post dose. Food does not affect the C_{max} of duloxetine, but delays the time to reach peak concentration from 6 to 10 hours and it marginally decreases the extent of absorption (AUC) by about 10%. There is a 3-hour delay in absorption and a one-third increase in apparent clearance of duloxetine after an evening dose as compared to a morning dose.
The apparent volume of distribution averages about 1640 L. Duloxetine is highly bound (>90%) to proteins in human plasma, binding primarily to albumin and α_1-acid glycoprotein. The interaction between duloxetine and other highly protein bound drugs has not been fully evaluated. Plasma protein binding of duloxetine is not affected by renal or hepatic impairment.
Metabolism and Elimination—Biotransformation and disposition of duloxetine in humans have been determined following oral administration of ^{14}C-labeled duloxetine. Duloxetine comprises about 3% of the total radiolabeled material in the plasma, indicating that it undergoes extensive metabolism to numerous metabolites. The major biotransformation pathways for duloxetine involve oxidation of the naphthyl ring followed by conjugation and further oxidation. Both CYP2D6 and CYP1A2 catalyze the oxidation of the naphthyl ring *in vitro*. Metabolites found in plasma include 4-hydroxy duloxetine glucuronide and 5-hydroxy, 6-methoxy duloxetine sulfate. Many additional metabolites have been identified in urine, some representing only minor pathways of elimination. Only trace (<1% of the dose) amounts of unchanged duloxetine are present in the urine. Most (about 70%) of the duloxetine dose appears in the urine as metabolites of duloxetine; about 20% is excreted in the feces.

Special Populations
Gender—Duloxetine's half-life is similar in men and women. Dosage adjustment based on gender is not necessary.
Age—The pharmacokinetics of duloxetine after a single dose of 40 mg were compared in healthy elderly females (65 to 77 years) and healthy middle-age females (32 to 50 years). There was no difference in the C_{max}, but the AUC of duloxetine was somewhat (about 25%) higher and the half-life about 4 hours longer in the elderly females. Population pharmacokinetic analyses suggest that the typical values for clearance decrease by approximately 1% for each year of age between 25 to 75 years of age; but age as a predictive factor only accounts for a small percentage of between-patient variability. Dosage adjustment based on the age of the patient is not necessary (*see* DOSAGE AND ADMINISTRATION).
Smoking Status—Duloxetine bioavailability (AUC) appears to be reduced by about one-third in smokers. Dosage modifications are not recommended for smokers.
Race—No specific pharmacokinetic study was conducted to investigate the effects of race.
Renal Insufficiency—Limited data are available on the effects of duloxetine in patients with end-stage renal disease (ESRD). After a single 60-mg dose of duloxetine, C_{max} and AUC values were approximately 100% greater in patients with end-stage renal disease receiving chronic intermittent hemodialysis than in subjects with normal renal function. The elimination half-life, however, was similar in both groups. The AUCs of the major circulating metabolites, 4-hydroxy duloxetine glucuronide and 5-hydroxy, 6-methoxy duloxetine sulfate, largely excreted in urine, were approximately 7- to 9-fold higher and would be expected to increase further with multiple dosing. For this reason, Cymbalta is not recommended for patients with end-stage renal disease (requiring dialysis) or severe renal impairment (estimated creatinine clearance [CrCl] <30 mL/min) (*see* DOSAGE AND ADMINISTRATION). Population PK analyses suggest that mild to moderate degrees of renal dysfunction (estimated CrCl 30–80 mL/min) have no significant effect on duloxetine apparent clearance.
Hepatic Insufficiency—Patients with clinically evident hepatic insufficiency have decreased duloxetine metabolism and elimination. After a single 20-mg dose of Cymbalta, 6 cirrhotic patients with moderate liver impairment (Child-Pugh Class B) had a mean plasma duloxetine clearance about 15% that of age- and gender-matched healthy subjects, with a 5-fold increase in mean exposure (AUC). Although C_{max} was similar to normals in the cirrhotic patients, the half-life was about 3 times longer (*see* PRECAUTIONS). It is recommended that duloxetine not be administered to patients with any hepatic insufficiency (*see* DOSAGE AND ADMINISTRATION).

Drug-Drug Interactions (also *see* PRECAUTIONS , Drug Interactions)
Potential for Other Drugs to Affect Duloxetine
Both CYP1A2 and CYP2D6 are responsible for duloxetine metabolism.
Inhibitors of CYP1A2—When duloxetine was co-administered with fluvoxamine, a potent CYP1A2 inhibitor, to male subjects (n=14) the AUC was increased over 5-fold, the C_{max} was increased about 2.5-fold, and duloxetine $t_{1/2}$ was increased approximately 3-fold. Other drugs that inhibit CYP1A2 metabolism include cimetidine and quinolone antimicrobials such as ciprofloxacin and enoxacin.
Inhibitors of CYP2D6—Because CYP2D6 is involved in duloxetine metabolism, concomitant use of duloxetine with potent inhibitors of CYP2D6 would be expected to, and does, result in higher concentrations of duloxetine (*see* PRECAUTIONS, Drug Interactions).
Studies with Benzodiazepines
Lorazepam—Under steady-state conditions for duloxetine (60 mg Q 12 hours) and lorazepam (2 mg Q 12 hours), the pharmacokinetics of duloxetine were not affected by co-administration.
Temazepam—Under steady-state conditions for duloxetine (20 mg qhs) and temazepam (30 mg qhs), the pharmacokinetics of duloxetine were not affected by co-administration.
Potential for Duloxetine to Affect Other Drugs
Drugs Metabolized by CYP1A2—*In vitro* drug interaction studies demonstrate that duloxetine does not induce CYP1A2 activity. Therefore, an increase in the metabolism of CYP1A2 substrates (e.g., theophylline, caffeine) resulting from induction is not anticipated, although clinical studies of induction have not been performed. Although duloxetine is an inhibitor of the CYP1A2 isoform in *in vitro* studies, the pharmacokinetics of theophylline, a CYP1A2 substrate, were not significantly affected by co-administration with duloxetine (60 mg BID). Duloxetine is thus unlikely to have a clinically significant effect on the metabolism of CYP1A2 substrates.
Drugs Metabolized by CYP2D6—Duloxetine is a moderate inhibitor of CYP2D6 and increases the AUC and C_{max} of drugs metabolized by CYP2D6 (*see* PRECAUTIONS). Therefore, co-administration of Cymbalta with other drugs that are extensively metabolized by this isozyme and that have a narrow therapeutic index should be approached with caution (*see* PRECAUTIONS, Drug Interactions).
Drugs Metabolized by CYP2C9—Duloxetine does not inhibit the *in vitro* enzyme activity of CYP2C9. Inhibition of the metabolism of CYP2C9 substrates is therefore not anticipated, although clinical studies have not been performed.
Drugs Metabolized by CYP3A—Results of *in vitro* studies demonstrate that duloxetine does not inhibit or induce CYP3A activity. Therefore, an increase or decrease in the metabolism of CYP3A substrates (e.g., oral contraceptives and other steroidal agents) resulting from induction or inhibition is not anticipated, although clinical studies have not been performed.
Drugs Metabolized by CYP2C19—Results of *in vitro* studies demonstrate that duloxetine does not inhibit CYP2C19 activity at therapeutic concentrations. Inhibition of the metabolism of CYP2C19 substrates is therefore not anticipated, although clinical studies have not been performed.
Studies with Benzodiazepines
Lorazepam—Under steady-state conditions for duloxetine (60 mg Q 12 hours) and lorazepam (2 mg Q 12 hours), the pharmacokinetics of lorazepam were not affected by co-administration.
Temazepam—Under steady-state conditions for duloxetine (20 mg qhs) and temazepam (30 mg qhs), the pharmacokinetics of temazepam were not affected by co-administration.
Drugs Highly Bound to Plasma Protein—Because duloxetine is highly bound to plasma protein, administration of Cymbalta to a patient taking another drug that is

highly protein bound may cause increased free concentrations of the other drug, potentially resulting in adverse events.

CLINICAL STUDIES

Major Depressive Disorder

The efficacy of Cymbalta as a treatment for depression was established in 4 randomized, double-blind, placebo-controlled, fixed-dose studies in adult outpatients (18 to 83 years) meeting DSM-IV criteria for major depression. In 2 studies, patients were randomized to Cymbalta 60 mg once daily (N=123 and N=128, respectively) or placebo (N=122 and N=139, respectively) for 9 weeks; in the third study, patients were randomized to Cymbalta 20 or 40 mg twice daily (N=86 and N=91, respectively) or placebo (N=89) for 8 weeks; in the fourth study, patients were randomized to Cymbalta 40 or 60 mg twice daily (N=95 and N=93, respectively) or placebo (N=93) for 8 weeks. There is no evidence that doses greater than 60 mg/day confer any additional benefit.

In all 4 studies, Cymbalta demonstrated superiority over placebo as measured by improvement in the 17-item Hamilton Depression Rating Scale (HAMD-17) total score.

Analyses of the relationship between treatment outcome and age, gender, and race did not suggest any differential responsiveness on the basis of these patient characteristics.

Diabetic Peripheral Neuropathic Pain

The efficacy of Cymbalta for the management of neuropathic pain associated with diabetic peripheral neuropathy (DPN) was established in 2 randomized, 12-week, double-blind, placebo-controlled, fixed-dose studies in adult patients having diabetic peripheral neuropathy for at least 6 months. Study 1 and 2 enrolled a total of 791 patients of whom 592 (75%) completed the studies. Patients enrolled had Type I or II diabetes mellitus with a diagnosis of painful distal symmetrical sensorimotor polyneuropathy for at least 6 months. The patients had a baseline pain score of ≥4 on an 11-point scale ranging from 0 (no pain) to 10 (worst possible pain). Patients were permitted up to 4 g of acetaminophen per day as needed for pain, in addition to Cymbalta. Patients recorded their pain daily in a diary.

Both studies compared Cymbalta 60 mg once daily or 60 mg twice daily with placebo. Study 1 additionally compared Cymbalta 20 mg with placebo. A total of 457 patients (342 Cymbalta, 115 placebo) were enrolled in Study 1 and a total of 334 patients (226 Cymbalta, 108 placebo) were enrolled in Study 2. Treatment with Cymbalta 60 mg one or two times a day statistically significantly improved the endpoint mean pain scores from baseline and increased the proportion of patients with at least a 50% reduction in pain score from baseline. For various degrees of improvement in pain from baseline to study endpoint, Figures 1 and 2 show the fraction of patients achieving that degree of improvement. The figures are cumulative, so that patients whose change from baseline is, for example, 50%, are also included at every level of improvement below 50%. Patients who did not complete the study were assigned 0% improvement. Some patients experienced a decrease in pain as early as Week 1, which persisted throughout the study.

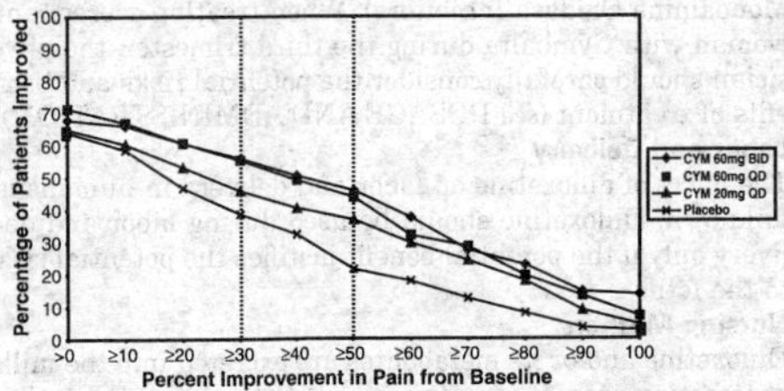

Figure 1: Percentage of Patients Achieving Various Levels of Pain Relief as Measured by 24-Hour Average Pain Severity - Study 1

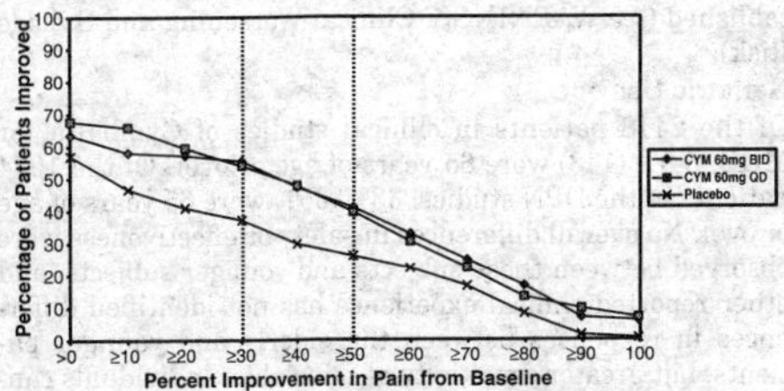

Figure 2: Percentage of Patients Achieving Various Levels of Pain Relief as Measured by 24-Hour Average Pain Severity - Study 2

INDICATIONS AND USAGE

Major Depressive Disorder

Cymbalta is indicated for the treatment of major depressive disorder (MDD).

The efficacy of Cymbalta has been established in 8- and 9-week placebo-controlled trials of outpatients who met DSM-IV diagnostic criteria for major depressive disorder (*see* CLINICAL STUDIES).

A major depressive episode (DSM-IV) implies a prominent and relatively persistent (nearly every day for at least 2 weeks) depressed or dysphoric mood that usually interferes with daily functioning, and includes at least 5 of the following 9 symptoms: depressed mood, loss of interest in usual activities, significant change in weight and/or appetite, insomnia or hypersomnia, psychomotor agitation or retardation, increased fatigue, feelings of guilt or worthlessness, slowed thinking or impaired concentration, or a suicide attempt or suicidal ideation.

The effectiveness of Cymbalta in hospitalized patients with major depressive disorder has not been studied.

The effectiveness of Cymbalta in long-term use for major depressive disorder, that is, for more than 9 weeks, has not been systematically evaluated in controlled trials. The physician who elects to use Cymbalta for extended periods should periodically evaluate the long-term usefulness of the drug for the individual patient.

Diabetic Peripheral Neuropathic Pain

Cymbalta is indicated for the management of neuropathic pain associated with diabetic peripheral neuropathy (*see* CLINICAL STUDIES).

CONTRAINDICATIONS

Hypersensitivity

Cymbalta is contraindicated in patients with a known hypersensitivity to duloxetine or any of the inactive ingredients.

Monoamine Oxidase Inhibitors

Concomitant use in patients taking monoamine oxidase inhibitors (MAOIs) is contraindicated (*see* WARNINGS).

Uncontrolled Narrow-Angle Glaucoma

In clinical trials, Cymbalta use was associated with an increased risk of mydriasis; therefore, its use should be avoided in patients with uncontrolled narrow-angle glaucoma.

WARNINGS

Clinical Worsening and Suicide Risk—Patients with major depressive disorder, both adult and pediatric, may experience worsening of their depression and/or the emergence of suicidal ideation and behavior (suicidality), whether or not they are taking antidepressant medications, and this risk may persist until significant remission occurs. Although there has been a long-standing concern that antidepressants may have a role in inducing worsening of depression and the emergence of suicidality in certain patients, a causal role for antidepressants in inducing such behaviors has not been established. **Nevertheless, patients being treated with antidepressants should be observed closely for clinical worsening and suicidality, especially at the beginning of a course of drug therapy, or at the time of dose changes, either increases or decreases.** Consideration should be given to changing the therapeutic regimen, including possibly discontinuing the medication, in patients whose depression is persistently worse or whose emergent suicidality is severe, abrupt in onset, or was not part of the patient's presenting symptoms.

Because of the possibility of co-morbidity between major depressive disorder and other psychiatric and nonpsychiatric disorders, the same precautions observed when treating patients with major depressive disorder should be observed when treating patients with other psychiatric and nonpsychiatric disorders.

The following symptoms - anxiety, agitation, panic attacks, insomnia, irritability, hostility (aggressiveness), impulsivity, akathisia (psychomotor restlessness), hypomania, and mania - have been reported in adult and pediatric patients being treated with antidepressants for major depressive disorder as well as for other indications, both psychiatric and nonpsychiatric. Although a causal link between the emergence of such symptoms and either the worsening of depression and/or the emergence of suicidal impulses has not been established, consideration should be given to changing the therapeutic regimen, including possibly discontinuing the medication, in patients for whom such symptoms are severe, abrupt in onset, or were not part of the patient's presenting symptoms.

Families and caregivers of patients being treated with antidepressants for major depressive disorder or other indications, both psychiatric and nonpsychiatric, should be alerted about the need to monitor patients for the emergence of agitation, irritability, and the other symptoms described above, as well as the emergence of suicidality, and to report such symptoms immediately to health care providers. Prescriptions for Cymbalta should be written for the smallest quantity of capsules consistent with good patient management, in order to reduce the risk of overdose.

If the decision has been made to discontinue treatment, medication should be tapered, as rapidly as is feasible, but with recognition that abrupt discontinuation can be associated with certain symptoms (*see* PRECAUTIONS *and* DOSAGE AND ADMINISTRATION, Discontinuing Cymbalta, for a description of the risks of discontinuation of Cymbalta).

A major depressive episode may be the initial presentation of bipolar disorder. It is generally believed (though not established in controlled trials) that treating such an episode with an antidepressant alone may increase the likelihood of precipitation of a mixed/manic episode in patients at risk for bipolar disorder. Whether any of the symptoms described above represent such a conversion is unknown. However, prior to initiating treatment with an antidepressant, patients should be adequately screened to determine if they are at risk for bipolar disorder; such screening should include a detailed psychiatric history, including a family history of suicide, bipolar disorder, and depression. It should be noted that Cymbalta is not approved for use in treating bipolar depression.

Monoamine Oxidase Inhibitors (MAOI)—In patients receiving a serotonin reuptake inhibitor in combination with a monoamine oxidase inhibitor, there have been reports of serious, sometimes fatal, reactions including hyperthermia, rigidity, myoclonus, autonomic instability with possible rapid fluctuations of vital signs, and mental status changes that include extreme agitation progressing to delirium and coma. These reactions have also been reported in patients who have recently discontinued serotonin reuptake inhibitors and are then started on an MAOI. Some cases presented with features resembling neuroleptic malignant syndrome. The effects of combined use of Cymbalta and MAOIs have not been evaluated in humans or animals. Therefore, because Cymbalta is an inhibitor of both serotonin and norepinephrine reuptake, it is recommended that Cymbalta not be used in combination with an MAOI, or within at least 14 days of discontinuing treatment with an MAOI. Based on the half-life of Cymbalta, at least 5 days should be allowed after stopping Cymbalta before starting an MAOI.

PRECAUTIONS

General

Hepatotoxicity—Cymbalta increases the risk of elevation of serum transaminase levels. Liver transaminase elevations resulted in the discontinuation of 0.4% (31/8454) of Cymbalta-treated patients. In these patients, the median time to detection of the transaminase elevation was about two months. In controlled trials in MDD, elevations of alanine transaminase (ALT) to >3 times the upper limit of normal occurred in 0.9% (8/930) of Cymbalta-treated patients and in 0.3% (2/652) of placebo-treated patients. In controlled trials in DPN, elevations of ALT to >3 times the upper limit of normal occurred in 1.68% (8/477) of Cymbalta-treated patients and in 0% (0/187) of placebo-treated patients. In the full cohort of placebo-controlled trials in any indication, 1% (39/3732) of Cymbalta-treated patients had a >3 times the upper limit of normal elevation of ALT compared to 0.2% (6/2568) of placebo-treated patients. In placebo-controlled studies using a fixed-dose design, there was evidence of a dose-response relationship for ALT and AST elevation of >3 times the upper limit of normal and >5 times the upper limit of normal, respectively.

The combination of transaminase elevations and elevated bilirubin, without evidence of obstruction, is generally recognized as an important predictor of severe liver injury. Three Cymbalta patients had elevations of transaminases and bilirubin, but also had elevation of alkaline phosphatase, suggesting an obstructive process; in these patients, there was evidence of heavy alcohol use and this may have contributed to the abnormalities seen. Two placebo-treated patients also had transaminase elevations with elevated bilirubin. Because it is possible that duloxetine and alcohol may interact to cause liver injury, Cymbalta should ordinarily not be prescribed to patients with substantial alcohol use.

Effect on Blood Pressure—In MDD clinical trials, Cymbalta treatment was associated with mean increases in blood pressure, averaging 2 mm Hg systolic and 0.5 mm Hg diastolic and an increase in the incidence of at least one measurement of systolic blood pressure over 140 mm Hg compared to placebo.

Blood pressure should be measured prior to initiating treatment and periodically measured throughout treatment (*see* ADVERSE REACTIONS, Vital Sign Changes).

Activation of Mania/Hypomania—In placebo-controlled trials in patients with major depressive disorder, activation of mania or hypomania was reported in 0.1% (1/1139) of Cymbalta-treated patients and 0.1% (1/777) of placebo-treated patients. Activation of mania/hypomania has been reported in a small proportion of patients with mood disorders who were treated with other marketed drugs effective in the treatment of major depressive disorder. As with these other agents, Cymbalta should be used cautiously in patients with a history of mania.

Seizures—Cymbalta has not been systematically evaluated in patients with a seizure disorder, and such patients were excluded from clinical studies. In placebo-controlled clinical trials in patients with major depressive disorder, seizures occurred in 0.1% (1/1139) of patients treated with Cymbalta and 0% (0/777) of patients treated with placebo. In placebo-controlled clinical trials in patients with diabetic peripheral neuropathy, seizures did not occur in any patients treated with either Cymbalta or placebo. Cymbalta should be prescribed with care in patients with a history of a seizure disorder.

Controlled Narrow-Angle Glaucoma—In clinical trials, Cymbalta was associated with an increased risk of mydriasis; therefore, it should be used cautiously in patients with controlled narrow-angle glaucoma (*see* CONTRAINDICATIONS, Uncontrolled Narrow-Angle Glaucoma).

Discontinuation of Treatment with Cymbalta—Discontinuation symptoms have been systematically evaluated in patients taking Cymbalta. Following abrupt discontinuation in MDD placebo-controlled clinical trials of up to 9-weeks duration, the following symptoms occurred at a rate greater than or equal to 2% and at a significantly higher rate in Cymbalta-treated patients compared to those discontinuing from placebo: dizziness; nausea; headache; paresthesia; vomiting; irritability; and nightmare.

During marketing of other SSRIs and SNRIs (serotonin and norepinephrine reuptake inhibitors), there have been spontaneous reports of adverse events occurring upon discontinuation of these drugs, particularly when abrupt, including the following: dysphoric mood, irritability, agitation,

Continued on next page

Cymbalta—Cont.

dizziness, sensory disturbances (e.g., paresthesias such as electric shock sensations), anxiety, confusion, headache, lethargy, emotional lability, insomnia, hypomania, tinnitus, and seizures. Although these events are generally self-limiting, some have been reported to be severe.

Patients should be monitored for these symptoms when discontinuing treatment with Cymbalta. A gradual reduction in the dose rather than abrupt cessation is recommended whenever possible. If intolerable symptoms occur following a decrease in the dose or upon discontinuation of treatment, then resuming the previously prescribed dose may be considered. Subsequently, the physician may continue decreasing the dose but at a more gradual rate (*see* DOSAGE AND ADMINISTRATION).

Use in Patients with Concomitant Illness—Clinical experience with Cymbalta in patients with concomitant systemic illnesses is limited. There is no information on the effect that alterations in gastric motility may have on the stability of Cymbalta's enteric coating. As duloxetine is rapidly hydrolyzed in acidic media to naphthol, caution is advised in using Cymbalta in patients with conditions that may slow gastric emptying (e.g., some diabetics).

Cymbalta has not been systematically evaluated in patients with a recent history of myocardial infarction or unstable coronary artery disease. Patients with these diagnoses were generally excluded from clinical studies during the product's premarketing testing. However, the electrocardiograms of 321 patients who received Cymbalta in MDD placebo-controlled clinical trials and had qualitatively normal ECGs at baseline were evaluated; Cymbalta was not associated with the development of clinically significant ECG abnormalities (*see* ADVERSE REACTIONS, Electrocardiogram Changes).

In DPN placebo-controlled clinical trials, Cymbalta-treated patients did not develop abnormal ECGs at a rate different from that in placebo-treated patients (*see* ADVERSE REACTIONS, Electrocardiogram Changes).

In clinical trials of Cymbalta for the management of neuropathic pain associated with diabetic peripheral neuropathy, the mean duration of diabetes was approximately 11 years, the mean baseline fasting blood glucose was 163 mg/dL, and the mean baseline hemoglobin $A1_c$ (HbA_{1c}) was 7.8%. In these studies, small increases in fasting blood glucose were observed in Cymbalta-treated patients compared to placebo at 12 weeks and routine care at 52 weeks. The increase was similar at both time points. Overall diabetic control did not worsen as evidenced by stable HbA_{1c} values and by no differences in incidence of serious and non-serious diabetes-related adverse events relative to placebo or routine care.

Increased plasma concentrations of duloxetine, and especially of its metabolites, occur in patients with end-stage renal disease (requiring dialysis). For this reason, Cymbalta is not recommended for patients with end-stage renal disease or severe renal impairment (creatinine clearance <30 mL/min) (*see* CLINICAL PHARMACOLOGY *and* DOSAGE AND ADMINISTRATION).

Markedly increased exposure to duloxetine occurs in patients with hepatic insufficiency and Cymbalta should not be administered to these patients (*see* CLINICAL PHARMACOLOGY *and* DOSAGE AND ADMINISTRATION).

Information for Patients

Physicians are advised to discuss the following issues with patients for whom they prescribe Cymbalta.

Patients and their families should be encouraged to be alert to the emergence of anxiety, agitation, panic attacks, insomnia, irritability, hostility, impulsivity, akathisia, hypomania, mania, worsening of depression, and suicidal ideation, especially early during antidepressant treatment. Such symptoms should be reported to the patient's physician, especially if they are severe, abrupt in onset, or were not part of the patient's presenting symptoms.

Cymbalta should be swallowed whole and should not be chewed or crushed, nor should the contents be sprinkled on food or mixed with liquids. All of these might affect the enteric coating.

Any psychoactive drug may impair judgment, thinking, or motor skills. Although in controlled studies Cymbalta has not been shown to impair psychomotor performance, cognitive function, or memory, it may be associated with sedation. Therefore, patients should be cautioned about operating hazardous machinery including automobiles, until they are reasonably certain that Cymbalta therapy does not affect their ability to engage in such activities.

Patients should be advised to inform their physicians if they are taking, or plan to take, any prescription or over-the-counter medications, since there is a potential for interactions.

Although Cymbalta does not increase the impairment of mental and motor skills caused by alcohol, use of Cymbalta concomitantly with heavy alcohol intake may be associated with severe liver injury. For this reason, Cymbalta should ordinarily not be prescribed for patients with substantial alcohol use.

Patients should be advised to notify their physician if they become pregnant or intend to become pregnant during therapy.

Patients should be advised to notify their physician if they are breast-feeding.

While patients with MDD may notice improvement with Cymbalta therapy in 1 to 4 weeks, they should be advised to continue therapy as directed.

Laboratory Tests

No specific laboratory tests are recommended.

Drug Interactions (also *see* CLINICAL PHARMACOLOGY, Drug-Drug Interactions)

Potential for Other Drugs to Affect Cymbalta

Both CYP1A2 and CYP2D6 are responsible for duloxetine metabolism.

Inhibitors of CYP1A2—Concomitant use of duloxetine with fluvoxamine, an inhibitor of CYP1A2, results in approximately a 6-fold increase in AUC and about a 2.5-fold increase in C_{max} of duloxetine. Some quinolone antibiotics would be expected to have similar effects and these combinations should be avoided.

Inhibitors of CYP2D6—Because CYP2D6 is involved in duloxetine metabolism, concomitant use of duloxetine with potent inhibitors of CYP2D6 may result in higher concentrations of duloxetine. Paroxetine (20 mg QD) increased the concentration of duloxetine (40 mg QD) by about 60%, and greater degrees of inhibition are expected with higher doses of paroxetine. Similar effects would be expected with other potent CYP2D6 inhibitors (e.g., fluoxetine, quinidine).

Potential for Duloxetine to Affect Other Drugs

Drugs Metabolized by CYP1A2—*In vitro* drug interaction studies demonstrate that duloxetine does not induce CYP1A2 activity, and it is unlikely to have a clinically significant effect on the metabolism of CYP1A2 substrates (*see* CLINICAL PHARMACOLOGY, Drug Interactions).

Drugs Metabolized by CYP2D6—Duloxetine is a moderate inhibitor of CYP2D6. When duloxetine was administered (at a dose of 60 mg BID) in conjunction with a single 50-mg dose of desipramine, a CYP2D6 substrate, the AUC of desipramine increased 3-fold. Therefore, co-administration of Cymbalta with other drugs that are extensively metabolized by this isozyme and which have a narrow therapeutic index, including certain antidepressants (tricyclic antidepressants [TCAs], such as nortriptyline, amitriptyline, and imipramine), phenothiazines and Type 1C antiarrhythmics (e.g., propafenone, flecainide), should be approached with caution. Plasma TCA concentrations may need to be monitored and the dose of the TCA may need to be reduced if a TCA is co-administered with Cymbalta. Because of the risk of serious ventricular arrhythmias and sudden death potentially associated with elevated plasma levels of thioridazine, Cymbalta and thioridazine should not be co-administered.

Drugs Metabolized by CYP3A—Results of *in vitro* studies demonstrate that duloxetine does not inhibit or induce CYP3A activity (*see* CLINICAL PHARMACOLOGY, Drug Interactions).

Cymbalta May Have a Clinically Important Interaction with the Following Other Drugs:

Alcohol—When Cymbalta and ethanol were administered several hours apart so that peak concentrations of each would coincide, Cymbalta did not increase the impairment of mental and motor skills caused by alcohol.

In the Cymbalta clinical trials database, three Cymbalta-treated patients had liver injury as manifested by ALT and total bilirubin elevations, with evidence of obstruction. Substantial intercurrent ethanol use was present in each of these cases, and this may have contributed to the abnormalities seen (*see* PRECAUTIONS, Hepatotoxicity).

CNS Acting Drugs—Given the primary CNS effects of Cymbalta, it should be used with caution when it is taken in combination with or substituted for other centrally acting drugs, including those with a similar mechanism of action.

Potential for Interaction with Drugs that Affect Gastric Acidity—Cymbalta has an enteric coating that resists dissolution until reaching a segment of the gastrointestinal tract where the pH exceeds 5.5. In extremely acidic conditions, Cymbalta, unprotected by the enteric coating, may undergo hydrolysis to form naphthol. Caution is advised in using Cymbalta in patients with conditions that may slow gastric emptying (e.g., some diabetics). Drugs that raise the gastrointestinal pH may lead to an earlier release of duloxetine. However, co-administration of Cymbalta with aluminum- and magnesium-containing antacids (51 mEq) or Cymbalta with famotidine, had no significant effect on the rate or extent of duloxetine absorption after administration of a 40-mg oral dose. It is unknown whether the concomitant administration of proton pump inhibitors affects duloxetine absorption.

Monoamine Oxidase Inhibitors—*See* CONTRAINDICATIONS *and* WARNINGS.

Carcinogenesis, Mutagenesis, Impairment of Fertility

Carcinogenesis—Duloxetine was administered in the diet to mice and rats for 2 years.

In female mice receiving duloxetine at 140 mg/kg/day (11 times the maximum recommended human dose [MRHD, 60 mg/day] and 6 times the human dose of 120 mg/day on a mg/m^2 basis), there was an increased incidence of hepatocellular adenomas and carcinomas. The no-effect dose was 50 mg/kg/day (4 times the MRHD and 2 times the human dose of 120 mg/day on a mg/m^2 basis). Tumor incidence was not increased in male mice receiving duloxetine at doses up to 100 mg/kg/day (8 times the MRHD and 4 times the human dose of 120 mg/day on a mg/m^2 basis).

In rats, dietary doses of duloxetine up to 27 mg/kg/day in females (4 times the MRHD and 2 times the human dose of 120 mg/day on a mg/m^2 basis) and up to 36 mg/kg/day in males (6 times the MRHD and 3 times the human dose of 120 mg/day on a mg/m^2 basis) did not increase the incidence of tumors.

Mutagenesis—Duloxetine was not mutagenic in the *in vitro* bacterial reverse mutation assay (Ames test) and was not clastogenic in an *in vivo* chromosomal aberration test in mouse bone marrow cells. Additionally, duloxetine was not genotoxic in an *in vitro* mammalian forward gene mutation assay in mouse lymphoma cells or in an *in vitro* unscheduled DNA synthesis (UDS) assay in primary rat hepatocytes, and did not induce sister chromatid exchange in Chinese hamster bone marrow *in vivo*.

Impairment of Fertility—Duloxetine administered orally to either male or female rats prior to and throughout mating at doses up to 45 mg/kg/day (7 times the maximum recommended human dose of 60 mg/day and 4 times the human dose of 120 mg/day on a mg/m^2 basis) did not alter mating or fertility.

Pregnancy

Pregnancy Category C—In animal reproduction studies, duloxetine has been shown to have adverse effects on embryo/fetal and postnatal development.

When duloxetine was administered orally to pregnant rats and rabbits during the period of organogenesis, there was no evidence of teratogenicity at doses up to 45 mg/kg/day (7 times the maximum recommended human dose [MRHD, 60 mg/day] and 4 times the human dose of 120 mg/day on a mg/m^2 basis, in rat; 15 times the MRHD and 7 times the human dose of 120 mg/day on a mg/m^2 basis in rabbit). However, fetal weights were decreased at this dose, with a no-effect dose of 10 mg/kg/day (2 times the MRHD and ≈1 times the human dose of 120 mg/day on a mg/m^2 basis in rat; 3 times the MRHD and 2 times the human dose of 120 mg/day on a mg/m^2 basis in rabbits).

When duloxetine was administered orally to pregnant rats throughout gestation and lactation, the survival of pups to 1 day postpartum and pup body weights at birth and during the lactation period were decreased at a dose of 30 mg/kg/day (5 times the MRHD and 2 times the human dose of 120 mg/day on a mg/m^2 basis); the no-effect dose was 10 mg/kg/day. Furthermore, behaviors consistent with increased reactivity, such as increased startle response to noise and decreased habituation of locomotor activity, were observed in pups following maternal exposure to 30 mg/kg/day. Post-weaning growth and reproductive performance of the progeny were not affected adversely by maternal duloxetine treatment.

There are no adequate and well-controlled studies in pregnant women; therefore, duloxetine should be used during pregnancy only if the potential benefit justifies the potential risk to the fetus.

Nonteratogenic Effects—Neonates exposed to SSRIs or serotonin and norepinephrine reuptake inhibitors (SNRIs), late in the third trimester have developed complications requiring prolonged hospitalization, respiratory support, and tube feeding. Such complications can arise immediately upon delivery. Reported clinical findings have included respiratory distress, cyanosis, apnea, seizures, temperature instability, feeding difficulty, vomiting, hypoglycemia, hypotonia, hypertonia, hyperreflexia, tremor, jitteriness, irritability, and constant crying. These features are consistent with either a direct toxic effect of SSRIs and SNRIs or, possibly, a drug discontinuation syndrome. It should be noted that, in some cases, the clinical picture is consistent with serotonin syndrome (*see* WARNINGS, Monoamine Oxidase Inhibitors). When treating a pregnant woman with Cymbalta during the third trimester, the physician should carefully consider the potential risks and benefits of treatment (*see* DOSAGE AND ADMINISTRATION).

Labor and Delivery

The effect of duloxetine on labor and delivery in humans is unknown. Duloxetine should be used during labor and delivery only if the potential benefit justifies the potential risk to the fetus.

Nursing Mothers

Duloxetine and/or its metabolites are excreted into the milk of lactating rats. It is unknown whether or not duloxetine and/or its metabolites are excreted into human milk, but nursing while on Cymbalta is not recommended.

Pediatric Use

Safety and efficacy in pediatric patients have not been established (*see* WARNINGS, Clinical Worsening and Suicide Risk).

Geriatric Use

Of the 2418 patients in clinical studies of Cymbalta for MDD, 5.9% (143) were 65 years of age or over. Of the 1074 patients in the DPN studies, 33% (357) were 65 years of age or over. No overall differences in safety or effectiveness were observed between these subjects and younger subjects, and other reported clinical experience has not identified differences in responses between the elderly and younger patients, but greater sensitivity of some older individuals cannot be ruled out.

ADVERSE REACTIONS

Cymbalta has been evaluated for safety in 2418 patients diagnosed with major depressive disorder who participated in multiple-dose premarketing trials, representing 1099 patient-years of exposure. Among these 2418 Cymbalta-treated patients, 1139 patients participated in eight 8- or 9-week, placebo-controlled trials at doses ranging from 40 to 120 mg/day, while the remaining 1279 patients were followed for up to 1 year in an open-label safety study using flexible doses from 80 to 120 mg/day. Two placebo-controlled studies with doses of 80 and 120 mg/day had 6-month maintenance extensions. Of these 2418 patients, 993 Cymbalta-treated patients were exposed for at least 180 days and 445 Cymbalta-treated patients were exposed for at least 1 year. Cymbalta has also been evaluated for safety in 1074 patients with diabetic peripheral neuropathy representing 472 patient-years of exposure. Among these 1074 Cymbalta-treated patients, 568 patients participated in two 12- to 13-week, placebo-controlled trials at doses ranging from 20 to 120 mg/day. An additional 449 patients were enrolled in an open-label safety study using 120 mg/day for a duration of 6 months. Another 57 patients, originally treated with placebo, were exposed to Cymbalta for up to 12 months at 60 mg twice daily in an extension phase. Among these 1074 patients, 484 had 6 months of exposure to Cymbalta, and 220 had 12 months of exposure.

For both MDD and DPN clinical trials, adverse reactions were assessed by collecting adverse events, results of physical examinations, vital signs, weights, laboratory analyses, and ECGs.

Clinical investigators recorded adverse events using descriptive terminology of their own choosing. To provide a meaningful estimate of the proportion of individuals experiencing adverse events, grouping similar types of events into a smaller number of standardized event categories is necessary. In the tables and tabulations that follow, MedDRA terminology has been used to classify reported adverse events.

The stated frequencies of adverse events represent the proportion of individuals who experienced, at least once, a treatment-emergent adverse event of the type listed. An event was considered treatment-emergent if it occurred for the first time or worsened while receiving therapy following baseline evaluation. Events reported during the studies were not necessarily caused by the therapy, and the frequencies do not reflect investigator impression (assessment) of causality.

The cited figures provide the prescriber with some basis for estimating the relative contribution of drug and non-drug factors to the adverse event incidence rate in the population studied. The prescriber should be aware that the figures in the tables and tabulations cannot be used to predict the incidence of adverse events in the course of usual medical practice where patient characteristics and other factors differ from those that prevailed in the clinical trials. Similarly, the cited frequencies cannot be compared with figures obtained from other clinical investigations involving different treatments, uses, and investigators.

Adverse Events Reported as Reasons for Discontinuation of Treatment in Placebo-Controlled Trials

Major Depressive Disorder

Approximately 10% of the 1139 patients who received Cymbalta in the MDD placebo-controlled trials discontinued treatment due to an adverse event, compared with 4% of the 777 patients receiving placebo. Nausea (Cymbalta 1.4%, placebo 0.1%) was the only common adverse event reported as reason for discontinuation and considered to be drug-related (i.e., discontinuation occurring in at least 1% of the Cymbalta-treated patients and at a rate of at least twice that of placebo).

Diabetic Peripheral Neuropathic Pain

Approximately 14% of the 568 patients who received Cymbalta in the DPN placebo-controlled trials discontinued treatment due to an adverse event, compared with 7% of the 223 patients receiving placebo. Nausea (Cymbalta 3.5%, placebo 0.4%), dizziness (Cymbalta 1.6%, placebo 0.4%), somnolence (Cymbalta 1.6%, placebo 0%) and fatigue (Cymbalta 1.1%, placebo 0%) were the common adverse events reported as reasons for discontinuation and considered to be drug-related (i.e., discontinuation occurring in at least 1% of the Cymbalta-treated patients and at a rate of at least twice that of placebo).

Adverse Events Occurring at an Incidence of 2% or More Among Cymbalta-Treated Patients in Placebo-Controlled Trials

Major Depressive Disorder

Table 1 gives the incidence of treatment-emergent adverse events that occurred in 2% or more of patients treated with Cymbalta in the acute phase of MDD placebo-controlled trials and with an incidence greater than placebo. The most commonly observed adverse events in Cymbalta-treated MDD patients (incidence of 5% or greater and at least twice the incidence in placebo patients) were: nausea; dry mouth; constipation; decreased appetite; fatigue; somnolence; and increased sweating (*see* Table 1).

[See table 1 above]

Table 1: Treatment-Emergent Adverse Events Incidence in MDD Placebo-Controlled Trials[1]

System Organ Class / Adverse Event	Percentage of Patients Reporting Event	
	Cymbalta (N=1139)	Placebo (N=777)
Gastrointestinal Disorders		
Nausea	20	7
Dry mouth	15	6
Constipation	11	4
Diarrhea	8	6
Vomiting	5	3
Metabolism and Nutrition Disorders		
Appetite decreased[2]	8	2
Investigations		
Weight decreased	2	1
General Disorders and Administration Site Conditions		
Fatigue	8	4
Nervous System Disorders		
Dizziness	9	5
Somnolence	7	3
Tremor	3	1
Skin and Subcutaneous Tissue Disorders		
Sweating increased	6	2
Vascular Disorders		
Hot flushes	2	1
Eye Disorders		
Vision blurred	4	1
Psychiatric Disorders		
Insomnia[3]	11	6
Anxiety	3	2
Libido decreased	3	1
Orgasm abnormal[4]	3	1
Reproductive System and Breast Disorders		
Erectile dysfunction[5]	4	1
Ejaculation delayed[5]	3	1
Ejaculatory dysfunction[5,6]	3	1

[1] Events reported by at least 2% of patients treated with Cymbalta and more often with placebo. The following events were reported by at least 2% of patients treated with Cymbalta for MDD and had an incidence equal to or less than placebo: upper abdominal pain, palpitations, dyspepsia, back pain, arthralgia, headache, pharyngitis, cough, nasopharyngitis, and upper respiratory tract infection.
[2] Term includes anorexia.
[3] Term includes middle insomnia.
[4] Term includes anorgasmia.
[5] Male patients only.
[6] Term includes ejaculation disorder and ejaculation failure.

Diabetic Peripheral Neuropathic Pain

Table 2 gives the incidence of treatment-emergent adverse events that occurred in 2% or more of patients treated with Cymbalta in the acute phase of DPN placebo-controlled trials (doses of 20 to 120 mg/day) and with an incidence greater than placebo. The most commonly observed adverse events in Cymbalta-treated DPN patients (incidence of 5% or greater and at least twice the incidence in placebo patients) were: nausea; somnolence; dizziness; constipation; dry mouth; hyperhidrosis; decreased appetite; and asthenia (*see* Table 2)

[See table 2 at top of next page]

Adverse events seen in men and women were generally similar except for effects on sexual function (described below). Clinical studies of Cymbalta did not suggest a difference in adverse event rates in people over or under 65 years of age. There were too few non-Caucasian patients studied to determine if these patients responded differently from Caucasian patients.

Effects on Male and Female Sexual Function

Although changes in sexual desire, sexual performance and sexual satisfaction often occur as manifestations of a psychiatric disorder, they may also be a consequence of pharmacologic treatment. Reliable estimates of the incidence and severity of untoward experiences involving sexual desire, performance and satisfaction are difficult to obtain, however, in part because patients and physicians may be reluctant to discuss them. Accordingly, estimates of the incidence of untoward sexual experience and performance cited in product labeling are likely to underestimate their actual incidence. Table 3 displays the incidence of sexual side effects spontaneously reported by at least 2% of either male or female patients taking Cymbalta in MDD placebo-controlled trials.

[See table 3 on next page]

Because adverse sexual events are presumed to be voluntarily underreported, the Arizona Sexual Experience Scale (ASEX), a validated measure designed to identify sexual side effects, was used prospectively in 4 MDD placebo-controlled trials. In these trials, as shown in Table 4 below, patients treated with Cymbalta experienced significantly more sexual dysfunction, as measured by the total score on the ASEX, than did patients treated with placebo. Gender analysis showed that this difference occurred only in males. Males treated with Cymbalta experienced more difficulty with ability to reach orgasm (ASEX Item 4) than males treated with placebo. Females did not experience more sexual dysfunction on Cymbalta than on placebo as measured by ASEX total score. These studies did not, however, include an active control drug with known effects on female sexual dysfunction, so that there is no evidence that its effects differ from other antidepressants. Negative numbers signify an improvement from a baseline level of dysfunction, which is commonly seen in depressed patients. Physicians should routinely inquire about possible sexual side effects.

[See table 4 on next page]

Urinary Hesitation

Cymbalta is in a class of drugs known to affect urethral resistance. If symptoms of urinary hesitation develop during treatment with Cymbalta, consideration should be given to the possibility that they might be drug-related.

Laboratory Changes

Cymbalta treatment, for up to 9-weeks in MDD or 13-weeks in DPN placebo-controlled clinical trials, was associated with small mean increases from baseline to endpoint in ALT, AST, CPK, and alkaline phosphatase; infrequent, modest, transient, abnormal values were observed for these analytes in Cymbalta-treated patients when compared with placebo-treated patients (*see* PRECAUTIONS).

Vital Sign Changes

Cymbalta treatment, for up to 9-weeks in MDD placebo-controlled clinical trials of 40 to 120 mg daily doses caused increases in blood pressure, averaging 2 mm Hg systolic and 0.5 mm Hg diastolic compared to placebo and an increase in the incidence of at least one measurement of systolic blood pressure over 140 mm Hg (*see* PRECAUTIONS).

Cymbalta treatment, for up to 9-weeks in MDD placebo-controlled clinical trials and for up to 13-weeks in DPN placebo-controlled trials caused a small increase in heart rate compared to placebo of about 2 beats per minute.

Weight Changes

In MDD placebo-controlled clinical trials, patients treated with Cymbalta for up to 9-weeks experienced a mean weight loss of approximately 0.5 kg, compared with a mean weight gain of approximately 0.2 kg in placebo-treated patients.

In DPN placebo-controlled clinical trials, patients treated with Cymbalta for up to 13-weeks experienced a mean weight loss of approximately 1.1 kg, compared with a mean weight gain of approximately 0.2 kg in placebo-treated patients.

Electrocardiogram Changes

Electrocardiograms were obtained from 321 Cymbalta-treated patients with major depressive disorder and 169 placebo-treated patients in clinical trials lasting up to 8-weeks. The rate-corrected QT (QTc) interval in Cymbalta-treated patients did not differ from that seen in placebo-treated patients. No clinically significant differences were observed for QT, PR, and QRS intervals between Cymbalta-treated and placebo-treated patients.

Electrocardiograms were obtained from 528 Cymbalta-treated patients with DPN and 205 placebo-treated patients in clinical trials lasting up to 13-weeks. The rate-corrected QT (QTc) interval in Cymbalta-treated patients did not differ from that seen in placebo-treated patients. No clinically significant differences were observed for QT, PR, QRS, or QTc measurements between Cymbalta-treated and placebo-treated patients.

Other Adverse Events Observed During the Premarketing Evaluation of Cymbalta for MDD and the Pain of DPN

Following is a list of modified MedDRA terms that reflect treatment-emergent adverse events as defined in the introduction to the ADVERSE REACTIONS section reported by

Continued on next page

Cymbalta—Cont.

patients treated with Cymbalta at multiple doses throu[illegible] out the dose range studied during any phase o[illegible]ed are within the premarketing database. The events [illegible]RSE REACTIONS and not considered in the [illegible]NINGS and PRECAUTIONS sections, that we[illegible]eported with an incidence of greater than or equal [illegible].05% and by more than one patient, are not com[illegible] as background events and were considered pos[illegible]y drug related (e.g., because of the drug's pharmacology) or potentially important.

It is important to emphasize that, although the events reported occurred during treatment with Cymbalta, they were not necessarily caused by it. Events are further categorized by body system and listed in order of decreasing frequency according to the following definitions: frequent adverse events are those occurring in at least 1/100 patients (only those not already listed in the tabulated results from placebo-controlled trials appear in this listing); infrequent adverse events are those occurring in 1/100 to 1/1000 patients; rare events are those occurring in fewer than 1/1000 patients.

Blood and Lymphatic System Disorders—*Infrequent:* anemia, leukopenia, increased white blood cell count, lymphadenopathy, and thrombocytopenia.

Cardiac Disorders—*Infrequent:* atrial fibrillation, bundle branch block right, cardiac failure, cardiac failure congestive, coronary artery disease, and myocardial infarction.

Eye Disorders—*Infrequent:* diplopia, glaucoma, keroconjunctivitis sicca, macular degeneration, maculopathy, photopsia, and retinal detachment.

Gastrointestinal Disorders—*Frequent:* gastritis; *Infrequent:* apthous stomatitis, blood in stool, colitis, diverticulitis, dysphagia, esophageal stenosis acquired, gastric irritation, gastric ulcer, gingivitis, impaired gastric emptying, irritable bowel syndrome, lower abdominal pain, and melena.

General Disorders and Administration Site Conditions—*Frequent:* rigors; *Infrequent:* edema, feeling jittery, influenza-like illness, and thirst.

Hepato-biliary Disorders—*Infrequent:* hepatic steatosis.

Investigations—*Frequent:* weight increased; *Infrequent:* blood cholesterol increased, blood creatinine increased, and urine output decreased.

Metabolism and Nutrition Disorders—*Frequent:* hypoglycemia and increased appetite; *Infrequent:* dehydration, dyslipidemia, hypercholesterolemia, hyperlipidemia, and hypertriglyceridemia.

Musculoskeletal and Connective Tissue Disorders—*Infrequent:* muscular weakness.

Nervous System Disorders—*Frequent:* hypoesthesia; *Infrequent:* ataxia and dysarthria.

Psychiatric Disorders—*Frequent:* initial insomnia, irritability, lethargy, nervousness, nightmare, restlessness, and sleep disorder; *Infrequent:* completed suicide, mania, mood swings, pressure of speech, sluggishness, and suicide attempt.

Renal and Urinary Disorders—*Frequent:* dysuria; *Infrequent:* micturition urgency, nephropathy, urinary hesitation, urinary incontinence, urinary retention, and urine flow decreased.

Respiratory, Thoracic and Mediastinal Disorders—*Infrequent:* oropharyngeal swelling.

Skin and Subcutaneous Tissue Disorders—*Frequent:* night sweats, pruritus, rash, and skin ulcer; *Infrequent:* acne, alopecia, cold sweat, ecchymosis, eczema, erythema, erythematous rash, exfoliative dermatitis, face edema, hyperkeratosis, increased tendency to bruise, photosensitivity reaction, and pruritic rash.

Vascular Disorders—*Infrequent:* hypertensive crisis, peripheral edema, and phlebitis.

DRUG ABUSE AND DEPENDENCE

Controlled Substance Class

Duloxetine is not a controlled substance.

Physical and Psychological Dependence

In animal studies, duloxetine did not demonstrate barbiturate-like (depressant) abuse potential. In drug dependence studies, duloxetine did not demonstrate dependence-producing potential in rats.

While Cymbalta has not been systematically studied in humans for its potential for abuse, there was no indication of drug-seeking behavior in the clinical trials. However, it is not possible to predict on the basis of premarketing experience the extent to which a CNS active drug will be misused, diverted, and/or abused once marketed. Consequently, physicians should carefully evaluate patients for a history of drug abuse and follow such patients closely, observing them for signs of misuse or abuse of Cymbalta (e.g., development of tolerance, incrementation of dose, drug-seeking behavior).

OVERDOSAGE

There is limited clinical experience with Cymbalta overdose in humans. In premarketing clinical trials, as of October 2003, no cases of fatal acute overdose of Cymbalta have been reported. Four non-fatal acute ingestions of Cymbalta (300 to 1400 mg), alone or in combination with other drugs, have been reported.

Management of Overdose

There is no specific antidote to Cymbalta. In case of acute overdose, treatment should consist of those general measures employed in the management of overdose with any drug.

[illegible]able 2: Treatment-Emergent Adverse Events Incidence in DPN Placebo-Controlled Trials[1]

System Organ Class/ Adverse Event	Percentage of Patients Reporting Event			
	Cymbalta 60 mg BID (N=225)	Cymbalta 60 mg QD (N=228)	Cymbalta 20 mg QD (N=115)	Placebo (N=223)
Gastrointestinal Disorders				
Nausea	30	22	14	9
Constipation	15	11	5	3
Diarrhea	7	11	13	6
Dry mouth	12	7	5	4
Vomiting	5	5	6	4
Dyspepsia	4	4	4	3
Loose stools	2	3	2	1
General Disorders and Administration Site Conditions				
Fatigue	12	10	2	5
Asthenia	8	4	2	1
Pyrexia	3	1	2	1
Infections and Infestations				
Nasopharyngitis	9	7	9	5
Metabolism and Nutrition Disorders				
Decreased appetite	11	4	3	<1
Anorexia	5	3	3	<1
Musculoskeletal and Connective Tissue Disorders				
Muscle cramp	4	4	5	3
Myalgia	4	1	3	<1
Nervous System Disorders				
Somnolence	21	15	7	5
Headache	15	13	13	10
Dizziness	17	14	6	6
Tremor	5	1	0	0
Psychiatric Disorders				
Insomnia	13	8	9	7
Renal and Urinary Disorders				
Pollakiuria	5	1	3	2
Reproductive System and Breast Disorders				
Erectile dysfunction[2]	4	1	0	0
Respiratory, Thoracic and Mediastinal Disorders				
Cough	5	3	6	4
Pharyngolaryngeal pain	6	1	3	1
Skin and Subcutaneous Tissue Disorders				
Hyperhidrosis	8	6	6	2

[1] Events reported by at least 2% of patients treated with Cymbalta and more often than placebo. The following events were reported by at least 2% of patients treated with Cymbalta for DPN and had an incidence equal to or less than placebo: edema peripheral, influenza, upper respiratory tract infection, back pain, arthralgia, pain in extremity, and pruritus.

[2] Male patients only.

Table 3: Treatment-Emergent Sexual Dysfunction-Related Adverse Events Incidence in MDD Placebo-Controlled Trials[1]

Adverse Event	Percentage of Patients Reporting Event			
	% Male Patients		% Female Patients	
	Cymbalta (N=378)	Placebo (N=247)	Cymbalta (N=761)	Placebo (N=530)
Orgasm abnormal[2]	4	1	2	0
Ejaculatory dysfunction[3]	3	1	NA	NA
Libido decreased	6	2	1	0
Erectile dysfunction	4	1	NA	N/
Ejaculation delayed	3	1	NA	N

[1] Events reported by at least 2% of patients treated with Cymbalta and more often than with placebo.
[2] Term includes anorgasmia.
[3] Term includes ejaculation disorder and ejaculation failure.
NA=Not applicable.

Table 4: Mean Change in ASEX Scores by Gender in MDD Placebo-Controlled Trials

	Male Patients		Female Patient	
	Cymbalta (n=175)	Placebo (n=83)	Cymbalta (n=241)	lacebo n=126)
ASEX Total (Items 1–5)	0.56*	-1.07	-1.15	-1.07
Item 1—Sex drive	-0.07	-0.12	-0.32	-0.24
Item 2—Arousal	0.01	-0.26	-0.21	-0.18
Item 3—Ability to achieve erection (men); Lubrication (women)	0.03	-0.25	-0.17	-0.18
Item 4—Ease of reaching orgasm	0.40**	-0.24	-0.09	-0.13
Item 5—Orgasm satisfaction	0.09	-0.13	-0.11	-0.17

n=Number of patients with non-missing change score for ASEX total.
* p=0.013 versus placebo.
**p<0.001 versus placebo.

An adequate airway, oxygenation, and ventilation should be assured, and cardiac rhythm and vital signs should be monitored. Induction of emesis is not recommended. Gastric lavage with a large-bore orogastric tube with ppropriate airway protection, if needed, may be indicat if performed soon after ingestion or in symptomatic patits.

Activated charcoal may be useful in limiting absorption of duloxetine from the gastrointestinal tract. Administration of activated charcoal has been shown to decrease AUC and C_{max} by an average of one-third, although some subjects had a limited effect of activated charcoal. Due to the large volume of distribution of this drug, forced diuresis, dialysis, hemoperfusion, and exchange transfusion are unlikely to be beneficial.

In managing overdose, the possibility of multiple drug involvement should be considered. A specific caution involves patients who are taking or have recently taken Cymbalta and might ingest excessive quantities of a TCA. In such a case, decreased clearance of the parent tricyclic and/or its active metabolite may increase the possibility of clinically significant sequelae and extend the time needed for close medical observation (*see* PRECAUTIONS, Drug Interactions). The physician should consider contacting a poison control center for additional information on the treatment of any overdose. Telephone numbers for certified poison control centers are listed in the *Physicians' Desk Reference* (PDR).

DOSAGE AND ADMINISTRATION

Initial Treatment

Major Depressive Disorder

Cymbalta should be administered at a total dose of 40 mg/day (given as 20 mg BID) to 60 mg/day (given either once a day or as 30 mg BID) without regard to meals.

There is no evidence that doses greater than 60 mg/day confer any additional benefits.

Diabetic Peripheral Neuropathic Pain

Cymbalta should be administered at a total dose of 60 mg/day given once a day, without regard to meals.

While a 120 mg/day dose was shown to be safe and effective, there is no evidence that doses higher than 60 mg confer additional significant benefit, and the higher dose is clearly less well tolerated. For patients for whom tolerability is a concern, a lower starting dose may be considered. Since diabetes is frequently complicated by renal disease, a lower starting dose and gradual increase in dose should be considered for patients with renal impairment (*see* CLINICAL PHARMACOLOGY, Special Populations *and* below).

Maintenance/Continuation/Extended Treatment

Major Depressive Disorder

It is generally agreed that acute episodes of major depression require several months or longer of sustained pharmacologic therapy. There is insufficient [illegible] answer the question of how long a patient [illegible] available to to be treated with Cymbalta. Patients should be p[illegible]ntinue reassessed to determine the need for maintenance [illegible]ment and the appropriate dose for such treatment.

Diabetic Peripheral Neuropathic Pain

As the progression of diabetic peripheral neuropathy is highly variable and management of pain is empirical, the effectiveness of Cymbalta must be assessed individually. Efficacy beyond 12 weeks has not been systematically studied in placebo-controlled trials, but a one-year open-label safety study was conducted.

Special Populations

Dosage for Renally Impaired Patients—Cymbalta is not recommended for patients with end-stage renal disease (requiring dialysis) or in severe renal impairment (estimated creatinine clearance <30 mL/min) (*see* CLINICAL PHARMACOLOGY).

Dosage for Hepatically Impaired Patients—It is recommended that Cymbalta not be administered to patients with any hepatic insufficiency (*see* CLINICAL PHARMACOLOGY *and* PRECAUTIONS).

Dosage for Elderly Patients—No dose adjustment is recommended for elderly patients on the basis of age. As with any drug, caution should be exercised in treating the elderly. When individualizing the dosage in elderly patients, extra care should be taken when increasing the dose.

Treatment of Pregnant Women During the Third Trimester—Neonates exposed to SSRIs or SNRIs, late in the third trimester have developed complications requiring prolonged hospitalization, respiratory support, and tube feeding (*see* PRECAUTIONS). When treating pregnant women with Cymbalta during the third trimester, the physician should carefully consider the potential risks and benefits of treatment. The physician may consider tapering Cymbalta in the third trimester.

Discontinuing Cymbalta

Symptoms associated with discontinuation of Cymbalta and other SSRIs and SNRIs have been reported (*see* PRECAUTIONS). Patients should be monitored for these symptoms when discontinuing treatment. A gradual reduction in the dose rather than abrupt cessation is recommended whenever possible. If intolerable symptoms occur following a decrease in the dose or upon discontinuation of treatment, then resuming the previously prescribed dose may be considered. Subsequently, the physician may continue decreasing the dose but at a more gradual rate.

Switching Patients to or from a Monoamine Oxidase I[illegible]

At [illegible] days should elapse between discontinuation of an MAO[illegible] initiation of therapy with Cymbalta. In addition, at least [illegible] should be allowed after stopping Cymbalta before start[illegible] MAOI (*see* CONTRAINDICATIONS *and* WARNINGS).

HOW SUPPLIED

Cymbalta® (duloxetine hydrochloride) Dela[illegible]d-release Capsules are available in 20, 30, and 60 mg strengths.

The 20 mg* capsule has an opaque green body and cap, and is imprinted with "20 mg" on the body and "LILLY 3235" on the cap:

NDC 0002-3235-60 (PU3235) — Bottles of 60
NDC 0002-3235-33 (PU3235) — (ID†100) Blisters

The 30 mg* capsule has an opaque white body and opaque blue cap, and is imprinted with "30 mg" on the body and "LILLY 3240" on the cap:

NDC 0002-3240-30 (PU3240) — Bottles of 30
NDC 0002-3240-90 (PU3240) — Bottles of 90
NDC 0002-3240-04 (PU3240) — Bottles of 1000
NDC 0002-3240-33 (PU3240) — (ID†100) Blisters

The 60 mg* capsule has an opaque green body and opaque blue cap, and is imprinted with "60 mg" on the body and "LILLY 3237" on the cap:

NDC 0002-3237-30 (PU3237) — Bottles of 30
NDC 0002-3237-90 (PU3237) — Bottles of 90
NDC 0002-3237-04 (PU3237) — Bottles of 1000
NDC 0002-3237-33 (PU3237) — (ID†100) Blisters

*equivalent to duloxetine base.
†Identi-Dose® (unit dose medication, Lilly).

Store at 25°C (77°F); excursions permitted to 15–30°C (59–86°F) [see USP Controlled Room Temperature].

Literature revised September 3, 2004

Eli Lilly and Company
Indianapolis, IN 46285, USA
www.Cymbalta.com

PV 3601 AMP PRINTED IN USA

DIAGNOSTIC PRODUCT INFORMATION

This section is made possible through the courtesy of the manufacturers whose products appear on the following pages. The information concerning each product has been prepared, edited, and approved by the medical department, medical director, and/or medical counsel of its manufacturer.

When a product appearing in *Physicians' Desk Reference* has an official package circular, its description must be in full compliance with Food and Drug Administration (FDA) regulations pertaining to labeling for prescription drugs. These regulations require that in *PDR* "indications, effects, dosages, routes, methods, and frequency and duration of administration, and any relevant warnings, hazards, contraindications, side effects, and precautions" must be *"same in language and emphasis"* as the approved labeling for the product. The FDA regards the words *"same in language and emphasis"* as requiring VERBATIM use of the approved labeling providing such information. Furthermore, information that is emphasized in the approved labeling by the use of type set in a box, or in capitals, boldface, or italics, must be given the same emphasis in *PDR*.

For products that do not have official package circulars, *PDR* has asked manufacturers to provide comprehensive product information to help physicians make the most informed decisions possible.

The product descriptions in *PDR* include all information made available to *PDR* by the manufacturer. The publisher does not warrant or guarantee any product, and does not perform any independent analysis of the information provided. Inclusion of a product in *PDR* does not represent an endorsement, and the publisher does not necessarily advocate the use of any product listed.

This edition of *PDR* contains the latest information available when the book went to press. As new drugs are released and new research data and clinical findings become available throughout the year, the information in the *PDR* database is revised accordingly. These revisions are published twice annually in the *PDR* Supplements. To be certain that you have the most current data, always consult the supplements before prescribing or administering any product described in the following pages.

Baxter Healthcare Corporation Anesthesia & Critical Care

95 SPRING ST
NEW PROVIDENCE, NJ 07974

Direct Inquiries to:
Professional Services D[...]partment
(800) ANA DRU[...]
(800) 26[...]784

For Medical Information Contact:
In Emergencies:
Paula Dimopoulos PharmD
Director Medical Affairs
(800) ANA-DRUG
(800) 262-3784

Sales and Ordering:
To place an order, call or fax:
(800) 667-0959
Fax 877-702-3580

FACTREL ℞

[*făc 'trel*]
(gonadorelin hydrochloride, USP)
Synthetic Luteinizing Hormone Releasing Hormone (LH-RH)
DIAGNOSTIC USE ONLY

DESCRIPTION

An agent for use in evaluating hypothalamic-pituitary gonadotropic function. FACTREL (gonadorelin hydrochloride, USP) injectable is available as a sterile lyophilized powder for reconstitution and administration by subcutaneous or intravenous routes.

Chemical Name: 5-oxo-L-prolyl-L-histidyl-L-tryptophyl-L-seryl-L-tyrosyl-glycyl-L-leucyl-L-arginyl-L-prolyl glycinamide hydrochloride
[See chemical structure below]

FACTREL is $C_{55}H_{75}N_{17}O_{13}HCl$, as the mono- or dihydrochloride, or their mixture. The gonadorelin base has a molecular weight of 1182.33. It is a white powder, soluble in alcohol and water, hygroscopic and moisture-sensitive, and stable at room temperature. The synthetic decapeptide, FACTREL, has a chemical composition and structure identical to the natural hormone, identified from porcine or ovine hypothalami.

Each vial of FACTREL contains 100 mcg gonadorelin hydrochloride, USP (with up to 7.0% Water Content) with 100 mg lactose, USP.

Each ampul of sterile diluent contains 2% benzyl alcohol in sterile water.

HOW SUPPLIED

Lyophilized Powder—in single-dose vial containing 100 mcg gonadorelin hydrochloride, USP (with up to 7.0% Water Content) with 100 mg lactose USP (NDC 60977-103-93). Each vial is accompanied by one ampul containing 2 mL sterile diluent of 2% benzyl alcohol in sterile water.

DIRECTIONS

Store at room temperature (approximately 25°C).
Reconstitute 100 mcg vial with 1 mL of the accompanying sterile diluent.
Prepare solution immediately before use. After reconstitution, store at room temperature and use within 1 day.
Discard unused reconstituted solution and diluent.

Factrel is a trademark of Baxter International Inc.
Baxter Healthcare Corporation
Deerfield, IL 60015 USA

Structural Formula

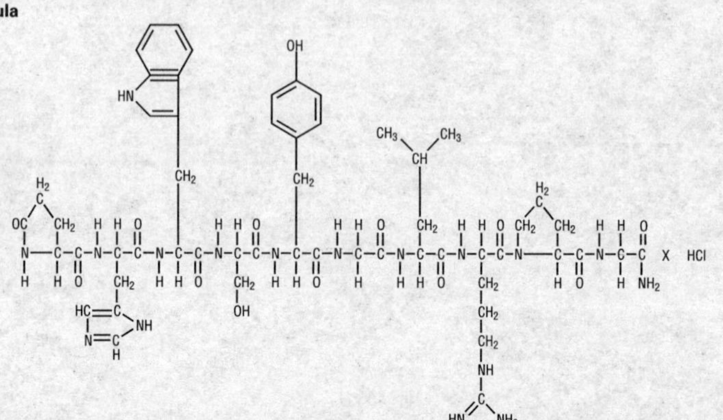

[...]g Pharmaceuticals Inc.

[...]0 RELLA BOULEVARD SUITE #300
SUFFERN, NY 10901

Direct Inquiries to:
Ferring Pharmaceuticals Inc.
Customer Service Department
400 Rella Boulevard, Suite 300
Suffern, NY 10901
1-(888)-FERRING (337-7464)

For Medical Information Contact:
In Emergencies:
Ferring Pharmaceuticals Inc.
Professional Services Department
400 Rella Boulevard, Suite 300
Suffern, NY 10901
1-(800)-822-8214

ACTHREL® ℞

(corticorelin ovine triflutate for injection)
For intravenous injection only
DIAGNOSTIC USE ONLY

DESCRIPTION

ACTHREL® (corticorelin ovine triflutate for injection) is a sterile, nonpyrogenic, lyophilized white cake powder, containing corticorelin ovine triflutate, a trifluoroacetate salt of a synthetic peptide that is used for the determination of pituitary corticotroph responsiveness. Corticorelin ovine has an amino acid sequence identical to ovine corticotropin-releasing hormone (oCRH). Corticorelin ovine is an analogue of the naturally occurring human CRH (hCRH) peptide. Both peptides are potent stimulators of adrenocorticotropic hormone (ACTH) release from the anterior pituitary. ACTH stimulates cortisol production from the adrenal cortex. The structural formula for corticorelin ovine triflutate is described below:

Ser-Gln-Glu-Pro-Pro-Ile-Ser-Leu-Asp-Leu-Thr-Phe-His-Leu-Leu-Arg-Glu-Val-Leu-Glu-Met-Thr-Lys-Ala-Asp-Gln-Leu-Ala-Gln-Gln-Ala-His-Ser-Asn-Arg-Lys-Leu-Leu-Asp-Ile-Ala-NH_2 • xCF_3COOH

whereas x=4 - 8.

The empirical formula of corticorelin ovine is $C_{205}H_{339}N_{59}O_{63}S$ with a molecular weight of 4670.35 Daltons.

ACTHREL® for injection is available in vials containing 100 mcg corticorelin ovine (as the trifluoroacetate), 0.88 mg ascorbic acid, 10 mg lactose, and 26 mg cysteine hydrochloride monohydrate. Trace amounts of chloride ion may be present from the manufacturing process. The preparation is intended for intravenous administration.

CLINICAL PHARMACOLOGY

Pharmacodynamics: In normal subjects, intravenous administration of corticorelin results in a rapid and sustained increase of plasma ACTH levels and a near parallel increase of plasma cortisol. In addition, intravenous administration of corticorelin to normal subjects causes a concomitant and prolonged release of the related proopiomelanocortin peptides β- and γ-lipotropins (β-and γ-LPH) and β-endorphin (β-END). A number of dose-response studies have been performed on normal subjects using a range of corticorelin doses. In one study, doses of corticorelin ranging from 0.001 to 30 mcg/kg body weight were administered to 29 healthy volunteers. Blood samples were taken over a 2-hour period for determination of plasma ACTH and cortisol concentrations. There was a direct dose-dependent relationship that was more pronounced for ACTH than for cortisol. The threshold dose was 0.03 mcg/kg, the half-maximal dose was 0.3-1.0 mcg/kg and the maximally effective dose was 3-10 mcg/kg.

Plasma ACTH levels in normal subjects increased 2 minutes after injection of corticorelin doses of ≥0.3 mcg/kg and reached peak levels after 10-15 minutes. Plasma cortisol levels increased within 10 minutes and reached peak levels at 30 to 60 minutes. As the dose of corticorelin was increased, the rises in plasma ACTH and cortisol were more sustained, showing a biphasic response with a second lower peak at 2-3 hours after injection. Similar results were found in another study using 0.3, 3.0, and 30 mcg/kg doses. The duration of mean plasma ACTH increase after injection of 0.3, 3.0, and 30 mcg/kg was 4, 7, and 8 hours, respectively. The effect on plasma cortisol was similar, but more prolonged. Because there are differences in basal levels and peak response levels following a.m. or p.m. administration, it is recommended that subsequent evaluations in the same patient using the corticorelin stimulation test be carried out at the same time of day as the original evaluation.

Baseline ACTH and cortisol levels are usually higher in the morning. Pooled ACTH values from normal unstressed subjects (n=119) were 25 ± 7 pg/mL in the a.m. and 10 ± 3 in the p.m.; similar pooled cortisol values (n=170) were 11 ± 3 mcg/dL in the a.m. and 4 ± 2 mcg/dL in the p.m. The normal unstressed person has about seven to ten secretory episodes of ACTH each day. Most of them occur in the early morning hours and are responsible for the morning plasma cortisol surge. The following figure shows the daily circadian rhythm of ACTH and cortisol secretions in a normal unstressed person. Insulin, plasma renin activity, prolactin, and growth hormone release are not affected by corticorelin administration in humans.

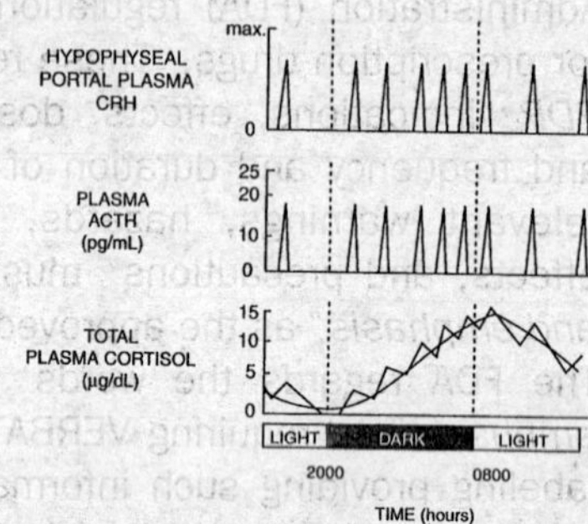

Continuous 24-hour infusion of corticorelin (0.5, 1.0, and 3.0 mcg/kg/hr) increased plasma ACTH concentrations to a plateau of 15-20 pg/mL by the third hour and urinary-free cortisol reaches 173 ± 43 mcg/dL by 24 hours, comparable to those levels observed in patients with major depression, but less than levels noted in Cushing's disease. Continuous infusion did not abolish the circadian rhythm of plasma ACTH and cortisol, but did appear to desensitize the corticotroph. Intermittent doses of corticorelin (25 mcg every 4 hours for 72 hours), however, continued to elicit the expected ACTH and cortisol responses.

Intravenous administration of 1 mcg/kg corticorelin in combination with 10 pressor units intramuscular vasopressin had a synergistic effect on ACTH and a less marked synergistic effect on cortisol secretion.

The basal and peak response levels of ACTH and cortisol to a 1 mcg/kg or 100 mcg dose of corticorelin administered to normal volunteers in the morning and the evening are given below. These values were obtained by combining the results from 9 clinical trials conducted in the a.m. and 4 clinical trials conducted in the p.m.

The following table is to be used only as a general guide.
[See table at top of next page]

Pharmokinetics: Following a single intravenous injection of 1 mcg/kg of corticorelin to normal men, the disappearance of immunoreactive corticorelin (IR-corticorelin) from plasma follows a biexponential decay curve. Plasma half-lives for IR-corticorelin are 11.6 ±1.5 minutes (mean ± SE) for the fast component and 73 ± 8 minutes for the slow component. The mean volume of distribution for IR-corticorelin is 6.2 ± 0.5 L with an approximate metabolic clearance rate of 95 ± 11 L/m²/day. Graded intravenous doses of corticorelin (0.01, 0.03, 0.1, 0.3, 1, 3, 10, 30 mcg/kg) produced a linear increase in plasma IR-corticorelin. Corticorelin does not appear to be bound specifically by a circulating plasma protein.

INDICATIONS AND USAGE

ACTHREL® is indicated for use in differentiating pituitary and ectopic production of ACTH in patients with ACTH-dependent Cushing's syndrome.

Differential Diagnosis: There are two forms of Cushing's syndrome:

(a) ACTH-dependent (83%), in which hypercortisolism is due either to pituitary hypersecretion of ACTH (Cushing's disease) resulting from an adenoma (40%, usually microadenomas) or nonadenomatous hyperplasia, possibly of hypothalamic origin (28%), or to hypercortisolism that is secondary to ectopic secretion of ACTH (15%) and,

(b) ACTH- independent (17%), in which hypercortisolism is due to autonomous cortisol secretion by an adrenal tumor (9% adenomas, 8% carcinomas),

After the establishment of hypercortisolism consistent with the presence of Cushing's syndrome, and following the elimination of autonomous adrenal hyperfunction as its cause, the corticorelin test is used to aid in establishing the source of excessive ACTH secretion.

The corticorelin stimulation test helps to differentiate between the etiologies of ACTH-dependent hypercortisolism as follows:

Basal Concentrations and Peak Responses of ACTH and Cortisol in Normal Subjects after 1 mcg/kg or 100 mcg of ACTHREL®

Time of Day	No. of Subjects	ACTH Concentration mean (range) pg/mL		Cortisol Concentration mean (range) mcg/dL	
		Basal	Peak	Basal	Peak
a.m.	143	28 (16-65)	68 (39-114)	11 (8-13)	21 (17-25)
p.m.	70	9 (8-13)	30 (25-42)	4 (2-6)	16 (15-18)

1. High basal plasma ACTH plus high basal plasma cortisol (20 - 40 mcg/dL).
   ACTHREL® injection (1 mcg/kg) results in:
   a. Increased plasma ACTH levels
   b. Increased plasma cortisol levels
   Diagnosis: Cushing's disease (ACTH of pituitary origin)
2. High basal plasma ACTH (may be very high) plus high basal plasma cortisol (20 - 40 mcg/dL).
   ACTHREL® injection (1 mcg/kg) results in:
   a. Little or no response of plasma ACTH levels
   b. Little or no response of plasma cortisol levels
   Diagnosis: Ectopic ACTH syndrome

Test Methodology: To evaluate the status of the pituitary-adrenal axis in the differentiation of a pituitary source from an ectopic source of excessive ACTH secretion, a corticorelin test procedure requires a minimum of five blood samples.

Procedure

1. Venous blood samples should be drawn 15 minutes before and immediately prior to ACTHREL® administration. The ACTH baseline is obtained by averaging the values of the two samples.
2. Administer ACTHREL® as an intravenous infusion over a 30- to 60- second interval at a dose of 1 mcg/kg body weight. Higher doses are not recommended (see **PRECAUTIONS** and **ADVERSE REACTIONS**).
3. Draw venous blood samples at 15, 30, and 60 minutes after administration.
4. Blood samples should be handled as recommended by the laboratory that will determine their ACTH content. It is extremely important to recognize that the reliability of the ACTHREL® test is directly related to the inter-assay and intra-assay variability of the laboratory performing the assay.

Cortisol determinations may be performed on the same blood samples for the same time points as outlined above. The blood sample handling precautions noted for ACTH should be followed for cortisol.

Interpretation of Test Results: The interpretation of the ACTH and cortisol responses following ACTHREL® administration requires a knowledge of the clinical status of the individual patient, understanding of hypothalamic-pituitary-adrenal physiology, and familiarity with the normal hormonal ranges and the standards used by the laboratory that performs the ACTH and cortisol assays.

Cushing's Disease

The results of challenge with corticorelin injection have been reported in approximately 300 patients with Cushing's disease. Although the ACTH and cortisol responses were variable, a hyper-response to corticorelin was seen in a majority of patients, despite high basal cortisol levels. This response pattern indicates an impairment of the negative feedback of cortisol on the pituitary. Patients with pituitary-dependent Cushing's disease tested with corticorelin do not show the negative correlation between basal and stimulated levels of ACTH and cortisol that is found in normal subjects. A positive correlation between basal ACTH levels and maximum ACTH increments after corticorelin administration has been found in Cushing's disease patients.

Ectopic ACTH Secretion

Patients with Cushing's syndrome due to ectopic ACTH secretion (N=32) were found to have very high basal levels of ACTH and cortisol, which were not further stimulated by corticorelin. However, there have been rare instances of patients with ectopic sources of ACTH that have responded to the corticorelin test.

SUMMARY OF ACTH RESPONSES IN PATIENTS WITH HIGH BASAL CORTISOL

	High ACTH Response	Low ACTH Response
High Basal ACTH	Cushing's Disease	Ectopic ACTH Secretion

CUSHING'S DISEASE ACTH RESPONSES
(mean of 181 patients)
Basal ACTH 63 ± 72 pg/mL (mean ± SD)
Peak ACTH 189 ± 262 pg/mL (mean ± SD)
Mean of individual change from baseline + 227%

ECTOPIC ACTH SECRETION RESPONSES
(mean for 31 patients)
Basal ACTH 266 ± 464 pg/mL (mean ± SD)
Peak ACTH 276 ± 466 pg/mL (mean ± SD)
Mean of individual change from baseline + 15%

False negative responses to the corticorelin test in Cushing's disease patients occur approximately 5 to 10% of the time, which may lead the clinician to an incorrect diagnosis of ectopic production of ACTH at that frequency. (See **INDICATIONS AND USAGE, Differential Diagnosis**)

PRECAUTIONS

General: The severity of adverse effects to a corticorelin injection appear to be dose-dependent. Dosages above 1 mcg/kg are not recommended. While few adverse effects have been observed at the 1 mcg/kg or 100 mcg dose, higher doses have been associated with transient tachycardia, decreased blood pressure, loss of consciousness, and asystole (see **ADVERSE REACTIONS**). These symptoms can be substantially reduced by administering the drug as a 30-second intravenous infusion instead of a bolus injection. At a dose of 200 mcg corticorelin, 4 of 60 volunteers and patients with disturbances of the hypothalamic-pituitary-adrenal (HPA) axis were reported to have had decreased blood pressures. One patient had a severe hypotensive reaction with asystole. Three other patients had an "absence-like" loss of consciousness lasting approximately 5 minutes. In subsequent investigations by the same researchers over a 3-year period using 100 mcg of corticorelin, one patient in approximately 150 to 200 experienced a severe drop in blood pressure and loss of sinus rhythm after receiving 55 mcg of corticorelin, which may have been due to interaction with heparin. (See **Drug Interactions**)

Drug Interactions: The plasma ACTH response to corticorelin injection is inhibited or blunted in normal subjects pretreated with dexamethasone. The use of a heparin solution to maintain i.v. cannula patency during the corticorelin test is not recommended. A possible interaction between corticorelin and heparin may have been responsible for a major hypotensive reaction that occurred after corticorelin administration. (See **ADVERSE REACTIONS**)

Carcinogenesis, Mutagenesis, Impairment of Fertility: Animal studies have not been conducted with corticorelin to evaluate carcinogenic potential, mutagenicity, or effect on fertility.

Pregnancy (Pregnancy Category C): Animal reproduction studies have not been conducted with corticorelin. It is also not known whether corticorelin can cause fetal harm when administered to a pregnant woman or can affect reproductive capacity. ACTHREL® should be given to a pregnant woman only if clearly needed.

Nursing Mothers: It is not known whether corticorelin is secreted in human milk. Because many drugs are excreted in human milk, caution should be exercised when ACTHREL® is administered to a nursing woman.

PEDIATRIC USE

Only a few tests have been performed on children. Dosages were 1 mcg/kg body weight. Patient studies have involved only children with multiple hypothalamic and/or pituitary hormone deficiencies, or tumors. Only two studies with normal pediatric subjects have been conducted. No differences in response to the corticorelin test have been reported in the children studied.

ADVERSE REACTIONS

Adverse effects reported with 1 mcg/kg or 100 mcg/patient include flushing of the face, neck, and upper chest (16%; 45/276), beginning almost immediately and lasting 3 to 5 minutes. Recipients have also reported an urge to take a deep breath (6%; 3/49), which occurs with a timing similar to, but less frequently than, that of flushing. Higher doses (≥3mcg/kg) are associated with more prolonged flushing, tachycardia, hypotension, dyspnea, and "chest compression" or tightness. In addition, at doses of ≥ 5 mcg/kg, significant increases in heart rate and decreases in blood pressure were observed. The cardiovascular effects occurred 2-3 minutes after injection and lasted for 30-60 minutes. The facial flushing was more prolonged, lasting up to 4 hours in some subjects. All signs and symptoms could be reduced by administering the drug as a 30-second infusion instead of by bolus injection.

Total doses of up to 200 mcg of corticorelin were administered as a bolus injection to 60 men and women, including both healthy normal subjects and patients with endocrine disorders. In most cases, only minor adverse effects, such as transient flushing and feelings of dyspnea, were noted. However, a few patients with disorders of the pituitary-adrenal axis had major symptoms. One patient had a precipitous fall in blood pressure and pulse rate and developed asystole, which required resuscitation. In two patients with Cushing's disease and in one with secondary adrenal insufficiency, an "absence-like" loss of consciousness occurred, which started within a few seconds after injection of corticorelin and lasted from 10 seconds to 5 minutes. This was accompanied by a slight fall in blood pressure. One patient with a well documented seizure diathesis experienced a grand mal epileptic seizure following ACTHREL® administration. The patient had discontinued anti-convulsant therapy the day of the procedure. (See **PRECAUTIONS** and **Drug Interactions**)

OVERDOSAGE

Symptoms of overdose include severe facial flushing, cardiovascular effects, and dyspnea. In the event of toxic overdose (see **ADVERSE REACTIONS**), adverse effects should be treated symptomatically.

DOSAGE AND ADMINISTRATION

Dosage: A single intravenous dose of ACTHREL® at 1 mcg/kg is recommended for the testing of pituitary corticotrophin function. A dose of 1 mcg/kg is the lowest dose that produces maximal cortisol responses and significant (though apparently sub-maximal) ACTH responses. Doses above 1 mcg/kg are not recommended. (See **PRECAUTIONS** and **ADVERSE REACTIONS**)

At a dose of 1 mcg/kg, the ACTH and cortisol responses to ACTHREL® are prolonged and remain elevated for up to 2 hours. The maximum increment in plasma ACTH occurs between 15 and 60 minutes after ACTHREL® administration, whereas the maximum increment in plasma cortisol occurs between 30 and 120 minutes. In a clinical study of 30 normal healthy men, the peak plasma ACTH and cortisol responses to ACTHREL® administration in the early afternoon occurred at 42 ± 29 minutes and 65 ± 26 minutes (average ± SD), respectively. **If a repeated evaluation using the corticorelin stimulation test with ACTHREL® is needed, it is recommended that the repeat test be carried out at the same time of day as the original test because there are differences in basal levels and peak response levels following a.m. or p.m. administration to normal humans.**

Administration: ACTHREL® is to be reconstituted aseptically with 2 mL of Sodium Chloride injection, USP (0.9% sodium chloride), at the time of use by injecting 2 mL of the saline diluent into the lyophilized drug product cake. To avoid bubble formation, DO NOT SHAKE the vial; instead, roll the vial to dissolve the product. The sterile solution containing 50 mcg corticorelin/mL is then ready for injection by the intravenous route. The dosage to be administered is determined by the patient's weight (1 mcg corticorelin/kg). Some of the adverse effects can be reduced by administering the drug as an infusion over 30 seconds instead of as a bolus injection.

Parenteral drug products should be inspected visually for particulate matter and discoloration prior to administration, whenever solution and container permit.

HOW SUPPLIED

ACTHREL® is supplied as a sterile, nonpyrogenic, lyophilized, white cake containing 100 mcg corticorelin ovine (as the trifluoroacetate), 0.88 mg ascorbic acid, 10 mg lactose, and 26 mg cysteine hydrochloride monohydrate. Trace amounts of chloride ion may be present from the manufacturing process. The package provides a single-dose, rubber-capped, 5 mL, brown-glass vial (NDC 55566-0302-1) containing 100 mcg corticorelin ovine (as the trifluoroacetate). ACTHREL® is stable in the lyophilized form when stored refrigerated at 2°C to 8°C (36°F to 46°F) and protected from light. The reconstituted solution is stable up to 8 hours under refrigerated conditions. Discard unused reconstituted solution.

Manufactured for:
Ferring Pharmaceuticals Inc.
Suffern, NY 10901
By:
Ben Venue Laboratories, Inc.
Bedford, OH 44146
Rx only
3/03 6011-03

Serono, Inc.
ONE TECHNOLOGY PLACE
ROCKLAND, MA 02370

Direct Inquiries to:
Customer Service, Sales and Ordering
(888) 398-4567
(781) 982-9000

For Medical Information or to report Adverse Drug Experiences Contact the U.S. Medical Information or U.S. Product Surveillance Department at
(888) 275-7376
(781) 982-9000
www.howkidsgrow.com
www.novantrone.com
www.rebif.com
www.seronofertility.com
www.seronousa.com
www.serostim.com
www.zorbtive.com

GEREF® DIAGNOSTIC ℞
[*gĕr ĕf*]
(sermorelin acetate for injection)
For intravenous injection only
FOR DIAGNOSTIC USE ONLY

Continued on next page

Geref Diagnostic—Cont.

DESCRIPTION

Geref® Diagnostic (sermorelin acetate for in[illegible] is a sterile, nonpyrogenic, lyophilized prepara[illegible]ontaining 50 mcg sermorelin (as the acetate), 5 [illegible]nnitol, 0.66 mg monobasic sodium phosphate, an[illegible] mg dibasic sodium phosphate. Sermorelin aceta[illegible] an acetate salt of a synthetic, 29-amino acid [illegible]peptide that is the amino-terminal segment of th[illegible]naturally occurring human growth hormone-releas[illegible] hormone (GHRH or GRH) consisting of 44 amino acid residues. The structural formula for sermorelin acetate is presented below:

[illegible]a-Ile-Phe-Thr-Asn-Ser-Tyr-
Tyr-[illegible]Val-Leu-Gly-Gln-Leu-Ser-Ala-Arg-
[illegible]s-Leu-Leu-Gln-Asp-Ile-Met-Ser-Arg-NH_2 • $(C_2H_4O_2)_{3\text{-}6}$

The free base of sermorelin has the empirical formula $C_{149}H_{246}N_{44}O_{42}S_1$ and a molecular weight of 3,358 daltons. Sermorelin appears to be equivalent to GRH (1–44) in its ability to stimulate growth hormone secretion in humans. It has also been called GRH (1–29) and GHRH (1–29).

HOW SUPPLIED

Geref® Diagnostic is supplied in sterile, nonpyrogenic, lyophilized form in ampules containing 50 mcg sermorelin (as the acetate).

The following package combination is available:

NDC 44087-4050-1
1 ampule containing 50 mcg sermorelin (as the acetate) and 1 vial containing 2 mL 0.9% Sodium Chloride Injection, USP

The lyophilized product must be stored refrigerated (2°-8°C/36°-46°F). Use immediately after reconstitution. Discard unused material.

℞ only

References available on request.

Manufactured for:
SERONO, INC.
Rockland, MA 02376 USA
Revised January 2003

U.S. Department of Health and Human Services

Form Approved: OMB No. 0910-0291, Expires: 03/31/05
See OMB statement on reverse.

MEDWATCH

The FDA Safety Information and Adverse Event Reporting Program

For VOLUNTARY reporting of adverse events and product problems

Page ____ of ____

FDA USE ONLY

Triage unit sequence #

A. PATIENT INFORMATION

1. Patient Identifier — In confidence
2. Age at Time of Event: ______ or Date of Birth:
3. Sex ☐ Female ☐ Male
4. Weight ______ lbs or ______ kgs

B. ADVERSE EVENT OR PRODUCT PROBLEM

1. ☐ Adverse Event and/or ☐ Product Problem *(e.g., defects/malfunctions)*
2. Outcomes Attributed to Adverse Event *(Check all that apply)*
   - ☐ Death: ______ *(mo/day/yr)*
   - ☐ Life-threatening
   - ☐ Hospitalization - initial or prolonged
   - ☐ Disability
   - ☐ Congenital Anomaly
   - ☐ Required Intervention to Prevent Permanent Impairment/Damage
   - ☐ Other: ______
3. Date of Event *(mo/day/year)*
4. Date of This Report *(mo/day/year)*
5. Describe Event or Problem
6. Relevant Tests/Laboratory Data, Including Dates
7. Other Relevant History, Including Preexisting Medical Conditions *(e.g., allergies, race, pregnancy, smoking and alcohol use, hepatic/renal dysfunction, etc.)*

PLEASE TYPE OR USE BLACK INK

C. SUSPECT MEDICATION(S)

1. Name *(Give labeled strength & mfr/labeler, if known)*
   #1
   #2
2. Dose, Frequency & Route Used
   #1
   #2
3. Therapy Dates *(If unknown, give duration) from/to (or best estimate)*
   #1
   #2
4. Diagnosis for Use *(Indication)*
   #1
   #2
5. Event Abated After Use Stopped or Dose Reduced?
   #1 ☐ Yes ☐ No ☐ Doesn't Apply
   #2 ☐ Yes ☐ No ☐ Doesn't Apply
6. Lot # *(if known)*
   #1
   #2
7. Exp. Date *(if known)*
   #1
   #2
8. Event Reappeared After Reintroduction?
   #1 ☐ Yes ☐ No ☐ Doesn't Apply
   #2 ☐ Yes ☐ No ☐ Doesn't Apply
9. NDC# *(For product problems only)*
   \- -
10. Concomitant Medical Products and Therapy Dates *(Exclude treatment of event)*

D. SUSPECT MEDICAL DEVICE

1. Brand Name
2. Type of Device
3. Manufacturer Name, City and State
4. Model #
   Lot #
   Catalog #
   Expiration Date *(mo/day/yr)*
   Serial #
   Other #
5. Operator of Device
   - ☐ Health Professional
   - ☐ Lay User/Patient
   - ☐ Other:
6. If Implanted, Give Date *(mo/day/yr)*
7. If Explanted, Give Date *(mo/day/yr)*
8. Is this a Single-use Device that was Reprocessed and Reused on a Patient?
   ☐ Yes ☐ No
9. If Yes to Item No. 8, Enter Name and Address of Reprocessor
10. Device Available for Evaluation? *(Do not send to FDA)*
    ☐ Yes ☐ No ☐ Returned to Manufacturer on: ______ *(mo/day/yr)*
11. Concomitant Medical Products and Therapy Dates *(Exclude treatment of event)*

E. REPORTER *(See confidentiality section on back)*

1. Name and Address
   Phone #
2. Health Professional? ☐ Yes ☐ No
3. Occupation
4. Also Reported to:
   - ☐ Manufacturer
   - ☐ User Facility
   - ☐ Distributor/Importer
5. If you do NOT want your identity disclosed to the manufacturer, place an "X" in this box: ☐

FDA

Mail to: MEDWATCH
5600 Fishers Lane
Rockville, MD 20852-9787

-or-

FAX to:
1-800-FDA-0178

FORM FDA 3500 (12/03) **Submission of a report does not constitute an admission that medical personnel or the product caused or contributed to the event.**

ADVICE ABOUT VOLUNTARY REPORTING

Report adverse experiences with:

- Medications *(drugs or biologics)*
- Medical devices *(including in-vitro diagnostics)*
- Special nutritional products *(dietary supplements, medical foods, infant formulas)*
- Cosmetics
- Medication errors

Report product problems - quality, performance or safety concerns such as:

- Suspected counterfeit product
- Suspected contamination
- Questionable stability
- Defective components
- Poor packaging or labeling
- Therapeutic failures

Report SERIOUS adverse events. An event is serious when the patient outcome is:

- Death
- Life-threatening *(real risk of dying)*
- Hospitalization *(initial or prolonged)*
- Disability *(significant, persistent or permanent)*
- Congenital anomaly
- Required intervention to prevent permanent impairment or damage

Report even if:

- You're not certain the product caused the event
- You don't have all the details

-Fold Here-

How to report:

- Just fill in the sections that apply to your report
- Use section C for all products except medical devices
- Attach additional blank pages if needed
- Use a separate form for each patient
- Report either to FDA or the manufacturer *(or both)*

Confidentiality: The patient's identity is held in strict confidence by FDA and protected to the fullest extent of the law. FDA will not disclose the reporter's identity in response to a request from the public, pursuant to the Freedom of Information Act. The reporter's identity, including the identity of a self-reporter, may be shared with the manufacturer unless requested otherwise.

If your report involves a serious adverse event with a device and it occurred in a facility outside a doctor's office, that facility may be legally required to report to FDA and/or the manufacturer. Please notify the person in that facility who would handle such reporting.

-Fold Here-

Important numbers:

- 1-800-FDA-0178 -- To FAX report
- 1-800-FDA-1088 -- To report by phone or for more information
- 1-800-822-7967 -- For a VAERS form for vaccines

To Report via the Internet:

http://www.fda.gov/medwatch/report.htm

The public reporting burden for this collection of information has been estimated to average 30 minutes per response, including the time for reviewing instructions, searching existing data sources, gathering and maintaining the data needed, and completing and reviewing the collection of information. Send comments regarding this burden estimate or any other aspect of this collection of information, including suggestions for reducing this burden to:

Department of Health and Human Services
Food and Drug Administration
MedWatch; HFD-410
5600 Fishers Lane
Rockville, MD 20857

Please DO NOT RETURN this form to this address.

OMB statement:
"An agency may not conduct or sponsor, and a person is not required to respond to, a collection of information unless it displays a currently valid OMB control number."

U.S. DEPARTMENT OF HEALTH AND HUMAN SERVICES
Food and Drug Administration

FORM FDA 3500 (12/03) (Back) **Please Use Address Provided Below -- Fold in Thirds, Tape and Mail**

DEPARTMENT OF HEALTH & HUMAN SERVICES

Public Health Service
Food and Drug Administration
Rockville, MD 20857

Official Business
Penalty for Private Use $300

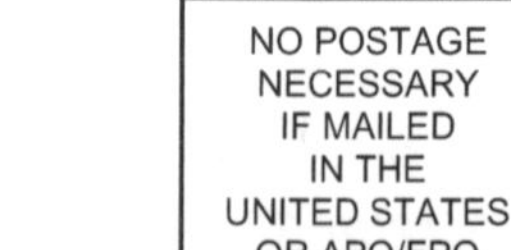

NO POSTAGE NECESSARY IF MAILED IN THE UNITED STATES OR APO/FPO

BUSINESS REPLY MAIL

FIRST CLASS MAIL PERMIT NO. 946 ROCKVILLE MD

POSTAGE WILL BE PAID BY FOOD AND DRUG ADMINISTRATION

MEDWATCH
The FDA Safety Information and Adverse Event Reporting Program
Food and Drug Administration
5600 Fishers Lane
Rockville, MD 20852-9787

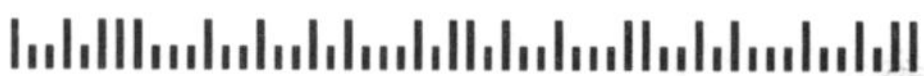

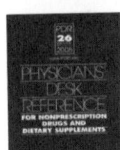

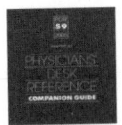

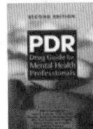

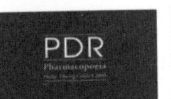

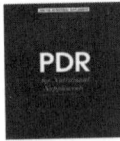

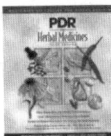

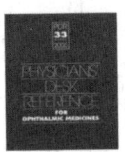

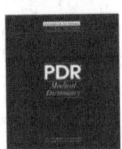

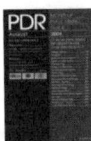

Announcing the new PDR® for Herbal Medicines *3rd Edition.*

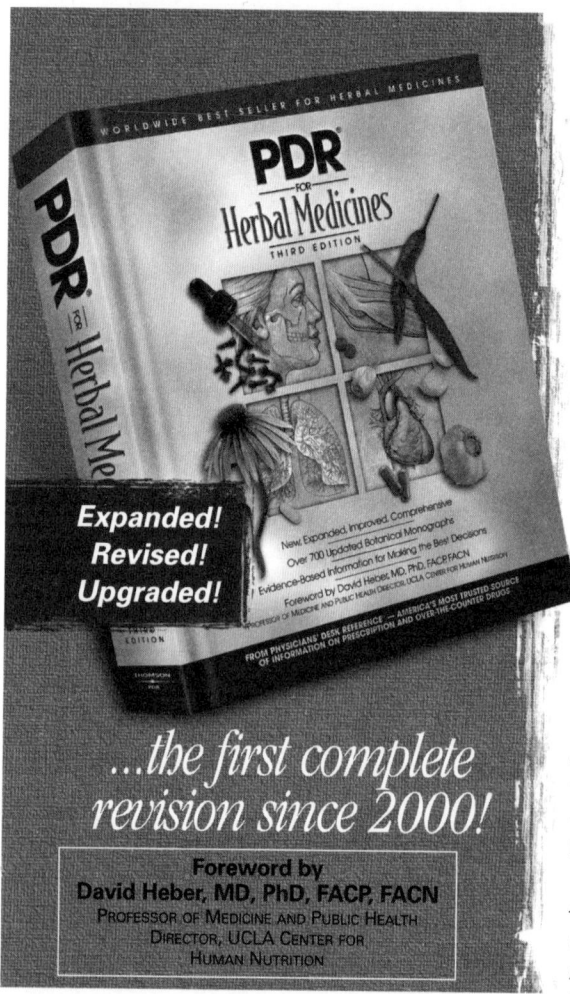

Patients who use herbals — prescribed or otherwise — are a daily reality for virtually every physician. But the herbal's contribution to a patient's health can be unclear and hard to assess. To make the best call for your patient, you need an authoritative, trustworthy reference that answers all your questions. It's here — the new updated PDR for Herbal Medicines *3rd Edition*.

Respected, comprehensive and current!

This new *3rd Edition* is the definitive guide to current herbal practices. With more than 700 monographs, a new section on the most popular nutritional supplements, and new information on clinical management of interactions, this edition is the ultimate source for accurate, evidence-based, trustworthy herbal information.

New interactions added

When herbal mixes with prescription, concerns over interactions are paramount. This new edition offers the most current, exhaustive interaction data available for the most extensive list of herbals assembled in one reference.

The most popular nutritional supplements added

Consumption of nutritional supplements has increased in the last decade as well. Therefore monographs of some of the most popular supplements make a logical addition to this guide.

New clinical management of interactions

At last, there's evidence-based guidance for managing herbal medicines with the most frequently prescribed drugs. This important section helps you make thoroughly informed decisions.

An herbal guide you can trust

In a field where scientific standards are not always applicable, a guide's source information is even more important. Here are three reasons why the PDR for Herbal Medicines *3rd Edition* is the world's most authoritative herbal reference:

1. The foundation for this edition continues to be the extensive herbal database of the **PhytoPharm U.S. Institute of Phytopharmaceuticals.** This resource provides extensive pharmacological and indication details that are generally not available from other sources.

2. The findings of the **German Regulatory Authority (Commission E)** are recognized for their expert consensus in the herbal field. Their widely accepted conclusions add an additional valuable dimension for physicians looking for the best counsel.

3. Finally, this edition is assembled by the same **PDR Editorial Team** that produces all the PDR reference guides. Only after their standards had been met was the PDR for Herbal Medicines *3rd Edition* ready for publication.

A typical monograph covers these critical aspects:

- herbs are listed by common name followed by its scientific name
- a thorough description of the herb is provided, including its medicinal parts (e.g., flower and fruit, etc,); unique characteristics, and additional common names and synonyms
- a detailed summary of the active compounds and the herb's clinical effects
- indications and usage — where applicable — under five categories: Commission E Approved; Chinese Medicine; Indian Medicine; Homeopathic; Unproven
- clinical studies are cited for many monographs
- drug/herb interactions and clinical management of those interactions
- precautions, adverse reactions, and dosage information provide a comprehensive overview
- a unique bibliography of the literature

HERBAL MONOGRAPHS — ARNICA / 41

Arnica

Arnica montana

DESCRIPTION

Medicinal Parts: The medicinal parts of Arnica are the ethereal oil of the flowers, the dried flowers, the leaves collected before flowering and dried, the roots, and the dried rhizome and roots.

Flower and Fruit: The terminal composite flower is found in the leaf axils of the upper pair of leaves. They have a diameter of 6 to 8 cm, are usually egg yolk-yellow to orange-yellow, but occasionally light yellow. The receptacle and epicalyx are hairy. The 10 to 20 female ray flowers are lingui-form. In addition, there are about 100 disc flowers, which are tubular. The 5-ribbed fruit is black-brown and has a bristly tuft of hair.

Leaves, Stem and Root: Arnica is a herbaceous plant growing 20 to 50 cm high. The brownish rhizome is 0.5 cm thick by 10 cm long, usually unbranched, 3-sectioned and sympodial. The rhizome may also be 3-headed with many yellow-brown secondary roots. Leaves are in basal rosettes. They are in 2 to 3 crossed opposite pairs and are obovate and entire-margined with 5 protruding vertical ribs. The glandular-haired stem has 2 to 6 smaller leaves, which are ovate to lanceolate, entire-margined or somewhat dentate.

Characteristics: The flower heads are aromatic; the taste is bitter and irritating.

Habitat: Arnica is found in Europe from Scandinavia to southern Europe. It is also found in southern Russia and central Asia.

Production: Arnica flower consists of the fresh or dried inflorescence of Arnica montana or Arnica chamissonis. The flower should be dried quickly at 45° to 50°C.

Not to be Confused With: Other yellow-flowering Asteracea.

Other Names: Arnica Flowers, Arnica Root, Leopard's

Sesquiterpene lactones ... ticularly esters of the helenalin- and 11,13-dihydrohelenalin with short-chained fatty acids such as acetic acid, isobutyric acid, 2- methyl-butyric acid, methylacrylic acid, isovaleric acid or tiglic acid

Volatile oil: with thymol, thymol esters, free fatty acids

Caffeic acid derivatives: including chlorogenic acid, 1,5-dicaffeoyl quinic acid

Flavonoids: numerous flavone and flavonol glycosides and their aglycones

EFFECTS

Arnica preparations have an antiphlogistic, analgesic and antiseptic effect when applied topically, due to the sesquiterpene lactone componant. The flavonoid bonds, essential oils and polyynes may also be involved. In cases of inflammation, Arnica preparations also show analgesic and antiseptic activity. The sesquiterpenes (helenalin) in the drug have an antimicrobial effect in vitro and an antiphlogistic effect in animal tests. A respiratory-analeptic, uterine tonic and cardiovascular effect (increase of contraction amplitude with simultaneous increase in frequency, i.e. positive inotropic effect) was demonstrated.

INDICATIONS AND USAGE

Approved by Commission E:

- Fever and colds
- Inflammation of the skin
- Cough/bronchitis
- Inflammation of the mouth and pharynx
- Rheumatism
- Common cold
- Blunt injuries
- Tendency to infection

Unproven Uses: External folk medicine uses include conse quences of injury such as traumatic edema, hematoma contusions, as well as rheumatic muscle and joint problems Other applications are inflammation of the oral and throa region, furunculosis, inflammation caused by insect bites ar phlebitis. In Russian folk medicine, the drug is used to tre uterine hemorrhaging. Furthermore, the drug is used f myocarditis, arteriosclerosis, angina pectoris, exhaustio cardiac insufficiency, sprains, contusions and for hair lo due to psychological causes. While some uses are plausib most are unproven.

luted tincture, as well as ... nevertheless lead to sensitization.

Allergy-related skin rashes with itching, blister forma ulcers and superficial necroses can result from repe contact with, among other things, cosmetics contai ... other composites (for example t

G-14/PDR FOR HERBAL MEDICINES

HENBANE — HIBISCUS — HOLLY

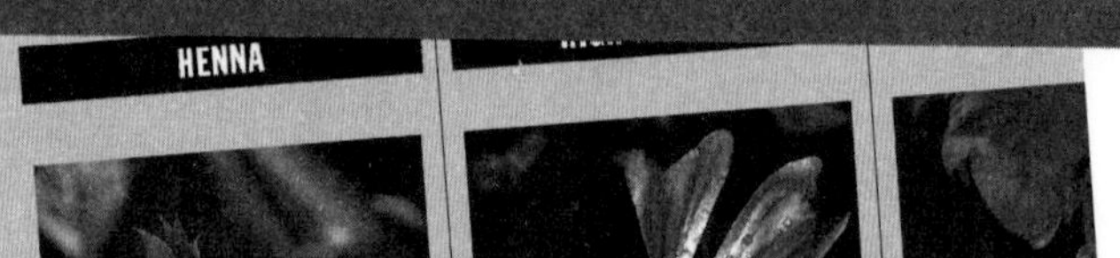

See other side for ordering information